D1682120

EUROPEAN PHARMACOPOEIA

5th Edition

published 15 June 2004

replaces the 4th Edition on 1 January 2005

Volumes 1 and 2 of this publication 5.0 constitute the 5th Edition of the European Pharmacopoeia. They will be complemented by **non-cumulative supplements** that are to be kept for the duration of the 5th Edition. 2 supplements will be published in 2004 and 3 supplements in each of the years 2005 and 2006. A cumulative list of reagents will be published in supplements 5.4 and 5.7.

If you are using the 5th Edition at any time later than 1 April 2005, make sure that you have all the published supplements and consult the index of the most recent supplement to ensure that you use the latest versions of the monographs and general chapters.

EUROPEAN PHARMACOPOEIA ELECTRONIC VERSION

The 5th Edition is also available in an electronic format (CD-ROM and internet version) with all the monographs and general chapters contained in the book. With the publication of each supplement the electronic version is replaced by a new fully updated cumulative version.

PHARMEUROPA

Quarterly Forum Publication

Pharmeuropa contains preliminary drafts of all new and revised monographs proposed for inclusion in the European Pharmacopoeia and gives an opportunity for all interested parties to comment on the specifications before they are finalised. Pharmeuropa also contains information on the work programme and on certificates of suitability to monographs of the European Pharmacopoeia issued by the EDQM, scientific articles on pharmacopoeial matters and other articles of general interest. Pharmeuropa is available on subscription from the EDQM.

INTERNATIONAL HARMONISATION

Refer to information given in chapter *5.8. Pharmacopoeial Harmonisation.*

WEBSITE

http://www.pheur.org
http://book.pheur.org (for prices and orders)

KEY TO MONOGRAPHS

Version date of the text

01/2005:0884

corrected

Text reference number

Modification to be taken into account from the publication date of volume 5.0

CARBIMAZOLE

Carbimazolum

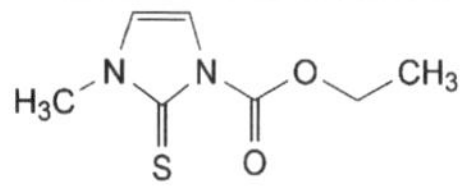

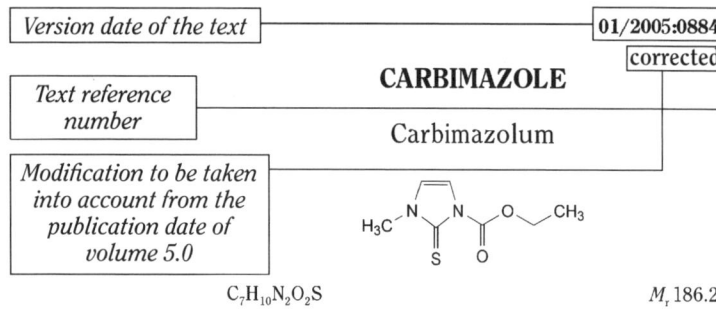

$C_7H_{10}N_2O_2S$ M_r 186.2

Chemical name in accordance with IUPAC nomenclature rules

DEFINITION

Ethyl 3-methyl-2-thioxo-2,3-dihydro-1*H*-imidazole-1-carboxylate.

Content: 98.0 per cent to 102.0 per cent (dried substance).

CHARACTERS

Appearance: white or yellowish-white, crystalline powder.

Solubility: slightly soluble in water, soluble in acetone and in alcohol.

Application of the first and second identification is defined in the General Notices (chapter 1)

IDENTIFICATION

First identification: B.

Second identification: A, C, D.

A. Melting point (*2.2.14*): 122 °C to 125 °C.

B. Infrared absorption spectrophotometry (*2.2.24*).

Preparation: discs.

Comparison: *carbimazole CRS*.

Chemical reference substance available from the Secretariat (see www.pheur.org)

C. Thin-layer chromatography (*2.2.27*).

Test solution. Dissolve 10 mg of the substance to be examined in *methylene chloride R* and dilute to 10 ml with the same solvent.

Reference solution. Dissolve 10 mg of *carbimazole CRS* in *methylene chloride R* and dilute to 10 ml with the same solvent.

Plate: *TLC silica gel GF_{254} plate R.*

Mobile phase: *acetone R*, *methylene chloride R* (20:80 *V/V*).

Reagents described in chapter 4

Application: 10 µl.

Development: over a path of 15 cm.

Drying: in air for 30 min.

Detection: examine in ultraviolet light at 254 nm.

Results: the principal spot in the chromatogram obtained with the test solution is similar in position and size to the principal spot in the chromatogram obtained with the reference solution.

D. Dissolve about 10 mg in a mixture of 50 ml of *water R* and 0.05 ml of *dilute hydrochloric acid R*. Add 1 ml of *potassium iodobismuthate solution R*. A red precipitate is formed.

TESTS

Impurity A and other related substances. Liquid chromatography (*2.2.29*).

Reference to a general chapter

Test solution. Dissolve 5.0 mg of the substance to be examined in 10.0 ml of a mixture of 20 volumes of *acetonitrile R* and 80 volumes of *water R*. Use this solution within 5 min of preparation.

Reference solution (a). Dissolve 5 mg of *thiamazole R* and 0.10 g of *carbimazole CRS* in a mixture of 20 volumes of *acetonitrile R* and 80 volumes of *water R* and dilute to 100.0 ml with the same mixture of solvents. Dilute 1.0 ml of this solution to 10.0 ml with a mixture of 20 volumes of *acetonitrile R* and 80 volumes of *water R*.

Reference solution (b). Dissolve 5.0 mg of *thiamazole R* in a mixture of 20 volumes of *acetonitrile R* and 80 volumes of *water R* and dilute to 10.0 ml with the same mixture of solvents. Dilute 1.0 ml of this solution to 100.0 ml with a mixture of 20 volumes of *acetonitrile R* and 80 volumes of *water R*.

Column:

- *size*: l = 0.15 m, Ø = 3.9 mm,
- *stationary phase*: *octadecylsilyl silica gel for chromatography R* (5 µm).

Mobile phase: *acetonitrile R*, *water R* (10:90 *V/V*).

Flow rate: 1 ml/min.

Detection: spectrophotometer at 254 nm.

Injection: 10 µl.

Run time: 1.5 times the retention time of carbimazole.

Retention time: carbimazole = about 6 min.

System suitability: reference solution (a):

- *resolution*: minimum 5.0 between the peaks due to impurity A and carbimazole.

Limits:

- *impurity A*: not more than half the area of the principal peak in the chromatogram obtained with reference solution (b) (0.5 per cent),
- *any other impurity*: not more than 0.1 times the area of the principal peak in the chromatogram obtained with reference solution (b) (0.1 per cent).

Loss on drying (*2.2.32*): maximum 0.5 per cent, determined on 1.000 g by drying in a desiccator over *diphosphorus pentoxide R* at a pressure not exceeding 0.7 kPa for 24 h.

Sulphated ash (*2.4.14*): maximum 0.1 per cent, determined on 1.0 g.

ASSAY

Dissolve 50.0 mg in *water R* and dilute to 500.0 ml with the same solvent. To 10.0 ml add 10 ml of *dilute hydrochloric acid R* and dilute to 100.0 ml with *water R*. Measure the absorbance (*2.2.25*) at the maximum at 291 nm. Calculate the content of $C_7H_{10}N_2O_2S$ taking the specific absorbance to be 557.

IMPURITIES

Specified impurities: A.

Other detectable impurities: B.

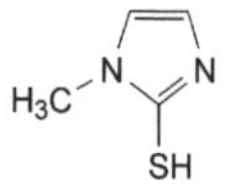

A. 1-methyl-1*H*-imidazole-2-thiol (thiamazole).

List of impurities detected by the tests (see the general monograph Substances for pharmaceutical use (2034) and chapter 5.10. Control of impurities in substances for pharmaceutical use)

See the information section on general monographs (cover pages)

General Notices (1) apply to all monographs and other texts

IMPORTANT NOTICE
GENERAL MONOGRAPHS

The European Pharmacopoeia contains a number of general monographs covering classes of products. These general monographs give requirements that are applicable to all products in the given class or, in some cases, to any product in the given class for which there is a specific monograph in the Pharmacopoeia (see *1. General Notices*, General monographs). Where no restriction on scope of a general monograph is given in a preamble, it is applicable to all products in the class defined, irrespective of whether there is an individual monograph for the product in the Pharmacopoeia.

Whenever a monograph is used, it is essential to ascertain whether there is a general monograph applicable to the product in question. The general monographs listed below are published in the section General Monographs (unless otherwise stated). This list is updated where necessary and republished in each Supplement.

Allergen products (1063)

Dosage Forms monographs
(published in the Dosage Forms section)

Extracts (0765)

Herbal drug preparations (1434)

Herbal drugs (1433)

Herbal drugs for homoeopathic preparations (2045)
(published in the Homoeopathy section)

Herbal teas (1435)

Homoeopathic preparations (1038)
(published in the Homoeopathy section)

Immunosera for human use, animal (0084)

Immunosera for veterinary use (0030)

Mother tinctures for homoeopathic preparations (2029)
(published in the Homoeopathy section)

Products of fermentation (1468)

Products with risk of transmitting agents of
animal spongiform encephalopathies (1483)

Radiopharmaceutical preparations (0125)

Recombinant DNA technology, products of (0784)

Substances for pharmaceutical use (2034)

Vaccines for human use (0153)

Vaccines for veterinary use (0062)

Vegetable fatty oils (1579)

Members of the European Pharmacopoeia Commission: Austria, Belgium, Bosnia and Herzegovina, Croatia, Cyprus, Czech Republic, Denmark, Estonia, Finland, France, Germany, Greece, Hungary, Iceland, Ireland, Italy, Latvia, Luxembourg, Netherlands, Norway, Portugal, Romania, Serbia and Montenegro, Slovak Republic, Slovenia, Spain, Sweden, Switzerland, "The former Yugoslav Republic of Macedonia", Turkey, United Kingdom and the European Union.

Observers to the European Pharmacopoeia Commission: Albania, Algeria, Australia, Bulgaria, Canada, China, Georgia, Lithuania, Malaysia, Malta, Morocco, Poland, Senegal, Syria, Tunisia, Ukraine and WHO (World Health Organisation).

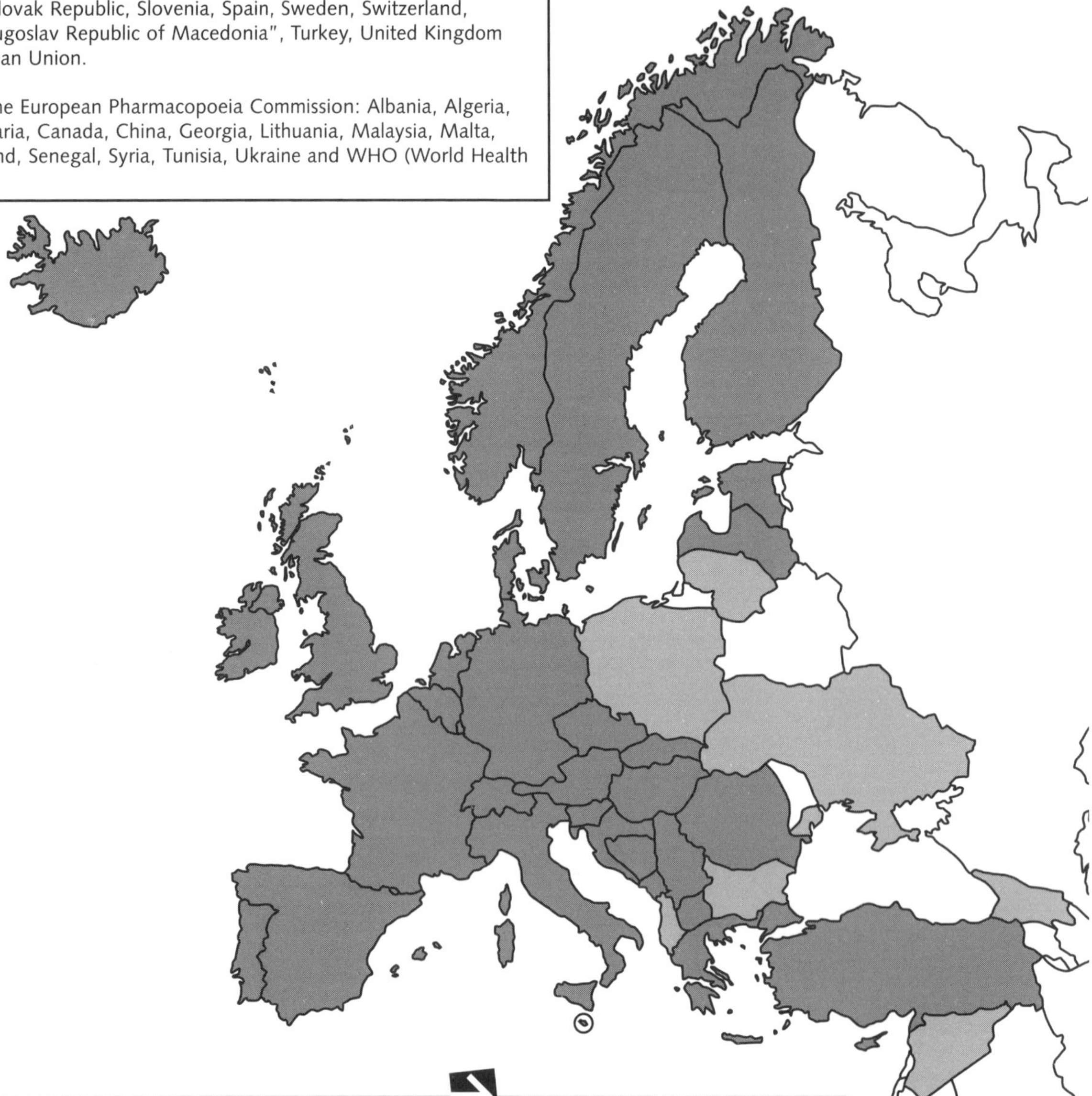

How to contact us

Information and orders **Internet : http://www.pheur.org**

European Directorate for the Quality of Medicines
Council of Europe - 226 avenue de Colmar BP 907
F-67029 STRASBOURG Cedex 1, FRANCE
Tel: +33 (0)3 88 41 30 30*
Fax: +33 (0)3 88 41 27 71*

	E-mail
CD-ROM	cdromtech@pheur.org
Certification	certification@pheur.org
Monographs	monographs@pheur.org
Publications	publications@pheur.org
Reference substances	crs@pheur.org
Conferences	publicrelations@pheur.org
All other correspondence	info@pheur.org

*: Do not dial 0 if calling from outside France.
All reference substances required for application of the monographs are available from the EDQM. A catalogue of reference substances is available on request; the catalogue is included in the Pharmeuropa subscription; it can also be consulted on the EDQM internet site.

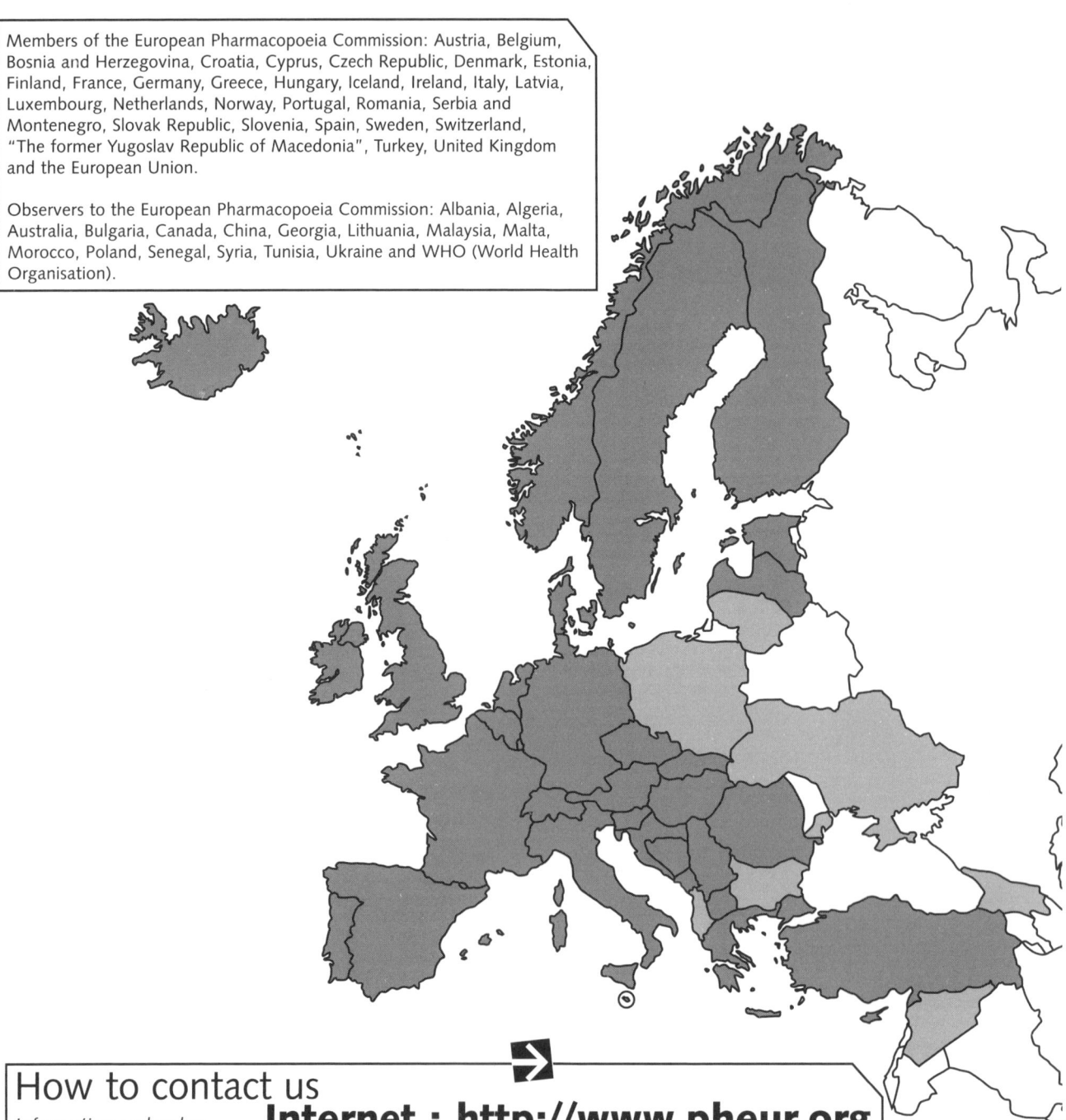

EUROPEAN PHARMACOPOEIA

FIFTH EDITION

Volume 2

EUROPEAN PHARMACOPOEIA

FIFTH EDITION

Volume 2

Published in accordance with the
Convention on the Elaboration of a European Pharmacopoeia
(European Treaty Series No. 50)

Council of Europe
Strasbourg

The European Pharmacopoeia is published by the Directorate for the Quality of Medicines of the Council of Europe (EDQM).

ISBN: 92-871-5281-0

Printed in France by Aubin, Ligugé

CONTENTS

VOLUME 1

VOLUME 2

Note : on the first page of each chapter/section there is a list of contents.

A

01/2005:0307

ACACIA

Acaciae gummi

DEFINITION

Acacia is the air-hardened, gummy exudate flowing naturally from or obtained by incision of the trunk and branches of *Acacia senegal* L. Willdenow, other species of *Acacia* of African origin and *Acacia seyal Del.*

CHARACTERS

Acacia is almost completely but very slowly soluble, after about 2 h, in twice its mass of water leaving only a very small residue of vegetable particles; the liquid obtained is colourless or yellowish, dense, viscous, adhesive, translucent and weakly acid to blue litmus paper. Acacia is practically insoluble in alcohol.

It has the macroscopic and microscopic characters described under identification tests A and B.

IDENTIFICATION

A. Acacia occurs as yellowish-white, yellow or pale amber, sometimes with a pinkish tint, friable, opaque, spheroidal, oval or reniform pieces (tears) of a diameter from about 1 cm to 3 cm, frequently with a cracked surface, easily broken into irregular, whitish or slightly yellowish angular fragments with conchoidal fracture and a glassy and transparent appearance. In the centre of an unbroken tear there is sometimes a small cavity.

B. Reduce to a powder (355). The powder is white or yellowish-white. Examine under a microscope using *glycerol R* (50 per cent *V/V*). The powder presents angular, irregular, colourless, transparent fragments. Only traces of starch or vegetable tissues are visible. No stratified membrane is apparent.

C. Examine the chromatograms obtained in the test for glucose and fructose. The chromatogram obtained with the test solution shows three zones due to galactose, arabinose and rhamnose. No other important zones are visible, particularly in the upper part of the chromatogram.

D. Dissolve 1 g of the powdered drug (355) in 2 ml of *water R* by stirring frequently for 2 h. Add 2 ml of *alcohol R*. After shaking, a white, gelatinous mucilage is formed which becomes fluid on adding 10 ml of *water R*.

TESTS

Solution S. Dissolve 3.0 g of the powdered drug (355) in 25 ml of *water R* by stirring for 30 min. Allow to stand for 30 min and dilute to 30 ml with *water R*.

Insoluble matter. To 5.0 g of the powdered drug (355) add 100 ml of *water R* and 14 ml of *dilute hydrochloric acid R*, boil gently for 15 min, shaking frequently, and filter while hot through a tared sintered-glass filter. Wash with hot *water R* and dry at 100-105 °C. The residue weighs not more than 25 mg (0.5 per cent).

Glucose and fructose. Examine by thin-layer chromatography (*2.2.27*), using a *TLC silica gel plate R*.

Test solution. To 0.100 g of the powdered drug (355) in a thick-walled centrifuge tube add 2 ml of a 100 g/l solution of *trifluoroacetic acid R*, shake vigorously to dissolve the forming gel, stopper the tube and heat the mixture at 120 °C for 1 h. Centrifuge the hydrolysate, transfer the clear supernatant carefully into a 50 ml flask, add 10 ml of *water R* and evaporate the solution to dryness under reduced pressure. To the resulting clear film add 0.1 ml of *water R* and 0.9 ml of *methanol R*. Centrifuge to separate the amorphous precipitate. Dilute the supernatant, if necessary, to 1 ml with *methanol R*.

Reference solution. Dissolve 10 mg of *arabinose R*, 10 mg of *galactose R*, 10 mg of *glucose R*, 10 mg of *rhamnose R* and 10 mg of *xylose R* in 1 ml of *water R* and dilute to 10 ml with *methanol R*.

Apply to the plate as bands 10 µl of each solution. Develop over a path of 10 cm using a mixture of 10 volumes of a 16 g/l solution of *sodium dihydrogen phosphate R*, 40 volumes of *butanol R* and 50 volumes of *acetone R*. Dry the plate in a current of warm air for a few minutes and develop again over a path of 15 cm using the same mobile phase. Dry the plate at 110 °C for 10 min, spray with *anisaldehyde solution R* and heat again at 110 °C for 10 min. The chromatogram obtained with the reference solution shows five clearly separated coloured zones due to galactose (greyish-green to green), glucose (grey), arabinose (yellowish-green) xylose (greenish-grey to yellowish-grey) and rhamnose (yellowish-green), in order of increasing R_f value. The chromatogram obtained with the test solution shows no grey zone and no greyish-green zone between the zones corresponding to galactose and arabinose in the chromatogram obtained with the reference solution.

Starch, dextrin and agar. To 10 ml of solution S previously boiled and cooled add 0.1 ml of *0.05 M iodine*. No blue or reddish-brown colour develops.

Sterculia gum

A. Place 0.2 g of the powdered drug (355) in a 10 ml ground-glass-stoppered cylinder graduated in 0.1 ml. Add 10 ml of *alcohol (60 per cent V/V) R* and shake. Any gel formed occupies not more than 1.5 ml.

B. To 1.0 g of the powdered drug (355) add 100 ml of *water R* and shake. Add 0.1 ml of *methyl red solution R*. Not more than 5.0 ml of *0.01 M sodium hydroxide* is required to change the colour of the indicator.

Tannins. To 10 ml of solution S add 0.1 ml of *ferric chloride solution R1*. A gelatinous precipitate is formed, but neither the precipitate nor the liquid shows a dark blue colour.

Tragacantha. Examine the chromatograms obtained in the test for glucose and fructose. The chromatogram obtained with the test solution shows no greenish-grey to yellowish-grey zone corresponding to the zone of xylose in the chromatogram obtained with the reference solution.

Loss on drying (*2.2.32*). Not more than 15.0 per cent, determined on 1.000 g of the powdered drug (355) by drying in an oven at 100-105 °C.

Total ash (*2.4.16*). Not more than 4.0 per cent.

Microbial contamination. Total viable aerobic count (*2.6.12*) not more than 10^4 micro-organisms per gram, determined by plate count. It complies with the test for *Escherichia coli* (*2.6.13*).

01/2005:0308

ACACIA, SPRAY-DRIED

Acaciae gummi dispersione desiccatum

DEFINITION

Spray-dried acacia is obtained from a solution of acacia.

CHARACTERS

It dissolves completely and rapidly, after about 20 min, in twice its mass of water. The liquid obtained is colourless or yellowish, dense, viscous, adhesive, translucent and weakly acid to blue litmus paper. Spray-dried acacia is practically insoluble in alcohol.

IDENTIFICATION

A. Examined under a microscope, in *alcohol R*, the powder is seen to consist predominantly of spheroidal particles about 4 µm to 40 µm in diameter, with a central cavity containing one or several air-bubbles; a few minute flat fragments are present. Only traces of starch granules are visible. No vegetable tissue is seen.

B. Examine the chromatograms obtained in the test for glucose and fructose. The chromatogram obtained with the test solution shows 3 zones due to galactose, arabinose and rhamnose. No other important zones are visible, particularly in the upper part of the chromatogram.

C. Dissolve 1 g of the drug to be examined in 2 ml of *water R* by stirring frequently for 20 min. Add 2 ml of *alcohol R*. After shaking a white gelatinous mucilage is formed which becomes fluid on adding 10 ml of *water R*.

TESTS

Solution S. Dissolve 3.0 g of the drug to be examined in 25 ml of *water R* by stirring for 10 min. Allow to stand for 20 min and dilute to 30 ml with *water R*.

Glucose and fructose. Examine by thin-layer chromatography (*2.2.27*), using a *TLC silica gel plate R*.

Test solution. To 0.100 g in a thick-walled centrifuge tube add 2 ml of a 100 g/l solution of *trifluoroacetic acid R*, shake vigorously to dissolve the forming gel, stopper the tube and heat the mixture at 120 °C for 1 h. Centrifuge the hydrolysate, transfer the clear supernatant carefully into a 50 ml flask, add 10 ml of *water R* and evaporate the solution to dryness under reduced pressure. To the resulting clear film add 0.1 ml of *water R* and 0.9 ml of *methanol R*. Centrifuge to separate the amorphous precipitate. Dilute the supernatant, if necessary, to 1 ml with *methanol R*.

Reference solution. Dissolve 10 mg of *arabinose R*, 10 mg of *galactose R*, 10 mg of *glucose R*, 10 mg of *rhamnose R* and 10 mg of *xylose R* in 1 ml of *water R* and dilute to 10 ml with *methanol R*.

Apply to the plate as bands 10 µl of each solution. Develop over a path of 10 cm using a mixture of 10 volumes of a 16 g/l solution of *sodium dihydrogen phosphate R*, 40 volumes of *butanol R* and 50 volumes of *acetone R*. Dry the plate in a current of warm air for a few minutes and develop again over a path of 15 cm using the same mobile phase. Dry the plate at 110 °C for 10 min, spray with *anisaldehyde solution R* and heat again at 110 °C for 10 min. The chromatogram obtained with the reference solution shows 5 clearly separated coloured zones due to galactose (greyish-green to green), glucose (grey), arabinose (yellowish-green) xylose (greenish-grey to yellowish-grey) and rhamnose (yellowish-green), in order of increasing R_f value. The chromatogram obtained with the test solution shows no grey zone and no greyish-green zone between the zones corresponding to galactose and arabinose in the chromatogram obtained with the reference solution.

Starch, dextrin and agar. To 10 ml of solution S previously boiled and cooled add 0.1 ml of *0.05 M iodine*. No blue or reddish-brown colour develops.

Sterculia gum

A. Place 0.2 g in a 10 ml ground-glass-stoppered cylinder graduated in 0.1 ml. Add 10 ml of *alcohol (60 per cent V/V) R* and shake. Any gel formed occupies not more than 1.5 ml.

B. To 1.0 g add 100 ml of *water R* and shake. Add 0.1 ml of *methyl red solution R*. Not more than 5.0 ml of *0.01 M sodium hydroxide* is required to change the colour of the indicator.

Tannins. To 10 ml of solution S add 0.1 ml of *ferric chloride solution R1*. A gelatinous precipitate is formed, but neither the precipitate nor the liquid shows a dark blue colour.

Tragacantha. Examine the chromatograms obtained in the test for Glucose and fructose. The chromatogram obtained with the test solution shows no greenish-grey to yellowish-grey zone corresponding to the zone of xylose in the chromatogram obtained with the reference solution.

Loss on drying (*2.2.32*). Not more than 10.0 per cent, determined on 1.000 g by drying in an oven at 100-105 °C.

Total ash (*2.4.16*). Not more than 4.0 per cent.

Microbial contamination. Total viable aerobic count (*2.6.12*) not more than 10^4 micro-organisms per gram, determined by plate count. It complies with the test for *Escherichia coli* (*2.6.13*).

01/2005:1585

ACAMPROSATE CALCIUM

Acamprosatum calcium

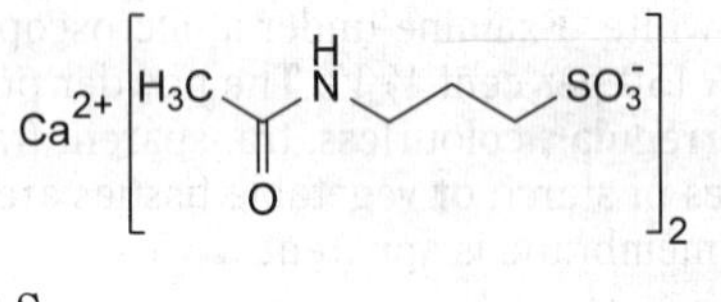

$C_{10}H_{20}CaN_2O_8S_2$ M_r 400.5

DEFINITION

Calcium bis[3-(acetylamino)propane-1-sulphonate].

Content: 98.0 per cent to 102.0 per cent (dried substance).

CHARACTERS

Appearance: white powder.

Solubility: freely soluble in water, practically insoluble in alcohol and in methylene chloride.

IDENTIFICATION

A. Infrared absorption spectrophotometry (*2.2.24*).

Comparison: *Ph. Eur. reference spectrum of acamprosate calcium.*

B. It gives reaction (a) of calcium (*2.3.1*).

TESTS

Solution S. Dissolve 5.0 g in *carbon dioxide-free water R* and dilute to 100 ml with the same solvent.

Appearance of solution. Solution S is clear (*2.2.1*) and colourless (*2.2.2, Method II*).

pH (*2.2.3*): 5.5 to 7.0 for solution S.

Impurity A. Liquid chromatography (*2.2.29*).

Test solution. Dissolve 0.40 g of the substance to be examined in *distilled water R* and dilute to 20.0 ml with the same solvent. Dilute 10.0 ml of this solution to 100.0 ml with *borate buffer solution pH 10.4 R*. Place 3.0 ml of the solution obtained in a 25 ml ground-glass-stoppered tube. Add 0.15 ml of a freshly prepared 5 g/l solution of *fluorescamine R* in *acetonitrile R*. Shake immediately and vigorously for 30 s. Place in a water-bath at 50 °C for 30 min. Cool under a stream of cold water. Centrifuge and filter the supernatant through a suitable membrane filter (0.45 μm), 25 mm in diameter.

Reference solution. Dissolve 50 mg of *acamprosate impurity A CRS* in *distilled water R* and dilute to 200.0 ml with the same solvent. Dilute 0.4 ml of the solution to 100.0 ml with *borate buffer solution pH 10.4 R*. Treat 3.0 ml of this solution in the same way as the test solution

Column:

- *size*: l = 0.15 m, Ø = 4.6 mm,
- *stationary phase*: *spherical octadecylsilyl silica gel for chromatography R* (5 μm) with a specific surface area of 170 m^2/g and a pore size of 12 nm.

Mobile phase: *acetonitrile R, methanol R, 0.1 M phosphate buffer solution pH 6.5 R* (10:10:80 *V/V/V*).

Flow rate: 1 ml/min.

Detection: spectrophotometer at 261 nm.

Injection: 20 μl.

Run time: 6 times the retention time of impurity A

Retention times: fluorescamine = about 4 min; impurity A = about 8 min; acamprosate is not detected by this system.

Limits:

- *impurity A*: not more than the area of the corresponding peak in the chromatogram obtained with the reference solution (0.05 per cent).

Heavy metals (*2.4.8*): maximum 10 ppm. Dissolve 2.0 g in *distilled water R* and dilute to 20 ml with the same solvent. 12 ml of the solution complies with limit test A. Prepare the standard using 10 ml of *lead standard solution (1 ppm Pb) R*.

Loss on drying (*2.2.32*): maximum 0.4 per cent, determined on 1.000 g by drying in an oven at 100-105 °C.

ASSAY

To 4 g of *cation exchange resin R* (75-150 μm) add 20 ml of *distilled water R* and stir magnetically for 10 min. Introduce this suspension into a glass column, 45 cm long and 2.2 cm in internal diameter, equipped with a polytetrafluoroethylene flow cap covered by a glass-wool plug. Allow a few millilitres of this solution to flow, then place a plug of glass wool over the resin. Pass 50 ml of *1 M hydrochloric acid* through the column. The pH of the eluate is close to 1. Wash with 3 quantities, each of 200 ml, of *distilled water R* to obtain an eluate at pH 6. Dissolve 0.100 g of the substance to be examined in 15 ml of *distilled water R*. Pass through the column and wash with 3 quantities, each of 25 ml, of *distilled water R*, collecting the eluate. Allow to elute until an eluate at pH 6 is obtained. Titrate the solution obtained with *0.1 M sodium hydroxide*, determining the end-point potentiometrically (*2.2.20*).

1 ml of *0.1 M sodium hydroxide* corresponds to 20.02 mg of $C_{10}H_{20}CaN_2O_8S_2$.

IMPURITIES

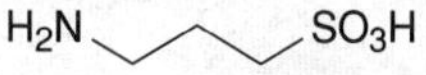

A. 3-aminopropane-1-sulphonic acid (homotaurine).

01/2005:0871

ACEBUTOLOL HYDROCHLORIDE

Acebutololi hydrochloridum

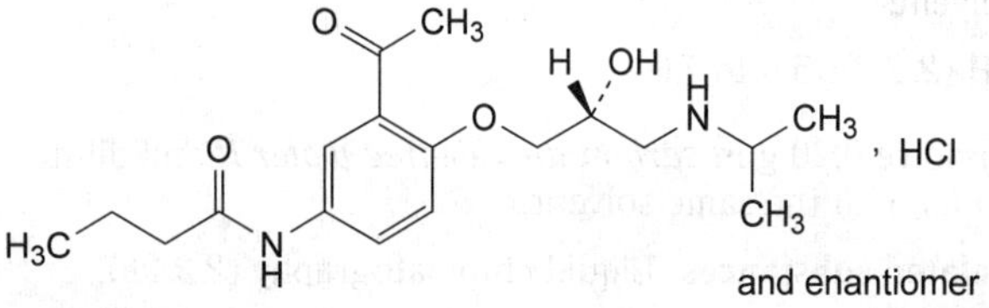

$C_{18}H_{29}ClN_2O_4$ M_r 372.9

DEFINITION

N-[3-Acetyl-4-[(2*RS*)-2-hydroxy-3-[(1-methylethyl)amino]propoxy]phenyl]butanamide hydrochloride.

Content: 99.0 per cent to 101.0 per cent (dried substance).

CHARACTERS

Appearance: white or almost white, crystalline powder.

Solubility: freely soluble in water and in alcohol, very slightly soluble in acetone and in methylene chloride.

mp: about 143 °C.

IDENTIFICATION

First identification: *B, D.*

Second identification: *A, C, D.*

A. Dissolve 20.0 mg in a 0.1 per cent *V/V* solution of *hydrochloric acid R* and dilute to 100.0 ml with the same acid solution. Dilute 5.0 ml to 100.0 ml with a 0.1 per cent *V/V* solution of *hydrochloric acid R*. Examined between 220 nm and 350 nm (*2.2.25*), the solution shows 2 absorption maxima, at 233 nm and 322 nm. The specific absorbance at the maximum at 233 nm is 555 to 605.

B. Infrared absorption spectrophotometry (*2.2.24*).

Preparation: discs.

Comparison: *acebutolol hydrochloride CRS*.

C. Thin-layer chromatography (*2.2.27*).

Test solution. Dissolve 20 mg of the substance to be examined in *methanol R* and dilute to 20 ml with the same solvent.

Reference solution (a). Dissolve 20 mg of *acebutolol hydrochloride CRS* in *methanol R* and dilute to 20 ml with the same solvent.

Reference solution (b). Dissolve 20 mg of *pindolol CRS* in *methanol R* and dilute to 20 ml with the same solvent. To 1 ml add 1 ml of reference solution (a).

Plate: *TLC silica gel F_{254} plate R.*

Mobile phase: *perchloric acid R, methanol R, water R* (5:395:600 *V/V/V*).

Application: 10 μl.

Development: over 3/4 of the plate.

Drying: in air.

Detection: examine in ultraviolet light at 254 nm.

System suitability: the chromatogram obtained with reference solution (b) shows 2 clearly separated principal spots.

Results: the principal spot in the chromatogram obtained with the test solution is similar in position and size to the principal spot in the chromatogram obtained with reference solution (a).

D. It gives reaction (a) of chlorides (*2.3.1*).

TESTS

Appearance of solution. The solution is not more opalescent than reference suspension II (*2.2.1*) and not more intensely coloured than reference solution BY_5 (*2.2.2, Method II*).

Dissolve 0.5 g in *water R* and dilute to 10 ml with the same solvent.

pH (*2.2.3*): 5.0 to 7.0.

Dissolve 0.20 g in *carbon dioxide-free water R* and dilute to 20 ml with the same solvent.

Related substances. Liquid chromatography (*2.2.29*).

Test solution. Dissolve 0.100 g of the substance to be examined in mobile phase A and dilute to 50.0 ml with mobile phase A.

Reference solution (a). Dissolve 20.0 mg of the substance to be examined in mobile phase A and dilute to 100.0 ml with mobile phase A. Dilute 0.5 ml to 50.0 ml with mobile phase A.

Reference solution (b). Dissolve 5.0 mg of *acebutolol impurity I CRS* in 10.0 ml of *acetonitrile R* and dilute to 25.0 ml with mobile phase A. Dilute 1.0 ml to 50.0 ml with mobile phase A.

Reference solution (c). Mix 2.0 ml of reference solution (a) and 1.0 ml of reference solution (b) and dilute to 10.0 ml with mobile phase A.

Reference solution (d). Dissolve 5.0 mg of *acebutolol impurity C CRS* in 10 ml of *acetonitrile R* and dilute to 25.0 ml with mobile phase A. Dilute 0.5 ml to 50.0 ml with mobile phase A.

Reference solution (e). Dissolve 5.0 mg of *acebutolol impurity B CRS* in 10.0 ml of *acetonitrile R* and dilute to 25.0 ml with mobile phase A. Dilute 1.0 ml to 50.0 ml with mobile phase A.

Column:

- *size*: l = 0.125 m, Ø = 4 mm,
- *stationary phase*: *end-capped octadecylsilyl silica gel for chromatography R* (5 µm),
- *temperature*: 40 °C.

Mobile phase:

- *mobile phase A*: mix 2.0 ml of *phosphoric acid R*, and 3.0 ml of *triethylamine R* and dilute to 1000 ml with *water R*,
- *mobile phase B*: mix equal volumes of *acetonitrile R* and mobile phase A,

Time (min)	Mobile phase A (per cent V/V)	Mobile phase B (per cent V/V)
0 - 2	98	2
2 - 30.5	98 → 10	2 → 90
30.5 - 41	10	90
41 - 42	10 → 98	90 → 2
42 - 50	98	2

Flow rate: 1.2 ml/min.

Detection: spectrophotometer at 240 nm.

Injection: 25 µl.

System suitability: reference solution (c):

- *resolution*: minimum 7.0 between the peaks due to impurity I and acebutolol.

Limits:

- *impurity B*: not more than the area of the principal peak in the chromatogram obtained with reference solution (e) (0.2 per cent),
- *impurity C*: not more than the area of the principal peak in the chromatogram obtained with reference solution (d) (0.1 per cent),
- *impurity I*: not more than the area of the principal peak in the chromatogram obtained with reference solution (b) (0.2 per cent),
- *any other impurity*: not more than the area of the principal peak in the chromatogram obtained with reference solution (a) (0.1 per cent),
- *total of impurities*: not more than 5 times the area of the principal peak in the chromatogram obtained with reference solution (a) (0.5 per cent),
- *disregard limit*: half the area of the principal peak in the chromatogram obtained with reference solution (a) (0.05 per cent).

Heavy metals (*2.4.8*): maximum 20 ppm.

Dissolve 0.50 g of the substance to be examined in 20.0 ml of *water R*. The solution complies with limit test E. Prepare the standard by diluting 10.0 ml of *lead standard solution (1 ppm Pb) R* to 20.0 ml with *water R*.

Loss on drying (*2.2.32*): maximum 0.5 per cent, determined on 1.000 g by drying in an oven at 100-105 °C for 3 h.

Sulphated ash (*2.4.14*): maximum 0.1 per cent, determined on 1.0 g.

ASSAY

Dissolve 0.300 g in 50 ml of *alcohol R* and add 1 ml of *0.1 M hydrochloric acid*. Carry out a potentiometric titration (*2.2.20*), using *0.1 M sodium hydroxide*. Read the volume added between the 2 points of inflexion.

1 ml of *0.1 M sodium hydroxide* is equivalent to 37.29 mg of $C_{18}H_{29}ClN_2O_4$.

STORAGE

Protected from light.

IMPURITIES

Specified impurities: *A, B, C, D, E, F, G, H, I, J, K*.

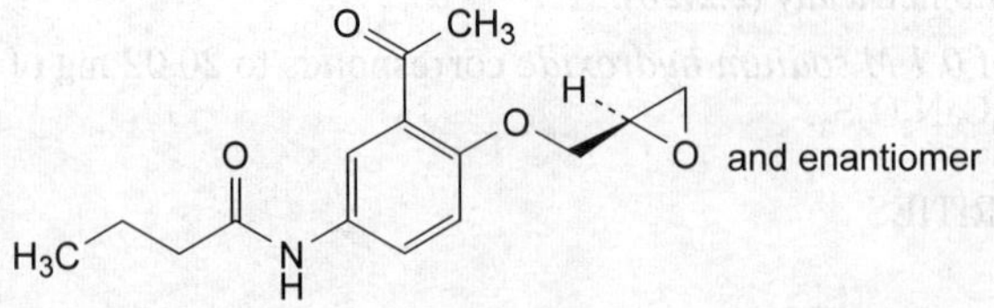

A. *N*-[3-acetyl-4-[(2*RS*)-oxiran-2-ylmethoxy]phenyl]butanamide,

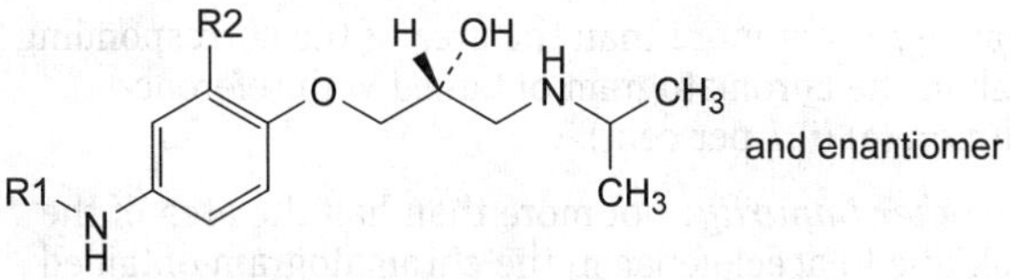

B. R1 = R2 = CO-CH_3: *N*-[3-acetyl-4-[(2*RS*)-2-hydroxy-3-[(1-methylethyl)amino]propoxy]phenyl]acetamide (diacetolol),

D. R1 = H, R2 = CO-CH_3: 1-[5-amino-2-[(2*RS*)-2-hydroxy-3-[(1-methylethyl)amino]propoxy]phenyl]ethanone,

E. R1 = CO-CH_2-CH_2-CH_3, R2 = H: *N*-[4-[(2*RS*)-2-hydroxy-3-[(1-methylethyl)amino]propoxy]phenyl]butanamide,

J. R1 = CO-CH_2-CH_3, R2 = CO-CH_3: *N*-[3-acetyl-4-[(2*RS*)-2-hydroxy-3-[(1-methylethyl)amino]propoxy]phenyl]propanamide,

K. R1 = R2 = CO-CH_2-CH_2-CH_3: *N*-[3-butanoyl-4-[(2*RS*)-2-hydroxy-3-[(1-methylethyl)amino]propoxy]phenyl]butanamide,

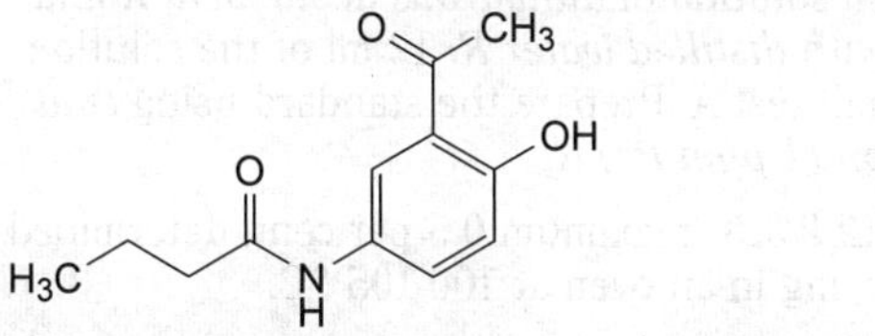

C. *N*-(3-acetyl-4-hydroxyphenyl)butanamide,

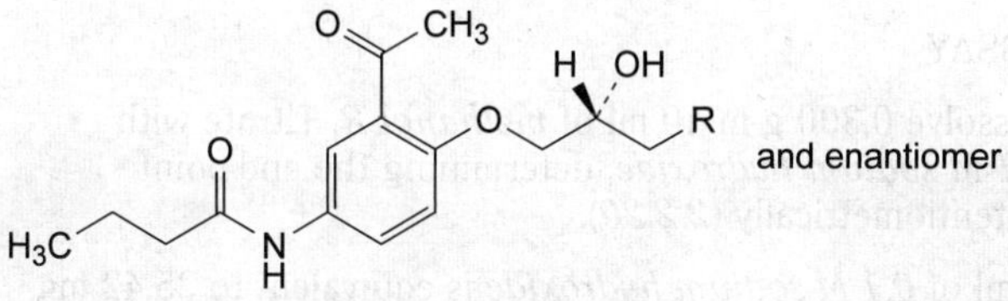

F. R = OH: *N*-[3-acetyl-4-[(2*RS*)-2,3-dihydroxypropoxy]phenyl]butanamide,

I. R = NH-CH_2-CH_3: *N*-[3-acetyl-4-[(2*RS*)-3-(ethylamino)-2-hydroxypropoxy]phenyl]butanamide,

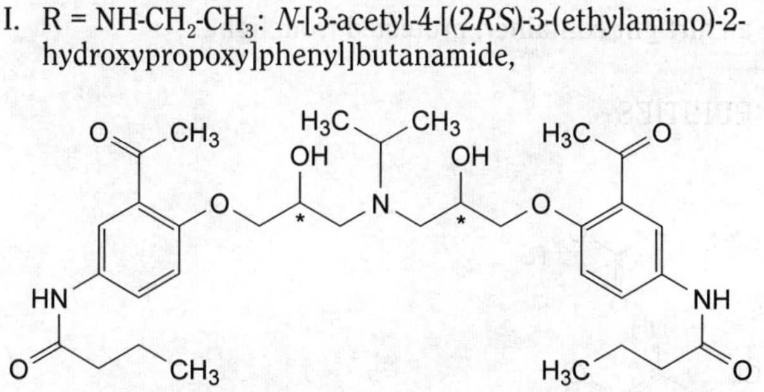

G. *N*,*N'*-[[(1-methylethyl)imino]bis[(2-hydroxypropane-1,3-diyl)oxy(3-acetyl-1,4-phenylene)]]dibutanamide (biamine),

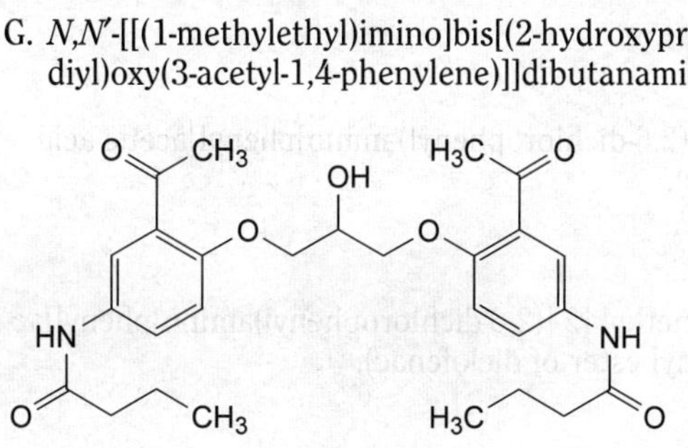

H. *N*,*N'*-[(2-hydroxypropane-1,3-diyl)bis[oxy(3-acetyl-1,4-phenylene)]]dibutanamide.

01/2005:1281

ACECLOFENAC

Aceclofenacum

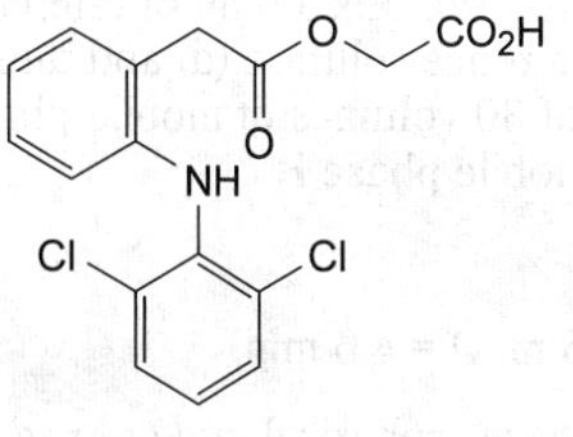

$C_{16}H_{13}Cl_2NO_4$ M_r 354.2

DEFINITION

[[[2-[(2,6-Dichlorophenyl)amino]phenyl]acetyl]oxy]acetic acid.

Content: 99.0 per cent to 101.0 per cent (dried substance).

CHARACTERS

Appearance: white or almost white, crystalline powder.

Solubility: practically insoluble in water, freely soluble in acetone, soluble in alcohol.

IDENTIFICATION

First identification: B.

Second identification: A, C.

A. Dissolve 50.0 mg in *methanol R* and dilute to 100.0 ml with the same solvent. Dilute 2.0 ml of the solution to 50.0 ml with *methanol R.* Examined between 220 nm and 370 nm (*2.2.25*), the solution shows an absorption maximum at 275 nm. The specific absorbance at the absorption maximum is 320 to 350.

B. Infrared absorption spectrophotometry (*2.2.24*).
Comparison: Ph. Eur. reference spectrum of aceclofenac.

C. Dissolve about 10 mg in 10 ml of *alcohol R*. To 1 ml of the solution, add 0.2 ml of a mixture, prepared immediately before use, of equal volumes of a 6 g/l solution of *potassium ferricyanide R* and a 9 g/l solution of *ferric chloride R*. Allow to stand protected from light for 5 min. Add 3 ml of a 10.0 g/l solution of *hydrochloric acid R*. Allow to stand protected from light for 15 min. A blue colour develops and a precipitate is formed.

TESTS

Related substances. Liquid chromatography (*2.2.29*). *Prepare the solutions immediately before use.*

Test solution. Dissolve 50.0 mg of the substance to be examined in a mixture of 30 volumes of mobile phase A and 70 volumes of mobile phase B and dilute to 25.0 ml with the same mixture of solvents.

Reference solution (a). Dissolve 21.6 mg of *diclofenac sodium CRS* in a mixture of 30 volumes of mobile phase A and 70 volumes of mobile phase B and dilute to 50.0 ml with the same mixture of solvents.

Reference solution (b). Dilute 2.0 ml of the test solution to 10.0 ml with a mixture of 30 volumes of mobile phase A and 70 volumes of mobile phase B.

Reference solution (c). Mix 1.0 ml of reference solution (a) and 1.0 ml of reference solution (b) and dilute to 100.0 ml with a mixture of 30 volumes of mobile phase A and 70 volumes of mobile phase B.

Reference solution (d). Dissolve 4.0 mg of *aceclofenac impurity F CRS*, 2.0 mg of *aceclofenac impurity H CRS* and 2.0 mg of *diclofenac impurity A CRS* (aceclofenac impurity I) in a mixture of 30 volumes of mobile phase A and 70 volumes of mobile phase B and dilute to 10.0 ml with the same mixture of solvents.

Reference solution (e). Mix 1.0 ml of reference solution (b) and 1.0 ml of reference solution (d) and dilute to 100.0 ml with a mixture of 30 volumes of mobile phase A and 70 volumes of mobile phase B.

Column:

- *size*: l = 0.25 m, Ø = 4.6 mm,
- *stationary phase*: spherical *end-capped octadecylsilyl silica gel for chromatography R* (5 µm) with a pore size of 10 nm and a carbon loading of 19 per cent,
- *temperature*: 40 °C.

Mobile phase:

- *mobile phase A*: 1.12 g/l solution of *phosphoric acid R* adjusted to pH 7.0 using a 42 g/l solution of *sodium hydroxide R*,
- *mobile phase B*: *water R, acetonitrile R* (1:9 *V/V*),

Time (min)	Mobile phase A (per cent *V/V*)	Mobile phase B (per cent *V/V*)
0 - 25	70 → 50	30 → 50
25 - 30	50 → 20	50 → 80
30 - 50	20	80
50 - 52	20 → 70	80 → 30
52 - 65	70	30

Flow rate: 1.0 ml/min.

Detection: spectrophotometer at 275 nm.

Injection: 10 µl; inject the test solution and reference solutions (c) and (e).

Relative retention with reference to aceclofenac (retention time = about 14 min): impurity A = about 0.8; impurity G = about 1.3; impurity H = about 1.5; impurity I = about 2.3; impurity D = about 2.6; impurity B = about 2.7; impurity E = about 2.8; impurity C = about 3.0; impurity F = about 3.2.

System suitability: reference solution (c):

- *resolution*: minimum 5.0 between the peaks due to aceclofenac and to impurity A.

Limits:

- *impurity A*: not more than the area of the corresponding peak in the chromatogram obtained with reference solution (c) (0.2 per cent),
- *impurities B, C, D, E, G*: for each impurity, not more than the area of the peak due to aceclofenac in the chromatogram obtained with reference solution (e) (0.2 per cent),
- *impurity F*: not more than the area of the corresponding peak in the chromatogram obtained with reference solution (e) (0.2 per cent),
- *impurity H*: not more than the area of the corresponding peak in the chromatogram obtained with reference solution (e) (0.1 per cent),
- *impurity I*: not more than the area of the corresponding peak in the chromatogram obtained with reference solution (e) (0.1 per cent),
- *any other impurity*: not more than half the area of the peak due to aceclofenac in the chromatogram obtained with reference solution (e) (0.1 per cent),
- *total*: not more than 0.7 per cent,
- *disregard limit*: 0.1 times the area of the peak due to aceclofenac in the chromatogram obtained with reference solution (e) (0.02 per cent).

Heavy metals (*2.4.8*): maximum 10 ppm.

To 2.0 g in a silica crucible, add 2 ml of *sulphuric acid R* to wet the substance. Heat progressively to ignition and continue heating until an almost white or at most a greyish residue is obtained. Carry out the ignition at a temperature not exceeding 800 °C. Allow to cool. Add 3 ml of *hydrochloric acid R* and 1 ml of *nitric acid R*. Heat and evaporate slowly to dryness. Cool and add 1 ml of a 100 g/l solution of *hydrochloric acid R* and 10.0 ml of *distilled water R*. Neutralise with a 1.0 g/l solution of *ammonia R* using 0.1 ml of *phenolphthalein solution R* as indicator. Add 2.0 ml of a 60 g/l solution of *anhydrous acetic acid R* and dilute to 20 ml with *distilled water R*. 12 ml of the solution complies with limit test A. Prepare the standard using *lead standard solution (1 ppm Pb) R*.

Loss on drying (*2.2.32*): maximum 0.5 per cent, determined on 1.000 g by drying in an oven at 100-105 °C.

Sulphated ash (*2.4.14*): maximum 0.1 per cent, determined on 1.0 g.

ASSAY

Dissolve 0.300 g in 40 ml of *methanol R*. Titrate with *0.1 M sodium hydroxide*, determining the end-point potentiometrically (*2.2.20*).

1 ml of *0.1 M sodium hydroxide* is equivalent to 35.42 mg of $C_{16}H_{13}Cl_2NO_4$.

STORAGE

In an airtight container, protected from light.

IMPURITIES

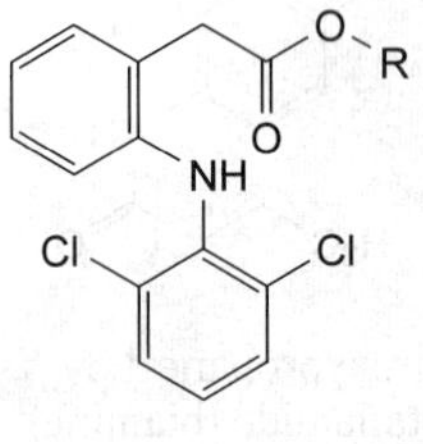

A. R = H: [2-[(2,6-dichlorophenyl)amino]phenyl]acetic acid (diclofenac),

B. R = CH_3: methyl [2-[(2,6-dichlorophenyl)amino]phenyl]acetate (methyl ester of diclofenac),

C. R = C_2H_5: ethyl [2-[(2,6-dichlorophenyl)amino]phenyl]acetate (ethyl ester of diclofenac),

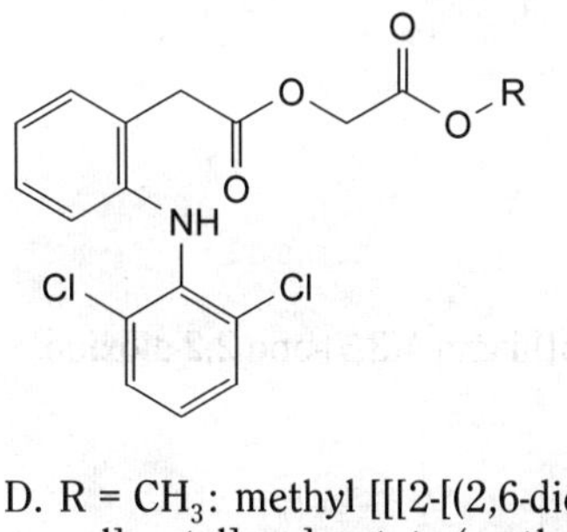

D. R = CH_3: methyl [[[2-[(2,6-dichlorophenyl)amino]phenyl]acetyl]oxy]acetate (methyl ester of aceclofenac),

E. R = C_2H_5: ethyl [[[2-[(2,6-dichlorophenyl)amino]phenyl]acetyl]oxy]acetate (ethyl ester of aceclofenac),

F. R = CH_2-C_6H_5: benzyl [[[2-[(2,6-dichlorophenyl)amino]phenyl]acetyl]oxy]acetate (benzyl ester of aceclofenac),

G. R = CH_2-CO_2H: [[[[[2-[(2,6-dichlorophenyl)amino]phenyl]acetyl]oxy]acetyl]oxy]acetic acid (acetic aceclofenac),

H. R = CH_2-CO-O-CH_2-CO_2H: [[[[[[[2-[(2,6-dichlorophenyl)amino]phenyl]acetyl]oxy]acetyl]oxy]acetyl]oxy]acetic acid (diacetic aceclofenac),

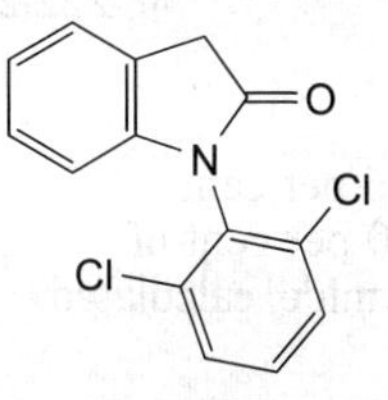

I. 1-(2,6-dichlorophenyl)-1,3-dihydro-2*H*-indol-2-one.

01/2005:1282

ACESULFAME POTASSIUM

Acesulfamum kalicum

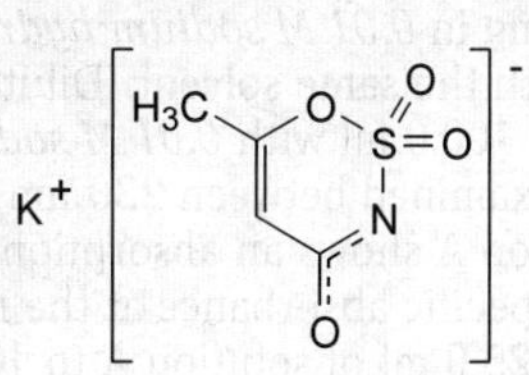

$C_4H_4KNO_4S$ M_r 201.2

DEFINITION

Acesulfame potassium contains not less than 99.0 per cent and not more than the equivalent of 101.0 per cent of potassium 6-methyl-1,2,3-oxathiazin-4-olate 2,2-dioxide, calculated with reference to the dried substance.

CHARACTERS

A white, crystalline powder or colourless crystals, soluble in water, very slightly soluble in acetone and in alcohol.

IDENTIFICATION

First identification: A, C.

Second identification: B, C.

A. Examine by infrared absorption spectrophotometry (*2.2.24*), comparing with the spectrum obtained with *acesulfame potassium CRS*. Examine the substances prepared as discs.

B. Examine by thin-layer chromatography (*2.2.27*), using *cellulose for chromatography R* as the coating substance.

Test solution. Dissolve 5 mg of the substance to be examined in *water R* and dilute to 5 ml with the same solvent.

Reference solution (a). Dissolve 5 mg of *acesulfame potassium CRS* in *water R* and dilute to 5 ml with the same solvent.

Reference solution (b). Dissolve 5 mg of *acesulfame potassium CRS* and 5 mg of *saccharin sodium R* in *water R* and dilute to 5 ml with the same solvent.

Apply to the plate as bands 5 µl of each solution. Develop twice over a path of 15 cm using a mixture of 10 volumes ofconcentrated *ammonia R*, 60 volumes of *acetone R* and 60 volumes of *ethyl acetate R*. Dry the plate in a current of warm air and examine in ultraviolet light at 254 nm. The principal band in the chromatogram obtained with the test solution is similar in position and size to the principal band in the chromatogram obtained with reference solution (a). The test is not valid unless the chromatogram obtained with reference solution (b) shows two clearly separated bands.

C. 0.5 ml of solution S (see Tests) gives reaction (b) of potassium (*2.3.1*).

TESTS

Solution S. Dissolve 10.0 g in *carbon dioxide-free water R* and dilute to 50 ml with the same solvent.

Appearance of solution. Solution S is clear (*2.2.1*) and colourless (*2.2.2, Method II*).

Acidity or alkalinity. To 20 ml of solution S add 0.1 ml of *bromothymol blue solution R1*. Not more than 0.2 ml of *0.01 M hydrochloric acid* or *0.01 M sodium hydroxide* is required to change the colour of the indicator.

Acetylacetamide. Examine by thin-layer chromatography (*2.2.27*), using a suitable silica gel as the coating substance.

Test solution. Dissolve 0.80 g of the substance to be examined in *water R* and dilute to 10 ml with the same solvent.

Reference solution (a). Dissolve 50 mg of *acetylacetamide R* in *water R* and dilute to 25 ml with the same solvent. To 5 ml of the solution add 45 ml of *water R* and dilute to 100 ml with *methanol R*.

Reference solution (b). To 10 ml of reference solution (a) add 1 ml of the test solution and dilute to 20 ml with *methanol R*.

Apply separately to the plate 5 µl of each solution. Develop over a path of 15 cm using a mixture of 2 volumes of *water R*, 15 volumes of *alcohol R* and 74 volumes of *ethyl acetate R*. Allow the plate to dry in air until the solvents are completely removed. Spray the plate with *vanillin phosphoric solution R* and heat at 120 °C for about 10 min. Examine in daylight. Any spot corresponding to acetylacetamide in the chromatogram obtained with the test solution, is not more intense than the spot in the chromatogram obtained with reference solution (a) (0.125 per cent). The test is not valid unless the chromatogram obtained with reference solution (a) shows a clearly visible spot and the chromatogram obtained with reference solution (b) shows two clearly separated spots.

Impurity B and related substances. Examine by liquid chromatography (*2.2.29*).

Test solution. Dissolve 0.100 g of the substance to be examined in *water R* and dilute to 10.0 ml with the same solvent.

Reference solution (a). Dissolve 20.0 mg of *acesulfame potassium impurity B CRS* in *water R* and dilute to 500.0 ml with the same solvent. Dilute 0.5 ml of this solution to 100.0 ml with *water R*.

Reference solution (b). Dissolve 10.0 mg of *acesulfame potassium impurity B CRS* and 10.0 mg of *acesulfame potassium CRS* in *water R* and dilute to 500.0 ml with the same solvent. Dilute 5.0 ml of this solution to 100.0 ml with *water R.*

The chromatographic procedure may be carried out using:

- a stainless steel column 0.25 m long and 4.6 mm in internal diameter packed with *octadecylsilyl silica gel for chromatography R* (3 μm),
- as mobile phase at a flow rate of 1 ml/min a mixture of 40 volumes of *acetonitrile R* and 60 volumes of a 3.3 g/l solution of *tetrabutylammonium hydrogen sulphate R,*
- as detector a spectrophotometer set at 234 nm.

Inject 20 μl of reference solution (b). Adjust the sensitivity of the system so that the height of the two principal peaks is at least 50 per cent of the full scale of the recorder. The test is not valid unless the resolution between the two peaks due to acesulfame and impurity B is at least 3.0.

Inject 20 μl of the test solution and 20 μl of reference solution (a). Continue the chromatography of the test solution for at least three times the retention time of the principal peak. In the chromatogram obtained with the test solution the area of any peak apart from the principal peak is not greater than the area of the principal peak in the chromatogram obtained with reference solution (a) (20 ppm).

Fluorides. Not more than 3 ppm of F, determined potentiometrically (*2.2.36, Method I*) using as indicator electrode a fluoride selective-membrane electrode and as reference electrode a silver-silver chloride electrode.

Test solution. Dissolve 3.000 g of the substance to be examined in *distilled water R,* add 15.0 ml of *total ionic strength adjustment buffer R1* and dilute to 50.0 ml with *distilled water R.*

Reference solutions. To 0.5 ml, 1.0 ml, 1.5 ml and 3.0 ml of *fluoride standard solution (10 ppm F) R* add 15.0 ml of *total ionic strength adjustment buffer R1* and dilute to 50.0 ml with *distilled water R.*

Carry out the measurements of each solution.

Heavy metals (*2.4.8*). 12 ml of solution S complies with the limit test A for heavy metals (5 ppm). Prepare the standard using *lead standard solution (1 ppm Pb) R.*

Loss on drying (*2.2.32*). Not more than 1.0 per cent, determined on 1.000 g by drying in an oven at 100 °C to 105 °C for 3 h.

ASSAY

Dissolve 0.150 g in 50 ml of *anhydrous acetic acid R.* Titrate with *0.1 M perchloric acid,* determining the end-point potentiometrically (*2.2.20*).

1 ml of *0.1 M perchloric acid* is equivalent to 20.12 mg of $C_4H_4KNO_4S$.

IMPURITIES

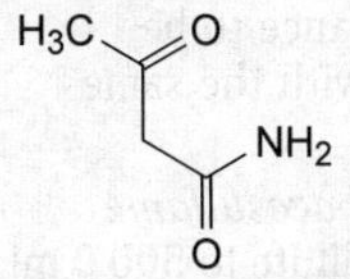

A. 3-oxobutanamide (acetylacetamide),

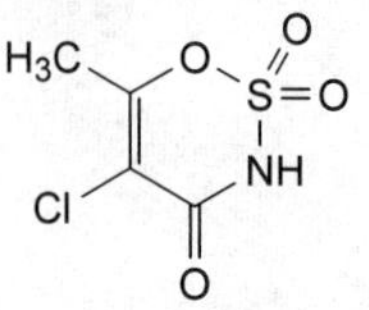

B. 5-chloro-6-methyl-1,2,3-oxathiazin-4(3*H*)-one 2,2-dioxide.

01/2005:0454

ACETAZOLAMIDE

Acetazolamidum

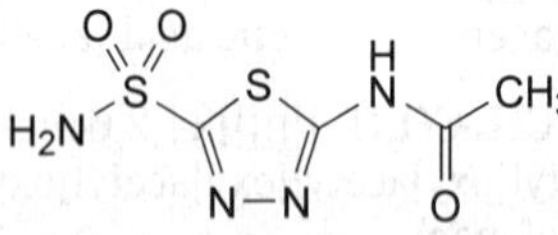

$C_4H_6N_4O_3S_2$ M_r 222.2

DEFINITION

Acetazolamide contains not less than 98.5 per cent and not more than the equivalent of 101.0 per cent of *N*-(5-sulphamoyl-1,3,4-thiadiazol-2-yl)acetamide, calculated with reference to the dried substance.

CHARACTERS

A white or almost white, crystalline powder, very slightly soluble in water, slightly soluble in alcohol. It dissolves in dilute solutions of alkali hydroxides.

IDENTIFICATION

First identification: A, B.

Second identification: A, C, D.

A. Dissolve 30.0 mg in *0.01 M sodium hydroxide* and dilute to 100.0 ml with the same solvent. Dilute 10.0 ml of the solution to 100.0 ml with *0.01 M sodium hydroxide* (solution A). Examined between 230 nm and 260 nm (*2.2.25*), solution A shows an absorption maximum at 240 nm. The specific absorbance at the maximum is 162 to 176. Dilute 25.0 ml of solution A to 100.0 ml with *0.01 M sodium hydroxide.* Examined between 260 nm and 350 nm, the solution shows an absorption maximum at 292 nm. The specific absorbance at the maximum is 570 to 620.

B. Examine by infrared absorption spectrophotometry (*2.2.24*), comparing with the spectrum obtained with *acetazolamide CRS.* If the spectra obtained in the solid state with the substance to be examined and the reference substance show differences, dissolve separately the substance to be examined and the reference substance in *alcohol R,* evaporate to dryness, prepare new discs and record the spectra.

C. Introduce about 20 mg into a test-tube and add 4 ml of *dilute hydrochloric acid R* and 0.2 g of *zinc powder R.* Immediately place a piece of *lead acetate paper R* over the mouth of the tube. The paper shows a brownish-black colour.

D. Dissolve about 25 mg in a mixture of 0.1 ml of *dilute sodium hydroxide solution R* and 5 ml of *water R.* Add 0.1 ml of *copper sulphate solution R.* A greenish-blue precipitate is formed.

TESTS

Appearance of solution. Dissolve 1.0 g in 10 ml of *1 M sodium hydroxide.* The solution is not more opalescent than reference suspension II (*2.2.1*) and not more intensely coloured than reference solution Y_5 or BY_5 (*2.2.2, Method II*).

Related substances. Examine by thin-layer chromatography (*2.2.27*), using *silica gel GF_{254} R* as the coating substance.

Test solution. Dissolve 50 mg of the substance to be examined in a mixture of equal volumes of *alcohol R* and *ethyl acetate R* and dilute to 10 ml with the same mixture of solvents.

Reference solution. Dilute 1 ml of the test solution to 100 ml with a mixture of equal volumes of *alcohol R* and *ethyl acetate R.*

Apply separately to the plate 20 µl of each solution. Use the tank without lining the walls and allow to saturate for 1 h before development. Develop over a path of 15 cm using a freshly prepared mixture of 20 volumes of *concentrated ammonia R,* 30 volumes of *ethyl acetate R* and 50 volumes of *2-propanol R.* Allow the plate to dry in air and examine in ultraviolet light at 254 nm. Any spot in the chromatogram obtained with the test solution, apart from the principal spot, is not more intense than the spot in the chromatogram obtained with the reference solution (1 per cent).

Sulphates (*2.4.13*). To 0.4 g add 20 ml of *distilled water R* and dissolve by heating to boiling. Allow to cool with frequent shaking and filter. 15 ml of the filtrate complies with the limit test for sulphates (500 ppm).

Heavy metals (*2.4.8*). 1.0 g complies with limit test C for heavy metals (20 ppm). Prepare the standard using 2 ml of *lead standard solution (10 ppm Pb) R.*

Loss on drying (*2.2.32*). Not more than 0.5 per cent, determined on 1.000 g by drying in an oven at 100 °C to 105 °C.

Sulphated ash (*2.4.14*). Not more than 0.1 per cent, determined on 1.0 g.

ASSAY

Dissolve 0.200 g in 25 ml of *dimethylformamide R.* Titrate with *0.1 M ethanolic sodium hydroxide,* determining the end-point potentiometrically (*2.2.20*).

1 ml of *0.1 M ethanolic sodium hydroxide* is equivalent to 22.22 mg of $C_4H_6N_4O_3S_2$.

01/2005:0590

ACETIC ACID, GLACIAL

Acidum aceticum glaciale

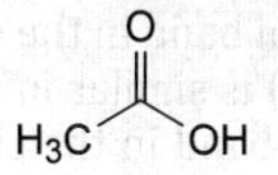

$C_2H_4O_2$ M_r 60.1

DEFINITION

Glacial acetic acid contains not less than 99.0 per cent *m/m* and not more than the equivalent of 100.5 per cent *m/m* of $C_2H_4O_2$.

CHARACTERS

A crystalline mass or a clear, colourless, volatile liquid, miscible with water, with alcohol and with methylene chloride.

IDENTIFICATION

A. A 100 g/l solution is strongly acid (*2.2.4*).

B. To 0.03 ml add 3 ml of *water R* and neutralise with *dilute sodium hydroxide solution R.* The solution gives reaction (b) of acetates (*2.3.1*).

TESTS

Solution S. Dilute 20 ml to 100 ml with *distilled water R.*

Appearance. It is clear (*2.2.1*) and colourless (*2.2.2, Method II*).

Freezing point (*2.2.18*). Not less than 14.8 °C.

Reducing substances. To 5.0 ml add 10.0 ml of *water R* and mix. To 5.0 ml of the solution add 6 ml of *sulphuric acid R,* cool and add 2.0 ml of *0.0167 M potassium dichromate.* Allow to stand for 1 min and add 25 ml of *water R* and 1 ml of a freshly prepared 100 g/l solution of *potassium iodide R.* Titrate with *0.1 M sodium thiosulphate,* using 1.0 ml of *starch solution R* as indicator. Not less than 1.0 ml of *0.1 M sodium thiosulphate* solution is required.

Chlorides (*2.4.4*). 10 ml of solution S diluted to 15 ml with *water R* complies with the limit test for chlorides (25 mg/l).

Sulphates (*2.4.13*). 15 ml of solution S complies with the limit test for sulphates (50 mg/l).

Iron (*2.4.9*). 5.0 ml of solution (a) obtained in the test for heavy metals diluted to 10.0 ml with *water R* complies with the limit test for iron (5 ppm).

Heavy metals (*2.4.8*). Dissolve the residue obtained in the test for residue on evaporation by heating with two quantities, each of 15 ml, of *water R* and dilute to 50.0 ml (solution (a)). 12 ml of solution (a) complies with limit test A for heavy metals (5 ppm). Prepare the standard using *lead standard solution (2 ppm Pb) R.*

Residue on evaporation. Evaporate 20 g to dryness on a water-bath and dry at 100 °C to 105 °C. The residue weighs not more than 2.0 mg (0.01 per cent).

ASSAY

Weigh accurately a conical flask with a ground-glass stopper containing 25 ml of *water R.* Add 1.0 ml of the substance to be examined and weigh again accurately. Add 0.5 ml of *phenolphthalein solution R* and titrate with *1 M sodium hydroxide.*

1 ml of *1 M sodium hydroxide* is equivalent to 60.1 mg of $C_2H_4O_2$.

STORAGE

Store in an airtight container.

01/2005:0872

ACETONE

Acetonum

C_3H_6O M_r 58.08

DEFINITION

Acetone is propan-2-one.

CHARACTERS

A volatile clear, colourless liquid, miscible with water and with alcohol. The vapour is flammable.

IDENTIFICATION

A. To 1 ml, add 3 ml of *dilute sodium hydroxide solution R* and 0.3 ml of a 25 g/l solution of *sodium nitroprusside R*. An intense red colour is produced which becomes violet with the addition of 3.5 ml of *acetic acid R*.

B. To 10 ml of a 0.1 per cent *V/V* solution in *alcohol (50 per cent V/V) R*, add 1 ml of a 10 g/l solution of *nitrobenzaldehyde R* in the same solvent and 0.5 ml of *strong sodium hydroxide solution R*. Allow to stand for about 2 min and acidify with *acetic acid R*. A greenish-blue colour is produced.

TESTS

Appearance of solution. To 10 ml add 10 ml of *water R*. The solution is clear (*2.2.1*) and colourless (*2.2.2, Method II*).

Acidity or alkalinity. To 5 ml add 5 ml of *carbon dioxide-free water R*, 0.15 ml of *phenolphthalein solution R* and 0.5 ml of *0.01 M sodium hydroxide*. The solution is pink. Add 0.7 ml of *0.01 M hydrochloric acid* and 0.05 ml of *methyl red solution R*. The solution is red or orange.

Relative density (*2.2.5*). 0.790 to 0.793.

Related substances. Examine by gas chromatography (*2.2.28*).

Test solution. The substance to be examined.

Reference solution. To 0.5 ml of *methanol R* add 0.5 ml of *2-propanol R* and dilute to 100.0 ml with the test solution. Dilute 1.0 ml to 10.0 ml with the test solution.

The chromatographic procedure may be carried out using:

– a fused-silica column 50 m long and 0.3 mm in internal diameter coated with a film (0.5 µm) of *macrogol 20 000 R*,
– *helium for chromatography R* as the carrier gas with a split ratio of about 50:1 and at a linear flow of 21 cm/s,
– a flame-ionisation detector,

maintaining the temperature of the column at 45 °C until injection, then raising the temperature at a rate of 5 °C per minute to 100 °C and maintaining the temperature of the injection port at 150 °C and that of the detector at 250 °C.

Inject 1 µl of the test solution and 1 µl of the reference solution.

When the chromatograms are recorded in the conditions described above, the substances are eluted in the following order: acetone, methanol, 2-propanol.

Continue the chromatography for three times the retention time of acetone (which is about 5.3 min).

The test is not valid unless, in the chromatogram obtained with the reference solution, the resolution between the peaks corresponding to methanol and 2-propanol is at least 1.0.

In the chromatogram obtained with the test solution: the area of any peak corresponding to methanol or 2-propanol is not greater than the difference between the areas of the corresponding peaks in the chromatogram obtained with the reference solution and the areas of the corresponding peaks in the chromatogram obtained with the test solution (0.05 per cent *V/V* for each impurity); the area of any peak, apart from the principal peak and any peaks corresponding to methanol and 2-propanol, is not greater than the difference between the area of the methanol peak in the chromatogram obtained with the reference solution and the area of the corresponding peak in the chromatogram obtained with the test solution (0.05 per cent *V/V* for each of the additional impurities).

Matter insoluble in water. To 1 ml add 19 ml of *water R*. The solution is clear (*2.2.1*).

Reducing substances. To 30 ml add 0.1 ml of *0.02 M potassium permanganate* and allow to stand in the dark for 2 h. The mixture is not completely decolourised.

Residue on evaporation. Evaporate 20.0 g to dryness on a water-bath and dry at 100 °C to 105 °C. The residue weighs not more than 1 mg (50 ppm).

Water (*2.5.12*). Not more than 3 g/l, determined on 10.0 ml by the semi-micro determination of water. Use 20 ml of *anhydrous pyridine R* as solvent.

STORAGE

Store protected from light.

IMPURITIES

A. CH_3-OH: methanol,

B. propan-2-ol.

01/2005:1485
corrected

ACETYLCHOLINE CHLORIDE

Acetylcholini chloridum

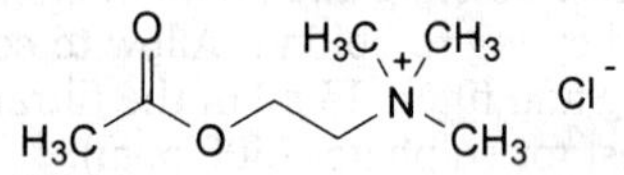

$C_7H_{16}ClNO_2$ M_r 181.7

DEFINITION

2-(Acetyloxy)-*N,N,N*-trimethylethanaminium chloride.

Content: 98.5 per cent to 101.5 per cent (dried substance).

CHARACTERS

Appearance: white or almost white crystalline powder or colourless crystals, very hygroscopic.

Solubility: very soluble in water, freely soluble in alcohol, slightly soluble in methylene chloride.

IDENTIFICATION

First identification: B, E.

Second identification: A, C, D, E.

A. Melting point (*2.2.14*): 149 °C to 152 °C.
Introduce the substance to be examined into a capillary tube. Dry in an oven at 100-105 °C for 3 h. Seal the tube and determine the melting point.

B. Infrared absorption spectrophotometry (*2.2.24*).
Comparison: *acetylcholine chloride CRS.*

C. Examine the chromatograms obtained in the test for related substances.
Results: the principal band in the chromatogram obtained with test solution (b) is similar in position, colour and size to the principal band in the chromatogram obtained with reference solution (b).

D. To 15 mg add 10 ml of *dilute sodium hydroxide solution R*, 2 ml of *0.02 M potassium permanganate* and heat. The vapours formed change the colour of *red litmus paper R* to blue.

E. 0.5 ml of solution S (see Tests) gives reaction (a) of chlorides (*2.3.1*).

TESTS

Solution S. Dissolve 5.0 g in *carbon dioxide-free water R* and dilute to 50 ml with the same solvent.

Appearance of solution. Solution S is clear (*2.2.1*) and not more intensely coloured than reference solution Y_6 or BY_6 (*2.2.2, Method II*).

Acidity. Dilute 1 ml of solution S to 10 ml with *carbon dioxide-free water R*. Add 0.05 ml of *phenolphthalein solution R*. Not more than 0.4 ml of *0.01 M sodium hydroxide* is required to change the colour of the indicator to pink.

Related substances. Thin-layer chromatography (*2.2.27*). *Prepare the solutions immediately before use.*

Test solution (a). Dissolve 0.30 g of the substance to be examined in *methanol R* and dilute to 3.0 ml with the same solvent.

Test solution (b). Dilute 1 ml of test solution (a) to 10 ml with *methanol R*.

Reference solution (a). Dilute 1 ml of test solution (a) to 100 ml with *methanol R*.

Reference solution (b). Dissolve 20.0 mg of *acetylcholine chloride CRS* in *methanol R* and dilute to 2.0 ml with the same solvent.

Reference solution (c). Dissolve 20 mg of *choline chloride R* in *methanol R*, add 0.4 ml of test solution (a) and dilute to 2.0 ml with *methanol R*.

Plate: *TLC silica gel plate R*.

Mobile phase: mix 20 volumes of a 40 g/l solution of *ammonium nitrate R*, 20 volumes of *methanol R* and 60 volumes of *acetonitrile R*.

Application: 5 µl as bands of 10 mm by 2 mm.

Development: over 2/3 of the plate.

Detection: spray with *potassium iodobismuthate solution R3*.

System suitability: the chromatogram obtained with reference solution (c) shows 2 clearly separated bands.

Limits:

– *any impurity*: any bands in the chromatogram obtained with test solution (a), apart from the principal band, are not more intense than the principal band in the chromatogram obtained with reference solution (a) (1 per cent).

Trimethylamine. Dissolve 0.1 g in 10 ml of *sodium carbonate solution R* and heat to boiling. No vapours appear which turn *red litmus paper R* blue.

Heavy metals (*2.4.8*): maximum 10 ppm.

12 ml of solution S complies with limit test A. Prepare the standard using *lead standard solution (1 ppm Pb) R*.

Loss on drying (*2.2.32*): maximum 1.0 per cent, determined on 1.000 g by drying in an oven at 100-105 °C for 3 h.

Sulphated ash (*2.4.14*): maximum 0.1 per cent, determined on the residue obtained in the test for loss on drying.

ASSAY

Dissolve 0.200 g in 20 ml of *carbon dioxide-free water R*. Neutralise with *0.01 M sodium hydroxide* using 0.15 ml of *phenolphthalein solution R* as indicator. Add 20.0 ml of *0.1 M sodium hydroxide* and allow to stand for 30 min. Titrate with *0.1 M hydrochloric acid*.

1 ml of *0.1 M sodium hydroxide* is equivalent to 18.17 mg of $C_7H_{16}ClNO_2$.

STORAGE

In ampoules, protected from light.

IMPURITIES

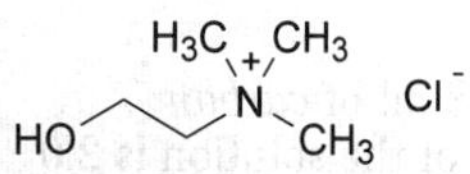

A. 2-hydroxy-*N,N,N*-trimethylethanaminium chloride (choline chloride),

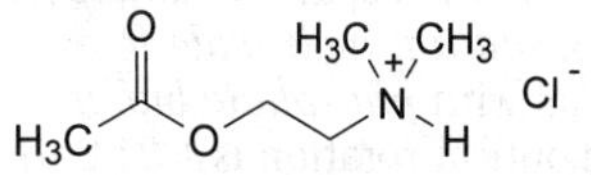

B. 2-(acetyloxy)-*N,N*-dimethylethanaminium chloride,

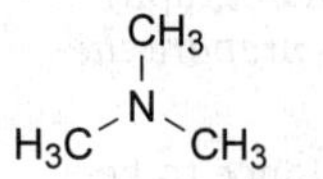

C. *N,N*-dimethylmethanamine.

01/2005:0967 corrected

ACETYLCYSTEINE

Acetylcysteinum

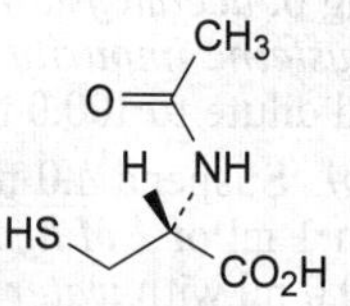

$C_5H_9NO_3S$ M_r 163.2

DEFINITION

Acetylcysteine contains not less than 98.0 per cent and not more than the equivalent of 101.0 per cent of (2*R*)-2-(acetylamino)-3-sulfanylpropanoic acid, calculated with reference to the dried substance.

CHARACTERS

A white, crystalline powder or colourless crystals, freely soluble in water and in alcohol, practically insoluble in methylene chloride.

IDENTIFICATION

First identification: A, C.

Second identification: A, B, D, E.

A. It complies with the test for specific optical rotation (see Tests).

B. Melting point (*2.2.14*): 104 °C to 110 °C.

C. Examine by infrared absorption spectrophotometry (*2.2.24*), comparing with the spectrum obtained with *acetylcysteine CRS*. Examine the substances prepared as discs using *potassium bromide R*.

D. Examine the chromatograms obtained in the test for related substances. The retention time and size of the principal peak in the chromatogram obtained with test solution (b) are approximately the same as those of the principal peak in the chromatogram obtained with reference solution (b).

E. To 0.5 ml of solution S (see Tests) add 0.05 ml of a 50 g/l solution of *sodium nitroprusside R* and 0.05 ml of *concentrated ammonia R*. A dark violet colour develops.

TESTS

Solution S. Dissolve 1.0 g in *carbon dioxide-free water R* and dilute to 20 ml with the same solvent.

Appearance of solution. Solution S is clear (*2.2.1*) and colourless (*2.2.2, Method II*).

pH (*2.2.3*). To 2 ml of solution S add 8 ml of *carbon dioxide-free water R* and mix. The pH of the solution is 2.0 to 2.8.

Specific optical rotation (*2.2.7*). In a 25 ml volumetric flask, mix 1.25 g with 1 ml of a 10 g/l solution of *sodium edetate R*. Add 7.5 ml of a 40 g/l solution of *sodium hydroxide R*, mix and dissolve. Dilute to 25.0 ml with *phosphate buffer solution pH 7.0 R2*. The specific optical rotation is + 21.0 to + 27.0, calculated with reference to the dried substance.

Related substances. Examine by liquid chromatography (*2.2.29*). *Except where otherwise prescribed, prepare the solutions immediately before use.*

Test solution (a). Suspend 0.80 g of the substance to be examined in 1 ml of *1 M hydrochloric acid* and dilute to 100.0 ml with *water R*.

Test solution (b). Dilute 5.0 ml of test solution (a) to 100.0 ml with *water R*. Dilute 5.0 ml of the solution to 50.0 ml with *water R*.

Test solution (c). Use test solution (a) after storage for at least 1 h.

Reference solution (a). Suspend 4.0 mg of *acetylcysteine CRS*, 4.0 mg of *L-cystine R*, 4.0 mg of *L-cysteine R*, 4.0 mg of *acetylcysteine impurity C CRS* and 4.0 mg of *acetylcysteine impurity D CRS* in 1 ml of *1 M hydrochloric acid* and dilute to 100.0 ml with *water R*.

Reference solution (b). Suspend 4.0 mg of *acetylcysteine CRS* in 1 ml of *1 M hydrochloric acid* and dilute to 100.0 ml with *water R*.

The chromatographic procedure may be carried out using:

- a stainless steel column 0.25 m long and 4 mm in internal diameter packed with *octadecylsilyl silica gel for chromatography R* (5 µm),
- as mobile phase at a flow rate at 1.0 ml/min a mixture prepared as follows: stir 3 volumes of *acetonitrile R* and 97 volumes of *water R* in a beaker; adjust to pH 3.0 with *phosphoric acid R*,
- as detector a spectrophotometer set at 220 nm.

When the chromatograms are recorded in the prescribed conditions, the retention times are: L-cystine, about 2.2 min; L-cysteine, about 2.4 min; 2-methyl-2-thiazoline-4-carboxylic acid, originating in test solution (c), about 3.3 min; acetylcysteine, about 6.4 min; acetylcysteine impurity C, about 12 min; acetylcysteine impurity D, about 14 min. Inject 20 µl of reference solution (a). The test is not valid unless:

- in the chromatogram obtained with reference solution (a), the resolution between the peaks due to L-cystine and L-cysteine is at least 1.5,
- in the chromatogram obtained with reference solution (a), the resolution between the peaks due to acetylcysteine impurity C and acetylcysteine impurity D is at least 2.0.

Inject 20 µl of *0.01 M hydrochloric acid* as a blank. Inject three times 20 µl of reference solution (a), 20 µl of reference solution (b) and 20 µl of each test solution. Continue the chromatography for five times the retention time of acetylcysteine which is about 30 min.

From the chromatogram obtained with test solution (a), calculate the percentage content of the known impurities and the unknown impurities using the following expressions:

$$\text{known impurity} = \frac{A_1 \times m_2 \times 100}{A_2 \times m_1}$$

$$\text{unknown impurity} = \frac{A_3 \times m_3 \times 100}{A_4 \times m_1}$$

A_1 = peak area of individual impurity (L-cystine, L-cysteine, acetylcysteine impurity C and acetylcysteine impurity D) in the chromatogram obtained with test solution (a),

A_2 = peak area of the corresponding individual impurity (L-cystine, L-cysteine, acetylcysteine impurity C and acetylcysteine impurity D) in the chromatogram obtained with reference solution (a),

A_3 = peak area of unknown impurity in the chromatogram obtained with test solution (a),

A_4 = peak area of acetylcysteine in the chromatogram obtained with reference solution (b),

m_1 = mass of the substance to be examined in test solution (a),

m_2 = mass of the individual impurity in reference solution (a),

m_3 = mass of acetylcysteine in reference solution (b).

The percentage content of each known impurity and of each unknown impurity is not greater than 0.5 per cent. The sum of the calculated percentage contents of known and unknown impurities is not greater than 0.5 per cent Disregard any peak due to the solvent, any peak appearing at retention time of about 3.3 min corresponding to 2-methyl-2-thiazoline-4-carboxylic acid and any peak with an area less than 0.1 times that of the principal peak in the chromatogram obtained with reference solution (b).

Heavy metals (*2.4.8*). 2.0 g complies with limit test C for heavy metals (10 ppm). Prepare the standard using 2 ml of *lead standard (10 ppm Pb) R*.

Zinc. Not more than 10 ppm of Zn, determined by atomic absorption spectrometry (*2.2.23, Method II*).

Test solution. Dissolve 1.00 g in *0.001 M hydrochloric acid* and dilute to 50.0 ml with the same acid.

Reference solutions. Prepare the reference solutions using *zinc standard solution (5 mg/ml Zn) R*, diluted with *0.001 M hydrochloric acid.*

Measure the absorbance at 213.8 nm using a zinc hollow-cathode lamp as the source of radiation, an air-acetylene flame and a correction procedure for non-specific absorption.

Loss on drying (*2.2.32*). Not more than 1.0 per cent, determined on 1.000 g by drying in an oven *in vacuo* at 70 °C for 3 h.

Sulphated ash (*2.4.14*). Not more than 0.2 per cent, determined on 1.0 g.

ASSAY

Dissolve 0.140 g in 60 ml of *water R* and add 10 ml of *dilute hydrochloric acid R*. After cooling in iced water, add 10 ml of *potassium iodide solution R* and titrate with *0.05 M iodine*, using 1 ml of *starch solution R* as indicator.

1 ml of *0.05 M iodine* is equivalent to 16.32 mg of $C_5H_9NO_3S$.

STORAGE

Store protected from light.

IMPURITIES

A. L-cystine,

B. L-cysteine,

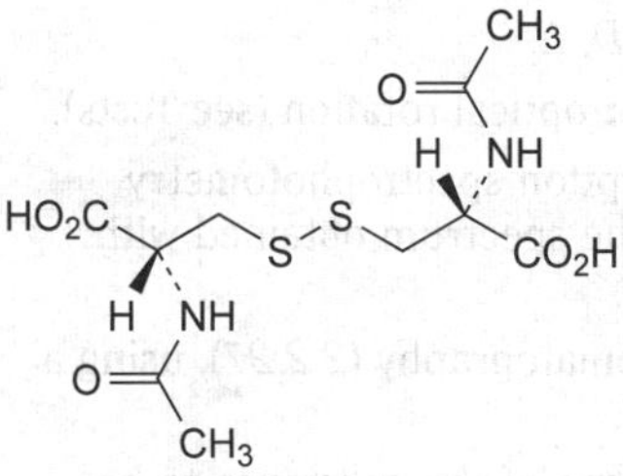

C. *N,N'*-diacetyl-L-cystine,

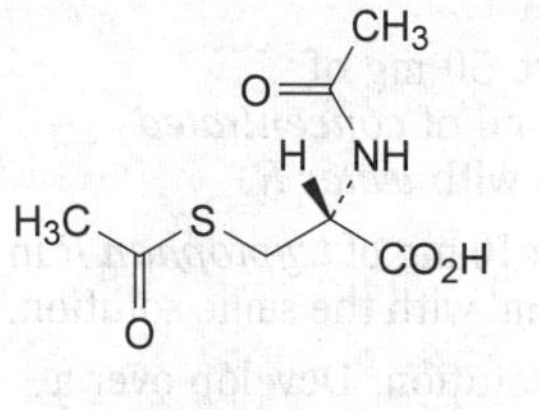

D. *N,S*-diacetyl-L-cysteine.

01/2005:0309

ACETYLSALICYLIC ACID

Acidum acetylsalicylicum

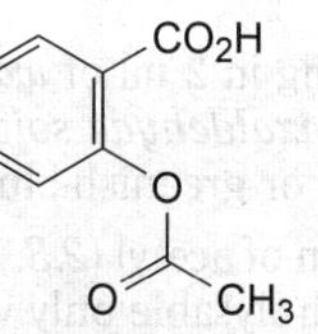

$C_9H_8O_4$ M_r 180.2

DEFINITION

Acetylsalicylic acid contains not less than 99.5 per cent and not more than the equivalent of 101.0 per cent of 2-(acetyloxy)benzoic acid, calculated with reference to the dried substance.

CHARACTERS

A white, crystalline powder or colourless crystals, slightly soluble in water, freely soluble in alcohol.

It melts at about 143 °C (instantaneous method).

IDENTIFICATION

First identification: A, B.

Second identification: B, C, D.

A. Examine by infrared absorption spectrophotometry (*2.2.24*), comparing with the spectrum obtained with *acetylsalicylic acid CRS*.

B. To 0.2 g add 4 ml of *dilute sodium hydroxide solution R* and boil for 3 min. Cool and add 5 ml of *dilute sulphuric acid R*. A crystalline precipitate is formed. Filter, wash the precipitate and dry at 100 °C to 105 °C. The melting point (*2.2.14*) is 156 °C to 161 °C.

C. In a test tube mix 0.1 g with 0.5 g of *calcium hydroxide R*. Heat the mixture and expose to the fumes produced a piece of filter paper impregnated with 0.05 ml of *nitrobenzaldehyde solution R*. A greenish-blue or greenish-yellow colour develops on the paper. Moisten the paper with *dilute hydrochloric acid R*. The colour becomes blue.

D. Dissolve with heating about 20 mg of the precipitate obtained in identification test B in 10 ml of *water R* and cool. The solution gives reaction (a) of salicylates (*2.3.1*).

TESTS

Appearance of solution. Dissolve 1.0 g in 9 ml of *alcohol R*. The solution is clear (*2.2.1*) and colourless (*2.2.2, Method II*).

Related substances. Examine by liquid chromatography (*2.2.29*). *Prepare the solutions immediately before use.*

Test solution. Dissolve 0.10 g of the substance to be examined in *acetonitrile for chromatography R* and dilute to 10.0 ml with the same solvent.

Reference solution (a). Dissolve 50.0 mg of *salicylic acid R* in the mobile phase and dilute to 50.0 ml with the mobile phase. Dilute 1.0 ml of this solution to 100.0 ml with the mobile phase.

Reference solution (b). Dissolve 10.0 mg of *salicylic acid R* in the mobile phase and dilute to 10.0 ml with the mobile phase. To 1.0 ml of this solution add 0.2 ml of the test solution and dilute to 100.0 ml with the mobile phase.

The chromatographic procedure may be carried out using:

– a stainless steel column 0.25 m long and 4.6 mm in internal diameter packed with *octadecylsilyl silica gel for chromatography R* (5 μm),

– as mobile phase at a flow rate of 1 ml/min a mixture of 2 volumes of *phosphoric acid R*, 400 volumes of *acetonitrile for chromatography R* and 600 volumes of *water R*,

– as detector a spectrophotometer set at 237 nm.

Inject 10 μl of each solution. Continue the chromatography of the test solution for seven times the retention time of acetylsalicylic acid. The test is not valid unless in the chromatogram obtained with reference solution (b), the resolution between the two principal peaks is at least 6.0. In the chromatogram obtained with the test solution the area of any peak, apart from the principal peak, is not greater than the area of the principal peak in the chromatogram obtained with reference solution (a) (0.1 per cent); the sum of the areas of all the peaks is not greater than 2.5 times the area of the principal peak in the chromatogram obtained with reference solution (a) (0.25 per cent). Disregard any peak with an area less than 0.25 times the area of the principal peak in the chromatogram obtained with reference solution (a).

Heavy metals (*2.4.8*). Dissolve 1.0 g in 12 ml of *acetone R* and dilute to 20 ml with *water R*. 12 ml of this solution complies with limit test B for heavy metals (20 ppm). Prepare the standard using lead standard solution (1 ppm Pb) obtained by diluting *lead standard solution (100 ppm Pb) R* with a mixture of 6 volumes of *water R* and 9 volumes of *acetone R*.

Loss on drying (*2.2.32*). Not more than 0.5 per cent, determined on 1.000 g by drying *in vacuo*.

Sulphated ash (*2.4.14*). Not more than 0.1 per cent, determined on 1.0 g.

ASSAY

In a flask with a ground-glass stopper, dissolve 1.000 g in 10 ml of *alcohol R*. Add 50.0 ml of *0.5 M sodium hydroxide*. Close the flask and allow to stand for 1 h. Using 0.2 ml of *phenolphthalein solution R* as indicator, titrate with *0.5 M hydrochloric acid*. Carry out a blank titration.

1 ml of *0.5 M sodium hydroxide* is equivalent to 45.04 mg of $C_9H_8O_4$.

STORAGE

Store in an airtight container.

IMPURITIES

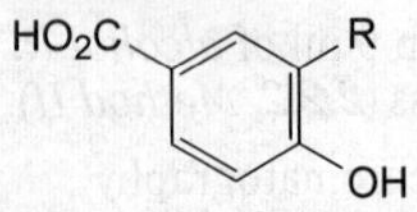

A. R = H: 4-hydroxybenzoic acid,

B. R = CO_2H: 4-hydroxybenzene-1,3-dicarboxylic acid (4-hydroxyisophthalic acid),

C. salicylic acid,

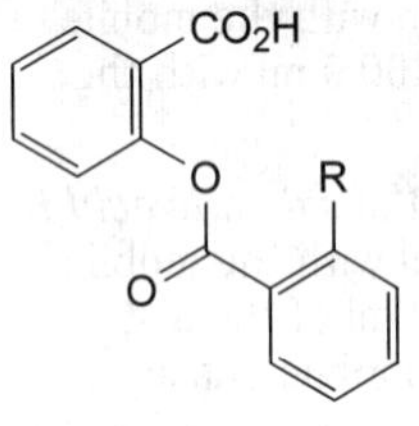

D. R = O-CO-CH_3: 2-[[2-(acetyloxy)benzoyl]oxy]benzoic acid (acetylsalicylsalicylic acid),

E. R = OH: 2-[(2-hydroxybenzoyl)oxy]benzoic acid (salicylsalicylic acid),

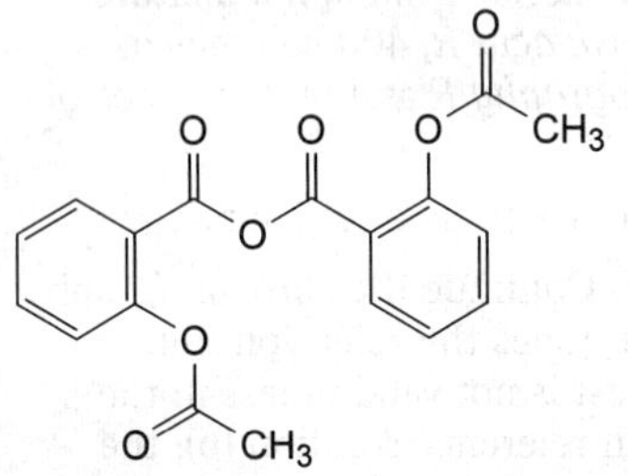

F. 2-(acetyloxy)benzoic anhydride (acetylsalicylic anhydride).

01/2005:1383

N-ACETYLTRYPTOPHAN

N-Acetyltryptophanum

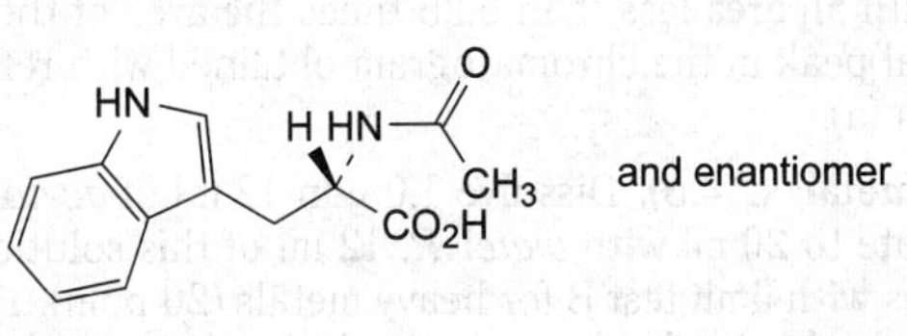

$C_{13}H_{14}N_2O_3$ M_r 246.3

DEFINITION

N-Acetyltryptophan contains not less than 99.0 per cent and not more than the equivalent of 101.0 per cent of (*RS*)-2-acetylamino-3-(1*H*-indol-3-yl)propanoic acid, calculated with reference to the dried substance.

PRODUCTION

Tryptophan used for the production of *N*-acetyltryptophan complies with the test for 1,1′-ethylidenebistryptophan and other related substances in the monograph on *Tryptophan (1272)*.

CHARACTERS

A white or almost white, crystalline powder, or colourless crystals, slightly soluble in water, very soluble in alcohol. It dissolves in dilute solutions of alkali hydroxides.

It melts at about 205 °C.

IDENTIFICATION

First identification: A, B.

Second identification: A, C, D, E.

A. It complies with the test for optical rotation (see Tests).

B. Examine by infrared absorption spectrophotometry (*2.2.24*), comparing with the spectrum obtained with *N-acetyltryptophan CRS*.

C. Examine by thin-layer chromatography (*2.2.27*), using a *TLC silica gel F_{254} plate R*.

Test solution. Dissolve 50 mg of the substance to be examined in 0.2 ml of *concentrated ammonia R* and dilute to 10 ml with *water R*.

Reference solution (a). Dissolve 50 mg of *N-acetyltryptophan CRS* in 0.2 ml of *concentrated ammonia R* and dilute to 10 ml with *water R*.

Reference solution (b). Dissolve 10 mg of *tryptophan R* in the test solution and dilute to 2 ml with the same solution.

Apply to the plate 2 µl of each solution. Develop over a path of 10 cm using a mixture of 25 volumes of *glacial acetic acid R*, 25 volumes of *water R* and 50 volumes of *butanol R*. Dry the plate in an oven at 100-105 °C for 15 min and examine in ultraviolet light at 254 nm. The principal spot in the chromatogram obtained with the test solution is similar in position and size to the principal spot in the chromatogram obtained with reference solution (a). The test is not valid unless the chromatogram obtained with reference solution (b) shows two clearly separated spots.

D. Dissolve about 2 mg in 2 ml of *water R*. Add 2 ml of *dimethylaminobenzaldehyde solution R6*. Heat on a water-bath. A blue or greenish-blue colour develops.

E. It gives the reaction of acetyl (*2.3.1*). Proceed as described for substances hydrolysable only with difficulty.

TESTS

Appearance of solution. Dissolve 1.0 g in a 40 g/l solution of *sodium hydroxide R* and dilute to 100 ml with the same alkaline solution. The solution is clear (*2.2.1*) and not more intensely coloured than reference solution Y_7 or GY_7 (*2.2.2, Method II*).

Optical rotation (*2.2.7*). Dissolve 2.50 g in a 40 g/l solution of *sodium hydroxide R* and dilute to 25.0 ml with the same alkaline solution. The angle of optical rotation is − 0.1° to + 0.1°.

Related substances. Examine by liquid chromatography (*2.2.29*).

Buffer solution pH 2.3. Dissolve 3.90 g of *sodium dihydrogen phosphate R* in 1000 ml of *water R*. Add about 700 ml of a 2.9 g/l solution of *phosphoric acid R* and adjust the pH to 2.3 with the same acidic solution.

Prepare the solutions immediately before use.

Test solution. Dissolve 0.10 g of the substance to be examined in a mixture of 50 volumes of *acetonitrile R* and 50 volumes of *water R* and dilute to 20.0 ml with the same mixture of solvents.

Reference solution (a). Dilute 1.0 ml of the test solution to 100.0 ml with a mixture of 10 volumes of *acetonitrile R* and 90 volumes of *water R*.

Reference solution (b). Dissolve 1.0 mg of *1,1′-ethylidenebis(tryptophan) CRS* in a mixture of 10 volumes of *acetonitrile R* and 90 volumes of *water R* and dilute to 100.0 ml with the same mixture of solvents.

Reference solution (c). To 4.0 ml of reference solution (a), add 20.0 ml of reference solution (b) and dilute to 100.0 ml with a mixture of 10 volumes of *acetonitrile R* and 90 volumes of *water R*.

The chromatographic procedure may be carried out using:

– a stainless steel column 0.25 m long and 4.6 mm in internal diameter packed with *octadecylsilyl silica gel for chromatography R* (5 µm),

– as mobile phase at a flow rate of 0.7 ml/min:

Mobile phase A. A mixture of 115 volumes of *acetonitrile R* and 885 volumes of buffer solution pH 2.3,

Mobile phase B. A mixture of 350 volumes of *acetonitrile R* and 650 volumes of buffer solution pH 2.3,

Time (min)	Mobile phase A (per cent *V/V*)	Mobile phase B (per cent *V/V*)	Comment
	100	0	equilibration
0 - 10	100	0	isocratic
10 - 45	100 → 0	0 → 100	linear gradient
45 - 65	0	100	isocratic
65 - 66	0 → 100	100 → 0	linear gradient
66 - 80	100	0	re-equilibration

– as detector a spectrophotometer set at 220 nm,

maintaining the temperature of the column at 40 °C.

When the chromatograms are recorded in the prescribed conditions, the retention times are about 29 min for *N*-acetyltryptophan and about 34 min for 1,1′-ethylidenebis(tryptophan). Adjust the sensitivity of the system so that the height of the peak due to *N*-acetyltryptophan in the chromatogram obtained with reference solution (a) is at least 50 per cent of the full scale of the recorder.

Inject 20 µl of reference solution (c). The test is not valid unless in the chromatogram obtained, the resolution between the peaks corresponding to *N*-acetyltryptophan and 1,1′-ethylidenebis(tryptophan) is at least 8.0. If necessary, adjust the time programme for the elution gradient. An increase in the duration of elution with mobile phase A produces longer retention times and a better resolution.

Inject 20 µl of the test solution and 20 µl of reference solution (a). Continue the chromatography of the test solution for 1.8 times the retention time of *N*-acetyltryptophan. In the chromatogram obtained with the test solution: the area of any peak, apart from the principal peak, is not greater than 0.25 times the area of the principal peak in the chromatogram obtained with reference solution (a) (0.25 per cent); the sum of the areas of all the peaks, apart from the principal peak, is not greater than 0.5 times the area of the principal peak in the chromatogram obtained with reference solution (a) (0.5 per cent). Disregard any peak due to the solvent and any peak with an area less than 0.01 times that of the peak due to *N*-acetyltryptophanin the chromatogram obtained with reference solution (a).

Ammonium (*2.4.1*). 0.10 g complies with limit test B for ammonium (200 ppm). Prepare the standard using 0.2 ml of *ammonium standard solution (100 ppm NH_4) R*.

Iron (*2.4.9*). Dissolve 1.0 g in 50 ml of *hydrochloric acid R1*, with heating at 50 °C. Allow to cool. In a separating funnel, shake with three quantities, each of 10 ml, of *methyl isobutyl ketone R1*, shaking for 3 min each time. To the combined organic layers add 10 ml of *water R* and shake for 3 min. The aqueous layer complies with the limit test for iron (10 ppm).

Heavy metals (*2.4.8*). 2.0 g complies with limit test C for heavy metals (10 ppm). Prepare the standard using 2 ml of *lead standard solution (10 ppm Pb) R*.

Loss on drying (*2.2.32*). Not more than 0.5 per cent, determined on 1.000 g by drying in an oven at 100-105 °C.

Sulphated ash (*2.4.14*). Not more than 0.1 per cent, determined on 1.0 g.

ASSAY

Dissolve 0.200 g in 5 ml of *methanol R*. Add 50 ml of *ethanol R*. Titrate with *0.1 M sodium hydroxide*, determining the end-point potentiometrically (*2.2.20*).

1 ml of *0.1 M sodium hydroxide* is equivalent to 24.63 mg of $C_{13}H_{14}N_2O_3$.

STORAGE

Store protected from light.

IMPURITIES

A. tryptophan,

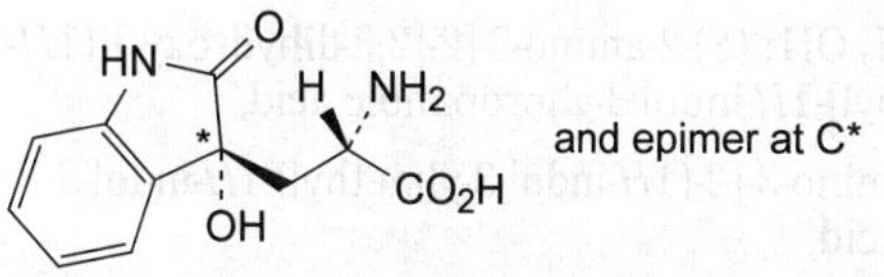

B. (*S*)-2-amino-3-[(3*RS*)-3-hydroxy-2-oxo-2,3-dihydro-1*H*-indol-3-yl]propanoic acid (dioxyindolylalanine),

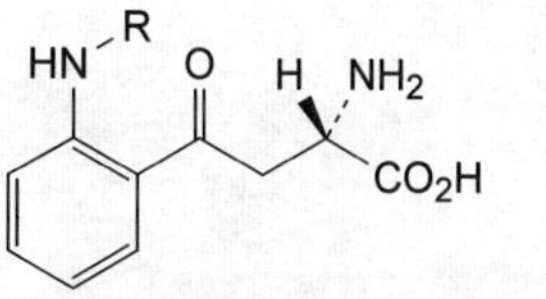

C. R = H: (*S*)-2-amino-4-(2-aminophenyl)-4-oxobutanoic acid (kynurenine),

E. R = CHO: (*S*)-2-amino-4-[2-(formylamino)phenyl]-4-oxobutanoic acid (*N*-formylkynurenine),

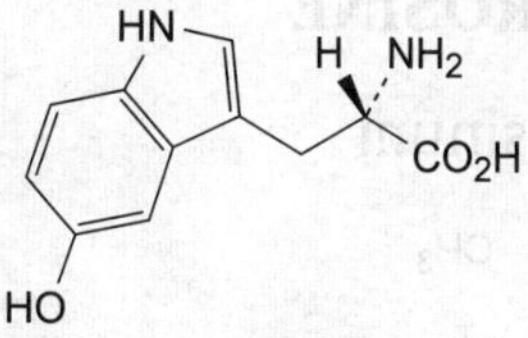

D. (*S*)-2-amino-3-(5-hydroxy-1*H*-indol-3-yl)propanoic acid (5-hydroxytryptophan),

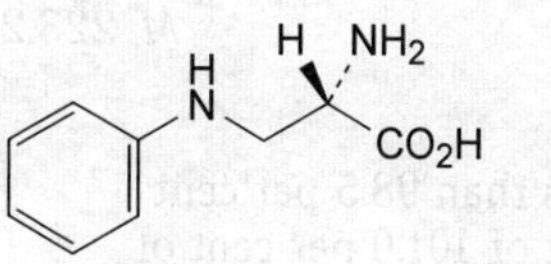

F. (*S*)-2-amino-3-(phenylamino)propanoic acid (3-phenylaminoalanine),

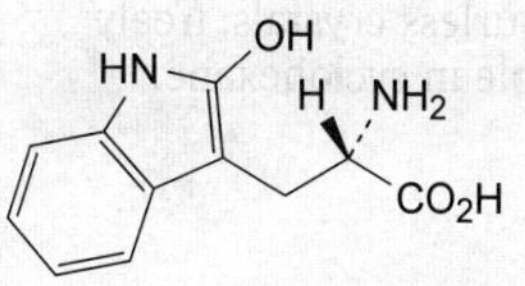

G. (*S*)-2-amino-3-(2-hydroxy-1*H*-indol-3-yl)propanoic acid (2-hydroxytryptophan),

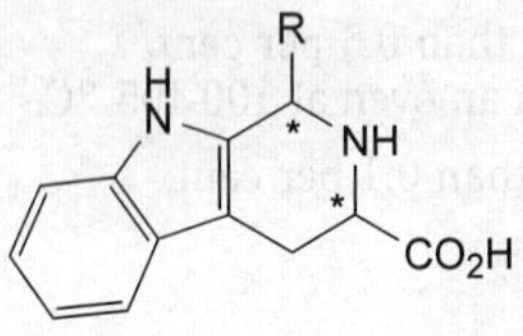

H. R = H: (3*RS*)-1,2,3,4-tetrahydro-9*H*-β-carboline-3-carboxylic acid,

I. R = CH_3: 1-methyl-1,2,3,4-tetrahydro-9*H*-β-carboline-3-carboxylic acid,

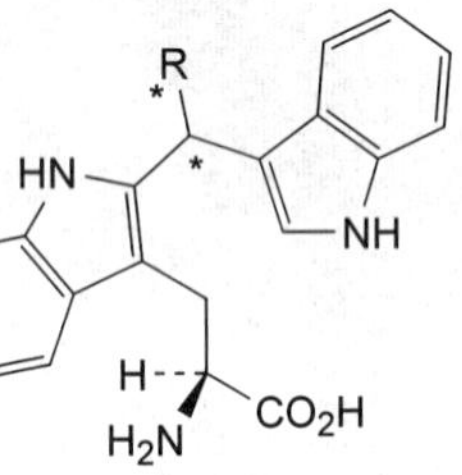

J. R = CHOH-CH_2-OH: (*S*)-2-amino-3-[2-[2,3-dihydroxy-1-(1*H*-indol-3-yl)propyl]-1*H*-indol-3-yl]propanoic acid,

K. R = H: (*S*)-2-amino-3-[2-(1*H*-indol-3-ylmethyl)-1*H*-indol-3-yl]propanoic acid,

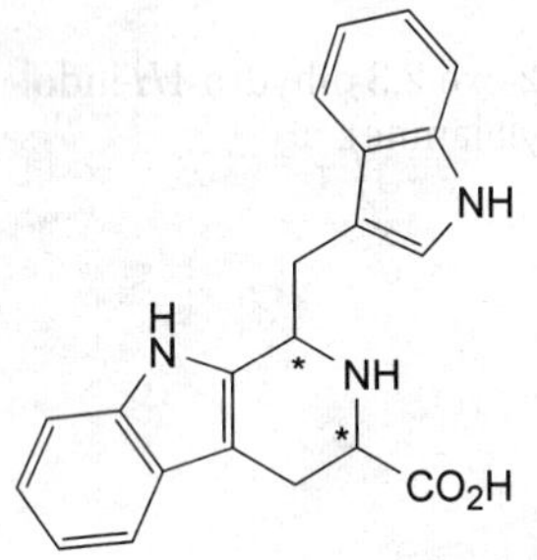

L. 1-(1*H*-indol-3-ylmethyl)-1,2,3,4-tetrahydro-9*H*-β-carboline-3-carboxylic acid.

01/2005:1384

N-ACETYLTYROSINE

N-Acetyltyrosinum

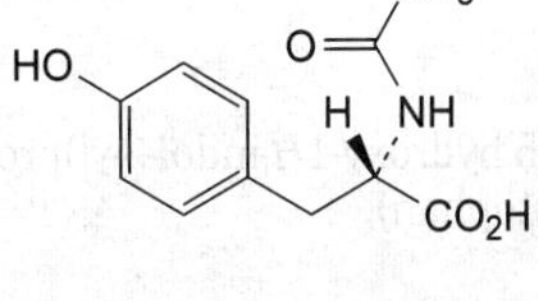

$C_{11}H_{13}NO_4$ M_r 223.2

DEFINITION

N-Acetyltyrosine contains not less than 98.5 per cent and not more than the equivalent of 101.0 per cent of (2*S*)-2-(acetylamino)-3-(4-hydroxyphenyl)propanoic acid, calculated with reference to the dried substance.

CHARACTERS

A white, crystalline powder or colourless crystals, freely soluble in water, practically insoluble in cyclohexane.

IDENTIFICATION

First identification: A, B.

Second identification: A, C, D.

A. It complies with the test for specific optical rotation (see Tests).

B. Examine by infrared absorption spectrophotometry (*2.2.24*), comparing with the spectrum obtained with *N-acetyltyrosine CRS*. Examine the substances prepared as discs.

C. Examine the chromatograms obtained in the test for related substances in ultraviolet light at 254 nm. The principal spot obtained with test solution (b) is similar in position and size to the principal spot in the chromatogram obtained with reference solution (a).

D. Solution S (see Tests) is strongly acid (*2.2.4*).

TESTS

Solution S. Dissolve 2.50 g in *water R* and dilute to 100.0 ml with the same solvent.

Appearance of solution. Solution S is clear (*2.2.1*) and colourless (*2.2.2, Method II*).

Specific optical rotation (*2.2.7*). Dilute 10.0 ml of solution S to 25.0 ml with *water R*. The specific optical rotation is + 46 to + 49, calculated with reference to the dried substance.

Related substances. Examine by thin-layer chromatography (*2.2.27*), using a *TLC silica gel F_{254} plate R*.

Test solution (a). Dissolve 0.80 g of the substance to be examined in 6 ml of a mixture of equal volumes of *glacial acetic acid R* and *water R* and dilute to 10 ml with *ethanol R*.

Test solution (b). Dilute 1 ml of test solution (a) to 10 ml with *ethanol R*.

Reference solution (a). Dissolve 80 mg of *N-acetyltyrosine CRS* in a mixture of 3 volumes of *water R*, 3 volumes of *glacial acetic acid R* and 94 volumes of *ethanol R* and dilute to 10 ml with the same mixture of solvents.

Reference solution (b). Dilute 0.5 ml of test solution (b) to 10 ml with *ethanol R*.

Reference solution (c). Dissolve 40 mg of *tyrosine CRS* in 20 ml of a mixture of equal volumes of *water R* and *glacial acetic acid R* and dilute to 50 ml with *ethanol R*.

Apply separately to the plate 5 µl of each solution. Develop over a path of 10 cm using a mixture of 10 volumes of *water R*, 15 volumes of *glacial acetic acid R* and 75 volumes of *ethyl acetate R*. Allow the plate to dry in air. Examine in ultraviolet light at 254 nm. Any spot in the chromatogram obtained with test solution (a), apart from the principal spot, is not more intense than the spot in the chromatogram obtained with reference solution (b) (0.5 per cent). Spray with *ninhydrin solution R* and heat at 100 °C to 105 °C for 10 min. Examine in daylight. Any spot corresponding to tyrosine is not more intense that the spot in the chromatogram obtained with reference solution (c) (1 per cent).

Chlorides (*2.4.4*). Dilute 10 ml of solution S to 15 ml with *water R*. The solution complies with the limit test for chlorides (200 ppm).

Sulphates (*2.4.13*). Dissolve 1.0 g in *distilled water R* and dilute to 20 ml with the same solvent. The solution complies with the limit test for sulphates (200 ppm).

Ammonium. Prepare a cell consisting of two watch-glasses 60 mm in diameter placed edge to edge. To the inner wall of the upper watch-glass stick a piece of *red litmus paper R* 5 mm square and wetted with a few drops of *water R*. Finely powder the substance to be examined, place 50 mg in the lower watch-glass and dissolve in 0.5 ml of *water R*. To the solution add 0.30 g of *heavy magnesium oxide R*. Briefly triturate with a glass rod. Immediately close the cell by putting the two watch-glasses together. Heat at 40 °C for 15 min. The litmus paper is not more intensely blue coloured than a standard prepared at the same time and in the same manner using 0.1 ml of *ammonium standard solution (100 ppm NH_4) R*, 0.5 ml of *water R* and 0.30 g of *heavy magnesium oxide R* (200 ppm).

Iron (*2.4.9*). In a separating funnel, dissolve 0.5 g in 10 ml of *dilute hydrochloric acid R*. Shake with three quantities, each of 10 ml, of *methyl isobutyl ketone R1*, shaking for 3 min each time. To the combined organic layers add 10 ml of *water R* and shake for 3 min. The aqueous layer complies with the limit test for iron (20 ppm).

Heavy metals (*2.4.8*). Dissolve 2.0 g in *water R* and dilute to 20 ml with the same solvent. 12 ml of the solution complies with limit test A for heavy metals (10 ppm). Prepare the standard using *lead standard solution (1 ppm Pb) R*.

Loss on drying (*2.2.32*). Not more than 0.5 per cent, determined on 1.000 g by drying in an oven at 100-105 °C.

Sulphated ash (*2.4.14*). Not more than 0.1 per cent, determined on 1.0 g.

Pyrogens (*2.6.8*). If intended for use in the manufacture of parenteral dosage forms without a further appropriate procedure for the removal of pyrogens, it complies with the test for pyrogens. Inject per kilogram of the rabbit's mass 1.0 ml of a freshly prepared solution in *water for injections R* containing per millilitre 10.0 mg of the substance to be examined and 9.0 mg of pyrogen-free *sodium chloride R*.

ASSAY

Dissolve 0.180 g in 50 ml of *carbon dioxide-free water R*. Titrate with *0.1 M sodium hydroxide*, determining the end-point potentiometrically (*2.2.20*).

1 ml of *0.1 M sodium hydroxide* is equivalent to 22.32 mg of $C_{11}H_{13}NO_4$.

STORAGE

Store protected from light. If the substance is sterile, store in a sterile, airtight, tamper-proof container.

LABELLING

The label states, where applicable, that the substance is apyrogenic.

IMPURITIES

A. tyrosine,

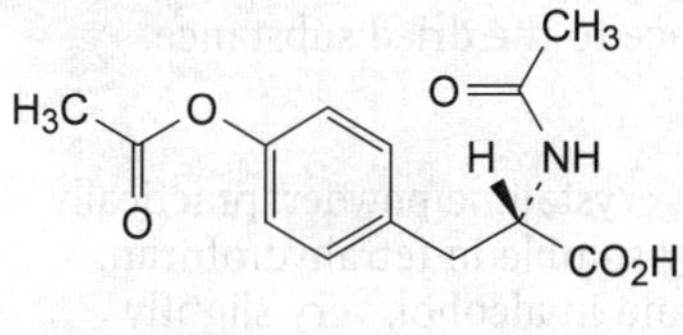

B. (2*S*)-2-(acetylamino)-3-[4-(acetoxy)phenyl]propanoic acid (diacetyltyrosine).

01/2005:0968

ACICLOVIR

Aciclovirum

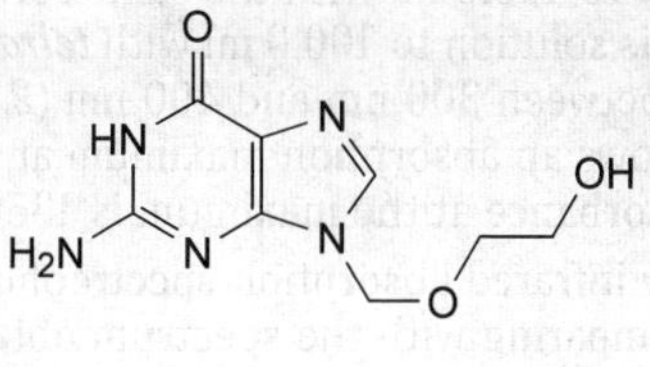

$C_8H_{11}N_5O_3$ M_r 225.2

DEFINITION

Aciclovir contains not less than 98.5 per cent and not more than the equivalent of 101.0 per cent of 2-amino-9-[(2-hydroxyethoxy)methyl]-1,9-dihydro-6*H*-purin-6-one, calculated with reference to the anhydrous substance.

CHARACTERS

A white or almost white, crystalline powder, slightly soluble in water, freely soluble in dimethyl sulphoxide, very slightly soluble in alcohol. It dissolves in dilute solutions of mineral acids and alkali hydroxides.

IDENTIFICATION

Examine by infrared absorption spectrophotometry (*2.2.24*), comparing with the spectrum obtained with *aciclovir CRS*.

TESTS

Appearance of solution. Dissolve 0.25 g in *0.1 M sodium hydroxide* and dilute to 25 ml with the same solvent. The solution is clear (*2.2.1*) and not more intensely coloured than reference solution Y_7 (*2.2.2, Method II*).

Related substances.

A. Examine by thin-layer chromatography (*2.2.27*), using *silica gel* GF_{254} *R* as the coating substance.

Prepare the solutions immediately before use.

Test solution. Dissolve 0.1 g of the substance to be examined in *dimethyl sulphoxide R* and dilute to 10 ml with the same solvent.

Reference solution. Dissolve 10 mg of *aciclovir impurity A CRS* in *dimethyl sulphoxide R* and dilute to 20 ml with the same solvent. Dilute 1 ml of the solution to 10 ml with *dimethyl sulphoxide R*.

Apply to the plate 10 µl of each solution. Keep the spots compact by drying in a current of warm air. Allow the plate to cool and develop over a path of 10 cm with a mixture of 2 volumes of *concentrated ammonia R*, 20 volumes of *methanol R* and 80 volumes of *methylene chloride R*. Allow the plate to dry in air and examine in ultraviolet light at 254 nm. In the chromatogram obtained with the test solution, any spot with an R_f value greater than that of the principal spot is not more intense than the spot in the chromatogram obtained with the reference solution (0.5 per cent).

B. Examine by liquid chromatography (*2.2.29*).

Test solution. Dissolve 50.0 mg of the substance to be examined in 10 ml of a mixture of 20 volumes of *glacial acetic acid R* and 80 volumes of *water R* and dilute to 100.0 ml with the mobile phase.

Reference solution (a). Dilute 1.0 ml of the test solution to 200.0 ml with the mobile phase.

Reference solution (b). Dissolve 20 mg of *aciclovir CRS* and 20 mg of *aciclovir impurity A CRS* in a mixture of 20 volumes of *glacial acetic acid R* and 80 volumes of *water R* and dilute to 100.0 ml with the same mixture of solvents. Dilute 1.0 ml of the solution to 10.0 ml with the mobile phase.

Reference solution (c). Dissolve 7 mg of *guanine R* in *0.1 M sodium hydroxide* and dilute to 100.0 ml with the same solution. Dilute 1.0 ml to 20.0 ml with the mobile phase.

The chromatographic procedure may be carried out using:

- a stainless steel column 0.10 m long and 4.6 mm in internal diameter packed with *octadecylsilyl silica gel for chromatography R* (3 µm),
- as mobile phase at a flow rate of 2 ml/min a mixture prepared as follows: dissolve 6.0 g of *sodium dihydrogen phosphate R* and 1.0 g of *sodium decanesulphonate R* in 900 ml of *water R* and adjust to pH 3 ± 0.1 with *phosphoric acid R*; add 40 ml of *acetonitrile R* and dilute to 1 litre with *water R*,
- as detector a spectrophotometer set at 254 nm,
- a loop injector.

Inject 20 µl of each solution. Record the chromatograms for seven times the retention time of aciclovir. The test is not valid unless in the chromatogram obtained with reference solution (b), the number of theoretical plates calculated for the peak due to aciclovir impurity A is at least 1500 and its mass distribution ratio is at least 7 (V_0 can be calculated using *dimethyl sulphoxide R*). In the chromatogram obtained with the test solution: the area of any peak corresponding to guanine is not greater than that of the peak in the chromatogram obtained with reference solution (c) (0.7 per cent); the area of any peak apart from the principal peak and any peak corresponding to guanine is not greater than the area of the peak in the chromatogram obtained with reference solution (a) (0.5 per cent) and the sum of the areas of such peaks is not greater than twice the area of the peak in the chromatogram obtained with reference solution (a) (1 per cent). Disregard any peak with an area less than 0.05 times that of the principal peak in the chromatogram obtained with reference solution (a).

Water (*2.5.12*). Not more than 6.0 per cent, determined on 0.500 g by the semi-micro determination of water.

Sulphated ash (*2.4.14*). Not more than 0.1 per cent, determined on 1.0 g.

ASSAY

Dissolve 0.150 g in 60 ml of *anhydrous acetic acid R*. Titrate with *0.1 M perchloric acid*, determining the end-point potentiometrically (*2.2.20*). Carry out a blank titration.

1 ml of *0.1 M perchloric acid* is equivalent to 22.52 mg of $C_8H_{11}N_5O_3$.

IMPURITIES

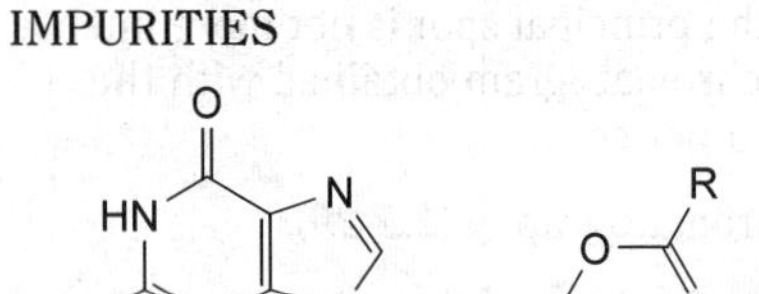

A. R = CH_3: 2-[(2-amino-6-oxo-1,6-dihydro-9*H*-purin-9-yl)methoxy]ethyl acetate,

D. R = C_6H_5: 2-[(2-amino-6-oxo-1,6-dihydro-9*H*-purin-9-yl)methoxy]ethyl benzoate,

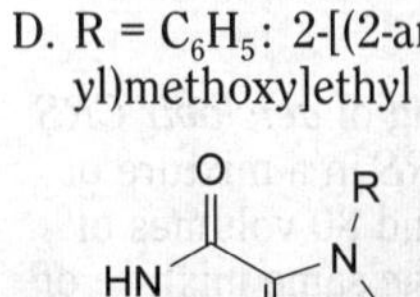

B. R = H: 2-amino-1,7-dihydro-6*H*-purin-6-one (guanine),

C. R = CH_2-O-CH_2-CH_2-OH: 2-amino-7-[(2-hydroxyethoxy)methyl]-1,7-dihydro-6*H*-purin-6-one,

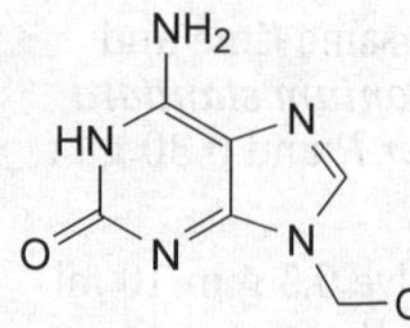

E. 6-amino-9-[(2-hydroxyethoxy)methyl]-1,9-dihydro-2*H*-purin-2-one,

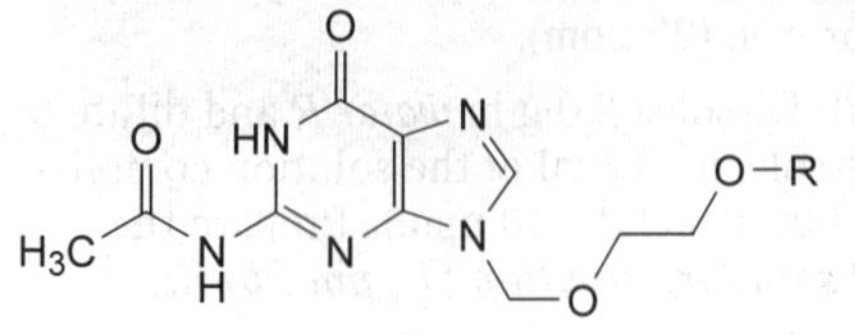

F. R = H: *N*-[9-[(2-hydroxyethoxy)methyl]-6-oxo-6,9-dihydro-1*H*-purin-2-yl]acetamide,

G. R = CO-CH_3: 2-[[2-(acetylamino)-6-oxo-1,6-dihydro-9*H*-purin-9-yl]methoxy]ethyl acetate,

H. R = CO-C_6H_5: 2-[[2-(acetylamino)-6-oxo-1,6-dihydro-9*H*-purin-9-yl]methoxy]ethyl benzoate.

01/2005:1385
corrected

ACITRETIN

Acitretinum

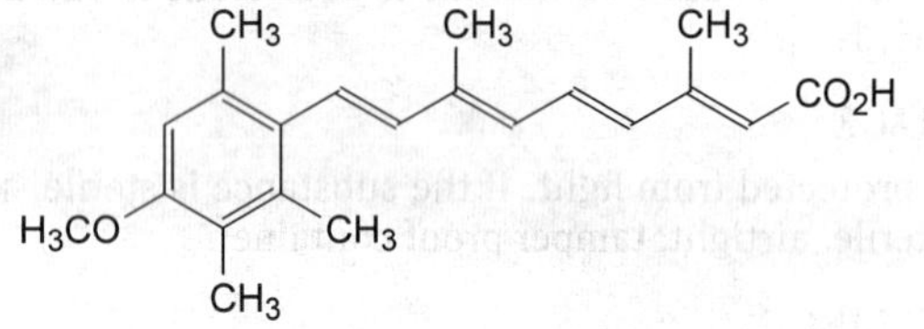

$C_{21}H_{26}O_3$ M_r 326.4

DEFINITION

Acitretin contains not less than 98.0 per cent and not more than the equivalent of 102.0 per cent of (all-*E*)-9-(4-methoxy-2,3,6-trimethylphenyl)-3,7-dimethylnona-2,4,6,8-tetraenoic acid, calculated with reference to the dried substance.

CHARACTERS

A yellow or greenish-yellow, crystalline powder, practically insoluble in water, sparingly soluble in tetrahydrofuran, slightly soluble in acetone and in alcohol, very slightly soluble in cyclohexane. It is sensitive to air, heat and light, especially in solution.

Carry out all operations as rapidly as possible and avoid exposure to actinic light; use freshly prepared solutions.

IDENTIFICATION

First identification: B.

Second identification: A, C.

A. Dissolve 15.0 mg in 10 ml of *tetrahydrofuran R* and dilute immediately to 100.0 ml with the same solvent. Dilute 2.5 ml of this solution to 100.0 ml with *tetrahydrofuran R*. Examined between 300 nm and 400 nm (*2.2.25*), the solution shows an absorption maximum at 358 nm. The specific absorbance at the maximum is 1350 to 1475.

B. Examine by infrared absorption spectrophotometry (*2.2.24*), comparing with the spectrum obtained with *acitretin CRS*. Examine the substances prepared as discs.

C. Examine the chromatograms obtained in the assay. The principal peak in the chromatogram obtained with the test solution has a retention time similar to that of the principal peak in the chromatogram obtained with reference solution (a).

TESTS

Related substances. Examine by liquid chromatography (*2.2.29*) as described under Assay.

Inject 10 µl each of reference solutions (b) and (c) and of the test solution (a). Adjust the sensitivity of the system so that the height of the principal peak in the chromatogram obtained with reference solution (b) is not less than 40 per cent of the full scale of the recorder. The test is not valid unless the resolution between the peaks due to acitretin and tretinoin in the chromatogram obtained with reference solution (b) is at least 2.0. If necessary, adjust the concentration of *ethanol R*. Continue the chromatography of the test solution (a) for 2.5 times the retention time of the principal peak. In the chromatogram obtained with the test solution (a), the area of any peak, apart from the principal peak, is not greater than the area of the peak due to acitretin in the chromatogram obtained with reference solution (c) (0.3 per cent); the sum of the areas of any peaks, apart from the principal peak, is not greater than the area of the peak due to acitretin in the chromatogram obtained with reference solution (b) (1.0 per cent). Disregard any peak with an area less than 0.1 times that of the principal peak in the chromatogram obtained with reference solution (c).

Heavy metals (*2.4.8*). 2.0 g complies with limit test C (20 ppm). Prepare the standard using 2 ml of *lead standard solution (10 ppm Pb) R*.

Palladium. Not more than 10 ppm of Pd, determined by atomic absorption spectrometry (*2.2.23, Method I*).

Test solution. Introduce 2.0 g of the substance to be examined into a quartz beaker and add 3 ml of *magnesium nitrate solution R*. Heat in a muffle furnace to 350 °C at a rate of 40 °C/min to incinerate the content. Ignite at about 450 °C for 8 h and then at 550 °C for a further hour. Dissolve the residue in a mixture of 0.75 ml of *hydrochloric acid R* and 0.25 ml of *nitric acid R* warming gently. Cool, transfer the solution into a volumetric flask with *water R* and dilute to 50.0 ml with the same solvent.

Reference solution. Dissolve 0.163 g of *heavy magnesium oxide R* in a mixture of 0.5 ml of *nitric acid R*, 1.5 ml of *hydrochloric acid R* and 50 ml of *water R*, add 2.0 ml of *palladium standard solution (20 ppm Pd R)* and dilute to 100.0 ml with *water R*.

Measure the absorbance at 247.6 nm using a palladium hollow-cathode lamp as source of radiation and an air-acetylene flame.

Loss on drying (*2.2.32*). Not more than 0.5 per cent, determined on 1.000 g by drying *in vacuo* at 100 °C for 4 h.

Sulphated ash (*2.4.14*). Not more than 0.1 per cent, determined on 1.0 g.

ASSAY

Carry out the assay protected from light, use amber volumetric flasks and prepare the solutions immediately before use.

Examine by liquid chromatography (*2.2.29*).

Test solution (a). Dissolve 25.0 mg of the substance to be examined in 5 ml of *tetrahydrofuran R* and dilute immediately to 100.0 ml with *ethanol R*.

Test solution (b). Dilute 10.0 ml of test solution (a) to 25.0 ml with *ethanol R*.

Reference solution (a). Dissolve 25.0 mg of *acitretin CRS* in 5 ml of *tetrahydrofuran R* and dilute immediately to 100.0 ml with *ethanol R*. Dilute 10.0 ml to 25.0 ml with *ethanol R*.

Reference solution (b). Dissolve 1.0 mg of *tretinoin CRS* in *ethanol R* and dilute to 20.0 ml with the same solvent. Mix 5.0 ml of the solution with 2.5 ml of reference solution (a) and dilute to 100.0 ml with *ethanol R*.

Reference solution (c). Dilute 2.5 ml of reference solution (a) to 50.0 ml with *ethanol R*. Dilute 3.0 ml of the solution to 20.0 ml with *ethanol R*.

The chromatographic procedure may be carried out using:

- a stainless steel column 0.25 m long and 4 mm in internal diameter packed with microparticulate *octadecylsilyl silica gel for chromatography R* (5 µm), with a carbon loading of 20 per cent, a specific surface area of 200 m^2/g and a pore size of 15 nm,
- as mobile phase at a flow rate of 0.6 ml/min a 0.3 per cent *V/V* solution of *glacial acetic acid R* in a mixture of 8 volumes of *water R* and 92 volumes of *ethanol R*,
- as detector a spectrophotometer set at 360 nm,
- a sampler kept at 4 °C,

maintaining the temperature of the column at 25 °C.

When the chromatograms are recorded in the prescribed conditions, the retention times are: impurity A about 4.8 min, tretinoin about 5.2 min, acitretin about 6.2 min and impurity B about 10.2 min.

Inject 10 µl of reference solution (a) 6 times. The test is not valid unless the relative standard deviation of the peak area for acitretin is at most 1.0 per cent. If necessary, adjust the integration parameters. Inject alternately the test solution (b) and reference solution (a).

STORAGE

In an airtight container, protected from light, at a temperature of 2 °C to 8 °C.

It is recommended that the contents of an opened container be used as soon as possible and any unused part be protected by an atmosphere of inert gas.

IMPURITIES

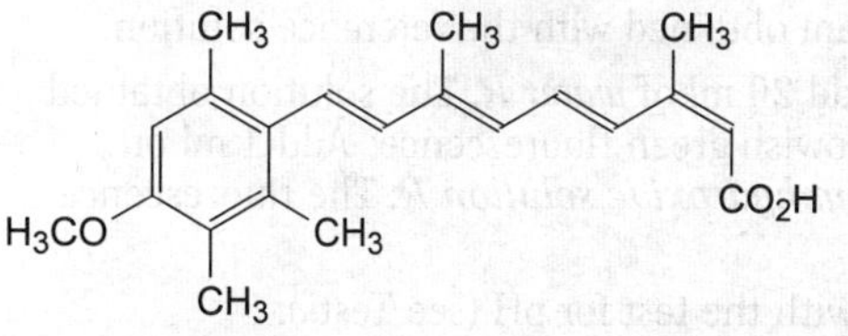

A. (2*Z*,4*E*,6*E*,8*E*)-9-(4-methoxy-2,3,6-trimethylphenyl)-3,7-dimethylnona-2,4,6,8-tetraenoic acid,

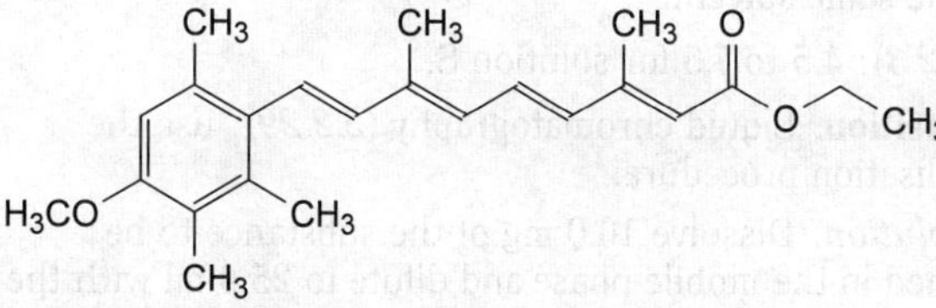

B. ethyl (all-*E*)-9-(4-methoxy-2,3,6-trimethylphenyl)-3,7-dimethylnona-2,4,6,8-tetraenoate.

01/2005:2043

ACRIFLAVINIUM MONOCHLORIDE

Acriflavinii monochloridum

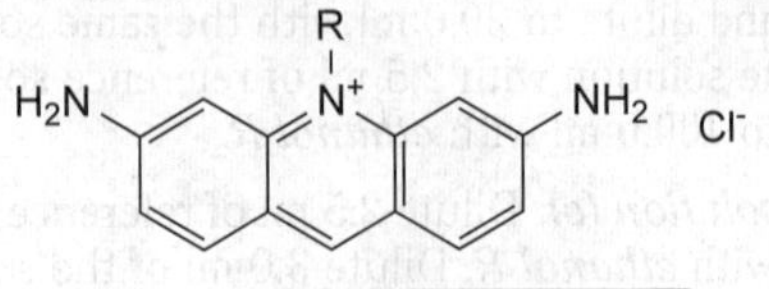

R	Mol. Formula	M_r
H	$C_{13}H_{12}ClN_3$	245.7
CH_3	$C_{14}H_{14}ClN_3$	259.7

DEFINITION

Mixture of 3,6-diamino-10-methylacridinium chloride and 3,6-diaminoacridine hydrochloride.

Content: 95.0 per cent to 105.0 per cent (anhydrous substance).

CHARACTERS

Appearance: reddish-brown powder, hygroscopic.

Solubility: freely soluble in water, sparingly soluble in alcohol, very slightly soluble in methylene chloride.

IDENTIFICATION

A. Thin-layer chromatography (*2.2.27*).

Test solution. Dilute 0.5 ml of solution S (see Tests) to 10 ml with *alcohol R*.

Reference solution. Dissolve 10 mg of *acriflavinium monochloride CRS* in *alcohol R* and dilute to 10 ml with the same solvent.

Plate: *TLC silica gel plate R*.

Mobile phase: *glacial acetic acid R, water R, butanol R* (1:1:4 *V/V/V*).

Application: 5 µl.

Development: over 2/3 of the plate.

Drying: at 100-105 °C.

Detection: examine in ultraviolet light at 365 nm.

Results: the 2 principal spots in the chromatogram obtained with the test solution are similar in position, fluorescence and size to the principal spots in the chromatogram obtained with the reference solution.

B. To 0.1 mg add 20 ml of *water R*. The solution obtained shows a yellowish-green fluorescence. Add 1 ml of *dilute sodium hydroxide solution R*. The fluorescence disappears.

C. It complies with the test for pH (see Tests).

TESTS

Solution S. Dissolve with heating 0.500 g in 15 ml of *carbon dioxide-free water R*; allow to cool and dilute to 25.0 ml with the same solvent.

pH (*2.2.3*): 4.5 to 7.5 for solution S.

Composition. Liquid chromatography (*2.2.29*): use the normalisation procedure.

Test solution. Dissolve 10.0 mg of the substance to be examined in the mobile phase and dilute to 25.0 ml with the mobile phase.

Reference solution (a). Dilute 1.0 ml of the test solution to 100.0 ml with the mobile phase.

Reference solution (b). Dilute 1.0 ml of reference solution (a) to 10.0 ml with the mobile phase.

Column:

- *size*: *l* = 0.25 m, Ø = 4.6 mm,
- *stationary phase*: *octadecylsilyl silica gel for chromatography R* (5 µm).

Mobile phase: dissolve 1.0 g of *sodium octanesulphonate R* and 5 ml of *triethylamine R* in a mixture of 400 ml of *acetonitrile R* and 600 ml of *phosphate buffer solution pH 2.8 R*.

Flow rate: 1 ml/min.

Detection: spectrophotometer at 262 nm.

Injection: 10 µl.

Run time: 30 min.

System suitability: reference solution (a):

- *resolution*: minimum 3.5 between the 2 principal peaks.

Limits:

- *first principal peak*: 30.0 per cent to 40.0 per cent,
- *second principal peak*: 50.0 per cent to 60.0 per cent,
- *any other peak*: maximum 6.0 per cent and not more than 2 such peaks have a peak area of more than 2.0 per cent,
- *disregard limit*: 0.5 times the area of the peak in the chromatogram obtained with reference solution (b) (0.05 per cent).

Heavy metals (*2.4.8*): maximum 40 ppm.

0.5 g complies with limit test D. Prepare the standard using 2 ml of *lead standard solution (10 ppm Pb) R*.

Water (*2.5.12*): maximum 10.0 per cent, determined on 0.250 g.

Sulphated ash (*2.4.14*): maximum 3.5 per cent, determined on 1.0 g.

ASSAY

Prepare the solutions immediately before use and protected from light.

Determine the water content immediately before the assay.

Dissolve 0.100 g in 500.0 ml of *water R*. Dilute 5.0 ml of the solution to 250.0 ml with *0.1 M hydrochloric acid*. Measure the absorbance (*2.2.25*) at the maximum at 262 nm.

Calculate the content of the sum of $C_{14}H_{14}ClN_3$ and $C_{13}H_{12}ClN_3$ taking the specific absorbance to be 1820.

STORAGE

In an airtight container, protected from light.

01/2005:0800

ADENINE

Adeninum

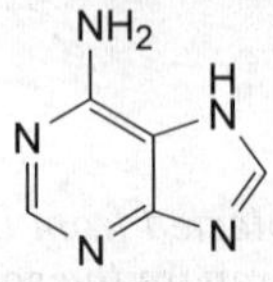

$C_5H_5N_5$ M_r 135.1

DEFINITION

Adenine contains not less than 98.5 per cent and not more than the equivalent of 101.0 per cent of 7*H*-purin-6-amine, calculated with reference to the dried substance.

CHARACTERS

A white powder, very slightly soluble in water and in alcohol. It dissolves in dilute mineral acids and in dilute solutions of alkali hydroxides.

IDENTIFICATION

First identification: A.

Second identification: B, C.

A. Examine by infrared absorption spectrophotometry (*2.2.24*), comparing with the spectrum obtained with *adenine CRS*. Examine the substances prepared as discs.

B. Examine the chromatograms obtained in the test for related substances. The principal spot in the chromatogram obtained with test solution (b) is similar in position and size to the principal spot in the chromatogram obtained with reference solution (a).

C. To 1 g add 3.5 ml of *propionic anhydride R* and boil for 15 min with stirring. Cool. To the resulting crystalline mass add 15 ml of *light petroleum R* and heat to boiling with vigorous stirring. Cool and filter. Wash the precipitate with two quantities, each of 5 ml, of *light petroleum R*. Dissolve the precipitate in 10 ml of *water R* and boil for 1 min. Filter the mixture at 30 °C to 40 °C. Allow to cool. Filter, and dry the precipitate at 100 °C to 105 °C for 1 h. The melting point (*2.2.14*) of the precipitate is 237 °C to 241 °C.

TESTS

Solution S. Suspend 2.5 g in 50 ml of *distilled water R* and boil for 3 min. Cool and dilute to 50 ml with *distilled water R*. Filter. Use the filtrate as solution S.

Appearance of solution. Dissolve 0.5 g in *dilute hydrochloric acid R* and dilute to 50 ml with the same acid. The solution is clear (*2.2.1*) and colourless (*2.2.2, Method II*).

Acidity or alkalinity. To 10 ml of solution S add 0.1 ml of *bromothymol blue solution R1* and 0.2 ml of *0.01 M sodium hydroxide*. The solution is blue. Add 0.4 ml of *0.01 M hydrochloric acid*. The solution is yellow.

Related substances. Examine by thin-layer chromatography (*2.2.27*), using *silica gel GF_{254} R* as the coating substance.

Test solution (a). Dissolve 0.10 g of the substance to be examined in *dilute acetic acid R*, with heating if necessary, and dilute to 10 ml with the same acid.

Test solution (b). Dilute 1 ml of test solution (a) to 10 ml with *dilute acetic acid R*.

Reference solution (a). Dissolve 10 mg of *adenine CRS* in *dilute acetic acid R*, with heating if necessary, and dilute to 10 ml with the same acid.

Reference solution (b). Dilute 1 ml of test solution (b) to 20 ml with *dilute acetic acid R*.

Reference solution (c). Dissolve 10 mg of *adenine CRS* and 10 mg of *adenosine R* in *dilute acetic acid R*, with heating if necessary, and dilute to 10 ml with the same acid.

Apply to the plate 5 µl of each solution. Develop over a path of 12 cm using a mixture of 20 volumes of *concentrated ammonia R*, 40 volumes of *ethyl acetate R* and 40 volumes of *propanol R*. Dry the plate in a current of warm air and examine in ultraviolet light at 254 nm. Any spot in the chromatogram obtained with test solution (a), apart from the principal spot, is not more intense than the spot in the chromatogram obtained with reference solution (b) (0.5 per cent). The test is not valid unless the chromatogram obtained with reference solution (c) shows two clearly separated spots.

Chlorides (*2.4.4*). To 10 ml of solution S add 1 ml of *concentrated ammonia R* and 3 ml of *silver nitrate solution R2*. Filter. Wash the precipitate with a little *water R* and dilute the filtrate to 15 ml with *water R*. The solution complies with the limit test for chlorides (100 ppm). When carrying out the test, add 2 ml of *dilute nitric acid R* instead of 1 ml of *dilute nitric acid R*.

Sulphates (*2.4.13*). Dilute 10 ml of solution S to 15 ml with *distilled water R*. The solution complies with the limit test for sulphates (300 ppm).

Ammonium. Prepare a cell consisting of two watch-glasses 60 mm in diameter placed edge to edge. To the inner wall of the upper watch-glass stick a piece of *red litmus paper R* 5 mm square and wetted with a few drops of *water R*. Finely powder the substance to be examined, place 0.5 g in the lower watch-glass and suspend in 0.5 ml of *water R*. To the suspension add 0.30 g of *heavy magnesium oxide R*. Briefly triturate with a glass rod. Immediately close the cell by putting the two watch-glasses together. Heat at 40 °C for 15 min. The litmus paper is not more intensely blue coloured than a standard prepared at the same time and in the same manner using 0.05 ml of *ammonium standard solution (100 ppm NH_4) R*, 0.5 ml of *water R* and 0.30 g of *heavy magnesium oxide R* (10 ppm).

Heavy metals (*2.4.8*). 1.0 g complies with limit test C for heavy metals (20 ppm). Prepare the standard using 2 ml of *lead standard solution (10 ppm Pb) R*.

Loss on drying (*2.2.32*). Not more than 0.5 per cent, determined on 1.000 g by drying in an oven at 100 °C to 105 °C.

Sulphated ash (*2.4.14*). Not more than 0.1 per cent, determined on 1.0 g.

ASSAY

Dissolve 0.100 g in a mixture of 20 ml of *acetic anhydride R* and 30 ml of *anhydrous acetic acid R*. Titrate with *0.1 M perchloric acid*, determining the end-point potentiometrically (*2.2.20*).

1 ml of *0.1 M perchloric acid* is equivalent to 13.51 mg of $C_5H_5N_5$.

01/2005:1486

ADENOSINE

Adenosinum

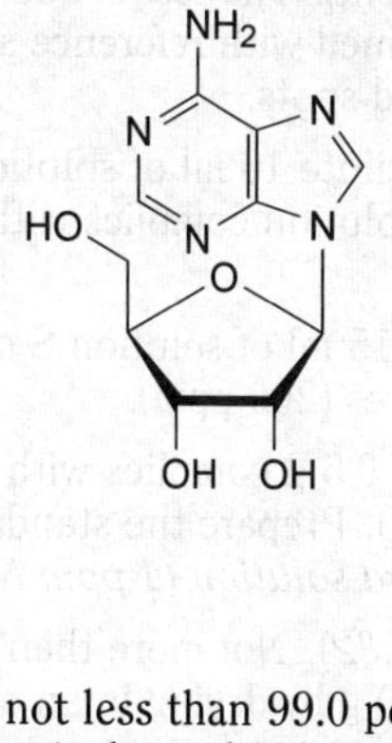

$C_{10}H_{13}N_5O_4$ M_r 267.2

DEFINITION

Adenosine contains not less than 99.0 per cent and not more than the equivalent of 101.0 per cent of 9-β-D-ribofuranosyl-9*H*-purin-6-amine, calculated with reference to the dried substance.

CHARACTERS

A white, crystalline powder slightly soluble in water, soluble in hot water, practically insoluble in alcohol and in methylene chloride. It dissolves in dilute mineral acids.

It melts at about 234 °C.

IDENTIFICATION

Examine by infrared absorption spectrophotometry (*2.2.24*), comparing with the spectrum obtained with *adenosine CRS*.

TESTS

Solution S. Suspend 5.0 g in 100 ml of *distilled water R* and heat to boiling. Allow to cool, filter with the aid of vacuum and dilute to 100 ml with *distilled water R*.

Appearance of solution. Solution S is colourless (*2.2.2, Method II*).

Acidity or alkalinity. To 10 ml of solution S, add 0.1 ml of *bromocresol purple solution R* and 0.1 ml of *0.01 M hydrochloric acid*. The solution is yellow. Add 0.4 ml of *0.01 M sodium hydroxide*, the solution is violet-blue.

Specific optical rotation (*2.2.7*). Dissolve 1.25 g in *1 M hydrochloric acid* and dilute to 50.0 ml with the same acid. Determined within 10 min and calculated with reference to the dried substance, the specific optical rotation is − 45 to − 49.

Related substances. Examine by thin-layer chromatography (*2.2.27*), using a *TLC silica gel F_{254} plate R*.

Test solution. Dissolve 0.20 g of the substance to be examined in *dilute acetic acid R* with slight heating and dilute to 5 ml with the same acid.

Reference solution (a). Dilute 1 ml of the test solution to 100 ml with *water R*.

Reference solution (b). Dissolve 10 mg of *adenosine CRS* and 10 mg of *adenine CRS* in *dilute acetic acid R*, with heating if necessary, and dilute to 10 ml with the same acid.

Apply to the plate 5 µl of each solution. Develop over a path of 12 cm using a mixture of 10 volumes of *water R*, 30 volumes of *concentrated ammonia R* and 60 volumes of *propanol R*. Allow the plate to dry in a current of warm air and examine in ultraviolet light at 254 nm. Any spot in the chromatogram obtained with the test solution, apart from the principal spot, is not more intense than the spot in the chromatogram obtained with reference solution (a) (1 per cent). Spray with a 5 g/l solution of *potassium permanganate R* in *1 M sodium hydroxide*. Allow the plate to dry in a current of warm air and examine in daylight. Any spot in the chromatogram obtained with the test solution, apart from the principal spot, is not more intense than the spot in the chromatogram obtained with reference solution (a) (1 per cent). The test is not valid unless the chromatogram obtained with reference solution (b) shows two clearly separated spots.

Chlorides (*2.4.4*). Dilute 10 ml of solution S to 15 ml with *water R*. The solution complies with the limit test for chlorides (100 ppm).

Sulphates (*2.4.13*). 15 ml of solution S complies with the limit test for sulphates (200 ppm).

Ammonium (*2.4.1*). 0.5 g complies with limit test B for ammonium (10 ppm). Prepare the standard using 5 ml of *ammonium standard solution (1 ppm NH_4) R*.

Loss on drying (*2.2.32*). Not more than 0.5 per cent, determined on 1.000 g by drying in an oven at 100 °C to 105 °C.

Sulphated ash (*2.4.14*). Not more than 0.1 per cent, determined on 1.0 g.

ASSAY

Dissolve 0.200 g, warming slightly if necessary, in a mixture of 20 ml of *acetic anhydride R* and 30 ml of *anhydrous acetic acid R*. Titrate with *0.1 M perchloric acid*, determining the end-point potentiometrically (*2.2.20*).

1 ml of *0.1 M perchloric acid* is equivalent to 26.72 mg of $C_{10}H_{13}N_5O_4$.

IMPURITIES

A. adenine,

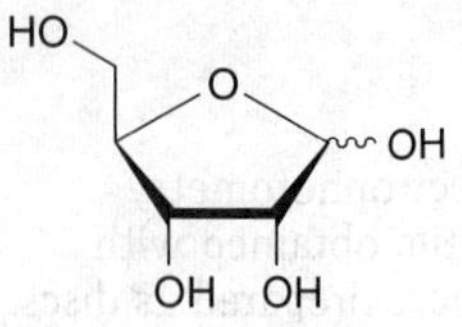

B. D-ribose,

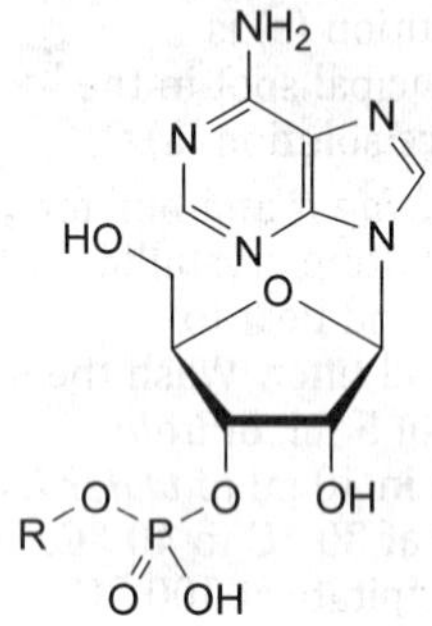

C. R = H: adenosine 3′-(dihydrogen phosphate),

D. R = PO_3H_2: adenosine 3′-(trihydrogen diphosphate),

E. R = PO_2H-O-PO_3H_2: adenosine 3′-(tetrahydrogen triphosphate).

01/2005:1586

ADIPIC ACID

Acidum adipicum

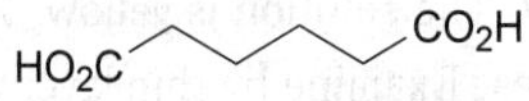

$C_6H_{10}O_4$ M_r 146.1

DEFINITION

Hexanedioic acid.

Content: 99.0 per cent to 101.0 per cent (dried substance).

CHARACTERS

Appearance: white, crystalline powder.

Solubility: sparingly soluble in water, soluble in boiling water, freely soluble in alcohol and in methanol, soluble in acetone.

IDENTIFICATION

A. Melting point (*2.2.14*): 151 °C to 154 °C.

B. Infrared absorption spectrophotometry (*2.2.24*).

Comparison: *adipic acid CRS*.

TESTS

Solution S. Dissolve 5.0 g with heating in *distilled water R* and dilute to 50 ml with the same solvent. Allow to cool and to crystallise. Filter through a sintered-glass filter (40). Wash the filter with *distilled water R*. Collect the filtrate and the washings until a volume of 50 ml is obtained.

Appearance of solution. The solution is clear (*2.2.1*) and colourless (*2.2.2, Method II*).

Dissolve 1.0 g in *methanol R* and dilute to 20 ml with the same solvent.

Related substances. Liquid chromatography (*2.2.29*).

Test solution. Dissolve 0.20 g of the substance to be examined in the mobile phase and dilute to 10.0 ml with the mobile phase.

Reference solution (a). Dissolve 20 mg of *glutaric acid R* in 1.0 ml of the test solution and dilute to 10.0 ml with the mobile phase.

Reference solution (b). Dilute 1.0 ml of the test solution to 100.0 ml with the mobile phase, dilute 1.0 ml of the solution to 10.0 ml with the mobile phase.

Column:

- *size*: l = 0.125 m, Ø = 4.0 mm,
- *stationary phase*: spherical *octadecylsilyl silica gel for chromatography R* (5 µm) with a specific surface area of 350 m^2/g and a pore size of 10 nm,
- *temperature*: 30 °C.

Mobile phase: mix 3 volumes of *acetonitrile R* and 97 volumes of a 24.5 g/l solution of *dilute phosphoric acid R*.

Flow rate: 1 ml/min.

Detection: spectrophotometer at 209 nm.

Injection: 20 µl.

Run time: 3 times the retention time of adipic acid.

System suitability: reference solution (a):

- *resolution*: minimum 9.0 between the peaks due to glutaric acid and adipic acid.

Limits:

- *any impurity*: not more than the area of the principal peak in the chromatogram obtained with reference solution (b) (0.1 per cent),
- *total*: not more than 5 times the area of the principal peak in the chromatogram obtained with reference solution (b) (0.5 per cent),
- *disregard limit*: 0.5 times the area of the principal peak in the chromatogram obtained with reference solution (b) (0.05 per cent).

Chlorides (*2.4.4*): maximum 200 ppm.

2.5 ml of solution S diluted to 15 ml with *water R* complies with the limit test for chlorides.

Nitrates: maximum 30 ppm.

To 1 ml of solution S add 2 ml of *concentrated ammonia R*, 0.5 ml of a 10 g/l solution of *manganese sulphate R*, 1 ml of a 10 g/l solution of *sulfanilamide R* and dilute to 20 ml with *water R*. Add 0.10 g of *zinc powder R* and cool in iced water for 30 min; shake from time to time. Filter and cool 10 ml of the filtrate in iced water. Add 2.5 ml of *hydrochloric acid R1* and 1 ml of a 10 g/l solution of *naphthylethylenediamine dihydrochloride R*. Allow to stand at room temperature. After 15 min the mixture is not more intensely coloured than a standard prepared at the same time and in the same manner, using 1.5 ml of *nitrate standard solution (2 ppm NO_3) R* instead of 1 ml of solution S. The test is invalid if a blank solution prepared at the same time and in the same manner, using 1 ml of *water R* instead of 1 ml of solution S, is more intensely coloured than a 2 mg/l solution of *potassium permanganate R*.

Sulphates (*2.4.13*): maximum 500 ppm.

3 ml of solution S diluted to 15 ml with *distilled water R* complies with the limit test for sulphates.

Iron (*2.4.9*): maximum 10 ppm.

10 ml of solution S complies with the limit test for iron.

Heavy metals (*2.4.8*): maximum 10 ppm.

12 ml of solution S complies with limit test A. Prepare the standard using *lead standard solution (1 ppm Pb) R*.

Loss on drying (*2.2.32*): maximum 0.2 per cent, determined on 1.000 g by drying in an oven at 100-105 °C.

Sulphated ash (*2.4.14*): maximum 0.1 per cent.

Melt 1.0 g completely over a gas burner, then ignite the melted substance with the burner. After ignition, lower or remove the flame in order to prevent the substance from boiling and keep it burning until completely carbonised. Carry out the test for sulphated ash using the residue.

ASSAY

Dissolve 60.0 mg in 50 ml of *water R*. Add 0.2 ml of *phenolphthalein solution R* and titrate with *0.1 M sodium hydroxide*.

1 ml of *0.1 M sodium hydroxide* is equivalent to 7.31 mg of $C_6H_{10}O_4$.

IMPURITIES

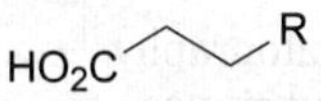

A. R = CH_2-CO_2H: pentanedioic acid (glutaric acid),

B. R = CO_2H: butanedioic acid (succinic acid),

C. R = $[CH_2]_3$-CO_2H: heptanedioic acid (pimelic acid).

01/2005:0254

ADRENALINE TARTRATE

Adrenalini tartras

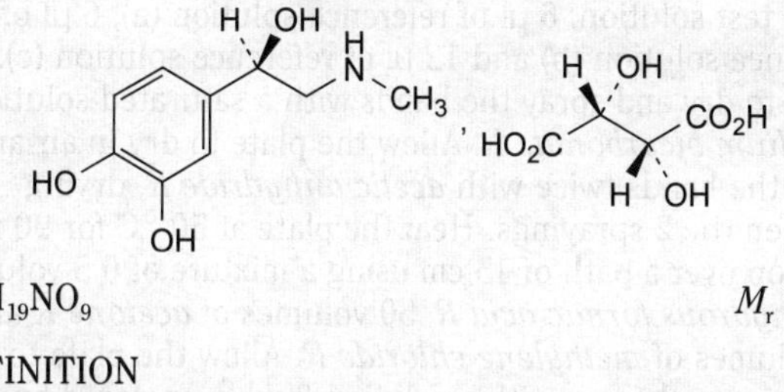

$C_{13}H_{19}NO_9$ M_r 333.3

DEFINITION

Adrenaline tartrate contains not less than 98.5 per cent and not more than the equivalent of 101.0 per cent of (1*R*)-1-(3,4-dihydroxyphenyl)-2-(methylamino)ethanol hydrogen (2*R*,3*R*)-2,3-dihydroxybutanedioate, calculated with reference to the dried substance.

CHARACTERS

A white or greyish-white, crystalline powder, freely soluble in water, slightly soluble in ethanol (96 per cent).

IDENTIFICATION

A. Dissolve 2 g in 20 ml of a 5 g/l solution of *sodium metabisulphite R* and make alkaline by addition of *ammonia R*. Keep the mixture in iced water for 1 h and filter. Reserve the filtrate for identification test C. Wash the precipitate with 3 quantities, each of 2 ml, of *water R*, with 5 ml of *ethanol (96 per cent) R* and finally with 5 ml of *ether R*. Dry *in vacuo* for 3 h. The specific optical rotation (*2.2.7*) of the precipitate (adrenaline base) is − 50 to − 54, determined using a 20.0 g/l solution in *0.5 M hydrochloric acid*.

B. Examine by infrared absorption spectrophotometry (*2.2.24*), comparing with the spectrum obtained with adrenaline base prepared by the same method from a suitable amount of *adrenaline tartrate CRS*. Use adrenaline base prepared as described under identification test A. Examine the substances prepared as discs.

C. 0.2 ml of the filtrate obtained in identification test A gives reaction (b) of tartrates (*2.3.1*).

TESTS

Appearance of solution. Dissolve 0.5 g in *water R* and dilute to 10 ml with the same solvent. Examine the solution immediately. The solution is not more opalescent than reference suspension II (*2.2.1*) and is not more intensely coloured than reference solution BY_5 (*2.2.2, Method II*).

Adrenalone. Dissolve 50.0 mg in *0.01 M hydrochloric acid* and dilute to 25.0 ml with the same acid. The absorbance (*2.2.25*) of the solution measured at 310 nm is not greater than 0.10.

Noradrenaline. Examine by thin-layer chromatography (*2.2.27*), using *silica gel G R* as the coating substance.

Test solution. Dissolve 0.25 g of the substance to be examined in *water R* and dilute to 10 ml with the same solvent. Prepare immediately before use.

Reference solution (a). Dissolve 12.5 mg of *noradrenaline tartrate CRS* in *water R* and dilute to 10 ml with the same solvent. Prepare immediately before use.

Reference solution (b). Dilute 2 ml of reference solution (a) to 10 ml with *water R*.

Reference solution (c). Mix 2 ml of the test solution with 2 ml of reference solution (b).

Apply separately to the plate as bands 20 mm by 2 mm 6 µl of the test solution, 6 µl of reference solution (a), 6 µl of reference solution (b) and 12 µl of reference solution (c). Allow to dry and spray the bands with a saturated solution of *sodium bicarbonate R*. Allow the plate to dry in air and spray the bands twice with *acetic anhydride R*, drying between the 2 sprayings. Heat the plate at 50 °C for 90 min. Develop over a path of 15 cm using a mixture of 0.5 volumes of *anhydrous formic acid R*, 50 volumes of *acetone R* and 50 volumes of *methylene chloride R*. Allow the plate to dry in air and spray with a solution freshly prepared by mixing 2 volumes of *ethylenediamine R* and 8 volumes of *methanol R* and adding 2 volumes of a 5 g/l solution of *potassium ferricyanide R*. Dry the plate at 60 °C for 10 min and examine in ultraviolet light at 254 nm and 365 nm. In the chromatogram obtained with the test solution, any zone situated between the 2 most intense zones is not more intense than the corresponding zone in the chromatogram obtained with reference solution (b) (1.0 per cent). The test is not valid unless the chromatogram obtained with reference solution (c) shows between the 2 most intense zones a clearly separated zone corresponding to the most intense zone in the chromatogram obtained with reference solution (a).

Loss on drying (*2.2.32*). Not more than 0.5 per cent, determined on 1.00 g by drying *in vacuo* for 18 h.

Sulphated ash (*2.4.14*). Not more than 0.1 per cent, determined on 1.0 g.

ASSAY

Dissolve 0.300 g in 50 ml of *anhydrous acetic acid R*, heating gently if necessary. Titrate with *0.1 M perchloric acid* until a bluish-green colour is obtained using 0.1 ml of *crystal violet solution R* as indicator.

1 ml of *0.1 M perchloric acid* is equivalent to 33.33 mg of $C_{13}H_{19}NO_9$.

STORAGE

In an airtight container, or preferably in a sealed tube under vacuum or under an inert gas, protected from light.

01/2005:0310

AGAR

Agar

DEFINITION

Agar consists of the polysaccharides from various species of Rhodophyceae mainly belonging to the genus *Gelidium*. It is prepared by treating the algae with boiling water; the extract is filtered whilst hot, concentrated and dried.

CHARACTERS

Agar has a mucilaginous taste.

It occurs in the form of a powder or in crumpled strips 2 mm to 5 mm wide or sometimes in flakes, colourless to pale yellow, translucent, somewhat tough and difficult to break, becoming more brittle on drying.

It has the microscopic characters described under identification test A.

IDENTIFICATION

A. Examine under a microscope. When mounted in *0.005 M iodine*, the strips or flakes are partly stained brownish-violet. Magnified 100 times, they show numerous minute, colourless, ovoid or rounded grains on an amorphous background; occasional brown, round to ovoid spores with a reticulated surface, measuring up to 60 µm, may be present. Reduce to a powder, if necessary. The powder is yellowish-white. Examine under a microscope using *0.005 M iodine*. The powder presents angular fragments with numerous grains similar to those seen in the strips and flakes; some of the fragments are stained brownish-violet.

B. Dissolve 0.1 g with heating in 50 ml of *water R*. Cool. To 1 ml of the mucilage carefully add 3 ml of *water R* so as to form two separate layers. Add 0.1 ml of *0.05 M iodine*. A dark brownish-violet colour appears at the interface. Mix. The liquid becomes pale yellow.

C. Heat 5 ml of the mucilage prepared for identification test B on a water-bath with 0.5 ml of *hydrochloric acid R* for 30 min. Add 1 ml of *barium chloride solution R1*. A white turbidity develops within 30 min.

D. Heat 0.5 g with 50 ml of *water R* on a water-bath until dissolved. Only a few fragments remain insoluble. During cooling, the solution gels between 35 °C and 30 °C. Heat the gel thus obtained on a water-bath; it does not liquefy below 80 °C.

TESTS

Swelling index (*2.8.4*). The swelling index, determined on the powdered drug (355), is not less than 10 and is within 10 per cent of the value stated on the label.

Insoluble matter. To 5.00 g of the powdered drug (355) add 100 ml of *water R* and 14 ml of *dilute hydrochloric acid R*. Boil gently for 15 min with frequent stirring. Filter the hot liquid through a tared, sintered-glass filter (160), rinse the filter with hot *water R* and dry at 100 °C to 105 °C. The residue weighs not more than 50 mg (1.0 per cent).

Gelatin. To 1.00 g add 100 ml of *water R* and heat on a water-bath until dissolved. Allow to cool to 50 °C. To 5 ml of the solution add 5 ml of *picric acid solution R*. No turbidity appears within 10 min.

Loss on drying (*2.2.32*). Not more than 20.0 per cent, determined on 1.000 g of the powdered drug (355) by drying in an oven at 100 °C to 105 °C.

Total ash (*2.4.16*). Not more than 5.0 per cent.

Microbial contamination. Total viable aerobic count (*2.6.12*) not more than 10^3 micro-organisms per gram, determined by plate-count. It complies with the tests for *Escherichia coli* and *Salmonella* (*2.6.13*).

LABELLING

The label states the swelling index.

01/2005:1587

AGRIMONY

Agrimoniae herba

DEFINITION

Dried flowering tops of *Agrimonia eupatoria* L.

Content: minimum 2.0 per cent of tannins, expressed as pyrogallol ($C_6H_6O_3$; M_r 126.1) (dried drug).

CHARACTERS

Macroscopic and microscopic characters described under identification tests A and B.

IDENTIFICATION

A. The stem is green or, more usually, reddish, cylindrical and infrequently branched. It is covered with long, erect or tangled hairs. The leaves are compound imparipennate with 3 or 6 opposite pairs of leaflets, with 2 or 3 smaller leaflets between. The leaflets are deeply dentate to serrate, dark green on the upper surface, greyish and densely tormentose on the lower face. The flowers are small and form a terminal spike. They are pentamerous and borne in the axils of hairy bracts, the calyces closely surrounded by numerous terminal hooked spires, which occur on the rim of the hairy receptacle. The petals are free, yellow and deciduous. Fruit-bearing obconical receptacles, with deep furrows and hooked bristles, are usually present at the base of the inflorescence.

B. Reduce to a powder (355). The powder is yellowish-green to grey. Examine under a microscope using *chloral hydrate solution R*. The powder shows numerous straight of bent, unicellular, long thick-walled (about 500 µm) trichomes finely warty and sometimes spiraly marked; fragments of parenchyma with prisms and cluster crystals of calcium oxalate; fragments of leaf epidermis with sinuous walls, those of the lower epidermis with abundant stomata, mostly anomocytic but occasionally anisocytic; ovoid to subspherical-pollen grains, with 3 pores and a smooth exine; fragments of glandular trichomes with a multicellular uniseriate stalk and a spherical unicellular or quadricellular head; groups of fibres and spiral and bardered-fitted vessels from the stem.

C. Thin-layer chromatography (*2.2.27*).

Test solution. To 2.0 g of the powdered drug (355) add 20 ml of *methanol R*. Heat with shaking at 40 °C for 10 min. Filter.

Reference solution. Dissolve 1.0 mg of *rutin R* and 1.0 mg of *isoquercitroside R* in 2 ml of *methanol R*.

Plate: *TLC silica gel plate R*.

Mobile phase: *anhydrous formic acid R, water R, ethyl acetate R* (10:10:80 *V/V/V*).

Application: 10 µl, as bands.

Development: over a path of 12 cm.

Drying: at 100-105 °C.

Detection: spray the still warm plate with a 10 g/l solution of *diphenylboric acid aminoethyl ester R* in *methanol R* and then with a 50 g/l solution of *macrogol 400 R* in *methanol R*. Allow the plate to dry in air for 30 min. Examine in ultraviolet light at 365 nm

Results: see below the sequence of the zones present in the chromatograms obtained with the reference and test solutions.

Top of the plate	
	An orange fluorescent zone may be present (quercitroside)
Isoquercitroside: an orange fluorescent zone	An orange fluorescent zone (isoquercitroside)
	An orange fluorescent zone (hyperoside)
Rutin: an orange fluorescent zone	An orange fluorescent zone (rutin)
Reference solution	**Test solution**

TESTS

Foreign matter (*2.8.2*): it complies with the test for foreign matter.

Loss on drying (*2.2.32*): maximum 10.0 per cent, determined on 1.000 g of the powdered drug (355) by drying in an oven at 100-105 °C for 2 h.

Total ash (*2.4.16*): maximum 10.0 per cent.

ASSAY

Carry out the determination of tannins in herbal drugs (*2.8.14*). Use a 1.000 g of powdered drug (180).

01/2005:1238
corrected

AIR, MEDICINAL

Aer medicinalis

DEFINITION

Compressed ambient air.

Content: 20.4 per cent *V/V* to 21.4 per cent *V/V* of oxygen (O_2).

CHARACTERS

A colourless, odourless gas.

Solubility: at a temperature of 20 °C and a pressure of 101 kPa, 1 volume dissolves in about 50 volumes of water.

PRODUCTION

Carbon dioxide: maximum 500 ppm *V/V*, determined using an infrared analyser (*2.5.24*).

Gas to be examined. Use the substance to be examined. It must be filtered to avoid stray light phenomena.

Reference gas (a). Use a mixture of 79 per cent *V/V* of *nitrogen R1* and 21 per cent *V/V* of *oxygen R* containing less than 1 ppm *V/V* of *carbon dioxide R1*.

Reference gas (b). Use a mixture of 79 per cent *V/V* of *nitrogen R1* and 21 per cent *V/V* of *oxygen R* containing 500 ppm *V/V* of *carbon dioxide R1*.

Calibrate the apparatus and set the sensitivity using reference gases (a) and (b). Measure the content of carbon dioxide in the gas to be examined.

Carbon monoxide: maximum 5 ppm *V/V*, determined using an infrared analyser (*2.5.25*).

Gas to be examined. Use the substance to be examined. It must be filtered to avoid stray light phenomena.

Reference gas (a). Use a mixture of 79 per cent *V/V* of *nitrogen R1* and 21 per cent *V/V* of *oxygen R* containing less than 1 ppm *V/V* of *carbon monoxide R.*

Reference gas (b). Use a mixture of 79 per cent *V/V* of *nitrogen R1* and 21 per cent *V/V* of *oxygen R* containing 5 ppm *V/V* of *carbon monoxide R.*

Calibrate the apparatus and set the sensitivity using reference gases (a) and (b). Measure the content of carbon monoxide in the gas to be examined.

Sulphur dioxide: maximum 1 ppm *V/V*, determined using an ultraviolet fluorescence analyser (Figure 1238.-1).

The apparatus consists of the following:

- a system generating ultraviolet radiation with a wavelength of 210 nm, made up of an ultraviolet lamp, a collimator, and a selective filter; the beam is blocked periodically by a chopper rotating at high speeds;
- a reaction chamber, through which flows the gas to be examined;
- a system that detects radiation emitted at a wavelength of 350 nm, made up of a selective filter, a photomultiplier tube and an amplifier.

Gas to be examined. Use the substance to be examined. It must be filtered.

Reference gas (a). Use a mixture of 79 per cent *V/V* of *nitrogen R1* and 21 per cent *V/V* of *oxygen R.*

Reference gas (b). Use a mixture of 79 per cent *V/V* of *nitrogen R1* and 21 per cent *V/V* of *oxygen R* containing 0.5 ppm *V/V* to 2 ppm *V/V* of *sulphur dioxide R1.*

Calibrate the apparatus and set the sensitivity using reference gases (a) and (b). Measure the content of sulphur dioxide in the gas to be examined.

Oil: maximum 0.1 mg/m^3 calculated for atmospheric pressure and at 0 °C, determined using a measuring system such as described in Figure 1238.-2.

The apparatus consists of the following:

- an on-off valve (1),
- a three-way valve (2),
- an oil cone (3),
- a bypass line (4),
- a pressure-regulator (5),
- a flow-metering device (6).

All of the apparatus is cleaned beforehand, using trichlorotrifluoroethane R free from oil and grease.

Place a micro fibre-glass filter in the oil cone (3); this filter has the following characteristics: 100 per cent borosilicate glass without binder; resistant to heat treatment at 500 °C (to eliminate organic traces); 99.999 per cent retention efficiency for NaCl particles with a diameter of 0.6 µm. Close the on-off valve (1); the substance to be examined enters the bypass line (4) and purges the three-way valve (2), the pressure-regulator (5) and the flow-metering device (6). Close the inlet valve of the compression and filtration system: open the on-off valve (1) and set the three-way valve (2) to the position allowing passage between the oil

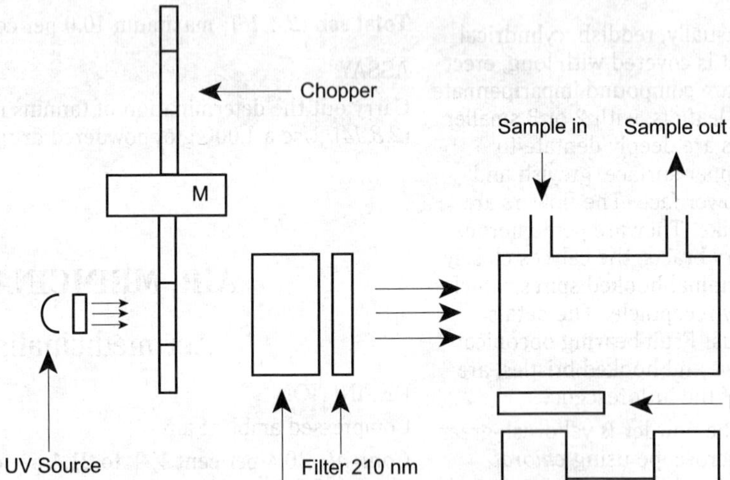

Figure 1238.-1. – *UV fluorescence analyser*

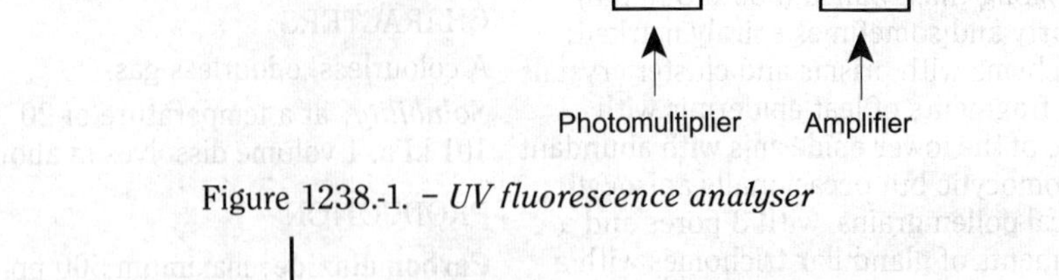

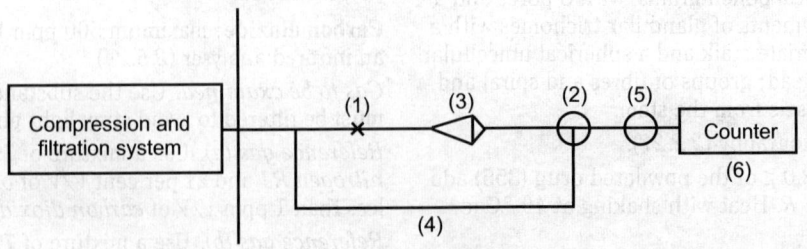

Figure 1238.-2. – *Measuring system for oil*

cone and the pressure-regulator. Open the inlet valve and set the pressure-regulator (5) so that the flow indicated by the flow-metering device (6) is 20 litres/min. Pass 100.0 litres of the substance to be examined through the system.

Test solution. Remove the micro fibre-glass filter and place in an airtight container. Carefully cut up the micro fibre-glass filter and place the pieces in 25.0 ml of *trichlorotrifluoroethane R.*

Reference solutions. Prepare the reference solutions with quantities of oil (used for the lubrication of the compression system) ranging from 0.05 μg/ml to 0.5 μg/ml in *trichlorotrifluoroethane R.*

Measure the absorbance of the test solution and the reference solutions, using an appropriate infrared spectrophotometer, at 2960.3 cm^{-1}, 2927.7 cm^{-1} and 2855.0 cm^{-1}. The sum of the 3 absorbances gives the absorbance of the oil. Use potassium bromide cells with a pathlength of several centimetres.

Plot the calibration curve from the absorbances obtained with the reference solutions and determine the quantity of oil from this curve.

Nitrogen monoxide and nitrogen dioxide: maximum 2 ppm *V/V* in total, determined using a chemiluminescence analyser (*2.5.26*).

Gas to be examined. Use the substance to be examined.

Reference gas (a). Use a mixture of 79 per cent *V/V* of *nitrogen R1* and 21 per cent *V/V* of *oxygen R* containing less than 0.05 ppm *V/V* of nitrogen monoxide and nitrogen dioxide.

Reference gas (b). Use a mixture of 2 ppm *V/V* of *nitrogen monoxide R* in *nitrogen R1.*

Calibrate the apparatus and set the sensitivity using reference gases (a) and (b). Measure the content of nitrogen monoxide and nitrogen dioxide in the gas to be examined.

Water: maximum 67 ppm *V/V*, determined using an electrolytic hygrometer (*2.5.28*), except where the competent authority decides that the following limit applies to medicinal air generated on-site and distributed in pipe-line systems operating at a pressure not greater than 10 bars and a temperature not less than 5 °C: maximum 870 ppm *V/V*, determined using an electrolytic hygrometer (*2.5.28*).

Assay. Determine the concentration of oxygen in air using a paramagnetic analyser (*2.5.27*).

IDENTIFICATION

First identification: C.

Second identification: A, B.

A. In a conical flask containing the substance to be examined, place a glowing wood splinter. The splinter remains glowing.

B. Use a gas burette (Figure 1238.-3) of 25 ml capacity in the form of a chamber in the middle of which is a tube graduated in 0.2 per cent between 19.0 per cent and 23.0 per cent, and isolated at each end by a tap with a conical barrel. The lower tap is joined to a tube with an olive-shaped nozzle and is used to introduce the gas into the apparatus. A cylindrical funnel above the upper tap is used to introduce the absorbent solution. Wash the burette with *water R* and dry. Open the 2 taps. Connect the nozzle to the source of the substance to be examined and set the flow rate to 1 litre/min. Flush the burette by passing the substance to be examined through it for 1 min. Close the lower tap of the burette and immediately afterwards the upper tap. Rapidly disconnect the burette from the source of the substance to be examined. Rapidly give a half turn to the upper tap to eliminate any excess pressure in the burette. Keeping the burette vertical, fill the funnel with a freshly prepared mixture of 21 ml of a 560 g/l solution of *potassium hydroxide R* and 130 ml of a 200 g/l solution of *sodium dithionite R.* Open the upper tap slowly. The solution absorbs the oxygen and enters the burette. Allow to stand for 10 min without shaking. Read the level of the liquid meniscus on the graduated part of the burette. This figure represents the percentage *V/V* of oxygen. The value read is 20.4 to 21.4.

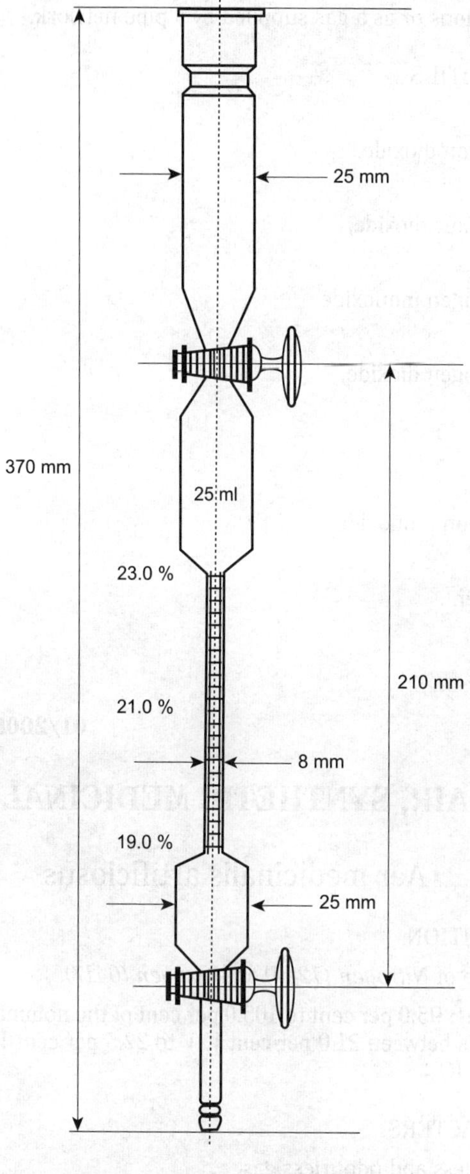

Figure 1238.-3. – *Gas burette*

C. It complies with the limits of the assay.

TESTS

Carbon dioxide: maximum 500 ppm *V/V*, determined using a carbon dioxide detector tube (*2.1.6*).

Sulphur dioxide: maximum 1 ppm *V/V*, determined using a sulphur dioxide detector tube (*2.1.6*).

Oil: maximum 0.1 mg/m^3, determined using an oil detector tube (*2.1.6*).

Nitrogen monoxide and nitrogen dioxide: maximum 2 ppm *V/V*, determined using a nitrogen monoxide and nitrogen dioxide detector tube (*2.1.6*).

Carbon monoxide: maximum 5 ppm *V/V*, determined using a carbon monoxide detector tube (*2.1.6*).

Water vapour: maximum 67 ppm *V/V*, determined using a water vapour detector tube (*2.1.6*), except where the competent authority decides that the following limit applies to medicinal air generated on-site and distributed in pipe-line systems operating at a pressure not greater than 10 bars and a temperature not less than 5 °C: maximum 870 ppm *V/V*, determined using a water vapour detector tube (*2.1.6*).

STORAGE

As a gas, in suitable containers complying with the legal regulations or as a gas supplied by a pipe network.

IMPURITIES

A. carbon dioxide,

B. sulphur dioxide,

C. nitrogen monoxide,

D. nitrogen dioxide,

E. oil,

F. carbon monoxide,

G. water.

01/2005:1684

AIR, SYNTHETIC MEDICINAL

Aer medicinalis artificiosus

DEFINITION

Mixture of *Nitrogen (1247)* and *Oxygen (0417)*.

Content: 95.0 per cent to 105.0 per cent of the nominal value which is between 21.0 per cent *V/V* to 22.5 per cent *V/V* of oxygen (O_2).

CHARACTERS

Colourless and odourless gas.

Solubility: at a temperature of 20 °C and a pressure of 101 kPa, 1 volume dissolves in about 50 volumes of water.

PRODUCTION

Water (*2.5.28*): maximum 67 ppm *V/V*.

Assay (*2.5.27*). Carry out the determination of oxygen in gases.

IDENTIFICATION

First identification: C.

Second identification: A, B.

A. In a conical flask containing the substance to be examined, place a glowing splinter of wood. The splinter remains glowing.

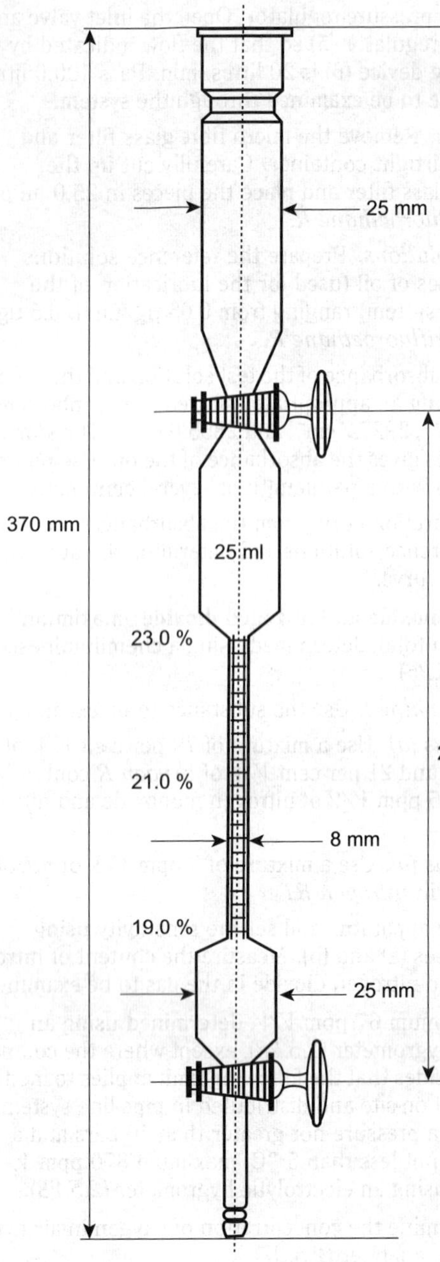

Figure 1684.-1.– *Gas burette*

B. Use a gas burette (Figure 1684.-1) of 25 ml capacity in the form of a chamber, in the middle of which is a tube graduated in 0.2 per cent between 19.0 per cent and 23.0 per cent, and isolated at each end by a tap with a conical barrel. The lower tap is joined to a tube with an olive-shaped nozzle and is used to introduce the gas into the apparatus. A cylindrical funnel above the upper tap is used to introduce the absorbent solution. Wash the burette with *water R* and dry. Open both taps. Connect the nozzle to the source of the substance to be examined and set the flow rate to 1 litre/min. Flush the burette by passing the substance to be examined through it for 1 min. Close the lower tap of the burette and immediately afterwards the upper tap. Rapidly disconnect the burette from the source of the substance to be examined. Rapidly give a half turn of the upper tap to eliminate any excess pressure in the burette. Keeping the burette vertical, fill the funnel with a freshly prepared mixture of 21 ml of a 560 g/l solution of *potassium hydroxide R* and 130 ml of a 200 g/l solution of *sodium dithionite R*. Open the upper tap slowly. The solution absorbs the oxygen and enters the burette. Allow to stand for 10 min without shaking. Read the level of the liquid meniscus on the graduated part of the burette. This figure represents the percentage *V/V* of oxygen. The value read is 95.0 per cent to 105.0 per cent of the nominal value.

C. It complies with the limits of the assay.

TESTS

Water vapour: maximum 67 ppm *V/V*, determined using a water vapour detector tube (*2.1.6*).

STORAGE

As a compressed gas in suitable containers complying with the legal regulations or as a compressed gas supplied by a pipe network, after mixing of the components.

LABELLING

The label states the nominal content of O_2 in per cent *V/V*.

IMPURITIES

A. water.

01/2005:0752

ALANINE

Alaninum

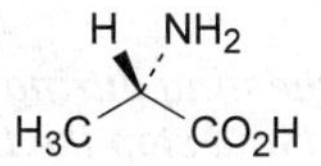

$C_3H_7NO_2$ M_r 89.1

DEFINITION

Alanine contains not less than 98.5 per cent and not more than the equivalent of 101.0 per cent of (*S*)-2-aminopropanoic acid, calculated with reference to the dried substance.

CHARACTERS

White or almost white, crystalline powder or colourless crystals, freely soluble in water, very slightly soluble in alcohol.

IDENTIFICATION

First identification: A, B.

Second identification: A, C, D.

A. It complies with the test for specific optical rotation (see Tests).

B. Examine by infrared absorption spectrophotometry (*2.2.24*), comparing with the spectrum obtained with *alanine CRS*. Examine the substances prepared as discs.

C. Examine the chromatograms obtained in the test for ninhydrin-positive substances. The principal spot in the chromatogram obtained with test solution (b) is similar in position, colour and size to the principal spot in the chromatogram obtained with reference solution (a).

D. Dissolve 0.5 g in a mixture of 1 ml of *water R*, 0.5 ml of a 100 g/l solution of *sodium nitrite R* and 0.25 ml of *hydrochloric acid R1*. Shake. Gas is given off. Add 2 ml of *dilute sodium hydroxide solution R*, followed by 0.25 ml of *iodinated potassium iodide solution R*. After about 30 min, a yellow precipitate with a characteristic odour is formed.

TESTS

Solution S. Dissolve 2.5 g in *distilled water R* and dilute to 50 ml with the same solvent.

Appearance of solution. Dilute 10 ml of solution S to 20 ml with *water R*. The solution is clear (*2.2.1*) and not more intensely coloured than reference solution BY_6 (*2.2.2, Method II*).

Specific optical rotation (*2.2.7*). Dissolve 2.50 g in *hydrochloric acid R1* and dilute to 25.0 ml with the same acid. The specific optical rotation is + 13.5 to + 15.5, calculated with reference to the dried substance.

Ninhydrin-positive substances. Examine by thin-layer chromatography (*2.2.27*), using a *TLC silica gel plate R*.

Test solution (a). Dissolve 0.10 g in *water R* and dilute to 10 ml with the same solvent.

Test solution (b). Dilute 1 ml of test solution (a) to 50 ml with *water R*.

Reference solution (a). Dissolve 10 mg of *alanine CRS* in *water R* and dilute to 50 ml with the same solvent.

Reference solution (b). Dilute 5 ml of test solution (b) to 20 ml with *water R*.

Reference solution (c). Dissolve 10 mg of *alanine CRS* and 10 mg of *glycine CRS* in *water R* and dilute to 25 ml with the same solvent.

Apply separately to the plate 5 µl of each solution. Allow the plate to dry in air. Develop over a path of 15 cm with a mixture of 20 volumes of *glacial acetic acid R*, 20 volumes of *water R* and 60 volumes of *butanol R*. Allow the plate to dry in air. Spray with *ninhydrin solution R*. Heat the plate at 100 °C to 105 °C for 15 min. Any spot in the chromatogram obtained with test solution (a), apart from the principal spot, is not more intense than the spot in the chromatogram obtained with reference solution (b) (0.5 per cent). The test is not valid unless the chromatogram obtained with reference solution (c) shows two clearly separated spots.

Chlorides (*2.4.4*). Dilute 5 ml of solution S to 15 ml with *water R*. The solution complies with the limit test for chlorides (200 ppm).

Sulphates (*2.4.13*). Dilute 10 ml of solution S to 15 ml with *distilled water R*. The solution complies with the limit test for sulphates (300 ppm).

Ammonium (*2.4.1*). 50 mg complies with limit test B for ammonium (200 ppm). Prepare the standard using 0.1 ml of *ammonium standard solution (100 ppm* NH_4*) R*.

Iron (*2.4.9*). In a separating funnel, dissolve 1.0 g in 10 ml of *dilute hydrochloric acid R*. Shake with three quantities, each of 10 ml, of *methyl isobutyl ketone R1*, shaking for 3 min each time. To the combined organic layers add 10 ml of *water R* and shake for 3 min. The aqueous layer complies with the limit test for iron (10 ppm).

Heavy metals (*2.4.8*). Dissolve 2.0 g in *water R* and dilute to 20 ml with the same solvent. 12 ml of the solution complies with limit test A for heavy metals (10 ppm). Prepare the standard using *lead standard solution (1 ppm Pb) R*.

Loss on drying (*2.2.32*). Not more than 0.5 per cent, determined on 1.000 g by drying in an oven at 100 °C to 105 °C.

Sulphated ash (*2.4.14*). Not more than 0.1 per cent, determined on 1.0 g.

ASSAY

Dissolve 80.0 mg in 3 ml of *anhydrous formic acid R*. Add 30 ml of *anhydrous acetic acid R*. Using 0.1 ml of *naphtholbenzein solution R* as indicator, titrate with *0.1 M perchloric acid*, until the colour changes from brownish-yellow to green.

1 ml of *0.1 M perchloric acid* is equivalent to 8.91 mg of $C_3H_7NO_2$.

STORAGE

Store protected from light.

01/2005:1386

ALBENDAZOLE

Albendazolum

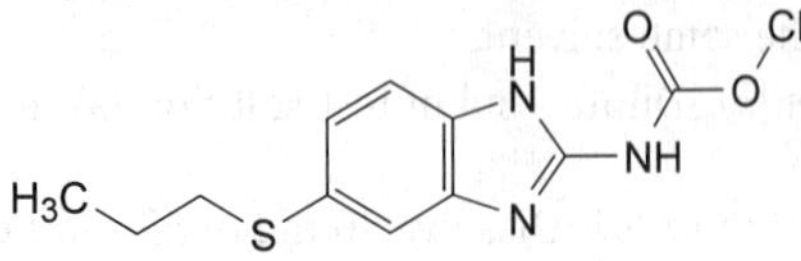

$C_{12}H_{15}N_3O_2S$ M_r 265.3

DEFINITION

Albendazole contains not less than 98.0 per cent and not more than the equivalent of 102.0 per cent of methyl [5-(propylsulphanyl)-1*H*-benzimidazol-2-yl]carbamate, calculated with reference to the dried substance.

CHARACTERS

A white or faintly yellowish powder, practically insoluble in water, freely soluble in anhydrous formic acid, very slightly soluble in methylene chloride, practically insoluble in alcohol.

IDENTIFICATION

Examine by infrared absorption spectrophotometry (*2.2.24*), comparing with the spectrum obtained with *albendazole CRS*. Examine the substances prepared as discs.

TESTS

Appearance of solution. Dissolve 0.10 g in a mixture of 1 volume of *anhydrous formic acid R* and 9 volumes of *methylene chloride R* and dilute to 10 ml with the same mixture of solvents. The solution is clear (*2.2.1*) and not more intensely coloured than reference solution BY_6 (*2.2.2, Method II*).

Related substances. Examine by liquid chromatography (*2.2.29*).

Test solution. Dissolve 25.0 mg of the substance to be examined in 5 ml of *methanol R* containing 1 per cent *V/V* of *sulphuric acid R* and dilute to 50.0 ml with the mobile phase.

Reference solution (a). Dissolve 10.0 mg of the substance to be examined in 10 ml of *methanol R* containing 1 per cent *V/V* of *sulphuric acid R* and dilute to 100.0 ml with the mobile phase. Dilute 0.5 ml of this solution to 20.0 ml with the mobile phase.

Reference solution (b). Dissolve 50.0 mg of the substance to be examined and 50 mg of *oxybendazole CRS* in 5 ml of *methanol R* containing 1 per cent *V/V* of *sulphuric acid R* and dilute to 100.0 ml with the mobile phase.

The chromatographic procedure may be carried out using:

- a stainless steel column 0.25 m long and 4.6 mm in internal diameter packed with spherical *end-capped octadecylsilyl silica gel for chromatography R* (5 µm) with a pore size of 10 nm and a carbon loading of 19 per cent,
- as the mobile phase at a flow rate of 0.7 ml/min a mixture of 300 volumes of a 1.67 g/l solution of *ammonium dihydrogen phosphate R* and 700 volumes of *methanol R*,
- as detector a spectrophotometer set at 254 nm.

Inject 20 µl of reference solution (a). Adjust the sensitivity of the system so that the height of the principal peak in the chromatogram obtained is at least 50 per cent of the full scale of the recorder. Inject 20 µl of reference solution (b). The test is not valid unless the resolution between the peaks corresponding to albendazole and oxybendazole is at least 3.0.

Inject 20 µl of the test solution. Continue the chromatography for 1.5 times the retention time of albendazole. When the chromatograms are recorded in the prescribed conditions, the approximate relative retention times are: 0.80 for impurity A, 0.43 for impurities B and C, 0.40 for impurity D, 0.47 for impurity E and 0.57 for impurity F. In the chromatogram obtained with the test solution the area of any peak, apart from the principal peak, is not greater than 1.5 times the area of the principal peak in the chromatogram obtained with reference solution (a) (0.75 per cent) and the sum of the areas of any such peaks is not greater than 3 times the area of the principal peak in the chromatogram obtained with reference solution (a) (1.5 per cent). Disregard any peak with an area less than 0.1 times the area of the principal peak in the chromatogram obtained with reference solution (a).

Loss on drying (*2.2.32*). Not more than 0.5 per cent, determined on 1.000 g by drying in an oven at 100-105 °C for 4 h.

Sulphated ash (*2.4.14*). Not more than 0.2 per cent, determined on 1.0 g.

ASSAY

In order to avoid overheating during the titration, mix thoroughly throughout and stop the titration immediately after the end-point has been reached.

Dissolve 0.250 g in 3 ml of *anhydrous formic acid R* and add 40 ml of *anhydrous acetic acid R*. Titrate with *0.1 M perchloric acid*, determining the end-point potentiometrically (*2.2.20*).

1 ml of *0.1 M perchloric acid* is equivalent to 26.53 mg of $C_{12}H_{15}N_3O_2S$.

STORAGE

Store protected from light.

IMPURITIES

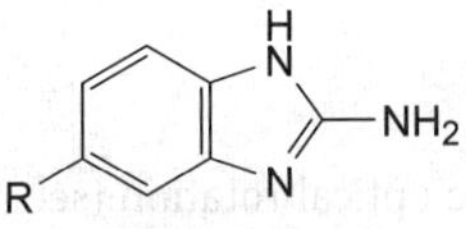

A. R = $S\text{-}CH_2\text{-}CH_2\text{-}CH_3$: 5-(propylsulphanyl)-1*H*-benzimidazol-2-amine,

D. R = $SO_2\text{-}CH_2\text{-}CH_2\text{-}CH_3$: 5-(propylsulphonyl)-1*H*-benzimidazol-2-amine,

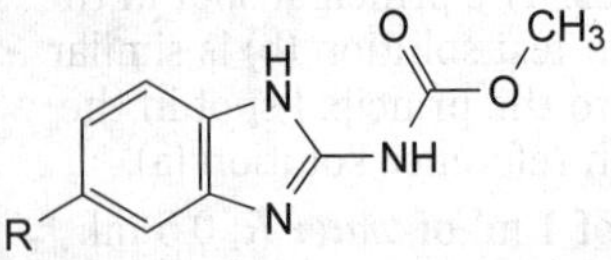

B. R = $SO\text{-}CH_2\text{-}CH_2\text{-}CH_3$: methyl [5-(propylsulphinyl)-1*H*-benzimidazol-2-yl]carbamate,

C. R = $SO_2\text{-}CH_2\text{-}CH_2\text{-}CH_3$: methyl [5-(propylsulphonyl)-1*H*-benzimidazol-2-yl]carbamate,

E. R = H: methyl (1*H*-benzimidazol-2-yl)carbamate,

F. R = $S\text{-}CH_3$: methyl [5-(methylsulphanyl)-1*H*-benzimidazol-2-yl]carbamate.

01/2005:1387

ALCHEMILLA

Alchemillae herba

DEFINITION

Alchemilla consists of the whole or cut, dried, flowering, aerial parts of *Alchemilla vulgaris* L. *sensu latiore.* It contains not less than 6.0 per cent of tannins, expressed as pyrogallol ($C_6H_6O_3$, M_r 126.1), calculated with reference to the dried drug.

CHARACTERS

It has the macroscopic and microscopic characters described under identification tests A and B.

IDENTIFICATION

A. The greyish-green, partly brownish-green, radical leaves which are the main part of the drug are reniform to slightly semicircular with a diameter generally up to 8 cm, seldom up to 11 cm and have 7 to 9, or 11 lobes and a long petiole. The smaller, cauline leaves, which have a pair of large stipules at the base, have 5 to 9 lobes and a shorter petiole or they are sessile. The leaves are densely pubescent especially on the lower surface and have a coarsely serrated margin. Young leaves are folded with a whitish-silvery pubescence; older leaves are slightly pubescent and have a finely meshed venation, prominent on the lower surface. The greyish-green to yellowish-green petiole is pubescent, about 1 mm in diameter, with an adaxial groove. The apetalous flowers are yellowish-green to light green and about 3 mm in diameter. The calyx is double with 4 small segments of the epicalyx alternating with 4 larger sepals, subacute to triangular. They are 4 short stamens and a single carpel with a capitate stigma. The greyish-green to yellowish-green stem is pubescent, more or less longitudinally wrinkled and hollow.

B. Reduce to a powder (355). The powder is greyish-green. Examine under a microscope, using *chloral hydrate solution R*. The powder shows unicellular, narrow trichomes up to 1 mm long partly tortuous, acuminate, and bluntly pointed at the apex, with thick lignified walls, somewhat enlarged and pitted at the base; fragments of leaves with 2 layers of palisade parenchyma, the upper layer of which is 2 to 3 times longer than the lower layer and with spongy parenchyma, containing scattered cluster crystals of calcium oxalate, up to 25 µm in diameter; leaf fragments in surface view with sinuous to wavy epidermal cells, the anticlinal walls unevenly thickened and beaded, anomocytic stomata (*2.8.3*); groups of vascular tissue and lignified fibres from the petioles and stems, the vessels spirally thickened or with bordered pits; occasional thin-walled conical trichomes, about 300 µm long; thin-walled parenchyma containing cluster crystals of calcium oxalate; spherical pollen grains, about 15 µm in diameter, with 3 distinct pores and a granular exine; occasional fragments of the ovary wall with cells containing a single crystal of calcium oxalate.

C. Thin-layer chromatography (*2.2.27*).

Test solution. To 0.5 g of the powdered drug (355) add 5 ml of *methanol R* and heat in a water-bath at 70 °C under a reflux condenser for 5 min. Cool and filter.

Reference solution. Dissolve 1.0 mg of *caffeic acid R* and 1.0 mg of *chlorogenic acid R* in 10 ml of *methanol R*.

Plate: *TLC silica gel plate R.*

Mobile phase: *anhydrous formic acid R, water R, ethyl acetate R* (8:8:84 *V/V/V*).

Application: 20 µl as bands for the test solution, 10 µl as bands for the reference solution.

Development: over a path of 10 cm.

Drying: at 100-105 °C for 5 min.

Detection: spray with a 10 g/l solution of *diphenylboric acid aminoethyl ester R* in *methanol R*. Subsequently spray with a 50 g/l solution of *macrogol 400 R* in *methanol R*. Allow the plate to dry in air for about 30 min. Examine in ultraviolet light at 365 nm.

Results: see below the sequence of the zones present in the chromatograms obtained with the reference solution and the test solution. Furthermore, other fluorescent zones may be present in the chromatogram obtained with the test solution.

Top of the plate	
	Two red fluorescent zones (chlorophyll)
Caffeic acid: a light blue florescent zone	One or two intense light blue fluorescent zones
	One or several intense green to greenish yellow fluorescent zone
———	———
Chlorogenic acid: a light blue fluorescent zone	An intense yellow to orange fluorescent zone
———	———
Reference solution	**Test solution**

TESTS

Foreign matter (*2.8.2*): maximum 2 per cent.

Loss on drying (*2.2.32*): maximum 10.0 per cent, determined on 1.000 g of powdered drug (355) by drying in an oven at 100-105 °C for 2 h.

Total ash (*2.4.16*): maximum 12.0 per cent.

ASSAY

Carry out the determination of tannins in herbal drugs (*2.8.14*). Use 0.50 g of the powdered drug (355).

01/2005:1285

ALCURONIUM CHLORIDE

Alcuronii chloridum

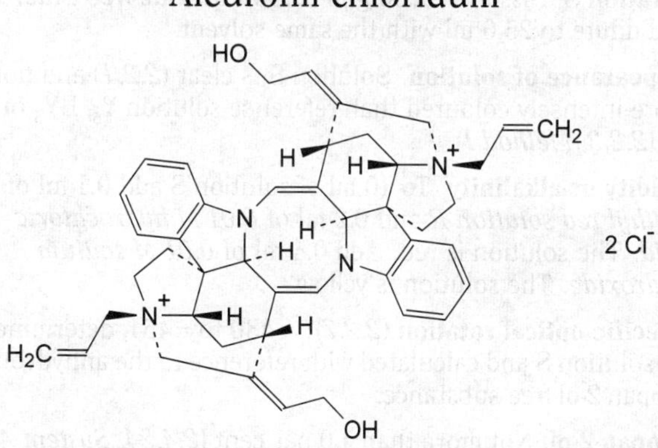

$C_{44}H_{50}Cl_2N_4O_2$ M_r 738

DEFINITION

Alcuronium chloride contains not less than 98.0 per cent and not more than the equivalent of 102.0 per cent of (1*R*,3a*S*,10*S*,11a*S*,12*R*,14a*S*,19a*S*,20b*S*,21*S*,22a*S*,23*E*,26*E*)-23,26-bis(2-hydroxyethylidene)-1,12-bis(prop-2-enyl)-2,3,11,11a,13,14,22,22a-octahydro-10*H*,21*H*-1,21:10,12-diethano-19a*H*,20b*H*-[1,5]diazocino[1,2,3-*lm*:5,6,7-

l'm]dipyrrolo[2′,3′-*d*:2″,3″:*d*]dicarbazolediium dichloride (4,4′-didesmethyl-4,4′-bis(prop-2-enyl)toxi- ferin I dichloride), calculated with reference to the anhydrous, propan-2-ol-free substance.

CHARACTERS

A white or slightly greyish-white, crystalline powder, freely soluble in water and in methanol, soluble in alcohol, practically insoluble in cyclohexane.

Carry out the identification, tests and assay as rapidly as possible avoiding exposure to actinic light.

IDENTIFICATION

First identification: A, C.

Second identification: B, C.

A. Examine by infrared absorption spectrophotometry (*2.2.24*), comparing with the spectrum obtained with *alcuronium chloride CRS.*

B. Examine by thin-layer chromatography (*2.2.27*) using a *TLC silica gel plate R.*

Test solution. Dissolve 10 mg of the substance to be examined in *methanol R* and dilute to 10 ml with the same solvent.

Reference solution. Dissolve 10 mg of *alcuronium chloride CRS* in *methanol R* and dilute to 10 ml with the same solvent.

Apply to the plate 10 µl of each solution. Develop over a path of 15 cm using a mixture of 15 volumes of a 58.4 g/l solution of *sodium chloride R*, 35 volumes of *dilute ammonia R2* and 50 volumes of *methanol R*. Allow the plate to dry in air for 10 min and then spray with *0.1 M ammonium and cerium nitrate*. The principal spot in the chromatogram obtained with the test solution is similar in position, colour and size to the principal spot in the chromatogram obtained with the reference solution.

C. It gives reaction (a) of chlorides (*2.3.1*).

TESTS

Solution S. Dissolve 0.250 g in *carbon dioxide-free water R* and dilute to 25.0 ml with the same solvent.

Appearance of solution. Solution S is clear (*2.2.1*) and not more intensely coloured than reference solution Y_6, BY_6 or B_6 (*2.2.2, Method I*).

Acidity or alkalinity. To 10 ml of solution S add 0.1 ml of *methyl red solution R* and 0.2 ml of *0.01 M hydrochloric acid*. The solution is red. Add 0.4 ml of *0.01 M sodium hydroxide*. The solution is yellow.

Specific optical rotation (*2.2.7*): − 430 to − 451, determined on solution S and calculated with reference to the anhydrous, propan-2-ol-free substance.

Propan-2-ol. Not more than 1.0 per cent (*2.4.24, System A*).

Related substances. Examine by liquid chromatography (*2.2.29*).

Solvent mixture. Mix 100 ml of *methanol R*, 200 ml of *acetonitrile R* and 200 ml of a 6.82 g/l solution of *potassium dihydrogen phosphate R*. Dissolve 1.09 g of *sodium laurylsulphonate for chromatography R* in the mixture and adjust the apparent pH to 8.0 with a 100 g/l solution of *sodium hydroxide R*.

Test solution. Dissolve 0.20 g of the substance to be examined in the solvent mixture and dilute to 100.0 ml with the solvent mixture.

Reference solution (a). Dilute 0.5 ml of the test solution to 100.0 ml with the solvent mixture.

Reference solution (b). Dilute 4.0 ml of reference solution (a) to 10.0 ml with the solvent mixture.

Reference solution (c). Dilute 1.0 ml of reference solution (a) to 10.0 ml with the solvent mixture.

Reference solution (d). To 5.0 ml of the test solution add 5.0 mg of *allylstrychnine bromide CRS*, dissolve in the solvent mixture and dilute to 100.0 ml with the solvent mixture.

The chromatographic procedure may be carried out using:

– a stainless steel column 0.25 m long and 4 mm in internal diameter packed with *octylsilyl silica gel for chromatography R* (5 µm),

– as mobile phase at a flow rate of 1.2 ml/min a solution prepared as follows: mix 200 ml of *methanol R*, 400 ml of *acetonitrile R* and 400 ml of a 6.82 g/l solution of *potassium dihydrogen phosphate R*. Dissolve 2.18 g of *sodium laurylsulphonate for chromatography R* in the mixture and adjust the apparent pH to 5.4 with a 100 g/l solution of *phosphoric acid R*,

– as detector a spectrophotometer set at 254 nm.

Inject 10 µl of reference solution (b). Adjust the sensitivity of the system so that the height of the peak due to alcuronium is at least 10 per cent of the full scale of the recorder. Inject 10 µl of reference solution (d). The test is not valid unless the resolution between the peak corresponding to *N*-allylstrychnine and alcuronium is at least 4.0. Inject 10 µl of the test solution, 10 µl of reference solution (a) and 10 µl of reference solution (c). Continue the chromatography of the test solution for twice the retention time of the peak corresponding to alcuronium. In the chromatogram obtained with the test solution the area of any peak, apart from the principal peak, is not greater than the area of the principal peak in the chromatogram obtained with reference solution (a) (0.5 per cent) and not more than one such peak has an area greater than the area of the principal peak in the chromatogram obtained with reference solution (b) (0.2 per cent); the sum of the areas of all the peaks, apart from the principal peak, is not greater than twice the area of the principal peak in the chromatogram obtained with reference solution (a) (1 per cent). Disregard any peak with an area less than the area of the principal peak in the chromatogram obtained with reference solution (c) (0.05 per cent).

Water (*2.5.12*). Not more than 5.0 per cent, determined on 0.500 g by the semi-micro determination of water.

Sulphated ash (*2.4.14*). Not more than 0.1 per cent, determined on 1.0 g.

ASSAY

Dissolve 0.300 g by stirring in 70 ml of *acetic anhydride R* for 1 min. Titrate with*0.1 M perchloric acid* until the colour changes from violet-blue to greenish-blue, using 0.1 ml of *crystal violet solution R* as indicator.

1 ml of *0.1 M perchloric acid* is equivalent to 36.9 mg of $C_{44}H_{50}Cl_2N_4O_2$.

STORAGE

Store in an airtight container under nitrogen, protected from light, at a temperature of 2 °C to 8 °C.

IMPURITIES

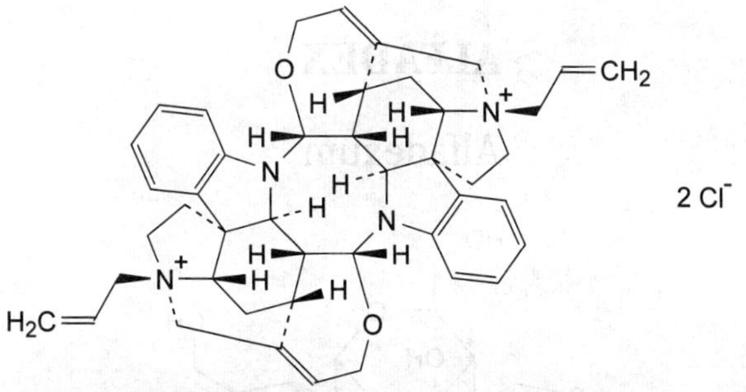

A. (1*R*,3a*S*,9*R*,9a*R*,10*R*,11a*S*,12*R*,14a*S*,19a*S*,20*R*,20a*R*,20b*S*,21*R*,22a*S*)-1,12-bis(prop-2-enyl)-2,3,9a,11,11a,13,14,19a,20a,21,22,22a-dodecahydro-10*H*,20b*H*-1,23:12,27-dimethano-9,10:20,21-bis(epoxyprop[2]eno)-9*H*,20*H*-[1,5]diazocino[1,2,3-*lm*:5,6,7-*l′m′*]dipyrrolo[2′,3′-*d*:2″,3″:*d′*]dicarbazolediium dichloride (4,4′-diallylcaracurin V dichloride),

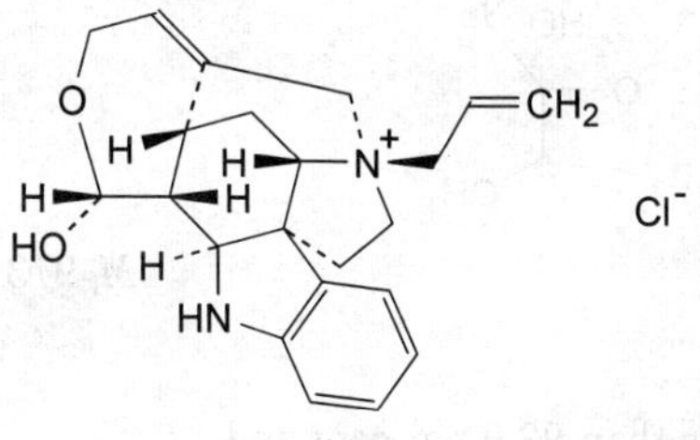

B. (4b*S*,7*R*,7a*S*,8a*R*,13*R*,13a*R*,13b*S*)-13-hydroxy-7-(prop-2-enyl)-5,6,7a,8,8a,11,13,13a,13b,14-decahydro-7,9-methano-7*H*-oxepino[3,4-*a*]pyrrolo[2,3-*d*]carbazolium chloride ((4*R*,17*R*)-4-allyl-17,18-epoxy-17-hydroxy-19,20-didehydrocuranium chloride).

01/2005:1286

ALFACALCIDOL

Alfacalcidolum

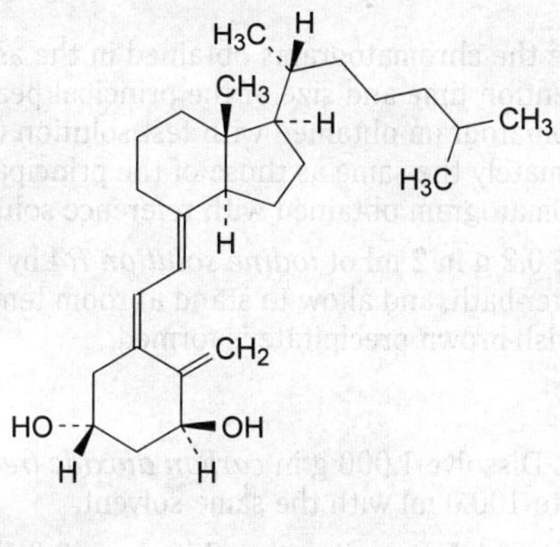

$C_{27}H_{44}O_2$ M_r 400.6

DEFINITION

Alfacalcidol contains not less that 97.0 per cent and not more than the equivalent of 102.0 per cent of (5*Z*,7*E*)-9,10-secocholesta-5,7,10(19)-triene-1α,3β-diol.

CHARACTERS

White or almost white crystals, practically insoluble in water, freely soluble in alcohol, soluble in fatty oils. It is sensitive to air, heat and light.

A reversible isomerisation to pre-alfacalcidol takes place in solution, depending on temperature and time. The activity is due to both compounds.

IDENTIFICATION

A. Examine by infrared absorption spectrophotometry (*2.2.24*), comparing with the *Ph. Eur. reference spectrum of alfacalcidol.*

B. Examine the chromatograms obtained in the assay. The principal peak in the chromatogram obtained with the test solution is similar in retention time and size to the principal peak in the chromatogram obtained with reference solution (a).

TESTS

Related substances. Examine by liquid chromatography (*2.2.29*) as described under Assay. Calculate the percentage content of related substances, apart from pre-alfacalcidol, that are eluted within twice the retention time of alfacalcidol from the areas of the peaks in the chromatogram obtained with the test solution by the normalisation procedure. The content of any individual related substance is not greater than 0.5 per cent and the sum of the related substances is not greater than 1.0 per cent. Disregard any peak below 0.1 per cent.

ASSAY

Carry out the assay as rapidly as possible, avoiding exposure to actinic light and air.

Examine by liquid chromatography (*2.2.29*).

Test solution. Dissolve 1.0 mg of the substance to be examined without heating in 10.0 ml of the mobile phase.

Reference solution (a). Dissolve 1.0 mg of *alfacalcidol CRS* without heating in 10.0 ml of the mobile phase.

Reference solution (b). Dilute reference solution (a) 100 times with the mobile phase.

Reference solution (c). Heat 2 ml of reference solution (a) in a water-bath at 80 °C under a reflux condenser for 2 h and cool.

The chromatographic procedure may be carried out using:

– a column 0.25 m long and 4.0 mm in internal diameter packed with *octadecylsilyl silica gel for chromatography R2* (5 μm),
– as mobile phase at a flow rate of 2.0 ml/min a mixture of 1 volume of *ammonia R*, 200 volumes of *water R* and 800 volumes of *acetonitrile R*,
– as detector a spectrophotometer set at 265 nm,
– a loop injector.

Inject 100 μl of reference solution (c) and record the chromatogram. Make a total of six injections. When the chromatograms are recorded in the prescribed conditions, the retention time for pre-alfacalcidol, relative to alfacalcidol, is about 1.3. The assay is not valid unless the relative standard deviation of the response for alfacalcidol is at most 1 per cent and the resolution between the peaks due to pre-alfacalcidol and alfacalcidol is at least 4.0; adjust the proportions of the constituents of the mobile phase, if necessary, to obtain this resolution.

Inject 100 μl of reference solution (a) and 100 μl of reference solution (b) and record the chromatograms. Inject 100 μl of the test solution and record the chromatogram in the same manner, continuing the chromatography for twice the retention time of the principal peak.

STORAGE

Store under nitrogen, in an airtight container, protected from light, at a temperature of 2 °C to 8 °C.

The contents of an opened container are to be used immediately.

IMPURITIES

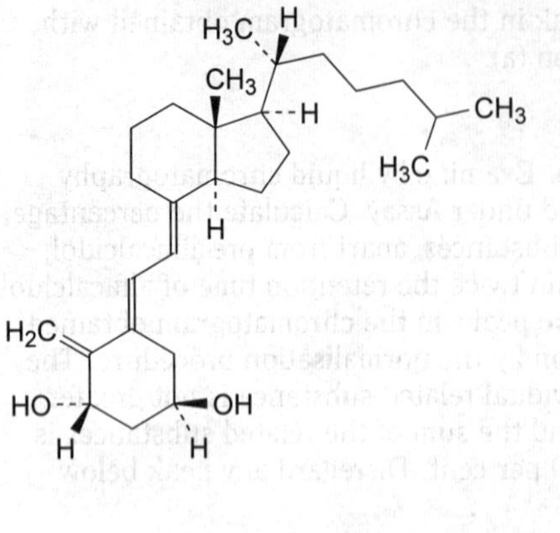

A. (5*E*,7*E*)-9,10-secocholesta-5,7,10(19)-triene-1α,3β-diol (*trans*-alfacalcidol),

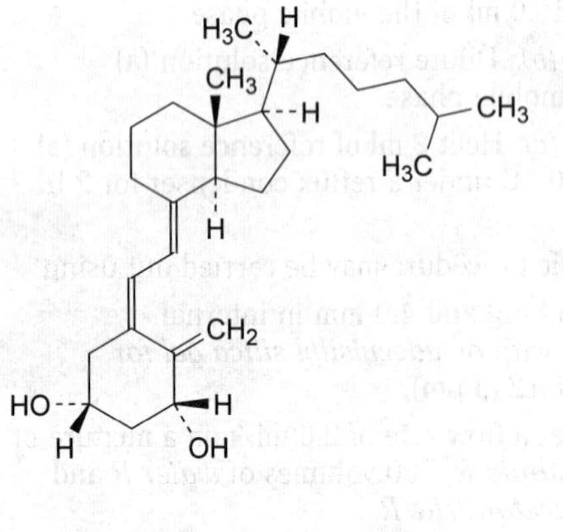

B. (5*Z*,7*E*)-9,10-secocholesta-5,7,10(19)-triene-1β,3β-diol (1β-calcidol),

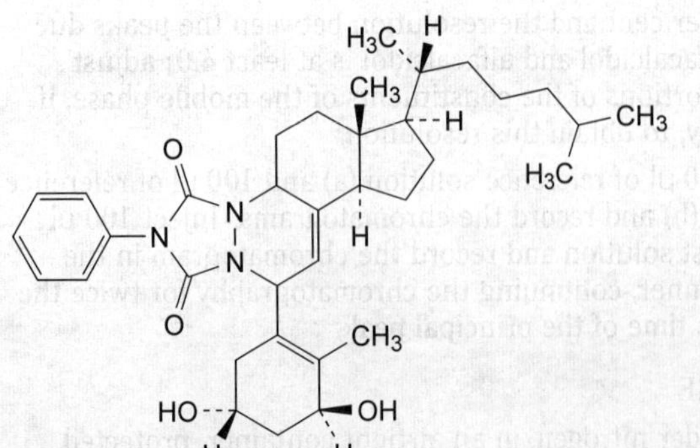

C. triazoline adduct of pre-alfacalcidol.

01/2005:1487

ALFADEX

Alfadexum

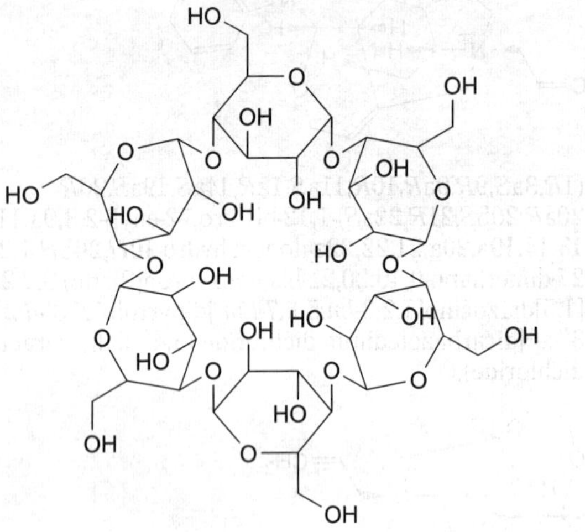

$[C_6H_{10}O_5]_6$ M_r 973

DEFINITION

Alfadex contains not less than 98.0 per cent and not more than the equivalent of 101.0 per cent of cyclohexakis-(1→4)-(α-D-glucopyranosyl) (cyclomaltohexaose or α-cyclodextrin), calculated with reference to the dried substance.

CHARACTERS

A white or almost white, amorphous or crystalline powder, freely soluble in water and in propylene glycol, practically insoluble in ethanol and in methylene chloride.

IDENTIFICATION

A. It complies with the test for specific optical rotation (see Tests).

B. Examine the chromatograms obtained in the assay. The retention time and size of the principal peak in the chromatogram obtained with test solution (b) are approximately the same as those of the principal peak in the chromatogram obtained with reference solution (c).

C. Dissolve 0.2 g in 2 ml of *iodine solution R4* by warming on a water-bath, and allow to stand at room temperature; a yellowish-brown precipitate is formed.

TESTS

Solution S. Dissolve 1.000 g in *carbon dioxide-free water R* and dilute to 100.0 ml with the same solvent.

Appearance of solution. Solution S is clear (*2.2.1*).

pH (*2.2.3*). The pH of a mixture of 30 ml of solution S and 1 ml of a 223.6 g/l solution of *potassium chloride R* is 5.0 to 8.0.

Specific optical rotation (*2.2.7*): + 147 to + 152, determined on solution S and calculated with reference to the dried substance.

Reducing sugars

Test solution. To 1 ml of solution S add 1 ml of *cupri-tartaric solution R4.* Heat on a water-bath for 10 min, cool to room temperature. Add 10 ml of *ammonium molybdate reagent R1* and allow to stand for 15 min.

Reference solution. Prepare a reference solution at the same time and in the same manner as the test solution, using 1 ml of a 0.02 g/l solution of *glucose R*.

Measure the absorbance of the test solution and the reference solution (*2.2.25*) at the maximum at 740 nm using *water R* as the compensation liquid. The absorbance of the test solution is not greater than that of the reference solution (0.2 per cent).

Light-absorbing impurities. Examine solution S between 230 nm and 750 nm (*2.2.25*). Between 230 nm and 350 nm, the absorbance is not greater than 0.10. Between 350 nm and 750 nm, the absorbance is not greater than 0.05.

Related substances. Examine by liquid chromatography (*2.2.29*) as described under Assay. Inject test solution (a) and reference solution (b). In the chromatogram obtained with test solution (a): the areas of any peaks corresponding to betadex or gammacyclodextrin are not greater than half of the area of the corresponding peaks in the chromatogram obtained with reference solution (b) (0.25 per cent); the sum of the areas of all the peaks, apart from the principal peak and any peaks corresponding to betadex or gammacyclodextrin, is not greater than half of the area of the peak corresponding to alfadex in the chromatogram obtained with reference solution (b) (0.5 per cent).

Heavy metals (*2.4.8*). 2.0 g complies with limit test C for heavy metals (10 ppm). Prepare the standard using 2 ml of *lead standard solution (10 ppm Pb) R*.

Loss on drying (*2.2.32*). Not more than 11 per cent, determined on 1.000 g by drying in an oven at 120 °C for 2 h.

Sulphated ash (*2.4.14*). Not more than 0.1 per cent, determined on 1.0 g.

ASSAY

Examine by liquid chromatography (*2.2.29*).

Test solution (a). Dissolve 0.25 g of the substance to be examined in *water R* with heating, cool and dilute to 25.0 ml with the same solvent.

Test solution (b). Dilute 5.0 ml of test solution (a) to 50.0 ml with *water R*.

Reference solution (a). Dissolve 25.0 mg of *betadex CRS*, 25.0 mg of *gammacyclodextrin CRS* and 50.0 mg of *alfadex CRS* in *water R* and dilute to 50.0 ml with the same solvent.

Reference solution (b). Dilute 5.0 ml of reference solution (a) to 50.0 ml with *water R*.

Reference solution (c). Dissolve 25.0 mg of *alfadex CRS* in *water R* and dilute to 25.0 ml with the same solvent.

The chromatographic procedure may be carried out using:

- a stainless steel column 0.25 m long and 4.6 mm in internal diameter packed with *octadecylsilyl silica gel for chromatography R* (10 μm),
- as mobile phase at a flow rate of 1.5 ml/min a mixture of 10 volumes of *methanol R* and 90 volumes of *water R*,
- as detector a differential refractometer,
- a 50 μl loop injector.

Equilibrate the column with the mobile phase at a flow rate of 1.5 ml/min for about 3 h. Inject reference solution (a) 5 times and record the chromatograms for 3.5 times the retention time of alfadex. Adjust the sensitivity of the system so that the height of the peak corresponding to gammacyclodextrin is 55 per cent to 75 per cent of the full scale of the recorder. The retention time of alfadex is about 10 min, the relative retention of gammacyclodextrin is about 0.7 and that of betadex is about 2.2. The test is not valid unless the resolution between the peaks corresponding to gammacyclodextrin and alfadex is at least 1.5 and the relative standard deviation for the area of the peak corresponding to alfadex is less than 2.0 per cent. If necessary, adjust the concentration of methanol in the mobile phase to achieve the required resolution. Inject alternately test solution (b) and reference solution (c). Calculate the percentage content of $[C_6H_{10}O_5]_6$ from the area of the principal peak in each of the chromatograms obtained and from the declared content of *alfadex CRS*.

STORAGE

Store in an airtight container.

IMPURITIES

A. betadex,

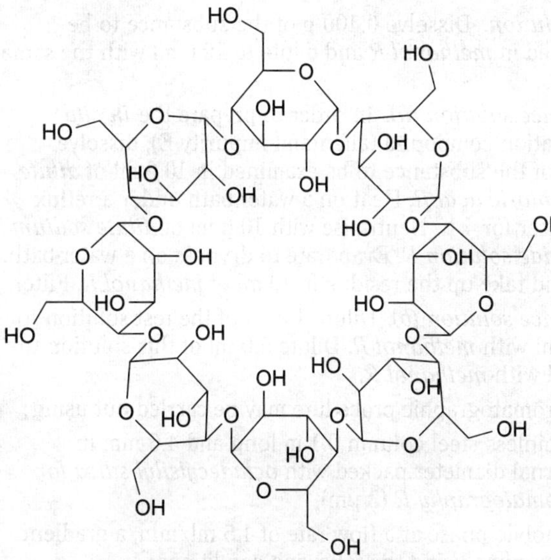

B. cyclooctakis-(1→4)-(α-D-glucopyranosyl) (cyclomaltooctaose or γ-cyclodextrin).

01/2005:1062

ALFENTANIL HYDROCHLORIDE

Alfentanili hydrochloridum

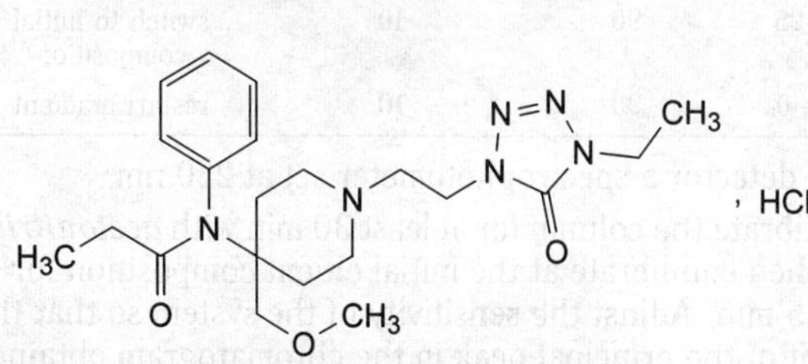

$C_{21}H_{33}ClN_6O_3$ M_r 453.0

DEFINITION

Alfentanil hydrochloride contains not less than 98.5 per cent and not more than the equivalent of 101.5 per cent of *N*-[1-[2-(4-ethyl-4,5-dihydro-5-oxo-1*H*-tetrazol-1-yl)ethyl]-4-(methoxymethyl)piperidin-4-yl]-*N*-phenylpropanamide hydrochloride, calculated with reference to the anhydrous substance.

CHARACTERS

A white or almost white powder, freely soluble in water, in alcohol and in methanol.

It melts at about 140 °C, with decomposition.

IDENTIFICATION

A. Examine by infrared absorption spectrophotometry (*2.2.24*), comparing with the *Ph. Eur. reference spectrum of alfentanil hydrochloride.*

B. Dissolve 50 mg in a mixture of 0.4 ml of *ammonia R* and 2 ml of *water R*. Mix, allow to stand for 5 min and filter. Acidify the filtrate with *dilute nitric acid R*. It gives reaction (a) of chlorides (*2.3.1*).

TESTS

Appearance of solution. Dissolve 0.2 g in *water R* and dilute to 20 ml with the same solvent. The solution is clear (*2.2.1*) and colourless (*2.2.2, Method II*).

Related substances. Examine by liquid chromatography (*2.2.29*).

Test solution. Dissolve 0.100 g of the substance to be examined in *methanol R* and dilute to 10.0 ml with the same solvent.

Reference solution (a). In order to prepare the *in situ* degradation compound (alfentanil impurity E), dissolve 10 mg of the substance to be examined in 10.0 ml of *dilute hydrochloric acid R*. Heat on a water-bath under a reflux condenser for 4 h. Neutralise with 10.0 ml of *dilute sodium hydroxide solution R*. Evaporate to dryness on a water-bath. Cool and take up the residue in 10 ml of *methanol R*. Filter.

Reference solution (b). Dilute 1.0 ml of the test solution to 100.0 ml with *methanol R*. Dilute 5.0 ml of this solution to 20.0 ml with *methanol R*.

The chromatographic procedure may be carried out using:

– a stainless steel column 0.1 m long and 4.6 mm in internal diameter packed with *octadecylsilyl silica for chromatography R* (3 µm),

– as mobile phase at a flow rate of 1.5 ml/min, a gradient programme using the following conditions:

Mobile phase A. A 5 g/l solution of *ammonium carbonate R* in a mixture of 10 volumes of *tetrahydrofuran R* and 90 volumes of *water R*,

Mobile phase B. Acetonitrile R,

Time (min)	Mobile phase A (per cent *V/V*)	Mobile phase B (per cent *V/V*)	Comment
0 - 15	90 → 40	10 → 60	linear gradient
15 - 20	40	60	isocratic elution
20 - 25	90	10	switch to initial composition
25 = 0	90	10	restart gradient

– as detector a spectrophotometer set at 220 nm.

Equilibrate the column for at least 30 min with *acetonitrile R* and then equilibrate at the initial eluent composition for at least 5 min. Adjust the sensitivity of the system so that the height of the principal peak in the chromatogram obtained with 10 µl of reference solution (b) is at least 50 per cent of the full scale of the recorder.

Inject 10 µl of reference solution (a). When the chromatograms are recorded in the prescribed conditions the retention times are: alfentanil impurity E about 6 min and alfentanil hydrochloride about 7 min. Disregard any other peak. The test is not valid unless the resolution between the peaks corresponding to alfentanil hydrochloride and alfentanil impurity E is at least 4.0. If necessary, adjust the concentration of acetonitrile in the mobile phase or adjust the time programme for the linear-gradient elution.

Inject 10 µl of *methanol R* as a blank, 10 µl of the test solution and 10 µl of reference solution (b). In the chromatogram obtained with the test solution: the area of any peak, apart from the principal peak, is not greater than the area of the principal peak in the chromatogram obtained with reference solution (b) (0.25 per cent); the sum of the areas of all such peaks is not greater than twice the area of the principal peak in the chromatogram obtained with reference solution (b) (0.5 per cent). Disregard any peak obtained with the blank-run, and any peak with an area less than 0.2 times the area of the principal peak in the chromatogram obtained with reference solution (b) (0.05 per cent).

Water (*2.5.12*): 3.0 per cent to 4.0 per cent, determined on 0.500 g by the semi-micro determination of water.

ASSAY

Dissolve 0.350 g in 50 ml of a mixture of 1 volume of *alcohol R* and 4 volumes of *water R* and add 5.0 ml of *0.01 M hydrochloric acid.* Titrate with *0.1 M sodium hydroxide*, determining the end-point potentiometrically (*2.2.20*). Read the volume added between the two points of inflexion.

1 ml of *0.1 M sodium hydroxide* is equivalent to 45.30 mg of $C_{21}H_{33}ClN_6O_3$.

STORAGE

Store protected from light.

IMPURITIES

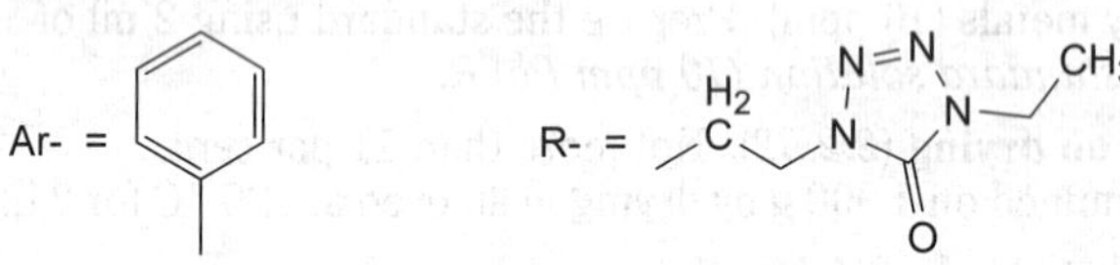

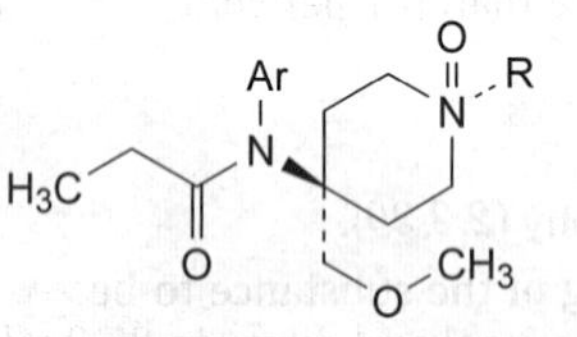

A. *cis*-*N*-[1-[2-(4-ethyl-4,5-dihydro-5-oxo-1*H*-tetrazol-1-yl)ethyl]-4-(methoxymethyl)piperidin-4-yl]-*N*-phenylpropanamide *N*-oxide,

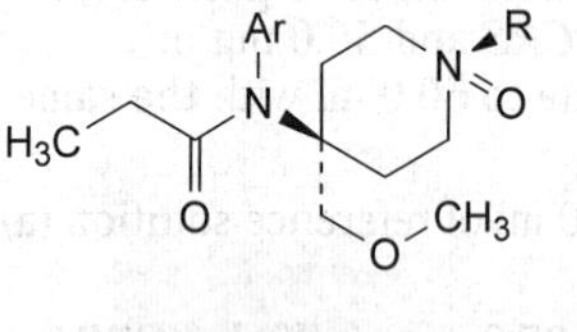

B. *trans*-*N*-[1-[2-(4-ethyl-4,5-dihydro-5-oxo-1*H*-tetrazol-1-yl)ethyl]-4-(methoxymethyl)piperidin-4-yl]-*N*-phenylpropanamide *N*-oxide,

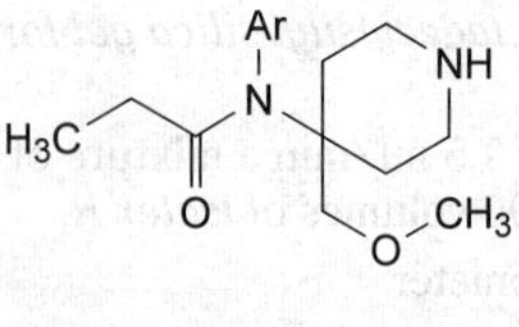

C. *N*-[4-(methoxymethyl)piperidin-4-yl]-*N*-phenylpropanamide,

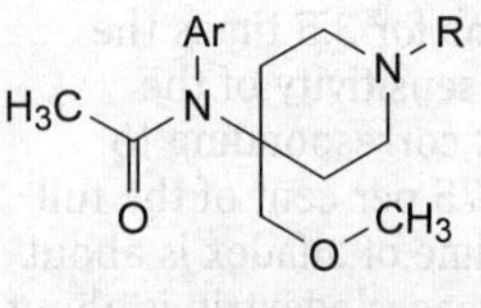

D. *N*-[1-[2-(4-ethyl-4,5-dihydro-5-oxo-1*H*-tetrazol-1-yl)ethyl]-4-(methoxymethyl)piperidin-4-yl]-*N*-phenylacetamide,

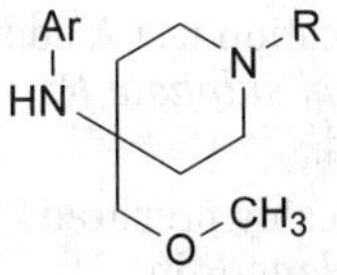

E. 1-ethyl-1,4-dihydro-4-[2-[[4-(methoxymethyl)-4-phenylamino]piperidin-1-yl]ethyl]-5*H*-tetrazol-5-one,

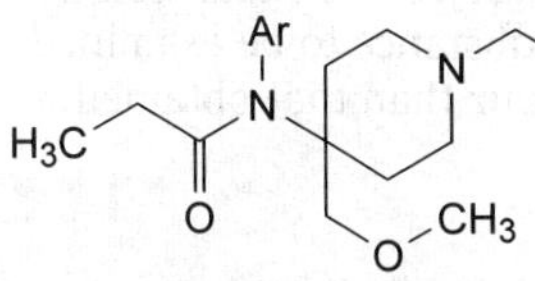

F. *N*-[1-(2-hydroxyethyl)-4-(methoxymethyl)piperidin-4-yl]-*N*-phenylpropanamide,

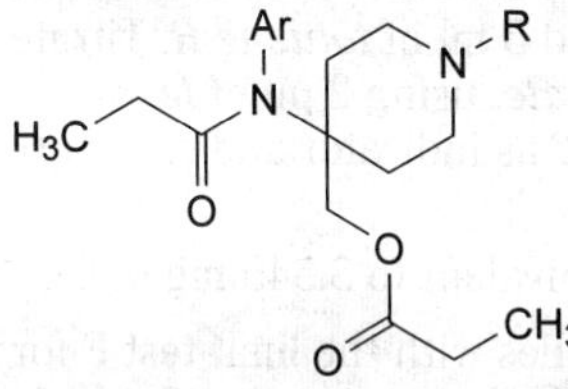

G. *N*-[1-[2-(4-ethyl-4,5-dihydro-5-oxo-1*H*-tetrazol-1-yl)ethyl]-4-(propanoyloxymethyl)piperidin-4-yl]-*N*-phenylpropanamide,

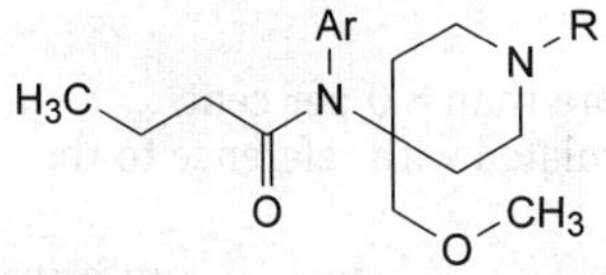

H. *N*-[1-[2-(4-ethyl-4,5-dihydro-5-oxo-1*H*-tetrazol-1-yl)ethyl]-4-(methoxymethyl)piperidin-4-yl]-*N*-phenylbutanamide.

01/2005:1287

ALFUZOSIN HYDROCHLORIDE

Alfuzosini hydrochloridum

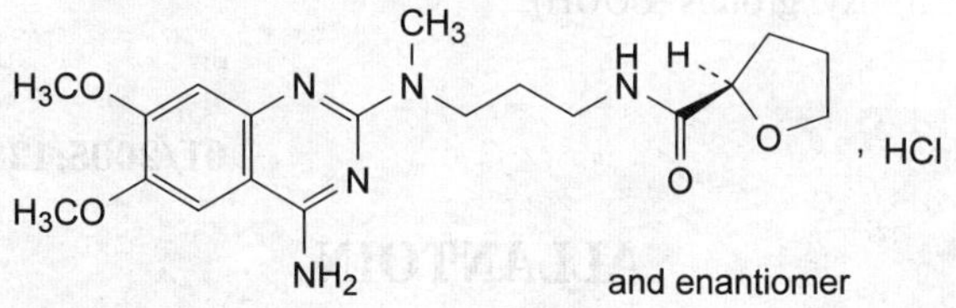

$C_{19}H_{28}ClN_5O_4$ M_r 425.9

DEFINITION

Alfuzosin hydrochloride contains not less than 98.5 per cent and not more than the equivalent of 101.0 per cent of (*RS*)-*N*-[3-[(4-amino-6,7-dimethoxyquinazolin-2-yl)(methyl)amino]propyl]tetrahydrofuran-2-carboxamide hydrochloride, calculated with reference to the anhydrous substance.

CHARACTERS

A white or almost white, crystalline powder, slightly hygroscopic, freely soluble in water, sparingly soluble in alcohol, practically insoluble in methylene chloride.

IDENTIFICATION

A. Examine by infrared absorption spectrophotometry (*2.2.24*), comparing with the spectrum obtained with *alfuzosin hydrochloride CRS*. Examine the substances prepared as discs.

B. To 1 ml of solution S (see Tests) add 1 ml of *water R*. The solution gives reaction (a) of chlorides (*2.3.1*).

TESTS

Solution S. Dissolve 0.500 g in *carbon dioxide-free water R* and dilute to 25.0 ml with the same solvent.

pH (*2.2.3*). The pH of freshly prepared solution S is 4.0 to 6.0.

Optical rotation (*2.2.7*). The angle of optical rotation, determined on solution S, is − 0.10° to + 0.10°.

Related substances. Examine by liquid chromatography (*2.2.29*).

Test solution. Dissolve 20.0 mg of the substance to be examined in the mobile phase and dilute to 100.0 ml with the mobile phase.

Reference solution (a). Dilute 1.0 ml of the test solution to 50.0 ml with the mobile phase. Dilute 5.0 ml of the solution to 20.0 ml with the mobile phase.

Reference solution (b). Dissolve 5 mg of *alfuzosin impurity A CRS* in the mobile phase and dilute to 25 ml with the mobile phase. To 1 ml of the solution, add 1 ml of the test solution and dilute to 100 ml with the mobile phase.

The chromatographic procedure may be carried out using:

– a stainless steel column 0.15 m long and 4.6 mm in internal diameter packed with microparticulate *octadecylsilyl silica gel for chromatography R* (5 μm), with a carbon loading of 18.5 per cent, a specific surface area of 320 m^2/g, a pore size of 15 nm, and end-capped with hexamethyldisilane,
– as mobile phase at a flow rate of 1.5 ml/min a mixture of 1 volume of *tetrahydrofuran R*, 20 volumes of *acetonitrile R* and 80 volumes of a solution of sodium perchlorate prepared as follows: dilute 5.0 ml of *perchloric acid R* in 900 ml of *water R*, adjust to pH 3.5 with *dilute sodium hydroxide solution R* and dilute to 1000 ml with *water R*,
– as detector a spectrophotometer set at 254 nm.

Inject 20 μl of reference solution (b). Adjust the sensitivity of the system so that the height of the two peaks in the chromatogram obtained is at least 50 per cent of the full scale of the recorder. The test is not valid unless the resolution between the peaks corresponding to alfuzosin and alfuzosin impurity A is at least 3.0. Inject 20 μl of the test solution and 20 μl of reference solution (a). In the chromatogram obtained with the test solution: the area of any peak, apart from the principal peak, is not greater than 0.6 times the area of the principal peak in the chromatogram obtained with reference solution (a) (0.3 per cent); the sum of the areas of all the peaks, apart from the principal peak, is not greater than the area of the principal peak in the chromatogram obtained with reference solution (a) (0.5 per cent). Disregard any peak with an area less than 0.025 times that of the principal peak in the chromatogram obtained with reference solution (a).

Water (*2.5.12*). Not more than 2.0 per cent, determined on 0.500 g by the semi-micro determination of water.

Sulphated ash (*2.4.14*). Not more than 0.1 per cent, determined on 1.0 g.

ASSAY

Dissolve 0.300 g in a mixture of 40 ml of *anhydrous acetic acid R* and 40 ml of *acetic anhydride R*. Titrate with *0.1 M perchloric acid*, determining the end-point potentiometrically (*2.2.20*).

1 ml of *0.1 M perchloric acid* is equivalent to 42.59 mg of $C_{19}H_{28}ClN_5O_4$.

STORAGE

Store in an airtight container, protected from light.

IMPURITIES

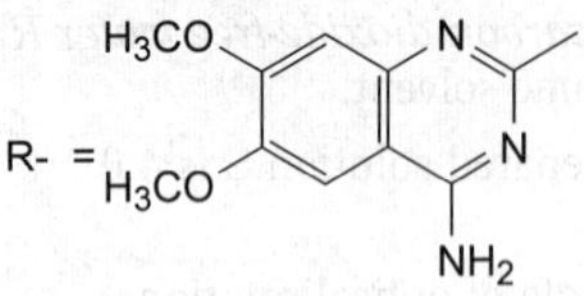

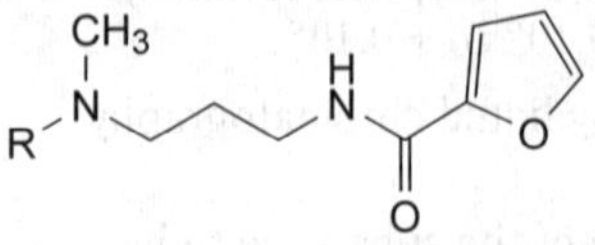

A. *N*-[3-[(4-amino-6,7-dimethoxyquinazolin-2-yl)(methyl)amino]propyl]furan-2-carboxamide,

B. R-Cl: 2-chloro-6,7-dimethoxyquinazolin-4-amine,

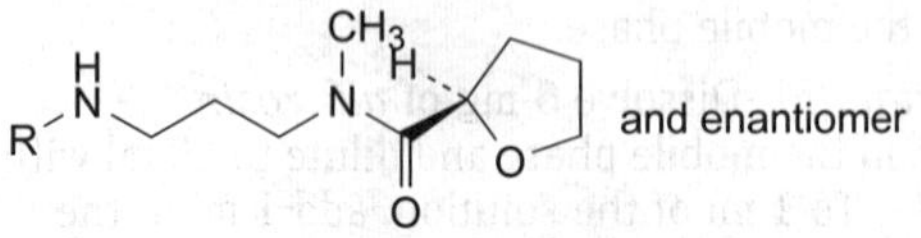

C. (*RS*)-*N*-[3-[(4-amino-6,7-dimethoxyquinazolin-2-yl)amino]propyl]-*N*-methyltetrahydrofuran-2-carboxamide,

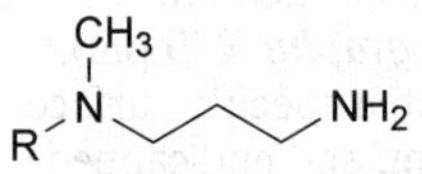

D. *N*-(4-amino-6,7-dimethoxyquinazolin-2-yl)-*N*-methylpropane-1,3-diamine,

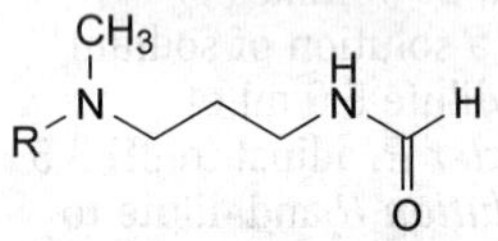

E. *N*-[3-[(4-amino-6,7-dimethoxyquinazolin-2-yl)(methyl)amino]propyl]formamide.

01/2005:0591

ALGINIC ACID

Acidum alginicum

DEFINITION

Alginic acid is a mixture of polyuronic acids $[(C_6H_8O_6)_n]$ composed of residues of D-mannuronic and L-guluronic acid and is obtained mainly from algae belonging to the Phaeophyceae. A small proportion of the carboxyl groups may be neutralised. It contains not less than 19.0 per cent and not more than 25.0 per cent of carboxyl groups (COOH), calculated with reference to the dried substance.

CHARACTERS

A white or pale yellowish-brown, crystalline or amorphous powder, very slightly soluble or practically insoluble in alcohol, practically insoluble in organic solvents. It swells in water but does not dissolve; it dissolves in solutions of alkali hydroxides.

IDENTIFICATION

A. To 0.2 g add 20 ml of *water R* and 0.5 ml of *sodium carbonate solution R*. Shake and filter. To 5 ml of the filtrate add 1 ml of *calcium chloride solution R*. A voluminous gelatinous mass is formed.

B. To 5 ml of the filtrate obtained in identification test A add 0.5 ml of a 123 g/l solution of *magnesium sulphate R*. No voluminous gelatinous mass is formed.

C. To 5 mg add 5 ml of *water R*, 1 ml of a freshly prepared 10 g/l solution of *1,3-dihydroxynaphthalene R* in *alcohol R* and 5 ml of *hydrochloric acid R*. Boil gently for 3 min, cool, add 5 ml of *water R*, and shake with 15 ml of *di-isopropyl ether R*. Carry out a blank test. The upper layer obtained with the substance to be examined exhibits a deeper bluish-red colour than that obtained with the blank.

TESTS

Chlorides. Not more than 1.0 per cent. To 2.50 g add 50 ml of *dilute nitric acid R*, shake for 1 h and dilute to 100.0 ml with *dilute nitric acid R*. Filter. To 50.0 ml of the filtrate add 10.0 ml of *0.1 M silver nitrate* and 5 ml of *toluene R*. Titrate with *0.1 M ammonium thiocyanate*, using 2 ml of *ferric ammonium sulphate solution R2* as indicator and shaking vigorously towards the end point.

1 ml of *0.1 M silver nitrate* is equivalent to 3.545 mg of Cl.

Heavy metals (*2.4.8*). 1.0 g complies with the limit test F for heavy metals (20 ppm). Prepare the standard using 2 ml of *lead standard solution (10 ppm Pb) R*.

Loss on drying (*2.2.32*). Not more than 15.0 per cent, determined on 0.1000 g by drying in an oven at 100 °C to 105 °C for 4 h.

Sulphated ash (*2.4.14*). Not more than 8.0 per cent, determined on 0.100 g and calculated with reference to the dried substance.

Microbial contamination. Total viable aerobic count (*2.6.12*) not more than 10^2 micro-organisms per gram, determined by plate-count. It complies with the tests for *Escherichia coli* and *Salmonella* (*2.6.13*).

ASSAY

To 0.2500 g add 25 ml of *water R*, 25.0 ml of *0.1 M sodium hydroxide* and 0.2 ml of *phenolphthalein solution R*. Titrate with *0.1 M hydrochloric acid*.

1 ml of *0.1 M sodium hydroxide* is equivalent to 4.502 mg of carboxyl groups (COOH).

01/2005:1288

ALLANTOIN

Allantoinum

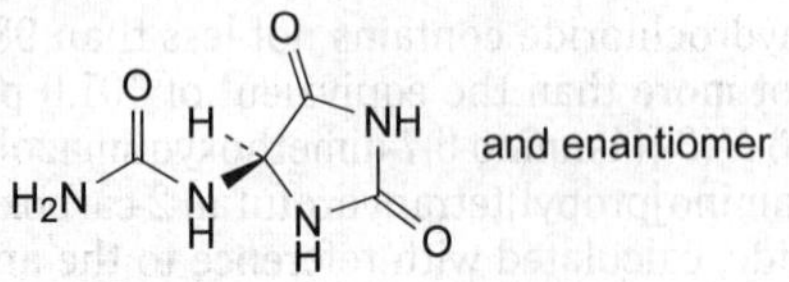

$C_4H_6N_4O_3$ M_r 158.1

DEFINITION

Allantoin contains not less than 98.5 per cent and not more than the equivalent of 101.0 per cent of (*RS*)-(2,5-dioxoimidazolidin-4-yl)urea.

CHARACTERS

A white, crystalline powder, slightly soluble in water, very slightly soluble in alcohol.

It melts at about 225 °C, with decomposition.

IDENTIFICATION

First identification: A.

Second identification: B, C, D.

A. Examine by infrared absorption spectrophotometry (*2.2.24*), comparing with the spectrum obtained with *allantoin CRS.*

B. Examine the chromatograms obtained in the test for related substances. The principal spot in the chromatogram obtained with test solution (b) is similar in position, colour and size to the principal spot in the chromatogram obtained with reference solution (a).

C. Boil 20 mg with a mixture of 1 ml of *dilute sodium hydroxide solution R* and 1 ml of *water R*. Allow to cool. Add 1 ml of *dilute hydrochloric acid R*. To 0.1 ml of the solution add 0.1 ml of a 100 g/l solution of *potassium bromide R*, 0.1 ml of a 20 g/l solution of *resorcinol R* and 3 ml of *sulphuric acid R*. Heat for 5 min to 10 min on a water-bath. A dark blue colour develops, which becomes red after cooling and pouring into about 10 ml of *water R*.

D. Heat about 0.5 g. Ammonia vapour is evolved, which turns *red litmus paper R* blue.

TESTS

Solution S. Dissolve 0.5 g in *carbon dioxide-free water R*, with heating if necessary, and dilute to 100 ml with the same solvent.

Acidity or alkalinity. To 5 ml of solution S add 5 ml of *carbon dioxide-free water R*, 0.1 ml of *methyl red solution R* and 0.2 ml of *0.01 M sodium hydroxide.* The solution is yellow. Add 0.4 ml of *0.01 M hydrochloric acid.* The solution is red.

Optical rotation (*2.2.7*). The angle of optical rotation, determined on solution S, is − 0.10° to + 0.10°.

Reducing substances. Shake 1.0 g with 10 ml of *water R* for 2 min. Filter. Add 1.5 ml of *0.02 M potassium permanganate.* The solution must remain violet for at least 10 min.

Related substances. Examine by thin-layer chromatography (*2.2.27*), using a suitable *cellulose for chromatography R* as the coating substance.

Test solution (a). Dissolve 0.10 g of the substance to be examined in 5.0 ml of *water R* with heating. Allow to cool. Dilute to 10 ml with *methanol R. Use the solution immediately after preparation.*

Test solution (b). Dilute 1 ml of test solution (a) to 10 ml with a mixture of 1 volume of *methanol R* and 1 volume of *water R.*

Reference solution (a). Dissolve 10 mg of *allantoin CRS* in a mixture of 1 volume of *methanol R* and 1 volume of *water R* and dilute to 10 ml with the same mixture of solvents.

Reference solution (b). Dissolve 10 mg of *urea R* in 10 ml of *water R*. Dilute 1 ml of this solution to 10 ml with *methanol R*.

Reference solution (c). Mix 1 ml of reference solution (a) and 1 ml of reference solution (b).

Apply to the plate 10 µl of test solution (a) and 5 µl each of test solution (b), reference solution (a), reference solution (b) and reference solution (c). Develop over a path of 10 cm using a mixture of 15 volumes of *glacial acetic acid R*, 25 volumes of *water R* and 60 volumes of *butanol R.* Allow the plate to dry in air. Spray the plate with a 5 g/l solution of *dimethylaminobenzaldehyde R* in a mixture of 1 volume of *hydrochloric acid R* and 3 volumes of *methanol R.* Dry the plate in a current of hot air. Examine in daylight after 30 min. Any spot in the chromatogram obtained with test solution (a), apart from the principal spot, is not more intense than the spot in the chromatogram obtained with reference solution (b) (0.5 per cent). The test is not valid unless the chromatogram obtained with reference solution (c) shows two clearly separated principal spots.

Loss on drying (*2.2.32*). Not more than 0.1 per cent, determined on 1.000 g by drying in an oven at 100-105 °C.

Sulphated ash (*2.4.14*). Not more than 0.1 per cent, determined on 1.0 g.

ASSAY

Dissolve 120.0 mg in 40 ml of *water R*. Titrate with *0.1 M sodium hydroxide,* determining the end-point potentiometrically (*2.2.20*).

1 ml of *0.1 M sodium hydroxide* is equivalent to 15.81 mg of $C_4H_6N_4O_3$.

IMPURITIES

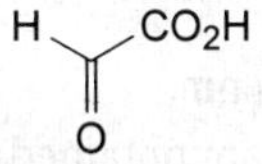

A. glyoxylic acid,

B. urea.

01/2005:0576

ALLOPURINOL

Allopurinolum

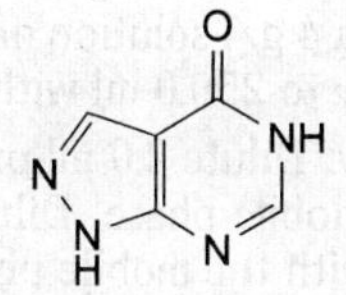

$C_5H_4N_4O$ M_r 136.1

DEFINITION

1,5-Dihydro-4*H*-pyrazolo[3,4-*d*]pyrimidin-4-one.

Content: 98.0 per cent to 102.0 per cent (dried substance).

CHARACTERS

Appearance: white or almost white powder.

Solubility: very slightly soluble in water and in alcohol. It dissolves in dilute solutions of alkali hydroxides.

IDENTIFICATION

First identification: B.

Second identification: A, C, D.

A. Dissolve 10 mg in 1 ml of a 4 g/l solution of *sodium hydroxide R* and dilute to 100.0 ml with a 10.3 g/l solution of *hydrochloric acid R.* Dilute 10.0 ml of this solution to 100.0 ml with a 10.3 g/l solution of *hydrochloric acid R.* Examined between 220 nm and 350 nm (*2.2.25*), the solution shows an absorption maximum at 250 nm and an absorption minimum at 231 nm. The ratio of the absorbance measured at the absorption minimum at 231 nm to that measured at the absorption maximum at 250 nm is 0.52 to 0.62.

B. Infrared absorption spectrophotometry (*2.2.24*).

Preparation: discs.

Comparison: *allopurinol CRS.*

C. Dissolve 0.3 g in 2.5 ml of *dilute sodium hydroxide solution R* and add 50 ml of *water R*. Add slowly and with shaking 5 ml of *silver nitrate solution R1*. A white precipitate is formed which does not dissolve on the addition of 5 ml of *ammonia R*.

D. Thin-layer chromatography (*2.2.27*).

Test solution. Dissolve 20 mg of the substance to be examined in *concentrated ammonia R* and dilute to 10 ml with the same solvent.

Reference solution. Dissolve 20 mg of *allopurinol CRS* in *concentrated ammonia R* and dilute to 10 ml with the same solvent.

Plate: *TLC silica gel F_{254} plate R*.

Mobile phase: *ethanol R, methylene chloride R* (40:60 *V/V*).

Application: 10 µl.

Development: over 2/3 of the plate.

Drying: in air.

Detection: examine in ultraviolet light at 254 nm.

Results: the principal spot in the chromatogram obtained with the test solution is similar in position and size to the principal spot in the chromatogram obtained with the reference solution.

TESTS

Related substances. Liquid chromatography (*2.2.29*). *Prepare the solutions immediately before use.* Store them and inject them at 8 °C using a cooled autosampler.

Test solution (a). Dissolve 25.0 mg of the substance to be examined in 2.5 ml of a 4 g/l solution of *sodium hydroxide R* and dilute immediately to 50.0 ml with the mobile phase.

Test solution (b). Dissolve 20.0 mg of the substance to be examined in 5.0 ml of a 4 g/l solution of *sodium hydroxide R* and dilute immediately to 250.0 ml with the mobile phase.

Reference solution (a). Dilute 2.0 ml of test solution (a) to 100.0 ml with the mobile phase. Dilute 5.0 ml of this solution to 100.0 ml with the mobile phase.

Reference solution (b). Dissolve 5.0 mg of *allopurinol impurity A CRS*, 5.0 mg of *allopurinol impurity B CRS* and 5.0 mg of *allopurinol impurity C CRS* in 5.0 ml of a 4 g/l solution of *sodium hydroxide R* and dilute immediately to 100.0 ml with the mobile phase. Dilute 1.0 ml of this solution to 100.0 ml with the mobile phase.

Reference solution (c). Dissolve 20.0 mg of *allopurinol CRS* in 5.0 ml of a 4 g/l solution of *sodium hydroxide R* and dilute immediately to 250.0 ml with the mobile phase.

Column:

- *size*: l = 0.25 m, Ø = 4.6 mm,
- *stationary phase*: *octadecylsilyl silica gel for chromatography R* (5 µm).

Mobile phase: 1.25 g/l solution of *potassium dihydrogen phosphate R*.

Flow rate: 1.4 ml/min.

Detection: spectrophotometer at 230 nm.

Injection: 20 µl of test solution (a) and reference solutions (a) and (b).

Run time: twice the retention time of allopurinol.

Elution order: impurity A, impurity B, impurity C, allopurinol.

Retention time: allopurinol = about 10 min.

System suitability: reference solution (b):

- *resolution*: minimum 1.1 between the peaks due to impurity B and impurity C.

Limits:

- *impurity A*: not more than twice the area of the principal peak in the chromatogram obtained with reference solution (a) (0.2 per cent),
- *impurity B*: not more than the area of the principal peak in the chromatogram obtained with reference solution (a) (0.1 per cent),
- *impurity C*: not more than the area of the corresponding peak in the chromatogram obtained with reference solution (b) (0.1 per cent),
- *any other impurity*: for each impurity, not more than the area of the principal peak in the chromatogram obtained with reference solution (a) (0.1 per cent),
- *sum of impurities other than A, B and C*: not more than 3 times the area of the principal peak in the chromatogram obtained with reference solution (a) (0.3 per cent),
- *disregard limit*: 0.5 times the area of the principal peak in the chromatogram obtained with reference solution (a) (0.05 per cent).

Impurities D and E. Liquid chromatography (*2.2.29*). *Prepare the solutions immediately before use.* Store them and inject them at 8 °C using a cooled autosampler.

Solution A: 1.25 g/l solution of *potassium dihydrogen phosphate R*.

Test solution. Dissolve 50.0 mg of the substance to be examined in 5.0 ml of a 4 g/l solution of *sodium hydroxide R* and dilute immediately to 100.0 ml with solution A.

Reference solution. Dissolve 5.0 mg of *allopurinol impurity D CRS* and 5.0 mg of *allopurinol impurity E CRS* in 5.0 ml of a 4 g/l solution of *sodium hydroxide R* and dilute immediately to 100.0 ml with solution A. Dilute 1.0 ml of this solution to 100.0 ml with solution A.

Column:

- *size*: l = 0.05 m, Ø = 4.6 mm,
- *stationary phase*: *base-deactivated octadecylsilyl silica gel for chromatography R* (3 µm).

Mobile phase: *methanol R*, 1.25 g/l solution of *potassium dihydrogen phosphate R* (10:90 *V/V*).

Flow rate: 2 ml/min.

Detection: spectrophotometer at 230 nm.

Injection: 20 µl.

Run time: 1.5 times the retention time of impurity E.

Retention times: impurity D = about 3.6 min; impurity E = about 4.5 min.

System suitability: reference solution:

- *resolution*: minimum 2.0 between the peaks due to impurity D and impurity E.

Limits:

- *impurity D*: not more than the area of the corresponding peak in the chromatogram obtained with the reference solution (0.1 per cent),
- *impurity E*: not more than the area of the corresponding peak in the chromatogram obtained with the reference solution (0.1 per cent).

Heavy metals (*2.4.8*): maximum 20 ppm.

1.0 g complies with limit test C. Prepare the standard using 2 ml of *lead standard solution (10 ppm Pb) R*.

Loss on drying (*2.2.32*): maximum 0.5 per cent, determined on 1.000 g by drying in an oven at 100-105 °C.

Sulphated ash (*2.4.14*): maximum 0.1 per cent, determined on 1.0 g.

ASSAY

Liquid chromatography (*2.2.29*) as described in the test for related substances with the following modification.

Injection: test solution (b) and reference solution (c).

Calculate the percentage content of $C_5H_4N_4O$ from the areas of the peaks and the declared content of *allopurinol CRS*.

IMPURITIES

Specified impurities: A, B, C, D, E.

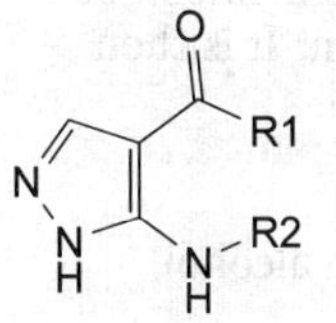

A. R1 = NH_2, R2 = H: 5-amino-1*H*-pyrazole-4-carboxamide,

B. R1 = NH_2, R2 = CHO: 5-(formylamino)-1*H*-pyrazole-4-carboxamide,

D. R1 = O-CH_2-CH_3, R2 = H: ethyl 5-amino-1*H*-pyrazole-4-carboxylate,

E. R1 = O-CH_2-CH_3, R2 = CHO: ethyl 5-(formylamino)-1*H*-pyrazole-4-carboxylate,

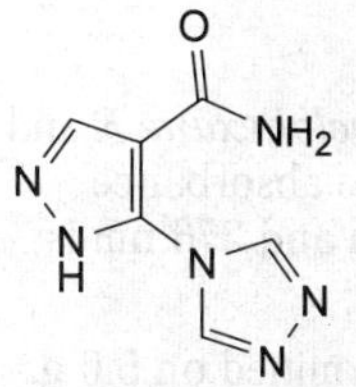

C. 5-(4*H*-1,2,4-triazol-4-yl)-1*H*-pyrazole-4-carboxamide.

01/2005:2010 corrected

ALMAGATE

Almagatum

$Al_2Mg_6C_2O_{20}H_{14},4H_2O$ M_r 630

DEFINITION

Hydrated aluminium magnesium hydroxycarbonate.

Content:

- aluminium: 15.0 per cent to 17.0 per cent (calculated as Al_2O_3),
- magnesium: 36.0 per cent to 40.0 per cent (calculated as MgO),
- carbonic acid: 12.5 per cent to 14.5 per cent (calculated as CO_2).

CHARACTERS

Appearance: white or almost white, fine crystalline powder.

Solubility: practically insoluble in water, in alcohol and in methylene chloride. It dissolves with effervescence and heating in dilute mineral acids.

IDENTIFICATION

A. Infrared absorption spectrophotometry (*2.2.24*).

Comparison: *Ph. Eur. reference spectrum of almagate.*

B. Dissolve 150 mg in *dilute hydrochloric acid R* and dilute to 20 ml with the same acid. 2 ml of the solution gives the reaction of aluminium (*2.3.1*).

C. 2 ml of the solution prepared under identification test B gives the reaction of magnesium (*2.3.1*).

TESTS

pH (*2.2.3*): 9.1 to 9.7.

Disperse 4.0 g in 100 ml of *carbon dioxide-free water R*, stir for 2 min and filter.

Neutralising capacity. *Carry out the test at 37 °C.* Disperse 0.5 g in 100 ml of *water R*, heat, add 100.0 ml of *0.1 M hydrochloric acid*, previously heated and stir continuously; the pH (*2.2.3*) of the solution between 5 min and 20 min is not less than 3.0 and not greater than 4.5. Add 10.0 ml of *0.5 M hydrochloric acid*, previously heated, stir continuously for 1 h and titrate with *0.1 M sodium hydroxide* to pH 3.5; not more than 20.0 ml of *0.1 M sodium hydroxide* is required.

Chlorides (*2.4.4*): maximum 0.1 per cent.

Dissolve 0.33 g in 5 ml of *dilute nitric acid R* and dilute to 100 ml with *water R*. 15 ml of the solution complies with the limit test for chlorides. Prepare simultaneously the standard by diluting 0.7 ml of *dilute nitric acid R* to 5 ml with *water R* and adding 10 ml of *chloride standard solution (5 ppm Cl) R.*

Sulphates (*2.4.13*): maximum 0.4 per cent.

Dissolve 0.25 g in 5 ml of *dilute hydrochloric acid R* and dilute to 100 ml with *distilled water R*. 15 ml of the solution complies with the limit test for sulphates. Prepare simultaneously the standard by adding 0.8 ml of *dilute hydrochloric acid R* to 15 ml of *sulphate standard solution (10 ppm SO_4) R*.

Sodium: maximum 150 ppm.

Atomic absorption spectrometry (*2.2.23, Method I*).

Test solution. Dissolve 0.25 g in 50 ml of a 103 g/l solution of *hydrochloric acid R*.

Reference solutions. Prepare the reference solutions using *sodium standard solution (200 ppm Na) R*, diluted as necessary with a 103 g/l solution of *hydrochloric acid R*.

Heavy metals (*2.4.8*): maximum 20 ppm.

Dissolve 1.0 g in *dilute hydrochloric acid R* and dilute to 20.0 ml with the same acid. 12 ml of the solution complies with limit test A. Prepare the standard using *lead standard solution (1 ppm Pb) R*.

Loss on ignition: 43.0 per cent to 49.0 per cent, determined on 1.000 g by ignition at 900 °C.

Microbial contamination. Total viable aerobic count (*2.6.12*) not more than 10^3 micro-organisms per gram determined by plate count. It complies with the tests for *Escherichia coli* and *Pseudomonas aeruginosa* (*2.6.13*).

ASSAY

Aluminium. Dissolve 1.000 g in 5 ml of *hydrochloric acid R*, heating if necessary. Allow to cool to room temperature and dilute to 100.0 ml with *water R* (solution A). Introduce 10.0 ml of solution A into a 250 ml conical flask, add 25.0 ml of *0.05 M sodium edetate*, 20 ml of *buffer solution pH 3.5 R*, 40 ml of *ethanol R* and 2 ml of a freshly prepared 0.25 g/l solution of *dithizone R* in *ethanol R*. Titrate the excess of sodium edetate with *0.05 M zinc sulphate* until the colour changes from greenish-violet to pink.

1 ml of *0.05 M sodium edetate* is equivalent to 2.549 mg of Al_2O_3.

Magnesium. Introduce 10.0 ml of solution A prepared in the assay of aluminium into a 500 ml conical flask, add 200 ml of *water R*, 20 ml of *triethanolamine R* with shaking, 10 ml of *ammonium chloride buffer solution pH 10.0 R* and 50 mg of *mordant black 11 triturate R*. Titrate with *0.05 M sodium edetate* until the colour changes from violet to pure blue.

1 ml of *0.05 M sodium edetate* is equivalent to 2.015 mg of MgO.

Carbonic acid: 12.5 per cent to 14.5 per cent.

Test sample. Place 7.00 mg of the substance to be examined in a tin capsule. Seal the capsule.

Reference sample. Place 7.00 mg of *almagate CRS* in a tin capsule. Seal the capsule.

Introduce separately the test sample and the reference sample into a combustion chamber of a CHN analyser purged with *helium for chromatography R* and maintained at a temperature of 1020 °C. Simultaneously, introduce *oxygen R* at a pressure of 276 kPa and a flow rate of 20 ml/min and allow complete combustion of the sample. Sweep the combustion gases through a reduction reactor and separate the gases formed by gas chromatography (*2.2.28*).

Column:

– *size*: l = 2 m, Ø = 4 mm,

– *stationary phase*: *ethylvinylbenzene-divinylbenzene copolymer R1*.

Carrier gas: *helium for chromatography R*.

Flow rate: 100 ml/min.

Temperature:

– *column*: 65 °C,

– *detector*: 190 °C.

Detection: thermal conductivity.

Run time: 16 min.

System suitability:

– average percentage of carbon in 5 reference samples must be within ± 0.2 per cent of the value assigned to the CRS. The difference between the upper and the lower values of the percentage of carbon in these samples must be below 0.2 per cent.

Calculate the percentage content of carbonic acid in the test sample according to the following formula:

$$C \times K \times \frac{A}{m}$$

C = percentage content of carbonic acid in the reference sample,

K = mean value for the 5 reference samples of the ratio of the mass in milligrams to the area of the peak due to carbonic acid,

A = area of the peak due to carbonic acid in the chromatogram obtained with the test sample,

m = sample mass, in milligrams.

STORAGE

In an airtight container.

01/2005:1064

ALMOND OIL, REFINED

Amygdalae oleum raffinatum

DEFINITION

Refined almond oil is the fatty oil from the ripe seeds of *Prunus dulcis* (Miller) D.A. Webb var. *dulcis* or *Prunus dulcis* (Miller) D.A. Webb var. *amara* (D.C.) Buchheim or a mixture of both varieties by cold expression. It is then refined. A suitable antioxidant may be added.

CHARACTERS

A pale yellow, clear liquid, slightly soluble in alcohol, miscible with light petroleum.

It solidifies at about – 18 °C and has a relative density of about 0.916.

IDENTIFICATION

A. Carry out the identification of fatty oils by thin-layer chromatography (*2.3.2*). The chromatogram obtained is comparable with the type chromatogram for almond oil.

B. It complies with the test for composition of fatty acids (see Tests).

TESTS

Absorbance (*2.2.25*). Dissolve 0.100 g in *cyclohexane R* and dilute to 10.0 ml with the same solvent. The absorbance measured at the maximum between 264 nm and 276 nm is 0.2 to 6.0.

Acid value (*2.5.1*). Not more than 0.5, determined on 5.0 g.

Peroxide value (*2.5.5*). Not more than 5.0.

Unsaponifiable matter (*2.5.7*). Not more than 0.7 per cent, determined on 5.0 g.

Composition of fatty acids (*2.4.22, Method A*). The fatty acid fraction of the oil has the following composition:

– *saturated fatty acids of chain length less than* C_{16}: not more than 0.1 per cent,
– *palmitic acid*: 4.0 per cent to 9.0 per cent,
– *palmitoleic acid* (equivalent chain length on polyethyleneglycol adipate 16.3): not more than 0.6 per cent,
– *margaric acid*: not more than 0.2 per cent,
– *stearic acid*: not more than 3.0 per cent,
– *oleic acid* (equivalent chain length on polyethyleneglycol adipate 18.3): 62.0 per cent to 86.0 per cent,
– *linoleic acid* (equivalent chain length on polyethyleneglycol adipate 18.9): 20.0 per cent to 30.0 per cent,
– *linolenic acid* (equivalent chain length on polyethyleneglycol adipate 19.7): not more than 0.4 per cent,
– *arachidic acid*: not more than 0.2 per cent,
– *eicosenoic acid* (equivalent chain length on polyethyleneglycol adipate 20.3): not more than 0.3 per cent,
– *behenic acid*: not more than 0.2 per cent,
– *erucic acid* (equivalent chain length on polyethyleneglycol adipate 22.3): not more than 0.1 per cent.

Sterols. Carry out the test for sterols in fatty oils (*2.4.23*). The sterol fraction of the oil has the following composition:

– *cholesterol*: not more than 0.7 per cent,
– *campesterol*: not more than 5.0 per cent,

- *stigmasterol*: not more than 4.0 per cent,
- *β-sitosterol*: 73.0 per cent to 87.0 per cent,
- *Δ5-avenasterol*: at least 5.0 per cent,
- *Δ7-avenasterol*: not more than 3.0 per cent,
- *Δ7-stigmastenol*: not more than 3.0 per cent,
- *brassicasterol*: not more than 0.3 per cent.

Water (*2.5.32*). If intended for use in the manufacture of parenteral dosage forms, not more than 0.1 per cent, determined on 5.00 g by the micro-determination of water.

STORAGE

Store in a well-filled container, protected from light.

LABELLING

The label states:

- where applicable, that the substance is suitable for use in the manufacture of parenteral dosage forms,
- the name and concentration of any added antioxidant.

01/2005:0261

ALMOND OIL, VIRGIN

Amygdalae oleum virginale

DEFINITION

Virgin almond oil is the fatty oil obtained by cold expression from the ripe seeds of *Prunus dulcis* (Miller) D.A. Webb var. *dulcis* or *Prunus dulcis* (Miller) D.A. Webb var. *amara* (D.C.) Buchheim or a mixture of both varieties.

CHARACTERS

A yellow, clear, liquid, slightly soluble in alcohol, miscible with light petroleum.

It solidifies at about − 18 °C and has a relative density of about 0.916.

IDENTIFICATION

First identification: A, C.

Second identification: A, B.

A. It complies with the test for absorbance (see Tests).

B. Carry out the identification of fatty oils by thin-layer chromatography (*2.3.2*). The chromatogram obtained is comparable with the type chromatogram for almond oil.

C. It complies with the test for composition of fatty acids (see Tests).

TESTS

Absorbance (*2.2.25*). Dissolve 0.100 g in *cyclohexane R* and dilute to 10.0 ml with the same solvent. The absorbance measured at the maximum between 264 nm and 276 nm is not greater than 0.2. The ratio of the absorbance at 232 nm to that at 270 nm is greater than 7.

Acid value (*2.5.1*). Not more than 2.0, determined on 5.0 g.

Peroxide value (*2.5.5*). Not more than 15.0.

Unsaponifiable matter (*2.5.7*). Not more than 0.7 per cent, determined on 5.0 g.

Composition of fatty acids (*2.4.22, Method A*). The fatty acid fraction of the oil has the following composition:

- *saturated fatty acids of chain length less than C_{16}*: not more than 0.1 per cent,
- *palmitic acid*: 4.0 per cent to 9.0 per cent,
- *palmitoleic acid* (equivalent chain length on polyethyleneglycol adipate 16.3): not more than 0.6 per cent,
- *margaric acid*: not more than 0.2 per cent,
- *stearic acid*: not more than 3.0 per cent,
- *oleic acid* (equivalent chain length on polyethyleneglycol adipate 18.3): 62.0 per cent to 86.0 per cent,
- *linoleic acid* (equivalent chain length on polyethyleneglycol adipate 18.9): 20.0 per cent to 30.0 per cent,
- *linolenic acid* (equivalent chain length on polyethyleneglycol adipate 19.7): not more than 0.4 per cent,
- *arachidic acid*: not more than 0.2 per cent,
- *eicosenoic acid* (equivalent chain length on polyethyleneglycol adipate 20.3): not more than 0.3 per cent,
- *behenic acid*: not more than 0.2 per cent,
- *erucic acid* (equivalent chain length on polyethyleneglycol adipate 22.3): not more than 0.1 per cent.

Sterols. Carry out the test for sterols in fatty oils (*2.4.23*). The sterol fraction of the oil has the following composition:

- *cholesterol*: not more than 0.7 per cent,
- *campesterol*: not more than 4.0 per cent,
- *stigmasterol*: not more than 3.0 per cent,
- *β-sitosterol*: 73.0 per cent to 87.0 per cent,
- *Δ5-avenasterol*: at least 10.0 per cent,
- *Δ7-avenasterol*: not more than 3.0 per cent,
- *Δ7-stigmastenol*: not more than 3.0 per cent,
- *brassicasterol*: not more than 0.3 per cent.

STORAGE

Store in a well-filled container, protected from light.

01/2005:0257

ALOES, BARBADOS

Aloe barbadensis

DEFINITION

Barbados aloes consists of the concentrated and dried juice of the leaves of *Aloe barbadensis* Miller. It contains not less than 28.0 per cent of hydroxyanthracene derivatives, expressed as barbaloin ($C_{21}H_{22}O_9$; M_r 418.4) and calculated with reference to the dried drug.

CHARACTERS

Dark brown masses, slightly shiny or opaque with a conchoidal fracture, or a brown powder, soluble in hot alcohol, partly soluble in boiling water.

IDENTIFICATION

A. Examine by thin-layer chromatography (*2.2.27*), using *silica gel G R* as the coating substance.

Test solution. To 0.25 g of the powdered drug add 20 ml of *methanol R* and heat to boiling in a water-bath. Shake for a few minutes and decant the solution. Store at about 4 °C and use within 24 h.

Reference solution. Dissolve 25 mg of *barbaloin R* in *methanol R* and dilute to 10 ml with the same solvent.

Apply separately to the plate as bands 20 mm by not more than 3 mm 10 µl of each solution. Develop over a path of 10 cm using a mixture of 13 volumes of *water R*, 17 volumes of *methanol R* and 100 volumes of *ethyl acetate R*. Allow the plate to dry in air, spray with a 100 g/l solution of *potassium hydroxide R* in *methanol R* and examine in ultraviolet light at 365 nm.

The chromatogram obtained with the test solution shows in the central part a zone of yellow fluorescence (barbaloin) similar in position to the zone corresponding to barbaloin in the chromatogram obtained with the reference solution and in the lower part a zone of light-blue fluorescence (aloesine). Heat the plate at 110 °C for 5 min. In the chromatogram obtained with the test solution, a zone of violet fluorescence appears just below the zone corresponding to barbaloin.

B. Shake 1 g of the powdered drug with 100 ml of boiling *water R*. Cool, add 1 g of *talc R* and filter. To 10 ml of the filtrate add 0.25 g of *disodium tetraborate R* and heat to dissolve. Pour 2 ml of the solution into 20 ml of *water R*. Yellowish-green fluorescence appears which is particularly marked in ultraviolet light at 365 nm.

C. To 5 ml of the filtrate obtained in identification test B add 1 ml of freshly prepared *bromine water R*. A brownish-yellow precipitate is formed and the supernatant liquid is violet.

TESTS

Loss on drying (*2.2.32*). Not more than 12.0 per cent, determined on 1.000 g of the powdered drug by drying in an oven at 100 °C to 105 °C.

Total ash (*2.4.16*). Not more than 2.0 per cent.

ASSAY

Carry out the assay protected from bright light.

Introduce 0.300 g of powdered drug (180) into a 250 ml conical flask. Moisten with 2 ml of *methanol R*, add 5 ml of *water R* warmed to about 60 °C, mix, add a further 75 ml of *water R* at about 60 °C and shake for 30 min. Cool, filter into a volumetric flask, rinse the conical flask and filter with 20 ml of *water R*, add the rinsings to the volumetric flask and dilute to 1000.0 ml with *water R*. Transfer 10.0 ml of this solution to a 100 ml round-bottomed flask containing 1 ml of a 600 g/l solution of *ferric chloride R* and 6 ml of *hydrochloric acid R*. Heat in a water-bath under a reflux condenser for 4 h, with the water level above that of the liquid in the flask. Allow to cool, transfer the solution to a separating funnel, rinse the flask successively with 4 ml of *water R*, 4 ml of *1 M sodium hydroxide* and 4 ml of *water R* and add the rinsings to the separating funnel. Shake the contents of the separating funnel with three quantities, each of 20 ml, of *ether R*. Wash the combined ether layers with two quantities, each of 10 ml, of *water R*. Discard the washings and dilute the organic phase to 100.0 ml with *ether R*. Evaporate 20.0 ml carefully to dryness on a water-bath and dissolve the residue in 10.0 ml of a 5 g/l solution of *magnesium acetate R* in *methanol R*. Measure the absorbance (*2.2.25*) at 512 nm using *methanol R* as the compensation liquid.

Calculate the percentage content of hydroxyanthracene derivatives, as barbaloin, from the expression:

$$\frac{A \times 19.6}{m}$$

i.e. taking the specific absorbance of barbaloin to be 255.

A = absorbance at 512 nm,

m = mass of the substance to be examined in grams.

STORAGE

Store in an airtight container, protected from light.

01/2005:0258

ALOES, CAPE

Aloe capensis

DEFINITION

Cape aloes consists of the concentrated and dried juice of the leaves of various species of *Aloe*, mainly *Aloe ferox* Miller and its hybrids. It contains not less than 18.0 per cent of hydroxyanthracene derivatives, expressed as barbaloin ($C_{21}H_{22}O_9$; M_r 418.4) and calculated with reference to the dried drug.

CHARACTERS

Dark brown masses tinged with green and having a shiny conchoidal fracture, or a greenish-brown powder, soluble in hot alcohol, partly soluble in boiling water.

IDENTIFICATION

A. Examine the chromatograms obtained in the test for Barbados aloes. The chromatogram obtained with the test solution shows in the central part a zone of yellow fluorescence (barbaloin) similar in position to the zone corresponding to barbaloin in the chromatogram obtained with the reference solution and in the lower part two zones of yellow fluorescence (aloinosides A and B) and a zone of blue fluorescence (aloesine).

B. Shake 1 g of the powdered drug with 100 ml of boiling *water R*. Cool, add 1 g of *talc R* and filter. To 10 ml of the filtrate add 0.25 g of *disodium tetraborate R* and heat to dissolve. Pour 2 ml of the solution into 20 ml of *water R*. A yellowish-green fluorescence appears which is particularly marked in ultraviolet light at 365 nm.

C. To 5 ml of the filtrate obtained in identification test B add 1 ml of freshly prepared *bromine water R*. A yellow precipitate is formed. The supernatant liquid is not coloured violet.

TESTS

Barbados aloes. Examine by thin-layer chromatography (*2.2.27*), using *silica gel G R* as the coating substance.

Test solution. To 0.25 g of the powdered drug add 20 ml of *methanol R* and heat to boiling in a water-bath. Shake for a few minutes and decant the solution. Store at about 4 °C and use within 24 h.

Reference solution. Dissolve 25 mg of *barbaloin R* in *methanol R* and dilute to 10 ml with the same solvent.

Apply separately to the plate as bands 20 mm by not more than 3 mm 10 µl of each solution. Develop over a path of 10 cm using a mixture of 13 volumes of *water R*, 17 volumes of *methanol R* and 100 volumes of *ethyl acetate R*. Allow the plate to dry in air, spray with a 100 g/l solution of *potassium hydroxide R* in *methanol R*. Heat the plate at 110 °C for 5 min and examine in ultraviolet light at 365 nm. The chromatogram obtained with the test solution shows no zone of violet fluorescence just below the zone corresponding to barbaloin.

Loss on drying (*2.2.32*). Not more than 10.0 per cent, determined on 1.000 g of the powdered drug by drying in an oven at 100 °C to 105 °C.

Total ash (*2.4.16*). Not more than 2.0 per cent.

ASSAY

Carry out the assay protected from bright light.

Introduce 0.400 g of powdered drug (180) into a 250 ml conical flask. Moisten with 2 ml of *methanol R*, add 5 ml of *water R* warmed to about 60 °C, mix, add a further 75 ml of *water R* at about 60 °C and shake for 30 min. Cool, filter into a volumetric flask, rinse the conical flask and filter with 20 ml of *water R*, add the rinsings to the volumetric flask and dilute to 1000.0 ml with *water R*. Transfer 10.0 ml of this solution to a 100 ml round-bottomed flask containing 1 ml of a 600 g/l solution of *ferric chloride R* and 6 ml of *hydrochloric acid R*. Heat in a water-bath under a reflux condenser for 4 h, with the water level above that of the liquid in the flask. Allow to cool, transfer the solution to a separating funnel, rinse the flask successively with 4 ml of *water R*, 4 ml of *1 M sodium hydroxide* and 4 ml of *water R* and add the rinsings to the separating funnel. Shake the contents of the separating funnel with three quantities, each of 20 ml, of *ether R*. Wash the combined ether layers with two quantities, each of 10 ml, of *water R*. Discard the washings and dilute the organic phase to 100.0 ml with *ether R*. Evaporate 20.0 ml carefully to dryness on a water-bath and dissolve the residue in 10.0 ml of a 5 g/l solution of *magnesium acetate R* in *methanol R*. Measure the absorbance (*2.2.25*) at 512 nm using *methanol R* as the compensation liquid.

Calculate the percentage content of barbaloin from the expression:

$$\frac{A \times 19.6}{m}$$

i.e. taking the specific absorbance of hydroxyanthracene derivatives, as barbaloin, to be 255.

A = absorbance at 512 nm,

m = mass of the substance to be examined in grams.

STORAGE

Store in an airtight container, protected from light.

01/2005:0259

ALOES DRY EXTRACT, STANDARDISED

Aloes extractum siccum normatum

DEFINITION

Standardised aloes dry extract is prepared from Barbados aloes or Cape aloes, or a mixture of the two, by treatment with boiling water. It is adjusted, if necessary, to contain not less than 19.0 per cent and not more than 21.0 per cent of hydroxyanthracene derivatives, expressed as barbaloin ($C_{21}H_{22}O_9$; M_r 418.4) and calculated with reference to the dried extract.

CHARACTERS

A brown or yellowish-brown powder, sparingly soluble in boiling water.

IDENTIFICATION

A. Examine by thin-layer chromatography (*2.2.27*), using *silica gel G R* as the coating substance.

Test solution. To 0.25 g of the preparation to be examined add 20 ml of *methanol R* and heat to boiling in a water-bath. Shake for a few minutes and decant the solution. Store at about 4 °C and use within 24 h.

Reference solution. Dissolve 25 mg of *barbaloin R* in *methanol R* and dilute to 10 ml with the same solvent.

Apply separately to the plate as bands 20 mm by not more than 3 mm 10 µl of each solution. Develop over a path of 10 cm using a mixture of 13 volumes of *water R*, 17 volumes of *methanol R* and 100 volumes of *ethyl acetate R*. Allow the plate to dry in air, spray with a 100 g/l solution of *potassium hydroxide R* in *methanol R* and examine in ultraviolet light at 365 nm. The chromatogram obtained with the test solution shows in the central part a zone of yellow fluorescence (barbaloin) similar in position to the zone corresponding to barbaloin in the chromatogram obtained with the reference solution and in the lower part there is a zone of light blue fluorescence (aloesine). In the lower part of the chromatogram obtained with the test solution two zones of yellow fluorescence (aloinosides A and B)(Cape aloes) and one zone of violet fluorescence just below the zone corresponding to barbaloin (Barbados aloes) may be present.

B. Shake 1 g of the preparation to be examined with 100 ml of boiling *water R*. Cool, add 1 g of *talc R* and filter. To 10 ml of the filtrate add 0.25 g of *disodium tetraborate R* and heat to dissolve. Pour 2 ml of the solution into 20 ml of *water R*. A yellowish-green fluorescence appears which is particularly marked in ultraviolet light at 365 nm.

TESTS

Loss on drying (*2.8.17*): maximum 4.0 per cent *m/m*.

Total ash (*2.4.16*). Not more than 2.0 per cent.

ASSAY

Carry out the assay protected from bright light.

Introduce 0.400 g into a 250 ml conical flask. Moisten with 2 ml of *methanol R*, add 5 ml of *water R* warmed to about 60 °C, mix, add a further 75 ml of *water R* at about 60 °C and shake for 30 min. Cool, filter into a volumetric flask, rinse the conical flask and filter with 20 ml of *water R*, add the rinsings to the volumetric flask and dilute to 1000.0 ml with *water R*. Transfer 10.0 ml of this solution to a 100 ml round-bottomed flask containing 1 ml of a 600 g/l solution of *ferric chloride R* and 6 ml of *hydrochloric acid R*. Heat in a water-bath under a reflux condenser for 4 h, with the water level above that of the liquid in the flask. Allow to cool, transfer the solution to a separating funnel, rinse the flask successively with 4 ml of *water R*, 4 ml of *1 M sodium hydroxide* and 4 ml of *water R*, and add the rinsings to the separating funnel. Shake the contents of the separating funnel with three quantities, each of 20 ml, of *ether R*. Wash the combined ether layers with two quantities, each of 10 ml, of *water R*. Discard the washings and dilute the organic phase to 100.0 ml with *ether R*. Evaporate 20.0 ml carefully to dryness on a water-bath and dissolve the residue in 10.0 ml of a 5 g/l solution of *magnesium acetate R* in *methanol R*. Measure the absorbance (*2.2.25*) at 512 nm using *methanol R* as the compensation liquid.

Calculate the percentage content of hydroxyanthracene derivatives, as barbaloin, from the expression:

$$\frac{A \times 19.6}{m}$$

i.e. taking the specific absorbance of barbaloin to be 255.

A = absorbance at 512 nm,

m = mass of the substance to be examined in grams.

01/2005:1065

ALPRAZOLAM

Alprazolamum

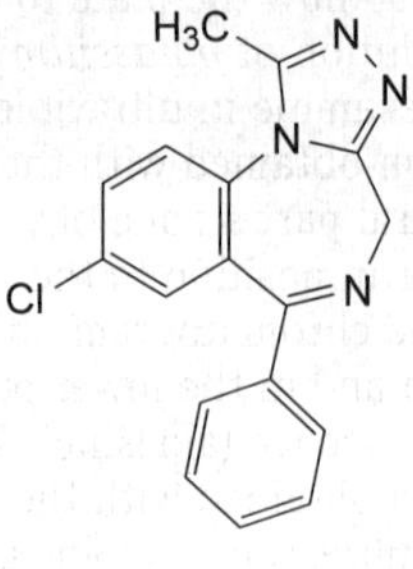

$C_{17}H_{13}ClN_4$ M_r 308.8

DEFINITION

Alprazolam contains not less than 99.0 per cent and not more than the equivalent of 101.0 per cent of 8-chloro-1-methyl-6-phenyl-4*H*-[1,2,4]triazolo[4,3-*a*][1,4]benzodiazepine, calculated with reference to the dried substance.

CHARACTERS

A white, crystalline powder, practically insoluble in water, freely soluble in methylene chloride sparingly soluble in acetone and in alcohol.

It shows polymorphism.

IDENTIFICATION

First identification: B.

Second identification: A, C.

A. Dissolve the substance to be examined in the smallest necessary quantity of *ethyl acetate R* and evaporate to dryness on a water-bath. Thoroughly mix 5.0 mg of the substance to be examined with 5.0 mg of *alprazolam CRS*. The melting point (*2.2.14*) of the mixture does not deviate from the melting point of the substance to be examined by more than 2 °C.

B. Examine by infrared absorption spectrophotometry (*2.2.24*), comparing with the spectrum obtained with *alprazolam CRS*. If the spectra obtained in the solid state show differences, dissolve the substance to be examined and the reference substance separately in the minimum volume of *ethyl acetate R*, evaporate to dryness on a water-bath and record new spectra using the residues. Examine the substances prepared as discs.

C. Examine by thin-layer chromatography (*2.2.27*), using *silica gel* GF_{254} *R* as the coating substance.

Test solution. Dissolve 10 mg of the substance to be examined in *methanol R* and dilute to 10 ml with the same solvent.

Reference solution (a). Dissolve 10 mg of *alprazolam CRS* in *methanol R* and dilute to 10 ml with the same solvent.

Reference solution (b). Dissolve 10 mg of *alprazolam CRS* and 10 mg of *midazolam CRS* in *methanol R* and dilute to 10 ml with the same solvent.

Apply separately to the plate 5 µl of each solution. Develop over a path or 12 cm using a mixture of 2 volumes of *glacial acetic acid R*, 15 volumes of *water R*, 20 volumes of *methanol R* and 80 volumes of *ethyl acetate R*. Allow the plate to dry in air and examine in ultraviolet light at 254 nm. The principal spot in the chromatogram obtained with the test solution is similar in position and size to the principal spot in the chromatogram obtained with reference solution (a). The test is not valid unless the chromatogram obtained with reference solution (b) shows two clearly separately spots.

TESTS

Related substances. Examine by liquid chromatography (*2.2.29*).

Test solution. Dissolve 0.100 g of the substance to be examined in *dimethylformamide R* and dilute to 10.0 ml with the same solvent.

Reference solution (a). Dissolve 2 mg of *alprazolam CRS* and 2 mg of *triazolam CRS* in *dimethylformamide R* and dilute to 100.0 ml with the same solvent.

Reference solution (b). Dilute 5.0 ml of the test solution to 100.0 ml with *dimethylformamide R*. Dilute 0.5 ml of this solution to 10.0 ml with *dimethylformamide R*.

The chromatographic procedure may be carried out using:

– a stainless steel column 0.25 m long and 4.6 mm in internal diameter packed with *phenylsilyl silica gel for chromatography R1* (5 µm),

– as mobile phase at a flow rate of 2 ml/min and at a temperature of 40 °C a gradient programme using the following conditions:

Mobile phase A. A mixture of 44 volumes of buffer solution and 56 volumes of *methanol R*.

Mobile phase B. A mixture of 5 volumes of buffer solution and 95 volumes of *methanol R*.

Buffer solution. Dissolve 7.7 g of *ammonium acetate R* in 1000 ml of *water R* and adjust to pH 4.2 with *glacial acetic acid R*,

Time (min)	Mobile phase A (per cent *V/V*)	Mobile phase B (per cent *V/V*)	Comment
0	98	2	isocratic
15	98	2	begin linear gradient
35	1	99	begin isocratic
40	1	99	end chromatogram and switch to initial equilibration
41	98	2	begin equilibration
50 = 0	98	2	end equilibration

– as detector a spectrophotometer set at 254 nm.

Equilibrate the column for at least 30 min with the initial eluent composition. For subsequent chromatograms, use the conditions described from 40 min to 50 min. Adjust the sensitivity of the system so that the height of the principal peak in the chromatogram obtained with reference solution (b) is at least 50 per cent of the full scale of the recorder.

Inject 10 µl of reference solution (a). When the chromatogram is recorded in the prescribed conditions the retention times are: triazolam, about 9 min and alprazolam, about 10 min. The test is not valid unless the resolution between the peaks corresponding to alprazolam and triazolam is at least 1.5.

Inject separately 10 µl of *dimethylformamide R* as a blank, 10 µl of the test solution and 10 µl of reference solution (b). In the chromatogram obtained with the test solution, the sum of the areas of the peaks, apart from the principal peak, is not greater than the area of the principal peak in the chromatogram obtained with reference solution (b) (0.25 per cent). Disregard any peak in the chromatogram obtained with the blank and any peak with an area less than 0.2 times the area of the principal peak in the chromatogram obtained with reference solution (b).

Loss on drying (*2.2.32*). Not more than 0.5 per cent, determined on 1.000 g by drying in an oven at 100 °C to 105 °C.

Sulphated ash (*2.4.14*). Not more than 0.1 per cent, determined on 1.0 g.

ASSAY

Dissolve 0.140 g in 50 ml of a mixture of 3 volumes of *anhydrous acetic acid R* and 2 volumes of *acetic anhydride R*. Titrate with *0.1 M perchloric acid*, determining the end-point potentiometrically (*2.2.20*). Titrate to the second point of inflexion.

1 ml of *0.1 M perchloric acid* is equivalent to 15.44 mg of $C_{17}H_{13}ClN_4$.

STORAGE

Store protected from light.

IMPURITIES

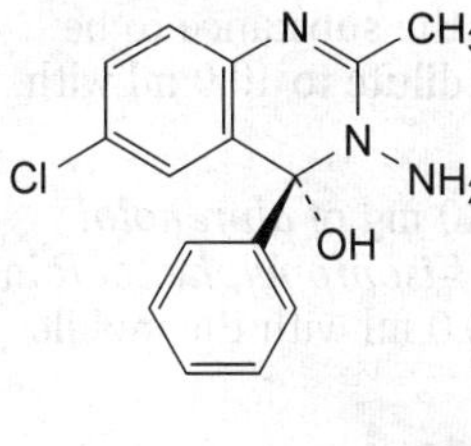

and enantiomer

A. (4*RS*)-3-amino-6-chloro-2-methyl-4-phenyl-3,4-dihydroquinazolin-4-ol,

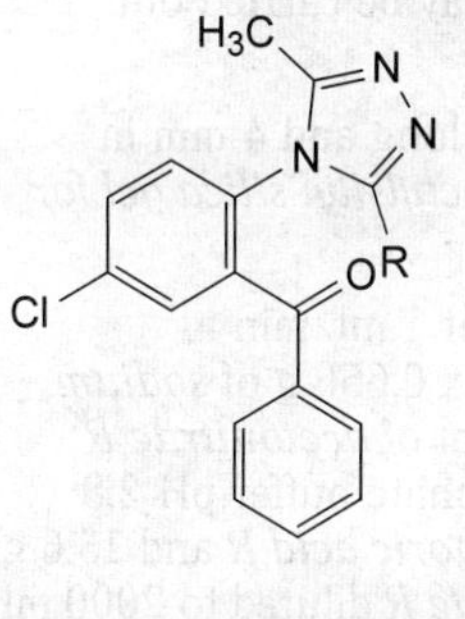

B. R = CH_2OH: [5-chloro-2-[3-(hydroxymethyl)-5-methyl-4*H*-1,2,4-triazol-4-yl]phenyl]phenylmethanone,

C. R = H: [5-chloro-2-[3-methyl-4*H*-1,2,4-triazol-4-yl]phenyl]phenylmethanone,

F. R = CH_2Cl: [5-chloro-2-[3-(chloromethyl)-5-methyl-4*H*-1,2,4-triazol-4-yl]phenyl]phenylmethanone,

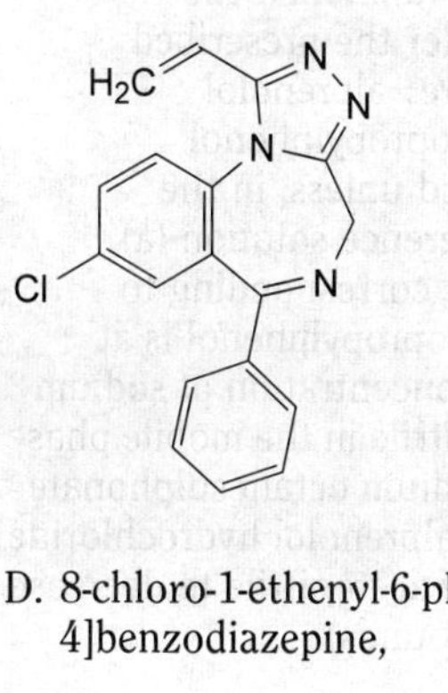

D. 8-chloro-1-ethenyl-6-phenyl-4*H*-[1,2,4]triazolo[4,3-*a*][1,4]benzodiazepine,

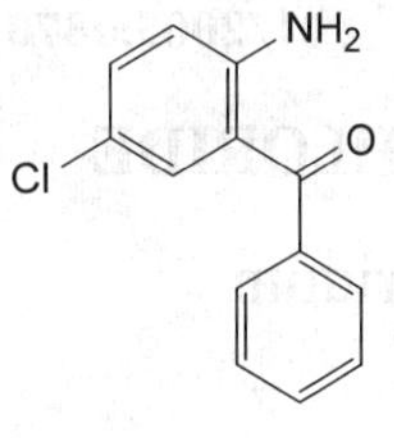

E. (2-amino-5-chlorophenyl)phenylmethanone,

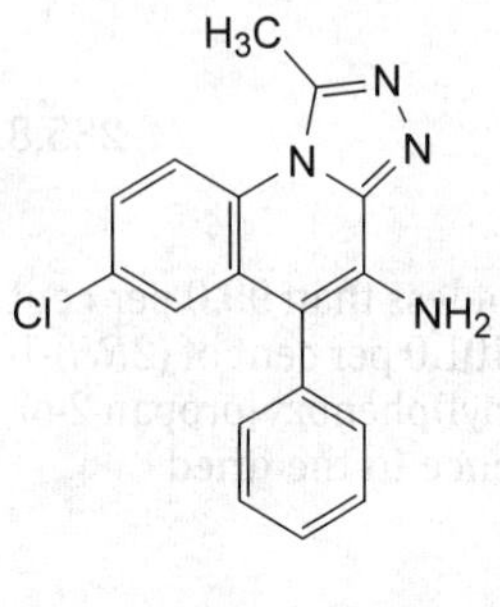

G. 7-chloro-1-methyl-5-phenyl[1,2,4]triazolo[4,3-*a*]quinolin-4-amine,

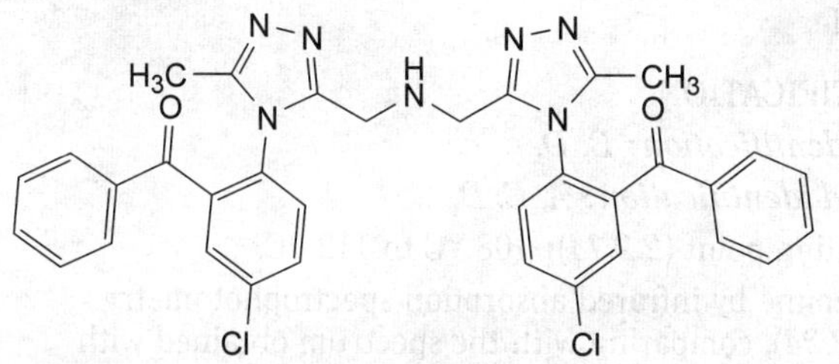

H. bis[[4-(2-benzoyl-4-chlorophenyl)-5-methyl-4*H*-1,2,4-triazol-3-yl]methyl]amine,

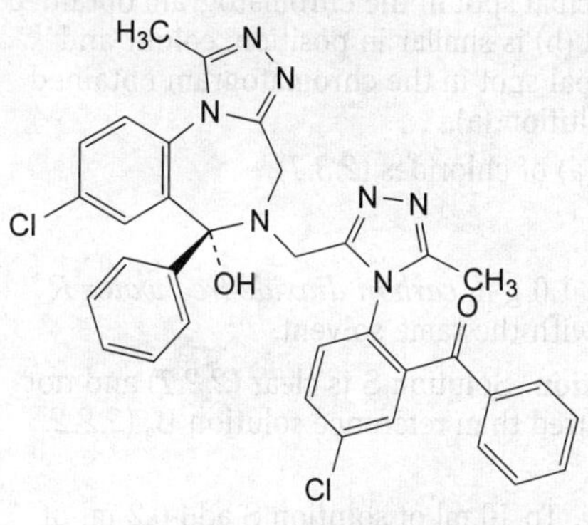

and enantiomer

I. [5-chloro-2-[3-[[(6*RS*)-8-chloro-6-hydroxy-1-methyl-6-phenyl-4*H*-[1,2,4]triazolo[4,3-*a*][1,4]benzodiazepin-5(6*H*)-yl]methyl]-5-methyl-4*H*-1,2,4-triazol-4-yl]phenyl]phenylmethanone,

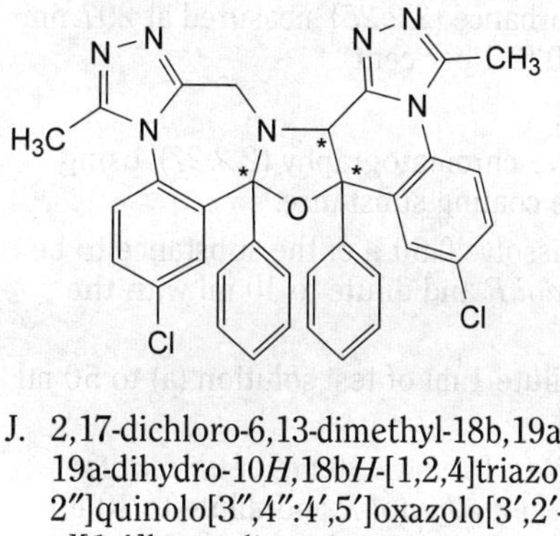

J. 2,17-dichloro-6,13-dimethyl-18b,19a-diphenyl-8b,19a-dihydro-10*H*,18b*H*-[1,2,4]triazolo[4‴,3‴:1″,2″]quinolo[3″,4″:4′,5′]oxazolo[3′,2′-*d*]-1,2,4-triazolo[4,3-*a*][1,4]benzodiazepine.

01/2005:0876

ALPRENOLOL HYDROCHLORIDE

Alprenololi hydrochloridum

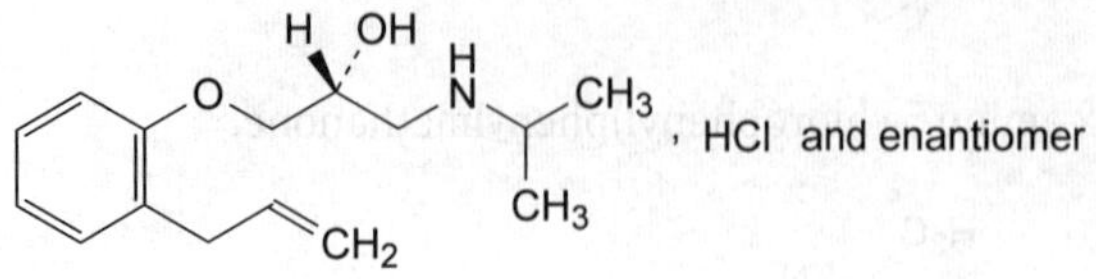

$C_{15}H_{24}ClNO_2$ M_r 285.8

DEFINITION

Alprenolol hydrochloride contains not less than 99.0 per cent and not more than the equivalent of 101.0 per cent of (2*RS*)-1-[(1-methylethyl)amino]-3-[2-(prop-2-enyl)phenoxy]propan-2-ol hydrochloride, calculated with reference to the dried substance.

CHARACTERS

A white, crystalline powder or colourless crystals, very soluble in water, freely soluble in alcohol and in methylene chloride.

IDENTIFICATION

First identification: B, D.

Second identification: A, C, D.

A. Melting point (*2.2.14*): 108 °C to 112 °C.

B. Examine by infrared absorption spectrophotometry (*2.2.24*), comparing with the spectrum obtained with *alprenolol hydrochloride CRS*.

C. Examine the chromatograms obtained in test A for related substances in daylight, after exposure to iodine vapour for 30 min. The principal spot in the chromatogram obtained with test solution (b) is similar in position, colour and size to the principal spot in the chromatogram obtained with reference solution (a).

D. It gives reaction (a) of chlorides (*2.3.1*).

TESTS

Solution S. Dissolve 1.0 g in *carbon dioxide-free water R* and dilute to 50 ml with the same solvent.

Appearance of solution. Solution S is clear (*2.2.1*) and not more intensely coloured than reference solution B_9 (*2.2.2, Method II*).

Acidity or alkalinity. To 10 ml of solution S add 0.2 ml of *methyl red solution R* and 0.2 ml of *0.01 M hydrochloric acid*. The solution is red. Add 0.4 ml of *0.01 M sodium hydroxide*. The solution is yellow.

1-Isopropylamino-3-(2-prop-1-enylphenoxy)propan-2-ol. Dissolve 0.25 g in *alcohol R* and dilute to 25 ml with the same solvent. The absorbance (*2.2.25*) measured at 297 nm is not greater than 0.20 (0.1 per cent).

Related substances

A. Examine by thin-layer chromatography (*2.2.27*), using *silica gel G R* as the coating substance.

Test solution (a). Dissolve 0.50 g of the substance to be examined in *methanol R* and dilute to 10 ml with the same solvent.

Test solution (b). Dilute 1 ml of test solution (a) to 50 ml with *methanol R*.

Reference solution (a). Dissolve 10 mg of *alprenolol hydrochloride CRS* in *methanol R* and dilute to 10 ml with the same solvent.

Reference solution (b). Dissolve 10 mg of *alprenolol hydrochloride CRS* and 10 mg of *oxprenolol hydrochloride CRS* in *methanol R* and dilute to 10 ml with the same solvent.

Reference solution (c). Dilute 5 ml of test solution (b) to 50 ml with *methanol R*.

Place two beakers each containing 30 ml of *ammonia R* at the bottom of the chamber which is saturated with the mobile phase and *ammonia R* for at least 1 h before use. Apply separately to the plate 5 µl of each solution. Develop over a path of 15 cm using a mixture of 5 volumes of *methanol R* and 95 volumes of *ethyl acetate R*. Dry the plate at 100 °C for 15 min. Expose the plate to iodine vapour for up to 6 h. In the chromatogram obtained with test solution (a) any spot with an R_f value higher than that of the principal spot is not more intense than the spot in the chromatogram obtained with reference solution (c). The test is not valid unless the chromatogram obtained with reference solution (b) shows two clearly separated spots.

B. Examine by liquid chromatography (*2.2.29*).

Test solution. Dissolve 20.0 mg of the substance to be examined in the mobile phase and dilute to 10.0 ml with the mobile phase.

Reference solution (a). Dissolve 4.0 mg of *alprenolol hydrochloride CRS* and 0.8 mg of *4-isopropylphenol R* in the mobile phase and dilute to 100.0 ml with the mobile phase.

Reference solution (b). Dilute 4.0 ml of the test solution to 100.0 ml with the mobile phase. Dilute 1.0 ml of the solution to 10.0 ml with the mobile phase.

The chromatographic procedure may be carried out using:

– a stainless steel column 0.15 m long and 4 mm in internal diameter packed with *octylsilyl silica gel for chromatography R* (5 µm),

– as mobile phase at a flow rate of 1 ml/min a mixture prepared as follows: mix 0.656 g of *sodium octanesulphonate R* with 150 ml of *acetonitrile R* and dilute to 500 ml with phosphate buffer pH 2.8 (prepared from 1.78 g of *phosphoric acid R* and 15.6 g of *sodium dihydrogen phosphate R* diluted to 2000 ml with *water R*),

– as detector a spectrophotometer set at 280 nm.

Equilibrate the column with the mobile phase at a flow rate of 1 ml/min for about 1 h.

Adjust the sensitivity of the system so that the height of the principal peak in the chromatogram obtained with 20 µl of reference solution (b) is at least 50 per cent of the full scale of the recorder.

Inject 20 µl of reference solution (a). When the chromatograms are recorded under the prescribed conditions, the retention times are: alprenolol hydrochloride about 11 min; 4-isopropylphenol about 18 min. The test is not valid unless, in the chromatogram obtained with reference solution (a), the resolution between the peaks corresponding to alprenolol hydrochloride and 4-isopropylphenol is at least 5; if necessary, adjust the concentration of sodium octanesulphonate and/or acetonitrile in the mobile phase (increase the concentration of sodium octanesulphonate to increase the retention time of alprenolol hydrochloride and increase the concentration of acetonitrile to decrease the retention times of both compounds).

Inject separately 20 µl of the test solution and 20 µl of reference solution (b). Continue the chromatography for twice the retention time of the principal peak. In the chromatogram obtained with the test solution, the sum of the areas of any peaks apart from the principal peak is not greater than the area of the principal peak in the chromatogram obtained with reference solution (b) (0.4 per cent). Disregard any peak with an area less than 0.1 times the area of the principal peak in the chromatogram obtained with reference solution (b).

Heavy metals (*2.4.8*). Dissolve 2.0 g in 20 ml of *water R*. 12 ml of the solution complies with limit test A for heavy metals (10 ppm). Prepare the standard using *lead standard solution (1 ppm Pb) R*.

Loss on drying (*2.2.32*). Not more than 0.5 per cent, determined on 1.000 g by drying over *diphosphorus pentoxide R* at a pressure not exceeding 2.7 kPa.

Sulphated ash (*2.4.14*). Not more than 0.1 per cent, determined on 1.0 g.

ASSAY

Dissolve 0.400 g in 25 ml of a mixture of equal volumes of *ethanol R* and *water R*. Add 10 ml of *0.01 M hydrochloric acid*. Carry out a potentiometric titration (*2.2.20*), using *0.1 M sodium hydroxide*. Read the volume added between the two points of inflexion.

1 ml of *0.1 M sodium hydroxide* is equivalent to 28.58 mg of $C_{15}H_{24}ClNO_2$.

STORAGE

Store protected from light.

IMPURITIES

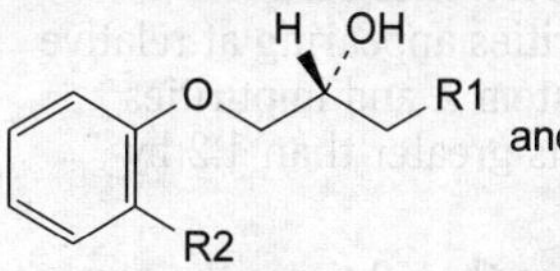

and enantiomer

A. R1 = OH, R2 = CH_2-CH=CH_2: (2*RS*)-3-[2-(prop-2-enyl)phenoxy]propan-1,2-diol,

C. R1 = NH-CH$(CH_3)_2$, R2 = CH=CH-CH_3: (2*RS*)-1-[(1-methylethyl)amino]-3-[2-(prop-1-enyl)phenoxy]propan-2-ol,

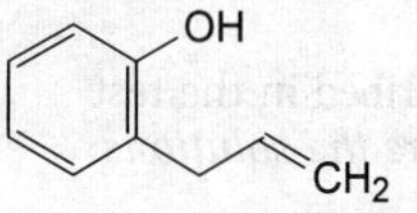

B. 2-(prop-2-enyl)phenol,

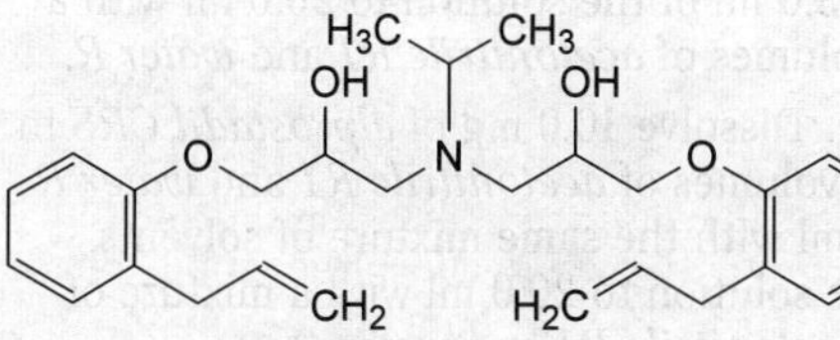

D. 1,1′-[(1-methylethyl)imino]bis[3-[2-(prop-2-enyl)phenoxy]propan-2-ol].

01/2005:1488

ALPROSTADIL

Alprostadilum

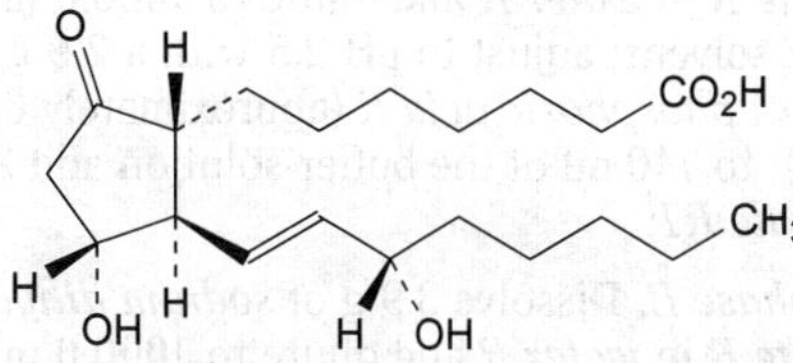

$C_{20}H_{34}O_5$ M_r 354.5

DEFINITION

7-[(1*R*,2*R*,3*R*)-3-Hydroxy-2-[(1*E*,3*S*)-3-hydroxyoct-1-enyl]-5-oxocyclopentyl]heptanoic acid.

Content: 95.0 per cent to 102.5 per cent (anhydrous substance).

CHARACTERS

Appearance: white or slightly yellowish, crystalline powder.

Solubility: practically insoluble in water, freely soluble in alcohol, soluble in acetone, slightly soluble in ethyl acetate.

IDENTIFICATION

A. Specific optical rotation (*2.2.7*): − 60 to − 70 (anhydrous substance).

Immediately before use, dissolve 50 mg in *alcohol R* and dilute to 10.0 ml with the same solvent.

B. Infrared absorption spectrophotometry (*2.2.24*).

Preparation: discs.

Comparison: *alprostadil CRS*.

C. Examine the chromatograms obtained in the assay.

Results: the principal peak in the chromatogram obtained with the test solution is similar in retention time and size to the principal peak in the chromatogram obtained with the reference solution.

TESTS

Related substances. Liquid chromatography (*2.2.29*). *Prepare the solutions protected from light.*

Test solution. Dissolve 10.0 mg of the substance to be examined in a mixture of equal volumes of *acetonitrile R1* and *water R* and dilute to 10.0 ml with the same mixture of solvents.

Reference solution (a). Dilute 100 µl of the test solution to 20.0 ml with a mixture of equal volumes of *acetonitrile R1* and *water R*.

Reference solution (b). Dissolve 1.0 mg of *dinoprostone impurity C CRS* (alprostadil impurity H) and 1.0 mg of *alprostadil CRS* in a mixture of equal volumes of *acetonitrile R1* and *water R* and dilute to 20.0 ml with the same mixture of solvents.

Reference solution (c). In order to prepare *in situ* the degradation compounds (impurity A and impurity B), dissolve 1 mg of the substance to be examined in 100 µl of *1 M sodium hydroxide* (the solution becomes brownish-red), wait for 3 min and add 100 µl of *1 M phosphoric acid* (yellowish-white opalescent solution); dilute to 5.0 ml with a mixture of equal volumes of *acetonitrile R1* and *water R*.

System A

Column:

– *size*: *l* = 0.25 m, Ø = 4.0 mm,

– *stationary phase*: *octylsilyl base-deactivated silica gel for chromatography R* (4 µm) with a pore size of 6 nm,
– *temperature*: 35 °C.

Mobile phase:
– *mobile phase A.* Dissolve 3.9 g of *sodium dihydrogen phosphate R* in *water R* and dilute to 1000.0 ml with the same solvent; adjust to pH 2.5 with a 2.9 g/l solution of *phosphoric acid R* (approximately 600 ml is required); to 740 ml of the buffer solution add 260 ml of *acetonitrile R1*;
– *mobile phase B.* Dissolve 3.9 g of *sodium dihydrogen phosphate R* in *water R* and dilute to 1000.0 ml with the same solvent; adjust to pH 2.5 with a 2.9 g/l solution of *phosphoric acid R* (approximately 600 ml is required); to 200 ml of the buffer solution add 800 ml of *acetonitrile R1*;

Time (min)	Mobile phase A (per cent V/V)	Mobile phase B (per cent V/V)
0 - 75	100	0
75 - 76	100 → 0	0 → 100
76 - 86	0	100
86 - 87	0 → 100	100 → 0
87 - 102	100	0

Flow rate: 1 ml/min.

Detection: spectrophotometer at 200 nm.

Injection: 20 µl loop injector.

System suitability:
– *retention time*: alprostadil = about 63 min,
– *resolution*: minimum of 1.5 between the peaks due to impurity H and alprostadil in the chromatogram obtained with reference solution (b).

System B

Use the same conditions as for system A with the following mobile phase and elution programme:
– *mobile phase A.* Dissolve 3.9 g of *sodium dihydrogen phosphate R* in *water R* and dilute to 1000.0 ml with the same solvent; adjust to pH 2.5 with a 2.9 g/l solution of *phosphoric acid R* (approximately 600 ml is required); to 600 ml of the buffer solution add 400 ml of *acetonitrile R1*;
– *mobile phase B.* Use mobile phase B as described under system A;

Time (min)	Mobile phase A (per cent V/V)	Mobile phase B (per cent V/V)
0 - 50	100	0
50 - 51	100 → 0	0 → 100
51 - 61	0	100
61 - 62	0 → 100	100 → 0
62 - 72	100	0

System suitability:
– *relative retentions* with reference to alprostadil (retention time = about 7 min): impurity A = about 2.4; impurity B = about 2.6,
– *resolution*: minimum of 1.5 between the peaks due to impurity A and impurity B in the chromatogram obtained with reference solution (c).

Carry out the test according to system A and B.

Limits:
– *correction factors*: multiply the areas of the corresponding peaks using the correction factors in Table 1488.-1 to obtain the corrected areas,

Table 1488.-1

Impurity	Relative retention (system A)	Relative retention (system B)	Correction factor
impurity G	0.80	-	0.7
impurity F	0.88	-	0.8
impurity D	0.90	-	1.0
impurity H	0.96	-	0.7
impurity E	1.10	-	0.7
impurity C	-	1.36	1.9
impurity K	-	1.85	0.06
impurity A	-	2.32	0.7
impurity B	-	2.45	1.5
impurity I	-	4.00	1.0
impurity J	-	5.89	1.0

– *impurity A (corrected area)*: not more than 3 times the area of the principal peak in the chromatogram obtained with reference solution (a) (1.5 per cent),
– *impurity B (corrected area)*: not more than the area of the principal peak in the chromatogram obtained with reference solution (a) (0.5 per cent),
– *any other impurity (corrected area)*: not more than 1.8 times the area of the principal peak in the chromatogram obtained with reference solution (a) (0.9 per cent), and not more than 1 such peak has an area greater than the area of the principal peak in the chromatogram obtained with reference solution (a) (0.5 per cent). Evaluate impurities appearing at relative retentions less than 1.2 by system A and impurities appearing at relative retentions greater than 1.2 by system B,
– *total (corrected area)*: not more than 3 times the area of the principal peak in the chromatogram obtained with reference solution (a) (1.5 per cent),
– *disregard limit*: 0.1 times the area of the principal peak in the chromatogram obtained with reference solution (a) (0.05 per cent).

Water (*2.5.32*): maximum 0.5 per cent, determined on 50 mg.

ASSAY

Liquid chromatography (*2.2.29*) as described in the test for related substances, system A. *Prepare the solutions protected from light.*

Test solution. Dissolve 10.0 mg of the substance to be examined in a mixture of equal volumes of *acetonitrile R1* and *water R* and dilute to 25.0 ml with the same mixture of solvents. Dilute 3.0 ml of the solution to 20.0 ml with a mixture of equal volumes of *acetonitrile R1* and *water R*.

Reference solution. Dissolve 10.0 mg of *alprostadil CRS* in a mixture of equal volumes of *acetonitrile R1* and *water R* and dilute to 25.0 ml with the same mixture of solvents. Dilute 3.0 ml of the solution to 20.0 ml with a mixture of equal volumes of *acetonitrile R1* and *water R*.

Injection: 20 µl.

Calculate the percentage content of $C_{20}H_{34}O_5$.

STORAGE

At a temperature of 2 °C to 8 °C.

IMPURITIES

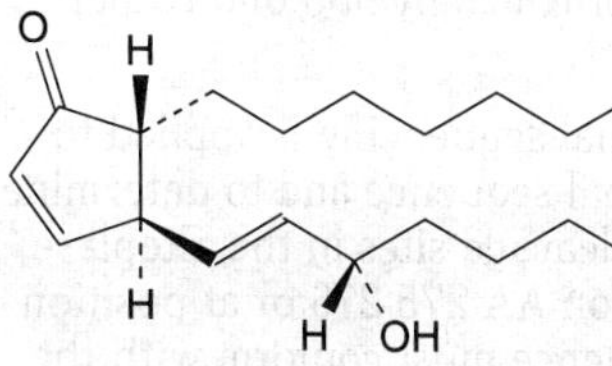

A. 7-[(1*R*,2*S*)-2-[(1*E*,3*S*)-3-hydroxyoct-1-enyl]-5-oxocyclopent-3-enyl]heptanoic acid (prostaglandin A_1),

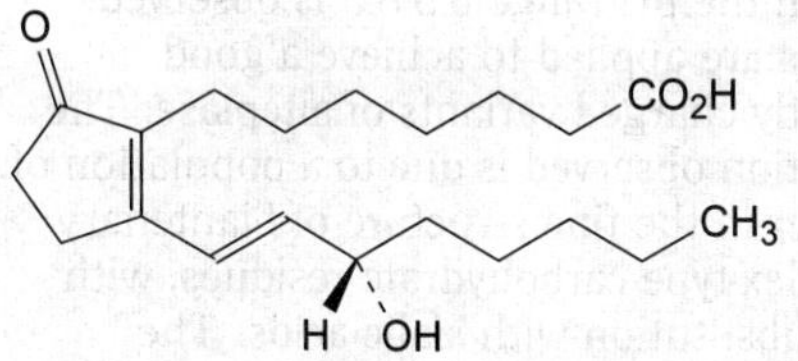

B. 7-[2-[(1*E*,3*S*)-3-hydroxyoct-1-enyl]-5-oxocyclopent-1-enyl]heptanoic acid (prostaglandin B_1),

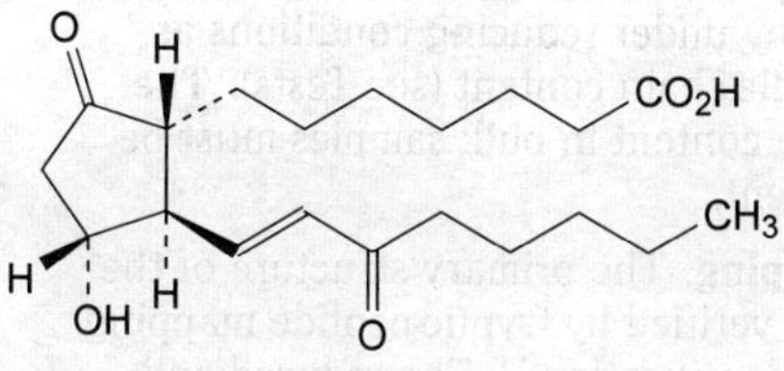

C. 7-[(1*R*,2*R*,3*R*)-3-hydroxy-2-[(1*E*)-3-oxooct-1-enyl]-5-oxocyclopentyl]heptanoic acid (15-oxoprostaglandin E_1),

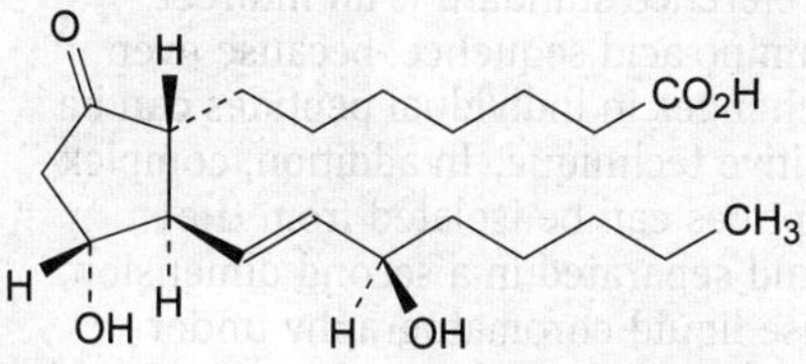

D. 7-[(1*R*,2*R*,3*R*)-3-hydroxy-2-[(1*E*,3*R*)-3-hydroxyoct-1-enyl]-5-oxocyclopentyl]heptanoic acid (15-epiprostaglandin E_1),

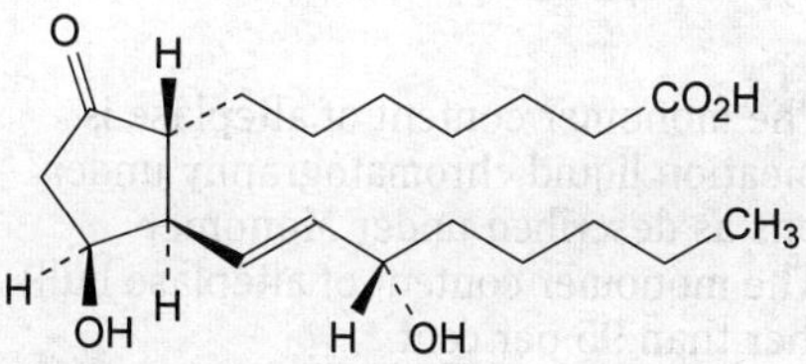

E. 7-[(1*R*,2*R*,3*S*)-3-hydroxy-2-[(1*E*,3*S*)-3-hydroxyoct-1-enyl]-5-oxocyclopentyl]heptanoic acid (11-epiprostaglandin E_1),

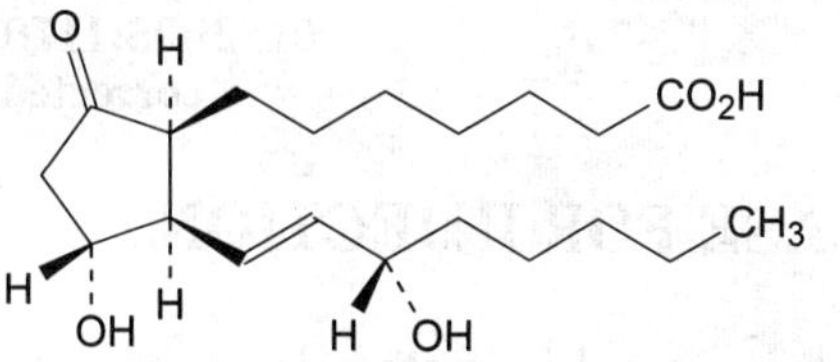

F. 7-[(1*S*,2*R*,3*R*)-3-hydroxy-2-[(1*E*,3*S*)-3-hydroxyoct-1-enyl]-5-oxocyclopentyl]heptanoic acid (8-epiprostaglandin E_1),

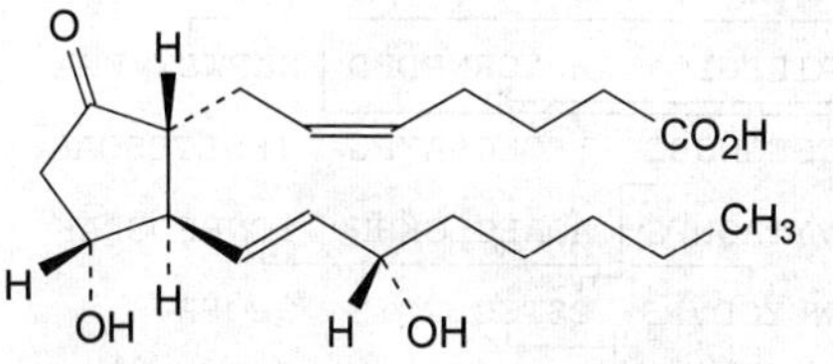

G. (5*Z*)-7-[(1*R*,2*R*,3*R*)-3-hydroxy-2-[(1*E*,3*S*)-3-hydroxyoct-1-enyl]-5-oxocyclopentyl]hept-5-enoic acid (dinoprostone),

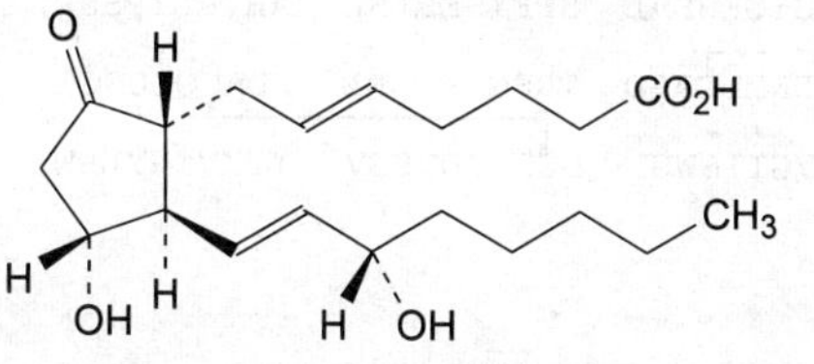

H. (5*E*)-7-[(1*R*,2*R*,3*R*)-3-hydroxy-2-[(1*E*,3*S*)-3-hydroxyoct-1-enyl]-5-oxocyclopentyl]hept-5-enoic acid ((5*E*)-prostaglandin E_2),

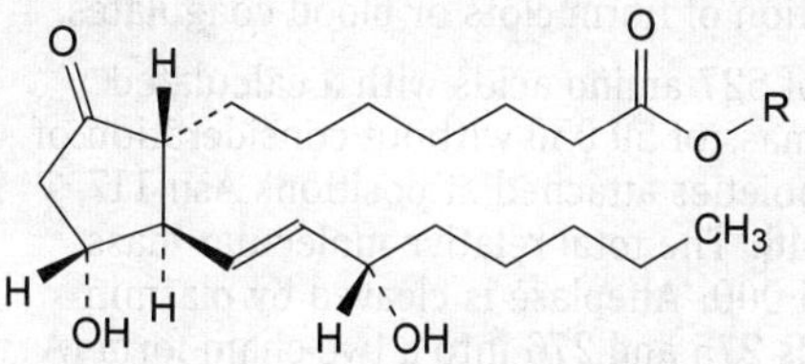

I. R = CH_2-CH_3: ethyl 7-[(1*R*,2*R*,3*R*)-3-hydroxy-2-[(1*E*,3*S*)-3-hydroxyoct-1-enyl]-5-oxocyclopentyl]heptanoate (prostaglandin E_1, ethyl ester),

J. R = $CH(CH_3)_2$: 1-methylethyl 7-[(1*R*,2*R*,3*R*)-3-hydroxy-2-[(1*E*,3*S*)-3-hydroxyoct-1-enyl]-5-oxocyclopentyl]heptanoate (prostaglandin E_1, isopropyl ester),

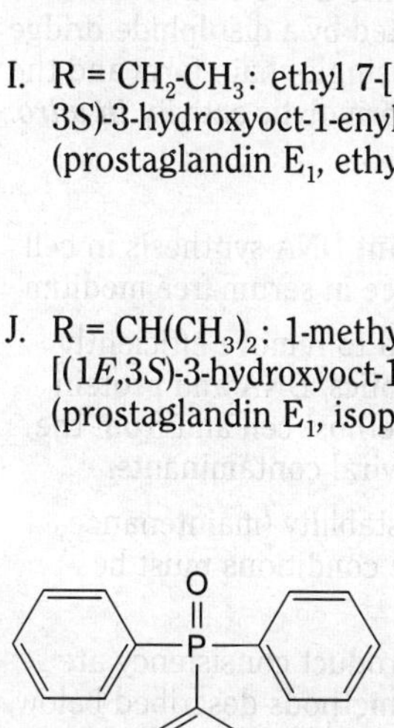

K. triphenylphosphine oxide.

01/2005:1170
corrected

ALTEPLASE FOR INJECTION

Alteplasum ad iniectabile

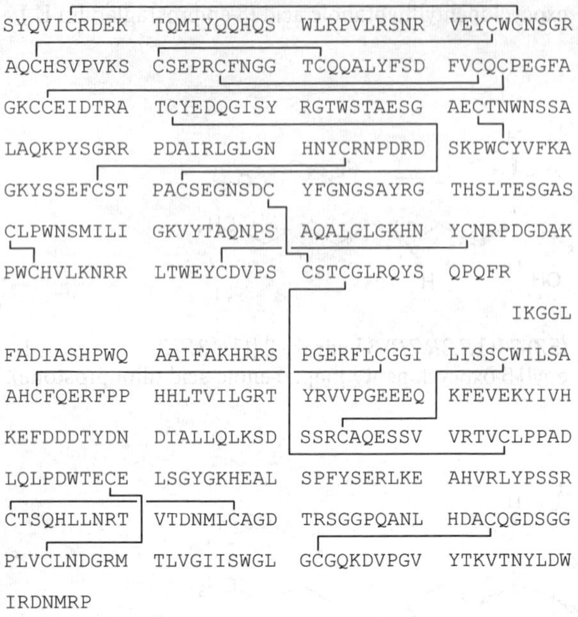

DEFINITION

Alteplase for injection is a sterile, freeze-dried preparation of alteplase, a tissue plasminogen activator produced by recombinant DNA technology. It has a potency of not less than 500 000 IU per milligram of protein.

Tissue plasminogen activator binds to fibrin clots and activates plasminogen, leading to the generation of plasmin and to the degradation of fibrin clots or blood coagulates.

Alteplase consists of 527 amino acids with a calculated relative molecular mass of 59 050 without consideration of the carbohydrate moieties attached at positions Asn 117, Asn 184 and Asn 448. The total relative molecular mass is approximately 65 000. Alteplase is cleaved by plasmin between amino-acids 275 and 276 into a two-chain form (A chain and B chain) that are connected by a disulphide bridge between Cys 264 and Cys 395. The single-chain form and the two-chain form show comparable fibrinolytic activity *in vitro*.

PRODUCTION

Alteplase is produced by recombinant DNA synthesis in cell culture; the fermentation takes place in serum-free medium.

The purification process is designed to remove efficiently potential impurities, such as antibiotics, DNA and protein contaminants derived both from the host cell and from the production medium, and potential viral contaminants.

If alteplase is stored in bulk form, stability (maintenance of potency) in the intended storage conditions must be demonstrated.

The production, purification and product consistency are checked by a number of analytical methods described below, carried out routinely as in-process controls.

Protein content. The protein concentration of alteplase solutions is determined by measuring the absorbance (*2.2.25*) of the protein solution at 280 nm and at 320 nm, using formulation buffer as the compensation liquid. If dilution of alteplase samples is necessary, the samples are diluted in formulation buffer. For the calculation of the alteplase concentration the absorbance value ($A_{280} - A_{320}$) is divided by the specific absorption coefficient for alteplase of 1.9.

Potency. The potency of alteplase is determined in an *in-vitro* clot-lysis assay as described under Assay. The specific activity of bulk alteplase is approximately 580 000 IU per milligram of alteplase.

***N*-terminal sequence**. *N*-terminal sequencing is applied to determine the correct *N*-terminal sequence and to determine semiquantitatively additional cleavage sites in the alteplase molecule, for example at position AA 275-276 or at position AA 27-28. The *N*-terminal sequence must conform with the sequence of human tissue plasminogen activator.

Isoelectric focusing. The consistency in the microheterogeneity of glycosylation of the alteplase molecule can be demonstrated by isoelectric focusing (IEF). A complex banding pattern with ten major and several minor bands in the pH range 6.5-8.5 is observed. Denaturing conditions are applied to achieve a good separation of differently charged variants of alteplase. The broad charge distribution observed is due to a population of molecules, which differ in the fine structure of biantenary and triantenary complex-type carbohydrate residues, with different degrees of substitution with sialic acids. The banding pattern of alteplase test samples must be consistent with the pattern of alteplase reference standard.

Single-chain alteplase content. The alteplase produced by CHO (Chinese hamster ovary) cells in serum-free medium is predominantly single-chain alteplase. The single-chain form can be separated from the two-chain form by gel-permeation liquid chromatography under reducing conditions as described under Single-chain content (see Tests). The single-chain alteplase content in bulk samples must be higher than 60 per cent.

Tryptic-peptide mapping. The primary structure of the alteplase molecule is verified by tryptic-peptide mapping as described under Identification B. The reduced and carboxymethylated molecule is cleaved by trypsin into about fifty peptides, which are separated by reverse-phase liquid chromatography. A characteristic chromatogram (fingerprint) is obtained. The identity of the tryptic-peptide map of a given alteplase sample with the profile of a well-characterised reference standard is an indirect confirmation of the amino-acid sequence, because even single amino-acid exchanges in individual peptides can be detected by this sensitive technique. In addition, complex peaks of the glycopeptides can be isolated from the tryptic-peptide map and separated in a second dimension, either by reverse-phase liquid chromatography under modified conditions or by capillary electrophoresis. By this two-dimensional separation of glycopeptide variants, lot-to-lot consistency of the microheterogeneity of glycosylation can be demonstrated.

The tryptic-peptide map of alteplase samples must be consistent with the tryptic-peptide map of alteplase reference standard.

Monomer content. The monomer content of alteplase is measured by gel-permeation liquid chromatography under non-reduced conditions as described under Monomer content (see Tests). The monomer content of alteplase bulk samples must be higher than 95 per cent.

Type I/Type II alteplase content. CHO cells produce two glycosylation variants of alteplase. Type I alteplase contains one polymannose-type glycosylation at position Asn 117 and two complex-type glycosylation sites at positions Asn 184 and Asn 448. Type II alteplase is only glycosylated at positions Asn 117 and Asn 448.

The ratio of Type I/Type II alteplase is constant in the range of 45 to 65 per cent of Type I and 35 to 55 per cent of Type II. The content of alteplase Type I and Type II can be determined by a densitometric scan of SDS-PAGE (sodium dodecyl sulphate polyacrylamide gel electrophoresis) gel. Plasmin-treated samples of alteplase, which are reduced and carboxymethylated before loading on the gel, are separated into three bands: Type I alteplase A-chain (AA 1-275), Type II alteplase A-chain (AA 1-275) and alteplase B-chain (AA 276-527). The ratio of Type I/Type II alteplase is determined from a calibration curve, which is obtained by a densitometric scan of defined mixtures of purified Type I alteplase and Type II alteplase standards.

SDS-PAGE. SDS-PAGE (silver staining) is used to demonstrate purity of the alteplase bulk material and the integrity of the alteplase molecule. For alteplase bulk samples, no additional protein bands compared to reference standard or degradation products must occur in SDS-PAGE gels at a loading amount of 2.5 µg alteplase protein per lane and a limit of detection of 5 ng per protein (BSA) band.

Bacterial endotoxins (*2.6.14*): less than 1 IU per milligram of alteplase.

Sialic acids. Dialyse samples and alteplase reference standard against enzyme buffer (8.9 g/l *sodium chloride R*, 4.1 g/l *sodium acetate R*, pH 5.5) using a membrane with a cut-off point corresponding to a relative molecular mass of 10 000 for globular proteins. After dialysis, determine the protein concentration. Add 5 µl of calcium chloride solution (19.98 per cent *m/m calcium chloride R*) to 1 ml of protein solution. Add 10 milliunits of neuraminidase per milligram of protein. Incubate this solution at 37 °C for about 17 h.

Prepare standard dilutions between 1.56 mg/ml and 25.0 mg/ml from an *N-acetylneuraminic acid R* reference stock solution with a concentration of 50 mg/ml. Pipette 0.2 ml of the sample and of the protein reference standard in duplicate into reagent tubes. Pipette also 0.2 ml of the standard dilutions into reagent tubes. Add 0.25 ml of periodate reagent (5.4 g/l solution of *sodium periodate R* in a 1.25 per cent *V/V* solution of *sulphuric acid R*), mix and incubate for 30 min at 37 °C. Add 0.2 ml of arsenite reagent (20 g/l solution of *sodium arsenite R* in a 1.55 per cent *V/V* solution of *hydrochloric acid R*) and mix. A yellowish-brown colour develops and disappears. Add 2.0 ml of a 28.9 g/l solution of *thiobarbituric acid R* and mix. Heat the closed tubes in boiling water for 7.5 min and then cool them in an ice-bath for 5 min. Add 2.0 ml of a mixture of *butanol R* and *hydrochloric acid R* (95:5) and mix. Centrifuge the tubes at 3000 r/min for 3 min. Measure the absorbance of the butanol-HCl layer at 552 nm within 30 min using the butanol-HCl mixture as the compensation solution. Perform a linear-regression analysis for the *N*-acetylneuraminic acid standard. The molar content of *N*-acetylneuraminic acid for the samples and for alteplase reference standard is calculated from the calibration curve. The sialic acids content for the test samples must be within the range 70 to 130 per cent of alteplase reference standard, which contains about 3 moles of sialic acids per mole of alteplase.

Neutral sugars. Dilute alteplase samples and the reference standard in the assay buffer, containing 34.8 g/l of *arginine R*, 0.1 g/l of *polysorbate 80 R* and adjusted to pH 7.4 with *phosphoric acid R*, to a protein concentration of 50 µg/ml. Prepare the following concentrations of mannose in the same assay buffer for a calibration curve: 20, 30, 40, 50 and 60 µg/ml. Pipette 2 ml of alteplase samples and reference standard, as well as 2 ml of each mannose concentration in duplicate in reagent tubes. Add 50 µl of *phenol R*, followed by 5 ml of *sulphuric acid R* in each reagent tube. Incubate the mixture for 30 min at room temperature. Measure the absorbance at 492 nm for each tube. Read the content of neutral sugars from the mannose calibration curve. The neutral sugar content is expressed in moles of neutral sugar per mole of alteplase, taking into account the dilution factor for alteplase samples and reference standard and using a relative molecular mass of 180.2 for mannose and a relative molecular mass of 59 050 for the alteplase protein moiety. The neutral sugar content of the alteplase samples must be in the range of 70 to 130 per cent compared to alteplase reference standard, which contains about 12 moles of neutral sugar per mole of alteplase.

CHARACTERS

A white or slightly yellow powder or solid friable mass.

Reconstitute the preparation as stated on the label immediately before carrying out the Identification, Tests (except those for solubility and water) and Assay.

IDENTIFICATION

A. The assay serves also to identify the preparation.

B. Tryptic-peptide mapping. Examine by liquid chromatography (*2.2.29*).

Test solution. Dilute the preparation to be examined with *water R* to obtain a solution containing about 1 mg of alteplase per millilitre. Dialyse about 2.5 ml of the solution for at least 12 h into a solution containing 480 g/l of *urea R*, 44 g/l of *tris(hydroxymethyl)aminomethane R* and 1.5 g/l of *disodium edetate R* and adjusted to pH 8.6, using a membrane with a cut-off point corresponding to a relative molecular mass of 10 000 for globular proteins. Measure the volume of the solution, transfer it to a clean test-tube and add per millilitre 10 µl of a 156 g/l solution of *dithiothreitol R*. Allow to stand for 4 h, cool in iced water and add per millilitre of solution 25 µl of a freshly prepared 190 g/l solution of *iodoacetic acid R*. Allow to stand in the dark for 30 min. Add per millilitre 50 µl of dithiothreitol solution to stop the reaction. Dialyse for 24 h against an 8 g/l solution of *ammonium hydrogen carbonate R*. Add 1 part of *trypsin for peptide mapping R* to 100 parts of the protein and allow to stand for 6 h to 8 h. Repeat the addition of trypsin and allow to stand for a total of 24 h.

Reference solution. Prepare as for the test solution using *alteplase CRS* instead of the preparation to be examined.

The chromatographic procedure may be carried out using:

– a column 0.1 m long and 4.6 mm in internal diameter packed with *octadecylsilyl silica gel for chromatography R* (5 µm to 10 µm),

  Mobile phase A. A 8 g/l solution of *sodium dihydrogen phosphate R*, adjusted to pH 2.85 with *phosphoric acid R*, filtered and degassed,

  Mobile phase B. *Acetonitrile R* 75 per cent *V/V* in mobile phase A,

– as detector a spectrophotometer set at 210 nm.

Equilibrate the system with mobile phase A at a flow rate of 1 ml/min. After injection of the solution, increase the proportion of mobile phase B at a rate of 0.44 per cent per minute until the ratio of mobile phase A to mobile phase B is 60:40 and then increase the proportion of mobile phase B at a rate of 1.33 per cent per minute until the ratio of mobile phase A to mobile phase B is 20:80

and then continue elution with this mixture for a further 10 min. Record the chromatogram for the reference solution: the test is not valid unless the resolution of peaks 6 (peptides 268-275) and 7 (peptides 1-7) is at least 1.5; $b_{0.5a}$ and $b_{0.5b}$ are not more than 0.4 min. Inject about 100 µl of the test solution and record the chromatogram. Verify the identity of the peaks by comparison with the chromatograms of the reference solution. There should not be any additional significant peaks or shoulders, a significant peak or shoulder being defined as one with an area response equal to or greater than 5 per cent of peak 19 (peptides 278-296); no significant peak is missing. A type chromatogram for identification of the peaks cited is given at the end of the monograph (see Figure 1170.-1).

TESTS

Appearance of solution. The reconstituted preparation is clear (*2.2.1*) and not more intensely coloured than reference solution Y_7 (*2.2.2, Method II*).

pH (*2.2.3*): 7.1 to 7.5.

Solubility. Add the volume of the liquid stated on the label. The preparation dissolves completely within 2 min at 20 °C to 25 °C.

Protein content. Prepare a solution of the substance to be examined with an accurately known concentration of about 1 g/l. Using a 34.8 g/l solution of *arginine R* adjusted to pH 7.3 with *phosphoric acid R*, dilute an accurately measured volume of the solution of the substance to be examined so that the absorbance measured at the maximum at about 280 nm is 0.5 to 1.0 (*test solution*). Measure the absorbance (*2.2.25*) of the solution at the maximum at about 280 nm and at 320 nm using the arginine solution as the compensation liquid. Calculate the protein content in the portion of alteplase taken from the expression:

$$\frac{V\,(A_{280} - A_{320})}{1.9}$$

in which V is the volume of arginine solution required to prepare the test solution, A_{280} is the absorbance at the maximum at about 280 nm and A_{320} is the absorbance at 320 nm.

Single-chain content. Examine by liquid chromatography(*2.2.29*).

Test solution. Dissolve the preparation to be examined in *water R* to obtain a solution containing about 1 mg of alteplase per millilitre. Place about 1 ml of the solution in a tube, add 3 ml of a 3 g/l solution of *dithiothreitol R* in the mobile phase, place a cap on the tube and heat at about 80 °C for 3 min to 5 min.

The chromatographic procedure may be carried out using:

- a column 0.6 m long and 7.5 mm in internal diameter packed with silica-based rigid, hydrophilic gel with spherical particles 10 µm to 13 µm in diameter, suitable for size-exclusion chromatography,
- as mobile phase at a flow rate of 0.5 ml/min a solution containing 30 g/l of *sodium dihydrogen phosphate R* and 1 g/l of *sodium dodecyl sulphate R*, adjusted to pH 6.8 with *dilute sodium hydroxide solution R*,
- as detector a spectrophotometer set at 214 nm.

Inject about 50 µl of the test solution and record the chromatogram. The chromatogram shows two major peaks corresponding to single-chain and two-chain alteplase. Calculate the relative amount of single-chain alteplase from the peak area values.

The test is not valid unless: the number of theoretical plates calculated on the basis of the single-chain alteplase peak is at least 1000. The content of single-chain alteplase is not less than 60 per cent of the total amount of alteplase-related substances found.

Monomer content. Examine by liquid chromatography (*2.2.29*).

Test solution. Reconstitute the preparation to be examined to obtain a solution containing about 1 mg per millilitre.

The chromatographic procedure may be carried out using:

- a column 0.6 m long and 7.5 mm in internal diameter packed with silica-based rigid, hydrophilic gel with spherical particles 10 µm to 13 µm in diameter, suitable for size-exclusion chromatography,
- as mobile phase at a flow rate of 0.5 ml/min a solution containing 30 g/l of *sodium dihydrogen phosphate R* and 1 g/l of *sodium dodecyl sulphate R*, adjusted to pH 6.8 with *dilute sodium hydroxide solution R*,
- as detector a spectrophotometer set at 214 nm.

Inject the test solution and record the chromatogram. The test is not valid unless the number of theoretical plates calculated for the alteplase monomer peak is at least 1000. Measure the response for all peaks, i.e. peaks corresponding to alteplase species of different molecular masses. Calculate the relative content of monomer from the area values of these peaks. The monomer content for alteplase must be at least 95 per cent.

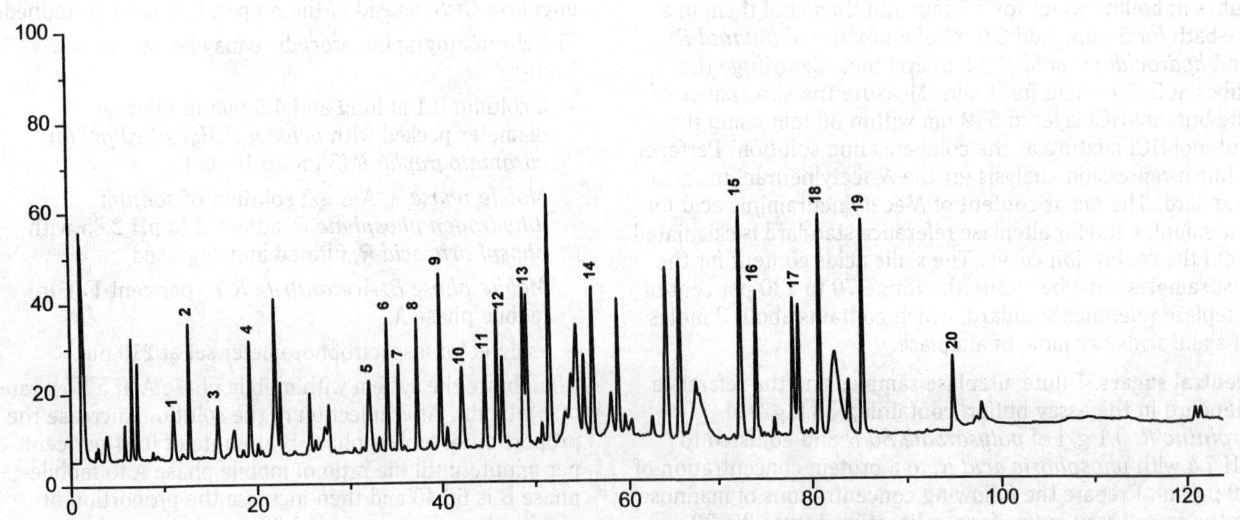

Figure 1170.-1. – *Chromatogram for tryptic-peptide mapping of alteplase*

Water (*2.5.12*). Not more than 4.0 per cent, determined by the semi-micro determination of water.

Bacterial endotoxins (*2.6.14*): less than 1 IU per milligram of protein.

Sterility (*2.6.1*). It complies with the test for sterility.

ASSAY

The potency of alteplase is determined by comparing its ability to activate plasminogen to form plasmin with the same capacity of a reference preparation calibrated in International Units. The formation of plasmin is measured by the determination of the lysis time of a fibrin clot in given conditions.

The International Unit is the activity of a stated quantity of the International Standard of alteplase. The equivalence in International Units of the International Standard is stated by the World Health Organisation.

Solvent buffer. A solution containing 1.38 g/l of *sodium dihydrogen phosphate monohydrate R*, 7.10 g/l of *anhydrous disodium hydrogen phosphate R*, 0.20 g/l of *sodium azide R* and 0.10 g/l of *polysorbate 80 R*.

Human thrombin solution. A solution of *human thrombin R* containing 33 IU/ml in solvent buffer.

Human fibrinogen solution. A 2 g/l solution of *fibrinogen R* in solvent buffer.

Human plasminogen solution. A 1 g/l solution of *human plasminogen R* in solvent buffer.

Test solutions. Using a solution of the substance to be examined containing 1 g/l, prepare serial dilutions using solvent buffer, for example 1:5000, 1:10 000, 1:20 000.

Reference solutions. Using a solution of *alteplase CRS* having an accurately known concentration of about 1 g/l (580 000 IU of alteplase per millilitre), prepare five serial dilutions using *water R* to obtain reference solutions having known concentrations in the range 9.0 IU/ml to 145 IU/ml.

To each of a set of labelled glass test-tubes, add 0.5 ml of human thrombin solution. Allocate each test and reference solution to a separate tube and add to each tube 0.5 ml of the solution allocated to it. To each of a second set of labelled glass tubes, add 20 µl of human plasminogen solution, and 1 ml of human fibrinogen solution, mix and store on ice. Beginning with the reference/thrombin mixture containing the lowest number of International Units per millilitre, record the time and separately add 200 µl of each of the thrombin mixtures to the test tubes containing the plasminogen-fibrinogen mixture. Using a vortex mixture, intermittently mix the contents of each tube for a total of 15 s and carefully place in a rack in a circulating water-bath at 37 °C. A visibly turbid clot forms within 30 s and bubbles subsequently form within the clot. Record the clot-lysis time as the time between the first addition of alteplase solution and the moment when the last bubble rises to the surface. Using a least-squares fit, determine the equation of the line using the logarithms of the concentrations of the reference preparation in International Units per millilitre versus the logarithms of the values of their clot-lysis times in seconds, according to the equation:

$$\log t = a + b\,(\log U_s)$$

in which t is the clot-lysis time, U_S the activity in International Units per millilitre of the reference preparation, b is the slope and a the y-intercept of the line. The test is not valid unless the correlation coefficient is − 0.9900 to − 1.0000. From the line equation and the clot-lysis time for the test solution, calculate the logarithm of the activity U_A from the equation:

$$\log U_A = \frac{[(\log t) - a]}{b}$$

Calculate the alteplase activity in International Units per millilitre from the expression:

$$D \times U_A$$

in which D is the dilution factor for the test solution. Calculate the specific activity in the portion of the substance to be examined from the expression:

$$\frac{U_A}{P}$$

in which P is the concentration of protein obtained in the test for protein content.

The estimated potency is not less than 90 per cent and not more than 110 per cent of the stated potency.

STORAGE

Store in a colourless, glass container, under vacuum or under an inert gas, protected from light, at a temperature between 2 °C and 30 °C.

LABELLING

The label states:

– the number of International Units per container,
– the amount of protein per container.

01/2005:0006

ALUM

Alumen

$AlK(SO_4)_2,12H_2O$ M_r 474.4

DEFINITION

Alum contains not less than 99.0 per cent and not more than the equivalent of 100.5 per cent of $AlK(SO_4)_2,12H_2O$.

CHARACTERS

A granular powder or colourless, transparent, crystalline masses, freely soluble in water, very soluble in boiling water, soluble in glycerol, practically insoluble in alcohol.

IDENTIFICATION

A. Solution S (see Tests) gives the reactions of sulphates (*2.3.1*).

B. Solution S gives the reaction of aluminium (*2.3.1*).

C. Shake 10 ml of solution S with 0.5 g of *sodium bicarbonate R* and filter. The filtrate gives reaction (a) of potassium (*2.3.1*).

TESTS

Solution S. Dissolve 2.5 g in *water R* and dilute to 50 ml with the same solvent.

Appearance of solution. Solution S is clear (*2.2.1*) and colourless (*2.2.2, Method II*).

pH (*2.2.3*). Dissolve 1.0 g in *carbon dioxide-free water R* and dilute to 10 ml with the same solvent. The pH of the solution is 3.0 to 3.5.

Ammonium (*2.4.1*). To 1 ml of solution S add 4 ml of *water R*. Dilute 0.5 ml of the solution to 14 ml with the same solvent. The solution complies with the limit test for ammonium (0.2 per cent).

Iron (*2.4.9*). 2 ml of solution S diluted to 10 ml with *water R* complies with the limit test for iron (100 ppm). Use in this test 0.3 ml of *thioglycollic acid R*.

Heavy metals (*2.4.8*). 12 ml of solution S complies with limit test A for heavy metals (20 ppm). Prepare the standard using *lead standard solution (1 ppm Pb) R*.

ASSAY

Dissolve 0.900 g in 20 ml of *water R* and carry out the complexometric titration of aluminium (*2.5.11*).

1 ml of *0.1 M sodium edetate* is equivalent to 47.44 mg of $AlK(SO_4)_2,12H_2O$.

01/2005:0971

ALUMINIUM CHLORIDE HEXAHYDRATE

Aluminii chloridum hexahydricum

$AlCl_3,6H_2O$ M_r 241.4

DEFINITION

Aluminium chloride hexahydrate contains not less than 95.0 per cent and not more than the equivalent of 101.0 per cent of $AlCl_3,6H_2O$.

CHARACTERS

A white or slightly yellow, crystalline powder or colourless crystals, deliquescent, very soluble in water, freely soluble in alcohol, soluble in glycerol.

IDENTIFICATION

A. Dilute 0.1 ml of solution S2 (see Tests) to 2 ml with *water R*. The solution gives reaction (a) of chlorides (*2.3.1*).

B. Dilute 0.3 ml of solution S2 to 2 ml with *water R*. The solution gives the reaction of aluminium (*2.3.1*).

TESTS

Solution S1. Dissolve 10.0 g in *distilled water R* and dilute to 100 ml with the same solvent.

Solution S2. Dilute 50 ml of solution S1 to 100 ml with *water R*.

Appearance of solution. Solution S2 is clear (*2.2.1*) and not more intensely coloured than reference solution B_7 (*2.2.2, Method II*).

Sulphates (*2.4.13*). 15 ml of solution S1 complies with the limit test for sulphates (100 ppm).

Iron (*2.4.9*). 10 ml of solution S1 complies with the limit test for iron (10 ppm).

Alkali and alkaline-earth metals. To 20 ml of solution S2 add 100 ml of *water R* and heat to boiling. To the hot solution add 0.2 ml of *methyl red solution R*. Add *dilute ammonia R1* until the colour of the indicator changes to yellow and dilute to 150 ml with *water R*. Heat to boiling and filter. Evaporate 75 ml of the filtrate to dryness on a water-bath and ignite to constant mass. The residue weighs not more than 2.5 mg (0.5 per cent).

Heavy metals (*2.4.8*). 12 ml of solution S1 complies with limit test A for heavy metals (20 ppm). Prepare the standard using *lead standard solution (2 ppm Pb) R*.

Water (*2.5.12*): 42.0 per cent to 48.0 per cent, determined on 50.0 mg by the semi-micro determination of water.

ASSAY

Dissolve 0.500 g in 25.0 ml of *water R*. Carry out the complexometric titration of aluminium (*2.5.11*). Titrate with *0.1 M zinc sulphate* until the colour of the indicator changes from greyish-green to pink. Carry out a blank titration.

1 ml of *0.1 M sodium edetate* is equivalent to 24.14 mg of $AlCl_3,6H_2O$.

STORAGE

Store in an airtight container.

01/2005:1664

ALUMINIUM HYDROXIDE, HYDRATED, FOR ADSORPTION

Aluminii hydroxidum hydricum ad adsorptionem

$[AlO(OH)],nH_2O$

DEFINITION

Content: 90.0 per cent to 110.0 per cent of the content of aluminium stated on the label.

NOTE: shake the gel vigorously for at least 30 s immediately before examining.

CHARACTERS

Appearance: white or almost white, translucent, viscous, colloidal gel. A supernatant may be formed upon standing.

Solubility: a clear or almost clear solution is obtained with alkali hydroxide solutions and mineral acids.

IDENTIFICATION

Solution S (see Tests) gives the reaction of aluminium.

To 10 ml of solution S add about 0.5 ml of *dilute hydrochloric acid R* and about 0.5 ml of *thioacetamide reagent R*. No precipitate is formed. Add dropwise 5 ml of *dilute sodium hydroxide solution R*. Allow to stand for 1 h. A gelatinous white precipitate is formed which dissolves upon addition of 5 ml of *dilute sodium hydroxide solution R*. Gradually add 5 ml of *ammonium chloride solution R* and allow to stand for 30 min. The gelatinous white precipitate is re-formed.

TESTS

Solution S. Add 1 g to 4 ml of *hydrochloric acid R*. Heat at 60 °C for 1 h, cool, dilute to 50 ml with *distilled water R* and filter if necessary.

pH (*2.2.3*): 5.5 to 8.5.

Adsorption power. Dilute the substance to be examined with *distilled water R* to obtain an aluminium concentration of 5 mg/ml. Prepare *bovine albumin R* solutions with the following concentrations of bovine albumin: 0.5 mg/ml, 1 mg/ml, 2 mg/ml, 3 mg/ml, 5 mg/ml and 10 mg/ml. If necessary, adjust the gel and the *bovine albumin R* solutions to pH 6.0 with *dilute hydrochloric acid R* or *dilute sodium hydroxide solution R*.

For adsorption, mix 1 part of the diluted gel with 4 parts of each of the solutions of *bovine albumin R* and allow to stand at room temperature for 1 h. During this time shake the mixture vigorously at least 5 times. Centrifuge or filter through a non-protein-retaining filter. Immediately determine the protein content (*2.5.33, Method 2*) of either the supernatant or the filtrate.

It complies with the test if no bovine albumin is detectable in the supernatant or filtrate of the 2 mg/ml *bovine albumin R* solution (maximum level of adsorption) and in the supernatant or filtrate of *bovine albumin R* solutions of lower concentrations. Those containing 3 mg/ml, 5 mg/ml and 10 mg/ml *bovine albumin R* solutions may show bovine albumin in the supernatant or filtrate, proportional to the amount of bovine albumin in the solutions.

Sedimentation. If necessary, adjust the substance to be examined to pH 6.0 using *dilute hydrochloric acid R* or dilute *sodium hydroxide solution R*. Dilute with *distilled water R* to obtain an aluminium concentration of approximately 5 mg/ml. If the aluminium content of the substance to be examined is lower than 5 mg/ml, adjust to pH 6.0 and dilute with a 9 g/l solution of *sodium chloride R* to obtain an aluminium concentration of about 1 mg/ml. After shaking for at least 30 s, place 25 ml of the preparation in a 25 ml graduated cylinder and allow to stand for 24 h.

It complies with the test if the volume of the clear supernatant is less than 5 ml for the gel with an aluminium content of about 5 mg/ml.

It complies with the test if the volume of the clear supernatant is less than 20 ml for the gel with an aluminium content of about 1 mg/ml.

Chlorides (*2.4.4*): maximum 0.33 per cent.

Dissolve 0.5 g in 10 ml of *dilute nitric acid R* and dilute to 500 ml with *water R*.

Nitrates: maximum 100 ppm.

Place 5 g in a test-tube immersed in ice-water, add 0.4 ml of a 100 g/l solution of *potassium chloride R*, 0.1 ml of *diphenylamine solution R* and, dropwise with shaking, 5 ml of *sulphuric acid R*. Transfer the tube to a water-bath at 50 °C. After 15 min, any blue colour in the solution is not more intense than that in a standard prepared at the same time and in the same manner using 5 ml of *nitrate standard solution (100 ppm NO_3) R*.

Sulphates (*2.4.13*): maximum 0.5 per cent.

Dilute 2 ml of solution S to 20 ml with *water R*.

Ammonium (*2.4.1*): maximum 50 ppm.

1.0 g complies with limit test B. Prepare the standard using 0.5 ml of *ammonium standard solution (100 ppm NH_4) R*.

Arsenic (*2.4.2, Method A*): maximum 1 ppm, determined on 1 g.

Iron (*2.4.9*): maximum 10 ppm, determined on 1 g.

Heavy metals (*2.4.8*): maximum 20 ppm.

Dissolve 2.0 g in 10 ml of *dilute nitric acid R* and dilute to 20 ml with *water R*. The solution complies with limit test A. Prepare the standard using *lead standard solution (2 ppm Pb) R*.

Bacterial endotoxins (*2.6.14*): less than 5 IU of endotoxin per milligram of aluminium, if intended for use in the manufacture of an adsorbed product without a further appropriate procedure for the removal of bacterial endotoxins.

ASSAY

Dissolve 10.00 g in 10 ml of *hydrochloric acid R1*, heating on a water-bath. Cool and dilute to 20 ml with *water R*. To 10 ml of the solution, add *dilute ammonia R1* until a precipitate is obtained. Add the smallest quantity of *dilute hydrochloric acid R* needed to dissolve the precipitate and dilute to 20 ml with *water R*. Carry out the complexometric titration of aluminium (*2.5.11*). Carry out a blank titration.

STORAGE

At a temperature not exceeding 30 °C. Do not allow to freeze. If the substance is sterile, store in a sterile, airtight, tamper-proof container.

LABELLING

The label states:

– where applicable, that the substance is free from bacterial endotoxins,

– the declared content of aluminium.

01/2005:1388

ALUMINIUM MAGNESIUM SILICATE

Aluminii magnesii silicas

DEFINITION

Aluminium magnesium silicate is a mixture of particles with colloidal particle size of montmorillonite and saponite, free from grit and nonswellable ore. It contains not less than 95.0 per cent and not more than 105.0 per cent of the amount of aluminium and magnesium stated on the label.

CHARACTERS

Almost white powder, granules or plates, practically insoluble in water and in organic solvents.

It swells in water to produce a colloidal dispersion.

IDENTIFICATION

A. Fuse 1 g with 2 g of *anhydrous sodium carbonate R*. Warm the residue with *water R* and filter. Acidify the filtrate with *hydrochloric acid R* and evaporate to dryness on a water-bath. 0.25 g of the residue gives the reaction of silicates (*2.3.1*).

B. Dissolve the remainder of the residue obtained in identification test A in a mixture of 5 ml of *dilute hydrochloric acid R* and 10 ml of *water R*. Filter and add *ammonium chloride buffer solution pH 10.0 R*. A white, gelatinous precipitate is formed. Centrifuge, keep the supernatant for identification C. Dissolve the remaining precipitate in *dilute hydrochloric acid R*. The solution gives the reaction of aluminium (*2.3.1*).

C. The supernatant liquid obtained after centrifugation in identification test B gives the reaction of magnesium (*2.3.1*).

TESTS

pH (*2.2.3*). Disperse 5.0 g in 100 ml of *carbon dioxide-free water R*. The pH of the dispersion is 9.0 to 10.0.

Arsenic (*2.4.2*). Transfer 16.6 g to a 250 ml beaker containing 100 ml of *dilute hydrochloric acid R*. Mix, cover with a watch glass and boil gently, with occasional stirring, for 15 min. Allow the insoluble matter to settle and decant the supernatant liquid through a rapid-flow filter paper into a 250 ml volumetric flask, retaining as much sediment as possible in the beaker. To the residue in the beaker add 25 ml of hot *dilute hydrochloric acid R*, stir, heat to boiling, allow the insoluble matter to settle and decant the supernatant liquid through the filter into the volumetric flask. Repeat the extraction with four additional quantities, each of 25 ml, of hot *dilute hydrochloric acid R*, decanting each supernatant liquid through the filter into the volumetric flask. At the last extraction, transfer as much of the insoluble matter as possible onto the filter. Allow to cool the combined filtrates to room temperature and dilute to 250.0 ml with *dilute* *hydrochloric acid R*. Dilute 5.0 ml of the solution to 25.0 ml with *dilute hydrochloric acid R*. The solution complies with limit test A for arsenic (3 ppm).

Lead. Not more than 15 ppm of Pb, determined by atomic absorption spectrometry (*2.2.23, Method I*).

Test solution. Transfer 10.0 g to a 250 ml beaker containing 100 ml of *dilute hydrochloric acid R*. Mix, cover with a watch glass and boil for 15 min. Allow to cool to room temperature and allow the insoluble matter to settle. Decant the supernatant liquid through a rapid-flow filter paper into a 400 ml beaker. To the insoluble matter in the 250 ml beaker add 25 ml of hot *water R*. Stir, allow the insoluble matter to settle and decant the supernatant liquid through the filter into the 400 ml beaker. Repeat the extraction with two additional quantities, each of 25 ml, of *water R*, decanting each supernatant liquid through the filter into the 400 ml beaker. Wash the filter with 25 ml of hot *water R*, collecting this filtrate in the 400 ml beaker. Concentrate the combined filtrates by gently boiling to about 20 ml. If a precipitate appears, add about 0.1 ml of *nitric acid R*, heat to boiling and allow to cool to room temperature. Filter the concentrated extracts through a rapid-flow filter paper into a 50 ml volumetric flask. Transfer the remaining contents of the 400 ml beaker through the filter paper and into the flask with *water R*. Dilute to 50.0 ml with *water R*.

Reference solutions. Prepare the reference solutions using *lead standard solution (10 ppm Pb) R*, diluted if necessary with *water R*.

Measure the absorbance at 217 nm, using a lead hollow-cathode lamp as source of radiation and an oxidising air-acetylene flame.

Loss on drying (*2.2.32*). Not more than 8.0 per cent, determined on 1.000 g by drying in an oven at 100 °C to 105 °C.

Microbial contamination. Total viable aerobic count (*2.6.12*) not more than 10^3 micro-organisms per gram determined by plate count. It complies with the test for *Escherichia coli* (*2.6.13*).

ASSAY

Aluminium. Determine by atomic absorption spectrometry (*2.2.23, Method I*).

Test solution. In a platinum crucible mix 0.200 g with 1.0 g of *lithium metaborate R*. Heat slowly at first and ignite at 1000 °C to 1200 °C for 15 min. Cool, place the crucible in a 100 ml beaker containing 25 ml of *dilute nitric acid R* and add an additional 50 ml of *dilute nitric acid R*, filling and submerging the crucible. Place a polytetrafluoroethylene coated magnetic stirring bar in the crucible and stir gently with a magnetic stirrer until dissolution is complete. Pour the contents into a 250 ml beaker and remove the crucible. Warm the solution and transfer through a rapid-flow filter paper into a 250 ml volumetric flask, wash the filter and beaker with *water R* and dilute to 250.0 ml with *water R* (solution A). To 20.0 ml of this solution add 20 ml of a 10 g/l solution of *sodium chloride R* and dilute to 100.0 ml with *water R*.

Reference solutions. Dissolve 1.000 g of *aluminium R* in a mixture of 10 ml of *hydrochloric acid R* and 10 ml of *water R* by gentle heating. Cool and dilute to 1000.0 ml with *water R* (1 mg of aluminium per millilitre). Into three identical volumetric flasks, each containing 0.20 g of *sodium chloride R*, introduce 2.0 ml, 5.0 ml and 10.0 ml of the solution, respectively and dilute to 100.0 ml with *water R*.

Measure the absorbance at 309 nm using an aluminium hollow-cathode lamp as the source of radiation and an oxidising acetylene-nitrous oxide flame.

Calculate the content of aluminium in the substance to be examined.

Magnesium. Determine by atomic absorption spectrometry (*2.2.23, Method I*).

Test solution. Dilute 25.0 ml of solution A, prepared in the assay for aluminium, to 50.0 ml with *water R*. To 5.0 ml of this solution add 20.0 ml of *lanthanum nitrate solution R* and dilute to 100.0 ml with *water R*.

Reference solutions. Place 1.000 g of *magnesium R* in a 250 ml beaker containing 20 ml of *water R* and carefully add 20 ml of *hydrochloric acid R*, warming if necessary to dissolve. Transfer the solution to a volumetric flask and dilute to 1000.0 ml with *water R* (1 mg of magnesium per millilitre). Dilute 5.0 ml of the solution to 250.0 ml with *water R*. Into four identical volumetric flasks, introduce 5.0 ml, 10.0 ml, 15.0 ml and 20.0 ml of the solution, respectively. To each flask add 20.0 ml of *lanthanum nitrate solution R* and dilute to 100.0 ml with *water R*.

Measure the absorbance at 285 nm using a magnesium hollow-cathode lamp as source of radiation and a reducing air-acetylene flame.

Calculate the content of magnesium in the substance to be examined.

LABELLING

The label states the content of aluminium and magnesium.

01/2005:0311

ALUMINIUM OXIDE, HYDRATED

Aluminii oxidum hydricum

DEFINITION

Hydrated aluminium oxide contains the equivalent of not less than 47.0 per cent and not more than 60.0 per cent of Al_2O_3 (M_r 102.0).

CHARACTERS

A white, amorphous powder, practically insoluble in water. It dissolves in dilute mineral acids and in solutions of alkali hydroxides.

IDENTIFICATION

Solution S (see Tests) gives the reaction of aluminium (*2.3.1*).

TESTS

Solution S. Dissolve 2.5 g in 15 ml of *hydrochloric acid R*, heating on a water-bath. Dilute to 100 ml with *distilled water R*.

Appearance of solution. Solution S is not more opalescent than reference suspension II (*2.2.1*) and not more intensely coloured than reference solution GY_6 (*2.2.2, Method II*).

Alkaline impurities. Shake 1.0 g with 20 ml of *carbon dioxide-free water R* for 1 min and filter. To 10 ml of the filtrate add 0.1 ml of *phenolphthalein solution R*. Any pink colour disappears on the addition of 0.3 ml of *0.1 M hydrochloric acid*.

Neutralising capacity. *Carry out the test at 37 °C*. Disperse 0.5 g in 100 ml of *water R*, heat, add 100.0 ml of *0.1 M hydrochloric acid*, previously heated, and stir continuously; the pH (*2.2.3*) of the solution after 10 min, 15 min and 20 min is not less than 1.8, 2.3 and 3.0 respectively and is at no time greater than 4.5. Add 10.0 ml of *0.5 M hydrochloric acid*, previously heated, stir continuously for 1 h and titrate with *0.1 M sodium hydroxide* to pH 3.5; not more than 35.0 ml of *0.1 M sodium hydroxide* is required.

Chlorides (*2.4.4*). Dissolve 0.1 g with heating in 10 ml of *dilute nitric acid R* and dilute to 100 ml with *water R*. 5 ml of the solution diluted to 15 ml with *water R* complies with the limit test for chlorides (1 per cent).

Sulphates (*2.4.13*). Dilute 4 ml of solution S to 100 ml with *distilled water R*. 15 ml of the solution complies with the limit test for sulphates (1 per cent).

Arsenic (*2.4.2*). 10 ml of solution S complies with limit test A for arsenic (4 ppm).

Heavy metals (*2.4.8*). Neutralise 20 ml of solution S with *concentrated ammonia R*, using *metanil yellow solution R* as an external indicator. Filter, if necessary, and dilute to 30 ml with *water R*. 12 ml of the solution complies with limit test A for heavy metals (60 ppm). Prepare the standard using 10 ml of *lead standard solution (1 ppm Pb) R*.

Microbial contamination. Total viable aerobic count (*2.6.12*) not more than 10^3 micro-organisms per gram, determined by plate count. It complies with the tests for enterobacteria and certain other gram-negative bacteria and with the test for *Escherichia coli* (*2.6.13*).

ASSAY

Dissolve 0.800 g in 10 ml of *hydrochloric acid R1*, heating on a water-bath. Cool and dilute to 50.0 ml with *water R*. To 10.0 ml of the solution, add *dilute ammonia R1* until a precipitate begins to appear. Add the smallest quantity of *dilute hydrochloric acid R* needed to dissolve the precipitate and dilute to 20 ml with *water R*. Carry out the complexometric titration of aluminium (*2.5.11*).

1 ml of *0.1 M sodium edetate* is equivalent to 5.098 mg of Al_2O_3.

STORAGE

Store in an airtight container, at a temperature below 30 °C.

01/2005:1598

ALUMINIUM PHOSPHATE, HYDRATED

Aluminii phosphas hydricus

$AlPO_4$,x H_2O — M_r 122.0 (anhydrous substance)

DEFINITION

Content: 94.0 per cent to 102.0 per cent of $AlPO_4$ (M_r 122.0) (ignited substance).

CHARACTERS

Appearance: white or almost white powder.

Solubility: very slightly soluble in water, practically insoluble in alcohol. It dissolves in dilute solutions of mineral acids and alkali hydroxides.

IDENTIFICATION

A. Solution S (see Tests) gives reaction (b) of phosphates (*2.3.1*).

B. Solution S gives the reaction of aluminium (*2.3.1*).

TESTS

Solution S. Dissolve 2.00 g in *dilute hydrochloric acid R* and dilute to 100 ml with the same acid.

Appearance of solution. Solution S is clear (*2.2.1*) and colourless (*2.2.2, Method II*).

pH (*2.2.3*): 5.5 to 7.2

Shake 4.0 g with *carbon dioxide-free water R* and dilute to 100 ml with the same solvent.

Chlorides (*2.4.4*): maximum 1.3 per cent.

Dissolve 50.0 mg in 10 ml of *dilute nitric acid R* and dilute to 200 ml with *water R*. 15 ml of the solution complies with the limit test for chlorides.

Soluble phosphates: maximum 1.0 per cent, calculated as PO_4^{3-}.

Test solution. Stir 5.0 g with 150 ml of *water R* for 2 h. Filter and wash the filter with 50 ml of *water R*. Combine the filtrate and the washings and dilute to 250.0 ml with *water R*. Dilute 10.0 ml of this solution to 100.0 ml with *water R*.

Reference solution (a). Dissolve 2.86 g of *potassium dihydrogen phosphate R* in *water R* and dilute to 100 ml with the same solvent.

Reference solution (b). Dilute 1 ml of reference solution (a) to 5 ml with *water R*.

Reference solution (c). Dilute 3 ml of reference solution (a) to 5 ml with *water R*.

Treat each solution as follows. To 5.0 ml add 4 ml of *dilute sulphuric acid R*, 1 ml of *ammonium molybdate solution R*, 5 ml of *water R* and 2 ml of a solution containing 0.10 g of *4-methylaminophenol sulphate R*, 0.5 g of *anhydrous sodium sulphite R* and 20.0 g of *sodium metabisulphite R* in 100 ml of *water R*. Shake and allow to stand for 15 min. Dilute to 25.0 ml with *water R* and allow to stand for a further 15 min. Measure the absorbance (*2.2.25*) at 730 nm. Calculate the content of soluble phosphates from a calibration curve prepared using reference solutions (a), (b) and (c) after treatment.

Sulphates (*2.4.13*): maximum 0.6 per cent.

Dilute 8 ml of solution S to 100 ml with *distilled water R*. 15 ml of the solution complies with the limit test for sulphates.

Arsenic (*2.4.2*): maximum 1 ppm.

1.0 g complies with limit test A.

Heavy metals (*2.4.8*): maximum 20 ppm.

Dissolve 1.0 g in *dilute hydrochloric acid R* and dilute to 20 ml with the same acid. 12 ml of the solution complies with limit test A. Prepare the standard using *lead standard solution (1 ppm Pb) R*.

Loss on ignition. 10.0 per cent to 20.0 per cent, determined on 1.000 g at 800 °C.

Neutralising capacity. Add 0.50 g to 30 ml of *0.1 M hydrochloric acid* previously heated to 37 °C and maintain at this temperature for 15 min while stirring. The pH (*2.2.3*) of the mixture after 15 min at 37 °C is 2.0 to 2.5.

ASSAY

Dissolve 0.400 g in 10 ml of *dilute hydrochloric acid R* and dilute to 100.0 ml with *water R*. To 10.0 ml of the solution, add 10.0 ml of *0.1 M sodium edetate* and 30 ml of a mixture of equal volumes of *ammonium acetate solution R* and *dilute acetic acid R*. Boil for 3 min, then cool. Add 25 ml of *alcohol R* and 1 ml of a freshly prepared 0.25 g/l solution of *dithizone R* in *alcohol R*. Titrate the excess of sodium edetate with *0.1 M zinc sulphate* until the colour changes to pink.

1 ml of *0.1 M sodium edetate* is equivalent to 12.20 mg of $AlPO_4$.

STORAGE

In an airtight container.

Monographs

01/2005:0165

ALUMINIUM SULPHATE

Aluminii sulfas

DEFINITION

Aluminium sulphate contains not less than 51.0 per cent and not more than the equivalent of 59.0 per cent of $Al_2(SO_4)_3$ (M_r 342.1). It contains a variable quantity of water of crystallisation.

CHARACTERS

Colourless, lustrous crystals or crystalline masses, soluble in cold water, freely soluble in hot water, practically insoluble in alcohol.

IDENTIFICATION

A. Solution S (see Tests) gives reaction (a) of sulphates (*2.3.1*).

B. Solution S gives the reaction of aluminium (*2.3.1*).

TESTS

Solution S. Dissolve 2.5 g in *water R* and dilute to 50 ml with the same solvent.

Appearance of solution. Solution S is not more opalescent than reference suspension III (*2.2.1*) and is colourless (*2.2.2, Method II*).

pH (*2.2.3*). Dissolve 0.5 g in *carbon dioxide-free water R* and dilute to 25 ml with the same solvent. The pH of the solution is 2.5 to 4.0.

Alkali and alkaline-earth metals. To 20 ml of solution S add 100 ml of *water R*, heat and add 0.1 ml of *methyl red solution R*. Add *dilute ammonia R1* until the colour of the indicator changes to yellow. Dilute to 150 ml with *water R*, heat to boiling and filter. Evaporate 75 ml of the filtrate to dryness on a water-bath and ignite. The residue weighs not more than 2 mg (0.4 per cent).

Ammonium (*2.4.1*). 0.4 ml of solution S diluted to 14 ml with *water R* complies with the limit test for ammonium (500 ppm).

Iron (*2.4.9*). 2 ml of solution S diluted to 10 ml with *water R* complies with the limit test for iron (100 ppm). Use 0.3 ml of *thioglycollic acid R* in this test.

Heavy metals (*2.4.8*). Dilute 8 ml of solution S to 20 ml with *water R*. 12 ml of the solution complies with limit test A for heavy metals (50 ppm). Prepare the standard using *lead standard solution (1 ppm Pb) R*.

ASSAY

Dissolve 0.500 g in 20 ml of *water R*. Carry out the complexometric titration of aluminium (*2.5.11*).

1 ml of *0.1 M sodium edetate* is equivalent to 17.11 mg of $Al_2(SO_4)_3$.

STORAGE

Store in an airtight container.

01/2005:0463
corrected

AMANTADINE HYDROCHLORIDE

Amantadini hydrochloridum

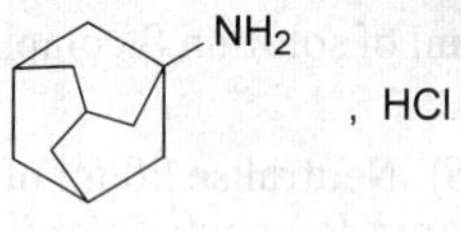

$C_{10}H_{18}ClN$ M_r 187.7

DEFINITION

Amantadine hydrochloride contains not less than 98.5 per cent and not more than the equivalent of 101.0 per cent of tricyclo[3.3.1.1^{3,7}]decan-1-amine hydrochloride, calculated with reference to the anhydrous substance.

CHARACTERS

A white or almost white, crystalline powder, freely soluble in water and in alcohol. It sublimes on being heated.

IDENTIFICATION

First identification: A, D.

Second identification: B, C, D.

A. Examine by infrared absorption spectrophotometry (*2.2.24*), comparing with the spectrum obtained with *amantadine hydrochloride CRS*. Examine the substances prepared as discs.

B. To 0.1 g add 1 ml of *pyridine R*, mix and add 0.1 ml of *acetic anhydride R*. Heat to boiling for about 10 s. Pour the hot solution into 10 ml of *dilute hydrochloric acid R*, cool to 5 °C and filter. The precipitate, washed with *water R* and dried *in vacuo* at 60 °C for 1 h, melts (*2.2.14*) at 147 °C to 151 °C.

C. Dissolve 0.2 g in 1 ml of *0.1 M hydrochloric acid*. Add 1 ml of a 500 g/l solution of *sodium nitrite R*. A white precipitate is formed.

D. 1 ml of solution S (see Tests) gives reaction (a) of chlorides (*2.3.1*).

TESTS

Solution S. Dissolve 2.5 g in *carbon dioxide-free water R* and dilute to 25 ml with the same solvent.

Appearance of solution. Solution S is clear (*2.2.1*) and not more intensely coloured than reference solution Y_7 (*2.2.2, Method II*).

Acidity or alkalinity. Dilute 2 ml of solution S to 10 ml with *carbon dioxide-free water R*. Add 0.1 ml of *methyl red solution R* and 0.2 ml of *0.01 M sodium hydroxide*. The solution is yellow. Add 0.4 ml of *0.01 M hydrochloric acid*. The solution is red.

Related substances. Examine by gas chromatography (*2.2.28*).

Test solution. Dissolve 0.10 g of the substance to be examined in 2 ml of *water R*. Add 2 ml of a 200 g/l solution of *sodium hydroxide R* and 2 ml of *chloroform R*. Shake for 10 min. Separate the chloroform layer, dry over *anhydrous sodium sulphate R* and filter.

The chromatographic procedure may be carried out using:

– a glass column 1.8 m long and 2 mm in internal diameter with a packing prepared as follows: mix 19.5 g of *silanised diatomaceous earth for gas chromatography R* with 60 ml of a 3.3 g/l solution of *potassium hydroxide R* in *methanol R* and evaporate the solvent under reduced pressure while rotating the mixture slowly (support); dissolve 0.4 g of *low-vapour-pressure hydrocarbons (type L) R* in 60 ml of *toluene R* (dissolution requires up to 5 h), add this solution to the support and evaporate the solvent under reduced pressure while rotating the mixture slowly,

- *nitrogen for chromatography R* as the carrier gas at a flow rate of 30 ml/min,
- a flame-ionisation detector.

Programme the temperature of the column linearly at a rate of 6 °C per minute from 100 °C to 200 °C. Maintain the temperature of the injection port at 220 °C and that of the detector at 300 °C. Inject 1 μl or the chosen volume of the test solution. Continue the chromatography for a period at least 2.5 times the retention time of the principal peak. In the chromatogram the sum of the area of any peaks apart from that corresponding to amantadine does not exceed 1 per cent of the total area of the peaks; no peak, apart from that corresponding to amantadine, has an area exceeding 0.3 per cent of the total area. Disregard the peak corresponding to the solvent during the evaluation.

Heavy metals (*2.4.8*). 12 ml of solution S complies with limit test A for heavy metals (20 ppm). Prepare the standard using *lead standard solution (2 ppm Pb) R*.

Water (*2.5.12*). Not more than 0.5 per cent, determined on 2.000 g by the semi-micro determination of water.

Sulphated ash (*2.4.14*). Not more than 0.1 per cent, determined on 1.0 g.

ASSAY

Dissolve 0.150 g in a mixture of 5.0 ml of *0.01 M hydrochloric acid* and 50 ml of *alcohol R*. Carry out a potentiometric titration (*2.2.20*), using *0.1 M sodium hydroxide*. Read the volume added between the two points of inflexion.

1 ml of *0.1 M sodium hydroxide* is equivalent to 18.77 mg of $C_{10}H_{18}ClN$.

01/2005:1489

AMBROXOL HYDROCHLORIDE

Ambroxoli hydrochloridum

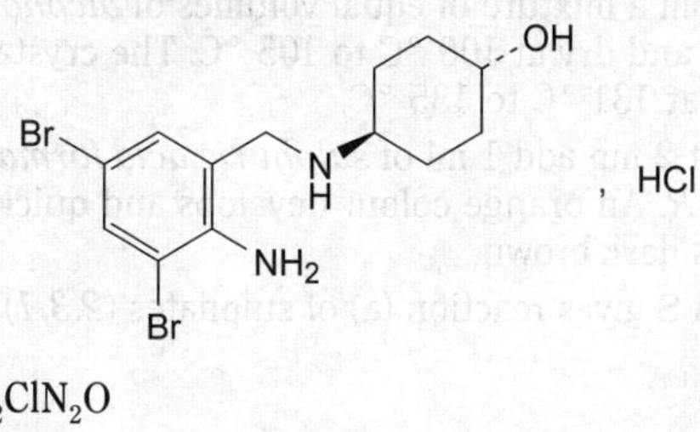

$C_{13}H_{19}Br_2ClN_2O$ M_r 414.6

DEFINITION

trans-4-[(2-Amino-3,5-dibromobenzyl)amino]cyclohexanol hydrochloride.

Content: 99.0 per cent to 101.0 per cent (dried substance).

CHARACTERS

Appearance: white or yellowish crystalline powder.

Solubility: sparingly soluble in water, soluble in methanol, practically insoluble in methylene chloride.

IDENTIFICATION

First identification: B, D.

Second identification: A, C, D.

A. Dissolve 20.0 mg in *0.05 M sulphuric acid* and dilute to 100.0 ml with the same acid. Dilute 2.0 ml of the solution to 10.0 ml with *0.05 M sulphuric acid*. Examined between 200 nm and 350 nm (*2.2.25*), the solution shows two absorption maxima at 245 nm and 310 nm. The ratio of the absorbance measured at 245 nm to that measured at 310 nm is 3.2 to 3.4.

B. Infrared absorption spectrophotometry (*2.2.24*).

Comparison: *ambroxol hydrochloride CRS*.

C. Examine by thin-layer chromatography (*2.2.27*).

Test solution. Dissolve 50 mg of the substance to be examined in *methanol R* and dilute to 5 ml with the same solvent.

Reference solution. Dissolve 50 mg of *ambroxol hydrochloride CRS* in *methanol R* and dilute to 5 ml with the same solvent.

Plate: *TLC silica gel F_{254} plate R.*

Mobile phase: *concentrated ammonia R, 1-propanol R, ethyl acetate R, hexane R* (1:10:20:70 *V/V/V/V*).

Application: 10 μl.

Development: over 2/3 of the plate.

Drying: in air.

Detection: examine in ultraviolet light at 254 nm.

Results: the principal spot in the chromatogram obtained with the test solution is similar in position and size to the principal spot in the chromatogram obtained with the reference solution.

D. Dissolve 25 mg in 2.5 ml of *water R*, mix with 1.0 ml of *dilute ammonia R1* and allow to stand for 5 min. Filter and acidify the filtrate with *dilute nitric acid R*. The filtrate gives reaction (a) of chlorides (*2.3.1*).

TESTS

Solution S. Dissolve 0.75 g in *methanol R* and dilute to 15 ml with the same solvent.

Appearance of solution. Solution S is clear (*2.2.1*) and not more intensely coloured than reference solution Y_6 (*2.2.2, Method II*).

pH (*2.2.3*): 4.5 to 6.0.

Dissolve 0.2 g in *carbon dioxide-free water R* and dilute to 20 ml with the same solvent.

Related substances. Liquid chromatography (*2.2.29*). *Prepare the solutions immediately before use.*

Test solution. Dissolve 50.0 mg of the substance to be examined in *water R* and dilute to 50.0 ml with the same solvent.

Reference solution (a). Dilute 5.0 ml of the test solution to 250.0 ml with *water R*. Dilute 1.0 ml of this solution to 20.0 ml with the mobile phase.

Reference solution (b). Dissolve 5 mg of the substance to be examined in 0.2 ml of *methanol R* and add 0.04 ml of a mixture of 1 volume of *formaldehyde solution R* and 99 volumes of *water R*. Heat at 60 °C for 5 min. Evaporate to dryness under a current of nitrogen. Dissolve the residue in 5 ml of *water R* and dilute to 20 ml with the mobile phase.

Column:

- *size*: *l* = 0.25 m, Ø = 4.0 mm,
- *stationary phase*: *octadecylsilyl silica gel for chromatography R* (5 μm).

Mobile phase: a mixture of equal volumes of *acetonitrile R* and a solution prepared as follows: dissolve 1.32 g of *ammonium phosphate R* in 900 ml of *water R*, adjust to pH 7.0 with *phosphoric acid R* and dilute to 1000 ml with *water R*.

Flow rate: 1 ml/min.

Detection: spectrophotometer at 248 nm.

Injection: 20 µl.

Sensitivity: reference solution (a).

Run time: 3 times the retention time of the principal peak in the chromatogram obtained with the test solution.

System suitability:

- *resolution*: minimum of 4.0 between the peaks due to impurity B and ambroxol in the chromatogram obtained with reference solution (b).

Limits:

- *any impurity*: not more than the area of the principal peak in the chromatogram obtained with reference solution (a) (0.1 per cent),
- *total*: not more than 3 times the area of the principal peak in the chromatogram obtained with reference solution (a) (0.3 per cent),
- *disregard limit*: 0.1 times the area of the principal peak in the chromatogram obtained with reference solution (a).

Heavy metals (*2.4.8*): maximum 20 ppm.

1.0 g complies with limit test C. Prepare the standard using 2 ml of *lead standard solution (10 ppm Pb) R*.

Loss on drying (*2.2.32*): maximum 0.5 per cent, determined on 1.000 g by drying in an oven at 100-105 °C.

Sulphated ash (*2.4.14*): maximum 0.1 per cent, determined on 1.0 g.

ASSAY

Dissolve 0.300 g in 70 ml of *alcohol R* and add 5 ml of *0.01 M hydrochloric acid*. Carry out a potentiometric titration (*2.2.20*), using *0.1 M sodium hydroxide*. Read the volume added between the two points of inflexion.

1 ml of *0.1 M sodium hydroxide* is equivalent to 41.46 mg of $C_{13}H_{19}Br_2ClN_2O$.

STORAGE

Store protected from light.

IMPURITIES

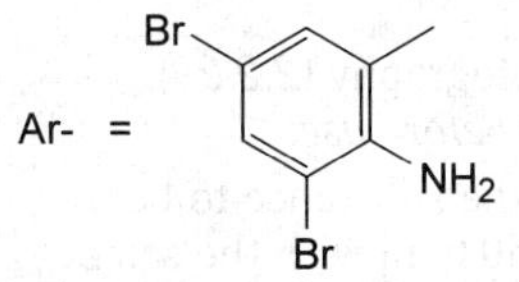

A. Ar-CH$_2$OH: (2-amino-3,5-dibromophenyl)methanol,

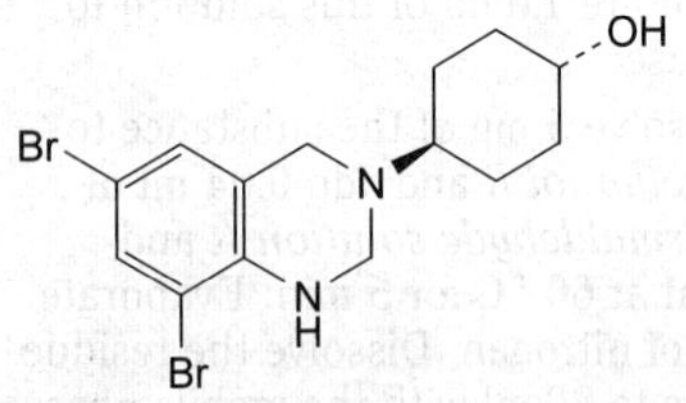

B. *trans*-4-(6,8-dibromo-1,4-dihydroquinazolin-3(2*H*)-yl)cyclohexanol,

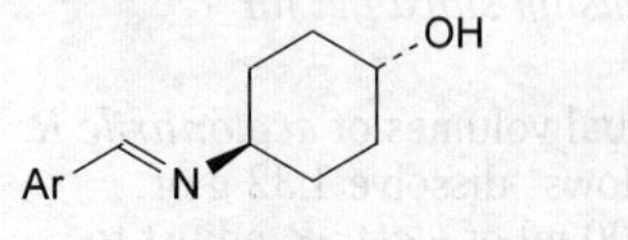

C. *trans*-4-[[(*E*)-2-amino-3,5-dibromobenzyliden]amino]cyclohexanol,

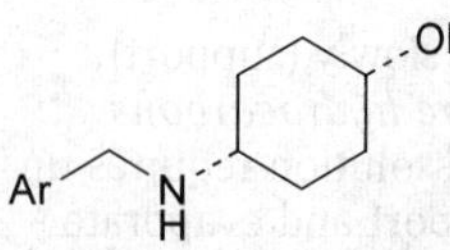

D. *cis*-4-[(2-amino-3,5-dibromobenzyl)amino]cyclohexanol,

E. Ar-CH=O: 2-amino-3,5-dibromobenzaldehyde.

01/2005:0368

AMFETAMINE SULPHATE

Amfetamini sulfas

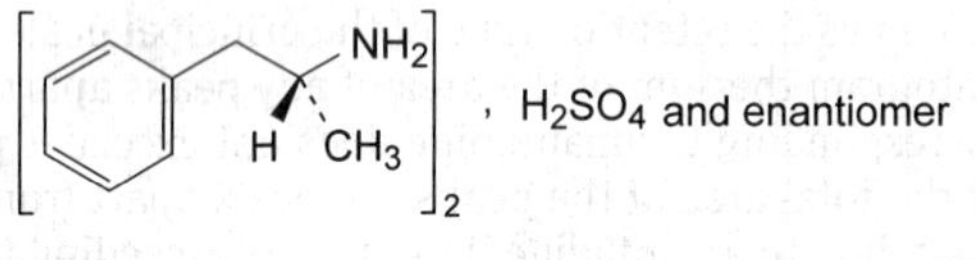

$C_{18}H_{28}N_2O_4S$ M_r 368.5

DEFINITION

Amfetamine sulphate contains not less than 99.0 per cent and not more than the equivalent of 100.5 per cent of bis[(2*RS*)-1-phenylpropan-2-amine] sulphate, calculated with reference to the dried substance.

CHARACTERS

A white powder, freely soluble in water, slightly soluble in alcohol.

IDENTIFICATION

First identification: A, B, E.

Second identification: A, C, D, E.

A. The angle of optical rotation (*2.2.7*) of solution S (see Tests), measured in a 2 dm tube, is − 0.04 to + 0.04.

B. Examine by infrared absorption spectrophotometry (*2.2.24*), comparing with the *Ph. Eur. reference spectrum of amfetamine sulphate.* Examine as a mull in *liquid paraffin R.*

C. To 50 ml of solution S add 5 ml of *strong sodium hydroxide solution R* and 0.5 ml of *benzoyl chloride R* and shake. Continue to add *benzoyl chloride R* in portions of 0.5 ml until no further precipitate is formed. Filter, wash the precipitate with *water R* and recrystallise twice from a mixture of equal volumes of *alcohol R* and *water R* and dry at 100 °C to 105 °C. The crystals melt (*2.2.14*) at 131 °C to 135 °C.

D. To about 2 mg add 1 ml of *sulphuric acid-formaldehyde reagent R.* An orange colour develops and quickly becomes dark-brown.

E. Solution S gives reaction (a) of sulphates (*2.3.1*).

TESTS

Solution S. Dissolve 2.0 g in *carbon dioxide-free water R* and dilute to 100 ml with the same solvent.

Appearance of solution. Solution S is clear (*2.2.1*) and colourless (*2.2.2, Method II*).

Acidity or alkalinity. To 25 ml of solution S add 0.1 ml of *methyl red solution R.* Not more than 0.1 ml of *0.01 M hydrochloric acid* or *0.01 M sodium hydroxide* is required to change the colour of the indicator.

Loss on drying (*2.2.32*). Not more than 1.0 per cent, determined on 1.00 g by drying in an oven at 100 °C to 105 °C.

Sulphated ash (*2.4.14*). Not more than 0.1 per cent, determined on 1.0 g.

ASSAY

Dissolve 0.300 g in 30 ml of *anhydrous acetic acid R*. Titrate with *0.1 M perchloric acid*, determining the end-point potentiometrically (*2.2.20*).

1 ml of *0.1 M perchloric acid* is equivalent to 36.85 mg of $C_{18}H_{28}N_2O_4S$.

STORAGE

Store protected from light.

01/2005:0873

AMIDOTRIZOIC ACID DIHYDRATE

Acidum amidotrizoicum dihydricum

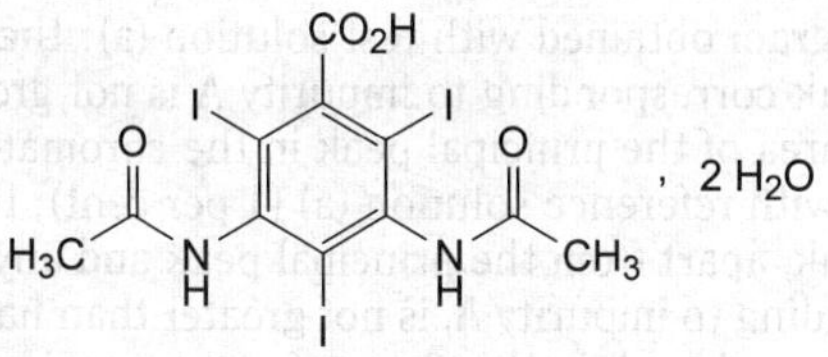

$C_{11}H_9I_3N_2O_4,2H_2O$ M_r 650

DEFINITION

Amidotrizoic acid dihydrate contains not less than 98.5 per cent and not more than the equivalent of 101.0 per cent of 3,5-bis(acetylamino)-2,4,6-triiodobenzoic acid, calculated with reference to the dried substance.

CHARACTERS

A white or almost white, crystalline powder, very slightly soluble in water and in alcohol. It dissolves in dilute solutions of alkali hydroxides.

IDENTIFICATION

First identification: A.

Second identification: B, C.

A. Examine by infrared absorption spectrophotometry (*2.2.24*), comparing with the spectrum obtained with *amidotrizoic acid dihydrate CRS*.

B. Examine the chromatograms obtained in the test for related substances (see Tests). The principal spot in the chromatogram obtained with test solution (b) is similar in position and size to the principal spot in the chromatogram obtained with reference solution (b).

C. Heat 50 mg gently in a small porcelain dish over a naked flame. Violet vapour is evolved.

TESTS

Appearance of solution. Dissolve 1.0 g in *dilute sodium hydroxide solution R* and dilute to 20 ml with the same solvent. The solution is clear (*2.2.1*) and colourless (*2.2.2, Method II*).

Related substances. Examine by thin-layer chromatography (*2.2.27*), using *silica gel GF_{254} R* as the coating substance.

Test solution (a). Dissolve 0.50 g of the substance to be examined in a 3 per cent *V/V* solution of *ammonia R* in *methanol R* and dilute to 10 ml with the same solvent.

Test solution (b). Dilute 1 ml of test solution (a) to 10 ml with a 3 per cent *V/V* solution of *ammonia R* in *methanol R*.

Reference solution (a). Dilute 1 ml of test solution (b) to 50 ml with a 3 per cent *V/V* solution of *ammonia R* in *methanol R*.

Reference solution (b). Dissolve 50 mg of *amidotrizoic acid dihydrate CRS* in a 3 per cent *V/V* solution of *ammonia R* in *methanol R* and dilute to 10 ml with the same solvent.

Apply separately to the plate 2 µl of each solution. Develop over a path of 15 cm using a mixture of 20 volumes of *anhydrous formic acid R*, 25 volumes of *methyl ethyl ketone R* and 60 volumes of *toluene R*. Allow the plate to dry until the solvents have evaporated and examine in ultraviolet light at 254 nm. Any spot in the chromatogram obtained with test solution (a), apart from the principal spot, is not more intense than the spot in the chromatogram obtained with reference solution (a) (0.2 per cent).

Halides. Dissolve 0.55 g in a mixture of 4 ml of *dilute sodium hydroxide solution R* and 15 ml of *water R*. Add 6 ml of *dilute nitric acid R* and filter. 15 ml of the filtrate complies with the limit test for chlorides (*2.4.4*) (150 ppm expressed as chloride).

Free aromatic amines. *Maintain the solutions and reagents in iced water protected from bright light.* To 0.50 g in a 50 ml volumetric flask add 15 ml of *water R*. Shake and add 1 ml of *dilute sodium hydroxide solution R*. Cool in iced water, add 5 ml of a freshly prepared 5 g/l solution of *sodium nitrite R* and 12 ml of *dilute hydrochloric acid R*. Shake gently and allow to stand for exactly 2 min after adding the hydrochloric acid. Add 10 ml of a 20 g/l solution of *ammonium sulphamate R*. Allow to stand for 5 min, shaking frequently, and add 0.15 ml of a 100 g/l solution of *α-naphthol R* in *alcohol R*. Shake and allow to stand for 5 min. Add 3.5 ml of *buffer solution pH 10.9 R*, mix and dilute to 50.0 ml with *water R*. The absorbance (*2.2.25*), measured within 20 min at 485 nm using as the compensation liquid a solution prepared at the same time and in the same manner but omitting the substance to be examined, is not greater than 0.30.

Heavy metals (*2.4.8*). Dissolve 2.0 g in 4 ml of *dilute sodium hydroxide solution R* and dilute to 20 ml with *water R*. 12 ml of this solution complies with limit test A for heavy metals (20 ppm). Prepare the standard using *lead standard solution (2 ppm Pb) R*.

Loss on drying (*2.2.32*): 4.5 per cent to 7.0 per cent, determined on 0.500 g by drying in an oven at 100 °C to 105 °C.

Sulphated ash (*2.4.14*). Not more than 0.1 per cent, determined on 1.0 g.

ASSAY

To 0.150 g in a 250 ml round-bottomed flask add 5 ml of *strong sodium hydroxide solution R*, 20 ml of *water R*, 1 g of *zinc powder R* and a few glass beads. Boil under a reflux condenser for 30 min. Allow to cool and rinse the condenser with 20 ml of *water R*, adding the rinsings to the flask. Filter through a sintered-glass filter and wash the filter with several quantities of *water R*. Collect the filtrate and washings. Add 40 ml of *dilute sulphuric acid R* and titrate immediately with *0.1 M silver nitrate*. Determine the end-point potentiometrically (*2.2.20*), using a suitable electrode system such as silver-mercurous sulphate.

1 ml of *0.1 M silver nitrate* is equivalent to 20.47 mg of $C_{11}H_9I_3N_2O_4$.

STORAGE

Store protected from light.

IMPURITIES

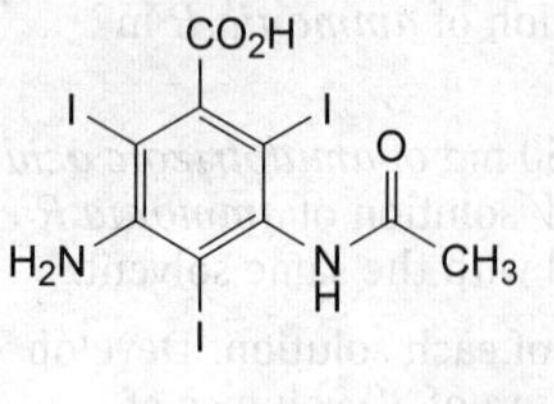

A. 3-(acetylamino)-5-amino-2,4,6-triiodobenzoic acid.

01/2005:1289

AMIKACIN

Amikacinum

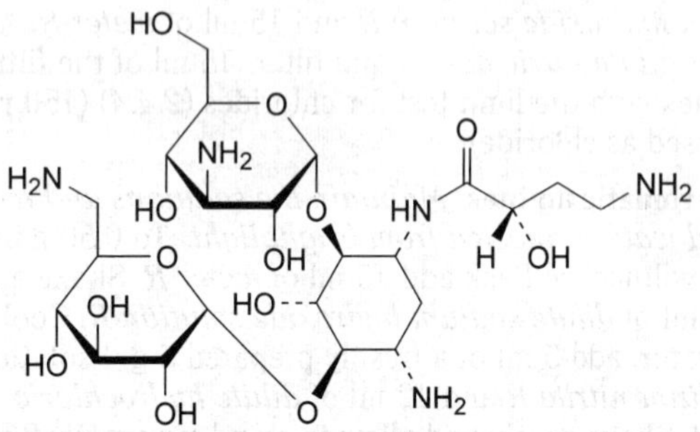

$C_{22}H_{43}N_5O_{13}$ *M*r 585.6

DEFINITION

Amikacin is 6-*O*-(3-amino-3-deoxy-α-D-glucopyranosyl)-4-*O*-(6-amino-6-deoxy-α-D-glucopyranosyl)-1-*N*-[(2*S*)-4-amino-2-hydroxybutanoyl]-2-deoxy-D-streptamine, an antimicrobial substance obtained from kanamycin A. It contains not less than 96.5 per cent and not more than the equivalent of 102.5 per cent of $C_{22}H_{43}N_5O_{13}$, calculated with reference to the anhydrous substance.

CHARACTERS

A white or almost white powder, sparingly soluble in water, slightly soluble in methanol, practically insoluble in acetone and in alcohol.

IDENTIFICATION

A. Examine by infrared absorption spectrophotometry (*2.2.24*), comparing with the spectrum of *amikacin CRS*.

B. Examine by thin-layer chromatography (*2.2.27*) using a *TLC silica gel plate R*.

Test solution. Dissolve 25 mg of the substance to be examined in *water R* and dilute to 10 ml with the same solvent.

Reference solution (a). Dissolve 25 mg of *amikacin CRS* in *water R* and dilute to 10 ml with the same solvent.

Reference solution (b). Dissolve 5 mg of *kanamycin monosulphate CRS* in 1 ml of the test solution and dilute to 10 ml with *water R*.

Apply to the plate 5 µl of each solution. Develop over a path of 15 cm using the lower layer of a mixture of equal volumes of *concentrated ammonia R*, *methanol R* and *methylene chloride R*. Allow the plate to dry in air and spray with *ninhydrin solution R1*. Heat at 110 °C for 5 min. The principal spot in the chromatogram obtained with the test solution is similar in position, colour and size to the principal spot in the chromatogram obtained with the reference solution (a). The identification test is not valid unless the chromatogram obtained with reference solution (b) shows two clearly separated spots.

TESTS

pH (*2.2.3*). Dissolve 0.1 g in *carbon dioxide-free water R* and dilute to 10 ml with the same solvent. The pH of the solution is 9.5 to 11.5.

Specific optical rotation (*2.2.7*). Dissolve 0.50 g in *water R* and dilute to 25.0 ml with the same solvent. The specific optical rotation is + 97 to + 105, calculated with reference to the anhydrous substance.

Related substances. Examine by liquid chromatography (*2.2.29*), as prescribed under Assay.

Inject 20 µl of reference solution (a). Adjust the sensitivity of the system so that the height of the principal peak in the chromatogram obtained is at least 50 per cent of the full scale of the recorder. Inject 20 µl of reference solution (c). The test is not valid unless, in the chromatogram obtained, the resolution between the peaks corresponding to amikacin and impurity A is at least 3.5 (see Figure 1289.-1). Inject 20 µl of test solution (a). Continue the chromatography for four times the retention time of amikacin. In the chromatogram obtained with test solution (a): the area of any peak corresponding to impurity A is not greater than the area of the principal peak in the chromatogram obtained with reference solution (a) (1 per cent); the area of any peak, apart from the principal peak and any peak corresponding to impurity A, is not greater than half the area of the principal peak in the chromatogram obtained with reference solution (a) (0.5 per cent); the sum of the areas of any such peaks is not greater than 1.5 times the area of the principal peak in the chromatogram obtained with reference solution (a) (1.5 per cent). Disregard any peak due to the blank and any peak with an area less than 0.1 times that of the principal peak in the chromatogram obtained with reference solution (a).

Water (*2.5.12*). Not more than 8.5 per cent, determined on 0.200 g by the semi-micro determination of water.

Sulphated ash (*2.4.14*). Not more than 0.5 per cent, determined on 1.0 g.

ASSAY

Examine by liquid chromatography (*2.2.29*).

Test solution (a). Dissolve 0.100 g of the substance to be examined in *water R* and dilute to 10.0 ml with the same solvent. In a round-glass-stoppered vial, add 0.2 ml of this solution to 2.0 ml of a 10 g/l solution of *2,4,6-trinitrobenzene sulphonic acid R*. Then add 3.0 ml of *pyridine R* and close the vial tightly. Shake vigorously for 30 s and heat in a water-bath at 75 °C for 45 min. Cool in cold water for 2 min and add 2 ml of *glacial acetic acid R*. Shake vigorously for 30 s.

Test solution (b). Dissolve 50.0 mg of the substance to be examined in *water R* and dilute to 50.0 ml with the same solvent. Then prepare as prescribed for test solution (a).

Reference solution (a). Dissolve 10.0 mg of *amikacin impurity A CRS* in *water R* and dilute to 100.0 ml with the same solvent. Then prepare as prescribed for test solution (a).

Reference solution (b). Dissolve 50.0 mg of *amikacin CRS* in *water R* and dilute to 50.0 ml with the same solvent. Then prepare as prescribed for test solution (a).

Reference solution (c). Dissolve 5 mg of *amikacin CRS* and 5 mg of *amikacin impurity A CRS* in *water R* and dilute to 50 ml with the same solvent. Then prepare as prescribed for test solution (a).

Blank solution. Prepare as described for test solution (a) using 0.2 ml of *water R*.

The chromatographic procedure may be carried out using:

- a stainless steel column 0.25 m long and 4.6 mm in internal diameter packed with *octadecylsilyl silica gel for chromatography R* (5 µm),
- as mobile phase at a flow rate of 1 ml/min a mixture of 30 volumes of a 2.7 g/l solution of *potassium dihydrogen phosphate R* adjusted to pH 6.5 with a 22 g/l solution of *potassium hydroxide R* and 70 volumes of *methanol R*,
- as detector a spectrophotometer set at 340 nm,

maintaining the temperature of the column at 30 °C and that of the solutions to be examined at 10 °C.

Inject 20 µl of reference solution (b). Adjust the sensitivity of the system so that the height of the principal peak is at least 50 per cent of the full scale of the recorder. Inject reference solution (b) six times. The assay is not valid unless the relative standard deviation of the peak area for amikacin is 2.0 per cent. Inject test solution (b) and reference solution (b).

IMPURITIES

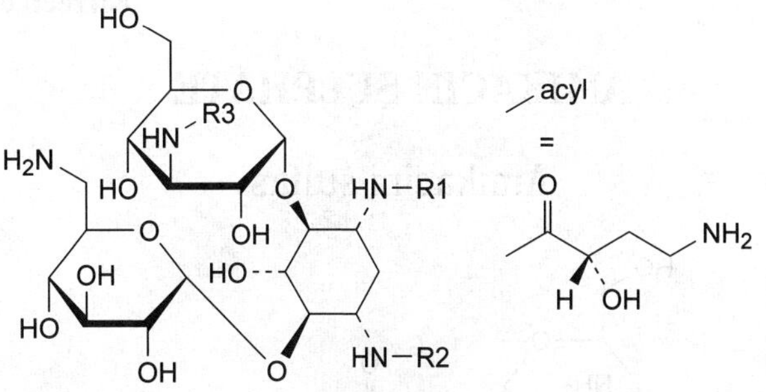

A. R1 = R3 = H, R2 = acyl: 4-*O*-(3-amino-3-deoxy-α-D-glucopyranosyl)-6-*O*-(6-amino-6-deoxy-α-D-glucopyranosyl)-1-*N*-[(2*S*)-4-amino-2-hydroxybutanoyl]-2-deoxy-L-streptamine,

B. R1 = R2 = acyl, R3 = H: 4-*O*-(3-amino-3-deoxy-α-D-glucopyranosyl)-6-*O*-(6-amino-6-deoxy-α-D-glucopyranosyl)-1,3-*N*-bis[(2*S*)-4-amino-2-hydroxybutanoyl]-2-deoxy-L-streptamine,

C. R1 = R2 = H, R3 = acyl: 4-*O*-(6-amino-6-deoxy-α-D-glucopyranosyl)-6-*O*-[3-[[(2*S*)-4-amino-2-hydroxybutanoyl]amino]-3-deoxy-α-D-glucopyranosyl]-2-deoxy-D-streptamine,

D. R1 = R2 = R3 = H: kanamycin.

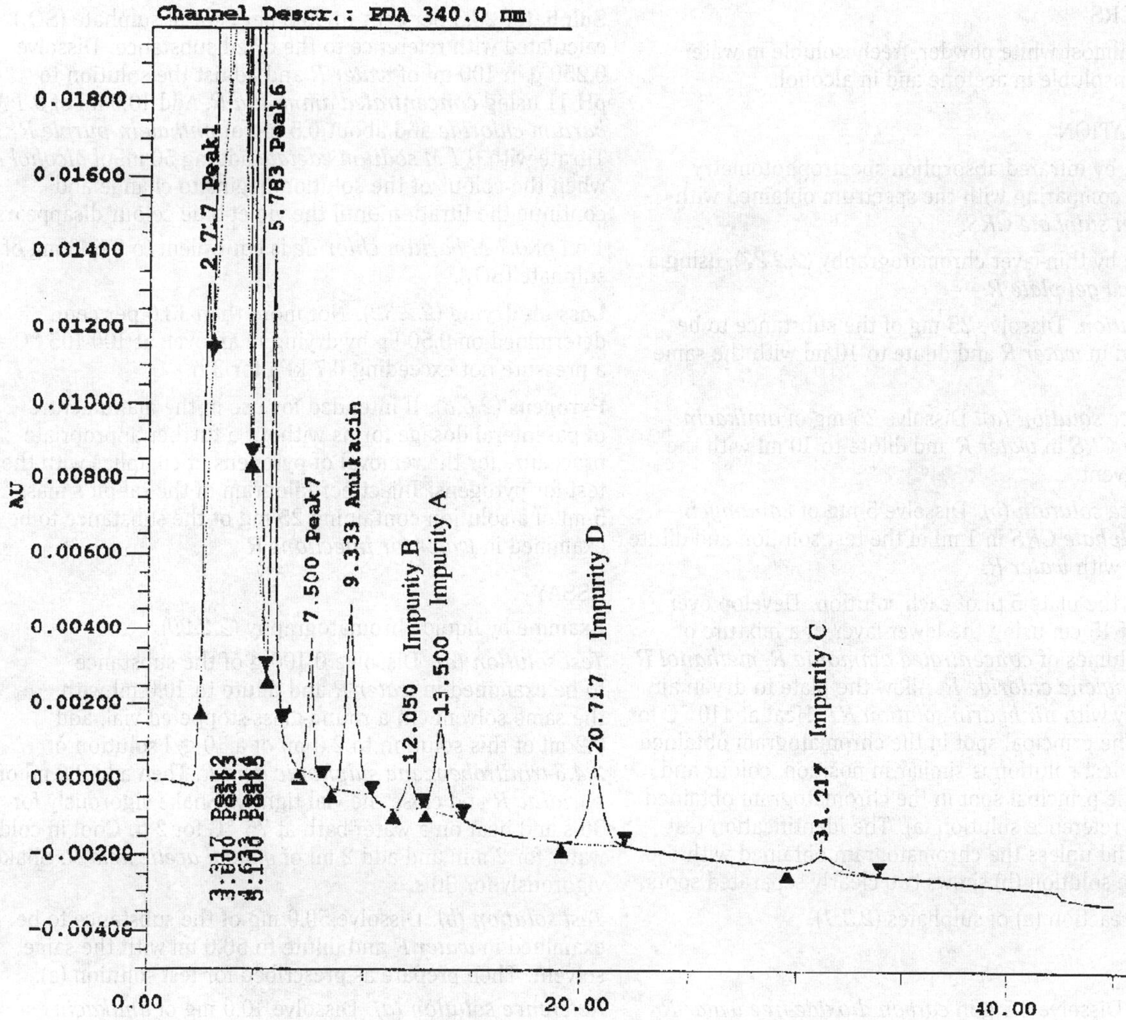

Figure 1289.-1. – *Chromatogram for the test for related substances of amikacin*

01/2005:1290
corrected

AMIKACIN SULPHATE

Amikacini sulfas

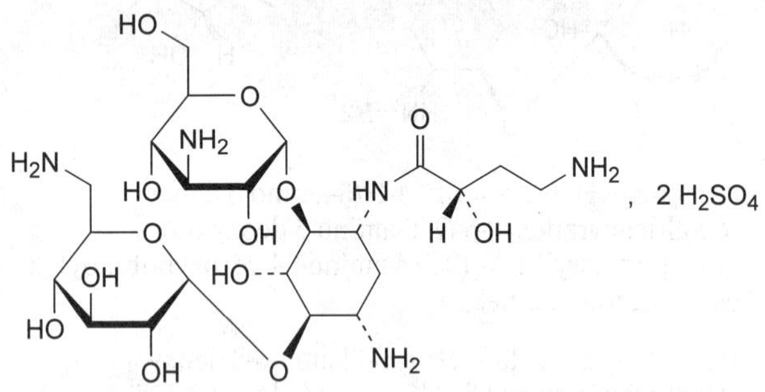

$C_{22}H_{47}N_5O_{21}S_2$ M_r 782

DEFINITION

Amikacin sulphate is 6-*O*-(3-amino-3-deoxy-α-D-glucopyranosyl)-4-*O*-(6-amino-6-deoxy-α-D-glucopyranosyl)-1-*N*-[(2*S*)-4-amino-2-hydroxybutanoyl]-2-deoxy-D-streptamine sulphate, an antimicrobial substance obtained from kanamycin A. It contains not less than 72.3 per cent and not more than the equivalent of 76.8 per cent of $C_{22}H_{43}N_5O_{13}$, calculated with reference to the dried substance.

CHARACTERS

A white or almost white powder, freely soluble in water, practically insoluble in acetone and in alcohol.

IDENTIFICATION

A. Examine by infrared absorption spectrophotometry (*2.2.24*), comparing with the spectrum obtained with *amikacin sulphate CRS*.

B. Examine by thin-layer chromatography (*2.2.27*), using a *TLC silica gel plate R*.

Test solution. Dissolve 25 mg of the substance to be examined in *water R* and dilute to 10 ml with the same solvent.

Reference solution (a). Dissolve 25 mg of *amikacin sulphate CRS* in *water R* and dilute to 10 ml with the same solvent.

Reference solution (b). Dissolve 5 mg of *kanamycin monosulphate CRS* in 1 ml of the test solution and dilute to 10 ml with *water R*.

Apply to the plate 5 µl of each solution. Develop over a path of 15 cm using the lower layer of a mixture of equal volumes of *concentrated ammonia R*, *methanol R* and *methylene chloride R*. Allow the plate to dry in air and spray with *ninhydrin solution R1*. Heat at 110 °C for 5 min. The principal spot in the chromatogram obtained with the test solution is similar in position, colour and size to the principal spot in the chromatogram obtained with the reference solution (a). The identification test is not valid unless the chromatogram obtained with reference solution (b) shows two clearly separated spots.

C. It gives reaction (a) of sulphates (*2.3.1*).

TESTS

pH (*2.2.3*). Dissolve 0.1 g in *carbon dioxide-free water R* and dilute to 10 ml with the same solvent. The pH of the solution is 2.0 to 4.0.

Specific optical rotation (*2.2.7*). Dissolve 0.50 g in *water R* and dilute to 25.0 ml with the same solvent. The specific optical rotation is + 76 to + 84, calculated with reference to the dried substance.

Related substances. Examine by liquid chromatography (*2.2.29*), as prescribed under Assay.

Inject 20 µl of reference solution (a). Adjust the sensitivity of the system so that the height of the principal peak in the chromatogram obtained is at least 50 per cent of the full scale of the recorder. Inject 20 µl of reference solution (c). The test is not valid unless in the chromatogram obtained, the resolution between the peaks corresponding to amikacin and impurity A is at least 3.5 (see Figure 1290.-1). Inject 20 µl of test solution (a). Continue the chromatography for four times the retention time of amikacin. In the chromatogram obtained with test solution (a): the area of any peak corresponding to impurity A is not greater than the area of the principal peak in the chromatogram obtained with reference solution (a) (1 per cent); the area of any peak, apart from the principal peak and any peak corresponding to impurity A, is not greater than half the area of the principal peak in the chromatogram obtained with reference solution (a) (0.5 per cent); the sum of the areas of any such peaks is not greater than 1.5 times the area of the principal peak in the chromatogram obtained with reference solution (a) (1.5 per cent). Disregard any peak due to the blank, any peak eluting before the principal peak and any peak with an area less than 0.1 times that of the principal peak in the chromatogram obtained with reference solution (a).

Sulphate: 23.3 per cent to 25.8 per cent of sulphate (SO_4), calculated with reference to the dried substance. Dissolve 0.250 g in 100 ml of *water R* and adjust the solution to pH 11 using *concentrated ammonia R*. Add 10.0 ml of *0.1 M barium chloride* and about 0.5 mg of *phthalein purple R*. Titrate with *0.1 M sodium edetate* adding 50 ml of *alcohol R* when the colour of the solution begins to change and continue the titration until the violet-blue colour disappears.

1 ml of *0.1 M barium chloride* is equivalent to 9.606 mg of sulphate (SO_4).

Loss on drying (*2.2.32*). Not more than 13.0 per cent, determined on 0.500 g by drying in an oven at 100-105 °C at a pressure not exceeding 0.7 kPa for 3 h.

Pyrogens (*2.6.8*). If intended for use in the manufacture of parenteral dosage forms without a further appropriate procedure for the removal of pyrogens, it complies with the test for pyrogens. Inject per kilogram of the rabbit's mass 5 ml of a solution containing 25 mg of the substance to be examined in *water for injections R*.

ASSAY

Examine by liquid chromatography (*2.2.29*).

Test solution (a). Dissolve 0.100 g of the substance to be examined in *water R* and dilute to 10.0 ml with the same solvent. In a round-glass-stoppered vial, add 0.2 ml of this solution to 2.0 ml of a 10 g/l solution of *2,4,6-trinitrobenzene sulphonic acid R*. Then add 3.0 ml of *pyridine R* and close the vial tightly. Shake vigorously for 30 s and heat on a water-bath at 75 °C for 2 h. Cool in cold water for 2 min and add 2 ml of *glacial acetic acid R*. Shake vigorously for 30 s.

Test solution (b). Dissolve 50.0 mg of the substance to be examined in *water R* and dilute to 50.0 ml with the same solvent. Then prepare as prescribed for test solution (a).

Reference solution (a). Dissolve 10.0 mg of *amikacin impurity A CRS* in *water R* and dilute to 100.0 ml with the same solvent. Then prepare as prescribed for test solution (a).

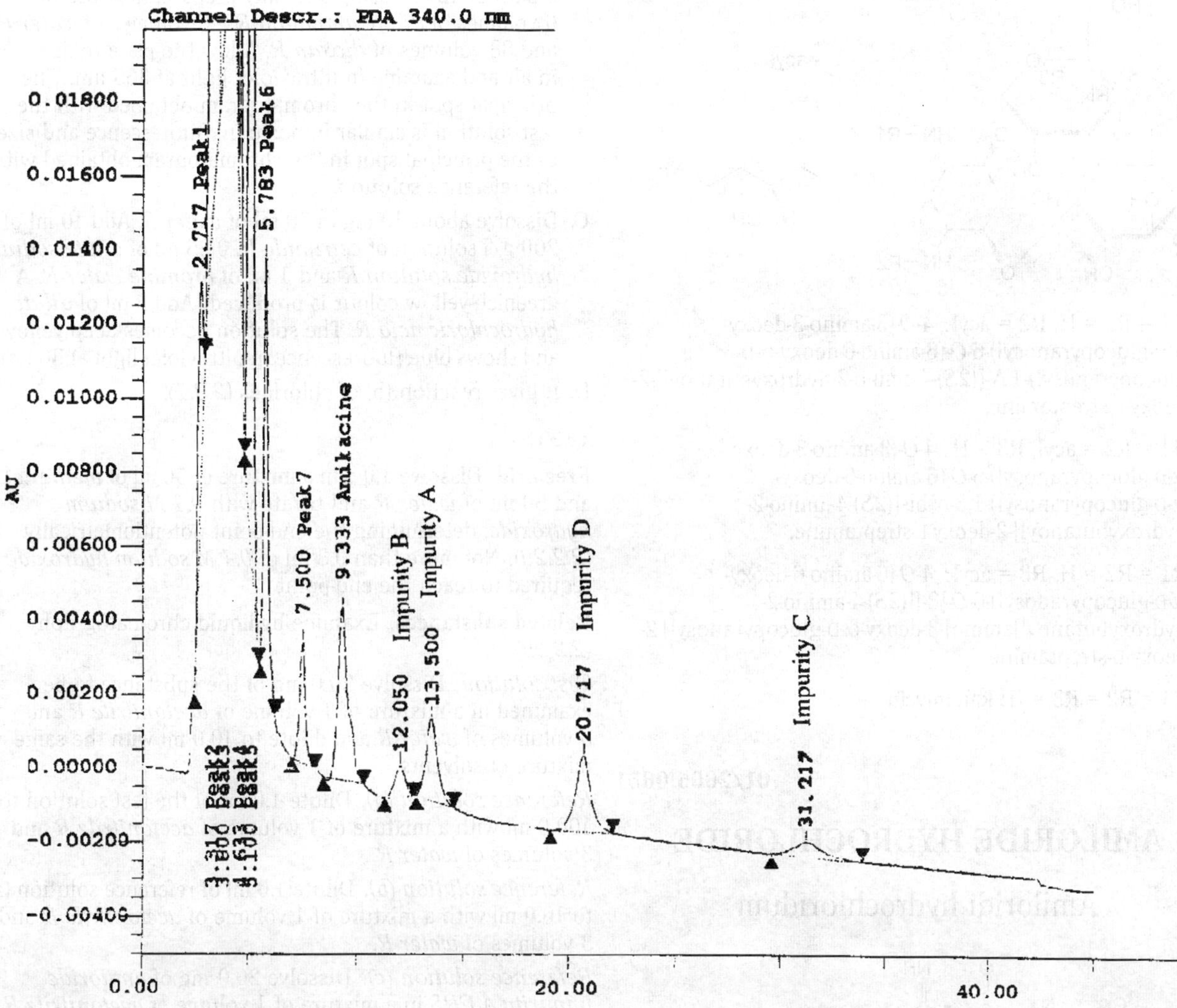

Figure 1290.-1. – *Chromatogram for the test for related substances of amikacin sulphate*

Reference solution (b). Dissolve 50.0 mg of *amikacin sulphate CRS* in *water R* and dilute to 50.0 ml with the same solvent. Then prepare as prescribed for test solution (a).

Reference solution (c). Dissolve 5 mg of *amikacin sulphate CRS* and 5 mg of *amikacin impurity A CRS* in *water R* and dilute to 50 ml with the same solvent. Then prepare as prescribed for test solution (a).

Blank solution. Prepare as described for test solution (a) using 0.2 ml of *water R*.

The chromatographic procedure may be carried out using:

– a stainless steel column 0.25 m long and 4.6 mm in internal diameter packed with *octadecylsilyl silica gel for chromatography R* (5 μm),

– as mobile phase at a flow rate of 1 ml/min a mixture of 30 volumes of a 2.7 g/l solution of *potassium dihydrogen phosphate R* adjusted to pH 6.5 with a 22 g/l solution of *potassium hydroxide R* and 70 volumes of *methanol R*,

– as detector a spectrophotometer set at 340 nm,

maintaining the temperature of the column at 30 °C and that of the solutions to be examined at 10 °C.

Inject 20 μl of reference solution (b). Adjust the sensitivity of the system so that the height of the principal peak is at least 50 per cent of the full scale of the recorder. Inject reference solution (b) six times. The assay is not valid unless the relative standard deviation of the peak area for amikacin is 2.0 per cent. Inject test solution (b) and reference solution (b).

STORAGE

If the substance is sterile, store in a sterile, airtight, tamper-proof container.

LABELLING

The label states, where applicable, that the substance is apyrogenic.

IMPURITIES

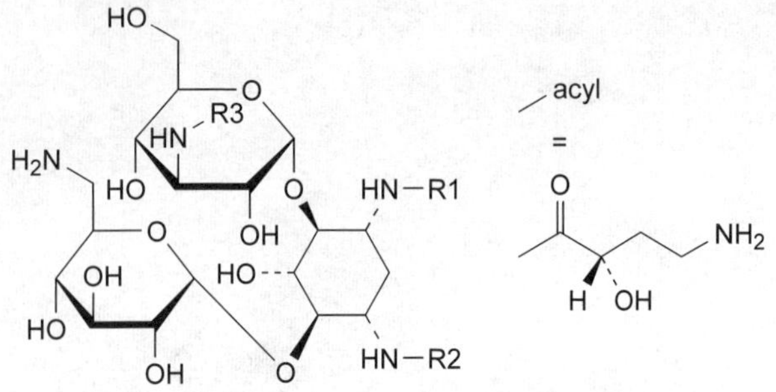

A. R1 = R3 = H, R2 = acyl: 4-*O*-(3-amino-3-deoxy-α-D-glucopyranosyl)-6-*O*-(6-amino-6-deoxy-α-D-glucopyranosyl)-1-*N*-[(2*S*)-4-amino-2-hydroxybutanoyl]-2-deoxy-L-streptamine,

B. R1 = R2 = acyl, R3 = H: 4-*O*-(3-amino-3-deoxy-α-D-glucopyranosyl)-6-*O*-(6-amino-6-deoxy-α-D-glucopyranosyl)-1,3-*N*-bis[(2*S*)-4-amino-2-hydroxybutanoyl]-2-deoxy-L-streptamine,

C. R1 = R2 = H, R3 = acyl: 4-*O*-(6-amino-6-deoxy-α-D-glucopyranosyl)-6-*O*-[3-[[(2*S*)-4-amino-2-hydroxybutanoyl]amino]-3-deoxy-α-D-glucopyranosyl]-2-deoxy-D-streptamine,

D. R1 = R2 = R3 = H: kanamycin.

01/2005:0651

AMILORIDE HYDROCHLORIDE

Amiloridi hydrochloridum

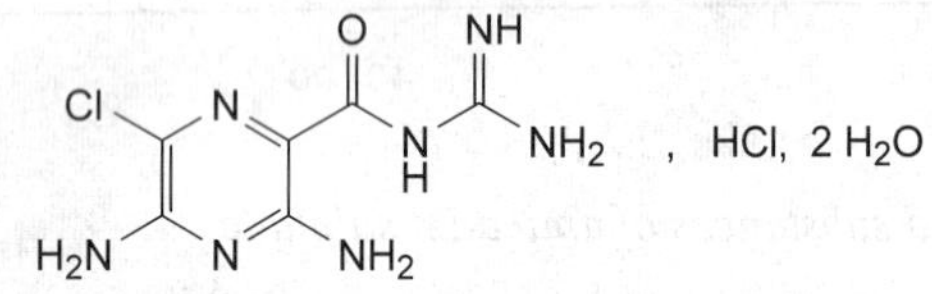

$C_6H_9Cl_2N_7O,2H_2O$ M_r 302.1

DEFINITION

Amiloride hydrochloride contains not less than 98.0 per cent and not more than the equivalent of 101.0 per cent of 3,5-diamino-*N*-carbamimidoyl-6-chloropyrazine-2-carboxamide, calculated with reference to the anhydrous substance.

CHARACTERS

A pale-yellow to greenish-yellow powder, slightly soluble in water and in ethanol.

IDENTIFICATION

First identification: A, D.

Second identification: B, C, D.

A. Examine by infrared absorption spectrophotometry (*2.2.24*), comparing with the spectrum obtained with *amiloride hydrochloride CRS.*

B. Examine by thin-layer chromatography (*2.2.27*), using a suitable silica gel as the coating substance.

Test solution. Dissolve 40 mg of the substance to be examined in *methanol R* and dilute to 10 ml with the same solvent.

Reference solution. Dissolve 40 mg of *amiloride hydrochloride CRS* in *methanol R* and dilute to 10 ml with the same solvent.

Apply to the plate 5 μl of each solution. Develop over a path of 12 cm using a freshly prepared mixture of 6 volumes of *dilute ammonia R1,* 6 volumes of *water R* and 88 volumes of *dioxan R.* Allow the plate to dry in air and examine in ultraviolet light at 365 nm. The principal spot in the chromatogram obtained with the test solution is similar in position, fluorescence and size to the principal spot in the chromatogram obtained with the reference solution.

C. Dissolve about 10 mg in 10 ml of *water R.* Add 10 ml of a 200 g/l solution of *cetrimide R,* 0.25 ml of *dilute sodium hydroxide solution R* and 1 ml of *bromine water R.* A greenish-yellow colour is produced. Add 2 ml of *dilute hydrochloric acid R.* The solution becomes deep yellow and shows blue fluorescence in ultraviolet light at 365 nm.

D. It gives reaction (b) of chlorides (*2.3.1*).

TESTS

Free acid. Dissolve 1.0 g in a mixture of 50 ml of *methanol R* and 50 ml of *water R* and titrate with *0.1 M sodium hydroxide,* determining the end-point potentiometrically (*2.2.20*). Not more than 0.3 ml of *0.1 M sodium hydroxide* is required to reach the end-point.

Related substances. Examine by liquid chromatography (*2.2.29*).

Test solution. Dissolve 20.0 mg of the substance to be examined in a mixture of 1 volume of *acetonitrile R* and 3 volumes of *water R* and dilute to 10.0 ml with the same mixture of solvents.

Reference solution (a). Dilute 1.0 ml of the test solution to 100.0 ml with a mixture of 1 volume of *acetonitrile R* and 3 volumes of *water R.*

Reference solution (b). Dilute 1.0 ml of reference solution (a) to 10.0 ml with a mixture of 1 volume of *acetonitrile R* and 3 volumes of *water R.*

Reference solution (c). Dissolve 20.0 mg of *amiloride impurity A CRS* in a mixture of 1 volume of *acetonitrile R* and 3 volumes of *water R* and dilute to 20.0 ml with the same mixture of solvents. Dilute 1.0 ml of the solution to 100.0 ml with a mixture of 1 volume of *acetonitrile R* and 3 volumes of *water R.*

The chromatographic procedure may be carried out using:

- a stainless steel column 0.25 m long and 4.6 mm in internal diameter packed with *octadecylsilyl silica gel for chromatography R* (5 μm),
- as mobile phase at a flow rate of 1 ml/min a mixture of 5 volumes of *tetramethylammonium hydroxide solution R,* 250 volumes of *acetonitrile R* and 745 volumes of *water R*; adjust to pH 7.0 using a mixture of 1 volume of *phosphoric acid R* and 9 volumes of *water R,*
- as detector a spectrophotometer set at 254 nm.

Inject 20 μl of reference solution (c). Adjust the concentration of acetonitrile in the mobile phase so that the retention time of impurity A is 5 min to 6 min (an increase in the concentration of acetonitrile results in a shorter retention time). Inject 20 μl of reference solution (a). Adjust the concentration of tetramethylammonium hydroxide and of phosphoric acid keeping the pH at 7.0 so that the retention time of amiloride is 9 min to 12 min (an increase in the concentration results in a shorter retention time for amiloride). Inject 20 μl of reference solution (b). The test is not valid unless the signal-to-noise ratio for the peak due to amiloride is at least 5.0.

Inject 20 μl of the test solution and 20 μl of reference solution (c). Record the chromatograms for five times the retention time of amiloride. In the chromatogram obtained with the test solution, the sum of the areas of the peaks, apart from the peak corresponding to amiloride, is not greater than the area of the peak corresponding to impurity A in the chromatogram obtained with reference solution (c) (0.5 per cent). Disregard any peak with an area less than 10 per cent of the area of the peak corresponding to impurity A in the chromatogram obtained with reference solution (c).

Water (*2.5.12*): 11.0 per cent to 13.0 per cent, determined on 0.200 g by the semi-micro determination of water.

Sulphated ash (*2.4.14*). Not more than 0.1 per cent, determined on 1.0 g.

ASSAY

Dissolve 0.200 g in a mixture of 5.0 ml of *0.01 M hydrochloric acid* and 50 ml of *alcohol R*. Carry out a potentiometric titration (*2.2.20*), using *0.1 M sodium hydroxide.* Read the volume added between the two points of inflexion.

1 ml of *0.1 M sodium hydroxide* is equivalent to 26.61 mg of $C_6H_9Cl_2N_7O$.

STORAGE

Store protected from light.

IMPURITIES

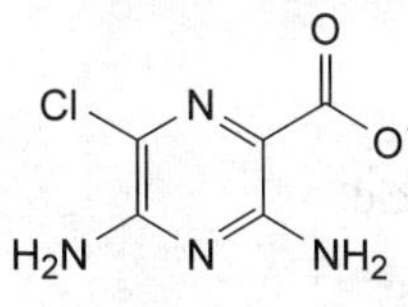

A. methyl 3,5-diamino-6-chloropyrazine-2-carboxylate.

01/2005:1687

4-AMINOBENZOIC ACID

Acidum 4-aminobenzoicum

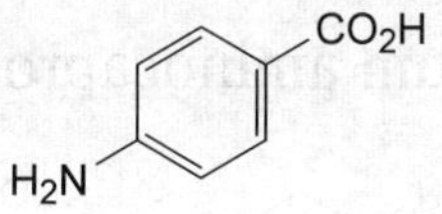

$C_7H_7NO_2$ M_r 137.1

DEFINITION

4-Aminobenzoic acid.

Content: 99.0 per cent to 101.0 per cent (anhydrous substance).

CHARACTERS

Appearance: white or slightly yellow, crystalline powder.

Solubility: slightly soluble in water, freely soluble in alcohol. It dissolves in dilute solutions of alkali hydroxides.

IDENTIFICATION

First identification: B.

Second identification: A, C.

A. Melting point (*2.2.14*): 186 °C to 189 °C.

B. Infrared absorption spectrophotometry (*2.2.24*).

Comparison: *4-aminobenzoic acid CRS.*

C. Thin-layer chromatography (*2.2.27*).

Test solution. Dissolve 20 mg of the substance to be examined in *methanol R* and dilute to 20 ml with the same solvent.

Reference solution (a). Dissolve 20 mg of *4-aminobenzoic acid CRS* in *methanol R* and dilute to 20 ml with the same solvent.

Reference solution (b). Dissolve 10 mg of *4-nitrobenzoic acid R* in 10 ml of reference solution (a).

Plate: suitable silica gel with a fluorescent indicator having an optimal intensity at 254 nm as the coating substance.

Mobile phase: *glacial acetic acid R, hexane R, methylene chloride R* (5:20:75 *V/V/V*).

Application: 1 µl.

Development: over a path of 10 cm.

Drying: in air.

Detection: examine in ultraviolet light at 254 nm.

System suitability: the chromatogram obtained with reference solution (b) shows 2 clearly separated spots.

Results: the principal spot in the chromatogram obtained with the test solution is similar in position and size to the principal spot in the chromatogram obtained with reference solution (a).

TESTS

Appearance of solution. The solution is clear (*2.2.1*) and not more intensely coloured than reference solution B_5 (*2.2.2, Method II*).

Dissolve 1.0 g in *alcohol R* and dilute to 20 ml with the same solvent.

Related substances. Liquid chromatography (*2.2.29*).

Test solution. Dissolve 25.0 mg of the substance to be examined in the mobile phase and dilute to 100.0 ml with the mobile phase.

Reference solution. Dissolve 25.0 mg of *4-nitrobenzoic acid R* and 25.0 mg of *benzocaine R* in *methanol R* and dilute to 100.0 ml with the same solvent. Dilute 1.0 ml to 50.0 ml with the mobile phase. Dilute 1.0 ml of this solution to 10.0 ml with the mobile phase.

Column:

- *size*: *l* = 0.12 m, Ø = 4.0 mm,
- *stationary phase*: *octylsilyl silica gel for chromatography R* (5 µm).

Mobile phase: mix 20 volumes of a mixture of 70 volumes of *acetonitrile R* and 80 volumes of *methanol R,* and 80 volumes of a solution containing 1.5 g/l of *potassium dihydrogen phosphate R* and 2.5 g/l of *sodium octanesulphonate R* adjusted to pH 2.2 with *phosphoric acid R.*

Flow rate: 1.0 ml/min.

Detection: spectrophotometer at 270 nm.

Injection: 20 µl.

Run time: 11 times the retention time of 4-aminobenzoic acid.

Relative retention with reference to 4-aminobenzoic acid (retention time = about 3 min): impurity A = about 4; impurity B = about 9.

Limits:

- *impurity A*: not more than the area of the corresponding peak in the chromatogram obtained with the reference solution (0.2 per cent),
- *impurity B*: not more than the area of the corresponding peak in the chromatogram obtained with the reference solution (0.2 per cent),
- *any other impurity*: not more than 0.5 times the area of the peak due to impurity A in the chromatogram obtained with the reference solution (0.1 per cent),
- *total*: not more than 2.5 times the area of the peak due to impurity A in the chromatogram obtained with the reference solution (0.5 per cent),

- *disregard limit*: 0.1 times the area of the peak due to impurity A in the chromatogram obtained with the reference solution (0.02 per cent).

Impurity C and impurity D. Gas chromatography (*2.2.28*).

Internal standard solution. Dissolve 20.0 mg of *lauric acid R* in *methylene chloride R* and dilute to 100.0 ml with the same solvent.

Test solution. Dissolve 1.000 g of the substance to be examined in 10.0 ml of an 84 g/l solution of *sodium hydroxide R* and extract with 2 quantities, each of 10 ml, of *methylene chloride R*. Combine and wash with 5 ml of *water R*; filter through *anhydrous sodium sulphate R*. Wash the filter with *methylene chloride R*. Evaporate in a water-bath at 50-60 °C to obtain a volume of about 1-5 ml. Add 1.0 ml of the internal standard solution and dilute to 10.0 ml with *methylene chloride R*.

Reference solution (a). Dissolve 20.0 mg of *aniline R* in *methylene chloride R* and dilute to 100.0 ml with the same solvent.

Reference solution (b). Dissolve 20.0 mg of *p-toluidine R* in *methylene chloride R* and dilute to 100.0 ml with the same solvent.

Reference solution (c). Dilute 0.50 ml of reference solution (a), 0.50 ml of reference solution (b) and 10.0 ml of the internal standard solution to 100.0 ml with *methylene chloride R*.

Column:
- *material*: fused silica,
- *size*: l = 30 m, Ø = 0.32 mm,
- *stationary phase*: *poly[methyl(95)phenyl(5)] siloxane R* (film thickness 0.5 μm).

Carrier gas: *helium for chromatography R*.

Flow rate: 1.0 ml/min.

Split ratio: 1:10.

Temperature:

	Time (min)	Temperature (°C)
Column	0 - 4	130
	4 - 6.5	130 → 180
	6.5 - 11.5	180
Injection port		280
Detector		300

Detection: flame ionisation.

Injection: 2 μl; inject the test solution and reference solution (c).

Retention time: internal standard = about 9.5 min.

Limits:
- *impurity C*: calculate the ratio (R) of the area of the peak due to impurity C to the area of the peak due to the internal standard from the chromatogram obtained with reference solution (c); calculate the ratio of the area of the peak due to impurity C to the area of the peak due to the internal standard from the chromatogram obtained with the test solution: this ratio is not greater than R (10 ppm),
- *impurity D*: calculate the ratio (R) of the area of the peak due to impurity D to the area of the peak due to the internal standard from the chromatogram obtained with reference solution (c); calculate the ratio of the area of the peak due to impurity D to the area of the peak due to the internal standard from the chromatogram obtained with the test solution: this ratio is not greater than R (10 ppm).

Iron (*2.4.9*): maximum 40 ppm.

Dissolve 0.250 g in 3 ml of *alcohol R* and dilute to 10.0 ml with *water R*.

Heavy metals (*2.4.8*): maximum 20 ppm.

1.0 g complies with limit test C. Prepare the standard using 2 ml of *lead standard solution (10 ppm Pb) R*.

Water (*2.5.12*): maximum 0.2 per cent, determined on 1.00 g.

Sulphated ash (*2.4.14*): maximum 0.1 per cent, determined on 1.0 g.

ASSAY

Dissolve 0.100 g with heating in 50 ml of *carbon dioxide-free water R*. Titrate with *0.1 M sodium hydroxide* determining the end-point potentiometrically (*2.2.20*).

1 ml of *0.1 M sodium hydroxide* is equivalent to 13.71 mg of $C_7H_7NO_2$.

STORAGE

Protected from light.

IMPURITIES

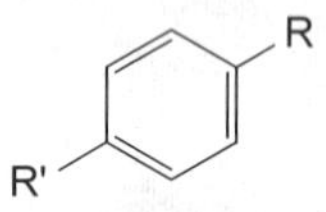

A. R = CO_2H, R′ = NO_2: 4-nitrobenzoic acid,

B. R = $CO\text{-}O\text{-}C_2H_5$, R′ = NH_2: benzocaine,

C. R = H, R′ = NH_2: aniline,

D. R = CH_3, R′ = NH_2: 4-methylaniline (*p*-toluidine).

01/2005:0874

AMINOCAPROIC ACID

Acidum aminocaproicum

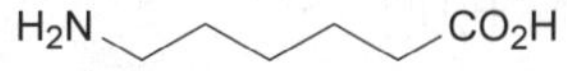

$C_6H_{13}NO_2$ M_r 131.2

DEFINITION

Aminocaproic acid contains not less than 98.5 per cent and not more than the equivalent of 101.0 per cent of 6-aminohexanoic acid, calculated with reference to the dried substance.

CHARACTERS

A white, crystalline powder or colourless crystals, freely soluble in water, slightly soluble in alcohol.

It melts at about 205 °C with decomposition.

IDENTIFICATION

First identification: A.

Second identification: B, C, D.

A. Examine by infrared absorption spectrophotometry (*2.2.24*), comparing with the spectrum obtained with *aminocaproic acid CRS*. Examine the substances prepared as discs.

B. Examine the chromatograms obtained in the test for ninhydrin-positive substances. The principal spot in the chromatogram obtained with the test solution (b) is similar in position, colour and size to the principal spot in the chromatogram obtained with reference solution (a).

C. Dissolve 0.5 g in 4 ml of a mixture of equal volumes of *dilute hydrochloric acid R* and *water R*. Evaporate to dryness by heating on a water-bath. Dry the residue in a desiccator. Dissolve the residue in about 2 ml of boiling *ethanol R*. Allow to cool and maintain at 4 °C to 8 °C for 3 h. Filter under reduced pressure. The residue washed with about 10 ml of *acetone R* and dried at 60 °C for 30 min, melts (*2.2.14*) at 131 °C to 133 °C.

D. Dissolve about 5 mg in 0.5 ml of *distilled water R*. Add 3 ml of *dimethylformamide R* and 2 ml of *ascorbic acid solution R*. Heat on a water-bath. An orange colour develops.

TESTS

Solution S. dissolve 10.0 g in *carbon dioxide-free water R* and dilute to 50.0 ml with the same solvent.

Appearance of solution. Solution S is colourless (*2.2.2, Method II*) and remains clear (*2.2.1*) on standing for 24 h.

pH (*2.2.3*). The pH of solution S is 7.5 to 8.0.

Absorbance (*2.2.25*).

A. The absorbance of solution S at 287 nm is not more than 0.10 and at 450 nm is not more than 0.03.

B. Place 2.0 g in an even layer in a shallow dish 9 cm in diameter, cover and allow to stand at 98 °C to 102 °C for 72 h. Dissolve in *water R* and dilute to 10.0 ml with the same solvent. The absorbance of the solution at 287 nm is not more than 0.15 and at 450 nm is not more than 0.03.

Ninhydrin-positive substances. Examine by thin-layer chromatography (*2.2.27*), using a suitable silica gel as the coating substance.

Test solution (a). Dissolve 0.10 g of the substance to be examined in *water R* and dilute to 10 ml with the same solvent.

Test solution (b). Dilute 1 ml of test solution (a) to 50 ml with *water R*.

Reference solution (a). Dissolve 10 mg of *aminocaproic acid CRS* in *water R* and dilute to 50 ml with the same solvent.

Reference solution (b). Dilute 5 ml of test solution (b) to 20 ml with *water R*.

Reference solution (c). Dissolve 10 mg of *aminocaproic acid CRS* and 10 mg of *leucine CRS* in *water R* and dilute to 25 ml with the same solvent.

Apply separately to the plate 5 µl of each solution. Allow the plate to dry in air. Develop over a path of 15 cm using a mixture of 20 volumes of *glacial acetic acid R*, 20 volumes of *water R* and 60 volumes of *butanol R*. Dry the plate in a current of warm air. Spray with *ninhydrin solution R* and heat at 100 °C to 105 °C for 15 min. Any spot in the chromatogram obtained with the test solution (a), apart from the principal spot, is not more intense than the spot in the chromatogram obtained with reference solution (b) (0.5 per cent). The test is not valid unless the chromatogram obtained with reference solution (c) shows two clearly separated principal spots.

Heavy metals (*2.4.8*). 12 ml of solution S complies with limit test A for heavy metals (10 ppm). Prepare the standard using *lead standard solution (2 ppm Pb) R*.

Loss on drying (*2.2.32*). Not more than 0.5 per cent, determined on 1.000 g by drying in an oven at 100 °C to 105 °C.

Sulphated ash (*2.4.14*). Not more than 0.1 per cent, determined on 1.0 g.

ASSAY

Dissolve 0.100 g in 20 ml of *anhydrous acetic acid R*. Using 0.1 ml of *crystal violet solution R* as indicator, titrate with *0.1 M perchloric acid* until the colour changes from bluish-violet to bluish-green.

1 ml of *0.1 M perchloric acid* is equivalent to 13.12 mg of $C_6H_{13}NO_2$.

01/2005:1291

AMINOGLUTETHIMIDE

Aminoglutethimidum

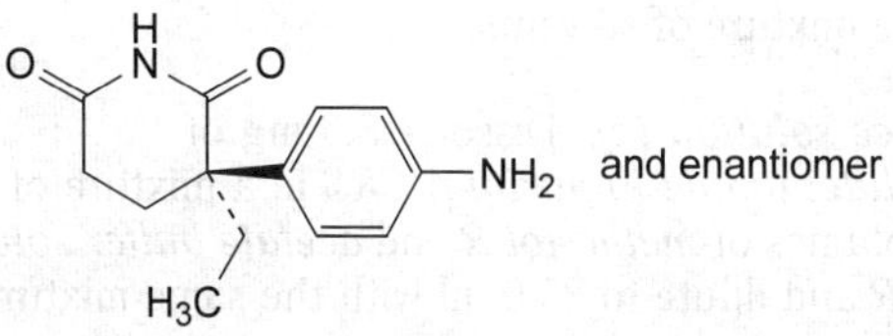

$C_{13}H_{16}N_2O_2$ M_r 232.3

DEFINITION

Aminoglutethimide contains not less than 98.0 per cent and not more than the equivalent of 101.5 per cent of (3*RS*)-3-(4-aminophenyl)-3-ethylpiperidine-2,6-dione, calculated with reference to the dried substance.

CHARACTERS

A white or slightly yellow, crystalline powder, practically insoluble in water, freely soluble in acetone, soluble in methanol.

IDENTIFICATION

First identification: B.

Second identification: A, C.

A. Melting point (*2.2.14*). 150 °C to 154 °C.

B. Examine by infrared absorption spectrophotometry (*2.2.24*), comparing with the spectrum obtained with *aminoglutethimide CRS*. Examine the substances prepared as discs.

C. Examine by thin-layer chromatography (*2.2.27*), using as the coating substance a suitable silica gel with a fluorescent indicator having an optimal intensity at 254 nm.

Test solution. Dissolve 25 mg of the substance to be examined in *acetone R* and dilute to 5 ml with the same solvent.

Reference solution (a). Dissolve 25 mg of *aminoglutethimide CRS* in *acetone R* and dilute to 5 ml with the same solvent.

Reference solution (b). Dissolve 25 mg of *aminoglutethimide CRS* and 25 mg of *glutethimide CRS* in *acetone R* and dilute to 5 ml with the same solvent.

Apply to the plate 5 µl of each solution. Develop over a path of 15 cm using a mixture of 0.5 volumes of *glacial acetic acid R*, 15 volumes of *methanol R* and 85 volumes of *ethyl acetate R*. Allow the plate to dry in air and examine in ultraviolet light at 254 nm. The principal spot in the chromatogram obtained with the test solution is similar in position and size to the principal spot in the chromatogram obtained with reference solution (a). The identification is not valid unless the chromatogram obtained with reference solution (b) shows two clearly separated spots.

TESTS

Solution S. Dissolve 1.0 g in *methanol R* and dilute to 20.0 ml with the same solvent.

Appearance of solution. Solution S is clear (*2.2.1*) and not more intensely coloured than reference solution Y_7 (*2.2.2, Method II*).

Optical rotation (*2.2.7*). The angle of optical rotation, determined on solution S, is − 0.10° to + 0.10°.

3-Aminoglutethimide and other related substances. Examine by liquid chromatography (*2.2.29*).

Test solution. Dissolve 0.10 g of the substance to be examined in a mixture of equal volumes of *methanol R* and *acetate buffer solution pH 5.0 R* and dilute to 50.0 ml with the same mixture of solvents.

Reference solution (a). Dissolve 5.0 mg of *aminoglutethimide impurity A CRS* in a mixture of equal volumes of *methanol R* and *acetate buffer solution pH 5.0 R* and dilute to 25.0 ml with the same mixture of solvents.

Reference solution (b). Dilute 1.0 ml of reference solution (a) to 10.0 ml with a mixture of equal volumes of *methanol R* and *acetate buffer solution pH 5.0 R*.

Reference solution (c). Dilute 1.0 ml of the test solution to 100.0 ml with a mixture of equal volumes of *methanol R* and *acetate buffer solution pH 5.0 R*.

Reference solution (d). Dilute 1.0 ml of the test solution to 10.0 ml with reference solution (a).

The chromatographic procedure may be carried out using:

– a stainless steel column 0.15 m long and 3.9 mm in internal diameter packed with *octadecylsilyl silica gel for chromatography R* (4 µm),

– as mobile phase at a flow rate of 1.3 ml/min a mixture of 27 volumes of *methanol R* and 73 volumes of *acetate buffer solution pH 5.0 R*,

– as detector a spectrophotometer set at 240 nm,

maintaining the temperature of the column at 40 °C.

Inject 10 µl of reference solution (d). When the chromatograms are recorded in the prescribed conditions, the retention times are: aminoglutethimide about 9 min and impurity A about 12 min. Adjust the sensitivity of the system so that the height of the principal peak in the chromatogram obtained with reference solution (d) is at least 60 per cent of the full scale of the recorder. The test is not valid unless in the chromatogram obtained with reference solution (d), the resolution between the peaks corresponding to aminoglutethimide and impurity A is at least 2.0.

Inject 10 µl of the test solution, 10 µl of reference solution (b) and 10 µl of reference solution (c). Continue the chromatography of the test solution for four times the retention time of the principal peak. In the chromatogram obtained with the test solution: the area of any peak due to impurity A is not greater than twice the area of the principal peak in the chromatogram obtained with reference solution (b) (2 per cent); the sum of the areas of any peaks apart from the principal peak and the peak due to impurity A is not greater than the area of the principal peak in the chromatogram obtained with reference solution (c) (1 per cent); the sum of the contents of all the impurities is not greater than 2.0 per cent. Disregard any peak with an area less than 0.05 times that of the principal peak in the chromatogram obtained with reference solution (c).

Azoglutethimide. Not more than 300 ppm, determined by liquid chromatography (*2.2.29*). *Carry out the test protected from light. Use shaking, not sonication or heat, to dissolve the reference substance and the substance to be examined.*

Test solution. Dissolve 0.100 g of the substance to be examined in *dimethyl sulphoxide R* and dilute to 100.0 ml with the same solvent.

Reference solution. Dissolve 3.0 mg of *aminoglutethimide impurity D CRS* in *dimethyl sulphoxide R* and dilute to 100.0 ml with the same solvent. Dilute 1.0 ml of this solution to 100.0 ml with *dimethyl sulphoxide R*.

The chromatographic procedure may be carried out using:

– a stainless steel column 0.12 m long and 4 mm in internal diameter packed with *octadecylsilyl silica gel for chromatography R* (5 µm),

– as mobile phase at a flow of 1.0 ml/min a mixture prepared as follows: dissolve 0.285 g of *sodium edetate R* in *water R*, add 7.5 ml of *dilute acetic acid R* and 50 ml of *0.1 M potassium hydroxide* and dilute to 1000 ml with *water R*; adjust to pH 5.0 with *glacial acetic acid R*; mix 350 ml of this solution with 650 ml of *methanol R*,

– as detector a spectrophotometer set at 328 nm.

Inject 10 µl of each solution. The test is not valid unless: in the chromatogram obtained with the test solution the number of theoretical plates calculated for the principal peak is at least 3300; the mass distribution ratio of the principal peak is 2.0 to 5.0 and the symmetry factor of the principal peak is less than 1.2. The area of the peak due to impurity D in the chromatogram obtained with the test solution is not greater than that of the principal peak in the chromatogram obtained with the reference solution.

Sulphates (*2.4.13*). Dilute 6 ml of solution S to 15 ml with *distilled water R*. The solution complies with the limit test for sulphates (500 ppm).

Heavy metals (*2.4.8*). Dissolve 2.0 g in 15 ml of *acetone R* and dilute to 20 ml with *water R*. 12 ml of the solution complies with limit test B for heavy metals (10 ppm). Prepare the standard using lead standard solution (1 ppm Pb) obtained by diluting *lead standard solution (100 ppm Pb) R* with a mixture of 15 ml of *acetone R* and 5 ml of *water R*.

Loss on drying (*2.2.32*). Not more than 0.5 per cent, determined on 1.000 g by drying in an oven at 100 °C to 105 °C.

Sulphated ash (*2.4.14*). Not more than 0.1 per cent, determined on 1.0 g.

ASSAY

Dissolve 0.180 g in 50 ml of *anhydrous acetic acid R* and titrate with *0.1 M perchloric acid*, determining the end-point potentiometrically (*2.2.20*).

1 ml of *0.1 M perchloric acid* is equivalent to 23.23 mg of $C_{13}H_{16}N_2O_2$.

IMPURITIES

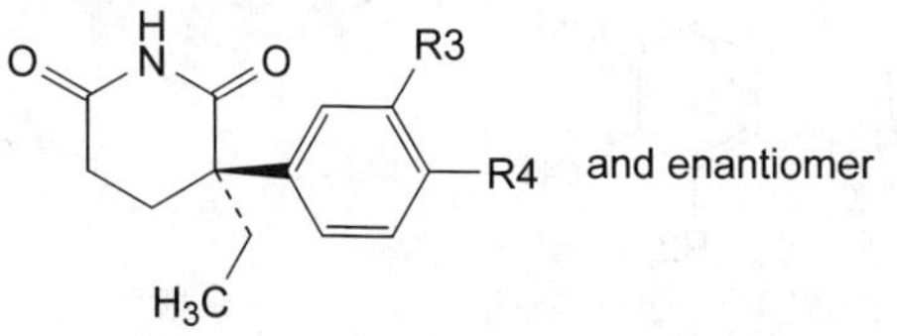

A. R3 = NH_2, R4 = H: (3*RS*)-3-(3-aminophenyl)-3-ethylpiperidine-2,6-dione (3-aminoglutethimide),

B. R3 = NO_2, R4 = H: (3*RS*)-3-ethyl-3-(3-nitrophenyl)piperidine-2,6-dione,

C. R3 = H, R4 = NO_2: (3*RS*)-3-ethyl-3-(4-nitrophenyl)piperidine-2,6-dione,

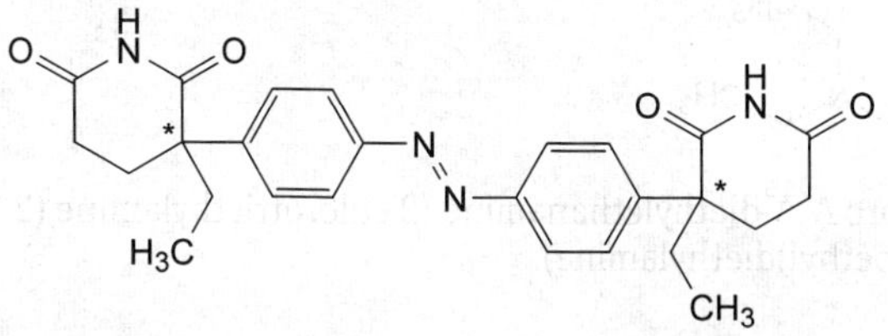

D. 3,3′-[diazenediylbis(4,1-phenylene)]bis(3-ethylpiperidine-2,6-dione) (azoglutethimide).

01/2005:0803

AMIODARONE HYDROCHLORIDE

Amiodaroni hydrochloridum

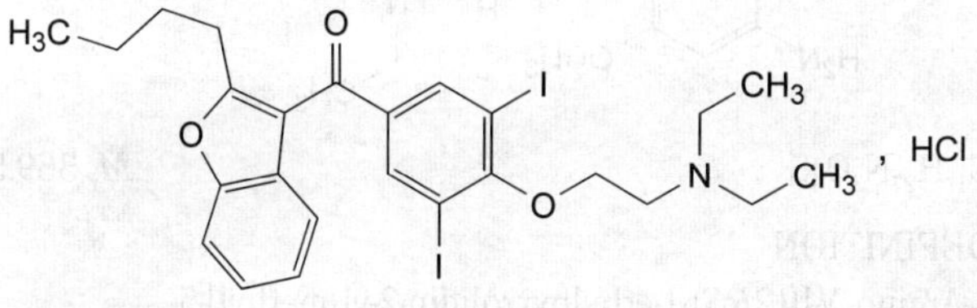

$C_{25}H_{30}ClI_2NO_3$ M_r 682

DEFINITION

(2-Butylbenzofuran-3-yl)[4-[2-(diethylamino)ethoxy]-3,5-diiodophenyl]methanone hydrochloride.

Content: 98.5 per cent to 101.0 per cent (dried substance).

CHARACTERS

Appearance: white or almost white, fine crystalline powder.

Solubility: very slightly soluble in water, freely soluble in methylene chloride, soluble in methanol, sparingly soluble in alcohol.

IDENTIFICATION

A. Infrared absorption spectrophotometry (*2.2.24*).
Comparison: *amiodarone hydrochloride CRS*.

B. It gives reaction (b) of chlorides (*2.3.1*).

TESTS

Appearance of solution. The solution is clear (*2.2.1*) and not more intensely coloured than reference solution GY_5 or BY_5 (*2.2.2, Method II*).

Dissolve 1.0 g in *methanol R* and dilute to 20 ml with the same solvent.

pH (*2.2.3*): 3.2 to 3.8.

Dissolve 1.0 g in *carbon dioxide-free water R*, heating at 80 °C, cool and dilute to 20 ml with the same solvent.

Impurity H. Thin-layer chromatography (*2.2.27*). *Prepare the solutions immediately before use and keep protected from bright light.*

Test solution. Dissolve 0.5 g of the substance to be examined in *methylene chloride R* and dilute to 5.0 ml with the same solvent.

Reference solution. Dissolve 10 mg of *(2-chloroethyl)diethylamine hydrochloride R* in *methylene chloride R* and dilute to 50.0 ml with the same solvent.

Plate: *TLC silica gel F_{254} plate R.*

Mobile phase: *anhydrous formic acid R, methanol R, methylene chloride R* (5:10:85 *V/V/V*).

Application: 5 µl.

Development: over a path of 15 cm.

Drying: in a current of cold air until the odour of solvents is no longer perceptible.

Detection: spray with *potassium iodobismuthate solution R1* and then with *dilute hydrogen peroxide solution R*. Examine immediately in daylight.

Limit:

– *impurity H*: any spot corresponding to impurity H is not more intense than the spot in the chromatogram obtained with the reference solution (0.2 per cent).

Related substances. Liquid chromatography (*2.2.29*).

Buffer solution pH 4.9. To 800 ml of *water R*, add 3.0 ml of *glacial acetic acid R*, adjust to pH 4.9 with *dilute ammonia R1* and dilute to 1000 ml with *water R*.

Test solution. Dissolve 0.125 g of the substance to be examined in a mixture of equal volumes of *acetonitrile R* and *water R* and dilute to 25.0 ml with the same mixture of solvents.

Reference solution. Dissolve 10 mg of *amiodarone impurity D CRS*, 10 mg of *amiodarone impurity E CRS* and 10.0 mg of *amiodarone hydrochloride CRS* in *methanol R* and dilute to 50.0 ml with the same solvent. Dilute 1.0 ml of the solution to 20.0 ml with a mixture of equal volumes of *acetonitrile R* and *water R*.

Column:

– *size*: *l* = 0.15 m, Ø = 4.6 mm,

– *stationary phase*: *octadecylsilyl silica gel for chromatography R* (5 µm),

– *temperature*: 30 °C.

Mobile phase: buffer solution pH 4.9, *methanol R, acetonitrile R* (30:30:40 *V/V/V*).

Flow rate: 1 ml/min.

Detection: spectrophotometer at 240 nm.

Injection: 10 µl.

Run time: twice the retention time of amiodarone.

Relative retention with reference to amiodarone (retention time = about 24 min): impurity A = about 0.26; impurity D = about 0.29; impurity E = about 0.37; impurity B = about 0.49; impurity C = about 0.55; impurity G = about 0.62; impurity F = about 0.69.

System suitability: reference solution:

– *resolution*: minimum 3.5 between the peaks due to impurity D and impurity E.

Limits:

– *any impurity*: not more than the area of the peak due to amiodarone in the chromatogram obtained with the reference solution (0.2 per cent),

– *total*: not more than 2.5 times the area of the peak due to amiodarone in the chromatogram obtained with the reference solution (0.5 per cent),

– *disregard limit*: 0.1 times the area of the peak due to amiodarone in the chromatogram obtained with the reference solution (0.02 per cent).

Iodides: maximum 150 ppm.

Prepare the test and reference solutions simultaneously.

Solution A. Add 1.50 g of the substance to be examined to 40 ml of *water R* at 80 °C and shake until completely dissolved. Cool and dilute to 50.0 ml with *water R*.

Test solution. To 15.0 ml of solution A add 1.0 ml of *0.1 M hydrochloric acid* and 1.0 ml of *0.05 M potassium iodate*. Dilute to 20.0 ml with *water R*. Allow to stand protected from light for 4 h.

Reference solution. To 15.0 ml of solution A add 1.0 ml of *0.1 M hydrochloric acid*, 1.0 ml of a 88.2 mg/l solution of *potassium iodide R* and 1.0 ml of *0.05 M potassium iodate*. Dilute to 20.0 ml with *water R*. Allow to stand protected from light for 4 h.

Measure the absorbances (*2.2.25*) of the solutions at 420 nm, using as the compensation liquid a mixture of 15.0 ml of solution A and 1.0 ml of *0.1 M hydrochloric acid* diluted to 20.0 ml with *water R*. The absorbance of the test solution is not greater than half the absorbance of the reference solution.

Heavy metals (*2.4.8*): maximum 20 ppm.

1.0 g complies with limit test C. Prepare the standard using 2 ml of *lead standard solution (10 ppm Pb) R*.

Loss on drying (*2.2.32*): maximum 0.5 per cent, determined on 1.000 g by drying at 50 °C at a pressure not exceeding 0.3 kPa for 4 h.

Sulphated ash (*2.4.14*): maximum 0.1 per cent, determined on 1.0 g.

ASSAY

Dissolve 0.600 g in a mixture of 5.0 ml of *0.01 M hydrochloric acid* and 75 ml of *alcohol R*. Carry out a potentiometric titration (*2.2.20*), using *0.1 M sodium hydroxide*. Read the volume added between the 2 points of inflexion.

1 ml of *0.1 M sodium hydroxide* is equivalent to 68.18 mg of $C_{25}H_{30}ClI_2NO_3$.

STORAGE

Protected from light, at a temperature not exceeding 30 °C.

IMPURITIES

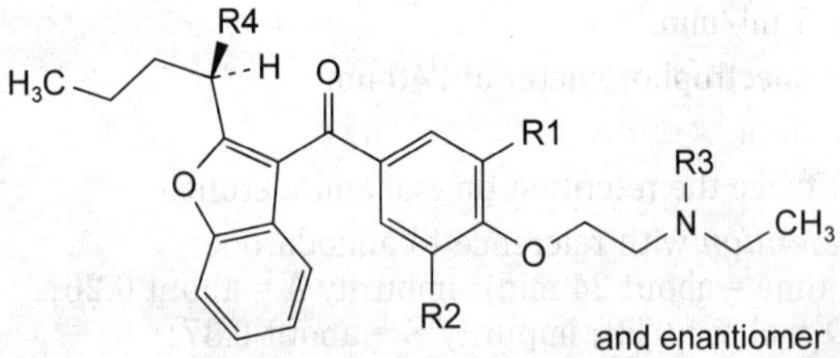

A. R1 = R2 = R4 = H, R3 = C_2H_5: (2-butylbenzofuran-3-yl)[4-[2-(diethylamino)ethoxy]phenyl]methanone,

B. R1 = R2 = I, R3 = R4 = H: (2-butylbenzofuran-3-yl)[4-[2-(ethylamino)ethoxy]-3,5-diiodophenyl]methanone,

C. R1 = I, R2 = R4 = H, R3 = C_2H_5: (2-butylbenzofuran-3-yl)[4-[2-(diethylamino)ethoxy]-3-iodophenyl]methanone,

G. R1 = R2 = I, R3 = C_2H_5, R4 = OCH_3: [2-[(1*RS*)-1-methoxybutyl]benzofuran-3-yl][4-[2-(diethylamino)ethoxy]-3,5-diiodophenyl]methanone,

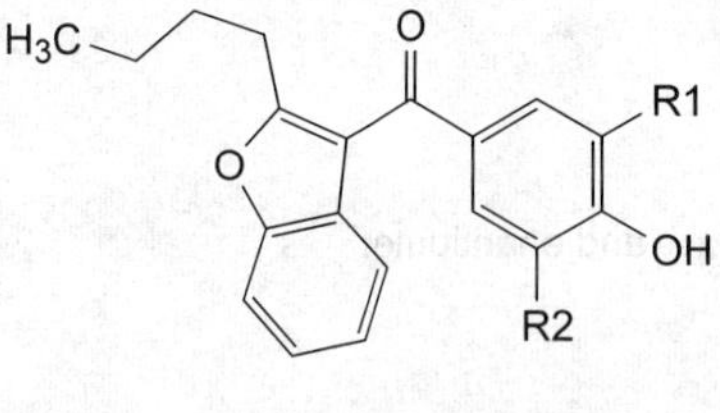

D. R1 = R2 = I: (2-butylbenzofuran-3-yl)(4-hydroxy-3,5-diiodophenyl)methanone,

E. R1 = R2 = H: (2-butylbenzofuran-3-yl)(4-hydroxyphenyl)methanone,

F. R1 = I, R2 = H: (2-butylbenzofuran-3-yl)(4-hydroxy-3-iodophenyl)methanone,

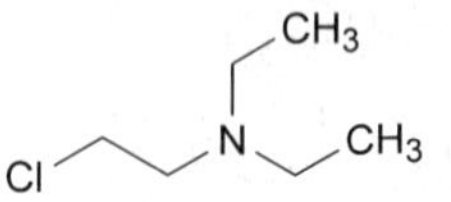

H. 2-chloro-*N*,*N*-diethylethanamine (2-chlorotriethylamine,(2-chloroethyl)diethylamine).

01/2005:1490

AMISULPRIDE

Amisulpridum

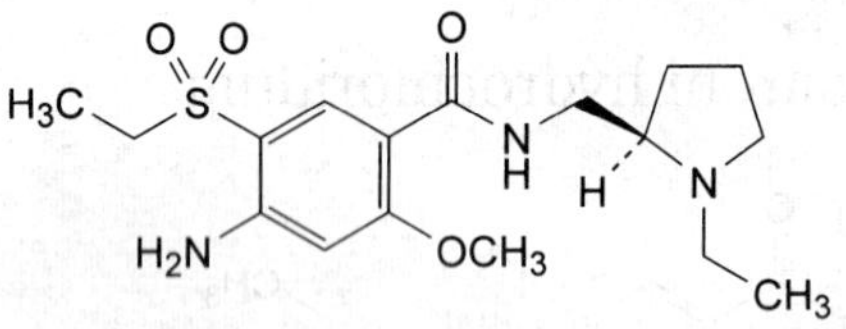

and enantiomer

$C_{17}H_{27}N_3O_4S$ M_r 369.5

DEFINITION

4-Amino-*N*-[[(2*RS*)-1-ethylpyrrolidin-2-yl]methyl]-5-(ethylsulphonyl)-2-methoxybenzamide.

Content: 99.0 per cent to 101.0 per cent (dried substance).

CHARACTERS

Appearance: white or almost white, crystalline powder.

Solubility: practically insoluble in water, freely soluble in methylene chloride, sparingly soluble in ethanol.

mp: about 126 °C.

IDENTIFICATION

Infrared absorption spectrophotometry (*2.2.24*).

Comparison: *amisulpride CRS*.

TESTS

Appearance of solution. The solution is not more opalescent than reference suspension II (*2.2.1*) and not more intensely coloured than reference solution Y_6 (*2.2.2, Method II*).

Dissolve 1.0 g in 3 ml of a mixture of 1 volume of *acetic acid R* and 4 volumes of *water R* and dilute to 20 ml with *water R*.

Optical rotation (*2.2.7*): − 0.10° to + 0.10°.

Dissolve 5.0 g in *dimethylformamide R* and dilute to 50.0 ml with the same solvent.

Impurity A. Thin-layer chromatography (*2.2.27*).

Test solution. Dissolve 0.20 g in *methanol R* and dilute to 10 ml with the same solvent.

Reference solution (a). Dissolve 20 mg of *amisulpride impurity A CRS* in *methanol R* and dilute to 100 ml with the same solvent. Dilute 2 ml of the solution to 20 ml with *methanol R.*

Reference solution (b). Dilute 1 ml of the test solution to 10 ml with reference solution (a).

Plate: *TLC silica gel G plate R.*

Mobile phase: the upper layer obtained after shaking a mixture of a 50 per cent *V/V* solution of *concentrated ammonia R, ethanol R* and *di-isopropyl ether R* (10:25:65 *V/V/V*).

Application: 10 µl.

Development: over a path of 12 cm.

Drying: in air.

Detection: spray with *ninhydrin solution R* and heat at 100-105 °C for 15 min.

System suitability: the chromatogram obtained with reference solution (b) shows 2 clearly separated spots.

Limit:

- *impurity A*: any spot corresponding to impurity A is not more intense than the spot in the chromatogram obtained with reference solution (a) (0.1 per cent).

Related substances. Examine by liquid chromatography (*2.2.29*).

Test solution. Dissolve 0.10 g in 30 ml of *methanol R* and dilute to 100.0 ml with mobile phase B.

Reference solution (a). Dilute 5.0 ml of the test solution to 100.0 ml with a mixture of 30 volumes of mobile phase A and 70 volumes of mobile phase B. Dilute 1.0 ml of the solution to 25.0 ml with a mixture of 30 volumes of mobile phase A and 70 volumes of mobile phase B.

Reference solution (b). Dissolve 5 mg of *amisulpride impurity B CRS* in 5 ml of the test solution and dilute to 50 ml with a mixture of 30 volumes of mobile phase A and 70 volumes of mobile phase B. Dilute 1 ml of the solution to 10 ml with a mixture of 30 volumes of mobile phase A and 70 volumes of mobile phase B.

Column:

- *size*: *l* = 0.25 m, Ø = 4.6 mm,
- *stationary phase*: *octylsilyl silica gel for chromatography R* (5 µm) with a carbon loading of 16 per cent, a specific surface area of 330 m²/g and a pore size of 7.5 nm.

Mobile phase:

- *mobile phase A*: *methanol R,*
- *mobile phase B*: a 0.7 g/l solution of *sodium octanesulphonate R* in a 0.25 per cent *V/V* solution of *dilute sulphuric acid R,*

Time (min)	Mobile phase A (per cent *V/V*)	Mobile phase B (per cent *V/V*)
0 - 18	30 → 36	70 → 64
18 - 35	36 → 52	64 → 48
35 - 45	52	48
45 - 46	52 → 30	48 → 70
46 - 56	30	70

Flow rate: 1.5 ml/min.

Detection: spectrophotometer at 225 nm.

Injection: 10 µl.

System suitability: reference solution (b):

- *resolution*: minimum 2.0 between the peaks due to amisulpride and impurity B.

Limits:

- *any impurity*: not more than 0.5 times the area of the principal peak in the chromatogram obtained with reference solution (a) (0.1 per cent),
- *total*: not more than 1.5 times the area of the principal peak in the chromatogram obtained with reference solution (a) (0.3 per cent),
- *disregard limit*: 0.1 times the area of the principal peak in the chromatogram obtained with reference solution (a) (0.02 per cent).

Chlorides (*2.4.4*): maximum 200 ppm.

Shake 0.5 g with 30 ml of *water R* for 10 min. Filter. 15 ml of the filtrate complies with the limit test for chlorides.

Heavy metals (*2.4.8*): maximum 10 ppm.

Dissolve 4.0 g by gently heating in 5 ml of *dilute acetic acid R.* Allow to cool and dilute to 20 ml with *water R.* 12 ml of the solution complies with limit test A. Prepare the standard using *lead standard solution (2 ppm Pb) R.*

Loss on drying (*2.2.32*): maximum 0.5 per cent, determined on 1.000 g by drying in an oven at 100-105 °C for 3 h.

Sulphated ash (*2.4.14*): maximum 0.1 per cent, determined on 1.0 g.

ASSAY

Dissolve 0.300 g with shaking in a mixture of 5 ml of *acetic anhydride R* and 50 ml of *anhydrous acetic acid R.* Titrate with *0.1 M perchloric acid,* determining the end-point potentiometrically (*2.2.20*).

1 ml of *0.1 M perchloric acid* is equivalent to 36.95 mg of $C_{17}H_{27}N_3O_4S$.

IMPURITIES

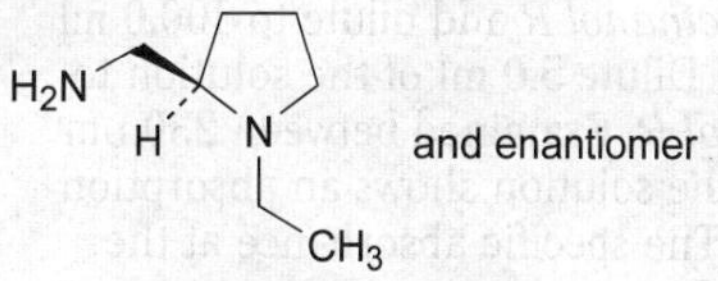

A. [(2*RS*)-1-ethylpyrrolidin-2-yl]methanamine,

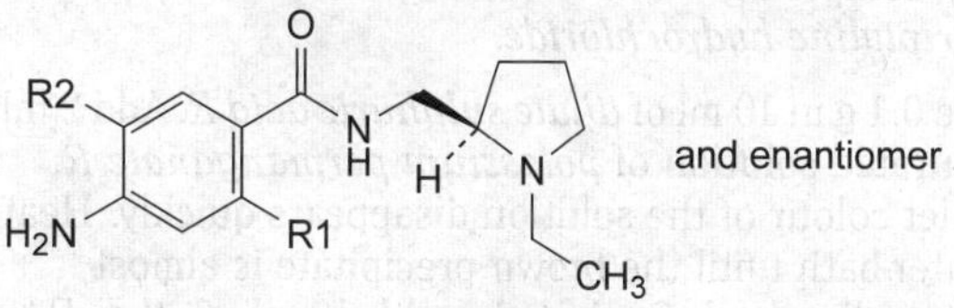

B. R1 = OH, R2 = SO_2-CH_2-CH_3: 4-amino-*N*-[[(2*RS*)-1-ethylpyrrolidin-2-yl]methyl]-5-(ethylsulphonyl)-2-hydroxybenzamide,

C. R1 = OCH_3, R2 = I: 4-amino-*N*-[[(2*RS*)-1-ethylpyrrolidin-2-yl]methyl]-5-iodo-2-methoxybenzamide,

D. R1 = OCH_3, R2 = SO_2-CH_3: 4-amino-*N*-[[(2*RS*)-1-ethylpyrrolidin-2-yl]methyl]-2-methoxy-5-(methylsulphonyl)benzamide,

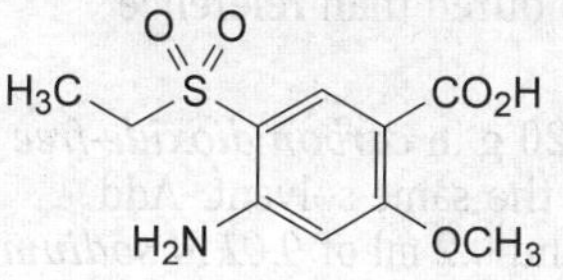

E. 4-amino-5-(ethylsulphonyl)-2-methoxybenzoic acid.

01/2005:0464

AMITRIPTYLINE HYDROCHLORIDE

Amitriptylini hydrochloridum

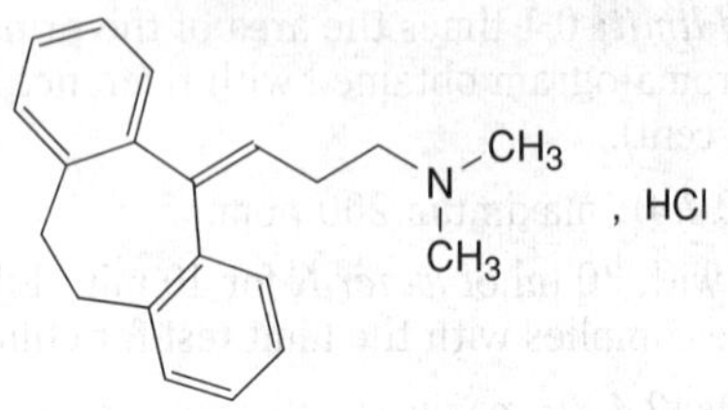

$C_{20}H_{24}ClN$ M_r 313.9

DEFINITION

Amitriptyline hydrochloride contains not less than 99.0 per cent and not more than the equivalent of 101.0 per cent of 3-(10,11-dihydro-5*H*-dibenzo[*a,d*][7]annulen-5-ylidene)-*N*,*N*-dimethylpropan-1-amine hydrochloride, calculated with reference to the dried substance.

CHARACTERS

A white or almost white powder or colourless crystals, freely soluble in water, in alcohol and in methylene chloride.

IDENTIFICATION

First identification: C, E.

Second identification: A, B, D, E.

A. Melting point (*2.2.14*): 195 °C to 199 °C.

B. Dissolve 25.0 mg in *methanol R* and dilute to 100.0 ml with the same solvent. Dilute 5.0 ml of the solution to 100.0 ml with *methanol R*. Examined between 230 nm and 350 nm (*2.2.25*), the solution shows an absorption maximum at 239 nm. The specific absorbance at the maximum is 435 to 475.

C. Examine by infrared absorption spectrophotometry (*2.2.24*), comparing with the *Ph. Eur. reference spectrum of amitriptyline hydrochloride.*

D. Dissolve 0.1 g in 10 ml of *dilute sulphuric acid R*. Add 2 ml of a saturated solution of *potassium permanganate R*. The violet colour of the solution disappears quickly. Heat on a water-bath until the brown precipitate is almost completely dissolved. Cool, shake with 15 ml of *ether R* to remove the white turbidity and discard the ether layer. To the aqueous layer add 5 ml of *concentrated ammonia R* and shake for 2 min. Add 3 ml of *methylene chloride R* and shake again. A violet-red colour is produced in the lower layer.

E. 50 mg gives reaction (b) of chlorides (*2.3.1*).

TESTS

Appearance of solution. Dissolve 1.25 g in *water R* and dilute to 25 ml with the same solvent. The solution is clear (*2.2.1*) and not more intensely coloured than reference solution B_7 (*2.2.2, Method II*).

Acidity or alkalinity. Dissolve 0.20 g in *carbon dioxide-free water R* and dilute to 10 ml with the same solvent. Add 0.1 ml of *methyl red solution R* and 0.2 ml of *0.01 M sodium hydroxide.* The solution is yellow. Add 0.4 ml of *0.01 M hydrochloric acid.* The solution is red.

Related substances. Examine by thin-layer chromatography (*2.2.27*), using a *TLC silica gel plate R. Prepare the solutions in subdued light and develop the chromatograms protected from light.*

Test solution. Dissolve 0.20 g of the substance to be examined in *alcohol R* and dilute to 10 ml with the same solvent.

Reference solution (a). Dissolve 10 mg of *dibenzosuberone CRS* in *alcohol R* and dilute to 10 ml with the same solvent. Dilute 1 ml of the solution to 100 ml with *alcohol R.*

Reference solution (b). Dissolve 10 mg of *cyclobenzaprine hydrochloride CRS* in *alcohol R* and dilute to 10 ml with the same solvent. Dilute 2 ml of the solution to 50 ml with *alcohol R.*

Apply to the plate 5 µl of each solution. Develop in an unsaturated tank over a path of 14 cm using a mixture of 3 volumes of *diethylamine R*, 15 volumes of *ethyl acetate R* and 85 volumes of *cyclohexane R*. Heat the plate at 100-105 °C for 10 min and spray with a freshly prepared mixture of 4 volumes of *formaldehyde solution R* and 96 volumes of *sulphuric acid R*. Heat at 100-105 °C for 10 min and examine immediately in ultraviolet light at 365 nm and at 254 nm. In the chromatogram obtained with the test solution: any spots corresponding to dibenzosuberone and cyclobenzaprine hydrochloride are not more intense than the spots in the chromatograms obtained with reference solutions (a) (0.05 per cent) and (b) (0.2 per cent), respectively; any spot, apart from the principal spot and any spots corresponding to dibenzosuberone and cyclobenzaprine hydrochloride, is not more intense than the spot in the chromatogram obtained with reference solution (b) (0.2 per cent).

Heavy metals (*2.4.8*). 1.0 g complies with limit test F (20 ppm). Prepare the standard using 2 ml of *lead standard solution (10 ppm Pb) R.*

Loss on drying (*2.2.32*). Not more than 0.5 per cent, determined on 1.000 g by drying in an oven at 100-105 °C for 2 h.

Sulphated ash (*2.4.14*). Not more than 0.1 per cent, determined on 1.0 g.

ASSAY

Dissolve 0.250 g in 30 ml of *alcohol R*. Titrate with *0.1 M sodium hydroxide,* determining the end-point potentiometrically (*2.2.20*).

1 ml of *0.1 M sodium hydroxide* is equivalent to 31.39 mg of $C_{20}H_{24}ClN$.

STORAGE

Store protected from light.

IMPURITIES

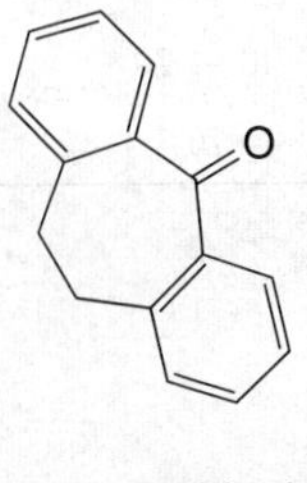

A. 10,11-dihydro-5*H*-dibenzo[*a,d*][7]annulen-5-one (dibenzosuberone),

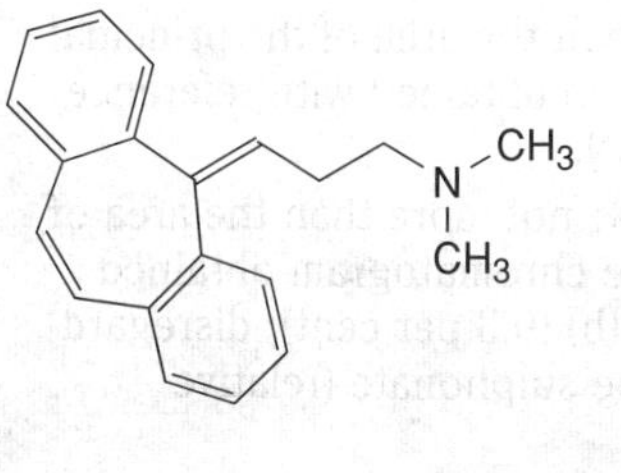

B. 3-(5*H*-dibenzo[*a,d*][7]annulen-5-ylidene)-*N,N*-dimethylpropan-1-amine (cyclobenzaprine),

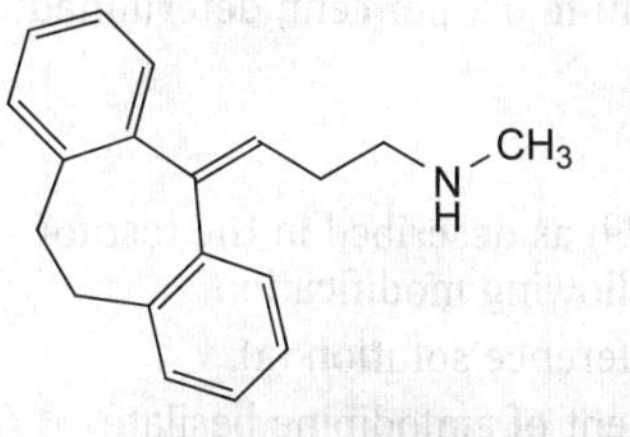

C. 3-(10,11-dihydro-5*H*-dibenzo[*a,d*][7]annulen-5-ylidene)-*N*-methylpropan-1-amine,

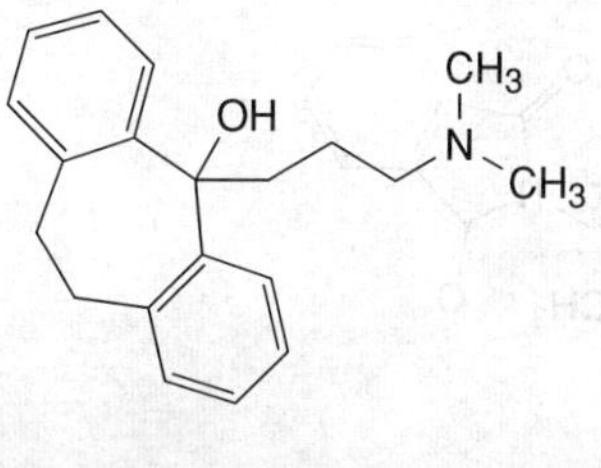

D. 5-[3-(dimethylamino)propyl]-10,11-dihydro-5*H*-dibenzo[*a,d*][7]annulen-5-ol,

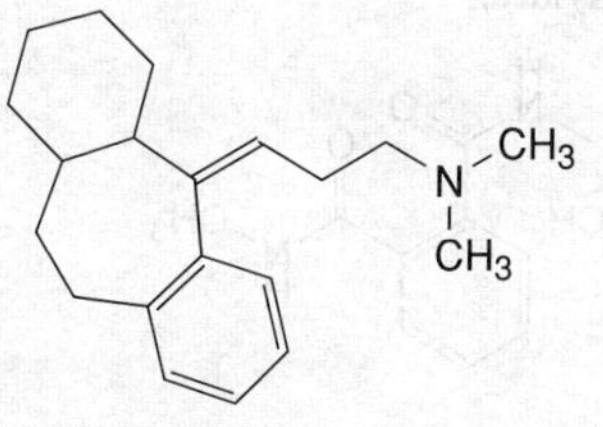

E. 3-(1,2,3,4,4a,10,11,11a-octahydro-5*H*-dibenzo[*a,d*][7]annulen-5-ylidene)-*N,N*-dimethylpropan-1-amine,

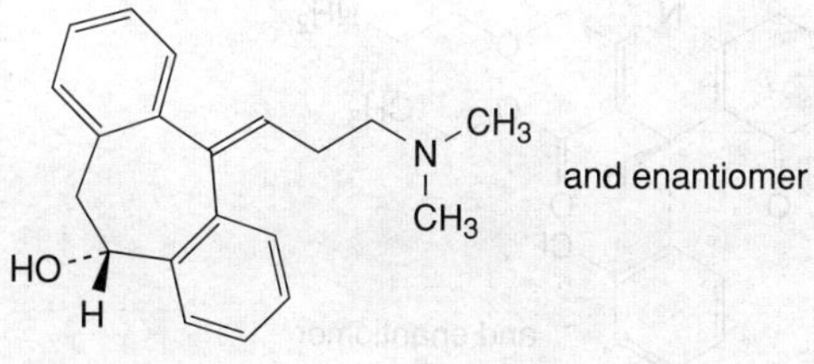

F. (10*RS*)-5-[3-(dimethylamino)propylidene]-10,11-dihydro-5*H*-dibenzo[*a,d*][7]annulen-10-ol.

01/2005:1491

AMLODIPINE BESILATE

Amlodipini besilas

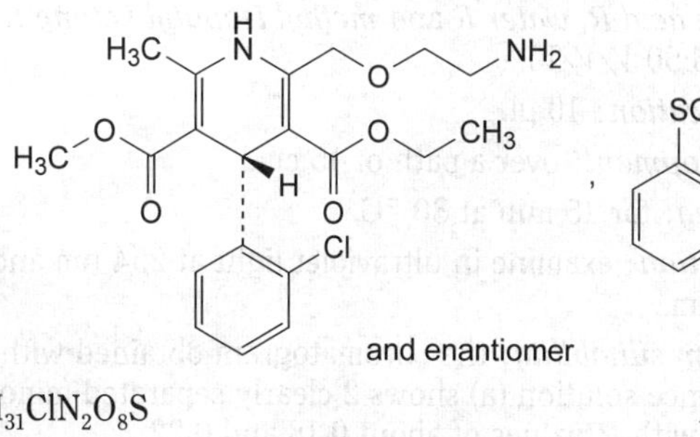

$C_{26}H_{31}ClN_2O_8S$ M_r 567.1

DEFINITION

3-Ethyl 5-methyl (4*RS*)-2-[(2-aminoethoxy)methyl]-4-(2-chlorophenyl)-6-methyl-1,4-dihydropyridine-3,5-dicarboxylate benzenesulphonate.

Content: 97.0 per cent to 102.0 per cent (anhydrous substance).

CHARACTERS

Appearance: white or almost white powder.

Solubility: slightly soluble in water, freely soluble in methanol, sparingly soluble in ethanol, slightly soluble in 2-propanol.

IDENTIFICATION

First identification: A.

Second identification: B, C.

A. Infrared absorption spectrophotometry (*2.2.24*).

Comparison: *amlodipine besilate CRS.*

Preparation: mulls.

B. Examine the chromatograms obtained in test A for related substances in ultraviolet light at 366 nm.

Results: the principal spot in the chromatogram obtained with test solution (b) is similar in position, colour and size to the principal spot in the chromatogram obtained with reference solution (b).

C. Dissolve 5.0 mg in a 1 per cent *V/V* solution of *0.1 M hydrochloric acid* in *methanol R* and dilute to 100.0 ml with the same acid solution. Examined between 300 nm and 400 nm (*2.2.25*), the solution shows an absorption maximum at 360 nm. The specific absorbance at the maximum is 113 to 121.

TESTS

Optical rotation (*2.2.7*): − 0.10° to + 0.10°.

Dissolve 0.250 g in *methanol R* and dilute to 25.0 ml with the same solvent.

Related substances

A. Thin-layer chromatography (*2.2.27*).

Test solution (a). Dissolve 0.140 g of the substance to be examined in *methanol R* and dilute to 2.0 ml with the same solvent.

Test solution (b). Dilute 1.0 ml of test solution (a) to 10.0 ml with *methanol R.*

Reference solution (a). Dissolve 70.0 mg of *amlodipine besilate CRS* in 1.0 ml of *methanol R.*

Reference solution (b). Dilute 1 ml of reference solution (a) to 10 ml with *methanol R.*

Reference solution (c). Dilute 3.0 ml of test solution (b) to 100.0 ml with *methanol R*.

Reference solution (d). Dilute 1.0 ml of test solution (b) to 100.0 ml with *methanol R*.

Plate: *TLC silica gel F_{254} plate R.*

Mobile phase: the upper layer of a mixture of *glacial acetic acid R*, *water R* and *methyl isobutyl ketone R* (25:25:50 *V/V/V*).

Application: 10 μl.

Development: over a path of 15 cm.

Drying: for 15 min at 80 °C.

Detection: examine in ultraviolet light at 254 nm and 366 nm.

System suitability: the chromatogram obtained with reference solution (a) shows 2 clearly separated minor spots with R_f values of about 0.18 and 0.22.

Limits: in the chromatogram obtained with test solution (a):

- *any impurity*: any spot, apart from the principal spot, is not more intense than the spot in the chromatogram obtained with reference solution (c) (0.3 per cent) and at most 2 spots are more intense than the spot in the chromatogram obtained with reference solution (d) (0.1 per cent).

B. Liquid chromatography (*2.2.29*).

Test solution (a). Dissolve 50.0 mg of the substance to be examined in the mobile phase and dilute to 50.0 ml with the mobile phase.

Test solution (b). Dilute 5.0 ml of test solution (a) to 100.0 ml with the mobile phase.

Reference solution (a). Dissolve 50.0 mg of *amlodipine besilate CRS* in the mobile phase and dilute to 50.0 ml with the mobile phase. Dilute 5.0 ml of the solution to 100.0 ml with the mobile phase.

Reference solution (b). Dilute 3.0 ml of test solution (a) to 100.0 ml with the mobile phase and dilute 5.0 ml of the solution to 50.0 ml with the mobile phase.

Reference solution (c). Dissolve 5 mg of the substance to be examined in 5 ml of *strong hydrogen peroxide solution R*. Heat at 70 °C for 45 min.

Column:

- *size*: *l* = 0.15 m, Ø = 3.9 mm,
- *stationary phase*: *octadecylsilyl silica gel for chromatography R* (5 μm).

Mobile phase: mix 15 volumes of *acetonitrile R*, 35 volumes of *methanol R* and 50 volumes of a solution prepared as follows: dissolve 7.0 ml of *triethylamine R* in 1 litre of *water R* and adjust to pH 3.0 ± 0.1 with *phosphoric acid R*.

Flow rate: 1.0 ml/min.

Detection: spectrophotometer at 237 nm.

Injection: 10 μl; inject test solution (a) and reference solutions (b) and (c).

Run time: 3 times the retention time of amlodipine.

Relative retention with reference to amlodipine (retention time = about 7 min): impurity D = about 0.5.

System suitability: reference solution (c):

- *resolution*: minimum 4.5 between the peaks corresponding to amlodipine and impurity D.

Limits:

- *correction factor*: for the calculation of content, multiply the peak area of impurity D by 2,
- *impurity D*: not more than the area of the principal peak in the chromatogram obtained with reference solution (b) (0.3 per cent),
- *total of other impurities*: not more than the area of the principal peak in the chromatogram obtained with reference solution (b) (0.3 per cent); disregard any peak due to benzene sulphonate (relative retention = about 0.2),
- *disregard limit*: 0.1 times the area of the principal peak in the chromatogram obtained with reference solution (b) (0.03 per cent).

Water (*2.5.12*): maximum 0.5 per cent, determined on 3.000 g.

Sulphated ash (*2.4.14*): maximum 0.2 per cent, determined on 1.0 g.

ASSAY

Liquid chromatography (*2.2.29*) as described in the test for related substances with the following modification.

Injection: test solution (b), reference solution (a).

Calculate the percentage content of amlodipine besilate from the areas of the peaks and the declared content of $C_{26}H_{31}ClN_2O_8S$ in *amlodipine besilate CRS*.

STORAGE

In an airtight container, protected from light.

IMPURITIES

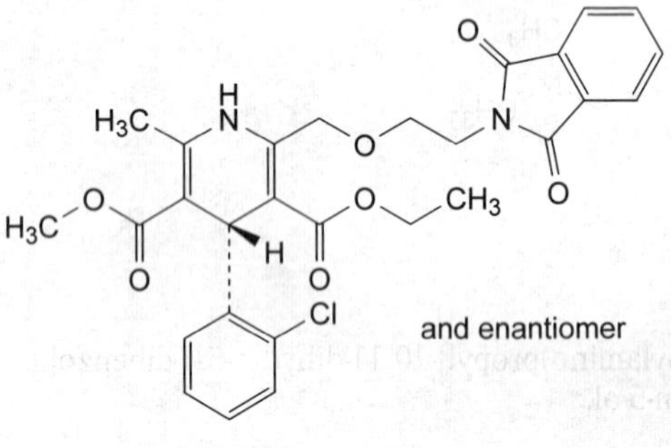

A. 3-ethyl 5-methyl (4*RS*)-4-(2-chlorophenyl)-2-[[2-(1,3-dioxo-1,3-dihydro-2*H*-isoindol-2-yl)ethoxy]methyl]-6-methyl-1,4-dihydropyridine-3,5-dicarboxylate,

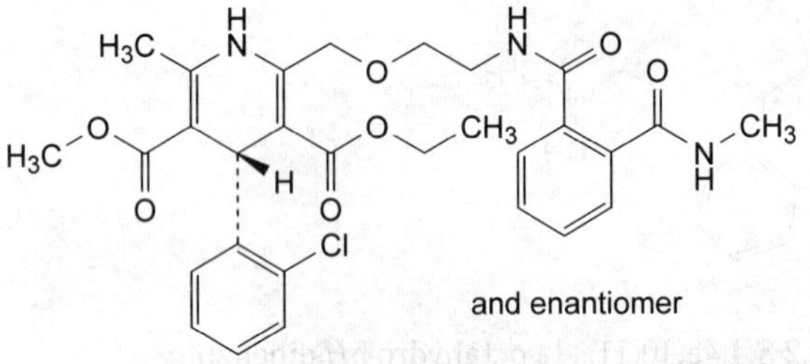

B. 3-ethyl 5-methyl (4*RS*)-4-(2-chlorophenyl)-6-methyl-2-[[2-[[2-(methylcarbamoyl)benzoyl]amino]ethoxy]methyl]-1,4-dihydropyridine-3,5-dicarboxylate,

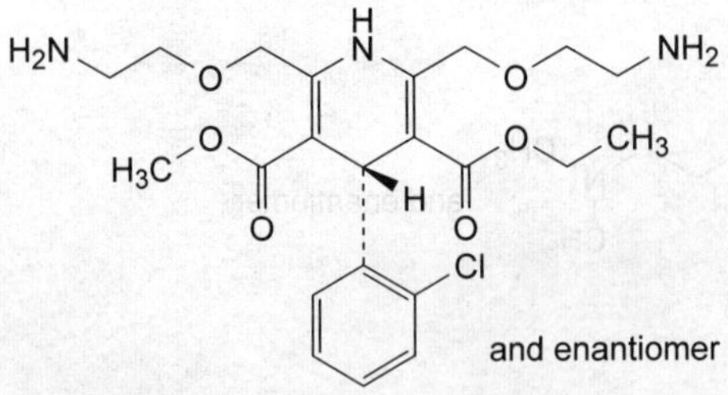

C. ethyl methyl (4*RS*)-2,6-bis[(2-aminoethoxy)methyl]-4-(2-chlorophenyl)-1,4-dihydropyridine-3,5-dicarboxylate,

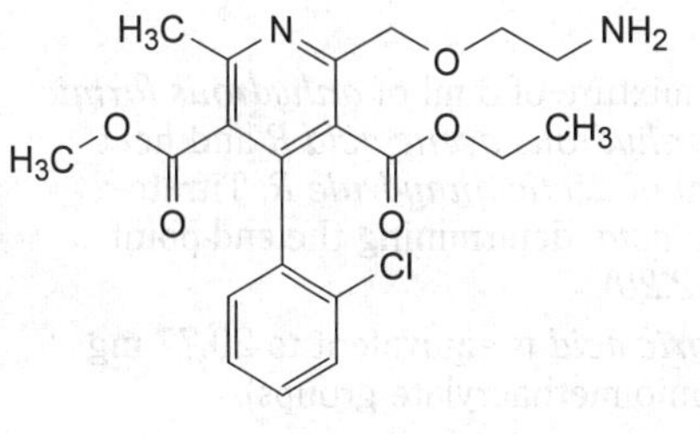

D. 3-ethyl 5-methyl 2-[(2-aminoethoxy)methyl]-4-(2-chlorophenyl)-6-methylpyridine-3,5-dicarboxylate.

01/2005:0877

AMMONIA SOLUTION, CONCENTRATED

Ammoniae solutio concentrata

DEFINITION

Concentrated ammonia solution contains not less than 25.0 per cent *m/m* and not more than 30.0 per cent *m/m* of ammonia (NH_3; M_r 17.03).

CHARACTERS

A clear, colourless liquid, very caustic, miscible with water and with alcohol.

IDENTIFICATION

A. Relative density (*2.2.5*): 0.892 to 0.910.

B. It is strongly alkaline (*2.2.4*).

C. To 0.5 ml add 5 ml of *water R*. Bubble air through the solution and lead the gaseous mixture obtained over the surface of a solution containing 1 ml of *0.1 M hydrochloric acid* and 0.05 ml of *methyl red solution R*. The colour changes from red to yellow. Add 1 ml of *sodium cobaltinitrite solution R*. A yellow precipitate is formed.

TESTS

Solution S. Evaporate 220 ml almost to dryness on a water-bath. Cool, add 1 ml of *dilute acetic acid R* and dilute to 20 ml with *distilled water R*.

Appearance of solution. To 2 ml add 8 ml of *water R*. The solution is clear (*2.2.1*) and colourless (*2.2.2, Method II*).

Oxidisable substances. Cautiously add, whilst cooling, 8.8 ml to 100 ml of *dilute sulphuric acid R*. Add 0.75 ml of *0.002 M potassium permanganate*. Allow to stand for 5 min. The solution remains faintly pink.

Pyridine and related substances. Measure the absorbance (*2.2.25*) at 252 nm using *water R* as the compensation liquid. The absorbance is not greater than 0.06 (2 ppm calculated as pyridine).

Carbonates. To 10 ml in a test-tube with a ground-glass neck add 10 ml of *calcium hydroxide solution R*. Stopper immediately and mix. Any opalescence in the solution is not more intense than that in a standard prepared at the same time and in the same manner using 10 ml of a 0.1 g/l solution of *anhydrous sodium carbonate R* (60 ppm).

Chlorides (*2.4.4*). Dilute 5 ml of solution S to 15 ml with *water R*. The solution complies with the limit test for chlorides (1 ppm).

Sulphates (*2.4.13*). Dilute 3 ml of solution S to 15 ml with *distilled water R*. The solution complies with the limit test for sulphates (5 ppm).

Iron (*2.4.9*). Dilute 4 ml of solution S to 10 ml with *water R*. The solution complies with the limit test for iron (0.25 ppm).

Heavy metals (*2.4.8*). Dilute 4 ml of solution S to 20 ml with *water R*. 12 ml of the solution complies with limit test A for heavy metals (1 ppm). Prepare the standard using *lead standard solution (2 ppm Pb) R*.

Residue on evaporation. Evaporate 50 ml to dryness on a water-bath and dry at 100 °C to 105 °C for 1 h. The residue weighs not more than 1 mg (0.02 g/l).

ASSAY

Weigh accurately a flask with a ground-glass neck containing 50.0 ml of *1 M hydrochloric acid*. Add 2 ml of the substance to be examined and re-weigh. Add 0.1 ml of *methyl red solution R* as indicator. Titrate with *1 M sodium hydroxide* until the colour changes from red to yellow.

1 ml of *1 M hydrochloric acid* is equivalent to 17.03 mg of NH_3.

STORAGE

Store protected from air, at a temperature not exceeding 20 °C.

01/2005:2081

AMMONIO METHACRYLATE COPOLYMER (TYPE A)

Ammonio methacrylatis copolymerum A

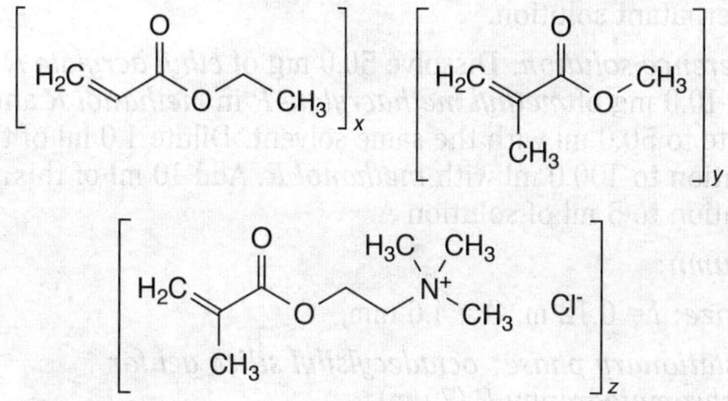

DEFINITION

Poly(ethyl propenoate-co-methyl 2-methylpropenoate-co-2-(trimethylammonio)ethyl 2-methylpropenoate) chloride having a mean relative molecular mass of about 150 000. The ratio of ethyl propenoate groups to methyl 2-methylpropenoate groups to 2-(trimethylammonio)ethyl 2-methylpropenoate groups is about 1:2:0.2.

Content of ammonio methacrylate groups: 8.9 per cent to 12.3 per cent (dried substance).

CHARACTERS

Appearance: colourless to white or almost white granules or powder.

Solubility: practically insoluble in water, freely soluble in ethanol and in methylene chloride giving clear to cloudy solutions. Due to the polymeric nature of the substance, a stirring time of up to 5 h may be necessary.

IDENTIFICATION

A. Infrared absorption spectrophotometry (*2.2.24*).

Preparation: drop solution S (see Tests) on a disc of *potassium bromide R* and dry *in vacuo* at 70 °C for 2 h.

Comparison: *Ph. Eur. reference spectrum of ammonio methacrylate copolymer (type A)*.

B. It complies with the test for viscosity (see Tests).

C. It complies with the limits of the assay.

TESTS

Solution S. Dissolve a quantity of the substance to be examined corresponding to 12.5 g of the dried substance in a mixture of 35.0 g of *acetone R* and 52.5 g of *2-propanol R.*

Viscosity (*2.2.10*): maximum 15 mPa·s, determined on solution S.

Apparatus: rotating viscosimeter.

Dimensions:

- *spindle*: diameter = 25.15 mm; height = 90.74 mm; shaft diameter = 4.0 mm;
- *cylinder*: diameter = 27.62 mm; height = 0.135 m.

Stirring speed: 30 r/min.

Volume of solution: 16 ml of solution S.

Temperature: 20 °C.

Appearance of a film. Spread 2 ml of solution S evenly on a glass plate. Upon drying a clear film is formed.

Monomers. Liquid chromatography (*2.2.29*).

Solution A. Dissolve 3.5 g of *sodium perchlorate R* in *water for chromatography R* and dilute to 100 ml with the same solvent.

Test solution. Dissolve 5.00 g of the substance to be examined in *methanol R* and dilute to 50.0 ml with the same solvent. To 10.0 ml of this solution add 5.0 ml of solution A, dropwise while continuously stirring. Remove the precipitated polymer by centrifugation. Use the clear supernatant solution.

Reference solution. Dissolve 50.0 mg of *ethyl acrylate R* and 10.0 mg of *methyl methacrylate R* in *methanol R* and dilute to 50.0 ml with the same solvent. Dilute 1.0 ml of the solution to 100.0 ml with *methanol R*. Add 10 ml of this solution to 5 ml of solution A.

Column:

- *size*: l = 0.12 m, Ø = 4.6 mm,
- *stationary phase*: *octadecylsilyl silica gel for chromatography R* (7 µm).

Mobile phase: dilute *phosphoric acid R* with *water for chromatography R* to obtain a solution at pH 2.0; mix 800 ml of this solution and 200 ml of *methanol R*, filter and degas.

Flow rate: 2.0 ml/min.

Detection: spectrophotometer at 202 nm.

Injection: 50 µl.

System suitability: reference solution:

- *resolution*: minimum 1.5 between the peaks due to impurity A and impurity B.

Limits:

- *impurity A*: not more than the area of the corresponding peak in the chromatogram obtained with the reference solution (100 ppm),
- *impurity B*: not more than 2.5 times the area of the corresponding peak in the chromatogram obtained with the reference solution (50 ppm).

Methanol (*2.4.24, System A*): maximum 1.5 per cent.

Heavy metals (*2.4.8*): maximum 20 ppm.

1.0 g complies with limit test C. Prepare the standard using 2.0 ml of *lead standard solution (10 ppm Pb) R*.

Loss on drying (*2.2.32*): maximum 3.0 per cent, determined on 1.000 g by drying *in vacuo* at 80 °C for 5 h.

ASSAY

Dissolve 1.000 g in a mixture of 3 ml of *anhydrous formic acid R* and 30 ml of *anhydrous acetic acid R* and heat to dissolve. Add 20 ml of *acetic anhydride R*. Titrate with *0.1 M perchloric acid*, determining the end-point potentiometrically (*2.2.20*).

1 ml of *0.1 M perchloric acid* is equivalent to 20.77 mg of $C_9H_{18}O_2NCl$ (ammonio methacrylate groups).

IMPURITIES

Specified impurities: A, B.

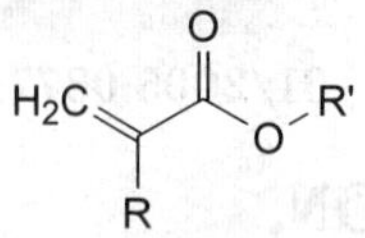

A. R = H, R′ = C_2H_5: ethyl propenoate (ethyl acrylate),

B. R = R′ = CH_3: methyl 2-methylpropenoate (methyl methacrylate).

01/2005:2082

AMMONIO METHACRYLATE COPOLYMER (TYPE B)

Ammonio methacrylatis copolymerum B

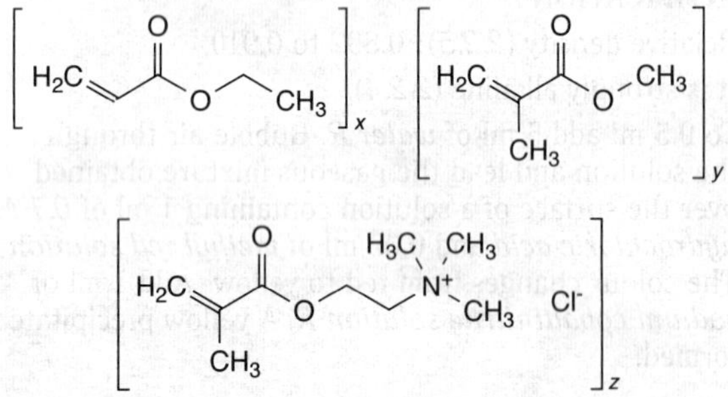

DEFINITION

Poly(ethyl propenoate-co-methyl 2-methylpropenoate-co-2-(trimethylammonio)ethyl 2-methylpropenoate) chloride having a mean relative molecular mass of about 150 000.

The ratio of ethyl propenoate groups to methyl 2-methylpropenoate groups to 2-(trimethylammonio)ethyl 2-methylpropenoate groups is about 1:2:0.1.

Content of ammonio methacrylate groups: 4.5 per cent to 7.0 per cent (dried substance).

CHARACTERS

Appearance: colourless to white or almost white granules or powder.

Solubility: practically insoluble in water, freely soluble in ethanol and in methylene chloride giving clear to cloudy solutions. Due to the polymeric nature of the substance, a stirring time of up to 5 h may be necessary.

IDENTIFICATION

A. Infrared absorption spectrophotometry (*2.2.24*).

Preparation: drop solution S (see Tests) on a disc of *potassium bromide R* and dry *in vacuo* at 70 °C for 2 h.

Comparison: *Ph. Eur. reference spectrum of ammonio methacrylate copolymer (type B).*

B. It complies with the test for viscosity (see Tests).

C. It complies with the limits of the assay.

TESTS

Solution S. Dissolve a quantity of the substance to be examined corresponding to 12.5 g of the dried substance in a mixture of 35.0 g of *acetone R* and 52.5 g of *2-propanol R.*

Viscosity (*2.2.10*): maximum 15 mPa·s, determined on solution S.

Apparatus: rotating viscosimeter.

Dimensions:

- *spindle*: diameter = 25.15 mm; height = 90.74 mm; shaft diameter = 4.0 mm;
- *cylinder*: diameter = 27.62 mm; height = 0.135 m.

Stirring speed: 30 r/min.

Volume of solution: 16 ml of solution S.

Temperature: 20 °C.

Appearance of a film. Spread 2 ml of solution S evenly on a glass plate. Upon drying a clear film is formed.

Monomers. Liquid chromatography (*2.2.29*).

Solution A. Dissolve 3.5 g of *sodium perchlorate R* in *water for chromatography R* and dilute to 100 ml with the same solvent.

Test solution. Dissolve 5.00 g of the substance to be examined in *methanol R* and dilute to 50.0 ml with the same solvent. To 10.0 ml of this solution add 5.0 ml of solution A, dropwise while continuously stirring. Remove the precipitated polymer by centrifugation. Use the clear supernatant solution.

Reference solution. Dissolve 50.0 mg of *ethyl acrylate R* and 10.0 mg of *methyl methacrylate R* in *methanol R* and dilute to 50.0 ml with the same solvent. Dilute 1.0 ml of the solution to 100.0 ml with *methanol R*. Add 10 ml of this solution to 5 ml of solution A.

Column:

- *size*: *l* = 0.12 m, Ø = 4.6 mm,
- *stationary phase*: *octadecylsilyl silica gel for chromatography R* (7 µm).

Mobile phase: dilute *phosphoric acid R* with *water for chromatography R* to obtain a solution at pH 2.0; mix 800 ml of this solution and 200 ml of *methanol R*, filter and degas.

Flow rate: 2.0 ml/min.

Detection: spectrophotometer at 202 nm.

Injection: 50 µl.

System suitability: reference solution:

- *resolution*: minimum 1.5 between the peaks due to impurity A and impurity B.

Limits:

- *impurity A*: not more than the area of the corresponding peak in the chromatogram obtained with the reference solution (100 ppm),
- *impurity B*: not more than 2.5 times the area of the corresponding peak in the chromatogram obtained with the reference solution (50 ppm).

Methanol (*2.4.24, System A*): maximum 1.5 per cent.

Heavy metals (*2.4.8*): maximum 20 ppm.

1.0 g complies with limit test C. Prepare the standard using 2.0 ml of *lead standard solution (10 ppm Pb) R*.

Loss on drying (*2.2.32*): maximum 3.0 per cent, determined on 1.000 g by drying *in vacuo* at 80 °C for 5 h.

ASSAY

Dissolve 2.000 g in a mixture of 3 ml of *anhydrous formic acid R* and 30 ml of *anhydrous acetic acid R* and heat to dissolve. Add 20 ml of *acetic anhydride R.* Titrate with *0.1 M perchloric acid*, determining the end-point potentiometrically (*2.2.20*).

1 ml of *0.1 M perchloric acid* is equivalent to 20.77 mg of $C_9H_{18}O_2NCl$ (ammonio methacrylate groups).

IMPURITIES

Specified impurities: A, B.

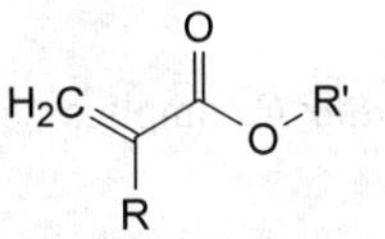

A. R = H, R′ = C_2H_5: ethyl propenoate (ethyl acrylate),

B. R = R′ = CH_3: methyl 2-methylpropenoate (methyl methacrylate).

01/2005:1389

AMMONIUM BROMIDE

Ammonii bromidum

NH_4Br M_r 97.9

DEFINITION

Content: 98.5 per cent to 100.5 per cent (dried substance).

CHARACTERS

Appearance: white or almost white, crystalline powder or colourless crystals, hygroscopic.

Solubility: freely soluble in water, sparingly soluble in alcohol.

It becomes yellow when exposed to light or air.

IDENTIFICATION

A. It gives reaction (a) of bromides (*2.3.1*).

B. 10 ml of solution S (see Tests) gives the reaction of ammonium salts (*2.3.1*).

TESTS

Solution S. Dissolve 10.0 g in *carbon dioxide-free water R* prepared from *distilled water R* and dilute to 100 ml with the same solvent.

Appearance of solution. Solution S is clear (*2.2.1*) and colourless (*2.2.2, Method II*).

Acidity or alkalinity. To 10 ml of solution S add 0.05 ml of *methyl red solution R*. Not more than 0.5 ml of *0.01 M hydrochloric acid* or *0.01 M sodium hydroxide* is required to change the colour of the indicator.

Bromates. To 10 ml of solution S add 1 ml of *starch solution R*, 0.1 ml of a 100 g/l solution of *potassium iodide R* and 0.25 ml of *0.5 M sulphuric acid* and allow to stand protected from light for 5 min. No blue or violet colour develops.

Chlorides: maximum 0.6 per cent.

In a conical flask, dissolve 1.000 g in 20 ml of *dilute nitric acid R*. Add 5 ml of *strong hydrogen peroxide solution R* and heat on a water-bath until the solution is completely decolorised. Wash down the sides of the flask with a little *water R* and heat on a water-bath for 15 min. Allow to cool, dilute to 50 ml with *water R* and add 5.0 ml of *0.1 M silver nitrate* and 1 ml of *dibutyl phthalate R*. Shake and titrate with *0.1 M ammonium thiocyanate* using 5 ml of *ferric ammonium sulphate solution R2* as indicator. Not more than 1.7 ml of *0.1 M silver nitrate* is used. Note the volume of *0.1 M silver nitrate* used (see Assay). Carry out a blank test.

Iodides. To 5 ml of solution S add 0.15 ml of *ferric chloride solution R1* and 2 ml of *methylene chloride R*. Shake and allow to separate. The lower layer is colourless (*2.2.2, Method I*).

Sulphates (*2.4.13*): maximum 100 ppm.

15 ml of solution S complies with the limit test for sulphates.

Iron (*2.4.9*): maximum 20 ppm.

5 ml of solution S diluted to 10 ml with *water R* complies with the limit test for iron.

Magnesium and alkaline-earth metals (*2.4.7*): maximum 200 ppm, calculated as Ca.

10.0 g complies with the limit test for magnesium and alkaline-earth metals. The volume of *0.01 M sodium edetate* used does not exceed 5.0 ml.

Heavy metals (*2.4.8*): maximum 10 ppm.

12 ml of solution S complies with limit test A. Prepare the standard using *lead standard solution (1 ppm Pb) R*.

Loss on drying (*2.2.32*): maximum 1.0 per cent, determined on 1.000 g by drying in an oven at 100-105 °C.

Sulphated ash (*2.4.14*): maximum 0.1 per cent, determined on 1.0 g.

ASSAY

Dissolve 1.500 g in *water R* and dilute to 100.0 ml with the same solvent. To 10.0 ml of the solution add 50 ml of *water R*, 5 ml of *dilute nitric acid R*, 25.0 ml of *0.1 M silver nitrate* and 2 ml of *dibutyl phthalate R*. Shake. Titrate with *0.1 M ammonium thiocyanate* using 2 ml of *ferric ammonium sulphate solution R2* as indicator and shaking vigorously towards the end-point.

1 ml of *0.1 M silver nitrate* is equivalent to 9.794 mg of NH_4Br.

Calculate the percentage content of NH_4Br from the expression:

$$a - 2.763\,b$$

a = percentage content of NH_4Br and NH_4Cl obtained in the assay and calculated as NH_4Br,

b = percentage content of Cl obtained in the test for chlorides.

STORAGE

In an airtight container, protected from light.

01/2005:0007

AMMONIUM CHLORIDE

Ammonii chloridum

NH_4Cl M_r 53.49

DEFINITION

Ammonium chloride contains not less than 99.0 per cent and not more than the equivalent of 100.5 per cent of NH_4Cl, calculated with reference to the dried substance.

CHARACTERS

A white, crystalline powder or colourless crystals, freely soluble in water.

IDENTIFICATION

A. It gives the reactions of chlorides (*2.3.1*).

B. 10 ml of solution S (see Tests) gives the reaction of ammonium salts (*2.3.1*).

TESTS

Solution S. Dissolve 10.0 g in *carbon dioxide-free water R* prepared from *distilled water R* and dilute to 100 ml with the same solvent.

Appearance of solution. Solution S is clear (*2.2.1*) and colourless (*2.2.2, Method II*).

Acidity or alkalinity. To 10 ml of solution S add 0.05 ml of *methyl red solution R*. Not more than 0.5 ml of *0.01 M hydrochloric acid* or *0.01 M sodium hydroxide* is required to change the colour of the indicator.

Bromides and iodides. To 10 ml of solution S add 0.1 ml of *dilute hydrochloric acid R* and 0.05 ml of *chloramine solution R*. After 1 min, add 2 ml of *chloroform R* and shake vigorously. The chloroform layer remains colourless (*2.2.2, Method I*).

Sulphates (*2.4.13*). 10 ml of solution S diluted to 15 ml with *distilled water R* complies with the limit test for sulphates (150 ppm).

Calcium (*2.4.3*). 5 ml of solution S diluted to 15 ml with *distilled water R* complies with the limit test for calcium (200 ppm).

Iron (*2.4.9*). 5 ml of solution S diluted to 10 ml with *water R* complies with the limit test for iron (20 ppm).

Heavy metals (*2.4.8*). 12 ml of solution S complies with limit test A (10 ppm). Prepare the standard using *lead standard solution (1 ppm Pb) R*.

Loss on drying (*2.2.32*). Not more than 1.0 per cent, determined on 1.00 g by drying in an oven at 100-105 °C for 2 h.

Sulphated ash (*2.4.14*). Not more than 0.1 per cent, determined on 2.0 g.

ASSAY

Dissolve 1.000 g in 20 ml of *water R* and add a mixture of 5 ml of *formaldehyde solution R*, previously neutralised to *phenolphthalein solution R*, and 20 ml of *water R*. After 1 min to 2 min, titrate slowly with *1 M sodium hydroxide*, using a further 0.2 ml of the same indicator.

1 ml of *1 M sodium hydroxide* is equivalent to 53.49 mg of NH_4Cl.

01/2005:1772

AMMONIUM GLYCYRRHIZATE

Ammonii glycyrrhizas

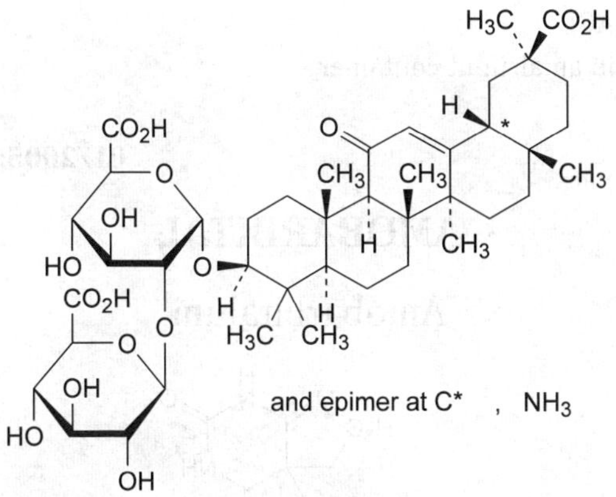

$C_{42}H_{65}NO_{16}$ M_r 840

DEFINITION

Mixture of ammonium 18α- and 18β-glycyrrhizate (ammonium salt of (20β)-3β-[[2-*O*-(β-D-glucopyranosyluronic acid)-α-D-glucopyranosyluronic acid]oxy]-11-oxoolean-12-en-29-oic acid), the 18β-isomer being the main component.

Content: 98.0 per cent to 102.0 per cent (anhydrous substance).

CHARACTERS

Appearance: white or yellowish-white, hygroscopic powder.

Solubility: slightly soluble in water, very slightly soluble in anhydrous ethanol, practically insoluble in acetone. It dissolves in dilute solutions of acids and of alkali hydroxides.

IDENTIFICATION

A. Infrared absorption spectrophotometry (*2.2.24*).
Comparison: *ammonium glycyrrhizate CRS.*

B. Dissolve 0.1 g in 20 ml of *water R,* add 2 ml of *dilute sodium hydroxide solution R* and heat cautiously. On heating, the solution gives off vapours that may be identified by the alkaline reaction of wet litmus paper (*2.3.1*).

TESTS

Appearance of solution. The solution is clear (*2.2.1*) and not more intensely coloured than reference solution BY_7 (*2.2.2, Method I*).

Dissolve 1.0 g in *ethanol (20 per cent V/V) R* and dilute to 100.0 ml with the same solvent.

Specific optical rotation (*2.2.7*): + 49.0 to + 54.0 (anhydrous substance).

Dissolve 0.5 g in *ethanol (50 per cent V/V) R* and dilute to 50.0 ml with the same solvent.

Related substances. Liquid chromatography (*2.2.29*).

Test solution. Dissolve 0.100 g of the substance to be examined in the mobile phase and dilute to 100.0 ml with the mobile phase.

Reference solution (a). Dilute 1.0 ml of the test solution to 20.0 ml with the mobile phase.

Reference solution (b). Dissolve 50 mg of *ammonium glycyrrhizate CRS* in the mobile phase and dilute to 50.0 ml with the mobile phase. Dilute 1.0 ml of the solution to 20.0 ml with the mobile phase.

Column:

- *size*: *l* = 0.25 m, Ø = 4.0 mm,
- *stationary phase*: *octadecylsilyl silica gel for chromatography R* (5-10 µm).

Mobile phase: *glacial acetic acid R, acetonitrile R, water R* (6:380:614 *V/V/V*).

Flow rate: 1.2 ml/min.

Detection: spectrophotometer at 254 nm.

Injection: 10 µl.

Run time: 3 times the retention time of 18β-glycyrrhizic acid.

Relative retention with reference to 18β-glycyrrhizic acid (retention time = about 8 min): impurity A = about 0.8; 18α-glycyrrhizic acid = about 1.2.

System suitability: reference solution (b):

- *resolution*: minimum 2.0 between the peaks due to 18β-glycyrrhizic acid and 18α-glycyrrhizic acid.

Limits:

- *18α-glycyrrhizic acid*: not more than twice the sum of the areas of the peaks in the chromatogram obtained with reference solution (a) (10.0 per cent),
- *impurity A*: not more than the sum of the areas of the peaks in the chromatogram obtained with reference solution (a) (5.0 per cent),
- *any other impurity*: for each impurity, not more than 0.4 times the sum of the areas of the peaks in the chromatogram obtained with reference solution (a) (2.0 per cent),
- *total of other impurities*: not more than 1.4 times the sum of the areas of the peaks in the chromatogram obtained with reference solution (a) (7.0 per cent),
- *disregard limit*: 0.04 times the sum of the areas of the peaks in the chromatogram obtained with reference solution (a) (0.2 per cent).

Heavy metals (*2.4.8*): maximum 20 ppm.

1.0 g complies with limit test C. Prepare the reference solution using 2 ml of *lead standard solution (10 ppm Pb) R.*

Water (*2.5.12*): maximum 6.0 per cent, determined on 0.250 g.

Sulphated ash (*2.4.14*): maximum 0.2 per cent, determined on 1.0 g.

ASSAY

Dissolve 0.600 g in 60 ml of *acetic acid R* heating at 80 °C if necessary. Cool. Titrate with *0.1 M perchloric acid,* determining the end-point potentiometrically (*2.2.20*).

1 ml of *0.1 M perchloric acid* is equivalent to 84.0 mg of $C_{42}H_{65}NO_{16}$.

STORAGE

In an airtight container.

IMPURITIES

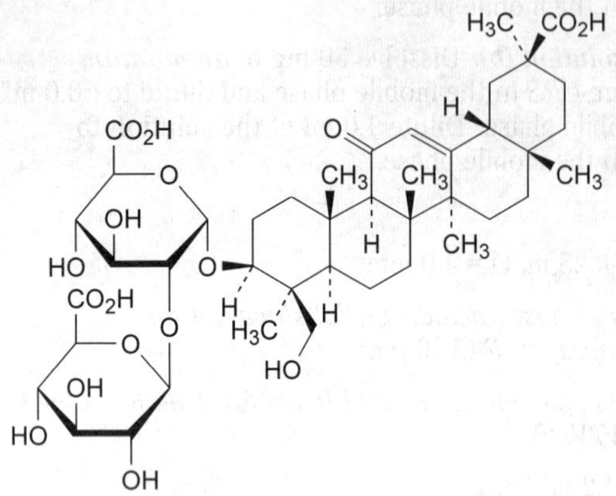

A. (4β,20β)-3β-[[2-*O*-(β-D-glucopyranosyluronic acid)-α-D-glucopyranosyluronic acid]oxy]-23-hydroxy-11-oxoolean-12-en-29-oic acid (24-hydroxyglycyrrhizinic acid).

01/2005:1390

AMMONIUM HYDROGEN CARBONATE

Ammonii hydrogenocarbonas

NH_4HCO_3 M_r 79.1

DEFINITION

Ammonium hydrogen carbonate contains not less than 98.0 per cent and not more than 101.0 per cent of the equivalent of ammonium hydrogen carbonate.

CHARACTERS

A fine, white, crystalline powder or white crystals, slightly hygroscopic, freely soluble in water, practically insoluble in alcohol.

It volatilises rapidly at 60 °C. The volatilisation takes place slowly at ambient temperatures if the substance is slightly moist. It is in a state of equilibrium with ammonium carbamate.

IDENTIFICATION

A. It gives the reaction of carbonates and bicarbonates (*2.3.1*).

B. Dissolve 50 mg in 2 ml of *water R*. The solution gives the reaction of ammonium salts (*2.3.1*).

TESTS

Solution S. Dissolve 14.0 g in 100 ml of *distilled water R*. Boil to remove the ammonia, allow to cool and dilute to 100.0 ml with *distilled water R*.

Chlorides (*2.4.4*). Dilute 5 ml of solution S to 15 ml with *water R*. The solution complies with the limit test for chlorides (70 ppm).

Sulphates (*2.4.13*). 15 ml of solution S complies with the limit test for sulphates (70 ppm).

Iron (*2.4.9*). Dilute 1.8 ml of solution S to 10 ml with *water R*. The solution complies with the limit test for iron (40 ppm).

Heavy metals (*2.4.8*). Dissolve cautiously 2.5 g in 25 ml of *1 M hydrochloric acid*. 12 ml of the solution complies with limit test A for heavy metals (10 ppm). Prepare the standard using *lead standard solution (1 ppm Pb) R*.

ASSAY

Dissolve cautiously 1.0 g in 20.0 ml of *0.5 M sulphuric acid* and dilute to 50 ml with *water R*. Boil, cool and titrate the excess of acid with *1 M sodium hydroxide*, using 0.1 ml of *methyl red solution R* as indicator.

1 ml of *0.5 M sulphuric acid* is equivalent to 79.1 mg of NH_4HCO_3.

STORAGE

Store in an airtight container.

01/2005:0594

AMOBARBITAL

Amobarbitalum

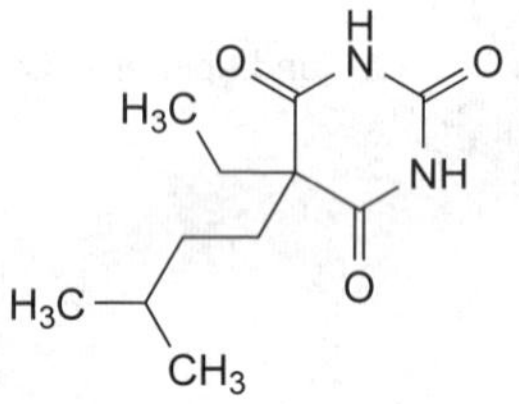

$C_{11}H_{18}N_2O_3$ M_r 226.3

DEFINITION

Amobarbital contains not less than 99.0 per cent and not more than the equivalent of 101.0 per cent of 5-ethyl-5-(3-methylbutyl)pyrimidin-2,4,6(1*H*,3*H*,5*H*)-trione, calculated with reference to the dried substance.

CHARACTERS

A white, crystalline powder, very slightly soluble in water, freely soluble in alcohol, soluble in methylene chloride. It forms water-soluble compounds with alkali hydroxides and carbonates and with ammonia.

IDENTIFICATION

First identification: A, B.

Second identification: A, C, D.

A. Determine the melting point (*2.2.14*) of the substance to be examined. Mix equal parts of the substance to be examined and *amobarbital CRS* and determine the melting point of the mixture. The difference between the melting points (which are about 157 °C) is not greater than 2 °C.

B. Examine by infrared absorption spectrophotometry (*2.2.24*), comparing with the spectrum obtained with *amobarbital CRS*.

C. Examine by thin-layer chromatography (*2.2.27*), using *silica gel GF_{254} R* as the coating substance.

Test solution. Dissolve 0.1 g of the substance to be examined in *alcohol R* and dilute to 100 ml with the same solvent.

Reference solution. Dissolve 0.1 g of *amobarbital CRS* in *alcohol R* and dilute to 100 ml with the same solvent.

Apply separately to the plate 10 µl of each solution. Develop over a path of 18 cm using the lower layer from a mixture of 5 volumes of *concentrated ammonia R*, 15 volumes of *alcohol R* and 80 volumes of *chloroform R*. Examine immediately in ultraviolet light at 254 nm. The principal spot in the chromatogram obtained with the test solution is similar in position and size to the principal spot in the chromatogram obtained with the reference solution.

D. It gives the reaction of non-nitrogen substituted barbiturates (*2.3.1*).

TESTS

Appearance of solution. Dissolve 1.0 g in a mixture of 4 ml of *dilute sodium hydroxide solution R* and 6 ml of *water R*. The solution is clear (*2.2.1*) and not more intensely coloured than reference solution Y_6 (*2.2.2, Method II*).

Acidity or alkalinity. To 1.0 g add 50 ml of *water R* and boil for 2 min. Allow to cool and filter. To 10 ml of the filtrate add 0.15 ml of *methyl red solution R* and 0.1 ml of *0.01 M sodium hydroxide*. The solution is yellow. Add 0.2 ml of *0.01 M hydrochloric acid*. The solution is red.

Related substances. Examine by thin-layer chromatography (*2.2.27*), using *silica gel GF_{254} R* as the coating substance.

Test solution. Dissolve 1.0 g of the substance to be examined in *alcohol R* and dilute to 100 ml with the same solvent.

Reference solution. Dilute 0.5 ml of the test solution to 100 ml with *alcohol R*.

Apply separately to the plate 20 µl of each solution. Develop over a path of 15 cm using the lower layer from a mixture of 5 volumes of *concentrated ammonia R*, 15 volumes of *alcohol R* and 80 volumes of *chloroform R*. Examine the plate immediately in ultraviolet light at 254 nm. Any spot in the chromatogram obtained with the test solution, apart from the principal spot, is not more intense than the spot in the chromatogram obtained with the reference solution. Spray with *diphenylcarbazone mercuric reagent R*. Allow the plate to dry in air and spray with freshly prepared *alcoholic potassium hydroxide solution R* diluted 1 in 5 with *aldehyde-free alcohol R*. Heat at 100 °C to 105 °C for 5 min and examine immediately. Any spot in the chromatogram obtained with the test solution, apart from the principal spot, is not more intense than the spot in the chromatogram obtained with the reference solution (0.5 per cent).

Loss on drying (*2.2.32*). Not more than 0.5 per cent, determined on 1.000 g by drying in an oven at 100 °C to 105 °C.

Sulphated ash (*2.4.14*). Not more than 0.1 per cent, determined on 1.0 g.

ASSAY

Dissolve 0.100 g in 5 ml of *pyridine R*. Add 0.5 ml of *thymolphthalein solution R* and 10 ml of *silver nitrate solution in pyridine R*. Titrate with *0.1 M ethanolic sodium hydroxide* until a pure blue colour is obtained. Carry out a blank titration.

1 ml of *0.1 M ethanolic sodium hydroxide* is equivalent to 11.31 mg of $C_{11}H_{18}N_2O_3$.

01/2005:0166

AMOBARBITAL SODIUM

Amobarbitalum natricum

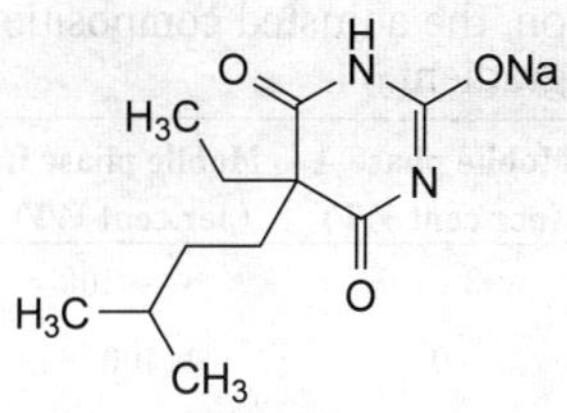

$C_{11}H_{17}N_2NaO_3$ M_r 248.3

DEFINITION

Amobarbital sodium contains not less than 98.5 per cent and not more than the equivalent of 102.0 per cent of sodium derivative of 5-ethyl-5-(3-methylbutyl)pyrimidin-2,4,6(1*H*,3*H*,5*H*)-trione, calculated with reference to the dried substance.

CHARACTERS

A white, granular powder, hygroscopic, very soluble in carbon dioxide-free water (a small fraction may be insoluble), freely soluble in alcohol.

IDENTIFICATION

First identification: A, B, E.

Second identification: A, C, D, E.

A. Acidify 10 ml of solution S (see Tests) with *dilute hydrochloric acid R* and shake with 20 ml of *ether R*. Separate the ether layer, wash with 10 ml of *water R*, dry over *anhydrous sodium sulphate R* and filter. Evaporate the filtrate to dryness and dry the residue at 100 °C to 105 °C (test residue). Repeat the operations using 0.1 g of *amobarbital sodium CRS* (reference residue). Determine the melting point (*2.2.14*) of the test residue. Mix equal parts of the test residue and the reference residue and determine the melting point of the mixture. The difference between the melting points (which are about 157 °C) is not greater than 2 °C.

B. Examine by infrared absorption spectrophotometry (*2.2.24*), comparing the spectrum obtained with the reference residue prepared from *amobarbital sodium CRS* with that obtained with the test residue (see identification test A).

C. Examine by thin-layer chromatography (*2.2.27*), using *silica gel GF_{254} R* as the coating substance.

Test solution. Dissolve 0.1 g of the substance to be examined in *alcohol R* and dilute to 100 ml with the same solvent.

Reference solution. Dissolve 0.1 g of *amobarbital sodium CRS* in *alcohol R* and dilute to 100 ml with the same solvent.

Apply separately to the plate 10 µl of each solution. Develop over a path of 18 cm using the lower layer of a mixture of 5 volumes of *concentrated ammonia R*, 15 volumes of *alcohol R* and 80 volumes of *chloroform R*. Examine immediately in ultraviolet light at 254 nm. The principal spot in the chromatogram obtained with the test solution is similar in position and size to the principal spot in the chromatogram obtained with the reference solution.

D. It gives the reaction of non-nitrogen substituted barbiturates (*2.3.1*).

E. It gives reaction (a) of sodium (*2.3.1*).

TESTS

Solution S. Dissolve 5.0 g in *alcohol (50 per cent V/V) R* and dilute to 50 ml with the same solvent.

Appearance of solution. Solution S is clear (*2.2.1*) and not more intensely coloured than reference solution Y_7 (*2.2.2, Method II*).

pH (*2.2.3*). Dissolve 5.0 g in *carbon dioxide-free water R* and dilute to 50 ml with the same solvent. Disregard any slight residue. The pH of the solution is not more than 11.0.

Related substances. Examine by thin-layer chromatography (*2.2.27*), using *silica gel GF_{254} R* as the coating substance.

Test solution. Dissolve 1.0 g of the substance to be examined in *alcohol R* and dilute to 100 ml with the same solvent.

Reference solution. Dilute 0.5 ml of the test solution to 100 ml with *alcohol R*.

Apply separately to the plate 20 µl of each solution. Develop over a path of 15 cm using the lower layer of a mixture of 5 volumes of *concentrated ammonia R*, 15 volumes of *alcohol R* and 80 volumes of *chloroform R*. Examine the plate immediately in ultraviolet light at 254 nm. Spray with *diphenylcarbazone mercuric reagent R*. Allow the plate to dry in air and spray with freshly prepared *alcoholic potassium hydroxide solution R* diluted 1 in 5 with *aldehyde-free alcohol R*. Heat at 100 °C to 105 °C for 5 min and examine immediately. When examined in ultraviolet light and after spraying, any spot in the chromatogram obtained with the test solution, apart from the principal spot, is not more intense than the spot in the chromatogram obtained with the reference solution (0.5 per cent). Disregard any spot at the starting-point.

Loss on drying (*2.2.32*). Not more than 3.0 per cent, determined on 0.50 g by drying in an oven at 130 °C.

ASSAY

Dissolve 0.200 g in 5 ml of *ethanol R*. Add 0.5 ml of *thymolphthalein solution R* and 10 ml of *silver nitrate solution in pyridine R*. Titrate with *0.1 M ethanolic sodium hydroxide* until a pure blue colour is obtained. Carry out a blank titration.

1 ml of *0.1 M ethanolic sodium hydroxide* is equivalent to 24.83 mg of $C_{11}H_{17}N_2NaO_3$.

STORAGE

Store in an airtight container.

01/2005:0577
corrected

AMOXICILLIN SODIUM

Amoxicillinum natricum

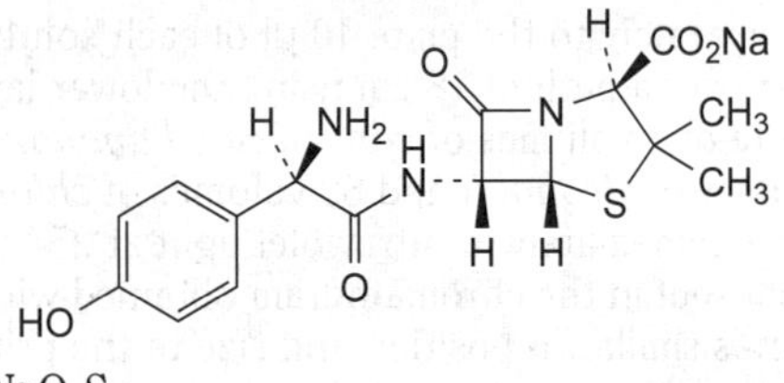

$C_{16}H_{18}N_3NaO_5S$ M_r 387.4

DEFINITION

Amoxicillin sodium contains not less than 89.0 per cent and not more than the equivalent of 102.0 per cent of sodium (2*S*,5*R*,6*R*)-6-[[(2*R*)-2-amino-2-(4-hydroxyphenyl)acetyl]amino]-3,3-dimethyl-7-oxo-4-thia-1-azabicyclo[3.2.0]heptane-2-carboxylate, calculated with reference to the anhydrous substance.

CHARACTERS

A white or almost white powder, very hygroscopic, very soluble in water, sparingly soluble in ethanol, very slightly soluble in acetone.

IDENTIFICATION

First identification: A, D.

Second identification: B, C, D.

A. Dissolve 0.250 g in 5 ml of *water R*, add 0.5 ml of *dilute acetic acid R*, swirl and allow to stand for 10 min in iced water. Filter the crystals and wash with 2 ml to 3 ml of a mixture of 1 volume of *water R* and 9 volumes of *acetone R*, then dry in an oven at 60 °C for 30 min. Examine by infrared absorption spectrophotometry (*2.2.24*), comparing with the spectrum obtained with *amoxicillin trihydrate CRS*.

B. Examine by thin-layer chromatography (*2.2.27*), using a *TLC silanised silica gel plate R*.

Test solution. Dissolve 25 mg of the substance to be examined in 10 ml of *sodium hydrogen carbonate solution R*.

Reference solution (a). Dissolve 25 mg of *amoxicillin trihydrate CRS* in 10 ml of *sodium hydrogen carbonate solution R*.

Reference solution (b). Dissolve 25 mg of *amoxicillin trihydrate CRS* and 25 mg of *ampicillin trihydrate CRS* in 10 ml of *sodium hydrogen carbonate solution R*.

Apply to the plate 1 µl of each solution. Develop over a path of 15 cm using a mixture of 10 volumes of *acetone R* and 90 volumes of a 154 g/l solution of *ammonium acetate R*, the pH of which has been adjusted to 5.0 with *glacial acetic acid R*. Allow the plate to dry in air and expose it to iodine vapour until the spots appear. Examine in daylight. The principal spot in the chromatogram obtained with the test solution is similar in position, colour and size to the principal spot in the chromatogram obtained with reference solution (a). The test is not valid unless the chromatogram obtained with reference solution (b) shows 2 clearly separated spots.

C. Place about 2 mg in a test-tube about 150 mm long and 15 mm in diameter. Moisten with 0.05 ml of *water R* and add 2 ml of *sulphuric acid-formaldehyde reagent R*. Mix the contents of the tube by swirling; the solution is practically colourless. Place the test-tube in a water-bath for 1 min; a dark yellow colour develops.

D. It gives reaction (a) of sodium (*2.3.1*).

TESTS

Appearance of solution. Dissolve 1.0 g in *water R* and dilute to 10.0 ml with the same solvent. Immediately after dissolution, the solution is not more opalescent than reference suspension II (*2.2.1*). The solution may show an initial, but transient, pink colour. After 5 min, the absorbance measured at 430 nm (*2.2.25*) is not greater than 0.20.

pH (*2.2.3*). Dissolve 2.0 g in *carbon dioxide-free water R* and dilute to 20 ml with the same solvent. The pH of the solution is 8.0 to 10.0.

Specific optical rotation (*2.2.7*). Dissolve 62.5 mg in a 4 g/l solution of *potassium hydrogen phthalate R* and dilute to 25.0 ml with the same solution. The specific optical rotation is + 240 to + 290, calculated with reference to the anhydrous substance.

Related substances. Examine by liquid chromatography (*2.2.29*) as described under Assay. Inject 50 µl of reference solution (d) and elute isocratically until elution of the amoxicillin peak. Inject 50 µl of test solution (b) and start the elution isocratically. Immediately after elution of the amoxicillin peak start the following linear gradient. If the mobile phase composition has been adjusted to achieve the required resolution, the adjusted composition will apply at time zero in the gradient.

Time (min)	Mobile phase A (per cent *V/V*)	Mobile phase B (per cent *V/V*)	Comment
0 - 25	92 → 0	8 → 100	linear gradient
25 - 40	0	100	isocratic
40 - 55	92	8	re-equilibration

Inject mobile phase A and use the same elution pattern to obtain a blank. Inject reference solution (e). The 3 principal peaks eluted after the main peak correspond to amoxicillin diketopiperazine, amoxicillin dimer (impurity J; *n* = 1) and amoxicillin trimer (impurity J; *n* = 2) and, compared to the principal peak they have a relative retention time of about 3.4, 4.1 and 4.5, respectively. In the chromatogram obtained with test solution (b): the area of any peak corresponding to amoxicillin dimer is not greater than 3 times the area of the principal peak in the chromatogram obtained with reference solution (d) (3 per cent); the area of any peak, apart from the principal peak and any peak corresponding to amoxicillin dimer, is not greater than twice the area of the principal peak in the chromatogram obtained with reference solution (d) (2 per cent); the sum of the areas of all the peaks, apart from the principal peak, is not greater than 9 times the area of the principal peak in the chromatogram obtained with reference solution (d) (9 per cent). Disregard any peak with an area less than 0.1 times that of the principal peak in the chromatogram obtained with reference solution (d).

***N,N*-Dimethylaniline** (*2.4.26, Method A or B*). Not more than 20 ppm.

2-Ethylhexanoic acid (*2.4.28*). Not more than 0.8 per cent *m/m*.

Heavy metals (*2.4.8*). 1.0 g complies with limit test C for heavy metals (20 ppm). Prepare the standard using 2 ml of *lead standard solution (10 ppm Pb) R*.

Water (*2.5.12*). Not more than 3.0 per cent, determined on 0.400 g by the semi-micro determination of water.

Bacterial endotoxins (*2.6.14*): less than 0.25 IU/mg, if intended for use in the manufacture of parenteral dosage forms without a further appropriate procedure for the removal of bacterial endotoxins.

ASSAY

Examine by liquid chromatography (*2.2.29*).

Test solution (a). Dissolve 30.0 mg of the substance to be examined in mobile phase A and dilute to 50.0 ml with the same mobile phase.

Test solution (b). Prepare immediately before use. Dissolve 30.0 mg of the substance to be examined in mobile phase A and dilute to 20.0 ml with the same mobile phase.

Reference solution (a). Dissolve 30.0 mg of *amoxicillin trihydrate CRS* in mobile phase A and dilute to 50.0 ml with the same mobile phase.

Reference solution (b). Dissolve 4.0 mg of *cefadroxil CRS* in mobile phase A and dilute to 50 ml with the same mobile phase. To 5.0 ml of this solution add 5.0 ml of reference solution (a) and dilute to 100 ml with mobile phase A.

Reference solution (c). Dilute 1.0 ml of reference solution (a) to 20.0 ml with mobile phase A. Dilute 1.0 ml of the solution to 50.0 ml with mobile phase A.

Reference solution (d). Dilute 2.0 ml of reference solution (a) to 20.0 ml with mobile phase A. Dilute 5.0 ml of the solution to 20.0 ml with mobile phase A.

Reference solution (e). To 0.20 g of *amoxicillin trihydrate R* add 1.0 ml of *water R*. Shake and add dropwise *dilute sodium hydroxide solution R* to obtain a solution. The pH of the solution is about 8.5. Store the solution at room temperature for 4 h. Dilute 0.5 ml of the solution to 50.0 ml with mobile phase A.

The chromatographic procedure may be carried out using:

– a column 0.25 m long and 4.6 mm in internal diameter packed with *octadecylsilyl silica gel for chromatography R* (5 µm),

– as mobile phase at a flow rate of 1.0 ml/min:

  Mobile phase A. Mix 1 volume of *acetonitrile R* and 99 volumes of a 25 per cent *V/V* solution of *0.2 M potassium dihydrogen phosphate R* adjusted to pH 5.0 with *dilute sodium hydroxide solution R*,

  Mobile phase B. Mix 20 volumes of *acetonitrile R* and 80 volumes of a 25 per cent *V/V* solution of *0.2 M potassium dihydrogen phosphate R* adjusted to pH 5.0 with *dilute sodium hydroxide solution R*,

– as detector a spectrophotometer set at 254 nm.

Equilibrate the column with a mobile phase ratio A:B of 92:8. Inject 50 µl of reference solution (b). The test is not valid unless in the chromatogram obtained, the resolution between the peaks corresponding to amoxicillin and cefadroxil is at least 2.0 (if necessary, adjust the ratio A:B of the mobile phase) and the mass distribution ratio for the first peak (amoxicillin) is 1.3 to 2.5. Inject reference solution (c). Adjust the system to obtain a peak with a signal-to-noise ratio of at least 3. Inject reference solution (a) 6 times. The test is not valid unless the relative standard deviation for the area of the principal peak is at most 1.0 per cent. Inject test solution (a) and reference solution (a).

Calculate the percentage content of amoxicillin sodium by multiplying the percentage content of amoxicillin by 1.060.

STORAGE

Store in an airtight container. If the substance is sterile, store in a sterile, airtight, tamper-proof container.

LABELLING

The label states, where applicable, that the substance is free from bacterial endotoxins.

IMPURITIES

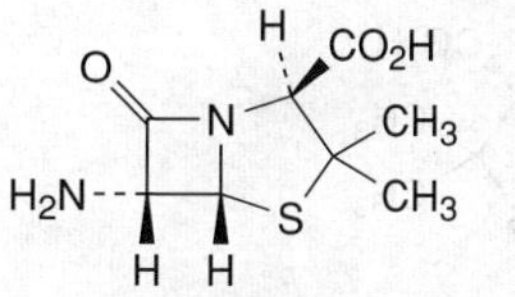

A. (2*S*,5*R*,6*R*)-6-amino-3,3-dimethyl-7-oxo-4-thia-1-azabicyclo[3.2.0]heptane-2-carboxylic acid (6-aminopenicillanic acid),

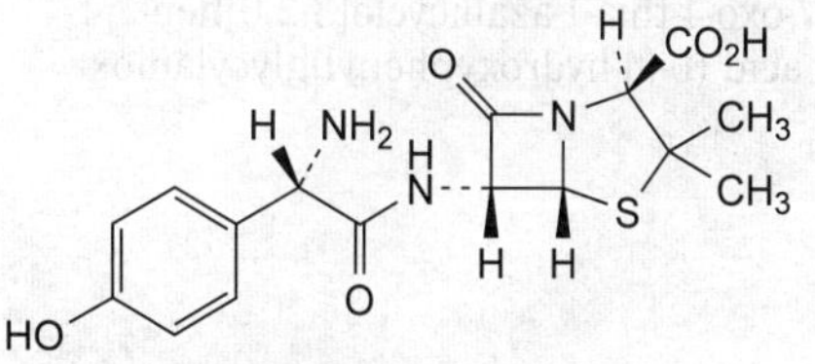

B. (2*S*,5*R*,6*R*)-6-[[(2*S*)-2-amino-2-(4-hydroxyphenyl)acetyl]amino]-3,3-dimethyl-7-oxo-4-thia-1-azabicyclo[3.2.0]heptane-2-carboxylic acid (L-amoxicillin),

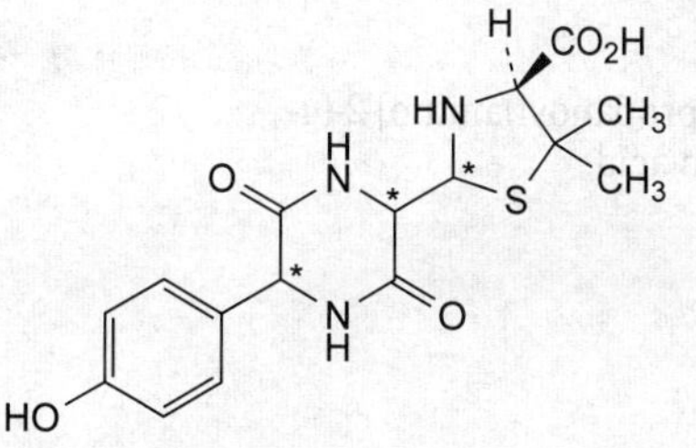

C. (4*S*)-2-[5-(4-hydroxyphenyl)-3,6-dioxopiperazin-2-yl]-5,5-dimethylthiazolidine-4-carboxylic acid (amoxicillin diketopiperazines),

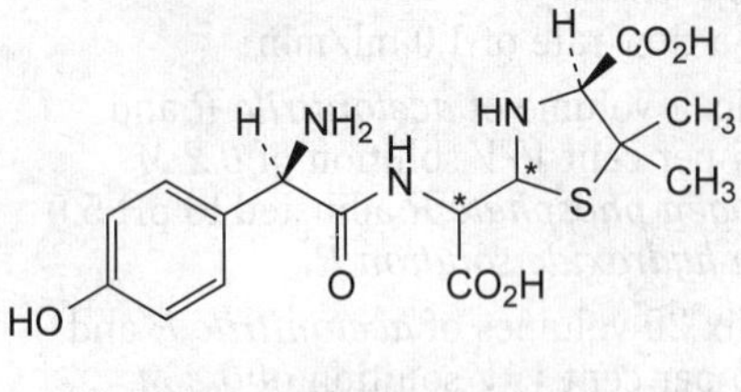

D. (4*S*)-2-[[[(2*R*)-2-amino-2-(4-hydroxyphenyl)acetyl]amino]carboxymethyl]-5,5-dimethylthiazolidine-4-carboxylic acid (penicilloic acids of amoxicillin),

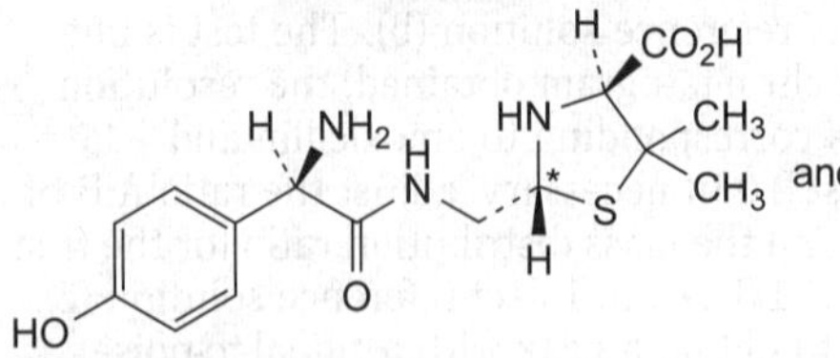

E. (2*RS*,4*S*)-2-[[[(2*R*)-2-amino-2-(4-hydroxyphenyl)acetyl]amino]methyl]-5,5-dimethylthiazolidine-4-carboxylic acid (penilloic acids of amoxicillin),

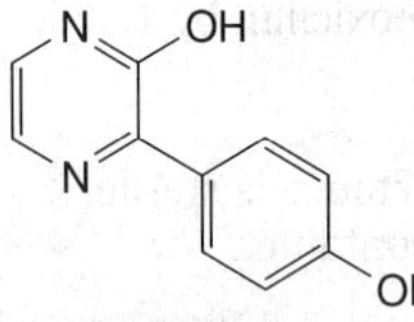

F. 3-(4-hydroxyphenyl)pyrazin-2-ol,

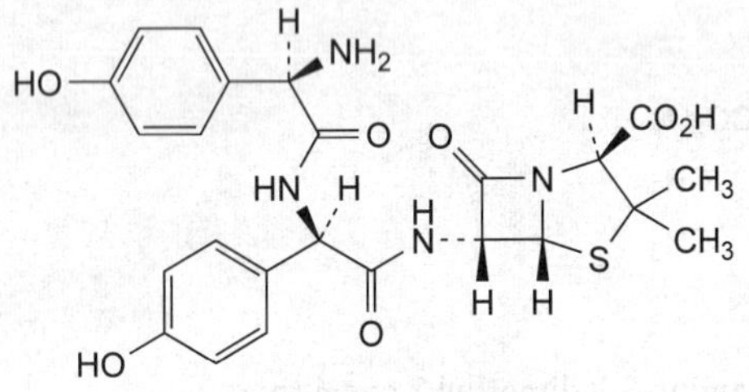

G. (2*S*,5*R*,6*R*)-6-[[(2*R*)-2-[[(2*R*)-2-amino-2-(4-hydroxyphenyl)acetyl]amino]-2-(4-hydroxyphenyl)acetyl]amino]-3,3-dimethyl-7-oxo-4-thia-1-azabicyclo[3.2.0]heptane-2-carboxylic acid (D-(4-hydroxyphenyl)glycylamoxicillin),

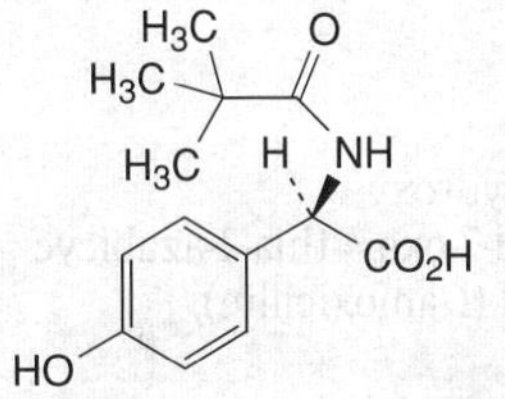

H. (2*R*)-2-[(2,2-dimethylpropanoyl)amino]-2-(4-hydroxyphenyl)acetic acid,

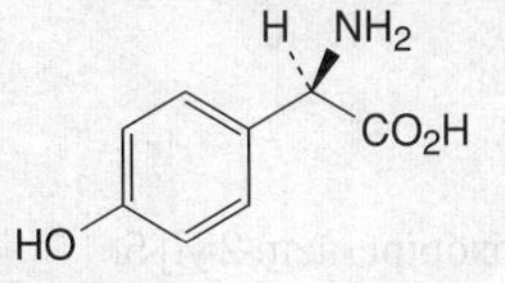

I. (2*R*)-2-amino-2-(4-hydroxyphenyl)acetic acid,

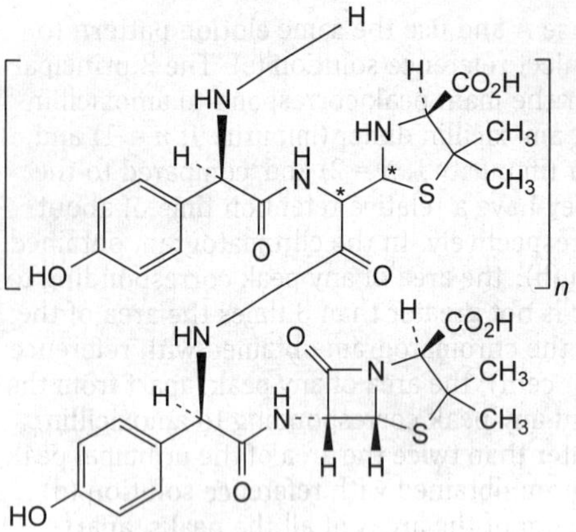

J. co-oligomers of amoxicillin and penicilloic acids of amoxicillin,

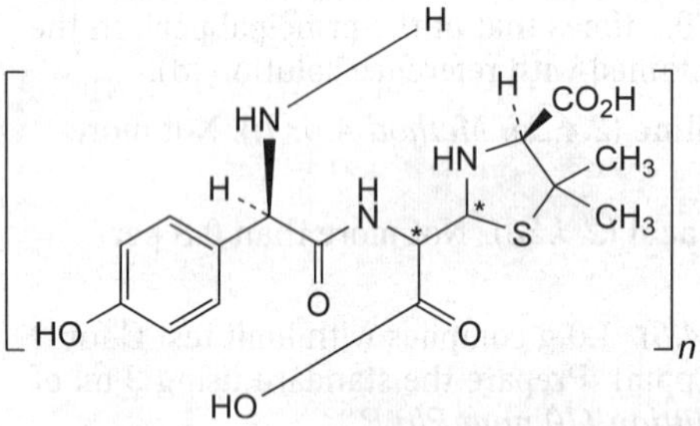

K. oligomers of penicilloic acids of amoxicillin.

01/2005:0260

AMOXICILLIN TRIHYDRATE

Amoxicillinum trihydricum

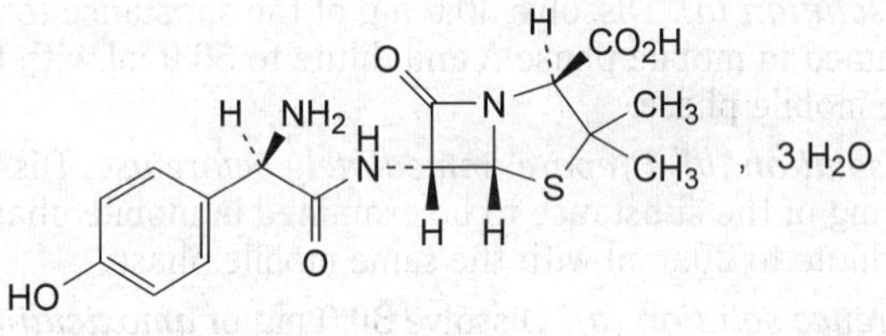

$C_{16}H_{19}N_3O_5S,3H_2O$ M_r 419.4

DEFINITION

Amoxicillin trihydrate contains not less than 95.0 per cent and not more than the equivalent of 102.0 per cent of (2*S*,5*R*,6*R*)-6-[[(2*R*)-2-amino-2-(4-hydroxyphenyl)acetyl]amino]-3,3-dimethyl-7-oxo-4-thia-1-azabicyclo[3.2.0]heptane-2-carboxylic acid, calculated with reference to the anhydrous substance.

CHARACTERS

A white or almost white, crystalline powder, slightly soluble in water, very slightly soluble in alcohol, practically insoluble in fatty oils. It dissolves in dilute acids and dilute solutions of alkali hydroxides.

IDENTIFICATION

First identification: A.

Second identification: B, C.

A. Examine by infrared absorption spectrophotometry (*2.2.24*), comparing with the spectrum obtained with *amoxicillin trihydrate CRS*.

B. Examine by thin-layer chromatography (*2.2.27*), using *silanised silica gel H R* as the coating substance.

Test solution. Dissolve 25 mg of the substance to be examined in 10 ml of *sodium hydrogen carbonate solution R.*

Reference solution (a). Dissolve 25 mg of *amoxicillin trihydrate CRS* in 10 ml of *sodium hydrogen carbonate solution R.*

Reference solution (b). Dissolve 25 mg of *amoxicillin trihydrate CRS* and 25 mg of *ampicillin trihydrate CRS* in 10 ml of *sodium hydrogen carbonate solution R.*

Apply to the plate 1 µl of each solution. Develop over a path of 15 cm using a mixture of 10 volumes of *acetone R* and 90 volumes of a 154 g/l solution of *ammonium acetate R,* the pH of which has been adjusted to 5.0 with *glacial acetic acid R.* Allow the plate to dry in air and expose it to iodine vapour until the spots appear. Examine in daylight. The principal spot in the chromatogram obtained with the test solution is similar in position, colour and size to the principal spot in the chromatogram obtained with reference solution (a). The test is not valid unless the chromatogram obtained with reference solution (b) shows 2 clearly separated spots.

C. Place about 2 mg in a test-tube about 150 mm long and 15 mm in diameter. Moisten with 0.05 ml of *water R* and add 2 ml of *sulphuric acid-formaldehyde reagent R.* Mix the contents of the tube by swirling; the solution is practically colourless. Place the test-tube in a water-bath for 1 min; a dark yellow colour develops.

TESTS

Solution S. With the aid of ultrasound or gentle heating, dissolve 0.100 g in *carbon dioxide-free water R* and dilute to 50.0 ml with the same solvent.

Appearance of solution. Dissolve 1.0 g in 10 ml of *0.5 M hydrochloric acid.* Dissolve separately 1.0 g in 10 ml of *dilute ammonia R2.* Immediately after dissolution, the solutions are not more opalescent than reference suspension II (*2.2.1*).

pH (*2.2.3*). The pH of solution S is 3.5 to 5.5.

Specific optical rotation (*2.2.7*): + 290 to + 315, determined on solution S and calculated with reference to the anhydrous substance.

Related substances. Examine by liquid chromatography (*2.2.29*) adjusting the ratio A:B of the mobile phase and the attenuation as described under Assay. Inject reference solution (d). Inject a freshly prepared test solution (b) and start the elution isocratically with the chosen mobile phase. Immediately after elution of the amoxicillin peak start a linear gradient elution to reach a mobile phase A:B of 0:100 over a period of 25 min. Continue the chromatography with mobile phase B for 15 min, then equilibrate the column for 15 min with the mobile phase chosen originally. Inject mobile phase A and use the same elution gradient to obtain a blank. In the chromatogram obtained with test solution (b), the area of any peak, apart from the principal peak and any peak observed in the blank chromatogram, is not greater than the area of the principal peak in the chromatogram obtained with reference solution (d) (1 per cent).

***N,N*-Dimethylaniline** (*2.4.26, Method A or B*). Not more than 20 ppm.

Water (*2.5.12*): 11.5 per cent to 14.5 per cent, determined on 0.100 g by the semi-micro determination of water.

Sulphated ash (*2.4.14*). Not more than 1.0 per cent, determined on 1.0 g.

ASSAY

Examine by liquid chromatography (*2.2.29*).

Test solution (a). Dissolve 30.0 mg of the substance to be examined in mobile phase A and dilute to 50.0 ml with the same mobile phase.

Test solution (b). Dissolve 30.0 mg of the substance to be examined in mobile phase A and dilute to 20.0 ml with the same mobile phase.

Reference solution (a). Dissolve 30.0 mg of *amoxicillin trihydrate CRS* in mobile phase A and dilute to 50.0 ml with the same mobile phase.

Reference solution (b). Dissolve 4.0 mg of *cefadroxil CRS* in mobile phase A and dilute to 50 ml with the same mobile phase. To 5.0 ml of this solution add 5.0 ml of reference solution (a) and dilute to 100 ml with mobile phase A.

Reference solution (c). Dilute 1.0 ml of reference solution (a) to 20.0 ml with mobile phase A. Dilute 1.0 ml of this solution to 50.0 ml with mobile phase A.

Reference solution (d). Dilute 2.0 ml of reference solution (a) to 20.0 ml with mobile phase A. Dilute 5.0 ml of this solution to 20.0 ml with mobile phase A.

The chromatographic procedure may be carried out using:

– a stainless steel column 0.25 m long and 4.6 mm in internal diameter packed with *octadecylsilyl silica gel for chromatography R* (5 µm),

– as mobile phase at a flow rate of 1.0 ml/min:

Mobile phase A. A mixture of 1 volume of *acetonitrile R* and 99 volumes of buffer solution pH 5.0,

Mobile phase B. A mixture of 20 volumes of *acetonitrile R* and 80 volumes of buffer solution pH 5.0,

Prepare the buffer solution as follows: to 250 ml of *0.2 M potassium dihydrogen phosphate R* add *dilute sodium hydroxide solution R* to pH 5.0 and dilute to 1000.0 ml with *water R,*

– as detector a spectrophotometer set at 254 nm,

– a 50 µl loop injector.

Equilibrate the column with a mobile phase with ratio A:B of 92:8. Inject reference solution (b). The assay is not valid unless the resolution between the 2 principal peaks is at least 2.0. If necessary, adjust the ratio A:B of the mobile phase. The mass distribution ratio for the first peak (amoxicillin) is 1.3 to 2.5. Inject reference solution (c). Adjust the system to obtain a peak with a signal-to-noise ratio of at least 3. Inject reference solution (a) 6 times. The test is not valid unless the relative standard deviation for the area of the principal peak is at most 1.0 per cent. Inject alternately test solution (a) and reference solution (a).

STORAGE

Store in an airtight container.

IMPURITIES

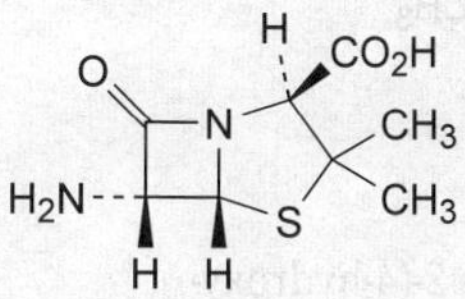

A. (2*S*,5*R*,6*R*)-6-amino-3,3-dimethyl-7-oxo-4-thia-1-azabicyclo[3.2.0]heptane-2-carboxylic acid (6-aminopenicillanic acid),

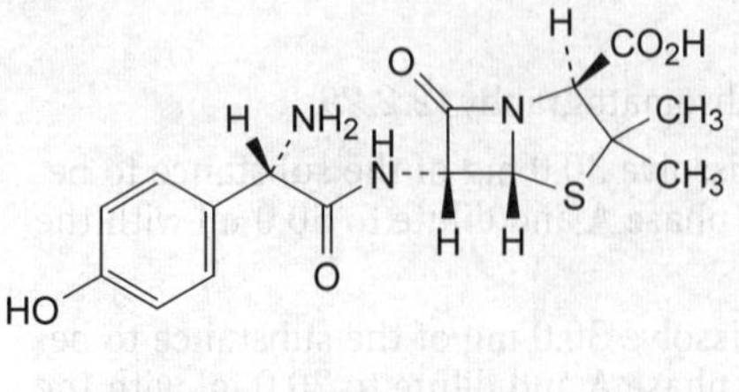

B. (2*S*,5*R*,6*R*)-6-[[(2*S*)-2-amino-2-(4-hydroxyphenyl)acetyl]amino]-3,3-dimethyl-7-oxo-4-thia-1-azabicyclo[3.2.0]heptane-2-carboxylic acid (L-amoxicillin),

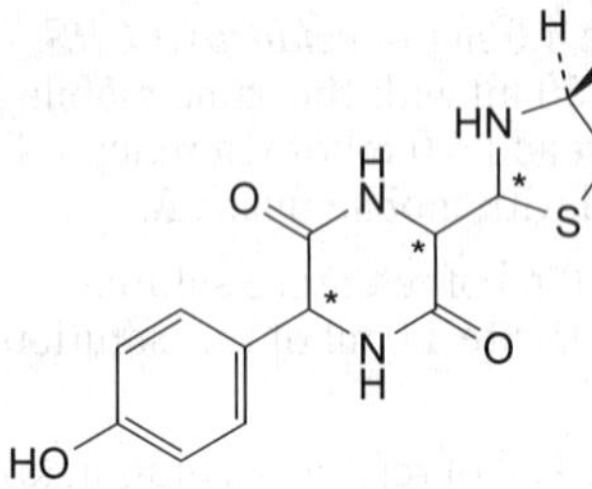

C. (4*S*)-2-[5-(4-hydroxyphenyl)-3,6-dioxopiperazin-2-yl]-5,5-dimethylthiazolidine-4-carboxylic acid (amoxicillin diketopiperazines),

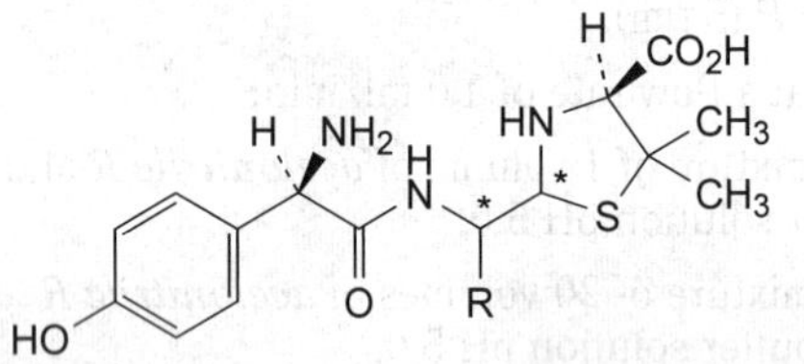

D. R = CO_2H: (4S)-2-[[[(2R)-2-amino-2-(4-hydroxyphenyl)acetyl]amino]carboxymethyl]-5,5-dimethylthiazolidine-4-carboxylic acid (penicilloic acids of amoxicillin),

E. R = H: (2*RS*,4*S*)-2-[[[(2*R*)-2-amino-2-(4-hydroxyphenyl)acetyl]amino]methyl]-5,5-dimethylthiazolidine-4-carboxylic acid (penilloic acids of amoxicillin),

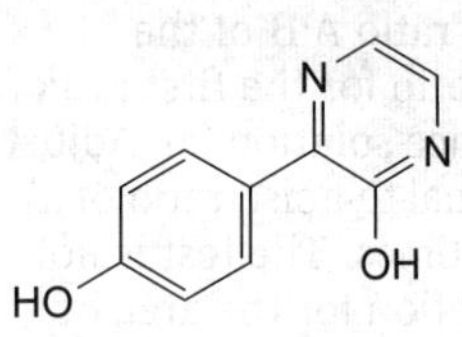

F. 3-(4-hydroxyphenyl)pyrazin-2-ol,

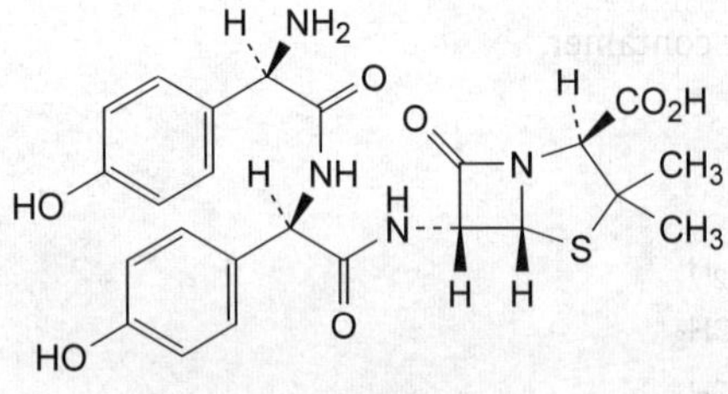

G. (2*S*,5*R*,6*R*)-6-[[(2*R*)-2-[[(2*R*)-2-amino-2-(4-hydroxyphenyl)acetyl]amino]-2-(4-hydroxyphenyl)acetyl]amino]-3,3-dimethyl-7-oxo-4-thia-1-azabicyclo[3.2.0]heptane-2-carboxylic acid (D-(4-hydroxyphenyl)glycylamoxicillin),

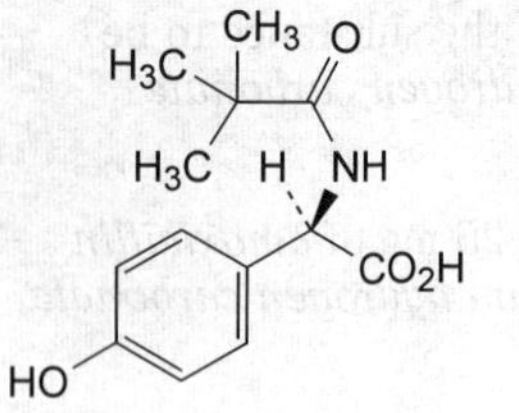

H. (2*R*)-2-[(2,2-dimethylpropanoyl)amino]-2-(4-hydroxyphenyl)acetic acid,

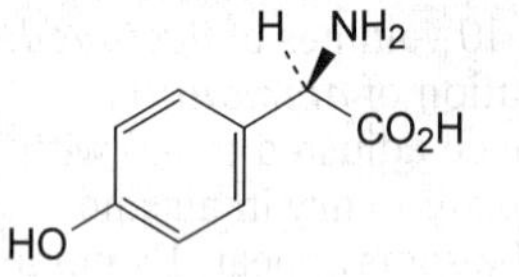

I. (2*R*)-2-amino-2-(4-hydroxyphenyl)acetic acid,

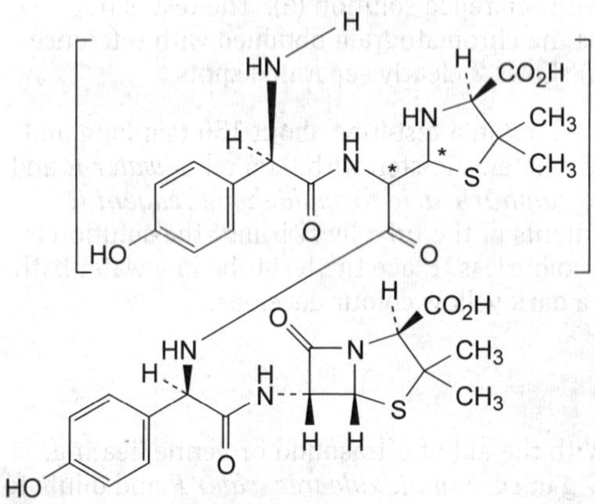

J. co-oligomers of amoxicillin and of penicilloic acids of amoxicillin,

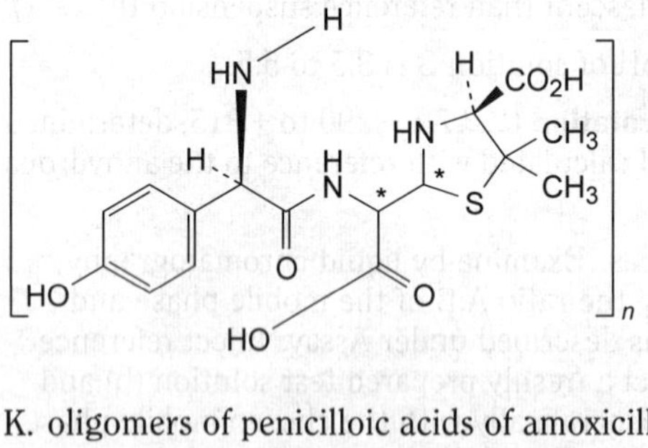

K. oligomers of penicilloic acids of amoxicillin,

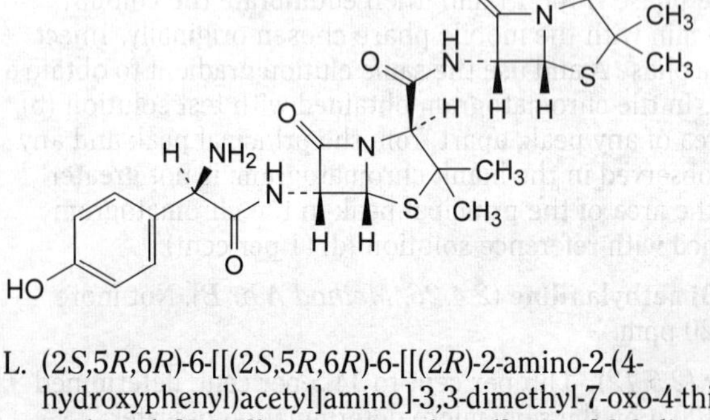

L. (2*S*,5*R*,6*R*)-6-[[(2*S*,5*R*,6*R*)-6-[[(2*R*)-2-amino-2-(4-hydroxyphenyl)acetyl]amino]-3,3-dimethyl-7-oxo-4-thia-1-azabicyclo[3.2.0]heptane-2-carbonyl]amino]-3,3-dimethyl-7-oxo-4-thia-1-azabicyclo[3.2.0]heptane-2-carboxylic acid (6-APA amoxicillin amide).

01/2005:1292

AMPHOTERICIN B

Amphotericinum B

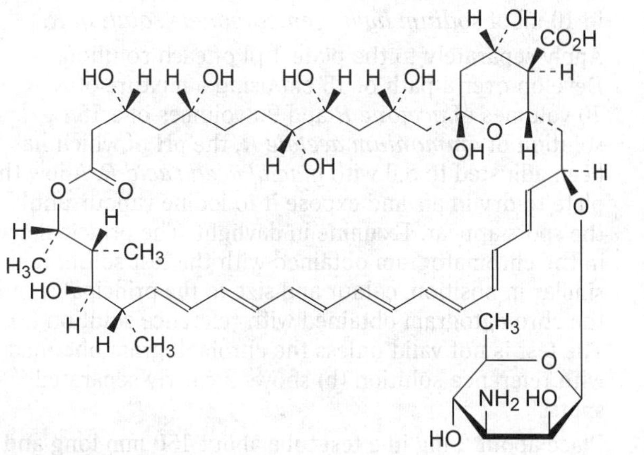

$C_{47}H_{73}NO_{17}$ M_r 924

DEFINITION

Amphotericin B is a mixture of antifungal polyenes produced by the growth of certain strains of *Streptomyces nodosus* or by any other means.

It consists mainly of amphotericin B which is (1*R*,3*S*,5*R*,6*R*,9*R*,11*R*,15*S*,16*R*,17*R*,18*S*,19*E*,21*E*,23*E*, 25*E*, 27*E*,29*E*,31*E*,33*R*,35*S*,36*R*,37*S*)-33-[(3-amino-3,6-dideoxy-β-D-mannopyranosyl)oxy]-1,3,5,6,9,11,17,37-octahydroxy-15,16, 18-trimethyl-13-oxo-14,39-dioxabicyclo[33.3.1]nonatriaconta-19,21,23,25,27,29,31-heptaene-36-carboxylic acid. The potency is not less than 750 IU/mg, calculated with reference to the dried substance.

CHARACTERS

A yellow or orange powder, practically insoluble in water, soluble in dimethyl sulphoxide and in propylene glycol, slightly soluble in dimethylformamide, very slightly soluble in methanol, practically insoluble in alcohol.

It is sensitive to light in dilute solutions and is inactivated at low pH values.

IDENTIFICATION

A. Dissolve 25 mg in 5 ml of *dimethyl sulphoxide R* and dilute to 50 ml with *methanol R*. Dilute 2 ml of the solution to 200 ml with *methanol R*. Examined between 300 nm and 450 nm (*2.2.25*), the solution shows 3 absorption maxima at 362 nm, 381 nm and 405 nm. The ratio of the absorbance measured at 362 nm to that measured at 381 nm is 0.57 to 0.61. The ratio of the absorbance measured at 381 nm to that measured at 405 nm is 0.87 to 0.93.

B. Examine by infrared absorption spectrophotometry (*2.2.24*), comparing with the spectrum obtained with *amphotericin B CRS*. If the spectra obtained show differences dry the substance to be examined at 60 °C at a pressure not exceeding 0.7 kPa for 1 h and prepare a new spectrum.

C. To 1 ml of a 0.5 g/l solution in *dimethyl sulphoxide R*, add 5 ml of *phosphoric acid R* to form a lower layer, avoiding mixing the 2 liquids. A blue ring is immediately produced at the junction of the liquids. Mix, an intense blue colour is produced. Add 15 ml of *water R* and mix; the solution becomes pale yellow.

TESTS

Content of tetraenes. Not more than 10.0 per cent and not more than 5.0 per cent if intended for use in the manufacture of parenteral dosage forms, determined by the following method.

Test solution. Dissolve 50.0 mg in 5 ml of *dimethyl sulphoxide R* and dilute to 50.0 ml with *methanol R*. Dilute 4.0 ml of the solution to 50.0 ml with *methanol R*.

Reference solution (a). Dissolve 50.0 mg of *amphotericin B CRS* in 5 ml of *dimethyl sulphoxide R* and dilute to 50.0 ml with *methanol R*. Dilute 4.0 ml of the solution to 50.0 ml with *methanol R*.

Reference solution (b). Dissolve 25.0 mg of *nystatin CRS* in 25 ml of *dimethyl sulphoxide R* and dilute to 250.0 ml with *methanol R*. Dilute 4.0 ml of the solution to 50.0 ml with *methanol R*.

Measure the absorbances (*2.2.25*) of the test solution and of reference solutions (a) and (b) at the maxima at 282 nm and 304 nm respectively, using a 0.8 per cent *V/V* solution of *dimethyl sulphoxide R* in *methanol R* as the compensation liquid. Calculate the specific absorbance of the substance being examined, of *nystatin CRS* and of *amphotericin B CRS* at both wavelengths, each with reference to the dried substance, and calculate the percentage content of tetraenes using the following expression:

$$F + \frac{100\,(B_1S_2 - B_2S_1)}{(N_2B_1 - N_1B_2)}$$

S_1 and S_2 = specific absorbances of the substance to be examined at 282 nm and 304 nm respectively,

N_1 and N_2 = specific absorbance of *nystatin CRS* at 282 nm and 304 nm respectively,

B_1 and B_2 = specific absorbance of *amphotericin B CRS* at 282 nm and 304 nm respectively,

F = declared content of tetraenes in *amphotericin B CRS*.

Loss on drying (*2.2.32*). Not more than 5.0 per cent, determined on 1.000 g by drying in an oven at 60 °C at a pressure not exceeding 0.7 kPa.

Sulphated ash (*2.4.14*). Not more than 3.0 per cent and not more than 0.5 per cent if intended for use in the manufacture of parenteral dosage forms, determined on 1.0 g.

Bacterial endotoxins (*2.6.14*): less than 1.0 IU/mg, if intended for use in the manufacture of parenteral dosage forms without a further appropriate procedure for the removal of bacterial endotoxins.

ASSAY

Protect all solutions from light throughout the assay. Dissolve 25.0 mg in *dimethyl sulphoxide R* and dilute, with shaking, to 25.0 ml with the same solvent. Under constant stirring of this stock solution, dilute with *dimethyl sulphoxide R* to obtain solutions of appropriate concentrations (the following concentrations have been found suitable: 44.4, 66.7 and 100 IU/ml). Final solutions are prepared by diluting 1 to 20 with 0.2 M phosphate buffer solution pH 10.5 so that they all contain 5 per cent *V/V* of dimethyl sulphoxide. Prepare the reference and the test solutions simultaneously. Carry out the microbiological assay of antibiotics (*2.7.2*).

STORAGE

Store protected from light, at a temperature of 2 °C to 8 °C. If the substance is sterile, store in a sterile, airtight, tamper-proof container.

LABELLING

The label states:
- where applicable, that the substance is free from bacterial endotoxins,
- where applicable, that the substance is suitable for use in the manufacture of parenteral dosage forms.

IMPURITIES

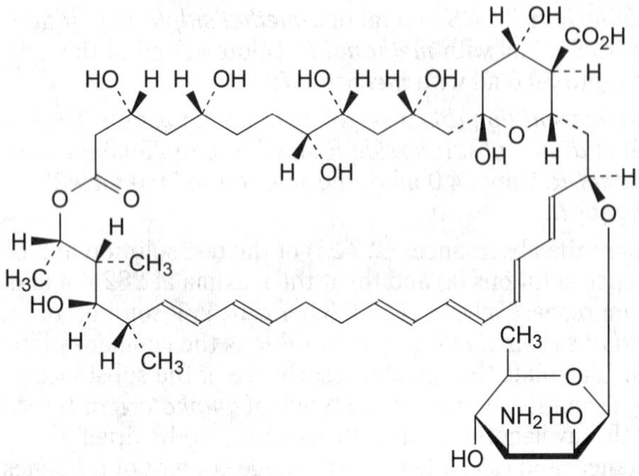

A. amphotericin A (tetraene).

01/2005:0167

AMPICILLIN, ANHYDROUS

Ampicillinum anhydricum

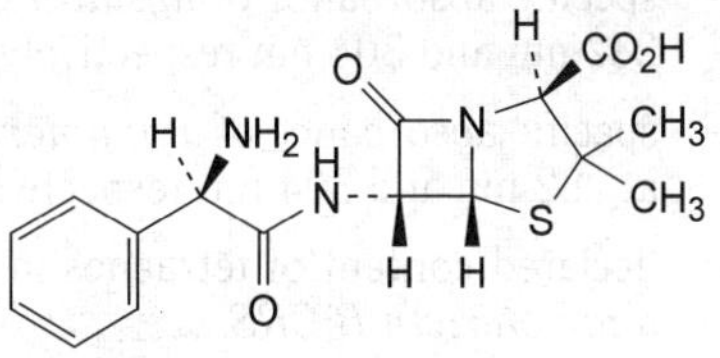

$C_{16}H_{19}N_3O_4S$ M_r 349.4

DEFINITION

Anhydrous ampicillin contains not less than 96.0 per cent and not more than the equivalent of 100.5 per cent of (2*S*,5*R*,6*R*)-6-[[(2*R*)-2-amino-2-phenylacetyl]amino]-3,3-dimethyl-7-oxo-4-thia-1-azabicyclo[3.2.0]heptane-2-carboxylic acid, calculated with reference to the anhydrous substance.

CHARACTERS

A white, crystalline powder, sparingly soluble in water, practically insoluble in acetone, in alcohol and in fatty oils. It dissolves in dilute solutions of acids and of alkali hydroxides. It shows polymorphism.

IDENTIFICATION

First identification: A, D.

Second identification: B, C, D.

A. Examine by infrared absorption spectrophotometry (*2.2.24*), comparing with the spectrum obtained with *anhydrous ampicillin CRS*. Examine the substances prepared as discs using *potassium bromide R*.

B. Examine by thin-layer chromatography (*2.2.27*), using *silanised silica gel H R* as the coating substance.

Test solution. Dissolve 25 mg of the substance to be examined in 10 ml of *sodium hydrogen carbonate solution R*.

Reference solution (a). Dissolve 25 mg of *anhydrous ampicillin CRS* in 10 ml of *sodium hydrogen carbonate solution R*.

Reference solution (b). Dissolve 25 mg of *amoxicillin trihydrate CRS* and 25 mg of *anhydrous ampicillin CRS* in 10 ml of *sodium hydrogen carbonate solution R*.

Apply separately to the plate 1 µl of each solution. Develop over a path of 15 cm using a mixture of 10 volumes of *acetone R* and 90 volumes of a 154 g/l solution of *ammonium acetate R*, the pH of which has been adjusted to 5.0 with *glacial acetic acid R*. Allow the plate to dry in air and expose it to iodine vapour until the spots appear. Examine in daylight. The principal spot in the chromatogram obtained with the test solution is similar in position, colour and size to the principal spot in the chromatogram obtained with reference solution (a). The test is not valid unless the chromatogram obtained with reference solution (b) shows 2 clearly separated spots.

C. Place about 2 mg in a test-tube about 150 mm long and 15 mm in diameter. Moisten with 0.05 ml of *water R* and add 2 ml of *sulphuric acid-formaldehyde reagent R*. Mix the contents of the tube by swirling; the solution is practically colourless. Place the test-tube in a water-bath for 1 min; a dark yellow colour develops.

D. It complies with the test for water (see Tests).

TESTS

Appearance of solution. Dissolve 1.0 g in 10 ml of *1 M hydrochloric acid*. Separately dissolve 1.0 g in 10 ml of *dilute ammonia R2*. Immediately after dissolution, the solutions are not more opalescent than reference suspension II (*2.2.1*).

pH (*2.2.3*). Dissolve 0.1 g in *carbon dioxide-free water R* and dilute to 40 ml with the same solvent. The pH of the solution is 3.5 to 5.5.

Specific optical rotation (*2.2.7*). Dissolve 62.5 mg in *water R* and dilute to 25.0 ml with the same solvent. The specific optical rotation is + 280 to + 305, calculated with reference to the anhydrous substance.

Related substances. Examine by liquid chromatography (*2.2.29*) as described under Assay. Inject reference solution (c) and elute isocratically. Inject freshly prepared test solution (b) and start the elution isocratically. Immediately after elution of the ampicillin peak start the following linear gradient. If the mobile phase composition has been adjusted to achieve the required resolution, the adjusted composition will apply at time zero in the gradient.

Time (min)	Mobile phase A (per cent *V/V*)	Mobile phase B (per cent *V/V*)
0	85	15
30	0	100
45	0	100

Equilibrate the column with the originally chosen mobile phase for 15 min. Inject mobile phase A and use the same elution gradient to obtain a blank. In the chromatogram obtained with test solution (b), the area of any peak, apart from the principal peak and any peak observed in the blank chromatogram, is not greater than the area of the principal peak in the chromatogram obtained with reference solution (c) (1.0 per cent).

***N,N*-Dimethylaniline** (*2.4.26, Method B*). Not more than 20 ppm.

Water (*2.5.12*). Not more than 2.0 per cent, determined on 0.300 g by the semi-micro determination of water.

Sulphated ash (*2.4.14*). Not more than 0.5 per cent, determined on 1.0 g.

ASSAY

Examine by liquid chromatography (*2.2.29*).

Test solution (a). Dissolve 27.0 mg of the substance to be examined in mobile phase A and dilute to 50.0 ml with the same solvent.

Test solution (b). Dissolve 27.0 mg of the substance to be examined in mobile phase A and dilute to 10.0 ml with the same solvent.

Reference solution (a). Dissolve 27.0 mg of *anhydrous ampicillin CRS* in mobile phase A and dilute to 50.0 ml with the same solvent.

Reference solution (b). Dissolve 2.0 mg of *cefradine CRS* in mobile phase A and dilute to 50 ml with the same solvent. To 5.0 ml of this solution add 5.0 ml of reference solution (a).

Reference solution (c). Dilute 1.0 ml of reference solution (a) to 20.0 ml with mobile phase A.

Reference solution (d). Dilute 1.0 ml of reference solution (c) to 25.0 ml with mobile phase A.

The chromatographic procedure may be carried out using:

- a column 0.25 m long and 4.6 mm in internal diameter packed with *octadecylsilyl silica gel for chromatography R* (5 µm),
- as mobile phase at a flow rate of 1.0 ml/min:
  Mobile phase A. A mixture of 0.5 ml of *dilute acetic acid R*, 50 ml of *0.2 M potassium dihydrogen phosphate R* and 50 ml of *acetonitrile R*, diluted to 1000 ml with *water R*,
  Mobile phase B. A mixture of 0.5 ml of *dilute acetic acid R*, 50 ml of *0.2 M potassium dihydrogen phosphate R* and 400 ml of *acetonitrile R*, diluted to 1000 ml with *water R*,
- as detector a spectrophotometer set at 254 nm,
- a 50 µl loop injector.

Equilibrate the column with a mobile phase with ratio A:B of 85:15. Inject reference solution (b). The test is not valid unless the resolution between the two principal peaks is at least 3.0. If necessary, adjust the ratio A:B of the mobile phase. The mass distribution ratio for the first peak (ampicillin) is 2.0 to 2.5. Inject reference solution (d). Adjust the system to obtain a peak with a signal-to-noise ratio of at least 3. Inject reference solution (a) 6 times. The test is not valid unless the relative standard deviation for the area of the principal peak is at most 1.0 per cent. Inject alternately test solution (a) and reference solution (a).

Calculate the percentage content of ampicillin.

STORAGE

Store in an airtight container, at a temperature not exceeding 30 °C.

IMPURITIES

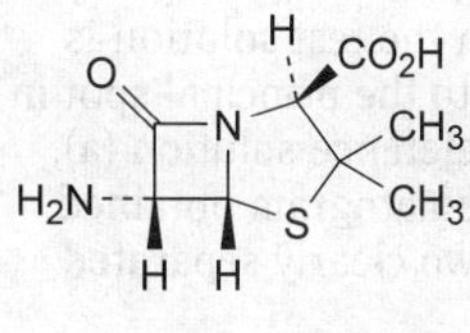

A. (2*S*,5*R*,6*R*)-6-amino-3,3-dimethyl-7-oxo-4-thia-1-azabicyclo[3.2.0]heptane-2-carboxylic acid (6-aminopenicillanic acid),

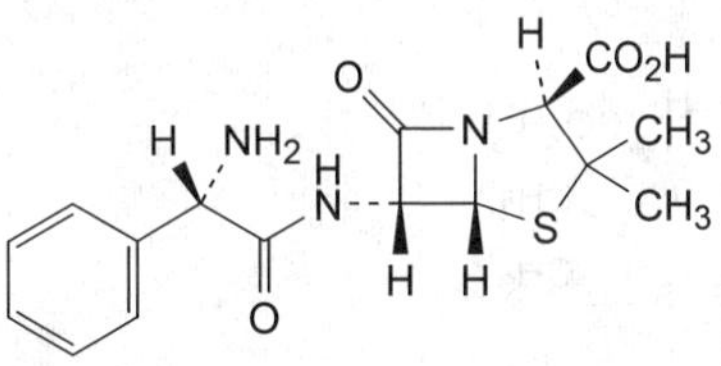

B. (2*S*,5*R*,6*R*)-6-[[(2*S*)-2-amino-2-phenylacetyl]amino]-3,3-dimethyl-7-oxo-4-thia-1-azabicyclo[3.2.0]heptane-2-carboxylic acid (L-ampicillin),

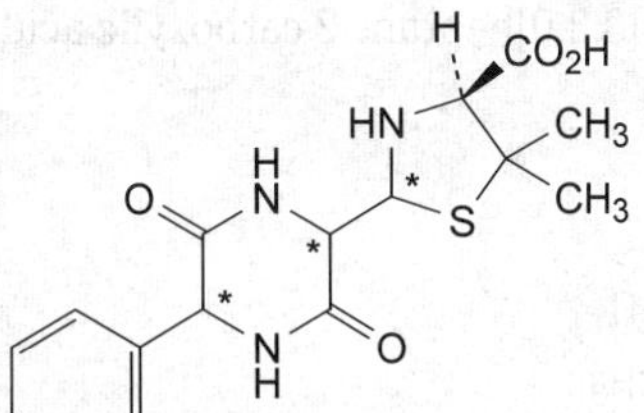

C. (4*S*)-2-(3,6-dioxo-5-phenylpiperazin-2-yl)-5,5-dimethylthiazolidine-4-carboxylic acid (diketopiperazines of ampicillin),

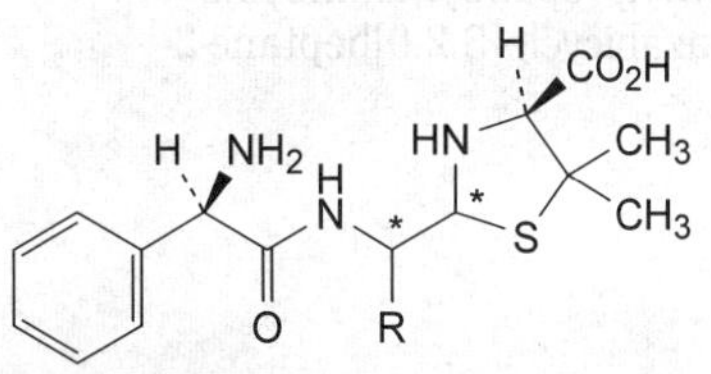

D. R = CO_2H: (4*S*)-2-[[[(2*R*)-2-amino-2-phenylacetyl]amino]carboxymethyl]-5,5-dimethylthiazolidine-4-carboxylic acid (penicilloic acids of ampicillin),

F. R = H: (2*RS*,4*S*)-2-[[[(2*R*)-2-amino-2-phenylacetyl]amino]methyl]-5,5-dimethylthiazolidine-4-carboxylic acid (penilloic acids of ampicillin),

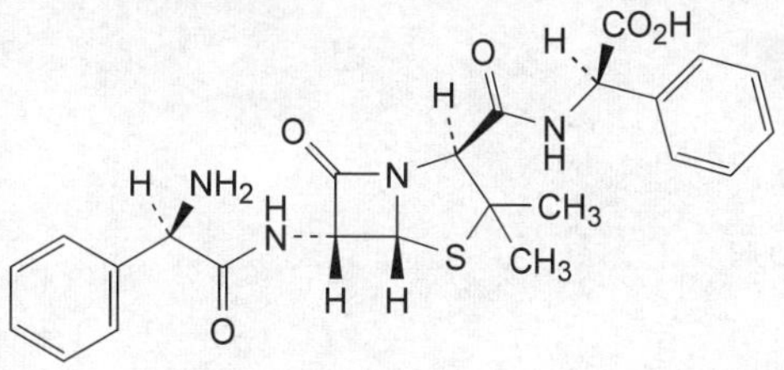

E. (2*R*)-2-[[[(2*S*,5*R*,6*R*)-6-[[(2*R*)-2-amino-2-phenylacetyl]amino]-3,3-dimethyl-7-oxo-4-thia-1-azabicyclo[3.2.0]hept-2-yl]carbonyl]amino]-2-phenylacetic acid (ampicillinyl-D-phenylglycine),

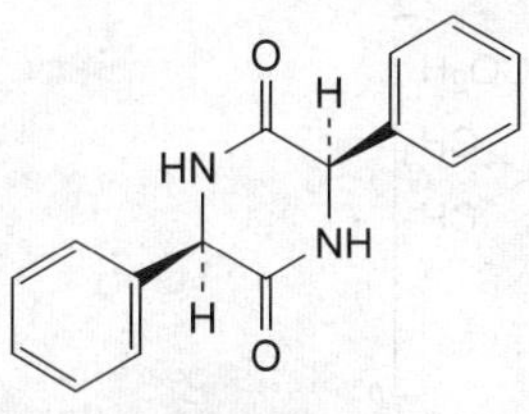

G. (3*R*,6*R*)-3,6-diphenylpiperazine-2,5-dione,

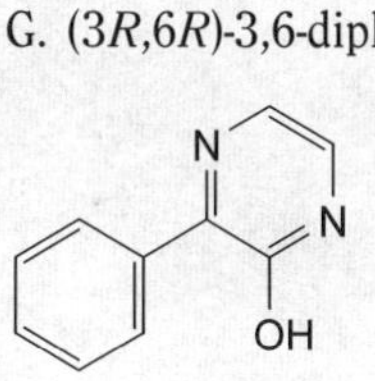

H. 3-phenylpyrazin-2-ol,

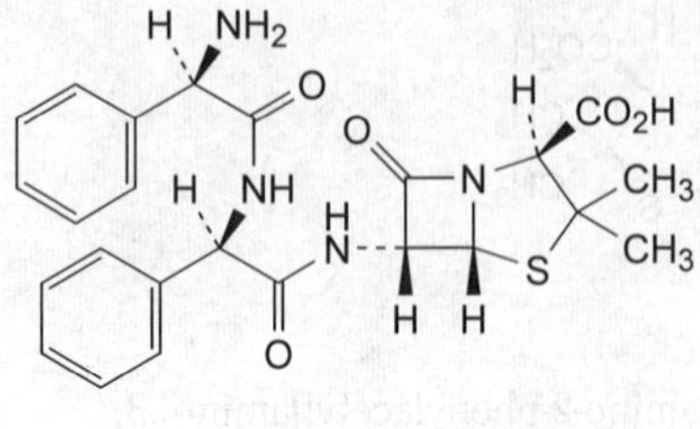

I. (2*S*,5*R*,6*R*)-6-[[(2*R*)-2-[[(2*R*)-2-amino-2-phenylacetyl]amino]-2-phenylacetyl]amino]-3,3-dimethyl-7-oxo-4-thia-1-azabicyclo[3.2.0]heptane-2-carboxylic acid (D-phenylglycylampicillin),

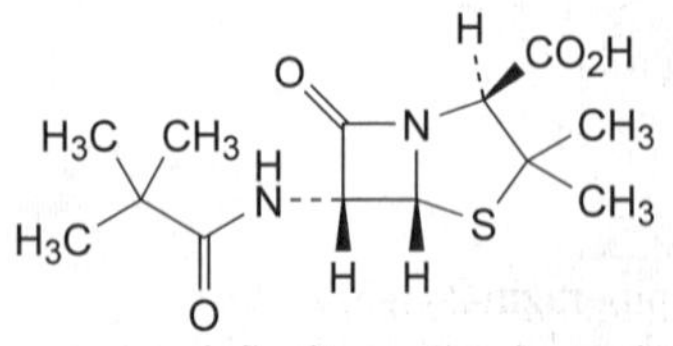

J. (2*S*,5*R*,6*R*)-6-[(2,2-dimethylpropanoyl)amino]-3,3-dimethyl-7-oxo-4-thia-1-azabicyclo[3.2.0]heptane-2-carboxylic acid,

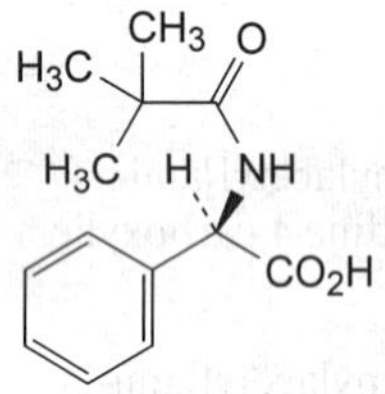

K. (2*R*)-2-[(2,2-dimethylpropanoyl)amino]-2-phenylacetic acid,

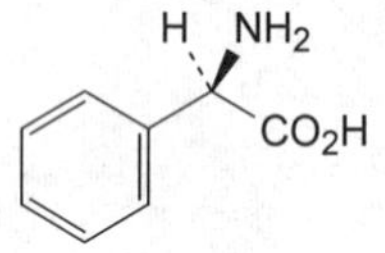

L. (2*R*)-2-amino-2-phenylacetic acid (D-phenylglycine),

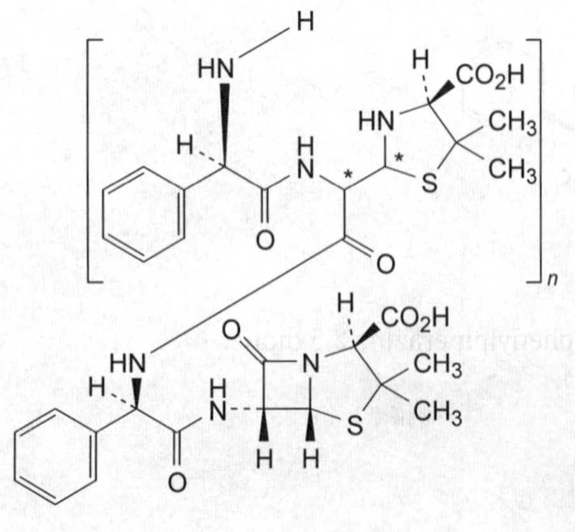

M. co-oligomers of ampicillin and of penicilloic acids of ampicillin.

01/2005:0578
corrected

AMPICILLIN SODIUM

Ampicillinum natricum

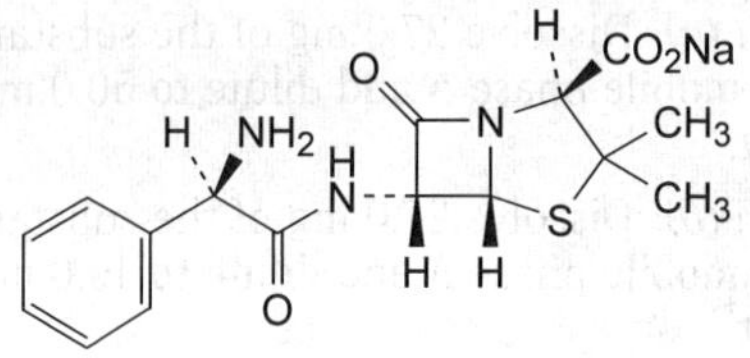

$C_{16}H_{18}N_3NaO_4S$ M_r 371.4

DEFINITION

Ampicillin sodium contains not less than 91.0 per cent and not more than the equivalent of 100.5 per cent of sodium (2*S*,5*R*,6*R*)-6-[[(2*R*)-2-amino-2-phenylacetyl]amino]-3,3-dimethyl-7-oxo-4-thia-1-azabicyclo[3.2.0]heptane-2-carboxylate, calculated with reference to the anhydrous substance.

CHARACTERS

A white or almost white powder, hygroscopic, freely soluble in water, sparingly soluble in acetone, practically insoluble in fatty oils and in liquid paraffin.

IDENTIFICATION

First identification: A, D.

Second identification: B, C, D.

A. Dissolve 0.250 g in 5 ml of *water R*, add 0.5 ml of *dilute acetic acid R*, swirl and allow to stand for 10 min in iced water. Filter the crystals through a small sintered-glass filter (40), applying suction, wash with 2 ml to 3 ml of a mixture of 1 volume of *water R* and 9 volumes of *acetone R* and dry in an oven at 60 °C for 30 min. Examine the crystals by infrared absorption spectrophotometry (*2.2.24*), comparing with the spectrum obtained with *ampicillin trihydrate CRS*.

B. Examine by thin-layer chromatography (*2.2.27*), using *silanised silica gel H R* as the coating substance.
Test solution. Dissolve 25 mg of the substance to be examined in 10 ml of *sodium hydrogen carbonate solution R*.
Reference solution (a). Dissolve 25 mg of *ampicillin trihydrate CRS* in 10 ml of *sodium hydrogen carbonate solution R*.
Reference solution (b). Dissolve 25 mg of *amoxicillin trihydrate CRS* and 25 mg of *ampicillin trihydrate CRS* in 10 ml of *sodium hydrogen carbonate solution R*.
Apply separately to the plate 1 µl of each solution. Develop over a path of 15 cm using a mixture of 10 volumes of *acetone R* and 90 volumes of a 154 g/l solution of *ammonium acetate R*, the pH of which has been adjusted to 5.0 with *glacial acetic acid R*. Allow the plate to dry in air and expose it to iodine vapour until the spots appear. Examine in daylight. The principal spot in the chromatogram obtained with the test solution is similar in position, colour and size to the principal spot in the chromatogram obtained with reference solution (a). The test is not valid unless the chromatogram obtained with reference solution (b) shows two clearly separated spots.

C. Place about 2 mg in a test-tube about 150 mm long and 15 mm in diameter. Moisten with 0.05 ml of *water R* and add 2 ml of *sulphuric acid-formaldehyde reagent R*.

Mix the contents of the tube by swirling; the solution is practically colourless. Place the test-tube in a water-bath for 1 min; a dark yellow colour develops.

D. It gives reaction (a) of sodium (*2.3.1*).

TESTS

Appearance of solution. Place 1.0 g in a conical flask and add slowly and with continuous swirling 10 ml of *1 M hydrochloric acid*. Separately dissolve 1.0 g in *water R* and dilute to 10.0 ml with the same solvent. Immediately after dissolution, the solutions are not more opalescent than reference suspension II (*2.2.1*). The absorbance (*2.2.25*) of the solution in watermeasured at 430 nm is not greater than 0.15.

pH (*2.2.3*). Dissolve 2.0 g in *carbon dioxide-free water R* and dilute to 20 ml with the same solvent. The pH of the solution, measured 10 min after dissolution, is 8.0 to 10.0.

Specific optical rotation (*2.2.7*). Dissolve 62.5 mg in a 4 g/l solution of *potassium hydrogen phthalate R* and dilute to 25.0 ml with the same solvent. The specific optical rotation is + 258 to + 287, calculated with reference to the anhydrous substance.

Related substances. Examine by liquid chromatography (*2.2.29*) as described under Assay. Inject 50 µl of reference solution (d) and elute isocratically until elution of the ampicillin peak. Inject 50 µl of test solution (b) and start the elution isocratically. Immediately after elution of the ampicillin peak start the following linear gradient. If the mobile phase composition has been adjusted to achieve the required resolution, the adjusted composition will apply at time zero in the gradient.

Time (min)	Mobile phase A (per cent *V/V*)	Mobile phase B (per cent *V/V*)	Comment
0 - 30	85 → 0	15 → 100	linear gradient
30 - 45	0	100	isocratic
45 - 60	85	15	re-equilibration

Inject mobile phase A and use the same elution pattern to obtain a blank. Inject reference solution (e) and use the same elution pattern. The chromatogram obtained with reference solution (e), shows an ampicillin peak and a dimer peak, with a retention time of 2.8 relative to ampicillin. In the chromatogram obtained with test solution (b), the area of any peak corresponding to ampicillin dimer is not greater than 4.5 times the area of the principal peak in the chromatogram obtained with reference solution (d) (4.5 per cent); the area of any peak, apart from the principal peak and any peak corresponding to ampicillin dimer, is not greater than twice the area of the principal peak in the chromatogram obtained with reference solution (d) (2 per cent). Disregard any peak due to the blank.

***N,N*-Dimethylaniline** (*2.4.26, Method B*). Not more than 20 ppm.

2-Ethylhexanoic acid (*2.4.28*). Not more than 0.8 per cent *m/m*.

Methylene chloride. Not more than 0.2 per cent *m/m*, determined by gas chromatography (*2.2.28*), using *ethylene chloride R* as the internal standard.

Internal standard solution. Dissolve 1.0 ml of *ethylene chloride R* in *water R* and dilute to 500.0 ml with the same solvent.

Test solution (a). Dissolve 1.0 g of the substance to be examined in *water R* and dilute to 10.0 ml with the same solvent.

Test solution (b). Dissolve 1.0 g of the substance to be examined in *water R*, add 1.0 ml of the internal standard solution and dilute to 10.0 ml with *water R*.

Reference solution. Dissolve 1.0 ml of *methylene chloride R* in *water R* and dilute to 500.0 ml with the same solvent. To 1.0 ml of the solution add 1.0 ml of the internal standard solution and dilute to 10.0 ml with *water R*.

The chromatographic procedure may be carried out using:

- a glass column 1.5 m long and 4 mm in internal diameter packed with *diatomaceous earth for gas chromatography R* impregnated with 10 per cent *m/m* of *macrogol 1000 R*,
- *nitrogen for chromatography R* as the carrier gas at a flow rate of 40 ml/min,
- a flame-ionisation detector,

maintaining the temperature of the column at 60 °C, that of the injection port at 100 °C and that of the detector at 150 °C. Calculate the content of methylene chloride taking its density at 20 °C to be 1.325 g/ml.

Heavy metals (*2.4.8*). 1.0 g complies with limit test C for heavy metals (20 ppm). Prepare the standard using 2 ml of *lead standard solution (10 ppm Pb) R*.

Water (*2.5.12*). Not more than 2.0 per cent, determined on 0.300 g by the semi-micro determination of water.

Bacterial endotoxins (*2.6.14*): less than 0.15 IU/mg, if intended for use in the manufacture of parenteral dosage forms without a further appropriate procedure for the removal of bacterial endotoxins.

ASSAY

Examine by liquid chromatography (*2.2.29*).

Test solution (a). Dissolve 31.0 mg of the substance to be examined in mobile phase A and dilute to 50.0 ml with mobile phase A.

Test solution (b). Prepare immediately before use. Dissolve 31.0 mg of the substance to be examined in mobile phase A and dilute to 10.0 ml with mobile phase A.

Reference solution (a). Dissolve 27.0 mg of *anhydrous ampicillin CRS* in mobile phase A and dilute to 50.0 ml with mobile phase A.

Reference solution (b). Dissolve 2.0 mg of *cefradine CRS* in mobile phase A and dilute to 50 ml with mobile phase A. To 5.0 ml of the solution add 5.0 ml of reference solution (a).

Reference solution (c). Dilute 1.0 ml of reference solution (a) to 20.0 ml with mobile phase A. Dilute 1.0 ml of the solution to 25.0 ml with mobile phase A.

Reference solution (d). Dilute 1.0 ml of reference solution (a) to 20.0 ml with mobile phase A.

Reference solution (e). To 0.20 g of the substance to be examined add 1.0 ml of *water R*. Heat the solution at 60 °C for 1 h. Dilute 0.5 ml of the solution to 50.0 ml with mobile phase A.

The chromatographic procedure may be carried out using:

- a column 0.25 m long and 4.6 mm in internal diameter packed with *octadecylsilyl silica gel for chromatography R* (5 µm),
- as mobile phase at a flow rate of 1.0 ml/min:

  Mobile phase A. A mixture of 0.5 ml of *dilute acetic acid R*, 50 ml of *0.2 M potassium dihydrogen phosphate R* and 50 ml of *acetonitrile R*, diluted to 1000 ml with *water R*,

  Mobile phase B. A mixture of 0.5 ml of *dilute acetic acid R*, 50 ml of *0.2 M potassium dihydrogen phosphate R* and 400 ml of *acetonitrile R*, diluted to 1000 ml with *water R*,
- as detector a spectrophotometer set at 254 nm.

Equilibrate the column with a mobile phase with A:B ratio of 85:15. Inject 50 µl of reference solution (b). The assay is not valid unless in the chromatogram obtained, the resolution between the two principal peaks is at least 3.0. If necessary, adjust the A:B ratio of the mobile phase. The mass distribution ratio for the first peak (ampicillin) is 2.0 to 2.5. Inject 50 µl of reference solution (c). Adjust the system to obtain a peak with a signal-to-noise ratio of at least 3. Inject reference solution (a) six times. The test is not valid unless the relative standard deviation for the area of the principal peak is at most 1.0 per cent. Inject alternately test solution (a) and reference solution (a).

Calculate the percentage content of ampicillin sodium by multiplying the percentage content of ampicillin by 1.063.

STORAGE

Store in an airtight container. If the substance is sterile, store in a sterile, airtight, tamper-proof container.

LABELLING

The label states, where applicable, that the substance is free from bacterial endotoxins.

IMPURITIES

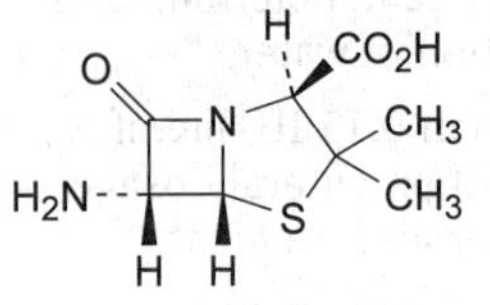

A. (2*S*,5*R*,6*R*)-6-amino-3,3-dimethyl-7-oxo-4-thia-1-azabicyclo[3.2.0]heptane-2-carboxylic acid (6-aminopenicillanic acid),

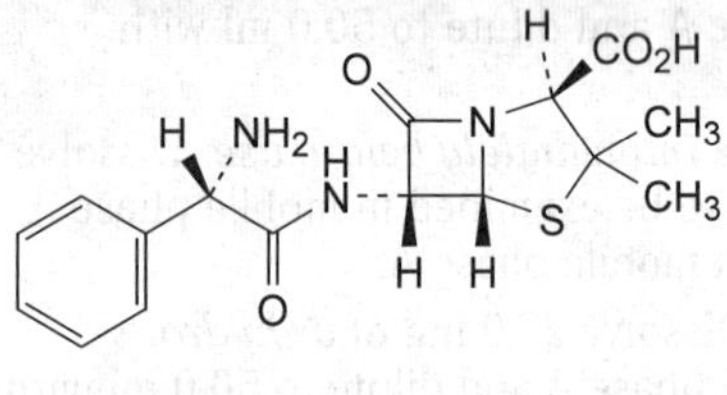

B. (2*S*,5*R*,6*R*)-6-[[(2*S*)-2-amino-2-phenylacetyl]amino]-3,3-dimethyl-7-oxo-4-thia-1-azabicyclo[3.2.0]heptane-2-carboxylic acid (L-ampicillin),

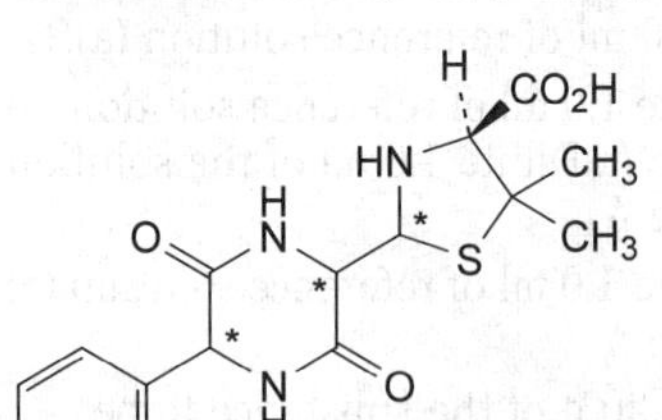

C. (4*S*)-2-(3,6-dioxo-5-phenylpiperazin-2-yl)-5,5-dimethylthiazolidine-4-carboxylic acid (diketopiperazines of ampicillin),

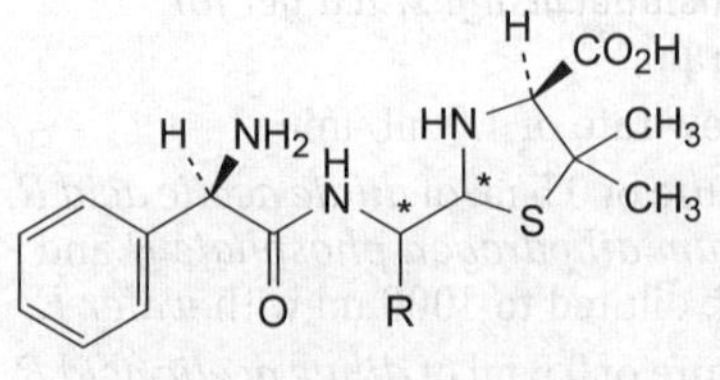

D. R = CO_2H: (4*S*)-2-[[[(2*R*)-2-amino-2-phenylacetyl]amino]carboxymethyl]-5,5-dimethylthiazolidine-4-carboxylic acid (penicilloic acids of ampicillin),

F. R = H: (2*RS*,4*S*)-2-[[[(2*R*)-2-amino-2-phenylacetyl]amino]methyl]-5,5-dimethylthiazolidine-4-carboxylic acid (penilloic acids of ampicillin),

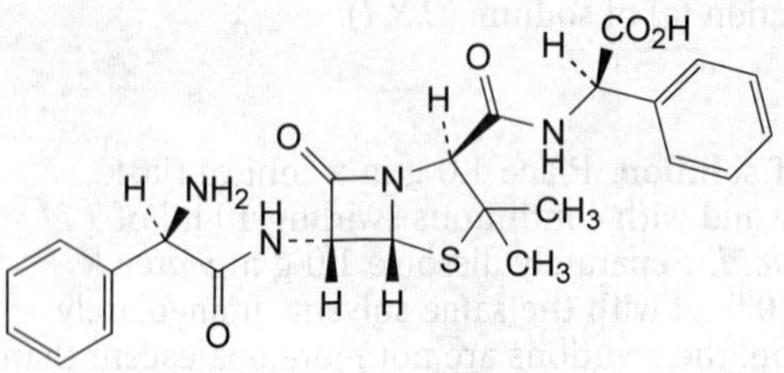

E. (2*R*)-2-[[[(2*S*,5*R*,6*R*)-6-[[(2*R*)-2-amino-2-phenylacetyl]amino]-3,3-dimethyl-7-oxo-4-thia-1-azabicyclo[3.2.0]hept-2-yl]carbonyl]amino]-2-phenylacetic acid (ampicillinyl-D-phenylglycine),

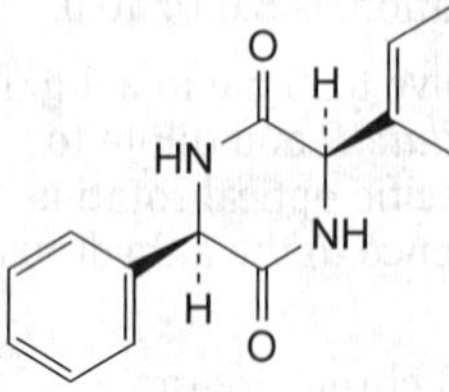

G. (3*R*,6*R*)-3,6-diphenylpiperazine-2,5-dione,

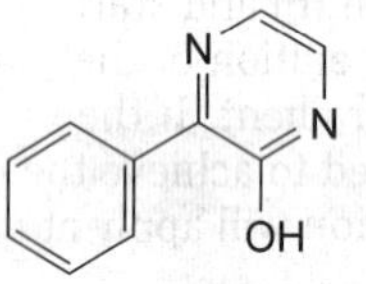

H. 3-phenylpyrazin-2-ol,

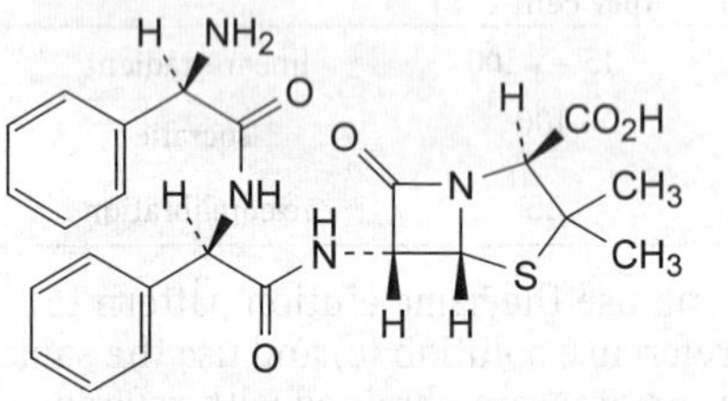

I. (2*S*,5*R*,6*R*)-6-[[(2*R*)-2-[[(2*R*)-2-amino-2-phenylacetyl]amino]-2-phenylacetyl]amino]-3,3-dimethyl-7-oxo-4-thia-1-azabicyclo[3.2.0]heptane-2-carboxylic acid (D-phenylglycylampicillin),

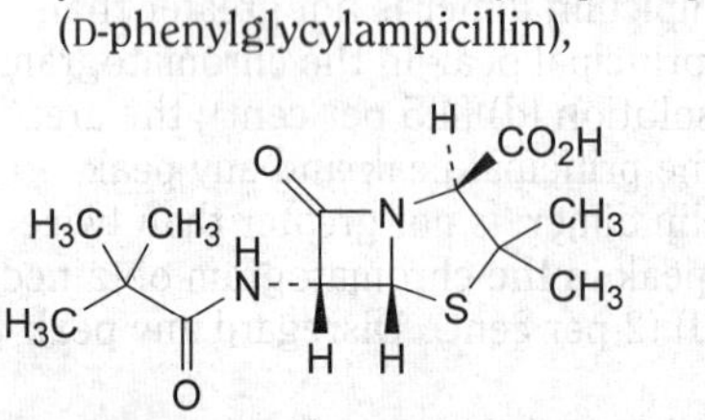

J. (2*S*,5*R*,6*R*)-6-[(2,2-dimethylpropanoyl)amino]-3,3-dimethyl-7-oxo-4-thia-1-azabicyclo[3.2.0]heptane-2-carboxylic acid,

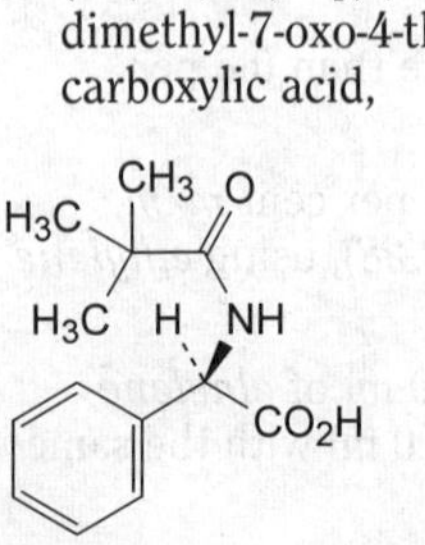

K. (2*R*)-2-[(2,2-dimethylpropanoyl)amino]-2-phenylacetic acid,

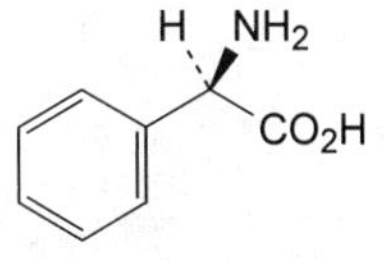

L. (2*R*)-2-amino-2-phenylacetic acid (D-phenylglycine),

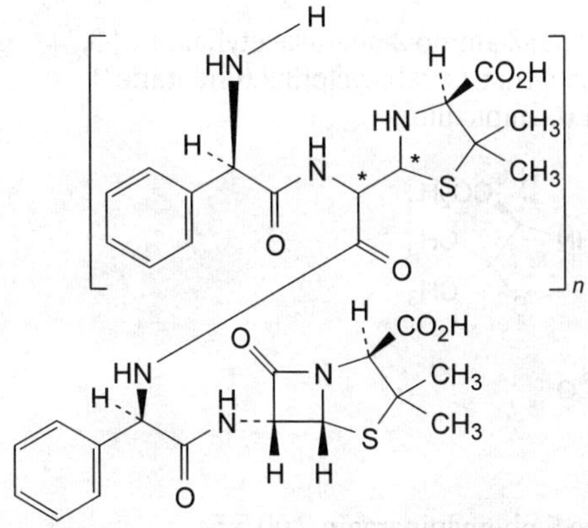

M. co-oligomers of ampicillin and of penicilloic acids of ampicillin,

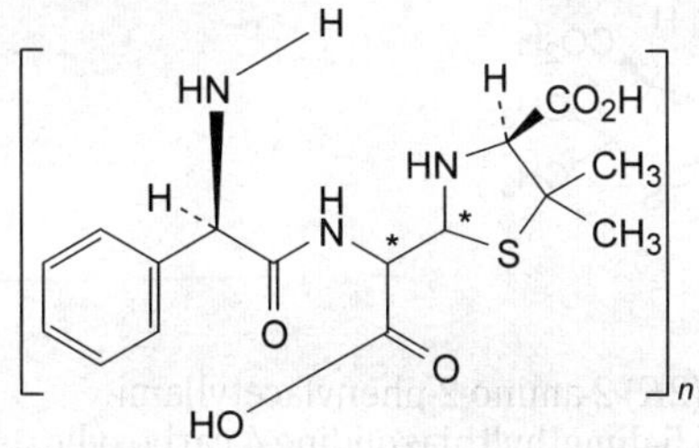

N. oligomers of penicilloic acids of ampicillin.

01/2005:0168

AMPICILLIN TRIHYDRATE

Ampicillinum trihydricum

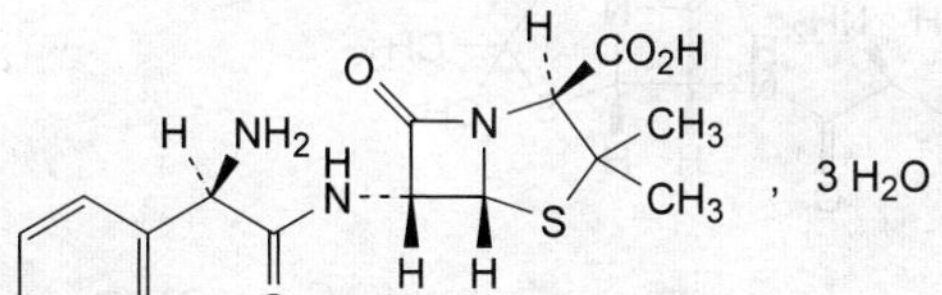

$C_{16}H_{19}N_3O_4S,3H_2O$ M_r 403.5

DEFINITION

Ampicillin trihydrate contains not less than 96.0 per cent and not more than the equivalent of 100.5 per cent of (2*S*,5*R*,6*R*)-6-[[(2*R*)-2-amino-2-phenylacetyl]amino]-3,3-dimethyl-7-oxo-4-thia-1-azabicyclo[3.2.0]heptane-2-carboxylic acid, calculated with reference to the anhydrous substance.

CHARACTERS

A white, crystalline powder, slightly soluble in water, practically insoluble in alcohol and in fatty oils. It dissolves in dilute solutions of acids and of alkali hydroxides.

IDENTIFICATION

First identification: A, D.

Second identification: B, C, D.

A. Examine by infrared absorption spectrophotometry (*2.2.24*), comparing with the spectrum obtained with *ampicillin trihydrate CRS.*

B. Examine by thin-layer chromatography (*2.2.27*), using *silanised silica gel H R* as the coating substance.

Test solution. Dissolve 25 mg of the substance to be examined in 10 ml of *sodium hydrogen carbonate solution R.*

Reference solution (a). Dissolve 25 mg of *ampicillin trihydrate CRS* in 10 ml of *sodium hydrogen carbonate solution R.*

Reference solution (b). Dissolve 25 mg of *amoxicillin trihydrate CRS* and 25 mg of *ampicillin trihydrate CRS* in 10 ml of *sodium hydrogen carbonate solution R.*

Apply separately to the plate 1 µl of each solution. Develop over a path of 15 cm using a mixture of 10 volumes of *acetone R* and 90 volumes of a 154 g/l solution of *ammonium acetate R*, the pH of which has been adjusted to 5.0 with *glacial acetic acid R.* Allow the plate to dry in air and expose it to iodine vapour until the spots appear. Examine in daylight. The principal spot in the chromatogram obtained with the test solution is similar in position, colour and size to the principal spot in the chromatogram obtained with reference solution (a). The test is not valid unless the chromatogram obtained with reference solution (b) shows 2 clearly separated spots.

C. Place about 2 mg in a test-tube about 150 mm long and 15 mm in diameter. Moisten with 0.05 ml of *water R* and add 2 ml of *sulphuric acid-formaldehyde reagent R.* Mix the contents of the tube by swirling; the solution is practically colourless. Place the test-tube in a water-bath for 1 min; a dark yellow colour develops.

D. It complies with the test for water (see Tests).

TESTS

Appearance of solution. Dissolve 1.0 g in 10 ml of *1 M hydrochloric acid.* Separately dissolve 1.0 g in 10 ml of *dilute ammonia R2.* Immediately after dissolution, the solutions are not more opalescent than reference suspension II (*2.2.1*).

pH (*2.2.3*). Dissolve 0.1 g in *carbon dioxide-free water R* and dilute to 40 ml with the same solvent. The pH of the solution is 3.5 to 5.5.

Specific optical rotation (*2.2.7*). Dissolve 62.5 mg in *water R* and dilute to 25.0 ml with the same solvent. The specific optical rotation is + 280 to + 305, calculated with reference to the anhydrous substance.

Related substances. Examine by liquid chromatography (*2.2.29*) as described under Assay. Inject reference solution (c) and elute isocratically. Inject freshly prepared test solution (b) and start the elution isocratically. Immediately after elution of the ampicillin peak start the following linear gradient. If the mobile phase composition has been adjusted to achieve the required resolution, the adjusted composition will apply at time zero in the gradient.

Time (min)	Mobile phase A (per cent *V/V*)	Mobile phase B (per cent *V/V*)
0	85	15
30	0	100
45	0	100

Equilibrate the column with the originally chosen mobile phase for 15 min. Inject mobile phase A and use the same elution gradient to obtain a blank. In the chromatogram obtained with test solution (b), the area of any peak, apart from the principal peak and any peak observed in the blank chromatogram, is not greater than the area of the principal peak in the chromatogram obtained with reference solution (c) (1.0 per cent).

***N,N*-Dimethylaniline** (*2.4.26, Method B*). Not more than 20 ppm.

Water (*2.5.12*). 12.0 per cent to 15.0 per cent, determined on 0.100 g by the semi-micro determination of water.

Sulphated ash (*2.4.14*). Not more than 0.5 per cent, determined on 1.0 g.

ASSAY

Examine by liquid chromatography (*2.2.29*).

Test solution (a). Dissolve 31.0 mg of the substance to be examined in mobile phase A and dilute to 50.0 ml with the same solvent.

Test solution (b). Dissolve 31.0 mg of the substance to be examined in mobile phase A and dilute to 10.0 ml with the same solvent.

Reference solution (a). Dissolve 27.0 mg of *anhydrous ampicillin CRS* in mobile phase A and dilute to 50.0 ml with the same solvent.

Reference solution (b). Dissolve 2.0 mg of *cefradine CRS* in mobile phase A and dilute to 50 ml with the same solvent. To 5.0 ml of this solution add 5.0 ml of reference solution (a).

Reference solution (c). Dilute 1.0 ml of reference solution (a) to 20.0 ml with mobile phase A.

Reference solution (d). Dilute 1.0 ml of reference solution (c) to 25.0 ml with mobile phase A.

The chromatographic procedure may be carried out using:

- a column 0.25 m long and 4.6 mm in internal diameter packed with *octadecylsilyl silica gel for chromatography R* (5 µm),
- as mobile phase at a flow rate of 1.0 ml/min:

  Mobile phase A. A mixture of 0.5 ml of *dilute acetic acid R*, 50 ml of *0.2 M potassium dihydrogen phosphate R*, 50 ml of *acetonitrile R* diluted to 1000 ml with *water R*,

  Mobile phase B. A mixture of 0.5 ml of *dilute acetic acid R*, 50 ml of *0.2 M potassium dihydrogen phosphate R* and 400 ml of *acetonitrile R* diluted to 1000 ml with *water R*,
- as detector a spectrophotometer set at 254 nm,
- a 50 µl loop injector.

Equilibrate the column with a mobile phase with ratio A:B of 85:15. Inject reference solution (b). The test is not valid unless the resolution between the two principal peaks is at least 3.0. If necessary, adjust the ratio A:B of the mobile phase. The mass distribution ratio for the first peak (ampicillin) is 2.0 to 2.5. Inject reference solution (d). Adjust the system to obtain a peak with a signal-to-noise ratio of at least 3. Inject reference solution (a) 6 times. The test is not valid unless the relative standard deviation for the area of the principal peak is at most 1.0 per cent. Inject alternately test solution (a) and reference solution (a).

Calculate the percentage content of ampicillin.

STORAGE

Store in an airtight container, at a temperature not exceeding 30 °C.

IMPURITIES

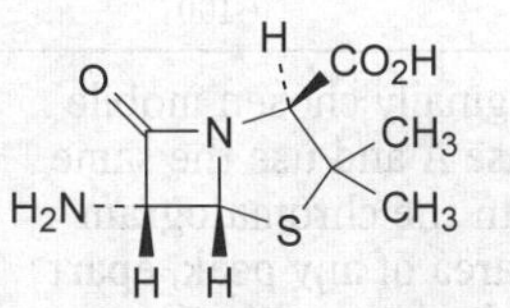

A. (2*S*,5*R*,6*R*)-6-amino-3,3-dimethyl-7-oxo-4-thia-1-azabicyclo[3.2.0]heptane-2-carboxylic acid (6-aminopenicillanic acid),

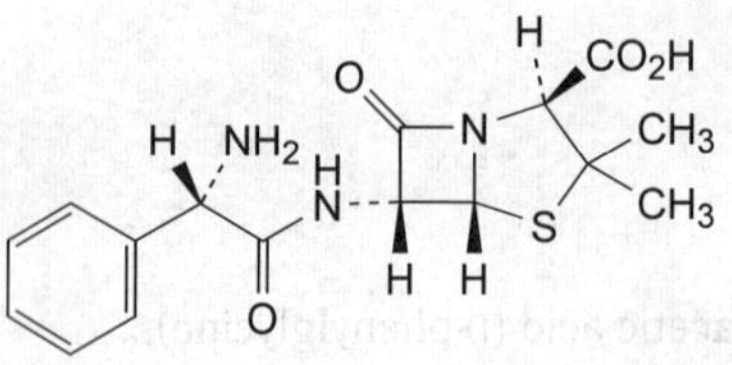

B. (2*S*,5*R*,6*R*)-6-[[(2*S*)-2-amino-2-phenylacetyl]amino]-3,3-dimethyl-7-oxo-4-thia-1-azabicyclo[3.2.0]heptane-2-carboxylic acid (L-ampicillin),

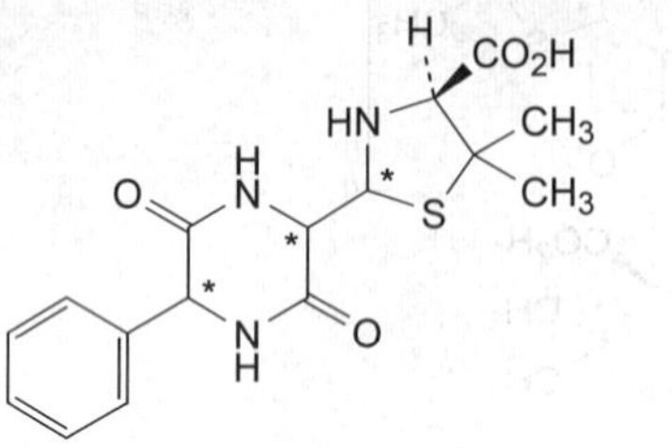

C. (4*S*)-2-(3,6-dioxo-5-phenylpiperazin-2-yl)-5,5-dimethylthiazolidine-4-carboxylic acid (diketopiperazines of ampicillin),

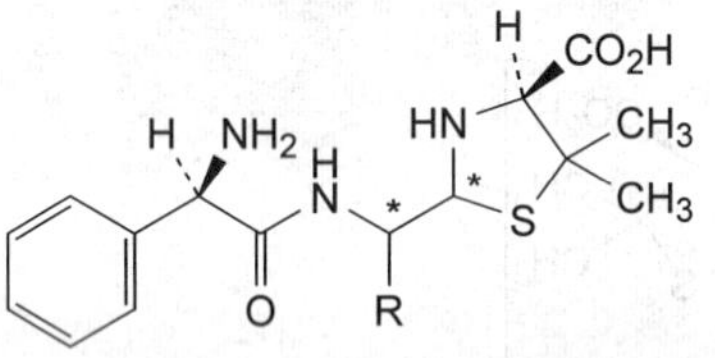

D. R = CO_2H: (4*S*)-2-[[[(2*R*)-2-amino-2-phenylacetyl]amino]carboxymethyl]-5,5-dimethylthiazolidine-4-carboxylic acid (penicilloic acids of ampicillin),

F. R = H: (2*RS*,4*S*)-2-[[[(2*R*)-2-amino-2-phenylacetyl]amino]methyl]-5,5-dimethylthiazolidine-4-carboxylic acid (penilloic acids of ampicillin),

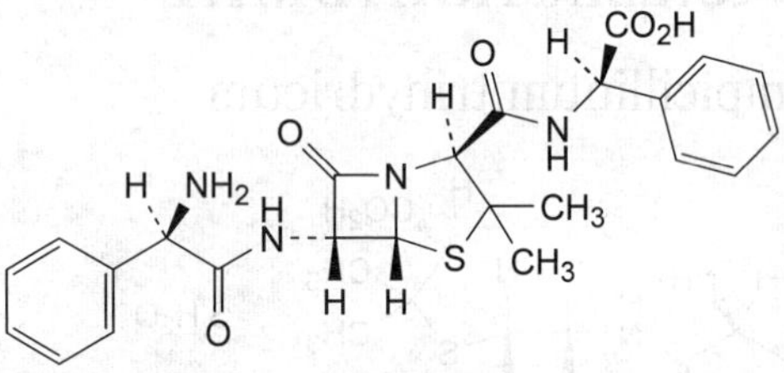

E. (2*R*)-2-[[[(2*S*,5*R*,6*R*)-6-[[(2*R*)-2-amino-2-phenylacetyl]amino]-3,3-dimethyl-7-oxo-4-thia-1-azabicyclo[3.2.0]hept-2-yl]carbonyl]amino]-2-phenylacetic acid (ampicillinyl-D-phenylglycine),

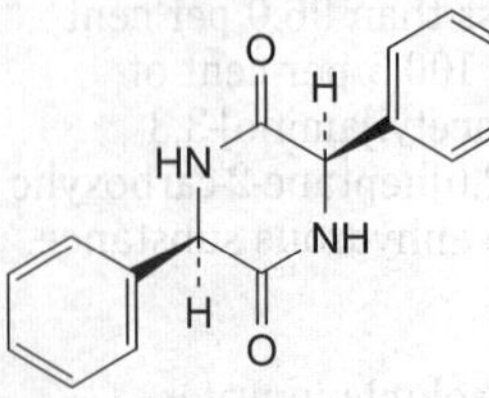

G. (3*R*,6*R*)-3,6-diphenylpiperazine-2,5-dione,

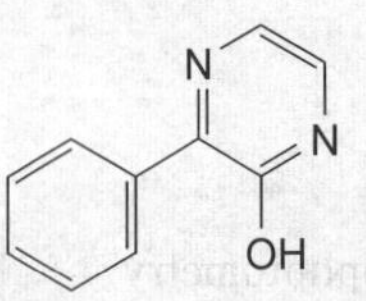

H. 3-phenylpyrazin-2-ol,

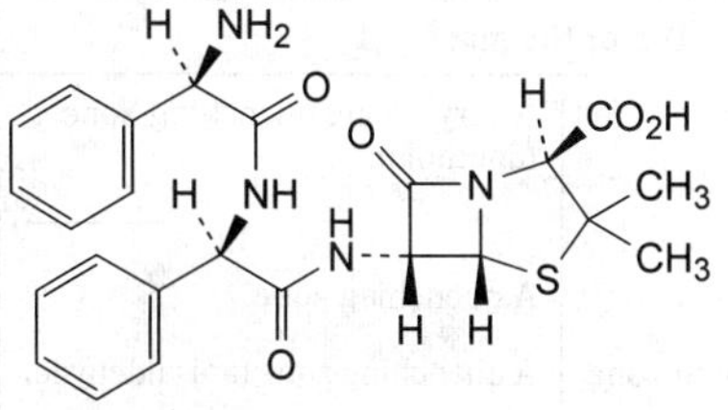

I. (2*S*,5*R*,6*R*)-6-[[(2*R*)-2-[[(2*R*)-2-amino-2-phenylacetyl]amino]-2-phenylacetyl]amino]-3,3-dimethyl-7-oxo-4-thia-1-azabicyclo[3.2.0]heptane-2-carboxylic acid (D-phenylglycylampicillin),

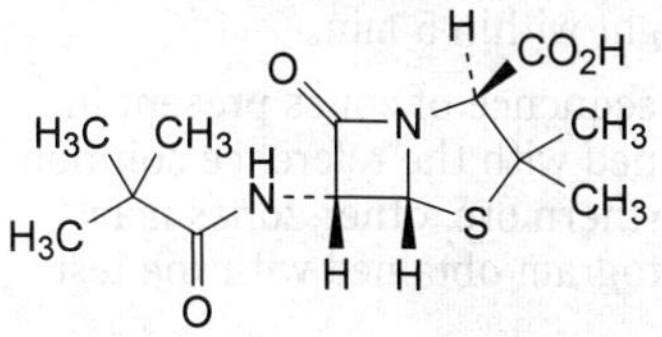

J. (2*S*,5*R*,6*R*)-6-[(2,2-dimethylpropanoyl)amino]-3,3-dimethyl-7-oxo-4-thia-1-azabicyclo[3.2.0]heptane-2-carboxylic acid,

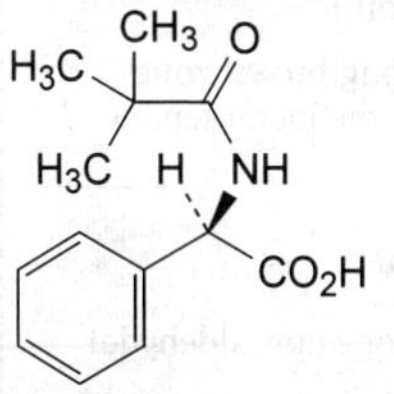

K. (2*R*)-2-[(2,2-dimethylpropanoyl)amino]-2-phenylacetic acid,

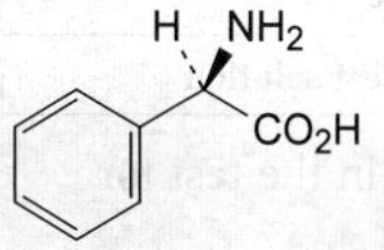

L. (2*R*)-2-amino-2-phenylacetic acid (D-phenylglycine),

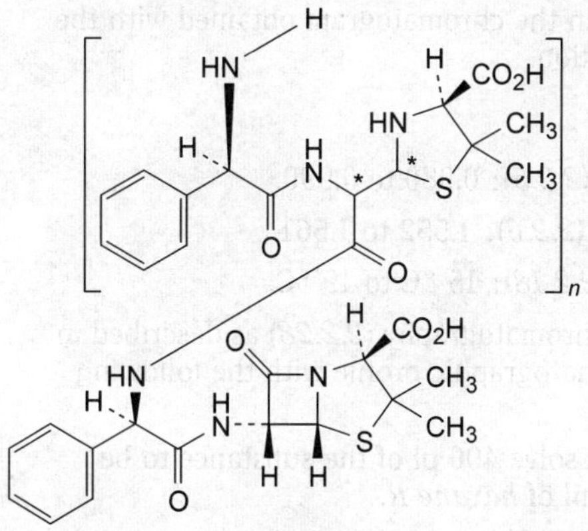

M. co-oligomers of ampicillin and of penicilloic acids of ampicillin.

01/2005:1857

ANGELICA ROOT

Angelicae radix

DEFINITION

Whole or cut, carefully dried rhizome and root of *Angelica archangelica* L. (*Archangelica officinalis Haffm.*).

Content: minimum 2.0 ml/kg of essential oil (dried drug).

CHARACTERS

Bitter taste.

Macroscopic and microscopic characters described under identification tests A and B.

IDENTIFICATION

A. The rhizome is greyish-brown or reddish-brown, transversely annulated. The base bears greyish-brown or reddish-brown, cylindrical, longitudinally furrowed, occasionally branched roots often with incompletely encircling, transverse ridges. The apex sometimes shows remnants of stem and leaf bases. The fracture is uneven. The transversely cut surface shows a greyish-white, spongy, distinctly radiate bark, in which the secretory channels are visible as brown spots, and a bright yellow to greyish-yellow wood which, in the rhizome, surrounds the greyish or brownish-white pith.

B. Reduce to a powder (355). The powder is brownish-white. Examine under a microscope using *chloral hydrate solution R*. The powder shows: fragments of cork consisting of several layers of thin-walled greyish-brown or reddish-brown cells; fragments of large, yellowish-brown secretory channels; fragments of medullary rays 2 to 4 cells wide; fragments of xylem with medullary rays and radially arranged, lignified vessels with reticulate thickening. Examine under a microscope using a 50 per cent *V/V* solution of *glycerol R*. The powder shows numerous, simple starch granules 2 µm to 4 µm in diameter.

C. Examine the chromatograms obtained in the test for lovage root.

Results: see below the sequence of the zones present in the chromatograms obtained with the reference solution and the test solution.

Top of the plate	
_______	
Eugenol: (marked at 254 nm)	
Coumarin: (marked at 254 nm)	
_______	
	An intense blue fluorescent zone
	Yellow fluorescent zones
	A blue fluorescent zone
	A yellow fluorescent zone
	An intense blue fluorescent zone
Reference solution	**Test solution**

TESTS

Lovage root. Thin-layer chromatography (*2.2.27*).

Test solution. To 1.0 g of the freshly powdered drug (355) add 5 ml of *methanol R* and boil for 30 s. Cool and filter.

Reference solution. Dissolve 5 mg of *coumarin R* and 25 µl of *eugenol R* in 10 ml of *methanol R*.

Plate: *TLC silica gel F_{254} plate R.*

Mobile phase: *methylene chloride R, toluene R* (50:50 *V/V*).

Application: 20 µl, as bands.

Development: twice over a path of 10 cm.

Drying: in air.

Detection: examine in ultraviolet light at 254 nm. Mark the quenching zones due to coumarin and eugenol on the chromatogram obtained with the reference solution. Examine in ultraviolet light at 365 nm.

Results: the chromatogram obtained with the test solution shows no pale blue to white fluorescent zone between the zones of coumarin and eugenol in the chromatogram obtained with the reference solution.

Foreign matter (*2.8.2*): maximum 5 per cent of leaf bases and stem bases, maximum 5 per cent of discoloured pieces and maximum 1 per cent of other foreign matter.

Loss on drying (*2.2.32*): maximum 10.0 per cent, determined on 1.000 g of the powdered drug (355) by drying in an oven at 100-105 °C for 2 h.

Total ash (*2.4.16*): maximum 10.0 per cent.

Ash insoluble in hydrochloric acid (*2.8.1*): maximum 2.0 per cent.

ASSAY

Carry out the determination of essential oils in vegetable drugs (*2.8.12*). Reduce the drug to a powder (500) and immediately use 40.0 g for the determination. Use a 2 litre round-bottomed flask, 10 drops of *liquid paraffin R*, 500 ml of *water R* as distillation liquid and 0.50 ml of *xylene R* in the graduated tube. Distil at a rate of 2-3 ml/min for 4 h.

01/2005:0804
corrected

ANISE OIL

Anisi aetheroleum

DEFINITION

Essential oil obtained by steam distillation from the dry ripe fruits of *Pimpinella anisum* L.

CHARACTERS

Appearance: clear, colourless or pale yellow liquid.

IDENTIFICATION

First identification: B.

Second identification: A.

A. Thin-layer chromatography (*2.2.27*).

Test solution. Dissolve 1 g of the substance to be examined in *toluene R* and dilute to 10 ml with the same solvent.

Reference solution. Dissolve 10 µl of *linalol R*, 30 µl of *anisaldehyde R* and 200 µl of *anethole R* in *toluene R* and dilute to 15 ml with the same solvent. Dilute 1 ml of this solution to 5 ml with *toluene R*.

Plate: *TLC silica gel F_{254} plate R.*

Mobile phase: *ethyl acetate R, toluene R* (7:93 *V/V*).

Application: 5 µl as bands of 10 mm (for normal TLC plates) or 2 µl as bands of 10 mm (for fine particle size plates).

Development: over a path of 15 cm (for normal TLC plates) or over a path of 6 cm (for fine particle size plates).

Drying: in air.

Detection A: examine in ultraviolet light at 254 nm.

Results A: see below the sequence of zones present in the chromatograms obtained with the reference solution and the test solution. Furthermore, other zones may be present in the chromatogram obtained with the test solution.

Top of the plate	
Anethole: a quenching zone	A very strong quenching zone (anethole)
_______	_______
	A quenching zone
Anisaldehyde: a quenching zone	A quenching zone (anisaldehyde)
_______	_______
Reference solution	**Test solution**

Detection B: spray with *methyl 4-acetylbenzoate reagent R* and heat at 100-105 °C for 10 min; examine the still hot plate in daylight within 5 min.

Results B: see below the sequence of zones present in the chromatograms obtained with the reference solution and the test solution. Furthermore, other zones may be present in the chromatogram obtained with the test solution.

Top of the plate	
	A violet-brown zone (monoterpene hydrocarbons) (solvent front)
Anethole: a brown zone	A very strong brown zone (anethole), distinctly separated
_______	_______
	A grey zone
Anisaldehyde: a yellow zone	A yellow zone (anisaldehyde)
_______	_______
Linalol: a grey zone	A grey zone (linalol)
	A grey zone
Reference solution	**Test solution**

B. Examine the chromatograms obtained in the test for chromatographic profile.

Results: the characteristic peaks in the chromatogram obtained with the test solution are similar in retention time to those in the chromatogram obtained with the reference solution.

TESTS

Relative density (*2.2.5*): 0.980 to 0.990.

Refractive index (*2.2.6*): 1.552 to 1.561.

Freezing point (*2.2.18*): 15 °C to 19 °C.

Fenchone. Gas chromatography (*2.2.28*) as described in the test for chromatographic profile with the following modifications.

Test solution. Dissolve 400 µl of the substance to be examined in 2.0 ml of *hexane R*.

Reference solution (a). Dilute 10 µl of *fenchone R* to 1.2 g with *hexane R*.

Reference solution (b). Dilute 100 µl of reference solution (a) to 100 ml with *hexane R*.

System suitability: reference solution (b):

- *signal-to-noise ratio*: minimum 10 for the principal peak.

Limit:

- *fenchone*: maximum 0.01 per cent.

Foeniculin. Gas chromatography (*2.2.28*) as described in the test for chromatographic profile with the following modifications.

Test solution. The substance to be examined.

Reference solution (a). Dilute 10 mg of the test solution to 1.000 g with *hexane R*. Dilute 0.5 ml of this solution to 100 ml with *hexane R*.

Reference solution (b). Foeniculin for peak identification CRS.

System suitability:

– the chromatogram obtained with reference solution (b) is similar to the chromatogram provided with *foeniculin for peak identification CRS*,
– *signal-to-noise ratio*: minimum 10 for the principal peak in the chromatogram obtained with reference solution (a).

Limit: locate the peak due to foeniculin by comparison with the chromatogram provided with *foeniculin for peak identification CRS.*

– *foeniculin*: maximum 0.01 per cent.

Fatty oils and resinified essential oils (*2.8.7*). It complies with the test for fatty oils and resinified essential oils.

Chromatographic profile. Gas chromatography (*2.2.28*): use the normalisation procedure.

Test solution. Dissolve 200 μl of the substance to be examined in 1.0 ml of *hexane R*.

Reference solution. To 1.0 ml of *hexane R*, add 20 μl of *linalol R*, 20 μl of *estragole R*, 20 μl of *α-terpineol R*, 60 μl of *anethole R* and 30 μl of *anisaldehyde R*.

Column:

– *material*: fused silica,
– *size*: *l* = 30 m, Ø = 0.25 mm,
– *stationary phase*: *macrogol 20 000 R* (film thickness 0.25 μm).

Carrier gas: *helium for chromatography R.*

Flow rate: 1.0 ml/min.

Split ratio: 1:100.

Temperature:

	Time (min)	Temperature (°C)
Column	0 - 5	60
	5 - 80	60 → 210
	80 - 95	210
Injection port		200
Detector		220

Detection: flame ionisation.

Injection: 0.2 μl.

Elution order: order indicated in the composition of the reference solution. Record the retention times of these substances.

System suitability: reference solution:

– *resolution*: minimum 1.5 between the peaks due to estragole and α-terpineol.

Using the retention times determined from the chromatogram obtained with the reference solution, locate the components of the reference solution in the chromatogram obtained with the test solution and locate *cis*-anethole and pseudoisoeugenyl 2-methylbutyrate using the chromatogram shown in Figure 0804.-1 (disregard any peak due to hexane). Determine the percentage content of these components. The percentages are within the following ranges:

– *linalol*: less than 1.5 per cent,
– *estragole*: 0.5 per cent to 5.0 per cent,
– *α-terpineol*: less than 1.2 per cent,
– *cis-anethole*: 0.1 per cent to 0.4 per cent,
– *trans-anethole*: 87 per cent to 94 per cent,
– *anisaldehyde*: 0.1 per cent to 1.4 per cent,
– *pseudoisoeugenyl 2-methylbutyrate*: 0.3 per cent to 2.0 per cent.

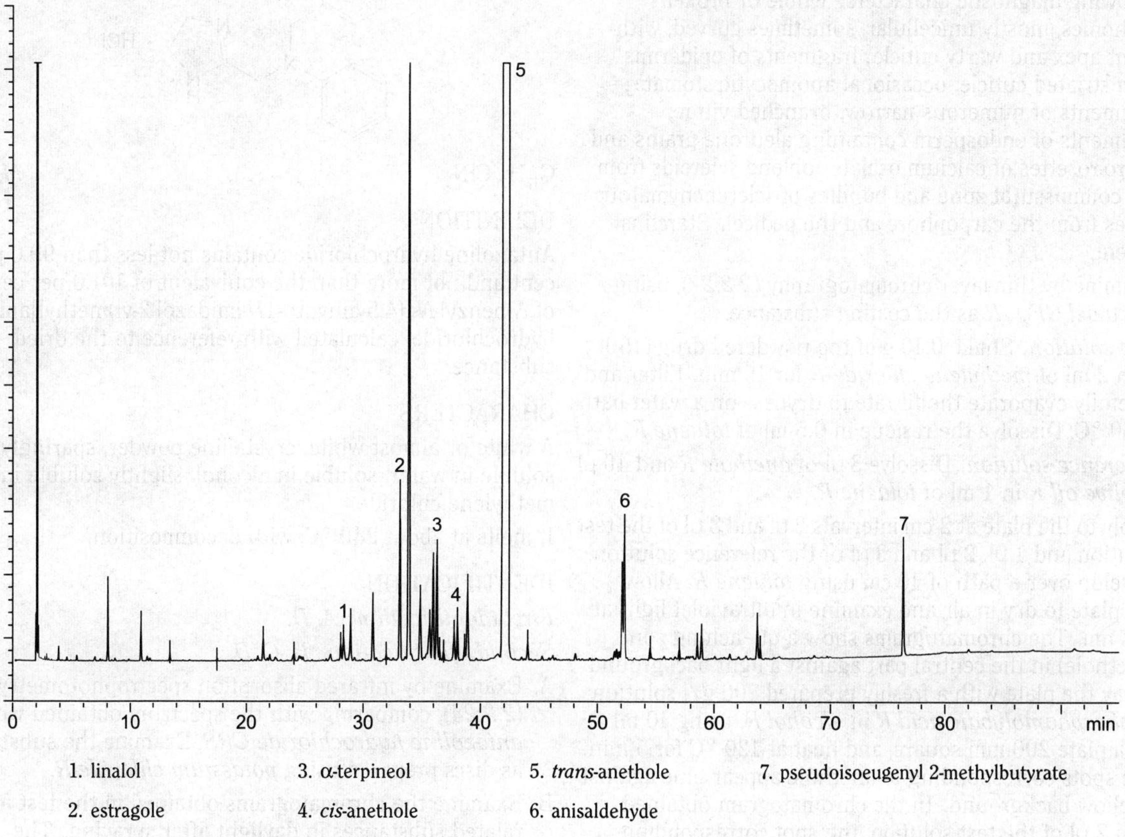

1. linalol
2. estragole
3. α-terpineol
4. *cis*-anethole
5. *trans*-anethole
6. anisaldehyde
7. pseudoisoeugenyl 2-methylbutyrate

Figure 0804.-1. – *Chromatogram for the test for chromatographic profile of anise oil*

STORAGE

In a well-filled, airtight container, protected from light and at a temperature not exceeding 25 °C.

01/2005:0262

ANISEED

Anisi fructus

DEFINITION

Aniseed consists of the whole dry cremocarp of *Pimpinella anisum* L. It contains not less than 20 ml/kg of essential oil.

CHARACTERS

Aniseed has an odour reminiscent of anethole.

The fruit is a cremocarp and generally entire; a small fragment of the thin, rigid, slightly curved pedicel is frequently attached.

It has the macroscopic and microscopic characters described under identification tests A and B.

IDENTIFICATION

A. The cremocarp is ovoid or pyriform and slightly compressed laterally, yellowish-green or greenish-grey, 3 mm to 5 mm long and up to 3 mm wide, surmounted by a stylopod with 2 short, reflexed stylar points. The mericarps are attached by their tops to the carpophore with a plane commissural surface and a convex dorsal surface, the latter being covered with short, warty trichomes visible using a lens; the fruit shows 5 primary ridges, running longitudinally, comprising 3 dorsal ridges and 2 lateral ridges, non-prominent, and lighter in colour.

B. Reduce to a powder (355). The powder is greenish-yellow to brownish-green. Examine under a microscope using *chloral hydrate solution R*. The powder shows the following diagnostic characters: whole or broken trichomes, mostly unicellular, sometimes curved, with blunt apex and warty cuticle; fragments of epidermis with striated cuticle, occasional anomocytic stomata; fragments of numerous narrow, branched vittae, fragments of endosperm containing aleurone grains and micro-rosettes of calcium oxalate; oblong sclereids from the commissural zone and bundles of sclerenchymatous fibres from the carpophore and the pedicel. Starch is absent.

C. Examine by thin-layer chromatography (*2.2.27*), using *silica gel GF_{254} R* as the coating substance.

Test solution. Shake 0.10 g of the powdered drug (1500) with 2 ml of *methylene chloride R* for 15 min. Filter and carefully evaporate the filtrate to dryness on a water-bath at 60 °C. Dissolve the residue in 0.5 ml of *toluene R*.

Reference solution. Dissolve 3 μl of *anethole R* and 40 μl of *olive oil R* in 1 ml of *toluene R*.

Apply to the plate at 2 cm intervals 2 μl and 3 μl of the test solution and 1 μl, 2 μl and 3 μl of the reference solution. Develop over a path of 10 cm using *toluene R*. Allow the plate to dry in air and examine in ultraviolet light at 254 nm. The chromatograms show a quenching zone (anethole) in the central part against a light background. Spray the plate with a freshly prepared 200 g/l solution of *phosphomolybdic acid R* in *alcohol R*, using 10 ml for a plate 200 mm square, and heat at 120 °C for 5 min. The spots corresponding to anethole appear blue against a yellow background. In the chromatogram obtained with 2 μl of the test solution, the spot corresponding to anethole is intermediate in size between the spots corresponding to anethole in the chromatograms obtained with 1 μl and 3 μl of the reference solution. The chromatograms obtained with the test solution show in the lower third a blue spot (triglycerides) similar in position to the spot in the lower third of the chromatograms obtained with the reference solution (triglycerides of olive oil).

TESTS

Foreign matter (*2.8.2*). It complies with the test for foreign matter.

Water (*2.2.13*). Not more than 70 ml/kg, determined by distillation on 20.0 g of the powdered drug.

Total ash (*2.4.16*). Not more than 12.0 per cent.

Ash insoluble in hydrochloric acid (*2.8.1*). Not more than 2.5 per cent.

ASSAY

Carry out the determination of essential oils in vegetable drugs (*2.8.12*). Use a 250 ml round-bottomed flask, 100 ml of *water R* as the distillation liquid and 0.50 ml of *xylene R* in the graduated tube. Reduce the drug to a coarse powder and immediately use 10.0 g for the determination. Distil at a rate of 2.5-3.5 ml/min for 2 h.

STORAGE

Store protected from light.

01/2005:0972

ANTAZOLINE HYDROCHLORIDE

Antazolini hydrochloridum

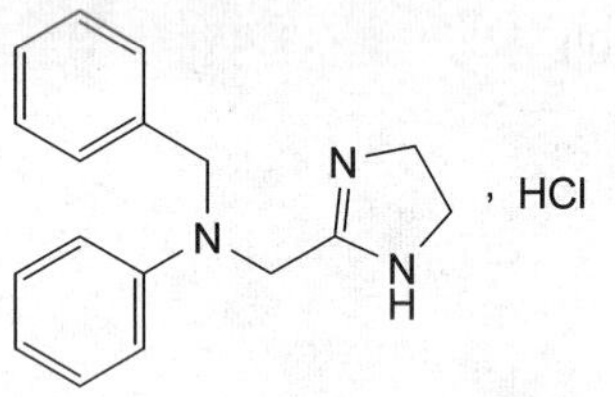

$C_{17}H_{20}ClN_3$ M_r 301.8

DEFINITION

Antazoline hydrochloride contains not less than 99.0 per cent and not more than the equivalent of 101.0 per cent of *N*-benzyl-*N*-[(4,5-dihydro-1*H*-imidazol-2-yl)methyl]aniline hydrochloride, calculated with reference to the dried substance.

CHARACTERS

A white or almost white, crystalline powder, sparingly soluble in water, soluble in alcohol, slightly soluble in methylene chloride.

It melts at about 240 °C, with decomposition.

IDENTIFICATION

First identification: A, D.

Second identification: B, C, D.

A. Examine by infrared absorption spectrophotometry (*2.2.24*), comparing with the spectrum obtained with *antazoline hydrochloride CRS*. Examine the substances as discs prepared using *potassium chloride R*.

B. Examine the chromatograms obtained in the test for related substances in daylight after spraying. The principal spot in the chromatogram obtained with test solution (b) is similar in position, colour and size to the principal spot in the chromatogram obtained with reference solution (b).

C. To 5 ml of solution S (see Tests) add, drop by drop, *dilute sodium hydroxide solution R* until an alkaline reaction is produced. Filter. The precipitate, washed with two quantities, each of 10 ml, of *water R* and dried in a desicator under reduced pressure, melts (*2.2.14*) at 119 °C to 123 °C.

D. It gives reaction (a) of chlorides (*2.3.1*).

TESTS

Solution S. Dissolve 2.0 g in *carbon dioxide-free water R* prepared from *distilled water R*, heating at 60 °C if necessary. Allow to cool and dilute to 100 ml with the same solvent.

Appearance of solution. Solution S is clear (*2.2.1*) and not more intensely coloured than reference solution Y_7 (*2.2.2, Method II*).

Acidity or alkalinity. To 10 ml of solution S add 0.2 ml of *methyl red solution R*. Not more than 0.1 ml of *0.01 M hydrochloric acid* or *0.01 M sodium hydroxide* is required to change the colour of the indicator.

Related substances. Examine by thin-layer chromatography (*2.2.27*), using *silica gel GF_{254} R* as the coating substance. Heat the plate at 110 °C for 15 min before using.

Test solution (a). Dissolve 0.10 g of the substance to be examined in *methanol R* and dilute to 5 ml with the same solvent.

Test solution (b). Dilute 1 ml of test solution (a) to 5 ml with *methanol R*.

Reference solution (a). Dilute 0.5 ml of test solution (a) to 100 ml with *methanol R*.

Reference solution (b). Dissolve 20 mg of *antazoline hydrochloride CRS* in *methanol R* and dilute to 5 ml with the same solvent.

Reference solution (c). Dissolve 20 mg of *xylometazoline hydrochloride CRS* in 1 ml of test solution (a) and dilute to 5 ml with *methanol R*.

Apply to the plate 5 µl of each solution. Develop over a path of 15 cm using a mixture of 5 volumes of *diethylamine R*, 10 volumes of *methanol R* and 85 volumes of *ethyl acetate R*. Dry the plate in a current of warm air for 15 min. Examine in ultraviolet light at 254 nm. The test is not valid unless the chromatogram obtained with reference solution (c) shows two clearly separated principal spots. Spray with a mixture of equal volumes of a 200 g/l solution of *ferric chloride R* and a 5 g/l solution of *potassium ferricyanide R*. Examine immediately in daylight. Any spot in the chromatogram obtained with test solution (a), apart from the principal spot, is not more intense than the spot in the chromatogram obtained with reference solution (a) (0.5 per cent).

Heavy metals (*2.4.8*). 1.0 g complies with limit test C for heavy metals (20 ppm). Prepare the standard using 2 ml of *lead standard solution (10 ppm Pb) R*.

Loss on drying (*2.2.32*). Not more than 0.5 per cent, determined on 1.000 g by drying in an oven at 100 °C to 105 °C for 3 h.

Sulphated ash (*2.4.14*). Not more than 0.1 per cent, determined on the residue obtained in the test for loss on drying.

ASSAY

Dissolve 0.250 g in 100 ml of *alcohol R*. Add 0.1 ml of *phenolphthalein solution R1*. Titrate with *0.1 M alcoholic potassium hydroxide*.

1 ml of *0.1 M alcoholic potassium hydroxide* is equivalent to 30.18 mg of $C_{17}H_{20}ClN_3$.

IMPURITIES

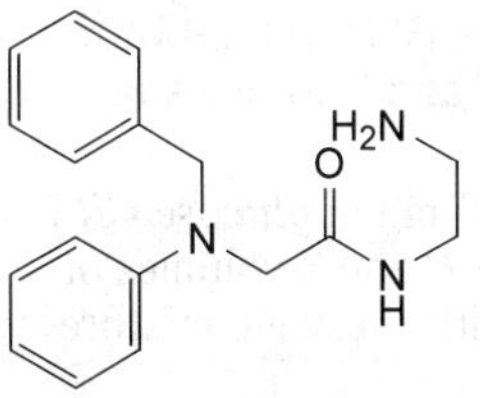

A. *N*-(2-aminoethyl)-2-(benzylphenylamino)acetamide.

01/2005:0209

ANTICOAGULANT AND PRESERVATIVE SOLUTIONS FOR HUMAN BLOOD

Solutiones anticoagulantes et sanguinem humanum conservantes

DEFINITION

Anticoagulant and preservative solutions for human blood are sterile and pyrogen-free solutions prepared with water for injections, filtered, distributed in the final containers and sterilised. The content of sodium citrate ($C_6H_5Na_3O_7,2H_2O$), glucose monohydrate ($C_6H_{12}O_6,H_2O$) or anhydrous glucose ($C_6H_{12}O_6$) and sodium dihydrogen phosphate dihydrate ($NaH_2PO_4,2H_2O$) is not less than 95.0 per cent and not more than 105.0 per cent of that stated in the formulae below. The content of citric acid monohydrate ($C_6H_8O_7,H_2O$) or anhydrous citric acid ($C_6H_8O_7$) is not less than 90.0 per cent and not more than 110.0 per cent of that stated in the formulae below. Subject to agreement by the competent authority, other substances, such as red-cell preservatives, may be included in the formula provided that their name and concentration are stated on the label.

Anticoagulant and preservative solutions for human blood are presented in airtight, tamper-proof containers of glass (*3.2.1*) or plastic (*3.2.3*).

Anticoagulant acid-citrate-glucose solutions (ACD)

	A	B
Sodium citrate (0412)	22.0 g	13.2 g
Citric acid monohydrate (0456)	8.0 g	4.8 g
or *Citric acid, anhydrous (0455)*	7.3 g	4.4 g
*Glucose monohydrate (0178)**	24.5 g	14.7 g
or *Glucose, anhydrous (0177)**	22.3 g	13.4 g
Water for injections (0169) to	1000.0 ml	1000.0 ml
Volume to be used per 100 ml of blood	15.0 ml	25.0 ml

*The competent authority may require that the substances comply with the test for pyrogens given in the monographs on *Glucose monohydrate (0178)* and *Glucose, anhydrous (0177)*, respectively.

CHARACTERS

A colourless or faintly yellow, clear liquid, practically free from particles.

IDENTIFICATION

A. Examine by thin-layer chromatography (*2.2.27*), using *silica gel G R* as the coating substance.

Test solution. Dilute 2 ml of the solution to be examined (for formula A) or 3 ml (for formula B) to 100 ml with a mixture of 2 volumes of *water R* and 3 volumes of *methanol R*.

Reference solution (a). Dissolve 10 mg of *glucose CRS* in a mixture of 2 volumes of *water R* and 3 volumes of *methanol R* and dilute to 20 ml with the same mixture of solvents.

Reference solution (b). Dissolve 10 mg each of *glucose CRS, lactose CRS, fructose CRS* and *sucrose CRS* in a mixture of 2 volumes of *water R* and 3 volumes of *methanol R* and dilute to 20 ml with the same mixture of solvents.

Apply separately to the plate 2 µl of each solution and thoroughly dry the starting points. Develop over a path of 15 cm using a mixture of 10 volumes of *water R*, 15 volumes of *methanol R*, 25 volumes of *anhydrous acetic acid R* and 50 volumes of *ethylene chloride R*. The volumes of solvents have to be measured accurately since a slight excess of water produces cloudiness. Dry the plate in a current of warm air. Repeat the development immediately, after renewing the mobile phase. Dry the plate in a current of warm air and spray evenly with a solution of 0.5 g of *thymol R* in a mixture of 5 ml of *sulphuric acid R* and 95 ml of *alcohol R*. Heat at 130 °C for 10 min. The principal spot in the chromatogram obtained with the test solution is similar in position, colour and size to the principal spot in the chromatogram obtained with reference solution (a). The test is not valid unless the chromatogram obtained with reference solution (b) shows 4 clearly separated spots.

B. To 2 ml add 5 ml of *cupri-citric solution R*. Heat to boiling. An orange precipitate is formed and the solution becomes yellow.

C. To 2 ml (for formula A) add 3 ml of *water R* or to 4 ml (for formula B) add 1 ml of *water R*. The solution gives the reaction of citrates (*2.3.1*).

D. 0.5 ml gives reaction (b) of sodium (*2.3.1*).

TESTS

pH (*2.2.3*). The pH of the solution to be examined is 4.7 to 5.3.

Hydroxymethylfurfural. To 2.0 ml add 5.0 ml of a 100 g/l solution of *p-toluidine R* in *2-propanol R* containing 10 per cent *V/V* of *glacial acetic acid R* and 1.0 ml of a 5 g/l solution of *barbituric acid R*. The absorbance (*2.2.25*), determined at 550 nm after allowing the mixture to stand for 2 min to 3 min, is not greater than that of a standard prepared at the same time in the same manner using 2.0 ml of a solution containing 5 ppm of *hydroxymethylfurfural R* for formula A or 3 ppm of *hydroxymethylfurfural R* for formula B.

Sterility (*2.6.1*). They comply with the test for sterility.

Pyrogens (*2.6.8*). They comply with the test for pyrogens. Dilute with a pyrogen-free, 9 g/l solution of *sodium chloride R* to obtain a solution containing approximately 5 g/l of sodium citrate. Inject 10 ml of the diluted solution per kilogram of the rabbit's mass.

ASSAY

Citric acid. To 10.0 ml (for formula A) or to 20.0 ml (for formula B) add 0.1 ml of *phenolphthalein solution R1*. Titrate with *0.2 M sodium hydroxide* until a pink colour is obtained.

1 ml of *0.2 M sodium hydroxide* is equivalent to 14.01 mg of $C_6H_8O_7,H_2O$ or to 12.81 mg of $C_6H_8O_7$.

Sodium citrate. Prepare a chromatography column 0.10 m long and 10 mm in internal diameter and filled with *strongly acidic ion-exchange resin R* (300 µm to 840 µm). Maintain a 1 cm layer of liquid above the resin at all times. Wash the column with 50 ml of de-ionised *water R* at a flow rate of 12-14 ml/min.

Dilute 10.0 ml of the solution to be examined (for formula A) or 15.0 ml (for formula B) to about 40 ml with de-ionised *water R* in a beaker and transfer to the column reservoir, washing the beaker 3 times with a few millilitres of de-ionised *water R*. Allow the solution to run through the column at a flow rate of 12-14 ml/min and collect the eluate. Wash the column with 2 quantities, each of 30 ml, and with one quantity of 50 ml, of de-ionised *water R*. The column can be used for 3 successive determinations before regeneration with 3 times its volume of *dilute hydrochloric acid R*. Titrate the combined eluate and washings (about 150 ml) with *0.2 M sodium hydroxide*, using 0.1 ml of *phenolphthalein solution R1* as indicator.

Calculate the content of sodium citrate in grams per litre from the following expressions:

For formula A: $1.961n - 1.40C$

or $1.961n - 1.53C'$

For formula B: $1.307n - 1.40C$

or $1.307n - 1.53C'$

n = number of millilitres of *0.2 M sodium hydroxide* used in the titration,

C = content of citric acid monohydrate in grams per litre determined as prescribed above,

C' = content of anhydrous citric acid in grams per litre determined as prescribed above.

Reducing sugars. Dilute 5.0 ml (for formula A) or 10.0 ml (for formula B) to 100.0 ml with *water R*. Introduce 25.0 ml of the solution into a 250 ml conical flask with ground-glass neck and add 25.0 ml of *cupri-citric solution R1*. Add a few pieces of porous material, attach a reflux condenser, heat so that boiling begins within 2 min and boil for exactly 10 min. Cool and add 3 g of *potassium iodide R* dissolved in 3 ml of *water R*. Add 25 ml of a 25 per cent *m/m* solution of *sulphuric acid R* with caution and in small quantities. Titrate with *0.1 M sodium thiosulphate* using 0.5 ml of *starch solution R*, added towards the end of the titration, as indicator (n_1 ml). Carry out a blank titration using 25.0 ml of *water R* (n_2 ml).

Calculate the content of reducing sugars as anhydrous glucose or as glucose monohydrate, as appropriate, from the Table 0209.-1.

Table 0209.-1

Volume of *0.1 M sodium thiosulphate* ($n_2 - n_1$ ml)	**Anhydrous glucose in milligrams**	**Glucose monohydrate in milligrams**
8	19.8	21.6
9	22.4	24.5
10	25.0	27.2
11	27.6	30.2
12	30.3	33.1
13	33.0	36.1
14	35.7	39.0
15	38.3	42.1
16	41.3	45.2

STORAGE

Store in an airtight, tamper-proof container, protected from light.

LABELLING

The label states:

- the composition and volume of the solution,
- the maximum amount of blood to be collected in the container.

Anticoagulant citrate-phosphate-glucose solution (CPD)

Sodium citrate (0412)	26.3 g
Citric acid monohydrate (0456)	3.27 g
or *Citric acid, anhydrous (0455)*	2.99 g
*Glucose monohydrate (0178)**	25.5 g
or *Glucose, anhydrous (0177)**	23.2 g
Sodium dihydrogen phosphate dihydrate (0194)	2.51 g
Water for injections (0169) to	1000.0 ml
Volume to be used per 100 ml of blood	14.0 ml

*The competent authority may require that the substances comply with the test for pyrogens given in the monographs on *Glucose monohydrate (0178)* and *Glucose, anhydrous (0177)*, respectively.

CHARACTERS

A colourless or faintly yellow, clear liquid, practically free from particles.

IDENTIFICATION

A. Examine by thin-layer chromatography (*2.2.27*), using *silica gel G R* as the coating substance.

Test solution. Dilute 2 ml of the solution to be examined to 100 ml with a mixture of 2 volumes of *water R* and 3 volumes of *methanol R*.

Reference solution (a). Dissolve 10 mg of *glucose CRS* in a mixture of 2 volumes of *water R* and 3 volumes of *methanol R* and dilute to 20 ml with the same mixture of solvents.

Reference solution (b). Dissolve 10 mg each of *glucose CRS, lactose CRS, fructose CRS* and *sucrose CRS* in a mixture of 2 volumes of *water R* and 3 volumes of *methanol R* and dilute to 20 ml with the same mixture of solvents.

Apply separately to the plate 2 µl of each solution and thoroughly dry the starting points. Develop over a path of 15 cm using a mixture of 10 volumes of *water R*, 15 volumes of *methanol R*, 25 volumes of *anhydrous acetic acid R* and 50 volumes of *ethylene chloride R*. The volumes of solvents have to be measured accurately since a slight excess of water produces cloudiness. Dry the plate in a current of warm air. Repeat the development immediately, after renewing the mobile phase. Dry the plate in a current of warm air and spray evenly with a solution of 0.5 g of *thymol R* in a mixture of 5 ml of *sulphuric acid R* and 95 ml of *alcohol R*. Heat at 130 °C for 10 min. The principal spot in the chromatogram obtained with the test solution is similar in position, colour and size to the principal spot in the chromatogram obtained with reference solution (a). The test is not valid unless the chromatogram obtained with reference solution (b) shows 4 clearly separated spots.

B. To 2 ml add 5 ml of *cupri-citric solution R*. Heat to boiling. An orange precipitate is formed and the solution becomes yellow.

C. To 2 ml add 3 ml of *water R*. The solution gives the reaction of citrates (*2.3.1*).

D. 1 ml gives reaction (b) of phosphates (*2.3.1*).

E. 0.5 ml gives reaction (b) of sodium (*2.3.1*).

TESTS

pH (*2.2.3*). The pH of the solution is 5.3 to 5.9.

Hydroxymethylfurfural. To 2.0 ml add 5.0 ml of a 100 g/l solution of *p-toluidine R* in *2-propanol R* containing 10 per cent *V/V* of *glacial acetic acid R* and 1.0 ml of a 5 g/l solution of *barbituric acid R*. The absorbance (*2.2.25*), determined at 550 nm after allowing the mixture to stand for 2 min to 3 min, is not greater than that of a standard prepared at the same time in the same manner using 2.0 ml of a solution containing 5 ppm of *hydroxymethylfurfural R*.

Sterility (*2.6.1*). They comply with the test for sterility.

Pyrogens (*2.6.8*). They comply with the test for pyrogens. Dilute with a pyrogen-free, 9 g/l solution of *sodium chloride R* to obtain a solution containing approximately 5 g/l of sodium citrate. Inject 10 ml of the diluted solution per kilogram of the rabbit's mass.

ASSAY

Sodium dihydrogen phosphate. Dilute 10.0 ml to 100.0 ml with *water R*. To 10.0 ml of this solution add 10.0 ml of *nitro-vanado-molybdic reagent R*. Mix and allow to stand at 20 °C to 25 °C for 30 min. At the same time and in the same manner, prepare a reference solution using 10.0 ml of a standard solution containing 0.219 g of *potassium dihydrogen phosphate R* per litre. Measure the absorbance (*2.2.25*) of the 2 solutions at 450 nm using as the compensation liquid a solution prepared in the same manner using 10 ml of *water R*. Calculate the content of sodium dihydrogen phosphate dihydrate (*P*) in grams per litre from the expression:

$$\frac{11.46 \times C \times A_1}{A_2}$$

C = concentration of *potassium dihydrogen phosphate R* in the standard solution in grams per litre,

A_1 = absorbance of the test solution,

A_2 = absorbance of the reference solution.

Citric acid. To 20.0 ml add 0.1 ml of *phenolphthalein solution R1* and titrate with *0.2 M sodium hydroxide.*

Calculate the content of citric acid monohydrate (*C*), or anhydrous citric acid (*C'*), in grams per litre from the equations:

$$C = 0.7005n - 0.4490P$$

$$C' = 0.6404n - 0.4105P$$

n = number of millilitres of *0.2 M sodium hydroxide* used in the titration,

P = content of sodium dihydrogen phosphate dihydrate in grams per litre determined as prescribed above.

Sodium citrate. Prepare a chromatography column 0.10 m long and 10 mm in internal diameter and filled with *strongly acidic ion-exchange resin R* (300 µm to 840 µm). Maintain a 1 cm layer of liquid above the resin at all times. Wash the column with 50 ml of de-ionised *water R* at a flow rate of 12-14 ml/min.

Dilute 10.0 ml of the solution to be examined to about 40 ml with de-ionised *water R* in a beaker and transfer to the column reservoir, washing the beaker 3 times with a few millilitres of de-ionised *water R*. Allow the solution to run through the column at a flow rate of 12-14 ml/min and collect the eluate. Wash the column with 2 quantities, each of 30 ml, and with one quantity of 50 ml, of de-ionised *water R*. The column can be used for 3 successive determinations before regeneration with 3 times its volume of *dilute hydrochloric acid R*. Titrate the combined eluate and washings (about 150 ml) with *0.2 M sodium hydroxide*, using 0.1 ml of *phenolphthalein solution R1* as indicator.

Calculate the content of sodium citrate in grams per litre from the following expressions:

$$1.961n - 1.257P - 1.40C$$

$$1.961n - 1.257P - 1.53C'$$

n = number of millilitres of *0.2 M sodium hydroxide* used in the titration,

P = content of sodium dihydrogen phosphate dihydrate in grams per litre determined as prescribed above,

C = content of citric acid monohydrate in grams per litre determined as prescribed above,

C' = content of anhydrous citric acid in grams per litre determined as prescribed above.

Reducing sugars. Dilute 5.0 ml to 100.0 ml with *water R*. Introduce 25.0 ml of the solution into a 250 ml conical flask with ground-glass neck and add 25.0 ml of *cupri-citric solution R1*. Add a few pieces of porous material, attach a reflux condenser, heat so that boiling begins within 2 min and boil for exactly 10 min. Cool and add 3 g of *potassium iodide R* dissolved in 3 ml of *water R*. Add 25 ml of a 25 per cent *m/m* solution of *sulphuric acid R* with caution and in small quantities. Titrate with *0.1 M sodium thiosulphate* using 0.5 ml of *starch solution R*, added towards the end of the titration, as indicator (n_1 ml). Carry out a blank titration using 25.0 ml of *water R* (n_2 ml).

Calculate the content of reducing sugars as anhydrous glucose or as glucose monohydrate, as appropriate, from the Table 0209.-1.

STORAGE

Store in an airtight, tamper-proof container, protected from light.

LABELLING

The label states:

- the composition and volume of the solution,
- the maximum amount of blood to be collected in the container.

01/2005:1928

ANTI-T LYMPHOCYTE IMMUNOGLOBULIN FOR HUMAN USE, ANIMAL

Immunoglobulinum anti-T lymphocytorum ex animale ad usum humanum

DEFINITION

Anti-T lymphocyte animal immunoglobulin for human use is a liquid or freeze-dried preparation containing immunoglobulins, obtained from serum or plasma of animals, mainly rabbits or horses, immunised with human lymphocytic antigens.

The immunoglobulin has the property of diminishing the number and function of immunocompetent cells, in particular T-lymphocytes. The preparation contains principally immunoglobulin G. It may contain antibodies against other lymphocyte subpopulations and against other cells. The preparation is intended for intravenous administration, after dilution with a suitable diluent where applicable.

Applicable provisions of the monograph on *Immunosera for human use, animal (0084)* are stated below.

PRODUCTION

GENERAL PROVISIONS

The production method has been shown to yield consistently immunoglobulins of acceptable safety, potency in man and stability.

Any reagent of biological origin used in production shall be free of contamination with bacteria, fungi and viruses. The method of preparation includes a step or steps that have been shown to remove or inactivate known agents of infection.

During development studies, it shall be demonstrated that the production method yields a product that:

- does not transmit infectious agents,
- is characterised by a defined pattern of immunological activity, notably: antigen binding, complement-dependent and independent cytotoxicity, cytokine release, induction of T-cell activation, cell death,
- does not contain antibodies that cross-react with human tissues to a degree that would impair clinical safety,
- has a defined maximum content of anti-thrombocyte antibody activity,
- has a defined maximum content of haemoglobin.

The product has been shown, by suitable tests in animals and evaluation during clinical trials, to be well tolerated.

Reference preparation. A batch shown to be suitable for checking the validity of the assay and whose efficacy has been demonstrated in clinical trials, or a batch representative thereof.

ANIMALS

The animals used are of a species approved by the competent authority, are healthy and exclusively reserved for production of anti-T lymphocyte immunoglobulin. They are tested and shown to be free from a defined list of infectious agents. The introduction of animals into a closed herd follows specified procedures, including definition of quarantine measures. Where appropriate, tests for additional specific agents are considered depending on the geographical localisation of the establishment used for the breeding and production of the animals. The feed originates from a controlled source and no animal proteins are added. The suppliers of animals are certified by the competent authority.

If the animals are treated with antibiotics, a suitable withdrawal period is allowed before collection of blood or plasma. The animals are not treated with penicillin antibiotics. If a live vaccine is administered, a suitable waiting period is imposed between vaccination and collection of serum or plasma for immunoglobulin production.

The species, origin and identification number of the animals are specified.

IMMUNISATION

The antigens used are identified and characterised, where appropriate. They are identified by their names and a batch number; information on the source and preparation are recorded.

The selected animals are isolated for at least 1 week before being immunised according to a defined schedule with booster injections at suitable intervals. Adjuvants may be used.

Animals are kept under general health surveillance and specific antibody production is controlled at each cycle of immunisation.

Animals are thoroughly examined before collection of blood or plasma. If an animal shows any pathological lesion not related to the immunisation process, it is not used, nor are any other of the animals in the group concerned, unless it is evident that their use will not impair the safety of the product.

Human antigens such as continuously growing T-lymphocyte cell lines or thymocytes are used to immunise the animals. Cells may be subjected to a sorting procedure. The immunising antigens are shown to be free from infectious agents by validated methods for relevant blood-borne pathogens, notably hepatitis B virus (HBV), hepatitis C virus (HCV) and human immunodeficiency virus (HIV) and other relevant adventitious agents originating from the preparation of the antigen. The cells used comply with defined requirements for purity of the cell population and freedom from adventitious agents.

COLLECTION OF BLOOD OR PLASMA

Collection of blood is made by venepuncture or plasmapheresis. The puncture area is shaved, cleaned and disinfected. The animals may be anaesthetised under conditions that do not influence the quality of the product.

No antimicrobial preservative is added to the plasma and serum samples. The blood or plasma is collected in such a manner as to maintain sterility of the product. The blood or plasma collection is conducted at a site separate from the area where the animals are kept or bred and the area where the immunoglobulin is purified. If the serum or plasma is stored before further processing, precautions are taken to avoid microbial contamination.

Several single plasma or serum samples may be pooled before purification. The single or pooled samples are tested before purification for the following tests.

Tests for contaminating viruses. Each pool is tested for contaminating viruses by suitable *in vitro* tests including inoculation to cell cultures capable of detecting a wide range of viruses relevant for the particular product. Where applicable, *in vitro* tests for contaminating viruses are carried out on the adsorbed pool, after the last production stage that may introduce viral contaminants.

PURIFICATION AND VIRAL INACTIVATION

The immunoglobulins are concentrated and purified by fractional precipitation, chromatography, immuno-adsorption or by other suitable chemical or physical methods. The methods are selected and validated to avoid contamination at all steps of processing and to avoid formation of protein aggregates that effect immunobiological characteristics of the product.

Unless otherwise justified and authorised, validated procedures are applied for removal and/or inactivation of viruses.

After purification and treatment for removal and/or inactivation of viruses, a stabiliser may be added to the intermediate product, which may be stored for a period defined in the light of stability data.

Only an intermediate product that complies with the following requirements may be used in the preparation of the final bulk.

If the method of preparation includes a step for adsorption of cross-reacting anti-human antibodies using material from human tissues and/or red blood cells, the human materials are submitted to a validated procedure for inactivation of infectious agents, unless otherwise justified and authorised. If erythrocytes are used for adsorption, the donors for such materials comply with the requirements for donors of blood and plasma of the monograph on *Human plasma for fractionation (0853)*. If other human material is used, it is shown by validated methods to be free from relevant blood-borne pathogens, notably HBV, HCV and HIV. If substances are used for inactivation or removal of viruses, it shall have been shown that any residues present in the final product have no adverse effects on the patients treated with the anti-T lymphocyte immunoglobulin.

FINAL BULK

The final bulk is prepared from a single intermediate product or from a pool of intermediate products obtained from animals of the same species. A stabiliser may be added. No antimicrobial preservative is added either during the manufacturing procedure or for preparation of the final bulk solution. During manufacturing, the solution is passed through a bacteria-retentive filter.

FINAL LOT

The final bulk of anti-T-lymphocyte immunoglobulin is distributed aseptically into sterile, tamper-proof containers. The containers are closed as to prevent contamination.

Only a final lot that complies with the requirements prescribed below under Identification, Tests and Assay may be released for use.

CHARACTERS

The liquid preparation is clear or slightly opalescent and colourless or pale yellow. The freeze-dried preparation is a white or slightly yellow powder or solid friable mass, which after reconstitution gives a liquid preparation corresponding to the description above.

IDENTIFICATION

A. Using a suitable range of species-specific antisera, carry out precipitation tests on the preparation to be examined. It is recommended that the test be carried

out using antisera specific to the plasma proteins of each species of domestic animal commonly used in the preparation of materials of biological origin in the country concerned and antisera specific to human plasma proteins. The preparation is shown to contain proteins originating from the animal used for the anti-T lymphocyte immunoglobulin production.

B. Examine by a suitable immunoelectrophoresis technique. Using antiserum to normal serum of the animal used for production, compare this serum and the preparation to be examined, both diluted to a concentration that will allow a clear gammaglobulin precipitation arc to be obtained on the gel. The main component of the preparation to be examined corresponds to the IgG component of normal serum of the animal used for production.

C. The preparation complies with the assay.

TESTS

Solubility. To a container of the preparation to be examined, add the volume of the liquid for reconstitution stated on the label. The preparation dissolves completely within the time stated on the label.

Extractable volume (*2.9.17*). It complies with the requirement for extractable volume.

pH (*2.2.3*). The pH is within the limits approved for the particular product.

Osmolality (*2.2.35*): minimum 240 mosmol/kg after dilution, where applicable.

Proteins (*2.5.33*): 90 per cent to 110 per cent of the amount stated on the label.

Stabiliser. Determine the amount of stabiliser by a suitable physico-chemical method. The preparation contains not less than 80 per cent and not more than 120 per cent of the quantity stated on the label.

Distribution of molecular size. Size exclusion chromatography (*2.2.30*).

Test solution. Dilute the preparation to be examined with a 9 g/l solution of *sodium chloride R* to a concentration suitable for the chromatographic system used. A concentration in the range 2-20 g/l is usually suitable.

Reference solution. Dilute *human immunoglobulin BRP* with a 9 g/l solution of *sodium chloride R* to the same protein concentration as the test solution.

Column:

– *size*: l = 0.6 m, Ø = 7.5 mm,

– *stationary phase*: *silica gel for size-exclusion chromatography R*, a grade suitable for fractionation of globular proteins in the molecular mass range of 20 000 to 200 000.

Mobile phase: dissolve 4.873 g of *disodium hydrogen phosphate dihydrate R*, 1.741 g of *sodium dihydrogen phosphate monohydrate R* and 11.688 g of *sodium chloride R* in 1 litre of *water R*.

Flow rate: 0.5 ml/min.

Detection: spectrophotometer at 280 nm.

Injection: 50-600 µg of protein.

Retention time: identify the peaks in the chromatogram obtained with the test solution by comparison with the chromatogram obtained with the reference solution; any peak with a retention time shorter than that of dimer corresponds to polymers and aggregates.

System suitability:

– *reference solution*: the principal peak corresponds to IgG monomer and there is a peak corresponding to dimer with a retention time relative to monomer of 0.85 ± 0.05,

– *test solution*: the relative retentions of monomer and dimer are 1 ± 0.05 with reference to the corresponding peaks in the chromatogram obtained with the reference solution.

Limits:

– *total monomer and dimer*: at least 95 per cent of the total area of the peaks,

– *total polymers and aggregates*: maximum 5 per cent of the total area of the peaks.

Purity. Polyacrylamide gel electrophoresis (*2.2.31*), under non-reducing and reducing conditions.

Resolving gel. Non-reducing conditions: 8 per cent acrylamide; reducing conditions: 12 per cent acrylamide.

Test solution. Dilute the preparation to be examined to a protein concentration of 0.5-2 mg/ml.

Reference solution. Dilute the reference preparation to the same protein concentration as the test solution.

Application: 10 µl.

Detection: Coomassie staining.

Results: compared with the electropherogram of the reference solution, no additional bands are found in the electropherogram of the test solution.

Anti-A and anti-B haemagglutinins (*2.6.20*). The 1 to 64 dilution does not show agglutination.

Where applicable, dilute the preparation to be examined as prescribed for use before preparing the dilutions for the test.

Haemolysins. Prepare a 1 to 64 dilution of the preparation to be examined, diluted if necessary as stated on the label. Take 6 aliquots of the 1 to 64 dilution. To 1 volume of 3 of the aliquots, add 1 volume of a 10 per cent *V/V* suspension of group A1, group B and group O erythrocytes in a 9 g/l solution of *sodium chloride R*, respectively. To 1 volume of the remaining 3 aliquots, add 1 volume of a 10 per cent *V/V* suspension of group A1, group B and group O erythrocytes in a 9 g/l solution of *sodium chloride R*, respectively, and to each aliquot 1 volume of fresh group AB serum (as a source of complement). Mix and incubate at 37 °C for 1 h. Examine the supernatant liquids for haemolysis. No signs of haemolysis are present.

Thrombocyte antibodies. Examined by a suitable method, the level of thrombocyte antibodies is shown to be below that approved for the specific product.

Water (*2.5.12*): maximum 3 per cent.

Sterility (*2.6.1*). It complies with the test for sterility.

Pyrogens (*2.6.8*). Unless otherwise justified and authorised, it complies with the test for pyrogens. Unless otherwise prescribed, inject 1 ml per kilogram of the rabbit's body mass.

ASSAY

The biological activity is determined by measuring the complement-dependent cytotoxicity on target cells. Flow cytometry is performed with read-out of dead cells stained using propidium iodide. The activity is expressed as the concentration of anti-T lymphocyte immunoglobulin in milligrams per millilitre which mediates 50 per cent cytotoxicity.

Lymphocyte separation medium. Commercial separation media with low viscosity and a density of 1.077 g/ml.

Complement. Commercial complement is suitable.

Buffered salt solution pH 7.2. Dissolve 8.0 g of *sodium chloride R*, 0.2 g of *potassium chloride R*, 3.18 g of *disodium hydrogen phosphate R* and 0.2 g of *potassium dihydrogen phosphate R* in *water R* and dilute to 1000.0 ml with the same solvent.

Buffer solution for flow cytometry. Add 40 ml of 0.1 per cent *V/V sodium azide R* and 10 ml of foetal calf serum to 440 ml of buffered salt solution pH 7.2. The foetal calf serum is inactivated at 56 °C for 30 min prior to use. Store at 4 °C.

Propidium iodide solution. Dissolve *propidium iodide R* in buffered salt solution pH 7.2, to a concentration of 1 mg/ml. Store this stock solution at 2-8 °C and use within 1 month. For the assay, dilute this solution with buffer solution for flow cytometry, to obtain a concentration of 5 µg/ml. Store at 2-8 °C and use within 3 h.

Microtitre plates. Plates used to prepare immunoglobulin dilutions are U- or V-bottomed polystyrene or poly(vinyl chloride) plates without surface treatment.

Micronic tubes. Suitable for flow cytometry measurement.

Cell suspension. Collect blood in anticoagulant from at least one healthy donor. Immediately isolate the peripheral blood mononuclear cells (PBMC) by gradient centrifugation in lymphocyte separation medium so that the PBMC form a visible clean interface between the plasma and the separation medium. Collect the layer containing the cells and dispense into centrifuge tubes containing buffered salt solution pH 7.2. Centrifuge at 400 *g* at 2-8 °C for 10 min. Discard the supernatant. Suspend the cell pellet in buffer solution for flow cytometry. Repeat the centrifugation and resuspension procedure of the cells twice. After the third centrifugation, resuspend the cell pellet in 1 ml of buffer solution for flow cytometry. Determine the number and vitality of the cells using a haemocytometer. Cell viability of at least 90 per cent is required. Adjust the cell number to 7 × 10^6/ml by adding buffer solution for flow cytometry. Store the cell suspension at 4 °C and use within 12 h.

If necessary, the first PBMC pellet may be resuspended in buffered salt solution pH 7.2 containing 20 per cent fœtal calf serum and stored overnight at 2 °C. Centrifuge at 400 *g* at 2-8 °C for 10 min. Discard the supernatant. Suspend the cell pellet in buffer solution for flow cytometry. Determine the number and vitality of the cells using a haemocytometer. Cell viability of at least 90 per cent is required. Adjust the cell number to 7 × 10^6/ml by adding buffer solution for flow cytometry.

It is also possible for cells to be immediately frozen and stored in nitrogen using the following method.

Buffer solution for freezing. To 20 ml of cell culture medium, add 25 ml of fœtal calf serum and 5 ml of dimethyl sulphoxide (DMSO). Store this solution at 2-8 °C and use within 3 h.

20 × 10^6 cells per ampoule are frozen. These ampoules are stored in liquid nitrogen.

Buffer solution for thawing. To 450 ml of cell culture medium, add 50 ml of foetal calf serum. Store this solution at 2-8 °C and use within 3 h.

Each ampoule is thawed in a water-bath at 37 °C with shaking. Cell suspension is repeated in a buffer solution for thawing. Centrifuge at 200 *g* at 2-8 °C for 10 min. Discard the supernatant. Suspend the cell pellet in buffer solution for flow cytometry. Repeat the procedure for centrifugation and resuspension of cells once. After the second centrifugation, resuspend the cells pellet in 1 ml of buffer solution for flow cytometry. Determine the number and vitality of the cells using a haemocytometer. Cell viability of at least 90 per cent is required. Adjust the cell number to 7 × 10^6/ml by adding buffer solution for flow cytometry. Store the cell suspension at 4 °C and use within 3 h.

Test solutions. For freeze-dried preparations, reconstitute as stated on the label. Prepare 3 independent series of not fewer than 7 dilutions using buffer solution for flow cytometry as diluent.

Reference solutions. For freeze-dried preparations, reconstitute according to the instructions for use. Prepare 3 independent dilution series of not fewer than 7 dilutions using buffer solution for flow cytometry as diluent.

Distribute 75 µl of each of the dilutions of the test solution or reference solution to each of a series of wells of a microtitre plate. Add 25 µl of the cell suspension of PBMC into each well. Add 25 µl of rabbit complement to each of the wells. Incubate at 37 °C for 30 min.

Centrifuge the plates at 200 *g* at 4 °C for 8 min, discard the supernatant and keep the plate on ice. Preparation for flow cytometry measurement is done step-wise by using a certain number of wells in order to allow labelling with *propidium iodide R* solution and measurement within a defined time period. Resuspend carefully the cell pellet of a certain number of wells with 200 µl of propidium iodide solution. Transfer the suspension into tubes. Incubate at 25 °C for 10 min then place immediately on ice.

Proceed with fluorescence measurement in a flow cytometer. Define a region including all propidium iodide-positive cells on the basis of Forward-Scattered, light (FSC) and flourescence (FL2 or FL3 for propidium iodide). Measure the percentage of propidium iodide-positive cells, without gating but excluding debris. Analyse at least 3000 cells for each of the test and reference solutions.

Use the percentages of dead cells to estimate the potency as the concentration in milligrams per millilitre of the preparation to be examined necessary to induce 50 per cent of cytotoxicity by fitting a sigmoidal dose response curve to the data obtained with the test and the reference preparations and by using a 4-parameter logistic model (see, for example, chapter *5.3*) and suitable software. The test is not valid unless the percentage of propidium iodide-positive cells at the lower asymptote of the curve is less then 15 per cent and the percentage of propidium iodide-positive cells at the upper asymptote of the curve is at least 80 per cent.

The estimated activity is 70 per cent to 130 per cent of the activity approved for the particular product.

The confidence limits ($P = 0.95$) are not less than 80 per cent and not more than 125 per cent of the estimated potency.

STORAGE

Protected from light at the temperature stated on the label.

Expiry date. The expiry date is calculated from the beginning of the assay.

LABELLING

The label states:

- for liquid preparations, the volume of the preparation in the container and the protein content,
- for freeze-dried preparations:
  - the name and the volume of the reconstitution liquid to be added,
  - the quantity of protein in the container,
  - that the immunoserum is to be used immediately after reconstitution,
  - the time required for complete dissolution,
- the animal species of origin,

– the name and amount of stabiliser, where applicable,
– the dilution to be made before use of the product.

01/2005:0136

APOMORPHINE HYDROCHLORIDE

Apomorphini hydrochloridum

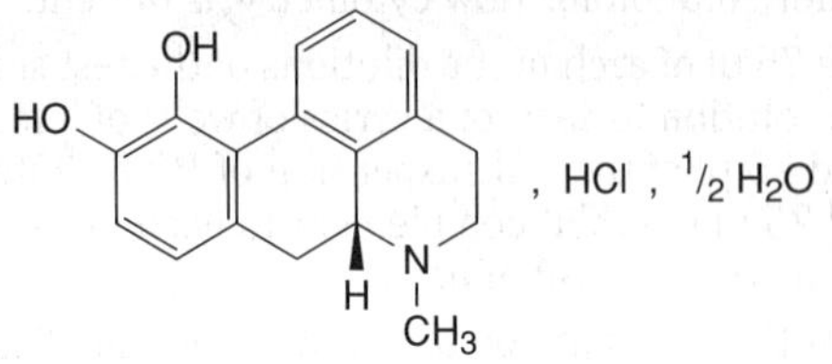

$C_{17}H_{18}ClNO_2,1/2H_2O$ M_r 312.8

DEFINITION

(6a*R*)-6-Methyl-5,6,6a,7-tetrahydro-4*H*-dibenzo[*de*,*g*]quinoline-10,11-diol hydrochloride hemihydrate.

Content: 99.0 per cent to 101.0 per cent (dried substance).

CHARACTERS

Appearance: white or slightly yellowish-brown or green-tinged greyish, crystalline powder or crystals; on exposure to air and light, the green tinge becomes more pronounced.

Solubility: sparingly soluble in water and in alcohol, practically insoluble in toluene.

IDENTIFICATION

First identification: *B, D*.

Second identification: *A, C, D*.

A. Dissolve 10.0 mg in *0.1 M hydrochloric acid* and dilute to 100.0 ml with the same acid. Dilute 10.0 ml of the solution to 100.0 ml with *0.1 M hydrochloric acid*. Examined between 230 nm and 350 nm (*2.2.25*), the solution shows an absorption maximum at 273 nm and a shoulder at 300 nm to 310 nm. The specific absorbance at the maximum is 530 to 570.

B. Infrared absorption spectrophotometry (*2.2.24*).
Comparison: *Ph. Eur. reference spectrum of apomorphine hydrochloride*.

C. To 5 ml of solution S (see Tests) add a few millilitres of *sodium hydrogen carbonate solution R* until a permanent, white precipitate is formed. The precipitate slowly becomes greenish. Add 0.25 ml of *0.05 M iodine* and shake. The precipitate becomes greyish-green. Collect the precipitate. The precipitate dissolves in *ether R* giving a purple solution, in *methylene chloride R* giving a violet-blue solution and in *alcohol R* giving a blue solution.

D. To 2 ml of solution S add 0.1 ml of *nitric acid R*. Mix and filter. The filtrate gives reaction (a) of chlorides (*2.3.1*).

TESTS

Solution S. Dissolve 0.25 g without heating in *carbon dioxide-free water R* and dilute to 25 ml with the same solvent.

Appearance of solution. Solution S is clear (*2.2.1*) and not more intensely coloured than reference solution BY_5 or GY_5(*2.2.2, Method II*).

pH (*2.2.3*): 4.0 to 5.0 for solution S.

Specific optical rotation (*2.2.7*): − 48 to − 52 (dried substance).

Dissolve 0.25 g in *0.02 M hydrochloric acid* and dilute to 25.0 ml with the same acid.

Related substances. Liquid chromatography (*2.2.29*).

Test solution. Dissolve 0.25 g of the substance to be examined in a 1 per cent *V/V* solution of *glacial acetic acid R* and dilute to 100.0 ml with the same solution.

Reference solution (a). Dilute 1.0 ml of the test solution to 10.0 ml with a 1 per cent *V/V* solution of *glacial acetic acid R*. Dilute 1.0 ml to 100.0 ml with a 1 per cent *V/V* solution of *glacial acetic acid R*.

Reference solution (b). Dissolve 25 mg of *boldine R* in a 1 per cent *V/V* solution of *glacial acetic acid R* and dilute to 10.0 ml with the same solvent. To 1 ml of this solution, add 1 ml of the test solution and dilute to 10.0 ml with a 1 per cent *V/V* solution of *glacial acetic acid R*.

Column:
– *size*: *l* = 0.15 m, Ø = 4.6 mm,
– *stationary phase*: *octadecylsilyl silica gel for chromatography R* (5 µm),
– *temperature*: 35 °C.

Mobile phase:
– *mobile phase A*: 1.1 g/l solution of *sodium octanesulphonate R*, adjusted to pH 2.2 using a 50 per cent *m/m* solution of *phosphoric acid R*,
– *mobile phase B*: *acetonitrile R*,

Time (min)	Mobile phase A (per cent *V/V*)	Mobile phase B (per cent *V/V*)
0 - 30	85 → 68	15 → 32
30 - 35	68	32
35 - 45	68 → 85	32 → 15

Flow rate: 1.5 ml/min.

Detection: spectrophotometer at 280 nm.

Injection: 10 µl.

System suitability: reference solution (b):
– *resolution*: minimum 2.5 between the peaks due to boldine and apomorphine.

Limits:
– *any impurity*: not more than twice the area of the principal peak in the chromatogram obtained with reference solution (a) (0.2 per cent),
– *total*: not more than 8 times the area of the principal peak in the chromatogram obtained with reference solution (a) (0.8 per cent),
– *disregard limit*: 0.2 times the area of the principal peak in the chromatogram obtained with reference solution (a) (0.02 per cent).

Heavy metals (*2.4.8*): maximum 20 ppm.

1.0 g complies with limit test C. Prepare the standard using 2 ml of *lead standard solution (10 ppm Pb) R*.

Loss on drying (*2.2.32*): 2.5 per cent to 4.2 per cent, determined on 1.000 g by drying in an oven at 100-105 °C.

Sulphated ash (*2.4.14*): maximum 0.1 per cent, determined on 1.0 g.

ASSAY

Dissolve 0.250 g in a mixture of 5.0 ml of *0.01 M hydrochloric acid* and 50 ml of *alcohol R*. Carry out a potentiometric titration (*2.2.20*), using *0.1 M sodium hydroxide*. Read the volume added between the first 2 points of inflexion.

1 ml of *0.1 M sodium hydroxide* is equivalent to 30.38 mg of $C_{17}H_{18}ClNO_2$.

STORAGE

In an airtight container, protected from light.

IMPURITIES

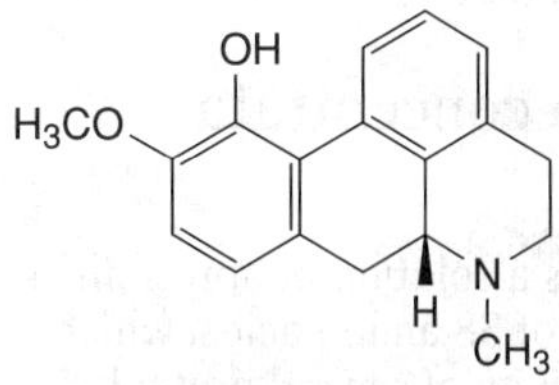

A. (6a*R*)-10-methoxy-6-methyl-5,6,6a,7-tetrahydro-4*H*-dibenzo[*de,g*]quinolin-11-ol (apocodeine),

B. morphine.

01/2005:0580

APROTININ

Aprotininum

DEFINITION

Aprotinin is a polypeptide consisting of a chain of 58 amino acids. It inhibits stoichiometrically the activity of several proteolytic enzymes such as chymotrypsin, kallikrein, plasmin and trypsin. It contains not less than 3.0 Ph. Eur. U. of aprotinin activity per milligram, calculated with reference to the dried substance.

PRODUCTION

The animals from which aprotinin is derived must fulfil the requirements for the health of animals suitable for human consumption to the satisfaction of the competent authority.

The manufacturing process is validated to demonstrate suitable inactivation or removal of any contamination by viruses or other infectious agents.

The method of manufacture is validated to demonstrate that the product, if tested, would comply with the following tests.

Abnormal toxicity (*2.6.9*). Inject into each mouse a quantity of the substance to be examined containing 2 Ph. Eur. U. dissolved in a sufficient quantity of *water for injections R* to give a volume of 0.5 ml.

Histamine (*2.6.10*): maximum 0.2 µg of histamine base per 3 Ph. Eur. U.

CHARACTERS

Appearance: almost white powder, hygroscopic.

Solubility: soluble in water and in isotonic solutions, practically insoluble in organic solvents.

IDENTIFICATION

A. Thin-layer chromatography (*2.2.27*).

Test solution. Solution S (see Tests).

Reference solution. Aprotinin solution BRP.

Plate: *TLC silica gel G plate R.*

Mobile phase: *water R, glacial acetic acid R* (80:100 *V/V*) containing 100 g/l of *sodium acetate R.*

Application: 10 µl.

Development: over a path of 12 cm.

Drying: in air.

Detection: spray with a solution of 0.1 g of *ninhydrin R* in a mixture of 6 ml of a 10 g/l solution of *cupric chloride R*, 21 ml of *glacial acetic acid R* and 70 ml of *ethanol R*. Dry the plate at 60 °C.

Results: the principal spot in the chromatogram obtained with the test solution is similar in position, colour and size to the principal spot in the chromatogram obtained with the reference solution.

B. Determine the ability of the substance to be examined to inhibit trypsin activity using the method described below.

Test solution. Dilute 1 ml of solution S to 50 ml with *buffer solution pH 7.2 R.*

Trypsin solution. Dissolve 10 mg of *trypsin BRP* in *0.002 M hydrochloric acid* and dilute to 100 ml with the same acid.

Casein solution. Dissolve 0.2 g of *casein R* in *buffer solution pH 7.2 R* and dilute to 100 ml with the same buffer solution.

Precipitating solution. Mix 1 volume of *glacial acetic acid R*, 49 volumes of *water R* and 50 volumes of *ethanol R.*

Mix 1 ml of the test solution with 1 ml of the trypsin solution. Allow to stand for 10 min and add 1 ml of the casein solution. Incubate at 35 °C for 30 min. Cool in iced water and add 0.5 ml of the precipitating solution. Shake and allow to stand at room temperature for 15 min. The solution is cloudy. Carry out a blank test under the same conditions using *buffer solution pH 7.2 R* instead of the test solution. The solution is not cloudy.

TESTS

Solution S. Prepare a solution of the substance to be examined containing 15 Ph. Eur. U./ml, calculated from the activity stated on the label.

Appearance of solution. Solution S is clear (*2.2.1*).

Absorbance (*2.2.25*): maximum 0.80 by measuring at the absorption maximum at 277 nm.

Prepare a solution of the substance to be examined containing 3.0 Ph. Eur. U./ml.

Protein impurities of higher molecular mass. Size-exclusion chromatography (*2.2.30*).

Use *cross-linked dextran for chromatography R2.* Use a 180 g/l solution of *anhydrous acetic acid R* to swell the gel and as the eluent. Prepare a column of gel 0.8 m to 1.0 m long and 25 mm in diameter, taking care to avoid the introduction of air bubbles. Place at the top of the column a quantity of the substance to be examined containing 300 Ph. Eur. U. dissolved in 1 ml of a 180 g/l solution of *anhydrous acetic acid R* and allow to elute. Collect the eluate in fractions of 2 ml. Measure the absorbance (*2.2.25*) of each fraction at the absorption maximum at 277 nm and plot the values on a graph. The chromatogram obtained does not present an absorption maximum before the elution of the aprotinin.

Loss on drying (*2.2.32*): maximum 6.0 per cent, determined on 0.100 g by drying *in vacuo.*

Bacterial endotoxins (*2.6.14*): less than 0.14 IU per European Pharmacopoeia Unit of aprotinin, if intended for use in the manufacture of parenteral dosage forms without a further appropriate procedure for the removal of bacterial endotoxins.

ASSAY

The activity of aprotinin is determined by measuring its inhibitory action on a solution of trypsin of known activity. The inhibiting activity of the aprotinin is calculated from the difference between the initial activity and the residual activity of the trypsin.

The inhibiting activity of aprotinin is expressed in European Pharmacopoeia Units. 1 Ph. Eur. U. inhibits 50 per cent of the enzymatic activity of 2 microkatals of trypsin.

Use a reaction vessel with a capacity of about 30 ml and provided with:

- a device that will maintain a temperature of 25 ± 0.1 °C;
- a stirring device, such as a magnetic stirrer;
- a lid with 5 holes for accommodating the electrodes, the tip of a burette, a tube for the admission of nitrogen and the introduction of the reagents.

An automatic or manual titration apparatus may be used. In the latter case the burette is graduated in 0.05 ml and the pH-meter is provided with a wide reading scale and glass and calomel electrodes.

Test solution. Prepare a solution of the substance to be examined in *0.0015 M borate buffer solution pH 8.0 R* expected to contain 1.67 Ph. Eur. U./ml (about 0.6 mg (m mg) per millilitre).

Trypsin solution. Prepare a solution of *trypsin BRP* containing about 0.8 microkatals per millilitre (about 1 mg/ml), using *0.001 M hydrochloric acid* as the solvent. Use a freshly prepared solution and keep in iced water.

Trypsin and aprotinin solution. To 4.0 ml of the trypsin solution add 1.0 ml of the test solution. Dilute immediately to 40.0 ml with *0.0015 M borate buffer solution pH 8.0 R*. Allow to stand at room temperature for 10 min and then keep in iced water. Use within 6 h of preparation.

Dilute trypsin solution. Dilute 0.5 ml of the trypsin solution to 10.0 ml with *0.0015 M borate buffer solution pH 8.0 R*. Allow to stand at room temperature for 10 min and then keep in iced water.

Maintain an atmosphere of nitrogen in the reaction flask and stir continuously; introduce 9.0 ml of *0.0015 M borate buffer solution pH 8.0 R* and 1.0 ml of a freshly prepared 6.9 g/l solution of *benzoylarginine ethyl ester hydrochloride R*. Adjust to pH 8.0 with *0.1 M sodium hydroxide*. When the temperature has reached equilibrium at 25 ± 0.1 °C, add 1.0 ml of the trypsin and aprotinin solution and start a timer. Maintain at pH 8.0 by the addition of *0.1 M sodium hydroxide* and note the volume added every 30 s. Continue the reaction for 6 min. Determine the number of millilitres of *0.1 M sodium hydroxide* used per second (n_1 ml). Carry out, under the same conditions, a titration using 1.0 ml of the dilute trypsin solution. Determine the number of millilitres of *0.1 M sodium hydroxide* used per second (n_2 ml).

Calculate the aprotinin activity in European Pharmacopoeia Units per milligram from the expression:

$$\frac{4000\,(2n_2 - n_1)}{m}$$

The estimated activity is not less than 90 per cent and not more than 110 per cent of the activity stated on the label.

STORAGE

In an airtight, tamper-proof container, protected from light.

LABELLING

The label states:

- the number of European Pharmacopoeia Units of aprotinin activity per milligram,
- where applicable, that the substance is free from bacterial endotoxins.

01/2005:0579

APROTININ CONCENTRATED SOLUTION

Aprotinini solutio concentrata

DEFINITION

Aprotinin concentrated solution is a solution of aprotinin, a polypeptide consisting of a chain of 58 amino acids, which inhibits stoichiometrically the activity of several proteolytic enzymes such as chymotrypsin, kallikrein, plasmin and trypsin. It contains not less than 15.0 Ph. Eur. U. of aprotinin activity per millilitre.

PRODUCTION

The animals from which aprotinin is derived must fulfil the requirements for the health of animals suitable for human consumption to the satisfaction of the competent authority.

The manufacturing process is validated to demonstrate suitable inactivation or removal of any contamination by viruses or other infectious agents.

The method of manufacture is validated to demonstrate that the product, if tested, would comply with the following tests.

Abnormal toxicity (*2.6.9*). Inject into each mouse a quantity of the preparation to be examined containing 2 Ph. Eur. U. diluted with a sufficient quantity of *water for injections R* to give a volume of 0.5 ml.

Histamine (*2.6.10*): maximum 0.2 µg of histamine base per 3 Ph. Eur. U.

CHARACTERS

Appearance: clear and colourless liquid.

IDENTIFICATION

A. Thin-layer chromatography (*2.2.27*).

Test solution. Solution S (see Tests).

Reference solution. *Aprotinin solution BRP*.

Plate: *TLC silica gel G plate R*.

Mobile phase: *water R, glacial acetic acid R* (80:100 *V/V*) containing 100 g/l of *sodium acetate R*).

Application: 10 µl.

Development: over a path of 12 cm.

Drying: in air.

Detection: spray with a solution of 0.1 g of *ninhydrin R* in a mixture of 6 ml of a 10 g/l solution of *cupric chloride R*, 21 ml of *glacial acetic acid R* and 70 ml of *ethanol R*. Dry the plate at 60 °C.

Results: the principal spot in the chromatogram obtained with the test solution is similar in position, colour and size to the principal spot in the chromatogram obtained with the reference solution.

B. Determine the ability of the preparation to be examined to inhibit trypsin activity using the method described below.

Test solution. Dilute 1 ml of solution S to 50 ml with *buffer solution pH 7.2 R*.

Trypsin solution. Dissolve 10 mg of *trypsin BRP* in *0.002 M hydrochloric acid* and dilute to 100 ml with the same acid.

Casein solution. Dissolve 0.2 g of *casein R* in *buffer solution pH 7.2 R* and dilute to 100 ml with the same buffer solution.

Precipitating solution. Mix 1 volume of *glacial acetic acid R*, 49 volumes of *water R* and 50 volumes of *ethanol R*.

Mix 1 ml of the test solution with 1 ml of the trypsin solution. Allow to stand for 10 min and add 1 ml of the casein solution. Incubate at 35 °C for 30 min. Cool in iced water and add 0.5 ml of the precipitating solution. Shake and allow to stand at room temperature for 15 min. The solution is cloudy. Carry out a blank test under the same conditions using *buffer solution pH 7.2 R* instead of the test solution. The solution is not cloudy.

TESTS

Solution S. Prepare a solution containing 15 Ph. Eur. U./ml, if necessary by dilution on the basis of the activity stated on the label.

Appearance of solution. Solution S is clear (*2.2.1*).

Absorbance (*2.2.25*): maximum 0.80 by measuring at the absorption maximum at 277 nm.

Prepare from the concentrated solution a dilution containing 3.0 Ph. Eur. U./ml.

Protein impurities of higher molecular mass. Size-exclusion chromatography (*2.2.30*).

Freeze-dry the preparation to be examined using a pressure of 2.7 Pa and a temperature of − 30 °C; the operation, including freeze-drying and a period of drying at 15-25 °C, takes 6-12 h.

Use *cross-linked dextran for chromatography R2*. Use a 180 g/l solution of *anhydrous acetic acid R* to swell the gel and as the eluent. Prepare a column of gel 0.8 m to 1.0 m long and 25 mm in diameter, taking care to avoid the introduction of air bubbles. Place at the top of the column a quantity of the preparation to be examined containing 300 Ph. Eur. U. dissolved in 1 ml of a 180 g/l solution of *anhydrous acetic acid R* and allow to elute. Collect the eluate in fractions of 2 ml. Measure the absorbance (*2.2.25*) of each fraction at the absorption maximum at 277 nm and plot the values on a graph. The chromatogram obtained does not present an absorption maximum before the elution of the aprotinin.

Specific activity of the dry residue: minimum 3.0 Ph. Eur. U. of aprotinin activity per milligram of dry residue.

Evaporate 25.0 ml to dryness in a water-bath, dry the residue at 110 °C for 15 h and weigh. From the mass of the residue and the activity determined as described below, calculate the number of European Pharmacopoeia Units per milligram of dry residue.

Bacterial endotoxins (*2.6.14*): less than 0.14 IU per European Pharmacopoeia Unit of aprotinin, if intended for use in the manufacture of parenteral dosage forms without a further appropriate procedure for the removal of bacterial endotoxins.

ASSAY

The activity of aprotinin is determined by measuring its inhibitory action on a solution of trypsin of known activity. The inhibiting activity of the aprotinin is calculated from the difference between the initial activity and the residual activity of the trypsin.

The inhibiting activity of aprotinin is expressed in European Pharmacopoeia Units. 1 Ph. Eur. U. inhibits 50 per cent of the enzymatic activity of 2 microkatals of trypsin.

Use a reaction vessel with a capacity of about 30 ml and provided with:

- a device that will maintain a temperature of 25 ± 0.1 °C;
- a stirring device, such as a magnetic stirrer;
- a lid with 5 holes for accommodating the electrodes, the tip of a burette, a tube for the admission of nitrogen and the introduction of the reagents.

An automatic or manual titration apparatus may be used. In the latter case the burette is graduated in 0.05 ml and the pH-meter is provided with a wide reading scale and glass and calomel electrodes.

Test solution. With *0.0015 M borate buffer solution pH 8.0 R* prepare an appropriate dilution (*D*) of the concentrated solution expected on the basis of the stated potency to contain 1.67 Ph. Eur. U./ml.

Trypsin solution. Prepare a solution of *trypsin BRP* containing about 0.8 microkatals per millilitre (about 1 mg/ml), using *0.001 M hydrochloric acid* as the solvent. Use a freshly prepared solution and keep in iced water.

Trypsin and aprotinin solution. To 4.0 ml of the trypsin solution add 1.0 ml of the test solution. Dilute immediately to 40.0 ml with *0.0015 M borate buffer solution pH 8.0 R*. Allow to stand at room temperature for 10 min and then keep in iced water. Use within 6 h of preparation.

Dilute trypsin solution. Dilute 0.5 ml of the trypsin solution to 10.0 ml with *0.0015 M borate buffer solution pH 8.0 R*. Allow to stand at room temperature for 10 min and then keep in iced water.

Maintain an atmosphere of nitrogen in the reaction flask and stir continuously; introduce 9.0 ml of *0.0015 M borate buffer solution pH 8.0 R* and 1.0 ml of a freshly prepared 6.9 g/l solution of *benzoylarginine ethyl ester hydrochloride R*. Adjust to pH 8.0 with *0.1 M sodium hydroxide*. When the temperature has reached equilibrium at 25 ± 0.1 °C, add 1.0 ml of the trypsin and aprotinin solution and start a timer. Maintain at pH 8.0 by the addition of *0.1 M sodium hydroxide* and note the volume added every 30 s. Continue the reaction for 6 min. Determine the number of millilitres of *0.1 M sodium hydroxide* used per second (n_1 ml). Carry out, under the same conditions, a titration using 1.0 ml of the dilute trypsin solution. Determine the number of millilitres of *0.1 M sodium hydroxide* used per second (n_2 ml).

Calculate the aprotinin activity in European Pharmacopoeia Units per millilitre from the expression:

$$4000\,(2n_2 - n_1) \times D$$

D = dilution factor of the aprotinin concentrated solution to be examined in order to obtain a solution containing 1.67 Ph. Eur. U./ml.

The estimated activity is not less than 90 per cent and not more than 110 per cent of the activity stated on the label.

STORAGE

In an airtight, tamper-proof container, protected from light.

LABELLING

The label states:

- the number of European Pharmacopoeia Units of aprotinin activity per millilitre.
- where applicable, that the solution is free from bacterial endotoxins.

Monographs A

01/2005:1171

ARACHIS OIL, HYDROGENATED

Arachidis oleum hydrogenatum

DEFINITION

Hydrogenated arachis oil is the product obtained by refining, bleaching, hydrogenating and deodorising oil obtained from the shelled seeds of *Arachis hypogaea* L. Each type of hydrogenated arachis oil is characterised by its nominal drop point.

CHARACTERS

A white or faintly yellowish, soft mass which melts to a clear, pale yellow liquid when heated, practically insoluble in water, freely soluble in methylene chloride and in light petroleum (bp: 65 °C to 70 °C), very slightly soluble in alcohol.

IDENTIFICATION

First identification: A, B.

Second identification: A, C.

A. It complies with the test for drop point (see Tests).

B. Carry out the identification of fatty oils by thin-layer chromatography (*2.3.2*). The chromatogram obtained is similar to the typical chromatogram for arachis oil.

C. It complies with the test for composition of fatty acids.

TESTS

Drop point (*2.2.17*): 32 °C to 43 °C. Within this range the drop point does not differ by more than 3 °C from the nominal value.

Acid value (*2.5.1*). Not more than 0.5. Dissolve 10.0 g in 50 ml of the prescribed solvent by heating on a water-bath.

Peroxide value (*2.5.5*). Not more than 5.0. Dissolve 5.0 g in 30 ml of the prescribed solvent by heating on a water-bath.

Unsaponifiable matter (*2.5.7*). Not more than 1.0 per cent.

Alkaline impurities (*2.4.19*). It complies with the test for alkaline impurities in fatty oils.

Composition of fatty acids (*2.4.22, Method A*).

The chromatographic procedure may be carried out using:

- a capillary fused-silica column 25 m long and 0.25 mm in internal diameter coated with *poly(cyanopropyl)siloxane R* (film thickness 0.2 μm),
- *helium for chromatography R* as the carrier gas at a flow rate of 0.7 ml/min,
- a flame-ionisation detector,
- a split injector (1:100),

maintaining the temperature of the column at 180 °C for 20 min and that of the injection port and of the detector at 250 °C.

The fatty acid fraction of the oil has the following composition:

- *saturated fatty acids of chain length less than* C_{14}: not more than 0.5 per cent,
- *myristic acid*: not more than 0.5 per cent,
- *palmitic acid*: 7.0 per cent to 16.0 per cent,
- *stearic acid*: 3.0 per cent to 19.0 per cent,
- *oleic acid and isomers* ($C_{18:1}$, *equivalent chain length on poly(cyanopropyl)siloxane 18.5 to 18.8)*: 54.0 per cent to 78.0 per cent,
- *linoleic acid and isomers* ($C_{18:2}$, *equivalent chain length on poly(cyanopropyl)siloxane 19.4 to 19.8)*: not more than 10.0 per cent,
- *arachidic acid*: 1.0 per cent to 3.0 per cent,
- *eicosenoic acids* ($C_{20:1}$, *equivalent chain length on poly(cyanopropyl)siloxane 20.4 to 20.7)*: not more than 2.1 per cent,
- *behenic acid*: 1.0 per cent to 5.0 per cent,
- *erucic acid and isomers* ($C_{22:1}$, *equivalent chain length on poly(cyanopropyl)siloxane 22.4 to 22.6)*: not more than 0.5 per cent,
- *lignoceric acid*: 0.5 per cent to 3.0 per cent.

Nickel. Not more than 1 ppm of Ni, determined by atomic absorption spectrometry (*2.2.23, Method II*).

Test solution. Into a platinum or silica crucible previously tared after ignition introduce 5.0 g. Cautiously heat and introduce into the substance a wick formed from twisted ashless filter paper. Ignite the wick. When the substance has ignited stop heating. After combustion, ignite in a muffle furnace at about 600 °C. Continue ignition until white ash is obtained. After cooling, take up the residue with two quantities, each of 2 ml, of *dilute hydrochloric acid R* and transfer into a 25 ml graduated flask. Add 0.3 ml of *nitric acid R* and dilute to 25.0 ml with *water R*.

Reference solutions. Prepare three reference solutions by adding 1.0 ml, 2.0 ml and 4.0 ml of *nickel standard solution (0.2 ppm Ni) R* to 2.0 ml of the test solution and diluting to 10.0 ml with *water R*.

Measure the absorbance at 232 nm using a nickel hollow-cathode lamp as a source of radiation, a graphite furnace as an atomic generator and *argon R* as the carrier gas.

Water (*2.5.12*). Not more than 0.3 per cent, determined on 1.000 g by the semi-micro determination of water.

STORAGE

Store protected from light.

LABELLING

The label states the nominal drop point.

01/2005:0263

ARACHIS OIL, REFINED

Arachidis oleum raffinatum

DEFINITION

The refined fatty oil obtained from the shelled seeds of *Arachis hypogaea* L. A suitable antioxidant may be added.

CHARACTERS

Appearance: clear, yellowish, viscous liquid.

Solubility: very slightly soluble in alcohol, miscible with light petroleum.

Relative density: about 0.915.

It solidifies at about 2 °C.

IDENTIFICATION

It complies with the identification test for fatty oils by thin-layer chromatography (*2.3.2*). The chromatogram obtained is similar to the typical chromatogram for arachis oil.

TESTS

Acid value (*2.5.1*): maximum 0.5, determined on 10.0 g.

Peroxide value (*2.5.5*): maximum 5.0.

Unsaponifiable matter (*2.5.7*): maximum 1.0 per cent, determined on 5.0 g.

Alkaline impurities (*2.4.19*). It complies with the test for alkaline impurities in fatty oils.

Composition of fatty acids. Gas chromatography (*2.4.22, Method A*).

Reference solution (a). Prepare 0.50 g of a mixture of the calibrating substances as indicated in Table 0263-1. Dissolve in *heptane R* and dilute to 50 ml with the same solvent.

Table 0263.-1

Calibrating substances	**Composition (per cent *m/m*)**
Methyl palmitate R	10
Methyl stearate R	5
Methyl oleate R	40
Methyl linoleate R	25
Methyl linolenate R	2
Methyl arachidate R	5
Methyl eicosenoate R	3
Methyl behenate R	5
Methyl erucate R	2
Methyl lignocerate R	3

Composition of the fatty acid fraction of the oil:

- *saturated fatty acids of chain length less than* C_{16}: maximum 0.4 per cent,
- *palmitic acid*: 7.0 per cent to 16.0 per cent,
- *stearic acid*: 1.3 per cent to 6.5 per cent,
- *oleic acid* (equivalent chain length on polyethyleneglycol adipate 18.3): 35.0 per cent to 72.0 per cent,
- *linoleic acid* (equivalent chain length on polyethyleneglycol adipate 18.9): 13.0 per cent to 43.0 per cent,
- *linolenic acid* (equivalent chain length on polyethyleneglycol adipate 19.7): maximum 0.6 per cent,
- *arachidic acid*: 0.5 per cent to 3.0 per cent,
- *eicosenoic acid* (equivalent chain length on polyethyleneglycol adipate 20.3): 0.5 per cent to 2.1 per cent,
- *behenic acid*: 1.0 per cent to 5.0 per cent,
- *erucic acid* (equivalent chain length on polyethyleneglycol adipate 22.3): maximum 0.5 per cent,
- *lignoceric acid*: 0.5 per cent to 3.0 per cent.

Water (*2.5.12*): maximum 0.3 per cent, determined on 3.00 g, if intended for use in the manufacture of parenteral dosage forms.

STORAGE

In a well-filled container, protected from light.

LABELLING

The label states:

- where applicable, that the substance is suitable for use in the manufacture of parenteral dosage forms,
- the name and concentration of any added antioxidant.

01/2005:0806

ARGININE

Argininum

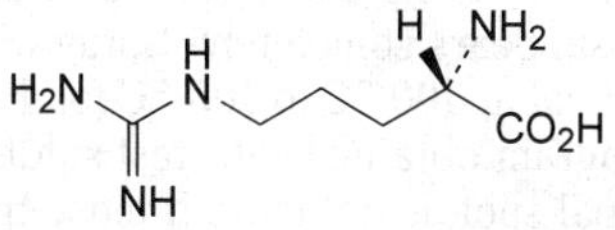

$C_6H_{14}N_4O_2$ M_r 174.2

DEFINITION

Arginine contains not less than 98.5 per cent and not more than the equivalent of 101.0 per cent of (*S*)-2-amino-5-guanidinopentanoic acid, calculated with reference to the dried substance.

CHARACTERS

A white or almost white, crystalline powder or colourless crystals, freely soluble in water, very slightly soluble in alcohol.

IDENTIFICATION

First identification: A, C.

Second identification: A, B, D, E.

A. It complies with the test for specific optical rotation (see Tests).

B. Solution S (see Tests) is strongly alkaline (*2.2.4*).

C. Examine by infrared absorption spectrophotometry (*2.2.24*), comparing with the spectrum obtained with *arginine CRS*. Examine the substances prepared as discs.

D. Examine the chromatograms obtained in the test for ninhydrin-positive substances. The principal spot in the chromatogram obtained with test solution (b) is similar in position, colour and size to the principal spot in the chromatogram obtained with reference solution (a).

E. Dissolve about 25 mg in 2 ml of *water R*. Add 1 ml of *α-naphthol solution R* and 2 ml of a mixture of equal volumes of *strong sodium hypochlorite solution R* and water. A red colour develops.

TESTS

Solution S. Dissolve 2.5 g in *distilled water R* and dilute to 50 ml with the same solvent.

Appearance of solution. Solution S is clear (*2.2.1*) and not more intensely coloured than reference solution BY_6 (*2.2.2, Method II*).

Specific optical rotation (*2.2.7*). Dissolve 2.00 g in *hydrochloric acid R1* and dilute to 25.0 ml with the same acid. The specific optical rotation is + 25.5 to + 28.5, calculated with reference to the dried substance.

Ninhydrin-positive substances. Examine by thin-layer chromatography (*2.2.27*), using a *TLC silica gel plate R*.

Test solution (a). Dissolve 0.10 g of the substance to be examined in *dilute hydrochloric acid R* and dilute to 10 ml with the same acid.

Test solution (b). Dilute 1 ml of test solution (a) to 50 ml with *water R*.

Reference solution (a). Dissolve 10 mg of *arginine CRS* in *0.1 M hydrochloric acid* and dilute to 50 ml with the same acid.

Reference solution (b). Dilute 5 ml of test solution (b) to 20 ml with *water R*.

Reference solution (c). Dissolve 10 mg of *arginine CRS* and 10 mg of *lysine hydrochloride CRS* in *0.1 M hydrochloric acid* and dilute to 25 ml with the same acid.

Apply to the plate 5 µl of each solution. Allow the plate to dry in air. Develop over a path of 15 cm using a mixture of 30 volumes of *concentrated ammonia R* and 70 volumes of *2-propanol R*. Dry the plate at 100 °C to 105 °C until the ammonia disappears completely. Spray with *ninhydrin solution R* and heat at 100 °C to 105 °C for 15 min. Any spot in the chromatogram obtained with test solution (a), apart from the principal spot, is not more intense than the spot in the chromatogram obtained with reference solution (b) (0.5 per cent). The test is not valid unless the chromatogram obtained with reference solution (c) shows two clearly separated spots.

Chlorides (*2.4.4*). To 5 ml of solution S add 0.5 ml of *dilute nitric acid R* and dilute to 15 ml with *water R*. The solution complies with the limit test for chlorides (200 ppm).

Sulphates (*2.4.13*). To 10 ml of solution S, add 1.7 ml of *dilute hydrochloric acid R* and dilute to 15 ml with *distilled water R*. The solution complies with the limit test for sulphates (300 ppm).

Ammonium (*2.4.1*). 50 mg complies with limit test B for ammonium (200 ppm). Prepare the standard using 0.1 ml of *ammonium standard solution (100 ppm* NH_4*) R*.

Iron (*2.4.9*). In a separating funnel, dissolve 1.0 g in 10 ml of *dilute hydrochloric acid R*. Shake with three quantities, each of 10 ml, of *methyl isobutyl ketone R1*, shaking for 3 min each time. To the combined organic layers add 10 ml of *water R* and shake for 3 min. The aqueous layer complies with the limit test for iron (10 ppm).

Heavy metals (*2.4.8*). Dissolve 2.0 g in *water R* and dilute to 20 ml with the same solvent. 12 ml of the solution complies with limit test A for heavy metals (10 ppm). Prepare the standard using *lead standard solution (1 ppm Pb) R*.

Loss on drying (*2.2.32*). Not more than 0.5 per cent, determined on 1.000 g by drying in an oven at 100 °C to 105 °C.

Sulphated ash (*2.4.14*). Not more than 0.1 per cent, determined on 1.0 g.

ASSAY

Dissolve 0.150 g in 50 ml of *water R*. Using 0.2 ml of *methyl red mixed solution R* as indicator, titrate with *0.1 M hydrochloric acid* until the colour changes from green to violet-red.

1 ml of *0.1 M hydrochloric acid* is equivalent to 17.42 mg of $C_6H_{14}N_4O_2$.

STORAGE

Store protected from light.

01/2005:2096

ARGININE ASPARTATE

Arginini aspartas

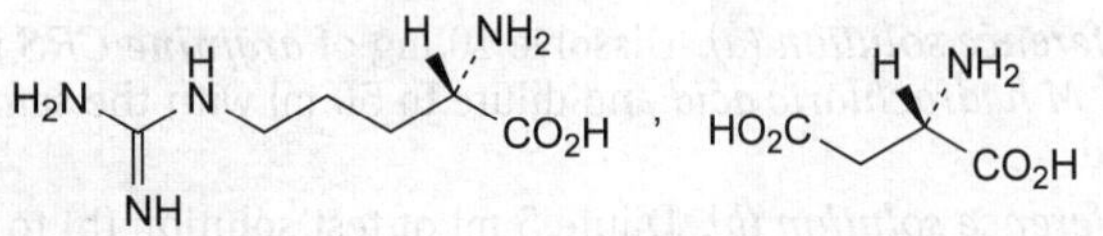

$C_{10}H_{21}N_5O_6$ M_r 307.3

DEFINITION

(2*S*)-2-Amino-5-guanidinopentanoic acid (2*S*)-2-aminobutanedioate.

Content: 99.0 per cent to 101.0 per cent (dried substance).

CHARACTERS

Appearance: white granules or powder.

Solubility: very soluble in water, practically insoluble in alcohol and in methylene chloride.

IDENTIFICATION

A. It complies with the test for specific optical rotation (see Tests).

B. Infrared absorption spectrophotometry (*2.2.24*).

Comparison: *arginine aspartate CRS*.

C. Examine the chromatograms obtained in the test for ninhydrin-positive substances.

Results: the 2 principal spots in the chromatogram obtained with test solution (b) are similar in position, colour and size to the 2 principal spots in the chromatogram obtained with reference solution (a).

TESTS

Solution S. Dissolve 5.0 g in *carbon dioxide-free water R* and dilute to 50 ml with the same solvent.

Appearance of solution. Solution S is clear (*2.2.1*) and not more intensely coloured than reference solution Y_7 (*2.2.2, Method II*).

pH (*2.2.3*): 6.0 to 7.0 for solution S.

Specific optical rotation (*2.2.7*): + 25 to + 27 (dried substance).

Dissolve 2.50 g in *dilute hydrochloric acid R* and dilute to 25.0 ml with the same acid.

Ninhydrin-positive substances. Thin-layer chromatography (*2.2.27*).

Test solution (a). Dissolve 0.20 g of the substance to be examined in *water R* and dilute to 10 ml with the same solvent.

Test solution (b). Dilute 1 ml of test solution (a) to 10 ml with *water R*.

Reference solution (a). Dissolve 25 mg of *arginine R* and 25 mg of *aspartic acid R* in *water R* and dilute to 25 ml with the same solvent.

Reference solution (b). Dilute 2 ml of reference solution (a) to 50 ml with *water R*.

Plate: *TLC silica gel G plate R*.

Mobile phase: *ammonia R, propanol R* (36:64 *V/V*).

Application: 5 µl.

Development: over 2/3 of the plate.

Drying: at 100-105 °C for 10 min.

Detection: spray with *ninhydrin solution R* and heat at 100-105 °C for 10 min.

System suitability: reference solution (b):

– the chromatogram shows 2 clearly separated principal spots.

Limit: test solution (a):

– *any impurity*: any spots, apart from the 2 principal spots, are not more intense than each of the 2 principal spots in the chromatogram obtained with reference solution (b) (0.2 per cent).

Chlorides (*2.4.4*): maximum 200 ppm.

Dilute 2.5 ml of solution S to 15 ml with *water R*.

Sulphates (*2.4.13*): maximum 300 ppm.

To 0.5 g add 2.5 ml of *dilute hydrochloric acid R* and dilute to 15 ml with *distilled water R*. Examine after 30 min.

Ammonium (*2.4.1*): maximum 100 ppm, determined on 100 mg.

Heavy metals (*2.4.8*): maximum 20 ppm.

12 ml of solution S complies with limit test A. Prepare the standard using *lead standard solution (2 ppm Pb) R*.

Loss on drying (*2.2.32*): maximum 0.5 per cent, determined on 1.000 g by drying in an oven at 60 °C for 24 h.

Sulphated ash (*2.4.14*): maximum 0.1 per cent, determined on 1.0 g.

ASSAY

Dissolve 80.0 mg in 2 ml of *anhydrous formic acid R*. Add 50 ml of *anhydrous acetic acid R*. Titrate with *0.1 M perchloric acid*, determining the end-point potentiometrically (*2.2.20*).

1 ml of *0.1 M perchloric acid* is equivalent to 10.24 mg of $C_{10}H_{21}N_5O_6$.

01/2005:0805

ARGININE HYDROCHLORIDE

Arginini hydrochloridum

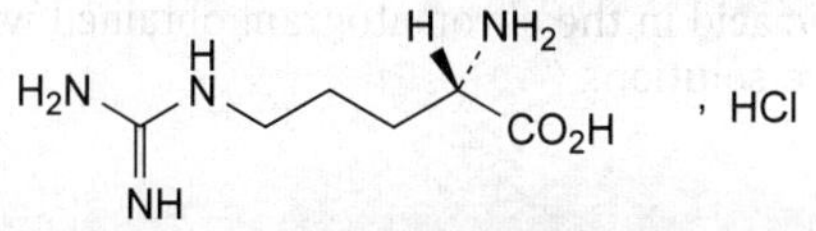

$C_6H_{15}ClN_4O_2$ M_r 210.7

DEFINITION

Arginine hydrochloride contains not less than 98.5 per cent and not more than the equivalent of 101.0 per cent of the hydrochloride of (*S*)-2-amino-5-guanidinopentanoic acid, calculated with reference to the dried substance.

CHARACTERS

A white or almost white, crystalline powder or colourless crystals, freely soluble in water, very slightly soluble in alcohol.

IDENTIFICATION

First identification: A, B, E.

Second identification: A, C, D, E.

A. It complies with the test for specific optical rotation (see Tests).

B. Examine by infrared absorption spectrophotometry (*2.2.24*), comparing with the spectrum obtained with *arginine hydrochloride CRS*. Examine the substances prepared as discs.

C. Examine the chromatograms obtained in the test for ninhydrin-positive substances. The principal spot in the chromatogram obtained with test solution (b) is similar in position, colour and size to the principal spot in the chromatogram obtained with reference solution (a).

D. Dissolve about 25 mg in 2 ml of *water R*. Add 1 ml of *α-naphthol solution R* and 2 ml of a mixture of equal volumes of *strong sodium hypochlorite solution R* and *water R*. A red colour develops.

E. About 20 mg gives reaction (a) of chlorides (*2.3.1*).

TESTS

Solution S. Dissolve 2.5 g in *distilled water R* and dilute to 50 ml with the same solvent.

Appearance of solution. Solution S is clear (*2.2.1*) and not more intensely coloured than reference solution BY_6 (*2.2.2, Method II*).

Specific optical rotation (*2.2.7*). Dissolve 2.00 g in *hydrochloric acid R1* and dilute to 25.0 ml with the same acid. The specific optical rotation is + 21.0 to + 23.5, calculated with reference to the dried substance.

Ninhydrin-positive substances. Examine by thin-layer chromatography (*2.2.27*), using a *TLC silica gel plate R*.

Test solution (a). Dissolve 0.10 g of the substance to be examined in *water R* and dilute to 10 ml with the same solvent.

Test solution (b). Dilute 1 ml of test solution (a) to 50 ml with *water R*.

Reference solution (a). Dissolve 10 mg of *arginine hydrochloride CRS* in *water R* and dilute to 50 ml with the same solvent.

Reference solution (b). Dilute 5 ml of test solution (b) to 20 ml with *water R*.

Reference solution (c). Dissolve 10 mg of *arginine hydrochloride CRS* and 10 mg of *lysine hydrochloride CRS* in *water R* and dilute to 25 ml with the same solvent.

Apply to the plate 5 µl of each solution. Allow the plate to dry in air. Develop over a path of 15 cm using a mixture of 30 volumes of *concentrated ammonia R* and 70 volumes of *2-propanol R*. Dry the plate at 100 °C to 105 °C until the ammonia disappears completely. Spray with *ninhydrin solution R* and heat at 100 °C to 105 °C for 15 min. Any spot in the chromatogram obtained with test solution (a), apart from the principal spot, is not more intense than the spot in the chromatogram obtained with reference solution (b) (0.5 per cent). The test is not valid unless the chromatogram obtained with reference solution (c) shows two clearly separated spots.

Sulphates (*2.4.13*). Dilute 10 ml of solution S to 15 ml with *distilled water R*. The solution complies with the limit test for sulphates (300 ppm).

Ammonium (*2.4.1*). 50 mg complies with limit test B for ammonium (200 ppm). Prepare the standard using 0.1 ml of *ammonium standard solution (100 ppm NH_4) R*.

Iron (*2.4.9*). In a separating funnel, dissolve 1.0 g in 10 ml of *dilute hydrochloric acid R*. Shake with three quantities, each of 10 ml, of *methyl isobutyl ketone R1*, shaking for 3 min each time. To the combined organic layers add 10 ml of *water R* and shake for 3 min. The aqueous layer complies with the limit test for iron (10 ppm).

Heavy metals (*2.4.8*). Dissolve 2.0 g in *water R* and dilute to 20 ml with the same solvent. 12 ml of the solution complies with limit test A for heavy metals (10 ppm). Prepare the standard using *lead standard solution (1 ppm Pb) R*.

Loss on drying (*2.2.32*). Not more than 0.5 per cent, determined on 1.000 g by drying in an oven at 100 °C to 105 °C.

Sulphated ash (*2.4.14*). Not more than 0.1 per cent, determined on 1.0 g.

ASSAY

Dissolve 0.180 g in 3 ml of *anhydrous formic acid R*. Add 30 ml of *anhydrous acetic acid R*. Using 0.1 ml of *naphtholbenzein solution R* as indicator, titrate with *0.1 M perchloric acid* until the colour changes from brownish-yellow to green.

1 ml of *0.1 M perchloric acid* is equivalent to 21.07 mg of $C_6H_{15}ClN_4O_2$.

STORAGE

Store protected from light.

01/2005:1391

ARNICA FLOWER

Arnicae flos

DEFINITION

Arnica flower consists of the whole or partially broken, dried flower-heads of *Arnica montana* L. It contains not less than 0.40 per cent *m/m* of total sesquiterpene lactones expressed as dihydrohelenalin tiglate, calculated with reference to the dried drug.

CHARACTERS

It has an aromatic odour.

The capitulum when spread out, is about 20 mm in diameter and about 15 mm deep, and has a peduncle of 2 cm to 3 cm in length. The involucre consists of eighteen to twenty-four elongated lanceolate bracts, with acute apices, arranged in one or two rows: the bracts, 8 mm to about 10 mm long, are green with yellowish-green external hairs visible under a lens. The receptacle, about 6 mm in diameter, is convex, alveolate and covered with hairs. Its periphery bears about twenty ligulate florets 20 mm to 30 mm long; the disc bears a greater number of tubular florets about 15 mm long. The ovary, 4 mm to 8 mm long, is crowned by a pappus of whitish bristles 4 mm to 8 mm long. Some brown achenes, crowned or not by a pappus, may be present.

It has the macroscopic and microscopic characters described under identification tests A and B.

IDENTIFICATION

A. The involucre consists of elongated oval bracts with acute apices; the margin is ciliated. The ligulate floret has a reduced calyx crowned by fine, shiny, whitish bristles, bearing small coarse trichomes. The orange-yellow corolla bears seven to ten parallel veins and ends in three small lobes. The stamens, with free anthers, are incompletely developed. The narrow, brown ovary bears a stigma divided into two branches curving outwards. The tubular floret is actinomorphic. The ovary and the calyx are similar to those of the ligulate floret. The short corolla has five reflexed triangular lobes; the five fertile stamens are fused at the anthers.

B. Separate the capitulum into its different parts. Reduce to a powder (355). Examine under a microscope using *chloral hydrate solution R*. The powder shows the following characteristics. The epidermises of the bracts of the involucre have stomata and trichomes, which are more abundant on the outer (abaxial) surface. There are several different types of trichomes: uniseriate multicellular covering trichomes, varying in length from 50 µm to 500 µm, particularly abundant on the margins of the bract; secretory trichomes with uni- or biseriate multicellular stalks and with multicellular, globular heads, about 300 µm long, abundant on the outer surface of the bract; secretory trichomes with uniseriate multicellular stalks and with multicellular, globular heads, about 80 µm long, abundant on the inner surface of the bract. The epidermis of the ligulate corolla consists of lobed or elongated cells, a few stomata and trichomes of different types: covering trichomes, with very sharp ends, whose length may exceed 500 µm, consisting of one to three proximal cells with thickened walls and two to four distal cells with thin walls; secretory trichomes with biseriate multicellular heads; secretory trichomes with multicellular stalks and multicellular globular heads. The ligule ends in rounded papillose cells. The epidermis of the ovary is covered with trichomes: secretory trichomes with short stalks and multicellular globular heads; twinned covering trichomes usually consisting of two longitudinally united cells, with common punctuated walls; their ends are sharp and sometimes bifid. The epidermises of the calyx consist of elongated cells bearing short, unicellular, covering trichomes pointing towards the upper end of the bristle. The pollen grains have a diameter of about 30 µm and are rounded, with a spiny exine; they have three germinal pores.

C. Examine the chromatograms obtained in the test for *Calendula officinalis* L. - *Heterotheca inuloides*. The chromatogram obtained with the test solution shows, in the middle, a fluorescent blue zone corresponding to the zone due to chlorogenic acid in the chromatogram obtained with the reference solution; it shows, above this zone, three fluorescent yellowish-brown to orange-yellow zones, and above these three zones a fluorescent greenish-yellow zone corresponding to astragalin. The zone located below the astragalin zone corresponds to isoquercitroside; the zone located just below this zone corresponds to luteolin-7-glucoside. It also shows a fluorescent greenish-blue zone below the zone due to caffeic acid in the chromatogram obtained with the reference solution.

TESTS

Foreign matter (*2.8.2*). Not more than 5.0 per cent.

Calendula officinalis* L. - *Heterotheca inuloides. Examine by thin-layer chromatography (*2.2.27*), using a *TLC silica gel plate R*.

Test solution. To 2.00 g of the powdered drug (710) add 10 ml of *methanol R*. Heat in a water-bath at 60 °C for 5 min with shaking. Cool and filter.

Reference solution. Dissolve 2.0 mg of *caffeic acid R*, 2.0 mg of *chlorogenic acid R* and 5.0 mg of *rutin R* in *methanol R* and dilute to 30 ml with the same solvent.

Apply separately to the plate, as bands, 15 µl of each solution. Develop over a path of 15 cm using a mixture of 10 volumes of *anhydrous formic acid R*, 10 volumes of *water R*, 30 volumes of *methyl ethyl ketone R* and 50 volumes of *ethyl acetate R*. Allow the plate to dry in air for a few minutes. Spray with a 10 g/l solution of *diphenylboric acid aminoethyl ester R* in *methanol R* and then with a 50 g/l solution of *macrogol 400 R* in *methanol R*. Heat for 5 min at 100 °C to 105 °C. Allow the plate to dry in air and examine in ultraviolet light at 365 nm. The chromatogram obtained with the reference solution shows in the lower part an orange-yellow fluorescent zone (rutin), in the middle part a fluorescent zone due to chlorogenic acid and in the upper part a light bluish fluorescent zone (caffeic acid). The chromatogram obtained with the test solution does not show a fluorescent orange-yellow zone corresponding to rutin in the chromatogram obtained with the reference solution, nor does it show a zone below the zone corresponding to rutin.

Loss on drying (*2.2.32*). Not more than 10.0 per cent, determined on 1.000 g of the powdered drug (355) by drying in an oven at 100 °C to 105 °C for 2 h.

Total ash (*2.4.16*). Not more than 10.0 per cent.

ASSAY

Examine by liquid chromatography (*2.2.29*), using *santonin R* as the internal standard.

Internal standard solution. Dissolve immediately before use 0.010 g of *santonin R* accurately weighed in 10.0 ml of *methanol R.*

Test solution. In a 250 ml round-bottomed flask introduce 1.00 g of the powdered drug (355), add 50 ml of a mixture of equal volumes of *methanol R* and *water R* and heat under a reflux condenser in a water-bath at 50 °C to 60 °C for 30 min, shaking frequently. Allow to cool and filter through a paper filter. Add the paper filter, cut in pieces, to the residue in the round-bottomed flask, add 50 ml of a mixture of equal volumes of *methanol R* and *water R* and heat under a reflux condenser in a water-bath at 50 °C to 60 °C for 30 min, shaking frequently. Repeat this procedure twice. To the combined filtrate add 3.00 ml of the internal standard solution and evaporate to 18 ml under reduced pressure. Rinse the round-bottomed flask with *water R* and dilute, with the washings, to 20.0 ml. Transfer the solution to a chromatography column about 0.15 m long and about 30 mm in internal diameter containing 15 g of *kieselguhr for chromatography R*. Allow to stand for 20 min. Elute with 200 ml of a mixture of equal volumes of *ethyl acetate R* and *methylene chloride R*. Evaporate the eluate to dryness in a 250 ml round-bottomed flask. Dissolve the residue in 10.0 ml of *methanol R* and add 10.0 ml of *water R*. Add 7.0 g of *neutral aluminium oxide R*, shake for 120 s, centrifuge (at 5000 *g* for 10 min) and filter through a paper filter. Evaporate 10.0 ml of the filtrate to dryness. Dissolve the residue in 3.0 ml of a mixture of equal volumes of *methanol R* and *water R* and filter.

The chromatographic procedure may be carried out using:

– a stainless steel column 0.12 m long and 4 mm in internal diameter packed with *octadecylsilyl silica gel for chromatography R* (4 µm),
– as mobile phase at a flow rate of 1.2 ml/min:
Mobile phase A. Water R,
Mobile phase B. Methanol R,

Time (min)	Mobile phase A (per cent V/V)	Mobile phase B (per cent V/V)	Comment
0 - 3	62	38	isocratic
3 - 20	62 → 55	38 → 45	linear gradient
20 - 30	55	45	isocratic
30 - 55	55 → 45	45 → 55	linear gradient
55 - 57	45 → 0	55 → 100	linear gradient
57 - 70	0	100	isocratic
70 - 90	62	38	isocratic

– as detector a spectrophotometer set at 225 nm,
– a 20 µl loop injector.

Calculate the percentage of total sesquiterpene lactones, expressed as dihydrohelenalin tiglate, from the expression:

$$\frac{S_{LS} \times C \times V \times 1.187 \times 100}{S_S \times m \times 1000}$$

S_{LS} = area of all peaks corresponding to sesquiterpene lactones appearing after the santonin peak in the chromatogram obtained with the test solution,

S_S = area of the peak corresponding to santonin in the chromatogram obtained with the test solution,

m = mass of the drug to be examined, in grams,

C = concentration of santonin in the internal standard solution used for the test solution, in milligrams per millilitre,

V = volume of the internal standard solution used for the test solution, in millilitres,

1.187 = peak correlation factor between dihydrohelenalin tiglate and santonin.

STORAGE

Store protected from light.

01/2005:1688

ARTICAINE HYDROCHLORIDE

Articaini hydrochloridum

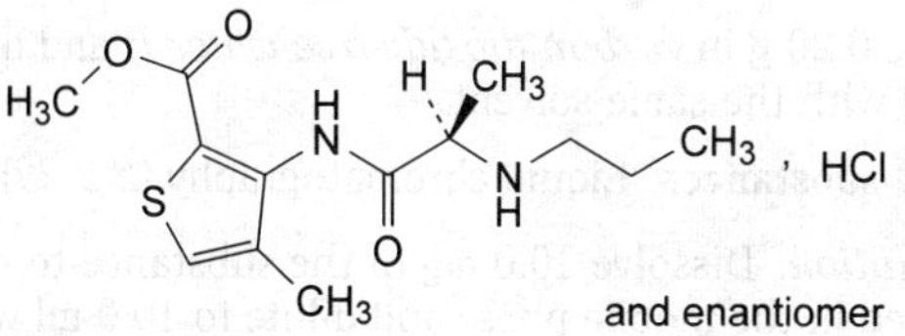

$C_{13}H_{21}ClN_2O_3S$ M_r 320.8

DEFINITION

Methyl 4-methyl-3-[[(2*RS*)-2-(propylamino)propanoyl]amino]thiophene-2-carboxylate hydrochloride.

Content: 98.5 per cent to 101.0 per cent (dried substance).

CHARACTERS

Appearance: white or almost white, crystalline powder.

Solubility: freely soluble in water and in alcohol.

IDENTIFICATION

First identification: B, D.

Second identification: A, C, D.

A. Dissolve 50.0 mg in a 1 g/l solution of *hydrochloric acid R* and dilute to 100.0 ml with the same acid. Dilute 5.0 ml of the solution to 100.0 ml with a 1 g/l solution of *hydrochloric acid R*. Examined between 200 nm and 350 nm (*2.2.25*), the solution shows an absorption maximum at 272 nm. The specific absorbance at the maximum is 290 to 320.

B. Infrared absorption spectrophotometry (*2.2.24*).
Preparation: place dropwise 20 µl of the test solution on 300 mg discs.
Test solution. Dissolve 0.1 g in 5 ml of *water R*, add 3 ml of a saturated solution of *sodium hydrogen carbonate R* and shake twice with 2 ml of *methylene chloride R*. Combine the methylene chloride layers, dilute to 5.0 ml with *methylene chloride R* and dry over *anhydrous sodium sulphate R*.
Comparison: *articaine hydrochloride CRS*.

C. Thin-layer chromatography (*2.2.27*).
Test solution. Dissolve 20 mg of the substance to be examined in 5 ml of *alcohol R*.
Reference solution. Dissolve 20 mg of *articaine hydrochloride CRS* in 5 ml of *alcohol R*.
Plate: *TLC silica gel F_{254} plate R*.
Mobile phase: *triethylamine R, ethyl acetate R, heptane R* (10:35:65 *V/V/V*).
Application: 5 µl.

Development: over a path of 15 cm.

Drying: in air.

Detection: examine in ultraviolet light at 254 nm.

Results: the principal spot in the chromatogram obtained with the test solution is similar in position and size to the principal spot in the chromatogram obtained with the reference solution.

D. It gives reaction (a) of chlorides (*2.3.1*).

TESTS

Solution S. Dissolve 0.50 g in *water R* and dilute to 10 ml with the same solvent.

Appearance of solution. Solution S is clear (*2.2.1*) and not more intensely coloured than reference solution BY_6 (*2.2.2, Method I*).

pH (*2.2.3*): 4.2 to 5.2.

Dissolve 0.20 g in *carbon dioxide-free water R* and dilute to 20.0 ml with the same solvent.

Related substances. Liquid chromatography (*2.2.29*).

Test solution. Dissolve 10.0 mg of the substance to be examined in the mobile phase and dilute to 10.0 ml with the mobile phase.

Reference solution (a). Dilute 1.0 ml of the test solution to 100.0 ml with the mobile phase. Dilute 1.0 ml of this solution to 10.0 ml with the mobile phase.

Reference solution (b). Dissolve 10.0 mg of *articaine impurity A CRS* and 5.0 mg of *articaine impurity E CRS* in the mobile phase and dilute to 100.0 ml with the mobile phase.

Reference solution (c). Add 1.0 ml of reference solution (b) to 50.0 mg of *articaine hydrochloride CRS* and dilute to 50 ml with the mobile phase.

Reference solution (d). Dilute 1.0 ml of reference solution (b) to 50.0 ml with the mobile phase.

Column:

- *size*: l = 0.25 m, Ø = 4.6 mm,
- *stationary phase*: spherical *end-capped octadecylsilyl silica gel for chromatography R* (5 µm) with a specific surface area of 335 m^2/g and a carbon loading of 19 per cent,
- *temperature*: 45 °C.

Mobile phase: mix 25 volumes of *acetonitrile R* and 75 volumes of a solution prepared as follows: dissolve 2.02 g of *sodium heptanesulphonate R* and 4.08 g of *potassium dihydrogen phosphate R* in *water R* and dilute to 1000 ml with the same solvent. Adjust to pH 2.0 with *phosphoric acid R*.

Flow rate: 1 ml/min.

Detection: spectrophotometer at 276 nm.

Injection: 10 µl; inject the test solution and reference solutions (a), (c) and (d).

Run time: 5 times the retention time of articaine.

Relative retentions with reference to articaine (retention time = about 9.3 min): impurity B = about 0.6; impurity D = about 0.7; impurity A = about 0.8; impurity E = about 0.86; impurity F = about 0.9; impurity G = about 1.7; impurity H = about 2.1; impurity I = about 2.6; impurity C = about 3.6; impurity J = about 4.0.

System suitability: reference solution (c):

- *resolution*: minimum 1.2 between the peaks due to impurity A and impurity E.

Limits:

- *impurity A*: not more than the area of the corresponding peak in the chromatogram obtained with reference solution (d) (0.2 per cent),
- *any other impurity*: not more than the area of the principal peak in the chromatogram obtained with reference solution (a) (0.1 per cent),
- *total of other impurities*: not more than 5 times the area of the principal peak in the chromatogram obtained with reference solution (a) (0.5 per cent),
- *disregard limit*: half the area of the principal peak in the chromatogram obtained with reference solution (a) (0.05 per cent).

Heavy metals (*2.4.8*): maximum 5 ppm.

Dissolve 4.0 g in 20.0 ml of *water R*. 12 ml of the solution complies with limit test A. Prepare the standard using *lead standard solution (1 ppm Pb) R*.

Loss on drying (*2.2.32*): maximum 0.5 per cent, determined on 1.000 g by drying in an oven at 100-105 °C for 5 h.

Sulphated ash (*2.4.14*): maximum 0.1 per cent, determined on 1.0 g.

ASSAY

Dissolve 0.250 g in a mixture of 5.0 ml of *0.01 M hydrochloric acid* and 50 ml of *alcohol R*. Carry out a potentiometric titration (*2.2.20*) using *0.1 M sodium hydroxide*. Read the volume added between the 2 points of inflexion.

1 ml of *0.1 M sodium hydroxide* is equivalent to 32.08 mg of $C_{13}H_{21}ClN_2O_3S$.

STORAGE

Protected from light.

IMPURITIES

Specified impurities: A, B, C.

Other detectable impurities: D, E, F, G, H, I, J.

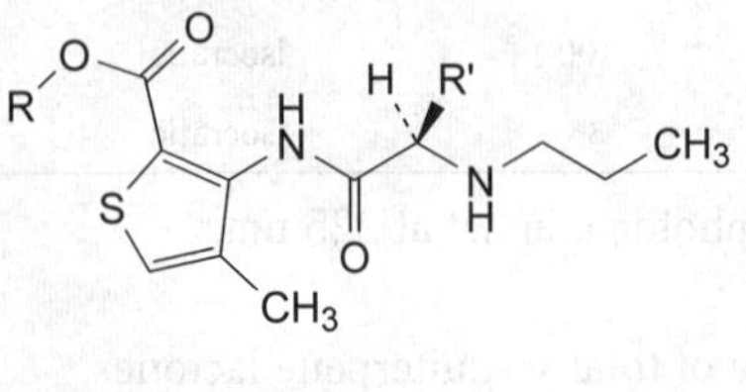

and enantiomer

A. R = CH_3, R′ = H: methyl 3-[[2-(propylamino)acetyl]amino]-4-methylthiophene-2-carboxylate (acetamidoarticaine),

B. R = H, R′ = CH_3: 4-methyl-3-[[(2*RS*)-2-(propylamino)propanoyl]amino]thiophene-2-carboxylic acid (articaine acid),

C. R = $CH(CH_3)_2$, R′ = CH_3: 1-methylethyl 4-methyl-3-[[(2*RS*)-2-(propylamino)propanoyl]amino]thiophene-2-carboxylate (articaine isopropyl ester),

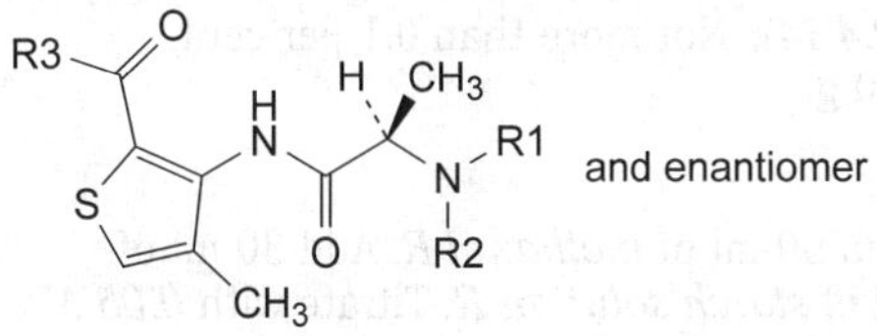

D. R1 = CH_2-CH_3, R2 = H, R3 = OCH_3: methyl 3-[[(2*RS*)-2-(ethylamino)propanoyl]amino]-4-methylthiophene-2-carboxylate (ethylarticaine),

E. R1 = $CH(CH_3)_2$, R2 = H, R3 = OCH_3: methyl 4-methyl-3-[[(2*RS*)-2-[(1-methylethyl)amino]propanoyl]amino]thiophene-2-carboxylate (isopropylarticaine),

F. R1 = CH_2-CH_2-CH_3, R2 = H, R3 = NH-CH_2-CH_2-CH_3: 4-methyl-*N*-propyl-3-[[(2*RS*)-2-(propylamino)propanoyl]amino]thiophene-2-carboxamide (articaine acid propionamide),

G. R1 = $(CH_2)_3$-CH_3, R2 = H, R3 = OCH_3: methyl 3-[[(2*RS*)-2-(butylamino)propanoyl]amino]-4-methylthiophene-2-carboxylate (butylarticaine),

H. R1 = R2 = CH_2-CH_2-CH_3, R3 = OCH_3: methyl 3-[[(2*RS*)-2-(dipropylamino)propanoyl]amino]-4-methylthiophene-2-carboxylate (dipropylarticaine),

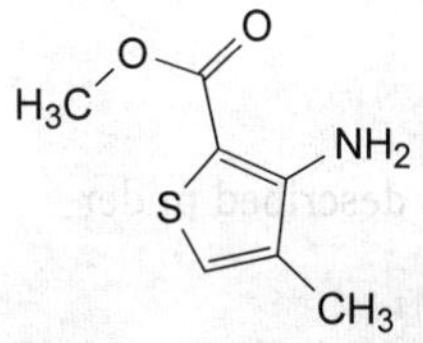

I. methyl 3-amino-4-methylthiophene-2-carboxylate (3-aminoarticaine),

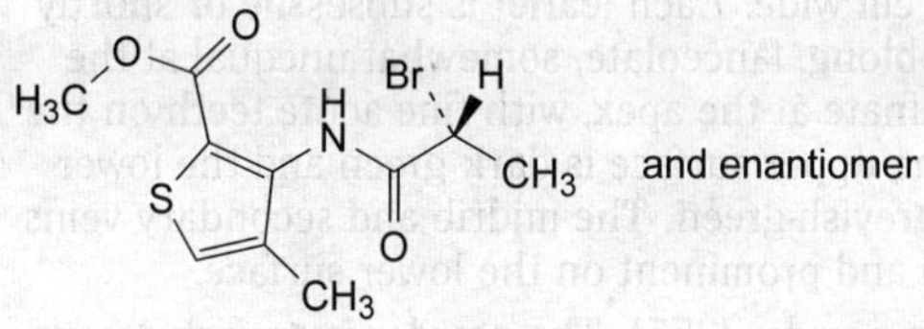

J. methyl 3-[[(2*RS*)-2-bromopropanoyl]amino]-4-methylthiophene-2-carboxylate (bromo compound).

01/2005:0253

ASCORBIC ACID

Acidum ascorbicum

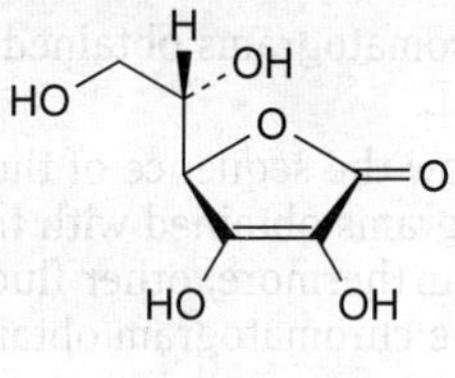

$C_6H_8O_6$ M_r 176.1

DEFINITION

Ascorbic acid contains not less than 99.0 per cent and not more than the equivalent of 100.5 per cent of (5*R*)-5-[(1*S*)-1,2-dihydroxyethyl]-3,4-dihydroxyfuran-2(5*H*)-one.

CHARACTERS

A white or almost white, crystalline powder or colourless crystals, becoming discoloured on exposure to air and moisture, freely soluble in water, soluble in alcohol.

It melts at about 190 °C, with decomposition.

IDENTIFICATION

First identification: B, C.

Second identification: A, C, D.

A. Dissolve 0.10 g in *water R* and dilute immediately to 100.0 ml with the same solvent. To 10 ml of *0.1 M hydrochloric acid*, add 1.0 ml of the solution and dilute to 100.0 ml with *water R*. Measure the absorbance (*2.2.25*) at the maximum at 243 nm immediately after dissolution. The specific absorbance at the maximum is 545 to 585.

B. Examine by infrared absorption spectrophotometry (*2.2.24*), comparing with the spectrum obtained with *ascorbic acid CRS*. Examine the substance prepared as discs containing 1 mg.

C. The pH (*2.2.3*) of solution S (see Tests) is 2.1 to 2.6.

D. To 1 ml of solution S add 0.2 ml of *dilute nitric acid R* and 0.2 ml of *silver nitrate solution R2*. A grey precipitate is formed.

TESTS

Solution S. Dissolve 1.0 g in *carbon dioxide-free water R* and dilute to 20 ml with the same solvent.

Appearance of solution. Solution S is clear (*2.2.1*) and not more intensely coloured than reference solution BY_7 (*2.2.2, Method II*).

Specific optical rotation (*2.2.7*). Dissolve 2.50 g in *water R* and dilute to 25.0 ml with the same solvent. The specific optical rotation is + 20.5 to + 21.5.

Oxalic acid. Dissolve 0.25 g in 5 ml of *water R*. Neutralise to *red litmus paper R* using *dilute sodium hydroxide solution R* and add 1 ml of *dilute acetic acid R* and 0.5 ml of *calcium chloride solution R* (test solution). Prepare a reference solution as follows: dissolve 70 mg of *oxalic acid R* in *water R* and dilute to 500 ml with the same solvent; to 5 ml of this solution add 1 ml of *dilute acetic acid R* and 0.5 ml of *calcium chloride solution R* (reference solution). Allow the solutions to stand for 1 h. Any opalescence in the test solution is not more intense than that in the reference solution (0.2 per cent).

Copper. Not more than 5 ppm of Cu, determined by atomic absorption spectrometry (*2.2.23, Method I*).

Test solution. Dissolve 2.0 g of the substance to be examined in *0.1 M nitric acid* and dilute to 25.0 ml with the same acid.

Reference solutions. Prepare reference solutions containing 0.2 ppm, 0.4 ppm and 0.6 ppm of Cu by diluting *copper standard solution (10 ppm Cu) R* with *0.1 M nitric acid.*

Measure the absorbance at 324.8 nm using a copper hollow-cathode lamp as a source of radiation and an air-acetylene flame. Adjust the zero of the apparatus using *0.1 M nitric acid.*

Iron. Not more than 2 ppm of Fe, determined by atomic absorption spectrometry (*2.2.23, Method I*).

Test solution. Dissolve 5.0 g of the substance to be examined in *0.1 M nitric acid* and dilute to 25.0 ml with the same acid.

Reference solutions. Prepare reference solutions containing 0.2 ppm, 0.4 ppm and 0.6 ppm of Fe by diluting *iron standard solution (20 ppm Fe) R* with *0.1 M nitric acid.*

Measure the absorbance at 248.3 nm using an iron hollow-cathode lamp as a source of radiation and an air-acetylene flame. Adjust the zero of the apparatus using *0.1 M nitric acid.*

Heavy metals (*2.4.8*). Dissolve 2.0 g in *water R* and dilute to 20 ml with the same solvent. 12 ml of the solution complies with limit test A for heavy metals (10 ppm). Prepare the standard using *lead standard solution (1 ppm Pb) R*.

Sulphated ash (*2.4.14*). Not more than 0.1 per cent, determined on 1.0 g.

ASSAY

Dissolve 0.150 g in a mixture of 10 ml of *dilute sulphuric acid R* and 80 ml of *carbon dioxide-free water R*. Add 1 ml of *starch solution R*. Titrate with *0.05 M iodine* until a persistent violet-blue colour is obtained.

1 ml of *0.05 M iodine* is equivalent to 8.81 mg of $C_6H_8O_6$.

STORAGE

Store in a non-metallic container, protected from light.

01/2005:0807

ASCORBYL PALMITATE

Ascorbylis palmitas

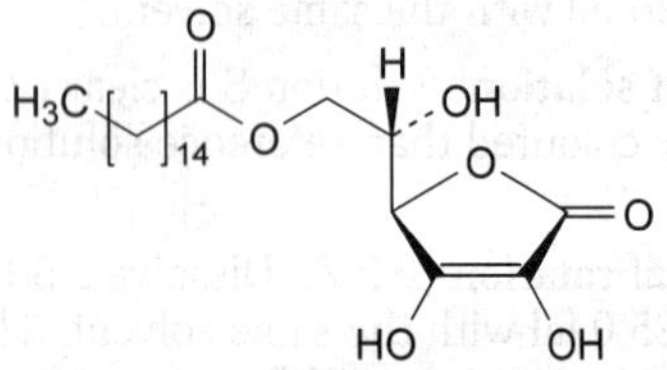

$C_{22}H_{38}O_7$ M_r 414.5

DEFINITION

Ascorbyl palmitate contains not less than 98.0 per cent and not more than the equivalent of 100.5 per cent of (2*S*)-2-[(5*R*)-3,4-dihydroxy-5-oxo-2,5-dihydrofuran-2-yl]-2-hydroxyethyl hexadecanoate, calculated with reference to the dried substance.

CHARACTERS

A white or yellowish-white powder, practically insoluble in water, freely soluble in alcohol and in methanol, practically insoluble in methylene chloride and in fatty oils.

IDENTIFICATION

A. It complies with the test for specific optical rotation (see Tests).

B. Examine by infrared absorption spectrophotometry (*2.2.24*), comparing with the *Ph. Eur. reference spectrum of ascorbyl palmitate*.

C. Dissolve about 10 mg in 5 ml of *methanol R*. The solution decolourises *dichlorophenolindophenol standard solution R*.

TESTS

Solution S. Dissolve 2.50 g in *methanol R* and dilute to 25.0 ml with the same solvent.

Appearance of solution. Solution S is clear (*2.2.1*) and not more intensely coloured than reference solution BY_4 (*2.2.2, Method I*).

Specific optical rotation (*2.2.7*): + 21 to + 24, determined on solution S and calculated with reference to the dried substance.

Heavy metals (*2.4.8*). 2.0 g complies with limit test C for heavy metals (10 ppm). Prepare the standard using 2 ml of *lead standard solution (10 ppm Pb) R*.

Loss on drying (*2.2.32*). Not more than 1.0 per cent, determined on 1.000 g by drying *in vacuo* at 60 °C for 5 h.

Sulphated ash (*2.4.14*). Not more than 0.1 per cent, determined on 1.0 g.

ASSAY

Dissolve 0.160 g in 50 ml of *methanol R*. Add 30 ml of *water R* and 1 ml of *starch solution R*. Titrate with *0.05 M iodine* until a persistent violet-blue colour is obtained.

1 ml of *0.05 M iodine* is equivalent to 20.73 mg of $C_{22}H_{38}O_7$.

STORAGE

Store in an airtight container, protected from light, at a temperature of 8 °C to 15 °C.

01/2005:1600

ASH LEAF

Fraxini folium

DEFINITION

Dried leaf of *Fraxinus excelsior* L. or *Fraxinus oxyphylla* M. Bieb.

Content: minimum 2.5 per cent of total hydroxycinnamic acid derivatives expressed as chlorogenic acid ($C_{16}H_{18}O_9$; M_r 354.3) (dried drug).

CHARACTERS

Macroscopic and microscopic characters described under identification tests A and B.

IDENTIFICATION

A. The leaf consists of leaflets which are sometimes detached and separated from the rachis. The leaflet is about 6 cm long and 3 cm wide. Each leaflet is subsessile or shortly petiolate, oblong, lanceolate, somewhat unequal at the base, acuminate at the apex, with fine acute teeth on the margins, the upper surface is dark green and the lower surface is greyish-green. The midrib and secondary veins are whitish and prominent on the lower surface.

B. Reduce to a powder (355). The powder is greyish-green. Examined under a microscope, using *chloral hydrate solution R*. The powder shows fragments of the lamina in surface view, with the lower epidermis showing numerous anomocytic stomata (*2.8.3.*) and some of the cells of the upper epidermis with cuticular striations; occasional uniseriate, conical covering trichomes composed of 1 or 2 cells with thick walls and a striated cuticle; rare peltate glands with a unicellular stalk and a shield-like glandular head composed of 8 radiating cells; groups of fibres and fragments of vascular tissue from the veins.

C. Examine the chromatograms obtained in the test for *Fraxinus ornus* L.

Results: see below the sequence of the zones present in the chromatograms obtained with the reference and test solutions. Furthermore, other fluorescent zones are present in the chromatogram obtained with the test solution.

Top of the plate	
	A light blue fluorescence zone
	An intense blue fluorescent zone (acteoside)
Chlorogenic acid: a blue fluorescent zone	A blue fluorescent zone (chlorogenic acid)
Rutin: an orange fluorescent zone	An orange fluorescent zone (rutin)
Reference solution	**Test solution**

TESTS

Foreign matter (*2.8.2*): maximum 3.0 per cent of stems and 2.0 per cent of other foreign matter.

Fraxinus ornus **L.** Thin-layer chromatography (*2.2.27*).

Test solution. To 1 g of the powdered drug (355) add 20 ml of *methanol R*. Heat with shaking at 40 °C for 10 min. Filter.

Reference solution. Dissolve 5.0 mg of *rutin R* and 5.0 mg of *chlorogenic acid R* in 10 ml of *methanol R.*

Plate: *TLC silica gel plate R.*

Mobile phase: *anhydrous formic acid R, water R, ethyl acetate R* (10:10:80 *V/V/V*).

Application: 10 µl as bands.

Development: over a path of 10 cm.

Drying: in air.

Detection: spray with a solution containing 10 g/l of *diphenylboric acid aminoethyl ester R* and 50 g/l of *macrogol 400 R* in *methanol R*. Examine in ultraviolet light at 365 nm.

Results: in the case of a substitution by F. *ornus*, the chromatogram obtained with the test solution does not show the zones of acteoside, chlorogenic acid and rutin.

Loss on drying (*2.2.32*): maximum 10.0 per cent, determined on 1.000 g of the powdered drug (355) by drying in an oven at 100-105 °C for 2 h.

Total ash (*2.4.16*): maximum 12.0 per cent.

ASSAY

Test solution (a). To 0.300 g of the powdered drug (355) add 95 ml of *alcohol (50 per cent V/V) R*. Boil in a water-bath under a reflux condenser for 30 min. Allow to cool and filter. Rinse the filter with 5 ml of *alcohol (50 per cent V/V) R*. Combine the filtrate and the rinsings in a volumetric flask and dilute to 100.0 ml with *alcohol (50 per cent V/V) R.*

Test solution (b). To 1.0 ml of test solution (a) in a test tube, add 2 ml of *0.5 M hydrochloric acid*, 2 ml of a solution prepared by dissolving 10 g of *sodium nitrite R* and 10 g of *sodium molybdate R* in 100 ml of *water R*, then add 2 ml of *dilute sodium hydroxide solution R* and dilute to 10.0 ml with *water R*; mix.

Immediately measure the absorbance (*2.2.25*) of test solution (b) at 525 nm, using as compensation liquid a solution prepared as follows: mix 1.0 ml of test solution (a), 2 ml of *0.5 M hydrochloric acid* and 2 ml of *dilute sodium hydroxide solution R* and dilute to 10.0 ml with *water R.*

Calculate the percentage content of total hydroxycinnamic acid derivatives expressed as chlorogenic acid, from the expression:

$$\frac{A \times 5.3}{m}$$

taking the specific absorbance of chlorogenic acid at 525 nm to be 188.

A = absorbance at 525 nm,

m = mass of the test sample in grams.

01/2005:2086

ASPARAGINE MONOHYDRATE

Asparaginum monohydricum

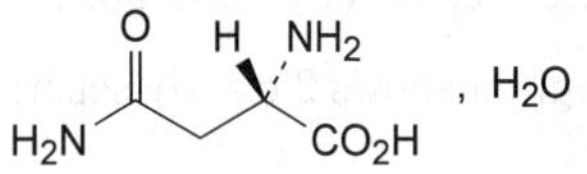

$C_4H_8N_2O_3,H_2O$ M_r 150.1

DEFINITION

(2*S*)-2,4-Diamino-4-oxobutanoic acid monohydrate.

Content: 99.0 per cent to 101.0 per cent (dried substance).

CHARACTERS

Appearance: white, crystalline powder or colourless crystals.

Solubility: slightly soluble in water, practically insoluble in alcohol and in methylene chloride.

IDENTIFICATION

First identification: *A, B.*

Second identification: *A, C.*

A. It complies with the test for specific optical rotation (see Tests).

B. Infrared absorption spectrophotometry (*2.2.24*).
Comparison: *asparagine monohydrate CRS.*

C. Examine the chromatograms obtained in the test for ninhydrin-positive substances.
Results: the principal spot in the chromatogram obtained with test solution (b) is similar in position, colour and size to the principal spot in the chromatogram obtained with reference solution (c).

TESTS

Solution S. Dissolve with heating 2.0 g in *carbon dioxide-free water R* and dilute to 100 ml with the same solvent.

Appearance of solution. Solution S is clear (*2.2.1*) and colourless (*2.2.2, Method II*).

pH (*2.2.3*): 4.0 to 6.0 for solution S.

Specific optical rotation (*2.2.7*): + 33.7 to + 36.0 (dried substance).

Dissolve 2.50 g in a 309.0 g/l solution of *hydrochloric acid R* and dilute to 25.0 ml with the same acid.

Ninhydrin-positive substances. Thin-layer chromatography (*2.2.27*).

Test solution (a). Dissolve 0.25 g of the substance to be examined in *water R*, heating to not more than 40 °C, and dilute to 10 ml with the same solvent.

Test solution (b). Dilute 1 ml of test solution (a) to 10 ml with *water R.*

Reference solution (a). Dilute 1.0 ml of test solution (a) to 200 ml with *water R.*

Reference solution (b). Dissolve 25 mg of *glutamic acid R* in *water R*, add 1 ml of test solution (a) and dilute to 10 ml with *water R.*

Reference solution (c). Dissolve 25 mg of *asparagine monohydrate CRS* in *water R* and dilute to 10 ml with the same solvent.

Plate: *TLC silica gel G plate R.*

Mobile phase: *glacial acetic acid R, water R, butanol R* (25:25:50 *V/V/V*).

Application: 5 µl.

Development: over half of the plate.

Drying: at 110 °C for 15 min.

Detection: spray with *ninhydrin solution R* and heat at 110 °C for 10 min.

System suitability: reference solution (b):

– the chromatogram shows 2 clearly separated principal spots.

Limit: test solution (a):

– *any impurity*: any spot, apart from the principal spot, is not more intense than the principal spot in the chromatogram obtained with reference solution (a) (0.5 per cent).

Chlorides (*2.4.4*): maximum 200 ppm.

Dilute 12.5 ml of solution S to 15 ml with *water R*.

Sulphates (*2.4.13*): maximum 200 ppm.

To 0.75 g add 2.5 ml of *dilute hydrochloric acid R* and dilute to 15 ml with *distilled water R*. Examine after 30 min.

Ammonium (*2.4.1, Method B*): maximum 0.1 per cent, determined on 10 mg.

Iron (*2.4.9*): maximum 10 ppm.

Dissolve 1.0 g in *dilute hydrochloric acid R* and dilute to 10 ml with the same acid. Shake 3 times with 10 ml of *methyl isobutyl ketone R1* for 3 min. Wash the combined organic phases with 10 ml of *water R* for 3 min. The aqueous phase complies with the limit test for iron.

Heavy metals (*2.4.8*): maximum 10 ppm.

Dissolve 2.0 g in a mixture of 3 ml of *dilute hydrochloric acid R* and 15 ml of *water R* with gentle warming if necessary. Dilute to 20 ml with *water R*. 12 ml of the solution complies with limit test A. Prepare the standard using *lead standard solution (1 ppm Pb) R*.

Loss on drying (*2.2.32*): 10.5 per cent to 12.5 per cent, determined on 1.000 g by drying in an oven at 60 °C for 24 h.

Sulphated ash (*2.4.14*): maximum 0.1 per cent, determined on 1.0 g.

ASSAY

Dissolve 0.110 g in 5 ml of *anhydrous formic acid R*. Add 50 ml of *anhydrous acetic acid R*. Titrate with *0.1 M perchloric acid*, determining the end-point potentiometrically (*2.2.20*).

1 ml of *0.1 M perchloric acid* is equivalent to 13.21 mg of $C_4H_8N_2O_3$.

IMPURITIES

Specified impurities: A, B.

A. aspartic acid,

B. glutamic acid.

01/2005:0973
corrected

ASPARTAME

Aspartamum

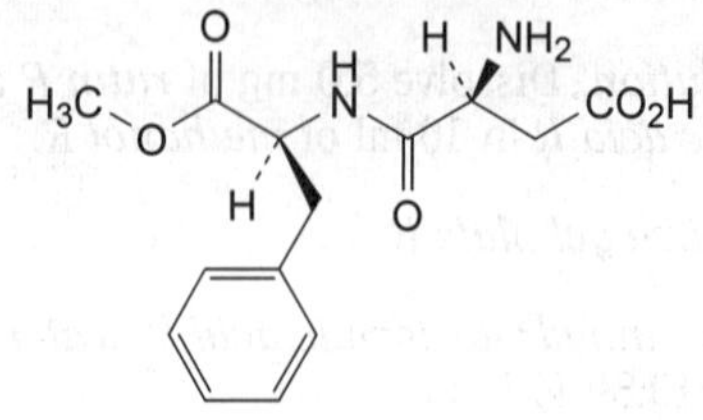

$C_{14}H_{18}N_2O_5$ M_r 294.3

DEFINITION

Aspartame contains not less than 98.0 per cent and not more than the equivalent of 102.0 per cent of (3*S*)-3-amino-4-[[(1*S*)-1-benzyl-2-methoxy-2-oxoethyl]amino]-4-oxobutanoic acid, calculated with reference to the dried substance.

CHARACTERS

A white, crystalline powder, slightly hygroscopic, sparingly soluble or slightly soluble in water and in alcohol, practically insoluble in hexane and in methylene chloride.

IDENTIFICATION

First identification: B.

Second identification: A, C, D.

A. Dissolve 0.1 g in *alcohol R* and dilute to 100 ml with the same solvent. Examined between 230 nm and 300 nm (*2.2.25*), the solution shows absorption maxima at 247 nm, 252 nm, 258 nm and 264 nm.

B. Examine by infrared absorption spectrophotometry (*2.2.24*), comparing with the spectrum obtained with *aspartame CRS*. Examine the substances prepared as discs.

C. Examine by thin-layer chromatography (*2.2.27*), using *silica gel G R* as the coating substance.

Test solution. Dissolve 15 mg of the substance to be examined in 2.5 ml of *water R* and dilute to 10 ml with *acetic acid R*.

Reference solution. Dissolve 15 mg of *aspartame CRS* in 2.5 ml of *water R* and dilute to 10 ml with *acetic acid R*.

Apply to the plate 20 µl of each solution. Develop over a path of 15 cm using a mixture of 2 volumes of *water R*, 4 volumes of *anhydrous formic acid R*, 30 volumes of *methanol R* and 64 volumes of *methylene chloride R*. Allow the plate to dry in air. Spray with *ninhydrin solution R* and heat at 100 °C to 105 °C for 15 min. The spot in the chromatogram obtained with the test solution is similar in position, colour and size to the spot in the chromatogram obtained with the reference solution.

D. Dissolve about 20 mg in 5 ml of *methanol R* and add 1 ml of *alkaline hydroxylamine solution R1*. Heat on a water-bath for 15 min. Allow to cool and adjust to about pH 2 with *dilute hydrochloric acid R*. Add 0.1 ml of *ferric chloride solution R1*. A brownish-red colour is produced.

TESTS

Solution S. Dissolve 0.8 g in *carbon dioxide-free water R* and dilute to 100 ml with the same solvent.

Appearance of solution. Solution S is clear (*2.2.1*) and not more intensely coloured than reference solution GY_6 (*2.2.2, Method II*).

Conductivity (*2.2.38*). Not more than 30 µS·cm^{-1}. Dissolve 0.80 g in *carbon dioxide-free water R* prepared from *distilled water R* and dilute to 100.0 ml with the same solvent. Measure the conductivity of the solution (C_1) and that of the water used for preparing the solution (C_2). The readings must be stable within 1 per cent over a period of 30 s. Calculate the conductivity of the solution of the substance to be examined from the expression:

$$C_1 - 0.992\,C_2$$

Specific optical rotation (*2.2.7*). Dissolve 2.00 g in a 690 g/l solution of *anhydrous formic acid R* and dilute to 50.0 ml with the same solution. The specific optical rotation is + 14.5 to + 16.5, measured within 30 min of preparation of the solution and calculated with reference to the dried substance.

Related substances. Examine by liquid chromatography (*2.2.29*).

Test solution. Dissolve 0.60 g of the substance to be examined in a mixture of 1.5 volumes of *glacial acetic acid R* and 98.5 volumes of *water R* and dilute to 100.0 ml with the same mixture of solvents.

Reference solution (a). Dissolve 4.5 mg of *aspartame impurity A CRS* in a mixture of 1.5 volumes of *glacial acetic acid R* and 98.5 volumes of *water R* and dilute to 50.0 ml with the same mixture of solvents.

Reference solution (b). Dissolve 30.0 mg of *phenylalanine R* in a mixture of 15 volumes of *glacial acetic acid R* and 85 volumes of *water R* and dilute to 100.0 ml with the same mixture of solvents. Dilute 1.0 ml of the solution to 10.0 ml with *water R*.

Reference solution (c). Dilute 5.0 ml of the test solution to 10.0 ml with *water R*. Dilute 3.0 ml of the solution to 100.0 ml with *water R*.

Reference solution (d). Dissolve 30.0 mg of *L-aspartyl-L-phenylalanine R* in a mixture of 15 volumes of *glacial acetic acid R* and 85 volumes of *water R* and dilute to 100.0 ml with the same mixture of solvents. Dilute 1.0 ml of the solution to 10.0 ml with *water R*. Mix 1.0 ml of this solution with 1.0 ml of reference solution (b).

The chromatographic procedure may be carried out using:

- a stainless steel column 0.25 m long and 4.0 mm in internal diameter packed with *octadecylsilyl silica gel for chromatography R* (5 µm to 10 µm),
- as mobile phase at a flow rate of 1 ml/min a mixture of 10 volumes of *acetonitrile R* and 90 volumes of a 6.8 g/l solution of *potassium dihydrogen phosphate R* previously adjusted to pH 3.7 with *phosphoric acid R*,
- as detector a spectrophotometer set at 220 nm.

Inject 20 µl of reference solution (c). Adjust the sensitivity of the system so that the height of the principal peak in the chromatogram obtained is not less than 50 per cent of the full scale of the recorder. Inject 20 µl of reference solution (d). The test is not valid unless in the chromatogram obtained, the resolution between the peaks due to phenylalanine and L-aspartyl-L-phenylalanine is at least 3.5. Inject separately 20 µl of each solution. Continue the chromatography for twice the retention time of aspartame. In the chromatogram obtained with the test solution: the area of any peak corresponding to aspartame impurity A is not greater than the area of the principal peak in the chromatogram obtained with reference solution (a) (1.5 per cent); the area of any peak corresponding to phenylalanine is not greater than the area of the principal peak in the chromatogram obtained with reference solution (b) (0.5 per cent); the sum of the areas of any other peaks, apart from the principal peak, is not greater than the area of the principal peak in the chromatogram obtained with reference solution (c) (1.5 per cent). Disregard any peak due to the solvent.

Heavy metals (*2.4.8*). 1.0 g complies with limit test C for heavy metals (10 ppm). Prepare the standard using 1 ml of *lead standard solution (10 ppm Pb) R*.

Loss on drying (*2.2.32*). Not more than 4.5 per cent, determined on 1.000 g by drying in an oven at 100 °C to 105 °C.

Sulphated ash (*2.4.14*). Not more than 0.2 per cent, determined on 1.0 g.

ASSAY

Dissolve 0.250 g in 1.5 ml of *anhydrous formic acid R* and 60 ml of *anhydrous acetic acid R*. Titrate immediately with *0.1 M perchloric acid*, determining the end-point potentiometrically (*2.2.20*).

1 ml of *0.1 M perchloric acid* is equivalent to 29.43 mg of $C_{14}H_{18}N_2O_5$.

STORAGE

Store in an airtight container.

IMPURITIES

A. 2-(5-benzyl-3,6-dioxopiperazin-2-yl)acetic acid (diketopiperazine),

B. L-aspartyl-L-phenylalanine,

C. phenylalanine.

01/2005:0797

ASPARTIC ACID

Acidum asparticum

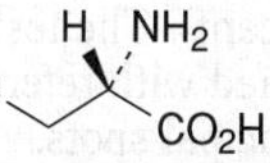

$C_4H_7NO_4$ M_r 133.1

DEFINITION

Aspartic acid contains not less than 98.5 per cent and not more than the equivalent of 101.5 per cent of (2*S*)-2-aminobutanedioic acid, calculated with reference to the dried substance.

CHARACTERS

A white or almost white, crystalline powder or colourless crystals, slightly soluble in water, practically insoluble in alcohol. It dissolves in dilute mineral acids and in dilute solutions of alkali hydroxides.

IDENTIFICATION

First identification: A, C.

Second identification: A, B, D.

A. It complies with the test for specific optical rotation (see Tests).

B. A suspension of 1 g in 10 ml of *water R* is strongly acid (*2.2.4*).

C. Examine by infrared absorption spectrophotometry (*2.2.24*), comparing with the spectrum obtained with *aspartic acid CRS*. Examine the substances prepared as discs.

D. Examine the chromatograms obtained in the test for ninhydrin-positive substances. The principal spot in the chromatogram obtained with test solution (b) is similar in position, colour and size to the principal spot in the chromatogram obtained with reference solution (a).

TESTS

Appearance of solution. Dissolve 0.5 g in *1 M hydrochloric acid* and dilute to 10 ml with the same acid. The solution is clear (*2.2.1*) and not more intensely coloured than reference solution BY_6 (*2.2.2, Method II*).

Specific optical rotation (*2.2.7*). Dissolve 2.000 g in *hydrochloric acid R1* and dilute to 25.0 ml with the same acid. The specific optical rotation is + 24.0 to + 26.0, calculated with reference to the dried substance.

Ninhydrin-positive substances. Examine by thin-layer chromatography (*2.2.27*), using a *TLC silica gel plate R*.

Test solution (a). Dissolve 0.10 g of the substance to be examined in 2 ml of *ammonia R* and dilute to 10 ml with *water R*.

Test solution (b). Dilute 1 ml of test solution (a) to 50 ml with *water R*.

Reference solution (a). Dissolve 10 mg of *aspartic acid CRS* in 2 ml of *dilute ammonia R1* and dilute to 50 ml with *water R*.

Reference solution (b). Dilute 5 ml of test solution (b) to 20 ml with *water R*.

Reference solution (c). Dissolve 10 mg of *aspartic acid CRS* and 10 mg of *glutamic acid CRS* in 2 ml of *dilute ammonia R1* and dilute to 25 ml with *water R*.

Apply separately to the plate 5 µl of each solution. Allow the plate to dry in air. Develop over a path of 15 cm using a mixture of 20 volumes of *glacial acetic acid R*, 20 volumes of *water R* and 60 volumes of *butanol R*. Allow the plate to dry in air, spray with *ninhydrin solution R*. Heat at 100-105 °C for 15 min. Any spot in the chromatogram obtained with test solution (a), apart from the principal spot, is not more intense than the spot in the chromatogram obtained with reference solution (b) (0.5 per cent). The test is not valid unless the chromatogram obtained with reference solution (c) shows 2 clearly separated principal spots.

Chlorides (*2.4.4*). Dissolve 0.25 g in 3 ml of *dilute nitric acid R* and dilute to 15 ml with *water R*. The solution, to which 1 ml of *water R* is added instead of *dilute nitric acid R*, complies with the limit test for chlorides (200 ppm).

Sulphates (*2.4.13*). Dissolve 0.5 g in 4 ml of *hydrochloric acid R* and dilute to 15 ml with *distilled water R*. The solution complies with the limit test for sulphates (300 ppm). Carry out the evaluation of the test after 30 min.

Ammonium.(*2.4.1*) 50 mg complies with limit test B (200 ppm). Prepare the standard using 0.1 ml of *ammonium standard solution (100 ppm NH_4) R*.

Iron (*2.4.9*). In a separating funnel, dissolve 1.0 g in 10 ml of *dilute hydrochloric acid R*. Shake with 3 quantities, each of 10 ml, of *methyl isobutyl ketone R1*, shaking for 3 min each time. To the combined organic layers add 10 ml of *water R* and shake for 3 min. The aqueous layer complies with the limit test for iron (10 ppm).

Heavy metals (*2.4.8*). 2.0 g complies with limit test D (10 ppm). Prepare the standard using 2 ml of *lead standard solution (10 ppm Pb) R*.

Loss on drying (*2.2.32*). Not more than 0.5 per cent, determined on 1.000 g by drying in an oven at 100-105 °C.

Sulphated ash (*2.4.14*). Not more than 0.1 per cent, determined on 1.0 g.

ASSAY

Dissolve 0.100 g in 50 ml of *carbon dioxide-free water R*, with slight heating if necessary. Cool and add 0.1 ml of *bromothymol blue solution R1*. Titrate with *0.1 M sodium hydroxide* until the colour changes from yellow to blue.

1 ml of *0.1 M sodium hydroxide* is equivalent to 13.31 mg of $C_4H_7NO_4$.

STORAGE

Protected from light.

01/2005:1067

ASTEMIZOLE

Astemizolum

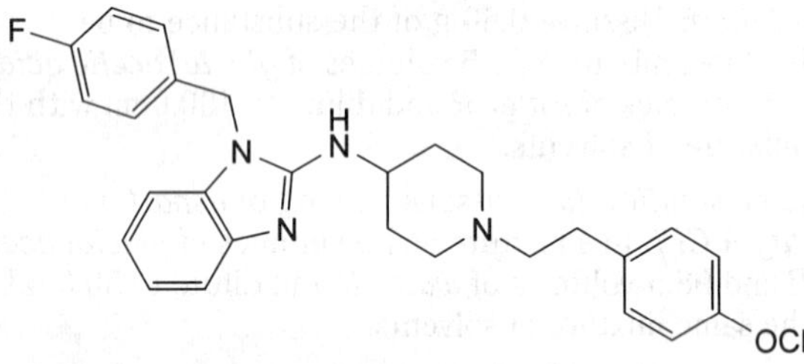

$C_{28}H_{31}FN_4O$ M_r 458.6

DEFINITION

Astemizole contains not less than 99.0 per cent and not more than the equivalent of 101.0 per cent of 1-(4-fluorobenzyl)-*N*-[1-[2-(4-methoxyphenyl)ethyl]piperidin-4-yl]-1*H*-benzimidazol-2-amine, calculated with reference to the dried substance.

CHARACTERS

A white or almost white powder, practically insoluble in water, freely soluble in methylene chloride and in methanol, soluble in alcohol.

IDENTIFICATION

First identification: A, B.

Second identification: A, C, D.

A. Melting point (*2.2.14*): 175 °C to 178 °C.

B. Examine by infrared absorption spectrophotometry (*2.2.24*), comparing with the spectrum obtained with *astemizole CRS*. Examine the substances prepared as discs.

C. Examine by thin layer chromatography (*2.2.27*), using a suitable octadecylsilyl silica gel as the coating substance.

Test solution. Dissolve 30 mg of the substance to be examined in *methanol R* and dilute to 5 ml with the same solvent.

Reference solution (a). Dissolve 30 mg of *astemizole CRS* in *methanol R* and dilute to 5 ml with the same solvent.

Reference solution (b). Dissolve 30 mg of *astemizole CRS* and 30 mg of *ketoconazole CRS* in *methanol R* and dilute to 5 ml with the same solvent.

Apply separately to the plate 5 µl of each solution. Develop over a path of 15 cm using a mixture of 20 volumes of *ammonium acetate solution R*, 40 volumes of *dioxan R* and 40 volumes of *methanol R*. Dry the plate in a current of warm air for 15 min and expose it to iodine vapour until the spots appear. Examine in daylight. The principal spot in the chromatogram obtained with the test solution is similar in position and size to the principal spot in the chromatogram obtained with reference solution (a). The test is not valid unless the chromatogram obtained with reference solution (b) shows two clearly separated spots.

D. Mix about 5 mg with 45 mg of *heavy magnesium oxide R* and ignite in a crucible until an almost white residue is obtained (usually less than 5 min). Allow to cool, add 1 ml of *water R*, 0.05 ml of *phenolphthalein solution R1* and about 1 ml of *dilute hydrochloric acid R* to render the solution colourless. Filter. To a freshly prepared mixture of 0.1 ml of *alizarin S solution R* and 0.1 ml of *zirconyl nitrate solution R*, add 1 ml of the filtrate. Mix, allow to stand for 5 min and compare the colour of the solution with that of a blank prepared in the same manner. The test solution is yellow and the blank is red.

TESTS

Appearance of solution. Dissolve 0.2 g in *methanol R* and dilute to 20 ml with the same solvent. The solution is clear (*2.2.1*) and is not more intensely coloured than reference solution Y_7 (*2.2.2, Method II*).

Related substances. Examine by liquid chromatography (*2.2.29*). *Prepare the solutions immediately before use.*

Test solution. Dissolve 0.100 g of the substance to be examined in *methanol R* and dilute to 10.0 ml with the same solvent.

Reference solution (a). Dissolve 2.5 mg of *astemizole CRS* and 25 mg of *ketoconazole CRS* in *methanol R* and dilute to 100.0 ml with the same solvent.

Reference solution (b). Dilute 1.0 ml of the test solution to 100.0 ml with *methanol R*. Dilute 5.0 ml of this solution to 20.0 ml with *methanol R*.

The chromatographic procedure may be carried out using:

- a stainless steel column 0.1 m long and 4.6 mm in internal diameter packed with *base-deactivated octadecylsilyl silica gel for chromatography R* (3 µm),
- as mobile phase at a flow rate of 1.5 ml/min, a linear gradient programme as follows:

  Mobile phase A. A 17 g/l solution of *tetrabutylammonium hydrogen sulphate R*,

  Mobile phase B. Acetonitrile R,

Time (min)	Mobile phase A (per cent V/V)	Mobile phase B (per cent V/V)	Comment
0	95	5	start gradient
15	80	20	end gradient
18	0	100	purge time
23	95	5	switch to initial equilibration
28 = 0	95	5	start of next chromatogram

- as detector a spectrophotometer set at 278 nm.

Equilibrate the column for at least 30 min with *acetonitrile R* and then equilibrate the initial elution composition for at least 5 min.

Adjust the sensitivity of the system so that the height of the principal peak in the chromatogram obtained with 10 µl of reference solution (b) is at least 50 per cent of the full scale of the recorder.

Inject 10 µl of reference solution (a). When the chromatograms are recorded in the prescribed conditions the retention times are: ketoconazole, about 8 min and astemizole, about 9 min. The test is not valid unless the resolution between the peaks corresponding to ketoconazole and astemizole is a least 1.5. If necessary, adjust the final concentration of acetonitrile or the percentage of tetrabutylammonium hydrogen sulphate in the mobile phase or adjust the time programme for the linear gradient elution.

Inject separately 10 µl of *methanol R* as a blank, 10 µl of the test solution and 10 µl of reference solution (b). In the chromatogram obtained with the test solution: the area of any peak, apart from the principal peak, is not greater than the area of the principal peak in the chromatogram obtained with reference solution (b) (0.25 per cent); the sum of the areas of all the peaks, apart from the principal peak, is not greater than twice the area of the principal peak in the chromatogram obtained with reference solution (b) (0.5 per cent). Disregard any peak obtained with the blank and any peak with an area less than 0.2 times the area of the principal peak in the chromatogram obtained with reference solution (b).

Loss on drying (*2.2.32*). Not more than 0.5 per cent, determined on 1.000 g by drying in an oven at 100 °C to 105 °C.

Sulphated ash (*2.4.14*). Not more than 0.1 per cent, determined on 1.0 g.

ASSAY

Dissolve 0.200 g in 50 ml of a mixture of 1 volume of *anhydrous acetic acid R* and 7 volumes of *methyl ethyl ketone R*. Titrate with *0.1 M perchloric acid*, using 0.2 ml of *naphtholbenzein solution R* as indicator.

1 ml of *0.1 M perchloric acid* is equivalent to 22.93 mg of $C_{28}H_{31}FN_4O$.

STORAGE

Store protected from light.

IMPURITIES

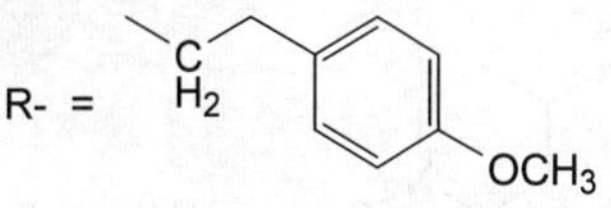

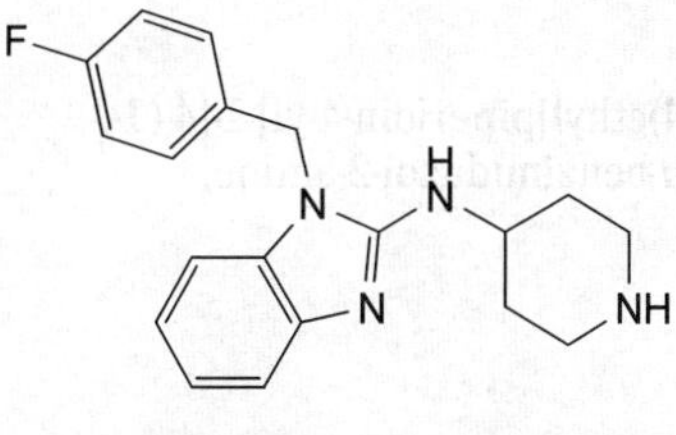

A. 1-(4-fluorobenzyl)-*N*-(piperidin-4-yl)-1*H*-benzimidazol-2-amine,

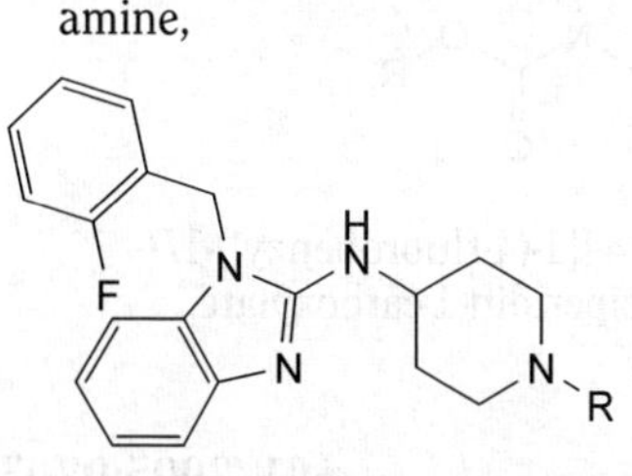

B. 1-(2-fluorobenzyl)-*N*-[1-[2-(4-methoxyphenyl)ethyl]piperidin-4-yl]-1*H*-benzimidazol-2-amine,

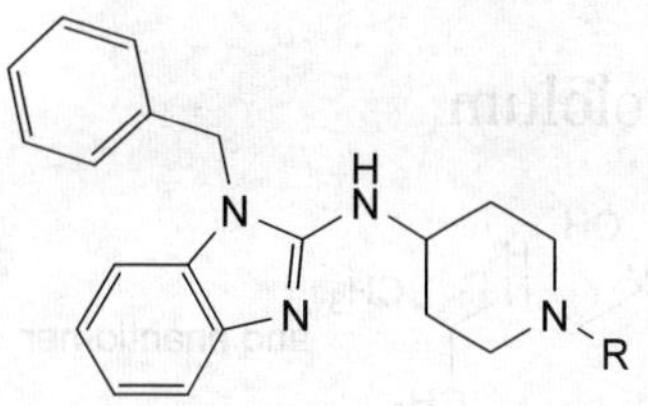

C. 1-benzyl-*N*-[1-[2-(4-methoxyphenyl)ethyl]piperidin-4-yl]-1*H*-benzimidazol-2-amine,

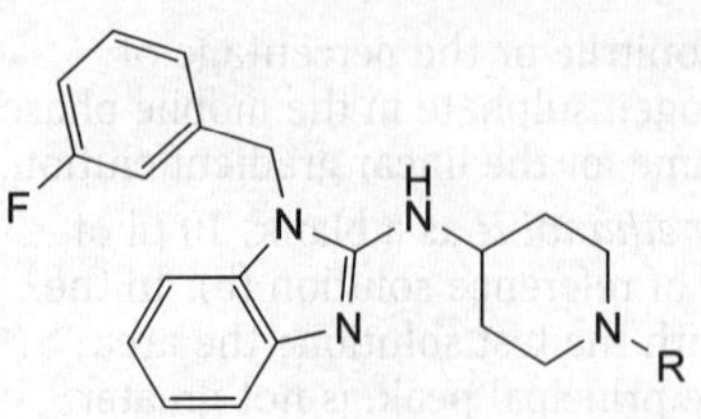

D. 1-(3-fluorobenzyl)-*N*-[1-[2-(4-methoxyphenyl)ethyl]piperidin-4-yl]-1*H*-benzimidazol-2-amine,

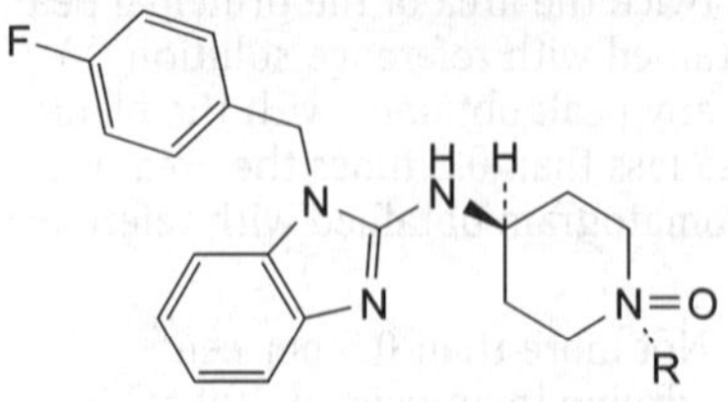

E. 1-(4-fluorobenzyl)-*N*-[*cis*-1-[2-(4-methoxyphenyl)ethyl]piperidin-4-yl 1-oxide]-1*H*-benzimidazol-2-amine,

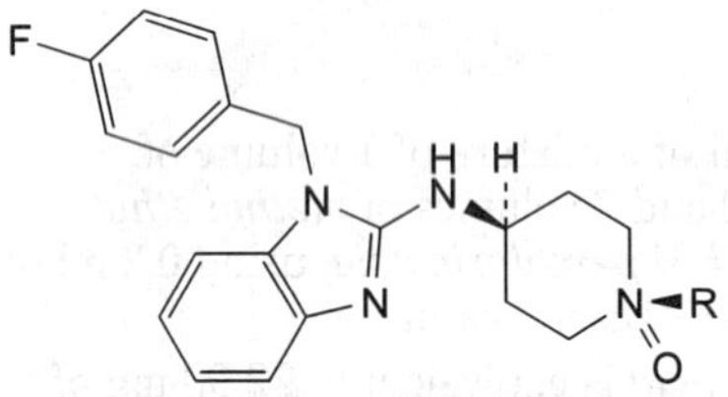

F. 1-(4-fluorobenzyl)-*N*-[*trans*-1-[2-(4-methoxyphenyl)ethyl]piperidin-4-yl 1-oxide]-1*H*-benzimidazol-2-amine,

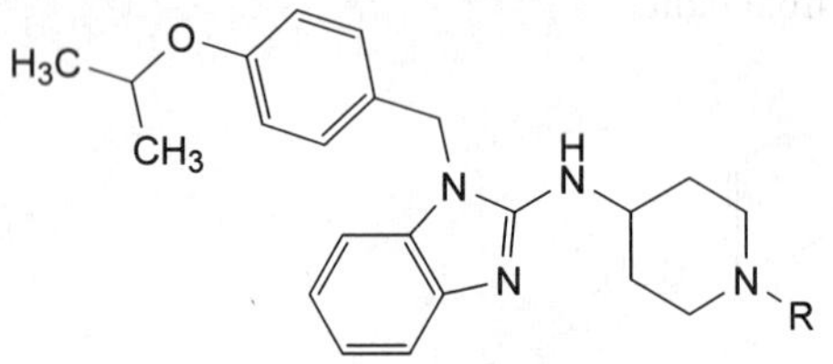

G. *N*-[1-[2-(4-methoxyphenyl)ethyl]piperidin-4-yl]-1-[4-(1-methylethoxy)benzyl]-1*H*-benzimidazol-2-amine,

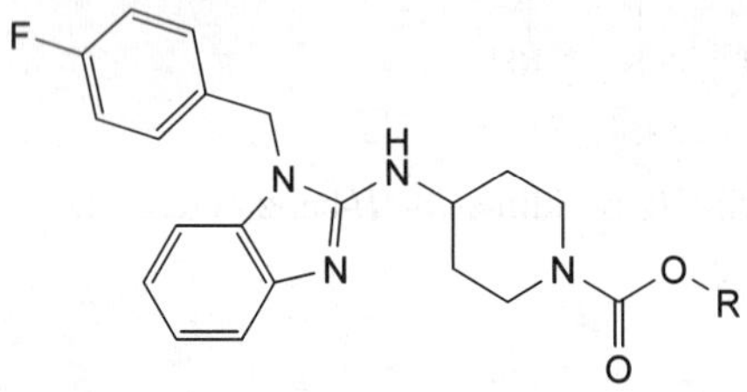

H. 2-(4-methoxyphenyl)ethyl 4-[[1-(4-fluorobenzyl)-1*H*-benzimidazol-2-yl]amino]piperidin-1-carboxylate.

01/2005:0703

ATENOLOL

Atenololum

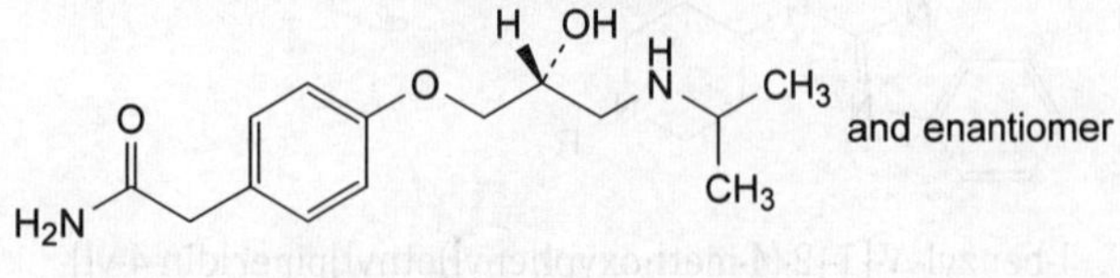

$C_{14}H_{22}N_2O_3$ M_r 266.3

DEFINITION

Atenolol contains not less than 99.0 per cent and not more than the equivalent of 101.0 per cent of 2-[4-[(2*RS*)-2-hydroxy-3-[(1-methylethyl)amino]propoxy]phenyl]acetamide, calculated with reference to the dried substance.

CHARACTERS

A white or almost white powder, sparingly soluble in water, soluble in ethanol, slightly soluble in methylene chloride.

IDENTIFICATION

First identification: C.

Second identification: A, B, D.

A. Melting point (*2.2.14*): 152 °C to 155 °C.

B. Dissolve 0.100 g in *methanol R* and dilute to 100 ml with the same solvent. Dilute 10.0 ml of this solution to 100 ml with *methanol R*. Examined between 230 nm and 350 nm (*2.2.25*), the solution shows two absorption maxima, at 275 nm and 282 nm. The ratio of the absorbance measured at the maximum at 275 nm to that measured at the maximum at 282 nm is 1.15 to 1.20.

C. Examine by infrared absorption spectrophotometry (*2.2.24*), comparing with the spectrum obtained with *atenolol CRS*.

D. Examine by thin-layer chromatography (*2.2.27*), using *silica gel* GF_{254} *R* as the coating substance.

Test solution. Dissolve 10 mg of the substance to be examined in 1 ml of *methanol R*.

Reference solution. Dissolve 10 mg of *atenolol CRS* in 1 ml of *methanol R*.

Apply separately to the plate 10 µl of each solution. Develop over a path of 15 cm using a mixture of 1 volume of *concentrated ammonia R1* and 99 volumes of *methanol R*. Allow the plate to dry in air and examine in ultraviolet light at 254 nm. The principal spot in the chromatogram obtained with the test solution is similar in position and size to the principal spot in the chromatogram obtained with the reference solution.

TESTS

Solution S. Dissolve 0.10 g in *water R* and dilute to 10 ml with the same solvent.

Appearance of solution. Solution S is clear (*2.2.1*) and not more intensely coloured than degree 6 of the range of reference solutions of the most appropriate colour (*2.2.2, Method II*).

Optical rotation (*2.2.7*). Determined on solution S, the angle of optical rotation is + 0.10° to − 0.10°.

Related substances. Examine by liquid chromatography (*2.2.29*).

Test solution (a). Dissolve 50.0 mg of the substance to be examined in 20 ml of the mobile phase and dilute to 25.0 ml with the mobile phase.

Test solution (b). Dissolve 50.0 mg of the substance to be examined in 0.1 ml of *dimethyl sulphoxide R*, if necessary applying gentle heat by placing the containing vessel in a water-bath for a few seconds, and dilute to 25.0 ml with the mobile phase.

Reference solution (a). Dilute 0.5 ml of test solution (a) to 100.0 ml with the mobile phase.

Reference solution (b). Dissolve 50.0 mg of *atenolol for column validation CRS* in 0.1 ml of *dimethyl sulphoxide R*, if necessary applying gentle heat by placing the containing vessel in a water-bath for a few seconds, and dilute to 25.0 ml with the mobile phase.

The chromatographic procedure may be carried out using:
- a stainless steel column 0.15 m long and 4.6 mm in internal diameter packed with *octadecylsilyl silica gel for chromatography R* (5 µm),
- as mobile phase at a flow rate of 1.0 ml/min a mixture prepared as follows: dissolve 1.0 g of *sodium octanesulphonate R* and 0.4 g of *tetrabutylammonium hydrogen sulphate R* in 1 litre of a mixture of 20 volumes of *tetrahydrofuran R*, 180 volumes of *methanol R* and 800 volumes of a 3.4 g/l solution of *potassium dihydrogen phosphate R*; adjust to pH 3.0 with *phosphoric acid R*,
- as detector a spectrophotometer set at 226 nm.

Equilibrate the column with the mobile phase at a flow rate of 1.0 ml/min for about 30 min.

Adjust the sensitivity of the system so that the height of the principal peak in the chromatogram obtained with 10 µl of reference solution (a) is at least 50 per cent of the full scale of the recorder.

Inject 10 µl of reference solution (b). The resulting chromatogram is similar to that of the specimen chromatogram provided with *atenolol for column validation CRS* in that the peak due to bis-ether precedes and is separated from that due to tertiary amine which normally appears as a doublet. If necessary, adjust the concentration of sodium octanesulphonate in the mobile phase. Increasing the concentration of sodium octanesulphonate increases the retention time of the tertiary amine.

Inject separately 10 µl of test solution (a) and reference solution (a). Continue the chromatography for four times the retention time of the principal peak. In the chromatogram obtained with test solution (a): the area of any peak apart from the principal peak is not greater than half the area of the principal peak in the chromatogram obtained with reference solution (a) (0.25 per cent); the sum of the areas of all the peaks, apart from the principal peak, is not greater than the area of the principal peak in the chromatogram obtained with reference solution (a) (0.5 per cent). Disregard any peak with an area less than 0.1 times of that of the principal peak in the chromatogram obtained with reference solution (a).

If the substance to be examined is found to contain more than 0.15 per cent of bis-ether, its compliance is confirmed by repeating the chromatography using 10 µl of test solution (b).

Chlorides (*2.4.4*). Dissolve 50 mg in a mixture of 1 ml of *dilute nitric acid R* and 15 ml of *water R*. The solution, without further addition of *dilute nitric acid R*, complies with the limit test for chlorides (0.1 per cent).

Loss on drying (*2.2.32*). Not more than 0.5 per cent, determined on 1.000 g by drying in an oven at 100 °C to 105 °C.

Sulphated ash (*2.4.14*). Not more than 0.1 per cent, determined on 1.0 g.

ASSAY

Dissolve 0.200 g in 80 ml of *anhydrous acetic acid R*. Titrate with *0.1 M perchloric acid*, determining the end-point potentiometrically (*2.2.20*).

1 ml of *0.1 M perchloric acid* is equivalent to 26.63 mg of $C_{14}H_{22}N_2O_3$.

IMPURITIES

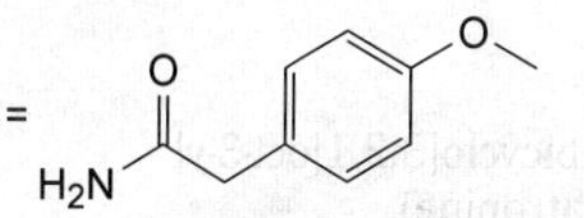

A. R-H: 2-(4-hydroxyphenyl)acetamide,

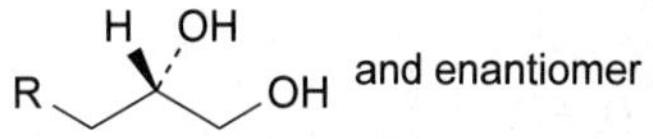

B. 2-[4-[(2*RS*)-2,3-dihydroxypropoxy]phenyl]acetamide,

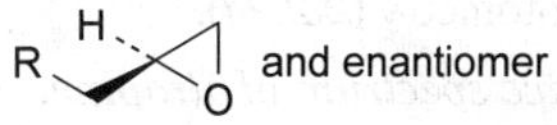

C. 2-[4-[[(2*RS*)-oxiran-2-yl]methoxy]phenyl]acetamide,

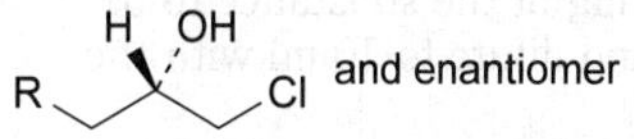

D. 2-[4-[(2*RS*)-3-chloro-2-hydroxypropoxy]phenyl]acetamide,

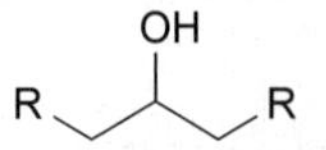

E. 2,2′-[2-hydroxypropan-1,3-diylbis(oxy-4,1-phenylene)]diacetamide,

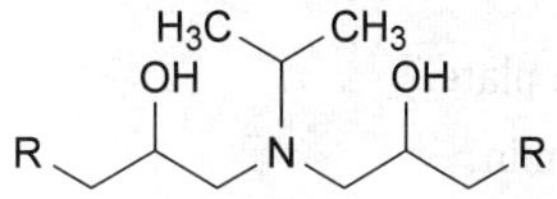

F. 2,2′-[(1-methylethyl)iminobis(2-hydroxypropan-3,1-diyloxy-4,1-phenylene)]diacetamide,

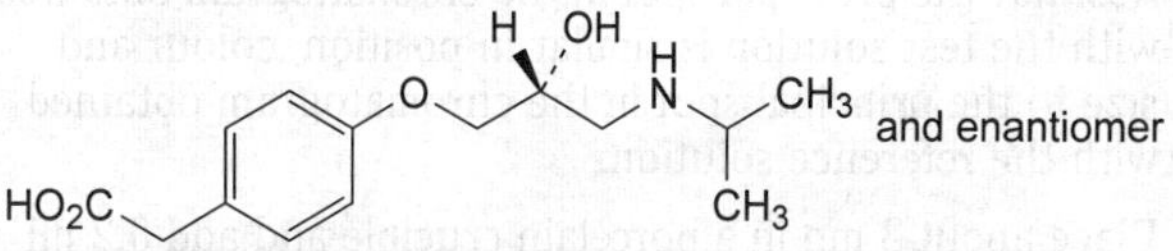

G. 2-[4-[(2*RS*)-2-hydroxy-3-[(1-methylethyl)amino]propoxy]phenyl]acetic acid,

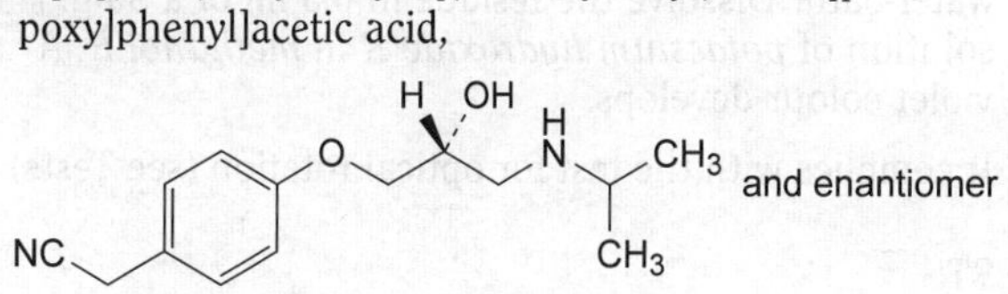

H. 2-[4-[(2*RS*)-2-hydroxy-3-[(1-methylethyl)amino]propoxy]phenyl]acetonitrile.

01/2005:2056

ATROPINE

Atropinum

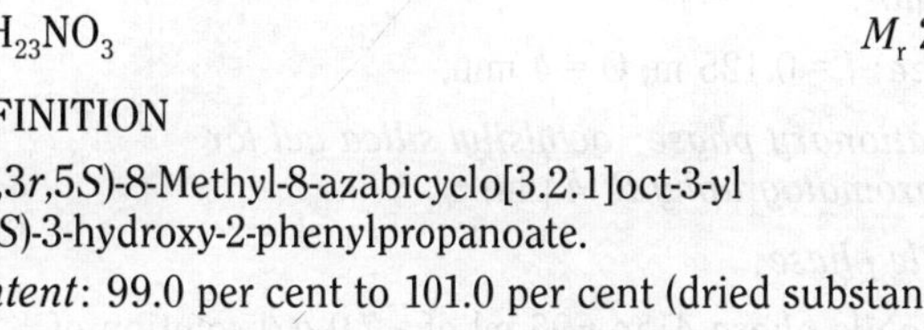

$C_{17}H_{23}NO_3$ M_r 289.4

DEFINITION

(1*R*,3*r*,5*S*)-8-Methyl-8-azabicyclo[3.2.1]oct-3-yl (2*RS*)-3-hydroxy-2-phenylpropanoate.

Content: 99.0 per cent to 101.0 per cent (dried substance).

CHARACTERS

Appearance: white, crystalline powder or colourless crystals.

Solubility: very slightly soluble in water, freely soluble in alcohol and in methylene chloride.

IDENTIFICATION

First identification: A, B, E.

Second identification: A, C, D, E.

A. Melting point (*2.2.14*): 115 °C to 119 °C.

B. Infrared absorption spectrophotometry (*2.2.24*).

Comparison: *Ph. Eur. reference spectrum of atropine.*

C. Thin-layer chromatography (*2.2.27*).

Test solution. Dissolve 10 mg of the substance to be examined in *methanol R* and dilute to 10 ml with the same solvent.

Reference solution. Dissolve 10 mg of *atropine sulphate CRS* in *methanol R* and dilute to 10 ml with the same solvent.

Plate: *TLC silica gel plate R.*

Mobile phase: *concentrated ammonia R, water R, acetone R* (3:7:90 *V/V/V*).

Application: 10 µl.

Development: over half of the plate.

Drying: at 100-105 °C for 15 min.

Detection: after cooling, spray with *dilute potassium iodobismuthate solution R.*

Results: the principal spot in the chromatogram obtained with the test solution is similar in position, colour and size to the principal spot in the chromatogram obtained with the reference solution.

D. Place about 3 mg in a porcelain crucible and add 0.2 ml of *fuming nitric acid R.* Evaporate to dryness on a water-bath. Dissolve the residue in 0.5 ml of a 30 g/l solution of *potassium hydroxide R* in *methanol R.* A violet colour develops.

E. It complies with the test for optical rotation (see Tests).

TESTS

Optical rotation (*2.2.7*): − 0.70° to + 0.05°.

Dissolve 1.25 g in *alcohol R* and dilute to 25.0 ml with the same solvent. Measure in a 2 dm tube.

Related substances. Liquid chromatography (*2.2.29*).

Test solution. Dissolve 50 mg of the substance to be examined in mobile phase A and dilute to 50 ml with mobile phase A. Dilute 10 ml of the solution to 50 ml with mobile phase A.

Reference solution (a). Dilute 1.0 ml of the test solution to 100.0 ml with mobile phase A. Dilute 1.0 ml of this solution to 10.0 ml with mobile phase A.

Reference solution (b). Dissolve 5 mg of *atropine for system suitability CRS* in mobile phase A and dilute to 25 ml with mobile phase A.

Column:

– *size*: l = 0.125 m, Ø = 4 mm,

– *stationary phase*: *octylsilyl silica gel for chromatography R* (4 µm).

Mobile phase:

– *mobile phase A*: to 606 ml of a 7.0 g/l solution of *potassium dihydrogen phosphate R* adjusted to pH 3.3 with *0.05 M phosphoric acid,* add 3.5 g of *sodium dodecyl sulphate R* and 320 ml of *acetonitrile R,*

– *mobile phase B*: *acetonitrile R,*

Time (min)	Mobile phase A (per cent *V/V*)	Mobile phase B (per cent *V/V*)
0 - 12	100	0
12 - 25	100 → 70	0 → 30
25 - 26	70 → 100	30 → 0
26 - 30	100	0

Flow rate: 1 ml/min.

Detection: spectrophotometer at 210 nm.

Injection: 10 µl.

System suitability: reference solution (b):

– the chromatogram obtained is similar to the chromatogram supplied with *atropine for system suitability CRS,*

– *peak-to-valley ratio*: minimum 20, where H_p = height above the baseline of the peak due to impurity B and H_v = height above the baseline of the lowest point of the curve separating this peak from the peak due to atropine.

Limits: locate the impurities by comparing with the chromatogram obtained with reference solution (b) and with the chromatogram supplied with *atropine for system suitability CRS*:

– *impurity B*: not more than 3 times the area of the principal peak in the chromatogram obtained with reference solution (a) (0.3 per cent),

– *impurity A*: not more than 4 times the area of the principal peak in the chromatogram obtained with reference solution (a) (0.4 per cent),

– *any other impurity*: not more than twice the area of the principal peak in the chromatogram obtained with reference solution (a) (0.2 per cent),

– *total*: not more than 15 times the area of the principal peak in the chromatogram obtained with reference solution (a) (1.5 per cent),

– *disregard limit*: the area of the principal peak in the chromatogram obtained with reference solution (a) (0.1 per cent); disregard peaks due to the blank.

Loss on drying (*2.2.32*): maximum 0.2 per cent, determined on 1.000 g by drying in an oven at 100-105 °C for 2 h.

ASSAY

Dissolve 0.250 g in 40 ml of *anhydrous acetic acid R* and heat if necessary. Allow the solution to cool. Titrate with *0.1 M perchloric acid,* determining the end-point potentiometrically (*2.2.20*).

1 ml of *0.1 M perchloric acid* is equivalent to 28.94 mg of $C_{17}H_{23}NO_3$.

STORAGE

Protected from light.

IMPURITIES

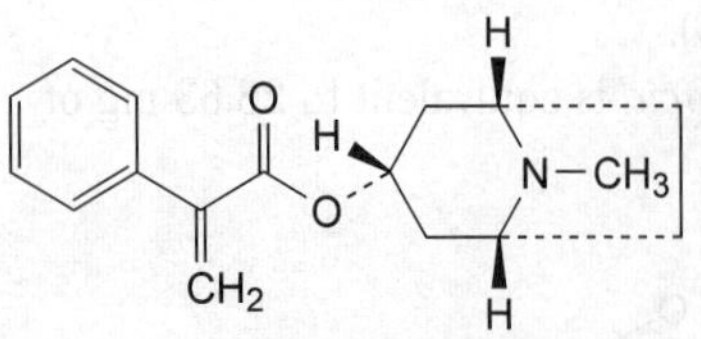

A. (1*R*,3*r*,5*S*)-8-methyl-8-azabicyclo[3.2.1]oct-3-yl 2-phenylpropenoate (apoatropine),

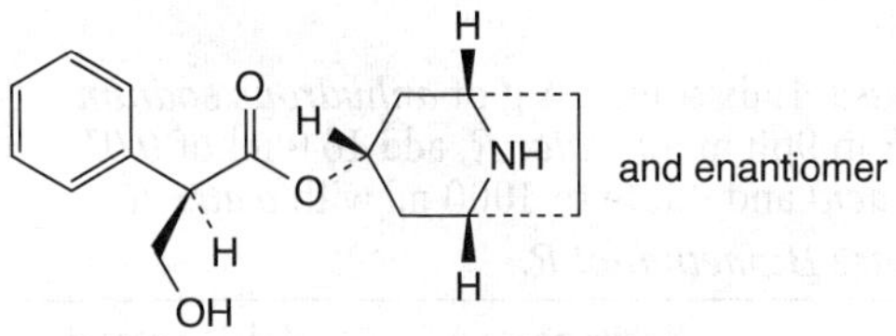

B. (1*R*,3*r*,5*S*)-8-azabicyclo[3.2.1]oct-3-yl (2*RS*)-3-hydroxy-2-phenylpropanoate (noratropine),

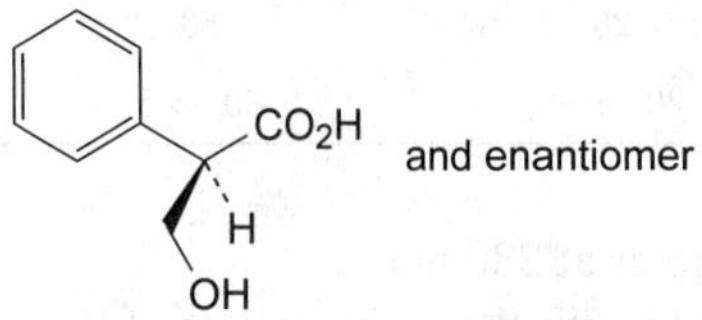

C. (2*RS*)-3-hydroxy-2-phenylpropanoic acid (tropic acid),

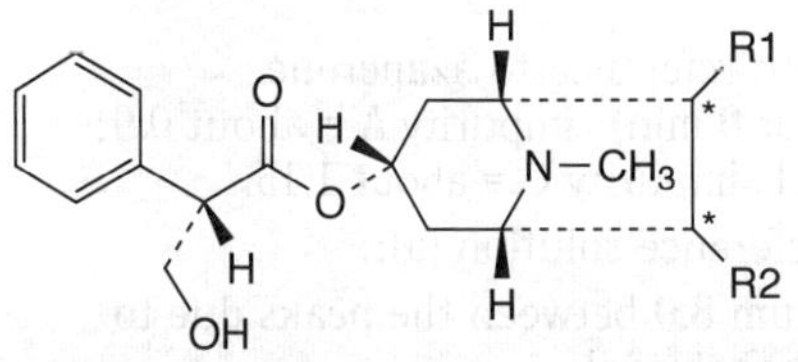

D. R1 = OH, R2 = H: (1*R*,3*S*,5*R*,6*RS*)-6-hydroxy-8-methyl-8-azabicyclo[3.2.1]oct-3-yl (2*S*)-3-hydroxy-2-phenylpropanoate (6-hydroxyhyoscyamine),

E. R1 = H, R2 = OH: (1*S*,3*R*,5*S*,6*RS*)-6-hydroxy-8-methyl-8-azabicyclo[3.2.1]oct-3-yl (2*S*)-3-hydroxy-2-phenylpropanoate (7-hydroxyhyoscyamine),

F. hyoscine,

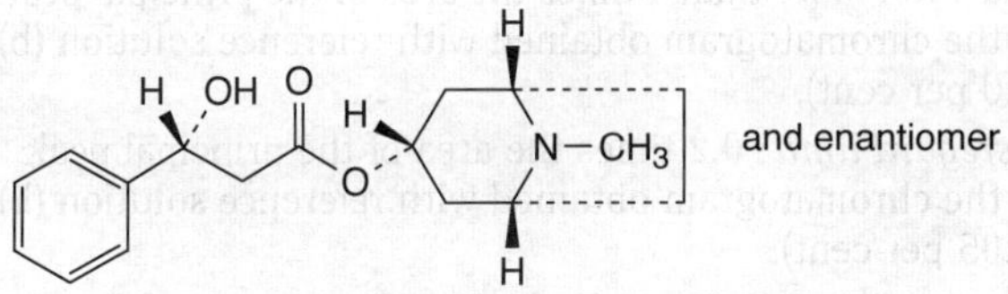

G. (1*R*,3*r*,5*S*)-8-methyl-8-azabicyclo[3.2.1]oct-3-yl (3*RS*)-3-hydroxy-3-phenylpropanoate (isolittorine).

01/2005:0068

ATROPINE SULPHATE

Atropini sulfas

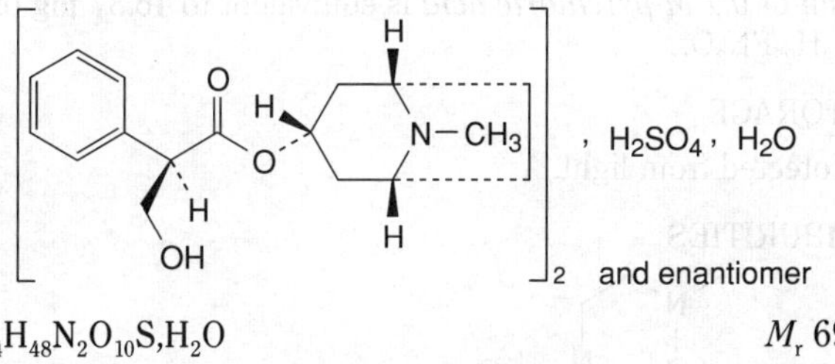

$C_{34}H_{48}N_2O_{10}S,H_2O$ M_r 695

DEFINITION

Atropine sulphate contains not less than 99.0 per cent and not more than the equivalent of 101.0 per cent of bis[(1*R*,3*r*,5*S*)-8-methyl-8-azabicyclo[3.2.1]oct-3-yl (2*RS*)-3-hydroxy-2-phenylpropanoate] sulphate, calculated with reference to the anhydrous substance.

CHARACTERS

A white, crystalline powder or colourless crystals, very soluble in water, freely soluble in alcohol.

It melts at about 190 °C with decomposition, determined on the substance dried at 135 °C for 15 min.

IDENTIFICATION

First identification: A, B, E.

Second identification: C, D, E, F.

A. An aqueous solution shows almost no optical rotation (see Tests).

B. Examine by infrared absorption spectrophotometry (*2.2.24*), comparing with the spectrum obtained with *atropine sulphate CRS*.

C. Dissolve about 50 mg in 5 ml of *water R* and add 5 ml of *picric acid solution R*. The precipitate, washed with *water R* and dried at 100 °C to 105 °C for 2 h, melts (*2.2.14*) at 174 °C to 179 °C.

D. To about 1 mg add 0.2 ml of *fuming nitric acid R* and evaporate to dryness in a water-bath. Dissolve the residue in 2 ml of *acetone R* and add 0.1 ml of a 30 g/l solution of *potassium hydroxide R* in *methanol R*. A violet colour develops.

E. It gives the reactions of sulphates (*2.3.1*).

F. It gives the reaction of alkaloids (*2.3.1*).

TESTS

pH (*2.2.3*). Dissolve 0.6 g in *carbon dioxide-free water R* and dilute to 30 ml with the same solvent. The pH of the solution is 4.5 to 6.2.

Optical rotation (*2.2.7*). Dissolve 2.50 g in *water R* and dilute to 25.0 ml with the same solvent. The angle of optical rotation measured in a 2 dm tube is − 0.50° to + 0.05°.

Foreign alkaloids and decomposition products. Examine by thin-layer chromatography (*2.2.27*), using *silica gel G R* as the coating substance.

Test solution. Dissolve 0.2 g of the substance to be examined in *methanol R* and dilute to 10 ml with the same solvent.

Reference solution (a). Dilute 1 ml of the test solution to 100 ml with *methanol R*.

Reference solution (b). Dilute 5 ml of reference solution (a) to 10 ml with *methanol R*.

Apply separately to the plate 10 µl of each solution. Develop over a path of 10 cm using a mixture of 90 volumes of *acetone R*, 7 volumes of *water R* and 3 volumes of *concentrated ammonia R*. Dry the plate at 100 °C to 105 °C for 15 min. Allow to cool and spray with *dilute potassium iodobismuthate solution R* until the spots appear. Any spot in the chromatogram obtained with the test solution, apart from the principal spot, is not more intense than the spot in the chromatogram obtained with reference solution (a) (1.0 per cent) and not more than one such spot is more intense than the spot in the chromatogram obtained with reference solution (b) (0.5 per cent).

Apoatropine. Dissolve 0.10 g in *0.01 M hydrochloric acid* and dilute to 100.0 ml with the same acid. Determine the absorbance (*2.2.25*) at 245 nm. The specific absorbance is not greater than 4.0, calculated with reference to the anhydrous substance (about 0.5 per cent).

Water (*2.5.12*). 2.0 per cent to 4.0 per cent, determined on 0.50 g by the semi-micro determination of water.

Sulphated ash (*2.4.14*). Not more than 0.1 per cent, determined on 1.0 g.

ASSAY

Dissolve 0.500 g in 30 ml of *anhydrous acetic acid R*, warming if necessary. Cool the solution. Titrate with *0.1 M perchloric acid* and determining the end-point potentiometrically (*2.2.20*).

1 ml of *0.1 M perchloric acid* is equivalent to 67.68 mg of $C_{34}H_{48}N_2O_{10}S$.

STORAGE

Store protected from light.

01/2005:1708

AZAPERONE FOR VETERINARY USE

Azaperonum ad usum veterinarium

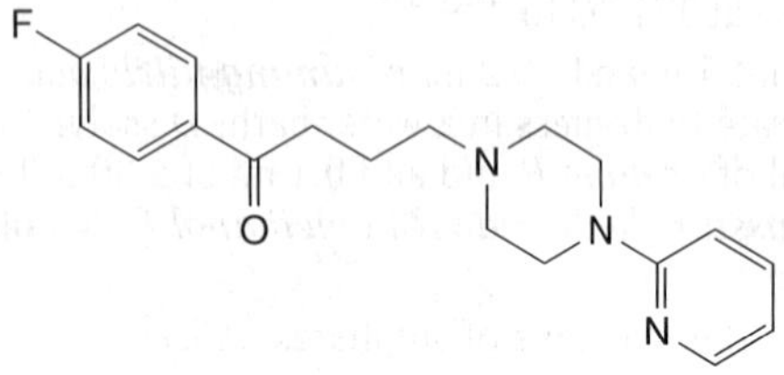

$C_{19}H_{22}FN_3O$ M_r 327.4

DEFINITION

1-(4-Fluorophenyl)-4-[4-(pyridin-2-yl)piperazin-1-yl]butan-1-one.

Content: 99.0 per cent to 101.0 per cent (dried substance).

CHARACTERS

Appearance: white or almost white powder.

Solubility: practically insoluble in water, freely soluble in acetone and in methylene chloride, soluble in alcohol.

It shows polymorphism.

IDENTIFICATION

Infrared absorption spectrophotometry (*2.2.24*).

Preparation: discs.

Comparison: *azaperone CRS*.

If the spectra obtained show differences, dissolve the substance to be examined and the reference substance separately in *acetone R*, evaporate to dryness and record new spectra using the residues.

TESTS

Appearance of solution. The solution is clear (*2.2.1*) and not more intensely coloured than reference solution Y_6 (*2.2.2, Method II*).

Dissolve 1.0 g in 25 ml of a 14 g/l solution of *tartaric acid R*.

Related substances. Liquid chromatography (*2.2.29*).

Test solution. Dissolve 0.100 g of the substance to be examined in *methanol R* and dilute to 10.0 ml with the same solvent.

Reference solution (a). Dissolve 5.0 mg of *azaperone CRS* and 6.0 mg of *benperidol CRS* in *methanol R* and dilute to 200.0 ml with the same solvent.

Reference solution (b). Dilute 1.0 ml of the test solution to 100.0 ml with *methanol R*. Dilute 5.0 ml of the solution to 20.0 ml with *methanol R*.

Column:

- *size*: l = 0.10 m, Ø = 4.6 mm,
- *stationary phase*: *base-deactivated octadecylsilyl silica gel for chromatography R* (3 µm),
- *temperature*: 25 °C.

Mobile phase:

- *mobile phase A*: dissolve 1.4 g of *anhydrous sodium sulphate R* in 900 ml of *water R*, add 16.0 ml of *0.01 M sulphuric acid* and dilute to 1000 ml with *water R*,
- *mobile phase B*: *methanol R*.

Time (min)	Mobile phase A (per cent *V/V*)	Mobile phase B (per cent *V/V*)
0 - 15	95 → 20	5 → 80
15 - 20	20	80
20 - 21	20 → 95	80 → 5

Flow rate: 1.5 ml/min.

Detection: spectrophotometer at 230 nm.

Equilibration: at least 4 min with the mobile phase at the initial composition.

Injection: 10 µl.

Relative retention with reference to azaperone (retention time = about 9 min): impurity A = about 0.9; impurity B = about 1.1; impurity C = about 1.15.

System suitability: reference solution (a):

- *resolution*: minimum 8.0 between the peaks due to azaperone and to benperidol.

Limits:

- *impurity A*: not more than the area of the principal peak in the chromatogram obtained with reference solution (b) (0.25 per cent),
- *total of impurities B and C*: not more than 3 times the area of the principal peak in the chromatogram obtained with reference solution (b) (0.75 per cent),
- *total*: not more than 4 times the area of the principal peak in the chromatogram obtained with reference solution (b) (1.0 per cent),
- *disregard limit*: 0.2 times the area of the principal peak in the chromatogram obtained with reference solution (b) (0.05 per cent).

Loss on drying (*2.2.32*): maximum 0.5 per cent, determined on 1.000 g by drying *in vacuo* at 60 °C for 4 h.

Sulphated ash (*2.4.14*): maximum 0.1 per cent, determined on 1.0 g.

ASSAY

Dissolve 0.130 g in 70 ml of a mixture of 1 volume of *anhydrous acetic acid R* and 7 volumes of *methyl ethyl ketone R*. Titrate with *0.1 M perchloric acid*, using 0.2 ml of *naphtholbenzein solution R* as indicator.

1 ml of *0.1 M perchloric acid* is equivalent to 16.37 mg of $C_{19}H_{22}FN_3O$.

STORAGE

Protected from light.

IMPURITIES

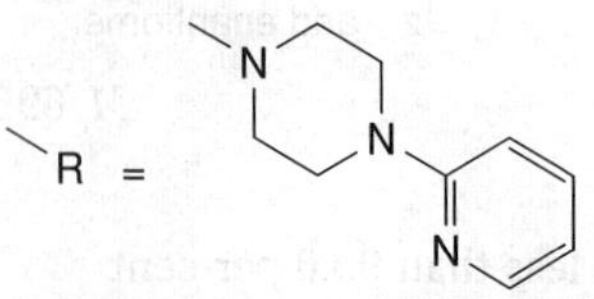

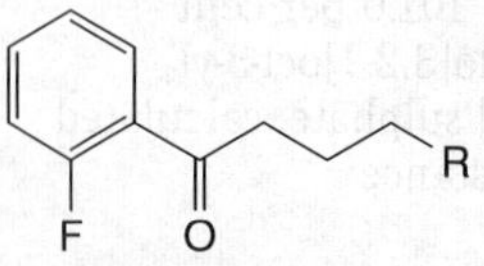

A. 1-(2-fluorophenyl)-4-[4-(pyridin-2-yl)piperazin-1-yl]butan-1-one,

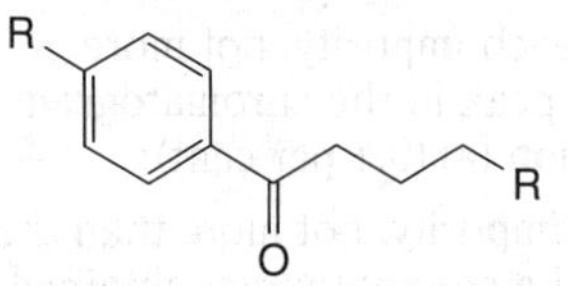

B. 4-[4-(pyridin-2-yl)piperazin-1-yl]-1-[4-[4-(pyridin-2-yl)piperazin-1-yl]phenyl]butan-1-one,

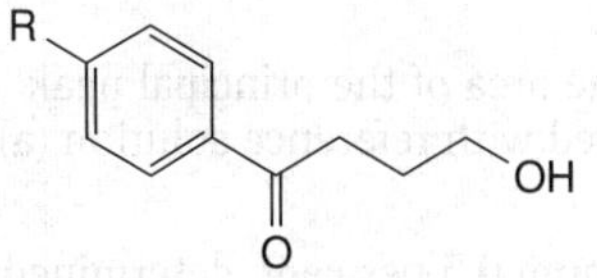

C. 4-hydroxy-1-[4-[4-(pyridin-2-yl)piperazin-1-yl]phenyl]butan-1-one.

01/2005:0369

AZATHIOPRINE

Azathioprinum

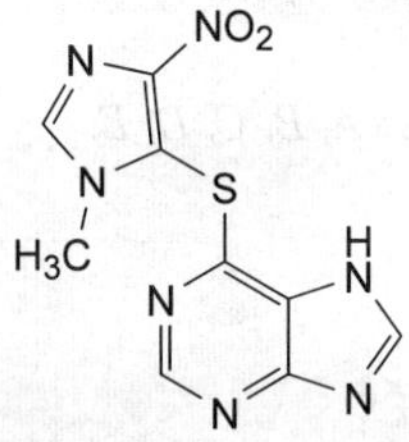

$C_9H_7N_7O_2S$ M_r 277.3

DEFINITION

Azathioprine contains not less than 98.5 per cent and not more than the equivalent of 101.0 per cent of 6-[(1-methyl-4-nitro-1*H*-imidazol-5-yl)sulfanyl]-7*H*-purine, calculated with reference to the dried substance.

CHARACTERS

A pale-yellow powder, practically insoluble in water and in alcohol. It is soluble in dilute solutions of alkali hydroxides and sparingly soluble in dilute mineral acids.

IDENTIFICATION

A. Dissolve 0.150 g in 30 ml of *dimethyl sulphoxide R* and dilute to 500.0 ml with *0.1 M hydrochloric acid.* Dilute 25.0 ml of the solution to 1000.0 ml with *0.1 M hydrochloric acid.* Examined between 230 nm and 350 nm (*2.2.25*), the solution shows an absorption maximum at 280 nm. The specific absorbance at the maximum is 600 to 660.

B. Examine by infrared absorption spectrophotometry (*2.2.24*), comparing with the spectrum obtained with *azathioprine CRS.*

C. To about 20 mg add 100 ml of *water R,* heat and filter. To 5 ml of the filtrate add 1 ml of *hydrochloric acid R* and about 10 mg of *zinc powder R.* Allow to stand for 5 min. The solution becomes yellow. Filter, cool in iced water, add 0.1 ml of *sodium nitrite solution R* and 0.1 g of *sulphamic acid R* and shake until the bubbles disappear. Add 1 ml of *β-naphthol solution R.* A pale-pink precipitate is formed.

TESTS

Acidity or alkalinity. To 0.5 g add 25 ml of *carbon dioxide-free water R,* shake for 15 min and filter. To 20 ml of the filtrate add 0.1 ml of *methyl red solution R.* Not more than 0.2 ml of *0.01 M hydrochloric acid* or *0.01 M sodium hydroxide* is required to change the colour of the indicator.

Chloromethylnitroimidazole and mercaptopurine. Examine by thin-layer chromatography (*2.2.27*), using *cellulose for chromatography F_{254} R* as the coating substance.

Test solution. Dissolve 0.2 g of the substance to be examined in *dilute ammonia R1* and dilute to 10 ml with the same solvent. Prepare immediately before use.

Reference solution (a). Dissolve 10 mg of *chloromethylnitroimidazole CRS* in *dilute ammonia R1* and dilute to 50 ml with the same solvent. Prepare immediately before use.

Reference solution (b). Dissolve 10 mg of *mercaptopurine R* in *dilute ammonia R1* and dilute to 50 ml with the same solvent. Prepare immediately before use.

Apply separately to the plate 5 µl of each solution. Develop over a path of 15 cm using *butanol R* saturated with *dilute ammonia R1.* Dry the plate at 50 °C and examine in ultraviolet light at 254 nm. In the chromatogram obtained with the test solution, any spots corresponding to chloromethyl-nitroimidazole and mercaptopurine are not more intense than the spots in the chromatograms obtained with reference solution (a) (1.0 per cent) and reference solution (b) (1.0 per cent), respectively.

Loss on drying (*2.2.32*). Not more than 1.0 per cent, determined on 0.50 g by drying in an oven at 100 °C to 105 °C.

Sulphated ash (*2.4.14*). Not more than 0.1 per cent, determined on 1.0 g.

ASSAY

Dissolve 0.250 g in 25 ml of *dimethylformamide R.* Titrate with *0.1 M tetrabutylammonium hydroxide,* determining the end-point potentiometrically (*2.2.20*).

1 ml of *0.1 M tetrabutylammonium hydroxide* is equivalent to 27.73 mg of $C_9H_7N_7O_2S$.

STORAGE

Store protected from light.

01/2005:1633
corrected

AZELASTINE HYDROCHLORIDE

Azelastini hydrochloridum

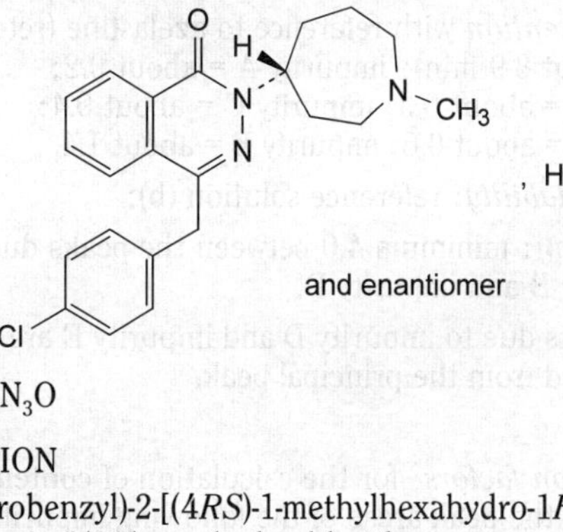

$C_{22}H_{25}Cl_2N_3O$ M_r 418.4

DEFINITION

4-(4-Chlorobenzyl)-2-[(4*RS*)-1-methylhexahydro-1*H*-azepin-4-yl]phthalazin-1(2*H*)-one hydrochloride.

Content: 99.0 per cent to 101.0 per cent (dried substance).

CHARACTERS

Appearance: white or almost white, crystalline powder.

Solubility: sparingly soluble in water, soluble in ethanol and in methylene chloride.

IDENTIFICATION

A. Infrared absorption spectrophotometry (*2.2.24*).

Comparison: *azelastine hydrochloride CRS*.

B. Solution S (see Tests) gives reaction (a) of chlorides (*2.3.1*).

TESTS

Solution S. Dissolve 1.0 g in *carbon dioxide-free water R* and dilute to 100 ml with the same solvent.

Appearance of solution. Solution S is clear (*2.2.1*) and colourless (*2.2.2, Method II*).

Acidity or alkalinity. To 10 ml of solution S add 0.2 ml of *bromothymol blue solution R1*. Not more than 0.1 ml of *0.01 M hydrochloric acid* or *0.01 M sodium hydroxide* is required to change the colour of the solution.

Related substances. Liquid chromatography (*2.2.29*).

Solvent mixture: *acetonitrile for chromatography R, water R* (45:55 *V/V*).

Test solution. Dissolve 0.125 g of the substance to be examined in the solvent mixture and dilute to 50.0 ml with the solvent mixture.

Reference solution (a). Dilute 1.0 ml of the test solution to 100.0 ml with the solvent mixture. Dilute 1.0 ml of this solution to 10.0 ml with the solvent mixture.

Reference solution (b). Dissolve 1 mg of *azelastine impurity B CRS*, 1 mg of *azelastine impurity D CRS* and 1 mg of *azelastine impurity E CRS* in the test solution and dilute to 20 ml with the test solution.

Column:

- *size*: *l* = 0.25 m, Ø = 4.6 mm,
- *stationary phase*: *nitrile silica gel for chromatography R* (10 µm),
- *temperature*: 30°C.

Mobile phase: dissolve 2.16 g of *sodium octanesulphonate R* and 0.68 g of *potassium dihydrogen phosphate R* in 740 ml of *water for chromatography R*, adjust to pH 3.0-3.1 with *dilute phosphoric acid R*, add 260 ml of *acetonitrile for chromatography R* and mix.

Flow rate: 2.0 ml/min.

Detection: spectrophotometer at 210 nm.

Injection: 10 µl.

Run time: twice the retention time of azelastine.

Relative retention with reference to azelastine (retention time = about 8-9 min): impurity A = about 0.2; impurity B = about 0.3; impurity C = about 0.4; impurity D = about 0.6; impurity E = about 1.4.

System suitability: reference solution (b):

- *resolution*: minimum 4.0 between the peaks due to impurity B and impurity D,
- the peaks due to impurity D and impurity E are baseline separated from the principal peak.

Limits:

- *correction factors*: for the calculation of contents, multiply the peak areas of the following impurities by the corresponding correction factor: impurity B = 3.6; impurity D = 0.7; impurity E = 2.1;
- *impurities A, B, C, D, E*: for each impurity, not more than the area of the principal peak in the chromatogram obtained with reference solution (a) (0.1 per cent);
- *any other impurity*: for each impurity, not more than the area of the principal peak in the chromatogram obtained with reference solution (a) (0.1 per cent);
- *total*: not more than twice the area of the principal peak in the chromatogram obtained with reference solution (a) (0.2 per cent);
- *disregard limit*: 0.5 times the area of the principal peak in the chromatogram obtained with reference solution (a) (0.05 per cent).

Loss on drying (*2.2.32*): maximum 0.5 per cent, determined on 1.000 g by drying in an oven at 100-105 °C.

ASSAY

In order to avoid overheating in the reaction medium, mix thoroughly throughout and stop the titration immediately after the end-point has been reached.

Dissolve 0.300 g in 5 ml of *anhydrous formic acid R*. Add 30 ml of *acetic anhydride R*. Titrate quickly with *0.1 M perchloric acid*, determining the end-point potentiometrically (*2.2.20*).

1.0 ml of *0.1 M perchloric acid* is equivalent to 41.84 mg of $C_{22}H_{25}Cl_2N_3O$.

IMPURITIES

Specified impurities: A, B, C, D, E.

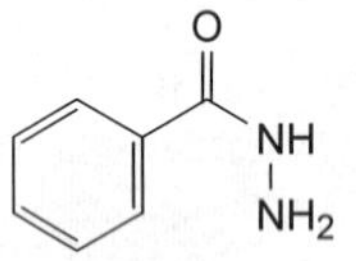

A. benzoyldiazane (benzohydrazide),

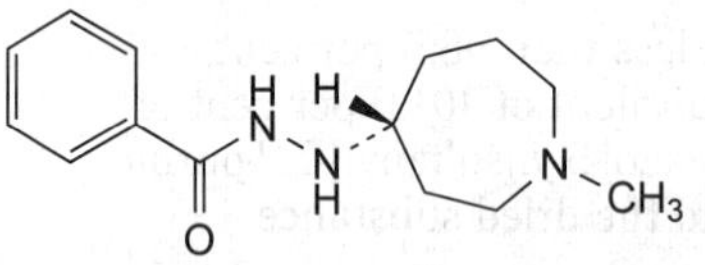

and enantiomer

B. 1-benzoyl-2-[(4*RS*)-1-methylhexahydro-1*H*-azepin-4-yl]diazane,

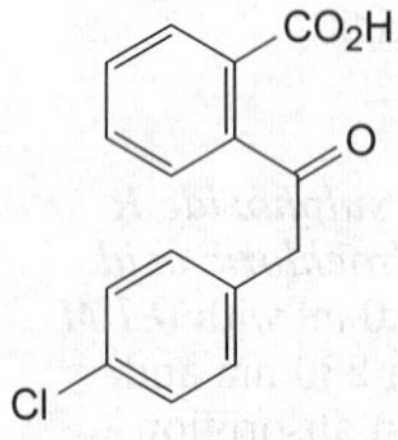

C. 2-[(4-chlorophenyl)acetyl]benzoic acid,

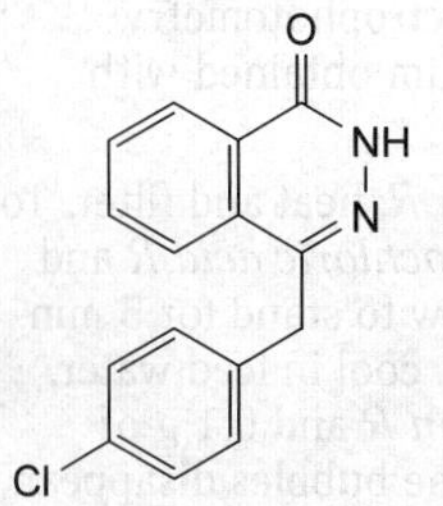

D. 4-(4-chlorobenzyl)phthalazin-1(2*H*)-one,

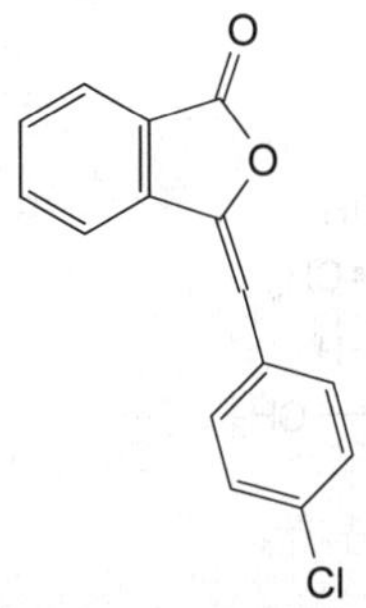

E. 3-(4-chlorobenzylidene)isobenzofuran-1(3*H*)-one.

01/2005:1649
corrected

AZITHROMYCIN

Azithromycinum

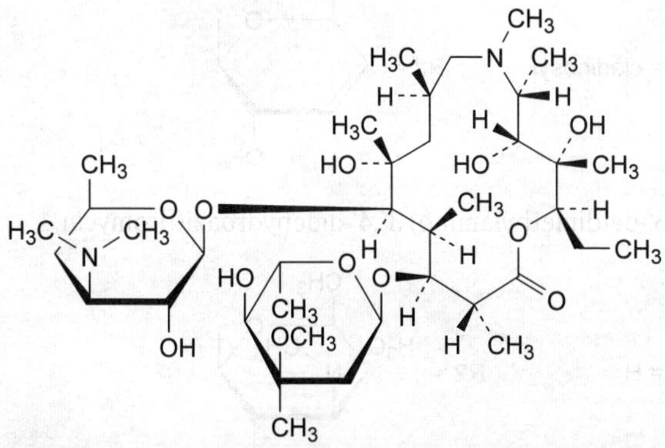

$C_{38}H_{72}N_2O_{12}$ M_r 749

DEFINITION

(2*R*,3*S*,4*R*,5*R*,8*R*,10*R*,11*R*,12*S*,13*S*,14*R*)-13-[(2,6-Dideoxy-3-*C*-methyl-3-*O*-methyl-α-L-*ribo*-hexopyranosyl)oxy]-2-ethyl-3,4,10-trihydroxy-3,5,6,8,10,12,14-heptamethyl-11-[[3,4,6-trideoxy-3-(dimethylamino)-β-D-*xylo*-hexopyranosyl]oxy]-1-oxa-6-azacyclopentadecan-15-one.

Content: 94.0 per cent to 102.0 per cent (anhydrous substance).

CHARACTERS

Appearance: white or almost white powder.

Solubility: practically insoluble in water, freely soluble in ethanol and in methylene chloride.

IDENTIFICATION

A. Infrared absorption spectrophotometry (*2.2.24*).
Comparison: *azithromycin CRS*.
If the spectra obtained show differences, prepare further spectra using 90 g/l solutions in *methylene chloride R*.

B. Examine the chromatograms obtained in the assay.
Results: the principal peak in the chromatogram obtained with test solution (b) is similar in retention time and size to the principal peak in the chromatogram obtained with reference solution (a).

TESTS

Solution S. Dissolve 0.500 g in *ethanol R* and dilute to 50.0 ml with the same solvent.

Appearance of solution. Solution S is clear (*2.2.1*) and colourless (*2.2.2, Method II*).

pH (*2.2.3*): 9.0 to 11.0.

Dissolve 0.100 g in 25.0 ml of *methanol R* and dilute to 50.0 ml with *carbon dioxide-free water R*.

Specific optical rotation (*2.2.7*): − 45 to − 49 (anhydrous substance), determined on solution S.

Related substances. Liquid chromatography (*2.2.29*). *Prepare the solutions immediately before use.*

Solvent mixture: *acetonitrile R, water R* (40:60 *V/V*).

Test solution (a). Dissolve 0.100 g of the substance to be examined in the solvent mixture and dilute to 25.0 ml with the solvent mixture.

Test solution (b). Dilute 5.0 ml of test solution (a) to 20.0 ml with the solvent mixture.

Reference solution (a). Dissolve 50.0 mg of *azithromycin CRS* in the solvent mixture and dilute to 50.0 ml with the solvent mixture.

Reference solution (b). Dilute 1.0 ml of test solution (a) to 100.0 ml with the solvent mixture.

Reference solution (c). Dissolve 5.0 mg of *azithromycin CRS* and 5.0 mg of *azithromycin impurity A CRS* in the solvent mixture and dilute to 50 ml with the solvent mixture.

Reference solution (d). Dissolve 2 mg of *azithromycin impurity B CRS* in the solvent mixture and dilute to 50 ml with the solvent mixture. Use this solution only for identification of the peak due to impurity B.

Column:
- *size*: *l* = 0.25 m, Ø = 4.6 mm,
- *stationary phase*: *end-capped polar-embedded octadecylsilyl amorphous organosilica polymer R* (5 µm),
- *temperature*: 70 °C.

Mobile phase: mix 10 volumes of a 34.84 g/l solution of *dipotassium hydrogen phosphate R* adjusted to pH 6.5 with *phosphoric acid R*, 35 volumes of *acetonitrile R* and 55 volumes of *water R*.

Flow rate: 1.0 ml/min.

Detection: spectrophotometer at 215 nm.

Injection: 100 µl; inject test solution (a) and reference solutions (b), (c) and (d).

Run time: 4.5 times the retention time of azithromycin.

Relative retention with reference to azithromycin (retention time = about 26 min): impurity D = about 0.37; impurity J = about 0.39; impurity A = about 0.42; impurity I = about 0.5; impurity C = about 0.65; impurity K = about 0.9; impurity F = about 1.6; impurity B = about 1.7; impurity G = about 2.8.

System suitability: reference solution (c):
- *resolution*: minimum 7.0 between the peaks due to impurity A and azithromycin.

Limits:
- *impurity B*: not more than twice the area of the principal peak in the chromatogram obtained with reference solution (b) (2.0 per cent),
- *any other impurity*: for each impurity, not more than the area of the principal peak in the chromatogram obtained with reference solution (b) (1.0 per cent),
- *total*: not more than 5 times the area of the principal peak in the chromatogram obtained with reference solution (b) (5.0 per cent),
- *disregard limit*: 0.1 times the area of the principal peak in the chromatogram obtained with reference solution (b) (0.1 per cent).

Heavy metals (*2.4.8*): maximum 25 ppm.

Dissolve 2.0 g in a mixture of 15 volumes of *water R* and 85 volumes of *ethanol R* and dilute to 20 ml with the same mixture of solvents. 12 ml of the solution complies with limit test B. Prepare the standard using lead standard solution (2.5 ppm Pb) obtained by diluting *lead standard solution (100 ppm Pb) R* with a mixture of 15 volumes of *water R* and 85 volumes of *ethanol R*.

Water (*2.5.12*): 1.8 per cent to 6.5 per cent, determined on 0.20 g.

Sulphated ash (*2.4.14*): maximum 0.2 per cent, determined on 1.0 g.

ASSAY

Liquid chromatography (*2.2.29*) as described in the test for related substances, with the following modifications.

Injection: 25 µl; inject test solution (b) and reference solution (a).

Calculate the percentage content of $C_{38}H_{72}N_2O_{12}$ using the declared content of *azithromycin CRS*.

STORAGE

In an airtight container.

IMPURITIES

Specified impurities: A, B, C, D, E, F, G, H, I, J, K.

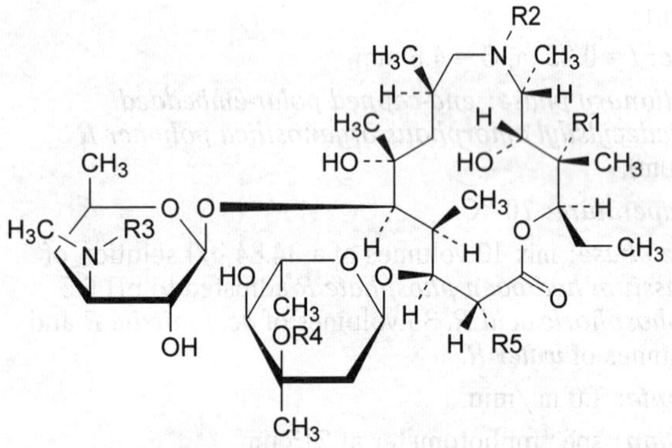

A. R1 = OH, R2 = H, R3 = R4 = R5 = CH_3: 6-demethylazithromycin,

B. R1 = H, R2 = R3 = R4 = R5 = CH_3: 3-deoxyazithromycin (azithromycin B),

C. R1 = OH, R2 = R3 = R5 = CH_3, R4 = H: 3′-*O*-demethylazithromycin (azithromycin C),

D. R1 = OH, R2 = R3 = R4 = CH_3, R5 = CH_2OH: 14-demethyl-14-(hydroxymethyl)azithromycin (azithromycin F),

F. R1 = OH, R2 = R4 = R5 = CH_3, R3 = CHO: 3′-*N*-demethyl-3′-*N*-formylazithromycin,

G. R1 = OH, R2 = R4 = R5 = CH_3, R3 = SO_2-C_6H_4-CH_3: 3′-*N*-demethyl-3′-*N*-[(4-methylphenyl)sulphonyl]azithromycin,

I. R1 = OH, R2 = R4 = R5 = CH_3, R3 = H: 3′-*N*-demethylazithromycin,

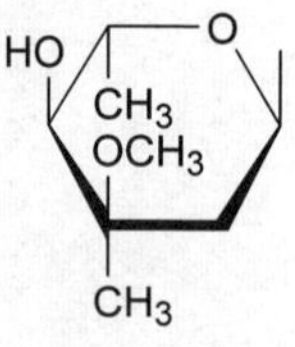

cladinosyl

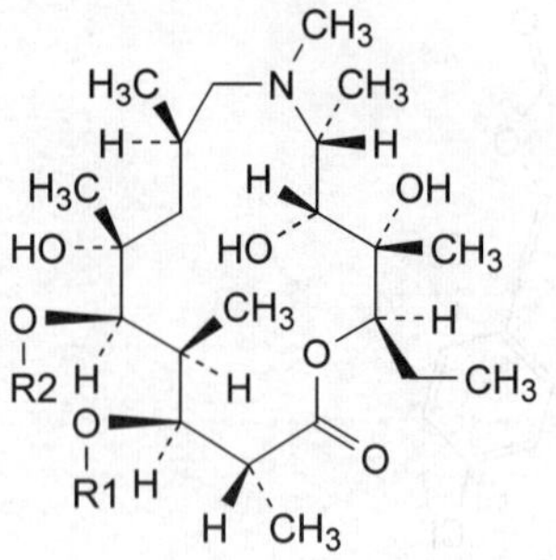

R1 = cladinosyl R2 =

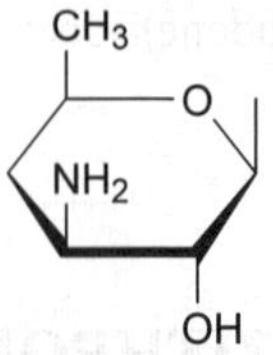

E. 3′-(*N,N*-didemethyl)azithromycin (aminoazithromycin),

R1 = cladinosyl R2 =

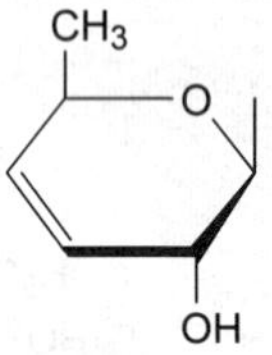

H. 3′-de(dimethylamino)-3′,4′-didehydroazithromycin,

R1 = H R2 =

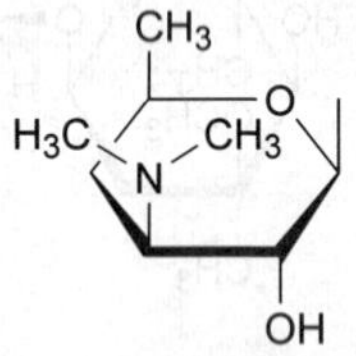

J. decladinosylazithromycin,

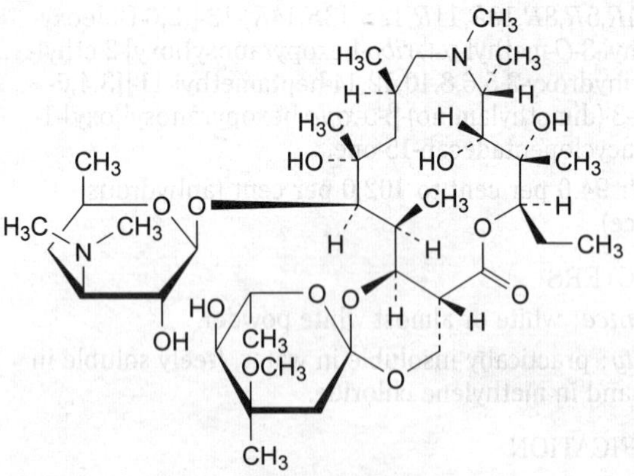

K. (2*S*,4′*R*,4a*R*,5′*S*,6′*S*,7*R*,8*S*,9*R*,10*R*,13*R*,15*R*,16*R*,17*S*,17a*S*)-7-ethyl-5′,8,9,15-tetrahydroxy-4′-methoxy-4′,6′,8,10,11,13,15,17-octamethyl-16-[[3,4,6-trideoxy-3-(dimethylamino)-β-D-*xylo*-hexopyranosyl]oxy]octadecahydro-5*H*-spiro[1,3-dioxino[4,5-*m*][1,6]oxazacyclopentadecine-2,2′-[2*H*]pyran]-5-one (azithromycin E).

B

01/2005:0808

BACAMPICILLIN HYDROCHLORIDE

Bacampicillini hydrochloridum

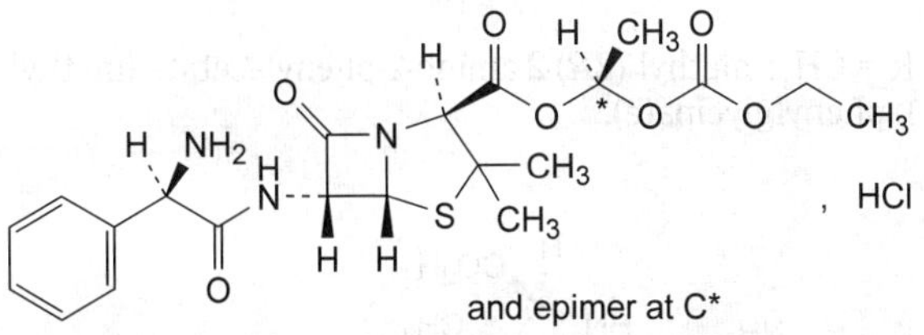

$C_{21}H_{28}ClN_3O_7S$ M_r 502.0

DEFINITION

Bacampicillin hydrochloride contains not less than 95.0 per cent and not more than the equivalent of 102.0 per cent of (1*RS*)-1-[(ethoxycarbonyl)oxy]ethyl (2*S*,5*R*,6*R*)-6-[[(2*R*)-2-amino-2-phenylacetyl]amino]-3,3-dimethyl-7-oxo-4-thia-1-azabicyclo[3.2.0]heptane-2-carboxylate hydrochloride, calculated with reference to the anhydrous, solvent-free substance.

PRODUCTION

If manufactured by a process that may leave residues of dimethylaniline in the substance and/or by a process using starting materials or intermediates which contain residues of dimethylaniline, it complies with the following test:

N,N-Dimethylaniline (*2.4.26, Method A*). Not more than 20 ppm.

CHARACTERS

A white or almost white powder or granules, hygroscopic, soluble in water, freely soluble in alcohol, soluble in methylene chloride.

IDENTIFICATION

First identification: A, D.

Second identification: B, C, D.

A. Examine by infrared absorption spectrophotometry (*2.2.24*), comparing with the spectrum obtained with *bacampicillin hydrochloride CRS*.

B. Examine by thin-layer chromatography (*2.2.27*), using a *TLC silanised silica gel plate R*.

Test solution. Dissolve 10 mg of the substance to be examined in 2 ml of *methanol R*.

Reference solution (a). Dissolve 10 mg of *bacampicillin hydrochloride CRS* in 2 ml of *methanol R*.

Reference solution (b). Dissolve 10 mg each of *bacampicillin hydrochloride CRS, talampicillin hydrochloride CRS* and *pivampicillin CRS* in 2 ml of *methanol R*.

Apply to the plate 1 µl of each solution. Develop over a path of 15 cm using a mixture of 10 volumes of a 272 g/l solution of *sodium acetate R*, the pH of which has been adjusted to 5.0 with *glacial acetic acid R*, 40 volumes of *water R* and 50 volumes of *alcohol R*. Dry the plate in a current of warm air, then spray with *ninhydrin solution R1* and heat at 60 °C for 10 min. The principal spot in the chromatogram obtained with the test solution is similar in position, colour and size to the principal spot in the chromatogram obtained with reference solution (a). The test is not valid unless the chromatogram obtained with reference solution (b) shows three clearly separated spots.

C. Place about 2 mg in a test-tube about 150 mm long and 15 mm in diameter. Moisten with 0.05 ml of *water R* and add 2 ml of *sulphuric acid-formaldehyde reagent R*. Mix the contents of the tube by swirling; the solution is practically colourless. Place the test-tube on a water-bath for 1 min; a dark yellow colour develops.

D. Dissolve about 25 mg in 2 ml of *water R*. Add 2 ml of *dilute sodium hydroxide solution R* and shake. Wait a few minutes and add 3 ml of *dilute nitric acid R* and 0.5 ml of *silver nitrate solution R1*. A white precipitate is formed. Add 0.5 ml of *concentrated ammonia R*. The precipitate dissolves.

TESTS

Appearance of solution. Dissolve 0.200 g in 20 ml of *water R*; the solution is not more opalescent than reference suspension II (*2.2.1*). Dissolve 0.500 g in 10 ml of *water R*; the absorbance (*2.2.25*) of the solution measured at 430 nm is not greater than 0.10.

pH (*2.2.3*). Dissolve 1.0 g in *carbon dioxide-free water R* and dilute to 50 ml with the same solvent. The pH of the solution is 3.0 to 4.5.

Specific optical rotation (*2.2.7*). Dissolve 0.250 g in *water R* and dilute to 25.0 ml with the same solvent. The specific optical rotation is + 175 to + 195, calculated with reference to the anhydrous, solvent-free substance.

Butyl acetate and ethyl acetate. Not more than 2.0 per cent *m/m* of butyl acetate, not more than 4.0 per cent *m/m* of ethyl acetate and not more than 5.0 per cent *m/m* for the sum determined by head-space gas chromatography (*2.2.28*), using the method of standard additions.

Sample solution. Dissolve 50.0 mg of the substance to be examined in *water R* and dilute to 10.0 ml with the same solvent.

The chromatographic procedure may be carried out using System A of the test for residual solvents (*2.4.24*) and the following static head-space injection conditions:

- equilibration temperature: 60 °C,
- equilibration time: 20 min.

Related substances. Examine by liquid chromatography (*2.2.29*) as prescribed in the Assay. Inject 20 µl of reference solution (b). Adjust the sensitivity of the system so that the height of the principal peak in the chromatogram obtained is at least 50 per cent of the full scale of the recorder. Inject 20 µl of reference solution (d). The test is not valid unless in the chromatogram obtained, the peak corresponding to ampicillin is separated from the peaks due to the solvent. Inject 20 µl of the test solution and continue the chromatography for 3.5 times the retention time of the principal peak. In the chromatogram obtained with the test solution: the area of any peak, apart from the principal peak, is not greater than 1.5 times the area of the principal peak in the chromatogram obtained with reference solution (b) (1.5 per cent); the sum of the areas of all the peaks, apart from the principal peak, is not greater than three times the area of the principal peak in the chromatogram obtained with reference solution (b) (3 per cent). Disregard any peak with an area less than 0.1 times the area of the principal peak in the chromatogram obtained with reference solution (b).

Water (*2.5.12*). Not more than 0.8 per cent, determined on 0.300 g by the semi-micro determination of water.

Sulphated ash (*2.4.14*). Not more than 1.5 per cent, determined on 1.0 g.

ASSAY

Examine by liquid chromatography (*2.2.29*). *Prepare the test solution and reference solutions (a), (b) and (d) immediately before use.*

Phosphate buffer A. Dissolve 1.4 g of *sodium dihydrogen phosphate monohydrate R* in *water R* and dilute to about 800 ml with the same solvent. Adjust to pH 3.0 with *dilute phosphoric acid R* and dilute to 1000.0 ml with *water R.*

Phosphate buffer B. Dissolve 2.75 g of *sodium dihydrogen phosphate monohydrate R* and 2.3 g of *disodium hydrogen phosphate dihydrate R* in *water R* and dilute to about 1800 ml with the same solvent. Adjust to pH 6.8, if necessary, using *dilute phosphoric acid R* or *dilute sodium hydroxide solution R* and dilute to 2000.0 ml with *water R.*

Test solution. Dissolve 30.0 mg of the substance to be examined in phosphate buffer A and dilute to 100.0 ml with the same solution.

Reference solution (a). Dissolve 30.0 mg of *bacampicillin hydrochloride CRS* in phosphate buffer A and dilute to 100.0 ml with the same solution.

Reference solution (b). Dilute 1.0 ml of reference solution (a) to 100.0 ml with phosphate buffer A.

Reference solution (c). Dissolve 30 mg of the substance to be examined in phosphate buffer B and dilute to 100 ml with the same solution. Heat the solution at 80 °C for about 30 min.

Reference solution (d). Dissolve 20 mg of *ampicillin trihydrate CRS* in phosphate buffer A and dilute to 250 ml with the same solution. Dilute 5 ml of the solution to 100 ml with phosphate buffer A.

The chromatographic procedure may be carried out using:

– a column 0.05 m long and 3.9 mm in internal diameter packed with *octadecylsilyl silica gel for chromatography R* (5 µm),
– as mobile phase at a flow rate of 1.0 ml/min a mixture of 30 volumes of *acetonitrile R* and 70 volumes of a 0.06 per cent *m/m* solution of *tetrahexylammonium hydrogen sulphate R* in phosphate buffer B,
– as detector a spectrophotometer set at 220 nm.

Inject 20 µl of reference solution (a). Adjust the sensitivity of the system so that the height of the principal peak in the chromatogram obtained is at least 50 per cent of the full scale of the recorder. Inject 20 µl of reference solution (c). The test is not valid unless, in the chromatogram obtained, the retention time of a degradation product eluting just after bacampicillin is 1.12 to 1.38 relative to bacampicillin. If necessary adjust the concentration of tetrahexylammonium hydrogen sulphate in the mobile phase. Inject reference solution (a) six times. The test is not valid unless the relative standard deviation of the peak area for bacampicillin is at most 1.0 per cent. Inject alternately the test solution and reference solution (a). Calculate the percentage content of bacampicillin hydrochloride.

STORAGE

Store in an airtight container.

IMPURITIES

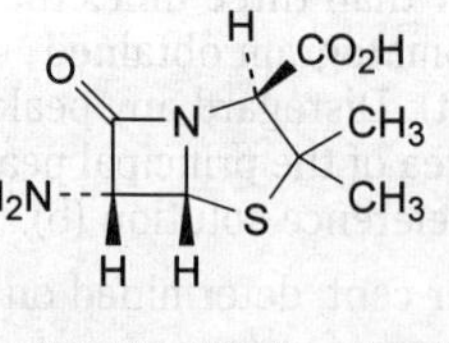

A. (2*S*,5*R*,6*R*)-6-amino-3,3-dimethyl-7-oxo-4-thia-1-azabicyclo[3.2.0]heptane-2-carboxylic acid (6-aminopenicillanic acid),

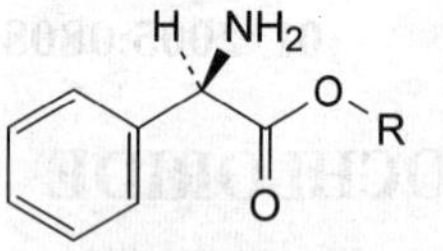

B. R = H: (2*R*)-2-amino-2-phenylacetic acid (D-phenylglycine),

G. R = CH_3: methyl (2*R*)-2-amino-2-phenylacetate (methyl D-phenylglycinate),

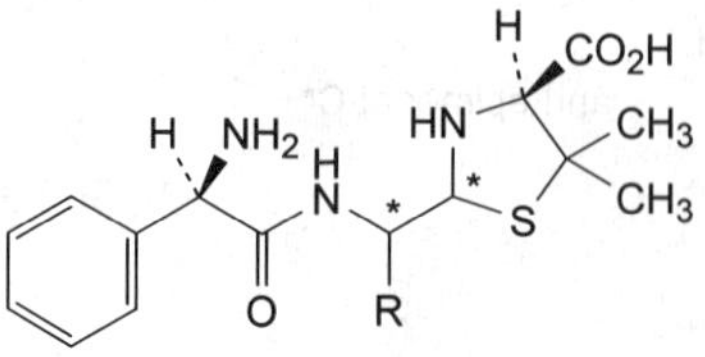

C. R = H: (2*RS*,4*S*)-2-[[[(2*R*)-2-amino-2-phenylacetyl]amino]methyl]-5,5-dimethylthiazolidine-4-carboxylic acid (penilloic acids of ampicillin),

D. R = CO_2H: (4*S*)-2-[[[(2*R*)-2-amino-2-phenylacetyl]amino]carboxymethyl]-5,5-dimethylthiazolidine-4-carboxylic acid (penicilloic acids of ampicillin),

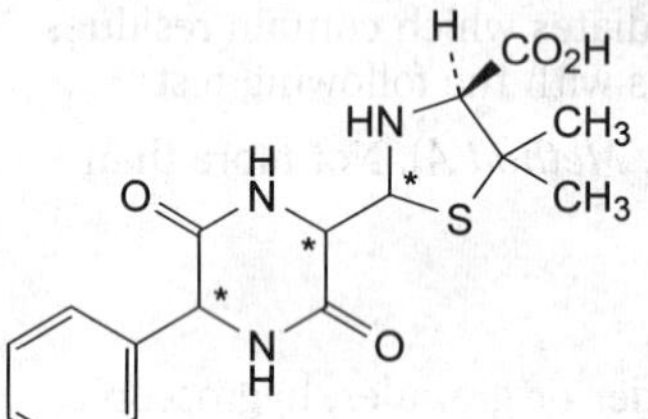

E. (4*S*)-2-(3,6-dioxo-5-phenylpiperazin-2-yl)-5,5-dimethylthiazolidine-4-carboxylic acid (diketopiperazines of ampicillin),

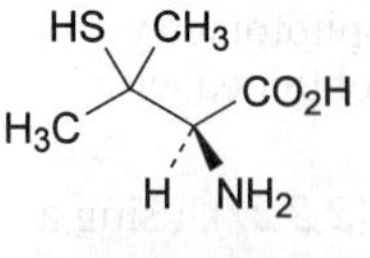

and enantiomer

F. (2*RS*)-2-amino-3-methyl-3-sulphanylbutanoic acid (DL-penicillamine),

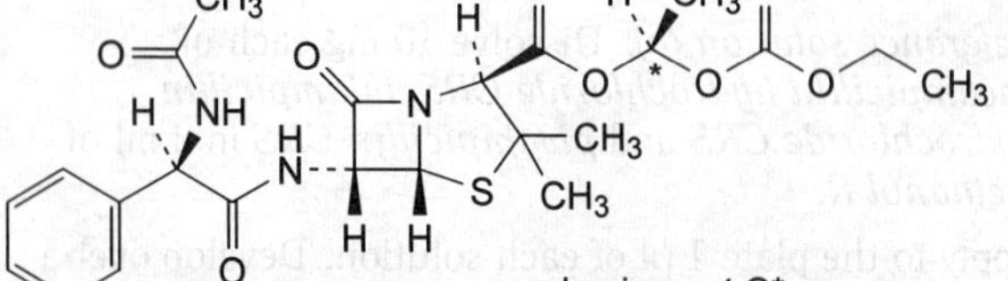

and epimer at C*

H. (1*RS*)-1-[(ethoxycarbonyl)oxy]ethyl (2*S*,5*R*,6*R*)-6-[[(2*R*)-2-(acetylamino)-2-phenylacetyl]amino]-3,3-dimethyl-7-oxo-4-thia-1-azabicyclo[3.2.0]heptane-2-carboxylate (*N*-acetylbacampicillin),

I. ampicillin.

01/2005:0465

BACITRACIN

Bacitracinum

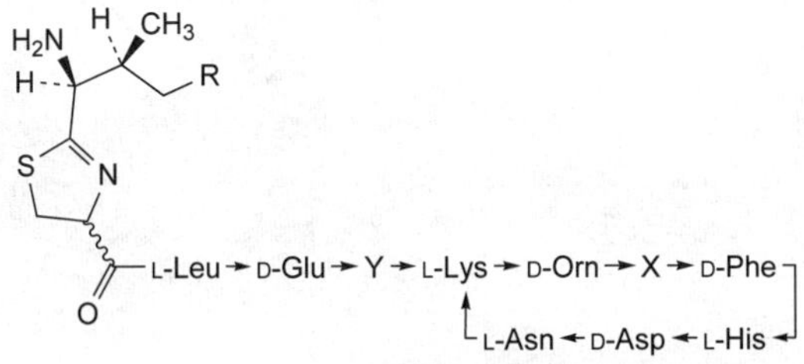

Name	Mol. Formula	X	Y	R
Bacitracin A	$C_{66}H_{103}N_{17}O_{16}S$	L-Ile	L-Ile	CH_3
Bacitracin B1	$C_{65}H_{101}N_{17}O_{16}S$	L-Ile	L-Ile	H
Bacitracin B2	$C_{65}H_{101}N_{17}O_{16}S$	L-Val	L-Ile	CH_3
Bacitracin B3	$C_{65}H_{101}N_{17}O_{16}S$	L-Ile	L-Val	CH_3

DEFINITION

Mixture of antimicrobial polypeptides produced by certain strains of *Bacillus licheniformis* or *Bacillus subtilis*, the main components being bacitracins A, B1, B2 and B3.

Content: minimum 60 IU/mg (dried substance).

CHARACTERS

Appearance: white or almost white powder, hygroscopic.

Solubility: freely soluble in water and in alcohol.

IDENTIFICATION

First identification: B, C.

Second identification: A, C.

A. Thin-layer chromatography (*2.2.27*).

Test solution. Dissolve 10 mg of the substance to be examined in a 3.4 g/l solution of *hydrochloric acid R* and dilute to 1.0 ml with the same solution.

Reference solution. Dissolve 10 mg of *bacitracin zinc CRS* in a 3.4 g/l solution of *hydrochloric acid R* and dilute to 1.0 ml with the same solution.

Plate: *TLC silica gel plate R*.

Mobile phase: *glacial acetic acid R, water R, butanol R* (1:2:4 *V/V/V*).

Application: 10 µl.

Development: over half of the plate.

Drying: at 100-105 °C.

Detection: spray with *ninhydrin solution R1* and heat at 110 °C for 5 min.

Results: the spots in the chromatogram obtained with the test solution are similar in position, size and colour to the spots in the chromatogram obtained with the reference solution.

B. It complies with the test for composition (see Tests).

C. Ignite 0.2 g. An insignificant residue remains which is not yellow at high temperature. Allow to cool. Dissolve the residue in 0.1 ml of *dilute hydrochloric acid R*. Add 5 ml of *water R* and 0.2 ml of *strong sodium hydroxide solution R*. No white precipitate is formed.

TESTS

Solution S. Dissolve 0.25 g in *carbon dioxide-free water R* and dilute to 25 ml with the same solvent.

Appearance of solution. Solution S is clear (*2.2.1*).

pH (*2.2.3*): 6.0 to 7.0 for solution S.

Composition. Liquid chromatography (*2.2.29*): use the normalisation procedure. *Prepare the solutions immediately before use.*

Test solution. Dissolve 0.100 g of the substance to be examined in 50.0 ml of the mobile phase.

Reference solution (a). Suspend 20.0 mg of *bacitracin zinc CRS* in *water R*, add 0.2 ml of *dilute hydrochloric acid R* and dilute to 10.0 ml with *water R*.

Reference solution (b). Dilute 5.0 ml of the test solution to 100.0 ml with the mobile phase.

Reference solution (c). Dilute 1.0 ml of reference solution (b) to 10.0 ml with the mobile phase.

Reference solution (d). Dissolve 50.0 mg of the substance to be examined in 25.0 ml of a 40 g/l solution of *sodium edetate R* adjusted to pH 7.0 with *dilute sodium hydroxide R*. Heat in a boiling water-bath for 30 min. Cool to room temperature.

Blank solution. A 40 g/l solution of *sodium edetate R* adjusted to pH 7.0 with *dilute sodium hydroxide R*.

Column:
- *size*: l = 0.25 m, Ø = 4.6 mm,
- *stationary phase*: *end-capped octadecylsilyl silica gel for chromatography R* (5 µm).

Mobile phase: add 520 volumes of *methanol R1*, 40 volumes of *acetonitrile R* and 300 volumes of *water R* to 100 volumes of a 34.8 g/l solution of *dipotassium hydrogen phosphate R* adjusted to pH 6.0 with a 27.2 g/l solution of *potassium dihydrogen phosphate R*.

Flow rate: 1.0 ml/min.

Detection: spectrophotometer at 254 nm.

Injection: 100 µl; inject the blank, the test solution and reference solutions (a) and (c).

Run time: 3 times the retention time of bacitracin A.

Relative retention with reference to bacitracin A (retention time = 15 min to 25 min): bacitracin B1 = about 0.6; bacitracin B3 = about 0.8; impurity E = about 2.5.

If necessary, adjust the composition of the mobile phase by changing the amount of organic modifier whilst keeping the ratio constant between methanol and acetonitrile.

System suitability: reference solution (a):
- *peak-to-valley ratio*: minimum of 1.2, where H_p = height above the baseline of the peak due to bacitracin B1 and H_v = height above the baseline of the lowest point of the curve separating this peak from the peak due to bacitracin B2.

Limits:
- *bacitracin A*: minimum 40.0 per cent,
- *sum of bacitracins A, B1, B2 and B3*: minimum 70.0 per cent,
- *disregard limit*: the area of the peak due to bacitracin A in the chromatogram obtained with reference solution (c) (0.5 per cent); disregard any peak observed in the blank run.

Related peptides. Liquid chromatography (*2.2.29*) as described in the test for composition.

See Figure 0465.-1.

Limit:
- *sum of the areas of all peaks eluting before the peak due to bacitracin B1*: maximum 20.0 per cent.

Impurity E. Liquid chromatography (*2.2.29*) as described in the test for composition.

See Figure 0465.-2.

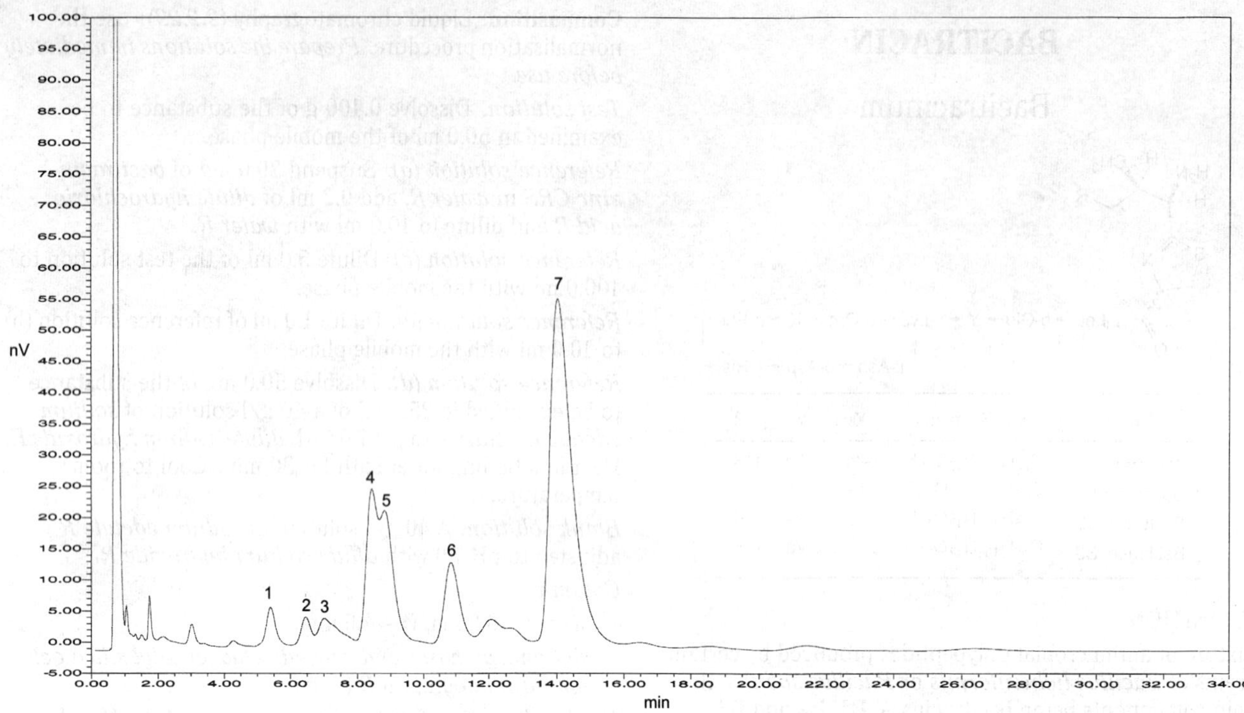

1. impurity A
2. impurity B
3. impurity C
4. bacitracin B1
5. bacitracin B2
6. bacitracin B3
7. bacitracin A

Figure 0465.-1. – *Chromatogram of the test for composition in bacitracin obtained with the test solution at 254 nm*

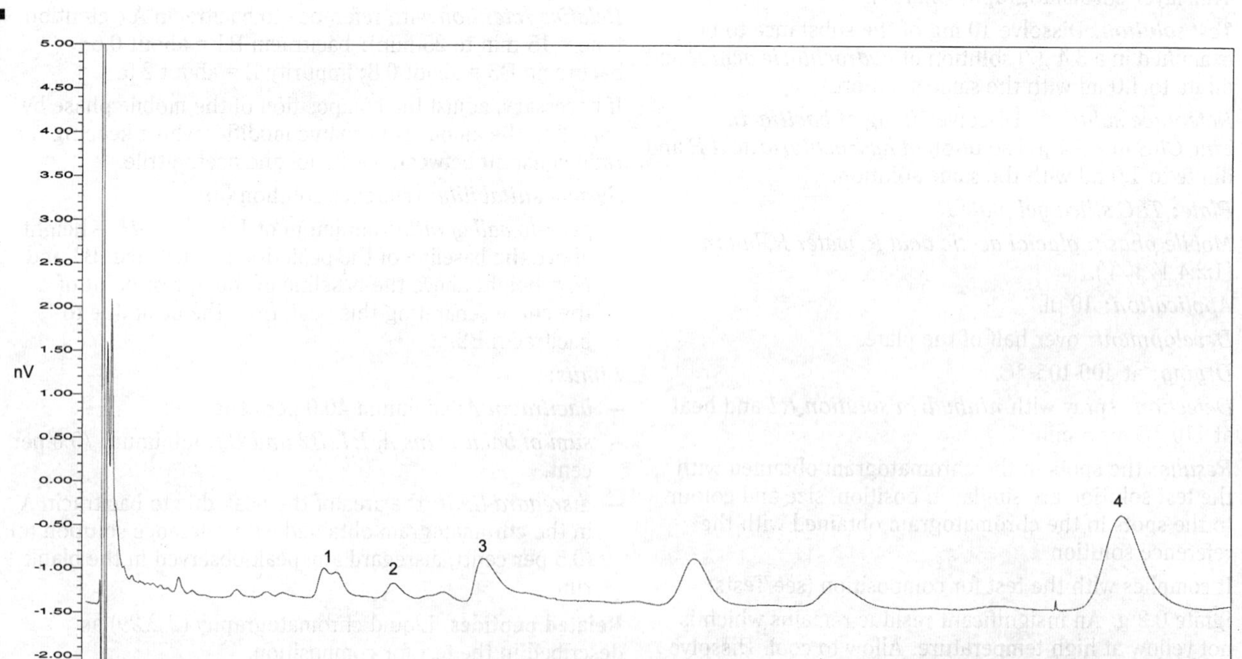

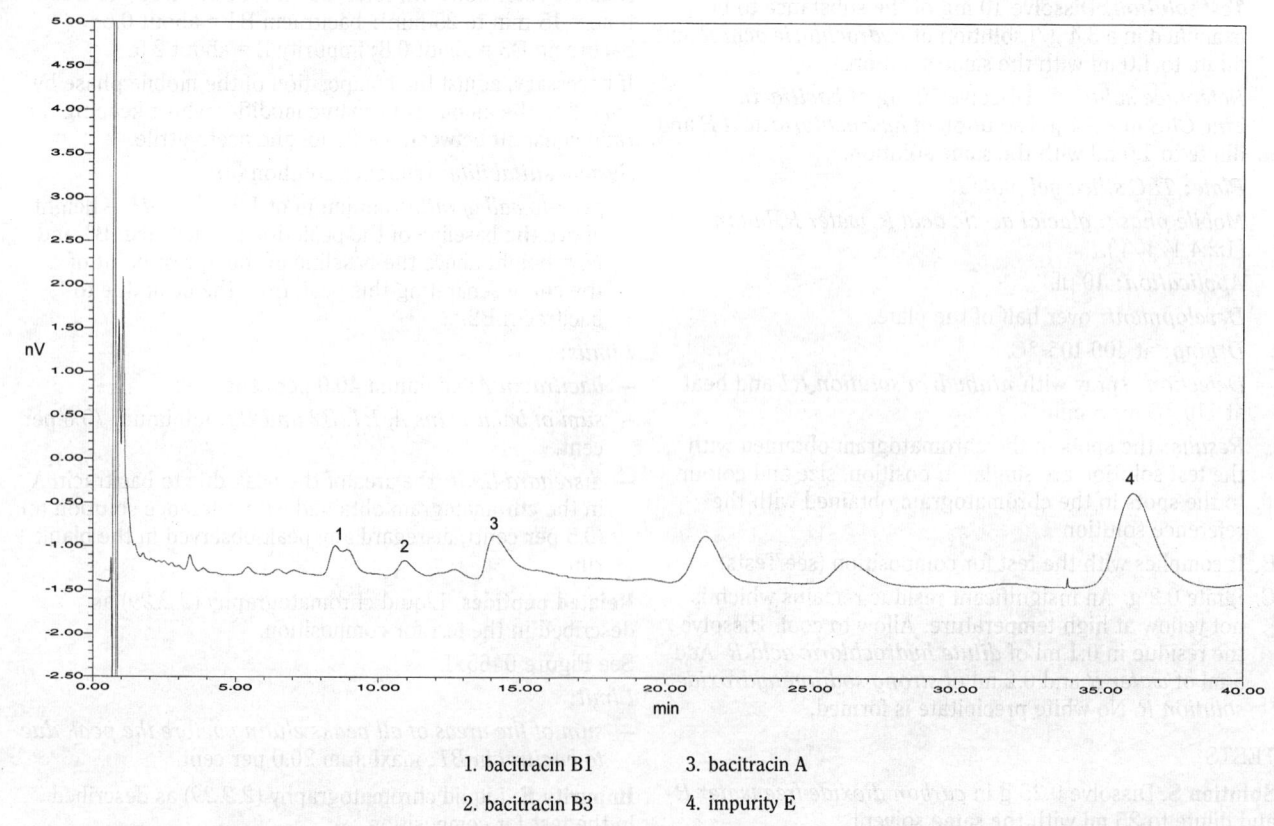

1. bacitracin B1
2. bacitracin B3
3. bacitracin A
4. impurity E

Figure 0465.-2. – *Chromatogram of the test for impurity E in bacitracin obtained with reference solution (d) at 300 nm*

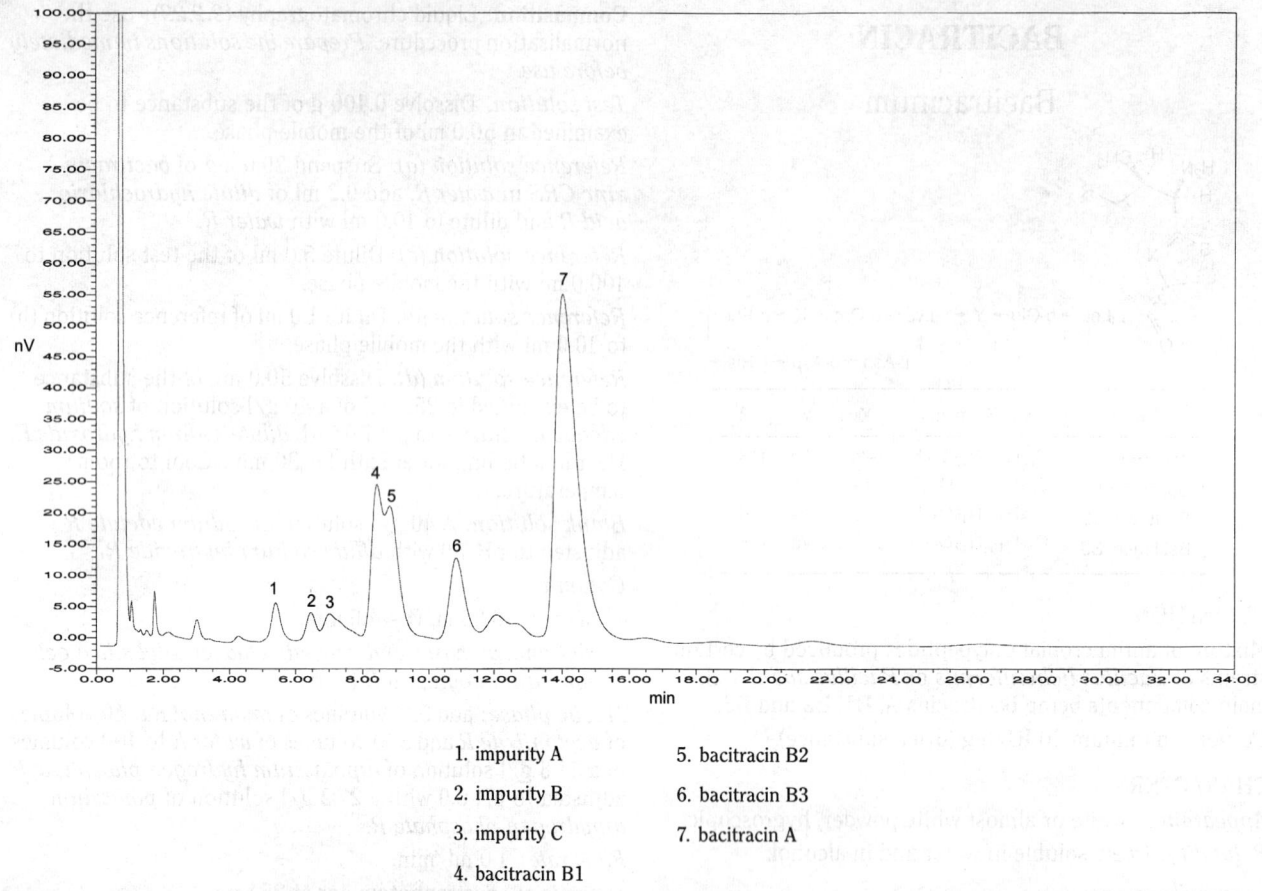

Detection: spectrophotometer at 254 nm; spectrophotometer at 300 nm for reference solution (d).

Injection: test solution and reference solutions (b) and (d).

Limit:

– *impurity E*: not more than 1.2 times the area of the principal peak in the chromatogram obtained with reference solution (b) (6.0 per cent).

Loss on drying (*2.2.32*): maximum 5.0 per cent, determined on 1.000 g by drying at 60 °C over *diphosphorus pentoxide R* at a pressure not exceeding 0.1 kPa for 3 h.

Sulphated ash (*2.4.14*): maximum 1.0 per cent, determined on 1.0 g.

Sterility (*2.6.1*). If intended for the preparation of ophthalmic dosage forms without a further appropriate sterilisation procedure, it complies with the test for sterility.

Bacterial endotoxins (*2.6.14*): less than 0.8 IU/mg, if intended for use in the manufacture of ophthalmic dosage forms without a further appropriate procedure for the removal of bacterial endotoxins.

ASSAY

Carry out the microbiological assay of antibiotics (*2.7.2*). Use *bacitracin zinc CRS* as the reference substance.

STORAGE

In an airtight container at 2 °C to 8 °C. If the substance is sterile, store in a sterile, airtight, tamper-proof container.

LABELLING

The label states, where applicable:

– that the substance is sterile,

– that the substance is free from bacterial endotoxins.

IMPURITIES

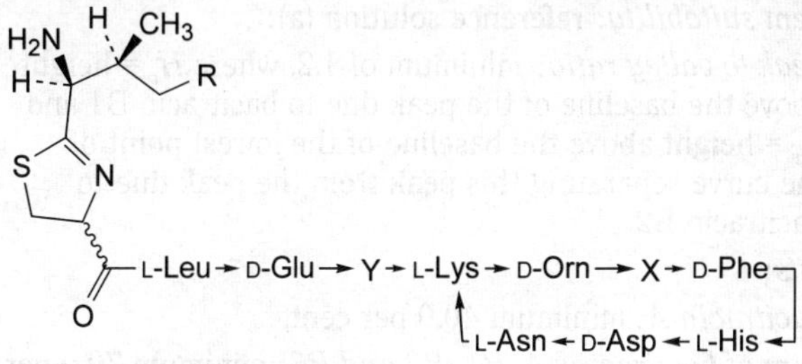

A. X = L-Val, Y = L-Ile, R = H: bacitracin C1,

B. X = L-Ile, Y = L-Val, R = H: bacitracin C2,

C. X = Y = L-Val, R = CH_3: bacitracin C3,

D. X = Y = L-Val, R = H: bacitracin E,

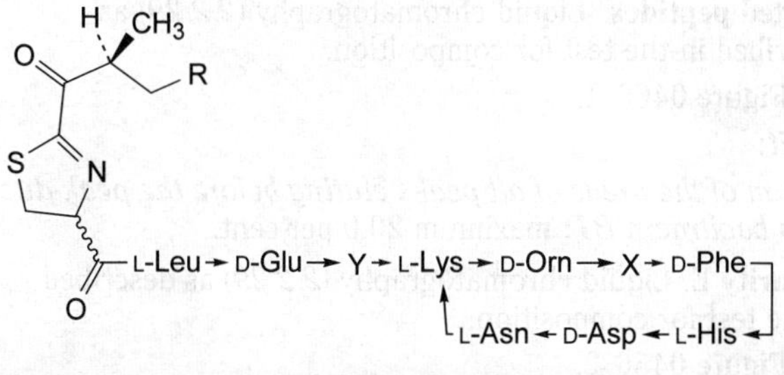

E. X = Y = L-Ile, R = CH_3: bacitracin F,

F. X = Y = L-Ile, R = H: bacitracin H1,

G. X = L-Val, Y = L-Ile, R = CH_3: bacitracin H2,

H. X = L-Ile, Y = L-Val, R = CH_3: bacitracin H3,

I. X = L-Val, Y = L-Ile, R = H: bacitracin I1,

J. X = L-Ile, Y = L-Val, R = H: bacitracin I2,

K. X = Y = L-Val, R = CH_3: bacitracin I3.

01/2005:0466

BACITRACIN ZINC

Bacitracinum zincum

DEFINITION

Zinc complex of bacitracin, which consists of a mixture of antimicrobial polypeptides produced by certain strains of *Bacillus licheniformis* or *Bacillus subtilis*, the main components being bacitracins A, B1, B2 and B3.

Content: minimum 60 IU/mg (dried substance).

CHARACTERS

Appearance: white or light yellowish-grey powder, hygroscopic.

Solubility: slightly soluble in water and in alcohol.

IDENTIFICATION

First identification: B, C.

Second identification: A, C.

A. Thin-layer chromatography (*2.2.27*).

Test solution. Dissolve 10 mg of the substance to be examined in 0.5 ml of *dilute hydrochloride acid R* and dilute to 1.0 ml with *water R*.

Reference solution. Dissolve 10 mg of *bacitracin zinc CRS* in 0.5 ml of *dilute hydrochloric acid R* and dilute to 1.0 ml with *water R*.

Plate: *TLC silica gel plate R*.

Mobile phase: *glacial acetic acid R, water R, butanol R* (1:2:4 *V/V/V*).

Application: 10 µl.

Development: over half of the plate.

Drying: at 100-105 °C.

Detection: spray with *ninhydrin solution R1* and heat at 110 °C for 5 min.

Results: the spots in the chromatogram obtained with the test solution are similar in position, size and colour to the spots in the chromatogram obtained with the reference solution.

B. It complies with the test for composition (see Tests).

C. Ignite about 0.15 g, allow to cool and dissolve the residue in 1 ml of *dilute hydrochloric acid R*. Add 4 ml of *water R*. The solution gives the reaction of zinc (*2.3.1*).

TESTS

pH (*2.2.3*): 6.0 to 7.5.

Shake 1.0 g for about 1 min with 10 ml of *carbon dioxide-free water R* and filter.

Composition. Liquid chromatography (*2.2.29*): use the normalisation procedure. *Prepare the solutions immediately before use.*

Test solution. Dissolve 0.100 g of the substance to be examined in 50.0 ml of a 40 g/l solution of *sodium edetate R* adjusted to pH 7.0 with *dilute sodium hydroxide R*.

Reference solution (a). Dissolve 20.0 mg of *bacitracin zinc CRS* in 10.0 ml of a 40 g/l solution of *sodium edetate R* adjusted to pH 7.0 with *dilute sodium hydroxide R*.

Reference solution (b). Dilute 5.0 ml of the test solution to 100.0 ml with *water R*.

Reference solution (c). Dilute 1.0 ml of reference solution (b) to 10.0 ml with *water R*.

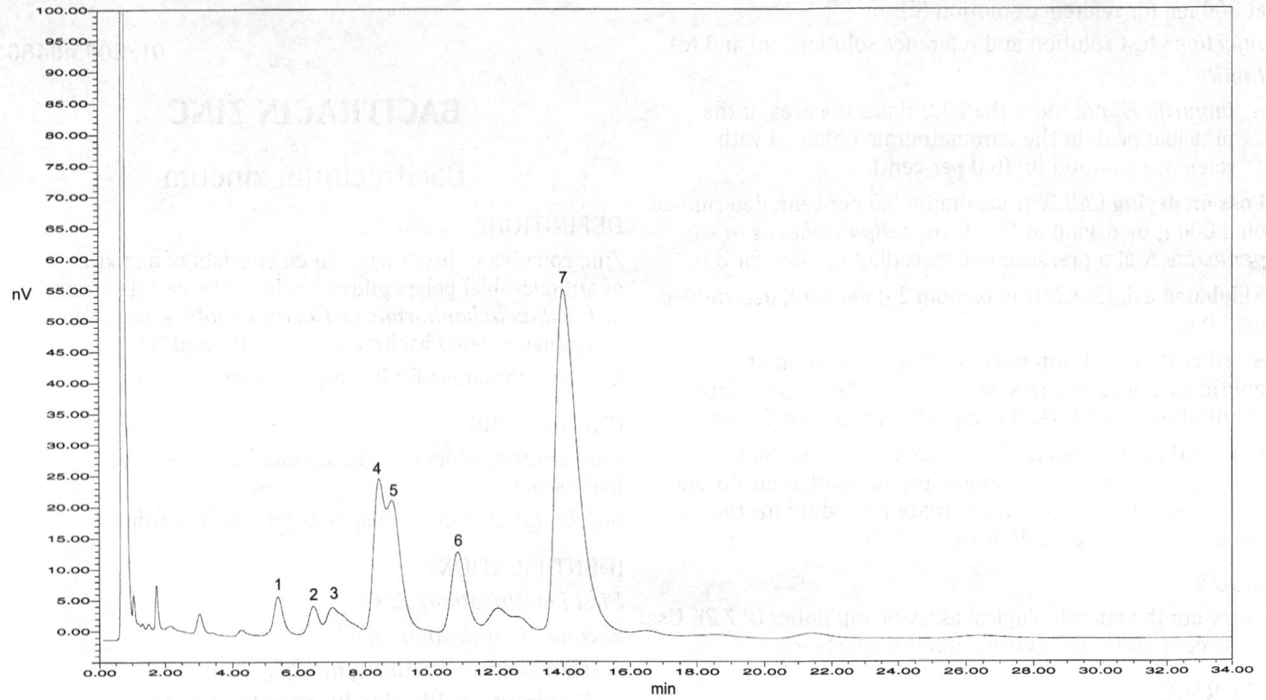

1. impurity A
2. impurity B
3. impurity C
4. bacitracin B1
5. bacitracin B2
6. bacitracin B3
7. bacitracin A

Figure 0466.-1. – *Chromatogram of the test for composition in bacitracin zinc obtained with the test solution at 254 nm*

Reference solution (d). Dissolve 50.0 mg of the substance to be examined in 25.0 ml of a 40 g/l solution of *sodium edetate R* adjusted to pH 7.0 with *dilute sodium hydroxide R*. Heat in a boiling water-bath for 30 min. Cool to room temperature.

Blank solution. A 40 g/l solution of *sodium edetate R* adjusted to pH 7.0 with dilute *sodium hydroxide R*.

Column:

– *size*: *l* = 0.25 m, Ø = 4.6 mm,

– *stationary phase*: *end-capped octadecylsilyl silica gel for chromatography R* (5 µm).

Mobile phase: add 520 volumes of *methanol R1*, 40 volumes of *acetonitrile R* and 300 volumes of *water R* to 100 volumes of a 34.8 g/l solution of *dipotassium hydrogen phosphate R*, adjusted to pH 6.0 with a 27.2 g/l solution of *potassium dihydrogen phosphate R*.

Flow rate: 1.0 ml/min.

Detection: spectrophotometer at 254 nm.

Injection: 100 µl; inject the blank, the test solution and reference solutions (a) and (c).

Run time: 3 times the retention time of bacitracin A.

Relative retention with reference to bacitracin A (retention time = 15 min to 25 min): bacitracin B1 = about 0.6; bacitracin B3 = about 0.8; impurity E = about 2.5.

If necessary, adjust the composition of the mobile phase by changing the amount of organic modifier whilst keeping the ratio constant between methanol and acetonitrile.

System suitability: reference solution (a):

– *peak-to-valley ratio*: minimum of 1.2, where H_p = height above the baseline of the peak due to bacitracin B1 and H_v = height above the baseline of the lowest point of the curve separating this peak from the peak due to bacitracin B2.

Limits:

– *bacitracin A*: minimum 40.0 per cent,

– *sum of bacitracins A, B1, B2 and B3*: minimum 70.0 per cent.

– *disregard limit*: the area of the peak due to bacitracin A in the chromatogram obtained with reference solution (c) (0.5 per cent); disregard any peak observed in the blank run.

Related peptides. Liquid chromatography (*2.2.29*) as described in the test for composition.

See Figure 0466.-1.

Limit:

– *sum of the areas of all peaks eluting before the peak due to bacitracin B1*: maximum 20.0 per cent.

Impurity E. Liquid chromatography (*2.2.29*) as described in the test for composition.

See Figure 0466.-2.

Detection: spectrophotometer at 254 nm; spectrophotometer at 300 nm for reference solution (d).

Injection: test solution and reference solutions (b) and (d).

Limit:

– *impurity E*: not more than 1.2 times the area of the principal peak in the chromatogram obtained with reference solution (b) (6.0 per cent).

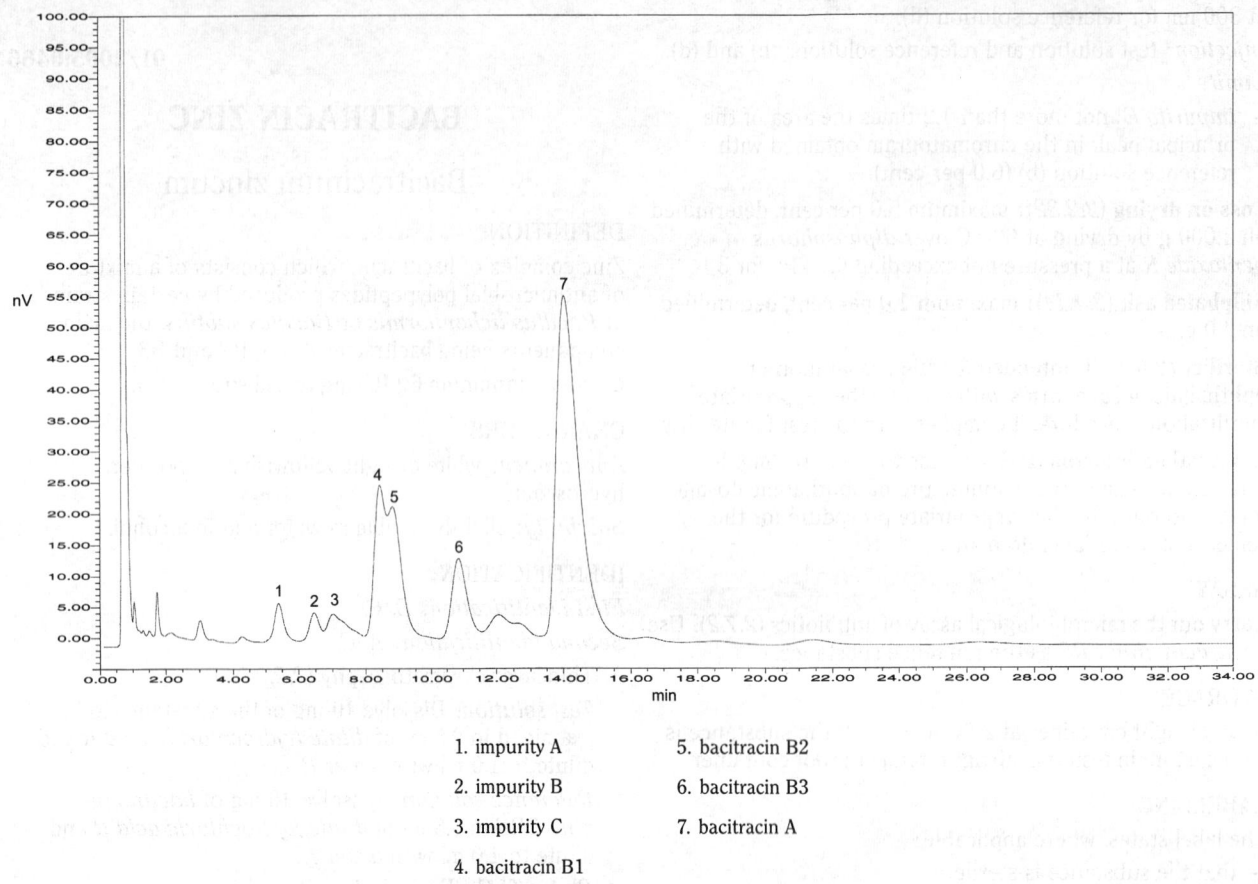

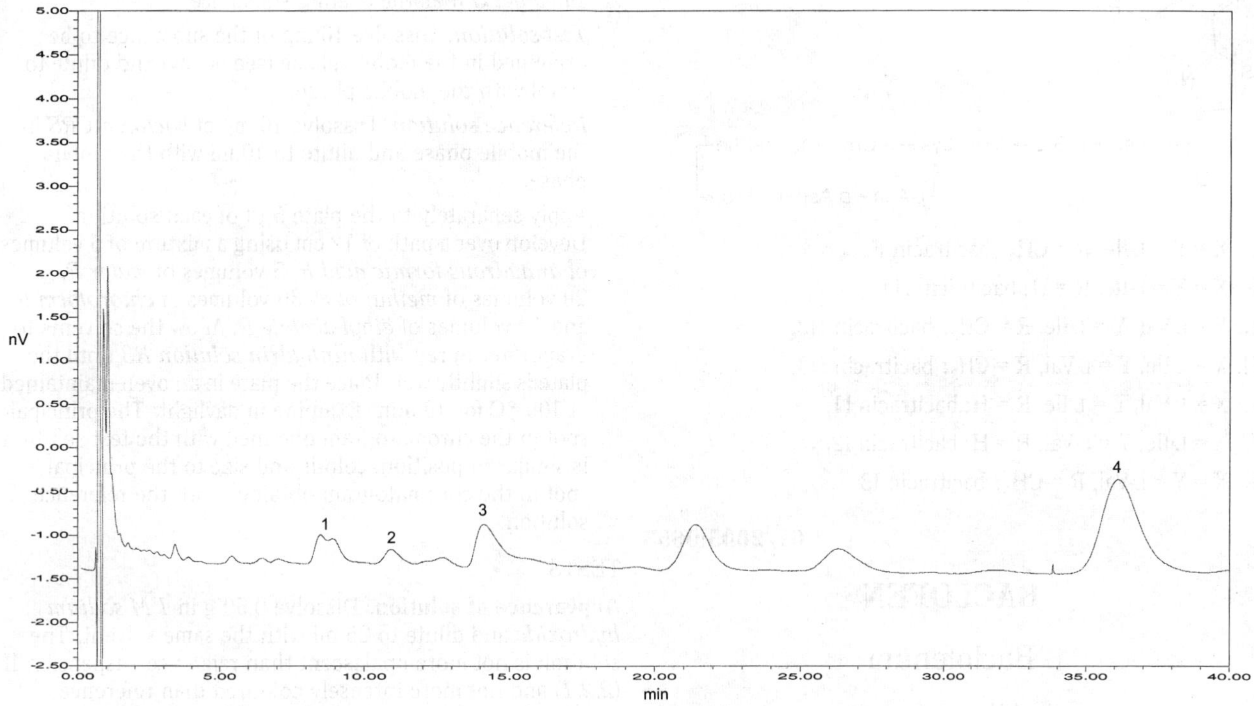

1. bacitracin B1
2. bacitracin B3
3. bacitracin A
4. impurity E

Figure 0466.-2. – *Chromatogram of the test for impurity E in bacitracin zinc obtained with reference solution (d) at 300 nm*

Zinc: 4.0 per cent to 6.0 per cent (dried substance).

Dissolve 0.200 g in a mixture of 2.5 ml of *dilute acetic acid R* and 2.5 ml of water. Add 50 ml of *water R*, 50 mg of *xylenol orange triturate R* and sufficient *hexamethylenetetramine R* to produce a red colour. Add 2 g of *hexamethylenetetramine R* in excess. Titrate with *0.01 M sodium edetate* until a yellow colour is obtained.

1 ml of *0.01 M sodium edetate* is equivalent to 0.654 mg of Zn.

Loss on drying (*2.2.32*): maximum 5.0 per cent, determined on 1.000 g by drying at 60 °C over *diphosphorus pentoxide R* at a pressure not exceeding 0.1 kPa for 3 h.

Sterility (*2.6.1*). If intended for administration by spraying into internal body cavities without a further appropriate sterilisation procedure, it complies with the test for sterility.

Pyrogens (*2.6.8*). If intended for administration by spraying into internal body cavities without a further appropriate procedure for the removal of pyrogens, it complies with the test for pyrogens. Inject per kilogram of the rabbit's mass 1 ml of the supernatant liquid obtained by centrifuging a suspension containing 11 mg per millilitre in a 9 g/l solution of *sodium chloride R*.

ASSAY

Suspend 50.0 mg in 5 ml of *water R*, add 0.5 ml of *dilute hydrochloric acid R* and dilute to 100.0 ml with *water R*. Allow the solution to stand for 30 min. Carry out the microbiological assay of antibiotics (*2.7.2*).

STORAGE

In an airtight container. If the substance is sterile, store in a sterile, airtight, tamper-proof container.

LABELLING

The label states, where applicable:

– that the substance is sterile,
– that the substance is apyrogenic.

IMPURITIES

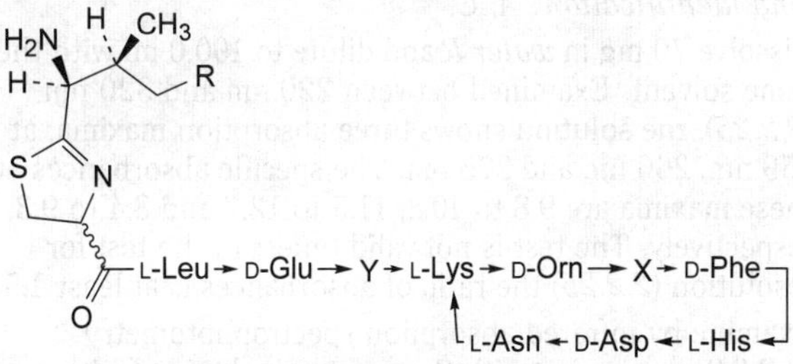

A. X = L-Val, Y = L-Ile, R = H: bacitracin C1,

B. X = L-Ile, Y = L-Val, R = H: bacitracin C2,

C. X = Y = L-Val, R = CH_3: bacitracin C3,

D. X = Y = L-Val, R = H: bacitracin E,

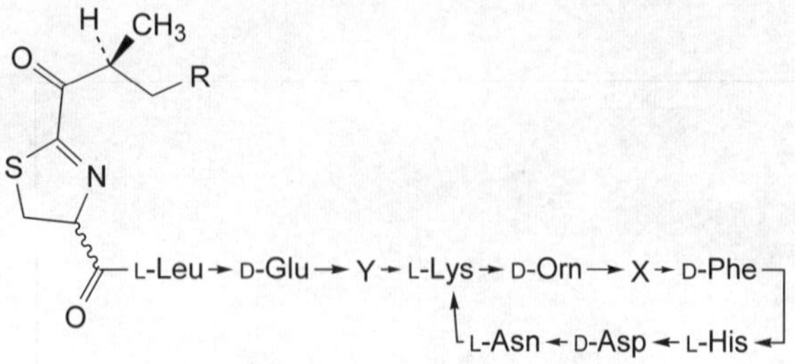

E. X = Y = L-Ile, R = CH_3: bacitracin F,

F. X = Y = L-Ile, R = H: bacitracin H1,

G. X = L-Val, Y = L-Ile, R = CH_3: bacitracin H2,

H. X = L-Ile, Y = L-Val, R = CH_3: bacitracin H3,

I. X = L-Val, Y = L-Ile, R = H: bacitracin I1,

J. X = L-Ile, Y = L-Val, R = H: bacitracin I2,

K. X = Y = L-Val, R = CH_3: bacitracin I3.

01/2005:0653

BACLOFEN

Baclofenum

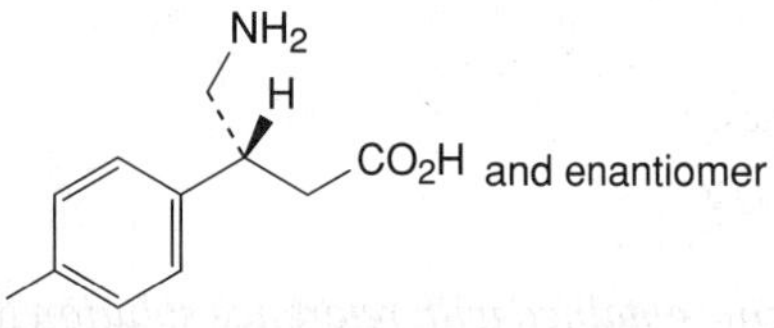

$C_{10}H_{12}ClNO_2$ M_r 213.7

DEFINITION

Baclofen contains not less than 98.0 per cent and not more than the equivalent of 101.0 per cent of (3*RS*)-4-amino-3-(4-chlorophenyl)butanoic acid, calculated with reference to the anhydrous substance.

CHARACTERS

A white or almost white powder, slightly soluble in water, very slightly soluble in alcohol, practically insoluble in acetone. It dissolves in dilute mineral acids and in dilute solutions of alkali hydroxides.

It shows polymorphism.

IDENTIFICATION

First identification: B.

Second identification: A, C.

A. Dissolve 70 mg in *water R* and dilute to 100.0 ml with the same solvent. Examined between 220 nm and 320 nm (*2.2.25*), the solution shows three absorption maxima, at 259 nm, 266 nm and 275 nm. The specific absorbances at these maxima are 9.8 to 10.8, 11.5 to 12.7 and 8.4 to 9.3, respectively. The test is not valid unless in the test for resolution (*2.2.25*) the ratio of absorbances is at least 1.5.

B. Examine by infrared absorption spectrophotometry (*2.2.24*), comparing with the spectrum obtained with *baclofen CRS*. Examine as discs prepared using 3 mg of substance and 300 mg of *potassium bromide R*. If the spectra obtained with the substance to be examined and the reference substance show differences, dissolve 0.1 g of each of the substances separately in 1 ml of *dilute sodium hydroxide solution R* and add 10 ml of *alcohol R* and 1 ml of *dilute acetic acid R*. Allow to stand for 1 h. Filter, wash the precipitate with *alcohol R* and dry *in vacuo*. Prepare new discs and record the spectra.

C. Examine by thin-layer chromatography (*2.2.27*), using *silica gel G R* as the coating substance.

Test solution. Dissolve 10 mg of the substance to be examined in the mobile phase (see below) and dilute to 10 ml with the mobile phase.

Reference solution. Dissolve 10 mg of *baclofen CRS* in the mobile phase and dilute to 10 ml with the mobile phase.

Apply separately to the plate 5 µl of each solution. Develop over a path of 12 cm using a mixture of 5 volumes of *anhydrous formic acid R*, 5 volumes of *water R*, 20 volumes of *methanol R*, 30 volumes of *chloroform R* and 40 volumes of *ethyl acetate R*. Allow the solvents to evaporate. Spray with *ninhydrin solution R3* until the plate is slightly wet. Place the plate in an oven maintained at 100 °C for 10 min. Examine in daylight. The principal spot in the chromatogram obtained with the test solution is similar in position, colour and size to the principal spot in the chromatogram obtained with the reference solution.

TESTS

Appearance of solution. Dissolve 0.50 g in *1 M sodium hydroxide* and dilute to 25 ml with the same solvent. The solution is not more opalescent than reference suspension II (*2.2.1*) and not more intensely coloured than reference solution BY_5 (*2.2.2, Method II*).

Related substances. Examine by liquid chromatography (*2.2.29*).

Test solution. Dissolve 25.0 mg of the substance to be examined in the mobile phase and dilute to 10.0 ml with the mobile phase.

Reference solution (a). Dissolve 25.0 mg of *baclofen impurity A CRS* in the mobile phase and dilute to 10.0 ml with the mobile phase.

Reference solution (b). Dilute 1.0 ml of reference solution (a) to 100.0 ml with the mobile phase.

Reference solution (c). Dilute 2.0 ml of the test solution to 100.0 ml with the mobile phase.

Reference solution (d). Dilute 2.0 ml of the test solution and 2.0 ml of reference solution (a) to 100.0 ml with the mobile phase.

The chromatographic procedure may be carried out using:

- a stainless steel column 0.25 m long and 4.0 mm in internal diameter packed with *octadecylsilyl silica gel for chromatography R* (10 µm),
- as mobile phase at a flow-rate of 2.0 ml/min a mixture prepared as follows: dissolve 1.822 g of *sodium hexanesulphonate R* in 1 litre of a mixture of 560 volumes of *water R*, 440 volumes of *methanol R* and 5 volumes of *glacial acetic acid R*,
- as detector a spectrophotometer set at 266 nm.

Adjust the sensitivity of the system so that the height of the principal peak in the chromatogram obtained with 20 µl of reference solution (c) is at least 50 per cent of the full scale of the recorder. Inject 20 µl of reference solution (d). The test is not valid unless the resolution between the peaks corresponding to baclofen and baclofen impurity A is at least 2.0. Inject separately 20 µl of the test solution, reference solution (b) and reference solution (c). Continue the chromatography for five times the retention time of the principal peak. In the chromatogram obtained with the test solution: the area of the peak corresponding to baclofen impurity A is not greater than the area of the principal peak in the chromatogram obtained with reference solution (b) (1.0 per cent); the sum of the areas of all the peaks, apart from the principal peak, is not greater than the area of the principal peak in the chromatogram obtained with reference solution (c) (2.0 per cent).

Water (*2.5.12*). Not more than 1.0 per cent, determined on 1.000 g by the semi-micro determination of water.

Sulphated ash (*2.4.14*). Not more than 0.1 per cent, determined on 1.0 g.

ASSAY

Dissolve 0.1500 g in 50 ml of *anhydrous acetic acid R*. Titrate with *0.1 M perchloric acid*, determining the end-point potentiometrically (*2.2.20*).

1 ml of *0.1 M perchloric acid* is equivalent to 21.37 mg of $C_{10}H_{12}ClNO_2$.

IMPURITIES

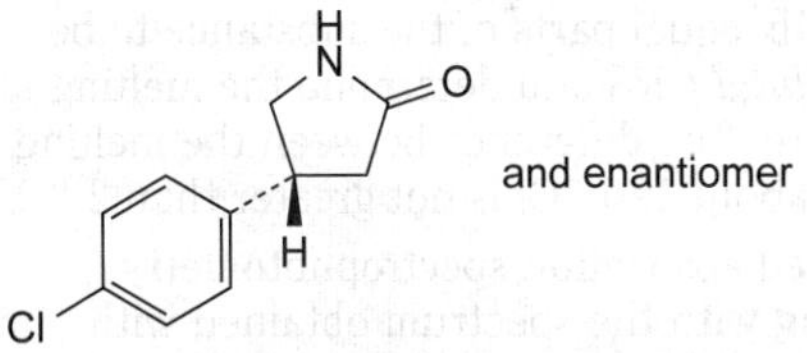

A. (4*RS*)-4-(4-chlorophenyl)pyrrolidin-2-one,

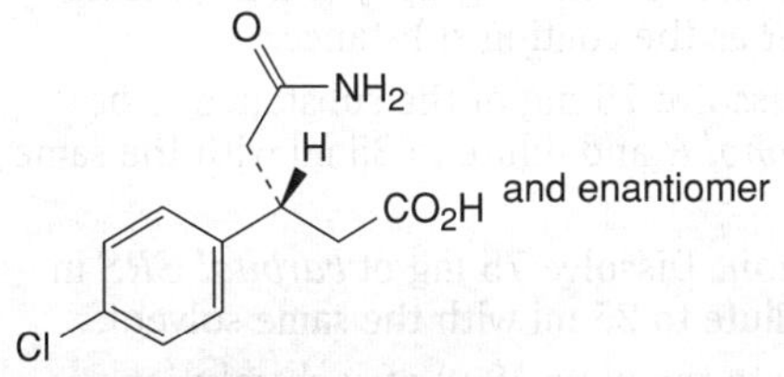

B. (3*RS*)-5-amino-3-(4-chlorophenyl)-5-oxopentanoic acid.

01/2005:1293

BAMBUTEROL HYDROCHLORIDE

Bambuteroli hydrochloridum

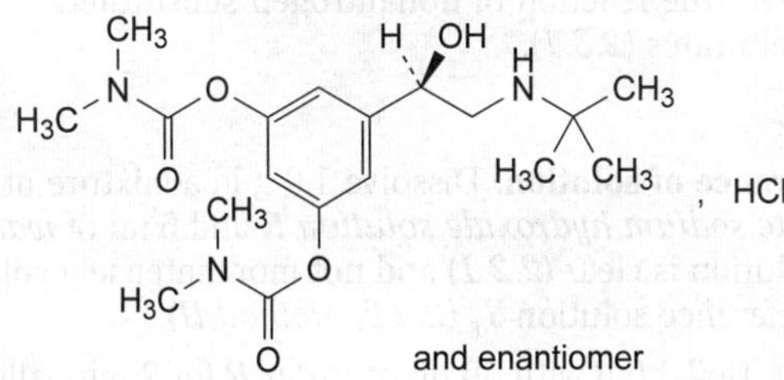

$C_{18}H_{30}ClN_3O_5$ M_r 403.9

DEFINITION

Bambuterol hydrochloride contains not less than 98.5 per cent and not more than the equivalent of 101.5 per cent of 5-[(1*RS*)-2-[(1,1-dimethylethyl)amino]-1-hydroxyethyl]-1,3-phenylene bis(dimethylcarbamate) hydrochloride, calculated with reference to the anhydrous substance.

CHARACTERS

A white or almost white, crystalline powder, freely soluble in water, soluble in alcohol.

It shows polymorphism.

IDENTIFICATION

A. Examine by infrared absorption spectrophotometry (*2.2.24*), comparing with the spectrum obtained with *bambuterol hydrochloride CRS*. Examine the substances prepared as discs. If the spectra obtained show differences, dissolve the substance to be examined and the reference substance in a mixture of 1 volume of *water R* and 6 volumes of *acetone R*, cool in ice to precipitate and dry both precipitates *in vacuo* at 50 °C to constant weight. Record new spectra using the residues.

B. It gives reaction (a) of chlorides (*2.3.1*).

TESTS

Solution S. Dissolve 4.0 g in *carbon dioxide-free water R* and dilute to 20.0 ml with the same solvent.

Acidity or alkalinity. To 10 ml of solution S add 0.2 ml of *methyl red solution R* and 0.2 ml of *0.01 M hydrochloric acid*. The solution is red. Add 0.4 ml of *0.01 M sodium hydroxide*. The solution is yellow.

Optical rotation (*2.2.7*). Dilute 1 ml of solution S to 10 ml with *carbon dioxide-free water R*. The angle of optical rotation is − 0.10° to + 0.10°.

Related substances. Examine by liquid chromatography (*2.2.29*).

Test solution. Dissolve 5.0 mg of the substance to be examined in the mobile phase and dilute to 10.0 ml with the mobile phase.

Reference solution (a). Dissolve 1.0 mg of *formoterol fumarate dihydrate CRS* in the mobile phase and dilute to 10.0 ml with the mobile phase. Mix 0.8 ml of the solution with 0.4 ml of the test solution and dilute to 100.0 ml with the mobile phase.

Reference solution (b). Dilute 1.0 ml of the test solution to 50.0 ml with the mobile phase. Dilute 2.0 ml of the solution to 20.0 ml with the mobile phase.

The chromatographic procedure may be carried out using:

– a stainless steel column 0.15 m long and 4.6 mm in internal diameter packed with *base-deactivated octadecylsilyl silica gel for chromatography R* (5 µm),

– as mobile phase at a flow rate of 1.5 ml/min a mixture prepared as follows: dissolve 1.3 g of *sodium octanesulphonate R* in 430 ml of a mixture of 25 volumes of *acetonitrile R1* and 75 volumes of *methanol R*; then mix this solution with 570 ml of 0.050 M phosphate buffer pH 3.0 (dissolve 6.90 g of *sodium dihydrogen phosphate monohydrate R* in *water R* and dilute to 1000 ml with *water R*, adjust the pH to 3.0 with a 50 g/l solution of *dilute phosphoric acid R*),

– as detector a spectrophotometer set at 214 nm.

Adjust the sensitivity of the system so that the height of the principal peak in the chromatogram obtained with 20 µl of reference solution (b) is about 50 per cent of the full scale of the recorder.

Inject 20 µl of reference solution (a). When the chromatograms are recorded under the prescribed conditions, the retention times are: formoterol about 7 min and bambuterol about 9 min. The test is not valid unless the resolution between the peaks corresponding to bambuterol and formoterol is at least 5.0. Continue the chromatography of the test solution for 1.5 times the retention time of bambuterol. If necessary adjust the composition of the mobile phase. Increase the content of phosphate buffer to increase the retention time.

Inject separately 20 µl of the mobile phase, 20 µl of the test solution and 20 µl of reference solution (b). In the chromatogram obtained with the test solution the area of any peak, apart from the principal peak, is not greater than the area of the principal peak obtained with reference solution (b) (0.2 per cent); the sum of the areas of all the peaks, apart from the principal peak, is not greater than three times the area of the principal peak in the chromatogram obtained with reference solution (b) (0.6 per cent). Disregard any peak due to the mobile phase and any peak with an area less than 0.25 times the area of the principal peak obtained with reference solution (b).

Water (*2.5.12*). Not more than 0.5 per cent, determined on 0.500 g by the semi-micro determination of water.

Sulphated ash (*2.4.14*). Not more than 0.1 per cent, determined on 1.0 g.

ASSAY

Dissolve 0.320 g in 50 ml of *alcohol R* and add 5 ml of *0.01 M hydrochloric acid.* Carry out a potentiometric titration (*2.2.20*), using *0.1 M sodium hydroxide.* Read the volume added between the two points of inflexion.

1 ml of *0.1 M sodium hydroxide* is equivalent to 40.39 mg of $C_{18}H_{30}ClN_3O_5$.

IMPURITIES

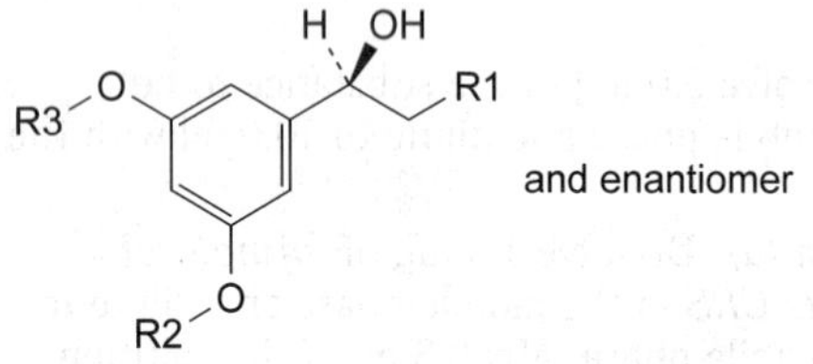

A. R1 = NH-C(CH_3)$_3$, R2 = R3 = H: (1*RS*)-1-(3,5-dihydroxyphenyl)-2-[(1,1-dimethylethyl)amino]ethanol (terbutaline),

B. R1 = OH, R2 = R3 = CO-N(CH_3)$_2$: 5-[(1*RS*)-1,2-dihydroxyethyl]-1,3-phenylene bis(dimethylcarbamate),

C. R1 = NH-C(CH_3)$_3$, R2 = H, R3 = CO-N(CH_3)$_2$: 3-[(1*RS*)-2-[(1,1-dimethylethyl)amino]-1-hydroxyethyl]-5-hydroxyphenyl dimethylcarbamate,

D. R1 = H, R2 = R3 = CO-N(CH_3)$_2$: 5-[(1*RS*)-1-hydroxyethyl]-1,3-phenylene bis(dimethylcarbamate),

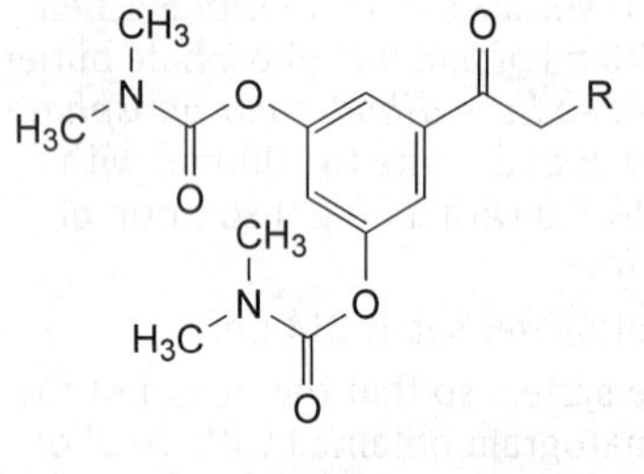

E. R = H: 5-acetyl-1,3-phenylene bis(dimethylcarbamate),

F. R = NH-C(CH_3)$_3$: 5-[[(1,1-dimethylethyl)amino]acetyl]-1,3-phenylene bis(dimethylcarbamate).

01/2005:0170

BARBITAL

Barbitalum

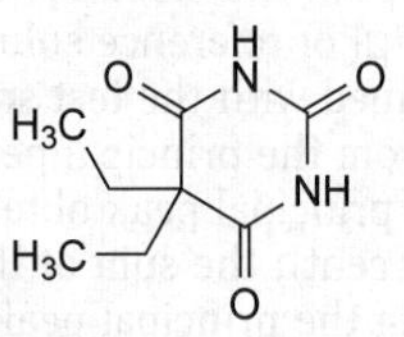

$C_8H_{12}N_2O_3$ M_r 184.2

DEFINITION

Barbital contains not less than 99.0 per cent and not more than the equivalent of 101.0 per cent of 5,5-diethylpyrimidine-2,4,6(1*H*,3*H*,5*H*)-trione, calculated with reference to the dried substance.

CHARACTERS

A white, crystalline powder or colourless crystals, slightly soluble in water, soluble in boiling water and in alcohol. It forms water-soluble compounds with alkali hydroxides and carbonates and with ammonia.

IDENTIFICATION

First identification: A, B.

Second identification: A, C, D.

A. Determine the melting point (*2.2.14*) of the substance to be examined. Mix equal parts of the substance to be examined and *barbital CRS* and determine the melting point of the mixture. The difference between the melting points (which are about 190 °C) is not greater than 2 °C.

B. Examine by infrared absorption spectrophotometry (*2.2.24*), comparing with the spectrum obtained with *barbital CRS.*

C. Examine by thin-layer chromatography (*2.2.27*), using *silica gel GF_{254} R* as the coating substance.

Test solution. Dissolve 75 mg of the substance to be examined in *alcohol R* and dilute to 25 ml with the same solvent.

Reference solution. Dissolve 75 mg of *barbital CRS* in *alcohol R* and dilute to 25 ml with the same solvent.

Apply separately to the plate 10 µl of each solution. Develop over a path of 18 cm using the lower layer of a mixture of 5 volumes of *concentrated ammonia R,* 15 volumes of *alcohol R* and 80 volumes of *chloroform R.* Examine immediately in ultraviolet light at 254 nm. The principal spot in the chromatogram obtained with the test solution is similar in position and size to the principal spot in the chromatogram obtained with the reference solution.

D. It gives the reaction of non-nitrogen substituted barbiturates (*2.3.1*).

TESTS

Appearance of solution. Dissolve 1.0 g in a mixture of 4 ml of *dilute sodium hydroxide solution R* and 6 ml of *water R.* The solution is clear (*2.2.1*) and not more intensely coloured than reference solution Y_6 (*2.2.2, Method II*).

Acidity. Boil 1.0 g with 50 ml of *water R* for 2 min, allow to cool and filter. To 10 ml of the filtrate add 0.15 ml of *methyl red solution R.* The solution is orange-yellow. Not more than 0.1 ml of *0.1 M sodium hydroxide* is required to produce a pure yellow colour.

Related substances. Examine by thin-layer chromatography (*2.2.27*), using *silica gel GF_{254} R* as the coating substance.

Test solution. Dissolve 1.0 g of the substance to be examined in *alcohol R* and dilute to 100 ml with the same solvent.

Reference solution. Dilute 0.5 ml of the test solution to 100 ml with *alcohol R.*

Apply separately to the plate 20 µl of each solution. Develop over a path of 15 cm using the lower layer of a mixture of 5 volumes of *concentrated ammonia R,* 15 volumes of *alcohol R* and 80 volumes of *chloroform R.* Examine immediately in ultraviolet light at 254 nm. Spray with *diphenylcarbazone mercuric reagent R.* Allow the plate to dry in air and spray with freshly prepared *alcoholic potassium hydroxide solution R* diluted 1 in 5 with *aldehyde-free alcohol R*. Heat at 100 °C to 105 °C for 5 min and examine immediately. When examined in ultraviolet light and after spraying, any spot in the chromatogram obtained with the test solution, apart from the principal spot, is not more intense than the spot in the chromatogram obtained with the reference solution (0.5 per cent).

Loss on drying (*2.2.32*). Not more than 0.5 per cent, determined on 1.00 g by drying in an oven at 100 °C to 105 °C.

Sulphated ash (*2.4.14*). Not more than 0.1 per cent, determined on 1.0 g.

ASSAY

Dissolve 85.0 mg in 5 ml of *pyridine R*. Add 0.5 ml of *thymolphthalein solution R* and 10 ml of *silver nitrate solution in pyridine R*. Titrate with *0.1 M ethanolic sodium hydroxide* until a pure blue colour is obtained. Carry out a blank titration.

1 ml of *0.1 M ethanolic sodium hydroxide* is equivalent to 9.21 mg of $C_8H_{12}N_2O_3$.

01/2005:0010

BARIUM SULPHATE

Barii sulfas

$BaSO_4$ M_r 233.4

CHARACTERS

A fine, heavy, white powder, free from gritty particles, practically insoluble in water and in organic solvents. It is very slightly soluble in acids and in solutions of alkali hydroxides.

IDENTIFICATION

A. Boil 0.2 g with 5 ml of a 500 g/l solution of *sodium carbonate R* for 5 min, add 10 ml of *water R*, filter and acidify a part of the filtrate with *dilute hydrochloric acid R*. The solution gives the reactions of sulphates (*2.3.1*).

B. Wash the residue collected in the preceding test with three successive small quantities of *water R*. To the residue add 5 ml of *dilute hydrochloric acid R*, filter and add to the filtrate 0.3 ml of *dilute sulphuric acid R*. A white precipitate is formed that is insoluble in *dilute sodium hydroxide solution R*.

TESTS

Solution S. To 20.0 g add 40 ml of *distilled water R* and 60 ml of *dilute acetic acid R*. Boil for 5 min, filter and dilute the cooled filtrate to 100 ml with *distilled water R*.

Acidity or alkalinity. Heat 5.0 g with 20 ml of *carbon dioxide-free water R* on a water-bath for 5 min and filter. To 10 ml of the filtrate add 0.05 ml of *bromothymol blue solution R1*. Not more than 0.5 ml of *0.01 M hydrochloric acid* or *0.01 M sodium hydroxide* is required to change the colour of the indicator.

Acid-soluble substances. Evaporate 25 ml of solution S to dryness on a water-bath and dry to constant mass at 100-105 °C. The residue weighs not more than 15 mg (0.3 per cent).

Oxidisable sulphur compounds. Shake 1.0 g with 5 ml of *water R* for 30 s and filter. To the filtrate add 0.1 ml of *starch solution R*, dissolve 0.1 g of *potassium iodide R* in the mixture, add 1.0 ml of a freshly prepared 3.6 mg/l solution of *potassium iodate R* and 1 ml of *1 M hydrochloric acid* and shake well. The colour of the solution is more intense than that of a standard prepared at the same time and in the same manner omitting the potassium iodate.

Soluble barium salts. To 10 ml of solution S add 1 ml of *dilute sulphuric acid R*. After 1 h, any opalescence in the solution is not more intense than that in a mixture of 10 ml of solution S and 1 ml of *distilled water R*.

Phosphates. To 1.0 g add a mixture of 3 ml of *dilute nitric acid R* and 7 ml of *water R*. Heat on a water-bath for 5 min, filter and dilute the filtrate to 10 ml with *water R*. Add 5 ml of *molybdovanadic reagent R*. After 5 min, any yellow colour in the test solution is not more intense than that in a standard prepared at the same time and in the same manner using 10 ml of *phosphate standard solution (5 ppm PO_4) R* (50 ppm).

Arsenic (*2.4.2*). In a small long-necked combustion flask, shake 0.5 g with 2 ml of *nitric acid R* and 30 ml of *water R*, insert a small funnel in the neck of the flask, heat in an inclined position on a water-bath for 2 h, allow to cool, adjust to the original volume with *water R* and filter. Wash the residue by decantation with three quantities, each of 5 ml, of *water R*. Combine the filtrate and washings, add 1 ml of *sulphuric acid R*, evaporate to dryness on a water-bath, and heat until copious white fumes are evolved. Dissolve the residue in 10 ml of *dilute sulphuric acid R* and add 10 ml of *water R*. The solution complies with limit test A for arsenic (2 ppm).

Heavy metals (*2.4.8*). Dilute 10 ml of solution S to 20 ml with *water R*, 12 ml of this solution complies with limit test A for heavy metals (10 ppm). Prepare the standard using *lead standard solution (1 ppm Pb) R*.

Loss on ignition. Not more than 2.0 per cent, determined on 1.0 g at 600 °C.

Sedimentation. Place 5.0 g in a glass-stoppered, 50 ml graduated cylinder having the 50 ml graduation mark 14 cm from the base. Add *water R* to 50 ml, shake the mixture for 5 min and allow to stand for 15 min. The barium sulphate does not settle below the 15 ml mark.

01/2005:1975

BASIC BUTYLATED METHACRYLATE COPOLYMER

Copolymerum methacrylatis butylati basicum

DEFINITION

Copolymer of 2-(dimethylamino)ethyl methacrylate, butyl methacrylate and methyl methacrylate having a mean relative molecular mass of about 150 000. The ratio of 2-dimethylaminoethyl methacrylate groups to butyl methacrylate and methyl methacrylate groups is about 2:1:1.

Content of dimethylaminoethyl groups: 20.8 per cent to 25.5 per cent (dried substance).

CHARACTERS

Appearance: colourless or yellowish granules or white powder, slightly hygroscopic.

Solubility: practically insoluble in water, freely soluble in methylene chloride. It dissolves slowly in alcohol.

IDENTIFICATION

A. Infrared absorption spectrophotometry (*2.2.24*).

Comparison: *Ph. Eur. reference spectrum of basic butylated methacrylate copolymer*.

Monographs B

B. It complies with the limits of the assay.

TESTS

Solution S. Dissolve 12.5 g in a mixture of 35.0 g of *acetone R* and 52.5 g of *2-propanol R*.

Viscosity (*2.2.10*): 3 mPa·s to 6 mPa·s, determined on solution S.

Apparatus: rotating viscosimeter.

Dimensions:

- *spindle*: diameter = 25.15 mm, height = 90.74 mm, shaft diameter = 4 mm,
- *cylinder*: diameter = 27.62 mm, height = 0.135 m.

Stirring speed: 30 r/min.

Volume of solution: 16 ml of solution S.

Temperature: 20 °C.

Absorbance (*2.2.25*): maximum 0.30 at 420 nm, determined on solution S.

Appearance of film. Spread evenly 1.0 ml of solution S on a glass plate. Upon drying a clear film is formed.

Monomers: maximum 0.3 per cent, for the sum of contents of butyl methacrylate, methyl methacrylate and 2-dimethylaminoethyl methacrylate calculated by procedures A and B.

A. Butyl methacrylate and methyl methacrylate. Liquid chromatography (*2.2.29*).

Test solution. Dissolve 1.00 g of the substance to be examined in *phosphate buffer solution pH 2.0 R* and dilute to 50.0 ml with the same buffer solution.

Reference solution. Dissolve 10.0 mg of *butyl methacrylate R* and 10.0 mg of *methyl methacrylate R* in 10.0 ml of *acetonitrile R* and dilute to 50.0 ml with *water R*. Dilute 1.0 ml of the solution to 50.0 ml with *water R*.

Column:

- *size*: l = 0.125 m, Ø = 4.6 mm,
- *stationary phase*: *octadecylsilyl silica gel for chromatography R* (7 μm).

Mobile phase: *phosphate buffer solution pH 2.0 R*, *methanol R* (45:55 *V/V*).

Flow rate: 2.0 ml/min.

Detection: spectrophotometer at 205 nm.

Injection: 50 μl.

B. 2-Dimethylaminoethyl methacrylate. Liquid chromatography (*2.2.29*).

Test solution. Dissolve 1.00 g of the substance to be examined in *tetrahydrofuran R* and dilute to 50.0 ml with the same solvent.

Reference solution. Dissolve 10.0 mg of *2-(dimethylamino)ethyl methacrylate R* in *tetrahydrofuran R* and dilute to 50.0 ml with the same solvent. Dilute 2.0 ml of the solution to 50.0 ml with *tetrahydrofuran R*.

Column:

- *size*: l = 0.125 m, Ø = 4.6 mm,
- *stationary phase*: *aminopropylsilyl silica gel for chromatography R* (10 μm).

Mobile phase: mix 25 volumes of a 3.404 g/l solution of *potassium dihydrogen phosphate R* and 75 volumes of *tetrahydrofuran R*.

Flow rate: 2.0 ml/min.

Detection: spectrophotometer at 215 nm.

Injection: 50 μl.

Heavy metals (*2.4.8*): maximum 20 ppm.

2.0 g complies with limit test C. Prepare the standard using 4.0 ml of *lead standard solution (10 ppm Pb) R*.

Loss on drying (*2.2.32*): maximum 2.0 per cent, determined on 1.000 g by drying in an oven at 110 °C for 3 h.

Sulphated ash (*2.4.14*): maximum 0.1 per cent, determined on 1.0 g.

ASSAY

Dissolve 0.200 g in a mixture of 4 ml of *water R* and 96 ml of *anhydrous acetic acid R*. Titrate with *0.1 M perchloric acid*, determining the end-point potentiometrically (*2.2.20*).

1 ml of *0.1 M perchloric acid* is equivalent to 7.21 mg of $C_4H_{10}N$.

STORAGE

In an airtight container.

IMPURITIES

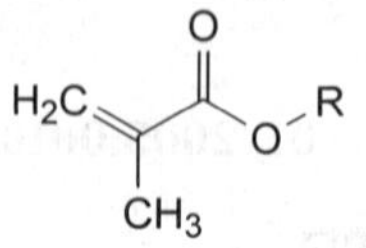

A. R = $[CH_2]_3$-CH_3: butyl methacrylate,

B. R = CH_3: methyl methacrylate,

C. R = CH_2-CH_2-$N(CH_3)_2$: 2-(dimethylamino)ethyl methacrylate.

01/2005:1054

BEARBERRY LEAF

Uvae ursi folium

DEFINITION

Whole or cut, dried leaf of *Arctostaphylos uva-ursi* (L.) Spreng.

Content: minimum 7.0 per cent of anhydrous arbutin ($C_{12}H_{16}O_7$; M_r 272.3) (dried drug).

CHARACTERS

Macroscopic and microscopic characters described under identification tests A and B.

IDENTIFICATION

A. The leaf, shiny and dark green on the adaxial surface, lighter on the abaxial surface, is normally 7 mm to 30 mm long and 5 mm to 12 mm wide. The entire leaf is obovate with smooth margins, somewhat reflexed downwards, narrowing at the base into a short petiole. The leaf is obtuse or retuse at its apex. The lamina is thick and coriaceous. The venation, pinnate and finely reticulate, is clearly visible on both surfaces. The adaxial surface is marked with sunken veinlets, giving it a characteristic grainy appearance. Only the young leaf has ciliated margins. Old leaves are glabrous.

B. Reduce to a powder (355). The powder is green to greenish-grey or yellowish-green. Examine under a microscope using *chloral hydrate solution R*. The powder consists of fragments of epidermises which, seen in surface view, show polygonal cells covered by a thick smooth cuticle, and with straight, thick and irregularly pitted walls; anomocytic stomata (*2.8.3*), surrounded by 5 to 11 subsidiary cells and scars of hair bases only on the abaxial epidermis; fragments of palisade parenchyma, with 3 or 4 layers of cells of unequal lengths, and spongy parenchyma; groups of lignified fibres from the pericycle, with rows of cells containing prisms of calcium oxalate; occasional conical, unicellular covering trichomes.

C. Thin-layer chromatography (*2.2.27*).

Test solution. To 0.5 g of the powdered drug (355) add 5 ml of a mixture of equal volumes of *methanol R* and *water R*, and heat under a reflux condenser for 10 min. Filter whilst hot. Wash the flask and the filter with a mixture of equal volumes of *methanol R* and *water R* and dilute to 5 ml with the same mixture of solvents.

Reference solution. Dissolve 25 mg of *arbutin R*, 25 mg of *gallic acid R* and 25 mg of *hydroquinone R* in *methanol R* and dilute to 10.0 ml with the same solvent.

Plate: *TLC silica gel G plate R.*

Mobile phase: *anhydrous formic acid R, water R, ethyl acetate R* (6:6:88 *V/V/V*).

Application: 10 µl of the reference solution and 20 µl of the test solution, as bands.

Development: over a path of 15 cm.

Drying: at 105-110 °C until the mobile phase has evaporated.

Detection: spray with a 10 g/l solution of *dichloroquinonechlorimide R* in *methanol R*. Next spray with a 20 g/l solution of *anhydrous sodium carbonate R*.

Results: see below the sequence of the zones present in the chromatograms obtained with the reference solution and the test solution. Furthermore, 2 or 3 blue bands and several brown or brownish-grey bands may be present in the chromatogram obtained with the test solution.

Top of the plate	
Hydroquinone: a blue zone	A blue zone
Gallic acid: a brownish zone	A brownish zone
_______	_______
Arbutin: a light blue zone	A light blue zone (arbutin)
Reference solution	**Test solution**

TESTS

Foreign matter (*2.8.2*): maximum 5 per cent of stems and maximum 3 per cent of other foreign matter.

Leaves of different colour: maximum 10 per cent, determined in the same manner as foreign matter (*2.8.2*).

Loss on drying (*2.2.32*): maximum 10.0 per cent, determined on 1.000 g of the powdered drug (355) by drying in an oven at 100-105 °C for 2 h.

Total ash (*2.4.16*): maximum 5.0 per cent.

ASSAY

Liquid chromatography (*2.2.29*).

Test solution. In a 100 ml flask with a ground-glass neck, place 0.800 g of the powdered drug (250). Add 20 ml of *water R* and heat under a reflux condenser on a water-bath for 30 min. Allow to cool and filter the liquid through a plug of absorbent cotton. Add the absorbent cotton to the residue in the 100 ml flask and extract with 20 ml of *water R* under a reflux condenser on a water-bath for 30 min. Allow to cool and filter through a paper filter. Combine the filtrates and dilute to 50.0 ml with *water R*. Filter the liquid through a paper filter. Discard the first 10 ml of the filtrate.

Reference solution. Dissolve 50.0 mg of *arbutin R* in the mobile phase and dilute to 50.0 ml with the mobile phase.

Column:

– *size*: l = 0.25 m, Ø = 4 mm,

– *stationary phase*: *base-deactivated octadecylsilyl silica gel for chromatography R* (5 µm).

Mobile phase: *methanol R, water R* (10:90 *V/V*).

Flow rate: 1.2 ml/min.

Detection: spectrophotometer at 280 nm.

Calculate the percentage content of arbutin using the following expression:

$$\frac{F_1 \times m_2 \times 100}{F_2 \times m_1}$$

F_1 = area of the peak due to arbutin in the chromatogram obtained with the test solution,

F_2 = area of the peak due to arbutin in the chromatogram obtained with the reference solution,

m_1 = mass of the drug to be examined, in grams,

m_2 = mass of *arbutin R* in the reference solution, in grams.

01/2005:0654

BECLOMETASONE DIPROPIONATE

Beclometasoni dipropionas

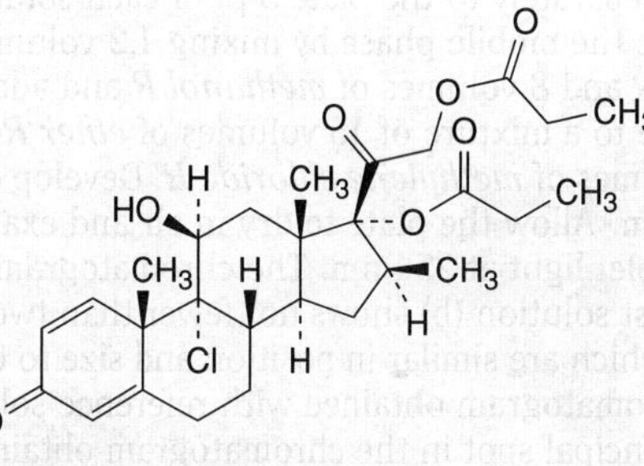

$C_{28}H_{37}ClO_7$ M_r 521.1

DEFINITION

Beclometasone dipropionate contains not less than 96.0 per cent and not more than the equivalent of 103.0 per cent of 9-chloro-11β,17,21-trihydroxy-16β-methylpregna-1,4-diene-3,20-dione 17,21-dipropionate, calculated with reference to the dried substance.

CHARACTERS

A white or almost white, crystalline powder, practically insoluble in water, freely soluble in acetone, sparingly soluble in alcohol.

It melts at about 210 °C, with decomposition.

IDENTIFICATION

First identification: *A, D.*

Second identification: *B, C, D.*

A. Examine by infrared absorption spectrophotometry (*2.2.24*), comparing with the spectrum obtained with *beclometasone dipropionate CRS*. If the spectra obtained in the solid state with the substance to be examined and the reference substance show differences, record further spectra using 50 g/l solutions in *chloroform R*.

B. Examine by thin-layer chromatography (*2.2.27*), using as the coating substance a suitable silica gel with a fluorescent indicator having an optimal intensity at 254 nm.

Test solution (a). Dissolve 25 mg of the substance to be examined in *methanol R* with gentle heating and dilute to 5 ml with the same solvent. (This solution is also used to prepare test solution (b)). Dilute 2 ml of the solution to 10 ml with *chloroform R.*

Test solution (b). Transfer 2 ml of the solution obtained during preparation of test solution (a) to a 15 ml glass tube with a ground-glass stopper or a polytetrafluoroethylene cap. Add 10 ml of *saturated methanolic potassium hydrogen carbonate solution R* and immediately pass a stream of *nitrogen R* briskly through the solution for 5 min. Stopper the tube. Heat in a water-bath at 45 °C, protected from light, for 3 h. Allow to cool.

Reference solution (a). Dissolve 25 mg of *beclometasone dipropionate CRS* in *methanol R* with gentle heating and dilute to 5 ml with the same solvent. (This solution is also used to prepare reference solution (b)). Dilute 2 ml of the solution to 10 ml with *chloroform R.*

Reference solution (b). Transfer 2 ml of the solution obtained during preparation of reference solution (a) to a 15 ml glass tube with a ground-glass stopper or a polytetrafluoroethylene cap. Add 10 ml of *saturated methanolic potassium hydrogen carbonate solution R* and immediately pass a stream of *nitrogen R* briskly through the solution for 5 min. Stopper the tube. Heat in a water-bath at 45 °C, protected from light, for 3 h. Allow to cool.

Apply separately to the plate 5 µl of each solution. Prepare the mobile phase by mixing 1.2 volumes of *water R* and 8 volumes of *methanol R* and adding the mixture to a mixture of 15 volumes of *ether R* and 77 volumes of *methylene chloride R.* Develop over a path of 15 cm. Allow the plate to dry in air and examine in ultraviolet light at 254 nm. The chromatogram obtained with test solution (b) shows not fewer than two distinct spots which are similar in position and size to the spots in the chromatogram obtained with reference solution (b). The principal spot in the chromatogram obtained with test solution (a) is similar in position and size to the principal spot in the chromatogram obtained with reference solution (a). Spray with *alcoholic solution of sulphuric acid R.* Heat at 120 °C for 10 min or until the spots appear. Allow to cool. Examine the plate in daylight and in ultraviolet light at 365 nm. The chromatogram obtained with test solution (b) shows not fewer than two distinct spots, similar in position, colour in daylight, fluorescence in ultraviolet light at 365 nm and size to the spots in the chromatogram obtained with reference solution (b). The principal spot in the chromatogram obtained with test solution (a) is similar in position, colour in daylight, fluorescence in ultraviolet light at 365 nm and size to the principal spot in the chromatogram obtained with reference solution (a). The principal spots in the chromatograms obtained with test solution (b) and reference solution (b) have R_f values distinctly lower than the principal spots in the chromatograms obtained with test solution (a) and reference solution (a).

C. Add about 2 mg to 2 ml of *sulphuric acid R* and shake to dissolve. Within 5 min, a deep reddish-brown colour develops. Add the solution to 10 ml of *water R* and mix. The colour is discharged and a clear solution remains.

D. Treat 25 mg by the oxygen-flask method (*2.5.10*). Use a mixture of 1 ml of *1 M sodium hydroxide* and 20 ml of *water R* to absorb the combustion products. The solution gives reaction (a) of chlorides (*2.3.1*).

TESTS

Specific optical rotation (*2.2.7*). Dissolve 0.250 g in *dioxan R* and dilute to 25.0 ml with the same solvent. The specific optical rotation is + 88 to + 94, calculated with reference to the dried substance.

Absorbance (*2.2.25*). Dissolve 50.0 mg in *alcohol R* and dilute to 100.0 ml with the same solvent. Dilute 2.0 ml of the solution to 50.0 ml with *alcohol R.* The specific absorbance at the maximum at 238 nm is 284 to 302, calculated with reference to the dried substance.

Related substances. Examine by liquid chromatography (*2.2.29*).

Test solution. Dissolve 62.5 mg of the substance to be examined in the mobile phase and dilute to 25.0 ml with the mobile phase.

Reference solution (a). Dissolve 2 mg of *beclometasone 17-propionate CRS* and 2 mg of *beclometasone 21-propionate CRS* in the mobile phase and dilute to 50.0 ml with the mobile phase.

Reference solution (b). Dilute 1.0 ml of the test solution to 50.0 ml with the mobile phase.

The chromatographic procedure may be carried out using:

- a stainless steel column 0.25 m long and 4.6 mm in internal diameter packed with *octadecylsilyl silica gel for chromatography R* (5 µm),
- as mobile phase at a flow rate of 1 ml/min a mixture prepared as follows: mix 600 ml of *acetonitrile R* and 350 ml of *water R,* allow to cool, dilute to 1000 ml with *water R* and mix again,
- as detector a spectrophotometer set at 254 nm and with the sensitivity adjusted so that the height of the principal peak in the chromatogram obtained with reference solution (b) is 70 per cent to 90 per cent of the full scale.

Equilibrate the column with the mobile phase at a flow rate of 1 ml/min for about 45 min. When the chromatograms are recorded in the conditions described above, the retention times are: beclometasone 17-propionate, about 6.2 min; beclometasone 21-propionate, about 6.7 min; beclometasone dipropionate, 13 min to 14 min. Inject 20 µl of reference solution (a). The system is not suitable unless the resolution between the peaks corresponding to beclometasone 17-propionate and beclometasone 21-propionate is at least 1.4; if this resolution is not achieved, adjust the concentration of acetonitrile in the mobile phase. Verify the repeatability by making five separate injections of 20 µl of reference solution (b); the system is not suitable unless the relative standard deviation for the area of the principal peak in the chromatograms obtained with reference solution (b) is less than 2.0 per cent.

Inject separately 20 µl of the test solution and 20 µl of reference solution (b). Continue the chromatography for twice the retention time of the principal peak. In the chromatogram obtained with the test solution: the area of any peak, apart from the principal peak, is not greater than the area of the principal peak in the chromatogram obtained with reference solution (b) (2.0 per cent) and not more than one such peak has an area greater than half the area of the principal peak in the chromatogram obtained with reference solution (b) (1.0 per cent); the sum of the areas of all the peaks, apart from the principal peak, is not greater than 1.25 times the area of the principal peak in the chromatogram obtained with reference solution (b) (2.5 per cent). Disregard any peak due to the solvent and any peak with an area less than 0.025 times the area of the principal peak in the chromatogram obtained with reference solution (b).

Loss on drying (*2.2.32*). Not more than 0.5 per cent, determined on 1.000 g by drying in an oven at 100 °C to 105 °C for 3 h.

ASSAY

Protect the solutions from light throughout the assay. The coloured reaction products tend to adsorb to the surface of glassware. To avoid low results, it is recommended that the glassware be treated with the coloured reaction products before use and that the treated glassware be reserved for this assay and washed only with water R between assays.

Dissolve an accurately weighed quantity in sufficient *aldehyde-free alcohol R* to produce a solution containing 340 µg to 360 µg in 10.0 ml. Prepare a reference solution at the same time and in the same manner, using *beclometasone dipropionate CRS*. Into two 25 ml volumetric flasks, introduce respectively 10.0 ml of each solution. Into a third identical flask, introduce 10 ml of *aldehyde-free alcohol R*. To each flask add 2.0 ml of *triphenyltetrazolium chloride solution R*. Displace the air from the flasks using *oxygen-free nitrogen R*, immediately add 2.0 ml of *dilute tetramethylammonium hydroxide solution R* and again displace the air with *oxygen-free nitrogen R*. Stopper the flasks, mix the contents by gentle swirling and allow to stand in a water-bath at 35 °C for 2 h. Cool rapidly and dilute to 25.0 ml with *aldehyde-free alcohol R*. Immediately measure the absorbance (*2.2.25*) of the test solution and of the reference solution at the maximum at 485 nm, using a closed 1 cm cell and as the compensation liquid the solution prepared from 10 ml of *aldehyde-free alcohol R*. Treat the test solution and the reference solution in such a manner that the period of time that elapses between the addition of the *dilute tetramethylammonium hydroxide solution R* and measurement of the absorbance is exactly the same for each solution.

Calculate the content of $C_{28}H_{37}ClO_7$ from the absorbances measured and the concentrations of the solutions.

STORAGE

Store protected from light.

01/2005:0069

BEESWAX, WHITE

Cera alba

DEFINITION

Wax obtained by bleaching yellow beeswax.

CHARACTERS

Appearance: white or yellowish-white pieces or plates, translucent when thin, with a fine-grained, matt and non-crystalline fracture; when warmed in the hand they become soft and malleable.

It has an odour similar to that of yellow beeswax, though fainter and never rancid. It is tasteless and does not stick to the teeth.

Solubility: practically insoluble in water, partially soluble in hot alcohol (90 per cent *V/V*) and completely soluble in fatty and essential oils.

Relative density: about 0.960.

TESTS

Drop point (*2.2.17*): 61 °C to 66 °C.

Melt the beeswax by heating on a water-bath, pour onto a glass plate and allow to cool to a semi-solid mass. Fill the metal cup by inserting the wider end into the beeswax and repeating the procedure until beeswax extrudes from the narrow opening. Remove the excess with a spatula and insert the thermometer immediately. Remove the beeswax displaced. Allow to stand at room temperature for at least 12 h before determining the drop point.

Acid value: 17.0 to 24.0.

To 2.00 g (*m* g), in a 250 ml conical flask fitted with a reflux condenser, add 40 ml of *xylene R* and a few glass beads. Heat until the substance is dissolved. Add 20 ml of *alcohol R* and 0.5 ml of *phenolphthalein solution R1* and titrate the hot solution with *0.5 M alcoholic potassium hydroxide* until a red colour persists for at least 10 s (n_1 ml). Carry out a blank test (n_2 ml).

$$\text{Acid value} = \frac{28.05\,(n_1 - n_2)}{m}$$

Ester value (*2.5.2*): 70 to 80.

Saponification value: 87 to 104.

To 2.00 g (*m* g), in a 250 ml conical flask fitted with a reflux condenser, add 30 ml of a mixture of equal volumes of *alcohol R* and *xylene R* and a few glass beads. Heat until the substance is dissolved. Add 25.0 ml of *0.5 M alcoholic potassium hydroxide* and heat under a reflux condenser for 3 h. Titrate the hot solution immediately with *0.5 M hydrochloric acid*, using 1 ml of *phenolphthalein solution R1* as indicator (n_1 ml). Reheat the solution to boiling several times during the course of the titration. Carry out a blank test (n_2 ml).

$$\text{Saponification value} = \frac{28.05\,(n_2 - n_1)}{m}$$

Ceresin, paraffins and certain other waxes. To 3.0 g, in a 100 ml round-bottomed flask, add 30 ml of a 40 g/l solution of *potassium hydroxide R* in *aldehyde-free alcohol R* and boil gently under a reflux condenser for 2 h. Remove the condenser and immediately insert a thermometer. Place the flask in a water-bath at 80 °C and allow to cool, swirling the solution continuously. No precipitate is formed until 65 °C, although the solution may be slightly opalescent. Above 65 °C, the solution may become cloudy and precipitates may be formed. At 59 °C, the solution is cloudy.

Glycerol and other polyols: maximum 0.5 per cent *m/m*, calculated as glycerol.

To 0.20 g add 10 ml of *alcoholic potassium hydroxide solution R* and heat on a water-bath under a reflux condenser for 30 min. Add 50 ml of *dilute sulphuric acid R*, cool and filter. Rinse the flask and the filter with *dilute sulphuric acid R*. Combine the filtrate and washings and dilute to 100.0 ml with *dilute sulphuric acid R*. Place 1.0 ml of the solution in a test-tube, add 0.5 ml of a 10.7 g/l solution of *sodium periodate R*, mix and allow to stand for 5 min. Add 1.0 ml of *decolorised fuchsin solution R* and mix. Any precipitate disappears. Place the tube in a beaker containing water at 40 °C. During cooling observe for 10-15 min. Any violet-blue colour in the solution is not more intense than that in a standard prepared at the same time and in the same manner using 1.0 ml of a 10 mg/l solution of *glycerol R* in *dilute sulphuric acid R*.

Monographs B

01/2005:0070

BEESWAX, YELLOW

Cera flava

DEFINITION

Wax obtained by melting the walls of the honeycomb made by the honey-bee, *Apis mellifera* L., with hot water and removing foreign matter.

CHARACTERS

Appearance: yellow or light brown pieces or plates with a fine-grained, matt and non-crystalline fracture; when warmed in the hand they become soft and malleable.

It has a faint odour, characteristic of honey. It is tasteless and does not stick to the teeth.

Solubility: practically insoluble in water, partially soluble in hot alcohol (90 per cent *V/V*) and completely soluble in fatty and essential oils.

Relative density: about 0.960.

TESTS

Drop point (*2.2.17*): 61 °C to 66 °C.

Melt the beeswax by heating on a water-bath, pour onto a glass plate and allow to cool to a semi-solid mass. Fill the metal cup by inserting the wider end into the beeswax and repeating the procedure until beeswax extrudes from the narrow opening. Remove the excess with a spatula and insert the thermometer immediately. Remove the beeswax displaced. Allow to stand at room temperature for at least 12 h before determining the drop point.

Acid value: 17.0 to 22.0.

To 2.00 g (*m* g), in a 250 ml conical flask fitted with a reflux condenser, add 40 ml of *xylene R* and a few glass beads. Heat until the substance is dissolved. Add 20 ml of *alcohol R* and 0.5 ml of *phenolphthalein solution R1* and titrate the hot solution with *0.5 M alcoholic potassium hydroxide* until a red colour persists for at least 10 s (n_1 ml). Carry out a blank test (n_2 ml).

$$\text{Acid value} = \frac{28.05\,(n_1 - n_2)}{m}$$

Ester value (*2.5.2*): 70 to 80.

Saponification value: 87 to 102.

To 2.00 g (*m* g), in a 250 ml conical flask fitted with a reflux condenser, add 30 ml of a mixture of equal volumes of *alcohol R* and *xylene R* and a few glass beads. Heat until the substance is dissolved. Add 25.0 ml of *0.5 M alcoholic potassium hydroxide* and heat under a reflux condenser for 3 h. Titrate the hot solution immediately with *0.5 M hydrochloric acid*, using 1 ml of *phenolphthalein solution R1* as indicator (n_1 ml). Reheat the solution to boiling several times during the course of the titration. Carry out a blank test (n_2 ml).

$$\text{Saponification value} = \frac{28.05\,(n_2 - n_1)}{m}$$

Ceresin, paraffins and certain other waxes. To 3.0 g, in a 100 ml round-bottomed flask, add 30 ml of a 40 g/l solution of *potassium hydroxide R* in *aldehyde-free alcohol R* and boil gently under a reflux condenser for 2 h. Remove the condenser and immediately insert a thermometer. Place the flask in a water-bath at 80 °C and allow to cool, swirling the solution continuously. No precipitate is formed until 65 °C, although the solution may be slightly opalescent. Above 65 °C, the solution may become cloudy and precipitates may be formed. At 59 °C, the solution is cloudy.

Glycerol and other polyols: maximum 0.5 per cent *m/m*, calculated as glycerol.

To 0.20 g add 10 ml of *alcoholic potassium hydroxide solution R* and heat on a water-bath under a reflux condenser for 30 min. Add 50 ml of *dilute sulphuric acid R*, cool and filter. Rinse the flask and the filter with *dilute sulphuric acid R*. Combine the filtrate and washings and dilute to 100.0 ml with *dilute sulphuric acid R*. Place 1.0 ml of the solution in a test-tube, add 0.5 ml of a 10.7 g/l solution of *sodium periodate R*, mix and allow to stand for 5 min. Add 1.0 ml of *decolorised fuchsin solution R* and mix. Any precipitate disappears. Place the tube in a beaker containing water at 40 °C. During cooling observe for 10-15 min. Any violet-blue colour in the solution is not more intense than that in a standard prepared at the same time and in the same manner using 1.0 ml of a 10 mg/l solution of *glycerol R* in *dilute sulphuric acid R*.

01/2005:0221

BELLADONNA LEAF

Belladonnae folium

DEFINITION

Belladonna leaf consists of the dried leaf or of the dried leaf and flowering, and occasionally fruit-bearing, tops of *Atropa belladonna* L. It contains not less than 0.30 per cent of total alkaloids, calculated as hyoscyamine (M_r 289.4) with reference to the drug dried at 100 °C to 105 °C. The alkaloids consist mainly of hyoscyamine together with small quantities of hyoscine (scopolamine).

CHARACTERS

Belladonna leaf has a slightly nauseous odour.

It has the macroscopic and microscopic characters described under identification tests A and B.

IDENTIFICATION

A. The leaves are green to brownish-green, slightly darker on the upper surface, often crumpled and rolled and partly matted together in the drug. The leaf is petiolate and the base of the lamina is acute and decurrent and the margin entire. The flowering stems are flattened and bear at each node a pair of leaves unequal in size, in the axils of which occur singly the flowers or occasionally fruits. The flowers have a gamosepalous calyx and campanulate corolla. The fruits are globular berries, green to brownish-black and surrounded by the persistent calyx with widely spread lobes.

B. Reduce to a powder (355). The powder is dark green. Examine under a microscope, using *chloral hydrate solution R*. The powder shows the following diagnostic characters: fragments of leaf lamina showing sinuous-walled epidermal cells, a striated cuticle and numerous stomata predominantly present on the lower epidermis (anisocytic and also some anomocytic); multicellular uniseriate covering trichomes with smooth cuticle, glandular trichomes with unicellular heads and multicellular, uniseriate stalks or with multicellular heads and unicellular stalks; parenchyma cells including rounded cells containing microsphenoidal crystals of calcium oxalate; annular and spirally thickened vessels. The powdered drug may also show the following: fibres and reticulately thickened vessels from the stems; subspherical pollen grains, 40 µm to 50 µm in diameter, with three germinal pores, three furrows and an extensively pitted exine; fragments of the corolla, with a papillose epidermis or bearing numerous covering or glandular trichomes of the types previously described; brownish-yellow seed fragments containing irregularly sclerified and pitted cells of the testa.

C. Shake 1 g of powdered drug with 10 ml of *0.05 M sulphuric acid* for 2 min. Filter and add to the filtrate 1 ml of *concentrated ammonia R* and 5 ml of *water R*. Shake cautiously with 15 ml of *ether R*, avoiding formation of an emulsion. Separate the ether layer and dry over *anhydrous sodium sulphate R*. Filter and evaporate the ether in a porcelain dish. Add 0.5 ml of *fuming nitric acid R* and evaporate to dryness on a water-bath. Add 10 ml of *acetone R* and, dropwise, a 30 g/l solution of *potassium hydroxide R* in *alcohol R*. A deep violet colour develops.

D. Examine the chromatogram obtained in the chromatography test. The principal zones in the chromatogram obtained with the test solution are similar in position, colour and size to the principal zones in the chromatogram obtained with the same volume of the reference solution.

TESTS

Chromatography. Examine by thin-layer chromatography (*2.2.27*), using *silica gel G R* as the coating substance.

Test solution. To 0.6 g of powdered drug (180) add 15 ml of *0.05 M sulphuric acid*, shake for 15 min and filter. Wash the filter with *0.05 M sulphuric acid* until 20 ml of filtrate is obtained. To the filtrate add 1 ml of *concentrated ammonia R* and shake with two quantities, each of 10 ml, of *peroxide-free ether R*. If necessary, separate by centrifugation. Dry the combined ether layers over *anhydrous sodium sulphate R*, filter and evaporate to dryness on a water-bath. Dissolve the residue in 0.5 ml of *methanol R*.

Reference solution. Dissolve 50 mg of *hyoscyamine sulphate R* in 9 ml of *methanol R*. Dissolve 15 mg of *hyoscine hydrobromide R* in 10 ml of *methanol R*. Mix 1.8 ml of the hyoscine hydrobromide solution and 8 ml of the hyoscyamine sulphate solution.

Apply separately to the plate as bands 20 mm by 3 mm 10 µl and 20 µl of each solution, leaving 1 cm between the bands. Develop over a path of 10 cm using a mixture of 3 volumes of *concentrated ammonia R*, 7 volumes of *water R* and 90 volumes of *acetone R*. Dry the plate at 100 °C to 105 °C for 15 min, allow to cool and spray with *potassium iodobismuthate solution R2*, using about 10 ml for a plate 200 mm square, until the orange or brown zones become visible against a yellow background. The zones in the chromatograms obtained with the test solution are similar to those in the chromatograms obtained with the reference solution with respect to their position (hyoscyamine in the lower third, hyoscine in the upper third of the chromatogram) and their colour. The zones in the chromatograms obtained with the test solution are at least equal in size to the corresponding zones in the chromatogram obtained with the same volume of the reference solution. Faint secondary zones may appear, particularly in the middle of the chromatogram obtained with 20 µl of the test solution or near the starting-point in the chromatogram obtained with 10 µl of the test solution. Spray the plate with *sodium nitrite solution R* until the coating is transparent. Examine after 15 min. The zones corresponding to hyoscyamine in the chromatograms obtained with the test solution and the reference solution change from brown to reddish-brown but not to greyish-blue (atropine) and any secondary zones disappear.

Foreign matter (*2.8.2*). Not more than 3 per cent of stem having a diameter exceeding 5 mm.

Total ash (*2.4.16*). Not more than 16.0 per cent.

Ash insoluble in hydrochloric acid (*2.8.1*). Not more than 4.0 per cent

ASSAY

Take about 50 g of drug and completely reduce it to a powder (180). Using the powder, determine the loss on drying and the total alkaloids.

a) Determine the loss on drying (*2.2.32*) on 2.000 g, by drying in an oven at 100 °C to 105 °C.

b) Moisten 10.00 g of powder with a mixture of 5 ml of *ammonia R*, 10 ml of *alcohol R* and 30 ml of *peroxide-free ether R* and mix thoroughly. Transfer the mixture to a suitable percolator, if necessary with the aid of the extracting mixture. Allow to macerate for 4 h and percolate with a mixture of 1 volume of *chloroform R* and 3 volumes of *peroxide-free ether R* until the alkaloids are completely extracted. Evaporate to dryness a few millilitres of the liquid flowing from the percolator, dissolve the residue in *0.25 M sulphuric acid* and verify the absence of alkaloids using *potassium tetraiodomercurate solution R*. Concentrate the percolate to about 50 ml by distilling on a water-bath and transfer it to a separating funnel, rinsing with *peroxide-free ether R*. Add a quantity of *peroxide-free ether R* equal to at least 2.1 times the volume of the percolate to produce a liquid of a density well below that of water. Shake the solution with no fewer than three quantities, each of 20 ml, of *0.25 M sulphuric acid*, separate the two layers by centrifugation if necessary and transfer the acid layers to a second separating funnel. Make the acid layer alkaline with *ammonia R* and shake with three quantities, each of 30 ml, of *chloroform R*. Combine the chloroform layers, add 4 g of *anhydrous sodium sulphate R* and allow to stand for 30 min with occasional shaking. Decant the chloroform and wash the sodium sulphate with three quantities, each of 10 ml, of *chloroform R*. Add the washings to the chloroform extract, evaporate to dryness on a water-bath and heat in an oven at 100 °C to 105 °C for 15 min. Dissolve the residue in a few millilitres of *chloroform R*, add 20.0 ml of *0.01 M sulphuric acid* and remove the chloroform by evaporation on a water-bath. Titrate the excess of acid with *0.02 M sodium hydroxide* using *methyl red mixed solution R* as indicator.

Calculate the percentage content of total alkaloids, expressed as hyoscyamine, from the expression:

$$\frac{57.88 \times (20 - n)}{(100 - d) \times m}$$

d = loss on drying as a percentage,

n = volume of *0.02 M sodium hydroxide* used in millilitres,

m = mass of drug used in grams.

STORAGE

Store protected from light.

Monographs B

01/2005:1294

BELLADONNA LEAF DRY EXTRACT, STANDARDISED

Belladonnae folii extractum siccum normatum

DEFINITION

Standardised belladonna leaf dry extract is produced from *Belladonna leaf (0221)*. It contains not less than 0.95 per cent and not more than 1.05 per cent of total alkaloids, calculated as hyoscyamine ($C_{17}H_{23}NO_3$, M_r 289.4), with reference to the dried extract.

PRODUCTION

The extract is produced from the drug and ethanol (70 per cent *V/V*) using an appropriate procedure.

CHARACTERS

A hygroscopic brown or greenish powder.

IDENTIFICATION

A. Examine by thin-layer chromatography (*2.2.27*), using a suitable silica gel as the coating substance.

Test solution. To 1 g of the extract to be examined add 5.0 ml of *methanol R*. Shake for 2 min and filter.

Reference solution. Dissolve 1.0 mg of *chlorogenic acid R* and 2.5 mg of *rutin R* in 10 ml of *methanol R*.

Apply to the plate, as bands, 20 µl of each solution. Develop over a path of 15 cm using a mixture of 10 volumes of *anhydrous formic acid R*, 10 volumes of *water R*, 30 volumes of *methyl ethyl ketone R* and 50 volumes of *ethyl acetate R*. Dry the plate at 100 °C to 105 °C and spray the warm plate with a 10 g/l solution of *diphenylboric acid aminoethyl ester R* in *methanol R*. Subsequently spray the plate with a 50 g/l solution of *macrogol 400 R* in *methanol R*. Allow the plate to dry in air for 30 min and examine in ultraviolet light at 365 nm. The chromatograms obtained with the reference solution and the test solution show in the central part a light blue fluorescent zone (chlorogenic acid) and in the lower part a yellowish-brown fluorescent zone (rutin). Furthermore, the chromatogram obtained with the test solution shows a little above the start a yellowish-brown fluorescent zone and directly above a yellow fluorescent zone, a yellow or yellowish-brown fluorescent zone between the zone due to rutin and the zone due to chlorogenic acid. Further zones may be present.

B. Examine the chromatogram obtained in the test for atropine. The principal zones in the chromatogram obtained with the test solution are similar in position and colour to the principal zones in the chromatogram obtained with the reference solution.

TESTS

Atropine. Examine by thin-layer chromatography (*2.2.27*), using a suitable silica gel as the coating substance.

Test solution. To 0.20 g of the extract to be examined add 10.0 ml of *0.05 M sulphuric acid*, shake for 2 min and filter. Add 1.0 ml of *concentrated ammonia R* and shake with two quantities, each of 10 ml, of *peroxide-free ether R*. If necessary, separate by centrifugation. Dry the combined ether layers over about 2 g of *anhydrous sodium sulphate R*, filter and evaporate to dryness on a water-bath. Dissolve the residue in 0.5 ml of *methanol R*.

Reference solution. Dissolve 50 mg of *hyoscyamine sulphate R* in 9 ml of *methanol R*. Dissolve 15 mg of *hyoscine hydrobromide R* in 10 ml of *methanol R*. Mix 1.8 ml of the hyoscine hydrobromide solution and 8 ml of the hyoscyamine sulphate solution.

Apply to the plate, as bands, 20 µl of each solution. Develop over a path of 10 cm using a mixture of 3 volumes of *concentrated ammonia R*, 7 volumes of *water R* and 90 volumes of *acetone R*. Dry the plate at 100 °C to 105 °C for 15 min, allow to cool and spray with *potassium iodobismuthate solution R2*, until the orange or brown zones become visible against a yellow background. The zones in the chromatogram obtained with the test solution are similar to those in the chromatogram obtained with the reference solution with respect to their position (hyoscyamine in the lower third, hyoscine in the upper third of the chromatogram) and their colour. Other faint zones may be present in the chromatogram obtained with the test solution. Spray the plate with *sodium nitrite solution R* until the coating is transparent. Examine after 15 min. The zones corresponding to hyoscyamine in the chromatograms obtained with the test solution and the reference solution change from orange or brown to reddish-brown but not to greyish-blue (atropine).

Loss on drying (*2.8.17*): maximum 5.0 per cent.

Microbial contamination. Total viable aerobic count (*2.6.12*) not more than 10^4 micro-organisms per gram of which not more than 10^2 fungi per gram, determined by plate count. It complies with the tests for *Escherichia coli* and for *Salmonella* (*2.6.13*).

ASSAY

At each extraction stage it is necessary to check that the alkaloids have been completely extracted. If the extraction is into the organic phase this is done by evaporating to dryness a few millilitres of the last organic layer, dissolving the residue in *0.25 M sulphuric acid* and verifying the absence of alkaloids using *potassium tetraiodomercurate solution R*. If the extraction is into the acid aqueous phase, this is done by taking a few millilitres of the last acid aqueous phase and verifying the absence of alkaloids using *potassium tetraiodomercurate solution R*.

Disperse 3.00 g in a mixture of 5 ml of *ammonia R* and 15 ml of *water R*. Shake with no fewer than three quantities, each of 40 ml of a mixture of 1 volume of *methylene chloride R* and 3 volumes of *peroxide-free ether R* until the alkaloids are completely extracted. Concentrate the combined organic layers to about 50 ml by distilling on a water-bath and transfer the resulting liquid to a separating funnel, rinsing with *peroxide-free ether R*. Add a quantity of *peroxide-free ether R* equal to at least 2.1 times the volume of the liquid to produce a layer having a density well below that of water. Shake the resulting solution with no fewer than three quantities, each of 20 ml, of *0.25 M sulphuric acid* until the alkaloids are completely extracted. Separate the layers by centrifugation, if necessary and transfer the acid layers to a second separating funnel. Make the combined acid layers alkaline with *ammonia R* and shake with no fewer than three quantities, each of 30 ml, of *methylene chloride R* until the alkaloids are completely extracted. Combine the organic layers, add 4 g of *anhydrous sodium sulphate R* and allow to stand for 30 min with occasional shaking. Decant the methylene chloride and wash the sodium sulphate with three quantities, each of 10 ml, of *methylene chloride R*. Combine the organic extracts, evaporate to dryness on a water-bath. Heat the residue in an oven at 100 °C to 105 °C for 15 min. Dissolve the residue in a few millilitres of *methylene chloride R*, evaporate to dryness on a water-bath and again heat the residue in an oven at 100 °C to 105 °C for 15 min. Dissolve the residue in a few millilitres of *methylene chloride R*, add 20.0 ml of *0.01 M sulphuric acid* and remove the methylene chloride by evaporation on a water-bath. Titrate the excess of acid with *0.02 M sodium hydroxide* using *methyl red mixed solution R* as indicator.

Calculate the percentage content of total alkaloids, expressed as hyoscyamine, from the expression:

$$\frac{57.88 \times (20 - n)}{100 \times m}$$

n = volume of *0.02 M sodium hydroxide* used, in millilitres,

m = mass of the substance to be examined, in grams.

STORAGE

Store in an airtight container, protected from light.

01/2005:1812

BELLADONNA LEAF TINCTURE, STANDARDISED

Belladonnae folii tinctura normata

DEFINITION

Tincture produced from *Belladonna leaf (0221)*.

Content: 0.027 per cent to 0.033 per cent of total alkaloids, calculated as hyoscyamine ($C_{17}H_{23}NO_3$; M_r 289.4). The alkaloids consist mainly of hyoscyamine together with small quantities of hyoscine.

PRODUCTION

The tincture is produced from 1 part of the powdered drug (355) and 10 parts of ethanol (70 per cent *V/V*) by a suitable procedure.

IDENTIFICATION

A. Thin-layer chromatography (*2.2.27*).

Test solution. Evaporate to dryness 10.0 ml of the tincture to be examined in a water-bath at 40 °C under reduced pressure. Dissolve the residue in 1.0 ml of *methanol R*.

Reference solution. Dissolve 1.0 mg of *chlorogenic acid R* and 2.5 mg of *rutin R* in 10 ml of *methanol R*.

Plate: *TLC silica gel plate R.*

Mobile phase: *anhydrous formic acid R, water R, methyl ethyl ketone R, ethyl acetate R* (10:10:30:50 *V/V/V/V*).

Application: 40 µl, as bands.

Development: over a path of 15 cm.

Drying: at 100-105 °C.

Detection: spray the warm plate with a 10 g/l solution of *diphenylboric acid aminoethyl ester R* in *methanol R*; subsequently spray the plate with a 50 g/l solution of *macrogol 400 R* in *methanol R*; allow the plate to dry in air for 30 min and examine in ultraviolet light at 365 nm.

Results: see below the sequence of zones present in the chromatograms obtained with the reference solution and the test solution. Furthermore, other fluorescent zones may be present in the chromatogram obtained with the test solution.

Top of the plate	
———	———
Chlorogenic acid: a light blue fluorescent zone	A light blue fluorescent zone (chlorogenic acid) A yellow or yellowish-brown fluorescent zone
———	———
Rutin: a yellowish-brown fluorescent zone	A bluish-grey fluorescent zone A yellow fluorescent zone A yellowish-brown fluorescent zone
Reference solution	**Test solution**

B. Examine the chromatograms obtained in the test for atropine, detection A.

Results A: see below the sequence of zones present in the chromatograms obtained with the reference solution and the test solution. Faint secondary zones may appear, particularly in the middle of the chromatogram obtained with 40 µl of the test solution or near the starting point in the chromatogram obtained with 20 µl of the test solution.

Top of the plate	
Hyoscine: a brownish-orange zone	A brownish-orange zone (hyoscine)
	———
	Faint secondary zones
Hyoscyamine: a brownish-orange zone	A brownish-orange zone (hyoscyamine) Faint secondary zones
Reference solution	**Test solution**

TESTS

Atropine. Thin-layer chromatography (*2.2.27*).

Test solution. To 15.0 ml of the tincture to be examined add 15 ml of *0.05 M sulphuric acid*. Filter. Add 1 ml of *concentrated ammonia R* to the filtrate and shake with 2 quantities, each of 10 ml, of *peroxide-free ether R*. Separate by centrifugation if necessary. Dry the combined ether layers over *anhydrous sodium sulphate R*. Filter and evaporate to dryness on a water-bath. Dissolve the residue in 0.5 ml of *methanol R*.

Reference solution. Dissolve 50 mg of *hyoscyamine sulphate R* in 9 ml of *methanol R*. Dissolve 15 mg of *hyoscine hydrobromide R* in 10 ml of *methanol R*. Mix 1.8 ml of the hyoscine hydrobromide solution and 8 ml of the hyoscyamine sulphate solution.

Plate: *TLC silica gel plate R.*

Mobile phase: *concentrated ammonia R, water R, acetone R* (3:7:90 *V/V/V*).

Application: 20 µl and 40 µl of each solution, as bands.

Development: over a path of 10 cm.

Drying: at 100-105 °C for 15 min.

Detection A: spray with *potassium iodobismuthate solution R2.*

Detection B: spray with *sodium nitrite solution R* until the plate is transparent. Examine after 15 min.

Results B: the zones due to hyoscyamine in the chromatograms obtained with the test solution and the reference solution change from brownish-orange to reddish-brown but not to greyish-blue (atropine) and any secondary zones disappear.

Ethanol (*2.9.10*): 64 per cent *V/V* to 69 per cent *V/V*.

ASSAY

Evaporate 50.0 g of the tincture to be examined to a volume of about 10 ml. Transfer quantitatively to a separating funnel, with the minimum volume of *alcohol (70 per cent V/V) R*. Add 5 ml of *ammonia R* and 15 ml of *water R*. Shake with not fewer than 3 quantities each of 40 ml of a mixture of 1 volume of *methylene chloride R* and 3 volumes of *peroxide-free ether R*, carefully to avoid emulsion, until the alkaloids are completely extracted. Combine the organic layers and concentrate the solution to a volume of about 50 ml by distilling on a water-bath. Transfer the resulting solution quantitatively to a separating funnel, rinsing with *peroxide-free ether R*. Add a quantity of *peroxide-free ether R* equal to at least 2.1 times the volume of the solution to produce a layer having a density well below that of water. Shake the resulting solution with not fewer than 3 quantities each of 20 ml of *0.25 M sulphuric acid* until the alkaloids are completely extracted. Separate the layers by centrifugation if necessary and transfer the layers to a separating funnel. Make the combined layers alkaline with *ammonia R* and shake with not fewer than 3 quantities each of 30 ml of *methylene chloride R* until the alkaloids are completely extracted. Combine the organic layers, add 4 g of *anhydrous sodium sulphate R* and allow to stand for 30 min with occasional shaking. Decant the methylene chloride and filter. Wash the sodium sulphate with 3 quantities each of 10 ml of *methylene chloride R*. Combine the organic extracts, evaporate to dryness on a water-bath. Heat the residue in an oven at 100-105 °C for 15 min. Dissolve the residue in a few millilitres of *methylene chloride R*, evaporate to dryness on a water-bath and heat the residue in an oven at 100-105 °C for 15 min again. Dissolve the residue in a few millilitres of *methylene chloride R*. Add 20.0 ml of *0.01 M sulphuric acid* and remove the methylene chloride by evaporation on a water-bath. Titrate the excess of acid with *0.02 M sodium hydroxide* using *methyl red mixed solution R* as indicator.

Calculate the percentage content of total alkaloids, expressed as hyoscyamine, from the expression:

$$\frac{57.88 \times (20 - n)}{100 \times m}$$

n = volume of *0.02 M sodium hydroxide* used, in millilitres,

m = mass of drug used, in grams.

01/2005:0222

BELLADONNA, PREPARED

Belladonnae pulvis normatus

DEFINITION

Prepared belladonna is belladonna leaf powder (180) adjusted if necessary by adding powdered lactose or belladonna leaf powder with a lower alkaloidal content to contain 0.28 per cent to 0.32 per cent of total alkaloids, calculated as hyoscyamine (M_r 289.4) with reference to the dried drug.

CHARACTERS

Slightly nauseous odour.

IDENTIFICATION

A. The powder is dark green. Examine under a microscope, using *chloral hydrate solution R*. The powder shows the following diagnostic characters: fragments of leaf lamina showing sinuous-walled epidermal cells, a striated cuticle and numerous stomata predominantly present on the lower epidermis (anisocytic and also some anomocytic); multicellular uniseriate covering trichomes with smooth cuticle, glandular trichomes with unicellular heads and multicellular, uniseriate stalks or with multicellular heads and unicellular stalks; parenchyma cells including rounded cells containing microsphenoidal crystals of calcium oxalate; annular and spirally thickened vessels. The powdered drug may also show the following: fibres and reticulately thickened vessels from the stems; subspherical pollen grains, 40 µm to 50 µm in diameter, with three germinal pores, three furrows and an extensively pitted exine; fragments of the corolla, with a papillose epidermis or bearing numerous covering or glandular trichomes of the types previously described; brownish-yellow seed fragments containing irregularly sclerified and pitted cells of the testa. Examined in *glycerol (85 per cent) R*, it may be seen to contain lactose crystals.

B. Shake 1 g with 10 ml of *0.05 M sulphuric acid* for 2 min. Filter and add to the filtrate 1 ml of *concentrated ammonia R* and 5 ml of *water R*. Shake cautiously with 15 ml of *ether R*, avoiding formation of an emulsion. Separate the ether layer and dry over *anhydrous sodium sulphate R*. Filter and evaporate the ether in a porcelain dish. Add 0.5 ml of *fuming nitric acid R* and evaporate to dryness on a water-bath. Add 10 ml of *acetone R* and, dropwise, a 30 g/l solution of *potassium hydroxide R* in *alcohol R*. A deep violet colour develops.

C. Examine the chromatogram obtained in the chromatography test. The principal zones in the chromatogram obtained with the test solution are similar in position, colour and size to the principal zones in the chromatogram obtained with the same volume of the reference solution.

TESTS

Chromatography. Examine by thin-layer chromatography (*2.2.27*), using *silica gel G R* as the coating substance.

Test solution. To 0.6 g add 15 ml of *0.05 M sulphuric acid*, shake for 15 min and filter. Wash the filter with *0.05 M sulphuric acid* until 20 ml of filtrate is obtained. To the filtrate add 1 ml of *concentrated ammonia R* and shake with two quantities, each of 10 ml, of *peroxide-free ether R*. If necessary, separate by centrifugation. Dry the combined ether layers over *anhydrous sodium sulphate R*, filter and evaporate to dryness on a water-bath. Dissolve the residue in 0.5 ml of *methanol R*.

Reference solution. Dissolve 50 mg of *hyoscyamine sulphate R* in 9 ml of *methanol R*. Dissolve 15 mg of *hyoscine hydrobromide R* in 10 ml of *methanol R*. Mix 1.8 ml of the hyoscine hydrobromide solution and 8 ml of the hyoscyamine sulphate solution.

Apply separately to the plate as bands 20 mm by 3 mm 10 µl and 20 µl of each solution, leaving 1 cm between the bands. Develop over a path of 10 cm using a mixture of 3 volumes of *concentrated ammonia R*, 7 volumes of *water R* and 90 volumes of *acetone R*. Dry the plate at 100 °C to 105 °C for 15 min, allow to cool and spray with *potassium iodobismuthate solution R2*, using about

10 ml for a plate 200 mm square, until the orange or brown zones become visible against a yellow background. The zones in the chromatograms obtained with the test solution are similar to those in the chromatograms obtained with the reference solution with respect to their position (hyoscyamine in the lower third, hyoscine in the upper third of the chromatogram) and their colour. The zones in the chromatograms obtained with the test solution are at least equal in size to the corresponding zones in the chromatogram obtained with the same volume of the reference solution. Faint secondary zones may appear, particularly in the middle of the chromatogram obtained with 20 µl of the test solution or near the starting-point in the chromatogram obtained with 10 µl of the test solution. Spray the plate with *sodium nitrite solution R* until the coating is transparent. Examine after 15 min. The zones corresponding to hyoscyamine in the chromatograms obtained with the test solution and the reference solution change from brown to reddish-brown but not to greyish-blue (atropine) and any secondary zones disappear.

Loss on drying (*2.2.32*). Not more than 5.0 per cent, determined on 1.000 g by drying in an oven at 100 °C to 105 °C.

Total ash (*2.4.16*). Not more than 16.0 per cent.

Ash insoluble in hydrochloric acid (*2.8.1*). Not more than 4.0 per cent.

ASSAY

a) Determine the loss on drying (*2.2.32*) on 2.000 g, by drying in an oven at 100 °C to 105 °C.

b) Moisten 10.00 g with a mixture of 5 ml of *ammonia R*, 10 ml of *alcohol R* and 30 ml of *peroxide-free ether R* and mix thoroughly. Transfer the mixture to a suitable percolator, if necessary with the aid of the extracting mixture. Allow to macerate for 4 h and percolate with a mixture of 1 volume of *chloroform R* and 3 volumes of *peroxide-free ether R* until the alkaloids are completely extracted. Evaporate to dryness a few millilitres of the liquid flowing from the percolator, dissolve the residue in *0.25 M sulphuric acid* and verify the absence of alkaloids using *potassium tetraiodomercurate solution R*. Concentrate the percolate to about 50 ml by distilling on a water-bath and transfer it to a separating funnel, rinsing with *peroxide-free ether R*. Add a quantity of *peroxide-free ether R* equal to at least 2.1 times the volume of the percolate to produce a liquid of a density well below that of water. Shake the solution with no fewer than three quantities, each of 20 ml, of *0.25 M sulphuric acid*, separate the two layers by centrifugation if necessary and transfer the acid layers to a second separating funnel. Make the acid layer alkaline with *ammonia R* and shake with three quantities, each of 30 ml, of *chloroform R*. Combine the chloroform layers, add 4 g of *anhydrous sodium sulphate R* and allow to stand for 30 min with occasional shaking. Decant the chloroform and wash the sodium sulphate with three quantities, each of 10 ml, of *chloroform R*. Add the washings to the chloroform extract, evaporate to dryness on a water-bath and heat in an oven at 100 °C to 105 °C for 15 min. Dissolve the residue in a few millilitres of *chloroform R*, add 20.0 ml of *0.01 M sulphuric acid* and remove the chloroform by evaporation on a water-bath. Titrate the excess of acid with *0.02 M sodium hydroxide* using *methyl red mixed solution R* as indicator.

Calculate the percentage content of total alkaloids, expressed as hyoscyamine, from the expression:

$$\frac{57.88 \times (20 - n)}{(100 - d) \times m}$$

d = loss on drying as a percentage,

n = volume of *0.02 M sodium hydroxide* used in millilitres,

m = mass of drug used in grams.

STORAGE

Store in an airtight container, protected from light.

01/2005:0370

BENDROFLUMETHIAZIDE

Bendroflumethiazidum

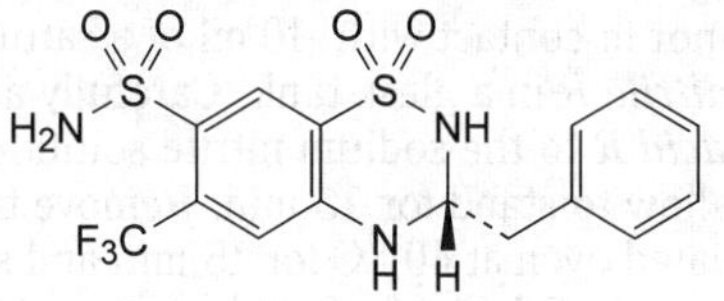

and enantiomer

$C_{15}H_{14}F_3N_3O_4S_2$ M_r 421.4

DEFINITION

Bendroflumethiazide contains not less than 98.0 per cent and not more than the equivalent of 102.0 per cent of 3-benzyl-3,4-dihydro-6-(trifluoromethyl)-2*H*-1,2,4-benzothiadiazine-7-sulphonamide 1,1-dioxide, calculated with reference to the dried substance.

CHARACTERS

A white or almost white, crystalline powder, practically insoluble in water, freely soluble in acetone, soluble in alcohol.

IDENTIFICATION

First identification: A.

Second identification: B, C, D.

A. Examine by infrared absorption spectrophotometry (*2.2.24*), comparing with the spectrum obtained with *bendroflumethiazide CRS*. Examine the substances prepared in the form of discs.

B. Examine the chromatograms obtained in the test for related substances. The principal spot in the chromatogram obtained with 4 µl of the test solution is similar in position, colour and size to the principal spot in the chromatogram obtained with reference solution (a).

C. In a test-tube, heat 0.5 ml of a saturated solution of *chromic acid cleansing mixture R* in a naked flame until white fumes appear in the upper part of the tube. The solution wets the side of the tube and there is no appearance of greasiness. Add about 2 mg of the substance to be examined and heat again in a naked flame until white fumes appear. The solution does not wet the side of the tube and does not pour easily from the tube.

D. Heat about 5 mg with a mixture of 5 ml of *potassium permanganate solution R* and 1 ml of *sulphuric acid R*. An odour of benzaldehyde is produced.

TESTS

Related substances. Examine by thin-layer chromatography (*2.2.27*), using *silica gel G R* as the coating substance.

Test solution. Dissolve 25 mg of the substance to be examined in *acetone R* and dilute to 5 ml with the same solvent.

Reference solution (a). Dissolve 25 mg of *bendroflumethiazide CRS* in *acetone R* and dilute to 5 ml with the same solvent.

Reference solution (b). Dilute 1 ml of reference solution (a) to 100 ml with *acetone R.*

Apply separately to the plate 4 µl and 20 µl of the test solution, 4 µl of reference solution (a) and 20 µl of reference solution (b). Develop over a path of 15 cm using *ethyl acetate R.* Dry the plate in a current of air for 10 min and spray with a mixture of equal volumes of *alcoholic solution of sulphuric acid R* and *alcohol R*; use about 10 ml for a plate 200 mm square and spray in small portions, allowing the solvent to evaporate each time to avoid excessive wetting. Heat at 100 °C to 105 °C for 30 min and immediately place the plate above, but not in contact with, 10 ml of a saturated solution of *sodium nitrite R* in a glass tank. Carefully add 0.5 ml of *sulphuric acid R* to the sodium nitrite solution, close the tank, and allow to stand for 15 min. Remove the plate, heat in a ventilated oven at 40 °C for 15 min and spray with three quantities, each of 5 ml, of a freshly prepared 5 g/l solution of *naphthylethylenediamine dihydrochloride R* in *alcohol R.* Examine the plate by transmitted light. Any spot in the chromatogram obtained with 20 µl of the test solution, apart from the principal spot, is not more intense than the spot in the chromatogram obtained with reference solution (b) (1.0 per cent).

Loss on drying (*2.2.32*). Not more than 0.5 per cent, determined on 1.00 g by drying in an oven at 100 °C to 105 °C.

Sulphated ash (*2.4.14*). Not more than 0.1 per cent, determined on 1.0 g

ASSAY

Dissolve 0.200 g in 50 ml of *anhydrous pyridine R.* Titrate with *0.1 M tetrabutylammonium hydroxide,* determining the end-point potentiometrically at the second point of inflexion (*2.2.20*). Carry out a blank titration.

1 ml of *0.1 M tetrabutylammonium hydroxide* is equivalent to 21.07 mg of $C_{15}H_{14}F_3N_3O_4S_2$.

01/2005:1601
corrected

BENFLUOREX HYDROCHLORIDE

Benfluorexi hydrochloridum

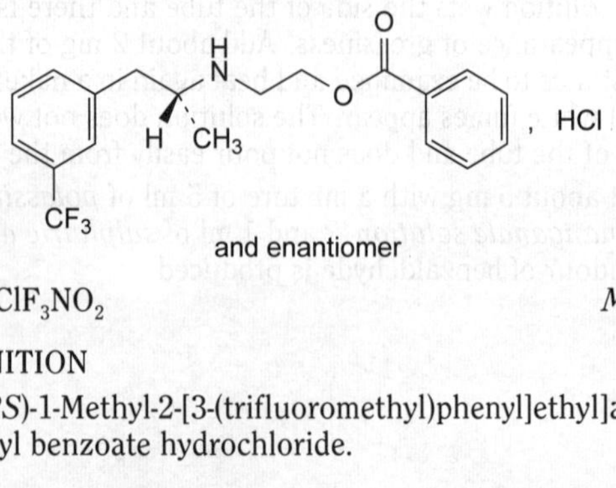

and enantiomer

$C_{19}H_{21}ClF_3NO_2$ M_r 387.8

DEFINITION

2-[[(1*RS*)-1-Methyl-2-[3-(trifluoromethyl)phenyl]ethyl]amino]ethyl benzoate hydrochloride.

Content: 98.5 per cent to 101.0 per cent (dried substance).

CHARACTERS

Appearance: white or almost white powder.

Solubility: slightly soluble in water, freely soluble in methanol, soluble in methylene chloride, sparingly soluble or soluble in alcohol.

It shows polymorphism.

IDENTIFICATION

A. Infrared absorption spectrophotometry (*2.2.24*).

Preparation: mulls in *liquid paraffin R.*

Comparison: *benfluorex hydrochloride CRS.*

If the spectra obtained show differences, heat the substance to be examined and the reference substance separately in an oven at 150 °C for 3 h and record new spectra.

B. It gives reaction (a) of chlorides (*2.3.1*).

TESTS

Optical rotation (*2.2.7*): − 0.10° to + 0.10°.

Dissolve 0.2 g in *ethanol R* and dilute to 20.0 ml with the same solvent.

Impurity B. Gas chromatography (*2.2.28*): use the normalisation procedure.

Test solution. Dissolve 0.30 g of the substance to be examined in *methylene chloride R* and dilute to 20 ml with the same solvent. Transfer to a separating funnel, add 10 ml of a 40 g/l solution of *sodium hydroxide R.* Shake the flask vigorously and allow the phases to separate. Collect the organic layer.

Reference solution. Dissolve 0.30 g of *benfluorex hydrochloride for system suitability CRS* in *methylene chloride R* and dilute to 20 ml with the same solvent. Transfer to a separating funnel and add 10 ml of a 40 g/l solution of *sodium hydroxide R.* Shake the flask vigorously and allow the phases to separate. Collect the organic layer.

Column:

- *material*: fused silica,
- *size*: l = 25 m, Ø = 0.32 mm,
- *stationary phase*: macrogol 20 000 R (film thickness 0.2 µm).

Carrier gas: *hydrogen for chromatography R.*

Linear velocity: 75 cm/s.

Split ratio: 1:35.

Temperature:

- *column*: 220 °C,
- *injection port and detector*: 250 °C.

Detection: flame ionisation.

Injection: 1 µl.

Run time: 1.5 times the retention time of benfluorex.

Relative retention with reference to benfluorex (retention time = about 4.5 min): impurity B = about 1.1.

System suitability:

- *peak-to-valley ratio*: minimum 2.5, where H_p = height above the baseline of the peak due to impurity B, and H_v = height above the baseline of the lowest point of the curve separating this peak from the peak due to benfluorex.

Limit:

- *impurity B*: maximum 0.1 per cent.

Related substances, other than impurity B. Liquid chromatography (*2.2.29*).

Test solution. Dissolve 60.0 mg of the substance to be examined in 50 ml of *acetonitrile R* and dilute to 100.0 ml with *water R.*

Reference solution (a). Dissolve 60.0 mg of *benfluorex hydrochloride for system suitability CRS* in 50 ml of *acetonitrile R* and dilute to 100.0 ml with *water R.*

Reference solution (b). Dilute 1.0 ml of the test solution to 100.0 ml with a mixture of equal volumes of *acetonitrile R* and *water R*. Dilute 5.0 ml of this solution to 50.0 ml with the same mixture of solvents.

Column:
- *size*: l = 0.15 m, Ø = 4.6 mm,
- *stationary phase*: silica gel bonded with alkylamide groups (5 µm),
- *temperature*: 60 °C.

Mobile phase: a mixture of equal volumes of *acetonitrile R* and a solution containing 2.18 g/l of *potassium dihydrogen phosphate R* adjusted to pH 2.5 with *phosphoric acid R* and 6.5 g/l of *sodium decyl sulphate R.*

Flow rate: 1.4 ml/min.

Detection: spectrophotometer at 210 nm.

Injection: 10 µl.

Run time: 3 times the retention time of benfluorex.

Relative retention with reference to benfluorex (retention time = about 5 min): impurity A = about 0.9.

System suitability:
- *signal-to-noise ratio*: minimum 20 for the principal peak in the chromatogram obtained with reference solution (b),
- *peak-to-valley ratio*: minimum 2.5, where H_p = height above the baseline of the peak due to impurity A, and H_v = height above the baseline of the lowest point of the curve separating this peak from the peak due to benfluorex in the chromatogram obtained with reference solution (a).

Limits:
- *any impurity*: not more than the area of the principal peak in the chromatogram obtained with reference solution (b) (0.1 per cent),
- *total*: not more than twice the area of the principal peak in the chromatogram obtained with reference solution (b) (0.2 per cent),
- *disregard limit*: 0.5 times the area of the principal peak in the chromatogram obtained with reference solution (b) (0.05 per cent).

Heavy metals (*2.4.8*): maximum 20 ppm.

1.0 g complies with limit test C. Prepare the standard using 2 ml of *lead standard solution (10 ppm Pb) R.*

Loss on drying (*2.2.32*): maximum 0.5 per cent, determined on 1.000 g by drying in an oven at 100-105 °C.

Sulphated ash (*2.4.14*): maximum 0.1 per cent, determined on 1.0 g.

ASSAY

In order to avoid overheating in the reaction medium, mix thoroughly throughout and stop the titration immediately after the end-point has been reached.

Dissolve 0.250 g rapidly in 2.0 ml of *anhydrous formic acid R* and add 50.0 ml of *acetic anhydride R*. Titrate immediately with *0.1 M perchloric acid,* determining the end-point potentiometrically (*2.2.20*).

1 ml of *0.1 M perchloric acid* is equivalent to 38.78 mg of $C_{19}H_{21}ClF_3NO_2$.

IMPURITIES

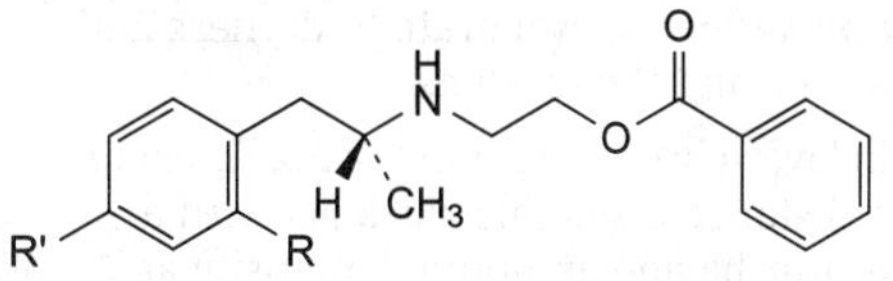

and enantiomer

A. R = CF_3, R′ = H: 2-[[(1*RS*)-1-methyl-2-[2-(trifluoromethyl)phenyl]ethyl]amino]ethyl benzoate,

B. R = H, R′ = CF_3: 2-[[(1*RS*)-1-methyl-2-[4-(trifluoromethyl)phenyl]ethyl]amino]ethyl benzoate,

C. benzoic acid,

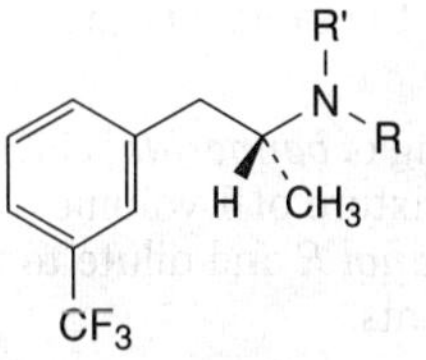

and enantiomer

D. R = CH_2-CH_2-OH, R′ = H: 2-[[(1*RS*)-1-methyl-2-[3-(trifluoromethyl)phenyl]ethyl]amino]ethanol,

E. R = CH_2-CH_2-OH, R′ = CO-C_6H_5: *N*-(2-hydroxyethyl)-*N*-[(1*RS*)-1-methyl-2-[3-(trifluoromethyl)phenyl]ethyl]benzamide,

F. R = CH_2-CH_2-O-CO-C_6H_5, R′ = CO-C_6H_5: 2-[benzoyl[(1*RS*)-1-methyl-2-[3-(trifluoromethyl)phenyl]ethyl]amino]ethyl benzoate.

01/2005:1172

BENPERIDOL

Benperidolum

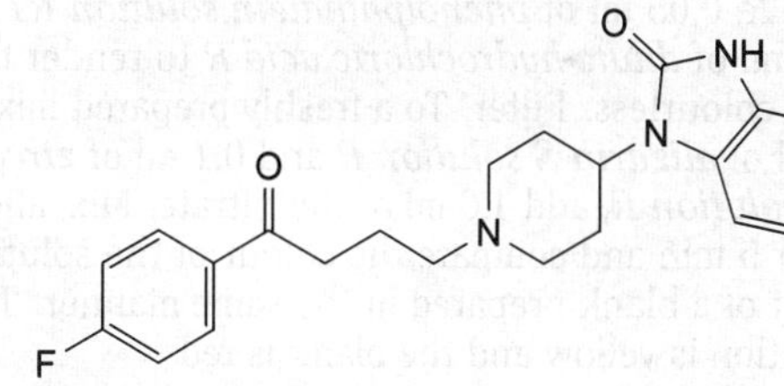

$C_{22}H_{24}FN_3O_2$ M_r 381.4

DEFINITION

Benperidol contains not less than 99.0 per cent and not more than the equivalent of 101.0 per cent of 1-[1-[4-(4-fluorophenyl)-4-oxobutyl]piperidin-4-yl]-1,3-dihydro-2*H*-benzimidazol-2-one, calculated with reference to the dried substance.

CHARACTERS

A white or almost white powder, practically insoluble in water, freely soluble in dimethylformamide, soluble in methylene chloride, slightly soluble in alcohol.

It shows polymorphism.

IDENTIFICATION

First identification: A.

Second identification: B, C, D.

A. Examine by infrared absorption spectrophotometry (*2.2.24*), comparing with the spectrum obtained with *benperidol CRS.* Examine the substances prepared as discs. If the spectra obtained in the solid state show differences, dissolve the substance to be examined and the reference substance separately in the minimum volume of *methyl isobutyl ketone R*, evaporate to dryness and record new spectra using the residues.

B. Examine by thin-layer chromatography (*2.2.27*), using as the coating substance a suitable silica gel with a fluorescent indicator having an optimal intensity at 254 nm.

Test solution. Dissolve 30 mg of the substance to be examined in a mixture of 1 volume of *acetone R* and 9 volumes of *methanol R* and dilute to 10 ml with the same mixture of solvents.

Reference solution (a). Dissolve 30 mg of *benperidol CRS* in a mixture of 1 volume of *acetone R* and 9 volumes of *methanol R* and dilute to 10 ml with the same mixture of solvents.

Reference solution (b). Dissolve 30 mg of *benperidol CRS* and 30 mg of *droperidol CRS* in a mixture of 1 volume of *acetone R* and 9 volumes of *methanol R* and dilute to 10 ml with the same mixture of solvents.

Apply to the plate 10 µl of each solution. Develop over a path of 15 cm using a mixture of 1 volume of *acetone R* and 9 volumes of *methanol R*. Allow the plate to dry in air and examine in ultraviolet light at 254 nm. The principal spot in the chromatogram obtained with the test solution is similar in position and size to the principal spot in the chromatogram obtained with reference solution (a). The test is not valid unless the chromatogram obtained with reference solution (b) shows two clearly separated spots.

C. Dissolve about 10 mg in 5 ml of *ethanol R*. Add 0.5 ml of *dinitrobenzene solution R* and 0.5 ml of *2 M alcoholic potassium hydroxide R*. A violet colour is produced which becomes brownish-red after 20 min.

D. Mix about 5 mg with 45 mg of *heavy magnesium oxide R* and ignite in a crucible until an almost white residue is obtained (usually less than 5 min). Allow to cool, add 1 ml of *water R*, 0.05 ml of *phenolphthalein solution R1* and about 1 ml of *dilute hydrochloric acid R* to render the solution colourless. Filter. To a freshly prepared mixture of 0.1 ml of *alizarin S solution R* and 0.1 ml of *zirconyl nitrate solution R*, add 1.0 ml of the filtrate. Mix, allow to stand for 5 min and compare the colour of the solution with that of a blank prepared in the same manner. The test solution is yellow and the blank is red.

TESTS

Related substances. Examine by liquid chromatography (*2.2.29*). *Prepare the solutions immediately before use.*

Test solution. Dissolve 0.10 g of the substance to be examined in *dimethylformamide R* and dilute to 10.0 ml with the same solvent.

Reference solution (a). Dissolve 2.5 mg of *benperidol CRS* and 2.5 mg of *droperidol CRS* in *dimethylformamide R* and dilute to 100.0 ml with the same solvent.

Reference solution (b). Dilute 1.0 ml of the test solution to 100.0 ml with *dimethylformamide R*. Dilute 5.0 ml of this solution to 20.0 ml with *dimethylformamide R*.

The chromatographic procedure may be carried out using:

- a stainless steel column 0.1 m long and 4.6 mm in internal diameter packed with *base-deactivated octadecylsilyl silica gel for chromatography R* (3 µm),
- as mobile phase at a flow rate of 1.5 ml/min:

  Mobile phase A. A 10 g/l solution of *tetrabutylammonium hydrogen sulphate R*,

  Mobile phase B. Acetonitrile R,

Time (min)	Mobile phase A (per cent *V/V*)	Mobile phase B (per cent *V/V*)	Comment
0 - 15	100 → 60	0 → 40	linear gradient
15 - 20	60	40	isocratic elution
20 - 25	100	0	switch to initial eluent composition
25 = 0	100	0	restart gradient

- as detector a spectrophotometer set at 275 nm.

Equilibrate the column for at least 30 min with *acetonitrile R* and then equilibrate with the initial eluent composition for at least 5 min.

Adjust the sensitivity of the system so that the height of the principal peak in the chromatogram obtained with 10 µl of reference solution (b) is at least 50 per cent of the full scale of the recorder.

Inject 10 µl of reference solution (a). When the chromatogram is recorded in the prescribed conditions, the retention times are: benperidol about 6.5 min and droperidol about 7 min. The test is not valid unless the resolution between the peaks corresponding to benperidol and droperidol is at least 2.0. If necessary, adjust the concentration of acetonitrile in the mobile phase or adjust the time programme for the linear gradient.

Inject 10 µl of *dimethylformamide R* as a blank, 10 µl of the test solution and 10 µl of reference solution (b). In the chromatogram obtained with the test solution: the area of any peak, apart from the principal peak, is not greater than the area of the principal peak in the chromatogram obtained with reference solution (b) (0.25 per cent); the sum of the areas of all the peaks, apart from the principal peak, is not greater than twice the area of the principal peak in the chromatogram obtained with reference solution (b) (0.5 per cent). Disregard any peak obtained with the blank and any peak with an area less than 0.2 times the area of the principal peak in the chromatogram obtained with reference solution (b).

Loss on drying (*2.2.32*). Not more than 0.5 per cent, determined on 1.000 g by drying in an oven at 100 °C to 105 °C.

Sulphated ash (*2.4.14*). Not more than 0.1 per cent, determined on 1.0 g in a platinum crucible.

ASSAY

Dissolve 0.300 g in 50 ml of a mixture of 1 volume of *anhydrous acetic acid R* and 7 volumes of *methyl ethyl ketone R* and titrate with *0.1 M perchloric acid*, using 0.2 ml of *naphtholbenzein solution R* as indicator.

1 ml of *0.1 M perchloric acid* is equivalent to 38.14 mg of $C_{22}H_{24}FN_3O_2$.

STORAGE

Store protected from light.

IMPURITIES

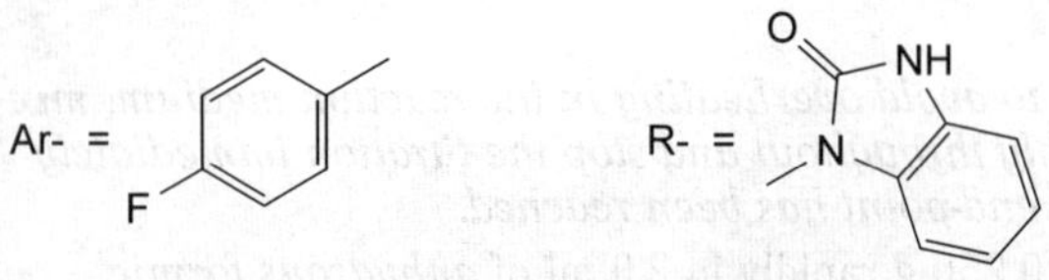

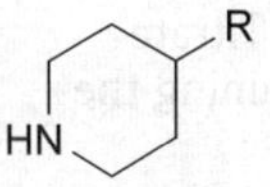

A. 1-(piperidin-4-yl)-1,3-dihydro-2*H*-benzimidazol-2-one,

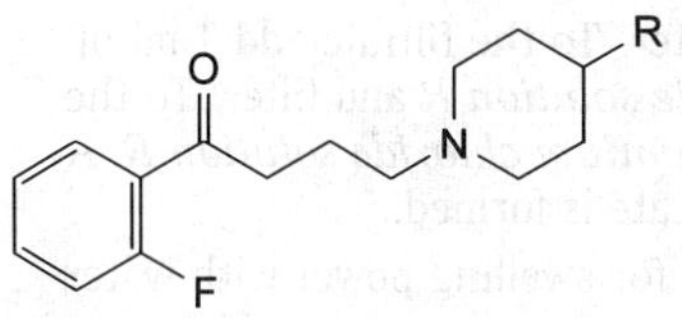

B. 1-[1-[4-(2-fluorophenyl)-4-oxobutyl]piperidin-4-yl]-1,3-dihydro-2*H*-benzimidazol-2-one,

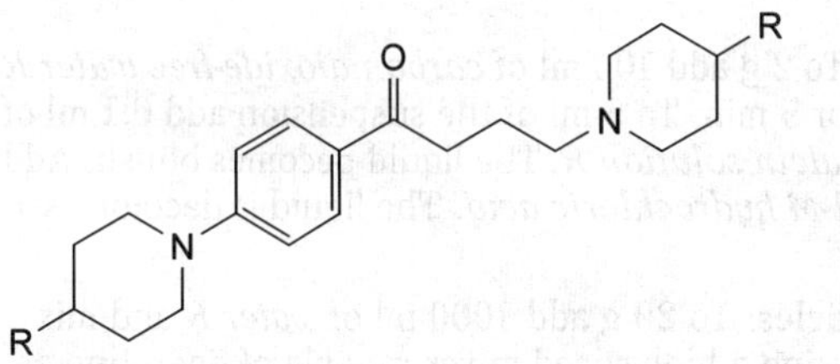

C. 1-[1-[4-oxo-4-[4-[4-(2-oxo-2,3-dihydro-1*H*-benzimidazol-1-yl)piperidin-1-yl]phenyl]butyl]piperidin-4-yl]-1,3-dihydro-2*H*-benzimidazol-2-one,

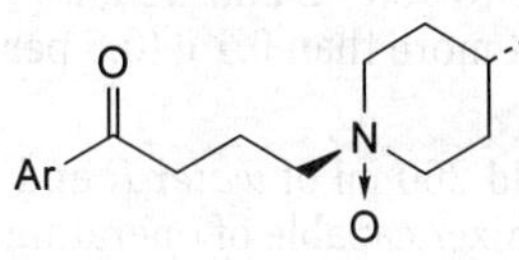

D. *cis*-1-[1-[4-(4-fluorophenyl)-4-oxobutyl]piperidin-4-yl 1-oxide]-1,3-dihydro-2*H*-benzimidazol-2-one,

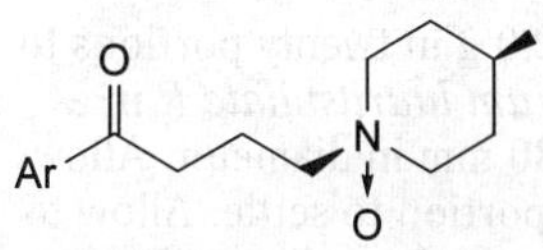

E. *trans*-1-[1-[4-(4-fluorophenyl)-4-oxobutyl]piperidin-4-yl 1-oxide]-1,3-dihydro-2*H*-benzimidazol-2-one.

01/2005:1173

BENSERAZIDE HYDROCHLORIDE

Benserazidi hydrochloridum

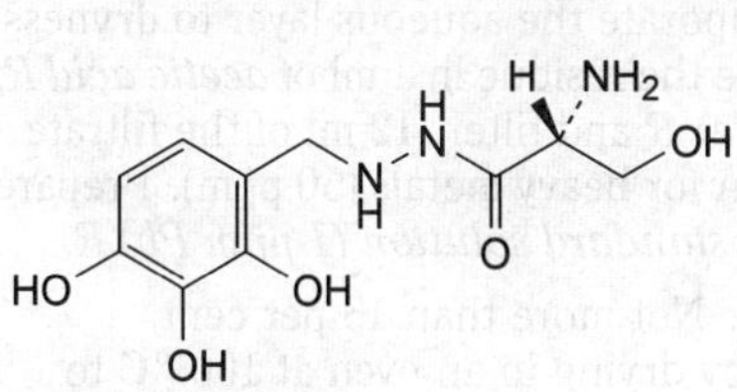

and enantiomer , HCl

$C_{10}H_{16}ClN_3O_5$ M_r 293.7

DEFINITION

Benserazide hydrochloride contains not less than 98.5 per cent and not more than the equivalent of 101.0 per cent of (*RS*)-2-amino-3-hydroxy-2′-(2,3,4-trihydroxybenzyl)propanohydrazide hydrochloride, calculated with reference to the anhydrous substance.

CHARACTERS

A white or yellowish-white or orange-white, crystalline powder, freely soluble in water, very slightly soluble in ethanol, practically insoluble in acetone.

It shows polymorphism.

IDENTIFICATION

A. Examine by infrared absorption spectrophotometry (*2.2.24*), comparing with the spectrum obtained with *benserazide hydrochloride CRS*. Examine the substances prepared as discs. If the spectra obtained show differences, dissolve the substance to be examined and the reference substance separately in hot *methanol R*, evaporate to dryness and record new spectra using the residues.

B. Solution S (see Tests) gives reaction (b) of chlorides (*2.3.1*).

TESTS

Solution S. Dissolve 1.0 g in *carbon dioxide-free water R* and dilute to 100 ml with the same solvent.

Appearance of solution. Solution S is clear (*2.2.1*) and not more intensely coloured than reference solution BY_6 (*2.2.2, Method II*).

pH (*2.2.3*). The pH of solution S is 4.0 to 5.0.

Optical rotation (*2.2.7*). The angle of optical rotation, determined on solution S, is − 0.05 to + 0.05.

Related substances. Examine by liquid chromatography (*2.2.29*).

Prepare the solutions using the mobile phase cooled to 4 °C and inject immediately.

Test solution. Dissolve 0.10 g of the substance to be examined in the mobile phase and dilute to 100.0 ml with the mobile phase.

Reference solution. Dissolve 5.0 mg of *benserazide impurity A CRS* and 5.0 mg of *benserazide hydrochloride CRS* in the mobile phase and dilute to 50.0 ml with the mobile phase. Dilute 5.0 ml of the solution to 100.0 ml with the mobile phase.

The chromatographic procedure may be carried out using:

- a stainless steel column 0.125 m long and4 mm in internal diameter packed with *octylsilyl silica gel for chromatography R* (5 µm),
- as mobile phase at a flow rate of 1.2 ml/min a mixture prepared as follows: dissolve 4.76 g of *potassium dihydrogen phosphate R* in 800 ml of *water R*; add 200 ml of *acetonitrile R* and 1.22 g of *sodium decanesulphonate R*; adjust to pH 3.5 with *phosphoric acid R*,
- as detector a spectrophotometer set at 220 nm.

Inject 20 µl of the reference solution. The test is not valid unless the resolution between the peaks corresponding to impurity A (first peak) and benserazide (second peak) is at least 2.0.

Inject 20 µl of the test solution. Continue the chromatography for nine times the retention time of benserazide. In the chromatogram obtained with the test solution: the area of any peak due to impurity A is not greater than the area of the corresponding peak in the chromatogram obtained with the reference solution (0.5 per cent); the area of any peak, apart from the principal peak and any peak due to impurity A, is not greater than the area of the peak due to benserazide in the chromatogram obtained with the reference solution (0.5 per cent); the sum of the areas of any such peaks is not greater than twice the area of the peak due to benserazide in the chromatogram obtained with the reference solution (1 per cent). Disregard any peak with an area less than 0.1 times that of the peak due to benserazide in the chromatogram obtained with the reference solution.

Heavy metals (*2.4.8*). 1.0 g complies with limit test C for heavy metals (20 ppm). Prepare the standard using 2 ml of *lead standard solution (10 ppm Pb) R*.

Water (*2.5.12*). Not more than 1.0 per cent, determined on 0.500 g by the semi-micro determination of water.

Sulphated ash (*2.4.14*). Not more than 0.1 per cent, determined on 1.0 g.

ASSAY

In order to avoid overheating during the titration, mix thoroughly throughout and stop the titration immediately after the end-point has been reached.

Dissolve 0.250 g in 5 ml of *anhydrous formic acid R*. Add 70 ml of *anhydrous acetic acid R*. Titrate immediately with *0.1 M perchloric acid*, determining the end-point potentiometrically (*2.2.20*).

1 ml of *0.1 M perchloric acid* is equivalent to 29.37 mg of $C_{10}H_{16}ClN_3O_5$.

STORAGE

Store protected from light.

IMPURITIES

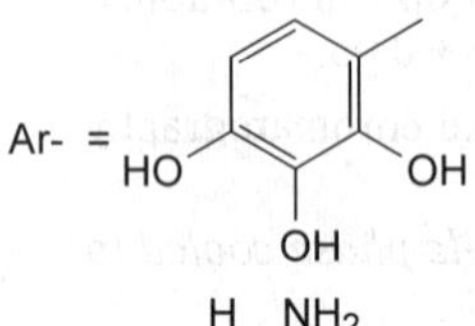

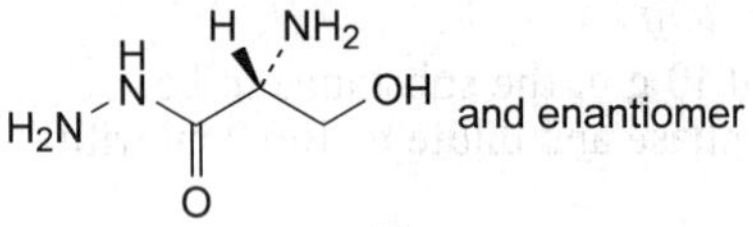

A. (*RS*)-2-amino-3-hydroxypropanohydrazide,

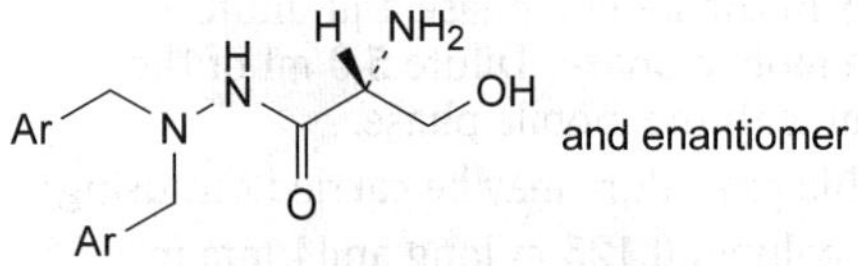

B. (*RS*)-2-amino-3-hydroxy-2′,2′-bis(2,3,4-trihydroxybenzyl)propanohydrazide,

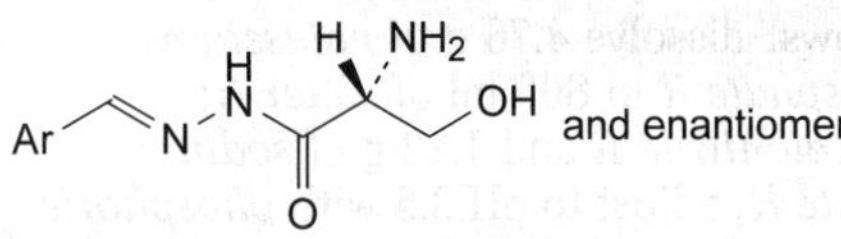

C. (*RS*)-2-amino-3-hydroxy-2′-(2,3,4-trihydroxybenzylidene)propanohydrazide.

01/2005:0467

BENTONITE

Bentonitum

DEFINITION

Bentonite is a natural clay containing a high proportion of montmorillonite, a native hydrated aluminium silicate in which some aluminium and silicon atoms may be replaced by other atoms such as magnesium and iron.

CHARACTERS

A very fine, homogeneous, greyish-white powder with a more or less yellowish or pinkish tint, practically insoluble in water and in aqueous solutions. It swells with a little water forming a malleable mass.

IDENTIFICATION

A. To 0.5 g in a metal crucible add 1 g of *potassium nitrate R* and 3 g of *sodium carbonate R* and heat until the mixture melts. Allow to cool. To the residue add 20 ml of boiling *water R*, mix and filter. Wash the residue with 50 ml of *water R*. To the residue add 1 ml of *hydrochloric acid R* and 5 ml of *water R*. Filter. To the filtrate add 1 ml of *strong sodium hydroxide solution R* and filter. To the filtrate add 3 ml of *ammonium chloride solution R*. A gelatinous white precipitate is formed.

B. It complies with the test for swelling power with water (see Tests).

C. 0.25 g gives the reaction of silicates (*2.3.1*).

TESTS

Alkalinity. To 2 g add 100 ml of *carbon dioxide-free water R* and shake for 5 min. To 5 ml of the suspension add 0.1 ml of *thymolphthalein solution R*. The liquid becomes bluish. Add 0.1 ml of *0.1 M hydrochloric acid*. The liquid is decolourised within 5 min.

Coarse particles. To 20 g add 1000 ml of *water R* and mix for 15 min using a high-speed mixer capable of operating at not less than 5000 r/min. Transfer to a wet sieve (75), tared after drying at 100 °C to 105 °C. Wash with three quantities, each of 500 ml, of *water R*, ensuring that any agglomerates have been dispersed. Dry at 100 °C to 105 °C and weigh. The particles on the sieve weigh not more than 0.1 g (0.5 per cent).

Sedimentation volume. To 6.0 g add 200 ml of *water R* and mix for 20 min using a high-speed mixer capable of operating at 10 000 r/min. Transfer 100 ml of the suspension to a graduated cylinder. Allow to stand for 24 h. The volume of the clear supernatant liquid is not greater than 2 ml.

Swelling power with water. Add 2.0 g in twenty portions to 100 ml of a 10 g/l solution of *sodium laurilsulfate R* in a 100 ml graduated cylinder about 30 mm in diameter. Allow 2 min between additions for each portion to settle. Allow to stand for 2 h. The apparent volume of the sediment is not less than 22 ml.

Heavy metals (*2.4.8*). To 5.0 g add 7.5 ml of *dilute hydrochloric acid R* and 27.5 ml of *water R*. Boil for 5 min. Centrifuge and filter the supernatant liquid. Wash the centrifugation residue with *water R* and filter. Dilute the combined filtrates to 50.0 ml with *water R*. To 5 ml of the solution add 5 ml of *water R*, 10 ml of *hydrochloric acid R* and 25 ml of *methyl isobutyl ketone R* and shake for 2 min. Separate the layers. Evaporate the aqueous layer to dryness on a water-bath. Dissolve the residue in 1 ml of *acetic acid R*, dilute to 25 ml with *water R* and filter. 12 ml of the filtrate complies with limit test A for heavy metals (50 ppm). Prepare the standard using *lead standard solution (1 ppm Pb) R*.

Loss on drying (*2.2.32*). Not more than 15 per cent, determined on 1.000 g by drying in an oven at 100 °C to 105 °C.

Microbial contamination. Total viable aerobic count (*2.6.12*) not more than 10^3 micro-organisms per gram, determined by plate-count.

01/2005:0372

BENZALKONIUM CHLORIDE

Benzalkonii chloridum

DEFINITION

Benzalkonium chloride is a mixture of alkylbenzyldimethylammonium chlorides, the alkyl groups having chain lengths of C_8 to C_{18}. It contains not less than 95.0 per cent and not more than the equivalent of 104.0 per cent of alkylbenzyldimethylammonium chlorides, calculated as $C_{22}H_{40}ClN$ (M_r 354.0) with reference to the anhydrous substance.

CHARACTERS

A white or yellowish-white powder or gelatinous, yellowish-white fragments, hygroscopic, soapy to the touch, very soluble in water and in alcohol. On heating it forms a clear molten mass. An aqueous solution froths copiously when shaken.

IDENTIFICATION

A. Dissolve 80 mg in *water R* and dilute to 100 ml with the same solvent. Examined between 220 nm and 350 nm (*2.2.25*), the solution shows three absorption maxima, at 257 nm, 263 nm and 269 nm, and a shoulder at about 250 nm.

B. To 2 ml of solution S (see Tests) add 0.1 ml of *glacial acetic acid R* and, dropwise, 1 ml of *sodium tetraphenylborate solution R*. A white precipitate is formed. Filter. Dissolve the precipitate in a mixture of 1 ml of *acetone R* and 5 ml of *alcohol R*, heating to not more than 70 °C. Add *water R* dropwise to the warm solution until a slight opalescence forms. Heat gently until the solution is clear and allow to cool. White crystals separate. Filter, wash with three quantities, each of 10 ml, of *water R* and dry *in vacuo* over *diphosphorus pentoxide R* or *anhydrous silica gel R* at a temperature not exceeding 50 °C. The crystals melt (*2.2.14*) at 127 °C to 133 °C.

C. To 5 ml of *dilute sodium hydroxide solution R* add 0.1 ml of *bromophenol blue solution R1* and 5 ml of *chloroform R* and shake. The chloroform layer is colourless. Add 0.1 ml of solution S and shake. The chloroform layer becomes blue.

D. To 2 ml of solution S add 1 ml of *dilute nitric acid R*. A white precipitate is formed which dissolves on the addition of 5 ml of *alcohol R*. The solution gives reaction (a) of chlorides (*2.3.1*).

TESTS

Solution S. Dissolve 1.0 g in *carbon dioxide-free water R* and dilute to 100 ml with the same solvent.

Appearance of solution. Solution S is clear (*2.2.1*) and not more intensely coloured than reference solution Y_6 (*2.2.2, Method II*).

Acidity or alkalinity. To 50 ml of solution S add 0.1 ml of *bromocresol purple solution R*. Not more than 0.1 ml of *0.1 M hydrochloric acid* or *0.1 M sodium hydroxide* is required to change the colour of the indicator.

Amines and amine salts. Dissolve 5.0 g with heating in 20 ml of a mixture of 3 volumes of *1 M hydrochloric acid* and 97 volumes of *methanol R* and add 100 ml of *2-propanol R*. Pass a stream of *nitrogen R* slowly through the solution. Gradually add 12.0 ml of *0.1 M tetrabutylammonium hydroxide* and record the potentiometric titration curve (*2.2.20*). If the curve shows two points of inflexion, the volume of titrant added between the two points is not greater than 5.0 ml. If the curve shows no point of inflexion, the substance to be examined does not comply with the test. If the curve shows one point of inflexion, repeat the test but add 3.0 ml of a 25.0 g/l solution of *dimethyldecylamine R* in *2-propanol R* before the titration. If the titration curve after addition of 12.0 ml of the titrant shows only one point of inflexion, the substance to be examined does not comply with the test.

Water (*2.5.12*). Not more than 10 per cent, determined on 0.300 g by the semi-micro determination of water.

Sulphated ash (*2.4.14*). Not more than 0.1 per cent, determined on 1.0 g.

ASSAY

Dissolve 2.00 g in *water R* and dilute to 100.0 ml with the same solvent. Transfer 25.0 ml of the solution to a separating funnel, add 25 ml of *chloroform R*, 10 ml of *0.1 M sodium hydroxide* and 10.0 ml of a freshly prepared 50 g/l solution of *potassium iodide R*. Shake well, allow to separate and discard the chloroform layer. Shake the aqueous layer with three quantities, each of 10 ml, of *chloroform R* and discard the chloroform layers. To the aqueous layer add 40 ml of *hydrochloric acid R*, allow to cool and titrate with *0.05 M potassium iodate* until the deep-brown colour is almost discharged. Add 2 ml of *chloroform R* and continue the titration, shaking vigorously, until the chloroform layer no longer changes colour. Carry out a blank titration on a mixture of 10.0 ml of the freshly prepared 50 g/l solution of *potassium iodide R*, 20 ml of *water R* and 40 ml of *hydrochloric acid R*.

1 ml of *0.05 M potassium iodate* is equivalent to 35.4 mg of $C_{22}H_{40}ClN$.

01/2005:0371

BENZALKONIUM CHLORIDE SOLUTION

Benzalkonii chloridi solutio

DEFINITION

Benzalkonium chloride solution is an aqueous solution of a mixture of alkylbenzyldimethylammonium chlorides, the alkyl groups having chain lengths of C_8 to C_{18}. Benzalkonium chloride solution contains not less than 475 g/l and not more than 525 g/l of alkylbenzyldimethylammonium chlorides, calculated as $C_{22}H_{40}ClN$ (M_r 354.0). The solution may contain alcohol.

CHARACTERS

A clear, colourless or slightly yellowish liquid, miscible with water and with alcohol. It froths copiously when shaken.

IDENTIFICATION

A. Dilute 0.3 ml to 100 ml with *water R*. Examined between 220 nm and 350 nm (*2.2.25*), the solution shows three absorption maxima, at 257 nm, 263 nm and 269 nm, and a shoulder at about 250 nm.

B. To 0.05 ml add 2 ml of *water R*, 0.1 ml of *glacial acetic acid R* and, dropwise, 1 ml of *sodium tetraphenylborate solution R*. A white precipitate is formed. Filter. Dissolve the precipitate in a mixture of 1 ml of *acetone R* and 5 ml of *alcohol R*, heating to not more than 70 °C. Add *water R* dropwise to the warm solution until a slight opalescence forms. Heat gently until the solution is clear and allow to cool. White crystals separate. Filter, wash with three quantities, each of 10 ml, of *water R* and dry *in vacuo* over *diphosphorus pentoxide R* or *anhydrous silica gel R* at a temperature not exceeding 50 °C. The crystals melt (*2.2.14*) at 127 °C to 133 °C.

C. To 5 ml of *dilute sodium hydroxide solution R* add 0.1 ml of *bromophenol blue solution R1* and 5 ml of *chloroform R* and shake. The chloroform layer is colourless. Add 0.05 ml of the solution to be examined and shake. The chloroform layer becomes blue.

D. To 0.05 ml add 1 ml of *dilute nitric acid R*. A white precipitate is formed which dissolves on the addition of 5 ml of *alcohol R*. The solution gives reaction (a) of chlorides (*2.3.1*).

TESTS

Solution S. Dilute 2.0 g to 100 ml with *carbon dioxide-free water R*.

Appearance of solution. Solution S is clear (*2.2.1*) and not more intensely coloured than reference solution Y_6 (*2.2.2, Method II*).

Acidity or alkalinity. To 50 ml of solution S add 0.1 ml of *bromocresol purple solution R*. Not more than 0.1 ml of *0.1 M hydrochloric acid* or *0.1 M sodium hydroxide* is required to change the colour of the indicator.

Amines and amine salts. Mix 10.0 g, while heating, with 20 ml of a mixture of 3 volumes of *1 M hydrochloric acid* and 97 volumes of *methanol R* and add 100 ml of *2-propanol R*. Pass a stream of *nitrogen R* slowly through the solution. Gradually add 12.0 ml of *0.1 M tetrabutylammonium hydroxide* and record the potentiometric titration curve (*2.2.20*). If the curve shows two points of inflexion, the volume of titrant added between the two points is not greater than 5.0 ml. If the curve shows no point of inflexion, the solution to be examined does not comply with the test. If the curve shows one point of inflexion, repeat the test but add 3.0 ml of a 25.0 g/l solution of *dimethyldecylamine R* in *2-propanol R* before the titration. If the titration curve after the addition of 12.0 ml of the titrant shows only one point of inflexion, the solution to be examined does not comply with the test.

Sulphated ash (*2.4.14*). Not more than 0.1 per cent, determined on 1.0 g.

ASSAY

Determine the density (*2.2.5*) of the solution to be examined. Dilute 4.00 g to 100.0 ml with *water R*. Transfer 25.0 ml of the solution to a separating funnel, add 25 ml of *chloroform R*, 10 ml of *0.1 M sodium hydroxide* and 10.0 ml of a freshly prepared 50 g/l solution of *potassium iodide R*. Shake well, allow to separate and discard the chloroform layer. Shake the aqueous layer with three quantities, each of 10 ml, of *chloroform R* and discard the chloroform layers. To the aqueous layer add 40 ml of *hydrochloric acid R*, allow to cool and titrate with *0.05 M potassium iodate* until the deep-brown colour is almost discharged. Add 2 ml of *chloroform R* and continue the titration, shaking vigorously, until the chloroform layer no longer changes colour. Carry out a blank titration on a mixture of 10.0 ml of the freshly prepared 50 g/l solution of *potassium iodide R*, 20 ml of *water R* and 40 ml of *hydrochloric acid R*.

1 ml of *0.05 M potassium iodate* is equivalent to 35.4 mg of $C_{22}H_{40}ClN$.

LABELLING

The label states the content of alcohol, if any.

01/2005:1393

BENZBROMARONE

Benzbromaronum

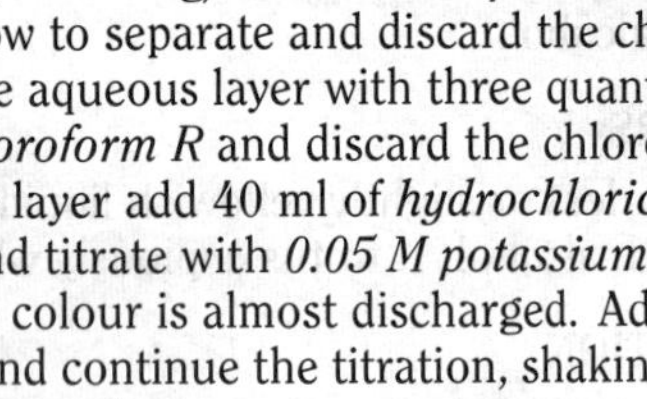

$C_{17}H_{12}Br_2O_3$ M_r 424.1

DEFINITION

Benzbromarone contains not less than 98.0 and not more than the equivalent of 101.0 per cent of (3,5-dibromo-4-hydroxyphenyl)(2-ethylbenzofuran-3-yl)methanone, calculated with reference to the dried substance.

CHARACTERS

A white or almost white, crystalline powder, practically insoluble in water, freely soluble in acetone and in methylene chloride, sparingly soluble in alcohol.

It melts at about 152 °C.

IDENTIFICATION

A. Examine by infrared absorption spectrophotometry (*2.2.24*), comparing with the *Ph. Eur. reference spectrum of benzbromarone*.

B. By means of a copper wire, previously ignited, introduce a small amount of the substance into the non-illuminated part of a flame. The colour of the flame becomes green.

TESTS

Appearance of solution. Dissolve 1.25 g in *dimethylformamide R* and dilute to 25 ml with the same solvent. The solution is clear (*2.2.1*) and not more intensely coloured than reference solution Y_5 (*2.2.2, Method II*).

Acidity or alkalinity. Shake 0.5 g with 10 ml of *carbon dioxide-free water R* for 1 min and filter. To 2.0 ml of the filtrate add 0.1 ml of *methyl red solution R* and 0.1 ml of *0.01 M hydrochloric acid*. The solution is red. Add 0.3 ml of *0.01 M sodium hydroxide*. The solution is yellow.

Related substances. Examine by liquid chromatography (*2.2.29*).

Test solution. Dissolve 0.125 g of the substance in 30 ml of *methanol R* and dilute to 50.0 ml with the mobile phase.

Reference solution (a). Dilute 1.0 ml of the test solution to 100 ml with the mobile phase. Dilute 1 ml of this solution to 10 ml with the mobile phase.

Reference solution (b). Dissolve 10 mg of *benzarone CRS* in the mobile phase and dilute to 20 ml with the mobile phase.

Reference solution (c). To 5 ml of reference solution (b) add 1 ml of the test solution and dilute to 100 ml with the mobile phase.

The chromatographic procedure may be carried out using:

– a stainless steel column 0.25 m long and 4.6 mm in internal diameter packed with *octadecylsilyl silica gel for chromatography R* (5 µm),

– as mobile phase at a flow rate of 1.5 ml/min a mixture of 5 volumes of *glacial acetic acid R*, 25 volumes of *acetonitrile R*, 300 volumes of *water R* and 990 volumes of *methanol R*,

– as detector a spectrophotometer set at 231 nm.

Inject 20 µl of reference solution (c). Adjust the sensitivity of the system so that the heights of the principal peaks in the chromatogram obtained are at least 50 per cent of the full scale of the recorder. The test is not valid unless the resolution between the first peak (impurity C) and the second peak (benzbromarone) is at least 10.0.

Inject 20 µl of the test solution and 20 µl of reference solution (a). Continue the chromatography of the test solution for 2.5 times the retention time of benzbromarone. If peaks other than the principal peak are observed in the chromatogram obtained with the test solution, these may be due to impurity A or to impurity B. When the chromatograms are recorded in the prescribed conditions, the relative retention times are: impurity A about 0.6 and impurity B about 2.

In the chromatogram obtained with the test solution: the area of the peak corresponding to impurity A is not greater than four times the area of the principal peak in the chromatogram obtained with reference solution (a) (0.4 per cent); the area of the peak corresponding to impurity B is not greater than ten times the area of the principal peak in the chromatogram obtained with reference solution (a) (1 per cent); the area of any peak, apart from the principal peak and the peaks corresponding to impurity A and impurity B, is not greater than the area of the principal peak in the chromatogram obtained with reference solution (a) (0.1 per cent); the sum of the areas of any such peaks is not greater than twice the area of the principal peak in the chromatogram obtained with reference solution (a) (0.2 per cent). Disregard any peak with an area less than 0.2 times that of the principal peak in the chromatogram obtained with reference solution (a).

Halides expressed as chlorides (*2.4.4*). Shake 1.25 g of the substance to be examined with a mixture of 5 ml of *dilute nitric acid R* and 15 ml of *water R*. Filter. Rinse the filter with *water R* and dilute the filtrate to 25 ml with the same solvent. Dilute 2.5 ml to 15 ml with *water R*. The solution obtained complies with the limit test for chlorides (400 ppm).

Iron (*2.4.9*). Moisten the residue obtained in the test for sulphated ash with 2 ml of *hydrochloric acid R* and evaporate to dryness on a water-bath. Add 0.05 ml of *hydrochloric acid R* and 10 ml of *water R* and heat until boiling for 1 min. Allow to cool. Rinse the crucible with *water R*, collect the rinsings and dilute to 25 ml with *water R*. Dilute 2 ml of this solution to 10 ml with *water R*. The solution complies with the limit test for iron (125 ppm).

Heavy metals (*2.4.8*). 0.5 g complies with limit test C for heavy metals (20 ppm). Prepare the standard using 1 ml of *lead standard solution (10 ppm Pb) R*.

Loss on drying (*2.2.32*). Not more than 0.5 per cent, determined on 1.000 g by drying in an oven *in vacuo* at 50 °C for 4 h.

Sulphated ash (*2.4.14*). Not more than 0.1 per cent, determined on 1.0 g.

ASSAY

Dissolve 0.300 g in 60 ml of *methanol R*. Stir until completely dissolved and add 10 ml of *water R*. Titrate with *0.1 M sodium hydroxide*, determining the end-point potentiometrically (*2.2.20*).

1 ml of *0.1 M sodium hydroxide* is equivalent to 42.41 mg of $C_{17}H_{12}Br_2O_3$.

STORAGE

Store protected from light.

IMPURITIES

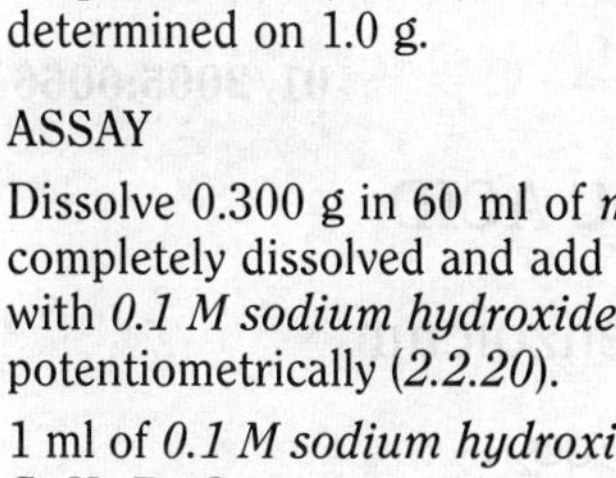

A. R1 = R2 = H, R3 = Br: (3-bromo-4-hydroxyphenyl)(2-ethylbenzofuran-3-yl)methanone,

B. R1 = R2 = R3 = Br: (6-bromo-2-ethylbenzofuran-3-yl)(3,5-dibromo-4-hydroxyphenyl)methanone,

C. R1 = R2 = R3 = H: (2-ethylbenzofuran-3-yl)(4-hydroxyphenyl)methanone (benzarone).

01/2005:0974

BENZETHONIUM CHLORIDE

Benzethonii chloridum

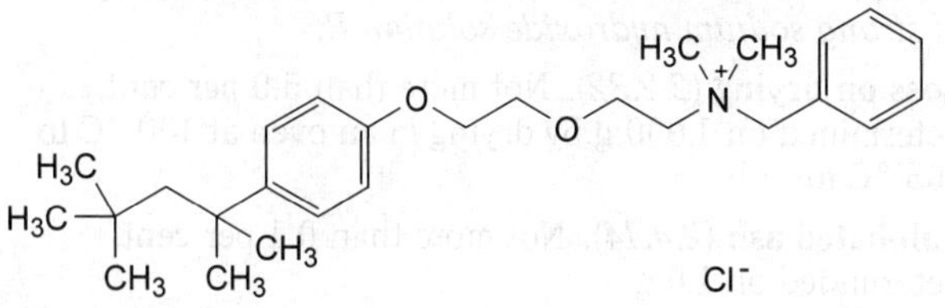

$C_{27}H_{42}ClNO_2$ M_r 448.1

DEFINITION

Benzethonium chloride contains not less than 97.0 per cent and not more than the equivalent of 103.0 per cent of *N*-benzyl-*N*,*N*-dimethyl-2-[2-[4-(1,1,3,3-tetramethylbutyl)phenoxy]ethoxy]ethanaminium chloride, calculated with reference to the dried substance.

CHARACTERS

A white or yellowish-white powder, very soluble in water and in alcohol, freely soluble in methylene chloride.

An aqueous solution froths copiously when shaken.

IDENTIFICATION

A. Melting point (*2.2.14*): 158 °C to 164 °C, after drying at 105 °C for 4 h.

B. Examine by thin-layer chromatography (*2.2.27*), using as the coating substance a suitable silica gel with a fluorescent indicator having an optimal intensity at 254 nm.

Test solution. Dissolve 25 mg of the substance to be examined in *water R* and dilute to 5 ml with the same solvent.

Reference solution. Dissolve 25 mg of *benzethonium chloride CRS* in *water R* and dilute to 5 ml with the same solvent.

Apply to the plate 20 µl of each solution. Develop over a path of 12 cm using a mixture of 5 volumes of *water R*, 5 volumes of *glacial acetic acid R* and 100 volumes of *methanol R*. Dry the plate in a current of warm air and examine in ultraviolet light at 254 nm. The principal spot in the chromatogram obtained with the test solution is similar in position and size to the principal spot in the chromatogram obtained with the reference solution.

C. To 5 ml of *dilute sodium hydroxide solution R* add 0.1 ml of *bromophenol blue solution R1* and 5 ml of *methylene chloride R* and shake. The lower layer is colourless. Add 0.1 ml of solution S (see Tests) and shake. A blue colour develops in the lower layer.

D. To 2 ml of solution S add 1 ml of *dilute nitric acid R*. A white precipitate is formed which dissolves upon addition of 5 ml of *alcohol R*. The solution gives reaction (a) of chlorides (*2.3.1*).

TESTS

Solution S. Dissolve 5.0 g in *carbon dioxide-free water R* and dilute to 50 ml with the same solvent.

Appearance of solution. Solution S is clear (*2.2.1*) and not more intensely coloured than reference solution Y_6 (*2.2.2, Method II*).

Acidity or alkalinity. To 25 ml of solution S add 0.1 ml of *phenolphthalein solution R*. The solution is colourless. Add 0.3 ml of *0.01 M sodium hydroxide*. The solution is pink. Add 0.1 ml of *methyl red solution R* and 0.5 ml of *0.01 M hydrochloric acid*. The solution is orange-red.

Volatile bases and salts of volatile bases (*2.4.1*). 0.20 g complies with limit test B for ammonium (50 ppm). Prepare the standard using 0.1 ml of *ammonium standard solution (100 ppm* NH_4*) R*. Replace heavy magnesium oxide by 2.0 ml of *strong sodium hydroxide solution R*.

Loss on drying (*2.2.32*). Not more than 5.0 per cent, determined on 1.000 g by drying in an oven at 100 °C to 105 °C for 4 h.

Sulphated ash (*2.4.14*). Not more than 0.1 per cent, determined on 1.0 g.

ASSAY

Dissolve 2.000 g in *water R* and dilute to 100.0 ml with the same solvent. Transfer 25.0 ml of the solution to a separating funnel, add 10 ml of a 4 g/l solution of *sodium hydroxide R*, 10.0 ml of a freshly prepared 50 g/l solution of *potassium iodide R* and 25 ml of *methylene chloride R*. Shake vigorously, allow to separate and discard the lower layer. Shake the upper layer with three quantities, each of 10 ml, of *methylene chloride R* and discard the lower layers. To the upper layer add 40 ml of *hydrochloric acid R*, allow to cool and titrate with *0.05 M potassium iodate* until the deep brown colour is almost discharged. Add 4 ml of *methylene chloride R* and continue the titration, shaking vigorously, until the lower layer is no longer brown. Carry out a blank titration using a mixture of 10.0 ml of a freshly prepared 50 g/l solution of *potassium iodide R*, 20 ml of *water R* and 40 ml of *hydrochloric acid R*.

1 ml of *0.05 M potassium iodate* is equivalent to 44.81 mg of $C_{27}H_{42}ClNO_2$.

STORAGE

Store protected from light.

01/2005:0011

BENZOCAINE

Benzocainum

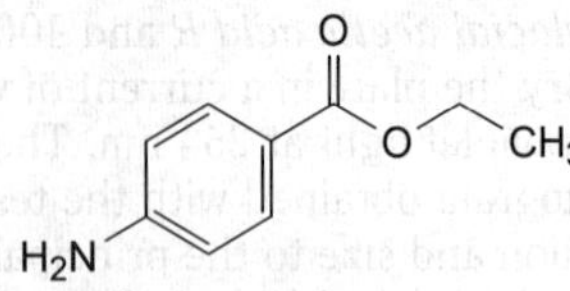

$C_9H_{11}NO_2$ M_r 165.2

DEFINITION

Benzocaine contains not less than 99.0 per cent and not more than the equivalent of 101.0 per cent of ethyl 4-aminobenzoate, calculated with reference to the dried substance.

CHARACTERS

A white, crystalline powder or colourless crystals, very slightly soluble in water, freely soluble in alcohol.

IDENTIFICATION

First identification: A, B.

Second identification: A, C, D.

A. Melting point (*2.2.14*): 89 °C to 92 °C.

B. Examine by infrared absorption spectrophotometry (*2.2.24*), comparing with the spectrum obtained with *benzocaine CRS*.

C. To about 50 mg in a test-tube add 0.2 ml of a 500 g/l solution of *chromium trioxide R*. Cover the mouth of the tube with a piece of filter paper moistened with a freshly prepared mixture of equal volumes of a 50 g/l solution of *sodium nitroprusside R* and a 200 g/l solution of *piperazine hydrate R*. Boil gently for at least 30 s. A blue colour develops on the filter paper.

D. Dissolve about 50 mg in *alcohol R* and dilute to 100 ml with the same solvent. 2 ml of the solution gives the reaction of primary aromatic amines (*2.3.1*).

TESTS

Appearance of solution. Dissolve 1.0 g in *alcohol R* and dilute to 20 ml with the same solvent. The solution is clear (*2.2.1*) and colourless (*2.2.2, Method II*).

Acidity or alkalinity. Dissolve 0.5 g in 10 ml of *alcohol R* previously neutralised to 0.05 ml of *phenolphthalein solution R*. Add 10 ml of *carbon dioxide-free water R*. The solution remains colourless and not more than 0.5 ml of *0.01 M sodium hydroxide* is required to change the colour of the indicator.

Loss on drying (*2.2.32*). Not more than 0.5 per cent, determined on 1.00 g by drying *in vacuo*.

Sulphated ash (*2.4.14*). Not more than 0.1 per cent, determined on 1.0 g.

ASSAY

Dissolve 0.400 g in a mixture of 25 ml of *hydrochloric acid R* and 50 ml of *water R*. Carry out the determination of primary aromatic amino-nitrogen (*2.5.8*).

1 ml of *0.1 M sodium nitrite* is equivalent to 16.52 mg of $C_9H_{11}NO_2$.

STORAGE

Store protected from light.

01/2005:0066

BENZOIC ACID

Acidum benzoicum

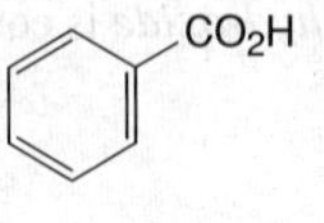

$C_7H_6O_2$ M_r 122.1

DEFINITION

Benzoic acid contains not less than 99.0 per cent and not more than the equivalent of 100.5 per cent of benzenecarboxylic acid.

CHARACTERS

A white, crystalline powder or colourless crystals, odourless or with a very slight characteristic odour, slightly soluble in water, soluble in boiling water, freely soluble in alcohol and in fatty oils.

IDENTIFICATION

A. Melting point (*2.2.14*): 121 °C to 124 °C.

B. Solution S (see Tests) gives reaction (a) of benzoates (*2.3.1*).

TESTS

Solution S. Dissolve 5.0 g in *alcohol R* and dilute to 100 ml with the same solvent.

Appearance of solution. Solution S is clear (*2.2.1*) and colourless (*2.2.2, Method II*).

Carbonisable substances. Dissolve 0.5 g with shaking in 5 ml of *sulphuric acid R*. After 5 min, the solution is not more intensely coloured than reference solution Y_5 (*2.2.2, Method I*).

Oxidisable substances. Dissolve 0.2 g in 10 ml of boiling *water R*. Cool, shake and filter. To the filtrate add 1 ml of *dilute sulphuric acid R* and 0.2 ml of *0.02 M potassium permanganate*. After 5 min, the solution is still coloured pink.

Halogenated compounds and halides.

All glassware used must be chloride-free and may be prepared by soaking overnight in a 500 g/l solution of nitric acid R, rinsed with water R and stored full of water R. It is recommended that glassware be reserved for this test.

Solution (a). Dissolve 6.7 g of the substance to be examined in a mixture of 40 ml of *1 M sodium hydroxide* and 50 ml of *alcohol R* and dilute to 100.0 ml with *water R*. To 10.0 ml of this solution add 7.5 ml of *dilute sodium hydroxide solution R* and 0.125 g of *nickel-aluminium alloy R* and heat on a water-bath for 10 min. Allow to cool to room temperature, filter into a 25 ml volumetric flask and wash with three quantities, each of 2 ml, of *alcohol R*. Dilute the filtrate and washings to 25.0 ml with *water R*. This solution is used to prepare solution A.

Solution (b). In the same manner, prepare a similar solution without the substance to be examined. This solution is used to prepare solution B.

In four 25 ml volumetric flasks, place separately 10 ml of solution (a), 10 ml of solution (b), 10 ml of *chloride standard solution (8 ppm Cl) R* (used to prepare solution C) and 10 ml of *water R*. To each flask add 5 ml of *ferric ammonium sulphate solution R5*, mix and add dropwise and with swirling 2 ml of *nitric acid R* and 5 ml of *mercuric thiocyanate solution R*. Shake. Dilute the contents of each flask to 25.0 ml with *water R* and allow the solutions to stand in a water-bath at 20 °C for 15 min. Measure at 460 nm the absorbance (*2.2.25*) of solution A using solution B as the compensation liquid, and the absorbance of solution C using the solution obtained with 10 ml of *water R* as the compensation liquid. The absorbance of solution A is not greater than that of solution C (300 ppm).

Heavy metals (*2.4.8*). 12 ml of solution S complies with limit test B for heavy metals (10 ppm). Prepare the standard using a mixture of 5 ml of *lead standard solution (1 ppm Pb) R* and 5 ml of *alcohol R*.

Sulphated ash (*2.4.14*). Not more than 0.1 per cent, determined on 1.0 g.

ASSAY

Dissolve 0.200 g in 20 ml of *alcohol R* and titrate with *0.1 M sodium hydroxide*, using 0.1 ml of *phenol red solution R* as indicator, until the colour changes from yellow to violet-red.

1 ml of *0.1 M sodium hydroxide* is equivalent to 12.21 mg of $C_7H_6O_2$.

01/2005:0704

BENZOYL PEROXIDE, HYDROUS

Benzoylis peroxidum cum aqua

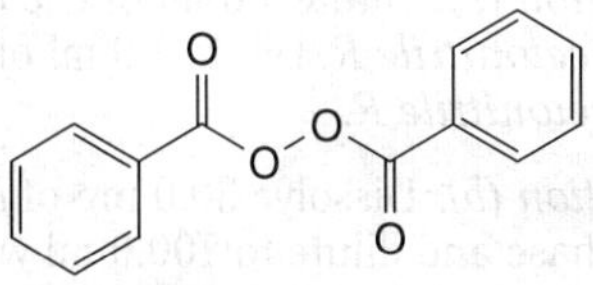

$C_{14}H_{10}O_4$ M_r 242.2

DEFINITION

Content:

– dibenzoyl peroxide: 70.0 per cent to 77.0 per cent,

– water: minimum 20.0 per cent.

CHARACTERS

Appearance: white, amorphous or granular powder.

Solubility: practically insoluble in water, soluble in acetone, soluble in methylene chloride with the separation of water, slightly soluble in alcohol.

It loses water rapidly on exposure to air with a risk of explosion.

Mix the entire sample thoroughly before carrying out the following tests.

IDENTIFICATION

First identification: B

Second identification: A, C, D.

A. Dissolve 80.0 mg in *alcohol R* and dilute to 100.0 ml with the same solvent. Dilute 10.0 ml of the solution to 100.0 ml with *alcohol R* (solution A). Dilute 10.0 ml of solution A to 100.0 ml with *alcohol R* (solution B). Examined between 250 nm and 300 nm (*2.2.25*), solution A shows an absorption maximum at 274 nm and a shoulder at about 282 nm. Examined between 220 nm and 250 nm, solution B shows an absorption maximum at 235 nm. The ratio of the absorbance at the maximum at 235 nm (solution B) to that at the maximum at 274 nm (solution A) is 1.17 to 1.21.

B. Infrared absorption spectrophotometry (*2.2.24*).

Comparison: *Ph. Eur. reference spectrum of hydrous benzoyl peroxide.*

C. Dissolve about 25 mg in 2 ml of *acetone R*. Add 1 ml of a 10 g/l solution of *diethylphenylenediamine sulphate R* and mix. A red colour develops which quickly darkens and becomes dark violet within 5 min.

D. To 1 g add 5 ml of *alcohol R*, 5 ml of *dilute sodium hydroxide solution R* and 10 ml of *water R*. Boil the mixture under reflux for 20 min. Cool. The solution gives reaction (c) of benzoates (*2.3.1*).

TESTS

Acidity. Dissolve a quantity of the substance to be examined containing the equivalent of 1.0 g of dibenzoyl peroxide in 25 ml of *acetone R*, add 75 ml of *water R* and filter. Wash the residue with two quantities, each of 10 ml, of *water R*. Combine the filtrate and the washings and add 0.25 ml of *phenolphthalein solution R1*. Not more than 1.25 ml of *0.1 M sodium hydroxide* is required to change the colour of the indicator. Carry out a blank test.

Related substances. Liquid chromatography (*2.2.29*). *Prepare the solutions immediately before use.*

Test solution. Dissolve a quantity of the substance to be examined containing the equivalent of 0.10 g of dibenzoyl peroxide in *acetonitrile R* and dilute to 50 ml with the same solvent.

Reference solution (a). Dilute 1.0 ml of the test solution to 100.0 ml with *acetonitrile R*. Dilute 1.0 ml of this solution to 10.0 ml with *acetonitrile R.*

Reference solution (b). Dissolve 30.0 mg of *benzoic acid R* in the mobile phase and dilute to 100.0 ml with the mobile phase. Dilute 1.0 ml of the solution to 10.0 ml with the mobile phase.

Reference solution (c). Dissolve 50.0 mg of *ethyl benzoate R* in the mobile phase and dilute to 100.0 ml with the mobile phase. Dilute 1.0 ml of the solution to 100.0 ml with the mobile phase.

Reference solution (d). Dissolve 50.0 mg of *benzaldehyde R* in the mobile phase and dilute to 100.0 ml with the mobile phase. Dilute 1.0 ml of the solution to 100.0 ml with the mobile phase.

Reference solution (e). Dissolve 30.0 mg of *benzoic acid R* and 30.0 mg of *benzaldehyde R* in the mobile phase and dilute to 100.0 ml with the mobile phase. Dilute 1.0 ml of the solution to 10.0 ml with the mobile phase.

Column:

- *size*: l = 0.25 m, Ø = 4.6 mm,
- *stationary phase*: *octadecylsilyl silica gel for chromatography R* (10 µm),

Mobile phase: *glacial acetic acid R, acetonitrile R, water R* (1:500:500 *V/V/V*).

Flow rate: 1 ml/min.

Detection: spectrophotometer at 235 nm.

Injection: 20 µl loop injector.

Run time: 2 times the retention time of dibenzoyl peroxide.

Relative retention with reference to dibenzoyl peroxide (retention time = about 28.4 min): impurity B = about 0.15; impurity A = about 0.2; impurity C = about 0.4.

System suitability: reference solution (e):

- *resolution*: minimum 6 between the peaks corresponding to benzoic acid and benzaldehyde.

Limits:

- *impurity A*: not more than the area of the principal peak in the chromatogram obtained with reference solution (d) (0.25 per cent),
- *impurity B*: not more than the area of the principal peak in the chromatogram obtained with reference solution (b) (1.5 per cent),
- *impurity C*: not more than the area of the principal peak in the chromatogram obtained with reference solution (c) (0.25 per cent),
- *any other impurity*: not more than the area of the principal peak in the chromatogram obtained with reference solution (a) (0.1 per cent),
- *disregard limit*: 0.2 times the area of the principal peak in the chromatogram obtained with reference solution (a) (0.02 per cent).

Chlorides (*2.4.4*): maximum 0.4 per cent.

Dissolve a quantity of the substance to be examined containing the equivalent of 0.5 g of dibenzoyl peroxide in 15 ml of *acetone R*. Add, while stirring, 50 ml of *0.05 M nitric acid.* Allow to stand for 10 min and filter. Wash the residue with 2 quantities, each of 10 ml, of *0.05 M nitric acid.* Combine the filtrate and the washings and dilute to 100 ml with *0.05 M nitric acid*. 2.5 ml of the solution diluted to 15.0 ml with *water R* complies with the limit test for chlorides.

ASSAY

Solution (a). Dissolve 2.500 g immediately before use in 75 ml of *dimethylformamide R* and dilute to 100.0 ml with the same solvent.

Dibenzoyl peroxide. To 5.0 ml of solution (a) add 20 ml of *acetone R* and 3 ml of a 500 g/l solution of *potassium iodide R* and mix. Allow to stand for 1 min. Titrate with *0.1 M sodium thiosulphate* using 1 ml of *starch solution R,* added towards the end of the titration, as indicator. Carry out a blank titration.

1 ml of *0.1 M sodium thiosulphate* is equivalent to 12.11 mg of $C_{14}H_{10}O_4$.

Water (*2.5.12*). Carry out the semi-micro determination of water, using 5.0 ml of solution (a). Use as the solvent a mixture of 20.0 ml of *anhydrous methanol R* and 3.0 ml of a 100 g/l solution of *potassium iodide R* in *dimethylformamide R.* After adding solution (a), stir for 5 min before starting the titration. Carry out a blank determination.

Calculate the percentage content of water using the expression:

$$\frac{(n_1 - n_2) \times w \times 2}{m} + (p \times 0.0744)$$

n_1 = number of millilitres of *iodosulphurous reagent R* used in the sample determination,

n_2 = number of millilitres of *iodosulphurous reagent R* used in the blank determination,

w = water equivalent of *iodosulphurous reagent R* in milligrams of water per millilitre of reagent,

m = mass of the substance to be examined used for the preparation of solution (a) in grams,

p = percentage content of dibenzoyl peroxide.

STORAGE

In a container that has been treated to reduce static discharge and that has a device for release of excess pressure, at a temperature of 2 °C to 8 °C, protected from light.

IMPURITIES

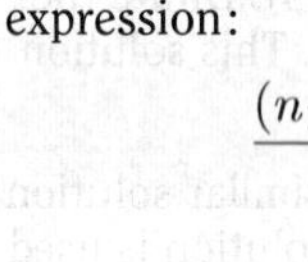

A. R = H: benzaldehyde,

B. R = OH: benzoic acid,

C. R = O-CH_2-CH_3: ethyl benzoate.

01/2005:0256
corrected

BENZYL ALCOHOL

Alcohol benzylicus

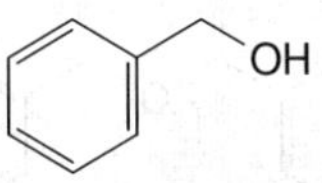

C_7H_8O M_r 108.1

DEFINITION

Phenylmethanol.

Content: 98.0 per cent to 100.5 per cent.

CHARACTERS

Appearance: clear, colourless, oily liquid.

Solubility: soluble in water, miscible with alcohol and with fatty and essential oils.

Relative density: 1.043 to 1.049.

IDENTIFICATION

Infrared absorption spectrophotometry (*2.2.24*).

Comparison: *Ph. Eur. reference spectrum of benzyl alcohol.*

TESTS

Appearance of solution. Shake 2.0 ml with 60 ml of *water R*. It dissolves completely. The solution is clear (*2.2.1*) and colourless (*2.2.2, Method II*).

Acidity. To 10 ml add 10 ml of *alcohol R* and 1 ml of *phenolphthalein solution R*. Not more than 1 ml of *0.1 M sodium hydroxide* is required to change the colour of the indicator to pink.

Refractive index (*2.2.6*): 1.538 to 1.541.

Peroxide value (*2.5.5*): maximum 5.

Benzaldehyde and other related substances. Gas chromatography (*2.2.28*).

Test solution. The substance to be examined.

Standard solution (a). Dissolve 0.100 g of *ethylbenzene R* in the test solution and dilute to 10.0 ml with the same solution. Dilute 2.0 ml of this solution to 20.0 ml with the test solution.

Standard solution (b). Dissolve 2.000 g of *dicyclohexyl R* in the test solution and dilute to 10.0 ml with the same solution. Dilute 2.0 ml of this solution to 20.0 ml with the test solution.

Reference solution (a). Dissolve 0.750 g of *benzaldehyde R* and 0.500 g of *cyclohexylmethanol R* in the test solution and dilute to 25.0 ml with the test solution. Add 1.0 ml of this solution to a mixture of 2.0 ml of standard solution (a) and 3.0 ml of standard solution (b) and dilute to 20.0 ml with the test solution.

Reference solution (b). Dissolve 0.250 g of *benzaldehyde R* and 0.500 g of *cyclohexylmethanol R* in the test solution and dilute to 25.0 ml with the test solution. Add 1.0 ml of this solution to a mixture of 2.0 ml of standard solution (a) and 2.0 ml of standard solution (b) and dilute to 20.0 ml with the test solution.

Column:
- *material*: fused silica,
- *size*: l = 30 m, Ø = 0.32 mm,
- *stationary phase*: *macrogol 20 000 R* (film thickness 0.5 µm).

Carrier gas: *helium for chromatography R.*

Linear velocity: 25 cm/s.

Temperature:

	Time (min)	Temperature (°C)
Column	0 - 34	50 → 220
	34 - 69	220
Injection port		200
Detector		310

Detection: flame ionisation.

Benzyl alcohol not intended for parenteral use.

Injection: without air-plug, 0.1 µl of the test solution and 0.1 µl of reference solution (a).

Relative retention with reference to benzyl alcohol (retention time = about 26 min): ethylbenzene = about 0.28; dicyclohexyl = about 0.59; benzaldehyde = about 0.68; cyclohexylmethanol = about 0.71.

System suitability: reference solution (a):
- *resolution*: minimum 3.0 between the peaks corresponding to benzaldehyde and to cyclohexylmethanol.

In the chromatogram obtained with the test solution, verify that there are no peaks with the same retention time as the standards.

Limits:
- *benzaldehyde*: not more than the difference between the area of the peak due to benzaldehyde in the chromatogram obtained with reference solution (a) and the area of the peak due to benzaldehyde in the chromatogram obtained with the test solution (0.15 per cent).
- *cyclohexylmethanol*: not more than the difference between the area of the peak due to cyclohexylmethanol in the chromatogram obtained with reference solution (a) and the area of the peak due to cyclohexylmethanol in the chromatogram obtained with the test solution (0.10 per cent).
- *total of other peaks with a relative retention less than that of benzyl alcohol*: not more than 4 times the area of the peak due to ethylbenzene in the chromatogram obtained with reference solution (a) (0.04 per cent).
- *total of peaks with a relative retention greater than that of benzyl alcohol*: not more than the area of the peak due to dicyclohexyl in the chromatogram obtained with reference solution (a) (0.3 per cent).
- *disregard limit*: 0.01 times the area of the peak due to ethylbenzene in the chromatogram obtained with reference solution (a) (0.0001 per cent).

Benzyl alcohol intended for parenteral use.

Injection: without air-plug, 0.1 µl of the test solution and 0.1 µl of reference solution (b).

Relative retention with reference to benzyl alcohol (retention time = about 26 min): ethylbenzene = about 0.28; dicyclohexyl = about 0.59; benzaldehyde = about 0.68; cyclohexylmethanol = about 0.71.

System suitability: reference solution (b):
- *resolution*: minimum 3.0 between the peaks corresponding to benzaldehyde and to cyclohexylmethanol.

In the chromatogram obtained with the test solution, verify that there are no peaks with the same retention time as the standards.

Limits:

- *benzaldehyde*: not more than the difference between the area of the peak due to benzaldehyde in the chromatogram obtained with reference solution (b) and the area of the peak due to benzaldehyde in the chromatogram obtained with the test solution (0.05 per cent).
- *cyclohexylmethanol*: not more than the difference between the area of the peak due to cyclohexylmethanol in the chromatogram obtained with reference solution (b) and the area of the peak due to cyclohexylmethanol in the chromatogram obtained with the test solution (0.10 per cent).
- *total of other peaks with a relative retention less than that of benzyl alcohol*: not more than twice the area of the peak due to ethylbenzene in the chromatogram obtained with reference solution (b) (0.02 per cent).
- *total of peaks with a relative retention greater than that of benzyl alcohol*: not more than the area of the peak due to dicyclohexyl in the chromatogram obtained with reference solution (b) (0.2 per cent).
- *disregard limit*: 0.01 times the area of the peak due to ethylbenzene in the chromatogram obtained with reference solution (b) (0.0001 per cent).

Residue on evaporation: maximum 0.05 per cent.

After ensuring that the substance to be examined complies with the test for peroxide value, evaporate 10.0 g to dryness on a water-bath, dry at 100-105 °C for 1 h and allow to cool in a desiccator. The residue weighs a maximum of 5 mg.

ASSAY

To 0.900 g (*m* g) add 15.0 ml of a freshly prepared mixture of 1 volume of *acetic anhydride R* and 7 volumes of *pyridine R* and boil under a reflux condenser for 30 min. Cool and add 25 ml of *water R*. Using 0.25 ml of *phenolphthalein solution R* as indicator, titrate with *1 M sodium hydroxide* (n_1 ml). Carry out a blank titration (n_2 ml).

Calculate the percentage content of C_7H_8O from the expression:

$$\frac{10.81\,(n_2 - n_1)}{m}$$

STORAGE

In an airtight container, under nitrogen, protected from light at a temperature between 2 °C and 8 °C.

LABELLING

The label states, where applicable, that the substance is suitable for use in the manufacture of parenteral dosage forms.

01/2005:0705

BENZYL BENZOATE

Benzylis benzoas

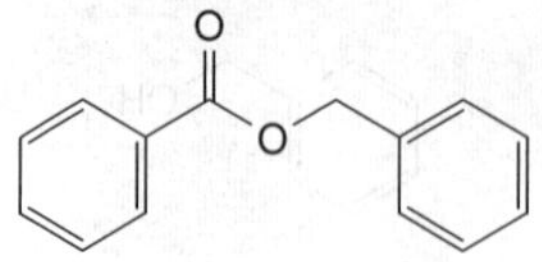

$C_{14}H_{12}O_2$ M_r 212.2

DEFINITION

Benzyl benzoate contains not less than 99.0 per cent and not more than the equivalent of 100.5 per cent of phenylmethyl benzoate.

CHARACTERS

Colourless or almost colourless crystals or a colourless or almost colourless, oily liquid, practically insoluble in water, miscible with alcohol, with methylene chloride and with fatty and essential oils.

It boils at about 320 °C.

IDENTIFICATION

First identification: A.

Second identification: B, C.

A. Examine by infrared absorption spectrophotometry (*2.2.24*), comparing with the *Ph. Eur. reference spectrum of benzyl benzoate.*

B. To 2 g add 25 ml of *alcoholic potassium hydroxide solution R* and boil under a reflux condenser for 2 h. Remove the ethanol on a water-bath, add 50 ml of *water R* and distil; collect about 25 ml of distillate and use it for identification test C. Acidify the liquid remaining in the distillation flask with *dilute hydrochloric acid R*; a white precipitate is formed, which, when washed with *water R* and dried *in vacuo*, melts (*2.2.14*) at 121 °C to 124 °C.

C. To the distillate obtained in identification test B add 2.5 g of *potassium permanganate R* and 5 ml of *dilute sodium hydroxide solution R*. Boil under a reflux condenser for 15 min, cool and filter. Acidify the filtrate with *dilute hydrochloric acid R*; a white precipitate is formed which, when washed with *water R* and dried *in vacuo*, melts (*2.2.14*) at 121 °C to 124 °C.

TESTS

Acidity. Dissolve 2.0 g in *alcohol R* and dilute to 10 ml with the same solvent. Titrate with *0.1 M sodium hydroxide* using *phenolphthalein solution R* as indicator. Not more than 0.2 ml is required to change the colour of the indicator to pink.

Relative density (*2.2.5*): 1.118 to 1.122.

Refractive index (*2.2.6*): 1.568 to 1.570.

Freezing point (*2.2.18*). Not less than 17.0 °C.

Sulphated ash (*2.4.14*). Not more than 0.1 per cent, determined on 1.0 g.

ASSAY

To 2.000 g add 50.0 ml of *0.5 M alcoholic potassium hydroxide* and boil gently under a reflux condenser for 1 h. Titrate the hot solution with *0.5 M hydrochloric acid* using 1 ml of *phenolphthalein solution R* as indicator. Carry out a blank determination.

1 ml of *0.5 M alcoholic potassium hydroxide* is equivalent to 106.1 mg of $C_{14}H_{12}O_2$.

STORAGE

Store in an airtight, well-filled container, protected from light.

01/2005:0373

BENZYLPENICILLIN, BENZATHINE

Benzylpenicillinum benzathinum

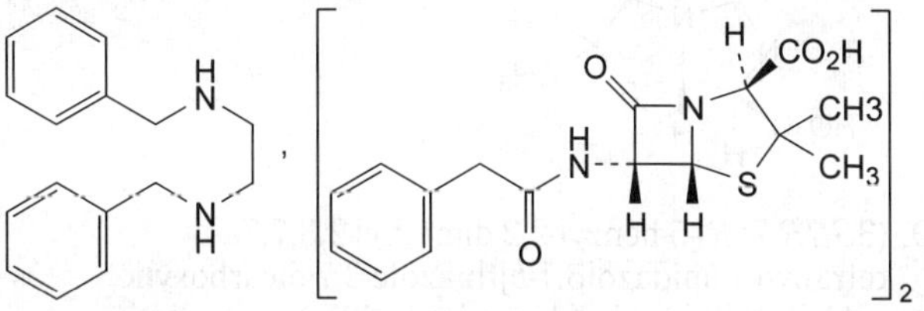

$C_{48}H_{56}N_6O_8S_2$ M_r 909

DEFINITION

Benzathine benzylpenicillin is *N,N'*-dibenzylethane-1,2-diamine compound (1:2) with (2*S*,5*R*,6*R*)-3,3-dimethyl-7-oxo-6-[(phenylacetyl)amino]-4-thia-1-azabicyclo[3.2.0]heptane-2-carboxylic acid. It contains not less than 96.0 per cent and not more than the equivalent of 102.0 per cent of benzathine benzylpenicillin and not less than 24.0 per cent and not more than 27.0 per cent of *N,N'*-dibenzylethylenediamine (benzathine $C_{16}H_{20}N_2$; M_r 240.3), both calculated with reference to the anhydrous substance. It contains a variable quantity of water. Dispersing or suspending agents may be added.

CHARACTERS

A white powder, very slightly soluble in water, freely soluble in dimethylformamide and in formamide, slightly soluble in alcohol.

IDENTIFICATION

First identification: A.

Second identification: B, C, D.

A. Examine by infrared absorption spectrophotometry (*2.2.24*), comparing with the spectrum obtained with *benzathine benzylpenicillin CRS*.

B. Examine by thin-layer chromatography (*2.2.27*), using a *TLC silanised silica gel plate R*.

Test solution. Dissolve 25 mg of the substance to be examined in 5 ml of *methanol R*.

Reference solution. Dissolve 25 mg of *benzathine benzylpenicillin CRS* in 5 ml of *methanol R*.

Apply to the plate 1 µl of each solution. Develop over a path of 15 cm using a mixture of 30 volumes of *acetone R* and 70 volumes of a 154 g/l solution of *ammonium acetate R*, the pH of which has been adjusted to 7.0 with *ammonia R*. Allow the plate to dry in air and expose it to iodine vapour until the spots appear. Examine in daylight. The two principal spots in the chromatogram obtained with the test solution are similar in position, colour and size to the two principal spots in the chromatogram obtained with the reference solution. The test is not valid unless the chromatogram obtained with the reference solution shows two clearly separated spots.

C. Place about 2 mg in a test-tube about 150 mm long and 15 mm in diameter. Moisten with 0.05 ml of *water R* and add 2 ml of *sulphuric acid-formaldehyde reagent R*. Mix the contents of the tube by swirling; the solution is practically colourless. Place the test-tube on a water-bath for 1 min; a reddish-brown colour develops.

D. To 0.1 g add 2 ml of *1 M sodium hydroxide* and shake for 2 min. Shake the mixture with two quantities, each of 3 ml, of *ether R*. Evaporate the combined ether layers to dryness and dissolve the residue in 1 ml of *alcohol (50 per cent V/V) R*. Add 5 ml of *picric acid solution R*, heat at 90 °C for 5 min and allow to cool slowly. Separate the crystals and recrystallise from *alcohol (25 per cent V/V) R* containing 10 g/l of *picric acid R*. The crystals melt (*2.2.14*) at about 214 °C.

TESTS

Acidity or alkalinity. To 0.50 g add 100 ml of *carbon dioxide-free water R* and shake for 5 min. Filter through a sintered-glass filter. To 20 ml of the filtrate add 0.1 ml of *bromothymol blue solution R1*. The solution is green or yellow. Not more than 0.2 ml of *0.02 M sodium hydroxide* is required to change the colour of the indicator to blue.

Related substances. Liquid chromatography (*2.2.29*). *Prepare the solutions immediately before use, using sonication (for about 2 min) to dissolve the samples. Avoid any over heating during the sample preparation.*

Test solution. Dissolve 70.0 mg of the substance to be examined in 25 ml of *methanol R* and dilute to 50.0 ml with a solution containing 6.8 g/l of *potassium dihydrogen phosphate R* and 1.02 g/l of *disodium hydrogen phosphate R*.

Reference solution (a). Dissolve 70.0 mg of *benzathine benzylpenicillin CRS* in 25 ml of *methanol R* and dilute to 50.0 ml with a solution containing 6.8 g/l of *potassium dihydrogen phosphate R* and 1.02 g/l of *disodium hydrogen phosphate R*.

Reference solution (b). Dilute 1.0 ml of reference solution (a) to 100.0 ml with mobile phase A.

Column:

- *size*: *l* = 0.25 m, Ø = 4.0 mm,
- *stationary phase*: *end-capped octadecylsilyl silica gel for chromatography R* (5 µm),
- *temperature*: 40 °C.

Mobile phase:

- *mobile phase A*: mix 10 volumes of a 34 g/l solution of *potassium dihydrogen phosphate R* adjusted to pH 3.5 with *phosphoric acid R*, 30 volumes of *methanol R* and 60 volumes of *water R*,
- *mobile phase B*: mix 10 volumes of a 34 g/l solution of *potassium dihydrogen phosphate R* adjusted to pH 3.5 with *phosphoric acid R*, 30 volumes of *water R* and 60 volumes of *methanol R*,

Time (min)	Mobile phase A (per cent *V/V*)	Mobile phase B (per cent *V/V*)
0 - 10	75	25
10 - 20	75 → 0	25 → 100
20 - 55	0	100
55 - 70	75	25

Flow rate: 1 ml/min.

Detection: spectrophotometer at 220 nm.

Injection: 20 µl; inject the test solution and the reference solutions.

System suitability: reference solution (a)

– *relative retention* with reference to benzylpenicillin: benzathine = 0.3 to 0.4; impurity C = about 2.4. If necessary, adjust the concentration of methanol in the mobile phase.

Limits:

– *impurity C*: not more than twice the sum of the areas of the 2 principal peaks in the chromatogram obtained with reference solution (b) (2 per cent),
– *any other impurity*: not more than the sum of the areas of the 2 principal peaks in the chromatogram obtained with reference solution (b) (1 per cent),
– *disregard limit*: 0.05 times the sum of the areas of the 2 principal peaks in the chromatogram obtained with reference solution (b) (0.05 per cent).

Water (*2.5.12*): 5.0 per cent to 8.0 per cent, determined on 0.300 g by the semi-micro determination of water.

Bacterial endotoxins (*2.6.14, Method E*). Suspend 20 mg of the substance to be examined in 20 ml of a solution of *0.1 M sodium hydroxide* diluted 1 to 100, shake thoroughly and centrifuge. The supernatant contains less than 0.13 IU/ml, if intended for use in the manufacture of parenteral dosage forms without a further appropriate procedure for the removal of bacterial endotoxins.

ASSAY

Liquid chromatography (*2.2.29*) as described in the test for related substances.

Mobile phase: *phosphate buffer solution pH 3.5 R, methanol R, water R* (10:35:55 *V/V/V*).

Injection: 20 µl; inject the test solution and reference solution (a).

Calculate the percentage contents of benzathine and of benzathine benzylpenicillin. Calculate the latter by multiplying the percentage content of benzylpenicillin by 1.36.

STORAGE

Store in an airtight container. If the substance is sterile, store in a sterile, airtight, tamper-proof container.

LABELLING

The label states:

– where applicable, the name and quantity of any added dispersing or suspending agent,
– where applicable, that the substance is free from bacterial endotoxins.

IMPURITIES

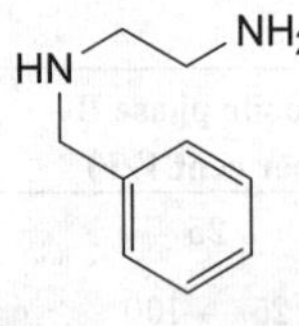

A. monobenzylethylenediamine,

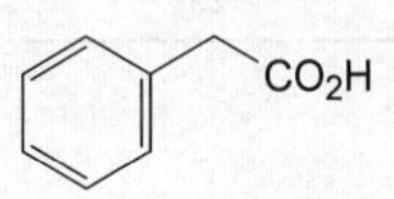

B. phenylacetic acid,

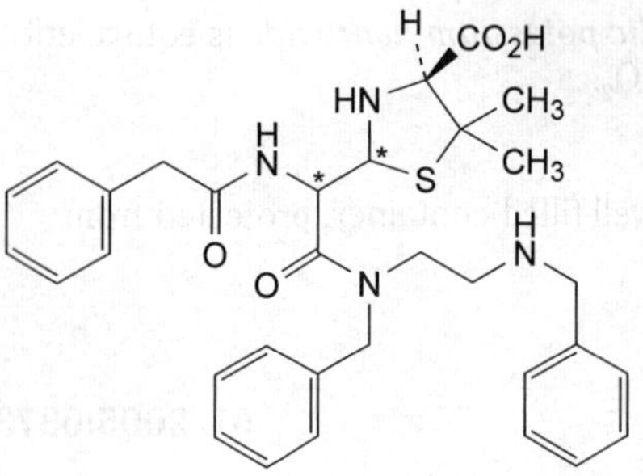

C. benzylpenicilloic acids benzathide,

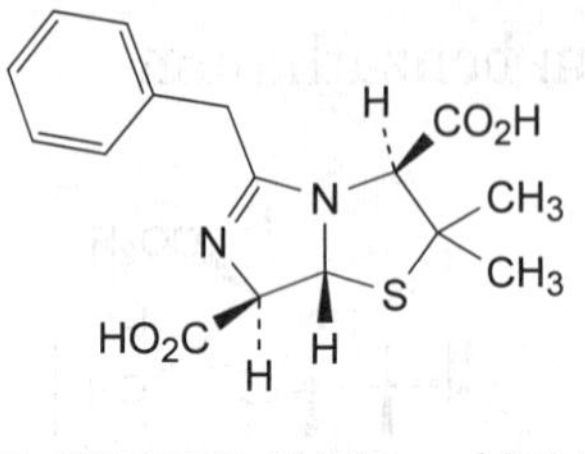

D. (3*S*,7*R*,7a*R*)-5-benzyl-2,2-dimethyl-2,3,7,7a-tetrahydroimidazo[5,1-*b*]thiazole-3,7-dicarboxylic acid (penillic acid of benzylpenicillin),

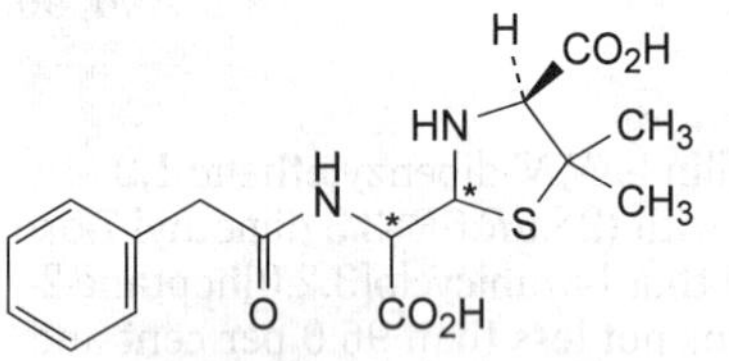

E. (4*S*)-2-[carboxy[(phenylacetyl)amino]methyl]-5,5-dimethylthiazolidine-4-carboxylic acid (penicilloic acids of benzylpenicillin),

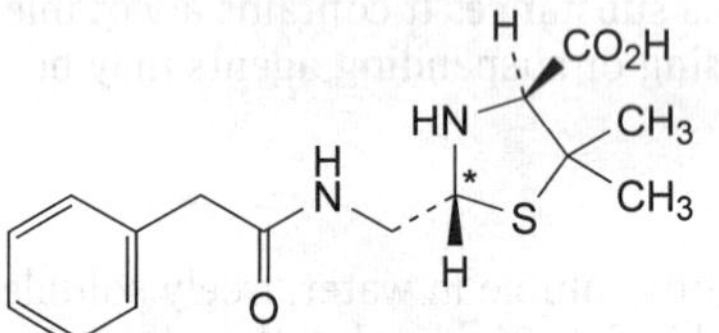

and epimer at C*

F. (2*RS*,4*S*)-2-[[(phenylacetyl)amino]methyl]-5,5-dimethylthiazolidine-4-carboxylic acid (penilloic acids of benzylpenicillin).

01/2005:0113

BENZYLPENICILLIN POTASSIUM

Benzylpenicillinum kalicum

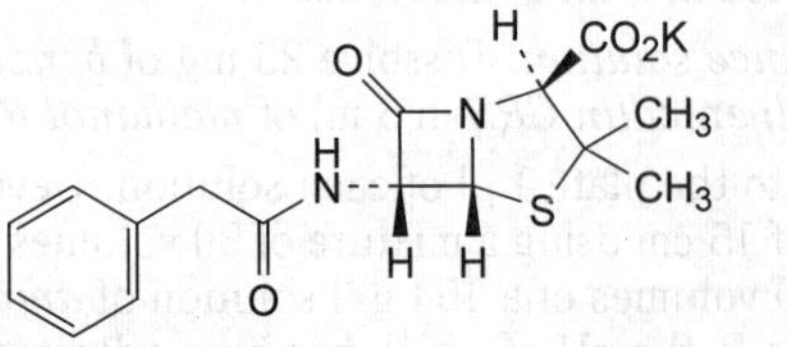

$C_{16}H_{17}KN_2O_4S$ M_r 372.5

DEFINITION

Benzylpenicillin potassium is potassium (2*S*,5*R*,6*R*)-3,3-dimethyl-7-oxo-6-[(phenylacetyl)amino]-4-thia-1-azabicyclo[3.2.0]heptane-2-carboxylate, a substance produced by the growth of certain strains of *Penicillium notatum* or related organisms, or obtained by any other means. It contains not less than 96.0 per cent and not more than the equivalent of 102.0 per cent of benzylpenicillin potassium, calculated with reference to the dried substance.

CHARACTERS

A white or almost white, crystalline powder, very soluble in water, practically insoluble in fatty oils and in liquid paraffin.

IDENTIFICATION

First identification: A, D.

Second identification: B, C, D.

A. Examine by infrared absorption spectrophotometry (*2.2.24*), comparing with the spectrum obtained with *benzylpenicillin potassium CRS.*

B. Examine by thin-layer chromatography (*2.2.27*), using a *TLC silanised silica gel plate R.*

Test solution. Dissolve 25 mg of the substance to be examined in 5 ml of *water R.*

Reference solution (a). Dissolve 25 mg of *benzylpenicillin potassium CRS* in 5 ml of *water R.*

Reference solution (b). Dissolve 25 mg of *benzylpenicillin potassium CRS* and 25 mg of *phenoxymethylpenicillin potassium CRS* in 5 ml of *water R.*

Apply to the plate 1 µl of each solution. Develop over a path of 15 cm using a mixture of 30 volumes of *acetone R* and 70 volumes of a 154 g/l solution of *ammonium acetate R*, the pH of which has been adjusted to 5.0 with *glacial acetic acid R.* Allow the plate to dry in air and expose it to iodine vapour until the spots appear. Examine in daylight. The principal spot in the chromatogram obtained with the test solution is similar in position, colour and size to the principal spot in the chromatogram obtained with reference solution (a). The test is not valid unless the chromatogram obtained with reference solution (b) shows 2 clearly separated spots.

C. Place about 2 mg in a test-tube about 150 mm long and 15 mm in diameter. Moisten with 0.05 ml of *water R* and add 2 ml of *sulphuric acid-formaldehyde reagent R.* Mix the contents of the tube by swirling; the solution is practically colourless. Place the test-tube on a water-bath for 1 min; a reddish-brown colour develops.

D. It gives reaction (a) of potassium (*2.3.1*).

TESTS

pH (*2.2.3*). Dissolve 2.0 g in *carbon dioxide-free water R* and dilute to 20 ml with the same solvent. The pH of the solution is 5.5 to 7.5.

Specific optical rotation (*2.2.7*). Dissolve 0.500 g in *carbon dioxide-free water R* and dilute to 25.0 ml with the same solvent. The specific optical rotation is + 270 to + 300, calculated with reference to the dried substance.

Absorbance (*2.2.25*). Dissolve 94.0 mg in *water R* and dilute to 50.0 ml with the same solvent. Measure the absorbance of the solution at 325 nm, 280 nm and at the maximum at 264 nm, diluting the solution, if necessary, for the measurement at 264 nm. The absorbances at 325 nm and 280 nm do not exceed 0.10 and that at the maximum at 264 nm is 0.80 to 0.88, calculated on the basis of the undiluted (1.88 g/l) solution. Verify the resolution of the apparatus (*2.2.25*); the ratio of the absorbances is at least 1.7.

Related substances. Examine by liquid chromatography (*2.2.29*) as described under Assay. Inject 20 µl of reference solution (d) and elute isocratically with the chosen mobile phase. Inject 20 µl of test solution (b) and start the elution isocratically. Immediately after elution of the benzylpenicillin peak start the following linear gradient:

Time (min)	Mobile phase A (per cent *V/V*)	Mobile phase B (per cent *V/V*)	Comment
0 - 20	70 → 0	30 → 100	linear gradient
20 - 35	0	100	isocratic
35 - 50	70	30	re-equilibration

Inject *water R* and use the same elution pattern to obtain a blank. In the chromatogram obtained with test solution (b), the area of any peak, apart from the principal peak, is not greater than the area of the principal peak in the chromatogram obtained with reference solution (d) (1 per cent).

Loss on drying (*2.2.32*). Not more than 1.0 per cent, determined on 1.000 g by drying in an oven at 100-105 °C.

Bacterial endotoxins (*2.6.14, Method E*): less than 0.16 IU/mg, if intended for use in the manufacture of parenteral dosage forms without a further appropriate procedure for the removal of bacterial endotoxins.

ASSAY

Examine by liquid chromatography (*2.2.29*). *Prepare the solutions immediately before use.*

Test solution (a). Dissolve 50.0 mg of the substance to be examined in *water R* and dilute to 50.0 ml with the same solvent.

Test solution (b). Dissolve 80.0 mg of the substance to be examined in *water R* and dilute to 20.0 ml with the same solvent.

Reference solution (a). Dissolve 50.0 mg of *benzylpenicillin sodium CRS* in *water R* and dilute to 50.0 ml with the same solvent.

Reference solution (b). Dissolve 10 mg of *benzylpenicillin sodium CRS* and 10 mg of *phenylacetic acid CRS* in *water R* and dilute to 50 ml with the same solvent.

Reference solution (c). Dilute 1.0 ml of reference solution (a) to 20.0 ml with *water R.* Dilute 1.0 ml of the solution to 50.0 ml with *water R.*

Reference solution (d). Dilute 4.0 ml of reference solution (a) to 100.0 ml with *water R.*

The chromatographic procedure may be carried out using:

- a column 0.25 m long and 4.6 mm in internal diameter packed with *octadecylsilyl silica gel for chromatography R* (5 µm),
- as mobile phase at a flow rate of 1.0 ml/min:

  Mobile phase A. Mix 10 volumes of a 68 g/l solution of *potassium dihydrogen phosphate R* adjusted to pH 3.5 with a 500 g/l solution of *dilute phosphoric acid R,* 30 volumes of *methanol R* and 60 volumes of *water R,*

  Mobile phase B. Mix 10 volumes of a 68 g/l solution of *potassium dihydrogen phosphate R* adjusted to pH 3.5 with a 500 g/l solution of *dilute phosphoric acid R,* 40 volumes of *water R* and 50 volumes of *methanol R,*
- as detector a spectrophotometer set at 225 nm.

Equilibrate the column with a mobile phase ratio A:B of 70:30. Inject 20 µl of reference solution (b). The test is not valid unless the resolution between the 2 principal peaks is at least 6.0 (if necessary, adjust the ratio A:B of the mobile phase) and the mass distribution ratio for the second peak (benzylpenicillin) is 4.0 to 6.0. Inject 20 µl of reference solution (c). Adjust the system to obtain a peak with a signal-to-noise ratio of at least 3.

Monographs B

Calculate the percentage content of benzylpenicillin potassium by multiplying the percentage content of benzylpenicillin sodium by 1.045.

STORAGE

Store in an airtight container. If the substance is sterile, store in a sterile, airtight, tamper-proof container.

LABELLING

The label states, where applicable, that the substance is free from bacterial endotoxins.

IMPURITIES

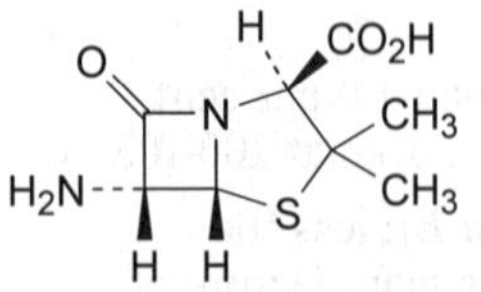

A. (2*S*,5*R*,6*R*)-6-amino-3,3-dimethyl-7-oxo-4-thia-1-azabicyclo[3.2.0]heptane-2-carboxylic acid (6-aminopenicillanic acid),

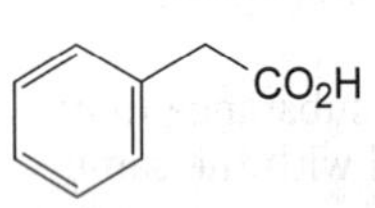

B. phenylacetic acid,

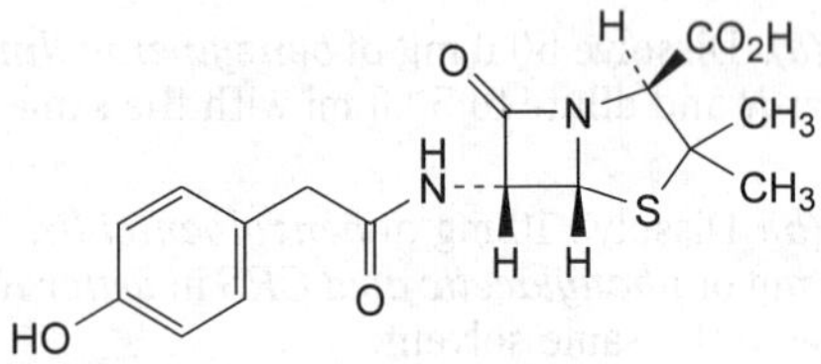

C. (2*S*,5*R*,6*R*)-6-[[(4-hydroxyphenyl)acetyl]amino]-3,3-dimethyl-7-oxo-4-thia-1-azabicyclo[3.2.0]heptane-2-carboxylic acid,

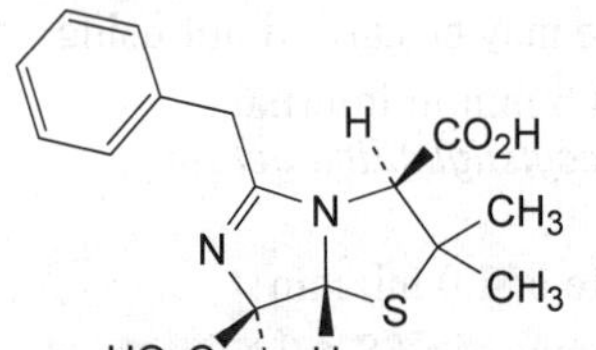

D. (3*S*,7*R*,7a*R*)-5-benzyl-2,2-dimethyl-2,3,7,7a-tetrahydroimidazo[5,1-*b*]thiazole-3,7-dicarboxylic acid (penillic acid of benzylpenicillin),

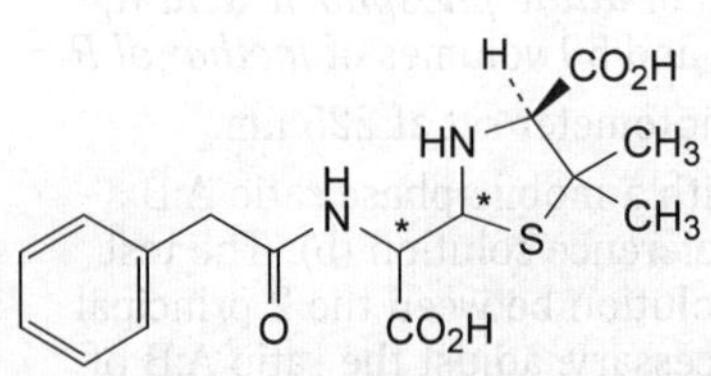

E. (4*S*)-2-[carboxy[(phenylacetyl)amino]methyl]-5,5-dimethylthiazolidine-4-carboxylic acid (penicilloic acids of benzylpenicillin),

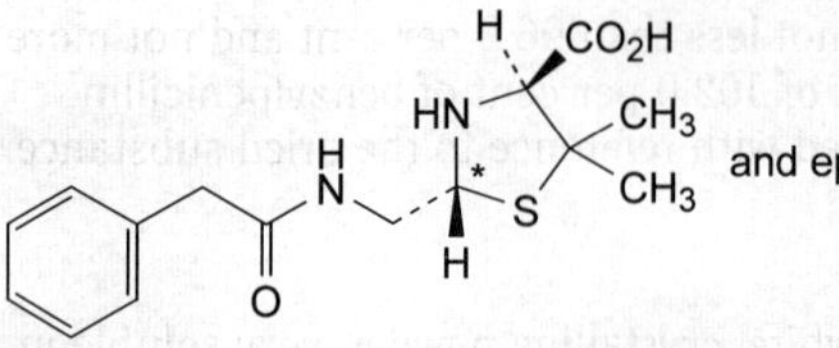

F. (2*RS*,4*S*)-2-[[(phenylacetyl)amino]methyl]-5,5-dimethylthiazolidine-4-carboxylic acid (penilloic acids of benzylpenicillin).

01/2005:0115

BENZYLPENICILLIN, PROCAINE

Benzylpenicillinum procainum

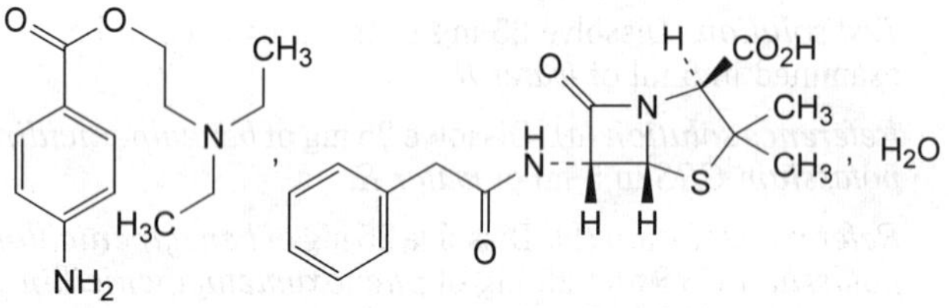

$C_{29}H_{38}N_4O_6S,H_2O$ M_r 588.7

DEFINITION

Procaine benzylpenicillin is the monohydrate of the (2*S*,5*R*,6*R*)-3,3-dimethyl-7-oxo-6-[(phenylacetyl)amino]-4-thia-1-azabicyclo[3.2.0]heptane-2-carboxylic acid compound with 2-(diethylamino)ethyl 4-aminobenzoate. It contains not less than 96.0 per cent and not more than the equivalent of 102.0 per cent of procaine benzylpenicillin and not less than 39.0 per cent and not more than 42.0 per cent of procaine ($C_{13}H_{20}N_2O_2$; M_r 236.3), both calculated with reference to the anhydrous substance. Dispersing or suspending agents (for example, lecithin and polysorbate 80) may be added.

CHARACTERS

A white, crystalline powder, slightly soluble in water, sparingly soluble in alcohol.

IDENTIFICATION

First identification: A.

Second identification: B, C, D.

A. Examine by infrared absorption spectrophotometry (*2.2.24*), comparing with the spectrum obtained with *procaine benzylpenicillin CRS*.

B. Examine by thin-layer chromatography (*2.2.27*), using a *TLC silanised silica gel plate R*.

Test solution. Dissolve 25 mg of the substance to be examined in 5 ml of *acetone R*.

Reference solution. Dissolve 25 mg of *procaine benzylpenicillin CRS* in 5 ml of *acetone R*.

Apply to the plate 1 µl of each solution. Develop over a path of 15 cm using a mixture of 30 volumes of *acetone R* and 70 volumes of a 154 g/l solution of *ammonium acetate R*, the pH of which has been adjusted to 7.0 with *ammonia R*. Allow the plate to dry in air and expose it to iodine vapour until the spots appear. Examine in daylight. The 2 principal spots in the chromatogram obtained with the test solution are similar in position, colour and size to the 2 principal spots in the chromatogram obtained with the reference solution. The test is not valid unless the chromatogram obtained with the reference solution shows 2 clearly separated spots.

C. Place about 2 mg in a test-tube about 150 mm long and 15 mm in diameter. Moisten with 0.05 ml of *water R* and add 2 ml of *sulphuric acid-formaldehyde reagent R*. Mix the contents of the tube by swirling; the solution is practically colourless. Place the test-tube on a water-bath for 1 min; a reddish-brown colour develops.

D. Dissolve 0.1 g in 2 ml of *dilute hydrochloric acid R* and use the solution which may be turbid. The solution gives the reaction of primary aromatic amines (*2.3.1*).

TESTS

pH (*2.2.3*). Dissolve 50 mg in *carbon dioxide-free water R* and dilute to 15 ml with the same solvent. Shake until dissolution is complete. The pH of the solution is 5.0 to 7.5.

Specific optical rotation (*2.2.7*). Dissolve 0.250 g in a mixture of 2 volumes of *water R* and 3 volumes of *acetone R* and dilute to 25.0 ml with the same mixture of solvents. The specific optical rotation is + 165 to + 180, calculated with reference to the anhydrous substance.

Related substances. Examine by liquid chromatography (*2.2.29*) as prescribed under Assay. Inject 10 µl of reference solution (c). Adjust the sensitivity of the system so that the height of the peak due to benzylpenicillin is at least 50 per cent of the full scale of the recorder. Inject 10 µl of test solution (a) and continue the chromatography for 1.5 times the retention time of the benzylpenicillin peak. In the chromatogram obtained with test solution (a): the area of any peak corresponding to 4-aminobenzoic acid is not greater than the area of the corresponding peak in the chromatogram obtained with reference solution (c) (0.024 per cent); the area of any peak, apart from the 2 principal peaks and any peak corresponding to 4-aminobenzoic acid, is not greater than the area of the peak corresponding to benzylpenicillin in the chromatogram obtained with reference solution (c) (1 per cent).

Water (*2.5.12*). 2.8 per cent to 4.2 per cent, determined on 0.500 g by the semi-micro determination of water.

Bacterial endotoxins (*2.6.14, Method E*): less than 0.10 IU/mg, if intended for use in the manufacture of parenteral dosage forms without a further appropriate procedure for the removal of bacterial endotoxins.

ASSAY

Examine by liquid chromatography (*2.2.29*). *Prepare the solutions immediately before use.*

Test solution (a). Dissolve 70.0 mg of the substance to be examined in the mobile phase and dilute to 50.0 ml with the mobile phase.

Test solution (b). Dissolve 70.0 mg of the substance to be examined in the mobile phase and dilute to 100.0 ml with the mobile phase.

Reference solution (a). Dissolve 70.0 mg of *procaine benzylpenicillin CRS* in the mobile phase and dilute to 100.0 ml with the mobile phase.

Reference solution (b). Dissolve 4 mg of *4-aminobenzoic acid R* in reference solution (a) and dilute to 25 ml with the same solution.

Reference solution (c). Dissolve 16.8 mg of *4-aminobenzoic acid R* in *water R* and dilute to 50.0 ml with the same solvent. Dilute 1.0 ml of the solution to 10.0 ml with *water R*. To 1.0 ml of this solution, add 1.0 ml of test solution (a) and dilute to 100.0 ml with the mobile phase.

The chromatographic procedure may be carried out using:

– a stainless steel column 0.25 m long and 4.6 mm in internal diameter packed with *octadecylsilyl silica gel for chromatography R* (5 µm),

– as mobile phase at a flow rate of 1.75 ml/min a mixture prepared as follows: mix 250 ml of *acetonitrile R*, 250 ml of *water R* and 500 ml of a solution containing 14 g/l of *potassium dihydrogen phosphate R* and 6.5 g/l of *tetrabutylammonium hydroxide solution (400 g/l) R* adjusted to pH 7.0 with *1 M potassium hydroxide*; adjust the mixture to pH 7.2 with *dilute phosphoric acid R*, if necessary,

– as detector a spectrophotometer set at 225 nm.

Inject 10 µl of reference solution (b). When the chromatogram is recorded in the prescribed conditions, the substances elute in the following order: 4-aminobenzoic acid, procaine, benzylpenicillin. Adjust the sensitivity of the system so that the height of the peak corresponding to 4-aminobenzoic acid is at least 50 per cent of the full scale of the recorder. The test is not valid unless, the resolution between the first peak (4-aminobenzoic acid) and the second peak (procaine) is at least 2.0. If necessary, adjust the concentration of acetonitrile in the mobile phase. Inject reference solution (a) 6 times. The test is not valid unless the relative standard deviation for the areas of the 2 peaks is at most 1.0 per cent. Inject alternately test solution (b) and reference solution (a).

Calculate the percentage contents of procaine and procaine benzylpenicillin.

STORAGE

Store in an airtight container. If the substance is sterile, store in a sterile, airtight, tamper-proof container.

LABELLING

The label states:

– where applicable, the name and quantity of any added dispersing or suspending agents,

– where applicable, that the substance is free from bacterial endotoxins.

IMPURITIES

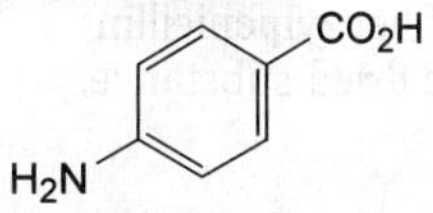

A. 4-aminobenzoic acid,

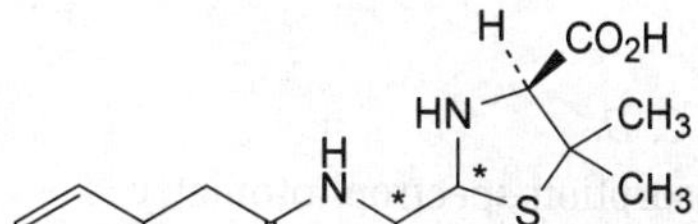

B. (4*S*)-2-[carboxy[(phenylacetyl)amino]methyl]-5,5-dimethylthiazolidine-4-carboxylic acid (penicilloic acids of benzylpenicillin),

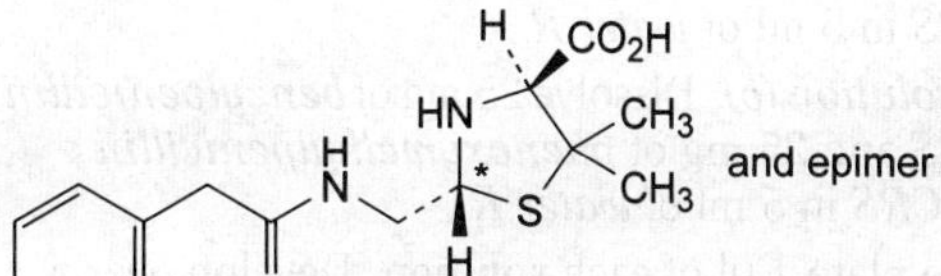

C. (2*RS*,4*S*)-2-[[(phenylacetyl)amino]methyl]-5,5-dimethylthiazolidine-4-carboxylic acid (penilloic acids of benzylpenicillin),

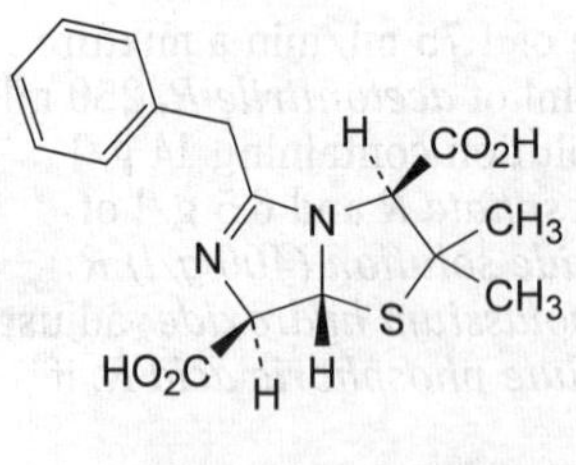

D. (3*S*,7*R*,7a*R*)-5-benzyl-2,2-dimethyl-2,3,7,7a-tetrahydroimidazo[5,1-*b*]thiazole-3,7-dicarboxylic acid (penillic acid of benzylpenicillin),

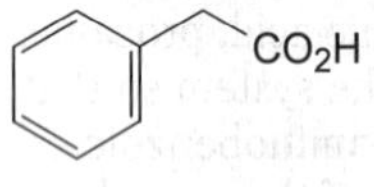

E. phenylacetic acid.

01/2005:0114

BENZYLPENICILLIN SODIUM

Benzylpenicillinum natricum

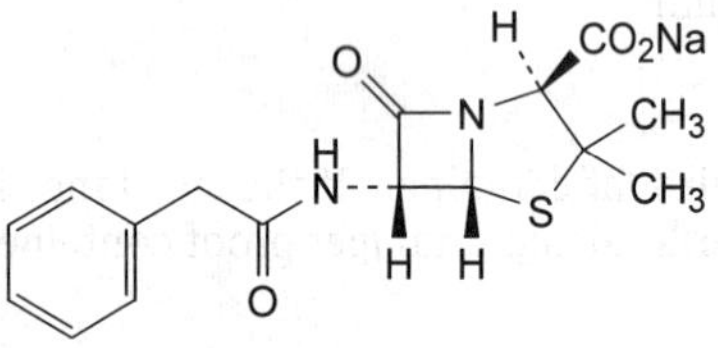

$C_{16}H_{17}N_2NaO_4S$ M_r 356.4

DEFINITION

Benzylpenicillin sodium is sodium (2*S*,5*R*,6*R*)-3,3-dimethyl-7-oxo-6-[(phenylacetyl)amino]-4-thia-1-azabicyclo[3.2.0]heptane-2-carboxylate, a substance produced by the growth of certain strains of *Penicillium notatum* or related organisms, or obtained by any other means. It contains not less than 96.0 per cent and not more than the equivalent of 102.0 per cent of benzylpenicillin sodium, calculated with reference to the dried substance.

CHARACTERS

A white or almost white, crystalline powder, very soluble in water, practically insoluble in fatty oils and in liquid paraffin.

IDENTIFICATION

First identification: A, D.

Second identification: B, C, D.

A. Examine by infrared absorption spectrophotometry (*2.2.24*), comparing with the spectrum obtained with *benzylpenicillin sodium CRS*.

B. Examine by thin-layer chromatography (*2.2.27*), using a *TLC silanised silica gel plate R*.

Test solution. Dissolve 25 mg of the substance to be examined in 5 ml of *water R*.

Reference solution (a). Dissolve 25 mg of *benzylpenicillin sodium CRS* in 5 ml of *water R*.

Reference solution (b). Dissolve 25 mg of *benzylpenicillin sodium CRS* and 25 mg of *phenoxymethylpenicillin potassium CRS* in 5 ml of *water R*.

Apply to the plate 1 µl of each solution. Develop over a path of 15 cm using a mixture of 30 volumes of *acetone R* and 70 volumes of a 154 g/l solution of *ammonium acetate R*, the pH of which has been adjusted to 5.0 with *glacial acetic acid R*. Allow the plate to dry in air and expose it to iodine vapour until the spots appear. Examine in daylight. The principal spot in the chromatogram obtained with the test solution is similar in position, colour and size to the principal spot in the chromatogram obtained with reference solution (a). The test is not valid unless the chromatogram obtained with reference solution (b) shows 2 clearly separated spots.

C. Place about 2 mg in a test-tube about 150 mm long and 15 mm in diameter. Moisten with 0.05 ml of *water R* and add 2 ml of *sulphuric acid-formaldehyde reagent R*. Mix the contents of the tube by swirling; the solution is practically colourless. Place the test-tube on a water-bath for 1 min; a reddish-brown colour develops.

D. It gives reaction (a) of sodium (*2.3.1*).

TESTS

pH (*2.2.3*). Dissolve 2.0 g in *carbon dioxide-free water R* and dilute to 20 ml with the same solvent. The pH of the solution is 5.5 to 7.5.

Specific optical rotation (*2.2.7*). Dissolve 0.500 g in *carbon dioxide-free water R* and dilute to 25.0 ml with the same solvent. The specific optical rotation is + 285 to + 310, calculated with reference to the dried substance.

Absorbance (*2.2.25*). Dissolve 90.0 mg in *water R* and dilute to 50.0 ml with the same solvent. Measure the absorbance of the solution at 325 nm, at 280 nm and at the maximum at 264 nm, diluting the solution, if necessary, for the measurement at 264 nm. The absorbances at 325 nm and 280 nm are not greater than 0.10 and the absorbance at the maximum at 264 nm is 0.80 to 0.88, calculated on the basis of the undiluted (1.80 g/l) solution. Verify the resolution of the apparatus (*2.2.25*); the ratio of the absorbances is at least 1.7.

Related substances. Liquid chromatography (*2.2.29*) as described under Assay. Inject 20 µl of reference solution (d) and elute isocratically with the chosen mobile phase. Inject 20 µl of test solution (b) and start the elution isocratically. Immediately after elution of the benzylpenicillin peak start the following linear gradient:

Time (min)	Mobile phase A (per cent *V/V*)	Mobile phase B (per cent *V/V*)	Comment
0 - 20	70 → 0	30 → 100	linear gradient
20 - 35	0	100	isocratic
35 - 50	70	30	re-equilibration

Inject *water R* and use the same elution pattern to obtain a blank. In the chromatogram obtained with test solution (b), the area of any peak, apart from the principal peak, is not greater than the area of the principal peak in the chromatogram obtained with reference solution (d) (1 per cent).

2-Ethylhexanoic acid (*2.4.28*). Not more than 0.5 per cent *m/m*.

Loss on drying (*2.2.32*). Not more than 1.0 per cent, determined on 1.000 g by drying in an oven at 100-105 °C.

Bacterial endotoxins (*2.6.14, Method E*): less than 0.16 IU/mg, if intended for use in the manufacture of parenteral dosage forms without a further appropriate procedure for the removal of bacterial endotoxins.

ASSAY

Liquid chromatography (*2.2.29*). *Prepare the solutions immediately before use.*

Test solution (a). Dissolve 50.0 mg of the substance to be examined in *water R* and dilute to 50.0 ml with the same solvent.

Test solution (b). Dissolve 80.0 mg of the substance to be examined in *water R* and dilute to 20.0 ml with the same solvent.

Reference solution (a). Dissolve 50.0 mg of *benzylpenicillin sodium CRS* in *water R* and dilute to 50.0 ml with the same solvent.

Reference solution (b). Dissolve 10 mg of *benzylpenicillin sodium CRS* and 10 mg of *phenylacetic acid CRS* in *water R* and dilute to 50 ml with the same solvent.

Reference solution (c). Dilute 1.0 ml of reference solution (a) to 20.0 ml with *water R*. Dilute 1.0 ml of the solution to 50.0 ml with *water R*.

Reference solution (d). Dilute 4.0 ml of reference solution (a) to 100.0 ml with *water R*.

The chromatographic procedure may be carried out using:

- a column 0.25 m long and 4.6 mm in internal diameter packed with *octadecylsilyl silica gel for chromatography R* (5 µm),
- as mobile phase at a flow rate of 1.0 ml/min:

  Mobile phase A. Mix 10 volumes of a 68 g/l solution of *potassium dihydrogen phosphate R* adjusted to pH 3.5 with a 500 g/l solution of *dilute phosphoric acid R*, 30 volumes of *methanol R* and 60 volumes of *water R*.

  Mobile phase B. Mix 10 volumes of a 68 g/l solution of *potassium dihydrogen phosphate R* adjusted to pH 3.5 with a 500 g/l solution of *dilute phosphoric acid R*, 40 volumes of *water R* and 50 volumes of *methanol R*.
- as detector a spectrophotometer set at 225 nm.

Equilibrate the column with a mobile phase ratio A:B of 70:30. Inject 20 µl of reference solution (b). The test is not valid unless the resolution between the 2 principal peaks is at least 6.0 (if necessary, adjust the ratio A:B of the mobile phase) and the mass distribution ratio for the second peak (benzylpenicillin) is 4.0 to 6.0. Inject 20 µl of reference solution (c). Adjust the system to obtain a peak with a signal-to-noise ratio of at least 3.

STORAGE

Store in an airtight container. If the substance is sterile, store in a sterile, airtight, tamper-proof container.

LABELLING

The label states, where applicable, that the substance is free from bacterial endotoxins.

IMPURITIES

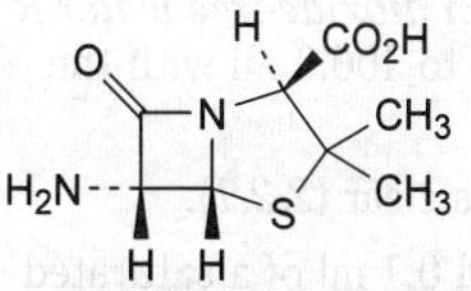

A. (2*S*,5*R*,6*R*)-6-amino-3,3-dimethyl-7-oxo-4-thia-1-azabicyclo[3.2.0]heptane-2-carboxylic acid (6-aminopenicillanic acid),

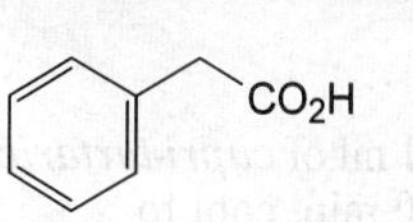

B. phenylacetic acid,

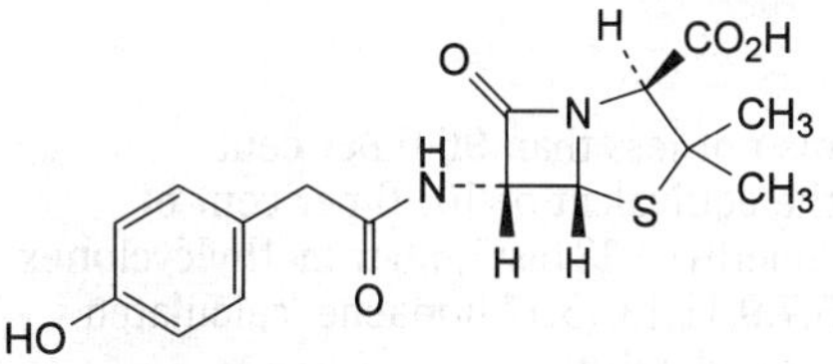

C. (2*S*,5*R*,6*R*)-6-[[(4-hydroxyphenyl)acetyl]amino]-3,3-dimethyl-7-oxo-4-thia- 1-azabicyclo[3.2.0]heptane-2-carboxylic acid,

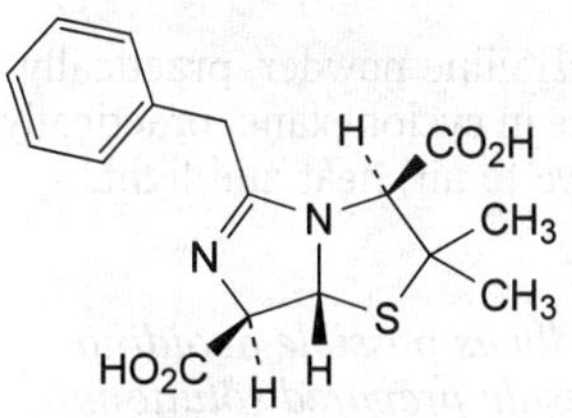

D. (3*S*,7*R*,7a*R*)-5-benzyl-2,2-dimethyl-2,3,7,7a-tetrahydroimidazo[5,1-*b*]thiazole-3,7-dicarboxylic acid (penillic acid of benzylpenicillin),

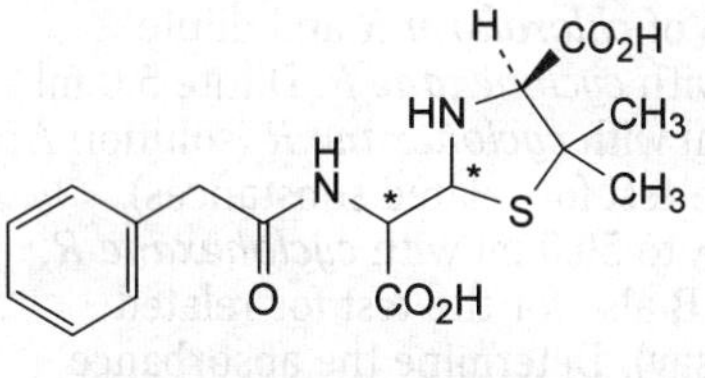

E. (4*S*)-2-[carboxy[(phenylacetyl)amino]methyl]-5,5-dimethylthiazolidine-4-carboxylic acid (penicilloic acids of benzylpenicillin),

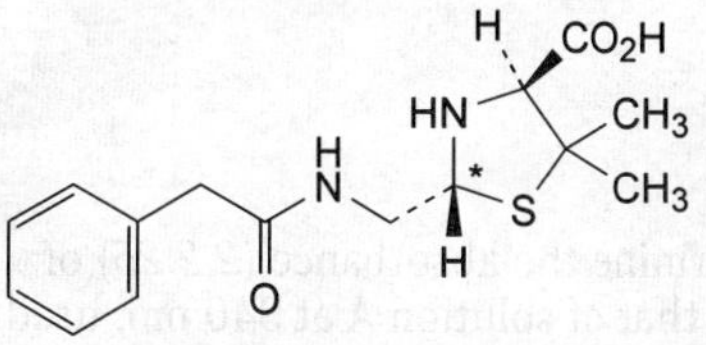

and epimer at C*

F. (2*RS*,4*S*)-2-[[(phenylacetyl)amino]methyl]-5,5-dimethylthiazolidine-4-carboxylic acid (penilloic acids of benzylpenicillin).

01/2005:1069

BETACAROTENE

Betacarotenum

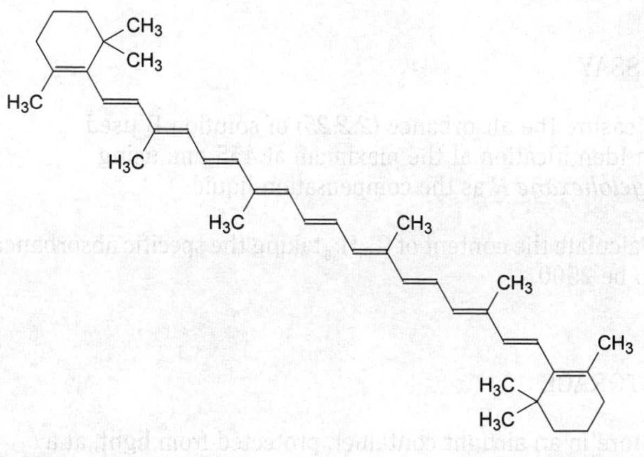

$C_{40}H_{56}$ M_r 536.9

Monographs R

DEFINITION

Betacarotene contains not less than 96.0 per cent and not more than the equivalent of 101.0 per cent of (all-*E*)-3,7,12,16-Tetramethyl-1,18-bis(2,6,6-trimethylcyclohex-1-enyl)octadeca-1,3,5,7,9,11,13,15,17-nonaene, calculated with reference to the dried substance.

CHARACTERS

A brown-red or brownish-red, crystalline powder, practically insoluble in water, slightly soluble in cyclohexane, practically insoluble in ethanol. It is sensitive to air, heat and light, especially in solution.

Carry out all operations as rapidly as possible avoiding exposure to actinic light; use freshly prepared solutions.

IDENTIFICATION

Dissolve 50.0 mg in 10 ml of *chloroform R* and dilute immediately to 100.0 ml with *cyclohexane R*. Dilute 5.0 ml of this solution to 100.0 ml with *cyclohexane R* (solution A; use solution A also for the test for related substances). Dilute 5.0 ml of solution A to 50.0 ml with *cyclohexane R*. (Solution B; use solution B also for the test for related substances and for the assay). Determine the absorbance (*2.2.25*) of solution B at 455 nm and at 483 nm using *cyclohexane R* as the compensation liquid. The ratio of the absorbance at 455 nm to that at 483 nm is between 1.14 and 1.18.

TESTS

Related substances. Determine the absorbance (*2.2.25*) of solution B at 455 nm and that of solution A at 340 nm, used in Identification. The ratio of the absorbance at 455 nm to that at 340 nm is not less than 1.5.

Heavy metals (*2.4.8*). 2.0 g complies with limit test D for heavy metals (10 ppm). Prepare the standard using 2 ml of *lead standard solution (10 ppm Pb) R*.

Loss on drying (*2.2.32*). Not more than 0.2 per cent, determined on 1.000 g by drying *in vacuo* over *diphosphorus pentoxide R* at 40 °C for 4 h.

Sulphated ash (*2.4.14*). Not more than 0.2 per cent, determined on 1.0 g, moistened with a mixture of 2 ml of *dilute sulphuric acid R* and 5 ml of *alcohol R*.

ASSAY

Measure the absorbance (*2.2.25*) of solution B used in Identification at the maximum at 455 nm, using *cyclohexane R* as the compensation liquid.

Calculate the content of $C_{40}H_{56}$ taking the specific absorbance to be 2500.

STORAGE

Store in an airtight container, protected from light, at a temperature not exceeding 25 °C.

01/2005:1070

BETADEX

Betadexum

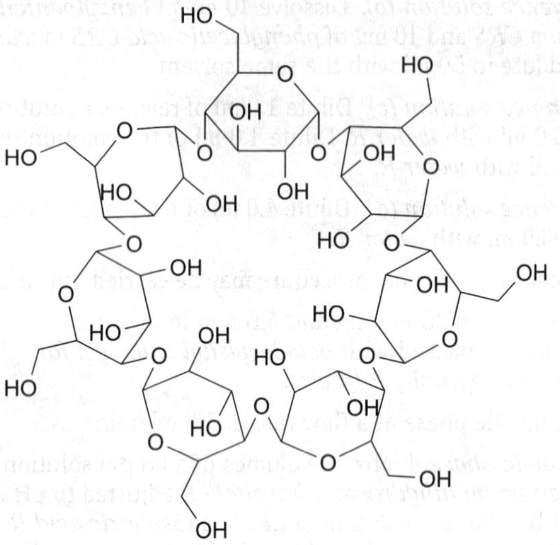

$[C_6H_{10}O_5]_7$ M_r 1135

DEFINITION

Betadex (betacyclodextrin) contains not less than 98.0 per cent and not more than the equivalent of 101.0 per cent of cyclo-α-(1→4)-D-heptaglucopyranoside, calculated with reference to the dried substance.

CHARACTERS

A white or almost white, amorphous or crystalline powder, sparingly soluble in water, freely soluble in propylene glycol, practically insoluble in ethanol and in methylene chloride.

IDENTIFICATION

A. It complies with the test for specific optical rotation (see Tests).

B. Examine the chromatograms obtained in the assay. The retention time and size of the principal peak in the chromatogram obtained with test solution (b) are approximately the same as those of the principal peak in the chromatogram obtained with reference solution (c).

C. Dissolve 0.2 g in 2 ml of *iodine solution R4* by warming on a water-bath, and allow to stand at room temperature. A yellowish-brown precipitate is formed.

TESTS

Solution S. Dissolve 1.000 g in *carbon dioxide-free water R* with heating, allow to cool and dilute to 100.0 ml with the same solvent.

Appearance of solution. Solution S is clear (*2.2.1*).

pH (*2.2.3*). To 10 ml of solution S add 0.1 ml of a saturated solution of *potassium chloride R*. The pH of the solution is 5.0 to 8.0.

Specific optical rotation (*2.2.7*): + 160 to + 164, determined on solution S and calculated with reference to the dried substance.

Reducing sugars

Test solution. To 1 ml of solution S add 1 ml of *cupri-tartaric solution R4*. Heat on a water-bath for 10 min, cool to room temperature. Add 10 ml of *ammonium molybdate reagent R1* and allow to stand for 15 min.

Reference solution. Prepare a reference solution at the same time and in the same manner as the test solution, using 1 ml of a 0.02 g/l solution of *glucose R*.

Measure the absorbance of the test solution and the reference solution (*2.2.25*) at the maximum at 740 nm using *water R* as the compensation liquid. The absorbance of the test solution is not greater than that of the reference solution (0.2 per cent).

Light-absorbing impurities. Examine solution S between 230 nm and 750 nm (*2.2.25*). Between 230 nm and 350 nm, the absorbance is not greater than 0.10. Between 350 nm and 750 nm, the absorbance is not greater than 0.05.

Related substances. Examine by liquid chromatography (*2.2.29*), as described under Assay. Inject separately test solution (a) and reference solution (b). In the chromatogram obtained with test solution (a): the areas of any peaks corresponding to gammacyclodextrin and alphacyclodextrin are not greater than half of the area of the corresponding peaks in the chromatogram obtained with reference solution (b) (0.25 per cent); the sum of the areas of all the peaks, apart from the principal peak and any peaks corresponding to alphacyclodextrin and gammacyclodextrin, is not greater than half of the area of the peak corresponding to betadex in the chromatogram obtained with reference solution (b) (0.5 per cent).

Residual solvents. Not more than 10 ppm of trichloroethylene and not more than 10 ppm of toluene. Examine by head-space gas chromatography (*2.2.28*), using the standard additions method and *ethylene chloride R* as the internal standard.

Test solutions. In each of four identical 20 ml flasks, dissolve 500 mg of the substance to be examined in *water R* and add 0.10 g of *calcium chloride R* and 30 µl of *α-amylase solution R*. Add 1 ml of reference solutions (a), (b), (c) and (d), adding a different solution to each flask. Dilute to 10 ml with *water R*.

Reference solutions. Prepare reference solution (a) containing 10 µl of *ethylene chloride R* per litre. From reference solution (a), prepare reference solutions (b), (c) and (d) containing per litre: 5 µl, 10 µl and 15 µl each of *trichloroethylene R* and of *toluene R*.

The chromatographic procedure may be carried out using:

- a fused-silica column 25 m long and 0.32 mm in internal diameter coated with a layer about 1 µm thick of *macrogol 20 000 R*,
- *helium for chromatography R* as the carrier gas,
- a flame-ionisation detector,

maintaining the temperature of the column at 50 °C, that of the injection port at 140 °C and that of the detector at 280 °C. Place the samples in a thermostated chamber at 45 °C for 2 h. Inject 200 µl of the head-space of each flask and repeat each test at least three times. The retention time of toluene is about 10 min. The test is not valid unless: the resolutions between the peaks corresponding to trichloroethylene and toluene and between the peaks corresponding to toluene and ethylene chloride are greater than 1.1 and the relative standard deviations of the ratios of the areas of the peaks corresponding to trichloroethylene and toluene to that of the peak corresponding to ethylene chloride are less than 5 per cent.

Calculate the content of trichloroethylene and of toluene taking their relative densities to be 1.46 and 0.87, respectively.

Heavy metals (*2.4.8*). 1.0 g complies with limit test C for heavy metals (10 ppm). Prepare the standard using 1 ml of *lead standard solution (10 ppm Pb) R*.

Loss on drying (*2.2.32*). Not more than 16.0 per cent, determined on 1.000 g by drying in an oven at 120 °C for 2 h.

Sulphated ash (*2.4.14*). Not more than 0.1 per cent, determined on 1.0 g.

ASSAY

Examine by liquid chromatography (*2.2.29*).

Test solution (a). Dissolve 0.25 g of the substance to be examined in *water R* with heating, cool and dilute to 25.0 ml with the same solvent.

Test solution (b). Dilute 5.0 ml of test solution (a) to 50.0 ml with *water R*.

Reference solution (a). Dissolve 25.0 mg of *alfadex CRS*, 25.0 mg of *gammacyclodextrin CRS* and 50.0 mg of *betadex CRS* in *water R* and dilute to 50.0 ml with the same solvent.

Reference solution (b). Dilute 5.0 ml of reference solution (a) to 50.0 ml with *water R*.

Reference solution (c). Dissolve 25.0 mg of *betadex CRS* in *water R* and dilute to 25.0 ml with the same solvent.

The chromatographic procedure may be carried out using:

- a stainless steel column 0.25 m long and 4.6 mm in internal diameter packed with *octadecylsilyl silica gel for chromatography R* (10 µm),
- as mobile phase at a flow rate of 1.5 ml/min a mixture of 10 volumes of *methanol R* and 90 volumes of *water R*,
- as detector a differential refractometer,
- a 50 µl loop injector.

Equilibrate the column with the mobile phase at a flow rate of 1.5 ml/min for about 3 h. Inject each solution. Record the chromatograms for 1.5 times the retention time of betadex. Adjust the sensitivity of the detector so that the height of the peak corresponding to gammacyclodextrin, in the chromatogram obtained with reference solution (a), is 55 per cent to 75 per cent of the full scale of the recorder. The retention time of betadex is about 10 min, the relative retention time of gammacyclodextrin is about 0.3 and that of alfadex is about 0.45. The test is not valid unless the resolution between the peaks corresponding to gammacyclodextrin and alfadex is not less than 1.5, and the relative standard deviation of the area of the peak corresponding to betadex is less than 2.0 per cent. If necessary, adjust the concentration of methanol in the mobile phase to achieve the required resolution. Calculate the percentage content of $[C_6H_{10}O_5]_7$ from the area of the principal peak in each of the chromatograms obtained with test solution (b) and reference solution (c) and the declared content of *betadex CRS*.

STORAGE

Store in an airtight container.

IMPURITIES

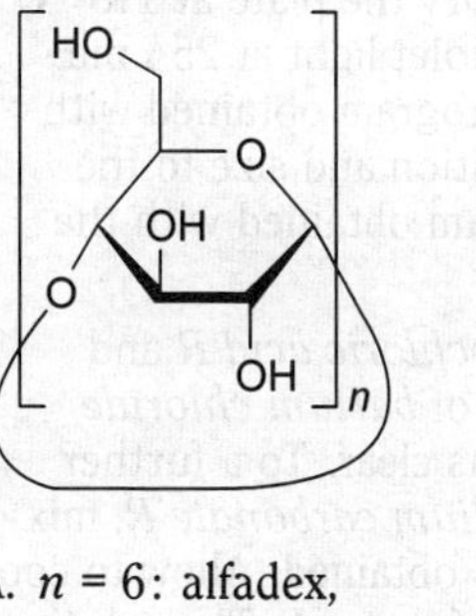

A. n = 6: alfadex,

B. n = 8: gammacyclodextrin.

01/2005:1071

BETAHISTINE MESILATE

Betahistini mesilas

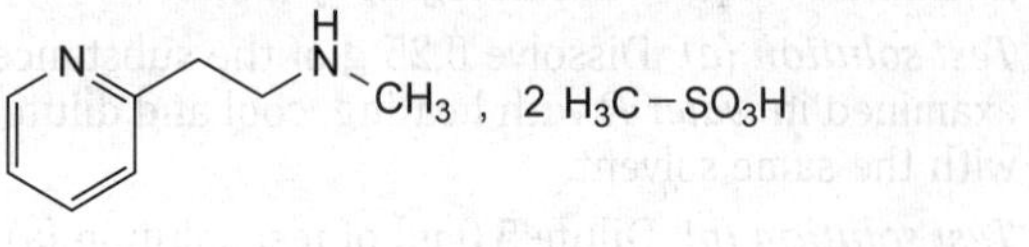

$C_{10}H_{20}N_2O_6S_2$ M_r 328.4

DEFINITION

Betahistine mesilate contains not less than 98.0 per cent and not more than the equivalent of 101.0 per cent of *N*-methyl-2-(pyridin-2-yl)ethanamine bis(methanesulphonate), calculated with reference to the anhydrous, 2-propanol-free substance.

PRODUCTION

The production method must be evaluated to determine the potential for formation of alkyl mesilates, which is particularly likely to occur if the reaction medium contains lower alcohols. Where necessary, the production method is validated to demonstrate that alkyl mesilates are not detectable in the final product.

CHARACTERS

A white, crystalline powder, very hygroscopic, very soluble in water, freely soluble in alcohol, very slightly soluble in 2-propanol.

IDENTIFICATION

First identification: B.

Second identification: A, C, D.

A. Melting point (*2.2.14*): 108 °C to 112 °C.

B. Examine by infrared absorption spectrophotometry (*2.2.24*), comparing with the spectrum obtained with *betahistine mesilate CRS*. Examine the substances prepared as discs.

C. Examine by thin-layer chromatography (*2.2.27*), using a suitable silica gel with a fluorescent indicator having an optimal intensity at 254 nm as the coating substance.

Test solution. Dissolve 10 mg of the substance to be examined in *alcohol R* and dilute to 2 ml with the same solvent.

Reference solution. Dissolve 10 mg of *betahistine mesilate CRS*, in *alcohol R* and dilute to 2 ml with the same solvent.

Apply to the plate 2 µl of each solution. Develop over a path of 15 cm using a mixture of 0.75 volumes of *concentrated ammonia R*, 15 volumes of *ethyl acetate R* and 30 volumes of *methanol R*. Dry the plate at 110 °C for 10 min and examine in ultraviolet light at 254 nm. The principal spot in the chromatogram obtained with the test solution is similar in position and size to the principal spot in the chromatogram obtained with the reference solution.

D. To 0.1 g add 5 ml of *dilute hydrochloric acid R* and shake for about 5 min. Add 1 ml of *barium chloride solution R1*. The solution remains clear. To a further 0.1 g add 0.5 g of *anhydrous sodium carbonate R*, mix and ignite until a white residue is obtained. Allow to cool and dissolve the residue in 7 ml of *water R*. The solution gives reaction (a) of sulphates (*2.3.1*).

TESTS

Solution S. Dissolve 5.0 g in *carbon dioxide-free water R* prepared from *distilled water R*, and dilute to 50 ml with the same solvent.

Appearance of solution. Solution S is clear (*2.2.1*) and colourless (*2.2.2, Method II*).

pH (*2.2.3*). The pH of solution S is 2.0 to 3.0.

Related substances. Examine by liquid chromatography (*2.2.29*).

Test solution. Dissolve 50 mg of the substance to be examined in the mobile phase and dilute to 10.0 ml with the mobile phase.

Reference solution (a). Dissolve 10 mg of *betahistine mesilate CRS* and 10 mg of *2-vinylpyridine R* in the mobile phase and dilute to 50.0 ml with the mobile phase. Dilute 2.0 ml of the solution to 50.0 ml with the mobile phase.

Reference solution (b). Dilute 1.0 ml of the test solution to 100.0 ml with the mobile phase.

Reference solution (c). Dilute 2.0 ml of reference solution (b) to 10.0 ml with the mobile phase.

The chromatographic procedure may be carried out using:

– a stainless steel column 0.25 m long and 4.6 mm in internal diameter packed with *octadecylsilyl silica gel for chromatography R* (5 µm),

– as mobile phase at a flow rate of 1 ml/min a mixture prepared as follows: dissolve 2.0 g of *sodium dodecyl sulphate R* in a mixture of 15 volumes of a 10 per cent *V/V* solution of *sulphuric acid R*, 35 volumes of a 17 g/l solution of *tetrabutylammoniumhydrogen sulphate R* and 650 volumes of *water R*; adjust to pH 3.3 using *dilute sodium hydroxide solution R* and mix with 300 volumes of *acetonitrile R*,

– as detector a spectrophotometer set at 260 nm.

Inject 20 µl of reference solution (a). When using a recorder, adjust the sensitivity of the system so that the height of the first peak in the chromatogram obtained with reference solution (a) is not less than 70 per cent of the full scale of the recorder. The test is not valid unless: in the chromatogram obtained with reference solution (a), the resolution between the peaks corresponding to 2-vinylpyridine and betahistine mesilate is at least 3.5.

Inject 20 µl of the test solution and of reference solutions (b) and (c). Continue the chromatography for 3 times the retention time of betahistine mesilate (which is about 8 min). In the chromatogram obtained with the test solution the area of any peak, apart from the principal peak, is not greater than the area of the principal peak in the chromatogram obtained with reference solution (c) (0.2 per cent); the sum of the areas of any peaks, apart from the principal peak, is not greater than half of the area of the principal peak in the chromatogram obtained with reference solution (b) (0.5 per cent).

Disregard any peak with an area less than 0.025 times that of the principal peak in the chromatogram obtained with reference solution (b).

2-Propanol. Not more than 0.5 per cent, determined by the test for residual solvents (*2.4.24*).

Chlorides (*2.4.4*). To 14 ml of solution S add 1 ml of *water R*. The solution complies with the limit test for chlorides (35 ppm).

Sulphates (*2.4.13*). Dilute 6 ml of solution S to 15 ml with *distilled water R*. The solution complies with the limit test for sulphates (250 ppm).

Heavy metals (*2.4.8*). 12 ml of solution S complies with limit test A for heavy metals (20 ppm). Prepare the standard using *lead standard solution (2 ppm Pb) R*.

Water (*2.5.12*). Not more than 2.0 per cent, determined on 0.50 g by the semi-micro determination of water.

ASSAY

Dissolve 0.140 g in 50 ml of a mixture of 1 volume of *anhydrous acetic acid R* and 7 volumes of *acetic anhydride R*. Titrate with *0.1 M perchloric acid*, determining the end-point potentiometrically (*2.2.20*).

1 ml of *0.1 M perchloric acid* is equivalent to 16.42 mg of $C_{10}H_{20}N_2O_6S_2$.

STORAGE

Store in an airtight container.

IMPURITIES

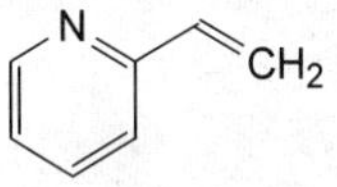

A. 2-ethenylpyridine.

01/2005:0312

BETAMETHASONE

Betamethasonum

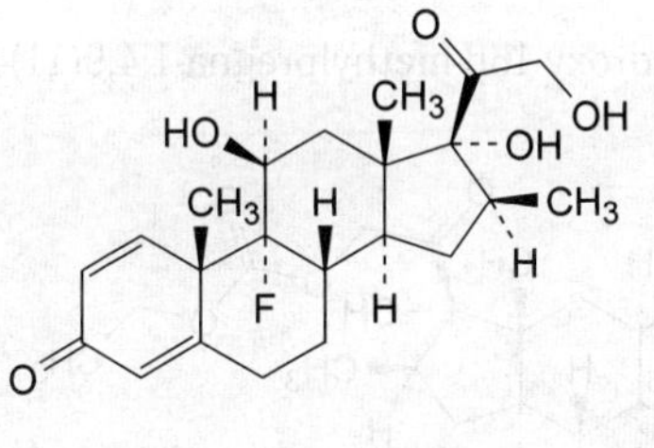

$C_{22}H_{29}FO_5$ M_r 392.5

DEFINITION

Betamethasone contains not less than 97.0 per cent and not more than the equivalent of 103.0 per cent of 9-fluoro-11β,17,21-trihydroxy-16β-methylpregna-1,4-diene-3,20-dione, calculated with reference to the dried substance.

CHARACTERS

A white or almost white, crystalline powder, practically insoluble in water, sparingly soluble in ethanol, very slightly soluble in methylene chloride.

IDENTIFICATION

First identification: B, C.

Second identification: A, C, D, E.

A. Dissolve 10.0 mg in *ethanol R* and dilute to 100.0 ml with the same solvent. Place 2.0 ml of the solution in a stoppered tube, add 10.0 ml of *phenylhydrazine-sulphuric acid solution R*, mix and heat in a water-bath at 60 °C for 20 min. Cool immediately. The absorbance (*2.2.25*) of the solution measured at 419 nm is not greater than 0.10.

B. Examine by infrared absorption spectrophotometry (*2.2.24*), comparing with the spectrum obtained with *betamethasone CRS*. If the spectra obtained in the solid state with the substance to be examined and the reference substance show differences, dissolve the substance to be examined and the reference substance separately in the smallest necessary quantity of *methylene chloride R* and evaporate to dryness on a water-bath. Using the residues, record the spectra again.

C. Examine by thin-layer chromatography (*2.2.27*), using as the coating substance a suitable silica gel with a fluorescent indicator having an optimal intensity at 254 nm.

Test solution. Dissolve 10 mg of the substance to be examined in a mixture of 1 volume of *methanol R* and 9 volumes of *methylene chloride R* and dilute to 10 ml with the same mixture of solvents.

Reference solution (a). Dissolve 20 mg of *betamethasone CRS* in a mixture of 1 volume of *methanol R* and 9 volumes of *methylene chloride R* and dilute to 20 ml with the same mixture of solvents.

Reference solution (b). Dissolve 10 mg of *dexamethasone CRS* in reference solution (a) and dilute to 10 ml with the same solution.

Apply separately to the plate 5 µl of each solution. Develop over a path of 15 cm using a mixture of 5 volumes of *butanol R* saturated with *water R*, 10 volumes of *toluene R* and 85 volumes of *ether R*. Allow the plate to dry in air and examine in ultraviolet light at 254 nm. The principal spot in the chromatogram obtained with the test solution is similar in position and size to the principal spot in the chromatogram obtained with reference solution (a). Spray with *alcoholic solution of sulphuric acid R*. Heat at 120 °C for 10 min or until the spots appear. Allow to cool. Examine the chromatograms in daylight and in ultraviolet light at 365 nm. The principal spot in the chromatogram obtained with the test solution is similar in position, colour in daylight, fluorescence in ultraviolet light at 365 nm and size to the principal spot in the chromatogram obtained with reference solution (a). The test is not valid unless the chromatogram obtained with reference solution (b) shows two spots which may however not be completely separated.

D. Mix about 5 mg with 45 mg of *heavy magnesium oxide R* and ignite in a crucible until an almost white residue is obtained (usually less than 5 min). Allow to cool, add 1 ml of *water R*, 0.05 ml of *phenolphthalein solution R1* and about 1 ml of *dilute hydrochloric acid R* to render the solution colourless. Filter. Add 1.0 ml of the filtrate to a freshly prepared mixture of 0.1 ml of *alizarin S solution R* and 0.1 ml of *zirconyl nitrate solution R*. Mix, allow to stand for 5 min and compare the colour of the solution with that of a blank prepared in the same manner. The test solution is yellow and the blank is red.

E. Add about 2 mg to 2 ml of *sulphuric acid R* and shake to dissolve. Within 5 min, a deep reddish-brown colour develops. Add the solution to 10 ml of *water R* and mix. The colour is discharged and a clear solution remains.

TESTS

Specific optical rotation (*2.2.7*). Dissolve 0.125 g in *methanol R* and dilute to 25.0 ml with the same solvent. The specific optical rotation is + 118 to + 126, calculated with reference to the dried substance.

Related substances. Examine by liquid chromatography (*2.2.29*).

Test solution. Dissolve 25.0 mg of the substance to be examined in a mixture of equal volumes of *acetonitrile R* and *methanol R* and dilute to 10.0 ml with the same solvent.

Reference solution (a). Dissolve 2 mg of *betamethasone CRS* and 2 mg of *methylprednisolone CRS* in mobile phase A and dilute to 100.0 ml with the same mobile phase.

Reference solution (b). Dilute 1.0 ml of the test solution to 100.0 ml with mobile phase A.

The chromatographic procedure may be carried out using:

– a stainless steel column 0.25 m long and 4.6 mm in internal diameter packed with *octadecylsilyl silica gel for chromatography R* (5 µm),

– as mobile phase at a flow rate of 2.5 ml/min, a linear-gradient programme using the following conditions:

Mobile phase A. In a 1000 ml volumetric flask mix 250 ml of *acetonitrile R* with 700 ml of *water R* and allow to equilibrate; adjust the volume to 1000 ml with *water R* and mix again,

Mobile phase B. Acetonitrile R,

Time (min)	Mobile phase A (per cent V/V)	Mobile phase B (per cent V/V)	Comment
0	100	0	isocratic
15	100	0	begin linear gradient
40	0	100	end chromatogram, return to 100A
41	100	0	begin equilibration with A
46 = 0	100	0	end equilibration, begin next chromatogram

– as detector a spectrophotometer set at 254 nm,

maintaining the temperature of the column at 45 °C.

Equilibrate the column with mobile phase B at a flow rate of 2.5 ml/min for at least 30 min and then with mobile phase A for 5 min. For subsequent chromatograms, use the conditions described from 40 min to 46 min.

Adjust the sensitivity of the system so that the height of the principal peak in the chromatogram obtained with 20 µl of reference solution (b) is not less than 50 per cent of the full scale of the recorder.

Inject 20 µl of reference solution (a). When the chromatograms are recorded in the conditions described above, the retention times are: methylprednisolone, about 11.5 minutes and betamethasone, about 12.5 minutes. The test is not valid unless the resolution between the peaks corresponding to methylprednisolone and betamethasone is at least 1.5; if necessary, adjust the concentration of acetonitrile in mobile phase A.

Inject separately 20 µl of the mixture of equal volumes of *acetonitrile R* and *methanol R* as a blank, 20 µl of the test solution and 20 µl of reference solution (b). In the chromatogram obtained with the test solution: the area of any peak, apart from the principal peak, is not greater than the area of the principal peak in the chromatogram obtained with reference solution (b) (1.0 per cent) and not more than one such peak has an area greater than half the area of the principal peak in the chromatogram obtained with reference solution (b) (0.5 per cent); the sum of the areas of all the peaks, apart from the principal peak, is not greater than twice the area of the principal peak in the chromatogram obtained with reference solution (b) (2.0 per cent). Disregard any peak due to the blank and any peak with an area less than 0.05 times the area of the principal peak in the chromatogram obtained with reference solution (b).

Loss on drying (*2.2.32*). Not more than 0.5 per cent, determined on 0.500 g by drying in an oven at 100 °C to 105 °C.

ASSAY

Dissolve 0.100 g in *alcohol R* and dilute to 100.0 ml with the same solvent. Dilute 2.0 ml of the solution to 100.0 ml with *alcohol R*. Measure the absorbance (*2.2.25*) at the maximum at 238.5 nm.

Calculate the content of $C_{22}H_{29}FO_5$ taking the specific absorbance to be 395.

STORAGE

Store protected from light.

IMPURITIES

A. dexamethasone,

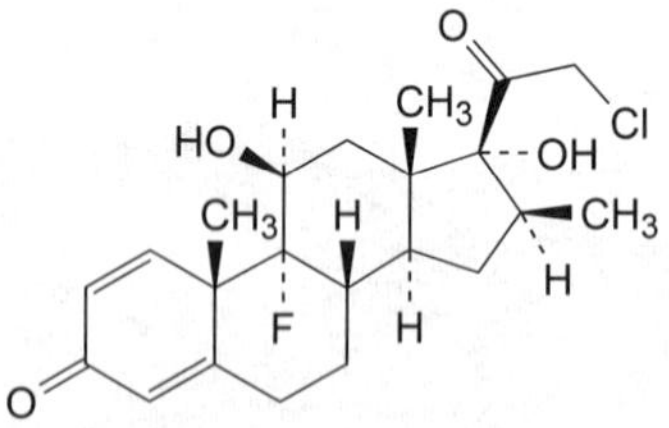

B. 21-chloro-9-fluoro-11β,17-dihydroxy-16β-methylpregna-1,4-diene-3,20-dione,

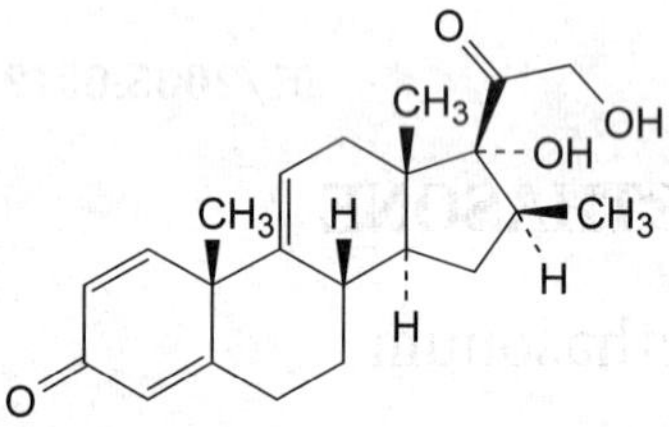

C. 17,21-dihydroxy-16β-methylpregna-1,4,9(11)-triene-3,20-dione,

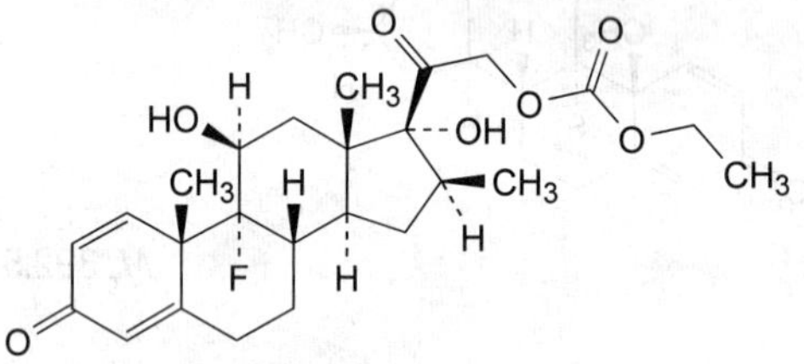

D. 9-fluoro-11β,17-dihydroxy-16β-methyl-3,20-dioxopregna-1,4-dien-21-yl ethoxycarboxylate,

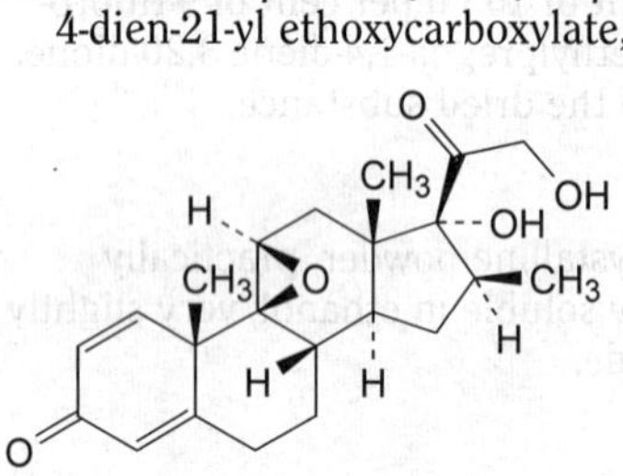

E. 9,11β-epoxy-17,21-dihydroxy-16β-methyl-9β-pregna-1,4-diene-3,20-dione,

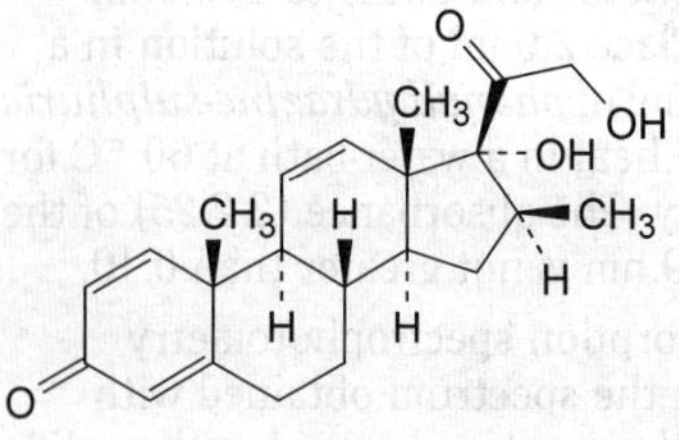

F. 17,21-dihydroxy-16β-methylpregna-1,4,11-triene-3,20-dione,

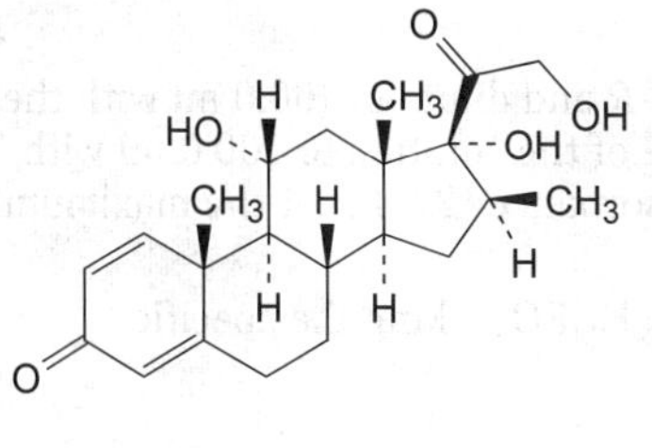

G. 11α,17,21-trihydroxy-16β-methylpregna-1,4-diene-3,20-dione,

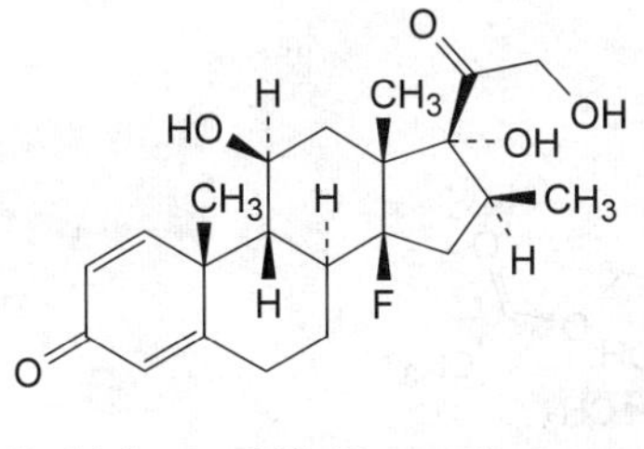

H. 14-fluoro-11β,17,21-trihydroxy-16β-methyl-8α,9β,14β-pregna-1,4-diene-3,20-dione,

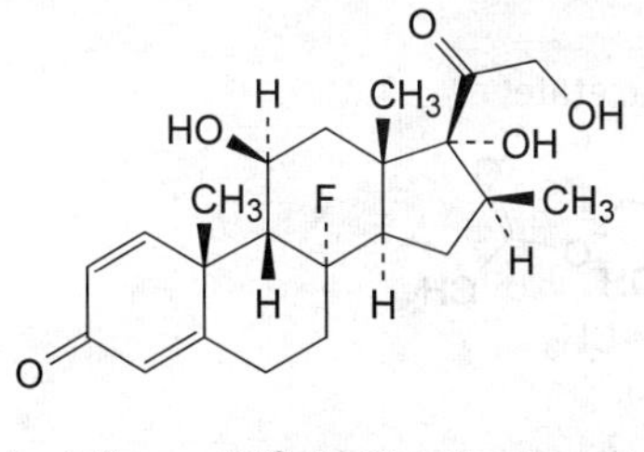

I. 8-fluoro-11β,17,21-trihydroxy-16β-methyl-8α,9β-pregna-1,4-diene-3,20-dione,

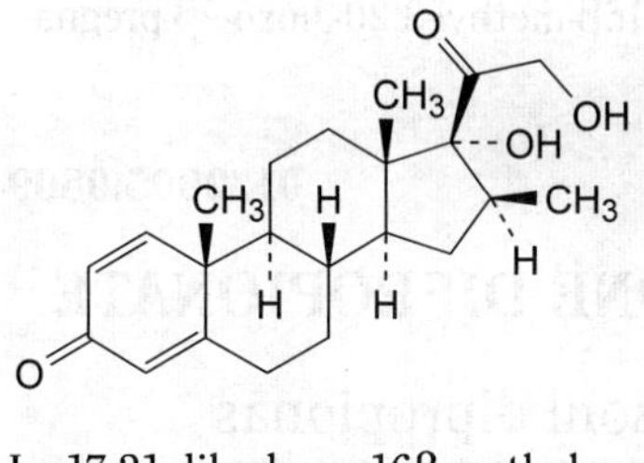

J. 17,21-dihydroxy-16β-methylpregna-1,4-diene-3,20-dione.

01/2005:0975

BETAMETHASONE ACETATE

Betamethasoni acetas

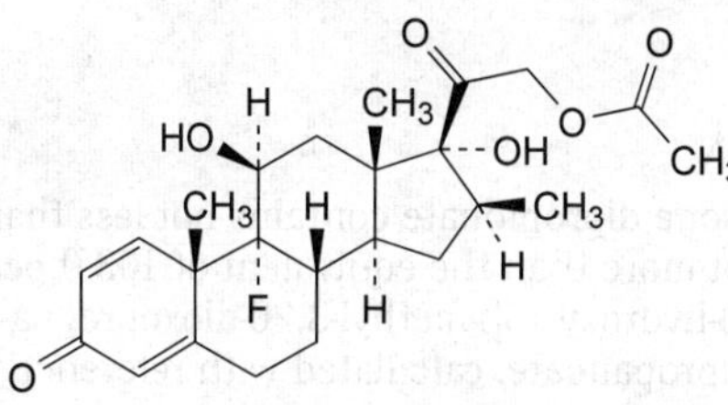

$C_{24}H_{31}FO_6$ M_r 434.5

DEFINITION

Betamethasone acetate contains not less than 97.0 per cent and not more than the equivalent of 103.0 per cent of 9-fluoro-11β,17-dihydroxy-16β-methyl-3,20-dioxopregna-1,4-diene-21-yl acetate, calculated with reference to the anhydrous substance.

CHARACTERS

A white or almost white, crystalline powder, practically insoluble in water, freely soluble in acetone, soluble in alcohol and in methylene chloride.

It shows polymorphism.

IDENTIFICATION

First identification: B, C.

Second identification: A, C, D, E, F.

A. Dissolve 10.0 mg in *ethanol R* and dilute to 100.0 ml with the same solvent. Place 2.0 ml of this solution in a ground-glass-stoppered tube, add 10.0 ml of *phenylhydrazine-sulphuric acid solution R*, mix and heat in a water-bath at 60 °C for 20 min. Cool immediately. The absorbance (*2.2.25*) of the solution measured at 419 nm is not more than 0.10.

B. Examine by infrared absorption spectrophotometry (*2.2.24*), comparing with the spectrum obtained with *betamethasone acetate CRS*. If the spectra obtained in the solid state show differences, dissolve the substance to be examined and the reference substance separately in the minimum volume of *methanol R*, evaporate to dryness on a water-bath and record new spectra using the residues.

C. Examine by thin-layer chromatography (*2.2.27*), using as the coating substance a suitable silica gel with a fluorescent indicator having an optimal intensity at 254 nm.

Test solution. Dissolve 10 mg of the substance to be examined in a mixture of 1 volume of *methanol R* and 9 volumes of *methylene chloride R* and dilute to 10 ml with the same mixture of solvents.

Reference solution (a). Dissolve 20 mg of *betamethasone acetate CRS* in a mixture of 1 volume of *methanol R* and 9 volumes of *methylene chloride R* and dilute to 20 ml with the same mixture of solvents.

Reference solution (b). Dissolve 10 mg of *prednisolone acetate CRS* in reference solution (a) and dilute to 10 ml with the same solution.

Apply to the plate 5 µl of each solution. Prepare the mobile phase by adding a mixture of 1.2 volumes of *water R* and 8 volumes of *methanol R* to a mixture of 15 volumes of *ether R* and 77 volumes of *methylene chloride R*. Develop over a path of 15 cm. Allow the plate to dry in air and examine in ultraviolet light at 254 nm. The principal spot in the chromatogram obtained with the test solution is similar in position and size to the principal spot in the chromatogram obtained with reference solution (a). Spray with *alcoholic solution of sulphuric acid R*. Heat at 120 °C for 10 min or until the spots appear. Allow to cool. Examine the plate in daylight and in ultraviolet light at 365 nm. The principal spot in the chromatogram obtained with the test solution is similar in position, colour in daylight, fluorescence in ultraviolet light at 365 nm and size to the principal spot in the chromatogram obtained with reference solution (a). The test is not valid unless the chromatogram obtained with reference solution (b) shows two clearly separated spots.

D. Add about 2 mg to 2 ml of *sulphuric acid R* and shake to dissolve. Within 5 min, a deep reddish-brown colour develops. Add the solution to 10 ml of *water R* and mix. The colour is discharged and a clear solution remains.

E. Mix about 5 mg with 45 mg of *heavy magnesium oxide R* and ignite in a crucible until an almost white residue is obtained (usually less than 5 min). Allow to cool, add 1 ml of *water R*, 0.05 ml of *phenolphthalein solution R1* and about 1 ml of *dilute hydrochloric acid R* to render the solution colourless. Filter. To a freshly prepared mixture of 0.1 ml of *alizarin S solution R* and 0.1 ml of *zirconyl nitrate solution R*, add 1.0 ml of the filtrate. Mix, allow to stand for 5 min and compare the colour of the solution with that of a blank prepared in the same manner. The test solution is yellow and the blank is red.

F. About 10 mg gives the reaction of acetyl (*2.3.1*).

TESTS

Specific optical rotation (*2.2.7*). Dissolve 0.250 g in *dioxan R* and dilute to 25.0 ml with the same solvent. The specific optical rotation is + 120 to + 128, calculated with reference to the anhydrous substance.

Related substances. Examine by liquid chromatography (*2.2.29*).

Test solution. Dissolve 25.0 mg of the substance to be examined in 4 ml of *acetonitrile R* and dilute to 10.0 ml with the same solvent.

Reference solution (a). Dissolve 2 mg of *betamethasone acetate CRS* and 2 mg of *dexamethasone acetate CRS* in the mobile phase and dilute to 100.0 ml with the mobile phase.

Reference solution (b). Dilute 1.0 ml of the test solution to 100.0 ml with the mobile phase.

The chromatographic procedure may be carried out using:

- a stainless steel column 0.25 m long and 4.6 mm in internal diameter packed with *octadecylsilyl silica gel for chromatography R* (5 µm),
- as mobile phase at a flow rate of 1 ml/min a mixture prepared as follows: in a 1000 ml volumetric flask mix 380 ml of *acetonitrile R* with 550 ml of *water R* and allow to equilibrate; dilute to 1000 ml with *water R* and mix again,
- as detector a spectrophotometer set at 254 nm.

Equilibrate the column with the mobile phase at a flow rate of 1 ml/min for about 30 min.

Adjust the sensitivity of the system so that the height of the principal peak in the chromatogram obtained with 20 µl of reference solution (b) is at least 50 per cent of the full scale of the recorder.

Inject 20 µl of reference solution (a).When the chromatograms are recorded in the prescribed conditions, the retention times are: betamethasone acetate about 19 min and dexamethasone acetate about 22 min. The test is not valid unless the resolution between the peaks due to betamethasone acetate and dexamethasone acetate is at least 3.3; if necessary, adjust slightly the concentration of acetonitrile in the mobile phase.

Inject 20 µl of the test solution and 20 µl of reference solution (b). Continue the chromatography for 2.5 times the retention time of the principal peak in the chromatogram obtained with the test solution. In the chromatogram obtained with the test solution: the area of any peak, apart from the principal peak, is not greater than half the area of the principal peak in the chromatogram obtained with reference solution (b) (0.5 per cent); the sum of the areas of all the peaks, apart from the principal peak, is not greater than 1.25 times the area of the principal peak in the chromatogram obtained with reference solution (b) (1.25 per cent). Disregard any peak with an area less than 0.05 times the area of the principal peak in the chromatogram obtained with reference solution (b).

Water (*2.5.12*). Not more than 4.0 per cent, determined on 0.100 g by the semi-micro determination of water.

ASSAY

Dissolve 0.100 g in *alcohol R* and dilute to 100.0 ml with the same solvent. Dilute 2.0 ml of the solution to 100.0 ml with *alcohol R*. Measure the absorbance (*2.2.25*) at the maximum at 240 nm.

Calculate the content of $C_{24}H_{31}FO_6$ taking the specific absorbance to be 350.

STORAGE

Store protected from light.

IMPURITIES

A. betamethasone,

B. dexamethasone acetate,

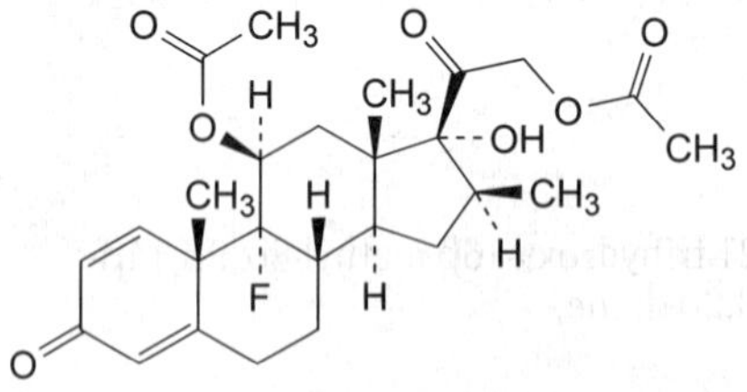

C. betamethasone 11,21-diacetate,

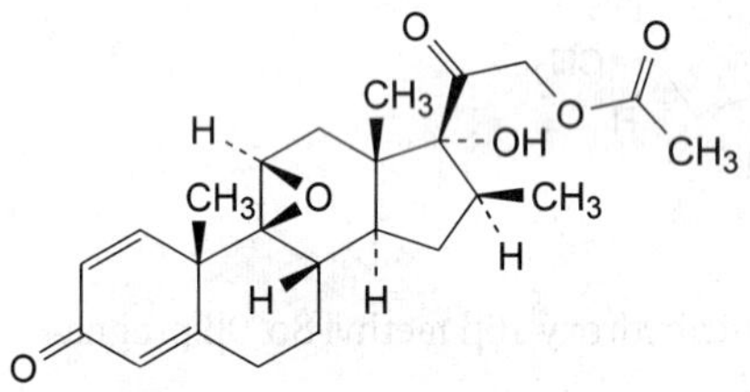

D. 9,11β-epoxy-17-hydroxy-16β-methyl-3,20-dioxo-9β-pregna-1,4-diene-21-yl acetate.

01/2005:0809

BETAMETHASONE DIPROPIONATE

Betamethasoni dipropionas

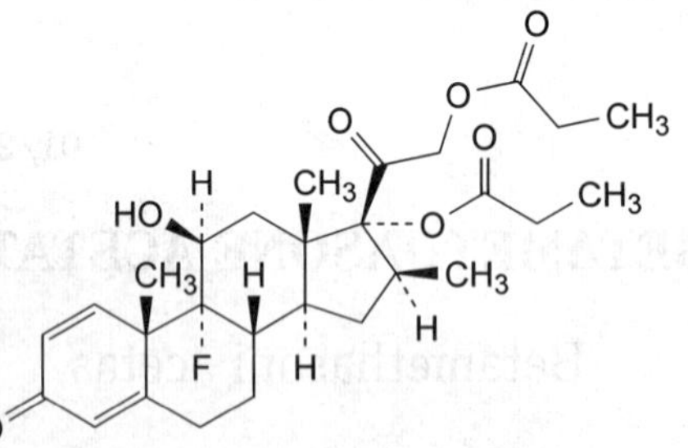

$C_{28}H_{37}FO_7$ M_r 504.6

DEFINITION

Betamethasone dipropionate contains not less than 97.0 per cent and not more than the equivalent of 103.0 per cent of 9-fluoro-11β-hydroxy-16β-methyl-3,20-dioxopregna-1,4-diene-17,21-diyl dipropanoate, calculated with reference to the dried substance.

CHARACTERS

A white or almost white, crystalline powder, practically insoluble in water, freely soluble in acetone and in methylene chloride, sparingly soluble in alcohol.

IDENTIFICATION

First identification: B, C.

Second identification: A, D, E, F.

A. Dissolve 10.0 mg in *ethanol R* and dilute to 100.0 ml with the same solvent. Place 2.0 ml of this solution in a ground-glass-stoppered tube, add 10.0 ml of *phenylhydrazine-sulphuric acid solution R,* mix and heat in a water-bath at 60 °C for 20 min. Cool immediately. The absorbance (*2.2.25*) of the solution measured at 419 nm is not more than 0.10.

B. Examine by infrared absorption spectrophotometry (*2.2.24*), comparing with the spectrum obtained with *betamethasone dipropionate CRS.*

C. Examine by thin-layer chromatography (*2.2.27*), using as the coating substance a suitable silica gel with a fluorescent indicator having an optimal intensity at 254 nm.

Test solution. Dissolve 10 mg of the substance to be examined in a mixture of 1 volume of *methanol R* and 9 volumes of *methylene chloride R* and dilute to 10 ml with the same mixture of solvents.

Reference solution (a). Dissolve 10 mg of *betamethasone dipropionate CRS* in a mixture of 1 volume of *methanol R* and 9 volumes of *methylene chloride R* and dilute to 10 ml with the same mixture of solvents.

Reference solution (b). Dissolve 10 mg of *desoxycortone acetate CRS* in a mixture of 1 volume of *methanol R* and 9 volumes of *methylene chloride R* and dilute to 10 ml with the same mixture of solvents. Dilute 5 ml of this solution to 10 ml with reference solution (a).

Apply to the plate 5 µl of each solution. Prepare the mobile phase by adding a mixture of 1.2 volumes of *water R* and 8 volumes of *methanol R* to a mixture of 15 volumes of *ether R* and 77 volumes of *methylene chloride R.* Develop over a path of 15 cm. Allow the plate to dry in air and examine in ultraviolet light at 254 nm. The principal spot in the chromatogram obtained with the test solution is similar in position and size to the principal spot in the chromatogram obtained with reference solution (a). Spray the plate with *alcoholic solution of sulphuric acid R.* Heat at 120 °C for 10 min or until the spots appear. Allow to cool. Examine in daylight and in ultraviolet light at 365 nm. The principal spot in the chromatogram obtained with the test solution is similar in position, colour in daylight, fluorescence in ultraviolet light at 365 nm and size to the principal spot in the chromatogram obtained with reference solution (a). The test is not valid unless the chromatogram obtained with reference solution (b) shows two clearly separated spots.

D. Examine by thin-layer chromatography (*2.2.27*), using as the coating substance a suitable silica gel with a fluorescent indicator having an optimal intensity at 254 nm.

Test solution (a). Dissolve 25 mg of the substance to be examined in *methanol R* with gentle heating and dilute to 5 ml with the same solvent. This solution is also used to prepare test solution (b). Dilute 2 ml of the solution to 10 ml with *methylene chloride R.*

Test solution (b). Transfer 2 ml of the solution obtained during preparation of test solution (a) to a 15 ml glass tube with a ground-glass stopper or a polytetrafluoroethylene cap. Add 10 ml of *saturated methanolic potassium hydrogen carbonate solution R* and immediately pass a current of *nitrogen R* briskly through the solution for 5 min. Stopper the tube. Heat in a water-bath at 45 °C, protected from light, for 2 h. Allow to cool.

Reference solution (a). Dissolve 25 mg of *betamethasone dipropionate CRS* in *methanol R* with gentle heating and dilute to 5 ml with the same solvent. This solution is also used to prepare reference solution (b). Dilute 2 ml of the solution to 10 ml with *methylene chloride R.*

Reference solution (b). Transfer 2 ml of the solution obtained during preparation of reference solution (a) to a 15 ml glass tube with a ground-glass stopper or a polytetrafluoroethylene cap. Add 10 ml of *saturated methanolic potassium hydrogen carbonate solution R* and immediately pass a current of *nitrogen R* briskly through the solution for 5 min. Stopper the tube. Heat in a water-bath at 45 °C, protected from light, for 2 h. Allow to cool.

Apply to the plate 5 µl of each solution. Prepare the mobile phase by adding a mixture of 1.2 volumes of *water R* and 8 volumes of *methanol R* to a mixture of 15 volumes of *ether R* and 77 volumes of *methylene chloride R.* Develop over a path of 15 cm. Allow the plate to dry in air and examine in ultraviolet light at 254 nm. The principal spot in each of the chromatograms obtained with the test solutions is similar in position and size to the principal spot in the chromatogram obtained with the corresponding reference solution. Spray the plate with *alcoholic solution of sulphuric acid R.* Heat at 120 °C for 10 min or until the spots appear. Allow to cool. Examine in daylight and in ultraviolet light at 365 nm. The principal spot in each of the chromatograms obtained with the test solutions is similar in position, colour in daylight, fluorescence in ultraviolet light at 365 nm and size to the principal spot in the chromatogram obtained with the corresponding reference solution. The principal spot in each of the chromatograms obtained with test solution (b) and reference solution (b) has an R_f value distinctly lower than that of the principal spots in each of the chromatograms obtained with test solution (a) and reference solution (a).

E. Add about 2 mg to 2 ml of *sulphuric acid R* and shake to dissolve. Within 5 min, a deep reddish-brown colour develops. Add the solution to 10 ml of *water R* and mix. The colour is discharged and a clear solution remains.

F. Mix about 5 mg with 45 mg of *heavy magnesium oxide R* and ignite in a crucible until an almost white residue is obtained (usually less than 5 min). Allow to cool, add 1 ml of *water R,* 0.05 ml of *phenolphthalein solution R1* and about 1 ml of *dilute hydrochloric acid R* to render the solution colourless. Filter. Add 1.0 ml of the filtrate to a freshly prepared mixture of 0.1 ml of *alizarin S solution R* and 0.1 ml of *zirconyl nitrate solution R.* Mix, allow to stand for 5 min and compare the colour of the solution with that of a blank prepared in the same manner. The test solution is yellow and the blank is red.

TESTS

Specific optical rotation (*2.2.7*). Dissolve 0.250 g in *dioxan R* and dilute to 25.0 ml with the same solvent. The specific optical rotation is + 63 to + 70, calculated with reference to the dried substance.

Related substances. Examine by liquid chromatography (*2.2.29*).

Test solution. Dissolve 62.5 mg of the substance to be examined in the mobile phase and dilute to 25.0 ml with the mobile phase.

Reference solution (a). Dissolve 2.5 mg of *betamethasone dipropionate CRS* and 2.5 mg of *beclometasone dipropionate CRS* in the mobile phase and dilute to 50.0 ml with the same solvent.

Reference solution (b). Dilute 1.0 ml of the test solution to 50.0 ml with the mobile phase.

The chromatographic procedure may be carried out using:

- a stainless steel column 0.25 m long and 4.6 mm in internal diameter packed with *octadecylsilyl silica gel for chromatography R* (5 µm),
- as mobile phase at a flow rate of 1 ml/min a mixture prepared as follows: mix carefully 350 ml of *water R* with 600 ml of *acetonitrile R* and allow to equilibrate; adjust the volume to 1000 ml with *water R* and mix again,
- as detector a spectrophotometer set at 254 nm.

Adjust the sensitivity so that the height of the principal peak in the chromatogram obtained with reference solution (b) is 70 per cent to 90 per cent of the full scale of the recorder.

Equilibrate the column with the mobile phase at a flow rate of 1 ml/min for about 45 min. Inject 20 µl of reference solution (a). When the chromatograms are recorded in the prescribed conditions, the retention times are: betamethasone dipropionate, about 9 min; beclometasone dipropionate, about 10.7 min. The test is not valid unless the resolution between the peaks corresponding to betamethasone dipropionate and beclometasone dipropionate is at least 2.5; if necessary, adjust the concentration of acetonitrile in the mobile phase.

Inject separately 20 µl of the test solution and 20 µl of reference solution (b). Continue the chromatography for 2.5 times the retention time of the principal peak. In the chromatogram obtained with the test solution: the area of any peak apart from the principal peak is not greater than 0.75 times the area of the principal peak in the chromatogram obtained with reference solution (b) (1.5 per cent) and not more than one such peak has an area greater than half the area of the principal peak in the chromatogram obtained with reference solution (b) (1 per cent); the sum of the areas of all the peaks, apart from the principal peak, is not greater than 1.25 times the area of the principal peak in the chromatogram obtained with reference solution (b) (2.5 per cent). Disregard any peak with an area less than 0.025 times the area of the principal peak in the chromatogram obtained with reference solution (b).

Loss on drying (*2.2.32*). Not more than 1.0 per cent, determined on 0.500 g by drying in an oven at 100-105 °C.

ASSAY

Dissolve 50.0 mg in *alcohol R* and dilute to 100.0 ml with the same solvent. Dilute 2.0 ml of the solution to 50.0 ml with *alcohol R*. Measure the absorbance (*2.2.25*) at the maximum at 240 nm.

Calculate the content of $C_{28}H_{37}FO_7$ taking the specific absorbance to be 305.

STORAGE

Store protected from light.

01/2005:0810

BETAMETHASONE SODIUM PHOSPHATE

Betamethasoni natrii phosphas

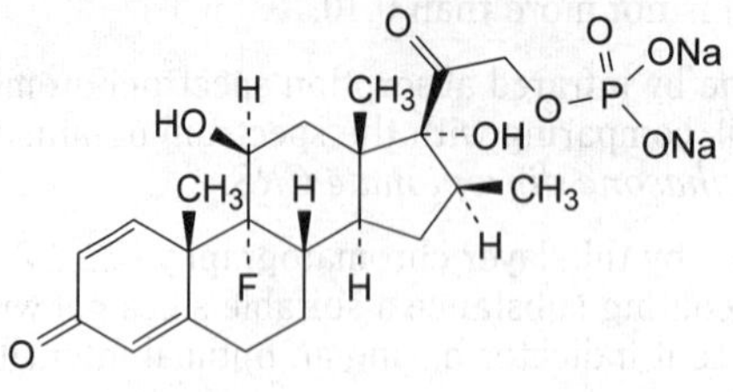

$C_{22}H_{28}FNa_2O_8P$ M_r 516.4

DEFINITION

Betamethasone sodium phosphate contains not less than 96.0 per cent and not more than the equivalent of 103.0 per cent of 9-fluoro-11β,17-dihydroxy-16β-methyl-3,20-dioxopregna-1,4-diene-21-yl disodium phosphate, calculated with reference to the anhydrous substance.

CHARACTERS

A white or almost white powder, very hygroscopic, freely soluble in water, slightly soluble in alcohol, practically insoluble in methylene chloride.

IDENTIFICATION

First identification: B, C.

Second identification: A, C, D, E, F.

A. Dissolve 10.0 mg in 5 ml of *water R* and dilute to 100.0 ml with *ethanol R*. Place 2.0 ml of this solution in a ground-glass-stoppered tube, add 10.0 ml of *phenylhydrazine-sulphuric acid solution R*, mix and heat in a water-bath at 60 °C for 20 min. Cool immediately. The absorbance (*2.2.25*) of the solution measured at the maximum at 450 nm is not more than 0.10.

B. Examine by infrared absorption spectrophotometry (*2.2.24*), comparing with the spectrum obtained with *betamethasone sodium phosphate CRS*. If the spectra obtained in the solid state show differences, dissolve the substance to be examined and the reference substance separately in the minimum volume of *alcohol R*, evaporate to dryness on a water-bath and record new spectra using the residues.

C. Examine by thin-layer chromatography (*2.2.27*), using as the coating substance a suitable silica gel with a fluorescent indicator having an optimal intensity at 254 nm.

Test solution. Dissolve 10 mg of the substance to be examined in *methanol R* and dilute to 10 ml with the same solvent.

Reference solution (a). Dissolve 10 mg of *betamethasone sodium phosphate CRS* in *methanol R* and dilute to 10 ml with the same solvent.

Reference solution (b). Dissolve 10 mg of *prednisolone sodium phosphate CRS* in *methanol R* and dilute to 10 ml with the same solvent. Dilute 5 ml of this solution to 10 ml with reference solution (a).

Apply to the plate 5 µl of each solution. Develop over a path of 15 cm using a mixture of 20 volumes of *glacial acetic acid R*, 20 volumes of *water R* and 60 volumes of *butanol R*. Allow the plate to dry in air and examine in ultraviolet light at 254 nm. The principal spot in the chromatogram obtained with the test solution is similar in position and size to the principal spot in the chromatogram obtained with reference solution (a). Spray the plate with *alcoholic solution of sulphuric acid R*. Heat at 120 °C for 10 min or until the spots appear. Allow to cool. Examine in daylight and in ultraviolet light at 365 nm. The principal spot in the chromatogram obtained with the test solution is similar in position, colour in daylight, fluorescence in ultraviolet light at 365 nm and size to the principal spot in the chromatogram obtained with reference solution (a). The test is not valid unless the chromatogram obtained with reference solution (b) shows two spots which may however not be completely separated.

D. Add about 2 mg to 2 ml of *sulphuric acid R* and shake to dissolve. Within 5 min, an intense reddish-brown colour develops. Add the solution to 10 ml of *water R* and mix. The colour is discharged and a clear solution remains.

E. Mix about 5 mg with 45 mg of *heavy magnesium oxide R* and ignite in a crucible until an almost white residue is obtained (usually less than 5 min). Allow to cool, add 1 ml of *water R*, 0.05 ml of *phenolphthalein solution R1* and about 1 ml of *dilute hydrochloric acid R* to render the solution colourless. Filter. Add 1.0 ml of the filtrate to a freshly prepared mixture of 0.1 ml of *alizarin S solution R* and 0.1 ml of *zirconyl nitrate solution R*. Mix, allow to stand for 5 min and compare the colour of the solution with that of a blank prepared in the same manner. The test solution is yellow and the blank is red.

F. To about 40 mg add 2 ml of *sulphuric acid R* and heat gently until white fumes are evolved. Add *nitric acid R* dropwise, continue the heating until the solution is almost colourless and cool. Add 2 ml of *water R*, heat until white fumes are again evolved, cool, add 10 ml of *water R* and neutralise to *red litmus paper R* with *dilute ammonia R1*. The solution gives reaction (a) of sodium (*2.3.1*) and reaction (b) of phosphates (*2.3.1*).

TESTS

Solution S. Dissolve 1.0 g in *carbon dioxide-free water R* and dilute to 20 ml with the same solvent.

Appearance of solution. Solution S is clear (*2.2.1*) and not more intensely coloured than reference solution B_7 (*2.2.2, Method II*).

pH (*2.2.3*). Dilute 1 ml of solution S to 5 ml with *carbon dioxide-free water R*. The pH of the solution is 7.5 to 9.0.

Specific optical rotation(*2.2.7*). Dissolve 0.250 g in *water R* and dilute to 25.0 ml with the same solvent. The specific optical rotation is + 98 to + 104, calculated with reference to the anhydrous substance.

Related substances. Examine by liquid chromatography (*2.2.29*).

Test solution. Dissolve 62.5 mg of the substance to be examined in the mobile phase and dilute to 25.0 ml with the mobile phase.

Reference solution (a). Dissolve 25 mg of *betamethasone sodium phosphate CRS* and 25 mg of *dexamethasone sodium phosphate CRS* in the mobile phase and dilute to 25.0 ml with the mobile phase. Dilute 1.0 ml of this solution to 25.0 ml with the mobile phase.

Reference solution (b). Dilute 1.0 ml of the test solution to 50.0 ml with the mobile phase.

The chromatographic procedure may be carried out using:

- a stainless steel column 0.25 m long and 4.6 mm in internal diameter packed with *octadecylsilyl silica gel for chromatography R* (5 µm),
- as mobile phase at a flow rate of 1 ml/min a mixture prepared as follows: in a 250 ml conical flask, weigh 1.360 g of *potassium dihydrogen phosphate R* and 0.600 g of *hexylamine R*, mix and allow to stand for 10 min and then dissolve in 185 ml of *water R*; add 65 ml of *acetonitrile R*, mix and filter (0.45 µm),
- as detector a spectrophotometer set at 254 nm.

Equilibrate the column with the mobile phase at a flow rate of 1 ml/min for about 45 min.

Adjust the sensitivity of the system so that the height of the principal peak in the chromatogram obtained with reference solution (b) is 70 per cent to 90 per cent of the full scale of the recorder.

Inject 20 µl of reference solution (a). When the chromatograms are recorded in the conditions described above, the retention times are: betamethasone sodium phosphate about 14 min; dexamethasone sodium phosphate about 15.5 min. The test is not valid unless the resolution between the peaks corresponding to betamethasone sodium phosphate and dexamethasone sodium phosphate is at least 2.0; if necessary, increase the concentration of acetonitrile or increase the concentration of water in the mobile phase.

Inject 20 µl of the test solution and 20 µl of reference solution (b). Continue the chromatography for twice the retention time of the principal peak. In the chromatogram obtained with the test solution: the area of any peak, apart from the principal peak, is not greater than the area of the principal peak in the chromatogram obtained with reference solution (b) (2 per cent) and not more than one such peak has an area greater than half the area of the principal peak in the chromatogram obtained with reference solution (b) (1 per cent); the sum of the areas of all the peaks, apart from the principal peak, is not greater than 1.5 times the area of the principal peak in the chromatogram obtained with reference solution (b) (3 per cent). Disregard any peak with an area less than 0.025 times the area of the principal peak in the chromatogram obtained with reference solution (b).

Inorganic phosphate. Dissolve 50 mg in *water R* and dilute to 100 ml with the same solvent. To 10 ml of this solution add 5 ml of *molybdovanadic reagent R*, mix and allow to stand for 5 min. Any yellow colour in the solution is not more intense than that in a standard prepared at the same time and in the same manner using 10 ml of *phosphate standard solution (5 ppm PO_4) R* (1 per cent).

Water (*2.5.12*). Not more than 8.0 per cent, determined on 0.200 g by the semi-micro determination of water.

ASSAY

Dissolve 0.100 g in *water R* and dilute to 100.0 ml with the same solvent. Dilute 5.0 ml of the solution to 250.0 ml with *water R*. Measure the absorbance (*2.2.25*) at the maximum at 241 nm.

Calculate the content of $C_{22}H_{28}FNa_2O_8P$ taking the specific absorbance to be 297.

STORAGE

Store in an airtight container, protected from light.

Monographs B

01/2005:0811

BETAMETHASONE VALERATE

Betamethasoni valeras

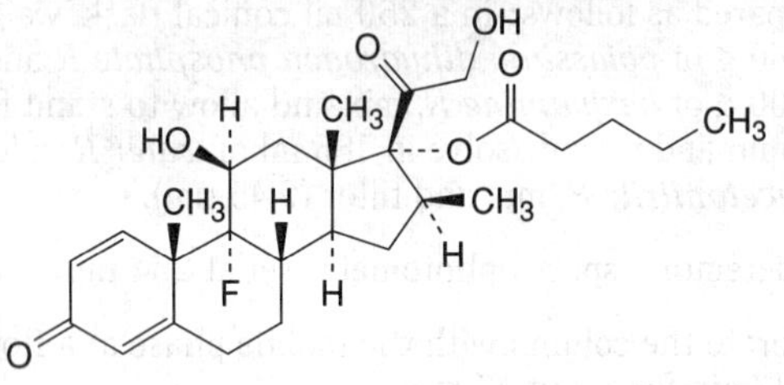

$C_{27}H_{37}FO_6$ M_r 476.6

DEFINITION

Betamethasone valerate contains not less than 97.0 per cent and not more than the equivalent of 103.0 per cent of 9-fluoro-11β,21-dihydroxy-16β-methyl-3,20-dioxopregna-1,4-dien-17-yl pentanoate, calculated with reference to the dried substance.

CHARACTERS

A white or almost white, crystalline powder, practically insoluble in water, freely soluble in acetone and in methylene chloride, soluble in alcohol.

It melts at about 192 °C, with decomposition.

IDENTIFICATION

First identification: C, D.

Second identification: A, B, E, F, G.

A. It complies with the test for specific optical rotation (see Tests).

B. Dissolve 10.0 mg in *ethanol R* and dilute to 100.0 ml with the same solvent. Place 2.0 ml of this solution in a ground-glass-stoppered tube, add 10.0 ml of *phenylhydrazine-sulphuric acid solution R*, mix and heat in a water-bath at 60 °C for 20 min. Cool immediately. The absorbance (*2.2.25*) of the solution measured at 419 nm is not more than 0.10.

C. Examine by infrared absorption spectrophotometry (*2.2.24*), comparing with the spectrum obtained with *betamethasone 17-valerate CRS*. If the spectra obtained in the solid state show differences, dissolve the substance to be examined and the reference substance separately in the minimum volume of *chloroform R*, evaporate to dryness on a water-bath and record new spectra using the residues.

D. Examine by thin-layer chromatography (*2.2.27*), using as the coating substance a suitable silica gel with a fluorescent indicator having an optimal intensity at 254 nm.

Test solution. Dissolve 10 mg of the substance to be examined in a mixture of 1 volume of *methanol R* and 9 volumes of *methylene chloride R* and dilute to 10 ml with the same mixture of solvents.

Reference solution (a). Dissolve 10 mg of *betamethasone 17-valerate CRS* in a mixture of 1 volume of *methanol R* and 9 volumes of *methylene chloride R* and dilute to 10 ml with the same mixture of solvents.

Reference solution (b). Dissolve 10 mg of *betamethasone 21-valerate CRS* in a mixture of 1 volume of *methanol R* and 9 volumes of *methylene chloride R* and dilute to 10 ml with the same mixture of solvents. Dilute 5 ml of this solution to 10 ml with reference solution (a).

Apply to the plate 5 µl of each solution. Prepare the mobile phase by adding a mixture of 1.2 volumes of *water R* and 8 volumes of *methanol R* to a mixture of 15 volumes of *ether R* and 77 volumes of *methylene chloride R*. Develop over a path of 15 cm. Allow the plate to dry in air and examine in ultraviolet light at 254 nm. The principal spot in the chromatogram obtained with the test solution is similar in position and size to the principal spot in the chromatogram obtained with reference solution (a). Spray the plate with *alcoholic solution of sulphuric acid R*. Heat at 120 °C for 10 min or until the spots appear. Allow to cool. Examine in daylight and in ultraviolet light at 365 nm. The principal spot in the chromatogram obtained with the test solution is similar in position, colour in daylight, fluorescence in ultraviolet light at 365 nm and size to the principal spot in the chromatogram obtained with reference solution (a). The test is not valid unless the chromatogram obtained with reference solution (b) shows two clearly separated spots.

E. Examine by thin-layer chromatography (*2.2.27*), using as the coating substance a suitable silica gel with a fluorescent indicator having an optimal intensity at 254 nm.

Test solution (a). Dissolve 25 mg of the substance to be examined in *methanol R* with gentle heating and dilute to 5 ml with the same solvent. This solution is also used to prepare test solution (b). Dilute 2 ml of the solution to 10 ml with *methylene chloride R*.

Test solution (b). Transfer 2 ml of the solution obtained during preparation of test solution (a) to a 15 ml glass tube with a ground-glass stopper or a polytetrafluoroethylene cap. Add 10 ml of *saturated methanolic potassium hydrogen carbonate solution R* and immediately pass a current of *nitrogen R* briskly through the solution for 5 min. Stopper the tube. Heat in a water-bath at 45 °C, protected from light, for 3 h. Allow to cool.

Reference solution (a). Dissolve 25 mg of *betamethasone 17-valerate CRS* in *methanol R* with gentle heating and dilute to 5 ml with the same solvent. This solution is also used to prepare reference solution (b). Dilute 2 ml of the solution to 10 ml with *methylene chloride R*.

Reference solution (b). Transfer 2 ml of the solution obtained during preparation of reference solution (a) to a 15 ml glass tube with a ground glass-stopper or a polytetrafluoroethylene cap. Add 10 ml of *saturated methanolic potassium hydrogen carbonate solution R* and immediately pass a current of *nitrogen R* briskly through the solution for 5 min. Stopper the tube. Heat in a water-bath at 45 °C, protected from light, for 3 h. Allow to cool.

Apply to the plate 5 µl of each solution. Prepare the mobile phase by adding a mixture of 1.2 volumes of *water R* and 8 volumes of *methanol R* to a mixture of 15 volumes of *ether R* and 77 volumes of *methylene chloride R*. Develop over a path of 15 cm. Allow the plate to dry in air and examine under ultraviolet light at 254 nm. The principal spot in each of the chromatograms obtained with the test solutions is similar in position and size to the principal spot in the chromatogram obtained with the corresponding reference solution. Spray with *alcoholic solution of sulphuric acid R*. Heat at 120 °C for 10 min or until the spots appear. Allow to cool. Examine in daylight and in ultraviolet light at 365 nm. The principal spot in each of the chromatograms obtained with the test solutions is similar in position, colour in daylight, fluorescence in ultraviolet light at 365 nm and size to the principal spot in the chromatograms obtained with the corresponding reference solution. The principal spot in each of the chromatograms obtained with test solution (b) and reference solution (b) has an R_f value distinctly lower than that of the principal spots in each of the chromatograms obtained with test solution (a) and reference solution (a).

F. Add about 2 mg to 2 ml of *sulphuric acid R* and shake to dissolve. Within 5 min, a deep reddish-brown colour develops. Add the solution to 10 ml of *water R* and mix. The colour is discharged and a clear solution remains.

G. Mix about 5 mg with 45 mg of *heavy magnesium oxide R* and ignite in a crucible until an almost white residue is obtained (usually less than 5 min). Allow to cool, add 1 ml of *water R*, 0.05 ml of *phenolphthalein solution R1* and about 1 ml of *dilute hydrochloric acid R* to render the solution colourless. Filter. Add 1.0 ml of the filtrate to a freshly prepared mixture of 0.1 ml of *alizarin S solution R* and 0.1 ml of *zirconyl nitrate solution R*. Mix, allow to stand for 5 min and compare the colour of the solution with that of a blank prepared in the same manner. The test solution is yellow and the blank is red.

TESTS

Specific optical rotation (*2.2.7*). Dissolve 0.250 g in *dioxan R* and dilute to 25.0 ml with the same solvent. The specific optical rotation is + 75 to + 82, calculated with reference to the dried substance.

Related substances. Examine by liquid chromatography (*2.2.29*).

Solution A. To 1000 ml of the mobile phase add 1 ml of *glacial acetic acid R* and mix carefully.

Test solution. Dissolve 62.5 mg of the substance to be examined in solution A and dilute to 25.0 ml with solution A.

Reference solution (a). Dissolve 2 mg of *betamethasone 17-valerate CRS* and 2 mg of *betamethasone 21-valerate CRS* in solution A and dilute to 50.0 ml with solution A.

Reference solution (b). Dilute 1.0 ml of the test solution to 50.0 ml with solution A.

The chromatographic procedure may be carried out using:

– a stainless steel column 0.25 m long and 4.6 mm in internal diameter packed with *octadecylsilyl silica gel for chromatography R* (5 µm),

– as mobile phase at a flow rate of 1 ml/min a mixture prepared as follows: mix 350 ml of *water R* with 600 ml of *acetonitrile R* and allow to equilibrate; adjust the volume to 1000 ml with *water R* and mix again,

– as detector a spectrophotometer set at 254 nm.

Equilibrate the column with the mobile phase for about 45 min.

Adjust the sensitivity so that the height of the principal peak in the chromatogram obtained with reference solution (b) is 70 per cent to 90 per cent of the full scale of the recorder.

Inject 20 µl of reference solution (a). When the chromatograms are recorded in the prescribed conditions, the retention times are: betamethasone 17-valerate, about 7 min; betamethasone 21-valerate, about 9 min. The test is not valid unless the resolution between the peaks corresponding to betamethasone 17-valerate and betamethasone 21-valerate is at least 5.0; if necessary, adjust the concentration of acetonitrile in the mobile phase.

Inject 20 µl of the test solution and 20 µl of reference solution (b). Continue the chromatography for 2.5 times the retention time of the principal peak. In the chromatogram obtained with the test solution: the area of any peak apart from the principal peak is not greater than 0.75 times the area of the principal peak in the chromatogram obtained with reference solution (b) (1.5 per cent) and not more than one such peak has an area greater than half the area of the principal peak in the chromatogram obtained with reference solution (b) (1.0 per cent); the sum of the areas of all the peaks, apart from the principal peak, is not greater than 1.5 times the area of the principal peak in the chromatogram obtained with reference solution (b) (3.0 per cent). Disregard any peak with an area less than 0.025 times the area of the principal peak in the chromatogram obtained with reference solution (b).

Loss on drying (*2.2.32*). Not more than 0.5 per cent, determined on 1.000 g by drying in an oven at 100-105 °C.

ASSAY

Dissolve 50.0 mg in *alcohol R* and dilute to 100.0 ml with the same solvent. Dilute 2.0 ml of the solution to 50.0 ml with *alcohol R*. Measure the absorbance (*2.2.25*) at the maximum at 240 nm.

Calculate the content of $C_{27}H_{37}FO_6$ taking the specific absorbance to be 325.

STORAGE

Store protected from light.

01/2005:1072

BETAXOLOL HYDROCHLORIDE

Betaxololi hydrochloridum

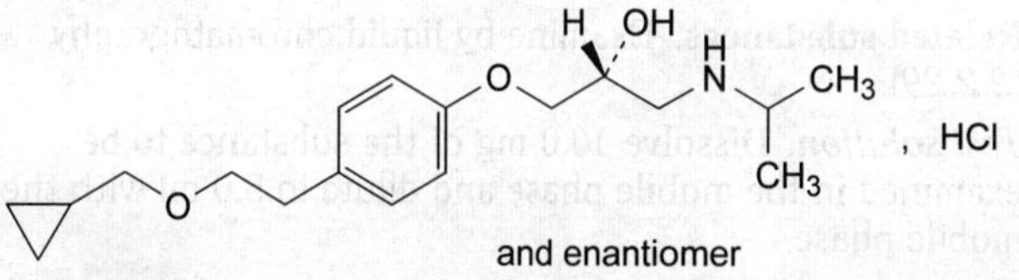

$C_{18}H_{30}ClNO_3$ M_r 343.9

DEFINITION

Betaxolol hydrochloride contains not less than 98.5 per cent and not more than the equivalent of 101.5 per cent of (2*RS*)-1-[4-[2-(cyclopropylmethoxy)ethyl]phenoxy]-3-[(1-methylethyl)amino]propan-2-ol hydrochloride, calculated with reference to the dried substance.

CHARACTERS

A white or almost white, crystalline powder, very soluble in water, freely soluble in alcohol, soluble in methylene chloride.

IDENTIFICATION

First identification: B, D.

Second identification: A, C, D.

A. Melting point (*2.2.14*): 113 °C to 117 °C.

B. Examine by infrared absorption spectrophotometry (*2.2.24*), comparing with the spectrum obtained with *betaxolol hydrochloride CRS*.

C. Examine by thin-layer chromatography (*2.2.27*), using as the coating substance *octadecylsilyl silica gel for chromatography R* with a fluorescent indicator having an optimal intensity at 254 nm.

Test solution. Dissolve 10 mg of the substance to be examined in 1 ml of *methanol R*.

Reference solution (a). Dissolve 20 mg of *betaxolol hydrochloride CRS* in 2 ml of *methanol R*.

Reference solution (b). Dissolve 10 mg of *oxprenolol hydrochloride CRS* in 1 ml of reference solution (a).

Apply separately to the plate 2 µl of each solution. Develop over a path of 10 cm using a mixture of 0.5 volumes of *perchloric acid R*, 50 volumes of *methanol R* and 50 volumes of *water R*. Allow the plate to dry in air and examine in ultraviolet light at 254 nm. The principal spot in the chromatogram obtained with the test solution is similar in position and size to the principal spot in the chromatogram obtained with reference solution (a). Spray the plate with a 50 g/l solution of *vanillin R* in a mixture of 5 volumes of *sulphuric acid R*, 10 volumes of *glacial acetic acid R* and 85 volumes of *methanol R*. Heat the plate at 100 °C to 105 °C until the colour of the spots reaches maximum intensity (10 min to 15 min). Examine in daylight. The principal spot in the chromatogram obtained with the test solution is similar in position, colour and size to the principal spot in the chromatogram obtained with reference solution (a). The test is not valid unless the chromatogram obtained with reference solution (b) shows two clearly separated spots.

D. It gives reaction (a) of chlorides (*2.3.1*).

TESTS

Appearance of solution. Dissolve 0.5 g in *water R* and dilute to 25 ml with the same solvent. The solution is clear (*2.2.1*) and colourless (*2.2.2, Method II*).

Acidity or alkalinity. Dissolve 0.20 g in *carbon dioxide-free water R* and dilute to 20 ml with the same solvent. Add 0.2 ml of *methyl red solution R* and 0.2 ml of *0.01 M hydrochloric acid*. The solution is red. Add 0.4 ml of *0.01 M sodium hydroxide*. The solution is yellow.

Related substances. Examine by liquid chromatography (*2.2.29*).

Test solution. Dissolve 10.0 mg of the substance to be examined in the mobile phase and dilute to 5.0 ml with the mobile phase.

Reference solution (a). Dissolve 8 mg of the substance to be examined and 4 mg of *betaxolol impurity A CRS* in 20.0 ml of the mobile phase.

Reference solution (b). Dilute 1.0 ml of the test solution to 100.0 ml with the mobile phase.

The chromatographic procedure may be carried out using:

- a stainless steel column 0.25 m long and 4 mm in internal diameter packed with *octylsilyl silica gel for chromatography R* (5 µm),
- as the mobile phase at a flow rate of 1.5 ml/min a mixture prepared as follows: mix 175 ml of *acetonitrile R* with 175 ml of *methanol R* and dilute the mixture to 1 litre with a 3.4 g/l solution of *potassium dihydrogen phosphate R*, previously adjusted to pH 3.0 with *phosphoric acid R*,
- as the detector a spectrophotometer set at 273 nm,
- a loop injector.

Inject 20 µl of each solution. Continue the chromatography for at least four times the retention time of the principal peak in the chromatogram obtained with the test solution. In the chromatogram obtained with the test solution: the area of any peak apart from the principal peak is not greater than 0.3 times the area of the peak in the chromatogram obtained with reference solution (b) (0.3 per cent) and the sum of the areas of such peaks is not greater than the area of the peak in the chromatogram obtained with reference solution (b) (1 per cent). The test is not valid unless the resolution between the peaks due to betaxolol impurity A and betaxolol in the chromatogram obtained with reference solution (a) is at least 2.0. Disregard any peak with an area less than 0.025 times that of the peak in the chromatogram obtained with reference solution (b).

Heavy metals (*2.4.8*). Dissolve 2.0 g in 20 ml of *water R*. 12 ml of the solution complies with limit test A for heavy metals (10 ppm). Prepare the standard using 10 ml of *lead standard solution (1 ppm Pb) R*.

Loss on drying (*2.2.32*). Not more than 0.5 per cent, determined on 1.000 g by drying in an oven at 100 °C to 105 °C.

Sulphated ash (*2.4.14*). Not more than 0.1 per cent, determined on 1.0 g.

ASSAY

Dissolve 0.300 g in a mixture of 10.0 ml of *0.01 M hydrochloric acid* and 50 ml of *alcohol R*. Carry out a potentiometric titration (*2.2.20*), using *0.1 M sodium hydroxide*. Read the volume added between the two points of inflexion.

1 ml of *0.1 M sodium hydroxide* is equivalent to 34.39 mg of $C_{18}H_{30}ClNO_3$.

STORAGE

Store protected from light.

IMPURITIES

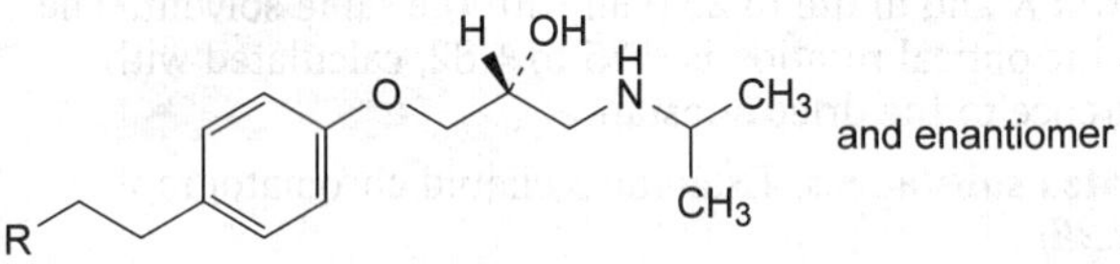

A. R = H: (2*RS*)-1-(4-ethylphenoxy)-3-[(1-methylethyl)amino]propan-2-ol,

B. R = OH: (2*RS*)-1-[4-(2-hydroxyethyl)phenoxy]-3-[(1-methylethyl)amino]propan-2-ol,

E. R = O-CH_2-CH_2-CH_2-CH_3: (2*RS*)-1-[4-(2-butoxyethyl)phenoxy]-3-[(1-methylethyl)amino]propan-2-ol,

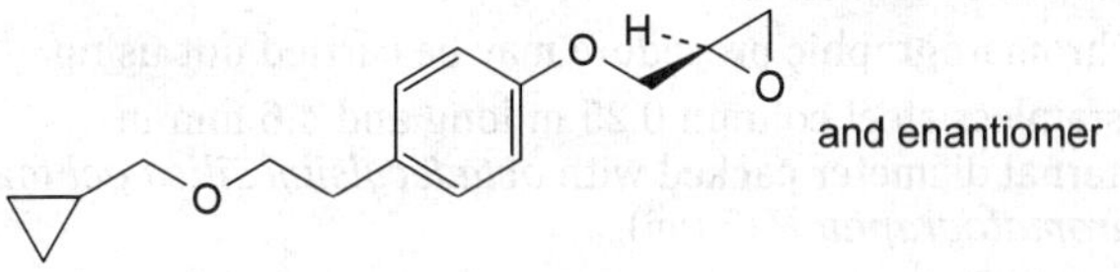

C. 2-[[4-[2-(cyclopropylmethoxy)ethyl]phenoxy]methyl]oxirane,

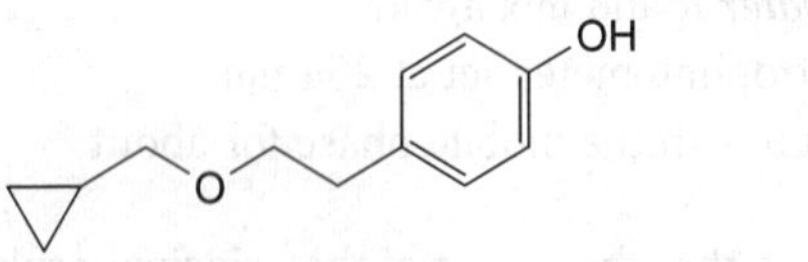

D. 4-[2-(cyclopropylmethoxy)ethyl]phenol.

01/2005:1394

BEZAFIBRATE

Bezafibratum

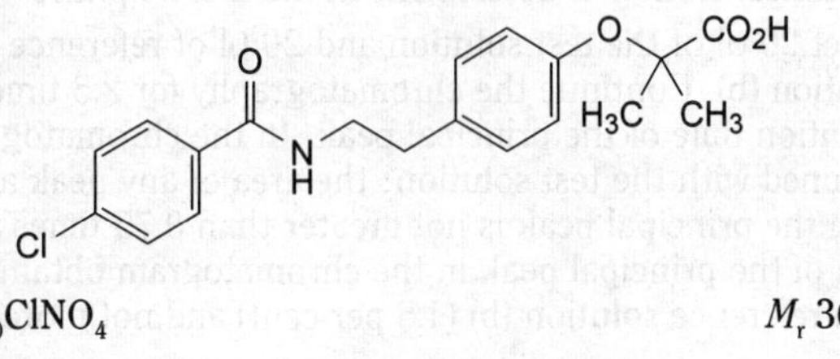

$C_{19}H_{20}ClNO_4$ M_r 361.8

DEFINITION

Bezafibrate contains not less than 98.0 per cent and not more than the equivalent of 102.0 per cent of 2-[4-[2-[(4-chlorobenzoyl)amino]ethyl]phenoxy]-2-methylpropanoic acid, calculated with reference to the dried substance.

CHARACTERS

A white or almost white crystalline powder, practically insoluble in water, freely soluble in dimethylformamide, sparingly soluble in acetone and in alcohol. It dissolves in dilute solutions of alkali hydroxides.

It shows polymorphism.

IDENTIFICATION

First identification: A, B.

Second identification: A, C.

A. Melting point (*2.2.14*): 181 °C to 185 °C.

B. Examine by infrared absorption spectrophotometry (*2.2.24*), comparing with the spectrum obtained with *bezafibrate CRS*. Examine the substances prepared as discs. If the spectra obtained show differences, dissolve the substance to be examined and the reference substance separately in *methanol R* and evaporate to dryness. Dry the residues *in vacuo* at 80 °C for 1 h and record new spectra using the residues.

C. Examine by thin-layer chromatography (*2.2.27*), using a *TLC silica gel* F_{254} *plate R*.

Test solution. Dissolve 10 mg of the substance to be examined in *methanol R* and dilute to 5 ml with the same solvent.

Reference solution. Dissolve 10 mg of *bezafibrate CRS* in *methanol R* and dilute to 5 ml with the same solvent.

Apply to the plate 5 µl of each solution. Develop over a path of 10 cm using a mixture of 2.7 volumes of *glacial acetic acid R*, 30 volumes of *methyl ethyl ketone R* and 60 volumes of *xylene R*. Dry the plate at 120 °C for at least 15 min and examine in ultraviolet light at 254 nm. The principal spot in the chromatogram obtained with the test solution is similar in position and size to the principal spot in the chromatogram obtained with the reference solution.

TESTS

Solution S. Dissolve 1.0 g in *dimethylformamide R* and dilute to 20 ml with the same solvent.

Appearance of solution. Solution S is clear (*2.2.1*) and not more intensely coloured than reference solution BY_5 (*2.2.2, Method II*).

Related substances. Examine by liquid chromatography (*2.2.29*).

Test solution. Dissolve 50.0 mg of the substance to be examined in the mobile phase and dilute to 100.0 ml with the mobile phase.

Reference solution (a). Dilute 10.0 ml of the test solution to 100.0 ml with the mobile phase. Dilute 5.0 ml of this solution to 100.0 ml with the mobile phase.

Reference solution (b). Dilute 5.0 ml of reference solution (a) to 50.0 ml with the mobile phase.

Reference solution (c). To 1 ml of the test solution, add 1 ml of *0.1 M hydrochloric acid* and evaporate to dryness on a hot plate. Dissolve the residue in 20 ml of the mobile phase.

The chromatographic procedure may be carried out using:

- a stainless steel column 0.125 m long and 4 mm in internal diameter packed with *octadecylsilyl silica gel for chromatography R* (5 µm),
- as mobile phase at a flow rate of 1 ml/min a mixture of 40 volumes of a 2.72 g/l solution of *potassium dihydrogen phosphate R* adjusted to pH 2.3 with *phosphoric acid R* and 60 volumes of *methanol R*,
- as detector a spectrophotometer set at 228 nm.

Inject separately 20 µl of the test solution and 20 µl of reference solutions (a), (b) and (c). When the chromatogram is recorded in the prescribed conditions, the retention times are: impurity A about 3 min, impurity B about 3.5 min, bezafibrate about 6.0 min, impurity C about 9 min, impurity D about 14 min and impurity E about 37 min. Continue the chromatography for the time necessary to detect the ester, which, depending on the route of synthesis, may be impurity C, D or E. The test is not valid unless: in the chromatogram obtained with reference solution (c) the resolution between the two principal peaks is at least 5.0 and the principal peak in the chromatogram obtained with reference solution (b) has a signal-to-noise ratio of at least 5. In the chromatogram obtained with the test solution: the area of any peak, apart from the principal peak, is not greater than the area of the principal peak in the chromatogram obtained with reference solution (a) (0.5 per cent); the sum of the areas of all the peaks, apart from the principal peak, is not greater than 1.5 times the area of the principal peak in the chromatogram obtained with reference solution (a) (0.75 per cent). Disregard any peak with an area less than 0.1 times the area of the principal peak in the chromatogram obtained with reference solution (a).

Chlorides (*2.4.4*). Dilute 10 ml of solution S to 50 ml with *water R*. Filter the resultant suspension through a wet filter previously washed with *water R* until free from chlorides. 15 ml of the filtrate complies with the limit test for chlorides (300 ppm). Prepare the standard using 9 ml of *chloride standard solution (5 ppm Cl) R* and 6 ml of *water R*.

Heavy metals (*2.4.8*). 2.0 g complies with limit test C for heavy metals (10 ppm). Prepare the standard using 2 ml of *lead standard solution (10 ppm Pb) R*.

Loss on drying (*2.2.32*). Not more than 0.5 per cent, determined on 1.000 g by drying in an oven at 100-105 °C.

Sulphated ash (*2.4.14*). Not more than 0.1 per cent, determined on 1.0 g.

ASSAY

Dissolve 0.300 g in 50 ml of a mixture of 25 volumes of *water R* and 75 volumes of *alcohol R*. Using 0.1 ml of *phenolphthalein solution R* as indicator, titrate with *0.1 M sodium hydroxide* until a pink colour is obtained. Carry out a blank titration.

1 ml of *0.1 M sodium hydroxide* is equivalent to 36.18 mg of $C_{19}H_{20}ClNO_4$.

IMPURITIES

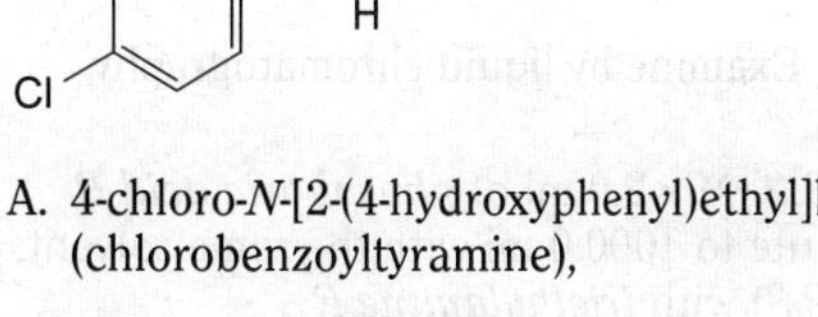

A. 4-chloro-*N*-[2-(4-hydroxyphenyl)ethyl]benzamide (chlorobenzoyltyramine),

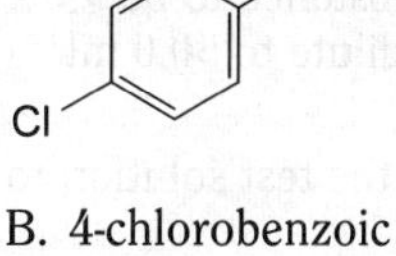

B. 4-chlorobenzoic acid,

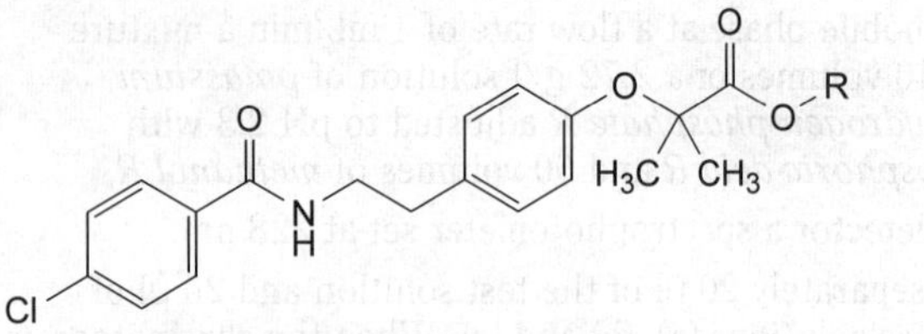

C. R = CH_3: methyl 2-[4-[2-[(4-chlorobenzoyl)amino]ethyl]phenoxy]-2 methylpropanoate,

D. R = CH_2-CH_3: ethyl 2-[4-[2-[(4-chlorobenzoyl)amino]ethyl]phenoxy]-2-methylpropanoate,

E. R = CH_2-CH_2-CH_2-CH_3: butyl 2-[4-[2-[(4-chlorobenzoyl)amino]ethyl]phenoxy]-2-methylpropanoate.

01/2005:1395

BIFONAZOLE

Bifonazolum

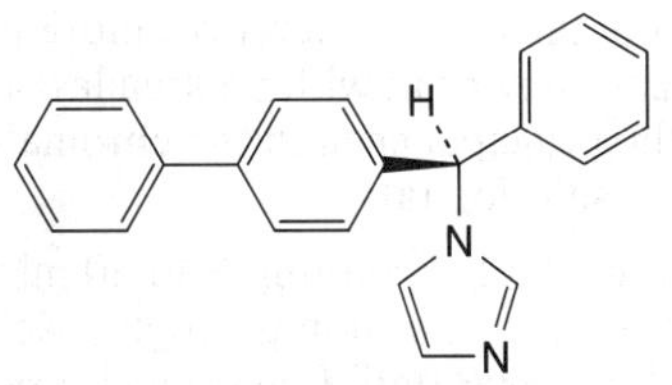

and enantiomer

$C_{22}H_{18}N_2$ M_r 310.4

DEFINITION

Bifonazole contains not less than 98.0 per cent and not more than the equivalent of 100.5 per cent of 1-[(*RS*)-(biphenyl-4-yl)phenylmethyl]-1*H*-imidazole, calculated with reference to the dried substance.

CHARACTERS

A white or almost white, crystalline powder, practically insoluble in water, sparingly soluble in ethanol.

It shows polymorphism.

IDENTIFICATION

Examine by infrared absorption spectrophotometry (*2.2.24*), comparing with the spectrum obtained with *bifonazole CRS*. If the spectra obtained in the solid state show differences, dissolve the substance to be examined and the reference substance separately in the minimum volume of *2-propanol R*, evaporate to dryness and record new spectra using the residues.

TESTS

Optical rotation (*2.2.7*). Dissolve 0.20 g in 20.0 ml of *methanol R*. The angle of optical rotation is − 0.10° to + 0.10°.

Related substances. Examine by liquid chromatography (*2.2.29*).

Buffer solution pH 3.2. Mix 2.0 ml of *phosphoric acid R* with *water R* and dilute to 1000.0 ml with the same solvent. Adjust to pH 3.2 (*2.2.3*) with *triethylamine R*.

Test solution. Dissolve 50.0 mg of the substance to be examined in 25 ml of *acetonitrile R* and dilute to 50.0 ml with buffer solution pH 3.2.

Reference solution (a). Dilute 0.25 ml of the test solution to 50.0 ml with buffer solution pH 3.2.

Reference solution (b). Dissolve 25.0 mg of *imidazole R* (impurity C) in *acetonitrile R* and dilute to 25.0 ml with the same solvent. Dilute 0.25 ml of the solution to 100.0 ml with buffer solution pH 3.2.

Reference solution (c). Dissolve 34.2 mg of *4-[(RS)-(biphenyl-4-yl)phenylmethyl]-1H-imidazole trifluoroacetate CRS* (corresponding to 25.0 mg of impurity B base) in *acetonitrile R* and dilute to 25.0 ml with the same solvent.

Reference solution (d). Dilute 0.25 ml of reference solution (c) to 50.0 ml with buffer solution pH 3.2.

Reference solution (e). Mix 0.25 ml of the test solution and 0.25 ml of reference solution (c) and dilute to 50.0 ml with buffer solution pH 3.2.

The chromatographic procedure may be carried out using:

– a stainless steel column 0.125 m long and 4.6 mm in internal diameter packed with *octadecylsilyl silica gel for chromatography R* (5 µm),

– as mobile phase at a flow rate of 1 ml/min a gradient programme using the following conditions:

Mobile phase A. A mixture of 20 volumes of *acetonitrile R* and 80 volumes of buffer solution pH 3.2,

Mobile phase B. A mixture of 20 volumes of buffer solution pH 3.2 and 80 volumes of *acetonitrile R*,

Time (min)	Mobile phase A (per cent *V/V*)	Mobile phase B (per cent *V/V*)	Comment
0 - 8	60	40	isocratic elution
8 - 12	60 → 10	40 → 90	linear gradient
12 - 30	10	90	isocratic elution
30 - 32	10 → 60	90 → 40	switch to initial eluent composition
32 - 40	60	40	equilibration
40 = 0	60	40	restart isocratic elution

– as detector a spectrophotometer set at 210 nm,

maintaining the column temperature at 40 °C.

Adjust the sensitivity of the system so that the height of the bifonazole peak in the chromatogram obtained with 50 µl of reference solution (e) is at least 50 per cent of the full scale of the recorder.

Inject 50 µl of reference solution (e). When the chromatogram is recorded in the prescribed conditions the retention times are: impurity B about 4 min and bifonazole about 4.5 min. The test is not valid unless the resolution between the peaks corresponding to impurity B and bifonazole is at least 2.5.

Inject 50 µl of the test solution and 50 µl each of reference solutions (a), (b) and (d). In the chromatogram obtained with the test solution: the area of any peak corresponding to impurity C is not greater than the corresponding peak in the chromatogram obtained with reference solution (b) (0.25 per cent); the area of any peak corresponding to impurity B is not greater than 3 times the area of the corresponding peak in the chromatogram obtained with reference solution (d) (1.5 per cent); none of the peaks, apart from the principal peak and the peaks corresponding to impurities B and C, has an area greater than the area of the peak in the chromatogram obtained with reference solution (a) (0.5 per cent); the sum of the areas of all the peaks, apart from the principal peak, is not greater than 4 times the area of the principal peak in the chromatogram obtained with reference solution (a) (2 per cent). Disregard any peak whose area is less than 0.1 times the area of the principal peak in the chromatogram obtained with reference solution (a).

Loss on drying (*2.2.32*). Not more than 0.5 per cent, determined on 1.000 g by drying in an oven at 100-105 °C.

Sulphated ash (*2.4.14*). Not more than 0.1 per cent, determined on 1.0 g.

ASSAY

Dissolve 0.250 g in 80 ml of *anhydrous acetic acid R*. Titrate with *0.1 M perchloric acid,* determining the end-point potentiometrically (*2.2.20*).

1 ml of *0.1 M perchloric acid* is equivalent to 31.04 mg of $C_{22}H_{18}N_2$.

IMPURITIES

R- = 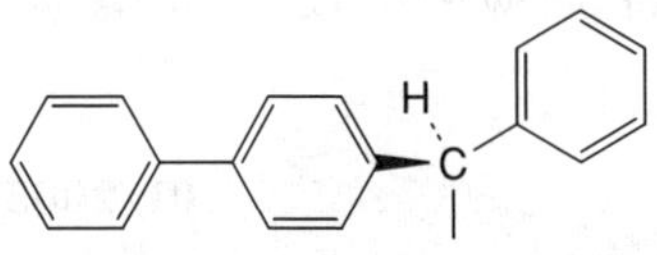 and enantiomer

A. R-OH: (*RS*)-(biphenyl-4-yl)phenylmethanol,

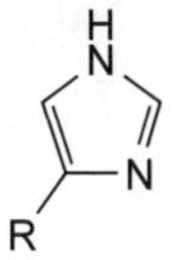

B. 4-[(*RS*)-(biphenyl-4-yl)phenylmethyl]-1*H*-imidazole,

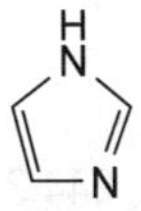

C. 1*H*-imidazole,

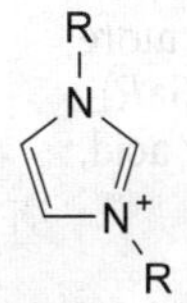

D. 1,3-bis[(biphenyl-4-yl)phenylmethyl]-1*H*-imidazolium ion.

01/2005:1588

BILBERRY FRUIT, DRIED

Myrtilli fructus siccus

DEFINITION

Dried ripe fruit of *Vaccinium myrtillus* L.

Content: minimum 1.0 per cent of tannins, expressed as pyrogallol ($C_6H_6O_3$; M_r 126.1) (dried drug).

CHARACTERS

Dried bilberry has a sweet and slightly astringent taste.

Macroscopic and microscopic characters described under identification tests A and B.

IDENTIFICATION

A. Dried bilberry is a dark blue, subglobular, shrunken berry about 5 mm in diameter, with a scar at the lower end and surmounted by the persistent calyx, which appears as a circular fold and the remains of the style. The deep violet, fleshy mesocarp contains numerous small, brown, ovoid seeds.

B. Reduce to a powder (355). The powder is violet-brown. Examine under a microscope using *chloral hydrate solution R.* The powder shows: violet-pink sclereids from the endocarp and the mesocarp, usually aggregated, with thick, channelled walls; reddish-brown fragments of the epicarp consisting of polygonal cells with moderately thickened walls; brownish-yellow fragments of the outer seed testa made up of elongated cells with U-shaped thickened walls; clusters and prisms crystals of various size of calcium oxalate.

C. Thin-layer chromatography (*2.2.27*)

Test solution. To 2 g of the powdered drug (355) add 20 ml of *methanol R*. Shake for 15 min and filter.

Reference solution. Dissolve 5 mg of *chrysanthemin R* in 10 ml of *methanol R*.

Plate: *TLC silica gel plate R.*

Mobile phase: *anhydrous formic acid R, water R, butanol R* (16:19:65 *V/V/V*).

Application: 10 µl, as bands.

Development: over a path of 10 cm.

Drying: in air.

Detection: examine in daylight.

Results: see below the sequence of the zones present in the chromatograms obtained with the reference and test solutions.

Top of the plate	
	A violet-red zone of low intensity
Chrysanthemin: a violet-red zone	A principal violet-red zone
	A compact set of other principal zones:
	– a violet-red zone
	– several violet-blue zones
Reference solution	**Test solution**

TESTS

Foreign matter (*2.8.2*): it complies with the test for foreign matter.

Loss on drying (*2.2.32*): maximum 12.0 per cent, determined on 1.000 g of the powdered drug by drying in an oven at 100-105 °C for 2 h.

Total ash (*2.4.16*): maximum 5.0 per cent.

ASSAY

Carry out the determination of tannins in herbal drugs (*2.8.14*). Use 1.500 g of the powdered drug (355).

01/2005:1602

BILBERRY FRUIT, FRESH

Myrtilli fructus recens

DEFINITION

Fresh or frozen ripe fruit of *Vaccinium myrtillus* L.

Content: minimum 0.30 per cent of anthocyanins, expressed as cyanidin-3-glucoside chloride (chrysanthemin, $C_{21}H_{21}ClO_{11}$; M_r 485.5) (dried drug).

CHARACTERS

Sweet and slightly astringent taste.

Macroscopic and microscopic characters described under identification tests A and B.

IDENTIFICATION

A. The fresh fruit is a blackish-blue globular berry about 5 mm in diameter. Its lower end shows a scar or, rarely, a fragment of the pedicel. The upper end is flattened and surmounted by the remains of the persistent style and of the calyx, which appears as a circular fold. The violet, fleshy mesocarp includes 4 to 5 locules containing numerous small, brown, ovoid seeds.

B. The crushed fresh fruit is violet-red. Examine under a microscope using *chloral hydrate solution R*. It shows violet-pink sclereids from the endocarp and the mesocarp, usually aggregated, with thick, channelled walls; reddish-brown fragments of the epicarp consisting of polygonal cells with moderately thickened walls; brownish-yellow fragments of the outer layer of the testa composed of elongated cells with U-shaped thickened walls; cluster crystals of calcium oxalate.

C. Thin-layer chromatography (*2.2.27*).

Test solution. To 5 g of the freshly crushed drug, add 20 ml of *methanol R*. Stir for 15 min and filter.

Reference solution. Dissolve 5 mg of *chrysanthemin R* in 10 ml of *methanol R*.

Plate: *TLC silica gel plate R*.

Mobile phase: *anhydrous formic acid R, water R, butanol R* (16:19:65 *V/V/V*).

Application: 10 µl, as bands.

Development: over a path of 10 cm.

Drying: in air.

Detection: examine in daylight.

Results: see below the sequence of the zones present in the chromatograms obtained with the reference solution and the test solution.

Top of the plate	
	A violet-red zone
Chrysanthemin: a violet-red zone	A principal violet-red zone
	A compact set of other principal zones:
	– a violet-red zone
	– several violet-blue zones
Reference solution	**Test solution**

TESTS

Total ash (*2.4.16*): maximum 0.6 per cent.

Foreign matter (*2.8.2*): it complies with the test for foreign matter.

Loss on drying (*2.2.32*): 80.0 per cent to 90.0 per cent, determined on 5.000 g of the freshly crushed drug by drying in an oven at 100-105 °C.

ASSAY

Crush 50 g extemporaneously. To about 5.00 g of the crushed, accurately weighed drug, add 95 ml of *methanol R*. Stir mechanically for 30 min. Filter into a 100.0 ml volumetric flask. Rinse the filter and dilute to 100.0 ml with *methanol R*. Prepare a 50-fold dilution of this solution in a 0.1 per cent *V/V* solution of *hydrochloric acid R* in *methanol R*.

Measure the absorbance (*2.2.25*) of the solution at 528 nm, using a 0.1 per cent *V/V* solution of *hydrochloric acid R* in *methanol R* as the compensation liquid.

Calculate the percentage content of anthocyanins, expressed as cyanidin-3-glucoside chloride, from the expression:

$$\frac{A \times 5000}{718 \times m}$$

718 = specific absorbance of cyanidin-3-glucoside chloride at 528 nm,

A = absorbance at 528 nm,

m = mass of the substance to be examined in grams.

STORAGE

When frozen, store at or below − 18 °C.

01/2005:1073

BIOTIN

Biotinum

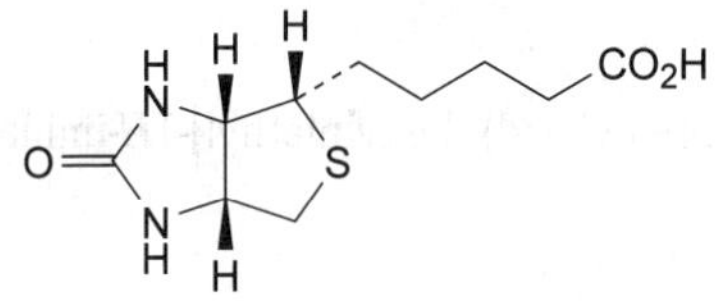

$C_{10}H_{16}N_2O_3S$ M_r 244.3

DEFINITION

Biotin contains not less than 98.5 per cent and not more than the equivalent of 101.0 per cent of 5-[(3a*S*,4*S*,6a*R*)-2-oxohexahydrothieno[3,4-*d*]imidazol-4-yl]pentanoic acid, calculated with reference to the dried substance.

CHARACTERS

A white, crystalline powder or colourless crystals, very slightly soluble in water and in alcohol, practically insoluble in acetone. It dissolves in dilute solutions of alkali hydroxides.

IDENTIFICATION

First identification: A.

Second identification: B, C.

A. Examine by infrared absorption spectrophotometry (*2.2.24*), comparing with the spectrum obtained with *biotin CRS*.

B. Examine the chromatograms obtained in the test for related substances (see Tests). The principal spot in the chromatogram obtained with test solution (b) is similar in position and size to the principal spot in the chromatogram obtained with reference solution (a).

C. Dissolve about 10 mg in 20 ml of *water R* with heating. Allow to cool. Add 0.1 ml of *bromine water R*. The bromine water is decolourised.

TESTS

Solution S. Dissolve 0.250 g in a 4 g/l solution of *sodium hydroxide R* and dilute to 25.0 ml with the same alkaline solution.

Appearance of solution. Solution S is clear (*2.2.1*) and colourless (*2.2.2, Method II*).

Specific optical rotation (*2.2.7*). The specific optical rotation is + 89 to + 93, determined on solution S and calculated with reference to the dried substance.

Related substances. Examine by thin-layer chromatography (*2.2.27*), using as the coating substance a suitable silica gel (5 µm). *Prepare the solutions immediately before use and keep protected from bright light.*

Test solution (a). Dissolve 50 mg of the substance to be examined in *glacial acetic acid R* and dilute to 10 ml with the same solvent.

Test solution (b). Dilute 1 ml of test solution (a) to 10 ml with *glacial acetic acid R*.

Reference solution (a). Dissolve 5 mg of *biotin CRS* in *glacial acetic acid R* and dilute to 10 ml with the same solvent.

Reference solution (b). Dilute 1 ml of test solution (b) to 20 ml with *glacial acetic acid R*.

Reference solution (c). Dilute 1 ml of test solution (b) to 40 ml with *glacial acetic acid R*.

Apply to the plate 10 µl of each solution. Develop over a path of 15 cm using a mixture of 5 volumes of *methanol R*, 25 volumes of *glacial acetic acid R* and 75 volumes of *toluene R*. Dry the plate in a current of warm air. Allow to cool and spray with *4-dimethylaminocinnamaldehyde solution R*. Examine immediately in daylight. Any spot in the chromatogram obtained with test solution (a), apart from the principal spot, is not more intense than the spot in the chromatogram obtained with reference solution (b) (0.5 per cent) and at most one such spot is more intense than the spot in the chromatogram obtained with reference solution (c) (0.25 per cent).

Heavy metals (*2.4.8*). 1.0 g complies with limit test C for heavy metals (10 ppm). Prepare the standard using 10 ml of *lead standard solution (1 ppm Pb) R*.

Loss on drying (*2.2.32*). Not more than 1.0 per cent, determined on 1.000 g by drying in an oven at 100 °C to 105 °C.

Sulphated ash (*2.4.14*). Not more than 0.1 per cent, determined on 1.0 g.

ASSAY

Suspend 0.200 g in 5 ml of *dimethylformamide R*. Heat until the substance has dissolved completely. Add 50 ml of *ethanol R* and titrate with *0.1 M tetrabutylammonium hydroxide*, determining the end-point potentiometrically (*2.2.20*).

1 ml of *0.1 M tetrabutylammonium hydroxide* is equivalent to 24.43 mg of $C_{10}H_{16}N_2O_3S$.

STORAGE

Store protected from light.

IMPURITIES

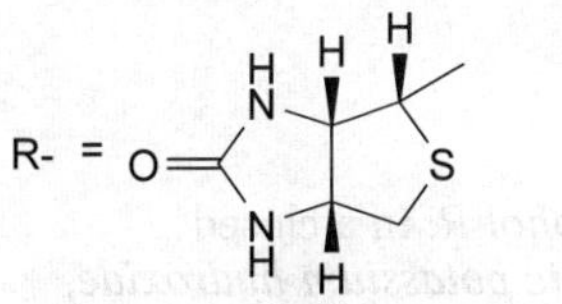

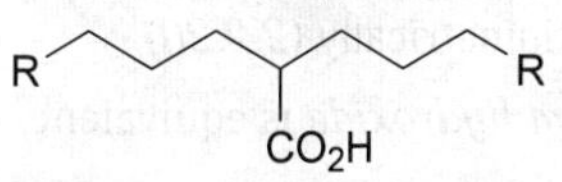

A. di[3-[(3a*S*,4*S*,6a*R*)-2-oxohexahydrothieno[3,4-*d*]imidazol-4-yl]propyl]acetic acid,

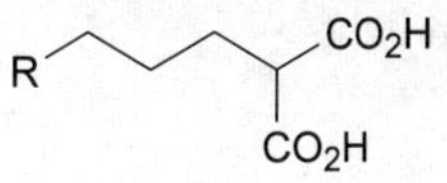

B. 4-[(3a*S*,4*S*,6a*R*)-2-oxohexahydrothieno[3,4-*d*]imidazol-4-yl]butane-1,1-dicarboxylic acid,

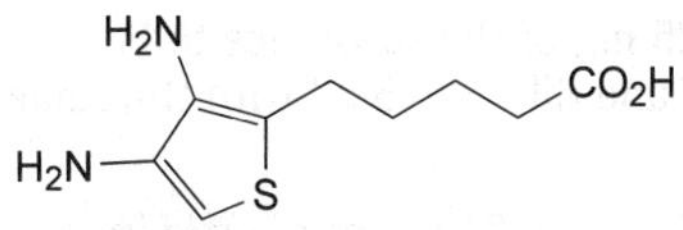

C. 5-(3,4-diamino-2-thienyl)pentanoic acid,

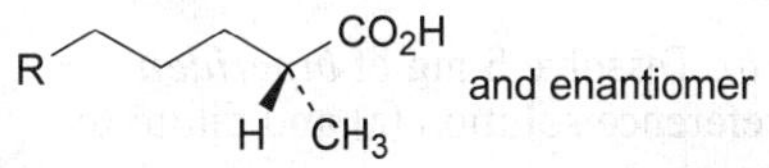

D. 2-methyl-5-[(3a*S*,4*S*,6a*R*)-2-oxohexahydrothieno[3,4-*d*]imidazol-4-yl]pentanoic acid,

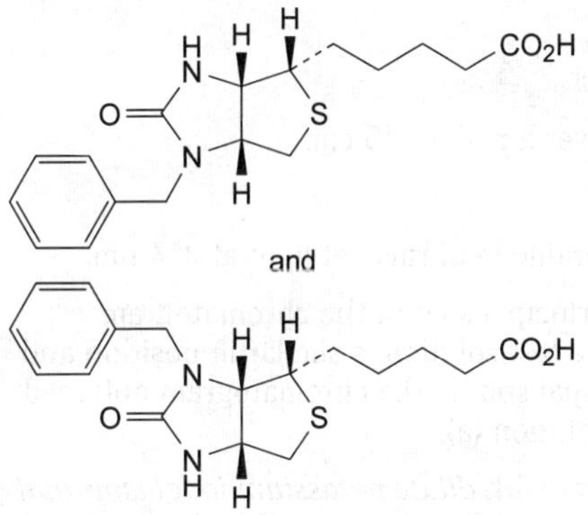

E. 5-[(3a*S*,4*S*,6a*R*)-3-benzyl-2-oxohexahydrothieno[3,4-*d*]imidazol-4-yl]pentanoic acid and 5-[(3a*S*,4*S*,6a*R*)-1-benzyl-2-oxohexahydrothieno[3,4-*d*]imidazol-4-yl]pentanoic acid.

01/2005:1074

BIPERIDEN HYDROCHLORIDE

Biperideni hydrochloridum

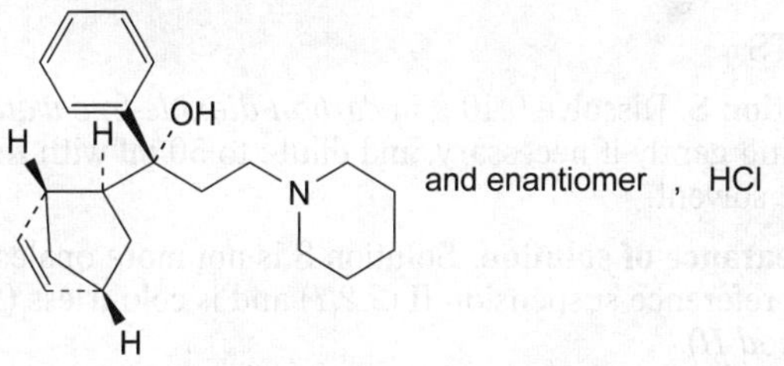

$C_{21}H_{30}ClNO$ M_r 347.9

DEFINITION

(1*RS*)-1-[(1*RS*,2*SR*,4*RS*)-Bicyclo[2.2.1]hept-5-en-2-yl]-1-phenyl-3-(piperidin-1-yl)propan-1-ol hydrochloride.

Content: 99.0 per cent to 101.0 per cent (dried substance).

CHARACTERS

Appearance: white, crystalline powder.

Solubility: slightly soluble in water and in alcohol, very slightly soluble in methylene chloride.

mp: about 280 °C, with decomposition.

IDENTIFICATION

First identification: A, D.

Second identification: B, C, D.

A. Infrared absorption spectrophotometry (*2.2.24*).

Comparison: *biperiden hydrochloride CRS.*

B. Thin-layer chromatography (*2.2.27*).

Test solution. Dissolve 25 mg of the substance to be examined in *methanol R* and dilute to 5 ml with the same solvent.

Reference solution (a). Dissolve 25 mg of *biperiden hydrochloride CRS* in *methanol R* and dilute to 5 ml with the same solvent.

Reference solution (b). Dissolve 5 mg of *biperiden impurity A CRS* in reference solution (a) and dilute to 2 ml with the same solution.

Plate: *TLC silica gel F_{254} plate R.*

Mobile phase: *diethylamine R, methanol R, toluene R* (1:1:20 *V/V/V*).

Application: 5 µl.

Development: over a path of 15 cm.

Drying: in air.

Detection A: examine in ultraviolet light at 254 nm.

Results A: the principal spot in the chromatogram obtained with the test solution is similar in position and size to the principal spot in the chromatogram obtained with reference solution (a).

Detection B: spray with *dilute potassium iodobismuthate solution R* and then with *sodium nitrite solution R* and examine in daylight.

Results B: the principal spot in the chromatogram obtained with the test solution is similar in position, colour and size to the principal spot in the chromatogram obtained with reference solution (a).

System suitability: reference solution (b):

– the chromatogram shows 2 clearly separated spots.

C. To about 20 mg add 5 ml of *phosphoric acid R*. A green colour develops.

D. It gives reaction (a) of chlorides (*2.3.1*).

TESTS

Solution S. Dissolve 0.10 g in *carbon dioxide-free water R*, heating gently if necessary, and dilute to 50 ml with the same solvent.

Appearance of solution. Solution S is not more opalescent than reference suspension II (*2.2.1*) and is colourless (*2.2.2, Method II*).

pH (*2.2.3*): 5.0 to 6.5 for solution S.

Related substances. Gas chromatography (*2.2.28*).

Test solution. Dissolve 0.10 g of the substance to be examined in *methanol R* and dilute to 10 ml with the same solvent.

Reference solution (a). Dilute 0.5 ml of the test solution to 100 ml with *methanol R*. Dilute 10 ml of this solution to 50 ml with *methanol R*.

Reference solution (b). Dissolve 5 mg of the substance to be examined and 5 mg of *biperiden impurity A CRS* in *methanol R* and dilute to 5 ml with the same solvent. Dilute 1 ml of the solution to 10 ml with *methanol R*.

Column:

– *material*: fused silica,
– *size*: l = 50 m, Ø = 0.25 mm,
– *stationary phase*: *poly(dimethyl)(diphenyl)(divinyl)siloxane R* (film thickness 0.25 µm).

Carrier gas: *nitrogen for chromatography R.*

Flow rate: 0.4 ml/min.

Split ratio: 1:250.

Temperature:

	Time (min)	Temperature (°C)
Column	0 - 5	200
	5 - 40	200 → 270
Injection port		250
Detector		300

Detection: flame ionisation.

Injection: 2 µl.

Run time: twice the retention time of biperiden.

Relative retention with reference to biperiden: impurities A, B and C = between 0.95 and 1.05.

System suitability:

– *resolution*: minimum 2.5 between the peak due to biperiden (1st peak) and the peak due to impurity A (2nd peak) in the chromatogram obtained with reference solution (b),
– *signal-to-noise ratio*: minimum 6 for the principal peak in the chromatogram obtained with reference solution (a).

Limits:

– *impurities A, B, C*: for each impurity, maximum 0.50 per cent of the area of the principal peak,
– *any other impurity*: for each impurity, maximum 0.10 per cent of the area of the principal peak,
– *total of impurities A, B and C*: maximum 1.0 per cent of the area of the principal peak,
– *total of impurities other than A, B and C*: maximum 0.50 per cent of the area of the principal peak,
– *disregard limit*: 0.05 per cent of the area of the principal peak.

Impurity F (*2.4.24*): maximum 2 ppm.

Heavy metals (*2.4.8*): maximum 20 ppm.

1.0 g complies with limit test D. Prepare the standard using 2 ml of *lead standard solution (10 ppm Pb) R*.

Loss on drying (*2.2.32*): maximum 0.5 per cent, determined on 1.000 g by drying in an oven at 100-105 °C for 2 h.

Sulphated ash (*2.4.14*): maximum 0.1 per cent, determined on 1.0 g.

ASSAY

Dissolve 0.200 g in 60 ml of *alcohol R*. In a closed vessel, titrate with *0.1 M alcoholic potassium hydroxide*, determining the end-point potentiometrically (*2.2.20*).

1 ml of *0.1 M alcoholic potassium hydroxide* is equivalent to 34.79 mg of $C_{21}H_{30}ClNO$.

STORAGE

In an airtight container, protected from light.

IMPURITIES

Specified impurities: A, B, C, F.

Other detectable impurities: D, E.

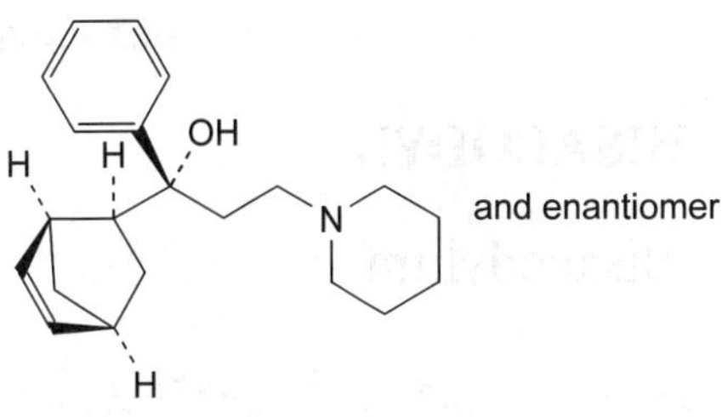

A. (1*RS*)-1-[(1*SR*,2*SR*,4*SR*)-bicyclo[2.2.1]hept-5-en-2-yl]-1-phenyl-3-(piperidin-1-yl)propan-1-ol (*endo* form),

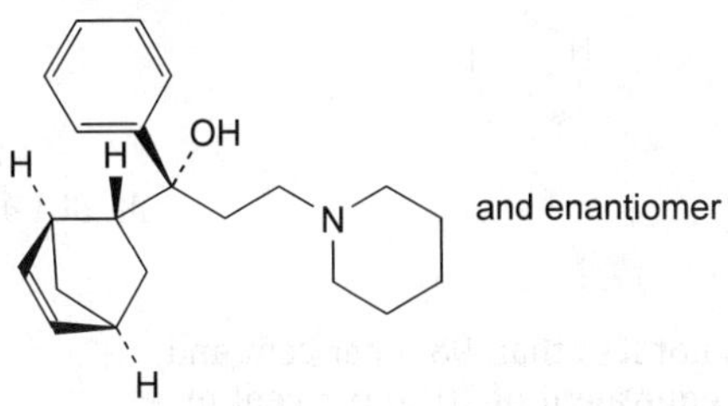

B. (1*RS*)-1-[(1*SR*,2*RS*,4*SR*)-bicyclo[2.2.1]hept-5-en-2-yl]-1-phenyl-3-(piperidin-1-yl)propan-1-ol,

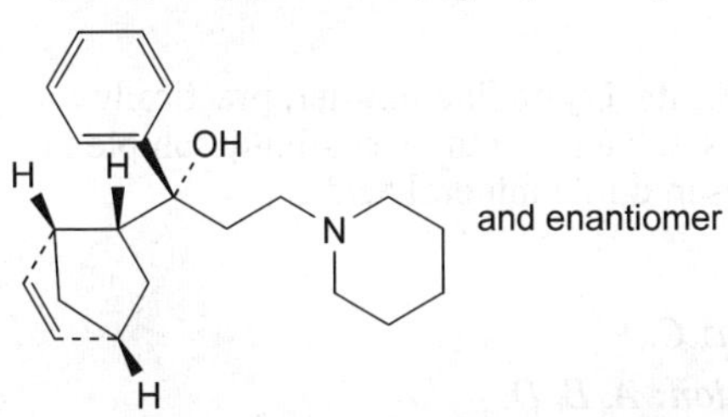

C. (1*RS*)-1-[(1*RS*,2*RS*,4*RS*)-bicyclo[2.2.1]hept-5-en-2-yl]-1-phenyl-3-(piperidin-1-yl)propan-1-ol,

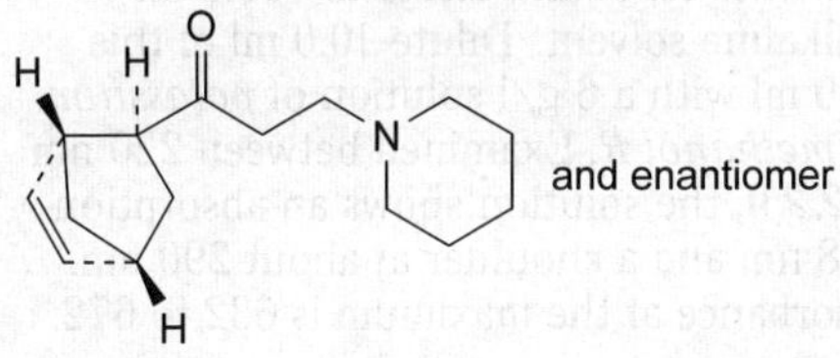

D. 1-[(1*RS*,2*SR*,4*RS*)-bicyclo[2.2.1]hept-5-en-2-yl]-3-(piperidin-1-yl)propan-1-one,

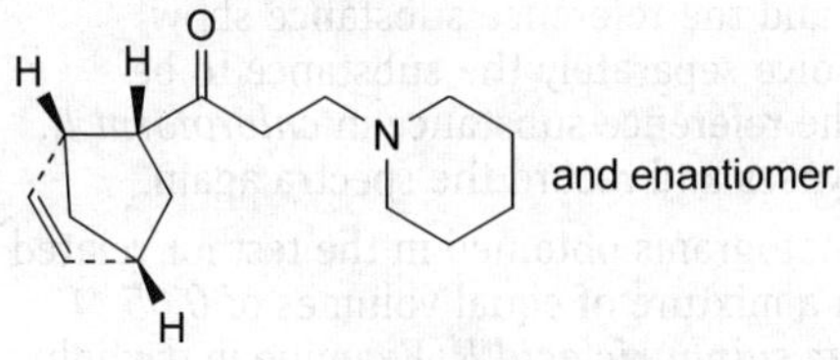

E. 1-[(1*RS*,2*RS*,4*RS*)-bicyclo[2.2.1]hept-5-en-2-yl]-3-(piperidin-1-yl)propan-1-one,

F. benzene.

01/2005:1174

BIRCH LEAF

Betulae folium

DEFINITION

Birch leaf consists of the whole or fragmented dried leaves of *Betula pendula* Roth and/or *Betula pubescens* Ehrh. as well as hybrids of both species. It contains not less than 1.5 per cent of flavonoids, calculated as hyperoside ($C_{21}H_{20}O_{12}$; M_r 464.4) with reference to the dried drug.

CHARACTERS

It has the macroscopic and microscopic characters described under identification tests A and B.

IDENTIFICATION

A. The leaves of both species are dark green on the adaxial surface and a lighter greenish-grey colour on the abaxial surface; they show a characteristic dense reticulate venation. The veins are light brown to almost white.

The leaves of *Betula pendula* are glabrous and show closely spaced glandular pits on both surfaces. The leaves of *Betula pendula* are 3 cm to 7 cm long and 2 cm to 5 cm wide; the petiole is long and the doubly dentate lamina is triangular to rhomboid and broadly cuneate or truncate at the base. The angle on each side is unrounded or slightly rounded, and the apex is long and acuminate.

The leaves of *Betula pubescens* show few glandular trichomes and are slightly pubescent on both surfaces. The abaxial surface shows small bundles of yellowish-grey trichomes at the branch points of the veins. The leaves of *Betula pubescens* are slightly smaller, oval to rhomboid and more rounded. They are more roughly and more regularly dentate. The apex is neither long nor acuminate.

B. Reduce to a powder (355). The powder is greenish-grey. Examine under a microscope using *chloral hydrate solution R*. The powder shows numerous fragments of lamina with straight-walled epidermal cells and cells of the lower epidermis surrounding anomocytic stomata (*2.8.3*). Peltate large glands usually measuring 100 µm to 120 µm are found on the upper and lower epidermises. The mesophyll fragments contain calcium oxalate crystals. Fragments of radial vascular bundles and sclerenchyma fibres are accompanied by crystal sheaths. If *Betula pubescens* is present, the powder also contains unicellular covering trichomes with very thick walls, about 80 µm to 600 µm long, usually between 100 µm and 200 µm.

C. Examine by thin-layer chromatography (*2.2.27*), using as the coating substance a suitable silica gel.

Test solution. To 1 g of the powdered drug (355) add 10 ml of *methanol R*. Heat in a water-bath at 60 °C for 5 min. Cool and filter the solution.

Reference solution. Dissolve 1 mg of *caffeic acid R* and 1 mg of *chlorogenic acid R*, 2.5 mg of *hyperoside R* and 2.5 mg of *rutin R* in 10 ml of *methanol R*.

Apply separately to the plates as bands, 10 µl of each solution. Develop over a path of 10 cm using a mixture of 10 volumes of *anhydrous formic acid R*, 10 volumes of *water R*, 30 volumes of *methyl ethyl ketone R* and 50 volumes of *ethyl acetate R*. Dry the plate in a current of warm air. Spray with a 10 g/l solution of *diphenylboric acid aminoethyl ester R* in *methanol R*. Subsequently spray the plate with a 50 g/l solution of *macrogol 400 R* in *methanol R*. Allow the plate to dry in air for 30 min and examine in ultraviolet light at 365 nm. The chromatogram obtained with the reference solution shows three zones in its lower half: in increasing order of R_f a yellowish-brown fluorescent zone (rutin), a light blue fluorescent zone (chlorogenic acid) and a yellowish-brown fluorescent zone (hyperoside), and in its upper third, a light blue fluorescent zone (caffeic acid).

The chromatogram obtained with the test solution shows three zones similar in position and fluorescence to the zones due to rutin, chlorogenic acid and hyperoside in the chromatogram obtained with the reference solution. The zone corresponding to rutin is very faint and the zone corresponding to hyperoside is intense. It also shows other yellowish-brown faint fluorescence zones between the zones corresponding to caffeic acid and chlorogenic acid in the chromatogram obtained with the reference solution. Near the solvent front, the red fluorescent zone due to chlorophylls is visible. In the chromatogram obtained with the test solution, between this zone and the zone corresponding to caffeic acid in the chromatogram obtained with the reference solution, there is a brownish-yellow zone corresponding to quercetin.

TESTS

Foreign matter (*2.8.2*). Not more than 3 per cent of fragments of female catkins and not more than 3 per cent of other foreign matter.

Loss on drying (*2.2.32*). Not more than 10.0 per cent, determined on 1.000 g of powered drug (355) by drying in an oven at 100 °C to 105 °C for 2 h.

Total ash (*2.4.16*). Not more than 5.0 per cent.

ASSAY

Stock solution. In a 100 ml round-bottomed flask introduce 0.200 g of the powdered drug (355), 1 ml of a 5 g/l solution of *hexamethylenetetramine R*, 20 ml of *acetone R* and 2 ml of *hydrochloric acid R1*. Boil the mixture under a reflux condenser for 30 min. Filter the liquid through a plug of absorbent cotton in a 100 ml flask. Add the absorbent cotton to the residue in the round-bottomed flask and extract with two quantities, each of 20 ml, of *acetone R*, each time boiling under a reflux condenser for 10 min. Allow to cool to room temperature, filter the liquid through a plug of absorbent cotton then filter the solution through a filter-paper in the volumetric flask, and dilute to 100.0 ml with *acetone R* by rinsing of the flask and filter. Introduce 20.0 ml of the solution into a separating funnel, add 20 ml of *water R* and extract the mixture with one quantity of 15 ml and then three quantities, each of 10 ml, of *ethyl acetate R*. Combine the ethyl acetate extracts in a separating funnel, rinse with two quantities, each of 50 ml, of *water R*, and filter the extract over 10 g of *anhydrous sodium sulphate R* into a 50 ml volumetric flask and dilute to 50.0 ml with *ethyl acetate R*.

Test solution. To 10.0 ml of the stock solution add 1 ml of *aluminium chloride reagent R* and dilute to 25.0 ml with a 5 per cent *V/V* solution of *glacial acetic acid R* in *methanol R*.

Compensation solution. Dilute 10.0 ml of the stock solution to 25.0 ml with a 5 per cent *V/V* solution of *glacial acetic acid R* in *methanol R*.

Measure the absorbance (*2.2.25*) of the test solution after 30 min, by comparison with the compensation solution at 425 nm.

Calculate the percentage content of flavonoids, calculated as hyperoside, from the expression:

$$\frac{A \times 1.25}{m}$$

i.e. taking the specific absorbance of hyperoside to be 500.

A = absorbance at 425 nm,

m = mass of the substance to be examined, in grams.

STORAGE

Store protected from light.

01/2005:0595

BISACODYL

Bisacodylum

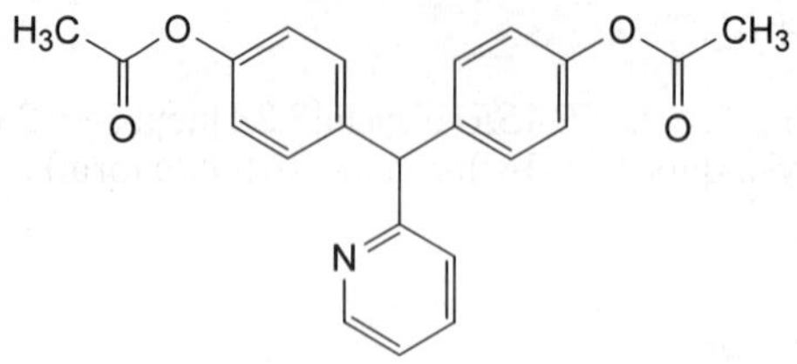

$C_{22}H_{19}NO_4$ M_r 361.4

DEFINITION

Bisacodyl contains not less than 98.0 per cent and not more than the equivalent of 101.0 per cent of 4,4′-(pyridin-2-ylmethylene)diphenyl diacetate, calculated with reference to the dried substance.

CHARACTERS

A white or almost white, crystalline powder, practically insoluble in water, soluble in acetone, sparingly soluble in alcohol. It dissolves in dilute mineral acids.

IDENTIFICATION

First identification: C.

Second identification: A, B, D.

A. Melting point (*2.2.14*): 131 °C to 135 °C.

B. Dissolve 10.0 mg in a 6 g/l solution of *potassium hydroxide R* in *methanol R* and dilute to 100.0 ml with the same alkaline solvent. Dilute 10.0 ml of this solution to 100.0 ml with a 6 g/l solution of *potassium hydroxide R* in *methanol R*. Examined between 220 nm and 350 nm (*2.2.25*), the solution shows an absorption maximum at 248 nm and a shoulder at about 290 nm. The specific absorbance at the maximum is 632 to 672.

C. Examine by infrared absorption spectrophotometry (*2.2.24*), comparing with the spectrum obtained with *bisacodyl CRS*. If the spectra obtained with the substance to be examined and the reference substance show differences, dissolve separately the substance to be examined and the reference substance in *chloroform R*, evaporate to dryness and record the spectra again.

D. Spray the chromatograms obtained in the test for related substances with a mixture of equal volumes of *0.05 M iodine* and *dilute sulphuric acid R*. Examine in daylight. The principal spot in the chromatogram obtained with test solution (b) is similar in position and size to the principal spot in the chromatogram obtained with reference solution (a).

TESTS

Acidity or alkalinity. To 1.0 g add 20 ml of *carbon dioxide-free water R*, shake, heat to boiling, cool and filter. Add 0.2 ml of *0.01 M sodium hydroxide* and 0.1 ml of *methyl red solution R*. The solution is yellow. Not more than 0.4 ml of *0.01 M hydrochloric acid* is required to change the colour of the indicator to red.

Related substances. Examine by thin-layer chromatography (*2.2.27*), using *silica gel GF_{254} R* as the coating substance.

Test solution (a). Dissolve 0.20 g of the substance to be examined in *acetone R* and dilute to 10 ml with the same solvent.

Test solution (b). Dilute 1 ml of test solution (a) to 10 ml with *acetone R*.

Reference solution (a). Dissolve 20 mg of *bisacodyl CRS* in *acetone R* and dilute to 10 ml with the same solvent.

Reference solution (b). Dilute 1 ml of test solution (a) to 100 ml with *acetone R*.

Reference solution (c). Dilute 5 ml of reference solution (b) to 10 ml with *acetone R*.

Apply separately to the plate 10 µl of each solution. Develop over a path of 10 cm using a mixture of 50 volumes of *xylene R* and 50 volumes of *methyl ethyl ketone R*. Allow the plate to dry in air, if necessary heating at 100 °C to 105 °C, and examine in ultraviolet light at 254 nm. Any spot in the chromatogram obtained with test solution (a), apart from the principal spot, is not more intense than the spot in the chromatogram obtained with reference solution (b) (1.0 per cent) and not more than one such spot is more intense than the spot in the chromatogram obtained with reference solution (c) (0.5 per cent).

Loss on drying (*2.2.32*). Not more than 0.5 per cent, determined on 0.500 g by drying in an oven at 100 °C to 105 °C.

Sulphated ash (*2.4.14*). Not more than 0.1 per cent, determined on 1.0 g.

ASSAY

Dissolve 0.300 g in 60 ml of *anhydrous acetic acid R*. Titrate with *0.1 M perchloric acid* determining the end-point potentiometrically (*2.2.20*).

1 ml of *0.1 M perchloric acid* is equivalent to 36.14 mg of $C_{22}H_{19}NO_4$.

STORAGE

Store protected from light.

01/2005:0012

BISMUTH SUBCARBONATE

Bismuthi subcarbonas

DEFINITION

Bismuth subcarbonate contains not less than 80.0 per cent and not more than 82.5 per cent of Bi (A_r 209.0), calculated with reference to the dried substance.

CHARACTERS

A white or almost white powder, practically insoluble in water and in alcohol. It dissolves with effervescence in mineral acids.

IDENTIFICATION

A. It gives the reaction of carbonates (*2.3.1*).

B. It gives the reactions of bismuth (*2.3.1*).

TESTS

Solution S. Shake 5.0 g with 10 ml of *water R* and add 20 ml of *nitric acid R*. Heat to dissolve, cool and dilute to 100 ml with *water R*.

Appearance of solution. Solution S is not more opalescent than reference suspension II (*2.2.1*) and is colourless (*2.2.2, Method II*).

Chlorides (*2.4.4*). To 6.6 ml of solution S add 4 ml of *nitric acid R* and dilute to 50 ml with *water R*. 15 ml of the solution complies with the limit test for chlorides (500 ppm).

Nitrates. To 0.25 g in a 125 ml conical flask, add 20 ml of *water R*, 0.05 ml of *indigo carmine solution R1* and then, as a single addition but with caution, 30 ml of *sulphuric acid R*. Titrate immediately with *indigo carmine solution R1* until a stable blue colour is obtained. Not more than *n* ml of the titrant is required, *n* ml being the volume corresponding to 1 mg of NO_3 (0.4 per cent).

Alkali and alkaline-earth metals. To 1.0 g add 10 ml of *water R* and 10 ml of *acetic acid R*. Boil for 2 min, cool and filter. Wash the residue with 20 ml of *water R*. To the combined filtrate and washings add 2 ml of *dilute hydrochloric acid R* and 20 ml of *water R*. Boil and pass *hydrogen sulphide R* through the boiling solution until no further precipitate is formed. Filter, wash the residue with *water R*, evaporate the combined filtrate and washings to dryness on a water-bath and add 0.5 ml of *sulphuric acid R*. Ignite gently and allow to cool. The residue weighs not more than 10 mg (1.0 per cent).

Arsenic (*2.4.2*). To 0.5 g in a distillation flask add 5 ml of *water R* and 7 ml of *sulphuric acid R*, allow to cool and add 5 g of *reducing mixture R* and 10 ml of *hydrochloric acid R*. Heat the contents of the flask to boiling gradually over 15 min to 30 min and continue heating at such a rate that the distillation proceeds steadily until the volume in the flask is reduced by half or until 5 min after the air-condenser has become full of steam. It is important that distillation be discontinued before fumes of sulphur trioxide appear. Collect the distillate in a tube containing 15 ml of *water R* cooled in ice-water. Wash down the condenser with *water R* and dilute the distillate to 25 ml with the same solvent. The solution complies with limit test A for arsenic (5 ppm). Prepare the standard using a mixture of 2.5 ml of *arsenic standard solution (1 ppm As) R* and 22.5 ml of *water R*.

Copper. To 5 ml of solution S, add 2 ml of *ammonia R* and dilute to 50 ml with *water R*. Filter. To 10 ml of the filtrate add 1 ml of a 1 g/l solution of *sodium diethyldithiocarbamate R*. The solution is not more intensely coloured than a standard prepared at the same time in the same manner using a mixture of 0.25 ml of *copper standard solution (10 ppm Cu) R* and 9.75 ml of *water R* instead of 10 ml of the filtrate (50 ppm).

Lead. Not more than 20 ppm of Pb, determined by atomic absorption spectrometry (*2.2.23, Method II*).

Test solution. Dissolve 12.5 g of the substance to be examined in 75 ml of a mixture of equal volumes of *lead-free nitric acid R* and *water R*. Boil for 1 min, cool and dilute to 100.0 ml with *water R*.

Reference solutions. Prepare the reference solutions using appropriate quantities of lead standard solution and a 37 per cent *V/V* solution of *lead-free nitric acid R*.

Measure the absorbance at 283.3 nm, using a hollow-cathode lamp as source of radiation and an air-acetylene flame. Depending on the apparatus, the line at 217.0 nm may be used.

Silver. To 2.0 g add 1 ml of *water R* and 4 ml of *nitric acid R*. Heat gently until dissolved and dilute to 11 ml with *water R*. Cool and add 2 ml of *1 M hydrochloric acid*. Allow to stand for 5 min, protected from light. Any opalescence in the solution is not more intense than that in a standard prepared at the same time in the same manner using a mixture of 10 ml of *silver standard solution (5 ppm Ag) R*, 1 ml of *nitric acid R* and 2 ml of *1 M hydrochloric acid* (25 ppm).

Loss on drying (*2.2.32*). Not more than 1.0 per cent, determined on 1.000 g by drying in an oven at 100-105 °C.

ASSAY

Dissolve 0.500 g in 3 ml of *nitric acid R* and dilute to 250 ml with *water R*. Carry out the complexometric titration of bismuth (*2.5.11*).

1 ml of *0.1 M sodium edetate* is equivalent to 20.90 mg of Bi.

STORAGE

Store protected from light.

01/2005:1493

BISMUTH SUBGALLATE

Bismuthi subgallas

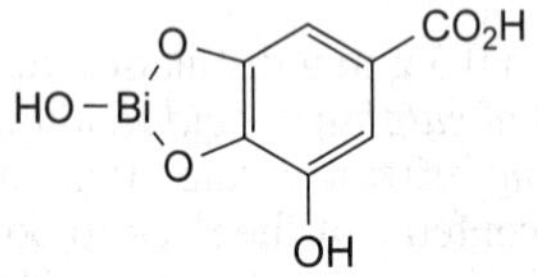

$C_7H_5BiO_6$ M_r 394.1

DEFINITION

Complex of bismuth and gallic acid.

Content: 48.0 per cent to 51.0 per cent of Bi (A_r 209.0) (dried substance).

CHARACTERS

Appearance: yellow powder.

Solubility: practically insoluble in water and in alcohol. It dissolves in mineral acids with decomposition and in solutions of alkali hydroxides, producing a reddish-brown liquid.

IDENTIFICATION

A. Mix 0.1 g with 5 ml of *water R* and 0.1 ml of *phosphoric acid R*. Heat to boiling and maintain boiling for 2 min. Cool and filter. To the filtrate, add 1.5 ml of *ferric chloride solution R1*, a blackish-blue colour develops.

B. It gives reaction (b) of bismuth (*2.3.1*).

TESTS

Solution S. In a porcelain or quartz dish, ignite 1.0 g, increasing the temperature very gradually. Heat in a muffle furnace at 600 ± 25 °C for 2 h. Cool and dissolve the residue with warming in 4 ml of a mixture of equal volumes of *lead-free nitric acid R* and *water R* and dilute to 20 ml with *water R*.

Acidity. Shake 1.0 g with 20 ml of *water R* for 1 min and filter. To the filtrate add 0.1 ml of *methyl red solution R*. Not more than 0.15 ml of *0.1 M sodium hydroxide* is required to change the colour of the indicator to yellow.

Chlorides (*2.4.4*): maximum 200 ppm.

To 0.5 g add 10 ml of *dilute nitric acid R*. Heat on a water-bath for 5 min and filter. Dilute 5 ml of the filtrate to 15 ml with *water R*.

Nitrates: maximum 0.2 per cent.

To 1.0 g add 25 ml of *water R* then 25 ml of a mixture of 2 volumes of *sulphuric acid R* and 9 volumes of *water R*. Heat at about 50 °C for 1 min with stirring and filter. To 10 ml of the filtrate, carefully add 30 ml of *sulphuric acid R*. The solution is not more intensely brownish-yellow coloured than a reference solution prepared at the same time as follows: to 0.4 g of *gallic acid R*, add 20 ml of *nitrate standard solution (100 ppm NO_3) R* and 30 ml of a mixture of 2 volumes of *sulphuric acid R* and 9 volumes of *water R*, then filter; to 10 ml of the filtrate, carefully add 30 ml of *sulphuric acid R*.

Copper: maximum 50 ppm.

Atomic absorption spectrometry (*2.2.23, Method I*).

Test solution. Solution S.

Reference solutions. Prepare the reference solutions using *copper standard solution (10 ppm Cu) R* and diluting with a 6.5 per cent *V/V* solution of *lead-free nitric acid R*.

Source: copper hollow-cathode lamp.

Wavelength: 324.7 nm.

Atomisation device: air-acetylene flame.

Lead: maximum 20 ppm.

Atomic absorption spectrometry (*2.2.23, Method II*).

Test solution. Solution S.

Reference solutions. Prepare the reference solutions using *lead standard solution (10 ppm Pb) R* and diluting with a 6.5 per cent *V/V* solution of *lead-free nitric acid R*.

Source: lead hollow-cathode lamp.

Wavelength: 283.3 nm (depending on the apparatus, the line at 217.0 nm may be used).

Atomisation device: air-acetylene flame.

Silver: maximum 25 ppm.

Atomic absorption spectrometry (*2.2.23, Method I*).

Test solution. Solution S.

Reference solutions. Prepare the reference solutions using *silver standard solution (5 ppm Ag) R* and diluting with a 6.5 per cent *V/V* solution of *lead-free nitric acid R*.

Source: silver hollow-cathode lamp.

Wavelength: 328.1 nm.

Atomisation device: air-acetylene flame.

Substances not precipitated by ammonia: maximum 1.0 per cent.

In a porcelain or quartz dish, ignite 2.0 g, increasing the temperature very gradually to 600 °C; allow to cool. Moisten the residue with 2 ml of *nitric acid R*, evaporate to dryness on a water-bath and carefully heat and ignite once more at 600 °C. After cooling, dissolve the residue in 5 ml of *nitric acid R* and dilute to 20 ml with *water R*. To 10 ml of this solution, add *concentrated ammonia R* until alkaline and filter. Wash the residue with *water R*, evaporate the combined filtrate and washings to dryness on a water-bath and add 0.3 ml of *dilute sulphuric acid R*. Ignite, the residue weighs a maximum of 10 mg.

Loss on drying (*2.2.32*): maximum 7.0 per cent, determined on 1.000 g by drying in an oven at 100-105 °C for 3 h.

ASSAY

To 0.300 g add 10 ml of a mixture of equal volumes of *nitric acid R* and *water R*, heat to boiling and maintain boiling for 2 min. Add 0.1 g of *potassium chlorate R*, heat to boiling and maintain boiling for 1 min. Add 10 ml of *water R* and heat until the solution becomes colourless. To the hot solution, add 200 ml of *water R* and 50 mg of *xylenol orange triturate R*. Titrate with *0.1 M sodium edetate* until a yellow colour is obtained.

1 ml of *0.1 M sodium edetate* is equivalent to 20.90 mg of Bi.

STORAGE

Protected from light.

01/2005:1494

BISMUTH SUBNITRATE, HEAVY

Bismuthi subnitras ponderosum

$4[BiNO_3(OH)_2],BiO(OH)$ M_r 1462

DEFINITION

Heavy bismuth subnitrate contains not less than 71.0 per cent and not more than 74.0 per cent of Bi (A_r 209.0), calculated with reference to the dried substance.

CHARACTERS

A white powder, practically insoluble in water and in alcohol. It dissolves in mineral acids with decomposition.

IDENTIFICATION

A. Dilute 1 ml of solution S1 (see Tests) to 5 ml with *water R*, add 0.3 ml of *potassium iodide solution R*. A black precipitate is formed which dissolves into an orange solution with the addition of 2 ml of *potassium iodide solution R*.

B. It gives reaction (b) of bismuth (*2.3.1*).

C. It gives the reaction of nitrates (*2.3.1*).

D. The pH (*2.2.3*) of solution S2 (see Tests) is not more than 2.0.

TESTS

Solution S1. Shake 5.0 g by gently heating in 10 ml of *water R*, add 20 ml of *nitric acid R*. Heat until dissolution, cool and dilute to 100 ml with *water R*.

Solution S2. Place 1.00 g in a 20 ml volumetric flask and add 2.0 ml of *lead-free nitric acid R*. Allow acid attack to take place without heating and if necessary warm slightly at the end to dissolve the test sample completely. Add 10 ml of *water R*, shake and add, in small fractions, 4.5 ml of *lead-free ammonia R*; shake, allow to cool, dilute to 20.0 ml with *water R*, shake again and allow the solids to settle. The clear supernatant solution is solution S2.

Acidity. Suspend 1.0 g in 15 ml of *water R* and shake several times. Allow to stand for 5 min and filter. To 10 ml of the filtrate, add 0.5 ml of *phenolphthalein solution R1*. Not more than 0.5 ml of *0.1 M sodium hydroxide* is required to change the colour of the indicator to pink.

Chlorides (*2.4.4*). To 5.0 ml of solution S1, add 3 ml of *nitric acid R* and dilute to 15 ml with *water R*. The solution complies with the limit test for chlorides (200 ppm).

Copper. Not more than 50 ppm of Cu, determined by atomic absorption spectrometry (*2.2.23, Method I*).

Test solution. Solution S2.

Reference solutions. Prepare the reference solutions using *copper standard solution (10 ppm Cu) R* and diluting with a 37 per cent *V/V* solution of *lead-free nitric acid R*.

Measure the absorbance at 324.7 nm using a copper hollow-cathode lamp as source of radiation and an air-acetylene flame.

Lead. Not more than 20 ppm of Pb, determined by atomic absorption spectrometry (*2.2.23, Method II*).

Test solution. Solution S2.

Reference solutions. Prepare the reference solutions using appropriate quantities of *lead standard solution (10 ppm Pb) R* and diluting with a 37 per cent *V/V* solution of *lead-free nitric acid R*.

Measure the absorbance at 283.3 nm, using a lead hollow-cathode lamp as source of radiation and an air-acetylene flame. Depending on the apparatus, the line at 217.0 nm may be used.

Silver. Not more than 25 ppm of Ag, determined by atomic absorption spectrometry (*2.2.23, Method I*).

Test solution. Solution S2.

Reference solutions. Prepare the reference solutions using *silver standard solution (5 ppm Ag) R* and diluting with a 37 per cent *V/V* solution of *lead-free nitric acid R*.

Measure the absorbance at 328.1 nm using a silver hollow-cathode lamp as source of radiation and an air-acetylene flame.

Substances not precipitated by ammonia. To 20 ml of solution S1, add *concentrated ammonia R* until alkaline and filter. Wash the residue with *water R*, and evaporate the combined filtrate and washings to dryness on a water-bath. Add 0.3 ml of *dilute sulphuric acid R* and ignite. The residue weighs not more than 10 mg (1.0 per cent).

Loss on drying (*2.2.32*). Not more than 3.0 per cent, determined on 1.000 g by drying in an oven at 100-105 °C.

ASSAY

Dissolve with heating 0.250 g in 10 ml of a mixture of 2 volumes of *perchloric acid R* and 5 volumes of *water R*. To the hot solution, add 200 ml of *water R* and 50 mg of *xylenol orange triturate R*. Titrate with *0.1 M sodium edetate* until a yellow colour is obtained.

1 ml of *0.1 M sodium edetate* is equivalent to 20.90 mg of Bi.

01/2005:1495

BISMUTH SUBSALICYLATE

Bismuthi subsalicylas

$C_7H_5BiO_4$ M_r 362.1

DEFINITION

Complex of bismuth and salicylic acid.

Content: 56.0 per cent to 59.4 per cent of Bi (A_r 209.0) (dried substance).

CHARACTERS

Appearance: white powder.

Solubility: practically insoluble in water and in alcohol. It dissolves in mineral acids with decomposition.

IDENTIFICATION

A. To 0.5 g add 10 ml of *hydrochloric acid R1*. Heat on a boiling water-bath for 5 min. Cool and filter. Retain the filtrate for identification test B. Wash the residue with *dilute hydrochloric acid R* and then with *water R*. Dissolve the residue in 0.5-1 ml of *dilute sodium hydroxide solution R*. Add 15 ml of *water R*. Neutralise with *dilute hydrochloric acid R*. The solution gives reaction (a) of salicylates (*2.3.1*).

B. The filtrate obtained in identification test A gives reaction (b) of bismuth (*2.3.1*).

TESTS

Solution S. In a porcelain or quartz dish, ignite 1.0 g, increasing the temperature very gradually. Heat in a muffle furnace at 600 ± 25 °C for 2 h. Cool and dissolve the residue with warming in 4 ml of a mixture of equal volumes of *lead-free nitric acid R* and *water R* and dilute to 20 ml with *water R*.

Monographs B

Acidity. Shake 2.0 g with 30 ml of *ether R* for 1 min and filter. To the filtrate add 30 ml of *alcohol R* and 0.1 ml of *thymol blue solution R*. Not more than 0.35 ml of *0.1 M sodium hydroxide* is required to change the colour of the indicator to blue.

Chlorides (*2.4.4*): maximum 200 ppm.

Dissolve 0.250 g in a mixture of 2 ml of *nitric acid R*, 5 ml of *water R* and 8 ml of *methanol R*.

Nitrates: maximum 0.4 per cent.

To 0.1 g add 10 ml of *water R* and, with caution, 20 ml of *sulphuric acid R* and stir. The solution is not more intensely yellow coloured than a reference solution prepared at the same time using 0.1 g of *salicylic acid R*, 6 ml of *water R*, 4 ml of *nitrate standard solution (100 ppm NO_3) R* and 20 ml of *sulphuric acid R*.

Copper: maximum 50 ppm.

Atomic absorption spectrometry (*2.2.23, Method I*).

Test solution. Solution S.

Reference solutions. Prepare the reference solutions using *copper standard solution (10 ppm Cu) R* and diluting with a 6.5 per cent *V/V* solution of *lead-free nitric acid R*.

Source: copper hollow-cathode lamp.

Wavelength: 324.7 nm.

Atomisation device: air-acetylene flame.

Lead: maximum 20 ppm.

Atomic absorption spectrometry (*2.2.23, Method II*).

Test solution. Solution S.

Reference solutions. Prepare the reference solutions using *lead standard solution (10 ppm Pb) R* and diluting with a 6.5 per cent *V/V* solution of *lead-free nitric acid R*.

Source: lead hollow-cathode lamp.

Wavelength: 283.3 nm (depending on the apparatus, the line at 217.0 nm may be used).

Atomisation device: air-acetylene flame.

Silver: maximum 25 ppm.

Atomic absorption spectrometry (*2.2.23, Method I*).

Test solution. Solution S.

Reference solutions. Prepare the reference solutions using *silver standard solution (5 ppm Ag) R* and diluting with a 6.5 per cent *V/V* solution of *lead-free nitric acid R*.

Source: silver hollow-cathode lamp.

Wavelength: 328.1 nm.

Atomisation device: air-acetylene flame.

Soluble bismuth: maximum 40 ppm.

Atomic absorption spectrometry (*2.2.23, Method I*).

Test solution. Suspend 5.0 g in 100 ml of *water R*. Stir constantly for 2 h at 20-23 °C. Filter through filter paper (slow filtration) then through a cellulose micropore membrane filter (0.1 µm). To 10.0 ml of clear filtrate, add 0.1 ml of *nitric acid R*.

Reference solutions. Prepare the reference solutions using *bismuth standard solution (100 ppm Bi) R* and diluting with a mixture of equal volumes of *dilute nitric acid R* and *water R*.

Source: bismuth hollow-cathode lamp.

Wavelength: 223.06 nm.

Atomisation device: air-acetylene flame.

Loss on drying (*2.2.32*): maximum 1.0 per cent, determined on 1.000 g by drying in an oven at 100-105 °C.

ASSAY

Dissolve with heating 0.300 g in 10 ml of a mixture of 2 volumes of *perchloric acid R* and 5 volumes of *water R*. To the hot solution, add 200 ml of *water R* and 50 mg of *xylenol orange triturate R*. Titrate with *0.1 M sodium edetate* until a yellow colour is obtained.

1 ml of *0.1 M sodium edetate* is equivalent to 20.90 mg of Bi.

STORAGE

Protected from light.

01/2005:1826

BITTER-FENNEL FRUIT OIL

Foeniculi amari fructus aetheroleum

DEFINITION

Essential oil obtained by steam distillation from the ripe fruits of *Foeniculum vulgare* Miller, ssp. *vulgare* var. *vulgare*.

Content:

- fenchone: 12.0 per cent to 25.0 per cent,
- *trans*-anethole: 55.0 per cent to 75.0 per cent.

CHARACTERS

Appearance: clear, colourless or pale yellow liquid.

It has a characteristic odour.

IDENTIFICATION

First identification: B.

Second identification: A.

A. Thin-layer chromatography (*2.2.27*).

Test solution. Dissolve 0.1 ml of the oil to be examined in 5 ml of *toluene R*.

Reference solution. Dissolve 10 µl of *fenchone R* and 80 µl of *anethole R* in 5 ml of *toluene R*.

Plate: *TLC silica gel plate R.*

Mobile phase: *ethyl acetate R, toluene R (5:95 V/V)*.

Application: 10 µl as bands.

Development: over a path of 15 cm.

Drying: in air.

Detection: spray with a freshly prepared 200 g/l solution of *phosphomolybdic acid R* in *ethanol (96 per cent) R* and heat at 150 °C for 15 min; examine in daylight.

Results: see below the sequence of the zones present in the chromatograms obtained with the reference solution and the test solution. Furthermore, other zones may be present in the chromatogram obtained with the test solution.

Top of the plate	
Anethole: a dark blue to dark violet zone	A dark blue to dark violet zone (anethole)
_______	_______
Fenchone: a blue or bluish-grey zone	A blue or bluish-grey zone (fenchone)
_______	
Reference solution	**Test solution**

B. Examine the chromatograms obtained in the test for chromatographic profile.

Results: the characteristic peaks in the chromatogram obtained with the test solution are similar in retention time to those in the chromatogram obtained with the reference solution.

TESTS

Relative density (*2.2.5*): 0.961 to 0.975.

Refractive index (*2.2.6*): 1.528 to 1.539.

Optical rotation (*2.2.7*): + 10.0° to + 24.0°.

Chromatographic profile. Gas chromatography (*2.2.28*): use the normalisation procedure.

Test solution. Dissolve 0.20 ml of the oil to be examined in *heptane R* and dilute to 10.0 ml with the same solvent.

Reference solution. Dissolve 20 µl of *α-pinene R*, 20 µl of *limonene R*, 50 µl of *fenchone R*, 20 µl of *estragole R*, 100 µl of *anethole R* and 20 µl of *anisaldehyde R* in *heptane R* and dilute to 10.0 ml with the same solvent.

Column:

- *material*: fused silica,
- *size*: *l* = 60 m, Ø = 0.25 mm,
- *stationary phase*: *macrogol 20 000 R* (film thickness 0.25 µm).

Carrier gas: *helium for chromatography R*.

Flow rate: 1 ml/min.

Split ratio: 1:200.

Temperature:

	Time (min)	Temperature (°C)
Column	0 - 4	60
	4 - 26	60 → 170
	26 - 41	170
Injection port		220
Detector		270

Detection: flame ionisation.

Injection: 1.0 µl.

Elution order: order indicated in the composition of the reference solution. Record the retention times of these substances.

System suitability: reference solution:

- *resolution*: minimum 5.0 between the peaks due to estragole and *trans*-anethole.

Using the retention times determined from the chromatogram obtained with the reference solution, locate the components of the reference solution on the chromatogram obtained with the test solution and locate *cis*-anethole using Figure 1826.-1. (Disregard the peak due to heptane).

Determine the percentage content of each of these components. The percentages are within the following ranges:

- *α-pinene*: 1.0 per cent to 10.0 per cent,
- *limonene*: 0.9 per cent to 5.0 per cent,
- *fenchone*: 12.0 per cent to 25.0 per cent,
- *estragole*: maximum 6.0 per cent,

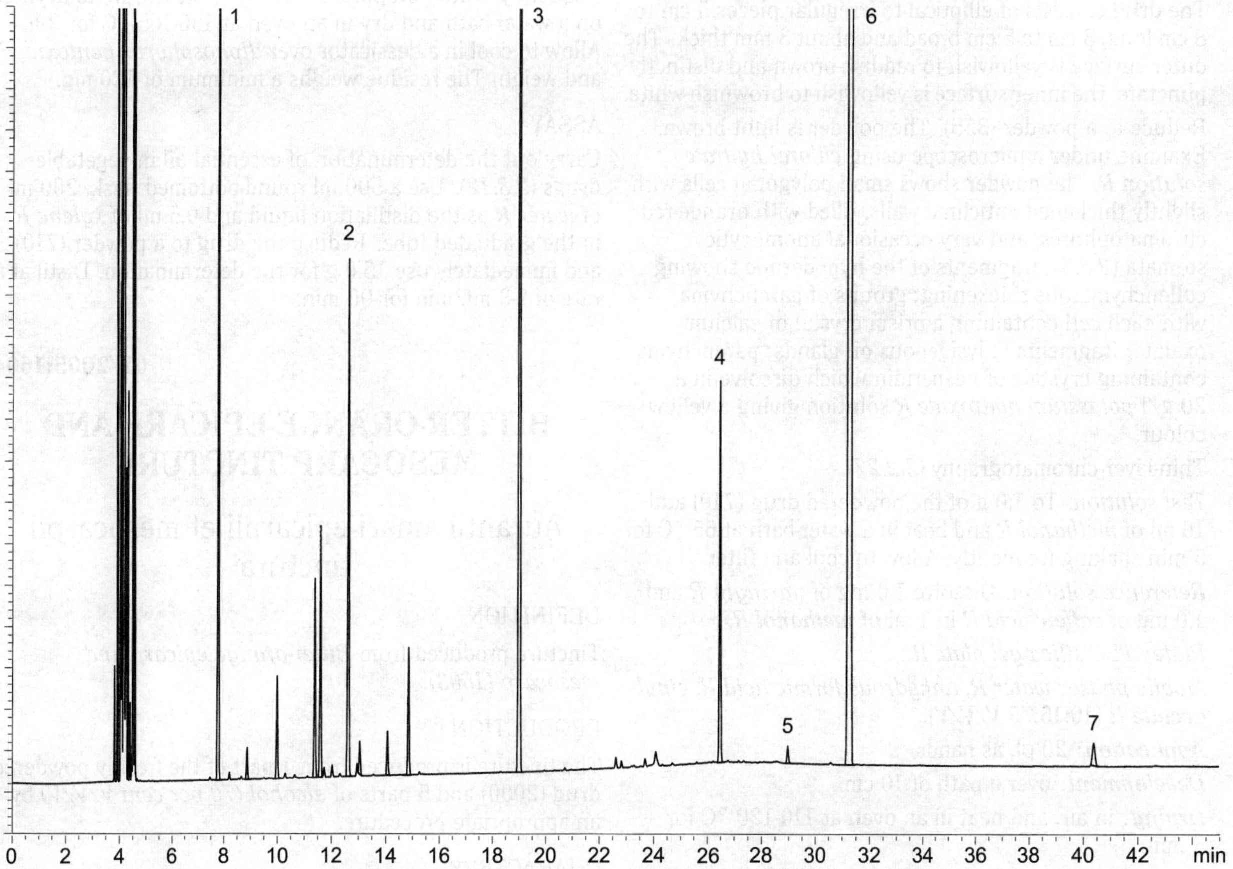

1. α-pinene 2. limonene 3. fenchone 4. estragole 5. *cis*-anethole 6. *trans*-anethole 7. anisaldehyde

Figure 1826.-1. – *Chromatogram for the test for chromatographic profile of bitter-fennel fruit oil*

Monographs B

- *cis-anethole*: maximum 0.5 per cent,
- *trans-anethole*: 55.0 per cent to 75.0 per cent,
- *anisaldehyde*: maximum 2.0 per cent.

The ratio of α-pinene content to limonene content is greater than 1.0.

STORAGE

In a well-filled, airtight container, protected from light and at a temperature not exceeding 25 °C.

01/2005:1603

BITTER-ORANGE EPICARP AND MESOCARP

Aurantii amari epicarpium et mesocarpium

DEFINITION

Dried epicarp and mesocarp of the ripe fruit of *Citrus aurantium* L. ssp. *aurantium* (*C. aurantium* L. ssp. *amara* Engl.) partly freed from the white spongy tissue of the mesocarp and endocarp.

Content: minimum 20 ml/kg of essential oil (anhydrous drug).

CHARACTERS

Aromatic odour and spicy bitter taste.

Macroscopic and microscopic characters described under identification A and B.

IDENTIFICATION

A. The drug consists of elliptical to irregular pieces 5 cm to 8 cm long, 3 cm to 5 cm broad and about 3 mm thick. The outer surface is yellowish to reddish-brown and distinctly punctate, the inner surface is yellowish to brownish-white.

B. Reduce to a powder (355). The powder is light brown. Examine under a microscope using *chloral hydrate solution R*. The powder shows small polygonal cells with slightly thickened anticlinal walls, filled with orange-red chromatophores, and very occasional anomocytic stomata (*2.8.3*); fragments of the hypodermic showing collenchymatous thickening; groups of parenchyma with each cell containing a prism crystal of calcium oxalate; fragments of lysigenous oil glands; parenchyma containing crystals of hesperidin which dissolve in a 20 g/l *potassium hydroxide R* solution giving a yellow colour.

C. Thin-layer chromatography (*2.2.27*).

Test solution. To 1.0 g of the powdered drug (710) add 10 ml of *methanol R* and heat in a water-bath at 65 °C for 5 min shaking frequently. Allow to cool and filter.

Reference solution. Dissolve 1.0 mg of *naringin R* and 1.0 mg of *caffeic acid R* in 1 ml of *methanol R*.

Plate: *TLC silica gel plate R.*

Mobile phase: *water R, anhydrous formic acid R, ethyl acetate R* (10:15:75 *V/V/V*).

Application: 20 µl, as bands.

Development: over a path of 10 cm.

Drying: in air, and heat in an oven at 110-120 °C for 5 min.

Detection: spray the warm plate with a 10 g/l solution of *diphenylboric acid aminoethyl ester R* in *methanol R* and then with a 50 g/l solution of *macrogol 400 R* in *methanol R*. After at least 1 h, examine in ultraviolet light at 365 nm.

Results: see below the sequence of the zones present in the chromatograms obtained with the reference and test solutions. Furthermore, other fluorescent zones are present in the chromatogram obtained with the test solution.

Top of the plate	
	A light blue fluorescent zone
	A light blue fluorescent zone
Caffeic acid: a light blue fluorescent zone	
	A light blue fluorescent zone
	A light blue fluorescent zone
Naringin: a dark green fluorescent zone	A dark green fluorescent zone (naringin)
	A red fluorescent zone (neoeriocitrin)
	An orange fluorescent zone
Reference solution	**Test solution**

TESTS

Foreign matter (*2.8.2*): it complies with the test for foreign matter.

Water (*2.2.13*): maximum 10.0 per cent, determined on 20.0 g of powdered drug (355) by distillation.

Total ash (*2.4.16*): maximum 7.0 per cent

Extractable matter: minimum 6.0 per cent.

To 2.000 g of the powdered drug (250) add a mixture of 3 ml of *water R* and 7 ml of *alcohol R* and extract for 2 h, shaking frequently. Filter, evaporate 2.000 g of the filtrate to dryness on a water-bath and dry in an oven at 100-105 °C for 3 h. Allow to cool in a dessicator over *diphosphorus pentoxide R* and weigh. The residue weighs a minimum of 120 mg.

ASSAY

Carry out the determination of essential oil in vegetable drugs (*2.8.12*). Use a 500 ml round-bottomed flask, 200 ml of *water R* as the distillation liquid and 0.5 ml of *xylene R* in the graduated tube. Reduce the drug to a powder (710) and immediately use 15.0 g for the determination. Distil at a rate of 2-3 ml/min for 90 min.

01/2005:1604

BITTER-ORANGE-EPICARP AND MESOCARP TINCTURE

Aurantii amari epicarpii et mesocarpii tinctura

DEFINITION

Tincture produced from *Bitter-orange epicarp and mesocarp (1603).*

PRODUCTION

The tincture is produced from 1 part of the freshly powdered drug (2000) and 5 parts of *alcohol (70 per cent V/V/V)* by an appropriate procedure.

CHARACTERS

Liquid with a bitter taste.

IDENTIFICATION

Examine by thin-layer chromatography (*2.2.27*).

Test solution. The tincture to be examined.

Reference solution. Dissolve 1.0 mg of *naringin R* and 1.0 mg of *caffeic acid R* in 1 ml of *methanol R.*

Plate: *TLC silica gel plate R.*

Mobile phase: *water R, anhydrous formic acid R, ethyl acetate R* (10:15:75 *V/V/V*).

Application: 20 µl, as bands.

Development: over a path of 10 cm.

Drying: in air, and heat in an oven at 110-120 °C for 5 min.

Detection: spray the warm plate with a 10 g/l solution of *diphenylboric acid aminoethyl ester R* in *methanol R* and then with a 50 g/l solution of *macrogol 400 R* in *methanol R*. After 1 h, examine in ultraviolet light at 365 nm.

Results: see below the sequence of the zones present in the chromatograms obtained with the reference and test solutions. Furthermore, other zones are present in the chromatogram obtained with the test solution.

Reference solution	Test solution
Top of the plate	
	A light blue fluorescent zone
	A light blue fluorescent zone
Caffeic acid: a light blue fluorescent zone	
	A light blue fluorescent zone
	A light blue fluorescent zone
Naringin: a dark green fluorescent zone	A dark green fluorescent zone (naringin)
	A red fluorescent zone (neoeriocitrin)
	An orange fluorescent zone

TESTS

Ethanol content (*2.9.10*): 63 per cent to 67 per cent *V/V*.

Methanol and 2-propanol (*2.9.11*): maximum 0.05 per cent *V/V* of methanol and maximum 0.05 per cent *V/V* of 2-propanol.

Dry residue: minimum 6.0 per cent *m/m*, determined on 2.00 g of tincture to be examined.

01/2005:1810

BITTER-ORANGE FLOWER

Aurantii amari flos

DEFINITION

Whole, dried, unopened flower of *Citrus aurantium* L. ssp. *aurantium* (*C. aurantium* L. ssp. *amara* Engl.).

Content: minimum 8.0 per cent of total flavonoids, expressed as naringin ($C_{27}H_{32}O_{14}$; M_r 580.5) (dried drug).

CHARACTERS

Macroscopic and microscopic characters described under identification tests A and B.

IDENTIFICATION

A. The flower buds are white or yellowish-white and may reach up to 25 mm in length. The dialypetalous corolla is composed of 5 thick, oblong and concave petals dotted with oil glands visible under a hand lens; the short, yellowish-green persistent gamosepalous calyx has 5 spreading sepals, connate at the base and forming a star-shaped structure attached to the yellowish-green peduncle which is about 5 mm to 10 mm long. The flower buds contain at least 20 stamens with yellow anthers and with filaments fused at the base into groups of 4 or 5; the ovary is superior, brownish-black and spherical, consists of 8 to 10 multi-ovular loculi and is surrounded at the base by an annular granular hypogynous disc; the thick, cylindrical style ends in a capitate stigma.

B. Reduce to a powder (355). The powder is brownish-yellow. Examine under a microscope using *chloral hydrate solution R*. The powder shows numerous spherical pollen grains, with a finely pitted exine and 3 to 5 germinal pores; fragments of the epidermis of the sepals with unicellular trichomes and with large prism crystals of calcium oxalate in the underlying mesophyll; fragments of the epidermis of the petals with a distinctly striated cuticle; fragments of large schizolysigenous oil glands which measure up to 100 µm in diameter, numerous anomocytic stomata (*2.8.3*). Examine under a microscope using a 300 g/l solution of *potassium hydroxide R*. The powder shows yellow crystals of hesperidin.

C. Examine the chromatograms obtained in the test for sweet-orange flower.

Results: see below the sequence of the zones present in the chromatograms obtained with the reference solution and the test solution.

Reference solution	Test solution
Top of the plate	
	A weak yellow fluorescent zone
	A weak yellow fluorescent zone
Hesperidin: a greenish-yellow fluorescent zone	A greenish-yellow fluorescent zone (hesperidin)
Naringin: a yellow fluorescent zone	A yellow fluorescent zone (naringin)
	A red fluorescent zone (neoeriocitrin)
	A yellow fluorescent zone (diosmin and neodiosmin)

TESTS

Sweet-orange flower. Thin-layer chromatography (*2.2.27*).

Test solution. To 0.5 g of the powdered drug (355), add 5 ml of *methanol R*. Heat with stirring at 40 °C for 10 min. Filter.

Reference solution. Dissolve 3.0 mg of *naringin R* and 3.0 mg of *hesperidin R* in 10 ml of *methanol R.*

Plate: *TLC silica gel plate R.*

Mobile phase: *water R, anhydrous formic acid R, ethyl acetate R* (10:15:75 *V/V/V*).

Application: 10 µl, as bands.

Development: over a path of 10 cm.

Drying: in air, then heat in an oven at 110-120 °C for 5 min.

Detection: spray the hot plate with a 10 g/l solution of *diphenylboric acid aminoethyl ester R* in *methanol R* and then with a 50 g/l solution of *macrogol 400 R* in *methanol R*. After at least 1 h, examine in ultraviolet light at 365 nm.

Results: the chromatogram obtained with the test solution shows a yellow zone similar in position to the zone of naringin in the chromatogram obtained with the reference solution and immediately below it a red zone (neoeriocitrin).

Foreign matter (*2.8.2*): maximum 2 per cent.

Loss on drying (*2.2.32*): maximum 11.0 per cent, determined on 1.000 g of the powdered drug (355) by drying in an oven at 100-105 °C.

Total ash (*2.4.16*): maximum 10.0 per cent.

Monographs B

ASSAY

Stock solution. To 0.175 g of the powdered drug (355) add 95 ml of *alcohol (50 per cent V/V) R.* Heat on a water-bath under a reflux condenser for 30 min. Allow to cool and filter through a sintered-glass filter. Rinse the filter with 5 ml of *alcohol (50 per cent V/V) R.* Combine the filtrate and the rinsings in a volumetric flask and dilute to 100.0 ml with *alcohol (50 per cent V/V) R.*

Test solution. Into a test tube (10 mm × 180 mm) introduce 0.150 g of powdered (250) *magnesium R,* a magnetic stirring bar 25 mm long and 2.00 ml of the stock solution. Maintain the test tube upright, centrifuge at 125 *g* and carefully add dropwise, especially at the beginning, 2.0 ml of *hydrochloric acid R,* and then 6.0 ml of *alcohol (50 per cent V/V) R.* Stopper the tube and mix by inverting.

Compensation solution. Into a second tube, introduce 2.00 ml of the stock solution and carefully add dropwise, especially at the beginning, 2.0 ml of *hydrochloric acid R* and then 6.0 ml of *alcohol (50 per cent V/V) R.*

After 10 min, measure the absorbance (*2.2.25*) of the test solution at 530 nm.

Calculate the percentage content of total flavonoids, expressed as naringin, from the expression:

$$\frac{A \times 9.62}{m}$$

i.e. taking the value of the specific absorbance of the reaction product of naringin to be 52.

A = absorbance at 530 nm,

m = mass of the substance to be examined, in grams.

01/2005:1175

BITTER-ORANGE-FLOWER OIL

Aurantii amari floris aetheroleum

DEFINITION

Bitter-orange-flower oil is obtained by steam distillation from the fresh flowers of *Citrus aurantium* L. subsp. *aurantium* (*C. aurantium* L. subsp. *amara* Engl.).

CHARACTERS

A clear, pale-yellow or dark-yellow liquid, with a characteristic odour reminiscent of bitter-orange flowers, miscible with alcohol, with light petroleum, with fatty oils and with liquid paraffin.

IDENTIFICATION

First identification: B.

Second identification: A.

A. Examine in ultraviolet light at 365 nm the chromatograms obtained in the test for bergapten. Before spraying with the reagent, the chromatogram obtained with the test solution shows a band similar in position and fluorescence to that corresponding to methyl anthranilate in the chromatogram obtained with the reference solution. Other bands may be visible. Examine in ultraviolet light at 365 nm after spraying with the reagent. The chromatogram obtained with the reference solution shows in the upper half a band of brownish-orange fluorescence corresponding to linalyl acetate, in the lower half a band of brownish-orange fluorescence corresponding to linalol and immediately below, a band of yellow-greenish fluorescence corresponding to bergapten. The chromatogram obtained with the test solution shows two bands similar in position and fluorescence to the bands corresponding to linalyl acetate and to linalol in the chromatogram obtained with the reference solution. Other bands may also be present.

B. Examine the chromatograms obtained in the test for chromatographic profile. The retention times of the principal peaks in the chromatogram obtained with the test solution are approximately the same as those of the peaks in the chromatogram obtained with the reference solution.

TESTS

Relative density (*2.2.5*): 0.866 to 0.880.

Refractive index (*2.2.6*): 1.468 to 1.474.

Optical rotation (*2.2.7*): + 1.5° to + 11.5°.

Acid value (*2.5.1*). Not more than 2.0.

Bergapten. Examine by thin-layer chromatography (*2.2.27*), using a suitable silica gel as the coating substance.

Test solution. Dissolve 0.1 g of the substance to be examined in *alcohol R* and dilute to 5.0 ml with the same solvent.

Reference solution. Dissolve 5 µl of *methyl anthranilate R,* 10 µl of *linalol R,* 20 µl of *linalyl acetate R* and 10 mg of *bergapten R* in *alcohol R* and dilute to 10.0 ml with the same solvent.

Apply separately to the plate, as bands, 10 µl of each solution. Develop over a path of 15 cm using a mixture of 15 volumes of *ethyl acetate R* and 85 volumes of *toluene R.* Allow the plate to dry in air and examine in ultraviolet light at 365 nm. The chromatogram obtained with the reference solution shows in the middle a band of blue fluorescence (methyl anthranilate) and below a band of greenish-yellow fluorescence (bergapten). Spray with *anisaldehyde solution R.* Heat the plate at 100 °C to 105 °C for 10 min. Examine in ultraviolet light at 365 nm. The chromatogram obtained with the test solution does not show a band corresponding to that due to bergapten (essential oil of bitter-orange peel) in the chromatogram obtained with the reference solution.

Chromatographic profile. Examine by gas chromatography (*2.2.28*).

Test solution. The substance to be examined.

Reference solution. Dissolve 20 µl of *β-pinene R,* 5 µl of *sabinene R,* 40 µl of *limonene R,* 40 µl of *linalol R,* 20 µl of *linalyl acetate R,* 5 µl of *α-terpineol R,* 5 µl of *neryl acetate R,* 5 µl of *geranyl acetate R,* 5 µl of *trans-nerolidol R* and 5 µl of *methyl anthranilate R* in 1 ml of *hexane R.*

The chromatographic procedure may be carried out using:

– a fused-silica capillary column 25 m to 60 m long and about 0.25 mm in internal diameter, impregnated with *macrogol 20 000 R* as the bonded phase,

– *helium for chromatography R* as the carrier gas at a flow rate of 1.5 ml/min,

– a flame-ionisation detector,

– a split ratio of 1:100,

maintaining the temperature of the column at 75 °C for 4 min, then raising the temperature at a rate of 4 °C/min to 230 °C and maintaining at 230 °C for 20 min, maintaining the temperature of the injection port and of the detector at 270 °C.

Inject about 0.1 µl of the reference solution. When the chromatograms are recorded in the prescribed conditions, the components elute in the order indicated in the composition of the reference solution. Record the retention times of these substances.

The test is not valid unless: the number of theoretical plates is not less than 30 000, calculated from the limonene peak at 110 °C; the resolution between the peaks due to β-pinene and to sabinene is not less than 1.5.

Inject about 0.2 µl of the substance to be examined. Using the retention times determined from the chromatogram obtained with the reference solution, locate the components of the reference solution on the chromatogram obtained with the test solution (disregard the peak due to hexane).

Determine the percentage content of each of these components by the normalisation procedure.

The percentages are within the following ranges:

- *β-pinene*: 7.0 per cent to 17.0 per cent,
- *limonene*: 9.0 per cent to 18.0 per cent,
- *linalol*: 18.0 per cent to 42.0 per cent,
- *linalyl acetate*: 3.0 per cent to 16.0 per cent,
- *α-terpineol*: 2.0 per cent to 7.0 per cent,
- *neryl acetate*: 1.0 per cent to 3.0 per cent,
- *geranyl acetate*: 1.5 per cent to 4.0 per cent,
- *trans-nerolidol*: 1.0 per cent to 9.0 per cent,
- *methyl anthranilate*: 0.1 per cent to 1.0 per cent.

STORAGE

Store in a well-filled, airtight container, protected from light and heat.

01/2005:1858

BLACK HOREHOUND

Ballotae nigrae herba

DEFINITION

Dried flowering tops of *Ballota nigra* L.

Content: minimum 1.5 per cent of total *ortho*-dihydroxycinnamic acid derivatives, expressed as acteoside ($C_{29}H_{36}O_{15}$; M_r 624.6) (dried drug).

CHARACTERS

Macroscopic and microscopic characters described under identification tests A and B.

IDENTIFICATION

A. Stems conspicuously four-angled, longitudinally striated, dark green or reddish-brown and more or less pubescent. Leaves greyish-green, petiolate, lamina ovate to orbicular, 2 cm to 4 cm wide, margin irregularly crenate, cuneate to cordate at the base; both surfaces covered with abundant whitish hairs; venation pinnate, prominent on the lower surface, slightly depressed on the upper. Flowers sessile or very shortly pedicellate, calyx infundibuliform, densely pubescent, with 10 prominent ribs and 5 subequal, broadly ovate teeth; corolla purple, tube slightly shorter than the calyx tube, bilabiate, the upper lip pubescent on the outer surface, the lower lip with 3 lobes, the middle lobe notched.

B. Reduce to a powder (355). The powder is greyish-green and slightly flocculent. Examine under a microscope using *chloral hydrate solution R*. The powder shows numerous long, uniseriate, multicellular covering trichomes consisting of 4 or more cells, thickened and swollen at the junctions, with slightly lignified and pitted walls; fewer glandular trichomes, some with a unicellular or multicellular stalk and a globose, uni- or bicellular head, others with a unicellular stalk and a multicellular head; fragments of the leaf epidermis with sinuous walls, those from the lower epidermis with numerous stomata, some diacytic (*2.8.3*) but the majority anomocytic; epidermis of the corolla composed of polygonal cells, those of the inner epidermis papillose; pollen grains subspherical with 3 pores and a smooth exine; groups of collenchyma and lignified, spirally thickened and bordered pitted vessels, from the stem.

C. Thin-layer chromatography (*2.2.27*).

Test solution. To 2 g of the powdered drug (355) add 100 ml of *methanol R*. Heat on a water-bath under a reflux condenser for 30 min. Allow to cool. Filter. Evaporate the filtrate under reduced pressure until a volume of about 10 ml is obtained.

Reference solution. Dissolve 2.5 mg of *rutin R* and 1 mg of *chlorogenic acid R* in 10 ml of *methanol R*.

Plate: *TLC silica gel plate R*.

Mobile phase: *anhydrous formic acid R, glacial acetic acid R, water R, ethyl acetate R* (7.5:7.5:18:67 *V/V/V/V*).

Application: 20 µl, as bands.

Development: over a path of 15 cm.

Drying: in air.

Detection: spray with a solution containing 10 g/l of *diphenylboric acid aminoethyl ester R* and 50 g/l of *macrogol 400 R* in *methanol R*. Allow to dry in a current of warm air. Examine in ultraviolet light at 365 nm after 30 min.

Results: see below the sequence of the zones present in the chromatogram obtained with the reference solution and the test solution. Furthermore, other fluorescent zones may be present in the chromatogram obtained with the test solution.

Top of the plate	
	A reddish fluorescent zone
	A faint yellow fluorescent zone
	A light blue fluorescent zone (caffeoylmalic acid)
	A greenish-blue fluorescent zone (acteoside)
	A yellow-brown fluorescent zone (luteolin 7-lactate)
Chlorogenic acid: a light blue fluorescent zone	
Rutin: an orange-yellow fluorescent zone	A greenish-blue fluorescent zone (forsythoside B)
	2 greenish-blue fluorescent zones (arenarioside)
	A yellow fluorescent zone (luteolin 7-lactate glucoside).
	A faint greenish-blue fluorescent zone (ballotetroside).
Reference solution	**Test solution**

TESTS

Foreign matter (*2.8.2*): maximum 2 per cent *m/m*.

Loss on drying (*2.2.32*): maximum 12.0 per cent, determined on 1.000 g of the powdered drug (355) in an oven at 100-105 °C for 2 h.

Total ash (*2.4.16*): maximum 13.0 per cent.

ASSAY

Stock solution. Place 1.000 g of the powdered drug (355) in a flask. Add 90 ml of *alcohol (50 per cent V/V) R*. Heat under a reflux condenser on a water-bath for 30 min. Allow to cool and filter collecting the filtrate into a 100 ml volumetric flask. Rinse the flask and the filter with 10 ml of *alcohol (50 per cent V/V) R*. Add the rinsings to the filtrate and dilute to 100.0 ml with *alcohol (50 per cent V/V) R*.

Test solution. In a 10 ml volumetric flask add successively, with shaking after each addition, 1.0 ml of the stock solution, 2 ml of *0.5 M hydrochloric acid*, 2 ml of a solution containing 100 g/l of *sodium nitrite R* and 100 g/l of *sodium molybdate R*, 2 ml of *dilute sodium hydroxide solution R* and dilute to 10.0 ml with *water R*.

Compensation liquid. In a 10 ml volumetric flask, add 1.0 ml of the stock solution, 2 ml of *0.5 M hydrochloric acid*, 2 ml of *dilute sodium hydroxide solution R* and dilute to 10.0 ml with *water R*.

Measure immediately the absorbance (*2.2.25*) of the test solution, by comparison with the compensation liquid at 525 nm.

Calculate the percentage content of total *ortho*-dihydroxycinnamic acid derivatives, calculated as acteoside, from the expression:

$$\frac{A \times 1000}{185 \times m}$$

i.e. taking the specific absorbance of acteoside to be 185 at 525 nm.

A = absorbance of the test solution at 525 nm,

m = mass of the substance to be examined, in grams.

01/2005:0976

BLEOMYCIN SULPHATE

Bleomycini sulfas

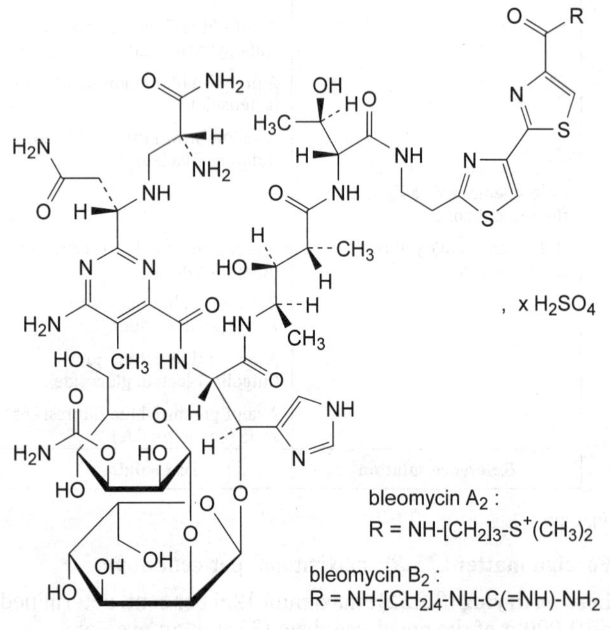

DEFINITION

Bleomycin sulphate is the sulphate of a mixture of glycopeptides produced by *Streptomyces verticillus* or by any other means; the two principal components of the mixture are *N*1-[3-(dimethylsulphonio)propyl]bleomycinamide (bleomycin A_2) and *N*1-4-(guanidobutyl)bleomycinamide (bleomycin B_2). The potency is not less than 1500 IU/mg, calculated with reference to the dried substance.

CHARACTERS

A white or yellowish-white powder, very hygroscopic, very soluble in water, slightly soluble in ethanol, practically insoluble in acetone.

IDENTIFICATION

A. Examine the chromatograms obtained in the test for composition. The retention times and sizes of the two principal peaks in the chromatogram obtained with the test solution are approximately the same as those of the two principal peaks in the chromatogram obtained with reference solution (a).

B. It gives the reactions of sulphates (*2.3.1*).

TESTS

Appearance of solution. Dissolve 0.200 g in *water R* and dilute to 10.0 ml with the same solvent. The solution is clear (*2.2.1*). The absorbance (*2.2.25*) measured at 430 nm is not greater than 0.10.

pH (*2.2.3*). Dissolve 50 mg in *carbon dioxide-free water R* and dilute to 10 ml with the same solvent. The pH of the solution is 4.5 to 6.0.

Composition. Examine by liquid chromatography (*2.2.29*).

Test solution. Dissolve 25.0 mg of the substance to be examined in *water R* and dilute to 50.0 ml with the same solvent.

Reference solution (a). Dissolve 25.0 mg of *bleomycin sulphate CRS* in *water R* and dilute to 50.0 ml with the same solvent.

Reference solution (b). Dilute 1.5 ml of reference solution (a) to 100.0 ml with *water R*.

The chromatographic procedure may be carried out using:

– a stainless steel column 0.25 m long and 4.6 mm in internal diameter packed with *octadecylsilyl silica gel for chromatography R* (7 µm),
– gradient elution at a flow rate of 1.2 ml/min with a mobile phase initially composed of 10 per cent *V/V* of *methanol R* and 90 per cent *V/V* of a mixture prepared as follows: dissolve 0.960 g of *sodium pentanesulphonate R* in 900 ml of acetic acid (4.8 g/l $C_2H_4O_2$), add 1.86 g of *sodium edetate R*, dilute to 1000 ml with the same solvent and adjust to pH 4.3 using *ammonia R*; increasing the proportion of *methanol R* to 40 per cent *V/V* over 60 min and continuing with the final mixture for about 20 min, until demethylbleomycin A_2 is eluted (retention time 1.5 to 2.5, relative to bleomycin A_2),
– as detector a spectrophotometer set at 254 nm,
– a 20 µl loop injector.

Inject reference solution (a). The test is not valid unless the resolution between the two principal peaks is at least 5. Inject reference solution (b). The test is not valid unless the signal-to-noise ratio calculated for the principal peak is at least 20.

Inject reference solution (a) six times. The test is not valid unless the relative standard deviation of the area of the principal peak is at most 2 per cent.

Inject the test solution. The composition, calculated by the normalisation procedure and disregarding any peak with an area less than 0.1 per cent of the total, is: bleomycin A_2 (first principal peak) 55 per cent to 70 per cent; bleomycin B_2 (second principal peak) 25 per cent to 32 per cent; sum of bleomycin A_2 and bleomycin B_2 not less than 85 per cent; demethylbleomycin A_2 (retention time relative to bleomycin A_2 1.5 to 2.5) not more than 5.5 per cent; other related substances not more than 9.5 per cent.

Copper. Not more than 200 ppm of Cu, determined by atomic absorption spectrometry (*2.2.23, Method I*).

Test solution. Dissolve 50 mg in *water R* and dilute to 10.0 ml with the same solvent.

Reference solution. Dilute 1.0 ml of *copper standard solution (10 ppm Cu) R* to 10.0 ml with *water R*.

Measure the absorbance at 324.7 nm using a copper hollow-cathode lamp as source of radiation and an air-acetylene flame.

Loss on drying (*2.2.32*). Not more than 3.0 per cent, determined on 50 mg by drying at 60 °C at a pressure not exceeding 670 Pa for 3 h.

Bacterial endotoxins (*2.6.14*): less than 5 IU/mg, if intended for use in the manufacture of parenteral dosage forms without a further appropriate procedure for the removal of bacterial endotoxins.

ASSAY

Carry out the microbiological assay of antibiotics (*2.7.2*), using the diffusion method. Use *bleomycin sulphate CRS* as the reference substance.

STORAGE

Store in an airtight container, at a temperature of 2 °C to 8 °C. If the substance is sterile, store in a sterile, aritight, tamper-proof container.

LABELLING

The label states, where applicable, that the substance is free from bacterial endotoxins.

IMPURITIES

A. R = OH: bleomycinic acid,

B. R = NH-$[CH_2]_3$-NH-$[CH_2]_4$-NH_2: bleomycin A_5,

C. R = NH-$[CH_2]_4$-NH-C(=NH)-NH-$[CH_2]_4$-NH-C(=NH)-NH_2: bleomycin B_4,

D. R = NH-$[CH_2]_3$-S-CH_3: demethylbleomycin A_2.

01/2005:1605

BOGBEAN LEAF

Menyanthidis trifoliatae folium

DEFINITION

Dried, entire or fragmented leaf of *Menyanthes trifoliata* L.

CHARACTERS

Very bitter and persistant taste.

Macroscopic and microscopic characters described under identification tests A and B.

IDENTIFICATION

A. The leaf is long-petiolated, trifoliate, with long sheaths from the base; the petiole is up to 5 mm in diameter and strongly striated longitudinally. The lamina is divided into equal leaflets, sessile, obovate up to 10 cm long and up to 5 cm wide, with an entire, occasionally sinuous margin with brownish or reddish hydathodes and a spathulate base; it is glabrous, dark green on the upper surface and paler green on the lower surface, with a wide, whitish, finely striated prominent midrib.

B. Reduce to a powder (355). The powder is yellowish-green. Examine under a microscope using *chloral hydrate solution R*. The powder shows fragments of upper epidermis with polyhedral cells and thin wavy walls; fragments of lower epidermis with sinuous walls; anomocytic stomata (*2.8.3*), on both surfaces, with the subsidiary cells showing radiating striations; epidermal cells from the veins straight walled and papillose; fragments of mesophyll parenchyma with large intercellular spaces (aerenchyma); irregular cells with rare sclereids; fragments of spiral or annular vessels.

C. Thin-layer chromatography (*2.2.27*).

Test solution. To 1.0 g of the powdered drug (355) add 10 ml of *methanol R*. Heat, with stirring, in a water-bath at 60 °C for 5 min. Allow to cool and filter. Evaporate to dryness under reduced pressure in a water-bath at 60 °C. Dissolve the residue in 2.0 ml of *methanol R*.

Reference solution. Dissolve 5 mg of *loganin R* in 15 ml of *methanol R*.

Plate: *TLC silica gel plate R*.

Mobile phase: *water R, methanol R, ethyl acetate R* (8:15:77 *V/V/V*).

Application: 30 µl, as bands.

Development: over a path of 15 cm.

Drying: in air.

Detection: spray with *vanillin reagent R*. Heat in an oven at 100-105 °C for 10 min. Examine in daylight.

Results: see below the sequence of the zones present in the chromatograms obtained with the reference and test solutions. Furthermore, other zones are present in the chromatogram obtained with the test solution.

Top of the plate	
	A violet zone
	An intense blue zone
Loganine: a greyish-violet zone	A violet to greyish-violet zone
	A grey to greyish-blue zone
	A brownish zone
Reference solution	**Test solution**

TESTS

Foreign matter (*2.8.2*): it complies with the test for foreign matter.

Loss on drying (*2.2.32*): maximum 10.0 per cent, determined on 1.000 g of the powdered drug (355) by drying in an oven at 100-105 °C for 2 h.

Total ash (*2.4.16*): maximum 10.0 per cent.

Bitterness value (*2.8.15*): minimum 3000.

01/2005:1396

BOLDO LEAF

Boldi folium

DEFINITION

Boldo leaf consists of the whole or fragmented dried leaf of *Peumus boldus* Molina. The whole drug contains not less than 20.0 ml/kg and not more than 40.0 ml/kg and the fragmented drug not less than 15.0 ml/kg of essential oil. It contains not less than 0.1 per cent of total alkaloids, expressed as boldine, ($C_{19}H_{21}NO_4$; M_r 327.4), calculated with reference to the anhydrous drug.

CHARACTERS

Boldo leaf has an aromatic odour especially when rubbed.

It has the microscopic and macroscopic characters described under Identification tests A and B.

Monographs B

IDENTIFICATION

A. The leaf is oval or elliptical usually 5 cm long with a short petiole, an obtuse or slightly emarginate or mucronate apex and an equal and rounded base; the margin is entire and slightly undulate and the thickened edges are more or less revolute. The lamina is greyish-green, thick, tough and brittle. The upper surface is rough with numerous prominent small protuberances and a depressed venation. The lower surface is finely pubescent, with the protuberances less well-marked, and a prominent, pinnate venation.

B. Reduce to a powder (355). The powder is greyish-green. Examine under a microscope, using *chloral hydrate solution R*. The powder shows fragments of the upper epidermis and underlying hypodermis with straight or slightly sinuous thickened and beaded walls, those of the lower epidermis with numerous stomata surrounded by four to seven subsidiary cells; solitary, bifurcated or stellate clustered unicellular covering trichomes with more or less thickened and lignified wall; fragments of the lamina showing a two-layered palisade; debris of the spongy mesophyll including numerous, large rounded oil cells and parenchyma containing fine needle-shaped crystals; thick walled fibres and lignified, pitted parenchymatous cells associated with vascular tissue from the veins.

C. Examine by thin-layer chromatography (*2.2.27*), using a *TLC silica gel plate R*.

Test solution. Add to 0.5 g of the powdered drug (355) a mixture of 1 ml of *dilute hydrochloric acid R* and 20 ml of *water R* and heat on a water-bath under reflux for 10 min. Cool and filter. Add to the filtrate 2 ml of *dilute ammonia R1* and extract with two quantities, each of 20 ml of *ether R* avoiding emulsifying. Combine the organic layers and evaporate the solvent on a water-bath. Dissolve the residue in 1.0 ml of *methanol R*.

Reference solution. Dissolve 2 mg of *boldine R* in 5 ml of *methanol R*.

Apply to the plate as bands 20 μl of the test solution and 10 μl of the reference solution. Develop over a path of 15 cm using a mixture of 10 volumes of *methanol R*, 10 volumes of *diethylamine R* and 80 volumes of *toluene R*. Allow the plate to dry in air. Spray the plate with *potassium iodobismuthate solution R2*. Allow the plate to dry in air for 5 min and then spray the plate with *sodium nitrite solution R*. Examine in daylight. The chromatograms show in the lower third the brown to reddish-brown zone of boldine. The chromatogram obtained with the test solution shows several brownish zones above and below the zone corresponding to boldine.

TESTS

Foreign matter (*2.8.2*). Not more than 4 per cent of twigs and 2 per cent of other foreign matter.

Water (*2.2.13*). Not more than 100 ml/kg determined by distillation of 20.0 g of the powdered drug (355).

Total ash (*2.4.16*). Not more than 13.0 per cent.

ASSAY

Essential oil. Carry out the determination of essential oils in vegetable drugs (*2.8.12*). Use 10.0 g of the freshly crushed drug, a 1000 ml flask and 300 ml of *water R* as the distillation liquid. Distil at a rate of 2 ml/min to 3 ml/min for 3 h.

Alkaloids. Examine by liquid chromatography (*2.2.29*).

Test solution. To 1.000 g (m_1) of the powdered drug (355) add 50 ml of *dilute hydrochloric acid R*. Shake in a water-bath at 80 °C for 30 min. Filter, take up the residue with 50 ml of *dilute hydrochloric acid R* and shake in a water-bath at 80 °C for 30 min. Filter and repeat the operation once on the residue obtained. Filter. Combine the cooled filtrates and shake with 100 ml of a mixture of equal volumes of *ethyl acetate R* and *hexane R*. Adjust the aqueous layer to pH 9.5 with *dilute ammonia R1*. Shake successively with 100 ml, 50 ml and 50 ml of *methylene chloride R* and combine the lower layers and evaporate to dryness under reduced pressure. In a 10.0 ml volumetric flask dilute the residue to 10.0 ml with the mobile phase.

Reference solution. In a 100.0 ml volumetric flask dissolve 12 mg (m_2) of *boldine R* in 100.0 ml of the mobile phase. Dilute 1.0 ml of the solution to 10.0 ml with the mobile phase.

The chromatographic procedure may be carried out using:

– a stainless steel column 0.25 m long and4.6 mm in internal diameter packed with *octadecylsilyl silica gel for chromatography R* (5 μm),

– as mobile phase at a flow rate of 1.5 ml/min a mixture of 16 volumes of solution A and 84 volumes of solution B,

Solution A. Mix 99.8 ml of *acetonitrile R* and 0.2 ml of *diethylamine R*,

Solution B. Mix 99.8 ml of *water R* and 0.2 ml of *diethylamine R*, adjusted to pH 3 with *formic acid R*,

– as detector a spectrophotometer set at 304 nm.

Inject 20 μl of each solution. When the chromatograms are recorded in the prescribed conditions, the retention times relative to boldine are: isoboldine about 0.9; isocorydine *N*-oxide about 1.8; laurotetanine about 2.2; isocorydine about 2.8 and *N*-methyllaurotetanine about 3.2. Additional peaks may be present.

Calculate the percentage content of total alkaloids expressed as boldine from the expression:

$$\frac{\sum A_1 \times m_2}{A_2 \times m_1}$$

m_1 = mass of the substance to be examined, in grams,

m_2 = mass of *boldine R*, in grams,

ΣA_1 = sum of the areas of the peaks due to the six alkaloids identified in the chromatogram obtained with the test solution,

A_2 = area of the peak due to boldine in the chromatogram obtained with the reference solution.

STORAGE

Store protected from light.

01/2005:0013

BORAX

Borax

$Na_2B_4O_7,10H_2O$ M_r 381.4

DEFINITION

Borax contains not less than 99.0 per cent and not more than the equivalent of 103.0 per cent of disodium tetraborate decahydrate.

CHARACTERS

A white, crystalline powder, colourless crystals or crystalline masses, efflorescent, soluble in water, very soluble in boiling water, freely soluble in glycerol.

IDENTIFICATION

A. To 1 ml of solution S (see Tests) add 0.1 ml of *sulphuric acid R* and 5 ml of *methanol R* and ignite. The flame has a green border.

B. To 5 ml of solution S add 0.1 ml of *phenolphthalein solution R*. The solution is red. On the addition of 5 ml of *glycerol (85 per cent) R* the colour disappears.

C. Solution S gives the reactions of sodium (*2.3.1*).

TESTS

Solution S. Dissolve 4.0 g in *carbon dioxide-free water R* prepared from *distilled water R* and dilute to 100 ml with the same solvent.

Appearance of solution. Solution S is clear (*2.2.1*) and colourless (*2.2.2, Method II*).

pH (*2.2.3*). The pH of solution S is 9.0 to 9.6.

Sulphates (*2.4.13*). 15 ml of solution S complies with the limit test for sulphates (50 ppm). Use 1.0 ml of *acetic acid R* instead of the 0.5 ml prescribed. Prepare the standard using a mixture of 3 ml of *sulphate standard solution (10 ppm SO_4) R* and 12 ml of *distilled water R*.

Ammonium (*2.4.1*). 6 ml of solution S diluted to 14 ml with *water R* complies with the limit test for ammonium (10 ppm). Prepare the standard using a mixture of 2.5 ml of *ammonium standard solution (1 ppm NH_4) R* and 7.5 ml of *water R*.

Arsenic (*2.4.2*). 5 ml of solution S complies with limit test A for arsenic (5 ppm).

Calcium (*2.4.3*). 15 ml of solution S complies with the limit test for calcium (100 ppm). Prepare the standard using a mixture of 6 ml of *calcium standard solution (10 ppm Ca) R* and 9 ml of *distilled water R*.

Heavy metals (*2.4.8*). 12 ml of solution S complies with limit test A for heavy metals (25 ppm). Prepare the standard using *lead standard solution (1 ppm Pb) R*.

ASSAY

Dissolve 20 g of *mannitol R* in 100 ml of *water R*, heating if necessary, cool, add 0.5 ml of *phenolphthalein solution R* and neutralise with *0.1 M sodium hydroxide* until a pink colour is obtained. To this solution add 3.00 g of the substance to be examined, heat until dissolution is complete, cool, and titrate with *1 M sodium hydroxide* until the pink colour reappears.

1 ml of *1 M sodium hydroxide* is equivalent to 0.1907 g of $Na_2B_4O_7,10H_2O$.

01/2005:0001

BORIC ACID

Acidum boricum

H_3BO_3 M_r 61.8

DEFINITION

Boric acid contains not less than 99.0 per cent and not more than the equivalent of 100.5 per cent of H_3BO_3.

CHARACTERS

A white, crystalline powder, colourless, shiny plates greasy to the touch, or white crystals, soluble in water and in alcohol, freely soluble in boiling water and in glycerol (85 per cent).

IDENTIFICATION

A. Dissolve 0.1 g by gently heating in 5 ml of *methanol R*, add 0.1 ml of *sulphuric acid R* and ignite the solution. The flame has a green border.

B. Solution S (see Tests) is acid (*2.2.4*).

TESTS

Solution S. Dissolve 3.3 g in 80 ml of boiling *distilled water R*, cool and dilute to 100 ml with *carbon dioxide-free water R* prepared from *distilled water R*.

Appearance of solution. Solution S is clear (*2.2.1*) and colourless (*2.2.2, Method II*).

pH (*2.2.3*). The pH of solution S is 3.8 to 4.8.

Solubility in alcohol. Dissolve 1.0 g in 10 ml of boiling *alcohol R*. The solution is not more opalescent than reference suspension II (*2.2.1*) and is colourless (*2.2.2, Method II*).

Organic matter. It does not darken on progressive heating to dull redness.

Sulphates (*2.4.13*). 10 ml of solution S diluted to 15 ml with *distilled water R* complies with the limit test for sulphates (450 ppm).

Heavy metals (*2.4.8*). 12 ml of solution S complies with limit test A for heavy metals (15 ppm). Prepare the standard using a mixture of 2.5 ml of *lead standard solution (2 ppm Pb) R* and 7.5 ml of *water R*.

ASSAY

Dissolve 1.000 g with heating in 100 ml of *water R* containing 15 g of *mannitol R*. Titrate with *1 M sodium hydroxide*, using 0.5 ml of *phenolphthalein solution R* as indicator, until a pink colour is obtained.

1 ml of *1 M sodium hydroxide* is equivalent to 61.8 mg of H_3BO_3.

01/2005:2113

BOTULINUM TOXIN TYPE A FOR INJECTION

Toxinum botulinicum typum A ad iniectabile

DEFINITION

Botulinum toxin type A for injection is a dried preparation containing purified botulinum neurotoxin type A which may be present in the form of a complex with haemagglutinins and non-toxic proteins. Botulinum neurotoxin type A or its haemagglutinin complex is prepared by a suitable purification process of the liquid supernatant from a broth-culture of a suitable strain of *Clostridium botulinum* type A.

The purified complexes consist of several proteins and can be of various sizes. The largest complex (relative molecular mass of about 900 000) consists of a 150 000 relative molecular mass neurotoxin, a 130 000 relative molecular mass non-toxic protein and various haemagglutinins ranging between relative molecular mass 14 000 and 43 000. The purified toxin moiety is composed of only the same 150 000 relative molecular mass neurotoxin as is found in the 900 000 relative molecular mass neurotoxin complex, which is initially produced as a single chain and further cleaved (nicked) by endogenous proteases into a fully active, disulphide-linked, 54 000 relative molecular mass light chain and a 97 000 relative molecular mass heavy chain.

The preparation is reconstituted before use, as stated on the label.

Monographs B

PRODUCTION

GENERAL PROVISIONS

Production of the toxin is based on seed cultures, managed in a defined seed-lot system in which the ability to produce toxin is conserved. The production method must be shown to yield consistently product of activity and profile comparable to that of lots shown in clinical studies to be of adequate safety and efficacy.

The production method is validated to demonstrate that the product, if tested, would comply with the general test of abnormal toxicity (*2.6.9*) using not less than the maximum human clinical dose, in the presence of a suitable amount of specific botulinum type A antitoxin used for neutralisation.

The production method and stability of the finished product and relevant intermediates are evaluated using the tests below. Such tests include the specific toxin activity per milligram of protein of purified toxin in an appropriate functional model of toxin activity and may be supported by tests confirming the presence of botulinum toxin type A, and, if appropriate, associated non-toxic proteins.

BACTERIAL SEED LOTS

A highly toxigenic strain of *C. botulinum* of known toxin type A and confirmed absence of genes encoding other botulinum toxins (particularly botulinum toxin type B), with known origin and history, is grown using suitable media. The bacterial strain, used for the master seed lot, shall be identified by historical records that include information on its origin and the tests used to characterise the strain. These will include morphological, cultural, biochemical, genetic and serological properties of the strain. The master seed lot and the working seed lot, where applicable, must be demonstrated to have identical profiles. Only a seed lot that complies with the following requirements may be used.

Identification. Each seed lot is identified as containing pure cultures of *C. botulinum* type A bacteria with no extraneous bacterial or fungal contamination.

Microbial purity. Each seed lot complies with the requirements for absence of contaminating micro-organisms. The purity of bacterial cultures is verified by methods of suitable sensitivity. These may include inoculation into suitable media and examination of colony morphology.

Phenotypic parameters. Each seed lot must have a known fatty acid profile, sugar fermentation profile (glucose, lactose, mannose, etc.) and proteolytic activity and must demonstrate relevant lipase, lecithinase and gelatinase activity.

Genetic purity. Each seed lot must have information on the toxin gene sequence and comply with requirements for the absence of other genes encoding other toxin serotypes.

Production of active toxin. A bacterial strain producing a high yield of active toxin, as determined by an acute toxicity assay, is suitable. Seed lots should demonstrate a capability of producing at least a minimum toxicity level appropriate for the manufacturing process and scale.

MANUFACTURER'S REFERENCE PREPARATIONS

During development, reference preparations are established for subsequent verification of batch consistency during production and for control of the bulk purified toxin and finished product. They are derived from representative batches of botulinum toxin type A that are characterised as described under Bulk Purified Toxin.

The reference preparations are suitably characterised for their intended purpose and are stored in suitably sized aliquots under conditions ensuring their suitability.

BULK PURIFIED TOXIN

C. botulinum type A strain is grown anaerobically, in suitable media, from which cultures are selected for step-up incubations under a suitably controlled anaerobic atmosphere through the seed culture and bulk fermentation stages to allow maximum production of toxin. The toxin is purified by suitable methods to remove nucleic acids and components likely to cause adverse reactions.

Only a purified toxin that complies with the following requirements may be used in the preparation of the final bulk. For each test and for each product, limits of acceptance are established and each new purified toxin must comply with these limits.

Residual reagents. Removal of residual reagents used in purification steps is confirmed by suitable limit tests or by validation of the process.

Nucleic acids. Removal of nucleic acids is confirmed by suitable limit tests or by validation of the process.

Immunological identity. The presence of specific type A toxin is confirmed by a suitable immunochemical method (*2.7.1*).

Specific activity. The specific activity is confirmed in a mouse model of toxicity or by *in vivo/ex vivo* methods validated with respect to the LD50 assay and expressed in mouse LD50 units per milligram of protein. Specific activity must not be less than 1×10^8 mouse LD50 units per milligram of protein for the 150 000 relative molecular mass neurotoxin and must not be less than 1×10^7 mouse LD50 units per milligram of protein for the 900 000 relative molecular mass neurotoxin complex.

Protein. The total protein concentration is determined by a suitable method. An acceptable value is established for the product and each batch must be shown to comply with the limits.

Protein profile. Identity and protein composition are determined by polyacrylamide gel electrophoresis (*2.2.31*) under reducing or non-reducing conditions or by other suitable physicochemical methods such as size-exclusion chromatography (*2.2.30*), comparing with suitable reference standards.

Total viable count. It complies with the limits approved for the particular product.

FINAL BULK

The final bulk is prepared by adding approved excipients to the bulk purified toxin. The solution is filtered through a bacteria-retentive filter. If human albumin is added, it complies with the monograph on *Human albumin solution (0255)*.

FINAL LOT

The final bulk is distributed aseptically into sterile, tamper-proof containers. Uniformity of fill is verified during filling and the test for uniformity of content (*2.9.6*) is not required. The containers are closed so as to prevent contamination.

Only a final lot that is within the limits approved for the particular product and is satisfactory with respect to each of the requirements given below under Identification, Tests and Assay may be released for use.

pH (*2.2.3*). The pH of the reconstituted product is within ± 0.5 pH units of the limit approved for the particular product.

Water: not more than the limit approved for the particular product.

IDENTIFICATION

The presence of botulinum toxin type A is confirmed by a suitable immunochemical method (*2.7.1*).

TESTS

Sterility (*2.6.1*). It complies with the test for sterility.

Bacterial endotoxins (*2.6.14*): less than 10 IU per vial.

ASSAY

The potency of the reconstituted product is determined by an LD50 assay in mice or by a method validated with respect to the LD50 assay. The potency is expressed in terms of the LD50 for mice or relative to the reference preparation.

For determination of the LD50, graded doses of the product are injected intraperitoneally into groups of mice and the LD50 is calculated by the usual statistical methods (*5.3*) from the mouse lethality in each group. A suitable reference preparation is assayed in parallel; the potency of the toxin is expressed relative to the reference or the value found for the reference is within suitable limits defined in terms of the assigned potency.

After validation with respect to the LD50 assay (reference method), the product may also be assayed by other methods that are preferable in terms of animal welfare, including 1 of the following:

1. endopeptidase assay *in vitro*;
2. *ex vivo* assay using the mouse phrenic nerve diaphragm;
3. mouse bioassay using paralysis as the end-point.

For these other methods, the potency is calculated with respect to a suitable reference preparation calibrated in mouse LD50 units.

The estimated potency is not less than 80 per cent and not more than 125 per cent of the stated potency. The confidence limits ($P = 0.95$) are not less than 80 per cent and not more than 125 per cent of the estimated potency.

The test may be repeated but when more than 1 test is performed, the results of all valid tests must be combined in the estimate of potency.

LABELLING

The label states:

– the number of units of toxin per vial with a statement that units are product specific and not applicable to other preparations containing botulinum toxin type A,

– the name and the volume of the diluent to be added for reconstitution of a dried product.

01/2005:0879

BROMAZEPAM

Bromazepamum

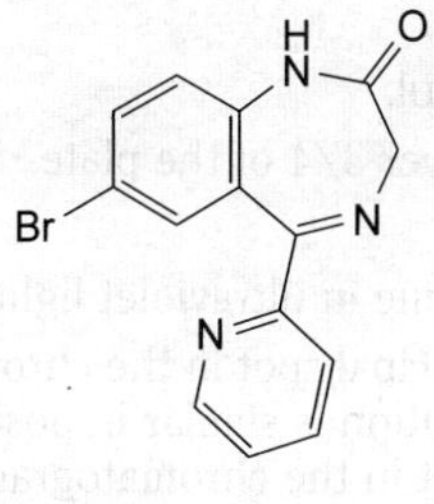

$C_{14}H_{10}BrN_3O$ M_r 316.2

DEFINITION

Bromazepam contains not less than 99.0 per cent and not more than the equivalent of 101.0 per cent of 7-bromo-5-(pyridin-2-yl)-1,3-dihydro-2*H*-1,4-benzodiazepin-2-one, calculated with reference to the dried substance.

CHARACTERS

A white or yellowish, crystalline powder, practically insoluble in water, sparingly soluble in alcohol and in methylene chloride.

IDENTIFICATION

First identification: B.

Second identification: A, C, D, E.

A. Dissolve 50.0 mg in *methanol R* and dilute to 100.0 ml with the same solvent. Dilute 1.0 ml of the solution to 100.0 ml with *methanol R*. Examined between 220 nm and 350 nm (*2.2.25*), the solution shows an absorption maximum at 233 nm and a shoulder at about 260 nm and may show a broad absorption maximum at about 325 nm. The specific absorbance at the maximum at 233 nm is 980 to 1080.

B. Examine by infrared absorption spectrophotometry (*2.2.24*), comparing with the spectrum obtained with *bromazepam CRS*. Examine the substances prepared as discs.

C. Examine by thin-layer chromatography (*2.2.27*), using as the coating substance a suitable silica gel with a fluorescent indicator having an optimal intensity at 254 nm.

Test solution. Dissolve 10 mg of the substance to be examined in a mixture of 1 volume of *methanol R* and 9 volumes of *methylene chloride R* and dilute to 10 ml with the same mixture of solvents.

Reference solution (a). Dissolve 10 mg of *bromazepam CRS* in a mixture of 1 volume of *methanol R* and 9 volumes of *methylene chloride R* and dilute to 10 ml with the same mixture of solvents.

Reference solution (b). Dissolve 10 mg of *bromazepam CRS* and 10 mg of *temazepam CRS* in a mixture of 1 volume of *methanol R* and 9 volumes of *methylene chloride R* and dilute to 10 ml with the same mixture of solvents.

Apply separately to the plate 5 µl of each solution. Develop over a path of 10 cm using a mixture of 30 volumes of *diethylamine R* and 70 volumes of *ether R*. Dry the plate in a current of air and examine in ultraviolet light at 254 nm. The principal spot in the chromatogram obtained with the test solution is similar in position and size to the principal spot in the chromatogram obtained with reference solution (a). The test is not valid unless the chromatogram obtained with reference solution (b) shows two clearly separated principal spots.

D. Dissolve about 20 mg in 5 ml of *methanol R*. Add 5 ml of *water R* and 1 ml of a 10 g/l solution of *ferrous ammonium sulphate R*. A violet colour develops.

E. To 0.15 g in a porcelain crucible add 0.5 g of *anhydrous sodium carbonate R*. Heat over an open flame for 10 min. Allow to cool. Take up the residue in 10 ml of *dilute nitric acid R* and filter. To 1 ml of the filtrate add 1 ml of *water R*. The solution gives reaction (a) of bromides (*2.3.1*).

TESTS

Appearance of solution. Dissolve 0.5 g in a mixture of 1 volume of *methanol R* and 4 volumes of *tetrahydrofuran R* and dilute to 20 ml with the same mixture of solvents. The solution is clear (*2.2.1*).

Related substances. Examine by thin-layer chromatography (*2.2.27*), using *silica gel GF_{254} R* as the coating substance. *Prepare the solutions immediately before use and carry out the test protected from light.*

Test solution. Dissolve 50 mg of the substance to be examined in a mixture of 1 volume of *methanol R* and 9 volumes of *methylene chloride R* and dilute to 5 ml with the same mixture of solvents.

Reference solution. Dilute 1 ml of the test solution to 20 ml with a mixture of 1 volume of *methanol R* and 9 volumes of *methylene chloride R*. Dilute 2 ml of the solution to 50 ml with a mixture of 1 volume of *methanol R* and 9 volumes of *methylene chloride R*.

Apply separately to the plate 5 µl of each solution. Develop over a path of 7.5 cm using a mixture of 5 volumes of *alcohol R*, 5 volumes of *triethylamine R*, 20 volumes of *methylene chloride R* and 70 volumes of *light petroleum R1*. Dry the plate in a current of air for 20 min and examine in ultraviolet light at 254 nm. Any spot in the chromatogram obtained with the test solution, apart from the principal spot, is not more intense than the spot in the chromatogram obtained with the reference solution (0.2 per cent).

Loss on drying (*2.2.32*). Not more than 0.2 per cent, determined on 1.000 g by drying at 80 °C at a pressure not exceeding 2.7 kPa for 4 h.

Sulphated ash (*2.4.14*). Not more than 0.1 per cent, determined on 1.0 g.

ASSAY

Dissolve 0.250 g in 20 ml of *anhydrous acetic acid R*. Add 50 ml of *acetic anhydride R*. Titrate with *0.1 M perchloric acid*, determining the end-point potentiometrically (*2.2.20*).

1 ml of *0.1 M perchloric acid* is equivalent to 31.62 mg of $C_{14}H_{10}BrN_3O$.

STORAGE

Store protected from light.

IMPURITIES

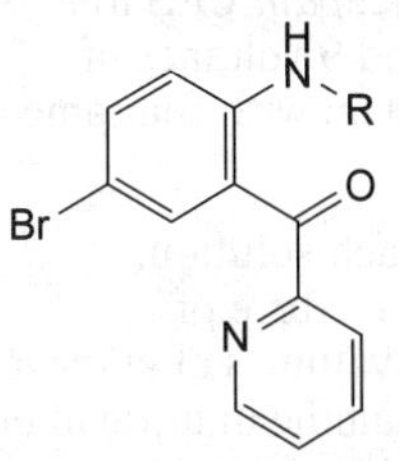

A. R = H: (2-amino-5-bromophenyl)(pyridin-2-yl)methanone,

B. R = CO-CH_2-Cl: *N*-[4-bromo-2-(pyridin-2-ylcarbonyl)phenyl]-2-chloroacetamide,

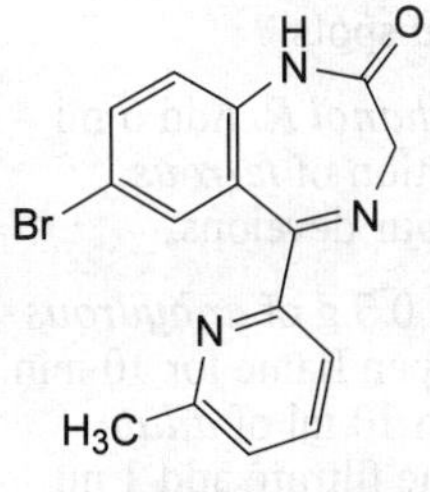

C. 7-bromo-5-(6-methylpyridin-2-yl)-1,3-dihydro-2*H*-1,4-benzodiazepin-2-one,

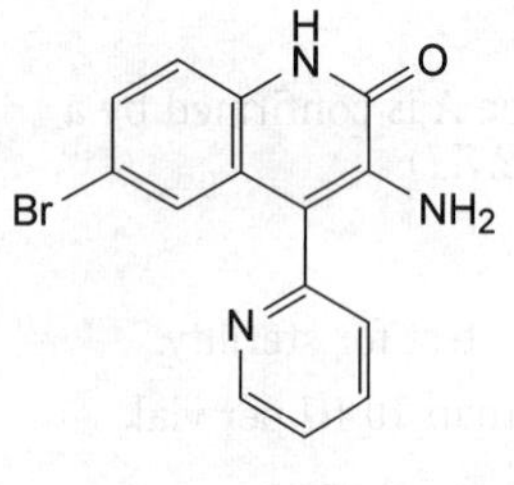

D. 3-amino-6-bromo-4-(pyridin-2-yl)quinolin-2(1*H*)-one.

01/2005:0706

BROMHEXINE HYDROCHLORIDE

Bromhexini hydrochloridum

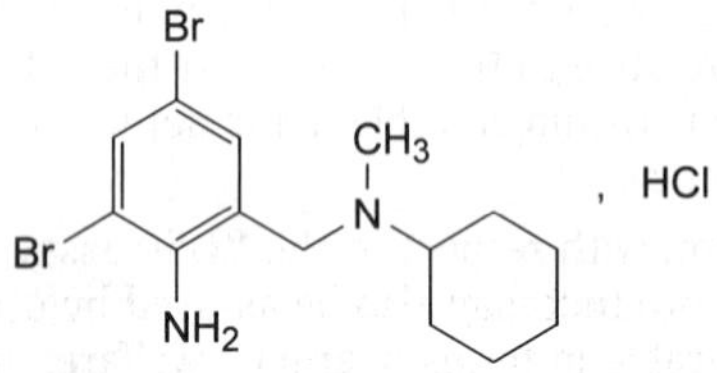

$C_{14}H_{21}Br_2ClN_2$ M_r 412.6

DEFINITION

N-(2-Amino-3,5-dibromobenzyl)-*N*-methylcyclohexanamine hydrochloride.

Content: 98.5 per cent to 101.5 per cent (dried substance).

CHARACTERS

Appearance: white or almost white, crystalline powder.

Solubility: very slightly soluble in water, slightly soluble in alcohol and in methylene chloride.

It shows polymorphism.

IDENTIFICATION

First identification: A, E.

Second identification: B, C, D, E.

A. Infrared absorption spectrophotometry (*2.2.24*).

Comparison: *bromhexine hydrochloride CRS*.

If the spectra obtained in the solid state show differences, dissolve the substance to be examined and the reference substance separately in *methanol R*, evaporate to dryness and record new spectra using the residues.

B. Thin-layer chromatography (*2.2.27*).

Test solution. Dissolve 20 mg of the substance to be examined in *methanol R* and dilute to 10 ml with the same solvent.

Reference solution. Dissolve 20 mg of *bromhexine hydrochloride CRS* in *methanol R* and dilute to 10 ml with the same solvent.

Plate: *TLC silica gel F_{254} plate R.*

Mobile phase: *glacial acetic acid R, water R, butanol R* (17:17:66 *V/V/V*).

Application: 20 µl.

Development: over 3/4 of the plate.

Drying: in air.

Detection: examine in ultraviolet light at 254 nm.

Results: the principal spot in the chromatogram obtained with the test solution is similar in position and size to the principal spot in the chromatogram obtained with the reference solution.

C. Dissolve about 25 mg in a mixture of 1 ml of *dilute sulphuric acid R* and 50 ml of *water R*. Add 2 ml of *methylene chloride R* and 5 ml of *chloramine solution R* and shake. A brownish-yellow colour develops in the lower layer.

D. Dissolve about 1 mg in 3 ml of *0.1 M hydrochloric acid*. The solution gives the reaction of primary aromatic amines (*2.3.1*).

E. Dissolve about 20 mg in 1 ml of *methanol R* and add 1 ml of *water R*. The solution gives reaction (a) of chlorides (*2.3.1*).

TESTS

Appearance of solution. The solution is clear (*2.2.1*) and not more intensely coloured than reference solution Y_6 (*2.2.2, Method II*).

Dissolve 0.6 g in *methanol R* and dilute to 20 ml with the same solvent.

Related substances. Liquid chromatography (*2.2.29*).

Test solution. Dissolve 50 mg of the substance to be examined in *methanol R* and dilute to 10.0 ml with the same solvent.

Reference solution (a). Dissolve 5 mg of *bromhexine impurity C CRS* in *methanol R*, add 1.0 ml of the test solution and dilute to 10.0 ml with the same solvent.

Reference solution (b). Dilute 1.0 ml of the test solution to 100.0 ml with *methanol R*. Dilute 1.0 ml of this solution to 10.0 ml with *methanol R*.

Column:

– *size*: l = 0.12 m, Ø = 4.6 mm,

– *stationary phase*: *end-capped octadecylsilyl silica gel for chromatography R* (3 µm).

Mobile phase: mix 0.50 ml of *phosphoric acid R* in 950 ml of *water R*, adjust to pH 7.0 with *triethylamine R* (about 1.5 ml) and dilute to 1000 ml with *water R*; mix 20 volumes of this solution with 80 volumes of *acetonitrile R*.

Flow rate: 1.0 ml/min.

Detection: spectrophotometer at 248 nm.

Injection: 10 µl.

Run time: 2.5 times the retention time of bromhexine.

Relative retention with reference to bromhexine (retention time = about 11 min): impurity A = about 0.1; impurity B = about 0.2; impurity C = about 0.4; impurity D = about 0.5.

System suitability: reference solution (a):

– *resolution*: minimum 12.0 between the peaks due to impurity C and bromhexine.

Limits:

– *any impurity*: not more than twice the area of the principal peak in the chromatogram obtained with reference solution (b) (0.2 per cent), and not more than 1 such peak has an area greater than the area of the principal peak in the chromatogram obtained with reference solution (b) (0.1 per cent),

– *total*: not more than 3 times the area of the principal peak in the chromatogram obtained with reference solution (b) (0.3 per cent),

– *disregard limit*: 0.5 times the area of the principal peak in the chromatogram obtained with reference solution (b) (0.05 per cent).

Loss on drying (*2.2.32*): maximum 1.0 per cent, determined on 1.000 g by drying in an oven at 100-105 °C.

Sulphated ash (*2.4.14*): maximum 0.1 per cent, determined on 1.0 g.

ASSAY

Dissolve 0.300 g in 70 ml of *alcohol R* and add 1 ml of *0.1 M hydrochloric acid*. Carry out a potentiometric titration (*2.2.20*), using *0.1 M sodium hydroxide*. Read the volume between the 2 points of inflexion.

1 ml of *0.1 M sodium hydroxide* is equivalent to 41.26 mg of $C_{14}H_{21}Br_2ClN_2$.

STORAGE

Protected from light.

IMPURITIES

Specified impurities: *A, B, C, D.*

Other detectable impurities: *E.*

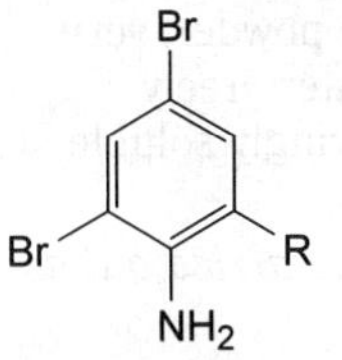

A. R = CH_2OH: (2-amino-3,5-dibromophenyl)methanol,

B. R = CHO: 2-amino-3,5-dibromobenzaldehyde,

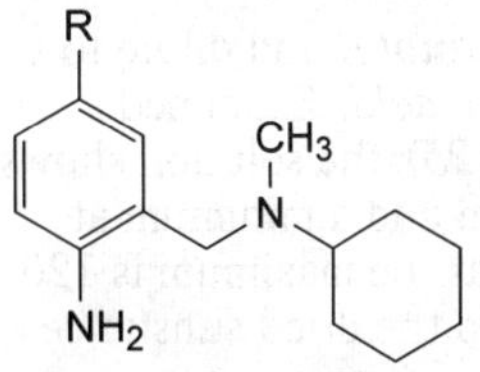

C. R = H: *N*-(2-aminobenzyl)-*N*-methylcyclohexanamine,

D. R = Br: *N*-(2-amino-5-bromobenzyl)-*N*-methylcyclohexanamine,

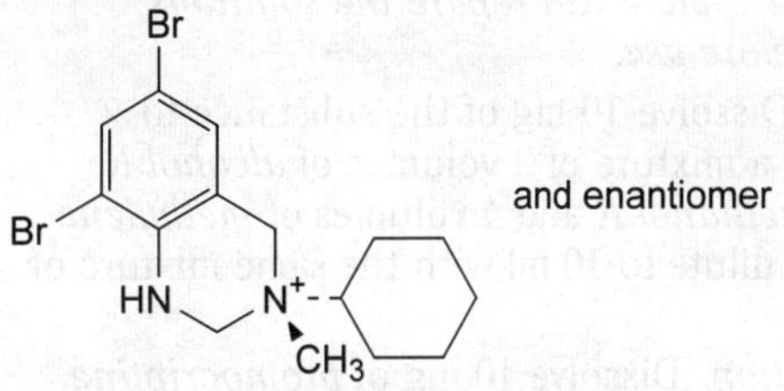

E. (3*RS*)-6,8-dibromo-3-cyclohexyl-3-methyl-1,2,3,4-tetrahydroquinazolin-3-ium.

01/2005:0596

BROMOCRIPTINE MESILATE

Bromocriptini mesilas

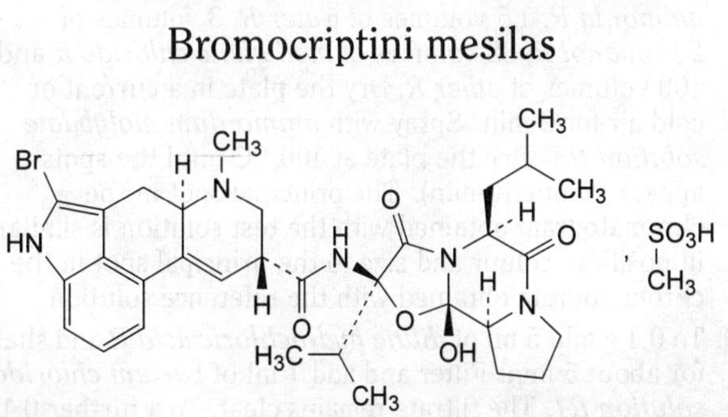

$C_{33}H_{44}BrN_5O_8S$ M_r 751

DEFINITION

Bromocriptine mesilate contains not less than 98.0 per cent and not more than the equivalent of 101.0 per cent of (6a*R*,9*R*)-5-bromo-*N*-[(2*R*,5*S*,10a*S*,10b*S*)-10b-hydroxy-

2-(1-methylethyl)-5-(2-methylpropyl)-3,6-dioxooctahydro-8*H*-oxazolo[3,2-*a*]pyrrolo[2,1-*c*]pyrazin-2-yl]-7-methyl-4,6,6a,7,8,9-hexahydroindolo[4,3-*fg*]quinoline-9-carboxamide monomethanesulphonate, calculated with reference to the dried substance.

PRODUCTION

The production method must be evaluated to determine the potential for formation of alkyl mesilates, which is particularly likely to occur if the reaction medium contains lower alcohols. Where necessary, the production method is validated to demonstrate that alkyl mesilates are not detectable in the final product.

CHARACTERS

A white or slightly coloured, fine crystalline powder, very sensitive to light, practically insoluble in water, freely soluble in methanol, soluble in alcohol, sparingly soluble in methylene chloride.

The identification, tests and assay are to be carried out as rapidly as possible, protected from light.

IDENTIFICATION

First identification: B.

Second identification: A, C, D, E.

A. Dissolve 10.0 mg in 10 ml of *methanol R* and dilute to 200.0 ml with *0.01 M hydrochloric acid.* Examined between 250 nm and 380 nm (*2.2.25*), the solution shows an absorption maximum at 305 nm and a minimum at 270 nm. The specific absorbance at the maximum is 120 to 135, calculated with reference to the dried substance.

B. Examine by infrared absorption spectrophotometry (*2.2.24*), comparing with the spectrum obtained with *bromocriptine mesilate CRS.*

C. Examine by thin-layer chromatography (*2.2.27*), using a *TLC silica gel G plate R. Prepare the solutions immediately before use.*

Test solution. Dissolve 10 mg of the substance to be examined in a mixture of 3 volumes of *alcohol R,* 3 volumes of *methanol R* and 4 volumes of *methylene chloride R* and dilute to 10 ml with the same mixture of solvents.

Reference solution. Dissolve 10 mg of *bromocriptine mesilate CRS* in a mixture of 3 volumes of *alcohol R,* 3 volumes of *methanol R* and 4 volumes of *methylene chloride R* and dilute to 10 ml with the same mixture of solvents.

Apply to the plate 10 µl of each solution. Develop immediately in an unsaturated tank over a path of 15 cm using a mixture of 0.1 volumes of *concentrated ammonia R,* 1.5 volumes of *water R,* 3 volumes of *2-propanol R,* 88 volumes of *methylene chloride R* and 100 volumes of *ether R.* Dry the plate in a current of cold air for 2 min. Spray with *ammonium molybdate solution R3.* Dry the plate at 100 °C until the spots appear (about 10 min). The principal spot in the chromatogram obtained with the test solution is similar in position, colour and size to the principal spot in the chromatogram obtained with the reference solution.

D. To 0.1 g add 5 ml of *dilute hydrochloric acid R* and shake for about 5 min. Filter and add 1 ml of *barium chloride solution R1.* The filtrate remains clear. To a further 0.1 g add 0.5 g of *anhydrous sodium carbonate R,* mix and ignite until a white residue is obtained. Allow to cool and dissolve the residue in 7 ml of *water R* (solution A). Solution A gives reaction (a) of sulphates (*2.3.1*).

E. Solution A obtained in identification test D gives reaction (a) of bromides (*2.3.1*).

TESTS

Appearance of solution. Dissolve 0.25 g in *methanol R* and dilute to 25 ml with the same solvent. The solution is clear (*2.2.1*) and not more intensely coloured than reference solution B_5, BY_5 or Y_5 (*2.2.2, Method II*).

pH (*2.2.3*). Dissolve 0.2 g in a mixture of 2 volumes of *methanol R* and 8 volumes of *carbon dioxide-free water R* and dilute to 20 ml with the same mixture of solvents. The pH of the solution is 3.1 to 3.8.

Specific optical rotation (*2.2.7*). Dissolve 0.100 g in a mixture of equal volumes of *methanol R* and *methylene chloride R* and dilute to 10.0 ml with the same mixture of solvents. The specific optical rotation is + 95 to + 105, calculated with reference to the dried substance.

Related substances. Examine by liquid chromatography (*2.2.29*).

Test solution. Dissolve 0.500 g of the substance to be examined in 5.0 ml of *methanol R* and dilute to 10.0 ml with *buffer solution pH 2.0 R.*

Reference solution (a). Dilute 1.0 ml of the test solution to 100.0 ml with a mixture of equal volumes of *buffer solution pH 2.0 R* and *methanol R.*

Reference solution (b). Dilute 1.0 ml of reference solution (a) to 10.0 ml with a mixture of equal volumes of *buffer solution pH 2.0 R* and *methanol R.*

Reference solution (c). Dissolve 5.0 mg of *bromocriptine impurity A CRS* in a mixture of equal volumes of *buffer solution pH 2.0 R* and *methanol R* and dilute to 5.0 ml with the same mixture of solvents.

Reference solution (d). Dissolve 5.0 mg of *bromocriptine impurity B CRS* in a mixture of equal volumes of *buffer solution pH 2.0 R* and *methanol R* and dilute to 5.0 ml with the same mixture of solvents.

Reference solution (e). Mix 0.5 ml of reference solution (c) and 0.5 ml of reference solution (d) and dilute to 10.0 ml with a mixture of equal volumes of *buffer solution pH 2.0 R* and *methanol R.*

Reference solution (f). Dilute 1.0 ml of reference solution (c) to 100.0 ml with a mixture of equal volumes of *buffer solution pH 2.0 R* and *methanol R.*

The chromatographic procedure may be carried out using:

– a stainless steel column 0.12 m long and 4 mm in internal diameter packed with *octadecylsilyl silica gel for chromatography R* (5 µm),

– as mobile phase at a flow rate of 2 ml/min:

Mobile phase A. A 0.791 g/l solution of *ammonium carbonate R,*

Mobile phase B. Acetonitrile R,

Time (min)	Mobile phase A (per cent *V/V*)	Mobile phase B (per cent *V/V*)	Comment
0 - 30	90 → 40	10 → 60	linear gradient
30 - 45	40	60	isocratic

– as detector a spectrophotometer set at 300 nm.

Inject 20 µl of reference solution (e) and adjust the sensitivity of the system so that the heights of the 2 peaks are about 20 per cent of the full scale of the recorder. The test is not valid unless the resolution between the peaks corresponding to impurity A and impurity B is at least 1.1.

Inject 20 µl of all other solutions. In the chromatogram obtained with the test solution: the area of the peak corresponding to impurity A is not greater than the area of the principal peak in the chromatogram obtained with reference solution (f) (0.02 per cent) and the area of the peak corresponding to impurity C, with a relative retention of about 1.2, is not greater than 4 times the area of the principal peak in the chromatogram obtained with reference solution (b) (0.4 per cent); the area of any peak, apart from the principal peak and the peak corresponding to impurity C, is not greater than twice the area of the principal peak in the chromatogram obtained with reference solution (b) (0.2 per cent) and not more than one such peak has an area greater than the area of the principal peak in the chromatogram obtained with reference solution (b) (0.1 per cent); the sum of the areas of all the peaks, apart from the principal peak, is not greater than 1.5 times the area of the principal peak in the chromatogram obtained with reference solution (a) (1.5 per cent). Disregard any peak, apart from the peak due to impurity A, with an area less than half the area of the principal peak in the chromatogram obtained with reference solution (b) (0.05 per cent).

Loss on drying (*2.2.32*). Not more than 3.0 per cent, determined on 0.500 g by drying *in vacuo* at 80 °C for 5 h.

ASSAY

Dissolve 0.500 g in 80 ml of a mixture of 10 volumes of *anhydrous acetic acid R* and 70 volumes of *acetic anhydride R*. Titrate with *0.1 M perchloric acid,* determining the end-point potentiometrically (*2.2.20*).

1 ml of *0.1 M perchloric acid* is equivalent to 75.1 mg of $C_{33}H_{44}BrN_5O_8S$.

STORAGE

Store in an airtight container, protected from light, at a temperature not exceeding − 15 °C.

IMPURITIES

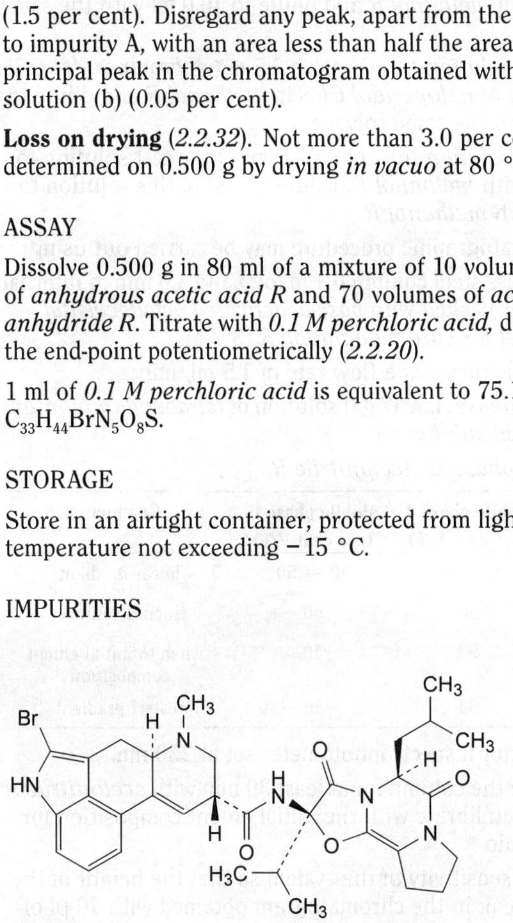

A. (6a*R*,9*R*)-5-bromo-*N*-[(2*R*,5*S*)-2-(1-methylethyl)-5-(2-methylpropyl)-3,6-dioxo-2,3,5,6,9,10-hexahydro-8*H*-oxazolo[3,2-*a*]pyrrolo[2,1-*c*]pyrazin-2-yl]-7-methyl-4,6,6a,7,8,9-hexahydroindolo[4,3-*fg*]quinoline-9-carboxamide (2-bromodehydro-α-ergocriptine),

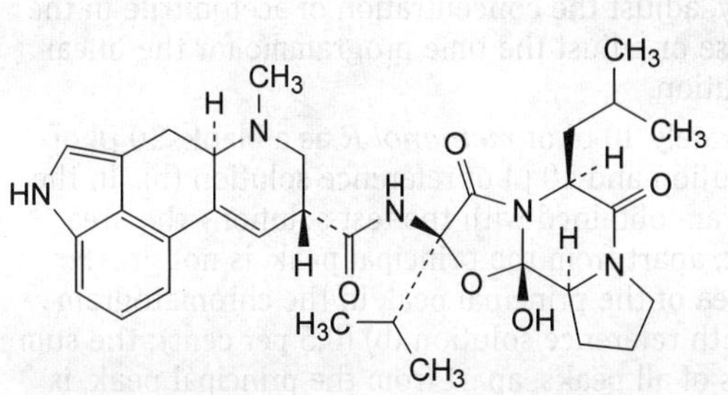

B. (6a*R*,9*R*)-*N*-[(2*R*,5*S*,10a*S*,10b*S*)-10b-hydroxy-2-(1-methylethyl)-5-(2-methylpropyl)-3,6-dioxooctahydro-8*H*-oxazolo[3,2-*a*]pyrrolo[2,1-*c*]pyrazin-2-yl]-7-methyl-4,6,6a,7,8,9-hexahydroindolo[4,3-*fg*]quinoline-9-carboxamide (α-ergocriptine),

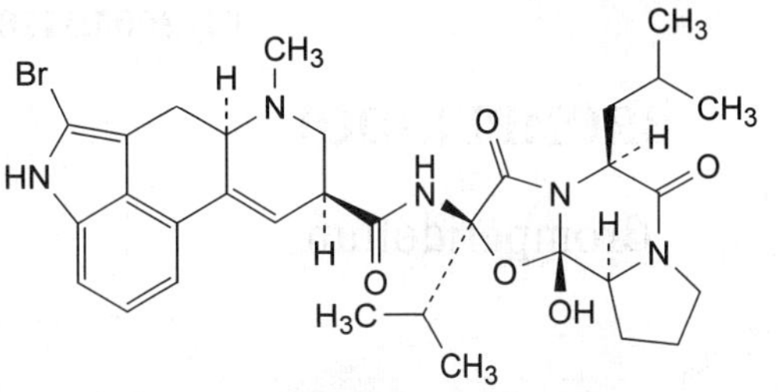

C. (6a*R*,9*S*)-5-bromo-*N*-[(2*R*,5*S*,10a*S*,10b*S*)-10b-hydroxy-2-(1-methylethyl)-5-(2-methylpropyl)-3,6-dioxooctahydro-8*H*-oxazolo[3,2-*a*]pyrrolo[2,1-*c*]pyrazin-2-yl]-7-methyl-4,6,6a,7,8,9-hexahydroindolo[4,3-*fg*]quinoline-9-carboxamide ((9*S*)-2-bromo-α-ergocriptine),

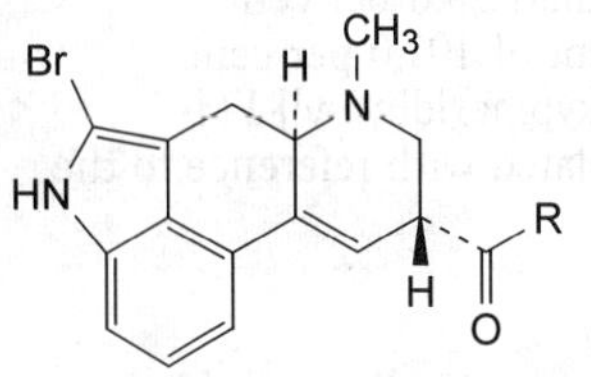

D. R = OH: (6a*R*,9*R*)-5-bromo-7-methyl-4,6,6a,7,8,9-hexahydroindolo[4,3-*fg*]quinoline-9-carboxylic acid,

E. R = NH_2: (6a*R*,9*R*)-5-bromo-7-methyl-4,6,6a,7,8,9-hexahydroindolo[4,3-*fg*]quinoline-9-carboxamide,

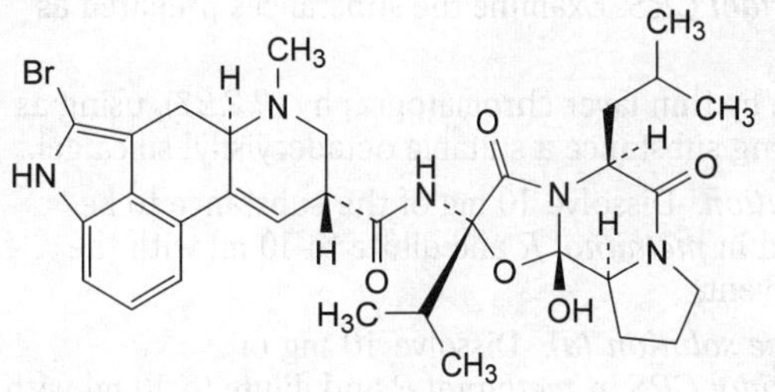

F. (6a*R*,9*R*)-5-bromo-*N*-[(2*S*,5*S*,10a*S*,10b*S*)-10b-hydroxy-2-(1-methylethyl)-5-(2-methylpropyl)-3,6-dioxooctahydro-8*H*-oxazolo[3,2-*a*]pyrrolo[2,1-*c*]pyrazin-2-yl]-7-methyl-4,6,6a,7,8,9-hexahydroindolo[4,3-*fg*]quinoline-9-carboxamide ((2′*S*)-2-bromo-α-ergocriptine),

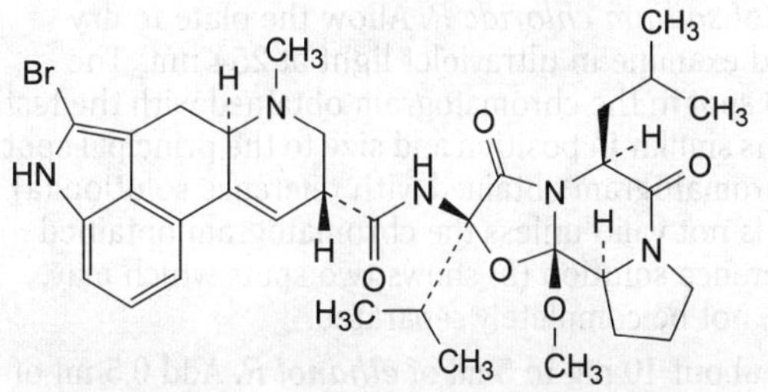

G. (6a*R*,9*R*)-5-bromo-*N*-[(2*R*,5*S*,10a*S*,10b*S*)-10b-methoxy-2-(1-methylethyl)-5-(2-methylpropyl)-3,6-dioxooctahydro-8*H*-oxazolo[3,2-*a*]pyrrolo[2,1-*c*]pyrazin-2-yl]-7-methyl-4,6,6a,7,8,9-hexahydroindolo[4,3-*fg*]quinoline-9-carboxamide (2-bromo-10′b-*O*-methyl-α-ergocriptine).

01/2005:1178

BROMPERIDOL

Bromperidolum

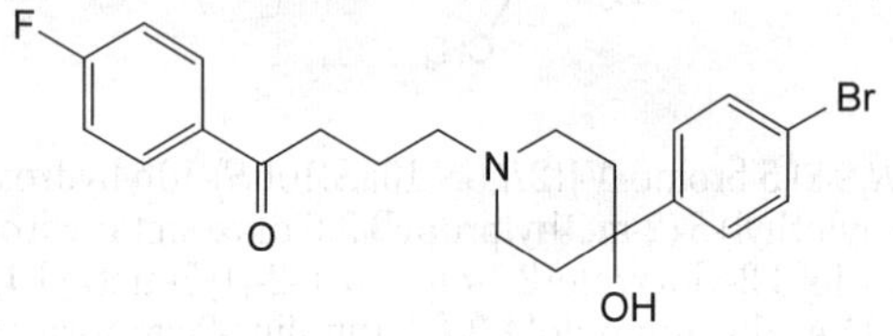

$C_{21}H_{23}BrFNO_2$ M_r 420.3

DEFINITION

Bromperidol contains not less than 99.0 per cent and not more than the equivalent of 101.0 per cent of 4-[4-(4-bromophenyl)-4-hydroxypiperidin-1-yl]-1-(4-fluorophenyl)butan-1-one, calculated with reference to the dried substance.

CHARACTERS

A white or almost white powder, practically insoluble in water, sparingly soluble in methanol and in methylene chloride, slightly soluble in alcohol.

IDENTIFICATION

First identification: B, E.

Second identification: A, C, D, E.

A. Melting point (*2.2.14*): 156 °C to 159 °C.

B. Examine by infrared absorption spectrophotometry (*2.2.24*), comparing with the spectrum obtained with *bromperidol CRS*. Examine the substances prepared as discs.

C. Examine by thin layer chromatography (*2.2.27*), using as the coating substance a suitable octadecylsilyl silica gel.

Test solution. Dissolve 10 mg of the substance to be examined in *methanol R* and dilute to 10 ml with the same solvent.

Reference solution (a). Dissolve 10 mg of *bromperidol CRS* in *methanol R* and dilute to 10 ml with the same solvent.

Reference solution (b). Dissolve 10 mg of *bromperidol CRS* and 10 mg of *haloperidol CRS* in *methanol R* and dilute to 10 ml with the same solvent.

Apply separately to the plate 1 µl of each solution. Develop in an unsaturated tank over a path of 15 cm using a mixture of 10 volumes of *tetrahydrofuran R*, 45 volumes of *methanol R* and 45 volumes of a 58 g/l solution of *sodium chloride R*. Allow the plate to dry in air and examine in ultraviolet light at 254 nm. The principal spot in the chromatogram obtained with the test solution is similar in position and size to the principal spot in the chromatogram obtained with reference solution (a). The test is not valid unless the chromatogram obtained with reference solution (b) shows two spots which may, however, not be completely separated.

D. Dissolve about 10 mg in 5 ml of *ethanol R*. Add 0.5 ml of *dinitrobenzene solution R* and 0.5 ml of *2 M alcoholic potassium hydroxide solution R*. A violet colour is produced that becomes brownish-red after 20 min.

E. To 0.1 g in a porcelain crucible add 0.5 g of *anhydrous sodium carbonate R*. Heat over an open flame for 10 min. Allow to cool. Take up the residue with 5 ml of *dilute nitric acid R* and filter. To 1 ml of the filtrate add 1 ml of *water R*. The solution gives reaction (a) of bromides (*2.3.1*).

TESTS

Appearance of solution. Dissolve 0.2 g in 20 ml of a 1 per cent *V/V* solution of *lactic acid R*. The solution is clear (*2.2.1*) and not more intensely coloured than reference solution Y_7 (*2.2.2, Method II*).

Related substances. Examine by liquid chromatography (*2.2.29*).

Test solution. Dissolve 0.100 g of the substance to be examined in *methanol R* and dilute to 10.0 ml with the same solvent.

Reference solution (a). Dissolve 2.5 mg of *bromperidol CRS* and 5.0 mg of *haloperidol CRS* in *methanol R* and dilute to 50.0 ml with the same solvent.

Reference solution (b). Dilute 5.0 ml of the test solution to 100.0 ml with *methanol R*. Dilute 1.0 ml of this solution to 10.0 ml with *methanol R*.

The chromatographic procedure may be carried out using:

– a stainless steel column 0.1 m long and 4.0 mm in internal diameter packed with *base-deactivated octadecylsilyl silica gel for chromatography R* (3 µm),

– as mobile phase at a flow rate of 1.5 ml/min:

Mobile phase A. A 17 g/l solution of *tetrabutylammonium hydrogen sulphate R*,

Mobile phase B. Acetonitrile R,

Time (min)	Mobile phase A (per cent *V/V*)	Mobile phase B (per cent *V/V*)	Comment
0 - 15	90 → 50	10 → 50	linear gradient
15 - 20	50	50	isocratic elution
20 - 25	90	10	switch to initial eluent composition
25 = 0	90	10	restart gradient

– as detector a spectrophotometer set at 230 nm.

Equilibrate the column for at least 30 min with *acetonitrile R* and then equilibrate with the initial eluent composition for at least 5 min.

Adjust the sensitivity of the system so that the height of the principal peak in the chromatogram obtained with 10 µl of reference solution (b) is at least 50 per cent of the full scale of the recorder.

Inject 10 µl of reference solution (a). When the chromatogram is recorded in the prescribed conditions, the retention times are: haloperidol, about 5.5 min and bromperidol about 6 min. The test is not valid unless the resolution between the peaks due to haloperidol and bromperidol is at least 3.0. If necessary, adjust the concentration of acetonitrile in the mobile phase or adjust the time programme for the linear gradient elution.

Inject separately 10 µl of *methanol R* as a blank, 10 µl of the test solution and 10 µl of reference solution (b). In the chromatogram obtained with the test solution: the area of any peak, apart from the principal peak, is not greater than the area of the principal peak in the chromatogram obtained with reference solution (b) (0.5 per cent); the sum of the areas of all peaks, apart from the principal peak, is not greater than twice the area of the principal peak in the chromatogram obtained with reference solution (b) (1 per cent). Disregard any peak obtained with the blank and any peak with an area less than 0.1 times the area of the principal peak in the chromatogram obtained with reference solution (b).

Loss on drying (*2.2.32*). Not more than 0.5 per cent, determined on 1.000 g by drying in an oven at 100-105 °C.

Sulphated ash (*2.4.14*). Not more than 0.1 per cent, determined on 1.0 g in a platinum crucible.

ASSAY

Dissolve 0.300 g in 50 ml of a mixture of 1 volume of *anhydrous acetic acid R* and 7 volumes of *methyl ethyl ketone R*. Titrate with *0.1 M perchloric acid*, using 0.2 ml of *naphtholbenzein solution R* as indicator.

1 ml of *0.1 M perchloric acid* is equivalent to 42.03 mg of $C_{21}H_{23}BrFNO_2$.

STORAGE

Store protected from light.

IMPURITIES

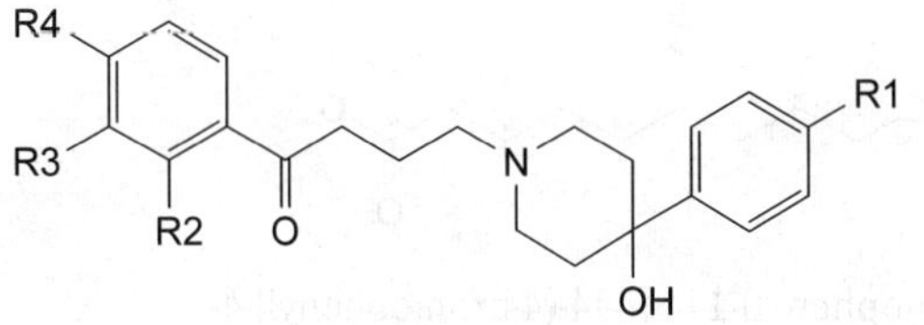

A. R1 = R2 = R3 = H, R4 = F: 1-(4-fluorophenyl)-4-(4-hydroxy-4-phenylpiperidin-1-yl)butan-1-one,

B. R1 = Br, R2 = F, R3 = R4 = H: 4-[4-(4-bromophenyl)-4-hydroxypiperidin-1-yl]-1-(2-fluorophenyl)butan-1-one,

C. R1 = C_6H_5, R2 = R3 = H, R4 = F: 4-[4-(biphenyl-4-yl)-4-hydroxypiperidin-1-yl]-1-(4-fluorophenyl)butan-1-one,

D. R1 = Br, R2 = H, R3 = C_2H_5, R4 = F: 4-[4-(4-bromophenyl)-4-hydroxypiperidin-1-yl]-1-(3-ethyl-4-fluorophenyl)butan-1-one,

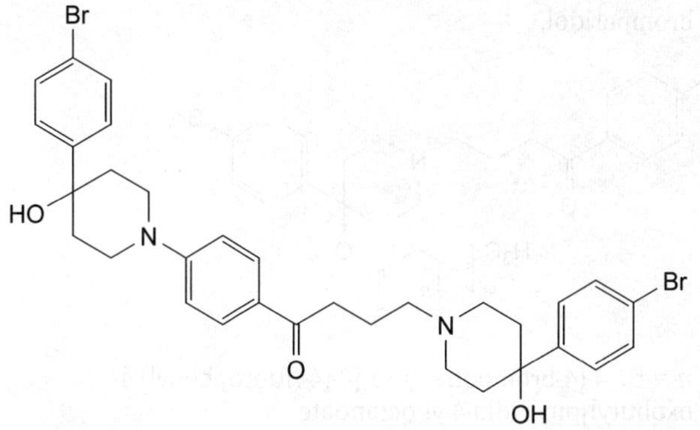

E. 4-[4-(4-bromophenyl)-4-hydroxypiperidin-1-yl]-1-[4-[4-(4-bromophenyl)-4-hydroxypiperidin-1-yl]phenyl]butan-1-one,

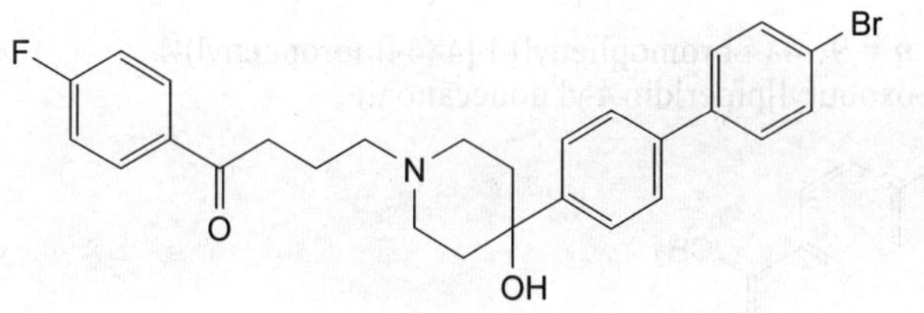

F. 4-[4-(4′-bromobiphenyl-4-yl)-4-hydroxypiperidin-1-yl]-1-(4-fluorophenyl)butan-1-one.

01/2005:1397

BROMPERIDOL DECANOATE

Bromperidoli decanoas

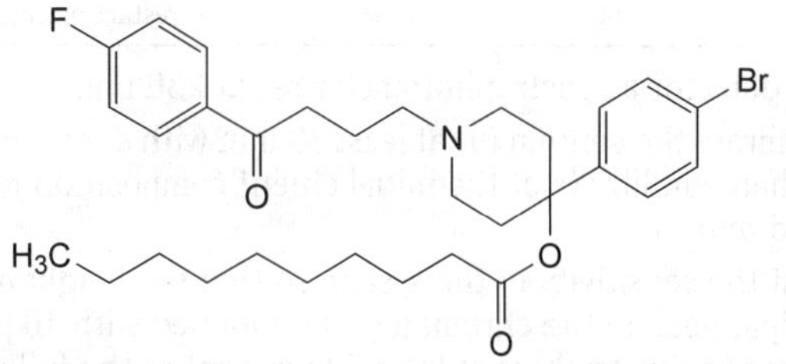

$C_{31}H_{41}BrFNO_3$ M_r 574.6

DEFINITION

Bromperidol decanoate contains not less than 98.5 per cent and not more than the equivalent of 101.0 per cent of 4-(4-bromophenyl)-1-[4-(4-fluorophenyl)-4-oxobutyl]piperidin-4-yl decanoate, calculated with reference to the dried substance.

CHARACTERS

A white or almost white powder, practically insoluble in water, very soluble in methylene chloride, soluble in alcohol.

It melts at about 60 °C.

IDENTIFICATION

A. Examine by infrared absorption spectrophotometry (*2.2.24*), comparing with the spectrum obtained with *bromperidol decanoate CRS*. Examine the substances prepared as mulls in *liquid paraffin R*.

B. To 0.1 g in a porcelain crucible add 0.5 g of *anhydrous sodium carbonate R*. Heat over an open flame for 10 min. Allow to cool. Take up the residue with 5 ml of *dilute nitric acid R* and filter. To 1 ml of the filtrate add 1 ml of *water R*. The solution gives reaction (a) of bromides (*2.3.1*).

TESTS

Appearance of solution. Dissolve 2.0 g in *methylene chloride R* and dilute to 20 ml with the same solvent. The solution is clear (*2.2.1*) and not more intensely coloured than reference solution B_5 (*2.2.2, Method II*).

Related substances. Examine by liquid chromatography (*2.2.29*). *Prepare the solutions immediately before use and protect from light.*

Test solution. Dissolve 0.100 g of the substance to be examined in *methanol R* and dilute to 10.0 ml with the same solvent.

Reference solution (a). Dissolve 2.5 mg of *bromperidol decanoate CRS* and 2.5 mg of *haloperidol decanoate CRS* in *methanol R* and dilute to 50.0 ml with the same solvent.

Reference solution (b). Dilute 5.0 ml of the test solution to 100.0 ml with *methanol R*. Dilute 1.0 ml of this solution to 10.0 ml with *methanol R*.

The chromatographic procedure may be carried out using:

– a stainless steel column 0.1 m long and 4.0 mm in internal diameter packed with *base-deactivated octadecylsilyl silica gel for chromatography R* (3 μm),

– as mobile phase at a flow rate of 1.5 ml/min:

Mobile phase A. A 27 g/l solution of *tetrabutylammonium hydrogen sulphate R*,

Mobile phase B. Acetonitrile R,

Time (min)	Mobile phase A (per cent V/V)	Mobile phase B (per cent V/V)	Comment
0 - 30	80 → 40	20 → 60	linear gradient
30 - 35	40	60	isocratic elution
35 - 40	40 → 80	60 → 20	switch to initial eluent composition
40 = 0	80	20	restart gradient

– as detector a spectrophotometer set at 230 nm.

Equilibrate the column for at least 30 min with *acetonitrile R* and then equilibrate at the initial eluent composition for at least 5 min.

Adjust the sensitivity of the system so that the height of the principal peak in the chromatogram obtained with 10 μl of reference solution (b) is at least 50 per cent of the full scale of the recorder.

Inject 10 μl of reference solution (a). When the chromatogram is recorded in the prescribed conditions, the retention times are: haloperidol decanoate about 24 min; bromperidol decanoate about 24.5 min. The test is not valid unless the resolution between the peaks due to haloperidol decanoate and bromperidol decanoate is at least 1.5. If necessary, adjust the gradient or the time programme for the linear gradient elution.

Inject separately 10 μl of *methanol R* as a blank, 10 μl of the test solution and 10 μl of reference solution (b). In the chromatogram obtained with the test solution: the area of any peak apart from the principal peak, is not greater than the area of the principal peak in the chromatogram obtained with reference solution (b) (0.5 per cent); the sum of the areas of all the peaks apart from the principal peak is not greater than three times the area of the principal peak in the chromatogram obtained with reference solution (b) (1.5 per cent). Disregard any peak due to the blank and any peak with an area less than 0.1 times the area of the principal peak in the chromatogram obtained with reference solution (b).

Loss on drying (*2.2.32*). Not more than 0.5 per cent, determined on 1.000 g by drying *in vacuo* at 30 °C.

Sulphated ash (*2.4.14*). Not more than 0.1 per cent, determined on 1.0 g in a platinum crucible.

ASSAY

Dissolve 0.450 g in 50 ml of a mixture of 1 volume of *anhydrous acetic acid R* and 7 volumes of *methyl ethyl ketone R*. Titrate with *0.1 M perchloric acid* using 0.2 ml of *naphtholbenzein solution R* as indicator.

1 ml of *0.1 M perchloric acid* is equivalent to 57.46 mg of $C_{31}H_{41}BrFNO_3$.

STORAGE

Store at a temperature below 25 °C, protected from light.

IMPURITIES

Specified impurities: A, B, C, D, E, F, G, H, I, J, K.

Other detectable impurities: L.

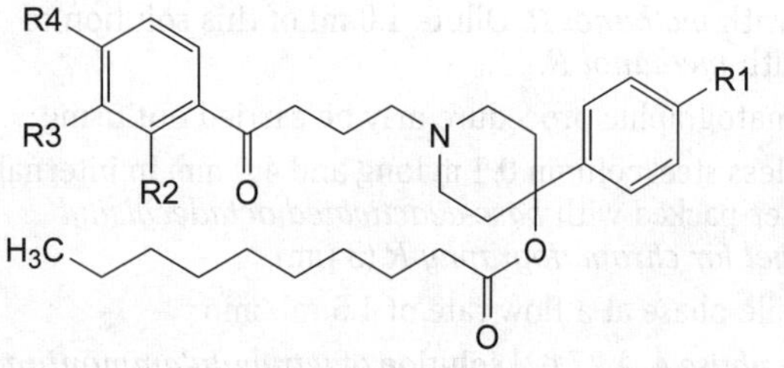

A. R1 = R2 = R3 = H, R4 = F: 1-[4-(4-fluorophenyl)-4-oxobutyl]-4-phenylpiperidin-4-yl decanoate,

B. R1 = Br, R2 = F, R3 = R4 = H: 4-(4-bromophenyl)-1-[4-(2-fluorophenyl)-4-oxobutyl]-piperidin-4-yl decanoate,

C. R1 = Br, R2 = H, R3 = C_2H_5, R4 = F: 4-(4-bromophenyl)-1-[4-(3-ethyl-4-fluorophenyl)-4-oxobutyl]-piperidin-4-yl decanoate,

F. R1 = C_6H_5, R2 = R3 = H, R4 = F: 4-(biphenyl-4-yl)-1-[4-(4-fluorophenyl)-4-oxobutyl]piperidin-4-yl decanoate,

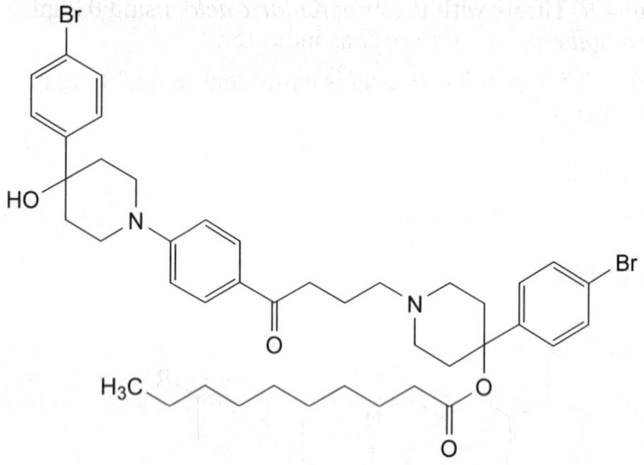

D. 4-(4-bromophenyl)-1-[4-[4-[4-(4-bromophenyl)-4-hydroxypiperidin-1-yl]phenyl]-4-oxobutyl]piperidin-4-yl decanoate,

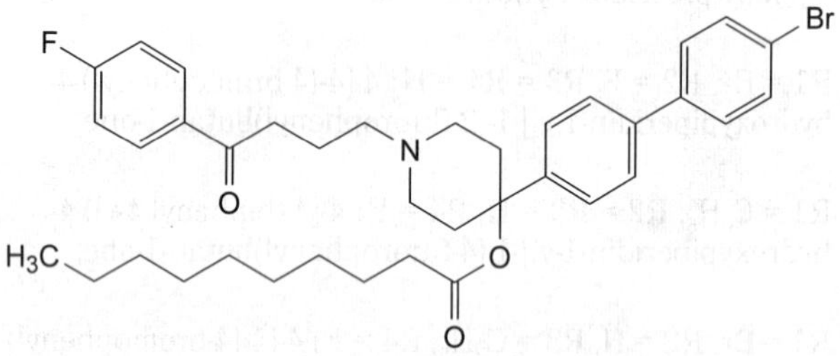

E. 4-(4′-bromobiphenyl-4-yl)-1-[4-(4-fluorophenyl)-4-oxobutyl]piperidin-4-yl decanoate,

G. bromperidol,

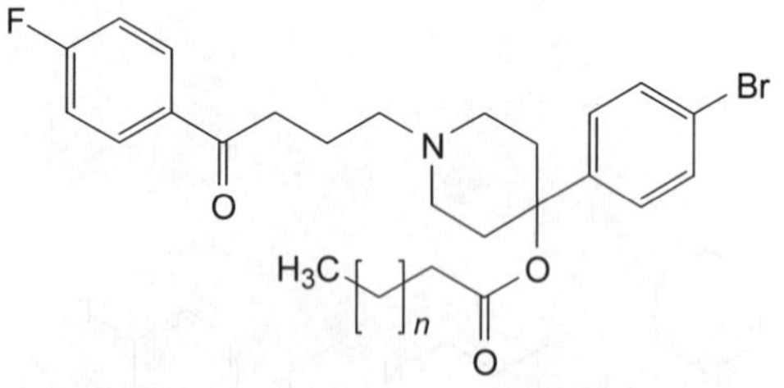

H. *n* = 5: 4-(4-bromophenyl)-1-[4-(4-fluorophenyl)-4-oxobutyl]piperidin-4-yl octanoate,

I. *n* = 6: 4-(4-bromophenyl)-1-[4-(4-fluorophenyl)-4-oxobutyl]piperidin-4-yl nonanoate,

J. *n* = 8: 4-(4-bromophenyl)-1-[4-(4-fluorophenyl)-4-oxobutyl]piperidin-4-yl undecanoate,

K. *n* = 9: 4-(4-bromophenyl)-1-[4-(4-fluorophenyl)-4-oxobutyl]piperidin-4-yl dodecanoate,

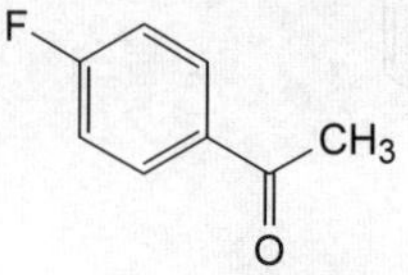

L. 1-(4-fluorophenyl)ethanone.

01/2005:0977

BROMPHENIRAMINE MALEATE

Brompheniramini maleas

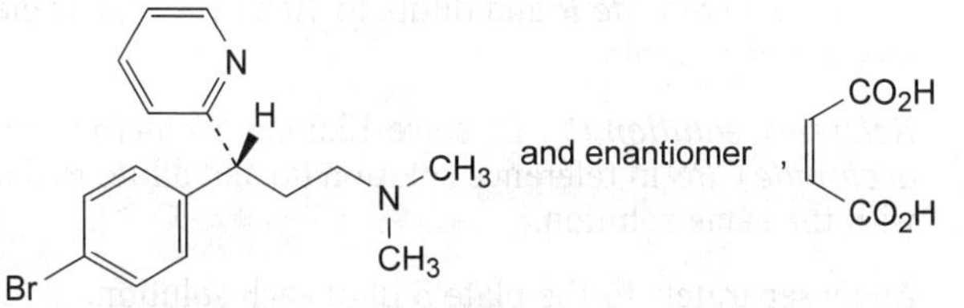

$C_{20}H_{23}BrN_2O_4$ M_r 435.3

DEFINITION

Brompheniramine maleate contains not less than 98.0 per cent and not more than the equivalent of 101.0 per cent of (3*RS*)-3-(4-bromophenyl)-*N*,*N*-dimethyl-3-(pyridin-2-yl)propan-1-amine (*Z*)-butenedioate, calculated with reference to the dried substance.

CHARACTERS

A white or almost white, crystalline powder, soluble in water, freely soluble in alcohol, in methanol and in methylene chloride.

IDENTIFICATION

First identification: A, B, C, D, E.

Second identification: A, B, E, F.

A. Melting point (*2.2.14*): 130 °C to 135 °C.

B. Dissolve 65 mg in *0.1 M hydrochloric acid* and dilute to 100.0 ml with the same acid. Dilute 5.0 ml of this solution to 100.0 ml with *0.1 M hydrochloric acid.* Examined between 220 nm and 320 nm (*2.2.25*), the solution shows an absorption maximum at 265 nm. The specific absorbance at the maximum is 190 to 210.

C. Examine by infrared absorption spectrophotometry (*2.2.24*), comparing with the spectrum obtained with *brompheniramine maleate CRS*. Examine the substances prepared as discs using *potassium bromide R*.

D. Examine the chromatograms obtained in the test for related substances. The retention time and size of the principal peak in the chromatogram obtained with the test solution are approximately the same as those of the principal peak in the chromatogram obtained with reference solution (a). The chromatogram obtained with reference solution (c) shows two principal peaks with retention times corresponding to the retention times of the peaks obtained with reference solutions (a) and (b).

E. Examine by thin-layer chromatography (*2.2.27*), using as the coating substance a suitable silica gel with a fluorescent indicator having an optimal intensity at 254 nm.

Test solution. Dissolve 0.10 g of the substance to be examined in *methanol R* and dilute to 5.0 ml with the same solvent.

Reference solution. Dissolve 56 mg of *maleic acid R* in *methanol R* and dilute to 10 ml with the same solvent.

Apply to the plate 5 µl of each solution. Develop over a path of 12 cm using a mixture of 3 volumes of *water R*, 7 volumes of *anhydrous formic acid R*, 20 volumes of *methanol R* and 70 volumes of *di-isopropyl ether R*. Allow the plate to dry in a current of air for a few minutes and examine in ultraviolet light at 254 nm. The chromatogram obtained with the test solution shows two clearly separated spots. The upper spot is similar in position and size to the spot in the chromatogram obtained with the reference solution.

F. To 0.15 g in a porcelain crucible add 0.5 g of *anhydrous sodium carbonate R*. Heat over an open flame for 10 min. Allow to cool. Take up the residue in 10 ml of *dilute nitric acid R* and filter. To 1 ml of the filtrate add 1 ml of *water R*. The solution gives reaction (a) of bromides (*2.3.1*).

TESTS

Appearance of solution. Dissolve 2.0 g in *methanol R* and dilute to 20 ml with the same solvent. The solution is clear (*2.2.1*) and not more intensely coloured than reference solution BY_6 (*2.2.2, Method II*).

pH (*2.2.3*). Dissolve 0.20 g in 20 ml of *carbon dioxide-free water R*. The pH of the solution is 4.0 to 5.0.

Optical rotation (*2.2.7*). Dissolve 2.5 g in *water R* and dilute to 25.0 ml with the same solvent. The angle of optical rotation measured in a 2 dm tube is − 0.2° to + 0.2°.

Related substances. Examine by gas chromatography (*2.2.28*).

Test solution. Dissolve 0.10 g of the substance to be examined in 10 ml of *methylene chloride R*.

Reference solution (a). Dissolve 10 mg of *brompheniramine maleate CRS* in *methylene chloride R* and dilute to 1 ml with the same solvent.

Reference solution (b). Dissolve 5 mg of *chlorphenamine maleate CRS* in *methylene chloride R* and dilute to 1 ml with the same solvent.

Reference solution (c). To 0.5 ml of the test solution add 0.5 ml of reference solution (b).

The chromatographic procedure may be carried out using:

- a glass column 2.3 m long and 2 mm in internal diameter packed with acid- and base-washed *silanised diatomaceous earth for gas chromatography R* (135-175 µm) impregnated with 3 per cent *m/m* of *polymethylphenylsiloxane R*,
- *nitrogen for chromatography R* as the carrier gas at a flow rate of 20 ml/min,
- a flame-ionisation detector,

maintaining the temperature of the column at 205 °C and that of the injection port and of the detector at 250 °C.

Inject 1 µl of each solution. The test is not valid unless, in the chromatogram obtained with reference solution (c), the resolution between the peaks corresponding to brompheniramine and chlorphenamine is at least 1.5. After injecting the test solution, continue the chromatography for at least 2.5 times the retention time of the principal peak. In the chromatogram obtained with the test solution: the sum of the areas of the peaks, apart from the principal peak, is not greater than 1 per cent of the area of the principal peak; none of the peaks, apart from the principal peak, has an area greater than 0.4 per cent of the area of the principal peak. Disregard any peak with an area less than 0.1 per cent of that of the peak corresponding to brompheniramine in the chromatogram obtained with the test solution.

Heavy metals (*2.4.8*). 1.0 g complies with limit test C for heavy metals (20 ppm). Prepare the standard using 2 ml of *lead standard solution (10 ppm Pb) R*.

Loss on drying (*2.2.32*). Not more than 0.5 per cent, determined on 1.000 g by drying in an oven at 100-105 °C for 3 h.

Sulphated ash (*2.4.14*). Not more than 0.1 per cent, determined on 1.0 g.

ASSAY

Dissolve 0.260 g in 50 ml of *anhydrous acetic acid R*. Titrate with *0.1 M perchloric acid*, determining the end-point potentiometrically (*2.2.20*).

1 ml of *0.1 M perchloric acid* is equivalent to 21.77 mg of $C_{20}H_{23}BrN_2O_4$.

STORAGE

Store protected from light.

IMPURITIES

A. chlorphenamine,

B. dexchlorpheniramine,

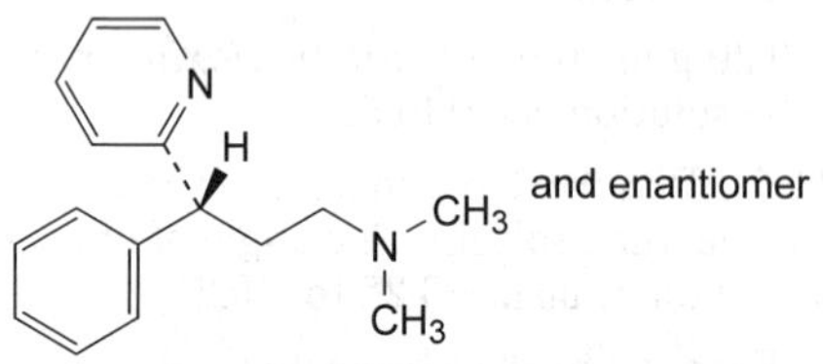

C. (3*RS*)-*N*,*N*-dimethyl-3-phenyl-3-(pyridin-2-yl)propan-1-amine (pheniramine).

01/2005:1075

BUDESONIDE

Budesonidum

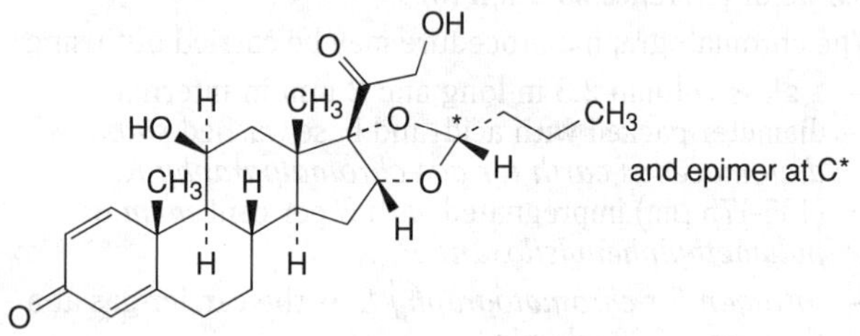

$C_{25}H_{34}O_6$ M_r 430.5

DEFINITION

Budesonide contains not less than 98.0 per cent and not more than the equivalent of 102.0 per cent of a mixture of the C-22*S* (epimer A) and the C-22*R* (epimer B) epimers of 16α,17-[(1*RS*)-butylidenebis(oxy)]-11β,21-dihydroxypregna-1,4-diene-3,20-dione, calculated with reference to the dried substance.

CHARACTERS

A white or almost white, crystalline powder, practically insoluble in water, freely soluble in methylene chloride, sparingly soluble in alcohol.

IDENTIFICATION

First identification: A.

Second identification: B, C, D.

A. Examine by infrared absorption spectrophotometry (*2.2.24*), comparing with the spectrum obtained with *budesonide CRS*. Examine the substances prepared as discs.

B. Examine by thin-layer chromatography (*2.2.27*), using as the coating substance a suitable silica gel with a fluorescent indicator having an optimal intensity at 254 nm.

Test solution. Dissolve 25 mg of the substance to be examined in a mixture of 1 volume of *methanol R* and 9 volumes of *methylene chloride R* and dilute to 10 ml with the same mixture of solvents.

Reference solution (a). Dissolve 25 mg *budesonide CRS* in a mixture of 1 volume of *methanol R* and 9 volumes of *methylene chloride R* and dilute to 10 ml with the same mixture of solvents.

Reference solution (b). Dissolve 12.5 mg *triamcinolone acetonide CRS* in reference solution (a) and dilute to 5 ml with the same solution.

Apply separately to the plate 5 µl of each solution. Prepare the mobile phase by adding a mixture of 1.2 volumes of *water R* and 8 volumes of *methanol R* to a mixture of 15 volumes of *ether R* and 77 volumes of *methylene chloride R*. Develop over a path of 15 cm. Allow the plate to dry in air and examine in ultraviolet light at 254 nm. The principal spot in the chromatogram obtained with the test solution is similar in position and size to the principal spot in the chromatogram obtained with reference solution (a). Spray with *alcoholic solution of sulphuric acid R*. Heat at 120 °C for 10 min or until spots appear. Allow to cool. Examine in daylight and in ultraviolet light at 365 nm. The principal spot in the chromatogram obtained with the test solution is similar in position, colour in daylight, fluorescence in ultraviolet light at 365 nm and size to the principal spot in the chromatogram obtained with the reference solution (a). The test is not valid unless the chromatogram obtained with reference solution (b) shows two clearly separated spots.

C. Dissolve about 2 mg in 2 ml of *sulphuric acid R*. Within 5 min, a yellow colour develops. Within 30 min, the colour changes to brown or reddish-brown. Add cautiously the solution to 10 ml of *water R* and mix. The colour fades and a clear solution remains.

D. Dissolve about 1 mg in 2 ml of a solution containing 2 g of *phosphomolybdic acid R* dissolved in a mixture of 10 ml of *dilute sodium hydroxide solution R*, 15 ml of *water R* and 25 ml of *glacial acetic acid R*. Heat for 5 min on a water-bath. Cool in iced water for 10 min and add 3 ml of *dilute sodium hydroxide solution R*. The solution is blue.

TESTS

Related substances. Examine by liquid chromatography (*2.2.29*) as described under Assay.

Inject 20 µl of reference solution (a). Adjust the sensitivity of the system so that the height of the peak corresponding to epimer B (the first of the two principal peaks) in the chromatogram obtained is not less than 50 per cent of the full scale of the recorder. Inject 20 µl of the test solution, 20 µl of reference solution (a) and 20 µl of reference solution (b). Continue the chromatography for 1.5 times the retention time of epimer B. In the chromatogram obtained with the test solution: the area of any peak, apart from the peaks corresponding to epimer A and epimer B, is not greater than the sum of the areas of the epimer peaks in the chromatogram obtained with reference solution (b) (0.5 per cent); the sum of the areas of any such peaks is not greater than the sum of the areas of the epimer peaks in the chromatogram obtained with reference solution (a) (1.5 per cent). Disregard any peak with an area less than 0.1 times the sum of the areas of the epimer peaks in the chromatogram obtained with reference solution (b).

Epimer A. Examine by liquid chromatography (*2.2.29*) as described under Assay.

Inject 20 µl of the test solution. The content of epimer A (second peak) is 40.0 per cent to 51.0 per cent of the sum of the areas of the two epimer peaks of budesonide.

Methanol. Not more than 0.1 per cent, determined by head-space gas chromatography using the standard addition method (*2.2.28*).

Test solution. Dissolve 2.000 g of the substance to be examined in *dimethylacetamide R* and dilute to 20.0 ml with the same solvent.

Reference solution. Dilute 0.500 g of *methanol R* in *dimethylacetamide R* and dilute to 100.0 ml with the same solvent.

The following head-space conditions may be used:

- equilibration temperature: 80 °C,
- equilibration time: 30 min,
- transfer-line temperature: 85 °C,
- pressurisation time: 10 s,
- injection time: 10 s.

The chromatographic procedure may be carried out using:

- a fused-silica capillary column 30 m long and 0.32 mm in internal diameter coated with *macrogol 20 000 R* (film thickness 1 µm),
- *nitrogen for chromatography R* as the carrier gas at a pressure of 55 kPa,
- a flame-ionisation detector,

maintaining the temperature of the column at 50 °C for 5 min, then raising the temperature at a rate of 30 °C per minute to 220 °C and maintaining at 220 °C for 2 min, and maintaining the temperature of the injection port at 250 °C and that of the detector at 300 °C.

Loss on drying (*2.2.32*). Not more than 0.5 per cent, determined on 1.000 g by drying in an oven at 100 °C to 105 °C.

ASSAY

Examine by liquid chromatography (*2.2.29*). *Protect the solutions from light throughout the assay.*

Test solution. Dissolve 25.0 mg of the substance to be examined in 15 ml of *acetonitrile R* and dilute to 50.0 ml with *phosphate buffer solution pH 3.2 R*. Allow to stand for at least 15 min before use.

Reference solution (a). Dilute 15.0 ml of the test solution to 100.0 ml with the mobile phase. Dilute 1.0 ml of the solution to 10.0 ml with the mobile phase.

Reference solution (b). Dilute 5.0 ml of the test solution to 100.0 ml with the mobile phase. Dilute 1.0 ml of the solution to 10.0 ml with the mobile phase.

Reference solution (c). Dissolve 25.0 mg of *budesonide CRS* in 15 ml of *acetonitrile R* and dilute to 50.0 ml with *phosphate buffer solution pH 3.2 R*.

The chromatographic procedure may be carried out using:

- a stainless steel column 0.12 m long and 4.6 mm in internal diameter packed with *octadecylsilyl silica gel for chromatography R* (5 µm),
- as mobile phase at a flow rate of 1.5 ml/min a mixture of 32 volumes of *acetonitrile R* and 68 volumes of *phosphate buffer solution pH 3.2 R*,
- as detector a spectrophotometer set at 240 nm.

Inject 20 µl of reference solution (c). Adjust the sensitivity of the system so that the height of the peak corresponding to epimer B (the first of the two principal peaks) in the chromatogram obtained is not less than 50 per cent of the full scale of the recorder. When the chromatograms are recorded in the prescribed conditions, the retention time for epimer B is about 16 min. If necessary, adjust the concentration of acetonitrile in the mobile phase (increasing the concentration to decrease the retention time). The test is not valid unless: in the chromatogram obtained with reference solution (c), the resolution between the peaks corresponding to epimer A and epimer B is not less than 1.5; the number of theoretical plates determined from the epimer B peak is at least 4000; the symmetry factor for the same peak is less than 1.5.

Inject 20 µl of reference solution (c) six times. The assay is not valid unless the relative standard deviation of the sum of the peak areas of the two epimers is at most 1.0 per cent. Inject alternatively the test solution and reference solution (c).

Calculate the percentage content of $C_{25}H_{34}O_6$ from the sum of the areas of the two epimer peaks.

IMPURITIES

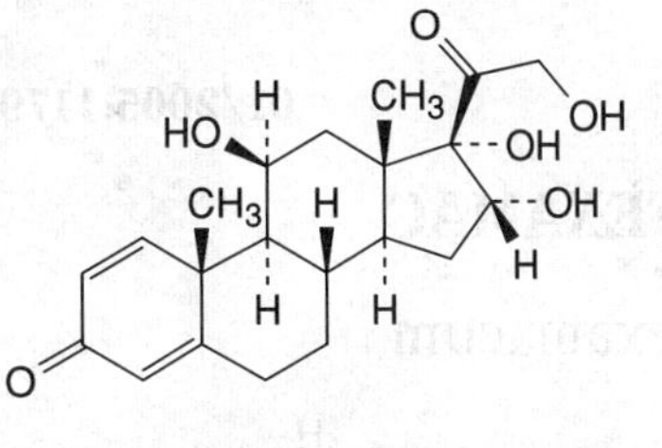

A. 11β,16α,17,21-tetrahydroxypregna-1,4-diene-3,20-dione,

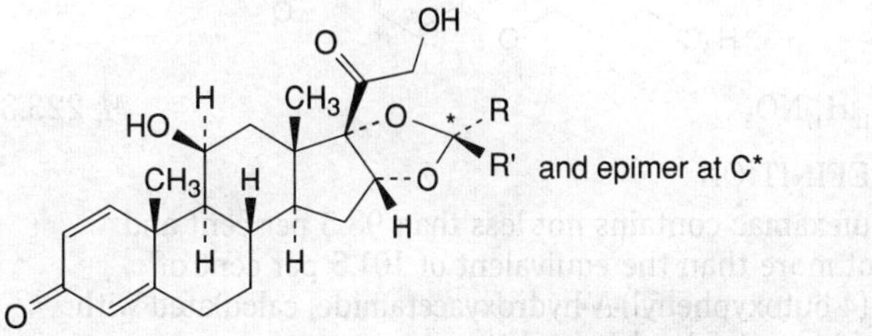

B. R = CH_3, R′ = H: 16α,17-[(1*RS*)-ethylidenebis(oxy)]-11β, 21-dihydroxypregna-1,4-diene-3,20-dione,

F. R = R′ = CH_3: 16α,17-[1-methylethylidenebis(oxy)]-11β, 21-dihydroxypregna-1,4-diene-3,20-dione,

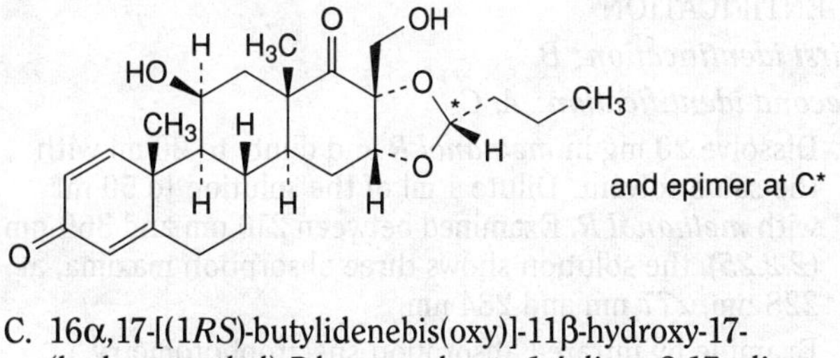

C. 16α,17-[(1*RS*)-butylidenebis(oxy)]-11β-hydroxy-17-(hydroxymethyl)-*D*-homoandrosta-1,4-diene-3,17a-dione,

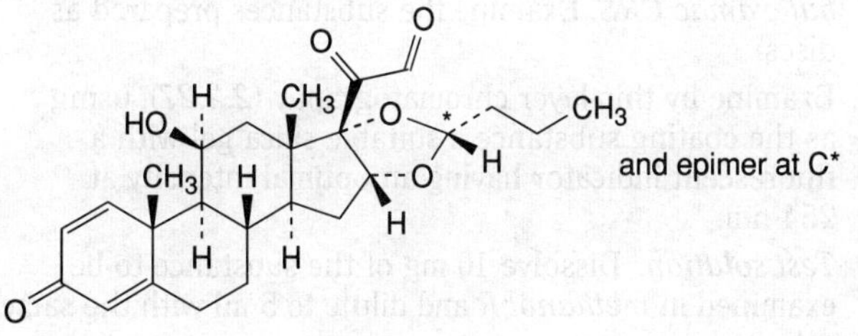

D. 16α,17-[(1*RS*)-butylidenebis(oxy)]-11β-hydroxy-3,20-dioxopregna-1,4-dien-21-al,

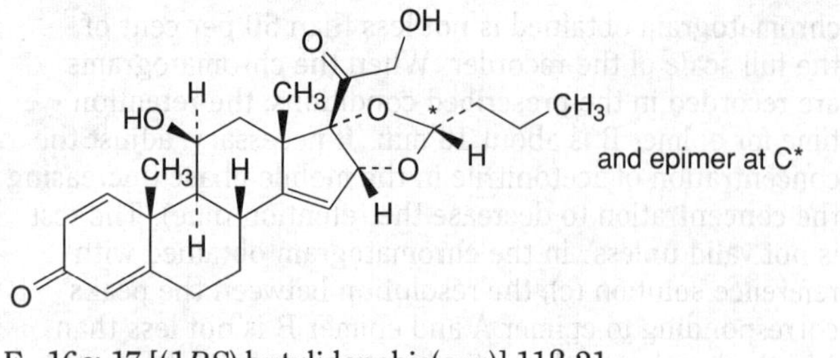

E. 16α,17-[(1*RS*)-butylidenebis(oxy)]-11β,21-dihydroxypregna-1,4,14-triene-3,20-dione,

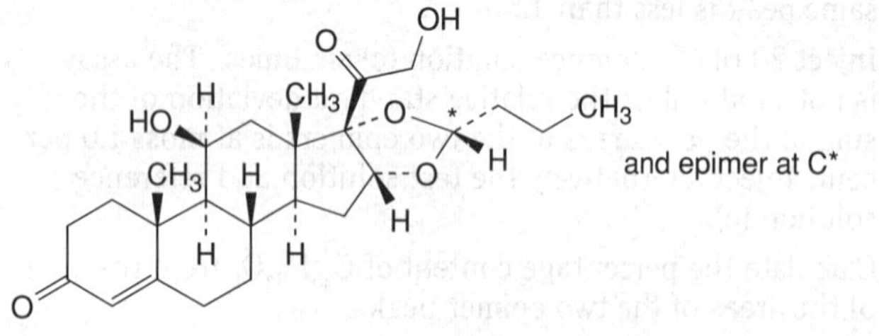

G. 16α,17-[(1*RS*)-butylidenebis(oxy)]-11β,21-dihydroxypregn-4-ene-3,20-dione.

01/2005:1179

BUFEXAMAC

Bufexamacum

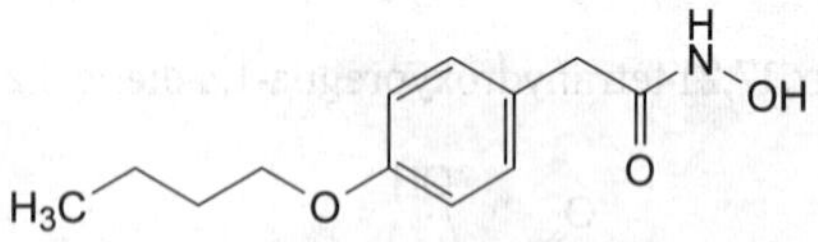

$C_{12}H_{17}NO_3$ M_r 223.3

DEFINITION

Bufexamac contains not less than 98.5 per cent and not more than the equivalent of 101.5 per cent of 2-(4-butoxyphenyl)-*N*-hydroxyacetamide, calculated with reference to the dried substance.

CHARACTERS

A white or almost white, crystalline powder, practically insoluble in water, soluble in dimethylformamide, slightly soluble in ethyl acetate and in methanol.

IDENTIFICATION

First identification: B.

Second identification: A, C.

A. Dissolve 20 mg in *methanol R* and dilute to 20 ml with the same solvent. Dilute 1 ml of the solution to 50 ml with *methanol R*. Examined between 210 nm and 360 nm (*2.2.25*), the solution shows three absorption maxima, at 228 nm, 277 nm and 284 nm.

B. Examine by infrared absorption spectrophotometry (*2.2.24*), comparing with the spectrum obtained with *bufexamac CRS*. Examine the substances prepared as discs.

C. Examine by thin-layer chromatography (*2.2.27*), using as the coating substance a suitable silica gel with a fluorescent indicator having an optimal intensity at 254 nm.

Test solution. Dissolve 10 mg of the substance to be examined in *methanol R* and dilute to 5 ml with the same solvent.

Reference solution (a). Dissolve 20 mg of *bufexamac CRS* in *methanol R* and dilute to 10 ml with the same solvent.

Reference solution (b). Dissolve 10 mg of *salicylic acid R* in reference solution (a) and dilute to 5 ml with the same solution.

Apply to the plate 10 μl of each solution. Develop over a path of 15 cm using a mixture of 4 volumes of *glacial acetic acid R*, 20 volumes of *dioxan R* and 90 volumes of *toluene R*. Dry the plate in a current of warm air and examine in ultraviolet light at 254 nm. The principal spot in the chromatogram obtained with the test solution is similar in position and size to the principal spot in the chromatogram obtained with reference solution (a). The test is not valid unless the chromatogram obtained with reference solution (b) shows two clearly separated spots.

TESTS

Related substances. Examine by liquid chromatography (*2.2.29*).

Test solution. Dissolve 50.0 mg of the substance to be examined in the mobile phase and dilute to 20.0 ml with the same solvent.

Reference solution (a). Dilute 5.0 ml of the test solution to 25.0 ml with the mobile phase. Dilute 1.0 ml of the solution to 100.0 ml with the mobile phase.

Reference solution (b). Dissolve 5 mg of *bufexamac CRS* and 5 mg of *salicylic acid R* in the mobile phase and dilute to 10 ml with the mobile phase. Dilute 1 ml of the solution to 10 ml with the mobile phase.

The chromatographic procedure may be carried out using:

- a stainless steel column 0.25 m long and 4.6 mm in internal diameter packed with *octadecylsilyl silica gel for chromatography R* (5 μm) having a specific surface area of 350 m^2/g and a pore size of 10 nm,
- as mobile phase at a flow rate of 1 ml/min a mixture of 30 volumes of a 1.4 g/l solution of *dipotassium hydrogen phosphate R* and 70 volumes of *methanol R* adjusted to pH 3.6 with *dilute phosphoric acid R*,
- as detector a spectrophotometer set at 275 nm.

Inject 20 μl of reference solution (a) and 20 μl of reference solution (b). Adjust the sensitivity of the system so that the height of the principal peak in the chromatogram obtained with reference solution (a) is at least 50 per cent of the full scale of the recorder. The test is not valid unless in the chromatogram obtained with reference solution (b) the resolution between the peaks corresponding to salicylic acid and to bufexamac is at least 2.0.

Inject 20 μl of the test solution. Continue the chromatography for four times the retention time of bufexamac. In the chromatogram obtained with the test solution: the area of any peak, apart from the principal peak is not greater than the area of the principal peak in the chromatogram obtained with reference solution (a) (0.2 per cent); the sum of the areas of all the peaks, apart from the principal peak, is not greater than 2.5 times the area of the principal peak in the chromatogram obtained with reference solution (a) (0.5 per cent). Disregard any peak due to the solvent and any peak with an area less than 0.05 times that of the principal peak in the chromatogram obtained with reference solution (a).

Loss on drying (*2.2.32*). Not more than 0.5 per cent, determined on 1.000 g by drying *in vacuo* at 80 °C for 3 h.

Sulphated ash (*2.4.14*). Not more than 0.1 per cent, determined on 1.0 g.

ASSAY

Dissolve 0.200 g in 50 ml of *dimethylformamide R*. Titrate with *0.1 M lithium methoxide*, determining the end-point potentiometrically (*2.2.20*).

1 ml of *0.1 M lithium methoxide* is equivalent to 22.33 mg of $C_{12}H_{17}NO_3$.

STORAGE

Store protected from light.

IMPURITIES

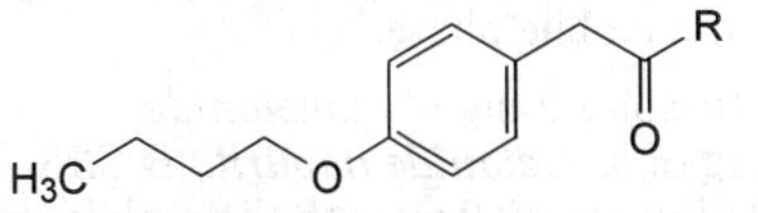

A. R = OH: 2-(4-butoxyphenyl)acetic acid,

B. R = OCH_3: methyl 2-(4-butoxyphenyl)acetate,

C. R = OC_4H_9: butyl 2-(4-butoxyphenyl)acetate,

D. R = NH_2: 2-(4-butoxyphenyl)acetamide.

01/2005:1398

BUFLOMEDIL HYDROCHLORIDE

Buflomedili hydrochloridum

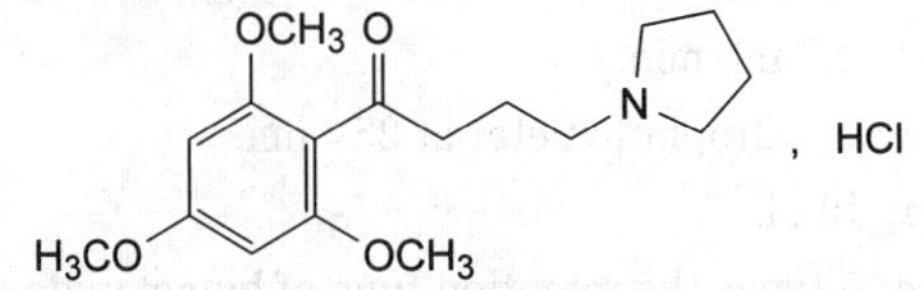

$C_{17}H_{26}ClNO_4$ M_r 343.9

DEFINITION

4-(Pyrrolidin-1-yl)-1-(2,4,6-trimethoxyphenyl)butan-1-one hydrochloride.

Content: 98.5 per cent to 101.5 per cent (dried substance).

CHARACTERS

Appearance: white or almost white, microcrystalline powder.

Solubility: freely soluble in water, soluble in alcohol, very slightly soluble in acetone.

mp: about 195 °C, with decomposition.

IDENTIFICATION

First identification: B, D.

Second identification: A, C, D.

A. Dissolve 25.0 mg in *alcohol R* and dilute to 50.0 ml with the same solvent. Dilute 2.0 ml to 20.0 ml with *alcohol R*. Examined between 220 nm and 350 nm (*2.2.25*), the solution shows an absorption maximum at 275 nm. The specific absorbance at the maximum is 143 to 149.

B. Infrared absorption spectrophotometry (*2.2.24*).

Preparation: discs.

Comparison: *buflomedil hydrochloride CRS*.

C. Thin-layer chromatography (*2.2.27*).

Test solution. Dissolve 40 mg of the substance to be examined in *methanol R* and dilute to 2 ml with the same solvent.

Reference solution. Dissolve 40 mg of *buflomedil hydrochloride CRS* in *methanol R* and dilute to 2 ml with the same solvent.

Plate: *TLC silica gel F_{254} plate R.*

Mobile phase: *triethylamine R, 2-propanol R, toluene R* (5:50:50 *V/V/V*).

Application: 10 µl.

Development: over a path of 15 cm.

Drying: in air.

Detection: examine in ultraviolet light at 254 nm.

Results: the principal spot in the chromatogram obtained with the test solution is similar in position and size to the principal spot in the chromatogram obtained with the reference solution.

D. It gives reaction (a) of chlorides (*2.3.1*).

TESTS

Solution S. Dissolve 2.5 g in *carbon dioxide-free water R* and dilute to 50 ml with the same solvent.

Appearance of solution. Solution S is clear (*2.2.1*) and colourless (*2.2.2, Method II*).

pH (*2.2.3*): 5.0 to 6.5 for solution S.

Related substances. Liquid chromatography (*2.2.29*).

Test solution. Dissolve 0.10 g of the substance to be examined in the mobile phase and dilute to 10.0 ml with the mobile phase.

Reference solution (a). Dilute 0.5 ml of the test solution to 100.0 ml with the mobile phase. Dilute 5.0 ml of this solution to 10.0 ml with the mobile phase.

Reference solution (b). Dissolve 2 mg of *buflomedil impurity B CRS* in the mobile phase. Add 0.5 ml of the test solution and dilute to 100 ml with the mobile phase.

Column:

- *size*: *l* = 0.25 m, Ø = 4.6 mm,
- *stationary phase*: *end-capped octadecylsilyl silica gel for chromatography R* (5 µm),
- *temperature*: 40 °C.

Mobile phase: mix 45 volumes of *acetonitrile R* and 55 volumes of a 9.25 g/l solution of *potassium dihydrogen phosphate R* adjusted to pH 2.5 with *phosphoric acid R*.

Flow rate: 1 ml/min.

Detection: spectrophotometer at 210 nm.

Injection: 10 µl.

Run time: twice the retention time of buflomedil.

Retention time: buflomedil = about 5 min.

System suitability: reference solution (b):

- *resolution*: minimum 5.0 between the peaks due to buflomedil and impurity B.

Limits:

- *any impurity*: not more than the area of the principal peak in the chromatogram obtained with reference solution (a) (0.25 per cent),
- *total*: not more than twice the area of the principal peak in the chromatogram obtained with reference solution (a) (0.5 per cent),
- *disregard limit*: 0.2 times the area of the principal peak in the chromatogram obtained with reference solution (a) (0.05 per cent).

Heavy metals (*2.4.8*): maximum 10 ppm.

2.0 g complies with limit test C. Prepare the standard using 2 ml of *lead standard solution (10 ppm Pb) R*.

Loss on drying (*2.2.32*): maximum 0.5 per cent, determined on 1.000 g by drying in an oven at 100-105 °C for 2 h.

Sulphated ash (*2.4.14*): maximum 0.1 per cent, determined on 1.0 g.

ASSAY

Dissolve 0.300 g in 15 ml of *anhydrous acetic acid R* and add 35 ml of *acetic anhydride R*. Titrate with *0.1 M perchloric acid*, determining the end-point potentiometrically (*2.2.20*).

1 ml of *0.1 M perchloric acid* is equivalent to 34.39 mg of $C_{17}H_{26}ClNO_4$.

IMPURITIES

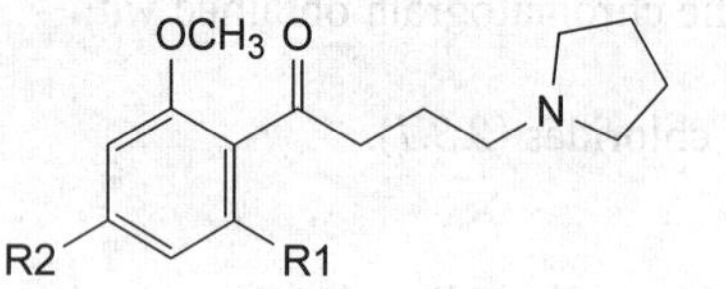

A. R1 = OH, R2 = OCH_3: 4-(pyrrolidin-1-yl)-1-(2-hydroxy-4,6-dimethoxyphenyl)butan-1-one,

B. R1 = OCH_3, R2 = OH: 4-(pyrrolidin-1-yl)-1-(4-hydroxy-2,6-dimethoxyphenyl)butan-1-one,

C. R1 = R2 = OH: 4-(pyrrolidin-1-yl)-1-(2,4-dihydroxy-6-methoxyphenyl)butan-1-one.

01/2005:1076

BUMETANIDE

Bumetanidum

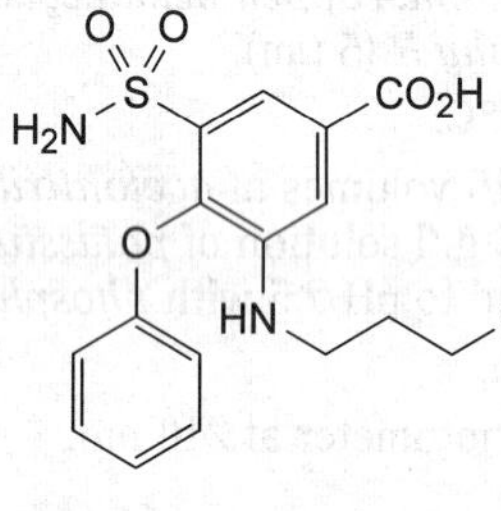

$C_{17}H_{20}N_2O_5S$ M_r 364.4

DEFINITION

3-(Butylamino)-4-phenoxy-5-sulphamoylbenzoic acid.

Content: 99.0 per cent to 101.0 per cent (dried substance).

CHARACTERS

Appearance: white, crystalline powder.

Solubility: practically insoluble in water, soluble in acetone and in alcohol, slightly soluble in methylene chloride. It dissolves in dilute solutions of alkali hydroxides.

It shows polymorphism.

mp: about 233 °C.

IDENTIFICATION

Infrared absorption spectrophotometry (*2.2.24*).

Comparison: *bumetanide CRS*.

If the spectra obtained in the solid state show differences, dissolve the substance to be examined and the reference substance separately in *acetone R*, evaporate to dryness and record new spectra using the residues.

TESTS

Appearance of solution. The solution is clear (*2.2.1*) and colourless (*2.2.2, Method II*).

Dissolve 0.1 g in a 6 g/l solution of *potassium hydroxide R* and dilute to 20 ml with the same solution.

Related substances. Liquid chromatography (*2.2.29*).

Test solution. Dissolve 50 mg of the substance to be examined in the mobile phase and dilute to 25.0 ml with the mobile phase.

Reference solution (a). Dilute 1.0 ml of the test solution to 100.0 ml with the mobile phase. Dilute 1.0 ml of this solution to 10.0 ml with the mobile phase.

Reference solution (b). Dissolve 2 mg of *bumetanide impurity A CRS* and 2 mg of *bumetanide impurity B CRS* in the mobile phase and dilute to 10.0 ml with the mobile phase. Dilute 1.0 ml of this solution to 100.0 ml with the mobile phase.

Column:

- *size*: l = 0.15 m, Ø = 4.6 mm,
- *stationary phase*: *end-capped octylsilyl silica gel for chromatography R* (3.5 μm).

Mobile phase: mix 70 volumes of *methanol R*, 25 volumes of *water for chromatography R* and 5 volumes of a 27.2 g/l solution of *potassium dihydrogen phosphate R* previously adjusted to pH 7.0 with a 280 g/l solution of *potassium hydroxide R*; add *tetrahexylammonium bromide R* to this mixture to obtain a concentration of 2.17 g/l.

Flow rate: 1.0 ml/min.

Detection: spectrophotometer at 254 nm.

Injection: 10 μl.

Run time: 5 times the retention time of bumetanide.

Relative retention with reference to bumetanide (retention time = about 6 min): impurity B = about 0.4; impurity A = about 0.6; impurity D = about 2.5; impurity C = about 4.4.

System suitability: reference solution (b):

- *resolution*: minimum 2.0 between the peaks due to impurity A and impurity B.

Limits:

- *impurities A, B, C, D*: for each impurity, not more than the area of the principal peak in the chromatogram obtained with reference solution (a) (0.1 per cent),
- *other impurities*: for each impurity, not more than the area of the principal peak in the chromatogram obtained with reference solution (a) (0.1 per cent),
- *total*: not more than twice the area of the principal peak in the chromatogram obtained with reference solution (a) (0.2 per cent),
- *disregard limit*: 0.5 times the area of the principal peak in the chromatogram obtained with reference solution (a) (0.05 per cent).

Loss on drying (*2.2.32*): maximum 0.5 per cent, determined on 1.000 g by drying in an oven at 100-105 °C for 4 h.

Sulphated ash (*2.4.14*): maximum 0.1 per cent, determined on 1.0 g.

ASSAY

Dissolve 0.300 g in 50 ml of *alcohol R*. Add 0.1 ml of *phenol red solution R*. Titrate with *0.1 M sodium hydroxide* until a violet-red colour is obtained. Carry out a blank titration.

1 ml of *0.1 M sodium hydroxide* is equivalent to 36.44 mg of $C_{17}H_{20}N_2O_5S$.

STORAGE

Protected from light.

IMPURITIES

Specified impurities: A, B, C, D.

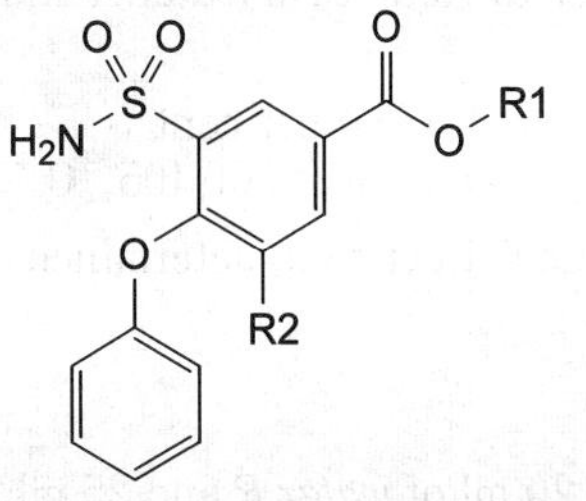

A. R1 = H, R2 = NO_2: 3-nitro-4-phenoxy-5-sulphamoylbenzoic acid,

B. R1 = H, R2 = NH_2: 3-amino-4-phenoxy-5-sulphamoylbenzoic acid,

C. R1 = C_4H_9, R2 = NH-C_4H_9: butyl 3-(butylamino)-4-phenoxy-5-sulphamoylbenzoate,

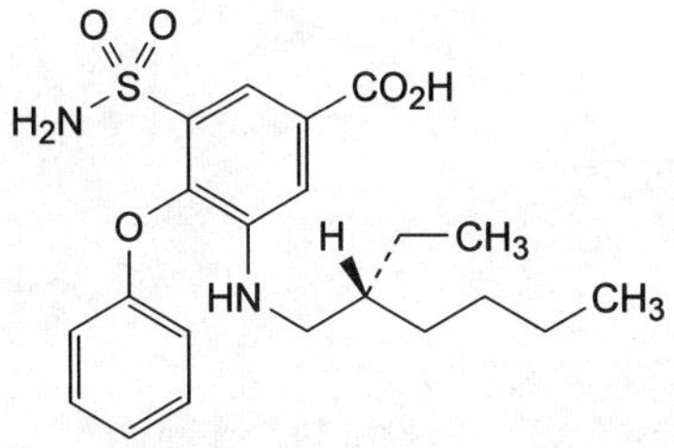

and enantiomer

D. 3-[[(2*RS*)-2-ethylhexyl]amino]-4-phenoxy-5-sulphamoylbenzoic acid.

01/2005:0541

BUPIVACAINE HYDROCHLORIDE

Bupivacaini hydrochloridum

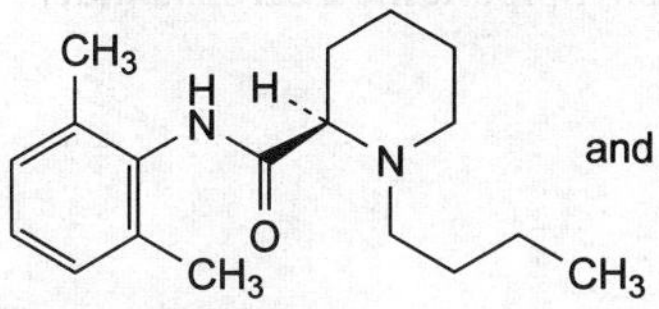

and enantiomer , HCl , H_2O

$C_{18}H_{29}ClN_2O,H_2O$ M_r 342.9

DEFINITION

(2*RS*)-1-Butyl-*N*-(2,6-dimethylphenyl)piperidine-2-carboxamide hydrochloride monohydrate.

Content: 98.5 per cent to 101.0 per cent (dried substance).

CHARACTERS

Appearance: white, crystalline powder or colourless crystals.

Solubility: soluble in water, freely soluble in alcohol.

mp: about 254 °C, with decomposition.

IDENTIFICATION

First identification: A, D.

Second identification: B, C, D.

A. Infrared absorption spectrophotometry (*2.2.24*).

Preparation: discs of *potassium bromide R*.

Comparison: *bupivacaine hydrochloride CRS*.

B. Thin-layer chromatography (*2.2.27*).

Test solution. Dissolve 25 mg of the substance to be examined in *methanol R* and dilute to 5 ml with the same solvent.

Reference solution. Dissolve 25 mg of *bupivacaine hydrochloride CRS* in *methanol R* and dilute to 5 ml with the same solvent.

Plate: *TLC silica gel G plate R.*

Mobile phase: *concentrated ammonia R, methanol R* (0.1:100 *V/V*).

Application: 5 µl.

Development: over a path of 10 cm.

Drying: in air.

Detection: spray with *dilute potassium iodobismuthate solution R.*

Results: the principal spot in the chromatogram obtained with the test solution is similar in position, colour and size to the principal spot in the chromatogram obtained with the reference solution.

C. Dissolve 0.1 g in 10 ml of *water R*, add 2 ml of *dilute sodium hydroxide solution R* and shake with 2 quantities, each of 15 ml, of *ether R*. Dry the combined ether layers over *anhydrous sodium sulphate R* and filter. Evaporate the ether, recrystallise the residue from *alcohol (90 per cent V/V) R* and dry under reduced pressure. The crystals melt (*2.2.14*) at 105 °C to 108 °C.

D. It gives reaction (a) of chlorides (*2.3.1*).

TESTS

Solution S. Dissolve 1.0 g in *carbon dioxide-free water R* and dilute to 50 ml with the same solvent.

Appearance of solution. Solution S is clear (*2.2.1*) and colourless (*2.2.2, Method II*).

Acidity or alkalinity. To 10 ml of solution S add 0.2 ml of *0.01 M sodium hydroxide*; the pH (*2.2.3*) is not less than 4.7. Add 0.4 ml of *0.01 M hydrochloric acid*; the pH is not greater than 4.7.

Related substances. Gas chromatography (*2.2.28*).

Internal standard solution. Dissolve 25 mg of *methyl behenate R* in *methylene chloride R* and dilute to 500 ml with the same solvent.

Test solution. Dissolve 50.0 mg of the substance to be examined in 2.5 ml of *water R*, add 2.5 ml of *dilute sodium hydroxide solution R* and extract with 2 quantities, each of 5 ml, of the internal standard solution. Filter the lower layer.

Reference solution (a). Dissolve 10 mg of the substance to be examined, 10 mg of *bupivacaine impurity B CRS* and 10 mg of *bupivacaine impurity E CRS* in 2.5 ml of *water R*, add 2.5 ml of *dilute sodium hydroxide solution R* and extract with 2 quantities, each of 5 ml, of the internal standard solution. Filter the lower layer and dilute to 20 ml with the internal standard solution.

Reference solution (b). Dilute 1.0 ml of the test solution to 100.0 ml with the internal standard solution.

Reference solution (c). Dilute 5.0 ml of reference solution (b) to 10.0 ml with the internal standard solution.

Reference solution (d). Dilute 1.0 ml of reference solution (b) to 10.0 ml with the internal standard solution.

Column:

- *material*: fused silica,
- *size*: *l* = 30 m, Ø = 0.32 mm,
- *stationary phase*: *poly(dimethyl)(diphenyl)siloxane R* (film thickness 0.25 µm).

Carrier gas: *helium for chromatography R.*

Flow rate: 2.5 ml/min.

Split ratio: 1:12.

Temperature:

	Time (min)	Temperature (°C)
Column	0	180
	0 - 10	180 → 230
	10 - 15	230
Injection port		250
Detector		250

Detection: flame ionisation.

Injection: 1 µl.

Relative retention with reference to bupivacaine (retention time = about 10 min): impurity C = about 0.5; impurity A = about 0.6; impurity B = about 0.7; impurity D = about 0.8; impurity E = about 1.1; internal standard = about 1.4.

System suitability: reference solution (a):

– *resolution*: minimum 3.0 between the peaks due to bupivacaine and impurity E.

Limits:

– *impurity B*: calculate the ratio (*R*) of the area of the principal peak to the area of the peak due to the internal standard from the chromatogram obtained with reference solution (c); from the chromatogram obtained with the test solution, calculate the ratio of the area of the peak due to impurity B to the area of the peak due to the internal standard: this ratio is not greater than *R* (0.5 per cent),

– *any other impurity*: calculate the ratio (*R*) of the area of the principal peak to the area of the peak due to the internal standard from the chromatogram obtained with reference solution (d); from the chromatogram obtained with the test solution, calculate the ratio of the area of any peak, apart from the principal peak, the peak due to impurity B and the peak due to the internal standard, to the area of the peak due to the internal standard: this ratio is not greater than *R* (0.1 per cent),

– *total*: calculate the ratio (*R*) of the area of the principal peak to the area of the peak due to the internal standard from the chromatogram obtained with reference solution (b); from the chromatogram obtained with the test solution, calculate the ratio of the sum of the areas of any peaks, apart from the principal peak and the peak due to the internal standard, to the area of the peak due to the internal standard: this ratio is not greater than *R* (1.0 per cent),

– *disregard limit*: ratio less than 0.01 times *R* (0.01 per cent).

2,6-Dimethylaniline: maximum 100 ppm.

Dissolve 0.50 g in *methanol R* and dilute to 10 ml with the same solvent. To 2 ml of the solution add 1 ml of a freshly prepared 10 g/l solution of *dimethylaminobenzaldehyde R* in *methanol R* and 2 ml of *glacial acetic acid R* and allow to stand for 10 min. Any yellow colour in the solution is not more intense than that in a standard prepared at the same time and in the same manner using 2 ml of a 5 mg/l solution of *2,6-dimethylaniline R* in *methanol R*.

Heavy metals (*2.4.8*): maximum 10 ppm.

Dissolve 2.0 g in a mixture of 15 volumes of *water R* and 85 volumes of *methanol R* and dilute to 20 ml with the same mixture of solvents. 12 ml of the solution complies with limit test B. Prepare the standard using lead standard solution (1 ppm Pb) obtained by diluting *lead standard solution (100 ppm Pb) R* with a mixture of 15 volumes of *water R* and 85 volumes of *methanol R*.

Loss on drying (*2.2.32*): 4.5 per cent to 6.0 per cent, determined on 1.000 g by drying in an oven at 100-105 °C.

Sulphated ash (*2.4.14*): maximum 0.1 per cent, determined on 1.0 g.

ASSAY

Dissolve 0.250 g in a mixture of 20 ml of *water R* and 25 ml of *alcohol R*. Add 5.0 ml of *0.01 M hydrochloric acid.* Carry out a potentiometric titration (*2.2.20*), using *0.1 M ethanolic sodium hydroxide*. Read the volume added between the 2 points of inflexion.

1 ml of *0.1 M ethanolic sodium hydroxide* is equivalent to 32.49 mg of $C_{18}H_{29}ClN_2O$.

STORAGE

Protected from light.

IMPURITIES

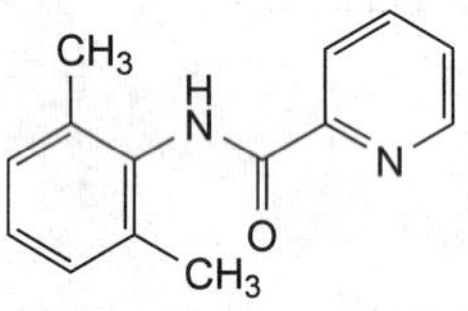

A. *N*-(2,6-dimethylphenyl)pyridine-2-carboxamide,

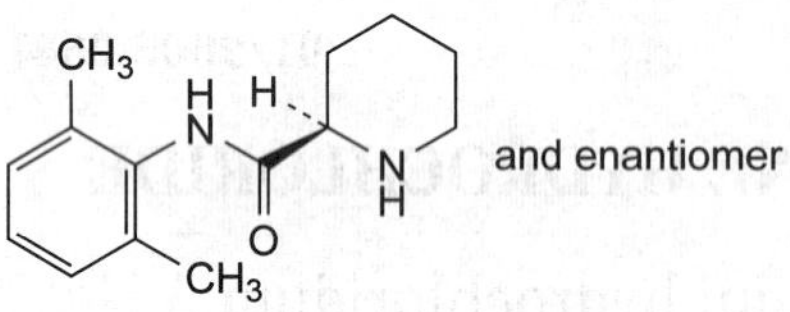

B. (2*RS*)-*N*-(2,6-dimethylphenyl)piperidine-2-carboxamide,

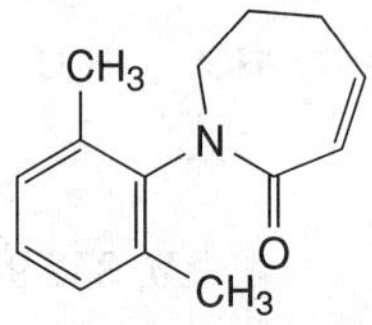

C. 1-(2,6-dimethylphenyl)-1,5,6,7-tetrahydro-2*H*-azepin-2-one,

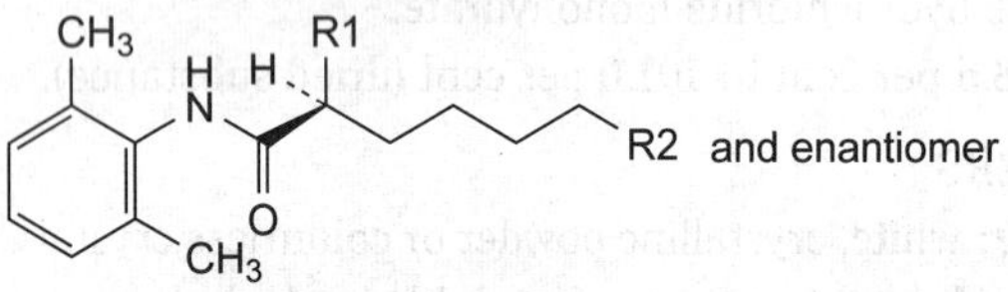

D. R1 = R2 = Cl: (2*RS*)-2,6-dichloro-*N*-(2,6-dimethylphenyl)hexanamide,

E. R1 = H, R2 = NH-$(CH_2)_3$-CH_3: 6-(butylamino)-*N*-(2,6-dimethylphenyl)hexanamide,

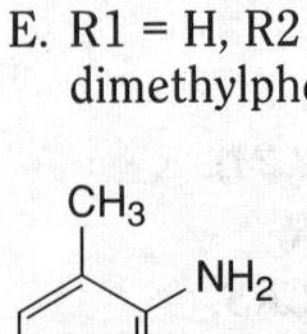

F. 2,6-dimethylaniline.

01/2005:1180

BUPRENORPHINE

Buprenorphinum

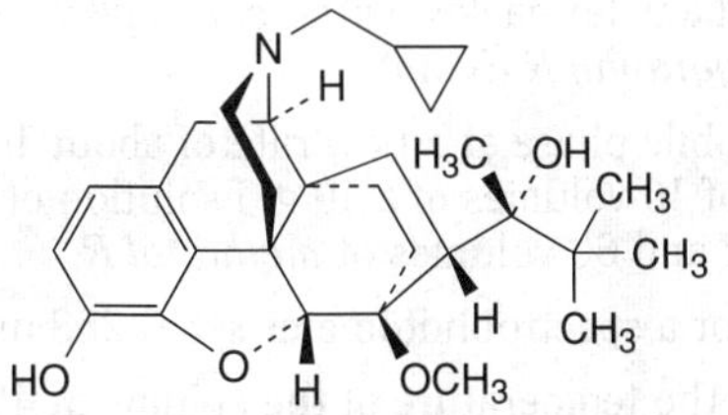

$C_{29}H_{41}NO_4$ M_r 467.6

DEFINITION

Buprenorphine contains not less than 98.5 per cent and not more than the equivalent of 101.0 per cent of (2*S*)-2-[17-(cyclopropylmethyl)-4,5α-epoxy-3-hydroxy-6-methoxy-6α,14-ethano-14α-morphinan-7α-yl]-3,3-dimethylbutan-2-ol, calculated with reference to the dried substance.

CHARACTERS

A white or almost white, crystalline powder, very slightly soluble in water, freely soluble in acetone, soluble in methanol, slightly soluble in cyclohexane. It dissolves in dilute solutions of acids.

It melts at about 217 °C.

IDENTIFICATION

Examine by infrared absorption spectrophotometry (*2.2.24*), comparing with the *Ph. Eur. reference spectrum of buprenorphine.*

TESTS

Solution S. Dissolve 0.250 g in *ethanol R* and dilute to 25.0 ml with the same solvent.

Appearance of solution. Solution S is clear (*2.2.1*) and colourless (*2.2.2, Method II*).

Specific optical rotation (*2.2.7*): − 103 to − 107, determined on solution S and calculated with reference to the dried substance.

Related substances. Examine by liquid chromatography (*2.2.29*).

Test solution. Dissolve 25.0 mg of the substance to be examined in the mobile phase and dilute to 10.0 ml with the mobile phase.

Reference solution (a). Dissolve 5.0 mg of the substance to be examined in 2.0 ml of *methanol R*. Add 0.25 ml of *2 M hydrochloric acid.*

Reference solution (b). Dilute 0.5 ml of the test solution to 200.0 ml with the mobile phase.

Reference solution (c). Dilute 0.65 ml of the test solution to 100.0 ml with the mobile phase.

Reference solution (d). Dilute 4.0 ml of reference solution (b) to 10.0 ml with the mobile phase.

The chromatographic procedure may be carried out using:

- a stainless steel column 0.25 m long and 4.6 mm in internal diameter packed with *octadecylsilyl silica gel for chromatography R* (5 µm),
- as mobile phase at a flow rate of about 1 ml/min, a mixture of 10 volumes of a 10 g/l solution of *ammonium acetate R* and 60 volumes of *methanol R*,
- as detector a spectrophotometer set at 288 nm, maintaining the temperature of the column at 40 °C.

Inject 20 µl of reference solution (a). Adjust the flow rate so that the retention time of the peak corresponding to buprenorphine is about 15 min. The test is not valid unless the chromatogram obtained with reference solution (a) presents 2 peaks, the first having a retention time of 0.93 relative to the second peak (buprenorphine). Inject 20 µl of each solution. Record the chromatogram of the test solution for 2.5 times the retention time of the principal peak. In the chromatogram obtained with the test solution: the area of any peak, apart from the principal peak, is not greater than the area of the principal peak in the chromatogram obtained with reference solution (b) (0.25 per cent); the sum of the areas of such peaks is not greater than the area of the peak in the chromatogram obtained with reference solution (c) (0.65 per cent). Disregard any peak with an area less than that of the principal peak in the chromatogram obtained with reference solution (d).

Loss on drying (*2.2.32*). Not more than 1.0 per cent, determined on 1.000 g by drying in an oven at 100-105 °C.

ASSAY

Dissolve 0.400 g in 40 ml of *anhydrous acetic acid R*. Titrate with *0.1 M perchloric acid* until the colour changes from violet-blue to green, using 0.1 ml of *crystal violet solution R* as indicator.

1 ml of *0.1 M perchloric acid* is equivalent to 46.76 mg of $C_{29}H_{41}NO_4$.

STORAGE

Store protected from light.

IMPURITIES

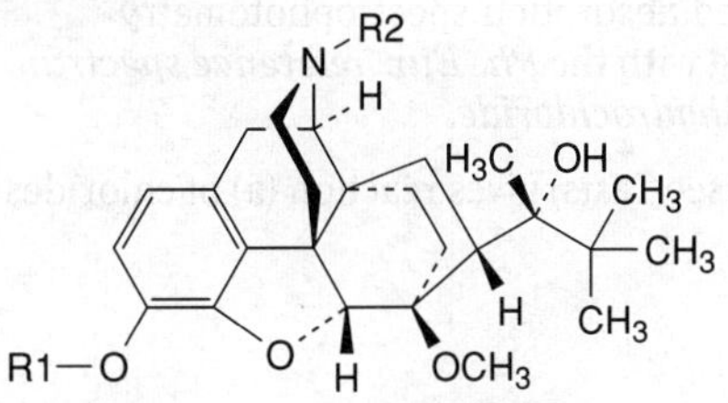

A. R1 = H, R2 = CH_2-CH_2-CH=CH_2: (2*S*)-2-[17-(but-3-enyl)-4,5α-epoxy-3-hydroxy-6-methoxy-6α,14-ethano-14α-morphinan-7α-yl]-3,3-dimethylbutan-2-ol,

B. R1 = R2 = H: (2*S*)-2-(4,5α-epoxy-3-hydroxy-6-methoxy-6α,14-ethano-14α-morphinan-7α-yl)-3,3-dimethylbutan-2-ol,

C. R1 = CH_3, R2 = CN: 4,5α-epoxy-7α-[(1*S*)-1-hydroxy-1,2,2-trimethylpropyl]-3,6-dimethoxy-6α,14-ethano-14α-morphinan-17-carbonitrile,

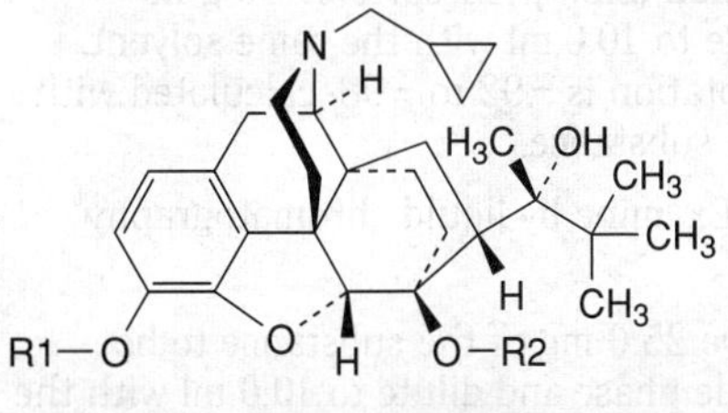

D. R1 = R2 = CH_3: (2*S*)-2-[17-(cyclopropylmethyl)-4,5α-epoxy-3,6-dimethoxy-6α,14-ethano-14α-morphinan-7α-yl]-3,3-dimethylbutan-2-ol (3-*O*-methylbuprenorphine),

E. R1 = R2 = H: (2*S*)-2-[17-(cyclopropylmethyl)-4,5α-epoxy-3,6-dihydroxy-6α,14-ethano-14α-morphinan-7α-yl]-3,3-dimethylbutan-2-ol (6-*O*-desmethylbuprenorphine).

01/2005:1181

BUPRENORPHINE HYDROCHLORIDE

Buprenorphini hydrochloridum

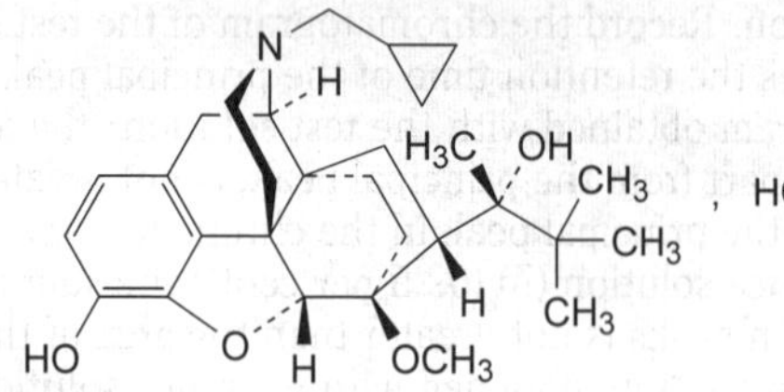

$C_{29}H_{42}ClNO_4$ M_r 504.1

DEFINITION

Buprenorphine hydrochloride contains not less than 98.5 per cent and not more than the equivalent of 101.0 per cent of (2*S*)-2-[17-(cyclopropylmethyl)-4,5α-epoxy-3-hydroxy-6-methoxy-6α,14-ethano-14α-morphinan-7α-yl]-3,3-dimethylbutan-2-ol hydrochloride, calculated with reference to the dried substance.

CHARACTERS

A white or almost white, crystalline powder, sparingly soluble in water, freely soluble in methanol, soluble in alcohol, practically insoluble in cyclohexane.

IDENTIFICATION

A. Examine by infrared absorption spectrophotometry (*2.2.24*), comparing with the *Ph. Eur. reference spectrum of buprenorphine hydrochloride.*

B. 3 ml of solution S (see Tests) gives reaction (a) of chlorides (*2.3.1*).

TESTS

Solution S. Dissolve 0.250 g in 5.0 ml of *methanol R* and while stirring dilute to 25.0 ml with *carbon dioxide-free water R.*

Appearance of solution. Solution S is clear (*2.2.1*) and colourless (*2.2.2, Method II*).

Acidity or alkalinity. To 10.0 ml of solution S add 0.05 ml of *methyl red solution R*. Not more than 0.2 ml of *0.02 M sodium hydroxide* or *0.02 M hydrochloric acid* is required to change the colour of the indicator.

Specific optical rotation (*2.2.7*). Dissolve 0.100 g in *methanol R* and dilute to 10.0 ml with the same solvent. The specific optical rotation is − 92 to − 98, calculated with reference to the dried substance.

Related substances. Examine by liquid chromatography (*2.2.29*).

Test solution. Dissolve 25.0 mg of the substance to be examined in the mobile phase and dilute to 10.0 ml with the mobile phase.

Reference solution (a). Dissolve 5 mg of the substance to be examined in 2.0 ml of *methanol R*. Add 0.25 ml of *2 M hydrochloric acid.*

Reference solution (b). Dilute 0.5 ml of the test solution to 200.0 ml with the mobile phase.

Reference solution (c). Dilute 0.65 ml of the test solution to 100.0 ml with the mobile phase.

Reference solution (d). Dilute 4.0 ml of reference solution (b) to 10.0 ml with the mobile phase.

The chromatographic procedure may be carried out using:

– a stainless steel column 0.25 m long and 4.6 mm in internal diameter packed with *octadecylsilyl silica gel for chromatography R* (5 µm),

– as the mobile phase at a flow rate of about 1 ml/min, a mixture of 10 volumes of a 10 g/l solution of *ammonium acetate R* and 60 volumes of *methanol R,*

– as detector a spectrophotometer set at 288 nm,

maintaining the temperature of the column at 40 °C.

Inject 20 µl of reference solution (a). Adjust the flow rate so that the retention time of the peak corresponding to buprenorphine is about 15 min. The test is not valid unless the chromatogram obtained with reference solution (a) presents two peaks, the first having a retention time of 0.93 relative to the second peak (buprenorphine). Inject separately 20 µl of each solution. Record the chromatogram of the test solution for 2.5 times the retention time of the main peak. In the chromatogram obtained with the test solution: the area of any peak, apart from the principal peak, is not greater than the area of the principal peak in the chromatogram obtained with reference solution (b) (0.25 per cent) and the sum of the areas of such peaks is not greater than the area of the peak in the chromatogram obtained with reference solution (c) (0.65 per cent). Disregard any peak with an area less than that of the principal peak in the chromatogram obtained with reference solution (d).

Loss on drying (*2.2.32*). Not more than 1.0 per cent, determined on 1.000 g by heating in an oven at 115-120 °C.

ASSAY

Dissolve 0.400 g in 40 ml of *anhydrous acetic acid R* and add 10 ml of *acetic anhydride R*. Titrate with *0.1 M perchloric acid*, determining the end-point potentiometrically (*2.2.20*).

1 ml of *0.1 M perchloric acid* is equivalent to 50.41 mg of $C_{29}H_{42}ClNO_4$.

STORAGE

Store protected from light.

IMPURITIES

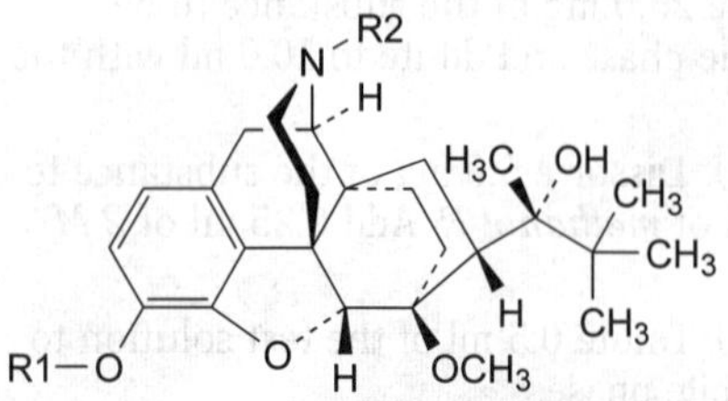

A. R1 = H, R2 = CH_2-CH_2-CH=CH_2: (2*S*)-2-[17-(but-3-enyl)-4,5α-epoxy-3-hydroxy-6-methoxy-6α,14-ethano-14α-morphinan-7α-yl]-3,3-dimethylbutan-2-ol,

B. R1 = H, R2 = H: (2*S*)-2-(4,5α-epoxy-3-hydroxy-6-methoxy-6α,14-ethano-14α-morphinan-7α-yl)-3,3-dimethylbutan-2-ol,

C. R1 = CH_3, R2 = CN: 4,5α-epoxy-7α-[(1*S*)-1-hydroxy-1,2,2-trimethylpropyl]-3,6-dimethoxy-6α,14-ethano-14α-morphinan-17-carbonitrile.

01/2005:1077

BUSERELIN

Buserelinum

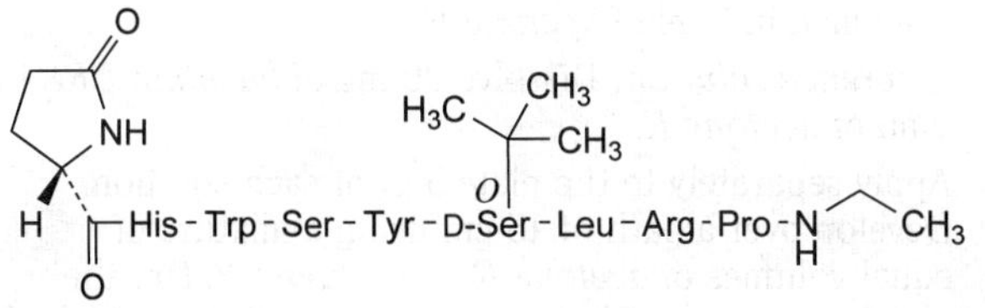

$C_{60}H_{86}N_{16}O_{13}$ M_r 1239

DEFINITION

5-Oxo-L-prolyl-L-histidyl-L-tryptophyl-L-seryl-L-tyrosyl-*O*-(1,1-dimethylethyl)-D-seryl-L-leucyl-L-arginyl-L-prolylethylamide.

Synthetic nonapeptide analogue of human gonadotrophin-releasing hormone GnRH with agonistic activity to gonadorelin. It is obtained by chemical synthesis and is available as an acetate.

Content: 95.0 per cent to 102.0 per cent (anhydrous, acetic acid-free substance).

CHARACTERS

Appearance: white or slightly yellowish powder, hygroscopic.

Solubility: sparingly soluble in water and in dilute acids.

IDENTIFICATION

A. Examine the chromatograms obtained in the assay.

Results: the principal peak in the chromatogram obtained with the test solution is similar in retention time and size to the principal peak in the chromatogram obtained with reference solution (b).

B. Nuclear magnetic resonance spectrometry (*2.2.33*).

Preparation: 4 mg/ml solution in a mixture of 20 volumes of *deuterated acetic acid R* and 80 volumes of *deuterium oxide R.*

Results: the ^1H NMR spectrum obtained is qualitatively similar to the *Ph. Eur. reference spectrum of buserelin.*

C. Amino acid analysis (*2.2.56*). For protein hydrolysis use Method 1 and for analysis use Method 1.

Express the content of each amino acid in moles. Calculate the relative proportions of the amino acids, taking one-sixth of the sum of the number of moles of glutamic acid, histidine, tyrosine, leucine, arginine, proline as equal to one. The values fall within the following limits: serine 1.4 to 2.0; proline 0.8 to 1.2; glutamic acid 0.9 to 1.1; leucine 0.9 to 1.1; tyrosine 0.9 to 1.1; histidine 0.9 to 1.1 and arginine 0.9 to 1.1. Not more than traces of other amino acids are present, with the exception of tryptophan.

TESTS

Appearance of solution. A 10 g/l solution is clear (*2.2.1*) and not more intensely coloured than reference solution Y_7 (*2.2.2, Method II*).

Specific optical rotation (*2.2.7*): − 49 to − 58 (anhydrous, acetic acid-free substance), determined on a 10 g/l solution.

Specific absorbance (*2.2.25*): 49 to 56 by measuring at the absorption maximum at 278 nm (anhydrous, acetic acid-free substance).

Dissolve 10.0 mg in 100.0 ml of *0.01 M hydrochloric acid.*

Related substances. Liquid chromatography (*2.2.29*).

Test solution. Dissolve 5.0 mg of the substance to be examined in 5.0 ml of the mobile phase.

Reference solution (a). Dissolve the contents of a vial of *D-His-buserelin CRS* in the mobile phase. Dilute an appropriate volume of this solution in the mobile phase to obtain a final concentration of 1 mg/ml. Add 1.0 ml of the test solution to 1.0 ml of this solution.

Reference solution (b). Dissolve the contents of a vial of *buserelin CRS* in the mobile phase. Dilute an appropriate volume of this solution in the mobile phase to obtain a final concentration of 1.0 mg/ml.

Reference solution (c). Dilute 1.0 ml of the test solution to 100.0 ml with the mobile phase.

Column:

- *size*: *l* = 0.25 m, Ø = 4 mm,
- *stationary phase*: *octadecylsilyl silica gel for chromatography R* (5 µm).

Mobile phase: mix 200 ml of *acetonitrile R* and 700 ml of an 11.2 g/l solution of *phosphoric acid R* and adjust to pH 2.5 with *triethylamine R.*

Flow rate: 0.8 ml/min.

Detection: spectrophotometer at 220 nm.

Injection: 10 µl of the test solution, reference solution (a) and reference solution (c).

Relative retention with reference to buserelin (retention time = about 36 min): impurity B = about 0.76; impurity C = about 0.83; impurity A = about 0.90; impurity D = about 0.94; impurity E = about 0.94.

System suitability: reference solution (a):

- *resolution*: minimum 1.5 between peaks due to impurity A and buserelin.

Limits:

- *sum of impurities D and E*: not more than 3 times the area of the principal peak in the chromatogram obtained with reference solution (c) (3 per cent),
- *any other impurity*: for each impurity, not more than 3 times the area of the principal peak in the chromatogram obtained with reference solution (c) (3 per cent),
- *total*: not more than 5 times the area of the principal peak in the chromatogram obtained with reference solution (c) (5 per cent),
- *disregard limit*: 0.1 times the area of the principal peak in the chromatogram obtained with reference solution (c) (0.1 per cent).

Acetic acid (*2.5.34*): 3.0 per cent to 7.0 per cent.

Test solution. Dissolve 20.0 mg of the substance to be examined in a mixture of 5 volumes of mobile phase B and 95 volumes of mobile phase A and dilute to 10.0 ml with the same mixture of solvents.

Water (*2.5.12*): maximum 4.0 per cent, determined on 80.0 mg.

Bacterial endotoxins (*2.6.14*): less than 55.5 IU/mg, if intended for use in the manufacture of parenteral dosage forms without a further appropriate procedure for the removal of bacterial endotoxins.

ASSAY

Liquid chromatography (*2.2.29*) as described in the test for related substances with the following modification.

Injection: 10 µl of the test solution and reference solution (b).

Calculate the content of buserelin ($C_{60}H_{86}N_{16}O_{13}$) using the areas of the peaks of the chromatograms obtained and the stated content of $C_{60}H_{86}N_{16}O_{13}$ in *buserelin CRS.*

STORAGE

In an airtight container, protected from light, at a temperature of 2 °C to 8 °C.

If the substance is sterile, store in an airtight, sterile, tamper-proof container.

LABELLING

The label states:

– the mass of peptide in the container,
– where applicable, that the substance is free from bacterial endotoxins.

IMPURITIES

Specified impurities: A, B, C, D, E.

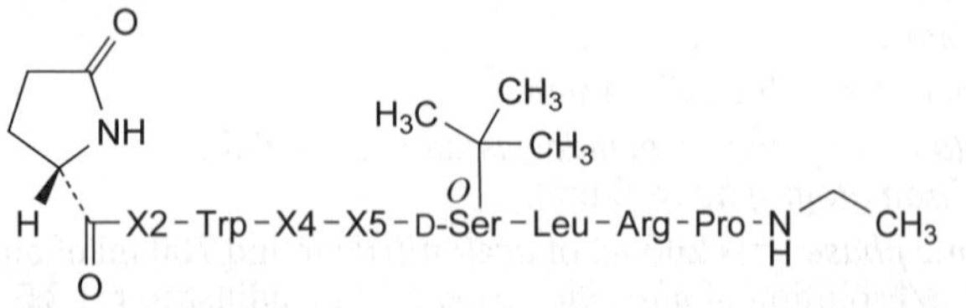

A. X2 = D-His, X4 = L-Ser, X5 = L-Tyr: [2-D-histidine]buserelin,

B. X2 = L-His, X4 = D-Ser, X5 = L-Tyr: [4-D-serine]buserelin,

D. X2 = L-His, X4 = L-Ser, X5 = D-Tyr: [5-D-tyrosine]buserelin,

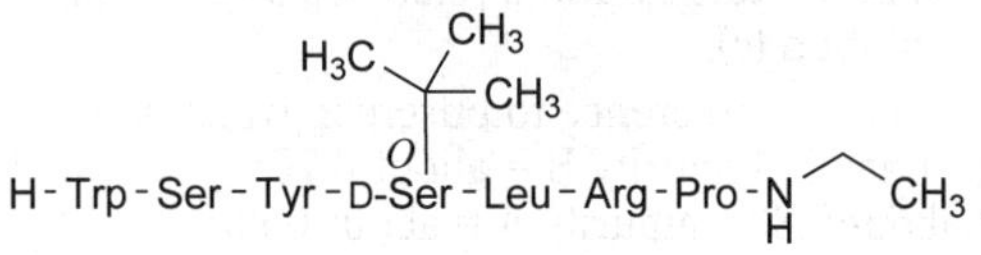

C. buserelin-(3-9)-peptide,

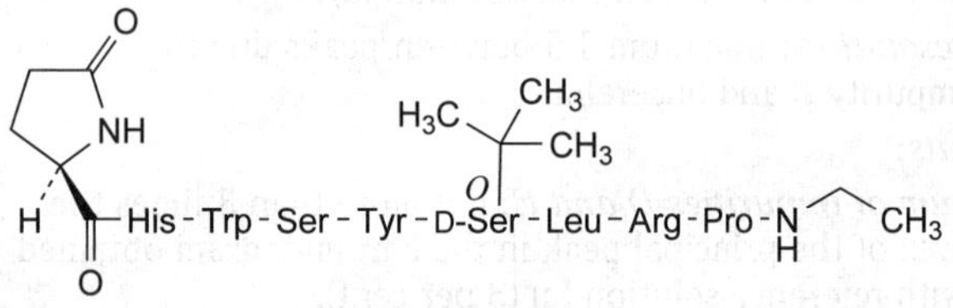

E. [1-(5-oxo-D-proline)]buserelin.

01/2005:0542

BUSULFAN

Busulfanum

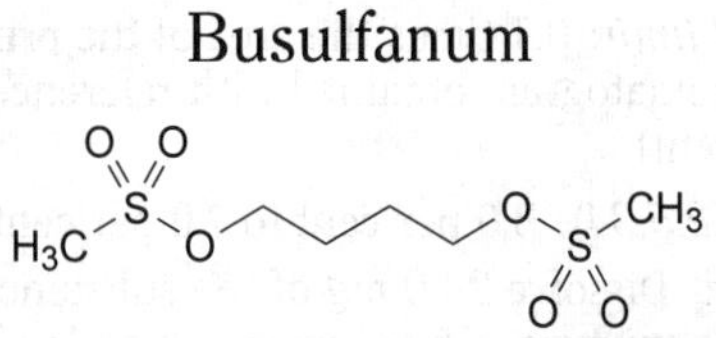

$C_6H_{14}O_6S_2$ M_r 246.3

DEFINITION

Busulfan contains not less than 99.0 per cent and not more than the equivalent of 100.5 per cent of butane-1,4-diyl di(methanesulphonate), calculated with reference to the dried substance.

CHARACTERS

A white or almost white, crystalline powder, very slightly soluble in water, freely soluble in acetone and in acetonitrile, very slightly soluble in alcohol.

It melts at about 116 °C.

IDENTIFICATION

First identification: A.

Second identification: B, C, D.

A. Examine by infrared absorption spectrophotometry (*2.2.24*), comparing with the spectrum obtained with *busulfan CRS*.

B. Examine by thin-layer chromatography (*2.2.27*), using *silica gel G R* as the coating substance.

Test solution. Dissolve 20 mg of the substance to be examined in 2 ml of *acetone R*.

Reference solution. Dissolve 20 mg of *busulfan CRS* in 2 ml of *acetone R*.

Apply separately to the plate 5 µl of each solution. Develop over a path of 15 cm using a mixture of equal volumes of *acetone R* and *toluene R*. Dry the plate in a stream of hot air and spray with *anisaldehyde solution R*. Heat the plate at 120 °C. The principal spot in the chromatogram obtained with the test solution is similar in position, colour and size to the principal spot in the chromatogram obtained with the reference solution.

C. To 0.1 g add 5 ml of *1 M sodium hydroxide*. Heat until a clear solution is obtained. Allow to cool. To 2 ml of the solution add 0.1 ml of *potassium permanganate solution R*. The colour changes from purple through violet to blue and finally to green. Filter and add 1 ml of *ammoniacal silver nitrate solution R*. A precipitate is formed.

D. To 0.1 g add 0.1 g of *potassium nitrate R* and 0.25 g of *sodium hydroxide R*, mix and heat to fusion. Allow to cool and dissolve the residue in 5 ml of *water R*. Adjust to pH 1 to 2 using *dilute hydrochloric acid R*. The solution gives reaction (a) of sulphates (*2.3.1*).

TESTS

Appearance of solution. Dissolve 0.25 g in 20 ml of *acetonitrile R*, dilute to 25 ml with *water R* and examine immediately. The solution is clear (*2.2.1*) and not more intensely coloured than reference solution B_7 (*2.2.2, Method II*).

Acidity. Dissolve 0.20 g with heating in 50 ml of *ethanol R*. Add 0.1 ml of *methyl red solution R*. Not more than 0.05 ml of *0.1 M sodium hydroxide* is required to change the colour of the indicator.

Loss on drying (*2.2.32*). Not more than 2.0 per cent, determined on 1.000 g by drying *in vacuo* at 60 °C.

Sulphated ash (*2.4.14*). Not more than 0.1 per cent, determined on 1.0 g.

ASSAY

To 0.250 g add 50 ml of *water R*. Shake. Boil under a reflux condenser for 30 min and, if necessary, make up to the initial volume with *water R*. Allow to cool. Using 0.3 ml of *phenolphthalein solution R* as indicator, titrate with *0.1 M sodium hydroxide* until a pink colour is obtained.

1 ml of *0.1 M sodium hydroxide* is equivalent to 12.32 mg of $C_6H_{14}O_6S_2$.

STORAGE

Store in an airtight container, protected from light.

01/2005:1847

BUTCHER'S BROOM

Rusci rhizoma

DEFINITION

Dried, whole or fragmented underground parts of *Ruscus aculeatus* L.

Content: minimum 1.0 per cent of total sapogenins, expressed as ruscogenins [mixture of neoruscogenin ($C_{27}H_{40}O_4$; M_r 428.6) and ruscogenin ($C_{27}H_{42}O_4$; M_r 430.6)] (dried drug).

CHARACTERS

Macroscopic and microscopic characters described under identification tests A and B.

IDENTIFICATION

A. The rhizome consists of yellowish, branched, articulated, somewhat knotty pieces, cylindrical or subconical, about 5 cm to 10 cm long and about 5 mm thick. The surface is marked with thin annulations about 1 mm to 3 mm wide, separated from one another; rounded scars of the aerial stems are present on the upper surface. On the lower surface numerous roots, or their scars, occur; the roots are about 2 mm in diameter and similar in colour to the rhizome. The outer layer is easily detached, revealing a yellowish-white, very hard central cylinder.

B. Reduce to a powder (355). The powder is yellowish. Examine under a microscope using *chloral hydrate solution R*. The powder shows groups of sclereids from the ground tissue of the rhizome, variously-shaped cells, ranging from rounded to elongated or rectangular; the walls are moderately thickened and distinctly beaded, with large, rounded to oval pits. Fragments of the endodermis composed of a single layer of irregularly-thickened cells. Groups of rounded parenchymatous cells, thickened at the corners, with small, triangular intercellular spaces; thin-walled parenchyma containing raphides of calcium oxalate. Groups of thick-walled fibres and small vessels, up to about 50 µm in diameter, the walls showing numerous small, slit-shaped pits.

C. Thin-layer chromatography (*2.2.27*).

Test solution. Introduce 1.0 g of the powdered drug (355) and 50 ml of *dilute hydrochloric acid R* into a 100 ml flask with a ground-glass neck. Heat on a water-bath under a reflux condenser for 40 min. Allow to cool and extract the unfiltered mixture with 3 quantities, each of 25 ml, of *methylene chloride R*. Combine the organic solutions and dry over *anhydrous sodium sulphate R*. Filter and evaporate to dryness. Dissolve the residue in 5 ml of *methanol R*.

Reference solution. Dissolve 1 mg of *ruscogenins R* and 1 mg of *stigmasterol R* in *methanol R* and dilute to 5 ml with the same solvent.

Plate: *TLC silica gel plate R*.

Mobile phase: *methanol R, methylene chloride R* (7:93 *V/V*).

Application: 10 µl, as bands.

Development: over a path of 15 cm.

Drying: in air.

Detection: spray with *vanillin reagent R*, dry the plate in an oven at 100-105 °C for 1 min and examine in daylight.

Results: see below the sequence of the zones present in the chromatograms obtained with the reference solution and the test solution. Furthermore, other weak zones may be present in the chromatogram obtained with the test solution.

Top of the plate	
	Several zones of various colours
Stigmasterol: a violet zone	A violet zone
_______	_______
	A violet zone
Ruscogenins: a yellow zone	A yellow zone (ruscogenins)
	Several zones of various colours
Reference solution	**Test solution**

TESTS

Foreign matter (*2.8.2*): maximum 5 per cent.

Loss on drying (*2.2.32*): maximum 12.0 per cent, determined on 1.000 g of the powdered drug (355) by drying in an oven at 100-105 °C for 2 h.

Total ash (*2.4.16*): maximum 12.0 per cent.

Ash insoluble in hydrochloric acid (*2.8.1*): maximum 5.0 per cent.

ASSAY

Liquid chromatography (*2.2.29*).

Test solution. To 2.000 g of the powdered drug (355), add 60 ml of *ethanol R*, 15 ml of *water R* and 0.2 g of *potassium hydroxide R*. Extract under reflux on a water-bath for 4 h. Allow to cool and filter into a 100 ml volumetric flask. Rinse the extraction flask and the residue in the filter with 3 quantities, each of 10 ml, of *ethanol R* and add the rinsings to the volumetric flask. Dilute to 100.0 ml with *ethanol R*. Introduce 25.0 ml of the solution into a round-bottomed flask fitted to a rotary evaporator and evaporate to dryness. Dissolve the residue in 10 ml of *butanol R*, add 3 ml of *hydrochloric acid R1* and 8 ml of *water R*. Heat under reflux on a water-bath for 1 h. Allow to cool and transfer the liquid into a separating funnel, rinse the round-bottomed flask with 2 quantities, each of 10 ml, of *butanol R*. Add the rinsings to the separating funnel. Extract with 3 quantities, each of 20 ml, of *butanol R* saturated with *water R*. Combine the butanolic extracts and evaporate to dryness using a rotary evaporator. Dissolve the residue in 20 ml of *methanol R* and transfer to a 100 ml volumetric flask. Rinse the extraction flask with 20 ml, 20 ml and 10 ml of *methanol R* and add the rinsings to the volumetric flask. Dilute to 100 ml with *methanol R*.

Reference solution. Dissolve 5.0 mg of *ruscogenins R* in 100 ml of *methanol R*.

Column:
- *size*: *l* = 0.25 m, Ø = 4.6 mm,
- *stationary phase*: *octadecylsilyl silica gel for chromatography R* (5 µm).

Mobile phase:
- *mobile phase A*: *water R*,
- *mobile phase B*: *acetonitrile for chromatography R*,

Time (min)	Mobile phase A (per cent *V/V*)	Mobile phase B (per cent *V/V*)
0 - 25	40	60
25 - 27	40 → 0	60 → 100
27 - 37	0	100
37 - 39	0 → 40	100 → 60
39 - 42	40	60

Flow rate: 1.2 ml/min.

Detection: spectrophotometer at 203 nm.

Injection: 20 µl.

Retention time with reference to neoruscogenin (retention time = about 16 min): ruscogenin = about 1.2.

System suitability: reference solution:

- *resolution*: minimum 1.5 between the peaks due to neoruscogenin and ruscogenin.

Calculate the percentage content of sapogenins expressed as ruscogenins (neoruscogenin and ruscogenin) in the test solution by comparing the areas of the peaks in the chromatograms obtained with the test solution and the reference solution.

01/2005:0881

BUTYL PARAHYDROXYBENZOATE

Butylis parahydroxybenzoas

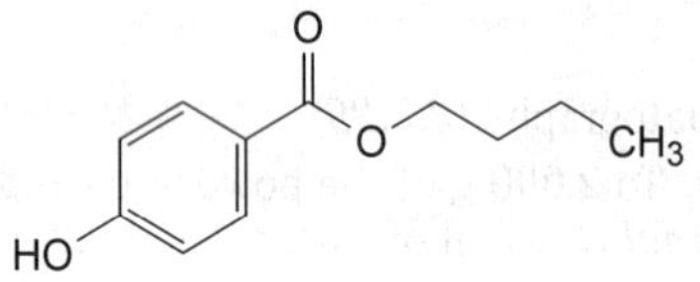

$C_{11}H_{14}O_3$ M_r 194.2

DEFINITION

Butyl 4-hydroxybenzoate.

Content: 98.0 per cent to 102.0 per cent.

CHARACTERS

Appearance: white or almost white, crystalline powder or colourless crystals.

Solubility: very slightly soluble in water, freely soluble in alcohol and in methanol.

IDENTIFICATION

First identification: A, B.

Second identification: A, C, D.

A. Melting point (*2.2.14*): 68 °C to 71 °C.

B. Infrared absorption spectrophotometry (*2.2.24*).

Comparison: *butyl parahydroxybenzoate CRS.*

C. Examine the chromatograms obtained in the test for related substances.

Results: the principal spot in the chromatogram obtained with test solution (b) is similar in position and size to the principal spot in the chromatogram obtained with reference solution (b).

D. To about 10 mg in a test-tube add 1 ml of *sodium carbonate solution R*, boil for 30 s and cool (solution A). To a further 10 mg in a similar test-tube add 1 ml of *sodium carbonate solution R*; the substance partly dissolves (solution B). Add at the same time to solution A and solution B 5 ml of *aminopyrazolone solution R* and 1 ml of *potassium ferricyanide solution R* and mix. Solution B is yellow to orange-brown. Solution A is orange to red, the colour being clearly more intense than any similar colour which may be obtained with solution B.

TESTS

Solution S. Dissolve 1.0 g in *alcohol R* and dilute to 10 ml with the same solvent.

Appearance of solution. Solution S is clear (*2.2.1*) and not more intensely coloured than reference solution BY_6 (*2.2.2, Method II*).

Acidity. To 2 ml of solution S add 3 ml of *alcohol R*, 5 ml of *carbon dioxide-free water R* and 0.1 ml of *bromocresol green solution R*. Not more than 0.1 ml of *0.1 M sodium hydroxide* is required to change the colour of the indicator to blue.

Related substances. Thin-layer chromatography (*2.2.27*).

Test solution (a). Dissolve 0.10 g of the substance to be examined in *acetone R* and dilute to 10 ml with the same solvent.

Test solution (b). Dilute 1 ml of test solution (a) to 10 ml with *acetone R*.

Reference solution (a). Dilute 0.5 ml of test solution (a) to 100 ml with *acetone R*.

Reference solution (b). Dissolve 10 mg of *butyl parahydroxybenzoate CRS* in *acetone R* and dilute to 10 ml with the same solvent.

Reference solution (c). Dissolve 10 mg of *propyl parahydroxybenzoate R* in 1 ml of test solution (a) and dilute to 10 ml with *acetone R*.

Plate: suitable octadecylsilyl silica gel with a fluorescent indicator having an optimal intensity at 254 nm as the coating substance.

Mobile phase: *glacial acetic acid R, water R, methanol R* (1:30:70 *V/V/V*).

Application: 2 µl.

Development: over a path of 15 cm.

Drying: in air.

Detection: examine in ultraviolet light at 254 nm.

System suitability: the chromatogram obtained with reference solution (c) shows 2 clearly separated principal spots.

Limits:

- *any impurity*: any spot in the chromatogram obtained with test solution (a), apart from the principal spot, is not more intense than the spot in the chromatogram obtained with reference solution (a) (0.5 per cent).

Sulphated ash (*2.4.14*): maximum 0.1 per cent, determined on 1.0 g.

ASSAY

To 1.000 g add 20.0 ml of *1 M sodium hydroxide*. Heat at about 70 °C for 1 h. Cool rapidly in an ice bath. Prepare a blank in the same manner. Carry out the titration on the solutions at room temperature. Titrate the excess sodium hydroxide with *0.5 M sulphuric acid*, continuing the titration until the second point of inflexion and determining the end-point potentiometrically (*2.2.20*).

1 ml of *1 M sodium hydroxide* is equivalent to 194.2 mg of $C_{11}H_{14}O_3$.

IMPURITIES

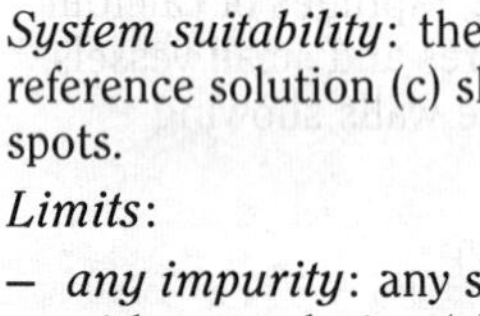

A. R = H: 4-hydroxybenzoic acid,

B. R = CH_3: methyl 4-hydroxybenzoate,

C. R = CH_2-CH_3: ethyl 4-hydroxybenzoate,

D. R = CH_2-CH_2-CH_3: propyl 4-hydroxybenzoate.

01/2005:0880

BUTYLHYDROXYANISOLE

Butylhydroxyanisolum

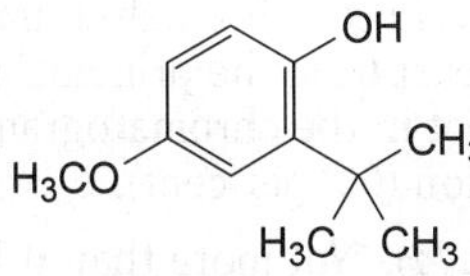

$C_{11}H_{16}O_2$ M_r 180.3

DEFINITION

Butylhydroxyanisole is 2-(1,1-dimethylethyl)-4-methoxyphenol containing not more than 10 per cent of 3-(1,1-dimethylethyl)-4-methoxyphenol.

CHARACTERS

A white, yellowish or slightly pinkish, crystalline powder, practically insoluble in water, very soluble in methylene chloride, freely soluble in alcohol and in fatty oils. It dissolves in dilute solutions of alkali hydroxides.

IDENTIFICATION

A. Examine the chromatograms obtained in the test for related substances. The principal spot in the chromatogram obtained with test solution (b) is similar in position, colour and size to the principal spot in the chromatogram obtained with reference solution (a).

B. To 0.5 ml of solution S (see Tests) add 10 ml of *aminopyrazolone solution R* and 1 ml of *potassium ferricyanide solution R*. Mix and add 10 ml of *methylene chloride R*. Shake vigorously. After separation, the organic layer is red.

C. Dissolve about 10 mg in 2 ml of *alcohol R*. Add 1 ml of a 1 g/l solution of *testosterone propionate R* in *alcohol R* and 2 ml of *dilute sodium hydroxide solution R*. Heat in a water-bath at 80 °C for 10 min and allow to cool. A red colour develops.

TESTS

Solution S. Dissolve 2.5 g in *alcohol R* and dilute to 25 ml with the same solvent.

Appearance of solution. Solution S is clear (*2.2.1*) and not more intensely coloured than intensity 5 of the range of reference solutions of the most appropriate colour (*2.2.2, Method II*).

Related substances. Examine by thin-layer chromatography (*2.2.27*), using *silica gel G R* as the coating substance.

Test solution (a). Dissolve 0.25 g of the substance to be examined in *methylene chloride R* and dilute to 10 ml with the same solvent.

Test solution (b). Dilute 1 ml of test solution (a) to 10 ml with *methylene chloride R*.

Reference solution (a). Dissolve 25 mg of *butylhydroxyanisole CRS* in *methylene chloride R* and dilute to 10 ml with the same solvent.

Reference solution (b). Dilute 1 ml of reference solution (a) to 20 ml with *methylene chloride R*.

Reference solution (c). Dissolve 50 mg of *hydroquinone R* in 5 ml of *alcohol R* and dilute to 100 ml with *methylene chloride R*. Dilute 1 ml of this solution to 10 ml with *methylene chloride R*.

Apply separately to the plate 5 µl of each solution. Develop over a path of 10 cm using *methylene chloride R*. Allow the plate to dry in air and spray with a freshly prepared mixture of 10 volumes of *potassium ferricyanide solution R*, 20 volumes of *ferric chloride solution R1* and 70 volumes of *water R*. In the chromatogram obtained with test solution (a): any violet-blue spot with an R_f value of about 0.35 (corresponding to 3-(1,1-dimethylethyl)-4-methoxyphenol) is not more intense than the principal spot in the chromatogram obtained with reference solution (a) (10 per cent); any spot corresponding to hydroquinone is not more intense than the principal spot in the chromatogram obtained with reference solution (c) (0.2 per cent); any spot, apart from the principal spot and any spots corresponding to 3-(1,1-dimethylethyl)-4-methoxyphenol and hydroquinone, is not more intense than the principal spot in the chromatogram obtained with reference solution (b) (0.5 per cent).

Heavy metals (*2.4.8*). 1.0 g complies with limit test C for heavy metals (10 ppm). Prepare the standard using 1 ml of *lead standard solution (10 ppm Pb) R*.

Sulphated ash (*2.4.14*). Not more than 0.1 per cent, determined on 1.0 g.

STORAGE

Store protected from light.

IMPURITIES

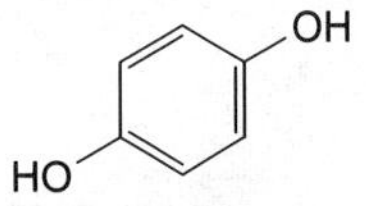

A. benzene-1,4-diol (hydroquinone).

01/2005:0581

BUTYLHYDROXYTOLUENE

Butylhydroxytoluenum

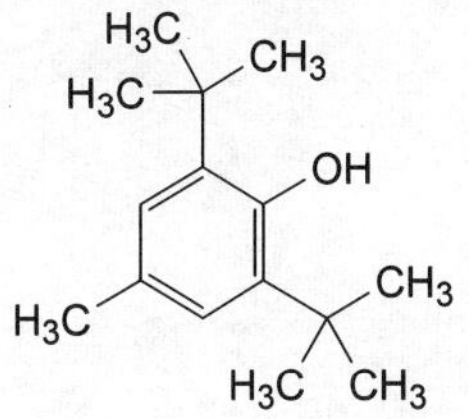

$C_{15}H_{24}O$ M_r 220.4

DEFINITION

Butylhydroxytoluene is 2,6-bis(1,1-dimethylethyl)-4-methylphenol.

CHARACTERS

A white or yellowish-white, crystalline powder, practically insoluble in water, very soluble in acetone, freely soluble in alcohol and in vegetable oils.

IDENTIFICATION

First identification: A, C.

Second identification: A, B, D.

A. It complies with the test for the freezing-point (see Tests).

B. Dissolve 0.500 g in *ethanol R* and dilute to 100.0 ml with the same solvent. Dilute 1.0 ml of this solution to 100.0 ml with *ethanol R*. Examined between 230 nm and 300 nm (*2.2.25*), the solution shows an absorption maximum at 278 nm. The specific absorbance at the maximum is 80 to 90.

C. Examine by infrared absorption spectrophotometry (*2.2.24*), comparing with the spectrum obtained with *butylhydroxytoluene CRS*.

D. Dissolve about 10 mg in 2 ml of *alcohol R*. Add 1 ml of a 1 g/l solution of *testosterone propionate R* in *alcohol R* and 2 ml of *dilute sodium hydroxide solution R*. Heat in a water-bath at 80 °C for 10 min and allow to cool. A blue colour develops.

TESTS

Appearance of solution. Dissolve 1.0 g in *methanol R* and dilute to 10 ml with the same solvent. The solution is clear (*2.2.1*) and not more intensely coloured than reference solution Y_5 or BY_5 (*2.2.2, Method II*).

Freezing-point (*2.2.18*): 69 °C to 70 °C.

Related substances. Examine by thin-layer chromatography (*2.2.27*), using *silica gel G R* as the coating substance.

Test solution. Dissolve 0.2 g of the substance to be examined in *methanol R* and dilute to 10.0 ml with the same solvent.

Reference solution. Dilute 1 ml of the test solution to 200 ml with *methanol R*.

Apply separately to the plate 10 µl of each solution. Develop over a path of 15 cm using *methylene chloride R*. Dry the plate in air and spray with a freshly prepared mixture of 10 volumes of *potassium ferricyanide solution R*, 20 volumes of *ferric chloride solution R1* and 70 volumes of *water R*. Any spot in the chromatogram obtained with the test solution, apart from the principal spot, is not more intense than the spot in the chromatogram obtained with the reference solution (0.5 per cent).

Sulphated ash (*2.4.14*). Not more than 0.1 per cent, determined on 1.0 g.

C

01/2005:0267

CAFFEINE

Coffeinum

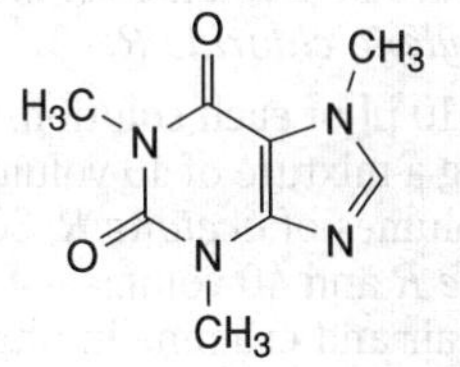

$C_8H_{10}N_4O_2$ M_r 194.2

DEFINITION

Caffeine contains not less than 98.5 per cent and not more than the equivalent of 101.5 per cent of 1,3,7-trimethyl-3,7-dihydro-1*H*-purine-2,6-dione, calculated with reference to the dried substance.

CHARACTERS

A white, crystalline powder or silky, white crystals, sublimes readily, sparingly soluble in water, freely soluble in boiling water, slightly soluble in ethanol. It dissolves in concentrated solutions of alkali benzoates or salicylates.

IDENTIFICATION

First identification: A, B, E.

Second identification: A, C, D, E, F.

A. Melting point (*2.2.14*): 234 °C to 239 °C.

B. Examine by infrared absorption spectrophotometry (*2.2.24*), comparing with the spectrum obtained with *caffeine CRS*.

C. To 2 ml of a saturated solution add 0.05 ml of *iodinated potassium iodide solution R*. The solution remains clear. Add 0.1 ml of *dilute hydrochloric acid R*. A brown precipitate is formed. Neutralise with *dilute sodium hydroxide solution R*. The precipitate dissolves.

D. In a glass-stoppered tube, dissolve about 10 mg in 0.25 ml of a mixture of 0.5 ml of *acetylacetone R* and 5 ml of *dilute sodium hydroxide solution R*. Heat in a water-bath at 80 °C for 7 min. Cool and add 0.5 ml of *dimethylaminobenzaldehyde solution R2*. Heat again in a water-bath at 80 °C for 7 min. Allow to cool and add 10 ml of *water R*. An intense blue colour develops.

E. It complies with the test for loss on drying (see Tests).

F. It gives the reaction of xanthines (*2.3.1*).

TESTS

Solution S. Dissolve 0.5 g with heating in 50 ml of *carbon dioxide-free water R* prepared from *distilled water R*, cool and dilute to 50 ml with the same solvent.

Appearance of solution. Solution S is clear (*2.2.1*) and colourless (*2.2.2, Method II*).

Acidity. To 10 ml of solution S add 0.05 ml of *bromothymol blue solution R1*. The solution is green or yellow. Not more than 0.2 ml of *0.01 M sodium hydroxide* is required to change the colour of the indicator to blue.

Related substances. Examine by thin-layer chromatography (*2.2.27*) using *silica gel* GF_{254} *R* as the coating substance.

Test solution. Dissolve 0.2 g of the substance to be examined in a mixture of 4 volumes of *methanol R* and 6 volumes of *methylene chloride R* and dilute to 10 ml with the same mixture of solvents.

Reference solution. Dilute 0.5 ml of the test solution to 100 ml with a mixture of 4 volumes of *methanol R* and 6 volumes of *methylene chloride R*.

Apply to the plate 10 µl of each solution. Develop over a path of 15 cm using a mixture of 10 volumes of *concentrated ammonia R*, 30 volumes of *acetone R*, 30 volumes of *methylene chloride R* and 40 volumes of *butanol R*. Allow the plate to dry in air and examine in ultraviolet light at 254 nm. Any spot in the chromatogram obtained with the test solution, apart from the principal spot, is not more intense than the spot in the chromatogram obtained with the reference solution (0.5 per cent).

Sulphates (*2.4.13*). 15 ml of solution S complies with the limit test for sulphates (500 ppm). Prepare the standard using a mixture of 7.5 ml of *sulphate standard solution (10 ppm* SO_4*) R* and 7.5 ml of *distilled water R*.

Heavy metals (*2.4.8*). 1.0 g complies with limit test C for heavy metals (20 ppm). Prepare the standard using 2 ml of *lead standard solution (10 ppm Pb) R*.

Loss on drying (*2.2.32*). Not more than 0.5 per cent, determined on 1.000 g by drying in an oven at 100-105 °C for 1 h.

Sulphated ash (*2.4.14*). Not more than 0.1 per cent, determined on 1.0 g.

ASSAY

Dissolve 0.170 g with heating in 5 ml of *anhydrous acetic acid R*. Allow to cool, add 10 ml of *acetic anhydride R* and 20 ml of *toluene R*. Titrate with *0.1 M perchloric acid*, determining the end-point potentiometrically (*2.2.20*).

1 ml of *0.1 M perchloric acid* is equivalent to 19.42 mg of $C_8H_{10}N_4O_2$.

IMPURITIES

Specified impurities: A.

Other detectable impurities: B, C.

A. theophylline,

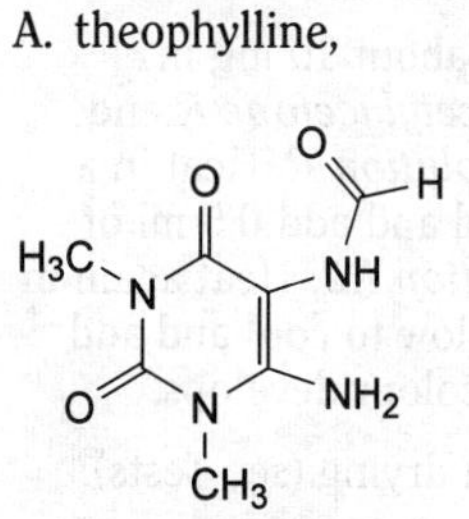

B. *N*-[6-amino-1,3-dimethyl-2,4(1*H*,3*H*)-dioxopyrimidin-5-yl]formamide,

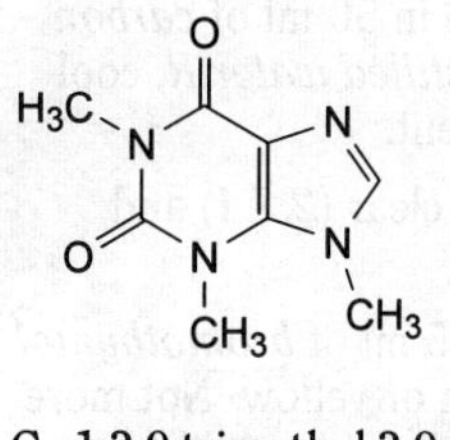

C. 1,3,9-trimethyl-3,9-dihydro-1*H*-purine-2,6-dione (isocaffeine).

01/2005:0268

CAFFEINE MONOHYDRATE

Coffeinum monohydricum

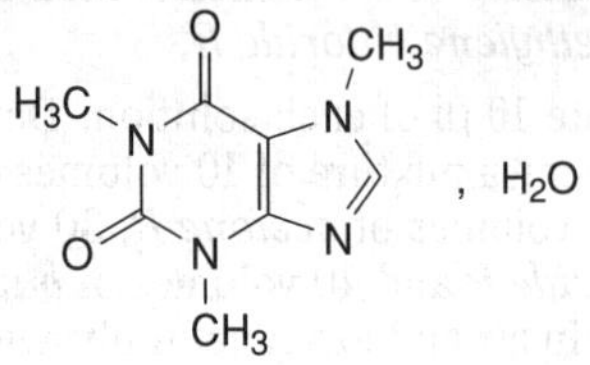

$C_8H_{10}N_4O_2,H_2O$ M_r 212.2

DEFINITION

Caffeine monohydrate contains not less than 98.5 per cent and not more than the equivalent of 101.5 per cent of 1,3,7-trimethyl-3,7-dihydro-1*H*-purine-2,6-dione, calculated with reference to the dried substance.

CHARACTERS

A white, crystalline powder or silky, white crystals, sublimes readily, sparingly soluble in water, freely soluble in boiling water, slightly soluble in ethanol. It dissolves in concentrated solutions of alkali benzoates or salicylates.

IDENTIFICATION

First identification: A, B, E.

Second identification: A, C, D, E, F.

A. Melting point (*2.2.14*): 234 °C to 239 °C, determined after drying at 100-105 °C.

B. Dry the substance to be examined at 100-105 °C. Examine by infrared absorption spectrophotometry (*2.2.24*), comparing with the spectrum obtained with *caffeine CRS.*

C. To 2 ml of a saturated solution add 0.05 ml of *iodinated potassium iodide solution R*. The solution remains clear. Add 0.1 ml of *dilute hydrochloric acid R*. A brown precipitate is formed. Neutralise with *dilute sodium hydroxide solution R*. The precipitate dissolves.

D. In a glass-stoppered tube, dissolve about 10 mg in 0.25 ml of a mixture of 0.5 ml of *acetylacetone R* and 5 ml of *dilute sodium hydroxide solution R*. Heat in a water-bath at 80 °C for 7 min. Cool and add 0.5 ml of *dimethylaminobenzaldehyde solution R2*. Heat again in a water-bath at 80 °C for 7 min. Allow to cool and add 10 ml of *water R*. An intense blue colour develops.

E. It complies with the test for loss on drying (see Tests).

F. It gives the reaction of xanthines (*2.3.1*).

TESTS

Solution S. Dissolve 0.5 g with heating in 50 ml of *carbon dioxide-free water R* prepared from *distilled water R*, cool and dilute to 50 ml with the same solvent.

Appearance of solution. Solution S is clear (*2.2.1*) and colourless (*2.2.2, Method II*).

Acidity. To 10 ml of solution S add 0.05 ml of *bromothymol blue solution R1*. The solution is green or yellow. Not more than 0.2 ml of *0.01 M sodium hydroxide* is required to change the colour of the indicator to blue.

Related substances. Examine by thin-layer chromatography (*2.2.27*) using *silica gel GF_{254} R* as the coating substance.

Test solution. Dissolve 0.2 g of the substance to be examined in a mixture of 4 volumes of *methanol R* and 6 volumes of *methylene chloride R* and dilute to 10 ml with the same mixture of solvents.

Reference solution. Dilute 0.5 ml of the test solution to 100 ml with a mixture of 4 volumes of *methanol R* and 6 volumes of *methylene chloride R.*

Apply to the plate 10 µl of each solution. Develop over a path of 15 cm using a mixture of 10 volumes of *concentrated ammonia R*, 30 volumes of *acetone R*, 30 volumes of *methylene chloride R* and 40 volumes of *butanol R*. Allow the plate to dry in air and examine in ultraviolet light at 254 nm. Any spot in the chromatogram obtained with the test solution, apart from the principal spot, is not more intense than the spot in the chromatogram obtained with the reference solution (0.5 per cent).

Sulphates (*2.4.13*). 15 ml of solution S complies with the limit test for sulphates (500 ppm). Prepare the standard using a mixture of 7.5 ml of *sulphate standard solution (10 ppm SO_4) R* and 7.5 ml of *distilled water R.*

Heavy metals (*2.4.8*). 1.0 g complies with limit test C for heavy metals (20 ppm). Prepare the standard using 2 ml of *lead standard solution (10 ppm Pb) R.*

Loss on drying (*2.2.32*). 5.0 per cent to 9.0 per cent, determined on 1.000 g by drying in an oven at 100-105 °C for 1 h.

Sulphated ash (*2.4.14*). Not more than 0.1 per cent, determined on 1.0 g.

ASSAY

Dissolve 0.170 g, previously dried at 100-105 °C, with heating in 5 ml of *anhydrous acetic acid R*. Allow to cool, add 10 ml of *acetic anhydride R* and 20 ml of *toluene R*. Titrate with *0.1 M perchloric acid*, determining the end-point potentiometrically (*2.2.20*).

1 ml of *0.1 M perchloric acid* is equivalent to 19.42 mg of $C_8H_{10}N_4O_2$.

IMPURITIES

Specified impurities: A.

Other detectable impurities: B, C.

A. theophylline,

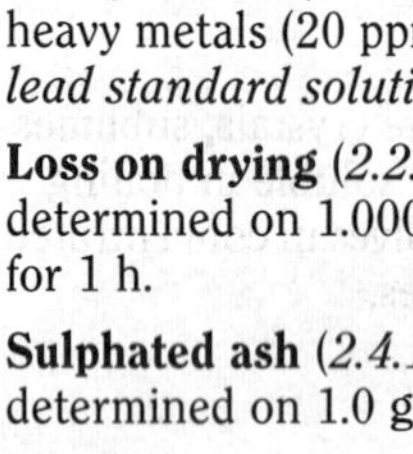

B. *N*-[6-amino-1,3-dimethyl-2,4(1*H*, 3*H*)-dioxopyrimidin-5-yl]formamide,

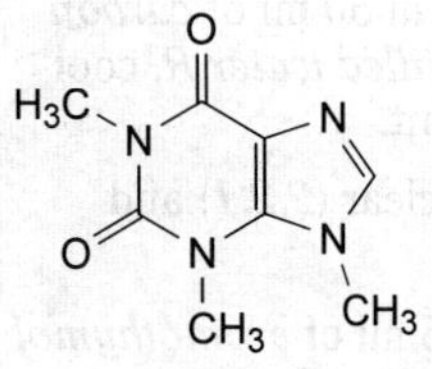

C. 1,3,9-trimethyl-3,9-dihydro-1*H*-purine-2,6-dione (isocaffeine).

01/2005:1295

CALCIFEDIOL

Calcifediolum

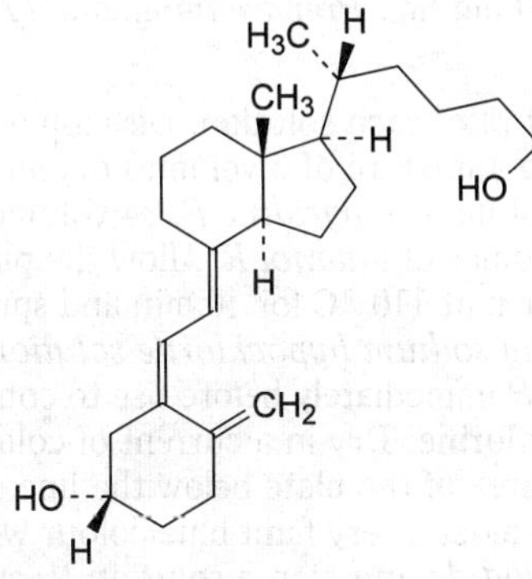

$C_{27}H_{44}O_2,H_2O$ M_r 418.7

DEFINITION

Calcifediol is the monohydrate of (5*Z*,7*E*)-9,10-secocholesta-5,7,10(19)-triene-3β,25-diol. It contains not less than 97.0 per cent and not more than the equivalent of 102.0 per cent of $C_{27}H_{44}O_2$, calculated with reference to the anhydrous substance.

CHARACTERS

White or almost white crystals, practically insoluble in water, freely soluble in alcohol, soluble in fatty oils. It is sensitive to air, heat and light.

A reversible isomerisation to pre-calcifediol takes place in solution, depending on temperature and time. The activity is due to both compounds.

IDENTIFICATION

A. Examine by infrared absorption spectrophotometry (*2.2.24*), comparing with the *Ph. Eur. reference spectrum of calcifediol*, prepared using 2 mg of the substance to be examined and 225 mg of *potassium bromide R*.

B. Examine the chromatograms obtained in the assay. The principal peak in the chromatogram obtained with the test solution is similar in retention time and approximate size to the principal peak in the chromatogram obtained with reference solution (a).

TESTS

Related substances. Examine by liquid chromatography (*2.2.29*) as described under Assay. Calculate the percentage content of related substances, apart from pre-calcifediol, that are eluted within twice the retention time of calcifediol from the areas of the peaks in the chromatogram obtained with the test solution by the normalisation procedure. The content of any individual related substance is not greater than 0.5 per cent and the sum of the related substances is not greater than 1.0 per cent. Disregard any peak below 0.1 per cent.

Water (*2.5.32*): 3.8 per cent to 5.0 per cent, determined on 10.0 mg by the micro determination of water.

ASSAY

Carry out the assay as rapidly as possible, avoiding exposure to actinic light and air.

Examine by liquid chromatography (*2.2.29*).

Test solution. Dissolve 1.0 mg of the substance to be examined without heating in 10.0 ml of the mobile phase.

Reference solution (a). Dissolve 1.0 mg of *calcifediol CRS* without heating in 10.0 ml of the mobile phase.

Reference solution (b). Dilute reference solution (a) 100 times with the mobile phase.

Reference solution (c). Heat 2 ml of reference solution (a) in a water-bath at 80 °C under a reflux condenser for 2 h and cool.

The chromatographic procedure may be carried out using:

- a column 0.15 m long and 4.6 mm in internal diameter packed with *octylsilyl silica gel for chromatography R1* (5 µm),
- as mobile phase at a flow rate of 1.5 ml/min a mixture of 200 volumes of *water R* and 800 volumes of *methanol R*,
- as detector a spectrophotometer set at 265 nm,
- a loop injector.

Inject 50 µl of reference solution (c) and record the chromatogram. Make a total of six injections. When the chromatograms are recorded in the prescribed conditions, the retention time for pre-calcifediol, relative to calcifediol, is about 1.3. The assay is not valid unless the relative standard deviation of the response for calcifediol is at most 1 per cent and the resolution between the peaks due to pre-calcifediol and calcifediol is at least 5.0; adjust the proportions of the constituents of the mobile phase, if necessary, to obtain this resolution.

Inject 50 µl of reference solution (a) and 50 µl of reference solution (b) and record the chromatograms. Inject 50 µl of the test solution and record the chromatogram in the same manner, continuing the chromatography for twice the retention time of the principal peak.

STORAGE

Store under nitrogen, in an airtight container, protected from light, at a temperature of 2 °C to 8 °C.

The contents of an opened container are to be used immediately.

IMPURITIES

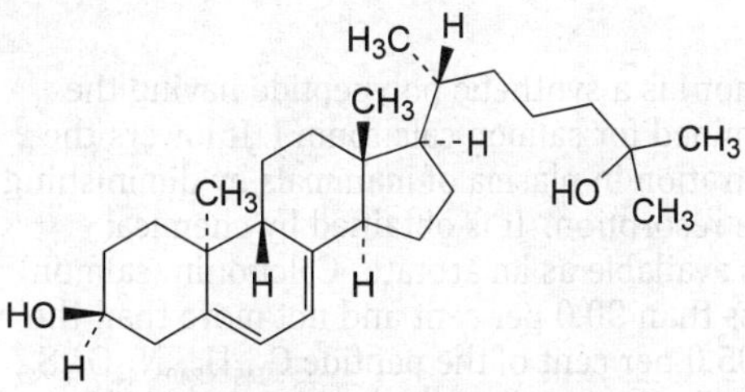

A. 9β,10α-cholesta-5,7-diene-3β,25-diol,

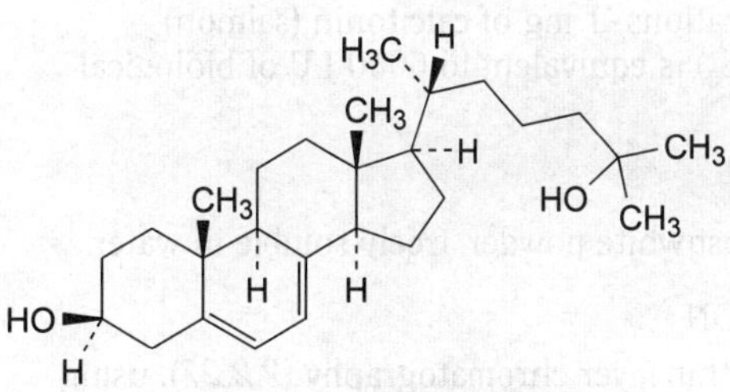

B. cholesta-5,7-diene-3β,25-diol,

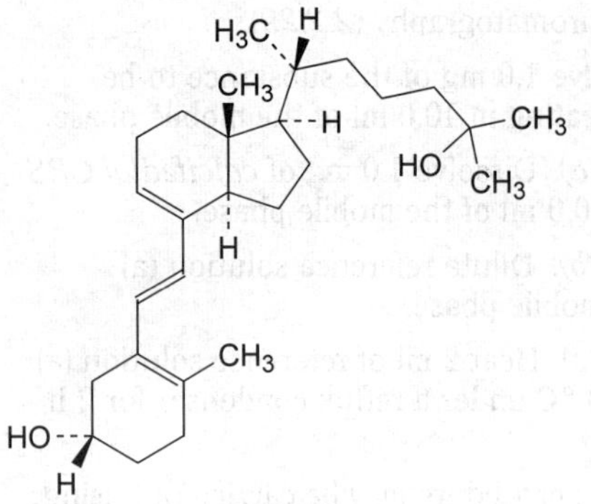

C. (6*E*)-9,10-secocholesta-5(10),6,8-triene-3β,25-diol,

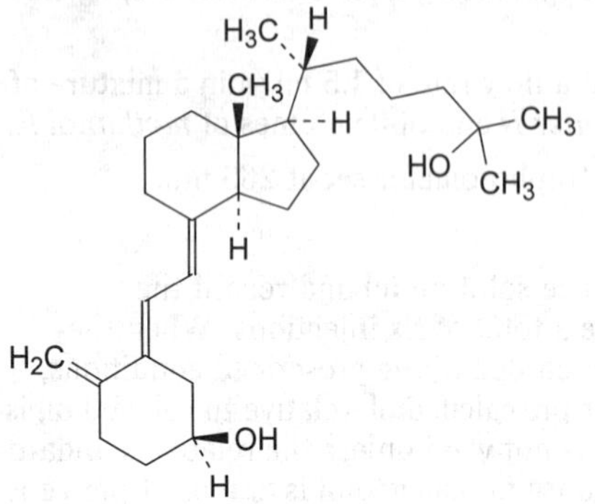

D. (5*E*,7*E*)-9,10-secocholesta-5,7,10(19)-triene-3β,25-diol.

01/2005:0471

CALCITONIN (SALMON)

Calcitoninum salmonis

H-Cys-Ser-Asn-Leu-Ser-Thr-Cys-Val-Leu-Gly-
Lys-Leu-Ser-Gln-Glu-Leu-His-Lys-Leu-Gln-
Thr-Tyr-Pro-Arg-Thr-Asn-Thr-Gly-Ser-Gly-
Thr-Pro-NH2

$C_{145}H_{240}N_{44}O_{48}S_2$ M_r 3432

DEFINITION

Calcitonin (salmon) is a synthetic polypeptide having the structure determined for salmon calcitonin I. It lowers the calcium concentration in plasma of mammals by diminishing the rate of bone resorption. It is obtained by chemical synthesis and is available as an acetate. Calcitonin (salmon) contains not less than 90.0 per cent and not more than the equivalent of 105.0 per cent of the peptide $C_{145}H_{240}N_{44}O_{48}S_2$, calculated with reference to the anhydrous, acetic acid-free substance.

By convention, for the purpose of labelling calcitonin (salmon) preparations, 1 mg of calcitonin (salmon) ($C_{145}H_{240}N_{44}O_{48}S_2$) is equivalent to 6000 I.U of biological activity.

CHARACTERS

A white or almost white powder, freely soluble in water.

IDENTIFICATION

A. Examine by thin-layer chromatography (*2.2.27*), using *cellulose for chromatography R1* as the coating substance.

Test solution. Dissolve 4 mg of the substance to be examined in 2 ml of a mixture of 2 volumes of *acetic acid R* and 98 volumes of *water R. Prepare immediately before use.*

Reference solution. Dissolve the contents of a vial of *calcitonin (salmon) CRS* in a mixture of 2 volumes of *acetic acid R* and 98 volumes of *water R* to obtain a concentration of 2.0 mg/ml. *Prepare immediately before use.*

Apply to the plate 1 µl of each solution. Develop over a path of 15 cm using a mixture of 6 volumes of *glacial acetic acid R*, 20 volumes of *pyridine R*, 24 volumes of *water R* and 30 volumes of *butanol R*. Allow the plate to dry in air for 1 h, heat at 110 °C for 10 min and spray the hot plate with *strong sodium hypochlorite solution R* diluted with *water R* immediately before use to contain 5 g/l of available chlorine. Dry in a current of cold air until a sprayed area of the plate below the line of application gives at most a very faint blue colour with a drop of *potassium iodide and starch solution R*; avoid prolonged exposure to cold air. Spray with *potassium iodide and starch solution R* until the spots are clearly visible. The principal spot in the chromatogram obtained with the test solution is similar in position, colour and size to the principal spot in the chromatogram obtained with the reference solution.

B. Examine the chromatograms obtained in the Assay. The retention time of the principal peak in the chromatogram obtained with the test solution is similar to that of the principal peak in the chromatogram obtained with the reference solution.

TESTS

Acetic acid (*2.5.34*): 4.0 per cent to 15.0 per cent.

Test solution. Dissolve 10.0 mg of the substance to be examined in a mixture of 5 volumes of mobile phase B and 95 volumes of mobile phase A and dilute to 10.0 ml with the same mixture of solvents.

Amino acids. Examine by means of an amino-acid analyser. Standardise the apparatus with a mixture containing equimolar amounts of ammonia, glycine and the L-form of the following amino acids:

lysine	histidine	arginine
serine	methionine	glutamic acid
isoleucine	proline	leucine
aspartic acid	alanine	tyrosine
threonine	valine	phenylalanine

together with half the equimolar amount of L-cystine. For the validation of the method, an appropriate internal standard, such as *DL-norleucine R*, is used.

Test solution. Place 1.0 mg of the substance to be examined in a rigorously cleaned hard-glass tube 100 mm long and 6 mm in internal diameter. Add a suitable amount of a 50 per cent *V/V* solution of *hydrochloric acid R*. Immerse the tube in a freezing mixture at − 5 °C, reduce the pressure to below 133 Pa and seal. Heat at 110 °C to 115 °C for 16 h. Cool, open the tube, transfer the contents to a 10 ml flask with the aid of five quantities, each of 0.2 ml, of *water R* and evaporate to dryness over *potassium hydroxide R* under reduced pressure. Take up the residue in *water R* and evaporate to dryness over *potassium hydroxide R* under reduced pressure; repeat these operations once. Take up the residue in a buffer solution suitable for the amino-acid analyser used and dilute to a suitable volume with the same buffer solution. Apply a suitable volume to the amino-acid analyser.

Express the content of each amino acid in moles. Calculate the relative proportions of the amino acids taking as equivalent to 1 the sum, divided by 20, of the number of moles of aspartic acid, glutamic acid, proline, glycine, valine, leucine, histidine, arginine and lysine. The values fall within the following limits: aspartic acid 1.8 to 2.2; glutamic acid 2.7 to 3.3; proline 1.7 to 2.3; glycine 2.7 to 3.3; valine 0.9 to 1.1; leucine 4.5 to 5.3; histidine 0.9 to 1.1; arginine 0.9 to 1.1; lysine 1.8 to 2.2; serine 3.2 to 4.2; threonine 4.2 to 5.2; tyrosine 0.7 to 1.1; half-cystine 1.4 to 2.1.

Related peptides. Examine by liquid chromatography (*2.2.29*) as described under Assay.

Inject 20 µl of the test solution. In the chromatogram obtained, the area of any peak apart from the principal peak is not greater than 3.0 per cent of the total area of the peaks. The sum of the areas of all the peaks, apart from the principal peak, is not greater than 5.0 per cent of the total area of the peaks. Disregard any peak due to the solvent and any peak with an area less than 0.1 per cent of that of the principal peak.

Water (*2.5.32*). Not more than 10.0 per cent, determined by the micro determination of water.

Acetic acid and water. Not more than 20 per cent, calculated by adding together the percentage contents of acetic acid and water determined by the methods described above.

Bacterial endotoxins (*2.6.14*): less than 1000 IU/mg, if intended for use in the manufacture of parenteral dosage forms without a further appropriate procedure for the removal of bacterial endotoxins.

ASSAY

Examine by liquid chromatography (*2.2.29*).

Test solution. Prepare a 1.0 mg/ml solution of the substance to be examined in mobile phase A.

Reference solution. Dissolve the contents of a vial of *calcitonin (salmon) CRS* in mobile phase A to obtain a concentration of 1.0 mg/ml.

Resolution solution. Dissolve the contents of a vial of *N-acetyl-cys[1]calcitonin CRS* in 400 µl of mobile phase A and add 100 µl of the test solution.

The chromatographic procedure may be carried out using:

- a stainless steel column 0.25 m long and 4.6 mm in internal diameter packed with *octadecylsilyl silica gel for chromatography R* (5 µm),
- as mobile phase at a flow rate of 1.0 ml/min:

  Mobile phase A. Dissolve 3.26 g of *tetramethylammonium hydroxide R* in 900 ml of *water R*, adjust the pH to 2.5 with *phosphoric acid R* and mix with 100 ml of *acetonitrile for chromatography R*; filter and degas,

  Mobile phase B. Dissolve 1.45 g of *tetramethylammonium hydroxide R* in 400 ml of *water R*, adjust the pH to 2.5 with *phosphoric acid R* and mix with 600 ml of *acetonitrile for chromatography R*; filter and degas,

Time (min)	Mobile phase A (per cent *V/V*)	Mobile phase B (per cent *V/V*)	Comment
0 - 30	72 → 48	28 → 52	linear gradient
30 - 32	48 → 72	52 → 28	switch to initial eluent composition
32 - 55	72	28	re-equilibration

- as detector a spectrophotometer set at 220 nm,

maintaining the temperature of the column at 65 °C.

Equilibrate the column with a mixture of 72 volumes of mobile phase A and 28 volumes of mobile phase B.

Inject 20 µl of the resolution solution. When the chromatogram is recorded in the prescribed conditions, the relative retention of *N*-acetyl-cys[1]calcitonin is about 1.15 relative to the principal peak. The test is not valid unless the resolution between the peaks corresponding to calcitonin and *N*-acetyl-cys[1]calcitonin is at least 5.0 and the symmetry factor for the *N*-acetyl-cys[1]calcitonin peak is not greater than 2.5. If necessary, adjust the initial A:B ratio of the mobile phase.

Inject 20 µl of the test solution and 20 µl of the reference solution.

Calculate the content of calcitonin (salmon) ($C_{145}H_{240}N_{44}O_{48}S_2$) from the peak areas in the chromatograms obtained with the test solution and the reference solution and the declared content of $C_{145}H_{240}N_{44}O_{48}S_2$ in *calcitonin (salmon) CRS*. Proceed with tangential integration of the peak areas.

STORAGE

Store protected from light at a temperature between 2 °C and 8 °C. If the substance is sterile, store in a sterile, airtight, tamper-proof container.

LABELLING

The label states:

- the calcitonin peptide content ($C_{145}H_{240}N_{44}O_{48}S_2$),
- where applicable, that the substance is free from bacterial endotoxins.

01/2005:0883

CALCITRIOL

Calcitriolum

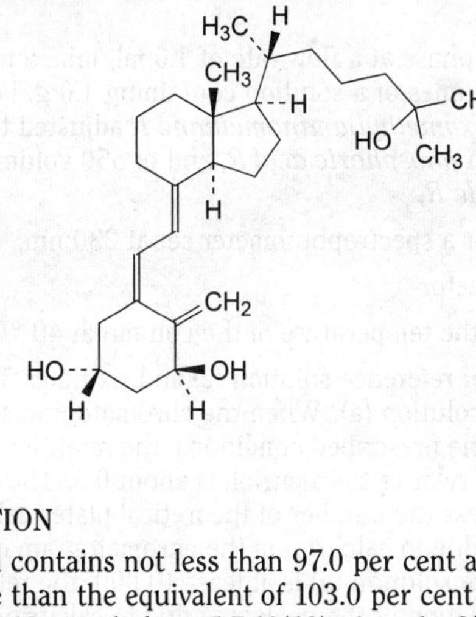

$C_{27}H_{44}O_3$ M_r 416.6

DEFINITION

Calcitriol contains not less than 97.0 per cent and not more than the equivalent of 103.0 per cent of (5*Z*,7*E*)-9,10-secocholesta-5,7,10(19)-triene-1α,3β,25-triol.

CHARACTERS

White or almost white crystals, practically insoluble in water, freely soluble in alcohol, soluble in fatty oils. It is sensitive to air, heat and light.

A reversible isomerisation to pre-calcitriol takes place in solution, depending on temperature and time. The activity is due to both compounds.

IDENTIFICATION

A. Examine by infrared absorption spectrophotometry (*2.2.24*), comparing with the *Ph. Eur. reference spectrum of calcitriol.*

B. Examine the chromatograms obtained in the assay. The retention time and size of the principal peak in the chromatogram obtained with the test solution are approximately the same as those of the principal peak in the chromatogram obtained with reference solution (a).

TESTS

Related substances. Examine by liquid chromatography (*2.2.29*) as described under Assay. Calculate the percentage content of related substances, apart from pre-calcitriol, that are eluted within twice the retention time of calcitriol from the areas of the peaks in the chromatogram obtained with the test solution by the normalisation procedure. The content of any individual related substance is not greater than 0.5 per cent and the sum of the related substances is not greater than 1.0 per cent. Disregard any peak with an area less than 0.1 times that of the peak in the chromatogram obtained with reference solution (b) (0.1 per cent).

ASSAY

Carry out the assay as rapidly as possible, avoiding exposure to actinic light and air.

Examine by liquid chromatography (*2.2.29*).

Test solution. Dissolve 1.000 mg of the substance to be examined without heating in 10.0 ml of the mobile phase.

Reference solution (a). Dissolve 1.000 mg of *calcitriol CRS* without heating in 10.0 ml of the mobile phase.

Reference solution (b). Dilute 1.0 ml of reference solution (a) to 100.0 ml with the mobile phase.

Reference solution (c). Keep 2 ml of reference solution (a) for 30 min at 80 °C.

The chromatographic procedure may be carried out using:

- a column 0.25 m long and 4.6 mm in internal diameter packed with *octylsilyl silica gel for chromatography R1* (5 µm),
- as mobile phase at a flow rate of 1.0 ml/min, a mixture of 450 volumes of a solution containing 1.0 g/l of *tris(hydroxymethyl)aminomethane R* adjusted to pH 7.0 to 7.5 with *phosphoric acid R*, and of 550 volumes of *acetonitrile R*,
- as detector a spectrophotometer set at 230 nm,
- a loop injector,

maintaining the temperature of the column at 40 °C.

Inject 50 µl of reference solution (c) and six times 50 µl of reference solution (a). When the chromatograms are recorded in the prescribed conditions, the retention time for pre-calcitriol, relative to calcitriol, is about 0.9. The assay is not valid unless the number of theoretical plates calculated for the peak due to calcitriol in the chromatogram obtained with reference solution (a) is at least 10 000, the relative standard deviation of the peak area due to calcitriol is at most 1 per cent and the resolution between the peaks due to calcitriol and pre-calcitriol is at least 3.5.

Inject 50 µl of reference solution (b) and 50 µl of the test solution. Continue the chromatography for twice the retention time of calcitriol.

Calculate the percentage content of calcitriol.

STORAGE

Store under nitrogen, in an airtight container, protected from light, at a temperature of 2 °C to 8 °C.

The contents of an opened container are to be used immediately.

IMPURITIES

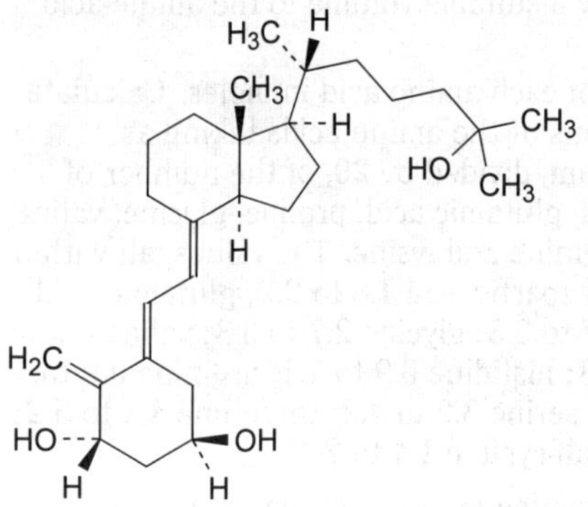

A. (5*E*,7*E*)-9,10-secocholesta-5,7,10(19)-triene-1α,3β,25-triol (*trans*-calcitriol),

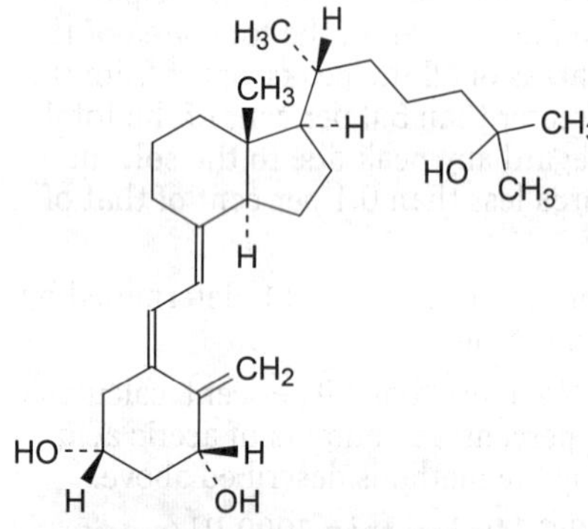

B. (5*Z*,7*E*)-9,10-secocholesta-5,7,10(19)-triene-1β,3β,25-triol (1β-calcitriol),

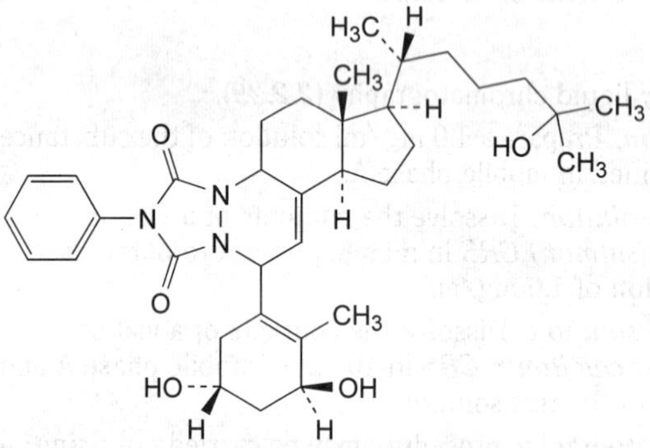

C. (6a*R*,7*R*,9a*R*)-11-[(3*S*,5*R*)-3,5-dihydroxy-2-methylcyclohex-1-enyl]-7-[(1*R*)-5-hydroxy-1,5-dimethylhexyl]-6a-methyl-2-phenyl-5,6,6a,7,8,9,9a,11-octahydro-1*H*,4a*H*-cyclopenta[*f*]1,2,4]triazolo[1,2-*a*]cinnoline-1,3(2*H*)-dione (triazoline adduct of pre-calcitriol).

01/2005:1182

CALCIUM ASCORBATE

Calcii ascorbas

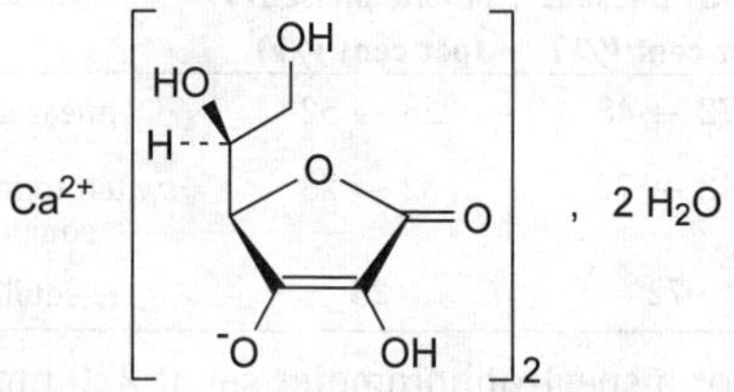

$C_{12}H_{14}CaO_{12},2H_2O$ M_r 426.3

DEFINITION

Calcium ascorbate contains not less than 99.0 per cent and not more than the equivalent of 100.5 per cent of calcium di[(*R*)-2-[(*S*)-1,2-dihydroxyethyl]-4-hydroxy-5-oxo-2*H*-furan-3-olate] dihydrate.

CHARACTERS

A white or slightly yellowish, crystalline powder, freely soluble in water, practically insoluble in alcohol.

IDENTIFICATION

First identification: A, B, E.

Second identification: A, C, D, E.

A. It complies with the test for specific optical rotation (see Tests).

B. Examine by infrared absorption spectrophotometry (*2.2.24*), comparing with the *Ph. Eur. reference spectrum of calcium ascorbate.*

C. Dilute 1 ml of solution S (see Tests) to 10 ml with *water R*. To 2 ml of the solution add 0.2 ml of a 100 g/l solution of *ferrous sulphate R*. A deep violet colour develops.

D. To 1 ml of solution S add 0.2 ml of *dilute nitric acid R* and 0.2 ml of *silver nitrate solution R2*. A grey precipitate is formed.

E. The substance gives reaction (b) of calcium (*2.3.1*).

TESTS

Solution S. Dissolve 5.00 g in *carbon dioxide-free water R* and dilute to 50.0 ml with the same solvent.

Appearance of solution. Solution S is clear (*2.2.1*) and not more intensely coloured than reference solution Y_6 (*2.2.2, Method II*). Examine the colour of the solution immediately after preparation of the solution.

pH (*2.2.3*). The pH of solution S is 6.8 to 7.4.

Specific optical rotation (*2.2.7*): + 95 to + 97, determined using freshly prepared solution S and calculated with reference to the dried substance.

Fluorides. Not more than 10 ppm of F, determined potentiometrically (*2.2.36, Method I*) using as indicator electrode a fluoride-selective electrode and as reference electrode a silver-silver chloride electrode.

Test solution. In a 50 ml volumetric flask, dissolve 1.000 g in a 10.3 g/l solution of *hydrochloric acid R*, add 5.0 ml of *fluoride standard solution (1 ppm F) R* and dilute to 50.0 ml with a 10.3 g/l solution of *hydrochloric acid R*. To 20.0 ml of the solution add 20.0 ml of *total-ionic-strength-adjustment buffer R* and 3 ml of an 82 g/l solution of *anhydrous sodium acetate R*. Adjust to pH 5.2 with *ammonia R* and dilute to 50.0 ml with *distilled water R*.

Reference solutions. To 0.25 ml, 0.5 ml, 1.0 ml, 2.0 ml and 5.0 ml of *fluoride standard solution (10 ppm F) R* add 20.0 ml of *total-ionic-strength-adjustment buffer R* and dilute to 50.0 ml with *distilled water R*.

Carry out the measurements for each solution. Calculate the concentration of fluorides using the calibration curve, taking into account the addition of fluoride to the test solution.

Copper. Not more than 5 ppm of Cu, determined by atomic absorption spectrometry (*2.2.23, Method I*).

Test solution. Dissolve 2.0 g of the substance to be examined in a 9.7 g/l solution of *nitric acid R* and dilute to 25.0 ml with the same acid solution.

Reference solutions. Prepare the reference solutions using *copper standard solution (10 ppm Cu) R*, diluting with a 9.7 g/l solution of *nitric acid R*.

Measure the absorbance at 324.8 nm using a copper hollow-cathode lamp as source of radiation and an air-acetylene flame.

Iron. Not more than 2 ppm of Fe, determined by atomic absorption spectrometry (*2.2.23, Method I*).

Test solution. Dissolve 5.0 g of the substance to be examined in a 9.7 g/l solution of *nitric acid R* and dilute to 25.0 ml with the same acid solution.

Reference solutions. Prepare the reference solutions using *iron standard solution (10 ppm Fe) R*, diluting with a 9.7 g/l solution of *nitric acid R*.

Measure the absorbance at 248.3 nm using an iron hollow-cathode lamp as the radiation source and an air-acetylene flame.

Heavy metals (*2.4.8*). 2.0 g complies with limit test D for heavy metals (10 ppm). Prepare the standard using 2.0 ml of *lead standard solution (10 ppm Pb) R*.

Loss on drying (*2.2.32*). Not more than 0.1 per cent, determined on 1.000 g by drying in an oven at 100-105 °C for 2 h.

ASSAY

Dissolve 80.0 mg in a mixture of 10 ml of *dilute sulphuric acid R* and 80 ml of *carbon dioxide-free water R*. Add 1 ml of *starch solution R*. Titrate with *0.05 M iodine* until a persistent violet-blue colour is obtained.

1 ml of *0.05 M iodine* is equivalent to 10.66 mg of $C_{12}H_{14}CaO_{12},2H_2O$.

STORAGE

Store in a non-metallic container, protected from light.

01/2005:0014

CALCIUM CARBONATE

Calcii carbonas

$CaCO_3$ M_r 100.1

DEFINITION

Calcium carbonate contains not less than 98.5 per cent and not more than the equivalent of 100.5 per cent of $CaCO_3$, calculated with reference to the dried substance.

CHARACTERS

A white powder, practically insoluble in water.

IDENTIFICATION

A. It gives the reaction of carbonates (*2.3.1*).

B. 0.2 ml of solution S (see Tests) gives the reactions of calcium (*2.3.1*).

TESTS

Solution S. Dissolve 5.0 g in 80 ml of *dilute acetic acid R*. When the effervescence ceases, boil the solution for 2 min, allow to cool, dilute to 100 ml with *dilute acetic acid R* and filter, if necessary, through a sintered-glass filter.

Substances insoluble in acetic acid. Wash any residue obtained during the preparation of solution S with four quantities, each of 5 ml, of hot *water R* and dry at 100-105 °C for 1 h. The residue weighs not more than 10 mg (0.2 per cent).

Chlorides (*2.4.4*). 3 ml of solution S diluted to 15 ml with *water R* complies with the limit test for chlorides (330 ppm).

Sulphates (*2.4.13*). 1.2 ml of solution S diluted to 15 ml with *distilled water R* complies with the limit test for sulphates (0.25 per cent).

Arsenic (*2.4.2*). 5 ml of solution S complies with limit test A for arsenic (4 ppm).

Barium. To 10 ml of solution S add 10 ml of *calcium sulphate solution R*. After at least 15 min, any opalescence in the solution is not more intense than that in a mixture of 10 ml of solution S and 10 ml of *distilled water R*.

Iron (*2.4.9*). Dissolve 50 mg in 5 ml of *dilute hydrochloric acid R* and dilute to 10 ml with *water R*. The solution complies with the limit test for iron (200 ppm).

Magnesium and alkali metals. Dissolve 1.0 g in 12 ml of *dilute hydrochloric acid R*. Boil the solution for about 2 min and add 20 ml of *water R*, 1 g of *ammonium chloride R* and 0.1 ml of *methyl red solution R*. Add *dilute ammonia R1* until the colour of the indicator changes and then 2 ml in excess. Heat to boiling and add 50 ml of hot *ammonium oxalate solution R*. Allow to stand for 4 h, dilute to 100 ml with *water R* and filter through a suitable filter. To 50 ml of the filtrate add 0.25 ml of *sulphuric acid R*. Evaporate to dryness on a water-bath and ignite to constant mass at 600 °C. The residue weighs not more than 7.5 mg (1.5 per cent).

Heavy metals (*2.4.8*). 12 ml of solution S complies with limit test A for heavy metals (20 ppm). Prepare the standard using *lead standard solution (1 ppm Pb) R*.

Loss on drying (*2.2.32*). Not more than 2.0 per cent, determined on 1.000 g by drying in an oven at 200 °C.

ASSAY

Dissolve 0.150 g in a mixture of 3 ml of *dilute hydrochloric acid R* and 20 ml of *water R*. Boil for 2 min, allow to cool and dilute to 50 ml with *water R*. Carry out the complexometric titration of calcium (*2.5.11*).

1 ml of *0.1 M sodium edetate* is equivalent to 10.01 mg of $CaCO_3$.

01/2005:0015

CALCIUM CHLORIDE DIHYDRATE

Calcii chloridum dihydricum

$CaCl_2,2H_2O$ M_r 147.0

DEFINITION

Content: 97.0 per cent to 103.0 per cent of $CaCl_2,2H_2O$.

CHARACTERS

Appearance: white, crystalline powder, hygroscopic.

Solubility: freely soluble in water, soluble in alcohol.

IDENTIFICATION

A. Solution S (see Tests) gives reaction (a) of chlorides (*2.3.1*).

B. It gives the reactions of calcium (*2.3.1*).

C. It complies with the limits of the assay.

TESTS

Solution S. Dissolve 10.0 g in *carbon dioxide-free water R* prepared from *distilled water R* and dilute to 100 ml with the same solvent.

Appearance of solution. Solution S is clear (*2.2.1*) and not more intensely coloured than reference solution Y_6 (*2.2.2, Method II*).

Acidity or alkalinity. To 10 ml of freshly prepared solution S add 0.1 ml of *phenolphthalein solution R*. If the solution is red, not more than 0.2 ml of *0.01 M hydrochloric acid* is required to discharge the colour and if the solution is colourless, not more than 0.2 ml of *0.01 M sodium hydroxide* is required to turn it red.

Sulphates (*2.4.13*): maximum 300 ppm.

5 ml of solution S diluted to 15 ml with *distilled water R* complies with the limit test for sulphates.

Aluminium. To 10 ml of solution S add 2 ml of *ammonium chloride solution R* and 1 ml of *dilute ammonia R1* and boil the solution. No turbidity or precipitate is formed.

If intended for use in the manufacture of dialysis solutions, it complies with the following test for aluminium (*2.4.17*) which replaces the test prescribed above: maximum 1 ppm.

Prescribed solution. Dissolve 4 g in 100 ml of *water R* and add 10 ml of *acetate buffer solution pH 6.0 R*.

Reference solution. Mix 2 ml of *aluminium standard solution (2 ppm Al) R*, 10 ml of *acetate buffer solution pH 6.0 R* and 98 ml of *water R*.

Blank solution. Mix 10 ml of *acetate buffer solution pH 6.0 R* and 100 ml of *water R*.

Barium. To 10 ml of solution S add 1 ml of *calcium sulphate solution R*. After at least 15 min, any opalescence in the solution is not more intense than that in a mixture of 10 ml of solution S and 1 ml of *distilled water R*.

Iron (*2.4.9*): maximum 10 ppm.

10 ml of solution S complies with the limit test for iron.

Magnesium and alkali metals: maximum 0.5 per cent.

To a mixture of 20 ml of solution S and 80 ml of *water R* add 2 g of *ammonium chloride R* and 2 ml of *dilute ammonia R1*, heat to boiling and pour into the boiling solution a hot solution of 5 g of *ammonium oxalate R* in 75 ml of *water R*. Allow to stand for 4 h, dilute to 200 ml with *water R* and filter through a suitable filter. To 100 ml of the filtrate add 0.5 ml of *sulphuric acid R*. Evaporate to dryness on a water-bath and ignite to constant mass at 600 °C. The residue weighs a maximum of 5 mg.

Heavy metals (*2.4.8*): maximum 20 ppm.

12 ml of solution S complies with limit test A. Prepare the standard using *lead standard solution (2 ppm Pb) R*.

ASSAY

Dissolve 0.280 g in 100 ml of *water R* and carry out the complexometric titration of calcium (*2.5.11*).

1 ml of *0.1 M sodium edetate* is equivalent to 14.70 mg of $CaCl_2,2H_2O$.

LABELLING

The label states, where applicable, that the substance is suitable for use in the manufacture of dialysis solutions.

STORAGE

In an airtight container.

01/2005:0707

CALCIUM CHLORIDE HEXAHYDRATE

Calcii chloridum hexahydricum

$CaCl_2,6H_2O$ M_r 219.1

DEFINITION

Calcium chloride hexahydrate contains not less than 97.0 per cent and not more than the equivalent of 103.0 per cent of $CaCl_2,6H_2O$.

CHARACTERS

A white, crystalline mass or colourless crystals, very soluble in water, freely soluble in alcohol.

It freezes at about 29 °C.

IDENTIFICATION

A. Solution S (see Tests) gives reaction (a) of chlorides (*2.3.1*).

B. It gives the reactions of calcium (*2.3.1*).

C. It complies with the limits of the assay.

TESTS

Solution S. Dissolve 15.0 g in *carbon dioxide-free water R* prepared from *distilled water R* and dilute to 100 ml with the same solvent.

Appearance of solution. Solution S is clear (*2.2.1*) and not more intensely coloured than reference solution Y_6 (*2.2.2, Method II*).

Acidity or alkalinity. To 10 ml of freshly prepared solution S add 0.1 ml of *phenolphthalein solution R*. If the solution is red, not more than 0.2 ml of *0.01 M hydrochloric acid* is required to discharge the colour and if the solution is colourless, not more than 0.2 ml of *0.01 M sodium hydroxide* is required to turn it red.

Sulphates (*2.4.13*). 5 ml of solution S diluted to 15 ml with *distilled water R* complies with the limit test for sulphates (200 ppm).

Aluminium. To 10 ml of solution S add 2 ml of *ammonium chloride solution R* and 1 ml of *dilute ammonia R1*. Heat to boiling. No turbidity or precipitate is formed.

If intended for use in the manufacture of dialysis solutions, it complies with the following test which replaces the test for aluminium prescribed above.

Dissolve 6 g in 100 ml of *water R* and add 10 ml of *acetate buffer solution pH 6.0 R*. The solution complies with the limit test for aluminium (1 ppm). Use as the reference solution a mixture of 2 ml of *aluminium standard solution (2 ppm Al) R*, 10 ml of *acetate buffer solution pH 6.0 R* and 98 ml of *water R*. To prepare the blank use a mixture of 10 ml of *acetate buffer solution pH 6.0 R* and 100 ml of *water R*.

Barium. To 10 ml of solution S add 1 ml of *calcium sulphate solution R*. After at least 15 min, any opalescence in the solution is not more intense than that in a mixture of 10 ml of solution S and 1 ml of *distilled water R*.

Iron (*2.4.9*). 10 ml of solution S complies with the limit test for iron (7 ppm).

Magnesium and alkali metals. To a mixture of 20 ml of solution S and 80 ml of *water R* add 2 g of *ammonium chloride R* and 2 ml of *dilute ammonia R1*, heat to boiling and pour into the boiling solution a hot solution of 5 g of *ammonium oxalate R* in 75 ml of *water R*. Allow to stand for 4 h, dilute to 200 ml with *water R* and filter through a suitable filter. To 100 ml of the filtrate add 0.5 ml of *sulphuric acid R*. Evapor-ate to dryness on a water-bath and ignite to constant mass at 600 °C. The residue weighs not more than 5 mg (0.3 per cent).

Heavy metals (*2.4.8*). 12 ml of solution S complies with limit test A for heavy metals (15 ppm). Prepare the standard using *lead standard solution (2 ppm Pb) R*.

ASSAY

Dissolve 0.200 g in 100 ml of *water R*. Carry out the complexometric titration of calcium (*2.5.11*).

1 ml of *0.1 M sodium edetate* is equivalent to 21.91 mg of $CaCl_2,6H_2O$.

LABELLING

The label states, where applicable, that the substance is suitable for use in the manufacture of dialysis solutions.

01/2005:1183

CALCIUM DOBESILATE MONOHYDRATE

Calcii dobesilas monohydricum

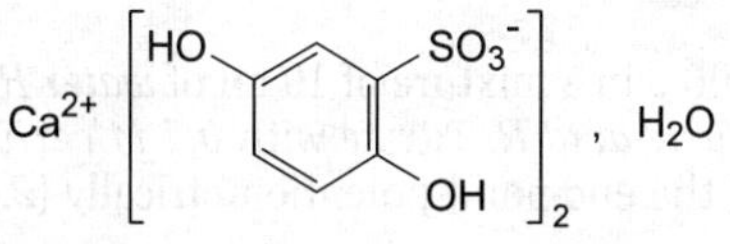

$C_{12}H_{10}CaO_{10}S_2,H_2O$ M_r 436.4

DEFINITION

Calcium dobesilate monohydrate contains not less than 99.0 per cent and not more than the equivalent of 102.0 per cent of calcium di(2,5-dihydroxybenzenesulphonate), calculated with reference to the anhydrous substance.

CHARACTERS

A white or almost white, hygroscopic powder, very soluble in water, freely soluble in ethanol, very slightly soluble in 2-propanol, practically insoluble in methylene chloride.

IDENTIFICATION

A. Dissolve 0.100 g in *water R* and dilute to 200.0 ml with the same solvent. Dilute 5.0 ml of the solution to 100.0 ml with *water R*. Examined between 210 nm and 350 nm (*2.2.25*), the solution shows two absorption maxima, at 221 nm and 301 nm. The specific absorbance at the maximum at 301 nm is 174 to 181.

B. Mix 1 ml of *ferric chloride solution R2*, 1 ml of a freshly prepared 10 g/l solution of *potassium ferricyanide R* and 0.1 ml of *nitric acid R*. To this mixture add 5 ml of freshly prepared solution S (see Tests): a blue colour and a precipitate are immediately produced.

C. 2 ml of freshly prepared solution S (see Tests) gives reaction (b) of calcium (*2.3.1*).

TESTS

Solution S. Dissolve 10.0 g in *carbon dioxide-free water R* and dilute to 100 ml with the same solvent.

Appearance of solution. Solution S, when freshly prepared, is clear (*2.2.1*) and colourless (*2.2.2, Method II*).

pH (*2.2.3*). The pH of solution S is 4.5 to 6.0.

Hydroquinone. Examine by thin-layer chromatography (*2.2.27*), using as the coating substance a suitable silica gel with a fluorescent indicator having an optimal intensity at 254 nm.

Test solution. Dissolve 2.0 g of the substance to be examined in *water R* and dilute to 10 ml with the same solvent.

Reference solution. Dissolve 10 mg of *hydroquinone R* in *water R* and dilute to 50 ml with the same solvent.

Apply to the plate 10 µl of each solution and dry the starting points in a current of cool air. Develop over a path of 15 cm using a mixture of 20 volumes of *methylene chloride R*, 30 volumes of *methyl acetate R* and 50 volumes of *ethyl acetate R*. Dry the plate in a current of hot air and examine in ultraviolet light at 254 nm. Any spot corresponding to hydroquinone in the chromatogram obtained with the test solution is not more intense than the principal spot in the chromatogram obtained with the reference solution (0.1 per cent).

Heavy metals (*2.4.8*). 1.0 g complies with limit test C for heavy metals (15 ppm). Prepare the standard using 1.5 ml of *lead standard solution (10 ppm Pb) R*.

Iron (*2.4.9*). 10 ml of solution S complies with the limit test for iron (10 ppm).

Water (*2.5.12*): 4.0 per cent to 6.0 per cent, determined on 0.500 g by the semi-micro determination of water.

ASSAY

Dissolve 0.200 g in a mixture of 10 ml of *water R* and40 ml of *dilute sulphuric acid R*. Titrate with *0.1 M cerium sulphate*, determining the end-point potentiometrically (*2.2.20*).

1 ml of *0.1 M cerium sulphate* is equivalent to 10.45 mg of $C_{12}H_{10}CaO_{10}S_2$.

STORAGE

Store in an airtight container, protected from light.

IMPURITIES

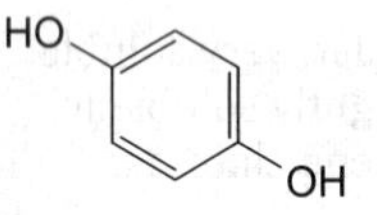

A. benzene-1,4-diol (hydroquinone).

01/2005:0978

CALCIUM FOLINATE

Calcii folinas

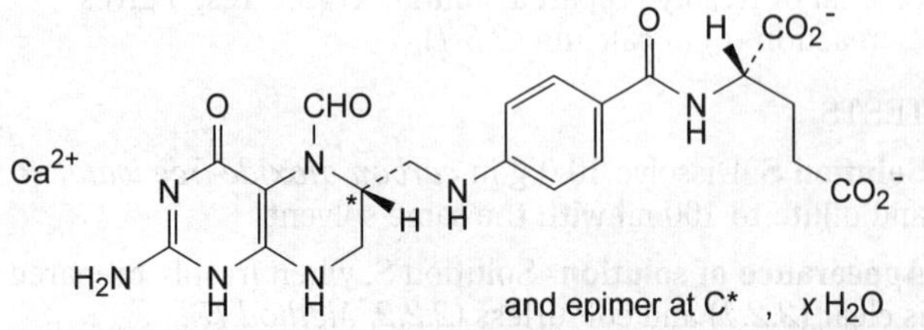

$C_{20}H_{21}CaN_7O_7,xH_2O$ M_r 511.5 (anhydrous substance)

DEFINITION

Calcium folinate contains not less than 97.0 per cent and not more than the equivalent of 102.0 per cent of calcium (2*S*)-2-[[4-[[[(6*RS*)-2-amino-5-formyl-4-oxo-1,4,5,6,7,8-hexahydropteridin-6-yl]methyl]amino]benzoyl]amino]pentanedioate and not less than 7.54 per cent and not more than the equivalent of 8.14 per cent of Ca, both calculated with reference to the anhydrous and solvent-free substance.

CHARACTERS

A white or light yellow, amorphous or crystalline powder, sparingly soluble in water, practically insoluble in acetone and in alcohol. The amorphous form may produce supersaturated solutions in water.

IDENTIFICATION

First identification: A, B, D.

Second identification: A, C, D.

A. It complies with the test for specific optical rotation (see Tests).

B. Examine by infrared absorption spectrophotometry (*2.2.24*), comparing with the spectrum obtained with *calcium folinate CRS*. Examine the substances prepared as discs. If the spectra obtained show differences, dissolve the substance to be examined and the reference substance separately in the minimum quantity of *water R* and add dropwise sufficient *acetone R* to produce sufficient precipitate. Allow to stand for 15 min, collect the precipitate by centrifugation, wash the precipitate with two small quantities of *acetone R* and dry. Record new spectra using the residues.

C. Examine by thin-layer chromatography (*2.2.27*), using *cellulose for chromatography F_{254} R* as the coating substance.
Test solution. Dissolve 15 mg of the substance to be examined in a 3 per cent *V/V* solution of *ammonia R* and dilute to 5 ml with the same solvent.
Reference solution. Dissolve 15 mg of *calcium folinate CRS* in a 3 per cent *V/V* solution of *ammonia R* and dilute to 5 ml with the same solvent.
Apply to the plate 5 µl of each solution. Develop over a path of 15 cm using the lower layer of a mixture of 1 volume of *isoamyl alcohol R* and 10 volumes of a 50 g/l solution of *citric acid R* previously adjusted to pH 8 with *ammonia R*. Allow the plate to dry in air and examine in ultraviolet light at 254 nm. The principal spot in the chromatogram obtained with the test solution is similar in position and size to the principal spot in the chromatogram obtained with the reference solution.

D. It gives reaction (b) of calcium (*2.3.1*).

Carry out the tests and the assay as rapidly as possible, protected from actinic light.

TESTS

Solution S. Dissolve 1.25 g in *carbon dioxide-free water R*, heating at 40 °C if necessary, and dilute to 50.0 ml with the same solvent.

Appearance of solution. Solution S is clear (*2.2.1*). The absorbance (*2.2.25*) of solution S, measured at 420 nm using *water R* as the compensation liquid, is not greater than 0.60.

pH (*2.2.3*). The pH of solution S is 6.8 to 8.0.

Specific optical rotation (*2.2.7*). The specific optical rotation is + 14.4 to + 18.0, determined on solution S and calculated with reference to the anhydrous and solvent-free substance.

Acetone, ethanol and methanol. Not more than 0.5 per cent of acetone, not more than 3.0 per cent of ethanol and not more than 0.5 per cent of methanol. Examine by head-space gas chromatography (*2.2.28*) using the standard additions method.

Test solution. Dissolve 0.25 g of the substance to be examined in *water R* and dilute to 10.0 ml with the same solvent.

Reference solution. Dilute 0.125 g of *acetone R,* 0.750 g of *ethanol R* and 0.125 g of *methanol R* in *water R* and dilute to 1000.0 ml with *water R.*

The chromatographic procedure may be carried out using:

- a fused-silica column 10 m long and 0.32 mm in internal diameter coated with *styrene-divinylbenzene copolymer R,*
- *nitrogen for chromatography R* as the carrier gas at a flow rate of 4 ml/min,
- a flame-ionisation detector,

raising the temperature of the column from 125 °C to 185 °C at a rate of 10 °C/min and maintaining at 185 °C until the total run time is 15 min. Maintain the temperature of the injection port at 250 °C and that of the detector at 250 °C. Place the samples in a thermostatically controlled chamber at 80 °C for 20 min and pressurise them for 30 s. Repeat the injections at least three times.

Related substances. Examine the chromatograms obtained in the Assay. In the chromatogram obtained with the test solution: the area of any peak corresponding to formylfolic acid is not greater than the area of the principal peak in the chromatogram obtained with reference solution (c) (1 per cent); the area of any peak, apart from the principal peak and any peak corresponding to formylfolic acid, is not greater than the area of the principal peak in the chromatogram obtained with reference solution (b) (1 per cent); the sum of the areas of all the peaks, apart from the principal peak, is not greater than 2.5 times the area of the principal peak in the chromatogram obtained with reference solution (b) (2.5 per cent). Disregard any peak with an area less than that of the principal peak in the chromatogram obtained with reference solution (d).

Chlorides (*2.4.4*). Dissolve 67 mg in 10 ml of *water R* and add 3 ml of *acetic acid R.* Filter and wash the precipitate with five quantities, each of 5 ml, of *water R.* Collect the filtrate and washings and dilute to 100 ml with *water R.* 15 ml of this solution complies with the limit test for chlorides (0.5 per cent).

Heavy metals (*2.4.8*). 1.0 g complies with limit test F for heavy metals (50 ppm). Prepare the standard using 5 ml of *lead standard solution (10 ppm Pb) R.*

Platinum. Not more than 20 ppm of Pt, determined by atomic absorption spectrometry (*2.2.23, Method II*).

Test solution. Dissolve 1.00 g in *water R* and dilute to 100.0 ml with the same solvent.

Reference solutions. Prepare the reference solutions using *platinum standard solution (30 ppm Pt) R,* diluted as necessary with a mixture of 1 volume of *nitric acid R* and 99 volumes of *water R.*

Measure the absorbance at 265.9 nm using a platinum hollow-cathode lamp as source of radiation.

Water (*2.5.12*). Not more than 17.0 per cent, determined on 0.200 g (ground to a very fine powder) by the semi-micro determination of water. Stir the substance to be examined in the titration solvent for about 6 min before titrating and use a suitable titrant that does not contain pyridine.

Bacterial endotoxins (*2.6.14*): less than 0.5 IU/mg, if intended for use in the manufacture of parenteral dosage forms without a further appropriate procedure for the removal of bacterial endotoxins.

ASSAY

Calcium. Dissolve 0.400 g in 150 ml of *water R* and dilute to 300 ml with the same solvent. Carry out the complexometric titration of calcium (*2.5.11*).

1 ml of *0.1 M sodium edetate* is equivalent to 4.008 mg of Ca.

Calcium folinate. Examine by liquid chromatography (*2.2.29*).

Test solution. Dissolve 10.0 mg of the substance to be examined in *water R* and dilute to 10.0 ml with the same solvent.

Reference solution (a). Dissolve 10.0 mg of *calcium folinate CRS* in *water R* and dilute to 10.0 ml with the same solvent.

Reference solution (b). Dilute 1.0 ml of reference solution (a) to 100.0 ml with *water R.*

Reference solution (c). Dissolve 10.0 mg of *formylfolic acid CRS* in the mobile phase and dilute to 100.0 ml with the mobile phase. Dilute 1.0 ml of this solution to 10.0 ml with *water R.*

Reference solution (d). Dilute 1.0 ml of reference solution (b) to 10.0 ml with *water R.*

Reference solution (e). Dilute 5.0 ml of reference solution (c) to 10.0 ml with reference solution (b).

The chromatographic procedure may be carried out using:

- a stainless steel column 0.25 m long and 4 mm in internal diameter packed with *octadecylsilyl silica gel for chromatography R* (5 µm),
- as mobile phase at a flow rate of 1 ml/min a mixture prepared as follows: mix 220 ml of *methanol R* and 780 ml of a solution containing 2.0 ml of *tetrabutylammonium hydroxide solution (400 g/l) R* and 2.2 g of *disodium hydrogen phosphate R* previously adjusted to pH 7.8 with *phosphoric acid R,*
- as detector a spectrophotometer set at 280 nm,

maintaining the temperature of the column at 40 °C.

Inject 10 µl of each solution. Continue the chromatography for 2.5 times the retention time of the principal peak in the chromatogram obtained with the test solution. The assay is not valid unless, in the chromatogram obtained with reference solution (e), the resolution between the peaks corresponding to calcium folinate and formylfolic acid is at least 2.2 and the relative standard deviation of the area of the principal peak for six replicate injections of reference solution (a) is at most 2.0 per cent.

Calculate the percentage content of $C_{20}H_{21}CaN_7O_7$ from the peak areas and the declared content of *calcium folinate CRS.*

STORAGE

Store in an airtight container, protected from light. If the substance is sterile, store in a sterile, airtight, tamper-proof container.

LABELLING

The label states, where applicable, that the substance is free from bacterial endotoxins.

IMPURITIES

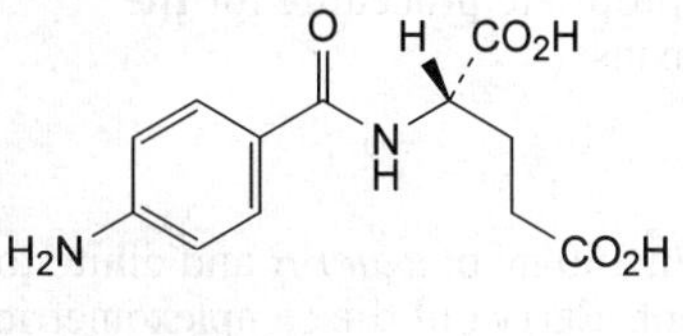

A. (2*S*)-2[(4-aminobenzoyl)amino]pentanedioic acid,

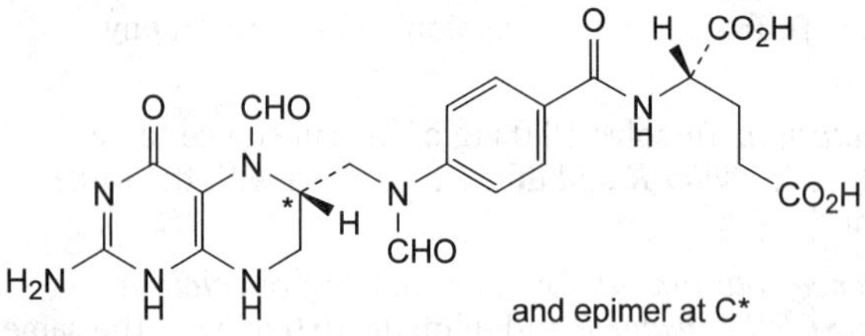

B. (2*S*)-2-[[4-[[[(6*RS*)-2-amino-5-formyl-4-oxo-1,4,5,6,7,8-hexahydropteridin-6-yl]methyl]formylamino]benzoyl]amino]pentanedioic acid (5,10-diformyltetrahydrofolic acid),

C. folic acid,

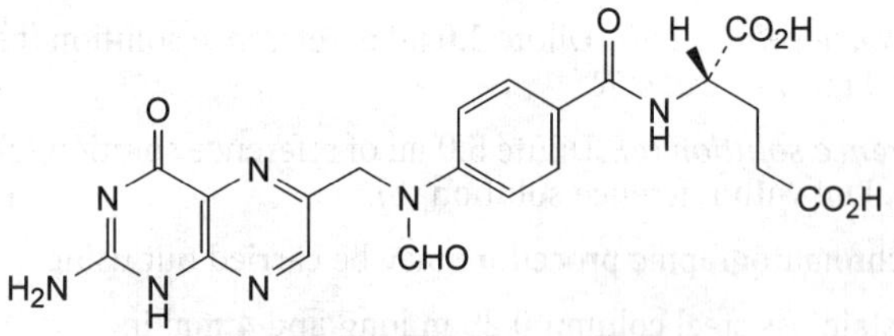

D. (2*S*)-2-[[4-[[(2-amino-4-oxo-1,4-dihydropteridin-6-yl)methyl]formylamino]benzoyl]amino]pentanedioic acid (10-formylfolic acid),

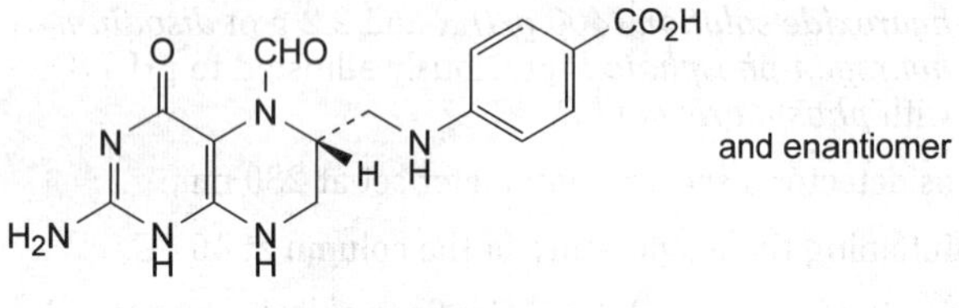

E. 4-[[[(6*RS*)-2-amino-5-formyl-4-oxo-1,4,5,6,7,8-hexahydropteridin-6-yl]methyl]amino]benzoic acid (5-formyltetrahydropteroic acid),

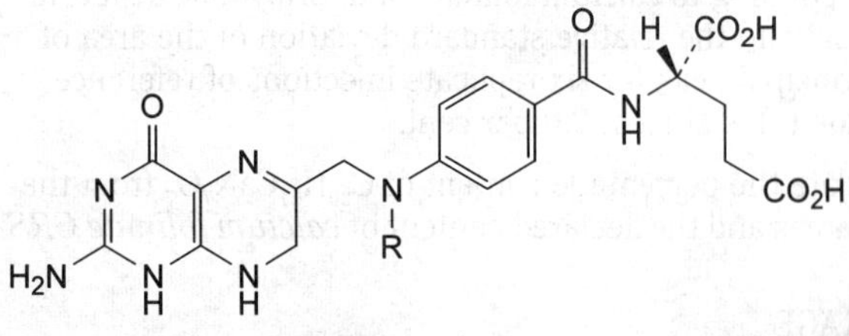

F. R = CHO: (2*S*)-2-[[4-[[(2-amino-4-oxo-1,4,7,8-tetrahydropteridin-6-yl)methyl]formylamino]benzoyl]amino]pentanedioic acid (10-formyldihydrofolic acid),

G. R = H: (2*S*)-2-[[4-[[(2-amino-4-oxo-1,4,7,8-tetrahydropteridin-6-yl)methyl]amino]benzoyl]amino]pentanedioic acid (dihydrofolic acid).

01/2005:1399

CALCIUM GLUCOHEPTONATE

Calcii glucoheptonas

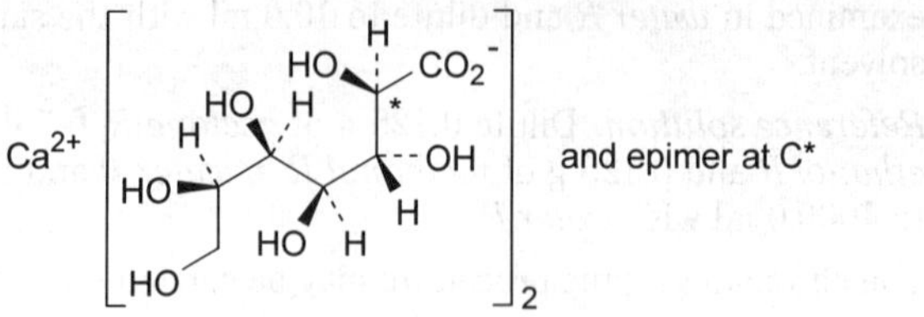

$C_{14}H_{26}CaO_{16}$ M_r 490.4

DEFINITION

Calcium glucoheptonate is a mixture, in variable proportions, of calcium di(D-*glycero*-D-*gulo*-heptonate) and calcium di(D-*glycero*-D-*ido*-heptonate). It contains not less than 98.0 per cent and not more than the equivalent of 102.0 per cent of calcium 2,3,4,5,6,7-hexahydroxyheptanoate, calculated with reference to the dried substance.

CHARACTERS

A white or very slightly yellow, amorphous powder, hygroscopic, very soluble in water, practically insoluble in acetone and in alcohol.

IDENTIFICATION

A. Examine by thin-layer chromatography (*2.2.27*), using *cellulose for chromatography R1* as the coating substance.

Test solution. Dissolve 20 mg of the substance to be examined in 1 ml of *water R*.

Reference solution (a). Dissolve 20 mg of *calcium glucoheptonate CRS* in 1 ml of *water R*.

Reference solution (b). Dissolve 10 mg of *calcium gluconate CRS* in 0.5 ml of the test solution and dilute to 1 ml with *water R*.

Apply separately to the plate, as bands 20 mm by 2 mm, 10 µl of each solution. Allow the tank to saturate for 10 min. Develop over a path of 12 cm using a freshly prepared mixture of 20 volumes of *anhydrous formic acid R*, 20 volumes of *water R*, 30 volumes of *acetone R* and 30 volumes of *butanol R*. Allow the plate to dry in air and spray with *0.02 M potassium permanganate*. The principal spot in the chromatogram obtained with the test solution is similar in position and size to the principal spot in the chromatogram obtained with reference solution (a). The test is not valid unless the chromatogram obtained with reference solution (b) shows two clearly separated spots.

B. 0.2 ml of solution S (see Tests) gives reaction (b) of calcium (*2.3.1*).

TESTS

Solution S. Dissolve 10.0 g in *carbon dioxide-free water R* prepared from *distilled water R* and dilute to 100 ml with the same solvent.

Appearance of solution. Solution S is clear (*2.2.1*) and not more intensely coloured than reference solution Y_6 (*2.2.2, Method II*).

pH (*2.2.3*). The pH of solution S is 6.0 to 8.0.

Reducing sugars. Dissolve 1.0 g in 5 ml of *water R* with the aid of gentle heat. Cool and add 20 ml of *cupri-citric solution R* and a few glass beads. Heat so that boiling begins after 4 min and maintain boiling for 3 min. Cool rapidly and add 100 ml of a 2.4 per cent *V/V* solution of *glacial acetic acid R* and 20.0 ml of *0.025 M iodine*. With continuous shaking, add 25 ml of a mixture of 6 volumes of *hydrochloric acid R* and 94 volumes of *water R* until the precipitate dissolves, titrate the excess of iodine with *0.05 M sodium thiosulphate* using 1 ml of *starch solution R* added towards the end of the titration, as indicator. Not less than 12.6 ml of *0.05 M sodium thiosulphate* is required (1 per cent expressed as glucose).

Cyanide. Dissolve 5.0 g in 50 ml of *water R* and add 2.0 g of *tartaric acid R*. Place this solution in a distillation apparatus (*2.2.11*). The plain bend adapter attached to the end of the condenser has a vertical part that is long enough to extend to 1 cm from the bottom of a 50 ml test-tube used as a receiver. Place 10 ml of *water R* and 2 ml of *0.1 M sodium hydroxide* into the receiver. Distil, collect 25 ml of distillate and dilute to 50 ml with *water R*. To 25 ml of this solution add 25 mg of *ferrous sulphate R* and boil for a short time. After cooling to about 70 °C add 10 ml of *hydrochloric acid R1*. After 30 min, filter the solution and wash the filter. A yellow spot appears on the filter; there is no blue or green spot.

Chlorides (*2.4.4*). To 5 ml of solution S, add 10 ml of *water R*. The solution complies with the limit test for chlorides (100 ppm).

Sulphates (*2.4.13*). 15 ml of solution S complies with the limit test for sulphates (100 ppm).

Iron (*2.4.9*). Dilute 2.5 ml of solution S to 10 ml with *water R*. The solution complies with the limit test for iron (40 ppm).

Heavy metals (*2.4.8*). Dissolve 2.0 g in 10 ml of *buffer solution pH 3.5 R* and dilute to 20 ml with *water R*. 12 ml of the solution complies with limit test A for heavy metals (10 ppm). Prepare the standard using *lead standard solution (1 ppm Pb) R*.

Loss on drying (*2.2.32*). Not more than 5.0 per cent, determined on 1.000 g by drying in an oven at 100 °C to 105 °C for 3 h.

Bacterial endotoxins (*2.6.14*): less than 167 IU/g, if intended for use in the manufacture of parenteral dosage forms without a further appropriate procedure for the removal of bacterial endotoxins.

ASSAY

Dissolve 0.800 g in a mixture of 150 ml of *water R* and 2 ml of *3 M hydrochloric acid*. While stirring, add 12.5 ml of *0.1 M sodium edetate*, 15 ml of *1 M sodium hydroxide* and 0.3 g of *hydroxynaphthol blue, sodium salt R*. Titrate with *0.1 M sodium edetate* until the colour changes from violet to pure blue.

1 ml of *0.1 M sodium edetate* is equivalent to 49.04 mg of $C_{14}H_{26}CaO_{16}$.

STORAGE

In an airtight container. If the substance is sterile, store in a sterile, airtight, tamper-proof container.

LABELLING

The label states, where applicable, that the substance is free from bacterial endotoxins.

01/2005:0172

CALCIUM GLUCONATE

Calcii gluconas

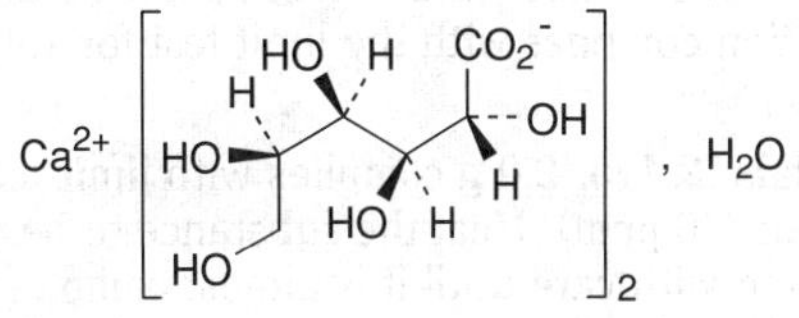

$C_{12}H_{22}CaO_{14},H_2O$ M_r 448.4

DEFINITION

Calcium gluconate contains not less than 98.5 per cent and not more than the equivalent of 102.0 per cent of calcium D-gluconate monohydrate.

CHARACTERS

A white, crystalline or granular powder, sparingly soluble in water, freely soluble in boiling water.

IDENTIFICATION

A. Examine by thin-layer chromatography (*2.2.27*), using *silica gel G R* as the coating substance.

Test solution. Dissolve 20 mg of the substance to be examined in 1 ml of *water R*, heating if necessary in a water-bath at 60 °C.

Reference solution. Dissolve 20 mg of *calcium gluconate CRS* in 1 ml of *water R*, heating if necessary in a water-bath at 60 °C.

Apply separately to the plate 5 µl of each solution. Develop over a path of 10 cm using a mixture of 10 volumes of *ethyl acetate R*, 10 volumes of *concentrated ammonia R*, 30 volumes of *water R* and 50 volumes of *alcohol R*. Dry the plate at 100 °C for 20 min. Allow to cool and spray with a 50 g/l solution of *potassium dichromate R* in a 40 per cent *m/m* solution of *sulphuric acid R*. After 5 min, the principal spot in the chromatogram obtained with the test solution is similar in position, colour and size to the principal spot in the chromatogram obtained with the reference solution.

B. Solution S (see Tests) gives the reactions of calcium (*2.3.1*).

TESTS

Solution S. Dissolve 1.0 g in *water R* heated to 60 °C and dilute to 50 ml with the same solvent.

Appearance of solution. At 60 °C, solution S is not more intensely coloured than reference solution Y_6 (*2.2.2, Method II*). After cooling, it is not more opalescent than reference suspension II (*2.2.1*).

Organic impurities and boric acid. Introduce 0.5 g into a porcelain dish previously rinsed with *sulphuric acid R* and placed in a bath of iced water. Add 2 ml of cooled *sulphuric acid R* and mix. No yellow or brown colour develops. Add 1 ml of *chromotrope II B solution R*. A violet colour develops and does not become dark blue. Compare the colour obtained with that of a mixture of 1 ml of *chromotrope II B solution R* and 2 ml of cooled *sulphuric acid R*.

Sucrose and reducing sugars. Dissolve 0.5 g in a mixture of 2 ml of *hydrochloric acid R1* and 10 ml of *water R*. Boil for 5 min, allow to cool, add 10 ml of *sodium carbonate solution R* and allow to stand. Dilute to 25 ml with *water R*

Monographs C

and filter. To 5 ml of the filtrate add 2 ml of *cupri-tartaric solution R* and boil for 1 min. Allow to stand for 2 min. No red precipitate is formed.

Chlorides (*2.4.4*). 12.5 ml of solution S diluted to 15 ml with *water R* complies with the limit test for chlorides (200 ppm).

Sulphates (*2.4.13*). Dissolve 10.0 g with heating in a mixture of 10 ml of *acetic acid R* and 90 ml of *distilled water R*. 15 ml of the solution complies with the limit test for sulphates (100 ppm).

Heavy metals (*2.4.8*). 2.0 g complies with limit test D for heavy metals (10 ppm). Heat the substance to be examined gradually and with care until it is almost completely transformed into a white mass and then ignite. Prepare the standard using 2 ml of *lead standard solution (10 ppm Pb) R*.

Magnesium and alkali metals. Dissolve 1.00 g in 100 ml of boiling *water R*, add 10 ml of *ammonium chloride solution R*, 1 ml of *ammonia R* and, dropwise, 50 ml of hot *ammonium oxalate solution R*. Allow to stand for 4 h, dilute to 200 ml with *water R* and filter. Evaporate 100 ml of the filtrate to dryness and ignite. The residue weighs not more than 2 mg (0.4 per cent).

Microbial contamination. Total viable aerobic count (*2.6.12*) not more than 10^3 micro-organisms per gram, determined by plate count.

ASSAY

Dissolve 0.8000 g in 20 ml of hot *water R*, allow to cool and dilute to 300 ml with *water R*. Carry out the complexometric titration of calcium (*2.5.11*).

1 ml of *0.1 M sodium edetate* is equivalent to 44.84 mg of $C_{12}H_{22}CaO_{14},H_2O$.

01/2005:0979

CALCIUM GLUCONATE FOR INJECTION

Calcii gluconas ad iniectabile

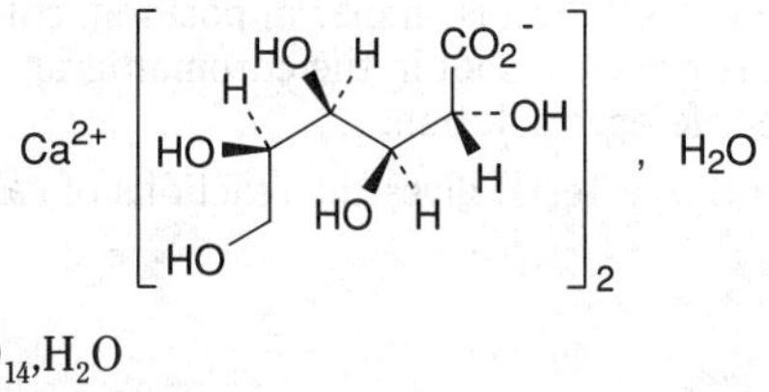

$C_{12}H_{22}CaO_{14},H_2O$ M_r 448.4

DEFINITION

Calcium gluconate for injection contains not less than 99.0 per cent and not more than the equivalent of 101.0 per cent of calcium D-gluconate monohydrate.

CHARACTERS

A white, crystalline or granular powder, sparingly soluble in water, freely soluble in boiling water.

IDENTIFICATION

A. Examine by thin-layer chromatography (*2.2.27*), using *silica gel G R* as the coating substance.

Test solution. Dissolve 20 mg of the substance to be examined in 1 ml of *water R*, heating if necessary in a water-bath at 60 °C.

Reference solution. Dissolve 20 mg of *calcium gluconate CRS* in 1 ml of *water R*, heating if necessary in a water-bath at 60 °C.

Apply to the plate 5 µl of each solution. Develop over a path of 10 cm using a mixture of 10 volumes of *concentrated ammonia R*, 10 volumes of *ethyl acetate R*, 30 volumes of *water R* and 50 volumes of *alcohol R*. Dry the plate at 100 °C for 20 min. Allow to cool and spray with a 50 g/l solution of *potassium dichromate R* in a 40 per cent *m/m* solution of *sulphuric acid R*. After 5 min, the principal spot in the chromatogram obtained with the test solution is similar in position, colour and size to the principal spot in the chromatogram obtained with the reference solution.

B. About 20 mg gives reaction (b) of calcium (*2.3.1*).

TESTS

Solution S. To 10.0 g add 90 ml of boiling *distilled water R* and boil with stirring, for not more than 10 s, until completely dissolved. Dilute to 100.0 ml with the same solvent.

Appearance of solution. Solution S at 60 °C is not more intensely coloured than reference solution B_7 (*2.2.2, Method II*). After cooling to 20 °C, it is not more opalescent than reference suspension II (*2.2.1*).

pH (*2.2.3*). Dissolve 1.0 g in 20 ml of *carbon dioxide-free water R*, heating on a water-bath. The pH of the solution is 6.4 to 8.3.

Organic impurities and boric acid. Introduce 0.5 g into a porcelain dish previously rinsed with *sulphuric acid R* and placed in a bath of iced water. Add 2 ml of cooled *sulphuric acid R* and mix. No yellow or brown colour develops. Add 1 ml of *chromotrope II B solution R*. A violet colour develops and does not become dark blue. The solution is not more intensely coloured than that of a mixture of 1 ml of *chromotrope II B solution R* and 2 ml of cooled *sulphuric acid R*.

Oxalate. Not more than 100 ppm, determined by liquid chromatography (*2.2.29*).

Test solution. Dissolve 1.00 g of the substance to be examined in *water for chromatography R* and dilute to 100.0 ml with the same solvent.

Reference solution. Dissolve 1.00 g of the substance to be examined in *water for chromatography R*, add 0.5 ml of a 0.152 g/l solution of *sodium oxalate R* in *water for chromatography R* and dilute to 100.0 ml with the same solvent.

The chromatographic procedure may be carried out using:

- a guard column 30 mm long and 4 mm in internal diameter packed with a suitable strong anion exchange resin (30 µm to 50 µm),
- two columns each 0.25 m long and 4 mm in internal diameter packed with a suitable strong anion exchange resin (30 µm to 50 µm),
- a micromembrane anion-suppressor column, connected in series with the guard and analytical columns; the anion-suppressor column is equipped with a micromembrane that separates the mobile phase from the suppressor regeneration solution, flowing countercurrent to the mobile phase at a rate of 4 ml/min,
- as mobile phase at a flow rate of 2 ml/min a solution prepared as follows: dissolve 0.212 g of *anhydrous sodium carbonate R* and 63 mg of *sodium hydrogen carbonate R* in *water for chromatography R* and dilute to 1000.0 ml with the same solvent,
- as suppressor regeneration solution a 1.23 g/l solution of *sulphuric acid R* in *water for chromatography R*,
- a conductance detector,
- a loop injector.

Inject 50 µl of the reference solution five times. The test is not valid unless the relative standard deviation of the peak area for oxalate in the chromatogram obtained with the reference solution is at most 2.0 per cent.

Inject 50 µl of each solution three times. Calculate the content of oxalate in parts per million using the following expression:

$$\frac{S_T \times 50}{S_R - S_T}$$

S_T = area of the oxalate peak in the chromatogram obtained with the test solution,

S_R = area of the oxalate peak in the chromatogram obtained with the reference solution.

Sucrose and reducing sugars. Dissolve 0.5 g in a mixture of 2 ml of *hydrochloric acid R1* and 10 ml of *water R*. Boil for 5 min, allow to cool, add 10 ml of *sodium carbonate solution R* and allow to stand for 10 min. Dilute to 25 ml with *water R* and filter. To 5 ml of the filtrate add 2 ml of *cupri-tartaric solution R* and boil for 1 min. Allow to stand for 2 min. No red precipitate is formed.

Chlorides (*2.4.4*). To 10 ml of previously filtered solution S add 5 ml of *water R*. The solution complies with the limit test for chlorides (50 ppm).

Phosphates (*2.4.11*). Dilute 1 ml of solution S to 100 ml with *water R*. The solution complies with the limit test for phosphates (100 ppm).

Sulphates (*2.4.13*). 15 ml of previously filtered solution S complies with the limit test for sulphates (50 ppm). Prepare the standard using a mixture of 7.5 ml of *sulphate standard solution (10 ppm SO_4) R* and 7.5 ml of *distilled water R*.

Iron. Not more than 5 ppm of Fe, determined by atomic absorption spectrometry (*2.2.23, Method I*).

Test solution. Introduce 2.0 g into a 100 ml polytetrafluoroethylene beaker and add 5 ml of *nitric acid R*. Boil, evaporating almost to dryness. Add 1 ml of *strong hydrogen peroxide solution R* and evaporate again almost to dryness. Repeat the hydrogen peroxide treatment until a clear solution is obtained. Using 2 ml of *nitric acid R*, transfer the solution into a 25 ml volumetric flask. Dilute to 25.0 ml with *dilute hydrochloric acid R*. In the same manner, prepare a compensation solution using 0.65 g of *calcium chloride R1* instead of the substance to be examined.

Reference solutions. Prepare the reference solutions from *iron solution (20 ppm Fe) R* diluted with *dilute hydrochloric acid R*.

Measure the absorbance at 248.3 nm, using an iron hollow-cathode lamp as source of radiation and an air-acetylene flame. Carry out a basic correction using a deuterium lamp.

Magnesium and alkali metals. To 0.50 g add a mixture of 1.0 ml of *dilute acetic acid R* and 10.0 ml of *water R* and rapidly boil, whilst shaking, until completely dissolved. To the boiling solution add 5.0 ml of *ammonium oxalate solution R* and allow to stand for at least 6 h. Filter through a sintered-glass filter (1.6) into a porcelain crucible. Carefully evaporate the filtrate to dryness and ignite. The residue weighs not more than 2 mg (0.4 per cent).

Heavy metals (*2.4.8*). 12 ml of solution S complies with limit test A for heavy metals (10 ppm). Prepare the standard using *lead standard solution (1 ppm Pb) R*.

Bacterial endotoxins (*2.6.14*): less than 167 IU/g.

Microbial contamination. Total viable aerobic count (*2.6.12*) not more than 10^2 micro-organisms per gram, determined by plate count. It complies with the tests for *Escherichia coli*, *Pseudomonas aeruginosa* and *Staphylococcus aureus* (*2.6.13*).

ASSAY

Dissolve 0.350 g in 20 ml of hot *water R*, allow to cool and dilute to 300 ml with *water R*. Carry out the complexometric titration of calcium (*2.5.11*). Use 50 mg of *calconecarboxylic acid triturate R*.

1 ml of *0.1 M sodium edetate* is equivalent to 44.84 mg of $C_{12}H_{22}CaO_{14},H_2O$.

Monographs C

01/2005:0980

CALCIUM GLYCEROPHOSPHATE

Calcii glycerophosphas

$C_3H_7CaO_6P$ M_r 210.1

DEFINITION

Calcium glycerophosphate is a mixture in variable proportions of calcium (*RS*)-2,3-dihydroxypropyl phosphate, and of calcium 2-hydroxy-1-(hydroxymethyl)ethyl phosphate, which may be hydrated. Calcium glycerophosphate contains not less than 18.6 per cent and not more than 19.4 per cent of Ca, calculated with reference to the dried substance.

CHARACTERS

A white powder, hygroscopic, sparingly soluble in water, practically insoluble in alcohol.

IDENTIFICATION

A. Mix 1 g with 1 g of *potassium hydrogen sulphate R* in a test tube fitted with a glass tube. Heat strongly and direct the white vapour towards a piece of filter paper impregnated with a freshly prepared 10 g/l solution of *sodium nitroprusside R*. The filter paper develops a blue colour in contact with *piperidine R*.

B. Ignite 0.1 g in a crucible. Take up the residue with 5 ml of *nitric acid R* and heat on a water-bath for 1 min. Filter. The filtrate gives reaction (b) of phosphates (*2.3.1*).

C. It gives reaction (b) of calcium (*2.3.1*).

TESTS

Solution S. Dissolve 1.5 g at room temperature in *carbon dioxide-free water R* prepared from *distilled water R* and dilute to 150 ml with the same solvent.

Appearance of solution. Solution S is not more opalescent than reference suspension III (*2.2.1*).

Acidity or alkalinity. To 100 ml of solution S add 0.1 ml of *phenolphthalein solution R*. Not more than 1.5 ml of *0.1 M hydrochloric acid* or 0.5 ml of *0.1 M sodium hydroxide* is required to change the colour of the indicator.

Citric acid. Shake 5.0 g with 20 ml of *carbon dioxide-free water R* and filter. To the filtrate add 0.15 ml of *sulphuric acid R* and filter again. To the filtrate add 5 ml of *mercuric sulphate solution R* and heat to boiling. Add 0.5 ml of a 3.2 g/l solution of *potassium permanganate R* and again heat to boiling. No precipitate is formed.

Glycerol and alcohol-soluble substances. Shake 1.000 g with 25 ml of *alcohol R* for 1 min. Filter. Evaporate the filtrate to dryness on a water-bath and dry the residue at 70 °C for 1 h. The residue weighs not more than 5 mg (0.5 per cent).

Chlorides (*2.4.4*). Dissolve 0.1 g in a mixture of 2 ml of *acetic acid R* and 8 ml of *water R* and dilute to 15 ml with *water R*. The solution complies with the limit test for chlorides (500 ppm).

Phosphates (*2.4.11*). Dilute 2.5 ml of solution S to 100 ml with *water R*. The solution complies with the limit test for phosphates (400 ppm).

Sulphates (*2.4.13*). 15 ml of solution S complies with the limit test for sulphates (0.1 per cent).

Arsenic (*2.4.2*). Dissolve 0.33 g in *water R* and dilute to 25 ml with the same solvent. The solution complies with limit test A for arsenic (3 ppm).

Iron (*2.4.9*). 0.20 g complies with the limit test for iron (50 ppm).

Heavy metals (*2.4.8*). Dissolve 2.0 g in 10 ml of *buffer solution pH 3.5 R* and dilute to 20 ml with *water R*. 12 ml of the solution complies with limit test A for heavy metals (20 ppm). Prepare the standard using *lead standard solution (2 ppm Pb) R*.

Loss on drying (*2.2.32*). Not more than 12.0 per cent, determined on 1.000 g by drying in an oven at 150 °C for 4 h.

ASSAY

Dissolve 0.200 g in *water R*. Carry out the complexometric titration of calcium (*2.5.11*).

1 ml of *0.1 M sodium edetate* is equivalent to 4.008 mg of Ca.

01/2005:0981
corrected

CALCIUM HYDROGEN PHOSPHATE, ANHYDROUS

Calcii hydrogenophosphas anhydricus

$CaHPO_4$ M_r 136.1

DEFINITION

Content: 98.0 per cent to 101.0 per cent (dried substance).

CHARACTERS

Appearance: white, crystalline powder, or colourless crystals.

Solubility: practically insoluble in water and in alcohol. It dissolves in dilute hydrochloric acid and in dilute nitric acid.

IDENTIFICATION

A. It complies with the limits of the assay.

B. Dissolve 0.1 g in a mixture of 5 ml of *dilute nitric acid R* and 5 ml of *water R*. The solution gives reaction (b) of phosphates (*2.3.1*).

C. Dissolve 5 mg in 5 ml of *acetic acid R*. The solution gives reaction (b) of calcium (*2.3.1*).

TESTS

Solution S. Dissolve 2.5 g in 20 ml of *dilute hydrochloric acid R*. Filter if necessary. Add *dilute ammonia R1* until a precipitate is formed. Dissolve by adding the minimum quantity needed of *dilute hydrochloric acid R* and dilute to 50 ml with *distilled water R*.

Carbonates. Shake 0.5 g with 5 ml of *carbon dioxide-free water R* and add 1 ml of *hydrochloric acid R*. No effervescence is produced.

Chlorides (*2.4.4*): maximum 330 ppm.

Dissolve 0.5 g in a mixture of 1 ml of *nitric acid R* and 10 ml of *water R* and dilute to 50 ml with *water R*. 15 ml of the solution complies with the limit test for chlorides.

Fluorides (*2.4.5*): maximum 100 ppm.

0.5 g complies with the limit test for fluorides.

Sulphates (*2.4.13*): maximum 0.5 per cent.

To 1 ml of solution S add 2 ml of *dilute hydrochloric acid R* and dilute to 25 ml with *distilled water R*. 15 ml of the solution complies with the limit test for sulphates.

Arsenic (*2.4.2*): maximum 10 ppm.

2 ml of solution S complies with limit test A.

Barium. To 10 ml of filtered solution S add 0.5 ml of *dilute sulphuric acid R*. Allow to stand for 15 min. Any opalescence in the solution is not more intense than that in a mixture of 10 ml of solution S and 0.5 ml of *distilled water R*.

Iron (*2.4.9*): maximum 400 ppm.

Dilute 0.5 ml of solution S to 10 ml with *water R*. The solution complies with the limit test for iron.

Heavy metals (*2.4.8*): maximum 40 ppm.

Dilute 10 ml of solution S to 20 ml with *water R*. 12 ml of the solution complies with limit test A. Prepare the standard using *lead standard solution (1 ppm Pb) R*.

Loss on drying (*2.2.32*): maximum 2.0 per cent, determined on 1.000 g by drying in an oven at 150 °C for 2 h.

ASSAY

Dissolve 0.250 g in a mixture of 1 ml of *hydrochloric acid R1* and 5 ml of *water R*. Add 25.0 ml of *0.1 M sodium edetate* and dilute to 200 ml with *water R*. Neutralise with *concentrated ammonia R*, add 10 ml of *ammonium chloride buffer solution pH 10.0 R* and about 50 mg of *mordant black 11 triturate R*. Titrate the excess of sodium edetate with *0.1 M zinc sulphate* until the colour changes from blue to violet. Carry out a blank titration.

1 ml of *0.1 M sodium edetate* is equivalent to 13.61 mg of $CaHPO_4$.

01/2005:0116

CALCIUM HYDROGEN PHOSPHATE DIHYDRATE

Calcii hydrogenophosphas dihydricus

$CaHPO_4,2H_2O$ M_r 172.1

DEFINITION

Content: 98.0 per cent to 105.0 per cent.

CHARACTERS

Appearance: white, crystalline powder.

Solubility: practically insoluble in cold water and in alcohol. It dissolves in dilute hydrochloric acid and in dilute nitric acid.

IDENTIFICATION

A. Dissolve 0.1 g in a mixture of 5 ml of *dilute nitric acid R* and 5 ml of *water R*. The solution gives reaction (b) of phosphates (*2.3.1*).

B. 5 mg gives reaction (b) of calcium (*2.3.1*).

C. It complies with the limits of the assay.

TESTS

Solution S. Dissolve 2.5 g in 20 ml of *dilute hydrochloric acid R*, filter if necessary and add *dilute ammonia R1* until a precipitate is formed. Add just sufficient *dilute hydrochloric acid R* to dissolve the precipitate and dilute to 50 ml with *distilled water R*.

Carbonates. Shake 0.5 g with 5 ml of *carbon dioxide-free water R* and add 1 ml of *hydrochloric acid R*. No effervescence is produced.

Chlorides (*2.4.4*): maximum 330 ppm.

Dissolve 0.5 g in a mixture of 1 ml of *nitric acid R* and 10 ml of *water R* and dilute to 50 ml with *water R*. 15 ml of the solution complies with the limit test for chlorides.

Fluorides (*2.4.5*): maximum 100 ppm.

0.5 g complies with the limit test for fluorides.

Sulphates (*2.4.13*): maximum 0.5 per cent.

To 1 ml of solution S add 2 ml of *dilute hydrochloric acid R* and dilute to 25 ml with *distilled water R*. 15 ml of the solution complies with the limit test for sulphates.

Arsenic (*2.4.2*): maximum 10 ppm.

2 ml of solution S complies with limit test A.

Barium. To 10 ml of solution S add 0.5 ml of *dilute sulphuric acid R*. After 15 min, any opalescence in the solution is not more intense than that in a mixture of 10 ml of solution S and 0.5 ml of *distilled water R*.

Iron (*2.4.9*): maximum 400 ppm.

0.5 ml of solution S diluted to 10 ml with *water R* complies with the limit test for iron.

Heavy metals (*2.4.8*): maximum 40 ppm.

Dilute 10 ml of solution S to 20 ml with *water R*. 12 ml of the solution complies with limit test A. Prepare the standard using *lead standard solution (1 ppm Pb) R*.

ASSAY

Dissolve 0.300 g in a mixture of 1 ml of *hydrochloric acid R1* and 5 ml of *water R*. Add 25.0 ml of *0.1 M sodium edetate* and dilute to 200 ml with *water R*. Neutralise with *concentrated ammonia R*, add 10 ml of *ammonium chloride buffer solution pH 10.0 R* and about 50 mg of *mordant black 11 triturate R*. Titrate the excess of sodium edetate with *0.1 M zinc sulphate* until the colour changes from blue to violet. Carry out a blank titration.

1 ml of *0.1 M sodium edetate* is equivalent to 17.21 mg of $CaHPO_4,2H_2O$.

01/2005:1078
corrected

CALCIUM HYDROXIDE

Calcii hydroxidum

$Ca(OH)_2$ M_r 74.1

DEFINITION

Calcium hydroxide contains not less than 95.0 per cent and not more than the equivalent of 100.5 per cent of $Ca(OH)_2$.

CHARACTERS

A white or almost white, fine powder, practically insoluble in water.

IDENTIFICATION

A. To 0.80 g in a mortar, add 10 ml of *water R* and 0.5 ml of *phenolphthalein solution R* and mix. The suspension turns red. On addition of 17.5 ml of *1 M hydrochloric acid*, the suspension becomes colourless without effervescing. The red colour occurs again when the mixture is triturated for 1 min. On addition of a further 6 ml of *1 M hydrochloric acid* and triturating, the solution becomes colourless.

B. Dissolve about 0.1 g in *dilute hydrochloric acid R* and dilute to 10 ml with *water R*. 5 ml of the solution give reaction (b) of calcium (*2.3.1*).

TESTS

Matter insoluble in hydrochloric acid. Dissolve 2.0 g in 30 ml of *hydrochloric acid R*. Boil the solution and filter. Wash the residue with hot *water R*. The residue weighs not more than 10 mg (0.5 per cent).

Carbonates. Not more than 5.0 per cent of $CaCO_3$.

Add 5.0 ml of *1 M hydrochloric acid* to the titrated solution obtained under Assay and titrate with *1 M sodium hydroxide* using 0.5 ml of *methyl orange solution R* as indicator.

1 ml of *1 M hydrochloric acid* is equivalent to 50.05 mg of $CaCO_3$.

Chlorides (*2.4.4*). Dissolve 0.30 g in a mixture of 2 ml of *nitric acid R* and 10 ml of *water R* and dilute to 30 ml with *water R*. 15 ml of the solution complies with the limit test for chlorides (330 ppm).

Sulphates (*2.4.13*). Dissolve 0.15 g in a mixture of 5 ml of *dilute hydrochloric acid R* and 10 ml of *distilled water R* and dilute to 60 ml with *distilled water R*. 15 ml of the solution complies with the limit test for sulphates (0.4 per cent).

Arsenic (*2.4.2*). Dissolve 0.50 g in 5 ml of *brominated hydrochloric acid R* and dilute to 50 ml with *water R*. 25 ml of the solution complies with the limit test A for arsenic (4 ppm).

Magnesium and alkali metals. Dissolve 1.0 g in a mixture of 10 ml of *hydrochloric acid R* and 40 ml of *water R*. Boil and add 50 ml of a 63 g/l solution of *oxalic acid R*. Neutralise with *ammonia R* and dilute to 200 ml with *water R*. Allow to stand for 1 h and filter through a suitable filter. To 100 ml of the filtrate, add 0.5 ml of *sulphuric acid R*. Cautiously evaporate to dryness and ignite. The residue weighs not more than 20 mg (4.0 per cent calculated as sulphates).

Heavy metals (*2.4.8*). Dissolve 1.0 g in 10 ml of *hydrochloric acid R1* and evaporate to dryness on a water-bath. Dissolve the residue in 20 ml of *water R* and filter. 12 ml of the filtrate complies with limit test A for heavy metals (20 ppm). Prepare the standard using *lead standard solution (1 ppm Pb) R*.

ASSAY

To 1.500 g in a mortar, add 20 ml to 30 ml of *water R* and 0.5 ml of *phenolphthalein solution R*. Titrate with *1 M hydrochloric acid* by triturating the substance until the red colour disappears. The final solution is used in the tests for carbonates.

1 ml of *1 M hydrochloric acid* is equivalent to 37.05 mg of $Ca(OH)_2$.

01/2005:0468

CALCIUM LACTATE PENTAHYDRATE

Calcii lactas pentahydricus

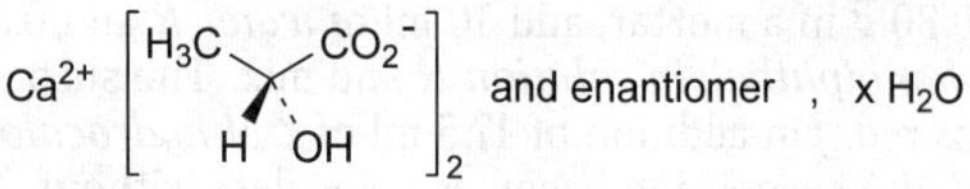

$C_6H_{10}CaO_6,xH_2O$ with $x \simeq 5$ M_r 218.2 (anhydrous substance)

DEFINITION

Calcium lactate pentahydrate contains not less than 98.0 per cent and not more than the equivalent of 102.0 per cent of calcium bis(2-hydroxypropanoate) or of a mixture of calcium (*R*)-, (*S*)- and (*RS*)-2-hydroxypropionates, calculated with reference to the dried substance. It contains not less than 22.0 per cent and not more than 27.0 per cent of water, determined by the loss on drying.

CHARACTERS

A white or almost white, crystalline or granular powder, slightly efflorescent, soluble in water, freely soluble in boiling water, very slightly soluble in alcohol.

IDENTIFICATION

A. It complies with the test for loss on drying (see Tests).

B. It gives the reaction of lactates (*2.3.1*).

C. It gives reaction (b) of calcium (*2.3.1*).

TESTS

Solution S. Dissolve 5.0 g with heating in *carbon dioxide-free water R* prepared from *distilled water R*, allow to cool and dilute to 100 ml with the same solvent.

Appearance of solution. Solution S is not more opalescent than reference suspension II (*2.2.1*) and not more intensely coloured than reference solution BY_6 (*2.2.2, Method II*).

Acidity or alkalinity. To 10 ml of solution S add 0.1 ml of *phenolphthalein solution R* and 0.5 ml of *0.01 M hydrochloric acid*. The solution is colourless. Not more than 2.0 ml of *0.01 M sodium hydroxide* is required to change the colour of the indicator to pink.

Volatile fatty acids. In a 100 ml ground-glass-stoppered flask stir 0.5 g with 1 ml of *phosphoric acid R*. Close the flask. Heat cautiously at 50 °C for 10 min. No unpleasant odour resembling that of the lower fatty acids is recognisable immediately after opening the flask.

Chlorides (*2.4.4*). 5 ml of solution S diluted to 15 ml with *water R* complies with the limit test for chlorides (200 ppm).

Sulphates (*2.4.13*). 7.5 ml of solution S diluted to 15 ml with *distilled water R* complies with the limit test for sulphates (400 ppm).

Barium. To 10 ml of solution S add 1 ml of *calcium sulphate solution R*. Allow to stand for 15 min. Any opalescence in the solution is not more intense than that in a mixture of 1 ml of *distilled water R* and 10 ml of solution S.

Heavy metals (*2.4.8*). 12 ml of solution S complies with limit test A for heavy metals (20 ppm). Prepare the standard using *lead standard solution (1 ppm Pb) R*.

Iron (*2.4.9*). 4 ml of solution S diluted to 10 ml with *water R* complies with the limit test for iron (50 ppm).

Magnesium and alkali salts. To 20 ml of solution S add 20 ml of *water R*, 2 g of *ammonium chloride R* and 2 ml of *dilute ammonia R1*. Heat to boiling and rapidly add 40 ml of hot *ammonium oxalate solution R*. Allow to stand for 4 h, dilute to 100.0 ml with *water R* and filter. To 50.0 ml of the filtrate add 0.5 ml of *sulphuric acid R*, evaporate to dryness and ignite the residue to constant mass at 600 °C. The residue weighs not more than 5 mg (1 per cent).

Loss on drying (*2.2.32*): 22.0 per cent to 27.0 per cent, determined on 0.500 g by drying in an oven at 125 °C.

ASSAY

Dissolve 0.200 g in *water R* and dilute to 300 ml with the same solvent. Carry out the complexometric titration of calcium (*2.5.11*).

1 ml of *0.1 M sodium edetate* is equivalent to 21.82 mg of $C_6H_{10}CaO_6$.

01/2005:0469

CALCIUM LACTATE TRIHYDRATE

Calcii lactas trihydricus

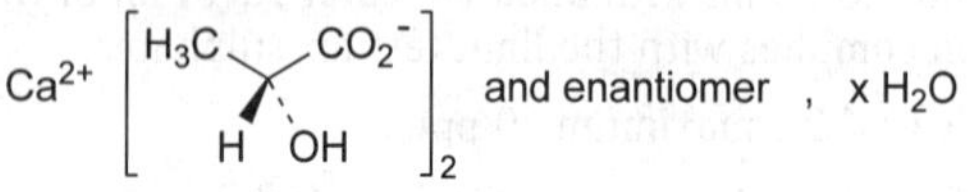

$C_6H_{10}CaO_6,xH_2O$ with $x \simeq 3$ M_r 218.2 (anhydrous substance)

DEFINITION

Calcium lactate trihydrate contains not less than 98.0 per cent and not more than the equivalent of 102.0 per cent of calcium bis(2-hydroxypropanoate) or of a mixture of calcium (*R*)-, (*S*)- and (*RS*)-2-hydroxypropionates, calculated with reference to the dried substance. It contains not less than 15.0 per cent and not more than 20.0 per cent of water, determined by the loss on drying.

CHARACTERS

A white or almost white, crystalline or granular powder, soluble in water, freely soluble in boiling water, very slightly soluble in alcohol.

IDENTIFICATION

A. It complies with the test for loss on drying (see Tests).

B. It gives the reaction of lactates (*2.3.1*).

C. It gives reaction (b) of calcium (*2.3.1*).

TESTS

Solution S. Dissolve 5.0 g with heating in *carbon dioxide-free water R* prepared from *distilled water R*, allow to cool and dilute to 100 ml with the same solvent.

Appearance of solution. Solution S is not more opalescent than reference suspension II (*2.2.1*) and not more intensely coloured than reference solution BY_6 (*2.2.2, Method II*).

Acidity or alkalinity. To 10 ml of solution S add 0.1 ml of *phenolphthalein solution R* and 0.5 ml of *0.01 M hydrochloric acid*. The solution is colourless. Not more than 2.0 ml of *0.01 M sodium hydroxide* is required to change the colour of the indicator to pink.

Volatile fatty acids. In a 100 ml ground-glass-stoppered flask stir 0.5 g with 1 ml of *phosphoric acid R*. Close the flask. Heat cautiously at 50 °C for 10 min. No unpleasant odour resembling that of the lower fatty acids is recognisable immediately after opening the flask.

Chlorides (*2.4.4*). 5 ml of solution S diluted to 15 ml with *water R* complies with the limit test for chlorides (200 ppm).

Sulphates (*2.4.13*). 7.5 ml of solution S diluted to 15 ml with *distilled water R* complies with the limit test for sulphates (400 ppm).

Monographs C

Barium. To 10 ml of solution S add 1 ml of *calcium sulphate solution R*. Allow to stand for 15 min. Any opalescence in the solution is not more intense than that in a mixture of 1 ml of *distilled water R* and 10 ml of solution S.

Heavy metals (*2.4.8*). 12 ml of solution S complies with limit test A for heavy metals (20 ppm). Prepare the standard using *lead standard solution (1 ppm Pb) R*.

Iron (*2.4.9*). 4 ml of solution S diluted to 10 ml with *water R* complies with the limit test for iron (50 ppm).

Magnesium and alkali salts. To 20 ml of solution S add 20 ml of *water R*, 2 g of *ammonium chloride R* and 2 ml of *dilute ammonia R1*. Heat to boiling and rapidly add 40 ml of hot *ammonium oxalate solution R*. Allow to stand for 4 h, dilute to 100.0 ml with *water R* and filter. To 50.0 ml of the filtrate add 0.5 ml of *sulphuric acid R*, evaporate to dryness and ignite the residue to constant mass at 600 °C. The residue weighs not more than 5 mg (1 per cent).

Loss on drying (*2.2.32*): 15.0 per cent to 20.0 per cent, determined on 0.500 g by drying in an oven at 125 °C.

ASSAY

Dissolve 0.200 g in *water R* and dilute to 300 ml with the same solvent. Carry out the complexometric titration of calcium (*2.5.11*).

1 ml of *0.1 M sodium edetate* is equivalent to 21.82 mg of $C_6H_{10}CaO_6$.

01/2005:1606

CALCIUM LEVOFOLINATE PENTAHYDRATE

Calcii levofolinas pentahydricus

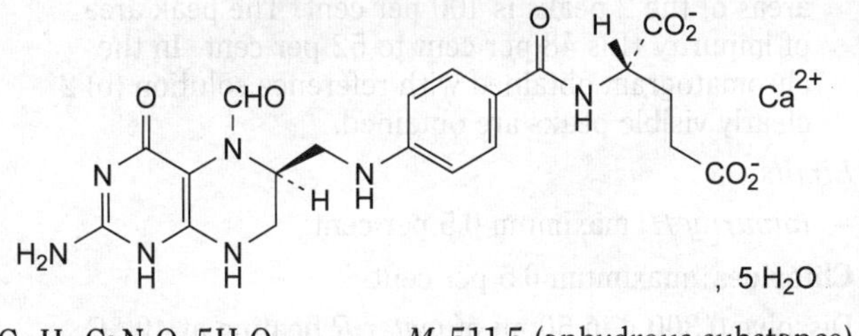

$C_{20}H_{21}CaN_7O_7,5H_2O$ M_r 511.5 (anhydrous substance)

DEFINITION

Calcium (2*S*)-2-[[4-[[[(6*S*)-2-amino-5-formyl-4-oxo-1,4,5,6,7,8-hexahydropteridin-6-yl]methyl]amino]benzoyl]amino]pentanedioate pentahydrate.

Content:

- calcium levofolinate ($C_{20}H_{21}CaN_7O_7$; M_r 511.5): 97.0 per cent to 102.0 per cent (anhydrous and solvent-free substance).
- calcium (Ca; A_r 40.08): 7.54 per cent to 8.14 per cent (anhydrous and solvent-free substance).

CHARACTERS

Appearance: white or light yellow, amorphous or crystalline powder, hygroscopic.

Solubility: slightly soluble in water, practically insoluble in acetone and in alcohol.

IDENTIFICATION

First identification: A, B, D.

Second identification: A, C, D.

A. It complies with the test for specific optical rotation (see Tests).

B. Infrared absorption spectrophotometry (*2.2.24*).

Preparation: discs.

Comparison: calcium folinate CRS.

If the spectra obtained show differences, dissolve the substance to be examined and the reference substance separately in the minimum quantity of *water R* and add dropwise sufficient *acetone R* to produce a precipitate. Allow to stand for 15 min, collect the precipitate by centrifugation, wash the precipitate twice with a minimum quantity of *acetone R* and dry. Record new spectra using the residues.

C. Thin-layer chromatography (*2.2.27*).

Test solution. Dissolve 15 mg of the substance to be examined in a 3 per cent *V/V* solution of *ammonia R* and dilute to 5 ml with the same solvent.

Reference solution. Dissolve 15 mg of *calcium folinate CRS* in a 3 per cent *V/V* solution of *ammonia R* and dilute to 5 ml with the same solvent.

Plate: *cellulose for chromatography F_{254} R.*

Mobile phase: the lower layer of a mixture of 1 volume of *isoamyl alcohol R* and 10 volumes of a 50 g/l solution of *citric acid R* previously adjusted to pH 8 with *ammonia R*.

Application: 5 µl.

Development: over a path of 15 cm.

Drying: in air.

Detection: examine in ultraviolet light at 254 nm.

Results: the principal spot in the chromatogram obtained with the test solution is similar in position and size to the principal spot in the chromatogram obtained with the reference solution.

D. It gives reaction (b) of calcium (*2.3.1*).

Carry out the tests and the assay as rapidly as possible, protected from bright light.

TESTS

Solution S. Dissolve 0.40 g in *carbon dioxide-free water R*, heating at 40 °C if necessary, and dilute to 50.0 ml with the same solvent.

Appearance of solution. Solution S is clear (*2.2.1*) and its absorbance (*2.2.25*) at 420 nm has a maximum of 0.25.

pH (*2.2.3*): 7.5 to 8.5 for solution S.

Specific optical rotation (*2.2.7*): − 10 to − 15 (anhydrous and solvent-free substance).

Dissolve 0.200 g in *tris(hydroxymethyl)aminomethane solution R* previously adjusted to pH 8.1 with *sodium hydroxide solution R* or *hydrochloric acid R1* and dilute to 20.0 ml with the same solvent.

Acetone and ethanol. Head-space gas chromatography (*2.2.28*): use the standard additions method.

Test solution. Dissolve 0.25 g of the substance to be examined in *water R* and dilute to 10.0 ml with the same solvent.

Reference solution. Dissolve 0.125 g of *acetone R* and 0.750 g of *ethanol R* in *water R* and dilute to 1000.0 ml with *water R*.

Column:

- *material*: fused silica,
- *size*: *l* = 10 m, Ø = 0.32 mm,
- *stationary phase*: *styrene-divinylbenzene copolymer R.*

Carrier gas: *nitrogen for chromatography R.*

Flow rate: 4 ml/min.

Static head-space conditions which may be used:

- *equilibration temperature*: 80 °C,

- *equilibration time*: 20 min,
- *pressurisation time*: 30 s.

Temperature:

	Time (min)	Temperature (°C)
Column	0 - 14	80 → 220
Injection port		110
Detector		270

Detection: flame ionisation.

Injection: at least 3 times.

Limits:

- *acetone*: maximum 0.5 per cent,
- *ethanol*: maximum 3.0 per cent.

Related substances. Liquid chromatography (*2.2.29*).

Test solution. Dissolve 10.0 mg of the substance to be examined in *water R* and dilute to 10.0 ml with the same solvent.

Reference solution (a). Dissolve 10.0 mg of *calcium folinate CRS* in *water R* and dilute to 10.0 ml with the same solvent.

Reference solution (b). Dilute 1.0 ml of reference solution (a) to 100.0 ml with *water R.*

Reference solution (c). Dissolve 10.0 mg of *formylfolic acid CRS* in the mobile phase and dilute to 100.0 ml with the mobile phase. Dilute 1.0 ml of this solution to 10.0 ml with *water R.*

Reference solution (d). Dilute 1.0 ml of reference solution (b) to 20.0 ml with *water R.*

Reference solution (e). Dilute 5.0 ml of reference solution (c) to 10.0 ml with reference solution (b).

Column:

- *size*: *l* = 0.25 m, Ø = 4 mm,
- *stationary phase*: *octadecylsilyl silica gel for chromatography R* (5 µm),
- *temperature*: 40 °C.

Mobile phase: mix 220 ml of *methanol R* and 780 ml of a solution containing 2.0 ml of *tetrabutylammonium hydroxide solution (400 g/l) R* and 2.2 g of *disodium hydrogen phosphate R* previously adjusted to pH 7.8 with *phosphoric acid R*. If necessary adjust the concentration of *methanol R* to achieve the prescribed resolution.

Flow rate: 1 ml/min.

Detection: spectrophotometer at 280 nm.

Injection: 10 µl.

Run time: 2.5 times the retention time of the principal peak in the chromatogram obtained with the test solution.

System suitability: reference solution (e):

- *resolution*: minimum of 2.2 between the peaks due to folinate and to impurity D.

Limits:

- *impurity D*: not more than 0.8 times the area of the principal peak in the chromatogram obtained with reference solution (c) (0.8 per cent),
- *any other impurity*: not more than 0.8 times the area of the principal peak in the chromatogram obtained with reference solution (b) (0.8 per cent),
- *total of other impurities*: not more than twice the area of the principal peak in the chromatogram obtained with reference solution (b) (2.0 per cent),
- *disregard limit*: area of the principal peak in the chromatogram obtained with reference solution (d) (0.05 per cent).

Impurity H. Liquid chromatography (*2.2.29*): use the normalisation procedure.

Test solution. Dissolve 50.0 mg of the substance to be examined in *water R* and dilute to 100.0 ml with the same solvent.

Reference solution (a). Dissolve 10.0 mg of *calcium folinate CRS* in *water R* and dilute to 20.0 ml with the same solvent.

Reference solution (b). Dilute 1.0 ml of reference solution (a) to 100.0 ml with *water R.*

Column:

- *size*: *l* = 0.15 m, Ø = 4 mm,
- *stationary phase*: *human albumin coated silica gel for chromatography R* (5 µm),
- *temperature*: 40 °C.

Mobile phase: dissolve 9.72 g of *sodium dihydrogen phosphate R* in 890 ml of *water R* and adjust to pH 5.0 with *sodium hydroxide solution R*. Add 100 ml of *2-propanol R* and 10 ml of *acetonitrile R.*

Flow rate: 1 ml/min.

Detection: spectrophotometer at 286 nm.

Injection: 10 µl.

Retention times: levofolinate = about 9 min; impurity H = about 19 min.

System suitability:

- *resolution*: minimum of 5.0 between the peaks due to levofolinate and to impurity H in the chromatogram obtained with reference solution (a). The sum of the areas of the 2 peaks is 100 per cent. The peak area of impurity H is 48 per cent to 52 per cent. In the chromatogram obtained with reference solution (b) 2 clearly visible peaks are obtained.

Limits:

- *impurity H*: maximum 0.5 per cent.

Chlorides: maximum 0.5 per cent.

Dissolve 0.300 g in 50 ml of *water R* heating at 40 °C if necessary. Add 10 ml of *2 M nitric acid* and titrate with *0.005 M silver nitrate* determining the end-point potentiometrically (*2.2.20*).

1 ml of *0.005 M silver nitrate* is equivalent to 0.177 mg of Cl.

Platinum: maximum 10 ppm.

Atomic absorption spectrometry (*2.2.23, Method II*).

Test solution. Dissolve 1.0 g in *water R* and dilute to 100.0 ml with the same solvent.

Reference solutions. Prepare the reference solutions using *platinum standard solution (30 ppm Pt) R*, diluted as necessary with a mixture of 1 volume of *nitric acid R* and 99 volumes of *water R.*

Source: platinum hollow-cathode lamp.

Wavelength: 265.9 nm.

Heavy metals (*2.4.8*): maximum 50 ppm.

1.0 g complies with limit test F. Prepare the standard using 5 ml of *lead standard solution (10 ppm Pb) R.*

Water (*2.5.12*): 10.0 per cent to 17.0 per cent, determined on 0.200 g (ground to a very fine powder). Stir the substance to be examined in the titration solvent for about 15 min before titrating and use *iodosulphurous reagent R* as titrant.

Bacterial endotoxins (*2.6.14*): less than 0.5 IU/mg, if intended for use in the manufacture of parenteral dosage forms without a further appropriate procedure for the removal of bacterial endotoxins.

ASSAY

Calcium. Dissolve 0.400 g in 150 ml of *water R* and dilute to 300 ml with the same solvent. Carry out the complexometric titration of calcium (*2.5.11*).

1 ml of *0.1 M sodium edetate* is equivalent to 4.008 mg of Ca.

Calcium folinate. Liquid chromatography (*2.2.29*) as described in the test for related substances.

Calculate the percentage content of $C_{20}H_{21}CaN_7O_7$ from the areas of the peaks in the chromatograms obtained with the test solution and reference solution (a) and the declared content of *calcium folinate CRS*.

STORAGE

In an airtight container, protected from light. If the substance is sterile, store in a sterile, airtight, tamper-proof container.

LABELLING

The label states, where applicable, that the substance is free from bacterial endotoxins.

IMPURITIES

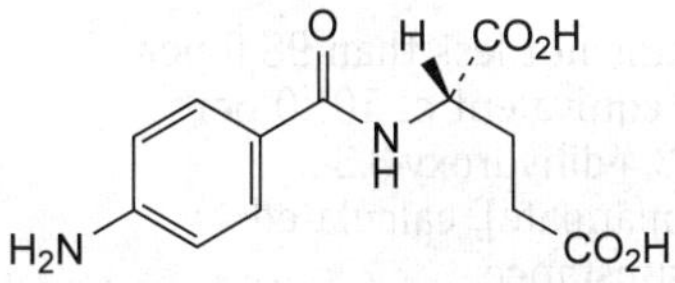

A. (2*S*)-2-[(4-aminobenzoyl)amino]pentanedioic acid,

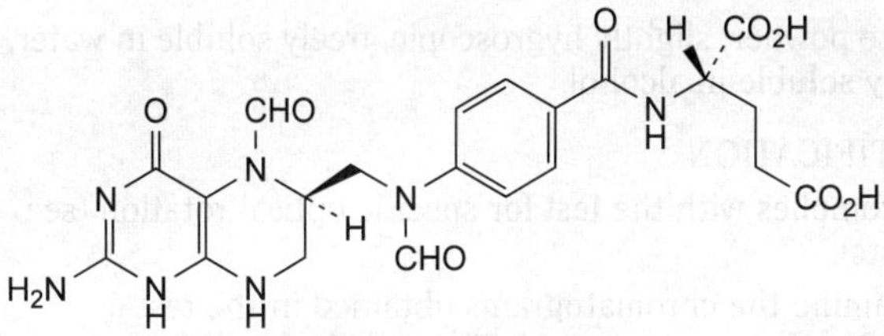

B. (2*S*)-2-[[4-[[[(6*R*)-2-amino-5-formyl-4-oxo-1,4,5,6,7,8-hexahydropteridin-6-yl]methyl]formylamino]benzoyl]amino]pentanedioic acid (5,10-diformyltetrahydrofolic acid),

C. folic acid,

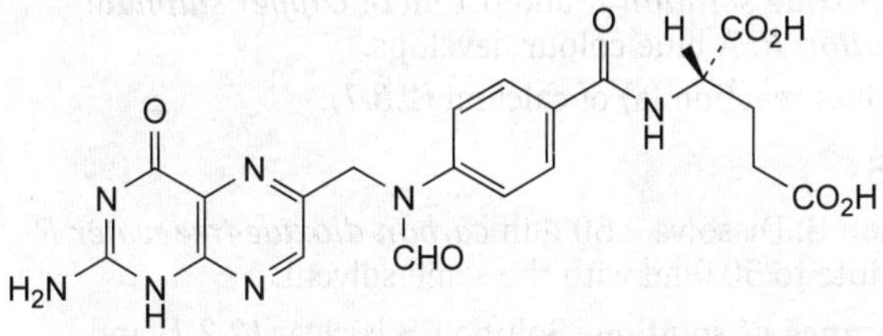

D. (2*S*)-2-[[4-[[(2-amino-4-oxo-1,4-dihydropteridin-6-yl)methyl]formylamino]benzoyl]amino]pentanedioic acid (10-formylfolic acid),

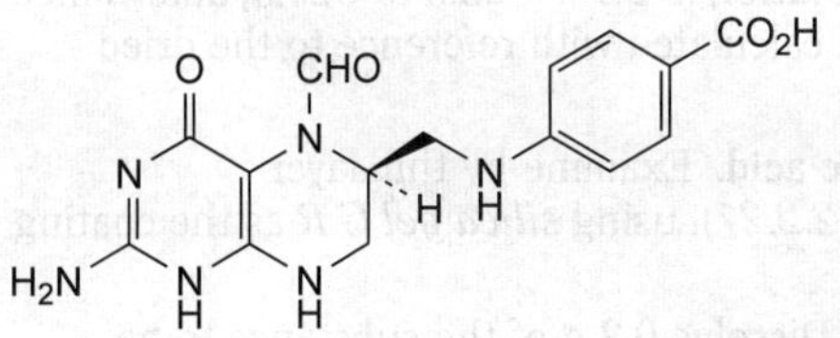

E. 4-[[[(6*S*)-2-amino-5-formyl-4-oxo-1,4,5,6,7,8-hexahydropteridin-6-yl]methyl]amino]benzoic acid (5-formyltetrahydropteroic acid),

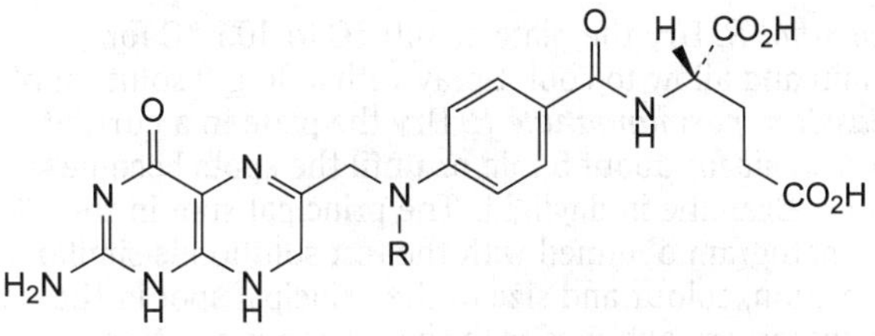

F. R = CHO: (2*S*)-2-[[4-[[(2-amino-4-oxo-1,4,7,8-tetrahydropteridin-6-yl)methyl]formylamino]benzoyl]amino]pentanedioic acid (10-formyldihydrofolic acid),

G. R = H: (2*S*)-2-[[4-[[(2-amino-4-oxo-1,4,7,8-tetrahydropteridin-6-yl)methyl]amino]benzoyl]amino]pentanedioic acid (dihydrofolic acid),

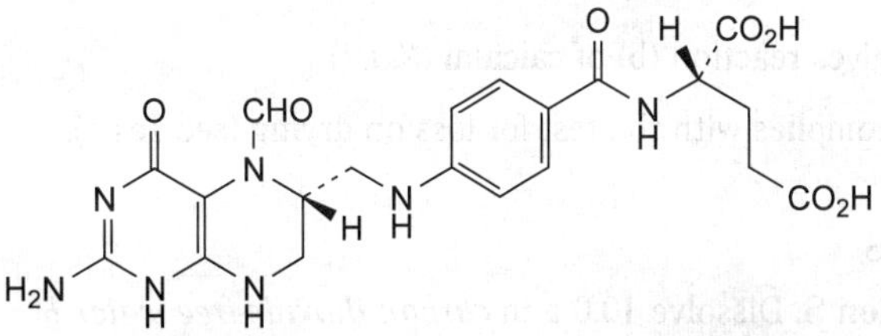

H. (2*S*)-2-[[4-[[[(6*R*)-2-amino-5-formyl-4-oxo-1,4,5,6,7,8-hexahydropteridin-6-yl]methyl]amino]benzoyl]amino]pentanedioic acid.

01/2005:1296

CALCIUM LEVULINATE DIHYDRATE

Calcii laevulinas dihydricum

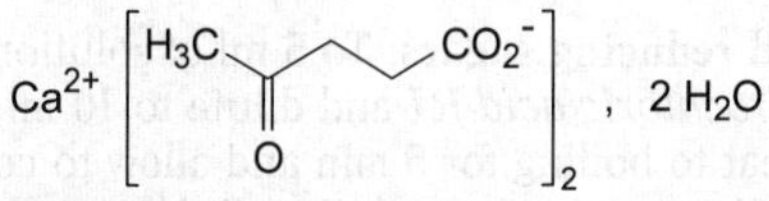

$C_{10}H_{14}CaO_6,2H_2O$ M_r 306.3

DEFINITION

Calcium levulinate dihydrate contains not less than 98.0 per cent and not more than the equivalent of 101.0 per cent of calcium di(4-oxopentanoate), calculated with reference to the dried substance.

CHARACTERS

A white or almost white, crystalline powder, freely soluble in water, very slightly soluble in alcohol, practically insoluble in methylene chloride.

IDENTIFICATION

First identification: A, D, E.

Second identification: B, C, D, E.

A. Examine by infrared absorption spectrophotometry (*2.2.24*), comparing with the spectrum obtained with *calcium levulinate dihydrate CRS*.

B. Examine by thin-layer chromatography (*2.2.27*), using a suitable silica gel as the coating substance.

Test solution. Dissolve 60 mg of the substance to be examined in *water R* and dilute to 1 ml with the same solvent.

Reference solution. Dissolve 60 mg of *calcium levulinate dihydrate CRS* in *water R* and dilute to 1 ml with the same solvent.

Apply separately to the plate 10 µl of each solution. Develop over a path of 10 cm using a mixture of 10 volumes of *concentrated ammonia R*, 10 volumes of *ethyl acetate R*, 30 volumes of *water R* and 50 volumes of *alcohol R*. Dry the plate at 100 °C to 105 °C for 20 min and allow to cool. Spray with a 30 g/l solution of *potassium permanganate R*. Dry the plate in a current of warm air for about 5 min or until the spots become yellow. Examine in daylight. The principal spot in the chromatogram obtained with the test solution is similar in position, colour and size to the principal spot in the chromatogram obtained with the reference solution.

C. To 1 ml of solution S (see Tests), add 20 ml of a 2.5 g/l solution of *dinitrophenylhydrazine R* in *dilute hydrochloric acid R*. Allow to stand for 15 min. Filter, wash the precipitate with *water R*. Dry the precipitate in an oven at 100 °C to 105 °C. The melting point (*2.2.14*) is 203 °C to 210 °C.

D. It gives reaction (b) of calcium (*2.3.1*).

E. It complies with the test for loss on drying (see Tests).

Monographs C

TESTS

Solution S. Dissolve 10.0 g in *carbon dioxide-free water R* prepared from *distilled water R* and dilute to 100.0 ml with the same solvent.

Appearance of solution. Solution S is clear (*2.2.1*) and not more intensely coloured than reference solution Y_6 (*2.2.2, Method II*).

pH (*2.2.3*). The pH of solution S is 6.8 to 7.8.

Oxidisable substances. To 1 ml of solution S, add 10 ml of *water R*, 1 ml of *dilute sulphuric acid R* and 0.25 ml of a 3.0 g/l solution of *potassium permanganate R*. Mix. After 5 min, the violet colour of the mixture is still visible.

Sucrose and reducing sugars. To 5 ml of solution S, add 2 ml of *hydrochloric acid R1* and dilute to 10 ml with *water R*. Heat to boiling for 5 min and allow to cool. Add 10 ml of *sodium carbonate solution R*. Allow to stand for 5 min, dilute to 25 ml with *water R* and filter. To 5 ml of the filtrate, add 2 ml of *cupri-tartaric solution R* and heat to boiling for 1 min. No red precipitate is formed.

Chlorides (*2.4.4*). Dilute 10 ml of solution S to 15 ml with *water R*. The solution complies with the limit test for chlorides (50 ppm).

Sulphates (*2.4.13*). Dilute 7.5 ml of solution S to 15 ml with *distilled water R*. The solution complies with the limit test for sulphates (200 ppm).

Magnesium and alkali metals. To 10 ml of solution S, add 80 ml of *water R*, 10 ml of *ammonium chloride solution R* and 1 ml of *ammonia R*. Heat to boiling. To the boiling solution, add dropwise 50 ml of warm *ammonium oxalate solution R*. Allow to stand for 4 h, then dilute to 200 ml with *water R* and filter. To 100 ml of the filtrate, add 0.5 ml of *sulphuric acid R*. Evaporate to dryness on a water-bath and ignite to constant mass at 600 °C. The residue weighs not more than 5.0 mg (1.0 per cent).

Heavy metals (*2.4.8*). 12 ml of solution S complies with limit test A for heavy metals (10 ppm). Prepare the standard using *lead standard solution (1 ppm Pb) R*.

Loss on drying (*2.2.32*): 11.0 per cent to 12.5 per cent, determined on 0.200 g by drying at 100 °C to 105 °C.

Pyrogens (*2.6.8*). If intended for use in the manufacture of parenteral dosage forms without a further appropriate procedure for the removal of pyrogens, it complies with the test for pyrogens. Inject per kilogram of the rabbit's mass 4 ml of a solution containing per millilitre 50 mg of the substance to be examined.

ASSAY

Dissolve 0.240 g in 50 ml of *water R*. Carry out the complexometric titration of calcium (*2.5.11*).

1 ml of *0.1 M sodium edetate* is equivalent to 27.03 mg of $C_{10}H_{14}CaO_6$.

STORAGE

Store protected from light.

LABELLING

The label states, where applicable, that the substance is apyrogenic.

01/2005:0470

CALCIUM PANTOTHENATE

Calcii pantothenas

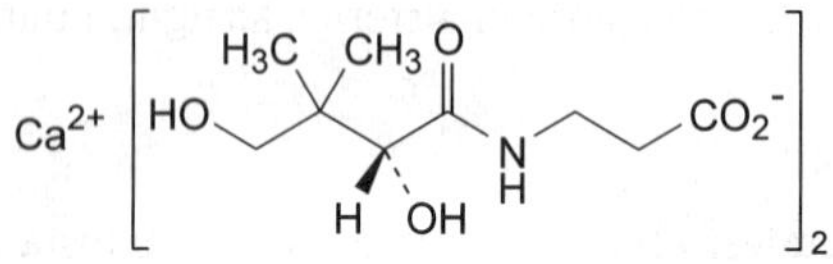

$C_{18}H_{32}CaN_2O_{10}$ M_r 476.5

DEFINITION

Calcium pantothenate contains not less than 98.0 per cent and not more than the equivalent of 101.0 per cent of calcium bis[3-[[(2*R*)-2,4-dihydroxy-3,3-dimethylbutanoyl]amino]propanoate], calculated with reference to the dried substance.

CHARACTERS

A white powder, slightly hygroscopic, freely soluble in water, slightly soluble in alcohol.

IDENTIFICATION

A. It complies with the test for specific optical rotation (see Tests).

B. Examine the chromatograms obtained in the test for 3-aminopropionic acid. The principal spot in the chromatogram obtained with test solution (b) is similar in position, colour and size to the principal spot in the chromatogram obtained with reference solution (a).

C. To 1 ml of solution S (see Tests) add 1 ml of *dilute sodium hydroxide solution R* and 0.1 ml of *copper sulphate solution R*. A blue colour develops.

D. It gives reaction (a) of calcium (*2.3.1*).

TESTS

Solution S. Dissolve 2.50 g in *carbon dioxide-free water R* and dilute to 50.0 ml with the same solvent.

Appearance of solution. Solution S is clear (*2.2.1*) and colourless (*2.2.2, Method II*).

pH (*2.2.3*). The pH of solution S is 6.8 to 8.0.

Specific optical rotation (*2.2.7*): + 25.5 to + 27.5, determined on solution S and calculated with reference to the dried substance.

3-Aminopropionic acid. Examine by thin-layer chromatography (*2.2.27*), using *silica gel G R* as the coating substance.

Test solution (a). Dissolve 0.2 g of the substance to be examined in *water R* and dilute to 5 ml with the same solvent.

Test solution (b). Dilute 1 ml of test solution (a) to 10 ml with *water R*.

Reference solution (a). Dissolve 20 mg of *calcium pantothenate CRS* in *water R* and dilute to 5 ml with the same solvent.

Reference solution (b). Dissolve 10 mg of *3-aminopropionic acid R* in *water R* and dilute to 50 ml with the same solvent.

Apply separately to the plate 5 µl of each solution. Develop over a path of 12 cm using a mixture of 35 volumes of *water R* and 65 volumes of *ethanol R*. Dry the plate in a current of air and spray with *ninhydrin solution R1*. Heat at 110 °C for 10 min. Any spot corresponding to 3-aminopropionic acid in the chromatogram obtained with test solution (a) is not more intense than the spot in the chromatogram obtained with reference solution (b) (0.5 per cent).

Chlorides (*2.4.4*). 5 ml of solution S diluted to 15 ml with *water R* complies with the limit test for chlorides (200 ppm).

Heavy metals (*2.4.8*). 12 ml of solution S complies with limit test A for heavy metals (20 ppm). Prepare the standard using *lead standard solution (1 ppm Pb) R*.

Loss on drying (*2.2.32*). Not more than 3.0 per cent, determined on 1.000 g by drying in an oven at 100 °C to 105 °C.

ASSAY

Dissolve 0.180 g in 50 ml of *anhydrous acetic acid R*. Titrate with *0.1 M perchloric acid* determining the end-point potentiometrically (*2.2.20*).

1 ml of *0.1 M perchloric acid* is equivalent to 23.83 mg of $C_{18}H_{32}CaN_2O_{10}$.

STORAGE

Store in an airtight container.

01/2005:1052

CALCIUM PHOSPHATE

Tricalcii phosphas

DEFINITION

Calcium phosphate consists of a mixture of calcium phosphates. It contains not less than 35.0 per cent and not more than the equivalent of 40.0 per cent of Ca (A_r 40.08).

CHARACTERS

A white or almost white powder, practically insoluble in water. It dissolves in dilute hydrochloric acid and in dilute nitric acid.

IDENTIFICATION

A. Dissolve 0.1 g in 5 ml of a 25 per cent *V/V* solution of *nitric acid R*. The solution gives reaction (b) of phosphates (*2.3.1*).

B. It gives reaction (b) of calcium (*2.3.1*). Filter before adding *potassium ferrocyanide solution R*.

C. It complies with the limits of the assay.

TESTS

Solution S. Dissolve 2.50 g in 20 ml of *dilute hydrochloric acid R*. If the solution is not clear, filter it. Add *dilute ammonia R1* dropwise until a precipitate is formed. Dissolve the precipitate by adding *dilute hydrochloric acid R* and dilute to 50 ml with *distilled water R*.

Chlorides (*2.4.4*). Dissolve 0.22 g in a mixture of 1 ml of *nitric acid R* and 10 ml of *water R* and dilute to 100 ml with *water R*. 15 ml of the solution complies with the limit test for chlorides (0.15 per cent).

Fluorides. Not more than 75 ppm of F, determined potentiometrically (*2.2.36, Method I*) using a fluoride-selective indicator electrode and a silver-silver chloride reference electrode.

Test solution. In a 50 ml volumetric flask, dissolve 0.250 g in *0.1 M hydrochloric acid*, add 5.0 ml of *fluoride standard solution (1 ppm F) R* and dilute to 50.0 ml with *0.1 M hydrochloric acid*. To 20.0 ml of the solution add 20.0 ml of *total-ionic-strength-adjustment buffer R* and 3 ml of an 82 g/l solution of *anhydrous sodium acetate R*. Adjust to pH 5.2 with *ammonia R* and dilute to 50.0 ml with *distilled water R*.

Reference solutions. To 5.0 ml, 2.0 ml, 1.0 ml, 0.5 ml and 0.25 ml of *fluoride standard solution (10 ppm F) R* add 20.0 ml of *total-ionic-strength-adjustment buffer R* and dilute to 50.0 ml with *distilled water R*.

Carry out the measurements on 20.0 ml of each solution. Calculate the concentration of fluorides using the calibration curve, taking into account the addition of fluoride to the test solution.

Sulphates (*2.4.13*). Dilute 1 ml of solution S to 25 ml with *distilled water R*. 15 ml of the solution complies with the limit test for sulphates (0.5 per cent).

Arsenic (*2.4.2*). 5 ml of solution S complies with limit test A for arsenic (4 ppm).

Iron (*2.4.9*). Dilute 0.5 ml of solution S to 10 ml with *water R*. The solution complies with the limit test for iron (400 ppm).

Heavy metals (*2.4.8*). Dilute 13 ml of solution S to 20 ml with *water R*. 12 ml of the solution complies with limit test A for heavy metals (30 ppm). Prepare the standard using *lead standard solution (1 ppm Pb) R*.

Acid-insoluble matter. Dissolve 5.0 g in a mixture of 10 ml of *hydrochloric acid R* and 30 ml of *water R*. Filter, wash the residue with *water R* and dry to constant mass at 100 °C to 105 °C. The residue weighs not more than 10 mg (0.2 per cent).

Loss on ignition. Not more than 8.0 per cent, determined on 1.000 g by ignition at 800 °C for 30 min.

ASSAY

Dissolve 0.200 g in a mixture of 1 ml of *hydrochloric acid R1* and 5 ml of *water R*. Add 25.0 ml of *0.1 M sodium edetate* and dilute to 200 ml with *water R*. Adjust to about pH 10 with *concentrated ammonia R*. Add 10 ml of *ammonium chloride buffer solution pH 10.0 R* and a few milligrams of *mordant black 11 triturate R*. Titrate the excess sodium edetate with *0.1 M zinc sulphate* until the colour changes from blue to violet.

1 ml of *0.1 M sodium edetate* is equivalent to 4.008 mg of Ca.

01/2005:0882

CALCIUM STEARATE

Calcii stearas

DEFINITION

Calcium stearate is a mixture of calcium salts of different fatty acids consisting mainly of stearic acid [$(C_{17}H_{35}COO)_2Ca$; M_r 607] and palmitic acid [$(C_{15}H_{31}COO)_2Ca$; M_r 550.9] with minor proportions of other fatty acids. It contains not less than 6.4 per cent and not more than 7.4 per cent of Ca (A_r 40.08), calculated with reference to the dried substance. The fatty acid fraction contains not less than 40.0 per cent of stearic acid and the sum of stearic acid and palmitic acid is not less than 90.0 per cent.

CHARACTERS

A fine, white or almost white, crystalline powder, practically insoluble in water and in alcohol.

IDENTIFICATION

First identification: C, D.

Second identification: A, B, D.

A. The residue obtained in the preparation of solution S (see Tests) has a freezing point (*2.2.18*) not lower than 53 °C.

B. The acid value of the fatty acids (*2.5.1*) is 195 to 210, determined on 0.200 g of the residue obtained in the preparation of solution S dissolved in 25 ml of the prescribed mixture of solvents.

C. Examine the chromatograms obtained in the test for fatty acid composition. The retention times of the principal peaks in the chromatogram obtained with the test solution are approximately the same as those of the principal peaks in the chromatogram obtained with the reference solution.

D. Neutralise 5 ml of solution S to *red litmus paper R* using *strong sodium hydroxide solution R*. The solution gives reaction (b) of calcium (*2.3.1*).

TESTS

Solution S. To 5.0 g add 50 ml of *peroxide-free ether R*, 20 ml of *dilute nitric acid R* and 20 ml of *distilled water R*. Boil under a reflux condenser until dissolution is complete. Allow to cool. In a separating funnel, separate the aqueous layer and shake the ether layer with 2 quantities, each of 5 ml, of *distilled water R*. Combine the aqueous layers, wash with 15 ml of *peroxide-free ether R* and dilute the aqueous layer to 50 ml with *distilled water R* (solution S). Evaporate the ether layer to dryness and dry the residue at 100-105 °C. Keep the residue for identification tests A and B.

Acidity or alkalinity. To 1.0 g add 20 ml of *carbon dioxide-free water R* and boil for 1 min with continuous shaking. Cool and filter. To 10 ml of the filtrate add 0.05 ml of *bromothymol blue solution R1*. Not more than 0.5 ml of *0.01 M hydrochloric acid* or *0.01 M sodium hydroxide* is required to change the colour of the indicator.

Chlorides (*2.4.4*). Dilute 0.5 ml of solution S to 15 ml with *water R*. The solution complies with the limit test for chlorides (0.1 per cent).

Sulphates (*2.4.13*). Dilute 0.5 ml of solution S to 15 ml with *distilled water R*. The solution complies with the limit test for sulphates (0.3 per cent).

Cadmium. Not more than 3 ppm of Cd, determined by atomic absorption spectrometry (*2.2.23, Method II*).

Test solution. Place 50.0 mg of the substance to be examined in a polytetrafluoroethylene digestion bomb and add 0.5 ml of a mixture of 1 volume of *hydrochloric acid R* and 5 volumes of *cadmium- and lead-free nitric acid R*. Allow to digest at 170 °C for 5 h. Allow to cool. Dissolve the residue in *water R* and dilute to 5.0 ml with the same solvent.

Reference solutions. Prepare the reference solutions using *cadmium standard solution (10 ppm Cd) R*, diluted if necessary with a 1 per cent *V/V* solution of *hydrochloric acid R*.

Measure the absorbance at 228.8 nm using a cadmium hollow-cathode lamp as source of radiation and a graphite furnace as atomic generator.

Lead. Not more than 10 ppm of Pb, determined by atomic absorption spectrometry (*2.2.23, Method II*).

Test solution. Use the solution described in the test for cadmium.

Reference solutions. Prepare the reference solutions using *lead standard solution (10 ppm Pb) R*, diluted if necessary with *water R*.

Measure the absorbance at 283.3 nm using a lead hollow-cathode lamp as source of radiation and a graphite furnace as atomic generator. Depending on the apparatus, the line at 217.0 nm may be used.

Nickel. Not more than 5 ppm of Ni, determined by atomic absorption spectrometry (*2.2.23, Method II*).

Test solution. Use the solution described in the test for cadmium.

Reference solutions. Prepare the reference solutions using *nickel standard solution (10 ppm Ni) R*, diluted if necessary with *water R*.

Measure the absorbance at 232.0 nm using a nickel hollow-cathode lamp as source of radiation and a graphite furnace as atomic generator.

Loss on drying (*2.2.32*). Not more than 6.0 per cent, determined on 1.000 g by drying in an oven at 100-105 °C.

Microbial contamination. Total viable aerobic count (*2.6.12*) not more than 10^3 micro-organisms per gram, determined by plate count. It complies with the test for *Escherichia coli* (*2.6.13*).

ASSAY

Calcium. To 0.500 g in a 250 ml conical flask add 50 ml of a mixture of equal volumes of *butanol R* and *ethanol R*, 5 ml of *concentrated ammonia R*, 3 ml of *ammonium chloride buffer solution pH 10.0 R*, 30.0 ml of *0.1 M sodium edetate* and 15 mg of *mordant black 11 triturate R*. Heat to 45-50 °C until the solution is clear. Cool and titrate with *0.1 M zinc sulphate* until the colour changes from blue to violet. Carry out a blank titration.

1 ml of *0.1 M sodium edetate* is equivalent to 4.008 mg of Ca.

Fatty acid composition. Examine by gas chromatography (*2.2.28*).

Test solution. In a conical flask fitted with a reflux condenser, dissolve 0.10 g of the substance to be examined in 5 ml of *boron trifluoride-methanol solution R*. Boil under a reflux condenser for 10 min. Add 4 ml of *heptane R* through the condenser and boil again under a reflux condenser for 10 min. Allow to cool. Add 20 ml of a *saturated sodium chloride solution R*. Shake and allow the layers to separate. Remove about 2 ml of the organic layer and dry over 0.2 g of *anhydrous sodium sulphate R*. Dilute 1.0 ml of the solution to 10.0 ml with *heptane R*.

Reference solution. Prepare the reference solution in the same manner as the test solution using 50.0 mg of *palmitic acid CRS* and 50.0 mg of *stearic acid CRS* instead of calcium stearate.

The chromatographic procedure may be carried out using:

– a fused-silica column 30 m long and 0.32 mm in internal diameter coated with *macrogol 20 000 R* (film thickness 0.5 µm),
– *helium for chromatography R* as the carrier gas at a flow rate of 2.4 ml/min,

– a flame-ionisation detector,

with the following temperature programme:

	Time (min)	Temperature (°C)	Rate (°C/min)	Comment
Column	0 - 2	70	-	isothermal
	2 - 36	70 → 240	5	linear gradient
	36 - 41	240	-	isothermal
Injection port		220		
Detector		260		

Inject 1 μl of the reference solution. When the chromatogram is recorded in the prescribed conditions, the retention time of methyl palmitate relative to that of methyl stearate is about 0.88. The test is not valid unless, in the chromatogram obtained with the reference solution, the resolution between the peaks corresponding to methyl stearate and methyl palmitate is at least 5.0.

Inject 1 μl of the test solution. Calculate the percentage content of stearic acid and palmitic acid from the areas of the peaks in the chromatogram obtained with the test solution by the normalisation procedure, disregarding the peak due to the solvent.

01/2005:0982

CALCIUM SULPHATE DIHYDRATE

Calcii sulfas dihydricus

$CaSO_4,2H_2O$ M_r 172.2

DEFINITION

Calcium sulphate dihydrate contains not less than 98.0 per cent and not more than the equivalent of 102.0 per cent of $CaSO_4,2H_2O$.

CHARACTERS

A white, fine powder, very slightly soluble in water, practically insoluble in alcohol.

IDENTIFICATION

A. It complies with the test for loss on ignition (see Tests).

B. Solution S (see Tests) gives reaction (a) of sulphates (*2.3.1*).

C. Solution S gives reaction (a) of calcium (*2.3.1*).

TESTS

Solution S. Dissolve 1.0 g in 50 ml of a 10 per cent *V/V* solution of *hydrochloric acid R* by heating at 50 °C for 5 min. Allow the solution to cool.

Acidity or alkalinity. Shake 1.5 g with 15 ml of *carbon dioxide-free water R* for 5 min. Allow to stand for 5 min and filter. To 10 ml of the filtrate, add 0.1 ml of *phenolphthalein solution R* and 0.25 ml of *0.01 M sodium hydroxide*. The solution is red. Add 0.30 ml of *0.01 M hydrochloric acid*. The solution is colourless. Add 0.2 ml of *methyl red solution R*. The solution is reddish-orange.

Chlorides (*2.4.4*). Shake 0.5 g with 15 ml of *water R* for 5 min. Allow to stand for 15 min and filter. Dilute 5 ml of the filtrate to 15 ml with *water R*. The solution complies with the limit test for chlorides (300 ppm).

Arsenic (*2.4.2*). 5 ml of solution S complies with limit test A for arsenic (10 ppm).

Iron (*2.4.9*). To 0.25 g add a mixture of 5 ml of *hydrochloric acid R* and 20 ml of *water R*. Heat to boiling, cool and filter. 10 ml of the filtrate complies with the limit test for iron (100 ppm).

Heavy metals (*2.4.8*). To 2.5 g add a mixture of 2 ml of *hydrochloric acid R* and 15 ml of *water R*. Heat to boiling. Cool and then add 0.5 ml of *phenolphthalein solution R*. Cautiously add *concentrated ammonia R* until the colour changes to pink. Add 0.5 ml of *glacial acetic acid R* and dilute to 25 ml with *water R*. Filter. 12 ml of the filtrate complies with limit test A for heavy metals (20 ppm). Prepare the standard using *lead standard solution (2 ppm Pb) R*.

Loss on ignition: 18.0 per cent to 22.0 per cent, determined on 1.000 g by ignition to constant mass at 800 °C.

ASSAY

Dissolve 0.150 g in 120 ml of *water R*. Carry out the complexometric titration of calcium (*2.5.11*).

1 ml of *0.1 M sodium edetate* is equivalent to 17.22 mg of $CaSO_4,2H_2O$.

01/2005:1297

CALENDULA FLOWER

Calendulae flos

DEFINITION

Calendula flower consists of the whole or cut, dried, and fully opened flowers which have been detached from the receptacle of the cultivated, double-flowered varieties of *Calendula officinalis* L. It contains not less than 0.4 per cent of flavonoids, calculated as hyperoside ($C_{21}H_{20}O_{12}$, M_r 464.4) with reference to the dried drug.

CHARACTERS

It has the macroscopic and microscopic characters described under identification tests A and B.

IDENTIFICATION

A. The ligulate florets consist of a yellow or orange-yellow ligule, about 3 mm to 5 mm wide and about 7 mm in the middle part, with a three toothed apex and a hairy, partly sickle-shaped yellowish-brown to orange-brown tube with a projecting style and a bifid stigma occasionally with a partly bent yellowish-brown to orange-brown ovary. The tubular florets, about 5 mm long, are present and consist of the yellow, orange-red or red-violet five lobed corolla and the yellowish-brown or orange-brown tube, hairy in its lower part, mostly with a partly bent yellowish-brown to orange-brown ovary.

B. Reduce to a powder (355). The powder is yellowish-brown. Examine under a microscope using *chloral hydrate solution R*. The powder shows fragments of the corollas containing light yellow oil droplets, some with fairly large anomocytic stomata (*2.8.3*), others containing prisms and very small cluster crystals of calcium oxalate; covering trichomes biseriate, multicellular and conical, glandular trichomes with a uniseriate or biseriate, multicellular biseriate stalk and a large, ovoid, biseriate and multicellular head; spherical pollen grains up to about 40 μm in diameter with a sharply spiny exine and three germinal pores; occasional fragments of the stigmas with short, bulbous papillae.

C. Examine by thin-layer chromatography (*2.2.27*), using a suitable silica gel as the coating substance.

Test solution. To 1.0 g of the powdered drug (500) add 10 ml of *methanol R* and heat on a water-bath under a reflux condenser for 10 min. Cool and filter.

Reference solution. Dissolve 1.0 mg of *caffeic acid R*, 1.0 mg of *chlorogenic acid R* and 2.5 mg of *rutin R* in 10 ml of *methanol R*.

Apply to the plate, as bands, 20 µl of the test solution and 10 µl of the reference solution. Develop over a path of 10 cm using a mixture of 10 volumes of *anhydrous formic acid R*, 10 volumes of *water R* and 80 volumes of *ethyl acetate R*. Allow the plate to dry at 100 °C to 105 °C and spray the still warm plate with a 10 g/l solution of *diphenylboric acid aminoethyl ester R* in *methanol R* and then spray with a 50 g/l solution of *macrogol 400 R* in *methanol R*. Allow the plate to dry in air for 30 min and examine in ultraviolet light at 365 nm. The chromatogram obtained with the reference solution shows in the lower part a yellowish-brown fluorescent zone (rutin), in the middle part a light bluish fluorescent zone (chlorogenic acid) and in the upper part a light bluish fluorescent zone (caffeic acid). The chromatogram obtained with the test solution shows a yellowish-brown fluorescent zone corresponding in position to the zone due to rutin in the chromatogram obtained with the reference solution, below and directly above it, it shows a yellowish-green fluorescent zone and a light bluish fluorescent zone corresponding to the zone due to chlorogenic acid in the chromatogram obtained with the reference solution, a yellowish-green fluorescent zone above it and a light bluish fluorescent zone shortly below the zone due to caffeic acid in the chromatogram obtained with the reference solution. Further zones are present.

Monographs C

TESTS

Foreign matter (*2.8.2*). Not more than 5 per cent of bracts and not more than 2 per cent of other foreign matter.

Loss on drying (*2.2.32*). Not more than 12.0 per cent, determined on 1.000 g of the powdered drug (500) by drying in an oven at 100 °C to 105 °C for 2 h.

Total ash (*2.4.16*). Not more than 10.0 per cent.

ASSAY

Stock solution. In a 100 ml round-bottomed flask introduce 0.800 g of the powdered drug (500), 1 ml of a 5 g/l solution of *hexamethylenetetramine R*, 20 ml of *acetone R* and 7 ml of *hydrochloric acid R1*. Boil the mixture under a reflux condenser for 30 min. Filter the liquid through a plug of absorbent cotton in a 100 ml flask. Add the absorbent cotton to the residue in the round-bottomed flask and extract with two quantities, each of 20 ml, of *acetone R*, each time boiling under a reflux condenser for 10 min. Allow to cool to room temperature, filter the liquid through a plug of absorbent cotton then filter the combined acetone solution through a filter-paper in the volumetric flask and dilute to 100.0 ml with *acetone R* by rinsing of the flask and the filter. Introduce 20.0 ml of the solution into a separating funnel, add 20 ml of *water R* and extract the mixture with one quantity of 15 ml and then three quantities, each of 10 ml, of *ethyl acetate R*. Combine the ethyl acetate extracts in a separating funnel, rinse with two quantities, each of 50 ml, of *water R*, filter the extract over 10 g of *anhydrous sodium sulphate R* in to a 50 ml volumetric flask and dilute to 50.0 ml with *ethyl acetate R*.

Test solution. To 10.0 ml of the stock solution add 1 ml of *aluminium chloride reagent R* and dilute to 25.0 ml with a 5 per cent *V/V* solution of *glacial acetic acid R* in *methanol R*.

Compensation solution. Dilute 10.0 ml of the stock solution to 25.0 ml with a 5 per cent *V/V* solution of *glacial acetic acid R* in *methanol R*.

Measure the absorbance (*2.2.25*) of the test solution after 30 min, by comparison with the compensation solution at 425 nm.

Calculate the percentage content of flavonoids, calculated as hyperoside, from the expression:

$$\frac{A \times 1.25}{m}$$

i.e. taking the specific absorbance of hyperoside to be 500.

A = absorbance at 425 nm,

m = mass of the substance to be examined in grams.

STORAGE

Store protected from light.

01/2005:1400

D-CAMPHOR

D-Camphora

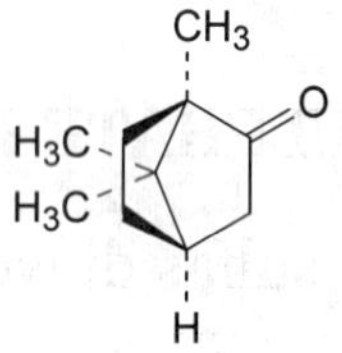

$C_{10}H_{16}O$ M_r 152.2

DEFINITION

(1*R*,4*R*)-1,7,7-Trimethylbicyclo[2.2.1]heptan-2-one.

CHARACTERS

Appearance: white, crystalline powder or friable, crystalline masses.

Highly volatile even at room temperature.

Solubility: slightly soluble in water, very soluble in alcohol and in light petroleum, freely soluble in fatty oils, very slightly soluble in glycerol.

IDENTIFICATION

First identification: A, C.

Second identification: A, B, D.

A. Specific optical rotation (see Tests).

B. Melting point (*2.2.14*): 175 °C to 179 °C.

C. Infrared absorption spectrophotometry (*2.2.24*).

Comparison: *racemic camphor CRS*.

D. Dissolve 1.0 g in 30 ml of *methanol R*. Add 1.0 g of *hydroxylamine hydrochloride R* and 1.0 g of *anhydrous sodium acetate R*. Boil under a reflux condenser for 2 h. Allow to cool and add 100 ml of *water R*. Filter, wash the precipitate obtained with 10 ml of *water R* and recrystallise from 10 ml of a mixture of 4 volumes of *alcohol R* and 6 volumes of *water R*. The crystals, dried *in vacuo*, melt (*2.2.14*) at 118 °C to 121 °C.

TESTS

Carry out the weighings and dissolution rapidly.

Solution S. Dissolve 2.50 g in 10 ml of *alcohol R* and dilute to 25.0 ml with the same solvent.

Appearance of solution. Solution S is clear (*2.2.1*) and colourless (*2.2.2, Method II*).

Acidity or alkalinity. To 10 ml of solution S add 0.1 ml of *phenolphthalein solution R1*. The solution is colourless. Not more than 0.2 ml of *0.1 M sodium hydroxide* is required to change the colour of the indicator.

Specific optical rotation (*2.2.7*): + 40.0 to + 43.0, determined on solution S.

Related substances. Gas chromatography (*2.2.28*).

Test solution. Dissolve 2.50 g of the substance to be examined in *heptane R* and dilute to 25.0 ml with the same solvent.

Reference solution (a). Dilute 1.0 ml of the test solution to 100.0 ml with *heptane R*.

Reference solution (b). Dilute 10.0 ml of reference solution (a) to 20.0 ml with *heptane R*.

Reference solution (c). Dissolve 0.50 g of *borneol R* in *heptane R* and dilute to 25.0 ml with the same solvent. Dilute 5.0 ml of the solution to 50.0 ml with *heptane R*.

Reference solution (d). Dissolve 50 mg of *linalol R* and 50 mg of *bornyl acetate R* in *heptane R* and dilute to 100.0 ml with the same solvent.

Column:
- *size*: l = 30 m, Ø = 0.25 mm,
- *stationary phase*: *macrogol 20 000 R* (0.25 µm).

Carrier gas: *helium for chromatography R*.

Split ratio: 1:70.

Flow rate: 45 cm/s.

Temperature:

	Time (min)	Temperature (°C)
Column	0 - 10	50
	10 - 35	50 → 100
	35 - 45	100 → 200
	45 - 55	200
Injection port		220
Detector		250

Detection: flame ionisation.

Injection: 1 µl.

System suitability: reference solution (d).
- *resolution*: minimum 3.0 between the peaks due to bornyl acetate and to linalol.

Limits:
- *borneol*: not more than the area of the principal peak in the chromatogram obtained with reference solution (c) (2.0 per cent),
- *any other impurity*: not more than half of the area of the principal peak in the chromatogram obtained with reference solution (a) (0.5 per cent),
- *total of other impurities*: not more than 4 times the area of the principal peak in the chromatogram obtained with reference solution (a) (4.0 per cent),
- *disregard limit*: 0.1 times the area of the principal peak in the chromatogram obtained with reference solution (b) (0.05 per cent).

Halogens: maximum 100 ppm.

Dissolve 1.0 g in 10 ml of *2-propanol R* in a distillation flask. Add 1.5 ml of *dilute sodium hydroxide solution R* and 50 mg of *nickel-aluminium alloy R*. Heat on a water-bath until the *2-propanol R* has evaporated. Allow to cool and add 5 ml of *water R*. Mix and filter through a wet filter previously washed with *water R* until free from chlorides. Dilute the filtrate to 10.0 ml with *water R*. To 5.0 ml of the solution, add *nitric acid R* dropwise until the precipitate which forms is redissolved and dilute to 15 ml with *water R*. The solution complies with the limit test for chlorides (*2.4.4*).

Residue on evaporation (*2.8.9*): maximum 0.05 per cent.

Evaporate 2.0 g on a water-bath and dry in an oven at 100-105 °C for 1 h. The residue weighs a maximum of 1 mg.

Water. Dissolve 1 g in 10 ml of *light petroleum R*. The solution is clear (*2.2.1*).

IMPURITIES

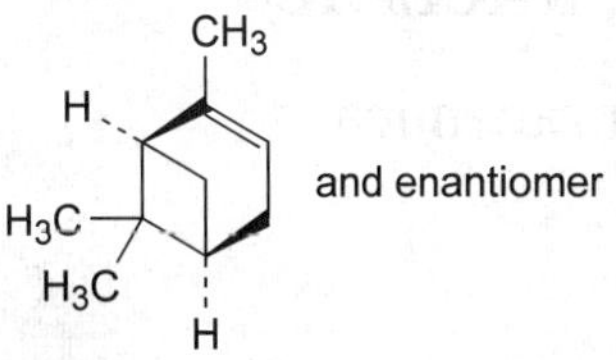

A. 2,6,6-trimethylbicyclo[3.1.1]hept-2-ene (α-pinene),

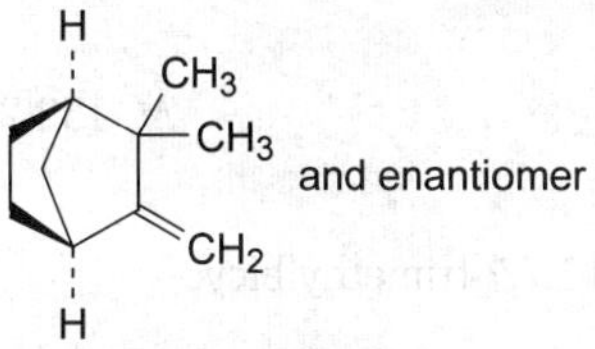

B. 2,2-dimethyl-3-methylenebicyclo[2.2.1]heptane (camphene),

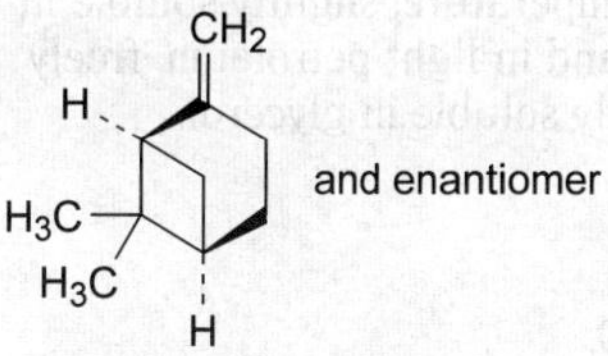

C. 6,6-dimethyl-2-methylenebicyclo[3.1.1]heptane (β-pinene),

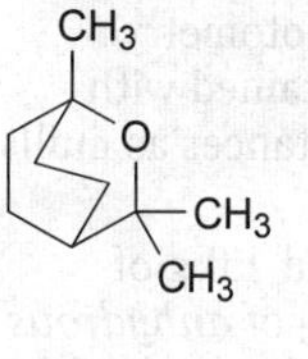

D. 3,3-dimethyl-2-oxabicyclo[2.2.2]octane (cineole),

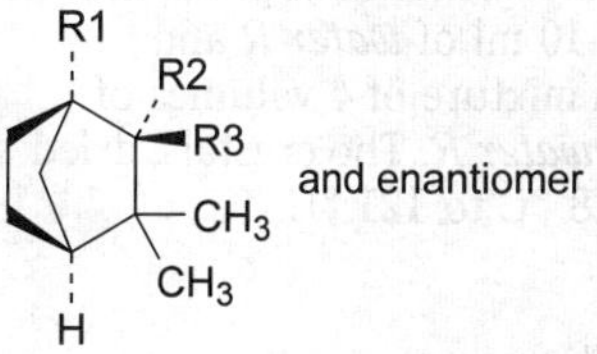

E. R1 = CH_3, R2 + R3 = O: 1,3,3-trimethylbicyclo[2.2.1]heptan-2-one (fenchone),

F. R1 = CH_3, R2 = OH, R3 = H: *exo*-1,3,3-trimethylbicyclo[2.2.1]heptan-2-ol (fenchol),

G. R1 = H, R2 = OH, R3 = CH_3: *exo*-2,3,3-trimethylbicyclo[2.2.1]heptan-2-ol (camphene hydrate),

H. R1 = H, R2 = CH_3, R3 = OH: *endo*-2,3,3-trimethylbicyclo[2.2.1]heptan-2-ol (methylcamphenilol),

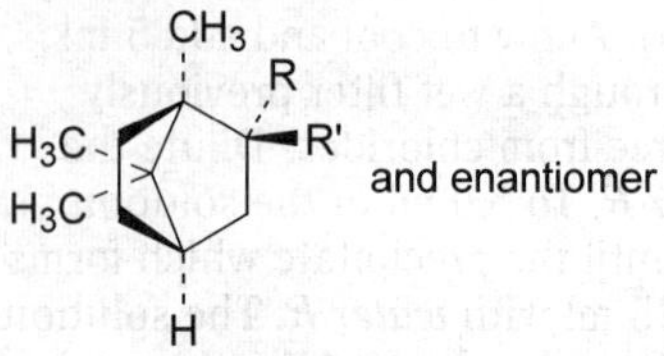

I. R = OH, R′ = H: *exo*-1,7,7-trimethylbicyclo[2.2.1]heptan-2-ol (*exo*-borneol),

J. R = H, R′ = OH: *endo*-1,7,7-trimethylbicyclo[2.2.1]heptan-2-ol (*endo*-borneol).

01/2005:0655

CAMPHOR, RACEMIC

Camphora racemica

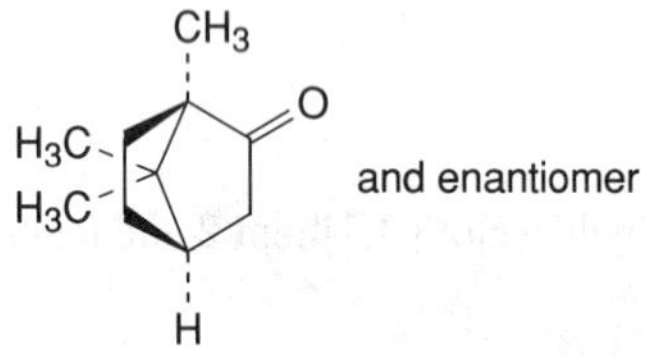

$C_{10}H_{16}O$ M_r 152.2

DEFINITION

Racemic camphor is (1*RS*,4*RS*)-1,7,7-trimethylbicyclo[2.2.1]heptan-2-one.

CHARACTERS

A white, crystalline powder or friable, crystalline masses, highly volatile even at room temperature, slightly soluble in water, very soluble in alcohol and in light petroleum, freely soluble in fatty oils, very slightly soluble in glycerol.

IDENTIFICATION

First identification: A, C.

Second identification: A, B, D.

A. It complies with the test for optical rotation (see Tests).

B. Melting point (*2.2.14*): 172 °C to 180 °C.

C. Examine by infrared absorption spectrophotometry (*2.2.24*), comparing with the spectrum obtained with *racemic camphor CRS*. Examine the substances as mulls in *liquid paraffin R*.

D. Dissolve 1.0 g in 30 ml of *methanol R*. Add 1.0 g of *hydroxylamine hydrochloride R* and 1.0 g of *anhydrous sodium acetate R*. Boil under a reflux condenser for 2 h. Allow to cool and add 100 ml of *water R*. A precipitate is formed. Filter, wash with 10 ml of *water R* and recrystallize from 10 ml of a mixture of 4 volumes of *alcohol R* and 6 volumes of *water R*. The crystals, dried *in vacuo*, melt (*2.2.14*) at 118 °C to 121 °C.

TESTS

Carry out the weighings rapidly.

Solution S. Dissolve 2.50 g in 10 ml of *alcohol R* and dilute to 25.0 ml with the same solvent.

Appearance of solution. Solution S is clear (*2.2.1*) and colourless (*2.2.2, Method II*).

Acidity or alkalinity. Dissolve 1.0 g in 10 ml of *alcohol R* and add 0.1 ml of *phenolphthalein solution R1*. The solution is colourless. Not more than 0.2 ml of *0.1 M sodium hydroxide* is required to change the colour of the indicator.

Optical rotation (*2.2.7*): + 0.15° to − 0.15°, determined on solution S.

Related substances. Examine by gas chromatography (*2.2.28*).

Test solution. Dissolve 50 mg of the substance to be examined in *hexane R* and dilute to 50.0 ml with the same solvent.

Reference solution (a). Dissolve 50 mg of the substance to be examined and 50 mg of *bornyl acetate R* in *hexane R* and dilute to 50.0 ml with the same solvent.

Reference solution (b). Dilute 1.0 ml of the test solution to 200.0 ml with *hexane R*.

The chromatographic procedure may be carried out using:

– a column 2 m long and 2 mm in internal diameter packed with *diatomaceous earth for gas chromatography R* impregnated with 10 per cent *m/m* of *macrogol 20 000 R*,

– *nitrogen for chromatography R* as the carrier gas at a flow rate of 30 ml/min,

– a flame-ionisation detector,

maintaining the temperature of the column at 130 °C and that of the injection port and the detector at 200 °C.

Inject 1 µl of each solution and adjust the sensitivity of the system so that the height of the principal peak in the chromatogram obtained with the test solution is about 80 per cent of the full scale of the recorder. Record the chromatograms for three times the retention time of camphor.

The test is not valid unless in the chromatogram obtained with reference solution (a), the resolution between the peaks corresponding to camphor and bornyl acetate is not less than 1.5; in the chromatogram obtained with reference solution (b), the principal peak has a signal-to-noise ratio of at least 5. In the chromatogram obtained with the test solution: the sum of the areas of the peaks, apart from the principal peak, is not greater than 4 per cent of the area of the principal peak; none of the peaks, apart from the principal peak, has an area greater than 2 per cent of the area of the principal peak. Disregard any peak with an area less than that of the peak in the chromatogram obtained with reference solution (b).

Halogens. Dissolve 1.0 g in 10 ml of *2-propanol R* in a distillation flask. Add 1.5 ml of *dilute sodium hydroxide solution R* and 50 mg of *nickel-aluminium alloy R*. Heat on a water-bath until the *2-propanol R* has evaporated. Allow to cool and add 5 ml of *water R*. Mix and filter through a wet filter previously washed with *water R* until free from chlorides. Dilute the filtrate to 10.0 ml with *water R*. To 5.0 ml of the solution, add *nitric acid R* dropwise until the precipitate which forms is redissolved and dilute to 15 ml with *water R*. The solution complies with the limit test for chlorides (*2.4.4*) (100 ppm).

Water. Dissolve 1 g in 10 ml of *light petroleum R*. The solution is clear (*2.2.1*).

Residue on evaporation. Evaporate 2.0 g on a water-bath and dry at 100 °C to 105 °C for 1 h. The residue weighs not more than 1 mg (0.05 per cent).

01/2005:1401

CAPRYLIC ACID

Acidum caprylicum

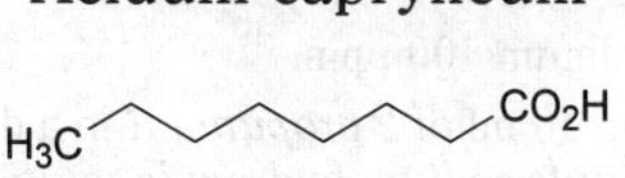

$C_8H_{16}O_2$ M_r 144.2

DEFINITION

Caprylic acid contains not less than 99.0 per cent and not more than the equivalent of 100.5 per cent of octanoic acid, calculated with reference to the anhydrous substance.

CHARACTERS

A clear, colourless or slightly yellowish, oily liquid, very slightly soluble in water, very soluble in acetone and in alcohol. It dissolves in dilute solutions of alkali hydroxides.

IDENTIFICATION

A. It complies with the test for relative density (see Tests).

B. Examine the chromatograms obtained in the test for related substances. The retention time and size of the principal peak in the chromatogram obtained with the test solution are approximately the same as those of the principal peak in the chromatogram obtained with reference solution (a).

TESTS

Appearance. The substance to be examined is clear (*2.2.1*) and not more intensely coloured than reference solution Y_5 (*2.2.2, Method II*).

Relative density (*2.2.5*): 0.909 to 0.912.

Related substances. Examine by gas chromatography (*2.2.28*).

Test solution. Dissolve 0.10 g of the substance to be examined in *ethyl acetate R* and dilute to 10.0 ml with the same solvent.

Reference solution (a). Dissolve 0.10 g of *caprylic acid CRS* in *ethyl acetate R* and dilute to 10.0 ml with the same solvent.

Reference solution (b). Dilute 1.0 ml of the test solution to 100.0 ml with *ethyl acetate R*. Dilute 5.0 ml of the solution to 50.0 ml with *ethyl acetate R*.

The chromatographic procedure may be carried out using:

- a fused-silica column 30 m long and 0.25 mm in internal diameter coated with *macrogol 20 000 2-nitroterephthalate R* (film thickness 0.25 µm),
- *helium for chromatography R* as the carrier gas at a flow rate of 1.5 ml/min,
- a flame-ionisation detector,
- a split ratio of 1:100,

with the following temperature programme:

	Time (min)	Temperature (°C)	Rate (°C/min)	Comment
Column	0 - 1	100	–	isothermal
	1 - 25	100 → 220	5	linear gradient
	25 - 35	220		isothermal
Injection port		250		
Detector		250		

Inject 1 µl of reference solution (b). The test is not valid unless in the chromatogram obtained the principal peak has a signal-to-noise ratio of at least 5.

Inject 1 µl of the test solution and 1 µl of reference solution (a). Calculate the percentage content of related substances from the areas of the peaks in the chromatogram obtained with the test solution by the normalisation procedure, disregarding any peaks with an area less than 0.5 times the area of the peak in the chromatogram obtained with reference solution (b). The content of any related substance is not greater than 0.3 per cent and the sum of the contents is not greater than 0.5 per cent.

Heavy metals (*2.4.8*). Dissolve 2.0 g in *alcohol R* and dilute to 20 ml with the same solvent. 12 ml of the solution complies with limit test B for heavy metals (10 ppm). Prepare the standard using 1 ml of *lead standard solution (10 ppm Pb) R* and 9 ml of *alcohol R*.

Water (*2.5.12*). Not more than 0.7 per cent, determined on 1.000 g by the semi-micro determination of water.

Sulphated ash (*2.4.14*). Not more than 0.1 per cent, determined on 1.0 g.

ASSAY

Dissolve 0.125 g in 25 ml of *alcohol R*. Titrate with *0.1 M sodium hydroxide*, determining the end-point potentiometrically (*2.2.20*).

1 ml of *0.1 M sodium hydroxide* is equivalent to 14.42 mg of $C_8H_{16}O_2$.

IMPURITIES

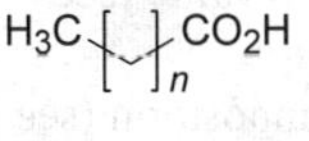

A. $n = 4$: hexanoic acid,

B. $n = 5$: heptanoic acid,

C. $n = 7$: nonanoic acid,

D. $n = 8$: decanoic acid,

E. valproic acid,

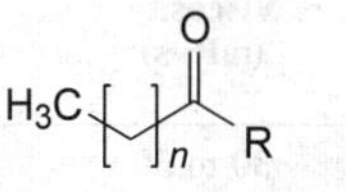

F. $R = OCH_3$, $n = 6$: methyl octanoate,

G. $R = OC_2H_5$, $n = 6$: ethyl octanoate,

H. $R = OCH_3$, $n = 8$: methyl decanoate,

I. $R = CH_3$, $n = 8$: undecan-2-one,

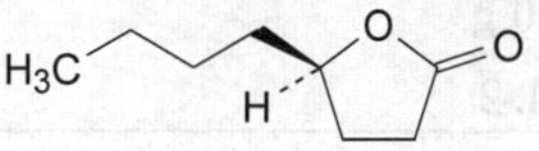

and enantiomer

J. 5-butyltetrahydrofuran-2-one (γ-hydroxyoctanoic acid lactone).

01/2005:1184

CAPRYLOCAPROYL MACROGOLGLYCERIDES

Macrogolglyceridorum caprylocaprates

DEFINITION

Caprylocaproyl macrogolglycerides are mixtures of monoesters, diesters and triesters of glycerol and monoesters and diesters of macrogols with a mean relative molecular mass between 200 and 400. They are obtained by partial alcoholysis of medium-chain triglycerides using macrogol or by esterification of glycerol and macrogol with caprylic acid and capric acid or a mixture of glycerol esters and condensates of ethylene oxide with caprylic acid (octanoic acid) and capric acid (decanoic acid). They may contain free macrogols.

CHARACTERS

Pale-yellow oily liquids, dispersible in hot water, freely soluble in methylene chloride.

The relative density at 20 °C is about 1.0, the refractive index at 20 °C is about 1.4.

IDENTIFICATION

A. Examine by thin-layer chromatography (*2.2.27*), using a suitable silica gel as the coating substance.

Test solution. Dissolve 1.0 g of the substance to be examined in *methylene chloride R* and dilute to 20 ml with the same solvent.

Apply to the plate 50 µl of the test solution. Develop over a path of 15 cm using a mixture of 30 volumes of *hexane R* and 70 volumes of *ether R*. Allow the plate to dry in air. Spray with a 0.1 g/l solution of *rhodamine B R* in *alcohol R* and examine in ultraviolet light at 365 nm. The chromatogram shows a spot corresponding to triglycerides with an R_f value of about 0.9 (R_{st} 1) and spots corresponding to 1,3-diglycerides (R_{st} 0.7), to 1,2-diglycerides (R_{st} 0.6), to monoglycerides (R_{st} 0.1) and to esters of macrogol (R_{st} 0).

B. They comply with the test for hydroxyl value (see Tests).

C. They comply with the test for saponification value (see Tests).

D. They comply with the test for fatty acid composition (see Tests).

TESTS

Viscosity (*2.2.9*). The ranges are presented in Table 1184.-1, determined at 20 ± 0.5 °C.

Table 1184.-1

Ethylene oxide units per molecule (nominal value)	Type of macrogol	Viscosity (mPa·s)
4	200	30 to 50
6	300	60 to 80
8	400	80 to 110

Acid value (*2.5.1*). Not more than 2.0, determined on 2.0 g.

Hydroxyl value (*2.5.3, Method A*). The ranges are presented in Table 1184.-2, determined on 1.0 g.

Table 1184.-2

Ethylene oxide units per molecule (nominal value)	Type of macrogol	Hydroxyl value
4	200	80 to 120
6	300	140 to 180
8	400	170 to 205

Peroxide value (*2.5.5*). Not more than 6.0, determined on 2.0 g.

Saponification value (*2.5.6*). The ranges are presented in Table 1184.-3, determined on 2.0 g.

Table 1184.-3

Ethylene oxide units per molecule (nominal value)	Type of macrogol	Saponification value
4	200	265 to 285
6	300	170 to 190
8	400	85 to 105

Alkaline impurities. Introduce into a test-tube 5.0 g and carefully add a mixture, neutralised if necessary with *0.01 M hydrochloric acid* or with *0.01 M sodium hydroxide*, of 0.05 ml of a 0.4 g/l solution of *bromophenol blue R* in *alcohol R*, 0.3 ml of *water R* and 10 ml of *alcohol R*. Shake and allow to stand. Not more than 1.0 ml of *0.01 M hydrochloric acid* is required to change the colour of the upper layer to yellow.

Free glycerol. Not more than 5.0 per cent. Dissolve 1.20 g in 25.0 ml of *methylene chloride R*. Heat if necessary. After cooling, add 100 ml of *water R*. Shake and add 25.0 ml of a 6 g/l solution of *periodic acid R*. Shake and allow to stand for 30 min. Add 40 ml of a 75 g/l solution of *potassium iodide R*. Allow to stand for 1 min. Add 1 ml of *starch solution R*. Titrate the iodine with *0.1 M sodium thiosulphate*. Carry out a blank titration.

1 ml of *0.1 M sodium thiosulphate* is equivalent to 2.3 mg of glycerol.

Fatty acid composition (*2.4.22, Method A*). The fatty acid fraction has the following composition:

- *caproic acid*: not more than 2.0 per cent,
- *caprylic acid*: 50.0 per cent to 80.0 per cent,
- *capric acid*: 20.0 per cent to 50.0 per cent,
- *lauric acid*: not more than 3.0 per cent,
- *myristic acid*: not more than 1.0 per cent.

Ethylene oxide and dioxan (*2.4.25*). Not more than 1 ppm of ethylene oxide and not more than 10 ppm of dioxan.

Heavy metals (*2.4.8*). 2.0 g complies with limit test C for heavy metals (10 ppm). Prepare the standard using 2 ml of *lead standard solution (10 ppm Pb) R*.

Water (*2.5.12*). Not more than 1.0 per cent, determined on 1.0 g by the semi-micro determination of water. Use a mixture of 30 volumes of *anhydrous methanol R* and 70 volumes of *methylene chloride R* as solvent.

Total ash (*2.4.16*). Not more than 0.1 per cent, determined on 1.0 g.

LABELLING

The label states the type of macrogol used (mean relative molecular mass) or the number of ethylene oxide units per molecule (nominal value).

01/2005:1859

CAPSICUM

Capsici fructus

DEFINITION

Dried ripe fruits of *Capsicum annuum* L. var. *minimum* (Miller) Heiser and small-fruited varieties of *Capsicum frutescens* L.

Content: minimum 0.4 per cent of total capsaicinoids expressed as capsaicin ($C_{18}H_{27}NO_3$; M_r 305.4) (dried drug).

CHARACTERS

Extremely pungent taste.

Macroscopic and microscopic characters described under identification tests A and B.

IDENTIFICATION

A. The fruit is yellowish-orange to reddish-brown, oblong conical with an obtuse apex, about 1 cm to 3 cm long and up to 1 cm in diameter at the widest part, occasionally attached to a 5-toothed inferior calyx and a straight pedicel. Pericarp somewhat shrivelled, glabrous, enclosing about 10 to 20 flat, reniform seeds 3 mm to 4 mm long, either loose or attached to a reddish dissepiment.

B. Reduce to a powder (355). The powder is orange. Examine under a microscope using *chloral hydrate solution R*. The powder shows the following diagnostic characters: fragments of the pericarp having an outer epicarp with cells often arranged in rows of 5 to

7, cuticle uniformly striated; parenchymatous cells frequently containing droplets of red oil, occasionally containing microsphenoidal crystals of calcium oxalate; endocarp with characteristic island groups of sclerenchymatous cells, the groups being separated by thin-walled parenchymatous cells. Fragments of the seeds having an episperm composed of large, greenish-yellow, sinuous-walled sclereids with thin outer walls and strongly and unevenly thickened radial and inner walls which are conspicuously pitted; endosperm parenchymatous cells with drops of fixed oil and aleurone grains 3 µm to 6 µm in diameter. Occasional fragments from the calyx having an outer epidermis with anisocytic stomata (*2.8.3*), inner epidermis with many trichomes but no stomata; trichomes glandular, with uniseriate stalks and multicellular heads; mesophyll with many idioblasts containing microsphenoidal crystals of calcium oxalate.

C. Thin-layer chromatography (*2.2.27*).

Test solution. To 0.50 g of the powdered drug (500) add 5.0 ml of *ether R*, shake for 5 min and filter.

Reference solution. Dissolve 2 mg of *capsaicin R* and 2 mg of *dihydrocapsaicin R* in 5.0 ml of *ether R*.

Plate: *TLC octadecylsilyl silica gel plate R.*

Mobile phase: *water R, methanol R (20:80 V/V).*

Application: 20 µl, as bands.

Development: over a path of 12 cm.

Drying: in air.

Detection: spray with a 5 g/l solution of *dichloroquinonechlorimide R* in *methanol R*. Expose the plate to ammonia vapour until blue zones appear. Examine in daylight.

Results: see below the sequence of the zones present in the chromatograms obtained with the reference solution and the test solution. Furthermore, other zones may be present in the chromatogram obtained with the test solution.

Top of the plate	
———	———
Capsaicin: a blue zone	A blue zone (capsaicin)
Dihydrocapsaicin: a blue zone	A blue zone (dihydrocapsaicin)
Reference solution	**Test solution**

TESTS

Nonivamide. Liquid chromatography (*2.2.29*).

Test solution. To 2.5 g of the powdered drug (500) add 100 ml of *methanol R*. Allow to macerate for 30 min. Place in an ultrasonic bath for 15 min. Filter into a 100 ml volumetric flask, rinse the flask and filter with *methanol R*. Dilute to 100.0 ml with *methanol R*.

Reference solution. Dissolve 20.0 mg of *capsaicin R* and 4.0 mg of *nonivamide R* in 100.0 ml of *methanol R*.

Column:
- *size*: l = 0.25 m, Ø = 4.6 mm,
- *stationary phase*: *phenylsilyl silica gel for chromatography R* (5 µm),
- *temperature*: 30 °C.

Mobile phase: mixture of 40 volumes of *acetonitrile R* and 60 volumes of a 1 g/l solution of *phosphoric acid R*.

Flow rate: 1.0 ml/min.

Detection: spectrophotometer at 225 nm.

Injection: 10 µl.

Elution order: elution order similar to that obtained in Figure 1859.-1.

System suitability: reference solution:
- *resolution*: minimum 3.0 between the peaks due to capsaicin and nonivamide.

Limit: calculate the percentage content of nonivamide from the expression:

$$\frac{F_1 \times m_2 \times p_1}{F_2 \times m_1}$$

F_1 = area of the peak corresponding to nonivamide in the chromatogram obtained with the test solution,

F_2 = area of the peak corresponding to nonivamide in the chromatogram obtained with the reference solution,

m_1 = mass of the drug to be examined in grams,

m_2 = mass of nonivamide used to prepare the reference solution in grams,

p_1 = percentage content of nonivamide in the reagent.

- *nonivamide*: maximum 5.0 per cent of the total capsaicinoid content.

Foreign matter (*2.8.2*): maximum 2 per cent *m/m*. Fruits of *C. annuum* L. var. *longum* (Sendtn.) are absent.

Loss on drying (*2.2.32*): maximum 11.0 per cent, determined on 1.000 g of the powdered drug (500) by drying in an oven at 100-105 °C for 2 h.

Total ash (*2.4.16*): maximum 10.0 per cent.

ASSAY

Liquid chromatography (*2.2.29*) as described in the test for nonivamide.

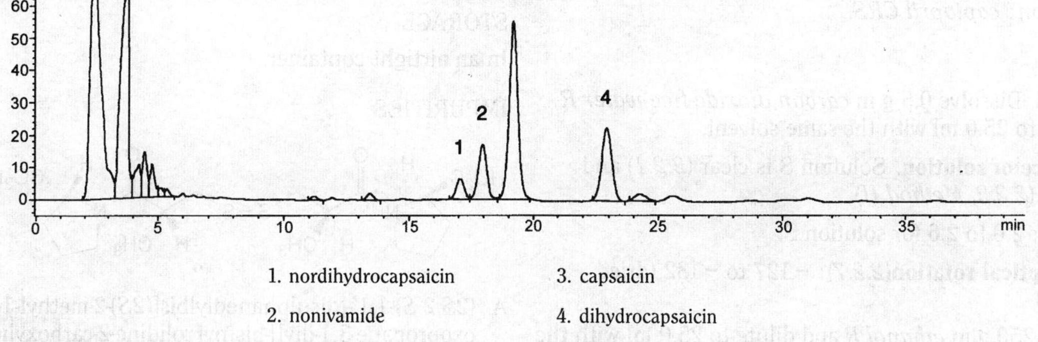

1. nordihydrocapsaicin
2. nonivamide
3. capsaicin
4. dihydrocapsaicin

Figure 1859.-1. – *Chromatogram for the test for nonivamide and the assay of capsicum*

Calculate the percentage content of capsaicinoids from the expression:

$$\frac{(F_3 + F_5 + F_6) \times m_4 \times p_2}{F_4 \times m_3}$$

F_3 = area of the peak corresponding to capsaicin in the chromatogram obtained with the test solution,

F_4 = area of the peak corresponding to capsaicin in the chromatogram obtained with the reference solution,

F_5 = area of the peak corresponding to dihydrocapsaicin in the chromatogram obtained with the test solution,

F_6 = area of the peak corresponding to nordihydrocapsaicin in the chromatogram obtained with the test solution,

m_3 = mass of the drug to be examined in grams,

m_4 = mass of capsaicin used to prepare the reference solution in grams,

p_2 = percentage content of capsaicin in the reagent.

01/2005:1079

CAPTOPRIL

Captoprilum

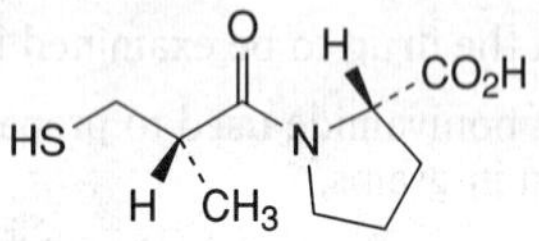

$C_9H_{15}NO_3S$ M_r 217.3

DEFINITION

(2*S*)-1-[(2*S*)-2-Methyl-3-sulphanylpropanoyl]pyrrolidine-2-carboxylic acid.

Content: 98.0 per cent to 101.5 per cent (dried substance).

CHARACTERS

Appearance: white or almost white crystalline powder.

Solubility: freely soluble in water, in methylene chloride and in methanol. It dissolves in dilute solutions of alkali hydroxides.

IDENTIFICATION

Infrared absorption spectrophotometry (*2.2.24*).

Comparison: *captopril CRS.*

TESTS

Solution S. Dissolve 0.5 g in *carbon dioxide-free water R* and dilute to 25.0 ml with the same solvent.

Appearance of solution. Solution S is clear (*2.2.1*) and colourless (*2.2.2, Method II*).

pH (*2.2.3*): 2.0 to 2.6 for solution S.

Specific optical rotation(*2.2.7*): − 127 to − 132 (dried substance).

Dissolve 0.250 g in *ethanol R* and dilute to 25.0 ml with the same solvent.

Related substances. Liquid chromatography (*2.2.29*).

Test solution. Dissolve 50 mg of the substance to be examined in the mobile phase and dilute to 100.0 ml with the mobile phase.

Reference solution (a). Dilute 2.0 ml of the test solution to 100.0 ml with the mobile phase.

Reference solution (b). Dissolve 10 mg of the substance to be examined in the mobile phase, add 1 ml of *0.05 M iodine* and dilute to 100.0 ml with the mobile phase. Dilute 10.0 ml of the solution to 100.0 ml with the mobile phase.

Column:

- *size*: l = 0.125 m, Ø = 4 mm,
- *stationary phase*: *octylsilyl silica gel for chromatography R* (5 μm).

Mobile phase: *phosphoric acid R, methanol R, water R* (0.05:50:50 *V/V/V*).

Flow rate: 1 ml/min.

Detection: spectrophotometer at 220 nm.

Injection: 20 μl.

Run time: 3 times the retention time of captopril.

System suitability: reference solution (b):

- the chromatogram shows 3 peaks,
- *resolution*: minimum of 2.0 between the last 2 eluting principal peaks,

Limits:

- *any impurity*: not more than half the area of the principal peak in the chromatogram obtained with reference solution (a) (1.0 per cent),
- *total*: not more than the area of the principal peak in the chromatogram obtained with reference solution (a) (2.0 per cent),
- *disregard limit*: 0.1 times the area of the principal peak in the chromatogram obtained with reference solution (a) (0.2 per cent). Disregard any peak with a retention time less than 1.4 min.

Heavy metals (*2.4.8*): maximum 20 ppm.

1.0 g complies with limit test C. Prepare the standard using 2 ml of *lead standard solution (10 ppm Pb) R.*

Loss on drying (*2.2.32*): maximum 1.0 per cent, determined on 1.000 g by drying under high vacuum at 60 °C for 3 h.

Sulphated ash (*2.4.14*): maximum 0.2 per cent, determined on 1.0 g.

ASSAY

Dissolve 0.150 g in 30 ml of *water R*. Titrate with *0.05 M iodine,* determining the end-point potentiometrically (*2.2.20*). Use a combined platinum electrode.

1 ml of *0.05 M iodine* is equivalent to 21.73 mg of $C_9H_{15}NO_3S$.

STORAGE

In an airtight container.

IMPURITIES

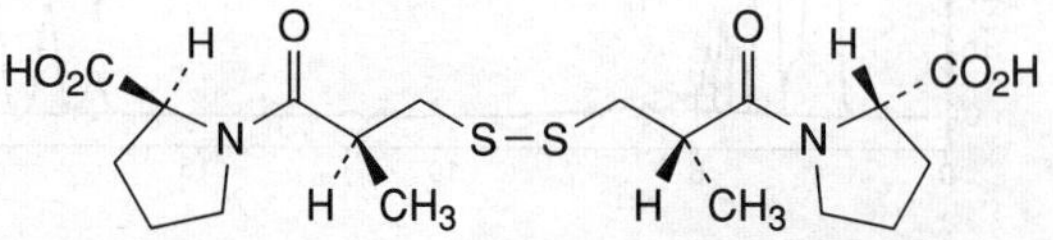

A. (2*S*,2′*S*)-1,1′-[disulphanediylbis[(2*S*)-2-methyl-1-oxopropane-3,1-diyl]]-bis[pyrrolidine-2-carboxylic] acid (captopril-disulphide).

01/2005:1080

CARAWAY FRUIT

Carvi fructus

DEFINITION

Caraway fruit consists of the whole, dry mericarp of *Carum carvi* L. It contains not less than 30 ml/kg of essential oil, calculated with reference to the anhydrous drug.

CHARACTERS

Caraway fruit has an odour reminiscent of carvone.

It has the macroscopic and microscopic characters described under identification tests A and B.

IDENTIFICATION

A. The fruit is a cremocarp of almost cylindrical shape. It is generally 3 mm to 6.5 mm long and 1 mm to 1.5 mm wide. The mericarps, usually free, are greyish-brown to brown, glabrous, mostly sickle-shaped, with both ends sharply terminated. Each bears five prominent narrow ridges. When cut transversely the profile shows an almost regular pentagon and four vittae on the dorsal surface and two on the commissural surface may be seen with a lens.

B. Reduce to a powder (355). The powder is yellowish-brown. Examine under a microscope using *chloral hydrate solution R*. The powder shows the following diagnostic characters: fragments of the secretory cells composed of yellowish-brown to brown, thin-walled, polygonal secretory cells, frequently associated with a layer of thin-walled transversely elongated cells, 8-12 µm wide; fragments of the epicarp with thick-walled cells and occasional anomocytic stomata (*2.8.3*); numerous endosperm fragments containing aleurone grains, droplets of fatty oil and microcrystals of calcium oxalate in rosette formation; spiral vessels accompanied by sclerenchymatous fibres; rarely some fibre bundles from the carpophore; groups of rectangular to sub-rectangular sclereids from the mesocarp with moderately thickened and pitted walls may be present.

C. Examine by thin-layer chromatography (*2.2.27*) using a suitable silica gel as the coating substance.

Test solution. Shake 0.5 g of the powdered drug (710) with 5.0 ml of *ethyl acetate R* for 2 min to 3 min. Filter over 2 g of *anhydrous sodium sulphate R*. Use the filtrate as the test solution.

Reference solution. Dissolve 2 µl of *carvone R* and 5 µl of *olive oil R* in 1.0 ml of *ethyl acetate R*.

Apply to the plate as bands 20 µl of the test solution and 10 µl of the reference solution. Develop over a path of 10 cm using a mixture of 5 volumes of *ethyl acetate R* and 95 volumes of *toluene R*. Allow the plate to dry in air and examine in ultraviolet light at 254 nm. The chromatograms of the test solution and of the reference solution show a quenching zone (carvone) in the central part against a light background. Spray with *anisaldehyde solution R* and heat under observation at 100 °C to 105 °C for 2 to 4 min. Examine in daylight. The zones corresponding to carvone appear strong orange-brown. The chromatogram obtained with the test solution shows above the zone corresponding to carvone a violet zone corresponding to triglycerides similar in position and colour to the zone in the chromatogram obtained with the reference solution (triglycerides of olive oil). The chromatogram obtained with the test solution shows close to the solvent front a weak violet zone corresponding to terpene hydrocarbons and in the lower part some weak, mostly violet-greyish and brownish zones.

TESTS

Foreign matter (*2.8.2*). It complies with the test for foreign matter.

Water (*2.2.13*). Not more than 100 ml/kg, determined on 10.0 g of powdered drug by distillation.

Total ash (*2.4.16*). Not more than 7.0 per cent.

ASSAY

Carry out the determination of essential oils in vegetable drugs (*2.8.12*). Use a 500 ml round-bottomed flask, 200 ml of *water R* as the distillation liquid and 0.50 ml of *xylene R* in the graduated tube. Reduce the drug to a powder (710) and immediately use 10.0 g for the determination. Distil at a rate of 2-3 ml/min for 90 min.

STORAGE

Store protected from light.

01/2005:1971

CARBACHOL

Carbacholum

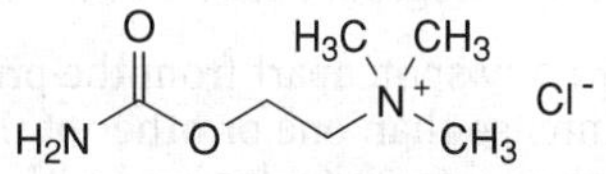

$C_6H_{15}ClN_2O_2$ M_r 182.7

DEFINITION

2-(Carbamoyloxy)-*N,N,N*-trimethylethanaminium chloride.

Content: 99.0 per cent to 101.5 per cent (dried substance).

CHARACTERS

Appearance: white, crystalline, hygroscopic powder.

Solubility: very soluble in water, sparingly soluble in alcohol, practically insoluble in acetone.

IDENTIFICATION

First identification: A, C.

Second identification: B, C.

A. Infrared absorption spectrophotometry (*2.2.24*).

Comparison: *carbachol CRS*.

B. Examine the chromatograms obtained in the test for related substances.

Results: the principal spot in the chromatogram obtained with test solution (b) is similar in position, colour and size to the principal spot in the chromatogram obtained with reference solution (a).

C. 0.5 ml of solution S (see Tests) gives reaction (a) of chlorides (*2.3.1*).

TESTS

Solution S. Dissolve 2.5 g in *carbon dioxide-free water R* and dilute to 25 ml with the same solvent.

Appearance of solution. Solution S is clear (*2.2.1*) and colourless (*2.2.2, Method II*).

Acidity or alkalinity. To 2.0 ml of solution S, add 0.05 ml of *methyl red mixed solution R*. Not more than 0.2 ml of *0.01 M hydrochloric acid* or *0.01 M sodium hydroxide* is required to change the colour of the indicator.

Related substances. Thin-layer chromatography (*2.2.27*).

Prepare the solutions immediately before use.

Test solution (a). Dissolve 0.20 g of the substance to be examined in *methanol R* and dilute to 5.0 ml with the same solvent.

Test solution (b). Dilute 2.0 ml of test solution (a) to 20.0 ml with *methanol R*.

Reference solution (a). Dissolve 20 mg of *carbachol CRS* in *methanol R* and dilute to 5.0 ml with the same solvent.

Reference solution (b). Dissolve 8 mg of *choline chloride R* and 8 mg of *acetylcholine chloride CRS* in *methanol R* and dilute to 10.0 ml with the same solvent. Dilute 5.0 ml to 10.0 ml with *methanol R*.

Plate: *cellulose for chromatography R* as the coating substance.

Mobile phase: *water R, methanol R* (10:90 *V/V*).

Application: 10 µl.

Development: over 2/3 of the plate.

Detection: spray with *potassium iodobismuthate solution R3.*

System suitability: the chromatogram obtained with reference solution (b) shows 2 clearly separated spots.

Limits: in the chromatogram obtained with test solution (a):

– *any impurity*: any spot, apart from the principal spot, is not more intense than one or other of the 2 principal spots in the chromatogram obtained with reference solution (b) (1 per cent). Compare the spots with the spot of the most appropriate colour in the chromatogram obtained with reference solution (b).

Heavy metals (*2.4.8*): maximum 20 ppm.

12 ml of solution S complies with limit test A. Prepare the standard using *lead standard solution (2 ppm Pb) R*.

Loss on drying (*2.2.32*): maximum 1.0 per cent, determined on 1.000 g by drying in an oven at 100-105 °C for 2 h.

Sulphated ash (*2.4.14*): maximum 0.1 per cent, determined on 1.0 g of the residue obtained in the test for loss on drying.

ASSAY

Dissolve 0.150 g in a mixture of 10 ml of *anhydrous acetic acid R* and 40 ml of *acetic anhydride R*. Titrate with *0.1 M perchloric acid*. Determine the end-point potentiometrically (*2.2.20*).

1 ml of *0.1 M perchloric acid* is equivalent to 18.27 mg of $C_6H_{15}ClN_2O_2$.

STORAGE

In an airtight container, protected from light.

IMPURITIES

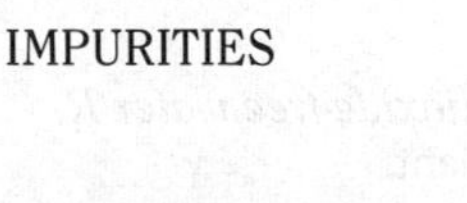

A. 2-hydroxy-*N,N,N*-trimethylethanaminium chloride (choline chloride).

01/2005:0543

CARBAMAZEPINE

Carbamazepinum

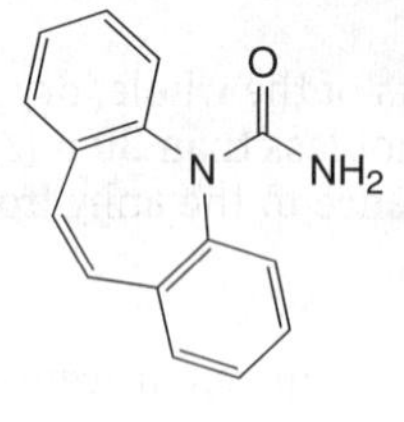

$C_{15}H_{12}N_2O$ M_r 236.3

DEFINITION

5*H*-dibenzo[*b,f*]azepine-5-carboxamide.

Content: 98.0 per cent to 102.0 per cent (dried substance).

CHARACTERS

Appearance: white or almost white crystalline powder.

Solubility: very slightly soluble in water, freely soluble in methylene chloride, sparingly soluble in acetone and in alcohol.

It shows polymorphism; the acceptable crystalline form corresponds to *carbamazepine CRS*.

IDENTIFICATION

A. Melting point (*2.2.14*): 189 °C to 193 °C.

B. Infrared absorption spectrophotometry (*2.2.24*).

Comparison: *carbamazepine CRS*.

Preparation: examine the substances as discs without prior treatment.

TESTS

Acidity or alkalinity. To 1.0 g add 20 ml of *carbon dioxide-free water R*, shake for 15 min and filter. To 10 ml of the filtrate add 0.05 ml of *phenolphthalein solution R1* and 0.5 ml of *0.01 M sodium hydroxide*; the solution is red. Add 1.0 ml of *0.01 M hydrochloric acid*; the solution is colourless. Add 0.15 ml of *methyl red solution R*; the solution is red.

Related substances. Liquid chromatography (*2.2.29*).

Test solution (a). Dissolve 0.150 g of the substance to be examined in *methanol R2* and dilute to 50.0 ml with the same solvent. Sonicate. Dilute 10.0 ml of this solution to 20.0 ml with *water R*.

Test solution (b). Dilute 10.0 ml of test solution (a) to 50.0 ml with a mixture of equal volumes of *methanol R2* and *water R*.

Reference solution (a). Dissolve 7.5 mg of *carbamazepine CRS*, 7.5 mg of *carbamazepine impurity A CRS* and 7.5 mg of *iminodibenzyl R* (impurity E) in *methanol R2* and dilute to 100.0 ml with the same solvent. Dilute 1.0 ml of this solution to 50.0 ml with a mixture of equal volumes of *methanol R2* and *water R*.

Reference solution (b). Dissolve 0.150 g of *carbamazepine CRS* in *methanol R2* and dilute to 50.0 ml with the same solvent. Dilute 5.0 ml of this solution to 50.0 ml with a mixture of equal volumes of *methanol R2* and *water R*.

Column:

– *size*: *l* = 0.25 m, Ø = 4.6 mm,

– *stationary phase*: *nitrile silica gel for chromatography R1* (10 µm).

Mobile phase: *tetrahydrofuran R, methanol R2, water R* (3:12:85 *V/V/V*). To 1000 ml of this solution add 0.2 ml of *anhydrous formic acid R* and 0.5 ml of *triethylamine R.*

Flow rate: 2.0 ml/min.

Detection: a spectrophotometer at 230 nm.

Injection: 20 µl; inject test solution (a) and reference solution (a).

Run time: 6 times the retention time of carbamazepine which is about 10 min.

Relative retention with reference to carbamazepine: impurity B = about 0.7; impurity A = about 0.9; impurity C = about 1.6; impurity D = about 3.5; impurity E = about 5.1.

System suitability:

– *resolution*: minimum of 1.7 between the peaks due to carbamazepine and impurity A in the chromatogram obtained with reference solution (a).

Limits:

– *impurity A*: not more than the area of the corresponding peak in the chromatogram obtained with reference solution (a) (0.1 per cent),

– *impurity E*: not more than the area of the corresponding peak in the chromatogram obtained with reference solution (a) (0.1 per cent),

– *any other impurity*: not more than the area of the peak due to carbamazepine in the chromatogram obtained with reference solution (a) (0.1 per cent),

– *total*: not more than 5 times the area of the peak due to carbamazepine in the chromatogram obtained with reference solution (a) (0.5 per cent),

– *disregard limit*: 0.5 times the area of the peak due to carbamazepine in the chromatogram obtained with reference solution (a) (0.05 per cent).

Chlorides (*2.4.4*): maximum 140 ppm.

Suspend 0.715 g in 20 ml of *water R* and boil for 10 min. Cool and dilute to 20 ml with *water R*. Filter through a membrane filter (nominal pore size: 0.8 µm). Dilute 10 ml of the filtrate to 15 ml with *water R*. This solution complies with the limit test for chlorides.

Heavy metals (*2.4.8*): maximum 20 ppm.

1.0 g complies with limit test C. Prepare the standard using 2 ml of *lead standard solution (10 ppm Pb) R*.

Loss on drying (*2.2.32*): maximum 0.5 per cent, determined on 1.000 g by drying in an oven at 100-105 °C for 2h.

Sulphated ash (*2.4.14*): maximum 0.1 per cent, determined on 1.0 g.

ASSAY

Liquid chromatography (*2.2.29*) as described in the test for related substances.

Injection: test solution (b) and reference solution (b).

System suitability:

– *repeatability*: reference solution (b).

Calculate the percentage content *m/m* of dried substance.

STORAGE

In an airtight container.

IMPURITIES

Specified impurities: A, B, C, D, E.

Other detectable impurities: F

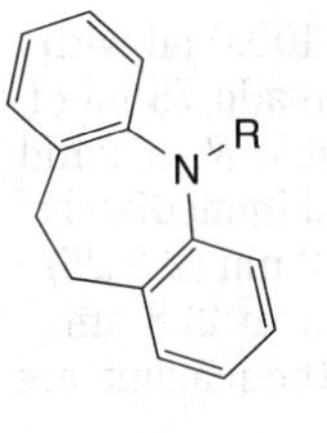

A. R = $CO\text{-}NH_2$: 10,11-dihydro-5*H*-dibenzo[*b,f*]azepine-5-carboxamide (10,11-dihydrocarbamazepine),

E. R = H: 10,11-dihydro-5*H*-dibenzo[*b,f*]azepine (iminodibenzyl),

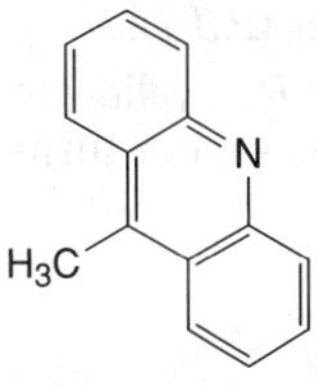

B. 9-methylacridine,

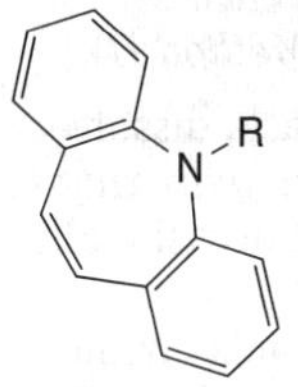

C. R = CO-NH-CO-NH_2: (5*H*-dibenzo[*b,f*]azepin-5-ylcarbonyl)urea (*N*-carbamoylcarbamazepine),

D. R = H: 5*H*-dibenzo[*b,f*]azepine (iminostilbene),

F. R = CO-Cl: 5*H*-dibenzo[*b,f*]azepine-5-carbonyl chloride (5-chlorocarbonyliminostilbene).

01/2005:1185

CARBASALATE CALCIUM

Carbasalatum calcicum

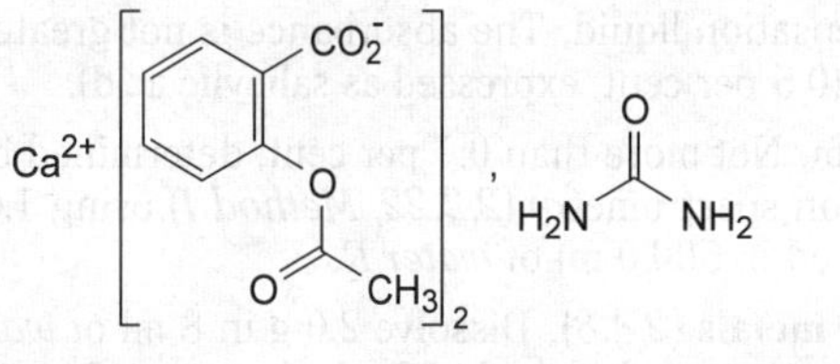

$C_{19}H_{18}CaN_2O_9$ M_r 458.4

DEFINITION

Carbasalate calcium contains not less than 99.0 per cent and not more than the equivalent of 101.0 per cent of an equimolecular compound of calcium di[2-(acetyloxy)benzoate] and urea, calculated with reference to the anhydrous substance.

CHARACTERS

A white, crystalline powder, freely soluble in water and dimethylformamide, practically insoluble in acetone and in anhydrous methanol.

Protect the substance from moisture during handling. Examination in aqueous solutions has to be performed immediately after preparation.

IDENTIFICATION

First identification: B, E.

Second identification: A, C, D, E.

A. Dissolve 0.250 g in *water R* and dilute to 100.0 ml with the same solvent. To 1.0 ml of the solution add 75 ml of *water R* and 5 ml of *dilute hydrochloric acid R*, mix and dilute with *water R* to 100.0 ml. Examined immediately after preparation between 220 nm and 350 nm (*2.2.25*), the solution shows two absorption maxima, at 228 nm and 276 nm. The specific absorbances at the maxima are 363 to 379 and 49 to 53, respectively.
B. Examine by infrared spectrophotometry (*2.2.24*), comparing with the *Ph. Eur. reference spectrum of carbasalate calcium*.
C. Dissolve 0.1 g in 10 ml of *water R*, boil for 2 min and cool. The solution gives reaction (a) of salicylates (*2.3.1*).
D. Heat 0.2 g with 0.2 g of *sodium hydroxide R*; a yellow to yellowish-brown colour is produced and the vapour turns *red litmus paper R* blue.
E. It gives reaction (a) of calcium (*2.3.1*).

TESTS

Appearance of solution. Dissolve 2.5 g in 50 ml of*water R*. The solution is not more opalescent than reference suspension II (*2.2.1*) and is colourless (*2.2.2, Method II*).

Related substances. In a 100 ml volumetric flask, dissolve 0.150 g in 10 ml of *0.1 M tetrabutylammonium hydroxide in 2-propanol*. Allow to stand for 10 min shaking occasionally. Add 8.0 ml of *0.1 M hydrochloric acid* and 20.0 ml of a 19 g/l solution of *disodium tetraborate R* and mix. While swirling continuously, add 2.0 ml of a 10 g/l solution of *aminopyrazolone R* and 2.0 ml of a 10 g/l solution of *potassium ferricyanide R*. Allow to stand for 2 min, dilute to 100.0 ml with *water R*, mix and allow to stand for 20 min. Measure the absorbance (*2.2.25*) of the solution at the maximum at 505 nm using *water R* as the compensation liquid. The absorbance is not greater than 0.125 (0.1 per cent, expressed as acetylsalicylsalicylic acid).

Salicylic acid. In a 100 ml volumetric flask, dissolve 0.200 g in 80 ml of *water R* and add 10 ml of a 10 g/l solution of *ferric nitrate R* in a 80 g/l solution of *dilute nitric acid R*. Dilute to 100.0 ml with *water R*. Immediately after preparation, measure the absorbance (*2.2.25*) of the solution at the maximum of 525 nm using *water R* as the compensation liquid. The absorbance is not greater than 0.115 (0.5 per cent, expressed as salicylic acid).

Sodium. Not more than 0.1 per cent, determined by atomic emission spectrometry (*2.2.22, Method I*) using 1.0 g dissolved in 500.0 ml of *water R*.

Heavy metals (*2.4.8*). Dissolve 2.0 g in 8 ml of *water R*, with heating, cool and add 12 ml of *acetone R*. 12 ml of the solution complies with limit test B for heavy metals (10 ppm). Prepare the standard using 10 ml of *lead standard solution (1 ppm Pb) R*.

Water (*2.5.12*). Not more than 0.1 per cent, determined on 1.000 g by the semi-micro determination of water. Use a mixture of 15 ml of *anhydrous methanol R* and 15 ml of *dimethylformamide R* as the solvent.

ASSAY

In a flask with a ground-glass stopper, dissolve 0.400 g in 25 ml of *water R*. Add 25.0 ml of *0.1 M sodium hydroxide*. Close the flask and allow to stand for 2 h. Titrate the excess of alkali with *0.1 M hydrochloric acid*, using 0.2 ml of *phenolphthalein solution R*. Carry out a blank titration.

1 ml of *0.1 M sodium hydroxide* is equivalent to 22.92 mg of $C_{19}H_{18}CaN_2O_9$.

STORAGE

Store in an airtight container.

IMPURITIES

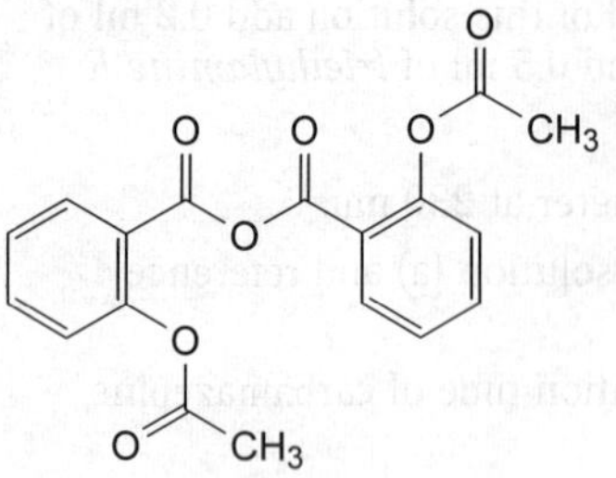

A. 2-(acetyloxy)benzoic anhydride,

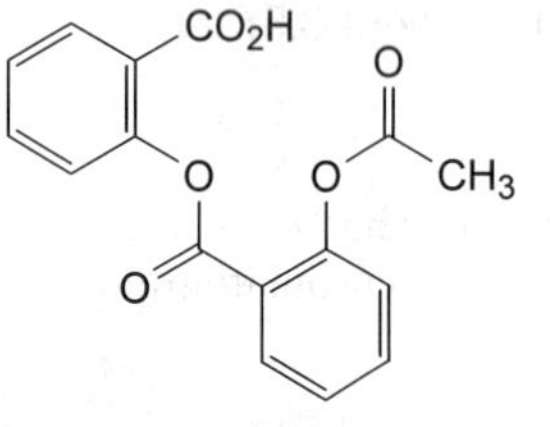

B. 2-[[2-(acetyloxy)benzoyl]oxy]benzoic acid (acetylsalicylsalicylic acid),

C. 2-hydroxybenzoic acid (salicylic acid).

01/2005:0755
corrected

CARBIDOPA

Carbidopum

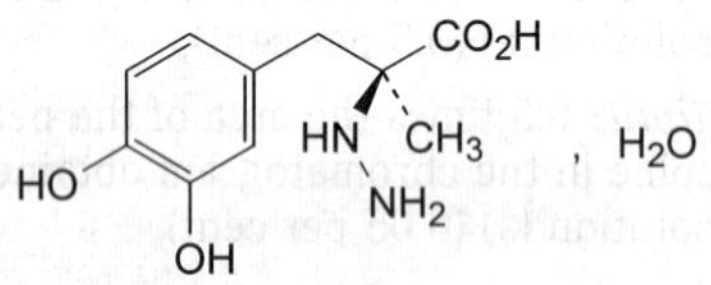

$C_{10}H_{14}N_2O_4,H_2O$ M_r 244.2

DEFINITION

Carbidopa contains not less than 98.5 per cent and not more than the equivalent of 101.0 per cent of (2*S*)-3-(3,4-dihydroxyphenyl)-2-hydrazino-2-methylpropanoic acid, calculated with reference to the dried substance.

CHARACTERS

A white or yellowish-white powder, slightly soluble in water, very slightly soluble in alcohol, practically insoluble in methylene chloride. It dissolves in dilute solutions of mineral acids.

IDENTIFICATION

First identification: A, C.

Second identification: A, B, D, E.

A. It complies with the test for specific optical rotation (see Tests).
B. Dissolve 50.0 mg in a 8.5 g/l solution of *hydrochloric acid R* in *methanol R* and dilute to 100.0 ml with the same acid. Dilute 10.0 ml of this solution to 100.0 ml with a 8.5 g/l solution of *hydrochloric acid R* in *methanol R*. Examined between 230 nm and 350 nm (*2.2.25*), the solution shows an absorption maximum at 283 nm. The specific absorbance at the maximum is 135 to 150, calculated with reference to the dried substance.
C. Examine by infrared absorption spectrophotometry (*2.2.24*), comparing with the spectrum obtained with *carbidopa CRS*. Examine the substances prepared as discs.

D. Shake vigorously about 5 mg with 10 ml of *water R* for 1 min and add 0.3 ml of *ferric chloride solution R2.* An intense green colour is produced, which quickly turns to reddish-brown.

E. Suspend about 20 mg in 5 ml of *water R* and add 5 ml of *cupri-tartaric solution R.* On heating, the colour of the solution changes to dark brown and a red precipitate is formed.

TESTS

Appearance of solution. Dissolve 0.25 g in 25 ml of *1 M hydrochloric acid.* The solution is clear (*2.2.1*) and not more intensely coloured than reference solution BY_6 or B_6 (*2.2.2, Method II*).

Specific optical rotation (*2.2.7*). With the aid of an ultrasonic bath, dissolve completely 0.250 g in *aluminium chloride solution R* and dilute to 25.0 ml with the same solution. The specific optical rotation is −22.5 to −26.5, calculated with reference to the dried substance.

Hydrazine. Examine by thin-layer chromatography (*2.2.27*), using *silanised silica gel H R* as the coating substance.

Test solution (a). Dissolve 0.50 g in *dilute hydrochloric acid R* and dilute to 2.0 ml with the same acid.

Test solution (b). Place 25 g of *strongly basic anion exchange resin R* into each of two conical flasks with ground-glass stoppers. To each, add 150 ml of *carbon dioxide-free water R* and shake from time to time during 30 min. Decant the liquid from both flasks and repeat the process with further quantities, each of 150 ml, of *carbon dioxide-free water R.*

Take two 100 ml measuring cylinders 3.5 cm to 4.5 cm in internal diameter and label these A and B. Into cylinder A, transfer as completely as possible the resin from one conical flask using 60 ml of *carbon dioxide-free water R*; into cylinder B, transfer the second quantity of resin, this time using 20 ml of *carbon dioxide-free water R.*

Into each cylinder, insert a gas-inlet tube, the end of which has an internal diameter of 2 mm to 3 mm and which reaches almost to the bottom of the cylinder. Pass a rapid stream of *nitrogen for chromatography R* through each mixture so that homogeneous suspensions are formed. After 30 min, without interrupting the gas flow, add 1.0 ml of test solution (a) to cylinder A; after 1 min stop the gas flow into cylinder A and transfer the contents, through a moistened filter paper, into cylinder B. After 1 min, stop the gas flow to cylinder B and pour the solution immediately through a moistened filter paper into a freshly prepared mixture of 1 ml of a 200 g/l solution of *salicylaldehyde R* in *methanol R* and 20 ml of *phosphate buffer solution pH 5.5 R* in a conical flask, shake thoroughly for 1 min and heat in a water-bath at 60 °C for 15 min. The liquid becomes clear. Allow to cool, add 2.0 ml of *toluene R* and shake vigorously for 2 min. Transfer the mixture into a centrifuge tube and centrifuge.

Separate the toluene layer in a 100 ml separating funnel and shake vigorously with two quantities, each of 20 ml, of a 200 g/l solution of *sodium metabisulphite R* and finally with two quantities, each of 50 ml, of *water R.* Separate the toluene layer.

Reference solution (a). Dissolve 10 mg of *hydrazine sulphate R* in *dilute hydrochloric acid R* and dilute to 50 ml with the same acid. Dilute 1.0 ml of this solution to 10.0 ml with *dilute hydrochloric acid R.*

Reference solution (b). Prepare the solution at the same time and in the same manner as described for test solution (b) using 1.0 ml of reference solution (a) in place of 1.0 ml of test solution (a).

Apply separately to the plate 10 µl of test solution (b) and 10 µl of reference solution (b). Develop over a path of 10 cm using a mixture of 1 volume of *water R* and 2 volumes of *methanol R.* Allow the plate to dry in air. Examine in ultraviolet light at 365 nm. Any spot in the chromatogram obtained with test solution (b) showing a yellow fluorescence is not more intense than the corresponding spot in the chromatogram obtained with reference solution (b) (20 ppm of hydrazine).

Methyldopa and methylcarbidopa. Examine by liquid chromatography (*2.2.29*).

Test solution. Dissolve 0.100 g of the substance to be examined in *0.1 M hydrochloric acid* and dilute to 10.0 ml with the same acid.

Reference solution (a). Dissolve the contents of a vial of *methylcarbidopa CRS* in *0.1 M hydrochloric acid,* add 1 mg of *methyldopa CRS* and dilute to 20.0 ml with the same acid.

Reference solution (b). Dissolve 5 mg of *carbidopa CRS* and 5 mg of *methyldopa CRS* in *0.1 M hydrochloric acid* and dilute to 10.0 ml with the same acid.

The chromatographic procedure may be carried out using:

- a stainless steel column 0.25 m long and 4.6 mm in internal diameter packed with *octylsilyl silica gel for chromatography R* (5 µm),
- as mobile phase at a flow rate of 1 ml/min a mixture of 2 volumes of *methanol R* and 98 volumes of a 14 g/l solution of *potassium dihydrogen phosphate R,*
- as detector a spectrophotometer set at 282 nm,
- a loop injector.

Inject 20 µl of each solution. The test is not valid unless the resolution between the peaks corresponding to methyldopa and carbidopa in the chromatogram obtained with reference solution (b) is greater than 4.0. In the chromatogram obtained with the test solution, the areas of any peaks corresponding to methyldopa and methylcarbidopa are not greater than the areas of the corresponding peaks in the chromatogram obtained with reference solution (a) (0.5 per cent).

Heavy metals (*2.4.8*). 1.0 g complies with limit test C for heavy metals (20 ppm). Prepare the standard using 2 ml of *lead standard solution (10 ppm Pb) R.*

Loss on drying (*2.2.32*): 6.9 per cent to 7.9 per cent, determined on 1.000 g by drying in an oven at 100 °C to 105 °C.

Sulphated ash (*2.4.14*). Not more than 0.1 per cent, determined on 1.0 g.

ASSAY

Dissolve 0.150 g with gentle heating in 75 ml of *anhydrous acetic acid R.* Titrate with *0.1 M perchloric acid,* determining the end-point potentiometrically (*2.2.20*).

1 ml of *0.1 M perchloric acid* is equivalent to 22.62 mg of $C_{10}H_{14}N_2O_4$.

STORAGE

Store protected from light.

Monographs C

01/2005:0884

CARBIMAZOLE

Carbimazolum

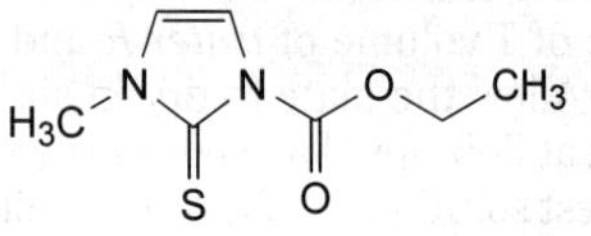

$C_7H_{10}N_2O_2S$ M_r 186.2

DEFINITION

Ethyl 3-methyl-2-thioxo-2,3-dihydro-1*H*-imidazole-1-carboxylate.

Content: 98.0 per cent to 102.0 per cent (dried substance).

CHARACTERS

Appearance: white or yellowish-white, crystalline powder.

Solubility: slightly soluble in water, soluble in acetone and in alcohol.

IDENTIFICATION

First identification: B.

Second identification: A, C, D.

A. Melting point (*2.2.14*): 122 °C to 125 °C.

B. Infrared absorption spectrophotometry (*2.2.24*).

Preparation: discs.

Comparison: *carbimazole CRS*.

C. Thin-layer chromatography (*2.2.27*).

Test solution. Dissolve 10 mg of the substance to be examined in *methylene chloride R* and dilute to 10 ml with the same solvent.

Reference solution. Dissolve 10 mg of *carbimazole CRS* in *methylene chloride R* and dilute to 10 ml with the same solvent.

Plate: *TLC silica gel GF_{254} plate R.*

Mobile phase: *acetone R, methylene chloride R* (20:80 *V/V*).

Application: 10 µl.

Development: over a path of 15 cm.

Drying: in air for 30 min.

Detection: examine in ultraviolet light at 254 nm.

Results: the principal spot in the chromatogram obtained with the test solution is similar in position and size to the principal spot in the chromatogram obtained with the reference solution.

D. Dissolve about 10 mg in a mixture of 50 ml of *water R* and 0.05 ml of *dilute hydrochloric acid R*. Add 1 ml of *potassium iodobismuthate solution R*. A red precipitate is formed.

TESTS

Impurity A and other related substances. Liquid chromatography (*2.2.29*).

Test solution. Dissolve 5.0 mg of the substance to be examined in 10.0 ml of a mixture of 20 volumes of *acetonitrile R* and 80 volumes of *water R*. Use this solution within 5 min of preparation.

Reference solution (a). Dissolve 5 mg of *thiamazole R* and 0.10 g of *carbimazole CRS* in a mixture of 20 volumes of *acetonitrile R* and 80 volumes of *water R* and dilute to 100.0 ml with the same mixture of solvents. Dilute 1.0 ml of this solution to 10.0 ml with a mixture of 20 volumes of *acetonitrile R* and 80 volumes of *water R*.

Reference solution (b). Dissolve 5.0 mg of *thiamazole R* in a mixture of 20 volumes of *acetonitrile R* and 80 volumes of *water R* and dilute to 10.0 ml with the same mixture of solvents. Dilute 1.0 ml of this solution to 100.0 ml with a mixture of 20 volumes of *acetonitrile R* and 80 volumes of *water R*.

Column:

- *size*: *l* = 0.15 m, Ø = 3.9 mm,
- *stationary phase*: *octadecylsilyl silica gel for chromatography R* (5 µm).

Mobile phase: *acetonitrile R, water R* (10:90 *V/V*).

Flow rate: 1 ml/min.

Detection: spectrophotometer at 254 nm.

Injection: 10 µl.

Run time: 1.5 times the retention time of carbimazole.

Retention time: carbimazole = about 6 min.

System suitability: reference solution (a):

- *resolution*: minimum 5.0 between the peaks due to impurity A and carbimazole.

Limits:

- *impurity A*: not more than half the area of the principal peak in the chromatogram obtained with reference solution (b) (0.5 per cent),
- *any other impurity*: not more than 0.1 times the area of the principal peak in the chromatogram obtained with reference solution (b) (0.1 per cent).

Loss on drying (*2.2.32*): maximum 0.5 per cent, determined on 1.000 g by drying in a desiccator over *diphosphorus pentoxide R* at a pressure not exceeding 0.7 kPa for 24 h.

Sulphated ash (*2.4.14*): maximum 0.1 per cent, determined on 1.0 g.

ASSAY

Dissolve 50.0 mg in *water R* and dilute to 500.0 ml with the same solvent. To 10.0 ml add 10 ml of *dilute hydrochloric acid R* and dilute to 100.0 ml with *water R*. Measure the absorbance (*2.2.25*) at the maximum at 291 nm. Calculate the content of $C_7H_{10}N_2O_2S$ taking the specific absorbance to be 557.

IMPURITIES

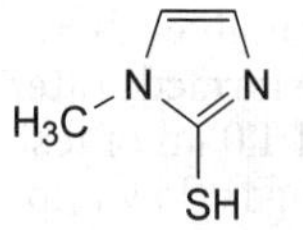

A. 1-methyl-1*H*-imidazole-2-thiol (thiamazole).

01/2005:0885

CARBOCISTEINE

Carbocisteinum

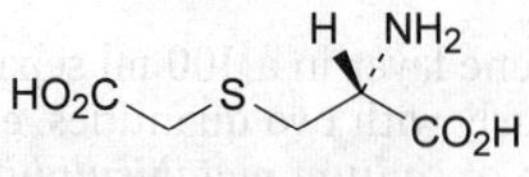

$C_5H_9NO_4S$ M_r 179.2

DEFINITION

Carbocisteine contains not less than 98.5 per cent and not more than the equivalent of 101.0 per cent of (2*R*)-2-amino-3-[(carboxymethyl)sulphanyl]propanoic acid, calculated with reference to the dried substance.

CHARACTERS

A white, crystalline powder, practically insoluble in water and in alcohol. It dissolves in dilute mineral acids and in dilute solutions of alkali hydroxides.

IDENTIFICATION

First identification: A, B.

Second identification: A, C, D.

A. It complies with the test for specific optical rotation (see Tests).

B. Examine by infrared absorption spectrophotometry (*2.2.24*), comparing with the spectrum obtained with *carbocisteine CRS*. Examine the substances prepared as discs.

C. Examine the chromatograms obtained in the test for ninhydrin-positive substances. The principal spot in the chromatogram obtained with test solution (b) is similar in position, colour and size to the principal spot in the chromatogram obtained with reference solution (a).

D. Dissolve 0.1 g in 4.5 ml of *dilute sodium hydroxide solution R*. Heat on a water-bath for 10 min. Cool and add 1 ml of a 25 g/l solution of *sodium nitroprusside R*. A dark red colour is produced, which changes to brown and then to yellow within a few minutes.

TESTS

Solution S. Disperse 5.00 g in 20 ml of *water R* and add dropwise with shaking 2.5 ml of *strong sodium hydroxide solution R*. Adjust to pH 6.3 with *1 M sodium hydroxide* and dilute to 50.0 ml with *water R*.

Appearance of solution. Solution S is clear (*2.2.1*) and colourless (*2.2.2, Method II*).

pH (*2.2.3*). Shake 0.2 g with 20 ml of *carbon dioxide-free water R*. The pH of the suspension is 2.8 to 3.0.

Specific optical rotation (*2.2.7*): − 32.5 to − 35.5, determined on solution S and calculated with reference to the dried substance.

Ninhydrin-positive substances. Examine by thin-layer chromatography (*2.2.27*), using a suitable silica gel as the coating substance.

Test solution (a). Dissolve 0.10 g of the substance to be examined in *dilute ammonia R2* and dilute to 10 ml with the same solvent.

Test solution (b). Dilute 1 ml of test solution (a) to 50 ml with *water R*.

Reference solution (a). Dissolve 10 mg of *carbocisteine CRS* in *dilute ammonia R2* and dilute to 50 ml with the same solvent.

Reference solution (b). Dilute 5 ml of test solution (b) to 20 ml with *water R*.

Reference solution (c). Dissolve 10 mg of *carbocisteine CRS* and 10 mg of *arginine hydrochloride CRS* in 5 ml of *dilute ammonia R2* and dilute to 25 ml with *water R*.

Apply separately to the plate 5 µl of each solution. Allow the plate to dry in air. Develop over a path of 15 cm using a mixture of 20 volumes of *glacial acetic acid R*, 20 volumes of *water R* and 60 volumes of *butanol R*. Dry the plate in a current of warm air. Spray with *ninhydrin solution R* and heat at 100 °C to 105 °C for 15 min. Any spot in the chromatogram obtained with test solution (a), apart from the principal spot, is not more intense than the spot in the chromatogram obtained with reference solution (b) (0.5 per cent). The test is not valid unless the chromatogram obtained with reference solution (c) shows two clearly separated principal spots.

Chlorides (*2.4.4*). Dissolve 33 mg in 5 ml of *dilute nitric acid R* and dilute to 15 ml with *water R*. The solution, without further addition of nitric acid, complies with the limit test for chlorides (0.15 per cent).

Sulphates (*2.4.13*). Dissolve 0.5 g in 5 ml of *dilute hydrochloric acid R* and dilute to 15 ml with *distilled water R*. The solution complies with the limit test for sulphates (300 ppm).

Heavy metals (*2.4.8*). 2.0 g complies with limit test D for heavy metals (10 ppm). Prepare the standard using 2 ml of *lead standard solution (10 ppm Pb) R*.

Loss on drying (*2.2.32*). Not more than 0.5 per cent, determined on 1.000 g by drying in an oven at 100 °C to 105 °C for 2 h.

Sulphated ash (*2.4.14*). Not more than 0.3 per cent, determined on 1.0 g.

ASSAY

Dissolve 0.150 g in 10 ml of *anhydrous formic acid R* with slight heating and shake until dissolution is complete. Add 50 ml of *anhydrous acetic acid R*. Titrate with *0.1 M perchloric acid*, determining the end-point potentiometrically (*2.2.20*).

1 ml of *0.1 M perchloric acid* is equivalent to 17.92 mg of $C_5H_9NO_4S$.

STORAGE

Store protected from light.

01/2005:1299

CARBOMERS

Carbomera

DEFINITION

High molecular mass polymers of acrylic acid cross-linked with polyalkenyl ethers of sugars or polyalcohols.

Content: 56.0 per cent to 68.0 per cent of carboxylic acid (-COOH) groups (dried substance).

CHARACTERS

Appearance: white, fluffy powder, hygroscopic.

Solubility: swells in water and in other polar solvents after dispersion and neutralisation with sodium hydroxide solution.

IDENTIFICATION

First identification: A, E.

Second identification: B, C, D, E.

A. Infrared absorption spectrophotometry (*2.2.24*).

Main bands: at 2960 cm^{-1}, 1720 cm^{-1}, 1455 cm^{-1}, 1415 cm^{-1}, 1250 cm^{-1}, 1175 cm^{-1} and 800 cm^{-1}, with the strongest band at 1720 cm^{-1}.

B. Adjust a 10 g/l dispersion to about pH 7.5 with *1 M sodium hydroxide*. A highly viscous gel is formed.

C. Add 2 ml of a 100 g/l solution of *calcium chloride R* with continuous stirring to 10 ml of the gel from test B. A white precipitate is immediately produced.

D. Add 0.5 ml of *thymol blue solution R* to 10 ml of a 10 g/l dispersion. An orange colour is produced. Add 0.5 ml of *cresol red solution R* to 10 ml of a 10 g/l dispersion. A yellow colour is produced.

E. It complies with the apparent nominal viscosity indicated on the label.

TESTS

Apparent viscosity: the nominal apparent viscosity is in the range 300 mPa·s to 115 000 mPa·s. For a product with a nominal apparent viscosity of 20 000 mPa·s or greater, the apparent viscosity is 70.0 per cent to 130.0 per cent of the value stated on the label; for a product with a nominal apparent viscosity less than 20 000 mPa·s, the apparent viscosity is 50.0 per cent to 150.0 per cent of the value stated on the label.

Dry the substance to be examined *in vacuo* at 80 °C for 1 h. Carefully add 2.50 g of the previously dried substance to be examined to 500 ml of *water R* in a 1000 ml beaker while stirring continuously at 1000 ± 50 r/min, with the stirrer shaft set at an angle of 60° to one side of the beaker. Add the previously dried substance over a period of 45-90 s, at a uniform rate, ensuring that loose aggregates of powder are broken up and continue stirring at 1000 ± 50 r/min for 15 min. Remove the stirrer, and place the beaker containing the dispersion in a water-bath at 25 ± 0.2 °C for 30 min. Insert the stirrer to a depth necessary to ensure that air is not drawn into the dispersion, and while stirring at 300 ± 25 r/min, titrate with a glass-calomel electrode system to pH 7.3-7.8 by adding a 180 g/l solution of *sodium hydroxide R* below the surface, determining the end-point potentiometrically (*2.2.20*). The total volume of the 180 g/l solution of *sodium hydroxide R* used is about 6.2 ml. Allow 2-3 min before the final pH determination. If the final pH exceeds 7.8, discard the preparation, and prepare another using a smaller amount of sodium hydroxide for titration. Return the neutralised preparation to the water-bath at 25 °C for 1 h, then perform the viscosity determination without delay to avoid slight viscosity changes that occur 75 min after neutralisation. Determine the viscosity (*2.2.10*) with a rotating viscometer with a spindle rotating at 20 r/min, using a spindle suitable for the expected apparent viscosity.

Free acrylic acid. Liquid chromatography (*2.2.29*).

Test solution. Mix 0.125 g of the substance to be examined with a 25 g/l solution of *aluminium potassium sulphate R* and dilute to 25.0 ml with the same solution. Heat the suspension at 50 °C for 20 min with shaking. Then shake the suspension at room temperature for 60 min. Centrifuge and use the clear supernatant solution as the test solution.

Reference solution. Dissolve 62.5 mg of *acrylic acid R* in a 25 g/l solution of *aluminium potassium sulphate R* and dilute to 100.0 ml with the same solution. Dilute 1.0 ml of this solution to 50.0 ml with a 25 g/l solution of *aluminium potassium sulphate R.*

Column:

- *size*: l = 0.12 m, Ø = 4.6 mm,
- *stationary phase*: *octadecylsilyl silica gel for chromatography R* (5 µm).

Mobile phase:

- *mobile phase A*: a 1.361 g/l solution of *potassium dihydrogen phosphate R*, adjusted to pH 2.5 using *dilute phosphoric acid R*,
- *mobile phase B*: equal volumes of a 1.361 g/l solution of *potassium dihydrogen phosphate R* and *acetonitrile for chromatography R.*

Time (min)	Mobile phase A (per cent *V/V*)	Mobile phase B (per cent *V/V*)
0 - 8	100	0
8 - 9	100 → 0	0 → 100
9 - 20	0	100
20 - 21	0 → 100	100 → 0
21 - 30	100	0

Flow rate: 1 ml/min.

Detection: spectrophotometer at 205 nm.

Injection: 20 µl.

Retention time: acrylic acid = about 6.0 min.

Limit:

- *acrylic acid*: not more than the area of the corresponding peak in the chromatogram obtained with the reference solution (0.25 per cent).

Benzene. Gas chromatography (*2.4.24, System A*).

Solvent solution. Dissolve 0.100 g of *benzene R* in *dimethyl sulphoxide R* and dilute to 100.0 ml with the same solvent. Dilute 1.0 ml of the solution to 100.0 ml with *water R*. Dilute 1.0 ml of this solution to 100.0 ml with *water R*.

Test solution. Weigh 50.0 mg of the substance to be examined into an injection vial and add 5.0 ml of *water R* and 1.0 ml of *dimethyl sulphoxide R.*

Reference solution. Weigh 50.0 mg of the substance to be examined into an injection vial and add 4.0 ml of *water R*, 1.0 ml of *dimethyl sulphoxide R* and 1.0 ml of the solvent solution.

Close the vials with a tight rubber membrane stopper coated with polytetrafluoroethylene and secure with an aluminium crimped cap. Shake to obtain a homogeneous dispersion.

Stratic head-space conditions which may be used:

- *equilibration temperature*: 80 °C,
- *equilibration time*: 60 min,
- *transfer line temperature*: 90 °C.

Injection: 1 ml of the gaseous phase of the test solution and 1 ml of the gaseous phase of the reference solution; repeat these injections twice more.

System suitability:

- *repeatability*: maximum relative standard deviation of the differences in area between the analyte peaks obtained from the 3 replicate pair injections of the reference solution and the test solution is 15 per cent.

Limit:

- *benzene*: the mean area of the peak corresponding to benzene in the chromatograms obtained with the test solution is not greater than half the mean area of the peak corresponding to benzene in the chromatograms obtained with the reference solution (2 ppm).

Heavy metals (*2.4.8*): maximum 20 ppm.

1.0 g complies with limit test C. Prepare the standard using 2 ml of *lead standard solution (10 ppm Pb) R.*

Loss on drying (*2.2.32*): maximum 3.0 per cent, determined on 1.000 g by drying *in vacuo* at 80 °C for 60 min.

Sulphated ash (*2.4.14*): maximum 4.0 per cent, determined on 1.0 g.

ASSAY

Slowly add 50 ml of *water R* to 0.120 g whilst stirring and heating at 60 °C for 15 min. Stop heating, add 150 ml of *water R* and continue stirring for 30 min. Add 2 g of *potassium chloride R* and titrate with *0.2 M sodium hydroxide*, determining the end-point potentiometrically (*2.2.20*).

1 ml of *0.2 M sodium hydroxide* is equivalent to 9.0 mg of carboxylic acid (-COOH) groups.

STORAGE

In an airtight container.

LABELLING

The label states the nominal apparent viscosity.

01/2005:0375

CARBON DIOXIDE

Carbonei dioxidum

CO_2 M_r 44.01

DEFINITION

Content: minimum 99.5 per cent *V/V* of CO_2 in the gaseous phase.

This monograph applies to carbon dioxide for medicinal use.

CHARACTERS

Appearance: colourless gas.

Solubility: at 20 °C and at a pressure of 101 kPa, 1 volume dissolves in about 1 volume of water.

PRODUCTION

Examine the gaseous phase.

If the test is performed on a cylinder of gas, keep the cylinder of the substance to be examined at room temperature for not less than 6 h before carrying out the tests. Keep the cylinder in the vertical position with the outlet valve uppermost.

Carbon monoxide. Gas chromatography (*2.2.28*).

Gas to be examined. The substance to be examined.

Reference gas. A mixture containing 5 ppm *V/V* of *carbon monoxide R* in *nitrogen R1.*

Column:

– *material*: stainless steel,

– *size*: *l* = 2 m, Ø = 4 mm,

– *stationary phase*: an appropriate molecular sieve for chromatography (0.5 nm).

Carrier gas: *helium for chromatography R.*

Flow rate: 60 ml/min.

Temperature:

– *column*: 50 °C,

– *injection port and detector*: 130 °C.

Detection: flame ionisation with methaniser.

Injection: loop injector.

Adjust the injected volumes and the operating conditions so that the height of the peak due to carbon monoxide in the chromatogram obtained with the reference gas is at least 35 per cent of the full scale of the recorder.

Limit:

– *carbon monoxide*: not more than the area of the corresponding peak in the chromatogram obtained with the reference gas (5 ppm *V/V*).

Nitrogen monoxide and nitrogen dioxide: maximum 2 ppm *V/V* in total, determined using a chemiluminescence analyser (*2.5.26*).

Gas to be examined. The substance to be examined.

Reference gas (a). Carbon dioxide R1.

Reference gas (b). A mixture containing 2 ppm *V/V* of *nitrogen monoxide R* in *carbon dioxide R1* or in *nitrogen R1.*

Calibrate the apparatus and set the sensitivity using reference gases (a) and (b). Measure the content of nitrogen monoxide and nitrogen dioxide in the gas to be examined.

If nitrogen is used instead of carbon dioxide in reference gas (b), multiply the result obtained by the quenching correction factor in order to correct the quenching effect on the analyser response caused by the carbon dioxide matrix effect.

The quenching correction factor is determined by applying a known reference mixture of nitrogen monoxide in carbon dioxide and comparing the actual content with the content indicated by the analyser which has been calibrated with a NO/N_2 reference mixture.

$$\text{Quenching correction factor} = \frac{\text{actual nitrogen monoxide content}}{\text{indicated nitrogen monoxide content}}$$

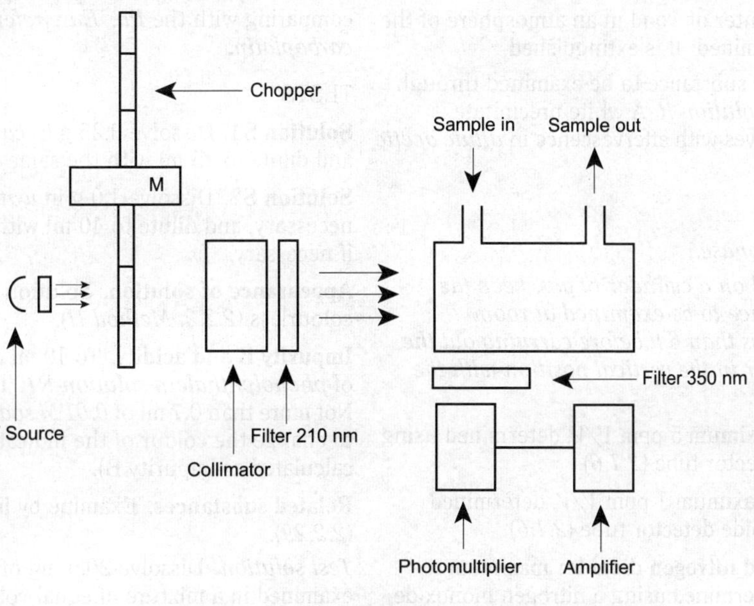

Figure 0375.-1.– *UV Fluorescence Analyser*

Total sulphur: maximum 1 ppm *V/V*, determined using an ultraviolet fluorescence analyser after oxidation of the sulphur compounds by heating at 1000 °C (Figure 0375.-1).

The apparatus consists of the following:

– a system generating ultraviolet radiation with a wavelength of 210 nm, made up of an ultraviolet lamp, a collimator, and a selective filter; the beam is blocked periodically by a chopper rotating at high speed,

– a reaction chamber through which flows the previously filtered gas to be examined,

– a system that detects radiation emitted at a wavelength of 350 nm, made up of a selective filter, a photomultiplier tube and an amplifier.

Gas to be examined. The substance to be examined.

Reference gas (a). Carbon dioxide R1.

Reference gas (b). A mixture containing between 0.5 ppm *V/V* and 2 ppm *V/V* of *hydrogen sulphide R1* in *carbon dioxide R1*.

Calibrate the apparatus and set the sensitivity using reference gases (a) and (b). Pass the gas to be examined through a quartz oven heated to 1000 °C. *Oxygen R* is circulated in the oven at a tenth of the flow rate of the gas to be examined. Measure the sulphur dioxide content in the gaseous mixture leaving the oven.

Water: maximum 67 ppm *V/V*, determined using an electrolytic hygrometer (*2.5.28*).

Assay. Infrared analyser (*2.5.24*).

Gas to be examined. The substance to be examined. It must be filtered to avoid stray light phenomena.

Reference gas (a). Carbon dioxide R1.

Reference gas (b). A mixture containing 95.0 per cent *V/V* of *carbon dioxide R1* and 5.0 per cent *V/V* of *nitrogen R1*.

Calibrate the apparatus and set the sensitivity using reference gases (a) and (b). Measure the content of carbon dioxide in the gas to be examined.

IDENTIFICATION

First identification: A.

Second identification: B, C.

A. Infrared absorption spectrophotometry (*2.2.24*).

   Comparison: *Ph. Eur. reference spectrum of carbon dioxide.*

B. Place a glowing splinter of wood in an atmosphere of the substance to be examined. It is extinguished.

C. Pass a stream of the substance to be examined through *barium hydroxide solution R*. A white precipitate is formed which dissolves with effervescence in *dilute acetic acid R*.

TESTS

Examine the gaseous phase.

If the test is performed on a cylinder of gas, keep the cylinder of the substance to be examined at room temperature for not less than 6 h before carrying out the tests. Keep the cylinder in the vertical position with the outlet valve uppermost.

Carbon monoxide: maximum 5 ppm *V/V*, determined using a carbon monoxide detector tube (*2.1.6*).

Hydrogen sulphide: maximum 1 ppm *V/V*, determined using a hydrogen sulphide detector tube (*2.1.6*).

Nitrogen monoxide and nitrogen dioxide: maximum 2 ppm *V/V* in total, determined using a nitrogen monoxide and nitrogen dioxide detector tube (*2.1.6*).

Sulphur dioxide: maximum 2 ppm *V/V*, determined using a sulphur dioxide detector tube (*2.1.6*).

Water vapour: maximum 67 ppm *V/V*, determined using a water vapour detector tube (*2.1.6*).

STORAGE

Store liquefied under pressure in suitable containers complying with the legal regulations.

IMPURITIES

A. nitrogen monoxide,

B. nitrogen dioxide,

C. carbon monoxide,

D. total sulphur,

E. water.

01/2005:1081

CARBOPLATIN

Carboplatinum

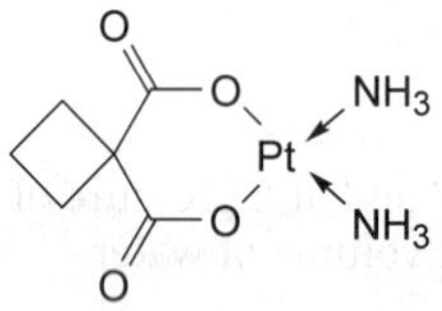

$C_6H_{12}N_2O_4Pt$ M_r 371.3

DEFINITION

Carboplatin contains not less than 98.0 per cent and not more than the equivalent of 102.0 per cent of (*SP*-4-2)-diammine[cyclobutan-1,1-dicarboxylato(2-)-*O,O′*]platin, calculated with reference to the dried substance.

CHARACTERS

A colourless, crystalline powder, sparingly soluble in water, very slightly soluble in acetone and in alcohol.

It melts at about 200 °C, with decomposition.

IDENTIFICATION

Examine by infrared absorption spectrophotometry (*2.2.24*), comparing with the *Ph. Eur. reference spectrum of carboplatin.*

TESTS

Solution S1. Dissolve 0.25 g in *carbon dioxide-free water R* and dilute to 25 ml with the same solvent.

Solution S2. Dissolve 1.0 g in *water R*, heating slightly if necessary, and dilute to 40 ml with the same solvent. Filter if necessary.

Appearance of solution. Solution S1 is clear (*2.2.1*) and colourless (*2.2.2, Method II*).

Impurity B and acidity. To 10 ml of solution S1 add 0.1 ml of *phenolphthalein solution R1*. The solution is colourless. Not more than 0.7 ml of *0.01 M sodium hydroxide* is required to change the colour of the indicator to pink (0.5 per cent calculated as impurity B).

Related substances. Examine by liquid chromatography (*2.2.29*).

Test solution. Dissolve 20.0 mg of the substance to be examined in a mixture of equal volumes of *acetonitrile R* and *water R* and dilute to 20.0 ml with the same mixture.

Reference solution. Dilute 0.5 ml of the test solution to 200.0 ml with the mobile phase.

The chromatographic procedure may be carried out using:

- a stainless steel column 0.25 m long and 4.6 mm in internal diameter packed with *aminopropylsilyl silica gel for chromatography R* (5 µm),
- as mobile phase at a flow rate of 2 ml/min a mixture of 130 volumes of *water R* and 870 volumes of *acetonitrile R*,
- a 10 µl loop injector,
- as detector a spectrophotometer set at 230 nm.

Inject the test solution. The test is not valid unless:

- the mass distribution ratio, D_m, is not less than 4.0,
- the number of theoretical plates, *n*, is not less than 5000,
- the symmetry factor is not more than 2.0.

If necessary adjust the concentration of acetonitrile in the mobile phase.

Inject the test solution and the reference solution. Continue the chromatography for 2.5 times the retention time of the principal peak. In the chromatogram obtained with the test solution; the area of any peak apart from the principal peak is not greater than the area of the principal peak in the chromatogram obtained with the reference solution (0.25 per cent); the sum of the areas of all the peaks apart from the principal peak is not greater than twice the area of the principal peak in the chromatogram obtained with the reference solution (0.5 per cent). Disregard any peak with an area less than 0.2 times the area of the principal peak in the chromatogram obtained with the reference solution.

Chlorides (*2.4.4*). Dilute 10 ml of solution S2 to 15 ml with *water R*. The solution complies with the limit test for chlorides (100 ppm). Prepare the standard using 5 ml of *chloride standard solution (5 ppm Cl) R*.

Ammonium (*2.4.1*). 0.20 g complies with the limit test B for ammonium (100 ppm). Prepare the standard using 0.2 ml of *ammonium standard solution (100 ppm NH_4) R*.

Silver. Not more than 10 ppm of Ag, determined by atomic emission spectrometry (*2.2.22, Method I*).

Test solution. Dissolve 0.50 g in a 1 per cent *V/V* solution of *nitric acid R* and dilute to 50.0 ml with the same acid.

Reference solutions. Prepare the reference solutions using *silver standard solution (5 ppm Ag) R*, diluted with a 1 per cent *V/V* solution of *nitric acid R*.

Measure the intensity emitted at 328.1 nm.

Soluble barium. Not more than 10 ppm of Ba, determined by atomic emission spectrometry (*2.2.22, Method I*).

Test solution. Use the solution described in the test for silver.

Reference solutions. Prepare the reference solutions using *barium standard solution (50 ppm Ba) R*, diluted with a 1 per cent *V/V* solution of *nitric acid R*.

Measure the intensity emitted at 455.4 nm.

Heavy metals (*2.4.8*). 12 ml of solution S2 complies with limit test A for heavy metals (20 ppm). Prepare the standard using 5 ml of *lead standard solution (1 ppm Pb R)*.

Loss on drying (*2.2.32*). Not more than 0.5 per cent, determined on 1.000 g by drying in an oven at 100 °C to 105 °C.

ASSAY

Use the residue obtained in the test for loss on drying.

Ignite 0.200 g of the residue to constant mass at 800 °C.

1 mg of the residue is equivalent to 1.903 mg of $C_6H_{12}N_2O_4Pt$.

STORAGE

Store protected from light.

IMPURITIES

A. cisplatin,

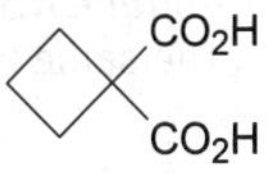

B. cyclobutane-1,1-dicarboxylic acid.

01/2005:1689

CARISOPRODOL

Carisoprodolum

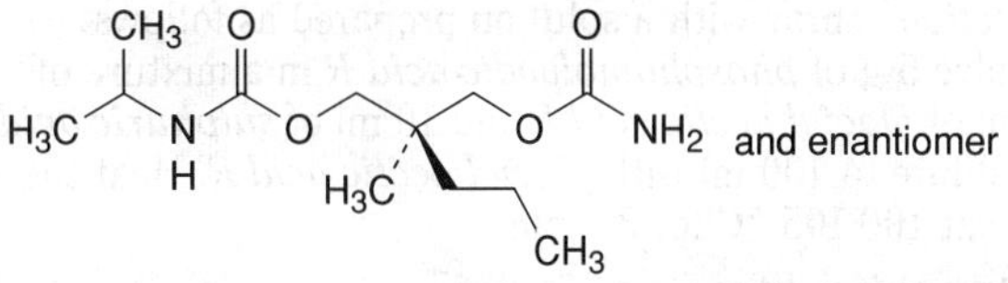

$C_{12}H_{24}N_2O_4$ M_r 260.3

DEFINITION

(2*RS*)-2-[(Carbamoyloxy)methyl]-2-methylpentyl (1-methylethyl)carbamate.

Content: 98.0 per cent to 102.0 per cent (dried substance).

CHARACTERS

Appearance: white or almost white, fine powder.

Solubility: very slightly soluble in water, freely soluble in acetone, in alcohol and in methylene chloride.

IDENTIFICATION

First identification: A, B.

Second identification: A, C, D.

A. Melting point (*2.2.14*): 92 °C to 95 °C.

B. Infrared absorption spectrophotometry (*2.2.24*).

   Comparison: *carisoprodol CRS*.

C. Examine the chromatograms obtained in the test for related substances.

   Results: the principal spot in the chromatogram obtained with test solution (b) is similar in position, colour and size to the principal spot in the chromatogram obtained with reference solution (d).

D. Dissolve 0.2 g in 15 ml of a 28 g/l solution of *potassium hydroxide R* in *alcohol R* and boil under a reflux condenser for 15 min. Add 0.5 ml of *glacial acetic acid R* and 1 ml of a 50 g/l solution of *cobalt nitrate R* in *ethanol R*. An intense blue colour develops.

TESTS

Optical rotation (*2.2.7*): − 0.10° to + 0.10°.

Dissolve 2.5 g in *alcohol R* and dilute to 25.0 ml with the same solvent.

Related substances. Thin-layer chromatography (*2.2.27*).

Test solution (a). Dissolve 0.20 g of the substance to be examined in *methylene chloride R* and dilute to 10 ml with the same solvent.

Test solution (b). Dilute 1 ml of test solution (a) to 10 ml with *methylene chloride R*.

Reference solution (a). Dissolve 5.0 mg of *meprobamate CRS* in *methylene chloride R* and dilute to 50 ml with the same solvent.

Reference solution (b). Dilute 1 ml of test solution (b) to 50 ml with *methylene chloride R*.

Monographs C

Reference solution (c). Dilute 5 ml of reference solution (b) to 10 ml with *methylene chloride R*.

Reference solution (d). Dissolve 20 mg of *carisoprodol CRS* in *methylene chloride R* and dilute to 10 ml with the same solvent.

Reference solution (e). Dissolve 10 mg of *carisoprodol impurity A CRS* in 5 ml of reference solution (d) and dilute to 50 ml with *methylene chloride R*.

Plate: *TLC silica gel plate R*.

Mobile phase: *acetone R, methylene chloride R* (20:80 *V/V*).

Application: 5 μl.

Development: over a path of 15 cm.

Drying: in air for 15 min.

Detection: spray with a solution prepared as follows: dissolve 5 g of *phosphomolybdic acid R* in a mixture of 50 ml of *glacial acetic acid R* and 10 ml of *sulphuric acid R*, and dilute to 100 ml with *glacial acetic acid R*. Heat the plate at 100-105 °C for 30 min.

System suitability:

- the chromatogram obtained with reference solution (c) shows 1 clearly visible spot,
- the chromatogram obtained with reference solution (e) shows 2 clearly separated spots.

Limits: in the chromatogram obtained with test solution (a):

- *impurity D*: any spot due to impurity D is not more intense than the spot in the chromatogram obtained with reference solution (a) (0.5 per cent),
- *any other impurity*: any spot, apart from the principal spot and any spot due to impurity D, is not more intense than the spot in the chromatogram obtained with reference solution (b) (0.2 per cent).

Heavy metals (*2.4.8*): maximum 10 ppm.

2.0 g complies with limit test C. Prepare the standard using 2 ml of *lead standard solution (10 ppm Pb) R*.

Loss on drying (*2.2.32*): maximum 0.5 per cent, determined on 1.000 g *in vacuo* at 60 °C for 3 h.

Sulphated ash (*2.4.14*): maximum 0.1 per cent, determined on 1.0 g.

ASSAY

Dissolve 0.100 g in 15 ml of a 25 per cent *V/V* solution of *sulphuric acid R* and boil under a reflux condenser for 3 h. Cool, dissolve by cautiously adding 30 ml of *water R*, cool again and place in a steam-distillation apparatus. Add 40 ml of *strong sodium hydroxide solution R* and distil immediately by passing steam through the mixture. Collect the distillate into 40 ml of a 40 g/l solution of *boric acid R* until the total volume in the receiver reaches about 200 ml. Add 0.25 ml of *methyl red mixed solution R*. Titrate with *0.1 M hydrochloric acid*, until the colour changes from green to violet. Carry out a blank titration.

1 ml of *0.1 M hydrochloric acid* is equivalent to 13.02 mg of $C_{12}H_{24}N_2O_4$.

IMPURITIES

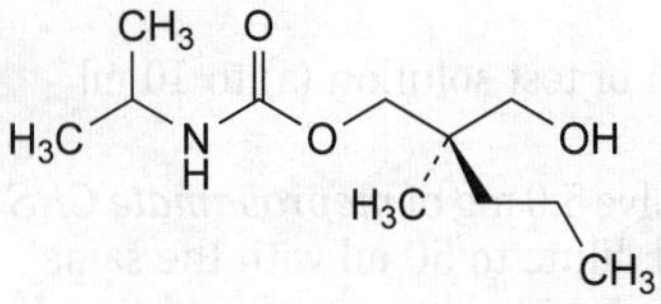

A. (2*RS*)-2-(hydroxymethyl)-2-methylpentyl (1-methylethyl)carbamate,

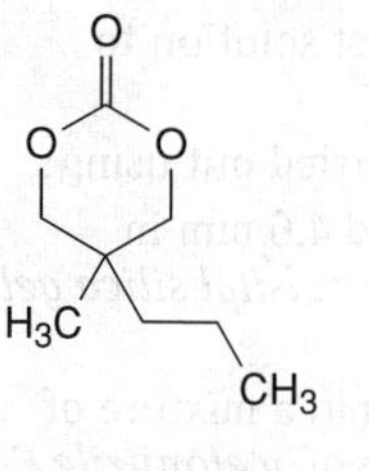

B. 5-methyl-5-propyl-1,3-dioxan-2-one,

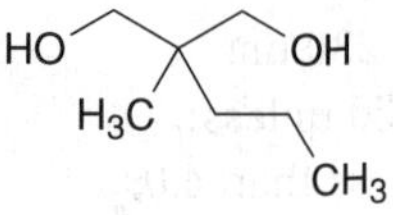

C. 2-methyl-2-propylpropane-1,3-diol,

D. meprobamate.

01/2005:0886

CARMELLOSE CALCIUM

Carmellosum calcicum

DEFINITION

Calcium salt of a partly *O*-carboxymethylated cellulose.

CHARACTERS

Appearance: white or yellowish-white powder, hygroscopic after drying.

Solubility: practically insoluble in acetone, in alcohol and in toluene. It swells with water to form a suspension.

IDENTIFICATION

A. Shake 0.1 g thoroughly with 10 ml of *water R*. Add 2 ml of *dilute sodium hydroxide solution R* and allow to stand for 10 min (solution A). Dilute 1 ml of solution A to 5 ml with *water R*. To 0.05 ml add 0.5 ml of a 0.5 g/l solution of *chromotropic acid, sodium salt R* in a 75 per cent *m/m* solution of *sulphuric acid R* and heat on a water-bath for 10 min. A reddish-violet colour develops.

B. Shake 5 ml of solution A obtained in identification test A with 10 ml of *acetone R*. A white, flocculent precipitate is produced.

C. Shake 5 ml of solution A obtained in identification test A with 1 ml of *ferric chloride solution R1*. A brown, flocculent precipitate is formed.

D. Ignite 1 g and dissolve the residue in a mixture of 5 ml of *acetic acid R* and 10 ml of *water R*. Filter if necessary and boil the filtrate for a few minutes. Cool and neutralise with *dilute ammonia R1*. The solution gives reaction (a) of calcium (*2.3.1*).

TESTS

Solution S. Shake 1.0 g with 50 ml of *distilled water R*, add 5 ml of *dilute sodium hydroxide solution R* and dilute to 100 ml with *distilled water R*.

Alkalinity. Shake 1.0 g thoroughly with 50 ml of *carbon dioxide-free water R* and add 0.05 ml of *phenolphthalein solution R*. No red colour develops.

Chlorides (*2.4.4*): maximum 0.36 per cent.

Heat 28 ml of solution S with 10 ml of *dilute nitric acid R* on a water-bath until a flocculent precipitate is produced. Cool, centrifuge and separate the supernatant liquid. Wash the precipitate with 3 quantities, each of 10 ml, of *water R*, centrifuging each time. Combine the supernatant liquid and the washings and dilute to 100 ml with *water R*. To 25 ml add 6 ml of *dilute nitric acid R* and dilute to 50 ml with *water R*. Dilute 10 ml of the solution to 15 ml with *water R*.

Sulphates (*2.4.13*): maximum 1 per cent.

Heat 20 ml of solution S with 1 ml of *hydrochloric acid R* on a water-bath until a flocculent precipitate is produced. Cool, centrifuge and separate the supernatant liquid. Wash the precipitate with 3 quantities, each of 10 ml, of *distilled water R*, centrifuging each time. Combine the supernatant liquid and the washings and dilute to 100 ml with *distilled water R*. To 25 ml add 1 ml of *dilute hydrochloric acid R* and dilute to 50 ml with *distilled water R*.

Heavy metals (*2.4.8*): maximum 20 ppm.

1.0 g complies with limit test D. Prepare the standard using 2 ml of *lead standard solution (10 ppm Pb) R*.

Loss on drying (*2.2.32*): maximum 10.0 per cent, determined on 1.000 g by drying in an oven at 100-105 °C for 4 h.

Sulphated ash (*2.4.14*): 10.0 per cent to 20.0 per cent, determined on 1.0 g in a platinum crucible.

STORAGE

In an airtight container.

01/2005:0472

CARMELLOSE SODIUM

Carmellosum natricum

DEFINITION

Carmellose sodium (carboxymethylcellulose sodium) is the sodium salt of a partly *O*-carboxymethylated cellulose. It contains not less than 6.5 per cent and not more than 10.8 per cent of sodium (Na), calculated with reference to the dried substance.

CHARACTERS

A white or almost white, granular powder, hygroscopic after drying, practically insoluble in acetone, in ethanol and in toluene. It is easily dispersed in water giving colloidal solutions.

IDENTIFICATION

A. To 10 ml of solution S (see Tests) add 1 ml of *copper sulphate solution R*. A blue, cotton-like precipitate is formed.

B. Boil 5 ml of solution S for a few minutes. No precipitate is formed.

C. The solution prepared from the sulphated ash in the test for heavy metals gives the reactions of sodium (*2.3.1*).

TESTS

Solution S. Sprinkle a quantity of the substance to be examined equivalent to 1.0 g of the dried substance onto 90 ml of *carbon dioxide-free water R* at 40 °C to 50 °C stirring vigorously. Continue stirring until a colloidal solution is obtained, cool and dilute to 100 ml with *carbon dioxide-free water R*.

Appearance of solution. Solution S is not more opalescent than reference suspension III (*2.2.1*) and not more intensely coloured than reference solution Y_6 (*2.2.2, Method II*).

pH (*2.2.3*). The pH of solution S is 6.0 to 8.0.

Apparent viscosity. While stirring, introduce a quantity of the substance to be examined equivalent to 2.00 g of the dried substance into 50 ml of *water R* heated to 90 °C. For a product of low viscosity, use if necessary, the quantity required to give the concentration indicated on the label. Allow to cool, dilute to 100.0 ml with *water R* and stir until dissolution is complete. Determine the viscosity (*2.2.10*) using a rotating viscometer at 20 °C and a shear rate of 10 s^{-1}. If it is impossible to obtain a shear rate of exactly 10 s^{-1}, use a shear rate slightly higher and a rate slightly lower and interpolate. The apparent viscosity is not less than 75 per cent and not more than 140 per cent of the value stated on the label.

Sodium glycollate. Place a quantity of the substance to be examined equivalent to 0.500 g of dried substance in a beaker. Add 5 ml of *acetic acid R* and 5 ml of *water R*. Stir until dissolution is complete (about 30 min). Add 80 ml of *acetone R* and 2 g of *sodium chloride R*. Filter through a fast filter paper impregnated with *acetone R* into a volumetric flask, rinse the beaker and filter with *acetone R* and dilute the filtrate to 100.0 ml with the same solvent. Allow to stand for 24 h without shaking. Use the clear supernatant liquid to prepare the test solution.

In a volumetric flask, dissolve 0.310 g of *glycollic acid R*, previously dried *in vacuo* over *diphosphorus pentoxide R*, in *water R* and dilute to 1000.0 ml with the same solvent. Place 5.0 ml of this solution in a volumetric flask, add 5 ml of *acetic acid R* and allow to stand for about 30 min. Add 80 ml of *acetone R* and 2 g of *sodium chloride R* and dilute to 100.0 ml with *acetone R*. Use this solution to prepare the reference solution.

Place 2.0 ml of each solution in a separate 25 ml volumetric flask. Heat on a water-bath to eliminate acetone. Cool to room temperature and add 5.0 ml of *2,7-dihydroxynaphthalene solution R* to each flask. Shake and add 15.0 ml of *2,7-dihydroxynaphthalene solution R*. Close the flasks with aluminium foil and heat on a water-bath for 20 min. Cool under running water and dilute to 25.0 ml with *sulphuric acid R*. Within 10 min, transfer 10.0 ml of each solution to a flat-bottomed tube. Examine the solutions viewing vertically. The test solution is not more intensely coloured than the reference solution (0.4 per cent).

Chlorides (*2.4.4*). Dilute 2 ml of solution S to 15 ml with *water R*. The solution complies with the limit test for chlorides (0.25 per cent).

Heavy metals (*2.4.8*). To the residue obtained in the determination of the sulphated ash, add 1 ml of *hydrochloric acid R* and evaporate on a water-bath. Take up the residue in 20 ml of *water R*. 12 ml of the solution complies with limit test A for heavy metals (20 ppm). Prepare the standard using *lead standard solution (1 ppm Pb) R*.

Loss on drying (*2.2.32*). Not more than 10.0 per cent, determined on 1.000 g by drying in an oven at 100 °C to 105 °C.

Sulphated ash (*2.4.14*): 20.0 per cent to 33.3 per cent, determined on 1.0 g using a mixture of equal volumes of *sulphuric acid R* and *water R* and calculated with reference to the dried substance. These limits correspond to a content of 6.5 per cent to 10.8 per cent of sodium (Na).

LABELLING

The label states the apparent viscosity in millipascal seconds for a 20 g/l solution; for a product of low viscosity, the label states the concentration of the solution to be used and the apparent viscosity in millipascal seconds.

01/2005:1186

CARMELLOSE SODIUM, LOW-SUBSTITUTED

Carmellosum natricum, substitutum humile

DEFINITION

Low-substituted carmellose sodium (sodium carboxymethylcellulose) is the sodium salt of a partly *O*-(carboxymethylated) cellulose. It contains not less than 2.0 per cent and not more than 4.5 per cent of sodium (Na), calculated with reference to the dried substance.

CHARACTERS

A white or almost white powder or short fibres, practically insoluble in acetone, in ethanol and in toluene. It swells in water to form a gel.

IDENTIFICATION

A. Shake 1 g with 100 ml of a 100 g/l solution of *sodium hydroxide R*. A suspension is produced.

B. Shake 1 g with 50 ml of *water R*. Transfer 1 ml of the mixture to a test tube, add 1 ml of *water R* and 0.05 ml of a freshly prepared 40 g/l solution of *α-naphthol R* in *methanol R*. Incline the test tube and add carefully 2 ml of *sulphuric acid R* down the side so that it forms a lower layer. A reddish-purple colour develops at the interface.

C. It complies with the test for sulphated ash (*2.4.14*) (see Tests).

D. The solution prepared from the sulphated ash for the test for heavy metals gives reaction (a) of sodium (*2.3.1*).

TESTS

pH (*2.2.3*). Shake 1 g with 100 ml of *carbon dioxide-free water R* for 5 min. Centrifuge. The pH of the suspension is 6.0 to 8.5.

Sodium chloride and sodium glycollate. The sum of the percentages of sodium chloride and sodium glycollate is not more than 0.5 per cent, calculated with reference to the dried substance.

Sodium chloride. Place 5.00 g in a 250 ml conical flask, add 50 ml of *water R* and 5 ml of *strong hydrogen peroxide solution R* and heat on a water bath for 20 min, stirring occasionally to ensure total hydration. Cool, add 100 ml of *water R* and 10 ml of *nitric acid R*. Titrate with *0.05 M silver nitrate* determining the end-point potentiometrically (*2.2.20*) using a silver-based indicator electrode and a double-junction reference electrode containing a 100 g/l solution of *potassium nitrate R* in the outer jacket and a standard filling solution in the inner jacket.

1 ml of *0.05 M silver nitrate* is equivalent to 2.922 mg of NaCl.

Sodium glycollate. Place a quantity of the substance to be examined equivalent to 0.500 g of the dried substance in a beaker. Add 5 ml of *glacial acetic acid R* and 5 ml of *water R* and stir to ensure total hydration (about 30 min). Add 80 ml of *acetone R* and 2 g of *sodium chloride R*. Stir for several minutes to ensure complete precipitation of the carboxymethylcellulose. Filter through a fast filter paper impregnated with *acetone R* into a volumetric flask, rinse the beaker and filter with *acetone R* and dilute the filtrate to 100.0 ml with the same solvent. Allow to stand for 24 h without shaking. Use the clear supernatant as the test solution.

Prepare the reference solutions as follows: in a 100 ml volumetric flask, dissolve 0.100 g of *glycollic acid R*, previously dried *in vacuo* over *diphosphorus pentoxide R*, in *water R* and dilute to 100.0 ml with the same solvent. Transfer 0.5 ml, 1.0 ml, 1.5 ml and 2.0 ml of the solution to separate volumetric flasks; dilute the contents of each flask to 5.0 ml with *water R*, add 5 ml of *glacial acetic acid R*, dilute to 100.0 ml with *acetone R* and mix.

Transfer 2.0 ml of the test solution and 2.0 ml of each of the reference solutions to separate 25 ml volumetric flasks. Heat the uncovered flasks in a water-bath to eliminate the acetone. Allow to cool and add 5.0 ml of *2,7-dihydroxynaphthalene solution R* to each flask. Mix, add a further 15.0 ml of *2,7-dihydroxynaphthalene solution R* and mix again. Close the flasks with aluminium foil and heat in a water-bath for 20 min. Cool and dilute to 25.0 ml with *sulphuric acid R*.

Measure the absorbance (*2.2.25*) of each solution at 540 nm. Prepare a blank using 2.0 ml of a solution containing 5 per cent *V/V* each of *glacial acetic acid R* and *water R* in *acetone R*. Prepare a standard curve using the absorbances obtained with the reference solutions. From the standard curve and the absorbance of the test solution, determine the mass *a*, in milligrams, of glycollic acid in the substance to be examined and calculate the content of sodium glycollate from the formula:

$$\frac{10 \times 1.29 \times a}{(100 - b)\, m}$$

1.29 = the factor converting glycollic acid to sodium glycollate,

b = the loss on drying as a percentage,

m = the mass of the substance to be examined, in grams.

Water-soluble substances. Not more than 70.0 per cent. Disperse 5.00 g in 400.0 ml of *water R* and stir for 1 min every 10 min during the first 30 min. Allow to stand for 1 h and centrifuge, if necessary. Decant 100.0 ml of the supernatant liquid onto a fast filter paper in a vacuum filtration funnel, apply vacuum and collect 75.0 ml of the filtrate. Evaporate to dryness and dry the residue at 100-105 °C for 4 h.

Heavy metals (*2.4.8*). To the residue obtained in the determination of the sulphated ash add 1 ml of *hydrochloric acid R* and evaporate on a water-bath. Take up the residue in 20 ml of *water R*. 12 ml of the solution complies with limit test A for heavy metals (20 ppm). Prepare the standard using *lead standard solution (1 ppm Pb) R*.

Loss on drying (*2.2.32*). Not more than 10.0 per cent, determined on 1.000 g by drying in an oven at 100-105 °C.

Sulphated ash (*2.4.14*): 6.5 per cent to 13.5 per cent, determined on 1.0 g using a mixture of equal volumes of *sulphuric acid R* and *water R* and calculated with reference to the dried substance. These limits correspond to a content of 2.0 per cent to 4.5 per cent of Na.

The following test concerning the pharmaco-technological properties may be carried out depending on the intended formulation. It is not a mandatory requirement.

Settling volume. In a 100 ml graduated cylinder, place 20 ml of *2-propanol R*, add 5.0 g of the substance to be examined and shake vigorously. Dilute to 30 ml with *2-propanol R* then to 50 ml with *water R* and shake vigorously. Within 15 min, repeat the shaking three times. Allow to stand for 4 h and determine the volume of the settled mass (15.0 ml to 35.0 ml).

01/2005:1187

CARMUSTINE

Carmustinum

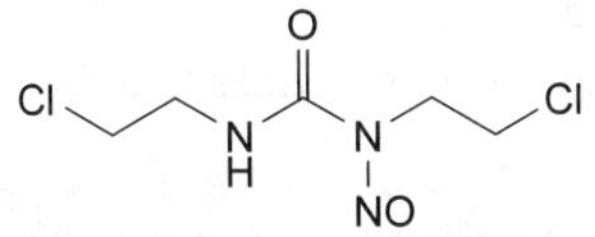

$C_5H_9Cl_2N_3O_2$ M_r 214.1

DEFINITION

Carmustine contains not less than 98.0 per cent and not more than the equivalent of 102.0 per cent of 1,3-bis(2-chloroethyl)-1-nitrosourea, calculated with reference to the anhydrous substance.

CHARACTERS

A yellowish, granular powder, very slightly soluble in water, very soluble in methylene chloride, freely soluble in ethanol.

It melts at about 31 °C with decomposition.

IDENTIFICATION

Examine by infrared absorption spectrophotometry(*2.2.24*), comparing with the *Ph. Eur. reference spectrum of carmustine.* Examine the melted substances prepared as films.

TESTS

1,3-bis(2-chloroethyl)urea (impurity A). Examine by thin-layer chromatography (*2.2.27*), using a suitable silica gel as the coating substance.

Test solution. Dissolve 0.10 g of the substance to be examined in *methylene chloride R* and dilute to 5 ml with the same solvent.

Reference solution (a). Dissolve 2 mg of *carmustine impurity A CRS* in *methylene chloride R* and dilute to 10 ml with the same solvent.

Reference solution (b). Dilute 1 ml of the test solution to 10 ml with *methylene chloride R.* To 5 ml of this solution, add 5 ml of reference solution (a).

Apply separately to the plate 2 µl of each solution. Develop over a path of 10 cm using a mixture of 10 volumes of *methanol R* and 90 volumes of *methylene chloride R.* Allow the plate to dry in air. Spray with *diethylamine R* and heat at 125 °C for 10 min. Allow to cool and spray with *silver nitrate solution R2.* Expose to ultraviolet light at 365 nm until brown to black spots appear. Any spot corresponding to carmustine impurity A in the chromatogram obtained with the test solution is not more intense than the spot in the chromatogram obtained with reference solution (a) (1 per cent). The test is not valid unless the chromatogram obtained with reference solution (b) shows two clearly separated spots.

Water (*2.5.12*). Not more than 1.0 per cent, determined on 0.50 g by the semi-micro determination of water.

ASSAY

Dissolve 0.100 g in 30 ml of *ethanol R* and dilute to 100.0 ml with *water R.* Dilute 3.0 ml of the solution to 100.0 ml with *water R.* Measure the absorbance (*2.2.25*) at the maximum at 230 nm.

Calculate the content of $C_5H_9Cl_2N_3O_2$ taking the specific absorbance to be 270.

STORAGE

Store in an airtight container, protected from light, at a temperature of 2 °C to 8 °C.

IMPURITIES

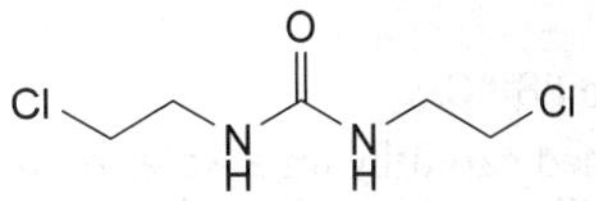

A. 1,3-bis(2-chloroethyl)urea.

01/2005:0597

CARNAUBA WAX

Cera carnauba

DEFINITION

Purified wax obtained from the leaves of *Copernicia cerifera* Mart.

CHARACTERS

Appearance: pale yellow or yellow powder, flakes or hard masses.

Solubility: practically insoluble in water, soluble on heating in ethyl acetate and in xylene, practically insoluble in alcohol.

Relative density: about 0.97.

IDENTIFICATION

Thin-layer chromatography (*2.2.27*).

Test solution. Dissolve 0.10 g of the substance to be examined with heating in 5 ml of *chloroform R.* Use the warm solution.

Reference solution. Dissolve 5 mg of *menthol R*, 5 µl of *menthyl acetate R* and 5 mg of *thymol R* in 10 ml of *toluene R.*

Plate: *TLC silica gel plate R.*

Mobile phase: *ethyl acetate R, chloroform R (2:98 V/V).*

Application: 30 µl of the test solution and 10 µl of the reference solution as bands 20 mm by 3 mm.

Development: over half of the plate.

Drying: in air.

Detection: spray with a freshly prepared 200 g/l solution of *phosphomolybdic acid R* in *alcohol R* (about 10 ml for a 20 cm plate). Heat at 100-105 °C for 10-15 min.

Results: the chromatogram obtained with the reference solution shows in the lower part a dark blue zone (menthol), above this zone a reddish zone (thymol) and in the upper part a dark blue zone (menthyl acetate). The chromatogram obtained with the test solution shows a large blue zone (triacontanol = melissyl alcohol) at a level between the thymol and menthol zones in the chromatogram obtained with the reference solution. Further blue zones are visible in the upper part of the chromatogram obtained with the test solution, at levels between those of the menthyl acetate and thymol zones in the chromatogram obtained with the reference solution; above these zones further zones are visible in the chromatogram obtained with the test solution; the zone with the highest R_f value is very pronounced. A number of faint zones are visible below the triacontanol zone and the starting point is coloured blue.

TESTS

Appearance of solution. The solution is clear (*2.2.1*) and not more intensely coloured than a 50 mg/l solution of *potassium dichromate R* (*2.2.2, Method II*).

Dissolve 0.10 g with heating in *chloroform R* and dilute to 10 ml with the same solvent.

Melting point (*2.2.15*): 80 °C to 88 °C.

Melt the substance to be examined carefully on a water-bath before introduction into the capillary tubes. Allow the tubes to stand in the refrigerator for 24 h or at 0 °C for 2 h.

Acid value: 2 to 7.

To 2.000 g (*m* g) in a 250 ml conical flask fitted with a reflux condenser add 40 ml of *xylene R* and a few glass beads. Heat with stirring until the substance is completely dissolved. Add 20 ml of *alcohol R* and 1 ml of *bromothymol blue solution R3* and titrate the hot solution with *0.5 M alcoholic potassium hydroxide* until a green colour persisting for at least 10 s is obtained (n_1 ml). Carry out a blank test (n_2 ml). Calculate the acid value from the expression:

$$\frac{28.05\,(n_1 - n_2)}{m}$$

Saponification value: 78 to 95.

To 2.000 g (*m* g) in a 250 ml conical flask fitted with a reflux condenser add 40 ml of *xylene R* and a few glass beads. Heat with stirring until the substance is completely dissolved. Add 20 ml of *alcohol R* and 20.0 ml of *0.5 M alcoholic potassium hydroxide*. Boil under a reflux condenser for 3 h. Add 1 ml of *phenolphthalein solution R1* and titrate the hot solution immediately with *0.5 M hydrochloric acid* until the red colour disappears. Repeat the heating and titration until the colour no longer reappears on heating (n_3 ml). Carry out a blank test (n_4 ml). Calculate the saponification value from the expression:

$$\frac{28.05\,(n_4 - n_3)}{m}$$

Total ash (*2.4.16*): maximum 0.25 per cent, determined on 2.0 g.

STORAGE

Protected from light.

01/2005:1972

CARTEOLOL HYDROCHLORIDE

Carteololi hydrochloridum

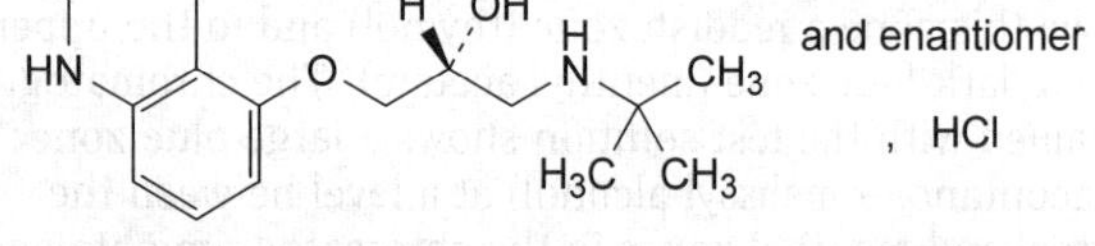

$C_{16}H_{25}N_2O_3Cl$ M_r 328.8

DEFINITION

5-[(2*RS*)-3-[(1,1-Dimethylethyl)amino]-2-hydroxypropoxy]-3,4-dihydroquinolin-2(1*H*)-one hydrochloride.

Content: 99.0 per cent to 101.0 per cent (dried substance).

CHARACTERS

Appearance: white crystals or crystalline powder.

Solubility: soluble in water, sparingly soluble in methanol, slightly soluble in alcohol, practically insoluble in methylene chloride.

IDENTIFICATION

A. Infrared absorption spectrophotometry (*2.2.24*).

Comparison: *Ph. Eur. reference spectrum of carteolol hydrochloride.*

B. It gives reaction (a) of chlorides (*2.3.1*).

TESTS

Appearance of solution. The solution is clear (*2.2.1*) and colourless (*2.2.2, Method II*).

Dissolve 0.300 g in *water R* and dilute to 10 ml with the same solvent.

pH (*2.2.3*): 5.0 to 6.0.

Dissolve 0.250 g in *carbon dioxide-free water R* and dilute to 25 ml with the same solvent.

Related substances. Liquid chromatography (*2.2.29*).

Test solution. Dissolve 20.0 mg of the substance to be examined in the mobile phase and dilute to 10.0 ml with the mobile phase.

Reference solution (a). Dilute 1.0 ml of the test solution to 100.0 ml with the mobile phase.

Reference solution (b). Dilute 1.0 ml of reference solution (a) to 10.0 ml with the mobile phase.

Reference solution (c). Dissolve 10 mg of *carteolol for system suitability CRS* in the mobile phase and dilute to 5 ml with the mobile phase.

Reference solution (d). Dilute 5.0 ml of reference solution (b) to 10.0 ml with the mobile phase.

Column:

- *size*: l = 0.25 m, Ø = 4.6 mm,
- *stationary phase*: *octadecylsilyl silica gel for chromatography R* (5 µm).

Mobile phase: mix 1 volume of *methanol R2*, 20 volumes of *acetonitrile R* and 79 volumes of a 2.82 g/l solution of *sodium hexanesulphonate R*.

Flow rate: 1 ml/min.

Detection: spectrophotometer at 252 nm.

Injection: 20 µl.

System suitability:

- the chromatogram obtained with reference solution (c) is similar to the chromatogram provided with *carteolol for system suitability CRS*; the peaks due to impurity H and carteolol show base-line separation,
- *signal-to-noise ratio*: minimum 10 for the principal peak in the chromatogram obtained with reference solution (d),
- *number of theoretical plates*: minimum 6000, calculated for the principal peak in the chromatogram obtained with reference solution (a).

Limits: locate impurity H by comparison with the chromatogram provided with *carteolol for system suitability CRS*,

- *impurity H*: not more than twice the area of the principal peak in the chromatogram obtained with reference solution (b) (0.2 per cent),
- *any other impurity*: not more than the area of the principal peak in the chromatogram obtained with reference solution (b) (0.1 per cent),
- *total*: not more than half the area of the principal peak in the chromatogram obtained with reference solution (a) (0.5 per cent),

– *disregard limit*: 0.2 times the area of the principal peak in the chromatogram obtained with reference solution (b) (0.02 per cent).

Loss on drying (*2.2.32*): maximum 0.5 per cent, determined on 1.000 g by drying in an oven at 100-105 °C for 3 h.

Sulphated ash (*2.4.14*): maximum 0.1 per cent, determined on 1.0 g.

ASSAY

Dissolve 0.250 g in 60 ml of *alcohol R*. Add 5.0 ml of *0.01 M hydrochloric acid.* Carry out a potentiometric titration (*2.2.20*), using *0.1 M sodium hydroxide*. Read the volume added between the 2 points of inflexion.

1 ml of *0.1 M sodium hydroxide* is equivalent to 32.88 mg of $C_{16}H_{25}N_2O_3Cl$.

STORAGE

In an airtight container.

IMPURITIES

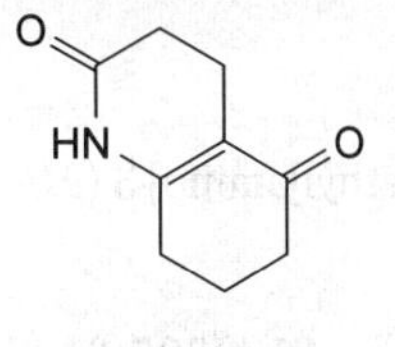

A. 4,6,7,8-tetrahydroquinoline-2,5(1*H*,3*H*)-dione,

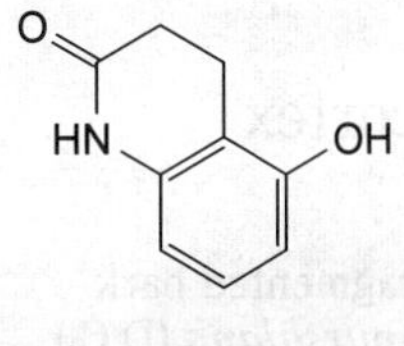

B. 5-hydroxy-3,4-dihydroquinolin-2(1*H*)-one,

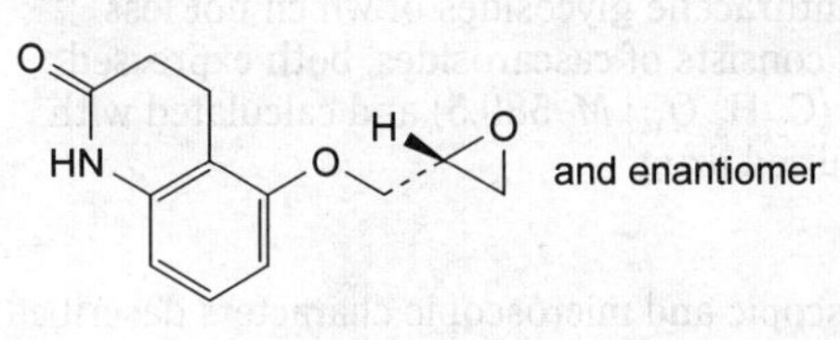

C. 5-[[(2*RS*)-oxiran-2-yl]methoxy]-3,4-dihydroquinolin-2(1*H*)-one,

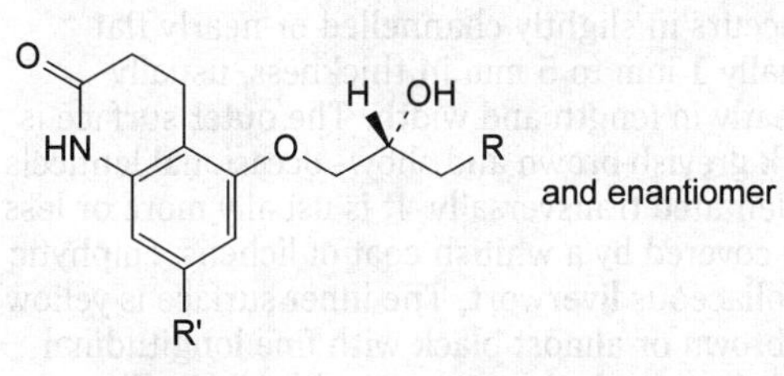

D. R = Cl, R′ = H: 5-[(2*RS*)-3-chloro-2-hydroxypropoxy]-3,4-dihydroquinolin-2(1*H*)-one,

F. R = OCH_3, R′ = H: 5-[(2*RS*)-2-hydroxy-3-methoxypropoxy]-3,4-dihydroquinolin-2(1*H*)-one,

G. R = OH, R′ = H: 5-[(2*RS*)-2,3-dihydroxypropoxy]-3,4-dihydroquinolin-2(1*H*)-one,

I. R = NH-C$(CH_3)_3$, R′ = Br: 7-bromo-5-[(2*RS*)-3-[(1,1-(dimethylethyl)amino]-2-hydroxypropoxy]-3,4-dihydroquinolin-2(1*H*)-one,

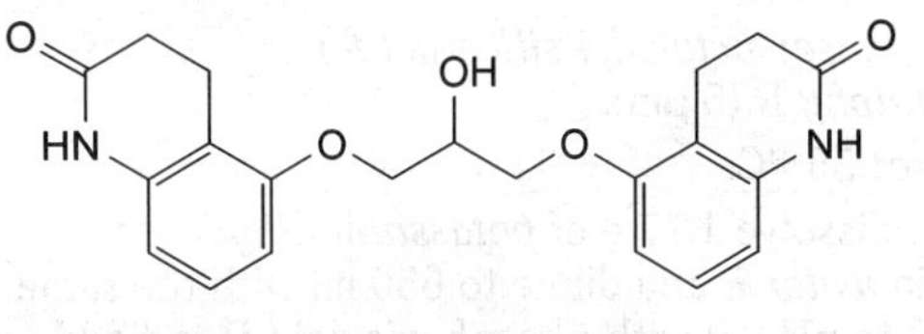

E. 5,5′-[(2-hydroxypropan-1,3-diyl)bis(oxy)]bis(3,4-dihydroquinolin-2(1*H*)-one),

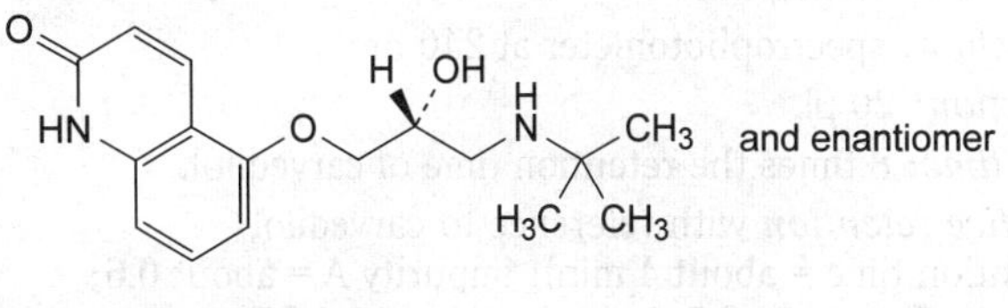

H. 5-[(2*RS*)-3-[(1,1-dimethylethyl)amino]-2-hydroxypropoxy]quinolin-2(1*H*)-one.

01/2005:1745

CARVEDILOL

Carvedilolum

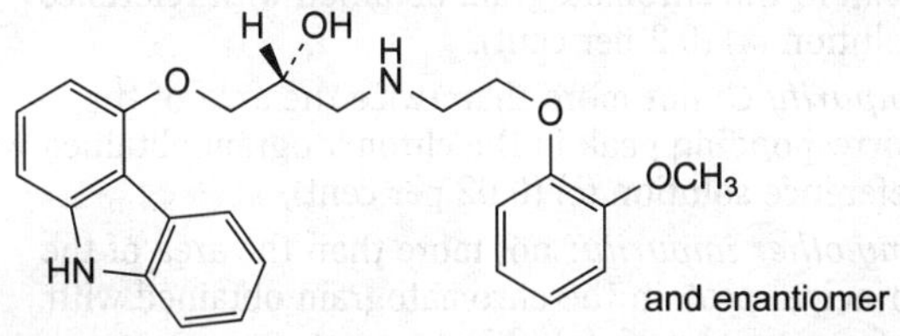

$C_{24}H_{26}N_2O_4$ *M_r* 406.5

DEFINITION

(2*RS*)-1-(9*H*-Carbazol-4-yloxy)-3-[[2-(2-methoxyphenoxy)ethyl]amino]propan-2-ol.

Content: 99.0 per cent to 101.0 per cent (dried substance).

CHARACTERS

Appearance: white or almost white, crystalline powder.

Solubility: practically insoluble in water, slightly soluble in alcohol, practically insoluble in dilute acids.

It shows polymorphism.

IDENTIFICATION

Infrared absorption spectrophotometry (*2.2.24*).

Comparison: *Ph. Eur. reference spectrum of carvedilol.*

If the spectrum obtained shows differences, dissolve the substance to be examined in *2-propanol R*, evaporate to dryness and record a new spectrum using the residue.

TESTS

Related substances. Liquid chromatography (*2.2.29*).

Test solution. Dissolve 25.0 mg of the substance to be examined in the mobile phase and dilute to 25.0 ml with the mobile phase.

Reference solution (a). Dilute 1.0 ml of the test solution to 100.0 ml with the mobile phase. Dilute 1.0 ml of this solution to 10.0 ml with the mobile phase.

Reference solution (b). Dissolve 5.0 mg of *carvedilol impurity C CRS* in 5.0 ml of the test solution and dilute to 100.0 ml with the mobile phase.

Reference solution (c). Dilute 1.0 ml of reference solution (b) to 100.0 ml with the mobile phase. Dilute 2.0 ml of this solution to 10.0 ml with the mobile phase.

Column:

– *size*: *l* = 0.125 m, Ø = 4.6 mm,

- *stationary phase*: *octylsilyl silica gel for chromatography R* (5 µm),
- *temperature*: 55 °C.

Mobile phase: dissolve 1.77 g of *potassium dihydrogen phosphate R* in *water R* and dilute to 650 ml with the same solvent; adjust to pH 2.0 with *phosphoric acid R* and add 350 ml of *acetonitrile R*.

Flow rate: 1.0 ml/min.

Detection: spectrophotometer at 240 nm.

Injection: 20 µl.

Run time: 8 times the retention time of carvedilol.

Relative retention with reference to carvedilol (retention time = about 4 min): impurity A = about 0.6; impurity C = about 3.5; impurity B = about 6.7.

System suitability: reference solution (b):
- *resolution*: minimum 17 between the peaks due to carvedilol and to impurity C.

Limits:
- *correction factor*: for the calculation of content, multiply the peak area of impurity A by 2,
- *impurity A*: not more than twice the area of the principal peak in the chromatogram obtained with reference solution (a) (0.2 per cent),
- *impurity C*: not more than twice the area of the corresponding peak in the chromatogram obtained with reference solution (c) (0.02 per cent),
- *any other impurity*: not more than the area of the principal peak in the chromatogram obtained with reference solution (a) (0.1 per cent),
- *total*: not more than 5 times the area of the principal peak in the chromatogram obtained with reference solution (a) (0.5 per cent),
- *disregard limit*: the area of the principal peak in the chromatogram obtained with reference solution (c) (0.01 per cent).

Heavy metals (*2.4.8*): maximum 10 ppm.

2.0 g complies with limit test C. Prepare the standard using 2.0 ml of *lead standard solution (10 ppm Pb) R*.

Loss on drying (*2.2.32*): maximum 0.5 per cent, determined on 1.000 g by drying in an oven at 100-105 °C.

Sulphated ash (*2.4.14*): maximum 0.1 per cent, determined on 1.0 g.

ASSAY

Dissolve 0.350 g in 60 ml of *anhydrous acetic acid R*. Titrate with *0.1 M perchloric acid*, determining the end-point potentiometrically (*2.2.20*).

1 ml of *0.1 M perchloric acid* is equivalent to 40.65 mg of $C_{24}H_{26}N_2O_4$.

IMPURITIES

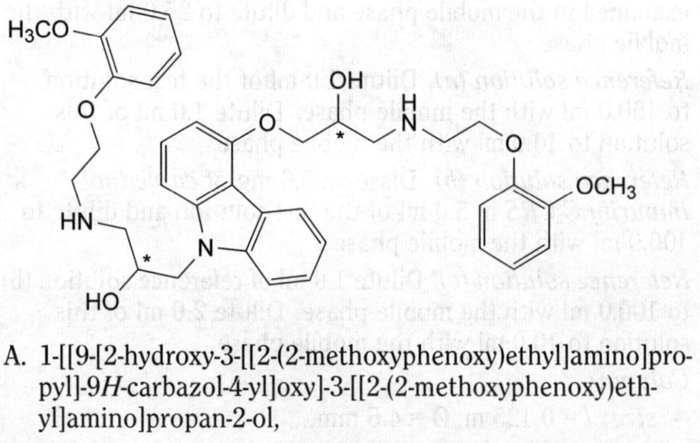

A. 1-[[9-[2-hydroxy-3-[[2-(2-methoxyphenoxy)ethyl]amino]propyl]-9*H*-carbazol-4-yl]oxy]-3-[[2-(2-methoxyphenoxy)ethyl]amino]propan-2-ol,

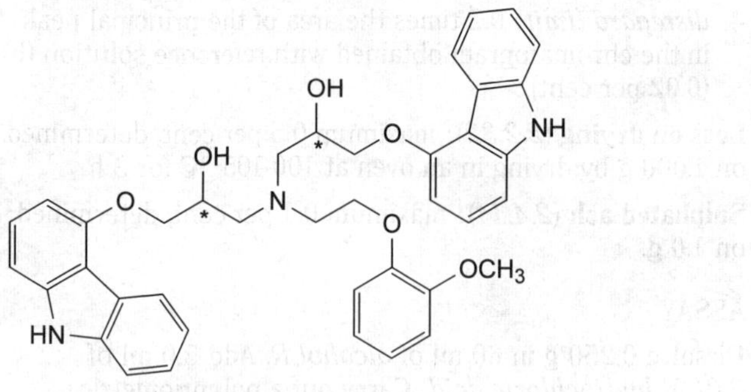

B. 1,1′-[[2-(2-methoxyphenoxy)ethyl]nitrilo]bis[3-(9*H*-carbazol-4-yloxy)propan-2-ol],

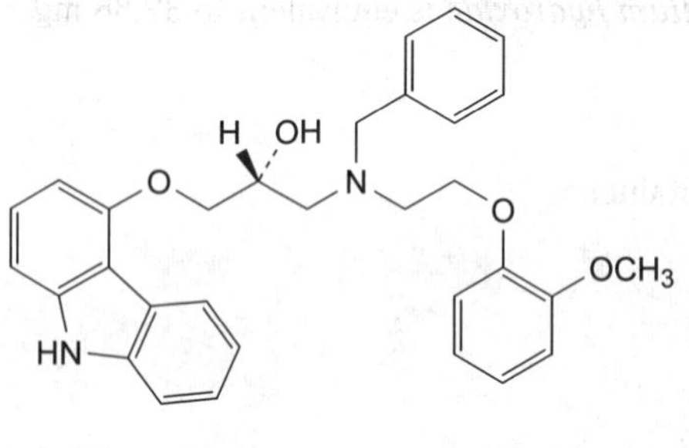

and enantiomer

C. (2*RS*)-1-[benzyl[2-(2-methoxyphenoxy)ethyl]amino]-3-(9*H*-carbazol-4-yloxy)propan-2-ol.

01/2005:0105

CASCARA

Rhamni purshianae cortex

DEFINITION

Cascara consists of the dried, whole or fragmented bark of *Rhamnus purshianus* D.C. (*Frangula purshiana* (D.C.) A. Gray ex J. C. Cooper). It contains not less than 8.0 per cent of hydroxyanthracene glycosides of which not less than 60 per cent consists of cascarosides, both expressed as cascaroside A ($C_{27}H_{32}O_{14}$; M_r 580.5) and calculated with reference to the dried drug.

CHARACTERS

It has the macroscopic and microscopic characters described under identification tests A and B.

IDENTIFICATION

A. The bark occurs in slightly channelled or nearly flat pieces, usually 1 mm to 5 mm in thickness, usually varying greatly in length and width. The outer surface is grey or dark greyish-brown and shows occasional lenticels that are orientated transversally. It is usually more or less completely covered by a whitish coat of lichens, epiphytic moss and foliaceous liverwort. The inner surface is yellow to reddish-brown or almost black with fine longitudinal striations; it turns red when treated with alkali. The yellow fracture is short and granular in the outer part and somewhat fibrous at the inner part.

B. Reduce to a powder (355). The powder is yellowish-brown. Examine under a microscope using *chloral hydrate solution R*. The powder shows: bundles of partly lignified phloem fibres accompanied by crystal sheaths containing prisms of calcium oxalate; groups of sclereids accompanied by crystal sheaths; cluster crystals of calcium oxalate; some parenchymatous cells contain a yellow substance which becomes deep red when treated with alkali; cork cells and, frequently, epiphytes; the latter may be liverworts, entire or in fragments, having a lamina one cell thick without a midrib and composed of isodiametric cells, or leaves of mosses, having a lamina one cell thick composed of elongated cells and possessing a midrib several cells thick.

C. Examine the chromatograms obtained in the test for "Other species of *Rhamnus*; anthrones" after spraying with a 50 g/l solution of *potassium hydroxide R* in *alcohol (50 per cent V/V) R* and heating. The chromatogram obtained with the test solution shows several reddish-brown zones with different intensities: there are four faint zones, three being situated at about the mid-point of the chromatogram and one in the lower third and there is a strong zone in the upper third of the chromatogram. Examine in ultraviolet light at 365 nm. The chromatogram obtained with the test solution shows several zones with the same fluorescence, situated above and particularly below (cascarosides) that corresponding to barbaloin in the chromatogram obtained with the reference solution.

D. Heat 0.2 g of the powdered drug (180) with 50 ml of *water R* on a water-bath for 15 min. Allow to cool and filter. To 10 ml of the filtrate add 20 ml of *hydrochloric acid R1* and heat on a water-bath for 15 min. Allow to cool, transfer to a separating funnel and shake with three quantities, each of 20 ml, of *ether R*. Reserve the aqueous layer (solution A).

(a) Combine the three ether extracts and shake with 10 ml of *dilute ammonia R2*. The aqueous layer becomes reddish-violet.

(b) Transfer solution A to a small flask, add 5 g of *ferric chloride R* and heat on a water-bath for 30 min. Allow to cool, transfer to a separating funnel and shake with 15 ml of *ether R*. Wash the ether layer with 10 ml of *water R*, discard the water and shake the ether layer with 5 ml of *dilute ammonia R2*. A red colour develops in the aqueous layer.

TESTS

Other species of *Rhamnus*; anthrones. Examine by thin-layer chromatography (*2.2.27*), using a suitable silica gel as the coating substance.

Test solution. To 0.5 g of the powdered drug (180) add 5 ml of *alcohol (70 per cent V/V) R* and heat to boiling. Cool and centrifuge. Decant the supernatant solution immediately and use within 30 min.

Reference solution. Dissolve 20 mg of *barbaloin R* in *alcohol (70 per cent V/V) R* and dilute to 10 ml with the same solvent.

Apply separately to the plate as bands 10 µl of each solution. Develop over a path of 10 cm using a mixture of 13 volumes of *water R*, 17 volumes of *methanol R* and 100 volumes of *ethyl acetate R*. Allow the plate to dry for 5 min, spray with about 10 ml of a 50 g/l solution of *potassium hydroxide R* in *alcohol (50 per cent V/V) R* and heat at 100 °C to 105 °C for 15 min. Examine the chromatograms immediately after heating. The chromatogram obtained with the reference solution shows, in the central part, a reddish-brown zone corresponding to barbaloin. Examine in ultraviolet light at 365 nm. The zone corresponding to barbaloin shows intense yellowish-brown fluorescence. In the chromatogram obtained with the test solution, no zone with orange-brown fluorescence is seen between the zone of barbaloin and the zones of cascarosides.

Apply to another plate as a band 10 µl of the test solution and develop as described above. Allow the plate to dry for not longer than 5 min and spray immediately with a 5 g/l solution of *nitrotetrazolium blue R* in *methanol R*. Examine the chromatogram immediately. No violet or greyish-blue zones appear.

Foreign matter (*2.8.2*). Not more than 1 per cent.

Loss on drying (*2.2.32*). Not more than 10.0 per cent, determined on 1.000 g of the powdered drug (180) by drying in an oven at 100 °C to 105 °C for 2 h.

Total ash (*2.4.16*). Not more than 7.0 per cent.

ASSAY

Carry out the assay protected from bright light in one day.

Stir 1.00 g of the powdered drug (180) into 100 ml of boiling *water R* and continue boiling and stirring for 5 min. Allow to cool, dilute to 100.0 ml with *water R*, shake, filter and discard the first 20 ml of filtrate. Transfer 10.0 ml of the filtrate to a separating funnel, add 0.1 ml of *1 M hydrochloric acid* and shake with two quantities, each of 20 ml, of a mixture of 1 volume of *ether R* and 3 volumes of *hexane R*. Wash the combined organic extracts with 5 ml of *water R*, discard the organic layer and return the rinsings to the aqueous layer. Shake the combined aqueous layers with four quantities, each of 30 ml, of *ethyl acetate R* freshly saturated with *water R*, (to 150 ml of *ethyl acetate R* add 15 ml of *water R*, shake for 3 min and allow to stand) on each occasion allowing separation to take place until the organic layer is clear. Combine the ethyl acetate extracts. Use the aqueous layer for the assay for cascarosides and the organic layer for the assay for hydroxyanthracene glycosides other than cascarosides.

Hydroxyanthracene glycosides other than cascarosides. Transfer the organic layer to a suitable flask and remove the solvent by distillation, evaporating almost to dryness. Dissolve the residue in 0.3 ml to 0.5 ml of *methanol R* and transfer to a volumetric flask, rinsing the first flask with warm *water R* and adding the rinsings to the methanolic solution. Allow to cool and dilute to 50.0 ml with *water R*. Transfer 20.0 ml of the solution to a 100 ml round-bottomed flask with a ground-glass neck and containing 2 g of *ferric chloride R* and 12 ml of *hydrochloric acid R*. Attach a reflux condenser and place the flask in a water-bath so that the level of the water is above that of the liquid in the flask and heat for 4 h. Allow to cool, transfer the solution to a separating funnel and rinse the flask successively with 3 ml to 4 ml of *1 M sodium hydroxide* and 3 ml to 4 ml of *water R*, adding the rinsings to the separating funnel. Shake the contents of the separating funnel with three quantities, each of 30 ml, of a mixture of 1 volume of *ether R* and 3 volumes of *hexane R*. Wash the combined organic layers with two quantities, each of 10 ml, of *water R* and discard the rinsings. Dilute the organic phase to 100.0 ml with the mixture of ether and hexane. Take 20.0 ml, evaporate carefully to dryness on a water-bath and dissolve the residue in 10.0 ml of a 5 g/l solution of *magnesium acetate R* in *methanol R*. Measure the absorbance (*2.2.25*) at 515 nm using *methanol R* as the compensation liquid.

Calculate the percentage content of hydroxyanthracene glycosides, expressed as cascaroside A, from the expression:

$$\frac{A \times 6.95}{m}$$

i.e. taking the specific absorbance to be 180.

A = absorbance at 515 nm,

m = mass of the sample in grams.

Measure the absorbance of the test solution at 440 nm. If the ratio of the absorbance at 515 nm to that at 440 nm is less than 2.4, the assay is not valid and must be repeated.

Monographs C

Cascarosides. Dilute the aqueous layer reserved for this assay to 50.0 ml with *water R*. Treat 20.0 ml of the solution as described above in the assay of hydroxyanthracene glycosides other than cascarosides.

Measure the absorbance of the test solution at 440 nm. If the ratio of the absorbance at 515 nm to that at 440 nm is less than 2.4, the assay is not valid and must be repeated.

Calculate the percentage content of cascarosides, expressed as cascaroside A from the expression:

$$\frac{A \times 6.95}{m}$$

i.e. taking the specific absorbance to be 180.

A = absorbance at 515 nm,

m = mass of the sample in grams.

Measure the absorbance of the test solution at 440 nm. If the ratio of the absorbance at 515 nm to that at 440 nm is less than 2.7, the assay is not valid and must be repeated.

STORAGE

Store protected from light.

01/2005:1496

CASSIA OIL

Cinnamomi cassiae aetheroleum

DEFINITION

Cassia oil is obtained by steam distillation of the leaves and young branches of *Cinnamomum cassia* Blume (*C. aromaticum* Nees).

CHARACTERS

A clear, mobile, yellow to reddish-brown liquid, with a characteristic odour reminiscent of cinnamic aldehyde.

IDENTIFICATION

First identification: B.

Second identification: A.

A. Examine by thin-layer chromatography (*2.2.27*), using a *TLC silica gel plate R*.

Test solution. Dissolve 0.5 ml of the substance to be examined in *acetone R* and dilute to 10 ml with the same solvent.

Reference solution. Dissolve 50 µl of *trans-cinnamic aldehyde R*, 10 µl of *eugenol R* and 50 mg of *coumarin R* in *acetone R* and dilute to 10 ml with the same solvent.

Apply to the plate, as bands, 10 µl of each solution. Develop over a path of 15 cm using a mixture of 10 volumes of *methanol R* and 90 volumes of *toluene R*. Allow the plate to dry in air and examine in ultraviolet light at 365 nm. The zone of blue fluorescence in the chromatogram obtained with the test solution is similar in position and colour to the zone in the chromatogram obtained with the reference solution (coumarin). Spray the plate with *anisaldehyde solution R*. Examine in daylight while heating at 100-105 °C for 5-10 min. The chromatogram obtained with the reference solution shows in its upper part a violet zone (eugenol) and above this zone a greenish-blue zone (*trans*-cinnamic aldehyde). The chromatogram obtained with the test solution shows a zone similar in position and colour to the zone due to *trans*-cinnamic aldehyde in the chromatogram obtained with the reference solution and may show a very faint zone corresponding to eugenol. Other faint zones are present.

B. Examine the chromatograms obtained in the test for chromatographic profile. The retention times of the principal peaks in the chromatogram obtained with the test solution are similar to those in the chromatogram obtained with the reference solution. Eugenol may be absent from the chromatogram obtained with the test solution.

TESTS

Relative density (*2.2.5*): 1.052 to 1.070.

Refractive index (*2.2.6*): 1.600 to 1.614.

Optical rotation (*2.2.7*): − 1° to + 1°.

Chromatographic profile. Examine by gas chromatography (*2.2.28*).

Test solution. The substance to be examined.

Reference solution. Dissolve 100 µl of *trans-cinnamic aldehyde R*, 10 µl of *cinnamyl acetate R*, 10 µl of *eugenol R*, 20 mg of *coumarin R* and 10 µl of *trans-2-methoxycinnamaldehyde R* in 1 ml of *acetone R*.

The chromatographic procedure may be carried out using:

– a fused-silica column 60 m long and about 0.25 mm in internal diameter coated with *macrogol 20 000 R* as the bonded phase,
– *helium for chromatography R* as the carrier gas at a flow rate of 1.5 ml/min,
– a flame-ionisation detector,
– a split ratio of 1:100,

with the following temperature programme:

	Time (min)	Temperature (°C)	Rate (°C/min)	Comment
Column	0 - 10	60	–	isothermal
	10 - 75	60 → 190	2	linear gradient
	75 - 160	190		isothermal
Injection port		200		
Detector		240		

Inject 0.2 µl of the reference solution. When the chromatogram is recorded in the prescribed conditions, the components elute in the order indicated in the composition of the reference solution. Depending on the operating conditions and the state of the column, coumarin may elute before or after *trans*-2-methoxycinnamaldehyde. Record the retention times of these substances.

The test is not valid unless the resolution between the peaks corresponding to coumarin and *trans*-2-methoxycinnamaldehyde is at least 1.5.

Inject 0.2 µl of the test solution. Using the retention times determined from the chromatogram obtained with the reference solution, locate the components of the reference solution in the chromatogram obtained with the test solution. Determine the percentage content of each of these components by the normalisation procedure.

The percentages are within the following ranges:

– *trans-cinnamic aldehyde*: 70 per cent to 90 per cent,
– *cinnamyl acetate*: 1.0 per cent to 6.0 per cent,
– *eugenol*: less than 0.5 per cent,
– *coumarin*: 1.5 per cent to 4.0 per cent,
– *trans-2-methoxycinnamaldehyde*: 3.0 per cent to 15 per cent.

STORAGE

Store in a well-filled, airtight container, protected from light and heat.

01/2005:1497
corrected

CASTOR OIL, HYDROGENATED

Ricini oleum hydrogenatum

DEFINITION

Hydrogenated castor oil is the oil obtained by hydrogenation of *Virgin Castor oil (0051)*. It consists mainly of the triglyceride of 12-hydroxystearic acid.

CHARACTERS

A fine, almost white or pale yellow powder or almost white or pale yellow masses or flakes, practically insoluble in water, freely soluble in methylene chloride, slightly soluble in light petroleum, very slightly soluble in ethanol.

IDENTIFICATION

A. Melting point (*2.2.14*): 83 °C to 88 °C.

B. It complies with the test for hydroxyl value (see Tests).

C. It complies with the test for composition of fatty acids (see Tests).

TESTS

Acid value (*2.5.1*). Not more than 4.0, determined on 10.0 g dissolved in 75 ml of hot *alcohol R*.

Hydroxyl value (*2.5.3, Method A*): 145 to 165, determined on a warm solution.

Iodine value (*2.5.4*). Not more than 5.0.

Alkaline impurities. Dissolve 1.0 g by gentle heating in a mixture of 1.5 ml of *alcohol R* and 3 ml of *toluene R*. Add 0.05 ml of a 0.4 g/l solution of *bromophenol blue R* in *alcohol R*. Not more than 0.2 ml of *0.01 M hydrochloric acid* is required to change the colour of the indicator to yellow.

Composition of fatty acids. Gas chromatography (*2.4.22*) with the following modifications.

Use the mixture of calibrating substances in Table 2.4.22.-3.

Test solution. Introduce 75 mg of the substance to be examined in a 10 ml centrifuge tube with a screw cap. Dissolve in 2 ml of *1,1-dimethylethyl methyl ether R1* by shaking and heat gently (50-60 °C). Add, when still warm, 1 ml of a 12 g/l solution of *sodium R* in *anhydrous methanol R*, prepared with the necessary precautions, and mix vigorously for at least 5 min. Add 5 ml of *distilled water R* and mix vigorously for about 30 s. Centrifuge for 15 min at 1500 *g*. Use the upper layer.

Reference solution. Dissolve 50 mg of *methyl 12-hydroxystearate CRS* and 50 mg of *methyl stearate CRS* in 10.0 ml of *1,1-dimethylethyl methyl ether R1*.

The chromatographic procedure may be carried out using:

- a fused-silica column 30 m long and 0.25 mm in internal diameter coated with *macrogol 20 000 R* (film thickness 0.25 µm),
- *helium for chromatography R* as the carrier gas at a flow rate of 0.9 ml/min,
- a flame-ionisation detector,
- a split injector (1:100),

maintaining the temperature of the column at 215 °C for 55 min and maintaining the temperature of the injection port and that of the detector at 250 °C.

Inject 1 µl of each solution.

Calculate the fraction of each fatty acid using the following expression:

$$A_{x,s,c} / \sum A_{x,s,c} \times 100 \text{ per cent } m/m$$

$A_{x,s,c}$ = corrected peak area of the fatty acid in the test solution:

$$A_{x,s,c} = A_{x,s} \times R_c$$

R_c = relative correction factor for the peak corresponding to methyl 12-hydroxystearate:

$$R_c = \frac{m_{1,r} \times A_{2,r}}{A_{1,r} \times m_{2,r}}$$

R_c = 1 for peaks corresponding to each of the other specified fatty acids or any unspecified fatty acid,

$m_{1,r}$ = mass of methyl 12-hydroxystearate in the reference solution,

$m_{2,r}$ = mass of methyl stearate in the reference solution,

$A_{1,r}$ = area of any peak corresponding to methyl 12-hydroxystearate in the chromatogram obtained with the reference solution,

$A_{2,r}$ = area of any peak corresponding to methyl stearate in the chromatogram obtained with the reference solution,

$A_{x,s}$ = area of the peaks corresponding to any specified or unspecified fatty acid methyl esters.

The fatty acid fraction of the oil has the following composition:

- *palmitic acid*: not more than 2.0 per cent,
- *stearic acid*: 7.0 per cent to 14.0 per cent,
- *arachidic acid*: not more than 1.0 per cent,
- *12-oxostearic acid* (equivalent chain length on macrogol 20 000: 22.7): not more than 5.0 per cent,
- *12-hydroxystearic acid* (equivalent chain length on macrogol 20 000: 23.9): 78.0 per cent to 91.0 per cent,
- *any other fatty acid*: not more than 3.0 per cent.

Nickel (*2.4.27*). Not more than 1 ppm of Ni.

STORAGE

Store in a well-filled container.

IMPURITIES

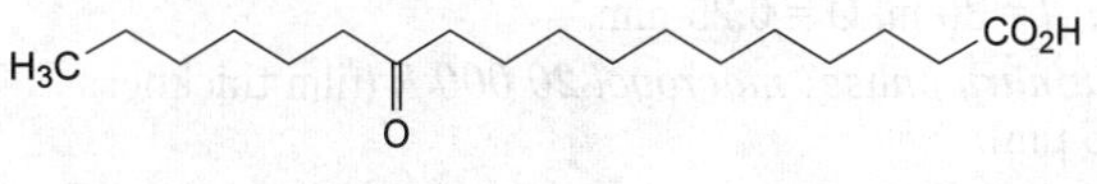

A. 12-oxostearic acid.

01/2005:0051
corrected

CASTOR OIL, VIRGIN

Ricini oleum virginale

DEFINITION

Fatty oil obtained by cold expression from the seeds of *Ricinus communis* L. A suitable antioxidant may be added.

CHARACTERS

Appearance: clear, almost colourless or slightly yellow, viscous, hygroscopic liquid.

Solubility: slightly soluble in light petroleum, miscible with alcohol and with glacial acetic acid.

Relative density: about 0.958.

Refractive index: about 1.479.

IDENTIFICATION

First identification: D.

Second identification: A, B, C.

A. It complies with the test for optical rotation (see Tests).

B. It complies with the test for hydroxyl value (see Tests).

C. Iodine value (*2.5.4*): 82 to 90.

D. It complies with the test for composition of fatty acids (see Tests).

TESTS

Optical rotation (*2.2.7*): + 3.5° to + 6.0°.

Specific absorbance (*2.2.25*): maximum 1.0, determined at the absorption maximum at 269 nm ± 1 nm.

To 1.0 g add *alcohol R* and dilute to 100.0 ml with the same solvent.

Acid value (*2.5.1*): maximum 2.0.

Dissolve 5.0 g in 25 ml of the prescribed mixture of solvents.

Hydroxyl value (*2.5.3, Method A*): minimum 150.

Peroxide value (*2.5.5*): maximum 10.0.

Unsaponifiable matter (*2.5.7*): maximum 0.8 per cent, determined on 5.0 g.

Composition of fatty acids. Gas chromatography (*2.4.22*) with the following modifications.

Use the mixture of calibrating substances in Table 2.4.22.-3.

Test solution. Introduce 75 mg of the substance to be examined into a 10 ml centrifuge tube with a screw cap. Dissolve in 2 ml of *1,1-dimethylethyl methyl ether R1* with shaking and heat gently (50-60 °C). Add, when still warm, 1 ml of a 12 g/l solution of *sodium R* in *anhydrous methanol R*, prepared with the necessary precautions, and mix vigorously for at least 5 min. Add 5 ml of *distilled water R* and mix vigorously for about 30 s. Centrifuge for 15 min at 1500 *g*. Use the upper layer.

Reference solution. Dissolve 50 mg of *methyl ricinoleate CRS* and 50 mg of *methyl stearate CRS* in 10.0 ml of *1,1-dimethylethyl methyl ether R1*.

Column:

– *material*: fused silica,

– *size*: *l* = 30 m, Ø = 0.25 mm,

– *stationary phase*: *macrogol 20 000 R* (film thickness 0.25 μm).

Carrier gas: *helium for chromatography R*.

Flow rate: 0.9 ml/min.

Split ratio: 1:100.

Temperature:

	Time (min)	Temperature (°C)
Column	0 - 55	215
Injection port		250
Detector		250

Detection: flame ionisation.

Injection: 1 μl.

Calculate the percentage content of each fatty acid by normalisation.

Correct the area of the peak due to methyl ricinoleate, multiplying by a factor *R* calculated using the following expression:

$$R = \frac{m_1 \times A_2}{A_1 \times m_2}$$

m_1 = mass of methyl ricinoleate in the reference solution,

m_2 = mass of methyl stearate in the reference solution,

A_1 = area of the peak due to methyl ricinoleate in the chromatogram obtained with the reference solution,

A_2 = area of the peak due to methyl stearate in the chromatogram obtained with the reference solution.

Composition of the fatty-acid fraction of the oil:

– *palmitic acid*: maximum 2.0 per cent,

– *stearic acid*: maximum 2.5 per cent,

– *oleic acid and isomers* (C18:1 equivalent chain length on macrogol 20 000: 18.3): 2.5 per cent to 6.0 per cent,

– *linoleic acid* (C18:2 equivalent chain length on macrogol 20 000: 18.8): 2.5 per cent to 7.0 per cent,

– *linolenic acid* (C18:3 equivalent chain length on macrogol 20 000: 19.2): maximum 1.0 per cent,

– *eicosenoic acid* (C20:1 equivalent chain length on macrogol 20 000: 20.2): maximum 1.0 per cent,

– *ricinoleic acid* (equivalent chain length on macrogol 20 000: 23.9): 85.0 per cent to 92.0 per cent,

– *any other fatty acid*: maximum 1.0 per cent.

Water (*2.5.12*): maximum 0.3 per cent, determined on 5.0 g.

STORAGE

In an airtight, well-filled container, protected from light.

LABELLING

The label states the name and concentration of any added antioxidant.

01/2005:0986
corrected

CEFACLOR

Cefaclorum

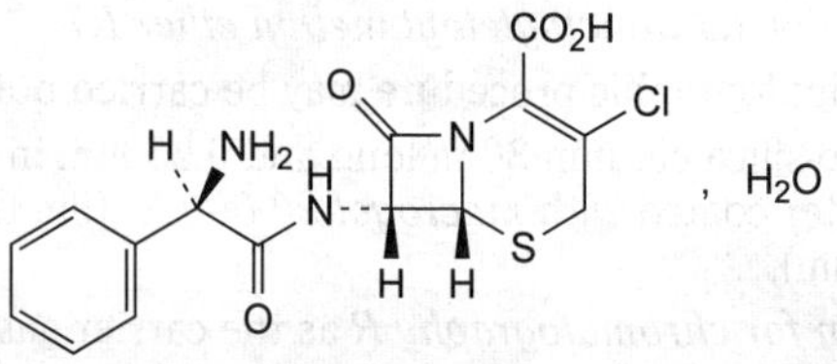

$C_{15}H_{14}ClN_3O_4S,H_2O$ M_r 385.8

DEFINITION

Cefaclor is the monohydrate of (6*R*,7*R*)-7-[[(2*R*)-2-amino-2-phenylacetyl]amino]-3-chloro-8-oxo-5-thia-1-azabicyclo[4.2.0]oct-2-ene-2-carboxylic acid. It contains not less than 96.0 per cent and not more than the equivalent of 102.0 per cent of $C_{15}H_{14}ClN_3O_4S$, calculated with reference to the anhydrous substance.

CHARACTERS

A white or slightly yellow powder, slightly soluble in water, practically insoluble in methanol and in methylene chloride.

IDENTIFICATION

Examine by infrared absorption spectrophotometry (*2.2.24*), comparing with the spectrum obtained with *cefaclor CRS*.

TESTS

pH (*2.2.3*). Suspend 0.250 g in *carbon dioxide-free water R* and dilute to 10 ml with the same solvent. The pH of the suspension is 3.0 to 4.5.

Specific optical rotation (*2.2.7*). Dissolve 0.250 g in a 10 g/l solution of *hydrochloric acid R* and dilute to 25.0 ml with the same solution. The specific optical rotation is + 101 to + 111, calculated with reference to the anhydrous substance.

Related substances. Examine by liquid chromatography (*2.2.29*).

Test solution. Dissolve 50.0 mg of the substance to be examined in 10.0 ml of a 2.7 g/l solution of *sodium dihydrogen phosphate R* adjusted to pH 2.5 with *phosphoric acid R*.

Reference solution (a). Dissolve 2.5 mg of *cefaclor CRS* and 5.0 mg of *delta-3-cefaclor CRS* in 100.0 ml of a 2.7 g/l solution of *sodium dihydrogen phosphate R* adjusted to pH 2.5 with *phosphoric acid R*.

Reference solution (b). Dilute 1.0 ml of the test solution to 100.0 ml with a 2.7 g/l solution of *sodium dihydrogen phosphate R* adjusted to pH 2.5 with *phosphoric acid R*.

The chromatographic procedure may be carried out using:

- a stainless steel column 0.25 m long and 4.6 mm in internal diameter packed with *end-capped octadecylsilyl silica gel for chromatography R* (5 µm),
- as mobile phase at a flow rate of 1.0 ml/min:

  Mobile phase A. Adjust a 7.8 g/l solution of *sodium dihydrogen phosphate R* to pH 4.0 with *phosphoric acid R*,

  Mobile phase B. Mix 450 ml of *acetonitrile R* with 550 ml of mobile phase A,
- as detector a spectrophotometer set at 220 nm,
- a 20 µl loop injector.

Equilibrate the column with a mixture of 5 volumes of mobile phase B and 95 volumes of mobile phase A for at least 15 min between each analysis. Inject the solutions. Operate by gradient elution increasing the concentration of mobile phase B continuously and linearly by 0.67 per cent *V/V* per minute for 30 min (25 per cent *V/V*). Then increase the concentration of mobile phase B continuously and linearly by 5 per cent *V/V* per minute for 15 min (100 per cent *V/V*). Finally elute with mobile phase B for 10 min. Change the composition to a mixture of 5 volumes of mobile phase B and 95 volumes of mobile phase A to re-equilibrate the column.

Inject reference solution (a). The test is not valid unless the resolution between the peaks due to cefaclor and delta-3-cefaclor is at least 2 and the symmetry factor of the cefaclor peak is at most 1.2. If necessary, adjust the acetonitrile content of the mobile phase.

Inject the test solution and reference solution (b). In the chromatogram obtained with the test solution: the area of any peak, apart from the principal peak and any peaks due to the mobile phase, is not greater than 0.5 times the area of the principal peak in the chromatogram obtained with reference solution (b) (0.5 per cent); and the sum of all such peaks is not more than twice the area of the principal peak in the chromatogram obtained with reference solution (b) (2 per cent). Disregard any peak with an area less than 0.1 times that of the principal peak in the chromatogram obtained with reference solution (b).

Heavy metals (*2.4.8*). 1.0 g complies with limit test C (30 ppm). Prepare the standard using 3 ml of *lead standard solution (10 ppm Pb) R*.

Water (*2.5.12*). 3.0 per cent to 6.5 per cent, determined on 0.200 g by the semi-micro determination of water.

ASSAY

Examine by liquid chromatography (*2.2.29*).

Test solution. Dissolve 15.0 mg of the substance to be examined in the mobile phase and dilute to 50.0 ml with the mobile phase.

Reference solution (a). Dissolve 15.0 mg of *cefaclor CRS* in the mobile phase and dilute to 50.0 ml with the mobile phase.

Reference solution (b). Dissolve 15.0 mg of *cefaclor CRS* and 15.0 mg of *delta-3-cefaclor CRS* in the mobile phase and dilute to 50.0 ml with the mobile phase.

The chromatographic procedure may be carried out using:

- a stainless steel column 0.25 m long and 4.6 mm in internal diameter packed with *octadecylsilyl silica gel for chromatography R* (5 µm),
- as mobile phase at a flow rate of 1.5 ml/min a mixture prepared by adding 220 ml of *methanol R* to a mixture of 780 ml of *water R*, 10 ml of *triethylamine R* and 1 g of *sodium pentanesulphonate R*, adjusted to pH 2.5 with *phosphoric acid R*,
- as detector a spectrophotometer set at 265 nm,
- a 20 µl loop injector.

Inject reference solution (b). The assay is not valid unless the resolution between the peaks due to cefaclor and delta-3-cefaclor is at least 2.5. Adjust the concentration of methanol in the mobile phase, if necessary. The assay is not valid unless the symmetry factor of the cefaclor peak is at most 1.5. Inject reference solution (a) six times. The assay is not valid unless the relative standard deviation of the peak area of cefaclor is at most 1.0 per cent. Inject alternately the test solution and reference solution (a).

IMPURITIES

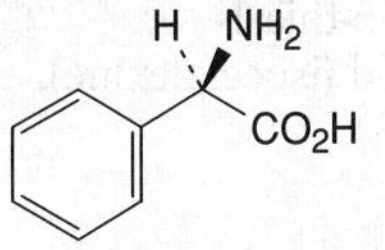

A. (2*R*)-2-amino-2-phenylacetic acid (phenylglycine),

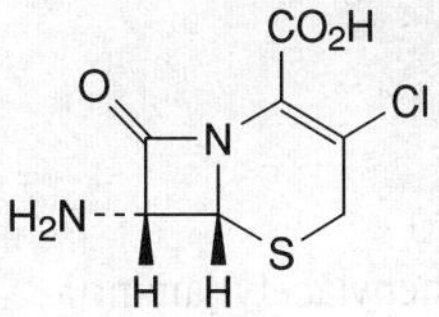

B. (6*R*,7*R*)-7-amino-3-chloro-8-oxo-5-thia-1-azabicyclo[4.2.0]oct-2-ene-2-carboxylic acid,

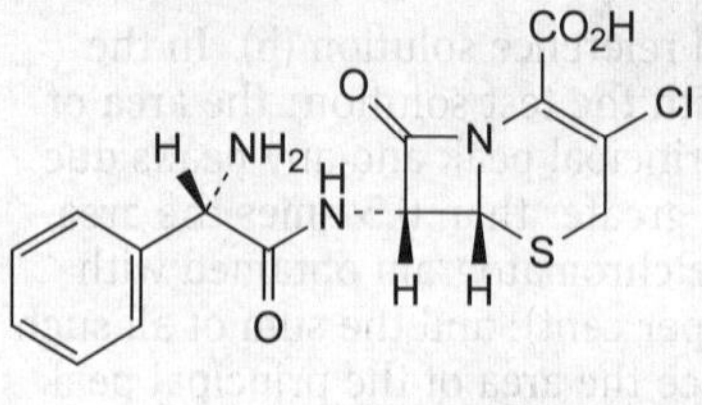

C. (6*R*,7*R*)-7-[[(2*S*)-2-amino-2-phenylacetyl]amino]-3-chloro-8-oxo-5-thia- 1-azabicyclo[4.2.0]oct-2-ene-2-carboxylic acid,

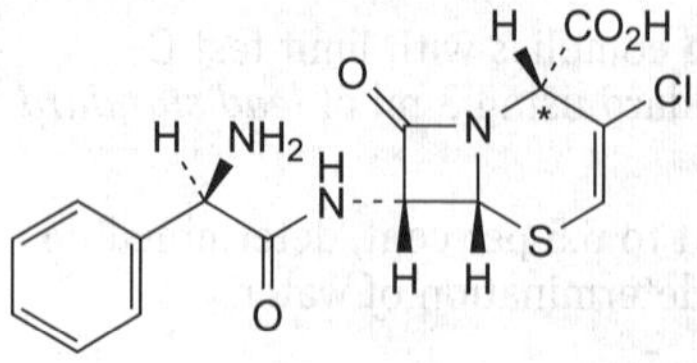

and epimer at C*

D. (2*R*,6*R*,7*R*)- and (2*S*,6*R*,7*R*)-7-[[(2*R*)-2-amino-2-phenylacetyl]amino]-3-chloro-8-oxo-5-thia-1-azabicyclo[4.2.0]oct-3-ene-2-carboxylic acid (delta-3-cefaclor),

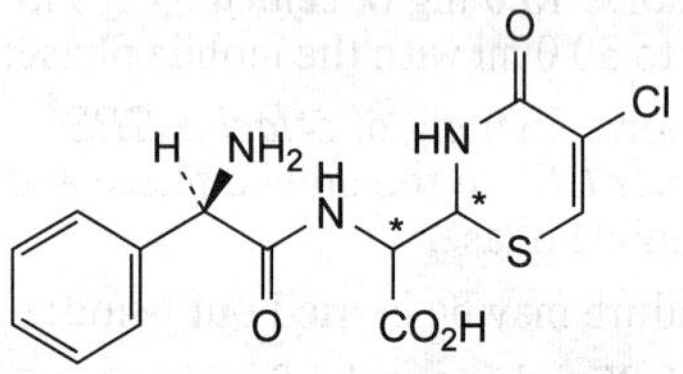

E. 2-[[(2*R*)-2-amino-2-phenylacetyl]amino]-2-(5-chloro-4-oxo-3,4-dihydro-2*H*-1,3-thiazin-2-yl)acetic acid,

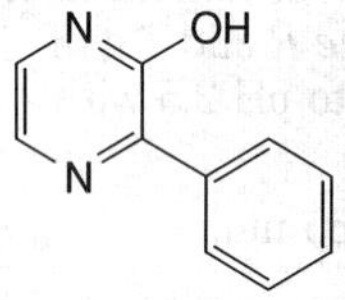

F. 3-phenylpyrazin-2-ol.

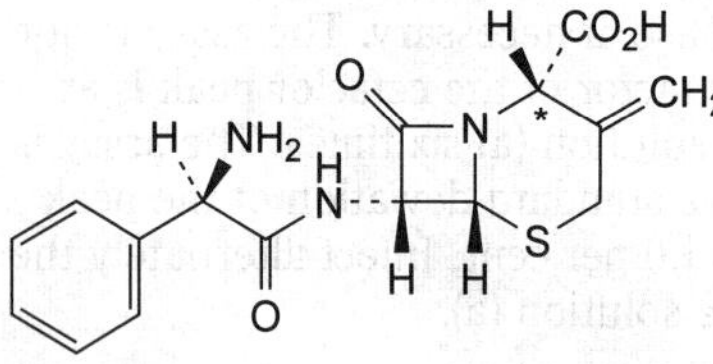

and epimer at C*

G. (2*R*,6*R*,7*R*)- and (2*S*,6*R*,7*R*)-7-[[(2*R*)-2-amino-2-phenylacetyl]amino]-3-methylene-8-oxo-5-thia-1-azabicyclo[4.2.0]octane-2-carboxylic acid (isocefalexine),

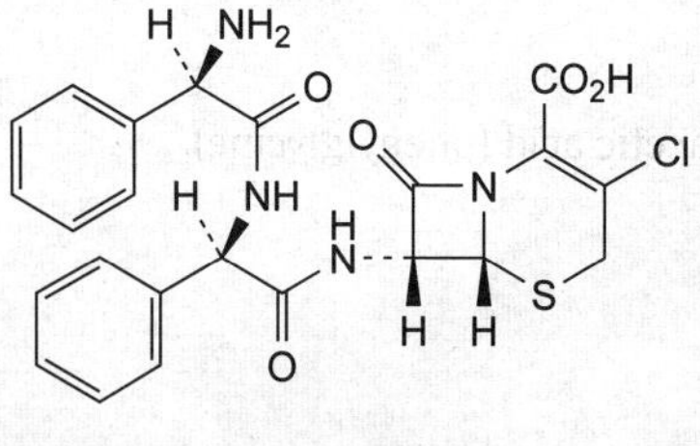

H. (6*R*,7*R*)-7-[[(2*R*)-2-[[(2*R*)-2-amino-2-phenylacetyl]amino]-2-phenylacetyl]amino]-3-chloro-8-oxo-5-thia-1-azabicyclo[4.2.0]oct-2-ene-2-carboxylic acid (*N*-phenylglycyl cefaclor).

01/2005:0813
corrected

CEFADROXIL MONOHYDRATE

Cefadroxilum monohydricum

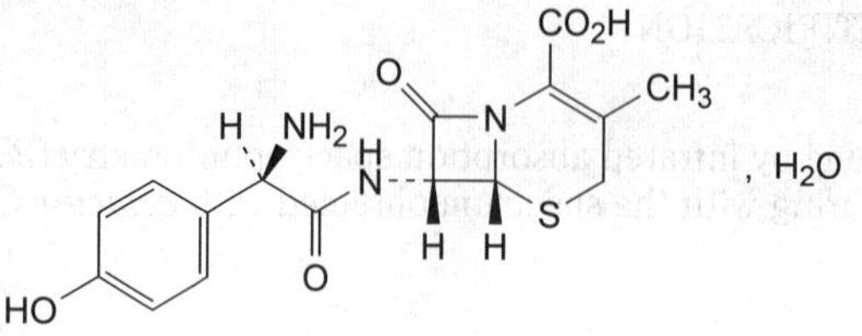

$C_{16}H_{17}N_3O_5S,H_2O$ M_r 381.4

DEFINITION

(6*R*,7*R*)-7-[[(2*R*)-2-Amino-2-(4-hydroxyphenyl)acetyl]amino]-3-methyl-8-oxo-5-thia-1-azabicyclo[4.2.0]oct-2-ene-2-carboxylic acid monohydrate.

Content: 95.0 per cent to 102.0 per cent (anhydrous substance).

CHARACTERS

Appearance: white or almost white powder.

Solubility: slightly soluble in water, very slightly soluble in alcohol.

IDENTIFICATION

Infrared absorption spectrophotometry (*2.2.24*).

TESTS

pH (*2.2.3*): 4.0 to 6.0.

Suspend 1.0 g in *carbon dioxide-free water R* and dilute to 20 ml with the same solvent.

Specific optical rotation (*2.2.7*): + 165 to + 178 (anhydrous substance).

Dissolve 0.500 g in *water R* and dilute to 50.0 ml with the same solvent.

Absorbance (*2.2.25*). Dissolve 20.0 mg in *phosphate buffer solution pH 6.0 R* and dilute to 100.0 ml with the same solvent. The absorbance of the solution determined at 330 nm is not greater than 0.05. Dilute 10.0 ml of the solution to 100.0 ml with *phosphate buffer solution pH 6.0 R*. Examined between 235 nm and 340 nm, the diluted solution shows an absorption maximum at 264 nm. The specific absorbance at this maximum is 225 to 250 (anhydrous substance).

Related substances. Liquid chromatography (*2.2.29*).

Test solution. Dissolve 50.0 mg of the substance to be examined in mobile phase A and dilute to 50.0 ml with mobile phase A.

Reference solution (a). Dissolve 10.0 mg of *D-α-(4-hydroxyphenyl)glycine CRS* (impurity A) in mobile phase A and dilute to 10.0 ml with mobile phase A.

Reference solution (b). Dissolve 10.0 mg of *7-aminodesacetoxycephalosporanic acid CRS* (impurity B) in *phosphate buffer solution pH 7.0 R5* and dilute to 10.0 ml with the same buffer solution.

Reference solution (c). Dilute 1.0 ml of reference solution (a) and 1.0 ml of reference solution (b) to 100.0 ml with mobile phase A.

Reference solution (d). Dissolve 10 mg of *dimethylformamide R* and 10 mg of *dimethylacetamide R* in mobile phase A and dilute to 10.0 ml with mobile phase A. Dilute 1.0 ml to 100.0 ml with mobile phase A.

Reference solution (e). Dilute 1.0 ml of reference solution (c) to 25.0 ml with mobile phase A.

Column:

- *size*: *l* = 0.10 m, Ø = 4.6 mm,
- *stationary phase*: spherical *octadecylsilyl silica gel for chromatography R* (5 µm).

Mobile phase:

- *mobile phase A*: *phosphate buffer solution pH 5.0 R,*
- *mobile phase B*: *methanol R2,*

Time (min)	Mobile phase A (per cent *V/V*)	Mobile phase B (per cent *V/V*)
0 - 1	98	2
1 - 20	98 → 70	2 → 30
20 - 23	70 → 98	30 → 2
23 - 30	98	2

Flow rate: 1.5 ml/min.

Detection: spectrophotometer at 220 nm.

Injection: 20 µl; inject the test solution and reference solutions (c), (d) and (e).

Relative retention with reference to cefadroxil (retention time = about 6 min): dimethylformamide = about 0.4; dimethylacetamide = about 0.75.

System suitability:

- *resolution*: minimum 5.0 between the peaks due to impurity A and to impurity B in the chromatogram obtained with reference solution (c),
- *signal-to-noise ratio*: minimum 10 for the second peak in the chromatogram obtained with reference solution (e).

Limits:

- *impurity A*: not more than the area of the first peak in the chromatogram obtained with reference solution (c) (1.0 per cent),
- *any other impurity*: not more than the area of the second peak in the chromatogram obtained with reference solution (c) (1.0 per cent),
- *total*: not more than 3 times the area of the second peak in the chromatogram obtained with reference solution (c) (3.0 per cent),
- *disregard limit*: 0.05 times the area of the second peak in the chromatogram obtained with reference solution (c) (0.05 per cent); disregard the peaks due to dimethylformamide and dimethylacetamide.

***N,N*-Dimethylaniline** (*2.4.26, Method B*): maximum 20 ppm.

Water (*2.5.12*): 4.0 per cent to 6.0 per cent, determined on 0.200 g.

Sulphated ash (*2.4.14*): maximum 0.5 per cent, determined on 1.0 g.

ASSAY

Liquid chromatography (*2.2.29*).

Test solution. Dissolve 50.0 mg of the substance to be examined in the mobile phase and dilute to 100.0 ml with the mobile phase.

Reference solution (a). Dissolve 50.0 mg of *cefadroxil CRS* in the mobile phase and dilute to 100.0 ml with the mobile phase.

Reference solution (b). Dissolve 5 mg of *cefadroxil CRS* and 50 mg of *amoxicillin trihydrate CRS* in the mobile phase and dilute to 100 ml with the mobile phase.

Column:

- *size*: *l* = 0.25 m, Ø = 4.6 mm,
- *stationary phase*: *octadecylsilyl silica gel for chromatography R* (5 µm).

Mobile phase: *acetonitrile R*, a 2.72 g/l solution of *potassium dihydrogen phosphate R* (4:96 *V/V*).

Flow rate: 1 ml/min.

Detection: spectrophotometer at 254 nm.

Injection: 20 µl.

System suitability: reference solution (b):

- *resolution*: minimum 5.0 between the peaks due to cefadroxil and to amoxicillin.

Calculate the percentage content of cefadroxil.

STORAGE

Protected from light.

IMPURITIES

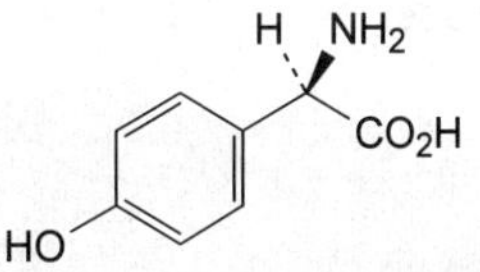

A. (2*R*)-2-amino-2-(4-hydroxyphenyl)acetic acid,

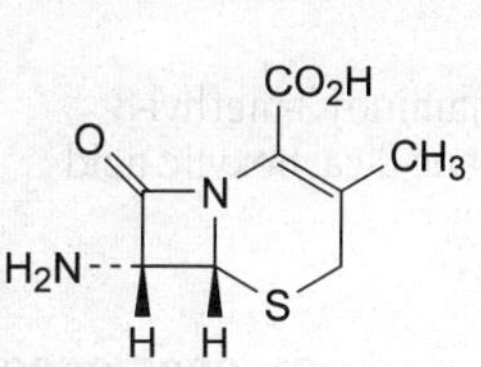

B. (6*R*,7*R*)-7-amino-3-methyl-8-oxo-5-thia-1-azabicyclo[4.2.0]oct-2-ene-2-carboxylic acid (7-ADCA),

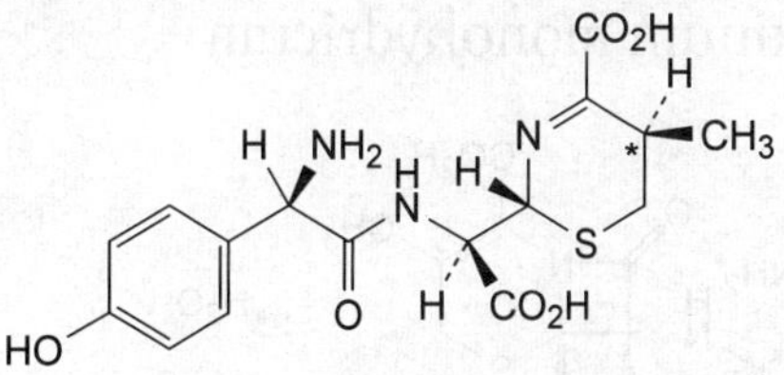

and epimer at C*

C. (2*R*,5*RS*)-2-[(*R*)-[[(2*R*)-2-amino-2-(4-hydroxyphenyl)acetyl]amino]carboxymethyl]-5-methyl-5,6-dihydro-2*H*-1,3-thiazine-4-carboxylic acid,

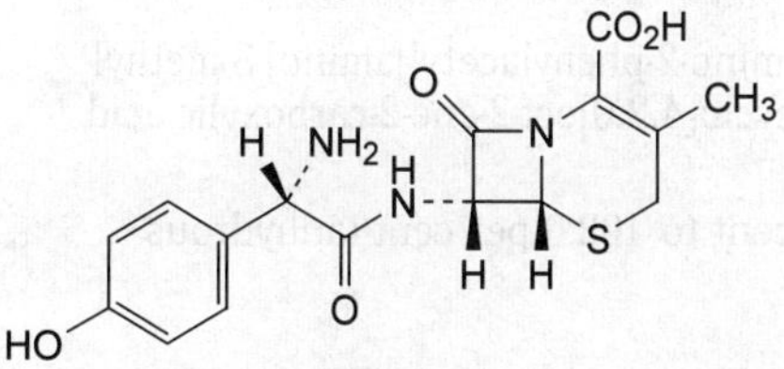

D. (6*R*,7*R*)-7-[[(2*S*)-2-amino-2-(4-hydroxyphenyl)acetyl]amino]-3-methyl-8-oxo-5-thia-1-azabicyclo[4.2.0]oct-2-ene-2-carboxylic acid (L-cefadroxil),

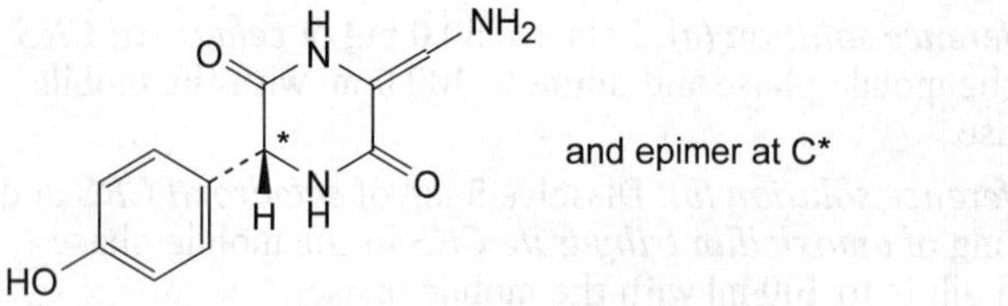

E. (6*RS*)-3-(aminomethylene)-6-(4-hydroxyphenyl)piperazine-2,5-dione,

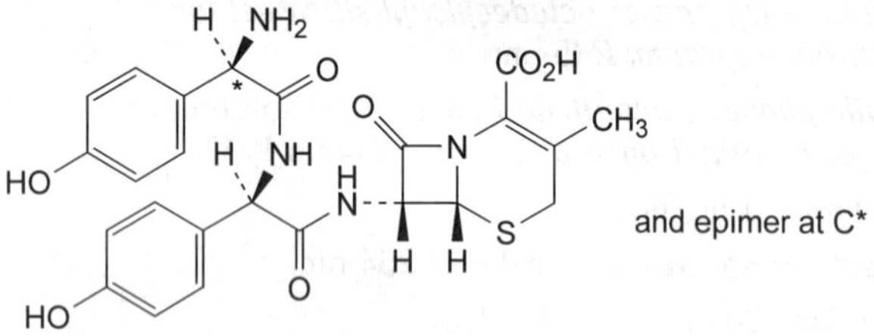

F. (6*R*,7*R*)-7-[[(2*R*)-2-[[(2*RS*)-2-amino-2-(4-hydroxyphenyl)acetyl]amino]-2-(4-hydroxyphenyl)acetyl]amino]-3-methyl-8-oxo-5-thia-1-azabicyclo[4.2.0]oct-2-ene-2-carboxylic acid,

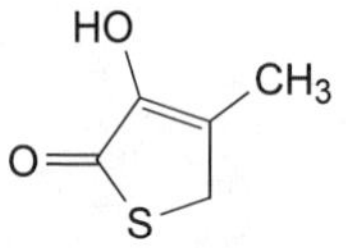

G. 3-hydroxy-4-methylthiophen-2(5*H*)-one,

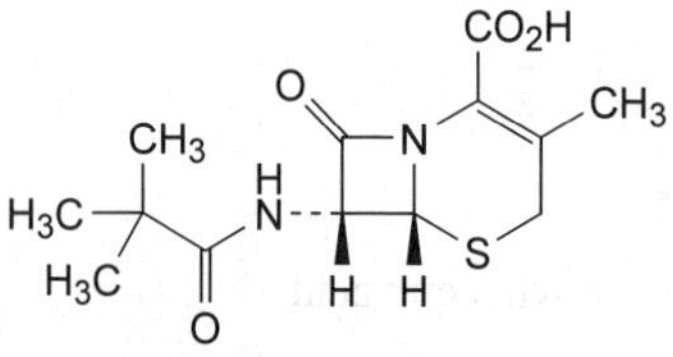

H. (6*R*,7*R*)-7-[(2,2-dimethylpropanoyl)amino]-3-methyl-8-oxo-5-thia-1-azabicyclo[4.2.0]oct-2-ene-2-carboxylic acid (7-ADCA pivalamide).

01/2005:0708

CEFALEXIN MONOHYDRATE

Cefalexinum monohydricum

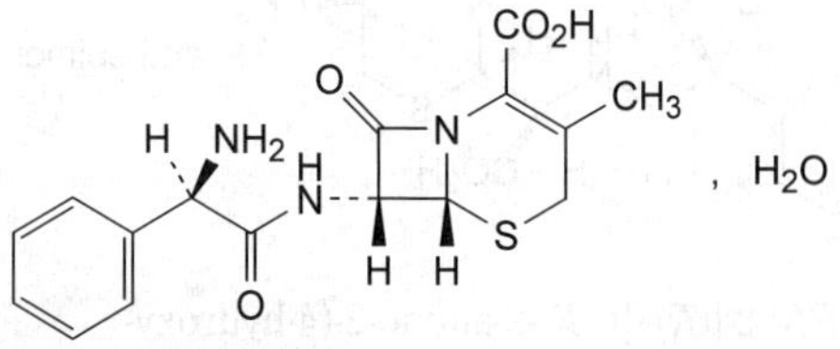

$C_{16}H_{17}N_3O_4S,H_2O$ — M_r 365.4

DEFINITION

(6*R*,7*R*)-7-[[(2*R*)-2-Amino-2-phenylacetyl]amino]-3-methyl-8-oxo-5-thia-1-azabicyclo[4.2.0]oct-2-ene-2-carboxylic acid monohydrate.

Content: 95.0 per cent to 102.0 per cent (anhydrous substance).

CHARACTERS

Appearance: white or almost white, crystalline powder.

Solubility: sparingly soluble in water, practically insoluble in alcohol.

IDENTIFICATION

Infrared absorption spectrophotometry (*2.2.24*).

Comparison: *cefalexin monohydrate CRS*.

TESTS

pH (*2.2.3*): 4.0 to 5.5.

Dissolve 50 mg in *carbon dioxide-free water R* and dilute to 10 ml with the same solvent.

Specific optical rotation (*2.2.7*): + 149 to + 158 (anhydrous substance).

Dissolve 0.125 g in *phthalate buffer solution pH 4.4 R* and dilute to 25.0 ml with the same solvent.

Absorbance (*2.2.25*). Dissolve 50 mg in *water R* and dilute to 100.0 ml with the same solvent. The absorbance of the solution determined at 330 nm is not greater than 0.05. Dilute 2.0 ml of the solution to 50.0 ml with *water R*. Examined between 220 nm and 300 nm, the diluted solution shows an absorption maximum at 262 nm. The specific absorbance at this maximum is 220 to 245, calculated with reference to the anhydrous substance.

Related substances. Liquid chromatography (*2.2.29*).

Test solution. Dissolve 50.0 mg of the substance to be examined in mobile phase A and dilute to 50.0 ml with mobile phase A.

Reference solution (a). Dissolve 10.0 mg of *D-phenylglycine R* in mobile phase A and dilute to 10.0 ml with mobile phase A.

Reference solution (b). Dissolve 10.0 mg of *7-aminodesacetoxycephalosporanic acid CRS* in *phosphate buffer solution pH 7.0 R5* and dilute to 10.0 ml with mobile phase A.

Reference solution (c). Dilute 1.0 ml of reference solution (a) and 1.0 ml of reference solution (b) to 100.0 ml with mobile phase A.

Reference solution (d). Dissolve 10 mg of *dimethylformamide R* and 10 mg of *dimethylacetamide R* in mobile phase A and dilute to 10.0 ml with mobile phase A. Dilute 1.0 ml to 100.0 ml with mobile phase A.

Reference solution (e). Dilute 1.0 ml of reference solution (c) to 20.0 ml with mobile phase A.

Reference solution (f). Dissolve 10 mg of *cefotaxime sodium CRS* in mobile phase A and dilute to 10.0 ml with mobile phase A. To 1.0 ml of the solution add 1.0 ml of the test solution and dilute to 100 ml with mobile phase A.

Column:

– *size*: *l* = 0.10 m, Ø = 4.6 mm,
– *stationary phase*: spherical *octadecylsilyl silica gel for chromatography R* (5 μm).

Mobile phase:

– *mobile phase A*: *phosphate buffer solution pH 5.0 R*,
– *mobile phase B*: *methanol R2*,

Time (min)	Mobile phase A (per cent *V/V*)	Mobile phase B (per cent *V/V*)
0 - 1	98	2
1 - 20	98 → 70	2 → 30
20 - 23	70 → 98	30 → 2
23 - 30	98	2

Flow rate: 1.5 ml/min.

Detection: spectrophotometer at 220 nm.

Injection: 20 μl; inject the test solution and reference solutions (c), (d), (e) and (f).

System suitability:

– *resolution*: minimum of 2.0 between the peaks due to impurity A and to impurity B in the chromatogram obtained with reference solution (c) and minimum of 1.5 between the peaks due to cefalexin and to cefotaxime in the chromatogram obtained with reference solution (f).

Limits:

– *impurity B*: not more than the area of the second peak in the chromatogram obtained with reference solution (c) (1.0 per cent),

– *any other impurity* (disregard the peaks due to dimethylformamide and dimethylacetamide): not more than the area of the first peak in the chromatogram obtained with reference solution (c) (1.0 per cent),

– *total*: not more than 3 times the area of the first peak in the chromatogram obtained with reference solution (c) (3.0 per cent),

– *disregard limit*: the area of the second peak in the chromatogram obtained with reference solution (e) (0.05 per cent).

***N,N*-Dimethylaniline** (*2.4.26, Method B*): maximum 20 ppm.

Water (*2.5.12*): 4.0 per cent to 8.0 per cent, determined on 0.300 g.

Sulphated ash (*2.4.14*): maximum 0.2 per cent, determined on 1.0 g.

ASSAY

Liquid chromatography (*2.2.29*).

Test solution. Dissolve 50.0 mg of the substance to be examined in *water R* and dilute to 100.0 ml with the same solvent.

Reference solution (a). Dissolve 50.0 mg of *cefalexin monohydrate CRS* in *water R* and dilute to 100.0 ml with the same solvent.

Reference solution (b). Dissolve 10 mg of *cefradine CRS* in 20 ml of reference solution (a) and dilute to 100 ml with *water R*.

Column:

– *size*: *l* = 0.25 m, Ø = 4.6 mm,

– *stationary phase*: *octadecylsilyl silica gel for chromatography R* (5 µm).

Mobile phase: *methanol R, acetonitrile R*, a 13.6 g/l solution of *potassium dihydrogen phosphate R, water R* (2:5:10:83 *V/V/V/V*).

Flow rate: 1.5 ml/min.

Detection: spectrophotometer at 254 nm.

Injection: 20 µl.

System suitability: reference solution (b):

– *resolution*: minimum 4.0 between the peaks due to cefalexin and to cefradine.

Calculate the percentage content of cefalexin monohydrate.

STORAGE

Protected from light.

IMPURITIES

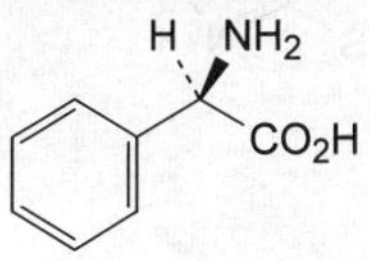

A. (2*R*)-2-amino-2-phenylacetic acid (D-phenylglycine),

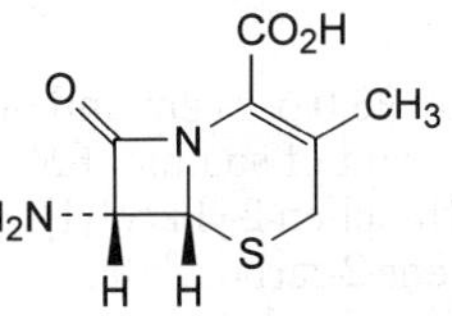

B. (6*R*,7*R*)-7-amino-3-methyl-8-oxo-5-thia-1-azabicyclo[4.2.0]oct-2-ene-2-carboxylic acid (7-aminodesacetoxycephalosporanic acid, 7-ADCA),

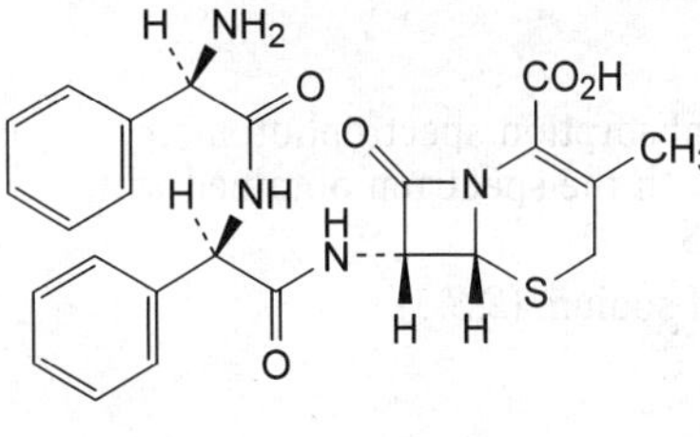

C. (6*R*,7*R*)-7-[[(2*R*)-2-[[(2*R*)-2-amino-2-phenylacetyl]amino]-2-phenylacetyl]amino]-3-methyl-8-oxo-5-thia-1-azabicyclo[4.2.0]oct-2-ene-2-carboxylic acid,

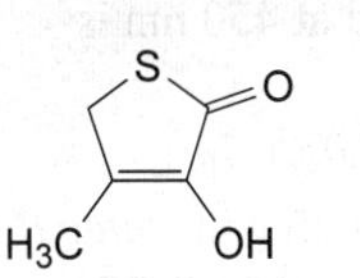

D. 3-hydroxy-4-methylthiophen-2(5*H*)-one,

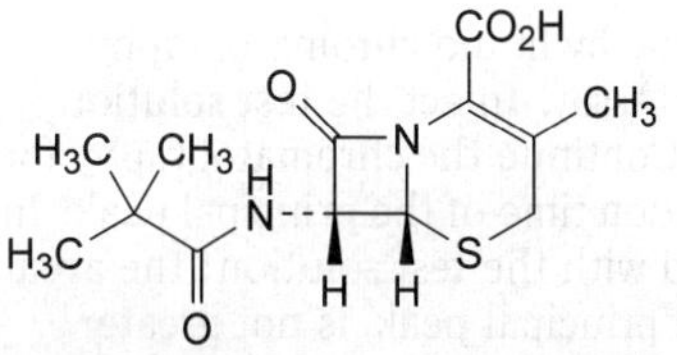

E. (6*R*,7*R*)-7-[(2,2-dimethylpropanoyl)amino]-3-methyl-8-oxo-5-thia-1-azabicyclo[4.2.0]oct-2-ene-2-carboxylic acid (7-ADCA pivalamide),

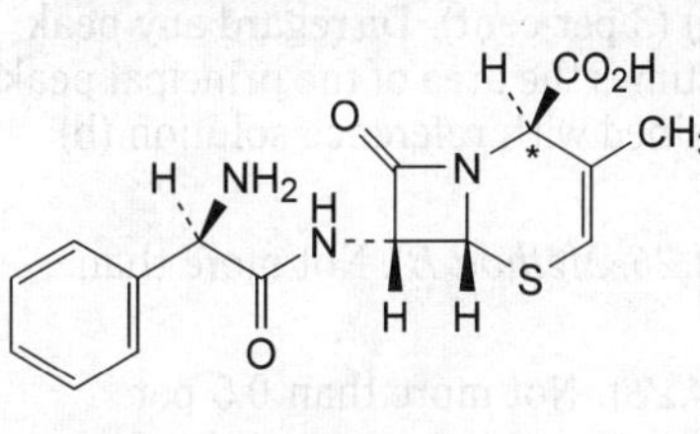

and epimer at C*

F. (2*RS*,6*R*,7*R*)-7-[[(2*R*)-2-amino-2-phenylacetyl]amino]-3-methyl-8-oxo-5-thia-1-azabicyclo[4.2.0]oct-3-ene-2-carboxylic acid (delta-2-cefalexin).

01/2005:0987

CEFALOTIN SODIUM

Cefalotinum natricum

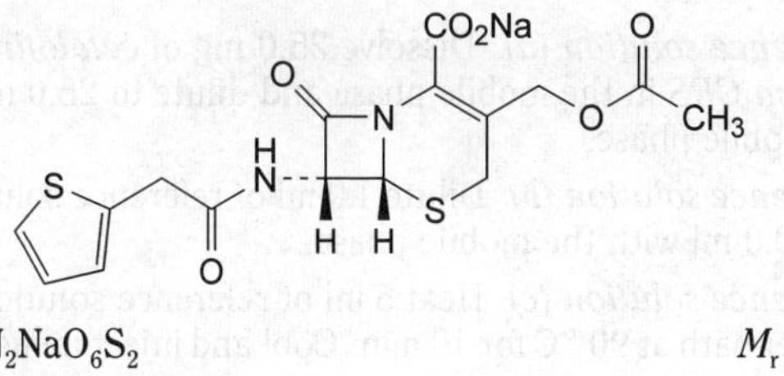

$C_{16}H_{15}N_2NaO_6S_2$ M_r 418.4

DEFINITION

Cefalotin sodium contains not less than 96.0 per cent and not more than the equivalent of 101.0 per cent of sodium (6*R*, 7*R*)-3-[(acetyloxy)methyl]-8-oxo-7-[[2-(thiophen-2-yl)acetyl]-amino]-5-thia-1-azabicyclo[4.2.0]oct-2-ene-2-carboxylate, calculated with reference to the anhydrous substance.

CHARACTERS

A white or almost white powder, freely soluble in water, slightly soluble in ethanol.

IDENTIFICATION

A. Examine by infrared absorption spectrophotometry (*2.2.24*), comparing with the spectrum obtained with *cefalotin sodium CRS*.

B. It gives reaction (a) of sodium (*2.3.1*).

TESTS

Solution S. Dissolve 2.50 g in *carbon dioxide-free water R* and dilute to 25.0 ml with the same solvent.

Appearance of solution. Solution S is clear (*2.2.1*). The absorbance (*2.2.25*) of solution S measured at 450 nm is not greater than 0.20.

pH (*2.2.3*). The pH of solution S is 4.5 to 7.0.

Specific optical rotation (*2.2.7*). Dissolve 1.25 g in *water R* and dilute to 25.0 ml with the same solvent. The specific optical rotation is + 124 to + 134, calculated with reference to the anhydrous substance.

Related substances. Examine by liquid chromatography (*2.2.29*) as described under Assay. Inject the test solution and reference solution (b). Continue the chromatography for at least four times the retention time of the principal peak. In the chromatogram obtained with the test solution: the area of any peak, apart from the principal peak, is not greater than the area of the principal peak in the chromatogram obtained with reference solution (b) (1 per cent) and the sum of the areas of any such peaks is not greater than three times the area of the principal peak in the chromatogram obtained with reference solution (b) (3 per cent). Disregard any peak with an area less than 0.1 times the area of the principal peak in the chromatogram obtained with reference solution (b) (0.1 per cent).

***N,N*-Dimethylaniline** (*2.4.26, Method B*). Not more than 20 ppm.

2-Ethylhexanoic acid (*2.4.28*). Not more than 0.5 per cent *m/m*.

Water (*2.5.12*). Not more than 1.5 per cent, determined on 0.500 g by the semi-micro determination of water.

Bacterial endotoxins (*2.6.14*): less than 0.13 IU/mg, if intended for use in the manufacture of parenteral dosage forms without a further appropriate procedure for the removal of bacterial endotoxins.

ASSAY

Examine by liquid chromatography (*2.2.29*).

Test solution. Dissolve 25.0 mg of the substance to be examined in the mobile phase and dilute to 25.0 ml with the mobile phase.

Reference solution (a). Dissolve 25.0 mg of *cefalotin sodium CRS* in the mobile phase and dilute to 25.0 ml with the mobile phase.

Reference solution (b). Dilute 1.0 ml of reference solution (a) to 100.0 ml with the mobile phase.

Reference solution (c). Heat 5 ml of reference solution (a) in a water-bath at 90 °C for 10 min. Cool and inject immediately.

The chromatographic procedure may be carried out using:

– a stainless steel column 0.25 m long and 4.6 mm in internal diameter packed with *octadecylsilyl silica gel for chromatography R* (5 µm),

– as mobile phase at a flow rate of 1.0 ml/min a solution prepared as follows: dissolve 17 g of *sodium acetate R* in 790 ml of *water R*, add 0.6 ml of *glacial acetic acid R* and adjust if necessary to pH 5.8 to 6.0 with *dilute sodium hydroxide solution R* or *glacial acetic acid R*, add 150 ml of *acetonitrile R* and 70 ml of *ethanol R* and mix,

– as detector a spectrophotometer set at 254 nm,

– a 10 µl loop injector,

maintaining the temperature of the column at 40 °C.

Inject reference solution (c). Adjust the sensitivity of the system to obtain peaks with a height corresponding to at least half the full scale of the recorder. The chromatogram obtained shows two principal peaks corresponding to cefalotin and desacetylcefalotin. The assay is not valid unless the resolution between these two peaks is at least 9.0. Adjust the concentration of acetonitrile in the mobile phase if necessary. The assay is not valid unless the symmetry factor of the cefalotin peak is at most 1.8. Inject reference solution (a) six times. The assay is not valid unless the relative standard deviation of the peak area for cefalotin is at most 1.0 per cent. Inject alternately the test solution and reference solution (a).

Calculate the percentage content of cefalotin sodium.

STORAGE

Store in an airtight container, protected from light. If the substance is sterile, store in a sterile, airtight, tamper-proof container.

LABELLING

The label states, where applicable, that the substance is free from bacterial endotoxins.

IMPURITIES

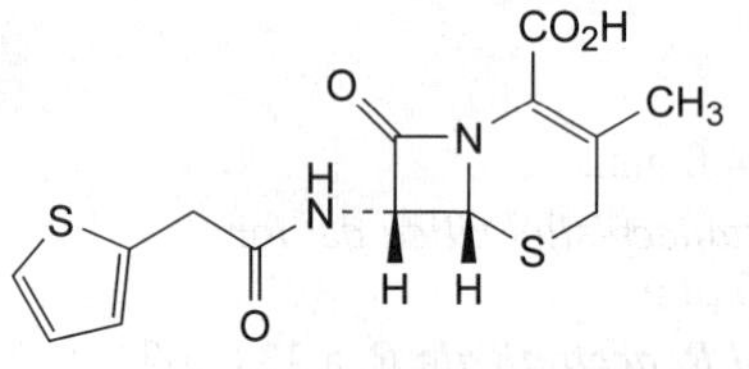

A. (6*R*,7*R*)-3-methyl-8-oxo-7-[[2-(thiophen-2-yl)acetyl]amino]-5-thia-1-azabicyclo[4.2.0]oct-2-ene- 2-carboxylic acid (desacetoxycefalotin).

01/2005:1402
corrected

CEFAMANDOLE NAFATE

Cefamandoli nafas

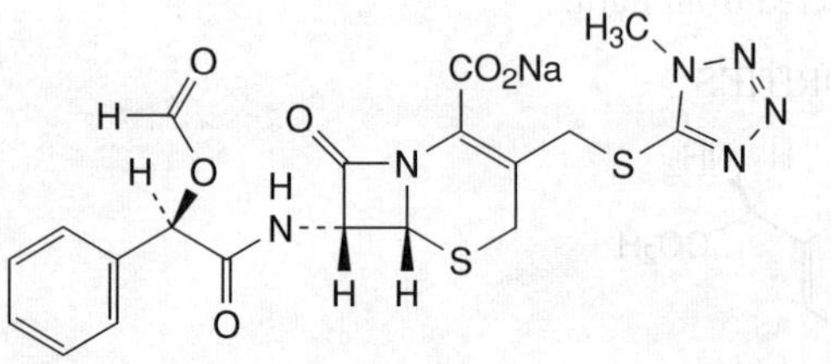

$C_{19}H_{17}N_6NaO_6S_2$ M_r 512.5

DEFINITION

Sodium (6*R*,7*R*)-7-[[(2*R*)-2-(formyloxy)-2-phenylacetyl]amino]-3-[[(1-methyl-1*H*-tetrazol-5-yl)sulphanyl]methyl]-8-oxo-5-thia-1-azabicyclo[4.2.0]oct-2-ene-2-carboxylate with sodium carbonate.

Content:

- cefamandole ($C_{18}H_{18}N_6O_5S_2$): 84.0 per cent to 93.0 per cent (anhydrous and sodium carbonate-free substance),
- sodium carbonate (Na_2CO_3): 4.8 per cent to 6.4 per cent.

CHARACTERS

Appearance: white or almost white powder.

Solubility: freely soluble in water, sparingly soluble in methanol.

IDENTIFICATION

A. Infrared absorption spectrophotometry (*2.2.24*).

Preparation: discs.

Comparison: *cefamandole nafate CRS*.

B. It gives reaction (a) of sodium (*2.3.1*).

TESTS

Solution S. Dissolve 2.5 g in *carbon dioxide-free water R* and dilute to 25 ml with the same solvent.

Appearance of solution. Solution S is clear (*2.2.1*) and its absorbance (*2.2.25*) at 475 nm has a maximum of 0.03.

pH: 6.0 to 8.0 for solution S, measured after 30 min.

Specific optical rotation (*2.2.7*): − 25.0 to − 33.0 (anhydrous and sodium carbonate-free substance).

Dissolve 1.00 g in *acetate buffer solution pH 4.7 R* and dilute to 10.0 ml with the same solvent.

Related substances. Liquid chromatography (*2.2.29*). *Prepare the solutions immediately before use.*

Solvent mixture. Mix 18 volumes of *acetonitrile R* and 75 volumes of a 10 per cent *V/V* solution of *triethylamine R* previously adjusted to pH 2.5 with *phosphoric acid R.*

Test solution. Dissolve 0.100 g of the substance to be examined in the solvent mixture and dilute to 10.0 ml with the solvent mixture.

Reference solution (a). Dilute 1 ml of the test solution to 10 ml with the solvent mixture, then heat the solution at 60 °C for 30 min.

Reference solution (b). Dilute 1.0 ml of the test solution to 100.0 ml with the solvent mixture.

Column:

- *size*: *l* = 0.25 m, Ø = 4.6 mm,
- *stationary phase: octadecylsilyl silica gel for chromatography R* (5 µm).

Mobile phase:

- *triethylamine phosphate solution*: dissolve 2.0 g of *sodium pentanesulphonate R* in 350 ml of *water R*, add 40 ml of *triethylamine R*, adjust to pH 2.5 with *phosphoric acid R* and dilute to 700 ml with *water R*,
- *mobile phase A*: mix 1 volume of triethylamine phosphate solution and 2 volumes of *water R*,
- *mobile phase B*: mix equal volumes of triethylamine phosphate solution, *methanol R* and *acetonitrile R*.

Time (min)	Mobile phase A (per cent *V/V*)	Mobile phase B (per cent *V/V*)
0 - 1	100	0
1 - 35	100 → 0	0 → 100
35 - 45	0	100
45 - 50	0 → 100	100 → 0

Flow rate: 1.5 ml/min.

Detection: spectrophotometer at 254 nm.

Injection: 20 µl loop injector.

System suitability: reference solution (a):

- *resolution*: minimum 5.0 between the peaks due to cefamandole and to cefamandole nafate.

Limits:

- *any impurity*: not more than the area of the principal peak in the chromatogram obtained with reference solution (b) (1 per cent),
- *total*: not more than 5 times the area of the principal peak in the chromatogram obtained with reference solution (b) (5 per cent),
- *disregard limit*: 0.1 times the area of the principal peak in the chromatogram obtained with reference solution (b) (0.1 per cent).

Cefamandole free acid: maximum 9.5 per cent (anhydrous and sodium carbonate-free substance), determined by liquid chromatography as described under Assay.

2-Ethylhexanoic acid (*2.4.28*): maximum 0.3 per cent *m/m*.

Heavy metals (*2.4.8*): maximum 20 ppm.

1.0 g complies with limit test C. Prepare the standard using 2 ml of *lead standard solution (10 ppm Pb) R.*

Water (*2.5.12*): maximum 2.0 per cent, determined on 0.500 g.

Bacterial endotoxins (*2.6.14*): less than 0.15 IU/mg, if intended for use in the manufacture of parenteral dosage forms without a further appropriate procedure for the removal of bacterial endotoxins.

ASSAY

Cefamandole. Liquid chromatography (*2.2.29*). *Prepare the solutions immediately before use.*

Test solution. Dissolve 50.0 mg of the substance to be examined in the mobile phase and dilute to 100.0 ml with the mobile phase.

Reference solution (a). Dissolve 50.0 mg of *cefamandole nafate CRS* in the mobile phase and dilute to 100.0 ml with the mobile phase.

Reference solution (b). Dilute 1 ml of the test solution to 10 ml with the mobile phase, then heat the solution at 60 °C for 30 min.

Column:

- *size*: *l* = 0.25 m, Ø = 4.6 mm,
- *stationary phase*: *octadecylsilyl silica gel for chromatography R* (5 µm).

Mobile phase: mix 25 volumes of *acetonitrile R* and 75 volumes of a 10 per cent *V/V* solution of *triethylamine R* previously adjusted to pH 2.5 with *phosphoric acid R*.

Flow rate: 1.0 ml/min.

Detection: spectrophotometer at 254 nm.

Injection: 20 µl loop injector.

System suitability:

- *resolution*: minimum of 7.0 between the 2 principal peaks in the chromatogram obtained with reference solution (b),

Monographs C

– *repeatability*: maximum relative standard deviation of 0.8 per cent after a series of single injections of a minimum 3 freshly prepared reference solutions (a).

Calculate the percentage content of cefamandole ($C_{18}H_{18}N_6O_5S_2$) from the sum of the contents of cefamandole nafate and cefamandole free acid using the declared contents of *cefamandole nafate CRS*. 1 mg of cefamandole nafate is equivalent to 0.9025 mg of cefamandole.

Sodium carbonate. Dissolve 0.500 g in 50 ml of *water R*. Titrate with *0.1 M hydrochloric acid*, determining the end-point potentiometrically (*2.2.20*).

1 ml of *0.1 M hydrochloric acid* is equivalent to 10.6 mg of Na_2CO_3.

STORAGE

In an airtight container, protected from light. If the substance is sterile, store in a sterile, airtight, tamper-proof container.

LABELLING

The label states:

– that the substance contains sodium carbonate,
– where applicable, that the substance is free from bacterial endotoxins.

IMPURITIES

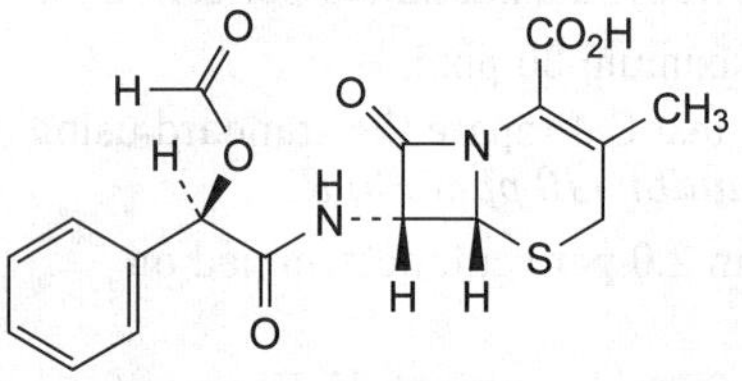

A. (6*R*,7*R*)-7-[[(2*R*)-2-(formyloxy)-2-phenylacetyl]amino]-3-methyl-8-oxo-5-thia-1-azabicyclo[4.2.0]oct-2-ene-2-carboxylic acid (formylmandeloyl-7-amino-desacetoxy-cephalosporanic acid),

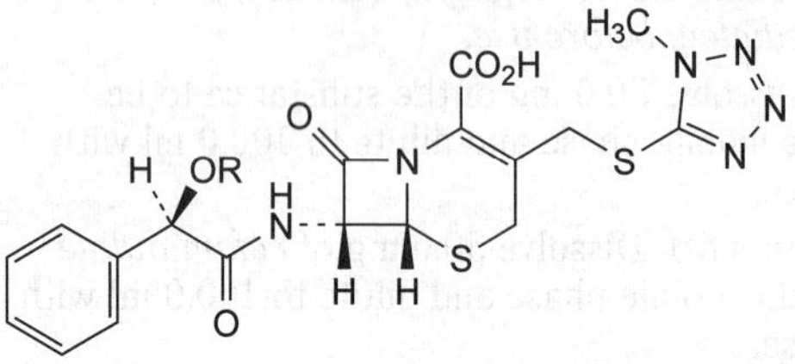

B. R = H: (6*R*,7*R*)-7-[[(2*R*)-2-hydroxy-2-phenylacetyl]amino]-3-[[(1-methyl-1*H*-tetrazol-5-yl)sulphanyl]methyl]-8-oxo-5-thia-1-azabicyclo[4.2.0]oct-2-ene-2-carboxylic acid (cefamandole),

C. R = CO-H_3C: (6*R*,7*R*)-7-[[(2*R*)-2-(acetyloxy)-2-phenylacetyl]amino]-3-[[(1-methyl-1*H*-tetrazol-5-yl)sulphanyl]methyl]-8-oxo-5-thia-1-azabicyclo[4.2.0]oct-2-ene-2-carboxylic acid (*O*-acetylcefamandole),

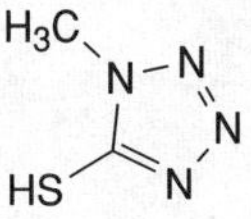

D. 1-methyl-1*H*-tetrazole-5-thiol,

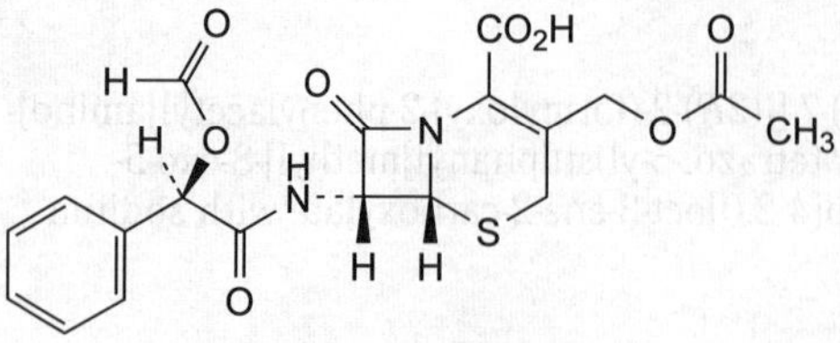

E. (6*R*,7*R*)-7-[[(2*R*)-2-(formyloxy)-2-phenylacetyl]amino]-3-[(acetyloxy)methyl]-8-oxo-5-thia-1-azabicyclo[4.2.0]oct-2-ene-2-carboxylic acid (formylmandeloyl-7-ACA).

01/2005:1650

CEFAPIRIN SODIUM

Cefapirinum natricum

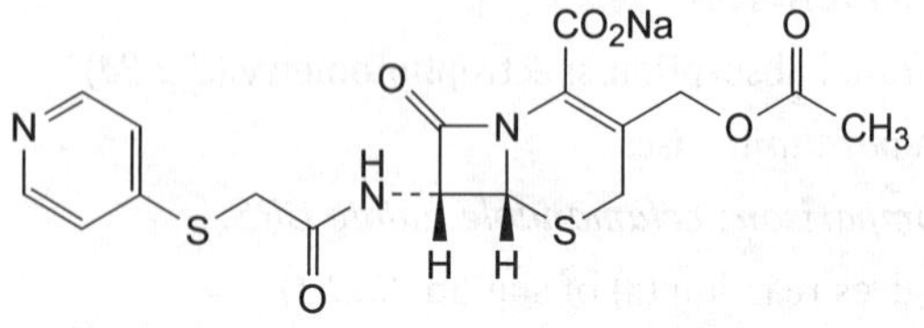

$C_{17}H_{16}N_3NaO_6S_2$ M_r 445.5

DEFINITION

Sodium (6*R*,7*R*)-3-[(acetyloxy)methyl]-8-oxo-7-[[[(pyridin-4-yl)sulphanyl]acetyl]amino]-5-thia-1-azabicyclo[4.2.0]oct-2-ene-2-carboxylate.

Content: 96.0 per cent to 102.0 per cent (anhydrous substance).

CHARACTERS

Appearance: white or pale yellow powder.

Solubility: soluble in water, practically insoluble in methylene chloride.

IDENTIFICATION

A. Infrared absorption spectrophotometry (*2.2.24*).

Comparison: *cefapirin sodium CRS*.

B. It gives reaction (a) of sodium (*2.3.1*).

TESTS

Appearance of solution. Dissolve 2.0 g in *water R* and dilute to 10.0 ml with the same solvent. The solution is clear (*2.2.1*). Dilute 5.0 ml to 10.0 ml with *water R*. The absorbance (*2.2.25*) of this solution at 450 nm is maximum 0.25.

pH (*2.2.3*): 6.5 to 8.5.

Dissolve 0.100 g in *carbon dioxide-free water R* and dilute to 10.0 ml with the same solvent.

Specific optical rotation (*2.2.7*): + 150 to + 165 (anhydrous substance).

Dissolve 0.500 g in *water R* and dilute to 25.0 ml with the same solvent.

Related substances. Liquid chromatography (*2.2.29*). *Prepare the solutions immediately before use.*

Test solution. Dissolve 42 mg of the substance to be examined in the mobile phase and dilute to 200.0 ml with the mobile phase.

Reference solution (a). Dissolve 42 mg of *cefapirin sodium CRS* in the mobile phase and dilute to 200.0 ml with the mobile phase.

Reference solution (b). Dilute 1.0 ml of the test solution to 100.0 ml with the mobile phase.

Reference solution (c). Dilute 1.0 ml of reference solution (b) to 20.0 ml with the mobile phase.

Reference solution (d). Mix 1 ml of the test solution, 8 ml of the mobile phase and 1 ml of *hydrochloric acid R1*. Heat at 60 °C for 10 min.

Column:

- *size*: *l* = 0.30 m, Ø = 4 mm,
- *stationary phase*: *octadecylsilyl silica gel for chromatography R* (10 µm).

Mobile phase: mix 80 ml of *dimethylformamide R*, 4.0 ml of *glacial acetic acid R* and 20 ml of a 4.5 per cent (*m/m*) solution of *potassium hydroxide R*. Dilute to 2 litres with *water R*.

Flow rate: 2.0 ml/min.

Detection: spectrophotometer at 254 nm.

Injection: 20 µl of the test solution and reference solutions (b), (c) and (d).

Run time: twice the retention time of cefapirin.

Relative retention with reference to cefapirin (retention time = about 13 min): impurity B = about 0.3; impurity C = about 0.5; impurity A = about 0.75.

System suitability: reference solution (d):

- *resolution*: minimum 2.0 between the peaks due to cefapirin and impurity A.

Limits:

- *any impurity*: for each impurity, not more than the area of the principal peak in the chromatogram obtained with reference solution (b) (1.0 per cent), and not more than 1 such peak has an area greater than 0.3 times the area of the principal peak in the chromatogram obtained with reference solution (b) (0.3 per cent),
- *total*: not more than twice the area of the principal peak in the chromatogram obtained with reference solution (b) (2.0 per cent),
- *disregard limit*: area of the principal peak in the chromatogram obtained with reference solution (c) (0.05 per cent).

***N,N*-Dimethylaniline** (*2.4.26, Method B*): maximum 20 ppm.

2-Ethylhexanoic acid (*2.4.28*): maximum 0.5 per cent.

Water (*2.5.12*): maximum 2.0 per cent, determined on 0.300 g.

Bacterial endotoxins (*2.6.14*): less than 0.17 IU/mg, if intended for use in the manufacture of parenteral dosage forms without a further appropriate procedure for the removal of bacterial endotoxins.

ASSAY

Liquid chromatography (*2.2.29*) as described in the test for related substances with the following modification.

Injection: test solution and reference solution (a).

Calculate the percentage content of $C_{17}H_{16}N_3NaO_6S_2$.

STORAGE

Protected from light. If the substance is sterile, store in a sterile, tamper-proof container.

LABELLING

The label states, where applicable, that the substance is free from bacterial endotoxins.

IMPURITIES

Specified impurities: A, B, C.

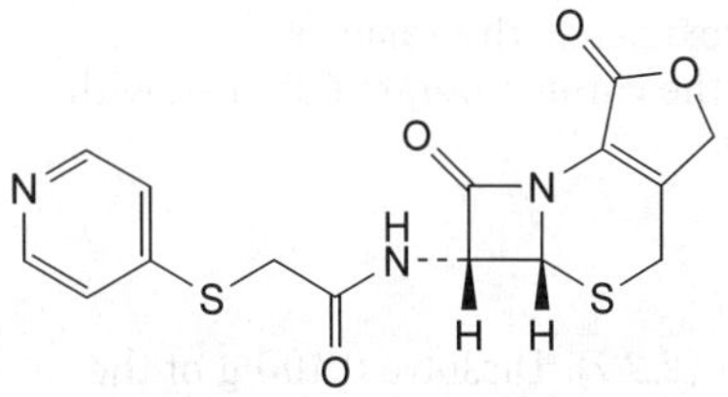

A. (5a*R*,6*R*)-6-[[[(pyridin-4-yl)sulphanyl]acetyl]amino]-5a,6-dihydro-3*H*,7*H*-azeto[2,1-*b*]furo[3,4-*d*][1,3]thiazine-1,7(4*H*)-dione (deacetylcefapirin lactone),

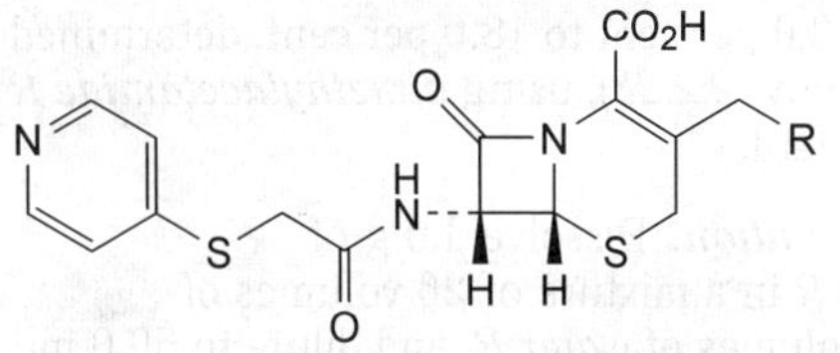

B. R = OH: (6*R*,7*R*)-3-(hydroxymethyl)-8-oxo-7-[[[(pyridin-4-yl)sulphanyl]acetyl]amino]-5-thia-1-azabicyclo[4.2.0]oct-2-ene-2-carboxylic acid (deacetylcefapirin),

C. R = H: (6*R*,7*R*)-3-methyl-8-oxo-7-[[[(pyridin-4-yl)sulphanyl]acetyl]amino]-5-thia-1-azabicyclo[4.2.0]oct-2-ene-2-carboxylic acid (deacetoxycefapirin).

01/2005:1403

CEFATRIZINE PROPYLENE GLYCOL

Cefatrizinum propylen glycolum

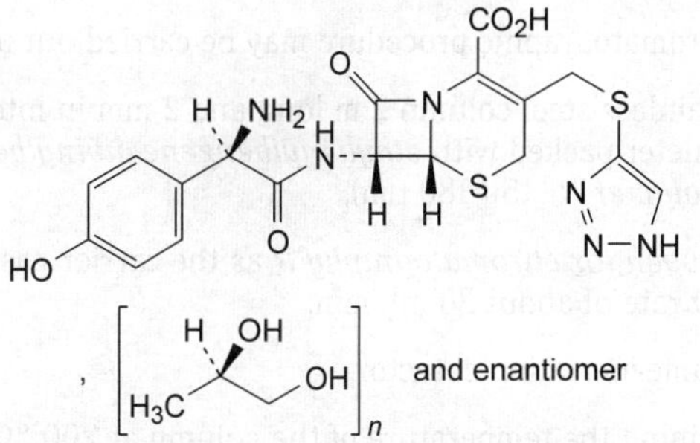

$C_{18}H_{18}N_6O_5S_2, (C_3H_8O_2)_n$ — M_r 462.5 (base)

DEFINITION

Cefatrizine propylene glycol contains not less than 95.0 per cent and not more than the equivalent of 102.0 per cent of (6*R*,7*R*)-7-[[(2*R*)-2-amino-2-(4-hydroxyphenyl)acetyl]amino]-8-oxo-3-[[(1*H*-1,2,3-triazol-4-yl)sulphanyl]methyl]-5-thia-1-azabicyclo[4.2.0]oct-2-ene-2-carboxylic acid, calculated with reference to the anhydrous and propylene glycol free substance. It consists of cefatrizine and propane-1,2-diol (molecular proportions about 1:1). It contains not less than 13.0 per cent and not more than 18.0 per cent of propylene glycol.

CHARACTERS

A white or almost white powder, slightly soluble in water, practically insoluble in alcohol and in methylene chloride.

IDENTIFICATION

A. Examine by infrared absorption spectrophotometry (*2.2.24*), comparing with the spectrum obtained with *cefatrizine propylene glycol CRS*.

B. Examine the chromatograms obtained in the test for propylene glycol. The retention time and size of the principal peak in the chromatogram obtained with the test solution are approximately the same as those of the principal peak in the chromatogram obtained with reference solution (b).

TESTS

Specific optical rotation (*2.2.7*). Dissolve 0.400 g of the substance to be examined in *1 M hydrochloric acid* and dilute to 20.0 ml with the same solvent. The specific optical rotation is + 63 to + 69, calculated with reference to the anhydrous, propylene glycol free substance.

Propylene glycol. 13.0 per cent to 18.0 per cent, determined by gas chromatography (*2.2.28*), using *dimethylacetamide R* as the internal standard.

Internal standard solution. Dissolve 1.0 g of *dimethylacetamide R* in a mixture of 20 volumes of *acetone R* and 80 volumes of *water R*, and dilute to 50.0 ml with the same mixture of solvents.

Test solution. Introduce 0.40 g of the substance to be examined into a ground-glass-stoppered test tube. Add 3.0 ml of the internal standard solution, 1.0 ml of a mixture of 20 volumes of *acetone R* and 80 volumes of *water R* and 2.0 ml of *hydrochloric acid R*. Seal the test tube and stir the solution.

Reference solution (a). Dissolve 2.0 g of *propylene glycol R* in a mixture of 20 volumes of *acetone R* and 80 volumes of *water R* and dilute to 100.0 ml with the same solvent.

Reference solution (b). Introduce into a ground-glass-stoppered test tube 1.0 ml of reference solution (a) and 1.0 ml of the internal standard solution.

The chromatographic procedure may be carried out using:

– a stainless steel column 2 m long and 2 mm in internal diameter packed with *ethylvinylbenzene-divinylbenzene copolymer R* (150-180 µm),

– *nitrogen for chromatography R* as the carrier gas at a flow rate of about 30 ml/min,

– a flame-ionisation detector,

maintaining the temperature of the column at 200 °C and that of the injection port and of the detector at 250 °C.

Inject separately 1 µl of the test solution and 1 µl of reference solution (b).

7-ACA triazole and other related substances. Examine by liquid chromatography (*2.2.29*) as described under Assay. Adjust the sensitivity of the system so that the height of the principal peak obtained with 20 µl of reference solution (c) is at least 50 per cent of the full scale of the recorder. Inject 20 µl of the test solution and continue the chromatography for at least twice the retention time of the principal peak. In the chromatogram obtained with the test solution: the area of any peak corresponding to cefatrizine impurity A is not greater than that of the peak due to cefatrizine impurity A in the chromatogram obtained with reference solution (d) (0.5 per cent); the area of any peak apart from the principal peak and any peak corresponding to cefatrizine impurity A is not greater than the area of the principal peak in the chromatogram obtained with reference solution (c) (0.6 per cent); the sum of the areas of any such peaks is not greater than 3.5 times the area of the principal peak in the chromatogram obtained with reference solution (c) (2.1 per cent). Disregard any peak with an area less than 0.05 times that of the principal peak in the chromatogram obtained with reference solution (c).

Water (*2.5.12*). Not more than 1.5 per cent, determined on 0.500 g by the semi-micro determination of water.

Sulphated ash (*2.4.14*). Not more than 0.1 per cent, determined on 1.0 g.

ASSAY

Examine by liquid chromatography (*2.2.29*).

Test solution. Dissolve 60.0 mg of the substance to be examined in the mobile phase and dilute to 100.0 ml with the mobile phase.

Reference solution (a). Dissolve 60.0 mg of *cefatrizine propylene glycol CRS* in the mobile phase and dilute to 100.0 ml with the mobile phase.

Reference solution (b). Dissolve 30.0 mg of *cefatrizine impurity A CRS* in *buffer solution pH 7.0 R* and dilute to 100.0 ml with the same buffer solution.

Reference solution (c). Dilute 0.6 ml of reference solution (a) to 100.0 ml with the mobile phase.

Reference solution (d). Dilute 1.0 ml of reference solution (b) to 100.0 ml with *buffer solution pH 7.0 R*.

Reference solution (e). To 1.0 ml of reference solution (a) add 1.0 ml of reference solution (b) and dilute to 10.0 ml with the mobile phase.

The chromatographic procedure may be carried out using:

– a stainless steel column 0.25 m long and 4 mm in internal diameter packed with *octadecylsilyl silica gel for chromatography R* (5 µm),

– as mobile phase at a flow rate of 2 ml/min a mixture of 5 volumes of *acetonitrile R* and 95 volumes of a 2.72 g/l solution of *potassium dihydrogen phosphate R* in *water R*,

– as detector a spectrophotometer set at 272 nm.

Adjust the sensitivity of the system so that the height of the principal peak obtained with 20 µl of reference solution (a) is at least 50 per cent of the full scale of the recorder. Inject 20 µl of reference solution (a) six times. The test is not valid unless the relative standard deviation is at most 1.0 per cent. Inject reference solution (e). The test is not valid unless the resolution between the peaks corresponding to cefatrizine and cefatrizine impurity A is at least 5.0.

Inject alternately 20 µl of the test solution and 20 µl of reference solution (a) and calculate the percentage content of cefatrizine using the chromatogram obtained with reference solution (a).

IMPURITIES

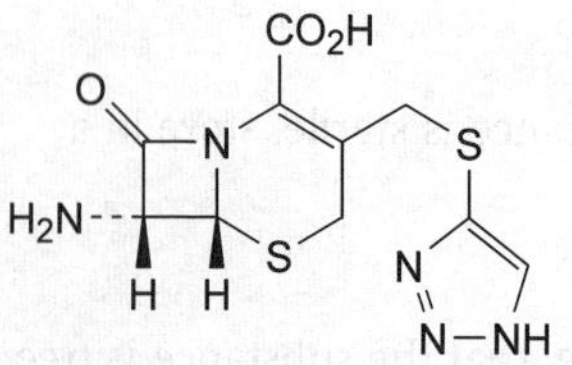

A. (6*R*,7*R*)-7-amino-8-oxo-3-[[(1*H*-1,2,3-triazol-4-yl)sulphanyl]methyl]-5-thia-1-azabicyclo[4.2.0]oct-2-ene-2-carboxylic acid (7-ACA triazole).

01/2005:0988

CEFAZOLIN SODIUM

Cefazolinum natricum

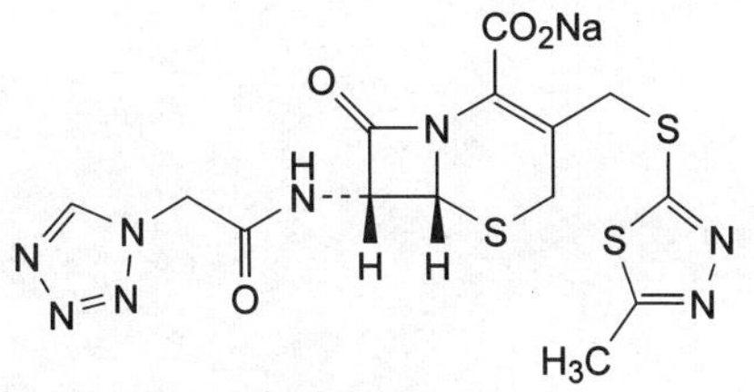

$C_{14}H_{13}N_8NaO_4S_3$ M_r 476.5

DEFINITION

Sodium (6*R*,7*R*)-3-[[(5-methyl-1,3,4-thiadiazol-2-yl)sulphanyl]methyl]-8-oxo-7-[(1*H*-tetrazol-1-ylacetyl)amino]-5-thia-1-azabicyclo[4.2.0]oct-2-ene-2-carboxylate.

Content: 95.0 per cent to 102.0 per cent (anhydrous substance).

CHARACTERS

Appearance: white or almost white powder, very hygroscopic.

Solubility: freely soluble in water, very slightly soluble in alcohol.

It shows polymorphism.

IDENTIFICATION

A. Infrared absorption spectrophotometry (*2.2.24*).

Preparation: dissolve 0.150 g in 5 ml of *water R*, add 0.5 ml of *dilute acetic acid R*, swirl and allow to stand for 10 min in iced water. Filter the precipitate and rinse with 1-2 ml of *water R*. Dissolve in a mixture of 1 volume of *water R* and 9 volumes of *acetone R*. Evaporate the solvent almost to dryness, then dry in an oven at 60 °C for 30 min.

Comparison: *cefazolin CRS*.

B. It gives reaction (a) of sodium (*2.3.1*).

TESTS

Solution S. Dissolve 2.50 g in *carbon dioxide-free water R* and dilute to 25.0 ml with the same solvent.

Appearance of solution. Solution S is clear (*2.2.1*) and its absorbance (*2.2.25*) at 430 nm has a maximum of 0.15.

pH (*2.2.3*): 4.0 to 6.0 for solution S.

Specific optical rotation (*2.2.7*): − 15 to − 24 (anhydrous substance).

Dissolve 1.25 g in *water R* and dilute to 25.0 ml with the same solvent.

Absorbance (*2.2.25*). Dissolve 0.100 g in *water R* and dilute to 100.0 ml with the same solvent. Dilute 2.0 ml of the solution to 100.0 ml with *sodium hydrogen carbonate solution R*. Examined between 220 nm and 350 nm, the solution shows an absorption maximum at 272 nm. The specific absorbance at the maximum is 260 to 300 (anhydrous substance).

Related substances. Liquid chromatography (*2.2.29*).

Test solution. Dissolve 50.0 mg of the substance to be examined in mobile phase A and dilute to 20.0 ml with the same mobile phase.

Reference solution (a). Dilute 1.0 ml of the test solution to 100.0 ml with mobile phase A.

Reference solution (b). Dissolve 20 mg of the substance to be examined in 10 ml of a 2 g/l solution of *sodium hydroxide R*. Allow to stand for 15-30 min. Dilute 1.0 ml of the solution to 20 ml with mobile phase A.

Column:

- *size*: *l* = 0.125 m, Ø = 4.0 mm,
- *stationary phase*: *octadecylsilyl silica gel for chromatography R* (3 µm),
- *temperature*: 45 °C.

Mobile phase:

- *mobile phase A*: solution containing 14.54 g/l of *disodium hydrogen phosphate R* and 3.53 g/l of *potassium dihydrogen phosphate R*,
- *mobile phase B*: *acetonitrile for chromatography R*,

Time (min)	Mobile phase A (per cent *V/V*)	Mobile phase B (per cent *V/V*)	λ (nm)
0 - 1	98	2	210
1 - 2	98	2	254
2 - 4	98 → 85	2 → 15	254
4 - 10	85 → 60	15 → 40	254
10 - 11.5	60 → 35	40 → 65	254
11.5 - 12	35	65	254
12 - 15	35 → 98	65 → 2	254
15 - 16	98	2	254
16 - 21	98	2	210

Flow rate: 1.2 ml/min.

Detection: spectrophotometer at 210 nm and at 254 nm (see table above).

Injection: 5 µl.

System suitability: reference solution (b):

- *resolution*: minimum 2.0 between the peaks due to cefazolin and to impurity I (see Figure 0988.-1).

Limits:

- *any impurity* (seen at 210 nm or 254 nm): not more than the area of the principal peak in the chromatogram obtained with reference solution (a) (1.0 per cent),
- *total*: not more than 3.5 times the area of the principal peak in the chromatogram obtained with reference solution (a) (3.5 per cent),
- *disregard limit*: 0.05 times the area of the principal peak in the chromatogram obtained with reference solution (a) (0.05 per cent).

***N,N*-Dimethylaniline** (*2.4.26, Method B*): maximum 20 ppm.

Water (*2.5.12*): maximum 6.0 per cent, determined on 0.300 g.

Bacterial endotoxins (*2.6.14*): less than 0.15 IU/mg, if intended for use in the manufacture of parenteral dosage forms without a further appropriate procedure for the removal of bacterial endotoxins.

ASSAY

Liquid chromatography (*2.2.29*).

Test solution. Dissolve 50.0 mg of the substance to be examined in the mobile phase and dilute to 50.0 ml with the mobile phase.

Reference solution (a). Dissolve 50.0 mg of *cefazolin CRS* in the mobile phase and dilute to 50.0 ml with the mobile phase.

Reference solution (b). Dissolve 5.0 mg of *cefuroxime sodium CRS* in 10.0 ml of reference solution (a) and dilute to 100.0 ml with the mobile phase.

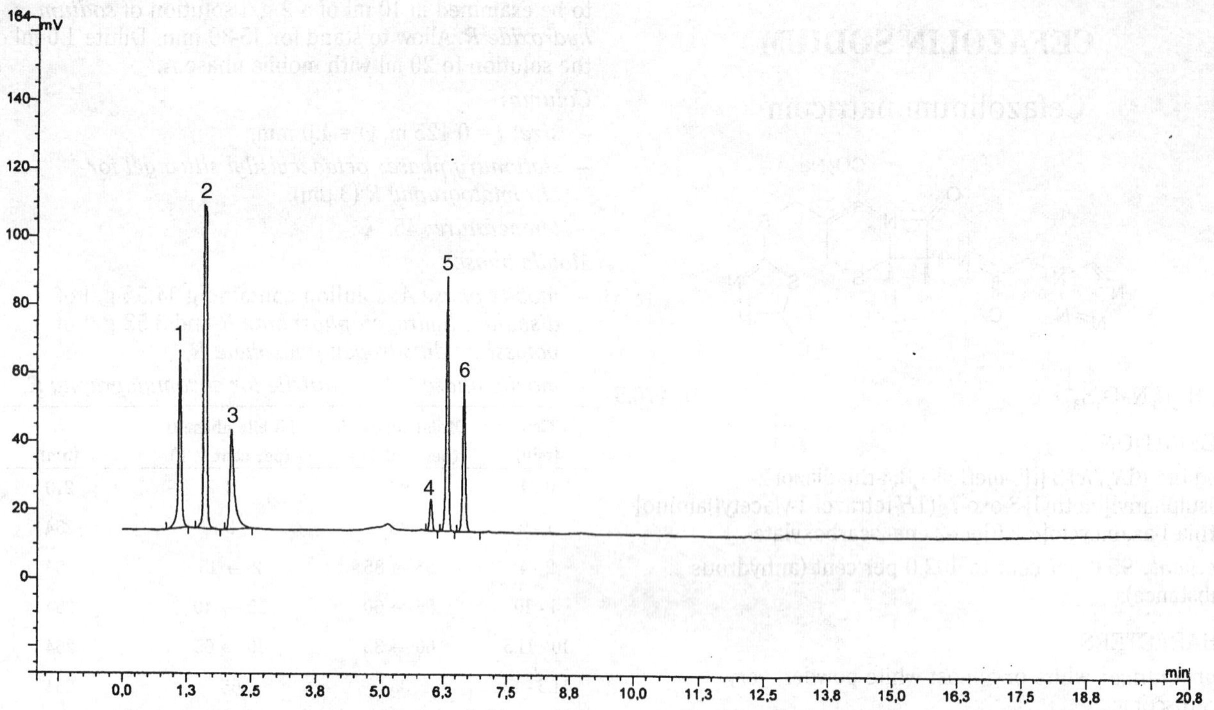

1. impurity F
2. impurity J
3. impurity E
4. unknown
5. cefazolin
6. impurity I

Figure 0988.-1. – *Chromatogram of reference solution (b) (in situ degradation) for the test for related substances of cefazolin sodium*

Column:

– *size*: l = 0.25 m, Ø = 4.6 mm,

– *stationary phase*: *octadecylsilyl silica gel for chromatography R* (5 µm).

Mobile phase: mix 10 volumes of *acetonitrile R* and 90 volumes of a solution containing 2.77 g/l of *disodium hydrogen phosphate R* and 1.86 g/l of *citric acid R.*

Flow rate: 1.0 ml/min.

Detection: spectrophotometer at 270 nm.

Injection: 20 µl.

System suitability: reference solution (b):

– *resolution*: minimum 2.0 between the peaks due to cefazolin and cefuroxime.

Calculate the percentage content of cefazolin sodium by multiplying the percentage content of cefazolin by 1.048.

STORAGE

In an airtight container, protected from light. If the substance is sterile, store in a sterile, airtight, tamper-proof container.

LABELLING

The label states, where applicable, that the substance is free from bacterial endotoxins.

IMPURITIES

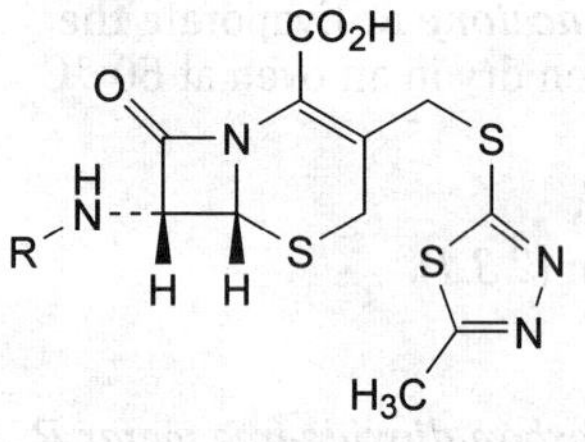

A. R = H: (6*R*,7*R*)-7-amino-3-[[(5-methyl-1,3,4-thiadiazol-2-yl)sulphanyl]methyl]-8-oxo-5-thia-1-azabicyclo[4.2.0]oct-2-ene-2-carboxylic acid,

B. R = CO-C(CH_3)$_3$: (6*R*,7*R*)-7-[(2,2-dimethylpropanoyl)amino]-3-[[(5-methyl-1,3,4-thiadiazol-2-yl)sulphanyl]methyl]-8-oxo-5-thia-1-azabicyclo[4.2.0]oct-2-ene-2-carboxylic acid,

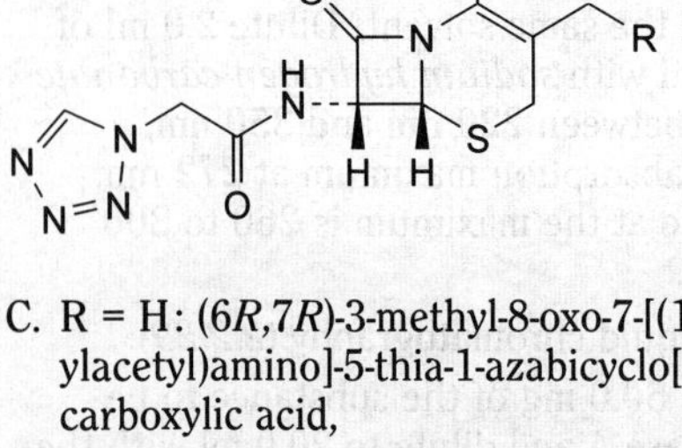

C. R = H: (6*R*,7*R*)-3-methyl-8-oxo-7-[(1*H*-tetrazol-1-ylacetyl)amino]-5-thia-1-azabicyclo[4.2.0]oct-2-ene-2-carboxylic acid,

D. R = O-CO-CH_3: (6*R*,7*R*)-3-[(acetyloxy)methyl]-8-oxo-7-[(1*H*-tetrazol-1-ylacetyl)amino]-5-thia-1-azabicyclo[4.2.0]oct-2-ene-2-carboxylic acid,

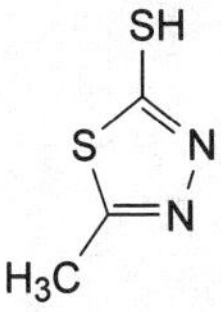

E. 5-methyl-1,3,4-thiadiazol-2-thiol (MMTD),

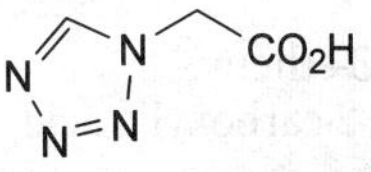

F. (1*H*-tetrazol-1-yl)acetic acid,

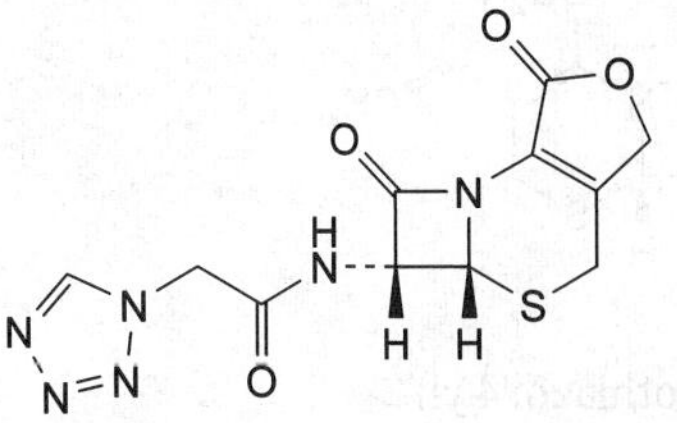

G. (5a*R*,6*R*)-6-[(1*H*-tetrazol-1-ylacetyl)amino]-5a,6-dihydro-3*H*,7*H*-azeto[2,1-*b*]furo[3,4-*d*][1,3]thiazine-1,7(4*H*)-dione,

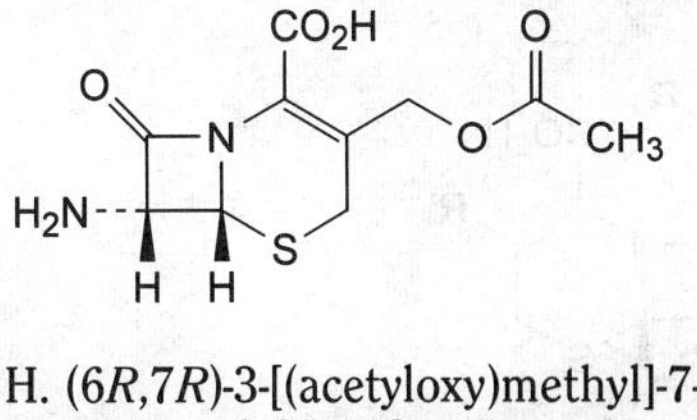

H. (6*R*,7*R*)-3-[(acetyloxy)methyl]-7-amino-8-oxo-5-thia-1-azabicyclo[4.2.0]oct-2-ene-2-carboxylic acid (7-ACA),

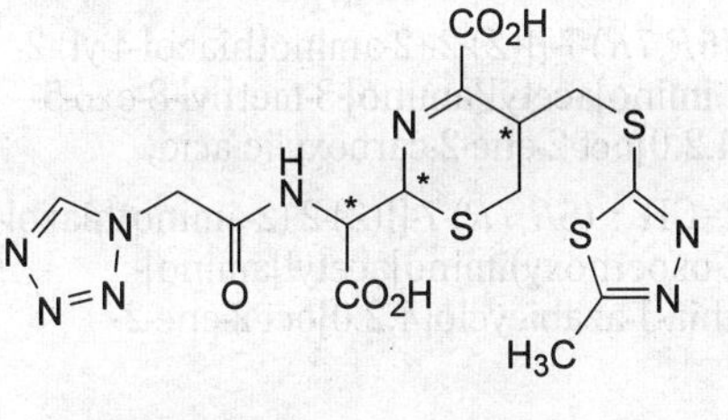

I. 2-[carboxy[(1*H*-tetrazol-1-ylacetyl)amino]methyl]-5-[[(5-methyl-1,3,4-thiadiazol-2-yl)sulphanyl]methyl]-5,6-dihydro-2*H*-1,3-thiazine-4-carboxylic acid (cefazoloic acid),

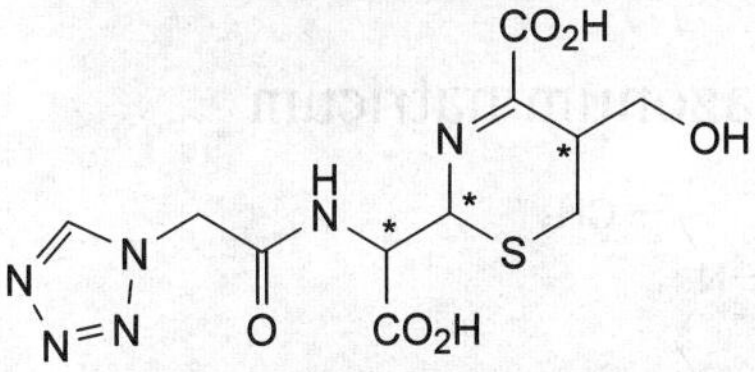

J. 2-[carboxy[(1*H*-tetrazol-1-ylacetyl)amino]methyl]-5-(hydroxymethyl)-5,6-dihydro-2*H*-1,3-thiazine-4-carboxylic acid (hydrolysed cefazoloic acid),

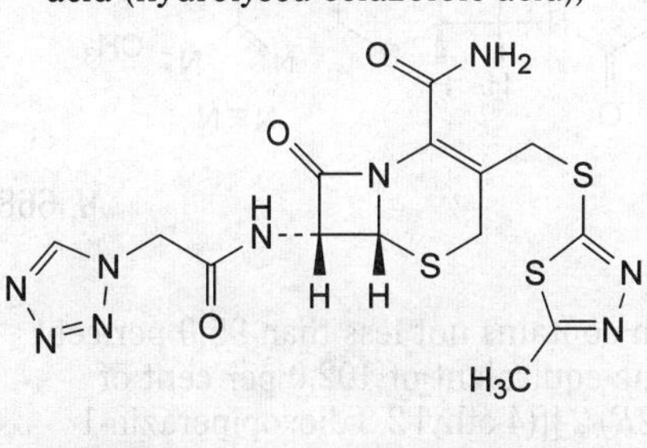

K. (6*R*,7*R*)-3-[[(5-methyl-1,3,4-thiadiazol-2-yl)sulphanyl]methyl]-8-oxo-7-[(1*H*-tetrazol-1-ylacetyl)amino]-5-thia-1-azabicyclo[4.2.0]oct-2-ene-2-carboxamide (cefazolinamide).

01/2005:1188
corrected

CEFIXIME

Cefiximum

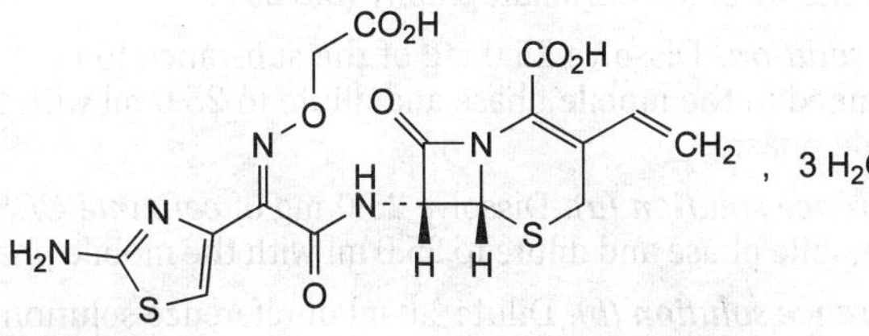

$C_{16}H_{15}N_5O_7S_2,3H_2O$ M_r 507.5

DEFINITION

Cefixime is (6*R*,7*R*)-7-[[(*Z*)-2-(2-aminothiazol-4-yl)-2-[(carboxymethoxy)imino]acetyl]amino]-3-ethenyl-8-oxo-5-thia-1-azabicyclo[4.2.0]oct-2-ene-2-carboxylic acid trihydrate. It contains not less than 95.0 per cent and not more than the equivalent of 101.0 per cent of $C_{16}H_{15}N_5O_7S_2$, calculated with reference to the anhydrous and ethanol-free substance.

CHARACTERS

A white or almost white powder, slightly hygroscopic, slightly soluble in water, soluble in methanol, sparingly soluble in ethanol, practically insoluble in ethyl acetate.

IDENTIFICATION

Examine by infrared absorption spectrophotometry (*2.2.24*), comparing with the spectrum obtained with *cefixime CRS*. If the spectra obtained show differences, dissolve the substance to be examined and the reference substance separately in *methanol R*, evaporate to dryness and record new spectra using the residues.

TESTS

pH (*2.2.3*). Suspend 0.5 g in *carbon dioxide-free water R* and dilute to 10 ml with the same solvent. The pH of the suspension is 2.6 to 4.1.

Related substances. Examine by liquid chromatography (*2.2.29*) as described under Assay. Inject reference solution (b). Adjust the sensitivity of the system so that the height of the principal peak in the chromatogram obtained is at least 50 per cent of the full scale of the recorder. Inject the test solution and continue the chromatography for 3 times the retention time of the principal peak. In the chromatogram obtained with the test solution: the area of any peak, apart from the principal peak, is not greater than half the area of the principal peak in the chromatogram obtained with reference solution (b) (0.5 per cent); the sum of the areas of all the peaks, apart from the principal peak, is not greater than 3 times the area of the principal peak in the chromatogram obtained with reference solution (b) (3 per cent). Disregard any peak with an area less than 0.1 times that of the principal peak in the chromatogram obtained with reference solution (b).

Ethanol (*2.4.24*). Not more than 1.0 per cent *m/m*, determined by head-space gas chromatography (*2.2.28*), using the standard additions method.

Sample solution. Dissolve 0.250 g of the substance to be examined in a mixture of 1 volume of *dimethylacetamide R* and 4 volumes of *water R* and dilute to 25.0 ml with the same mixture of solvents.

Water (*2.5.12*): 9.0 per cent to 12.0 per cent, determined on 0.200 g by the semi-micro determination of water.

Sulphated ash (*2.4.14*). Not more than 0.2 per cent, determined on 1.0 g.

ASSAY

Examine by liquid chromatography (*2.2.29*).

Test solution. Dissolve 25.0 mg of the substance to be examined in the mobile phase and dilute to 25.0 ml with the mobile phase.

Reference solution (a). Dissolve 25.0 mg of *cefixime CRS* in the mobile phase and dilute to 25.0 ml with the mobile phase.

Reference solution (b). Dilute 1.0 ml of reference solution (a) to 100.0 ml with the mobile phase.

Reference solution (c). Dissolve 10 mg of *cefixime CRS* in 10 ml of *water R*. Heat on a water-bath for 45 min. Cool and inject immediately.

The chromatographic procedure may be carried out using:

- a column 0.125 m long and 4 mm in internal diameter packed with *octadecylsilyl silica gel for chromatography R* (5 µm),
- as mobile phase at a flow rate of 1.0 ml/min a mixture of 250 volumes of *acetonitrile R* and 750 volumes of a tetrabutylammonium hydroxide solution prepared as follows: dissolve 8.2 g of *tetrabutylammonium hydroxide R* in *water R* and dilute to 800 ml with the same solvent; adjust to pH 6.5 with *dilute phosphoric acid R* and dilute to 1000 ml with *water R*,
- as detector a spectrophotometer set at 254 nm,
- a 10 µl loop injector,

maintaining the temperature of the column at 40 °C.

Inject reference solution (c). Adjust the sensitivity of the system so that the heights of the principal peaks are at least 20 per cent of the full scale of the recorder. The test is not valid unless the resolution between the 2 principal peaks (cefixime and *E*-isomer) is at least 2.0. If necessary, adjust the concentration of acetonitrile in the mobile phase. Inject reference solution (a) 6 times. The test is not valid unless the relative standard deviation of the peak area for cefixime is at most 1.0 per cent. Inject alternately the test solution and reference solution (a).

STORAGE

Store in an airtight container, protected from light.

IMPURITIES

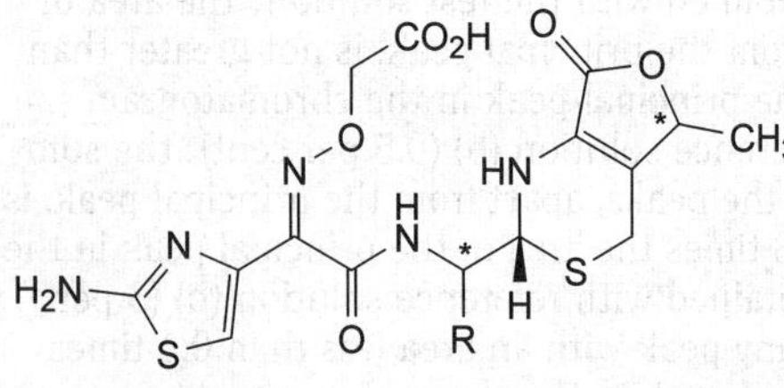

A. R = CO_2H: 2-[[(*Z*)-2-(2-aminothiazol-4-yl)-2-[(carboxymethoxy)imino]acetyl]amino]-2-[(2*R*)-5-methyl-7-oxo-1,2,5,7-tetrahydro-4*H*-furo[3,4-*d*][1,3]thiazin-2-yl]acetic acid,

B. R = H: 2-[[[(*Z*)-1-(2-aminothiazol-4-yl)-2-[[[(2*R*,5*RS*)-5-methyl-7-oxo-1,2,5,7-tetrahydro-4*H*-furo[3,4-*d*][1,3]thiazin-2-yl]methyl]amino]-2-oxoethylidene]amino]oxy]acetic acid,

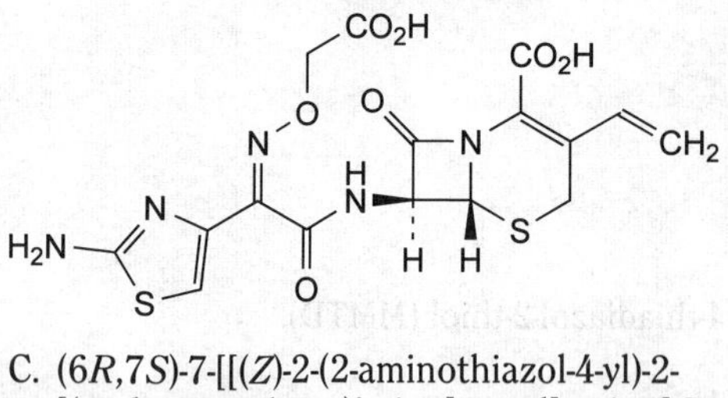

C. (6*R*,7*S*)-7-[[(*Z*)-2-(2-aminothiazol-4-yl)-2-[(carboxymethoxy)imino]acetyl]amino]-3-ethenyl-8-oxo-5-thia-1-azabicyclo[4.2.0]oct-2-ene-2-carboxylic acid (cefixime 7-epimer),

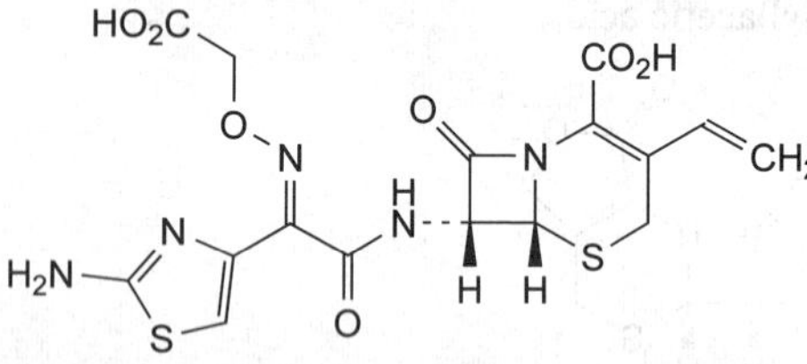

D. (6*R*,7*R*)-7-[[(*E*)-2-(2-aminothiazol-4-yl)-2-[(carboxymethoxy)imino]acetyl]amino]-3-ethenyl-8-oxo-5-thia-1-azabicyclo[4.2.0]oct-2-ene-2-carboxylic acid (cefixime *E*-isomer),

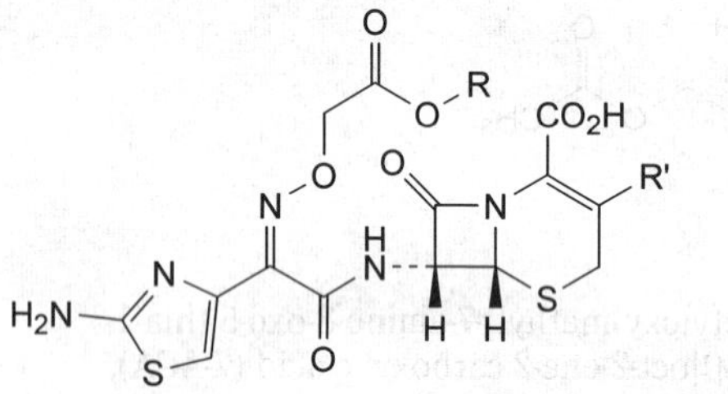

E. R = H, R′ = CH_3: (6*R*,7*R*)-7-[[(*Z*)-2-(2-aminothiazol-4-yl)-2-[(carboxymethoxy)imino]acetyl]amino]-3-methyl-8-oxo-5-thia-1-azabicyclo[4.2.0]oct-2-ene-2-carboxylic acid,

F. R = C_2H_5, R′ = $CH=CH_2$: (6*R*,7*R*)-7-[[(*Z*)-2-(2-aminothiazol-4-yl)-2-[(2-ethoxy-2-oxoethoxy)imino]acetyl]amino]-3-ethenyl-8-oxo-5-thia-1-azabicyclo[4.2.0]oct-2-ene-2-carboxylic acid.

01/2005:1404

CEFOPERAZONE SODIUM

Cefoperazonum natricum

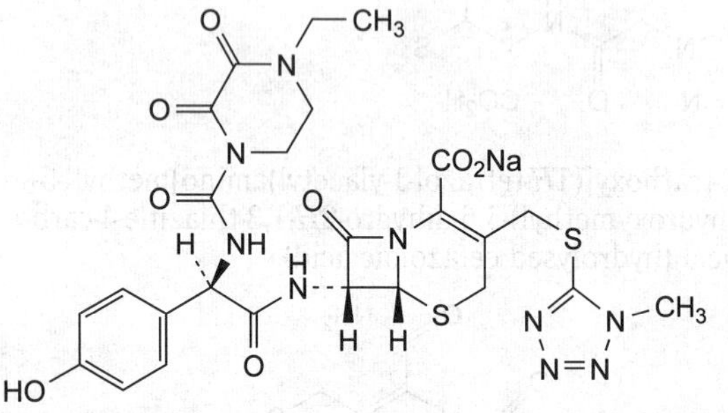

$C_{25}H_{26}N_9NaO_8S_2$ M_r 668

DEFINITION

Cefoperazone sodium contains not less than 95.0 per cent and not more than the equivalent of 102.0 per cent of sodium (6*R*,7*R*)-7-[[(2*R*)-2-[[(4-ethyl-2,3-dioxopiperazin-1-yl)carbonyl]amino]-2-(4-hydroxyphenyl)acetyl]amino]-3-[[(1-methyl-1*H*-tetrazol-5-yl)sulphanyl]methyl]-8-oxo-5-thia-1-azabicyclo[4.2.0]oct-2-ene-2-carboxylate, calculated with reference to the anhydrous and acetone-free substance.

CHARACTERS

A white or slightly yellow powder, hygroscopic, freely soluble in water, soluble in methanol, slightly soluble in alcohol.

If crystalline, it shows polymorphism.

IDENTIFICATION

A. Dissolve the substance to be examined in *methanol R* and evaporate to dryness. Examine by infrared absorption spectrophotometry (*2.2.24*), comparing with the *Ph. Eur. reference spectrum of cefoperazone sodium.*

B. Examine the chromatograms obtained in the assay. The retention time and size of the principal peak in the chromatogram obtained with test solution (a) are approximately the same as those of the principal peak in the chromatogram obtained with reference solution (a).

C. It gives reaction (a) of sodium (*2.3.1*).

TESTS

Appearance of solution. Dissolve 2.5 g in *water R* and dilute to 25.0 ml with the same solvent. The solution is clear (*2.2.1*). The absorbance of the solution measured at 430 nm (*2.2.25*) is not greater than 0.15.

pH (*2.2.3*). Dissolve 2.5 g in *carbon dioxide-free water R* and dilute to 10 ml with the same solvent. The pH of the solution is 4.5 to 6.5.

Related substances. Examine by liquid chromatography (*2.2.29*) as prescribed under Assay. Inject 20 µl of reference solution (b) and adjust the sensitivity of the system so that the height of the principal peak in the chromatogram obtained is at least 50 per cent of the full scale of the recorder. Inject 20 µl of test solution (b). Continue the chromatography for at least 2.5 times the retention time of the principal peak. In the chromatogram obtained with test solution (b): the area of any peak, apart from the principal peak, is not greater than 1.5 times the area of the principal peak in the chromatogram obtained with reference solution (b) (1.5 per cent); the sum of the areas of any such peaks is not greater than 4.5 times the area of the principal peak in the chromatogram obtained with reference solution (b) (4.5 per cent). Disregard any peak with an area less than 0.1 times the area of the principal peak in the chromatogram obtained with reference solution (b).

Acetone. Not more than 2.0 per cent, determined by head-space gas chromatography (*2.2.28*), using the method of standard additions.

Sample solution. Dissolve 0.500 g of the substance to be examined in *water R* and dilute to 10.0 ml with the same solvent.

Solvent solution. Dissolve 0.350 g of *acetone R* in *water R* and dilute to 100.0 ml with the same solvent. Dilute 10.0 ml of the solution to 100.0 ml with *water R*.

Prepare each of 4 injection vials as shown in the table below:

Vial No.	Sample solution (ml)	Solvent solution (ml)	*Water R* (ml)
1	1.0	0	4.0
2	1.0	1.0	3.0
3	1.0	2.0	2.0
4	1.0	3.0	1.0

The chromatographic procedure may be carried out using system B of the test for residual solvents (*2.4.24*) and the following static head-space injection conditions:

- equilibration time: 15 min,
- transfer-line temperature: 110 °C,

maintaining the temperature of the column at 40 °C for 10 min.

Heavy metals (*2.4.8*). 2.0 g complies with limit test C (5 ppm). Prepare the standard using 1 ml of *lead standard solution (10 ppm Pb) R.*

Water (*2.5.12*). Not more than 5.0 per cent, determined on 0.200 g.

Bacterial endotoxins (*2.6.14*): less than 0.20 IU/mg, if intended for use in the manufacture of parenteral dosage forms without a further appropriate procedure for the removal of bacterial endotoxins.

ASSAY

Examine by liquid chromatography (*2.2.29*). *Prepare the solutions immediately before use.*

Test solution (a). Dissolve 25.0 mg of the substance to be examined in the mobile phase and dilute to 250.0 ml with the mobile phase.

Test solution (b). Dissolve 25.0 mg of the substance to be examined in the mobile phase and dilute to 50.0 ml with the mobile phase.

Reference solution (a). Dissolve 25.0 mg of *cefoperazone dihydrate CRS* in the mobile phase and dilute to 250.0 ml with the mobile phase.

Reference solution (b). Dilute 5.0 ml of reference solution (a) to 100.0 ml with the mobile phase.

The chromatographic procedure may be carried out using:

- a stainless steel column 0.15 m long and 4.6 mm in internal diameter packed with *end-capped octadecylsilyl silica gel for chromatography R* (5 µm),
- as mobile phase at a flow rate of 1 ml/min a mixture of 884 volumes of *water R*; 110 volumes of *acetonitrile R*; 3.5 volumes of a 60 g/l solution of *acetic acid R*; 2.5 volumes of a triethylammonium acetate solution prepared by diluting 14 ml of *triethylamine R* and 5.7 ml of *glacial acetic acid R* to 100 ml with *water R*,
- as detector a spectrophotometer set at 254 nm.

Inject 20 µl of reference solution (a). When the chromatogram is recorded in the prescribed conditions, the retention time is about 15 min for cefoperazone. Adjust the sensitivity of the system so that the height of the principal peak in the chromatogram obtained is at least 50 per cent of the full scale of the recorder. The test is not valid unless in the chromatogram obtained with reference solution (a), the number of theoretical plates calculated for the principal peak is at least 5000 and its symmetry factor is at most 1.6. If necessary adjust the content of *acetonitrile R* in the mobile phase. Inject reference solution (a) 6 times. The test is not valid unless the relative standard deviation of the peak area is at most 1.0 per cent. Inject alternately test solution (a) and reference solution (a).

Calculate the percentage content of cefoperazone sodium by multiplying the percentage content of cefoperazone by 1.034.

STORAGE

In an airtight container, protected from light, at a temperature of 2 °C to 8 °C. If the substance is sterile, store in a sterile, airtight, tamper-proof container.

LABELLING

The label states, where applicable, that the substance is free from bacterial endotoxins.

IMPURITIES

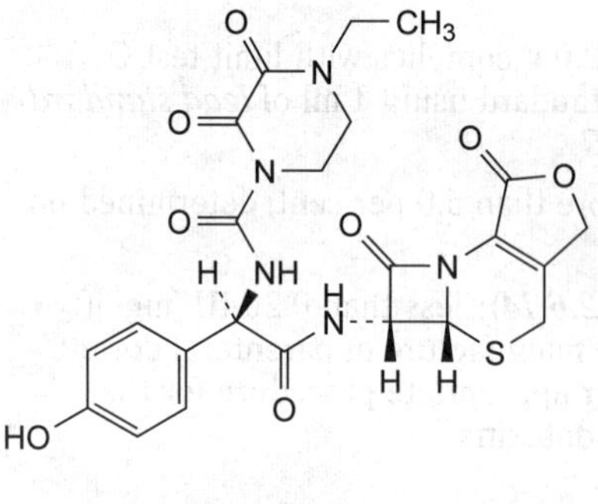

A. (5a*R*,6*R*)-6-[[(2*R*)-2-[[(4-ethyl-2,3-dioxopiperazin-1-yl)carbonyl]amino]-2-(4-hydroxyphenyl)acetyl]amino]-5a,6-dihydro-3*H*,7*H*-azeto[2,1-*b*]furo[3,4-*d*][1,3]thiazine-1,7(4*H*)-dione,

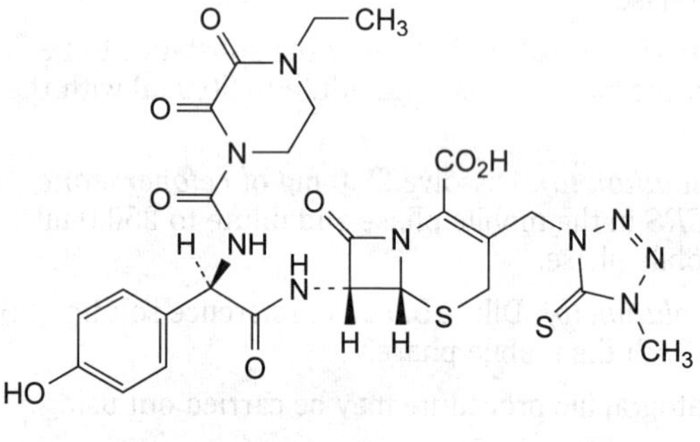

B. (6*R*,7*R*)-7-[[(2*R*)-2-[[(4-ethyl-2,3-dioxopiperazin-1-yl)carbonyl]amino]-2-(4-hydroxyphenyl)acetyl]amino]-3-[(4-methyl-5-thioxo-4,5-dihydro-1*H*-tetrazol-1-yl)methyl]-8-oxo-5-thia-1-azabicyclo[4.2.0]oct-2-ene-2-carboxylic acid,

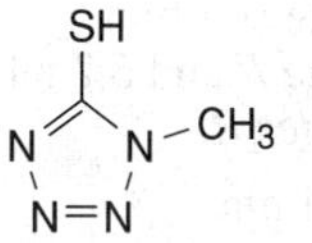

C. 1-methyl-1*H*-tetrazole-5-thiol,

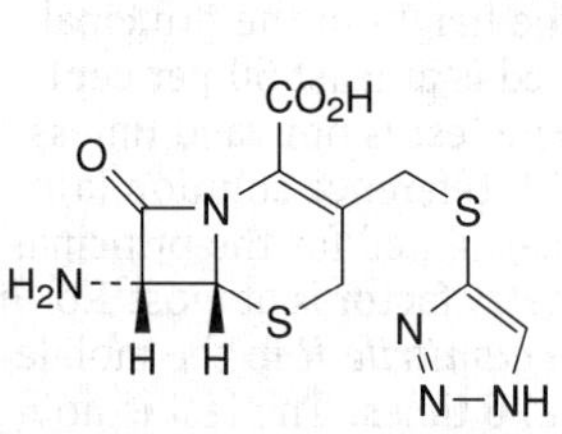

D. (6*R*,7*R*)-7-amino-8-oxo-3-[(1*H*-1,2,3-triazol-4-ylsulphanyl)methyl]-5-thia-1-azabicyclo[4.2.0]oct-2-ene-2-carboxylic acid (7-TACA),

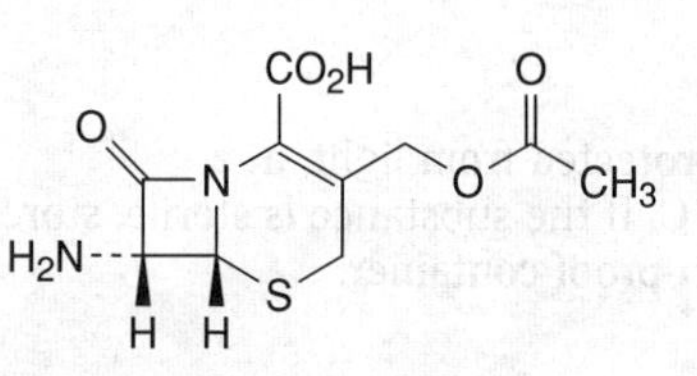

E. (6*R*,7*R*)-3-[(acetyloxy)methyl]-7-amino-8-oxo-5-thia-1-azabicyclo[4.2.0]oct-2-ene-2-carboxylic acid (7-ACA),

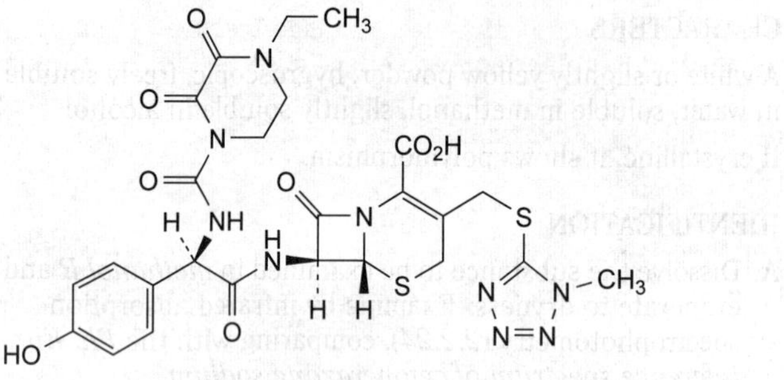

F. (6*R*,7*S*)-7-[[(2*R*)-2-[[(4-ethyl-2,3-dioxopiperazine-1-yl)carbonyl]amino]-2-(4-hydroxyphenyl)acetyl]amino]-3-[[(1-methyl-1*H*-tetrazol-5-yl)sulphanyl]methyl]-8-oxo-5-thia-1-azabicyclo[4.2.0]oct-2-ene-2-carboxylic acid.

01/2005:0989
corrected

CEFOTAXIME SODIUM

Cefotaximum natricum

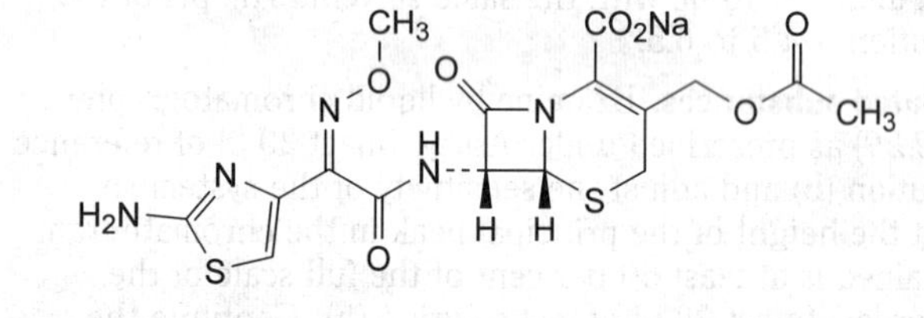

$C_{16}H_{16}N_5NaO_7S_2$ M_r 477.4

DEFINITION

Cefotaxime sodium contains not less than 96.0 per cent and not more than the equivalent of 101.0 per cent of sodium (6*R*,7*R*)-3-[(acetyloxy)methyl]-7-[[(*Z*)-2-(2-aminothiazol-4-yl)-2-(methoxyimino)acetyl]amino]-8-oxo-5-thia-1-azabicyclo[4.2.0]oct-2-ene-2-carboxylate, calculated with reference to the dried substance.

CHARACTERS

A white or slightly yellow powder, hygroscopic, freely soluble in water, sparingly soluble in methanol.

IDENTIFICATION

A. Examine by infrared absorption spectrophotometry (*2.2.24*), comparing with the spectrum obtained with *cefotaxime sodium CRS*.

B. It gives reaction (a) of sodium (*2.3.1*).

TESTS

Solution S. Dissolve 2.5 g in *carbon dioxide-free water R* and dilute to 25.0 ml with the same solvent.

Appearance of solution. Solution S is clear (*2.2.1*). Add 1 ml of *glacial acetic acid R* to 10 ml of solution S. The solution, examined immediately, is clear. The absorbance (*2.2.25*) of solution S measured at 430 nm is not greater than 0.20.

pH (*2.2.3*). The pH of solution S is 4.5 to 6.5.

Specific optical rotation (*2.2.7*). Dissolve 0.100 g in *water R* and dilute to 10.0 ml with the same solvent. The specific optical rotation is + 58 to + 64, calculated with reference to the dried substance.

Absorbance (*2.2.25*). Dissolve 20.0 mg in *water R* and dilute to 100.0 ml with the same solvent. Dilute 10.0 ml of this solution to 100.0 ml with *water R*. The specific absorbance determined at the maximum at 235 nm is 360 to 390, calculated with reference to the dried substance.

Related substances. Examine by liquid chromatography (*2.2.29*) as described under Assay.

Inject the test solution and reference solution (b). Continue the chromatography for at least eight times the retention time of the main peak. In the chromatogram obtained with the test solution: the area of any peak, apart from the principal peak, is not greater than the area of the principal peak in the chromatogram obtained with reference solution (b) (1 per cent); the sum of the areas of such peaks is at most three times the area of the principal peak in the chromatogram obtained with reference solution (b) (3 per cent).

***N,N*-Dimethylaniline** (*2.4.26, Method B*). Not more than 20 ppm.

2-Ethylhexanoic acid (*2.4.28*). Not more than 0.5 per cent *m/m*.

Loss on drying (*2.2.32*). Not more than 3.0 per cent, determined on 1.000 g by drying in an oven at 100 °C to 105 °C.

Bacterial endotoxins (*2.6.14*): less than 0.05 IU/mg, if intended for use in the manufacture of parenteral dosage forms without a further appropriate procedure for removal of bacterial endotoxins.

ASSAY

Examine by liquid chromatography (*2.2.29*).

Test solution. Dissolve 25.0 mg of the substance to be examined in the mobile phase and dilute to 25.0 ml with the same solvent.

Reference solution (a). Dissolve 25.0 mg of *cefotaxime sodium CRS* in the mobile phase and dilute to 25.0 ml with the same solvent.

Reference solution (b). Dilute 1.0 ml of reference solution (a) to 100.0 ml with the mobile phase.

Reference solution (c). Add 1.0 ml of *dilute hydrochloric acid R* to 4.0 ml of the test solution. Heat the solution at 40 °C for 2 h. Add 5.0 ml of *buffer solution pH 6.6 R* and 1.0 ml of *dilute sodium hydroxide solution R*.

The chromatographic procedure may be carried out using:

- a column 0.25 m long and 4.6 mm in internal diameter packed with *octadecylsilyl silica gel for chromatography R* (5 µm),
- as mobile phase at a flow rate of 1.0 ml/min a mixture prepared as follows: dissolve 3.5 g of *potassium dihydrogen phosphate R* and 11.6 g of *disodium hydrogen phosphate R* in 1000 ml of *water R* at pH 7.0 and add 180 ml of *methanol R*,
- as detector a spectrophotometer set at 235 nm,
- an injector with a fixed loop of 10 µl.

Inject reference solution (a) and reference solution (c). Adjust the attenuation to obtain principal peaks from reference solution (c) with a height of at least 50 per cent of the full-scale deflection of the recorder. The test is not valid unless cefotaxime is eluted as the second of the principal peaks and the resolution between the two principal peaks is at least 3.5. If necessary, use another stationary phase or adjust the methanol content of the mobile phase. The test is not valid if the symmetry factor of the cefotaxime peak is greater than 2.0. Inject reference solution (a) six times. The test is not valid unless the relative standard deviation of the area of the cefotaxime peak is at most 1.0 per cent. Inject alternately the test solution and reference solution (a).

STORAGE

Store in an airtight container, protected from light at a temperature not exceeding 30 °C. If the substance is sterile, store in an sterile, airtight, tamper-proof container.

LABELLING

The label states, where applicable, that the substance is free from bacterial endotoxins.

IMPURITIES

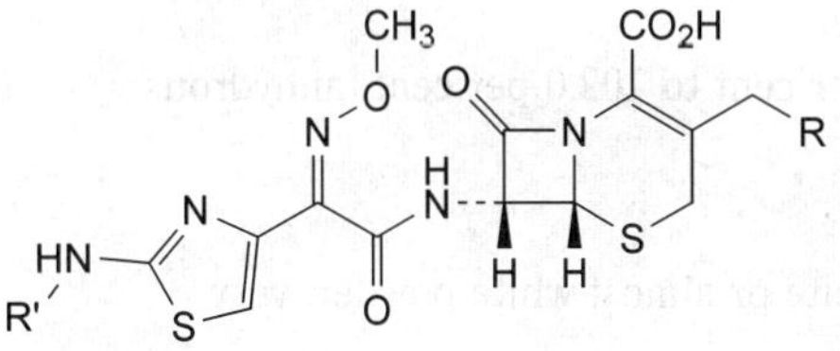

A. R = R′ = H: (6*R*,7*R*)-7-[[(*Z*)-2-(2-aminothiazol-4-yl)-2-methoxyimino)acetyl]amino]-3-methyl-8-oxo-5-thia-1-azabicyclo[4.2.0]oct-2-ene-2-carboxylic acid (desacetoxycefotaxime),

B. R = OH, R′ = H: (6*R*,7*R*)-7-[[(*Z*)-2-(2-aminothiazol-4-yl)-2-methoxyimino)acetyl]amino]-3-(hydroxymethyl)-8-oxo-5-thia-1-azabicyclo[4.2.0]oct-2-ene-2-carboxylic acid (desacetylcefotaxime),

C. R = O-CO-CH_3, R′ = CHO: (6*R*,7*R*)-3-[(acetyloxy)methyl]-7-[[(*Z*)-2-[2-(formylamino)thiazol-4-yl]-2-(methoxyimino)acetyl]amino]-8-oxo-5-thia-1-azabicyclo[4.2.0]oct-2-ene-2-carboxylic acid (*N*-formylcefotaxime),

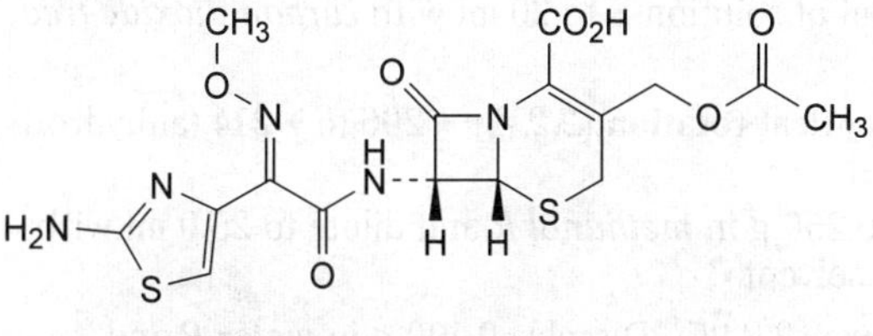

D. (6*R*,7*R*)-3-[(acetyloxy)methyl]-7-[[(*E*)-2-(2-aminothiazol-4-yl)-2-(methoxyimino)acetyl]amino]-8-oxo-5-thia-1-azabicyclo[4.2.0]oct-2-ene-2-carboxylic acid (*E*-cefotaxime),

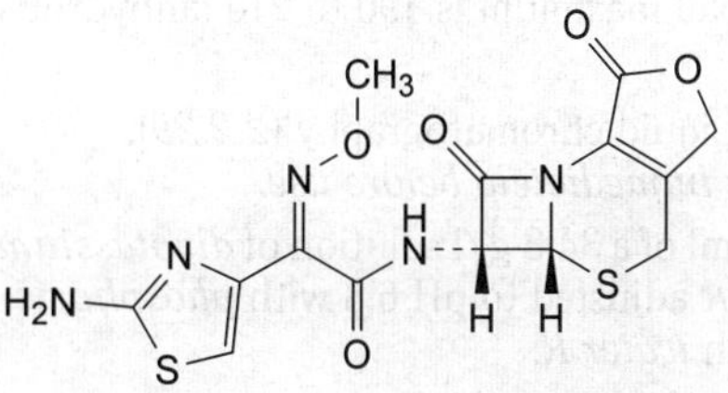

E. (5a*R*,6*R*)-6-[[(*Z*)-2-(2-aminothiazol-4-yl)-2-(methoxyimino)acetyl]amino]-5a,6-dihydro-3*H*,7*H*-azeto[2,1-*b*]furo[3,4-*d*][1,3]thiazine-1,7(4*H*)-dione (deacetylcefotaxime lactone).

01/2005:0990

CEFOXITIN SODIUM

Cefoxitinum natricum

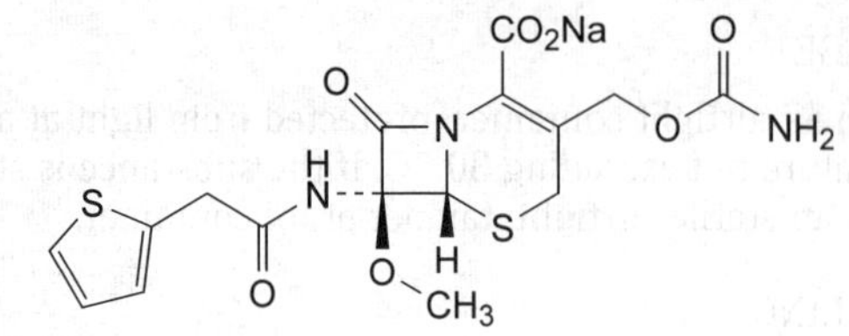

$C_{16}H_{16}N_3NaO_7S_2$ M_r 449.4

DEFINITION

Sodium (6*R*,7*S*)-3-[(carbamoyloxy)methyl]-7-methoxy-8-oxo-7-[[(thiophen-2-yl)acetyl]amino]-5-thia-1-azabicyclo[4.2.0]oct-2-ene-2-carboxylate.

Content: 95.0 per cent to 102.0 per cent (anhydrous substance).

CHARACTERS

Appearance: white or almost white powder, very hygroscopic.

Solubility: very soluble in water, sparingly soluble in alcohol.

IDENTIFICATION

A. Infrared absorption spectrophotometry (*2.2.24*).

Comparison: *cefoxitin sodium CRS*.

B. It gives reaction (a) of sodium (*2.3.1*).

TESTS

Solution S. Dissolve 2.50 g in *carbon dioxide-free water R* and dilute to 25 ml with the same solvent.

Appearance of solution. Solution S is clear (*2.2.1*) and not more intensely coloured than intensity 5 of the range of reference solutions of the most appropriate colour (*2.2.2, Method II*).

pH (*2.2.3*): 4.2 to 7.0.

Dilute 2 ml of solution S to 20 ml with *carbon dioxide-free water R*.

Specific optical rotation (*2.2.7*): + 206 to + 214 (anhydrous substance).

Dissolve 0.250 g in *methanol R* and dilute to 25.0 ml with the same solvent.

Absorbance (*2.2.25*). Dissolve 0.100 g in *water R* and dilute to 100.0 ml with the same solvent. Dilute 2.0 ml of the solution to 100.0 ml with *sodium hydrogen carbonate solution R*. Examined between 220 nm and 350 nm, the solution shows an absorption maximum at 236 nm and a broad absorption maximum at about 262 nm. The specific absorbance at this broad maximum is 190 to 210 (anhydrous substance).

Related substances. Liquid chromatography (*2.2.29*). *Prepare the solutions immediately before use.*

Solution A. Dilute 20 ml of a 34.8 g/l solution of *dipotassium hydrogen phosphate R* adjusted to pH 6.8 with *phosphoric acid R* to 1000 ml with *water R*.

Test solution. Dissolve 50.0 mg of the substance to be examined in solution A and dilute to 10.0 ml with the same solution.

Reference solution (a). Dilute 1.0 ml of the test solution to 100.0 ml with solution A.

Reference solution (b). To 1.0 ml of the test solution add 7.0 ml of *water R* and 2.0 ml of *methanol R*. Add 25 mg of *sodium carbonate R*, stir for 10 min at room temperature, then heat in a water-bath at 70 °C for 30 min. Allow to cool. Add 3 drops of *glacial acetic acid R* and 1 ml of the test solution and mix.

Column:

- *size*: *l* = 0.25 m, Ø = 4.6 mm,
- *stationary phase*: *phenylsilyl silica gel for chromatography R* (5 µm) with a specific surface area of 300 m^2/g and a pore size of 7 nm.

Mobile phase:

- *mobile phase A*: *water R* adjusted to pH 2.7 with *anhydrous formic acid R*,
- *mobile phase B*: *acetonitrile R*,

Time (min)	Mobile phase A (per cent *V/V*)	Mobile phase B (per cent *V/V*)
0 - 12	90	10
12 - 37	90 → 80	10 → 20
37 - 50	80 → 60	20 → 40
50 - 55	60 → 20	40 → 80
55 - 60	20	80
60 - 62	20 → 90	80 → 10
62 - 70	90	10

Flow rate: 1 ml/min.

Detection: spectrophotometer at 235 nm.

Injection: 50 µl.

Relative retentions with reference to cefoxitin (retention time = about 34 min): impurity A = about 0.82; impurity B = about 1.16; impurity C = about 1.27; impurity D = about 1.31.

System suitability: reference solution (b):

- *resolution*: minimum 5.0 between the 2 principal peaks.

Limits:

- *any impurity*: not more than half the area of the principal peak in the chromatogram obtained with reference solution (a) (0.5 per cent),
- *total*: not more than 4 times the area of the principal peak in the chromatogram obtained with reference solution (a) (4.0 per cent),
- *disregard limit*: 0.05 times the area of the principal peak in the chromatogram obtained with reference solution (a) (0.05 per cent).

Water (*2.5.12*): maximum 1.0 per cent, determined on 0.500 g.

Bacterial endotoxins (*2.6.14*): less than 0.13 IU/mg, if intended for use in the manufacture of parenteral dosage forms without a further appropriate procedure for the removal of bacterial endotoxins.

ASSAY

Liquid chromatography (*2.2.29*).

Test solution. Dissolve 25.0 mg of the substance to be examined in *water R* and dilute to 25.0 ml with the same solvent.

Reference solution (a). Dissolve 25.0 mg of *cefoxitin sodium CRS* in *water R* and dilute to 25.0 ml with the same solvent.

Reference solution (b). Dissolve 20.0 mg of *2-(2-thienyl)acetic acid R* in *water R* and dilute to 25.0 ml with the same solvent.

Reference solution (c). Mix 1.0 ml of reference solution (a) and 5.0 ml of reference solution (b).

Column:

- *size*: *l* = 0.25 m, Ø = 4.6 mm,
- *stationary phase*: *octadecylsilyl silica gel for chromatography R* (5 µm).

Mobile phase: *acetic acid R, acetonitrile R, water R* (1:19:81 *V/V/V*).

Flow rate: 1 ml/min.

Detection: spectrophotometer at 254 nm.

Injection: 20 µl; inject the test solution and reference solutions (a) and (c).

System suitability: reference solution (c):

- *resolution*: minimum 3.5 between the 2 principal peaks.

Calculate the percentage content of cefoxitin sodium.

STORAGE

In an airtight container. If the substance is sterile, store in a sterile, airtight, tamper-proof container.

LABELLING

The label states, where applicable, that the substance is free from bacterial endotoxins.

IMPURITIES

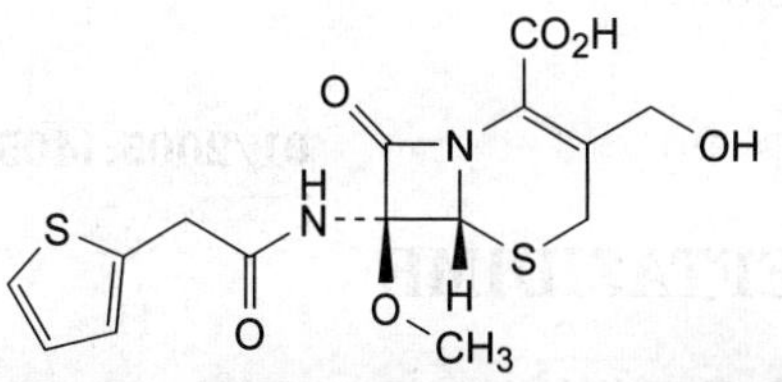

A. (6*R*,7*S*)-3-(hydroxymethyl)-7-methoxy-8-oxo-7-[[(thiophen-2-yl)acetyl]amino]-5-thia-1-azabicyclo[4.2.0]oct-2-ene-2-carboxylic acid (decarbamoylcefoxitin),

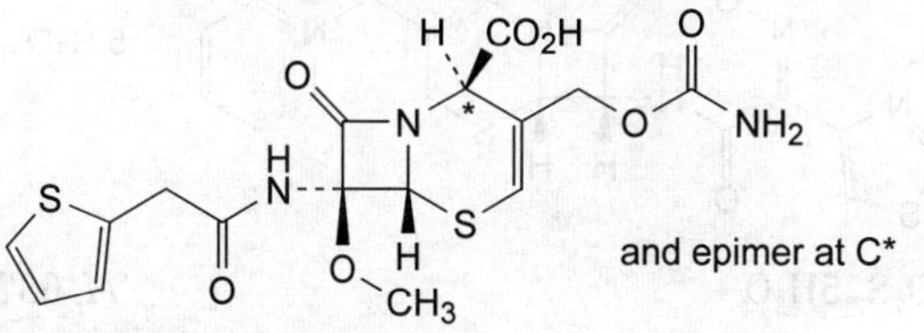

B. (2*RS*,6*R*,7*S*)-3-[(carbamoyloxy)methyl]-7-methoxy-8-oxo-7-[[(thiophen-2-yl)acetyl]amino]-5-thia-1-azabicyclo[4.2.0]oct-3-ene-2-carboxylic acid (delta-3-cefoxitin),

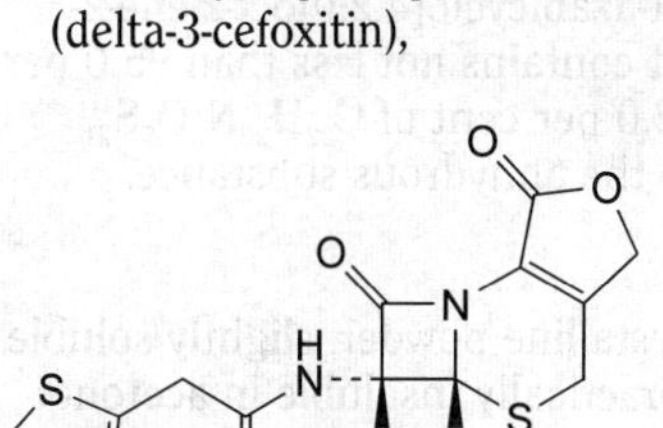

C. R = H: (5a*R*,6*R*)-6-[[(thiophen-2-yl)acetyl]amino]-5a,6-dihydro-3*H*,7*H*-azeto[2,1-*b*]furo[3,4-*d*][1,3]thiazine-1,7(4*H*)-dione (cefalotin lactone),

D. R = OCH_3: (5a*R*,6*S*)-6-methoxy-6-[[(thiophen-2-yl)acetyl]amino]-5a,6-dihydro-3*H*,7*H*-azeto[2,1-*b*]furo[3,4-*d*][1,3]thiazine-1,7(4*H*)-dione (cefoxitin lactone).

01/2005:0814
corrected

CEFRADINE

Cefradinum

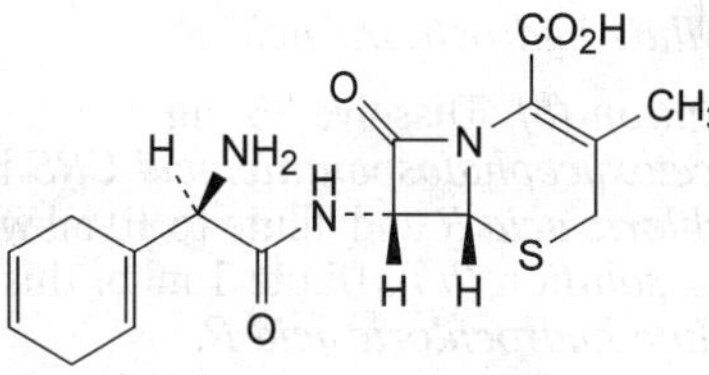

$C_{16}H_{19}N_3O_4S$ M_r 349.4

DEFINITION

Cefradine contains not less than 90.0 per cent of (6*R*,7*R*)-7-[[(2*R*)-2-amino-2-(cyclohexa-1,4-dienyl)acetyl]amino]-3-methyl-8-oxo-5-thia-1-azabicyclo[4.2.0]oct-2-ene-2-carboxylic acid, calculated with reference to the anhydrous substance. The sum of the percentage contents of $C_{16}H_{19}N_3O_4S$ and of cefalexin ($C_{16}H_{17}N_3O_4S$; M_r 347.4) is not less than 95.0 per cent and not more than the equivalent of 102.0 per cent, calculated with reference to the anhydrous substance.

CHARACTERS

A white or slightly yellow, hygroscopic powder, sparingly soluble in water, practically insoluble in alcohol.

IDENTIFICATION

Examine by infrared absorption spectrophotometry (*2.2.24*), comparing with the spectrum obtained with *cefradine CRS*. If the spectra obtained in the solid state show differences, dissolve 30 mg of the substance to be examined and of the reference substance separately in 10 ml of *methanol R*, evaporate to dryness at 40 °C at a pressure less than 2 kPa and record new spectra using the residues.

TESTS

Solution S. Dissolve 2.50 g in *sodium carbonate solution R* and dilute to 25.0 ml with the same solvent.

Appearance of solution. Solution S is not more opalescent than reference suspension II (*2.2.1*). Allow solution S to stand for 5 min. The absorbance of solution S measured at 450 nm (*2.2.25*) is not greater than 0.60.

pH (*2.2.3*). Dissolve 0.100 g in *carbon dioxide-free water R* and dilute to 10 ml with the same solvent. The pH of the solution is 3.5 to 6.0.

Specific optical rotation (*2.2.7*). Dissolve 0.250 g in *acetate buffer solution pH 4.6 R* and dilute to 25.0 ml with the same solvent. The specific optical rotation is + 80 to + 90, calculated with reference to the anhydrous substance.

Absorbance (*2.2.25*). Dissolve 50.0 mg in *water R* and dilute to 100.0 ml with the same solvent. The absorbance measured at 330 nm is not greater than 0.05. Dilute 2.0 ml of the solution to 50.0 ml with *water R*. Examined between 220 nm and 300 nm, the diluted solution shows an absorption maximum at 262 nm. The specific absorbance at this maximum is 215 to 240, calculated with reference to the anhydrous substance.

Related substances. Examine by thin-layer chromatography (*2.2.27*), using *silica gel G R* as the coating substance. Impregnate the plate by development with a 5 per cent *V/V* solution of *tetradecane R* in *hexane R*. Allow the solvent to evaporate and carry out the chromatography in the same direction as the impregnation.

Test solution. Dissolve 0.25 g of the substance to be examined in *dilute hydrochloric acid R* and dilute to 10 ml with the same acid.

Reference solution (a). Dilute 1 ml of the test solution to 100 ml with *dilute hydrochloric acid R*.

Reference solution (b). Dissolve 25 mg of *7-aminodesacetoxycephalosporanic acid CRS* in *dilute hydrochloric acid R* and dilute to 10 ml with the same acid (*reference solution (b')*). Dilute 1 ml of this solution to 10 ml with *dilute hydrochloric acid R*.

Reference solution (c). Dissolve 25 mg of *cyclohexa-1,4-dienylglycine CRS* in *dilute hydrochloric acid R* and dilute to 10 ml with the same acid (*reference solution (c')*). Dilute 1 ml of this solution to 10 ml with *dilute hydrochloric acid R*.

Reference solution (d). Dissolve 0.25 g of the substance to be examined in a mixture of 1 ml of reference solution (b′) and 1 ml of reference solution (c′) and dilute to 10 ml with *dilute hydrochloric acid R*.

Apply to the plate 5 µl of each solution. Develop over a path of 15 cm using a mixture of 3 volumes of *acetone R*, 80 volumes of a 72 g/l solution of *disodium hydrogen phosphate R* and 120 volumes of a 21 g/l solution of *citric acid R*. Dry the plate by heating at 90 °C for 3 min. Spray the hot plate with a 1 g/l solution of *ninhydrin R* in the mobile phase. Heat the plate at 90 °C for 15 min and allow to cool. In the chromatogram obtained with the test solution: any spot corresponding to 7-aminodesacetoxycephalosporanic acid is not more intense than the spot in the chromatogram obtained with reference solution (b) (1.0 per cent); any spot corresponding to cyclohexa-1,4-dienylglycine (the position of which is defined by comparison with the chromatogram obtained with reference solution (d)), is not more intense than the spot in the chromatogram obtained with reference solution (c) (1.0 per cent); any spot, apart from the principal spot and the spots corresponding to 7-aminodesacetoxycephalosporanic acid and to cyclohexa-1,4-dienylglycine, is not more intense than the principal spot in the chromatogram obtained with reference solution (a) (1.0 per cent). The test is not valid unless the chromatogram obtained with reference solution (d) shows 3 clearly separated spots.

Cefalexin. Not more than 5.0 per cent, calculated with reference to the anhydrous substance and determined by liquid chromatography (*2.2.29*), as prescribed under Assay. Inject separately the test solution and reference solution (b).

***N,N*-Dimethylaniline** (*2.4.26, Method B*). Not more than 20 ppm.

Water (*2.5.12*). Not more than 6.0 per cent, determined on 0.300 g by the semi-micro determination of water.

Sulphated ash (*2.4.14*). Not more than 0.2 per cent, determined on 1.0 g.

ASSAY

Examine by liquid chromatography (*2.2.29*).

Test solution. Dissolve 50.0 mg of the substance to be examined in the mobile phase and dilute to 100.0 ml with the mobile phase.

Reference solution (a). Dissolve 50.0 mg of *cefradine CRS* in the mobile phase and dilute to 100.0 ml with the mobile phase.

Reference solution (b). Dissolve 10.0 mg of *cefradine CRS* and 10.0 mg of *cefalexin CRS* in the mobile phase and dilute to 100.0 ml with the mobile phase.

The chromatographic procedure may be carried out using:

- a column 0.25 m long and 4.6 mm in internal diameter, packed with *octadecylsilyl silica gel for chromatography R* (5 µm or 10 µm),
- as mobile phase at a flow rate of 1.0 ml/min a mixture of 1 volume of *dilute acetic acid R*, 17 volumes of a 36.2 g/l solution of *sodium acetate R*, 200 volumes of *methanol R* and 782 volumes of *water R*,
- as detector a spectrophotometer set at 254 nm,
- a 20 µl loop injector.

Inject reference solution (b). Adjust the sensitivity of the detector so that the height of the peaks is at least half the full scale of the recorder. The test is not valid unless the resolution between the peaks corresponding to cefalexin and cefradine is at least 4. If necessary, adjust the methanol content of the mobile phase. Inject reference solution (a) 6 times. The test is not valid unless the relative standard deviation of the peak area for cefradine is at most 1.0 per cent. Inject separately the test solution and reference solution (a).

Calculate the percentage content of cefradine and cefalexin.

STORAGE

Store in an airtight container, protected from light, at a temperature of 2 °C to 8 °C.

01/2005:1405

CEFTAZIDIME

Ceftazidimum

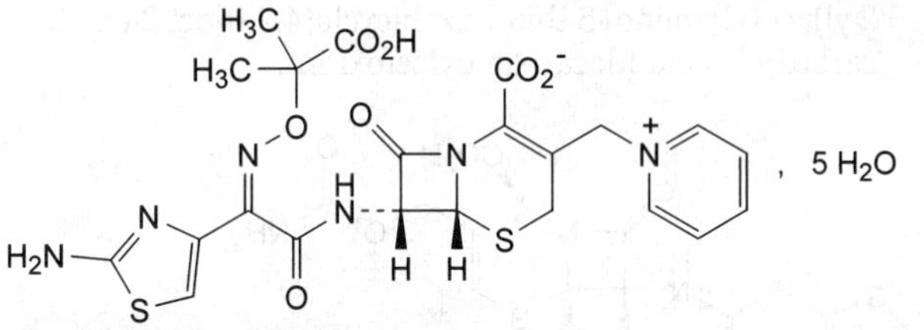

$C_{22}H_{22}N_6O_7S_2,5H_2O$ M_r 637

DEFINITION

Ceftazidime is (6*R*,7*R*)-7-[[(*Z*)-2-(2-aminothiazol-4-yl)-2-[(1-carboxy-1-methylethoxy)imino]acetyl]amino]-8-oxo-3-[(1-pyridinio)methyl]-5-thia-1-azabicyclo[4.2.0]oct-2-ene-2-carboxylate pentahydrate. It contains not less than 95.0 per cent and not more than 102.0 per cent of $C_{22}H_{22}N_6O_7S_2$, calculated with reference to the anhydrous substance.

CHARACTERS

A white or almost white, crystalline powder, slightly soluble in water and in methanol, practically insoluble in acetone and in alcohol. It dissolves in acid and alkali solutions.

IDENTIFICATION

Examine by infrared absorption spectrophotometry (*2.2.24*), comparing with the spectrum obtained with *ceftazidime CRS*.

TESTS

Solution S. Dissolve 0.25 g in *carbon dioxide-free water R* and dilute to 50 ml with the same solvent.

Appearance of solution. Solution S is clear (*2.2.1*) and colourless (*2.2.2, Method II*).

pH (*2.2.3*). The pH of solution S is 3.0 to 4.0.

Related substances

A. Examine by thin-layer chromatography (*2.2.27*), using a *TLC silica gel F_{254} plate R*.

Test solution. Dissolve 0.100 g of the substance to be examined in a 36 g/l solution of *disodium hydrogen phosphate R* and dilute to 2.0 ml with the same solution.

Reference solution. Dilute 1 ml of the test solution to 200 ml with a 36 g/l solution of *disodium hydrogen phosphate R*.

Apply to the plate 2 µl of each solution. Develop over a path of 15 cm using a mixture of 6 volumes of *butanol R*, 26 volumes of *sodium acetate buffer solution pH 4.5 R*, 32 volumes of *butyl acetate R* and 32 volumes of *glacial acetic acid R*. Dry the plate in a current of warm air and examine in ultraviolet light at 254 nm. Any spot with an R_f value greater than that of the principal spot in the chromatogram obtained with the test solution is not more intense than the spot in the chromatogram obtained with the reference solution (0.5 per cent).

B. Examine by liquid chromatography (*2.2.29*).

Test solution. Dissolve 0.100 g of the substance to be examined in the mobile phase and dilute to 20.0 ml with the mobile phase. Dilute 5.0 ml of the solution to 20.0 ml with the mobile phase.

Reference solution (a). Dissolve 5.0 mg of *ceftazidime impurity A CRS* in the mobile phase and dilute to 20.0 ml with the mobile phase. Dilute 1.0 ml of the solution to 20.0 ml with the mobile phase.

Reference solution (b). Dissolve 5 mg of *ceftazidime impurity A CRS* and 5 mg of *ceftazidime CRS* in the mobile phase and dilute to 20.0 ml with the mobile phase. Dilute 1.0 ml of the solution to 20.0 ml with the mobile phase.

The chromatographic procedure may be carried out using:

- a stainless steel column 0.25 m long and 4.6 mm in internal diameter packed with *octadecylsilyl silica gel for chromatography R* (5 µm),
- as mobile phase at a flow rate of 1.3 ml/min a mixture of 7 volumes of *acetonitrile R* and 93 volumes of a 22.6 g/l solution of *ammonium dihydrogen phosphate R*, adjusted to pH 3.9 with a 10 per cent *V/V* solution of *phosphoric acid R*,
- as detector a spectrophotometer set at 255 nm,

maintaining the temperature of the column at 35 °C.

Inject 20 µl of reference solution (b). Adjust the sensitivity of the system so that the heights of the 2 peaks in the chromatogram obtained are at least 50 per cent of the full scale of the recorder. The test is not valid unless in the chromatogram obtained, the resolution between the peaks corresponding to ceftazidime and impurity A is at least 5.9. Inject 20 µl of the test solution and 20 µl of reference solution (a). Continue the chromatography of the test solution for 3 times the retention time of ceftazidime. In the chromatogram obtained with the test solution: the area of any peak, apart from the principal peak, is not greater than half the area of the principal peak in the chromatogram obtained with reference solution (a) (0.5 per cent); the sum of the areas of all the peaks, apart from the principal peak, is not greater than twice the area of the principal peak in the chromatogram obtained with reference solution (a) (2 per cent). Disregard any peak with an area less than 0.1 times the area of the principal peak in the chromatogram obtained with reference solution (a).

Impurity F. Not more than 500 ppm, determined by liquid chromatography (*2.2.29*). *Prepare the solutions immediately before use.*

Test solution. Dissolve 0.500 g of the substance to be examined in a 10 per cent *V/V* solution of *phosphate buffer solution pH 7.0 R4* and dilute to 100.0 ml with the same solvent.

Reference solution (a). Dissolve 1.00 g of *pyridine R* in *water R* and dilute to 100.0 ml with the same solvent. Dilute 5.0 ml of the solution to 200.0 ml with *water R*. To 1.0 ml of the solution, add 10 ml of *phosphate buffer solution pH 7.0 R4* and dilute to 100.0 ml with *water R*.

Reference solution (b). Dilute 1.0 ml of the test solution to 200.0 ml with a 10 per cent *V/V* solution of *phosphate buffer solution pH 7.0 R4*. To 1.0 ml of the solution add 20 ml of reference solution (a) and dilute to 200 ml with a 10 per cent *V/V* solution of *phosphate buffer solution pH 7.0 R4*.

The chromatographic procedure may be carried out using:

- a stainless steel column 0.25 m long and 4.6 mm in internal diameter packed with *octadecylsilyl silica gel for chromatography R* (5 µm),
- as mobile phase at a flow rate of 1.0 ml/min a mixture of 8 volumes of a 28.8 g/l solution of *ammonium dihydrogen phosphate R* previously adjusted to pH 7.0 with *ammonia R*, 24 volumes of *acetonitrile R* and 68 volumes of *water R*,
- as detector a spectrophotometer set at 255 nm,

Inject 20 µl of reference solution (b). The test is not valid unless in the chromatogram obtained, the resolution between the peaks due to ceftazidime and to impurity F is at least 7.0.

Inject 20 µl of reference solution (a). Adjust the sensitivity of the system so that the height of the principal peak in the chromatogram obtained is at least 50 per cent of the full scale of the recorder. Inject reference solution (a) 6 times. The test is not valid unless the relative standard deviation of the area of the principal peak is at most 1.0 per cent. Inject alternately 20 µl of the test solution and 20 µl of reference solution (a).

Water (*2.5.12*): 13.0 per cent to 15.0 per cent, determined on 0.200 g by the semi-micro determination of water.

Bacterial endotoxins (*2.6.14*): less than 0.10 IU/mg, if intended for use in the manufacture of parenteral dosage forms without a further appropriate procedure for the removal of bacterial endotoxins.

ASSAY

Examine by liquid chromatography (*2.2.29*).

Test solution. Dissolve 25.0 mg of the substance to be examined in the mobile phase and dilute to 25.0 ml with the mobile phase.

Reference solution (a). Dissolve 25.0 mg of *ceftazidime CRS* in the mobile phase and dilute to 25.0 ml with the mobile phase.

Reference solution (b). Dissolve 5 mg of *ceftazidime impurity A CRS* in 5.0 ml of reference solution (a).

The chromatographic procedure may be carried out using:

- a column 0.15 m long and 4.6 mm in internal diameter packed with *hexylsilyl silica gel for chromatography R* (5 µm),

- as mobile phase at a flow rate of 2 ml/min a mixture prepared as follows: dissolve 4.26 g of *disodium hydrogen phosphate R* and 2.73 g of *potassium dihydrogen phosphate R* in 980 ml of *water R*, then add 20 ml of *acetonitrile R*,
- as detector a spectrophotometer set at 245 nm.

Inject 20 µl of reference solution (b). Adjust the sensitivity of the system so that the heights of the 2 principal peaks in the chromatogram obtained are at least 50 per cent of the full scale of the recorder. The test is not valid unless, in the chromatogram obtained, the resolution between the peaks corresponding to ceftazidime and impurity A is at least 1.0. Inject alternately the test solution and reference solution (a). Calculate the percentage content of ceftazidime.

STORAGE

Store in an airtight container. If the substance is sterile, store in a sterile, airtight, tamper-proof container.

LABELLING

The label states, where applicable, that the substance is free from bacterial endotoxins.

IMPURITIES

By liquid chromatography (related substances test): A, B, C.

By thin-layer chromatography (related substances test): D, E.

By liquid chromatography (impurity F test): F.

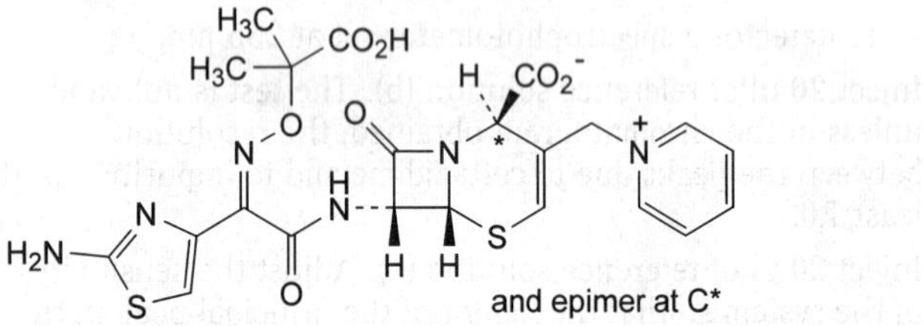

A. (2*RS*,6*R*,7*R*)-7-[[(*Z*)-2-(2-aminothiazol-4-yl)-2-[(1-carboxy-1-methylethoxy)imino]acetyl]amino]-8-oxo-3-[(1-pyridinio)methyl]-5-thia-1-azabicyclo[4.2.0]oct-3-ene-2-carboxylate (Δ-2-ceftazidime),

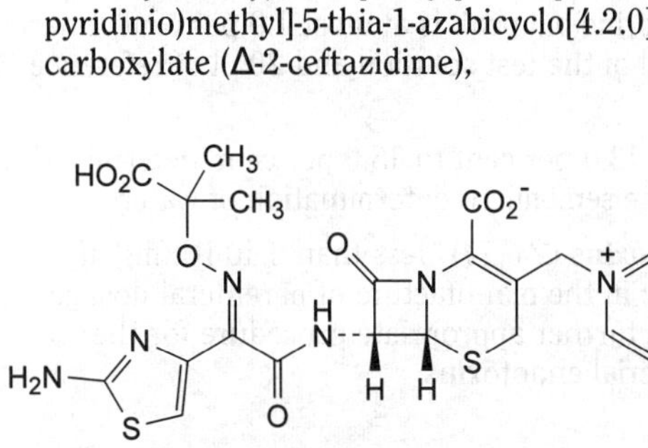

B. (6*R*,7*R*)-7-[[(*E*)-2-(2-aminothiazol-4-yl)-2-[(1-carboxy-1-methylethoxy)imino]acetyl]amino]-8-oxo-3-[(1-pyridinio)methyl]-5-thia-1-azabicyclo[4.2.0]oct-2-ene-2-carboxylate,

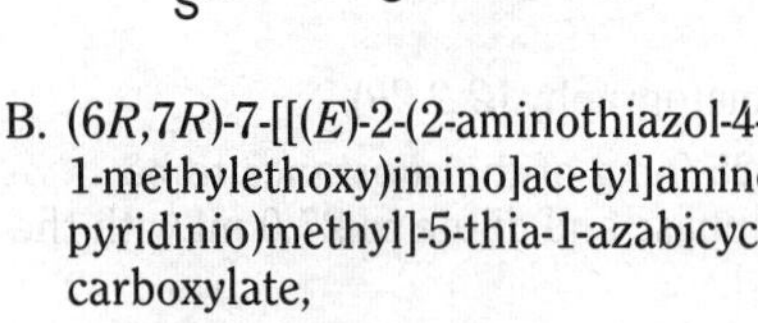

C. (6*R*,7*R*)-2-carboxy-8-oxo-3-(pyridiniomethyl)-5-thia-1-azabicyclo[4.2.0]oct-2-en-7-aminium dichloride,

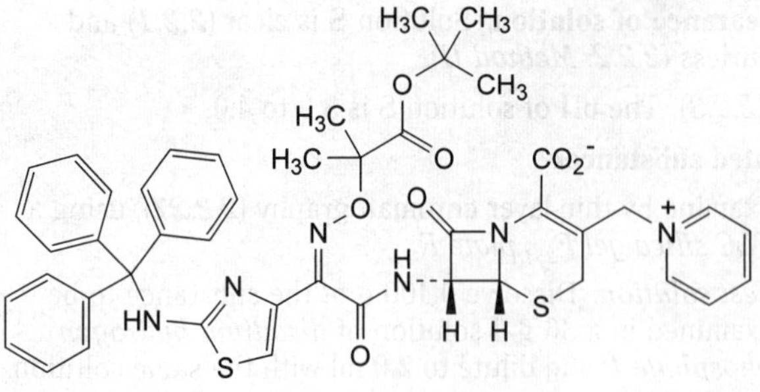

D. (6*R*,7*R*)-7-[[(*Z*)-2-[[2-(1,1-dimethylethoxy)-1,1-dimethyl-2-oxoethoxy]imino]-2-[2-[(triphenylmethyl)amino]thiazol-4-yl]acetyl]amino]-8-oxo-3-(pyridiniomethyl)-5-thia-1-azabicyclo[4.2.0]oct-2-ene-2-carboxylate,

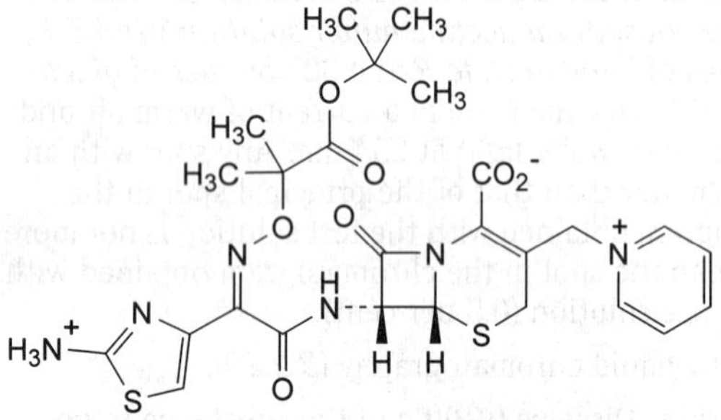

E. (6*R*,7*R*)-7-[[(*Z*)-2-(2-ammoniothiazol-4-yl)-2-[[2-(1,1-dimethylethoxy)-1,1-dimethyl-2-oxoethoxy]imino]acetyl]amino]-8-oxo-3-(pyridiniomethyl)-5-thia-1-azabicyclo[4.2.0]oct-2-ene-2-carboxylate chloride,

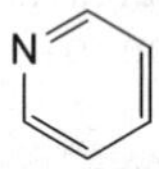

F. pyridine.

01/2005:0991

CEFTRIAXONE SODIUM

Ceftriaxonum natricum

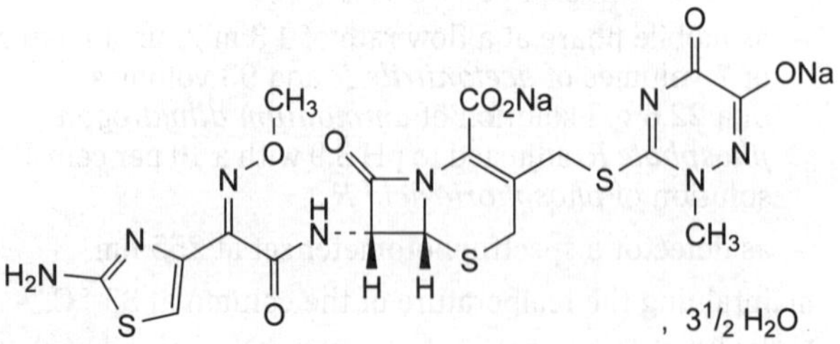

, $3^1/_2\ H_2O$

$C_{18}H_{16}N_8Na_2O_7S_3, 3^1/_2H_2O$ M_r 662

DEFINITION

Disodium (6*R*,7*R*)-7-[[(*Z*)-(2-aminothiazol-4-yl)(methoxyimino)acetyl]amino]-3-[[(2-methyl-6-oxido-5-oxo-2,5-dihydro-1,2,4-triazin-3-yl)sulphanyl]methyl]-8-oxo-5-thia-1-azabicyclo[4.2.0]oct-2-ene-2-carboxylate.

Content: 96.0 per cent to 102.0 per cent (anhydrous substance).

CHARACTERS

Appearance: almost white or yellowish, crystalline powder, slightly hygroscopic.

Solubility: freely soluble in water, sparingly soluble in methanol, very slightly soluble in ethanol.

IDENTIFICATION

A. Infrared absorption spectrophotometry (*2.2.24*).
Comparison: *ceftriaxone sodium CRS.*

B. It gives reaction (a) of sodium (*2.3.1*).

TESTS

Solution S. Dissolve 2.40 g in *carbon dioxide-free water R* and dilute to 20.0 ml with the same solvent.

Appearance of solution. The solution is clear (*2.2.1*) and not more intensely coloured than reference solution Y_5 or BY_5 (*2.2.2*).
Dilute 2 ml of solution S to 20 ml with *water R*.

pH (*2.2.3*): 6.0 to 8.0 for solution S.

Specific optical rotation (*2.2.7*): − 155 to − 170 (anhydrous substance).
Dissolve 0.250 g in *water R* and dilute to 25.0 ml with the same solvent.

Related substances. Liquid chromatography (*2.2.29*).
Test solution. Dissolve 30.0 mg of the substance to be examined in the mobile phase and dilute to 100.0 ml with the mobile phase.
Reference solution (a). Dissolve 30.0 mg of *ceftriaxone sodium CRS* in the mobile phase and dilute to 100.0 ml with the mobile phase.
Reference solution (b). Dissolve 5.0 mg of *ceftriaxone sodium CRS* and 5.0 mg of *ceftriaxone impurity A CRS* in the mobile phase and dilute to 100.0 ml with the mobile phase.
Reference solution (c). Dilute 1.0 ml of the test solution to 100.0 ml with the mobile phase.
Column:
- *size*: *l* = 0.25 m, Ø = 4.6 mm,
- *stationary phase*: *octadecylsilyl silica gel for chromatography R* (5 µm).

Mobile phase: dissolve 2.0 g of *tetradecylammonium bromide R* and 2.0 g of *tetraheptylammonium bromide R* in a mixture of 440 ml of *water R*, 55 ml of *0.067 M phosphate buffer solution pH 7.0 R*, 5.0 ml of citrate buffer solution pH 5.0 prepared by dissolving 20.17 g of *citric acid R* in 800 ml of *water R*, adjusting topH 5.0 with *strong sodium hydroxide solution R* and diluting to 1000.0 ml with *water R*, and 500 ml of *acetonitrile R*.
Flow rate: 1.5 ml/min.
Detection: spectrophotometer at 254 nm.
Injection: 20 µl; inject the test solution and reference solutions (b) and (c).
Run time: twice the retention time of ceftriaxone.
System suitability: reference solution (b):
- *resolution*: minimum of 3.0 between the peaks due to ceftriaxone and impurity A.

Limits:
- *any impurity*: not more than the area of the principal peak in the chromatogram obtained with reference solution (c) (1 per cent),
- *total*: not more than 4 times the area of the principal peak in the chromatogram obtained with reference solution (c) (4 per cent),
- *disregard limit*: 0.1 times the area of the principal peak in the chromatogram obtained with reference solution (c) (0.1 per cent).

***N,N*-Dimethylaniline** (*2.4.26, Method B*): maximum 20 ppm.

2-Ethylhexanoic acid (*2.4.28*): maximum 0.8 per cent *m/m*.

Water (*2.5.12*): 8.0 per cent to 11.0 per cent, determined on 0.100 g.

Bacterial endotoxins (*2.6.14*): less than 0.20 IU/mg, if intended for use in the manufacture of parenteral dosage forms without a further appropriate procedure for the removal of bacterial endotoxins.

ASSAY

Liquid chromatography (*2.2.29*) as described in the test for related substances.
Injection: test solution and reference solution (a).
Calculate the percentage content of ceftriaxone sodium.

STORAGE

In an airtight container protected from light. If the substance is sterile, store in a sterile, airtight, tamper-proof container.

LABELLING

The label states, where applicable, that the substance is free from bacterial endotoxins.

IMPURITIES

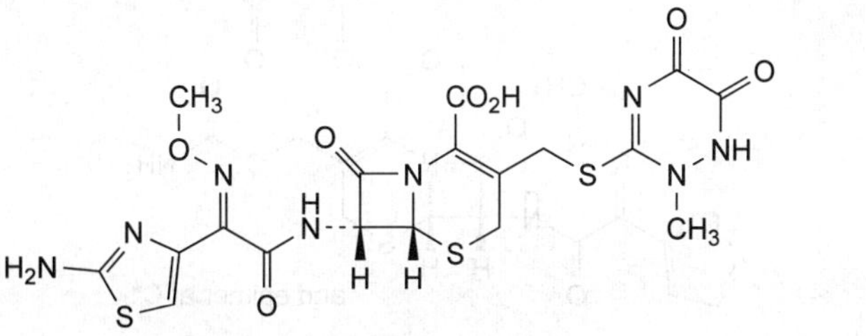

A. (6*R*,7*R*)-7-[[(*E*)-(2-aminothiazol-4-yl)(methoxyimino)acetyl]amino]-3-[[(2-methyl-5,6-dioxo-1,2,5,6-tetrahydro-1,2,4-triazin-3-yl)sulphanyl]methyl]-8-oxo-5-thia-1-azabicyclo[4.2.0]oct-2-ene-2-carboxylic acid (*E*-isomer),

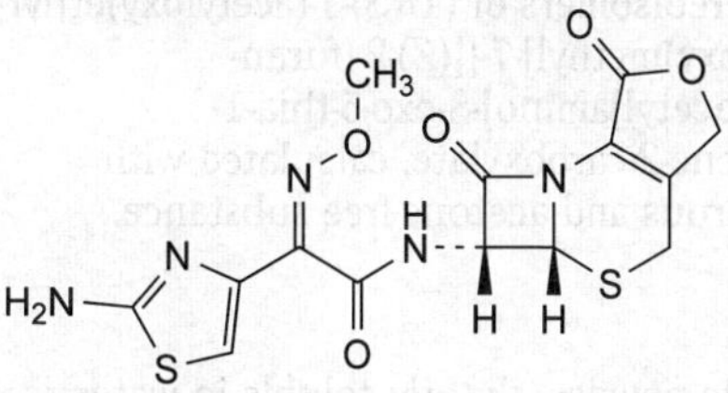

B. (5a*R*,6*R*)-6-[[(*Z*)-(2-aminothiazol-4-yl)(methoxyimino)acetyl]amino]-5a,6-dihydro-3*H*,7*H*-azeto[2,1-*b*]furo[3,4-*d*][1,3]thiazine-1,7(4*H*)-dione,

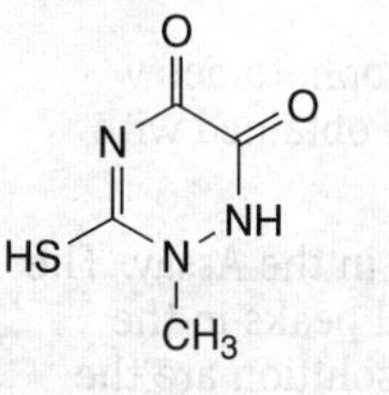

C. 2-methyl-3-sulphanyl-1,2-dihydro-1,2,4-triazin-5,6-dione,

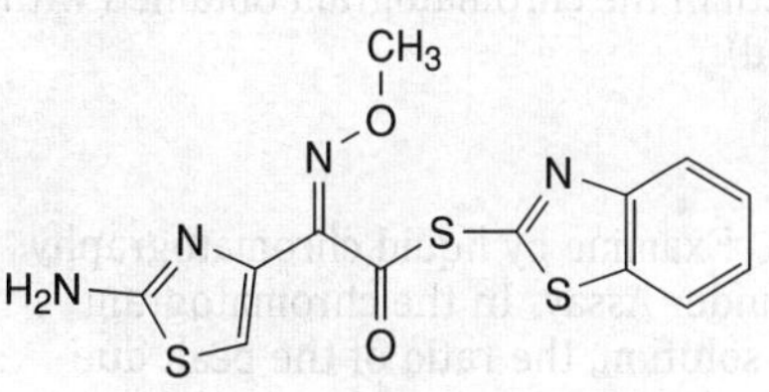

D. *S*-benzothiazol-2-yl (*Z*)-(2-aminothiazol-4-yl)(methoxyimino)thioacetate,

Monographs C

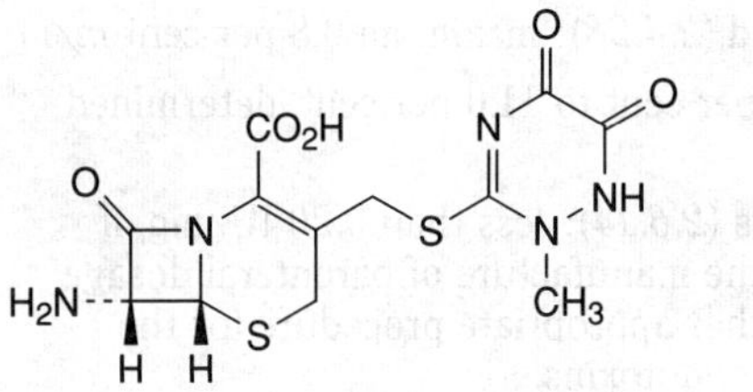

E. (6*R*,7*R*)-7-amino-3-[[(2-methyl-5,6-dioxo-1,2,5,6-tetrahydro-1,2,4-triazin-3-yl)sulphanyl]methyl]-8-oxo-5-thia-1-azabicyclo[4.2.0]oct-2-ene-2-carboxylic acid.

01/2005:1300

CEFUROXIME AXETIL

Cefuroximum axetili

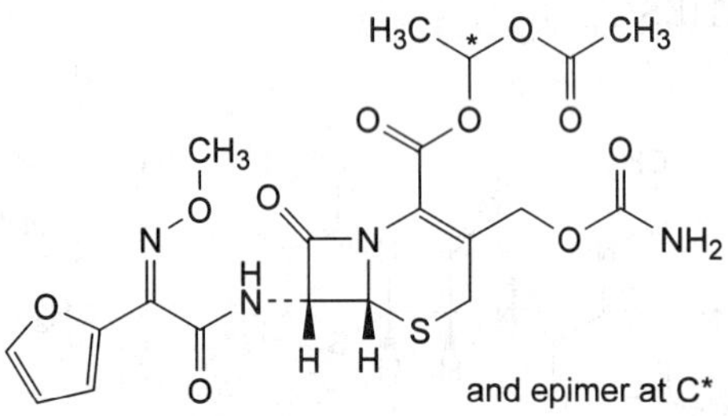

and epimer at C*

$C_{20}H_{22}N_4O_{10}S$ M_r 510.5

DEFINITION

Cefuroxime axetil contains not less than 96.0 per cent and not more than the equivalent of 102.0 per cent of a mixture of the 2 diastereoisomers of (1*RS*)-1-(acetyloxy)ethyl (6*R*,7*R*)-3-[(carbamoyloxy)methyl]-7-[[(*Z*)-2-(furan-2-yl)-2-(methoxyimino)acetyl]amino]-8-oxo-5-thia-1-azabicyclo[4.2.0]oct-2-ene-2-carboxylate, calculated with reference to the anhydrous and acetone-free substance.

CHARACTERS

A white or almost white powder, slightly soluble in water, soluble in acetone, in ethyl acetate and in methanol, slightly soluble in alcohol.

IDENTIFICATION

A. Examine by infrared absorption spectrophotometry (*2.2.24*), comparing with the spectrum obtained with *cefuroxime axetil CRS*.

B. Examine the chromatograms obtained in the Assay. The retention time and size of the principal peaks in the chromatogram obtained with the test solution are the same as those of the peaks due to diastereoisomers A and B of cefuroxime axetil in the chromatogram obtained with reference solution (d).

TESTS

Diastereoisomer ratio. Examine by liquid chromatography (*2.2.29*) as described under Assay. In the chromatogram obtained with the test solution, the ratio of the peak due to cefuroxime axetil diastereoisomer A to the sum of the peaks due to cefuroxime axetil diastereoisomers A and B is between 0.48 and 0.55 by the normalisation procedure.

Related substances. Examine by liquid chromatography (*2.2.29*) as described under Assay. Calculate the percentage content of related substances from the areas of the peaks in the chromatogram obtained with the test solution by the normalisation procedure, disregarding any peak with an area less than 0.05 times that of the 2 principal peaks in the chromatogram obtained with reference solution (a). The percentage sum of the pair of peaks corresponding to the *E*-isomers located by comparison with the chromatogram obtained with reference solution (c) is not greater than 1.0 per cent, the percentage sum of the pair of peaks corresponding to the Δ^3-isomers located by comparison with the chromatogram obtained with reference solution (b) is not greater than 1.5 per cent and the area of any other secondary peak is not greater than 0.5 per cent. The sum of related substances is not greater than 3.0 per cent.

Acetone (*2.4.24*). Not more than 1.1 per cent.

Water (*2.5.12*). Not more than 1.5 per cent, determined on 0.400 g by the semi-micro determination of water.

ASSAY

Examine by liquid chromatography (*2.2.29*).

Test solution. Prepare the solution immediately before use. Dissolve 10.0 mg of the substance to be examined in the mobile phase and dilute to 50.0 ml with the mobile phase.

Reference solution (a). Dilute 1.0 ml of the test solution to 100.0 ml with the mobile phase.

Reference solution (b). Heat 5 ml of the test solution at 60 °C for 1 h to generate the Δ^3-isomers.

Reference solution (c). Expose 5 ml of the test solution to ultraviolet light at 254 nm for 24 h to generate *E*-isomers.

Reference solution (d). Prepare the solution immediately before use. Dissolve 10.0 mg of *cefuroxime axetil CRS* in the mobile phase and dilute to 50.0 ml with the mobile phase.

The chromatographic procedure may be carried out using:

- a column 0.25 m long and 4.6 mm in internal diameter packed with *trimethylsilyl silica gel for chromatography R* (5 µm),
- as mobile phase at a flow rate of 1.0 ml/min a mixture of 38 volumes of *methanol R* and 62 volumes of a 23 g/l solution of *ammonium dihydrogen phosphate R*,
- as detector a spectrophotometer set at 278 nm.

Inject 20 µl each of reference solutions (a), (b), (c) and (d). When the chromatograms are recorded in the prescribed conditions the retention times relative to cefuroxime axetil diastereoisomer A (second peak) are approximately 0.9 for cefuroxime axetil diastereoisomer B, 1.2 for the cefuroxime axetil Δ^3-isomers and 1.7 and 2.1 for the *E*-isomers. The test is not valid unless in the chromatogram obtained with reference solution (d), the resolution between the peaks corresponding to cefuroxime axetil diastereoisomers A and B is at least 1.5. In the chromatogram obtained with reference solution (b), the resolution between the peaks corresponding to cefuroxime axetil diastereoisomer A and cefuroxime axetil Δ^3-isomer is at least 1.5.

Inject reference solution (d) solution 6 times. The assay is not valid unless the relative standard deviation of the sum of the peaks corresponding to cefuroxime axetil diastereoisomers A and B is at most 2.0 per cent.

Calculate the percentage content of $C_{20}H_{22}N_4O_{10}S$ from the sum of areas of the two diastereoisomer peaks and the declared content of $C_{20}H_{22}N_4O_{10}S$ in *cefuroxime axetil CRS*.

STORAGE

Store in an airtight container, protected from light.

IMPURITIES

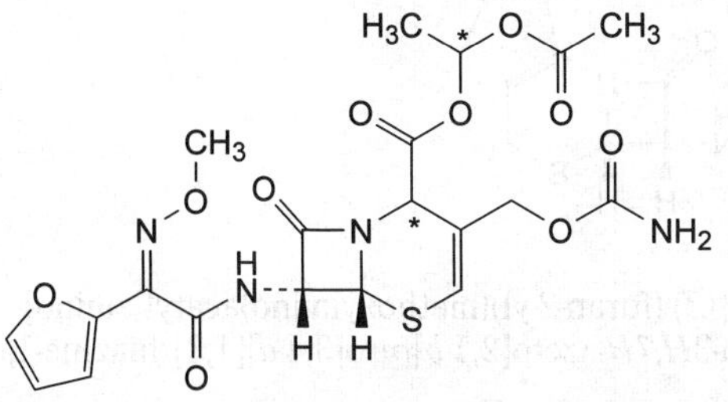

A. 1-(acetyloxy)ethyl (6R,7R)-3-[(carbamoyloxy)methyl]-7-[[(*Z*)-2-(furan-2-yl)-2-(methoxyimino)acetyl]amino]-8-oxo-5-thia-1-azabicyclo[4.2.0]oct-3-ene-2-carboxylate (Δ^3-isomers),

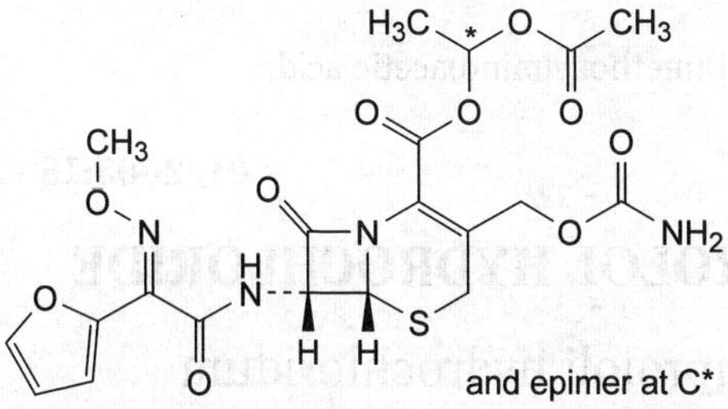

B. (1*RS*)-1-(acetyloxy)ethyl (6*R*,7*R*)-3-[(carbamoyloxy)methyl]-7-[[(*E*)-2-(furan-2-yl)-2-(methoxyimino)acetyl]amino]-8-oxo-5-thia-1-azabicyclo[4.2.0]oct-2-ene-2-carboxylate (*E*-isomers),

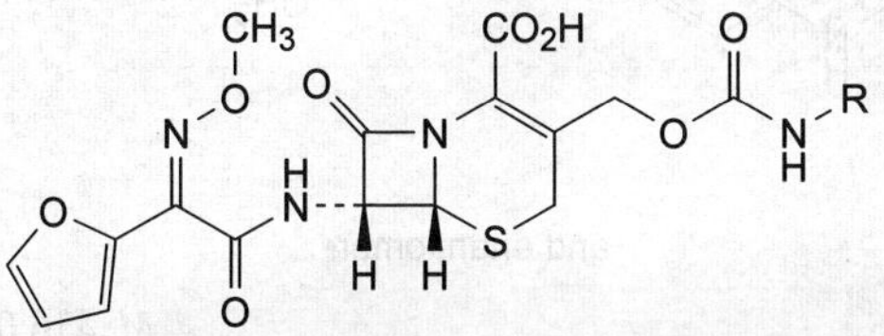

C. R = CO-CCl_3: (6*R*,7*R*)-7-[[(*Z*)-2-(furan-2-yl)-2-(methoxyimino)acetyl]amino]-8-oxo-3-[[[(trichloroacetyl)carbamoyl]oxy]methyl]-5-thia-1-azabicyclo[4.2.0]oct-2-ene-2-carboxylic acid,

D. R = H: cefuroxime.

01/2005:0992

CEFUROXIME SODIUM

Cefuroximum natricum

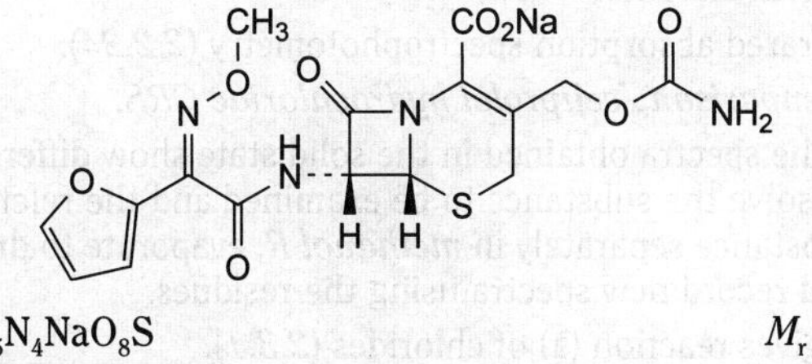

$C_{16}H_{15}N_4NaO_8S$ M_r 446.4

DEFINITION

Sodium (6*R*,7*R*)-3-[(carbamoyloxy)methyl]-7-[[(*Z*)-(furan-2-yl)(methoxyimino)acetyl]amino]-8-oxo-5-thia-1-azabicyclo[4.2.0]oct-2-ene-2-carboxylate.

Content: 96.0 per cent to 102.0 per cent (anhydrous substance).

CHARACTERS

Appearance: white or almost white powder, slightly hygroscopic.

Solubility: freely soluble in water, very slightly soluble in alcohol.

IDENTIFICATION

A. Infrared absorption spectrophotometry (*2.2.24*).
Comparison: *cefuroxime sodium CRS*.

B. It gives reaction (a) of sodium (*2.3.1*).

TESTS

Solution S. Dissolve 2.0 g in *carbon dioxide-free water R* and dilute to 20.0 ml with the same solvent.

Appearance of solution. Solution S is not more opalescent than reference suspension II (*2.2.1*). The absorbance (*2.2.25*) of solution S measured at 450 nm is not greater than 0.25.

pH (*2.2.3*): 5.5 to 8.5.

Dilute 2 ml of solution S to 20 ml with *carbon dioxide-free water R*.

Specific optical rotation (*2.2.7*): + 59 to + 66 (anhydrous substance).

Dissolve 0.500 g in *acetate buffer solution pH 4.6 R* and dilute to 25.0 ml with the same buffer solution.

Related substances. Liquid chromatography (*2.2.29*).

Test solution (a). Dissolve 25.0 mg of the substance to be examined in *water R* and dilute to 25.0 ml with the same solvent.

Test solution (b). Dilute 5.0 ml of test solution (a) to 50.0 ml with *water R*.

Reference solution (a). Dissolve 25.0 mg of *cefuroxime sodium CRS* in *water R* and dilute to 25.0 ml with the same solvent. Dilute 5.0 ml to 50.0 ml with *water R*.

Reference solution (b). Place 20 ml of reference solution (a) in a water-bath at 80 °C for 15 min. Cool and inject immediately.

Reference solution (c). Dilute 1.0 ml of test solution (a) to 100.0 ml with *water R*.

Column:

- *size*: *l* = 0.125 m, Ø = 4.6 mm,
- *stationary phase*: *hexylsilyl silica gel for chromatography R* (5 µm).

Mobile phase: mix 1 volume of *acetonitrile R* and 99 volumes of an acetate buffer solution pH 3.4, prepared by dissolving 6.01 g of *glacial acetic acid R* and 0.68 g of *sodium acetate R* in *water R* and diluting to 1000 ml with the same solvent.

Flow rate: 1.5 ml/min.

Detection: spectrophotometer at 273 nm.

Injection: 20 µl loop injector; inject test solution (a) and reference solutions (b) and (c).

Run time: 4 times the retention time of cefuroxime.

System suitability: reference solution (b):

- *resolution*: minimum of 2.0 between the peaks due to cefuroxime and to impurity A.

Limits:

- *impurity A*: not more than the area of the principal peak in the chromatogram obtained with reference solution (c) (1.0 per cent),
- *any other impurity*: not more than the area of the principal peak in the chromatogram obtained with reference solution (c) (1.0 per cent),
- *total*: not more than 3 times the area of the principal peak in the chromatogram obtained with reference solution (c) (3.0 per cent),

- *disregard limit*: 0.05 times the area of the principal peak in the chromatogram obtained with reference solution (c) (0.05 per cent).

***N,N*-Dimethylaniline** (*2.4.26, Method B*): maximum 20 ppm.

2-Ethylhexanoic acid (*2.4.28*): maximum 0.5 per cent *m/m*.

Water (*2.5.12*): maximum 3.5 per cent, determined on 0.400 g.

Bacterial endotoxins (*2.6.14*): less than 0.10 IU/mg, if intended for use in the manufacture of parenteral dosage forms without a further appropriate procedure for the removal of bacterial endotoxins.

ASSAY

Liquid chromatography (*2.2.29*) as described in the test for related substances with the following modification.

Injection: test solution (b) and reference solution (a).

Calculate the percentage content of cefuroxime sodium.

STORAGE

In an airtight container. If the substance is sterile, store in a sterile, airtight, tamper-proof container.

LABELLING

The label states, where applicable, that the substance is free from bacterial endotoxins.

IMPURITIES

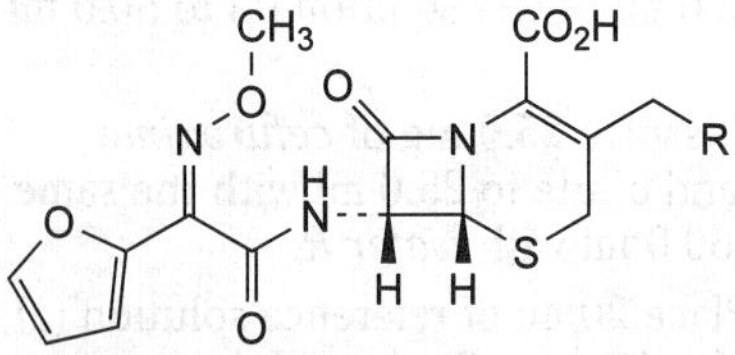

A. R = OH: (6*R*,7*R*)-7-[[(*Z*)-(furan-2-yl)(methoxyimino)acetyl]amino]-3-(hydroxymethyl)-8-oxo-5-thia-1-azabicyclo[4.2.0]oct-2-ene-2-carboxylic acid (descarbamoylcefuroxime),

B. R = O-CO-CH_3: (6*R*,7*R*)-3-[(acetyloxy)methyl]-7-[[(*Z*)-(furan-2-yl)(methoxyimino)acetyl]amino]-8-oxo-5-thia-1-azabicyclo[4.2.0]oct-2-ene-2-carboxylic acid,

C. R = H: (6*R*,7*R*)-7-[[(*Z*)-(furan-2-yl)(methoxyimino)acetyl]amino]-3-methyl-8-oxo-5-thia-1-azabicyclo[4.2.0]oct-2-ene-2-carboxylic acid,

D. R = O-CO-NH-CO-CCl_3: (6*R*,7*R*)-7-[[(*Z*)-(furan-2-yl)(methoxyimino)acetyl]amino]-8-oxo-3-[[[(trichloroacetyl)carbamoyl]oxy]methyl]-5-thia-1-azabicyclo[4.2.0]oct-2-ene-2-carboxylic acid,

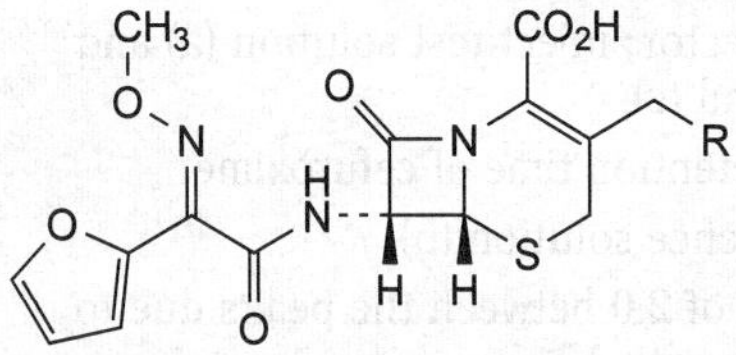

E. R = O-CO-NH_2: (6*R*,7*R*)-3-[(carbamoyloxy)methyl]-7-[[(*E*)-(furan-2-yl)(methoxyimino)acetyl]amino]-8-oxo-5-thia-1-azabicyclo[4.2.0]oct-2-ene-2-carboxylic acid (*trans*-cefuroxime),

F. R = OH: (6*R*,7*R*)-7-[[(*E*)-(furan-2-yl)(methoxyimino)acetyl]amino]-3-(hydroxymethyl)-8-oxo-5-thia-1-azabicyclo[4.2.0]oct-2-ene-2-carboxylic acid,

G. R = O-CO-CH_3: (6*R*,7*R*)-3-[(acetyloxy)methyl]-7-[[(*E*)-(furan-2-yl)(methoxyimino)acetyl]amino]-8-oxo-5-thia-1-azabicyclo[4.2.0]oct-2-ene-2-carboxylic acid,

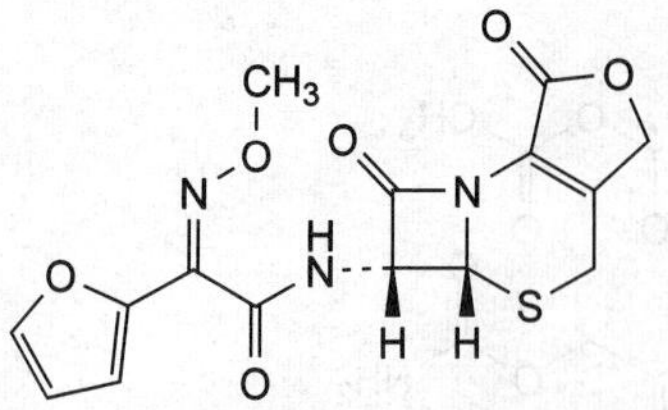

H. (5a*R*,6*R*)-6-[[(*Z*)-(furan-2-yl)(methoxyimino)acetyl]amino]-5a,6-dihydro-3*H*,7*H*-azeto[2,1-*b*]furo[3,4-*d*][1,3]thiazine-1,7(4*H*)-dione,

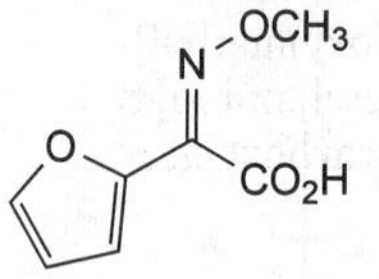

I. (*Z*)-(furan-2-yl)(methoxyimino)acetic acid.

01/2005:1632

CELIPROLOL HYDROCHLORIDE

Celiprololi hydrochloridum

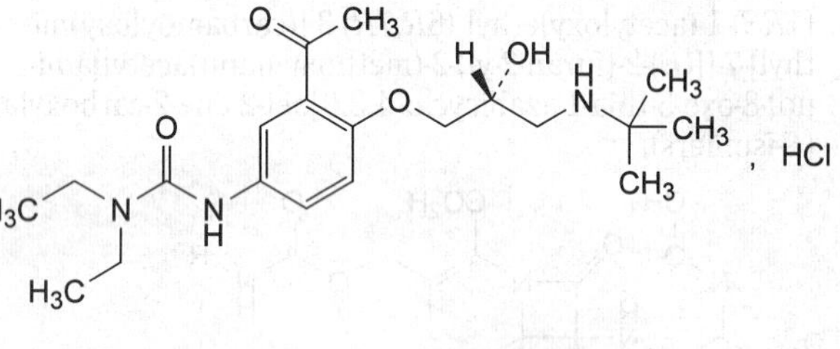

and enantiomer

$C_{20}H_{34}ClN_3O_4$ M_r 416.0

DEFINITION

3-[3-Acetyl-4-[(2*RS*)-3-[(1,1-dimethylethyl)amino]-2-hydroxypropoxy]phenyl]-1,1-diethylurea hydrochloride.

Content: 99.0 per cent to 101.0 per cent (dried substance).

CHARACTERS

Appearance: white or very slightly yellow, crystalline powder.

Solubility: freely soluble in water and in methanol, soluble in alcohol, very slightly soluble in methylene chloride.

It shows polymorphism.

IDENTIFICATION

A. Infrared absorption spectrophotometry (*2.2.24*).

Comparison: *celiprolol hydrochloride CRS*.

If the spectra obtained in the solid state show differences, dissolve the substance to be examined and the reference substance separately in *methanol R*, evaporate to dryness and record new spectra using the residues.

B. It gives reaction (a) of chlorides (*2.3.1*).

TESTS

Optical rotation (*2.2.7*): − 0.10° to + 0.10°.

Dissolve 1.0 g in *water R* and dilute to 10.0 ml with the same solvent.

Related substances. Liquid chromatography (*2.2.29*). *Prepare the solutions immediately before use.*

Test solution. Dissolve 0.100 g of the substance to be examined in mobile phase A and dilute to 20.0 ml with mobile phase A.

Reference solution (a). Dissolve 2 mg of the substance to be examined and 2 mg of *acebutolol hydrochloride R* in mobile phase A and dilute to 50.0 ml with mobile phase A.

Reference solution (b). Dissolve 10 mg of the substance to be examined in 2 ml of mobile phase A and allow to stand for 24 h (for identification of impurity A).

Reference solution (c). Dilute 1.0 ml of the test solution to 100.0 ml with mobile phase A. Dilute 1.0 ml of this solution to 10.0 ml with mobile phase A.

Reference solution (d). Dissolve 10 mg of *celiprolol for peak identification CRS* in mobile phase A and dilute to 2 ml with mobile phase A.

Reference solution (e). This solution is only prepared if required (see below) and is used to determine the identity of impurity I which co-elutes with impurity H (the 2 impurities originate from different synthesis routes). Dissolve 2 mg of *celiprolol impurity I CRS* in mobile phase A and dilute to 20 ml with mobile phase A. Dilute 1.0 ml of the solution to 10.0 ml with mobile phase A.

Column:

- *size*: l = 0.15 m, Ø = 4.6 mm,
- *stationary phase*: *octylsilyl silica gel for chromatography R* (5 µm),
- *temperature*: 30 °C.

Mobile phase:

- *mobile phase A*: mix 91 ml of *tetrahydrofuran R*, 63 ml of *acetonitrile R1*, 0.6 ml of *pentafluoropropanoic acid R* and 0.2 ml of *trifluoroacetic acid R*; dilute to 1000 ml with *water R*;
- *mobile phase B*: *acetonitrile R1*;

Time (min)	Mobile phase A (per cent *V/V*)	Mobile phase B (per cent *V/V*)
0 - 50	100 → 80	0 → 20
50 - 51	80 → 100	20 → 0
51 - 65	100	0

Flow rate: 1.4 ml/min.

Detection: spectrophotometer at 232 nm.

Injection: 10 µl.

Relative retention with reference to celiprolol (retention time = about 10 min): impurity A = about 0.3; impurity D = about 0.7; impurity G = about 1.2; impurity B = about 1.4; impurity F = about 1.6; impurity C = about 2.2; impurity H or I = about 2.5; impurity E = about 3.9.

System suitability: reference solution (a):

- *resolution*: minimum 4.0 between the peaks due to celiprolol and acebutolol.

Limits: use the chromatogram supplied with *celiprolol for peak identification CRS* and the chromatogram obtained with reference solution (d) to identify the peaks due to impurities B, E and F:

- *correction factors*: for the calculation of contents, multiply the peak areas of the following impurities by the corresponding correction factor: impurity A = 4.0; impurity B = 1.5; impurity E = 2.3; impurity F = 0.5; impurity I = 1.7;
- *any impurity*: not more than twice the area of the principal peak in the chromatogram obtained with reference solution (c) (0.2 per cent), and not more than 1 such peak has an area greater than the area of the principal peak in the chromatogram obtained with reference solution (c) (0.1 per cent);
- *total*: not more than 5 times the area of the principal peak in the chromatogram obtained with reference solution (c) (0.5 per cent);
- if any of the above limits are exceeded and if a peak occurs with a relative retention of about 2.5 (impurity H or I), the identity of this peak has to be clarified by use of a UV spectrum recorded with a diode array detector; if this spectrum is different from the one obtained with reference solution (e), no correction factor is applied;
- *disregard limit*: 0.5 times the area of the principal peak in the chromatogram obtained with reference solution (c) (0.05 per cent).

Loss on drying (*2.2.32*): maximum 0.5 per cent, determined on 1.000 g by drying in an oven at 100-105 °C for 3 h.

ASSAY

Dissolve 0.350 g under an atmosphere of nitrogen in 50 ml of *alcohol R* and add 1.0 ml of *0.1 M hydrochloric acid.* Carry out a potentiometric titration (*2.2.20*), using *0.1 M sodium hydroxide.* Read the volume added between the 2 points of inflexion.

1 ml of *0.1 M sodium hydroxide* is equivalent to 41.60 mg of $C_{20}H_{34}ClN_3O_4$.

STORAGE

Protected from light.

IMPURITIES

Specified impurities: A, B, C, D, E, F, G, H, I.

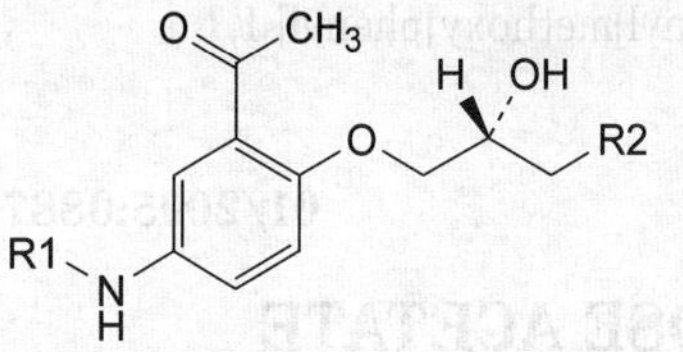

A. R1 = H, R2 = NH-C(CH_3)$_3$: 1-[5-amino-2-[(2*RS*)-3-[(1,1-dimethylethyl)amino]-2-hydroxypropoxy]phenyl]ethanone,

C. R1 = CO-NH-C(CH_3)$_3$, R2 = NH-C(CH_3)$_3$: 1-[3-acetyl-4-[(2*RS*)-3-[(1,1-dimethylethyl)amino]-2-hydroxypropoxy]phenyl]-3-(1,1-dimethylethyl)urea,

D. R1 = CO-N(C_2H_5)$_2$, R2 = N(C_2H_5)$_2$: 3-[3-acetyl-4-[(2*RS*)-3-(diethylamino)-2-hydroxypropoxy]phenyl]-1,1-diethylurea,

H. R1 = CO-N(C_2H_5)$_2$, R2 = Br: 3-[3-acetyl-4-[(2*RS*)-3-bromo-2-hydroxypropoxy]phenyl]-1,1-diethylurea (bromhydrin compound),

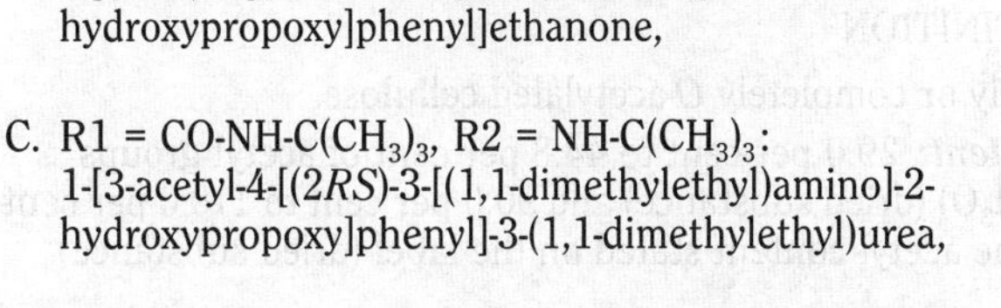

B. 1,3-bis[3-acetyl-4-[3-[(1,1-dimethylethyl)amino]-2-hydroxypropoxy]phenyl]urea,

Monographs C

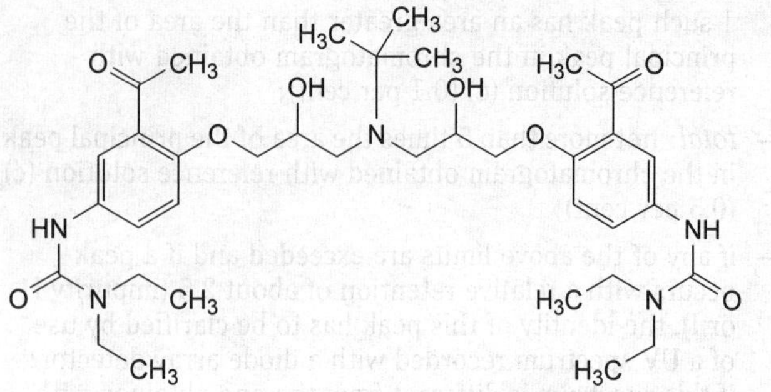

E. 1,1′-[[(1,1-dimethylethyl)imino]bis[(2-hydroxypropane-1,3-diyl)oxy(3-acetyl-1,4-phenylene)]]bis(3,3-diethylurea),

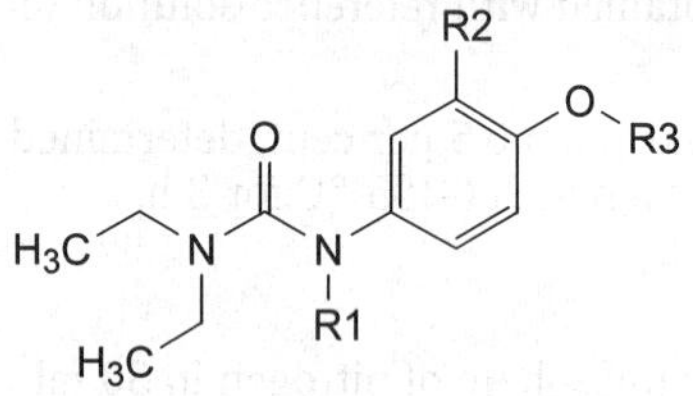

F. R1 = R3 = H, R2 = CO-CH_3: 3-(3-acetyl-4-hydroxyphenyl)-1,1-diethylurea,

I. R1 = CO-CH_3, R2 = H, R3 = C_2H_5: 1-acetyl-1-(4-ethoxyphenyl)-3,3-diethylurea,

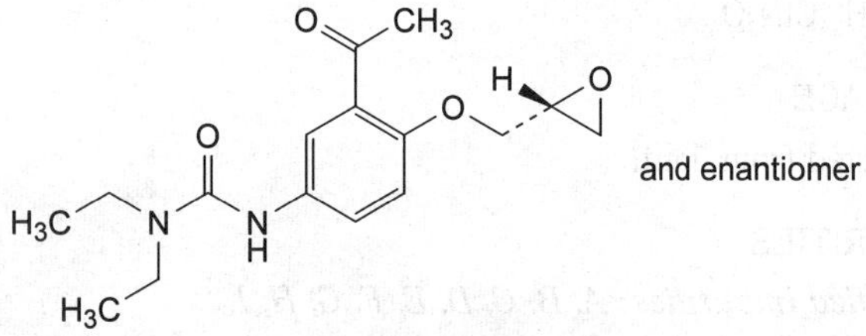

G. 3-[3-acetyl-4-[[(*RS*)-oxiranyl]methoxy]phenyl]-1,1-diethylurea.

01/2005:0887

CELLULOSE ACETATE

Cellulosi acetas

DEFINITION

Partly or completely *O*-acetylated cellulose.

Content: 29.0 per cent to 44.8 per cent of acetyl groups (C_2H_3O) (dried substance) and 90.0 per cent to 110.0 per cent of the acetyl content stated on the label (dried substance).

CHARACTERS

Appearance: white, yellowish-white or greyish-white powder or granules, hygroscopic.

Solubility: practically insoluble in water, soluble in acetone, in formic acid and in a mixture of equal volumes of methanol and methylene chloride, practically insoluble in alcohol.

IDENTIFICATION

Infrared absorption spectrophotometry (*2.2.24*).

Comparison: *Ph. Eur. reference spectrum of cellulose acetate.*

TESTS

Free acid: maximum 0.1 per cent, calculated as acetic acid (dried substance).

To 5.00 g in a 250 ml conical flask, add 150 ml of *carbon dioxide-free water R*, insert the stopper, swirl the suspension gently and allow to stand for 3 h. Filter, wash the flask and the filter with *carbon dioxide-free water R*. Combine the filtrate and washings. Add 0.1 ml of *phenolphthalein solution R1*. Titrate with *0.01 M sodium hydroxide* until a faint pink colour is obtained.

1 ml of *0.01 M sodium hydroxide* is equivalent to 0.6005 mg of free acid, calculated as acetic acid.

Heavy metals (*2.4.8*): maximum 10 ppm.

2.0 g complies with limit test D. Prepare the standard using 2 ml of *lead standard solution (10 ppm Pb) R*.

Loss on drying (*2.2.32*): maximum 5.0 per cent, determined on 1.000 g by drying in an oven at 100-105 °C for 3 h.

Sulphated ash (*2.4.14*): maximum 0.1 per cent, determined on 1.0 g.

Microbial contamination. Total viable aerobic count (*2.6.12*) not more than 10^3 micro-organisms per gram of which not more than 10^2 fungi per gram determined by plate count. It complies with the tests for *Escherichia coli* and *Salmonella* (*2.6.13*).

ASSAY

Cellulose acetate containing not more than 42.0 per cent of acetyl groups

To 2.000 g in a 500 ml conical flask add 100 ml of *acetone R* and 10 ml of *water R*. Close the flask and stir with a magnetic stirrer until dissolution is complete. Add 30.0 ml of *1 M sodium hydroxide* with constant stirring. Close the flask and stir with a magnetic stirrer for 30 min. Add 100 ml of *water R* at 80 °C, washing down the sides of the flask, stir for 2 min and cool to room temperature. Titrate with *0.5 M sulphuric acid*, using 0.1 ml of *phenolphthalein solution R* as indicator. Carry out a blank titration.

Calculate the percentage content of acetyl groups from the expression:

$$\frac{4.305\,(n_2 - n_1)}{(100 - d) \times m} \times 100$$

d = loss on drying as a percentage,

m = mass of the substance to be examined, in grams,

n_1 = number of millilitres of *0.5 M sulphuric acid* used in the test,

n_2 = number of millilitres of *0.5 M sulphuric acid* used in the blank titration.

Cellulose acetate containing more than 42.0 per cent of acetyl groups

To 2.000 g in a 500 ml conical flask add 30 ml of *dimethyl sulphoxide R* and 100 ml of *acetone R*. Close the flask and stir with a magnetic stirrer for 16 h. Add 30.0 ml of *1 M sodium hydroxide* with constant stirring. Close the flask and stir with a magnetic stirrer for 6 min. Allow to stand without stirring for 60 min. Add 100 ml of *water R* at 80 °C, washing down the sides of the flask, stir for 2 min and cool to room temperature. Titrate with *0.5 M hydrochloric acid*, using 0.1 ml of *phenolphthalein solution R*. Add 0.5 ml of *0.5 M hydrochloric acid* in excess, stir for 5 min and allow to stand for 30 min. Titrate with *0.5 M sodium hydroxide*, until a persistent pink colour is obtained, stirring with a magnetic stirrer. Calculate the net number of millimoles of *0.5 M sodium hydroxide* consumed, taking the mean of 2 blank titrations into consideration.

Calculate the percentage content of acetyl groups from the expression:

$$\frac{4.305 \times n}{(100 - d) \times m} \times 100$$

d = loss on drying as a percentage,

m = mass of the substance to be examined, in grams,

n = net number of millimoles of *0.5 M sodium hydroxide*.

STORAGE

In an airtight container.

LABELLING

The label states the nominal percentage content of acetyl groups.

01/2005:1406

CELLULOSE ACETATE BUTYRATE

Cellulosi acetas butyras

DEFINITION

Cellulose acetate butyrate is partly or completely *O*-acetylated and *O*-butyrated cellulose. It contains not less than 2.0 per cent and not more than 30.0 per cent of acetyl groups (C_2H_3O) and not less than 16.0 per cent and not more than 53.0 per cent of butyryl groups (C_4H_7O) calculated with reference to the dried substance. Both the acetyl content and the butyryl content are not less than 90.0 per cent and not more than 110.0 per cent of those stated on the label, calculated with reference to the dried substance.

CHARACTERS

A white, yellowish-white or greyish-white powder or granules, slightly hygroscopic, practically insoluble in water and in alcohol, soluble in acetone, in formic acid and in a mixture of equal volumes of methanol and methylene chloride.

IDENTIFICATION

A. Examine by infrared absorption spectrophotometry (*2.2.24*), comparing with the *Ph. Eur. reference spectrum of cellulose acetate butyrate*. The intensities of the bands may vary according to the degree of substitution.

B. It complies with the limits of the assay.

TESTS

Acidity. To 5.00 g in a 250 ml conical flask, add 150 ml of *carbon dioxide-free water R*, insert the stopper, swirl the suspension gently and allow to stand for 3 h. Filter, wash the flask and the filter with *carbon dioxide-free water R*. Combine the filtrate and washings. Add 0.1 ml of *phenolphthalein solution R1*. Not more than 3.0 ml of *0.01 M sodium hydroxide* is required to change the colour of the indicator.

Heavy metals (*2.4.8*). 1.0 g complies with limit test F for heavy metals (20 ppm). Prepare the standard using 2 ml of *lead standard solution (10 ppm Pb) R*.

Loss on drying (*2.2.32*). Not more than 2.0 per cent, determined on 1.000 g by drying in an oven at 100 °C to 105 °C for 3 h.

Total ash (*2.4.16*). Not more than 0.1 per cent, determined on 1.0 g.

ASSAY

Examine by liquid chromatography (*2.2.29*).

Test solution. To 1.000 g in a 500 ml conical flask, add 100 ml of *acetone R* and 10 ml of *water R*. Close the flask and stir with a magnetic stirrer until dissolution is complete. Add 30.0 ml of *1 M sodium hydroxide* with constant stirring. Close the flask and stir with a magnetic stirrer for 30 min. Add 100 ml of hot *water R* at 80 °C, washing down the sides of the flask and stir for 2 min. Cool, centrifuge or filter the suspension and wash the residue with *water R*. Combine the filtrate and washings, adjust the pH to 3 (*2.2.3*) using *dilute phosphoric acid R* and dilute to 500.0 ml with *water R*.

Reference solution. Dissolve 0.200 g of *glacial acetic acid R* and 0.400 g of *butyric acid R* in *water R*, adjust the pH to 3 (*2.2.3*) using *dilute phosphoric acid R* and dilute to 500.0 ml with *water R*.

The chromatographic procedure may be carried out using:

- a column 0.25 m long and 4.6 mm in internal diameter packed with *octadecylsilyl silica gel for chromatography R* (5 µm),
- as mobile phase at a flow rate of 1.2 ml/min a mixture of 5 volumes of *methanol R* and 95 volumes of *phosphate buffer solution pH 3.0 R1*, changing after 30 min, by linear gradient elution over 5 min, to a mixture of 20 volumes of *methanol R* and 80 volumes of *phosphate buffer solution pH 3.0 R1* and eluting for a further 25 min. Restore the initial solvent mixture for 1 min,
- as detector a spectrophotometer set at 210 nm.

Inject successively 20 µl of the reference solution and 20 µl of the test solution.

Calculate the percentage contents of acetic acid and butyric acid in the substance to be examined from the peak areas in the chromatograms obtained with the two solutions.

To calculate the percentage contents of acetyl (C_2H_3O) and of butyryl (C_4H_7O) groups, multiply the percentage contents of acetic acid and of butyric acid by 0.717 and 0.807, respectively.

STORAGE

Store in an airtight container.

LABELLING

The label states the nominal percentage content of acetyl and butyryl groups.

01/2005:0314

CELLULOSE ACETATE PHTHALATE

Cellulosi acetas phthalas

DEFINITION

Partly *O*-acetylated and *O*-phthalylated cellulose.

Content:

- phthaloyl groups ($C_8H_5O_3$, relative mass of the group 149.1): 30.0 per cent to 36.0 per cent (anhydrous and acid-free substance).
- acetyl groups (C_2H_3O, relative mass of the group 43.05): 21.5 per cent to 26.0 per cent (anhydrous and acid-free substance).

CHARACTERS

Appearance: white, free-flowing powder or colourless flakes, hygroscopic.

Solubility: practically insoluble in water, freely soluble in acetone, soluble in diethylene glycol, practically insoluble in ethanol and in methylene chloride. It dissolves in dilute solutions of alkalis.

IDENTIFICATION

Infrared absorption spectrophotometry (*2.2.24*).

Comparison: *Ph. Eur. reference spectrum of cellulose acetate phthalate.*

TESTS

Viscosity (*2.2.9*): 45 mPa·s to 90 mPa·s for the apparent viscosity determined at 25 °C.

Dissolve 15 g, calculated with reference to the anhydrous substance, in 85 g of a mixture of 1 part of *water R* and 249 parts of *acetone R*.

Free acid: maximum 3.0 per cent, calculated as phthalic acid (anhydrous substance).

Shake 3.0 g for 2 h with 100 ml of a 50 per cent *V/V* solution of *methanol R* and filter. Wash the flask and the filter with 2 quantities, each of 10 ml, of a mixture of a 50 per cent *V/V* solution of *methanol R*. Combine the filtrate and washings, add *phenolphthalein solution R* and titrate with *0.1 M sodium hydroxide* until a faint pink colour is obtained. Carry out a blank titration.

1 ml of *0.1 M sodium hydroxide* is equivalent to 8.3 mg of free acid, calculated as phthalic acid.

Heavy metals (*2.4.8*): maximum 10 ppm.

2.0 g complies with limit test C. Prepare the standard using 2 ml of *lead standard solution (10 ppm Pb) R*.

Water (*2.5.12*): maximum 5.0 per cent, determined on 0.500 g.

Carry out the test using a mixture of 2 volumes of *methylene chloride R* and 3 volumes of *ethanol R*.

Sulphated ash (*2.4.14*): maximum 0.1 per cent, determined on 1.0 g.

ASSAY

Phthaloyl groups. Dissolve 1.000 g in 50 ml of a mixture of 2 volumes of *acetone R* and 3 volumes of *alcohol R*. Add 0.1 ml of *phenolphthalein solution R* and titrate with *0.1 M sodium hydroxide* until a faint pink colour is obtained. Carry out a blank titration.

Calculate the percentage content of phthaloyl groups (P) from the expression:

$$\frac{14\,900n}{(100-a)(100-S)\,m}-\frac{179.5S}{(100-S)}$$

a = percentage content of water,

m = mass of the substance to be examined, in grams,

n = number of millilitres of *0.1 M sodium hydroxide* used,

S = percentage content of free acid (see Tests).

Acetyl groups. To 0.100 g add 25.0 ml of *0.1 M sodium hydroxide* and heat on a water-bath under a reflux condenser for 30 min. Cool, add 0.1 ml of *phenolphthalein solution R* and titrate with *0.1 M hydrochloric acid* until the colour is discharged. Carry out a blank titration.

Calculate the percentage content of acetyl groups from the expression:

$$\left[\frac{4300\,(n_2-n_1)}{(100-a)\,(100-S)\,m}-\frac{51.8S}{(100-S)}\right]-0.578P$$

a = percentage content of water,

m = mass of the substance to be examined, in grams,

n_1 = number of millilitres of *0.1 M hydrochloric acid* used in the test,

n_2 = number of millilitres of *0.1 M hydrochloric acid* used in the blank titration,

P = percentage content of phthaloyl groups,

S = percentage content of free acid (see Tests).

STORAGE

In an airtight container.

01/2005:0316

CELLULOSE, MICROCRYSTALLINE

Cellulosum microcristallinum

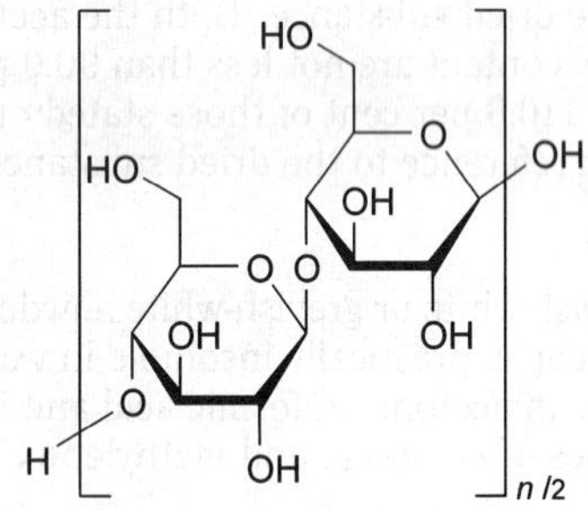

$C_{6n}H_{10n+2}O_{5n+1}$

DEFINITION

Purified, partly depolymerised cellulose prepared by treating alpha-cellulose, obtained as a pulp from fibrous plant material, with mineral acids.

CHARACTERS

Appearance: white or almost white, fine or granular powder.

Solubility: practically insoluble in water, in acetone, in ethanol, in toluene, in dilute acids and in a 50 g/l solution of sodium hydroxide.

IDENTIFICATION

A. Place about 10 mg on a watch-glass and disperse in 2 ml of *iodinated zinc chloride solution R*. The substance becomes violet-blue.

B. The degree of polymerisation is not more than 350. Transfer 1.300 g to a 125 ml conical flask. Add 25.0 ml of *water R* and 25.0 ml of *cupriethylenediamine hydroxide solution R*. Immediately purge the solution with *nitrogen R*, insert the stopper and shake until completely dissolved. Transfer 7.0 ml of the solution to a suitable capillary viscometer (*2.2.9*). Equilibrate the solution at 25 ± 0.1 °C for at least 5 min. Record the flow time t_1 in seconds, between the 2 marks on the viscometer. Calculate the kinematic viscosity ν_1 of the solution using the formula:

$$t_1 (k_1)$$

where k_1 is the viscometer constant.

Dilute a suitable volume of *cupriethylenediamine hydroxide solution R* with an equal volume of *water R* and measure the flow time t_2 using a suitable capillary viscometer. Calculate the kinematic viscosity ν_2 of the solvent using the formula:

$$t_2 (k_2)$$

where k_2 is the viscometer constant.

Determine the relative viscosity η_{rel} of the substance to be examined using the formula:

$$\nu_1/\nu_2$$

Determine the intrinsic viscosity $[\eta]_c$ by interpolation, using the intrinsic viscosity table (Table 0316.-1).

Calculate the degree of polymerisation P using the formula:

$$\frac{95\,[\eta]_c}{m\,[(100-b)/100]}$$

where m is the mass in grams of the substance to be examined and b is the loss on drying as a percentage.

TESTS

Solubility. Dissolve 50 mg in 10 ml of *ammoniacal solution of copper tetrammine R*. It dissolves completely, leaving no residue.

pH (*2.2.3*): 5.0 to 7.5 for the supernatant liquid.

Shake 5 g with 40 ml of *carbon dioxide-free water R* for 20 min and centrifuge.

Table 0316.-1. – *Intrinsic viscosity table*

Intrinsic viscosity $[\eta]_c$ at different values of relative viscosity η_{rel}										
					$[\eta]_c$					
η_{rel}	0.00	0.01	0.02	0.03	0.04	0.05	0.06	0.07	0.08	0.09
1.1	0.098	0.106	0.115	0.125	0.134	0.143	0.152	0.161	0.170	0.180
1.2	0.189	0.198	0.207	0.216	0.225	0.233	0.242	0.250	0.259	0.268
1.3	0.276	0.285	0.293	0.302	0.310	0.318	0.326	0.334	0.342	0.350
1.4	0.358	0.367	0.375	0.383	0.391	0.399	0.407	0.414	0.422	0.430
1.5	0.437	0.445	0.453	0.460	0.468	0.476	0.484	0.491	0.499	0.507
1.6	0.515	0.522	0.529	0.536	0.544	0.551	0.558	0.566	0.573	0.580
1.7	0.587	0.595	0.602	0.608	0.615	0.622	0.629	0.636	0.642	0.649
1.8	0.656	0.663	0.670	0.677	0.683	0.690	0.697	0.704	0.710	0.717
1.9	0.723	0.730	0.736	0.743	0.749	0.756	0.762	0.769	0.775	0.782
2.0	0.788	0.795	0.802	0.809	0.815	0.821	0.827	0.833	0.840	0.846
2.1	0.852	0.858	0.864	0.870	0.876	0.882	0.888	0.894	0.900	0.906
2.2	0.912	0.918	0.924	0.929	0.935	0.941	0.948	0.953	0.959	0.965
2.3	0.971	0.976	0.983	0.988	0.994	1.000	1.006	1.011	1.017	1.022
2.4	1.028	1.033	1.039	1.044	1.050	1.056	1.061	1.067	1.072	1.078
2.5	1.083	1.089	1.094	1.100	1.105	1.111	1.116	1.121	1.126	1.131
2.6	1.137	1.142	1.147	1.153	1.158	1.163	1.169	1.174	1.179	1.184
2.7	1.190	1.195	1.200	1.205	1.210	1.215	1.220	1.225	1.230	1.235
2.8	1.240	1.245	1.250	1.255	1.260	1.265	1.270	1.275	1.280	1.285
2.9	1.290	1.295	1.300	1.305	1.310	1.314	1.319	1.324	1.329	1.333
3.0	1.338	1.343	1.348	1.352	1.357	1.362	1.367	1.371	1.376	1.381
3.1	1.386	1.390	1.395	1.400	1.405	1.409	1.414	1.418	1.423	1.427
3.2	1.432	1.436	1.441	1.446	1.450	1.455	1.459	1.464	1.468	1.473
3.3	1.477	1.482	1.486	1.491	1.496	1.500	1.504	1.508	1.513	1.517
3.4	1.521	1.525	1.529	1.533	1.537	1.542	1.546	1.550	1.554	1.558
3.5	1.562	1.566	1.570	1.575	1.579	1.583	1.587	1.591	1.595	1.600
3.6	1.604	1.608	1.612	1.617	1.621	1.625	1.629	1.633	1.637	1.642
3.7	1.646	1.650	1.654	1.658	1.662	1.666	1.671	1.675	1.679	1.683

Intrinsic viscosity $[\eta]_c$ at different values of relative viscosity η_{rel}

	$[\eta]_c$									
η_{rel}	0.00	0.01	0.02	0.03	0.04	0.05	0.06	0.07	0.08	0.09
3.8	1.687	1.691	1.695	1.700	1.704	1.708	1.712	1.715	1.719	1.723
3.9	1.727	1.731	1.735	1.739	1.742	1.746	1.750	1.754	1.758	1.762
4.0	1.765	1.769	1.773	1.777	1.781	1.785	1.789	1.792	1.796	1.800
4.1	1.804	1.808	1.811	1.815	1.819	1.822	1.826	1.830	1.833	1.837
4.2	1.841	1.845	1.848	1.852	1.856	1.859	1.863	1.867	1.870	1.874
4.3	1.878	1.882	1.885	1.889	1.893	1.896	1.900	1.904	1.907	1.911
4.4	1.914	1.918	1.921	1.925	1.929	1.932	1.936	1.939	1.943	1.946
4.5	1.950	1.954	1.957	1.961	1.964	1.968	1.971	1.975	1.979	1.982
4.6	1.986	1.989	1.993	1.996	2.000	2.003	2.007	2.010	2.013	2.017
4.7	2.020	2.023	2.027	2.030	2.033	2.037	2.040	2.043	2.047	2.050
4.8	2.053	2.057	2.060	2.063	2.067	2.070	2.073	2.077	2.080	2.083
4.9	2.087	2.090	2.093	2.097	2.100	2.103	2.107	2.110	2.113	2.116
5.0	2.119	2.122	2.125	2.129	2.132	2.135	2.139	2.142	2.145	2.148
5.1	2.151	2.154	2.158	2.160	2.164	2.167	2.170	2.173	2.176	2.180
5.2	2.183	2.186	2.190	2.192	2.195	2.197	2.200	2.203	2.206	2.209
5.3	2.212	2.215	2.218	2.221	2.224	2.227	2.230	2.233	2.236	2.240
5.4	2.243	2.246	2.249	2.252	2.255	2.258	2.261	2.264	2.267	2.270
5.5	2.273	2.276	2.279	2.282	2.285	2.288	2.291	2.294	2.297	2.300
5.6	2.303	2.306	2.309	2.312	2.315	2.318	2.320	2.324	2.326	2.329
5.7	2.332	2.335	2.338	2.341	2.344	2.347	2.350	2.353	2.355	2.358
5.8	2.361	2.364	2.367	2.370	2.373	2.376	2.379	2.382	2.384	2.387
5.9	2.390	2.393	2.396	2.400	2.403	2.405	2.408	2.411	2.414	2.417
6.0	2.419	2.422	2.425	2.428	2.431	2.433	2.436	2.439	2.442	2.444
6.1	2.447	2.450	2.453	2.456	2.458	2.461	2.464	2.467	2.470	2.472
6.2	2.475	2.478	2.481	2.483	2.486	2.489	2.492	2.494	2.497	2.500
6.3	2.503	2.505	2.508	2.511	2.513	2.516	2.518	2.521	2.524	2.526
6.4	2.529	2.532	2.534	2.537	2.540	2.542	2.545	2.547	2.550	2.553
6.5	2.555	2.558	2.561	2.563	2.566	2.568	2.571	2.574	2.576	2.579
6.6	2.581	2.584	2.587	2.590	2.592	2.595	2.597	2.600	2.603	2.605
6.7	2.608	2.610	2.613	2.615	2.618	2.620	2.623	2.625	2.627	2.630
6.8	2.633	2.635	2.637	2.640	2.643	2.645	2.648	2.650	2.653	2.655
6.9	2.658	2.660	2.663	2.665	2.668	2.670	2.673	2.675	2.678	2.680
7.0	2.683	2.685	2.687	2.690	2.693	2.695	2.698	2.700	2.702	2.705
7.1	2.707	2.710	2.712	2.714	2.717	2.719	2.721	2.724	2.726	2.729
7.2	2.731	2.733	2.736	2.738	2.740	2.743	2.745	2.748	2.750	2.752
7.3	2.755	2.757	2.760	2.762	2.764	2.767	2.769	2.771	2.774	2.776
7.4	2.779	2.781	2.783	2.786	2.788	2.790	2.793	2.795	2.798	2.800
7.5	2.802	2.805	2.807	2.809	2.812	2.814	2.816	2.819	2.821	2.823
7.6	2.826	2.828	2.830	2.833	2.835	2.837	2.840	2.842	2.844	2.847
7.7	2.849	2.851	2.854	2.856	2.858	2.860	2.863	2.865	2.868	2.870
7.8	2.873	2.875	2.877	2.879	2.881	2.884	2.887	2.889	2.891	2.893

Intrinsic viscosity $[\eta]_c$ at different values of relative viscosity η_{rel}

	$[\eta]_c$									
η_{rel}	0.00	0.01	0.02	0.03	0.04	0.05	0.06	0.07	0.08	0.09
7.9	2.895	2.898	2.900	2.902	2.905	2.907	2.909	2.911	2.913	2.915
8.0	2.918	2.920	2.922	2.924	2.926	2.928	2.931	2.933	2.935	2.937
8.1	2.939	2.942	2.944	2.946	2.948	2.950	2.952	2.955	2.957	2.959
8.2	2.961	2.963	2.966	2.968	2.970	2.972	2.974	2.976	2.979	2.981
8.3	2.983	2.985	2.987	2.990	2.992	2.994	2.996	2.998	3.000	3.002
8.4	3.004	3.006	3.008	3.010	3.012	3.015	3.017	3.019	3.021	3.023
8.5	3.025	3.027	3.029	3.031	3.033	3.035	3.037	3.040	3.042	3.044
8.6	3.046	3.048	3.050	3.052	3.054	3.056	3.058	3.060	3.062	3.064
8.7	3.067	3.069	3.071	3.073	3.075	3.077	3.079	3.081	3.083	3.085
8.8	3.087	3.089	3.092	3.094	3.096	3.098	3.100	3.102	3.104	3.106
8.9	3.108	3.110	3.112	3.114	3.116	3.118	3.120	3.122	3.124	3.126
9.0	3.128	3.130	3.132	3.134	3.136	3.138	3.140	3.142	3.144	3.146
9.1	3.148	3.150	3.152	3.154	3.156	3.158	3.160	3.162	3.164	3.166
9.2	3.168	3.170	3.172	3.174	3.176	3.178	3.180	3.182	3.184	3.186
9.3	3.188	3.190	3.192	3.194	3.196	3.198	3.200	3.202	3.204	3.206
9.4	3.208	3.210	3.212	3.214	3.215	3.217	3.219	3.221	3.223	3.225
9.5	3.227	3.229	3.231	3.233	3.235	3.237	3.239	3.241	3.242	3.244
9.6	3.246	3.248	3.250	3.252	3.254	3.256	3.258	3.260	3.262	3.264
9.7	3.266	3.268	3.269	3.271	3.273	3.275	3.277	3.279	3.281	3.283
9.8	3.285	3.287	3.289	3.291	3.293	3.295	3.297	3.298	3.300	3.302
9.9	3.304	3.305	3.307	3.309	3.311	3.313	3.316	3.318	3.320	3.321

Intrinsic viscosity $[\eta]_c$ at different values of relative viscosity η_{rel}

	$[\eta]_c$									
η_{rel}	0.0	0.1	0.2	0.3	0.4	0.5	0.6	0.7	0.8	0.9
10	3.32	3.34	3.36	3.37	3.39	3.41	3.43	3.45	3.46	3.48
11	3.50	3.52	3.53	3.55	3.56	3.58	3.60	3.61	3.63	3.64
12	3.66	3.68	3.69	3.71	3.72	3.74	3.76	3.77	3.79	3.80
13	3.80	3.83	3.85	3.86	3.88	3.89	3.90	3.92	3.93	3.95
14	3.96	3.97	3.99	4.00	4.02	4.03	4.04	4.06	4.07	4.09
15	4.10	4.11	4.13	4.14	4.15	4.17	4.18	4.19	4.20	4.22
16	4.23	4.24	4.25	4.27	4.28	4.29	4.30	4.31	4.33	4.34
17	4.35	4.36	4.37	4.38	4.39	4.41	4.42	4.43	4.44	4.45
18	4.46	4.47	4.48	4.49	4.50	4.52	4.53	4.54	4.55	4.56
19	4.57	4.58	4.59	4.60	4.61	4.62	4.63	4.64	4.65	4.66

Conductivity (*2.2.38*). The conductivity of the test solution does not exceed the conductivity of the water by more than 75 µS·cm^{-1}.

Use as test solution the supernatant liquid obtained in the test for pH. Measure the conductivity of the supernatant liquid after a stable reading has been obtained and measure the conductivity of the water used to prepare the test solution.

Ether-soluble substances: maximum 0.05 per cent (5 mg) for the difference between the weight of the residue and the weight obtained from a blank determination.

Place 10.0 g in a column about 20 mm in internal diameter and pass 50 ml of *peroxide-free ether R* through the column. Evaporate the eluate to dryness and weigh. Carry out a blank determination under the same conditions.

Water-soluble substances: maximum 0.25 per cent (12.5 mg) for the difference between the weight of the residue and the weight obtained from a blank determination.

Shake 5.0 g with 80 ml of *water R* for 10 min. Filter with the aid of vacuum into a tared flask. Evaporate to dryness on a water-bath. Dry at 100-105 °C for 1 h and weigh. Carry out a blank determination under the same conditions.

Heavy metals (*2.4.8*): maximum 10 ppm.

2.0 g complies with limit test C. Prepare the standard using 2 ml of *lead standard solution (10 ppm Pb) R*.

Loss on drying (*2.2.32*): maximum 7.0 per cent, determined on 1.000 g by drying in an oven at 100-105 °C for 3 h.

Sulphated ash (*2.4.14*): maximum 0.1 per cent, determined on 1.0 g.

Microbial contamination. Total viable aerobic count (*2.6.12*) not more than 10^3 micro-organisms per gram and with a limit for fungi of 10^2 per gram, determined by plate count. It complies with the tests for *Escherichia coli*, for *Pseudomonas aeruginosa*, for *Staphylococcus aureus* and for *Salmonella* (*2.6.13*).

01/2005:0315

CELLULOSE, POWDERED

Cellulosi pulvis

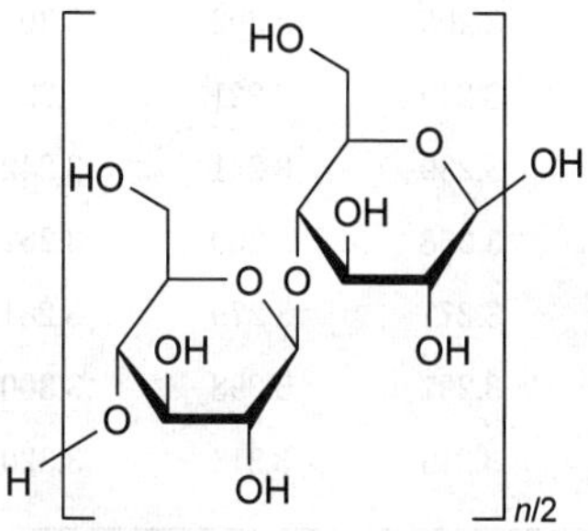

$C_{6n}H_{10n+2}O_{5n+1}$

DEFINITION

Purified, mechanically disintegrated cellulose prepared by processing alpha-cellulose obtained as a pulp from fibrous plant material.

CHARACTERS

Appearance: white or almost white, fine or granular powder.

Solubility: practically insoluble in water, slightly soluble in a 50 g/l solution of sodium hydroxide, practically insoluble in acetone, in ethanol, in toluene, in dilute acids and in most organic solvents.

IDENTIFICATION

A. Place about 10 mg on a watch-glass and disperse in 2 ml of *iodinated zinc chloride solution R*. The substance becomes violet-blue.

B. The degree of polymerisation is 440 to 2250.

Transfer 0.250 g to a 125 ml conical flask. Add 25.0 ml of *water R* and 25.0 ml of *cupriethylenediamine hydroxide solution R*. Immediately purge the solution with *nitrogen R*, insert the stopper and shake until completely dissolved. Transfer 7.0 ml of the solution to a suitable capillary viscometer (*2.2.9*). Equilibrate the solution at 25 ± 0.1 °C for at least 5 min. Record the flow time t_1 in seconds, between the 2 marks on the viscometer. Calculate the kinematic viscosity ν_1 of the solution using the formula:

$$t_1\,(k_1)$$

where k_1 is the viscometer constant.

Dilute a suitable volume of *cupriethylenediamine hydroxide solution R* with an equal volume of *water R* and measure the flow time t_2 using a suitable capillary viscometer. Calculate the kinematic viscosity ν_2 of the solvent using the formula:

$$t_2\,(k_2)$$

where k_2 is the viscometer constant.

Determine the relative viscosity η_{rel} of the substance to be examined using the formula:

$$\nu_1/\nu_2$$

Determine the intrinsic viscosity $[\eta]_c$ by interpolation, using the intrinsic viscosity table (Table 0315.-1).

Calculate the degree of polymerisation, *P*, using the formula:

$$\frac{95\,[\eta]_c}{m\,[(100-b)/100]}$$

where *m* is the mass in grams of the substance to be examined and *b* is the loss on drying as a percentage.

Table 0315.-1. – *Intrinsic viscosity table*

Intrinsic viscosity $[\eta]_c$ at different values of relative viscosity η_{rel}										
					$[\eta]_c$					
η_{rel}	0.00	0.01	0.02	0.03	0.04	0.05	0.06	0.07	0.08	0.09
1.1	0.098	0.106	0.115	0.125	0.134	0.143	0.152	0.161	0.170	0.180
1.2	0.189	0.198	0.207	0.216	0.225	0.233	0.242	0.250	0.259	0.268
1.3	0.276	0.285	0.293	0.302	0.310	0.318	0.326	0.334	0.342	0.350
1.4	0.358	0.367	0.375	0.383	0.391	0.399	0.407	0.414	0.422	0.430
1.5	0.437	0.445	0.453	0.460	0.468	0.476	0.484	0.491	0.499	0.507
1.6	0.515	0.522	0.529	0.536	0.544	0.551	0.558	0.566	0.573	0.580
1.7	0.587	0.595	0.602	0.608	0.615	0.622	0.629	0.636	0.642	0.649
1.8	0.656	0.663	0.670	0.677	0.683	0.690	0.697	0.704	0.710	0.717
1.9	0.723	0.730	0.736	0.743	0.749	0.756	0.762	0.769	0.775	0.782

Intrinsic viscosity $[\eta]_c$ at different values of relative viscosity η_{rel}

	$[\eta]_c$									
η_{rel}	0.00	0.01	0.02	0.03	0.04	0.05	0.06	0.07	0.08	0.09
2.0	0.788	0.795	0.802	0.809	0.815	0.821	0.827	0.833	0.840	0.846
2.1	0.852	0.858	0.864	0.870	0.876	0.882	0.888	0.894	0.900	0.906
2.2	0.912	0.918	0.924	0.929	0.935	0.941	0.948	0.953	0.959	0.965
2.3	0.971	0.976	0.983	0.988	0.994	1.000	1.006	1.011	1.017	1.022
2.4	1.028	1.033	1.039	1.044	1.050	1.056	1.061	1.067	1.072	1.078
2.5	1.083	1.089	1.094	1.100	1.105	1.111	1.116	1.121	1.126	1.131
2.6	1.137	1.142	1.147	1.153	1.158	1.163	1.169	1.174	1.179	1.184
2.7	1.190	1.195	1.200	1.205	1.210	1.215	1.220	1.225	1.230	1.235
2.8	1.240	1.245	1.250	1.255	1.260	1.265	1.270	1.275	1.280	1.285
2.9	1.290	1.295	1.300	1.305	1.310	1.314	1.319	1.324	1.329	1.333
3.0	1.338	1.343	1.348	1.352	1.357	1.362	1.367	1.371	1.376	1.381
3.1	1.386	1.390	1.395	1.400	1.405	1.409	1.414	1.418	1.423	1.427
3.2	1.432	1.436	1.441	1.446	1.450	1.455	1.459	1.464	1.468	1.473
3.3	1.477	1.482	1.486	1.491	1.496	1.500	1.504	1.508	1.513	1.517
3.4	1.521	1.525	1.529	1.533	1.537	1.542	1.546	1.550	1.554	1.558
3.5	1.562	1.566	1.570	1.575	1.579	1.583	1.587	1.591	1.595	1.600
3.6	1.604	1.608	1.612	1.617	1.621	1.625	1.629	1.633	1.637	1.642
3.7	1.646	1.650	1.654	1.658	1.662	1.666	1.671	1.675	1.679	1.683
3.8	1.687	1.691	1.695	1.700	1.704	1.708	1.712	1.715	1.719	1.723
3.9	1.727	1.731	1.735	1.739	1.742	1.746	1.750	1.754	1.758	1.762
4.0	1.765	1.769	1.773	1.777	1.781	1.785	1.789	1.792	1.796	1.800
4.1	1.804	1.808	1.811	1.815	1.819	1.822	1.826	1.830	1.833	1.837
4.2	1.841	1.845	1.848	1.852	1.856	1.859	1.863	1.867	1.870	1.874
4.3	1.878	1.882	1.885	1.889	1.893	1.896	1.900	1.904	1.907	1.911
4.4	1.914	1.918	1.921	1.925	1.929	1.932	1.936	1.939	1.943	1.946
4.5	1.950	1.954	1.957	1.961	1.964	1.968	1.971	1.975	1.979	1.982
4.6	1.986	1.989	1.993	1.996	2.000	2.003	2.007	2.010	2.013	2.017
4.7	2.020	2.023	2.027	2.030	2.033	2.037	2.040	2.043	2.047	2.050
4.8	2.053	2.057	2.060	2.063	2.067	2.070	2.073	2.077	2.080	2.083
4.9	2.087	2.090	2.093	2.097	2.100	2.103	2.107	2.110	2.113	2.116
5.0	2.119	2.122	2.125	2.129	2.132	2.135	2.139	2.142	2.145	2.148
5.1	2.151	2.154	2.158	2.160	2.164	2.167	2.170	2.173	2.176	2.180
5.2	2.183	2.186	2.190	2.192	2.195	2.197	2.200	2.203	2.206	2.209
5.3	2.212	2.215	2.218	2.221	2.224	2.227	2.230	2.233	2.236	2.240
5.4	2.243	2.246	2.249	2.252	2.255	2.258	2.261	2.264	2.267	2.270
5.5	2.273	2.276	2.279	2.282	2.285	2.288	2.291	2.294	2.297	2.300
5.6	2.303	2.306	2.309	2.312	2.315	2.318	2.320	2.324	2.326	2.329
5.7	2.332	2.335	2.338	2.341	2.344	2.347	2.350	2.353	2.355	2.358
5.8	2.361	2.364	2.367	2.370	2.373	2.376	2.379	2.382	2.384	2.387
5.9	2.390	2.393	2.396	2.400	2.403	2.405	2.408	2.411	2.414	2.417
6.0	2.419	2.422	2.425	2.428	2.431	2.433	2.436	2.439	2.442	2.444

Intrinsic viscosity $[\eta]_c$ at different values of relative viscosity η_{rel}

η_{rel}	$[\eta]_c$ 0.00	0.01	0.02	0.03	0.04	0.05	0.06	0.07	0.08	0.09
6.1	2.447	2.450	2.453	2.456	2.458	2.461	2.464	2.467	2.470	2.472
6.2	2.475	2.478	2.481	2.483	2.486	2.489	2.492	2.494	2.497	2.500
6.3	2.503	2.505	2.508	2.511	2.513	2.516	2.518	2.521	2.524	2.526
6.4	2.529	2.532	2.534	2.537	2.540	2.542	2.545	2.547	2.550	2.553
6.5	2.555	2.558	2.561	2.563	2.566	2.568	2.571	2.574	2.576	2.579
6.6	2.581	2.584	2.587	2.590	2.592	2.595	2.597	2.600	2.603	2.605
6.7	2.608	2.610	2.613	2.615	2.618	2.620	2.623	2.625	2.627	2.630
6.8	2.633	2.635	2.637	2.640	2.643	2.645	2.648	2.650	2.653	2.655
6.9	2.658	2.660	2.663	2.665	2.668	2.670	2.673	2.675	2.678	2.680
7.0	2.683	2.685	2.687	2.690	2.693	2.695	2.698	2.700	2.702	2.705
7.1	2.707	2.710	2.712	2.714	2.717	2.719	2.721	2.724	2.726	2.729
7.2	2.731	2.733	2.736	2.738	2.740	2.743	2.745	2.748	2.750	2.752
7.3	2.755	2.757	2.760	2.762	2.764	2.767	2.769	2.771	2.774	2.776
7.4	2.779	2.781	2.783	2.786	2.788	2.790	2.793	2.795	2.798	2.800
7.5	2.802	2.805	2.807	2.809	2.812	2.814	2.816	2.819	2.821	2.823
7.6	2.826	2.828	2.830	2.833	2.835	2.837	2.840	2.842	2.844	2.847
7.7	2.849	2.851	2.854	2.856	2.858	2.860	2.863	2.865	2.868	2.870
7.8	2.873	2.875	2.877	2.879	2.881	2.884	2.887	2.889	2.891	2.893
7.9	2.895	2.898	2.900	2.902	2.905	2.907	2.909	2.911	2.913	2.915
8.0	2.918	2.920	2.922	2.924	2.926	2.928	2.931	2.933	2.935	2.937
8.1	2.939	2.942	2.944	2.946	2.948	2.950	2.952	2.955	2.957	2.959
8.2	2.961	2.963	2.966	2.968	2.970	2.972	2.974	2.976	2.979	2.981
8.3	2.983	2.985	2.987	2.990	2.992	2.994	2.996	2.998	3.000	3.002
8.4	3.004	3.006	3.008	3.010	3.012	3.015	3.017	3.019	3.021	3.023
8.5	3.025	3.027	3.029	3.031	3.033	3.035	3.037	3.040	3.042	3.044
8.6	3.046	3.048	3.050	3.052	3.054	3.056	3.058	3.060	3.062	3.064
8.7	3.067	3.069	3.071	3.073	3.075	3.077	3.079	3.081	3.083	3.085
8.8	3.087	3.089	3.092	3.094	3.096	3.098	3.100	3.102	3.104	3.106
8.9	3.108	3.110	3.112	3.114	3.116	3.118	3.120	3.122	3.124	3.126
9.0	3.128	3.130	3.132	3.134	3.136	3.138	3.140	3.142	3.144	3.146
9.1	3.148	3.150	3.152	3.154	3.156	3.158	3.160	3.162	3.164	3.166
9.2	3.168	3.170	3.172	3.174	3.176	3.178	3.180	3.182	3.184	3.186
9.3	3.188	3.190	3.192	3.194	3.196	3.198	3.200	3.202	3.204	3.206
9.4	3.208	3.210	3.212	3.214	3.215	3.217	3.219	3.221	3.223	3.225
9.5	3.227	3.229	3.231	3.233	3.235	3.237	3.239	3.241	3.242	3.244
9.6	3.246	3.248	3.250	3.252	3.254	3.256	3.258	3.260	3.262	3.264
9.7	3.266	3.268	3.269	3.271	3.273	3.275	3.277	3.279	3.281	3.283
9.8	3.285	3.287	3.289	3.291	3.293	3.295	3.297	3.298	3.300	3.302
9.9	3.304	3.305	3.307	3.309	3.311	3.313	3.316	3.318	3.320	3.321

Intrinsic viscosity $[\eta]_c$ at different values of relative viscosity η_{rel}

	$[\eta]_c$									
η_{rel}	0.0	0.1	0.2	0.3	0.4	0.5	0.6	0.7	0.8	0.9
10	3.32	3.34	3.36	3.37	3.39	3.41	3.43	3.45	3.46	3.48
11	3.50	3.52	3.53	3.55	3.56	3.58	3.60	3.61	3.63	3.64
12	3.66	3.68	3.69	3.71	3.72	3.74	3.76	3.77	3.79	3.80
13	3.80	3.83	3.85	3.86	3.88	3.89	3.90	3.92	3.93	3.95
14	3.96	3.97	3.99	4.00	4.02	4.03	4.04	4.06	4.07	4.09
15	4.10	4.11	4.13	4.14	4.15	4.17	4.18	4.19	4.20	4.22
16	4.23	4.24	4.25	4.27	4.28	4.29	4.30	4.31	4.33	4.34
17	4.35	4.36	4.37	4.38	4.39	4.41	4.42	4.43	4.44	4.45
18	4.46	4.47	4.48	4.49	4.50	4.52	4.53	4.54	4.55	4.56
19	4.57	4.58	4.59	4.60	4.61	4.62	4.63	4.64	4.65	4.66

TESTS

Solubility. Dissolve 50 mg in 10 ml of *ammoniacal solution of copper tetrammine R*. It dissolves completely, leaving no residue.

pH (*2.2.3*): 5.0 to 7.5 for the supernatant liquid.

Mix 10 g with 90 ml of *carbon dioxide-free water R* and allow to stand with occasional stirring for 1 h.

Ether-soluble substances: maximum 0.15 per cent (15 mg) for the difference between the weight of the residue and the weight obtained from a blank determination.

Place 10.0 g in a column about 20 mm in internal diameter and pass 50 ml of *peroxide-free ether R* through the column. Evaporate the eluate to dryness and weigh. Carry out a blank determination under the same conditions.

Water-soluble substances: maximum 1.5 per cent (75.0 mg) for the difference between the weight of the residue and the weight obtained from a blank determination.

Shake 5.0 g with 80 ml of *water R* for 10 min. Filter with the aid of vacuum into a tared flask. Evaporate to dryness on a water-bath. Dry at 100-105 °C for 1 h and weigh. Carry out a blank determination under the same conditions.

Heavy metals (*2.4.8*): maximum 10 ppm.

2.0 g complies with limit test C. Prepare the standard using 2 ml of *lead standard solution (10 ppm Pb) R*.

Loss on drying (*2.2.32*): maximum 6.5 per cent, determined on 1.000 g by drying in an oven at 100-105 °C for 3 h.

Sulphated ash (*2.4.14*): maximum 0.3 per cent, determined on 1.0 g.

Microbial contamination. Total viable aerobic count (*2.6.12*) not more than 10^3 micro-organisms per gram and with a limit for fungi of 10^2 per gram, determined by plate count. It complies with the tests for *Escherichia coli*, for *Pseudomonas aeruginosa*, for *Staphylococcus aureus* and for *Salmonella* (*2.6.13*).

01/2005:1301

CENTAURY

Centaurii herba

DEFINITION

Centaury consists of the whole or cut dried flowering aerial parts of *Centaurium erythraea* Rafn (*C. minus* Moench, *C. umbellatum* Gilib., *Erythraea centaurium* (L.) Pers.).

CHARACTERS

Centaury has a very bitter taste.

It has the macroscopic and microscopic characters described under identification tests A and B.

IDENTIFICATION

A. The hollow cylindrical, light green to dark brown stem has longitudinal ridges, and is branched only in its upper part. The sessile leaves are entire, decussately arranged, and have an ovate to lanceolate lamina, up to about 3 cm long. Both surfaces are glabrous and green to brownish-green. The inflorescence is diaxially branched. The tubular calyx is green and has five lanceolate, acuminate teeth. The corolla consists of a whitish tube divided in five elongated lanceolate pink lobes, about 5 mm to 8 mm long. Five stamens are present attached to the top of the corolla tube. The ovary is superior and has a short style, a broad bifid stigma and numerous ovules. Cylindrical capsules, about 7 mm to 10 mm long, with small brown markedly rough seeds are frequently present.

B. Reduce to a powder (355). The powder is greenish-yellow to brownish. Examine under a microscope, using *chloral hydrate solution R*. The powder shows numerous fragments of stem containing sclerenchymatous fibres and narrow vessels with bordered pits or spiral of reticulate thickening, as well as rectangular pitted cells of the pith and medullary rays; fragments of leaves with sinuous epidermal cells and striated cuticle, especially over the margins and surrounding the stomata, anisocytic stomata (*2.8.3*) and cells of the mesophyll with crystals of calcium oxalate of various types; fragments of calyx and corolla, those of the calyx with straight-walled epidermal cells, epidermis of the corolla with obtuse papillae and radially striated cuticle; parts of the endothecium with reticulate or ridge-shaped wall thickenings; triangularly rounded to elliptical, yellow pollen grains, about 30 µm in diameter, with a finely grained exine and three germinal pores; fragments of the wall of the fruit capsule composed of crossed layers of fusiform cells; small yellowish-brown seeds with a raised reticulate, dark brown structure formed by the coarse lateral walls of their epidermis.

C. Examine by thin-layer chromatography (*2.2.27*), using a *TLC silica gel F_{254} plate R*.

Test solution. To 1.0 g of the powdered drug (355) add 20 ml of *methanol R* and heat under a reflux condenser for 10 min. Cool and filter.

Reference solution. Dissolve 10 mg of *rutin R* in 10 ml of *methanol R*.

Apply to the plate as bands 30 µl of the test solution and 10 µl of the reference solution. Develop over a path of 12 cm using a mixture of 16 volumes of *anhydrous acetic acid R*, 16 volumes of *water R* and 68 volumes of *ethyl acetate R*. Allow the plate to dry in a current of cold air and develop again in the same manner. Allow the plate to dry in a current of cold air. Examine the plate in ultraviolet light at 254 nm. The chromatogram obtained with the test solution shows as the main quenching zone a strong zone (swertiamarin) similar in position to the quenching zone of rutin in the chromatogram obtained with the reference solution; further weaker quenching zones may also be present. Spray the plate with *anisaldehyde solution R*. Examine in daylight whilst heating at 100 °C to 105 °C for 5 min to 10 min. The chromatogram obtained with the reference solution shows a yellowish-brown zone (rutin). The chromatogram obtained with the test solution shows: a violet-brown zone (swertiamarin); a little above this zone, a faint yellowish-brown zone; and above this a few, very faint, mostly grey zones leading to a reddish-violet zone at the solvent front. Examine the plate in ultraviolet light at 365 nm. The chromatogram obtained with the test solution shows: a strong brown to brownish-yellow fluorescent zone (swertiamarin); a little above this zone, a blue to yellowish-green fluorescent zone; and above this a few faint blue to yellow fluorescent zones, leading to a faint reddish-violet fluorescent zone at the solvent front. Below the zone due to swertiamarin occur zones of intense light green to yellowish-green fluorescence as well as a number of faint brown fluorescent zones.

TESTS

Foreign matter (*2.8.2*). Not more than 3 per cent.

Bitterness value. Not less than 2000. The bitterness value is determined by comparison with quinine hydrochloride, the bitterness value of which is set at 200 000; the bitterness value is the reciprocal of the dilution that still has a bitter taste.

Quinine hydrochloride stock solution. Dissolve 0.100 g of *quinine hydrochloride R* in *water R* and dilute to 100.0 ml with the same solvent. Dilute 1.0 ml of the solution to 100.0 ml with *water R*.

Centaury extract. To 1.0 g of powdered drug (355) add 1000 ml of boiling *water R*. Heat on a water-bath for 30 min, stirring continuously. Allow to cool and dilute to 1000 ml with *water R*. Shake vigorously and filter, discarding the first 20 ml of filtrate.

Prepare a series of dilutions by placing in the first tube 4.2 ml of quinine hydrochloride stock solution and increasing the volume by 0.2 ml in each subsequent tube to a total of 5.8 ml; dilute the contents of each tube to 10.0 ml with *water R*. Determine as follows the dilution with the lowest concentration that still has a bitter taste. Take 10.0 ml of the weakest solution into the mouth and pass it from side to side over the back of the tongue for 30 s. If the solution is not found to be bitter, spit it out and wait for 1 min. Rinse the mouth with *water R*. After 10 min, use the next dilution in order of increasing concentration.

Calculate the correction factor k from the expression:

$$\frac{5.00}{n}$$

n = number of millilitres of quinine hydrochloride stock solution in the dilution of lowest concentration that is bitter.

Dilute $10/k$ ml of the centaury extract to 20.0 ml with *water R*. 10.0 ml of this dilution has a bitter taste.

Loss on drying (*2.2.32*). Not more than 10.0 per cent, determined on 1.000 g of powdered drug (355) by drying in an oven at 100 °C to 105 °C for 2 h.

Total ash (*2.4.16*). Not more than 6.0 per cent.

STORAGE

Store protected from light.

01/2005:1498

CENTELLA

Centellae asiaticae herba

DEFINITION

Centella consists of the dried, fragmented aerial parts of *Centella asiatica* (L.) Urban. It contains not less than 6.0 per cent of total triterpenoid derivatives, expressed as asiaticoside ($C_{48}H_{78}O_{19}$; M_r 959.15), calculated with reference to the dried drug.

CHARACTERS

It has the macroscopic and microscopic characters described under identification tests A and B.

The leaves are very variable in size; the petiole is usually 5 to 10, sometimes 15, times longer than the lamina, which is 10 mm to 40 mm long and 20 mm to 40 mm, sometimes up to 70 mm, wide.

IDENTIFICATION

A. The leaves are alternate, sometimes grouped together at the nodes, reniform or orbicular or oblong-elliptic and have palmate nervation, usually with seven veins, and a crenate margin. Young leaves show a few trichomes on the lower surface while adult leaves are glabrous. The inflorescence, if present, is a single umbel which usually consists of three flowers, rarely two or four; the flowers are very small (about 2 mm) pentamerous and have an inferior ovary; the fruit, a brownish-grey, orbicular cremocarp, up to 5 mm long, is very flattened laterally and has seven to nine prominent curved ridges.

B. Reduce the drug to a powder (355). The powder is greenish-grey. Examine under a microscope using *chloral hydrate solution R*. The powder shows numerous fragments of leaf epidermis with polygonal cells having an irregularly striated cuticle, and paracytic stomata (*2.8.3*) that are more numerous in the lower epidermis; fragments of petiole epidermis with elongated cells; uniseriate, long, flexuous unicellular covering trichomes, occasionally multicellular; young leaves; spiral vessels; resiniferous canals; calcium oxalate prisms and macles up to 40 µm in diameter; bundles of narrow septate fibres from the stem; fragments of the fruit: layers of wide cells in a parquetry arrangement, annular vessels, parenchyma cells containing simple or compound starch granules.

C. Examine by thin-layer chromatography (*2.2.27*), using a *TLC silica gel G plate R*.

Test solution. To 5.0 g of the powdered drug (355) add 50 ml of *alcohol (30 per cent V/V) R*; heat to boiling under a reflux condenser and centrifuge.

Reference solution. Dissolve 5 mg of *asiaticoside R* in *methanol R* and dilute to 10 ml with the same solvent.

Apply to the plate as bands 10 µl of each solution. Develop over a path of 15 cm using a mixture of 11 volumes of *acetic acid R*, 11 volumes of *formic acid R*, 27 volumes of *water R* and 100 volumes of *ethyl acetate R*. Allow the plate to dry in air. Spray with *anisaldehyde solution R* and heat at 100 °C to 105 °C. Examine in daylight. The chromatograms obtained with the reference and the test solutions show in the lower third a greenish-blue zone (asiaticoside). The chromatogram obtained with the test solution shows also below this zone a violet zone (madecassoside); near the solvent front it shows a light blue zone (asiatic acid) and just below a pinkish-violet zone (madecassic acid); in the lower half it shows brown, grey and brownish-green zones between the starting point and the zone due to madecassoside, and other brownish-yellow or light yellow zones above the zone due to asiaticoside.

TESTS

Foreign matter (*2.8.2*). Not more than 7 per cent of which not more than 5 per cent of underground organs and not more than 2 per cent of other foreign matter.

Loss on drying (*2.2.32*). Not more than 10.0 per cent, determined on 1.000 g of the powdered drug by drying in an oven at 100 °C to 105 °C for 2 h.

Total ash (*2.4.16*). Not more than 12.0 per cent.

ASSAY

Examine by liquid chromatography (*2.2.29*).

Test solution. Place 5.0 g of the powdered drug (355) in a cellulose fingerstall in a continuous extraction apparatus (Soxhlet type). Add 100 ml of *methanol R* and heat for 8 h. Cool and dilute the extract to 100.0 ml with *methanol R*. Filter through a 0.45 µm filter. Dilute 2.0 ml of the filtrate and dilute to 20.0 ml with *methanol R*.

Reference solution. Dissolve 20.0 mg of *asiaticoside R* in *methanol R*, if necessary using sonication, and dilute to 20.0 ml with the same solvent. Dilute 2.0 ml of the solution to 100.0 ml with *methanol R*.

The chromatographic procedure may be carried out using:

– a stainless steel column 0.25 m long and 4 mm in internal diameter packed with *octadecylsilyl silica gel for chromatography R* (5 µm),

– as mobile phase at a flow rate of 1.0 ml/min:
Mobile phase A. Acetonitrile for chromatography R,
Mobile phase B. Dilute 3 ml of *phosphoric acid R* to 1000 ml with water R,

Time (min)	Mobile phase A (per cent *V/V*)	Mobile phase B (per cent *V/V*)
0 - 65	22	78
65 - 66	55	45
66 - 76	95	5
76 - 85	22	78

– as detector a spectrophotometer set at 200 nm.

Inject 20 µl of each solution.

Calculate the response factor of asiaticoside from the expression:

$$R_f = \frac{A_1 \times V_1 \times 100}{m_1 \times HPLC_P}$$

A_1 = area of the peak corresponding to asiaticoside in the chromatogram obtained with the reference solution,

V_1 = volume of the reference solution, in millilitres,

m_1 = mass of asiaticoside in the reference solution, in milligrams,

$HPLC_P$ = purity determined for asiaticoside.

Calculate the mean response factor for asiaticoside from the expression:

$$\overline{R_f} = \frac{\sum_{i=1}^{N} R_{fi}}{N}$$

$\sum_{i=1}^{N} R_{fi}$ = sum of response factors of asiaticoside for the chromatograms obtained with the reference solution,

N = number of injections of reference solution (N = 4, at least).

Calculate the percentage content of total triterpenoid derivatives, expressed as asiaticoside from the expression:

$$\frac{V}{m}\left[\frac{A + (B \times 1.017) + (C \times 0.526) + (D \times 0.509)}{\overline{R_f}}\right]$$

V = volume of the test solution, in millilitres,

m = mass of the substance to be examined in the test solution, in milligrams,

A = area of the peak corresponding to asiaticoside in the chromatogram with the test solution,

B = area of the peak corresponding to madecassoside in the chromatogram with the test solution,

C = area of the peak corresponding to madecassic acid in the chromatogram with the test solution,

D = area of the peak corresponding to asiatic acid in the chromatogram with the test solution,

$\overline{R_f}$ = mean response factor of asiaticoside.

Relative retention with reference to the solvent: madecassoside = about 5.8; asiaticoside = about 8.1; madecassic acid = about 17.6; asiatic acid = about 21.7.

STORAGE

Store protected from light.

01/2005:1084

CETIRIZINE DIHYDROCHLORIDE

Cetirizini dihydrochloridum

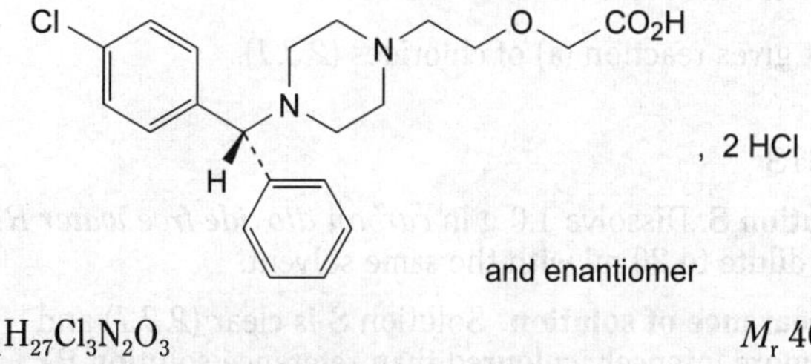

$C_{21}H_{27}Cl_3N_2O_3$ M_r 461.8

DEFINITION

(*RS*)-2-[2-[4-[(4-Chlorophenyl)phenylmethyl]piperazin-1-yl]ethoxy]acetic acid dihydrochloride.

Content: 99.0 per cent to 100.5 per cent (dried substance).

CHARACTERS

Appearance: white or almost white powder.

Solubility: freely soluble in water, practically insoluble in acetone and in methylene chloride.

IDENTIFICATION

First identification: B, D.

Second identification: A, C, D.

A. Dissolve 20.0 mg in 50 ml of a 10.3 g/l solution of *hydrochloric acid R* and dilute to 100.0 ml with the same acid. Dilute 10.0 ml of the solution to 100.0 ml with a 10.3 g/l solution of *hydrochloric acid R*. Examined between 210 nm and 350 nm (*2.2.25*), the solution shows an absorption maximum at 231 nm. The specific absorbance at the maximum is 359 to 381.

B. Infrared absorption spectrophotometry (*2.2.24*).

Preparation: discs.

Comparison: *cetirizine dihydrochloride CRS.*

C. Thin-layer chromatography (*2.2.27*).

Test solution. Dissolve 10 mg of the substance to be examined in *water R* and dilute to 5 ml with the same solvent.

Reference solution (a). Dissolve 10 mg of *cetirizine dihydrochloride CRS* in *water R* and dilute to 5 ml with the same solvent.

Reference solution (b). Dissolve 10 mg of *chlorphenamine maleate CRS* in *water R* and dilute to 5 ml with the same solvent. To 1 ml of the solution add 1 ml of reference solution (a).

Plate: *TLC silica gel GF_{254} plate R.*

Mobile phase: *ammonia R, methanol R, methylene chloride R* (1:10:90 *V/V/V*).

Application: 5 µl.

Development: over 2/3 of the plate.

Drying: in a current of cold air.

Detection: examine in ultraviolet light at 254 nm.

System suitability: reference solution (b):

– the chromatogram obtained shows 2 clearly separated spots.

Results: the principal spot in the chromatogram obtained with the test solution is similar in position and size to the principal spot in the chromatogram obtained with reference solution (a).

D. It gives reaction (a) of chlorides (*2.3.1*).

TESTS

Solution S. Dissolve 1.0 g in *carbon dioxide-free water R* and dilute to 20 ml with the same solvent.

Appearance of solution. Solution S is clear (*2.2.1*) and not more intensely coloured than reference solution BY_7 (*2.2.2, Method II*).

pH (*2.2.3*): 1.2 to 1.8 for solution S.

Related substances. Liquid chromatography (*2.2.29*).

Test solution. Dissolve 20.0 mg of the substance to be examined in the mobile phase and dilute to 100.0 ml with the mobile phase.

Reference solution (a). Dissolve 5.0 mg of *cetirizine dihydrochloride CRS* and 5.0 mg of *cetirizine impurity A CRS* in the mobile phase and dilute to 25.0 ml with the mobile phase. Dilute 1.0 ml of the solution to 100.0 ml with the mobile phase.

Reference solution (b). Dilute 2.0 ml of the test solution to 50.0 ml with the mobile phase. Dilute 5.0 ml of this solution to 100.0 ml with the mobile phase.

Column:

– *size*: *l* = 0.25 m, Ø = 4.6 mm,

– *stationary phase*: *silica gel for chromatography R* (5 µm).

Mobile phase: *dilute sulphuric acid R, water R, acetonitrile R* (0.4:6.6:93 *V/V/V*).

Flow rate: 1 ml/min.

Detection: spectrophotometer at 230 nm.

Injection: 20 µl.

Run time: 3 times the retention time of cetirizine.

System suitability: reference solution (a):

– *resolution*: minimum 3 between the peaks due to cetirizine and impurity A,

– *symmetry factors*: maximum 2.0.

Limits:

– *impurities A, B, C, D, E, F*: for each impurity, not more than 0.5 times the area of the principal peak in the chromatogram obtained with reference solution (b) (0.1 per cent),

– *any other impurity*: for each impurity, not more than 0.5 times the area of the principal peak in the chromatogram obtained with reference solution (b) (0.1 per cent),

– *total*: not more than 1.5 times the area of the principal peak in the chromatogram obtained with reference solution (b) (0.3 per cent),

– *disregard limit*: 0.1 times the area of the principal peak in the chromatogram obtained with reference solution (b) (0.02 per cent).

Loss on drying (*2.2.32*): maximum 0.5 per cent, determined on 1.000 g by drying in an oven at 100-105 °C.

Sulphated ash (*2.4.14*): maximum 0.2 per cent, determined on 1.0 g.

ASSAY

Dissolve 0.100 g in 70 ml of a mixture of 30 volumes of *water R* and 70 volumes of *acetone R*. Titrate with *0.1 M sodium hydroxide* to the second point of inflexion. Determine the end-point potentiometrically (*2.2.20*). Carry out a blank titration.

1 ml of *0.1 M sodium hydroxide* is equivalent to 15.39 mg of $C_{21}H_{27}Cl_3N_2O_3$.

STORAGE

Protected from light.

IMPURITIES

Specified impurities: A, B, C, D, E, F.

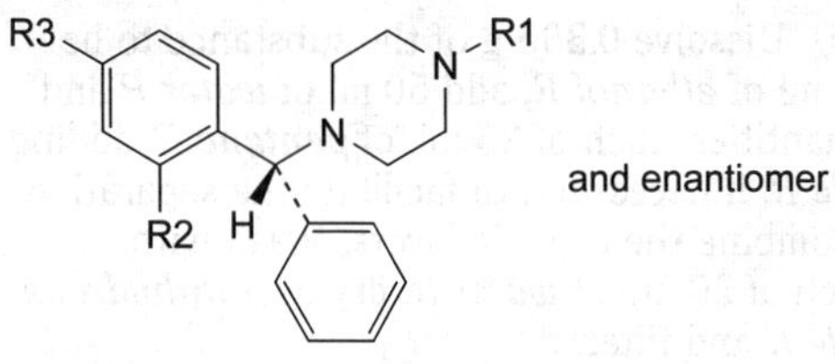

A. R1 = R2 = H, R3 = Cl: (*RS*)-1-[(4-chlorophenyl)phenylmethyl]piperazine,

B. R1 = CH_2-CO_2H, R2 = H, R3 = Cl: (*RS*)-2-[4-[(4-chlorophenyl)phenylmethyl]piperazin-1-yl]acetic acid,

C. R1 = CH_2-CH_2-O-CH_2-CO_2H, R2 = Cl, R3 = H: (*RS*)-2-[2-[4-[(2-chlorophenyl)phenylmethyl]piperazin-1-yl]ethoxy]acetic acid,

E. R1 = CH_2-[CH_2-O-CH_2]$_2$-CO_2H, R2 = H, R3 = Cl: (*RS*)-2-[2-[2-[4-[(4-chlorophenyl)phenylmethyl]piperazin-1-yl]ethoxy]ethoxy]acetic acid (ethoxycetirizine),

F. R1 = CH_2-CH_2-O-CH_2-CO_2H, R2 = R3 = H: [2-[4-(diphenylmethyl)piperazin-1-yl]ethoxy]acetic acid,

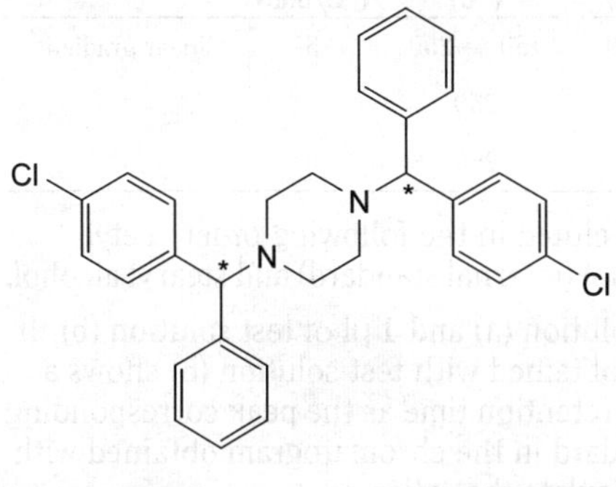

D. 1,4-bis[(4-chlorophenyl)phenylmethyl]piperazine.

01/2005:0702

CETOSTEARYL ALCOHOL

Alcohol cetylicus et stearylicus

DEFINITION

Cetostearyl alcohol is a mixture of solid aliphatic alcohols. It contains not less than 40.0 per cent of stearyl alcohol ($C_{18}H_{38}O$; M_r 270.5) and the sum of the contents of cetyl alcohol ($C_{16}H_{34}O$; M_r 242.4) and of stearyl alcohol is not less than 90.0 per cent.

CHARACTERS

White or pale yellow, wax-like mass, plates, flakes or granules, practically insoluble in water, soluble in alcohol (90 per cent *V/V*) and in light petroleum; when melted, it is miscible with fatty oils, with liquid paraffin and with melted wool fat.

IDENTIFICATION

Examine the chromatograms obtained in the assay. The 2 principal peaks in the chromatogram obtained with the test solution have similar retention times to the principal peaks in the chromatograms obtained with reference solution (a) and reference solution (b), respectively.

TESTS

Appearance of solution. Dissolve 0.50 g in 20 ml of boiling *alcohol R*. The solution is clear (*2.2.1*) and not more intensely coloured than reference solution B_6 (*2.2.2, Method II*).

Melting point (*2.2.14*): 49 °C to 56 °C.

Acid value (*2.5.1*). Not more than 1.0.

Hydroxyl value (*2.5.3, Method A*): 208 to 228.

Iodine value (*2.5.4*). Not more than 2.0, determined on 2.00 g, dissolved in 25 ml of *chloroform R*.

Saponification value (*2.5.6*). Not more than 2.0.

ASSAY

Examine by gas chromatography (*2.2.28*).

Test solution. Dissolve 0.100 g of the substance to be examined in *ethanol R* and dilute to 10.0 ml with the same solvent.

Reference solution (a). Dissolve 60.0 mg of *cetyl alcohol CRS* in *ethanol R* and dilute to 10.0 ml with the same solvent.

Reference solution (b) Dissolve 40.0 mg of *stearyl alcohol CRS* in *ethanol R* and dilute to 10.0 ml with the same solvent.

Reference solution (c). Mix 1 ml of reference solution (a) and 1 ml of reference solution (b) and dilute to 10.0 ml with *ethanol R*.

The chromatographic procedure may be carried out using:

- a stainless steel column 3 m long and 4 mm in internal diameter packed with *diatomaceous earth for gas chromatography R* impregnated with 10 per cent *m/m* of *poly(dimethyl)siloxane R*,
- *nitrogen for chromatography R* as the carrier gas at a flow rate of 30 ml/min,
- a flame-ionisation detector,

maintaining the temperature of the column at 200 °C and that of the injection port and the detector at 250 °C.

Inject separately 2 µl of each solution. Adjust the flow rate so that the resolution between the 2 principal peaks in the chromatogram obtained with the test solution is not less than 1.25. The test is not valid unless the chromatogram obtained with reference solution (c) shows 2 principal peaks with a signal-to-noise ratio of at least 5. Determine the content of cetyl alcohol and of stearyl alcohol from the chromatogram obtained with the test solution, using the normalisation procedure and identifying the peaks by comparison with the chromatograms obtained with reference solution (a) and reference solution (b), respectively.

01/2005:0801

CETOSTEARYL ALCOHOL (TYPE A), EMULSIFYING

Alcohol cetylicus et stearylicus emulsificans A

DEFINITION

Emulsifying cetostearyl alcohol (type A) is a mixture which contains not less than 80.0 per cent of cetostearyl alcohol and not less than 7.0 per cent of sodium cetostearyl sulphate, both calculated with reference to the anhydrous substance. A suitable buffer may be added.

CHARACTERS

White or pale yellow, wax-like mass, plates, flakes or granules, soluble in hot water giving an opalescent solution, practically insoluble in cold water, slightly soluble in alcohol.

IDENTIFICATION

First identification: B, C, D.

Second identification: A, C.

A. Examine by thin-layer chromatography (*2.2.27*), using a *TLC silanised silica gel plate R*.

Test solution (a). Dissolve 0.1 g of the substance to be examined in 10 ml of *trimethylpentane R*, heating on a water-bath. Shake with 2 ml of *alcohol (70 per cent V/V) R* and allow to separate. Use the lower layer as test solution (b). Dilute 1 ml of the upper layer to 8 ml with *trimethylpentane R*.

Test solution (b). Use the lower layer obtained in the preparation of test solution (a).

Reference solution (a). Dissolve 40 mg of *cetostearyl alcohol R* in 10 ml of *trimethylpentane R*.

Reference solution (b). Dissolve 20 mg of *sodium cetostearyl sulphate R* in 10 ml of *alcohol (70 per cent V/V) R*, heating on a water-bath.

Apply to the plate 2 µl of each solution. Develop over a path of 12 cm using a mixture of 20 volumes of *water R*, 40 volumes of *acetone R* and 40 volumes of *methanol R*. Allow the plate to dry in air and spray with a 50 g/l solution of *phosphomolybdic acid R* in *alcohol R*. Heat at 120 °C until spots appear (about 3 h). The 2 principal spots in the chromatogram obtained with test solution (a) are similar in position and colour to the principal spots in the chromatogram obtained with reference solution (a). 2 of the spots in the chromatogram obtained with test solution (b) are similar in position and colour to the principal spots in the chromatogram obtained with reference solution (b).

B. Examine the chromatograms obtained in the assay. The retention times of the 2 principal peaks in the chromatogram obtained with test solution (b) are similar to those of the 2 principal peaks in the chromatogram obtained with the reference solution.

C. It gives a yellow colour to a non-luminous flame.

D. To 0.3 g add 20 ml of *ethanol R* and heat on a water-bath with shaking. Filter the mixture immediately, evaporate to dryness and take up the residue in 7 ml of *water R*. To 1 ml of the solution add 0.1 ml of a 1 g/l solution of *methylene blue R*, 2 ml of *dilute sulphuric acid R* and 2 ml of *methylene chloride R* and shake. A blue colour develops in the lower layer.

TESTS

Acid value (*2.5.1*). Not more than 2.0.

Iodine value (*2.5.4*). Not more than 3.0, determined on 2.00 g dissolved in 25 ml of *methylene chloride R*.

Saponification value (*2.5.6*). Not more than 2.0.

Water (*2.5.12*). Not more than 3.0 per cent, determined on 2.50 g by the semi-micro determination of water.

ASSAY

Cetostearyl alcohol. Examine by gas chromatography (*2.2.28*).

Internal standard solution. Dissolve 0.60 g of *heptadecanol CRS* in *ethanol R* and dilute to 150 ml with the same solvent.

Test solution (a). Dissolve 0.300 g of the substance to be examined in 50 ml of the internal standard solution, add 50 ml of *water R* and shake with 4 quantities, each of 25 ml, of *pentane R*, adding *sodium chloride R*, if necessary, to facilitate the separation of the layers. Combine the organic layers. Wash with 2 quantities, each of 30 ml, of *water R*, dry over *anhydrous sodium sulphate R* and filter.

Test solution (b). Dissolve 0.300 g of the substance to be examined in 50 ml of *ethanol R*, add 50 ml of *water R* and shake with 4 quantities, each of 25 ml, of *pentane R*, adding *sodium chloride R*, if necessary, to facilitate the separation of the layers. Combine the organic layers. Wash with 2 quantities, each of 30 ml, of *water R*, dry over *anhydrous sodium sulphate R* and filter.

Reference solution. Dissolve 50 mg of *cetyl alcohol CRS* and 50 mg of *stearyl alcohol CRS* in *ethanol R* and dilute to 10 ml with the same solvent.

The chromatographic procedure may be carried out using:

- a fused-silica column 25 m long and 0.25 mm in internal diameter coated with *poly(dimethyl)siloxane R*,
- *nitrogen for chromatography R* as the carrier gas at a flow rate of 1 ml/min,
- a flame-ionisation detector,
- a split ratio of 1:100,

with the following temperature programme:

	Time (min)	Temperature (°C)	Rate (°C/min)	Comment
Column	0 - 20	150 → 250	5	linear gradient
Injection port		250		
Detector		250		

The substances are eluted in the following order: cetyl alcohol, heptadecanol (internal standard) and stearyl alcohol.

Inject 1 µl of test solution (a) and 1 µl of test solution (b). If the chromatogram obtained with test solution (b) shows a peak with the same retention time as the peak corresponding to the internal standard in the chromatogram obtained with test solution (a), calculate the ratio:

$$r = \frac{S_{ci}}{S_i}$$

S_{ci} = area of the peak corresponding to cetyl alcohol in the chromatogram obtained with test solution (b),

S_i = area of the peak with the same retention time as the peak corresponding to the internal standard in the chromatogram obtained with test solution (a).

If r is less than 300, calculate the corrected area $S_{Ha(corr)}$ of the peak corresponding to the internal standard in the chromatogram obtained with test solution (a):

$$S_{Ha(corr)} = S'_{Ha} - \frac{S_i \times S_c}{S_{ci}}$$

S'_{Ha} = area of the peak corresponding to the internal standard in the chromatogram obtained with test solution (a),

S_c = area of the peak corresponding to cetyl alcohol in the chromatogram obtained with test solution (a).

Inject, under the same conditions, equal volumes of the reference solution and of test solution (a). Identify the peaks in the chromatogram obtained with test solution (a) by comparing their retention times with those of the peaks in the chromatogram obtained with the reference solution and determine the area of each peak.

Calculate the percentage content of cetyl alcohol using the expression:

$$S_A \frac{100 \times m_H}{S_{Ha(coor)} \times m}$$

S_A = area of the peak corresponding to cetyl alcohol in the chromatogram obtained with test solution (a),

m_H = mass of the internal standard in test solution (a), in milligrams,

$S_{Ha(corr)}$ = corrected area of the peak corresponding to the internal standard in the chromatogram obtained with test solution (a),

m = mass of the substance to be examined in test solution (a), in milligrams.

Calculate the percentage content of stearyl alcohol using the expression:

$$S_B \frac{100 \times m_H}{S_{Ha(coor)} \times m}$$

S_B = area of the peak corresponding to stearyl alcohol in the chromatogram obtained with test solution (a).

The percentage content of cetostearyl alcohol corresponds to the sum of the percentage content of cetyl alcohol and of stearyl alcohol.

Sodium cetostearyl sulphate. Disperse 0.300 g in 25 ml of *methylene chloride R*. Add 50 ml of *water R* and 10 ml of *dimidium bromide-sulphan blue mixed solution R*. Titrate with *0.004 M benzethonium chloride*, using sonication and heating and allowing the layers to separate before each addition, until the colour of the lower layer changes from pink to grey.

1 ml of *0.004 M benzethonium chloride* is equivalent to 1.434 mg of sodium cetostearyl sulphate.

LABELLING

The label states, where applicable, the name and concentration of any added buffer.

01/2005:0802

CETOSTEARYL ALCOHOL (TYPE B), EMULSIFYING

Alcohol cetylicus et stearylicus emulsificans B

DEFINITION

Emulsifying cetostearyl alcohol (type B) is a mixture which contains not less than 80.0 per cent of cetostearyl alcohol and not less than 7.0 per cent of sodium laurilsulfate, both calculated with reference to the anhydrous substance. A suitable buffer may be added.

CHARACTERS

White or pale yellow, wax-like mass, plates, flakes or granules, soluble in hot water giving an opalescent solution, practically insoluble in cold water, slightly soluble in alcohol.

IDENTIFICATION

First identification: B, C, D.

Second identification: A, C.

A. Examine by thin-layer chromatography (*2.2.27*), using a *TLC silanised silica gel plate R*.

Test solution (a). Dissolve 0.1 g of the substance to be examined in 10 ml of *trimethylpentane R*, heating on a water-bath. Shake with 2 ml of *alcohol (70 per cent V/V) R* and allow to separate. Use the lower layer as test solution (b). Dilute 1 ml of the upper layer to 8 ml with *trimethylpentane R*.

Test solution (b). Use the lower layer obtained in the preparation of test solution (a).

Reference solution (a). Dissolve 40 mg of *cetostearyl alcohol R* in 10 ml of *trimethylpentane R*.

Reference solution (b). Dissolve 20 mg of *sodium laurilsulfate R* in 10 ml of *alcohol (70 per cent V/V) R*, heating on a water-bath.

Apply to the plate 2 µl of each solution. Develop over a path of 12 cm using a mixture of 20 volumes of *water R*, 40 volumes of *acetone R* and 40 volumes of *methanol R*. Allow the plate to dry in air and spray with a 50 g/l solution of *phosphomolybdic acid R* in *alcohol R*. Heat at 120 °C until spots appear (about 3 h). The 2 principal spots in the chromatogram obtained with test solution (a) are similar in position and colour to the principal spots in the chromatogram obtained with reference solution (a). 1 of the spots in the chromatogram obtained with test solution (b) is similar in position and colour to the principal spot in the chromatogram obtained with reference solution (b).

B. Examine the chromatograms obtained in the assay. The retention times of the 2 principal peaks in the chromatogram obtained with test solution (b) are similar to those of the 2 principal peaks in the chromatogram obtained with the reference solution.

C. It gives a yellow colour to a non-luminous flame.

D. To 0.3 g add 20 ml of *ethanol R* and heat to boiling on a water-bath with shaking. Filter the mixture immediately, evaporate to dryness and take up the residue in 7 ml of *water R*. To 1 ml of the solution add 0.1 ml of a 1 g/l solution of *methylene blue R*, 2 ml of *dilute sulphuric acid R* and 2 ml of *methylene chloride R* and shake. A blue colour develops in the lower layer.

TESTS

Acid value (*2.5.1*). Not more than 2.0.

Iodine value (*2.5.4*). Not more than 3.0, determined on 2.00 g dissolved in 25 ml of *methylene chloride R*.

Saponification value (*2.5.6*). Not more than 2.0.

Water (*2.5.12*). Not more than 3.0 per cent, determined on 2.50 g by the semi-micro determination of water.

ASSAY

Cetostearyl alcohol. Examine by gas chromatography (*2.2.28*).

Internal standard solution. Dissolve 0.60 g of *heptadecanol CRS* in *ethanol R* and dilute to 150 ml with the same solvent.

Test solution (a). Dissolve 0.300 g of the substance to be examined in 50 ml of the internal standard solution, add 50 ml of *water R* and shake with 4 quantities, each of 25 ml, of *pentane R*, adding *sodium chloride R*, if necessary, to facilitate the separation of the layers. Combine the organic layers. Wash with 2 quantities, each of 30 ml, of *water R*, dry over *anhydrous sodium sulphate R* and filter.

Test solution (b). Dissolve 0.300 g of the substance to be examined in 50 ml of *ethanol R*, add 50 ml of *water R* and shake with 4 quantities, each of 25 ml, of *pentane R*, adding *sodium chloride R*, if necessary, to facilitate the separation of the layers. Combine the organic layers. Wash with 2 quantities, each of 30 ml, of *water R*, dry over *anhydrous sodium sulphate R* and filter.

Monographs C

Reference solution. Dissolve 50 mg of *cetyl alcohol CRS* and 50 mg of *stearyl alcohol CRS* in *ethanol R* and dilute to 10 ml with the same solvent.

The chromatographic procedure may be carried out using:

- a fused-silica column 25 m long and 0.25 mm in internal diameter coated with *poly(dimethyl)siloxane R*,
- *nitrogen for chromatography R* as the carrier gas at a flow rate of 1 ml/min,
- a flame-ionisation detector,
- a split ratio of 1:100,

with the following temperature programme:

	Time (min)	Temperature (°C)	Rate (°C/min)	Comment
Column	0 - 20	150 → 250	5	linear gradient
Injection port		250		
Detector		250		

The substances are eluted in the following order: cetyl alcohol, heptadecanol (internal standard) and stearyl alcohol.

Inject 1 µl of test solution (a) and 1 µl of test solution (b). If the chromatogram obtained with test solution (b) shows a peak with the same retention time as the peak corresponding to the internal standard in the chromatogram obtained with test solution (a), calculate the ratio:

$$r = \frac{S_{ci}}{S_i}$$

S_{ci} = area of the peak corresponding to cetyl alcohol in the chromatogram obtained with test solution (b),

S_i = area of the peak with the same retention time as the peak corresponding to the internal standard in the chromatogram obtained with test solution (a).

If r is less than 300, calculate the corrected area $S_{Ha(corr)}$ of the peak corresponding to the internal standard in the chromatogram obtained with test solution (a):

$$S_{Ha(corr)} = S'_{Ha} - \frac{S_i \times S_c}{S_{ci}}$$

S'_{Ha} = area of the peak corresponding to the internal standard in the chromatogram obtained with test solution (a),

S_c = area of the peak corresponding to cetyl alcohol in the chromatogram obtained with test solution (a).

Inject, under the same conditions, equal volumes of the reference solution and of test solution (a). Identify the peaks in the chromatogram obtained with test solution (a) by comparing their retention times with those of the peaks in the chromatogram obtained with the reference solution and determine the area of each peak.

Calculate the percentage content of cetyl alcohol using the expression:

$$S_A \frac{100 \times m_H}{S_{Ha(corr)} \times m}$$

S_A = area of the peak corresponding to cetyl alcohol in the chromatogram obtained with test solution (a),

m_H = mass of the internal standard in test solution (a), in milligrams,

$S_{Ha(corr)}$ = corrected area of the peak corresponding to the internal standard in the chromatogram obtained with test solution (a),

m = mass of the substance to be examined in test solution (a), in milligrams.

Calculate the percentage content of stearyl alcohol using the expression:

$$S_B \frac{100 \times m_H}{S_{Ha(corr)} \times m}$$

S_B = area of the peak corresponding to stearyl alcohol in the chromatogram obtained with test solution (a).

The percentage content of cetostearyl alcohol corresponds to the sum of the percentage content of cetyl alcohol and of stearyl alcohol.

Sodium laurilsulfate. Disperse 0.300 g in 25 ml of *methylene chloride R*. Add 50 ml of *water R* and 10 ml of *dimidium bromide-sulphan blue mixed solution R*. Titrate with *0.004 M benzethonium chloride*, using sonication and heating, and allowing the layers to separate before each addition, until the colour of the lower layer changes from pink to grey.

1 ml of *0.004 M benzethonium chloride* is equivalent to 1.154 mg of sodium laurilsulfate.

LABELLING

The label states, where applicable, the name and concentration of any added buffer.

01/2005:1085

CETOSTEARYL ISONONANOATE

Cetostearylis isononanoas

DEFINITION

Cetostearyl isononanoate is a mixture of esters of cetostearyl alcohol with isononanoic acid, mainly 3,5,5-trimethylhexanoic acid.

CHARACTERS

A clear, colourless or slightly yellowish liquid, practically insoluble in water, soluble in alcohol and in light petroleum, miscible with fatty oils and with liquid paraffins.

It has a viscosity of 15 mPa·s to 30 mPa·s, a relative density of 0.85 to 0.86 and a refractive index of 1.44 to 1.45.

IDENTIFICATION

A. On cooling, turbidity occurs below 15 °C.

B. It complies with the test for saponification value (see Tests).

C. Examine by infrared absorption spectrophotometry (*2.2.24*), comparing with the *Ph. Eur. reference spectrum of cetostearyl isononanoate*.

TESTS

Appearance. The substance to be examined is clear (*2.2.1*) and not more intensely coloured than reference solution Y_6 (*2.2.2, Method I*).

Acid value (*2.5.1*). Not more than 1.0, determined on 5.0 g.

Hydroxyl value (*2.5.3, Method A*). Not more than 5.0.

Iodine value (*2.5.4*). Not more than 1.0.

Saponification value (*2.5.6*): 135 to 148, determined on 1.0 g.

Heavy metals (*2.4.8*). 2.0 g complies with limit test D for heavy metals (10 ppm). Prepare the standard using 2 ml of *lead standard solution (10 ppm Pb) R*.

Water (*2.5.12*). Not more than 0.2 per cent, determined on 10.0 g by the semi-micro determination of water.

Total ash (*2.4.16*). Not more than 0.2 per cent, determined on 2.0 g.

01/2005:0378

CETRIMIDE

Cetrimidum

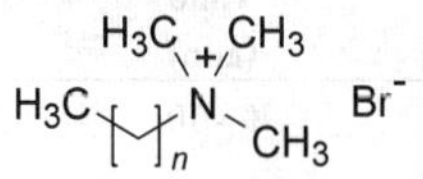

DEFINITION

Cetrimide consists of trimethyltetradecylammonium bromide and may contain smaller amounts of dodecyl- and hexadecyl-trimethylammonium bromides.

Content: 96.0 per cent to 101.0 per cent of alkyltrimethylammonium bromides, calculated as $C_{17}H_{38}BrN$ (M_r 336.4) (dried substance).

CHARACTERS

Appearance: white or almost white, voluminous, free-flowing powder.

Solubility: freely soluble in water and in alcohol.

IDENTIFICATION

A. Dissolve 0.25 g in *alcohol R* and dilute to 25.0 ml with the same solvent. At wavelengths from 260 nm to 280 nm, the absorbance (*2.2.25*) of the solution has a maximum of 0.05.

B. Dissolve about 5 mg in 5 ml of *buffer solution pH 8.0 R*. Add about 10 mg of *potassium ferricyanide R*. A yellow precipitate is formed. Prepare a blank in the same manner but omitting the substance to be examined: a yellow solution is observed but no precipitate is formed.

C. Solution S (see Tests) froths copiously when shaken.

D. Thin-layer chromatography (*2.2.27*).

Test solution. Dissolve 0.10 g of the substance to be examined in *water R* and dilute to 5 ml with the same solvent.

Reference solution. Dissolve 0.10 g of *trimethyltetradecylammonium bromide CRS* in *water R* and dilute to 5 ml with the same solvent.

Plate: *TLC silica gel F_{254} silanised plate R*.

Mobile phase: *acetone R*, 270 g/l solution of *sodium acetate R*, *methanol R* (20:35:45 *V/V/V*).

Application: 1 µl.

Development: over a path of 12 cm.

Drying: in a current of hot air.

Detection: allow to cool; expose the plate to iodine vapour and examine in daylight.

Result: the principal spot in the chromatogram obtained with the test solution is similar in position, colour and size to the principal spot in the chromatogram obtained with the reference solution.

E. It gives reaction (a) of bromides (*2.3.1*).

TESTS

Solution S. Dissolve 2.0 g in *carbon dioxide-free water R* and dilute to 100 ml with the same solvent.

Appearance of solution. Solution S is clear (*2.2.1*) and colourless (*2.2.2, Method II*).

Acidity or alkalinity. To 50 ml of solution S add 0.1 ml of *bromocresol purple solution R*. Not more than 0.1 ml of *0.1 M hydrochloric acid* or *0.1 M sodium hydroxide* is required to change the colour of the indicator.

Amines and amine salts. Dissolve 5.0 g in 30 ml of a mixture of 1 volume of *1 M hydrochloric acid* and 99 volumes of *methanol R* and add 100 ml of *2-propanol R*. Pass a stream of *nitrogen R* slowly through the solution. Gradually add 15.0 ml of *0.1 M tetrabutylammonium hydroxide* and record the potentiometric titration curve (*2.2.20*). If the curve shows 2 points of inflexion, the volume of titrant added between the 2 points is not greater than 2.0 ml.

Loss on drying (*2.2.32*): maximum 2.0 per cent, determined on 1.000 g by drying in an oven at 100-105 °C for 2 h.

Sulphated ash (*2.4.14*): maximum 0.5 per cent, determined on 1.0 g.

ASSAY

Dissolve 2.000 g in *water R* and dilute to 100.0 ml with the same solvent. Transfer 25.0 ml of the solution to a separating funnel, add 25 ml of *chloroform R*, 10 ml of *0.1 M sodium hydroxide* and 10.0 ml of a freshly prepared 50 g/l solution of *potassium iodide R*. Shake, allow to separate and discard the chloroform layer. Shake the aqueous layer with 3 quantities, each of 10 ml, of *chloroform R* and discard the chloroform layers. Add 40 ml of *hydrochloric acid R*, allow to cool and titrate with *0.05 M potassium iodate* until the deep brown colour is almost discharged. Add 2 ml of *chloroform R* and continue the titration, shaking vigorously, until the colour of the chloroform layer no longer changes. Carry out a blank titration on a mixture of 10.0 ml of the freshly prepared 50 g/l solution of *potassium iodide R*, 20 ml of *water R* and 40 ml of *hydrochloric acid R*.

1 ml of *0.05 M potassium iodate* is equivalent to 33.64 mg of $C_{17}H_{38}BrN$.

01/2005:0540

CETYL ALCOHOL

Alcohol cetylicus

DEFINITION

Cetyl alcohol is a mixture of solid alcohols consisting mainly of hexadecanol (CH_3-$(CH_2)_{14}$-CH_2OH; M_r 242.4).

CHARACTERS

White, unctuous mass, powder, flakes or granules, practically insoluble in water, freely to sparingly soluble in alcohol; when melted, it is miscible with vegetable and animal oils, with liquid paraffin and with melted wool fat.

IDENTIFICATION

A. Melting point (*2.2.14*): 46 °C to 52 °C.

B. Hydroxyl value (*2.5.3, Method A*): 218 to 238.

TESTS

Appearance of solution. Dissolve 0.5 g in boiling *alcohol R*, allow to cool and dilute to 20 ml with the same solvent. The solution is clear (*2.2.1*) and not more intensely coloured than reference solution B_6 (*2.2.2, Method II*).

Acid value (*2.5.1*). Not more than 1.0.

Iodine value (*2.5.4*). Not more than 2.0, determined on 2.00 g dissolved in 25 ml of *chloroform R*.

Saponification value (*2.5.6*). Not more than 2.0.

01/2005:1906

CETYL PALMITATE

Cetylis palmitas

DEFINITION

Mixture of C_{14}-C_{18} esters of lauric, myristic, palmitic and stearic acids ("Cetyl esters wax").

Content (expressed as hexadecyl hexadecanoate): 10.0 per cent to 20.0 per cent for Cetyl palmitate 15, 60.0 per cent to 70.0 per cent for Cetyl palmitate 65 and not less than 90.0 per cent for Cetyl palmitate 95.

CHARACTERS

Appearance: white, waxy plates, flakes or powder.

Solubility: practically insoluble in water, soluble in boiling ethanol and in methylene chloride, slightly soluble in light petroleum, practically insoluble in ethanol.

mp: about 45 °C for Cetyl palmitate 15 and Cetyl palmitate 65 and about 52 °C for Cetyl palmitate 95.

IDENTIFICATION

A. It complies with the limits of the assay and the chromatogram obtained with the test solution shows the typical main peak(s).

B. It complies with the test for saponification value (see Tests).

TESTS

Appearance of solution. The solution is not more intensely coloured than reference solution Y_6 (*2.2.2, Method II*).

Dissolve 4.0 g in *methylene chloride R* and dilute to 20 ml with the same solvent.

Acid value (*2.5.1*): maximum 4.0.

Dissolve 10.0 g in 50 ml of the solvent mixture described by heating under reflux on a water-bath for 5 min.

Hydroxyl value (*2.5.3, Method A*): maximum 20.0.

Iodine value (*2.5.4*): maximum 2.0.

Saponification value (*2.5.6*): 105 to 120.

Heat under reflux for 2 h.

Alkaline impurities. Dissolve with gentle heating 2.0 g in a mixture of 1.5 ml of *alcohol R* and 3 ml of *toluene R*. Add 0.05 ml of a 0.4 g/l solution of *bromophenol blue R* in *alcohol R*. Not more than 0.4 ml of *0.01 M hydrochloric acid* is required to change the colour of the solution to yellow.

Nickel (*2.4.27*): maximum 1 ppm.

Water (*2.5.12*): maximum 0.3 per cent, determined on 1.0 g using a mixture of equal volumes of *anhydrous methanol R* and *methylene chloride R* as solvent.

Total ash (*2.4.16*): maximum 0.2 per cent, determined on 1.0 g.

ASSAY

Gas chromatography (*2.2.28*): use the normalisation procedure.

Test solution. Dissolve 20.0 mg of the substance to be examined in *hexane R* and dilute to 20.0 ml with the same solvent.

Reference solution (a). Dissolve 20.0 mg of *cetyl palmitate 95 CRS* in *hexane R* and dilute to 20.0 ml with the same solvent.

Reference solution (b). Dissolve 20.0 mg of *cetyl palmitate 15 CRS* in *hexane R* and dilute to 20.0 ml with the same solvent.

Column:

- *material*: stainless steel,
- *size*: l = 10 m, Ø = 0.53 mm,
- *stationary phase*: *poly(dimethyl)siloxane R* (film thickness: 2.65 μm).

Carrier gas: *helium for chromatography R*.

Flow rate: 6.5 ml/min.

Split ratio: 1:10.

Temperature:

	Time (min)	Temperature (°C)
Column	0 - 10	100 → 300
	10 - 15	300
Injection port		350
Detector		350

Detection: flame ionisation.

Injection: 1 μl.

Relative retention with reference to cetyl palmitate (retention time = about 9 min): cetyl alcohol = about 0.3; palmitic acid = about 0.4; lauric ester = about 0.8; myristic ester = about 0.9; stearic ester = about 1.1.

System suitability: reference solution (b):

- *resolution*: minimum of 1.5 between the peaks due to cetyl palmitate and cetyl stearate.

STORAGE

At a temperature not exceeding 25 °C.

LABELLING

The label states the type of cetyl palmitate.

01/2005:0379

CETYLPYRIDINIUM CHLORIDE

Cetylpyridinii chloridum

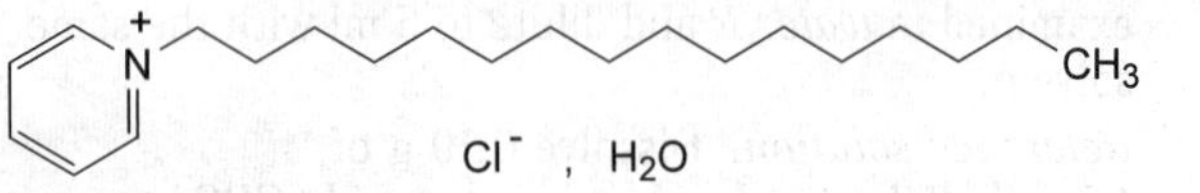

$C_{21}H_{38}ClN,H_2O$ M_r 358.0

DEFINITION

Cetylpyridinium chloride contains not less than 96.0 per cent and not more than the equivalent of 101.0 per cent of 1-hexadecylpyridinium chloride, calculated with reference to the anhydrous substance.

CHARACTERS

A white powder, slightly soapy to the touch, soluble in water and in alcohol. An aqueous solution froths copiously when shaken.

IDENTIFICATION

First identification: B, D.

Second identification: A, C, D.

A. Dissolve 0.10 g in *water R* and dilute to 100.0 ml with the same solvent. Dilute 5.0 ml of this solution to 100.0 ml with *water R*. Examined between 240 nm and 300 nm (*2.2.25*), the solution shows an absorption maximum at 259 nm and 2 shoulders at about 254 nm and at about 265 nm. The specific absorbance at the maximum is 126 to 134, calculated with reference to the anhydrous substance.

B. Examine by infrared absorption spectrophotometry (*2.2.24*), comparing with the spectrum obtained with *cetylpyridinium chloride CRS*. Examine the substances in the solid state.

C. To 5 ml of *dilute sodium hydroxide solution R* add 0.1 ml of *bromophenol blue solution R1* and 5 ml of *chloroform R* and shake. The chloroform layer is colourless. Add 0.1 ml of solution S (see Tests) and shake. The chloroform layer becomes blue.

D. Solution S gives reaction (a) of chlorides (*2.3.1*).

TESTS

Solution S. Dissolve 1.0 g in *carbon dioxide-free water R* and dilute to 100 ml with the same solvent.

Appearance of solution. Solution S is not more opalescent than reference suspension II (*2.2.1*) and is colourless (*2.2.2, Method II*).

Acidity. To 50 ml of solution S add 0.1 ml of *phenolphthalein solution R*. Not more than 2.5 ml of *0.02 M sodium hydroxide* is required to change the colour of the indicator.

Amines and amine salts. Dissolve 5.0 g with heating in 20 ml of a mixture of 3 volumes of *1 M hydrochloric acid* and 97 volumes of *methanol R* and add 100 ml of *2-propanol R*. Pass a stream of *nitrogen R* slowly through the solution. Gradually add 12.0 ml of *0.1 M tetrabutylammonium hydroxide* and record the potentiometric titration curve (*2.2.20*). If the curve shows 2 points of inflexion, the volume of titrant added between the two points is not greater than 5.0 ml. If the curve shows no point of inflexion, the substance to be examined does not comply with the test. If the curve shows one point of inflexion, repeat the test but add 3.0 ml of a 25.0 g/l solution of *dimethyldecylamine R* in *2-propanol R* before the titration. If the titration curve after the addition of 12.0 ml of the titrant shows only one point of inflexion, the substance to be examined does not comply with the test.

Water (*2.5.12*): 4.5 per cent to 5.5 per cent, determined on 0.300 g by the semi-micro determination of water.

Sulphated ash (*2.4.14*). Not more than 0.2 per cent, determined on 1.0 g.

ASSAY

Dissolve 2.00 g in *water R* and dilute to 100.0 ml with the same solvent. Transfer 25.0 ml of the solution to a separating funnel, add 25 ml of *chloroform R*, 10 ml of *0.1 M sodium hydroxide* and 10.0 ml of a freshly prepared 50 g/l solution of *potassium iodide R*. Shake well, allow to separate and discard the chloroform layer. Shake the aqueous layer with three quantities, each of 10 ml, of *chloroform R* and discard the chloroform layers. To the aqueous layer add 40 ml of *hydrochloric acid R*, allow to cool and titrate with *0.05 M potassium iodate* until the deep-brown colour is almost discharged. Add 2 ml of *chloroform R* and continue the titration, shaking vigorously, until the chloroform layer no longer changes colour. Carry out a blank titration on a mixture of 10.0 ml of the freshly prepared 50 g/l solution of *potassium iodide R*, 20 ml of *water R* and 40 ml of *hydrochloric acid R*.

1 ml of *0.05 M potassium iodate* is equivalent to 34.0 mg of $C_{21}H_{38}ClN$.

01/2005:0380

CHAMOMILE FLOWER, ROMAN

Chamomillae romanae flos

DEFINITION

Roman chamomile flower consists of the dried flower-heads of the cultivated double variety of *Chamaemelum nobile* (L.) All. (*Anthemis nobilis* L.). It contains not less than 7 ml/kg of essential oil.

CHARACTERS

It consists of flower-heads with a white to yellowish-grey colour, being composed of solitary hemispherical capitula, made up of a solid conical receptacle bearing the florets, each subtended by a transparent small palea.

It has a strong and characteristic odour.

It has the macroscopic and microscopic characters described under identification tests A and B.

IDENTIFICATION

A. The capitula have a diameter of 8 mm to 20 mm; the receptacle is solid; the base of the receptacle is surrounded by an involucre consisting of 2 or 3 rows of compact and imbricated bracts with scarious margins. Most florets are ligulate, but a few pale yellow tubular florets occur in the central region. Ligulate florets are white, dull, lanceolate and reflexed with a dark brown, inferior ovary, a filiform style and a bifid stigma; tubular florets have a five-toothed corolla tube, 5 syngenesious, epipetalous stamens and a gynoecium similar to that of the ligulate florets.

B. Separate the capitulum into its different parts. Examine under a microscope using *chloral hydrate solution R*. All parts of the flower-heads are covered with numerous small yellow glistening glandular trichomes. The involucral bracts and paleae have epidermal cells in longitudal rows, sclerified at the base and they are covered with conical trichomes, about 500 µm long, each composed of 3 or 4 very short base cells and a long, bent, terminal cell about 20 µm wide. The corolla of the ligulate flowers consists of papillary cells with cuticular striations. The ovaries of both kinds of florets have at their base a sclerous ring consisting of a single row of cells. The receptacle and the ovaries contain small clusters of calcium oxalate. The pollen grains have a diameter of about 35 µm and are rounded and triangular with 3 germinal pores and a spiny exine.

C. Examine by thin-layer chromatography (*2.2.27*), using a suitable silica gel as the coating substance.

Test solution. To 0.5 g of the powdered drug (710) add 10 ml of *methanol R* and heat with shaking in a water-bath at 60 °C for 5 min. Allow to cool and filter.

Reference solution. Dissolve 2.5 mg of *apigenin R* and 2.5 mg of *apigenin-7-glucoside R* in 10 ml of *methanol R*.

Apply to the plate as bands 10 µl of each solution. Develop over a path of 10 cm using a mixture of 17 volumes of *glacial acetic acid R*, 17 volumes of *water R* and 66 volumes of *butanol R*. Dry the plate at 100-105 °C for 5 min and spray the warm plate with a 10 g/l solution of *diphenylboric acid aminoethyl ester R* in *methanol R*, using about 10 ml for a plate 200 mm square. Spray the plate with the same volume of a 50 g/l solution of *macrogol 400 R* in *methanol R*. Allow to stand for about

30 min and examine in ultraviolet light at 365 nm. The chromatogram obtained with the reference solution shows in the upper third a zone of yellowish-green fluorescence (apigenin) and in the middle third a zone of yellowish fluorescence (apigenin-7-glucoside). The chromatogram obtained with the test solution shows a zone of yellowish-green fluorescence corresponding in position and fluorescence to the zone due to apigenin and a zone of yellowish fluorescence corresponding in position and fluorescence to the zone due to apigenin-7-glucoside in the chromatogram obtained with the reference solution; above the apigenin-7-glucoside zone there is a zone of brownish fluorescence (luteolin); immediately below the apigenin-7-glucoside zone there is a zone of light brownish fluorescence (apiin); immediately below the apiin zone there is a zone of bright blue fluorescence and below this zone a zone of bright blue fluorescence; other faint zones may be present.

Monographs C

TESTS

Diameter of the flower-heads. Not more than 3 per cent of flower-heads have a diameter smaller than 8 mm.

Deteriorated flower-heads. Brown or darkened flower-heads are absent.

Loss on drying (*2.2.32*): maximum 11.0 per cent, determined on 1.000 g of the powdered drug (355) by drying in an oven at 100-105 °C for 2 h.

Total ash (*2.4.16*). Not more than 8.0 per cent.

ASSAY

Carry out the determination of essential oils in vegetable drugs (*2.8.12*). Use 20.0 g of whole drug, a 500 ml round-bottomed flask, 250 ml of *water R* as the distillation liquid and 0.50 ml of *xylene R* in the graduated tube. Distil at a rate of 3-3.5 ml/min for 3 h.

STORAGE

Store protected from light.

01/2005:0313

CHARCOAL, ACTIVATED

Carbo activatus

DEFINITION

Activated charcoal is obtained from vegetable matter by suitable carbonisation processes intended to confer a high adsorption power.

CHARACTERS

A black, light powder free from grittiness, practically insoluble in all usual solvents.

IDENTIFICATION

A. When heated to redness it burns slowly without a flame.

B. It complies with the test for adsorption power (see Tests).

TESTS

Solution S. To 2.0 g in a conical flask with a ground-glass neck add 50 ml of *dilute hydrochloric acid R*. Boil gently under a reflux condenser for 1 h, filter and wash the filter with *dilute hydrochloric acid R*. Evaporate the combined filtrate and washings to dryness on a water-bath, dissolve the residue in *0.1 M hydrochloric acid* and dilute to 50.0 ml with the same acid.

Acidity or alkalinity. To 2.0 g add 40 ml of *water R* and boil for 5 min. Cool, restore to the original mass with *carbon dioxide-free water R* and filter. Reject the first 20 ml of the filtrate. To 10 ml of the filtrate add 0.25 ml of *bromothymol blue solution R1* and 0.25 ml of *0.02 M sodium hydroxide*. The solution is blue. Not more than 0.75 ml of *0.02 M hydrochloric acid* is required to change the colour of the indicator to yellow.

Acid-soluble substances. To 1.0 g add 25 ml of *dilute nitric acid R* and boil for 5 min. Filter whilst hot through a sintered-glass filter (10) and wash with 10 ml of hot *water R*. Evaporate the combined filtrate and washings to dryness on a water-bath, add to the residue 1 ml of *hydrochloric acid R*, evaporate to dryness again and dry the residue to constant mass at 100 °C to 105 °C. The residue weighs not more than 30 mg (3 per cent).

Alkali-soluble coloured substances. To 0.25 g add 10 ml of *dilute sodium hydroxide solution R* and boil for 1 min. Cool, filter and dilute the filtrate to 10 ml with *water R*. The solution is not more intensely coloured than reference solution GY_4 (*2.2.2, Method II*).

Alcohol-soluble substances. To 2.0 g add 50 ml of *alcohol R* and boil under a reflux condenser for 10 min. Filter immediately, cool, and dilute to 50 ml with *alcohol R*. The filtrate is not more intensely coloured than reference solution Y_6 or BY_6 (*2.2.2, Method II*). Evaporate 40 ml of the filtrate to dryness and dry to constant mass at 100 °C to 105 °C. The residue weighs not more than 8 mg (0.5 per cent).

Fluorescent substances. In an intermittent-extraction apparatus, treat 10.0 g with 100 ml of *cyclohexane R1* for 2 h. Collect the liquid and dilute to 100 ml with *cyclohexane R1*. Examine in ultraviolet light at 365 nm. The fluorescence of the solution is not more intense than that of a solution of 83 µg of *quinine R* in 1000 ml of *0.005 M sulphuric acid* examined in the same manner.

Sulphides. To 1.0 g in a conical flask add 5 ml of *hydrochloric acid R1* and 20 ml of *water R*. Heat to boiling. The fumes released do not turn *lead acetate paper R* brown.

Copper. Not more than 25 ppm of Cu, determined by atomic absorption spectrometry (*2.2.23, Method I*).

Test solution. Use solution S.

Reference solutions. Prepare the reference solutions using *copper standard solution (0.1 per cent Cu) R* and diluting with *0.1 M hydrochloric acid*.

Measure the absorbance at 325.0 nm using a copper hollow-cathode lamp as source of radiation and an air-acetylene flame.

Lead. Not more than 10 ppm of Pb, determined by atomic absorption spectrometry (*2.2.23, Method I*).

Test solution. Use solution S.

Reference solutions. Prepare the reference solutions using *lead standard solution (100 ppm Pb) R* and diluting with *0.1 M hydrochloric acid*.

Measure the absorbance at 283.3 nm using a lead hollow-cathode lamp as source of radiation and an air-acetylene flame. Depending on the apparatus the line at 217.0 nm may be used.

Zinc. Not more than 25 ppm of Zn, determined by atomic absorption spectrometry (*2.2.23, Method I*).

Test solution. Use solution S.

Reference solutions. Prepare the reference solutions using *zinc standard solution (100 ppm Zn) R* and diluting with *0.1 M hydrochloric acid*.

Measure the absorbance at 214.0 nm using a zinc hollow-cathode lamp as source of radiation and an air-acetylene flame.

Loss on drying (*2.2.32*). Not more than 15 per cent, determined on 1.00 g by drying in an oven at 120 °C for 4 h.

Sulphated ash (*2.4.14*). Not more than 5.0 per cent, determined on 1.0 g.

Adsorption power. To 0.300 g in a 100 ml ground-glass-stoppered conical flask add 25.0 ml of a freshly prepared solution of 0.5 g of *phenazone R* in 50 ml of *water R*. Shake thoroughly for 15 min. Filter and reject the first 5 ml of filtrate. To 10.0 ml of the filtrate add 1.0 g of *potassium bromide R* and 20 ml of *dilute hydrochloric acid R*. Using 0.1 ml of *methyl red solution R* as indicator, titrate with *0.0167 M potassium bromate* until the red colour is discharged. Titrate slowly (1 drop every 15 s) towards the end of the titration. Carry out a blank titration using 10.0 ml of the phenazone solution.

Calculate the quantity of phenazone adsorbed per 100 g of activated charcoal from the expression:

$$\frac{2.353\,(a - b)}{m}$$

a = number of millilitres of *0.0167 M potassium bromate* used for the blank,

b = number of millilitres of *0.0167 M potassium bromate* used for the test,

m = mass in grams of the substance to be examined.

Not less than 40 g of phenazone is adsorbed per 100 g of activated charcoal, calculated with reference to the dried substance.

Microbial contamination. Total viable aerobic count (*2.6.12*) not more than 10^3 micro-organisms per gram, determined by plate count.

STORAGE

Store in an airtight container.

01/2005:1189

CHENODEOXYCHOLIC ACID

Acidum chenodeoxycholicum

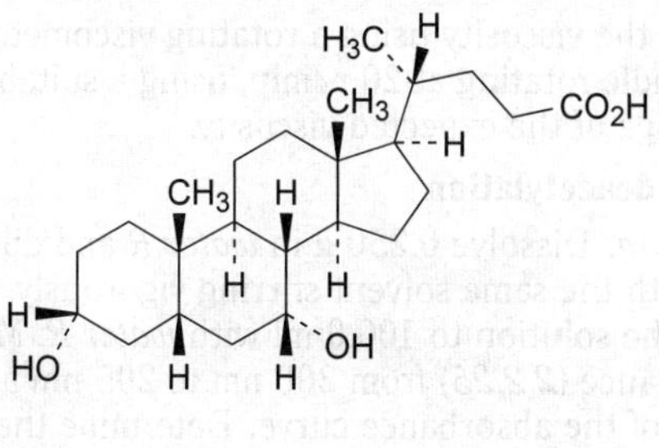

$C_{24}H_{40}O_4$ M_r 392.6

DEFINITION

Chenodeoxycholic acid contains not less than 99.0 per cent and not more than the equivalent of 101.0 per cent of 3α,7α-dihydroxy-5β-cholan-24-oic acid, calculated with reference to the dried substance.

CHARACTERS

A white or almost white powder, very slightly soluble in water, freely soluble in alcohol, soluble in acetone, slightly soluble in methylene chloride.

IDENTIFICATION

First identification: A.

Second identification: B, C.

A. Examine by infrared absorption spectrophotometry (*2.2.24*), comparing with the spectrum obtained with *chenodeoxycholic acid CRS*. Examine the substances prepared as discs using *potassium bromide R*.

B. Examine the chromatograms obtained in the test for related substances. The principal spot in the chromatogram obtained with test solution (b) is similar in position, colour and size to the principal spot in the chromatogram obtained with reference solution (a).

C. Dissolve about 10 mg in 1 ml of *sulphuric acid R*. Add 0.1 ml of *formaldehyde solution R* and allow to stand for 5 min. Add 5 ml of *water R*. The suspension obtained is greenish-blue.

TESTS

Specific optical rotation (*2.2.7*). Dissolve 0.500 g in *methanol R* and dilute to 25.0 ml with the same solvent. The specific optical rotation is + 11.0 to + 13.0, calculated with reference to the dried substance.

Related substances. Examine by thin-layer chromatography (*2.2.27*), using a suitable silica gel as the coating substance.

Test solution (a). Dissolve 0.40 g of the substance to be examined in a mixture of 1 volume of *water R* and 9 volumes of *acetone R* and dilute to 10 ml with the same mixture of solvents.

Test solution (b). Dilute 1 ml of test solution (a) to 10 ml with a mixture of 1 volume of *water R* and 9 volumes of *acetone R*.

Reference solution (a). Dissolve 40 mg of *chenodeoxycholic acid CRS* in a mixture of 1 volume of *water R* and 9 volumes of *acetone R* and dilute to 10 ml with the same mixture of solvents.

Reference solution (b). Dissolve 20 mg of *lithocholic acid CRS* in a mixture of 1 volume of *water R* and 9 volumes of *acetone R* and dilute to 10 ml with the same mixture of solvents. Dilute 2 ml of the solution to 100 ml with a mixture of 1 volume of *water R* and 9 volumes of *acetone R*.

Reference solution (c). Dissolve 20 mg of *ursodeoxycholic acid CRS* in a mixture of 1 volume of *water R* and 9 volumes of *acetone R* and dilute to 50 ml with the same mixture of solvents.

Reference solution (d). Dissolve 20 mg of *cholic acid CRS* in a mixture of 1 volume of *water R* and 9 volumes of *acetone R* and dilute to 100 ml with the same mixture of solvents.

Reference solution (e). Dilute 0.5 ml of test solution (a) to 20 ml with a mixture of 1 volume of *water R* and 9 volumes of *acetone R*. Dilute 1 ml of the solution to 10 ml with a mixture of 1 volume of *water R* and 9 volumes of *acetone R*.

Reference solution (f). Dissolve 10 mg of *chenodeoxycholic acid CRS* in reference solution (c) and dilute to 25 ml with the same solution.

Apply separately to the plate 5 µl of each solution. Develop in an unsaturated tank over a path of 15 cm using a mixture of 1 volume of *glacial acetic acid R*, 30 volumes of *acetone R* and 60 volumes of *methylene chloride R*. Dry the plate at 120 °C for 10 min. Spray the plate immediately with a 47.6 g/l solution of *phosphomolybdic acid R* in a mixture of 1 volume of *sulphuric acid R* and 20 volumes of *glacial acetic acid R* and heat again at 120 °C until blue spots appear on a lighter background. In the chromatogram obtained with test solution (a): any spot corresponding to lithocholic acid is not more intense than the principal spot in the chromatogram obtained with reference solution (b)

(0.1 per cent); any spot corresponding to ursodeoxycholic acid is not more intense than the principal spot in the chromatogram obtained with reference solution (c) (1 per cent); any spot corresponding to cholic acid is not more intense than the principal spot in the chromatogram obtained with reference solution (d) (0.5 per cent); any spot apart from the principal spot and any spots corresponding to lithocholic acid, ursodeoxycholic acid and cholic acid, is not more intense than the principal spot in the chromatogram obtained with reference solution (e) (0.25 per cent). The test is not valid unless the chromatogram obtained with reference solution (f) shows two clearly separated principal spots.

Heavy metals (*2.4.8*). 1.0 g complies with limit test C for heavy metals (20 ppm). Prepare the standard using 2 ml of *lead standard solution (10 ppm Pb) R*.

Loss on drying (*2.2.32*). Not more than 1.5 per cent, determined on 1.000 g by drying in an oven at 100 °C to 105 °C.

Sulphated ash (*2.4.14*). Not more than 0.1 per cent, determined on 1.0 g.

ASSAY

Dissolve 0.350 g in 50 ml of *alcohol R*, previously neutralised to 0.2 ml of *phenolphthalein solution R*. Add 50 ml of *water R* and titrate with *0.1 M sodium hydroxide* until a pink colour is obtained.

1 ml of *0.1 M sodium hydroxide* is equivalent to 39.26 mg of $C_{24}H_{40}O_4$.

IMPURITIES

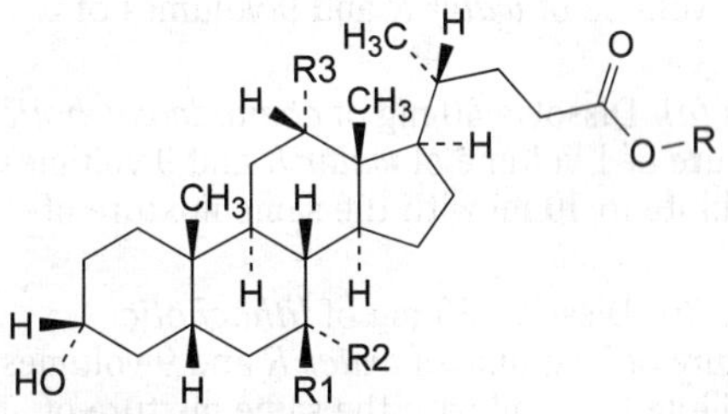

A. R = H, R1 = OH, R2 = H, R3 = H: ursodeoxycholic acid,

B. R = H, R1 = H, R2 = OH, R3 = OH: 3α,7α,12α-trihydroxy-5β-cholan-24-oic acid (cholic acid),

C. R = H, R1 = H, R2 = H, R3 = H: 3α-hydroxy-5β-cholan-24-oic acid (lithocholic acid),

D. R = H, R1 = OH, R2 = H, R3 = OH: 3α,7β,12α-trihydroxy-5β-cholan-24-oic acid (ursocholic acid),

E. R = H, R1 = H, R2 = H, R3 = OH: 3α,12α-dihydroxy-5β-cholan-24-oic acid (deoxycholic acid),

F. R = H, R1+R2 = = O, R3 = H: 3α-hydroxy-7-oxo-5β-cholan-24-oic acid,

G. R = CH_3, R1 = OH, R2 = H, R3 = H: methyl 3α,7β-dihydroxy-5β-cholan-24-oate.

01/2005:1774

CHITOSAN HYDROCHLORIDE

Chitosani hydrochloridum

DEFINITION

Chitosan hydrochloride is the chloride salt of an unbranched binary heteropolysaccharide consisting of the two units *N*-acetyl-D-glucosamine and D-glucosamine, obtained by partial deacetylation of chitin normally leading to a degree of deacetylation of 70.0 per cent to 95.0 per cent. Chitin is extracted from the shells of shrimp and crab.

PRODUCTION

The animals from which chitosan hydrochloride is derived must fulfil the requirements for the health of animals suitable for human consumption to the satisfaction of the competent authority. It must have been shown to what extent the method of production allows inactivation or removal of any contamination by viruses or other infectious agents.

CHARACTERS

Appearance: white or almost white fine powder.

Solubility: sparingly soluble in water, practically insoluble in ethanol.

IDENTIFICATION

A. Infrared absorption spectrophotometry (*2.2.24*).
   Preparation: discs.
   Comparison: *chitosan hydrochloride CRS*.

B. It gives reaction (a) of chlorides (*2.3.1*).

C. Dilute 50 ml of solution S (see Tests) to 250 ml with a 25 per cent *V/V* solution of *ammonia R*. A voluminous gelatinous mass is formed.

D. To 10 ml of solution S add 90 ml of *acetone R*. A voluminous gelatinous mass is formed.

TESTS

Solution S. Dissolve 1.0 g in 100 ml of *water R* and stir vigorously for 20 min with a mechanical stirrer.

Appearance of solution. Solution S is not more opalescent than reference suspension II (*2.2.1*) and not more intensely coloured than reference solution BY_5 (*2.2.2, Method II*).

Matter insoluble in water: maximum 0.5 per cent.

Add 2.00 g to 400.0 ml of *water R* while stirring until no further dissolution takes place. Transfer the solution to a 2 litre beaker, add 200 ml of *water R*. Boil the solution gently for 2 h, covering the beaker during the operation. Filter through a sintered-glass filter (40) wash the residue with water and dry to constant weight in an oven at 100-105 °C. The residue weighs a maximum of 10 mg.

pH (*2.2.3*): 4.0 to 6.0 for solution S.

Viscosity (*2.2.10*): 80 per cent to 120 per cent of the value stated on the label, determined on solution S.

Determine the viscosity using a rotating viscometer at 20 °C with a spindle rotating at 20 r/min, using a suitable spindle for the range of the expected viscosity.

Degree of deacetylation

Test solution. Dissolve 0.250 g in *water R* and dilute to 50.0 ml with the same solvent stirring vigorously. Dilute 1.0 ml of the solution to 100.0 ml with *water R*. Measure the absorbance (*2.2.25*) from 200 nm to 205 nm as the first derivative of the absorbance curve. Determine the pH of the solution.

Reference solutions. Prepare solutions of 1.0 µg/ml, 5.0 µg/ml, 15.0 µg/ml and 35.0 µg/ml of *N-acetylglucosamine R* in *water R*. Measure the absorbance (*2.2.25*) from 200 nm to 205 nm of each solution as first derivative of the absorption curve. Make a standard curve by plotting the first derivative at 202 nm as a function of the concentration of *N*-acetylglucosamine, and calculate the slope of the curve by least squares linear regression. Use the standard curve to determine the equivalent amount of *N*-acetylglucosamine for the substance to be examined.

Calculate the degree of deacetylation (molar) using the expression:

$$\frac{100 \times M_1 \times (C_1 - C_2)}{(M_1 \times C_1) - [(M_1 - M_3) \times C_2]}$$

C_1 = concentration of chitosan hydrochloride in the test solution in micrograms per millilitre,

C_2 = concentration of *N*-acetylglucosamine in the test solution, as determined from the standard curve prepared using the reference solution in micrograms per millilitre,

M_1 = 203 (relative molecular mass of *N*-acetylglucosamine unit ($C_8H_{13}NO_5$) in polymer),

M_3 = relative molecular mass of chitosan hydrochloride.

M_3 is calculated from the pH in solution, assuming a pKa value of 6.8, using the following expressions:

$$M_3 = f \times M_2 + (1 - f) \times (M_2 + 36.5)$$

$$f = \frac{p}{1+p}$$

$$p = 10^{(\mathrm{pH}-\mathrm{pKa})}$$

M_2 = 161 (relative molecular mass of deacetylated unit (glucosamine) ($C_6H_{11}NO_4$) in polymer).

Chlorides: 10.0 per cent to 20.0 per cent.

Introduce 0.200 g into a 250 ml borosilicate flask fitted with a reflux condenser. Add 40 ml of a mixture of 1 volume of *nitric acid R* and 2 volumes of *water R*. Boil gently under a reflux condenser for 5 min. Cool and add 25 ml of *water R* through the condenser. Add 16.0 ml of *0.1 M silver nitrate*, shake vigorously and titrate with *0.1 M ammonium thiocyanate*, using 1 ml of *ferric ammonium sulphate solution R2* as indicator, and shaking vigorously towards the end-point. Carry out a blank titration.

1 ml of *0.1 M silver nitrate* is equivalent to 3.55 mg of Cl.

Heavy metals (*2.4.8*): maximum 40 ppm.

1.0 g complies with limit test F. Prepare the standard using 4 ml of *lead standard solution (10 ppm Pb) R*.

Loss on drying (*2.2.32*): maximum 10 per cent, determined on 1.000 g by drying in an oven at 100-105 °C.

Sulphated ash (*2.4.14*): maximum 1.0 per cent, determined on 1.0 g.

STORAGE

At a temperature of 2-8 °C, protected from moisture and light.

LABELLING

The label states the nominal viscosity in millipascal seconds for a 10 g/l solution in *water R*.

01/2005:0265

CHLORAL HYDRATE

Chlorali hydras

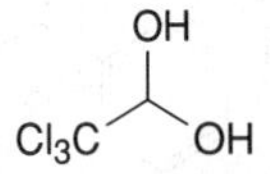

$C_2H_3Cl_3O_2$ M_r 165.4

DEFINITION

Chloral hydrate contains not less than 98.5 per cent and not more than the equivalent of 101.0 per cent of 2,2,2-trichloroethane-1,1-diol.

CHARACTERS

Colourless, transparent crystals, very soluble in water, freely soluble in alcohol.

IDENTIFICATION

A. To 10 ml of solution S (see Tests) add 2 ml of *dilute sodium hydroxide solution R*. The mixture becomes cloudy and, when heated, gives off an odour of chloroform.

B. To 1 ml of solution S add 2 ml of *sodium sulphide solution R*. A yellow colour develops which quickly becomes reddish-brown. On standing for a short time, a red precipitate may be formed.

TESTS

Solution S. Dissolve 3.0 g in *carbon dioxide-free water R* and dilute to 30 ml with the same solvent.

Appearance of solution. Solution S is clear (*2.2.1*) and colourless (*2.2.2, Method II*).

pH (*2.2.3*). The pH of solution S is 3.5 to 5.5.

Chloral alcoholate. Warm 1.0 g with 10 ml of *dilute sodium hydroxide solution R*, filter the supernatant solution and add *0.05 M iodine* dropwise until a yellow colour is obtained. Allow to stand for 1 h. No precipitate is formed.

Chlorides (*2.4.4*). 5 ml of solution S diluted to 15 ml with *water R* complies with the limit test for chlorides (100 ppm).

Heavy metals (*2.4.8*). 10 ml of solution S diluted to 20 ml with *water R* complies with limit test A for heavy metals (20 ppm). Prepare the standard using *lead standard solution (1 ppm Pb) R*.

Non-volatile residue. Evaporate 2.000 g on a water-bath. The residue weighs not more than 2 mg (0.1 per cent).

ASSAY

Dissolve 4.000 g in 10 ml of *water R* and add 40.0 ml of *1 M sodium hydroxide*. Allow to stand for exactly 2 min and titrate with *0.5 M sulphuric acid*, using 0.1 ml of *phenolphthalein solution R* as indicator. Titrate the neutralised solution with *0.1 M silver nitrate*, using 0.2 ml of *potassium chromate solution R* as indicator. Calculate the number of millilitres of *1 M sodium hydroxide* used by deducting from the volume of *1 M sodium hydroxide*, added at the beginning of the titration, the volume of *0.5 M sulphuric acid* used in the first titration and two-fifteenths of the volume of *0.1 M silver nitrate* used in the second titration.

1 ml of *1 M sodium hydroxide* is equivalent to 0.1654 g of $C_2H_3Cl_3O_2$.

STORAGE

Store in an airtight container.

01/2005:0137

CHLORAMBUCIL

Chlorambucilum

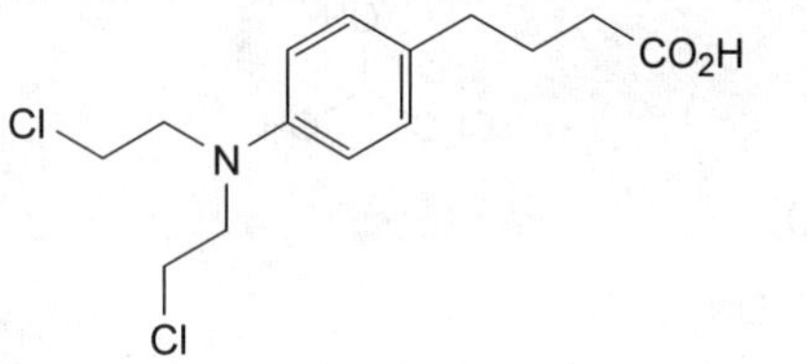

$C_{14}H_{19}Cl_2NO_2$ M_r 304.2

DEFINITION

Chlorambucil contains not less than 98.5 per cent and not more than the equivalent of 101.0 per cent of 4-4-[di(2-chloroethyl)amino]phenylbutyric acid, calculated with reference to the anhydrous substance.

CHARACTERS

A white, crystalline powder, practically insoluble in water, freely soluble in acetone and in alcohol.

IDENTIFICATION

First identification: A, B.

Second identification: A, C, D.

A. Melting point (*2.2.14*): 64 °C to 67 °C.

B. Examine by infrared absorption spectrophotometry (*2.2.24*), comparing with the spectrum obtained with *chlorambucil CRS*.

C. To 0.4 g add 10 ml of *dilute hydrochloric acid R*, mix and allow to stand for 30 min, shaking from time to time. Filter and wash the precipitate with 2 quantities, each of 10 ml, of *water R*. To 10 ml of the combined filtrate and washings add 0.5 ml of *potassium tetraiodomercurate solution R*. A pale-brown precipitate is formed. To another 10 ml of the combined filtrate and washings add 0.2 ml of *potassium permanganate solution R*. The colour of the latter is discharged immediately.

D. Dissolve 50 mg in 5 ml of *acetone R* and dilute to 10 ml with *water R*. Add 0.05 ml of *dilute nitric acid R* and 0.2 ml of *silver nitrate solution R2*. No opalescence is produced immediately. Heat the solution on a water-bath; an opalescence develops.

TESTS

Related substances. Examine by thin-layer chromatography (*2.2.27*), using *silica gel* GF_{254} *R* as the coating substance. *Carry out all operations as rapidly as possible protected from light. Prepare the solutions immediately before use.*

Test solution. Dissolve 0.2 g of the substance to be examined in *acetone R* and dilute to 10 ml with the same solvent.

Reference solution (a). Dilute 1 ml of the test solution to 50 ml with *acetone R*.

Reference solution (b). Dilute 25 ml of reference solution (a) to 100 ml with *acetone R*.

Apply separately to the plate 5 µl of each solution. Develop over a path of 10 cm using a mixture of 20 volumes of *methyl ethyl ketone R*, 20 volumes of *heptane R*, 25 volumes of *methanol R* and 40 volumes of *toluene R*. Examine in ultraviolet light at 254 nm. Any spot in the chromatogram obtained with the test solution, apart from the principal spot, is not more intense than the spot in the chromatogram obtained with reference solution (a) (2.0 per cent) and at most 1 such spot is more intense than the spot in the chromatogram obtained with reference solution (b) (0.5 per cent).

Water (*2.5.12*). Not more than 0.5 per cent, determined on 1.000 g by the semi-micro determination of water.

Sulphated ash (*2.4.14*). Not more than 0.1 per cent, determined on 1.0 g.

ASSAY

Dissolve 0.200 g in 10 ml of *acetone R* and add 10 ml of *water R*. Titrate with *0.1 M sodium hydroxide*, using 0.1 ml of *phenolphthalein solution R* as indicator.

1 ml of *0.1 M sodium hydroxide* is equivalent to 30.42 mg of $C_{14}H_{19}Cl_2NO_2$.

STORAGE

Store protected from light.

01/2005:0071

CHLORAMPHENICOL

Chloramphenicolum

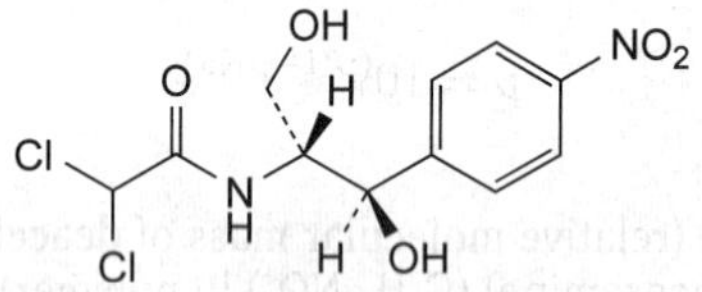

$C_{11}H_{12}Cl_2N_2O_5$ M_r 323.1

DEFINITION

Chloramphenicol is 2,2-dichloro-*N*-[(1*R*,2*R*)-2-hydroxy-1-(hydroxymethyl)-2-(4-nitrophenyl)ethyl]acetamide, produced by the growth of certain strains of *Streptomyces venezuelae* in a suitable medium. It is normally prepared by synthesis. It contains not less than 98.0 per cent and not more than the equivalent of 102.0 per cent of $C_{11}H_{12}Cl_2N_2O_5$, calculated with reference to the dried substance.

CHARACTERS

A white, greyish-white or yellowish-white, fine, crystalline powder or fine crystals, needles or elongated plates, slightly soluble in water, freely soluble in alcohol and in propylene glycol.

A solution in ethanol is dextrorotatory and a solution in ethyl acetate is laevorotatory.

IDENTIFICATION

First identification: A, B.

Second identification: A, C, D, E.

A. Melting point (*2.2.14*): 149 °C to 153 °C.

B. Examine by infrared absorption spectrophotometry (*2.2.24*), comparing with the spectrum obtained with *chloramphenicol CRS*.

C. Examine the chromatograms obtained in the test for related substances. The principal spot in the chromatogram obtained with 1 µl of the test solution is similar in position and size to the principal spot in the chromatogram obtained with reference solution (a).

D. Dissolve about 10 mg in 1 ml of *alcohol (50 per cent V/V) R*, add 3 ml of a 10 g/l solution of *calcium chloride R* and 50 mg of *zinc powder R* and heat on a water-bath for 10 min. Filter the hot solution and allow to cool. Add 0.1 ml of *benzoyl chloride R* and shake for

1 min. Add 0.5 ml of *ferric chloride solution R1* and 2 ml of *chloroform R* and shake. The aqueous layer is coloured light violet-red to purple.

E. To 50 mg in a porcelain crucible add 0.5 g of *anhydrous sodium carbonate R*. Heat over an open flame for 10 min. Allow to cool. Take up the residue with 5 ml of *dilute nitric acid R* and filter. To 1 ml of the filtrate add 1 ml of *water R*. The solution gives reaction (a) of chlorides (*2.3.1*).

TESTS

Acidity or alkalinity. To 0.1 g add 20 ml of *carbon dioxide-free water R*, shake and add 0.1 ml of *bromothymol blue solution R1*. Not more than 0.1 ml of *0.02 M hydrochloric acid* or *0.02 M sodium hydroxide* is required to change the colour of the indicator.

Specific optical rotation (*2.2.7*). Dissolve 1.50 g in *ethanol R* and dilute to 25.0 ml with the same solvent. The specific optical rotation is + 18.5 to + 20.5.

Related substances. Examine by thin-layer chromatography (*2.2.27*), using *silica gel* GF_{254} *R* as the coating substance.

Test solution. Dissolve 0.10 g of the substance to be examined in *acetone R* and dilute to 10 ml with the same solvent.

Reference solution (a). Dissolve 0.10 g of *chloramphenicol CRS* in *acetone R* and dilute to 10 ml with the same solvent.

Reference solution (b). Dilute 0.5 ml of reference solution (a) to 100 ml with *acetone R*.

Apply separately to the plate 1 µl and 20 µl of the test solution, 1 µl of reference solution (a) and 20 µl of reference solution (b). Develop over a path of 15 cm using a mixture of 1 volume of *water R*, 10 volumes of *methanol R* and 90 volumes of *chloroform R*. Allow the plate to dry in air and examine in ultraviolet light at 254 nm. Any spot in the chromatogram obtained with 20 µl of the test solution, apart from the principal spot, is not more intense than the spot in the chromatogram obtained with reference solution (b) (0.5 per cent).

Chlorides (*2.4.4*). To 1.00 g add 20 ml of *water R* and 10 ml of *nitric acid R* and shake for 5 min. Filter through a filter paper previously washed by filtering 5 ml portions of *water R* until 5 ml of filtrate no longer becomes opalescent on addition of 0.1 ml of *nitric acid R* and 0.1 ml of *silver nitrate solution R1*. 15 ml of the filtrate complies with the limit test for chlorides (100 ppm).

Loss on drying (*2.2.32*). Not more than 0.5 per cent, determined on 1.000 g by drying in an oven at 100 °C to 105 °C.

Sulphated ash (*2.4.14*). Not more than 0.1 per cent, determined on 2.0 g.

Pyrogens (*2.6.8*). If intended for use in the manufacture of a parenteral dosage form without a further appropriate procedure for the removal of pyrogens, it complies with the test for pyrogens. Inject per kilogram of the rabbit's mass 2.5 ml of a solution containing per millilitre 2 mg of the substance to be examined.

ASSAY

Dissolve 0.100 g in *water R* and dilute to 500.0 ml with the same solvent. Dilute 10.0 ml of this solution to 100.0 ml with *water R*. Measure the absorbance (*2.2.25*) at the maximum at 278 nm.

Calculate the content of $C_{11}H_{12}Cl_2N_2O_5$ taking the specific absorbance to be 297.

STORAGE

Store protected from light. If the substance is sterile, store in a sterile, airtight, tamper-proof container.

LABELLING

The label states, where applicable, that the substance is apyrogenic.

01/2005:0473

CHLORAMPHENICOL PALMITATE

Chloramphenicoli palmitas

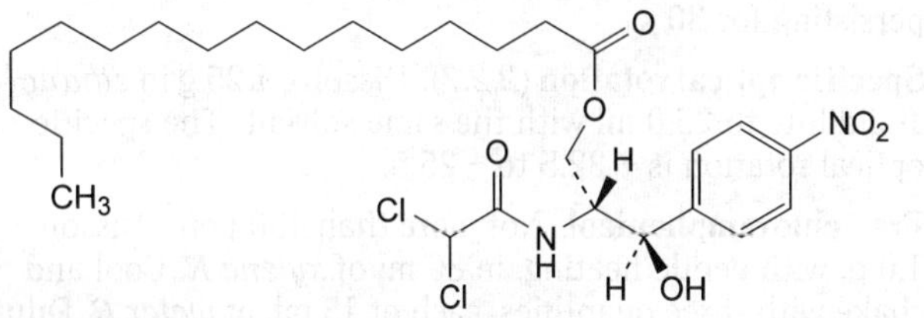

$C_{27}H_{42}Cl_2N_2O_6$ M_r 561.6

DEFINITION

Chloramphenicol palmitate contains not less than 98.0 per cent and not more than the equivalent of 102.0 per cent of (2*R*,3*R*)-2-[(dichloroacetyl)amino]-3-hydroxy-3-(4-nitrophenyl)propyl hexadecanoate, calculated with reference to the dried substance.

CHARACTERS

A white or almost white, fine, unctuous powder, practically insoluble in water, freely soluble in acetone, sparingly soluble in alcohol, very slightly soluble in hexane.

It melts at 87 °C to 95 °C.

It shows polymorphism and the thermodynamically stable form has low bioavailability following oral administration.

IDENTIFICATION

A. Examine by thin-layer chromatography (*2.2.27*), using *silanised silica gel H R* as the coating substance.

Test solution. Dissolve 50 mg of the substance to be examined in a mixture of 1 ml of *1 M sodium hydroxide* and 5 ml of *acetone R* and allow to stand for 30 min. Add 1.1 ml of *1 M hydrochloric acid* and 3 ml of *acetone R*.

Reference solution (a). Dissolve 10 mg of *chloramphenicol CRS* in *acetone R* and dilute to 5 ml with the same solvent.

Reference solution (b). Dissolve 10 mg of *palmitic acid R* in *acetone R* and dilute to 5 ml with the same solvent.

Reference solution (c). Dissolve 10 mg of the substance to be examined in *acetone R* and dilute to 5 ml with the same solvent.

Apply to the plate 4 µl of each solution. Develop over a path of 15 cm using a mixture of 30 volumes of a 100 g/l solution of *ammonium acetate R* and 70 volumes of *alcohol R*. Allow the plate to dry in air and spray with a solution containing 0.2 g/l of *dichlorofluorescein R* and 0.1 g/l of *rhodamine B R* in *alcohol R*. Allow the plate to dry in air and examine in ultraviolet light at 254 nm. The chromatogram obtained with the test solution shows three spots corresponding in position to the principal spots in the chromatograms obtained with reference solutions (a), (b) and (c).

B. Dissolve 0.2 g in 2 ml of *pyridine R*, add 2 ml of a 100 g/l solution of *potassium hydroxide R* and heat on a water-bath. A red colour is produced.

Monographs C

C. Dissolve 10 mg in 5 ml of *alcohol R* and add 4.5 ml of *dilute sulphuric acid R* and 50 mg of *zinc powder R*. Allow to stand for 10 min and if necessary decant the supernatant liquid or filter. Cool the solution in iced water and add 0.5 ml of *sodium nitrite solution R*. Allow to stand for 2 min and add 1 g of *urea R*, 2 ml of *strong sodium hydroxide solution R* and 1 ml of *β-naphthol solution R*. A red colour develops.

TESTS

Acidity. Dissolve 1.0 g in 5 ml of a mixture of equal volumes of *alcohol R* and *ether R*, warming to 35 °C. Add 0.2 ml of *phenolphthalein solution R*. Not more than 0.4 ml of *0.1 M sodium hydroxide* is required to produce a pink colour persisting for 30 s.

Specific optical rotation (*2.2.7*). Dissolve 1.25 g in *ethanol R* and dilute to 25.0 ml with the same solvent. The specific optical rotation is + 22.5 to + 25.5.

Free chloramphenicol. Not more than 450 ppm. Dissolve 1.0 g, with gentle heating, in 80 ml of *xylene R*. Cool and shake with three quantities, each of 15 ml, of *water R*. Dilute the combined aqueous extracts to 50 ml with *water R* and shake with 10 ml of *toluene R*. Allow to separate and discard the toluene layer. Centrifuge a portion of the aqueous layer and measure the absorbance (*A*) (*2.2.25*) at the maximum at 278 nm using as the compensation liquid a blank solution having an absorbance not greater than 0.05.

Calculate the content of free chloramphenicol in parts per million from the expression:

$$\frac{A \times 10^4}{5.96}$$

Related substances. Examine by thin-layer chromatography (*2.2.27*), using *silica gel GF$_{254}$ R* as the coating substance.

Test solution. Dissolve 0.1 g of the substance to be examined in *acetone R* and dilute to 10 ml with the same solvent.

Reference solution (a). Dissolve 20 mg of *chloramphenicol palmitate isomer CRS* in *acetone R* and dilute to 10 ml with the same solvent. Dilute 1 ml of this solution to 10 ml with *acetone R*.

Reference solution (b). Dissolve 20 mg of *chloramphenicol dipalmitate CRS* in *acetone R* and dilute to 10 ml with the same solvent. Dilute 1 ml of this solution to 10 ml with *acetone R*.

Reference solution (c). Dissolve 5 mg of *chloramphenicol CRS* in *acetone R* and dilute to 10 ml with the same solvent. Dilute 1 ml of this solution to 10 ml with *acetone R*.

Apply to the plate 10 µl of each solution. Develop over a path of 15 cm using a mixture of 10 volumes of *methanol R*, 40 volumes of *chloroform R* and 50 volumes of *cyclohexane R*. Allow the plate to dry in air and examine in ultraviolet light at 254 nm. In the chromatogram obtained with the test solution, any spots corresponding to chloramphenicol palmitate isomer and chloramphenicol dipalmitate are not more intense than the corresponding spots in the chromatograms obtained with reference solutions (a) and (b) respectively (2.0 per cent) and any spot, apart from the principal spot and the spots corresponding to chloramphenicol palmitate isomer and chloramphenicol dipalmitate, is not more intense than the principal spot in the chromatogram obtained with reference solution (c) (0.5 per cent).

Loss on drying (*2.2.32*). Not more than 0.5 per cent, determined on 1.000 g by heating at 80 °C over *diphosphorus pentoxide R* at a pressure not exceeding 0.1 kPa for 3 h.

Sulphated ash (*2.4.14*). Not more than 0.1 per cent, determined on 1.0 g.

ASSAY

Dissolve 90.0 mg in *alcohol R* and dilute to 100.0 ml with the same solvent. Dilute 10.0 ml of this solution to 250.0 ml with *alcohol R*. Measure the absorbance (*2.2.25*) of the solution at the maximum at 271 nm.

Calculate the content of $C_{27}H_{42}Cl_2N_2O_6$ taking the specific absorbance to be 178.

STORAGE

Store protected from light.

IMPURITIES

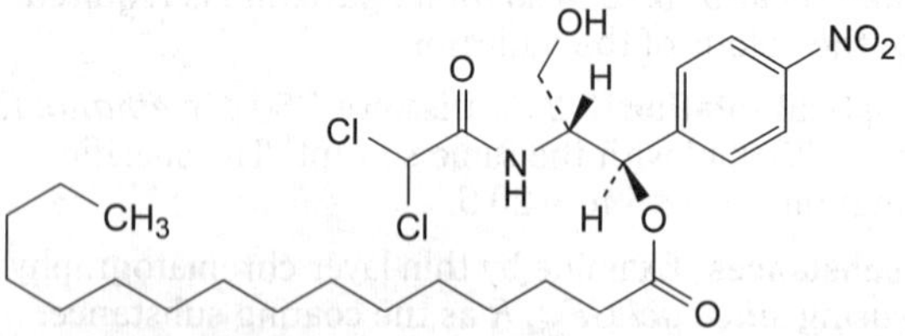

A. (1*R*,2*R*)-2-[(dichloroacetyl)amino]-3-hydroxy-1-(4-nitrophenyl)propyl hexadecanoate (chloramphenicol palmitate isomer),

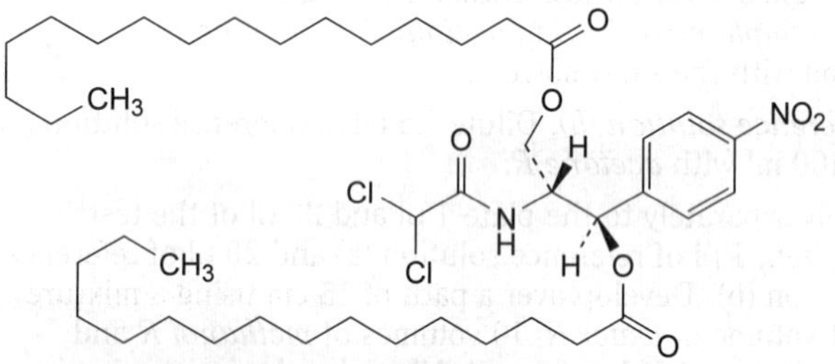

B. (1*R*,2*R*)-2-[(dichloroacetyl)amino]-1-(4-nitrophenyl)propane-1,3-diyl bishexadecanoate (chloramphenicol dipalmitate).

01/2005:0709

CHLORAMPHENICOL SODIUM SUCCINATE

Chloramphenicoli natrii succinas

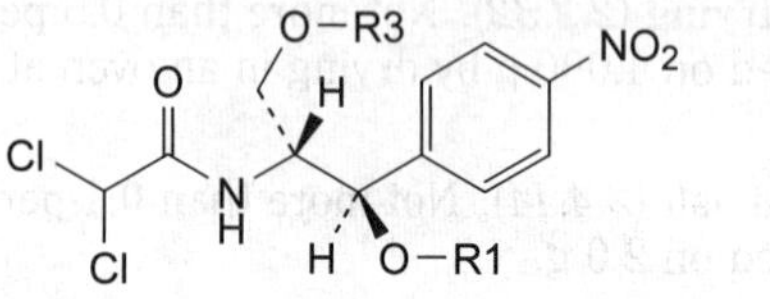

1 isomer : R1 = CO-CH2-CH2-CO2Na, R3 = H
3 isomer : R1 = H, R3 = CO-CH2-CH2-CO2Na

$C_{15}H_{15}Cl_2N_2NaO_8$ M_r 445.2

DEFINITION

Chloramphenicol sodium succinate, a mixture in variable proportions of sodium (2*R*,3*R*)-2-[(dichloroacetyl)amino]-3-hydroxy-3-(4-nitrophenyl)propyl butanedioate (3 isomer) and of sodium (1*R*,2*R*)-2-[(dichloroacetyl)amino]-3-hydroxy-1-(4-nitrophenyl)propyl butanedioate (1 isomer), contains not less than 98.0 per cent and not more than the equivalent of 102.0 per cent of $C_{15}H_{15}Cl_2N_2NaO_8$, calculated with reference to the anhydrous substance.

CHARACTERS

A white or yellowish-white powder, hygroscopic, very soluble in water, freely soluble in alcohol.

IDENTIFICATION

A. Examine by thin-layer chromatography (*2.2.27*), using *silica gel* GF_{254} *R* as the coating substance.

Test solution. Dissolve 20 mg of the substance to be examined in 2 ml of *acetone R*.

Reference solution (a). Dissolve 20 mg of *chloramphenicol sodium succinate CRS* in 2 ml of *acetone R*.

Reference solution (b). Dissolve 20 mg of *chloramphenicol CRS* in 2 ml of *acetone R*.

Apply separately to the plate 2 µl of each solution. Develop over a path of 15 cm using a mixture of 1 volume of *dilute acetic acid R*, 14 volumes of *methanol R* and 85 volumes of *chloroform R*. Allow the plate to dry in air and examine in ultraviolet light at 254 nm. The two principal spots in the chromatogram obtained with the test solution are similar in position and size to those in the chromatogram obtained with reference solution (a). Their positions are different from that of the principal spot in the chromatogram obtained with reference solution (b).

B. Dissolve about 10 mg in 1 ml of *alcohol (50 per cent V/V) R*, add 3 ml of a 10 g/l solution of *calcium chloride R* and 50 mg of *zinc powder R* and heat on a water-bath for 10 min. Filter the hot solution and allow to cool. Add 0.1 ml of *benzoyl chloride R* and shake for 1 min. Add 0.5 ml of *ferric chloride solution R1* and 2 ml of *chloroform R* and shake. The upper layer is light violet-red to purple.

C. Dissolve 50 mg in 1 ml of *pyridine R*. Add 0.5 ml of *dilute sodium hydroxide solution R* and 1.5 ml of *water R*. Heat in a water-bath for 3 min. A red colour develops. Add 2 ml of *nitric acid R* and cool under running water. Add 1 ml of *0.1 M silver nitrate*. A white precipitate is formed slowly.

D. It gives reaction (a) of sodium (*2.3.1*).

TESTS

pH (*2.2.3*). Dissolve 2.50 g in *carbon dioxide-free water R* and dilute to 10 ml with the same solvent. The pH of the solution is 6.4 to 7.0.

Specific optical rotation (*2.2.7*). Dissolve 0.50 g in *water R* and dilute to 10.0 ml with the same solvent. The specific optical rotation is + 5.0 to + 8.0, calculated with reference to the anhydrous substance.

Chloramphenicol and chloramphenicol disodium disuccinate. Examine by liquid chromatography (*2.2.29*).

Test solution. Dissolve 25.0 mg of the substance to be examined in the mobile phase and dilute to 100.0 ml with the mobile phase.

Reference solution (a). Dissolve 10.0 mg of *chloramphenicol CRS* in the mobile phase and dilute to 100.0 ml with the mobile phase (*solution a'*). Dilute 5.0 ml of this solution to 100.0 ml with the mobile phase.

Reference solution (b). Dissolve 10.0 mg of *chloramphenicol disodium disuccinate CRS* in the mobile phase and dilute to 100.0 ml with the mobile phase (*solution b'*). Dilute 5.0 ml of this solution to 100.0 ml with the mobile phase.

Reference solution (c). Dissolve 25 mg of the substance to be examined in the mobile phase, add 5 ml of solution (a′) and 5 ml of solution (b′) and dilute to 100 ml with the mobile phase.

The chromatographic procedure may be carried out using:

– a column 0.25 m long and 4.6 mm in internal diameter packed with *octadecylsilyl silica gel for chromatography R* (5 µm),

– as mobile phase at a flow rate of 1.0 ml/min a mixture of 5 volumes of a 20 g/l solution of *phosphoric acid R*, 40 volumes of *methanol R* and 55 volumes of *water R*,

– as detector a spectrophotometer set at 275 nm,

– a 20 µl fixed-loop injector.

Inject the test solution and each of the reference solutions. The test is not valid unless, in the chromatogram obtained with reference solution (c), the two peaks corresponding to those in the chromatograms obtained with reference solutions (a) and (b) are clearly separated from the peaks corresponding to the two principal peaks in the chromatogram obtained with the test solution. If necessary, adjust the methanol content of the mobile phase.

In the chromatogram obtained with the test solution, the area of any peak corresponding to chloramphenicol is not greater than the area of the principal peak in the chromatogram obtained with reference solution (a) (2.0 per cent); the area of any peak corresponding to chloramphenicol disodium disuccinate is not greater than the area of the principal peak in the chromatogram obtained with reference solution (b) (2.0 per cent).

Water (*2.5.12*). Not more than 2.0 per cent, determined on 0.500 g by the semi-micro determination of water.

Pyrogens (*2.6.8*). If intended for use in the manufacture of a parenteral dosage form without a further appropriate procedure for removal of pyrogens, it complies with the test for pyrogens. Inject per kilogram of the rabbit's mass 2.5 ml of a solution in *water for injections R* containing 2 mg of the substance to be examined per millilitre.

ASSAY

Dissolve 0.200 g in *water R* and dilute to 500.0 ml with the same solvent. Dilute 5.0 ml of this solution to 100.0 ml with *water R*. Measure the absorbance (*2.2.25*) at the maximum at 276 nm.

Calculate the content of $C_{15}H_{15}Cl_2N_2NaO_8$, taking the specific absorbance to be 220.

STORAGE

Store in an airtight container, protected from light. If the substance is sterile, store in a sterile, airtight, tamper-proof container, protected from light.

LABELLING

The label states, where applicable, that the substance is apyrogenic.

01/2005:1086

CHLORCYCLIZINE HYDROCHLORIDE

Chlorcyclizini hydrochloridum

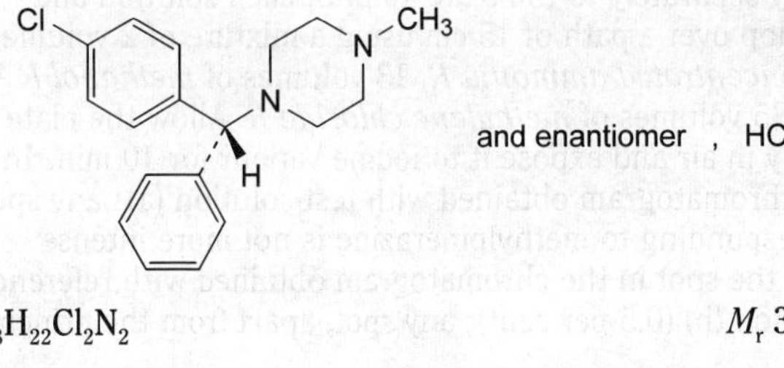

$C_{18}H_{22}Cl_2N_2$ M_r 337.3

DEFINITION

Chlorcyclizine hydrochloride contains not less than 99.0 per cent and not more than the equivalent of 101.0 per cent of (*RS*)-1-[(4-chlorophenyl)phenylmethyl]-4-methylpiperazine hydrochloride, calculated with reference to the dried substance.

CHARACTERS

A white, crystalline powder, freely soluble in water and in methylene chloride, soluble in alcohol.

IDENTIFICATION

First identification: B, D.

Second identification: A, C, D.

A. Dissolve 10.0 mg in a 5 g/l solution of *sulphuric acid R* and dilute to 100.0 ml with the same acid. Dilute 10.0 ml of the solution to 100.0 ml with a 5 g/l solution of *sulphuric acid R*. Examined between 215 nm and 300 nm (*2.2.25*), the solution shows an absorption maximum at 231 nm. The specific absorbance at the maximum is 475 to 525, calculated with reference to the dried substance.

B. Examine by infrared absorption spectrophotometry (*2.2.24*), comparing with the spectrum obtained with *chlorcyclizine hydrochloride CRS*. Examine the substances prepared as discs.

C. Examine the chromatograms obtained in the test for related substances (see Tests). The principal spot in the chromatogram obtained with test solution (b) is similar in position and size to the principal spot in the chromatogram obtained with reference solution (a).

D. It gives reaction (a) of chlorides (*2.3.1*).

TESTS

Appearance of solution. Dissolve 0.5 g in *water R* and dilute to 10 ml with the same solvent. The solution is clear (*2.2.1*) and colourless (*2.2.2, Method II*).

pH (*2.2.3*). Dissolve 0.10 g in *carbon dioxide-free water R* and dilute to 10 ml with the same solvent. The pH of the solution is 5.0 to 6.0.

Related substances. Examine by thin-layer chromatography (*2.2.27*), using a plate coated with a suitable silica gel.

Test solution (a). Dissolve 0.20 g of the substance to be examined in *methanol R* and dilute to 10 ml with the same solvent.

Test solution (b). Dilute 5 ml of test solution (a) to 100 ml with *methanol R*.

Reference solution (a). Dissolve 10 mg of *chlorcyclizine hydrochloride CRS* in *methanol R* and dilute to 10 ml with the same solvent.

Reference solution (b). Dissolve 5 mg of *methylpiperazine R* in *methanol R* and dilute to 50 ml with the same solvent.

Reference solution (c). Dilute 1 ml of test solution (b) to 25 ml with *methanol R*.

Reference solution (d). Dissolve 10 mg of *hydroxyzine hydrochloride CRS* and 10 mg of *chlorcyclizine hydrochloride CRS* in *methanol R* and dilute to 10 ml with the same solvent.

Apply separately to the plate 10 µl of each solution and develop over a path of 15 cm using a mixture of 2 volumes of *concentrated ammonia R*, 13 volumes of *methanol R* and 85 volumes of *methylene chloride R*. Allow the plate to dry in air and expose it to iodine vapour for 10 min. In the chromatogram obtained with test solution (a): any spot corresponding to methylpiperazine is not more intense than the spot in the chromatogram obtained with reference solution (b) (0.5 per cent); any spot, apart from the principal spot and any spot corresponding to methylpiperazine, is not more intense than the spot in the chromatogram obtained with reference solution (c) (0.2 per cent). The test is not valid unless the chromatogram obtained with reference solution (d) shows two clearly separated spots.

Loss on drying (*2.2.32*). Not more than 1.0 per cent, determined on 1.000 g by drying in an oven at 130 °C.

Sulphated ash (*2.4.14*). Not more than 0.1 per cent, determined on 1.0 g.

ASSAY

Dissolve 0.200 g in a mixture of 1 ml of *0.1 M hydrochloric acid* and 50 ml of *methanol R*. Carry out a potentiometric titration (*2.2.20*), using *0.1 M sodium hydroxide*. Read the volume added between the two points of inflexion.

1 ml of *0.1 M sodium hydroxide* is equivalent to 33.73 mg of $C_{18}H_{22}Cl_2N_2$.

STORAGE

Store protected from light.

IMPURITIES

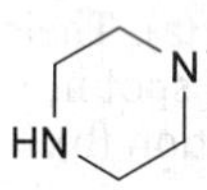

A. *N*-methylpiperazine.

01/2005:0656

CHLORDIAZEPOXIDE

Chlordiazepoxidum

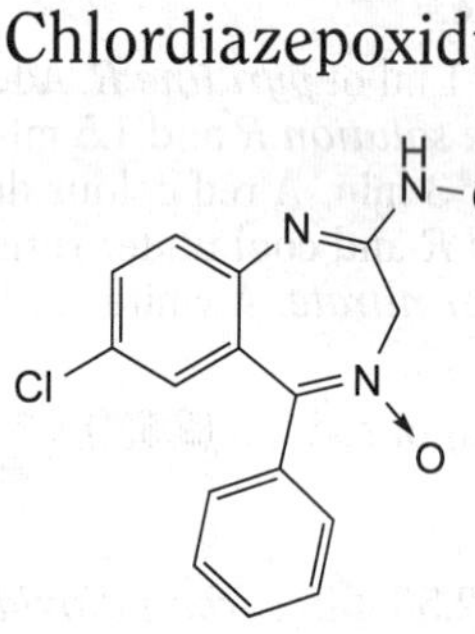

$C_{16}H_{14}ClN_3O$ M_r 299.8

DEFINITION

7-Chloro-*N*-methyl-5-phenyl-3*H*-1,4-benzodiazepin-2-amine 4-oxide.

Content: 99.0 per cent to 101.0 per cent (dried substance).

CHARACTERS

Appearance: almost white or light yellow, crystalline powder.

Solubility: practically insoluble in water, sparingly soluble in alcohol.

IDENTIFICATION

Infrared absorption spectrophotometry (*2.2.24*).

Comparison: *chlordiazepoxide CRS*.

TESTS

Related substances. Liquid chromatography (*2.2.29*). *Carry out the test protected from bright light and prepare the solutions immediately before use.*

Test solution. Dissolve 20.0 mg of the substance to be examined in the mobile phase and dilute to 100.0 ml with the mobile phase.

Reference solution (a). Dilute 1.0 ml of the test solution to 100.0 ml with the mobile phase. Dilute 2.0 ml of this solution to 10.0 ml with the mobile phase.

Reference solution (b). Dissolve 5 mg of *nitrazepam R* in the mobile phase, add 25.0 ml of the test solution and dilute to 100.0 ml with the mobile phase. Dilute 2.0 ml of this solution to 50.0 ml with the mobile phase.

Reference solution (c). Dissolve 4.0 mg of *aminochlorobenzophenone R* in the mobile phase and dilute to 100.0 ml with the mobile phase. Dilute 1.0 ml of the solution to 100.0 ml with the mobile phase.

Column:

- *size*: *l* = 0.15 m, Ø = 4.6 mm,
- *stationary phase*: *octadecylsilyl silica gel for chromatography R* (5 µm).

Mobile phase: *acetonitrile R, water R* (50:50 *V/V*).

Flow rate: 1.0 ml/min.

Detection: spectrophotometer at 254 nm.

Injection: 10 µl.

Run time: 6 times the retention time of chlordiazepoxide.

Retention time: nitrazepam = about 3.1 min; chlordiazepoxide = about 3.6 min.

Relative retention with reference to chlordiazepoxide: impurity A = about 0.7; impurity B = about 2.3; impurity C = about 3.9.

System suitability: reference solution (b):

- *resolution*: minimum 2.0 between the peaks due to nitrazepam and chlordiazepoxide.

Limits:

- *impurities A, B*: for each impurity, not more than the area of the principal peak in the chromatogram obtained with reference solution (a) (0.2 per cent),
- *impurity C*: not more than the area of the principal peak in the chromatogram obtained with reference solution (c) (0.2 per cent),
- *any other impurity*: not more than half the area of the principal peak in the chromatogram obtained with reference solution (a) (0.1 per cent),
- *total*: not more than 2.5 times the area of the principal peak in the chromatogram obtained with reference solution (a) (0.5 per cent),
- *disregard limit*: 0.25 times the area of the principal peak in the chromatogram obtained with reference solution (a) (0.05 per cent).

Loss on drying (*2.2.32*): maximum 0.5 per cent, determined on 1.000 g by drying in an oven at 100-105 °C.

Sulphated ash (*2.4.14*): maximum 0.1 per cent, determined on 1.0 g.

ASSAY

Dissolve 0.250 g, with heating if necessary, in 80 ml of *anhydrous acetic acid R*. Titrate with *0.1 M perchloric acid*, determining the end-point potentiometrically (*2.2.20*).

1 ml of *0.1 M perchloric acid* is equivalent to 29.98 mg of $C_{16}H_{14}ClN_3O$.

STORAGE

Protected from light.

IMPURITIES

Specified impurities: A, B, C.

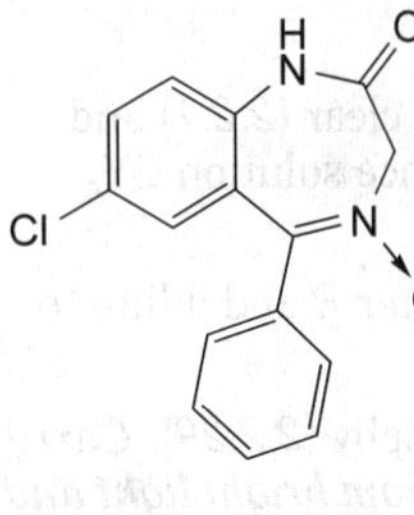

A. 7-chloro-5-phenyl-1,3-dihydro-2*H*-1,4-benzodiazepin-2-one 4-oxide,

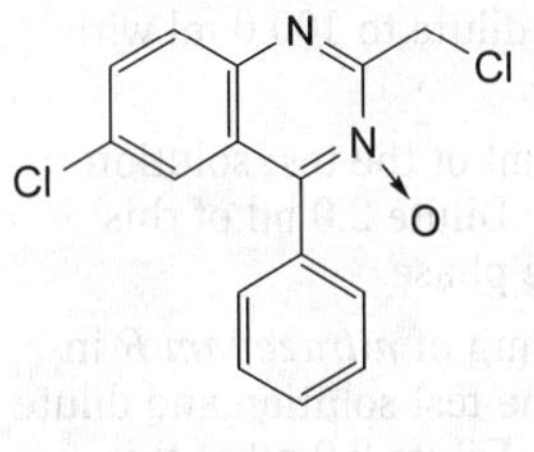

B. 6-chloro-2-(chloromethyl)-4-phenylquinazoline 3-oxide,

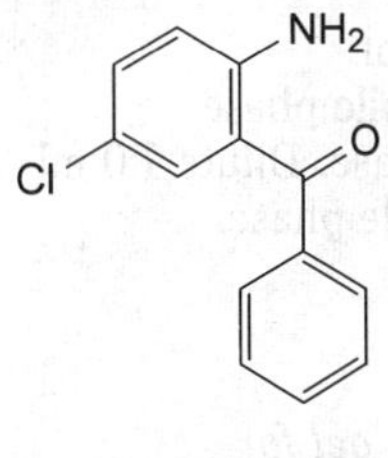

C. (2-amino-5-chlorophenyl)phenylmethanone (aminochlorobenzophenone).

01/2005:0474

CHLORDIAZEPOXIDE HYDROCHLORIDE

Chlordiazepoxidi hydrochloridum

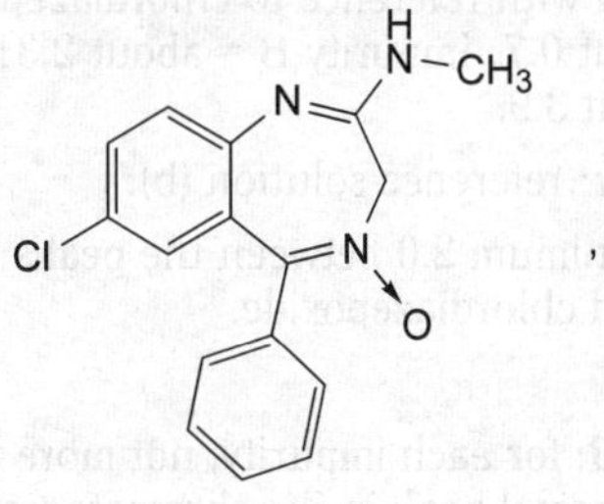

$C_{16}H_{15}Cl_2N_3O$ M_r 336.2

DEFINITION

7-Chloro-*N*-methyl-5-phenyl-3*H*-1,4-benzodiazepin-2-amine 4-oxide hydrochloride.

Content: 99.0 per cent to 101.0 per cent (dried substance).

CHARACTERS

Appearance: white or slightly yellow, crystalline powder, slightly hygroscopic.

Solubility: soluble in water, sparingly soluble in alcohol.

IDENTIFICATION

A. Infrared absorption spectrophotometry (*2.2.24*).

Comparison: *chlordiazepoxide hydrochloride CRS.*

B. Dissolve 50 mg in 5 ml of *water R*, add 1 ml of *dilute ammonia R1*, mix, allow to stand for 5 min and filter. Acidify the filtrate with *dilute nitric acid R*. The solution gives reaction (a) of chlorides (*2.3.1*).

TESTS

Appearance of solution. The solution is clear (*2.2.1*) and not more intensely coloured than reference solution GY_6 (*2.2.2, Method II*).

Dissolve 2.5 g in *carbon dioxide-free water R* and dilute to 25 ml with the same solvent.

Related substances. Liquid chromatography (*2.2.29*). *Carry out the following operations protected from bright light and prepare the solutions immediately before use.*

Test solution. Dissolve 20.0 mg of the substance to be examined in the mobile phase and dilute to 100.0 ml with the mobile phase.

Reference solution (a). Dilute 1.0 ml of the test solution to 100.0 ml with the mobile phase. Dilute 2.0 ml of this solution to 10.0 ml with the mobile phase.

Reference solution (b). Dissolve 5 mg of *nitrazepam R* in the mobile phase, add 25.0 ml of the test solution and dilute to 100.0 ml with the mobile phase. Dilute 2.0 ml of this solution to 50.0 ml with the mobile phase.

Reference solution (c). Dissolve 4.0 mg of *aminochlorobenzophenone R* in the mobile phase and dilute to 100.0 ml with the mobile phase. Dilute 1.0 ml of this solution to 100.0 ml with the mobile phase.

Column:

- *size*: *l* = 0.15 m, Ø = 4.6 mm,
- *stationary phase*: *octadecylsilyl silica gel for chromatography R* (5 µm).

Mobile phase: *acetonitrile R, water R* (50:50 *V/V*).

Flow rate: 1.0 ml/min.

Detection: spectrophotometer at 254 nm.

Injection: 10 µl.

Run time: 6 times the retention time of chlordiazepoxide.

Retention time: nitrazepam = about 3.1 min; chlordiazepoxide = about 3.6 min.

Relative retention with reference to chlordiazepoxide: impurity A = about 0.7; impurity B = about 2.3; impurity C = about 3.9.

System suitability: reference solution (b):

- *resolution*: minimum 2.0 between the peaks due to nitrazepam and chlordiazepoxide.

Limits:

- *impurities A, B*: for each impurity, not more than the area of the principal peak in the chromatogram obtained with reference solution (a) (0.2 per cent),
- *impurity C*: not more than the area of the principal peak in the chromatogram obtained with reference solution (c) (0.2 per cent),
- *any other impurity*: not more than half the area of the principal peak in the chromatogram obtained with reference solution (a) (0.1 per cent),
- *total*: not more than 2.5 times the area of the principal peak in the chromatogram obtained with reference solution (a) (0.5 per cent),
- *disregard limit*: 0.25 times the area of the principal peak in the chromatogram obtained with reference solution (a) (0.05 per cent).

Loss on drying (*2.2.32*): maximum 0.5 per cent, determined on 1.000 g by drying *in vacuo* at 60 °C for 4 h.

Sulphated ash (*2.4.14*): maximum 0.1 per cent, determined on 1.0 g.

ASSAY

Dissolve 0.250 g in 80 ml of *anhydrous acetic acid R,* heating if necessary. Cool and add 10 ml of *mercuric acetate solution R.* Titrate with *0.1 M perchloric acid,* determining the end-point potentiometrically (*2.2.20*).

1 ml of *0.1 M perchloric acid* is equivalent to 33.62 mg of $C_{16}H_{15}Cl_2N_3O$.

STORAGE

In an airtight container, protected from light.

IMPURITIES

Specified impurities: A, B, C.

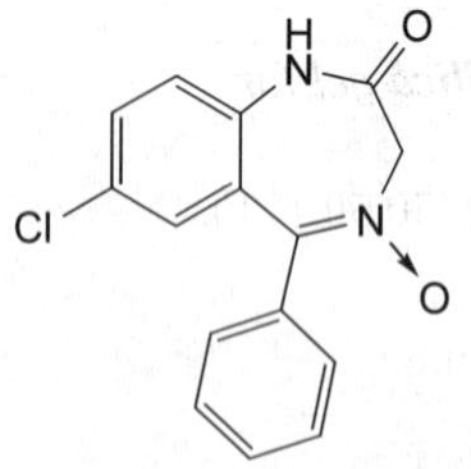

A. 7-chloro-5-phenyl-1,3-dihydro-2*H*-1,4-benzodiazepin-2-one 4-oxide,

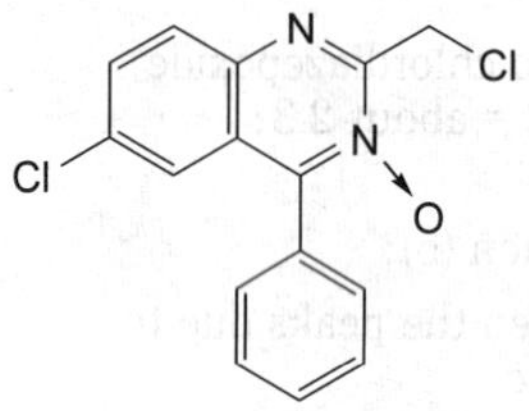

B. 6-chloro-2-(chloromethyl)-4-phenylquinazoline 3-oxide,

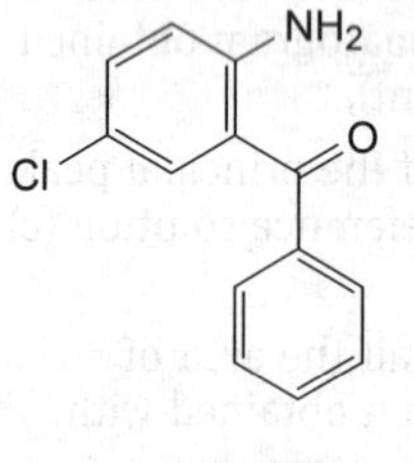

C. (2-amino-5-chlorophenyl)phenylmethanone (aminochlorobenzophenone).

01/2005:0657

CHLORHEXIDINE DIACETATE

Chlorhexidini diacetas

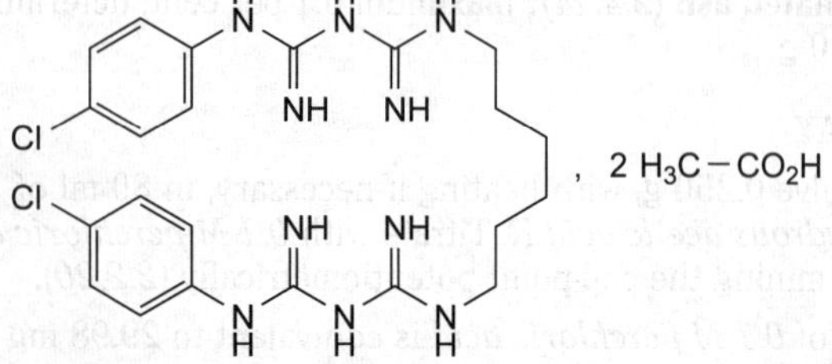

$C_{26}H_{38}Cl_2N_{10}O_4$ M_r 625.6

DEFINITION

Chlorhexidine diacetate contains not less than 98.0 per cent and not more than the equivalent of 101.0 per cent of 1,1′-(hexane-1,6-diyl)bis[5-(4-chlorophenyl)biguanide] diacetate, calculated with reference to the dried substance.

CHARACTERS

A white or almost white, microcrystalline powder, sparingly soluble in water, soluble in alcohol, slightly soluble in glycerol and in propylene glycol.

IDENTIFICATION

First identification: A.

Second identification: B, C, D.

A. Examine by infrared absorption spectrophotometry (*2.2.24*), comparing with the spectrum obtained with *chlorhexidine diacetate CRS.*

B. Dissolve about 5 mg in 5 ml of a warm 10 g/l solution of *cetrimide R* and add 1 ml of *strong sodium hydroxide solution R* and 1 ml of *bromine water R*. A deep red colour is produced.

C. Dissolve 0.3 g in 10 ml of a mixture of equal volumes of *hydrochloric acid R* and *water R*. Add 40 ml of *water R*, filter if necessary and cool in ice water. Make alkaline to *titan yellow paper R* by adding dropwise and with stirring *strong sodium hydroxide solution R* and add 1 ml in excess. Filter, wash the precipitate with *water R* until the washings are free from alkali and recrystallise from *alcohol (70 per cent V/V) R*. Dry at 100 °C to 105 °C. The residue melts (*2.2.14*) at 132 °C to 136 °C.

D. It gives reaction (a) of acetates (*2.3.1*).

TESTS

Chloroaniline. Dissolve 0.20 g of the substance to be examined in 25 ml of *water R* with shaking if necessary. Add 1 ml of *hydrochloric acid R* and dilute to 30 ml with *water R*. Add rapidly and with thorough mixing after each addition: 2.5 ml of *dilute hydrochloric acid R*, 0.35 ml of *sodium nitrite solution R*, 2 ml of a 50 g/l solution of *ammonium sulphamate R*, 5 ml of a 1.0 g/l solution of *naphthylethylenediamine dihydrochloride R* and 1 ml of *alcohol R*, dilute to 50.0 ml with *water R* and allow to stand for 30 min. Any reddish-blue colour in the solution is not more intense than that in a standard prepared at the same time in the same manner using a mixture of 10.0 ml of a 0.010 g/l solution of *chloroaniline R* in *dilute hydrochloric acid R* and 20 ml of *dilute hydrochloric acid R* instead of the solution of the substance to be examined (500 ppm).

Related substances. Examined by liquid chromatography (*2.2.29*).

Test solution. Dissolve 0.200 g of the substance to be examined in the mobile phase and dilute to 100 ml with the mobile phase.

Reference solution (a). Dissolve 15 mg of *chlorhexidine for performance test CRS* in the mobile phase and dilute to 10.0 ml with the mobile phase.

Reference solution (b). Dilute 2.5 ml of the test solution to 100 ml with the mobile phase.

Reference solution (c). Dilute 2.0 ml of reference solution (b) to 10 ml with the mobile phase. Dilute 1.0 ml of this solution to 10 ml with the mobile phase.

The chromatographic procedure may be carried out using:

– a stainless steel column 0.2 m long and 4 mm in internal diameter, packed with *octadecylsilyl silica gel for chromatography R* (5 µm),

– as mobile phase at a flow-rate of 1.0 ml/min, a solution of 2.0 g of *sodium octanesulphonate R* in a mixture of 120 ml of *glacial acetic acid R*, 270 ml of *water R* and 730 ml of *methanol R*,

– as detector a spectrophotometer set at 254 nm.

Equilibrate the column with the mobile phase for at least 1 h. Adjust the sensitivity of the system so that the height of the principal peak in the chromatogram obtained with 10 µl of reference solution (b) is at least 50 per cent of the full scale of the recorder.

Inject 10 µl of reference solution (a). The test is not valid unless the resulting chromatogram is similar to the specimen chromatogram provided with *chlorhexidine for performance test CRS* in that the peaks due to impurity-A and impurity-B precede that due to chlorhexidine. If necessary, adjust the concentration of acetic acid in the mobile phase (increasing the concentration decreases the retention times).

Inject separately 10 µl of the test solution and 10 µl each of reference solutions (b) and (c). Record the chromatograms of reference solutions (b) and (c) until the peak due to chlorhexidine has been eluted and record the chromatogram of the test solution for six times the retention time of the peak due to chlorhexidine. In the chromatogram obtained with the test solution, the sum of the areas of all the peaks, apart from the principal peak is not greater than the area of the principal peak in the chromatogram obtained with reference solution (b) (2.5 per cent). Disregard any peak with a with a relative retention time of 0.25 or less with respect to the principal peak and any peak whose area is less than that of the principal peak in the chromatogram obtained with reference solution (c).

Loss on drying (*2.2.32*). Not more than 3.5 per cent, determined on 1.000 g by drying in an oven at 100 °C to 105 °C.

Sulphated ash (*2.4.14*). Not more than 0.15 per cent, determined on 1.0 g.

ASSAY

Dissolve 0.140 g in 100 ml of *anhydrous acetic acid R* and titrate with *0.1 M perchloric acid*. Determine the end-point potentiometrically (*2.2.20*).

1 ml of *0.1 M perchloric acid* is equivalent to 15.64 mg of $C_{26}H_{38}Cl_2N_{10}O_4$.

IMPURITIES

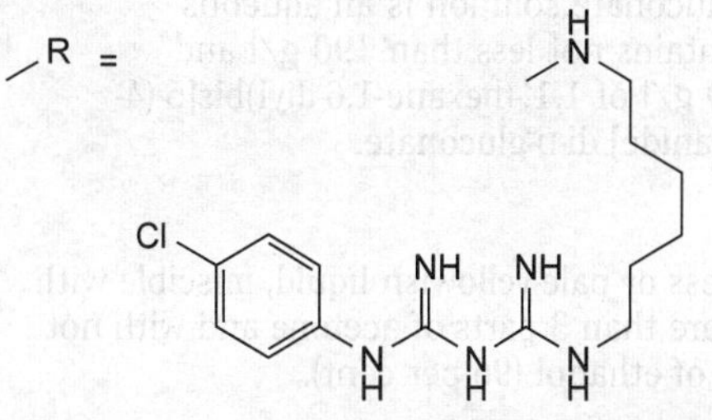

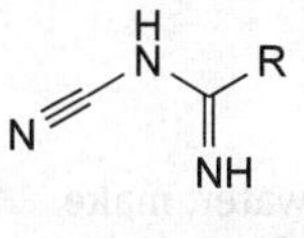

A. 1-(4-chlorophenyl)-5-[6-(3-cyanoguanidino)hexyl]biguanide,

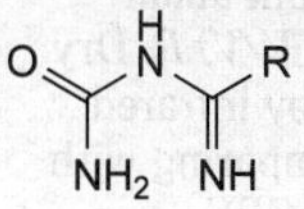

B. [[[6-[5-(4-chlorophenyl)guanidino]hexyl]amino]iminomethyl]urea,

Monographs C

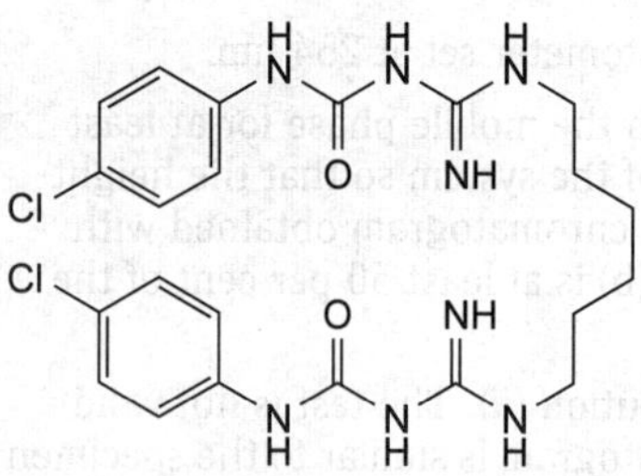

C. 1,1′-[hexane-1,6-diylbis[imino(iminocarbonyl)]]bis[3-(4-chlorophenyl)urea],

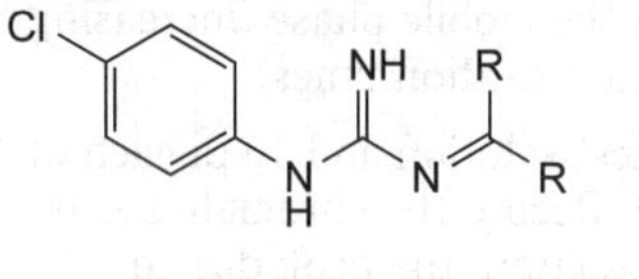

D. 1,1′-[[[[[(4-chlorophenyl)amino]iminomethyl]imino]methylene]bis[imino(hexane-1,6-diyl)]]bis[5-(4-chlorophenyl)biguanide].

01/2005:0658
corrected

CHLORHEXIDINE DIGLUCONATE SOLUTION

Chlorhexidini digluconatis solutio

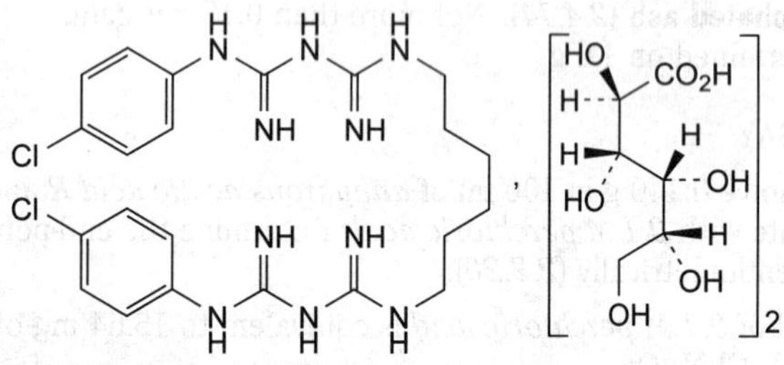

$C_{34}H_{54}Cl_2N_{10}O_{14}$ M_r 898

DEFINITION

Chlorhexidine digluconate solution is an aqueous solution which contains not less than 190 g/l and not more than 210 g/l of 1,1′-(hexane-1,6-diyl)bis[5-(4-chlorophenyl)biguanide] di-D-gluconate.

CHARACTERS

An almost colourless or pale-yellowish liquid, miscible with water, with not more than 3 parts of acetone and with not more than 5 parts of ethanol (96 per cent).

IDENTIFICATION

First identification: A, B.

Second identification: B, C, D.

A. To 1 ml add 40 ml of *water R*, cool in iced water, make alkaline to *titan yellow paper R* by adding dropwise and with stirring *strong sodium hydroxide solution R* and add 1 ml in excess. Filter, wash the precipitate with *water R* until the washings are free from alkali and recrystallise from *alcohol (70 per cent V/V) R*. Dry at 100 °C to 105 °C. Examine the residue by infrared absorption spectrophotometry (*2.2.24*), comparing with the spectrum obtained with *chlorhexidine CRS*.

B. Examine by thin-layer chromatography (*2.2.27*), using *silica gel G R* as the coating substance.

Test solution. Dilute 10.0 ml of the solution to be examined to 50 ml with *water R*.

Reference solution. Dissolve 25 mg of *calcium gluconate CRS* in 1 ml of *water R*.

Apply separately to the plate 5 µl of each solution. Develop over a path of 10 cm using a mixture of 10 volumes of *ethyl acetate R*, 10 volumes of *concentrated ammonia R*, 30 volumes of *water R* and 50 volumes of *alcohol R*. Dry the plate at 100 °C for 20 min, allow to cool and spray with a 50 g/l solution of *potassium dichromate R* in a 40 per cent *m/m* solution of *sulphuric acid R*. After 5 min, the principal spot in the chromatogram obtained with the test solution is similar in position, colour and size to the principal spot in the chromatogram obtained with the reference solution.

C. To 1 ml add 40 ml of *water R*, cool in iced water, make alkaline to *titan yellow paper R* by adding dropwise and with stirring *strong sodium hydroxide solution R* and add 1 ml in excess. Filter, wash the precipitate with *water R* until the washings are free from alkali and recrystallise from *alcohol (70 per cent V/V) R*. Dry at 100 °C to 105 °C. The residue melts (*2.2.14*) at 132 °C to 136 °C.

D. To 0.05 ml add 5 ml of a 10 g/l solution of *cetrimide R*, 1 ml of *strong sodium hydroxide solution R* and 1 ml of *bromine water R*; a deep red colour is produced.

TESTS

Relative density (*2.2.5*): 1.06 to 1.07.

pH (*2.2.3*). Dilute 5.0 ml to 100 ml with *carbon dioxide-free water R*. The pH of the solution is 5.5 to 7.0.

Chloroaniline. Dilute 2.0 ml to 100 ml with *water R*. To 10 ml of the solution add 2.5 ml of *dilute hydrochloric acid R* and dilute to 20 ml with *water R*. Add rapidly and with thorough mixing after each addition: 0.35 ml of *sodium nitrite solution R*, 2 ml of a 50 g/l solution of *ammonium sulphamate R*, 5 ml of a 1 g/l solution of *naphthylethylenediamine dihydrochloride R*, 1 ml of *alcohol R*, dilute to 50.0 ml with *water R* and allow to stand for 30 min. Any reddish-blue colour in the solution is not greater than that in a standard prepared at the same time in the same manner using a mixture of 10.0 ml of a 0.010 g/l solution of *chloroaniline R* in *dilute hydrochloric acid R* and 10 ml of *water R* instead of the dilution of the solution to be examined (0.25 per cent with reference to chlorhexidine digluconate at a nominal concentration of 200 g/l).

Related substances. Examined by liquid chromatography (*2.2.29*).

Test solution. Dilute 5.0 ml of the sample to be examined to 50.0 ml with the mobile phase. Dilute 5.0 ml of this solution to 50.0 ml with the mobile phase.

Reference solution (a). Dissolve 15 mg of *chlorhexidine for performance test CRS* in the mobile phase and dilute to 10.0 ml with the mobile phase.

Reference solution (b). Dilute 3.0 ml of the test solution to 100 ml with the mobile phase.

Reference solution (c). Dilute 1.0 ml of reference solution (b) to 50 ml with the mobile phase.

The chromatographic procedure may be carried out using:

– a stainless steel column 0.2 m long and 4 mm in internal diameter, packed with *octadecylsilyl silica gel for chromatography R* (5 µm),

– as mobile phase at a flow-rate of 1.0 ml/min, a solution of 2.0 g of *sodium octanesulphonate R* in a mixture of 120 ml of *glacial acetic acid R*, 270 ml of *water R* and 730 ml of *methanol R*,

– as detector a spectrophotometer set at 254 nm.

Equilibrate the column with mobile phase for at least 1 hour. Adjust the sensitivity of the system so that the height of the principal peak in the chromatogram obtained with 10 µl of reference solution (b) is at least 50 per cent of the full scale of the recorder.

Inject 10 µl of reference solution (a). The test is not valid unless the resulting chromatogram is similar to the specimen chromatogram provided with *chlorhexidine for performance test CRS* in that the peaks due to impurity A and impurity B precede that due to chlorhexidine. If necessary, adjust the concentration of acetic acid in the mobile phase (increasing the concentration decreases the retention times).

Inject separately 10 µl of the test solution and 10 µl each of reference solutions (b) and (c). Record the chromatograms of reference solutions (b) and (c) until the peak due to chlorhexidine has been eluted and record the chromatogram of the test solution for six times the retention time of the peak due to chlorhexidine. In the chromatogram obtained with the test solution, the sum of the areas of the peaks, apart from the principal peak is not greater than the area of the principal peak in the chromatogram obtained with reference solution (b) (3.0 per cent). Disregard any peak with a relative retention time of 0.25 or less with respect to the principal peak and any peak whose area is less than that of the principal peak in the chromatogram obtained with reference solution (c).

ASSAY

Determine the density (*2.2.5*) of the solution to be examined. Transfer 1.00 g to a 250 ml beaker and add 50 ml of *anhydrous acetic acid R*. Titrate with *0.1 M perchloric acid*. Determine the end-point potentiometrically (*2.2.20*).

1 ml of *0.1 M perchloric acid* is equivalent to 22.44 mg of $C_{34}H_{54}Cl_2N_{10}O_{14}$.

STORAGE

Store protected from light.

IMPURITIES

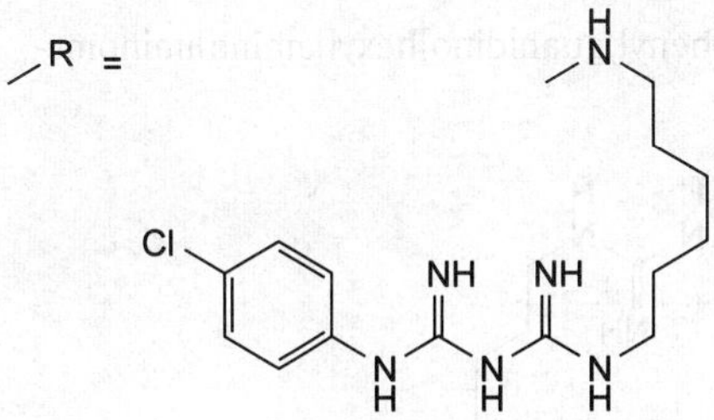

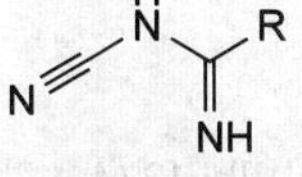

A. 1-(4-chlorophenyl)-5-[6-(3-cyanoguanidino)hexyl]biguanide,

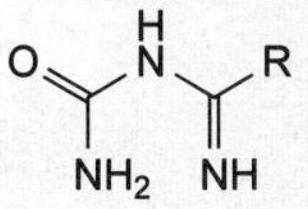

B. [[[6-[5-(4-chlorophenyl)guanidino]hexyl]amino]iminomethyl]urea,

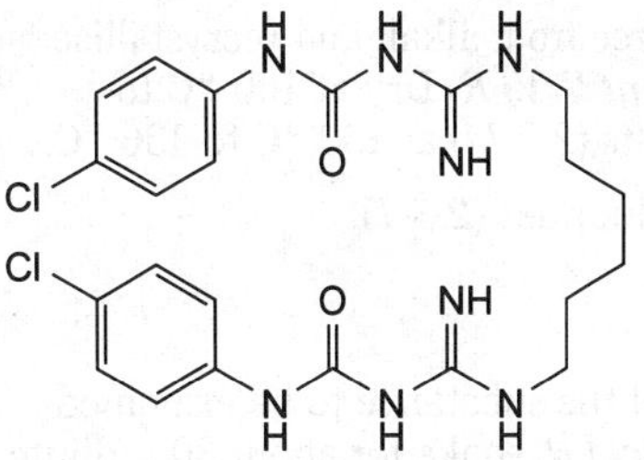

C. 1,1′-[hexane-1,6-diylbis[imino(iminocarbonyl)]]bis[3-(4-chlorophenyl)urea],

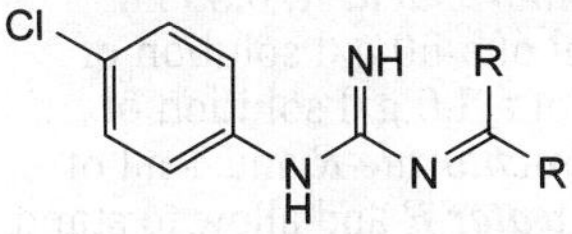

D. 1,1′-[[[[(4-chlorophenyl)amino]iminomethyl]imino]methylene]bis[imino(hexane-1,6-diyl)]]bis[5-(4-chlorophenyl)biguanide].

01/2005:0659

CHLORHEXIDINE DIHYDROCHLORIDE

Chlorhexidini dihydrochloridum

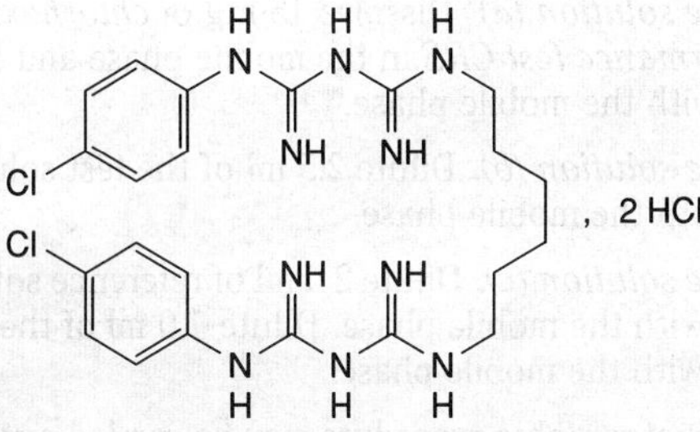

$C_{22}H_{32}Cl_4N_{10}$ M_r 578.4

DEFINITION

Chlorhexidine dihydrochloride contains not less than 98.0 per cent and not more than the equivalent of 101.0 per cent of 1,1'-(hexane-1,6-diyl)bis[5-(4-chlorophenyl)biguanide] dihydrochloride, calculated with reference to the dried substance.

CHARACTERS

A white or almost white, crystalline powder, sparingly soluble in water and in propylene glycol, very slightly soluble in alcohol.

IDENTIFICATION

First identification: A, D.

Second identification: B, C, D.

A. Examine by infrared absorption spectrophotometry (*2.2.24*), comparing with the spectrum obtained with *chlorhexidine dihydrochloride CRS*.

B. Dissolve about 5 mg in 5 ml of a warm 10 g/l solution of *cetrimide R* and add 1 ml of *strong sodium hydroxide solution R* and 1 ml of *bromine water R*. A dark red colour is produced.

C. Dissolve 0.3 g in 10 ml of a mixture of equal volumes of *hydrochloric acid R* and *water R*. Add 40 ml of *water R*, filter if necessary and cool in iced water. Make alkaline to *titan yellow paper R* by adding dropwise, and with stirring, *strong sodium hydroxide solution R* and add 1 ml in excess. Filter, wash the precipitate with *water R* until the washings are free from alkali and recrystallise from *alcohol (70 per cent V/V) R*. Dry at 100 °C to 105 °C. The residue melts (*2.2.14*) at 132 °C to 136 °C.

D. It gives reaction (a) of chlorides (*2.3.1*).

TESTS

Chloroaniline. To 0.20 g of the substance to be examined add 1 ml of *hydrochloric acid R*, shake for about 30 s, dilute to 30 ml with *water R* and shake until a clear solution is obtained. Add rapidly and with thorough mixing after each addition: 2.5 ml of *dilute hydrochloric acid R*, 0.35 ml of *sodium nitrite solution R*, 2 ml of a 50 g/l solution of *ammonium sulphamate R*, 5 ml of a 1.0 g/l solution of *naphthylethylenediamine dihydrochloride R* and 1 ml of *alcohol R*; dilute to 50.0 ml with *water R* and allow to stand for 30 min. Any reddish-blue colour in the solution is not more intense than that in a standard prepared at the same time and in the same manner using a mixture of 10.0 ml of a 0.010 g/l solution of *chloroaniline R* in *dilute hydrochloric acid R* and 20 ml of *dilute hydrochloric acid R* instead of the solution of the substance to be examined (500 ppm).

Related substances. Examine by liquid chromatography (*2.2.29*).

Test solution. Dissolve 0.200 g of the substance to be examined in the mobile phase and dilute to 100 ml with the mobile phase.

Reference solution (a). Dissolve 15 mg of *chlorhexidine for performance test CRS* in the mobile phase and dilute to 10.0 ml with the mobile phase.

Reference solution (b). Dilute 2.5 ml of the test solution to 100 ml with the mobile phase.

Reference solution (c). Dilute 2.0 ml of reference solution (b) to 10 ml with the mobile phase. Dilute 1.0 ml of the solution to 10 ml with the mobile phase.

The chromatographic procedure may be carried out using:

- a stainless steel column 0.2 m long and 4 mm in internal diameter, packed with *octadecylsilyl silica gel for chromatography R* (5 μm),
- as mobile phase at a flow rate of 1.0 ml/min, a solution of 2.0 g of *sodium octanesulphonate R* in a mixture of 120 ml of *glacial acetic acid R*, 270 ml of *water R* and 730 ml of *methanol R*,
- as detector a spectrophotometer set at 254 nm.

Equilibrate the column with the mobile phase for at least 1 h. Adjust the sensitivity of the system so that the height of the principal peak in the chromatogram obtained with 10 μl of reference solution (b) is at least 50 per cent of the full scale of the recorder.

Inject 10 μl of reference solution (a). The test is not valid unless the resulting chromatogram is similar to the specimen chromatogram provided with *chlorhexidine for performance test CRS* in that the peaks due to impurity A and impurity B precede that due to chlorhexidine. If necessary, adjust the concentration of acetic acid in the mobile phase (increasing the concentration decreases the retention times).

Inject 10 μl of the test solution and 10 μl each of reference solutions (b) and (c). Record the chromatograms of reference solutions (b) and (c) until the peak due to chlorhexidine is eluted and record the chromatogram of the test solution for six times the retention time of the peak due to chlorhexidine. In the chromatogram obtained with the test solution, the sum of the areas of the peaks, apart from the principal peak, is not greater than the area of the principal peak in the chromatogram obtained with reference solution (b) (2.5 per cent). Disregard any peak with a relative retention time of 0.25 or less, with respect to chlorhexidine, and any peak with an area less than that of the principal peak in the chromatogram obtained with reference solution (c).

Loss on drying (*2.2.32*). Not more than 1.0 per cent, determined on 1.000 g by drying in an oven at 100-105 °C.

Sulphated ash (*2.4.14*). Not more than 0.1 per cent, determined on 1.0 g.

ASSAY

Dissolve 100.0 mg in 5 ml of *anhydrous formic acid R* and add 70 ml of *acetic anhydride R*. Titrate with *0.1 M perchloric acid*, determining the end-point potentiometrically (*2.2.20*).

1 ml of *0.1 M perchloric acid* is equivalent to 14.46 mg of $C_{22}H_{32}Cl_4N_{10}$.

IMPURITIES

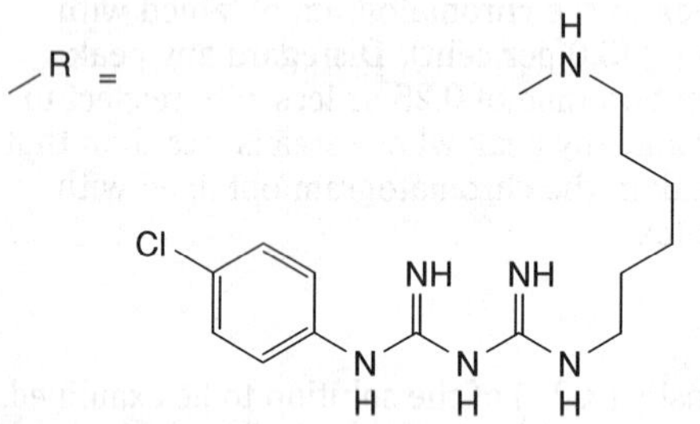

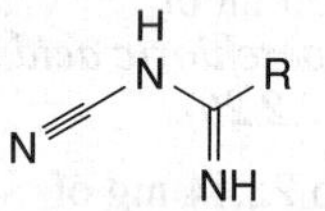

A. 1-(4-chlorophenyl)-5-[6-(3-cyanoguanidino)hexyl]biguanide,

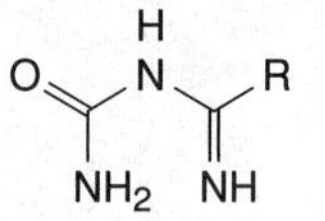

B. [[[6-[5-(4-chlorophenyl)guanidino]hexyl]amino]iminomethyl]urea,

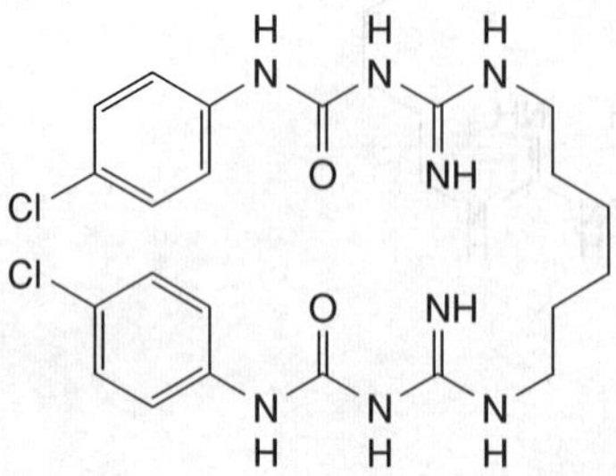

C. 1,1′-[hexane-1,6-diylbis[imino(iminocarbonyl)]]bis[3-(4-chlorophenyl)urea],

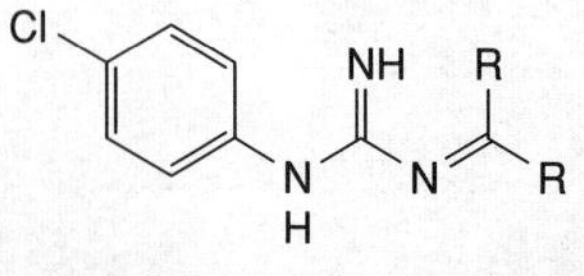

D. 1,1′-[[[[(4-chlorophenyl)amino]iminomethyl]imino]methylene]bis[imino(hexane-1,6-diyl)]]bis[5-(4-chlorophenyl)biguanide].

01/2005:0382

CHLOROBUTANOL, ANHYDROUS

Chlorobutanolum anhydricum

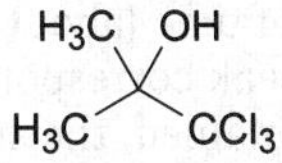

$C_4H_7Cl_3O$ M_r 177.5

DEFINITION

Anhydrous chlorobutanol contains not less than 98.0 per cent and not more than the equivalent of 101.0 per cent of 1,1,1-trichloro-2-methylpropan-2-ol, calculated with reference to the anhydrous substance.

CHARACTERS

A white, crystalline powder or colourless crystals, sublimes readily, slightly soluble in water, very soluble in alcohol, soluble in glycerol (85 per cent).

It melts at about 95 °C, determined without previous drying.

IDENTIFICATION

A. Add about 20 mg to a mixture of 1 ml of *pyridine R* and 2 ml of *strong sodium hydroxide solution R*. Heat in a water-bath and shake. Allow to stand. The pyridine layer becomes red.

B. Add about 20 mg to 5 ml of *ammoniacal silver nitrate solution R* and warm slightly. A black precipitate is formed.

C. To about 20 mg add 3 ml of *1 M sodium hydroxide* and shake to dissolve. Add 5 ml of *water R* and then, slowly, 2 ml of *iodinated potassium iodide solution R*. A yellowish precipitate is formed.

D. It complies with the test for water (see Tests).

TESTS

Solution S. Dissolve 5 g in *alcohol R* and dilute to 10 ml with the same solvent.

Appearance of solution. Solution S is not more opalescent than reference suspension II (*2.2.1*) and not more intensely coloured than reference solution BY_5 (*2.2.2, Method II*).

Acidity. To 4 ml of solution S add 15 ml of *alcohol R* and 0.1 ml of *bromothymol blue solution R1*. Not more than 1.0 ml of *0.01 M sodium hydroxide* is required to change the colour of the indicator to blue.

Chlorides (*2.4.4*). Dissolve 0.17 g in 5 ml of *alcohol R* and dilute to 15 ml with *water R*. The solution complies with the limit test for chlorides (300 ppm). When preparing the standard, replace the 5 ml of *water R* by 5 ml of *alcohol R*.

Water (*2.5.12*). Not more than 1.0 per cent, determined on 2.00 g by the semi-micro determination of water.

Sulphated ash (*2.4.14*). Not more than 0.1 per cent, determined on 1.0 g.

ASSAY

Dissolve 0.100 g in 20 ml of *alcohol R*. Add 10 ml of *dilute sodium hydroxide solution R*, heat in a water-bath for 5 min and cool. Add 20 ml of *dilute nitric acid R*, 25.0 ml of *0.1 M silver nitrate* and 2 ml of *dibutyl phthalate R* and shake vigorously. Add 2 ml of *ferric ammonium sulphate solution R2* and titrate with *0.1 M ammonium thiocyanate* until an orange colour is obtained.

1 ml of *0.1 M silver nitrate* is equivalent to 5.92 mg of $C_4H_7Cl_3O$.

STORAGE

In an airtight container.

01/2005:0383

CHLOROBUTANOL HEMIHYDRATE

Chlorobutanolum hemihydricum

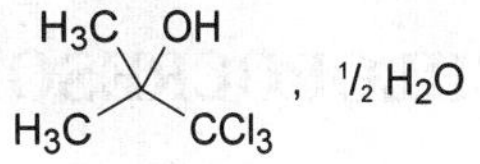

$C_4H_7Cl_3O,{}^1/_2H_2O$ M_r 186.5

DEFINITION

Chlorobutanol hemihydrate contains not less than 98.0 per cent and not more than the equivalent of 101.0 per cent of 1,1,1-trichloro-2-methylpropan-2-ol, calculated with reference to the anhydrous substance.

CHARACTERS

A white, crystalline powder or colourless crystals, sublimes readily, slightly soluble in water, very soluble in alcohol, soluble in glycerol (85 per cent).

It melts at about 78 °C, determined without previous drying.

IDENTIFICATION

A. Add about 20 mg to a mixture of 1 ml of *pyridine R* and 2 ml of *strong sodium hydroxide solution R*. Heat in a water-bath and shake. Allow to stand. The pyridine layer becomes red.

B. Add about 20 mg to 5 ml of *ammoniacal silver nitrate solution R* and warm slightly. A black precipitate is formed.

C. To about 20 mg add 3 ml of *1 M sodium hydroxide* and shake to dissolve. Add 5 ml of *water R* and then, slowly, 2 ml of *iodinated potassium iodide solution R*. A yellowish precipitate is formed.

D. It complies with the test for water (see Tests).

TESTS

Solution S. Dissolve 5 g in *alcohol R* and dilute to 10 ml with the same solvent.

Appearance of solution. Solution S is not more opalescent than reference suspension II (*2.2.1*) and not more intensely coloured than reference solution BY_5 (*2.2.2, Method II*).

Acidity. To 4 ml of solution S add 15 ml of *alcohol R* and 0.1 ml of *bromothymol blue solution R1*. Not more than 1.0 ml of *0.01 M sodium hydroxide* is required to change the colour of the indicator to blue.

Chlorides (*2.4.4*). To 1 ml of solution S add 4 ml of *alcohol R* and dilute to 15 ml with *water R*. The solution complies with the limit test for chlorides (100 ppm). When preparing the standard, replace the 5 ml of *water R* by 5 ml of *alcohol R*.

Water (*2.5.12*). 4.5 per cent to 5.5 per cent, determined on 0.300 g by the semi-micro determination of water.

Sulphated ash (*2.4.14*). Not more than 0.1 per cent, determined on 1.0 g.

ASSAY

Dissolve 0.100 g in 20 ml of *alcohol R*. Add 10 ml of *dilute sodium hydroxide solution R*, heat in a water-bath for 5 min and cool. Add 20 ml of *dilute nitric acid R*, 25.0 ml of *0.1 M silver nitrate* and 2 ml of *dibutyl phthalate R* and shake vigorously. Add 2 ml of *ferric ammonium sulphate solution R2* and titrate with *0.1 M ammonium thiocyanate* until an orange colour is obtained.

1 ml of *0.1 M silver nitrate* is equivalent to 5.92 mg of $C_4H_7Cl_3O$.

STORAGE

In an airtight container.

01/2005:0384

CHLOROCRESOL

Chlorocresolum

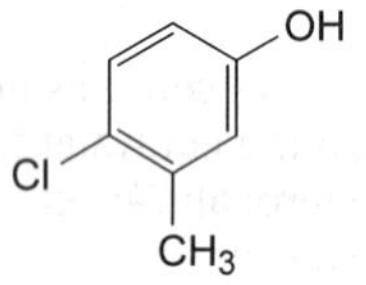

C_7H_7ClO M_r 142.6

DEFINITION

Chlorocresol contains not less than 98.0 per cent and not more than the equivalent of 101.0 per cent of 4-chloro-3-methylphenol.

CHARACTERS

A white or almost white, crystalline powder or compacted crystalline masses supplied as pellets or colourless or white crystals, slightly soluble in water, very soluble in alcohol, freely soluble in fatty oils. It dissolves in solutions of alkali hydroxides.

IDENTIFICATION

A. Melting point (*2.2.14*): 64 °C to 67 °C.

B. To 0.1 g add 0.2 ml of *benzoyl chloride R* and 0.5 ml of *dilute sodium hydroxide solution R*. Shake vigorously until a white, crystalline precipitate is formed. Add 5 ml of *water R* and filter. The precipitate, recrystallised from 5 ml of *methanol R* and dried at 70 °C, melts (*2.2.14*) at 85 °C to 88 °C.

C. To 5 ml of solution S (see Tests) add 0.1 ml of *ferric chloride solution R1*. A bluish colour is produced.

TESTS

Solution S. To 3.0 g, finely powdered, add 60 ml of *carbon dioxide-free water R*, shake for 2 min and filter.

Appearance of solution. Dissolve 1.25 g in *alcohol R* and dilute to 25 ml with the same solvent. The solution is clear (*2.2.1*) and not more intensely coloured than reference solution BY_6 (*2.2.2, Method II*).

Acidity. To 10 ml of solution S add 0.1 ml of *methyl red solution R*. The solution is orange or red. Not more than 0.2 ml of *0.01 M sodium hydroxide* is required to produce a pure yellow colour.

Related substances. Examine by gas chromatography (*2.2.28*).

Test solution. Dissolve 1.0 g of the substance to be examined in *acetone R* and dilute to 100 ml with the same solvent.

The chromatographic procedure may be carried out using:

– a glass column 1.80 m long and 3 mm to 4 mm in internal diameter packed with *silanised diatomaceous earth for gas chromatography R* impregnated with 3 per cent *m/m* to 5 per cent *m/m* of *polymethylphenylsiloxane R*,

– *nitrogen for chromatography R* as the carrier gas at a flow rate of 30 ml/min,

– a flame-ionisation detector,

maintaining the temperature of the column at 125 °C, that of the injection port at 210 °C and that of the detector at 230 °C. Continue the chromatography for three times the period of time (about 8 min) required for the appearance of the peak corresponding to chlorocresol. In the chromatogram obtained, the sum of the areas of the peaks apart from that corresponding to chlorocresol does not exceed 1 per cent of the total area of the peaks. Disregard the peak corresponding to the solvent.

Non-volatile matter. Evaporate 2.0 g to dryness on a water-bath and dry the residue at 100 °C to 105 °C. The residue weighs not more than 2 mg (0.1 per cent).

ASSAY

In a ground-glass-stoppered flask, dissolve 70.0 mg in 30 ml of *glacial acetic acid R*. Add 25.0 ml of *0.0167 M potassium bromate*, 20 ml of a 150 g/l solution of *potassium bromide R* and 10 ml of *hydrochloric acid R*. Allow to stand protected from light for 15 min. Add 1 g of *potassium iodide R* and 100 ml of *water R*. Titrate with *0.1 M sodium thiosulphate*, shaking vigorously and using 1 ml of *starch solution R*, added towards the end of the titration, as indicator. Carry out a blank titration.

1 ml of *0.0167 M potassium bromate* is equivalent to 3.565 mg of C_7H_7ClO.

STORAGE

Store protected from light.

01/2005:0544

CHLOROQUINE PHOSPHATE

Chloroquini phosphas

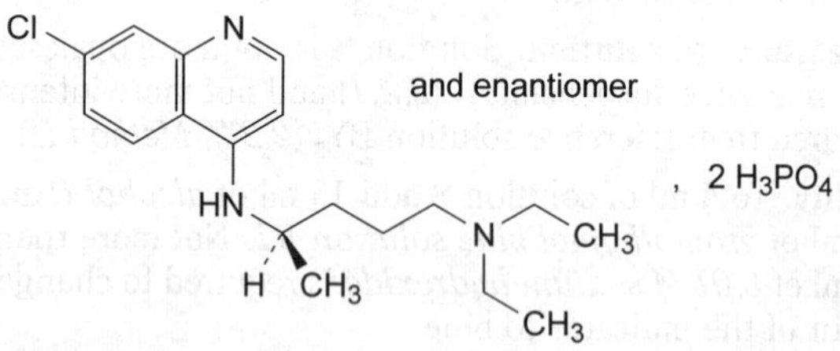

$C_{18}H_{32}ClN_3O_8P_2$ M_r 515.9

DEFINITION

Chloroquine phosphate contains not less than 98.5 per cent and not more than the equivalent of 101.0 per cent of N^4-(7-chloroquinolin-4-yl)-N^1,N^1-diethylpentane-1,4-diamine bis(dihydrogen phosphate), calculated with reference to the dried substance.

CHARACTERS

A white or almost white, crystalline powder, hygroscopic, freely soluble in water, very slightly soluble in alcohol and in methanol.

It exists in 2 forms, one of which melts at about 195 °C and the other at about 218 °C.

IDENTIFICATION

First identification: B, D.

Second identification: A, C, D.

A. Dissolve 0.100 g in *water R* and dilute to 100.0 ml with the same solvent. Dilute 1.0 ml of this solution to 100.0 ml with *water R*. Examined between 210 nm and 370 nm (*2.2.25*), the solution shows absorption maxima at 220 nm, 235 nm, 256 nm, 329 nm and 342 nm. The specific absorbances at the maxima are respectively 600 to 660, 350 to 390, 300 to 330, 325 to 355 and 360 to 390.

B. Examine by infrared absorption spectrophotometry (*2.2.24*), comparing with the spectrum obtained with the base isolated from *chloroquine sulphate CRS*. Record the spectra using solutions prepared as follows: dissolve separately 0.1 g of the substance to be examined and 80 mg of the reference substance in 10 ml of *water R*, add 2 ml of *dilute sodium hydroxide solution R* and shake with 2 quantities, each of 20 ml, of *methylene chloride R*; combine the organic layers, wash with *water R*, dry over *anhydrous sodium sulphate R*, evaporate to dryness and dissolve the residues separately, each in 2 ml of *methylene chloride R*.

C. Dissolve 25 mg in 20 ml of *water R* and add 8 ml of *picric acid solution R1*. The precipitate, washed with *water R*, with *alcohol R* and finally with *methylene chloride R*, melts (*2.2.14*) at 206-209 °C.

D. Dissolve 0.1 g in 10 ml of *water R*, add 2 ml of *dilute sodium hydroxide solution R* and shake with 2 quantities, each of 20 ml, of *methylene chloride R*. The aqueous layer, acidified by the addition of *nitric acid R*, gives reaction (b) of phosphates (*2.3.1*).

TESTS

Solution S. Dissolve 2.5 g in *carbon dioxide-free water R* and dilute to 25 ml with the same solvent.

Appearance of solution. Solution S is clear (*2.2.1*) and not more intensely coloured than reference solution BY_5 or GY_5 (*2.2.2, Method II*).

pH (*2.2.3*). The pH of solution S is 3.8 to 4.3.

Related substances. Examine by thin-layer chromatography (*2.2.27*), using *silica gel GF_{254} R* as the coating substance.

Test solution. Dissolve 0.50 g of the substance to be examined in *water R* and dilute to 10 ml with the same solvent.

Reference solution (a). Dilute 1 ml of the test solution to 100 ml with *water R*.

Reference solution (b). Dilute 5 ml of reference solution (a) to 10 ml with *water R*.

Apply to the plate 2 µl of each solution. Develop over a path of 12 cm using a mixture of 10 volumes of *diethylamine R*, 40 volumes of *cyclohexane R* and 50 volumes of *chloroform R*. Allow the plate to dry in air. Examine in ultraviolet light at 254 nm. Any spot in the chromatogram obtained with the test solution, apart from the principal spot, is not more intense than the spot in the chromatogram obtained with reference solution (a) (1.0 per cent) and not more than one such spot is more intense than the spot in the chromatogram obtained with reference solution (b) (0.5 per cent).

Heavy metals (*2.4.8*). Dissolve 2.0 gin 10 ml of *water R*. Add 5 ml of *concentrated ammonia R* and shake with 40 ml of *methylene chloride R*. Filter the aqueous layer and neutralise the filtrate with *glacial acetic acid R*. Heat on a water-bath to eliminate methylene chloride, allow to cool and dilute to 20.0 ml with *water R*. 12 ml of this solution complies with limit test A for heavy metals (20 ppm). Prepare the standard using *lead standard solution (2 ppm Pb) R*.

Loss on drying (*2.2.32*): maximum 2.0 per cent, determined on 1.000 g by drying in an oven at 100-105 °C.

ASSAY

Dissolve 0.200 g in 50 ml of *anhydrous acetic acid R*. Titrate with *0.1 M perchloric acid* determining the end-point potentiometrically (*2.2.20*).

1 ml of *0.1 M perchloric acid* is equivalent to 25.79 mg of $C_{18}H_{32}ClN_3O_8P_2$.

STORAGE

In an airtight container, protected from light.

01/2005:0545

CHLOROQUINE SULPHATE

Chloroquini sulfas

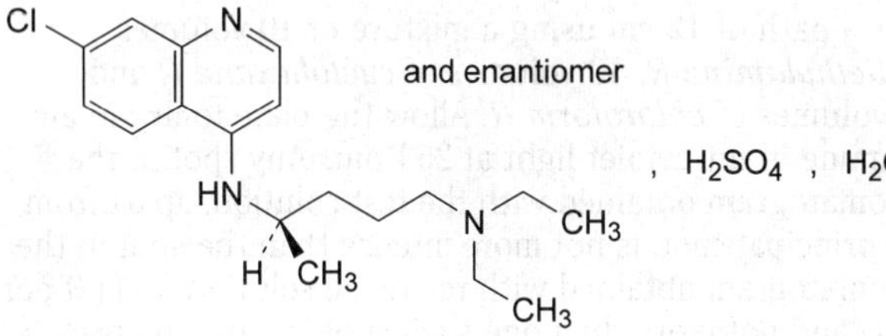

$C_{18}H_{28}ClN_3O_4S,H_2O$ M_r 436.0

DEFINITION

Chloroquine sulphate contains not less than 98.5 per cent and not more than the equivalent of 101.0 per cent of N^4-(7-chloroquinolin-4-yl)-N^1,N^1-diethylpentane-1,4-diamine sulphate, calculated with reference to the anhydrous substance.

CHARACTERS

A white or almost white, crystalline powder, freely soluble in water and in methanol, very slightly soluble in alcohol.

It melts at about 208 °C (instantaneous method).

IDENTIFICATION

First identification: B, D.

Second identification: A, C, D.

A. Dissolve 0.100 g in *water R* and dilute to 100.0 ml with the same solvent. Dilute 1.0 ml of this solution to 100.0 ml with *water R*. Examined between 210 nm and 370 nm (*2.2.25*), the solution shows absorption maxima at 220 nm, 235 nm, 256 nm, 329 nm and 342 nm. The specific absorbances at the maxima are respectively 730 to 810, 430 to 470, 370 to 410, 400 to 440 and 430 to 470.

B. Examine by infrared absorption spectrophotometry (*2.2.24*), comparing with the spectrum obtained with the base isolated from *chloroquine sulphate CRS*. Record the spectra using solutions prepared as follows: dissolve separately 0.1 g of the substance to be examined and of the reference substance in 10 ml of *water R*, add 2 ml of *dilute sodium hydroxide solution R* and shake with two quantities, each of 20 ml, of *chloroform R*; combine the chloroform layers, wash with *water R*, dry over *anhydrous sodium sulphate R*, evaporate to dryness and dissolve the residues separately each in 2 ml of *chloroform R*.

C. Dissolve 25 mg in 20 ml of *water R* and add 8 ml of *picric acid solution R1*. The precipitate, washed with *water R*, with *alcohol R* and finally with *ether R*, melts (*2.2.14*) at 206 °C to 209 °C.

D. It gives reaction (a) of sulphates (*2.3.1*).

Monographs C

TESTS

Solution S. Dissolve 2.0 g in *carbon dioxide-free water R* and dilute to 25 ml with the same solvent.

Appearance of solution. Solution S is clear (*2.2.1*) and not more intensely coloured than reference solution BY_5 or GY_5 (*2.2.2, Method II*).

pH (*2.2.3*). The pH of solution S is 4.0 to 5.0.

Related substances. Examine by thin-layer chromatography (*2.2.27*), using *silica gel GF_{254} R* as the coating substance.

Test solution. Dissolve 0.50 g of the substance to be examined in *water R* and dilute to 10 ml with the same solvent.

Reference solution (a). Dilute 1 ml of the test solution to 100 ml with *water R*.

Reference solution (b). Dilute 5 ml of reference solution (a) to 10 ml with *water R*.

Apply separately to the plate 2 µl of each solution. Develop over a path of 12 cm using a mixture of 10 volumes of *diethylamine R*, 40 volumes of *cyclohexane R* and 50 volumes of *chloroform R*. Allow the plate to dry in air. Examine in ultraviolet light at 254 nm. Any spot in the chromatogram obtained with the test solution, apart from the principal spot, is not more intense than the spot in the chromatogram obtained with reference solution (a) (1.0 per cent) and not more than one such spot is more intense than the spot in the chromatogram obtained with reference solution (b) (0.5 per cent).

Heavy metals (*2.4.8*). Dissolve 2.0 g in 10 ml of *water R*. Add 5 ml of *concentrated ammonia R* and shake with 40 ml of *ether R*. Filter the aqueous layer and neutralise the filtrate with *glacial acetic acid R*. Heat on a water-bath to eliminate ether, allow to cool and dilute to 20.0 ml with *water R*. 12 ml of this solution complies with limit test A for heavy metals (20 ppm). Prepare the standard using *lead standard solution (2 ppm Pb) R*.

Water (*2.5.12*): 3.0 per cent to 5.0 per cent, determined on 0.500 g by the semi-micro determination of water.

Sulphated ash (*2.4.14*). Not more than 0.1 per cent, determined on 1.0 g.

ASSAY

Dissolve 0.400 g in 50 ml of *anhydrous acetic acid R*. Titrate with *0.1 M perchloric acid* determining the end-point potentiometrically (*2.2.20*).

1 ml of *0.1 M perchloric acid* is equivalent to 41.8 mg of $C_{18}H_{28}ClN_3O_4S$.

STORAGE

Store in an airtight container, protected from light.

01/2005:0385

CHLOROTHIAZIDE

Chlorothiazidum

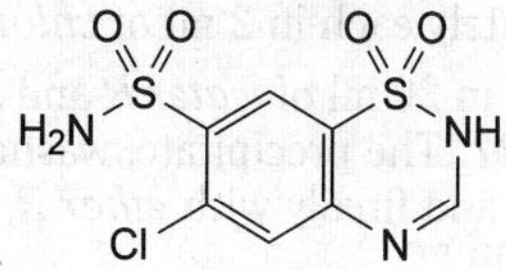

$C_7H_6ClN_3O_4S_2$ M_r 295.7

DEFINITION

Chlorothiazide contains not less than 98.0 per cent and not more than the equivalent of 102.0 per cent of 6-chloro-2*H*-1,2,4-benzothiadiazine-7-sulphonamide 1,1-dioxide, calculated with reference to the dried substance.

CHARACTERS

A white or almost white, crystalline powder, very slightly soluble in water, sparingly soluble in acetone, slightly soluble in alcohol. It dissolves in dilute solutions of alkali hydroxides.

IDENTIFICATION

First identification: B, C.

Second identification: A, C, D.

A. Dissolve 80.0 mg in 100 ml of *0.1 M sodium hydroxide* and dilute to 1000.0 ml with *water R*. Dilute 10.0 ml of the solution to 100.0 ml with *0.01 M sodium hydroxide*. Examined between 220 nm and 320 nm (*2.2.25*), the solution shows 2 absorption maxima, at 225 nm and 292 nm, and a shoulder at about 310 nm. The specific absorbances at the maxima are 725 to 800 and 425 to 455, respectively.

B. Examine by infrared absorption spectrophotometry (*2.2.24*), comparing with the spectrum obtained with *chlorothiazide CRS*.

C. Examine by thin-layer chromatography (*2.2.27*), using *silica gel GF_{254} R* as the coating substance.

Test solution. Dissolve 25 mg of the substance to be examined in *acetone R* and dilute to 5 ml with the same solvent.

Reference solution. Dissolve 25 mg of *chlorothiazide CRS* in *acetone R* and dilute to 5 ml with the same solvent.

Apply to the plate 2 µl of each solution. Develop over a path of 10 cm using *ethyl acetate R*. Dry the plate in a current of air and examine in ultraviolet light at 254 nm. The principal spot in the chromatogram obtained with the test solution is similar in position and size to the principal spot in the chromatogram obtained with the reference solution.

D. To 0.1 g add a pellet of *sodium hydroxide R* and heat strongly. Gas is evolved which turns *red litmus paper R* blue. After cooling, take up the residue with 10 ml of *dilute hydrochloric acid R*. Gas is evolved which turns *lead acetate paper R* black.

TESTS

Solution S. To 1.0 g of the powdered substance to be examined add 50 ml of *water R*, shake for 2 min and filter.

Acidity or alkalinity. To 10 ml of solution S add 0.2 ml of *0.01 M sodium hydroxide* and 0.15 ml of *methyl red solution R*. The solution is yellow. Not more than 0.4 ml of *0.01 M hydrochloric acid* is required to change the colour of the indicator to red.

Related substances. Examine by thin-layer chromatography (*2.2.27*), using *silica gel G R* as the coating substance.

Test solution. Dissolve 25 mg of the substance to be examined in *acetone R* and dilute to 5 ml with the same solvent.

Reference solution. Dilute 1 ml of the test solution to 100 ml with *acetone R*.

Apply to the plate 5 µl of each solution. Develop over a path of 15 cm using a mixture of 15 volumes of *2-propanol R* and 85 volumes of *ethyl acetate R*. Dry the plate in a current of air until the solvents have evaporated (about 10 min) and spray with a mixture of equal volumes of *alcoholic solution of sulphuric acid R* and *alcohol R*; use about 10 ml for a plate 200 mm square and spray in small portions, allowing the solvent to evaporate each time to avoid excessive wetting. Heat at 100-105 °C for 30 min and immediately place the plate above, but not in contact with, 10 ml of a saturated solution of *sodium nitrite R* in a glass tank. Carefully add 0.5 ml of *sulphuric acid R* to the sodium nitrite solution, close the tank, and allow to stand for 15 min. Remove the plate, heat in a ventilated oven at 40 °C for 15 min and spray with 3 quantities, each of 5 ml, of a freshly prepared 5 g/l solution of *naphthylethylenediamine dihydrochloride R* in *alcohol R*. Examine the plate by transmitted light. Any spot in the chromatogram obtained with the test solution, apart from the principal spot, is not more intense than the spot in the chromatogram obtained with the reference solution (1.0 per cent).

Chlorides (*2.4.4*). 15 ml of solution S complies with the limit test for chlorides (160 ppm).

Heavy metals (*2.4.8*). 1.0 g complies with limit test C for heavy metals (20 ppm). Prepare the standard using 2 ml of *lead standard solution (10 ppm Pb) R*.

Loss on drying (*2.2.32*). Not more than 1.0 per cent, determined on 1.000 g by drying in an oven at 100-105 °C.

Sulphated ash (*2.4.14*). Not more than 0.1 per cent, determined on 1.0 g.

ASSAY

Dissolve 0.250 g in 50 ml of *dimethylformamide R*. Titrate with *0.1 M tetrabutylammonium hydroxide in 2-propanol* determining the end-point potentiometrically (*2.2.20*) at the first point of inflexion. Carry out a blank titration.

1 ml of *0.1 M tetrabutylammonium hydroxide in 2-propanol* is equivalent to 29.57 mg of $C_7H_6ClN_3O_4S_2$.

01/2005:0386

CHLORPHENAMINE MALEATE

Chlorphenamini maleas

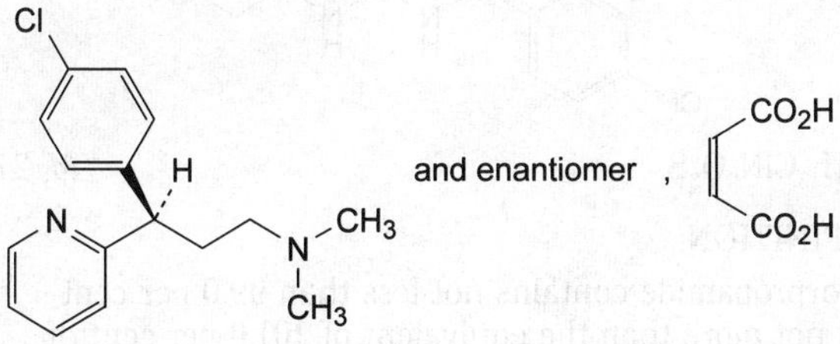

$C_{20}H_{23}ClN_2O_4$ M_r 390.9

DEFINITION

Chlorphenamine maleate contains not less than 98.0 per cent and not more than the equivalent of 101.0 per cent of (3*RS*)-3-(4-chlorophenyl)-*N*,*N*-dimethyl-3-(pyridin-2-yl)propan-1-amine hydrogen (*Z*)-butenedioate, calculated with reference to the dried substance.

CHARACTERS

A white, crystalline powder, freely soluble in water, soluble in alcohol.

IDENTIFICATION

First identification: A, C.

Second identification: A, B, D, E.

A. Melting point (*2.2.14*): 132 °C to 135 °C.

B. Dissolve 30.0 mg in *0.1 M hydrochloric acid* and dilute to 100.0 ml with the same acid. Dilute 10.0 ml of this solution to 100.0 ml with *0.1 M hydrochloric acid*. Examined between 230 nm and 350 nm (*2.2.25*), the solution shows an absorption maximum at 265 nm. The specific absorbance at the maximum is 200 to 220.

C. Examine by infrared absorption spectrophotometry (*2.2.24*), comparing with the spectrum obtained with *chlorphenamine maleate CRS*. Examine the substances prepared as discs.

D. Dissolve 0.1 g in 10 ml of *water R* and add dropwise and with shaking 25 ml of *picric acid solution R*. Collect the precipitate on a sintered-glass filter. The precipitate, washed with 3 ml of *alcohol R*, recrystallised from a mixture of equal volumes of *alcohol R* and *water R* and dried at 100 °C to 105 °C, melts (*2.2.14*) at 196 °C to 200 °C.

E. To 0.2 g add 3 ml of *water R* and 1 ml of *strong sodium hydroxide solution R*. Shake with three quantities, each of 5 ml, of *ether R*. To 0.1 ml of the aqueous layer add a solution of 10 mg of *resorcinol R* in 3 ml of *sulphuric acid R*. Heat on a water-bath for 15 min. No colour develops. To the remainder of the aqueous layer add 2 ml of *bromine solution R*. Heat in a water-bath for 15 min, heat to boiling and cool. To 0.2 ml of the solution add a solution of 10 mg of *resorcinol R* in 3 ml of *sulphuric acid R* and heat on a water-bath for 15 min. A blue colour develops.

TESTS

Solution S. Dissolve 2.0 g in *water R* and dilute to 20 ml with the same solvent.

Appearance of solution. Solution S is clear (*2.2.1*) and not more intensely coloured than reference solution BY_6 (*2.2.2, Method II*).

Related substances. Examine by thin-layer chromatography (*2.2.27*), using *silica gel GF_{254} R* as the coating substance.

Test solution. Dissolve 0.5 g of the substance to be examined in *chloroform R* and dilute to 10 ml with the same solvent.

Reference solution. Dilute 1 ml of the test solution to 50 ml with *chloroform R*. Dilute 1 ml of this solution to 10 ml with *chloroform R*.

Apply to the plate 10 µl of each solution. Develop over a path of 12 cm using a mixture of 10 volumes of *diethylamine R*, 40 volumes of *chloroform R* and 50 volumes of *cyclohexane R*. Allow the plate to dry in air and examine in ultraviolet light at 254 nm. Any spot in the chromatogram obtained with the test solution, apart from the principal spot, is not more intense than the spot in the chromatogram obtained with the reference solution (0.2 per cent). Disregard any spots remaining on the starting-line.

Heavy metals (*2.4.8*). 1.0 g complies with limit test C for heavy metals (20 ppm). Prepare the standard using 2 ml of *lead standard solution (10 ppm Pb) R*.

Loss on drying (*2.2.32*). Not more than 0.5 per cent, determined on 1.00 g by drying in an oven at 100 °C to 105 °C for 4 h.

Sulphated ash (*2.4.14*). Not more than 0.1 per cent, determined on 1.0 g.

ASSAY

Dissolve 0.150 g in 25 ml of *anhydrous acetic acid R*. Titrate with *0.1 M perchloric acid* determining the end-point potentiometrically (*2.2.20*).

1 ml of *0.1 M perchloric acid* is equivalent to 19.54 mg of $C_{20}H_{23}ClN_2O_4$.

STORAGE

Store protected from light.

01/2005:0475

CHLORPROMAZINE HYDROCHLORIDE

Chlorpromazini hydrochloridum

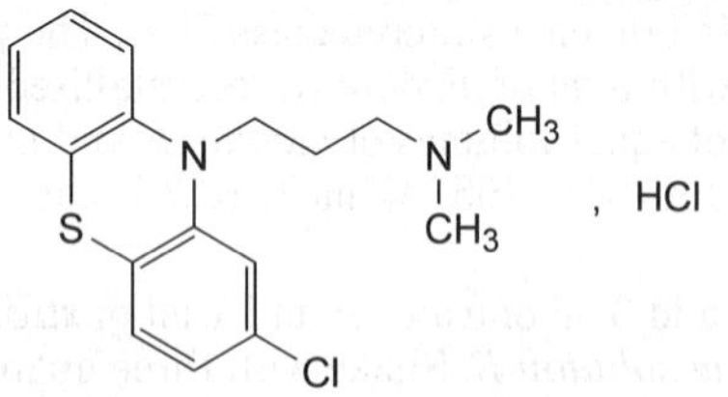

$C_{17}H_{20}Cl_2N_2S$ M_r 355.3

DEFINITION

Chlorpromazine hydrochloride contains not less than 99.0 per cent and not more than the equivalent of 101.0 per cent of 3-(2-chloro-10*H*-phenothiazin-10-yl)-*N*,*N*-dimethylpropan-1-amine hydrochloride, calculated with reference to the dried substance.

CHARACTERS

A white or almost white, crystalline powder, very soluble in water, freely soluble in alcohol. It decomposes on exposure to air and light.

It melts at about 196 °C.

IDENTIFICATION

First identification: B, C, D.

Second identification: A, C, D.

A. Prepare the solutions protected from bright light and measure the absorbances immediately. Dissolve 50.0 mg in *0.1 M hydrochloric acid* and dilute to 500.0 ml with the same acid. Dilute 5.0 ml of the solution to 100.0 ml with *0.1 M hydrochloric acid.* Examined between 230 nm and 340 nm (*2.2.25*), the solution shows two absorption maxima, at 254 nm and 306 nm respectively. The specific absorbance at the maximum at 254 nm is 890 to 960.

B. Examine by infrared absorption spectrophotometry (*2.2.24*), comparing with the spectrum obtained with *chlorpromazine hydrochloride CRS.* Examine the substances as 60 g/l solutions in *methylene chloride R* using a 0.1 mm cell.

C. It complies with the identification test for phenothiazines by thin-layer chromatography (*2.3.3*).

D. It gives reaction (b) of chlorides (*2.3.1*).

TESTS

pH (*2.2.3*). Dissolve 1.0 g in *carbon dioxide-free water R* and dilute to 10 ml with the same solvent. The pH of the freshly prepared solution is 3.5 to 4.5.

Related substances. *Carry out the test protected from bright light.*

Examine by thin-layer chromatography (*2.2.27*), using *silica gel GF_{254} R* as the coating substance.

Test solution. Dissolve 0.2 g of the substance to be examined in a mixture of 5 volumes of *diethylamine R* and 95 volumes of *methanol R* and dilute to 10 ml with the same mixture of solvents. Prepare immediately before use.

Reference solution. Dilute 1 ml of the test solution to 200 ml with a mixture of 5 volumes of *diethylamine R* and 95 volumes of *methanol R.*

Apply to the plate 10 µl of each solution. Develop over a path of 15 cm using a mixture of 10 volumes of *acetone R*, 10 volumes of *diethylamine R* and 80 volumes of *cyclohexane R.* Allow the plate to dry in air and examine in ultraviolet light at 254 nm. Any spot in the chromatogram obtained with the test solution, apart from the principal spot, is not more intense than the spot in the chromatogram obtained with the reference solution (0.5 per cent). Disregard any spot at the starting point.

Heavy metals (*2.4.8*). 1.0 g complies with limit test C for heavy metals (10 ppm). Prepare the standard using 1 ml of *lead standard solution (10 ppm Pb) R.*

Loss on drying (*2.2.32*). Not more than 0.5 per cent, determined on 1.000 g by drying in an oven at 100 °C to 105 °C.

Sulphated ash (*2.4.14*). Not more than 0.1 per cent, determined on 1.0 g.

ASSAY

Dissolve 0.250 g in a mixture of 5.0 ml of *0.01 M hydrochloric acid* and 50 ml of *alcohol R.* Carry out a potentiometric titration (*2.2.20*), using *0.1 M sodium hydroxide.* Read the volume of *0.1 M sodium hydroxide* added between the two points of inflexion.

1 ml of *0.1 M sodium hydroxide* is equivalent to 35.53 mg of $C_{17}H_{20}Cl_2N_2S$.

STORAGE

Store in an airtight container, protected from light.

01/2005:1087

CHLORPROPAMIDE

Chlorpropamidum

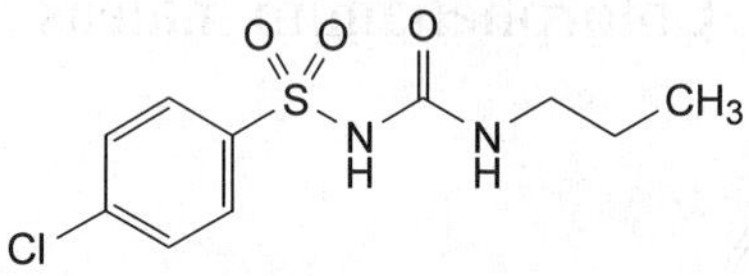

$C_{10}H_{13}ClN_2O_3S$ M_r 276.7

DEFINITION

Chlorpropamide contains not less than 99.0 per cent and not more than the equivalent of 101.0 per cent of 1-[(4-chlorophenyl)sulphonyl]-3-propylurea, calculated with reference to the dried substance.

CHARACTERS

A white, crystalline powder, practically insoluble in water, freely soluble in acetone and in methylene chloride, soluble in alcohol. It dissolves in dilute solutions of alkali hydroxides. It shows polymorphism.

IDENTIFICATION

First identification: C, D.

Second identification: A, B, D.

A. Melting point (*2.2.14*): 126 °C to 130 °C.

B. Dissolve 0.10 g in *methanol R* and dilute to 50.0 ml with the same solvent. Dilute 5.0 ml of the solution to 100.0 ml with *0.01 M hydrochloric acid.* Dilute 10.0 ml of the solution to 100.0 ml with *0.01 M hydrochloric acid*. Examined between 220 nm and 350 nm (*2.2.25*), the solution shows an absorption maximum at 232 nm. The specific absorption at the maximum is 570 to 630.

C. Examine by infrared absorption spectrophotometry (*2.2.24*), comparing with the spectrum obtained with *chlorpropamide CRS*. Examine the substances prepared as discs. If the spectra obtained show differences, dissolve the substance to be examined and the reference substance in *methylene chloride R*, evaporate to dryness and record the new spectra using the residues.

D. Heat 0.1 g with 2 g of *anhydrous sodium carbonate R* until a dull red colour appears for 10 min. Allow to cool, extract the residue with about 5 ml of *water R*, dilute to 10 ml with *water R* and filter. The solution gives the reaction (a) of chloride (*2.3.1*).

TESTS

Related substances. Examine by thin-layer chromatography (*2.2.27*), using a suitable silica gel as the coating substance.

Test solution. Dissolve 0.50 g of the substance to be examined in *acetone R* and dilute to 10 ml with the same solvent.

Reference solution (a). Dissolve 15 mg of *4-chlorobenzenesulphonamide R* (chlorpropamide impurity A) in *acetone R* and dilute to 100 ml with the same solvent.

Reference solution (b). Dissolve 15 mg of *chlorpropamide impurity B CRS* in *acetone R* and dilute to 100 ml with the same solvent.

Reference solution (c). Dilute 0.3 ml of the test solution to 100 ml with *acetone R*.

Reference solution (d). Dilute 5 ml of reference solution (c) to 15 ml with *acetone R*.

Reference solution (e). Dissolve 0.10 g of the substance to be examined, 5 mg of *4-chlorobenzenesulphonamide R* and 5 mg of *chlorpropamide impurity B CRS* in *acetone R* and dilute to 10 ml with the same solvent.

Apply to the plate 5 µl of each solution. Develop over a path of 15 cm using a mixture of 11.5 volumes of *concentrated ammonia R*, 30 volumes of *cyclohexane R*, 50 volumes of *methanol R* and 100 volumes of *methylene chloride R*. Allow the plate to dry in a current of cold air, heat at 110 °C for 10 min. At the bottom of a chromatographic tank, place an evaporating dish containing a mixture of 1 volume of *hydrochloric acid R*, 1 volume of *water R* and 2 volumes of a 50 g/l solution of *potassium permanganate R*, close the tank and allow to stand for 15 min. Place the dried hot plate in the tank and close the tank. Leave the plate in contact with the chlorine vapour for 2 min. Withdraw the plate and place it in a current of cold air until the excess of chlorine is removed and an area of coating below the points of application does not give a blue colour with a drop of *potassium iodide and starch solution R*. Spray with *potassium iodide and starch solution R*. In the chromatogram obtained with the test solution: any spot corresponding to impurity A is not more intense than the spot in the chromatogram obtained with reference solution (a) (0.3 per cent); any spot corresponding to impurity B is not more intense than the spot in the chromatogram obtained with reference solution (b) (0.3 per cent); any spot, apart from the principal spot and any spot corresponding to impurity A and B, is not more intense than the spot in the chromatogram obtained with reference solution (c) (0.3 per cent); not more than two such spots are more intense than the spot in the chromatogram obtained with reference solution (d) (0.1 per cent). The test is not valid unless the chromatogram obtained with reference solution (e) shows three clearly separated spots with approximate R_f values of 0.4, 0.6 and 0.9 corresponding to chlorpropamide, impurity A and impurity B respectively.

Heavy metals (*2.4.8*). Dissolve 2.0 g in a mixture of 15 volumes of *water R* and 85 volumes of *acetone R* and dilute to 20 ml with the same mixture of solvents. 12 ml of solution complies with limit test B for heavy metals (20 ppm). Prepare the standard using lead standard solution (2 ppm Pb) prepared by diluting *lead standard solution (100 ppm Pb) R* with a mixture of 15 volumes of *water R* and 85 volumes of *acetone R*.

Loss on drying (*2.2.32*). Not more than 0.5 per cent, determined on 1.000 g by drying in an oven at 100 °C to 105 °C.

Sulphated ash (*2.4.14*). Not more than 0.1 per cent, determined on 1.0 g.

ASSAY

Dissolve 0.250 g in 50 ml of *alcohol R* previously neutralised using *phenolphthalein solution R1* as indicator and add 25 ml of *water R*. Titrate with *0.1 M sodium hydroxide* until a pink colour is obtained.

1 ml of *0.1 M sodium hydroxide* is equivalent to 27.67 mg of $C_{10}H_{13}ClN_2O_3S$.

STORAGE

Store protected from light.

IMPURITIES

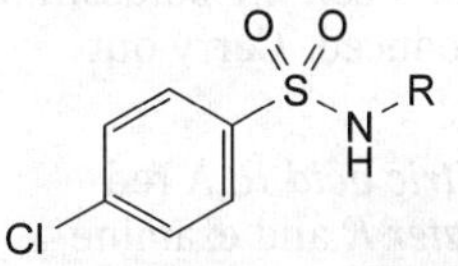

A. R = H: 4-chlorobenzenesulphonamide,

C. R = CO-NH_2: [(4-chlorophenyl)sulphonyl]urea.

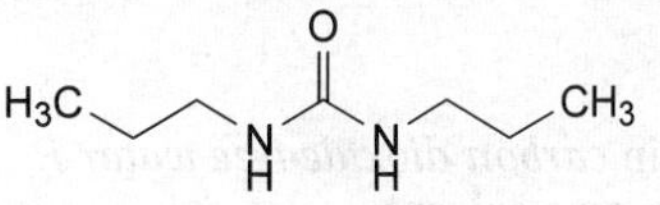

B. 1,3-dipropylurea,

01/2005:0815

CHLORPROTHIXENE HYDROCHLORIDE

Chlorprothixeni hydrochloridum

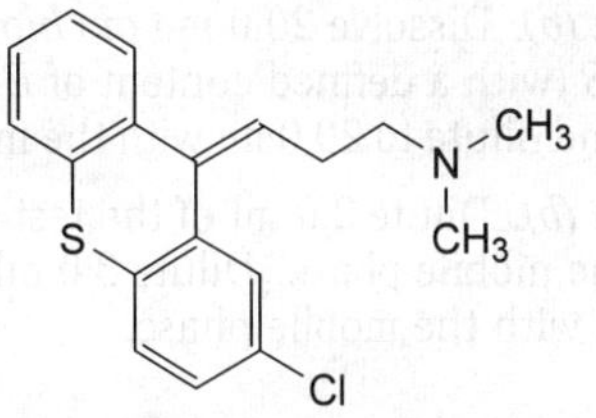

$C_{18}H_{19}Cl_2NS$ M_r 352.3

DEFINITION

(*Z*)-3-(2-Chloro-9*H*-thioxanthen-9-ylidene)-*N*,*N*-dimethylpropan-1-amine hydrochloride.

Content: 99.0 per cent to 101.0 per cent (dried substance).

CHARACTERS

Appearance: white or almost white, crystalline powder.

Solubility: soluble in water and in alcohol, slightly soluble in methylene chloride.

mp: about 220 °C.

IDENTIFICATION

First identification: A, E.

Second identification: B, C, D, E.

A. Infrared absorption spectrophotometry (*2.2.24*).
   Preparation: dissolve 0.25 g in 10 ml of *water R*. Add 1 ml of *dilute sodium hydroxide solution R*. Shake with 20 ml of *methylene chloride R*. Separate the organic layer and wash with 5 ml of *water R*. Evaporate the organic layer to dryness and dry the residue at 40-50 °C. Examine the residues prepared as discs.
   Comparison: *chlorprothixene hydrochloride CRS*.

B. Dissolve 0.2 g in a mixture of 5 ml of *dioxan R* and 5 ml of a 1.5 g/l solution of *sodium nitrite R*. Add 0.8 ml of *nitric acid R*. After 10 min add the solution to 20 ml of *water R*. 1 h later filter the precipate formed. The filtrate is used immediately for identification test C. Dissolve the precipitate by warming in about 15 ml of *alcohol R* and add the solution to 10 ml of *water R*. Filter and dry the precipitate at 100-105 °C for 2 h. The melting point (*2.2.14*) is 152 °C to 154 °C.

C. To 1 ml of the filtrate obtained in identification test B, add 0.2 ml of a suspension of 50 mg of *fast red B salt R* in 1 ml of *alcohol R*. Add 1 ml of *0.5 M alcoholic potassium hydroxide*. A dark red colour is produced. Carry out a blank test.

D. Dissolve about 20 mg in 2 ml of *nitric acid R*. A red colour is produced. Add 5 ml of *water R* and examine in ultraviolet light at 365 nm. The solution shows green fluorescence.

E. It gives reaction (a) of chlorides (*2.3.1*).

TESTS

Solution S. Dissolve 0.25 g in *carbon dioxide-free water R* and dilute to 25 ml with the same solvent.

Appearance of solution. Solution S is clear (*2.2.1*) and colourless (*2.2.2, Method II*).

pH (*2.2.3*): 4.4 to 5.2 for solution S.

Related substances. Liquid chromatography (*2.2.29*). *Carry out the test protected from bright light.*

Test solution. Dissolve 20.0 mg of the substance to be examined in the mobile phase and dilute to 20.0 ml with the mobile phase.

Reference solution (a). Dissolve 20.0 mg of *chlorprothixene hydrochloride CRS* (with a defined content of *E*-isomer) in the mobile phase and dilute to 20.0 ml with the mobile phase.

Reference solution (b). Dilute 2.0 ml of the test solution to 100.0 ml with the mobile phase. Dilute 3.0 ml of this solution to 20.0 ml with the mobile phase.

Column:

- *size*: *l* = 0.12 m, Ø = 4.0 mm,
- *stationary phase*: *base-deactivated octadecylsilyl silica gel for chromatography R* (3 μm or 5 μm).

Mobile phase: solution containing 6.0 g/l of *potassium dihydrogen phosphate R*, 2.9 g/l of *sodium laurilsulfate R* and 9 g/l of *tetrabutylammonium bromide R* in a mixture of 50 volumes of *methanol R*, 400 volumes of *acetonitrile R* and 550 volumes of *distilled water R*.

Flow rate: 1.5 ml/min.

Detection: spectrophotometer at 254 nm.

Equilibration: for about 30 min with the mobile phase.

Injection: 20 μl.

Run time: twice the retention time of chlorprothixene.

Relative retention with reference to chlorprothixene: impurity E = about 1.55.

System suitability: reference solution (a):

- *retention time*: chlorprothixene = about 10 min,
- *relative retention* with reference to chlorprothixene: *E*-isomer = about 1.35.

Limits:

- *E-isomer*: not more than 2.0 per cent, calculated from the area of the corresponding peak in the chromatogram obtained with reference solution (a) and taking into account the assigned content of this isomer in *chlorprothixene hydrochloride CRS*,
- *impurity E*: not more than 3 times the area of the principal peak in the chromatogram obtained with reference solution (b) (0.3 per cent taking into account a response factor of 3),
- *any other impurity*: not more than the area of the principal peak in the chromatogram obtained with reference solution (b) (0.3 per cent),
- *total of any other impurity*: not more than 2.33 times the area of the principal peak in the chromatogram obtained with reference solution (b) (0.7 per cent),
- *disregard limit*: 0.1 times the area of the principal peak in the chromatogram obtained with reference solution (b) (0.03 per cent).

Heavy metals (*2.4.8*): maximum 20 ppm.

1.0 g complies with limit test F. Prepare the standard using 2 ml of *lead standard solution (10 ppm Pb) R*.

Loss on drying (*2.2.32*): maximum 0.5 per cent, determined on 1.000 g by drying *in vacuo* at 60 °C for 3 h.

Sulphated ash (*2.4.14*): maximum 0.1 per cent, determined on 1.0 g.

ASSAY

Dissolve 0.300 g in a mixture of 5.0 ml of *0.01 M hydrochloric acid* and 50 ml of *alcohol R*. Carry out a potentiometric titration (*2.2.20*), using *0.1 M sodium hydroxide*. Read the volume added between the 2 points of inflexion.

1 ml of *0.1 M sodium hydroxide* is equivalent to 35.23 mg of $C_{18}H_{19}Cl_2NS$.

STORAGE

Protected from light.

IMPURITIES

Specified impurities: A, B, C, D, E, F.

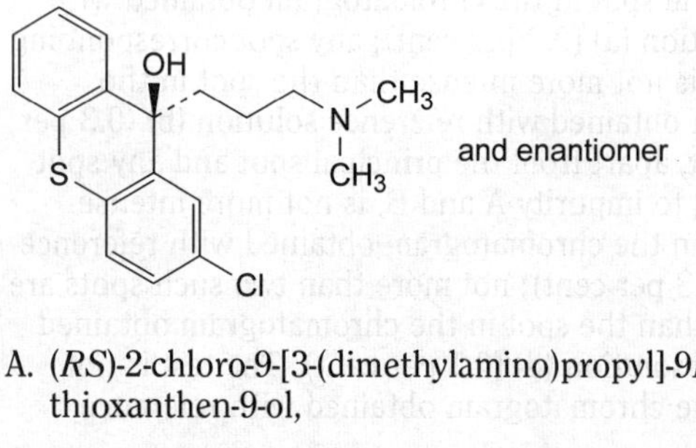

A. (*RS*)-2-chloro-9-[3-(dimethylamino)propyl]-9*H*-thioxanthen-9-ol,

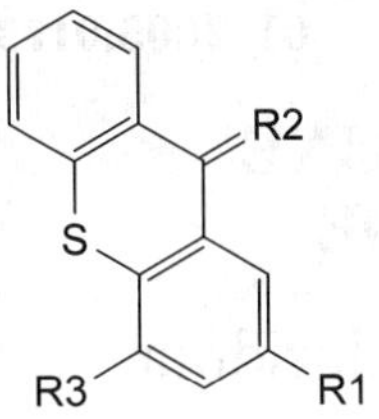

B. R1 = H, R2 = CH-CH_2-CH_2-N$(CH_3)_2$, R3 = H: *N,N*-dimethyl-3-(9*H*-thioxanthen-9-ylidene)propan-1-amine,

C. R1 = Cl, R2 = CH-CH_2-CH_2-NH-CH_3, R3 = H: (*Z*)-3-(2-chloro-9*H*-thioxanthen-9-ylidene)-*N*-methylpropan-1-amine,

D. R1 = H, R2 = CH-CH_2-CH_2-N$(CH_3)_2$, R3 = Cl: (*Z*)-3-(4-chloro-9*H*-thioxanthen-9-ylidene)-*N,N*-dimethylpropan-1-amine,

E. R1 = Cl, R2 = O, R3 = H: 2-chloro-9*H*-thioxanthen-9-one,

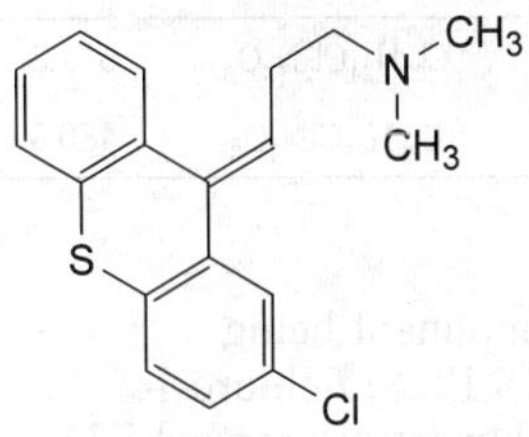

F. (*E*)-3-(2-chloro-9*H*-thioxanthen-9-ylidene)-*N,N*-dimethylpropan-1-amine (*E*-isomer).

01/2005:0546

CHLORTALIDONE

Chlortalidonum

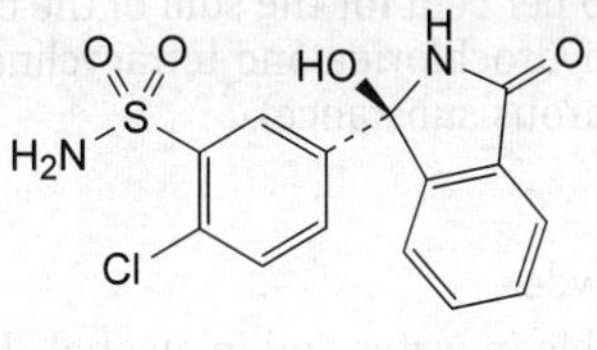

and enantiomer

$C_{14}H_{11}ClN_2O_4S$ M_r 338.8

DEFINITION

Chlortalidone contains not less than 98.0 per cent and not more than the equivalent of 102.0 per cent of 2-chloro-5-[(1*RS*)-1-hydroxy-3-oxo-2,3-dihydro-1*H*-isoindol-1-yl]benzenesulphonamide, calculated with reference to the dried substance.

CHARACTERS

A white or yellowish-white powder, practically insoluble in water, soluble in acetone and in methanol, slightly soluble in alcohol, practically insoluble in methylene chloride. It dissolves in dilute solutions of the alkali hydroxides.

It melts at about 220 °C, with decomposition.

IDENTIFICATION

First identification: B.

Second identification: A, C, D, E.

A. Dissolve 50.0 mg in *alcohol R* and dilute to 50.0 ml with the same solvent. Dilute 10.0 ml of this solution to 100.0 ml with *alcohol R*. Examined between 230 nm and 340 nm (*2.2.25*), the solution shows 2 absorption maxima, at 275 nm and 284 nm. The ratio of the absorbance measured at the absorption maximum at 284 nm to that measured at the absorption maximum at 275 nm is 0.73 to 0.88.

B. Examine by infrared absorption spectrophotometry (*2.2.24*), comparing with the spectrum obtained with *chlortalidone CRS*. Examine the substances prepared as discs using *potassium bromide R*.

C. Examine by thin-layer chromatography (*2.2.27*), using *silica gel GF* R as the coating substance.

Test solution. Dissolve 10 mg of the substance to be examined in *acetone R* and dilute to 10 ml with the same solvent.

Reference solution (a). Dissolve 10 mg of *chlortalidone CRS* in *acetone R* and dilute to 10 ml with the same solvent.

Reference solution (b). Dissolve 10 mg of *chlortalidone CRS* and 10 mg of *hydrochlorothiazide CRS* in *acetone R* and dilute to 10 ml with the same solvent.

Apply separately to the plate 5 µl of each solution. Develop over a path of 10 cm using a mixture of 1.5 volumes of *water R* and 98.5 volumes of *ethyl acetate R*. Allow the plate to dry in air and examine in ultraviolet light at 254 nm. The principal spot in the chromatogram obtained with the test solution is similar in position and size to the principal spot in the chromatogram obtained with reference solution (a). The test is not valid unless the chromatogram obtained with reference solution (b) shows 2 clearly separated spots.

D. Dissolve about 10 mg in 1 ml of *sulphuric acid R*. An intense yellow colour develops.

E. It complies with the test for optical rotation (see Tests).

TESTS

Appearance of solution. Dissolve 1.0 g in *dilute sodium hydroxide solution R* and dilute to 10 ml with the same solution. The solution is clear (*2.2.1*) and not more intensely coloured than intensity 6 of the range of reference solutions of the most appropriate colour (*2.2.2, Method II*).

Acidity. Dissolve 1.0 g with heating in a mixture of 25 ml of *acetone R* and 25 ml of *carbon dioxide-free water R*. Cool. Titrate with *0.1 M sodium hydroxide*, determining the end-point potentiometrically (*2.2.20*). Not more than 0.75 ml of *0.1 M sodium hydroxide* is required.

Optical rotation (*2.2.7*). Dissolve 0.20 g in *methanol R* and dilute to 20 ml with the same solvent. The angle of optical rotation is − 0.15° to + 0.15°.

Related substances. Examine by thin-layer chromatography (*2.2.27*), using as the coating substance a suitable silica gel with a fluorescent indicator having an optimal intensity at 254 nm.

Test solution. Dissolve 0.2 g of the substance to be examined in a mixture of 1 volume of *water R* and 4 volumes of *acetone R* and dilute to 5 ml with the same mixture of solvents.

Reference solution (a). Dissolve 20 mg of *chlortalidone impurity B CRS* and 20 mg of *chlortalidone CRS* in a mixture of 1 volume of *water R* and 4 volumes of *acetone R* and dilute to 50 ml with the same mixture of solvents.

Reference solution (b). Dilute 1 ml of the test solution to 200 ml with a mixture of 1 volume of *water R* and 4 volumes of *acetone R*.

Apply separately to the plate 5 µl of each solution. Develop over a path of 15 cm using a mixture of 5 volumes of *toluene R*, 10 volumes of *xylene R*, 20 volumes of *concentrated ammonia R*, 30 volumes of *dioxan R* and 30 volumes of *2-propanol R*. Allow the plate to dry in a current of warm air and examine in ultraviolet light at 254 nm. In the chromatogram obtained with the test solution: any spot corresponding to impurity B is not more intense than the corresponding spot in the chromatogram obtained with reference solution (a) (1 per cent); and any spot, apart from the principal spot and the spot corresponding to impurity B, is not more intense than the spot in the chromatogram obtained with reference solution (b) (0.5 per cent). The test is not valid unless the chromatogram obtained with reference solution (a) shows 2 clearly separated spots.

Chlorides (*2.4.4*). Triturate 0.3 g, add 30 ml of *water R*, shake for 5 min and filter. 15 ml of the filtrate complies with the limit test for chlorides (350 ppm). Prepare the standard using 10 ml of *chloride standard solution (5 ppm Cl) R*.

Loss on drying (*2.2.32*). Not more than 0.5 per cent, determined on 1.000 g by drying in an oven at 100-105 °C.

Sulphated ash (*2.4.14*). Not more than 0.1 per cent, determined on 1.0 g.

ASSAY

Dissolve 0.200 g in 50 ml of *acetone R*. In an atmosphere of nitrogen, titrate with *0.1 M tetrabutylammonium hydroxide*, determining the end-point potentiometrically (*2.2.20*). Carry out a blank titration.

1 ml of *0.1 M tetrabutylammonium hydroxide* is equivalent to 33.88 mg of $C_{14}H_{11}ClN_2O_4S$.

IMPURITIES

Specified impurities: A, B, C, D, E, F, G, H, I.

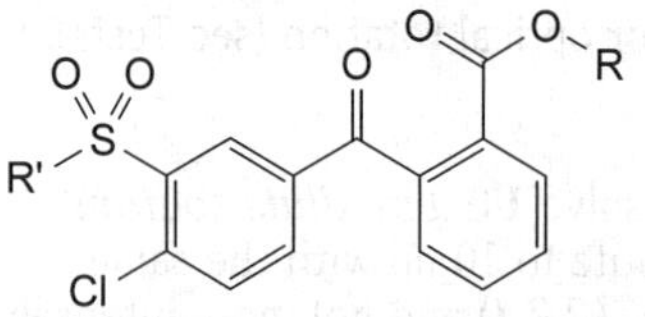

A. R = H, R′ = OH: 2-(4-chloro-3-sulphobenzoyl)benzoic acid,

B. R = H, R′ = NH_2: 2-(4-chloro-3-sulphamoylbenzoyl)benzoic acid,

C. R = C_2H_5, R′ = NH_2: ethyl 2-(4-chloro-3-sulphamoylbenzoyl)benzoate,

I. R = $CH(CH_3)_2$, R′ = NH_2: 1-methylethyl 2-(4-chloro-3-sulphamoylbenzoyl)benzoate,

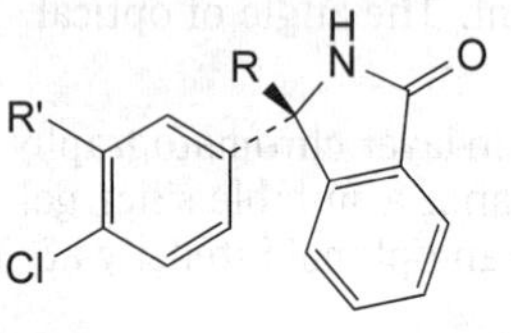

and enantiomer

D. R = OC_2H_5, R′ = SO_2-NH_2: 2-chloro-5-[(1*RS*)-1-ethoxy-3-oxo-2,3-dihydro-1*H*-isoindol-1-yl]benzenesulphonamide,

E. R = H, R′ = SO_2-NH_2: 2-chloro-5-[(1*RS*)-3-oxo-2,3-dihydro-1*H*-isoindol-1-yl]benzenesulphonamide,

G. R = OH, R′ = Cl: (3*RS*)-3-(3,4-dichlorophenyl)-3-hydroxy-2,3-dihydro-1*H*-isoindol-1-one,

H. R = $OCH(CH_3)_2$, R′ = SO_2-NH_2: 2-chloro-5-[(1*RS*)-1-(1-methylethoxy)-3-oxo-2,3-dihydro-1*H*-isoindol-1-yl]benzenesulphonamide,

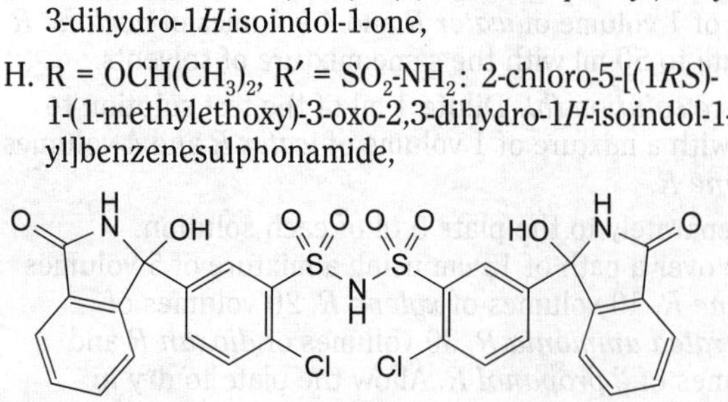

F. bis[2-chloro-5-(1-hydroxy-3-oxo-2,3-dihydro-1*H*-isoindol-1-yl)benzenesulphonyl]amine.

01/2005:0173

CHLORTETRACYCLINE HYDROCHLORIDE

Chlortetracyclini hydrochloridum

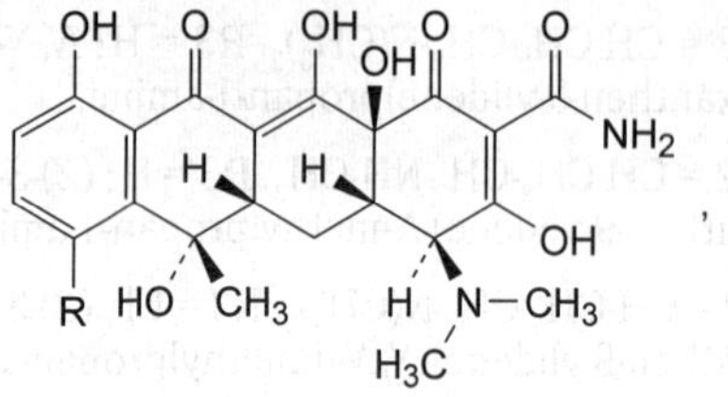

Compound	R	Molecular formula	M_r
Chlortetracycline hydrochloride	Cl	$C_{22}H_{24}Cl_2N_2O_8$	515.3
Tetracycline hydrochloride	H	$C_{22}H_{25}ClN_2O_8$	480.9

DEFINITION

Mixture of antibiotics, the main component being the hydrochloride of (4*S*,4a*S*,5a*S*,6*S*,12a*S*)-7-chloro-4-(dimethylamino)-3,6,10,12,12a-pentahydroxy-6-methyl-1,11-dioxo-1,4,4a,5,5a,6,11,12a-octahydrotetracene-2-carboxamide (chlortetracycline hydrochloride), a substance produced by the growth of certain strains of *Streptomyces aureofaciens* or obtained by any other means.

Content:

– $C_{22}H_{24}Cl_2N_2O_8$: minimum 89.5 per cent (anhydrous substance),

– $C_{22}H_{25}ClN_2O_8$: maximum 8.0 per cent (anhydrous substance),

– 94.5 per cent to 102.0 per cent for the sum of the contents of chlortetracycline hydrochloride and tetracycline hydrochloride (anhydrous substance).

CHARACTERS

Appearance: yellow powder.

Solubility: slightly soluble in water and in alcohol. It dissolves in solutions of alkali hydroxides and carbonates.

IDENTIFICATION

A. Thin-layer chromatography (*2.2.27*).

Test solution. Dissolve 5 mg of the substance to be examined in *methanol R* and dilute to 10 ml with the same solvent.

Reference solution (a). Dissolve 5 mg of *chlortetracycline hydrochloride CRS* in *methanol R* and dilute to 10 ml with the same solvent.

Reference solution (b). Dissolve 5 mg of *chlortetracycline hydrochloride CRS*, 5 mg of *doxycycline R* and 5 mg of *demeclocycline hydrochloride R* in *methanol R* and dilute to 10 ml with the same solvent.

Plate: *TLC octadecylsilyl silica gel F_{254} plate R.*

Mobile phase: mix 20 volumes of *acetonitrile R*, 20 volumes of *methanol R* and 60 volumes of a 63 g/l solution of *oxalic acid R* previously adjusted to pH 2 with *concentrated ammonia R*.

Application: 1 µl.

Development: over 3/4 of the plate.

Drying: in air.

Detection: examine in ultraviolet light at 254 nm.

System suitability: the chromatogram obtained with reference solution (b) shows 3 clearly separated spots.

Results: the principal spot in the chromatogram obtained with the test solution is similar in position and size to the principal spot in the chromatogram obtained with reference solution (a).

B. To about 2 mg add 5 ml of *sulphuric acid R*. A deep blue colour develops which becomes bluish-green. Add the solution to 2.5 ml of *water R*. The colour becomes brownish.

C. It gives reaction (a) of chlorides (*2.3.1*).

TESTS

pH (*2.2.3*): 2.3 to 3.3.

Dissolve 0.1 g in 10 ml of *carbon dioxide-free water R*, heating slightly.

Specific optical rotation (*2.2.7*): − 235 to − 250 (anhydrous substance).

Dissolve 0.125 g in *water R* and dilute to 50.0 ml with the same solvent.

Absorbance (*2.2.25*): maximum 0.40 at 460 nm.

Dissolve 0.125 g in *water R* and dilute to 25.0 ml with the same solvent.

Related substances. Liquid chromatography (*2.2.29*). *Prepare the solutions immediately before use.*

Test solution. Dissolve 25.0 mg of the substance to be examined in *0.01 M hydrochloric acid* and dilute to 25.0 ml with the same acid.

Reference solution (a). Dissolve 25.0 mg of *chlortetracycline hydrochloride CRS* in *0.01 M hydrochloric acid* and dilute to 25.0 ml with the same acid.

Reference solution (b). Dissolve 10.0 mg of *4-epichlortetracycline hydrochloride CRS* in *0.01 M hydrochloric acid* and dilute to 25.0 ml with the same acid.

Reference solution (c). Dissolve 20.0 mg of *tetracycline hydrochloride CRS* in *0.01 M hydrochloric acid* and dilute to 25.0 ml with the same acid.

Reference solution (d). Mix 5.0 ml of reference solution (a) and 10.0 ml of reference solution (b) and dilute to 25.0 ml with *0.01 M hydrochloric acid.*

Reference solution (e). Mix 5.0 ml of reference solution (b) and 5.0 ml of reference solution (c) and dilute to 50.0 ml with *0.01 M hydrochloric acid.*

Reference solution (f). Dilute 1.0 ml of reference solution (c) to 20.0 ml with *0.01 M hydrochloric acid.* Dilute 5.0 ml of this solution to 200.0 ml with *0.01 M hydrochloric acid.*

Column:

- *size*: *l* = 0.25 m, Ø = 4.6 mm,
- *stationary phase*: *octylsilyl silica gel for chromatography R* (5 µm),
- *temperature*: 35 °C.

Mobile phase: to 500 ml of *water R*, add 50 ml of *perchloric acid solution R*, shake and add 450 ml of *dimethyl sulphoxide R*,

Flow rate: 1 ml/min.

Detection: spectrophotometer at 280 nm.

Injection: 20 µl; inject the test solution and reference solutions (d), (e) and (f).

System suitability: reference solution (d):

- *resolution*: minimum 2.0 between the peaks due to impurity A and to chlortetracycline; if necessary, adjust the dimethyl sulphoxide content in the mobile phase,
- *symmetry factor*: maximum 1.3 for the peak due to chlortetracycline.

Limits:

- *impurity A*: not more than the area of the corresponding peak in the chromatogram obtained with reference solution (e) (4.0 per cent),
- *total of other impurities eluting between the solvent peak and the peak corresponding to chlortetracycline*: not more than 0.25 times the area of the peak due to impurity A in the chromatogram obtained with reference solution (e) (1.0 per cent),
- *disregard limit*: area of the principal peak in the chromatogram obtained with reference solution (f) (0.1 per cent).

Heavy metals (*2.4.8*): maximum 50 ppm.

0.5 g complies with limit test C. Prepare the standard using 2.5 ml of *lead standard solution (10 ppm Pb) R*.

Water (*2.5.12*): maximum 2.0 per cent, determined on 0.300 g.

Sulphated ash (*2.4.14*): maximum 0.5 per cent, determined on 1.0 g.

Bacterial endotoxins (*2.6.14*): less than 1 IU/mg, if intended for use in the manufacture of parenteral dosage forms without a further appropriate procedure for the removal of bacterial endotoxins.

ASSAY

Liquid chromatography (*2.2.29*) as described in the test for related substances with the following modification.

Injection: test solution and reference solutions (a) and (e).

Calculate the percentage content of $C_{22}H_{24}Cl_2N_2O_8$ using the chromatogram obtained with reference solution (a). Calculate the percentage content of $C_{22}H_{25}ClN_2O_8$ using the chromatogram obtained with reference solution (e).

STORAGE

Protected from light. If the substance is sterile, store in a sterile, airtight, tamper-proof container.

LABELLING

The label states, where applicable, that the substance is free from bacterial endotoxins.

IMPURITIES

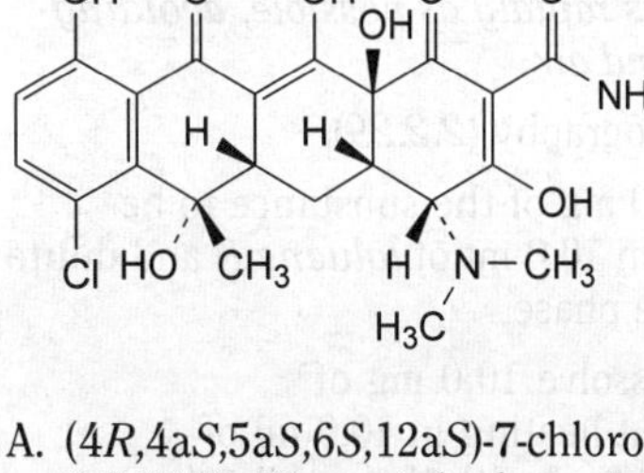

A. (4*R*,4a*S*,5a*S*,6*S*,12a*S*)-7-chloro-4-(dimethylamino)-3,6,10,12,12a-pentahydroxy-6-methyl-1,11-dioxo-1,4,4a,5,5a,6,11,12a-octahydrotetracene-2-carboxamide (4-epichlortetracycline),

B. demeclocycline.

Monographs C

01/2005:0072

CHOLECALCIFEROL

Cholecalciferolum

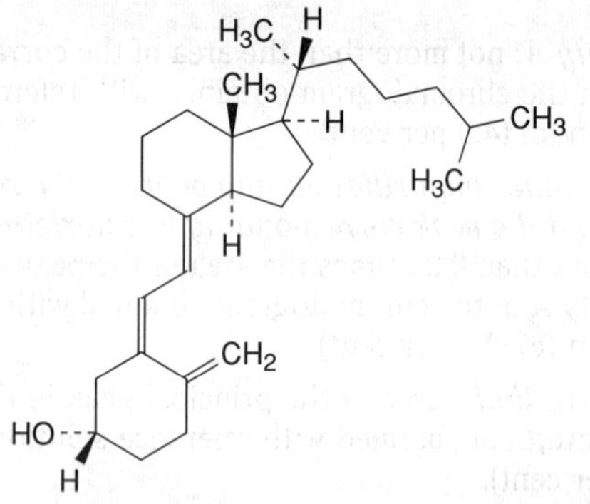

$C_{27}H_{44}O$ M_r 384.6

DEFINITION

Cholecalciferol contains not less than 97.0 per cent and not more than the equivalent of 103.0 per cent of (5*Z*,7*E*)-9,10-secocholesta-5,7,10(19)-trien-3β-ol.

1 milligram of cholecalciferol is equivalent to 40 000 IU of antirachitic activity (vitamin D) in rats.

CHARACTERS

White or almost white crystals, practically insoluble in water, freely soluble in alcohol, soluble in fatty oils. It is sensitive to air, heat and light. Solutions in volatile solvents are unstable and are to be used immediately.

A reversible isomerisation to pre-cholecalciferol takes place in solution, depending on temperature and time. The activity is due to both compounds.

IDENTIFICATION

Examine by infrared absorption spectrophotometry (*2.2.24*), comparing with the spectrum obtained with *cholecalciferol CRS*. Examine the substances prepared as discs.

TESTS

Specific optical rotation (*2.2.7*). Dissolve 0.200 g rapidly and without heating in *aldehyde-free alcohol R* and dilute to 25.0 ml with the same solvent. The specific optical rotation, determined within 30 min of preparing the solution, is + 105 to + 112.

ASSAY

Carry out the operations as rapidly as possible, avoiding exposure to actinic light and air.

Examine by liquid chromatography (*2.2.29*).

Test solution. Dissolve 10.0 mg of the substance to be examined without heating in 10.0 ml of *toluene R* and dilute to 100.0 ml with the mobile phase.

Reference solution (a). Dissolve 10.0 mg of *cholecalciferol CRS* without heating in 10.0 ml of *toluene R* and dilute to 100.0 ml with the mobile phase.

Reference solution (b). Dilute 1.0 ml of *cholecalciferol for performance test CRS* to 5.0 ml with the mobile phase. Heat in a water-bath at 90 °C under a reflux condenser for 45 min and cool.

The chromatographic procedure may be carried out using:

- a stainless steel column 0.25 m long and 4.6 mm in internal diameter packed with a suitable silica gel (5 μm),
- as mobile phase at a flow rate of 2 ml/min a mixture of 3 volumes of *pentanol R* and 997 volumes of *hexane R*,
- as detector a spectrophotometer set at 254 nm.

An automatic injection device or a sample loop is recommended. Inject a suitable volume of reference solution (b). Adjust the sensitivity of the system so that the height of the principal peak is at least 50 per cent of the full scale of the recorder. Inject reference solution (b) 6 times. When the chromatograms are recorded in the prescribed conditions, the approximate relative retention times with reference to cholecalciferol are 0.4 for pre-cholecalciferol and 0.5 for *trans*-cholecalciferol. The relative standard deviation of the response for cholecalciferol is not greater than 1 per cent and the resolution between the peaks due to pre-cholecalciferol and *trans*-cholecalciferol is not less than 1.0. If necessary adjust the proportions of the constituents and the flow rate of the mobile phase to obtain this resolution.

Inject a suitable volume of reference solution (a). Adjust the sensitivity of the system so that the height of the principal peak is at least 50 per cent of the full scale of the recorder. Inject the same volume of the test solution and record the chromatogram in the same manner.

Calculate the percentage content of cholecalciferol from the expression:

$$\frac{m'}{m} \times \frac{S_D}{S'_D} \times 100$$

m = mass of the substance to be examined in the test solution, in milligrams,

m' = mass of *cholecalciferol CRS* in reference solution (a), in milligrams,

S_D = area (or height) of the peak due to cholecalciferol in the chromatogram obtained with the test solution,

S'_D = area (or height) of the peak due to cholecalciferol in the chromatogram obtained with reference solution (a).

STORAGE

Store in an airtight container, under nitrogen, protected from light, at a temperature between 2 °C and 8 °C.

The contents of an opened container are to be used immediately.

IMPURITIES

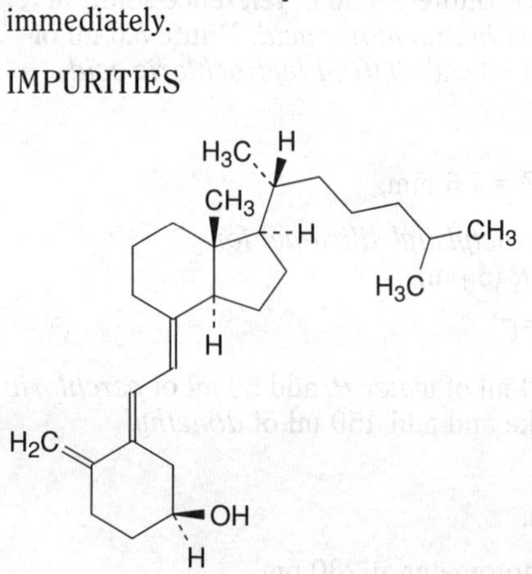

A. (5*E*,7*E*)-9,10-secocholesta-5,7,10(19)-trien-3β-ol (*trans*-cholecalciferol, *trans*-vitamin D_3),

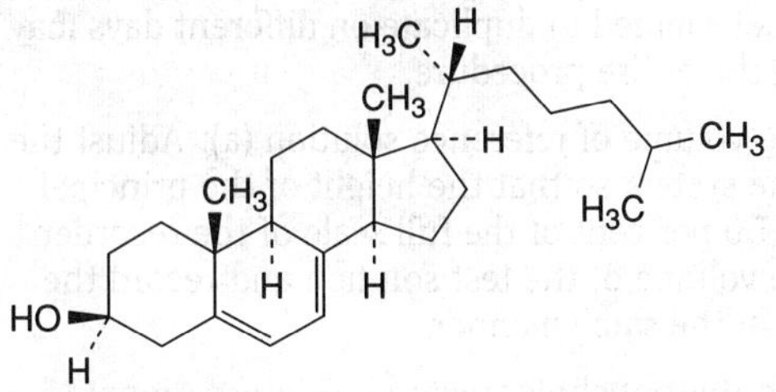

B. cholesta-5,7-dien-3β-ol (7,8-didehydrocholesterol, provitamin D_3),

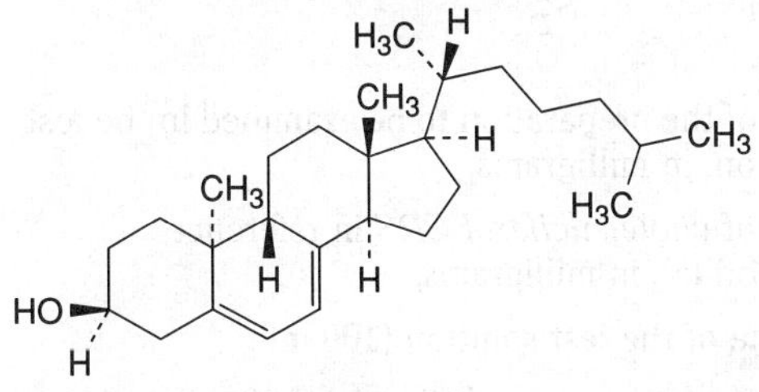

C. 9β,10α-cholesta-5,7-dien-3β-ol (lumisterol$_3$),

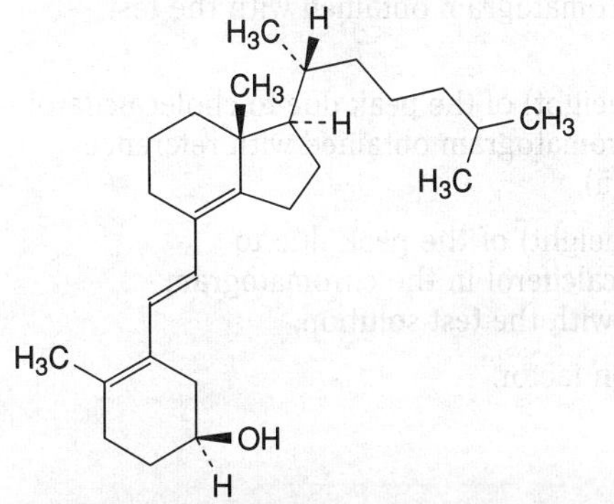

D. (6*E*)-9,10-secocholesta-5(10),6,8(14)-trien-3β-ol (iso-tachysterol$_3$),

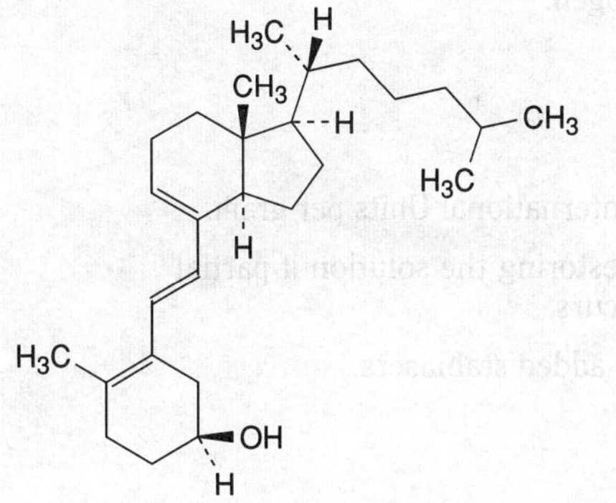

E. (6*E*)-9,10-secocholesta-5(10),6,8-trien-3β-ol (tachysterol$_3$).

01/2005:0575

CHOLECALCIFEROL CONCENTRATE (OILY FORM)

Cholecalciferolum densatum oleosum

DEFINITION

Cholecalciferol concentrate (oily form) consists of a solution of *Cholecalciferol (0072)* in a suitable vegetable fatty oil, authorised by the competent authority.

The content of cholecalciferol stated on the label is not less than 500 000 IU/g and the concentrate contains not less than 90.0 per cent and not more than 110.0 per cent of the content stated on the label. The concentrate may contain suitable stabilisers such as antioxidants.

CHARACTERS

A clear, yellow liquid, practically insoluble in water, slightly soluble in ethanol, miscible with solvents of fats.

Partial solidification may occur, depending on the temperature.

IDENTIFICATION

First identification: A, C.

Second identification: A, B.

A. Examine by thin-layer chromatography (*2.2.27*), using a *TLC silica gel G plate R*.

Test solution. Dissolve an amount of the substance to be examined corresponding to 400 000 IU in *ethylene chloride R* containing 10 g/l of *squalane R* and 0.1 g/l of *butylhydroxytoluene R* and dilute to 4 ml with the same solvent. Prepare immediately before use.

Reference solution (a). Dissolve 10 mg of *cholecalciferol CRS* in *ethylene chloride R* containing 10 g/l of *squalane R* and 0.1 g/l of *butylhydroxytoluene R* and dilute to 4 ml with the same solvent. Prepare immediately before use.

Reference solution (b). Dissolve 10 mg of *ergocalciferol CRS* in *ethylene chloride R* containing 10 g/l of *squalane R* and 0.1 g/l of *butylhydroxytoluene R* and dilute to 4 ml with the same solvent. Prepare immediately before use.

Apply to the plate 20 µl of each solution. Develop immediately, protected from light, over a path of 15 cm using a mixture of equal volumes of *cyclohexane R* and *peroxide-free ether R*, the mixture containing 0.1 g/l of *butylhydroxytoluene R*. Allow the plate to dry in air and spray with *sulphuric acid R*. Compare the principal spot in the chromatogram obtained with the test solution with the principal spot in each of the chromatograms obtained with reference solution (a) and reference solution (b), respectively. The chromatogram obtained with the test solution shows immediately a bright yellow principal spot which rapidly becomes orange-brown, then gradually greenish-grey and remains so for 10 min. This spot is similar in position, colour and size to the spot in the chromatogram obtained with reference solution (a). The chromatogram obtained with reference solution (b) shows immediately at the same level an orange principal spot which gradually becomes reddish-brown and remains so for 10 min.

B. Prepare a solution in *cyclohexane R* containing the equivalent of about 400 IU/ml. Examined between 250 nm and 300 nm (*2.2.25*), the solution shows an absorption maximum at 267 nm.

C. Examine the chromatograms obtained in the assay. The principal peak in the chromatogram obtained with the test solution has a similar retention time to the principal peak in the chromatogram obtained with reference solution (a).

TESTS

Acid value (*2.5.1*). Not more than 2.0, determined on 5.0 g dissolved in 25 ml of the prescribed mixture of solvents.

Peroxide value (*2.5.5*). Not more than 20.

ASSAY

Carry out the assay as rapidly as possible, avoiding exposure to actinic light and air.

Examine by liquid chromatography (*2.2.29*).

Test solution. Dissolve a quantity of the preparation to be examined, weighed with an accuracy of 0.1 per cent, equivalent to about 400 000 IU, in 10.0 ml of *toluene R* and dilute to 100.0 ml with the mobile phase.

Reference solution (a). Dissolve 10.0 mg of *cholecalciferol CRS* without heating in 10.0 ml of *toluene R* and dilute to 100.0 ml with the mobile phase.

Reference solution (b). Dilute 1.0 ml of *cholecalciferol for performance test CRS* to 5.0 ml with the mobile phase. Heat in a water-bath at 90 °C under a reflux condenser for 45 min and cool.

Reference solution (c). Dissolve 0.10 g of *cholecalciferol CRS* without heating in *toluene R* and dilute to 100.0 ml with the same solvent.

Reference solution (d). Dilute 5.0 ml of reference solution (c) to 50.0 ml with the mobile phase. Keep the solution in iced water.

Reference solution (e). Place 5.0 ml of reference solution (c) in a volumetric flask, add about 10 mg of *butylhydroxytoluene R* and displace air from the flask with *nitrogen R*. Heat in a water-bath at 90 °C under a reflux condenser protected from light and under *nitrogen R* for 45 min. Cool and dilute to 50.0 ml with the mobile phase.

The chromatographic procedure may be carried out using:

- a stainless steel column 0.25 m long and 4.6 mm in internal diameter packed with a suitable silica gel (5 μm),
- as mobile phase at a flow rate of 2 ml/min a mixture of 3 volumes of *pentanol R* and 997 volumes of *hexane R*,
- as detector a spectrophotometer set at 254 nm.

An automatic injection device or a sample loop is recommended. Inject a suitable volume of reference solution (b). Adjust the sensitivity of the system so that the height of the principal peak is at least 50 per cent of the full scale of the recorder. Inject reference solution (b) 6 times. When the chromatograms are recorded in the prescribed conditions, the approximate relative retention times with reference to cholecalciferol are 0.4 for pre-cholecalciferol and 0.5 for *trans*-cholecalciferol. The relative standard deviation of the response for cholecalciferol is not greater than 1 per cent and the resolution between the peaks due to pre-cholecalciferol and *trans*-cholecalciferol is not less than 1.0. If necessary adjust the proportions of the constituents and the flow rate of the mobile phase to obtain this resolution.

Inject a suitable volume of reference solution (d) and of reference solution (e).

Calculate the conversion factor (*f*) from the expression:

$$f = \frac{K - L}{M}$$

K = area (or height) of the peak due to cholecalciferol in the chromatogram obtained with reference solution (d),

L = area (or height) of the peak due to cholecalciferol in the chromatogram obtained with reference solution (e),

M = area (or height) of the peak due to pre-cholecalciferol in the chromatogram obtained with reference solution (e).

The value of *f* determined in duplicate on different days may be used during the entire procedure.

Inject a suitable volume of reference solution (a). Adjust the sensitivity of the system so that the height of the principal peak is at least 50 per cent of the full scale of the recorder. Inject the same volume of the test solution and record the chromatogram in the same manner.

Calculate the content of cholecalciferol in International Units per gram from the expression:

$$\frac{m'}{V'} \times \frac{V}{m} \times \frac{S_D + (f \times S_p)}{S'_D} \times 40\,000 \times 1000$$

m = mass of the preparation to be examined in the test solution, in milligrams,

m' = mass of *cholecalciferol CRS* in reference solution (a), in milligrams,

V = volume of the test solution (100 ml),

V' = volume of reference solution (a) (100 ml),

S_D = area (or height) of the peak due to cholecalciferol in the chromatogram obtained with the test solution,

S'_D = area (or height) of the peak due to cholecalciferol in the chromatogram obtained with reference solution (a),

S_p = area (or height) of the peak due to pre-cholecalciferol in the chromatogram obtained with the test solution,

f = conversion factor.

STORAGE

Store in an airtight, well-filled container, protected from light. The contents of an opened container are to be used as soon as possible; any unused part is to be protected by an atmosphere of nitrogen.

LABELLING

The label states:

- the number of International Units per gram,
- the method of restoring the solution if partial solidification occurs,
- the name of any added stabilisers.

IMPURITIES

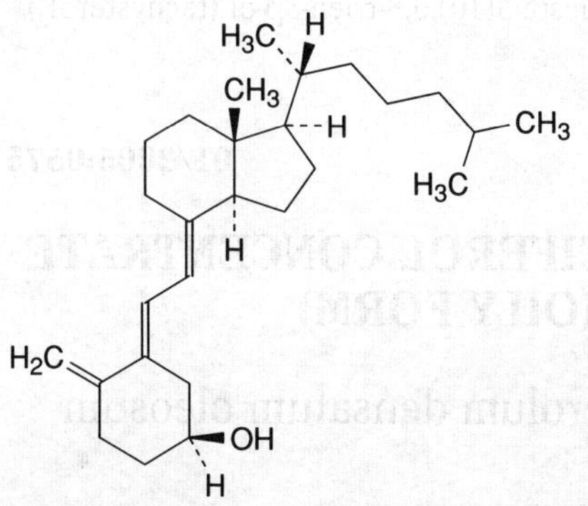

A. (5*E*,7*E*)-9,10-secocholesta-5,7,10(19)-trien-3β-ol (*trans*-cholecalciferol, *trans*-vitamin D_3),

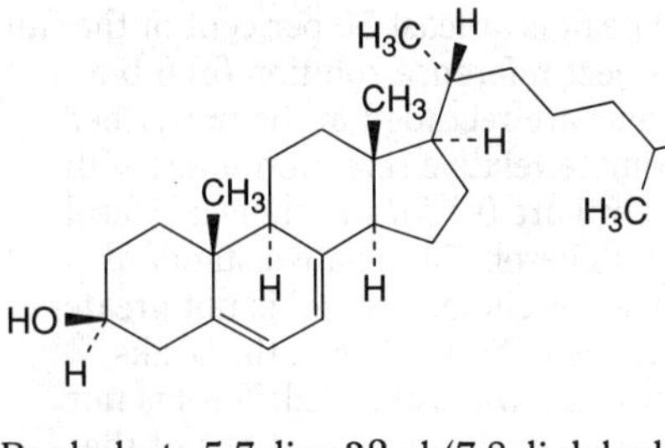

B. cholesta-5,7-dien-3β-ol (7,8-di dehydrocholesterol, provitamin D_3),

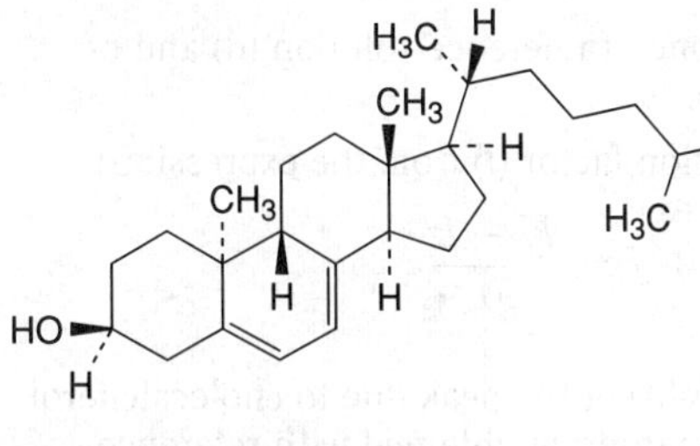

C. (9β,10α)-cholesta-5,7-dien-3β-ol (lumisterol$_3$),

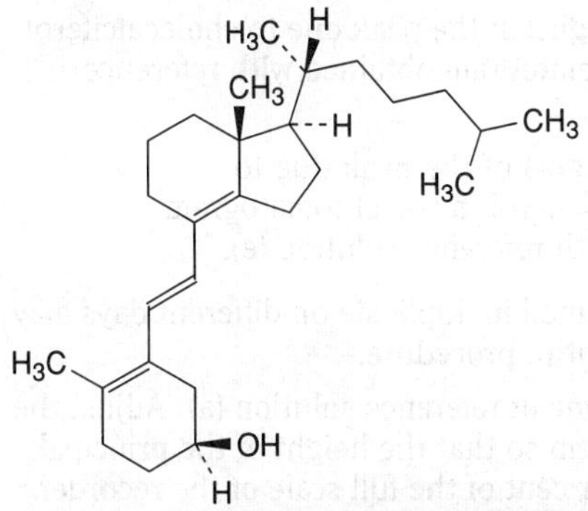

D. (6*E*)-9,10-secocholesta-5(10),6,8(14)-trien-3β-ol (iso-tachysterol$_3$),

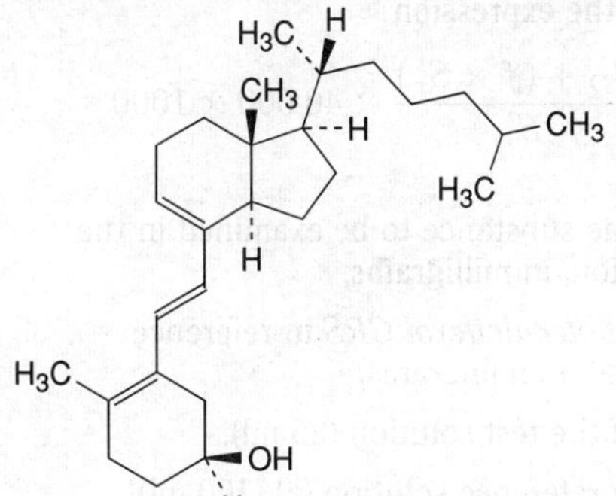

E. (6*E*)-9,10-secocholesta-5(10),6,8-trien-3β-ol (tachysterol$_3$).

01/2005:0574

CHOLECALCIFEROL CONCENTRATE (POWDER FORM)

Cholecalciferoli pulvis

DEFINITION

Cholecalciferol concentrate (powder form) is obtained by dispersing an oily solution of *Cholecalciferol (0072)* in an appropriate matrix which is usually based on a combination of gelatin and carbohydrates of suitable quality, authorised by the competent authority.

The declared content of cholecalciferol is not less than 100 000 IU/g and the concentrate contains not less than 90.0 per cent and not more than 110.0 per cent of the content stated on the label. The concentrate may contain suitable stabilisers such as antioxidants.

CHARACTERS

White or yellowish-white, small particles which, depending on their formulation, may be practically insoluble in water or may swell or form a dispersion.

IDENTIFICATION

First identification: A, C.

Second identification: A, B.

A. Examine by thin-layer chromatography (*2.2.27*), using a *TLC silica gel G plate R*.

Test solution. Place 10.0 ml of the test solution prepared for the assay in a suitable flask and evaporate to dryness under reduced pressure by swirling in a water-bath at 40 °C. Cool under running water and restore atmospheric pressure with *nitrogen R*. Dissolve the residue immediately in 0.4 ml of *ethylene chloride R* containing 10 g/l of *squalane R* and 0.1 g/l of *butylhydroxytoluene R*. Prepare immediately before use.

Reference solution (a). Dissolve 10 mg of *cholecalciferol CRS* in *ethylene chloride R* containing 10 g/l of *squalane R* and 0.1 g/l of *butylhydroxytoluene R* and dilute to 4 ml with the same solvent. Prepare immediately before use.

Reference solution (b). Dissolve 10 mg of *ergocalciferol CRS* in *ethylene chloride R* containing 10 g/l of *squalane R* and 0.1 g/l of *butylhydroxytoluene R* and dilute to 4 ml with the same solvent. Prepare immediately before use.

Apply to the plate 20 µl of each solution. Develop immediately, protected from light, over a path of 15 cm using a mixture of equal volumes of *cyclohexane R* and *peroxide-free ether R*, the mixture containing 0.1 g/l of *butylhydroxytoluene R*. Allow the plate to dry in air and spray with *sulphuric acid R*. Compare the principal spot in the chromatogram obtained with the test solution with the principal spot in each of the chromatograms obtained with reference solution (a) and reference solution (b), respectively. The chromatogram obtained with the test solution shows immediately a bright-yellow principal spot which rapidly becomes orange-brown, then gradually greenish-grey and remains so for 10 min. This spot is similar in position, colour and size to the spot in the chromatogram obtained with reference solution (a). The chromatogram obtained with reference solution (b) shows immediately at the same level an orange principal spot which gradually becomes reddish-brown and remains so for 10 min.

B. Place 5.0 ml of the test solution prepared for the assay in a suitable flask and evaporate to dryness under reduced pressure by swirling in a water-bath at 40 °C. Cool under running water and restore atmospheric pressure with *nitrogen R*. Dissolve the residue immediately in 50.0 ml of *cyclohexane R*. Examined between 250 nm and 300 nm (*2.2.25*), the solution shows an absorption maximum at 265 nm.

C. Examine the chromatograms obtained in the assay. The principal peak in the chromatogram obtained with the test solution has a similar retention time to the principal peak in the chromatogram obtained with reference solution (a).

ASSAY

Carry out the assay as rapidly as possible, avoiding exposure to actinic light and air.

Examine by liquid chromatography (*2.2.29*).

Test solution. Introduce into a saponification flask a quantity of the preparation to be examined, weighed with an accuracy of 0.1 per cent, equivalent to about 100 000 IU. Add 5 ml of *water R*, 20 ml of *ethanol R*, 1 ml of *sodium ascorbate solution R* and 3 ml of a freshly prepared 50 per cent *m/m* solution of *potassium hydroxide R*. Heat under a reflux condenser on a water-bath for 30 min. Cool rapidly under running water. Transfer the liquid to a separating funnel with the aid of two quantities, each of 15 ml, of *water R*, one quantity of 10 ml of *alcohol R* and two quantities, each of 50 ml, of *pentane R*. Shake vigorously for 30 s. Allow to stand until the two layers are clear. Transfer the lower aqueous-alcoholic layer to a second separating funnel and shake with a mixture of 10 ml of *alcohol R* and 50 ml of *pentane R*. After separation, transfer the aqueous-alcoholic layer to a third separating funnel and the pentane layer to the first separating funnel, washing the second separating funnel with two quantities, each of 10 ml, of *pentane R* and adding the washings to the first separating funnel. Shake the aqueous-alcoholic layer with 50 ml of *pentane R* and add the pentane layer to the first funnel. Wash the pentane layer with two quantities, each of 50 ml, of a freshly prepared 30 g/l solution of *potassium hydroxide R* in *alcohol (10 per cent V/V) R*, shaking vigorously, then wash with successive quantities, each of 50 ml, of *water R* until the washings are neutral to phenolphthalein. Transfer the washed pentane extract to a ground-glass-stoppered flask. Evaporate the contents of the flask to dryness under reduced pressure by swirling in a water-bath at 40 °C. Cool under running water and restore atmospheric pressure with *nitrogen R*. Dissolve the residue immediately in 5.0 ml of *toluene R* and add 20.0 ml of the mobile phase to obtain a solution containing about 4000 IU/ml.

Reference solution (a). Dissolve 10.0 mg of *cholecalciferol CRS* without heating in 10.0 ml of *toluene R* and dilute to 100.0 ml with the mobile phase.

Reference solution (b). Dilute 1.0 g of *cholecalciferol for performance test CRS* to 5.0 ml with the mobile phase. Heat in a water-bath at 90 °C under a reflux condenser for 45 min and cool.

Reference solution (c). Dissolve 0.10 g of *cholecalciferol CRS* without heating in *toluene R* and dilute to 100.0 ml with the same solvent.

Reference solution (d). Dilute 5.0 ml of reference solution (c) to 50.0 ml with the mobile phase. Keep the solution in iced water.

Reference solution (e). Place 5.0 ml of reference solution (c) in a volumetric flask, add about 10 mg of *butylhydroxytoluene R* and displace air from the flask with *nitrogen R*. Heat in a water-bath at 90 °C under a reflux condenser protected from light and under *nitrogen R* for 45 min. Cool and dilute to 50.0 ml with the mobile phase.

The chromatographic procedure may be carried out using:

– a stainless steel column 0.25 m long and 4.6 mm in internal diameter packed with a suitable silica gel (5 µm),
– as mobile phase at a flow rate of 2 ml/min, a mixture of 3 volumes of *pentanol R* and 997 volumes of *hexane R*,
– as detector a spectrophotometer set at 254 nm.

An automatic injection device or a sample loop is recommended. Inject a suitable volume of reference solution (b). Adjust the sensitivity of the system so that the height of the principal peak is at least 50 per cent of the full scale of the recorder. Inject reference solution (b) 6 times. When the chromatograms are recorded in the prescribed conditions, the approximate relative retention times with reference to cholecalciferol are 0.4 for pre-cholecalciferol and 0.5 for *trans*-cholecalciferol. The relative standard deviation of the response for cholecalciferol is not greater than 1 per cent and the resolution between the peaks due to pre-cholecalciferol and *trans*-cholecalciferol is not less than 1.0. If necessary adjust the proportions of the constituents and the flow rate of the mobile phase to obtain this resolution.

Inject a suitable volume of reference solution (d) and of reference solution (e).

Calculate the conversion factor (*f*) from the expression:

$$f = \frac{K - L}{M}$$

K = area (or height) of the peak due to cholecalciferol in the chromatogram obtained with reference solution (d),

L = area (or height) of the peak due to cholecalciferol in the chromatogram obtained with reference solution (e),

M = area (or height) of the peak due to pre-cholecalciferol in the chromatogram obtained with reference solution (e).

The value of *f* determined in duplicate on different days may be used during the entire procedure.

Inject a suitable volume of reference solution (a). Adjust the sensitivity of the system so that the height of the principal peak is at least 50 per cent of the full scale of the recorder. Inject the same volume of the test solution and record the chromatogram in the same manner.

Calculate the content of cholecalciferol in International Units per gram from the expression:

$$\frac{m'}{V'} \times \frac{V}{m} \times \frac{S_D + (f \times S_p)}{S'_D} \times 40\,000 \times 1000$$

m = mass of the substance to be examined in the test solution, in milligrams,

m' = mass of *cholecalciferol CRS* in reference solution (a), in milligrams,

V = volume of the test solution (25 ml),

V' = volume of reference solution (a) (100 ml),

S_D = area (or height) of the peak due to cholecalciferol in the chromatogram obtained with the test solution,

S'_D = area (or height) of the peak due to cholecalciferol in the chromatogram obtained with reference solution (a),

S_p = area (or height) of the peak due to pre-cholecalciferol in the chromatogram obtained with the test solution,

f = conversion factor.

STORAGE

Store in an airtight, well-filled container, protected from light. The contents of an opened container are to be used as soon as possible; any unused part is to be protected by an atmosphere of nitrogen.

LABELLING

The label states:

- the number of International Units per gram,
- the name of any added stabilisers.

IMPURITIES

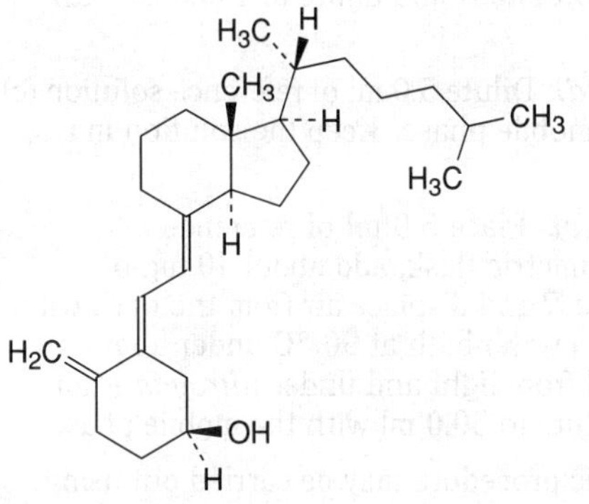

A. (5*E*,7*E*)-9,10-secocholesta-5,7,10(19)-trien-3β-ol (*trans*-cholecalciferol, *trans*-vitamin D_3),

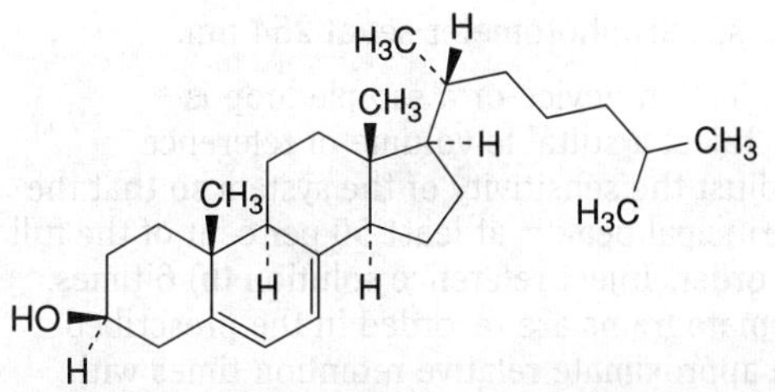

B. cholesta-5,7-dien-3β-ol (7,8-di dehydrocholesterol, provitamin D_3),

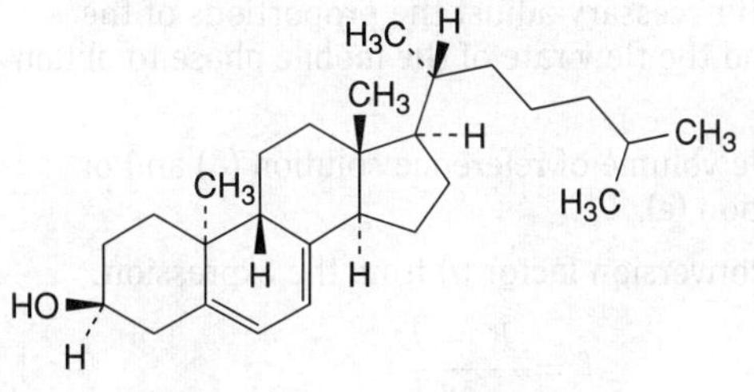

C. (9β,10α)-cholesta-5,7-dien-3β-ol (lumisterol$_3$),

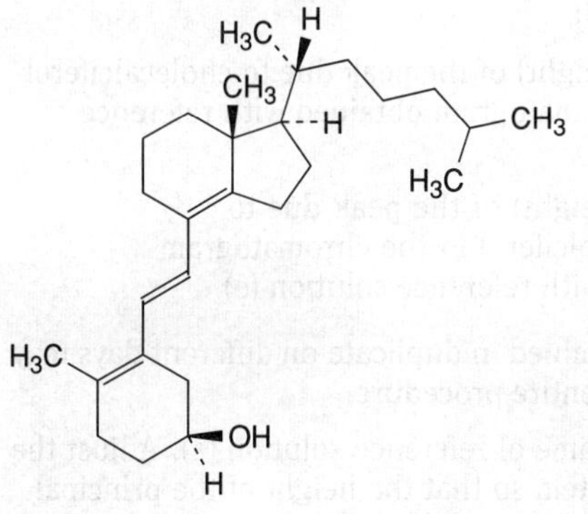

D. (6*E*)-9,10-secocholesta-5(10),6,8(14)-trien-3β-ol (iso-tachysterol$_3$),

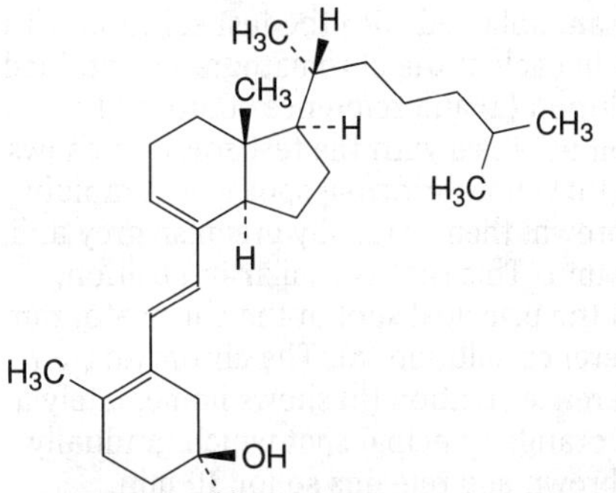

E. (6*E*)-9,10-secocholesta-5(10),6,8-trien-3β-ol (tachysterol$_3$).

01/2005:0598

CHOLECALCIFEROL CONCENTRATE (WATER-DISPERSIBLE FORM)

Cholecalciferolum in aqua dispergibile

DEFINITION

Cholecalciferol concentrate (water-dispersible form) consists of a solution of *Cholecalciferol (0072)* in a suitable vegetable fatty oil, authorised by the competent authority, to which suitable solubilisers have been added.

The declared content of cholecalciferol is not less than 100 000 IU/g and the concentrate contains not less than 90.0 per cent and not more than 115.0 per cent of the content stated on the label. The concentrate may contain suitable stabilisers such as antioxidants.

CHARACTERS

A slightly yellowish liquid of variable opalescence and viscosity. Highly concentrated solutions may become cloudy at low temperatures or form a gel at room temperature.

IDENTIFICATION

First identification: A, C, D.

Second identification: A, B, D.

A. Examine by thin-layer chromatography (*2.2.27*), using a *TLC silica gel G plate R*.

Test solution. Place 10.0 ml of the test solution prepared for the assay in a suitable flask and evaporate to dryness under reduced pressure by swirling in a water-bath at 40 °C. Cool under running water and restore atmospheric pressure with *nitrogen R*. Dissolve the residue immediately in 0.4 ml of *ethylene chloride R* containing 10 g/l of *squalane R* and 0.1 g/l of *butylhydroxytoluene R*. Prepare immediately before use.

Reference solution (a). Dissolve 10 mg of *cholecalciferol CRS* in *ethylene chloride R* containing 10 g/l of *squalane R* and 0.1 g/l of *butylhydroxytoluene R* and dilute to 4 ml with the same solvent. Prepare immediately before use.

Reference solution (b). Dissolve 10 mg of *ergocalciferol CRS* in *ethylene chloride R* containing 10 g/l of *squalane R* and 0.1 g/l of *butylhydroxytoluene R* and dilute to 4 ml with the same solvent. Prepare immediately before use.

Apply to the plate 20 μl of each solution. Develop immediately, protected from light, over a path of 15 cm using a mixture of equal volumes of *cyclohexane R* and *peroxide-free ether R*, the mixture containing 0.1 g/l of *butylhydroxytoluene R*. Allow the plate to dry in air and spray with *sulphuric acid R*. Compare the principal spot in the chromatogram obtained with the test solution with the principal spot in each of the chromatograms obtained with reference solution (a) and reference solution (b). The chromatogram obtained with the test solution shows immediately a bright-yellow principal spot which rapidly becomes orange-brown, then gradually greenish-grey and remains so for 10 min. This spot is similar in position, colour and size to the principal spot in the chromatogram obtained with reference solution (a). The chromatogram obtained with reference solution (b) shows immediately at the same level an orange principal spot which gradually becomes reddish-brown and remains so for 10 min.

B. Place 5.0 ml of the test solution prepared for the assay in a suitable flask and evaporate to dryness under reduced pressure by swirling in a water-bath at 40 °C. Cool under running water and restore atmospheric pressure with *nitrogen R*. Dissolve the residue immediately in 50.0 ml of *cyclohexane R*. Examined between 250 nm and 300 nm (*2.2.25*), the solution shows an absorption maximum at 265 nm.

C. Examine the chromatograms obtained in the assay. The principal peak in the chromatogram obtained with the test solution has a similar retention time to the principal peak in the chromatogram obtained with reference solution (a).

D. Mix about 1 g with 10 ml of *water R* previously warmed to 50 °C and cool to 20 °C. Immediately after cooling, a uniform, slightly opalescent and slightly yellow dispersion is obtained.

ASSAY

Carry out the assay as rapidly as possible, avoiding exposure to actinic light and air.

Examine by liquid chromatography (*2.2.29*).

Test solution. Introduce into a saponification flask a quantity of the preparation to be examined, weighed with an accuracy of 0.1 per cent, equivalent to about 100 000 IU. Add 5 ml of *water R*, 20 ml of *ethanol R*, 1 ml of *sodium ascorbate solution R* and 3 ml of a freshly prepared 50 per cent *m/m* solution of *potassium hydroxide R*. Heat under a reflux condenser on a water-bath for 30 min. Cool rapidly under running water. Transfer the liquid to a separating funnel with the aid of two quantities, each of 15 ml, of *water R*, one quantity of 10 ml of *alcohol R* and two quantities, each of 50 ml, of *pentane R*. Shake vigorously for 30 s. Allow to stand until the two layers are clear. Transfer the aqueous-alcoholic layer to a second separating funnel and shake with a mixture of 10 ml of *alcohol R* and 50 ml of *pentane R*. After separation, transfer the aqueous-alcoholic layer to a third separating funnel and the pentane layer to the first separating funnel, washing the second separating funnel with two quantities, each of 10 ml, of *pentane R* and adding the washings to the first separating funnel. Shake the aqueous-alcoholic layer with 50 ml of *pentane R* and add the pentane layer to the first funnel. Wash the pentane layer with two quantities, each of 50 ml, of a freshly prepared 30 g/l solution of *potassium hydroxide R* in *alcohol (10 per cent V/V) R*, shaking vigorously, and then wash with successive quantities, each of 50 ml, of *water R* until the washings are neutral to phenolphthalein. Transfer the washed pentane extract to a ground-glass-stoppered flask. Evaporate the contents of the flask to dryness under reduced pressure by swirling in a water-bath at 40 °C. Cool under running water and restore atmospheric pressure with *nitrogen R*. Dissolve the residue immediately in 5.0 ml of *toluene R* and add 20.0 ml of the mobile phase to obtain a solution containing about 4000 IU/ml.

Reference solution (a). Dissolve 10.0 mg of *cholecalciferol CRS* without heating in 10.0 ml of *toluene R* and dilute to 100.0 ml with the mobile phase.

Reference solution (b). Dilute 1.0 g of *cholecalciferol for performance test CRS* to 5.0 ml with the mobile phase. Heat in a water-bath at 90 °C under a reflux condenser for 45 min and cool.

Reference solution (c). Dissolve 0.10 g of *cholecalciferol CRS* without heating in *toluene R* and dilute to 100.0 ml with the same solvent.

Reference solution (d). Dilute 5.0 ml of reference solution (c) to 50.0 ml with the mobile phase. Keep the solution in iced water.

Reference solution (e). Place 5.0 ml of reference solution (c) in a volumetric flask, add about 10 mg of *butylhydroxytoluene R* and displace air from the flask with *nitrogen R*. Heat in a water-bath at 90 °C under a reflux condenser protected from light and under *nitrogen R* for 45 min. Cool and dilute to 50.0 ml with the mobile phase.

The chromatographic procedure may be carried out using:

- a stainless steel column 0.25 m long and 4.6 mm in internal diameter packed with a suitable silica gel (5 μm),
- as mobile phase at a flow rate of 2 ml/min a mixture of 3 volumes of *pentanol R* and 997 volumes of *hexane R*,
- as detector a spectrophotometer set at 254 nm.

An automatic injection device or a sample loop is recommended. Inject a suitable volume of reference solution (b). Adjust the sensitivity of the system so that the height of the principal peak is at least 50 per cent of the full scale of the recorder. Inject reference solution (b) 6 times. When the chromatograms are recorded in the prescribed conditions, the approximate relative retention times with reference to cholecalciferol are 0.4 for pre-cholecalciferol and 0.5 for *trans*-cholecalciferol. The relative standard deviation of the response for cholecalciferol is not greater than 1 per cent and the resolution between the peaks due to pre-cholecalciferol and *trans*-cholecalciferol is not less than 1.0. If necessary adjust the proportions of the constituents and the flow rate of the mobile phase to obtain this resolution.

Inject a suitable volume of reference solution (d) and of reference solution (e).

Calculate the conversion factor (f) from the expression:

$$f = \frac{K - L}{M}$$

K = area (or height) of the peak due to cholecalciferol in the chromatogram obtained with reference solution (d),

L = area (or height) of the peak due to cholecalciferol in the chromatogram obtained with reference solution (e),

M = area (or height) of the peak due to pre-cholecalciferol in the chromatogram obtained with reference solution (e).

The value of f determined in duplicate on different days may be used during the entire procedure.

Inject a suitable volume of reference solution (a). Adjust the sensitivity of the system so that the height of the principal peak is at least 50 per cent of the full scale of the recorder. Inject the same volume of the test solution and record the chromatogram in the same manner.

Calculate the content of cholecalciferol in International Units per gram from the expression:

$$\frac{m'}{V'} \times \frac{V}{m} \times \frac{S_D + (f \times S_p)}{S'_D} \times 40\,000 \times 1000$$

m = mass of the preparation to be examined in the test solution, in milligrams,

m' = mass of *cholecalciferol CRS* in reference solution (a), in milligrams,

V = volume of the test solution (25 ml),

V' = volume of reference solution (a) (100 ml),

S_D = area (or height) of the peak due to cholecalciferol in the chromatogram obtained with the test solution,

S'_D = area (or height) of the peak due to cholecalciferol in the chromatogram obtained with reference solution (a),

S_p = area (or height) of the peak due to pre-cholecalciferol in the chromatogram obtained with the test solution,

f = conversion factor.

STORAGE

Store in an airtight, well-filled container, protected from light, at the temperature stated on the label.
Once the container has been opened, its contents are to be used as soon as possible; any part of the contents not used at once is to be protected by an atmosphere of inert gas.

LABELLING

The label states:

- the number of International Units per gram,
- the name of the principal solubiliser or solubilisers used and the name of any added stabilisers,
- the storage temperature.

IMPURITIES

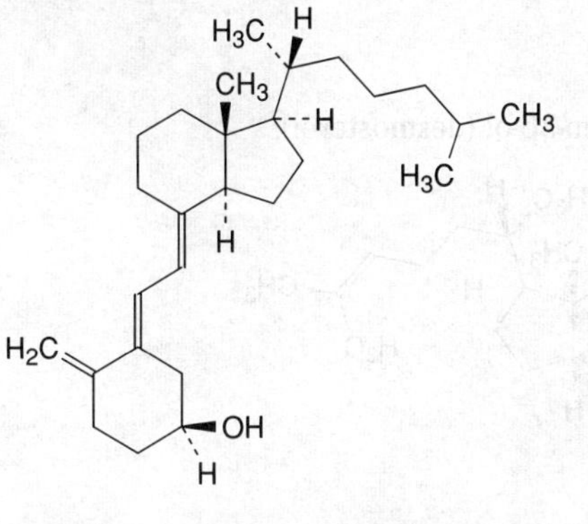

A. (5*E*,7*E*)-9,10-secocholesta-5,7,10(19)-trien-3β-ol (*trans*-cholecalciferol, *trans*-vitamin D_3),

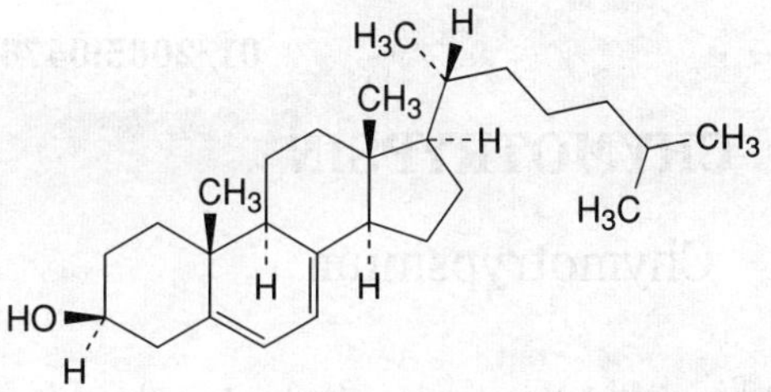

B. cholesta-5,7-dien-3β-ol (7,8-di dehydrocholesterol, provitamin D_3),

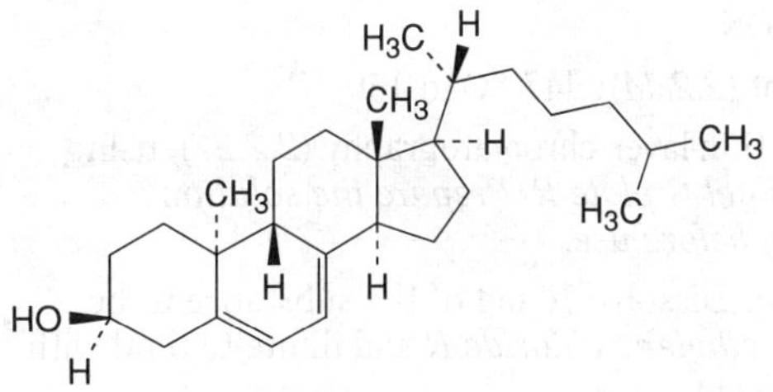

C. (9β,10α)-cholesta-5,7-dien-3β-ol (lumisterol$_3$),

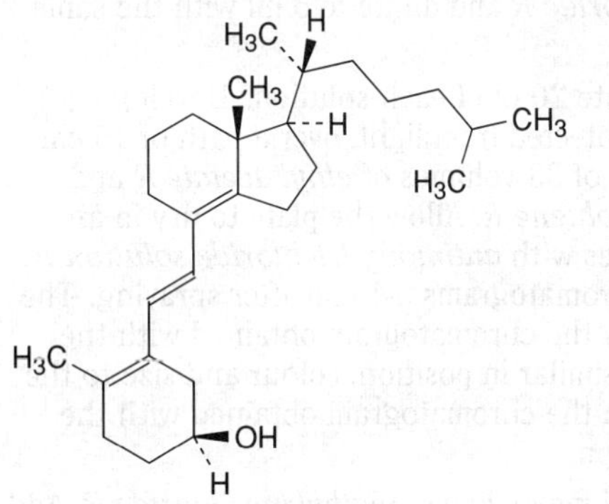

D. (6*E*)-9,10-secocholesta-5(10),6,8(14)-trien-3β-ol (iso-tachysterol$_3$),

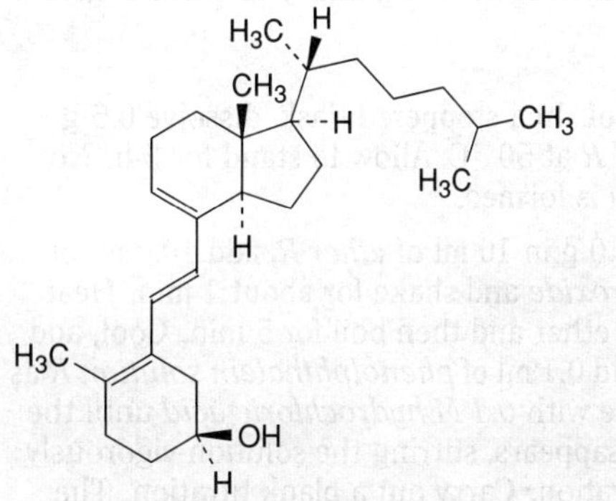

E. (6*E*)-9,10-secocholesta-5(10),6,8-trien-3β-ol (tachysterol$_3$).

01/2005:0993

CHOLESTEROL

Cholesterolum

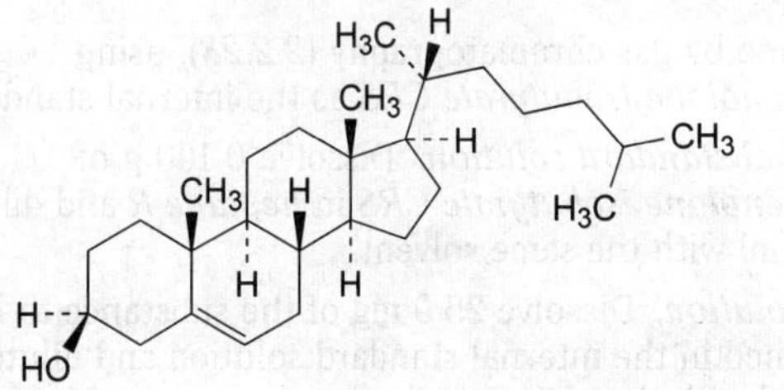

$C_{27}H_{46}O$ M_r 386.7

DEFINITION

Cholesterol contains not less than 95.0 per cent of cholest-5-en-3β-ol and not less than 97.0 per cent and not more than 103.0 per cent of total sterols, calculated with reference to the dried substance.

CHARACTERS

A white or almost white, crystalline powder, practically insoluble in water, sparingly soluble in acetone and in alcohol. It is sensitive to light.

IDENTIFICATION

A. Melting point (*2.2.14*): 147 °C to 150 °C.

B. Examine by thin-layer chromatography (*2.2.27*), using a *TLC silica gel G plate R. Prepare the solutions immediately before use.*

Test solution. Dissolve 10 mg of the substance to be examined in *ethylene chloride R* and dilute to 5 ml with the same solvent.

Reference solution. Dissolve 10 mg of *cholesterol CRS* in *ethylene chloride R* and dilute to 5 ml with the same solvent.

Apply to the plate 20 µl of each solution. Develop immediately, protected from light, over a path of 15 cm using a mixture of 33 volumes of *ethyl acetate R* and 66 volumes of *toluene R*. Allow the plate to dry in air and spray 3 times with *antimony trichloride solution R*. Examine the chromatograms 3-4 min after spraying. The principal spot in the chromatogram obtained with the test solution is similar in position, colour and size to the principal spot in the chromatogram obtained with the reference solution.

C. Dissolve about 5 mg in 2 ml of *methylene chloride R*. Add 1 ml of *acetic anhydride R*, 0.01 ml of *sulphuric acid R* and shake. A pink colour is produced which rapidly changes to red, then to blue and finally to brilliant green.

TESTS

Solubility in alcohol. In a stoppered flask, dissolve 0.5 g in 50 ml of *alcohol R* at 50 °C. Allow to stand for 2 h. No deposit or turbidity is formed.

Acidity. Dissolve 1.0 g in 10 ml of *ether R*, add 10.0 ml of *0.1 M sodium hydroxide* and shake for about 1 min. Heat gently to eliminate ether and then boil for 5 min. Cool, add 10 ml of *water R* and 0.1 ml of *phenolphthalein solution R* as indicator and titrate with *0.1 M hydrochloric acid* until the pink colour just disappears, stirring the solution vigorously throughout the titration. Carry out a blank titration. The difference between the volumes of *0.1 M hydrochloric acid* required to change the colour of the indicator in the blank and in the test is not more than 0.3 ml.

Loss on drying (*2.2.32*). Not more than 0.3 per cent, determined on 1.000 g by drying *in vacuo* at 60 °C for 4 h.

Sulphated ash (*2.4.14*). Not more than 0.1 per cent, determined on 1.0 g.

ASSAY

Examine by gas chromatography (*2.2.28*), using *pregnenolone isobutyrate CRS* as the internal standard.

Internal standard solution. Dissolve 0.100 g of *pregnenolone isobutyrate CRS* in *heptane R* and dilute to 100.0 ml with the same solvent.

Test solution. Dissolve 25.0 mg of the substance to be examined in the internal standard solution and dilute to 25.0 ml with the same solution.

Reference solution. Dissolve 25.0 mg of *cholesterol CRS* in the internal standard solution and dilute to 25.0 ml with the same solution.

The chromatographic procedure may be carried out using:

- a fused-silica column 30 m long and 0.25 mm in internal diameter coated with *poly(dimethyl)siloxane R* (film thickness 0.25 µm),
- *helium for chromatography R* as the carrier gas with a split ratio of 1:25 at a flow rate of 2 ml/min,
- a flame-ionisation detector,

maintaining the temperature of the column at 275 °C, that of the injection port at 285 °C and that of the detector at 300 °C.

Inject 1.0 µl of each solution. The assay is not valid unless the resolution between the peaks due to pregnenolone isobutyrate and cholest-5-en-3β-ol in the chromatogram obtained with the reference solution is at least 10.0.

Calculate the percentage content of cholest-5-en-3β-ol, using the declared content of cholest-5-en-3β-ol in *cholesterol CRS*. Calculate the percentage content of total sterols by adding together the contents of cholest-5-en-3β-ol and other substances with a retention time less than or equal to 1.5 times the retention time of cholest-5-en-3β-ol. Disregard the peaks due to the internal standard and the solvent.

STORAGE

Store protected from light.

LABELLING

The label states the source material for the production of cholesterol (for example bovine brain and spinal cord, wool fat or chicken eggs).

IMPURITIES

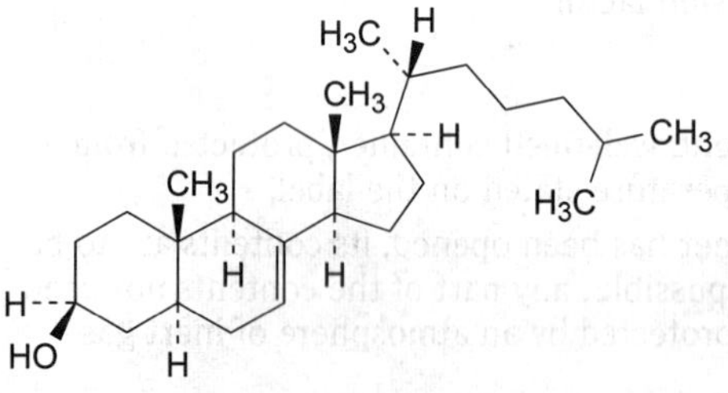

A. 5α-cholest-7-en-3β-ol (lathosterol),

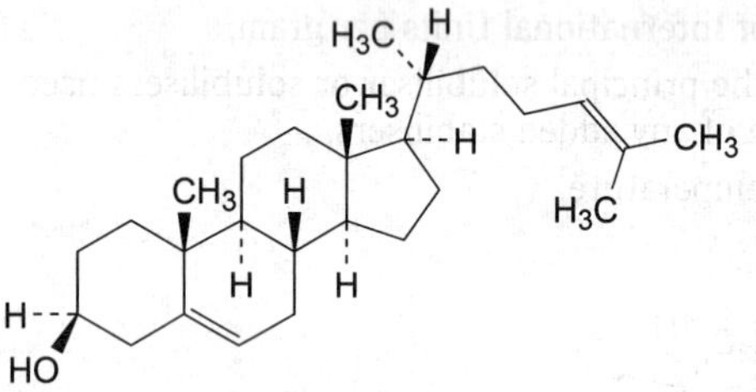

B. cholesta-5,24-dien-3β-ol (desmosterol),

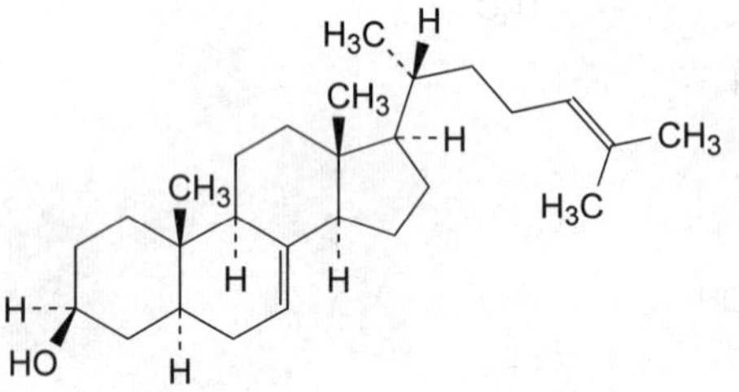

C. 5α-cholesta-7,24-dien-3β-ol.

01/2005:0476

CHYMOTRYPSIN

Chymotrypsinum

DEFINITION

Chymotrypsin is a proteolytic enzyme obtained by the activation of chrymotrypsinogen extracted from the pancreas of beef (*Bos taurus* L.). It has an activity not less than

5.0 microkatals per milligram. In solution it has maximal enzymic activity at about pH 8; the activity is reversibly inhibited at pH 3, at which pH it is most stable.

PRODUCTION

The animals from which chymotrypsin is derived must fulfil the requirements for the health of animals suitable for human consumption to the satisfaction of the competent authority; furthermore the tissues used shall not include any specified risk material as defined by any relevant international or, where appropriate, national legislation. It must have been shown to what extent the method of production allows inactivation or removal of any contamination by viruses or other infectious agents.

The method of manufacture is validated to demonstrate that the product, if tested, would comply with the following test:

Histamine (*2.6.10*). Not more than 1 μg (calculated as histamine base) per 5 microkatals of chymotrypsin activity. Before carrying out the test, heat the solution of the substance to be examined on a water-bath for 30 min.

CHARACTERS

A white, crystalline or amorphous powder, sparingly soluble in water; the amorphous form is hygroscopic.

IDENTIFICATION

A. Dilute 1 ml of solution S (see Tests) to 10 ml with *water R*. In a depression in a white spot plate, mix 0.05 ml of this solution with 0.2 ml of substrate solution. A purple colour develops.
Substrate solution. To 24.0 mg of *acetyltyrosine ethyl ester R* add 0.2 ml of *alcohol R*, and swirl until solution is effected. Add 2.0 ml of *0.067 M phosphate buffer solution pH 7.0 R* and 1 ml of *methyl red mixed solution R* and dilute to 10.0 ml with *water R*.

B. Dilute 0.5 ml of solution S to 5 ml with *water R*. Add 0.10 ml of a 20 g/l solution of *tosylphenylalanylchloromethane R* in *alcohol R*. Adjust to pH 7.0 and shake for 2 h. In a depression in a white spot plate, mix 0.05 ml of this solution with 0.2 ml of the substrate solution (see Identification test A). No colour develops within 3 min of mixing.

TESTS

Solution S. Dissolve 0.10 g in *carbon dioxide-free water R* and dilute to 10.0 ml with the same solvent.

Appearance of solution. Solution S is not more opalescent than reference suspension II (*2.2.1*).

pH (*2.2.3*). The pH of solution S is 3.0 to 5.0.

Absorbance (*2.2.25*). Dissolve 30.0 mg in *0.001 M hydrochloric acid* and dilute to 100.0 ml with the same acid. The solution shows an absorption maximum at 281 nm and a minimum at 250 nm. The specific absorbance at the maximum is 18.5 to 22.5 and that at the minimum is not greater than 8.

Trypsin. Transfer to a depression in a white spot plate 0.05 ml of *tris(hydroxymethyl)aminomethane buffer solution pH 8.1 R* and 0.1 ml of solution S. Add 0.2 ml of substrate solution (test solution). At the same time and in the same manner, prepare a reference solution using the substance to be examined to which not more than 1 per cent *m/m* of *trypsin BRP* has been added. Start a timer. No colour appears in the test solution within 3 min to 5 min after the addition of the substrate solution. A purple colour is produced in the control solution.

Substrate solution. To 98.5 mg of *tosylarginine methyl ester hydrochloride R*, suitable for assaying trypsin, add 5 ml of *tris(hydroxymethyl)aminomethane buffer solution pH 8.1 R* and swirl to dissolve. Add 2.5 ml of *methyl red mixed solution R* and dilute to 25.0 ml with *water R*.

Loss on drying (*2.2.32*). Not more than 5.0 per cent, determined on 0.100 g by drying at 60 °C at a pressure not exceeding 0.7 kPa for 2 h.

ASSAY

The activity of chymotrypsin is determined by comparing the rate at which it hydrolyses *acetyltyrosine ethyl ester R* with the rate at which *chymotrypsin BRP* hydrolyses the same substrate under the same conditions.

Apparatus. Use a reaction vessel of about 30 ml capacity provided with:

- a device that will maintain a temperature of 25.0 ± 0.1 °C,
- a stirring device, for example a magnetic stirrer,
- a lid with holes for the insertion of electrodes, the tip of a burette, a tube for the admission of nitrogen and the introduction of reagents.

An automatic or manual titration apparatus may be used. For the latter the burette is graduated in 0.005 ml and the pH meter is provided with a wide scale and glass-calomel electrodes.

Test solution. Dissolve 25.0 mg of the substance to be examined in *0.001 M hydrochloric acid* and dilute to 250.0 ml with the same acid.

Reference solution. Dissolve 25.0 mg of *chymotrypsin BRP* in *0.001 M hydrochloric acid* and dilute to 250.0 ml with the same acid.

Store the solutions at 0 °C to 5 °C. Warm 1 ml of each solution to about 25 °C over 15 min and use 50 μl of each solution (corresponding to about 25 nanokatals) for each titration. Carry out the titration in an atmosphere of nitrogen. Transfer 10.0 ml of *0.01 M calcium chloride solution R* to the reaction vessel and, while stirring, add 0.35 ml of *0.2 M acetyltyrosine ethyl ester solution R*. When the temperature is steady at 25.0 ± 0.1 °C (after about 5 min) adjust the pH to exactly 8.0 with *0.02 M sodium hydroxide*. Add 50 μl of the test solution (equivalent to about 5 μg of the substance to be examined) and start a timer. Maintain the pH at 8.0 by the addition of *0.02 M sodium hydroxide*, noting the volume added every 30 s. Calculate the volume of *0.02 M sodium hydroxide* used per second between 30 s and 210 s. Carry out a titration in the same manner using the reference solution and calculate the volume of *0.02 M sodium hydroxide* used per second.

Calculate the activity in microkatals per milligram using the expression:

$$\frac{m' \times V}{m \times V'} \times A$$

m = mass of the substance to be examined, in milligrams,

m' = mass of *chymotrypsin BRP*, in milligrams,

V = volume of *0.02 M sodium hydroxide* used per second by the test solution,

V' = volume of *0.02 M sodium hydroxide* used per second by the reference solution,

A = activity of *chymotrypsin BRP*, in microkatals per milligram.

STORAGE

Store in an airtight container at 2 °C to 8 °C, protected from light.

LABELLING

The label states:

- the quantity of chymotrypsin and the total activity in microkatals per container,
- for the amorphous substance, that it is hygroscopic.

01/2005:1407

CICLOPIROX

Ciclopiroxum

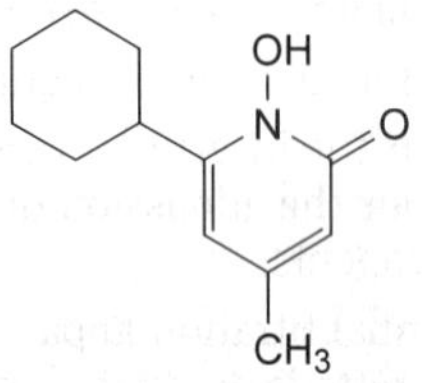

$C_{12}H_{17}NO_2$ M_r 207.3

DEFINITION

Ciclopirox contains not less than 98.0 per cent and not more than the equivalent of 101.0 per cent of 6-cyclohexyl-1-hydroxy-4-methylpyridin-2(1*H*)-one, calculated with reference to the dried substance.

CHARACTERS

A white or yellowish-white, crystalline powder, slightly soluble in water, freely soluble in ethanol and in methylene chloride.

IDENTIFICATION

First identification: B.

Second identification: A, C.

A. Melting point (*2.2.14*): 140 °C to 145 °C.

B. Examine by infrared absorption spectrophotometry (*2.2.24*), comparing with the spectrum obtained with *ciclopirox CRS*.

C. Examine by thin-layer chromatography (*2.2.27*), using a *TLC silica gel F_{254} plate R*.

Test solution. Dissolve 20 mg of the substance to be examined in *methanol R* and dilute to 10 ml with the same solvent.

Reference solution. Dissolve 20 mg of *ciclopirox CRS* in *methanol R* and dilute to 10 ml with the same solvent.

Before use predevelop the plate with a mixture of 10 volumes of *concentrated ammonia R*, 15 volumes of *water R* and 75 volumes of *alcohol R* until the solvent front has migrated to the top of the plate. Allow the plate to dry in air for 5 min.

Apply to the plate 10 µl of each solution. Develop over a path of 15 cm using a mixture of 10 volumes of *concentrated ammonia R*, 15 volumes of *water R* and 75 volumes of *alcohol R*. Allow the plate to dry in air for 10 min and examine in ultraviolet light at 254 nm. The principal spot in the chromatogram obtained with the test solution is similar in position and size to the principal spot in the chromatogram obtained with the reference solution. Spray the plate with a 20 g/l solution of *ferric chloride R* in *ethanol R*. The principal spot in the chromatogram obtained with the test solution is similar in position, colour and size to the principal spot in the chromatogram obtained with the reference solution.

TESTS

Appearance of solution. Dissolve 2.0 g in *methanol R* and dilute to 10 ml with the same solvent. The solution is clear (*2.2.1*) and not more intensely coloured than reference solution Y_5 (*2.2.2, Method II*).

Related substances. Examine by liquid chromatography (*2.2.29*). *Carry out the operations avoiding exposure to actinic light. All materials which are in direct contact with the substance to be examined like column materials, reagents, solvents and others should contain only very low amounts of extractable metal cations.*

Solvent mixture. Mix 1 volume of *acetonitrile R* and 9 volumes of the mobile phase.

Test solution. Dissolve 30.0 mg of the substance to be examined in 15 ml of the solvent mixture. If necessary, use an ultrasonic bath. Dilute to 20.0 ml with the solvent mixture.

Reference solution (a). Dissolve 15.0 mg of *ciclopirox impurity A CRS* and 15.0 mg of *ciclopirox impurity B CRS* in the solvent mixture and dilute to 10.0 ml with the same solvent mixture.

Reference solution (b). Dilute 1.0 ml of reference solution (a) to 200.0 ml with the solvent mixture.

Reference solution (c). Dilute 2.0 ml of reference solution (b) to 10.0 ml with the solvent mixture.

Reference solution (d). Mix 5 ml of reference solution (a) with 5 ml of the test solution.

The chromatographic procedure may be carried out using:

- a stainless steel column 80 mm long and 4 mm in internal diameter packed with *nitrile silica gel for chromatography R2* (5 µm),
- as rinsing solution a mixture of 1 volume of *glacial acetic acid R*, 1 volume of *acetylacetone R*, 500 volumes of *acetonitrile R* and 500 volumes of *water R*,
- as mobile phase at a flow rate of 0.7 ml/min a mixture of 0.1 ml of *glacial acetic acid R*, 230 ml of *acetonitrile R* and 770 ml of a 0.96 g/l solution of *sodium edetate R*. If the retention time of the principal peak in the chromatogram obtained with the test solution is not between 8 min and 11 min adjust the ratio of the 0.96 g/l solution of sodium edetate: acetonitrile accordingly,
- as detector a spectrophotometer set at 220 nm and 298 nm.

In order to ensure desorption of disruptive metal ions, every new column is to be rinsed with the rinsing solution over a period of not less than 15 h and then with the mobile phase for not less than 5 h at a flow rate of 0.2 ml/min.

Inject 10 µl each of the solvent mixture, the test solution and the reference solutions (b), (c) and (d) and record the chromatograms at 220 nm and 298 nm. Continue the chromatography of the test solution for 2.5 times the retention time of the principal peak.

The relative retention times are:

- impurity A: 0.5
- impurity C: 0.9
- ciclopirox: 1
- impurity B: 1.3

The test is not valid unless: in the chromatogram obtained with reference solution (d), the resolution between the peaks corresponding to impurity B and ciclopirox is not less than 2.0; the chromatogram obtained with reference solution (c) shows at 298 nm a peak corresponding to impurity B with a signal-to-noise ratio of not less than three; in the chromatogram obtained with the test solution the symmetry factor of the principal peak is between 0.8 and 2.0.

In the chromatogram obtained with the test solution at 220 nm, the area of the peak due to impurity A is not greater than the area of the corresponding peak in the chromatogram obtained with reference solution (b) at the same wavelength (0.5 per cent). In the chromatogram obtained with the test solution at 298 nm, the area of any peak apart from the principal peak is not greater than the area of the peak due to impurity B in the chromatogram obtained with reference solution (b) at the same wavelength (0.5 per cent); the sum of all peak areas at 298 nm, apart from the principal peak and any peak due to impurity B, is not greater than the area of the peak due to impurity B in the chromatogram obtained with reference solution (b) (0.5 per cent). At 298 nm disregard any peak due to the solvent and any peak with an area less than half the area of the peak due to impurity B in the chromatogram obtained with reference solution (c) at the same wavelength.

Heavy metals (*2.4.8*). 2.0 g complies with limit test C for heavy metals (10 ppm). Prepare the standard using 2 ml of *lead standard solution (10 ppm Pb) R*.

Loss on drying (*2.2.32*). Not more than 1.5 per cent, determined on 1.000 g by drying *in vacuo* at 60 °C over *diphosphorus pentoxide R*.

Sulphated ash (*2.4.14*). Not more than 0.1 per cent determined on 1.0 g.

ASSAY

Dissolve 0.150 g in 20 ml of *methanol R*. Add 20 ml of *water R* and titrate with *0.1 M sodium hydroxide*, determining the end-point potentiometrically (*2.2.20*). Carry out a blank titration.

1 ml of *0.1 M sodium hydroxide* is equivalent to 20.73 mg of $C_{12}H_{17}NO_2$.

STORAGE

Store protected from light.

IMPURITIES

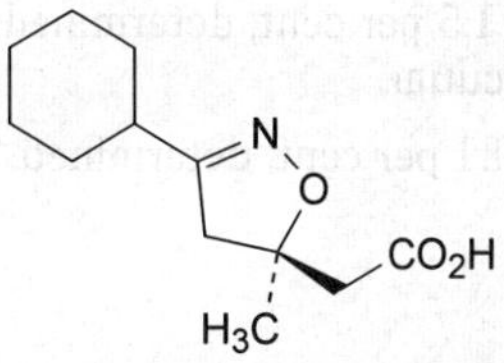

A. (*RS*)-2-(3-cyclohexyl-5-methyl-4,5-dihydroisoxazol-5-yl)acetic acid,

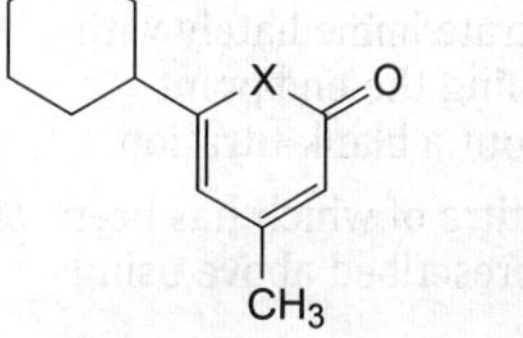

B. X = O: 6-cyclohexyl-4-methyl-2*H*-pyran-2-one,

C. X = NH: 6-cyclohexyl-4-methylpyridin-2(1*H*)-one.

01/2005:1302

CICLOPIROX OLAMINE

Ciclopirox olaminum

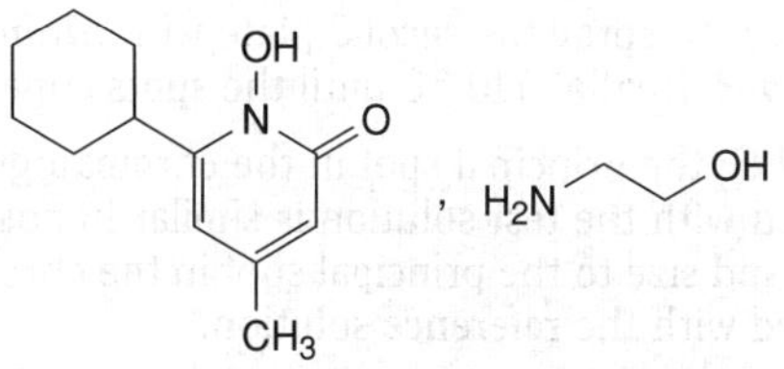

$C_{14}H_{24}N_2O_3$ M_r 268.4

DEFINITION

6-Cyclohexyl-1-hydroxy-4-methylpyridin-2(1*H*)-one and 2-aminoethanol.

Content:

- ciclopirox ($C_{12}H_{17}NO_2$; M_r 207.3): 76.0 per cent to 78.5 per cent (dried substance),
- 2-aminoethanol (C_2H_7NO; M_r 61.1): 22.2 per cent to 23.3 per cent (dried substance).

CHARACTERS

Appearance: white or pale yellow, crystalline powder.

Solubility: sparingly soluble in water, very soluble in alcohol and in methylene chloride, slightly soluble in ethyl acetate, practically insoluble in cyclohexane.

It shows polymorphism.

IDENTIFICATION

First identification: A.

Second identification: B.

A. Infrared absorption spectrophotometry (*2.2.24*).

Comparison: *ciclopirox olamine CRS*.

If the spectra obtained in the solid state show differences, dissolve the substance to be examined and the reference substance separately in the minimum volume of *ethyl acetate R*, evaporate to dryness on a water-bath and record new spectra using the residues.

B. Thin-layer chromatography (*2.2.27*).

Test solution. Dissolve 25 mg of the substance to be examined in *methanol R* and dilute to 10 ml with the same solvent.

Reference solution. Dissolve 25 mg of *ciclopirox olamine CRS* in *methanol R* and dilute to 10 ml with the same solvent.

Plate: *TLC silica gel* F_{254} *plate R*.

Before use wash 2 plates by allowing a mixture of 10 volumes of *concentrated ammonia R*, 15 volumes of *water R* and 75 volumes of *ethanol R* to migrate until the solvent front has reached the top of the plate. Allow the plates to dry in air for 5 min.

Mobile phase: *concentrated ammonia R*, *water R*, *ethanol R* (10:15:75 *V/V/V*).

Application: 10 µl.

Development: over a path of 15 cm.

Drying: in air for 10 min.

Detection A: examine in ultraviolet light at 254 nm.

Results A: the principal spot in the chromatogram obtained with the test solution is similar in position and size to the principal spot in the chromatogram obtained with the reference solution.

Detection B: spray one plate with *ferric chloride solution R3.*

Results B: the principal spot in the chromatogram obtained with the test solution is similar in position, colour and size to the principal spot in the chromatogram obtained with the reference solution.

Detection C: spray the second plate with *ninhydrin solution R.* Heat at 110 °C until the spots appear.

Results C: the principal spot in the chromatogram obtained with the test solution is similar in position, colour and size to the principal spot in the chromatogram obtained with the reference solution.

TESTS

Appearance of solution. The solution is clear (*2.2.1*) and not more intensely coloured than reference solution BY_7 (*2.2.2, Method II*).

Dissolve 2.0 g in *methanol R* and dilute to 20 ml with the same solvent.

pH (*2.2.3*): 8.0 to 9.0.

Dissolve 1.0 g in *carbon dioxide-free water R* and dilute to 100 ml with the same solvent.

Related substances. Liquid chromatography (*2.2.29*). *Carry out the operations avoiding exposure to actinic light. All materials which are in direct contact with the substance to be examined, such as column materials, reagents, solvents, etc. should contain only small amounts of extractable metal cations.*

Test solution. Dissolve 40.0 mg of the substance to be examined (corresponding to about 30 mg of ciclopirox) in a mixture of 20 µl of *anhydrous acetic acid R*, 2 ml of *acetonitrile R*, and 15 ml of the mobile phase. If necessary, use an ultrasonic bath. Dilute to 20.0 ml with the mobile phase.

Reference solution (a). Dissolve 15.0 mg of *ciclopirox impurity A CRS* and 15.0 mg of *ciclopirox impurity B CRS* in a mixture of 1 ml of *acetonitrile R* and 7 ml of the mobile phase. Dilute to 10.0 ml with the mobile phase.

Reference solution (b). Dilute 1.0 ml of reference solution (a) to 200.0 ml with a mixture of 1 volume of *acetonitrile R* and 9 volumes of the mobile phase.

Reference solution (c). Dilute 2.0 ml of reference solution (b) to 10.0 ml with a mixture of 1 volume of *acetonitrile R* and 9 volumes of the mobile phase.

Reference solution (d). Mix 5 ml of reference solution (a) with 5 ml of the test solution.

Column:

- *size*: l = 80 mm, Ø = 4 mm,
- *stationary phase*: *nitrile silica gel for chromatography R* (5 µm),
- *rinsing solution*: a mixture of 1 volume of *anhydrous acetic acid R*, 1 volume of *acetylacetone R*, 500 volumes of *acetonitrile R* and 500 volumes of *water R.*

Mobile phase: a mixture of 0.1 volumes of *anhydrous acetic acid R*, 230 volumes of *acetonitrile R* and 770 volumes of a 0.96 g/l solution of *sodium edetate R.* If the retention time of the principal peak in the chromatogram obtained with the test solution is not between 8 min and 11 min adjust the ratio of the 0.96 g/l solution of sodium edetate to acetonitrile accordingly.

Flow rate: 0.7 ml/min.

Detection: variable wavelength spectrophotometer capable of operating at 220 nm and 298 nm.

In order to ensure desorption of interfering metal ions, a new column is to be rinsed with the rinsing solution over a period of at least 15 h and then with the mobile phase for at least 5 h at a flow rate of 0.2 ml/min.

Injection: 10 µl; inject the test solution and reference solutions (b), (c) and (d).

Run time: 2.5 times the retention time of ciclopirox.

Relative retention with reference to ciclopirox: impurity A = about 0.5; impurity C = about 0.9; impurity B = about 1.3.

System suitability:

- *resolution*: minimum of 2.0 between the peaks corresponding to impurity B and ciclopirox in the chromatogram obtained with reference solution (d),
- *signal-to-noise ratio*: minimum of 10 for the peak corresponding to impurity B in the chromatogram obtained with reference solution (c) at 298 nm,
- *symmetry factor*: 0.8 to 2.0 for the principal peak in the chromatogram obtained with the test solution.

Limits:

- *impurity A at 220 nm*: not more than the area of the corresponding peak in the chromatogram obtained with reference solution (b) at the same wavelength (0.5 per cent),
- *any impurity at 298 nm*: not more than the area of the peak due to impurity B in the chromatogram obtained with reference solution (b) at the same wavelength (0.5 per cent),
- *total at 298 nm apart from impurity B*: not more than the area of the peak due to impurity B in the chromatogram obtained with reference solution (b) (0.5 per cent),
- *disregard limit at 298 nm*: area of the peak due to impurity B in the chromatogram obtained with reference solution (c) at the same wavelength (0.1 per cent).

Heavy metals (*2.4.8*): maximum 20 ppm.

1.0 g complies with limit test C. Prepare the standard using 2 ml of *lead standard solution (10 ppm Pb) R.*

Loss on drying (*2.2.32*): maximum 1.5 per cent, determined on 1.000 g by drying under high vacuum.

Sulphated ash (*2.4.14*): maximum 0.1 per cent, determined on 1.0 g.

ASSAY

2-Aminoethanol. Dissolve 0.250 g in 25 ml of *anhydrous acetic acid R*. Titrate with *0.1 M perchloric acid*, determining the end-point potentiometrically (*2.2.20*).

1 ml of *0.1 M perchloric acid* is equivalent to 6.108 mg of C_2H_7NO.

Ciclopirox. Dissolve 0.200 g in 2 ml of *methanol R.* Add 38 ml of *water R*, swirl and titrate immediately with *0.1 M sodium hydroxide*, determining the end-point potentiometrically (*2.2.20*). Carry out a blank titration.

Use *0.1 M sodium hydroxide*, the titre of which has been determined under the conditions prescribed above using 0.100 g of *benzoic acid RV.*

1 ml of *0.1 M sodium hydroxide* is equivalent to 20.73 mg of $C_{12}H_{17}NO_2$.

STORAGE

Protected from light.

IMPURITIES

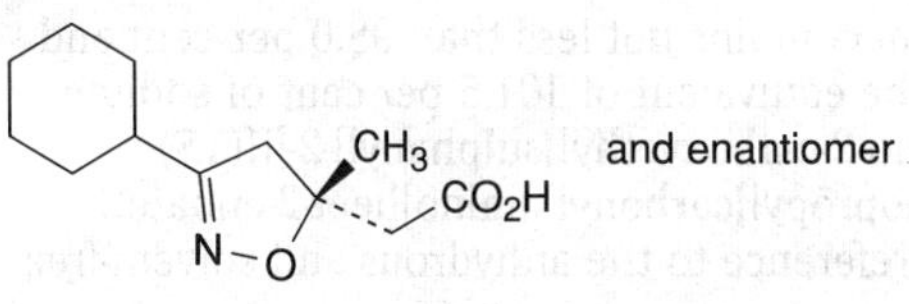

A. (*RS*)-2-(3-cyclohexyl-5-methyl-4,5-dihydroisoxazol-5-yl)acetic acid,

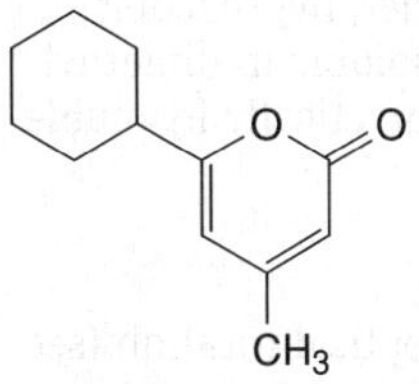

B. 6-cyclohexyl-4-methyl-2*H*-pyran-2-one,

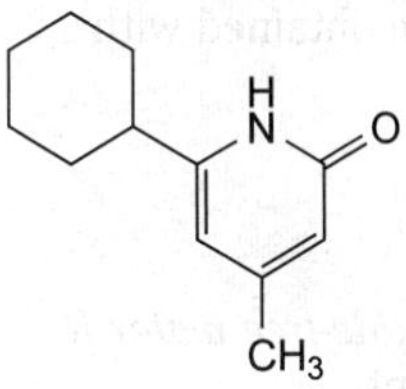

C. 6-cyclohexyl-4-methylpyridin-2(1*H*)-one.

01/2005:0994
corrected

CICLOSPORIN

Ciclosporinum

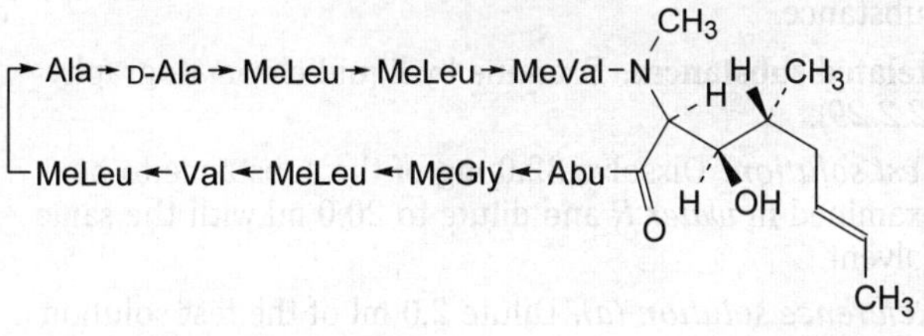

$C_{62}H_{111}N_{11}O_{12}$ M_r 1203

DEFINITION

Ciclosporin contains not less than 98.5 per cent and not more than the equivalent of 101.5 per cent of cyclo[[(2*S*,3*R*,4*R*,6*E*)-3-hydroxy-4-methyl-2-(methylamino)oct-6-enoyl]-L-2-aminobutanoyl-*N*-methylglycyl-*N*-methyl-L-leucyl-L-valyl-*N*-methyl-L-leucyl-L-alanyl-D-alanyl-*N*-methyl-L-leucyl-*N*-methyl-L-leucyl-*N*-methyl-L-valyl], calculated with reference to the dried substance. Ciclosporin is a substance produced by *Beauveria nivea (Tolypocladium inflatum Gams)* or obtained by any other means.

CHARACTERS

A white or almost white powder, practically insoluble in water, freely soluble in ethanol and in methylene chloride.

IDENTIFICATION

A. Examine by infrared absorption spectrophotometry (*2.2.24*), comparing with the spectrum obtained with *ciclosporin CRS.*

B. Examine the chromatograms obtained in the assay. The principal peak in the chromatogram obtained with the test solution is similar in retention time to the principal peak in the chromatogram obtained with reference solution (a).

TESTS

Appearance of solution. Dissolve 1.5 g in *ethanol R* and dilute to 15 ml with the same solvent. The solution is clear (*2.2.1*) and not more intensely coloured than reference solution Y_5, BY_5 or R_7 (*2.2.2, Method II*).

Specific optical rotation (*2.2.7*). Dissolve 0.125 g in *methanol R* and dilute to 25.0 ml with the same solvent. The specific optical rotation is − 185 to − 193, calculated with reference to the dried substance.

Related substances. Examine by liquid chromatography (*2.2.29*) as prescribed under Assay. Inject separately the test solution and reference solution (b). Continue the chromatography for 1.7 times the retention time of the principal peak. In the chromatogram obtained with the test solution: the area of any peak, apart from the principal peak, is not greater than 0.7 times the area of the principal peak in the chromatogram obtained with reference solution (b) (0.7 per cent); the sum of the areas of all the peaks, apart from the principal peak, is not greater than 1.5 times the area of the principal peak in the chromatogram obtained with reference solution (b) (1.5 per cent). Disregard any peak due to the solvent and any peak with an area less than 0.05 times that of the principal peak in the chromatogram with reference solution (b).

Heavy metals (*2.4.8*). The residue obtained in the test for loss on drying complies with limit test C for heavy metals (20 ppm). Prepare the standard using 2 ml of *lead standard solution (10 ppm Pb) R*.

Loss on drying (*2.2.32*). Not more than 2.0 per cent, determined on 1.000 g at 60 °C at a pressure not exceeding 15 Pa for 3 h.

Bacterial endotoxins (*2.6.14*): less than 0.84 IU/mg, if intended for use in the manufacture of parenteral dosage forms without a further appropriate procedure for the removal of bacterial endotoxins. Dissolve 50 mg of the substance to be examined in a mixture of 280 mg of *alcohol R* and 650 mg of *polyoxyethylated castor oil R* and dilute to the required concentration using water LAL.

ASSAY

Examine by liquid chromatography (*2.2.29*).

Test solution. Dissolve 30.0 mg of the substance to be examined in a mixture of equal volumes of *acetonitrile R* and *water R* and dilute to 25.0 ml with the same mixture of solvents.

Reference solution (a). Dissolve 30.0 mg of *ciclosporin CRS* in a mixture of equal volumes of *acetonitrile R* and *water R* and dilute to 25.0 ml with the same mixture of solvents.

Reference solution (b). Dilute 2.0 ml of reference solution (a) to 200.0 ml with a mixture of equal volumes of *acetonitrile R* and *water R.*

Reference solution (c). Dissolve the contents of a vial of *ciclosporin for system suitability CRS* in 5.0 ml of the mobile phase.

The chromatographic procedure may be carried out using:

- a stainless steel column 0.25 m long and 4 mm in internal diameter packed with *octadecylsilyl silica gel for chromatography R* (3 µm to 5 µm); the column is connected to the injection port by a steel capillary tube about 1 m long and having an internal diameter of 0.25 mm,
- as mobile phase at a flow rate of about 1.5 ml per minute a mixture of 1 volume of *phosphoric acid R*, 50 volumes of *1,1-dimethylethyl methyl ether R*, 430 volumes of *acetonitrile R* and 520 volumes of *water R,*
- as detector a spectrophotometer set at 210 nm,

– a 20 µl loop injector,

maintaining the temperature of the column and of the steel capillary tube at 80 °C.

Inject reference solution (c). The test is not valid unless the peak-to-valley ratio is minimum 1.4 where H_p = height above the baseline of the peak due to ciclosporin U and H_v = height above the baseline of the lowest point of the curve separating this peak from the peak due to ciclosporin. Adjust the ratio of 1,1 dimethylethylmethyl ether to acetonitrile, if necessary. The test is not valid unless the retention time of the principal peak is 25 min to 30 min. Adjust the ratio of acetonitrile to water, if necessary. Inject reference solution (a) 6 times. The test is not valid unless the relative standard deviation of the area of the principal peak is at most 1.0 per cent. Inject alternately the test solution and reference solution (a). Calculate the percentage content of ciclosporin.

STORAGE

Store in an airtight container, protected from light. If the substance is sterile, store in a sterile, airtight, tamper-proof container.

LABELLING

The label states, where applicable, that the substance is free from bacterial endotoxins.

IMPURITIES

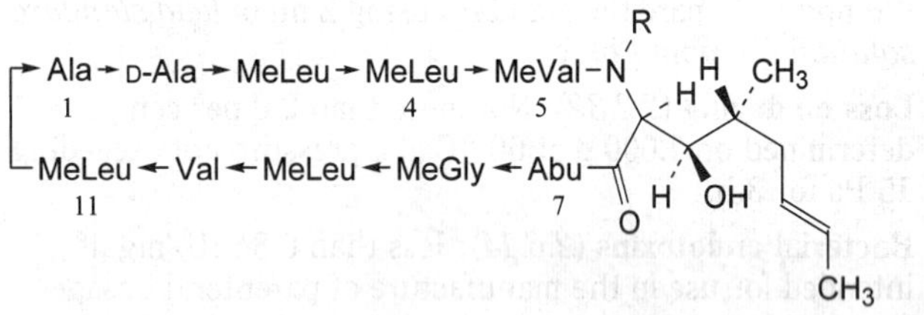

A. different ciclosporins [difference with ciclosporin (R = CH_3: ciclosporin A)]: ciclosporin B [7-L-Ala]; ciclosporin C [7-L-Thr]; ciclosporin D [7-L-Val]; ciclosporin E [5-L-Val]; ciclosporin G [7-(L-2-aminopentanoyl)]; ciclosporin H [5-D-MeVal]; ciclosporin L [R = H]; ciclosporin T [4-L-Leu]; ciclosporin U [11-L-Leu]; ciclosporin V [1-L-Abu],

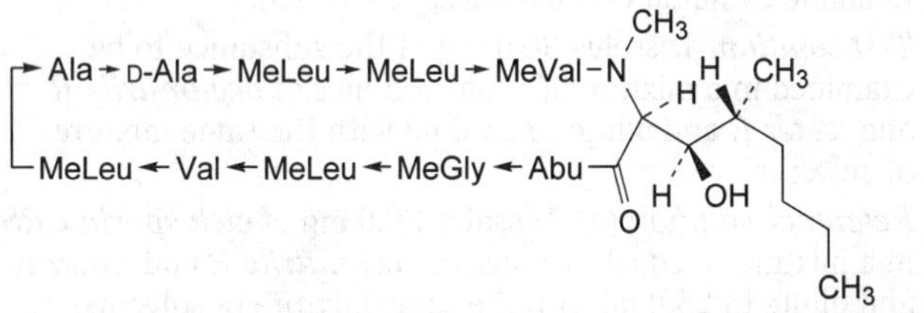

B. [6-[(2*S*,3*R*,4*R*)-3-hydroxy-4-methyl-2-(methylamino)octanoic acid]]ciclosporin A,

C. isociclosporin A.

01/2005:1408

CILASTATIN SODIUM

Cilastatinum natricum

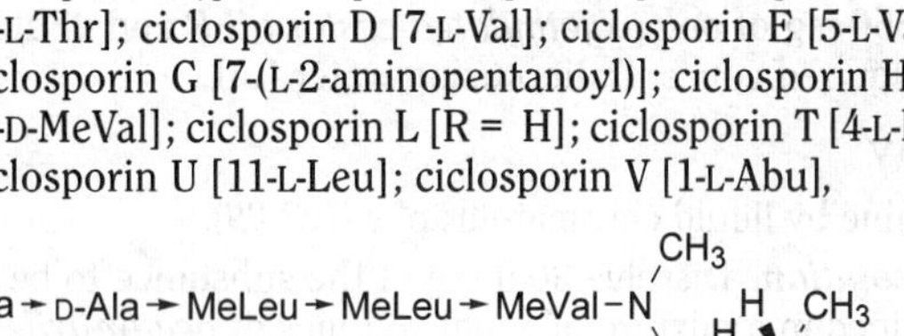

$C_{16}H_{25}N_2NaO_5S$ M_r 380.4

DEFINITION

Cilastatin sodium contains not less than 98.0 per cent and not more than the equivalent of 101.5 per cent of sodium (*Z*)-7-[[(*R*)-2-amino-2-carboxyethyl]sulphanyl]-2-[[[(1*S*)-2,2-dimethylcyclopropyl]carbonyl]amino]hept-2-enoate, calculated with reference to the anhydrous and solvent-free substance.

CHARACTERS

A white or light yellow amorphous powder, hygroscopic, very soluble in water and in methanol, soluble in dimethyl sulphoxide, slightly soluble in ethanol, practically insoluble in acetone and in methylene chloride.

IDENTIFICATION

A. It complies with the test for specific optical rotation (see Tests).

B. Examine by infrared absorption spectrophotometry (*2.2.24*), comparing with the spectrum obtained with *cilastatin sodium CRS*.

C. It gives reaction (a) of sodium (*2.3.1*).

TESTS

Solution S. Dissolve 1.0 g in *carbon dioxide-free water R* and dilute to 100 ml with the same solvent.

Appearance of solution. Solution S is clear (*2.2.1*) and not more intensely coloured than reference solution Y_6 (*2.2.2, Method II*).

pH (*2.2.3*). The pH of solution S is 6.5 to 7.5.

Specific optical rotation (*2.2.7*). Dissolve 0.250 g in a mixture of 1 volume of *hydrochloric acid R* and 120 volumes of *methanol R* and dilute to 25.0 ml with the same mixture of solvents. The specific optical rotation is + 41.5 to + 44.5, calculated with reference to the anhydrous and solvent-free substance.

Related substances. Examine by liquid chromatography (*2.2.29*).

Test solution. Dissolve 32.0 mg of the substance to be examined in *water R* and dilute to 20.0 ml with the same solvent.

Reference solution (a). Dilute 2.0 ml of the test solution to 100.0 ml with *water R*. Dilute 5.0 ml of this solution to 100.0 ml with *water R*.

Reference solution (b). Dilute 5.0 ml the test solution to 100.0 ml with *water R*. Dilute 2.0 ml of this solution to 20.0 ml with *water R*.

Reference solution (c). Dissolve 16 mg of the substance to be examined in *dilute hydrogen peroxide solution R* and dilute to 10.0 ml with the same solvent. Allow to stand for 30 min. Dilute 1 ml of this solution to 100 ml with *water R*.

Reference solution (d). Dissolve 32 mg of *mesityl oxide R* in 100 ml of *water R*. Dilute 1 ml of the solution to 50 ml with *water R*.

The chromatographic procedure may be carried out using:

– a stainless steel column 0.25 m long and 4.6 mm in internal diameter packed with *octadecylsilyl silica gel for chromatography R* (5 µm),

– as mobile phase at a flow rate of 2.0 ml/min, the following mixtures:

Mobile phase A. Prepare a mixture of 300 volumes of *acetonitrile R* and 700 volumes of a 0.1 per cent *V/V* solution of *phosphoric acid R* in *water R*,

Mobile phase B. A 0.1 per cent *V/V* solution of *phosphoric acid R* in *water R*,

Time (min)	Mobile phase A (per cent *V/V*)	Mobile phase B (per cent *V/V*)
	15	85
0 - 30	15 → 100	85 → 0
30 - 46	100	0
46 - 56	100 → 15	0 → 85

– as detector a spectrophotometer set at 210 nm,

– a 20 μl loop injector,

maintaining the temperature of the column at 50 °C.

Equilibrate the column with a mixture of 15 per cent *V/V* of mobile phase A and 85 per cent *V/V* of mobile phase B. Inject separately each solution. Adjust the sensitivity of the system so that the height of the principal peak in the chromatogram obtained with reference solution (b) is at least 15 per cent of the full scale of the recorder.

The test is not valid unless, the chromatogram obtained with reference solution (c) shows three principal peaks: the first two peaks (cilastatin impurity A) may elute without being completely resolved and the mass distribution ratio of the third peak (cilastatin) is at least ten; in the chromatogram obtained with reference solution (a), the principal peak has a signal-to-noise ratio of at least 5.0.

In the chromatogram obtained with the test solution, the area of any peak, apart from the principal peak, is not greater than the area of the principal peak in the chromatogram obtained with reference solution (b) (0.5 per cent); the sum of the areas of all peaks, apart from the principal peak, is not greater than twice the area of the principal peak in the chromatogram obtained with reference solution (b) (1 per cent). Disregard any peak due to the solvent, any peak with an area less than that of the principal peak in the chromatogram obtained with reference solution (a) and any peak corresponding to the principal peak in the chromatogram obtained with reference solution (d).

Mesityl oxide, acetone and methanol. Not more than 1.0 per cent *m/m* of acetone, 0.5 per cent *m/m* of methanol and 0.4 per cent *m/m* of mesityl oxide. Examine by gas chromatography (*2.2.28*) using *propanol R* as the internal standard.

Internal standard solution. Dissolve 0.5 ml of *propanol R* in *water R* and dilute to 1000 ml with the same solvent.

Test solution. Dissolve 0.200 g of the substance to be examined in *water R*, add 2.0 ml of the internal standard solution and dilute to 10.0 ml with *water R*.

Reference solution. Dissolve 2.0 ml of *acetone R*, 0.5 ml of *methanol R* and 0.5 ml of *mesityl oxide R* in *water R* and dilute to 1000 ml with the same solvent. To 2.0 ml of this solution add 2.0 ml of the internal standard solution and dilute to 10.0 ml with *water R*. This solution contains 316 μg of acetone, 79 μg of methanol and 86 μg of mesityl oxide per millilitre.

The chromatographic procedure may be carried out using:

– a fused-silica column 30 m long and 0.53 mm in internal diameter coated with *macrogol 20 000 R* (film thickness 1.0 μm),

– *helium for chromatography R* as the carrier gas at a flow rate of 9 ml/min,

– a flame-ionisation detector,

with the following temperature programme:

	Time (min)	Temperature (°C)	Rate (°C/min)	Comment
Column	0 - 2.5	50	–	isothermal
	2.5 - 5	50 → 70	8	linear gradient
	5 - 5.5	70		isothermal
Injection port		160		
Detector		220		

Inject 1 μl of the reference solution and then 1 μl of the test solution. Calculate the percentage contents of acetone, methanol and mesityl oxide using the following expression:

$$\left(\frac{C}{W}\right) \times \left(\frac{R_u}{R_s}\right)$$

in which C is the concentration in μg/ml of the solvent in the reference solution, W is the quantity in milligrams of cilastatin sodium in the test solution and R_u and R_s are the ratios of the corresponding solvent peak areas to the propanol peak area in the test solution and the reference solution, respectively.

Heavy metals (*2.4.8*). 1.0 g complies with limit test C for heavy metals (20 ppm). Prepare the standard using 2.0 ml of *lead standard solution (10 ppm Pb) R*.

Water (*2.5.12*). Not more than 2.0 per cent, determined on 0.50 g by the semi-micro determination of water.

Bacterial endotoxins (*2.6.14*): less than 0.17 IU/mg, if intended for use in the manufacture of parenteral dosage forms without a further appropriate procedure for the removal of bacterial endotoxins.

ASSAY

Dissolve 0.300 g in 30 ml of *methanol R* and add 5 ml of *water R*. Add *0.1 M hydrochloric acid* to a pH of about 3.0. Carry out a potentiometric titration (*2.2.20*), using *0.1 M sodium hydroxide*. Three jumps of potential are observed. Titrate to the third equivalence point.

1 ml of *0.1 M sodium hydroxide* is equivalent to 19.02 mg of $C_{16}H_{25}N_2NaO_5S$.

STORAGE

Store in an airtight container, at a temperature not exceeding 8 °C. If the substance is sterile, store in a sterile, airtight, tamper-proof container.

LABELLING

The label states, where applicable, that the substance is free from bacterial endotoxins.

IMPURITIES

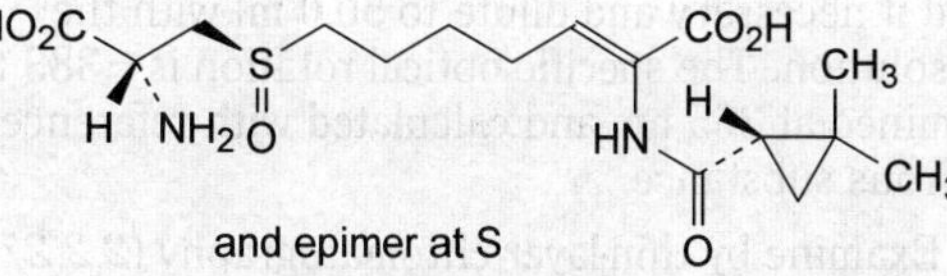

and epimer at S

A. (*Z*)-7-[(*RS*)-[(*R*)-2-amino-2-carboxyethyl]sulphinyl]-2-[[(1*S*)-2,2-dimethylcyclopropyl]carbonyl]amino]hept-2-enoic acid,

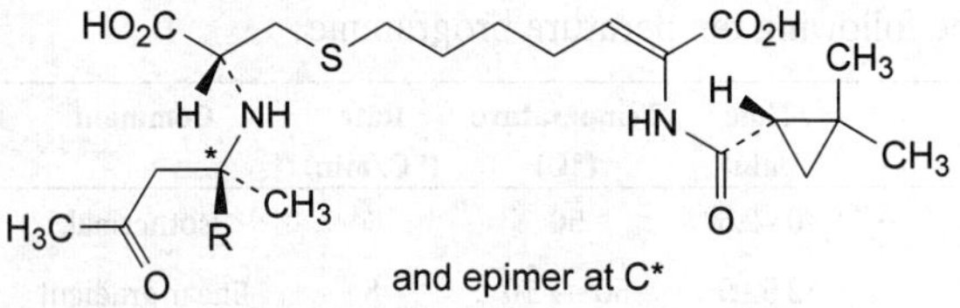

and epimer at C*

B. R = H: (*Z*)-7-[[(*R*)-2-[[(1*RS*)-1-methyl-3-oxobutyl]amino]-2-carboxyethyl]sulphanyl]-2-[[[(1*S*)-2,2-dimethylcyclopropyl]carbonyl]amino]hept-2-enoic acid,

C. R = CH_3: (*Z*)-7-[[(*R*)-2-[(1,1-dimethyl-3-oxobutyl)amino]-2-carboxyethyl]sulphanyl]-2-[[[(1*S*)-2,2-dimethylcyclopropyl]carbonyl]amino]hept-2-enoic acid,

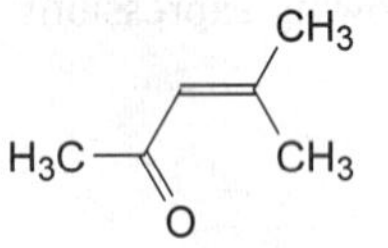

D. 4-methylpent-3-en-2-one (mesityl oxide).

01/2005:1499
corrected

CILAZAPRIL

Cilazaprilum

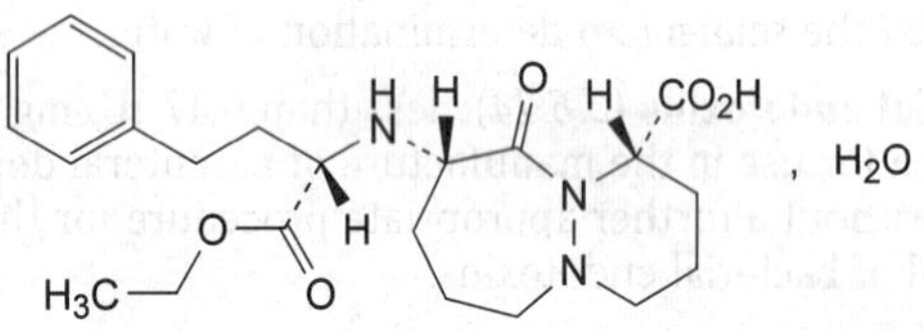

$C_{22}H_{31}N_3O_5,H_2O$ M_r 435.5

DEFINITION

Cilazapril contains not less than 98.5 per cent and not more than the equivalent of 101.5 per cent of (1*S*,9*S*)-9-[[(1*S*)-1-(ethoxycarbonyl)-3-phenylpropyl]amino]-10-oxooctahydro-6*H*-pyridazino[1,2-*a*][1,2]diazepine-1-carboxylic acid, calculated with reference to the anhydrous substance.

CHARACTERS

A white or almost white, crystalline powder, slightly soluble in water, freely soluble in methanol and in methylene chloride.

IDENTIFICATION

A. Examine by infrared absorption spectrophotometry (*2.2.24*), comparing with the spectrum obtained with *cilazapril CRS*.

B. It complies with the test for specific optical rotation (see Tests).

TESTS

Specific optical rotation (*2.2.7*). Dissolve 0.200 g in *0.067 M phosphate buffer solution pH 7.0 R*, with the aid of ultrasound if necessary and dilute to 50.0 ml with the same buffer solution. The specific optical rotation is − 383 to − 399, determined at 365 nm and calculated with reference to the anhydrous substance.

Impurity A. Examine by thin-layer chromatography (*2.2.27*), using a *TLC silica gel plate R*.

Test solution. Dissolve 0.20 g of the substance to be examined in *methanol R* and dilute to 5.0 ml with the same solvent.

Reference solution (a). Dissolve 2 mg of *cilazapril impurity A CRS* in *methanol R* and dilute to 50.0 ml with the same solvent.

Reference solution (b). Dissolve 5 mg of *cilazapril impurity A CRS* and 5 mg of the substance to be examined in *methanol R* and dilute to 10.0 ml with the same solvent.

Apply to the plate 5 µl of each solution. Develop over a path of 10 cm using a mixture of 5 volumes of *glacial acetic acid R*, 5 volumes of *water R*, 15 volumes of *hexane R*, 15 volumes of *methanol R* and 60 volumes of *ethyl acetate R*. Dry the plate in a current of cold air for 10 min. Spray the plate with a freshly prepared mixture of 1 volume of *potassium iodobismuthate solution R* and 10 volumes of *dilute acetic acid R* and then with *dilute hydrogen peroxide solution R*. Any spot corresponding to impurity A in the chromatogram obtained with the test solution is not more intense than the spot in the chromatogram obtained with reference solution (a) (0.1 per cent). The test is not valid unless the chromatogram obtained with reference solution (b) shows 2 clearly separated spots.

Other related substances. Examine by liquid chromatography (*2.2.29*).

Test solution. Dissolve 25.0 mg of the substance to be examined in the mobile phase and dilute to 50.0 ml with the mobile phase.

Reference solution (a). Dilute 1.0 ml of the test solution to 50.0 ml with the mobile phase. Dilute 5.0 ml of this solution to 20.0 ml with the mobile phase.

Reference solution (b). Dissolve 5.0 mg of *cilazapril impurity D CRS* in the test solution and dilute to 10.0 ml with the same solution.

The chromatographic procedure may be carried out using:

– a stainless steel column 0.25 m long and 4.6 mm in internal diameter packed with *octadecylsilyl silica gel for chromatography R* (5 µm),
– as mobile phase at a flow rate of 1.0 ml/min a mixture prepared as follows: mix 10 volumes of *triethylamine R* and 750 volumes of *water R*, adjust to pH 2.30 with *phosphoric acid R*, and add 200 volumes of *tetrahydrofuran R*,
– as detector a spectrophotometer set at 214 nm.

Inject 20 µl of reference solution (a) and 20 µl of reference solution (b). Adjust the sensitivity of the system so that the height of the principal peak in the chromatogram obtained with reference solution (a) is at least 50 per cent of the full scale of the recorder. The test is not valid unless the resolution between the peaks corresponding to cilazapril and impurity D in the chromatogram obtained with reference solution (b) is at least 2.5 and the symmetry factor of the peak due to cilazapril is not more than 3.0.

Inject 20 µl of the test solution and 20 µl of reference solution (a). Continue the chromatography for twice the retention time of the principal peak. When impurity A is present (relative retention time of 4 to 5), it may be necessary to continue the chromatography until it is eluted. When the chromatograms are recorded in the prescribed conditions, the retention times relative to cilazapril are: impurity B about 0.6; impurity D about 0.9; impurity C about 1.6. In the chromatogram obtained with the test solution: the area of any peak corresponding to impurity D is not greater than 0.4 times the area of the principal peak in the chromatogram obtained with reference solution (a) (0.2 per cent); the area of any peak corresponding to impurity B is not greater than the area of the principal peak in the chromatogram obtained with reference solution (a) (0.5 per cent); the area of any peak corresponding to impurity C is not greater than 0.2 times the area of the principal peak in the chromatogram obtained with reference solution (a) (0.1 per cent); the area of any peak, apart from the principal peak and the peaks corresponding to impurities B, C and D, is not greater than 0.2 times the area of the principal peak in the chromatogram obtained with reference solution (a) (0.1 per cent); the sum of the areas of all the peaks, apart from the principal peak, is not greater than twice the area of the principal peak in the chromatogram obtained with reference solution (a) (1 per cent). Disregard any peak with an area less than 0.1 times that of the principal peak in the chromatogram obtained with reference solution (a) and any peak due to impurity A.

Water (*2.5.12*): 3.5 per cent to 5.0 per cent, determined on 0.300 g by the semi-micro determination of water.

Sulphated ash (*2.4.14*). Not more than 0.1 per cent, determined on 1.0 g.

ASSAY

Dissolve 0.300 g in 10 ml of *ethanol R* and add 50 ml of *water R*. Titrate with *0.1 M sodium hydroxide*, determining the end-point potentiometrically (*2.2.20*). Carry out a blank titration.

1 ml of *0.1 M sodium hydroxide* is equivalent to 41.75 mg of $C_{22}H_{31}N_3O_5$.

STORAGE

Protected from light.

IMPURITIES

Specified impurities: A, B, C, D.

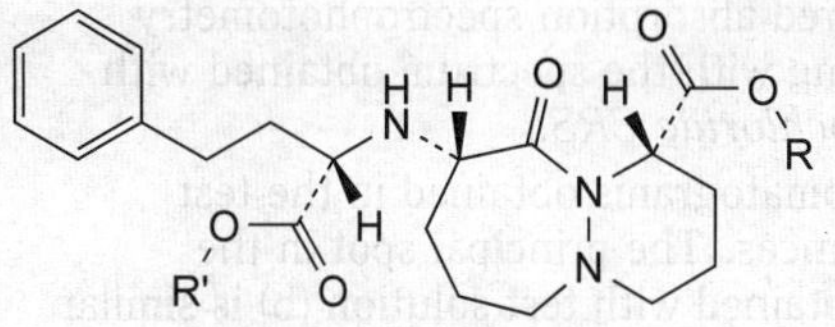

A. R = $C(CH_3)_3$, R′ = C_2H_5: 1,1-dimethylethyl (1*S*,9*S*)-9-[[(*S*)-1-(ethoxycarbonyl)-3-phenylpropyl]amino]-10-oxooctahydro-6*H*-pyridazino[1,2-*a*][1,2]diazepine-1-carboxylate,

B. R = R′ = H: (1*S*,9*S*)-9-[[(*S*)-1-carboxy-3-phenylpropyl]amino]-10-oxooctahydro-6*H*-pyridazino[1,2-*a*][1,2]diazepine-1-carboxylic acid,

C. R = R′ = C_2H_5: ethyl (1*S*,9*S*)-9-[[(*S*)-1-(ethoxycarbonyl)-3-phenylpropyl]amino]-10-oxooctahydro-6*H*-pyridazino[1,2-*a*][1,2]diazepine-1-carboxylate,

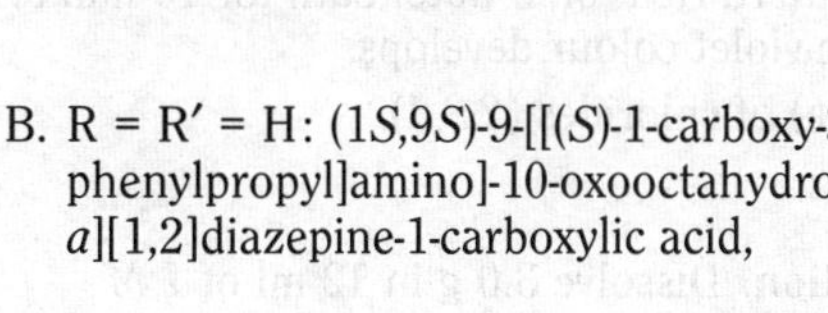

D. (1*S*,9*S*)-9-[[(*R*)-1-(ethoxycarbonyl)-3-phenylpropyl]amino]-10-oxooctahydro-6*H*-pyridazino-[1,2-*a*][1,2]diazepine-1-carboxylic acid.

01/2005:0756

CIMETIDINE

Cimetidinum

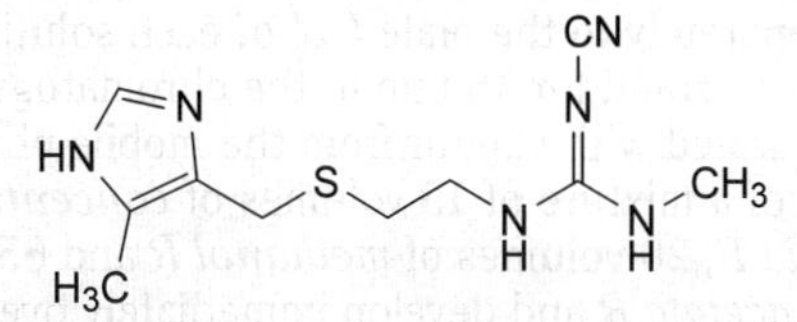

$C_{10}H_{16}N_6S$ M_r 252.3

DEFINITION

Cimetidine contains not less than 98.5 per cent and not more than the equivalent of 101.5 per cent of 2-cyano-1-methyl-3-[2-[[(5-methyl-1*H*-imidazol-4-yl)methyl]sulphanyl]ethyl]guanidine, calculated with reference to the dried substance.

CHARACTERS

A white or almost white powder, slightly soluble in water, soluble in alcohol, practically insoluble in methylene chloride. It dissolves in dilute mineral acids.

It shows polymorphism.

IDENTIFICATION

First identification: B.

Second identification: A, C, D.

A. Melting point (*2.2.14*): 139 °C to 144 °C. If necessary, dissolve the substance to be examined in *2-propanol R*, evaporate to dryness and determine the melting point again.

B. Examine by infrared absorption spectrophotometry (*2.2.24*), comparing with the spectrum obtained with *cimetidine CRS*. If the spectra obtained in the solid state show differences, dissolve the substance to be examined and the reference substance separately in *2-propanol R*, evaporate to dryness and record the spectra again.

C. Examine the chromatograms obtained in the test for related substances. The principal spot in the chromatogram obtained with test solution (b) is similar in position, colour and size to the principal spot in the chromatogram obtained with reference solution (d).

D. Dissolve about 1 mg in a mixture of 1 ml of *ethanol R* and 5 ml of a freshly prepared 20 g/l solution of *citric acid R* in *acetic anhydride R*. Heat in a water-bath for 10 min to 15 min. A reddish-violet colour develops.

TESTS

Appearance of solution. Dissolve 3.0 g in 12 ml of *1 M hydrochloric acid* and dilute to 20 ml with *water R*. The solution is clear (*2.2.1*) and not more intensely coloured than reference solution Y_5 (*2.2.2, Method II*).

Related substances. Examine by thin-layer chromatography (*2.2.27*), using *silica gel* GF_{254} *R* as the coating substance.

Test solution (a). Dissolve 0.50 g of the substance to be examined in *methanol R* and dilute to 10 ml with the same solvent.

Test solution (b). Dilute 1 ml of test solution (a) to 10 ml with *methanol R*.

Reference solution (a). Dilute 1 ml of test solution (a) to 100 ml with *methanol R*. Dilute 20 ml of this solution to 100 ml with *methanol R*.

Reference solution (b). Dilute 5 ml of reference solution (a) to 10 ml with *methanol R*.

Reference solution (c). Dilute 5 ml of reference solution (b) to 10 ml with *methanol R.*

Reference solution (d). Dissolve 10 mg of *cimetidine CRS* in 2 ml of *methanol R.*

A. Apply separately to the plate 4 µl of each solution. Allow the plate to stand for 15 min in the chromatographic tank saturated with vapour from the mobile phase which consists of a mixture of 15 volumes of *concentrated ammonia R,* 20 volumes of *methanol R* and 65 volumes of *ethyl acetate R* and develop immediately over a path of 15 cm using the same mixture of solvents. Dry the plate in a stream of cold air, expose to iodine vapour until maximum contrast of the spots has been obtained and examine in ultraviolet light at 254 nm. Any spot in the chromatogram obtained with test solution (a), apart from the principal spot, is not more intense than the principal spot in the chromatogram obtained with reference solution (a) (0.2 per cent) and not more than two such spots are more intense than the principal spot in the chromatogram obtained with reference solution (b) (0.1 per cent). The test is not valid unless the chromatogram obtained with reference solution (c) shows a clearly visible spot.

B. Apply separately to the plate 4 µl of each solution. Develop over a path of 15 cm using a mixture of 8 volumes of *concentrated ammonia R,* 8 volumes of *methanol R* and 84 volumes of *ethyl acetate R.* Dry the plate in a stream of cold air, expose to iodine vapour until maximum contrast of the spots has been obtained and examine in ultraviolet light at 254 nm. Any spot in the chromatogram obtained with the test solution (a), apart from the principal spot, is not more intense than the principal spot in the chromatogram obtained with reference solution (a) (0.2 per cent) and not more than two such spots are more intense than the principal spot in the chromatogram obtained with reference solution (b) (0.1 per cent). The test is not valid unless the chromatogram obtained with reference solution (c) shows a clearly visible spot.

Heavy metals (*2.4.8*). 1.0 g complies with limit test C for heavy metals (20 ppm). Prepare the standard using 2 ml of *lead standard solution (10 ppm Pb) R.*

Loss on drying (*2.2.32*). Not more than 0.5 per cent, determined on 1.000 g by drying in an oven at 100 °C to 105 °C.

Sulphated ash (*2.4.14*). Not more than 0.2 per cent, determined on 1.0 g.

ASSAY

Dissolve 0.200 g in 60 ml of *anhydrous acetic acid R.* Titrate with *0.1 M perchloric acid* determining the end-point potentiometrically (*2.2.20*).

1 ml of *0.1 M perchloric acid* is equivalent to 25.23 mg of $C_{10}H_{16}N_6S$.

STORAGE

Store in an airtight container, protected from light.

01/2005:1500

CIMETIDINE HYDROCHLORIDE

Cimetidini hydrochloridum

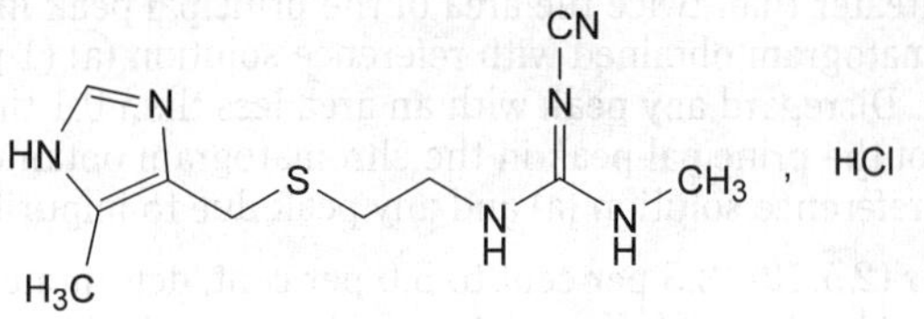

$C_{10}H_{17}ClN_6S$ M_r 288.8

DEFINITION

Cimetidine hydrochloride contains not less than 98.5 per cent and not more than the equivalent of 101.5 per cent of 2-cyano-1-methyl-3-[2-[[(5-methyl-1*H*-imidazol-4-yl)methyl]sulphanyl]ethyl]guanidine hydrochloride, calculated with reference to the dried substance.

CHARACTERS

A white or almost white, crystalline powder, freely soluble in water, sparingly soluble in ethanol.

IDENTIFICATION

First identification: B, E.

Second identification: A, C, D, E.

A. Dissolve 70 mg in *0.2 M sulphuric acid* and dilute to 100.0 ml with the same acid. Dilute 2.0 ml of the solution to 100.0 ml with *0.2 M sulphuric acid.* Measure the absorbance (*2.2.25*) at the absorption maximum at 218 nm. The specific absorbance at the maximum is 650 to 705.

B. Examine by infrared absorption spectrophotometry (*2.2.24*), comparing with the spectrum obtained with *cimetidine hydrochloride CRS.*

C. Examine the chromatograms obtained in the test for related substances. The principal spot in the chromatogram obtained with test solution (b) is similar in position, colour and size to the principal spot in the chromatogram obtained with reference solution (d).

D. Dissolve about 1 mg in a mixture of 1 ml of *ethanol R* and 5 ml of a freshly prepared 20 g/l solution of *citric acid R* in *acetic anhydride R.* Heat on a water-bath for 10 min to 15 min. A reddish-violet colour develops.

E. It gives reaction (a) of chlorides (*2.3.1*).

TESTS

Appearance of solution. Dissolve 3.0 g in 12 ml of *1 M hydrochloric acid* and dilute to 20 ml with *water R.* The solution is clear (*2.2.1*) and not more intensely coloured than reference solution Y_5 (*2.2.2, Method II*).

pH (*2.2.3*). Dissolve 100 mg in *carbon dioxide-free water R* and dilute to 10.0 ml with the same solvent. The pH of the solution is 4.0 to 5.0.

Related substances. Examine by thin-layer chromatography (*2.2.27*), using a *TLC silica gel GF_{254} plate R.*

Test solution (a). Dissolve 0.50 g of the substance to be examined in *methanol R* and dilute to 10 ml with the same solvent.

Test solution (b). Dilute 1 ml of test solution (a) to 10 ml with *methanol R.*

Reference solution (a). Dilute 2 ml of test solution (b) to 100 ml with *methanol R.*

Reference solution (b). Dilute 5 ml of reference solution (a) to 10 ml with *methanol R.*

Reference solution (c). Dilute 5 ml of reference solution (b) to 10 ml with *methanol R.*

Reference solution (d). Dissolve 10 mg of *cimetidine hydrochloride CRS* in 2 ml of *methanol R.*

A. Apply to the plate 4 µl of each solution. Allow the plate to stand for 15 min in a chromatographic tank saturated with vapour from the mobile phase, which consists of a mixture of 15 volumes of *concentrated ammonia R,* 20 volumes of *methanol R* and 65 volumes of *ethyl acetate R,* and develop immediately over a path of 15 cm using the same mixture of solvents. Dry the plate in a stream of cold air, expose to iodine vapour until maximum contrast of the spots has been obtained and examine in ultraviolet light at 254 nm. Any spot in the chromatogram obtained with test solution (a), apart from the principal spot, is not more intense than the principal spot in the chromatogram obtained with reference solution (a) (0.2 per cent) and at most two such spots are more intense than the principal spot in the chromatogram obtained with reference solution (b) (0.1 per cent). The test is not valid unless the chromatogram obtained with reference solution (c) shows a clearly visible spot.

B. Apply to the plate 4 µl of each solution. Develop over a path of 15 cm using a mixture of 8 volumes of *concentrated ammonia R,* 8 volumes of *methanol R* and 84 volumes of *ethyl acetate R.* Dry the plate in a stream of cold air, expose to iodine vapour until maximum contrast of the spots has been obtained and examine in ultraviolet light at 254 nm. Any spot in the chromatogram obtained with test solution (a), apart from the principal spot, is not more intense than the principal spot in the chromatogram obtained with reference solution (a) (0.2 per cent) and at most two such spots are more intense than the principal spot in the chromatogram obtained with reference solution (b) (0.1 per cent). The test is not valid unless the chromatogram obtained with reference solution (c) shows a clearly visible spot.

Heavy metals (*2.4.8*). 1.0 g complies with limit test C for heavy metals (20 ppm). Prepare the standard using 2 ml of *lead standard solution (10 ppm Pb) R.*

Loss on drying (*2.2.32*). Not more than 1.0 per cent, determined on 1.000 g by drying in an oven at 100 °C to 105 °C.

Sulphated ash (*2.4.14*). Not more than 0.2 per cent, determined on 1.0 g.

ASSAY

Dissolve 0.200 g of the substance to be examined in a mixture of 5 ml of *0.01 M hydrochloric acid* and 50 ml of *alcohol R.* Carry out a potentiometric titration (*2.2.20*), using *0.1 M sodium hydroxide.* Read the volume added between the two points of inflexion.

1 ml of *0.1 M sodium hydroxide* is equivalent to 28.88 mg of $C_{10}H_{17}ClN_6S$.

STORAGE

Store in an airtight container, protected from light.

IMPURITIES

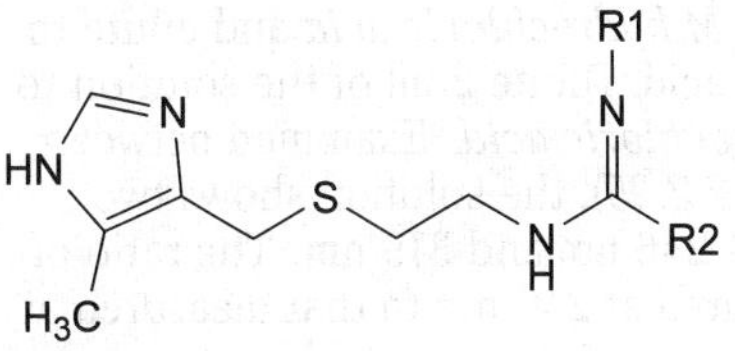

A. R1 = CN, R2 = SCH_3: 3-cyano-2-methyl-1-[2-[[(5-methyl-1*H*-imidazol-4-yl)methyl]sulphanyl]ethyl]isothiourea,

B. R1 = CN, R2 = OCH_3: 3-cyano-2-methyl-1-[2-[[(5-methyl-1*H*-imidazol-4-yl)methyl]sulphanyl]ethyl]isourea,

C. R1 = $CONH_2$, R2 = $NHCH_3$: 1-[(methylamino)[[2-[[(5-methyl-1*H*-imidazol-4-yl)methyl]sulphanyl]ethyl]amino]methylene]urea,

D. R1 = H, R2 = $NHCH_3$: 1-methyl-3-[2-[[(5-methyl-1*H*-imidazol-4-yl)methyl]sulphanyl]ethyl]guanidine,

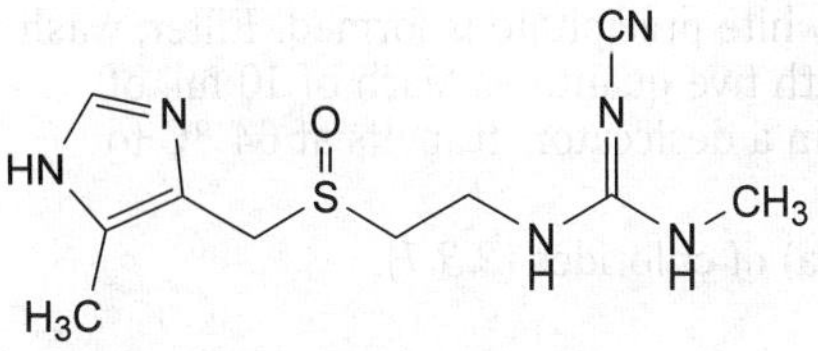

E. 2-cyano-1-methyl-3-[2-[[(5-methyl-1*H*-imidazol-4-yl)methyl]sulphinyl]ethyl]guanidine,

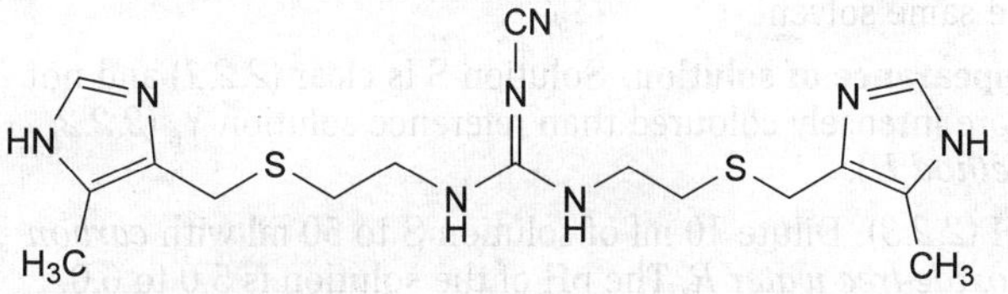

F. 2-cyano-1,3-bis[2-[[(5-methyl-1*H*-imidazol-4-yl)methyl]-sulphanyl]ethyl]guanidine.

01/2005:1088

CINCHOCAINE HYDROCHLORIDE

Cinchocaini hydrochloridum

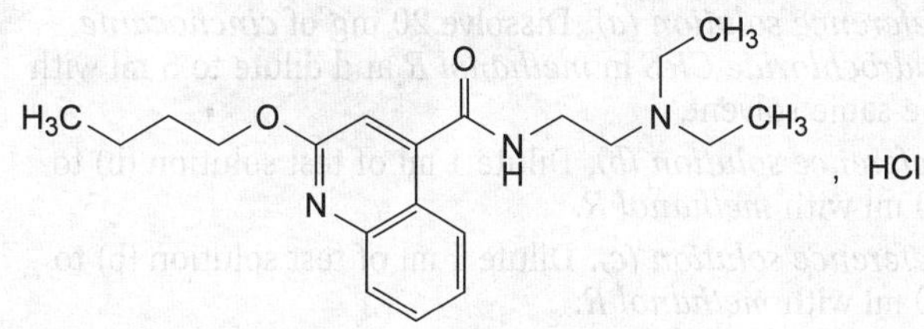

$C_{20}H_{30}ClN_3O_2$ M_r 379.9

DEFINITION

Cinchocaine hydrochloride contains not less than 98.5 per cent and not more than the equivalent of 101.0 per cent of 2-butoxy-*N*-[2-(diethylamino)ethyl]quinoline-4-carboxamide hydrochloride, calculated with reference to the dried substance.

CHARACTERS

A white or almost white, crystalline powder or colourless crystals, hygroscopic, very soluble in water, freely soluble in acetone, in alcohol and in methylene chloride. It agglomerates very easily.

IDENTIFICATION

First identification: B, E.

Second identification: A, C, D, E.

A. Dissolve 60.0 mg in *1 M hydrochloric acid* and dilute to 100 ml with the same acid. Dilute 2 ml of the solution to 100 ml with *1 M hydrochloric acid.* Examined between 220 nm and 350 nm (*2.2.25*), the solution shows two absorption maxima, at 246 nm and 319 nm. The ratio of the absorbance measured at 246 nm to that measured at 319 nm is 2.7 to 3.0.

B. Examine by infrared absorption spectrophotometry (*2.2.24*), comparing with the spectrum obtained with *cinchocaine hydrochloride CRS*. Examine the substances prepared as discs using *potassium chloride R*.

C. Examine the chromatograms obtained in the test for related substances. The principal spot in the chromatogram obtained with test solution (b) is similar in position and size to the principal spot in the chromatogram obtained with reference solution (a).

D. Dissolve 0.5 g in 5 ml of *water R*. Add 1 ml of *dilute ammonia R2*. A white precipitate is formed. Filter, wash the precipitate with five quantities, each of 10 ml, of *water R* and dry in a desiccator. It melts at 64 °C to 66 °C (*2.2.14*).

E. It gives reaction (a) of chlorides (*2.3.1*).

TESTS

Solution S. Dissolve 5.0 g in *carbon dioxide-free water R* prepared from *distilled water R,* and dilute to 50 ml with the same solvent.

Appearance of solution. Solution S is clear (*2.2.1*) and not more intensely coloured than reference solution Y_6 (*2.2.2, Method II*).

pH (*2.2.3*). Dilute 10 ml of solution S to 50 ml with *carbon dioxide-free water R*. The pH of the solution is 5.0 to 6.0.

Related substances. Examine by thin-layer chromatography (*2.2.27*), using as the coating substance a suitable silica gel with a fluorescent indicator having an optimal intensity at 254 nm.

Test solution (a). Dissolve 0.20 g of the substance to be examined in *methanol R* and dilute to 5 ml with the same solvent.

Test solution (b). Dilute 1 ml of test solution (a) to 10 ml with *methanol R.*

Reference solution (a). Dissolve 20 mg of *cinchocaine hydrochloride CRS* in *methanol R* and dilute to 5 ml with the same solvent.

Reference solution (b). Dilute 1 ml of test solution (b) to 20 ml with *methanol R.*

Reference solution (c). Dilute 1 ml of test solution (b) to 50 ml with *methanol R.*

Reference solution (d). Dissolve 20 mg of *benzocaine CRS* in *methanol R* and dilute to 5 ml with the same solvent. Dilute 1 ml of the solution and 1 ml of reference solution (a) to 20 ml with *methanol R.*

Apply separately to the plate 5 µl of each solution. Develop over a path of 15 cm using a mixture of 1 volume of *ammonia R,* 5 volumes of *methanol R,* 30 volumes of *acetone R* and 50 volumes of *toluene R.* Dry the plate in a current of warm air for 15 min. Examine in ultraviolet light at 254 nm. Any spot in the chromatogram obtained with test solution (a), apart from the principal spot, is not more intense than the principal spot in the chromatogram obtained with reference solution (b) (0.5 per cent) and at most one such spot is more intense than the spot in the chromatogram obtained with reference solution (c) (0.2 per cent). The test is not valid unless the chromatogram obtained with reference solution (d) shows two clearly separated spots.

Heavy metals (*2.4.8*). 12 ml of solution S complies with limit test A for heavy metals (20 ppm). Prepare the standard using *lead standard solution (2 ppm Pb) R.*

Loss on drying (*2.2.32*). Not more than 2.0 per cent, determined on 0.500 g by drying *in vacuo* at 60 °C.

Sulphated ash (*2.4.14*). Not more than 0.1 per cent, determined on 1.0 g.

ASSAY

Dissolve 0.300 g in a mixture of 15.0 ml of *0.01 M hydrochloric acid* and 50 ml of *alcohol R.* Carry out a potentiometric titration (*2.2.20*), using *0.1 M sodium hydroxide.* Read the volume added between the two points of inflexion.

1 ml of *0.1 M sodium hydroxide* is equivalent to 37.99 mg of $C_{20}H_{30}ClN_3O_2$.

STORAGE

Store in an airtight container, protected from light.

IMPURITIES

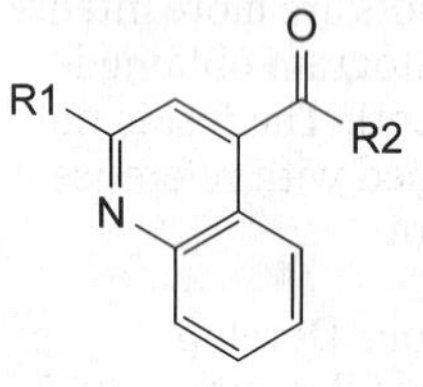

A. R1 = Cl, R2 = NH-$[CH_2]_2$-$N(C_2H_5)_2$: 2-chloro-*N*-[2-(diethylamino)ethyl]quinoline-4-carboxamide,

B. R1 = R2 = OH: 2-hydroxyquinoline-4-carboxylic acid,

C. R1 = OH, R2 = NH-$[CH_2]_2$-$N(C_2H_5)_2$: *N*-[2-(diethylamino)ethyl]-2-hydroxyquinoline-4-carboxamide,

D. R1 = O-$[CH_2]_3$-CH_3, R2 = OH: 2-butoxyquinoline-4-carboxylic acid.

01/2005:0174

CINCHONA BARK

Cinchonae cortex

DEFINITION

Whole or cut, dried bark of *Cinchona pubescens* Vahl (*Cinchona succirubra* Pavon), of *C. calisaya* (Weddell), of *C. ledgeriana* (Moens ex Trimen) or of its varieties or hybrids.

Content: minimum 6.5 per cent of total alkaloids, of which 30 per cent to 60 per cent consists of quinine-type alkaloids (dried drug).

CHARACTERS

Intense bitter, somewhat astringent taste.

Macroscopic and microscopic characters described under identification tests A and B.

IDENTIFICATION

A. The stem and branch bark is supplied in quilled or curved pieces 2 mm to 6 mm thick. The outer surface is dull brownish-grey or grey and frequently bears lichens; it is usually rough, marked with transverse fissures and longitudinally furrowed or wrinkled; exfoliation of the outer surface occurs in some varieties. The inner surface is striated and deep reddish-brown; the fracture is short in the outer part and fibrous in the inner part.

B. Reduce to a powder (355). The powder is reddish-brown. Examine under a microscope using *chloral hydrate solution R*. The powder shows the following diagnostic characters: thin-walled cork cells filled with reddish-brown contents; yellow, spindle-shaped striated phloem fibres up to 90 µm in diameter and up to 1300 µm in length, very thick-walled with an uneven lumen and with conspicuous, funnel-shaped pits; parenchymatous idioblasts filled with microprisms of calcium oxalate. Examine under a microscope using a 50 per cent *V/V* solution of *glycerol R*. The powder shows a few starch granules 6 µm to 10 µm in diameter; mostly simple but occasionally with 2 or 3 components.

C. Thin-layer chromatography (*2.2.27*).

Test solution. To 0.10 g of the powdered drug (180) in a test-tube add 0.1 ml of *concentrated ammonia R* and 5 ml of *methylene chloride R*. Shake vigorously occasionally during 30 min and filter. Evaporate the filtrate to dryness on a water-bath and dissolve the residue in 1 ml of *ethanol R*.

Reference solution. Dissolve 17.5 mg of *quinine R*, 2.5 mg of *quinidine R*, 10 mg of *cinchonine R* and 10 mg of *cinchonidine R* in 5 ml of *ethanol R*.

Plate: *TLC silica gel plate R*.

Mobile phase: *diethylamine R, ethyl acetate R, toluene R* (10:20:70 *V/V/V*).

Application: 10 µl, as bands.

Development: twice over a path of 15 cm.

Drying: at 100-105 °C then allow to cool.

Detection A: spray with *anhydrous formic acid R* and allow to dry in air. Examine in ultraviolet light at 365 nm.

Results A: see below the sequence of the zones present in the chromatograms obtained with the reference solution and the test solution. Furthermore, other fluorescent zones are present in the chromatogram obtained with the test solution.

Top of the plate	
___	___
Quinidine: a distinct blue fluorescent zone	A distinct blue fluorescent zone (quinidine)
___	___
Quinine: a distinct blue fluorescent zone	A distinct blue fluorescent zone (quinine)
Reference solution	**Test solution**

Detection B: spray with *iodoplatinate reagent R*.

Results B: see below the sequence of the zones present in the chromatograms obtained with the reference solution and the test solution. Furthermore, other zones are present in the chromatogram obtained with the test solution.

Top of the plate	
___	___
Cinchonine: a violet zone which becomes violet-grey	A violet zone, which becomes violet-grey (cinchonine)
Quinidine: a violet zone which becomes violet-grey	A violet zone, which becomes violet-grey (quinidine)
Cinchonidine: an intense dark blue zone	An intense dark blue zone (cinchonidine)
___	___
Quinine: a violet zone which becomes violet-grey	A violet zone, which becomes violet-grey (quinine)
Reference solution	**Test solution**

TESTS

Foreign matter (*2.8.2*): maximum 2 per cent *m/m*.

Total ash (*2.4.16*): maximum 6.0 per cent.

Loss on drying (*2.2.32*): maximum 10 per cent, determined on 1.000 g of the powdered drug (355) by drying in an oven at 100-105 °C for 2 h.

ASSAY

Test solution. In a 250 ml conical flask mix 1.000 g of the powdered drug (180) with 10 ml of *water R* and 7 ml of *dilute hydrochloric acid R*. Heat in a water-bath for 30 min, allow to cool and add 25 ml of *methylene chloride R*, 50 ml of *ether R* and 5 ml of a 200 g/l solution of *sodium hydroxide R*. Shake the mixture repeatedly for 30 min, add 3 g of powdered *tragacanth R* and shake until the mixture becomes clear. Filter through a plug of absorbent cotton and rinse the flask and the cotton with 5 quantities, each of 20 ml, of a mixture of 1 volume of *methylene chloride R* and 2 volumes of *ether R*. Combine the filtrate and washings, evaporate to dryness and dissolve the residue in 10.0 ml of *ethanol R*. Evaporate 5.0 ml of the solution to dryness, dissolve the residue in *0.1 M hydrochloric acid* and dilute to 1000.0 ml with the same acid.

Reference solutions. Dissolve separately 30.0 mg of *quinine R* and 30.0 mg of *cinchonine R* in *0.1 M hydrochloric acid* and dilute each solution to 1000.0 ml with the same acid.

Measure the absorbances (*2.2.25*) of the 3 solutions at 316 nm and 348 nm using *0.1 M hydrochloric acid* as the compensation liquid.

Calculate the percentage content of alkaloids from the following equations:

$$x = \frac{[A_{316} \times A_{348c}] - [A_{316c} \times A_{348}]}{[A_{316q} \times A_{348c}] - [A_{316c} \times A_{348q}]} \times \frac{100}{m} \times \frac{2}{1000}$$

$$y = \frac{[A_{316} \times A_{348q}] - [A_{316q} \times A_{348}]}{[A_{316c} \times A_{348q}] - [A_{316q} \times A_{348c}]} \times \frac{100}{m} \times \frac{2}{1000}$$

m = mass of the drug used, in grams,

x = percentage content of quinine-type alkaloids,

y = percentage content of cinchonine-type alkaloids,

A_{316} = absorbance of the test solution at 316 nm,

A_{348} = absorbance of the test solution at 348 nm,

A_{316c} = absorbance of the reference solution containing cinchonine at 316 nm, corrected to a concentration of 1 mg/1000 ml,

A_{316q} = absorbance of the reference solution containing quinine at 316 nm, corrected to a concentration of 1 mg/1000 ml,

A_{348c} = absorbance of the reference solution containing cinchonine at 348 nm, corrected to a concentration of 1 mg/1000 ml,

A_{348q} = absorbance of the reference solution containing quinine at 348 nm, corrected to a concentration of 1 mg/1000 ml.

Calculate the content of total alkaloids, ($x + y$), and the relative content of quinine-type alkaloids, from the following expression:

$$\frac{100x}{x + y}$$

01/2005:1973

CINEOLE

Cineolum

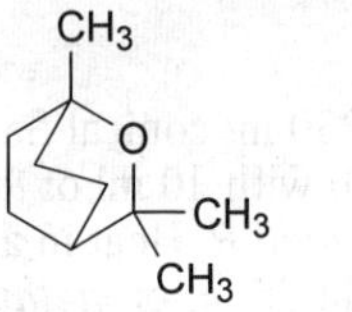

$C_{10}H_{18}O$ M_r 154.3

DEFINITION

1,3,3-Trimethyl-2-oxabicyclo[2.2.2]octane.

CHARACTERS

Appearance: clear colourless liquid.

Solubility: practically insoluble in water, miscible with alcohol and with methylene chloride.

It solidifies at about 0.5 °C.

IDENTIFICATION

A. It complies with the test for refractive index (see Tests).

B. Thin-layer chromatography (*2.2.27*).

Test solution. Dilute 1 ml of solution S (see Tests) to 25 ml with *alcohol R*.

Reference solution. Mix 80 mg of *cineole CRS* with *alcohol R* and dilute to 10 ml with the same solvent.

Plate: *TLC silica gel plate R*.

Mobile phase: *ethyl acetate R, toluene R* (10:90 *V/V*).

Application: 2 µl.

Development: over 2/3 of the plate.

Drying: in a current of cold air.

Detection: spray with *anisaldehyde solution R*, heat at 100-105 °C for 5 min.

Results: the principal spot in the chromatogram obtained with the test solution is similar in position, colour and size to the principal spot in the chromatogram obtained with the reference solution.

C. To 0.1 ml add 4 ml of *sulphuric acid R*. An orange-red colour develops. Add 0.2 ml of *formaldehyde solution R*. The colour changes to deep brown.

TESTS

Solution S. Dilute 2.00 g to 10.0 ml with *alcohol R*.

Appearance of solution. Solution S is clear (*2.2.1*) and colourless (*2.2.2, Method I*).

Chiral impurities. The optical rotation (*2.2.7*) of solution S is − 0.10° to + 0.10°.

Refractive index (*2.2.6*): 1.456 to 1.460.

Related substances. Gas chromatography (*2.2.28*).

Internal standard solution. Dissolve 1.0 g of *camphor R* in *heptane R* and dilute to 200 ml with the same solvent.

Test solution (a). Dissolve 2.5 g of the substance to be examined in *heptane R* and dilute to 25.0 ml with the same solvent.

Test solution (b). Dissolve 2.5 g of the substance to be examined in *heptane R*, add 5.0 ml of the internal standard solution and dilute to 25.0 ml with *heptane R*.

Reference solution (a). To 2.0 ml of test solution (a) add 20.0 ml of the internal standard solution and dilute to 100.0 ml with *heptane R*.

Reference solution (b). Dissolve 50 mg of *1,4-cineole R* and 50 mg of the substance to be examined in *heptane R* and dilute to 50.0 ml with the same solvent.

Column:

– *size*: *l* = 30 m, Ø = 0.25 mm,

– *stationary phase*: *macrogol 20 000 R* (film thickness 0.25 µm).

Carrier gas: *helium for chromatography R*.

Linear velocity: 45 cm/s.

Split-ratio: 1:70.

Temperature:

	Time (min)	Temperature (°C)
Column	0 - 10	50
	10 - 35	50 → 100
	35 - 45	100 → 200
	45 - 55	200
Injection port		220
Detector		250

Detection: flame ionisation.

Injection: 1 µl.

System suitability: reference solution (b):

– *resolution*: minimum 10 between the peaks due to impurity A and to cineole.

Limits:

– *total*: calculate the ratio (*R*) of the area of the peak due to cineole to the area of the peak due to the internal standard from the chromatogram obtained with reference solution (a); from the chromatogram obtained with test solution (b), calculate the ratio of the sum of the areas of any peaks, apart from the principal peak and the peak due to the internal standard, to the area of the peak due to internal standard: this ratio is not greater than *R* (2 per cent),

– *disregard limit*: 0.025 times the area of the principal peak in the chromatogram obtained with reference solution (a) (0.05 per cent).

Residue on evaporation: maximum 0.1 per cent.

To 2.0 g add 5 ml of *water R*, evaporate to dryness on a water-bath and dry at 100-105 °C for 1 h. The residue weighs a maximum of 2 mg.

STORAGE

In an airtight container, protected from light.

IMPURITIES

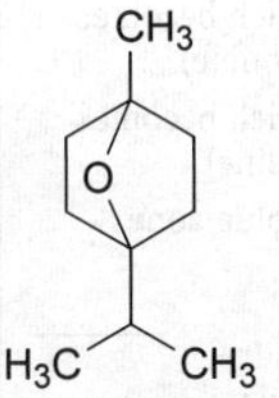

A. 1-methyl-4-(1-methylethyl)-7-oxabicyclo[2.2.1]heptane (1,4-cineole).

01/2005:0387

CINNAMON

Cinnamomi cortex

DEFINITION

Cinnamon consists of the dried bark, freed from the outer cork and the underlying parenchyma, of the shoots grown on cut stock of *Cinnamomum zeylanicum* Nees. It contains not less than 12 ml/kg of essential oil.

CHARACTERS

Cinnamon has a characteristic, aromatic odour.

It has the macroscopic and microscopic characters described under identification tests A and B.

IDENTIFICATION

A. The bark is about 0.2 mm to 0.8 mm thick and occurs in closely-packed compound quills made up of single or double quills. The outer surface is smooth, yellowish-brown with faint scars marking the position of leaves and axillary buds and has fine, whitish and wavy longitudinal striations. The inner surface is slightly darker and longitudinally striated. The fracture is short and fibrous.

B. Reduce to a powder (355). The powder is yellowish to reddish-brown. Examine under a microscope using *chloral hydrate solution R*. The powder shows the following diagnostic characters: groups of rounded sclereids with pitted, channelled and moderately thickened walls; numerous colourless single fibres, often whole with narrow lumen and thickened, lignified walls and few pits; small acicular crystals of calcium oxalate. Examine under a microscope using a 50 per cent *V/V* solution of *glycerol R*; the powder shows abundant starch granules. Cork fragments are absent or very rare.

C. Examine by thin-layer chromatography (*2.2.27*), using *silica gel* GF_{254} *R* as the coating substance.

Test solution. Shake 0.1 g of powdered drug (500) with 2 ml of *methylene chloride R* for 15 min. Filter and evaporate the filtrate carefully almost to dryness on a water-bath. Dissolve the residue in 0.4 ml of *toluene R*.

Reference solution. Dissolve 50 µl of *cinnamic aldehyde R* and 10 µl of *eugenol R* in *toluene R* and dilute to 10 ml with the same solvent.

Apply separately to the plate as bands 20 mm by 3 mm, 10 µl of each solution. Develop over a path of 10 cm using *methylene chloride R*. Allow the plate to dry in air, examine in ultraviolet light at 254 nm and mark the quenching zones. Examine the plate in ultraviolet light at 365 nm and mark the fluorescent zones. In ultraviolet light at 254 nm, the chromatograms obtained with the test and reference solutions show a quenching zone (cinnamaldehyde) in the median part and just above it a weaker quenching zone (eugenol). In ultraviolet light at 365 nm, the chromatogram obtained with the test solution shows a zone of light-blue fluorescence (*o*-methoxy-cinnamaldehyde) just below the zone corresponding to cinnamaldehyde. Spray with *phloroglucinol solution R*. The zone corresponding to cinnamaldehyde is yellowish-brown and the zone corresponding to *o*-methoxycinn-amaldehyde is violet.

TESTS

Total ash (*2.4.16*). Not more than 6.0 per cent.

ASSAY

Carry out the determination of essential oils in vegetable drugs (*2.8.12*). Use a 500 ml flask, 200 ml of *0.1 M hydrochloric acid* as the distillation liquid and 0.50 ml of *xylene R* in the graduated tube. Powder the drug (710) and proceed immediately with the determination, using 20.0 g. Distil at a rate of 2.5-3.5 ml/min for 3 h.

STORAGE

Store protected from light.

01/2005:1501

CINNAMON BARK OIL, CEYLON

Cinnamomi zeylanicii corticis aetheroleum

DEFINITION

Ceylon cinnamon bark oil is obtained by steam distillation of the bark of the shoots of *Cinnamomum zeylanicum* Nees (*C. Verum* J.S. Presl.).

CHARACTERS

A clear, mobile, light yellow liquid becoming reddish over time, with a characteristic odour reminiscent of cinnamic aldehyde.

IDENTIFICATION

First identification: B.

Second identification: A.

A. Examine by thin-layer chromatography (*2.2.27*), using a *TLC silica gel plate R*.

Test solution. Dissolve 1 ml of the substance to be examined in *acetone R* and dilute to 10 ml with the same solvent.

Reference solution. Dissolve 50 µl of *trans-cinnamic aldehyde R*, 10 µl of *eugenol R*, 10 µl of *linalol R* and 10 µl of *β-caryophyllene R* in *alcohol R* and dilute to 10 ml with the same solvent.

Apply to the plate, as bands, 10 µl of each solution. Develop over a path of 15 cm using a mixture of 10 volumes of *methanol R* and 90 volumes of *toluene R*. Allow the plate to dry in air and spray with *anisaldehyde solution R*. Examine in daylight while heating at 100-105 °C for 5-10 min. The chromatogram obtained with the test solution shows zones similar in position and colour to those in the chromatogram obtained with the reference solution.

B. Examine the chromatograms obtained in the test for chromatographic profile. The retention times of the principal peaks in the chromatogram obtained with the test solution are similar to those in the chromatogram obtained with the reference solution. Safrole, coumarin and cineole may be absent from the chromatogram obtained with the test solution.

TESTS

Relative density (*2.2.5*): 1.000 to 1.030.

Refractive index (*2.2.6*): 1.572 to 1.591.

Optical rotation (*2.2.7*): − 2° to + 1°.

Chromatographic profile. Examine by gas chromatography (*2.2.28*).

Test solution. The substance to be examined.

Monographs C

Reference solution. Dissolve 10 μl of *cineole R,* 10 μl of *linalol R,* 10 μl of *β-caryophyllene R,* 10 μl of *safrole R,* 100 μl of *trans-cinnamic aldehyde R,* 10 μl of *eugenol R,* 20 mg of *coumarin R,* 10 μl of *trans-2-methoxycinnamaldehyde R* and 10 μl of *benzyl benzoate R* in 1 ml of *acetone R.*

The chromatographic procedure may be carried out using:

– a fused-silica column 60 m long and about 0.25 mm in internal diameter coated with *macrogol 20 000 R* as the bonded phase,
– *helium for chromatography R* as the carrier gas at a flow rate of 1.5 ml/min,
– a flame-ionisation detector,
– a split ratio of 1:100,

with the following temperature programme:

	Time (min)	Temperature (°C)	Rate (°C/min)	Comment
Column	0 - 10	60		isothermal
	10 - 75	60 → 190	2	linear gradient
	75 - 200	190		isothermal
Injection port		200		
Detector		240		

Inject 0.2 μl of the reference solution. When the chromatogram is recorded in the prescribed conditions, the components elute in the order indicated in the composition of the reference solution. Depending on the operating conditions and the state of the column, coumarin may elute before or after *trans*-2-methoxycinnamaldehyde. Record the retention times of these substances.

The test is not valid unless the resolution between the peaks corresponding to linalol and β-caryophyllene is at least 1.5.

Inject 0.2 μl of the test solution. Using the retention times determined from the chromatogram obtained with the reference solution, locate the components of the reference solution in the chromatogram obtained with the test solution. Determine the percentage content of each of these components by the normalisation procedure.

The percentages are within the following ranges:

– *cineole*: less than 3.0 per cent,
– *linalol*: 1.0 per cent to 6.0 per cent,
– *β-caryophyllene*: 1.0 per cent to 4.0 per cent,
– *safrole*: less than 0.5 per cent,
– *trans-cinnamic aldehyde*: 55 per cent to 75 per cent,
– *eugenol*: less than 7.5 per cent,
– *coumarin*: less than 0.5 per cent,
– *trans-2-methoxycinnamaldehyde*: 0.1 per cent to 1.0 per cent,
– *benzyl benzoate*: less than 1.0 per cent.

STORAGE

Store in a well-filled, airtight container, protected from light and heat.

01/2005:1608

CINNAMON LEAF OIL, CEYLON

Cinnamomi zeylanici folii aetheroleum

DEFINITION

Oil obtained by steam distillation of the leaves of *Cinnamomum verum* J.S. Presl.

CHARACTERS

Clear, mobile, reddish-brown to dark brown liquid, with a characteristic odour reminiscent of eugenol.

IDENTIFICATION

First identification: B.

Second identification: A.

A. Thin-layer chromatography (*2.2.27*).

Test solution. Dilute 1 ml of the substance to be examined in *acetone R* and dilute to 10 ml with the same solvent.

Reference solution. Dilute about 50 μl of *trans-cinnamic aldehyde R,* 10 μl of *eugenol R,* 10 μl of *linalol R* and 10 μl of *β-caryophyllene R* in *alcohol R* and dilute to 10 ml with the same solvent.

Plate: *TLC silica gel plate R.*

Mobile phase: *methanol R, toluene R* (10:90 *V/V*).

Application: 10 μl, as bands.

Development: over a path of 15 cm.

Drying: in air.

Detection: spray with *anisaldehyde solution R.* Examine in day light while heating at 100-105 °C for 5-10 min.

Results: the zones in the chromatogram obtained with the test solution are similar in position and colour to those in the chromatogram obtained with the reference solution. The zone due to *trans*-cinnamic aldehyde may be very faint or absent.

B. Examine the chromatogram obtained in the test for chromatographic profile.

Results: the characteristic peaks in the chromatogram obtained with the test solution are similar in retention time to those in the chromatogram obtained with the reference solution. The peaks corresponding to cineole, safrole, *trans*-cinnamic aldehyde, cinnamyl acetate and coumarin may be absent in the chromatogram obtained with the test solution.

TESTS

Relative density (*2.2.5*): 1.030 to 1.059.

Refractive index (*2.2.6*): 1.527 to 1.540.

Optical rotation (*2.2.7*): −2.5° to + 2.0°.

Chromatographic profile. Gas chromatography (*2.2.28*): use the normalisation procedure.

Test solution. The substance to be examined.

Reference solution. Dissolve 10 μl of *cineole R,* 10 μl of *linalol R,* 10 μl of *β-caryophyllene R,* 10 μl of *safrole R,* 10 μl of *trans-cinnamic aldehyde R,* 10 μl of *cinnamyl acetate R,* 100 μl of *eugenol R* and 10 mg of *coumarin R* in 1 ml of *acetone R.*

Column:

– *material*: fused silica,
– *size*: *l* = 60 m, Ø = 0.25 mm,
– *stationary phase*: *macrogol 20 000 R.*

Carrier gas: *helium for chromatography R.*

Flow rate: 1.5 ml/min.

Split ratio: 1/100.

Temperature:

	Time (min)	Temperature (°C)
Column	0 - 10	45
	10 - 78	45 → 180
	78 - 88	180
Injection port		200
Detector		240

Detection: flame ionisation.

Injection: 0.2 μl.

Elution order: the order indicated in the composition of the reference solution. Record the retention times of these substances.

System suitability: reference solution:

– *resolution*: minimum of 1.5 between the peaks due to linalol and β-caryophyllene.

Using the retention times determined from the chromatogram obtained with the reference solution, locate the components of the reference solution in the chromatogram obtained with the test solution.

Determine the percentage content of these components. The percentages are within the following ranges:

– *cineole*: less than 1.0 per cent,
– *linalol*: 1.5 per cent to 3.5 per cent,
– *β-caryophyllene*: 1.5 per cent to 7.0 per cent,
– *safrole*: less than 3.0 per cent,
– *trans-cinnamic aldehyde*: less than 3.0 per cent,
– *cinnamyl acetate*: less than 2.0 per cent,
– *eugenol*: 70 per cent to 85 per cent,
– *coumarin*: less than 1.0 per cent.

STORAGE

In a well-filled, airtight container, protected from light and heat.

01/2005:1819

CINNAMON TINCTURE

Cinnamomi corticis tinctura

DEFINITION

Tincture produced from *Cinnamon (0387)*.

PRODUCTION

The tincture is produced from 1 part of the drug and 5 parts of ethanol (70 per cent *V/V*) by an appropriate procedure.

CHARACTERS

Appearance: clear, brownish-red liquid, with a characteristic odour.

IDENTIFICATION

Thin-layer chromatography (*2.2.27*).

Test solution. Place 10 ml of the tincture to be examined, 10 ml of *saturated sodium chloride solution R* and 5 ml of *toluene R* in a ground glass-stoppered tube. Shake for 2 min and centrifuge for 10 min. Use the organic layer.

Reference solution. Dissolve 5 μl of *eugenol R*, 25 μl of *trans-cinnamic aldehyde R* and 5 μl of *trans-2-methoxycinnamaldehyde R* in *toluene R* and dilute to 10 ml with the same solvent.

Plate: *TLC silica gel G plate R*.

Mobile phase: *methylene chloride R*.

Application: 20 μl, as bands.

Development: over a path of 10 cm.

Drying: in air.

Detection A: examine in ultraviolet light at 365 nm.

Results A: see below the sequence of the zones present in the chromatograms obtained with the reference solution and the test solution.

Top of the plate	
———	
Trans-2-methoxycinnamaldehyde: a light blue fluorescent zone	A light blue fluorescent zone (*trans*-2- methoxycinnamaldehyde)
———	
	A greenish fluorescent zone (above the starting line)
Reference solution	**Test solution**

Detection B: spray with a 200 g/l solution of *phosphomolybdic acid R* in *ethanol R*. Examine in daylight while heating at 100-105 °C for 5-10 min.

Results B: see below the sequence of the zones present in the chromatograms obtained with the reference solution and the test solution. Furthermore, other zones may be present in the chromatogram obtained with the test solution.

Top of the plate	
	1 blue zone (terpenhydrocarbons)
———	
Eugenol: a blue zone	A blue zone (eugenol)
Trans-cinnamic aldehyde: a blue zone	A blue zone (*trans*-cinnamic aldehyde)
Trans-2-methoxycinnamaldehyde: an orange-brown zone (the colour fades away)	A weak orange-brown zone (*trans*-2-methoxycinnamaldehyde)
———	———
	2 or 3 blue zones above the starting line
Reference solution	**Test solution**

TESTS

Ethanol (*2.9.10*): 64 per cent *V/V* to 70 per cent *V/V*.

Methanol and 2-propanol (*2.9.11*): maximum 0.05 per cent *V/V* of methanol and maximum 0.05 per cent *V/V* of 2-propanol.

Dry residue (*2.8.16*): minimum 1.5 per cent *m/m*, determined on 5.0 g.

01/2005:0816

CINNARIZINE

Cinnarizinum

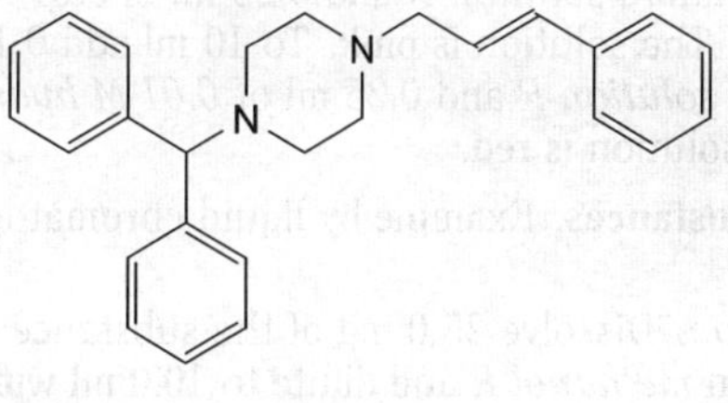

$C_{26}H_{28}N_2$ M_r 368.5

DEFINITION

Cinnarizine contains not less than 99.0 per cent and not more than the equivalent of 101.0 per cent of (*E*)-1-(diphenylmethyl)-4-(3-phenylprop-2-enyl)piperazine, calculated with reference to the dried substance.

CHARACTERS

A white or almost white powder, practically insoluble in water, freely soluble in methylene chloride, soluble in acetone, slightly soluble in alcohol and in methanol.

IDENTIFICATION

First identification: A, B.

Second identification: A, C, D.

A. Melting point (*2.2.14*): 118 °C to 122 °C.

B. Examine by infrared absorption spectrophotometry (*2.2.24*), comparing with the spectrum obtained with *cinnarizine CRS*. Examine the substances prepared as discs.

C. Examine by thin-layer chromatography (*2.2.27*), using as the coating substance a suitable octadecylsilyl silica gel with a fluorescent indicator having an optimal intensity at 254 nm.

Test solution. Dissolve 10 mg of the substance to be examined in *methanol R* and dilute to 20 ml with the same solvent.

Reference solution (a). Dissolve 10 mg of *cinnarizine CRS* in *methanol R* and dilute to 20 ml with the same solvent.

Reference solution (b). Dissolve 10 mg of *cinnarizine CRS* and 10 mg of *flunarizine dihydrochloride CRS* in *methanol R* and dilute to 20 ml with the same solvent.

Apply to the plate 5 µl of each solution. Develop in an unsaturated tank over a path of 15 cm using a mixture of 20 volumes of *1 M sodium chloride*, 30 volumes of *methanol R* and 50 volumes of *acetone R*. Allow the plate to dry in air and examine in ultraviolet light at 254 nm. The principal spot in the chromatogram obtained with the test solution is similar in position and size to the principal spot in the chromatogram obtained with reference solution (a). The test is not valid unless the chromatogram obtained with reference solution (b) shows two clearly separated spots.

D. Dissolve 0.2 g of *anhydrous citric acid R* in 10 ml of *acetic anhydride R* in a water-bath at 80 °C and maintain the temperature of the water-bath at 80 °C for 10 min. Add about 20 mg of the substance to be examined. A purple colour develops.

TESTS

Appearance of solution. Dissolve 0.5 g in *methylene chloride R* and dilute to 20 ml with the same solvent. The solution is clear (*2.2.1*) and not more intensely coloured than reference solution BY_7 (*2.2.2, Method II*).

Acidity or alkalinity. Suspend 0.5 g in 15 ml of *water R*. Boil for 2 min. Cool and filter. Dilute the filtrate to 20 ml with *carbon dioxide-free water R*. To 10 ml add 0.1 ml of *phenolphthalein solution R* and 0.25 ml of *0.01 M sodium hydroxide*. The solution is pink. To 10 ml add 0.1 ml of *methyl red solution R* and 0.25 ml of *0.01 M hydrochloric acid*. The solution is red.

Related substances. Examine by liquid chromatography (*2.2.29*).

Test solution. Dissolve 25.0 mg of the substance to be examined in *methanol R* and dilute to 10.0 ml with the same solvent.

Reference solution (a). Dissolve 12.5 mg of *cinnarizine CRS* and 15.0 mg of *flunarizine dihydrochloride CRS* in *methanol R* and dilute to 100.0 ml with the same solvent. Dilute 1.0 ml of this solution to 20.0 ml with *methanol R*.

Reference solution (b). Dilute 1.0 ml of the test solution to 100.0 ml with *methanol R*. Dilute 5.0 ml of this solution to 20.0 ml with *methanol R*.

The chromatographic procedure may be carried out using:

– a stainless steel column 0.1 m long and 4.0 mm in internal diameter packed with *base-deactivated octadecylsilyl silica gel for chromatography R* (3 µm),

– as mobile phase at a flow rate of 1.5 ml/min a gradient programme using the following conditions:

Mobile phase A. A 10 g/l solution of *ammonium acetate R*,

Mobile phase B. A 0.2 per cent *V/V* solution of *glacial acetic acid R* in *acetonitrile R*,

Time (min)	Mobile phase A (per cent *V/V*)	Mobile phase B (per cent *V/V*)	Comment
0 – 20	75 → 10	25 → 90	linear gradient
20 - 25	10	90	isocratic elution
25 - 30	75	25	switch to initial eluent composition
30 = 0	75	25	restart gradient

– as detector a spectrophotometer set at 230 nm.

Equilibrate the column for a least 30 min at the initial eluent composition.

Adjust the sensitivity of the system so that the height of the principal peak in the chromatogram obtained with 10 µl of reference solution (b) is at least 50 per cent of the full scale of the recorder. If necessary, adjust the concentration of glacial acetic acid in mobile phase B to obtain a horizontal base-line in the chromatogram.

Inject 10 µl of reference solution (a). When the chromatogram is recorded in the prescribed conditions, the retention times are: cinnarizine about 11 min and flunarizine about 11.5 min. The test is not valid unless the resolution between the peaks corresponding to cinnarizine and flunarizine is at least 5.0. If necessary, adjust the time programme for the gradient elution.

Inject 10 µl of *methanol R* as a blank, 10 µl of the test solution and 10 µl of reference solution (b). In the chromatogram obtained with the test solution: the area of any peak, apart from the principal peak, is not greater than the area of the principal peak in the chromatogram obtained with reference solution (b) (0.25 per cent); the sum of the areas of the peaks, apart from the principal peak, is not greater than twice the area of the principal peak in the chromatogram obtained with reference solution (b) (0.5 per cent). Disregard any peak due to the blank and any peak with an area less than 0.2 times the area of the principal peak in the chromatogram obtained with reference solution (b).

Heavy metals (*2.4.8*). Dissolve 1.0 g in a mixture of 15 volumes of *water R* and 85 volumes of *acetone R*. Add *dilute hydrochloric acid R* until dissolution is complete. Dilute to 20 ml with the same mixture of *water R* and *acetone R*. 12 ml of the solution complies with limit test B for heavy metals (20 ppm). Prepare the standard using 10 ml of lead standard solution (1 ppm Pb) obtained by diluting *lead standard solution (100 ppm Pb) R* with the mixture of *water R* and *acetone R*.

Loss on drying (*2.2.32*). Not more than 0.5 per cent, determined on 1.000 g by drying in an oven *in vacuo* at 60 °C for 4 h.

Sulphated ash (*2.4.14*). Not more than 0.1 per cent, determined on 1.0 g.

ASSAY

Dissolve 0.150 g in 50 ml of a mixture of 1 volume of *anhydrous acetic acid R* and 7 volumes of *ethyl methyl ketone R*. Titrate with *0.1 M perchloric acid*, using 0.2 ml of *naphtholbenzein solution R* as indicator.

1 ml of *0.1 M perchloric acid* is equivalent to 18.43 mg of $C_{26}H_{28}N_2$.

STORAGE

Store protected from light.

IMPURITIES

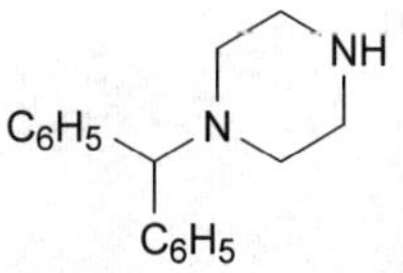

A. 1-(diphenylmethyl)piperazine,

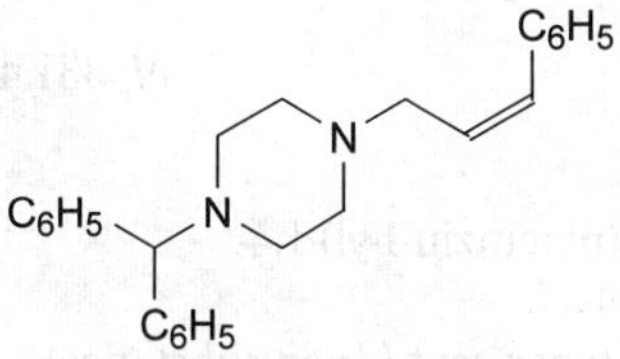

B. (*Z*)-1-(diphenylmethyl)-4-(3-phenylprop-2-enyl)piperazine,

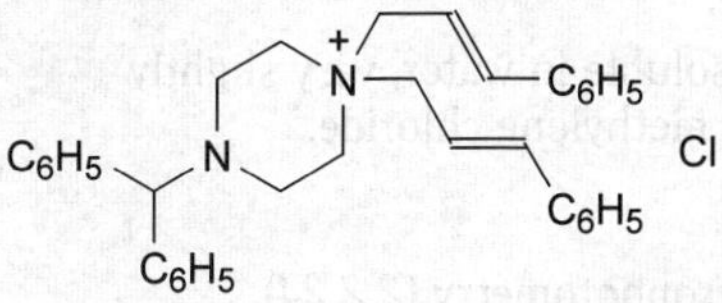

C. (4-(diphenylmethyl)-1,1-bis[(*E*)-3-phenylprop-2-enyl]piperazinium chloride,

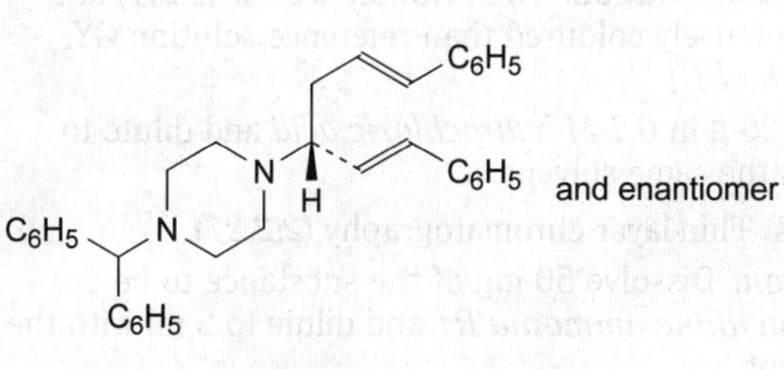

D. 1-(diphenylmethyl)-4-[(1*RS*,3*E*)-4-phenyl-1-[(*E*)-2-phenylethenyl]but-3-enyl]piperazine,

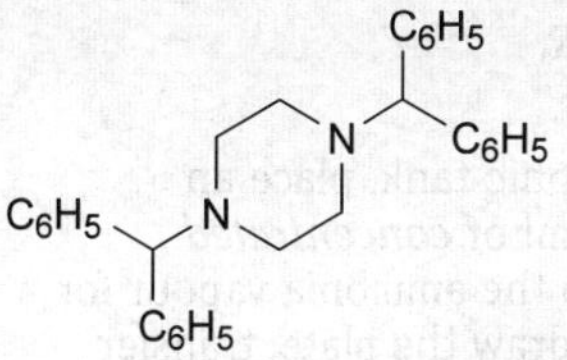

E. 1,4-bis(diphenylmethyl)piperazine.

01/2005:2013

CIPROFIBRATE

Ciprofibratum

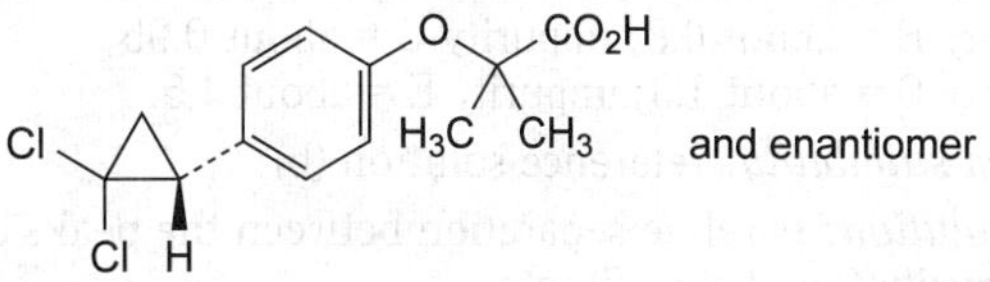

$C_{13}H_{14}Cl_2O_3$ M_r 289.2

DEFINITION

2-[4-[(1*RS*)-2,2-Dichlorocyclopropyl]phenoxy]-2-methylpropanoic acid.

Content: 99.0 per cent to 101.0 per cent (anhydrous substance).

CHARACTERS

Appearance: white or slightly yellow, crystalline powder.

Solubility: practically insoluble in water, freely soluble in anhydrous ethanol, soluble in toluene.

mp: about 115 °C.

IDENTIFICATION

Infrared absorption spectrophotometry (*2.2.24*).

Comparison: *ciprofibrate CRS*.

TESTS

Appearance of solution. The solution is clear (*2.2.1*) and not more intensely coloured than reference solution BY_4 (*2.2.2, Method II*).

Dissolve 1.0 g in *anhydrous ethanol R* and dilute to 10.0 ml with the same solvent.

Related substances. Liquid chromatography (*2.2.29*).

Test solution. Dissolve 0.125 g of the substance to be examined in a mixture of equal volumes of *acetonitrile R* and *water R* and dilute to 50 ml with the same mixture of solvents.

Reference solution (a). Dilute 1.0 ml of the test solution to 100.0 ml with a mixture of equal volumes of *acetonitrile R* and *water R*. Dilute 1.0 ml of this solution to 10.0 ml with a mixture of equal volumes of *acetonitrile R* and *water R*.

Reference solution (b). Dissolve the contents of a vial of *ciprofibrate for system suitability CRS* in 2.0 ml of a mixture of equal volumes of *acetonitrile R* and *water R*.

Column:

– *size*: l = 0.15 m, Ø = 4.6 mm,
– *stationary phase*: *octylsilyl silica gel for chromatography R* (5 µm).

Mobile phase:

– *mobile phase A*: 1.36 g/l solution of *potassium dihydrogen phosphate R* adjusted to pH 2.2 with *phosphoric acid R*,
– *mobile phase B*: *acetonitrile R*,

Time (min)	Mobile phase A (per cent *V/V*)	Mobile phase B (per cent *V/V*)
0 - 30	75 → 30	25 → 70
30 - 40	30	70
40 - 42	30 → 75	70 → 25

Flow rate: 1.5 ml/min.

Detection: spectrophotometer at 230 nm.

Injection: 10 µl.

Identification of impurities: use the chromatogram supplied with *ciprofibrate for system suitability CRS* to identify the peaks due to impurities A, B, C, D and E.

Relative retention with reference to ciprofibrate (retention time = about 18 min): impurity A = about 0.7; impurity B = about 0.8; impurity C = about 0.95; impurity D = about 1.3; impurity E = about 1.5.

System suitability: reference solution (b):

- *resolution*: baseline separation between the peaks due to impurity C and ciprofibrate.

Limits:

- *correction factor*: for the calculation of content, multiply the peak area of impurity A by 2.3,
- *impurities A, C, D*: for each impurity, not more than the area of the principal peak in the chromatogram obtained with reference solution (a) (0.1 per cent),
- *impurity B*: not more than twice the area of the principal peak in the chromatogram obtained with reference solution (a) (0.2 per cent),
- *impurity E*: not more than 8 times the area of the principal peak in the chromatogram obtained with reference solution (a) (0.8 per cent),
- *any other impurity*: for each impurity, not more than the area of the principal peak in the chromatogram obtained with reference solution (a) (0.1 per cent),
- *total of other impurities*: not more than 5 times the area of the principal peak in the chromatogram obtained with reference solution (a) (0.5 per cent),
- *disregard limit*: 0.5 times the area of the principal peak in the chromatogram obtained with reference solution (a) (0.05 per cent).

Chlorides (*2.4.4*): maximum 350 ppm.

To 0.190 g add 20 ml of *water R* and treat in an ultrasonic bath for 8 min. Filter. 15 ml of the filtrate complies with the test.

Water (*2.5.12*): maximum 0.5 per cent, determined on 1.000 g.

Sulphated ash (*2.4.14*): maximum 0.1 per cent, determined on 1.0 g.

ASSAY

Dissolve 0.250 g in a mixture of 20 ml of *water R* and 40 ml of *anhydrous ethanol R*. Titrate with *0.1 M sodium hydroxide*, determining the end-point potentiometrically (*2.2.20*).

1 ml of *0.1 M sodium hydroxide* is equivalent to 28.92 mg of $C_{13}H_{14}Cl_2O_3$.

STORAGE

In an airtight container, protected from light.

IMPURITIES

Specified impurities: A, B, C, D, E.

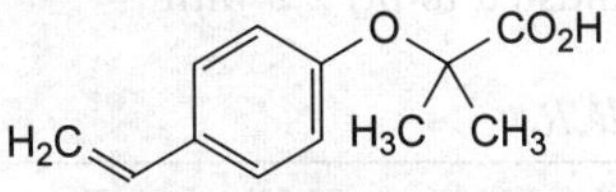

A. 2-(4-ethenylphenoxy)-2-methylpropanoic acid,

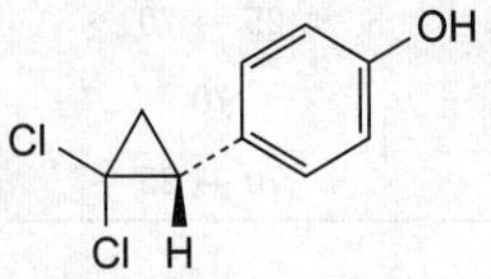

and enantiomer

B. 4-[(1*RS*)-2,2-dichlorocyclopropyl]phenol,

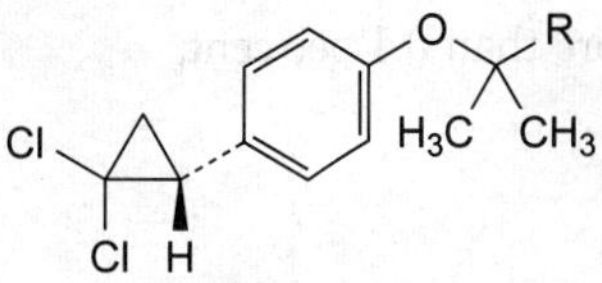

and enantiomer

C. R = CH_2OH: 2-[4-[(1*RS*)-2,2-dichlorocyclopropyl]phenoxy]-2-methylpropan-1-ol,

D. R = $CO\text{-}OCH_3$: methyl 2-[4-[(1*RS*)-2,2-dichlorocyclopropyl]phenoxy]-2-methylpropanoate,

E. R = $CO\text{-}OC_2H_5$: ethyl 2-[4-[(1*RS*)-2,2-dichlorocyclopropyl]phenoxy]-2-methylpropanoate.

01/2005:1089
corrected

CIPROFLOXACIN

Ciprofloxacinum

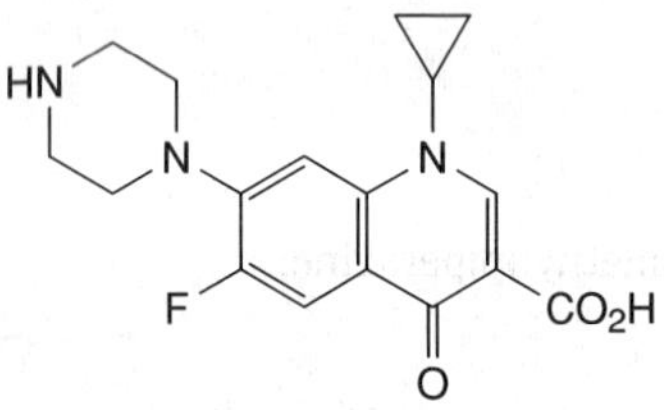

$C_{17}H_{18}FN_3O_3$ M_r 331.4

DEFINITION

1-Cyclopropyl-6-fluoro-4-oxo-7-(piperazin-1-yl)-1,4-dihydroquinoline-3-carboxylic acid.

Content: 99.0 per cent to 101.0 per cent (dried substance).

CHARACTERS

Appearance: almost white or pale yellow, crystalline powder, slightly hygroscopic.

Solubility: practically insoluble in water, very slightly soluble in ethanol and in methylene chloride.

IDENTIFICATION

Infrared absorption spectrophotometry (*2.2.24*).

Comparison: *ciprofloxacin CRS.*

TESTS

Appearance of solution. The solution is clear (*2.2.1*) and not more intensely coloured than reference solution GY_5 (*2.2.2, Method II*).

Dissolve 0.25 g in *0.1 M hydrochloric acid* and dilute to 20 ml with the same solvent.

Impurity A. Thin-layer chromatography (*2.2.27*).

Test solution. Dissolve 50 mg of the substance to be examined in *dilute ammonia R1* and dilute to 5 ml with the same solvent.

Reference solution. Dissolve 10 mg of *ciprofloxacin impurity A CRS* in a mixture of 0.1 ml of *dilute ammonia R1* and 90 ml of *water R* and dilute to 100 ml with *water R*. Dilute 2 ml of the solution to 10 ml with *water R*.

Plate: *TLC silica gel F_{254} plate R.*

Application: 5 µl.

At the bottom of a chromatographic tank, place an evaporating dish containing 50 ml of *concentrated ammonia R*. Expose the plate to the ammonia vapour for 15 min in the closed tank. Withdraw the plate, transfer to a second chromatographic tank and proceed with development.

Mobile phase: *acetonitrile R, concentrated ammonia R, methanol R, methylene chloride R* (10:20:40:40 *V/V/V/V*).

Development: over 3/4 of the plate.

Drying: in air.

Detection: examine in ultraviolet light at 254 nm.

Limit:

– *impurity A*: any spot corresponding to impurity A is not more intense than the principal spot in the chromatogram obtained with the reference solution (0.2 per cent).

Related substances. Liquid chromatography (*2.2.29*).

Test solution. To 25.0 mg of the substance to be examined add 0.2 ml of *dilute phosphoric acid R* and dilute to 50.0 ml with the mobile phase and treat in an ultrasonic bath until a clear solution is obtained.

Reference solution (a). Dilute 1.0 ml of the test solution to 100.0 ml with the mobile phase. Dilute 1.0 ml of this solution to 5.0 ml with the mobile phase.

Reference solution (b). Dissolve 5 mg of *ciprofloxacin hydrochloride for peak identification CRS* in the mobile phase and dilute to 10.0 ml with the mobile phase.

Column:

– *size*: l = 0.25 m, Ø = 4.6 mm;
– *stationary phase*: *base-deactivated octadecylsilyl silica gel for chromatography R* (5 µm);
– *temperature*: 40 °C.

Mobile phase: mix 13 volumes of *acetonitrile R* and 87 volumes of a 2.45 g/l solution of *phosphoric acid R*, previously adjusted to pH 3.0 with *triethylamine R*.

Flow rate: 1.5 ml/min.

Detection: spectrophotometer at 278 nm.

Injection: 50 µl.

Run time: twice the retention time of ciprofloxacin.

Relative retention with reference to ciprofloxacin (retention time = about 9 min): impurity E = about 0.4; impurity F = about 0.5; impurity B = about 0.6; impurity C = about 0.7; impurity D = about 1.2.

System suitability: reference solution (b):

– *resolution*: minimum 1.3 between the peaks due to impurity B and impurity C.

Limits:

– *correction factors*: for the calculation of contents, multiply the peak areas of the following impurities by the corresponding correction factor: impurity B = 0.7; impurity C = 0.6; impurity D = 1.4; impurity E = 6.7; use the chromatogram obtained with reference solution (b) and the type chromatogram supplied with the CRS to identify the corresponding peaks;
– *impurities B, C, D, E*: for each impurity, not more than the area of the principal peak in the chromatogram obtained with reference solution (a) (0.2 per cent);
– *any other impurity*: not more than half the area of the principal peak in the chromatogram obtained with reference solution (a) (0.1 per cent);
– *total*: not more than 2.5 times the area of the principal peak in the chromatogram obtained with reference solution (a) (0.5 per cent);
– *disregard limit*: 0.25 times the area of the principal peak in the chromatogram obtained with reference solution (a) (0.05 per cent).

Heavy metals (*2.4.8*): maximum 20 ppm.

Dissolve 0.5 g in *dilute acetic acid R* and dilute to 30 ml with the same solvent. Add 2 ml of *water R* instead of 2 ml of *buffer solution pH 3.5 R*. The filtrate complies with limit test E. Prepare the standard using 10 ml of *lead standard solution (1 ppm Pb) R*.

Loss on drying (*2.2.32*): maximum 1.0 per cent, determined on 1.000 g by drying under vacuum at 120 °C.

Sulphated ash (*2.4.14*): maximum 0.1 per cent, determined on 1.0 g in a platinum crucible.

ASSAY

Dissolve 0.300 g in 80 ml of *glacial acetic acid R*. Titrate with *0.1 M perchloric acid*, determining the end-point potentiometrically (*2.2.20*).

1 ml of *0.1 M perchloric acid* is equivalent to 33.14 mg of $C_{17}H_{18}FN_3O_3$.

STORAGE

In an airtight container, protected from light.

IMPURITIES

Specified impurities: *A, B, C, D, E.*

Other detectable impurities: *F.*

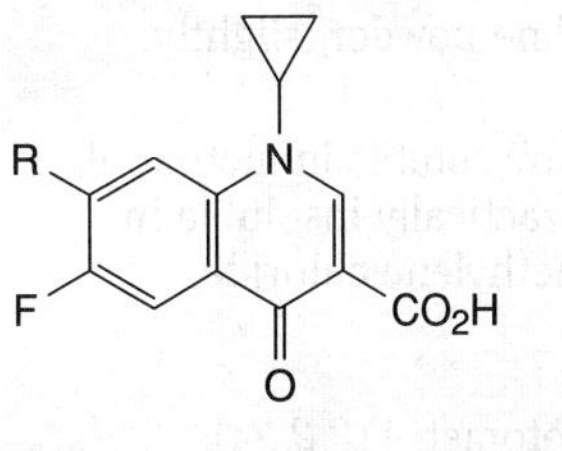

A. R = Cl: 7-chloro-1-cyclopropyl-6-fluoro-4-oxo-1,4-dihydroquinoline-3-carboxylic acid (fluoroquinolonic acid),

C. R = NH-$[CH_2]_2$-NH_2: 7-[(2-aminoethyl)amino]-1-cyclopropyl-6-fluoro-4-oxo-1,4-dihydroquinoline-3-carboxylic acid (ethylenediamine compound),

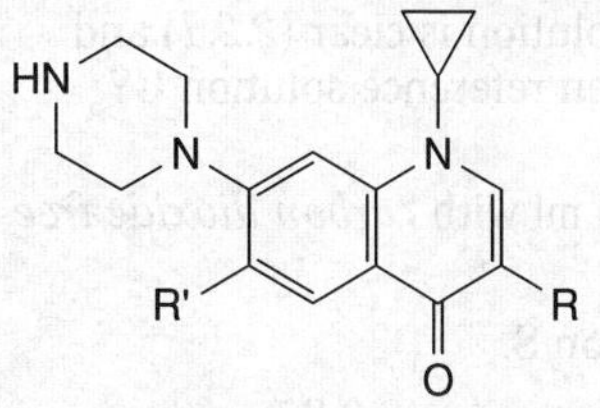

B. R = CO_2H, R′ = H: 1-cyclopropyl-4-oxo-7-(piperazin-1-yl)-1,4-dihydroquinoline-3-carboxylic acid (desfluoro compound),

E. R = H, R′ = F: 1-cyclopropyl-6-fluoro-7-(piperazin-1-yl)quinolin-4(1*H*)-one (decarboxylated compound),

F. R = CO_2H, R′ = OH: 1-cyclopropyl-6-hydroxy-4-oxo-7-(piperazin-1-yl)-1,4-dihydroquinoline-3-carboxylic acid,

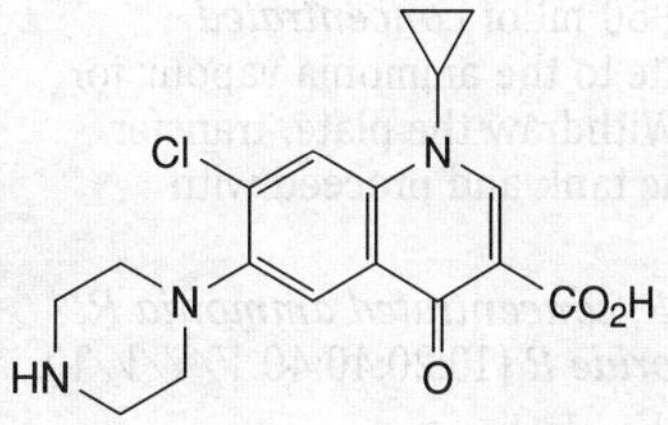

D. 7-chloro-1-cyclopropyl-4-oxo-6-(piperazin-1-yl)-1,4-dihydroquinoline-3-carboxylic acid.

Monographs C

01/2005:0888

CIPROFLOXACIN HYDROCHLORIDE

Ciprofloxacini hydrochloridum

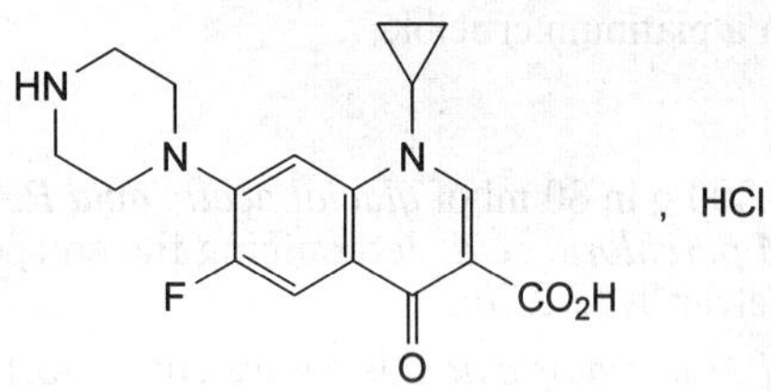

$C_{17}H_{19}ClFN_3O_3$ M_r 367.8

DEFINITION

1-Cyclopropyl-6-fluoro-4-oxo-7-(piperazin-1-yl)-1,4-dihydroquinoline-3-carboxylic acid hydrochloride.

Content: 98.0 per cent to 102.0 per cent (anhydrous substance).

CHARACTERS

Appearance: pale yellow, crystalline powder, slightly hygroscopic.

Solubility: soluble in water, slightly soluble in methanol, very slightly soluble in ethanol, practically insoluble in acetone, in ethyl acetate and in methylene chloride.

IDENTIFICATION

A. Infrared absorption spectrophotometry (*2.2.24*).

Preparation: discs.

Comparison: *ciprofloxacin hydrochloride CRS.*

B. 0.1 g gives reaction (b) of chlorides (*2.3.1*).

TESTS

Solution S. Dissolve 0.5 g in *carbon dioxide-free water R* and dilute to 20 ml with the same solvent.

Appearance of solution. The solution is clear (*2.2.1*) and not more intensely coloured than reference solution GY_5 (*2.2.2, Method II*).

Dilute 10 ml of solution S to 20 ml with *carbon dioxide-free water R.*

pH (*2.2.3*): 3.5 to 4.5 for solution S.

Impurity A. Thin-layer chromatography (*2.2.27*).

Test solution. Dissolve 50 mg of the substance to be examined in *water R* and dilute to 5 ml with the same solvent.

Reference solution. Dissolve 10 mg of *ciprofloxacin impurity A CRS* in a mixture of 0.1 ml of *dilute ammonia R1* and 90 ml of *water R* and dilute to 100 ml with *water R.* Dilute 2 ml of the solution to 10 ml with *water R.*

Plate: *TLC silica gel F_{254} plate R.*

Application: 5 µl.

At the bottom of a chromatographic tank, place an evaporating dish containing 50 ml of *concentrated ammonia R.* Expose the plate to the ammonia vapour for 15 min in the closed tank. Withdraw the plate, transfer to a second chromatographic tank and proceed with development.

Mobile phase: *acetonitrile R, concentrated ammonia R, methanol R, methylene chloride R* (10:20:40:40 *V/V/V/V*).

Development: over 3/4 of the plate.

Drying: in air.

Detection: examine in ultraviolet light at 254 nm.

Limit:

- *impurity A*: any spot corresponding to impurity A is not more intense than the principal spot in the chromatogram obtained with the reference solution (0.2 per cent).

Related substances. Liquid chromatography (*2.2.29*).

Test solution. Dissolve 25.0 mg of the substance to be examined in the mobile phase and dilute to 50.0 ml with the mobile phase.

Reference solution (a). Dissolve 25.0 mg of *ciprofloxacin hydrochloride CRS* in the mobile phase and dilute to 50.0 ml with the mobile phase.

Reference solution (b). Dissolve 5 mg of *ciprofloxacin hydrochloride for peak identification CRS* in the mobile phase and dilute to 10.0 ml with the mobile phase.

Reference solution (c). Dilute 1.0 ml of the test solution to 50.0 ml with the mobile phase. Dilute 1.0 ml of this solution to 10.0 ml with the mobile phase.

Column:

- *size*: l = 0.25 m, Ø = 4.6 mm;
- *stationary phase*: *base-deactivated octadecylsilyl silica gel for chromatography R* (5 µm);
- *temperature*: 40 °C.

Mobile phase: mix 13 volumes of *acetonitrile R* and 87 volumes of a 2.45 g/l solution of *phosphoric acid R,* previously adjusted to pH 3.0 with *triethylamine R.*

Flow rate: 1.5 ml/min.

Detection: spectrophotometer at 278 nm.

Injection: 50 µl.

Run time: twice the retention time of ciprofloxacin.

Relative retention with reference to ciprofloxacin (retention time = about 9 min): impurity E = about 0.4; impurity F = about 0.5; impurity B = about 0.6; impurity C = about 0.7; impurity D = about 1.2.

System suitability: reference solution (b):

- *resolution*: minimum 1.3 between the peaks due to impurity B and impurity C.

Limits:

- *correction factors*: for the calculation of contents, multiply the peak areas of the following impurities by the corresponding correction factor: impurity B = 0.7; impurity C = 0.6; impurity D = 1.4; impurity E = 6.7; use the chromatogram obtained with reference solution (b) and the type chromatogram supplied with the CRS to identify the corresponding peaks;
- *impurities B, C, D, E*: for each impurity, not more than the area of the principal peak in the chromatogram obtained with reference solution (c) (0.2 per cent);
- *any other impurity*: not more than half the area of the principal peak in the chromatogram obtained with reference solution (c) (0.1 per cent);
- *total*: not more than 2.5 times the area of the principal peak in the chromatogram obtained with reference solution (c) (0.5 per cent);
- *disregard limit*: 0.25 times the area of the principal peak in the chromatogram obtained with reference solution (c) (0.05 per cent).

Heavy metals (*2.4.8*): maximum 20 ppm.

Dissolve 0.25 g in *water R* and dilute to 30 ml with the same solvent. Carry out the prefiltration. The filtrate complies with limit test E. Prepare the standard using 5 ml of *lead standard solution (1 ppm Pb) R.*

Water (*2.5.12*): maximum 6.7 per cent, determined on 0.200 g.

Sulphated ash (*2.4.14*): maximum 0.1 per cent, determined on 1.0 g in a platinum crucible.

ASSAY

Liquid chromatography (*2.2.29*) as described in the test for related substances with the following modifications.

Injection: 10 µl; inject the test solution and reference solution (a).

Calculate the percentage content of $C_{17}H_{19}ClFN_3O_3$.

STORAGE

In an airtight container, protected from light.

IMPURITIES

Specified impurities: A, B, C, D, E.

Other detectable impurities: F.

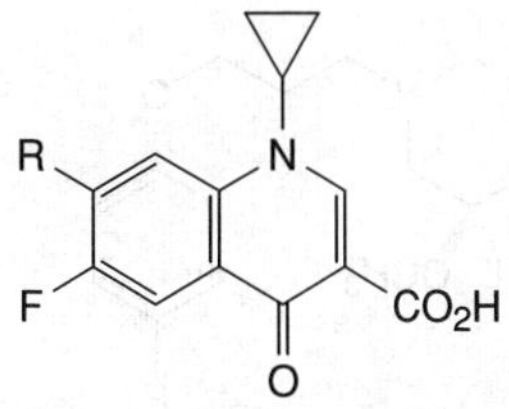

A. R = Cl: 7-chloro-1-cyclopropyl-6-fluoro-4-oxo-1,4-dihydroquinoline-3-carboxylic acid (fluoroquinolonic acid),

C. R = NH-$[CH_2]_2$-NH_2: 7-[(2-aminoethyl)amino]-1-cyclopropyl-6-fluoro-4-oxo-1,4-dihydroquinoline-3-carboxylic acid (ethylenediamine compound),

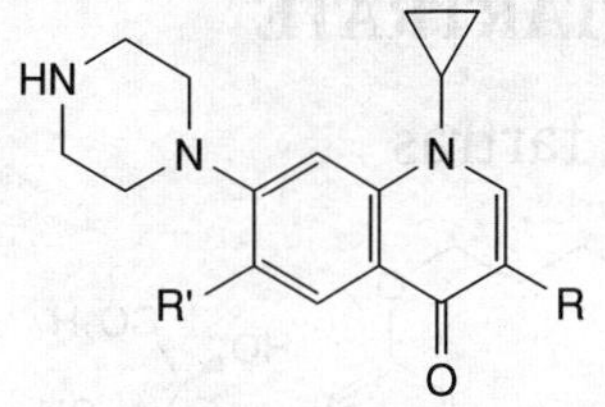

B. R = CO_2H, R′ = H: 1-cyclopropyl-4-oxo-7-(piperazin-1-yl)-1,4-dihydroquinoline-3-carboxylic acid (desfluoro compound),

E. R = H, R′ = F: 1-cyclopropyl-6-fluoro-7-(piperazin-1-yl)quinolin-4(1*H*)-one (decarboxylated compound),

F. R = CO_2H, R′ = OH: 1-cyclopropyl-6-hydroxy-4-oxo-7-(piperazin-1-yl)-1,4-dihydroquinoline-3-carboxylic acid,

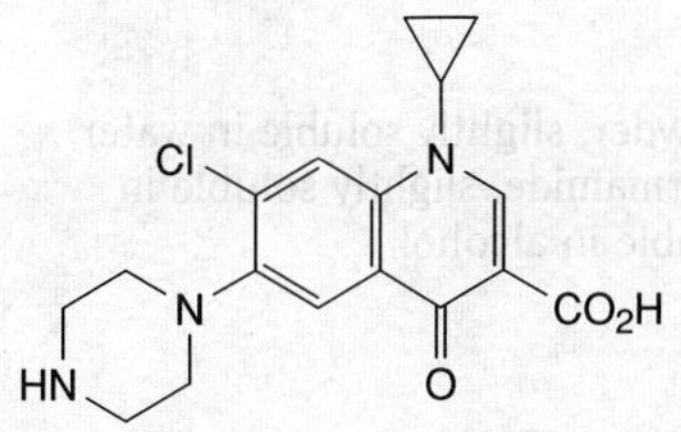

D. 7-chloro-1-cyclopropyl-4-oxo-6-(piperazin-1-yl)-1,4-dihydroquinoline-3-carboxylic acid.

01/2005:0995

CISAPRIDE MONOHYDRATE

Cisapridum monohydricum

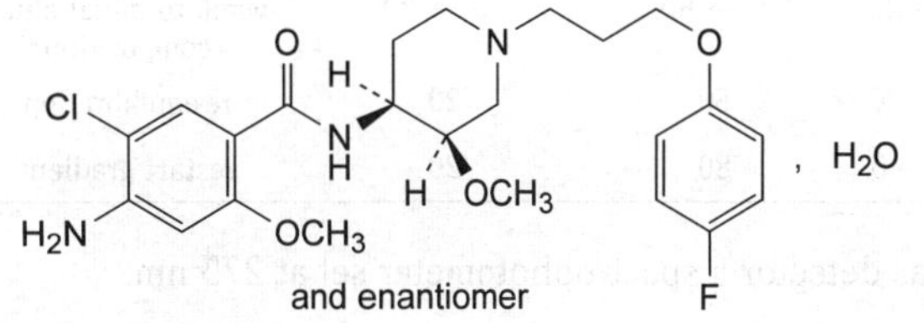

$C_{23}H_{29}ClFN_3O_4,H_2O$ M_r 484.0

DEFINITION

Cisapride monohydrate contains not less than 99.0 per cent and not more than the equivalent of 101.0 per cent of 4-amino-5-chloro-*N*-[(3*RS*,4*SR*)-1-[3-(4-fluorophenoxy)propyl]-3-methoxypiperidin-4-yl]-2-methoxybenzamide, calculated with reference to the anhydrous substance.

CHARACTERS

A white or almost white powder, practically insoluble in water, freely soluble in dimethylformamide, soluble in methylene chloride, sparingly soluble in methanol.

It shows polymorphism.

IDENTIFICATION

Examine by infrared absorption spectrophotometry (*2.2.24*), comparing with the spectrum obtained with *cisapride monohydrate CRS*. Examine the substances prepared as discs. If the spectra obtained show differences, dissolve the substance to be examined and the reference substance separately in the minimum volume of *methanol R*, evaporate to dryness in a current of air and record new spectra using the residues.

TESTS

Solution S. Dissolve 0.20 g in *methylene chloride R* and dilute to 20.0 ml with the same solvent.

Appearance of solution. Solution S is clear (*2.2.1*) and not more intensely coloured than reference solution BY_6 (*2.2.2, Method II*).

Optical rotation (*2.2.7*). The angle of optical rotation, determined on solution S, is − 0.1° to + 0.1°.

Related substances. Examine by liquid chromatography (*2.2.29*).

Test solution. Dissolve 0.100 g of the substance to be examined in *methanol R* and dilute to 10.0 ml with the same solvent.

Reference solution (a). Dissolve 5.0 mg of *cisapride monohydrate CRS* and 40.0 mg of *haloperidol CRS* in *methanol R* and dilute to 100.0 ml with the same solvent.

Reference solution (b). Dilute 5.0 ml of the test solution to 100.0 ml with *methanol R*. Dilute 1.0 ml of this solution to 10.0 ml with *methanol R*.

The chromatographic procedure may be carried out using:

– a stainless steel column 0.1 m long and 4.0 mm in internal diameter packed with *base-deactivated octadecylsilyl silica gel for chromatography R* (3 µm),

– as mobile phase at a flow rate of 1.2 ml/min:

Mobile phase A. A 20 g/l solution of *tetrabutylammonium hydrogen sulphate R*,

Mobile phase B. Methanol R,

Time (min)	Mobile phase A (per cent V/V)	Mobile phase B (per cent V/V)	Comment
0 - 20	80 → 55	20 → 45	linear gradient
20 - 21	55 → 5	45 → 95	switch to next step
21 - 25	5	95	isocratic
25 - 26	5 → 80	95 → 20	switch to initial eluent composition
26 - 30	80	20	re-equilibration
30 = 0	80	20	restart gradient

– as detector a spectrophotometer set at 275 nm.

Equilibrate the column with the initial mobile phase composition for at least 5 min.

Adjust the sensitivity of the system so that the height of the principal peak in the chromatogram obtained with 10 µl of reference solution (b) is at least 50 per cent of the full scale of the recorder.

Inject 10 µl of reference solution (a). When the chromatogram is recorded in the prescribed conditions, the retention times are: cisapride about 15 min and haloperidol about 16 min. The test is not valid unless the resolution between the peaks due to cisapride and haloperidol is at least 2.5. If necessary, adjust the concentration of methanol in the mobile phase or adjust the time programme for the linear gradient.

Inject separately 10 µl of *methanol R* as a blank, 10 µl of the test solution and 10 µl of reference solution (b). In the chromatogram obtained with the test solution: the area of any peak, apart from the principal peak, is not greater than the area of the principal peak in the chromatogram obtained with reference solution (b) (0.5 per cent); the sum of the areas of all the peaks, apart from the principal peak, is not greater than twice the area of the principal peak in the chromatogram obtained with reference solution (b) (1 per cent). Disregard any peak due to the solvent (blank) and any peak with an area less than 0.1 times the area of the principal peak in the chromatogram obtained with reference solution (b).

Water (*2.5.12*): 3.4 per cent to 4.0 per cent, determined on 0.500 g by the semi-micro determination of water.

Sulphated ash (*2.4.14*). Not more than 0.1 per cent, determined on 1.0 g in a platinum crucible.

ASSAY

Dissolve 0.350 g in 70 ml of a mixture of 1 volume of *anhydrous acetic acid R* and 7 volumes of *methyl ethyl ketone R* and titrate with *0.1 M perchloric acid*. Determine the end-point potentiometrically (*2.2.20*).

1 ml of *0.1 M perchloric acid* is equivalent to 46.60 mg of $C_{23}H_{29}ClFN_3O_4$.

STORAGE

Store protected from light.

IMPURITIES

Specified impurities: A, B, C, E.

Other detectable impurities: D.

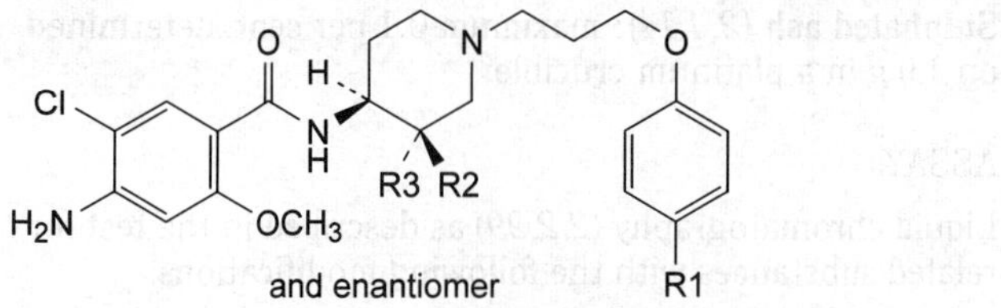

A. R1 = R3 = H, R2 = OCH_3: 4-amino-5-chloro-2-methoxy-*N*-[(3*RS*,4*SR*)-3-methoxy-1-(3-phenoxypropyl)piperidin-4-yl]benzamide,

B. R1 = F, R2 = R3 = H: 4-amino-5-chloro-*N*-[1-[3-(4-fluorophenoxy)propyl]piperidin-4-yl]-2-methoxybenzamide,

C. R1 = F, R2 = H, R3 = OCH_3: 4-amino-5-chloro-*N*-[(3*RS*,4*RS*)-1-[3-(4-fluorophenoxy)propyl]-3-methoxypiperidin-4-yl-2-methoxybenzamide,

E. R1 = F, R2 = OH, R3 = H: 4-amino-5-chloro-*N*-[(3*RS*,4*SR*)-1-[3-(4-fluorophenoxy)propyl]-3-hydroxypiperidin-4-yl]-2-methoxybenzamide,

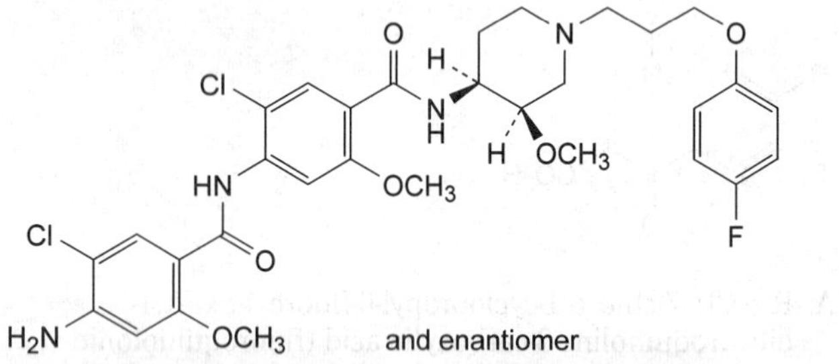

D. 4-[(4-amino-5-chloro-2-methoxybenzoyl)amino]-5-chloro-*N*-[(3*RS*,4*SR*)-1-[3-(4-fluorophenoxy)propyl]-3-methoxypiperidin-4-yl]-2-methoxybenzamide.

01/2005:1503

CISAPRIDE TARTRATE

Cisapridi tartras

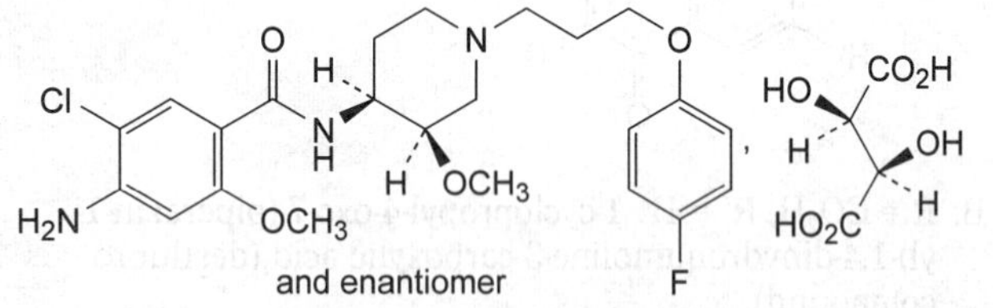

$C_{27}H_{35}ClFN_3O_{10}$ M_r 616.0

DEFINITION

Cisapride tartrate contains not less than 99.0 per cent and not more than the equivalent of 101.0 per cent of 4-amino-5-chloro-*N*-[(3*RS*,4*SR*)-1-[3-(4-fluorophenoxy)propyl]-3-methoxypiperidin-4-yl]-2-methoxybenzamide (2*R*,3*R*)-2,3-dihydroxybutanedioate, calculated with reference to the dried substance.

CHARACTERS

A white or almost white powder, slightly soluble in water, freely soluble in dimethylformamide, slightly soluble in methanol, very slightly soluble in alcohol.

It shows polymorphism.

IDENTIFICATION

A. Examine by infrared absorption spectrophotometry (*2.2.24*), comparing with the spectrum obtained with *cisapride tartrate CRS*. Examine the substances prepared as discs. If the spectra obtained show differences, dissolve the substance to be examined and the reference substance separately in the minimum volume of *alcohol R*, evaporate to dryness in a current of air and record new spectra using the residues.

B. It complies with the test for specific optical rotation (see Tests).

TESTS

Specific optical rotation (*2.2.7*). Dissolve 0.100 g in *methanol R* and dilute to 25.0 ml with the same solvent. The specific optical rotation is + 5.0 to + 10.0, calculated with reference to the dried substance.

Related substances. Examine by liquid chromatography (*2.2.29*).

Test solution. Dissolve 0.100 g of the substance to be examined in a mixture of 10 volumes of *water R* and 90 volumes of *methanol R*, with gentle warming if necessary, and dilute to 10.0 ml with the same mixture of solvents.

Reference solution (a). Dissolve 5.0 mg of *cisapride tartrate CRS* and 30.0 mg of *haloperidol CRS* in a mixture of 10 volumes of *water R* and 90 volumes of *methanol R* and dilute to 100.0 ml with the same mixture of solvents.

Reference solution (b). Dilute 1.0 ml of the test solution to 100.0 ml with a mixture of 10 volumes of *water R* and 90 volumes of *methanol R*. Dilute 5.0 ml of the solution to 20.0 ml with the same mixture of solvents.

The chromatographic procedure may be carried out using:

- a stainless steel column 0.1 m long and 4.0 mm in internal diameter packed with *base-deactivated octadecylsilyl silica gel for chromatography R* (3 µm),
- as mobile phase at a flow rate of 1.2 ml/min:
  Mobile phase A. A 20 g/l solution of *tetrabutylammonium hydrogen sulphate R*,
  Mobile phase B. Methanol R,

Time (min)	Mobile phase A (per cent *V/V*)	Mobile phase B (per cent *V/V*)	Comment
0 - 20	80 → 55	20 → 45	linear gradient
20 - 21	55 → 5	45 → 95	switch to next step
21 - 25	5	95	isocratic
25 - 26	5 → 80	95 → 20	switch to initial eluent composition
26 - 30	80	20	re-equilibration
30 = 0	80	20	restart gradient

- as detector a spectrophotometer set at 275 nm.

Equilibrate the column with the initial mobile phase composition for at least 5 min.

Adjust the sensitivity of the system so that the height of the principal peak in the chromatogram obtained with 10 µl of reference solution (b) is at least 50 per cent of the full scale of the recorder.

Inject 10 µl of reference solution (a). When the chromatogram is recorded in the prescribed conditions, the retention times are: cisapride about 15 min and haloperidol about 16 min. The test is not valid unless the resolution between the peaks due to cisapride and haloperidol is at least 2.5. If necessary, adjust the concentration of methanol in the mobile phase or adjust the time programme for the linear gradient.

Inject separately 10 µl of a mixture of 10 volumes of *water R* and 90 volumes of *methanol R* as a blank, 10 µl of the test solution and 10 µl of reference solution (b). In the chromatogram obtained with the test solution: the area of any peak, apart from the principal peak, is not greater than the area of the principal peak in the chromatogram obtained with reference solution (b) (0.25 per cent); the sum of the areas of all the peaks, apart from the principal peak, is not greater than twice the area of the principal peak in the chromatogram obtained with reference solution (b) (0.5 per cent). Disregard any peak due to the solvent (blank) and any peak with an area less than 0.2 times the area of the principal peak in the chromatogram obtained with reference solution (b).

Loss on drying (*2.2.32*). Not more than 0.5 per cent, determined on 1.000 g by drying in an oven at 100 °C to 105 °C.

Sulphated ash (*2.4.14*). Not more than 0.1 per cent, determined on 1.0 g in a platinum crucible.

Monographs C

ASSAY

Dissolve 0.500 g in 70 ml of *anhydrous acetic acid R* and titrate with *0.1 M perchloric acid*. Determine the end-point potentiometrically (*2.2.20*).

1 ml of *0.1 M perchloric acid* is equivalent to 61.60 mg of $C_{27}H_{35}ClFN_3O_{10}$.

STORAGE

Store protected from light.

IMPURITIES

Specified impurities: A, C.

Other detectable impurities: B, D, E.

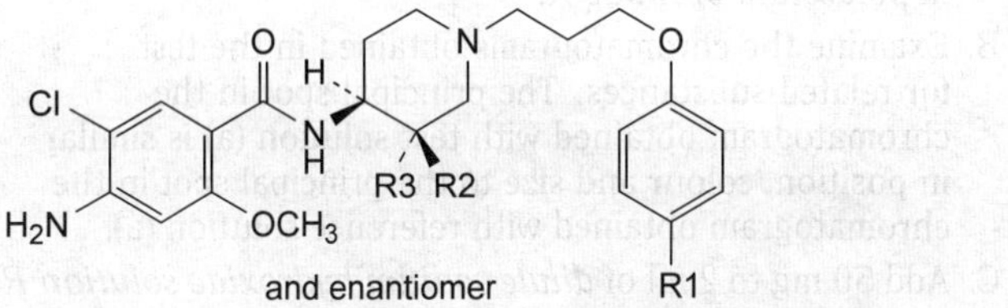

A. R1 = R3 = H, R2 = OCH_3: 4-amino-5-chloro-2-methoxy-*N*-[(3*RS*,4*SR*)-3-methoxy-1-(3-phenoxypropyl)piperidin-4-yl]benzamide,

B. R1 = F, R2 = R3 = H: 4-amino-5-chloro-*N*-[1-[3-(4-fluorophenoxy)propyl]piperidin-4-yl]-2-methoxybenzamide,

C. R1 = F, R2 = H, R3 = OCH_3: 4-amino-5-chloro-*N*-[(3*RS*,4*RS*)-1-[3-(4-fluorophenoxy)propyl]-3-methoxypiperidin-4-yl]-2-methoxybenzamide,

E. R1 = F, R2 = OH, R3 = H: 4-amino-5-chloro-*N*-[(3*RS*,4*SR*)-1-[3-(4-fluorophenoxy)propyl]-3-hydroxypiperidin-4-yl]-2-methoxybenzamide.

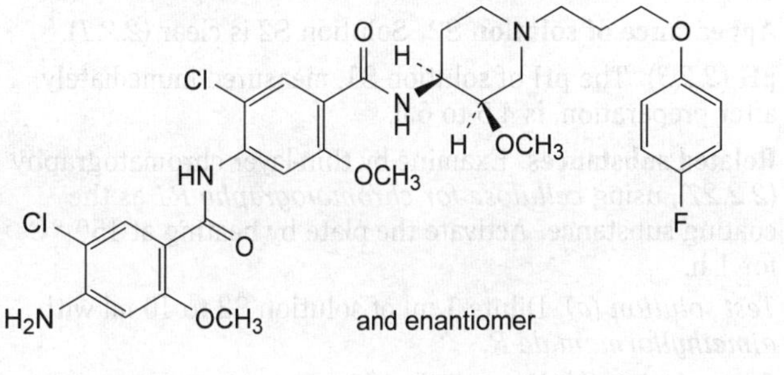

D. 4-[(4-amino-5-chloro-2-methoxybenzoyl)amino]-5-chloro-*N*-[(3*RS*,4*SR*)-1-[3-(4-fluorophenoxy)propyl]-3-methoxypiperidin-4-yl]-2-methoxybenzamide,

01/2005:0599

CISPLATIN

Cisplatinum

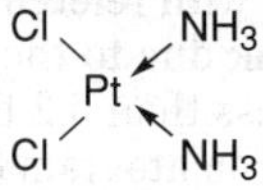

$[PtCl_2(NH_3)_2]$ M_r 300.0

DEFINITION

Cisplatin contains not less than 97.0 per cent and not more than the equivalent of 102.0 per cent of *cis*-diamminedi-chloroplatinum (II).

CHARACTERS

A yellow powder or yellow or orange-yellow crystals, slightly soluble in water, sparingly soluble in dimethylformamide, practically insoluble in alcohol.

It decomposes with blackening at about 270 °C.

Carry out identification test B, the tests (except that for silver) and the assay protected from light.

IDENTIFICATION

First identification: A, B.

Second identification: B, C.

A. Examine by infrared absorption spectrophotometry (*2.2.24*), comparing with the spectrum obtained with *cisplatin CRS*. Examine the substances prepared as discs in *potassium bromide R*.

B. Examine the chromatograms obtained in the test for related substances. The principal spot in the chromatogram obtained with test solution (a) is similar in position, colour and size to the principal spot in the chromatogram obtained with reference solution (a).

C. Add 50 mg to 2 ml of *dilute sodium hydroxide solution R* in a glass dish. Evaporate to dryness. Dissolve the residue in a mixture of 0.5 ml of *nitric acid R* and 1.5 ml of *hydrochloric acid R*. Evaporate to dryness. The residue is orange. Dissolve the residue in 0.5 ml of *water R* and add 0.5 ml of *ammonium chloride solution R*. A yellow, crystalline precipitate is formed.

TESTS

Solution S1. Dissolve 25 mg in a 9 g/l solution of *sodium chloride R* prepared with *carbon dioxide-free water R* and dilute to 25 ml with the same solvent.

Solution S2. Dissolve 0.20 g in *dimethylformamide R* and dilute to 10 ml with the same solvent.

Appearance of solution S1. Solution S1 is clear (*2.2.1*) and not more intensely coloured than reference solution GY_5 (*2.2.2, Method II*).

Appearance of solution S2. Solution S2 is clear (*2.2.1*).

pH (*2.2.3*). The pH of solution S1, measured immediately after preparation, is 4.5 to 6.0.

Related substances. Examine by thin-layer chromatography (*2.2.27*), using *cellulose for chromatography R1* as the coating substance. Activate the plate by heating at 150 °C for 1 h.

Test solution (a). Dilute 1 ml of solution S2 to 10 ml with *dimethylformamide R.*

Test solution (b). Use solution S2.

Reference solution (a). Dissolve 10 mg of *cisplatin CRS* in 5 ml of *dimethylformamide R.*

Reference solution (b). Dilute 1 ml of solution S2 to 50 ml with *dimethylformamide R.*

Apply separately to the plate 2.5 µl of test solution (a), 2.5 µl of reference solution (a), 5 µl of test solution (b) and 5 µl of reference solution (b). Develop over a path of 15 cm using a mixture of 10 volumes of *acetone R* and 90 volumes of *dimethylformamide R*. Allow the plate to dry in air and spray with a 50 g/l solution of *stannous chloride R* in a mixture of equal volumes of *dilute hydrochloric acid R* and *water R*. After 1 h, the chromatogram obtained with test solution (b) shows no spot with an R_f value less than that of the principal spot and any spot with an R_f value greater than that of the principal spot is not more intense than the spot in the chromatogram obtained with reference solution (b).

Silver. Not more than 250 ppm of Ag, determined by atomic absorption spectrometry (*2.2.23, Method I*).

Test solution. Dissolve 0.100 g of the substance to be examined in 15 ml of *nitric acid R*, heating to 80 °C. Cool and dilute to 25.0 ml with *water R*.

Reference solutions. To suitable volumes (10 ml to 30 ml) of *silver standard solution (5 ppm Ag) R* add 50 ml of *nitric acid R* and dilute to 100.0 ml with *water R*.

Measure the absorbance at 328 nm using a silver hollow-cathode lamp as source of radiation, a fuel-lean air-acetylene flame and, preferably, a spectral slit width of 0.5 nm. Carry out a blank determination.

ASSAY

Examine by liquid chromatography (*2.2.29*).

Test solution. Dissolve 50.0 mg of the substance to be examined in a 9 g/l solution of *sodium chloride R* and dilute to 100.0 ml with the same solvent.

Reference solution. Dissolve 50.0 mg of *cisplatin CRS* in a 9 g/l solution of *sodium chloride R* and dilute to 100.0 ml with the same solvent.

The chromatographic procedure may be carried out using:

- a column 0.25 m long and 4.6 mm in internal diameter packed with *strong-anion-exchange silica gel for chromatography R* (10 µm),
- as mobile phase at a flow rate of 1.2 ml/min a mixture of 10 volumes of a 9 g/l solution of *sodium chloride R* and 90 volumes of *methanol R,*
- as detector a spectrophotometer set at 220 nm.

Use a sample loop. Inject separately 20 µl of the test solution and 20 µl of the reference solution.

STORAGE

Store in an airtight container, protected from light.

01/2005:0455

CITRIC ACID, ANHYDROUS

Acidum citricum anhydricum

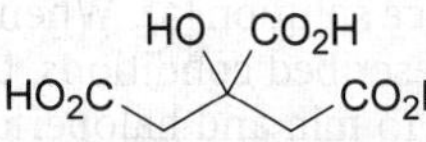

$C_6H_8O_7$ M_r 192.1

DEFINITION

Anhydrous citric acid contains not less than 99.5 per cent and not more than the equivalent of 100.5 per cent of 2-hydroxypropane-1,2,3-tricarboxylic acid, calculated with reference to the anhydrous substance.

CHARACTERS

A white, crystalline powder, colourless crystals or granules, very soluble in water, freely soluble in alcohol. It melts at about 153 °C with decomposition.

IDENTIFICATION

First identification: B, E.

Second identification: A, C, D, E.

A. Dissolve 1 g in 10 ml of *water R*. The solution is strongly acidic (*2.2.4*).

B. Examine by infrared absorption spectrophotometry (*2.2.24*), comparing with the spectrum obtained with *anhydrous citric acid CRS* after drying both the substance to be examined and the reference substance at 100-105 °C for 2 h.

C. Add about 5 mg to a mixture of 1 ml of *acetic anhydride R* and 3 ml of *pyridine R*. A red colour develops.

D. Dissolve 0.5 g in 5 ml of *water R*, neutralise using *1 M sodium hydroxide* (about 7 ml), add 10 ml of *calcium chloride solution R* and heat to boiling. A white precipitate is formed.

E. It complies with the test for water (see Tests).

TESTS

Appearance of solution. Dissolve 2.0 g in *water R* and dilute to 10 ml with the same solvent. The solution is clear (*2.2.1*) and not more intensely coloured than reference solution Y_7, BY_7 or GY_7 (*2.2.2, Method II*).

Readily carbonisable substances. To 1.0 g in a cleaned test tube add 10 ml of *sulphuric acid R* and immediately heat the mixture in a water-bath at 90 ± 1 °C for 60 min. Immediately cool rapidly. The solution is not more intensely coloured than a mixture of 1 ml of red primary solution and 9 ml of yellow primary solution (*2.2.2, Method I*).

Oxalic acid. Dissolve 0.80 g in 4 ml of *water R*. Add 3 ml of *hydrochloric acid R* and 1 g of *zinc R* in granules. Boil for 1 min. Allow to stand for 2 min. Transfer the supernatant liquid to a test-tube containing 0.25 ml of a 10 g/l solution of *phenylhydrazine hydrochloride R* and heat to boiling. Cool rapidly, transfer to a graduated cylinder and add an equal volume of *hydrochloric acid R* and 0.25 ml of a 50 g/l solution of *potassium ferricyanide R*. Shake and allow to stand for 30 min. Any pink colour in the solution is not more intense than that in a standard prepared at the same time in the same manner using 4 ml of a 0.1 g/l solution of *oxalic acid R* (360 ppm, calculated as anhydrous oxalic acid).

Sulphates (*2.4.13*). Dissolve 2.0 g in *distilled water R* and dilute to 30 ml with the same solvent. The solution complies with the limit test for sulphates (150 ppm).

Aluminium (*2.4.17*). If intended for use in the manufacture of dialysis solutions, it complies with the test for aluminium. Dissolve 20 g in 100 ml of *water R* and add 10 ml of *acetate buffer solution pH 6.0 R*. The solution complies with the limit test for aluminium (0.2 ppm). Use as the reference solution a mixture of 2 ml of *aluminium standard solution (2 ppm Al) R*, 10 ml of *acetate buffer solution pH 6.0 R* and 98 ml of *water R*. To prepare the blank use a mixture of 10 ml of *acetate buffer solution pH 6.0 R* and 100 ml of *water R*.

Heavy metals (*2.4.8*). Dissolve 5.0 g in several portions in 39 ml of *dilute sodium hydroxide solution R* and dilute to 50 ml with *distilled water R*. 12 ml complies with limit test A for heavy metals (10 ppm). Prepare the standard using *lead standard solution (1 ppm Pb) R*.

Water (*2.5.12*). Not more than 1.0 per cent, determined on 2.000 g by the semi-micro determination of water.

Sulphated ash (*2.4.14*). Not more than 0.1 per cent, determined on 1.0 g.

Bacterial endotoxins (*2.6.14*): less than 0.5 IU/mg, if intended for use in the manufacture of parenteral dosage forms without a further appropriate procedure for the removal of bacterial endotoxins.

ASSAY

Dissolve 0.550 g in 50 ml of *water R*. Titrate with *1 M sodium hydroxide*, using 0.5 ml of *phenolphthalein solution R* as indicator.

1 ml of *1 M sodium hydroxide* is equivalent to 64.03 mg of $C_6H_8O_7$.

LABELLING

The label states:

– where applicable, that the substance is free from bacterial endotoxins,

– where applicable, that the substance is intended for use in the manufacture of dialysis solutions.

01/2005:0456

CITRIC ACID MONOHYDRATE

Acidum citricum monohydricum

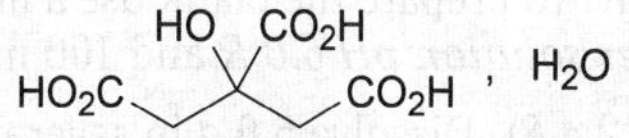

$C_6H_8O_7,H_2O$ M_r 210.1

DEFINITION

Citric acid monohydrate contains not less than 99.5 per cent and not more than the equivalent of 100.5 per cent of 2-hydroxypropane-1,2,3-tricarboxylic acid, calculated with reference to the anhydrous substance.

CHARACTERS

A white, crystalline powder, colourless crystals or granules, efflorescent, very soluble in water, freely soluble in alcohol.

IDENTIFICATION

First identification: B, E.

Second identification: A, C, D, E.

A. Dissolve 1 g in 10 ml of *water R*. The solution is strongly acidic (*2.2.4*).

B. Examine by infrared absorption spectrophotometry (*2.2.24*), comparing with the spectrum obtained with *citric acid monohydrate CRS* after drying both the substance to be examined and the reference substance at 100-105 °C for 2 h.

C. Add about 5 mg to a mixture of 1 ml of *acetic anhydride R* and 3 ml of *pyridine R*. A red colour develops.

D. Dissolve 0.5 g in 5 ml of *water R*, neutralise using *1 M sodium hydroxide* (about 7 ml), add 10 ml of *calcium chloride solution R* and heat to boiling. A white precipitate is formed.

E. It complies with the test for water (see Tests).

TESTS

Appearance of solution. Dissolve 2.0 g in *water R* and dilute to 10 ml with the same solvent. The solution is clear (*2.2.1*) and not more intensely coloured than reference solution Y_7, BY_7 or GY_7 (*2.2.2, Method II*).

Readily carbonisable substances. To 1.0 g in a cleaned test tube add 10 ml of *sulphuric acid R* and immediately heat the mixture in a water-bath at 90 ± 1 °C for 60 min. Immediately cool rapidly. The solution is not more intensely coloured than a mixture of 1 ml of red primary solution and 9 ml of yellow primary solution (*2.2.2, Method I*).

Oxalic acid. Dissolve 0.80 g in 4 ml of *water R*. Add 3 ml of *hydrochloric acid R* and 1 g of *zinc R* in granules. Boil for 1 min. Allow to stand for 2 min. Transfer the supernatant liquid to a test-tube containing 0.25 ml of a 10 g/l solution of *phenylhydrazine hydrochloride R* and heat to boiling. Cool rapidly, transfer to a graduated cylinder and add an equal volume of *hydrochloric acid R* and 0.25 ml of a 50 g/l solution of *potassium ferricyanide R*. Shake and allow to stand for 30 min. Any pink colour in the solution is not more intense than that in a standard prepared at the same time in the same manner using 4 ml of a 0.1 g/l solution of *oxalic acid R* (360 ppm, calculated as anhydrous oxalic acid).

Sulphates (*2.4.13*). Dissolve 2.0 g in *distilled water R* and dilute to 30 ml with the same solvent. The solution complies with the limit test for sulphates (150 ppm).

Aluminium (*2.4.17*). If intended for use in the manufacture of dialysis solutions, it complies with the test for aluminium. Dissolve 20 g in 100 ml of *water R* and add 10 ml of *acetate buffer solution pH 6.0 R*. The solution complies with the limit test for aluminium (0.2 ppm). Use as the reference solution a mixture of 2 ml of *aluminium standard solution (2 ppm Al) R*, 10 ml of *acetate buffer solution pH 6.0 R* and 98 ml of *water R*. To prepare the blank use a mixture of 10 ml of *acetate buffer solution pH 6.0 R* and 100 ml of *water R*.

Heavy metals (*2.4.8*). Dissolve 5.0 g in several portions in 39 ml of *dilute sodium hydroxide solution R* and dilute to 50 ml with *distilled water R*. 12 ml complies with limit test A for heavy metals (10 ppm). Prepare the standard using *lead standard solution (1 ppm Pb) R*.

Water (*2.5.12*): 7.5 per cent to 9.0 per cent, determined on 0.500 g by the semi-micro determination of water.

Sulphated ash (*2.4.14*). Not more than 0.1 per cent, determined on 1.0 g.

Bacterial endotoxins (*2.6.14*): less than 0.5 IU/mg, if intended for use in the manufacture of parenteral dosage forms without a further appropriate procedure for the removal of bacterial endotoxins.

ASSAY

Dissolve 0.550 g in 50 ml of *water R*. Titrate with *1 M sodium hydroxide*, using 0.5 ml of *phenolphthalein solution R* as indicator.

1 ml of *1 M sodium hydroxide* is equivalent to 64.03 mg of $C_6H_8O_7$.

STORAGE

In an airtight container.

LABELLING

The label states:

- where applicable, that the substance is free from bacterial endotoxins,
- where applicable, that the substance is intended for use in the manufacture of dialysis solutions.

01/2005:1609

CITRONELLA OIL

Citronellae aetheroleum

DEFINITION

Oil obtained by steam distillation from the fresh or partially dried aerial parts of *Cymbopogon winterianus* Jowitt.

CHARACTERS

Pale yellow to brown-yellow liquid, with a very strong odour of citronellal.

IDENTIFICATION

First identification: B.

Second identification: A.

A. Thin-layer chromatography (*2.2.27*).

Test solution. Dilute 0.1 g of citronella oil in 10.0 ml of *alcohol R*.

Reference solution. Dilute 20 µl of *citronellal R* in 10.0 ml of *alcohol R*.

Plate: *TLC silica gel plate R*.

Mobile phase: *ethyl acetate R, toluene R* (10:90 *V/V*).

Application: 5 µl, as bands.

Development: over a path of 15 cm.

Drying: in air.

Detection: spray with *anisaldehyde solution R* and heat at 100-105 °C for 10 min. Examine in ultraviolet light at 365 nm.

Result: see below the sequence of the zones present in the chromatograms obtained with the reference and test solutions. Furthermore, other zones are present in the chromatogram obtained with the test solution.

Top of the plate	
Citronellal: a violet zone	A zone similar in colour to the citronellal zone An orange zone (citronellol-geraniol)
Reference solution	**Test solution**

B. Examine the chromatograms obtained in the test for chromatographic profile.

Results: the characteristic peaks in the chromatogram obtained with the test solution are similar in retention time to those in the chromatogram obtained with the reference solution. Neral and geranial may be absent in the chromatogram obtained with the test solution.

TESTS

Relative density (*2.2.5*): 0.881 to 0.895.

Refractive index (*2.2.6*): 1.463 to 1.475.

Optical rotation (*2.2.7*): −4° to + 1.5°.

Chromatographic profile. Gas chromatography (*2.2.28*): use the normalisation procedure.

Test solution. The substance to be examined.

Reference solution. Dilute 25 µl of *limonene R*, 100 µl of *citronellal R*, 25 µl of *citronellyl acetate R*, 25 µl of *citral R*, 25 µl of *geranyl acetate R*, 25 µl of *citronellol R* and 100 µl of *geraniol R* in 5 ml of *hexane R*.

Column:

- *material*: fused silica,
- *size*: *l* = 60 m, Ø = 0.25 mm,
- *stationary phase*: *macrogol 20 000 R* (0.2 µm).

Carrier gas: *helium for chromatography R*.
Flow rate: 1.0 ml/min.
Split ratio: 1:100.
Temperature:

	Time (min)	Temperature (°C)
Column	0 - 2	80
	2 - 26	80 → 150
	26 - 42	150 → 185
	42 - 49	185 → 250
Injection port		260
Detector		260

Detection: flame ionisation.
Injection: 1 μl of the reference solution, 0.2 μl of the test solution.
Elution order: the order indicated in the composition of the reference solution. Record the retention times of these substances.
System suitability: reference solution:
- *resolution*: minimum of 1.2 between the peaks due to geranyl acetate and citronellol.

Using the retention times determined from the chromatogram obtained with the reference solution, locate the components of the reference solution in the chromatogram obtained with the test solution.
Determine the percentage content of each of these components.
The percentages are within the following values:
- *limonene*: 1.0 per cent to 5.0 per cent,
- *citronellal*: 30.0 per cent to 45.0 per cent,
- *citronellyl acetate*: 2.0 per cent to 4.0 per cent,
- *neral*: less than 2.0 per cent,
- *geranial*: less than 2.0 per cent,
- *geranyl acetate*: 3.0 per cent to 8.0 per cent,
- *citronellol*: 9.0 per cent to 15.0 per cent,
- *geraniol*: 20.0 per cent to 25.0 per cent.

STORAGE
In a well-filled container, protected from light.

01/2005:1651 corrected

CLARITHROMYCIN

Clarithromycinum

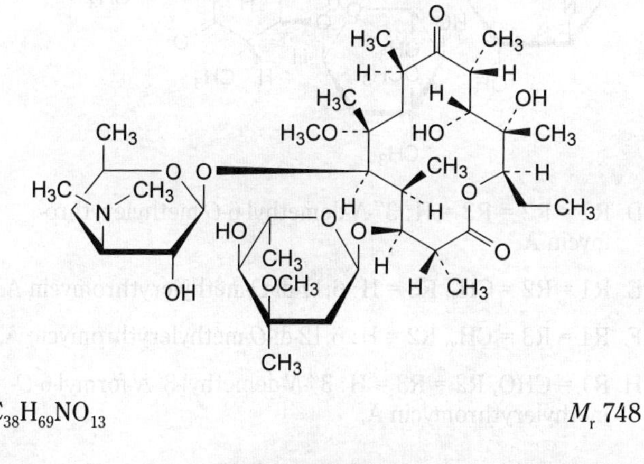

$C_{38}H_{69}NO_{13}$ M_r 748

DEFINITION
(3*R*,4*S*,5*S*,6*R*,7*R*,9*R*,11*R*,12*R*,13*S*,14*R*)-4-[(2,6-Dideoxy-3-*C*-methyl-3-*O*-methyl-α-L-*ribo*-hexopyranosyl)oxy]-14-ethyl-12,13-dihydroxy-7-methoxy-3,5,7,9,11,13-hexamethyl-6-[[3,4,6-trideoxy-3-(dimethylamino)-β-D-*xylo*-hexopyranosyl]oxy]oxacyclotetradecane-2,10-dione (6-*O*-methylerythromycin A).
Content: 96.0 per cent to 102.0 per cent (anhydrous substance).

CHARACTERS
Appearance: white or almost white, crystalline powder.
Solubility: practically insoluble in water, soluble in acetone and in methylene chloride, slightly soluble in methanol.

Monographs C

IDENTIFICATION
Infrared absorption spectrophotometry (*2.2.24*).
Comparison: *clarithromycin CRS*.

TESTS
Solution S. Dissolve 0.500 g in *methylene chloride R* and dilute to 50.0 ml with the same solvent.
Appearance of solution. Solution S is clear or not more opalescent than reference suspension II (*2.2.1*) and not more intensely coloured than reference solution Y_7 (*2.2.2, Method II*).
Specific optical rotation (*2.2.7*): − 94 to − 102 (anhydrous substance), determined on solution S.
Related substances. Liquid chromatography (*2.2.29*).
Test solution. Dissolve 75.0 mg of the substance to be examined in 25 ml of *acetonitrile R1* and dilute to 50.0 ml with *water R*.
Reference solution (a). Dissolve 75.0 mg of *clarithromycin CRS* in 25 ml of *acetonitrile R1* and dilute to 50.0 ml with *water R*.
Reference solution (b). Dilute 5.0 ml of reference solution (a) to 100.0 ml with a mixture of equal volumes of *acetonitrile R1* and *water R*.
Reference solution (c). Dilute 1.0 ml of reference solution (b) to 10.0 ml with a mixture of equal volumes of *acetonitrile R1* and *water R*.
Reference solution (d). Dissolve 15.0 mg of *clarithromycin for peak identification CRS* in 5.0 ml of *acetonitrile R1* and dilute to 10.0 ml with *water R*.
Blank solution. Dilute 25.0 ml of *acetonitrile R1* to 50.0 ml with *water R* and mix.
Column:
- *size*: *l* = 0.10 m, Ø = 4.6 mm,
- *stationary phase*: *octadecylsilyl silica gel for chromatography R* (3.5 μm),
- *temperature*: 40 °C.

Mobile phase:
- *mobile phase A*: a 4.76 g/l solution of *potassium dihydrogen phosphate R* adjusted to pH 4.4 with *dilute phosphoric acid R* or a 45 g/l solution of *potassium hydroxide R*, filtered through a C18 filtration kit,
- *mobile phase B*: *acetonitrile R1*,

Time (min)	Mobile phase A (per cent *V/V*)	Mobile phase B (per cent *V/V*)
0 - 32	75 → 40	25 → 60
32 - 34	40	60
34 - 36	40 → 75	60 → 25
36 - 42	75	25

Flow rate: 1.1 ml/min.

Detection: spectrophotometer at 205 nm.

Injection: 10 μl; inject the blank solution, the test solution and reference solutions (b), (c) and (d).

Relative retention with reference to clarithromycin (retention time = about 11 min): impurity I = about 0.38; impurity A = about 0.42; impurity J = about 0.63; impurity L = about 0.74; impurity B = about 0.79; impurity M = about 0.81; impurity C = about 0.89; impurity D = about 0.96; impurity N = about 1.15; impurity E = about 1.27; impurity O = about 1.31; impurity F = about 1.33; impurity P = about 1.35; impurity K = about 1.59; impurity G = about 1.72; impurity H = about 1.82.

System suitability:

- *symmetry factor*: maximum 1.7 for the peak due to clarithromycin in the chromatogram obtained with reference solution (b),
- *peak-to-valley ratio*: minimum 3.0, where H_p = height above the baseline of the peak due to impurity D and H_v = height above the baseline of the lowest point of the curve separating this peak from the peak due to clarithromycin in the chromatogram obtained with reference solution (d).

Limits:

- *correction factors*: for the calculation of contents, multiply the peak areas of the following impurities by the corresponding correction factor: impurity G = 0.27; impurity H = 0.15; use the chromatogram supplied with *clarithromycin for peak identification CRS* to identify the peaks;
- *any impurity*: not more than twice the area of the principal peak in the chromatogram obtained with reference solution (c) (1.0 per cent), and not more than 4 such peaks have an area greater than 0.8 times the area of the principal peak in the chromatogram obtained with reference solution (c) (0.4 per cent);
- *total*: not more than 7 times the area of the principal peak in the chromatogram obtained with reference solution (c) (3.5 per cent);
- *disregard limit*: 0.2 times the area of the principal peak in the chromatogram obtained with reference solution (c) (0.1 per cent); disregard the peaks eluting before impurity I and after impurity H.

Heavy metals (*2.4.8*): maximum 20 ppm.

Dissolve 1.0 g in a mixture of 15 volumes of *water R* and 85 volumes of *dioxan R* and dilute to 20 ml with the same mixture of solvents. 12 ml of the solution complies with limit test B. Prepare the standard using lead standard solution (1 ppm Pb) obtained by diluting *lead standard solution (100 ppm Pb) R* with a mixture of 15 volumes of *water R* and 85 volumes of *dioxan R*.

Water (*2.5.12*): maximum 2.0 per cent, determined on 0.500 g.

Sulphated ash (*2.4.14*): maximum 0.2 per cent, determined on 0.5 g.

ASSAY

Liquid chromatography (*2.2.29*) as described in the test for related substances with the following modifications.

Injection: test solution and reference solution (a).

Calculate the percentage content of $C_{38}H_{69}NO_{13}$.

IMPURITIES

Specified impurities: A, B, C, D, E, F, G, H, I, J, K, L, M, N, O, P.

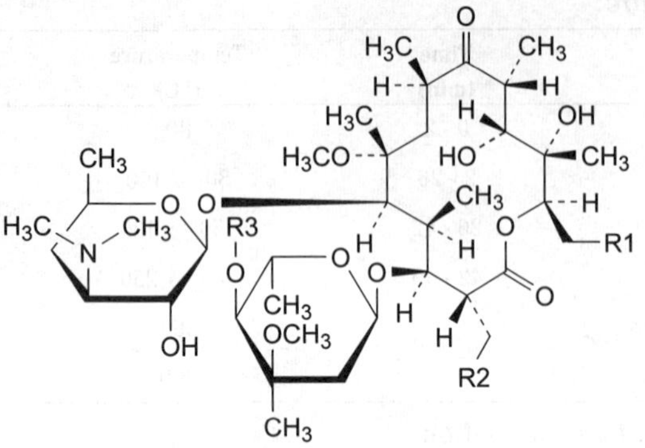

A. R1 = CH_3, R2 = OH, R3 = H: 2-demethyl-2-(hydroxymethyl)-6-*O*-methylerythromycin A (clarithromycin F),

B. R1 = R2 = R3 = H: 6-*O*-methyl-15-norerythromycin A,

P. R1 = R3 = CH_3, R2 = H: 4′,6-di-*O*-methylerythromycin A,

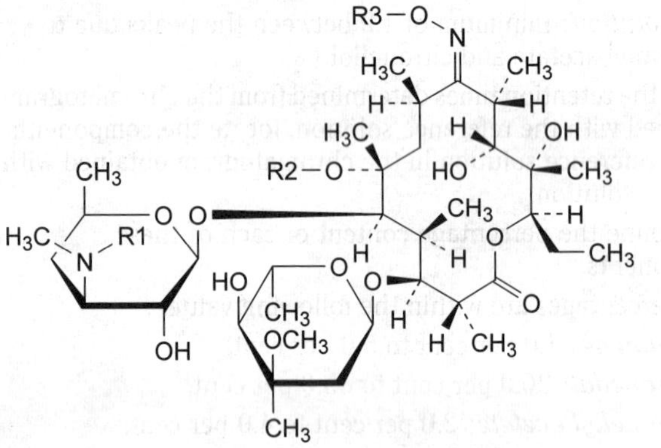

C. R1 = R2 = CH_3, R3 = H: 6-*O*-methylerythromycin A (*E*)-9-oxime,

G. R1 = R2 = R3 = CH_3: 6-*O*-methylerythromycin A (*E*)-9-(*O*-methyloxime),

J. R1 = CH_3, R2 = R3 = H: erythromycin A (*E*)-9-oxime,

M. R1 = R3 = H, R2 = CH_3: 3″-*N*-demethyl-6-*O*-methylerythromycin A (*E*)-9-oxime,

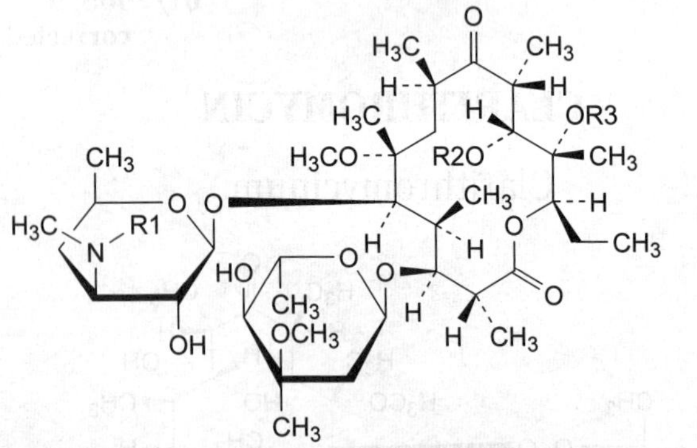

D. R1 = R2 = R3 = H: 3″-*N*-demethyl-6-*O*-methylerythromycin A,

E. R1 = R2 = CH_3, R3 = H: 6,11-di-*O*-methylerythromycin A,

F. R1 = R3 = CH_3, R2 = H: 6,12-di-*O*-methylerythromycin A,

H. R1 = CHO, R2 = R3 = H: 3″-*N*-demethyl-3′-*N*-formyl-6-*O*-methylerythromycin A,

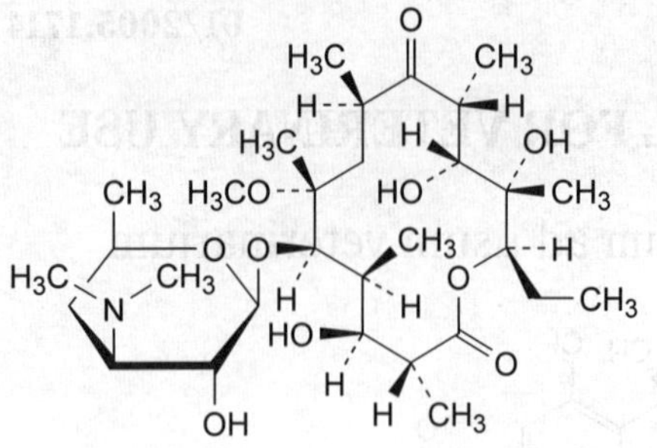

I. 3-*O*-decladinosyl-6-*O*-methylerythromycin A,

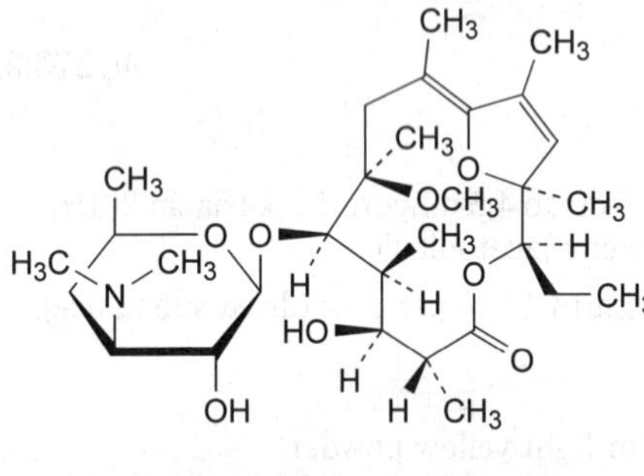

K. (1*S*,2*R*,5*R*,6*S*,7*S*,8*R*,9*R*,11*Z*)-2-ethyl-6-hydroxy-9-methoxy-1,5,7,9,11,13-hexamethyl-8-[[3,4,6-trideoxy-3-(dimethylamino)-β-D-*xylo*-hexopyranosyl]oxy]-3,15-dioxabicyclo[10.2.1]pentadeca-11,13-dien-4-one (3-*O*-decladinosyl-8,9:10,11-dianhydro-6-*O*-methylerythromycin A-9,12-hemiketal,

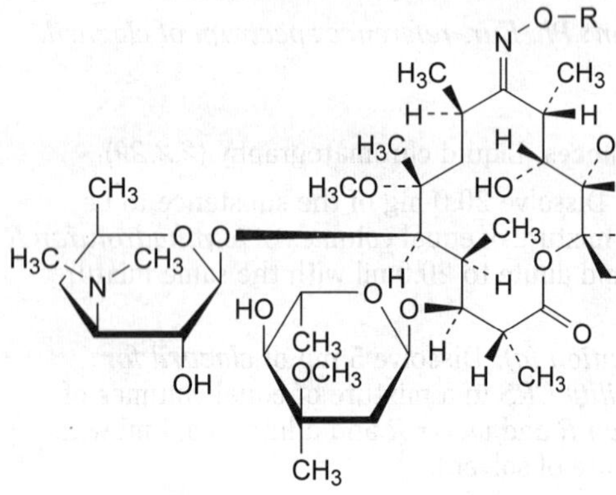

L. R = H: 6-*O*-methylerythromycin A (*Z*)-9-oxime,

O. R = CH_3: 6-*O*-methylerythromycin A (*Z*)-9-(*O*-methyloxime),

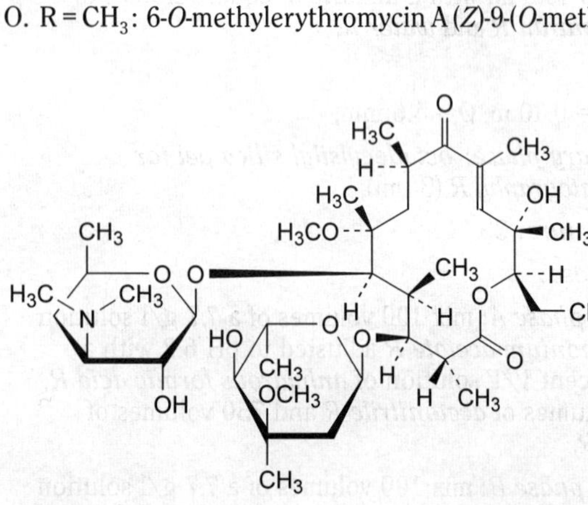

N. (10*E*)-10,11-didehydro-11-deoxy-6-*O*-methylerythromycin A.

01/2005:1850

CLARY SAGE OIL

Salviae sclareae aetheroleum

DEFINITION

Essential oil obtained by steam distillation from the fresh or dried flowering stems of *Salvia sclarea* L.

CHARACTERS

Appearance: colourless to brownish-yellow liquid, usually pale yellow, with a characteristic odour.

IDENTIFICATION

First identification: B.

Second identification: A.

A. Thin-layer chromatography (*2.2.27*).

Test solution. Dissolve 1 ml of the substance to be examined in *toluene R* and dilute to 10 ml with the same solvent.

Reference solution. Dissolve 60 µl of *linalol R*, 200 µl of *linalyl acetate R* and 60 µl of *α-terpineol R* in *toluene R* and dilute to 10 ml with the same solvent.

Plate: *TLC silica gel plate R.*

Mobile phase: *ethyl acetate R, toluene R* (5:95 *V/V*).

Application: 5 µl of the test solution and 10 µl of the reference solution, as bands.

Development: over a path of 15 cm.

Drying: in air.

Detection: spray with *vanillin reagent R* and heat at 100-105 °C for 5-10 min; examine in daylight within 5 min.

Results: see below the sequence of the zones present in the chromatograms obtained with the reference solution and the test solution. Furthermore, other faint zones are present in the chromatogram obtained with the test solution.

Top of the plate	
α-Terpineol: a dark violet zone	A dark violet zone
–––––	–––––
Linalyl acetate: a dark violet zone	A dark violet zone
–––––	–––––
Linalol: a dark violet zone	A dark violet zone
Reference solution	**Test solution**

B. Examine the chromatograms obtained in the test for chromatographic profile.

Results: the chromatogram obtained with the test solution shows 5 peaks similar in position to the 5 peaks in the chromatogram obtained with the reference solution. The 2 peaks corresponding to α- and β-thujone may be absent.

TESTS

Relative density (*2.2.5*): 0.890 to 0.908.

Refractive index (*2.2.6*): 1.456 to 1.466.

Optical rotation (*2.2.7*): − 26° to − 10°.

Acid value (*2.5.1*): maximum 1.0.

Chromatographic profile. Gas chromatography (*2.2.28*): use the normalisation procedure.

Test solution. The substance to be examined.

Reference solution. To 1 g of *hexane R,* add 5 µl of *thujone R,* 5 µl of *linalol R,* 100 µl of *linalyl acetate R,* 10 µl of *α-terpineol R* and 25 mg (± 20 per cent) of *sclareol R.* Mix thoroughly by stirring.

Column:

- *material*: fused silica,
- *size*: *l* = 30 m (a film thickness of 1 µm may be used) to 60 m (a film thickness of 0.2 µm may be used), Ø = 0.25-0.53 mm,
- *stationary phase*: *macrogol 20 000 R.*

Carrier gas: *helium for chromatography R.*

Split ratio: 1:100.

Temperature:

	Time (min)	Temperature (°C)
Column	0 - 10	60
	10 - 75	60 → 190
	75 - 120	190
Injection port		220
Detector		240

Detection: flame ionisation.

Injection: 0.2 µl.

Elution order: order indicated in the composition of the reference solution. Record the retention times of these substances.

System suitability: reference solution:

- *resolution*: minimum 1.5 between the peaks due to linalol and linalyl acetate,

Using the retention times determined from the chromatogram obtained with the reference solution, locate the components of the reference solution in the chromatogram obtained with the test solution (disregard any peak due to hexane). *Thujone R* is a mixture of α- and β-thujone. α-Thujone elutes before β-thujone under the described conditions.

Determine the percentage content of each of these components.

Also determine the percentage content of germacrene-D. The germacrene-D peak can be identified in the chromatogram obtained with the test solution by its relative retention of 1.23 with reference to linalol under the described operating conditions.

The percentages are within the following ranges:

- *α- and β-thujone*: less than 0.2 per cent,
- *linalol*: 6.5 per cent to 24 per cent,
- *linalyl acetate*: 56 per cent to 78 per cent,
- *α-terpineol*: less than 5.0 per cent,
- *germacrene-D*: 1.0 per cent to 12 per cent,
- *sclareol*: 0.4 per cent to 2.6 per cent.

STORAGE

In an airtight container, protected from light, at a temperature not exceeding 25 °C.

01/2005:1714

CLAZURIL FOR VETERINARY USE

Clazurilum ad usum veterinarium

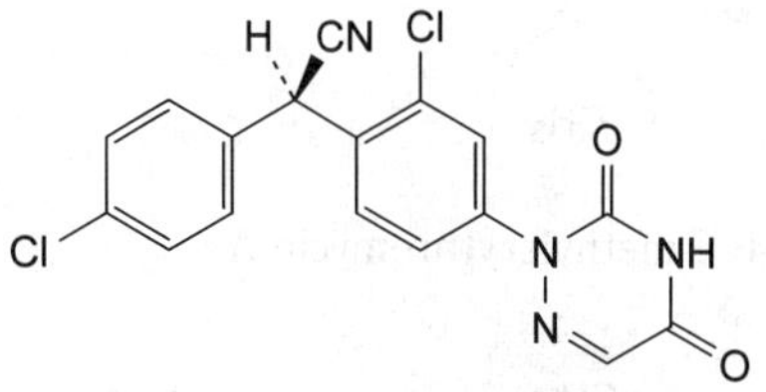

$C_{17}H_{10}Cl_2N_4O_2$ M_r 373.2

DEFINITION

(2*RS*)-[2-Chloro-4-(3,5-dioxo-4,5-dihydro-1,2,4-triazin-2(3*H*)-yl)phenyl](4-chlorophenyl)acetonitrile.

Content: 99.0 per cent to 101.0 per cent (dried substance).

CHARACTERS

Appearance: white or light yellow powder.

Solubility: practically insoluble in water, freely soluble in dimethylformamide, slightly soluble in alcohol and in methylene chloride.

IDENTIFICATION

A. Melting point (*2.2.14*): 199 °C to 203 °C.

B. Infrared absorption spectrophotometry (*2.2.24*).

Comparison: *Ph. Eur. reference spectrum of clazuril.*

TESTS

Related substances. Liquid chromatography (*2.2.29*).

Test solution. Dissolve 20.0 mg of the substance to be examined in a mixture of equal volumes of *tetrahydrofuran R* and *water R* and dilute to 20.0 ml with the same mixture of solvents.

Reference solution (a). Dissolve 5 mg of *clazuril for system suitability CRS* in a mixture of equal volumes of *tetrahydrofuran R* and *water R* and dilute to 5.0 ml with the same mixture of solvents.

Reference solution (b). Dilute 1.0 ml of the test solution to 100.0 ml with a mixture of equal volumes of *tetrahydrofuran R* and *water R.* Dilute 2.0 ml of this solution to 10.0 ml with a mixture of equal volumes of *tetrahydrofuran R* and *water R.*

Column:

- *size*: *l* = 0.10 m, Ø = 4.6 mm,
- *stationary phase*: *octadecylsilyl silica gel for chromatography R* (3 µm),
- *temperature*: 35 °C.

Mobile phase:

- *mobile phase A*: mix 100 volumes of a 7.7 g/l solution of *ammonium acetate R* adjusted to pH 6.2 with a 10 per cent *V/V* solution of *anhydrous formic acid R,* 150 volumes of *acetonitrile R* and 750 volumes of *water R,*
- *mobile phase B*: mix 100 volumes of a 7.7 g/l solution of *ammonium acetate R* adjusted to pH 6.2 with a 10 per cent *V/V* solution of *anhydrous formic acid R,* 850 volumes of *acetonitrile R* and 50 volumes of *water R,*

Time (min)	Mobile phase A (per cent V/V)	Mobile phase B (per cent V/V)
0 - 20	100 → 0	0 → 100
20 - 25	0	100
25 - 30	0 → 100	100 → 0
30 - 40	100	0

Flow rate: 1.0 ml/min.

Detection: spectrophotometer at 230 nm.

Injection: 5 μl.

System suitability: reference solution (a):

- *peak-to-valley ratio*: minimum 1.5, where H_p = height above the baseline of the peak due to impurity G and H_v = height above the baseline of the lowest point of the curve separating this peak from the peak due to clazuril,
- the chromatogram obtained is concordant with the chromatogram supplied with *clazuril for system suitability CRS*.

Limits:

- *correction factors*: for the calculation of contents, multiply the peak areas of the following impurities by the corresponding correction factor: impurity G = 1.4; impurity H = 0.8;
- *any impurity*: not more than the area of the principal peak in the chromatogram obtained with reference solution (b) (0.2 per cent);
- *total*: not more than 3 times the area of the principal peak in the chromatogram obtained with reference solution (b) (0.6 per cent);
- *disregard limit*: 0.25 times the area of the principal peak in the chromatogram obtained with reference solution (b) (0.05 per cent); disregard the peaks due to the solvents.

Loss on drying (*2.2.32*): maximum 0.5 per cent, determined on 1.000 g by drying in an oven at 100-105 °C for 4 h.

Sulphated ash (*2.4.14*): maximum 0.1 per cent, determined on 1.0 g.

ASSAY

Dissolve about 0.260 g in 35 ml of *tetrahydrofuran R* and add 35 ml of *water R*. Titrate with *0.1 M sodium hydroxide*, determining the end-point potentiometrically (*2.2.20*). Carry out a blank titration.

1 ml of *0.1 M sodium hydroxide* is equivalent to 37.32 mg of $C_{17}H_{10}Cl_2N_4O_2$.

STORAGE

Protected from light.

IMPURITIES

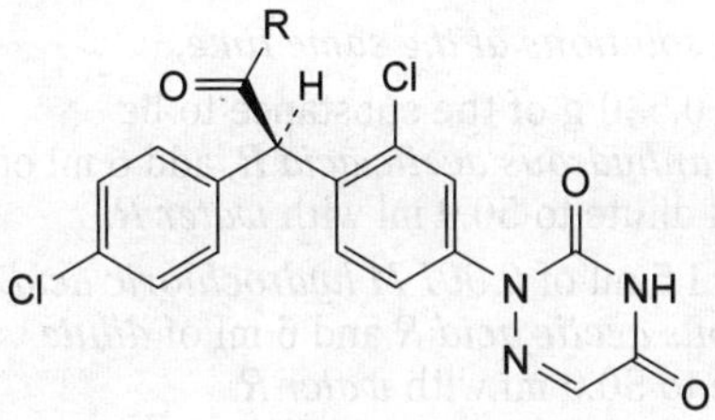

and enantiomer

A. R = OH: (2*RS*)-[2-chloro-4-(3,5-dioxo-4,5-dihydro-1,2,4-triazin-2(3*H*)-yl)phenyl](4-chlorophenyl)acetic acid,

C. R = NH_2: (2*RS*)-2-[2-chloro-4-(3,5-dioxo-4,5-dihydro-1,2,4-triazin-2(3*H*)-yl)phenyl]-2-(4-chlorophenyl)acetamide,

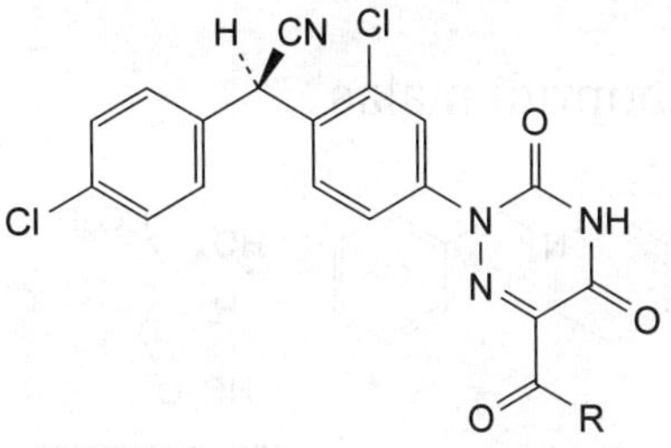

and enantiomer

B. R = NH_2: 2-[3-chloro-4-[(*RS*)-(4-chlorophenyl)cyanomethyl]phenyl]-3,5-dioxo-2,3,4,5-tetrahydro-1,2,4-triazine-6-carboxamide,

D. R = $N(CH_3)_2$: 2-[3-chloro-4-[(*RS*)-(4-chlorophenyl)cyanomethyl]phenyl]-*N*,*N*-dimethyl-3,5-dioxo-2,3,4,5-tetrahydro-1,2,4-triazine-6-carboxamide,

E. R = OCH_3: methyl 2-[3-chloro-4-[(*RS*)-(4-chlorophenyl)cyanomethyl]phenyl]-3,5-dioxo-2,3,4,5-tetrahydro-1,2,4-triazine-6-carboxylate,

F. R = OC_2H_5: ethyl 2-[3-chloro-4-[(*RS*)-(4-chlorophenyl)cyanomethyl]phenyl]-3,5-dioxo-2,3,4,5-tetrahydro-1,2,4-triazine-6-carboxylate,

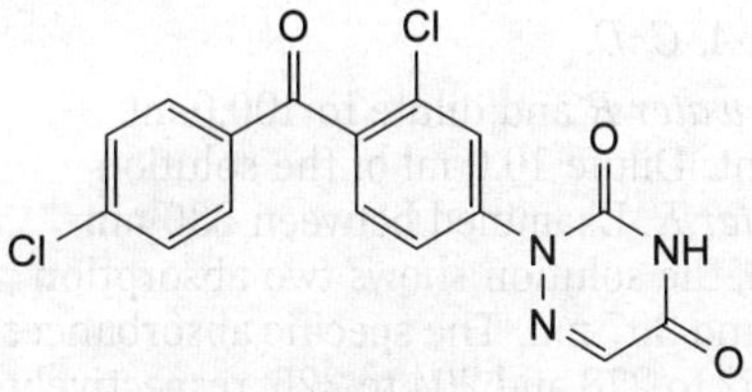

G. 2-[3-chloro-4-(4-chlorobenzoyl)phenyl]-1,2,4-triazine-3,5(2*H*,4*H*)-dione,

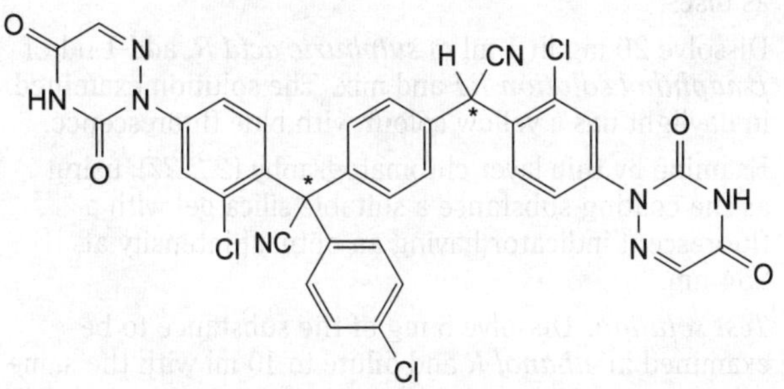

H. [2-chloro-4-(3,5-dioxo-4,5-dihydro-1,2,4-triazin-2(3*H*)-yl)phenyl][4-[[2-chloro-4-(3,5-dioxo-4,5-dihydro-1,2,4-triazin-2(3*H*)-yl)phenyl]cyanomethyl]phenyl](4-chlorophenyl)acetonitrile,

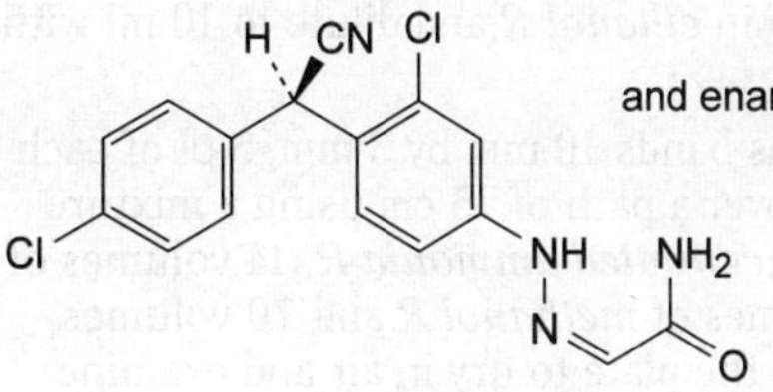

and enantiomer

I. (*Z*)-2-[[3-chloro-4-[(*RS*)-(4-chlorophenyl)cyanomethyl]phenyl]diazanylidene]acetamide.

01/2005:1303

CLEBOPRIDE MALATE

Clebopridi malas

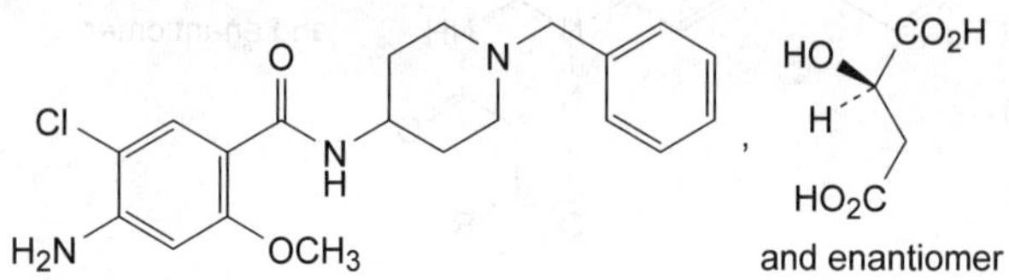

$C_{24}H_{30}ClN_3O_7$ M_r 508.0

DEFINITION

Clebopride malate contains not less than 98.5 per cent and not more than the equivalent of 101.0 per cent of 4-amino-*N*-(1-benzylpiperidin-4-yl)-5-chloro-2-methoxybenzamide acid (*RS*)-2-hydroxybutanedioate, calculated with reference to the dried substance.

CHARACTERS

A white or almost white, crystalline powder, sparingly soluble in water and in methanol, slightly soluble in ethanol, practically insoluble in methylene chloride.

It melts at about 164 °C, with decomposition.

IDENTIFICATION

First identification: B, C.

Second identification: A, C, D.

A. Dissolve 20.0 mg in *water R* and dilute to 100.0 ml with the same solvent. Dilute 10.0 ml of the solution to 100.0 ml with *water R*. Examined between 230 nm and 350 nm (*2.2.25*), the solution shows two absorption maxima, at 270 nm and 307 nm. The specific absorbances at the maxima are 252 to 278 and 204 to 226, respectively.

B. Examine by infrared absorption spectrophotometry (*2.2.24*), comparing with the spectrum obtained with *clebopride malate CRS*. Examine the substances prepared as discs.

C. Dissolve 20 mg in 1 ml of *sulphuric acid R*, add 1 ml of *β-naphthol solution R1* and mix. The solution examined in daylight has a yellow colour with blue fluorescence.

D. Examine by thin-layer chromatography (*2.2.27*), using as the coating substance a suitable silica gel with a fluorescent indicator having an optimal intensity at 254 nm.

Test solution. Dissolve 5 mg of the substance to be examined in *ethanol R* and dilute to 10 ml with the same solvent.

Reference solution (a). Dissolve 5 mg of *clebopride malate CRS* in *ethanol R* and dilute to 10 ml with the same solvent.

Reference solution (b). Dissolve 5 mg of *clebopride malate CRS* and 5 mg of *metoclopramide hydrochloride CRS* in *ethanol R* and dilute to 10 ml with the same solvent.

Apply to the plate as bands 10 mm by 3 mm, 5 μl of each solution. Develop over a path of 15 cm using a mixture of 2 volumes of *concentrated ammonia R*, 14 volumes of *acetone R*, 14 volumes of *methanol R* and 70 volumes of *toluene R*. Allow the plate to dry in air and examine in ultraviolet light at 254 nm. The principal band in the chromatogram obtained with the test solution is similar in position and size to the principal band in the chromatogram obtained with the reference solution (a). The identification is not valid unless the chromatogram obtained with reference solution (b) shows two clearly separated bands.

TESTS

Solution S. Dissolve 1.0 g in *carbon dioxide-free water R* and dilute to 100.0 ml with the same solvent.

Appearance of solution. Examined immediately after preparation, solution S is clear (*2.2.1*) and colourless (*2.2.2, Method I*).

pH (*2.2.3*). The pH of solution S is 3.8 to 4.2.

Related substances. Examine by liquid chromatography (*2.2.29*).

Test solution. Dissolve 0.10 g of the substance to be examined in the mobile phase and dilute to 100.0 ml with the mobile phase.

Reference solution (a). Dilute 1.0 ml of the test solution to 100.0 ml with the mobile phase. Dilute 1.0 ml of this solution to 10.0 ml with the mobile phase.

Reference solution (b). Dissolve 10.0 mg of *clebopride malate CRS* and 10.0 mg of *metoclopramide hydrochloride CRS* in the mobile phase and dilute to 100.0 ml with the mobile phase. Dilute 1.0 ml of this solution to 10.0 ml with the mobile phase.

The chromatographic procedure may be carried out using:

- a stainless steel column 0.12 m long and 4.0 mm in internal diameter packed with *octadecylsilyl silica gel for chromatography R* (5 μm),
- as mobile phase at a flow rate of 1 ml/min a mixture of 20 volumes of *acetonitrile R* and 80 volumes of a 1 g/l solution of *heptane sulphonate sodium R* adjusted to pH 2.5 with *phosphoric acid R*,
- as detector a spectrophotometer set at 215 nm.

Equilibrate the column with the mobile phase for 30 min. Inject 20 μl of reference solution (b). Adjust the sensitivity of the system so that the heights of the peaks in the chromatogram obtained are at least 30 per cent of the full scale of the recorder. The test is not valid unless the retention time of the second peak (clebopride) is about 15 min and the relative retention time of the first peak is about 0.45. Inject 20 μl of the test solution and 20 μl of reference solution (a). Continue the chromatography of the test solution for twice the retention time of the principal peak. In the chromatogram obtained with the test solution: the area of any peak, apart from the principal peak and the two peaks eluting within 2 min, is not greater than the area of the principal peak in the chromatogram obtained with reference solution (a) (0.1 per cent); the sum of the areas of all peaks, apart from the principal peak and the two peaks eluting within 2 min, is not greater than three times the area of the principal peak in the chromatogram obtained with reference solution (a) (0.3 per cent). Disregard any peak with an area less than 0.25 times that of the principal peak in the chromatogram obtained with reference solution (a).

Chlorides. *Prepare the solutions at the same time.*

Test solution. Dissolve 0.530 g of the substance to be examined in 20.0 ml of *anhydrous acetic acid R*, add 6 ml of *dilute nitric acid R* and dilute to 50.0 ml with *water R*.

Reference solution. To 1.5 ml of *0.001 M hydrochloric acid*, add 20.0 ml of *anhydrous acetic acid R* and 6 ml of *dilute nitric acid R* and dilute to 50.0 ml with *water R*.

Transfer separately both solutions recently prepared to test tubes. Add to each tube 1 ml of *silver nitrate solution R2*. Allow to stand for 5 min protected from light. Examine the tubes laterally against a black background. Any opalescence in the test solution is not more intense than that in the reference solution (100 ppm).

Sulphates. *Prepare the solutions at the same time.*

Test solution. Dissolve 3.00 g of the substance to be examined in 20.0 ml of *glacial acetic acid R,* heating gently if necessary. Allow to cool and dilute to 50.0 ml with *water R.*

Reference solution. To 9 ml of *sulphate standard solution (10 ppm SO_4) R1,* add 6 ml of *glacial acetic acid R.*

Into two test tubes introduce 1.5 ml of *sulphate standard solution (10 ppm SO_4) R1* and add 1 ml of a 250 g/l solution of *barium chloride R.* Shake and allow to stand for 1 min. To one of the tubes add 15 ml of the test solution and to the other one add 15 ml of the reference solution.

After 5 min, any opalescence in the tube containing the test solution is not more intense than that containing the reference solution (100 ppm).

Heavy metals (*2.4.8*). 1.0 g complies with limit test D for heavy metals (20 ppm). Prepare the standard using 2 ml of *lead standard solution (10 ppm Pb) R.*

Loss on drying (*2.2.32*). Not more than 0.5 per cent, determined on 1.000 g by drying in an oven at 100 °C to 105 °C.

Sulphated ash (*2.4.14*). Not more than 0.1 per cent, determined on 1.0 g.

ASSAY

Dissolve 0.400 g in 50 ml of *anhydrous acetic acid R.* Titrate with *0.1 M perchloric acid,* determining the end-point potentiometrically (*2.2.20*).

1 ml of *0.1 M perchloric acid* is equivalent to 50.80 mg of $C_{24}H_{30}ClN_3O_7$.

STORAGE

Store protected from light.

IMPURITIES

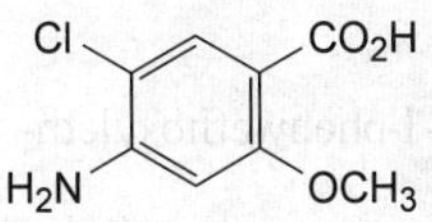

A. 4-amino-5-chloro-2-methoxybenzoic acid,

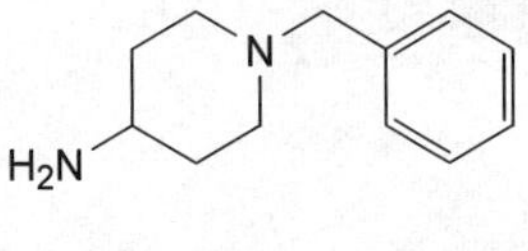

B. 1-benzylpiperidin-4-amine,

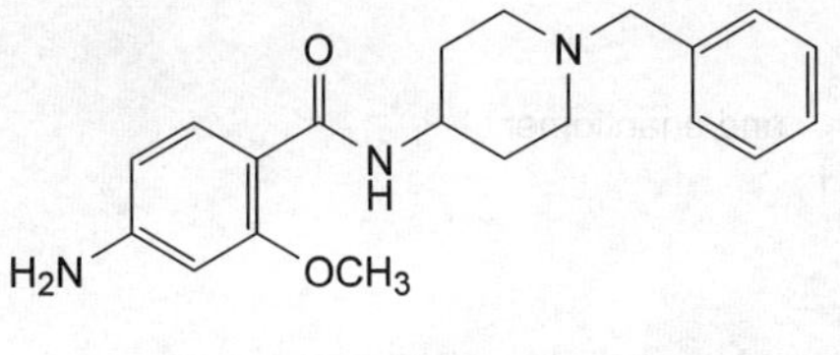

C. 4-amino-*N*-(1-benzylpiperidin-4-yl)-2-methoxybenzamide.

01/2005:1190

CLEMASTINE FUMARATE

Clemastini fumaras

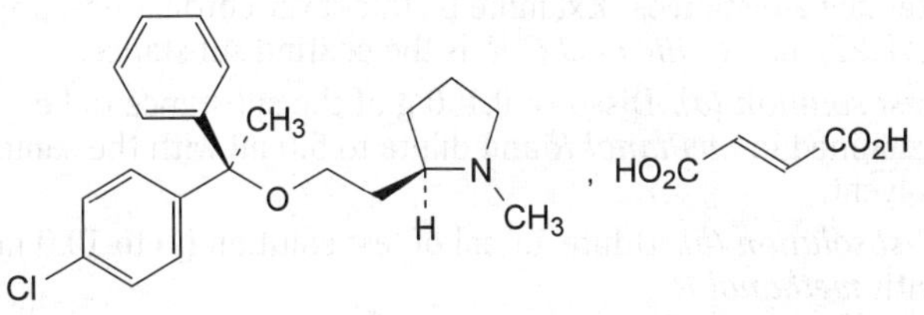

$C_{25}H_{30}ClNO_5$ M_r 460.0

DEFINITION

Clemastine fumarate contains not less than 98.5 per cent and not more than the equivalent of 101.0 per cent of (2*R*)-2-[2-[(*R*)-1-(4-chlorophenyl)-1-phenylethoxy]ethyl]-1-methylpyrrolidine (*E*)-butenedioate, calculated with reference to the dried substance.

CHARACTERS

A white or almost white, crystalline powder, very slightly soluble in water, sparingly soluble in alcohol (70 per cent *V/V*), slightly soluble in alcohol (50 per cent *V/V*) and in methanol.

IDENTIFICATION

First identification: A, B.

Second identification: A, C, D.

A. It complies with the test for specific optical rotation (see Tests).

B. Examine by infrared absorption spectrophotometry (*2.2.24*), comparing with the spectrum obtained with *clemastine fumarate CRS.*

C. Examine the chromatograms obtained in the test for related substances (see Tests). The principal spot in the chromatogram obtained with test solution (b) is similar in position, colour and size to the principal spot in the chromatogram obtained with reference solution (a).

D. Examine by thin-layer chromatography (*2.2.27*), using *silica gel G R* as the coating substance.

Test solution. Dissolve 40 mg of the substance to be examined in *methanol R* and dilute to 2 ml with the same solvent.

Reference solution. Dissolve 50 mg of *fumaric acid CRS* in *alcohol R* and dilute to 10 ml with the same solvent.

Apply separately to the plate 5 µl of each solution. Develop over a path of 15 cm using a mixture of 5 volumes of *water R,* 25 volumes of *anhydrous formic acid R* and 70 volumes of *di-isopropyl ether R.* Dry the plate at 100 °C to 105 °C for 30 min, allow to cool and spray with a 16 g/l solution of *potassium permanganate R.* Examine in daylight. In the chromatogram obtained with test solution the spot with the highest R_f value is similar in position, colour and size to the spot in the chromatogram obtained with the reference solution.

TESTS

Solution S. Dissolve 0.500 g of substance to be examined in *methanol R* and dilute to 50.0 ml with the same solvent.

Appearance of solution. Solution S is clear (*2.2.1*) and not more intensely coloured than reference solution BY_7 (*2.2.2, Method II*).

pH (*2.2.3*). Suspend 1.0 g of the substance to be examined in 10 ml of *carbon dioxide-free water R*. The pH of the suspension is 3.2 to 4.2.

Specific optical rotation (*2.2.7*). The specific optical rotation is + 15.0 to + 18.0, determined on solution S and calculated with reference to the dried substance.

Related substances. Examine by thin-layer chromatography (*2.2.27*), using *silica gel G R* as the coating substance.

Test solution (a). Dissolve 0.100 g of the substance to be examined in *methanol R* and dilute to 5.0 ml with the same solvent.

Test solution (b). Dilute 1.0 ml of test solution (a) to 10.0 ml with *methanol R*.

Reference solution (a). Dissolve 20.0 mg of *clemastine fumarate CRS* in *methanol R* and dilute to 10.0 ml with the same solvent.

Reference solution (b). Dilute 1.5 ml of test solution (b) to 50.0 ml with *methanol R*.

Reference solution (c). Dilute 0.5 ml of test solution (b) to 50.0 ml with *methanol R*.

Reference solution (d). Dissolve 10.0 mg of *diphenhydramine hydrochloride CRS* in 5.0 ml of reference solution (a).

Apply separately to the plate 5 µl of each solution. Develop over a path of 15 cm using a mixture of 1 volume of *concentrated ammonia R*, 20 volumes of *methanol R* and 80 volumes of *tetrahydrofuran R*. Dry the plate in a current of cold air for 5 min, spray with a freshly prepared mixture of 1 volume of *potassium iodobismuthate solution R* and 10 volumes of *dilute acetic acid R* and then with *dilute hydrogen peroxide solution R*. Cover the plate immediately with a glass plate of the same size and examine the chromatograms after 2 min. Any spot in the chromatogram obtained with test solution (a), apart from the principal spot, is not more intense than the spot in the chromatogram obtained with reference solution (b) (0.3 per cent) and at most four such spots are more intense than the spot in the chromatogram obtained with reference solution (c) (0.1 per cent). Disregard any spot remaining at the starting point (fumaric acid). The test is not valid unless the chromatogram obtained with reference solution (d) shows two clearly separated spots.

1-(4-Chlorophenyl)-1-phenylethanol. Examine by liquid chromatography (*2.2.29*).

Test solution. Dissolve 20 mg of the substance to be examined in a mixture of 25 volumes of *acetonitrile R* and 75 volumes of a 10 g/l solution of *ammonium dihydrogen phosphate R* and dilute to 100 ml with the same mixture of solvents.

Reference solution (a). Dissolve 6 mg of *1-(4-chlorophenyl)-1-phenylethanol CRS* in a mixture of 25 volumes of *acetonitrile R* and 75 volumes of a 10 g/l solution of *ammonium dihydrogen phosphate R* and dilute to 100 ml with the same mixture of solvents.

Reference solution (b). Dilute 1 ml of reference solution (a) to 100 ml with a mixture of 25 volumes of *acetonitrile R* and 75 volumes of a 10 g/l solution of *ammonium dihydrogen phosphate R*.

Reference solution (c). Dissolve 10 mg of the substance to be examined in a mixture of 25 volumes of *acetonitrile R* and 75 volumes of a 10 g/l solution of *ammonium dihydrogen phosphate R* and dilute to 100 ml with the same mixture of solvents. To 1 ml of the solution add 1 ml of reference solution (a) and dilute to 100 ml with a mixture of 25 volumes of *acetonitrile R* and 75 volumes of a 10 g/l solution of *ammonium dihydrogen phosphate R*.

The chromatographic procedure may be carried out using:

- a stainless steel column 0.1 m long and 4.6 mm in internal diameter packed with *octadecylsilyl silica gel for chromatography R* (5 µm),
- as mobile phase at a flow rate of 1 ml/min a mixture of 0.1 volumes of *phosphoric acid R*, 45 volumes of *acetonitrile R* and 55 volumes of a 10 g/l solution of *ammonium dihydrogen phosphate R*,
- as detector a spectrophotometer set at 220 nm.

Inject 100 µl of each solution. The test is not valid unless the resolution between the peaks due to clemastine and 1-(4-chlorophenyl)-1-phenylethanol in the chromatogram obtained with reference solution (c) is greater than 2.2. In the chromatogram obtained with the test solution: the area of any peak corresponding to 1-(4-chlorophenyl)-1-phenylethanol is not greater than the area of the peak in the chromatogram obtained with reference solution (b) (0.3 per cent).

Loss on drying (*2.2.32*). Not more than 0.5 per cent, determined on 1.000 g by drying in an oven at 100 °C to 105 °C for 6 h.

Sulphated ash (*2.4.14*). Not more than 0.1 per cent, determined on 1.0 g.

ASSAY

Dissolve 0.350 g of the substance to be examined in 60 ml of *anhydrous acetic acid R*. Titrate with *0.1 M perchloric acid*, determining the end-point potentiometrically (*2.2.20*).

1 ml of *0.1 M perchloric acid* is equivalent to 46.00 mg of $C_{25}H_{30}ClNO_5$.

IMPURITIES

Specified impurities: A, B, C.

Other detectable impurities: D.

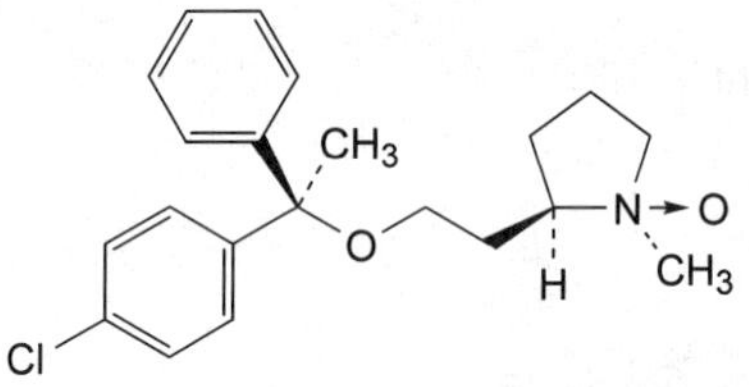

and epimer at N

A. (1*RS*,2*R*)-2-[2-[(*R*)-1-(4-chlorophenyl)-1-phenylethoxy]ethyl]-1-methylpyrrolidine 1-oxide,

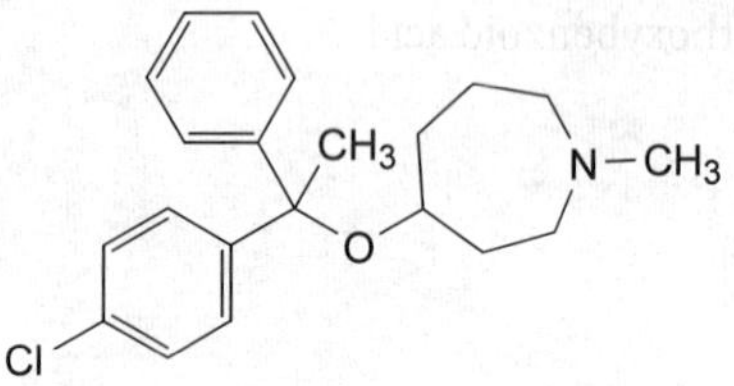

B. 4-[1-(4-chlorophenyl)-1-phenylethoxy]-1-methylazepane,

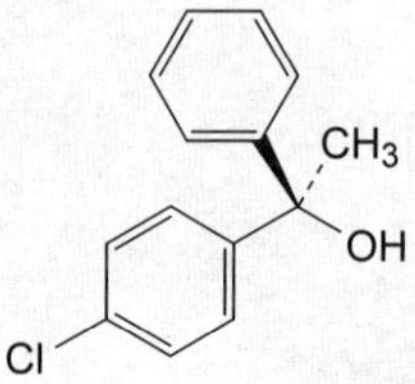

and enantiomer

C. (*RS*)-1-(4-chlorophenyl)-1-phenylethanol,

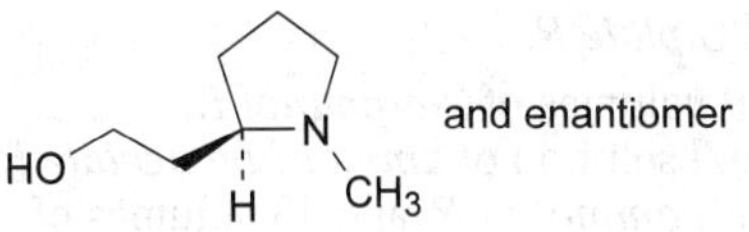

D. 2-[(2*RS*)-1-methylpyrrolidin-2-yl]ethanol.

01/2005:1409

CLENBUTEROL HYDROCHLORIDE

Clenbuteroli hydrochloridum

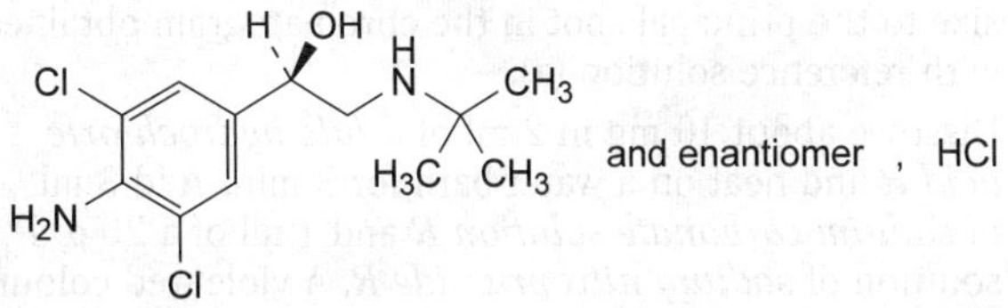

$C_{12}H_{19}Cl_3N_2O$ M_r 313.7

DEFINITION

Clenbuterol hydrochloride contains not less than 99.0 per cent and not more than the equivalent of 101.0 per cent of (*RS*)-1-(4-amino-3,5-dichlorophenyl)-2-[(1,1-dimethylethyl)amino]ethanol hydrochloride, calculated with reference to the anhydrous substance.

CHARACTERS

A white or almost white, crystalline powder, soluble in water and in alcohol, slightly soluble in acetone.

It melts at about 173 °C, with decomposition.

IDENTIFICATION

First identification: A, C.

Second identification: B, C.

A. Examine by infrared absorption spectrophotometry (*2.2.24*), comparing with the spectrum obtained with *clenbuterol hydrochloride CRS*.

B. Examine by thin-layer chromatography (*2.2.27*), using a *TLC silica gel F_{254} plate R*.

Test solution. Dissolve 10 mg of the substance to be examined in 10 ml of *methanol R*.

Reference solution. Dissolve 10 mg of *clenbuterol hydrochloride CRS* in 10 ml of *methanol R*.

Apply to the plate 10 µl of each solution. Develop over a path of 10 cm using a mixture of 0.15 volumes of *ammonia R*, 10 volumes of *ethanol R* and 15 volumes of *toluene R*. Allow the plate to dry in air. Spray with a 10 g/l solution of *sodium nitrite R* in *1 M hydrochloric acid* and dip after 10 min in a 4 g/l solution of *naphthylethylenediamine dihydrochloride R* in *methanol R*. Allow the plate to dry in air. The principal spot in the chromatogram obtained with the test solution is similar in position, colour and size to the principal spot in the chromatogram obtained with the reference solution.

C. It gives reaction (a) of chlorides (*2.3.1*).

TESTS

Solution S. Dissolve 0.5 g in 10 ml of *carbon dioxide-free water R*.

Appearance of solution. Solution S is not more opalescent than reference suspension II (*2.2.1*) and not more intensely coloured than reference solution Y_6 (*2.2.2, Method II*).

pH (*2.2.3*). The pH of solution S is 5.0 to 7.0.

Optical rotation (*2.2.7*). Dissolve 0.30 g in *water R* and dilute to 10.0 ml with the same solvent. If necessary filter. The angle of optical rotation is − 0.10° to + 0.10°.

Related substances. Examine by liquid chromatography (*2.2.29*).

Test solution. Disperse 100.0 mg of the substance to be examined in the mobile phase and dilute to 50.0 ml with the mobile phase.

Reference solution (a). Dilute 0.1 ml of the test solution to 100.0 ml with *water R*.

Reference solution (b). Dissolve 10 mg of *clenbuterol impurity B CRS* in 20 ml of the mobile phase, add 5 ml of the test solution and dilute to 50.0 ml with the mobile phase.

The chromatographic procedure may be carried out using:

– a stainless steel column 0.125 m long and 4 mm in internal diameter, packed with *end-capped octadecylsilyl silica gel for chromatography R* (5 µm),
– as mobile phase at a flow rate of 0.5 ml/min a mixture of 200 volumes of *acetonitrile R*, 200 volumes of *methanol R* and 600 volumes of a solution prepared as follows: dissolve 3.0 g of *sodium decanesulphonate R* and 5.0 g of *potassium dihydrogen phosphate R* in 900 ml of*water R*, adjust to pH 3.0 with *dilute phosphoric acid R* and dilute to 1000 ml with *water R*,
– as detector a spectrophotometer set at 215 nm,

maintaining the temperature of the column at 40 °C.

Inject 5 µl of reference solution (a) and 5 µl of reference solution (b). Adjust the sensitivity of the system so that the height of the principal peak in the chromatogram obtained with reference solution (a) is at least 50 per cent of the full scale of the recorder. When the chromatogram are recorded in the prescribed conditions, the retention time of clenbuterol is about 11 min. The test is not valid until in the chromatogram obtained with reference solution (b) the resolution between the peaks corresponding to impurity B and clenbuterol is at least 2.5.

Inject 5 µl of the test solution and continue the chromatography for 1.5 times the retention time of the principal peak. In the chromatogram obtained with the test solution: the area of any peak apart from the principal peak is not greater than the area of the principal peak in the chromatogram obtained with reference solution (a) (0.1 per cent) and the sum of the areas of all the peaks apart of the principal peak is not greater than 2 times the area of the principal peak in the chromatogram obtained with reference solution (a) (0.2 per cent). Disregard any peak with an area less than 0.1 times the area of the principal peak in the chromatogram obtained with reference solution (a).

Water (*2.5.12*). Not more than 1.0 per cent, determined on 0.500 g by the semi-micro determination of water.

Sulphated ash (*2.4.14*). Not more than 0.1 per cent, determined on 1.0 g.

ASSAY

Dissolve 0.250 g in 50 ml of *alcohol R* and add 5.0 ml of *0.01 M hydrochloric acid*. Titrate with *0.1 M sodium hydroxide*, determining the end-point potentiometrically (*2.2.20*). Read the volume added between the two points of inflexion.

1 ml of *0.1 M sodium hydroxide* is equivalent to 31.37 mg of $C_{12}H_{19}Cl_3N_2O$.

Monographs C

IMPURITIES

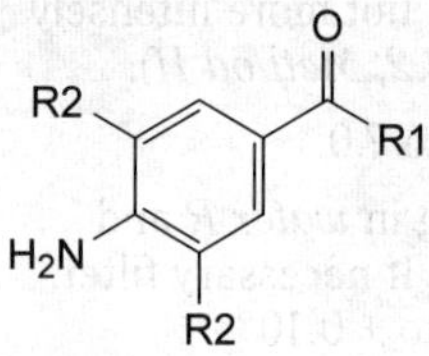

A. R1 = H, R2 = Cl: 4-amino-3,5-dichlorobenzaldehyde,

B. R1 = CH_2-NH-C(CH_3)$_3$, R2 = Cl: 1-(4-amino-3,5-dichlorophenyl)-2-[(1,1-dimethylethyl)amino]ethanone (clenbuterol-ketone),

C. R1 = CH_3, R2 = Cl: 1-(4-amino-3,5-dichlorophenyl)ethanone,

D. R1 = CH_3, R2 = H: 1-(4-aminophenyl)ethanone,

E. R1 = CH_2Br, R2 = Cl: 1-(4-amino-3,5-dichlorophenyl)-2-bromoethanone.

01/2005:0582

CLINDAMYCIN HYDROCHLORIDE

Clindamycini hydrochloridum

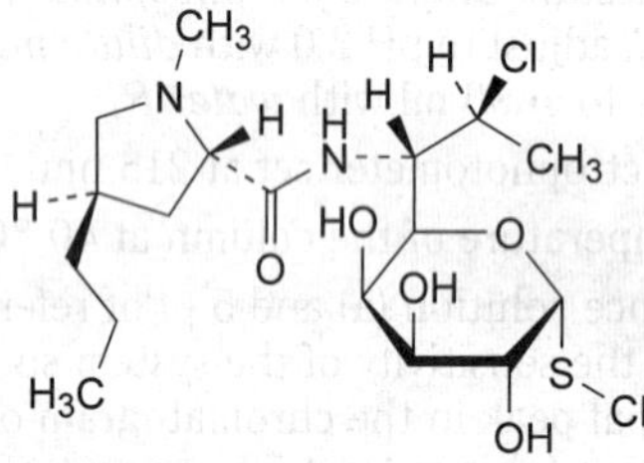

$C_{18}H_{34}Cl_2N_2O_5S$ M_r 461.5

DEFINITION

Methyl 7-chloro-6,7,8-trideoxy-6-[[[(2*S*,4*R*)-1-methyl-4-propylpyrrolidin-2-yl]carbonyl]amino]-1-thio-L-*threo*-α-D-*galacto*-octopyranoside hydrochloride. It contains a variable quantity of water.

Content: 84.0 per cent to 93.0 per cent of clindamycin ($C_{18}H_{33}ClN_2O_5S$) (anhydrous substance).

CHARACTERS

Appearance: white or almost white, crystalline powder.

Solubility: very soluble in water, slightly soluble in alcohol.

IDENTIFICATION

First identification: A, D.

Second identification: B, C, D.

A. Infrared absorption spectrophotometry (*2.2.24*).
Comparison: *clindamycin hydrochloride CRS.*

B. Thin-layer chromatography (*2.2.27*).
Test solution. Dissolve 10 mg of the substance to be examined in *methanol R* and dilute to 10 ml with the same solvent.
Reference solution (a). Dissolve 10 mg of *clindamycin hydrochloride CRS* in *methanol R* and dilute to 10 ml with the same solvent.
Reference solution (b). Dissolve 10 mg of *clindamycin hydrochloride CRS* and 10 mg of *lincomycin hydrochloride CRS* in *methanol R* and dilute to 10 ml with the same solvent.
Plate: *TLC silica gel G plate R.*
Mobile phase: mix 19 volumes of *2-propanol R*, 38 volumes of a 150 g/l solution of *ammonium acetate R* adjusted to pH 9.6 with *ammonia R*, and 43 volumes of *ethyl acetate R.*
Application: 5 µl.
Development: over a path of 15 cm using the upper layer of the mobile phase.
Drying: in air.
Detection: spray with a 1 g/l solution of *potassium permanganate R.*
System suitability: the chromatogram obtained with reference solution (b) shows 2 clearly separated spots.
Results: the principal spot in the chromatogram obtained with the test solution is similar in position, colour and size to the principal spot in the chromatogram obtained with reference solution (a).

C. Dissolve about 10 mg in 2 ml of *dilute hydrochloric acid R* and heat on a water-bath for 3 min. Add 3 ml of *sodium carbonate solution R* and 1 ml of a 20 g/l solution of *sodium nitroprusside R.* A violet-red colour develops.

D. Dissolve 0.1 g in *water R* and dilute to 10 ml with the same solvent. The solution gives reaction (a) of chlorides (*2.3.1*).

TESTS

pH (*2.2.3*): 3.0 to 5.0.

Dissolve 1.0 g in *carbon dioxide-free water R* and dilute to 10 ml with the same solvent.

Specific optical rotation (*2.2.7*): + 135 to + 150 (anhydrous substance).

Dissolve 1.000 g in *water R* and dilute to 25.0 ml with the same solvent.

Related substances. Liquid chromatography (*2.2.29*).

Test solution. Dissolve 50.0 mg of the substance to be examined in the mobile phase and dilute to 50.0 ml with the mobile phase.

Reference solution (a). Dissolve 50.0 mg of *clindamycin hydrochloride CRS* in the mobile phase and dilute to 50.0 ml with the mobile phase.

Reference solution (b). Dilute 2.0 ml of the test solution to 100.0 ml with the mobile phase.

Column:

– *size*: *l* = 0.25 m, Ø = 4.6 mm,
– *stationary phase*: *octadecylsilyl silica gel for chromatography R* (5 µm).

Mobile phase: mix 45 volumes of *acetonitrile R* and 55 volumes of a 6.8 g/l solution of *potassium dihydrogen phosphate R* adjusted to pH 7.5 with a 250 g/l solution of *potassium hydroxide R.*

Flow rate: 1 ml/min.

Detection: spectrophotometer at 210 nm.

Injection: 20 µl.

Run time: twice the retention time of clindamycin.

System suitability: reference solution (a):

– *relative retentions* with reference to clindamycin (retention time = about 10 min): impurity A = about 0.4; impurity B = about 0.65; impurity C = about 0.8.

Limits:

– *impurity B*: not more than the area of the principal peak in the chromatogram obtained with reference solution (b) (2.0 per cent),

– *impurity C*: not more than twice the area of the principal peak in the chromatogram obtained with reference solution (b) (4.0 per cent),
– *any other impurity*: not more than half the area of the principal peak in the chromatogram obtained with reference solution (b) (1 per cent),
– *total*: not more than 3 times the area of the principal peak in the chromatogram obtained with reference solution (b) (6.0 per cent),
– *disregard limit*: 0.025 times the area of the principal peak in the chromatogram obtained with reference solution (b) (0.05 per cent).

Water (*2.5.12*): 3.0 per cent to 6.0 per cent, determined on 0.500 g.

Sulphated ash (*2.4.14*): maximum 0.5 per cent, determined on 1.0 g.

ASSAY

Liquid chromatography (*2.2.29*) as described in the test for related substances with the following modifications.

Injection: 20 µl; inject the test solution and reference solution (a).

System suitability: reference solution (a):
– *repeatability*: maximum relative standard deviation of 0.85 per cent for 6 replicate injections.

STORAGE

In an airtight container.

IMPURITIES

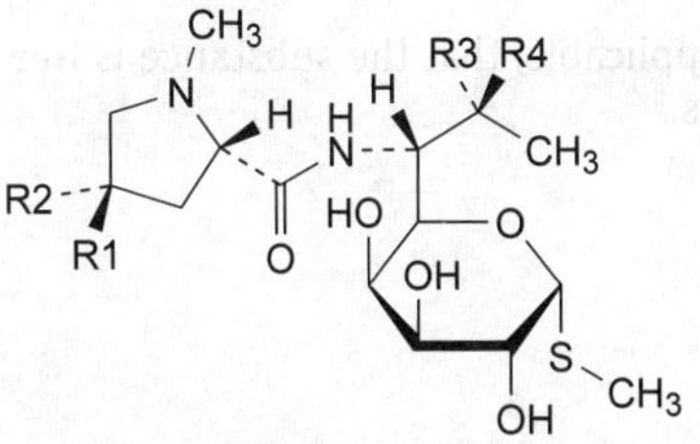

A. R1 = CH_2-CH_2-CH_3, R2 = R4 = H, R3 = OH: methyl 6,8-dideoxy-6-[[[(2*S*,4*R*)-1-methyl-4-propylpyrrolidin-2-yl]carbonyl]amino]-1-thio-D-*erythro*-α-D-*galacto*-octopyranoside (lincomycin),

B. R1 = R3 = H, R2 = C_2H_5, R4 = Cl: methyl 7-chloro-6,7,8-trideoxy-6-[[[(2*S*,4*S*)-4-ethyl-1-methylpyrrolidin-2-yl]carbonyl]amino]-1-thio-L-*threo*-α-D-*galacto*-octopyranoside (clindamycin B),

C. R1 = CH_2-CH_2-CH_3, R2 = R4 = H, R3 = Cl: methyl 7-chloro-6,7,8-trideoxy-6-[[[(2*S*,4*R*)-1-methyl-4-propylpyrrolidin-2-yl]carbonyl]amino]-1-thio-D-*erythro*-α-D-*galacto*-octopyranoside (7-epiclindamycin).

01/2005:0996

CLINDAMYCIN PHOSPHATE

Clindamycini phosphas

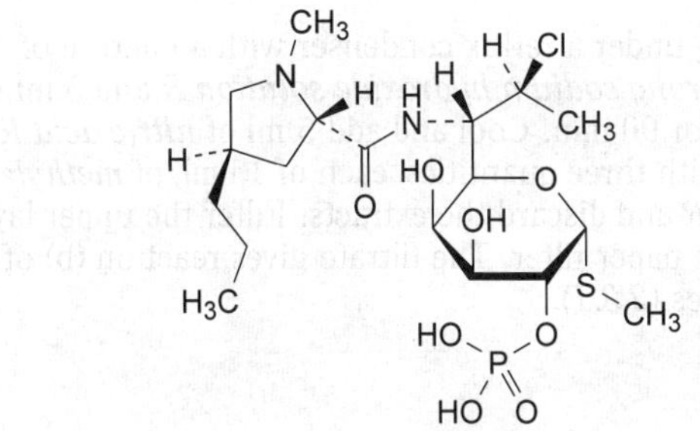

$C_{18}H_{34}ClN_2O_8PS$ M_r 505.0

DEFINITION

Clindamycin phosphate contains not less than 95.0 per cent and not more than the equivalent of 100.5 per cent of methyl 7-chloro-6,7,8-trideoxy-6-[[[(2*S*,4*R*)-1-methyl-4-propylpyrrolidin-2-yl]carbonyl]amino]-1-thio-L-*threo*-α-D-*galacto*-octopyranoside 2-(dihydrogen phosphate), calculated with reference to the anhydrous substance.

CHARACTERS

A white or almost white powder, slightly hygroscopic, freely soluble in water, very slightly soluble in alcohol, practically insoluble in methylene chloride.

It shows polymorphism.

IDENTIFICATION

First identification: A, D.

Second identification: B, C, D.

A. Examine by infrared spectrophotometry (*2.2.24*), comparing with the spectrum obtained with *clindamycin phosphate CRS*. In two separate tubes place 50 mg of the substance to be examined and 50 mg of *clindamycin phosphate CRS*. Add 0.2 ml of *water R* and heat until completely dissolved. Evaporate to dryness under reduced pressure and dry at 100 °C to 105 °C for 2 h. Examine the substances prepared as discs using *potassium bromide R*.

B. Examine by thin-layer chromatography (*2.2.27*), using *silica gel H R* as the coating substance.

Test solution. Dissolve 20 mg of the substance to be examined in *methanol R* and dilute to 10 ml with the same solvent.

Reference solution (a). Dissolve 20 mg of *clindamycin phosphate CRS* in *methanol R* and dilute to 10 ml with the same solvent.

Reference solution (b). Dissolve 10 mg of *lincomycin hydrochloride CRS* in 5 ml of reference solution (a).

Apply separately to the plate 5 µl of each solution. Develop over a path of 12 cm using a mixture of 20 volumes of *glacial acetic acid R*, 20 volumes of *water R* and 60 volumes of *butanol R*. Dry the plate at 100 °C to 105 °C for 30 min and spray with a 1 g/l solution of *potassium permanganate R*. The principal spot in the chromatogram obtained with the test solution is similar in position, colour and size to the principal spot in the chromatogram obtained with reference solution (a). The test is not valid unless the chromatogram obtained with reference solution (b) shows two principal spots.

C. Dissolve about 10 mg in 2 ml of *dilute hydrochloric acid R* and heat in a water-bath for 3 min. Add 4 ml of *sodium carbonate solution R* and 1 ml of a 20 g/l solution of *sodium nitroprusside R*. Prepare a standard in the same manner using *clindamycin phosphate CRS*. The colour in the test solution corresponds to that in the standard.

D. Boil 0.1 g under a reflux condenser with a mixture of 5 ml of *strong sodium hydroxide solution R* and 5 ml of *water R* for 90 min. Cool and add 5 ml of *nitric acid R*. Extract with three quantities, each of 15 ml, of *methylene chloride R* and discard the extracts. Filter the upper layer through a paper filter. The filtrate gives reaction (b) of phosphates (*2.3.1*).

TESTS

Solution S. Dissolve 1.00 g in *carbon dioxide-free water R*. Heat gently if necessary. Cool and dilute to 25.0 ml with *carbon dioxide-free water R*.

Appearance of the solution. Solution S is clear (*2.2.1*) and colourless (*2.2.2, Method II*).

pH (*2.2.3*). Dilute 5.0 ml of solution S to 20 ml with *carbon dioxide-free water R*. The pH of the solution is 3.5 to 4.5.

Specific optical rotation (*2.2.7*). Dissolve 0.250 g in *water R* and dilute to 25.0 ml with the same solvent. The specific optical rotation is + 115 to + 130, calculated with reference to the anhydrous substance.

Related substances. Examine by liquid chromatography (*2.2.29*), as described under Assay. Inject reference solution (c). Adjust the sensitivity of the detector so that the height of the principal peak is not less than 50 per cent of the full scale of the recorder. Inject the test solution and continue the chromatography for the retention time of clindamycin: the area of any peak, apart from the principal peak and any peak due to the solvent, is not greater than 2.5 times the area of the peak corresponding to clindamycin phosphate in the chromatogram obtained with reference solution (c) (2.5 per cent) and the sum of the areas of all the peaks, apart from the principal peak and any peak due to the solvent, is not greater than four times the area of the peak corresponding to clindamycin phosphate in the chromatogram obtained with reference solution (c) (4.0 per cent). Disregard any peak with an area less than 10.0 per cent of that of the principal peak in the chromatogram obtained with reference solution (c).

Water (*2.5.12*). Not more than 6.0 per cent, determined on 0.250 g by the semi-micro determination of water.

Bacterial endotoxins (*2.6.14*): less than 0.6 IU/mg, if intended for use in the manufacture of parenteral dosage forms without a further appropriate procedure for removal of bacterial endotoxins.

ASSAY

Examine by liquid chromatography (*2.2.29*).

Test solution. Dissolve 75.0 mg of the substance to be examined in the mobile phase and dilute to 25.0 ml with the mobile phase.

Reference solution (a). Dissolve 75.0 mg of *clindamycin phosphate CRS* in the mobile phase and dilute to 25.0 ml with the mobile phase.

Reference solution (b). Dissolve 5.0 mg of *lincomycin hydrochloride CRS* and 15.0 mg of *clindamycin hydrochloride CRS* in 5.0 ml of reference solution (a) and dilute to 100.0 ml with the mobile phase.

Reference solution (c). Dilute 1.0 ml of reference solution (a) to 100.0 ml with the mobile phase.

The chromatographic procedure may be carried out using:

- a stainless steel column 0.25 m long and 4.6 mm in internal diameter packed with *octylsilyl silica gel for chromatography R* (5 µm to 10 µm),
- as mobile phase at a flow rate of 1.0 ml/min a mixture of 200 ml of *acetonitrile R* and 800 ml of a 13.6 g/l solution of *potassium dihydrogen phosphate R*, previously adjusted to pH 2.5 with *phosphoric acid R*,
- as detector a spectrophotometer set at 210 nm,
- a 20 µl loop injector.

Inject reference solution (b). Adjust the sensitivity of the detector so that the height of the peaks is not less than 50 per cent of the full scale of the recorder. The assay is not valid unless the first peak (lincomycin) is clearly separated from the solvent peak and the resolution between the second peak (clindamycin phosphate) and the third peak (clindamycin) is at least 6.0. Adjust the concentration of acetonitrile in the mobile phase, if necessary. The assay is not valid unless the symmetry factor of the clindamycin phosphate peak is at most 1.5. Inject reference solution (a) six times. The test is not valid unless the relative standard deviation of the peak area for clindamycin phosphate is at most 1.0 per cent. If necessary adjust the integrator parameters. Inject alternately the test solution and reference solution (a).

Calculate the percentage content of clindamycin phosphate.

STORAGE

Store in an airtight container, at a temperature not exceeding 30 °C. If the substance is sterile, store in a sterile, airtight, tamper-proof container.

LABELLING

The label states, where applicable, that the substance is free from bacterial endotoxins.

IMPURITIES

A. lincomycin,

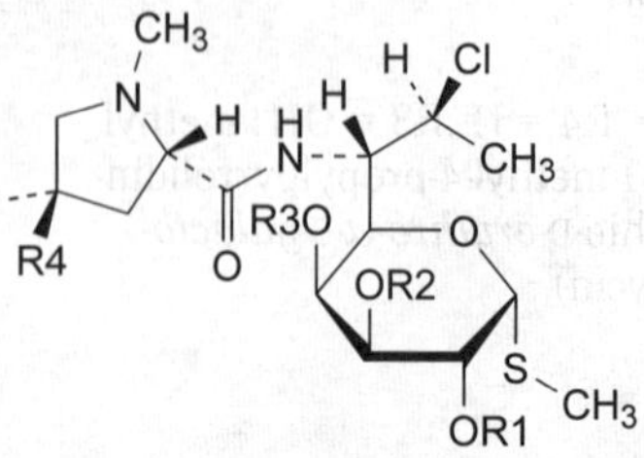

B. R1 = PO_3H_2, R2 = R3 = H, R4 = C_2H_5: clindamycin B 2-(dihydrogen phosphate),

C. R1 = R3 = H, R2 = PO_3H_2, R4 = C_3H_7: clindamycin 3-(dihydrogen phosphate),

D. R1 = R2 = H, R3 = PO_3H_2, R4 = C_3H_7: clindamycin 4-(dihydrogen phosphate),

E. R1 = R2 = R3 = H, R4 = C_3H_7: clindamycin.

01/2005:2111

CLIOQUINOL

Clioquinolum

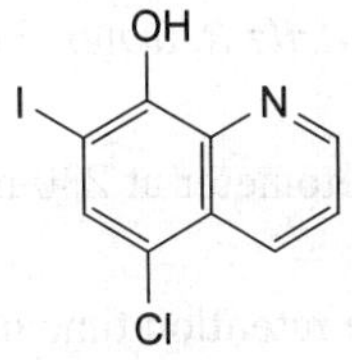

C_9H_5ClINO M_r 305.5

DEFINITION

5-Chloro-7-iodoquinolin-8-ol.

Content: 98.0 per cent to 102.0 per cent (dried substance).

CHARACTERS

Appearance: almost white, light yellow, brownish-yellow or yellowish-grey powder.

Solubility: practically insoluble in water, sparingly soluble in methylene chloride, very slightly soluble or slightly soluble in ethanol (96 per cent).

IDENTIFICATION

First identification: B.

Second identification: A, C, D.

A. Dissolve 40.0 mg in *methanol R* and dilute to 100.0 ml with the same solvent. Dilute 10.0 ml to 100.0 ml with *methanol R* (solution A). Examined between 280 nm and 350 nm (*2.2.25*), solution A shows an absorption maximum at 321 nm. Dilute 10.0 ml of solution A to 100.0 ml with *methanol R* (solution B). Examined between 230 nm and 280 nm, solution B shows an absorption maximum at 255 nm. The specific absorbance at this absorption maximum is 1530 to 1660.

B. Infrared absorption spectrophotometry (*2.2.24*).

Preparation: discs of *potassium bromide R*.

Comparison: *clioquinol CRS*.

C. When heated, violet fumes are produced.

D. Dissolve about 1 mg in 5 ml of *ethanol (96 per cent) R*. Add 0.05 ml of *ferric chloride solution R1*. A dark green colour develops.

TESTS

Acidity or alkalinity. Shake 0.5 g with 10 ml of *carbon dioxide-free water R* and filter. To the filtrate add 0.2 ml of *phenolphthalein solution R*. The solution is colourless. Not more than 0.5 ml of *0.01 M sodium hydroxide* is required to change the colour of the indicator to pink.

Related substances. Liquid chromatography (*2.2.29*).

Test solution. Dissolve 50.0 mg of the substance to be examined in *methanol R* and dilute to 50.0 ml with the same solvent, heating gently if necessary. Dilute 10.0 ml of the solution to 25.0 ml with the mobile phase.

Reference solution (a). Dissolve 20.0 mg of *5-chloroquinolin-8-ol R*, 10.0 mg of *5,7-dichloroquinolin-8-ol R*, 5 mg of the substance to be examined and 10.0 mg of *5,7-diiodoquinolin-8-ol R* in *methanol R*, heating gently if necessary and dilute to 20.0 ml with the same solvent. Dilute 4.0 ml of the solution to 50.0 ml with the mobile phase.

Reference solution (b). Dilute 1.0 ml of reference solution (a) to 10.0 ml with the mobile phase.

Reference solution (c). Dilute 1.0 ml of the test solution to 100.0 ml with the mobile phase. Dilute 1.0 ml of this solution to 20.0 ml with the mobile phase.

Column:

- *size*: l = 0.15 m, Ø = 3.9 mm,
- *stationary phase*: *octylsilyl silica gel for chromatography R* (5 µm).

Mobile phase: dissolve 0.50 g of *sodium edetate R* in 350 ml of *water R*, add 4.0 ml of *hexylamine R* and mix. Adjust to pH 3.0 with *phosphoric acid R*. Add 600 ml of *methanol R* and dilute to 1000 ml with *water R*.

Flow rate: 1.3 ml/min.

Detection: spectrophotometer at 254 nm.

Injection: 20 µl.

Run time: 4 times the retention time of clioquinol.

Relative retention with reference to clioquinol (retention time = about 10 min): impurity A = about 0.4; impurity B = about 0.7; impurity C = about 1.3.

System suitability: reference solution (a):

- *resolution*: minimum 3.0 between the peaks due to clioquinol and impurity C.

Limits:

- *impurity A*: not more than the area of the corresponding peak in the chromatogram obtained with reference solution (b) (2.0 per cent),
- *impurity B*: not more than the area of the corresponding peak in the chromatogram obtained with reference solution (b) (1.0 per cent),
- *impurity C*: not more than the area of the corresponding peak in the chromatogram obtained with reference solution (b) (1.0 per cent),
- *any other impurity*: for each impurity, not more than twice the area of the principal peak in the chromatogram obtained with reference solution (c) (0.1 per cent),
- *total of the nominal contents of impurities A, B, C and any other impurities*: maximum 3.0 per cent,
- *disregard limit*: the area of the principal peak in the chromatogram obtained with reference solution (c) (0.05 per cent).

Halides: maximum 140 ppm, expressed as chlorides. Shake 0.5 g with 25 ml of *water R* for 1 min and filter. To the filtrate add 0.5 ml of *dilute nitric acid R* and 0.5 ml of *silver nitrate solution R2*. Allow to stand for 5 min. Any opalescence is not more intense than that in a standard prepared at the same time by adding 0.5 ml of *silver nitrate solution R2* to 25 ml of *water R* containing 0.2 ml of *0.01 M hydrochloric acid* and 0.5 ml of *dilute nitric acid R*.

Loss on drying (*2.2.32*): maximum 0.5 per cent, determined on 1.000 g by drying over *diphosphorus pentoxide R* at a pressure not exceeding 0.7 kPa for 24 h.

Sulphated ash (*2.4.14*): maximum 0.1 per cent, determined on 1.0 g.

ASSAY

Dissolve 0.200 g in 20 ml of *acetic anhydride R* and add 30 ml of *glacial acetic acid R*. Titrate with *0.1 M perchloric acid*, determining the end-point potentiometrically (*2.2.20*).

1 ml of *0.1 M perchloric acid* is equivalent to 30.55 mg of total quinolines, calculated as clioquinol.

STORAGE

Protected from light.

Monographs C

IMPURITIES

Specified impurities: *A, B, C.*

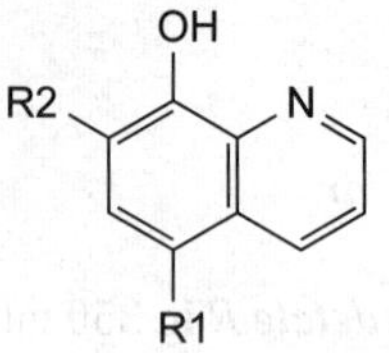

A. R1 = Cl, R2 = H: 5-chloroquinolin-8-ol,

B. R1 = R2 = Cl: 5,7-dichloroquinolin-8-ol,

C. R1 = R2 = I: 5,7-diiodoquinolin-8-ol.

01/2005:1974 corrected

CLOBAZAM

Clobazamum

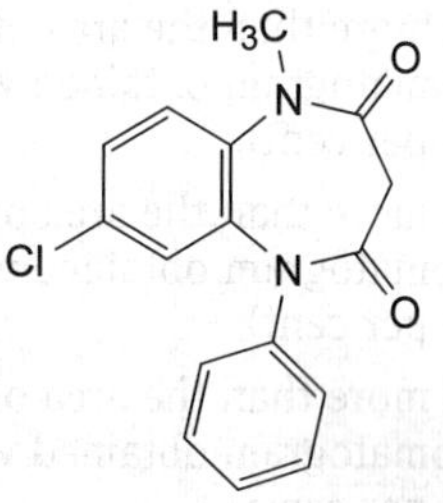

$C_{16}H_{13}ClN_2O_2$ M_r 300.7

DEFINITION

7-Chloro-1-methyl-5-phenyl-1,5-dihydro-3*H*-1,5-benzodiazepine-2,4-dione.

Content: 97.0 per cent to 103.0 per cent (dried substance).

CHARACTERS

Appearance: white or almost white, crystalline powder.

Solubility: slightly soluble in water, freely soluble in methylene chloride, sparingly soluble in alcohol.

IDENTIFICATION

Infrared absorption spectrophotometry (*2.2.24*).

Comparison: *Ph. Eur. reference spectrum of clobazam.*

TESTS

Related substances. Liquid chromatography (*2.2.29*).

Test solution. Dissolve 10.0 mg of the substance to be examined in the mobile phase and dilute to 50.0 ml with the mobile phase.

Reference solution (a). Dissolve 5.0 mg of *clobazam impurity A CRS* in the mobile phase and dilute to 50.0 ml with the mobile phase. Dilute 1.0 ml of the solution to 100.0 ml with the mobile phase.

Reference solution (b). Dissolve 5 mg of *chlordiazepoxide CRS* and 5 mg of *clonazepam CRS* in the mobile phase and dilute to 50 ml with the mobile phase. Dilute 1 ml of the solution to 100 ml with the mobile phase.

Reference solution (c). Dilute 1.0 ml of the test solution to 200.0 ml with the mobile phase.

Column:

- *size*: *l* = 0.25 m, Ø = 4.6 mm,
- *stationary phase*: *octadecylsilyl silica gel for chromatography R* (5 µm).

Mobile phase: *acetonitrile R, water R* (40:60 *V/V*).

Flow rate: 1 ml/min.

Detection: spectrophotometer at 230 nm.

Injection: 20 µl.

Run time: 5 times the retention time of clobazam.

Retention time: clobazam = about 15 min.

System suitability: reference solution (b):

- *resolution*: minimum 1.3 between the peaks due to chlordiazepoxide and clonazepam.

Limits:

- *impurity A*: not more than the area of the principal peak in the chromatogram obtained with reference solution (a) (0.5 per cent),
- *any other impurity*: not more than 0.4 times the area of the principal peak in the chromatogram obtained with reference solution (c) (0.2 per cent),
- *total of other impurities*: not more than twice the area of the principal peak in the chromatogram obtained with reference solution (c) (1.0 per cent),
- *disregard limit*: 0.1 times the area of the principal peak in the chromatogram obtained with reference solution (c) (0.05 per cent).

Loss on drying (*2.2.32*): maximum 0.5 per cent, determined on 1.000 g by drying in an oven at 100-105 °C.

Sulphated ash (*2.4.14*): maximum 0.1 per cent, determined on the residue obtained in the test for loss on drying.

ASSAY

Dissolve 50.0 mg in *alcohol R* and dilute to 100.0 ml with the same solvent. Dilute 2.0 ml of the solution to 250.0 ml with *alcohol R*. Measure the absorbance (*2.2.25*) at the maximum at 232 nm.

Calculate the content of $C_{16}H_{13}ClN_2O_2$ taking the specific absorbance to be 1380.

IMPURITIES

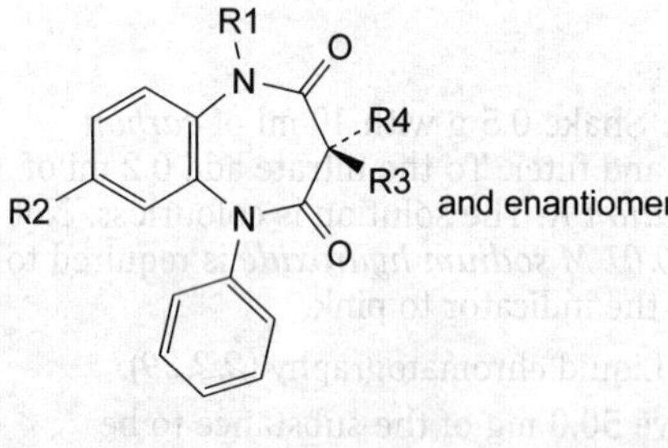

A. R1 = R3 = R4 = H, R2 = Cl: 7-chloro-5-phenyl-1,5-dihydro-3*H*-1,5-benzodiazepine-2,4-dione,

B. R1 = CH_3, R2 = R3 = R4 = H: 1-methyl-5-phenyl-1,5-dihydro-3*H*-1,5-benzodiazepine-2,4-dione,

C. R1 = R3 = CH_3, R2 = Cl, R4 = H: (3*RS*)-7-chloro-1,3-dimethyl-5-phenyl-1,5-dihydro-3*H*-1,5-benzodiazepine-2,4-dione,

D. R1 = R3 = R4 = CH_3, R2 = Cl: 7-chloro-1,3,3-trimethyl-5-phenyl-1,5-dihydro-3*H*-1,5-benzodiazepine-2,4-dione,

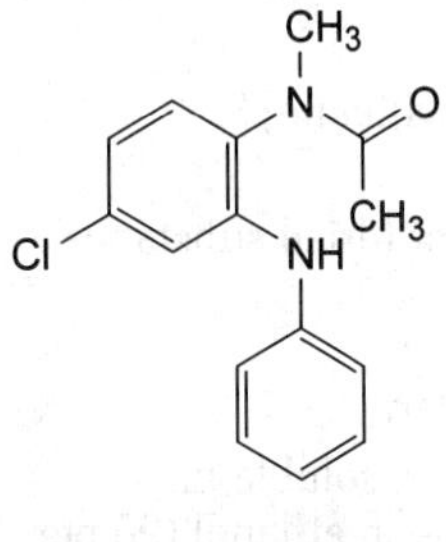

E. *N*-[4-chloro-2-(phenylamino)phenyl]-*N*-methylacetamide,

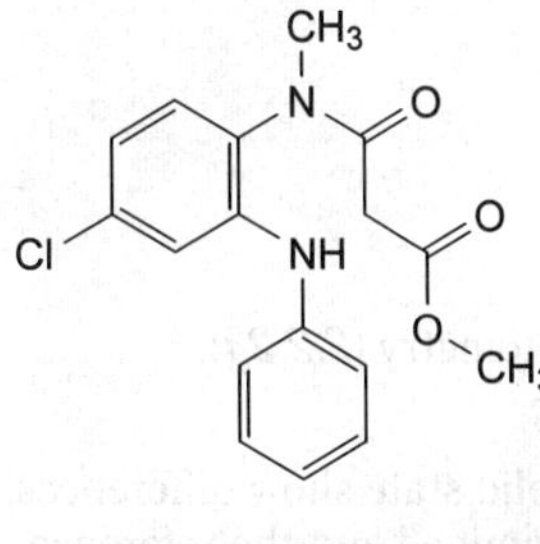

F. methyl 3-[[4-chloro-2-(phenylamino)phenyl]methylamino]-3-oxopropanoate.

01/2005:1090
corrected

CLOBETASONE BUTYRATE

Clobetasoni butyras

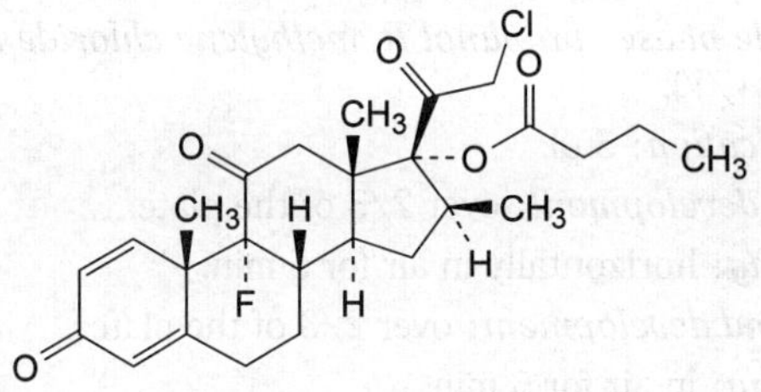

$C_{26}H_{32}ClFO_5$ M_r 479.0

DEFINITION

Clobetasone butyrate contains not less than 97.0 per cent and not more than the equivalent of 102.0 per cent of 21-chloro-9-fluoro-16β-methyl-3,11,20-trioxopregna-1,4-dien-17-yl butanoate, calculated with reference to the dried substance.

CHARACTERS

A white or almost white powder, practically insoluble in water, freely soluble in acetone and in methylene chloride, slightly soluble in alcohol.

It melts at about 178 °C.

IDENTIFICATION

A. Examine by infrared absorption spectrophotometry (*2.2.24*), comparing with the spectrum obtained with *clobetasone butyrate CRS*. Examine the substances prepared as discs.

B. Examine by thin-layer chromatography (*2.2.27*), using as the coating substance a suitable silica gel with a fluorescent indicator having an optimal intensity at 254 nm.

Test solution. Dissolve 10 mg of the substance to be examined in a mixture of equal volumes of *methanol R* and *methylene chloride R* and dilute to 10 ml with the same mixture of solvents.

Reference solution (a). Dissolve 10 mg of *clobetasone butyrate CRS* in a mixture of equal volumes of *methanol R* and *methylene chloride R* and dilute to 10 ml with the same mixture of solvents.

Reference solution (b). Dissolve 10 mg of *clobetasol propionate R* in a mixture of equal volumes of *methanol R* and *methylene chloride R* and dilute to 10 ml with the same mixture of solvents. Dilute 5 ml of this solution to 10 ml with reference solution (a).

Apply separately to the plate 5 µl of each solution. Develop over a path of 15 cm using a mixture of equal volumes of *cyclohexane R* and *methyl acetate R*. Allow the plate to dry in air and examine in ultraviolet light at 254 nm. The principal spot in the chromatogram obtained with the test solution is similar in position and size to the principal spot in the chromatogram obtained with reference solution (a). The test is not valid unless the chromatogram obtained with reference solution (b) shows two clearly separated spots.

C. Mix about 5 mg with 45 mg of *heavy magnesium oxide R* and ignite in a crucible until an almost white residue is obtained (usually less than 5 min). Allow to cool, add 1 ml of *water R*, 0.05 ml of *phenolphthalein solution R1* and about 1 ml of *dilute hydrochloric acid R* to render the solution colourless. Filter. To a freshly prepared mixture of 0.1 ml *alizarin S solution R* and 0.1 ml of *zirconyl nitrate solution R*, add 1.0 ml of the filtrate. Mix, allow to stand for 5 min and compare the colour of the solution with that of a blank prepared in the same manner. The colour of the test solution is yellow and that of the blank is red.

TESTS

Specific optical rotation (*2.2.7*). Dissolve 0.250 g in *dioxan R* and dilute to 25.0 ml with the same solvent. The specific optical rotation is + 127 to + 133, calculated with reference to the dried substance.

Related substances. *Prepare the solutions immediately before use.*

Examine by liquid chromatography (*2.2.29*).

Test solution. Dissolve 50.0 mg of the substance to be examined in 5.0 ml of *ethanol R* and dilute to 50.0 ml with the mobile phase.

Reference solution (a). Dissolve 2 mg of *clobetasone butyrate CRS* and 1.5 mg of *clobetasol propionate R* in 5 ml of *ethanol R* and dilute to 100 ml with the mobile phase.

Reference solution (b). Dilute 1.0 ml of the test solution to 100.0 ml with the mobile phase.

The chromatographic procedure may be carried out using:

- a stainless steel column 0.20 m long and 4.6 mm in internal diameter, packed with *octadecylsilyl silica gel for chromatography R* (5 µm),
- as mobile phase at a flow rate of 1 ml/min a mixture of 45 volumes of *ethanol R* and 55 volumes of *water R*,
- as detector a spectrophotometer set at 241 nm,

maintaining the temperature of the column at 60 °C. Inject 20 µl of reference solution (a). When using a recorder, adjust the sensitivity of the system so that the height of the two principal peaks are at least 50 per cent of the full scale of the recorder. The test is not valid unless the resolution between the first peak (clobetasol propionate) and the second peak (clobetasone butyrate) is at least five.

Inject 20 µl of the test solution and 20 µl of reference solution (b). Continue the chromatography for 2.5 times the retention time of the principal peak. In the chromatogram obtained with the test solution: the area of any peak, apart from the principal peak, is not greater than the area of the principal peak in the chromatogram obtained with reference solution (b) (1.0 per cent) and not more than one such peak has an area greater than half the area of the principal peak in the chromatogram obtained with reference solution (b) (0.5 per cent); the sum of the areas of all the peaks, apart from the principal peak, is not greater than 1.5 times the area of the principal peak in the chromatogram obtained with reference solution (b) (1.5 per cent). Disregard any peak with an area less than 0.05 times the area of the principal peak in the chromatogram obtained with reference solution (b).

Loss on drying (*2.2.32*). Not more than 0.5 per cent, determined on 1.000 g by drying in an oven at 100 °C to 105 °C.

ASSAY

Dissolve 20.0 mg in *alcohol R* and dilute to 100.0 ml with the same solvent. Dilute 5.0 ml of the solution to 50.0 ml with *alcohol R*. Measure the absorbance (*2.2.25*) at the maximum at 235 nm.

Calculate the content of $C_{26}H_{32}ClFO_5$, taking the specific absorbance to be 327.

STORAGE

Store protected from light.

IMPURITIES

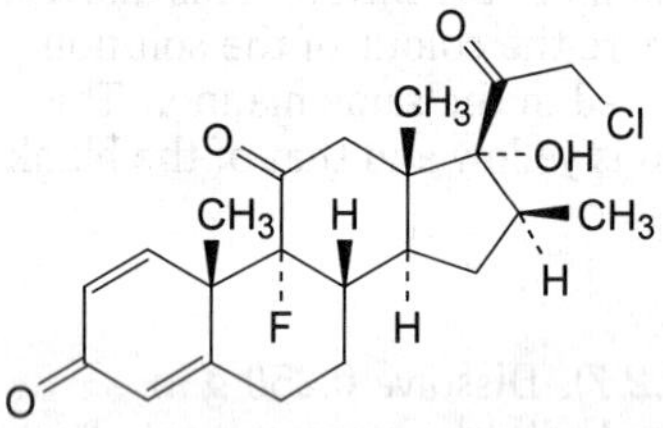

A. clobetasone,

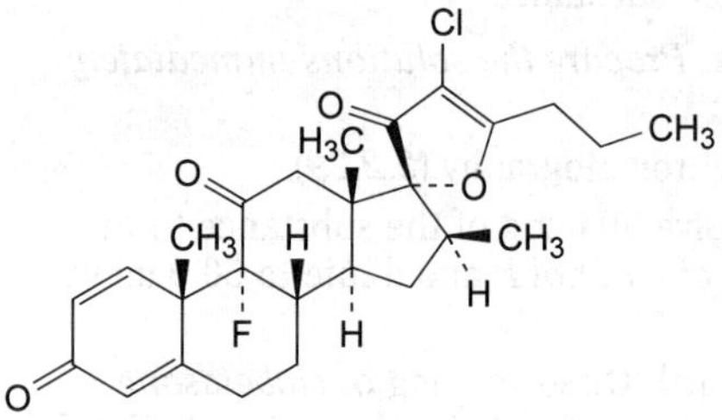

B. (17*R*)-4′-chloro-9-fluoro-16β-methyl-5′-propylspiro[androsta-1,4-diene-17,2′(3′*H*)furan]-3,3′,11-trione.

01/2005:2054

CLOFAZIMINE

Clofaziminum

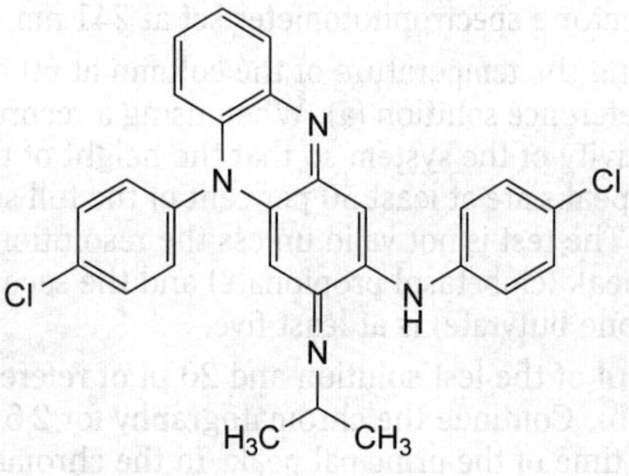

$C_{27}H_{22}Cl_2N_4$ M_r 473.4

DEFINITION

N,5-Bis(4-chlorophenyl)-3-[(1-methylethyl)imino]-3,5-dihydrophenazin-2-amine.

Content: 99.0 per cent to 101.0 per cent (dried substance).

CHARACTERS

Appearance: reddish-brown, fine powder.

Solubility: practically insoluble in water, soluble in methylene chloride, very slightly soluble in ethanol (96 per cent).

It shows polymorphism.

IDENTIFICATION

First identification: A.

Second identification: B, C.

A. Infrared absorption spectrophotometry (*2.2.24*).

Comparison: *clofazimine CRS.*

If the spectra obtained in the solid state show differences, dissolve the substance to be examined and the reference substance separately in *methylene chloride R*, evaporate to dryness and record new spectra using the residues.

B. Thin-layer chromatography (*2.2.27*).

Test solution. Dissolve 10 mg of the substance to be examined in *methylene chloride R* and dilute to 10 ml with the same solvent.

Reference solution. Dissolve 10 mg of *clofazimine CRS* in *methylene chloride R* and dilute to 10 ml with the same solvent.

Plate: *TLC silica gel GF_{254} plate R.*

Mobile phase: *propanol R, methylene chloride R* (6:85 *V/V*).

Application: 5 µl.

First development: over 2/3 of the plate.

Drying: horizontally in air for 5 min.

Second development: over 2/3 of the plate.

Drying: in air for 5 min.

Detection: examine in ultraviolet light at 254 nm.

Results: the principal spot in the chromatogram obtained with the test solution is similar in position and size to the principal spot in the chromatogram obtained with the reference solution.

C. Dissolve 2 mg in 3 ml of *acetone R* and add 0.1 ml of *hydrochloric acid R*. An intense violet colour is produced. Add 0.5 ml of a 200 g/l solution of *sodium hydroxide R*; the colour changes to orange-red.

TESTS

Related substances. Liquid chromatography (*2.2.29*). *Prepare the solutions immediately before use.*

Test solution. Dissolve 50 mg of the substance to be examined in the mobile phase and dilute to 100 ml with the mobile phase.

Reference solution (a). Dilute 1.0 ml of the test solution to 100.0 ml with the mobile phase. Dilute 1.0 ml of this solution to 10.0 ml with the mobile phase.

Reference solution (b). Dissolve 5.0 mg of *clofazimine for system suitability CRS* in the mobile phase and dilute to 10.0 ml with the mobile phase.

Column:

– *size*: *l* = 0.25 m, Ø = 4.6 mm,

– *stationary phase*: *octylsilyl silica gel for chromatography R* (5 µm).

Mobile phase: dissolve 2.25 g of *sodium laurilsulfate R*, 0.85 g of *tetrabutylammonium hydrogen sulphate R* and 0.885 g of *disodium hydrogen phosphate R* in *water R*. Adjust to pH 3.0 with *dilute phosphoric acid R* and dilute to 500 ml with *water R*. Mix 35 volumes of this solution and 65 volumes of *acetonitrile R*.

Flow rate: 1 ml/min.

Detection: spectrophotometer at 280 nm.

Injection: 20 µl.

Run time: 3 times the retention time of clofazimine.

Identification of impurities: use the chromatogram supplied with *clofazimine for system suitability CRS* to identify the peak due to impurity B.

Relative retention with reference to clofazimine (retention time = about 15 min): impurity A = about 0.7; impurity B = about 0.8.

System suitability: reference solution (b):

– *resolution*: baseline separation between the peaks due to impurity B and clofazimine.

Limits:

– *impurity A*: not more than the area of the principal peak in the chromatogram obtained with reference solution (a) (0.1 per cent),
– *impurity B*: not more than 3 times the area of the principal peak in the chromatogram obtained with reference solution (a) (0.3 per cent),
– *any other impurity*: for each impurity, not more than the area of the principal peak in the chromatogram obtained with reference solution (a) (0.1 per cent),
– *total*: not more than 5 times the area of the principal peak in the chromatogram obtained with reference solution (a) (0.5 per cent),
– *disregard limit*: 0.5 times the area of the principal peak in the chromatogram obtained with reference solution (a) (0.05 per cent).

Heavy metals (*2.4.8*): maximum 10 ppm.

2.0 g complies with limit test C. Prepare the reference solution using 2 ml of *lead standard solution (10 ppm Pb) R*.

Loss on drying (*2.2.32*): maximum 0.5 per cent, determined on 1.000 g by drying in an oven at 100-105 °C.

Sulphated ash (*2.4.14*): maximum 0.1 per cent, determined on 1.0 g.

ASSAY

Dissolve 0.400 g in 5 ml of *methylene chloride R* and add 20 ml of *acetone R* and 5 ml of *anhydrous acetic acid R*. Titrate with *0.1 M perchloric acid*, determining the end-point potentiometrically (*2.2.20*).

1 ml of *0.1 M perchloric acid* is equivalent to 47.34 mg of $C_{27}H_{22}Cl_2N_4$.

IMPURITIES

Specified impurities: A, B.

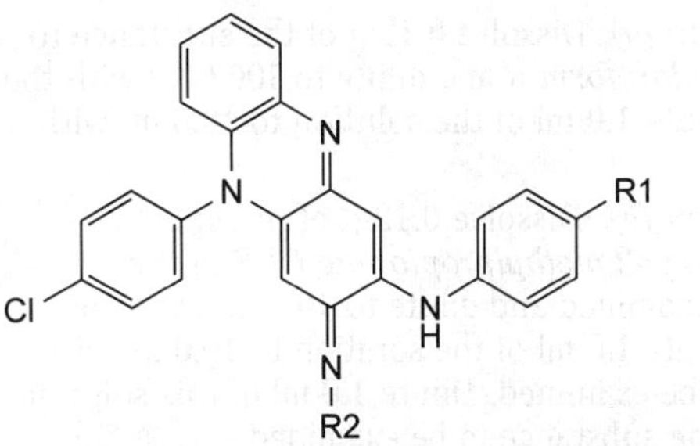

A. R1 = Cl, R2 = H: *N*,5-bis(4-chlorophenyl)-3-imino-3,5-dihydrophenazin-2-amine,

B. R1 = H, R2 = $CH(CH_3)_2$: 5-(4-chlorophenyl)-3-[(1-methylethyl)imino]-*N*-phenyl-3,5-dihydrophenazin-2-amine.

01/2005:0318

CLOFIBRATE

Clofibratum

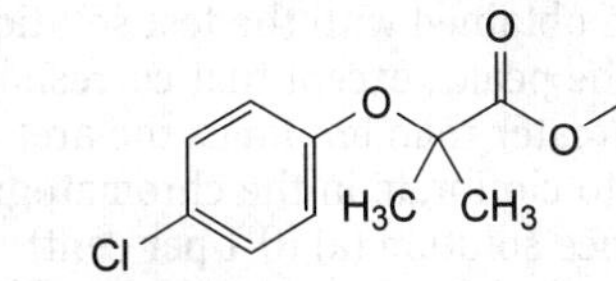

$C_{12}H_{15}ClO_3$ M_r 242.7

DEFINITION

Clofibrate is ethyl 2-(4-chlorophenoxy)-2-methylpropionate.

CHARACTERS

A clear, almost colourless liquid, very slightly soluble in water, miscible with alcohol.

IDENTIFICATION

A. Examine by infrared absorption spectrophotometry (*2.2.24*), comparing with the spectrum obtained with *clofibrate CRS*.

B. Dissolve 0.10 g in *methanol R* and dilute to 100.0 ml with the same solvent. Dilute 10.0 ml of the solution to 100.0 ml with *methanol R* (solution a). Examined between 250 nm and 350 nm (*2.2.25*), solution (a) shows two absorption maxima, at 280 nm and at 288 nm. The specific absorbances at the maxima are about 44 and 31, respectively. Dilute 10.0 ml of solution (a) to 100.0 ml with *methanol R*. Examined between 220 nm and 250 nm, the solution shows an absorption maximum at 226 nm. The specific absorbance at the maximum is about 460.

TESTS

Refractive index (*2.2.6*): 1.500 to 1.505.

Relative density (*2.2.5*): 1.138 to 1.147.

Acidity. To 1.0 g add 10 ml of *ethanol R* and 0.1 ml of *phenol red solution R*. Not more than 1.0 ml of *0.01 M sodium hydroxide* is required to change the colour of the indicator.

Volatile related substances. Examine by gas chromatography (*2.2.28*).

Test solution. To 10.0 g of the substance to be examined add a mixture of 10 ml of *dilute sodium hydroxide solution R* and 10 ml of *water R*. Shake, separate the lower (organic) layer, wash with 5 ml of *water R* and add the washings to the aqueous layer. Dry the organic layer with *anhydrous sodium sulphate R* and use as the test solution. Reserve the aqueous layer for the test for 4-chlorophenol.

Reference solution (a). Dissolve 0.12 g of the substance to be examined in *chloroform R* and dilute to 100.0 ml with the same solvent. Dilute 1.0 ml of the solution to 10.0 ml with *chloroform R.*

Reference solution (b). Dissolve 0.12 g of *methyl 2-(4-chlorophenoxy)-2-methylpropionate CRS* in the substance to be examined and dilute to 10.0 ml with the same solvent. Dilute 1.0 ml of the solution to 10.0 ml with the substance to be examined. Dilute 1.0 ml of this solution to 10.0 ml with the substance to be examined.

The chromatographic procedure may be carried out using:

- a column 1.5 m long and 4 mm in internal diameter packed with either: *silanised diatomaceous earth for gas chromatography R* (250 µm to 420 µm) impregnated with 30 per cent *m/m* of *poly(dimethyl)siloxane R*; or *silanised diatomaceous earth for gas chromatography R* (150 µm to 180 µm) impregnated with 10 per cent *m/m* of *poly(dimethyl)siloxane R,*
- *nitrogen for chromatography R* as the carrier gas,
- a flame-ionisation detector.

Maintain the temperature of the column at 185 °C. Inject 2 µl of each solution.

In the chromatogram obtained with the test solution, the sum of the areas of the peaks, except that corresponding to clofibrate, is not greater than ten times the area of the peak corresponding to clofibrate in the chromatogram obtained with reference solution (a) (0.1 per cent). In the chromatogram obtained with reference solution (b), measure from the baseline the height (*A*) of the peak corresponding to methyl 2-(4-chlorophenoxy)-2-methylpropionate and the height (*B*) of the lowest point of the curve separating this peak from the peak corresponding to clofibrate (see Figure 0318-1). The test is not valid unless *A* is equal to at least 30 per cent of the recorder-chart scale and *A* – *B* is greater than 75 per cent of *A.*

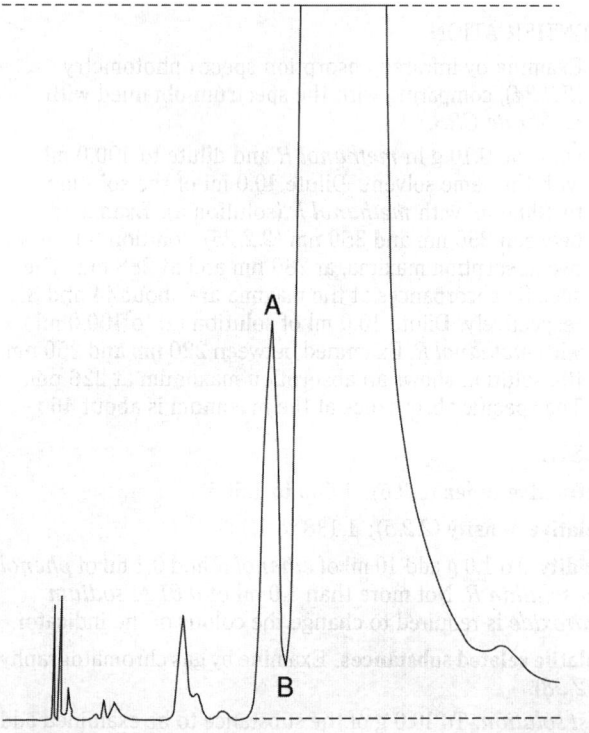

Figure 0318.-1. – *Typical chromatogram for the test for volatile related substances*

4-Chlorophenol. Examine by gas chromatography (*2.2.28*).

Test solution. Shake the aqueous layer reserved in the test for volatile related substances with two quantities, each of 5 ml, of *chloroform R* and discard the organic layers. Acidify the aqueous layer by the dropwise addition of *hydrochloric acid R.* Shake with three quantities, each of 3 ml, of *chloroform R.* Combine the organic layers and dilute to 10.0 ml with *chloroform R.*

Reference solution. Dissolve 0.25 g of *chlorophenol R* in *chloroform R* and dilute to 100.0 ml with the same solvent. Dilute 1.0 ml of the solution to 100.0 ml with *chloroform R.*

The chromatographic procedure may be carried out as described in the test for volatile related substances. Inject 2 µl of each solution.

The area of any peak corresponding to 4-chlorophenol in the chromatogram obtained with the test solution is not greater than the area of the peak corresponding to 4-chlorophenol in the chromatogram obtained with the reference solution (25 ppm).

01/2005:0997

CLOMIFENE CITRATE

Clomifeni citras

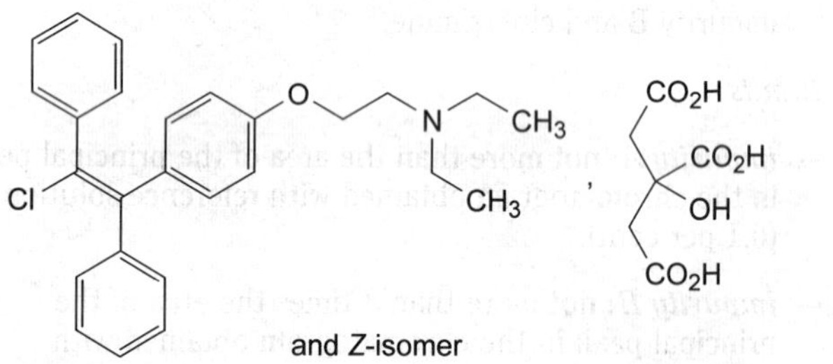

and *Z*-isomer

$C_{32}H_{36}ClNO_8$ M_r 598.1

DEFINITION

Clomifene citrate contains not less than 98.0 per cent and not more than the equivalent of 101.0 per cent of a mixture of the *E*- and *Z*-isomers of 2-[4-(2-chloro-1,2-diphenylethenyl)phenoxy]-*N,N*-diethylethanamine dihydrogen citrate, calculated with reference to the anhydrous substance.

CHARACTERS

A white or pale yellow, crystalline powder, slightly soluble in water, sparingly soluble in alcohol.

IDENTIFICATION

A. Examine by infrared absorption spectrophotometry (*2.2.24*), comparing with the spectrum obtained with *clomifene citrate CRS.* Examine the substances as discs prepared using *potassium bromide R.*

B. Dissolve about 5 mg in 5 ml of a mixture of 1 volume of *acetic anhydride R* and 5 volumes of *pyridine R* and heat in a water-bath. A deep red colour is produced.

TESTS

Prepare the solutions protected from light in brown-glass vessels. Ensure minimum exposure of the solutions to daylight until they are required for chromatography.

Related substances. Examine by liquid chromatography (*2.2.29*).

Test solution. Dissolve 12.5 mg of the substance to be examined in the mobile phase and dilute to 10.0 ml with the mobile phase.

Reference solution (a). Dissolve 12.5 mg of *clomifene citrate for performance test CRS* in the mobile phase and dilute to 10.0 ml with the mobile phase.

Reference solution (b). Dilute 1.0 ml of the test solution to 50.0 ml with the mobile phase.

The chromatographic procedure may be carried out using:

- a stainless steel column 0.25 m long and 4.6 mm internal diameter packed with *butylsilyl silica gel for chromatography R* (5 µm),
- as mobile phase at a flow rate of 1.2 ml/min a mixture prepared as follows: mix 400 ml of *acetonitrile R* with 600 ml of *water R* and add 8.0 ml of *diethylamine R*; adjust the the mixture to pH 6.2 by the addition of about 1 ml to 2 ml of *phosphoric acid R* taking care to reduce progressively the volume of each addition as the required pH is approached,
- as detector a spectrophotometer set at 233 nm.

Equilibrate the column with the mobile phase at a flow rate of 1.2 ml/min for about 1 h.

Adjust the sensitivity of the system so that the height of the principal peak in the chromatogram obtained with 10 µl of reference solution (b) is not less than 50 per cent of the full scale of the recorder.

Inject 10 µl of reference solution (a). Continue the chromatography for twice the retention time of the principal peak. Measure the height (*A*) above the base-line of the peak due to impurity A and the height (*B*) above the base-line of the lowest point of the curve separating this peak from the peak due to clomifene. The test is not valid unless *A* is greater than fifteen times *B* and the chromatogram obtained resembles the reference chromatogram. If necessary, adjust the concentration of acetonitrile in the mobile phase.

Inject separately 10 µl of the test solution and 10 µl of reference solution (b). Continue the chromatography for four times the retention time of the principal peak. In the chromatogram obtained with the test solution: the area of any peak due to impurity A is not greater than the area of the principal peak in the chromatogram obtained with reference solution (b) (2.0 per cent); the area of any other peak, apart from the principal peak, is not greater than half the area of the principal peak in the chromatogram obtained with reference solution (b) (1.0 per cent); the sum of the areas of all the peaks, apart from the principal peak, is not greater than 1.25 times the area of the principal peak in the chromatogram obtained with reference solution (b) (2.5 per cent). Disregard any peak with a retention time relative to the clomifene peak of 0.2 or less and any peak with an area less than 0.025 times the area of the principal peak in the chromatogram obtained with reference solution (b).

***Z*-isomer**: 30.0 per cent to 50.0 per cent, determined by liquid chromatography (*2.2.29*).

Test solution. Dissolve 25 mg of the substance to be examined in 25 ml of *0.1 M hydrochloric acid,* add 5 ml of *1 M sodium hydroxide* and shake with three quantities, each of 25 ml, of *ethanol-free chloroform R*. Wash the combined extracts with 10 ml of *water R*, dry over *anhydrous sodium sulphate R* and dilute to 100 ml with *ethanol-free chloroform R*. To 20 ml of the solution add 0.1 ml of *triethylamine R* and dilute to 100 ml with *hexane R*.

Reference solution. Dissolve 25 mg of *clomifene citrate CRS* in 25 ml of *0.1 M hydrochloric acid,* add 5 ml of *1 M sodium hydroxide* and shake with three quantities, each of 25 ml, of *ethanol-free chloroform R*. Wash the combined extracts with 10 ml of *water R*, dry over *anhydrous sodium sulphate R* and dilute to 100 ml with *ethanol-free chloroform R*. To 20 ml of the solution add 0.1 ml of *triethylamine R* and dilute to 100 ml with *hexane R*.

The chromatographic procedure may be carried out using:

- a stainless steel column 0.3 m long and 4 mm in internal diameter packed with *silica gel for chromatography R* (10 µm),
- as mobile phase at a flow rate of 2 ml/min a mixture of 1 volume of *triethylamine R*, 200 volumes of *ethanol-free chloroform R* and 800 volumes of *hexane R,*
- as detector a spectrophotometer set at 302 nm.

Equilibrate the column with the mobile phase for about 2 h. Inject 50 µl of the reference solution. The chromatogram obtained shows a peak due to the *E*-isomer just before a peak due to the *Z*-isomer. The test is not valid unless the resolution between the peaks corresponding to the *E*- and *Z*-isomers is at least 1.0. If necessary, adjust the relative proportions of ethanol-free chloroform and hexane in the mobile phase. Measure the area of the peak due to the *Z*-isomer in the chromatograms obtained with the test solution and the reference solution. Calculate the content of the *Z*-isomer as a percentage of the total clomifene citrate present using the declared content of *clomifene citrate CRS.*

Water (*2.5.12*). Not more than 1.0 per cent, determined on 1.000 g by the semi-micro determination of water.

ASSAY

Dissolve 0.500 g in 50 ml of *anhydrous acetic acid R*. Titrate with *0.1 M perchloric acid* determining the end-point potentiometrically (*2.2.20*).

1 ml of *0.1 M perchloric acid* is equivalent to 59.81 mg of $C_{32}H_{36}ClNO_8$.

STORAGE

Store protected from light.

IMPURITIES

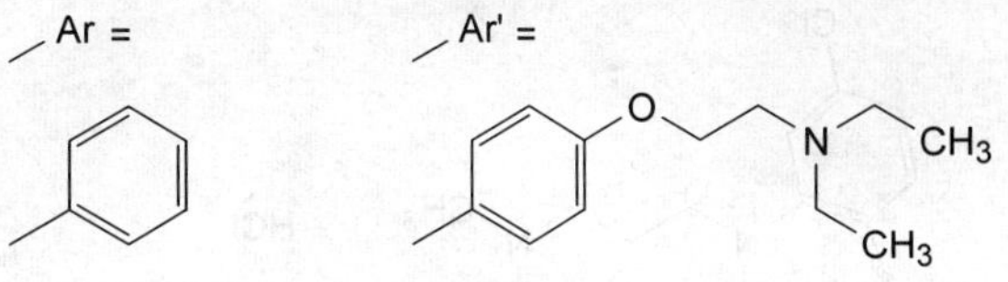

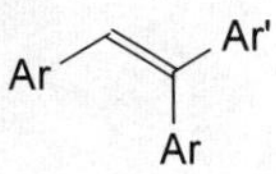

and Z-isomer

A. 2-[4-(1,2-diphenylethenyl)phenoxy]-*N*,*N*-diethylethanamine,

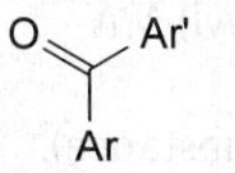

B. [4-[2-(diethylamino)ethoxy]phenyl]phenylmethanone,

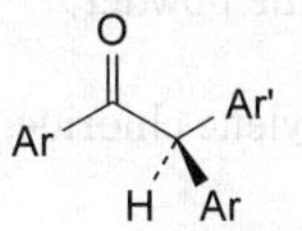

and enantiomer

C. (2*RS*)-2-[4-[2-(diethylamino)ethoxy]phenyl]-1,2-diphenylethanone,

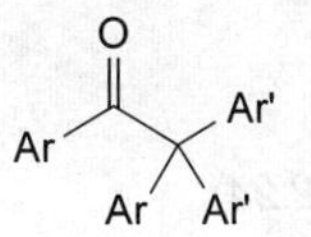

D. 2,2-bis[4-[2-(diethylamino)ethoxy]phenyl]-1,2-diphenylethanone,

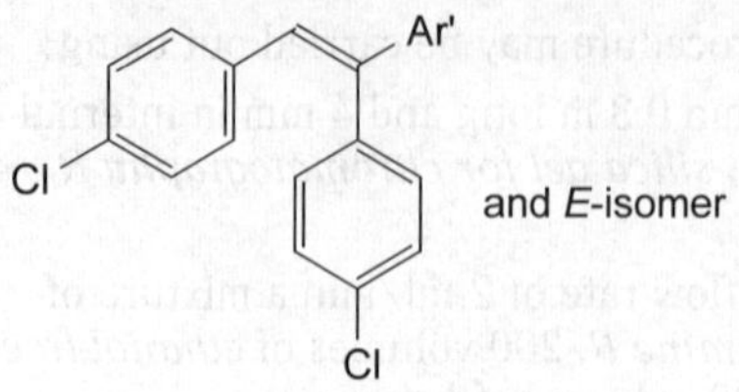

E. 2-[4-[1,2-bis(4-chlorophenyl)ethenyl]phenoxy]-*N*,*N*-diethylethanamine,

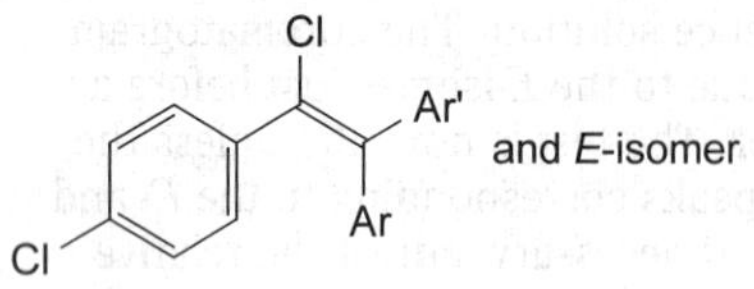

F. 2-[4-[2-chloro-2-(4-chlorophenyl)-1-phenylethenyl]phenoxy]-*N*,*N*-diethylethanamine,

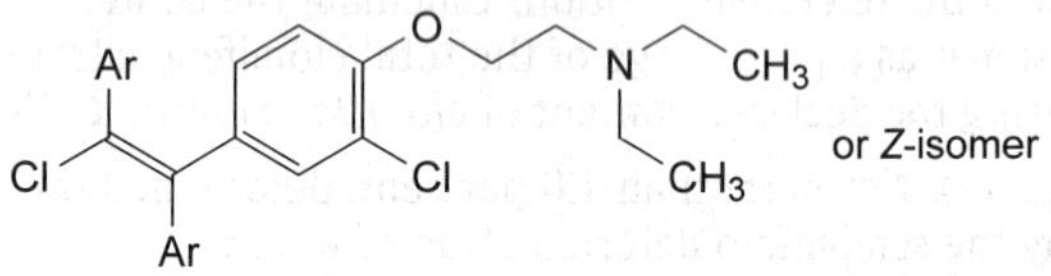

GH. 2-[2-chloro-4-(2-chloro-1,2-diphenylethenyl)phenoxy]-*N*,*N*-diethylethanamine (G. higher-melting point isomer; H. lower-melting point isomer).

01/2005:0889

CLOMIPRAMINE HYDROCHLORIDE

Clomipramini hydrochloridum

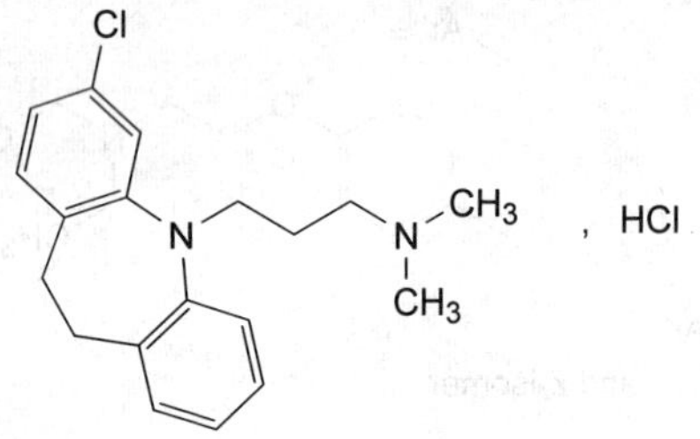

$C_{19}H_{24}Cl_2N_2$ M_r 351.3

DEFINITION

3-(3-Chloro-10,11-dihydro-5*H*-dibenzo[*b*,*f*]azepin-5-yl)-*N*,*N*-dimethylpropan-1-amine hydrochloride.

Content: 99.0 per cent to 101.0 per cent (dried substance).

CHARACTERS

Appearance: white or slightly yellow, crystalline powder, slightly hygroscopic.

Solubility: freely soluble in water and in methylene chloride, soluble in alcohol.

It shows polymorphism.

IDENTIFICATION

First identification: B, E.

Second identification: A, C, D, E.

A. Melting point (*2.2.14*): 191 °C to 195 °C.

B. Infrared absorption spectrophotometry (*2.2.24*).

Preparation: discs of *potassium bromide R*. The transmittance at about 2000 cm^{-1} (5 µm) is at least 65 per cent without compensation.

Comparison: *clomipramine hydrochloride CRS.*

C. Thin-layer chromatography (*2.2.27*). *Prepare the solutions immediately before use and protected from light.*

Test solution. Dissolve 20 mg of the substance to be examined in *methanol R* and dilute to 10 ml with the same solvent.

Reference solution. Dissolve 20 mg of *clomipramine hydrochloride CRS* in *methanol R* and dilute to 10 ml with the same solvent.

Plate: *TLC silica gel G plate R.*

Mobile phase: *concentrated ammonia R, acetone R, ethyl acetate R* (5:25:75 *V/V/V*).

Application: 5 µl.

Development: over a path of 15 cm.

Drying: in air.

Detection: spray with a 5 g/l solution of *potassium dichromate R* in a 20 per cent *V/V* solution of *sulphuric acid R*. Examine immediately.

Results: the principal spot in the chromatogram obtained with the test solution is similar in position, colour and size to the principal spot in the chromatogram obtained with the reference solution.

D. Dissolve about 5 mg in 2 ml of *nitric acid R*. An intense blue colour develops.

E. Dissolve about 50 mg in 5 ml of *water R* and add 1 ml of *dilute ammonia R1*. Mix, allow to stand for 5 min and filter. Acidify the filtrate with *dilute nitric acid R*. The solution gives reaction (a) of chlorides (*2.3.1*).

TESTS

Solution S. Dissolve 2.0 g in *carbon dioxide-free water R* and dilute to 20 ml with the same solvent.

Appearance of solution. Solution S is clear (*2.2.1*) and not more intensely coloured than reference solution Y_5 (*2.2.2, Method I*).

pH (*2.2.3*): 3.5 to 5.0 for solution S.

Related substances. Liquid chromatography (*2.2.29*). *Prepare the solutions immediately before use and protected from light.*

Test solution. Dissolve 20.0 mg of the substance to be examined in a mixture of 25 volumes of mobile phase B and 75 volumes of mobile phase A and dilute to 10.0 ml with the same mixture of mobile phases.

Reference solution (a). Dissolve 22.6 mg of *imipramine hydrochloride CRS,* 4.0 mg of *clomipramine impurity C CRS,* 4.0 mg of *clomipramine impurity D CRS* and 2.0 mg of *clomipramine impurity F CRS* in a mixture of 25 volumes of mobile phase B and 75 volumes of mobile phase A and dilute to 100.0 ml with the same mixture of mobile phases. Dilute 1.0 ml of this solution to 10.0 ml with a mixture of 25 volumes of mobile phase B and 75 volumes of mobile phase A.

Reference solution (b). Dilute 1.0 ml of the test solution to 100.0 ml with a mixture of 25 volumes of mobile phase B and 75 volumes of mobile phase A.

Reference solution (c). Dissolve 10.0 mg of *clomipramine hydrochloride CRS* and 3.0 mg of *clomipramine impurity C CRS* in a mixture of 25 volumes of mobile phase B and 75 volumes of mobile phase A and dilute to 20.0 ml with the same mixture of mobile phases. Dilute 1.0 ml of this solution to 10.0 ml with a mixture of 25 volumes of mobile phase B and 75 volumes of mobile phase A.

Column:

– *size*: l = 0.25 m, Ø = 4.6 mm,

- *stationary phase*: *cyanopropylsilyl silica gel for chromatography R* (5 μm),
- *temperature*: 30 °C.

Mobile phase:
- *mobile phase A*: dissolve 1.2 g of *sodium dihydrogen phosphate R* in *water R*, add 1.1 ml of *nonylamine R*, adjust to pH 3.0 with *phosphoric acid R* and dilute to 1000 ml with *water R*,
- *mobile phase B*: *acetonitrile R*.

Time (min)	Mobile phase A (per cent *V/V*)	Mobile phase B (per cent *V/V*)
0 - 10	75	25
10 - 20	75 → 65	25 → 35
20 - 32	65	35
32 - 34	65 → 75	35 → 25
34 - 44	75	25

Flow rate: 1.5 ml/min.

Detection: spectrophotometer at 254 nm.

Injection: 20 μl.

Relative retentions with reference to clomipramine (retention time = about 8 min): impurity A = about 0.5; impurity B = about 0.7; impurity C = about 0.9; impurity D = about 1.7; impurity E = about 2.5; impurity F = about 3.4; impurity G = about 4.3.

System suitability: reference solution (c):
- *resolution*: minimum 3.0 between the peaks due to clomipramine and to impurity C.

Limits:
- *impurity B*: not more than the area of the corresponding peak in the chromatogram obtained with reference solution (a) (1.0 per cent),
- *impurity C, D*: for each impurity, not more than the area of the corresponding peak in the chromatogram obtained with reference solution (a) (0.2 per cent),
- *impurity F*: not more than the area of the corresponding peak in the chromatogram obtained with reference solution (a) (0.1 per cent),
- *any other impurity*: not more than 0.1 times the area of the principal peak in the chromatogram obtained with reference solution (b) (0.1 per cent),
- *total of other impurities*: not more than 0.2 times the area of the principal peak in the chromatogram obtained with reference solution (b) (0.2 per cent),
- *total*: not more than the area of the principal peak in the chromatogram obtained with reference solution (b) (1.0 per cent),
- *disregard limit*: 0.01 times the area of the principal peak in the chromatogram obtained with reference solution (b) (0.01 per cent).

Heavy metals (*2.4.8*): maximum 20 ppm.

2.0 g complies with limit test C. Prepare the standard using 4 ml of *lead standard solution (10 ppm Pb) R*.

Loss on drying (*2.2.32*): maximum 0.5 per cent, determined on 1.000 g by drying in an oven at 100-105 °C.

Sulphated ash (*2.4.14*): maximum 0.1 per cent, determined on 1.0 g.

ASSAY

Dissolve 0.250 g in 50 ml of *alcohol R* and add 5.0 ml of *0.01 M hydrochloric acid*. Carry out a potentiometric titration (*2.2.20*), using *0.1 M sodium hydroxide*. Read the volume added between the 2 points of inflexion.

1 ml of *0.1 M sodium hydroxide* is equivalent to 35.13 mg of $C_{19}H_{24}Cl_2N_2$.

STORAGE

In an airtight container, protected from light.

IMPURITIES

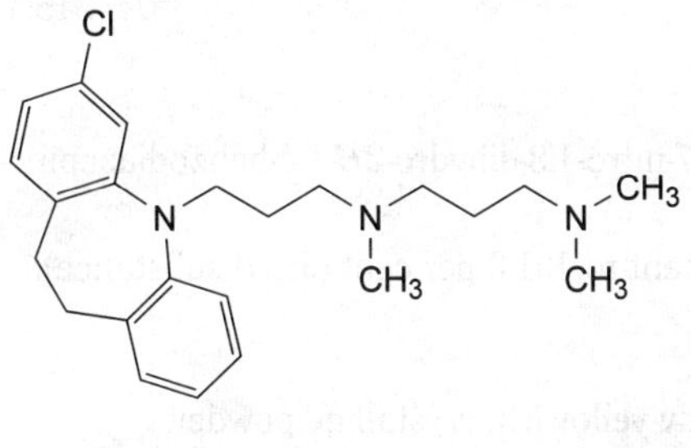

A. *N*-[3-(3-chloro-10,11-dihydro-5*H*-dibenzo[*b,f*]azepin-5-yl)propyl]-*N,N′,N′*-trimethylpropane-1,3-diamine,

B. imipramine,

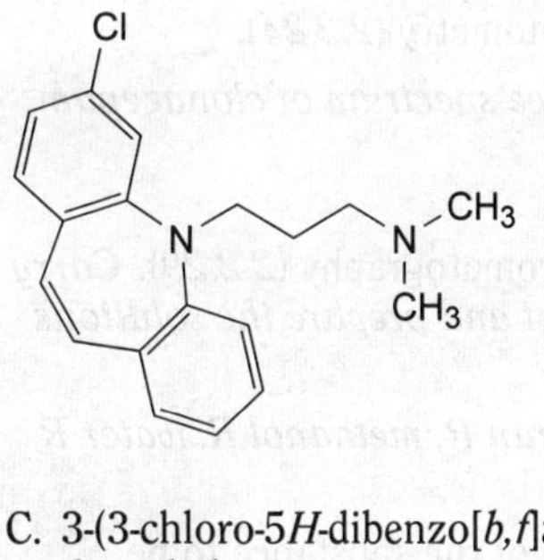

C. 3-(3-chloro-5*H*-dibenzo[*b,f*]azepin-5-yl)-*N,N*-dimethylpropan-1-amine,

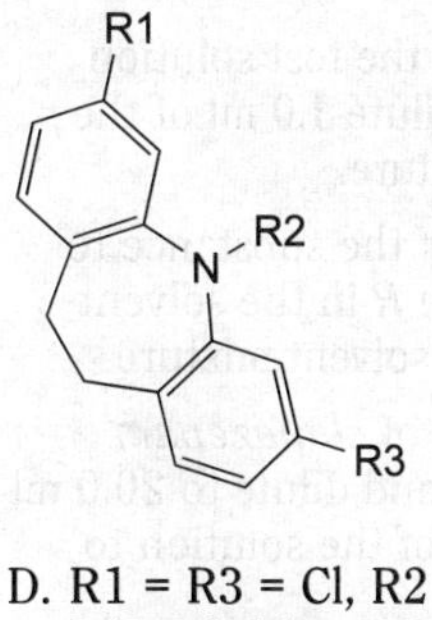

D. R1 = R3 = Cl, R2 = CH_2-CH_2-CH_2-$N(CH_3)_2$: 3-(3,7-dichloro-10,11-dihydro-5*H*-dibenzo[*b,f*]azepin-5-yl)-*N,N*-dimethylpropan-1-amine,

E. R1 = R2 = R3 = H: 10,11-dihydro-5*H*-dibenzo[*b,f*]azepine (iminodibenzyl),

F. R1 = Cl, R2 = R3 = H: 3-chloro-10,11-dihydro-5*H*-dibenzo[*b,f*]azepine,

G. R1 = Cl, R2 = CH_2-CH=CH_2, R3 = H: 3-chloro-5-(prop-2-enyl)-10,11-dihydro-5*H*-dibenzo[*b,f*]azepine.

01/2005:0890

CLONAZEPAM

Clonazepamum

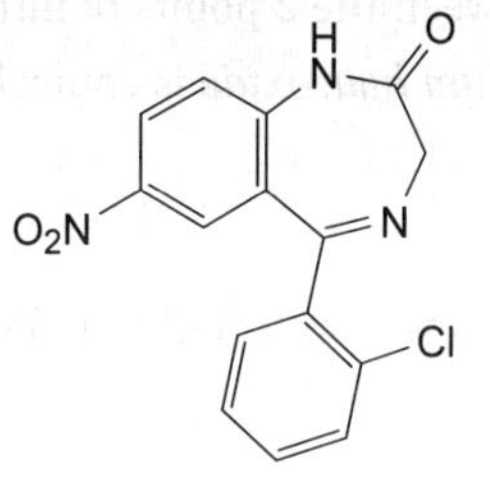

$C_{15}H_{10}ClN_3O_3$ M_r 315.7

DEFINITION

5-(2-Chlorophenyl)-7-nitro-1,3-dihydro-2*H*-1,4-benzodiazepin-2-one.

Content: 99.0 per cent to 101.0 per cent (dried substance).

CHARACTERS

Appearance: slightly yellowish, crystalline powder.

Solubility: practically insoluble in water, slightly soluble in alcohol and in methanol.

mp: about 239 °C.

IDENTIFICATION

Infrared absorption spectrophotometry (*2.2.24*).

Comparison: *Ph. Eur. reference spectrum of clonazepam.*

TESTS

Related substances. Liquid chromatography (*2.2.29*). *Carry out the test protected from light and prepare the solutions immediately before use.*

Solvent mixture: *tetrahydrofuran R, methanol R, water R* (10:42:48 *V/V/V*).

Test solution. Dissolve 0.100 g of the substance to be examined in *methanol R* and dilute to 20.0 ml with the same solvent. Dilute 1.0 ml to 10.0 ml with the solvent mixture.

Reference solution (a). Dilute 1.0 ml of the test solution to 100.0 ml with the solvent mixture. Dilute 1.0 ml of the solution to 10.0 ml with the solvent mixture.

Reference solution (b). Dissolve 5 mg of the substance to be examined and 5 mg of *flunitrazepam R* in the solvent mixture and dilute to 100.0 ml with the solvent mixture.

Reference solution (c). Dissolve 1.0 mg of *clonazepam impurity B CRS* in the solvent mixture and dilute to 20.0 ml with the solvent mixture. Dilute 1.0 ml of the solution to 100.0 ml with the solvent mixture.

Column:

- *size*: l = 0.15 m, Ø = 4.6 mm,
- *stationary phase*: *end-capped octylsilyl silica gel for chromatography R* (5 µm).

Mobile phase: mix 10 volumes of *tetrahydrofuran R*, 42 volumes of *methanol R* and 48 volumes of a 6.6 g/l solution of *ammonium phosphate R* previously adjusted to pH 8.0 with a 40 g/l solution of *sodium hydroxide R* or *dilute phosphoric acid R*.

Flow rate: 1.0 ml/min.

Detection: spectrophotometer at 254 nm.

Injection: 10 µl.

Run time: 3 times the retention time of clonazepam.

Relative retention with reference to clonazepam (retention time = about 7 min): impurity B = about 2.1; impurity A = about 2.4.

System suitability: reference solution (b):

- *resolution*: minimum 1.8 between the peaks due to flunitrazepam and to clonazepam.

Limits:

- *impurity A*: not more than the area of the principal peak in the chromatogram obtained with reference solution (a) (0.1 per cent),
- *impurity B*: not more than the area of the principal peak in the chromatogram obtained with reference solution (c) (0.1 per cent)
- *any other impurity*: for each impurity, not more than the area of the principal peak in the chromatogram obtained with reference solution (a) (0.1 per cent),
- *total*: not more than twice the area of the principal peak in the chromatogram obtained with reference solution (a) (0.2 per cent),
- *disregard limit*: 0.5 times the area of the principal peak in the chromatogram obtained with reference solution (a) (0.05 per cent).

Loss on drying (*2.2.32*): maximum 0.5 per cent, determined on 1.000 g by drying in an oven at 100-105 °C for 4 h.

Sulphated ash (*2.4.14*): maximum 0.1 per cent, determined on 1.0 g.

ASSAY

Dissolve 0.275 g in 50 ml of *acetic anhydride R*. Titrate with *0.1 M perchloric acid*, determining the end-point potentiometrically (*2.2.20*).

1 ml of *0.1 M perchloric acid* is equivalent to 31.57 mg of $C_{15}H_{10}ClN_3O_3$.

STORAGE

Protected from light.

IMPURITIES

Specified impurities: *A, B.*

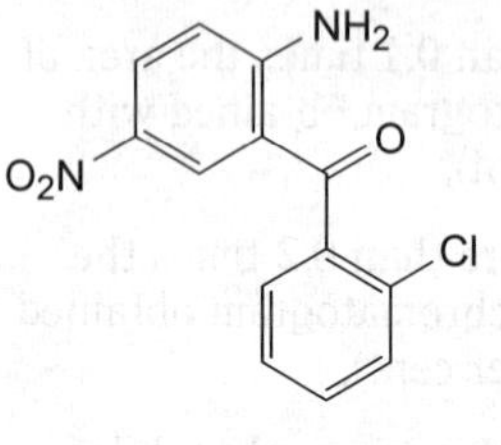

A. (2-amino-5-nitrophenyl)(2-chlorophenyl)methanone,

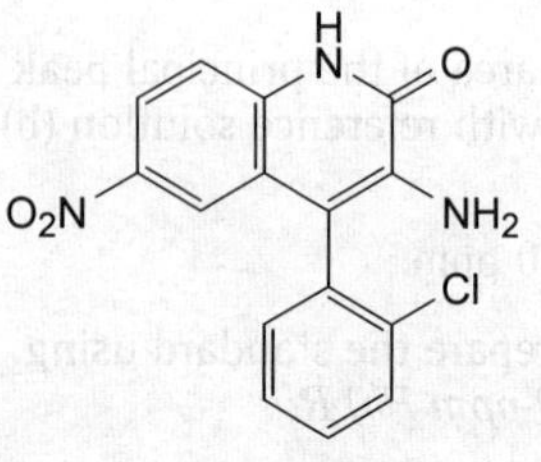

B. 3-amino-4-(2-chlorophenyl)-6-nitroquinolin-2(1*H*)-one.

01/2005:0477

CLONIDINE HYDROCHLORIDE

Clonidini hydrochloridum

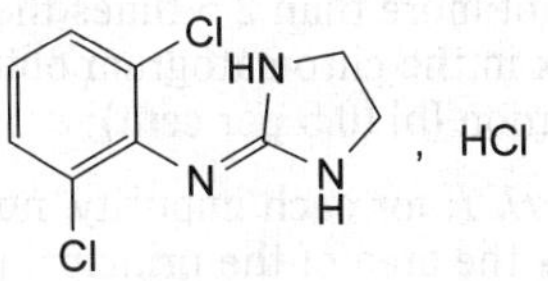

$C_9H_{10}Cl_3N_3$ M_r 266.6

DEFINITION

Clonidine hydrochloride contains not less than 98.5 per cent and not more than the equivalent of 101.0 per cent of 2,6-dichloro-*N*-(imidazolidin-2-ylidene)aniline, calculated with reference to the dried substance.

CHARACTERS

A white or almost white, crystalline powder, soluble in water and in ethanol.

IDENTIFICATION

First identification: B, D.

Second identification: A, C, D.

A. Dissolve 30.0 mg in *0.01 M hydrochloric acid* and dilute to 100.0 ml with the same acid. Examined between 245 nm and 350 nm (*2.2.25*), the solution shows two absorption maxima, at 272 nm and at 279 nm, and a point of inflexion at 265 nm. The specific absorbances at the maxima are about 18 and about 16, respectively.

B. Examine by infrared absorption spectrophotometry (*2.2.24*), comparing with the spectrum obtained with *clonidine hydrochloride CRS*.

C. Examine the chromatograms obtained in the test for related substances. The principal spot in the chromatogram obtained with test solution (b) is similar in position, colour and size to the principal spot in the chromatogram obtained with reference solution (a).

D. It gives reaction (a) of chlorides (*2.3.1*).

TESTS

Solution S. Dissolve 1.25 g in *carbon dioxide-free water R* and dilute to 25 ml with the same solvent.

Appearance of solution. Solution S is clear (*2.2.1*) and not more intensely coloured than reference solution Y_7 (*2.2.2, Method II*).

pH (*2.2.3*). The pH of solution S is 4.0 to 5.0.

Related substances. Examine by thin-layer chromatography (*2.2.27*), using *silica gel G R* as the coating substance.

Test solution (a). Dissolve 0.1 g of the substance to be examined in *methanol R* and dilute to 10 ml with the same solvent.

Test solution (b). Dilute 1 ml of test solution (a) to 10 ml with *methanol R*.

Reference solution (a). Dissolve 10 mg of *clonidine hydrochloride CRS* in *methanol R* and dilute to 10 ml with the same solvent.

Reference solution (b). Dilute 1 ml of test solution (a) to 10 ml with *methanol R*. Dilute 5 ml of this solution to 100 ml with *methanol R*.

Apply to the plate 10 µl of each solution. Shake a mixture of 10 volumes of *glacial acetic acid R*, 40 volumes of *butanol R* and 50 volumes of *water R*. Allow to separate. Filter the upper layer and use the filtrate as the mobile phase. Develop over a path of 15 cm. Allow the plate to dry in air and spray with *potassium iodobismuthate solution R2*. Allow the plate to dry in air for 1 h, spray again with *potassium iodobismuthate solution R2* and then immediately spray with a 50 g/l solution of *sodium nitrite R*. Any spot in the chromatogram obtained with test solution (a), apart from the principal spot, is not more intense than the spot in the chromatogram obtained with reference solution (b) (0.5 per cent).

Loss on drying (*2.2.32*). Not more than 0.5 per cent, determined on 1.000 g by drying in an oven at 100 °C to 105 °C.

Sulphated ash (*2.4.14*). Not more than 0.1 per cent, determined on 1.0 g.

ASSAY

Dissolve 0.200 g in 70 ml of *alcohol R*. Titrate with *0.1 M ethanolic sodium hydroxide* determining the end-point potentiometrically (*2.2.20*).

1 ml of *0.1 M sodium hydroxide* is equivalent to 26.66 mg of $C_9H_{10}Cl_3N_3$.

01/2005:1716

CLOSANTEL SODIUM DIHYDRATE FOR VETERINARY USE

Closantelum natricum dihydricum ad usum veterinarium

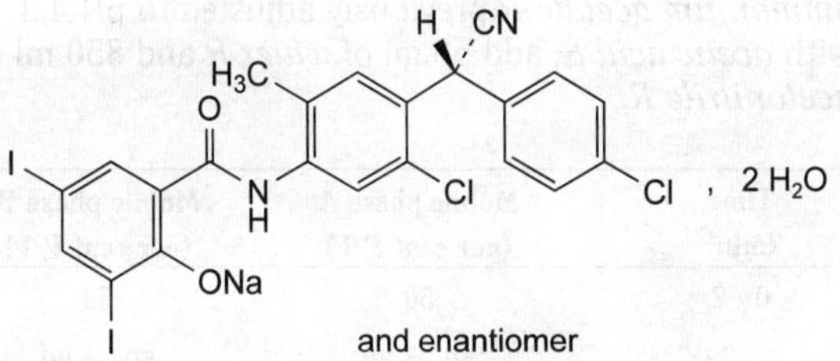

and enantiomer

$C_{22}H_{13}Cl_2I_2N_2NaO_2,2H_2O$ M_r 721

DEFINITION

N-[5-Chloro-4-[(*RS*)-(4-chlorophenyl)cyanomethyl]-2-methylphenyl]-2-hydroxy-3,5-diiodobenzamide sodium salt dihydrate.

Content: 98.5 per cent to 101.5 per cent (anhydrous substance).

CHARACTERS

Appearance: yellow powder, slightly hygroscopic.

Solubility: very slightly soluble in water, freely soluble in ethanol (96 per cent), soluble in methanol.

It shows polymorphism.

IDENTIFICATION

Infrared absorption spectrophotometry (*2.2.24*).

Preparation: discs without recrystallisation.

Comparison: *closantel sodium dihydrate CRS*.

TESTS

Appearance of solution. The solution is clear (*2.2.1*) and not more intensely coloured than reference solution GY_4 (*2.2.2, Method II*).

Dissolve 0.50 g in *ethanol (96 per cent) R* and dilute to 50 ml with the same solvent.

Monographs C

Related substances. Liquid chromatography (*2.2.29*). *Prepare the solutions immediately before use and protect from light.*

Test solution. Dissolve 0.100 g of the substance to be examined in *methanol R* and dilute to 10.0 ml with the same solvent.

Reference solution (a). Dissolve 10 mg of *closantel for system suitability CRS* (containing impurities A to J) in *methanol R* and dilute to 1.0 ml with the same solvent.

Reference solution (b). Dilute 1.0 ml of the test solution to 100.0 ml with *methanol R*. Dilute 5.0 ml of this solution to 25.0 ml with *methanol R*.

Column:

- *size*: *l* = 0.10 m, Ø = 4.6 mm,
- *stationary phase*: *base-deactivated octadecylsilyl silica gel for chromatography R* (3 µm),
- *temperature*: 35 °C.

Mobile phase:

- *mobile phase A*: to 100 ml of a 7.7 g/l solution of *ammonium acetate R* previously adjusted to pH 4.3 with *acetic acid R*, add 50 ml of *acetonitrile R* and 850 ml of *water R*,
- *mobile phase B*: to 100 ml of a 7.7 g/l solution of *ammonium acetate R* previously adjusted to pH 4.3 with *acetic acid R*, add 50 ml of *water R* and 850 ml of *acetonitrile R*,

Time (min)	Mobile phase A (per cent *V/V*)	Mobile phase B (per cent *V/V*)
0 - 2	50	50
2 - 22	50 → 20	50 → 80
22 - 27	20	80
27 - 28	20 → 50	80 → 50
28 - 32	50	50

Flow rate: 1.5 ml/min.

Detection: spectrophotometer at 240 nm.

Injection: 10 µl.

Relative retention with reference to closantel (retention time = about 16 min): impurity A = about 0.07; impurity B = about 0.48; impurity C = about 0.62; impurity D = about 0.65; impurity E = about 0.82; impurity F = about 0.89; impurity G = about 0.93; impurity H = about 1.13; impurity I = about 1.16; impurity J = about 1.55.

System suitability: reference solution (a):

- *resolution*: baseline separation between the peaks due to impurity G and closantel,
- the chromatogram obtained is similar to the chromatogram supplied with *closantel for system suitability CRS*.

Limits:

- *correction factors*: for the calculation of contents, multiply the peak areas of the following impurities by the corresponding correction factor: impurity A = 1.5; impurity B = 1.3;
- *impurity G*: not more than 2.5 times the area of the principal peak in the chromatogram obtained with reference solution (b) (0.5 per cent);
- *impurities F, H, I*: for each impurity, not more than 1.5 times the area of the principal peak in the chromatogram obtained with reference solution (b) (0.3 per cent);
- *impurities A, B, C, D, E, J*: for each impurity, not more than the area of the principal peak in the chromatogram obtained with reference solution (b) (0.2 per cent);
- *any other impurity*: for each impurity, not more than the area of the principal peak in the chromatogram obtained with reference solution (b) (0.2 per cent);
- *total*: not more than 7.5 times the area of the principal peak in the chromatogram obtained with reference solution (b) (1.5 per cent);
- *disregard limit*: 0.25 times the area of the principal peak in the chromatogram obtained with reference solution (b) (0.05 per cent).

Water (*2.5.12*): 4.8 per cent to 5.8 per cent, determined on 0.250 g.

Use a mixture of 1 volume of *dimethylformamide R* and 4 volumes of *methanol R* as the solvent.

ASSAY

Dissolve 0.500 g in 50 ml of a mixture of 1 volume of *anhydrous acetic acid R* and 7 volumes of *methyl ethyl ketone R*. Titrate with *0.1 M perchloric acid*, determining the end-point potentiometrically (*2.2.20*).

1 ml of *0.1 M perchloric acid* is equivalent to 68.5 mg of $C_{22}H_{13}Cl_2I_2N_2NaO_2$.

STORAGE

In an airtight container, protected from light.

IMPURITIES

Specified impurities: A, B, C, D, E, F, G, H, I, J.

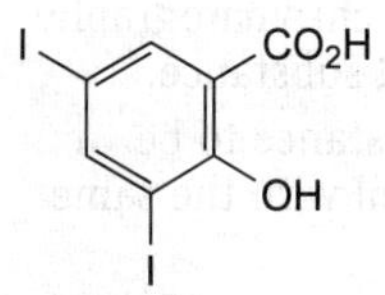

A. 2-hydroxy-3,5-diiodobenzoic acid,

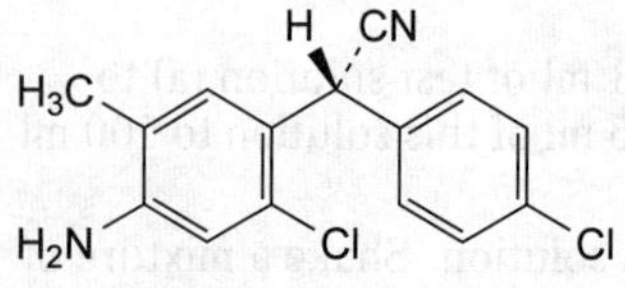

B. (2*RS*)-(4-amino-2-chloro-5-methylphenyl)(4-chlorophenyl)ethanenitrile,

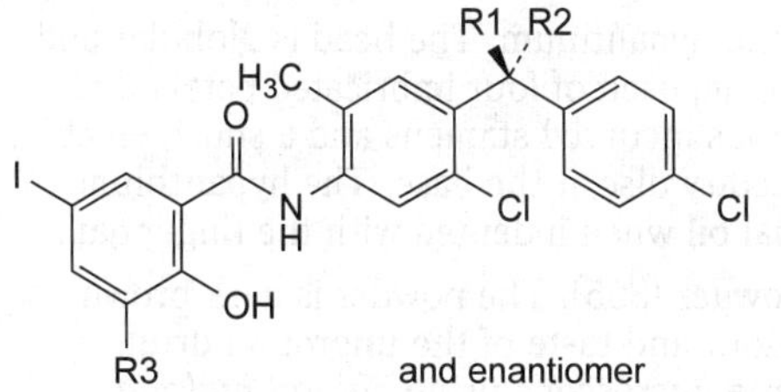

C. R1 = H, R2 = CO_2H, R3 = I: (2*RS*)-[2-chloro-4-[(2-hydroxy-3,5-diiodobenzoyl)amino]-5-methylphenyl](4-chlorophenyl)acetic acid,

D. R1 = H, R2 = $CONH_2$, R3 = I: *N*-[4-[(1*RS*)-2-amino-1-(4-chlorophenyl)-2-oxoethyl]-5-chloro-2-methylphenyl]-2-hydroxy-3,5-diiodobenzamide,

E. R1 = H, R2 = CN, R3 = Cl: 3-chloro-*N*-[5-chloro-4-[(*RS*)-(4-chlorophenyl)cyanomethyl]-2-methylphenyl]-2-hydroxy-5-iodobenzamide,

F. R1 + R2 = O, R3 = I: *N*-[5-chloro-4-(4-chlorobenzoyl)-2-methylphenyl]-2-hydroxy-3,5-diiodobenzamide,

G. R1 = H, R2 = C(=NH)OCH_3, R3 = I: methyl (2*RS*)-2-[2-chloro-4-[(2-hydroxy-3,5-diiodobenzoyl)amino]-5-methylphenyl]-2-(4-chlorophenyl)acetimidate,

H. R1 = H, R2 = CO-OCH_3, R3 = I: methyl (2*RS*)-[2-chloro-4-[(2-hydroxy-3,5-diiodobenzoyl)amino]-5-methylphenyl](4-chlorophenyl)acetate,

I. R1 = R3 = H, R2 = CN: *N*-[5-chloro-4-[(*RS*)-(4-chlorophenyl)cyanomethyl]-2-methylphenyl]-2-hydroxy-5-iodobenzamide,

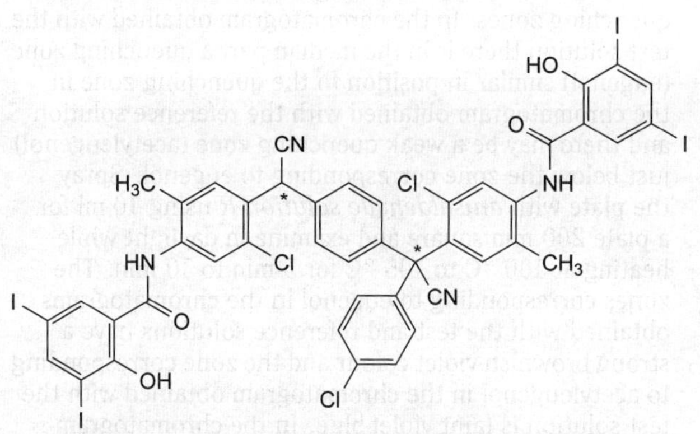

J. *N*-[5-chloro-4-[[4-[[2-chloro-4-[(2-hydroxy-3,5-diiodobenzoyl)amino]-5-methylphenyl]cyanomethyl]phenyl](4-chlorophenyl)cyanomethyl]-2-methylphenyl]-2-hydroxy-3,5-diiodobenzamide.

01/2005:0757

CLOTRIMAZOLE

Clotrimazolum

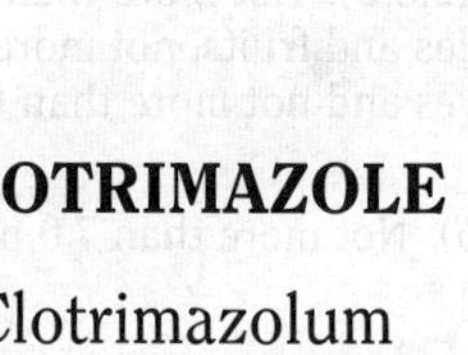

$C_{22}H_{17}ClN_2$ M_r 344.8

DEFINITION

Clotrimazole contains not less than 98.5 per cent and not more than the equivalent of 100.5 per cent of 1-[(2-chlorophenyl)diphenylmethyl]-1*H*-imidazole, calculated with reference to the dried substance.

CHARACTERS

A white or pale yellow, crystalline powder, practically insoluble in water, soluble in alcohol and in methylene chloride.

IDENTIFICATION

First identification: B.

Second identification: A, C, D.

A. Melting point (*2.2.14*): 141 °C to 145 °C.

B. Examine by infrared absorption spectrophotometry (*2.2.24*), comparing with the spectrum obtained with *clotrimazole CRS*.

C. Examine before spraying in ultraviolet light at 254 nm, the chromatograms obtained in the test for (2-chlorophenyl)diphenylmethanol. The principal spot in the chromatogram obtained with test solution (b) is similar in position and size to the principal spot in the chromatogram obtained with reference solution (a).

D. Dissolve about 10 mg in 3 ml of *sulphuric acid R*. The solution is pale yellow. Add 10 mg of *mercuric oxide R* and 20 mg of *sodium nitrite R*. Allow to stand with occasional shaking. An orange colour develops, becoming orange-brown.

TESTS

Appearance of solution. Dissolve 1.25 g in *alcohol R* and dilute to 25 ml with the same solvent. The solution is clear (*2.2.1*) and not more intensely coloured than reference solution BY_6 (*2.2.2, Method II*).

(2-Chlorophenyl)diphenylmethanol. Examine by thin-layer chromatography (*2.2.27*), using *silica gel GF_{254} R* as the coating substance.

Test solution (a). Dissolve 0.50 g of the substance to be examined in *alcohol R* and dilute to 5 ml with the same solvent.

Test solution (b). Dilute 1 ml of test solution (a) to 10 ml with *alcohol R*.

Reference solution (a). Dissolve 50 mg of *clotrimazole CRS* in *alcohol R* and dilute to 5 ml with the same solvent.

Reference solution (b). Dissolve 10 mg of *(2-chlorophenyl)diphenylmethanol CRS* in *alcohol R* and dilute to 5 ml with the same solvent. Dilute 1 ml of the solution to 10 ml with *alcohol R*.

Apply separately to the plate 10 µl of each solution. Develop over a path of 15 cm using a mixture of 0.5 volumes of *concentrated ammonia R1*, 10 volumes of *propanol R* and 90 volumes of *toluene R*. Allow the plate to dry in air. Spray with a 10 per cent *V/V* solution of *sulphuric acid R* in *alcohol R* and heat at 100 °C to 105 °C for 30 min. Any spot corresponding to (2-chlorophenyl)diphenylmethanol in the chromatogram obtained with test solution (a) is not more intense than the spot in the chromatogram obtained with reference solution (b) (0.2 per cent).

Imidazole. Examine by thin-layer chromatography (*2.2.27*), using *silica gel G R* as the coating substance.

Test solution. Dissolve 0.50 g of the substance to be examined in *alcohol R* and dilute to 10 ml with the same solvent.

Monographs C

Reference solution. Dissolve 10 mg of *imidazole R* in *alcohol R* and dilute to 10 ml with the same solvent. Dilute 1 ml of the solution to 10 ml with *alcohol R*.

Apply separately to the plate 10 µl of each solution. Develop over a path of 15 cm using a mixture of 0.5 volumes of *concentrated ammonia R1*, 10 volumes of *propanol R* and 90 volumes of *toluene R*. Allow the plate to dry in air. At the bottom of a chromatography tank, place an evaporating dish containing a mixture of 1 volume of *hydrochloric acid R1*, 1 volume of *water R* and 2 volumes of a 15 g/l solution of *potassium permanganate R*, close the tank and allow to stand for 15 min. Place the dried plate in the tank and close the tank. Leave the plate in contact with the chlorine vapour for 5 min. Withdraw the plate and place it in a current of cold air until the excess of chlorine is removed and an area of coating below the points of application does not give a blue colour with a drop of *potassium iodide and starch solution R*. Spray with *potassium iodide and starch solution R*. Any spot corresponding to imidazole in the chromatogram obtained with the test solution is not more intense than the spot in the chromatogram obtained with the reference solution (0.2 per cent).

Loss on drying (*2.2.32*). Not more than 0.5 per cent, determined on 1.000 g by drying in an oven at 100 °C to 105 °C.

Sulphated ash (*2.4.14*). Not more than 0.1 per cent, determined on 1.0 g.

ASSAY

Dissolve 0.300 g in 80 ml of *anhydrous acetic acid R*. Titrate with *0.1 M perchloric acid* using 0.3 ml of *naphtholbenzein solution R* as indicator until the colour changes from brownish-yellow to green.

1 ml of *0.1 M perchloric acid* is equivalent to 34.48 mg of $C_{22}H_{17}ClN_2$.

STORAGE

Store protected from light.

01/2005:0376

CLOVE

Caryophylli flos

DEFINITION

Clove consists of the whole flower buds of *Syzygium aromaticum* (L.) Merill et L. M. Perry (*Eugenia caryophyllus* (C. Spreng.) Bull. et Harr.) dried until they become reddish-brown. It contains not less than 150 ml/kg of essential oil.

CHARACTERS

Clove has a characteristic, aromatic odour.

It has the macroscopic and microscopic characters described under identification tests A and B.

IDENTIFICATION

A. The flower bud is reddish-brown and consists of a quadrangular stalked portion, the hypanthium, 10 mm to 12 mm long and 2 mm to 3 mm in diameter, surmounted by four divergent lobes of sepals which surround a globular head 4 mm to 6 mm in diameter. A bilocular ovary containing numerous ovules is situated in the upper part of the hypanthium. The head is globular and dome-shaped, composed of four imbricated petals that enclose numerous incurved stamens and a short, erect style with a nectary disc at the base. The hypanthium exudes essential oil when indented with the finger-nail.

B. Reduce to a powder (355). The powder is dark brown and has the odour and taste of the unground drug. Examine under a microscope using *chloral hydrate solution R*. The powder shows the following diagnostic characters: fragments of the hypanthium showing the epidermis and underlying parenchyma containing large oil glands; short fibres occurring singly or in small groups, with thickened, lignified walls and few pits; abundant fragments of parenchyma containing cluster crystals of calcium oxalate; numerous triangular pollen grains about 15 µm in diameter with three pores in the angles. Starch granules are absent.

C. Examine by thin-layer chromatography (*2.2.27*), using *silica gel* GF_{254} *R* as the coating substance.

Test solution. Shake 0.1 g of the powdered drug (500) with 2 ml of *methylene chloride R* for 15 min. Filter and carefully evaporate the filtrate to dryness on a water-bath. Dissolve the residue in 2 ml of *toluene R*.

Reference solution. Dissolve 20 µl of *eugenol R* in 2 ml of *toluene R*.

Apply to the plate as bands 20 mm by 3 mm, 10 µl of the reference solution and 20 µl of the test solution. Develop in an unsaturated tank over a path of 10 cm using *toluene R*. Allow the plate to stand for 5 min and develop again in the same manner. Allow the plate to dry in air, examine in ultraviolet light at 254 nm and mark the quenching zones. In the chromatogram obtained with the test solution there is in the median part a quenching zone (eugenol) similar in position to the quenching zone in the chromatogram obtained with the reference solution and there may be a weak quenching zone (acetyleugenol) just below the zone corresponding to eugenol. Spray the plate with *anisaldehyde solution R* using 10 ml for a plate 200 mm square and examine in daylight while heating at 100 °C to 105 °C for 5 min to 10 min. The zones corresponding to eugenol in the chromatograms obtained with the test and reference solutions have a strong brownish-violet colour and the zone corresponding to acetyleugenol in the chromatogram obtained with the test solution is faint violet-blue. In the chromatogram obtained with the test solution there are other coloured zones, particularly a faint red zone in the lower part and a reddish-violet zone (caryophyllene) in the upper part.

TESTS

Foreign matter (*2.8.2*). Not more than 6 per cent of peduncles, petioles and fruits, not more than 2 per cent of deteriorated cloves and not more than 0.5 per cent of other foreign matter.

Total ash (*2.4.16*). Not more than 7.0 per cent.

ASSAY

Carry out the determination of essential oils in vegetable drugs (*2.8.12*). Use a 250 ml flask, 100 ml of *water R* as the distillation liquid and 0.50 ml of *xylene R* in the graduated tube. Grind 5.0 g of the drug with 5.0 g of *diatomaceous earth R* to form a fine, homogeneous powder and proceed immediately with the determination using 4.0 g of the mixture. Distil at a rate of 2.5 ml/min to 3.5 ml/min for 2 h.

STORAGE

Store protected from light.

01/2005:1091

CLOVE OIL

Caryophylli floris aetheroleum

DEFINITION

Clove oil is obtained by steam distillation from the dried flower buds of *Syzygium aromaticum* (L.) Merill et L. M. Perry (*Eugenia caryophyllus* C. Spreng. Bull. et Harr.).

CHARACTERS

A clear, yellow liquid which becomes brown when exposed to air, miscible with methylene chloride, toluene and fatty oils.

IDENTIFICATION

First identification: B,

Second identification: A.

A. Examine by thin-layer chromatography (*2.2.27*) using a suitable silica gel with a fluorescent indicator having an optimal intensity at 254 nm as the coating substance.

Test solution. Dissolve 20 µl of the substance to be examined in 2.0 ml of *toluene R*.

Reference solution. Dissolve 15 µl of *eugenol R* and 15 µl of *acetyleugenol R* in 2.0 ml of *toluene R*.

Apply separately to the plate, as bands, 20 µl of the test solution and 15 µl of the reference solution. Develop in an unsaturated tank over a path of 10 cm using *toluene R*. Allow the plate to stand for 5 min and develop again in the same manner. Allow the plate to dry in air, examine in ultraviolet light at 254 nm and mark the quenching zones. The chromatogram obtained with the test solution shows in the medium part a quenching zone (eugenol) which corresponds in position to the quenching zone in the chromatogram obtained with the reference solution; there is a weak quenching zone (acetyleugenol) just below the quenching zone of eugenol which corresponds in position to the zone of acetyleugenol in the chromatogram obtained with the reference solution. Spray the plate with *anisaldehyde solution R* and examine in daylight while heating at 100 °C to 105 °C for 5 to 10 min. The zones corresponding to eugenol in the chromatogram obtained with the test and reference solutions have a strong brownish-violet colour and the zone corresponding to acetyleugenol in the chromatogram obtained with the test solution is faint violet-blue. In the chromatogram obtained with the test solution there are other coloured zones particularly a faint red zone in the lower part and a reddish-violet zone (β-caryophyllene) in the upper part.

B. Examine the chromatograms obtained in the test for chromatographic profile. The chromatogram obtained with the test solution shows three main peaks similar in retention time to the three peaks obtained with the reference solution.

TESTS

Relative density (*2.2.5*): 1.030 to 1.063.

Refractive index (*2.2.6*): 1.528 to 1.537.

Angle of optical rotation (*2.2.7*): 0° to −2°.

Fatty oils and resinified essential oils (*2.8.7*). It complies with the test for fatty oils and resinified oils.

Solubility in alcohol (*2.8.10*). 1.0 ml is soluble in 2.0 ml or more of *alcohol (70 per cent V/V) R*.

Chromatographic profile. Examine by gas chromatography (*2.2.28*).

Test solution. Dissolve 0.2 g of the substance to be examined in 10 g of *hexane R*.

Reference solution. Dissolve 7 mg of *β-caryophyllene R*, 80 mg of *eugenol R* and 4 mg of *acetyleugenol R* in 10 g of *hexane R*.

The chromatographic procedure may be carried out using:

- a fused silica capillary column 60 m long and about 0.25 mm in internal diameter, coated with *macrogol 20 000 R*,
- *helium for chromatography R* as the carrier gas at a flow rate of 1.5 ml per min,
- a flame-ionisation detector,
- a split ratio of 1/100,

maintaining the temperature of the column at 60 °C for 8 min, then raising the temperature at a rate of 3 °C per min to 180 °C and maintaining at 180 °C for 5 min and maintaining the temperature of the injection port and that of the detector at 270 °C.

Inject about 1.0 µl of the reference solution. Identify the eluted components following the order indicated in the composition of the reference solution. Record the retention times of these substances.

The test is not valid unless: the number of theoretical plates is at least 30 000, calculated from the β-caryophyllene peak at 110 °C and the resolution between the peak corresponding to eugenol and that corresponding to acetyleugenol is at least 1.5.

Inject about 1.0 µl of the substance to be examined. Using the retention times determined from the chromatogram obtained with the reference solution, locate the components of the reference solution on the chromatogram obtained with the test solution. Disregard the peak due to the solvent.

Determine the percentage content of each of the three components by the normalisation procedure. The contents are within the following ranges:

- *β-caryophyllene*: 5.0 per cent to 14.0 per cent,
- *eugenol*: 75.0 per cent to 88.0 per cent,
- *acetyleugenol*: 4.0 per cent to 15.0 per cent.

STORAGE

Store in a well-filled, airtight container, protected from light and heat.

01/2005:0661

CLOXACILLIN SODIUM

Cloxacillinum natricum

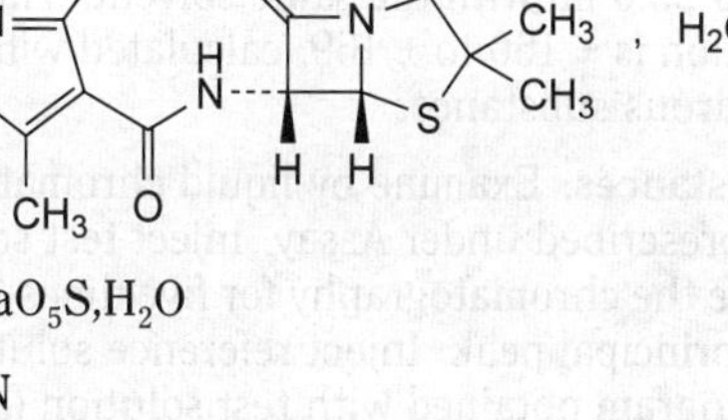

$C_{19}H_{17}ClN_3NaO_5S,H_2O$ M_r 475.9

DEFINITION

Cloxacillin sodium contains not less than 95.0 per cent and not more than the equivalent of 101.0 per cent of sodium (2*S*,5*R*,6*R*)-6-[[[3-(2-chlorophenyl)-5-

methylisoxazol-4-yl]carbonyl]amino]-3,3-dimethyl-7-oxo-4-thia-1-azabicyclo[3.2.0]heptane-2-carboxylate, calculated with reference to the anhydrous substance.

CHARACTERS

A white or almost white, crystalline powder, hygroscopic, freely soluble in water and in methanol, soluble in alcohol.

IDENTIFICATION

First identification: A, D.

Second identification: B, C, D.

A. Examine by infrared absorption spectrophotometry (*2.2.24*), comparing with the spectrum obtained with *cloxacillin sodium CRS*. Examine the substances prepared as discs.

B. Examine by thin-layer chromatography (*2.2.27*), using *silanised silica gel H R* as the coating substance.

Test solution. Dissolve 25 mg of the substance to be examined in 5 ml of *water R*.

Reference solution (a). Dissolve 25 mg of *cloxacillin sodium CRS* in 5 ml of *water R*.

Reference solution (b). Dissolve 25 mg of each of *cloxacillin sodium CRS, dicloxacillin sodium CRS* and *flucloxacillin sodium CRS* in 5 ml of *water R*.

Apply separately to the plate 1 µl of each solution. Develop over a path of 15 cm using a mixture of 30 volumes of *acetone R* and 70 volumes of a 154 g/l solution of *ammonium acetate R*, adjusted to pH 5.0 with *glacial acetic acid R*. Allow the plate to dry in air and expose it to iodine vapour until the spots appear. Examine in daylight. The principal spot in the chromatogram obtained with the test solution is similar in position, colour and size to the principal spot in the chromatogram obtained with reference solution (a). The test is not valid unless the chromatogram obtained with reference solution (b) shows three clearly separated spots.

C. Place about 2 mg in a test-tube about 150 mm long and 15 mm in diameter. Moisten with 0.05 ml of *water R* and add 2 ml of *sulphuric acid-formaldehyde reagent R*. Mix the contents of the tube by swirling; the colour of the solution is slightly greenish-yellow. Place the test-tube in a water-bath for 1 min; the solution becomes yellow.

D. It gives reaction (a) of sodium (*2.3.1*).

TESTS

Solution S. Dissolve 2.50 g in *carbon dioxide-free water R* and dilute to 25.0 ml with the same solvent.

Appearance of solution. Solution S is clear (*2.2.1*). The absorbance (*2.2.25*) of solution S measured at 430 nm is not greater than 0.04.

pH (*2.2.3*). The pH of solution S is 5.0 to 7.0.

Specific optical rotation (*2.2.7*). Dissolve 0.250 g in *water R* and dilute to 25.0 ml with the same solvent. The specific optical rotation is + 160 to + 169, calculated with reference to the anhydrous substance.

Related substances. Examine by liquid chromatography (*2.2.29*) as prescribed under Assay. Inject test solution (a) and continue the chromatography for five times the retention time of the principal peak. Inject reference solution (b). In the chromatogram obtained with test solution (a): the area of any peak, apart from the principal peak, is not greater than the area of the principal peak in the chromatogram obtained with reference solution (b) (1 per cent); the sum of the areas of all the peaks, apart from the principal peak, is not greater than five times the area of the principal peak in the chromatogram obtained with reference solution (b) (5 per cent). Disregard any peak with an area less than 0.05 times the area of the principal peak in the chromatogram obtained with reference solution (b).

***N,N*-Dimethylaniline** (*2.4.26, Method B*). Not more than 20 ppm.

2-Ethylhexanoic acid (*2.4.28*). Not more than 0.8 per cent *m/m*.

Water (*2.5.12*): 3.0 per cent to 4.5 per cent, determined on 0.300 g by the semi-micro determination of water.

Bacterial endotoxins (*2.6.14*): less than 0.40 IU/mg, if intended for use in the manufacture of parenteral dosage forms without a further appropriate procedure for the removal of bacterial endotoxins.

ASSAY

Examine by liquid chromatography (*2.2.29*).

Test solution (a). Dissolve 50.0 mg of the substance to be examined in the mobile phase and dilute to 50.0 ml with the mobile phase.

Test solution (b). Dilute 5.0 ml of test solution (a) to 50.0 ml with the mobile phase.

Reference solution (a). Dissolve 50.0 mg of *cloxacillin sodium CRS* in the mobile phase and dilute to 50.0 ml with the mobile phase. Dilute 5.0 ml of the solution to 50.0 ml with the mobile phase.

Reference solution (b). Dilute 5.0 ml of test solution (b) to 50.0 ml with the mobile phase.

Reference solution (c). Dissolve 5 mg of *flucloxacillin sodium CRS* and 5 mg of *cloxacillin sodium CRS* in the mobile phase and dilute to 50.0 ml with the mobile phase.

The chromatographic procedure may be carried out using:

- a stainless steel column 0.25 m long and 4 mm in internal diameter packed with *octadecylsilyl silica gel for chromatography R* (5 µm),
- as mobile phase at a flow rate of 1.0 ml/min a mixture of 25 volumes of *acetonitrile R* and 75 volumes of a 2.7 g/l solution of *potassium dihydrogen phosphate R* adjusted to pH 5.0 with *dilute sodium hydroxide solution R*,
- as detector a spectrophotometer set at 225 nm,
- a 20 µl loop injector.

Inject reference solution (c). Adjust the sensitivity of the system so that the heights of the principal peaks in the chromatogram obtained are at least 50 per cent of the full scale of the recorder. The test is not valid unless the resolution between the first peak (cloxacillin) and the second peak (flucloxacillin) is at least 2.5. Inject reference solution (a) six times. The test is not valid unless the relative standard deviation of the peak area for cloxacillin is at most 1.0 per cent. Inject alternately test solution (b) and reference solution (a).

STORAGE

Store in an airtight container, at a temperature not exceeding 25 °C. If the substance is sterile, store in a sterile, airtight, tamper-proof container.

LABELLING

The label states, where applicable, that the substance is free from bacterial endotoxins.

IMPURITIES

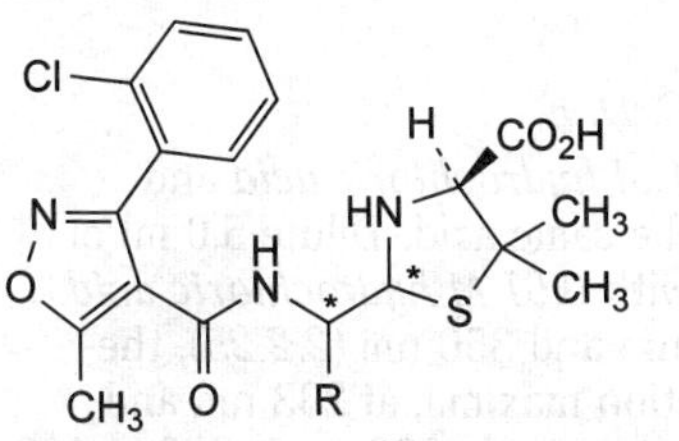

A. R = CO_2H: (4*S*)-2-[carboxy[[[3-(2-chlorophenyl)-5-methylisoxazol-4-yl]carbonyl]amino]methyl]-5,5-dimethylthiazolidine-4-carboxylic acid (penicilloic acids of cloxacillin),

B. R = H: (2*RS*,4*S*)-2-[[[[3-(2-chlorophenyl)-5-methylisoxazol-4-yl]carbonyl]amino]methyl]-5,5-dimethylthiazolidine-4-carboxylic acid (penilloic acids of cloxacillin),

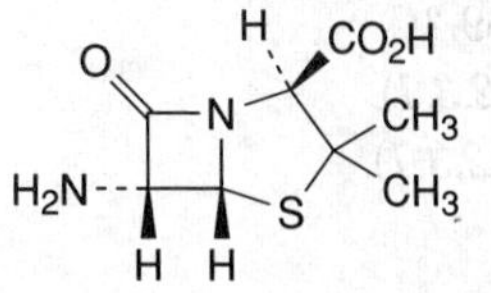

C. (2*S*,5*R*,6*R*)-6-amino-3,3-dimethyl-7-oxo-4-thia-1-azabicyclo[3.2.0]heptane-2-carboxylic acid (6-aminopenicillanic acid),

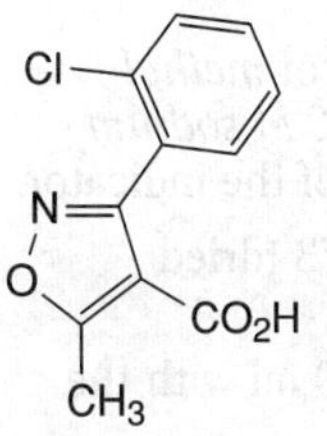

D. 3-(2-chlorophenyl)-5-methylisoxazole-4-carboxylic acid,

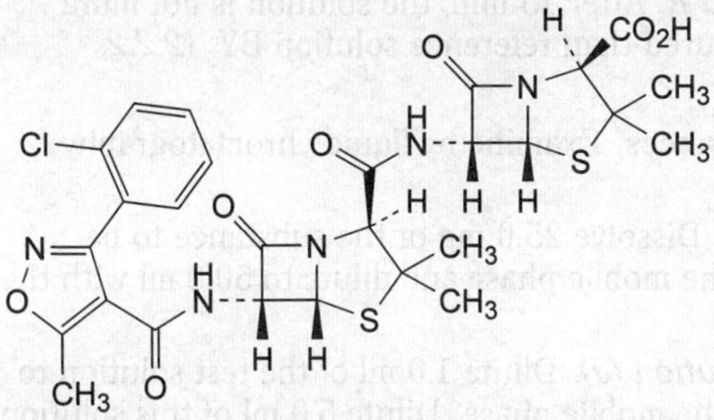

E. (2*S*,5*R*,6*R*)-6-[[(2*S*,5*R*,6*R*)-6-[[[3-(2-chlorophenyl)-5-methylisoxazol-4-yl]carbonyl]amino]-3,3-dimethyl-7-oxo-4-thia-1-azabicyclo[3.2.0]heptane-2-carbonyl]amino]-3,3-dimethyl-7-oxo-4-thia-1-azabicyclo[3.2.0]heptane-2-carboxylic acid (6-APA cloxacillin amide).

01/2005:1191

CLOZAPINE

Clozapinum

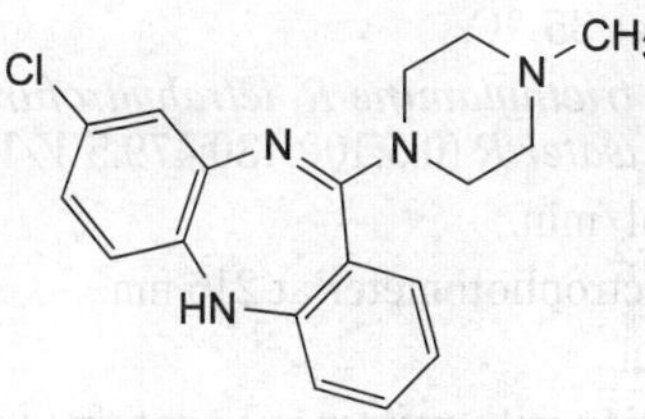

$C_{18}H_{19}ClN_4$ M_r 326.8

DEFINITION

Clozapine contains not less than 99.0 per cent and not more than the equivalent of 101.0 per cent of 8-chloro-11-(4-methylpiperazin-1-yl)-5*H*-dibenzo[*b*,*e*][1,4]diazepine, calculated with reference to the dried substance.

CHARACTERS

A yellow, crystalline powder, practically insoluble in water, freely soluble in methylene chloride, soluble in alcohol. It dissolves in dilute acetic acid.

IDENTIFICATION

A. Melting point (*2.2.14*): 182 °C to 186 °C.

B. Examine by infrared absorption spectrophotometry (*2.2.24*), comparing with the spectrum obtained with *clozapine CRS*. Examine the substances prepared as discs.

TESTS

Related substances. Examine by thin-layer chromatography (*2.2.27*), using as the coating substance a suitable silica gel with a fluorescent indicator having an optimal intensity at 254 nm. Before use, develop the plate with a mixture of 25 volumes of *methanol R* and 75 volumes of *methylene chloride R*. Allow the plate to dry in air for 15 min.

Test solution (a). Dissolve 0.20 g of the substance to be examined in *methylene chloride R* and dilute to 5 ml with the same solvent.

Test solution (b). Dilute 1 ml of test solution (a) to 10 ml with *methylene chloride R*.

Reference solution (a). Dissolve 20 mg of *clozapine CRS* in *methylene chloride R* and dilute to 5 ml with the same solvent.

Reference solution (b). Dilute 1.5 ml of test solution (b) to 50 ml with *methylene chloride R*.

Reference solution (c). Dilute 1 ml of test solution (b) to 50 ml with *methylene chloride R*.

Reference solution (d). Dilute 5 ml of reference solution (c) to 10 ml with *methylene chloride R*.

Reference solution (e). Dissolve 10 mg of *clozapine CRS* and 10 mg of *oxazepam CRS* in *methylene chloride R* and dilute to 5 ml with the same solvent.

Apply separately to the plate 5 µl of each solution. Develop over a path of 10 cm using a mixture of 25 volumes of *methanol R* and 75 volumes of *methylene chloride R*. Allow the plate to dry in air and examine in ultraviolet light at 254 nm. Any spot in the chromatogram obtained with test solution (a), apart from the principal spot, is not more intense than the spot in the chromatogram obtained with reference solution (b) (0.3 per cent); at most one such spot is more intense than the spot in the chromatogram obtained with reference solution (c) (0.2 per cent); and at most two such spots are more intense than the spot in the chromatogram obtained with reference solution (d) (0.1 per cent). The test is not valid unless the chromatogram obtained with reference solution (e) shows two clearly separated spots and the chromatogram obtained with reference solution (d) shows a clearly visible spot.

Heavy metals (*2.4.8*). 1.0 g complies with limit test C for heavy metals (20 ppm). Prepare the standard using 2 ml of *lead standard solution (10 ppm Pb) R*.

Loss on drying (*2.2.32*). Not more than 0.5 per cent, determined on 1.000 g by drying at 100 °C to 105 °C.

Sulphated ash (*2.4.14*). Not more than 0.1 per cent, determined on 1.0 g.

ASSAY

Dissolve 0.100 g in 50 ml of *anhydrous acetic acid R*. Titrate with *0.1 M perchloric acid*, determining the end-point potentiometrically (*2.2.20*).

1 ml of *0.1 M perchloric acid* is equivalent to 16.34 mg of $C_{18}H_{19}ClN_4$.

IMPURITIES

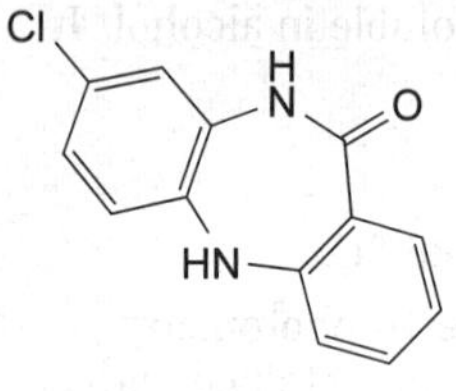

A. 8-chloro-5,10-dihydro-11*H*-dibenzo[*b*,*e*][1,4]diazepin-11-one,

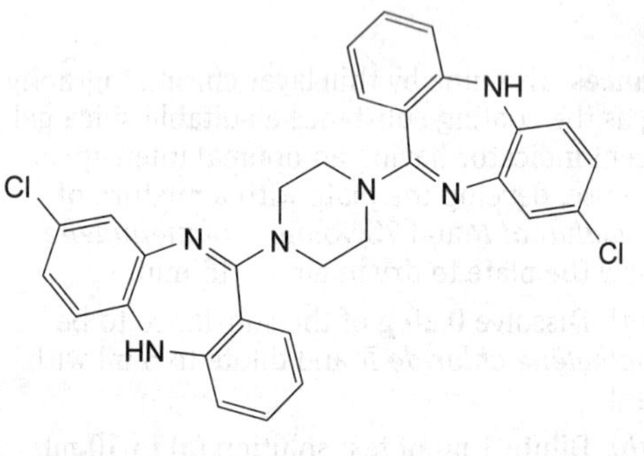

B. 11,11′-(piperazin-1,4-diyl)bis(8-chloro-5*H*-dibenzo[*b*,*e*][1,4]diazepine),

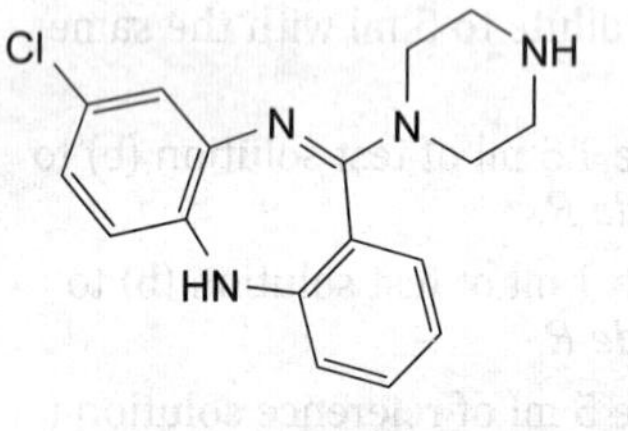

C. 8-chloro-11-(piperazin-1-yl)-5*H*-dibenzo[*b*,*e*][1,4]diazepine.

01/2005:0073

COCAINE HYDROCHLORIDE

Cocaini hydrochloridum

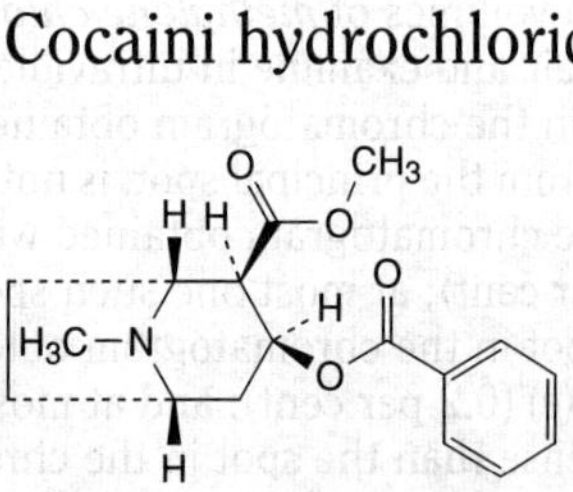

$C_{17}H_{22}ClNO_4$ M_r 339.8

DEFINITION

Methyl (1*R*,2*R*,3*S*,5*S*)-3-(benzoyloxy)-8-methyl-8-azabicyclo[3.2.1]octane-2-carboxylate hydrochloride.

Content: 98.5 per cent to 101.0 per cent (dried substance).

CHARACTERS

Appearance: white, crystalline powder or colourless crystals.

Solubility: very soluble in water, freely soluble in alcohol, slightly soluble in methylene chloride.

mp: about 197 °C, with decomposition.

IDENTIFICATION

First identification: B, D.

Second identification: A, C, D, E.

A. Dissolve 20.0 mg in *0.01 M hydrochloric acid* and dilute to 100.0 ml with the same acid. Dilute 5.0 ml of the solution to 50.0 ml with *0.01 M hydrochloric acid*. Examined between 220 nm and 350 nm (*2.2.25*), the solution shows 2 absorption maxima, at 233 nm and 273 nm. The specific absorbance at 233 nm is 378 to 402.

B. Infrared absorption spectrophotometry (*2.2.24*).
Comparison: *Ph. Eur. reference spectrum of cocaine hydrochloride.*

C. Dissolve 0.1 g in 5 ml of *water R* and add 1 ml of *dilute ammonia R2*. A white precipitate is formed. Initiate crystallisation by scratching the wall of the tube with a glass rod. The crystals, washed with *water R* and dried *in vacuo*, melt (*2.2.14*) at 96 °C to 99 °C.

D. It gives reaction (a) of chlorides (*2.3.1*).

E. It gives the reaction of alkaloids (*2.3.1*).

TESTS

Solution S. Dissolve 0.5 g in *water R* and dilute to 25 ml with the same solvent.

Appearance of solution. Solution S is clear (*2.2.1*) and colourless (*2.2.2, Method II*).

Acidity. To 10 ml of solution S add 0.05 ml of *methyl red solution R*. Not more than 0.2 ml of *0.02 M sodium hydroxide* is required to change the colour of the indicator.

Specific optical rotation (*2.2.7*): − 70 to − 73 (dried substance).

Dissolve 0.50 g in *water R* and dilute to 20.0 ml with the same solvent.

Readily carbonisable substances. To 0.2 g add 2 ml of *sulphuric acid R*. After 15 min, the solution is not more intensely coloured than reference solution BY_5 (*2.2.2, Method I*).

Related substances. Examine by liquid chromatography (*2.2.29*).

Test solution. Dissolve 25.0 mg of the substance to be examined in the mobile phase and dilute to 50.0 ml with the mobile phase.

Reference solution (a). Dilute 1.0 ml of the test solution to 50.0 ml with the mobile phase. Dilute 5.0 ml of this solution to 100.0 ml with the mobile phase.

Reference solution (b). Dissolve 25 mg of the substance to be examined in *0.01 M sodium hydroxide* and dilute to 10.0 ml with the same solvent. Dilute 1.0 ml of the solution to 10.0 ml with *0.01 M sodium hydroxide*. Allow the solution to stand for 15 min.

Column:

- *size*: l = 0.15 m, Ø = 4.6 mm,
- *stationary phase*: *end-capped octadecylsilyl silica gel for chromatography R* (5 µm) with a specific surface area of 335 m^2/g, a pore size of 10 nm and a carbon loading of 19.1 per cent,
- *temperature*: 35 °C.

Mobile phase: *triethylamine R, tetrahydrofuran R, acetonitrile R, water R* (0.5:100:430:479.5 *V/V/V/V*).

Flow rate: 1 ml/min.

Detection: spectrophotometer at 216 nm.

Injection: 20 µl.

Relative retention with reference to cocaine (retention time = about 7.4 min): degradation product = about 0.7.

System suitability: reference solution (b):

- *resolution*: minimum of 5 between the peaks due to cocaine and to the degradation product.

Limits:

- *any impurity eluting after the principal peak*: not more than the area of the principal peak in the chromatogram obtained with reference solution (a) (0.1 per cent),
- *total*: not more than 5 times the area of the principal peak in the chromatogram obtained with reference solution (a) (0.5 per cent),
- *disregard limit*: 0.5 times the area of the principal peak in the chromatogram obtained with reference solution (a) (0.05 per cent).

Loss on drying (*2.2.32*): maximum 0.5 per cent, determined on 1.000 g by drying in an oven at 100-105 °C.

Sulphated ash (*2.4.14*): maximum 0.1 per cent, determined on the residue from the test for loss on drying.

ASSAY

Dissolve 0.250 g in a mixture of 5.0 ml of *0.01 M hydrochloric acid* and 50 ml of *alcohol R*. Carry out a potentiometric titration (*2.2.20*), using *0.1 M sodium hydroxide*. Read the volume added between the 2 points of inflexion.

1 ml of *0.1 M sodium hydroxide* is equivalent to 33.98 mg of $C_{17}H_{22}ClNO_4$.

STORAGE

Protected from light.

IMPURITIES

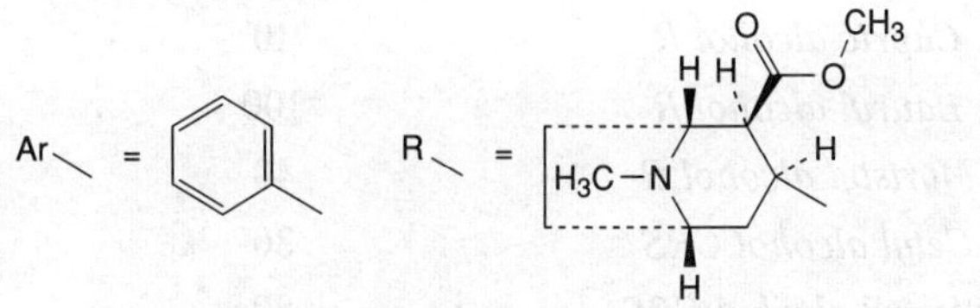

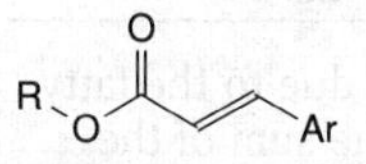

A. methyl (1*R*,2*R*,3*S*,5*S*)-8-methyl-3-[[(*E*)-3-phenylpropenoyl]oxy]-8-azabicyclo[3.2.1]octane-2-carboxylate (cinnamoylcocaine),

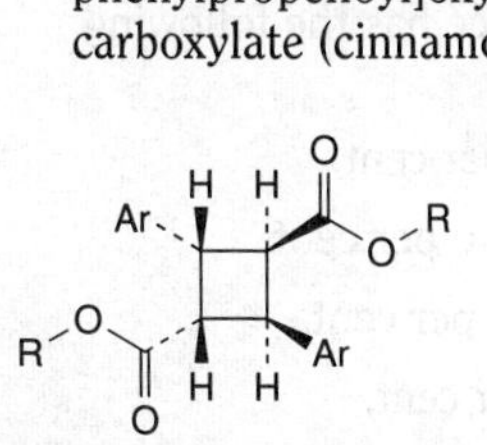

B. bis[(1*R*,2*R*,3*S*,5*S*)-2-(methoxycarbonyl)-8-methyl-8-azabicyclo[3.2.1]oct-3-yl] (1*r*,2*c*,3*t*,4*t*)-2,4-diphenylcyclobutane-1,3-dicarboxylate (α-truxilline),

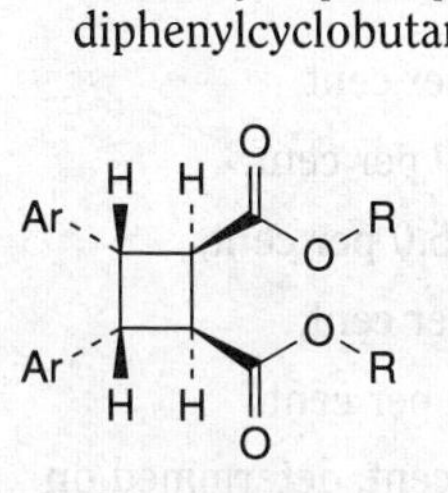

C. bis[(1*R*,2*R*,3*S*,5*S*)-2-(methoxycarbonyl)-8-methyl-8-azabicyclo[3.2.1]oct-3-yl] (1*r*,2*c*,3*t*,4*t*)-3,4-diphenylcyclobutane-1,2-dicarboxylate (β-truxilline).

01/2005:1410

COCONUT OIL, REFINED

Cocois oleum raffinatum

DEFINITION

Refined coconut oil is the fatty oil obtained from the dried, solid part of the endosperm of *Cocos nucifera* L., then refined.

CHARACTERS

A white or almost white, unctuous mass, practically insoluble in water, freely soluble in methylene chloride and in light petroleum (bp: 65 °C to 70 °C), very slightly soluble in alcohol.

The refractive index is about 1.449, determined at 40 °C.

IDENTIFICATION

A. It complies with the test for melting point (see Tests).

B. It complies with the test for composition of fatty acids (see Tests).

TESTS

Melting point (*2.2.14*): 23 °C to 26 °C.

Acid value (*2.5.1*). Not more than 0.5, determined on 20.0 g.

Peroxide value (*2.5.5*). Not more than 5.0.

Unsaponifiable matter (*2.5.7*). Not more than 1.0 per cent, determined on 5.0 g.

Alkaline impurities in fatty oils (*2.4.19*). It complies with the test for alkaline impurities in fatty oils.

Composition of fatty acids (*2.4.22, Method B*). Coconut oil is melted under gentle heating to a homogeneous liquid prior to sampling.

Reference solution. Dissolve 15.0 mg of *tricaproin CRS*, 80.0 mg of *tristearin CRS*, 0.150 g of *tricaprin CRS*, 0.200 g of *tricaprylin CRS*, 0.450 g of *trimyristin CRS* and 1.25 g of *trilaurin CRS* in a mixture of 2 volumes of *methylene chloride R* and 8 volumes of *heptane R* and dilute to 50 ml with the same mixture of solvents heating at 45 °C to 50 °C. Transfer 2 ml to a 10 ml centrifuge tube with a screw cap and evaporate the solvent in a current of *nitrogen R*. Dissolve with 1 ml of *heptane R* and 1 ml of *dimethyl carbonate R* and mix vigorously under gentle heating (50 °C to 60 °C). Add, while still warm, 1 ml of a 12 g/l solution of *sodium R* in *anhydrous methanol R*, prepared with the necessary precautions and mix vigorously for about 5 min. Add 3 ml of *distilled water R* and mix vigorously for about 30 s. Centrifuge for 15 min at 1500 *g*. Inject 1 µl of the organic phase.

Calculate the percentage content of each fatty acid using the following expression:

$$\frac{A_{x,s,c}}{\sum A_{x,s,c}} \times 100 \text{ per cent } m/m$$

$A_{x,s,c}$ is the corrected peak area of each fatty acid in the test solution:

$$A_{x,s,c} = A_{x,s} \times R_c$$

R_c is the relative correction factor:

$$R_c = \frac{m_{x,r} \times A_{1,r}}{A_{x,r} \times m_{1,r}}$$

for the peaks corresponding to caproic, caprylic, capric, lauric and myristic acid methyl esters.

$m_{x,r}$ = mass of tricaproin, tricaprylin, tricaprin, trilaurin or trimyristin in the reference solution, in milligrams,

$m_{1,r}$ = mass of tristearin in the reference solution, in milligrams,

$A_{x,r}$ = area of the peaks corresponding to caproic, caprylic, capric, lauric and myristic acid methyl esters in the reference solution,

$A_{1,r}$ = area of the peak corresponding to stearic acid methyl ester in the reference solution,

$A_{x,s}$ = area of peaks corresponding to any specified or unspecified fatty acid methyl esters,

R_c = 1 for peaks corresponding to each of the remaining specified fatty acid methyl esters or any unspecified fatty acid methyl ester.

The fatty acid fraction of the oil has the following composition:

- *caproic acid (R_{Rt} 0.11)*: not more than 1.5 per cent,
- *caprylic acid (R_{Rt} 0.23)*: 5.0 per cent to 11.0 per cent,
- *capric acid (R_{Rt} 0.56)*: 4.0 per cent to 9.0 per cent,
- *lauric acid (R_{Rt} 0.75)*: 40.0 per cent to 50.0 per cent,
- *myristic acid (R_{Rt} 0.85)*: 15.0 per cent to 20.0 per cent,
- *palmitic acid (R_{Rt} 0.93)*: 7.0 per cent to 12.0 per cent,
- *stearic acid (R_{Rt} 1.00)*: 1.5 per cent to 5.0 per cent,
- *oleic acid and isomers (R_{Rt} 1.01)*: 4.0 per cent to 10.0 per cent,
- *linoleic acid (R_{Rt} 1.03)*: 1.0 per cent to 3.0 per cent,
- *linolenic acid (R_{Rt} 1.06)*: not more than 0.2 per cent,
- *arachidic acid (R_{Rt} 1.10)*: not more than 0.2 per cent,
- *eicosenoic acid (R_{Rt} 1.11)*: not more than 0.2 per cent.

STORAGE

Store in a well-filled container, protected from light.

01/2005:1411

COCOYL CAPRYLOCAPRATE

Cocoylis caprylocapras

DEFINITION

Cocoyl caprylocaprate is a mixture of esters of saturated C_{12} to C_{18} alcohols with caprylic (octanoic) and capric (decanoic) acids obtained by the reaction of these acids with vegetable saturated fatty alcohols.

CHARACTERS

A slightly yellowish liquid, practically insoluble in water, miscible with alcohol and with liquid paraffin.

It has a relative density of about 0.86, a refractive index of about 1.445 and a viscosity of about 11 mPa·s.

IDENTIFICATION

A. Freezing point (*2.2.18*): not more than 15 °C.

B. Examine by infrared absorption spectrophotometry (*2.2.24*), comparing with the spectrum obtained with *cocoyl caprylocaprate CRS*.

C. It complies with the test for composition of fatty acids and fatty alcohols (see Tests).

TESTS

Appearance. The substance to be examined is not more intensely coloured than reference solution Y_5 (*2.2.2, Method I*).

Acid value (*2.5.1*). Not more than 0.5, determined on 5.0 g.

Hydroxyl value (*2.5.3, Method A*). Not more than 5.0.

Iodine value (*2.5.4*). Not more than 1.0.

Saponification value (*2.5.6*): 160 to 173.

Composition of fatty acids and fatty alcohols (*2.4.22, Method C*). Use the chromatogram obtained with the following reference solution for identification of the peaks corresponding to the fatty alcohols.

Reference solution. Dissolve the following amounts of the substances listed in Table 1411.-1 in 10 ml of *heptane R*.

Table 1411.-1

Substance	Amount (mg)
Methyl caproate R	10
Methyl caprylate R	90
Methyl caprate R	50
Methyl laurate R	20
Methyl myristate R	10
Methyl palmitate R	10
Methyl stearate R	10
Capric alcohol R	10
Lauryl alcohol R	100
Myristyl alcohol R	40
Cetyl alcohol CRS	30
Stearyl alcohol CRS	20

Consider the sum of the areas of the peaks due to the fatty acids listed below to be equal to 100 and the sum of the areas of the peaks due to the fatty alcohols listed below to be equal to 100.

The fatty-acid fraction of the substance has the following composition:

- *caproic acid*: not more than 2.0 per cent,
- *caprylic acid*: 50.0 per cent to 80.0 per cent,
- *capric acid*: 20.0 per cent to 50.0 per cent,
- *lauric acid*: not more than 3.0 per cent,
- *myristic acid*: not more than 1.0 per cent.

The fatty-alcohol fraction of the substance has the following composition:

- *capric alcohol*: not more than 3.0 per cent,
- *lauryl alcohol*: 48.0 per cent to 59.0 per cent,
- *myristyl alcohol*: 18.0 per cent to 25.0 per cent,
- *cetyl alcohol*: 6.0 per cent to 12.0 per cent,
- *stearyl alcohol*: 9.0 per cent to 16.0 per cent.

Water (*2.5.12*). Not more than 0.1 per cent, determined on 5.00 g by the semi-micro determination of water.

Total ash (*2.4.16*). Not more than 0.1 per cent, determined on 1.0 g.

01/2005:0076

CODEINE

Codeinum

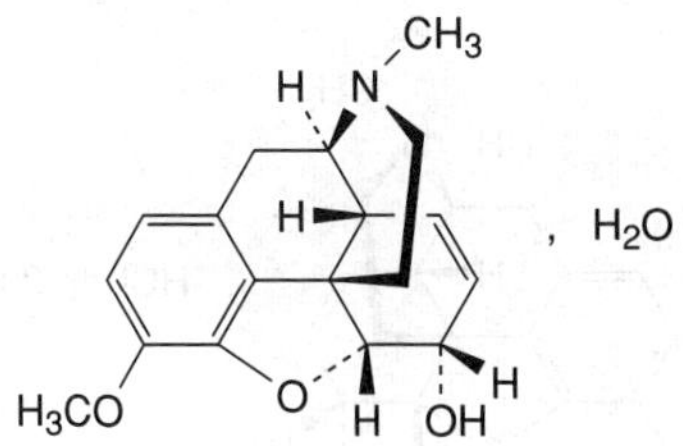

$C_{18}H_{21}NO_3,H_2O$ M_r 317.4

DEFINITION

7,8-Didehydro-4,5α-epoxy-3-methoxy-17-methylmorphinan-6α-ol.

Content: 99.0 per cent to 101.0 per cent (dried substance).

CHARACTERS

Appearance: white or almost white, crystalline powder or colourless crystals.

Solubility: soluble in boiling water, freely soluble in alcohol.

IDENTIFICATION

First identification: A, C.

Second identification: A, B, D, E.

A. Melting point (*2.2.14*): 155 °C to 159 °C.

B. To 2.0 ml of solution S (see Tests) add 50 ml of *water R* then 10 ml of *1 M sodium hydroxide* and dilute to 100.0 ml with *water R*. Examined between 250 nm and 350 nm (*2.2.25*), the solution shows only 1 absorption maximum at 284 nm. The specific absorbance at the absorption maximum is about 50 (dried substance).

C. Infrared absorption spectrophotometry (*2.2.24*).

Preparation: dried substance prepared as a disc of *potassium bromide R*.

Comparison: *Ph. Eur. reference spectrum of codeine.*

D. To about 10 mg add 1 ml of *sulphuric acid R* and 0.05 ml of *ferric chloride solution R2* and heat on a water-bath. A blue colour develops. Add 0.05 ml of *nitric acid R*. The colour changes to red.

E. It gives the reaction of alkaloids (*2.3.1*).

TESTS

Solution S. Dissolve 50 mg in *carbon dioxide-free water R* and dilute to 10.0 ml with the same solvent.

Appearance of solution. Solution S is clear (*2.2.1*) and colourless (*2.2.2, Method II*).

Specific optical rotation (*2.2.7*): − 142 to − 146 (dried substance).

Dissolve 0.50 g in *alcohol R* and dilute to 25.0 ml with the same solvent.

Related substances. Liquid chromatography (*2.2.29*).

Test solution. Dissolve 0.100 g of the substance to be examined and 0.100 g of *sodium octanesulphonate R* in the mobile phase and dilute to 10.0 ml with the mobile phase.

Reference solution (a). Dissolve 5.0 mg of *codeine impurity A CRS* in the mobile phase and dilute to 5.0 ml with the mobile phase.

Reference solution (b). Dilute 1.0 ml of reference solution (a) to 20.0 ml with the mobile phase.

Reference solution (c). Dilute 1.0 ml of the test solution to 50.0 ml with the mobile phase. Dilute 5.0 ml of this solution to 100.0 ml with the mobile phase.

Reference solution (d). Dilute 0.5 ml of the test solution to 5.0 ml with reference solution (a).

Column:

- *size*: l = 0.25 m, Ø = 4.6 mm,
- *stationary phase*: *end-capped octylsilyl silica gel for chromatography R* (5 µm).

Mobile phase: dissolve 1.08 g of *sodium octanesulphonate R* in a mixture of 20 ml of *glacial acetic acid R* and 250 ml of *acetonitrile R* and dilute to 1000 ml with *water R*.

Flow rate: 2 ml/min.

Detection: spectrophotometer at 245 nm.

Injection: 10 µl.

Run time: 10 times the retention time of codeine.

Relative retention with reference to codeine (retention time = about 6 min): impurity B = about 0.6; impurity E = about 0.7; impurity A = about 2.0; impurity C = about 2.3; impurity D = about 3.6.

System suitability: reference solution (d):

- *resolution*: minimum 3 between the peaks due to codeine and impurity A.

Limits:

- *correction factor*: for the calculation of content, multiply the peak area of impurity C by 0.25,
- *impurity A*: not more than twice the area of the principal peak in the chromatogram obtained with reference solution (b) (1.0 per cent),
- *impurities B, C, D, E*: for each impurity, not more than twice the area of the principal peak in the chromatogram obtained with reference solution (c) (0.2 per cent),
- *any other impurity*: for each impurity, not more than the area of the principal peak in the chromatogram obtained with reference solution (c) (0.1 per cent),
- *total of impurities other than A*: not more than 10 times the area of the principal peak in the chromatogram obtained with reference solution (c) (1.0 per cent),
- *disregard limit*: 0.5 times the area of the principal peak in the chromatogram obtained with reference solution (c) (0.05 per cent).

Loss on drying (*2.2.32*): 4.0 per cent to 6.0 per cent, determined on 1.000 g by drying in an oven at 100-105 °C.

Sulphated ash (*2.4.14*): maximum 0.1 per cent, determined on 1.0 g.

ASSAY

Dissolve 0.250 g in 10 ml of *anhydrous acetic acid R*. Add 20 ml of *dioxan R*. Titrate with *0.1 M perchloric acid* using 0.05 ml of *crystal violet solution R* as indicator.

1 ml of *0.1 M perchloric acid* is equivalent to 29.94 mg of $C_{18}H_{21}NO_3$.

STORAGE

Protected from light.

IMPURITIES

Specified impurities: A, B, C, D, E.

Other detectable impurities: F, G.

Monographs C

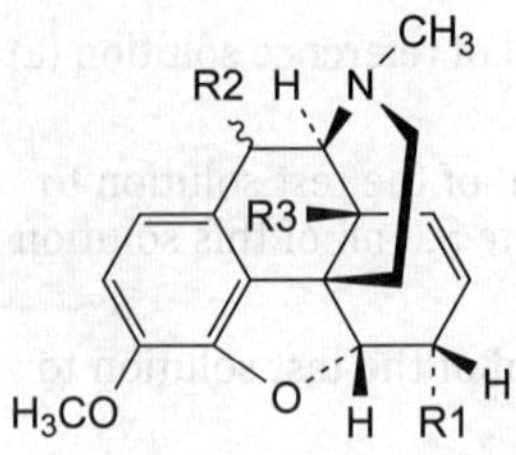

A. R1 = OCH_3, R2 = R3 = H: 7,8-didehydro-4,5α-epoxy-3,6α-dimethoxy-17-methylmorphinan (methylcodeine),

E. R1 = R2 = OH, R3 = H: 7,8-didehydro-4,5α-epoxy-3-methoxy-17-methylmorphinan-6α,10-diol,

F. R1 = R3 = OH, R2 = H: 7,8-didehydro-4,5α-epoxy-3-methoxy-17-methylmorphinan-6α,14-diol,

B. morphine,

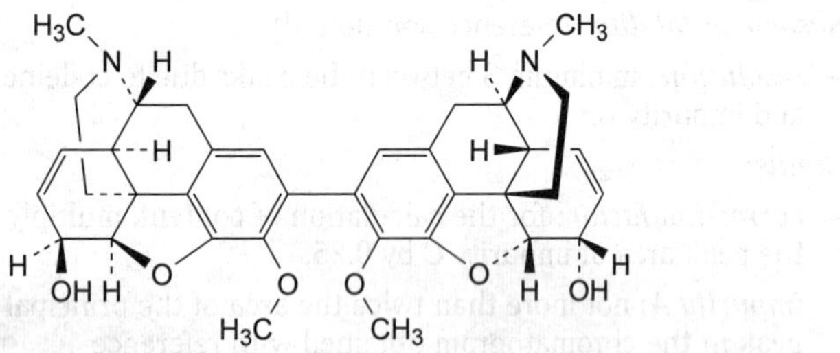

C. 7,7′,8,8′-tetradehydro-4,5α:4′,5′α-diepoxy-3,3′-dimethoxy-17,17′-dimethyl-2,2′-bimorphinanyl-6α,6′α-diol (codeine dimer),

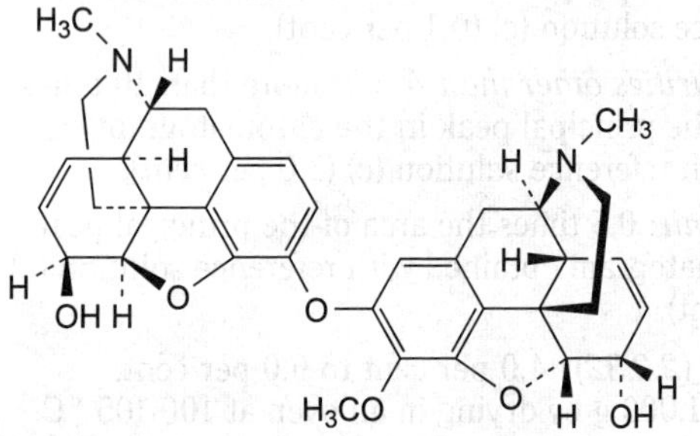

D. 7,8-didehydro-2-[(7,8-didehydro-4,5α-epoxy-6α-hydroxy-17-methylmorphinan-3-yl)oxy]-4,5α-epoxy-3-methoxy-17-methylmorphinan-6α-ol (3-O-(codein-2-yl)morphine),

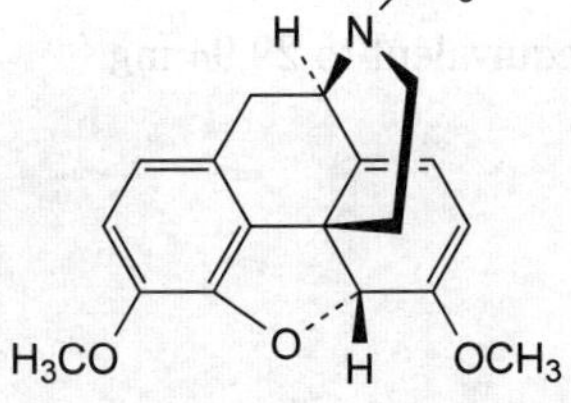

G. 6,7,8,14-tetradehydro-4,5α-epoxy-3,6-dimethoxy-17-methylmorphinan (thebaine).

01/2005:1412

CODEINE HYDROCHLORIDE DIHYDRATE

Codeini hydrochloridum dihydricum

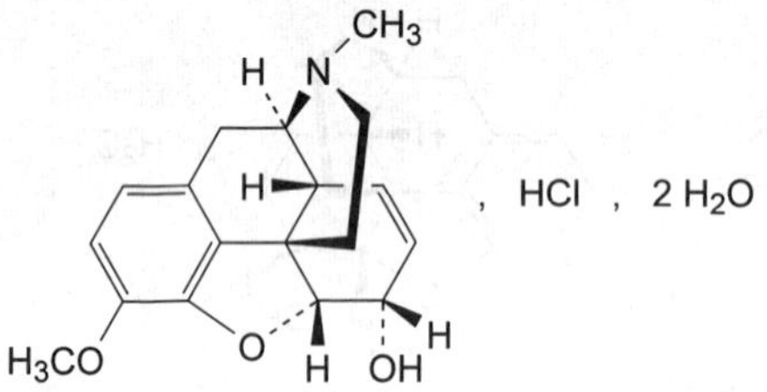

$C_{18}H_{22}ClNO_3,2H_2O$ M_r 371.9

DEFINITION

7,8-Didehydro-4,5α-epoxy-3-methoxy-17-methylmorphinan-6α-ol hydrochloride dihydrate.

Content: 99.0 per cent to 101.0 per cent (anhydrous substance).

CHARACTERS

Appearance: white or almost white, crystalline powder or small, colourless crystals.

Solubility: soluble in water, slightly soluble in ethanol, practically insoluble in cyclohexane.

IDENTIFICATION

First identification: A, D.

Second identification: B, C, D, E.

A. Infrared absorption spectrophotometry (*2.2.24*).
Comparison: *Ph. Eur. reference spectrum of codeine hydrochloride dihydrate.*

B. To 5 ml of solution S (see Tests) add 1 ml of a mixture of equal volumes of *strong sodium hydroxide solution R* and *water R* and initiate crystallisation, if necessary, by scratching the wall of the tube with a glass rod and cooling in iced water. Wash the precipitate with *water R* and dry at 100-105 °C. It melts (*2.2.15*) at 155 °C to 159 °C.

C. To about 10 mg add 1 ml of *sulphuric acid R* and 0.05 ml of *ferric chloride solution R2* and heat on a water-bath. A blue colour develops. Add 0.05 ml of *nitric acid R*. The colour changes to red.

D. Solution S gives reaction (a) of chlorides (*2.3.1*).

E. It gives the reaction of alkaloids (*2.3.1*).

TESTS

Solution S. Dissolve 2.00 g in *carbon dioxide-free water R* prepared from *distilled water R* and dilute to 50.0 ml with the same solvent.

Appearance of solution. Solution S is clear (*2.2.1*) and not more intensely coloured than reference solution Y_6 (*2.2.2, Method II*).

Acidity or alkalinity. To 5 ml of solution S add 5 ml of *carbon dioxide-free water R*. Add 0.05 ml of *methyl red solution R* and 0.2 ml of *0.02 M hydrochloric acid*; the solution is red. Add 0.4 ml of *0.02 M sodium hydroxide*; the solution becomes yellow.

Specific optical rotation (*2.2.7*): − 117 to − 121 (anhydrous substance).

Dilute 5.0 ml of solution S to 10.0 ml with *water R*.

Related substances. Liquid chromatography (*2.2.29*).

Test solution. Dissolve 0.100 g of the substance to be examined and 0.100 g of *sodium octanesulphonate R* in the mobile phase and dilute to 10.0 ml with the mobile phase.

Reference solution (a). Dissolve 5.0 mg of *codeine impurity A CRS* in the mobile phase and dilute to 5.0 ml with the mobile phase.

Reference solution (b). Dilute 1.0 ml of reference solution (a) to 20.0 ml with the mobile phase.

Reference solution (c). Dilute 1.0 ml of the test solution to 50.0 ml with the mobile phase. Dilute 5.0 ml of this solution to 100.0 ml with the mobile phase.

Reference solution (d). Dilute 0.5 ml of the test solution to 5.0 ml with reference solution (a).

Column:
- *size*: *l* = 0.25 m, Ø = 4.6 mm,
- *stationary phase*: *end-capped octylsilyl silica gel for chromatography R* (5 µm).

Mobile phase: dissolve 1.08 g of *sodium octanesulphonate R* in a mixture of 20 ml of *glacial acetic acid R* and 250 ml of *acetonitrile R* and dilute to 1000 ml with *water R*.

Flow rate: 2 ml/min.

Detection: spectrophotometer at 245 nm.

Injection: 10 µl.

Run time: 10 times the retention time of codeine.

Relative retention with reference to codeine (retention time = about 6 min): impurity B = about 0.6; impurity E = about 0.7; impurity A = about 2.0; impurity C = about 2.3; impurity D = about 3.6.

System suitability: reference solution (d):
- *resolution*: minimum 3 between the peaks due to codeine and impurity A.

Limits:
- *correction factor*: for the calculation of content, multiply the peak area of impurity C by 0.25,
- *impurity A*: not more than twice the area of the principal peak in the chromatogram obtained with reference solution (b) (1.0 per cent),
- *impurities B, C, D, E*: for each impurity, not more than twice the area of the principal peak in the chromatogram obtained with reference solution (c) (0.2 per cent),
- *any other impurity*: for each impurity, not more than the area of the principal peak in the chromatogram obtained with reference solution (c) (0.1 per cent),
- *total of impurities other than A*: not more than 10 times the area of the principal peak in the chromatogram obtained with reference solution (c) (1.0 per cent),
- *disregard limit*: 0.5 times the area of the principal peak in the chromatogram obtained with reference solution (c) (0.05 per cent).

Sulphates (*2.4.13*): maximum 0.1 per cent.

Dilute 5 ml of solution S to 20 ml with *distilled water R*. 15 ml of the solution complies with the limit test for sulphates.

Water (*2.5.12*): 8.0 per cent to 10.5 per cent, determined on 0.250 g.

ASSAY

Dissolve 0.300 g in a mixture of 5 ml of *0.01 M hydrochloric acid R* and 30 ml of *alcohol R*. Carry out a potentiometric titration (*2.2.20*), using *0.1 M sodium hydroxide*. Read the volume added between the 2 points of inflexion.

1 ml of *0.1 M sodium hydroxide* is equivalent to 33.59 mg of $C_{18}H_{22}ClNO_3$.

STORAGE

Protected from light.

IMPURITIES

Specified impurities: A, B, C, D, E.

Other detectable impurities: F, G.

Monographs C

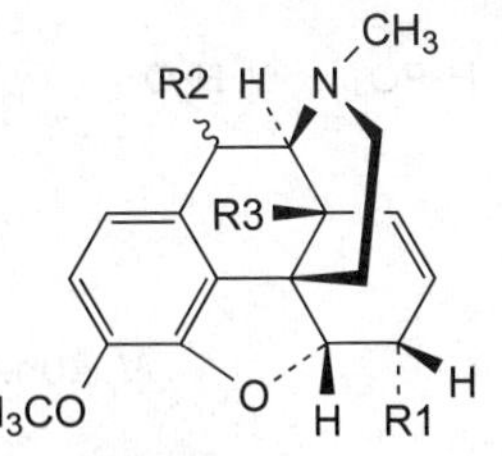

A. R1 = OCH_3, R2 = R3 = H: 7,8-didehydro-4,5α-epoxy-3,6α-dimethoxy-17-methylmorphinan (methylcodeine),

E. R1 = R2 = OH, R3 = H: 7,8-didehydro-4,5α-epoxy-3-methoxy-17-methylmorphinan-6α,10-diol,

F. R1 = R3 = OH, R2 = H: 7,8-didehydro-4,5α-epoxy-3-methoxy-17-methylmorphinan-6α,14-diol,

B. morphine,

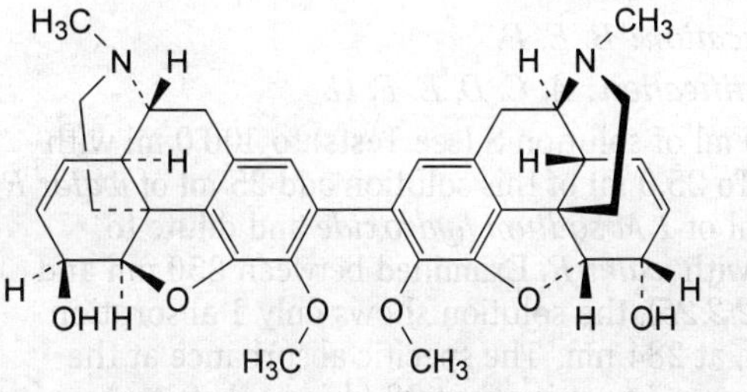

C. 7,7′,8,8′-tetradehydro-4,5α:4′,5′α-diepoxy-3,3′-dimethoxy-17,17′-dimethyl-2,2′-bimorphinanyl-6α,6′α-diol (codeine dimer),

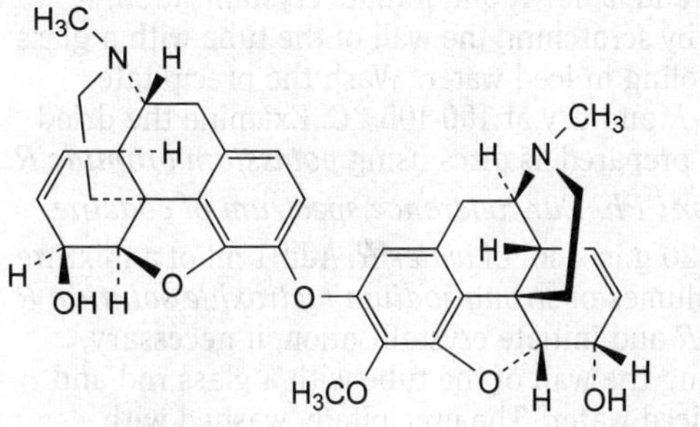

D. 7,8-didehydro-2-[(7,8-didehydro-4,5α-epoxy-6α-hydroxy-17-methylmorphinan-3-yl)oxy]-4,5α-epoxy-3-methoxy-17-methylmorphinan-6α-ol (3-*O*-(codein-2-yl)morphine),

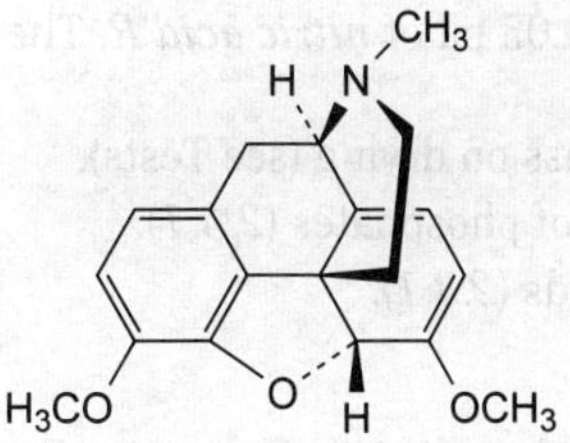

G. 6,7,8,14-tetradehydro-4,5α-epoxy-3,6-dimethoxy-17-methylmorphinan (thebaine).

01/2005:0074

CODEINE PHOSPHATE HEMIHYDRATE

Codeini phosphas hemihydricus

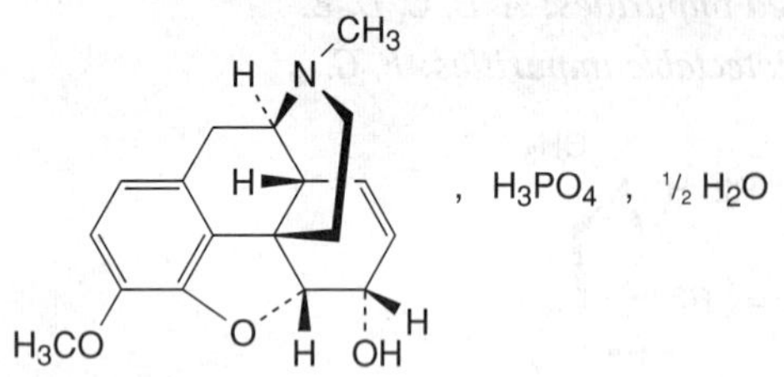

$C_{18}H_{24}NO_7P,{}^1/_2H_2O$ M_r 406.4

DEFINITION

7,8-Didehydro-4,5α-epoxy-3-methoxy-17-methylmorphinan-6α-ol phosphate hemihydrate.

Content: 98.5 per cent to 101.0 per cent (dried substance).

CHARACTERS

Appearance: white or almost white, crystalline powder or small, colourless crystals.

Solubility: freely soluble in water, slightly soluble or very slightly soluble in alcohol.

IDENTIFICATION

First identification: B, E, F.

Second identification: A, C, D, E, F, G.

A. Dilute 1.0 ml of solution S (see Tests) to 100.0 ml with *water R*. To 25.0 ml of this solution add 25 ml of *water R* then 10 ml of *1 M sodium hydroxide* and dilute to 100.0 ml with *water R*. Examined between 250 nm and 350 nm (*2.2.25*), the solution shows only 1 absorption maximum, at 284 nm. The specific absorbance at the absorption maximum is about 38 (dried substance).

B. Infrared absorption spectrophotometry (*2.2.24*).
Preparation: dissolve 0.20 g in 4 ml of *water R*. Add 1 ml of a mixture of equal volumes of *strong sodium hydroxide solution R* and *water R* and initiate crystallisation, if necessary, by scratching the wall of the tube with a glass rod and cooling in iced water. Wash the precipitate with *water R* and dry at 100-105 °C. Examine the dried precipitate prepared as discs using *potassium bromide R*.
Comparison: *Ph. Eur. reference spectrum of codeine.*

C. Dissolve 0.20 g in 4 ml of *water R*. Add 1 ml of a mixture of equal volumes of *strong sodium hydroxide solution R* and *water R* and initiate crystallisation, if necessary, by scratching the wall of the tube with a glass rod and cooling in iced water. The precipitate, washed with *water R* and dried at 100-105 °C, melts (*2.2.14*) at 155 °C to 159 °C.

D. To about 10 mg add 1 ml of *sulphuric acid R* and 0.05 ml of *ferric chloride solution R2* and heat on a water-bath. A blue colour develops. Add 0.05 ml of *nitric acid R*. The colour changes to red.

E. It complies with the test for loss on drying (see Tests).

F. Solution S gives reaction (a) of phosphates (*2.3.1*).

G. It gives the reaction of alkaloids (*2.3.1*).

TESTS

Solution S. Dissolve 1.00 g in *carbon dioxide-free water R* prepared from *distilled water R* and dilute to 25.0 ml with the same solvent.

pH (*2.2.3*): 4.0 to 5.0 for solution S.

Specific optical rotation (*2.2.7*): − 98 to − 102 (dried substance).

Dilute 5.0 ml of solution S to 10.0 ml with *water R*.

Related substances. Liquid chromatography (*2.2.29*).

Test solution. Dissolve 0.100 g of the substance to be examined and 0.100 g of *sodium octanesulphonate R* in the mobile phase and dilute to 10.0 ml with the mobile phase.

Reference solution (a). Dissolve 5.0 mg of *codeine impurity A CRS* in the mobile phase and dilute to 5.0 ml with the mobile phase.

Reference solution (b). Dilute 1.0 ml of reference solution (a) to 20.0 ml with the mobile phase.

Reference solution (c). Dilute 1.0 ml of the test solution to 50.0 ml with the mobile phase. Dilute 5.0 ml of this solution to 100.0 ml with the mobile phase.

Reference solution (d). Dilute 0.5 ml of the test solution to 5.0 ml with reference solution (a).

Column:
- *size*: *l* = 0.25 m, Ø = 4.6 mm,
- *stationary phase*: *end-capped octylsilyl silica gel for chromatography R* (5 µm).

Mobile phase: dissolve 1.08 g of *sodium octanesulphonate R* in a mixture of 20 ml of *glacial acetic acid R* and 250 ml of *acetonitrile R* and dilute to 1000 ml with *water R*.

Flow rate: 2 ml/min.

Detection: spectrophotometer at 245 nm.

Injection: 10 µl.

Run time: 10 times the retention time of codeine.

Relative retention with reference to codeine (retention time = about 6 min): impurity B = about 0.6; impurity E = about 0.7; impurity A = about 2.0; impurity C = about 2.3; impurity D = about 3.6.

System suitability: reference solution (d):
- *resolution*: minimum 3 between the peaks due to codeine and impurity A.

Limits:
- *correction factor*: for the calculation of content, multiply the peak area of impurity C by 0.25,
- *impurity A*: not more than twice the area of the principal peak in the chromatogram obtained with reference solution (b) (1.0 per cent),
- *impurities B, C, D, E*: for each impurity, not more than twice the area of the principal peak in the chromatogram obtained with reference solution (c) (0.2 per cent),
- *any other impurity*: for each impurity, not more than the area of the principal peak in the chromatogram obtained with reference solution (c) (0.1 per cent),
- *total of impurities other than A*: not more than 10 times the area of the principal peak in the chromatogram obtained with reference solution (c) (1.0 per cent),
- *disregard limit*: 0.5 times the area of the principal peak in the chromatogram obtained with reference solution (c) (0.05 per cent).

Sulphates (*2.4.13*): maximum 0.1 per cent.

Dilute 5 ml of solution S to 20 ml with *distilled water R*. 15 ml of the solution complies with the limit test for sulphates.

Loss on drying (*2.2.32*): 1.5 per cent to 3.0 per cent, determined on 1.000 g by drying in an oven at 100-105 °C.

ASSAY

Dissolve 0.350 g in a mixture of 10 ml of *anhydrous acetic acid R* and 20 ml of *dioxan R*. Titrate with *0.1 M perchloric acid* using 0.05 ml of *crystal violet solution R* as indicator.

1 ml of *0.1 M perchloric acid* is equivalent to 39.74 mg of $C_{18}H_{24}NO_7P$.

STORAGE

Protected from light.

IMPURITIES

Specified impurities: *A, B, C, D, E*.

Other detectable impurities: *F, G*.

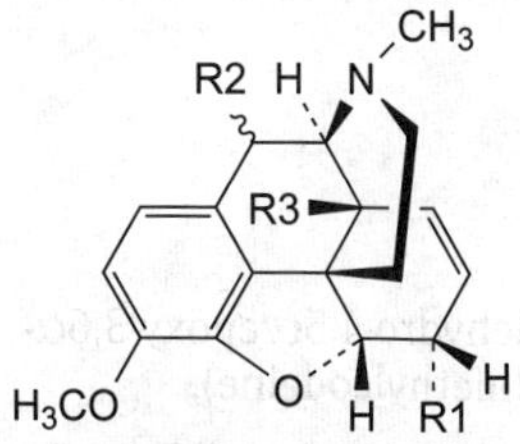

A. R1 = OCH_3, R2 = R3 = H: 7,8-didehydro-4,5α-epoxy-3,6α-dimethoxy-17-methylmorphinan (methylcodeine),

E. R1 = R2 = OH, R3 = H: 7,8-didehydro-4,5α-epoxy-3-methoxy-17-methylmorphinan-6α,10-diol,

F. R1 = R3 = OH, R2 = H: 7,8-didehydro-4,5α-epoxy-3-methoxy-17-methylmorphinan-6α,14-diol,

B. morphine,

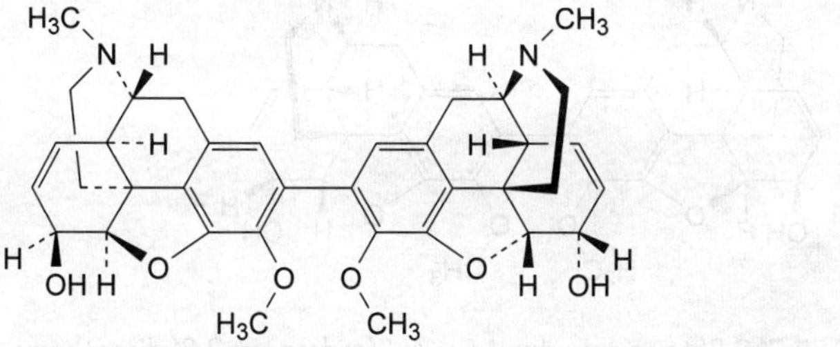

C. 7,7′,8,8′-tetradehydro-4,5α:4′,5′α-diepoxy-3,3′-dimethoxy-17,17′-dimethyl-2,2′-bimorphinanyl-6α,6′α-diol (codeine dimer),

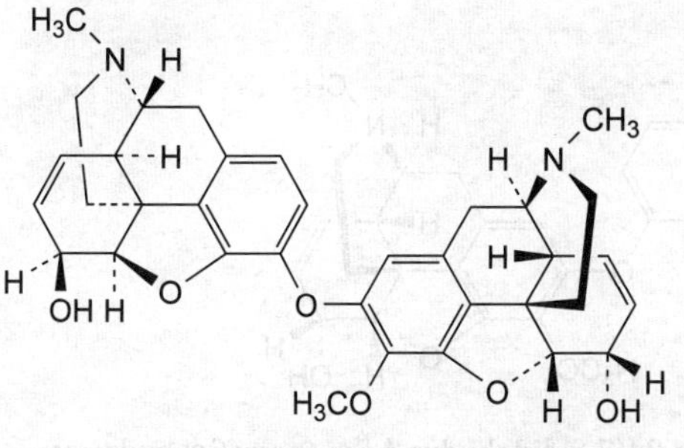

D. 7,8-didehydro-2-[(7,8-didehydro-4,5α-epoxy-6α-hydroxy-17-methylmorphinan-3-yl)oxy]-4,5α-epoxy-3-methoxy-17-methylmorphinan-6α-ol (3-*O*-(codein-2-yl)morphine),

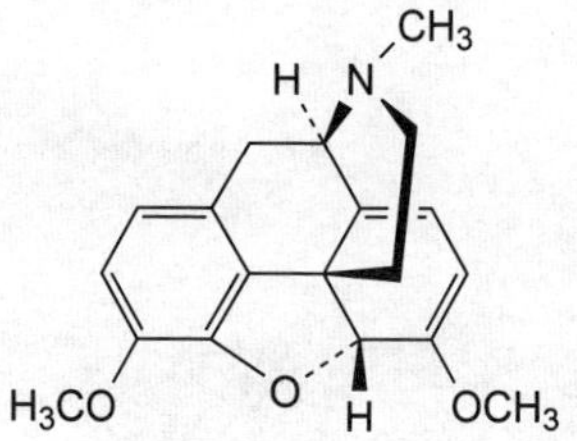

G. 6,7,8,14-tetradehydro-4,5α-epoxy-3,6-dimethoxy-17-methylmorphinan (thebaine).

01/2005:0075

CODEINE PHOSPHATE SESQUIHYDRATE

Codeini phosphas sesquihydricus

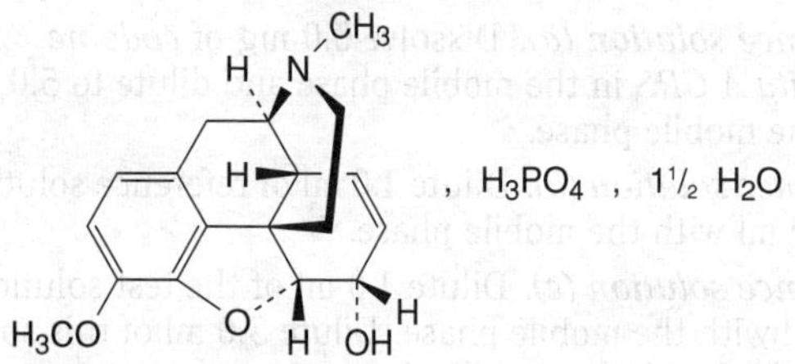

$C_{18}H_{24}NO_7P,1^1/_2H_2O$ — M_r 424.4

DEFINITION

7,8-Didehydro-4,5α-epoxy-3-methoxy-17-methylmorphinan-6α-ol phosphate sesquihydrate.

Content: 98.5 per cent to 101.0 per cent (dried substance).

CHARACTERS

Appearance: white or almost white, crystalline powder or small, colourless crystals.

Solubility: freely soluble in water, slightly soluble in alcohol.

IDENTIFICATION

First identification: *B, E, F*.

Second identification: *A, C, D, E, F, G*.

A. Dilute 1.0 ml of solution S (see Tests) to 100.0 ml with *water R*. To 25.0 ml of this solution add 25 ml of *water R* then 10 ml of *1 M sodium hydroxide* and dilute to 100.0 ml with *water R*. Examined between 250 nm and 350 nm (*2.2.25*), the solution shows only 1 absorption maximum, at 284 nm. The specific absorbance at the absorption maximum is about 38 (dried substance).

B. Infrared absorption spectrophotometry (*2.2.24*).

Preparation: dissolve 0.20 g in 4 ml of *water R*. Add 1 ml of a mixture of equal volumes of *strong sodium hydroxide solution R* and *water R* and initiate crystallisation, if necessary, by scratching the wall of the tube with a glass rod and cooling in iced water. Wash the precipitate with *water R* and dry at 100-105 °C. Examine the dried precipitate prepared as discs using *potassium bromide R*.

Comparison: *Ph. Eur. reference spectrum of codeine.*

C. Dissolve 0.20 g in 4 ml of *water R*. Add 1 ml of a mixture of equal volumes of *strong sodium hydroxide solution R* and *water R* and initiate crystallisation, if necessary, by scratching the wall of the tube with a glass rod and cooling in iced water. The precipitate, washed with *water R* and dried at 100-105 °C, melts (*2.2.14*) at 155 °C to 159 °C.

D. To about 10 mg add 1 ml of *sulphuric acid R* and 0.05 ml of *ferric chloride solution R2* and heat on a water-bath. A blue colour develops. Add 0.05 ml of *nitric acid R*. The colour changes to red.

E. It complies with the test for loss on drying (see Tests).

F. Solution S gives reaction (a) of phosphates (*2.3.1*).

G. It gives the reaction of alkaloids (*2.3.1*).

TESTS

Solution S. Dissolve 1.00 g in *carbon dioxide-free water R* prepared from *distilled water R* and dilute to 25.0 ml with the same solvent.

pH (*2.2.3*): 4.0 to 5.0 for solution S.

Specific optical rotation (*2.2.7*): − 98 to − 102 (dried substance).

Dilute 5.0 ml of solution S to 10.0 ml with *water R*.

Related substances. Liquid chromatography (*2.2.29*).

Test solution. Dissolve 0.100 g of the substance to be examined and 0.100 g of *sodium octanesulphonate R* in the mobile phase and dilute to 10.0 ml with the mobile phase.

Reference solution (a). Dissolve 5.0 mg of *codeine impurity A CRS* in the mobile phase and dilute to 5.0 ml with the mobile phase.

Reference solution (b). Dilute 1.0 ml of reference solution (a) to 20.0 ml with the mobile phase.

Reference solution (c). Dilute 1.0 ml of the test solution to 50.0 ml with the mobile phase. Dilute 5.0 ml of this solution to 100.0 ml with the mobile phase.

Reference solution (d). Dilute 0.5 ml of the test solution to 5.0 ml with reference solution (a).

Column:
- *size*: *l* = 0.25 m, Ø = 4.6 mm,
- *stationary phase*: *end-capped octylsilyl silica gel for chromatography R* (5 µm).

Mobile phase: dissolve 1.08 g of *sodium octanesulphonate R* in a mixture of 20 ml of *glacial acetic acid R* and 250 ml of *acetonitrile R* and dilute to 1000 ml with *water R*.

Flow rate: 2 ml/min.

Detection: spectrophotometer at 245 nm.

Injection: 10 µl.

Run time: 10 times the retention time of codeine.

Relative retention with reference to codeine (retention time = about 6 min): impurity B = about 0.6; impurity E = about 0.7; impurity A = about 2.0; impurity C = about 2.3; impurity D = about 3.6.

System suitability: reference solution (d):
- *resolution*: minimum 3 between the peaks due to codeine and impurity A.

Limits:
- *correction factor*: for the calculation of content, multiply the peak area of impurity C by 0.25,
- *impurity A*: not more than twice the area of the principal peak in the chromatogram obtained with reference solution (b) (1.0 per cent),
- *impurities B, C, D, E*: for each impurity, not more than twice the area of the principal peak in the chromatogram obtained with reference solution (c) (0.2 per cent),
- *any other impurity*: for each impurity, not more than the area of the principal peak in the chromatogram obtained with reference solution (c) (0.1 per cent),
- *total of impurities other than A*: not more than 10 times the area of the principal peak in the chromatogram obtained with reference solution (c) (1.0 per cent),
- *disregard limit*: 0.5 times the area of the principal peak in the chromatogram obtained with reference solution (c) (0.05 per cent).

Sulphates (*2.4.13*): maximum 0.1 per cent.

Dilute 5 ml of solution S to 20 ml with *distilled water R*. 15 ml of the solution complies with the limit test for sulphates.

Loss on drying (*2.2.32*): 5.0 per cent to 7.5 per cent, determined on 0.500 g by drying in an oven at 100-105 °C.

ASSAY

Dissolve 0.350 g in a mixture of 10 ml of *anhydrous acetic acid R* and 20 ml of *dioxan R*. Titrate with *0.1 M perchloric acid* using 0.05 ml of *crystal violet solution R* as indicator.

1 ml of *0.1 M perchloric acid* is equivalent to 39.74 mg of $C_{18}H_{24}NO_7P$.

STORAGE

Protected from light.

IMPURITIES

Specified impurities: A, B, C, D, E.

Other detectable impurities: F, G.

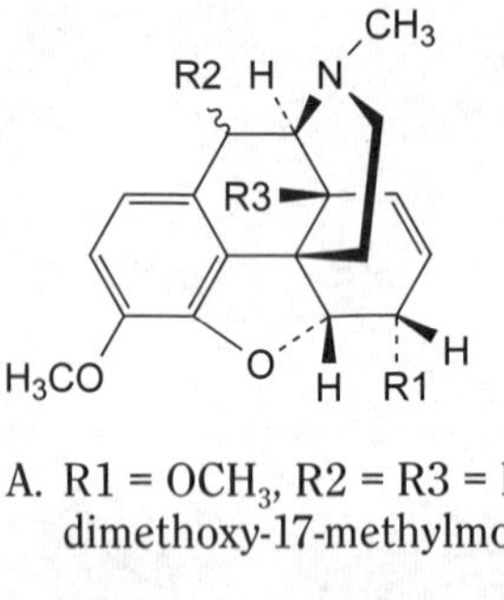

A. R1 = OCH_3, R2 = R3 = H: 7,8-didehydro-4,5α-epoxy-3,6α-dimethoxy-17-methylmorphinan (methylcodeine),

E. R1 = R2 = OH, R3 = H: 7,8-didehydro-4,5α-epoxy-3-methoxy-17-methylmorphinan-6α,10-diol,

F. R1 = R3 = OH, R2 = H: 7,8-didehydro-4,5α-epoxy-3-methoxy-17-methylmorphinan-6α,14-diol,

B. morphine,

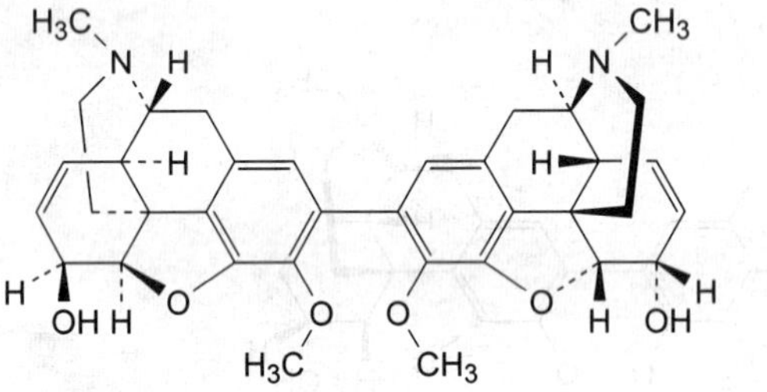

C. 7,7′,8,8′-tetradehydro-4,5α:4′,5′α-diepoxy-3,3′-dimethoxy-17,17′-dimethyl-2,2′-bimorphinanyl-6α,6′α-diol (codeine dimer),

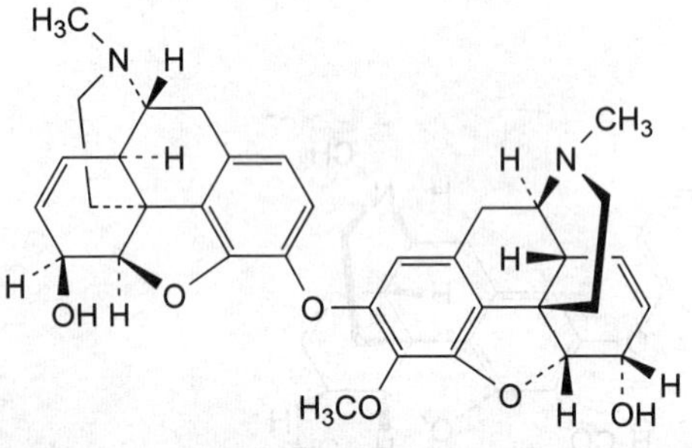

D. 7,8-didehydro-2-[(7,8-didehydro-4,5α-epoxy-6α-hydroxy-17-methylmorphinan-3-yl)oxy]-4,5α-epoxy-3-methoxy-17-methylmorphinan-6α-ol (3-*O*-(codein-2-yl)morphine),

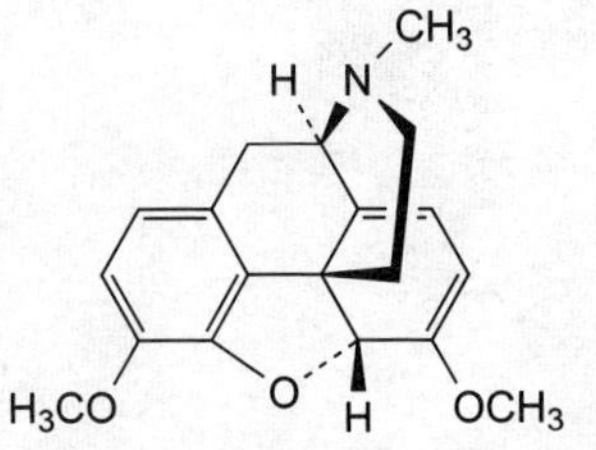

G. 6,7,8,14-tetradehydro-4,5α-epoxy-3,6-dimethoxy-17-methylmorphinan (thebaine).

01/2005:2060

CODERGOCRINE MESILATE

Codergocrini mesilas

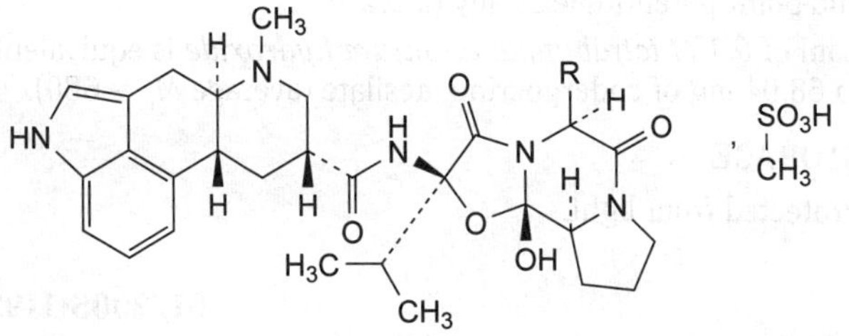

Name	Mol. Formula	M_r	R
dihydroergocornine mesilate	$C_{32}H_{45}N_5O_8S$	660	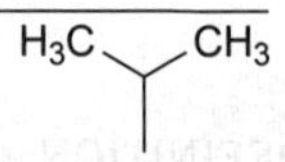
dihydroergocristine mesilate	$C_{36}H_{45}N_5O_8S$	708	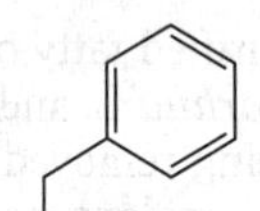
α-dihydroergocryptine mesilate	$C_{33}H_{47}N_5O_8S$	674	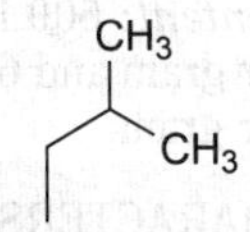
β-dihydroergocryptine mesilate	$C_{33}H_{47}N_5O_8S$	674	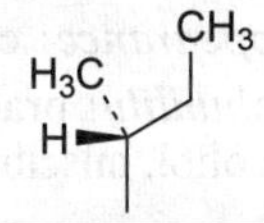

DEFINITION

A mixture of:

– (6a*R*,9*R*,10a*R*)-*N*-[(2*R*,5*S*,10a*S*,10b*S*)-10b-hydroxy-2,5-bis(1-methylethyl)-3,6-dioxooctahydro-8*H*-oxazolo[3,2-*a*]pyrrolo[2,1-c]pyrazin-2-yl]-7-methyl-4,6,6a,7,8,9,10,10a-octahydroindolo[4,3-*fg*]quinoline-9-carboxamide methanesulphonate (dihydroergocornine mesilate);

– (6a*R*,9*R*,10a*R*)-*N*-[(2*R*,5*S*,10a*S*,10b*S*)-5-benzyl-10b-hydroxy-2-(1-methylethyl)-3,6-dioxooctahydro-8*H*-oxazolo[3,2-*a*]pyrrolo[2,1-*c*]pyrazin-2-yl]-7-methyl-4,6,6a,7,8,9,10,10a-octahydroindolo[4,3-*fg*]quinoline-9-carboxamide methanesulphonate (dihydroergocristine mesilate);

– (6a*R*,9*R*,10a*R*)-*N*-[(2*R*,5*S*,10a*S*,10b*S*)-10b-hydroxy-2-(1-methylethyl)-5-(2-methylpropyl)-3,6-dioxooctahydro-8*H*-oxazolo[3,2-*a*]pyrrolo[2,1-*c*]pyrazin-2-yl]-7-methyl-4,6,6a,7,8,9,10,10a-octahydroindolo[4,3-*fg*]quinoline-9-carboxamide methanesulphonate (α-dihydroergocryptine mesilate);

– (6a*R*,9*R*,10a*R*)-*N*-[(2*R*,5*S*,10a*S*,10b*S*)-10b-hydroxy-2-(1-methylethyl)-5-[(1*RS*)-1-methylpropyl]-3,6-dioxooctahydro-8*H*-oxazolo[3,2-*a*]pyrrolo[2,1-*c*]pyrazin-2-yl]-7-methyl-4,6,6a,7,8,9,10,10a-octahydroindolo[4,3-*fg*]quinoline-9-carboxamide methanesulphonate (β-dihydroergocryptine mesilate or epicriptine mesilate).

Content: 98.0 per cent to 102.0 per cent (dried substance).

PRODUCTION

The production method must be evaluated to determine the potential for formation of alkyl mesilates, which is particularly likely to occur if the reaction medium contains lower alcohols. Where necessary, the production method is validated to demonstrate that alkyl mesilates are not detectable in the final product.

CHARACTERS

Appearance: white or yellowish powder.

Solubility: sparingly soluble in water, sparingly soluble to soluble in ethanol (96 per cent), slightly soluble in methylene chloride.

IDENTIFICATION

A. Thin-layer chromatography (*2.2.27*).

Test solution. Dissolve 0.20 g of the substance to be examined in a mixture of 1 volume of *methanol R* and 9 volumes of *methylene chloride R* and dilute to 5 ml with the same mixture of solvents.

Reference solution. Dissolve 0.20 g of *methanesulphonic acid R* in a mixture of 1 volume of *methanol R* and 9 volumes of *methylene chloride R* and dilute to 5 ml with the same mixture of solvents.

Plate: *TLC silica gel plate R*.

Mobile phase: *water R, concentrated ammonia R, butanol R, acetone R (5:10:20:65 V/V/V/V)*.

Application: 10 µl.

Development: over 2/3 of the plate.

Drying: in a current of cold air for not more than 1 min.

Detection: spray with a 1 g/l solution of *bromocresol purple R* in *methanol R*, adjusted to a violet-red colour with 0.05 ml of *dilute ammonia R1*.

Drying: in a current of hot air at 100 °C.

Results: the principal spot in the chromatogram obtained with the test solution is similar in position and colour to the principal spot in the chromatogram obtained with the reference solution.

B. Examine the chromatograms obtained in the test for composition.

Results: the 4 principal peaks in the chromatogram obtained with the test solution are similar in retention time and size to the 4 principal peaks in the chromatogram obtained with the reference solution.

TESTS

pH (*2.2.3*): 4.2 to 5.2.

Dissolve 0.10 g in *carbon dioxide-free water R* and dilute to 20 ml with the same solvent.

Composition. Liquid chromatography (*2.2.29*): use the normalisation procedure.

Test solution. Dissolve 20 mg of the substance to be examined in a mixture of 1 volume of *anhydrous ethanol R* and 2 volumes of a 10 g/l solution of *tartaric acid R* and dilute to 10 ml with the same mixture of solvents.

Reference solution. Dissolve 20 mg of *codergocrine mesilate CRS* in a mixture of 1 volume of *anhydrous ethanol R* and 2 volumes of a 10 g/l solution of *tartaric acid R* and dilute to 10 ml with the same mixture of solvents.

Column:

– *size*: *l* = 0.15 m, Ø = 4.6 mm,

– *stationary phase*: *octadecylsilyl silica gel for chromatography R* (5 µm).

Mobile phase: *triethylamine R, acetonitrile R, water R* (2.5:25:75 *V/V/V*).

Flow rate: 1.5 ml/min.

Detection: spectrophotometer at 280 nm.

Injection: 20 µl.

Run time: 20 min.
Elution order: dihydroergocornine, α-dihydroergocryptine, dihydroergocristine, β-dihydroergocryptine.
System suitability: test solution:
- *resolution*: minimum 3 between any 2 consecutive principal peaks.

Composition:
- *dihydroergocornine*: 30.0 per cent to 35.0 per cent,
- *α-dihydroergocryptine*: 20.0 per cent to 25.0 per cent,
- *dihydroergocristine*: 30.0 per cent to 35.0 per cent,
- *β-dihydroergocryptine*: 10.0 per cent to 13.0 per cent,
- *disregard limit*: 1.0 per cent.

Related substances. Thin-layer chromatography (*2.2.27*). *Perform the test as rapidly as possible and protected from direct light. Prepare the test solution last and immediately before application on the plate.*
Test solution. Dissolve 0.40 g of the substance to be examined in a mixture of 1 volume of *methanol R* and 9 volumes of *methylene chloride R* and dilute to 5.0 ml with the same mixture of solvents.
Reference solution (a). Dissolve 40 mg of *dihydroergocristine mesilate CRS* in a mixture of 1 volume of *methanol R* and 9 volumes of *methylene chloride R* and dilute to 10.0 ml with the same mixture of solvents. Dilute 3.0 ml of the solution to 50.0 ml with a mixture of 1 volume of *methanol R* and 9 volumes of *methylene chloride R.*
Reference solution (b). To 2.0 ml of reference solution (a), add 1.0 ml of a mixture of 1 volume of *methanol R* and 9 volumes of *methylene chloride R.*
Reference solution (c). To 1.0 ml of reference solution (a), add 2.0 ml of a mixture of 1 volume of *methanol R* and 9 volumes of *methylene chloride R.*
Reference solution (d). To 1.0 ml of reference solution (a), add 5.0 ml of a mixture of 1 volume of *methanol R* and 9 volumes of *methylene chloride R.*
Plate: *TLC silica gel plate R.*
Mobile phase: *concentrated ammonia R, methanol R, ethyl acetate R, methylene chloride R* (1:3:50:50 *V/V/V/V*).
Application: 10 μl.
Drying: in the dark for 2 min after the application of the last solution.
First development: in an unsaturated tank, over 2/3 of the plate.
Drying: in a current of cold air for not more than 1 min.
Second development: in an unsaturated tank, over 2/3 of the plate; use freshly prepared mobile phase.
Drying: in a current of cold air for not more than 1 min.
Detection: spray thoroughly with *dimethylaminobenzaldehyde solution R7* and dry in a current of hot air until the spot in the chromatogram obtained with reference solution (d) is clearly visible.
System suitability: test solution:
- the chromatogram shows at least 3 separated secondary spots.

Limits:
- *any impurity*: any spots, apart from the principal spot, are not more intense than the spot in the chromatogram obtained with reference solution (a) (0.3 per cent); not more than 4 such spots are more intense than the spot in the chromatogram obtained with reference solution (c) (0.1 per cent) and 2 of these may be more intense than the spot in the chromatogram obtained with reference solution (b) (0.2 per cent).

Loss on drying (*2.2.32*): maximum 5.0 per cent, determined on 0.500 g by drying at 120 °C under high vacuum.

ASSAY

Dissolve 0.500 g in 60 ml of *pyridine R*. Pass a stream of *nitrogen R* over the surface of the solution and titrate with *0.1 M tetrabutylammonium hydroxide,* determining the end-point potentiometrically (*2.2.20*).

1 ml of *0.1 M tetrabutylammonium hydroxide* is equivalent to 68.04 mg of codergocrine mesilate (average M_r = 680).

STORAGE

Protected from light.

01/2005:1192

COD-LIVER OIL (TYPE A)

Iecoris aselli oleum A

DEFINITION

Purified fatty oil obtained from the fresh livers of *Gadus morhua* L. and other species of *Gadidae,* solid substances being removed by cooling and filtering. A suitable antioxidant may be added.

Content: 600 IU (180 μg) to 2500 IU (750 μg) of vitamin A per gram and 60 IU (1.5 μg) to 250 IU (6.25 μg) of vitamin D_3 per gram.

CHARACTERS

Appearance: clear, yellowish, viscous liquid.
Solubility: practically insoluble in water, slightly soluble in alcohol, miscible with light petroleum.

IDENTIFICATION

First identification: A, B, C.
Second identification: C, D.

A. In the assay for vitamin A using method A, the test solution shows an absorption maximum (*2.2.25*) at 325 ± 2 nm. In the assay for vitamin A using method B, the chromatogram obtained with the test solution shows a peak corresponding to the peak of all-*trans*-retinol in the chromatogram obtained with the reference solution.
B. In the assay for vitamin D_3, the chromatogram obtained with test solution (a) shows a peak corresponding to the peak of cholecalciferol in the chromatogram obtained with reference solution (b).
C. It complies with the test for composition of fatty acids (see Tests).
D. To 0.1 g add 0.5 ml of *methylene chloride R* and 1 ml of *antimony trichloride solution R.* Mix. A deep blue colour develops in about 10 s.

TESTS

Colour: not more intensely coloured than a reference solution prepared as follows: to 3.0 ml of red primary solution add 25.0 ml of yellow primary solution and dilute to 50.0 ml with a 10 g/l solution of *hydrochloric acid R* (*2.2.2, Method II*).

Relative density (*2.2.5*): 0.917 to 0.930.

Refractive index (*2.2.6*): 1.477 to 1.484.

Acid value (*2.5.1*): maximum 2.0.

Anisidine value (*2.5.36*): maximum 30.0.

Iodine value (*2.5.4, Method B*): 150 to 180.
Use *starch solution R2.*

Peroxide value (*2.5.5, Method B*): maximum 10.0.

Unsaponifiable matter (*2.5.7*): maximum 1.5 per cent, determined on 2.0 g, and extracting with 3 quantities, each of 50 ml, of *peroxide-free ether R*.

Stearin. 10 ml remains clear after cooling in iced water for 3 h.

Composition of fatty acids. Gas chromatography (*2.2.28*).

Trivial name of fatty acid	Nomenclature	Lower limit area (per cent)	Upper limit area (per cent)
Saturated fatty acids:			
Myristic acid	14:0	2.0	6.0
Palmitic acid	16:0	7.0	14.0
Stearic acid	18:0	1.0	4.0
Mono-unsaturated fatty acids:			
Palmitoleic acid	16:1 n-7	4.5	11.5
cis-Vaccenic acid	18:1 n-7	2.0	7.0
Oleic acid	18:1 n-9	12.0	21.0
Gadoleic acid	20:1 n-11	1.0	5.5
Gondoic acid	20:1 n-9	5.0	17.0
Erucic acid	22:1 n-9	0	1.5
Cetoleic acid (22:1 n-11)	22:1 n-11+13	5.0	12.0
Poly-unsaturated fatty acids:			
Linoleic acid	18:2 n-6	0.5	3.0
α-Linolenic acid	18:3 n-3	0	2.0
Moroctic acid	18:4 n-3	0.5	4.5
Timnodonic (eicosapentaenoic) acid (EPA)	20:5 n-3	7.0	16.0
Cervonic (docosahexaenoic) acid (DHA)	22:6 n-3	6.0	18.0

Test solution. Introduce about 0.45 g of the substance to be examined into a 10 ml volumetric flask, dissolve in *hexane R* containing 50 mg of *butylhydroxytoluene R* per litre and dilute to 10.0 ml with the same solvent. Transfer 2.0 ml of the solution into a quartz tube and evaporate the solvent with a gentle current of *nitrogen R*. Add 1.5 ml of a 20 g/l solution of *sodium hydroxide R* in *methanol R*, cover with *nitrogen R*, cap tightly with a polytetrafluoroethylene lined cap, mix and heat in a water-bath for 7 min. Cool, add 2 ml of *boron trichloride-methanol solution R*, cover with *nitrogen R*, cap tightly, mix and heat in a water-bath for 30 min. Cool to 40-50 °C, add 1 ml of *trimethylpentane R*, cap and vortex or shake vigorously for at least 30 s. Immediately add 5 ml of *saturated sodium chloride solution R*, cover with *nitrogen R*, cap and vortex or shake thoroughly for at least 15 s. Allow the upper layer to become clear and transfer to a separate tube. Shake the methanol layer once more with 1 ml of *trimethylpentane R* and combine the trimethylpentane extracts. Wash the combined extracts with 2 quantities, each of 1 ml, of *water R* and dry over *anhydrous sodium sulphate R*. Prepare 2 solutions for each sample.

Column:

- *material*: fused silica,
- *size*: l = 30 m, Ø = 0.25 mm,
- *stationary phase*: *macrogol 20 000 R* (film thickness 0.25 μm).

Carrier gas: *hydrogen for chromatography R* or *helium for chromatography R*, where oxygen scrubber is applied.

Split ratio: 1:200.

Temperature:

	Time (min)	Temperature (°C)
Column	0 - 55	170 → 225
	55 - 75	225
Injection port		250
Detection		280

Detection: flame ionisation.

Injection: 1 μl, twice.

System suitability:

- the 15 fatty acids to be tested are satisfactorily identified from the chromatogram shown in Figure 1192.-1,
- injection of a mixture of equal amounts of *methyl palmitate R, methyl stearate R, methyl arachidate R* and *methyl behenate R* give area percentages of 24.4, 24.8, 25.2 and 25.6 (± 0.5 per cent), respectively,
- *resolution*: minimum of 1.3 between the peaks due to methyl oleate and methyl *cis*-vaccenate; the resolution between the pair due to methyl gadoleate and methyl gondoate is sufficient for purposes of identification and area measurement.

Calculate the area per cent for each fatty acid methyl ester from the expression:

$$\frac{A_x}{A_t} \times 100$$

A_x = peak area of fatty acid x,

A_t = sum of the peak areas (up to C22:6 n-3).

The calculation is not valid unless:

- the total area is based only on peaks due to solely fatty acids methyl esters,
- the number of fatty acid methyl ester peaks exceeding 0.05 per cent of the total area is at least 24,
- the 24 largest peaks of the methyl esters account for more than 90 per cent of the total area. (These correspond to, in common elution order: 14:0, 15:0, 16:0, 16:1 n-7, 16:4 n-1, 18:0, 18:1 n-9, 18:1 n-7, 18:2 n-6, 18:3 n-3, 18:4 n-3, 20:1 n-11, 20:1 n-9, 20:1 n-7, 20:2 n-6, 20:4 n-6, 20:3 n-3, 20:4 n-3, 20:5 n-3, 22:1 n-11, 22:1 n-9, 21:5 n-3, 22:5 n-3, 22:6 n-3).

ASSAY

Vitamin A. *Carry out the test as rapidly as possible, avoiding exposure to actinic light and air, oxidising agents, oxidation catalysts (for example, copper and iron) and acids.*

Use method A. If method A is found not to be valid, use method B.

METHOD A

Ultraviolet absorption spectrophotometry (*2.2.25*).

Test solution. To 1.00 g in a round-bottomed flask, add 3 ml of a freshly prepared 50 per cent *m/m* solution of *potassium hydroxide R* and 30 ml of *ethanol R*. Boil under reflux in a current of *nitrogen R* for 30 min. Cool rapidly and add 30 ml of *water R*. Extract with 50 ml of *ether R*. Repeat the extraction 3 times and discard the lower layer after complete separation. Wash the combined upper layers with 4 quantities, each of 50 ml, of *water R* and evaporate to dryness under a gentle current of *nitrogen R* at a temperature not exceeding 30 °C or in a rotary evaporator at a temperature not exceeding 30 °C under

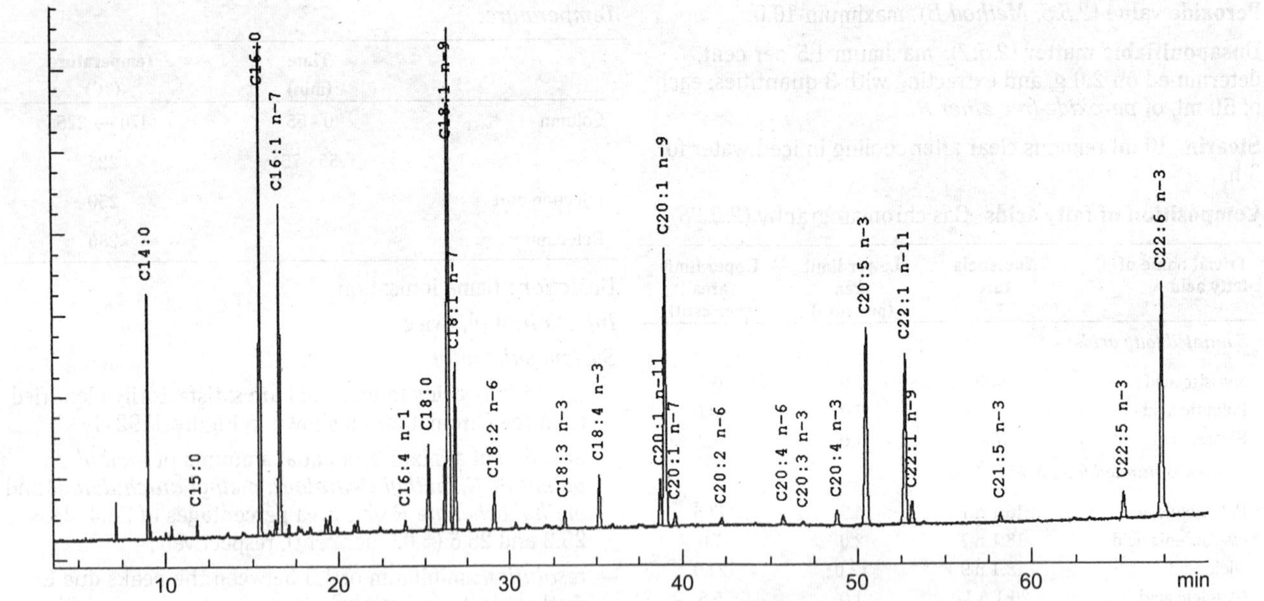

Figure 1192.-1. – *Chromatogram for the test for composition of fatty acids of cod-liver oil (type A)*

reduced pressure (water ejector). Dissolve the residue in sufficient *2-propanol R1* to give an expected concentration of vitamin A equivalent to 10-15 IU/ml.

Measure the absorbances of the solution at 300 nm, 310 nm, 325 nm and 334 nm and at the wavelength of maximum absorption with a suitable spectrophotometer in 1 cm specially matched cells, using *2-propanol R1* as the compensation liquid.

Calculate the content of vitamin A, as all-*trans*-retinol, in International Units per gram from the expression:

$$A_{325} \times \frac{1830}{100m} \times V$$

A_{325} = absorbance at 325 nm,

m = mass of the substance to be examined, in grams,

V = total volume of solution containing 10-15 IU of vitamin A per millilitre,

1830 = conversion factor for the specific absorbance of all-*trans*-retinol, in International Units.

The above expression can be used only if A_{325} has a value of not greater than $A_{325,corr}/0.970$ where $A_{325,corr}$ is the corrected absorbance at 325 nm and is given by the equation:

$$A_{325,\,corr} = 6.815A_{325} - 2.555A_{310} - 4.260A_{334}$$

A designates the absorbance at the wavelength indicated by the subscript.

If A_{325} has a value greater than $A_{325,corr}/0.970$, calculate the content of vitamin A from the following expression:

$$A_{325,\,corr} \times \frac{1830}{100m} \times V$$

The assay is not valid unless:

- the wavelength of maximum absorption lies between 323 nm and 327 nm,
- the absorbance at 300 nm relative to that at 325 nm is at most 0.73.

METHOD B

Liquid chromatography (*2.2.29*).

Test solution. To 2.00 g in a round-bottomed flask, add 5 ml of a freshly prepared 100 g/l solution of *ascorbic acid R* and 10 ml of a freshly prepared 800 g/l solution of *potassium hydroxide R* and 100 ml of *ethanol R*. Boil under a reflux condenser on a water-bath for 15 min. Add 100 ml of a 10 g/l solution of *sodium chloride R* and cool. Transfer the solution to a 500 ml separating funnel rinsing the round-bottomed flask with about 75 ml of a 10 g/l solution of *sodium chloride R* and then with 150 ml of a mixture of equal volumes of *light petroleum R1* and *ether R*. Shake for 1 min. When the layers have separated completely, discard the lower layer and wash the upper layer, first with 50 ml of a 30 g/l solution of *potassium hydroxide R* in a 10 per cent *V/V* solution of *ethanol R* and then with 3 quantities, each of 50 ml, of a 10 g/l solution of *sodium chloride R*. Filter the upper layer through 5 g of *anhydrous sodium sulphate R* on a fast filter paper into a 250 ml flask suitable for a rotary evaporator. Wash the funnel with 10 ml of fresh extraction mixture, filter and combine the upper layers. Distil them at a temperature not exceeding 30 °C under reduced pressure (water ejector) and fill with *nitrogen R* when evaporation is completed. Alternatively evaporate the solvent under a gentle current of *nitrogen R* at a temperature not exceeding 30 °C. Dissolve the residue in *2-propanol R*, transfer to a 25 ml volumetric flask and dilute to 25 ml with *2-propanol R*. Gentle heating in an ultrasonic bath may be required. (A large fraction of the white residue is cholesterol, constituting approximately 50 per cent of the unsaponifiable matter of cod-liver oil).

Reference solution (a). Prepare a solution of *retinol acetate CRS* in *2-propanol R1* so that 1 ml contains about 1000 IU of all-*trans*-retinol.

The exact concentration of reference solution (a) is assessed by ultraviolet absorption spectrophotometry (*2.2.25*). Dilute reference solution (a) with *2-propanol R1* to a presumed concentration of 10-15 IU/ml and measure the absorbance at 326 nm in matched 1 cm cells using *2-propanol R1* as the compensation liquid.

Calculate the content of vitamin A in International Units per millilitre of reference solution (a) from the following expression, taking into account the assigned content of *retinol acetate CRS*:

$$A_{326} \times \frac{1900 \times V_2}{100 \times V_1}$$

A_{326} = absorbance at 326 nm,

V_1 = volume of reference solution (a) used,

V_2 = volume of the diluted solution,

1900 = conversion factor for the specific absorbance of *retinol acetate CRS*, in International Units.

Reference solution (b). Proceed as described for the test solution but using 2.00 ml of reference solution (a) in place of the substance to be examined.

The exact concentration of reference solution (b) is assessed by ultraviolet absorption spectrophotometry (*2.2.25*). Dilute reference solution (b) with *2-propanol R1* to a presumed concentration of 10-15 IU/ml of all-*trans*-retinol and measure the absorbance at 325 nm in matched 1 cm cells using *2-propanol R1* as the compensation liquid.

Calculate the content of all-*trans*-retinol in International Units per millilitre of reference solution (b) from the expression:

$$A_{325} \times \frac{1830 \times V_3}{100 \times V_4}$$

A_{325} = absorbance at 325 nm,

V_3 = volume of the diluted solution,

V_4 = volume of reference solution (b) used,

1830 = conversion factor for the specific absorbance of all-*trans*-retinol, in International Units.

Column:

- *size*: l = 0.25 m, Ø = 4.6 mm,
- *stationary phase*: *octadecylsilyl silica gel for chromatography R* (film thickness 5-10 µm).

Mobile phase: *water R, methanol R* (3:97 *V/V*).

Flow rate: 1 ml/min.

Detection: spectrophotometer at 325 nm.

Injection: 10 µl; inject in triplicate the test solution and reference solution (b).

Retention time: all-*trans*-retinol = 5 ± 1 min.

System suitability:

- the chromatogram obtained with the test solution shows a peak due to that of all-*trans*-retinol in the chromatogram obtained with reference solution (b),
- when using the method of standard additions to the test solution there is greater than 95 per cent recovery of the added *retinol acetate CRS*,
- the recovery of all-*trans*-retinol in reference solution (b) as assessed by direct absorption spectrophotometry is greater than 95 per cent.

Calculate the content of vitamin A using the following expression:

$$A_1 \times \frac{C \times V}{A_2} \times \frac{1}{m}$$

A_1 = area of the peak due to all-*trans*-retinol in the chromatogram obtained with the test solution,

A_2 = area of the peak due to all-*trans*-retinol in the chromatogram obtained with reference solution (b),

C = concentration of *retinol acetate CRS* in reference solution (a) as assessed prior to the saponification, in International Units per millilitre (= 1000 IU/ml),

V = volume of reference solution (a) treated (2.00 ml),

m = mass of the substance to be examined in the test solution (2.00 g).

Vitamin D_3. Liquid chromatography (*2.2.29*). *Carry out the assay as rapidly as possible, avoiding exposure to actinic light and air.*

Internal standard solution. Dissolve 0.50 mg of *ergocalciferol CRS* in 100 ml of *ethanol R*.

Test solution (a). To 4.00 g in a round-bottomed flask, add 5 ml of a freshly prepared 100 g/l solution of *ascorbic acid R*, 10 ml of a freshly prepared 800 g/l solution of *potassium hydroxide R* and 100 ml of *ethanol R*. Boil under a reflux condenser on a water-bath for 30 min. Add 100 ml of a 10 g/l solution of *sodium chloride R* and cool the solution to room temperature. Transfer the solution to a 500 ml separating funnel rinsing the round-bottomed flask with about 75 ml of a 10 g/l solution of *sodium chloride R* and then with 150 ml of a mixture of equal volumes of *light petroleum R1* and *ether R*. Shake for 1 min. When the layers have separated completely, discard the lower layer and wash the upper layer, first with 50 ml of a 30 g/l solution of *potassium hydroxide R* in a 10 per cent *V/V* solution of *ethanol R*, and then with 3 quantities, each of 50 ml, of a 10 g/l solution of *sodium chloride R*. Filter the upper layer through 5 g of *anhydrous sodium sulphate R* on a fast filter paper into a 250 ml flask suitable for a rotary evaporator. Wash the funnel with 10 ml of fresh extraction mixture, filter and combine the upper layers. Distil them at a temperature not exceeding 30 °C under reduced pressure (water ejector) and fill with *nitrogen R* when evaporation is completed. Alternatively evaporate the solvent under a gentle current of *nitrogen R* at a temperature not exceeding 30 °C. Dissolve the residue in 1.5 ml of the mobile phase described under Purification. Gentle heating in an ultrasonic bath may be required. (A large fraction of the white residue is cholesterol, constituting approximately 50 per cent *m/m* of the unsaponifiable matter of cod-liver oil).

Test solution (b). To 4.00 g add 2.0 ml of the internal standard solution and proceed as described for test solution (a).

Reference solution (a). Dissolve 0.50 mg of *cholecalciferol CRS* in 100.0 ml of *ethanol R*.

Reference solution (b). In a round-bottomed flask, add 2.0 ml of reference solution (a) and 2.0 ml of the internal standard solution and proceed as described for test solution (a).

PURIFICATION

Column:

- *size*: l = 0.25 m, Ø = 4.6 mm,
- *stationary phase*: *nitrile silica gel for chromatography R* (film thickness 10 µm).

Mobile phase: *isoamyl alcohol R, hexane R* (1.6:98.4 *V/V*).

Flow rate: 1.1 ml/min.

Detection: spectrophotometer at 265 nm.

Inject 350 µl of reference solution (b). Collect the eluate from 2 min before until 2 min after the retention time of cholecalciferol, in a ground-glass-stoppered tube containing 1 ml of a 1 g/l solution of *butylhydroxytoluene R* in *hexane R*. Repeat the procedure with test solutions (a) and (b). Evaporate the eluates obtained from reference solution (b) and from test solutions (a) and (b), separately, to dryness at a temperature not exceeding 30 °C under a gentle current of *nitrogen R*. Dissolve each residue in 1.5 ml of *acetonitrile R*.

DETERMINATION

Column:

- *size*: l = 0.15 m, Ø = 4.6 mm,
- *stationary phase*: *octadecylsilyl silica gel for chromatography R* (film thickness 5 µm).

Mobile phase: *phosphoric acid R*, 96 per cent *V/V* solution of *acetonitrile R* (0.2:99.8 *V/V*).

Flow rate: 1.0 ml/min.

Detection: spectrophotometer at 265 nm.

Injection: 2 quantities not exceeding 200 µl of each of the 3 solutions obtained under Purification.

System suitability:

- *resolution*: minimum 1.4 between the peaks corresponding to ergocalciferol and cholecalciferol in the chromatogram obtained with reference solution (b),
- when using the method of standard additions to test solution (a) there is greater than 95 per cent recovery of the added *cholecalciferol CRS* when due consideration has been given to correction by the internal standard.

Calculate the content of vitamin D_3 in International Units per gram using the following expression, taking into account the assigned content of *cholecalciferol CRS*:

$$\frac{A_2}{A_6} \times \frac{A_3}{A_4 - \left[\frac{A_5}{A_1}\right] \times A_2} \times \frac{m_2}{m_1} \times \frac{V_2}{V_1} \times 40$$

m_1 = mass of the sample in test solution (b) in grams,

m_2 = total mass of *cholecalciferol CRS* used for the preparation of reference solution (a) in micrograms (500 µg),

A_1 = area (or height) of the peak due to cholecalciferol in the chromatogram obtained with test solution (a),

A_2 = area (or height) of the peak due to cholecalciferol in the chromatogram obtained with test solution (b),

A_3 = area (or height) of the peak due to ergocalciferol in the chromatogram obtained with reference solution (b),

A_4 = area (or height) of the peak due to ergocalciferol in the chromatogram obtained with test solution (b),

A_5 = area (or height) of a possible peak in the chromatogram obtained with test solution (a) with the same retention time as the peak co-eluting with ergocalciferol in test solution (b),

A_6 = area (or height) of the peak due to cholecalciferol in the chromatogram obtained with reference solution (b),

V_1 = total volume of reference solution (a) (100 ml),

V_2 = volume of reference solution (a) used for preparing reference solution (b) (2.0 ml).

STORAGE

In an airtight and well-filled container, protected from light. If no antioxidant is added, store under an inert gas. Once the container has been opened, its contents are used as soon as possible and any part of the contents not used at once is protected by an atmosphere of inert gas.

LABELLING

The label states:

- the number of International Units of vitamin A,
- the number of International Units of vitamin D_3,
- the name and concentration of any added antioxidant.

01/2005:1193

COD-LIVER OIL (TYPE B)

Iecoris aselli oleum B

DEFINITION

Purified fatty oil obtained from the fresh livers of *Gadus morhua* L. and other species of *Gadidae*, solid substances being removed by cooling and filtering. A suitable antioxidant may be added.

Content: 600 IU (180 µg) to 2500 IU (750 µg) of vitamin A per gram and 60 IU (1.5 µg) to 250 IU (6.25 µg) of vitamin D_3 per gram.

CHARACTERS

Appearance: clear, yellowish, viscous liquid.

Solubility: practically insoluble in water, slightly soluble in alcohol, miscible with light petroleum.

IDENTIFICATION

First identification: A, B, C.

Second identification: C, D.

A. In the assay for vitamin A using method A, the test solution shows an absorption maximum (*2.2.25*) at 325 ± 2 nm. In the assay for vitamin A using method B, the chromatogram obtained with the test solution shows a peak corresponding to the peak of all-*trans*-retinol in the chromatogram obtained with the reference solution.

B. In the assay for vitamin D_3, the chromatogram obtained with test solution (a) shows a peak corresponding to the peak of cholecalciferol in the chromatogram obtained with reference solution (b).

C. It complies with the test for composition of fatty acids (see Tests).

D. To 0.1 g add 0.5 ml of *methylene chloride R* and 1 ml of *antimony trichloride solution R*. Mix. A deep blue colour develops in about 10 s.

TESTS

Colour: not more intensely coloured than a reference solution prepared as follows: to 3.0 ml of red primary solution add 25.0 ml of yellow primary solution and dilute to 50.0 ml with a 10 g/l solution of *hydrochloric acid R* (*2.2.2, Method II*).

Relative density (*2.2.5*): 0.917 to 0.930.

Refractive index (*2.2.6*): 1.477 to 1.484.

Acid value (*2.5.1*): maximum 2.0.

Iodine value (*2.5.4, Method B*): 150 to 180.

Use *starch solution R2*.

Peroxide value (*2.5.5, Method B*): maximum 10.0.

Unsaponifiable matter (*2.5.7*): maximum 1.5 per cent, determined on 2.0 g and extracting with 3 quantities, each of 50 ml, of *peroxide-free ether R*.

Stearin. 10 ml remains clear after cooling in iced water for 3 h.

Composition of fatty acids. Gas chromatography (*2.2.28*).

Trivial name of fatty acid	Nomenclature	Lower limit area (per cent)	Upper limit area (per cent)
Saturated fatty acids:			
Myristic acid	14:0	2.0	6.0
Palmitic acid	16:0	7.0	14.0
Stearic acid	18:0	1.0	4.0
Mono-unsaturated fatty acids:			
Palmitoleic acid	16:1 n-7	4.5	11.5
cis-Vaccenic acid	18:1 n-7	2.0	7.0
Oleic acid	18:1 n-9	12.0	21.0
Gadoleic acid	20:1 n-11	1.0	5.5
Gondoic acid	20:1 n-9	5.0	17.0
Erucic acid	22:1 n-9	0	1.5
Cetoleic acid (22:1 n-11)	22:1 n-11+13	5.0	12.0
Poly-unsaturated fatty acids:			
Linoleic acid	18:2 n-6	0.5	3.0
α-Linolenic acid	18:3 n-3	0	2.0
Moroctic acid	18:4 n-3	0.5	4.5
Timnodonic (eicosapentaenoic) acid (EPA)	20:5 n-3	7.0	16.0
Cervonic (docosahexaenoic) acid (DHA)	22:6 n-3	6.0	18.0

Test solution. Introduce about 0.45 g of the substance to be examined into a 10 ml volumetric flask, dissolve in *hexane R* containing 50 mg of *butylhydroxytoluene R* per litre and dilute to 10.0 ml with the same solvent. Transfer 2.0 ml of the solution into a quartz tube and evaporate the solvent with a gentle current of *nitrogen R*. Add 1.5 ml of a 20 g/l solution of *sodium hydroxide R* in *methanol R*, cover with *nitrogen R*, cap tightly with a polytetrafluoroethylene lined cap, mix and heat in a water-bath for 7 min. Cool, add 2 ml of *boron trichloride-methanol solution R*, cover with *nitrogen R*, cap tightly, mix and heat in a water-bath for 30 min. Cool to 40-50 °C, add 1 ml of *trimethylpentane R*, cap and vortex or shake vigorously for at least 30 s. Immediately add 5 ml of *saturated sodium chloride solution R*, cover with *nitrogen R*, cap and vortex or shake thoroughly for at least 15 s. Allow the upper layer to become clear and transfer to a separate tube. Shake the methanol layer once more with 1 ml of *trimethylpentane R* and combine the trimethylpentane extracts. Wash the combined extracts with 2 quantities, each of 1 ml, of *water R* and dry over *anhydrous sodium sulphate R*. Prepare 2 solutions for each sample.

Column:

- *material*: fused silica,
- *size*: l = 30 m, Ø = 0.25 mm,
- *stationary phase*: *macrogol 20 000 R* (film thickness 0.25 µm).

Carrier gas: *hydrogen for chromatography R* or *helium for chromatography R*, where oxygen scrubber is applied.

Split ratio: 1:200.

Temperature:

	Time (min)	Temperature (°C)
Column	0 - 55	170 → 225
	55 - 75	225
Injection port		250
Detector		280

Detection: flame ionisation.

Injection: 1 µl, twice.

System suitability:

- the 15 fatty acids to be tested are satisfactorily identified from the chromatogram shown in Figure 1193.-1.
- injection of a mixture of equal amounts of *methyl palmitate R*, *methyl stearate R*, *methyl arachidate R*, and *methyl behenate R* give area percentages of 24.4, 24.8, 25.2 and 25.6 (± 0.5 per cent), respectively,
- *resolution*: minimum of 1.3 between the peaks due to methyl oleate and methyl *cis*-vaccenate; the resolution between the pair due to methyl gadoleate and methyl gondoate is sufficient for purposes of identification and area measurement.

Calculate the area per cent for each fatty acid methyl ester from the expression:

$$\frac{A_x}{A_t} \times 100$$

A_x = peak area of fatty acid x,

A_t = sum of the peak areas (up to C22:6 n-3).

The calculation is not valid unless:

- the total area is based only on peaks due to solely fatty acids methyl esters,
- the number of fatty acid methyl ester peaks exceeding 0.05 per cent of the total area is at least 24,
- the 24 largest peaks of the methyl esters account for more than 90 per cent of the total area. (These correspond to, in common elution order: 14:0, 15:0, 16:0, 16:1 n-7, 16:4 n-1, 18:0, 18:1 n-9, 18:1 n-7, 18:2 n-6, 18:3 n-3, 18:4 n-3, 20:1 n-11, 20:1 n-9, 20:1 n-7, 20:2 n-6, 20:4 n-6, 20:3 n-3, 20:4 n-3, 20:5 n-3, 22:1 n-11, 22:1 n-9, 21:5 n-3, 22:5 n-3, 22:6 n-3).

ASSAY

Vitamin A. *Carry out the test as rapidly as possible, avoiding exposure to actinic light and air, oxidising agents, oxidation catalysts (for example, copper and iron) and acids.*

Use method A. If method A is found not to be valid, use method B.

METHOD A

Ultraviolet absorption spectrophotometry (*2.2.25*).

Test solution. To 1.00 g in a round-bottomed flask, add 3 ml of a freshly prepared 50 per cent *m/m* solution of *potassium hydroxide R* and 30 ml of *ethanol R*. Boil under reflux in a current of *nitrogen R* for 30 min. Cool rapidly and add 30 ml of *water R*. Extract with 50 ml of *ether R*. Repeat the extraction 3 times and discard the lower layer after complete separation. Wash the combined upper layers with 4 quantities, each of 50 ml, of *water R* and evaporate to dryness under a gentle current of *nitrogen R* at a temperature not exceeding 30 °C or in a rotary evaporator at a temperature not exceeding 30 °C under

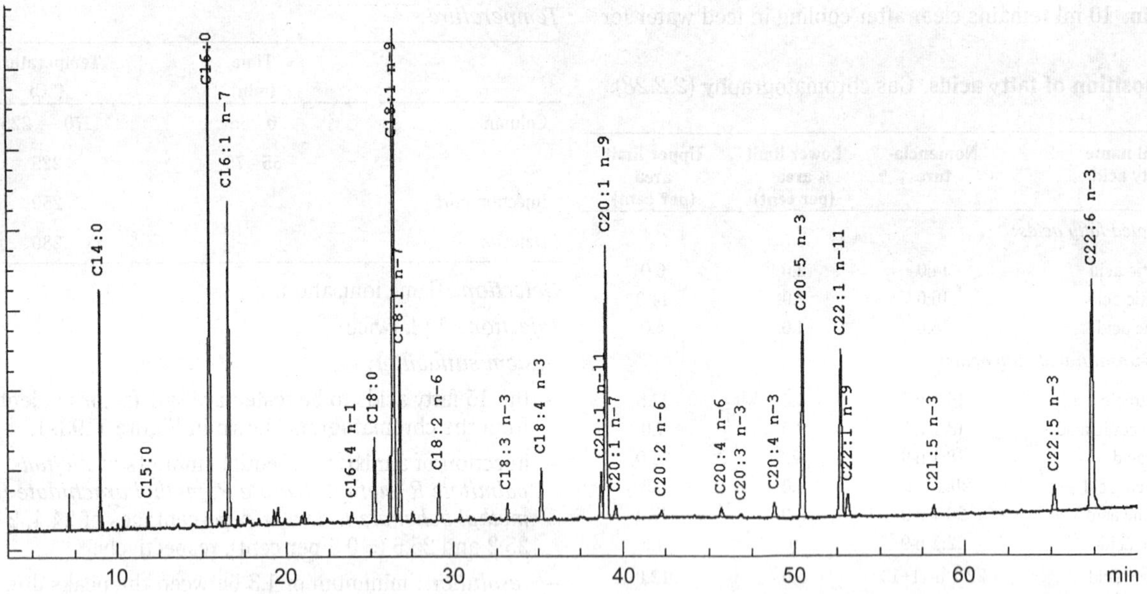

Figure 1193.-1. – *Chromatogram for the test for composition of fatty acids of cod-liver oil (type B)*

reduced pressure (water ejector). Dissolve the residue in sufficient *2-propanol R1* to give an expected concentration of vitamin A equivalent to 10-15 IU/ml.

Measure the absorbances of the solution at 300 nm, 310 nm, 325 nm and 334 nm and at the wavelength of maximum absorption with a suitable spectrophotometer in 1 cm specially matched cells, using *2-propanol R1* as the compensation liquid.

Calculate the content of vitamin A, as all-*trans*-retinol, in International Units per gram from the expression:

$$A_{325} \times \frac{1830}{100m} \times V$$

A_{325} = absorbance at 325 nm,

m = mass of the substance to be examined, in grams,

V = total volume of solution containing 10-15 IU of vitamin A per millilitre,

1830 = conversion factor for the specific absorbance of all-*trans*-retinol, in International Units.

The above expression can be used only if A_{325} has a value of not greater than $A_{325,corr}/0.970$ where $A_{325,corr}$ is the corrected absorbance at 325 nm and is given by the equation:

$$A_{325,\,corr} = 6.815A_{325} - 2.555A_{310} - 4.260A_{334}$$

A designates the absorbance at the wavelength indicated by the subscript.

If A_{325} has a value greater than $A_{325,corr}/0.970$, calculate the content of vitamin A from the expression:

$$A_{325,\,corr} \times \frac{1830}{100m} \times V$$

The assay is not valid unless:

– the wavelength of maximum absorption lies between 323 nm and 327 nm,
– the absorbance at 300 nm relative to that at 325 nm is at most 0.73.

METHOD B

Liquid chromatography (*2.2.29*).

Test solution. To 2.00 g in a round-bottomed flask, add 5 ml of a freshly prepared 100 g/l solution of *ascorbic acid R* and 10 ml of a freshly prepared 800 g/l solution of *potassium hydroxide R* and 100 ml of *ethanol R*. Boil under a reflux condenser on a water-bath for 15 min. Add 100 ml of a 10 g/l solution of *sodium chloride R* and cool. Transfer the solution to a 500 ml separating funnel rinsing the round-bottomed flask with about 75 ml of a 10 g/l solution of *sodium chloride R* and then with 150 ml of a mixture of equal volumes of *light petroleum R1* and *ether R*. Shake for 1 min. When the layers have separated completely, discard the lower layer and wash the upper layer, first with 50 ml of a 30 g/l solution of *potassium hydroxide R* in a 10 per cent *V/V* solution of *ethanol R* and then with 3 quantities, each of 50 ml, of a 10 g/l solution of *sodium chloride R*. Filter the upper layer through 5 g of *anhydrous sodium sulphate R* on a fast filter paper into a 250 ml flask suitable for a rotary evaporator. Wash the funnel with 10 ml of fresh extraction mixture, filter and combine the upper layers. Distil them at a temperature not exceeding 30 °C under reduced pressure (water ejector) and fill with *nitrogen R* when evaporation is completed. Alternatively evaporate the solvent under a gentle current of *nitrogen R* at a temperature not exceeding 30 °C. Dissolve the residue in *2-propanol R*, transfer to a 25 ml volumetric flask and dilute to 25 ml with *2-propanol R*. Gentle heating in an ultrasonic bath may be required. (A large fraction of the white residue is cholesterol, constituting approximately 50 per cent of the unsaponifiable matter of cod-liver oil).

Reference solution (a). Prepare a solution of *retinol acetate CRS* in *2-propanol R1* so that 1 ml contains about 1000 IU of all-*trans*-retinol.

The exact concentration of reference solution (a) is assessed by ultraviolet absorption spectrophotometry (*2.2.25*). Dilute reference solution (a) with *2-propanol R1* to a presumed concentration of 10-15 IU/ml and measure the absorbance at 326 nm in matched 1 cm cells using *2-propanol R1* as the compensation liquid.

Calculate the content of vitamin A in International Units per millilitre of reference solution (a) using the following expression, taking into account the assigned content of *retinol acetate CRS*:

$$A_{326} \times \frac{1900 \times V_2}{100 \times V_1}$$

A_{326} = absorbance at 326 nm,

V_1 = volume of reference solution (a) used,

V_2 = volume of the diluted solution,

1900 = conversion factor for the specific absorbance of *retinol acetate CRS*, in International Units.

Reference solution (b). Proceed as described for the test solution but using 2.00 ml of reference solution (a) in place of the substance to be examined.

The exact concentration of reference solution (b) is assessed by ultraviolet absorption spectrophotometry (*2.2.25*). Dilute reference solution (b) with *2-propanol R1* to a presumed concentration of 10-15 IU/ml of all-*trans*-retinol and measure the absorbance at 325 nm in matched 1 cm cells using *2-propanol R1* as the compensation liquid.

Calculate the content of all-*trans*-retinol in International Units per millilitre of reference solution (b) from the expression:

$$A_{325} \times \frac{1830 \times V_3}{100 \times V_4}$$

A_{325} = absorbance at 325 nm,

V_3 = volume of the diluted solution,

V_4 = volume of reference solution (b) used,

1830 = conversion factor for the specific absorbance of all-*trans*-retinol, in International Units.

Column:

- *size*: l = 0.25 m, Ø = 4.6 mm,
- *stationary phase*: *octadecylsilyl silica gel for chromatography R* (film thickness 5-10 µm).

Mobile phase: *water R, methanol R* (3:97 *V/V*).

Flow rate: 1 ml/min.

Detection: spectrophotometer at 325 nm.

Injection: 10 µl; inject in triplicate the test solution and reference solution (b).

Retention time: all-*trans*-retinol = 5 ± 1 min.

System suitability:

- the chromatogram obtained with the test solution shows a peak due to that of all-*trans*-retinol in the chromatogram obtained with reference solution (b),
- when using the method of standard additions to the test solution there is greater than 95 per cent recovery of the added *retinol acetate CRS*,
- the recovery of all-*trans*-retinol in reference solution (b) as assessed by direct absorption spectrophotometry is greater than 95 per cent.

Calculate the content of vitamin A using the following expression:

$$A_1 \times \frac{C \times V}{A_2} \times \frac{1}{m}$$

A_1 = area of the peak due to all-*trans*-retinol in the chromatogram obtained with the test solution,

A_2 = area of the peak due to all-*trans*-retinol in the chromatogram obtained with reference solution (b),

C = concentration of *retinol acetate CRS* in reference solution (a) as assessed prior to the saponification, in International Units per millilitre (= 1000 IU/ml),

V = volume of reference solution (a) treated (2.00 ml),

m = mass of the substance to be examined in the test solution (2.00 g).

Vitamin D_3. Liquid chromatography (*2.2.29*). *Carry out the assay as rapidly as possible, avoiding exposure to actinic light and air.*

Internal standard solution. Dissolve 0.50 mg of *ergocalciferol CRS* in 100 ml of *ethanol R*.

Test solution (a). To 4.00 g in a round-bottomed flask, add 5 ml of a freshly prepared 100 g/l solution of *ascorbic acid R*, 10 ml of a freshly prepared 800 g/l solution of *potassium hydroxide R* and 100 ml of *ethanol R*. Boil under a reflux condenser on a water-bath for 30 min. Add 100 ml of a 10 g/l solution of *sodium chloride R* and cool the solution to room temperature. Transfer the solution to a 500 ml separating funnel rinsing the round-bottomed flask with about 75 ml of a 10 g/l solution of *sodium chloride R* and then with 150 ml of a mixture of equal volumes of *light petroleum R1* and *ether R*. Shake for 1 min. When the layers have separated completely, discard the lower layer and wash the upper layer, first with 50 ml of a 30 g/l solution of *potassium hydroxide R* in a 10 per cent *V/V* solution of *ethanol R*, and then with 3 quantities, each of 50 ml, of a 10 g/l solution of *sodium chloride R*. Filter the upper layer through 5 g of *anhydrous sodium sulphate R* on a fast filter paper into a 250 ml flask suitable for a rotary evaporator. Wash the funnel with 10 ml of fresh extraction mixture, filter and combine the upper layers. Distil them at a temperature not exceeding 30 °C under reduced pressure (water ejector) and fill with *nitrogen R* when evaporation is completed. Alternatively evaporate the solvent under a gentle current of *nitrogen R* at a temperature not exceeding 30 °C. Dissolve the residue in 1.5 ml of the mobile phase described under Purification. Gentle heating in an ultrasonic bath may be required. (A large fraction of the white residue is cholesterol, constituting approximately 50 per cent *m/m* of the unsaponifiable matter of cod-liver oil).

Test solution (b). To 4.00 g add 2.0 ml of the internal standard solution and proceed as described for test solution (a).

Reference solution (a). Dissolve 0.50 mg of *cholecalciferol CRS* in 100.0 ml of *ethanol R*.

Reference solution (b). In a round-bottomed flask, add 2.0 ml of reference solution (a) and 2.0 ml of the internal standard solution and proceed as described for test solution (a).

PURIFICATION

Column:

- *size*: l = 0.25 m, Ø = 4.6 mm,
- *stationary phase*: *nitrile silica gel for chromatography R* (film thickness 10 µm).

Mobile phase: *isoamyl alcohol R, hexane R* (1.6:98.4 *V/V*).

Flow rate: 1.1 ml/min.

Detection: spectrophotometer at 265 nm.

Inject 350 µl of reference solution (b). Collect the eluate from 2 min before until 2 min after the retention time of cholecalciferol, in a ground-glass-stoppered tube containing 1 ml of a 1 g/l solution of *butylhydroxytoluene R* in *hexane R*. Repeat the procedure with test solutions (a) and (b). Evaporate the eluates obtained from reference solution (b) and from test solutions (a) and (b), separately, to dryness at a temperature not exceeding 30 °C under a gentle current of *nitrogen R*. Dissolve each residue in 1.5 ml of *acetonitrile R*.

DETERMINATION

Column:

- *size*: l = 0.15 m, Ø = 4.6 mm,
- *stationary phase*: *octadecylsilyl silica gel for chromatography R* (film thickness 5 µm).

Monographs C

Mobile phase: *phosphoric acid R*, a 96 per cent *V/V* solution of *acetonitrile R* (0.2:99.8 *V/V*).

Flow rate: 1.0 ml/min.

Detection: spectrophotometer at 265 nm.

Injection: 2 quantities not exceeding 200 µl of each of the 3 solutions obtained under Purification.

System suitability:
- *resolution*: minimum 1.4 between the peaks due to ergocalciferol and cholecalciferol in the chromatogram obtained with reference solution (b),
- when using the method of standard additions to test solution (a) there is greater than 95 per cent recovery of the added *cholecalciferol CRS* when due consideration has been given to correction by the internal standard.

Calculate the content of vitamin D_3 in International Units per gram using the following expression, taking into account the assigned content of *cholecalciferol CRS*:

$$\frac{A_2}{A_6} \times \frac{A_3}{A_4 - \left[\frac{A_5}{A_1}\right] \times A_2} \times \frac{m_2}{m_1} \times \frac{V_2}{V_1} \times 40$$

m_1 = mass of the sample in test solution (b) in grams,

m_2 = total mass of *cholecalciferol CRS* used for the preparation of reference solution (a) in micrograms (500 µg),

A_1 = area (or height) of the peak due to cholecalciferol in the chromatogram obtained with test solution (a),

A_2 = area (or height) of the peak due to cholecalciferol in the chromatogram obtained with test solution (b),

A_3 = area (or height) of the peak due to ergocalciferol in the chromatogram obtained with reference solution (b),

A_4 = area (or height) of the peak due to ergocalciferol in the chromatogram obtained with test solution (b),

A_5 = area (or height) of a possible peak in the chromatogram obtained with test solution (a) with the same retention time as the peak co-eluting with ergocalciferol in test solution (b),

A_6 = area (or height) of the peak due to cholecalciferol in the chromatogram obtained with reference solution (b),

V_1 = total volume of reference solution (a) (100 ml),

V_2 = volume of reference solution (a) used for preparing reference solution (b) (2.0 ml).

STORAGE

In an airtight and well-filled container, protected from light. If no antioxidant is added, store under an inert gas.

Once the container has been opened, its contents are used as soon as possible and any part of the contents not used at once is protected by an atmosphere of inert gas.

LABELLING

The label states:
- the number of International Units of vitamin A,
- the number of International Units of vitamin D_3,
- the name and concentration of any added antioxidant.

01/2005:1504

COLA

Colae semen

DEFINITION

Cola consists of the whole or fragmented dried seeds, freed from the testa, of *Cola nitida* (Vent.) Schott et Endl. (*C. vera* K. Schum.) and its varieties, as well as of *Cola acuminata* (P. Beauv.) Schott et Endl. (*Sterculia acuminata* P. Beauv.). It contains not less than 1.5 per cent of caffeine (M_r 194.2), calculated with reference to the dried drug.

CHARACTERS

It has the macroscopic and microscopic characters described under identification tests A and B.

IDENTIFICATION

A. The kernels have an oblong, somewhat obtuse, sub-tetragonal shape, with deformations resulting from mutual pressure inside the fruit; they vary in size and mass, ranging from 5 g to 15 g; the outside is hard, smooth and very dark brown, the inside is more reddish-brown. In *C. nitida* and its varieties, the kernels are divided in two parts, almost plano-convex, corresponding to the cotyledons and usually occurring separated in the commercial drug; the cotyledons are 3 cm to 4 cm long, 2 cm to 2.5 cm wide and 1 cm to 2 cm thick. In *C. acuminata*, the cotyledons are smaller and divided into four to six irregular parts.

B. Reduce to a powder (355). The powder is reddish-brown. Examine under a microscope using a 50 per cent *V/V* solution of *glycerol R*. The powder shows numerous ovoid or reniform starch granules, 5 µm to 25 µm in size, with concentric striations and a stellate, slightly eccentric hilum; fragments of cotyledon tissue showing large, thick-walled, reddish polygonal cells filled with starch granules; occasional fragments of the external epidermis of the cotyledons.

C. Examine by thin-layer chromatography (*2.2.27*), using a *TLC silica gel F_{254} plate R*.

Test solution. To 1.0 g of the powdered drug (355), add 5 ml of *alcohol (60 per cent V/V) R*. Shake mechanically at 40 °C for 30 min and filter.

Reference solution (a). Dissolve 25 mg of *caffeine R* in 10 ml of *alcohol (60 per cent V/V) R*.

Reference solution (b). Dissolve 50 mg of *theobromine R* in 10 ml of a mixture of 10 volumes of *water R*, 13 volumes of *methanol R* and 77 volumes of *ethyl acetate R*. Filter.

Apply to the plate as bands 20 µl of each solution. Develop over a path of 10 cm using a mixture of 10 volumes of *water R*, 13 volumes of *methanol R* and 77 volumes of *ethyl acetate R*. Allow the plate to dry in air for 5 min. Examine in ultraviolet light at 254 nm. The chromatogram obtained with the test solution shows two principal quenching zones which are similar in position to the zones in the chromatograms obtained with reference solutions (a) and (b), respectively. Spray the plates with a mixture of equal volumes of *alcohol R* and *hydrochloric acid R* and then with a solution prepared immediately before use by dissolving 1 g of *iodine R* and 1 g of *potassium iodide R* in 100 ml of *alcohol R*. The chromatogram obtained with the test solution shows a reddish-brown principal zone similar in position and colour to the zone in the chromatogram obtained with reference solution (a).

TESTS

Foreign matter (*2.8.2*). It complies with the test for foreign matter.

Loss on drying (*2.2.32*). Not more than 12.0 per cent, determined on 2.00 g of the powdered drug (355) by drying in an oven at 100-105 °C for 2 h.

Total ash (*2.4.16*). Not more than 9.0 per cent.

ASSAY

Examine by liquid chromatography (*2.2.29*).

Test solution. To 1.00 g (m_1) of the powdered drug (355), add 50 ml of *methanol R*. Heat the mixture under a reflux condenser on a water-bath for 30 min. Allow to cool and filter. Rinse the filter with 10 ml of *methanol R*. Take up the residue with 50 ml of *methanol R*. Proceed as before. Combine the filtrates and the washings in a 200.0 ml volumetric flask and dilute to 200.0 ml with *methanol R*. Transfer 20.0 ml of this solution into a round-bottomed flask and evaporate to dryness under reduced pressure. Take up the residue with the mobile phase, transfer to a 50.0 ml volumetric flask and dilute to 50.0 ml with the mobile phase.

Reference solution. In a 100.0 ml volumetric flask, dissolve 30.0 mg (m_2) of *caffeine R* and 15.0 mg of *theobromine R* in the mobile phase and dilute to 100.0 ml with the mobile phase. Transfer 10.0 ml of this solution to a 100.0 ml volumetric flask and dilute to 100.0 ml with the mobile phase.

The chromatographic procedure may be carried out using:

- a stainless steel column 0.25 m long and 4.6 mm in internal diameter packed with *octadecylsilyl silica gel for chromatography R* (5 µm),
- as mobile phase at a flow rate of 1 ml/min a mixture of 25 volumes of *methanol R* and 75 volumes of *water R*,
- as detector a spectrophotometer set at 272 nm,
- a loop injector.

Inject appropriate volumes of each solution. The test is not valid unless: in the chromatogram obtained with the reference solution, the resolution between the peaks corresponding respectively to cafeine and theobromine is at least 2.5. If necessary, adjust the volume of *water R* in the mobile phase.

Calculate the caffeine content using the expression:

$$\frac{m_2 \times A_1 \times 50}{m_1 \times A_2}$$

A_1 = area of the peak due to caffeine in the chromatogram obtained with the test solution,

A_2 = area of the peak due to caffeine in the chromatogram obtained with the reference solution,

m_1 = mass of the drug to be examined in the test solution, in grams,

m_2 = mass of *caffeine R* in the reference solution, in grams.

STORAGE

Store protected from light.

01/2005:0758

COLCHICINE

Colchicinum

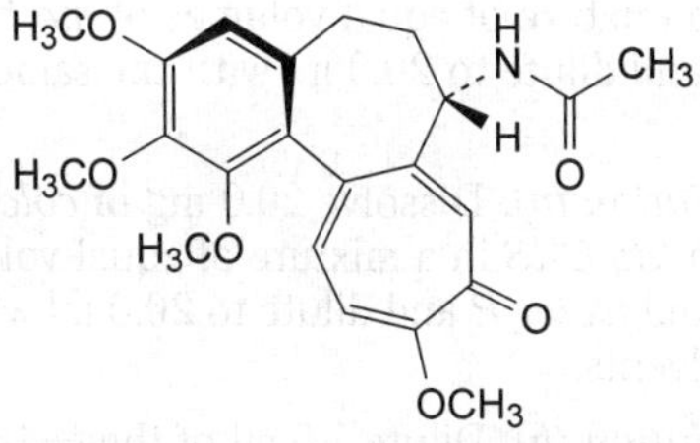

$C_{22}H_{25}NO_6$ M_r 399.4

DEFINITION

(-)-*N*-[(7*S*,12a*S*)-1,2,3,10-Tetramethoxy-9-oxo-5,6,7,9-tetrahydrobenzo[*a*]heptalen-7-yl]acetamide.

Content: 97.0 per cent to 102.0 per cent (anhydrous and ethyl acetate-free substance).

CHARACTERS

Appearance: yellowish-white, amorphous or crystalline powder.

Solubility: very soluble in water, rapidly recrystallising from concentrated solutions as the sesquihydrate, freely soluble in alcohol, practically insoluble in cyclohexane.

IDENTIFICATION

First identification: B.

Second identification: A, C, D.

A. Dissolve 5 mg in *alcohol R* and dilute to 100.0 ml with the same solvent. Dilute 5.0 ml of the solution to 25.0 ml with *alcohol R*. Examined between 230 nm and 400 nm (*2.2.25*), the solution shows 2 absorption maxima, at 243 nm and 350 nm. The ratio of the absorbance measured at 243 nm to that measured at 350 nm is 1.7 to 1.9.

B. Infrared absorption spectrophotometry (*2.2.24*).
Preparation: discs of *potassium bromide R*.
Comparison: *colchicine CRS*.

C. To 0.5 ml of solution S (see Tests) add 0.5 ml of *dilute hydrochloric acid R* and 0.15 ml of *ferric chloride solution R1*. The solution is yellow and becomes dark green on boiling for 30 s. Cool, add 2 ml of *methylene chloride R* and shake. The organic layer is greenish-yellow.

D. Dissolve about 30 mg in 1 ml of *alcohol R* and add 0.15 ml of *ferric chloride solution R1*. A brownish-red colour develops.

TESTS

Solution S. Dissolve 0.10 g in *water R* and dilute to 20 ml with the same solvent.

Appearance of solution. Solution S is clear (*2.2.1*) and not more intensely coloured than reference solution GY_3 (*2.2.2, Method II*).

Acidity or alkalinity. To 10 ml of solution S add 0.1 ml of *bromothymol blue solution R1*. Either the solution does not change colour or it becomes green. Not more than 0.1 ml of *0.01 M sodium hydroxide* is required to change the colour of the indicator to blue.

Specific optical rotation (*2.2.7*): − 235 to − 250 (anhydrous and ethyl acetate-free substance).

Dissolve 50.0 mg in *alcohol R* and dilute to 10.0 ml with the same solvent.

Related substances. Liquid chromatography (*2.2.29*).

Test solution. Dissolve 20.0 mg of the substance to be examined in a mixture of equal volumes of *methanol R* and *water R* and dilute to 20.0 ml with the same mixture of solvents.

Reference solution (a). Dissolve 20.0 mg of *colchicine for system suitability CRS* in a mixture of equal volumes of *methanol R* and *water R* and dilute to 20.0 ml with the same mixture of solvents.

Reference solution (b). Dilute 1.0 ml of the test solution to 100.0 ml with a mixture of equal volumes of *methanol R* and *water R*.

Reference solution (c). Dilute 1 ml of reference solution (b) to 20.0 ml with a mixture of equal volumes of *methanol R* and *water R*.

Column:

- *size*: *l* = 0.25 m, Ø = 4.6 mm,
- *stationary phase*: *octylsilyl silica gel for chromatography R1* (5 µm).

Mobile phase: mix 450 volumes of a 6.8 g/l solution of *potassium dihydrogen phosphate R* and 530 volumes of *methanol R*. After cooling to room temperature, adjust the volume to 1000 ml with *methanol R*. Adjust the apparent pH to 5.5 with *dilute phosphoric acid R*.

Flow rate: 1 ml/min.

Detection: spectrophotometer at 254 nm.

Injection: 20 µl.

Run time: 3 times the retention time of colchicine.

Relative retention with reference to colchicine (retention time = about 7 min): impurity D = about 0.4; impurity E = about 0.7; impurity B = about 0.8; impurity A = about 0.94; impurity C = about 1.2.

System suitability: reference solution (a):

Peak-to-valley ratio: minimum 2, where H_p = height above the baseline of the peak due to impurity A and H_v = height above the baseline of the lowest point of the curve separating this peak from the peak due to colchicine.

Limits:

- *impurity A*: not more than 3.5 times the area of the principal peak in the chromatogram obtained with reference solution (b) (3.5 per cent),
- *any other impurity*: not more than the area of the principal peak in the chromatogram obtained with reference solution (b) (1 per cent),
- *total*: not more than 5 times the area of the principal peak in the chromatogram obtained with reference solution (b) (5 per cent),
- *disregard limit*: area of the principal peak in the chromatogram obtained with reference solution (c) (0.05 per cent).

Colchiceine: maximum 0.2 per cent.

Dissolve 50 mg in *water R* and dilute to 5 ml with the same solvent. Add 0.1 ml of *ferric chloride solution R1*. The solution is not more intensely coloured than a mixture of 1 ml of red primary solution, 2 ml of yellow primary solution and 2 ml of blue primary solution (*2.2.2, Method II*).

Chloroform (*2.4.24*): maximum 500 ppm.

Ethyl acetate (*2.4.24*): maximum 6.0 per cent *m/m*.

Water (*2.5.12*): maximum 2.0 per cent, determined on 0.500 g.

Sulphated ash (*2.4.14*): maximum 0.1 per cent, determined on 0.5 g.

ASSAY

Dissolve 0.250 g with gentle heating in a mixture of 10 ml of *acetic anhydride R* and 20 ml of *toluene R*. Titrate with *0.1 M perchloric acid*, determining the end-point potentiometrically (*2.2.20*).

1 ml of *0.1 M perchloric acid* is equivalent to 39.94 mg of $C_{22}H_{25}NO_6$.

STORAGE

Protected from light.

IMPURITIES

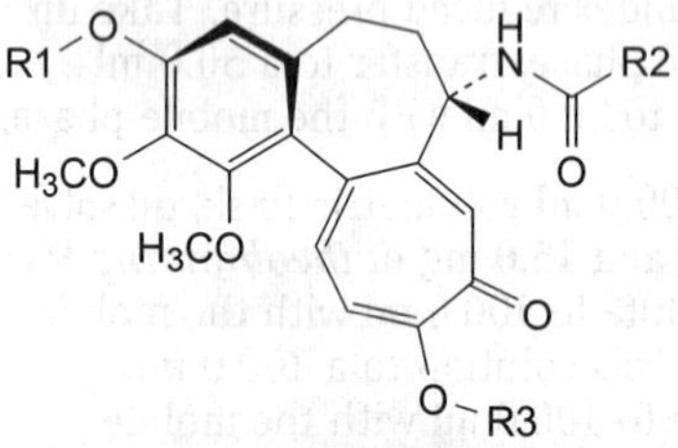

A. R1 = R3 = CH_3, R2 = H: *N*-[(7*S*,12a*S*)-1,2,3,10-tetramethoxy-9-oxo-5,6,7,9-tetrahydrobenzo[*a*]heptalen-7-yl]formamide (*N*-deacetyl-*N*-formylcolchicine),

E. R1 = H, R2 = R3 = CH_3: *N*-[(7*S*,12a*S*)-3-hydroxy-1,2,10-trimethoxy-9-oxo-5,6,7,9-tetrahydrobenzo[*a*]heptalen-7-yl]acetamide (3-*O*-demethylcolchicine),

F. R1 = R2 = CH_3, R3 = H: *N*-[(7*S*,12a*S*)-10-hydroxy-1,2,3-trimethoxy-9-oxo-5,6,7,9-tetrahydrobenzo[*a*]heptalen-7-yl]acetamide (colchiceine),

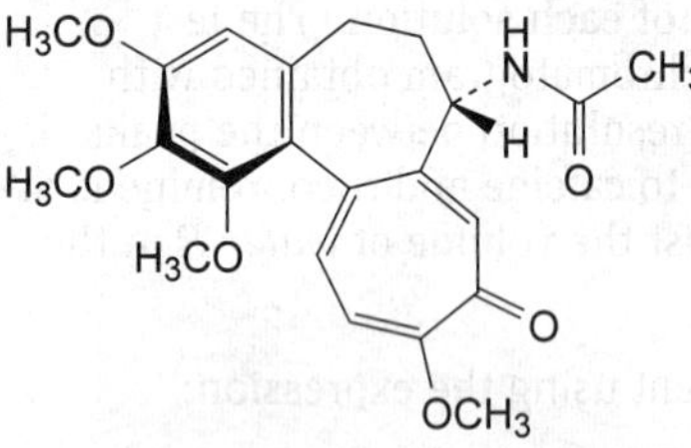

B. (-)-*N*-[(7*S*,12a*R*)-1,2,3,10-tetramethoxy-9-oxo-5,6,7,9-tetrahydrobenzo[*a*]heptalen-7-yl]acetamide (conformationnal isomer),

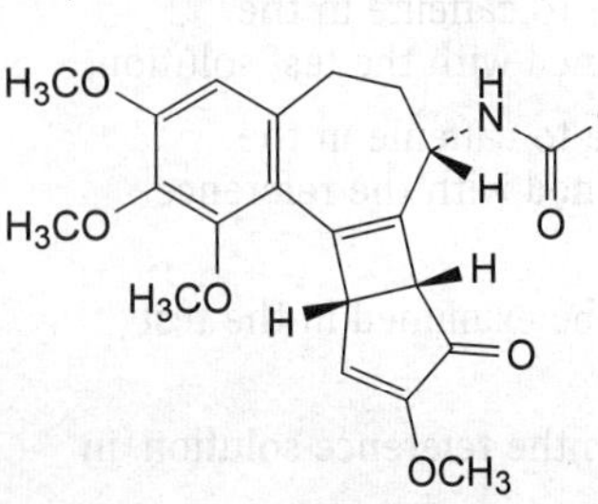

C. *N*-[(7*S*,7b*R*,10a*S*)-1,2,3,9-tetramethoxy-8-oxo-5,6,7,7b,8,10a-hexahydrobenzo[*a*]cyclopenta[3,4]-cyclobuta[1,2-*c*]cyclohepten-7-yl]acetamide (β-lumicolchicine),

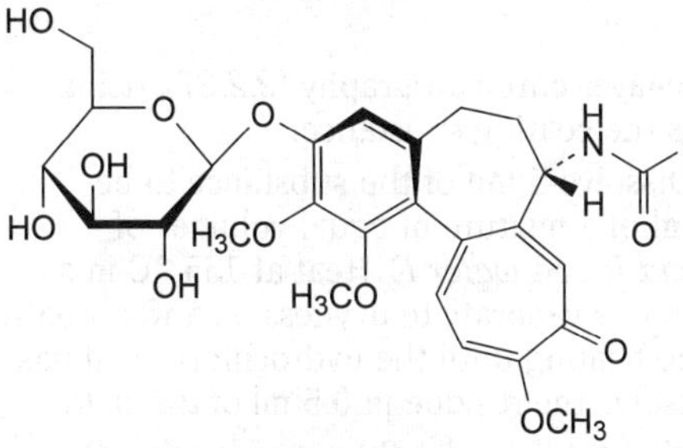

D. *N*-[(7*S*,12a*S*)-3-(β-D-glucopyranosyloxy)-1,2,10-trimethoxy-9-oxo-5,6,7,9-tetrahydrobenzo[*a*]heptalen-7-yl]acetamide (colchicoside).

01/2005:1775

COLESTYRAMINE

Colestyraminum

DEFINITION

Strongly basic anion-exchange resin in chloride form, consisting of styrene-divinylbenzene copolymer with quaternary ammonium groups.

Nominal exchange capacity: 1.8 g to 2.2 g of sodium glycocholate per gram (dried substance).

CHARACTERS

Appearance: white or almost white, fine powder, hygroscopic.

Solubility: insoluble in water, in methylene chloride and in ethanol (96 per cent).

IDENTIFICATION

A. Infrared absorption spectrophotometry (*2.2.24*).

Comparison: colestyramine CRS.

B. It complies with the test for chlorides (see Tests).

TESTS

pH (*2.2.3*): 4.0 to 6.0.

Suspend 0.100 g in 10 ml of *water R* and allow to stand for 10 min.

Dialysable quaternary amines: maximum 500 ppm, expressed as benzyltrimethylammonium chloride.

Test solution. Place a 25 cm piece of cellulose dialysis tubing having a molecular weight cut-off of 12 000-14 000 and an inflated diameter of 3-6 cm (flat width of 5-9 cm) in *water R* to hydrate until pliable, appropriately sealing one end. Introduce 2.0 g of the substance to be examined into the tube and add 10 ml of *water R*. Seal the tube and completely immerse it in 100 ml of *water R* in a suitable vessel and stir the liquid for 16 h to effect dialysis. Use the dialysate as test solution.

Reference solution. Prepare the reference solution in a similar manner but using 10 ml of a freshly prepared 0.1 g/l solution of *benzyltrimethylammonium chloride R* instead of the substance to be examined.

Transfer 5.0 ml of the test solution to a separating funnel and add 5 ml of a 3.8 g/l solution of *disodium tetraborate R*, 1 ml of a solution containing 1.5 g/l of *bromothymol blue R* and 4.05 g/l of *sodium carbonate R* and 10 ml of *chloroform R*. Shake the mixture vigourously for 1 min, allow the phases to separate and transfer the clear organic layer to a 25 ml volumetric flask. Repeat the extraction with a further 10 ml of *chloroform R*, combine the organic layers and dilute to 25 ml with *chloroform R*. Measure the absorbance (*2.2.25*) of the solution at the absorption maximum at 420 nm, using as compensation liquid a solution prepared in the same manner but using 5.0 ml of *water R* instead of the test solution. Repeat the operation using 5.0 ml of the reference solution. The absorbance obtained with the test solution is not greater than that obtained with the reference solution.

Impurity A. Liquid chromatography (*2.2.29*).

Test solution. Shake 5.0 g with 10 ml of *acetone R* for 30 min. Centrifuge and use the supernatant liquid.

Reference solution (a). Dissolve 5 mg of *styrene R* in *acetone R* and dilute to 100.0 ml with the same solvent. Dilute 1.0 ml to 100.0 ml with *acetone R*.

Reference solution (b). Dissolve 0.35 ml of *styrene R* in *acetone R* and dilute to 100.0 ml with the same solvent. Dilute 1.0 ml to 100.0 ml with *acetone R*.

Reference solution (c). Dissolve 0.35 ml of *toluene R* in *acetone R* and dilute to 100.0 ml with the same solvent.

Reference solution (d). Mix 1.0 ml of reference solution (b) and 1.0 ml of reference solution (c) with *acetone R* and dilute to 100.0 ml with the same solvent.

Column:

– *size*: l = 0.30 m, Ø = 3.9 mm,
– *stationary phase*: *octadecylsilyl silica gel for chromatography R* (10 µm) with a specific surface area of 330 m^2/g and a pore size of 12.5 nm.

Mobile phase: *acetonitrile R, water R* (50:50 *V/V*).

Flow rate: 2.0 ml/min.

Detection: spectrophotometer at 254 nm.

Injection: 20 µl of test solution, reference solutions (a) and (d).

System suitability: reference solution (d):

– *resolution*: minimum 1.5 between the peaks due to impurity A and toluene.

Limit:

– *impurity A*: not more than the area of the principal peak in the chromatogram obtained with reference solution (a) (1 ppm).

Chloride: 13.0 per cent to 17.0 per cent (dried substance).

To 0.2 g add 100 ml of *water R* and 50 mg of *potassium nitrate R*. Add, with stirring, 2 ml of *nitric acid R* and titrate with *0.1 M silver nitrate*, determining the end-point potentiometrically (*2.2.20*).

1 ml of *0.1 M silver nitrate* is equivalent to 3.55 mg of Cl.

Heavy metals (*2.4.8*): maximum 20 ppm.

1.0 g complies with limit test F. Prepare the reference solution using 2 ml of *lead standard solution (10 ppm Pb) R*.

Loss on drying (*2.2.32*): maximum 12 per cent, determined on 1.000 g by drying in an oven at 70 °C over *diphosphorus pentoxide R* at a pressure not exceeding 7 kPa for 16 h.

Sulphated ash (*2.4.14*): maximum 0.1 per cent, determined on 1.0 g.

ASSAY

Exchange capacity. Liquid chromatography (*2.2.29*).

Solution A. Dissolve 1.500 g of *sodium glycocholate R* in a solution containing 4 g/l of *potassium dihydrogen phosphate R* and 12 g/l of *dipotassium hydrogen phosphate R* and dilute to 100.0 ml with the same solution.

Test solution. Add 20.0 ml of solution A to a quantity of the substance to be examined equivalent to about 0.100 g of the dried substance. Shake mechanically for 2 h and centrifuge for 15 min. Dilute 5.0 ml of the supernatant liquid to 50.0 ml with *water R*.

Reference solution (a). Dilute 4.0 ml of solution A to 100.0 ml with *water R*.

Reference solution (b). Dissolve 60 mg of *sodium glycocholate R* and 30 mg of *sodium taurodeoxycholate R* in *water R* and dilute to 100 ml with the same solvent. Dilute 1 ml of the solution to 10 ml with *water R*.

Column:
- *size*: l = 0.25 m, Ø = 4.6 mm,
- *stationary phase*: *octadecylsilyl silica gel for chromatography R* (5 µm).

Mobile phase: mix 35 volumes of *acetonitrile R* and 65 volumes of a 10.9 g/l solution of *potassium dihydrogen phosphate R* adjusted to pH 3.0 with *phosphoric acid R*.

Flow rate: 1.5 ml/min.

Detection: spectrophotometer at 214 nm.

Injection: 50 µl.

Run time: twice the retention time of glycocholate.

System suitability: reference solution (b):
- *resolution*: minimum 1.5 between the peaks due to glycocholate and taurodeoxycholate.

Calculate the nominal exchange capacity using the following expression:

$$\frac{(2.5\, A_1 - A_2) \times m_1 \times 0.73}{12.5 \times A_1 \times m_2}$$

A_1 = area of the peak due to glycocholate in the chromatogram obtained with reference solution (a),

A_2 = area of the peak due to glycocholate in the chromatogram obtained with the test solution,

m_1 = mass, in milligrams, of *sodium glycocholate R* used in the preparation of solution A,

m_2 = mass, in milligrams, of the dried substance to be examined used in the preparation of the test solution,

0.73 = correction factor to convert the true exchange capacity to the conventionally used nominal exchange capacity.

STORAGE

In an airtight container.

IMPURITIES

Specified impurities: A.

A. styrene.

01/2005:0319

COLISTIMETHATE SODIUM

Colistimethatum natricum

DEFINITION

Colistimethate sodium is prepared from colistin by the action of formaldehyde and sodium hydrogen sulphite. The potency is not less than 11 500 IU/mg, calculated with reference to the dried substance.

CHARACTERS

A white or almost white powder, hygroscopic, very soluble in water, slightly soluble in alcohol, practically insoluble in acetone.

IDENTIFICATION

A. Examine by thin-layer chromatography (*2.2.27*), using *silica gel G R* as the coating substance.

Test solution. Dissolve 5 mg of the substance to be examined in 1 ml of a mixture of equal volumes of *hydrochloric acid R* and *water R*. Heat at 135 °C in a sealed tube for 5 h. Evaporate to dryness on a water-bath and continue the heating until the hydrochloric acid has evaporated. Dissolve the residue in 0.5 ml of *water R*.

Reference solution (a). Dissolve 20 mg of *leucine R* in *water R* and dilute to 10 ml with the same solvent.

Reference solution (b). Dissolve 20 mg of *threonine R* in *water R* and dilute to 10 ml with the same solvent.

Reference solution (c). Dissolve 20 mg of *phenylalanine R* in *water R* and dilute to 10 ml with the same solvent.

Reference solution (d). Dissolve 20 mg of *serine R* in *water R* and dilute to 10 ml with the same solvent.

Carry out the following procedures protected from light.

Apply to the plate as 10 mm bands 5 µl of each solution. Place the plate in the chromatographic tank so that it is not in contact with the mobile phase consisting of a mixture of 25 volumes of *water R* and 75 volumes of *phenol R*. Leave the plate to become impregnated with the vapour of the solvent for at least 12 h. Develop over a path of 12 cm using the same mobile phase. Dry the plate at 100-105 °C and spray with *ninhydrin solution R1*. Heat at 110 °C for 5 min. The chromatogram obtained with the test solution shows zones corresponding to those in the chromatograms obtained with reference solutions (a) and (b), but shows no zones corresponding to those in the chromatograms obtained with reference solutions (c) and (d). The chromatogram obtained with the test solution also shows a zone with a very low R_f value (2,4-diaminobutyric acid).

B. Dissolve about 5 mg in 3 ml of *water R*. Add 3 ml of *dilute sodium hydroxide solution R*. Shake and add 0.5 ml of a 10 g/l solution of *copper sulphate R*. A violet colour is produced.

C. Dissolve about 50 mg in 1 ml of *1 M hydrochloric acid* and add 0.5 ml of *0.01 M iodine*. The solution is decolourised and gives reaction (a) of sulphates (*2.3.1*).

D. It gives reaction (b) of sodium (*2.3.1*).

TESTS

Appearance of solution. Dissolve 0.16 g in 10 ml of *water R*. The solution is clear (*2.2.1*).

pH (*2.2.3*). Dissolve 0.1 g in *carbon dioxide-free water R* and dilute to 10 ml with the same solvent. The pH of the solution, measured after 30 min, is 6.5 to 8.5.

Specific optical rotation (*2.2.7*). Dissolve 1.25 g in *water R* and dilute to 25.0 ml with the same solvent. The specific optical rotation is − 46 to − 51, calculated with reference to the dried substance.

Free colistin. Dissolve 80 mg in 3 ml of *water R*. Add 0.1 ml of a 100 g/l solution of *silicotungstic acid R*; 10 s to 20 s after addition of the reagent, the solution is not more opalescent than reference suspension II (*2.2.1*).

Total sulphite. *Work in a fume cupboard.* Dissolve 0.100 g in 50 ml of *water R* and add 5 ml of a 100 g/l solution of *sodium hydroxide R* and 0.3 g of *potassium cyanide R*. Boil gently for 3 min and then cool. Neutralise with *0.5 M sulphuric acid* using 0.2 ml of *methyl orange solution R* as indicator. Add an excess of 0.5 ml of the acid and 0.2 g of *potassium iodide R*. Titrate with *0.05 M iodine* using 1 ml of *starch solution R* as indicator. The volume of *0.05 M iodine* used in the titration is 5.5 ml to 7.0 ml.

Loss on drying (*2.2.32*). Not more than 5.0 per cent, determined on 1.000 g by drying at 60 °C over *diphosphorus pentoxide R* at a pressure not exceeding 670 Pa for 3 h.

Sulphated ash (*2.4.14*). 16 per cent to 21 per cent, determined on 0.50 g.

Pyrogens (*2.6.8*). If intended for use in the manufacture of parenteral dosage forms without a further appropriate procedure for removal of pyrogens, it complies with the test for pyrogens. Inject per kilogram of the rabbit's mass 1 ml of a solution in *water for injections R* containing 2.5 mg of the substance to be examined per millilitre.

ASSAY

Carry out the microbiological assay of antibiotics (*2.7.2*).

STORAGE

Store in an airtight container, protected from light. If the substance is sterile, store in a sterile, airtight, tamper-proof container.

LABELLING

The label states, where applicable, that the substance is free from pyrogens.

01/2005:0320

COLISTIN SULPHATE

Colistini sulfas

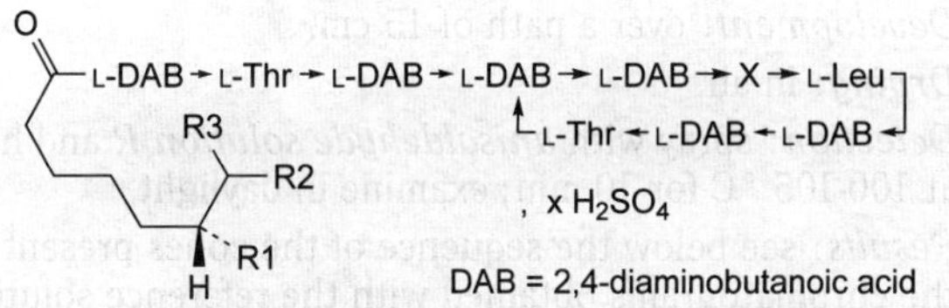

colistin	X	R1	R2	R3	Mol. Formula	M_r
E1	D-Leu	CH_3	CH_3	H	$C_{53}H_{100}N_{16}O_{13}$	1170
E2	D-Leu	CH_3	H	H	$C_{52}H_{98}N_{16}O_{13}$	1155
E3	D-Leu	H	CH_3	H	$C_{52}H_{98}N_{16}O_{13}$	1155
E1-I	D-Ile	CH_3	CH_3	H	$C_{53}H_{100}N_{16}O_{13}$	1170
E1-7MOA	D-Leu	H	CH_3	CH_3	$C_{53}H_{100}N_{16}O_{13}$	1170

DEFINITION

A mixture of the sulphates of polypeptides produced by certain strains of *Bacillus polymyxa* var. *colistinus* or obtained by any other means.

Content:

- sum of colistins E1, E2, E3, E1-I and E1-7MOA: minimum 77.0 per cent (dried substance),
- colistin E1-I: maximum 10.0 per cent (dried substance),
- colistin E1-7MOA: maximum 10.0 per cent (dried substance),
- colistin E3: maximum 10.0 per cent (dried substance).

CHARACTERS

Appearance: white or almost white powder, hygroscopic.

Solubility: freely soluble in water, slightly soluble in alcohol, practically insoluble in acetone.

IDENTIFICATION

First identification: B, E.

Second identification: A, C, D, E.

A. Thin-layer chromatography (*2.2.27*).

Test solution. Dissolve 5 mg of the substance to be examined in 1 ml of a mixture of equal volumes of *hydrochloric acid R* and *water R*. Heat at 135 °C in a sealed tube for 5 h. Evaporate to dryness on a water-bath and continue the heating until moistened *blue litmus paper R* does not turn red. Dissolve the residue in 0.5 ml of *water R*.

Reference solution (a). Dissolve 20 mg of *leucine R* in *water R* and dilute to 10 ml with the same solvent.

Reference solution (b). Dissolve 20 mg of *threonine R* in *water R* and dilute to 10 ml with the same solvent.

Reference solution (c). Dissolve 20 mg of *phenylalanine R* in *water R* and dilute to 10 ml with the same solvent.

Reference solution (d). Dissolve 20 mg of *serine R* in *water R* and dilute to 10 ml with the same solvent.

Plate: *TLC silica gel G plate R.*

Mobile phase: *water R, phenol R* (25:75 *V/V*).

Carry out the following procedures protected from light.

Application: 5 µl as 10 mm bands.

Preconditioning: place the plate in the chromatographic tank, so that it is not in contact with the mobile phase, and allow to become impregnated with the vapour of the mobile phase for at least 12 h.

Development: over a path of 12 cm.

Drying: at 100-105 °C.

Detection: spray with *ninhydrin solution R1* and heat at 110 °C for 5 min.

Results: the chromatogram obtained with the test solution shows zones corresponding to those in the chromatograms obtained with reference solutions (a) and (b), but shows no zones corresponding to those in the chromatograms obtained with reference solutions (c) and (d). The chromatogram obtained with the test solution also shows a zone with a very low R_f value (2,4-diaminobutyric acid).

B. Examine the chromatograms obtained in the assay.

Results: the peaks due to colistin E1 and colistin E2 in the chromatogram obtained with the test solution are similar in retention time to the corresponding peaks in the chromatogram obtained with reference solution (a).

C. Dissolve about 5 mg in 3 ml of *water R*. Add 3 ml of *dilute sodium hydroxide solution R*. Shake and add 0.5 ml of a 10 g/l solution of *copper sulphate R*. A violet colour is produced.

D. Dissolve about 50 mg in 1 ml of *1 M hydrochloric acid* and add 0.5 ml of *0.01 M iodine*. The solution remains coloured.

E. It gives reaction (a) of sulphates (*2.3.1*).

TESTS

pH (*2.2.3*): 4.0 to 6.0.

Dissolve 0.1 g in *carbon dioxide-free water R* and dilute to 10 ml with the same solvent.

Specific optical rotation (*2.2.7*): − 63 to − 73 (dried substance).

Dissolve 1.25 g in *water R* and dilute to 25.0 ml with the same solvent.

Related substances. Liquid chromatography (*2.2.29*): use the normalisation procedure.

Test solution. Dissolve 25.0 mg of the substance to be examined in 40 ml of *water R* and dilute to 50.0 ml with *acetonitrile R.*

Reference solution (a). Dissolve 25.0 mg of *colistin sulphate CRS* in 40 ml of *water R* and dilute to 50.0 ml with *acetonitrile R.*

Reference solution (b). Dilute 1.0 ml of reference solution (a) to 100.0 ml with a mixture of 20 volumes of *acetonitrile R* and 80 volumes of *water R.*

Column:

– *size*: l = 0.15 m, Ø = 4.6 mm,
– *stationary phase*: *end-capped octadecylsilyl silica gel for chromatography R* (3.5 μm),
– *temperature*: 30 °C.

Mobile phase: mix 22 volumes of *acetonitrile R* and 78 volumes of a solution prepared as follows: dissolve 4.46 g of *anhydrous sodium sulphate R* in 900 ml of *water R,* add 2.5 ml of *phosphoric acid R* and dilute to 1000 ml with *water R* (pH 2.3 to 2.5).

Flow rate: 1.0 ml/min.

Detection: spectrophotometer at 215 nm.

Injection: 20 μl.

Run time: 1.5 times the retention time of colistin E1.

Relative retention with reference to colistin E1 (retention time = about 16 min): colistin E2 = about 0.45; colistin E3 = about 0.5; colistin E1-I = about 0.8; colistin E1-7MOA = about 1.1.

System suitability: reference solution (a):

– *resolution*: minimum 8.0 between the peaks due to colistin E2 and colistin E1, minimum 6.0 between the peaks due to colistin E2 and colistin E1-I, minimum 2.5 between the peaks due to colistin E1-I and colistin E1, minimum 1.5 between the peaks due to colistin E1 and colistin E1-7MOA,
– the chromatogram obtained is concordant with the chromatogram supplied with *colistin sulphate CRS.*

Limits:

– *any impurity*: maximum 4.0 per cent,
– *total*: maximum 23.0 per cent,
– *disregard limit*: the area of the peak due to colistin E1 in the chromatogram obtained with reference solution (b); disregard the peaks due to colistin E2, E3, E1-I, E1 and E1-7MOA.

Sulphate: 16.0 per cent to 18.0 per cent (dried substance). Dissolve 0.250 g in 100 ml of *water R* and adjust to pH 11 using *concentrated ammonia R.* Add 10.0 ml of *0.1 M barium chloride* and about 0.5 mg of *phthalein purple R.* Titrate with *0.1 M sodium edetate,* adding 50 ml of *alcohol R* when the colour of the solution begins to change and continuing the titration until the violet-blue colour disappears.

1 ml of *0.1 M barium chloride* is equivalent to 9.606 mg of SO_4.

Loss on drying (*2.2.32*): maximum 3.5 per cent, determined on 1.000 g by drying at 60 °C over *diphosphorus pentoxide R* at a pressure not exceeding 670 Pa for 3 h.

Sulphated ash (*2.4.14*): maximum 1.0 per cent, determined on 1.0 g.

ASSAY

Liquid chromatography (*2.2.29*) as described in the test for related substances with the following modification.

Injection: test solution and reference solution (a).

Calculate the percentage content of the sum of colistins E2, E3, E1-I, E1 and E1-7MOA, the percentage content of colistin E3, the percentage content of colistin E1-I and the percentage content of colistin E1-7MOA using the chromatogram obtained with reference solution (a) and the declared contents of *colistin sulphate CRS.*

STORAGE

In an airtight container, protected from light.

01/2005:1862

COLOPHONY

Colophonium

DEFINITION

Residue remaining after distillation of the volatile oil from the oleoresin obtained from various species of *Pinus.*

CHARACTERS

Macroscopic characters described under identification A.

IDENTIFICATION

A. Translucent, pale yellow to brownish-yellow, angular, irregularly-shaped, brittle, glassy pieces of different sizes the surfaces of which bear conchoidal markings.

B. Thin-layer chromatography (*2.2.27*).

Test solution. Dissolve 1 g in 10 ml of *methanol R* by gently warming.

Reference solution. Dissolve 10 mg of *thymol R* and 10 mg of *linalol R* in 10 ml of *methanol R.*

Plate: *TLC silica gel plate R.*

Mobile phase: *methylene chloride R.*

Application: 10 μl, as bands.

Development: over a path of 15 cm.

Drying: in air.

Detection: spray with *anisaldehyde solution R* and heat at 100-105 °C for 10 min; examine in daylight.

Results: see below the sequence of the zones present in the chromatograms obtained with the reference solution and the test solution. Furthermore, other coloured zones are present in the chromatogram obtained with the test solution.

Top of the plate	
	A purple band
	A purple band
_______	_______
	2 purple bands
Thymol: an orange band	
_______	_______
Linalol: a purple band	Sequence of narrow purple bands
	Purple extended baseline band
Reference solution	**Test solution**

TESTS

Acid value (*2.5.1*): 145 to 180, determined on 1.0 g.

Foreign matter (*2.8.2*): maximum 2 per cent.

Total ash (*2.4.16*): maximum 0.2 per cent.

STORAGE

Do not reduce to a powder.

01/2005:0891

COPOVIDONE

Copovidonum

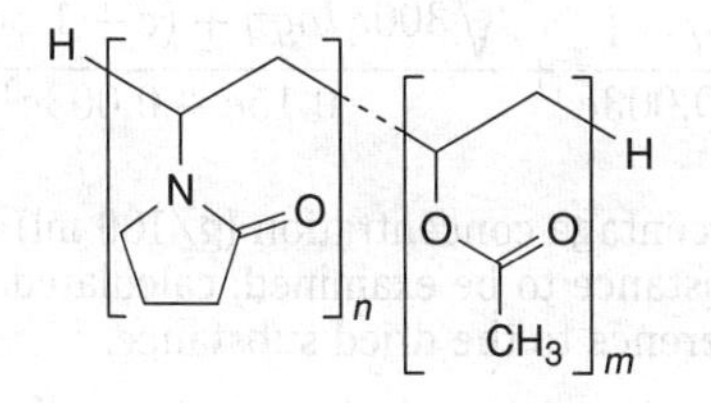

$n = 1.2m$

$(C_6H_9NO)_n, (C_4H_6O_2)_m$ M_r $(111.1)_n + (86.1)_m$

DEFINITION

Copovidone is a copolymer of 1-ethenylpyrrolidin-2-one and ethenyl acetate in the mass proportion 3:2.

Content:

- nitrogen (N; A_r 14.01): 7.0 per cent to 8.0 per cent (dried substance),
- ethenyl acetate $C_4H_6O_2$; M_r 86.10): 35.3 per cent to 42.0 per cent (dried substance).

K-value: 90.0 per cent to 110.0 per cent of the value stated on the label.

CHARACTERS

Aspect: white or yellowish-white powder or flakes, hygroscopic.

Solubility: freely soluble in water, in alcohol and in methylene chloride.

IDENTIFICATION

First identification: A.

Second identification: B, C.

A. Infrared absorption spectrophotometry (*2.2.24*).

Comparison: *Ph. Eur. reference spectrum of copovidone.*

B. To 1 ml of solution S (see Tests) add 5 ml of *water R* and 0.2 ml of *0.05 M iodine*. A red colour appears.

C. Dissolve 0.7 g of *hydroxylamine hydrochloride R* in 10 ml of *methanol R*, add 20 ml of a 40 g/l solution of *sodium hydroxide R* and filter if necessary. To 5 ml of the solution add 0.1 g of the substance to be examined and boil for 2 min. Transfer 50 µl to a filter paper and add 0.1 ml of a mixture of equal volumes of *ferric chloride solution R1* and *hydrochloric acid R*. A violet colour appears.

TESTS

Solution S. Dissolve 10 g in *water R* and dilute to 100 ml with the same solvent. Add the substance to be examined to the *water R* in small portions with constant stirring.

Appearance of solution. Solution S is not more opalescent than reference suspension III (*2.2.1*) and not more intensely coloured than reference solution B_5, R_5 or BY_5 (*2.2.2, Method II*).

Aldehydes: maximum 500 ppm, expressed as acetaldehyde.

Test solution. Dissolve 1.0 g of the substance to be examined in *phosphate buffer solution pH 9.0 R* and dilute to 100.0 ml with the same solvent. Stopper the flask and heat at 60 °C for 1 h. Allow to cool.

Reference solution. Dissolve 0.140 g of *acetaldehyde ammonia trimer trihydrate R* in *water R* and dilute to 200.0 ml with the same solvent. Dilute 1.0 ml of this solution to 100.0 ml with *phosphate buffer solution pH 9.0 R*.

Into 3 identical spectrophotometric cells with a path length of 1 cm, introduce separately 0.5 ml of the test solution, 0.5 ml of the reference solution and 0.5 ml of *water R* (blank). To each cell, add 2.5 ml of *phosphate buffer solution pH 9.0 R* and 0.2 ml of *nicotinamide-adenine dinucleotide solution R*. Mix and stopper tightly. Allow to stand at 22 ± 2 °C for 2-3 min and measure the absorbance (*2.2.25*) of each solution at 340 nm, using *water R* as the compensation liquid. To each cell, add 0.05 ml of *aldehyde dehydrogenase solution R*, mix and stopper tightly. Allow to stand at 22 ± 2 °C for 5 min. Measure the absorbance of each solution at 340 nm using *water R* as compensation liquid. Determine the content of aldehydes using the expression:

$$\frac{(A_{t2} - A_{t1}) - (A_{b2} - A_{b1})}{(A_{s2} - A_{s1}) - (A_{b2} - A_{b1})} \times \frac{100\,000 \times C}{m}$$

A_{t1} = absorbance of the test solution before the addition of aldehyde dehydrogenase,

A_{t2} = absorbance of the test solution after the addition of aldehyde dehydrogenase,

A_{s1} = absorbance of the reference solution before the addition of aldehyde dehydrogenase,

A_{s2} = absorbance of the reference solution after the addition of aldehyde dehydrogenase,

A_{b1} = absorbance of the blank before the addition of aldehyde dehydrogenase,

A_{b2} = absorbance of the blank after the addition of aldehyde dehydrogenase,

m = mass of povidone, in grams, calculated with reference to the dried substance,

C = concentration (mg/ml), of acetaldehyde in the reference solution, calculated from the weight of the acetaldehyde ammonia trimer trihydrate with the factor 0.72.

Peroxides: maximum 400 ppm, expressed as H_2O_2.

Dilute 10 ml of solution S to 25 ml with *water R*. Add 2 ml of *titanium trichloride-sulphuric acid reagent R* and allow to stand for 30 min. The absorbance (*2.2.25*) of the solution, measured at 405 nm using a mixture of 25 ml of a 40 g/l solution of the substance to be examined and 2 ml of a 13 per cent *V/V* solution of *sulphuric acid R* as the compensation liquid, is not greater than 0.35.

Hydrazine. Thin-layer chromatography (*2.2.27*). *Use freshly prepared solutions.*

Test solution. To 25 ml of solution S add 0.5 ml of a 50 g/l solution of *salicylaldehyde R* in *methanol R*, mix and heat in a water-bath at 60 °C for 15 min. Allow to cool, add 2.0 ml of *xylene R*, shake for 2 min and centrifuge. Use the clear supernatant layer.

Reference solution. Dissolve 9 mg of *salicylaldehyde azine R* in *xylene R* and dilute to 100 ml with the same solvent. Dilute 1 ml of this solution to 10 ml with *xylene R*.

Plate: *TLC silanised silica gel plate R.*

Mobile phase: *water R, methanol R* (20:80 *V/V*).

Application: 10 µl.

Development: over a path of 15 cm.

Drying: in air.

Detection: examine in ultraviolet light at 365 nm.

Monographs C

Limit:

- *hydrazine*: any spot corresponding to salicylaldehyde azine in the chromatogram obtained with the test solution is not more intense than the spot in the chromatogram obtained with the reference solution (1 ppm).

Monomers: maximum 0.1 per cent.

Dissolve 10.0 g in 30 ml of *methanol R* and add slowly 20.0 ml of *iodine bromide solution R*. Allow to stand for 30 min protected from light with repeated shaking. Add 10 ml of a 100 g/l solution of *potassium iodide R* and titrate with *0.1 M sodium thiosulphate* until a yellow colour is obtained. Continue titration dropwise until the solution becomes colourless. Carry out a blank titration. Not more than 1.8 ml of *0.1 M sodium thiosulphate* is used.

Impurity A. Liquid chromatography (*2.2.29*).

Test solution. Dissolve 100 mg of the substance to be examined in *water R* and dilute to 50.0 ml with the same solvent.

Reference solution. Dissolve 100 mg of *2-pyrrolidone R* in *water R* and dilute to 100 ml with the same solvent. Dilute 1.0 ml to 100.0 ml with *water R*.

Precolumn:

- *size*: *l* = 0.025 m, Ø = 4 mm,
- *stationary phase*: *end-capped octadecylsilyl silica gel for chromatography R* (5 µm).

Column:

- *size*: *l* = 0.25 m, Ø = 4 mm,
- *stationary phase*: spherical *aminohexadecylsilyl silica gel for chromatography R* (5 µm),
- *temperature*: 30 °C.

Mobile phase: *water R*, adjusted to pH 2.4 with *phosphoric acid R*.

Flow rate: 1 ml/min.

Detection: spectrophotometer at 205 nm. A detector is placed between the precolumn and the analytical column. A second detector is placed after the analytical column.

Injection: 10 µl. When impurity A has left the precolumn (after about 1.2 min) switch the flow directly from the pump to the analytical column. Before the next chromatogram is run, wash the precolumn by reversed flow.

Limit:

- *impurity A*: not more than the area of the principal peak obtained with the reference solution (0.5 per cent).

Heavy metals (*2.4.8*): maximum 20 ppm.

12 ml of solution S complies with limit test A. Prepare the standard using *lead standard solution (2 ppm Pb) R*.

Loss on drying (*2.2.32*): maximum 5.0 per cent, determined on 0.500 g by drying in an oven at 100-105 °C.

Sulphated ash (*2.4.14*): maximum 0.1 per cent, determined on 1.0 g.

Viscosity, expressed as *K*-value. Dilute 5.0 ml of solution S to 50.0 ml with *water R*. Allow to stand for 1 h and determine the viscosity (*2.2.9*) of the solution at 25 ± 0.1 °C using viscometer No. 1 with a minimum flow time of 100 s. Calculate the *K*-value from the expression:

$$\frac{1.5 \log \eta - 1}{0.15 + 0.003c} + \frac{\sqrt{300c \log \eta + (c + 1.5c \log \eta)^2}}{0.15c + 0.003c^2}$$

c = percentage concentration (g/100 ml) of the substance to be examined, calculated with reference to the dried substance,

η = viscosity of the solution relative to that of water.

ASSAY

Ethenyl acetate. Determine the saponification value (*2.5.6*) on 2.00 g of the substance to be examined. Multiply the result obtained by 0.1534 to obtain the percentage content of the ethenyl acetate component.

Nitrogen. Carry out the determination of nitrogen (*2.5.9*) using 30.0 mg of the substance to be examined and 1 g of a mixture of 3 parts of *copper sulphate R* and 997 parts of *dipotassium sulphate R*, heating until a clear, light green solution is obtained and then for a further 45 min.

STORAGE

In an airtight container.

LABELLING

The label states the *K*-value.

IMPURITIES

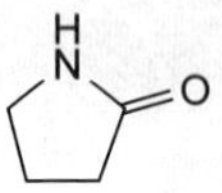

A. pyrrolidin-2-one (2-pyrrolidone).

01/2005:0893

COPPER SULPHATE, ANHYDROUS

Cupri sulfas anhydricus

$CuSO_4$ M_r 159.6

DEFINITION

Anhydrous copper sulphate contains not less than 99.0 per cent and not more than the equivalent of 101.0 per cent of $CuSO_4$, calculated with reference to the dried substance.

CHARACTERS

A greenish-grey powder, very hygroscopic, freely soluble in water, slightly soluble in methanol, practically insoluble in alcohol.

IDENTIFICATION

A. Add several drops of *dilute ammonia R2* to 1 ml of solution S (see Tests). A blue precipitate is formed on further addition of *dilute ammonia R2*, the precipitate dissolves and a dark blue colour is produced.

B. It complies with the test for loss on drying (see Tests).

C. Dilute 1 ml of solution S to 5 ml with *water R*. The solution gives reaction (a) of sulphates (*2.3.1*).

TESTS

Solution S. Dissolve 1.6 g in *water R* and dilute to 50 ml with the same solvent.

Appearance of solution. Solution S is clear (*2.2.1*).

Chlorides (*2.4.4*). Dilute 10 ml of solution S to 15 ml with *water R*. The solution complies with the limit test for chlor-ides (150 ppm). Examine the tubes laterally against a black background.

Iron. Not more than 150 ppm of Fe, determined by atomic absorption spectrometry (*2.2.23, Method I*).

Test solution. Dissolve 0.32 g in 10 ml of *water R*, add 2.5 ml of *lead-free nitric acid R* and dilute to 25.0 ml with *water R*.

Reference solutions. Prepare the reference solutions using *iron standard solution (20 ppm Fe) R*, adding 2.5 ml of *lead-free nitric acid R* and diluting to 25.0 ml with *water R*.

Measure the absorbance at 248.3 nm using an iron hollow-cathode lamp as a source of radiation and an air-butane flame.

Lead. Not more than 80 ppm of Pb, determined by atomic absorption spectrometry (*2.2.23, Method I*).

Test solution. Dissolve 1.6 g in 10 ml of *water R*, add 2.5 ml of *lead-free nitric acid R* and dilute to 25.0 ml with *water R*.

Reference solutions. Prepare the reference solutions using *lead standard solution (100 ppm Pb) R*, adding 2.5 ml of *lead-free nitric acid R* and diluting to 25.0 ml with *water R*.

Measure the absorbance at 217.0 nm using a lead hollow-cathode lamp as a source of radiation and an air-butane flame.

Loss on drying (*2.2.32*). Not more than 1.0 per cent, determined on 0.500 g by drying in an oven at 250 °C.

ASSAY

Dissolve 0.125 g in 50 ml of *water R*. Add 2 ml of *sulphuric acid R* and 3 g of *potassium iodide R*. Titrate with *0.1 M sodium thiosulphate*, using 1 ml of *starch solution R*, added towards the end of the titration, as indicator.

1 ml of *0.1 M sodium thiosulphate* is equivalent to 15.96 mg of $CuSO_4$.

STORAGE

Store in an airtight container.

01/2005:0894

COPPER SULPHATE PENTAHYDRATE

Cupri sulfas pentahydricus

$CuSO_4,5H_2O$ M_r 249.7

DEFINITION

Copper sulphate pentahydrate contains not less than 99.0 per cent and not more than the equivalent of 101.0 per cent of $CuSO_4,5H_2O$.

CHARACTERS

A blue, crystalline powder or transparent, blue crystals, freely soluble in water, soluble in methanol, practically insoluble in alcohol.

IDENTIFICATION

A. Add several drops of *dilute ammonia R2* to 1 ml of solution S (see Tests). A blue precipitate is formed on further addition of *dilute ammonia R2*, the precipitate dissolves and a dark blue colour is produced.

B. It complies with the test for loss on drying (see Tests).

C. Dilute 1 ml of solution S to 5 ml with *water R*. The solution gives reaction (a) of sulphates (*2.3.1*).

TESTS

Solution S. Dissolve 5 g in *water R* and dilute to 100 ml with the same solvent.

Appearance of solution. Solution S is clear (*2.2.1*).

Chlorides (*2.4.4*). Dilute 10 ml of solution S to 15 ml with *water R*. The solution complies with the limit test for chlorides (100 ppm). Examine the tubes laterally against a black background.

Iron. Not more than 100 ppm of Fe, determined by atomic absorption spectrometry (*2.2.23, Method I*).

Test solution. Dissolve 0.5 g in 10 ml of *water R*, add 2.5 ml of *lead-free nitric acid R* and dilute to 25.0 ml with *water R*.

Reference solutions. Prepare the reference solutions using *iron standard solution (20 ppm Fe) R*, adding 2.5 ml of *lead-free nitric acid R* and diluting to 25.0 ml with *water R*.

Measure the absorbance at 248.3 nm using an iron hollow-cathode lamp as a source of radiation and an air-butane flame.

Lead. Not more than 50 ppm of Pb, determined by atomic absorption spectrometry (*2.2.23, Method I*).

Test solution. Dissolve 2.5 g in 10 ml of *water R*, add 2.5 ml of *lead-free nitric acid R* and dilute to 25.0 ml with *water R*.

Reference solutions. Prepare the reference solutions using *lead standard solution (100 ppm Pb) R*, adding 2.5 ml of *lead-free nitric acid R* and diluting to 25.0 ml with *water R*.

Measure the absorbance at 217.0 nm using a lead hollow-cathode lamp as a source of radiation and an air-butane flame.

Loss on drying (*2.2.32*): 35.0 per cent to 36.5 per cent, determined on 0.500 g by drying in an oven at 250 °C.

ASSAY

Dissolve 0.200 g in 50 ml of *water R*. Add 2 ml of *sulphuric acid R* and 3 g of *potassium iodide R*. Titrate with *0.1 M sodium thiosulphate*, adding 1 ml of *starch solution R* towards the end of the titration.

1 ml *0.1 M sodium thiosulphate* is equivalent to 24.97 mg of $CuSO_4,5H_2O$.

01/2005:1304

CORIANDER

Coriandri fructus

DEFINITION

Coriander consists of the dried cremocarp of *Coriandrum sativum* L. It contains not less than 3 ml/kg of essential oil, calculated with reference to the dried drug.

CHARACTERS

The cremocarp is brown or light brown and is more or less spherical, about 1.5 mm to 5 mm in diameter, or oval form 2 mm to 6 mm long.

It has the macroscopic and microscopic characters described under identification tests A and B.

IDENTIFICATION

A. The mericarps are usually tightly connected. The cremocarp is glabrous and has ten wavy, slightly raised primary ridges and eight straight, more prominent

Monographs C

secondary ridges. The stylopod crowns the apex. The mericarps are concave on the internal surface. A small fragment of the pedicel may be present.

B. Reduce to a powder (355). The powder is brown. Examine under a microscope using *chloral hydrate solution R*. The powder shows numerous oil droplets; fragments of endosperm with small thick-walled regular cells containing microcrystals and microrosettes of calcium oxalate and oil droplets; fragments of endocarp with very narrow cells having a parquetry arrangement and usually associated with a layer of thin-walled rectangular sclereids of the mesocarp; fragments from the sclerenchymatous layer of the mesocarp with short, strongly thickened, pitted, fusiform cells occurring in layers with the cells of adjacent layers approximately at right angles to one another; fragments of parenchyma with small, thick-walled cells; occasional fragments of vascular bundles.

C. Examine by thin-layer chromatography (*2.2.27*), using a suitable silica gel as the coating substance.

Test solution. Shake 0.50 g of the freshly powdered drug (355) with 5.0 ml of *hexane R* for 2 min to 3 min and filter over 2 g of *anhydrous sodium sulphate R*.

Reference solution. Dissolve 15 µl of *linalol R* and 25 µl of *olive oil R* in 5.0 ml of *hexane R* immediately before use.

Apply to the plate as bands 20 µl of the test solution and 10 µl of the reference solution. Develop over a path of 10 cm using a mixture of 5 volumes of *ethyl acetate R* and 95 volumes of *toluene R*. Allow the plate to dry in air and develop again in the same conditions. Allow the plate to dry in air. Spray the plate with *anisaldehyde solution R* and examine in daylight while heating at 100 °C to 105 °C for 5 min to 10 min. The chromatogram obtained with the reference solution shows in the lower half a violet to greyish-violet zone (linalol) and in the upper half a bluish-violet zone (triglycerides). The chromatogram obtained with the test solution shows zones similar in position and colour to the zones in the chromatogram obtained with the reference solution. Several violet-grey to brownish zones, including the zone corresponding to geraniol, are between the starting point and the zone due to linalol in the chromatogram obtained with the reference solution. It may also show several faint violet-grey zones between the zone due to triglycerides and that due to linalol in the chromatogram obtained with the reference solution.

TESTS

Foreign matter (*2.8.2*). It complies with the test for foreign matter. None of the cremocarps show perforations due to animals.

Loss on drying (*2.2.32*). Not more than 10.0 per cent, determined on 1.000 g of the powdered drug (355) by drying in an oven at 100 °C to 105 °C for 2 h.

Total ash (*2.4.16*). Not more than 8.0 per cent.

ASSAY

Carry out the determination of essential oils in vegetable drugs (*2.8.12*). Use a 500 ml round-bottomed flask, 200 ml of *water R* as the distillation liquid and 0.5 ml of *xylene R* in the graduated tube. Reduce the drug to a coarse powder and immediately use 30.0 g for the determination. Distil at a rate of 2 ml/min to 3 ml/min for 2 h.

STORAGE

Store protected from light.

01/2005:1820

CORIANDER OIL

Coriandri aetheroleum

DEFINITION

Essential oil obtained by steam distillation from the fruits of *Coriandrum sativum* L.

CHARACTERS

Appearance: clear, colourless or pale yellow liquid.

It has a characteristic spicy odour.

IDENTIFICATION

First identification: B.

Second identification: A.

A. Examine by thin-layer chromatography (*2.2.27*).

Test solution. Dissolve 10 µl of the substance to be examined in 1.0 ml of *toluene R*.

Reference solution. Dissolve 10 µl *linalol R* and 2 µl of *geranyl acetate R* in 1.0 ml of *toluene R*.

Plate: *TLC silica gel plate R*.

Mobile phase: *ethyl acetate R, toluene R* (5:95 *V/V*).

Application: 10 µl as bands.

Development: over a path of 10 cm.

Drying: in air.

Detection: spray with *anisaldehyde solution R* and heat at 100-105 °C for 10-15 min. Examine immediately in daylight.

Results: see below the sequence of the zones present in the chromatograms obtained with the reference solution and the test solution.

Top of the plate	
—	—
Geranyl acetate: a violet-blue zone	A violet-blue zone (geranyl acetate)
—	—
Linalol: an intense violet zone	An intense violet zone (linalol)
	A violet-blue zone (geraniol)
Reference solution	**Test solution**

B. Examine the chromatograms obtained in the test for chromatographic profile.

Results: the characteristic peaks in the chromatogram obtained with the test solution are similar in retention time to those in the chromatogram obtained with the reference solution.

TESTS

Relative density (*2.2.5*): 0.860 to 0.880.

Refractive index (*2.2.6*): 1.462 to 1.470.

Optical rotation (*2.2.7*): + 7° to + 13°.

Acid value (*2.5.1*): maximum 3.0, determined on 5.00 g of the substance to be examined.

Chromatographic profile. Gas chromatography (*2.2.28*): use the normalisation procedure.

Test solution. The substance to be examined.

Reference solution (a). Dissolve 10 μl of *α-pinene R*, 10 μl of *limonene R*, 10 μl of *γ-terpinene R*, 10 μl of *p-cymene R*, 10 mg of *camphor R*, 20 μl of *linalol R*, 10 μl of *α-terpineol R*, 10 μl of *geranyl acetate R* and 10 μl of *geraniol R* in 1 ml of *hexane R*.

Reference solution (b). Dissolve 5 μl of *geraniol R* in *hexane R* and dilute to 10 ml with the same solvent.

Column:
- *material*: fused silica,
- *size*: *l* = 60 m, Ø = 0.25 mm,
- *stationary phase*: *macrogol 20 000 R* (film thickness 0.25 μm).

Carrier gas: *helium for chromatography R*.

Flow rate: 1 ml/min.

Split ratio: 1:65.

Temperature:

	Time (min)	Temperature (°C)
Column	0 - 10	60
	10 - 75	60 → 190
	75 - 120	190
Injection port		220
Detector		240

Detection: flame ionisation.

Injection: 0.2 μl.

Elution order: order indicated in the composition of reference solution (a). Record the retention times of these substances.

System suitability: reference solution (a):
- *resolution*: minimum 1.5 between the peaks due to linalol and camphor.

Using the retention times determined from the chromatogram obtained with reference solution (a), locate the components of reference solution (a) in the chromatogram obtained with the test solution.

Determine the percentage content of each of these components. The percentages are within the following ranges:
- *α-pinene*: 3.0 per cent to 7.0 per cent,
- *limonene*: 1.5 per cent to 5.0 per cent,
- *γ-terpinene*: 1.5 per cent to 8.0 per cent,
- *p-cymene*: 0.5 per cent to 4.0 per cent,
- *camphor*: 3.0 per cent to 6.0 per cent,
- *linalol*: 65.0 per cent to 78.0 per cent,
- *α-terpineol*: 0.1 per cent to 1.5 per cent,
- *geranyl acetate*: 0.5 per cent to 4.0 per cent,
- *geraniol*: 0.5 per cent to 3.0 per cent,
- *disregard limit*: area of the peak in the chromatogram obtained with reference solution (b) (0.05 per cent).

Chiral purity. Gas chromatography (*2.2.28*).

Test solution. Dissolve 0.02 g of the substance to be examined in *pentane R* and dilute to 10 ml with the same solvent.

Reference solution. Dissolve 10 μl of *linalol R* and 5 mg of *borneol R* in *pentane R* and dilute to 10 ml with the same solvent.

Column:
- *material*: fused silica,
- *size*: *l* = 25 m, Ø = 0.25 mm,
- *stationary phase*: *modified β-cyclodextrin for chiral chromatography R* (film thickness 0.25 μm).

Carrier gas: *helium for chromatography R*.

Flow rate: 1.3 ml/min.

Split ratio: 1:30.

Temperature:

	Time (min)	Temperature (°C)
Column	0 - 65	50 → 180
Injection port		230
Detector		230

Detection: flame ionisation.

Injection: 1 μl.

System suitability: reference solution:
- *resolution*: minimum 5.5 between the peaks due to (*R*)-linalol (1st peak) and (*S*)-linalol (2nd peak) and minimum 2.9 between the peaks due to (*S*)-linalol and borneol (3rd peak).

Limit: calculate the percentage content of (*R*)-linalol from the expression:

$$\frac{A_R}{A_S + A_R} \times 100$$

A_S = area of the peak due to (*S*)-linalol,

A_R = area of the peak due to (*R*)-linalol.

- *(R)-linalol*: maximum 14 per cent.

STORAGE

In a well-filled, airtight container, protected from light and at a temperature not exceeding 25 °C.

01/2005:0321

CORTISONE ACETATE

Cortisoni acetas

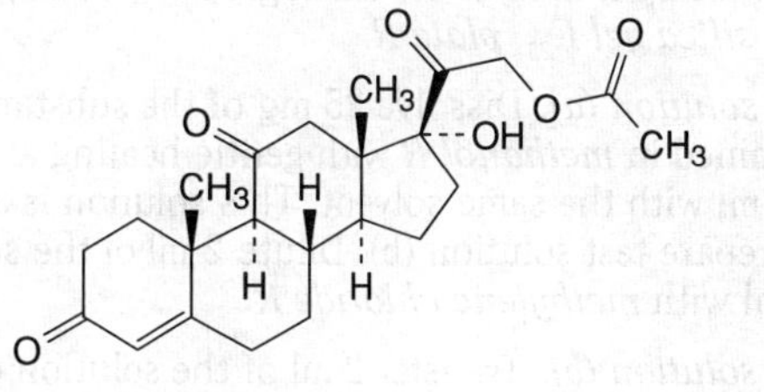

$C_{23}H_{30}O_6$ M_r 402.5

DEFINITION

Cortisone acetate contains not less than 97.0 per cent and not more than the equivalent of 103.0 per cent of 17-hydroxy-3,11,20-trioxopregn-4-en-21-yl acetate, calculated with reference to the dried substance.

CHARACTERS

A white or almost white, crystalline powder, practically insoluble in water, freely soluble in methylene chloride, soluble in dioxan, sparingly soluble in acetone, slightly soluble in alcohol and in methanol.

It shows polymorphism.

IDENTIFICATION

First identification: A, B.

Second identification: C, D, E.

A. Examine by infrared absorption spectrophotometry (*2.2.24*), comparing with the spectrum obtained with *cortisone acetate CRS*. If the spectra obtained in the solid state show differences, record new spectra using 50 g/l solutions of the substance to be examined and of the reference substance in *methylene chloride R* in a 0.2 mm cell.

B. Examine by thin-layer chromatography (*2.2.27*), using a *TLC silica gel* F_{254} *plate R*.

Test solution. Dissolve 10 mg of the substance to be examined in a mixture of 1 volume of *methanol R* and 9 volumes of *methylene chloride R* and dilute to 10 ml with the same mixture of solvents.

Reference solution (a). Dissolve 20 mg of *cortisone acetate CRS* in a mixture of 1 volume of *methanol R* and 9 volumes of *methylene chloride R* and dilute to 20 ml with the same mixture of solvents.

Reference solution (b). Dissolve 10 mg of *hydrocortisone acetate R* in reference solution (a) and dilute to 10 ml with reference solution (a).

Apply to the plate 5 µl of each solution. Prepare the mobile phase by adding a mixture of 1.2 volumes of *water R* and 8 volumes of *methanol R* to a mixture of 15 volumes of *ether R* and 77 volumes of *methylene chloride R*. Develop over a path of 15 cm. Allow the plate to dry in air and examine in ultraviolet light at 254 nm. The principal spot in the chromatogram obtained with the test solution is similar in position and size to the principal spot in the chromatogram obtained with reference solution (a). Spray with *alcoholic solution of sulphuric acid R*. Heat at 120 °C for 10 min or until the spots appear. Allow to cool. Examine the plate in daylight and in ultraviolet light at 365 nm. The principal spot in the chromatogram obtained with the test solution is similar in position, colour in daylight, fluorescence in ultraviolet light at 365 nm and size to the principal spot in the chromatogram obtained with reference solution (a). The test is not valid unless the chromatogram obtained with reference solution (b) shows two clearly separated spots.

C. Examine by thin-layer chromatography (*2.2.27*), using a *TLC silica gel* F_{254} *plate R*.

Test solution (a). Dissolve 25 mg of the substance to be examined in *methanol R* with gentle heating and dilute to 5 ml with the same solvent. This solution is also used to prepare test solution (b). Dilute 2 ml of the solution to 10 ml with *methylene chloride R*.

Test solution (b). Transfer 2 ml of the solution obtained during preparation of test solution (a) to a 15 ml glass tube with a ground-glass stopper or a polytetrafluoroethylene cap. Add 10 ml of *saturated methanolic potassium hydrogen carbonate solution R* and immediately pass a stream of *nitrogen R* briskly through the solution for 5 min. Stopper the tube. Heat in a water-bath at 45 °C protected from light for 2.5 h. Allow to cool.

Reference solution (a). Dissolve 25 mg of *cortisone acetate CRS* in *methanol R* with gentle heating and dilute to 5 ml with the same solvent. This solution is also used to prepare reference solution (b). Dilute 2 ml of the solution to 10 ml with *methylene chloride R*.

Reference solution (b). Transfer 2 ml of the solution obtained during preparation of reference solution (a) to a 15 ml glass tube with a ground-glass stopper or a polytetrafluoroethylene cap. Add 10 ml of *saturated methanolic potassium hydrogen carbonate solution R* and immediately pass a stream of *nitrogen R* briskly through the solution for 5 min. Stopper the tube. Heat in a water-bath at 45 °C protected from light for 2.5 h. Allow to cool.

Apply to the plate 5 µl of each solution. Prepare the mobile phase by adding a mixture of 1.2 volumes of *water R* and 8 volumes of *methanol R* to a mixture of 15 volumes of *ether R* and 77 volumes of *methylene chloride R*. Develop over a path of 15 cm. Allow the plate to dry in air and examine in ultraviolet light at 254 nm. The principal spot in each of the chromatograms obtained with the test solutions is similar in position and size to the principal spot in the chromatogram obtained with the corresponding reference solution. Spray with *alcoholic solution of sulphuric acid R* and heat at 120 °C for 10 min or until the spots appear. Allow to cool. Examine the plate in daylight and in ultraviolet light at 365 nm. The principal spot in each of the chromatograms obtained with the test solutions is similar in position, colour in daylight, fluorescence in ultraviolet light at 365 nm and size to the principal spot in the chromatogram obtained with the corresponding reference solution. The principal spots in the chromatograms obtained with test solution (b) and reference solution (b) have an R_f value distinctly lower than that of the principal spots in the chromatograms obtained with test solution (a) and reference solution (a).

D. Add about 2 mg to 2 ml of *sulphuric acid R* and shake to dissolve. Within 5 min, a faint yellow colour develops. Add the solution to 10 ml of *water R* and mix. The colour is discharged and a clear solution remains.

E. About 10 mg gives the reaction of acetyl (*2.3.1*).

TESTS

Specific optical rotation (*2.2.7*). Dissolve 0.250 g in *dioxan R* and dilute to 25.0 ml with the same solvent. The specific optical rotation is + 211 to + 220, calculated with reference to the dried substance.

Related substances. Examine by liquid chromatography (*2.2.29*). *Prepare the solutions immediately before use.*

Test solution. Dissolve 25.0 mg of the substance to be examined in *acetonitrile R* and dilute to 10.0 ml with the same solvent.

Reference solution (a). Dissolve 2 mg of *cortisone acetate CRS* and 2 mg of *hydrocortisone acetate CRS* in *acetonitrile R* and dilute to 100.0 ml with the same solvent.

Reference solution (b). Dilute 1.0 ml of the test solution to 100.0 ml with *acetonitrile R*.

The chromatographic procedure may be carried out using:

- a stainless steel column 0.25 m long and 4.6 mm in internal diameter packed with *octadecylsilyl silica gel for chromatography R* (5 µm),
- as mobile phase at a flow rate of 1 ml/min a mixture prepared as follows: in a 1000 ml volumetric flask mix 400 ml of *acetonitrile R* with 550 ml of *water R* and allow to equilibrate; adjust the volume to 1000 ml with *water R* and mix again,
- as detector a spectrophotometer set at 254 nm.

Equilibrate the column with the mobile phase at a flow rate of 1 ml/min for about 30 min.

Adjust the sensitivity of the system so that the height of the principal peak in the chromatogram obtained with 20 µl of reference solution (b) is at least 50 per cent of the full scale of the recorder.

Inject 20 µl of reference solution (a). When the chromatograms are recorded in the prescribed conditions the retention times are: hydrocortisone acetate about

10 min and cortisone acetate about 12 min. The test is not valid unless the resolution between the peaks due to hydrocortisone acetate and cortisone acetate is at least 4.2; if necessary, adjust the concentration of acetonitrile in the mobile phase.

Inject 20 µl of the test solution, 20 µl of reference solution (b) and 20 µl of acetonitrile as a blank. Continue the chromatography for twice the retention time of the principal peak. In the chromatogram obtained with the test solution: the area of any peak apart from the principal peak, is not greater than half the area of the principal peak in the chromatogram obtained with reference solution (b) (0.5 per cent); the sum of the areas of all the peaks apart from the principal peak, is not greater than 1.5 times the area of the principal peak in the chromatogram obtained with reference solution (b) (1.5 per cent). Disregard any peak with an area less than 0.05 times the area of the principal peak in the chromatogram obtained with reference solution (b).

Loss on drying (*2.2.32*). Not more than 0.5 per cent, determined on 0.500 g by drying in an oven at 100-105 °C.

ASSAY

Dissolve 0.100 g in *alcohol R* and dilute to 100.0 ml with the same solvent. Dilute 2.0 ml of the solution to 100.0 ml with *alcohol R*. Measure the absorbance (*2.2.25*) at the maximum of 237 nm.

Calculate the content of $C_{23}H_{30}O_6$ taking the specific absorbance to be 395.

STORAGE

Store protected from light.

IMPURITIES

A. hydrocortisone acetate.

01/2005:0036

COTTON, ABSORBENT

Lanugo gossypii absorbens

DEFINITION

Absorbent cotton consists of new fibres or good quality combers obtained from the seed-coat of various species of the genus *Gossypium* L., cleaned, purified, bleached and carefully carded. It may not contain any compensatory colouring matter.

CHARACTERS

It is white and is composed of fibres of average length not less than 10 mm, determined by a suitable method, and contains not more than traces of leaf residue, pericarp, seed-coat or other impurities. It offers appreciable resistance when pulled. It does not shed any appreciable quantity of dust when gently shaken.

IDENTIFICATION

A. Examined under a microscope, each fibre is seen to consist of a single cell, up to about 4 cm long and up to 40 µm wide, in the form of a flattened tube with thick and rounded walls and often twisted.

B. When treated with *iodinated zinc chloride solution R*, the fibres become violet.

C. To 0.1 g add 10 ml of *zinc chloride-formic acid solution R*. Heat to 40 °C and allow to stand for 2 h 30 min, shaking occasionally. It does not dissolve.

TESTS

Solution S. Place 15.0 g in a suitable vessel, add 150 ml of *water R*, close the vessel and allow to macerate for 2 h. Decant the solution, squeeze the residual liquid carefully from the sample with a glass rod and mix. Reserve 10 ml of the solution for the test for surface-active substances and filter the remainder.

Acidity or alkalinity. To 25 ml of solution S add 0.1 ml of *phenolphthalein solution R* and to another 25 ml add 0.05 ml of *methyl orange solution R*. Neither solution is pink.

Foreign fibres. Examined under a microscope, it is seen to consist exclusively of typical cotton fibres, except that occasionally a few isolated foreign fibres may be present.

Fluorescence. Examine a layer about 5 mm in thickness under ultraviolet light at 365 nm. It displays only a slight brownish-violet fluorescence and a few yellow particles. It shows no intense blue fluorescence, apart from that which may be shown by a few isolated fibres.

Neps. Spread about 1 g evenly between 2 colourless transparent plates each 10 cm square. Examine for neps by transmitted light and compare with *Absorbent cotton RM*. The product to be examined is not more neppy than the standard.

Absorbency

Apparatus. A dry cylindrical copper wire basket 8.0 cm high and 5.0 cm in diameter. The wire of which the basket is constructed is about 0.4 mm in diameter, the mesh is 1.5 cm to 2.0 cm wide and the mass of the basket is 2.7 ± 0.3 g.

Sinking time. Not more than 10 s. Weigh the basket to the nearest centigram (m_1). Take a total of 5.00 g in approximately equal quantities from 5 different places in the product to be examined, place loosely in the basket and weigh the filled basket to the nearest centigram (m_2). Fill a beaker 11 cm to 12 cm in diameter to a depth of 10 cm with water at about 20 °C. Hold the basket horizontally and drop it from a height of about 10 mm into the water. Measure with a stopwatch the time taken for the basket to sink below the surface of the water. Calculate the result as the average of 3 tests.

Water-holding capacity. Not less than 23.0 g of water per gram. After the sinking time has been measured, remove the basket from the water, allow it to drain for exactly 30 s suspended in a horizontal position over the beaker, transfer it to a tared beaker (m_3) and weigh to the nearest centigram (m_4). Calculate the water-holding capacity per gram of absorbent cotton using the following expression:

$$\frac{m_4 - (m_2 + m_3)}{m_2 - m_1}$$

Calculate the result as the average of 3 tests.

Ether-soluble substances. Not more than 0.50 per cent. In an extraction apparatus, extract 5.00 g with *ether R* for 4 h at a rate of at least 4 extractions per hour. Evaporate the ether extract and dry the residue to constant mass at 100 °C to 105 °C.

Extractable colouring matter. In a narrow percolator, slowly extract 10.0 g with *alcohol R* until 50 ml of extract is obtained. The liquid obtained is not more intensely coloured (*2.2.2, Method II*) than reference solution Y_5, GY_6 or a reference solution prepared as follows: to 3.0 ml of blue primary solution add 7.0 ml of hydrochloric acid (10 g/l HCl). Dilute 0.5 ml of this solution to 10.0 ml with hydrochloric acid (10 g/l HCl).

Monographs C

Surface-active substances. Introduce the 10 ml portion of solution S reserved before filtration into a 25 ml graduated ground-glass-stoppered cylinder with an external diameter of 20 mm and a wall thickness of not greater than 1.5 mm, previously rinsed 3 times with *sulphuric acid R* and then with *water R*. Shake vigorously 30 times in 10 s, allow to stand for 1 min and repeat the shaking. After 5 min, any foam present must not cover the entire surface of the liquid.

Water-soluble substances. Not more than 0.50 per cent. Boil 5.000 g in 500 ml of *water R* for 30 min, stirring frequently. Replace the water lost by evaporation. Decant the liquid, squeeze the residual liquid carefully from the sample with a glass rod and mix. Filter the liquid whilst hot. Evaporate 400 ml of the filtrate (corresponding to 4/5 of the mass of the sample taken) and dry the residue to constant mass at 100 °C to 105 °C.

Loss on drying (*2.2.32*). Not more than 8.0 per cent, determined on 5.000 g by drying in an oven at 100 °C to 105 °C.

Sulphated ash (*2.4.14*). Not more than 0.40 per cent. Introduce 5.00 g into a previously heated and cooled, tared crucible. Heat cautiously over a naked flame and then carefully to dull redness at 600 °C. Allow to cool, add a few drops of *dilute sulphuric acid R*, then heat and incinerate until all the black particles have disappeared. Allow to cool. Add a few drops of *ammonium carbonate solution R*. Evaporate and incinerate carefully, allow to cool and weigh again. Repeat the incineration for periods of 5 min to constant mass.

STORAGE

Store in a dust-proof package in a dry place.

01/2005:1305

COTTONSEED OIL, HYDROGENATED

Gossypii oleum hydrogenatum

DEFINITION

Hydrogenated cottonseed oil is the product obtained by refining and hydrogenation of oil obtained from seeds of cultivated plants of various varieties of *Gossypium hirsutum* L. or of other species of *Gossypium*. The product consists mainly of triglycerides of palmitic and stearic acids.

CHARACTERS

A white mass or powder which melts to a clear, pale yellow liquid when heated, practically insoluble in water, freely soluble in methylene chloride and in toluene, very slightly soluble in alcohol.

IDENTIFICATION

A. It complies with the test for melting point (see Tests).

B. It complies with the test for foreign fatty oils (see Tests).

TESTS

Melting point (*2.2.14*): 57 °C to 70 °C.

Acid value (*2.5.1*). Not more than 0.5, determined on 10.0 g. Dissolve the substance to be examined in 50 ml of a hot mixture of equal volumes of *alcohol R* and *toluene R*, previously neutralised with *0.1 M potassium hydroxide* using 0.5 ml of *phenolphthalein solution R1* as indicator. Titrate the solution immediately while still hot.

Peroxide value (*2.5.5*). Not more than 5.0.

Unsaponifiable matter (*2.5.7*). Not more than 1.0 per cent, determined on 5.0 g.

Alkaline impurities. Dissolve by gentle heating 2.0 g of the substance to be examined in a mixture of 1.5 ml of *alcohol R* and 3 ml of *toluene R*. Add 0.05 ml of a 0.4 g/l solution of *bromophenol blue R* in *alcohol R*. Not more than 0.4 ml of *0.01 M hydrochloric acid* is required to change the colour to yellow.

Composition of fatty acids (*2.4.22, Method A*).

The chromatographic procedure may be carried out using:

- a fused-silica capillary column 25 m long and 0.25 mm in internal diameter coated on the inner wall with *poly(cyanopropyl)siloxane R* (film thickness 0.2 µm),
- *helium for chromatography R* as the carrier gas at a flow rate of 0.65 ml/min,
- a flame-ionisation detector,
- a split injector (1:100),

maintaining the temperature of the column at 180 °C for 35 min and that of the injection port and the detector at 250 °C.

The fatty acid fraction of the oil has the following composition:

- *saturated fatty acids of chain length less than C_{14}*: not more than 0.2 per cent,
- *myristic acid*: not more than 1.0 per cent,
- *palmitic acid*: 19.0 per cent to 26.0 per cent,
- *stearic acid*: 68.0 per cent to 80.0 per cent,
- *oleic acid and isomers ($C_{18:1}$ equivalent chain length on poly(cyanopropyl)siloxane 18.5 to 18.8)*: not more than 4.0 per cent,
- *linoleic acid and isomers ($C_{18:2}$ equivalent chain length on poly(cyanopropyl)siloxane 19.4 to 19.8)*: not more than 1.0 per cent,
- *arachidic acid*: not more than 1.0 per cent,
- *behenic acid*: not more than 1.0 per cent,
- *lignoceric acid*: not more than 0.5 per cent.

Nickel. Not more than 1 ppm of Ni, determined by atomic absorption spectrometry (*2.2.23, Method II*).

Test solution. Introduce 5.0 g of the substance to be examined into a platinum or silica crucible tared after ignition. Cautiously heat and introduce into the substance a wick formed from twisted ashless filter paper. Ignite the wick. When the substance ignites, stop heating. After combustion, ignite in a muffle furnace at about 600 °C. Continue the incineration until white ash is obtained. After cooling, take up the residue with two quantities, each of 2 ml, of *dilute hydrochloric acid R* and transfer into a 25 ml graduated flask. Add 0.3 ml of *nitric acid R* and dilute to 25.0 ml with *distilled water R*.

Reference solutions. Prepare three reference solutions by adding 1.0 ml, 2.0 ml and 4.0 ml of *nickel standard solution (0.2 ppm Ni) R* to 2.0 ml portions of the test solution, diluting to 10.0 ml with *distilled water R*.

Measure the absorbance at 232 nm using a nickel hollow-cathode lamp as a source of radiation, a graphite furnace as an atomic generator and *argon R* as the carrier gas.

STORAGE

Store protected from light.

01/2005:1306

COUCH GRASS RHIZOME

Graminis rhizoma

DEFINITION

Whole or cut, washed and dried rhizome of *Agropyron repens* (L.) Beauv. (*Elymus repens* (L.) Gould); the adventitious roots are removed.

CHARACTERS

Ma croscopic and microscopic characters described under identification tests A and B.

IDENTIFICATION

A. The shiny yellowish, light brown or yellowish-brown pieces of the rhizome are 2 mm to 3 mm thick and longitudinally furrowed. At the nodes are the remains of very thin, more or less branched roots and whitish or brownish scale-like leaves; the internodes, up to 6 cm long, are furrowed and hollow inside. The transverse section of the nodes shows a yellowish medulla.

B. Reduce to a powder (355). The powder is whitish-yellow. Examine under a microscope, using *chloral hydrate solution R*. The powder shows the following diagnostic characters: fragments of the epidermis covered with a thick cuticle and composed of rectangular and elongated thick-walled cells with pitted slightly wavy walls which alternate with small rounded to almost square cells; U-shaped thickened endodermic cells; numerous fragments of moderately thickened fibres and groups of vessels with slit-shaped pits or with spiral and annular thickening.

TESTS

Cynodon dactilon, Imperata cylindrica. Examine under a microscope using *iodine solution R1*. No blue starch grains are visible.

Foreign matter (*2.8.2*): maximum 15 per cent of greyish-black pieces of rhizome in the cut drug.

Water-soluble extractive: minimum 25 per cent.

To 5.0 g of the powdered drug (355) add 200 ml of boiling *water R*. Allow to stand for 10 min, shaking occasionally. Allow to cool, dilute to 200.0 ml with *water R* and filter. Evaporate 20.0 ml of the filtrate to dryness on a water-bath. Dry the residue in an oven at 100-105 °C. The residue weighs a minimum of 0.125 g.

Loss on drying (*2.2.32*): maximum 12.0 per cent, determined on 1.000 g of the powdered drug (355) by drying in an oven at 100-105 °C for 2 h.

Total ash (*2.4.16*): maximum 5.0 per cent.

Ash insoluble in hydrochloric acid (*2.8.1*): maximum 1.5 per cent.

01/2005:1628

CRESOL, CRUDE

Cresolum crudum

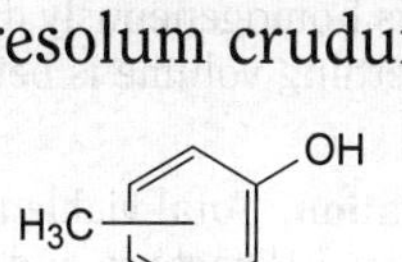

C_7H_8O M_r 108.1

DEFINITION

Mixture of 2-, 3- and 4-methylphenol.

CHARACTERS

Appearance: colourless or pale brown liquid.

Solubility: sparingly soluble in water, miscible with alcohol and with methylene chloride.

IDENTIFICATION

A. To 0.5 ml add 300 ml of *water R*, mix and filter. To 10 ml of the filtrate add 1 ml of *ferric chloride solution R1*. A blue colour is produced.

B. To 10 ml of the filtrate obtained in identification test A, add 1 ml of *bromine water R*. A pale yellow flocculent precipitate is produced.

C. It complies with the test for relative density (see Tests).

TESTS

Solution S. To 2.5 g of the substance to be examined add 50 ml of *water R*, shake for 1 min and filter through a moistened filter.

Acidity or alkalinity. To 10 ml of solution S add 0.1 ml of *methyl red solution R* and 0.2 ml of *0.01 M sodium hydroxide*. The solution is yellow. Add 0.3 ml of *0.01 M hydrochloric acid*. The solution is red.

Relative density (*2.2.5*): 1.029 to 1.044.

Distillation range (*2.2.11*): a maximum of 2.0 per cent *V/V* distils below 188 °C and a minimum of 80 per cent *V/V* distils between 195 °C and 205 °C.

Sulphur compounds. Place 20 ml in a small conical flask. Over the mouth of the flask fix a piece of filter paper moistened with *lead acetate solution R*. Heat on a water-bath for 5 min. Not more than a light yellow colour is produced on the filter paper.

Residue on evaporation: maximum 0.1 per cent.

Evaporate 2.0 g to dryness on a water-bath and dry at 100-105 °C for 1 h. The residue weighs not more than 2 mg.

STORAGE

Protected from light.

01/2005:0985

CROSCARMELLOSE SODIUM

Carmellosum natricum conexum

DEFINITION

Croscarmellose sodium (cross-linked sodium carboxymethylcellulose) is the sodium salt of a cross-linked, partly *O*-carboxymethylated cellulose.

CHARACTERS

A white or greyish-white powder, practically insoluble in acetone, in ethanol and in toluene.

IDENTIFICATION

A. Shake 1 g with 100 ml of a solution containing 4 ppm of *methylene blue R* and allow to settle. The substance to be examined absorbs the methylene blue and settles as a blue, fibrous mass.

B. Shake 1 g with 50 ml of *water R*. Transfer 1 ml of the mixture to a test-tube, add 1 ml of *water R* and 0.05 ml of a freshly prepared 40 g/l solution of *α-naphthol R* in *methanol R*. Incline the test-tube and add carefully 2 ml of *sulphuric acid R* down the side so that it forms a lower layer. A reddish-violet colour develops at the interface.

C. It gives reaction (a) of sodium (*2.3.1*).

TESTS

pH (*2.2.3*). Shake 1 g with 100 ml of *carbon dioxide-free water R* for 5 min. The pH of the suspension is 5.0 to 7.0.

Degree of substitution. Place 1.000 g in a 500 ml conical flask, add 300 ml of a 100 g/l solution of *sodium chloride R*, 25.0 ml of *0.1 M sodium hydroxide*, stopper the flask and allow to stand for 5 min, shaking occasionally. Add 0.05 ml of *m-cresol purple solution R* and about 15 ml of *0.1 M hydrochloric acid* from a burette. Insert the stopper and shake. If the solution is violet, add *0.1 M hydrochloric acid* in 1 ml portions until the solution becomes yellow, shaking after each addition. Titrate with *0.1 M sodium hydroxide* until the colour turns to violet.

Calculate the number of milliequivalents (M) of base required for the neutralisation equivalent to 1 g of dried substance.

Calculate the degree of acid carboxymethyl substitution (A) from the expression:

$$\frac{1150M}{(7102 - 412M - 80C)}$$

C = sulphated ash as a percentage.

Calculate the degree of sodium carboxymethyl substitution (S) from the expression:

$$\frac{(162 + 58A)\,C}{(7102 - 80C)}$$

The degree of substitution is the sum of $A + S$ and it is between 0.60 and 0.85, calculated with reference to the dried substance.

Sodium chloride and sodium glycollate. The sum of the percentage contents of sodium chloride and sodium glycollate is not more than 0.5 per cent, calculated with reference to the dried substance.

Sodium chloride. Place 5.00 g in a 250 ml conical flask, add 50 ml of *water R* and 5 ml of *strong hydrogen peroxide solution R* and heat on a water-bath for 20 min, stirring occasionally to ensure total hydration. Cool, add 100 ml of *water R* and 10 ml of *nitric acid R*. Titrate with *0.05 M silver nitrate* determining the end-point potentiometrically (*2.2.20*) using a silver indicator electrode and a double-junction reference electrode containing a 100 g/l solution of *potassium nitrate R* in the outer jacket and a standard filling solution in the inner jacket, and stirring constantly.

1 ml of *0.05 M silver nitrate* is equivalent to 2.922 mg of NaCl.

Sodium glycollate. Place a quantity of the substance to be examined equivalent to 0.500 g of the dried substance in a 100 ml beaker. Add 5 ml of *glacial acetic acid R* and 5 ml of *water R* and stir to ensure total hydration (about 15 min). Add 50 ml of *acetone R* and 1 g of *sodium chloride R*. Stir for several minutes to ensure complete precipitation of the carboxymethylcellulose. Filter through a fast filter paper impregnated with *acetone R* into a volumetric flask, rinse the beaker and filter with 30 ml of *acetone R* and dilute the filtrate to 100.0 ml with the same solvent. Allow to stand for 24 h without shaking. Use the clear supernatant to prepare the test solution.

Prepare the reference solutions as follows: in a 100 ml volumetric flask, dissolve 0.100 g of *glycollic acid R*, previously dried *in vacuo* over *diphosphorus pentoxide R*, in *water R* and dilute to 100.0 ml with the same solvent. Use the solution within 30 days. Transfer 1.0 ml, 2.0 ml, 3.0 ml and 4.0 ml of the solution to separate volumetric flasks; dilute the contents of each flask to 5.0 ml with *water R*, add 5 ml of *glacial acetic acid R*, dilute to 100.0 ml with *acetone R* and mix.

Transfer 2.0 ml of the test solution and 2.0 ml of each of the reference solutions to separate 25 ml volumetric flasks. Heat the uncovered flasks for 20 min on a water-bath to eliminate acetone. Allow to cool and add 5.0 ml of *2,7-dihydroxynaphthalene solution R* to each flask. Mix, add a further 15.0 ml of *2,7-dihydroxynaphthalene solution R* and mix again. Close the flasks with aluminium foil and heat on a water-bath for 20 min. Cool and dilute to 25.0 ml with *sulphuric acid R*.

Measure the absorbance (*2.2.25*) of each solution at 540 nm. Prepare a blank using 2.0 ml of a solution containing 5 per cent *V/V* each of *glacial acetic acid R* and *water R* in *acetone R*. Prepare a standard curve using the absorbances obtained with the reference solutions. From the standard curve and the absorbance of the test solution, determine the mass a, in milligrams, of glycollic acid in the substance to be examined, and calculate the content of sodium glycollate from the expression:

$$\frac{10 \times 1.29 \times a}{(100 - b)\,m}$$

1.29 = the factor converting glycollic acid to sodium glycollate,

b = loss on drying as a percentage,

m = mass of the substance to be examined, in grams.

Water-soluble substances. Not more than 10.0 per cent. Disperse 10.00 g in 800.0 ml of *water R* and stir for 1 min every 10 min during the first 30 min. Allow to stand for 1 h and centrifuge, if necessary. Decant 200.0 ml of the supernatant liquid onto a fast filter paper in a vacuum filtration funnel, apply vacuum and collect 150.0 ml of the filtrate. Evaporate to dryness and dry the residue at 100 °C to 105 °C for 4 h.

Heavy metals (*2.4.8*). To the residue obtained in the determination of the sulphated ash add 1 ml of *hydrochloric acid R* and evaporate on a water-bath. Take up the residue in 20 ml of *water R*. 12 ml of the solution complies with limit test A for heavy metals (10 ppm). Prepare the standard using *lead standard solution (1 ppm Pb) R*.

Loss on drying (*2.2.32*). Not more than 10.0 per cent, determined on 1.000 g by drying in an oven at 100 °C to 105 °C for 6 h.

Sulphated ash (*2.4.14*): 14.0 per cent to 28.0 per cent, determined on 2.000 g, using a mixture of equal volumes of *sulphuric acid R* and *water R*, and calculated with reference to the dried substance.

Settling volume. Place 75 ml of *water R* in a 100 ml graduated cylinder and add 1.5 g of the substance to be examined in 0.5 g portions, shaking vigorously after each addition. Dilute to 100.0 ml with *water R* and shake again until the substance is homogeneously distributed. Allow to stand for 4 h. The settling volume is between 10.0 ml and 30.0 ml.

Microbial contamination. Total viable aerobic count (*2.6.12*) not more than 10^3 bacteria and 10^2 fungi per gram, determined by plate count. It complies with the test for *Escherichia coli* (*2.6.13*).

01/2005:0892

CROSPOVIDONE

Crospovidonum

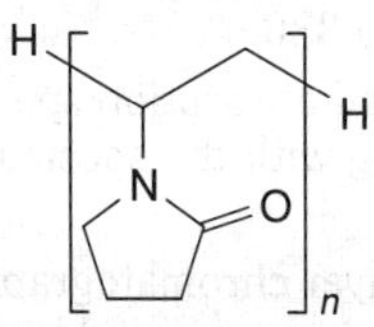

$(C_6H_9NO)_n$ M_r $(111.1)_n$

DEFINITION

Crospovidone is a cross-linked homopolymer of 1-ethenylpyrrolidin-2-one. It is available in different degrees of powder fineness (type A and type B).

Content: 11.0 per cent to 12.8 per cent of nitrogen (N; A_r 14.01) (dried substance).

CHARACTERS

Appearance: white or yellowish-white powder or flakes, hygroscopic.

Solubility: practically insoluble in water, in alcohol and in methylene chloride.

IDENTIFICATION

A. Infrared absorption spectrophotometry (*2.2.24*).
Comparison: *Ph. Eur. reference spectrum of crospovidone.*

B. Suspend 1 g in 10 ml of *water R*, add 0.1 ml of *0.05 M iodine* and shake for 30 s. Add 1 ml of *starch solution R* and shake. No blue colour develops within 30 s.

C. To 10 ml of *water R*, add 0.1 g and shake. A suspension is formed and no clear solution is obtained within 15 min.

D. Weigh a suitable quantity of the substance to be examined (for example 10 mg to 100 mg) and suspend it in 10.0 ml of *water R*, adding a wetting agent. Observe under a microscope at a suitable magnification using a calibrated ocular micrometer. If the majority of particles are in the range 50 µm to 300 µm, the product is classified as type A. If almost all the particles are below 50 µm, the product is classified as type B.

TESTS

Peroxides. Type A: maximum 400 ppm expressed as H_2O_2; type B: maximum 1000 ppm expressed as H_2O_2.

Suspend 2.0 g in 50 ml of *water R*. To 25 ml of this suspension add 2 ml of *titanium trichloride-sulphuric acid reagent R*. Allow to stand for 30 min and filter. The absorbance (*2.2.25*) of the filtrate, measured at 405 nm using a mixture of 25 ml of a filtered 40 g/l suspension of the substance to be examined and 2 ml of a 13 per cent *V/V* solution of *sulphuric acid R* as the compensation liquid has a maximum of 0.35.

For type B use 10 ml of the suspension diluted to 25 ml with *water R* for the test.

Water-soluble substances: maximum 1.0 per cent.

Transfer 25.0 g to a 400 ml beaker, add 200 ml of *water R* and stir for 1 h using a magnetic stirrer. Transfer the suspension to a 250.0 ml volumetric flask, rinsing with *water R*, and dilute to volume with the same solvent. Allow the bulk of the solids to settle. Filter about 100 ml of the almost clear supernatant liquid through a 0.45 µm membrane filter, protected by superimposing a 3 µm membrane filter. While filtering, stir the liquid above the filter manually or by means of a mechanical stirrer, taking care not to damage the filter. Transfer 50.0 ml of the clear filtrate to a tared 100 ml beaker, evaporate to dryness and dry at 105-110 °C for 3 h. The residue weighs a maximum of 50 mg.

Impurity A. Liquid chromatography (*2.2.29*).

Test solution. Suspend 1.250 g in 50.0 ml of *methanol R* and shake for 60 min. Leave the bulk to settle and filter through a 0.2 µm filter.

Reference solution (a). Dissolve 50 mg of *1-vinylpyrrolidin-2-one R* in *methanol R* and dilute to 100.0 ml with the same solvent. Dilute 1.0 ml of the solution to 100.0 ml with *methanol R*. Dilute 5.0 ml of this solution to 100.0 ml with the mobile phase.

Reference solution (b). Dissolve 10 mg of *1-vinylpyrrolidin-2-one R* and 0.50 g of *vinyl acetate R* in *methanol R* and dilute to 100 ml with the same solvent. Dilute 1.0 ml of the solution to 100.0 ml with the mobile phase.

Precolumn:
- *size*: l = 0.025 m, Ø = 4 mm,
- *stationary phase*: *octadecylsilyl silica gel for chromatography R* (5 µm).

Column:
- *size*: l = 0.25 m, Ø = 4 mm,
- *stationary phase*: *octadecylsilyl silica gel for chromatography R* (5 µm),
- *temperature*: 40 °C.

Mobile phase: *acetonitrile R, water R* (10:90 *V/V*).

Flow rate: adjusted so that the retention time of the peak corresponding to impurity A is about 10 min.

Detection: spectrophotometer at 235 nm.

Injection: 50 µl. After each injection of the test solution, wash the precolumn by passing the mobile phase backward, at the same flow rate as applied in the test, for 30 min.

System suitability:
- *resolution*: minimum of 2.0 between the peaks corresponding to impurity A and to vinyl acetate in the chromatogram obtained with reference solution (b),
- *repeatability*: maximum relative standard deviation of 2.0 per cent after 5 injections of reference solution (a).

Limits:
- *impurity A*: not more than the area of the principal peak in the chromatogram obtained with reference solution (a) (10 ppm).

Heavy metals (*2.4.8*): maximum 10 ppm.

2.0 g complies with limit test D. Prepare the standard using 2 ml of *lead standard solution (10 ppm Pb) R*.

Loss on drying (*2.2.32*): maximum 5.0 per cent, determined on 0.500 g by drying in an oven at 100-105 °C.

Sulphated ash (*2.4.14*): maximum 0.1 per cent, determined on 1.0 g.

ASSAY

Place 100.0 mg of the substance to be examined (*m* mg) in a combustion flask, add 5 g of a mixture of 1 g of *copper sulphate R*, 1 g of *titanium dioxide R* and 33 g of *dipotassium sulphate R*, and 3 glass beads. Wash any adhering particles from the neck into the flask with a small quantity of *water R*. Add 7 ml of *sulphuric acid R*, allowing it to run down the sides of the flask, and mix the contents by rotation. Close the mouth of the flask loosely, for example by means of a glass bulb with a short stem, to avoid excessive loss of sulphuric acid. Heat gradually at first, then increase the temperature until there is vigorous

Monographs C

boiling with condensation of sulphuric acid in the neck of the flask; precautions are to be taken to prevent the upper part of the flask from becoming overheated. Continue the heating for 45 min. Cool, dissolve the solid material by cautiously adding to the mixture 20 ml of *water R*, cool again and place in a steam-distillation apparatus. Add 30 ml of *strong sodium hydroxide solution R* through the funnel, rinse the funnel cautiously with 10 ml of *water R* and distil immediately by passing steam through the mixture. Collect 80-100 ml of distillate in a mixture of 30 ml of a 40 g/l solution of *boric acid R* and 0.05 ml of *bromocresol green-methyl red solution R* and enough *water R* to cover the tip of the condenser. Towards the end of the distillation lower the receiver so that the tip of the condenser is above the surface of the acid solution and rinse the end part of the condenser with a small quantity of *water R*. Titrate the distillate with *0.025 M sulphuric acid* until the colour of the solution changes from green through pale greyish-blue to pale greyish-red-purple (n_1 ml of *0.025 M sulphuric acid*).

Repeat the test using about 100 mg of *glucose R* in place of the substance to be examined (n_2 ml of *0.025 M sulphuric acid*).

$$\text{Percentage content of nitrogen} = \frac{0.7004\,(n_1 - n_2)}{m} \times 100$$

STORAGE

In an airtight container.

LABELLING

The label states the type (type A or type B).

IMPURITIES

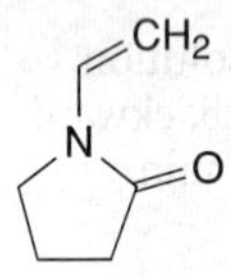

A. 1-ethenylpyrrolidin-2-one (1-vinylpyrrolidin-2-one).

01/2005:1194

CROTAMITON

Crotamitonum

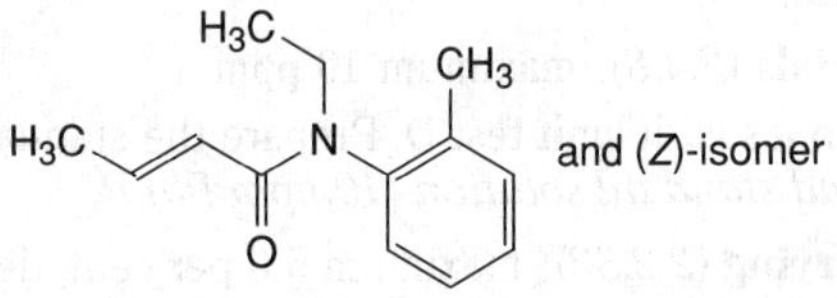

$C_{13}H_{17}NO$ — M_r 203.3

DEFINITION

Crotamiton contains not less than 96.0 per cent and not more than the equivalent of 102.0 per cent of *N*-ethyl-*N*-(2-methylphenyl)but-2-enamide, calculated as the sum of the *E*- and *Z*-isomers, and not more than 15.0 per cent of the *Z*-isomer.

CHARACTERS

A colourless or pale yellow, oily liquid, slightly soluble in water, miscible with alcohol. At low temperatures it may partly or completely solidify.

IDENTIFICATION

First identification: B.

Second identification: A, C, D.

A. Dissolve 25.0 mg in *cyclohexane R* and dilute to 100.0 ml with the same solvent. Dilute 1.0 ml of the solution to 10.0 ml with *cyclohexane R*. Examined between 220 nm and 300 nm (*2.2.25*), the solution shows an absorption maximum at 242 nm. The specific absorbance at the maximum is 300 to 330.

B. Examine by infrared absorption spectrophotometry (*2.2.24*), comparing with the spectrum obtained with *crotamiton CRS*.

C. Examine by thin-layer chromatography (*2.2.27*), using as the coating substance a suitable silica gel with a fluorescent indicator having an optimal intensity at 254 nm.

Test solution. Dissolve 25 mg of the substance to be examined in *ethanol R* and dilute to 10 ml with the same solvent.

Reference solution. Dissolve 25 mg of *crotamiton CRS* in *ethanol R* and dilute to 10 ml with the same solvent.

Apply separately to the plate 5 µl of each solution. Develop over a path of 15 cm using the mixture prepared as follows: shake 98 volumes of *methylene chloride R* with 2 volumes of *concentrated ammonia R*, dry over *anhydrous sodium sulphate R*, filter and mix 97 volumes of the filtrate with 3 volumes of *2-propanol R*. Allow the plate to dry in air and examine in ultraviolet light at 254 nm. The principal spot in the chromatogram obtained with the test solution is similar in position and size to the principal spot in the chromatogram obtained with the reference solution.

D. To 10 ml of a saturated solution add a few drops of a 3 g/l solution of *potassium permanganate R*. A brown colour is produced and a brown precipitate is formed on standing.

TESTS

Relative density (*2.2.5*): 1.006 to 1.011.

Refractive index (*2.2.6*): 1.540 to 1.542.

Free amines. Dissolve 5.00 g in 16 ml of *methylene chloride R* and add 4.0 ml of *glacial acetic acid R*. Add 0.1 ml of *metanil yellow solution R* and 1.0 ml of *0.02 M perchloric acid*. The solution is red-violet (500 ppm as ethylaminotoluene).

Chlorides. Boil 5.0 g under a reflux condenser for 1 h with 25 ml of *alcohol R* and 5 ml of a 200 g/l solution of *sodium hydroxide R*. Cool, add 5 ml of *water R* and shake with 25 ml of *ether R*. Dilute the lower layer to 20 ml with *water R*; add 5 ml of *nitric acid R*, dilute to 50 ml with *water R* and add 1 ml of a freshly prepared 50 g/l solution of *silver nitrate R*. Any opalescence in the solution is not more intense than that in a mixture of 1 ml of a freshly prepared 50 g/l solution of *silver nitrate R* and a solution prepared by diluting 5 ml of a 200 g/l solution of *sodium hydroxide R* to 20 ml with *water R* and adding 1.5 ml of *0.01 M hydrochloric acid*, 5 ml of *nitric acid R* and sufficient *water R* to produce 50 ml (100 ppm).

Related substances. Examine by liquid chromatography (*2.2.29*) as described under Assay.

Inject 20 µl each of test solution (a), reference solution (b) and reference solution (c). Continue the chromatography for 2.5 times the retention time of the principal peak. In the chromatogram obtained with test solution (a): the area of any peak corresponding to crotamiton impurity A is not greater than the area of the corresponding peak in the chromatogram obtained with reference solution (b) (3 per cent); the sum of the areas of any peaks, apart from the principal peak, the peak corresponding to the *Z*-isomer and any peak corresponding to crotamiton impurity A, is not greater than the sum of the areas of the peaks corresponding to the *Z*- and *E*-isomers in the chromatogram obtained with reference solution (c) (1 per cent). Disregard any peak with an area less than 0.02 times the area of the principal peak in the chromatogram obtained with reference solution (c).

Sulphated ash (*2.4.14*). Not more than 0.1 per cent, determined on 1.0 g.

ASSAY

Examine by liquid chromatography (*2.2.29*).

Test solution (a). Dissolve 50.0 mg of the substance to be examined in the mobile phase and dilute to 100.0 ml with the mobile phase.

Test solution (b). Dilute 1.0 ml of test solution (a) to 20.0 ml with the mobile phase.

Reference solution (a). Dissolve 50.0 mg of *crotamiton CRS* in the mobile phase and dilute to 100.0 ml with the mobile phase. Dilute 1.0 ml of the solution to 20.0 ml with the mobile phase.

Reference solution (b). Dissolve 15.0 mg of *crotamiton impurity A CRS* in the mobile phase and dilute to 20.0 ml with the mobile phase. Dilute 1.0 ml of the solution to 50.0 ml with the mobile phase.

Reference solution (c). Dilute 1.0 ml of test solution (a) to 100.0 ml with the mobile phase.

Reference solution (d). Dissolve 15 mg of *crotamiton impurity A CRS* in the mobile phase and dilute to 100 ml with the mobile phase. Dilute 1 ml of the solution to 10 ml with test solution (a).

The chromatographic procedure may be carried out using:

- a stainless steel column 0.25 m long and 4 mm in internal diameter packed with *silica gel for chromatography R* (5 µm),
- as mobile phase at a flow rate of 1.0 ml/min a mixture of 8 volumes of *tetrahydrofuran R* and 92 volumes of *cyclohexane R*,
- as detector a spectrophotometer set at 242 nm.

Inject 20 µl of reference solution (b) and 20 µl of reference solution (d). When the chromatograms are recorded in the prescribed conditions, the retention times relative to the principal peak (*E*-isomer) are: *Z*-isomer about 0.5 and crotamiton impurity A about 0.8. Adjust the sensitivity of the system so that the height of the principal peak in the chromatogram obtained with reference solution (b) is at least 70 per cent of the full scale of the recorder. The test is not valid unless, in the chromatogram obtained with reference solution (d), the resolution between the peaks corresponding to impurity A and the *E*-isomer is at least 4.5.

Inject alternately test solution (b) and reference solution (a). Calculate the percentage content of $C_{13}H_{17}NO$ from the sum of the areas of the peaks due to the *Z*- and *E*-isomers in the chromatograms obtained. Calculate the content of the *Z*-isomer, as a percentage of the total content of the *E*- and *Z*-isomers, from the chromatogram obtained with test solution (b).

STORAGE

Protected from light.

IMPURITIES

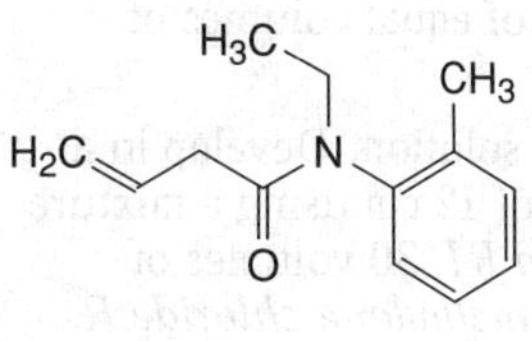

A. *N*-ethyl-*N*-(2-methylphenyl)but-3-enamide.

01/2005:0547

CYANOCOBALAMIN

Cyanocobalaminum

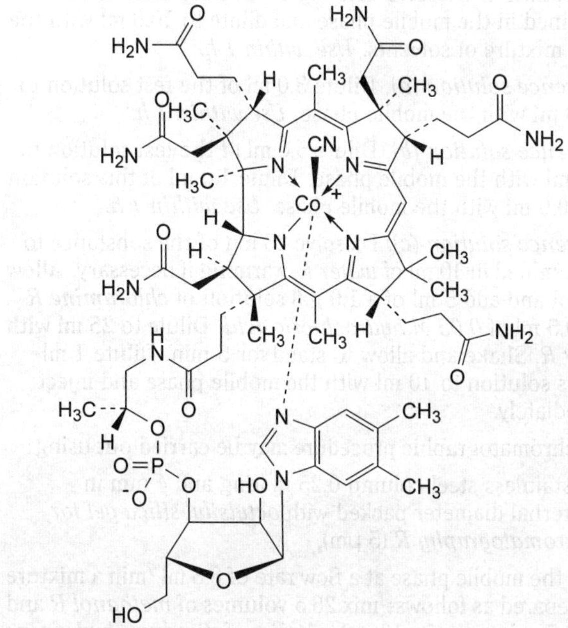

$C_{63}H_{88}CoN_{14}O_{14}P$ M_r 1355

DEFINITION

Cyanocobalamin contains not less than 96.0 per cent and not more than the equivalent of 102.0 per cent of α-(5,6-dimethylbenzimidazol-1-yl)cobamide cyanide, calculated with reference to the dried substance.

CHARACTERS

A dark-red, crystalline powder or dark-red crystals, sparingly soluble in water and in alcohol, practically insoluble in acetone. The anhydrous substance is very hygroscopic.

IDENTIFICATION

A. Dissolve 2.5 mg in *water R* and dilute to 100.0 ml with the same solvent. Examined between 260 nm and 610 nm (*2.2.25*), the solution shows 3 absorption maxima, at 278 nm, 361 nm and at 547 nm to 559 nm. The ratio of the absorbance at the maximum at 361 nm to that at the maximum at 547 nm to 559 nm is 3.15 to 3.45. The ratio of the absorbance at the maximum at 361 nm to that at the maximum at 278 nm is 1.70 to 1.90.

B. *Carry out the test protected from light.*

Examine by thin-layer chromatography (*2.2.27*), using *silica gel G R* as the coating substance.

Test solution. Dissolve 2 mg of the substance to be examined in 1 ml of a mixture of equal volumes of *alcohol R* and *water R*.

Reference solution. Dissolve 2 mg of *cyanocobalamin CRS* in 1 ml of a mixture of equal volumes of *alcohol R* and *water R*.

Apply to the plate 10 µl of each solution. Develop in a non-saturated tank over a path of 12 cm using a mixture of 9 volumes of *dilute ammonia R1*, 30 volumes of *methanol R* and 45 volumes of *methylene chloride R*. Allow the plate to dry in air. Examine in daylight. The principal spot in the chromatogram obtained with the test solution is similar in position, colour and size to the principal spot in the chromatogram obtained with the reference solution.

TESTS

Related substances. Examine by liquid chromatography (*2.2.29*).

Test solution. Dissolve 10.0 mg of the substance to be examined in the mobile phase and dilute to 10.0 ml with the same mixture of solvents. *Use within 1 h.*

Reference solution (a). Dilute 3.0 ml of the test solution to 100.0 ml with the mobile phase. *Use within 1 h.*

Reference solution (b). Dilute 5.0 ml of the test solution to 50.0 ml with the mobile phase. Dilute 1.0 ml of this solution to 100.0 ml with the mobile phase. *Use within 1 h.*

Reference solution (c). Dissolve 25 mg of the substance to be examined in 10 ml of *water R*, warming if necessary. Allow to cool and add 5 ml of a 1.0 g/l solution of *chloramine R* and 0.5 ml of *0.05 M hydrochloric acid.* Dilute to 25 ml with *water R.* Shake and allow to stand for 5 min. Dilute 1 ml of this solution to 10 ml with the mobile phase and inject immediately.

The chromatographic procedure may be carried out using:

- a stainless steel column 0.25 m long and 4 mm in internal diameter packed with *octylsilyl silica gel for chromatography R* (5 µm),
- as the mobile phase at a flow rate of 0.8 ml/min a mixture prepared as follows: mix 26.5 volumes of *methanol R* and 73.5 volumes of a 10 g/l solution of *disodium hydrogen phosphate R* adjusted to pH 3.5 using *phosphoric acid R* and use within 2 days,
- a spectrophotometer set at 361 nm as detector,
- a loop injector.

Inject separately 20 µl of each solution and continue the chromatography for 3 times the retention time of cyanocobalamin. In the chromatogram obtained with the test solution, the sum of the areas of any peaks apart from the principal peak is not greater than the area of the principal peak in the chromatogram obtained with reference solution (a) (3 per cent). Disregard any peak whose area is less than that of the principal peak in the chromatogram obtained with reference solution (b). The test is not valid unless the chromatogram obtained with reference solution (c) shows 2 principal peaks, the resolution between these peaks is not less than 2.5 and the chromatogram obtained with reference solution (b) shows one principal peak with a signal-to-noise ratio of not less than 5.

Loss on drying (*2.2.32*). Not more than 12.0 per cent, determined on 20.00 mg by drying *in vacuo* at 100-105 °C for 2 h.

ASSAY

Dissolve 25.00 mg in *water R* and dilute to 1000.0 ml with the same solvent. Measure the absorbance (*2.2.25*) of the solution at the maximum at 361 nm. Calculate the content of $C_{63}H_{88}CoN_{14}O_{14}P$, taking the specific absorbance to be 207.

STORAGE

Store in an airtight container, protected from light.

01/2005:1092

CYCLIZINE HYDROCHLORIDE

Cyclizini hydrochloridum

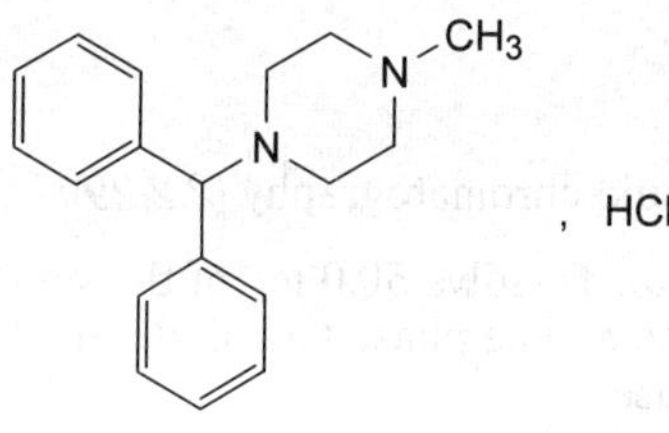

$C_{18}H_{23}ClN_2$ M_r 302.8

DEFINITION

Cyclizine hydrochloride contains not less than 98.5 per cent and not more than the equivalent of 101.0 per cent of 1-(diphenylmethyl)-4-methylpiperazine hydrochloride, calculated with reference to the dried substance.

CHARACTERS

A white, crystalline powder, slightly soluble in water and in alcohol.

IDENTIFICATION

First identification: B, E.

Second identification: A, C, D, E.

A. Dissolve 20.0 mg in a 5 g/l solution of *sulphuric acid R* and dilute to 100.0 ml with the same acid solution (solution A). Examined between 240 nm and 350 nm (*2.2.25*), solution A shows two absorption maxima, at 258 nm and 262 nm. The ratio of the absorbance measured at the maximum at 262 nm to that measured at the maximum at 258 nm is 1.0 to 1.1. Dilute 10.0 ml of solution A to 100.0 ml with a 5 g/l solution of *sulphuric acid R* (solution B). Examined between 210 nm and 240 nm, solution B shows an absorption maximum at 225 nm. The specific absorbance at the maximum is 370 to 410. Verify the resolution of the apparatus (*2.2.25*); the test is not valid unless the ratio of the absorbances is at least 1.7.

B. Examine by infrared absorption spectrophotometry (*2.2.24*), comparing with the spectrum obtained with *cyclizine hydrochloride CRS.* Examine the substances prepared as discs using *potassium chloride R.*

C. Examine the chromatograms obtained in the test for related substances. The principal spot in the chromatogram obtained with test solution (b) is similar in position, colour and size to the principal spot in the chromatogram obtained with reference solution (a).

D. Dissolve 0.5 g in 10 ml of *alcohol (60 per cent V/V) R* using heat, if necessary. Cool in iced water. Add 1 ml of *dilute sodium hydroxide solution R* and 10 ml of *water R.* Filter, wash the precipitate with *water R* and dry it at 60 °C at a pressure not exceeding 0.7 kPa for 2 h. The melting point (*2.2.14*) is 105 °C to 108 °C.

E. It gives reaction (a) of chlorides (*2.3.1*).

TESTS

pH (*2.2.3*). Dissolve 0.5 g in a mixture of 40 volumes of *alcohol R* and 60 volumes of *carbon dioxide-free water R* and dilute to 25 ml with the same mixture of solvents. The pH of the solution is 4.5 to 5.5.

Related substances. Examine by thin-layer chromatography (*2.2.27*), using a *TLC silica gel plate R*. *Prepare the solutions immediately before use.*

Test solution (a). Dissolve 0.20 g of the substance to be examined in *methanol R* and dilute to 10 ml with the same solvent.

Test solution (b). Dilute 5 ml of test solution (a) to 100 ml with *methanol R*.

Reference solution (a). Dissolve 10 mg of *cyclizine hydrochloride CRS* in *methanol R* and dilute to 10 ml with the same solvent.

Reference solution (b). Dissolve 5 mg of *methylpiperazine R* in *methanol R* and dilute to 50 ml with the same solvent.

Reference solution (c). Dilute 1 ml of test solution (b) to 10 ml with *methanol R*.

Reference solution (d). Dissolve 10 mg of *cyclizine hydrochloride CRS* and 10 mg of *hydroxyzine hydrochloride CRS* in *methanol R* and dilute to 10 ml with the same solvent.

Apply to the plate 20 µl of each solution. Develop over a path of 15 cm using a mixture of 2 volumes of *concentrated ammonia R*, 13 volumes of *methanol R* and 85 volumes of *methylene chloride R*. Allow the plate to dry in air for 30 min. Expose the plate to iodine vapour for 10 min. In the chromatogram obtained with test solution (a): any spot corresponding to 1-methylpiperazine is not more intense than the spot in the chromatogram obtained with reference solution (b) (0.5 per cent); any spot, apart from the principal spot and any spot corresponding to 1-methylpiperazine, is not more intense than the principal spot in the chromatogram obtained with reference solution (c) (0.5 per cent). The test is not valid unless the chromatogram obtained with reference solution (d) shows two clearly separated spots.

Loss on drying (*2.2.32*). Not more than 1.0 per cent, determined on 1.000 g by drying in an oven at 130 °C.

Sulphated ash (*2.4.14*). Not more than 0.1 per cent, determined on 1.0 g.

ASSAY

Dissolve 0.200 g in 15 ml of *anhydrous formic acid R* and add 40 ml of *acetic anhydride R*. Titrate with *0.1 M perchloric acid*, determining the end-point potentiometrically (*2.2.20*).

1 ml of *0.1 M perchloric acid* is equivalent to 15.14 mg of $C_{18}H_{23}ClN_2$.

STORAGE

Store protected from light.

IMPURITIES

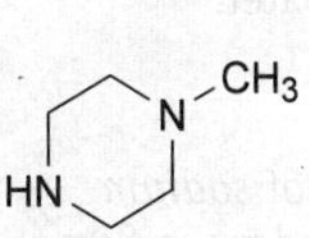

A. 1-methylpiperazine.

01/2005:1093

CYCLOPENTOLATE HYDROCHLORIDE

Cyclopentolati hydrochloridum

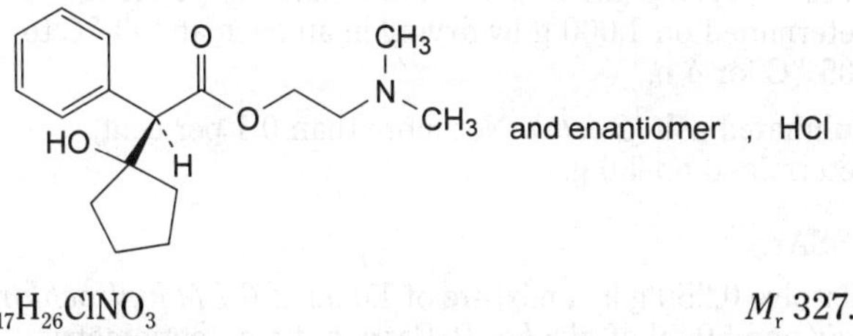

$C_{17}H_{26}ClNO_3$ M_r 327.9

DEFINITION

Cyclopentolate hydrochloride contains not less than 98.5 per cent and not more than the equivalent of 101.5 per cent of 2-(dimethylamino)ethyl (*RS*)-2-(1-hydroxycyclopentyl)-2-phenylacetate hydrochloride, calculated with reference to the dried substance.

CHARACTERS

A white, crystalline powder, very soluble in water, freely soluble in alcohol.

IDENTIFICATION

First identification: B, D.

Second identification: A, C, D.

A. Melting point (*2.2.14*): 135 °C to 141 °C.

B. Examine by infrared absorption spectrophotometry (*2.2.24*), comparing with the spectrum obtained with *cyclopentolate hydrochloride CRS*. Examine the substances as discs prepared using *potassium chloride R*. If the spectra obtained show differences, dissolve the substance to be examined and the reference substance separ-ately in *alcohol R*, evaporate to dryness and record new spectra using the residues.

C. Examine the chromatograms obtained in the test for related substances. The principal spot in the chromatogram obtained with test solution (b) is similar in position, fluorescence and size to the principal spot in the chromatogram obtained with reference solution (b).

D. It gives reaction (a) of chlorides (*2.3.1*).

TESTS

pH (*2.2.3*). Dissolve 0.2 g in *carbon dioxide-free water R* and dilute to 20 ml with the same solvent. The pH of the solution is 4.5 to 5.5.

Related substances. Examine by thin-layer chromatography (*2.2.27*), using a suitable silica gel as the coating substance.

Test solution (a). Dissolve 0.20 g of the substance to be examined in *alcohol R* and dilute to 5 ml with the same solvent.

Test solution (b). Dilute 1 ml of test solution (a) to 20 ml with *alcohol R*.

Reference solution (a). Dilute 1 ml of test solution (a) to 200 ml with *alcohol R*.

Reference solution (b). Dissolve 10 mg of *cyclopentolate hydrochloride CRS* in *alcohol R* and dilute to 5 ml with the same solvent.

Apply separately to the plate 10 µl of each solution. Develop over a path of 15 cm using a mixture of 5 volumes of *concentrated ammonia R*, 15 volumes of *water R*, 30 volumes of *butyl acetate R* and 50 volumes of *2-propanol R*. Allow the plate to dry in air. Spray with *analcoholic solution of sulphuric acid R* and heat the plate at 120 °C for 30 min. Examine in ultraviolet light at 365 nm. Any spot in the chromatogram obtained with test solution (a), apart from the principal spot, is not more intense than the spot in the chromatogram obtained with reference solution (a) (0.5 per cent).

Loss on drying (*2.2.32*). Not more than 0.5 per cent, determined on 1.000 g by drying in an oven at 100 °C to 105 °C for 4 h.

Sulphated ash (*2.4.14*). Not more than 0.1 per cent, determined on 1.0 g.

ASSAY

Dissolve 0.250 g in a mixture of 1.0 ml of *0.1 M hydrochloric acid* and 50 ml of *alcohol R*. Carry out a potentiometric titration (*2.2.20*), using *0.1 M sodium hydroxide*. Read the volume added between the two points of inflexion.

1 ml of *0.1 M sodium hydroxide* is equivalent to 32.79 mg of $C_{17}H_{26}ClNO_3$.

01/2005:0711

CYCLOPHOSPHAMIDE

Cyclophosphamidum

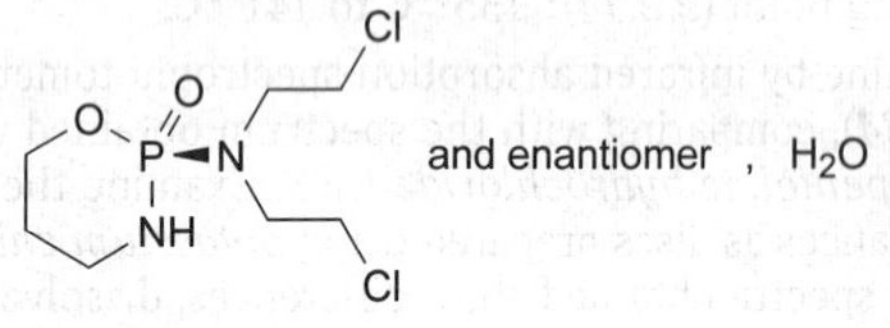

$C_7H_{15}Cl_2N_2O_2P,H_2O$ M_r 279.1

DEFINITION

Cyclophosphamide contains not less than 98.0 per cent and not more than the equivalent of 102.0 per cent of (2*RS*)-*N*,*N*-bis(2-chloroethyl)tetrahydro-2*H*-1,3,2-oxazaphosphorin-2-amine 2-oxide, calculated with reference to the anhydrous substance.

CHARACTERS

A white or almost white, crystalline powder, soluble in water, freely soluble in alcohol.

IDENTIFICATION

First identification: B.

Second identification: A, C, D.

A. Determine the melting point (*2.2.14*) of the substance to be examined. Mix equal parts of the substance to be examined and *cyclophosphamide CRS* and determine the melting point of the mixture. The difference between the melting points (which are about 51 °C) is not greater than 2 °C.

B. Examine by infrared absorption spectrophotometry (*2.2.24*), comparing with the spectrum obtained with *cyclophosphamide CRS*.

C. Examine the chromatograms obtained in the test for related substances. The principal spot in the chromatogram obtained with test solution (b) is similar in position, colour and size to the principal spot in the chromatogram obtained with reference solution (a).

D. Dissolve 0.1 g in 10 ml of *water R* and add 5 ml of *silver nitrate solution R1*; the solution remains clear. Boil, a white precipitate is formed which dissolves in *concentrated ammonia R* and is reprecipitated on the addition of *dilute nitric acid R*.

TESTS

Solution S. Dissolve 0.50 g in *carbon dioxide-free water R* and dilute to 25.0 ml with the same solvent.

Appearance of solution. Solution S is clear (*2.2.1*) and not more intensely coloured than reference solution Y_6 (*2.2.2, Method II*).

pH (*2.2.3*). The pH of solution S is 4.0 to 6.0, determined immediately after preparation of the solution.

Related substances. Examine by thin-layer chromatography (*2.2.27*), using *silica gel G R* as the coating substance.

Test solution (a). Dissolve 0.10 g of the substance to be examined in *alcohol R* and dilute to 5 ml with the same solvent.

Test solution (b). Dilute 1 ml of test solution (a) to 10 ml with *alcohol R*.

Reference solution (a). Dissolve 10 mg of *cyclophosphamide CRS* in *alcohol R* and dilute to 5 ml with the same solvent.

Reference solution (b). Dilute 0.1 ml of test solution (a) to 10 ml with *alcohol R*.

Apply separately to the plate 10 µl of each solution. Develop over a path of 15 cm using a mixture of 2 volumes of *anhydrous formic acid R*, 4 volumes of *acetone R*, 12 volumes of *water R* and 80 volumes of *methyl ethyl ketone R*. Dry the plate in a current of warm air and heat at 110 °C for 10 min. At the bottom of a chromatography tank, place an evaporating dish containing a 50 g/l solution of *potassium permanganate R* and add an equal volume of *hydrochloric acid R*. Place the plate whilst still hot in the tank and close the tank. Leave the plate in contact with the chlorine gas for 2 min. Withdraw the plate and place it in a current of cold air until the excess of chlorine is removed and an area of coating below the points of application gives at most a very faint blue colour with a drop of *potassium iodide and starch solution R*. Avoid prolonged exposure to cold air. Spray with *potassium iodide and starch solution R* and allow to stand for 5 min. Any spot in the chromatogram obtained with test solution (a), apart from the principal spot, is not more intense than the spot in the chromatogram obtained with reference solution (b) (1.0 per cent). Disregard any spot remaining at the starting-point.

Chlorides (*2.4.4*). Dissolve 0.15 g in *water R* and dilute to 15 ml with the same solvent. The freshly prepared solution complies with the limit test for chlorides (330 ppm).

Phosphates (*2.4.11*). Dissolve 0.10 g in *water R* and dilute to 100 ml with the same solvent. The solution complies with the limit test for phosphates (100 ppm).

Heavy metals (*2.4.8*). 1.0 g complies with limit test C for heavy metals (20 ppm). Prepare the standard using 2 ml of *lead standard solution (10 ppm Pb) R*.

Water (*2.5.12*): 6.0 per cent to 7.0 per cent, determined on 0.300 g by the semi-micro determination of water.

ASSAY

Dissolve 0.100 g in 50 ml of a 1 g/l solution of *sodium hydroxide R* in *ethylene glycol R* and boil under a reflux condenser for 30 min. Allow to cool and rinse the condenser with 25 ml of *water R*. Add 75 ml of *2-propanol R*, 15 ml of *dilute nitric acid R*, 10.0 ml of *0.1 M silver nitrate* and 2.0 ml of *ferric ammonium sulfate solution R2* and titrate with *0.1 M ammonium thiocyanate*.

1 ml of *0.1 M silver nitrate* is equivalent to 13.05 mg of $C_7H_{15}Cl_2N_2O_2P$.

01/2005:0817

CYPROHEPTADINE HYDROCHLORIDE

Cyproheptadini hydrochloridum

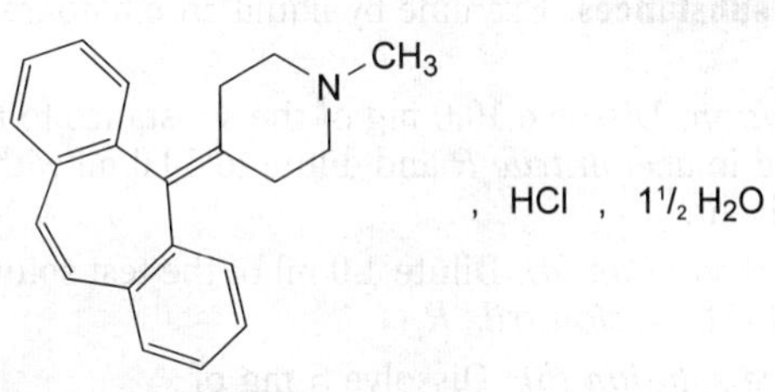

$C_{21}H_{22}ClN,1^1/_2\ H_2O$ M_r 350.9

DEFINITION

Cyproheptadine hydrochloride contains not less than 98.5 per cent and not more than the equivalent of 101.0 per cent of 4-(5*H*-dibenzo[*a,d*]cyclohepten-5-ylidene)-1-methylpiperidine hydrochloride, calculated with reference to the anhydrous substance.

CHARACTERS

A white or slightly yellow, crystalline powder, slightly soluble in water, freely soluble in methanol, sparingly soluble in alcohol.

IDENTIFICATION

First identification: B, D.

Second identification: A, C, D.

A. Dissolve 50.0 mg in *alcohol R* and dilute to 50.0 ml with the same solvent. Dilute 2.0 ml of the solution to 100.0 ml with *alcohol R*. Examined between 230 nm and 320 nm (*2.2.25*), the solution shows an absorption maximum at 286 nm. The specific absorbance at the maximum is 335 to 365, calculated with reference to the anhydrous substance.

B. Examine by infrared absorption spectrophotometry (*2.2.24*), comparing with the spectrum obtained with *cyproheptadine hydrochloride CRS*. Examine the substances as mulls in *liquid paraffin R*.

C. Examine by thin-layer chromatography (*2.2.27*), using *silica gel GF_{254} R* as the coating substance.

Test solution. Dissolve 25 mg of the substance to be examined in *methanol R* and dilute to 25 ml with the same solvent.

Reference solution (a). Dissolve 10 mg of *cyproheptadine hydrochloride CRS* in *methanol R* and dilute to 10 ml with the same solvent.

Reference solution (b). Dissolve 10 mg of *imipramine hydrochloride CRS* in *methanol R* and dilute to 10 ml with the same solvent. Dilute 1 ml to 2 ml with reference solution (a).

Apply to the plate 2 µl of each solution. Develop over a path of 15 cm using a mixture of 5 volumes of *diethylamine R*, 20 volumes of *ether R* and 75 volumes of *cyclohexane R*. Allow the plate to dry in air and examine in ultraviolet light at 254 nm. The principal spot in the chromatogram obtained with the test solution is similar in position and size to the principal spot in the chromatogram obtained with reference solution (a). The test is not valid unless the chromatogram obtained with reference solution (b) shows 2 clearly separated principal spots.

D. A saturated solution gives reaction (b) of chlorides (*2.3.1*).

TESTS

Acidity. Dissolve 0.10 g in *water R* and dilute to 25 ml with the same solvent. Add 0.1 ml of *methyl red solution R*. Not more than 0.15 ml of *0.01 M sodium hydroxide* is required to change the colour of the indicator.

Related substances. Examine by thin-layer chromatography (*2.2.27*), using *silica gel G R* as the coating substance.

Test solution. Dissolve 50 mg of the substance to be examined in a mixture of 1 volume of *methanol R* and 9 volumes of *methylene chloride R* and dilute to 5 ml with the same mixture of solvents.

Reference solution (a). Dissolve 10 mg of *dibenzocycloheptene CRS* (5*H*-dibenzo[*a,d*]cycloheptene) in a mixture of 1 volume of *methanol R* and 9 volumes of *methylene chloride R* and dilute to 50 ml with the same mixture of solvents. Dilute 1 ml to 10 ml with a mixture of 1 volume of *methanol R* and 9 volumes of *methylene chloride R*.

Reference solution (b). Dilute 1 ml of the test solution to 100 ml with a mixture of 1 volume of *methanol R* and 9 volumes of *methylene chloride R*. Dilute 1 ml to 10 ml with a mixture of 1 volume of *methanol R* and 9 volumes of *methylene chloride R*.

Apply to the plate 10 µl of each solution. Develop over a path of 15 cm using a mixture of 10 volumes of *methanol R* and 90 volumes of *methylene chloride R*. Allow the plate to dry in air and spray with *alcoholic solution of sulphuric acid R*. Heat at 110 °C for 30 min and examine in ultraviolet light at 365 nm while hot. In the chromatogram obtained with the test solution: any spot corresponding to dibenzocycloheptene is not more intense than the spot in the chromatogram obtained with reference solution (a) (0.2 per cent); any spot apart from the principal spot and any spot corresponding to dibenzocycloheptene is not more intense than the spot in the chromatogram obtained with reference solution (b) (0.1 per cent).

Water (*2.5.12*): 7.0 per cent to 9.0 per cent, determined on 0.200 g.

Sulphated ash (*2.4.14*). Not more than 0.1 per cent, determined on 1.0 g.

ASSAY

Dissolve 0.250 g in a mixture of 5.0 ml of *0.01 M hydrochloric acid* and 50 ml of *alcohol R*. Carry out a potentiometric titration (*2.2.20*), using *0.1 M sodium hydroxide*. Read the volume added between the 2 points of inflexion.

1 ml of *0.1 M sodium hydroxide* is equivalent to 32.39 mg of $C_{21}H_{22}ClN$.

STORAGE

Store protected from light.

IMPURITIES

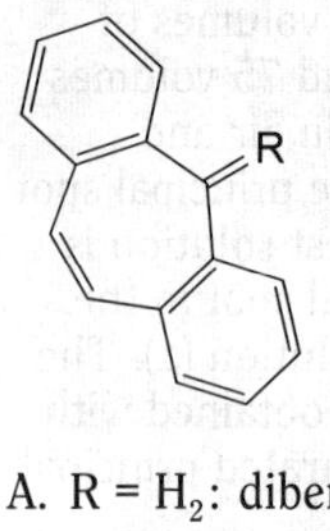

A. R = H_2: dibenzo[*a*,*d*]cycloheptene,

B. R = O: 5*H*-dibenzo[*a*,*d*]cyclohepten-5-one (dibenzosuberone).

01/2005:1094

CYPROTERONE ACETATE

Cyproteroni acetas

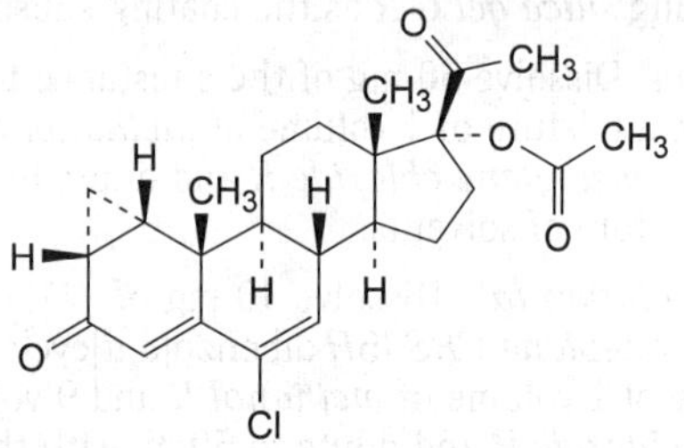

$C_{24}H_{29}ClO_4$ M_r 416.9

DEFINITION

Cyproterone acetate contains not less than 97.0 per cent and not more than the equivalent of 103.0 per cent of 6-chloro-3,20-dioxo-1β,2β-dihydro-3′*H*-cyclopropa[1,2]pregna-1,4,6-trien-17-yl acetate, calculated with reference to the dried substance.

CHARACTERS

A white or almost white, crystalline powder, practically insoluble in water, very soluble in methylene chloride, freely soluble in acetone, soluble in methanol, sparingly soluble in ethanol.

It melts at about 210 °C.

IDENTIFICATION

First identification: A.

Second identification: B, C, D, E.

A. Examine by infrared absorption spectrophotometry (*2.2.24*), comparing with the spectrum obtained with *cyproterone acetate CRS*.

B. Examine by thin-layer chromatography (*2.2.27*), using a *TLC silica gel F_{254} plate R*.

Test solution. Dissolve 20 mg of the substance to be examined in *methylene chloride R* and dilute to 10 ml with the same solvent.

Reference solution. Dissolve 10 mg of *cyproterone acetate CRS* in *methylene chloride R* and dilute to 5 ml with the same solvent.

Apply to the plate 5 µl of each solution. Develop over a path of 15 cm using a mixture of equal volumes of *cyclohexane R* and *ethyl acetate R*. Allow the plate to dry in air. Repeat the development. Allow the plate to dry in air. Examine in ultraviolet light at 254 nm. The principal spot in the chromatogram obtained with the test solution is similar in position and size to the principal spot in the chromatogram obtained with the reference solution.

C. To about 1 mg add 2 ml of *sulphuric acid R* and heat on a water-bath for 2 min. A red colour develops. Cool. Add the solution cautiously to 4 ml of *water R* and shake. The solution becomes violet.

D. Incinerate about 30 mg with 0.3 g of *anhydrous sodium carbonate R* over a naked flame for about 10 min. Cool and dissolve the residue in 5 ml of *dilute nitric acid R*. Filter. To 1 ml of the filtrate add 1 ml of *water R*. The solution gives reaction (a) of chlorides (*2.3.1*).

E. It gives the reaction of acetyl (*2.3.1*).

TESTS

Specific optical rotation (*2.2.7*). Dissolve 0.25 g in *acetone R* and dilute to 25.0 ml with the same solvent. The specific optical rotation is + 152 to + 157, calculated with reference to the dried substance.

Related substances. Examine by liquid chromatography (*2.2.29*).

Test solution. Dissolve 10.0 mg of the substance to be examined in *acetonitrile R* and dilute to 10.0 ml with the same solvent.

Reference solution (a). Dilute 1.0 ml of the test solution to 100.0 ml with *acetonitrile R*.

Reference solution (b). Dissolve 5 mg of *medroxyprogesterone acetate CRS* in *acetonitrile R* and dilute to 50.0 ml with the same solvent. Dilute 1.0 ml of the solution to 10.0 ml with reference solution (a).

The chromatographic procedure may be carried out using:

– a stainless steel column 0.125 m long and 4.6 mm in internal diameter packed with *octadecylsilyl silica gel for chromatography R* (3 µm),

– as mobile phase at a flow rate of 1.5 ml/min a mixture of 40 volumes of *acetonitrile R* and 60 volumes of *water R*,

– as detector a spectrophotometer set at 254 nm.

Inject 20 µl of reference solution (a) and 20 µl of reference solution (b). Adjust the sensitivity of the system so that the height of the principal peak in the chromatogram obtained with reference solution (a) is at least 50 per cent of the full scale of the recorder. The test is not valid unless, in the chromatogram obtained with reference solution (b), the resolution between the peak corresponding to cyproterone acetate and the peak corresponding to medroxyprogesterone acetate is at least 3.0.

Inject 20 µl of the test solution. Continue the chromatography for twice the retention time of cyproterone acetate. In the chromatogram obtained with the test solution, the sum of the areas of all the peaks, apart from the principal peak, is not greater than 0.5 times the area of the principal peak in the chromatogram obtained with reference solution (a) (0.5 per cent). Disregard any peak with an area less than 0.05 times that of the principal peak in the chromatogram obtained with reference solution (a).

Loss on drying (*2.2.32*). Not more than 0.5 per cent, determined on 1.000 g by drying at 80 °C at a pressure not exceeding 0.7 kPa.

Sulphated ash (*2.4.14*). Not more than 0.1 per cent, determined on 1.0 g.

ASSAY

Dissolve 50.0 mg in *methanol R* and dilute to 50.0 ml with the same solvent. Dilute 1.0 ml of the solution to 100.0 ml with *methanol R*. Measure the absorbance (*2.2.25*) at the maximum at 282 nm.

Calculate the content of $C_{24}H_{29}ClO_4$ taking the specific absorbance to be 414.

STORAGE

Store protected from light.

IMPURITIES

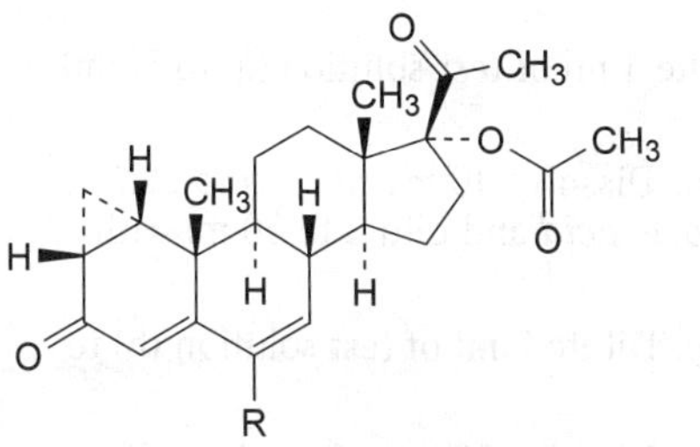

A. R = H: 3,20-dioxo-1β,2β-dihydro-3′*H*-cyclopropa[1,2]pregna-1,4,6-trien-17-yl acetate,

B. R = OCH_3: 6-methoxy-3,20-dioxo-1β,2β-dihydro-3′*H*-cyclopropa[1,2]pregna-1,4,6-trien-17-yl acetate.

01/2005:0895

CYSTEINE HYDROCHLORIDE MONOHYDRATE

Cysteini hydrochloridum monohydricum

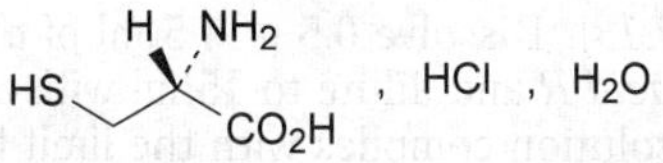

$C_3H_8ClNO_2S,H_2O$ M_r 175.6

DEFINITION

Cysteine hydrochloride monohydrate contains not less than 98.5 per cent and not more than the equivalent of 101.0 per cent of (2*R*)-2-amino-3-sulfanylpropanoic acid hydrochloride, calculated with reference to the dried substance.

CHARACTERS

A white, crystalline powder or colourless crystals, freely soluble in water, slightly soluble in alcohol.

IDENTIFICATION

First identification: A, B, E.

Second identification: A, C, D, E.

A. It complies with the test for specific optical rotation (see Tests).

B. Examine by infrared absorption spectrophotometry (*2.2.24*), comparing with the spectrum obtained with *cysteine hydrochloride monohydrate CRS*. Examine the substances prepared as discs.

C. Examine the chromatograms obtained in the test for ninhydrin-positive substances. The principal spot in the chromatogram obtained with test solution (b) is similar in position, colour, and size to the principal spot in the chromatogram obtained with reference solution (b).

D. Dissolve about 5 mg in 1 ml of *dilute sodium hydroxide solution R*. Add 1 ml of a 30 g/l solution of *sodium nitroprusside R*. An intense violet colour develops which becomes brownish-red and then orange. Add 1 ml of *hydrochloric acid R*. The solution becomes green.

E. It gives reaction (a) of chlorides (*2.3.1*).

TESTS

Solution S. Dissolve 2.5 g in *distilled water R* and dilute to 50 ml with the same solvent.

Appearance of solution. Dilute 10 ml of solution S to 20 ml with *water R*. The solution is clear (*2.2.1*) and not more intensely coloured than reference solution BY_6 (*2.2.2, Method II*).

Specific optical rotation (*2.2.7*). Dissolve 2.00 g in *hydrochloric acid R1* and dilute to 25.0 ml with the same acid. The specific optical rotation is + 5.5 to + 7.0, calculated with reference to the dried substance.

Ninhydrin-positive substances. Examine by thin-layer chromatography (*2.2.27*), using a *TLC silica gel plate R*.

Test solution (a). Dissolve 0.20 g of the substance to be examined in *water R* and dilute to 10 ml with the same solvent. To 5 ml of the solution add 5 ml of a 40 g/l solution of *N-ethylmaleimide R* in *alcohol R*. Allow to stand for 5 min.

Test solution (b). Dilute 1 ml of test solution (a) to 50 ml with *water R*.

Reference solution (a). Dissolve 20 mg of *cysteine hydrochloride monohydrate CRS* in *water R* and dilute to 10 ml with the same solvent. Add 10 ml of a 40 g/l solution of *N-ethylmaleimide R* in *alcohol R*. Allow to stand for 5 min.

Reference solution (b). Dilute 2 ml of reference solution (a) to 10 ml with *water R*.

Reference solution (c). Dilute 5 ml of test solution (b) to 20 ml with *water R*.

Reference solution (d). Dissolve 10 mg of *tyrosine CRS* in 10 ml of reference solution (a) and dilute to 25 ml with *water R*.

Apply separately to the plate 5 µl of each test solution and reference solutions (b), (c), and (d). Develop over a path of 15 cm using a mixture of 20 volumes of *glacial acetic acid R*, 20 volumes of *water R* and 60 volumes of *butanol R*. Dry the plate at 80 °C for 30 min. Spray with *ninhydrin solution R* and heat at 100 °C to 105 °C for 15 min. Any spot in the chromatogram obtained with test solution (a), apart from the principal spot, is not more intense than the spot in the chromatogram obtained with reference solution (c) (0.5 per cent). The test is not valid unless the chromatogram obtained with reference solution (d) shows 2 clearly separated principal spots.

Sulphates (*2.4.13*). Dilute 10 ml of solution S to 15 ml with *distilled water R*. The solution complies with the limit test for sulphates (300 ppm).

Ammonium (*2.4.1*). 50 mg complies with limit test B for ammonium (200 ppm). Prepare the standard using 0.1 ml of *ammonium standard solution (100 ppm NH_4) R*.

Iron (*2.4.9*). In a separating funnel, dissolve 0.50 g in 10 ml of *dilute hydrochloric acid R*. Shake with 3 quantities, each of 10 ml, of *methyl isobutyl ketone R1*, shaking for 3 min each time. To the combined organic layers add 10 ml of *water R* and shake for 3 min. The aqueous layer complies with the limit test for iron (20 ppm).

Heavy metals (*2.4.8*). Dissolve 2.0 g in *water R*. Adjust to pH 3 to 4 with *concentrated ammonia R* and dilute to 20 ml with *water R*. 12 ml of the solution complies with limit test A for heavy metals (10 ppm). Prepare the standard using *lead standard solution (1 ppm Pb) R*.

Loss on drying (*2.2.32*): 8.0 per cent to 12.0 per cent, determined on 1.000 g by drying at a pressure not exceeding 0.7 kPa for 24 h.

Sulphated ash (*2.4.14*). Not more than 0.1 per cent, determined on 1.0 g.

ASSAY

In a ground-glass stoppered flask dissolve 0.300 g of the substance to be examined and 4 g of *potassium iodide R* in 20 ml of *water R*. Cool the solution in iced water and add 3 ml of *hydrochloric acid R1* and 25.0 ml of *0.05 M iodine*. Stopper the flask and allow to stand in the dark for 20 min. Titrate with *0.1 M sodium thiosulphate* using 3 ml of *starch solution R*, added towards the end of the titration, as indicator. Carry out a blank titration.

1 ml of *0.05 M iodine* is equivalent to 15.76 mg of $C_3H_8ClNO_2S$.

STORAGE

Store protected from light.

01/2005:0998

CYSTINE

Cystinum

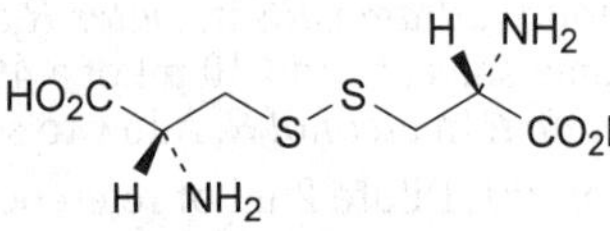

$C_6H_{12}N_2O_4S_2$ M_r 240.3

DEFINITION

Cystine contains not less than 98.5 per cent and not more than the equivalent of 101.0 per cent of 3,3′-disulfanediylbis[(2*R*)-2-aminopropanoic acid], calculated with reference to the dried substance.

CHARACTERS

A white, crystalline powder, practically insoluble in water and in alcohol. It dissolves in dilute solutions of alkali hydroxides.

IDENTIFICATION

First identification: A, B.

Second identification: A, C, D.

A. It complies with the test for specific optical rotation (see Tests).

B. Examine by infrared absorption spectrophotometry (*2.2.24*), comparing with the spectrum obtained with *cystine CRS*. Examine the substances prepared as discs.

C. Examine the chromatograms obtained in the test for ninhydrin-positive substances. The principal spot in the chromatogram obtained with test solution (b) is similar in position, colour and size to the principal spot in the chromatogram obtained with reference solution (a).

D. To 0.1 g carefully add 1 ml of *strong hydrogen peroxide solution R* and 0.1 ml of *ferric chloride solution R1*. Allow to cool. Add 1 ml of *dilute hydrochloric acid R* and 5 ml of *water R*. Add 1 ml of *barium chloride solution R1*. Turbidity or a white precipitate develops within 3 min.

TESTS

Appearance of solution. Dissolve 1.0 g in *dilute hydrochloric acid R* and dilute to 10 ml with the same acid. The solution is clear (*2.2.1*) and not more intensely coloured than reference solution Y_7 (*2.2.2, Method II*).

Specific optical rotation (*2.2.7*). Dissolve 0.50 g in *1 M hydrochloric acid* and dilute to 25.0 ml with the same acid. The specific optical rotation is − 218 to − 224, calculated with reference to the dried substance.

Ninhydrin-positive substances. Examine by thin-layer chromatography (*2.2.27*), using a *TLC silica gel plate R*.

Test solution (a). Dissolve 0.10 g of the substance to be examined in *1 M hydrochloric acid* and dilute to 10 ml with the same acid.

Test solution (b). Dilute 1 ml of test solution (a) to 50 ml with *water R*.

Reference solution (a). Dissolve 10 mg of *cystine CRS* in 1 ml of *1 M hydrochloric acid* and dilute to 50 ml with *water R*.

Reference solution (b). Dilute 2 ml of test solution (b) to 20 ml with *water R*.

Reference solution (c). Dissolve 10 mg of *cystine CRS* and 10 mg of *arginine hydrochloride CRS* in 1 ml of *1 M hydrochloric acid* and dilute to 25 ml with *water R*.

Apply separately to the plate 5 µl of each solution. Develop over a path of 15 cm using a mixture of 30 volumes of *concentrated ammonia R* and 70 volumes of *2-propanol R*. Allow the plate to dry in air. Spray with *ninhydrin solution R* and heat at 100 °C to 105 °C for 15 min. Any spot in the chromatogram obtained with test solution (a), apart from the principal spot, is not more intense than the spot in the chromatogram obtained with reference solution (b) (0.2 per cent). The test is not valid unless the chromatogram obtained with reference solution (c) shows two clearly separated spots.

Chlorides (*2.4.4*). Dissolve 0.25 g in 5 ml of *dilute nitric acid R* and dilute to 15 ml with *water R*. The solution, without further addition of nitric acid, complies with the limit test for chlorides (200 ppm).

Sulphates (*2.4.13*). Dissolve 0.5 g in 5 ml of *dilute hydrochloric acid R* and dilute to 15 ml with *distilled water R*. The solution complies with the limit test for sulphates (300 ppm).

Ammonium (*2.4.1*). 0.10 g complies with limit test B for ammonium (200 ppm). Prepare the standard using 0.2 ml of *ammonium standard solution (100 ppm NH_4) R*.

Iron (*2.4.9*). In a separating funnel, dissolve 1.0 g in 10 ml of *dilute hydrochloric acid R*. Shake with three quantities, each of 10 ml, of *methyl isobutyl ketone R1*, shaking for 3 min each time. To the combined organic layers add 10 ml of *water R* and shake for 3 min. The aqueous layer complies with the limit test for iron (10 ppm).

Heavy metals (*2.4.8*). 2.0 g complies with limit test D for heavy metals (10 ppm). Prepare the standard using 2 ml of *lead standard solution (10 ppm Pb) R*.

Loss on drying (*2.2.32*). Not more than 0.5 per cent, determined on 1.000 g by drying in an oven at 100 °C to 105 °C.

Sulphated ash (*2.4.14*). Not more than 0.1 per cent, determined on 1.0 g.

ASSAY

In a flask with a ground-glass stopper, dissolve 0.100 g in a mixture of 2 ml of *dilute sodium hydroxide solution R* and 10 ml of *water R*. Add 10 ml of a 200 g/l solution of *potassium bromide R*, 50.0 ml of *0.0167 M potassium bromate* and 15 ml of *dilute hydrochloric acid R*. Stopper the flask and cool in iced water. Allow to stand in the dark for 10 min. Add 1.5 g of *potassium iodide R*. After 1 min, titrate with *0.1 M sodium thiosulphate*, using 2 ml of *starch solution R*, added towards the end-point, as indicator. Carry out a blank titration.

1 ml of *0.0167 M potassium bromate* is equivalent to 2.403 mg of $C_6H_{12}N_2O_4S_2$.

STORAGE

Store protected from light.

01/2005:0760

CYTARABINE

Cytarabinum

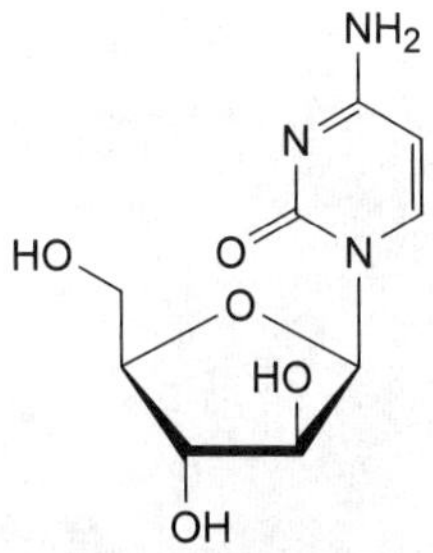

$C_9H_{13}N_3O_5$ M_r 243.2

DEFINITION

Cytarabine contains not less than 99.0 per cent and not more than the equivalent of 100.5 per cent of 4-amino-1-β-D-arabinofuranosylpyrimidin-2(1*H*)-one, calculated with reference to the dried substance.

CHARACTERS

A white or almost white, crystalline powder, freely soluble in water, very slightly soluble in alcohol and in methylene chloride.

It melts at about 215 °C.

IDENTIFICATION

A. Dissolve 20.0 mg in *0.1 M hydrochloric acid* and dilute to 100.0 ml with the same acid. Dilute 5.0 ml of the solution to 100.0 ml with *0.1 M hydrochloric acid*. Examined between 230 nm and 350 nm (*2.2.25*), the solution shows an absorption maximum at 281 nm. The specific absorbance at the maximum is 540 to 570.

B. Examine by infrared absorption spectrophotometry (*2.2.24*), comparing with the spectrum obtained with *cytarabine CRS*. Examine the substances prepared as discs.

C. Examine the chromatograms obtained in the test for related substances in ultraviolet light at 254 nm. The principal spot in the chromatogram obtained with test solution (b) is similar in position and size to the principal spot in the chromatogram obtained with reference solution (a).

TESTS

Appearance of solution. Dissolve 1.0 g in *water R* and dilute to 10 ml with the same solvent. The solution is clear (*2.2.1*) and not more intensely coloured than reference solution Y_5 (*2.2.2, Method II*).

Specific optical rotation (*2.2.7*). Dissolve 0.250 g in *water R* and dilute to 25.0 ml with the same solvent. The specific optical rotation is + 154 to + 160, calculated with reference to the dried substance.

Related substances. Examine by thin-layer chromatography (*2.2.27*), using *silica gel GF_{254} R* as the coating substance.

Test solution (a). Dissolve 0.25 g of the substance to be examined in *water R* and dilute to 5 ml with the same solvent.

Test solution (b). Dilute 2 ml of test solution (a) to 50 ml with *water R*.

Reference solution (a). Dissolve 10 mg of *cytarabine CRS* in *water R* and dilute to 5 ml with the same solvent.

Reference solution (b). Dilute 0.5 ml of test solution (a) to 100 ml with *water R*.

Reference solution (c). Dissolve 20 mg of *uridine R* and 20 mg of *uracil arabinoside CRS* in *methanol R* and dilute to 10 ml with the same solvent.

Apply separately to the plate 5 µl of each solution. Develop over a path of 15 cm using a mixture of 15 volumes of *water R*, 20 volumes of *acetone R* and 65 volumes of *methyl ethyl ketone R*. Allow the plate to dry in air and examine in ultraviolet light at 254 nm. Any spot in the chromatogram obtained with test solution (a), apart from the principal spot, is not more intense than the spot in the chromatogram obtained with reference solution (b) (0.5 per cent). The test is not valid unless the chromatogram obtained with reference solution (c) shows two clearly separated spots.

Loss on drying (*2.2.32*). Not more than 1.0 per cent, determined on 0.250 g by drying over *diphosphorus pentoxide R* at 60 °C at a pressure of 0.2 kPa to 0.7 kPa for 3 h.

Sulphated ash (*2.4.14*). Not more than 0.5 per cent, determined on 1.0 g.

ASSAY

Dissolve 0.200 g in 60 ml of *anhydrous acetic acid R*, warming if necessary. Titrate with *0.1 M perchloric acid* determining the end-point potentiometrically (*2.2.20*).

1 ml of *0.1 M perchloric acid* is equivalent to 24.32 mg of $C_9H_{13}N_3O_5$.

STORAGE

Store in an airtight container, protected from light.

IMPURITIES

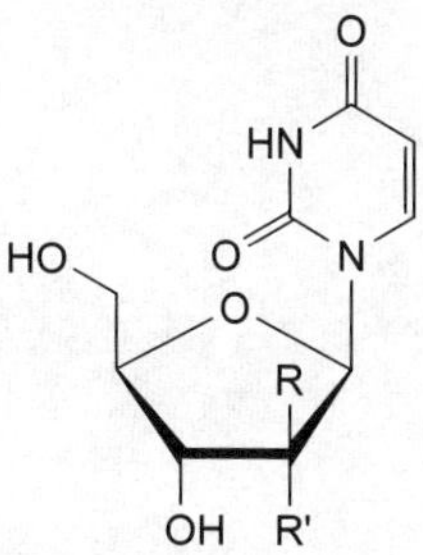

A. R = OH, R′ = H: 1-β-D-arabinofuranosylpyrimidine-2,4(1*H*,3*H*)-dione (uracil arabonoside),

B. R = H, R′ = OH: 1-β-D-ribofuranosylpyrimidine-2,4(1*H*,3*H*)-dione (uridine).

Monographs C

D

01/2005:1195

DALTEPARIN SODIUM

Dalteparinum natricum

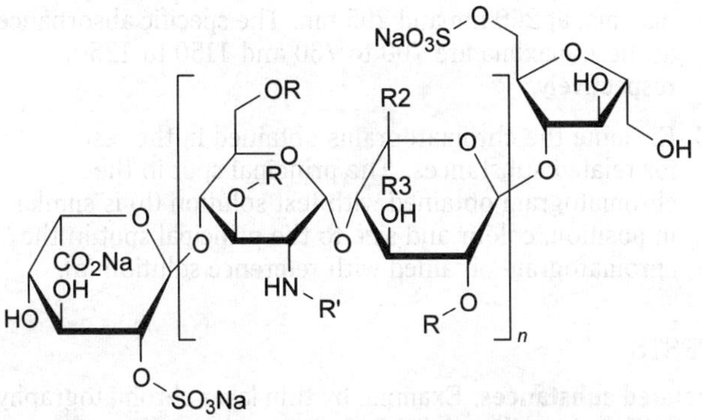

n = 3 to 20 , R = H or SO_3Na , R' = SO_3Na or $CO\text{-}CH_3$
R2 = H and R3 = CO_2Na or R2 = CO_2Na and R3 = H

DEFINITION

Dalteparin sodium is the sodium salt of a low-molecular-mass heparin that is obtained by nitrous acid depolymerisation of heparin from porcine intestinal mucosa. The majority of the components have a 2-*O*-sulpho-α-L-idopyranosuronic acid structure at the non-reducing end and a 6-*O*-sulpho-2,5-anhydro-D-mannitol structure at the reducing end of their chain.

Dalteparin sodium complies with the monograph on Low-molecular-mass heparins (0828) with the modifications and additional requirements below:

The mass-average molecular mass ranges between 5600 and 6400, with a characteristic value of about 6000.

The degree of sulphatation is 2.0 to 2.5 per disaccharide unit.

The potency is not less than 110 IU and not more than 210 IU of anti-factor Xa activity per milligram, calculated with reference to the dried substance. The anti-factor IIa activity is not less than 35 IU and not more than 100 IU/mg, calculated with reference to the dried substance. The ratio of anti-factor Xa activity to anti-factor IIa activity is between 1.9 and 3.2.

PRODUCTION

Dalteparin sodium is produced by a validated manufacturing and purification procedure under conditions designed to minimise the presence of N-NO groups.

The manufacturing procedure must have been shown to reduce any contamination by N-NO groups to approved limits using an appropriate, validated quantification method.

IDENTIFICATION

Carry out identification test C as described in the monograph on *Low-molecular-mass heparins (0828)*. The following requirements apply:

The mass-average molecular mass ranges between 5600 and 6400. The mass percentage of chains lower than 3000 is not more than 13.0 per cent. The mass percentage of chains higher than 8000 ranges between 15.0 per cent and 25.0 per cent.

TESTS

Appearance of solution. Dissolve 1 g in 10 ml of *water R*. The solution is clear (*2.2.1*) and not more intensely coloured than intensity 5 of the range of reference solutions of the most appropriate colour (*2.2.2, Method II*).

Nitrite. Not more than 5 ppm. Examine by liquid chromatography (*2.2.29*). *Rinse all volumetric flasks at least three times with water R before the preparation of the solutions.*

Test solution. Dissolve 80.0 mg of the substance to be examined in *water R* and dilute to 10.0 ml with the same solvent. Allow to stand for at least 30 min.

Reference solution (a). Dissolve 60.0 mg of *sodium nitrite R* in *water R* and dilute to 1000.0 ml with the same solvent.

For the preparation of reference solution (b), use a pipette previously rinsed with reference solution (a).

Reference solution (b). Dilute 1.00 ml of reference solution (a) to 50.0 ml with *water R.*

Before preparing reference solutions (c), (d) and (e), rinse all pipettes with reference solution (b).

Reference solution (c). Dilute 1.00 ml of reference solution (b) to 100.0 ml with *water R* (1 ppm nitrite).

Reference solution (d). Dilute 3.00 ml of reference solution (b) to 100.0 ml with *water R* (3 ppm nitrite).

Reference solution (e). Dilute 5.00 ml of reference solution (b) to 100.0 ml with *water R* (5 ppm nitrite).

The chromatographic procedure may be carried out using:

- a column 0.125 m long and 4.3 mm in internal diameter packed with a strong anion-exchange resin,
- as mobile phase at a flow rate of 1.0 ml/min a solution consisting of 13.61 g of *sodium acetate R* dissolved in *water R*, adjusted to pH 4.3 with *phosphoric acid R* and diluted to 1000 ml with *water R*,
- as detector an appropriate electrochemical device with the following characteristics and settings: a suitable working electrode, a detector potential of + 1.00 V versus Ag/AgCl reference electrode and a detector sensitivity of 0.1 µA full scale.

Inject 100 µl of reference solution (d). When the chromatograms are recorded in the prescribed conditions, the retention time for nitrite is 3.3 to 4.0 min. The test is not valid unless:

- the number of theoretical plates calculated for the nitrite peak is at least 7000 per metre per column (dalteparin sodium will block the binding sites of the stationary phase, which will cause shorter retention times and lower separation efficiency for the analyte; the initial performance of the column may be partially restored using a 58 g/l solution of *sodium chloride R* at a flow rate of 1.0 ml/min for 1 h; after regeneration the column is rinsed with 200 ml to 400 ml of *water R*),
- the symmetry factor for the nitrite peak is less than three,
- the relative standard deviation of the peak area for nitrite obtained from six injections is less than 3.0 per cent.

Inject 100 µl each of reference solutions (c) and (e). The test is not valid unless:

- the correlation factor for a linear relationship between concentration and response for reference solutions (c), (d) and (e) is at least 0.995,
- the signal-to-noise ratio for reference solution (c) is not less than 5 (if the noise level is too high, electrode recalibration is recommended),
- a blank injection of *water R* does not give rise to spurious peaks.

Inject 100 µl of the test solution. Calculate the content of nitrite from the peak areas in the chromatogram obtained with reference solutions (c), (d) and (e).

Boron. Not more than 1 ppm, determined by inductively coupled plasma atomic emission spectroscopy.

Boron is determined by measurement of the emission from an inductively coupled plasma (ICP) at a wavelength specific to boron. The emission line at 249.733 nm is used. Use an appropriate apparatus, whose settings have been optimised as directed by the manufacturer.

Test solution. Dissolve 0.2500 g of the substance to be examined in about 2 ml of *water for chromatography R*, add 100 µl of *nitric acid R* and dilute to 10.00 ml with the same solvent.

Reference solution (a). Prepare a 1 per cent *V/V* solution of *nitric acid R* in *water for chromatography R* (blank).

Reference solution (b). Prepare a 11.4 µg/ml solution of *boric acid R* in a 1 per cent *V/V* solution of *nitric acid R* in *water for chromatography R* (STD_{cal}).

Reference solution (c). Dissolve 0.2500 g of a reference dalteparin sodium with no detectable boron in about 2 ml of *water for chromatography R*, add 100 µl of *nitric acid R* and dilute to 10.00 ml with the same solvent (STD_0).

Reference solution (d). Dissolve 0.2500 g of a reference dalteparin sodium with no boron detected in about 2 ml of a 1 per cent *V/V* solution of *nitric acid R* in *water for chromatography R*, add 10 µl of a 5.7 mg/ml solution of *boric acid R* and dilute to 10.00 ml with the same solvent (STD_1). This solution contains 1 µg/ml of boron.

Calculate the content of boron in the substance to be examined, using the following correction factor:

$$f = \frac{(STD_1 - STD_0) \times 2}{(STD_{cal} - \text{blank})}$$

Loss on drying (*2.2.32*). Not more than 5.0 per cent, determined on 1.000 g by drying in an oven at 60 °C over *diphosphorus pentoxide R* at a pressure not exceeding 670 Pa for 3 h.

01/2005:0077

DAPSONE

Dapsonum

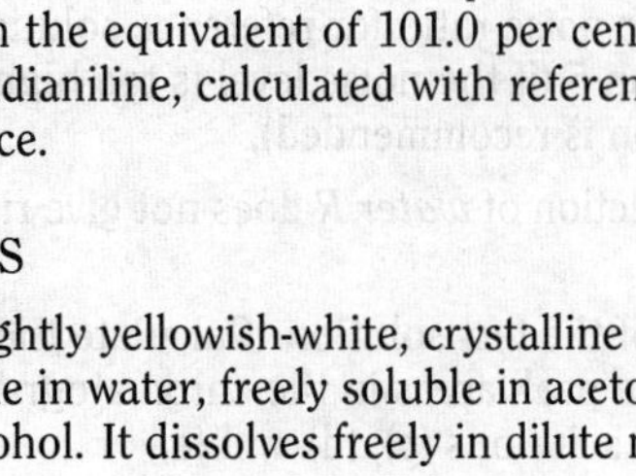

$C_{12}H_{12}N_2O_2S$ M_r 248.3

DEFINITION

Dapsone contains not less than 99.0 per cent and not more than the equivalent of 101.0 per cent of 4,4′-sulphonyldianiline, calculated with reference to the dried substance.

CHARACTERS

A white or slightly yellowish-white, crystalline powder, very slightly soluble in water, freely soluble in acetone, sparingly soluble in alcohol. It dissolves freely in dilute mineral acids.

IDENTIFICATION

A. Melting point (*2.2.14*): 175 °C to 181 °C.

B. Dissolve 50.0 mg in *methanol R* and dilute to 100.0 ml with the same solvent. Dilute 1.0 ml of this solution to 100.0 ml with *methanol R*. Examined between 230 nm and 350 nm (*2.2.25*), the solution shows 2 absorption maxima, at 260 nm and 295 nm. The specific absorbances at these maxima are 700 to 760 and 1150 to 1250, respectively.

C. Examine the chromatograms obtained in the test for related substances. The principal spot in the chromatogram obtained with test solution (b) is similar in position, colour and size to the principal spot in the chromatogram obtained with reference solution (a).

TESTS

Related substances. Examine by thin-layer chromatography (*2.2.27*), using *silica gel G R* as the coating substance.

Test solution (a). Dissolve 0.10 g of the substance to be examined in *methanol R* and dilute to 10 ml with the same solvent.

Test solution (b). Dilute 1 ml of test solution (a) to 10 ml with *methanol R*.

Reference solution (a). Dissolve 10 mg of *dapsone CRS* in *methanol R* and dilute to 10 ml with the same solvent.

Reference solution (b). Dilute 1 ml of test solution (b) to 10 ml with *methanol R*.

Reference solution (c). Dilute 2 ml of reference solution (b) to 10 ml with *methanol R*.

Apply separately to the plate 1 µl of test solution (b), 1 µl of reference solution (a), 10 µl of test solution (a), 10 µl of reference solution (b) and 10 µl of reference solution (c). Develop in an unsaturated tank over a path of 15 cm using a mixture of 1 volume of *concentrated ammonia R*, 6 volumes of *methanol R*, 20 volumes of *ethyl acetate R* and 20 volumes of *heptane R*. Allow the plate to dry in air. Spray the plate with a 1 g/l solution of *4-dimethylaminocinnamaldehyde R* in a mixture of 1 volume of *hydrochloric acid R* and 99 volumes of *alcohol R*. Examine in daylight. Any spot in the chromatogram obtained with test solution (a), apart from the principal spot, is not more intense than the spot in the chromatogram obtained with reference solution (b) (1.0 per cent) and not more than 2 such spots are more intense than the spot in the chromatogram obtained with reference solution (c) (0.2 per cent).

Loss on drying (*2.2.32*). Not more than 1.5 per cent, determined on 1.000 g by drying in an oven at 100 °C to 105 °C.

Sulphated ash (*2.4.14*). Not more than 0.1 per cent, determined on 1.0 g.

ASSAY

Dissolve 0.100 g in 50 ml of *dilute hydrochloric acid R*. Carry out the determination of primary aromatic amino-nitrogen (*2.5.8*).

1 ml of *0.1 M sodium nitrite* is equivalent to 12.42 mg of $C_{12}H_{12}N_2O_2S$.

STORAGE

Store protected from light.

Monographs D-E

01/2005:0662

DAUNORUBICIN HYDROCHLORIDE

Daunorubicini hydrochloridum

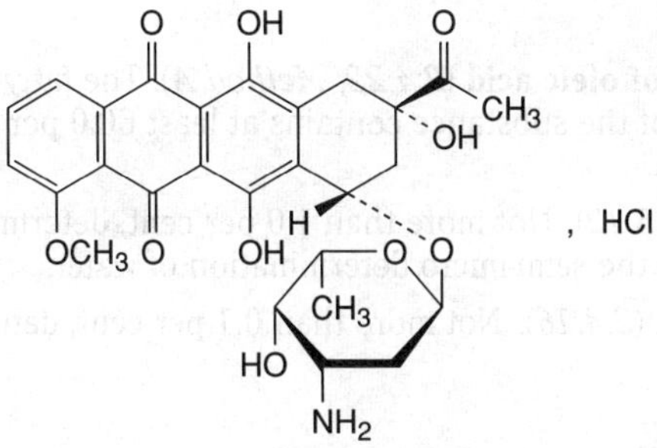

$C_{27}H_{30}ClNO_{10}$ M_r 564.0

DEFINITION

(8*S*,10*S*)-8-Acetyl-10-[(3-amino-2,3,6-trideoxy-α-L-*lyxo*-hexopyranosyl)oxy]-6,8,11-trihydroxy-1-methoxy-7,8,9,10-tetrahydrotetracene-5,12-dione hydrochloride.

Substance produced by certain strains of *Streptomyces coeruleorubidus* or of *Streptomyces peucetius* or obtained by any other means.

Content: 95.0 per cent to 102.0 per cent (anhydrous and solvent-free substance).

PRODUCTION

It is produced by methods of manufacture designed to eliminate or minimise the presence of histamine.

CHARACTERS

Appearance: crystalline, orange-red powder, hygroscopic.

Solubility: freely soluble in water and in methanol, slightly soluble in alcohol, practically insoluble in acetone.

IDENTIFICATION

A. Infrared absorption spectrophotometry (*2.2.24*).
Comparison: *daunorubicin hydrochloride CRS*.

B. Dissolve about 10 mg in 0.5 ml of *nitric acid R*, add 0.5 ml of *water R* and heat over a flame for 2 min. Allow to cool and add 0.5 ml of *silver nitrate solution R1*. A white precipitate is formed.

TESTS

pH (*2.2.3*): 4.5 to 6.5.

Dissolve 50 mg in *carbon dioxide-free water R* and dilute to 10 ml with the same solvent.

Related substances. Liquid chromatography (*2.2.29*). *Prepare the solutions immediately before use.*

Test solution. Dissolve 50.0 mg of the substance to be examined in the mobile phase and dilute to 50.0 ml with the mobile phase.

Reference solution (a). Dissolve 50.0 mg of *daunorubicin hydrochloride CRS* in the mobile phase and dilute to 50.0 ml with the mobile phase.

Reference solution (b). Dissolve 10 mg of *doxorubicin hydrochloride CRS* and 10 mg of *epirubicin hydrochloride CRS* in the mobile phase and dilute to 100.0 ml with the mobile phase. Dilute 1.0 ml of the solution to 10.0 ml with the mobile phase.

Reference solution (c). Dissolve 5.0 mg of *daunorubicinone CRS* and 5.0 mg of *doxorubicin hydrochloride CRS* in the mobile phase and dilute to 100.0 ml with the mobile phase. Dilute 1.0 ml of the solution to 10.0 ml with the mobile phase.

Reference solution (d). Dilute 1.0 ml of reference solution (a) to 200.0 ml with the mobile phase.

Column:

- *size*: *l* = 0.25 m, Ø = 4.0 mm,
- *stationary phase*: *end-capped octadecylsilyl silica gel for chromatography R* (5 µm).

Mobile phase: mixture of equal volumes of *acetonitrile R* and a solution containing 2.88 g/l of *sodium laurilsulfate R* and 2.25 g/l of *phosphoric acid R*.

Flow rate: 1 ml/min.

Detection: spectrophotometer at 254 nm.

Injection: 5 µl; inject the test solution and reference solutions (b), (c) and (d).

Run time: twice the retention time of daunorubicin.

Relative retention with reference to daunorubicin (retention time = about 15 min): impurity A = about 0.4; impurity D = about 0.5; epirubicin = about 0.6; impurity B = about 0.7.

System suitability: reference solution (b):

- *resolution*: minimum of 2.0 between the peaks due to impurity D and epirubicin.

Limits:

- *impurity A*: not more than the area of the corresponding peak in the chromatogram obtained with reference solution (c) (0.5 per cent),
- *impurity B*: not more than 3 times the area of the principal peak in the chromatogram obtained with reference solution (d) (1.5 per cent),
- *impurity D*: not more than the area of the corresponding peak in the chromatogram obtained with reference solution (c) (0.5 per cent),
- *any other impurity*: not more than the area of the principal peak in the chromatogram obtained with reference solution (d) (0.5 per cent),
- *total of other impurities*: not more than 5 times the area of the principal peak in the chromatogram obtained with reference solution (d) (2.5 per cent),
- *disregard limit*: 0.1 times the area of the principal peak in the chromatogram obtained with reference solution (d) (0.05 per cent).

Butanol (*2.4.24, System B*): maximum 1.0 per cent.

Water (*2.5.12*): maximum 3.0 per cent, determined on 0.100 g.

Bacterial endotoxins (*2.6.14*): less than 4.3 IU/mg, if intended for use in the manufacture of parenteral dosage forms without a further appropriate procedure for the removal of bacterial endotoxins.

ASSAY

Liquid chromatography (*2.2.29*) as described in the test for related substances.

Injection: test solution and reference solution (a).

Calculate the percentage content of $C_{27}H_{30}ClNO_{10}$.

STORAGE

In an airtight container, protected from light. If the substance is sterile, store in a sterile, airtight, tamper-proof container.

LABELLING

The label states, where applicable, that the substance is free from bacterial endotoxins.

IMPURITIES

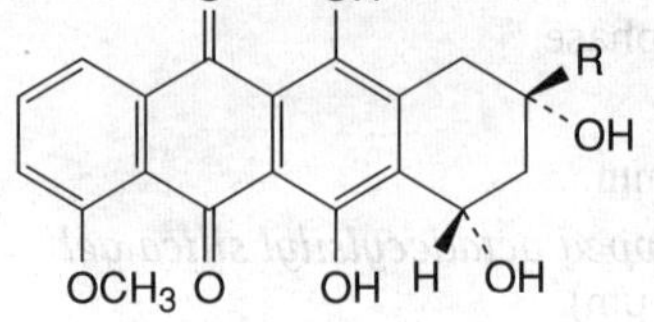

A. R = CO-CH_3: (8*S*,10*S*)-8-acetyl-6,8,10,11-tetrahydroxy-1-methoxy-7,8,9,10-tetrahydrotetracene-5,12-dione (daunorubicin aglycone, daunorubicinone),

E. R = CHOH-CH_3: (8*S*,10*S*)-6,8,10,11-tetrahydroxy-8-[(1*RS*)-1-hydroxyethyl]-1-methoxy-7,8,9,10-tetrahydrotetracene-5,12-dione (13-dihydrodaunorubicinone),

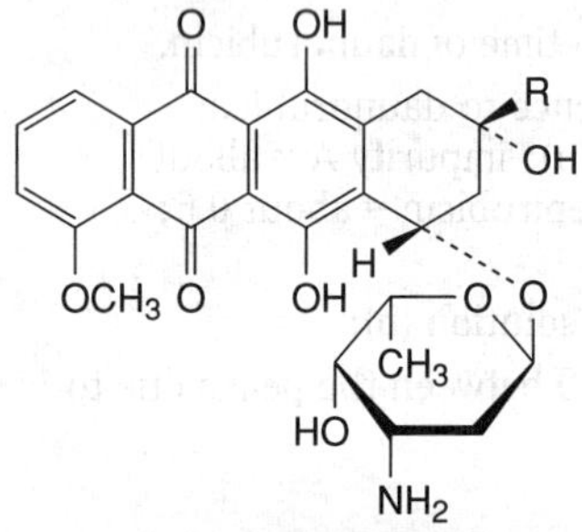

B. R = CHOH-CH_3: (8*S*,10*S*)-10-[(3-amino-2,3,6-trideoxy-α-L-*lyxo*-hexopyranosyl)oxy]-6,8,11-trihydroxy-8-[(1*RS*)-1-hydroxyethyl]-1-methoxy-7,8,9,10-tetrahydrotetracene-5,12-dione (daunorubicinol),

C. R = CH_2-CO-CH_3: (8*S*,10*S*)-10-[(3-amino-2,3,6-trideoxy-α-L-*lyxo*-hexopyranosyl)oxy]-6,8,11-trihydroxy-1-methoxy-8-(2-oxopropyl)-7,8,9,10-tetrahydrotetracene-5,12-dione (feudomycin B),

D. R = CO-CH_2-OH: doxorubicin,

F. R = CO-CH_2-CH_3: (8*S*,10*S*)-10-[(3-amino-2,3,6-trideoxy-α-L-*lyxo*-hexopyranosyl)oxy]-6,8,11-trihydroxy-1-methoxy-8-propanoyl-7,8,9,10-tetrahydrotetracene-5,12-dione (8-ethyldaunorubicin).

01/2005:1307

DECYL OLEATE

Decylis oleas

DEFINITION

Decyl oleate is a mixture consisting of decyl esters of fatty acids, mainly oleic acid. A suitable antioxidant may be added.

CHARACTERS

A clear, pale yellow or colourless liquid, practically insoluble in water, miscible with alcohol, with methylene chloride and with light petroleum (40 °C to 60 °C).

IDENTIFICATION

A. It complies with the test for relative density (see Tests).

B. It complies with the test for saponification value (see Tests).

C. It complies with the test for content of oleic acid (see Tests).

TESTS

Relative density (*2.2.5*): 0.860 to 0.870.

Acid value (*2.5.1*). Not more than 1.0, determined on 10.0 g.

Iodine value (*2.5.4*): 55 to 70.

Peroxide value (*2.5.5*). Not more than 10.0.

Saponification value (*2.5.6*): 130 to 140, determined on 2.0 g.

Content of oleic acid (*2.4.22, Method A*). The fatty acid fraction of the substance contains at least 60.0 per cent of oleic acid.

Water (*2.5.12*). Not more than 1.0 per cent, determined on 1.00 g by the semi-micro determination of water.

Total ash (*2.4.16*). Not more than 0.1 per cent, determined on 2.0 g.

STORAGE

Store protected from light.

LABELLING

The label states, where applicable, the name and concentration of any added antioxidant.

01/2005:0896

DEFEROXAMINE MESILATE

Deferoxamini mesilas

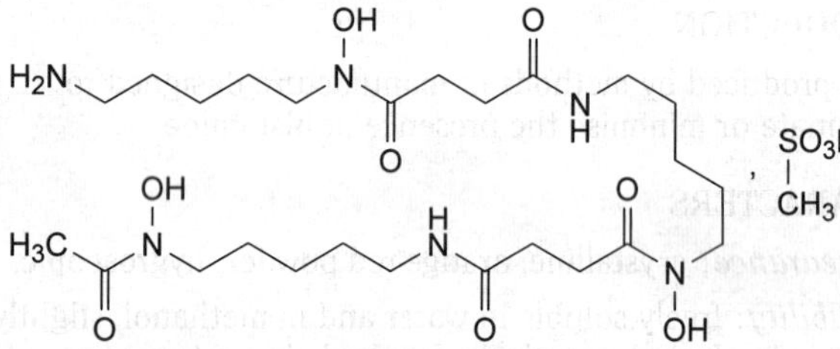

$C_{26}H_{52}N_6O_{11}S$ M_r 657

DEFINITION

Deferoxamine mesilate contains not less than 98.0 per cent and not more than the equivalent of 102.0 per cent expressed as *N'*-[5-[[4-[[5-(acetylhydroxyamino)pentyl]amino]-4-oxobutanoyl]hydroxyamino]pentyl]-*N*-(5-aminopentyl)-*N*-hydroxybutanediamide methanesulfonate, calculated with reference to the anhydrous substance.

PRODUCTION

The production method must be evaluated to determine the potential for formation of alkyl mesilates, which is particularly likely to occur if the reaction medium contains lower alcohols. Where necessary, the production method is validated to demonstrate that alkyl mesilates are not detectable in the final product.

CHARACTERS

A white or almost white powder, freely soluble in water, slightly soluble in methanol, very slightly soluble in alcohol.

IDENTIFICATION

First identification: A, D.

Second identification: B, C, D.

A. Examine by infrared absorption spectrophotometry (*2.2.24*), comparing with the spectrum obtained with *deferoxamine mesilate CRS*. Examine the substances prepared as discs. If the spectra obtained show differences, dissolve the substance to be examined and the reference substance separately in *alcohol R*, evaporate to dryness and record new spectra using the residues.

B. Dissolve about 5 mg in 5 ml of *water R*. Add 2 ml of a 5 g/l solution of *trisodium phosphate dodecahydrate R* and 0.5 ml of a 25 g/l solution of *sodium naphthoquinonesulphonate R*. A brownish-black colour develops.

C. The titrated solution obtained in the Assay (solution (a)) is brownish-red. To 10 ml of solution (a) add 3 ml of *ether R*. Shake. The organic layer is colourless. To 10 ml of solution (a) add 3 ml of *benzyl alcohol R*. Shake. The organic layer is brownish-red.

D. Dissolve 0.1 g in 5 ml of *dilute hydrochloric acid R*. Add 1 ml of *barium chloride solution R2*. The solution is clear. In a porcelain crucible, mix 0.1 g with 1 g of *anhydrous sodium carbonate R*, heat and ignite over a naked flame. Allow to cool. Dissolve the residue in 10 ml of *water R*, heating if necessary, and filter. The filtrate gives reaction (a) of sulphates (*2.3.1*).

TESTS

Solution S. Dissolve 2.5 g in *carbon dioxide-free water R* prepared from *distilled water R* and dilute to 25 ml with the same solvent.

Appearance of solution. Solution S is clear (*2.2.1*) and not more intensely coloured than reference solution Y_5 (*2.2.2, Method II*).

pH (*2.2.3*). The pH of freshly prepared solution S is 3.7 to 5.5.

Related substances. Examine by liquid chromatography (*2.2.29*). *Prepare the solutions immediately before use, protected from light.*

Test solution. Dissolve 50.0 mg of the substance to be examined in the mobile phase and dilute to 50.0 ml with the mobile phase.

Reference solution (a). Dissolve 10.0 mg of *deferoxamine mesilate CRS* in the mobile phase and dilute to 10.0 ml with the mobile phase.

Reference solution (b). Dilute 1.0 ml of the test solution to 25.0 ml with the mobile phase.

The chromatographic procedure may be carried out using:

- a stainless steel column 0.25 m long and 4.6 mm in internal diameter packed with *octadecylsilyl silica gel for chromatography R* (10 µm),
- as mobile phase at a flow rate of 2 ml/min a solution prepared as follows: dissolve 1.32 g of *ammonium phosphate R* and 0.37 g of *sodium edetate R* in 950 ml of *water R*; adjust to pH 2.8 with *phosphoric acid R* (about 3-4 ml) and add 55 ml of *tetrahydrofuran R*,
- as detector a spectrophotometer set at 220 nm.

Inject 20 µl of reference solution (a). If a recorder is used, adjust the sensitivity of the detector so that the height of the peak with a relative retention time of about 0.8 is not less than 15 per cent of the full scale of the recorder. The test is not valid unless the resolution between the peak with the relative retention time of about 0.8 and the principal peak is at least 1.0.

Inject 20 µl of the test solution and 20 µl of reference solution (b). Continue the chromatography for 3 times the retention time of deferoxamine. In the chromatogram obtained with the test solution: the area of any peak, apart from the principal peak, is not greater than the area of the principal peak in the chromatogram obtained with reference solution (b) (4.0 per cent); the sum of the area of any such peaks is not greater than 1.75 times the area of the principal peak in the chromatogram obtained with reference solution (b) (7.0 per cent). Disregard any peak with an area less than 0.02 times that of the principal peak in the chromatogram obtained with reference solution (b).

Chlorides (*2.4.4*). Dilute 2 ml of solution S to 20 ml with *water R*. 15 ml of the solution complies with the limit test for chlorides (330 ppm).

Sulphates (*2.4.13*). Dilute 5 ml of solution S to 20 ml with *distilled water R*. 15 ml of the solution complies with the limit test for sulphates (400 ppm).

Heavy metals (*2.4.8*). 2.0 g complies with limit test C for heavy metals (10 ppm). Prepare the standard using 2 ml of *lead standard solution (10 ppm Pb) R*.

Water (*2.5.12*). Not more than 2.0 per cent, determined on 1.000 g by the semi-micro determination of water.

Sulphated ash (*2.4.14*). Not more than 0.1 per cent, determined on 1.0 g.

Bacterial endotoxins (*2.6.14*): less than 0.025 IU/mg, if intended for use in the manufacture of parenteral dosage forms without a further appropriate procedure for the removal of bacterial endotoxins.

ASSAY

Dissolve 0.500 g in 25 ml of *water R*. Add 4 ml of *0.05 M sulphuric acid*. Titrate with *0.1 M ferric ammonium sulphate*. Towards the end of the titration, titrate uniformly and at a rate of about 0.2 ml/min. Determine the end-point potentiometrically (*2.2.20*) using a platinum indicator electrode and a calomel reference electrode. Retain the titrated solution for identification test C.

1 ml of *0.1 M ferric ammonium sulphate* is equivalent to 65.68 mg of $C_{26}H_{52}N_6O_{11}S$.

STORAGE

Store protected from light, at a temperature of 2 °C to 8 °C. If the substance is sterile, store in a sterile, airtight, tamper-proof container.

LABELLING

The label states, where applicable, that the substance is free from bacterial endotoxins.

IMPURITIES

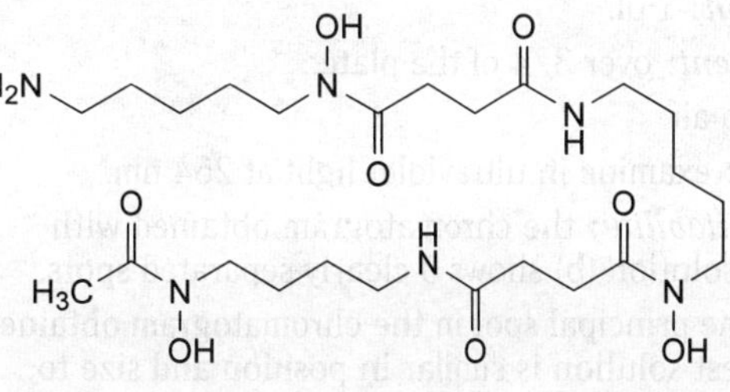

A. *N'*-[5-[[4-[[4-(acetylhydroxyamino)butyl]amino]-4-oxobutanoyl]hydroxyamino]pentyl]-*N*-(5-aminopentyl)-*N*-hydroxybutanediamide(desferrioxamine A_1),

B. other desferrioxamines.

01/2005:0176

DEMECLOCYCLINE HYDROCHLORIDE

Demeclocyclini hydrochloridum

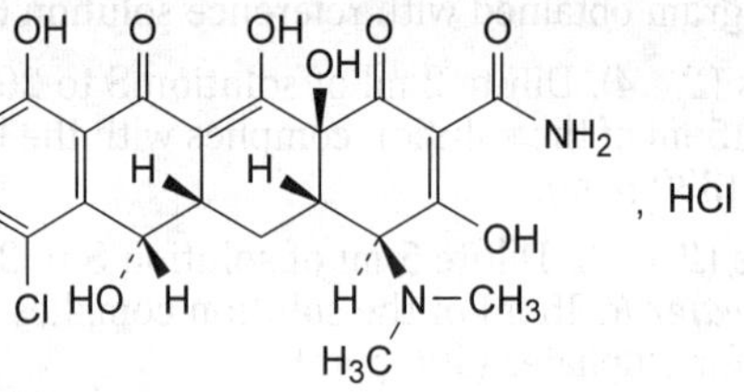

$C_{21}H_{22}Cl_2N_2O_8$ M_r 501.3

DEFINITION

(4*S*,4a*S*,5a*S*,6*S*,12a*S*)-7-Chloro-4-(dimethylamino)-3,6,10,12,12a-pentahydroxy-1,11-dioxo-1,4,4a,5,5a,6,11,12a-octahydrotetracene-2-carboxamide hydrochloride.

Substance produced by certain strains of *Streptomyces aureofaciens* or obtained by any other means.

Content: 89.5 per cent to 102.0 per cent (anhydrous substance).

CHARACTERS

Appearance: yellow powder.

Solubility: soluble or sparingly soluble in water, slightly soluble in alcohol, very slightly soluble in acetone. It dissolves in solutions of alkali hydroxides and carbonates.

IDENTIFICATION

A. Thin-layer chromatography (*2.2.27*).

Test solution. Dissolve 5 mg of the substance to be examined in *methanol R* and dilute to 10 ml with the same solvent.

Reference solution (a). Dissolve 5 mg of *demeclocycline hydrochloride CRS* in *methanol R* and dilute to 10 ml with the same solvent.

Reference solution (b). Dissolve 5 mg of *demeclocycline hydrochloride CRS*, 5 mg of *chlortetracycline hydrochloride R* and 5 mg of *tetracycline hydrochloride R* in *methanol R* and dilute to 10 ml with the same solvent.

Plate: *TLC octadecylsilyl silica gel F_{254} plate R*.

Mobile phase: mix 20 volumes of *acetonitrile R*, 20 volumes of *methanol R* and 60 volumes of a 63 g/l solution of *oxalic acid R* previously adjusted to pH 2 with *concentrated ammonia R*.

Application: 1 µl.

Development: over 3/4 of the plate.

Drying: in air.

Detection: examine in ultraviolet light at 254 nm.

System suitability: the chromatogram obtained with reference solution (b) shows 3 clearly separated spots.

Results: the principal spot in the chromatogram obtained with the test solution is similar in position and size to the principal spot in the chromatogram obtained with reference solution (a).

B. To about 2 mg add 5 ml of *sulphuric acid R*. A violet colour develops. Add the solution to 2.5 ml of *water R*. The colour becomes yellow.

C. It gives reaction (a) of chlorides (*2.3.1*).

TESTS

pH (*2.2.3*): 2.0 to 3.0.

Dissolve 0.1 g in *carbon dioxide-free water R* and dilute to 10 ml with the same solvent.

Specific optical rotation (*2.2.7*): − 248 to − 263 (anhydrous substance).

Dissolve 0.250 g in *0.1 M hydrochloric acid* and dilute to 25.0 ml with the same acid.

Specific absorbance (*2.2.25*): 340 to 370 determined at the maximum at 385 nm (anhydrous substance).

Dissolve 10.0 mg in *0.01 M hydrochloric acid* and dilute to 100.0 ml with the same acid. To 10.0 ml of the solution add 12 ml of *dilute sodium hydroxide solution R* and dilute to 100.0 ml with *water R*.

Related substances. Liquid chromatography (*2.2.29*). *Prepare the solutions immediately before use.*

Test solution. Dissolve 25.0 mg of the substance to be examined in *0.01 M hydrochloric acid* and dilute to 25.0 ml with the same acid.

Reference solution (a). Dissolve 25.0 mg of *demeclocycline hydrochloride CRS* in *0.01 M hydrochloric acid* and dilute to 25.0 ml with the same acid.

Reference solution (b). Dissolve 5.0 mg of *4-epidemeclocycline hydrochloride CRS* in *0.01 M hydrochloric acid* and dilute to 25.0 ml with the same acid.

Reference solution (c). Mix 1.0 ml of reference solution (a) and 5.0 ml of reference solution (b) and dilute to 25.0 ml with *0.01 M hydrochloric acid*.

Reference solution (d). Dilute 5.0 ml of reference solution (a) to 100.0 ml with *0.01 M hydrochloric acid*.

Column:

– *size*: *l* = 0.25 m, Ø = 4.6 mm,
– *stationary phase*: *styrene-divinylbenzene copolymer R* (8 µm),
– *temperature*: 60 °C,

Mobile phase: weigh 80.0 g of *2-methyl-2-propanol R* and transfer to a 1000 ml volumetric flask with the aid of 200 ml of *water R*; add 100 ml of a 35 g/l solution of *dipotassium hydrogen phosphate R* adjusted to pH 9.0 with *dilute phosphoric acid R*, 150 ml of a 10 g/l solution of *tetrabutylammonium hydrogen sulphate R* adjusted to pH 9.0 with *dilute sodium hydroxide solution R* and 10 ml of a 40 g/l solution of *sodium edetate R* adjusted to pH 9.0 with *dilute sodium hydroxide solution R*; dilute to 1000 ml with *water R*.

Flow rate: 1 ml/min.

Detection: spectrophotometer at 254 nm.

Injection: 20 µl; inject the test solution and reference solutions (c) and (d).

System suitability: reference solution (c):

– *resolution*: minimum of 2.8 between the peaks due to impurity B (1st peak) and demeclocycline (2nd peak); if necessary, adjust the 2-methyl-2-propanol content of the mobile phase or lower the pH of the mobile phase,
– *symmetry factor*: maximum 1.25 for the peak due to demeclocycline.

Limits:

– *any impurity*: not more than the area of the principal peak in the chromatogram obtained with reference solution (d) (5.0 per cent), and not more than 1 such peak has an area greater than 0.8 times the area of the principal peak in the chromatogram obtained with reference solution (d) (4.0 per cent),

– *total*: not more than twice the area of the principal peak in the chromatogram obtained with reference solution (d) (10.0 per cent),
– *disregard limit*: 0.02 times the area of the principal peak in the chromatogram obtained with reference solution (d) (0.1 per cent).

Heavy metals (*2.4.8*): maximum 50 ppm.

0.5 g complies with limit test C. Prepare the standard using 2.5 ml of *lead standard solution (10 ppm Pb) R*.

Water (*2.5.12*): maximum 3.0 per cent, determined on 1.000 g.

Sulphated ash (*2.4.14*): maximum 0.5 per cent, determined on 1.0 g.

ASSAY

Liquid chromatography (*2.2.29*) as described in the test for related substances with the following modification.

Injection: test solution and reference solution (a).

Calculate the percentage content of $C_{21}H_{22}Cl_2N_2O_8$.

STORAGE

Protected from light.

IMPURITIES

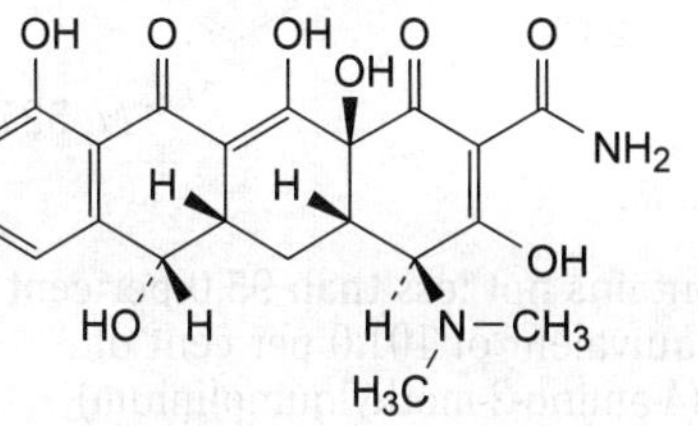

A. (4*S*,4a*S*,5a*S*,6*S*,12a*S*)-4-(dimethylamino)-3,6,10,12,12a-pentahydroxy-1,11-dioxo-1,4,4a,5,5a,6,11,12a-octahydrotetracene-2-carboxamide (demethyltetracycline),

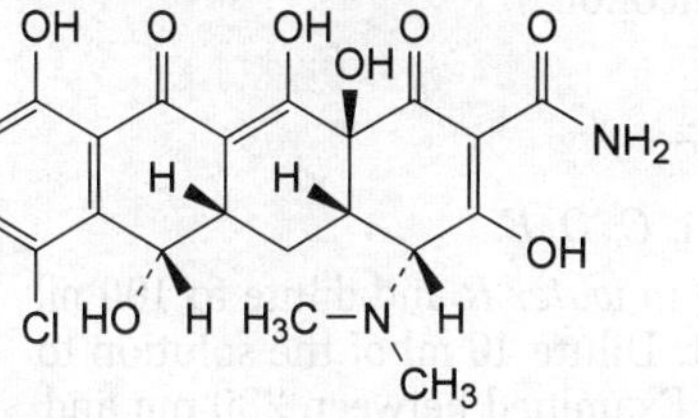

B. (4*R*,4a*S*,5a*S*,6*S*,12a*S*)-7-chloro-4-(dimethylamino)-3,6,10,12,12a-pentahydroxy-1,11-dioxo-1,4,4a,5,5a,6,11,12a-octahydrotetracene-2-carboxamide (4-epidemeclocycline).

01/2005:1308

DEPTROPINE CITRATE

Deptropini citras

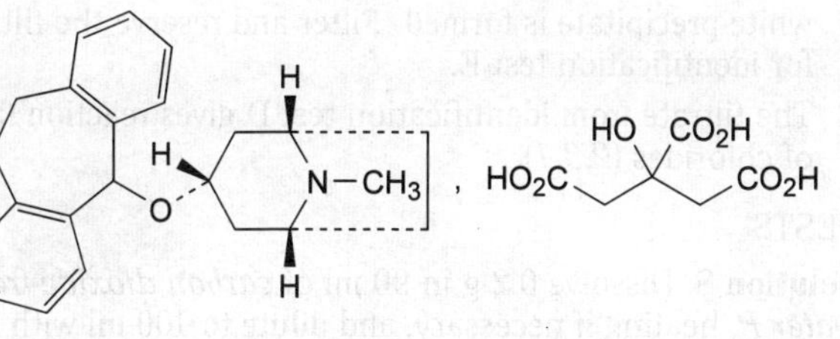

$C_{29}H_{35}NO_8$ M_r 525.6

DEFINITION

Deptropine citrate contains not less than 98.0 per cent and not more than the equivalent of 101.0 per cent of (1*R*,3*r*,5*S*)-3-(10,11-dihydro-5*H*-dibenzo[*a,d*][7]annulen-5-yloxy)-8-methyl-8-azabicyclo[3.2.1]octane dihydrogen citrate, calculated with reference to the dried substance.

CHARACTERS

A white or almost white, microcrystalline powder, very slightly soluble in water and in ethanol, practically insoluble in methylene chloride.

It melts at about 170 °C, with decomposition.

IDENTIFICATION

First identification: A.

Second identification: B, C, D, E.

A. Examine by infrared absorption spectrophotometry (*2.2.24*), comparing with the spectrum obtained with *deptropine citrate CRS*.

B. Examine the chromatograms obtained in the test for related substances. The principal spot in the chromatogram obtained with test solution (b) is similar in position, colour and size to the principal spot in the chromatogram obtained with reference solution (b).

C. To about 1 mg add 0.5 ml of *sulphuric acid R*. A stable red-orange colour develops.

D. Dissolve about 1 mg in 0.25 ml of *perchloric acid R* and warm gently until the solution becomes turbid. Add 5 ml of *glacial acetic acid R*; a pink colour with an intense green fluorescence appears.

E. To about 5 mg add 1 ml of *acetic anhydride R* and 5 ml of *pyridine R*. A purple colour develops.

TESTS

pH (*2.2.3*). Suspend 0.25 g in *carbon dioxide-free water R*, dilute to 25 ml with the same solvent and filter. The pH of the solution is 3.7 to 4.5.

Related substances. Examine by thin-layer chromatography (*2.2.27*), using as the coating substance a suitable silica gel with a fluorescent indicator having an optimal intensity at 254 nm.

Test solution (a). Dissolve 0.10 g of the substance to be examined in *methanol R* and dilute to 10 ml with the same solvent.

Test solution (b). Dilute 1 ml of test solution (a) to 10 ml with *methanol R*.

Reference solution (a). Dilute 1.0 ml of test solution (a) to 100.0 ml with *methanol R*.

Reference solution (b). Dissolve 20 mg of *deptropine citrate CRS* in *methanol R* and dilute to 2 ml with the same solvent. Dilute 1 ml of the solution to 10 ml with *methanol R*.

Reference solution (c). Dissolve 5 mg of *tropine CRS* in *methanol R* and dilute to 100.0 ml with the same solvent.

Reference solution (d). Dissolve 10 mg of *deptropine citrate CRS* and 10 mg of *tropine CRS* in *methanol R* and dilute to 25 ml with the same solvent.

Apply to the plate 40 µl of each solution. Develop over a path of 10 cm using a mixture of 8 volumes of *concentrated ammonia R* and 92 volumes of *butanol R*. Dry the plate at 100 °C to 105 °C until the ammonia has completely evaporated. Examine in ultraviolet light at 254 nm. Any spot in the chromatogram obtained with test solution (a), apart from the principal spot, is not more intense than the spot in the chromatogram obtained with reference solution (a) (1 per cent). Spray with *dilute potassium iodobismuthate solution R* and then with a 10 g/l solution of *sodium nitrite R*. Expose the plate to iodine vapours. Examine in daylight and in ultraviolet light at 254 nm. In the chromatogram obtained with test solution (a): any spot corresponding to tropine is not more intense than the spot in the chromatogram obtained with reference solution (c) (0.5 per cent); any spot, apart from the principal spot and any spot corresponding to tropine, is not more intense than the spot in the chromatogram obtained with reference solution (a) (1 per cent). The test is not valid unless the chromatogram obtained with reference solution (d) shows two clearly separated spots.

Heavy metals (*2.4.8*). 1.0 g complies with limit test C for heavy metals (20 ppm). Prepare the standard using 2 ml of *lead standard solution (10 ppm Pb) R*.

Loss on drying (*2.2.32*). Not more than 2.0 per cent, determined on 1.000 g by drying in an oven at 100-105 °C for 4 h.

Sulphated ash (*2.4.14*). Not more than 0.1 per cent, determined on 1.0 g.

ASSAY

Dissolve 0.400 g in 50 ml of *anhydrous acetic acid R*. Titrate with *0.1 M perchloric acid*, determining the end-point potentiometrically (*2.2.20*).

1 ml of *0.1 M perchloric acid* is equivalent to 52.56 mg of $C_{29}H_{35}NO_8$.

STORAGE

Store protected from light.

IMPURITIES

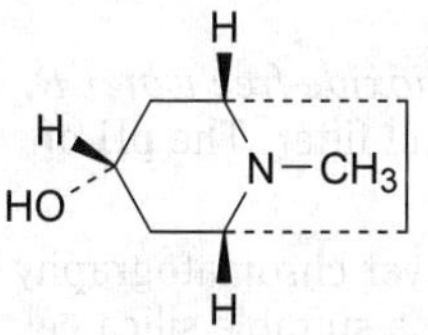

A. (1*R*,3*r*,5*S*)-8-methyl-8-azabicyclo[3.2.1]octan-3-ol (tropine),

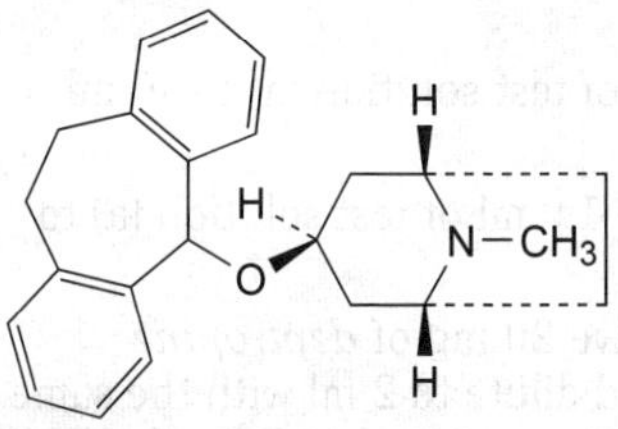

B. (1*R*,3*s*,5*S*)-3-(10,11-dihydro-5*H*-dibenzo[*a*,*d*][7]annulen-5-yloxy)-8-methyl-8-azabicyclo[3.2.1]octane (pseudodeptropine),

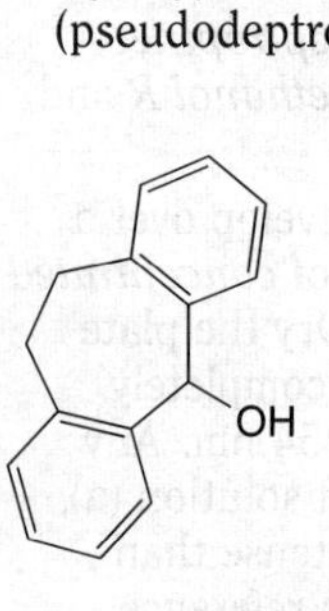

C. 10,11-dihydro-5*H*-dibenzo[*a*,*d*][7]annulen-5-ol (dibenzocycloheptadienol),

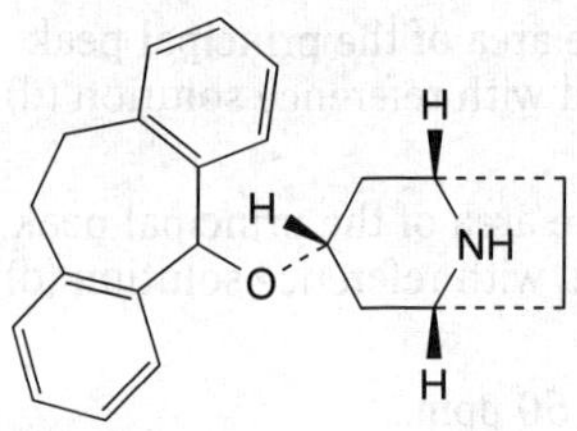

D. (1*R*,3*r*,5*S*)-3-(10,11-dihydro-5*H*-dibenzo[*a*,*d*][7]annulen-5-yloxy)-8-azabicyclo[3.2.1]octane (demethyldeptropine).

01/2005:1413

DEQUALINIUM CHLORIDE

Dequalinii chloridum

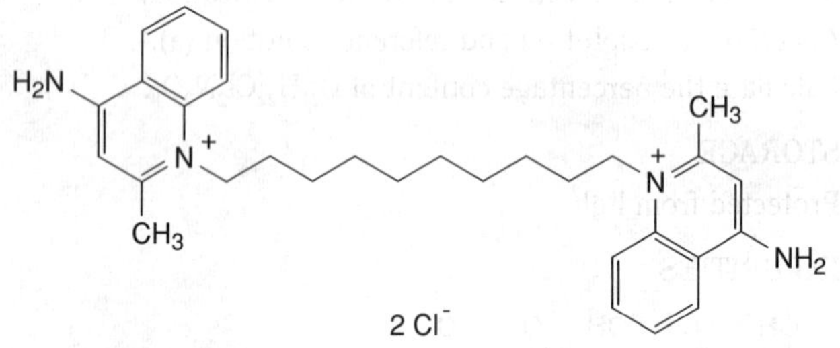

$C_{30}H_{40}Cl_2N_4$ M_r 527.6

DEFINITION

Dequalinium chloride contains not less than 95.0 per cent and not more than the equivalent of 101.0 per cent of 1,1′-(decane-1,10-diyl)bis(4-amino-2-methylquinolinium) dichloride, calculated with reference to the dried substance.

CHARACTERS

A white or yellowish-white powder, hygroscopic, slightly soluble in water and in alcohol.

IDENTIFICATION

First identification: B, E.

Second identification: A, C, D, E.

A. Dissolve about 10 mg in *water R* and dilute to 100 ml with the same solvent. Dilute 10 ml of the solution to 100 ml with *water R*. Examined between 230 nm and 350 nm (*2.2.25*), the solution shows 2 absorption maxima, at 240 nm and 326 nm and a shoulder at 336 nm. The ratio of the absorbance measured at the maximum at 240 nm to that measured at the maximum at 326 nm is 1.56 to 1.80 and the ratio of the absorbance measured at the maximum at 326 nm to that measured at the shoulder at 336 nm is 1.12 to 1.30.

B. Examine by infrared absorption spectrophotometry between 600 cm^{-1} and 2000 cm^{-1} (*2.2.24*), comparing with the spectrum obtained with *dequalinium chloride CRS*.

C. To 5 ml of solution S (see Tests) add 5 ml of *potassium ferricyanide solution R*. A yellow precipitate is formed.

D. To 10 ml of solution S add 1 ml of *dilute nitric acid R*. A white precipitate is formed. Filter and reserve the filtrate for identification test E.

E. The filtrate from identification test D gives reaction (a) of chlorides (*2.3.1*).

TESTS

Solution S. Dissolve 0.2 g in 90 ml of *carbon dioxide-free water R*, heating if necessary, and dilute to 100 ml with the same solvent.

Appearance of solution. Solution S is clear (*2.2.1*) and colourless (*2.2.2, Method II*).

Acidity or alkalinity. To 5 ml of solution S add 0.1 ml of *bromothymol blue solution R1*. Not more than 0.2 ml of *0.01 M hydrochloric acid* or *0.01 M sodium hydroxide* is required to change the colour of the indicator.

Related substances. Examine by liquid chromatography (*2.2.29*).

Test solution. Dissolve 10.0 mg of the substance to be examined in the mobile phase and dilute to 10.0 ml with the mobile phase.

Reference solution (a). Dissolve 10.0 mg of *dequalinium chloride for performance test CRS* in the mobile phase and dilute to 10.0 ml with the mobile phase.

Reference solution (b). Dissolve 10.0 mg of *dequalinium chloride CRS* in the mobile phase and dilute to 10.0 ml with the mobile phase. Dilute 1.0 ml to 50.0 ml with the mobile phase.

The chromatographic procedure may be carried out using:

– a stainless steel column 0.25 m long and 4.6 mm in internal diameter packed with an *end-capped octadecylsilyl silica gel for chromatography R*,
– as mobile phase at a flow rate of 1.5 ml/min the following solution: dissolve 2 g of *sodium hexanesulphonate R* in 300 ml of *water R*. Adjust to pH 4.0 with *acetic acid R* and add 700 ml of *methanol R*,
– as detector a spectrophotometer set at 240 nm.

Adjust the sensitivity of the system so that the height of the peak due to impurity B in the chromatogram obtained with 10 µl of reference solution (a) is at least 25 per cent of the full scale of the recorder. Measure the height (*A*) above the baseline of the peak due to impurity B and the height (*B*) above the baseline at the lowest point of the curve separating this peak from the peak due to dequalinium chloride. The test is not valid unless *A* is greater than twice *B*. If necessary, adjust the concentration of methanol in the mobile phase.

Inject 10 µl of the test solution and 10 µl of reference solution (b). Continue the chromatography of the test solution for 5 times the retention time of the peak due to dequalinium chloride. In the chromatogram obtained with the test solution: the area of any peak due to impurity A is not greater than half the area of the principal peak in the chromatogram obtained with reference solution (b) (1 per cent); and the sum of the areas of all the peaks, apart from the principal peak, is not greater than 5 times the area of the principal peak in the chromatogram obtained with reference solution (b) (10 per cent). Disregard any peak with an area less than 0.025 times the area of the principal peak in the chromatogram obtained with reference solution (b).

Readily carbonisable substances. Dissolve 20 mg in 2 ml of *sulphuric acid R*. After 5 min the solution is not more intensely coloured than reference solution BY_4 (*2.2.2, Method I*).

Loss on drying (*2.2.32*). Not more than 7.0 per cent, determined on 1.000 g by drying at 100-105 °C at a pressure not exceeding 0.7 kPa.

Sulphated ash (*2.4.14*). Not more than 0.1 per cent, determined on 1.0 g.

ASSAY

In order to avoid overheating in the reaction medium, mix thoroughly throughout and stop the titration immediately after the end-point has been reached.

Dissolve 0.200 g in 5 ml of *anhydrous formic acid R* and add 50 ml of *acetic anhydride R*. Titrate with *0.1 M perchloric acid*, determining the end-point potentiometrically (*2.2.20*).

1 ml of *0.1 M perchloric acid* is equivalent to 26.38 mg of $C_{30}H_{40}Cl_2N_4$.

STORAGE

In an airtight container.

IMPURITIES

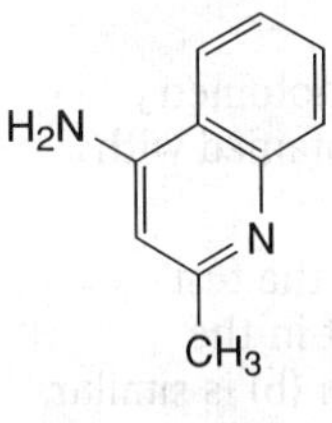

A. 2-methylquinolin-4-amine,

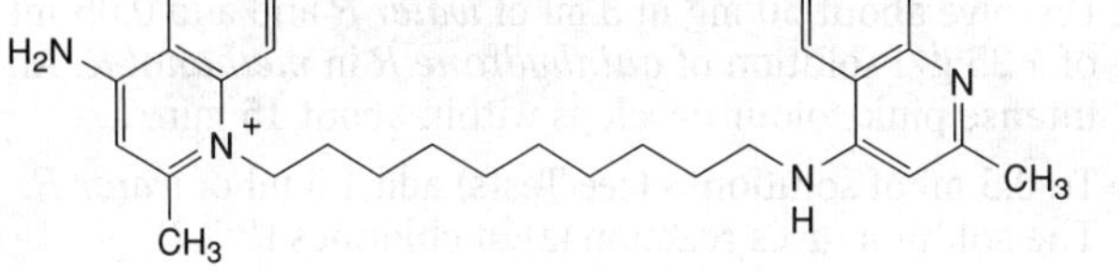

B. 4-amino-1-[10-[(2-methylquinolin-4-yl)amino]decyl]-2-methylquinolinium chloride,

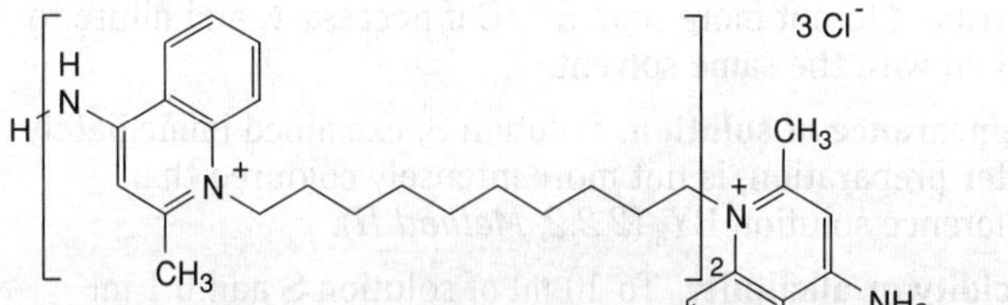

C. 1-[10-(4-amino-2-methylquinolinio)decyl]-4-[[10-(4-amino-2-methylquinolinio)decyl]amino]-2-methylquinolinium trichloride.

01/2005:0481

DESIPRAMINE HYDROCHLORIDE

Desipramini hydrochloridum

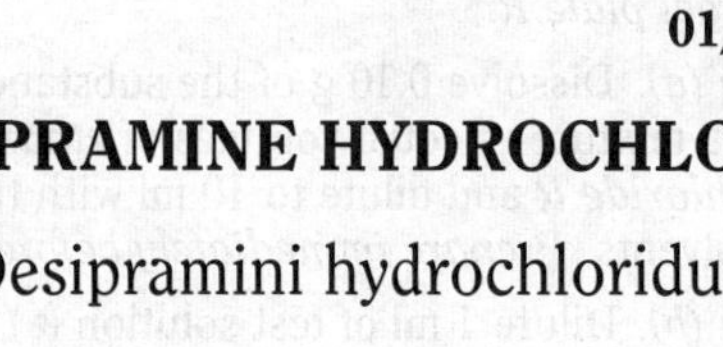

$C_{18}H_{23}ClN_2$ M_r 302.8

DEFINITION

Desipramine hydrochloride contains not less than 99.0 per cent and not more than the equivalent of 101.0 per cent of 3-(10,11-dihydro-5*H*-dibenzo[*b,f*]azepin-5-yl)-*N*-methylpropan-1-amine hydrochloride, calculated with reference to the dried substance.

CHARACTERS

A white or almost white, crystalline powder, soluble in water and in alcohol.

It melts at about 214 °C.

IDENTIFICATION

First identification: B, E.

Second identification: A, C, D, E.

A. Dissolve 40.0 mg in *0.01 M hydrochloric acid* and dilute to 100.0 ml with the same acid. Dilute 5.0 ml of the solution to 100.0 ml with *0.01 M hydrochloric acid.* Examined between 230 nm and 350 nm (*2.2.25*), the solution shows an absorption maximum at 251 nm and a shoulder at 270 nm. The specific absorbance at the maximum is 255 to 285.

B. Examine by infrared absorption spectrophotometry (*2.2.24*), comparing with the spectrum obtained with *desipramine hydrochloride CRS.*

C. Examine the chromatograms obtained in the test for related substances. The principal spot in the chromatogram obtained with test solution (b) is similar in position, colour and size to the principal spot in the chromatogram obtained with reference solution (a).

D. Dissolve about 50 mg in 3 ml of *water R* and add 0.05 ml of a 25 g/l solution of *quinhydrone R* in *methanol R*. An intense pink colour develops within about 15 min.

E. To 0.5 ml of solution S (see Tests) add 1.5 ml of *water R.* The solution gives reaction (a) of chlorides (*2.3.1*).

TESTS

Solution S. Dissolve 1.25 g in *carbon dioxide-free water R,* warming to not more than 30 °C if necessary, and dilute to 25 ml with the same solvent.

Appearance of solution. Solution S, examined immediately after preparation, is not more intensely coloured than reference solution BY_6 (*2.2.2, Method II*).

Acidity or alkalinity. To 10 ml of solution S add 0.1 ml of *methyl red solution R* and 0.3 ml of *0.01 M sodium hydroxide.* The solution is yellow. Not more than 0.5 ml of *0.01 M hydrochloric acid* is required to change the colour of the indicator to red.

Related substances. *Carry out the test protected from bright light.* Examine by thin-layer chromatography (*2.2.27*), using a *TLC silica gel plate R.*

Test solution (a). Dissolve 0.10 g of the substance to be examined in a mixture of equal volumes of *ethanol R* and *methylene chloride R* and dilute to 10 ml with the same mixture of solvents. *Prepare immediately before use.*

Test solution (b). Dilute 1 ml of test solution (a) to 10 ml with a mixture of equal volumes of *ethanol R* and *methylene chloride R.*

Reference solution (a). Dissolve 25 mg of *desipramine hydrochloride CRS* in a mixture of equal volumes of *ethanol R* and *methylene chloride R* and dilute to 25 ml with the same mixture of solvents. *Prepare immediately before use.*

Reference solution (b). Dilute 1 ml of reference solution (a) to 50 ml with a mixture of equal volumes of *ethanol R* and *methylene chloride R.*

Apply to the plate 5 µl of each solution. Develop over a path of 7 cm using a mixture of 1 volume of *water R,* 10 volumes of *anhydrous acetic acid R* and 10 volumes of *toluene R.* Dry the plate in a current of air for 10 min, spray with a 5 g/l solution of *potassium dichromate R* in a mixture of 1 volume of *sulphuric acid R* and 4 volumes of *water R* and examine immediately. Any spot in the chromatogram obtained with test solution (a), apart from the principal spot, is not more intense than the spot in the chromatogram obtained with reference solution (b) (0.2 per cent).

Heavy metals (*2.4.8*). 2.0 g complies with limit test C for heavy metals (20 ppm). Prepare the standard using 4 ml of *lead standard solution (10 ppm Pb) R.*

Loss on drying (*2.2.32*). Not more than 0.5 per cent, determined on 1.000 g by drying in an oven at 100 °C to 105 °C.

Sulphated ash (*2.4.14*). Not more than 0.1 per cent, determined on 1.0 g.

ASSAY

Dissolve 0.2500 g in a mixture of 5 ml of *0.01 M hydrochloric acid* and 50 ml of *alcohol R.* Carry out a potentiometric titration (*2.2.20*), using *0.1 M sodium hydroxide.* Read the volume added between the two points of inflexion.

1 ml of *0.1 M sodium hydroxide* is equivalent to 30.28 mg of $C_{18}H_{23}ClN_2$.

STORAGE

Store protected from light.

01/2005:0482

DESLANOSIDE

Deslanosidum

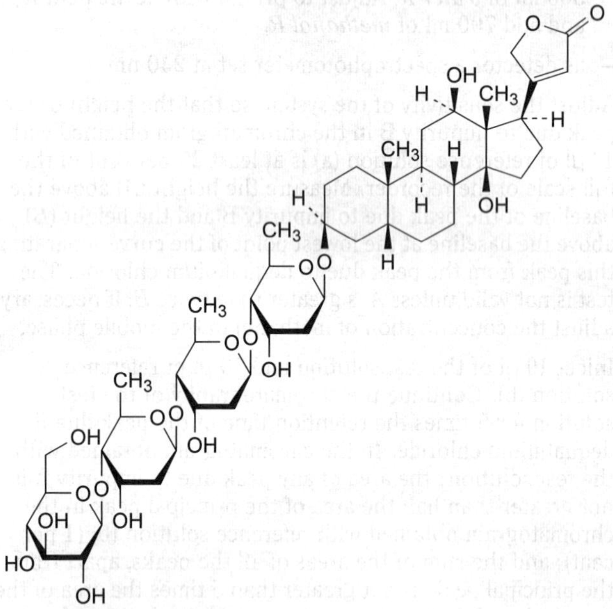

$C_{47}H_{74}O_{19}$ M_r 943

DEFINITION

Deslanoside contains not less than 95.0 per cent and not more than the equivalent of 105.0 per cent of 3β-[(*O*-β-D-glucopyranosyl-(1→4)-*O*-2,6-dideoxy-β-D-*ribo*-hexopyranosyl-(1→4)-*O*-2,6-dideoxy-β-D-*ribo*-hexopyranosyl-(1→4)-2,6-dideoxy-β-D-*ribo*-hexopyranosyl)oxy]-12β,14-dihydroxy-5β,14β-card-20(22)-enolide, calculated with reference to the dried substance.

CHARACTERS

A white, crystalline or finely crystalline powder, hygroscopic, practically insoluble in water, very slightly soluble in alcohol. In an atmosphere of low relative humidity, it loses water.

IDENTIFICATION

First identification: A.

Second identification: B, C, D.

A. Examine by infrared absorption spectrophotometry (*2.2.24*), comparing with the spectrum obtained with *deslanoside CRS*. When comparing the spectra, special attention is given to the absence of a distinct absorption maximum at about 1260 cm^{-1} and to the intensity of the absorption maximum at about 1740 cm^{-1}. Examine the substances in discs prepared by dissolving 1 mg of the substance to be examined or 1 mg of the reference substance in 0.3 ml of *methanol R* and triturating with about 0.4 g of dry, finely powdered *potassium bromide R* until the mixture is uniform and completely dry.

B. Examine the chromatograms obtained in the test for related substances. The principal band in the chromatogram obtained with test solution (b) is similar in position, colour and size to the principal band in the chromatogram obtained with reference solution (a).

C. Suspend about 0.5 mg in 0.2 ml of *alcohol (60 per cent V/V) R*. Add 0.1 ml of *dinitrobenzoic acid solution R* and 0.1 ml of *dilute sodium hydroxide solution R*. A violet colour develops.

D. Dissolve about 5 mg in 5 ml of *glacial acetic acid R* and add 0.05 ml of *ferric chloride solution R1*. Cautiously add 2 ml of *sulphuric acid R*, avoiding mixing the two liquids. Allow to stand; a brown but not reddish ring develops at the interface and a greenish-yellow, then bluish-green colour diffuses from it to the upper layer.

TESTS

Solution S. Dissolve 0.20 g in a mixture of equal volumes of *chloroform R* and *methanol R* and dilute to 10 ml with the same mixture of solvents.

Appearance of solution. Solution S is clear (*2.2.1*) and colourless (*2.2.2, Method II*).

Specific optical rotation (*2.2.7*). Dissolve 0.200 g in *anhydrous pyridine R* and dilute to 10.0 ml with the same solvent. The specific optical rotation is + 6.5 to + 8.5, calculated with reference to the dried substance.

Related substances. Examine by thin-layer chromatography (*2.2.27*), using *silica gel G R* as the coating substance.

Test solution (a). Use solution S.

Test solution (b). Dilute 1 ml of test solution (a) to 10 ml with a mixture of equal volumes of *chloroform R* and *methanol R*.

Reference solution (a). Dissolve 20 mg of *deslanoside CRS* in a mixture of equal volumes of *chloroform R* and *methanol R* and dilute to 10 ml with the same mixture of solvents.

Reference solution (b). Dilute 2.5 ml of reference solution (a) to 10 ml with a mixture of equal volumes of *chloroform R* and *methanol R*.

Reference solution (c). Dilute 1 ml of reference solution (a) to 10 ml with a mixture of equal volumes of *chloroform R* and *methanol R*.

Apply separately to the plate as 10 mm bands 5 µl of each solution. Develop immediately over a path of 15 cm using a mixture of 3 volumes of *water R*, 36 volumes of *methanol R* and 130 volumes of *methylene chloride R*. Dry the plate in a current of warm air, spray with a mixture of 5 volumes of *sulphuric acid R* and 95 volumes of *alcohol R* and heat at 140 °C for 15 min. Examine in daylight. In the chromatogram obtained with test solution (a), any band, apart from the principal band, is not more intense than the band in the chromatogram obtained with reference solution (b) (2.5 per cent) and at most two such bands are more intense than the band in the chromatogram obtained with reference solution (c) (1.0 per cent).

Loss on drying (*2.2.32*). Not more than 5.0 per cent, determined on 0.500 g by drying *in vacuo* at 100 °C to 105 °C.

Sulphated ash (*2.4.14*). Not more than 0.1 per cent, determined on the residue obtained in the test for loss on drying.

ASSAY

Dissolve 50.0 mg in *alcohol R* and dilute to 50.0 ml with the same solvent. Dilute 5.0 ml of this solution to 100.0 ml with *alcohol R*. Prepare a reference solution in the same manner, using 50.0 mg of *deslanoside CRS* (undried). To 5.0 ml of each solution add 3.0 ml of *alkaline sodium picrate solution R* and allow to stand protected from bright light in a water-bath at 20 ± 1 °C for 40 min. Measure the absorbance (*2.2.25*) of each solution at the maximum at 484 nm, using as the compensation liquid a mixture of 3.0 ml of *alkaline sodium picrate solution R* and 5.0 ml of *alcohol R* prepared at the same time.

Calculate the content of $C_{47}H_{74}O_{19}$ from the absorbances measured and the concentrations of the solutions.

STORAGE

Store in an airtight, glass container, protected from light, at a temperature below 10 °C.

01/2005:0712

DESMOPRESSIN

Desmopressinum

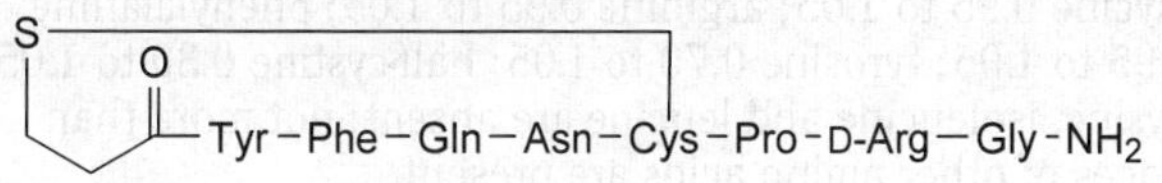

$C_{46}H_{64}N_{14}O_{12}S_2$ M_r 1069

DEFINITION

Desmopressin is a synthetic cyclic nonapeptide having an antidiuretic action. It contains not less than 95.0 per cent and not more than the equivalent of 105.0 per cent of the peptide $C_{46}H_{64}N_{14}O_{12}S_2$, calculated with reference to the anhydrous, acetic acid-free substance. It is available as an acetate.

CHARACTERS

A white, fluffy powder, soluble in water, in alcohol and in glacial acetic acid.

IDENTIFICATION

Examine the chromatograms obtained in the assay. The retention time and size of the principal peak in the chromatogram obtained with the test solution are approximately the same as those of the principal peak in the chromatogram obtained with the reference solution.

TESTS

Specific optical rotation (*2.2.7*). Dissolve 10.0 mg in a 1 per cent *V/V* solution of *glacial acetic acid R* and dilute to 5.0 ml with the same acid. The specific optical rotation is − 72 to − 82, calculated with reference to the anhydrous, acetic acid-free substance.

Amino acids. Examine by means of an amino-acid analyser. Standardise the apparatus with a mixture containing equimolar amounts of ammonia, glycine and the L-form of the following amino acids:

lysine	threonine	alanine	leucine
histidine	serine	valine	tyrosine
arginine	glutamic acid	methionine	phenylalanine
aspartic acid	proline	isoleucine	

together with half the equimolar amount of L-cystine. For the validation of the method, an appropriate internal standard, such as *DL-norleucine R*, is used.

Test solution. Place 1.0 mg of the substance to be examined in a rigorously cleaned hard-glass tube 100 mm long and 6 mm in internal diameter. Add a suitable amount of a 50 per cent *V/V* solution of *hydrochloric acid R*. Immerse the tube in a freezing mixture at −5 °C, reduce the pressure to below 133 Pa and seal. Heat at 110 °C to 115 °C for 16 h. Cool, open the tube, transfer the contents to a 10 ml flask with the aid of five quantities, each of 0.2 ml, of *water R* and evaporate to dryness over *potassium hydroxide R* under reduced pressure. Take up the residue in *water R* and evaporate to dryness over *potassium hydroxide R* under reduced pressure; repeat these operations once. Take up the residue in a buffer solution suitable for the amino-acid analyser used and dilute to a suitable volume with the same buffer solution. Apply a suitable volume to the amino-acid analyser.

Express the content of each amino acid in moles. Calculate the relative proportions of the amino acids, taking one-sixth of the sum of the number of moles of aspartic acid, glutamic acid, proline, glycine, arginine and phenylalanine as equal to one. The values fall within the following limits: aspartic acid 0.95 to 1.05; glutamic acid 0.95 to 1.05; proline 0.95 to 1.05; glycine 0.95 to 1.05; arginine 0.95 to 1.05; phenylalanine 0.95 to 1.05; tyrosine 0.70 to 1.05; half-cystine 0.30 to 1.05. Lysine, isoleucine and leucine are absent; not more than traces of other amino acids are present.

Related peptides. Examine by liquid chromatography (*2.2.29*) as described under Assay, following the elution conditions shown in the table below, at a flow rate of 1.5 ml/min:

Time (min)	Mobile phase A (per cent *V/V*)	Mobile phase B (per cent *V/V*)	Comment
0 - 4	76	24	isocratic
4 - 18	76 → 58	24 → 42	linear gradient
18 - 35	58 → 48	42 → 52	linear gradient
35 - 40	48 → 76	52 → 24	switch to initial eluent composition
40 - 50	76	24	re-equilibration

Inject 50 µl of the resolution solution and identify the peaks due to desmopressin and oxytocin (first and second peaks, respectively). If necessary, adjust the concentration of acetonitrile in the mobile phase to obtain a retention time of about 16 min for the desmopressin peak. The test is not valid unless the resolution between the peaks corresponding to desmopressin and oxytocin is at least 1.5.

Inject 50 µl of the test solution. In the chromatogram obtained the area of any peak, apart from the principal peak, is not greater than 0.5 per cent of the total area of the peaks; the sum of the areas of all the peaks, apart from the principal peak, is not greater than 1.5 per cent of the total area of the peaks. Disregard any peak due to the solvent and any peak with an area less than 0.05 per cent of that of the principal peak.

Acetic acid (*2.5.34*): 3.0 per cent to 8.0 per cent.

Test solution. Dissolve 20.0 mg of the substance to be examined in a mixture of 5 volumes of mobile phase B and 95 volumes of mobile phase A and dilute to 10.0 ml with the same mixture of solvents.

Water (*2.5.32*). Not more than 6.0 per cent, determined by the micro determination of water.

Bacterial endotoxins (*2.6.14*): less than 500 IU/mg, if intended for use in the manufacture of parenteral dosage forms without a further appropriate procedure for the removal of bacterial endotoxins.

ASSAY

Examine by liquid chromatography (*2.2.29*).

Test solution. Dissolve 1.0 mg of the substance to be examined in 2.0 ml of *water R*.

Reference solution. Dissolve the contents of a vial of *desmopressin CRS* in *water R* to obtain a concentration of 0.5 mg/ml.

Resolution solution. Dissolve the contents of a vial of *oxytocin/desmopressin validation mixture CRS* in 500 µl of *water R*.

The chromatographic procedure may be carried out using:

– a stainless steel column 0.12 m long and 4.0 mm in internal diameter packed with *octadecylsilyl silica gel for chromatography R* (5 µm),

– as mobile phase at a flow rate of 2.0 ml/min a mixture of 60 volumes of mobile phase A and 40 volumes of mobile phase B:

Mobile phase A. 0.067 M phosphate buffer solution pH 7.0 R; filter and degas,

Mobile phase B. Mix equal volumes of mobile phase A and of *acetonitrile for chromatography R*; filter and degas,

– as detector a spectrophotometer set at 220 nm.

Inject 50 µl of the resolution solution and identify the peaks due to desmopressin and oxytocin (first and second peaks, respectively). If necessary, adjust the concentration of acetonitrile in the mobile phase to obtain a retention time of about 5 min for the desmopressin peak. The test is not valid unless the resolution between the peaks corresponding to desmopression and oxytocin is at least 1.5.

Inject 50 µl of the test solution and 50 µl of the reference solution.

Calculate the content of desmopressin ($C_{46}H_{64}N_{14}O_{12}S_2$) from the peak areas in the chromatograms obtained with the test solution and the reference solution and the declared content of $C_{46}H_{64}N_{14}O_{12}S_2$ in *desmopressin CRS*.

STORAGE

Store in an airtight container, protected from light, at a temperature of 2 °C to 8 °C. If the substance is sterile, store in a sterile, airtight, tamper-proof container.

LABELLING

The label states:

– the mass of peptide per container,

– where applicable, that the substance is free from bacterial endotoxins.

01/2005:0322

DESOXYCORTONE ACETATE

Desoxycortoni acetas

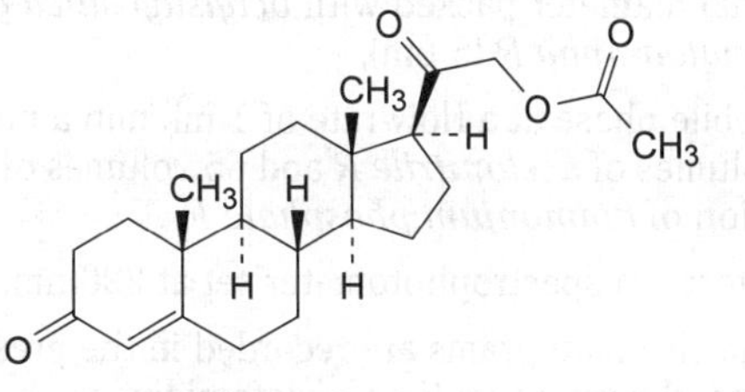

$C_{23}H_{32}O_4$ M_r 372.5

DEFINITION

Desoxycortone acetate contains not less than 97.0 per cent and not more than the equivalent of 103.0 per cent of 3,20-dioxopregn-4-en-21-yl acetate, calculated with reference to the dried substance.

CHARACTERS

A white or almost white, crystalline powder or colourless crystals, practically insoluble in water, freely soluble in methylene chloride, soluble in acetone, sparingly soluble in alcohol, slightly soluble in propylene glycol and in fatty oils.

IDENTIFICATION

First identification: B, C.

Second identification: A, C, D, E.

A. Melting point (*2.2.14*): 157 °C to 161 °C.

B. Examine by infrared absorption spectrophotometry (*2.2.24*), comparing with the spectrum obtained with *desoxycortone acetate CRS*.

C. Examine by thin-layer chromatography (*2.2.27*), using as the coating substance a suitable silica gel with a fluorescent indicator having an optimal intensity at 254 nm.

Test solution. Dissolve 10 mg of the substance to be examined in a mixture of 1 volume of *methanol R* and 9 volumes of *methylene chloride R* and dilute to 10 ml with the same mixture of solvents.

Reference solution (a). Dissolve 20 mg of *desoxycortone acetate CRS* in a mixture of 1 volume of *methanol R* and 9 volumes of *methylene chloride R* and dilute to 20 ml with the same mixture of solvents.

Reference solution (b). Dissolve 10 mg of *cortisone acetate R* in reference solution (a) and dilute to 10 ml with reference solution (a).

Apply separately to the plate 5 µl of each solution. Prepare the mobile phase by adding a mixture of 1.2 volumes of *water R* and 8 volumes of *methanol R* to a mixture of 15 volumes of *ether R* and 77 volumes of *methylene chloride R*. Develop over a path of 15 cm. Allow the plate to dry in air and examine in ultraviolet light at 254 nm. The principal spot in the chromatogram obtained with the test solution is similar in position and size to the principal spot in the chromatogram obtained with reference solution (a). Spray with *alcoholic solution of sulphuric acid R*. Heat at 120 °C for 10 min or until the spots appear. Allow to cool. Examine the plate in daylight and in ultraviolet light at 365 nm. The principal spot in the chromatogram obtained with the test solution is similar in position, colour in daylight, fluorescence in ultraviolet light at 365 nm and size to the principal spot in the chromatogram obtained with reference solution (a). The test is not valid unless the chromatogram obtained with reference solution (b) shows two clearly separated spots.

D. Add about 2 mg to 2 ml of *sulphuric acid R* and shake to dissolve. Within 5 min, a yellow colour develops. Add the solution to 2 ml of *water R* and shake. The resulting solution is dichroic showing an intense blue colour by transparency, and red fluorescence which is particularly intense in ultraviolet light at 365 nm.

E. About 10 mg gives the reaction of acetyl (*2.3.1*).

TESTS

Specific optical rotation (*2.2.7*). Dissolve 0.250 g in *dioxan R* and dilute to 25.0 ml with the same solvent. The specific optical rotation is + 171 to + 179, calculated with reference to the dried substance.

Related substances. Examine by liquid chromatography (*2.2.29*).

Test solution. Dissolve 25.0 mg of the substance to be examined in the mobile phase and dilute to 10.0 ml with the mobile phase.

Reference solution (a). Dissolve 2 mg of *desoxycortone acetate CRS* and 2 mg of *betamethasone 17-valerate CRS* in the mobile phase and dilute to 200.0 ml with the mobile phase.

Reference solution (b). Dilute 1.0 ml of the test solution to 200.0 ml with the mobile phase.

The chromatographic procedure may be carried out using:

– a stainless steel column 0.25 m long and 4.6 mm in internal diameter packed with *octadecylsilyl silica gel for chromatography R* (5 µm),

– as mobile phase at a flow rate of 1 ml/min a mixture prepared as follows: in a 1000 ml volumetric flask mix 350 ml of *water R* with 600 ml of *acetonitrile R* and allow to equilibrate; adjust the volume to 1000 ml with *water R* and mix again,

– as detector a spectrophotometer set at 254 nm.

Equilibrate the column with the mobile phase at a flow rate of 1 ml/min for about 30 min.

Adjust the sensitivity of the system so that the height of the principal peak in the chromatogram obtained with 20 µl of reference solution (b) is not less than 50 per cent of the full scale of the recorder.

Inject 20 µl of reference solution (a). When the chromatograms are recorded in the prescribed conditions, the retention times are: betamethasone 17-valerate, about 7.5 min and desoxycortone acetate, about 9.5 min. The test is not valid unless the resolution between the peaks due to betamethasone 17-valerate and desoxycortone acetate is at least 4.5; if necessary, adjust the concentration of acetonitrile in the mobile phase.

Inject separately 20 µl of the test solution and 20 µl of reference solution (b). Continue the chromatography for three times the retention time of the principal peak. In the chromatogram obtained with the test solution, the sum of the areas of all the peaks, apart from the principal peak, is not greater than the area of the principal peak in the chromatogram obtained with reference solution (b) (0.5 per cent). Disregard any peak with an area less than 0.1 times the area of the principal peak in the chromatogram obtained with reference solution (b).

Loss on drying (*2.2.32*). Not more than 0.5 per cent, determined on 0.500 g by drying in an oven at 100 °C to 105 °C.

ASSAY

Dissolve 0.100 g in *alcohol R* and dilute to 100.0 ml with the same solvent. Dilute 2.0 ml to 100.0 ml with *alcohol R*. Measure the absorbance (*2.2.25*) at the maximum at 240 nm.

Calculate the content of $C_{23}H_{32}O_4$ taking the specific absorbance to be 450.

STORAGE

Store protected from light.

Monographs D-E

01/2005:1414 corrected

DETOMIDINE HYDROCHLORIDE FOR VETERINARY USE

Detomidini hydrochloridum ad usum veterinarium

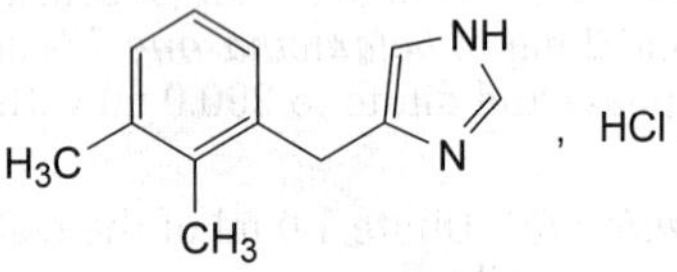

$C_{12}H_{15}ClN_2$ M_r 222.7

DEFINITION

Detomidine hydrochloride for veterinary use contains not less than 98.5 per cent and not more than the equivalent of 101.5 per cent of 4-(2,3-dimethylbenzyl)-1*H*-imidazole hydrochloride, calculated with reference to the dried substance.

CHARACTERS

A white or almost white, hygroscopic, crystalline powder, soluble in water, freely soluble in alcohol, very slightly soluble in methylene chloride, practically insoluble in acetone.

It melts at about 160 °C.

IDENTIFICATION

A. Examine by infrared absorption spectrophotometry (*2.2.24*), comparing with the spectrum obtained with *detomidine hydrochloride CRS*. Examine the substances prepared as discs. If the spectra obtained show differences, dry the substance to be examined and the reference substance in an oven at 100 °C to 105 °C and record new spectra.

B. It gives reaction (a) of chlorides (*2.3.1*).

TESTS

Appearance of solution. Dissolve 0.25 g in *water R* and dilute to 25 ml with the same solvent. The solution is clear (*2.2.1*) and colourless (*2.2.2, Method II*).

Related substances. Examine by liquid chromatography (*2.2.29*).

Test solution. Dissolve 25.0 mg of the substance to be examined in 20 ml of the mobile phase and dilute to 50.0 ml with the mobile phase.

Reference solution (a). Dilute 0.20 ml of the test solution to 100.0 ml with the mobile phase.

Reference solution (b). Dissolve 1 mg of *detomidine impurity B CRS* in the mobile phase and dilute to 100 ml with the mobile phase. Dilute 1 ml of the solution to 10 ml with reference solution (a).

The chromatographic procedure may be carried out using:

- a stainless steel column 0.15 m long and 4.6 mm in internal diameter packed with *octylsilyl silica gel for chromatography R* (5 µm),
- as mobile phase at a flow rate of 1 ml/min a mixture of 35 volumes of *acetonitrile R* and 65 volumes of a 2.64 g/l solution of *ammonium phosphate R*,
- as detector a spectrophotometer set at 220 nm.

When the chromatograms are recorded in the prescribed conditions, the retention time of detomidine is about 7 min and the relative retention times of impurities A, B and C with respect to detomidine are about 0.4, 2.0 and 3.0, respectively. Inject 20 µl of reference solution (a). Adjust the sensitivity of the system so that the height of the principal peak in the chromatogram obtained is at least 50 per cent of the full scale of the recorder. Inject 20 µl of reference solution (b). The test is not valid unless: the resolution between the peaks corresponding to detomidine and to impurity B is at least 5.

Inject 20 µl of the test solution. Continue the chromatography for four times the retention time of the principal peak. Multiply the area of any peak (corresponding to the impurity C and its diastereoisomer) eluting with a relative retention time of about 3, by the correction factor 2.7. The sum of the areas of such peaks is not greater than 2.5 times the area of the principal peak in the chromatogram obtained with reference solution (a) (0.5 per cent); the area of any other peak apart from the principal peak and the peak corresponding to the impurity C is not greater than the area of the principal peak in the chromatogram obtained with reference solution (a) (0.2 per cent); the sum of the areas of all the peaks apart from the principal peak is not greater than five times the area of the principal peak in the chromatogram obtained with reference solution (a) (1 per cent). Disregard any peak with an area less than 0.25 times the area of the principal peak in the chromatogram obtained with reference solution (a).

Loss on drying (*2.2.32*). Not more than 0.5 per cent, determined on 1.000 g by drying in oven at 100 °C to 105 °C.

Sulphated ash (*2.4.14*). Not more than 0.1 per cent, determined on 1.0 g.

ASSAY

Dissolve 0.170 g in 50 ml of *alcohol R*. Add 5.0 ml of *0.01 M hydrochloric acid.* Carry out a potentiometric titration (*2.2.20*), using *0.1 M sodium hydroxide.* Read the volume added between the two points of inflection.

1 ml of *0.1 M sodium hydroxide* corresponds to 22.27 mg of $C_{12}H_{15}ClN_2$.

STORAGE

Store in an airtight container.

IMPURITIES

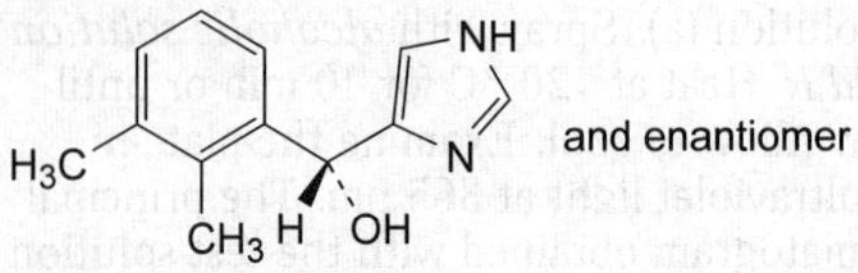

A. (*RS*)-(2,3-dimethylphenyl)(1*H*-imidazol-4-yl)methanol,

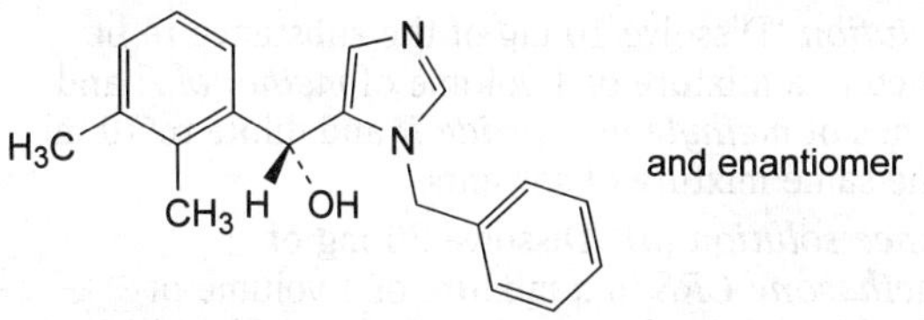

B. (*RS*)-(1-benzyl-1*H*-imidazol-5-yl)(2,3-dimethylphenyl)methanol,

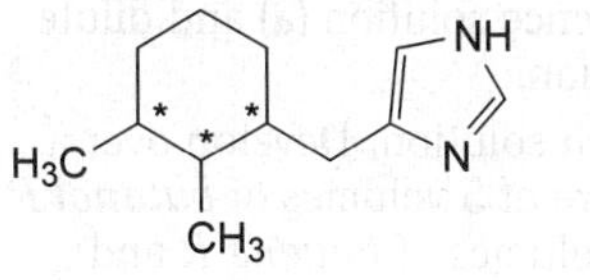

C. 4-[(2,3-dimethylcyclohexyl)methyl]-1*H*-imidazole.

01/2005:1095

DEVIL'S CLAW ROOT

Harpagophyti radix

DEFINITION

Devil's claw root consists of the cut and dried tuberous, secondary roots of *Harpagophytum procumbens* D.C. and/or *H. zeyheri* L. Decne. It contains not less than 1.2 per cent of harpagoside ($C_{24}H_{30}O_{11}$; M_r 494.5), calculated with reference to the dried drug.

CHARACTERS

Devil's claw root is greyish-brown to dark brown and it has a bitter taste.

It has the macroscopic and microscopic characters described in identification tests A and B.

IDENTIFICATION

A. It consists of thick, fan-shaped or rounded slices or of roughly crushed discs. The darker outer surface is traversed by tortuous longitudinal wrinkles. The paler cut surface shows a dark cambial zone and xylem bundles distinctly aligned in radial rows. The central cylinder shows fine concentric striations. Seen under a lens, the cut surface presents yellow to brownish-red granules.

B. Reduce to a powder (355). The powder is brownish-yellow. Examine under a microscope using *chloral hydrate solution R*. The powder shows the following diagnostic characters: fragments of cork layer consisting of yellowish-brown, thin-walled cells; fragments of cortical parenchyma consisting of large, thin-walled cells, sometimes containing reddish-brown granular inclusions and isolated yellow droplets; fragments of reticulately thickened vessels and tracheidal vessels with associated lignified parenchyma from the central cylinder; small needles and crystals of calcium oxalate are present in the parenchyma. The powder may show rectangular or polygonal pitted sclereids with dark reddish-brown contents. With a solution of phloroglucinol in hydrochloric acid, the parenchyma turns green.

C. Examine by thin-layer chromatography (*2.2.27*), using a suitable silica gel as the coating substance.

Test solution. Heat on a water-bath at 60 °C for 10 min 1.0 g of the powdered drug (355) with 10 ml of *methanol R*. Filter and reduce the filtrate to about 2 ml under reduced pressure at a temperature not exceeding 40 °C.

Reference solution. Dissolve 1 mg of *harpagoside R* in 1 ml of *methanol R*.

Apply to the plate as bands 20 µl of each solution. Develop over a path of 10 cm using a mixture of 8 volumes of *water R*, 15 volumes of *methanol R* and 77 volumes of *ethyl acetate R*. Dry the plate in a current of warm air. Examine in ultraviolet light at 254 nm. The chromatograms obtained with the test solution and the reference solution both show in the middle a quenching zone corresponding to harpagoside. The chromatogram obtained with the test solution shows other distinct bands, mainly above the zone corresponding to harpagoside. Spray with a 10 g/l solution of *phloroglucinol R* in *alcohol R* and then with *hydrochloric acid R*. Dry the plate at 80 °C for 5-10 min. In the chromatograms obtained with the reference solution and the test solution the zone corresponding to harpagoside is green. The chromatogram obtained with the test solution also shows several yellow to brown zones below and above the zone corresponding to harpagoside.

TESTS

Starch. Examine the powdered drug (355) under a microscope using *water R*. Add *iodine solution R1*. No blue colour develops.

Foreign matter (*2.8.2*). It complies with the test for foreign matter.

Loss on drying (*2.2.32*). Not more than 12.0 per cent, determined on 1.000 g of the powdered drug (355) by drying in an oven at 100-105 °C.

Total ash (*2.4.16*). Not more than 10.0 per cent.

ASSAY

Examine by liquid chromatography (*2.2.29*) using *methyl cinnamate R* as the internal standard.

Internal standard solution. Dissolve 0.130 g of *methyl cinnamate R* in 50 ml of *methanol R* and dilute to 100.0 ml with the same solvent.

Test solution. To 0.500 g of the powdered drug (355) add 50 ml of *methanol R*. Shake for 1 h and filter. Transfer the filter with the residue to a 100 ml flask, add 50 ml of *methanol R* and heat under a reflux condenser for 1 h. Cool and filter. Rinse the flask and the filter with 2 quantities, each of 5 ml, of *methanol R*. Combine the filtrate and the rinsing solution and evaporate to dryness under reduced pressure at a temperature not exceeding 40 °C. Take up the residue with 3 quantities, each of 5 ml, of *methanol R* and filter the extracts into a 25 ml volumetric flask. Whilst washing the filter, dilute to 25.0 ml with *methanol R*. To 10.0 ml of this solution add 1.0 ml of the internal standard solution and dilute to 25.0 ml with *methanol R*.

Reference solution. Dilute 0.5 ml of the reference solution described in Identification test C to 2.0 ml with *methanol R*.

The chromatographic procedure may be carried out using:

- a stainless steel column 0.10 m long and 4 mm in internal diameter packed with *octadecylsilyl silica gel for chromatography R* (5 µm),
- as mobile phase at a flow rate of 1.5 ml/min a mixture of equal volumes of *methanol R* and *water R*,
- as detector a spectrophotometer set at 278 nm,
- a 10 µl loop injector.

Inject the test solution. Adjust the sensitivity of the detector so that the height of the peak due to methyl cinnamate is about 50 per cent of the full scale of the recorder.

Determine the retention time of harpagoside using 10 µl of the reference solution examined under the same conditions as the test solution.

Calculate the percentage content of harpagoside from the expression:

$$\frac{m_2 \times F_1 \times 7.622}{F_2 \times m_1}$$

m_1 = mass of the drug, in grams,

m_2 = mass of *methyl cinnamate R*, in grams in the internal standard solution,

F_1 = area of the peak corresponding to harpagoside in the chromatogram obtained with the test solution,

F_2 = area of the peak corresponding to methyl cinnamate in the chromatogram obtained with the test solution.

STORAGE

Store protected from light.

01/2005:0388

DEXAMETHASONE

Dexamethasonum

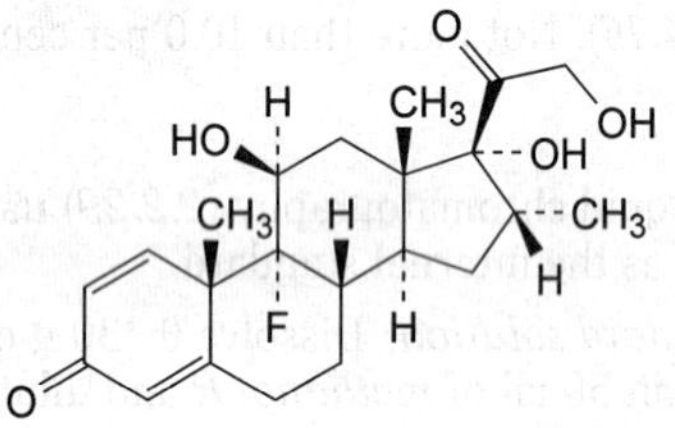

$C_{22}H_{29}FO_5$ M_r 392.5

DEFINITION

Dexamethasone contains not less than 97.0 per cent and not more than the equivalent of 103.0 per cent of 9-fluoro-11β,17,21-trihydroxy-16α-methylpregna-1,4-diene-3,20-dione, calculated with reference to the dried substance.

CHARACTERS

A white or almost white, crystalline powder, practically insoluble in water, sparingly soluble in ethanol, slightly soluble in methylene chloride.

IDENTIFICATION

First identification: B, C.

Second identification: A, C, D, E.

A. Dissolve 10.0 mg in *ethanol R* and dilute to 100.0 ml with the same solvent. Place 2.0 ml of the solution in a stoppered test tube, add 10.0 ml of *phenylhydrazine-sulphuric acid solution R*, mix and heat in a water-bath at 60 °C for 20 min. Cool immediately. The absorbance (*2.2.25*) of the solution at the maximum at 419 nm is not less than 0.4.

B. Examine by infrared absorption spectrophotometry (*2.2.24*), comparing with the spectrum obtained with *dexamethasone CRS*.

C. Examine by thin-layer chromatography (*2.2.27*), using as the coating substance a suitable silica gel with a fluorescent indicator having an optimal intensity at 254 nm.

Test solution. Dissolve 10 mg of the substance to be examined in a mixture of 1 volume of *methanol R* and 9 volumes of *methylene chloride R* and dilute to 10 ml with the same mixture of solvents.

Reference solution (a). Dissolve 20 mg of *dexamethasone CRS* in a mixture of 1 volume of *methanol R* and 9 volumes of *methylene chloride R* and dilute to 20 ml with the same mixture of solvents.

Reference solution (b). Dissolve 10 mg of *betamethasone CRS* in reference solution (a) and dilute to 10 ml with the same solution.

Apply to the plate 5 µl of each solution. Develop over a path of 15 cm, using a mixture of 5 volumes of *butanol R* saturated with *water R*, 10 volumes of *toluene R* and 85 volumes of *ether R*. Allow the plate to dry in air and examine in ultraviolet light at 254 nm. The principal spot in the chromatogram obtained with the test solution is similar in position and size to the principal spot in the chromatogram obtained with reference solution (a). Spray with *alcoholic solution of sulphuric acid R*. Heat at 120 °C for 10 min or until the spots appear. Allow to cool. Examine the chromatograms in daylight and in ultraviolet light at 365 nm. The principal spot in the chromatogram obtained with the test solution is similar in position, colour in daylight, fluorescence in ultraviolet light at 365 nm and size to the principal spot in the chromatogram obtained with reference solution (a). The test is not valid unless the chromatogram obtained with reference solution (b) shows 2 spots which may, however, not be completely separated.

D. Add about 2 mg to 2 ml of *sulphuric acid R* and shake to dissolve. Within 5 min, a faint reddish-brown colour develops. Add the solution to 10 ml of *water R* and mix. The colour is discharged.

E. Mix about 5 mg with 45 mg of *heavy magnesium oxide R* and ignite in a crucible until an almost white residue is obtained (usually less than 5 min). Allow to cool, add 1 ml of *water R*, 0.05 ml of *phenolphthalein solution R1* and about 1 ml of *dilute hydrochloric acid R* to render the solution colourless. Filter. To a freshly prepared mixture of 0.1 ml of *alizarin S solution R* and 0.1 ml of *zirconyl nitrate solution R*, add 1.0 ml of the filtrate. Mix, allow to stand for 5 min and compare the colour of the solution with that of a blank prepared in the same manner. The test solution is yellow and the blank is red.

TESTS

Specific optical rotation (*2.2.7*). Dissolve 0.250 g in *dioxan R* and dilute to 25.0 ml with the same solvent. The specific optical rotation is + 75 to + 80, calculated with reference to the dried substance.

Related substances. Examine by liquid chromatography (*2.2.29*).

Test solution. Place 25.0 mg of the substance to be examined in a 10.0 ml volumetric flask, add 1.5 ml of *acetonitrile R* and then 5 ml of mobile phase A. Mix with the aid of an ultrasonic bath until complete dissolution and dilute to 10.0 ml with mobile phase A.

Reference solution (a). Dissolve 2 mg of *dexamethasone CRS* and 2 mg of *methylprednisolone CRS* in mobile phase A and dilute to 100.0 ml with the same mobile phase.

Reference solution (b). Dilute 1.0 ml of the test solution to 100.0 ml with mobile phase A.

The chromatographic procedure may be carried out using:

– a stainless steel column 0.25 m long and 4.6 mm in internal diameter packed with *octadecylsilyl silica gel for chromatography R* (5 µm),

– as mobile phase at a flow rate of 2.5 ml/min a linear gradient programme using the following conditions:

Mobile phase A. In a 1000 ml volumetric flask, mix 250 ml of *acetonitrile R* with 700 ml of *water R* and allow to equilibrate; adjust the volume to 1000 ml with *water R* and mix again,

Mobile phase B. Acetonitrile R,

Time (min)	Mobile phase A (per cent *V/V*)	Mobile phase B (per cent *V/V*)	Comment
0	100	0	isocratic
15	100 → 0	0 → 100	begin linear gradient
40	0	100	end chromatogram, return to 100 A
41	100	0	begin equilibration with A
46 = 0	100	0	end equilibration, begin next chromatogram

– as detector a spectrophotometer set at 254 nm,

maintaining the temperature of the column at 45 °C.

Equilibrate the column for at least 30 min with mobile phase B at a flow rate of 2.5 ml/min and then with mobile phase A for 5 min. For subsequent chromatograms, use the conditions described from 40.0 min to 46.0 min.

Adjust the sensitivity of the system so that the height of the principal peak in the chromatogram obtained with 20 µl of reference solution (b) is at least 50 per cent of the full scale of the recorder.

Inject 20 µl of reference solution (a). When the chromatograms are recorded in the prescribed conditions, the retention times are: methylprednisolone about 11.5 min and dexamethasone about 13 min. The test is not valid unless the resolution between the peaks corresponding to methylprednisolone and dexamethasone is at least 2.8; if necessary, adjust the concentration of acetonitrile in mobile phase A.

Inject 20 µl of mobile phase A as a blank, 20 µl of the test solution and 20 µl of reference solution (b). Record the chromatogram of the test solution for twice the retention time of the principal peak. In the chromatogram obtained with the test solution: the area of any peak, apart from the principal peak, is not greater than 0.5 times the area of the principal peak in the chromatogram obtained with reference solution (b) (0.5 per cent); the sum of the areas of all the peaks, apart from the principal peak, is not greater than the area of the principal peak in the chromatogram obtained with reference solution (b) (1 per cent). Disregard any peak due to the blank and any peak with an area less than 0.05 times the area of the principal peak in the chromatogram obtained with reference solution (b).

Loss on drying (*2.2.32*). Not more than 0.5 per cent, determined on 0.500 g by drying in an oven at 100-105 °C.

ASSAY

Dissolve 0.100 g in *alcohol R* and dilute to 100.0 ml with the same solvent. Dilute 2.0 ml of the solution to 100.0 ml with *alcohol R*. Measure the absorbance (*2.2.25*) at the maximum at 238.5 nm.

Calculate the content of $C_{22}H_{29}FO_5$ taking the specific absorbance to be 394.

STORAGE

Protected from light.

01/2005:0548

DEXAMETHASONE ACETATE

Dexamethasoni acetas

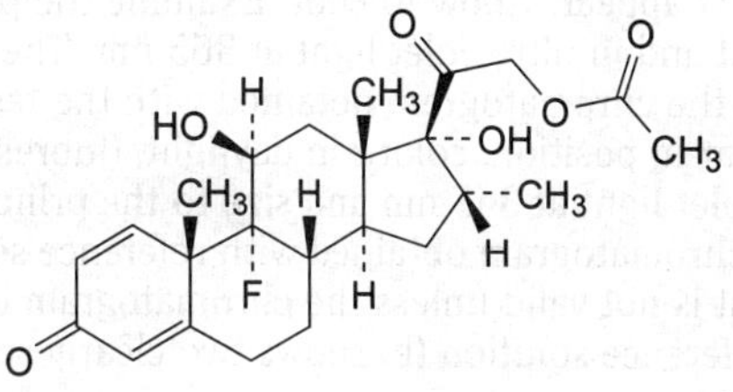

$C_{24}H_{31}FO_6$ M_r 434.5

DEFINITION

Dexamethasone acetate contains not less than 97.0 per cent and not more than the equivalent of 103.0 per cent of 9-fluoro-11β,17-dihydroxy-16α-methyl-3,20-dioxopregna-1,4-dien-21-yl acetate, calculated with reference to the dried substance.

CHARACTERS

A white or almost white, crystalline powder, practically insoluble in water, freely soluble in acetone and in alcohol, slightly soluble in methylene chloride.

Dexamethasone acetate shows polymorphism.

IDENTIFICATION

First identification: B, C.

Second identification: A, C, D, E, F.

A. Dissolve 10.0 mg in *ethanol R* and dilute to 100.0 ml with the same solvent. Place 2.0 ml of this solution in a ground-glass-stoppered tube, add 10.0 ml of *phenylhydrazine-sulphuric acid solution R*, mix and heat in a water-bath at 60 °C for 20 min. Cool immediately. The absorbance (*2.2.25*) of the solution at the maximum at 419 nm is not less than 0.35.

B. Examine by infrared absorption spectrophotometry (*2.2.24*), comparing with the spectrum obtained with *dexamethasone acetate CRS*. If the spectra obtained in the solid state with the substance to be examined and the reference substance show differences, record further spectra using saturated solutions (about 30 g/l) of the substance to be examined and of the reference substance in *chloroform R* in a 0.2 mm cell.

C. Examine by thin-layer chromatography (*2.2.27*), using as the coating substance a suitable silica gel with a fluorescent indicator having an optimal intensity at 254 nm.

Test solution. Dissolve 10 mg of the substance to be examined in a mixture of 1 volume of *methanol R* and 9 volumes of *methylene chloride R* and dilute to 10 ml with the same mixture of solvents.

Reference solution (a). Dissolve 20 mg of *dexamethasone acetate CRS* in a mixture of 1 volume of *methanol R* and 9 volumes of *methylene chloride R* and dilute to 20 ml with the same mixture of solvents.

Reference solution (b). Dissolve 10 mg of *cortisone acetate R* in reference solution (a) and dilute to 10 ml with the same solution.

Apply separately to the plate 5 µl of each solution. Prepare the mobile phase by adding a mixture of 1.2 volumes of *water R* and 8 volumes of *methanol R* to a mixture of 15 volumes of *ether R* and 77 volumes of *methylene chloride R*. Develop over a path of 15 cm.

Allow the plate to dry in air and examine in ultraviolet light at 254 nm. The principal spot in the chromatogram obtained with the test solution is similar in position and size to the principal spot in the chromatogram obtained with reference solution (a). Spray with *alcoholic solution of sulphuric acid R*. Heat at 120 °C for 10 min or until the spots appear. Allow to cool. Examine the plate in daylight and in ultraviolet light at 365 nm. The principal spot in the chromatogram obtained with the test solution is similar in position, colour in daylight, fluorescence in ultraviolet light at 365 nm and size to the principal spot in the chromatogram obtained with reference solution (a). The test is not valid unless the chromatogram obtained with reference solution (b) shows two clearly separated spots.

D. Add about 2 mg to 2 ml of *sulphuric acid R* and shake to dissolve. Within 5 min, a faint reddish-brown colour develops. Add the solution to 10 ml of *water R* and mix. The colour is discharged and a clear solution remains.

E. Mix about 5 mg with 45 mg of *heavy magnesium oxide R* and ignite in a crucible until an almost white residue is obtained (usually less than 5 min). Allow to cool, add 1 ml of *water R*, 0.05 ml of *phenolphthalein solution R1* and about 1 ml of *dilute hydrochloric acid R* to render the solution colourless. Filter. To a freshly prepared mixture of 0.1 ml of *alizarin S solution R* and 0.1 ml of *zirconyl nitrate solution R*, add 1.0 ml of the filtrate. Mix, allow to stand for 5 min and compare the colour of the solution with that of a blank prepared in the same manner. The test solution is yellow and the blank is red.

F. About 10 mg gives the reaction of acetyl (*2.3.1*).

TESTS

Specific optical rotation (*2.2.7*). Dissolve 0.250 g in *dioxan R* and dilute to 25.0 ml with the same solvent. The specific optical rotation is + 84 to + 90, calculated with reference to the dried substance.

Related substances. Examine by liquid chromatography (*2.2.29*).

Test solution. Dissolve 25.0 mg of the substance to be examined in about 4 ml of *acetonitrile R* and dilute to 10.0 ml with *water R*.

Reference solution (a). Dissolve 2 mg of *dexamethasone acetate CRS* and 2 mg of *betamethasone acetate CRS* in the mobile phase and dilute to 100.0 ml with the mobile phase.

Reference solution (b). Dilute 1.0 ml of the test solution to 100.0 ml with the mobile phase.

The chromatographic procedure may be carried out using:

– a stainless steel column 0.25 m long and 4.6 mm in internal diameter, packed with *octadecylsilyl silica gel for chromatography R* (5 µm),
– as mobile phase at a flow rate of 1 ml/min a mixture prepared as follows: in a 1000 ml volumetric flask mix 380 ml of *acetonitrile R* with 550 ml of *water R* and allow to equilibrate; dilute to 1000 ml with *water R* and mix again,
– as detector a spectrophotometer set at 254 nm.

Equilibrate the column with the mobile phase at a flow rate of 1 ml/min for about 30 min.

Adjust the sensitivity of the system so that the height of the principal peak in the chromatogram obtained with 20 µl of reference solution (b) is not less than 50 per cent of the full scale of the recorder.

Inject 20 µl of reference solution (a). When the chromatograms are recorded in the prescribed conditions, the retention times are: betamethasone acetate, about 19 min and dexamethasone acetate, about 22 min. The test is not valid unless the resolution between the peaks due to betamethasone acetate and dexamethasone acetate is at least 3.3; if necessary, adjust the concentration of acetonitrile in the mobile phase.

Inject separately 20 µl of the test solution and 20 µl of reference solution (b). Continue the chromatography for 1.5 times the retention time of the principal peak. In the chromatogram obtained with the test solution: the area of any peak, apart from the principal peak, is not greater than half the area of the principal peak in the chromatogram obtained with reference solution (b) (0.5 per cent); the sum of the areas of all such peaks is not greater than the area of the principal peak in the chromatogram obtained with reference solution (b) (1.0 per cent). Disregard any peak with an area less than 0.05 times the area of the principal peak in the chromatogram obtained with reference solution (b).

Loss on drying (*2.2.32*). Not more than 0.5 per cent, determined on 0.500 g by drying *in vacuo* in an oven at 100 °C to 105 °C.

ASSAY

Dissolve 0.100 g in *alcohol R* and dilute to 100.0 ml with the same solvent. Dilute 2.0 ml to 100.0 ml with *alcohol R*. Measure the absorbance (*2.2.25*) at the maximum at 238.5 nm.

Calculate the content of $C_{24}H_{31}FO_6$ taking the specific absorbance to be 357.

STORAGE

Store protected from light.

01/2005:0549

DEXAMETHASONE SODIUM PHOSPHATE

Dexamethasoni natrii phosphas

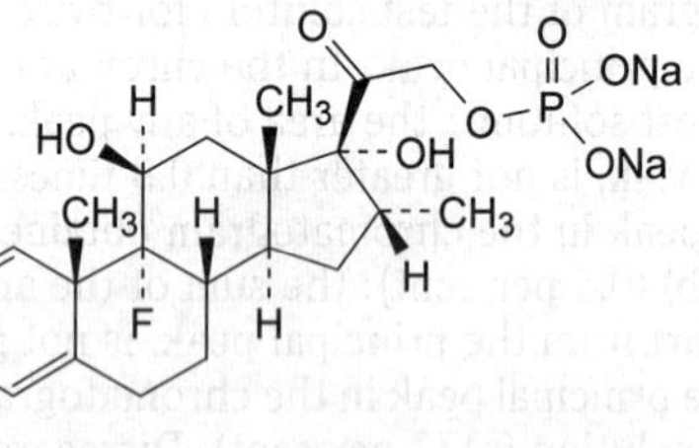

$C_{22}H_{28}FNa_2O_8P$ *M*r 516.4

DEFINITION

Dexamethasone sodium phosphate contains not less than 97.0 per cent and not more than the equivalent of 103.0 per cent of 9-fluoro-11β,17-dihydroxy-16α-methyl-3,20-dioxopregna-1,4-dien-21-yl disodium phosphate, calculated with reference to the anhydrous, ethanol-free substance.

CHARACTERS

A white or almost white powder, very hygroscopic, freely soluble in water, slightly soluble in alcohol, practically insoluble in methylene chloride.

It shows polymorphism.

IDENTIFICATION

First identification: B, C.

Second identification: A, C, D, E, F.

A. Dissolve 10.0 mg in 5 ml of *water R* and dilute to 100.0 ml with *ethanol R*. Place 2.0 ml of this solution in a ground-glass-stoppered tube, add 10.0 ml of *phenylhydrazine-sulphuric acid solution R*, mix and heat in a water-bath at 60 °C for 20 min. Cool immediately. The absorbance (*2.2.25*) of the solution measured at the maximum at 419 nm is at least 0.20.

B. Examine by infrared absorption spectrophotometry (*2.2.24*), comparing with the spectrum obtained with *dexamethasone sodium phosphate CRS*. If the spectra obtained in the solid state show differences, dissolve the substance to be examined and the reference substance separately in the minimum volume of *alcohol R*, evaporate to dryness on a water-bath and record new spectra using the residues.

C. Examine by thin-layer chromatography (*2.2.27*), using as the coating substance a suitable silica gel with a fluorescent indicator having an optimal intensity at 254 nm.

Test solution. Dissolve 10 mg of the substance to be examined in *methanol R* and dilute to 10 ml with the same solvent.

Reference solution (a). Dissolve 20 mg of *dexamethasone sodium phosphate CRS* in *methanol R* and dilute to 20 ml with the same solvent.

Reference solution (b). Dissolve 10 mg of *prednisolone sodium phosphate CRS* in reference solution (a) and dilute to 10 ml with the same solution.

Apply separately to the plate 5 µl of each solution. Develop over a path of 15 cm, using a mixture of 20 volumes of *glacial acetic acid R*, 20 volumes of *water R* and 60 volumes of *butanol R*. Allow the plate to dry in air and examine in ultraviolet light at 254 nm. The principal spot in the chromatogram obtained with the test solution is similar in position and size to the principal spot in the chromatogram obtained with reference solution (a). Spray with *alcoholic solution of sulphuric acid R*. Heat at 120 °C for 10 min or until the spots appear. Allow to cool. Examine in daylight and in ultraviolet light at 365 nm. The principal spot in the chromatogram obtained with the test solution is similar in position, colour in daylight, fluorescence in ultraviolet light at 365 nm and size to the principal spot in the chromatogram obtained with reference solution (a). The test is not valid unless the chromatogram obtained with reference solution (b) shows two spots which may, however, not be completely separated.

D. Add about 2 mg to 2 ml of *sulphuric acid R* and shake to dissolve. Within 5 min, a faint yellowish-brown colour develops. Add the solution to 10 ml of *water R* and mix. The colour fades and a clear solution remains.

E. Mix about 5 mg with 45 mg of *heavy magnesium oxide R* and ignite in a crucible until an almost white residue is obtained (usually less than 5 min). Allow to cool, add 1 ml of *water R*, 0.05 ml of *phenolphthalein solution R1* and about 1 ml of *dilute hydrochloric acid R* to render the solution colourless. Filter. To a freshly prepared mixture of 0.1 ml of *alizarin S solution R* and 0.1 ml of *zirconyl nitrate solution R*, add 1.0 ml of the filtrate. Mix, allow to stand for 5 min and compare the colour of the solution with that of a blank prepared in the same manner. The test solution is yellow and the blank is red.

F. To 40 mg add 2 ml of *sulphuric acid R* and heat gently until white fumes are evolved, add *nitric acid R* dropwise, continue the heating until the solution is almost colourless and cool. Add 2 ml of *water R*, heat until white fumes are again evolved, cool, add 10 ml of *water R* and neutralise to *red litmus paper R* with *dilute ammonia R1*. The solution gives reaction (a) of sodium (*2.3.1*) and reaction (b) of phosphates (*2.3.1*).

TESTS

Solution S. Dissolve 1.0 g in *carbon dioxide-free water R* and dilute to 20 ml with the same solvent.

Appearance of solution. Solution S is clear (*2.2.1*) and not more intensely coloured than reference solution B_7 (*2.2.2, Method II*).

pH (*2.2.3*). Dilute 1 ml of solution S to 5 ml with *carbon dioxide-free water R*. The pH of the solution is 7.5 to 9.5.

Specific optical rotation (*2.2.7*). Dissolve 0.250 g in *water R* and dilute to 25.0 ml with the same solvent. The specific optical rotation is + 75 to + 83, calculated with reference to the anhydrous, ethanol-free substance.

Related substances. Examine by liquid chromatography (*2.2.29*).

Test solution. Dissolve 25.0 mg of the substance to be examined in the mobile phase and dilute to 10.0 ml with the mobile phase.

Reference solution (a). Dissolve 2 mg of *dexamethasone sodium phosphate CRS* and 2 mg of *betamethasone sodium phosphate CRS* in the mobile phase and dilute to 100.0 ml with the mobile phase.

Reference solution (b). Dilute 1.0 ml of the test solution to 100.0 ml with the mobile phase.

The chromatographic procedure may be carried out using:

- a stainless steel column 0.25 m long and 4.6 mm in internal diameter packed with *octadecylsilyl silica gel for chromatography R* (5 µm),
- as mobile phase at a flow rate of 1 ml/min a mixture prepared as follows: in a 250 ml conical flask, weigh 1.360 g of *potassium dihydrogen phosphate R* and 0.600 g of *hexylamine R*, mix and allow to stand for 10 min and then dissolve in 182.5 ml of *water R*; add 67.5 ml of *acetonitrile R*, mix and filter (0.45 µm),
- as detector a spectrophotometer set at 254 nm.

Equilibrate the column with the mobile phase at a flow rate of 1 ml/min for about 45 min.

Adjust the sensitivity of the system so that the height of the principal peak in the chromatogram obtained with 20 µl of reference solution (b) is at least 50 per cent of the full scale of the recorder.

Inject 20 µl of reference solution (a). When the chromatograms are recorded in the prescribed conditions, the retention times are: betamethasone sodium phosphate, about 12.5 min and dexamethasone sodium phosphate about 14 min. The test is not valid unless the resolution between the peaks corresponding to betamethasone sodium phosphate and dexamethasone sodium phosphate is at least 2.2. If necessary, adjust slightly the concentration of acetonitrile or increase the concentration of water in the mobile phase.

Inject separately 20 µl of the test solution and 20 µl of reference solution (b). Continue the chromatography for twice the retention time of the principal peak. In the chromatogram obtained with the test solution: the area of any peak, apart from the principal peak, is not greater than half the area of the principal peak in the chromatogram obtained with reference solution (b) (0.5 per cent); the sum of the areas of all such peaks is not greater than the area of the principal peak in the chromatogram obtained with reference solution (b) (1 per cent). Disregard any peak with an area less than 0.05 times that of the principal peak in the chromatogram obtained with reference solution (b).

Inorganic phosphates. Dissolve 50 mg in *water R* and dilute to 100 ml with the same solvent. To 10 ml of this solution add 5 ml of *molybdovanadic reagent R*, mix and allow to stand for 5 min. Any yellow colour in the solution is not more intense than that in a standard prepared at the same time in the same manner using 10 ml of *phosphate standard solution (5 ppm PO_4) R* (1 per cent).

Ethanol. Not more than 3.0 per cent *m/m*, determined by gas chromatography (*2.2.28*), using *propanol R* as the internal standard.

Internal standard solution. Dilute 1.0 ml of *propanol R* to 100.0 ml with *water R*.

Test solution. Dissolve 0.50 g of the substance to be examined in 5.0 ml of the internal standard solution and dilute to 10.0 ml with *water R*.

Reference solution. Dilute 1.0 g of *ethanol R* to 100.0 ml with *water R*. To 2.0 ml of the solution add 5.0 ml of the internal standard solution and dilute to 10.0 ml with *water R*.

The chromatographic procedure may be carried out using:

– a column 1 m long and 3.2 mm in internal diameter packed with *ethylvinylbenzene-divinylbenzene copolymer R1* (150 µm to 180 µm),
– *nitrogen for chromatography R* as the carrier gas at a flow rate of 30 ml/min,
– a flame-ionisation detector,

maintaining the temperature of the column at 150 °C, that of the injection port at 250 °C and that of the detector at 280 °C. Inject 2 µl of each solution.

Ethanol and water. Determine the water content using 0.200 g by the semi-micro determination of water (*2.5.12*). Add the percentage content of water and the percentage content of ethanol obtained in the test for ethanol. The sum of the percentage contents of water and ethanol is not greater than 13.0 per cent *m/m*.

ASSAY

Dissolve 0.100 g in *water R* and dilute to 100.0 ml with the same solvent. Dilute 10.0 ml of the solution to 500.0 ml with *water R*. Measure the absorbance (*2.2.25*) at the maximum at 241.5 nm.

Calculate the content of $C_{22}H_{28}FNa_2O_8P$ taking the specific absorbance to be 303.

STORAGE

Store in an airtight container, protected from light.

IMPURITIES

A. dexamethasone,

B. betamethasone sodium phosphate.

01/2005:1196

DEXCHLORPHENIRAMINE MALEATE

Dexchlorpheniramini maleas

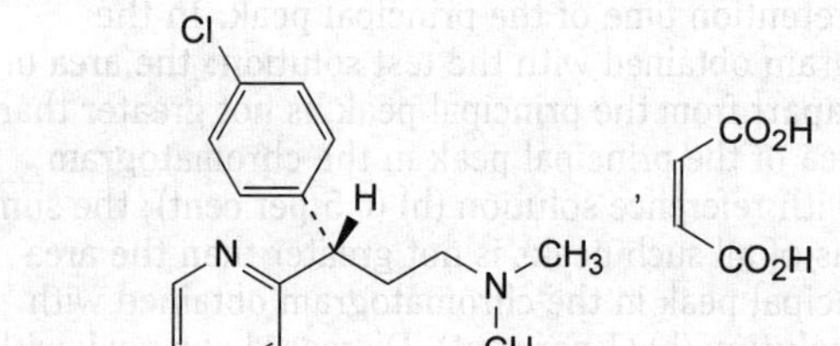

$C_{20}H_{23}ClN_2O_4$ M_r 390.9

DEFINITION

Dexchlorpheniramine maleate contains not less than 98.0 per cent and not more than the equivalent of 100.5 per cent of (3*S*)-3-(4-chlorophenyl)-*N*,*N*-dimethyl-3-(pyridin-2-yl)propan-1-amine (*Z*)-butanedioate, calculated with reference to the dried substance.

CHARACTERS

A white crystalline powder, very soluble in water, freely soluble in alcohol, in methanol and in methylene chloride.

IDENTIFICATION

First identification: A, C, E.

Second identification: A, B, D, E.

A. It complies with the test for specific optical rotation (see Tests).

B. Melting point (*2.2.14*): 110 °C to 115 °C.

C. Examine by infrared absorption spectrophotometry (*2.2.24*), comparing with the spectrum obtained with *dexchlorpheniramine maleate CRS*. Examine the substances prepared as discs using *potassium bromide R*.

D. Examine by thin-layer chromatography (*2.2.27*), using a *TLC silica gel F_{254} plate R*.

Test solution. Dissolve 0.10 g of the substance to be examined in *methanol R* and dilute to 5.0 ml with the same solvent.

Reference solution. Dissolve 56 mg of *maleic acid R* in *methanol R* and dilute to 10 ml with the same solvent.

Apply to the plate 5 µl of each solution. Develop over a path of 12 cm using a mixture of 3 volumes of *water R*, 7 volumes of *anhydrous formic acid R*, 20 volumes of *methanol R* and 70 volumes of *di-isopropyl ether R*. Allow the plate to dry in a current of air for a few minutes and examine in ultraviolet light at 254 nm. The chromatogram obtained with the test solution shows two clearly separated spots. The upper spot is similar in position and size to the spot in the chromatogram obtained with the reference solution.

E. To 0.15 g in a porcelain crucible add 0.5 g of *anhydrous sodium carbonate R*. Heat over an open flame for 10 min. Allow to cool. Take up the residue with 10 ml of *dilute nitric acid R* and filter. To 1 ml of the filtrate add 1 ml of *water R*. The solution gives reaction (a) of chlorides (*2.3.1*).

TESTS

Solution S. Dissolve 2.0 g in *water R* and dilute to 20.0 ml with the same solvent.

Appearance of solution. Solution S is clear (*2.2.1*) and not more intensely coloured than reference solution BY_6 (*2.2.2, Method II*).

pH (*2.2.3*). Dissolve 0.20 g in 20 ml of *water R*. The pH of the solution is 4.5 to 5.5.

Specific optical rotation (*2.2.7*): + 22 to + 23, determined on solution S and calculated with reference to the dried substance.

Related substances. Examine by gas chromatography (*2.2.28*).

Test solution. Dissolve 10.0 mg in 1.0 ml of *methylene chloride R*.

Reference solution. Dissolve 5.0 mg of *brompheniramine maleate CRS* in 0.5 ml of *methylene chloride R* and add 0.5 ml of the test solution. Dilute 0.5 ml of this solution to 50.0 ml with *methylene chloride R*.

The chromatographic procedure may be carried out using:

- a glass column 2.3 m long and 2 mm in internal diameter packed with acid- and base- washed *silanised diatomaceous earth for gas chromatography R* (135 μm to 175 μm) impregnated with 3 per cent *m/m* of a mixture of 50 per cent of poly(dimethyl)siloxane and 50 per cent of poly(diphenyl)siloxane,
- *nitrogen for chromatography R* as the carrier gas at a flow rate of 20 ml/min,
- a flame-ionisation detector,

maintaining the temperature of the column at 205 °C and that of the injection port and of the detector at 250 °C.

Inject 1 μl of the reference solution. The test is not valid unless, in the chromatogram obtained with the reference solution, the resolution between the two peaks corresponding to dexchlorpheniramine and brompheniramine is at least 1.5. Inject 1 μl of the test solution. Continue the chromatography for at least 2.5 times the retention time of the principal peak. In the chromatogram obtained with the test solution: none of the peaks, apart from the principal peak, has an area greater than 0.8 times the area of the peak corresponding to dexchlorpheniramine in the chromatogram obtained with the reference solution (0.4 per cent); the sum of the areas of all the peaks, apart from the principal peak, is not greater than twice the area of the peak corresponding to dexchlorpheniramine in the chromatogram obtained with the reference solution (1 per cent).

Enantiomeric purity. Examine by liquid chromatography (*2.2.29*).

Test solution. Dissolve 10.0 mg in 3 ml of *water R*. Add a few drops of *concentrated ammonia R* until an alkaline reaction is produced. Shake with 5 ml of *methylene chloride R*. Separate the layers. Evaporate the lower, methylene chloride layer to an oily residue on a water-bath. Dissolve the oily residue in *2-propanol R* and dilute to 10.0 ml with the same solvent.

Reference solution (a). Dissolve 10.0 mg of *dexchlorpheniramine maleate CRS* in 3 ml of *water R*. Add a few drops of *concentrated ammonia R* until an alkaline reaction is produced. Shake with 5 ml of *methylene chloride R*. Separate the layers. Evaporate the lower, methylene chloride layer to an oily residue on a water-bath. Dissolve the oily residue in *2-propanol R* and dilute to 10.0 ml with the same solvent.

Reference solution (b). Dissolve 10.0 mg of *chlorphenamine maleate CRS* in 3 ml of *water R*. Add a few drops of *concentrated ammonia R* until an alkaline reaction is produced. Shake with 5 ml of *methylene chloride R*. Separate the layers. Evaporate the lower, methylene chloride layer to an oily residue on a water-bath. Dissolve the oily residue in *2-propanol R* and dilute to 10.0 ml with the same solvent.

Reference solution (c). Dilute 1.0 ml of the test solution to 50 ml with *2-propanol R*.

The chromatographic procedure may be carried out using:

- a stainless steel column 0.25 m long and 4.6 mm in internal diameter packed with *amylose derivative of silica gel for chromatography R*,
- as mobile phase at a flow rate of 1 ml/min a mixture of 3 volumes of *diethylamine R*, 20 volumes of *2-propanol R* and 980 volumes of *hexane R*,
- as detector a spectrophotometer set at 254 nm.

Under these conditions the peak of the (*S*)-isomer appears first.

Inject 10 μl of each solution. The test is not valid unless: in the chromatogram obtained with reference solution (b), the resolution between the peaks corresponding to the (*R*)-enantiomer and to the (*S*)-enantiomer is at least 1.5; the retention times of the principal peaks in the chromatograms obtained with the test solution and reference solution (a) are identical ((*S*)-enantiomer). In the chromatogram obtained with the test solution, the area of the peak corresponding to the (*R*)-enantiomer is not greater than the area of the principal peak in the chromatogram obtained with reference solution (c) (2 per cent) and the area of any peak, apart from the principal peak and any peak corresponding to the (*R*)-enantiomer, is not greater than 0.25 times the area of the principal peak in the chromatogram obtained with reference solution (c) (0.5 per cent).

Heavy metals (*2.4.8*). 1.0 g complies with limit test C for heavy metals (20 ppm). Prepare the standard using 2 ml of *lead standard solution (10 ppm Pb) R*.

Loss on drying (*2.2.32*). Not more than 0.5 per cent, determined on 1.000 g by drying in an oven at 65 °C for 4 h.

Sulphated ash (*2.4.14*). Not more than 0.1 per cent, determined on 1.0 g.

ASSAY

Dissolve 0.150 g in 25 ml of *anhydrous acetic acid R*. Titrate with *0.1 M perchloric acid*, determining the end-point potentiometrically (*2.2.20*).

1 ml of *0.1 M perchloric acid* is equivalent to 19.54 mg of $C_{20}H_{23}ClN_2O_4$.

STORAGE

Store protected from light.

IMPURITIES

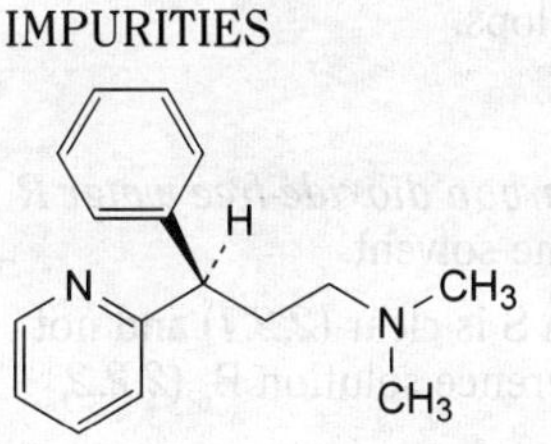

and enantiomer

A. (3*RS*)-*N*,*N*-dimethyl-3-phenyl-3-(pyridin-2-yl)propan-1-amine,

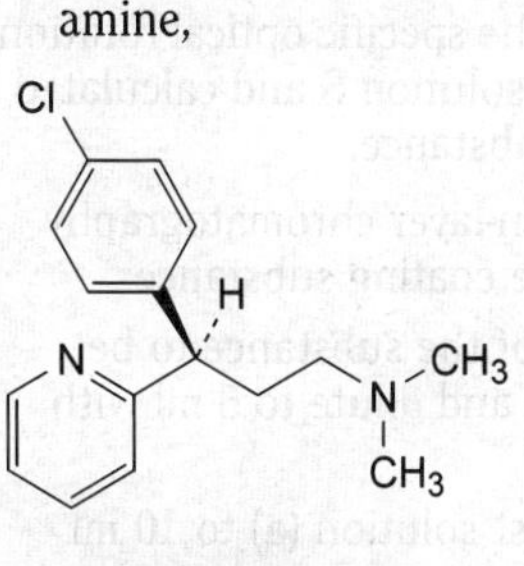

B. (3*R*)-3-(4-chlorophenyl)-*N*,*N*-dimethyl-3-(pyridin-2-yl)propan-1-amine.

01/2005:0761

DEXPANTHENOL

Dexpanthenolum

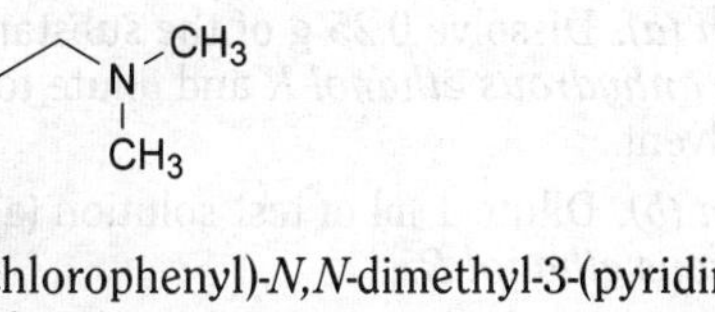

$C_9H_{19}NO_4$ M_r 205.3

DEFINITION

Dexpanthenol contains not less than 98.0 per cent and not more than the equivalent of 101.0 per cent of (2*R*)-2,4-dihydroxy-*N*-(3-hydroxypropyl)-3,3-dimethylbutanamide, calculated with reference to the anhydrous substance.

CHARACTERS

A colourless or slightly yellowish, viscous hygroscopic liquid, or a white or almost white, crystalline powder, very soluble in water, freely soluble in ethanol (96 per cent).

IDENTIFICATION

First identification: A, B.

Second identification: A, C, D.

A. It complies with the test for specific optical rotation (see Tests).

B. Examine by infrared absorption spectrophotometry (*2.2.24*), comparing with the spectrum obtained with *dexpanthenol CRS*. Examine the substances using discs prepared as follows: dissolve the substance to be examined and the reference substance separately in 1.0 ml of *anhydrous ethanol R* to obtain a concentration of 5 mg/ml. Place dropwise 0.5 ml of this solution on a disc of *potassium bromide R*. Dry the disc at 100-105 °C for 15 min.

C. Examine the chromatograms obtained in the test for 3-aminopropanol. The principal spot in the chromatogram obtained with test solution (b) is similar in position, colour and size to the principal spot in the chromatogram obtained with reference solution (a).

D. To 1 ml of solution S (see Tests) add 1 ml of *dilute sodium hydroxide solution R* and 0.1 ml of *copper sulphate solution R*. A blue colour develops.

TESTS

Solution S. Dissolve 2.500 g in *carbon dioxide-free water R* and dilute to 50.0 ml with the same solvent.

Appearance of solution. Solution S is clear (*2.2.1*) and not more intensely coloured than reference solution B_6 (*2.2.2, Method II*).

pH (*2.2.3*). The pH of solution S is not greater than 10.5.

Specific optical rotation (*2.2.7*). The specific optical rotation is + 29.0 to + 32.0, determined on solution S and calculated with reference to the anhydrous substance.

3-Aminopropanol. Examine by thin-layer chromatography (*2.2.27*), using *silica gel G R* as the coating substance.

Test solution (a). Dissolve 0.25 g of the substance to be examined in *anhydrous ethanol R* and dilute to 5 ml with the same solvent.

Test solution (b). Dilute 1 ml of test solution (a) to 10 ml with *anhydrous ethanol R*.

Reference solution (a). Dissolve the contents of a vial of *dexpanthenol CRS* in 1.0 ml of *anhydrous ethanol R* to obtain a concentration of 5 mg/ml.

Reference solution (b). Dissolve 25 mg of *3-aminopropanol R* in *anhydrous ethanol R* and dilute to 100 ml with the same solvent.

Apply separately to the plate 10 µl of each solution. Develop over a path of 15 cm using a mixture of 20 volumes of *concentrated ammonia R*, 25 volumes of *methanol R* and 55 volumes of *butanol R*. Allow the plate to dry in air, spray with a 100 g/l solution of *trichloroacetic acid R* in *methanol R* and heat at 150 °C for 10 min. Spray with a 1 g/l solution of *ninhydrin R* in *methanol R* and heat at 120 °C until a colour appears. Any spot due to 3-aminopropanol in the chromatogram obtained with test solution (a) is not more intense than the spot in the chromatogram obtained with reference solution (b) (0.5 per cent).

Heavy metals (*2.4.8*). 12 ml of solution S complies with limit test A for heavy metals (20 ppm). Prepare the reference solution using *lead standard solution (1 ppm Pb) R*.

Water (*2.5.12*). Not more than 1.0 per cent, determined on 1.000 g.

Sulphated ash (*2.4.14*). Not more than 0.1 per cent, determined on 1.0 g.

ASSAY

To 0.400 g add 50.0 ml of *0.1 M perchloric acid*. Boil under a reflux condenser for 5 h protected from humidity. Allow to cool. Add 50 ml of *dioxan R* by rinsing the condenser, protected from humidity. Add 0.2 ml of *naphtholbenzein solution R* and titrate with *0.1 M potassium hydrogen phthalate* until the colour changes from green to yellow. Carry out a blank titration.

1 ml of *0.1 M perchloric acid* is equivalent to 20.53 mg of $C_9H_{19}NO_4$.

STORAGE

In an airtight container.

01/2005:1506

DEXTRAN 1 FOR INJECTION

Dextranum 1 ad iniectabile

DEFINITION

Dextran 1 for injection is a low molecular weight fraction of dextran, consisting of a mixture of isomaltooligosaccharides. The average relative molecular mass is about 1000.

PRODUCTION

It is obtained by hydrolysis and fractionation of dextrans produced by fermentation of sucrose using *Leuconostoc mesenteroides* strain NRRL B-512 = CIP 78.59 or substrains thereof (for example *L. mesenteroides* B-512 F = NCTC 10817).

It is prepared in conditions designed to minimise the risk of microbial contamination.

CHARACTERS

A white or almost white powder, hygroscopic, very soluble in water, very slightly soluble in alcohol.

IDENTIFICATION

A. Dissolve 3.000 g in *water R*, heat on a water-bath and dilute to 100.0 ml with the same solvent. The specific optical rotation (*2.2.7*) is + 148 to + 164, calculated with reference to the dried substance. Dry an aliquot of the solution first on a water-bath and then to constant weight *in vacuo* at 70 °C. Calculate the dextran content after correction for the content of sodium chloride.

B. Examine by infrared absorption spectrophotometry (*2.2.24*), comparing with the spectrum obtained with *dextran 1 CRS*. Prepare the discs as follows: to 1-2 mg add one or a few drops of *water R*; grind in an agate mortar for 1-2 min; add about 300 mg of *potassium bromide R* and mix to a slurry (do not grind); dry *in vacuo* at 40 °C for 15 min, crush the residue (if it is not dry, dry for another 15 min). Prepare a disc using *potassium bromide R*. Run the infrared spectrum with a blank disc using *potassium bromide R* in the reference beam.

C. It complies with the test for molecular-mass distribution (see Tests).

TESTS

Solution S. Dissolve 7.5 g in *carbon dioxide-free water R*, heat on a water-bath and dilute to 50 ml with the same solvent.

Absorbance (*2.2.25*). Measure the absorbance of solution S at 375 nm. The absorbance is not more than 0.12.

Acidity or alkalinity. To 10 ml of solution S add 0.1 ml of *phenolphthalein solution R*. The solution is colourless. Add 0.2 ml of *0.01 M sodium hydroxide*. The solution is pink. Add 0.4 ml of *0.01 M hydrochloric acid*. The solution is colourless. Add 0.1 ml of *methyl red solution R*. The solution is red or orange.

Nitrogen-containing substances. Carry out the determination of nitrogen by sulphuric acid digestion (*2.5.9*), using 0.200 g and heating for 2 h. Collect the distillate in a mixture of 0.5 ml of *bromocresol green solution R*, 0.5 ml of *methyl red solution R* and 20 ml of *water R*. Titrate with *0.01 M hydrochloric acid*. Not more than 0.15 ml of *0.01 M hydrochloric acid* is required to change the colour of the indicator (110 ppm N).

Sodium chloride. Not more than 1.5 per cent. Accurately weigh 3-5 g and dissolve in 100 ml of *water R*. Add 0.3 ml of *potassium chromate solution R* and titrate with *0.1 M silver nitrate* until the yellowish-white colour changes to reddish-brown.

1 ml of *0.1 M silver nitrate* is equivalent to 5.844 mg of NaCl.

Molecular-mass distribution. The average molecular mass (M_w) is 850 to 1150. The fraction with less than 3 units of glucose is less than 15 per cent, the fraction with more than 9 units of glucose is less than 20 per cent.

Examine by size-exclusion chromatography (*2.2.30*).

Test solution. Dissolve 6.0-6.5 mg of the substance to be examined in 1.0 ml of the mobile phase.

Reference solution (a). Dissolve 6.0-6.5 mg of *dextran 1 CRS* in 1.0 ml of the mobile phase.

Reference solution (b). Dissolve the content of an ampoule of *isomaltooligosaccharide CRS* in 1 ml of the mobile phase, and mix. This corresponds to approximately 45 µg of isomaltotriose (3 glucose units), approximately 45 µg of isomaltononaose (9 glucose units), and approximately 60 µg of sodium chloride per 100 µl.

The chromatographic procedure may be carried out using:

– 2 columns, 30 cm long and 10 mm in internal diameter, in series, prepacked with a packing material of dextran covalently bound to highly cross-linked porous agarose beads, allowing resolution of oligosaccharides in the molecular mass range of 180 to 3000, kept at a temperature of 20-25 °C,

– as mobile phase at a flow rate of 0.07-0.08 ml/min maintained constant to ± 1 per cent, a 2.92 g/l solution of *sodium chloride R*,

– as detector a differential refractometer.

Inject 100 µl of reference solution (b) and record the chromatogram for definition of the positions of isomaltotriose, isomaltononaose and sodium chloride. Inject 100 µl of the test solution and 100 µl of reference solution (a) and record the chromatograms. Determine the peak areas. Disregard any peak due to sodium chloride.

Calculate the average relative molecular mass M_w and the amount of the fraction with less than 3 and more than 9 glucose units, of *dextran 1 CRS* and of the substance to be examined. The test is not valid unless the values obtained for *dextran 1 CRS* are within the values stated on the label.

$$M_w = \sum w_i \times m_i$$

M_w = average molecular mass of the dextran,

m_i = molecular mass of oligosaccharide *i*,

w_i = weight proportion of oligosaccharide *i*.

Use the following molecular mass values for the calculation:

Oligosaccharide *i*	m_i
glucose	180
isomaltose	342
isomaltotriose	504
isomaltotetraose	666
isomaltopentaose	828
isomaltohexaose	990
isomaltoheptaose	1152
isomaltooctaose	1314
isomaltononaose	1476
isomaltodecaose	1638
isomaltoundecaose	1800
isomaltododecaose	1962
isomaltotridecaose	2124
isomaltotetradecaose	2286
isomaltopentadecaose	2448
isomaltohexadecaose	2610
isomaltoheptadecaose	2772
isomaltooctadecaose	2934
isomaltononadecaose	3096

Heavy metals (*2.4.8*). Dilute 20 ml of solution S to 30 ml with *water R*. 12 ml of this solution complies with limit test A (10 ppm). Prepare the reference solution using *lead standard solution (1 ppm Pb) R*.

Loss on drying (*2.2.32*). Not more than 5.0 per cent, determined on 5.000 g by drying in an oven at 100-105 °C for 5 h.

Bacterial endotoxins (*2.6.14*): less than 25 IU/g.

Microbial contamination. Total viable aerobic count (*2.6.12*) not more than 10^2 micro-organisms per gram, determined by plate-count. It complies with the test for *Escherichia coli* (*2.6.13*).

01/2005:0999

DEXTRAN 40 FOR INJECTION

Dextranum 40 ad iniectabile

DEFINITION

Dextran 40 for injection is a mixture of polysaccharides, principally of the α-1,6-glucan type.

The average relative molecular mass is about 40 000.

Monographs D-E

PRODUCTION

It is obtained by hydrolysis and fractionation of dextrans produced by fermentation of sucrose using *Leuconostoc mesenteroides* strain NRRL B-512 = CIP 78.59 or substrains thereof (for example *L. mesenteroides* B-512F = NCTC 10817).

It is prepared in conditions designed to minimise the risk of microbial contamination.

CHARACTERS

A white or almost white powder, very soluble in water, very slightly soluble in alcohol.

IDENTIFICATION

A. Dissolve 1.0 g in *water R*, heating on a water-bath, and dilute to 50.0 ml with the same solvent. The specific optical rotation (*2.2.7*) of the solution is + 195 to + 201, calculated with reference to the dried substance.

B. Examine by infrared absorption spectrophotometry (*2.2.24*), comparing with the spectrum obtained with *dextran CRS*.

C. It complies with the test for molecular-mass distribution (see Tests).

TESTS

Solution S. Dissolve 5.0 g in *distilled water R*, heating on a water-bath, and dilute to 50 ml with the same solvent.

Appearance of solution. Solution S is clear (*2.2.1*) and colourless (*2.2.2, Method II*).

Acidity or alkalinity. To 10 ml of solution S add 0.1 ml of *phenolphthalein solution R*. The solution remains colourless. Add 0.2 ml of *0.01 M sodium hydroxide*. The solution is red. Add 0.4 ml of *0.01 M hydrochloric acid*. The solution is colourless. Add 0.1 ml of *methyl red solution R*. The solution is red or orange.

Nitrogen-containing substances. Carry out the determination of nitrogen by sulphuric acid digestion (*2.5.9*), using 0.200 g and heating for 2 h. Collect the distillate in a mixture of 0.5 ml of *bromocresol green solution R*, 0.5 ml of *methyl red solution R* and 20 ml of *water R*. Titrate with *0.01 M hydrochloric acid*. Not more than 0.15 ml of *0.01 M hydrochloric acid* is required to change the colour of the indicator (110 ppm N).

Residual solvents. Examine by gas chromatography (*2.2.28*), using *propanol R* as internal standard.

Test solution. Dissolve 5 g of the substance to be examined in 100 ml of *water R* and distil. Collect the first 45 ml of the distillate, add 1 ml of a 25 g/l solution of *propanol R* and dilute to 50 ml with *water R*.

Reference solution. Mix 0.5 ml of a 25 g/l solution of *ethanol R*, 0.5 ml of a 25 g/l solution of *propanol R* and 0.5 ml of a 2.5 g/l solution of *methanol R* and dilute to 25.0 ml with *water R*.

The chromatographic procedure may be carried out using:

- a stainless steel column 1.8 m long and 2 mm in internal diameter packed with *ethylvinylbenzene-divinylbenzene copolymer R* (125-150 μm),
- *nitrogen for chromatography R* as the carrier gas at a flow rate of 25 ml/min,
- a flame-ionisation detector,

maintaining the temperature of the column at 190 °C, that of the injection port at 240 °C and that of the detector at 210 °C. Inject the chosen volume of each solution. In the chromatogram obtained with the test solution, the area of any peak corresponding to ethanol or methanol is not greater than the area of the corresponding peak in the chromatogram obtained with the reference solution (0.5 per cent of ethanol and 0.05 per cent of methanol) and the sum of the areas of any peaks, apart from the peaks corresponding to ethanol, methanol and the internal standard, is not greater than the area of the peak corresponding to the internal standard (0.5 per cent calculated as propanol).

Molecular-mass distribution (*2.2.39*). The average molecular mass (M_w) is 35 000 to 45 000. The average molecular mass of the 10 per cent high fraction is not more than 110 000. The average molecular mass of the 10 per cent low fraction is not less than 7000.

Heavy metals (*2.4.8*). 12 ml of solution S complies with limit test A (10 ppm). Prepare the standard using *lead standard solution (1 ppm Pb) R*.

Loss on drying (*2.2.32*). Not more than 7.0 per cent, determined on 0.200 g by heating in an oven at 105 ± 2 °C for 5 h.

Sulphated ash (*2.4.14*). Not more than 0.3 per cent, determined on 0.50 g.

Bacterial endotoxins (*2.6.14*): less than 10 IU/g.

Microbial contamination. Total viable aerobic count (*2.6.12*) not more than 10^2 micro-organisms per gram, determined by plate-count. It complies with the test for *Escherichia coli* (*2.6.13*).

01/2005:1000

DEXTRAN 60 FOR INJECTION

Dextranum 60 ad iniectabile

DEFINITION

Dextran 60 for injection is a mixture of polysaccharides, principally of the α-1,6-glucan type.

The average relative molecular mass is about 60 000.

PRODUCTION

It is obtained by hydrolysis and fractionation of dextrans produced by fermentation of sucrose using *Leuconostoc mesenteroides* strain NRRL B-512 = CIP 78.59 or substrains thereof (for example *L. mesenteroides* B-512F = NCTC 10817).

It is prepared in conditions designed to minimise the risk of microbial contamination.

CHARACTERS

A white or almost white powder, very soluble in water, very slightly soluble in alcohol.

IDENTIFICATION

A. Dissolve 1.0 g in *water R*, heating on a water-bath, and dilute to 50.0 ml with the same solvent. The specific optical rotation (*2.2.7*) of the solution is + 195 to + 201, calculated with reference to the dried substance.

B. Examine by infrared absorption spectrophotometry (*2.2.24*), comparing with the spectrum obtained with *dextran CRS*.

C. It complies with the test for molecular-mass distribution (see Tests).

TESTS

Solution S. Dissolve 5.0 g in *distilled water R*, heating on a water-bath, and dilute to 50 ml with the same solvent.

Appearance of solution. Solution S is clear (*2.2.1*) and colourless (*2.2.2, Method II*).

Acidity or alkalinity. To 10 ml of solution S add 0.1 ml of *phenolphthalein solution R*. The solution remains colourless. Add 0.2 ml of *0.01 M sodium hydroxide*. The solution is red. Add 0.4 ml of *0.01 M hydrochloric acid*. The solution is colourless. Add 0.1 ml of *methyl red solution R*. The solution is red or orange.

Nitrogen-containing substances. Carry out the determination of nitrogen by sulphuric acid digestion (*2.5.9*), using 0.200 g and heating for 2 h. Collect the distillate in a mixture of 0.5 ml of *bromocresol green solution R*, 0.5 ml of *methyl red solution R* and 20 ml of *water R*. Titrate with *0.01 M hydrochloric acid*. Not more than 0.15 ml of *0.01 M hydrochloric acid* is required to change the colour of the indicator (110 ppm N).

Residual solvents. Examine by gas chromatography (*2.2.28*), using *propanol R* as internal standard.

Test solution. Dissolve 5 g of the substance to be examined in 100 ml of *water R* and distil. Collect the first 45 ml of the distillate, add 1 ml of a 25 g/l solution of *propanol R* and dilute to 50 ml with *water R*.

Reference solution. Mix 0.5 ml of a 25 g/l solution of *ethanol R*, 0.5 ml of a 25 g/l solution of *propanol R* and 0.5 ml of a 2.5 g/l solution of *methanol R* and dilute to 25.0 ml with *water R*.

The chromatographic procedure may be carried out using:

- a stainless steel column 1.8 m long and 2 mm in internal diameter packed with *ethylvinylbenzene-divinylbenzene copolymer R* (125-150 µm),
- *nitrogen for chromatography R* as the carrier gas at a flow rate of 25 ml/min,
- a flame-ionisation detector,

maintaining the temperature of the column at 190 °C, that of the injection port at 240 °C and that of the detector at 210 °C. Inject the chosen volume of each solution. In the chromatogram obtained with the test solution, the area of any peak corresponding to ethanol or methanol is not greater than the area of the corresponding peak in the chromatogram obtained with the reference solution (0.5 per cent of ethanol and 0.05 per cent of methanol) and the sum of the areas of any peaks, apart from the peaks corresponding to ethanol, methanol and the internal standard, is not greater than the area of the peak corresponding to the internal standard (0.5 per cent calculated as propanol).

Molecular-mass distribution (*2.2.39*). The average molecular mass (M_w) is 54 000 to 66 000. The average molecular mass of the 10 per cent high fraction is not more than 180 000. The average molecular mass of the 10 per cent low fraction is not less than 14 000.

Heavy metals (*2.4.8*). 12 ml of solution S complies with limit test A (10 ppm). Prepare the standard using *lead standard solution (1 ppm Pb) R*.

Loss on drying (*2.2.32*). Not more than 7.0 per cent, determined on 0.200 g by heating in an oven at 105 ± 2 °C for 5 h.

Sulphated ash (*2.4.14*). Not more than 0.3 per cent, determined on 0.50 g.

Bacterial endotoxins (*2.6.14*): less than 16 IU/g.

Microbial contamination. Total viable count (*2.6.12*) not more than 10^2 micro-organisms per gram, determined by plate-count. It complies with the test for *Escherichia coli* (*2.6.13*).

01/2005:1001

DEXTRAN 70 FOR INJECTION

Dextranum 70 ad iniectabile

DEFINITION

Dextran 70 for injection is a mixture of polysaccharides, principally of the α-1,6-glucan type.

The average relative molecular mass is about 70 000.

PRODUCTION

It is obtained by hydrolysis and fractionation of dextrans produced by fermentation of sucrose using *Leuconostoc mesenteroides* strain NRRL B-512 = CIP 78.59 or substrains thereof (for example *L. mesenteroides* B-512F = NCTC 10817).

It is prepared in conditions designed to minimise the risk of microbial contamination.

CHARACTERS

A white or almost white powder, very soluble in water, very slightly soluble in alcohol.

IDENTIFICATION

A. Dissolve 1.0 g in *water R*, heating on a water-bath, and dilute to 50.0 ml with the same solvent. The specific optical rotation (*2.2.7*) of the solution is + 195 to + 201, calculated with reference to the dried substance.

B. Examine by infrared absorption spectrophotometry (*2.2.24*), comparing with the spectrum obtained with *dextran CRS*.

C. It complies with the test for molecular-mass distribution (see Tests).

TESTS

Solution S. Dissolve 5.0 g in *distilled water R*, heating on a water-bath, and dilute to 50 ml with the same solvent.

Appearance of solution. Solution S is clear (*2.2.1*) and colourless (*2.2.2, Method II*).

Acidity or alkalinity. To 10 ml of solution S add 0.1 ml of *phenolphthalein solution R*. The solution remains colourless. Add 0.2 ml of *0.01 M sodium hydroxide*. The solution is red. Add 0.4 ml of *0.01 M hydrochloric acid*. The solution is colourless. Add 0.1 ml of *methyl red solution R*. The solution is red or orange.

Nitrogen-containing substances. Carry out the determination of nitrogen by sulphuric acid digestion (*2.5.9*), using 0.200 g and heating for 2 h. Collect the distillate in a mixture of 0.5 ml of *bromocresol green solution R*, 0.5 ml of *methyl red solution R* and 20 ml of *water R*. Titrate with *0.01 M hydrochloric acid*. Not more than 0.15 ml of *0.01 M hydrochloric acid* is required to change the colour of the indicator (110 ppm N).

Residual solvents. Examine by gas chromatography (*2.2.28*), using *propanol R* as internal standard.

Test solution. Dissolve 5 g of the substance to be examined in 100 ml of *water R* and distil. Collect the first 45 ml of the distillate, add 1 ml of a 25 g/l solution of *propanol R* and dilute to 50 ml with *water R*.

Reference solution. Mix 0.5 ml of a 25 g/l solution of *ethanol R*, 0.5 ml of a 25 g/l solution of *propanol R* and 0.5 ml of a 2.5 g/l solution of *methanol R* and dilute to 25.0 ml with *water R*.

The chromatographic procedure may be carried out using:
- a stainless steel column 1.8 m long and 2 mm in internal diameter packed with *ethylvinylbenzene-divinylbenzene copolymer R* (125-150 µm),
- *nitrogen for chromatography R* as the carrier gas at a flow rate of 25 ml/min,
- a flame-ionisation detector,

maintaining the temperature of the column at 190 °C, that of the injection port at 240 °C and that of the detector at 210 °C. Inject the chosen volume of each solution. In the chromatogram obtained with the test solution, the area of any peak corresponding to ethanol or methanol is not greater than the area of the corresponding peak in the chromatogram obtained with the reference solution (0.5 per cent of ethanol and 0.05 per cent of methanol) and the sum of the areas of any peaks, apart from the peaks corresponding to ethanol, methanol and the internal standard, is not greater than the area of the peak corresponding to the internal standard (0.5 per cent calculated as propanol).

Molecular-mass distribution (*2.2.39*). The average molecular mass (M_w) is 64 000 to 76 000. The average molecular mass of the 10 per cent high fraction is not more than 185 000. The average molecular mass of the 10 per cent low fraction is not less than 15 000.

Heavy metals (*2.4.8*). 12 ml of solution S complies with limit test A (10 ppm). Prepare the standard using *lead standard solution (1 ppm Pb) R*.

Loss on drying (*2.2.32*). Not more than 7.0 per cent, determined on 0.200 g by heating in an oven at 105 ± 2 °C for 5 h.

Sulphated ash (*2.4.14*). Not more than 0.3 per cent, determined on 0.50 g.

Bacterial endotoxins (*2.6.14*): less than 16 IU/g.

Microbial contamination. Total viable count (*2.6.12*) not more than 10^2 micro-organisms per gram, determined by plate-count. It complies with the test for *Escherichia coli* (*2.6.13*).

01/2005:1507

DEXTRIN

Dextrinum

DEFINITION

Dextrin is maize, potato or cassava starch partly hydrolysed and modified by heating with or without the presence of acids, alkalis or pH control agents.

CHARACTERS

White or almost white, free-flowing powder, very soluble in boiling water forming a mucilaginous solution, slowly soluble in cold water, practically insoluble in alcohol.

IDENTIFICATION

A. Suspend 1 g in 50 ml of *water R*, boil for 1 min and cool. To 1 ml of the solution add 0.05 ml of *iodine solution R1*. A dark blue to reddish-brown colour is produced which disappears on heating.

B. Centrifuge 5 ml of the mucilage obtained in identification test A. To the upper layer add 2 ml of *dilute sodium hydroxide solution R* and, dropwise with shaking, 0.5 ml of *copper sulphate solution R* and boil. A red precipitate is produced.

C. It is very soluble in boiling *water R*, forming a mucilaginous solution.

TESTS

pH (*2.2.3*). Disperse 5.0 g in 100 ml of *carbon dioxide-free water R*. The pH is 2.0 to 8.0.

Chlorides. Dissolve 2.5 g in 50 ml of boiling *water R*, dilute to 100 ml with *water R* and filter. Dilute 1 ml of the filtrate to 15 ml, add 1 ml of *dilute nitric acid R*, pour the mixture as a single addition into 1 ml of *silver nitrate solution R2* and allow to stand for 5 min protected from light. When viewed transversely against a black background any opalescence produced is not more intense than that obtained by treating a mixture of 10 ml of *chloride standard solution (5 ppm Cl) R* and 5 ml of *water R*, prepared in the same manner (0.2 per cent).

Reducing sugars. To a quantity of dextrin equivalent to 2.0 g (dried substance) add 100 ml of *water R*, shake for 30 min, dilute with *water R* to 200.0 ml and filter. To 10.0 ml of alkaline *cupri-tartaric solution R* add 20.0 ml of the filtrate, mix, and heat on a hot plate adjusted to bring the solution to boil within 3 min. Boil for 2 min, and cool immediately. Add 5 ml of a 300 g/l solution of *potassium iodide R* and 10 ml of *1 M sulphuric acid*, mix, and titrate immediately with *0.1 M sodium thiosulphate*, using *starch solution R*, added towards the end of the titration, as indicator. Repeat the procedure beginning with "To 10.0 ml of...", using, in place of the filtrate, 20.0 ml of a 1 g/l solution of *glucose R*, accurately prepared. Perform a blank titration. ($V_B - V_U$) is not greater than ($V_B - V_S$), in which V_B, V_U and V_S are the number of millilitres of *0.1 M sodium thiosulphate* consumed in the titrations of the blank, the dextrin and the glucose, respectively (10 per cent, calculated as glucose $C_6H_{12}O_6$).

Heavy metals (*2.4.8*). 1.0 g complies with limit test C for heavy metals (20 ppm). Prepare the standard using 2 ml of *lead standard solution (10 ppm Pb) R*.

Loss on drying (*2.2.32*). Not more than 13.0 per cent, determined on 1.000 g by drying at 130 °C to 135 °C for 90 min.

Sulphated ash (*2.4.14*). Not more than 0.5 per cent, determined on 1.0 g.

01/2005:0020

DEXTROMETHORPHAN HYDROBROMIDE

Dextromethorphani hydrobromidum

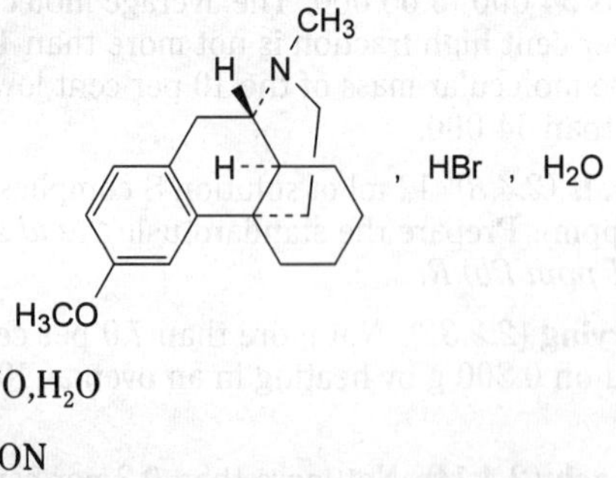

$C_{18}H_{26}BrNO,H_2O$ M_r 370.3

DEFINITION

ent-3-Methoxy-17-methylmorphinan hydrobromide monohydrate.

Content: 99.0 per cent to 101.0 per cent (anhydrous substance).

CHARACTERS

Appearance: almost white, crystalline powder.

Solubility: sparingly soluble in water, freely soluble in alcohol.

mp: about 125 °C, with decomposition.

IDENTIFICATION

First identification: A, B, D.

Second identification: A, C, D.

A. It complies with the test for specific optical rotation (see Tests).

B. Infrared absorption spectrophotometry (*2.2.24*).

Preparation: discs.

Comparison: *dextromethorphan hydrobromide CRS.*

C. Thin-layer chromatography (*2.2.27*).

Test solution. Dissolve 25 mg of the substance to be examined in *methanol R* and dilute to 10 ml with the same solvent.

Reference solution. Dissolve 25 mg of *dextromethorphan hydrobromide CRS* in *methanol R* and dilute to 10 ml with the same solvent.

Plate: *TLC silica gel G plate R.*

Mobile phase: *concentrated ammonia R, methylene chloride R, methanol R, ethyl acetate R, toluene R* (2:10:13:20:55 *V/V/V/V/V*).

Application: 5 µl.

Development: over 2/3 of the plate.

Drying: in air.

Detection: spray with *potassium iodobismuthate solution R2.*

Results: the principal spot in the chromatogram obtained with the test solution is similar in position and size to the principal spot in the chromatogram obtained with the reference solution.

D. It gives reaction (a) of bromides (*2.3.1*).

TESTS

Solution S. Dissolve 1.0 g in *alcohol R* and dilute to 20 ml with the same solvent.

Appearance of solution. Solution S is clear (*2.2.1*) and colourless (*2.2.2, Method II*).

Acidity or alkalinity. Dissolve 0.4 g in *carbon dioxide-free water R* with gentle heating, cool and dilute to 20 ml with the same solvent. Add 0.1 ml of *methyl red solution R* and 0.2 ml of *0.01 M sodium hydroxide.* The solution is yellow. Not more than 0.4 ml of *0.01 M hydrochloric acid* is required to change the colour of the indicator to red.

Specific optical rotation (*2.2.7*). + 28 to + 30 (anhydrous substance).

Dissolve 0.200 g in *0.1 M hydrochloric acid* and dilute to 10.0 ml with the same acid.

Related substances. Liquid chromatography (*2.2.29*).

Test solution. Dissolve 10.0 mg of the substance to be examined in the mobile phase and dilute to 10.0 ml with the mobile phase.

Reference solution (a). Dissolve 2 mg of *dextromethorphan impurity A CRS* in 2 ml of the test solution and dilute to 25.0 ml with the mobile phase.

Reference solution (b). Dilute 1.0 ml of the test solution to 200.0 ml with the mobile phase.

Column:

- *size*: *l* = 0.25 m, Ø = 4.6 mm,
- *stationary phase*: *octadecylsilyl silica gel for chromatography R* (5 µm).

Mobile phase: dissolve 3.11 g of *docusate sodium R* in a mixture of 400 ml of *water R* and 600 ml of *acetonitrile R.* Add 0.56 g of *ammonium nitrate R.* Adjust to apparent pH 2.0 with *glacial acetic acid R.*

Flow rate: 1.0 ml/min.

Detection: spectrophotometer at 280 nm.

Injection: 20 µl.

Run time: twice the retention time of dextromethorphan.

Relative retention with reference to dextromethorphan (retention time = about 21.9 min): impurity B = about 0.44; impurity C = about 0.85; impurity D = about 0.90; impurity A = about 1.13.

System suitability: reference solution (a):

- *resolution*: minimum 1.5 between the peaks due to impurity A and dextromethorphan.

Limits:

- *correction factor*: for the calculation of content, multiply the peak area of impurity C by 0.2,
- *any impurity*: not more than the area of the principal peak in the chromatogram obtained with reference solution (b) (0.5 per cent), and not more than 1 such peak has an area greater than half the area of the principal peak in the chromatogram obtained with reference solution (b) (0.25 per cent),
- *total*: not more than twice the area of the principal peak in the chromatogram obtained with reference solution (b) (1 per cent),
- *disregard limit*: 0.1 times the area of the principal peak in the chromatogram obtained with reference solution (b) (0.05 per cent).

***N,N*-Dimethylaniline**: maximum 10 ppm.

Dissolve 0.5 g with heating in 20 ml of *water R.* Allow to cool, add 2 ml of *dilute acetic acid R* and 1 ml of a 10 g/l solution of *sodium nitrite R* and dilute to 25 ml with *water R.* The solution is not more intensely coloured than a reference solution prepared at the same time in the same manner using 20 ml of a 0.25 mg/l solution of *dimethylaniline R.*

Water (*2.5.12*): 4.0 per cent to 5.5 per cent, determined on 0.200 g.

Sulphated ash (*2.4.14*): maximum 0.1 per cent, determined on 1.0 g.

ASSAY

Dissolve 0.300 g in a mixture of 5.0 ml of *0.01 M hydrochloric acid* and 20 ml of *alcohol R.* Titrate with *0.1 M sodium hydroxide,* determining the end-point potentiometrically (*2.2.20*). Read the volume added between the 2 points of inflexion.

1 ml of *0.1 M sodium hydroxide* is equivalent to 35.23 mg of $C_{18}H_{26}BrNO$.

STORAGE

Protected from light.

Monographs D-E

IMPURITIES

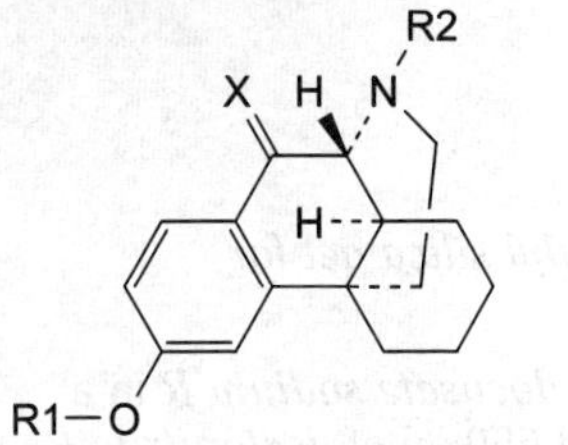

A. R1 = CH_3, R2 = H, X = H_2: *ent*-3-methoxymorphinan,

B. R1 = H, R2 = CH_3, X = H_2: *ent*-17-methylmorphinan-3-ol,

C. R1 = R2 = CH_3, X = O: *ent*-3-methoxy-17-methylmorphinan-10-one,

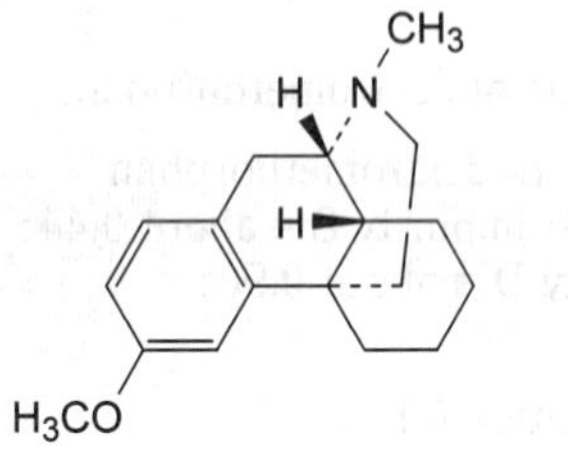

D. *ent*-(14*S*)-3-methoxy-17-methylmorphinan.

01/2005:0021

DEXTROMORAMIDE TARTRATE

Dextromoramidi tartras

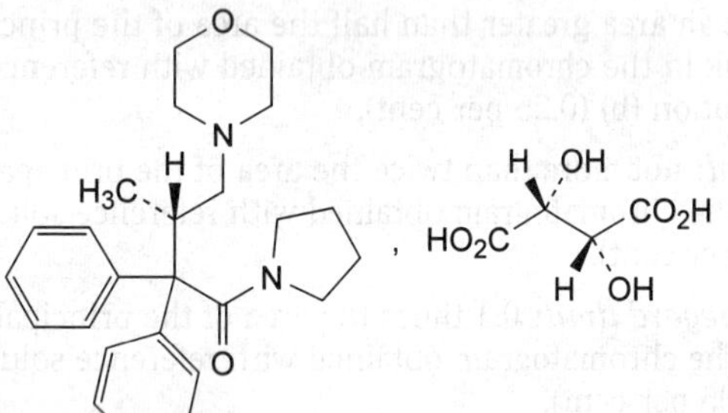

$C_{29}H_{38}N_2O_8$ M_r 542.6

DEFINITION

Dextromoramide tartrate contains not less than 98.0 per cent and not more than the equivalent of 101.0 per cent of 1-[(3*S*)-3-methyl-4-(morpholin-4-yl)-2,2-diphenylbutanoyl]pyrrolidine hydrogen (2*R*,3*R*)-2,3-dihydroxybutanedioate, calculated with reference to the dried substance.

CHARACTERS

A white, amorphous or crystalline powder, soluble in water, sparingly soluble in alcohol.

It melts at about 190 °C, with slight decomposition.

IDENTIFICATION

A. Dissolve 75 mg in *1 M hydrochloric acid* and dilute to 100.0 ml with the same acid. Examined between 230 nm and 350 nm (*2.2.25*), the solution shows 3 absorption maxima, at 254 nm, 259 nm and 264 nm. The specific absorbances at the maxima are about 6.9, 7.7 and 6.5, respectively.

B. Dissolve about 50 mg in *water R* and dilute to 10 ml with the same solvent. To 2 ml of the solution add 3 ml of *ammoniacal silver nitrate solution R* and heat on a water-bath. A grey or black precipitate is formed.

C. It gives reaction (b) of tartrates (*2.3.1*).

TESTS

pH (*2.2.3*). Dissolve 0.2 g in *carbon dioxide-free water R* and dilute to 20 ml with the same solvent. The pH of the solution is 3.0 to 4.0.

Specific optical rotation (*2.2.7*). Dissolve 0.50 g in *0.1 M hydrochloric acid* and dilute to 10.0 ml with the same acid. The specific optical rotation is + 21 to + 23.

Related substances. Examine by thin-layer chromatography (*2.2.27*), using *silica gel G R* as the coating substance.

Test solution. Dissolve 0.2 g of the substance to be examined in *methanol R* and dilute to 10 ml with the same solvent.

Reference solution. Dilute 1 ml of the test solution to 100 ml with *methanol R*.

Apply separately to the plate 10 µl of each solution. Develop over a path of 15 cm using *methanol R*. Allow the plate to dry in air and spray with *dilute potassium iodobismuthate solution R*. Any spot in the chromatogram obtained with the test solution, apart from the principal spot, is not more intense than the spot in the chromatogram obtained with the reference solution (1.0 per cent).

Loss on drying (*2.2.32*). Not more than 0.5 per cent, determined on 1.00 g by drying in an oven at 100 °C to 105 °C.

Sulphated ash (*2.4.14*). Not more than 0.1 per cent, determined on 1.0 g.

ASSAY

Dissolve 0.250 g in 30 ml of *anhydrous acetic acid R*. Titrate with *0.05 M perchloric acid* using 0.15 ml of *naphtholbenzein solution R* as indicator.

1 ml of *0.05 M perchloric acid* is equivalent to 27.13 mg of $C_{29}H_{38}N_2O_8$.

01/2005:0713

DEXTROPROPOXYPHENE HYDROCHLORIDE

Dextropropoxypheni hydrochloridum

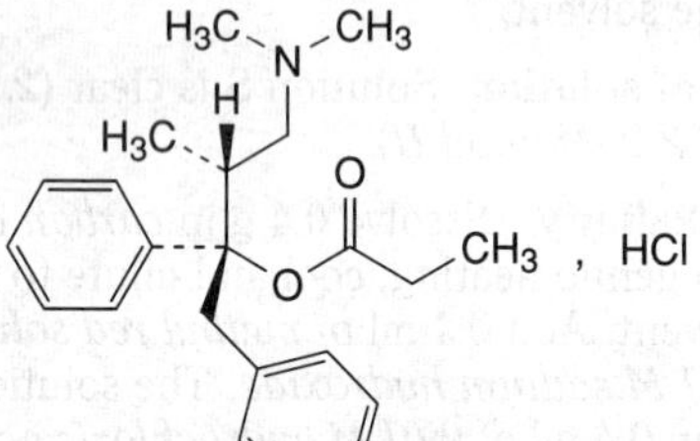

$C_{22}H_{30}ClNO_2$ M_r 375.9

DEFINITION

Dextropropoxyphene hydrochloride contains not less than 98.5 per cent and not more than the equivalent of 101.0 per cent of (1*S*,2*R*)-1-benzyl-3-(dimethylamino)-2-methyl-1-phenylpropyl propanoate hydrochloride, calculated with reference to the dried substance.

CHARACTERS

A white or almost white, crystalline powder, very soluble in water, freely soluble in alcohol.

It melts at about 165 °C.

IDENTIFICATION

First identification: A, C, D.

Second identification: A, B, D.

A. It complies with the test for specific optical rotation (see Tests).

B. Dissolve 50.0 mg in *0.01 M hydrochloric acid* and dilute to 100.0 ml with the same acid. Examined between 220 nm and 360 nm (*2.2.25*), the solution shows 3 absorption maxima, at 252 nm, 257 nm and 263 nm and 2 shoulders, at 240 nm and 246 nm. The ratio of the absorbance at the maximum at 257 nm to that at the maximum at 252 nm is 1.22 to 1.28. The ratio of the absorbance at the maximum at 257 nm to that at the maximum at 263 nm is 1.29 to 1.35. The test is not valid unless, in the test for resolution (*2.2.25*), the ratio of the absorbances is at least 1.5.

C. Examine by infrared absorption spectrophotometry (*2.2.24*), comparing with the *Ph. Eur. reference spectrum of dextropropoxyphene hydrochloride*.

D. Solution S (see Tests) gives reaction (a) of chlorides (*2.3.1*).

TESTS

Solution S. Dissolve 1.5 g in *carbon dioxide-free water R* and dilute to 30 ml with the same solvent.

Appearance of solution. Solution S is clear (*2.2.1*) and colourless (*2.2.2, Method II*).

Acidity or alkalinity. Dilute 10 ml of solution S to 25 ml with *carbon dioxide-free water R*. To 10 ml of this solution, add 0.1 ml of *methyl red solution R* and 0.2 ml of *0.01 M sodium hydroxide*. The solution is yellow. Add 0.4 ml of *0.01 M hydrochloric acid*. The solution is red.

Specific optical rotation (*2.2.7*). Dissolve 0.100 g in *water R* and dilute to 10.0 ml with the same solvent. The specific optical rotation is + 52 to + 57.

Related substances. Examine by liquid chromatography (*2.2.29*).

Test solution. Dissolve 50.0 mg of the substance to be examined in the mobile phase and dilute to 10.0 ml with the mobile phase.

Reference solution (a). Dilute 0.50 ml of the test solution to 100.0 ml with the mobile phase.

Reference solution (b). Dissolve 50.0 mg of the substance to be examined in 2.5 ml of *2 M alcoholic potassium hydroxide*. Add 2.5 ml of *water R* and boil under a reflux condenser for 30 min. Add 2.5 ml of *dilute hydrochloric acid R* and dilute to 50 ml with the mobile phase.

The chromatographic procedure may be carried out using:

- a column 0.125 m long and 4.6 mm in internal diameter packed with *silica gel for chromatography R* (5 µm),
- a guard column packed with a suitable silica gel, equilibrated with the mobile phase and placed between the column and the injection device,
- as mobile phase at a flow rate of 1.0 ml/min a mixture of 50 volumes of *0.2 M phosphate buffer solution pH 7.5 R*, 84 volumes of *tetrahydrofuran R*, 350 volumes of *methanol R* and 516 volumes of *water R*, containing 0.9 g/l of *cetyltrimethylammonium bromide R*,
- as detector a spectrophotometer set at 220 nm,
- a loop injector.

Equilibrate the chromatographic system by passage of the mobile phase for 16 h (the mobile phase may be recirculated after 6 h).

Inject 20 µl of each solution and record the chromatograms for twice the retention time of the principal peak. The test is not valid unless:

- the chromatogram obtained with reference solution (a) shows a peak with a signal-to-noise ratio of at least 5,
- the chromatogram obtained with reference solution (b) shows 2 peaks with a resolution of not less than 2.0.

In the chromatogram obtained with the test solution, the area of any peak, apart from the principal peak, is not greater than the area of the principal peak in the chromatogram obtained with reference solution (a) (0.5 per cent).

Heavy metals (*2.4.8*). 12 ml of solution S complies with limit test A (20 ppm). Prepare the standard using *lead standard solution (1 ppm Pb) R*.

Loss on drying (*2.2.32*). Not more than 1.0 per cent, determined on 1.000 g by drying in an oven at 100-105 °C.

Sulphated ash (*2.4.14*). Not more than 0.1 per cent, determined on 1.0 g.

ASSAY

Dissolve 0.270 g in 60 ml of *acetic anhydride R*. Titrate with *0.1 M perchloric acid*, determining the end-point potentiometrically (*2.2.20*).

1 ml of *0.1 M perchloric acid* is equivalent to 37.59 mg of $C_{22}H_{30}ClNO_2$.

STORAGE

Protected from light.

IMPURITIES

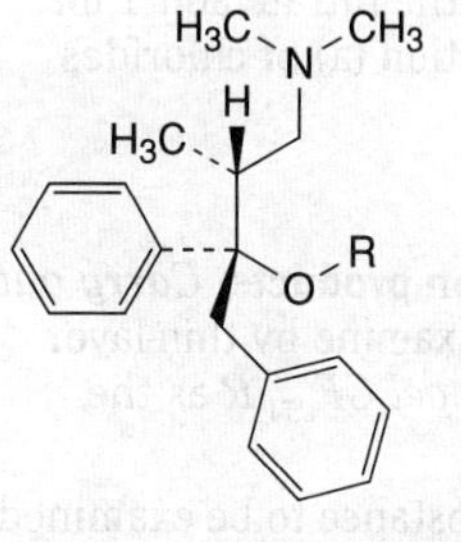

A. R = H: (2*S*,3*R*)-4-(dimethylamino)-1,2-diphenyl-3-methylbutan-2-ol,

B. R = CO-CH_3: (1*S*,2*R*)-1-benzyl-3-(dimethylamino)-2-methyl-1-phenylpropyl acetate.

01/2005:0022

DIAZEPAM

Diazepamum

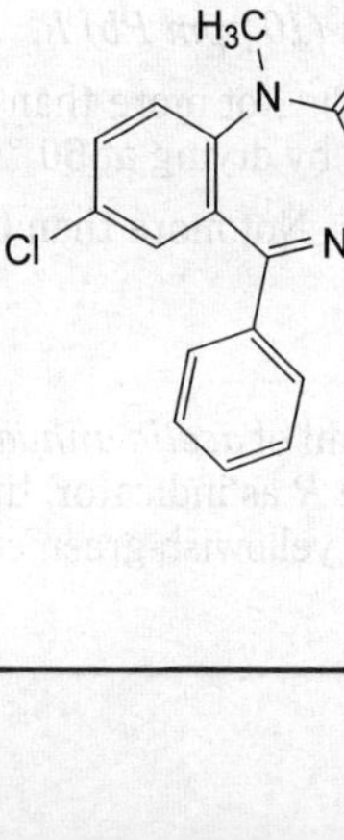

$C_{16}H_{13}ClN_2O$ M_r 284.7

DEFINITION

Diazepam contains not less than 99.0 per cent and not more than the equivalent of 101.0 per cent of 7-chloro-1-methyl-5-phenyl-1,3-dihydro-2*H*-1,4-benzodiazepin-2-one, calculated with reference to the dried substance.

CHARACTERS

A white or almost white, crystalline powder, very slightly soluble in water, soluble in alcohol.

IDENTIFICATION

A. Melting point (*2.2.14*): 131 °C to 135 °C.

B. *Protect the solutions from bright light and measure the absorbances immediately.* Dissolve 25 mg in a 5 g/l solution of *sulphuric acid R* in *methanol R* and dilute to 250.0 ml with the same acid solution (solution A). Dilute 5.0 ml of solution A to 100.0 ml with a 5 g/l solution of *sulphuric acid R* in *methanol R*. Examined between 230 nm and 330 nm (*2.2.25*), the solution shows 2 absorption maxima, at 242 nm and 285 nm. The specific absorbance at the maximum at 242 nm is about 1020. Dilute 25.0 ml of solution A to 100.0 ml with a 5 g/l solution of *sulphuric acid R* in *methanol R*. Examined between 325 nm and 400 nm, the solution shows a single absorption maximum at 366 nm. The specific absorbance at the maximum is 140 to 155.

C. Dissolve about 10 mg in 3 ml of *sulphuric acid R*. The solution shows greenish-yellow fluorescence in ultraviolet light at 365 nm.

D. To 80 mg in a porcelain crucible add 0.3 g of *anhydrous sodium carbonate R*. Heat over an open flame for 10 min. Allow to cool. Take up the residue with 5 ml of *dilute nitric acid R* and filter. To 1 ml of the filtrate add 1 ml of *water R*. The solution gives reaction (a) of chlorides (*2.3.1*).

TESTS

Related substances and decomposition products. *Carry out the test protected from bright light.* Examine by thin-layer chromatography (*2.2.27*), using *silica gel GF_{254} R* as the coating substance.

Test solution. Dissolve 1.0 g of the substance to be examined in *acetone R* and dilute to 10 ml with the same solvent. Prepare immediately before use.

Reference solution. Dilute 1 ml of the test solution to 100 ml with *acetone R*. Dilute 1 ml of this solution to 10 ml with *acetone R*.

Apply separately to the plate 5 µl of each solution. Develop over a path of 12 cm using a mixture of equal volumes of *ethyl acetate R* and *hexane R*. Allow the plate to dry and examine in ultraviolet light at 254 nm. Any spot in the chromatogram obtained with the test solution, apart from the principal spot, is not more intense than the spot in the chromatogram obtained with the reference solution (0.1 per cent).

Heavy metals (*2.4.8*). 2.0 g complies with limit test C for heavy metals (20 ppm). Prepare the standard using 4 ml of *lead standard solution (10 ppm Pb) R*.

Loss on drying (*2.2.32*). Not more than 0.5 per cent, determined on 1.000 g by drying at 60 °C *in vacuo* for 4 h.

Sulphated ash (*2.4.14*). Not more than 0.1 per cent, determined on 1.0 g.

ASSAY

Dissolve 0.500 g in 50 ml of *acetic anhydride R*. Using 0.3 ml of *Nile blue A solution R* as indicator, titrate with *0.1 M perchloric acid* until a yellowish-green colour is obtained.

1 ml of *0.1 M perchloric acid* is equivalent to 28.47 mg of $C_{16}H_{13}ClN_2O$.

STORAGE

Store protected from light.

01/2005:0550

DIAZOXIDE

Diazoxidum

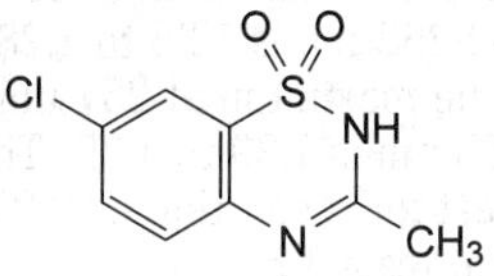

$C_8H_7ClN_2O_2S$ M_r 230.7

DEFINITION

Diazoxide contains not less than 98.0 per cent and not more than the equivalent of 101.0 per cent of 7-chloro-3-methyl-2*H*-1,2,4-benzothiadiazine 1,1-dioxide, calculated with reference to the dried substance.

CHARACTERS

A white or almost white, fine or crystalline powder, practically insoluble in water, freely soluble in dimethylformamide, slightly soluble in alcohol. It is very soluble in dilute solutions of the alkali hydroxides.

IDENTIFICATION

First identification: B.

Second identification: A, C, D.

A. Dissolve 50.0 mg in 5 ml of *1 M sodium hydroxide* and dilute to 50.0 ml with *water R*. Dilute 1.0 ml of this solution to 100.0 ml with *0.1 M sodium hydroxide*. Examined between 230 nm and 350 nm (*2.2.25*), the solution shows an absorption maximum at 280 nm and a shoulder at 304 nm. The specific absorbance at the maximum is 570 to 610.

B. Examine by infrared absorption spectrophotometry (*2.2.24*), comparing with the spectrum obtained with *diazoxide CRS*. Examine the substances prepared as discs using *potassium bromide R*.

C. Examine the chromatograms obtained in the test for related substances in ultraviolet light at 254 nm. The principal spot in the chromatogram obtained with test solution (b) is similar in position and size to the principal spot in the chromatogram obtained with reference solution (b).

D. Dissolve about 20 mg in a mixture of 5 ml of *hydrochloric acid R* and 10 ml of *water R*. Add 0.1 g of *zinc powder R*. Boil for 5 min, cool and filter. To the filtrate add 2 ml of a 1 g/l solution of *sodium nitrite R* and mix. Allow to stand for 1 min and add 1 ml of a 5 g/l solution of *naphthylethylenediamine dihydrochloride R*. A red or violet-red colour develops.

TESTS

Appearance of solution. Dissolve 0.4 g in 2 ml of *1 M sodium hydroxide* and dilute to 20 ml with *water R*. The solution is clear (*2.2.1*) and not more intensely coloured than reference solution Y_7 (*2.2.2, Method II*).

Acidity or alkalinity. To 0.5 g of the powdered substance to be examined add 30 ml of *carbon dioxide-free water R*, shake for 2 min and filter. To 10 ml of the filtrate add 0.2 ml of *0.01 M sodium hydroxide* and 0.15 ml of *methyl red*

Monographs D-E

solution R. The solution is yellow. Not more than 0.4 ml of *0.01 M hydrochloric acid* is required to change the colour of the indicator to red.

Related substances. Examine by thin-layer chromatography (*2.2.27*), using *silica gel GF_{254} R* as the coating substance.

Test solution (a). Dissolve 0.1 g of the substance to be examined in a mixture of 0.5 ml of *1 M sodium hydroxide* and 1 ml of *methanol R* and dilute to 5 ml with *methanol R.*

Test solution (b). Dilute 1 ml of test solution (a) to 5 ml with a mixture of 1 volume of *1 M sodium hydroxide* and 9 volumes of *methanol R.*

Reference solution (a). Dilute 0.5 ml of test solution (a) to 100 ml with a mixture of 1 volume of *1 M sodium hydroxide* and 9 volumes of *methanol R.*

Reference solution (b). Dissolve 20 mg of *diazoxide CRS* in a mixture of 0.5 ml of *1 M sodium hydroxide* and 1 ml of *methanol R* and dilute to 5 ml with *methanol R.*

Apply separately to the plate 5 µl of each solution. Develop over a path of 15 cm using a mixture of 7 volumes of *concentrated ammonia R,* 25 volumes of *methanol R* and 68 volumes of *chloroform R.* Allow the plate to dry in air and examine in ultraviolet light at 254 nm. Any spot in the chromatogram obtained with test solution (a), apart from the principal spot, is not more intense than the spot in the chromatogram obtained with reference solution (a) (0.5 per cent).

Loss on drying (*2.2.32*). Not more than 0.5 per cent, determined on 1.000 g by drying in an oven at 100 °C to 105 °C for 2 h.

Sulphated ash (*2.4.14*). Not more than 0.1 per cent, determined on 1.0 g.

ASSAY

Dissolve 0.200 g with gentle heating in 50 ml of a mixture of 1 volume of *water R* and 2 volumes of *dimethylformamide R.* Titrate with *0.1 M sodium hydroxide,* determining the end-point potentiometrically (*2.2.20*). Carry out a blank titration.

1 ml of *0.1 M sodium hydroxide* is equivalent to 23.07 mg of $C_8H_7ClN_2O_2S$.

01/2005:0762

DIBUTYL PHTHALATE

Dibutylis phthalas

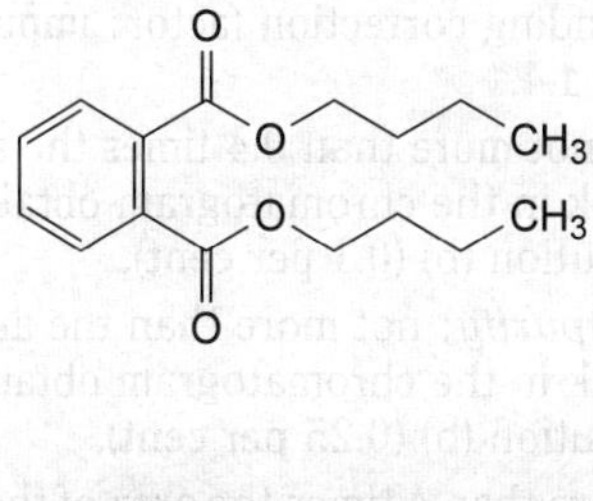

$C_{16}H_{22}O_4$ M_r 278.3

DEFINITION

Dibutyl phthalate contains not less than 99.0 per cent and not more than the equivalent of 101.0 per cent *m/m* of dibutyl benzene-1,2-dicarboxylate.

CHARACTERS

A clear, oily liquid, colourless or very slightly yellow, practically insoluble in water, miscible with alcohol.

IDENTIFICATION

First identification: B, C.

Second identification: A, D, E.

A. Relative density (*2.2.5*): 1.043 to 1.048.

B. Refractive index (*2.2.6*): 1.490 to 1.495.

C. Examine by infrared absorption spectrophotometry (*2.2.24*), comparing with the spectrum obtained with *dibutyl phthalate CRS.*

D. Examine by thin-layer chromatography (*2.2.27*), using *silica gel GF_{254} R* as the coating substance.

Test solution. Dissolve 50 mg of the substance to be examined in *ether R* and dilute to 10 ml with the same solvent.

Reference solution. Dissolve 50 mg of *dibutyl phthalate CRS* in *ether R* and dilute to 10 ml with the same solvent.

Apply separately to the plate 10 µl of each solution. Develop over a path of 15 cm using a mixture of 30 volumes of *heptane R* and 70 volumes of *ether R.* Allow the plate to dry in air and examine in ultraviolet light at 254 nm. The principal spot in the chromatogram obtained with the test solution is similar in position and size to the principal spot in the chromatogram obtained with the reference solution.

E. To about 0.1 ml add 0.25 ml of *sulphuric acid R* and 50 mg of *resorcinol R.* Heat in a water-bath for 5 min. Allow to cool. Add 10 ml of *water R* and 1 ml of *strong sodium hydroxide solution R.* The solution becomes yellow or brownish-yellow and shows a green fluorescence.

TESTS

Appearance. The substance to be examined is clear (*2.2.1*) and not more intensely coloured than reference solution Y_6 (*2.2.2, Method II*).

Acidity. Dissolve 20.0 g in 50 ml of *alcohol R* previously neutralised to *phenolphthalein solution R1.* Add 0.2 ml of *phenolphthalein solution R1.* Not more than 0.50 ml of *0.1 M sodium hydroxide* is required to change the colour of the indicator.

Related substances. Examine by gas chromatography (*2.2.28*), using *bibenzyl R* as internal standard.

Internal standard solution. Dissolve 60 mg of *bibenzyl R* in *methylene chloride R* and dilute to 20 ml with the same solvent.

Test solution (a). Dissolve 1.0 g of the substance to be examined in *methylene chloride R* and dilute to 20.0 ml with the same solvent.

Test solution (b). Dissolve 1.0 g of the substance to be examined in *methylene chloride R,* add 2.0 ml of the internal standard solution and dilute to 20.0 ml with *methylene chloride R.*

Reference solution. To 1.0 ml of test solution (a) add 10.0 ml of the internal standard solution and dilute to 100.0 ml with *methylene chloride R.*

The chromatographic procedure may be carried out using:

- a glass column 1.5 m long and 4 mm in internal diameter, packed with *silanised diatomaceous earth for gas chromatography R* (150 µm to 180 µm) impregnated with 3 per cent *m/m* of *polymethylphenylsiloxane R,*
- *nitrogen for chromatography R* as the carrier gas at a flow rate of 30 ml per minute,
- a flame-ionisation detector,

maintaining the temperature of the column at 190 °C and that of the injection port and of the detector at 225 °C.

Inject 1 µl of the reference solution. The substances elute in the following order: bibenzyl and dibutyl phthalate. Adjust the sensitivity of the detector so that the height of the bibenzyl peak is not less than 70 per cent of the full scale of the recorder. The test is not valid unless the resolution between the peaks corresponding to bibenzyl and dibutyl phthalate is at least 12.

Inject 1 µl of test solution (a). In the chromatogram obtained, verify that there is no peak with the same retention time as the internal standard.

Inject separately 1 µl of test solution (b) and the reference solution. Continue the chromatography for 3 times the retention time of dibutyl phthalate, which is about 12 min. From the chromatogram obtained with the reference solution, calculate the ratio (*R*) of the area of the peak due to dibutyl phthalate to the area of the peak due to the internal standard. From the chromatogram obtained with test solution (b), calculate the ratio of the sum of the areas of any peaks, apart from the principal peak, the peak due to the internal standard and the peak due to the solvent, to the area of the peak due to the internal standard: this ratio is not greater than *R* (1.0 per cent).

Water (*2.5.12*). Not more than 0.2 per cent, determined on 10.00 g by the semi-micro determination of water.

Sulphated ash (*2.4.14*). Not more than 0.1 per cent, determined on 1.0 g.

ASSAY

Introduce 0.750 g into a 250 ml borosilicate glass flask. Add 25.0 ml of *0.5 M alcoholic potassium hydroxide* and a few glass beads. Heat in a water-bath under a reflux condenser for 1 h. Add 1 ml of *phenolphthalein solution R1* and titrate immediately with *0.5 M hydrochloric acid* until the colour changes from red to colourless. Carry out a blank titration. Calculate the volume of potassium hydroxide used in the saponification.

1 ml of *0.5 M alcoholic potassium hydroxide* is equivalent to 69.59 mg of $C_{16}H_{22}O_4$.

STORAGE

Store in an airtight container.

01/2005:1718

DICLAZURIL FOR VETERINARY USE

Diclazurilum ad usum veterinarium

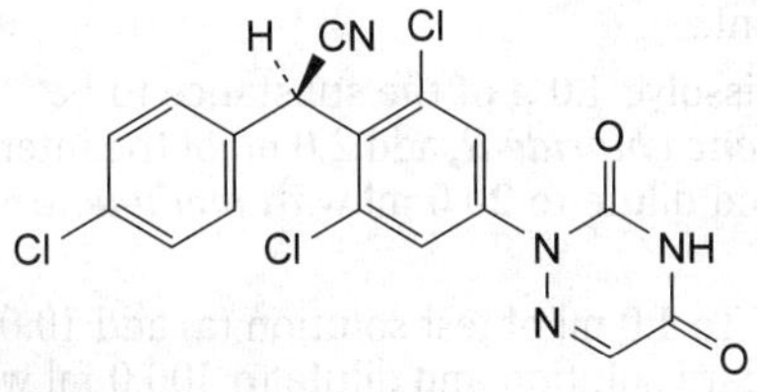

$C_{17}H_9Cl_3N_4O_2$ M_r 407.6

DEFINITION

(*RS*)-(4-Chlorophenyl)[2,6-dichloro-4-(3,5-dioxo-4,5-dihydro-1,2,4-triazin-2(3*H*)-yl)phenyl]acetonitrile.

Content: 99.0 per cent to 101.0 per cent (dried substance).

CHARACTERS

Appearance: white or light yellow powder.

Solubility: practically insoluble in water, sparingly soluble in dimethylformamide, practically insoluble in alcohol and methylene chloride.

IDENTIFICATION

Infrared absorption spectrophotometry (*2.2.24*).

Comparison: *Ph. Eur. reference spectrum of diclazuril.*

TESTS

Related substances. Liquid chromatography (*2.2.29*).

Test solution. Dissolve 20.0 mg of the substance to be examined in *dimethylformamide R* and dilute to 20.0 ml with the same solvent.

Reference solution (a). Dissolve 5 mg of *diclazuril for system suitability CRS* in *dimethylformamide R* and dilute to 5.0 ml with the same solvent.

Reference solution (b). Dilute 1.0 ml of the test solution to 100.0 ml with *dimethylformamide R*. Dilute 5.0 ml of the solution to 20.0 ml with *dimethylformamide R*.

Column:
- *size*: *l* = 0.10 m, Ø = 4.6 mm,
- *stationary phase*: *base-deactivated octadecylsilyl silica gel for chromatography R* (3 µm),
- *temperature*: 35 °C.

Mobile phase:
- *mobile phase A*: mix 10 volumes of a 6.3 g/l solution of *ammonium formate R* adjusted to pH 4.0 with *anhydrous formic acid R*, 15 volumes of *acetonitrile R* and 75 volumes of *water R*,
- *mobile phase B*: mix 10 volumes of a 6.3 g/l solution of *ammonium formate R* adjusted to pH 4.0 with *anhydrous formic acid* R, 85 volumes of *acetonitrile R* and 5 volumes of *water R*,

Time (min)	Mobile phase A (per cent *V/V*)	Mobile phase B (per cent *V/V*)
0 - 20	100 → 0	0 → 100
20 - 25	0	100
25 - 26	0 → 100	100 → 0
26 - 36	100	0

Flow rate: 1.0 ml/min.

Detection: spectrophotometer at 230 nm.

Injection: 5 µl.

System suitability: reference solution (a):
- *peak-to-valley ratio*: minimum of 1.5, where H_p = height above the baseline of the peak due to impurity D and H_v = height above the baseline of the lowest point of the curve separating this peak from the peak due to diclazuril.

Limits:
- *correction factors*: for the calculation of contents, multiply the peak areas of the following impurities by the corresponding correction factor: impurity D = 1.9; impurity H = 1.4,
- *impurity D*: not more than 0.4 times the area of the principal peak in the chromatogram obtained with reference solution (b) (0.1 per cent),
- *any other impurity*: not more than the area of the principal peak in the chromatogram obtained with reference solution (b) (0.25 per cent),
- *total*: not more than 4 times the area of the principal peak in the chromatogram obtained with reference solution (b) (1.0 per cent),
- *disregard limit*: 0.2 times the area of the principal peak in the chromatogram obtained with reference solution (b) (0.05 per cent).

Loss on drying (*2.2.32*): maximum 0.5 per cent, determined on 1.000 g by drying in an oven at 100-105 °C for 4 h.

Sulphated ash (*2.4.14*): maximum 0.1 per cent, determined on 1.0 g.

ASSAY

Dissolve 0.150 g in 75 ml of *dimethylformamide R*. Carry out a potentiometric titration (*2.2.20*), using *0.1 M tetrabutylammonium hydroxide*. Read the volume added at the second inflexion point. Carry out a blank titration.

1 ml of *0.1 M tetrabutylammonium hydroxide* is equivalent to 20.38 mg of $C_{17}H_9Cl_3N_4O_2$.

STORAGE

Protected from light.

IMPURITIES

Specified impurities: A, B, C, D, E, F, G, H, I.

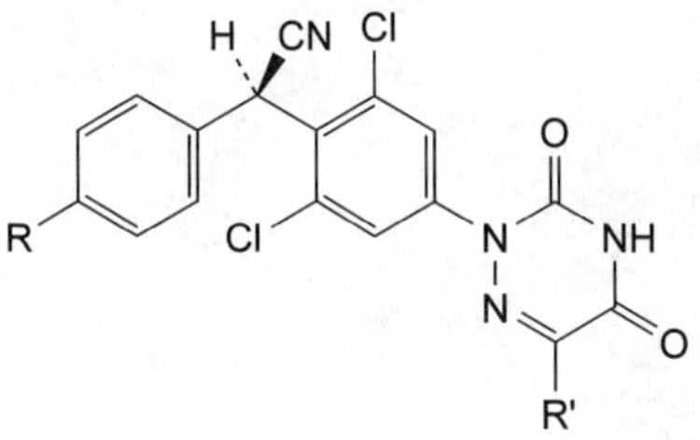

and enantiomer

A. R = Cl, R′ = CO_2H: 2-[3,5-dichloro-4-[(*RS*)-(4-chlorophenyl)cyanomethyl]phenyl]-3,5-dioxo-2,3,4,5-tetrahydro-1,2,4-triazine-6-carboxylic acid,

B. R = OH, R′ = H: (*RS*)-[2,6-dichloro-4-(3,5-dioxo-4,5-dihydro-1,2,4-triazin-2(3*H*)-yl)phenyl](4-hydroxyphenyl)acetonitrile,

C. R = Cl, R′ = $CONH_2$: 2-[3,5-dichloro-4-[(*RS*)-(4-chlorophenyl)cyanomethyl]phenyl]-3,5-dioxo-2,3,4,5-tetrahydro-1,2,4-triazine-6-carboxamide,

G. R = Cl, R′ = CO-O-$[CH_2]_3$-CH_3: butyl 2-[3,5-dichloro-4-[(*RS*)-(4-chlorophenyl)cyanomethyl]phenyl]-3,5-dioxo-2,3,4,5-tetrahydro-1,2,4-triazine-6-carboxylate,

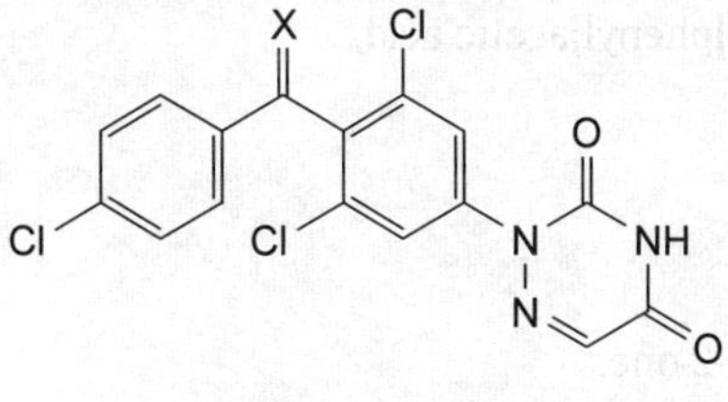

D. X = O: 2-[3,5-dichloro-4-(4-chlorobenzoyl)phenyl]-1,2,4-triazine-3,5(2*H*,4*H*)-dione,

F. X = H_2: 2-[3,5-dichloro-4-(4-chlorobenzyl)phenyl]-1,2,4-triazine-3,5(2*H*,4*H*)-dione,

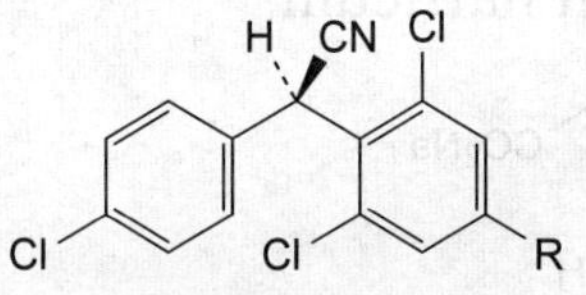

and enantiomer

E. R = NH_2: (*RS*)-(4-amino-2,6-dichlorophenyl)(4-chlorophenyl)acetonitrile,

H. R = H: (*RS*)-(4-chlorophenyl)(2,6-dichlorophenyl)acetonitrile,

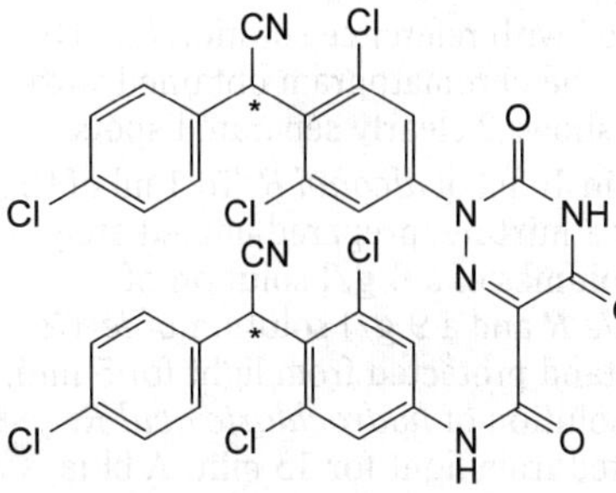

I. *N*,2-bis[3,5-dichloro-4-[(4-chlorophenyl)cyanomethyl]phenyl]-3,5-dioxo-2,3,4,5-tetrahydro-1,2,4-triazine-6-carboxamide.

01/2005:1508

DICLOFENAC POTASSIUM

Diclofenacum kalicum

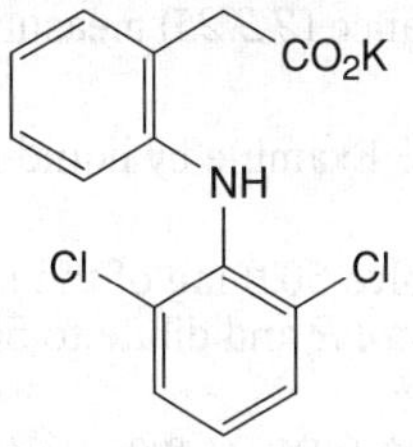

$C_{14}H_{10}Cl_2KNO_2$ M_r 334.2

DEFINITION

Potassium diclofenac contains not less than 99.0 per cent and not more than the equivalent of 101.0 per cent of potassium [2-[(2,6-dichlorophenyl)amino]phenyl]acetate, calculated with reference to the dried substance.

CHARACTERS

A white or slightly yellowish, crystalline powder, slightly hygroscopic, sparingly soluble in water, freely soluble in methanol, soluble in alcohol, slightly soluble in acetone.

IDENTIFICATION

First identification: A, D.

Second identification: B, C, D.

A. Examine by infrared absorption spectrophotometry (*2.2.24*), comparing with the spectrum obtained with *diclofenac potassium CRS*. Examine the substances prepared as discs.

B. Examine by thin-layer chromatography (*2.2.27*), using a *TLC silica gel GF_{254} plate R*.

Test solution. Dissolve 25 mg of the substance to be examined in *methanol R* and dilute to 5 ml with the same solvent.

Reference solution (a). Dissolve 25 mg of *diclofenac potassium CRS* in *methanol R* and dilute to 5 ml with the same solvent.

Reference solution (b). Dissolve 10 mg of *indometacin R* in reference solution (a) and dilute to 2 ml with the same solution.

Apply to the plate 5 µl of each solution. Develop over a path of 10 cm using a mixture of 10 volumes of *concentrated ammonia R*, 10 volumes of *methanol R* and 80 volumes of *ethyl acetate R*. Allow the plate to dry in air. Examine in ultraviolet light at 254 nm. The principal spot in the chromatogram obtained with the test solution is similar in position and size to the principal spot in the chromatogram obtained with reference solution (a). The test is not valid unless the chromatogram obtained with reference solution (b) shows 2 clearly separated spots.

C. Dissolve about 10 mg in 10 ml of *alcohol R*. To 1 ml of the solution add 0.2 ml of a mixture, prepared immediately before use, of equal volumes of a 6 g/l solution of *potassium ferricyanide R* and a 9 g/l solution of *ferric chloride R*. Allow to stand protected from light for 5 min. Add 3 ml of a 10 g/l solution of *hydrochloric acid R*. Allow to stand protected from light for 15 min. A blue colour develops and a precipitate is formed.

D. Suspend 0.5 g of the substance to be examined in 10 ml of *water R*. Stir, add *water R* until the substance is dissolved. Add 2 ml of *hydrochloric acid R1*, stir for 1 h and filter with the aid of vacuum. Neutralise the solution with *sodium hydroxide solution R*. The solution gives reaction (b) of potassium (*2.3.1*).

TESTS

Appearance of solution. Dissolve 1.25 g in *methanol R* and dilute to 25.0 ml with the same solvent. The solution is clear (*2.2.1*). The absorbance (*2.2.25*) measured at 440 nm is not greater than 0.05.

Related substances. Examine by liquid chromatography (*2.2.29*).

Test solution. Dissolve 50.0 mg of the substance to be examined in *methanol R* and dilute to 50.0 ml with the same solvent.

Reference solution (a). Dilute 2.0 ml of the test solution to 100.0 ml with *methanol R*. Dilute 1.0 ml of the solution to 10.0 ml with *methanol R*.

Reference solution (b). Dissolve 1.0 mg of *diclofenac impurity A CRS* in *methanol R*, add 1.0 ml of the test solution and dilute to 200.0 ml with *methanol R*.

The chromatographic procedure may be carried out using:

- a stainless steel column 0.25 m long and 4.6 mm in internal diameter packed with *end-capped octylsilyl silica gel for chromatography R* (5 µm),
- as mobile phase at a flow rate of 1 ml/min a mixture of 34 volumes of a solution containing 0.5 g/l of *phosphoric acid R* and 0.8 g/l of *sodium dihydrogen phosphate R* adjusted to pH 2.5 with *phosphoric acid R*, and 66 volumes of *methanol R*,
- as detector a spectrophotometer set at 254 nm.

Inject 20 µl of reference solution (b). When the chromatograms are recorded in the prescribed conditions, the retention times are: diclofenac, about 25 min and impurity A, about 12 min. Adjust the sensitivity of the system so that the height of the peaks in the chromatogram obtained is at least 50 per cent of the full scale of the recorder. The test is not valid unless in the chromatogram obtained the resolution between the peaks corresponding to diclofenac and impurity A is not less than 6.5.

Inject 20 µl of the test solution and 20 µl of reference solution (a). Continue the chromatography for 1.5 times the retention time of the principal peak in the chromatogram obtained with the test solution. In the chromatogram obtained with the test solution: the area of any peak, apart from the principal peak, is not greater than the area of the principal peak in the chromatogram obtained with reference solution (a) (0.2 per cent); the sum of the areas of all the peaks, apart from the principal peak, is not greater than 2.5 times that of the principal peak in the chromatogram obtained with reference solution (a) (0.5 per cent). Disregard any peak with an area less than 0.25 times the area of the principal peak in the chromatogram obtained with reference solution (a).

Heavy metals (*2.4.8*). 2.0 g complies with limit test C (10 ppm). Use a quartz crucible. Prepare the standard using 2 ml of *lead standard solution (10 ppm Pb) R*.

Loss on drying (*2.2.32*). Not more than 0.5 per cent, determined on 1.000 g by drying in an oven at 100-105 °C for 3 h.

ASSAY

Dissolve 0.250 g in 30 ml of *anhydrous acetic acid R*. Titrate with *0.1 M perchloric acid*, determining the end-point potentiometrically (*2.2.20*).

1 ml of *0.1 M perchloric acid* is equivalent to 33.42 mg of $C_{14}H_{10}Cl_2KNO_2$.

STORAGE

In an airtight container, protected from light.

IMPURITIES

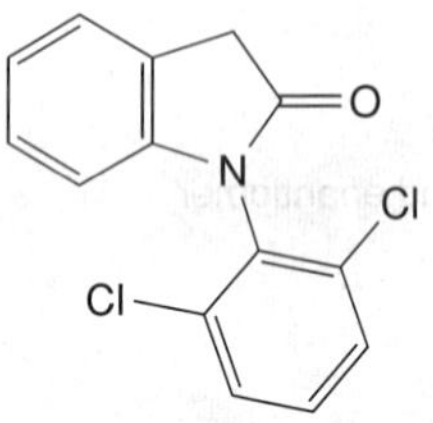

A. 1-(2,6-dichlorophenyl)-1,3-dihydro-2*H*-indol-2-one,

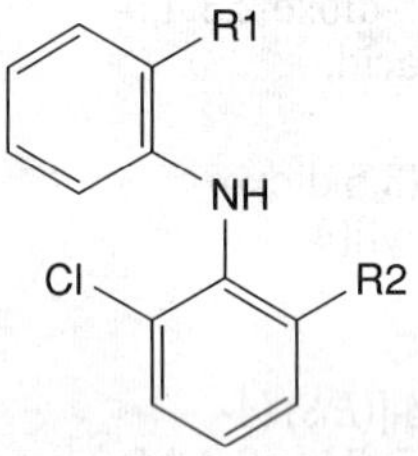

B. R1 = CHO, R2 = Cl: 2-[(2,6-dichlorophenyl)amino]benzaldehyde,

C. R1 = CH_2OH, R2 = Cl: [2-[(2,6-dichlorophenyl)amino]phenyl]methanol,

D. R1 = CH_2-CO_2H, R2 = Br: 2-[2-[(2-bromo-6-chlorophenyl)amino]phenyl]acetic acid,

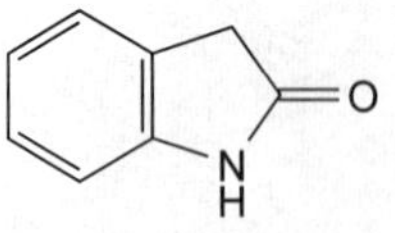

E. 1,3-dihydro-2*H*-indol-2-one.

01/2005:1002

DICLOFENAC SODIUM

Diclofenacum natricum

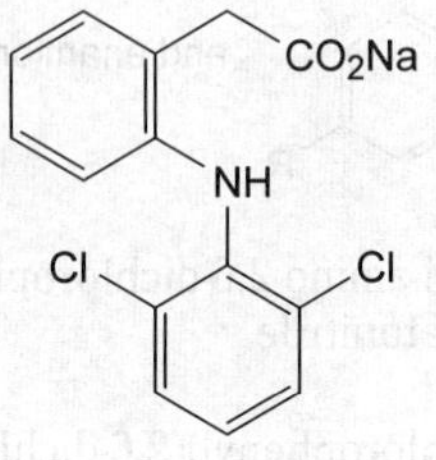

$C_{14}H_{10}Cl_2NNaO_2$ M_r 318.1

DEFINITION

Diclofenac sodium contains not less than 99.0 per cent and not more than the equivalent of 101.0 per cent of sodium 2-[(2,6-dichlorophenyl)amino]phenyl]acetate, calculated with reference to the dried substance.

CHARACTERS

A white or slightly yellowish, crystalline powder, slightly hygroscopic, sparingly soluble in water, freely soluble in methanol, soluble in alcohol, slightly soluble in acetone.

It melts at about 280 °C, with decomposition.

IDENTIFICATION

First identification: A, D.

Second identification: B, C, D.

A. Examine by infrared absorption spectrophotometry (*2.2.24*), comparing with the spectrum obtained with *diclofenac sodium CRS*. Examine the substances prepared as discs.

B. Examine by thin-layer chromatography (*2.2.27*), using a *TLC silica gel GF_{254} plate R*.

Test solution. Dissolve 25 mg of the substance to be examined in *methanol R* and dilute to 5 ml with the same solvent.

Reference solution (a). Dissolve 25 mg of *diclofenac sodium CRS* in *methanol R* and dilute to 5 ml with the same solvent.

Reference solution (b). Dissolve 10 mg of *indometacin R* in reference solution (a) and dilute to 2 ml with the same solution.

Apply to the plate 5 µl of each solution. Develop over a path of 10 cm using a mixture of 10 volumes of *concentrated ammonia R*, 10 volumes of *methanol R* and 80 volumes of *ethyl acetate R*. Allow the plate to dry in air. Examine in ultraviolet light at 254 nm. The principal spot in the chromatogram obtained with the test solution is similar in position and size to the principal spot in the chromatogram obtained with reference solution (a). The test is not valid unless the chromatogram obtained with reference solution (b) shows 2 clearly separated spots.

C. Dissolve about 10 mg in 10 ml of *alcohol R*. To 1 ml of the solution add 0.2 ml of a mixture, prepared immediately before use, of equal volumes of a 6 g/l solution of *potassium ferricyanide R* and a 9 g/l solution of *ferric chloride R*. Allow to stand protected from light for 5 min. Add 3 ml of a 10 g/l solution of *hydrochloric acid R*. Allow to stand, protected from light, for 15 min. A blue colour develops and a precipitate is formed.

D. Dissolve 60 mg in 0.5 ml of *methanol R* and add 0.5 ml of *water R*. The solution gives reaction (b) of sodium (*2.3.1*).

TESTS

Appearance of solution. Dissolve 1.25 g in *methanol R* and dilute to 25.0 ml with the same solvent. The solution is clear (*2.2.1*). The absorbance (*2.2.25*) measured at 440 nm is not greater than 0.05.

Related substances. Examine by liquid chromatography (*2.2.29*).

Test solution. Dissolve 50.0 mg of the substance to be examined in *methanol R* and dilute to 50.0 ml with the same solvent.

Reference solution (a). Dilute 2.0 ml of the test solution to 100.0 ml with *methanol R*. Dilute 1.0 ml of the solution to 10.0 ml with *methanol R*.

Reference solution (b). Dissolve 1.0 mg of *diclofenac impurity A CRS* in *methanol R*, add 1.0 ml of the test solution and dilute to 200.0 ml with *methanol R*.

The chromatographic procedure may be carried out using:

- a stainless steel column 0.25 m long and 4.6 mm in internal diameter packed with *end-capped octylsilyl silica gel for chromatography R* (5 µm),
- as mobile phase at a flow rate of 1 ml/min a mixture of 34 volumes of a solution containing 0.5 g/l of *phosphoric acid R* and 0.8 g/l of *sodium dihydrogen phosphate R* adjusted to pH 2.5 with *phosphoric acid R*, and 66 volumes of *methanol R*,
- as detector a spectrophotometer set at 254 nm.

Inject 20 µl of reference solution (b). When the chromatograms are recorded in the prescribed conditions, the retention times are about 25 min for diclofenac and about 12 min for impurity A. Adjust the sensitivity of the system so that the height of the peaks in the chromatogram obtained with reference solution (b) is not less than 50 per cent of the full scale of the recorder. Continue the chromatography for 1.5 times the retention time of diclofenac. The test is not valid unless in the chromatogram obtained the resolution between the peaks corresponding to diclofenac and impurity A is at least 6.5.

Inject 20 µl of the test solution and 20 µl of reference solution (a). In the chromatogram obtained with the test solution: the area of any peak, apart from the principal peak, is not greater than the area of the principal peak in the chromatogram obtained with reference solution (a) (0.2 per cent); the sum of the areas of all the peaks apart from the principal peak is not greater than 2.5 times that of the principal peak in the chromatogram obtained with reference solution (a) (0.5 per cent). Disregard any peak with an area less than 0.25 times the area of the principal peak in the chromatogram obtained with reference solution (a).

Heavy metals (*2.4.8*). 2.0 g complies with limit test C (10 ppm). Use a quartz crucible. Prepare the standard using 2 ml of *lead standard solution (10 ppm Pb) R*.

Loss on drying (*2.2.32*). Not more than 0.5 per cent, determined on 1.000 g by drying in an oven at 100-105 °C for 3 h.

ASSAY

Dissolve 0.250 g in 30 ml of *anhydrous acetic acid R*. Titrate with *0.1 M perchloric acid*, determining the end-point potentiometrically (*2.2.20*).

1 ml of *0.1 M perchloric acid* is equivalent to 31.81 mg of $C_{14}H_{10}Cl_2NNaO_2$.

STORAGE

In an airtight container, protected from light.

IMPURITIES

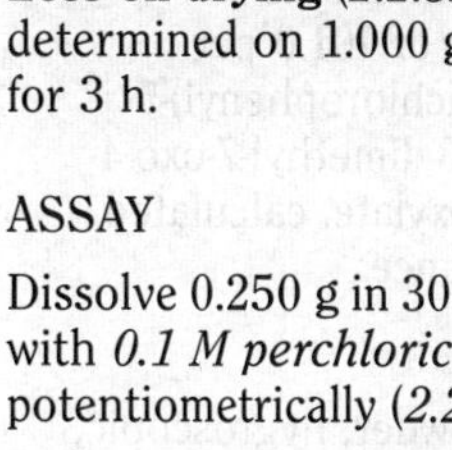

A. 1-(2,6-dichlorophenyl)-1,3-dihydro-2*H*-indol-2-one,

Monographs D-E

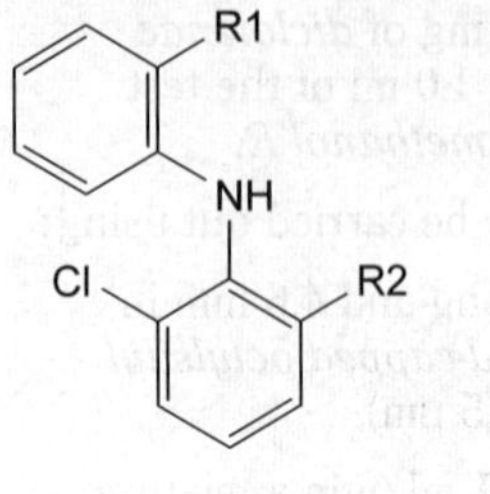

B. R1 = CHO, R2 = Cl: 2-[(2,6-dichlorophenyl)amino]benzaldehyde,

C. R1 = CH_2OH, R2 = Cl: [2-[(2,6-dichlorophenyl)amino]phenyl]methanol,

D. R1 = CH_2-CO_2H, R2 = Br: 2-[2-[(2-bromo-6-chlorophenyl)amino]phenyl]acetic acid,

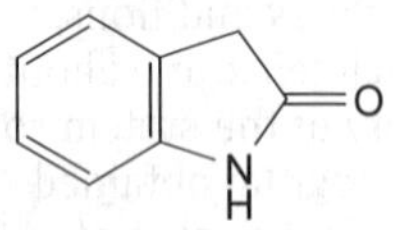

E. 1,3-dihydro-2*H*-indol-2-one.

01/2005:0663

DICLOXACILLIN SODIUM

Dicloxacillinum natricum

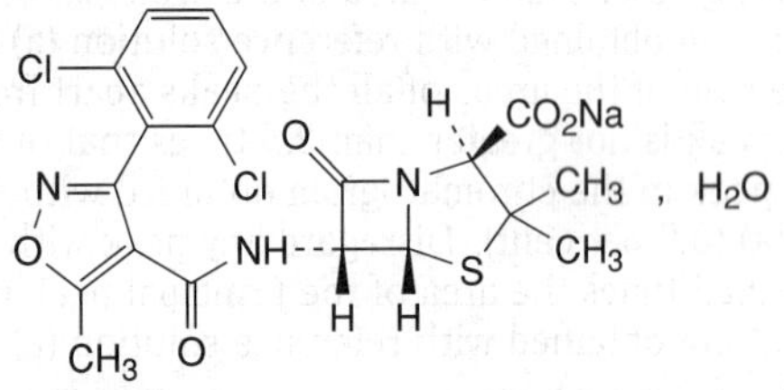

$C_{19}H_{16}Cl_2N_3NaO_5S,H_2O$ M_r 510.3

DEFINITION

Dicloxacillin sodium contains not less than 95.0 per cent and not more than the equivalent of 101.0 per cent of sodium (2*S*,5*R*,6*R*)-6-[[[3-(2,6-dichlorophenyl)-5-methylisoxazol-4-yl]carbonyl]amino]-3,3-dimethyl-7-oxo-4-thia-1-azabicyclo[3.2.0]heptane-2-carboxylate, calculated with reference to the anhydrous substance.

CHARACTERS

A white or almost white, crystalline powder, hygroscopic, freely soluble in water, soluble in alcohol and in methanol.

IDENTIFICATION

First identification: A, D.

Second identification: B, C, D.

A. Examine by infrared absorption spectrophotometry (*2.2.24*), comparing with the spectrum obtained with *dicloxacillin sodium CRS*. Examine the substances prepared as discs.

B. Examine by thin-layer chromatography (*2.2.27*), using *silanised silica gel H R* as the coating substance.

Test solution. Dissolve 25 mg of the substance to be examined in 5 ml of *water R*.

Reference solution (a). Dissolve 25 mg of *dicloxacillin sodium CRS* in 5 ml of *water R*.

Reference solution (b). Dissolve 25 mg each of *cloxacillin sodium CRS, dicloxacillin sodium CRS* and *flucloxacillin sodium CRS* in 5 ml of *water R*.

Apply to the plate 1 µl of each solution. Develop over a path of 15 cm using a mixture of 30 volumes of *acetone R* and 70 volumes of a 154 g/l solution of *ammonium acetate R* the pH of which has been adjusted to 5.0 with *glacial acetic acid R*. Allow the plate to dry in air and expose it to iodine vapour until the spots appear. Examine in daylight. The principal spot in the chromatogram obtained with the test solution is similar in position, colour and size to the principal spot in the chromatogram obtained with reference solution (a). The test is not valid unless the chromatogram obtained with reference solution (b) shows three clearly separated spots.

C. Place about 2 mg in a test-tube about 150 mm long and 15 mm in diameter. Moisten with 0.05 ml of *water R* and add 2 ml of *sulphuric acid-formaldehyde reagent R*. Mix the contents of the tube by swirling; the colour of the solution is slightly greenish-yellow. Place the test-tube in a water-bath for 1 min; a yellow colour develops.

D. It gives reaction (a) of sodium (*2.3.1*).

TESTS

Solution S. Dissolve 2.50 g in *carbon dioxide-free water R* and dilute to 25.0 ml with the same solvent.

Appearance of solution. Solution S is clear (*2.2.1*). The absorbance (*2.2.25*) of solution S measured at 430 nm is not greater than 0.04.

pH (*2.2.3*). The pH of solution S is 5.0 to 7.0.

Specific optical rotation (*2.2.7*). Dissolve 0.250 g in *water R* and dilute to 25.0 ml with the same solvent. The specific optical rotation is + 128 to + 143, calculated with reference to the anhydrous substance.

Related substances. Examine by liquid chromatography (*2.2.29*) as prescribed under Assay. Inject reference solution (b). Adjust the sensitivity of the system so that the height of the principal peak in the chromatogram obtained is at least 50 per cent of the full scale of the recorder. Inject test solution (a) and continue the chromatography for five times the retention time of the principal peak. In the chromatogram obtained with test solution (a): the area of any peak, apart from the principal peak, is not greater than the area of the principal peak in the chromatogram obtained with reference solution (b) (1 per cent); the sum of the areas of all peaks, apart from the principal peak, is not greater than five times the area of the principal peak in the chromatogram obtained with reference solution (b) (5 per cent). Disregard any peak with an area less than 0.05 times the area of the principal peak in the chromatogram obtained with reference solution (b).

***N,N*-Dimethylaniline** (*2.4.26, Method B*). Not more than 20 ppm.

2-Ethylhexanoic acid (*2.4.28*). Not more than 0.8 per cent *m/m*.

Water (*2.5.12*): 3.0 per cent to 4.5 per cent, determined on 0.300 g by the semi-micro determination of water.

Pyrogens (*2.6.8*). If intended for use in the manufacture of parenteral dosage forms without a further appropriate procedure for the removal of pyrogens, it complies with the test for pyrogens. Inject per kilogram of the rabbit's mass 1 ml of a solution in *water for injections R* containing 20 mg of the substance to be examined per millilitre.

ASSAY

Examine by liquid chromatography (*2.2.29*).

Test solution (a). Dissolve 50.0 mg of the substance to be examined in the mobile phase and dilute to 50.0 ml with the mobile phase.

Test solution (b). Dilute 5.0 ml of test solution (a) to 50.0 ml with the mobile phase.

Reference solution (a). Dissolve 50.0 mg of *dicloxacillin sodium CRS* in the mobile phase and dilute to 50.0 ml with the mobile phase. Dilute 5.0 ml of the solution to 50.0 ml with the mobile phase.

Reference solution (b). Dilute 5.0 ml of test solution (b) to 50.0 ml with the mobile phase.

Reference solution (c). Dissolve 5 mg of *flucloxacillin sodium CRS* and 5 mg of *dicloxacillin sodium CRS* in the mobile phase and dilute to 50.0 ml with the mobile phase.

The chromatographic procedure may be carried out using:

- a stainless steel column 0.25 m long and 4 mm in internal diameter packed with *octadecylsilyl silica gel for chromatography R* (5 µm),
- as mobile phase at a flow rate of 1.0 ml/min a mixture of 75 volumes of a 2.7 g/l solution of *potassium dihydrogen phosphate R* adjusted to pH 5.0 with *dilute sodium hydroxide solution R* and 25 volumes of *acetonitrile R*,
- as detector a spectrophotometer set at 225 nm,
- a 20 µl loop injector.

Inject reference solution (c). When the chromatograms are recorded in the prescribed conditions, the retention time of dicloxacillin is about 10 min. Adjust the sensitivity of the system so that the heights of the principal peaks in the chromatogram obtained are at least 50 per cent of the full scale of the recorder. The test is not valid unless in the chromatogram obtained, the resolution between the first peak (flucloxacillin) and the second peak (dicloxacillin) is at least 2.5. Inject reference solution (a) six times. The test is not valid unless the relative standard deviation of the peak area for dicloxacillin is at most 1.0 per cent. Inject alternately test solution (b) and reference solution (a).

STORAGE

Store in an airtight container, at a temperature not exceeding 25 °C. If the substance is sterile, store in a sterile, airtight, tamper-proof container.

LABELLING

The label states, where applicable, that the substance is apyrogenic.

IMPURITIES

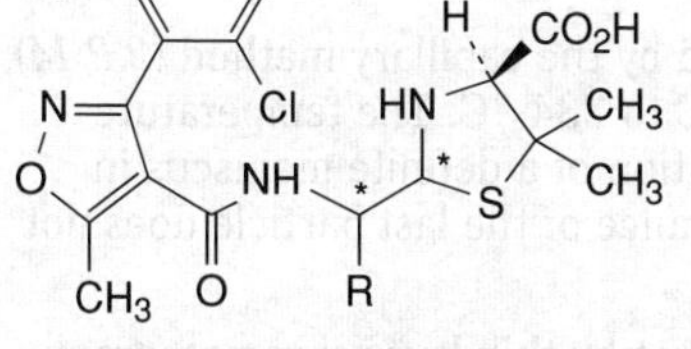

A. R = CO_2H: (4*S*)-2-[carboxy[[[3-(2,6-dichlorophenyl)-5-methylisoxazol-4-yl]carbonyl]amino]methyl]-5,5-dimethylthiazolidine-4-carboxylic acid (penicilloic acids of dicloxacillin),

B. R = H: (2*RS*,4*S*)-2-[[[[3-(2,6-dichlorophenyl)-5-methylisoxazol-4-yl]carbonyl]amino]methyl]-5,5-dimethylthiazolidine-4-carboxylic acid (penilloic acids of dicloxacillin),

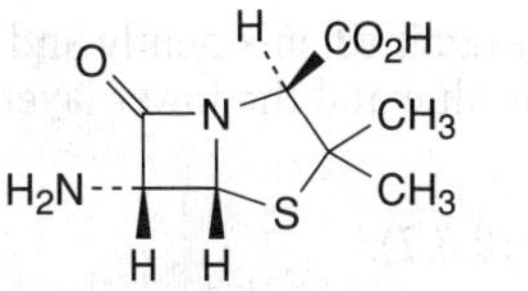

C. (2*S*,5*R*,6*R*)-6-amino-3,3-dimethyl-7-oxo-4-thia-1-azabicyclo[3.2.0]heptane-2-carboxylic acid (6-aminopenicillanic acid),

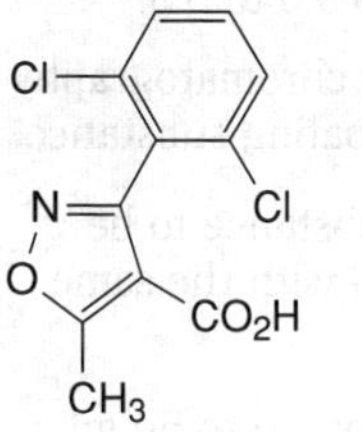

D. 3-(2,6-dichlorophenyl)-5-methylisoxazole-4-carboxylic acid.

01/2005:1197

DICYCLOVERINE HYDROCHLORIDE

Dicycloverini hydrochloridum

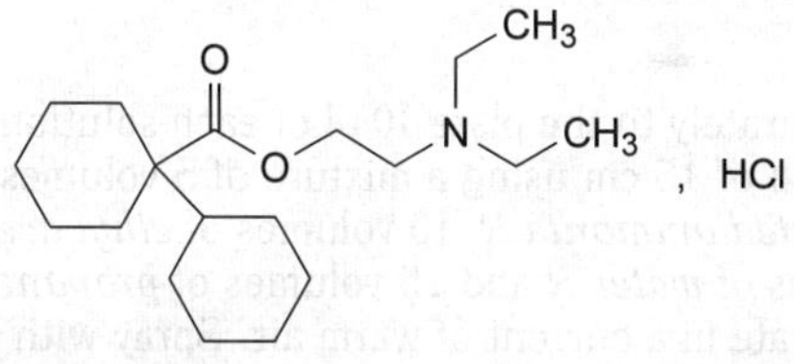

$C_{19}H_{36}ClNO_2$ M_r 346.0

DEFINITION

Dicycloverine hydrochloride contains not less than 99.0 per cent and not more than the equivalent of 101.0 per cent of 2-(diethylamino)ethyl bicyclohexyl-1-carboxylate hydrochloride, calculated with reference to the dried substance.

CHARACTERS

A white or almost white, crystalline powder, soluble in water, freely soluble in alcohol and in methylene chloride.

It shows polymorphism.

IDENTIFICATION

First identification: A, D.

Second identification: B, C, D.

A. Examine by infrared absorption spectrophotometry (*2.2.24*), comparing with the spectrum obtained with *dicycloverine hydrochloride CRS.* Examine the substances prepared as discs using *potassium chloride R.* If the spectra obtained show differences, dissolve the substance to be examined and the reference substance separately in *acetone R,* evaporate to dryness and record new spectra using the residues.

B. Examine the chromatograms obtained in the test for related substances. The principal spot in the chromatogram obtained with test solution (b) is similar in position, colour and size to the principal spot in the chromatogram obtained with reference solution (b).

C. To 3 ml of a 1.0 g/l solution of *sodium laurilsulfate R* add 5 ml of *methylene chloride R* and 0.05 ml of a 2.5 g/l solution of *methylene blue R,* mix gently and allow to stand; the lower layer is blue. Add 2 ml of a 20 g/l solution of the substance to be examined, mix gently and allow to stand; the upper layer is blue and the lower layer is colourless.

D. It gives reaction (a) of chlorides (*2.3.1*).

TESTS

pH (*2.2.3*). Dissolve 0.5 g in *water R* and dilute to 50 ml with the same solvent. The pH of the solution is 5.0 to 5.5.

Related substances. Examine by thin-layer chromatography (*2.2.27*), using a suitable silica gel as the coating substance.

Test solution (a). Dissolve 0.25 g to the substance to be examined in *methanol R* and dilute to 5 ml with the same solvent.

Test solution (b). Dilute 1 ml of test solution (a) to 50 ml with *methanol R*.

Reference solution (a). Dilute 1 ml of test solution (b) to 10 ml with *methanol R*.

Reference solution (b). Dissolve 10 mg of *dicycloverine hydrochloride CRS* in *methanol R* and dilute to 10 ml with the same solvent.

Reference solution (c). Dissolve 5 mg of *tropicamide CRS* in reference solution (b) and dilute to 5 ml with the same solution.

Apply separately to the plate 10 µl of each solution. Develop over a path of 15 cm using a mixture of 5 volumes of *concentrated ammonia R*, 10 volumes of *ethyl acetate R*, 10 volumes of *water R* and 75 volumes of *propanol R*. Dry the plate in a current of warm air. Spray with *dilute potassium iodobismuthate solution R*. Any spot in the chromatogram obtained with test solution (a), apart from the principal spot, is not more intense than the spot in the chromatogram obtained with reference solution (a) (0.2 per cent). The test is not valid unless the chromatogram obtained with reference solution (c) shows two clearly separated spots.

Loss on drying (*2.2.32*). Not more than 1.0 per cent, determined on 1.000 g by drying in an oven at 100 °C to 105 °C.

Sulphated ash (*2.4.14*). Not more than 0.1 per cent, determined on 1.0 g.

ASSAY

Dissolve 0.300 g in a mixture of 5.0 ml of *0.01 M hydrochloric acid* and 50 ml of *alcohol R*. Carry out a potentiometric titration (*2.2.20*), using *0.1 M sodium hydroxide*. Read the volume added between the two points of inflexion.

1 ml of *0.1 M sodium hydroxide* is equivalent to 34.60 mg of $C_{19}H_{36}ClNO_2$.

IMPURITIES

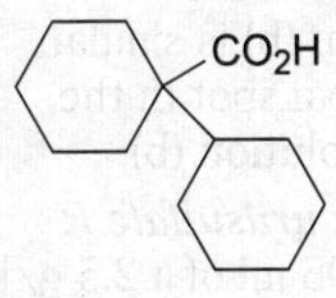

A. bicyclohexyl-1-carboxylic acid.

01/2005:0483

DIENESTROL

Dienestrolum

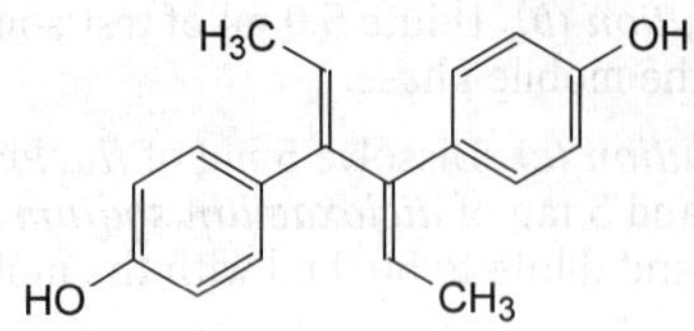

$C_{18}H_{18}O_2$ M_r 266.3

DEFINITION

Dienestrol contains not less than 98.5 per cent and not more than the equivalent of 101.5 per cent of (*E*,*E*)-4,4′-(1,2-diethylidene-ethylene)diphenol, calculated with reference to the dried substance.

CHARACTERS

A white or almost white, crystalline powder, practically insoluble in water, freely soluble in acetone and in alcohol. It dissolves in dilute solutions of the alkali hydroxides.

IDENTIFICATION

First identification: A, D.

Second identification: B, C, D.

A. Examine by infrared absorption spectrophotometry (*2.2.24*), comparing with the spectrum obtained with *dienestrol CRS*. Examine the substances prepared as discs.

B. Examine the chromatograms obtained in the test for related substances. The principal spot in the chromatogram obtained with test solution (b) is similar in position, colour and size to the spot in the chromatogram obtained with reference solution (a).

C. Dissolve about 1 mg in 5 ml of *glacial acetic acid R*, add 1 ml of a 1 per cent *V/V* solution of *bromine R* in *glacial acetic acid R* and heat in a water-bath for 2 min. Place 0.5 ml of this solution in a dry test-tube, add 0.5 ml of *ethanol R*, mix and add 10 ml of *water R*. A reddish-violet colour is produced. Add 5 ml of *chloroform R*, shake vigorously and allow to separate. The chloroform layer is red and the aqueous layer is almost colourless.

D. Dissolve about 0.5 mg in 0.2 ml of *glacial acetic acid R*, add 1 ml of *phosphoric acid R* and heat on a water-bath for 3 min. A reddish-violet colour is produced.

TESTS

Melting range. Determined by the capillary method (*2.2.14*), the melting point is 227 °C to 234 °C. The temperature interval between the formation of a definite meniscus in the melt and the disappearance of the last particle does not exceed 3 °C.

Related substances. Examine by thin-layer chromatography (*2.2.27*), using *silica gel G R* as the coating substance.

Test solution (a). Dissolve 0.2 g of the substance to be examined in 2 ml of *alcohol R*.

Test solution (b). Dilute 1 ml of test solution (a) to 20 ml with *alcohol R*.

Reference solution (a). Dissolve 25 mg of *dienestrol CRS* in *alcohol R* and dilute to 5 ml with the same solvent.

Reference solution (b). Dilute 1 ml of reference solution (a) to 10 ml with *alcohol R*.

Reference solution (c). Dissolve 10 mg of *diethylstilbestrol CRS* in 2 ml of *alcohol R*. To 1 ml of this solution add 1 ml of reference solution (a).

Apply separately to the plate 1 µl of each solution. Develop over a path of 15 cm using a mixture of 10 volumes of *diethylamine R* and 90 volumes of *toluene R*. Allow the plate to dry in air, spray with *alcoholic solution of sulphuric acid R* and heat at 120 °C for 10 min. Any spot in the chromatogram obtained with test solution (a), apart from the principal spot, is not more intense than the spot in the chromatogram obtained with reference solution (b) (0.5 per cent). The test is not valid unless the chromatogram obtained with reference solution (c) shows at least two clearly separated spots having approximately the same intensity.

Loss on drying (*2.2.32*). Not more than 0.5 per cent, determined on 1.000 g by drying in an oven at 100 °C to 105 °C.

Sulphated ash (*2.4.14*). Not more than 0.1 per cent, determined on 1.0 g.

ASSAY

Dissolve 25.0 mg in *ethanol R* and dilute to 100.0 ml with the same solvent. To 5.0 ml of this solution add 10 ml of *ethanol R* and dilute to 250.0 ml with *0.1 M sodium hydroxide*. Prepare a reference solution in the same manner using 25.0 mg of *dienestrol CRS*. Measure the absorbance (*2.2.25*) of the solutions at the maximum at 245 nm.

Calculate the content of $C_{18}H_{18}O_2$ from the measured absorbances and the concentrations of the solutions.

STORAGE

Store protected from light.

01/2005:0897

DIETHYL PHTHALATE

Diethylis phthalas

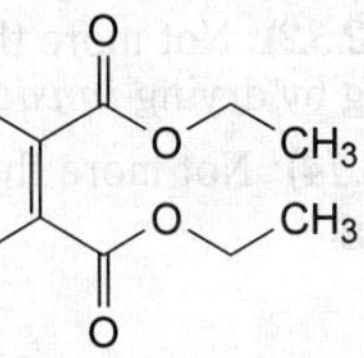

$C_{12}H_{14}O_4$ M_r 222.2

DEFINITION

Diethyl phthalate contains not less than 99.0 per cent and not more than the equivalent of 101.0 per cent *m/m* of diethyl benzene-1,2-dicarboxylate.

CHARACTERS

A clear, oily liquid, colourless or very slightly yellow, practically insoluble in water, miscible with alcohol.

IDENTIFICATION

First identification: B, C.

Second identification: A, D, E.

A. Relative density (*2.2.5*): 1.117 to 1.121.

B. Refractive index (*2.2.6*): 1.500 to 1.505.

C. Examine by infrared absorption spectrophotometry (*2.2.24*), comparing with the spectrum obtained with *diethyl phthalate CRS*. Examine as thin films.

D. Examine by thin-layer chromatography (*2.2.27*), using *silica gel GF_{254} R* as the coating substance.

Test solution. Dissolve 50 mg of the substance to be examined in *ether R* and dilute to 10 ml with the same solvent.

Reference solution. Dissolve 50 mg of *diethyl phthalate CRS* in *ether R* and dilute to 10 ml with the same solvent.

Apply separately to the plate 10 µl of each solution. Develop over a path of 15 cm using a mixture of 30 volumes of *heptane R* and 70 volumes of *ether R*. Allow the plate to dry in air and examine in ultraviolet light at 254 nm. The principal spot in the chromatogram obtained with the test solution is similar in position and size to the principal spot in the chromatogram obtained with the reference solution.

E. To about 0.1 ml add 0.25 ml of *sulphuric acid R* and 50 mg of *resorcinol R*. Heat on a water-bath for 5 min. Allow to cool. Add 10 ml of *water R* and 1 ml of *strong sodium hydroxide solution R*. The solution becomes yellow or brownish-yellow and shows green fluorescence.

TESTS

Appearance. The substance to be examined is clear (*2.2.1*) and not more intensely coloured than reference solution Y_6 (*2.2.2, Method II*).

Acidity. Dissolve 20.0 g in 50 ml of *alcohol R* previously neutralised to *phenolphthalein solution R1*. Add 0.2 ml of *phenolphthalein solution R1*. Not more than 0.1 ml of *0.1 M sodium hydroxide* is required to change the colour of the indicator to pink.

Related substances. Examine by gas chromatography (*2.2.28*), using *naphthalene R* as the internal standard.

Internal standard solution. Dissolve 60 mg of *naphthalene R* in *methylene chloride R* and dilute to 20 ml with the same solvent.

Test solution (a). Dissolve 1.0 g of the substance to be examined in *methylene chloride R* and dilute to 20.0 ml with the same solvent.

Test solution (b). Dissolve 1.0 g of the substance to be examined in *methylene chloride R*, add 2.0 ml of the internal standard solution and dilute to 20.0 ml with *methylene chloride R*.

Reference solution. To 1.0 ml of test solution (a) add 10.0 ml of the internal standard solution and dilute to 100.0 ml with *methylene chloride R*.

The chromatographic procedure may be carried out using:

– a glass column 2 m long and 2 mm in internal diameter packed with *silanised diatomaceous earth for gas chromatography R* (150 µm to 180 µm) impregnated with 3 per cent *m/m* of *polymethylphenylsiloxane R*,

– *nitrogen for chromatography R* as the carrier gas at a flow rate of 30 ml/min,

– a flame-ionisation detector,

maintaining the temperature of the column at 150 °C and that of the injection port and of the detector at 225 °C.

Inject 1 µl of the reference solution. The substances are eluted in the following order: naphthalene and diethyl phthalate. Adjust the sensitivity of the detector so that the height of the peak due to naphthalene is not less than 50 per cent of the full scale of the recorder. The test is not valid unless the resolution between the peaks corresponding to naphthalene and diethyl phthalate is at least 10.

Inject 1 µl of test solution (a). In the chromatogram obtained, verify that there is no peak with the same retention time as the internal standard.

Inject separately 1 µl of test solution (b) and 1 µl of the reference solution. Continue the chromatography for three times the retention time of diethyl phthalate. From the chromatogram obtained with the reference solution, calculate the ratio (*R*) of the area of the peak due to diethyl phthalate to the area of the peak due to the internal standard. From the chromatogram obtained with test solution (b), calculate the ratio of the sum of the areas of any peaks, apart from the principal peak and the peaks due to the internal standard and the solvent, to the area of the peak due to the internal standard; this ratio is not greater than *R* (1.0 per cent).

Water (*2.5.12*). Not more than 0.2 per cent, determined on 5.0 g by the semi-micro determination of water.

Sulphated ash (*2.4.14*). Not more than 0.1 per cent, determined on 1.0 g.

ASSAY

Introduce 0.750 g into a 250 ml borosilicate glass flask. Add 25.0 ml of *0.5 M alcoholic potassium hydroxide* and a few glass beads. Boil on a water-bath under a reflux condenser for 1 h. Add 1 ml of *phenolphthalein solution R1* and titrate immediately with *0.5 M hydrochloric acid.* Carry out a blank titration. Calculate the volume of *0.5 M alcoholic potassium hydroxide* used in the saponification.

1 ml of *0.5 M alcoholic potassium hydroxide* is equivalent to 55.56 mg of $C_{12}H_{14}O_4$.

STORAGE

Store in an airtight container.

01/2005:0271

DIETHYLCARBAMAZINE CITRATE

Diethylcarbamazini citras

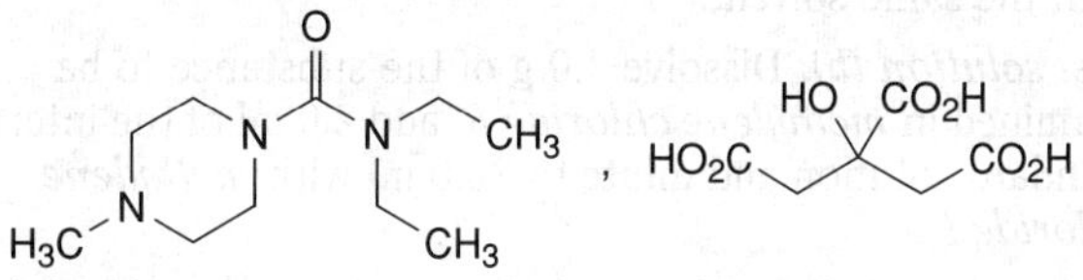

$C_{16}H_{29}N_3O_8$ M_r 391.4

DEFINITION

Diethylcarbamazine citrate contains not less than 98.0 per cent and not more than the equivalent of 101.0 per cent of *N,N*-diethyl-4-methylpiperazine-1-carboxamide dihydrogen 2-hydroxypropane-1,2,3-tricarboxylate, calculated with reference to the dried substance.

CHARACTERS

A white, crystalline powder, slightly hygroscopic, very soluble in water, soluble in alcohol, practically insoluble in acetone.

It melts at about 138 °C, with decomposition.

IDENTIFICATION

First identification: A, C.

Second identification: B, C.

A. Examine by infrared absorption spectrophotometry (*2.2.24*), comparing with the spectrum obtained with *diethylcarbamazine citrate CRS.*

B. Examine the chromatograms obtained in the test for dimethylpiperazine and methylpiperazine. The principal spot in the chromatogram obtained with the test solution corresponds in position, colour and size to the principal spot in the chromatogram obtained with reference solution (a).

C. Dissolve 0.1 g in 5 ml of *water R*. The solution gives the reaction of citrates (*2.3.1*).

TESTS

Solution S. Shake 2.5 g with *water R* until dissolved and dilute to 25 ml with the same solvent.

Appearance of solution. Solution S is not more opalescent than reference suspension II (*2.2.1*) and is not more intensely coloured than reference solution BY_6 (*2.2.2, Method II*).

Dimethylpiperazine and methylpiperazine. Examine by thin-layer chromatography (*2.2.27*), using *silica gel G R* as the coating substance.

Test solution. Dissolve 0.5 g of the substance to be examined in *methanol R* and dilute to 10 ml with the same solvent.

Reference solution (a). Dissolve 0.1 g of *diethylcarbamazine citrate CRS* in *methanol R* and dilute to 2.0 ml with the same solvent.

Reference solution (b). Dissolve 10 mg of *methylpiperazine R* in *methanol R* and dilute to 100 ml with the same solvent.

Reference solution (c). Dissolve 10 mg of *dimethylpiperazine R* in *methanol R* and dilute to 100 ml with the same solvent.

Apply to the plate 10 µl of each solution. Develop over a path of 12 cm using a mixture of 5 volumes of *concentrated ammonia R*, 30 volumes of *methyl ethyl ketone R* and 65 volumes of *methanol R*. Dry the plate at 100-105 °C and expose to iodine vapour for 30 min. In the chromatogram obtained with the test solution, any spots corresponding to methylpiperazine and dimethylpiperazine are not more intense than the spots in the chromatograms obtained with reference solutions (b) and (c) respectively (0.2 per cent).

Heavy metals (*2.4.8*). 12 ml of solution S complies with limit test A for heavy metals (20 ppm). Prepare the standard using 10 ml of *lead standard solution (2 ppm Pb) R.*

Loss on drying (*2.2.32*). Not more than 0.5 per cent, determined on 1.0 g by drying *in vacuo* at 60 °C for 4 h.

Sulphated ash (*2.4.14*). Not more than 0.1 per cent, determined on 1.0 g.

ASSAY

Dissolve 0.350 g in 25 ml of *anhydrous acetic acid R* and add 25 ml of *acetic anhydride R*. Using 0.2 ml of *crystal violet solution R* as indicator, titrate with *0.1 M perchloric acid* until a greenish-blue colour is obtained.

1 ml of *0.1 M perchloric acid* is equivalent to 39.14 mg of $C_{16}H_{29}N_3O_8$.

STORAGE

Store in an airtight container.

01/2005:1198

DIETHYLENE GLYCOL MONOETHYL ETHER

Diethylenglycoli monoethylicum aetherum

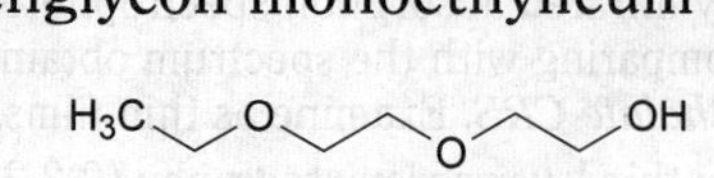

$C_6H_{14}O_3$ M_r 134.2

DEFINITION

2-(2-Ethoxyethoxy)ethanol, produced by condensation of ethylene oxide and alcohol, followed by distillation.

CHARACTERS

Appearance: clear, colourless, hygroscopic liquid.

Solubility: miscible with water, with acetone and with alcohol, miscible in certain proportions with vegetable oils, not miscible with mineral oils.

Relative density: about 0.991.

IDENTIFICATION

A. Refractive index (*2.2.6*): 1.426 to 1.428.

B. Infrared absorption spectrophotometry (*2.2.24*).

Comparison: *Ph. Eur. reference spectrum of diethylene glycol monoethyl ether.*

TESTS

Acid value (*2.5.1*): maximum 0.1.

Mix 30.0 ml with 30 ml of *alcohol R* previously neutralised with *0.1 M potassium hydroxide* using *phenolphthalein solution R* as indicator. Titrate with *0.01 M alcoholic potassium hydroxide.*

Peroxide value (*2.5.5*): maximum 8.0, determined on 2.00 g.

Related substances. Gas chromatography (*2.2.28*).

Internal standard solution. Dilute 1.00 g of *decane R* to 100.0 ml with *methanol R.*

Test solution. To 5.00 g of the substance to be examined, add 0.1 ml of the internal standard solution and dilute to 10.0 ml with *methanol R.*

Reference solution (a). Dilute 25.0 mg of *ethylene glycol monomethyl ether R*, 80.0 mg of *ethylene glycol monoethyl ether R*, 0.310 g of *ethylene glycol R* and 0.125 g of *diethylene glycol R* to 100.0 ml with *methanol R.* To 1.0 ml of this solution add 0.1 ml of the internal standard solution and dilute to 10.0 ml with *methanol R.*

Reference solution (b). Dilute 25.0 mg of *ethylene glycol monoethyl ether R* and 25.0 mg of *ethylene glycol R* to 100.0 ml with *methanol R.* Dilute 1.0 ml of this solution to 5.0 ml with *methanol R.*

Reference solution (c). Dilute 1.00 g of the substance to be examined to 100.0 ml with *methanol R.* To 1.0 ml of this solution add 0.1 ml of the internal standard solution and dilute to 10.0 ml with *methanol R.*

Column:

- *material*: fused silica,
- *size*: *l* = 30 m, Ø = 0.32 mm,
- *stationary phase*: *poly(cyanopropyl)(7)(phenyl)(7)methyl(86)siloxane R* (film thickness 1 µm).

Carrier gas: *nitrogen for chromatography R* or *helium for chromatography R.*

Flow rate: 2.0 ml/min.

Split ratio: 1:80.

Temperature:

	Time (min)	Temperature (°C)
Column	0 - 1	120
	1 - 10	120 → 225
	10 - 12	225
Injection port		275
Detector		250

Detection: flame ionisation.

Injection: 0.5 µl.

Relative retentions with reference to diethylene glycol monoethyl ether (retention time = about 4 min): ethylene glycol monomethyl ether = about 0.4; ethylene glycol monoethyl ether = about 0.5; ethylene glycol = about 0.55; diethylene glycol = about 1.1.

System suitability:

- *resolution*: minimum 3.0 between the peaks due to ethylene glycol monoethyl ether and to ethylene glycol in the chromatogram obtained with reference solution (b),
- *signal-to-noise ratio*: minimum 3.0 for the peak due to ethylene glycol monomethyl ether in the chromatogram obtained with reference solution (a),

Limits (take into account the impurity/internal standard peak area ratio):

- *ethylene glycol monomethyl ether*: not more than the area of the corresponding peak in the chromatogram obtained with reference solution (a) (50 ppm),
- *ethylene glycol monoethyl ether*: not more than the area of the corresponding peak in the chromatogram obtained with reference solution (a) (160 ppm),
- *ethylene glycol*: not more than the area of the corresponding peak in the chromatogram obtained with reference solution (a) (620 ppm),
- *diethylene glycol*: not more than the area of the corresponding peak in the chromatogram obtained with reference solution (a) (250 ppm),
- *total*: not more than the area of the principal peak in the chromatogram obtained with reference solution (c) (0.2 per cent).

Ethylene oxide. Head-space gas chromatography (*2.2.28*).

Test solution. To 1.00 g of the substance to be examined in a vial, add 50 µl of *water R.*

Reference solution. To 1.00 g of the substance to be examined in a vial, add 50 µl of *ethylene oxide solution R4* and close tightly.

Column:

- *material*: fused silica,
- *size*: *l* = 30 m, Ø = 0.32 mm,
- *stationary phase*: *poly(cyanopropyl)(7)(phenyl)(7)methyl(86)siloxane R* (film thickness 1 µm).

Carrier gas: *helium for chromatography R.*

Flow rate: 1.1 ml/min.

Static head-space conditions which may be used:

- *equilibration temperature*: 80 °C,
- *equilibration time*: 45 min,
- *transfer line temperature*: 110 °C,
- *pressurisation time*: 2 min,
- *injection time*: 12 s.

Temperature:

	Time (min)	Temperature (°C)
Column	0 - 5	40
	5 - 18	40 → 200
Injection port		150
Detector		250

Detection: flame ionisation.

Injection: 1.0 ml.

The peak due to ethylene oxide is identified by injecting solutions of ethylene oxide of increasing concentration.

Monographs D-E

Determine the content of ethylene oxide (ppm) in the substance to be examined using the following expression:

$$\frac{S_T \times C}{(S_S \times M_T) - (S_T \times M_S)}$$

S_T = area of the peak corresponding to ethylene oxide in the chromatogram obtained with the test solution,

S_S = area of the peak corresponding to ethylene oxide in the chromatogram obtained with the reference solution,

M_T = mass of the substance to be examined in the test solution, in grams,

M_S = mass of the substance to be examined in the reference solution, in grams,

C = mass of added ethylene oxide in the reference solution, in micrograms.

Limit:

– *ethylene oxide*: maximum 1 ppm.

Water (*2.5.12*): maximum 0.1 per cent, determined on 10.0 g.

STORAGE

Under an inert gas, in an airtight container.

LABELLING

The label states that the substance is stored under an inert gas.

Monographs D-E

01/2005:1415

DIETHYLENE GLYCOL MONOPALMITOSTEARATE

Diethylenglycoli monopalmitostearas

DEFINITION

Diethylene glycol monopalmitostearate is a mixture of diethylene glycol mono- and diesters of stearic and palmitic acids. It contains not less than 45.0 per cent of monoesters produced from the condensation of diethylene glycol and stearic acid 50 of vegetable or animal origin.

CHARACTERS

A white or almost white, waxy solid, practically insoluble in water, soluble in acetone and in hot alcohol.

IDENTIFICATION

A. It complies with the test for melting point (see Tests).

B. It complies with the test for composition of fatty acids (see Tests).

C. It complies with the assay (monoesters content).

TESTS

Melting point (*2.2.15*): 43 °C to 50 °C.

Acid value (*2.5.1*). Not more than 4.0, determined on 10.0 g.

Iodine value (*2.5.4*). Not more than 3.0.

Saponification value (*2.5.6*): 150 to 170, determined on 2.0 g.

Composition of fatty acids (*2.4.22, Method A*). The fatty acid fraction has the following composition:

– *stearic acid*: 40.0 per cent to 60.0 per cent,

– *sum of contents of palmitic acid and stearic acid*: not less than 90.0 per cent.

Free diethylene glycol. Not more than 8.0 per cent, determined as prescribed under Assay.

Total ash (*2.4.16*). Not more than 0.1 per cent, determined on 1.0 g.

ASSAY

Determine the free diethylene glycol content and monoesters content by size-exclusion chromatography (*2.2.30*).

Test solution. Into a 15 ml flask, weigh about 0.2 g (*m*), to the nearest 0.1 mg. Add 5.0 ml of *tetrahydrofuran R* and shake to dissolve. Heat gently, if necessary. Reweigh the flask and calculate the total mass of solvent and substance (*M*).

Reference solutions. Into four 15 ml flasks, respectively weigh, to the nearest 0.1 mg, about 2.5 mg, 5.0 mg, 10.0 mg and 20.0 mg of *diethylene glycol R*. Add 5.0 ml of *tetrahydrofuran R* and shake to dissolve. Weigh the flasks again and calculate the concentration of diethylene glycol in milligrams per gram for each reference solution.

The chromatographic procedure may be carried out using:

– a gel-permeation column 0.6 m long and 7 mm in internal diameter packed with *styrene-divinylbenzene copolymer R* (particle diameter 5 µm and pore size 10 nm),

– as mobile phase at a flow rate of 1 ml/min *tetrahydrofuran R*,

– a differential refractive index detector.

Inject 40 µl of each solution. When the chromatograms are recorded in the prescribed conditions, the retention times relative to diethylene glycol are about 0.84 for the monoesters and about 0.78 for the diesters. From the calibration curve obtained with the reference solutions determine the concentration (*C*) in milligrams per gram of diethylene glycol in the test solution.

Calculate the percentage content of free diethylene glycol in the substance to be examined using the following expression:

$$\frac{C \times M}{m \times 10}$$

From the peak area of the monoesters (*A*) and the diesters (*B*), calculate the percentage content of monoesters using the following expression:

$$\frac{A}{A + B} \times (100 - D)$$

D = the percentage content of free diethylene glycol and the percentage content of free fatty acids.

Calculate the percentage content of free fatty acids using the expression:

$$\frac{I_A \times 270}{561.1}$$

I_A = acid value.

STORAGE

Store protected from light.

01/2005:0484

DIETHYLSTILBESTROL

Diethylstilbestrolum

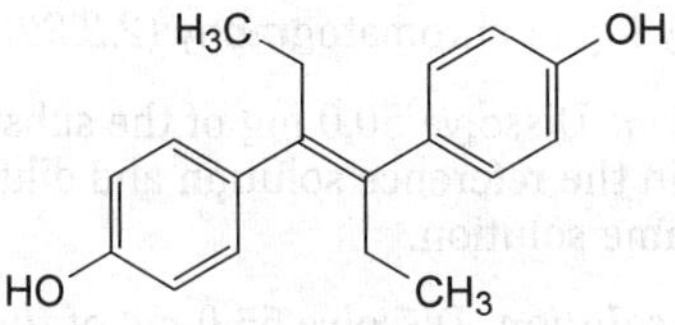

$C_{18}H_{20}O_2$ M_r 268.4

DEFINITION

Diethylstilbestrol contains not less than 97.0 per cent and not more than the equivalent of 101.0 per cent of (*E*)-4,4′-(1,2-diethylethene-1,2-diyl)diphenol, calculated with reference to the dried substance.

CHARACTERS

A white or almost white, crystalline powder, practically insoluble in water, freely soluble in alcohol. It dissolves in solutions of the alkali hydroxides.

It melts at about 172 °C.

IDENTIFICATION

First identification: B, D.

Second identification: A, C, D.

A. Examined between 230 nm and 450 nm (*2.2.25*), the irradiated solution of the substance to be examined prepared as prescribed in the assay shows two absorption maxima, at 292 nm and 418 nm.

B. Examine by infrared absorption spectrophotometry (*2.2.24*), comparing with the spectrum obtained with *diethylstilbestrol CRS*. Examine the substances prepared as discs.

C. Examine the chromatograms obtained in the test for mono-and dimethyl ethers. The principal spot in the chromatogram obtained with test solution (b) is similar in position, colour and size to the principal spot in the chromatogram obtained with reference solution (a).

D. Dissolve about 0.5 mg in 0.2 ml of *glacial acetic acid R*, add 1 ml of *phosphoric acid R* and heat on a water-bath for 3 min. A deep-yellow colour develops.

TESTS

4,4′-Dihydroxystilbene and related ethers. Dissolve 0.100 g in *ethanol R* and dilute to 10.0 ml with the same solvent. The absorbance (*2.2.25*) of the solution measured at 325 nm is not greater than 0.50.

Mono- and dimethyl ethers. Examine by thin-layer chromatography (*2.2.27*), using *silica gel G R* as the coating substance.

Test solution (a). Dissolve 0.2 g of the substance to be examined in 2 ml of *alcohol R*.

Test solution (b). Dilute 1 ml of test solution (a) to 20 ml with *alcohol R*.

Reference solution (a). Dissolve 10 mg of *diethylstilbestrol CRS* in 2 ml of *alcohol R*.

Reference solution (b). Dissolve 5 mg of *diethylstilbestrol monomethyl ether CRS* in *alcohol R* and dilute to 10 ml with the same solvent.

Reference solution (c). Dissolve 5 mg of *diethylstilbestrol dimethyl ether CRS* in *alcohol R* and dilute to 10 ml with the same solvent.

Reference solution (d). Dissolve 10 mg of *dienestrol CRS* in 2 ml of *alcohol R*. To 1 ml of this solution add 1 ml of reference solution (a).

Apply to the plate 1 µl of each solution. Develop over a path of 15 cm using a mixture of 10 volumes of *diethylamine R* and 90 volumes of *toluene R*. Allow the plate to dry in air, spray with *alcoholic solution of sulphuric acid R* and heat at 120 °C for 10 min. In the chromatogram obtained with test solution (a), any spots corresponding to diethylstilbestrol monomethyl ether and diethylstilbestrol dimethyl ether are not more intense than the spots in the chromatograms obtained with reference solutions (b) and (c) respectively (0.5 per cent). Diethylstilbestrol gives one or sometimes two spots. The test is not valid unless the chromatogram obtained with reference solution (d) shows at least two clearly separated spots having approximately the same intensity.

Loss on drying (*2.2.32*). Not more than 0.5 per cent, determined on 1.000 g by drying in an oven at 100 °C to 105 °C.

Sulphated ash (*2.4.14*). Not more than 0.1 per cent, determined on 1.0 g.

ASSAY

Dissolve 20.0 mg in *ethanol R* and dilute to 100.0 ml with the same solvent. Dilute 10.0 ml of the solution to 100.0 ml with *ethanol R*. To 25.0 ml of the resulting solution add 25.0 ml of a solution of 1 g of *dipotassium hydrogen phosphate R* in 55 ml of *water R*. Prepare in the same manner a reference solution using 20.0 mg of *diethylstilbestrol CRS*. Transfer an equal volume of each solution to separate 1 cm quartz cells and close the cells; place the two cells about 5 cm from a low-pressure, short-wave 2 W to 20 W mercury lamp and irradiate for about 5 min. Measure the absorbance (*2.2.25*) of the irradiated solutions at the maximum at 418 nm, using *water R* as the compensation liquid. Continue the irradiation for successive periods of 3 min to 15 min, depending on the power of the lamp, and repeat the measurement of the absorbances at 418 nm until the maximum absorbance (about 0.7) is obtained. If necessary, adjust the geometry of the irradiation apparatus to obtain a maximum, reproducible absorbance at 418 nm.

Calculate the content of $C_{18}H_{20}O_2$ from the measured absorbances and the concentrations of the solutions.

STORAGE

Store protected from light.

01/2005:0818

DIFLUNISAL

Diflunisalum

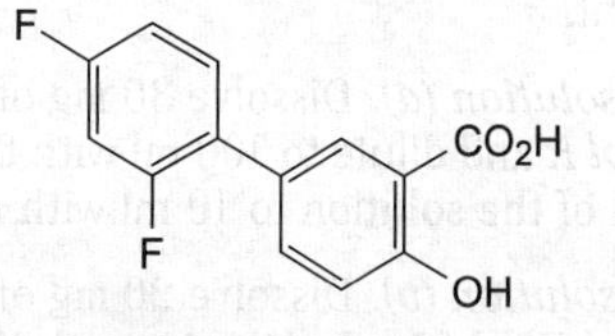

$C_{13}H_8F_2O_3$ M_r 250.2

DEFINITION

Diflunisal contains not less than 99.0 per cent and not more than the equivalent of 101.0 per cent of 2′,4′-difluoro-4-hydroxybiphenyl-3-carboxylic acid, calculated with reference to the dried substance.

CHARACTERS

A white or almost white, crystalline powder, practically insoluble in water, soluble in alcohol. It dissolves in dilute solutions of alkali hydroxides.

IDENTIFICATION

First identification: B.

Second identification: A, C, D.

A. Dissolve 10 mg in a 0.3 per cent *V/V* solution of *hydrochloric acid R* in *methanol R* and dilute to 100.0 ml with the same acid solution. Dilute 2.0 ml of the solution to 10.0 ml with a 0.3 per cent *V/V* solution of *hydrochloric acid R* in *methanol R*. Examined between 230 nm and 350 nm (*2.2.25*), the solution shows two absorption maxima, at 251 nm and 315 nm. The ratio of the absorbance measured at the maximum at 251 nm to that measured at the maximum at 315 nm is 4.2 to 4.6.

B. Examine by infrared absorption spectrophotometry (*2.2.24*), comparing with the spectrum obtained with *diflunisal CRS*. Examine the substances prepared as discs. If the spectra obtained show differences, dissolve the substance to be examined and the reference substance separately in *alcohol R*, evaporate to dryness and record new spectra using the residues.

C. Dissolve about 2 mg in 10 ml of *alcohol R* and add 0.1 ml of *ferric chloride solution R1*. A violet-red colour is produced.

D. Mix about 5 mg with 45 mg of *heavy magnesium oxide R* and ignite in a crucible until an almost white residue is obtained (usually less than 5 min). Allow to cool, add 1 ml of *water R*, 0.05 ml of *phenolphthalein solution R1* and about 1 ml of *dilute hydrochloric acid R* to render the solution colourless. Filter. Add 1.0 ml of the filtrate to a freshly prepared mixture of 0.1 ml of *alizarin S solution R* and 0.1 ml of *zirconyl nitrate solution R*. Mix, allow to stand for 5 min and compare the colour of the solution with that of a blank prepared in the same manner. The test solution is yellow and the blank is red.

TESTS

Appearance of solution. Dissolve 0.5 g in *alcohol R* and dilute to 50 ml with the same solvent. The solution is clear (*2.2.1*) and not more intensely coloured than reference solution Y_7 (*2.2.2, Method II*).

Related substances

A. Examine by thin-layer chromatography (*2.2.27*), using *silica gel* GF_{254} *R* as the coating substance.

Test solution. Dissolve 0.20 g of the substance to be examined in *methanol R* and dilute to 10 ml with the same solvent.

Reference solution (a). Dissolve 30 mg of *biphenyl-4-ol R* in *methanol R* and dilute to 100 ml with the same solvent. Dilute 1 ml of the solution to 10 ml with *methanol R*.

Reference solution (b). Dissolve 20 mg of *biphenyl-4-ol R* in *methanol R*, add 1 ml of the test solution and dilute to 10 ml with *methanol R*.

Apply to the plate 10 µl of each solution. Develop over a path of 15 cm using a mixture of 10 volumes of *glacial acetic acid R*, 20 volumes of *acetone R* and 70 volumes of *methylene chloride R*. Dry the plate in a current of warm air and examine in ultraviolet light at 254 nm. Any spot in the chromatogram obtained with the test solution, apart from the principal spot, is not more intense than the spot in the chromatogram obtained with reference solution (a) (0.15 per cent). The test is not valid unless the chromatogram obtained with reference solution (b) shows two clearly separated principal spots.

B. Examine by liquid chromatography (*2.2.29*).

Test solution. Dissolve 50.0 mg of the substance to be examined in the reference solution and dilute to 10.0 ml with the same solution.

Reference solution. Dissolve 55.0 mg of *fluoranthene R* in a mixture of 1 volume of *water R* and 4 volumes of *acetonitrile R* and dilute to 100.0 ml with the same mixture of solvents. Dilute 1.0 ml to 100.0 ml with a mixture of 1 volume of *water R* and 4 volumes of *acetonitrile R*.

The chromatographic procedure may be carried out using:

- a stainless steel column 0.25 m long and 4 mm in internal diameter packed with *octadecylsilyl silica gel for chromatography R* (10 µm),
- as mobile phase at a flow rate of 2 ml/min a mixture of 2 volumes of *glacial acetic acid R*, 25 volumes of *methanol R*, 55 volumes of *water R* and 70 volumes of *acetonitrile R*,
- as detector a spectrophotometer set at 254 nm.

Inject 20 µl of the reference solution and adjust the sensitivity of the detector so that the height of the principal peak in the chromatogram obtained is not less than 10 per cent of the full scale of the recorder. Inject separately 20 µl of the test solution and 20 µl of the reference solution. Continue the chromatography for three times the retention time of fluoranthene. In the chromatogram obtained with the test solution, the sum of the areas of any peaks, apart from the principal peak, with a retention time greater than that of fluoranthene is not greater than the area of the principal peak in the chromatogram obtained with the reference solution (0.1 per cent). Disregard any peak with an area less than 0.05 times that of the principal peak in the chromatogram obtained with the reference solution.

Heavy metals (*2.4.8*). 2.0 g complies with limit test C for heavy metals (10 ppm). Use a platinum crucible. Prepare the standard using 2 ml of *lead standard solution (10 ppm Pb) R*.

Loss on drying (*2.2.32*). Not more than 0.3 per cent, determined on 1.000 g by drying at 60 °C at a pressure not exceeding 700 Pa for 2 h.

Sulphated ash (*2.4.14*). Not more than 0.1 per cent, determined on 1.0 g in a platinum crucible.

ASSAY

Dissolve 0.200 g in 40 ml of *methanol R*. Add 5 ml of *water R* and 0.2 ml of *phenol red solution R*. Titrate with *0.1 M sodium hydroxide* until the colour changes from yellow to reddish-violet.

1 ml of *0.1 M sodium hydroxide* is equivalent to 25.02 mg of $C_{13}H_8F_2O_3$.

STORAGE

Store protected from light.

IMPURITIES

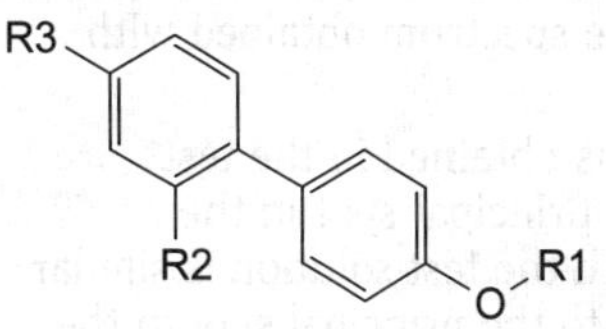

A. R1 = R2 = R3 = H: biphenyl-4-ol,

B. R1 = H, R2 = R3 = F: 2′,4′-difluorobiphenyl-4-ol,

C. R1 = CO-CH_3, R2 = R3 = F: 2′,4′-difluorobiphenyl-4-yl acetate,

D. condensation products.

01/2005:0117

DIGITALIS LEAF

Digitalis purpureae folium

DEFINITION

Digitalis leaf consists of the dried leaf of *Digitalis purpurea* L. It contains not less than 0.3 per cent of cardenolic glycosides, expressed as digitoxin (M_r 765), and calculated with reference to the drug dried at 100 °C to 105 °C.

CHARACTERS

Digitalis leaf has a faint but characteristic odour. The whole leaf is about 10 cm to 40 cm long and 4 cm to 15 cm wide. The lamina is ovate lanceolate to broadly ovate. The winged petiole is from one quarter as long as to equal in length to the lamina.

It has the macroscopic and microscopic characters described in identication tests A and B.

IDENTIFICATION

A. The leaf is brittle and often occurs broken. The upper surface is green and the lower surface is greyish-green. The apex is subacute and the margin is irregularly crenate, dentate or serrate. The base is decurrent. The venation is pinnate, the lateral veins being prominent especially on the lower surface, leaving the midrib at about 45° and anastomosing near the margin; a veinlet terminates in each tooth of the margin and the lower veins run down the winged petiole. The upper surface is rugose and pubescent; the lower surface shows a network of raised veinlets and is densely pubescent.

B. Reduce to a powder (355). Examine under a microscope using *chloral hydrate solution R*. The powder shows the following diagnostic characters: epidermal cells with anticlinal walls which are straight or slightly sinuous on the upper surface and markedly sinuous on the lower surface; the cuticle is smooth. Trichomes are of two types: uniseriate, bluntly pointed non-glandular, usually of three to five cells, often with one or more collapsed cells, walls mostly finely warty or faintly striated; glandular trichomes usually with a unicellular, sometimes a multicellular uniseriate stalk and a unicellular or bicellular or exceptionally tetracellular head. Anomocytic stomata (*2.8.3*) are absent or very rare on the upper surface, numerous on the lower surface. Calcium oxalate crystals and sclerenchyma are absent.

C. Examine by thin-layer chromatography (*2.2.27*), using *silica gel G R* as the coating substance.

Test solution. To 1.0 g of the powdered drug (180) add a mixture of 20 ml of *alcohol (50 per cent V/V) R* and 10 ml of *lead acetate solution R*. Boil for 2 min, allow to cool and centrifuge. Shake the supernatant solution with two quantities, each of 15 ml, of *chloroform R*; separate the two layers by centrifugation if necessary. Dry the chloroform layers over *anhydrous sodium sulphate R* and filter. Evaporate 10 ml of the solution to dryness on a water-bath and dissolve the residue in 1 ml of a mixture of equal volumes of *chloroform R* and *methanol R*.

Reference solution. Dissolve 5 mg of *purpureaglycoside A CRS*, 2 mg of *purpureaglycoside B CRS*, 5 mg of *digitoxin R* and 2 mg of *gitoxin R* in a mixture of equal volumes of *chloroform R* and *methanol R* and dilute to 10 ml with the same mixture of solvents.

Apply separately to the plate as bands 2 cm by 0.3 cm 20 µl of each solution. Develop over a path of 10 cm using a mixture of 7.5 volumes of *water R*, 10 volumes of *methanol R* and 75 volumes of *ethyl acetate R*. Allow the solvents to evaporate. Spray with a mixture of 2 volumes of a 10 g/l solution of *chloramine R* and 8 volumes of a 250 g/l solution of *trichloroacetic acid R* in *alcohol R*. Heat at 100 °C to 105 °C for 10 min. Examine in ultraviolet light at 365 nm. The chromatogram obtained with the reference solution shows a zone of light-blue fluorescence in the lower part of the chromatogram, corresponding to purpureaglycoside B, and just above it a zone of brownish-yellow fluorescence, corresponding to purpureaglycoside A. A zone of light-blue fluorescence, corresponding to gitoxin, appears in the middle of the chromatogram and above it a zone of brownish-yellow fluorescence, corresponding to digitoxin. The zones in the chromatogram obtained with the test solution are similar in position, colour and size to the zones in the chromatogram obtained with the reference solution. Other zones of fluorescence may also appear in the chromatogram obtained with the test solution.

D. Evaporate 5 ml of the chloroformic solution obtained in identification test C to dryness on a water-bath. To the residue add 2 ml of *dinitrobenzoic acid solution R* and 1 ml of *1 M sodium hydroxide*. A reddish-violet colour develops within 5 min.

E. Evaporate 5 ml of the chloroformic solution obtained in identification test C to dryness on a water-bath. To the residue add 3 ml of *xanthydrol solution R* and heat on a water-bath for 3 min. A red colour develops.

TESTS

Foreign matter (*2.8.2*). There are no leaves with few or no trichomes and epidermal cells showing, in surface view, beaded anticlinal walls (*Digitalis lanata*).

Loss on drying (*2.2.32*). Not more than 6.0 per cent, determined on 1.000 g of the powdered drug (355) by drying in an oven at 100 °C to 105 °C.

Total ash (*2.4.16*). Not more than 12.0 per cent.

Ash insoluble in hydrochloric acid (*2.8.1*). Not more than 5.0 per cent.

ASSAY

Shake 0.250 g of the powdered drug (180) with 50.0 ml of *water R* for 1 h. Add 5.0 ml of a 150 g/l solution of *lead acetate R*, shake and after a few minutes add 7.5 ml of a 40 g/l solution of *disodium hydrogen phosphate R*. Filter through a pleated filter paper. Heat 50.0 ml of the filtrate with 5 ml of hydrochloric acid (150 g/l HCl) under a reflux condenser on a water-bath for 1 h. Transfer to a separating funnel, rinse the flask with two quantities, each of 5 ml, of *water R* and shake with three quantities, each of 25 ml, of *chloroform R*. Dry the combined chloroform layers over *anhydrous sodium sulphate R* and dilute to 100.0 ml with *chloroform R*. Evaporate 40.0 ml of the chloroformic solution to dryness, dissolve the residue in 7 ml of *alcohol (50 per cent V/V) R* and add 2 ml of *dinitrobenzoic acid solution R* and 1 ml of *1 M sodium hydroxide*. At the same time prepare a reference solution as follows. Dissolve 50.0 mg of *digitoxin CRS* in *alcohol R* and dilute to 50.0 ml with the same solvent. Dilute 5.0 ml of the solution to 50.0 ml with *alcohol R*. To 5.0 ml of the resulting solution add 25 ml of *water R* and 3 ml of hydrochloric acid (150 g/l HCl). Heat the solution under a reflux condenser on a water-bath for 1 h and complete the preparation as described above. Measure the absorbance (*2.2.25*) of the two solutions at 540 nm several times during the first 12 min until the maximum is reached, using as the compensation liquid a mixture of 7 ml of *alcohol (50 per cent V/V) R*, 2 ml of *dinitrobenzoic acid solution R* and 1 ml of *1 M sodium hydroxide*.

From the absorbances measured and the concentrations of the solutions, calculate the content of cardenolic glycosides, expressed as digitoxin.

STORAGE

Store protected from light and moisture.

01/2005:0078

DIGITOXIN

Digitoxinum

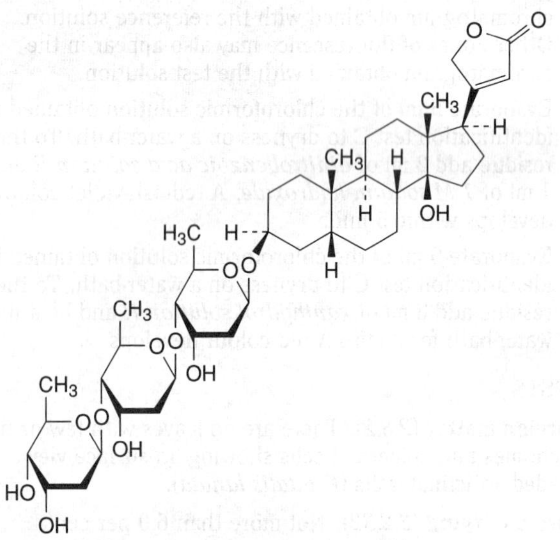

$C_{41}H_{64}O_{13}$ M_r 765

DEFINITION

Digitoxin contains not less than 95.0 per cent and not more than the equivalent of 103.0 per cent of 3β-[(*O*-2,6-dideoxy-β-D-*ribo*-hexopyranosyl-(1→4)-*O*-2,6-dideoxy-β-D-*ribo*-hexopyranosyl-(1→4)-2,6-dideoxy-β-D-*ribo*-hexopyranosyl)oxy]-14-hydroxy-5β,14β-card-20(22)-enolide, calculated with reference to the dried substance.

CHARACTERS

A white or almost white powder, practically insoluble in water, freely soluble in a mixture of equal volumes of methanol and methylene chloride, slightly soluble in alcohol and in methanol.

IDENTIFICATION

First identification: A.

Second identification: B, C, D.

A. Examine by infrared absorption spectrophotometry (*2.2.24*), comparing with the spectrum obtained with *digitoxin CRS*.

B. Examine the chromatograms obtained in the test for related substances. The principal spot in the chromatogram obtained with the test solution is similar in position, colour and size to the principal spot in the chromatogram obtained with reference solution (a).

C. Suspend about 0.5 mg in 0.2 ml of *alcohol (60 per cent V/V) R*. Add 0.1 ml of *dinitrobenzoic acid solution R* and 0.1 ml of *dilute sodium hydroxide solution R*. A violet colour develops.

D. Dissolve about 0.5 mg in 1 ml of *glacial acetic acid R*, heating gently, allow to cool and add 0.05 ml of *ferric chloride solution R1*. Cautiously add 1 ml of *sulphuric acid R*, avoiding mixing the two liquids. A brown ring develops at the interface and on standing a green, then blue colour passes to the upper layer.

TESTS

Appearance of solution. Dissolve 50 mg in a mixture of equal volumes of *methanol R* and *methylene chloride R* and dilute to 10 ml with the same mixture of solvents. The solution is clear (*2.2.1*) and colourless (*2.2.2, Method I*).

Specific optical rotation (*2.2.7*). Dissolve 0.25 g in *chloroform R* and dilute to 10.0 ml with the same solvent. The specific optical rotation is + 16.0 to + 18.5.

Related substances. Examine by thin-layer chromatography (*2.2.27*), using a *TLC silica gel G plate R*.

Test solution. Dissolve 20 mg of the substance to be examined in a mixture of equal volumes of *methanol R* and *methylene chloride R* and dilute to 2 ml with the same mixture of solvents.

Reference solution (a). Dissolve 20 mg of *digitoxin CRS* in a mixture of equal volumes of *methanol R* and *methylene chloride R* and dilute to 2 ml with the same mixture of solvents.

Reference solution (b). Dilute 0.5 ml of reference solution (a) to 50 ml with a mixture of equal volumes of *methanol R* and *methylene chloride R*.

Reference solution (c). Dissolve 10 mg of *gitoxin CRS* with stirring in a mixture of equal volumes of *methanol R* and *methylene chloride R* and dilute to 50 ml with the same mixture of solvents.

Reference solution (d). Dilute 1 ml of reference solution (b) to 2 ml with a mixture of equal volumes of *methanol R* and *methylene chloride R*.

Reference solution (e). Mix 1 ml of reference solution (a) and 1 ml of reference solution (c).

Apply to the plate 5 µl of each solution. Develop immediately over a path of 15 cm using a mixture of 15 volumes of *methanol R*, 40 volumes of *cyclohexane R* and 90 volumes of *methylene chloride R*. Dry the plate in a stream of cold air for 5 min. Repeat the development and dry the plate in a stream of cold air for 5 min. Spray with a mixture of 1 volume of *sulphuric acid R* and 9 volumes of *alcohol R* and heat at 130 °C for 15 min. Examine in daylight.

Gitoxin. Any spot corresponding to gitoxin in the chromatogram obtained with the test solution is not more intense than the spot in the chromatogram obtained with reference solution (c) (2.0 per cent).

Other glycosides. Any spot in the chromatogram obtained with the test solution, apart from the principal spot and the spot corresponding to gitoxin, is not more intense than the spot in the chromatogram obtained with reference solution (b) (1.0 per cent).

The test is not valid unless the chromatogram obtained with reference solution (e) shows clearly separated spots corresponding to digitoxin, gitoxin and other glycosides and the spot in the chromatogram obtained with reference solution (d) is clearly visible.

Loss on drying (*2.2.32*). Not more than 1.5 per cent, determined on 0.500 g by drying in an oven at 100 °C to 105 °C for 2 h.

Sulphated ash (*2.4.14*). Not more than 0.1 per cent, determined on the residue from the test for loss on drying.

ASSAY

Dissolve 40.0 mg in *alcohol R* and dilute to 50.0 ml with the same solvent. Dilute 5.0 ml of the solution to 100.0 ml with *alcohol R*. Prepare a reference solution in the same manner, using 40.0 mg of *digitoxin CRS*. To 5.0 ml of each solution add 3.0 ml of *alkaline sodium picrate solution R*, allow to stand protected from bright light for 30 min and measure the absorbance (*2.2.25*) of each solution at the maximum at 495 nm, using as the compensation liquid a mixture of 5.0 ml of *alcohol R* and 3.0 ml of *alkaline sodium picrate solution R* prepared at the same time.

Calculate the content of $C_{41}H_{64}O_{13}$ from the absorbances measured and the concentrations of the solutions.

STORAGE

Store protected from light.

01/2005:0079

DIGOXIN

Digoxinum

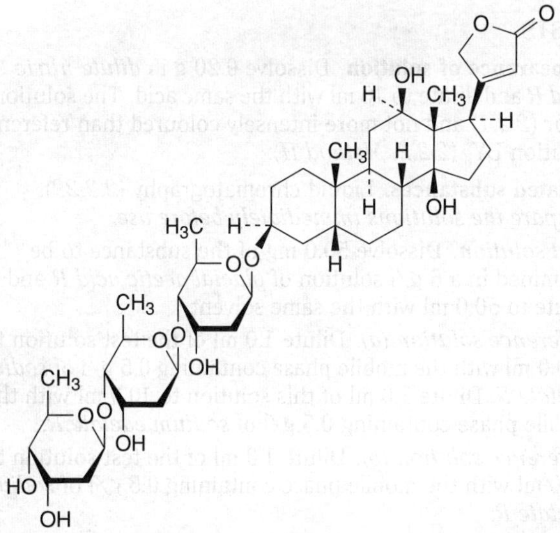

$C_{41}H_{64}O_{14}$ M_r 781

DEFINITION

Digoxin contains not less than 95.0 per cent and not more than the equivalent of 103.0 per cent of 3β-[(*O*-2,6-dideoxy-β-D-*ribo*-hexopyranosyl-(1→4)-*O*-2,6-dideoxy-β-D-*ribo*-hexopyranosyl-(1→4)-2,6-dideoxy-β-D-*ribo*-hexopyranosyl)oxy]-12β,14-dihydroxy-5β-card-20(22)-enolide, calculated with reference to the dried substance.

CHARACTERS

A white or almost white powder or colourless crystals, practically insoluble in water, freely soluble in a mixture of equal volumes of methanol and methylene chloride, slightly soluble in alcohol.

IDENTIFICATION

First identification: A.

Second identification: B, C, D.

A. Examine by infrared absorption spectrophotometry (*2.2.24*), comparing with the spectrum obtained with *digoxin CRS*.

B. Examine the chromatograms obtained in the test for related substances. The principal spot in the chromatogram obtained with the test solution is similar in position, colour and size to the principal spot in the chromatogram obtained with reference solution (a).

C. Suspend about 0.5 mg in 0.2 ml of *alcohol (60 per cent V/V) R*. Add 0.1 ml of *dinitrobenzoic acid solution R* and 0.1 ml of *dilute sodium hydroxide solution R*. A violet colour develops.

D. Dissolve about 0.5 mg in 1 ml of *glacial acetic acid R*, heating gently, allow to cool and add 0.05 ml of *ferric chloride solution R1*. Cautiously add 1 ml of *sulphuric acid R* avoiding mixing the two liquids. A brown ring develops at the interface and on standing a green, then blue colour passes to the upper layer.

TESTS

Appearance of solution. Dissolve 50 mg in a mixture of equal volumes of *methanol R* and *methylene chloride R* and dilute to 10 ml with the same mixture of solvents. The solution is clear (*2.2.1*) and colourless (*2.2.2, Method I*).

Specific optical rotation (*2.2.7*). Dissolve 0.20 g in *anhydrous pyridine R* and dilute to 10.0 ml with the same solvent. The specific optical rotation is + 10.0 to + 13.0, calculated with reference to the dried substance.

Related substances. Examine by thin-layer chromatography (*2.2.27*), using *kieselguhr G R* as the coating substance. Impregnate the plate by placing it in a closed chromatographic tank containing the necessary quantity of a mixture of 10 volumes of *formamide R* and 90 volumes of *acetone R* so that the plate dips about 5 mm into the liquid. When the impregnation mixture has risen at least 15 cm from the lower edge of the plate, remove the plate and allow the solvent to evaporate for 30 min. Use the plate immediately.

Test solution. Dissolve 50 mg of the substance to be examined in a mixture of equal volumes of *methanol R* and *methylene chloride R* and dilute to 5 ml with the same mixture of solvents.

Reference solution (a). Dissolve 20 mg of *digoxin CRS* in a mixture of equal volumes of *methanol R* and *methylene chloride R* and dilute to 2 ml with the same mixture of solvents.

Reference solution (b). Dilute 1 ml of reference solution (a) to 50 ml with a mixture of equal volumes of *methanol R* and *methylene chloride R*.

Reference solution (c). Dilute 2 ml of reference solution (b) to 4 ml with a mixture of equal volumes of *methanol R* and *methylene chloride R*.

Reference solution (d). Dissolve 5 mg of *digitoxin CRS* in a mixture of equal volumes of *methanol R* and *methylene chloride R* and dilute to 50 ml with the same mixture of solvents.

Reference solution (e). Dissolve 5 mg of *gitoxin CRS* in a mixture of equal volumes of *methanol R* and *methylene chloride R* and dilute to 25 ml with the same mixture of solvents.

Apply separately to the plate 2 µl of each solution. Develop over a path of 12 cm using a mixture of 4 volumes of *formamide R*, 50 volumes of *methyl ethyl ketone R* and 50 volumes of *xylene R*. Dry the plate in a current of cold air until only the lower edge is still visibly moist. Repeat the development and dry the plate at 115 °C for 20 min. Allow to cool, spray with a mixture of 1 volume of a freshly prepared 30 g/l solution of *chloramine R* and 15 volumes of a 250 g/l solution of *trichloroacetic acid R* in *alcohol R* and heat at 115 °C for 5 min. Examine in ultraviolet light at 365 nm. Any spot corresponding to digitoxin in the chromatogram obtained with the test solution is not more intense than the spot in the chromatogram obtained with reference solution (d) (1.0 per cent). Any spot corresponding to gitoxin in the chromatogram obtained with the test solution is not more intense than the spot in the chromatogram obtained with reference solution (e) (2.0 per cent). Any spot in the chromatogram obtained with the test solution, apart from the principal spot and spots corresponding to digitoxin and gitoxin, is not more intense than the spot in the chromatogram obtained with reference solution (b) (2.0 per cent) and at most one such spot is more intense than the spot in the chromatogram obtained with reference solution (c) (1.0 per cent).

Loss on drying (*2.2.32*). Not more than 1.0 per cent, determined on 0.500 g by drying *in vacuo*.

Sulphated ash (*2.4.14*). Not more than 0.1 per cent, determined on the residue from the test for loss on drying.

ASSAY

Dissolve 40.0 mg in *alcohol R*, heating if necessary, and dilute to 50.0 ml with the same solvent. Dilute 5.0 ml of the solution to 100.0 ml with *alcohol R*. Prepare a reference solution in the same manner, using 40.0 mg of *digoxin CRS*. To 5.0 ml of each solution add 3.0 ml of *alkaline sodium picrate solution R*, allow to stand protected from bright light for 30 min and measure the absorbance (*2.2.25*) of each solution at the maximum at 495 nm, using as the compensation liquid a mixture of 5.0 ml of *alcohol R* and 3.0 ml of *alkaline sodium picrate solution R* prepared at the same time.

Calculate the content of $C_{41}H_{64}O_{14}$ from the absorbances measured and the concentrations of the solutions.

STORAGE

Store protected from light.

IMPURITIES

A. digitoxin,

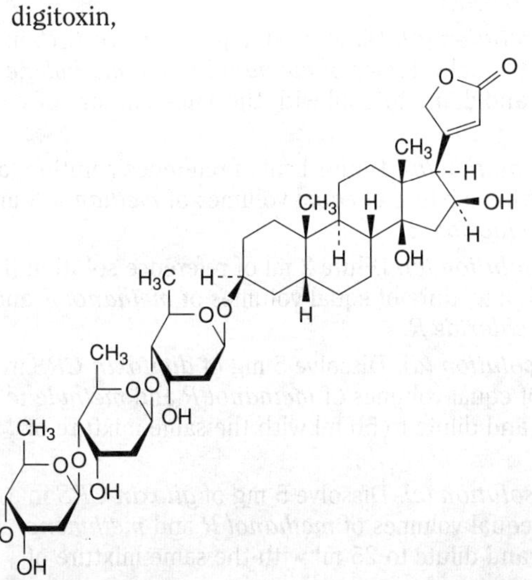

B. 3β-[(*O*-2,6-dideoxy-β-D-*ribo*-hexopyranosyl-(1→4)-*O*-2,6-dideoxy-β-D-*ribo*-hexopyranosyl-(1→4)-2,6-dideoxy-β-D-*ribo*-hexopyranosyl)oxy]-14,16β-dihydroxy-5β-card-20(22)-enolide (gitoxin).

01/2005:1310
corrected

DIHYDRALAZINE SULPHATE, HYDRATED

Dihydralazini sulfas hydricus

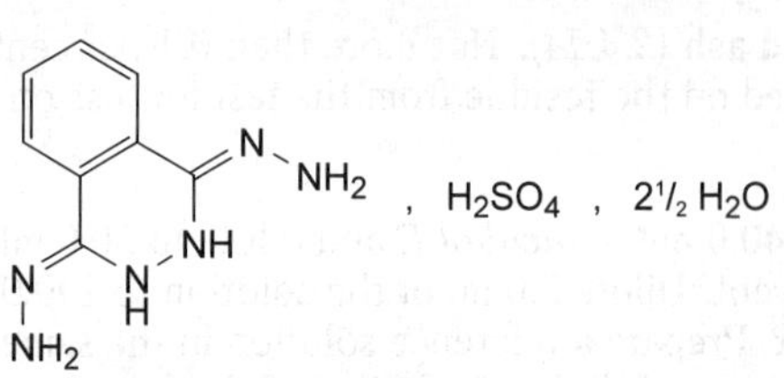

$C_8H_{12}N_6O_4S,2^1/_2H_2O$ M_r 333.3

DEFINITION

Hydrated dihydralazine sulphate contains not less than 98.0 per cent and not more than the equivalent of 102.0 per cent of (phthalazine-1,4(2*H*,3*H*)-diylidene)dihydrazine sulphate, calculated with reference to the dried substance.

CHARACTERS

A white or slightly yellow, crystalline powder, slightly soluble in water, practically insoluble in ethanol. It dissolves in dilute mineral acids.

IDENTIFICATION

A. Examine by infrared absorption spectrophotometry (*2.2.24*), comparing with the *Ph. Eur. reference spectrum of dihydralazine sulphate hydrated*.

B. Dissolve about 50 mg in 5 ml of *dilute hydrochloric acid R*. The solution gives reaction (a) of sulphates (*2.3.1*).

TESTS

Appearance of solution. Dissolve 0.20 g in *dilute nitric acid R* and dilute to 10 ml with the same acid. The solution is clear (*2.2.1*) and not more intensely coloured than reference solution BY_6 (*2.2.2, Method II*).

Related substances. Liquid chromatography (*2.2.29*). *Prepare the solutions immediately before use.*

Test solution. Dissolve 50.0 mg of the substance to be examined in a 6 g/l solution of *glacial acetic acid R* and dilute to 50.0 ml with the same solvent.

Reference solution (a). Dilute 1.0 ml of the test solution to 100.0 ml with the mobile phase containing 0.5 g/l of *sodium edetate R*. Dilute 1.0 ml of this solution to 10.0 ml with the mobile phase containing 0.5 g/l of *sodium edetate R*.

Reference solution (b). Dilute 1.0 ml of the test solution to 50.0 ml with the mobile phase containing 0.5 g/l of *sodium edetate R*.

Reference solution (c). Dissolve 5 mg of *dihydralazine for system suitability CRS* in a 6 g/l solution of *glacial acetic acid R* and dilute to 5.0 ml with the same solvent.

Column:

– *size*: *l* = 0.25 m, Ø = 4.6 mm,
– *stationary phase*: *nitrile silica gel for chromatography R* (5 µm).

Mobile phase: to 22 volumes of *acetonitrile R* add 78 volumes of a solution containing 1.44 g/l of *sodium laurilsulfate R* and 0.75 g/l of *tetrabutylammonium bromide R* and adjust to pH 3.0 with *0.05 M sulphuric acid*.

Flow rate: 1.5 ml/min.

Detection: spectrophotometer at 230 nm.

Injection: 20 µl.

Run time: twice the retention time of dihydralazine.
Relative retention with reference to dihydralazine: impurity A = about 0.8.
System suitability: reference solution (c):
- the peaks due to impurity A and dihydralazine are baseline separated as in the chromatogram supplied with *dihydralazine for system suitability CRS*.

Limits:
- *impurity A*: not more than the area of the principal peak in the chromatogram obtained with reference solution (b) (2 per cent),
- *impurity C*: not more than the area of the principal peak in the chromatogram obtained with reference solution (a) (0.1 per cent),
- *any other impurity*: for each impurity, not more than the area of the principal peak in the chromatogram obtained with reference solution (a) (0.1 per cent),
- *total of impurities other than A*: not more than 5 times the area of the principal peak in the chromatogram obtained with reference solution (a) (0.5 per cent),
- *disregard limit*: 0.1 times the area of the principal peak in the chromatogram obtained with reference solution (a).

Hydrazine. Examine by liquid chromatography (*2.2.29*). *Prepare the solutions immediately before use.*

Test solution. Dissolve 40.0 mg of *hydrazine sulphate R* in *water R* and dilute to 100.0 ml with the same solvent. Dilute 1.0 ml of the solution to 25.0 ml with *water R*. To 0.50 ml of the solution, add 0.200 g of the substance to be examined and dissolve in 6 ml of *dilute hydrochloric acid R*, then dilute to 10.0 ml with *water R*. In a centrifuge tube with a ground-glass stopper, place immediately 0.50 ml of the solution and 2.0 ml of a 60 g/l solution of *benzaldehyde R* in a mixture of equal volumes of *methanol R* and *water R*. Shake for 90 s. Add 1.0 ml of *water R* and 5.0 ml of *heptane R*. Shake for 1 min and centrifuge. Use the upper layer.

Reference solution. Dissolve 40.0 mg of *hydrazine sulphate R* in *water R* and dilute to 100.0 ml with the same solvent. Dilute 1.0 ml of the solution to 25.0 ml with *water R*. To 0.50 ml of the solution, add 6 ml of *dilute hydrochloric acid R* and dilute to 10.0 ml with *water R*. In a centrifuge tube with a ground-glass stopper, place 0.50 ml of the solution and 2.0 ml of a 60 g/l solution of *benzaldehyde R* in a mixture of equal volumes of *methanol R* and *water R*. Shake for 90 s. Add 1.0 ml of *water R* and 5.0 ml of *heptane R*. Shake for 1 min and centrifuge. Use the upper layer.

Blank solution. Prepare in the same manner as for the reference solution but replacing the 0.50 ml of hydrazine sulphate solution by 0.50 ml of *water R*.

The chromatographic procedure may be carried out using:
- a stainless steel column 0.25 m long and 4.6 mm in internal diameter packed with *octadecylsilyl silica gel for chromatography R* (5 µm),
- as mobile phase at a flow rate of 1 ml/min a mixture of 30 volumes of a 0.3 g/l solution of *sodium edetate R* and 70 volumes of *acetonitrile R*,
- as detector a spectrophotometer set at 305 nm.

Inject 20 µl each of the test solution, the reference solution and the blank solution. Comparing the chromatograms obtained with the reference solution and the blank solution, identify the peak of benzaldehyde azine (benzalazine) corresponding to hydrazine having a retention time relative to the principal peak (benzaldehyde) of about 1.8. In the chromatogram obtained with the test solution, the area of the peak corresponding to benzaldehyde azine is not greater than twice that of the corresponding peak in the chromatogram obtained with the reference solution (10 ppm of hydrazine).

Iron (*2.4.9*). To the residue obtained in the test for sulphated ash add 0.2 ml of *sulphuric acid R* and heat carefully until the acid is almost completely eliminated. Allow to cool and dissolve the residue with heating in 5.5 ml of *hydrochloric acid R1*. Filter the hot solution through a filter previously washed 3 times with *dilute hydrochloric acid R*. Wash the crucible and the filter with 5 ml of *water R*. Combine the filtrate and the washings and neutralise with about 3.5 ml of *strong sodium hydroxide solution R*. Adjust the pH to between 3 and 4 with *acetic acid R* and dilute to 20 ml with *water R*. The solution complies with the limit test for iron (20 ppm). Prepare the standard with 5 ml of *iron standard solution (2 ppm Fe) R* and 5 ml of *water R*.

Loss on drying (*2.2.32*): 13.0 per cent to 15.0 per cent, determined on 1.000 g by drying in an oven at 50 °C at a pressure not exceeding 0.7 kPa for 5 h.

Sulphated ash (*2.4.14*). Not more than 0.1 per cent, determined on 1.0 g.

ASSAY

Dissolve 60.0 mg in 25 ml of *water R*. Add 35 ml of *hydrochloric acid R* and titrate slowly with *0.05 M potassium iodate*, determining the end-point potentiometrically (*2.2.20*), using a calomel reference electrode and a platinum indicator electrode.

1 ml of *0.05 M potassium iodate* is equivalent to 7.208 mg of $C_8H_{12}N_6O_4S$.

IMPURITIES

Specified impurities: A, B, C.

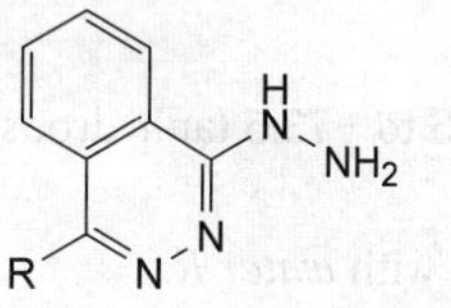

A. R = NH_2: 4-hydrazinophthalazin-1-amine,

C. R = H:(phthalazin-1-yl)hydrazine (hydralazine),

B. H_2N-NH_2: hydrazine.

01/2005:1776

DIHYDROCODEINE HYDROGEN TARTRATE

Dihydrocodeini hydrogenotartras

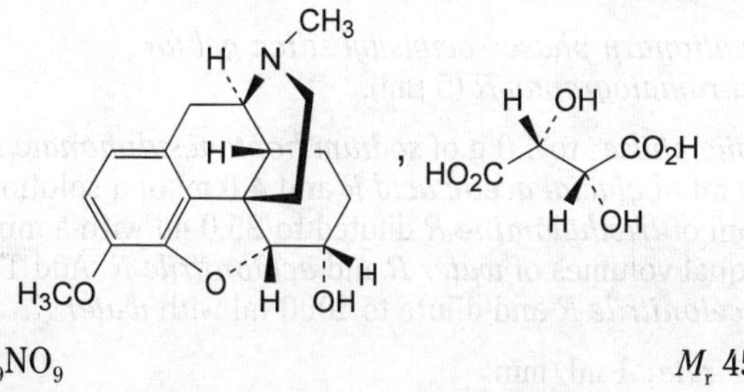

$C_{22}H_{29}NO_9$ M_r 451.5

DEFINITION

4,5α-Epoxy-3-methoxy-17-methylmorphinan-6α-ol hydrogen (2*R*,3*R*)-2,3-dihydroxybutanedioate.

Content: 98.5 per cent to 101.0 per cent (anhydrous substance).

Monographs D-E

CHARACTERS

Appearance: white or almost white, crystalline powder.

Solubility: freely soluble in water, sparingly soluble in alcohol, practically insoluble in cyclohexane.

IDENTIFICATION

First identification: A.

Second identification: B, C, D.

A. Infrared absorption spectrophotometry (*2.2.24*).

Comparison: *Ph. Eur. reference spectrum of dihydrocodeine hydrogen tartrate.*

B. To about 0.1 g add 1 ml of *sulphuric acid R* and 0.05 ml of *ferric chloride solution R1* and heat on a water-bath. A brownish-yellow colour develops. Add 0.05 ml of *dilute nitric acid R*. The colour does not become red.

C. To 1 ml of solution S (see Tests) add 5 ml of *picric acid solution R*. Heat on a water-bath until a clear solution is obtained. Allow to cool. A precipitate is formed. Filter, wash with 5 ml of *water R* and dry at 100-105 °C. The crystals melt (*2.2.14*) at 220 °C to 223 °C.

D. It gives reaction (b) of tartrates (*2.3.1*).

TESTS

Solution S. Dissolve 2.50 g in *carbon dioxide-free water R* and dilute to 25.0 ml with the same solvent.

Appearance of solution. Solution S is clear (*2.2.1*) and not more intensely coloured than reference solution BY_5 (*2.2.2, Method II*).

pH (*2.2.3*): 3.2 to 4.2 for solution S.

Specific optical rotation (*2.2.7*): − 70.5 to − 73.5 (anhydrous substance).

Dilute 10.0 ml of solution S to 20.0 ml with *water R*.

Related substances. Liquid chromatography (*2.2.29*).

Test solution. Dissolve 10.0 mg of the substance to be examined in the mobile phase and dilute to 10.0 ml with the mobile phase.

Reference solution (a). Dissolve 2.0 mg of *codeine phosphate R* in 2.0 ml of the test solution and dilute to 25.0 ml with the mobile phase.

Reference solution (b). Dilute 1.0 ml of the test solution to 200 ml with the mobile phase.

Column:

- *size*: *l* = 0.25 m, Ø = 4.6 mm,
- *stationary phase*: *octylsilyl silica gel for chromatography R* (5 µm).

Mobile phase: to 1.0 g of *sodium heptanesulphonate R*, add 10.0 ml of *glacial acetic acid R* and 4.0 ml of a solution of 5.0 ml of *triethylamine R* diluted to 25.0 ml with a mixture of equal volumes of *water R* and *acetonitrile R*. Add 170 ml of *acetonitrile R* and dilute to 1000 ml with *water R*.

Flow rate: 1 ml/min.

Detection: spectrophotometer at 284 nm.

Injection: 20 µl.

Run time: 5 times the retention time of dihydrocodeine.

Retention time: dihydrocodeine = about 14 min.

System suitability: reference solution (a):

- *resolution*: minimum of 2 between the peaks due to dihydrocodeine and to impurity A.

Limits:

- *impurity A*: not more than the area of the principal peak in the chromatogram obtained with reference solution (b) (0.5 per cent),
- *any other peak*: not more than 0.6 times the area of the principal peak in the chromatogram obtained with reference solution (b) (0.3 per cent),
- *total*: not more than twice the area of the principal peak in the chromatogram obtained with reference solution (b) (1 per cent); disregard any peak due to tartaric acid (relative retention with reference to dihydrocodeine = about 0.25),
- *disregard limit*: 0.1 times the area of the principal peak in the chromatogram obtained with reference solution (b) (0.05 per cent).

Water (*2.5.12*): maximum 0.7 per cent, determined on 1.00 g.

Sulphated ash (*2.4.14*): maximum 0.1 per cent, determined on 1.0 g.

ASSAY

Dissolve 0.350 g in 60 ml of *anhydrous acetic acid R*. Titrate with *0.1 M perchloric acid* determining the end-point potentiometrically (*2.2.20*).

1 ml of *0.1 M perchloric acid* is equivalent to 45.15 mg of $C_{22}H_{29}NO_9$.

STORAGE

Protected from light.

IMPURITIES

A. codeine,

B. morphine,

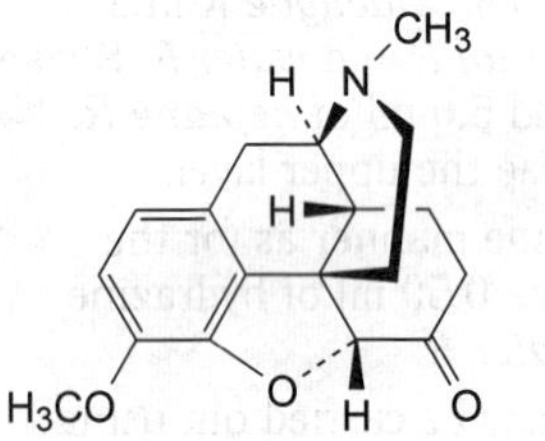

C. 4,5α-epoxy-3-methoxy-17-methylmorphinan-6-one (hydrocodone),

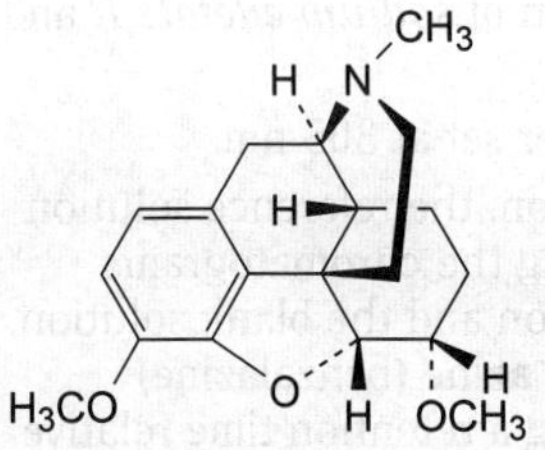

D. 4,5α-epoxy-3,6α-dimethoxy-17-methylmorphinan (tetrahydrothebaine).

01/2005:1416

DIHYDROERGOCRISTINE MESILATE

Dihydroergocristini mesilas

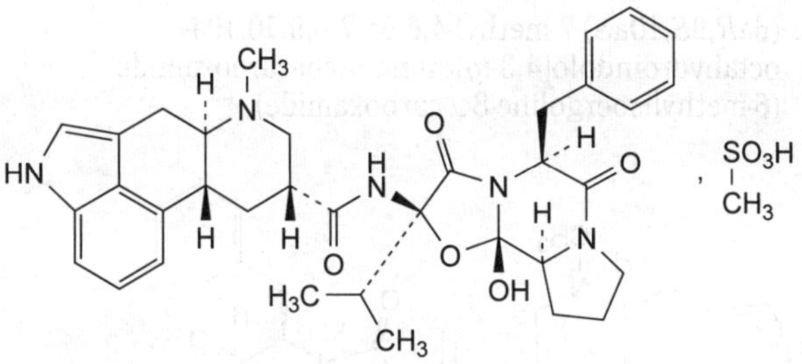

$C_{36}H_{45}N_5O_8S$ M_r 708

DEFINITION

(6a*R*,9*R*,10a*R*)-*N*-[(2*R*,5*S*,10a*S*,10b*S*)-5-Benzyl-10b-hydroxy-2-(1-methylethyl)-3,6-dioxo-octahydro-8*H*-oxazolo[3,2-*a*]pyrrolo[2,1-*c*]pyrazin-2-yl]-7-methyl-4,6,6a,7,8,9,10,10a-octahydroindolo[4,3-*fg*]quinoline-9-carboxamide methanesulphonate.

Content: 98.0 per cent to 102.0 per cent (dried substance).

PRODUCTION

The production method must be evaluated to determine the potential for formation of alkyl mesilates, which is particularly likely to occur if the reaction medium contains lower alcohols. Where necessary, the production method is validated to demonstrate that alkyl mesilates are not detectable in the final product.

CHARACTERS

Appearance: white or almost white, fine crystalline powder.

Solubility: slightly soluble in water, soluble in methanol.

IDENTIFICATION

A. Infrared absorption spectrophotometry (*2.2.24*).

Preparation: discs.

Comparison: *dihydroergocristine mesilate CRS.*

B. Thin-layer chromatography (*2.2.27*).

Test solution. Dissolve 0.10 g of the substance to be examined in a mixture of 1 volume of *methanol R* and 9 volumes of *methylene chloride R* and dilute to 5 ml with the same mixture of solvents.

Reference solution. Dissolve 0.10 g of *dihydroergocristine mesilate CRS* in a mixture of 1 volume of *methanol R* and 9 volumes of *methylene chloride R* and dilute to 5 ml with the same mixture of solvents.

Plate: *TLC silica gel F_{254} plate R.*

Mobile phase: *concentrated ammonia R*, *dimethylformamide R*, *ether R* (2:15:85 *V/V/V*).

Application: 5 µl.

Development: over 2/3 of the plate protected from light.

Drying: in a current of cold air for 5 min.

Detection: spray with *dimethylaminobenzaldehyde solution R7* and dry in a current of hot air for 2 min.

Results: the principal spot in the chromatogram obtained with the test solution is similar in position, colour and size to the principal spot in the chromatogram obtained with the reference solution.

C. Thin-layer chromatography (*2.2.27*).

Test solution. Dissolve 0.20 g of the substance to be examined in a mixture of 1 volume of *methanol R* and 9 volumes of *methylene chloride R* and dilute to 5 ml with the same mixture of solvents.

Reference solution. Dissolve 0.20 g of *methanesulphonic acid R* in a mixture of 1 volume of *methanol R* and 9 volumes of *methylene chloride R* and dilute to 5 ml with the same mixture of solvents. Dilute 1 ml of the solution to 10 ml with a mixture of 1 volume of *methanol R* and 9 volumes of *methylene chloride R.*

Plate: *TLC silica gel F_{254} plate R.*

Mobile phase: *water R*, *concentrated ammonia R*, *butanol R*, *acetone R* (5:10:20:65 *V/V/V/V*).

Application: 10 µl.

Development: over a path of 10 cm protected from light.

Drying: in a current of cold air for not more than 1 min.

Detection: spray with a 1 g/l solution of *bromocresol purple R* in *methanol R*, adjusting the colour to violet-red with one drop of *dilute ammonia R1* and dry the plate in a current of hot air at 100 °C.

Results: the principal spot in the chromatogram obtained with the test solution is similar in position, colour and size to the principal spot in the chromatogram obtained with the reference solution.

TESTS

Appearance of solution. The solution is clear (*2.2.1*) and not more intensely coloured than reference solution B_7 (*2.2.2, Method II*).

Dissolve 0.50 g in *methanol R* and dilute to 25.0 ml with the same solvent.

pH (*2.2.3*): 4.0 to 5.0.

Dissolve 0.10 g in *carbon dioxide-free water R* and dilute to 20 ml with the same solvent.

Specific optical rotation (*2.2.7*): − 37 to − 43 (dried substance).

Dissolve 0.250 g in *anhydrous pyridine R* and dilute to 25.0 ml with the same solvent.

Related substances. Liquid chromatography (*2.2.29*). *Carry out the test and preparation of the solutions protected from bright light.*

Test solution. Dissolve 75.0 mg of the substance to be examined in 10 ml of *acetonitrile R*. Add 10 ml of a 1.0 g/l solution of *phosphoric acid R* and dilute to 50.0 ml with *water R.*

Reference solution. Dissolve 20.0 mg of *codergocrine mesilate CRS* in 10 ml of *acetonitrile R*. Add 10 ml of a 1.0 g/l solution of *phosphoric acid R* and dilute to 50.0 ml with *water R*. Dilute 6.0 ml of the solution to 50.0 ml with a mixture of 20 volumes of *acetonitrile R*, 20 volumes of a 1.0 g/l solution of *phosphoric acid R* and 60 volumes of *water R.*

Column:

– *size*: *l* = 0.25 m, Ø = 4.6 mm,

– *stationary phase*: *octadecylsilyl silica gel for chromatography R* (5 µm) with a pore size of 10 nm and a carbon loading of 19 per cent.

Mobile phase:

– *mobile phase A*: mix 100 volumes of *acetonitrile R* with 900 volumes of *water R* and add 10 volumes of *triethylamine R*,

- *mobile phase B*: mix 100 volumes of *water R* with 900 volumes of *acetonitrile R* and add 10 volumes of *triethylamine R*.

Time (min)	Mobile phase A (per cent *V/V*)	Mobile phase B (per cent *V/V*)
0 - 5	75	25
5 - 20	75 → 25	25 → 75
20 - 22	25 → 75	75 → 25
22 - 30	75	25

Flow rate: 1.2 ml/min.

Detection: spectrophotometer at 280 nm.

Injection: 10 µl.

Relative retention with reference to dihydroergocristine (retention time = about 13.7 min): impurity F = about 0.8; impurity H = about 0.9; impurity I = about 1.02.

System suitability: reference solution:
- the chromatogram shows 4 peaks,
- *resolution*: minimum 1 between the peaks corresponding to dihydroergocristine and impurity I.

Limits:
- *any impurity*: not more than the area of the peak corresponding to dihydroergocristine in the chromatogram obtained with the reference solution (1 per cent),
- *total*: not more than twice the area of the peak corresponding to dihydroergocristine in the chromatogram obtained with the reference solution (2 per cent),
- *disregard limit*: 0.1 times the area of the peak corresponding to dihydroergocristine in the chromatogram obtained with the reference solution (0.1 per cent).

Loss on drying (*2.2.32*): maximum 3.0 per cent, determined on 0.500 g by drying under high vacuum at 80 °C.

ASSAY

Dissolve 0.300 g in 60 ml of *pyridine R*. Pass a stream of *nitrogen R* over the surface of the solution and titrate with *0.1 M tetrabutylammonium hydroxide*, determining the end-point potentiometrically (*2.2.20*). Note the volume used at the second point of inflexion.

1 ml of *0.1 M tetrabutylammonium hydroxide* is equivalent to 35.39 mg of $C_{36}H_{45}N_5O_8S$.

STORAGE

Store protected from light.

IMPURITIES

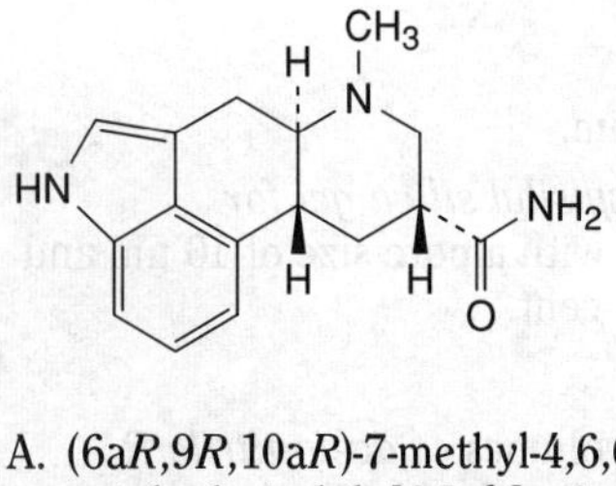

A. (6a*R*,9*R*,10a*R*)-7-methyl-4,6,6a,7,8,9,10,10a-octahydroindolo[4,3-*fg*]quinoline-9-carboxamide (6-methylergoline-8β-carboxamide),

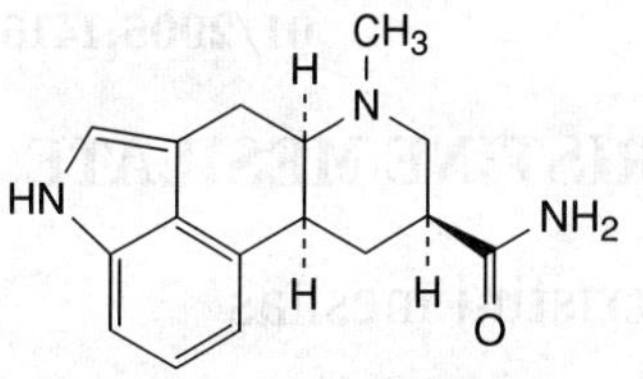

B. (6a*R*,9*S*,10a*S*)-7-methyl-4,6,6a,7,8,9,10,10a-octahydroindolo[4,3-*fg*]quinoline-9-carboxamide (6-methylisoergoline-8α-carboxamide),

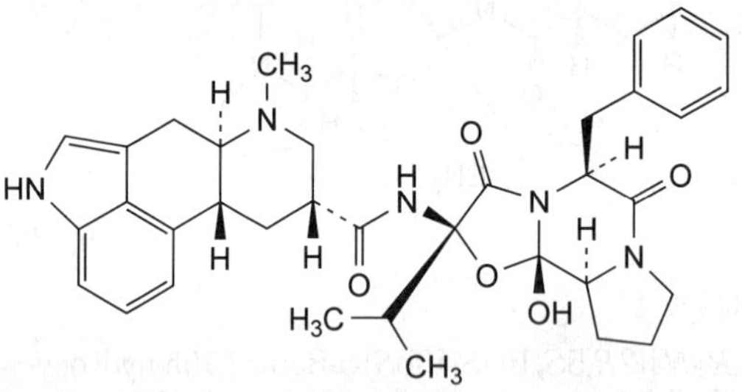

C. (6a*R*,9*R*,10a*R*)-*N*-[(2*S*,5*S*,10a*S*,10b*S*)-5-benzyl-10b-hydroxy-2-(1-methylethyl)-3,6-dioxooctahydro-8*H*-oxazolo[3,2-*a*]pyrrolo[2,1-*c*]pyrazin-2-yl]-7-methyl-4,6,6a,7,8,9,10,10a-octahydroindolo[4,3-*fg*]quinoline-9-carboxamide (2′-epidihydroergocristine),

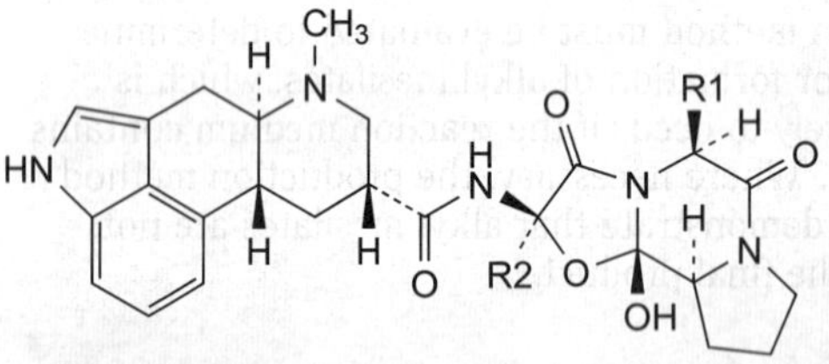

D. R1 = $CH(CH_3)_2$, R2 = CH_3: (6a*R*,9*R*,10a*R*)-*N*-[(2*R*,5*S*,10a*S*,10b*S*)-10b-hydroxy-2-methyl-5-(1-methylethyl)-3,6-dioxooctahydro-8*H*-oxazolo[3,2-*a*]pyrrolo[2,1-*c*]pyrazin-2-yl]-7-methyl-4,6,6a,7,8,9,10,10a-octahydroindolo[4,3-*fg*]quinoline-9-carboxamide (dihydroergosine),

E. R1 = CH_2-C_6H_5, R2 = CH_3: (6a*R*,9*R*,10a*R*)-*N*-[(2*R*,5*S*,10a*S*,10b*S*)-5-benzyl-10b-hydroxy-2-methyl-3,6-dioxooctahydro-8*H*-oxazolo[3,2-*a*]pyrrolo[2,1-*c*]pyrazin-2-yl]-7-methyl-4,6,6a,7,8,9,10,10a-octahydroindolo[4,3-*fg*]quinoline-9-carboxamide (dihydroergotamine),

F. R1 = R2 = $CH(CH_3)_2$: (6a*R*,9*R*,10a*R*)-*N*-[(2*R*,5*S*,10a*S*,10b*S*)10b-hydroxy-2,5-bis(1-methylethyl)-3,6-dioxooctahydro-8*H*-oxazolo[3,2-*a*]pyrrolo[2,1-*c*]pyrazin-2-yl]-7-methyl-4,6,6a,7,8,9,10,10a-octahydroindolo[4,3-*fg*]quinoline-9-carboxamide (dihydroergocornine),

G. R1 = CH_2-C_6H_5, R2 = CH_2-CH_3: (6a*R*,9*R*,10a*R*)-*N*-[(2*R*,5*S*,10a*S*,10b*S*)-5-benzyl-2-ethyl-10b-hydroxy-3,6-dioxooctahydro-8*H*-oxazolo[3,2-*a*]pyrrolo[2,1-*c*]pyrazin-2-yl]-7-methyl-4,6,6a,7,8,9,10,10a-octahydroindolo[4,3-*fg*]quinoline-9-carboxamide (dihydroergostine),

H. R1 = CH_2-$CH(CH_3)_2$, R2 = $CH(CH_3)_2$: (6a*R*,9*R*,10a*R*)-*N*-[(2*R*,5*S*,10a*S*,10b*S*)-10b-hydroxy-2-(1-methylethyl)-5-(2-methylpropyl)-3,6-dioxooctahydro-8*H*-oxazolo[3,2-*a*]pyrrolo[2,1-*c*]pyrazin-2-yl]-7-methyl-4,6,6a,7,8,9,10,10a-octahydroindolo[4,3-*fg*]quinoline-9-carboxamide (α-dihydroergocryptine),

I. R1 = C*H(CH_3)-CH_2-CH_3, R2 = CH(CH_3)$_2$: (6a*R*,9*R*,10a*R*)-*N*-[(2*R*,5*S*,10a*S*,10b*S*)-10b-hydroxy-2-(1-methylethyl)-5-[(1*RS*-1-methylpropyl]-3,6-dioxooctahydro-8*H*-oxazolo[3,2-*a*]pyrrolo[2,1-*c*]pyrazin-2-yl]-7-methyl-4,6,6a,7,8,9,10,10a-octahydroindolo[4,3-*fg*]quinoline-9-carboxamide (β-dihydroergocryptine or epicriptine),

J. R1 = CH_2-C_6H_5, R2 = C*H(CH_3)-CH_2-CH_3: (6a*R*,9*R*,10a*R*)-*N*-[(2*R*,5*S*,10a*S*,10b*S*)-5-benzyl-10b-hydroxy-2-[(1*RS*)-1-methylpropyl]-3,6-dioxooctahydro-8*H*-oxazolo[3,2-*a*]pyrrolo[2,1-*c*]pyrazin-2-yl]-7-methyl-4,6,6a,7,8,9,10,10a-octahydroindolo[4,3-*fg*]quinoline-9-carboxamide (dihydroergosedmine),

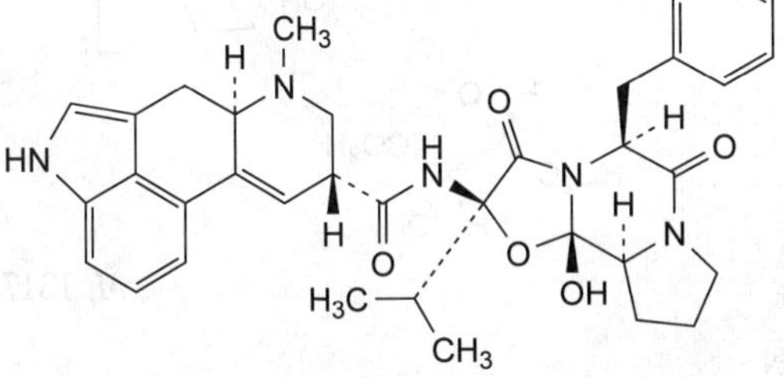

K. (6a*R*,9*R*,10a*R*)-*N*-[(2*R*,5*S*,10a*S*,10b*S*)-5-benzyl-10b-hydroxy-2-(1-methylethyl)-3,6-dioxooctahydro-8*H*-oxazolo[3,2-*a*]pyrrolo[2,1-*c*]pyrazin-2-yl]-7-methyl-4,6,6a,7,8,9-hexahydroindolo[4,3-*fg*]quinoline-9-carboxamide (ergocristine),

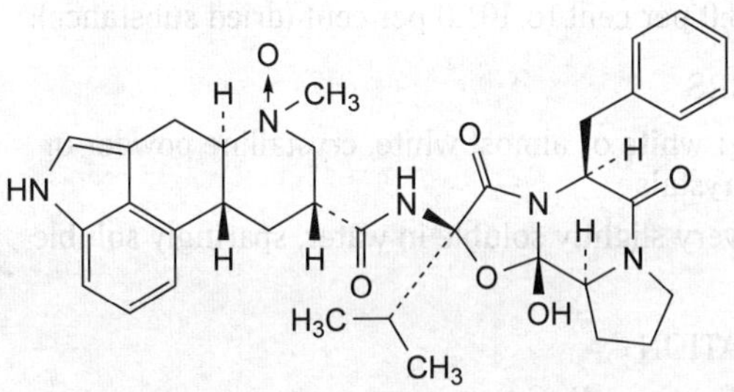

L. (6a*R*,7*RS*,9*R*,10a*R*)-*N*-[(2*R*,5*S*,10a*S*,10b*S*)-5-benzyl-10b-hydroxy-2-(1-methylethyl)-3,6-dioxooctahydro-8*H*-oxazolo[3,2-*a*]pyrrolo[2,1-*c*]pyrazin-2-yl]-7-methyl-4,6,6a,7,8,9,10,10a-octahydroindolo[4,3-*fg*]quinoline-9-carboxamide 7-oxide (dihydroergocristine 6-oxide).

01/2005:0551

DIHYDROERGOTAMINE MESILATE

Dihydroergotamini mesilas

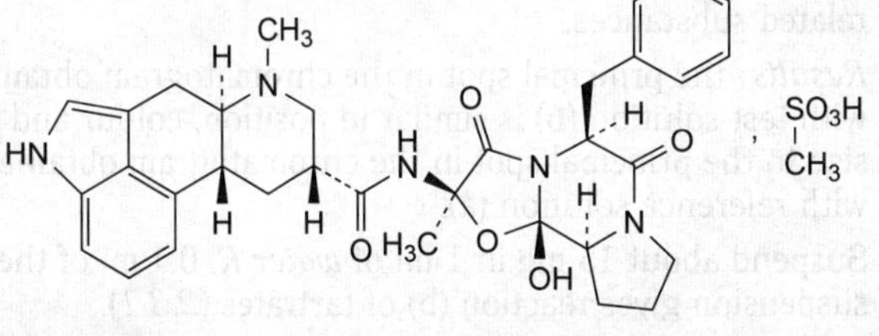

$C_{34}H_{41}N_5O_8S$ M_r 680

DEFINITION

(6a*R*,9*R*,10a*R*)-*N*-[(2*R*,5*S*,10a*S*,10b*S*)-5-Benzyl-10b-hydroxy-2-methyl-3,6-dioxooctahydro-8*H*-oxazolo[3,2-*a*]pyrrolo[2,1-*c*]pyrazin-2-yl]-7-methyl-4,6,6a,7,8,9,10,10a-octahydroindolo[4,3-*fg*]quinoline-9-carboxamide methanesulphonate.

Content: 98.0 per cent to 101.0 per cent (dried substance).

PRODUCTION

The production method must be evaluated to determine the potential for formation of alkyl mesilates, which is particularly likely to occur if the reaction medium contains lower alcohols. Where necessary, the production method is validated to demonstrate that alkyl mesilates are not detectable in the final product.

CHARACTERS

Appearance: white or almost white, crystalline powder or colourless crystals.

Solubility: slightly soluble in water, sparingly soluble in methanol, slightly soluble in alcohol.

IDENTIFICATION

First identification: B, C.

Second identification: A, C, D.

A. Dissolve 5.0 mg in *methanol R* and dilute to 100.0 ml with the same solvent. Examined between 250 nm and 350 nm (*2.2.25*), the solution shows 2 absorption maxima, at 281 nm and 291 nm, and a shoulder at 275 nm. Above 320 nm the absorbance is negligible. The specific absorbance at the absorption maximum at 281 nm is 95 to 105 (dried substance).

B. Infrared absorption spectrophotometry (*2.2.24*).
Preparation: discs.
Comparison: *dihydroergotamine mesilate CRS.*

C. Examine the chromatograms obtained in the test for related substances.
Results: the principal spot in the chromatogram obtained with test solution (b) is similar in position, colour and size to the principal spot in the chromatogram obtained with reference solution (a).

D. To 0.1 g add 5 ml of *dilute hydrochloric acid R* and shake for about 5 min. Filter and add 1 ml of *barium chloride solution R1*. The filtrate remains clear. Mix 0.1 g with 0.4 g of powdered *sodium hydroxide R*, heat to fusion and continue to heat for 1 min. Cool, add 5 ml of *water R*, boil and filter. Acidify the filtrate by the addition of *hydrochloric acid R1* and filter again. The filtrate gives reaction (a) of sulphates (*2.3.1*).

TESTS

Appearance of solution. The solution is clear (*2.2.1*) and not more intensely coloured than reference solution Y_7 or BY_7 (*2.2.2, Method II*).

Dissolve 0.10 g in a mixture of 0.1 ml of a 70 g/l solution of *methanesulphonic acid R* and 50 ml of *water R*.

pH (*2.2.3*): 4.4 to 5.4.

Dissolve 0.10 g in *carbon dioxide-free water R* and dilute to 100 ml with the same solvent.

Specific optical rotation (*2.2.7*): − 42 to − 47 (dried substance).

Dissolve 0.250 g in *anhydrous pyridine R* and dilute to 25.0 ml with the same solvent.

Related substances. Thin-layer chromatography (*2.2.27*). *Prepare the reference solutions and the test solutions immediately before use and in the order indicated below.*

Reference solution (a). Dissolve 10.0 mg of *dihydroergotamine mesilate CRS* in a mixture of 1 volume of *methanol R* and 9 volumes of *methylene chloride R* and dilute to 5 ml with the same mixture of solvents.

Monographs D-E

Reference solution (b). Dilute 2.5 ml of reference solution (a) to 50 ml with a mixture of 1 volume of *methanol R* and 9 volumes of *methylene chloride R.*

Reference solution (c). Dilute 2 ml of reference solution (b) to 5 ml with a mixture of 1 volume of *methanol R* and 9 volumes of *methylene chloride R.*

Test solution (a). Dissolve 0.10 g of the substance to be examined in a mixture of 1 volume of *methanol R* and 9 volumes of *methylene chloride R* and dilute to 5 ml with the same mixture of solvents.

Test solution (b). Dilute 1 ml of test solution (a) to 10 ml with a mixture of 1 volume of *methanol R* and 9 volumes of *methylene chloride R.*

Plate: *TLC silica gel G plate R.*

Mobile phase: *concentrated ammonia R, methanol R, ethyl acetate R, methylene chloride R* (1:6:50:50 *V/V/V/V*).

Application: 5 µl.

Development: protected from light over a path of 15 cm. Dry the plate in a current of cold air for not longer than 1 min. Repeat the development protected from light over a path of 15 cm using a freshly prepared amount of the mobile phase.

Drying: in a current of cold air.

Detection: spray abundantly with *dimethylaminobenzaldehyde solution R7* and dry in a current of hot air for about 2 min.

Limits: test solution (a):

– *any impurity*: any spot, apart from the principal spot, is not more intense than the principal spot in the chromatogram obtained with reference solution (b) (0.5 per cent) and not more than 2 such spots are more intense than the principal spot in the chromatogram obtained with reference solution (c) (0.2 per cent).

Loss on drying (*2.2.32*): maximum 4.0 per cent, determined on 0.500 g by drying at 100-105 °C at a pressure not exceeding 0.1 kPa for 5 h.

ASSAY

Dissolve 0.500 g in a mixture of 10 ml of *anhydrous acetic acid R* and 70 ml of *acetic anhydride R*. Titrate with *0.1 M perchloric acid,* determining the end-point potentiometrically (*2.2.20*).

1 ml of *0.1 M perchloric acid* is equivalent to 68.00 mg of $C_{34}H_{41}N_5O_8S$.

STORAGE

Protected from light.

01/2005:0600

DIHYDROERGOTAMINE TARTRATE

Dihydroergotamini tartras

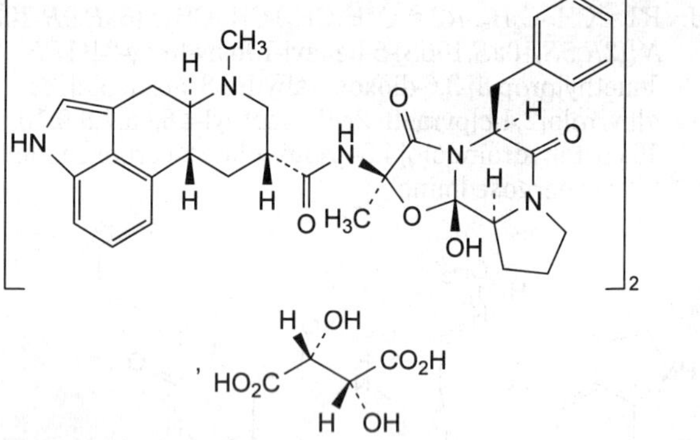

$C_{70}H_{80}N_{10}O_{16}$ M_r 1317

DEFINITION

Bis[(6a*R*,9*R*,10a*R*)-*N*-[(2*R*,5*S*,10a*S*,10b*S*)-5-benzyl-10b-hydroxy-2-methyl-3,6-dioxooctahydro-8*H*-oxazolo[3,2-*a*]pyrrolo[2,1-*c*]pyrazin-2-yl]-7-methyl-4,6,6a,7,8,9,10,10a-octahydroindolo[4,3-*fg*]quinoline-9-carboxamide] (2*R*,3*R*)-2,3-dihydroxybutanedioate.

Content: 98.0 per cent to 101.0 per cent (dried substance).

CHARACTERS

Appearance: white or almost white, crystalline powder or colourless crystals.

Solubility: very slightly soluble in water, sparingly soluble in alcohol.

IDENTIFICATION

First identification: B, C.

Second identification: A, C, D.

A. Dissolve 5.0 mg in *methanol R* and dilute to 100.0 ml with the same solvent. Examined between 250 nm and 350 nm (*2.2.25*), the solution shows 2 absorption maxima, at 281 nm and 291 nm, and a shoulder at 275 nm. Above 320 nm the absorbance is negligible. The specific absorbance at the maximum at 281 nm is 95 to 115 (dried substance).

B. Infrared absorption spectrophotometry (*2.2.24*).

Preparation: discs.

Comparison: *dihydroergotamine tartrate CRS.*

C. Examine the chromatograms obtained in the test for related substances.

Results: the principal spot in the chromatogram obtained with test solution (b) is similar in position, colour and size to the principal spot in the chromatogram obtained with reference solution (a).

D. Suspend about 15 mg in 1 ml of *water R*. 0.1 ml of the suspension gives reaction (b) of tartrates (*2.3.1*).

TESTS

Appearance of solution. The solution is clear (*2.2.1*) and not more intensely coloured than reference solution Y_7 or BY_7 (*2.2.2, Method II*).

Dissolve 0.1 g in *alcohol (85 per cent V/V) R* warming carefully in a water-bath at 40 °C and dilute to 50 ml with the same solvent.

pH (*2.2.3*): 4.0 to 5.5 for the clear supernatant.

Suspend 50 mg in 50 ml of *carbon dioxide-free water R* and shake for 10 min. Allow to stand.

Specific optical rotation (*2.2.7*): −52 to −57 (dried substance).

Dissolve 0.250 g in *anhydrous pyridine R* and dilute to 25.0 ml with the same solvent.

Related substances. Thin-layer chromatography (*2.2.27*). *Prepare the reference solutions and the test solutions immediately before use and in the order indicated.*

Reference solution (a). Dissolve 20 mg of *dihydroergotamine tartrate CRS* in a mixture of 1 volume of *methanol R* and 9 volumes of *chloroform R* and dilute to 10 ml with the same mixture of solvents.

Reference solution (b). Dilute 2.5 ml of reference solution (a) to 50 ml with a mixture of 1 volume of *methanol R* and 9 volumes of *chloroform R.*

Reference solution (c). Dilute 2 ml of reference solution (b) to 5 ml with a mixture of 1 volume of *methanol R* and 9 volumes of *chloroform R.*

Test solution (a). Dissolve 0.10 g of the substance to be examined in a mixture of 1 volume of *methanol R* and 9 volumes of *chloroform R* and dilute to 5 ml with the same mixture of solvents.

Test solution (b). Dilute 1 ml of test solution (a) to 10 ml with a mixture of 1 volume of *methanol R* and 9 volumes of *chloroform R.*

Plate: *TLC silica gel G plate R.*

Mobile phase: *concentrated ammonia R, methanol R, ethyl acetate R, methylene chloride R* (1:6:50:50 *V/V/V/V*).

Application: 5 µl.

Development: protected from light over a path of 15 cm. Dry the plate in a current of cold air for not longer than 1 min. Repeat the development protected from light over a path of 15 cm using a freshly prepared amount of the mobile phase.

Drying: in a current of cold air.

Detection: spray the plate abundantly with *dimethylaminobenzaldehyde solution R7* and dry in a current of hot air for about 2 min.

Limits: in the chromatogram obtained with test solution (a):

– *any impurity*: any spot, apart from the principal spot, is not more intense than the principal spot in the chromatogram obtained with reference solution (b) (0.5 per cent) and not more than 2 such spots are more intense than the principal spot in the chromatogram obtained with reference solution (c) (0.2 per cent).

Loss on drying (*2.2.32*): maximum 5.0 per cent, determined on 0.200 g by drying in an oven at 100-105 °C.

ASSAY

Dissolve 0.250 g in 50 ml of *anhydrous acetic acid R.* Titrate with *0.05 M perchloric acid,* determining the end-point potentiometrically (*2.2.20*).

1 ml of *0.05 M perchloric acid* is equivalent to 32.93 mg of $C_{70}H_{80}N_{10}O_{16}$.

STORAGE

Protected from light.

01/2005:0485

DIHYDROSTREPTOMYCIN SULPHATE FOR VETERINARY USE

Dihydrostreptomycini sulfas ad usum veterinarium

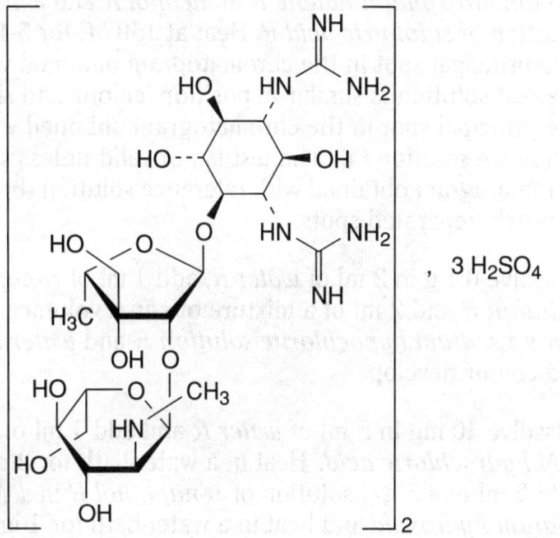

$C_{42}H_{88}N_{14}O_{36}S_3$ M_r 1461

DEFINITION

Dihydrostreptomycin sulphate for veterinary use is bis[*N,N'*-bis(aminoiminomethyl)-4-*O*-[5-deoxy-2-*O*-[2-deoxy-2-(methylamino)-α-L-glucopyranosyl]-3-*C*-(hydroxymethyl)-α-L-lyxofuranosyl]-D-streptamine] tris(sulphate), the sulphate of a substance obtained by catalytic hydrogenation of streptomycin or by any other means. Stabilisers may be added. The potency is not less than 730 IU/mg, calculated with reference to the dried substance.

PRODUCTION

The method of manufacture is validated to demonstrate that the product if tested would comply with the following test:

Abnormal toxicity (*2.6.9*). Inject into each mouse 1 mg dissolved in 0.5 ml of *water for injections R.*

CHARACTERS

A white or almost white powder, freely soluble in water, practically insoluble in acetone, in alcohol and in methanol. It may be hygroscopic.

IDENTIFICATION

A. Examine by thin-layer chromatography (*2.2.27*) using a plate coated with a 0.75 mm layer of the following mixture: mix 0.3 g of *carbomer R* with 240 ml of *water R* and allow to stand, with moderate shaking, for 1 h; adjust to pH 7 by the gradual addition, with continuous shaking, of *dilute sodium hydroxide solution R* and add 30 g of *silica gel H R.*

Heat the plate at 110 °C for 1 h, allow to cool and use immediately.

Test solution. Dissolve 10 mg of the substance to be examined in *water R* and dilute to 10 ml with the same solvent.

Reference solution (a). Dissolve 10 mg of *dihydrostreptomycin sulphate CRS* in *water R* and dilute to 10 ml with the same solvent.

Reference solution (b). Dissolve 10 mg of *dihydrostreptomycin sulphate CRS*, 10 mg of *kanamycin monosulphate CRS* and 10 mg of *neomycin sulphate CRS* in *water R* and dilute to 10 ml with the same solvent.

Apply separately to the plate 10 µl of each solution. Develop over a path of 15 cm using a 70 g/l solution of *potassium dihydrogen phosphate R*. Dry the plate in a current of warm air and spray with a mixture of equal volumes of a 2 g/l solution of *1,3-dihydroxynaphthalene R* in *alcohol R* and a 460 g/l solution of *sulphuric acid R*. Heat at 150 °C for 5-10 min. The principal spot in the chromatogram obtained with the test solution is similar in position, colour and size to the principal spot in the chromatogram obtained with reference solution (a). The test is not valid unless the chromatogram obtained with reference solution (b) shows 3 clearly separated spots.

B. Dissolve 0.1 g in 2 ml of *water R*, add 1 ml of *α-naphthol solution R* and 2 ml of a mixture of equal volumes of *strong sodium hypochlorite solution R* and *water R*. A red colour develops.

C. Dissolve 10 mg in 5 ml of *water R* and add 1 ml of *1 M hydrochloric acid*. Heat in a water-bath for 2 min. Add 2 ml of a 5 g/l solution of *α-naphthol R* in *1 M sodium hydroxide* and heat in a water-bath for 1 min. A violet-pink colour is produced.

D. It gives reaction (a) of sulphates (*2.3.1*).

Monographs D-E

TESTS

Solution S. Dissolve 2.5 g in *carbon dioxide-free water R* and dilute to 10 ml with the same solvent.

Appearance of solution. Solution S is not more intensely coloured than intensity 5 of the range of reference solutions of the most appropriate colour (*2.2.2, Method II*). Allow to stand protected from light at a temperature of about 20 °C for 24 h; solution S is not more opalescent than reference suspension II (*2.2.1*).

pH (*2.2.3*). The pH of solution S is 5.0 to 7.0.

Specific optical rotation (*2.2.7*). Dissolve 0.200 g in *water R* and dilute to 10.0 ml with the same solvent. The specific optical rotation is − 83 to − 91, calculated with reference to the dried substance.

Methanol. Not more than 0.2 per cent, determined by gas chromatography (*2.2.28*).

Test solution. Dissolve 1.00 g of the substance to be examined in *water R* and dilute to 25.0 ml with the same solvent.

Reference solution. Dilute 8.0 mg of *methanol R* to 100 ml with *water R*.

The chromatographic procedure may be carried out using:

- a column 1.5 m to 2.0 m long and 2.0 mm to 4.0 mm in internal diameter packed with *ethylvinylbenzene-divinylbenzene copolymer R* (150-180 µm),
- *nitrogen for chromatography R* as the carrier gas at a constant flow rate of 30-40 ml/min,
- a flame-ionisation detector.

Maintain the column at a constant temperature between 120 °C and 140 °C and the injection port and the detector at a temperature at least 50 °C higher than that of the column. The area of the peak corresponding to methanol in the chromatogram obtained with the test solution is not greater than the area of the peak in the chromatogram obtained with the reference solution.

Streptomycin. Dissolve 0.100 g in *water R* and dilute to 5.0 ml with the same solvent. Add 5.0 ml of *0.2 M sodium hydroxide* and heat in a water-bath for exactly 10 min. Cool in ice for exactly 5 min, add 3 ml of a 15 g/l solution of *ferric ammonium sulphate R* in *0.25 M sulphuric acid*, dilute to 25.0 ml with *water R* and mix (test solution). Prepare at the same time and in the same manner a reference solution using 10 mg of *streptomycin sulphate CRS* in 50 ml of *water R*. Using 5.0 ml of this solution, operate as for the test solution. Exactly 20 min after addition of the ferric ammonium sulphate solution, measure the absorbance (*2.2.25*) of each solution at the maximum at 525 nm in a 2 cm cell, using as the compensation liquid a solution prepared at the same time and in the same manner as the test solution but omitting the substance to be examined. The absorbance of the test solution is not greater than that of the reference solution (1 per cent).

Heavy metals (*2.4.8*). 1.0 g complies with limit test C for heavy metals (20 ppm). Prepare the standard using 2 ml of *lead standard solution (10 ppm Pb) R*.

Loss on drying (*2.2.32*). Not more than 5.0 per cent, determined on 1.000 g by drying at 60 °C over *diphosphorus pentoxide R* at a pressure not exceeding 0.1 kPa for 4 h.

Sulphated ash (*2.4.14*). Not more than 1.0 per cent, determined on 1.0 g.

Sulphate. 18.0 per cent to 21.5 per cent of sulphate (SO_4), calculated with reference to the dried substance. Dissolve 0.250 g in 100 ml of *water R* and adjust the solution to pH 11 using *concentrated ammonia R*. Add 10.0 ml of *0.1 M barium chloride* and about 0.5 mg of *phthalein purple R*. Titrate with *0.1 M sodium edetate*, adding 50 ml of *alcohol R* when the colour of the solution begins to change and continue the titration until the violet-blue colour disappears.

1 ml of *0.1 M barium chloride* is equivalent to 9.606 mg of sulphate (SO_4).

Bacterial endotoxins (*2.6.14*): less than 0.50 IU/mg, if intended for use in the manufacture of parenteral dosage forms without a further appropriate procedure for removal of bacterial endotoxins.

ASSAY

Carry out the microbiological assay of antibiotics (*2.7.2*).

STORAGE

In an airtight container, protected from light. If the substance is sterile, store in a sterile, airtight, tamper-proof container.

LABELLING

The label states:

- where applicable, the name and quantity of any added stabiliser,
- where applicable, that the substance is free from bacterial endotoxins.

01/2005:1004

DILTIAZEM HYDROCHLORIDE

Diltiazemi hydrochloridum

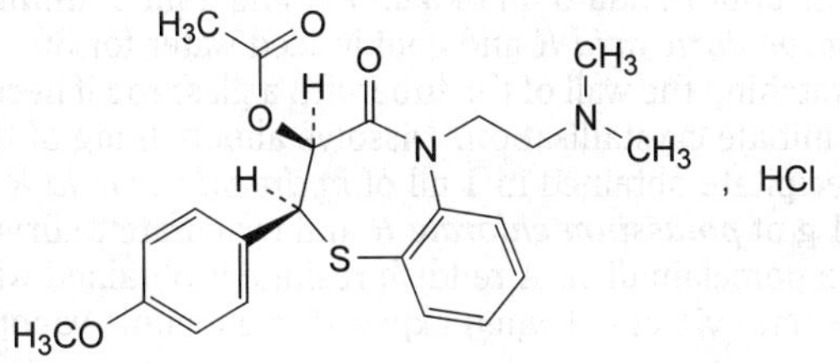

$C_{22}H_{27}ClN_2O_4S$ M_r 451.0

DEFINITION

Diltiazem hydrochloride contains not less than 98.5 per cent and not more than the equivalent of 101.0 per cent of (2*S*,3*S*)-5-[2-(dimethylamino)ethyl]-2-(4-methoxyphenyl)-4-oxo-2,3,4,5-tetrahydro-1,5-benzothiazepin-3-yl acetate hydrochloride, calculated with reference to the dried substance.

CHARACTERS

A white, crystalline powder, freely soluble in water, in methanol and in methylene chloride, slightly soluble in ethanol. It melts at about 213 °C with decomposition.

IDENTIFICATION

First identification: A, D.

Second identification: B, C, D.

A. Examine by infrared absorption spectrophotometry (*2.2.24*), comparing with the spectrum obtained with *diltiazem hydrochloride CRS*. Examine the substances prepared as discs.

B. Examine by thin-layer chromatography (*2.2.27*), using as the coating substance a suitable silica gel with a fluorescent indicator having an optimal intensity at 254 nm.

Test solution. Dissolve 0.10 g of the substance to be examined in *methylene chloride R* and dilute to 10 ml with the same solvent.

Reference solution. Dissolve 0.10 g of *diltiazem hydrochloride CRS* in *methylene chloride R* and dilute to 10 ml with the same solvent.

Apply to the plate 10 µl of each solution. Develop over a path of 10 cm using a mixture of 1 volume of *acetic acid R*, 3 volumes of *water R*, 10 volumes of *methylene chloride R* and 12 volumes of *ethanol R*. Allow the plate to dry in air and examine in ultraviolet light at 254 nm. The principal spot in the chromatogram obtained with the test solution is similar in position and size to the principal spot in the chromatogram obtained with the reference solution.

C. Dissolve 50 mg in 5 ml of *water R*. Add 1 ml of *ammonium reineckate solution R*. A pink precipitate is produced.

D. It gives reaction (a) of chlorides (*2.3.1*).

TESTS

Solution S. Dissolve 1.00 g in *carbon-dioxide free water R* and dilute to 20.0 ml with the same solvent.

Appearance of solution. Solution S is clear (*2.2.1*) and colourless (*2.2.2, Method II*).

pH (*2.2.3*). Dilute 2.0 ml of solution S to 10.0 ml with *carbon dioxide-free water R*. The pH of the solution is 4.3 to 5.3.

Specific optical rotation (*2.2.7*). Dilute 5.0 ml of solution S to 25.0 ml with *water R*. The specific optical rotation is + 115 to + 120, calculated with reference to the dried substance.

Related substances. Examine by liquid chromatography (*2.2.29*).

Test solution. Dissolve 50.0 mg of the substance to be examined in the mobile phase and dilute to 200.0 ml with the mobile phase.

Reference solution(a). Dissolve 50.0 mg of *diltiazem hydrochloride CRS* in the mobile phase and dilute to 200.0 ml with the mobile phase.

Reference solution (b). Dissolve 3 mg of *diltiazem impurity A CRS* in the mobile phase and dilute to 10 ml with the mobile phase. To 1 ml of this solution, add 1.2 ml of reference solution (a) and dilute to 100.0 ml with the mobile phase.

Reference solution(c). Dilute 0.3 ml of the test solution to 100.0 ml with the mobile phase.

The chromatographic procedure may be carried out using:

– a stainless steel column 0.10 m long and 4.6 mm in internal diameter packed with *octadecylsilyl silica gel for chromatography R* (3 µm),
– as mobile phase at a flow rate of 1.5 ml/min a mixture of 5 volumes of *ethanol R*, 25 volumes of *acetonitrile R* and 70 volumes of a solution containing, in 1 litre, 6.8 g of *potassium dihydrogen phosphate R* and 0.1 ml of *N,N-dimethyloctylamine R*, adjusted to pH 4.5 using *dilute phosphoric acid R*,
– as detector a spectrophotometer set at 240 nm,
– a loop injector.

Inject separately 20 µl of each solution. Adjust the sensitivity of the detector so that the height of the principal peak in the chromatogram obtained with reference solution (c) is at least 10 per cent of the full scale of the recorder. Continue the chromatography for five times the retention time of the principal peak. The test is not valid unless in the chromatogram obtained with reference solution (b), the resolution between the peaks due to diltiazem impurity A and diltiazem is at least 4.0 and the symmetry factors are not more than 2.0. If necessary, adjust the concentration of *N,N*-dimethyloctylamine in the mobile phase. In the chromatogram obtained with the test solution, the sum of the areas of any peaks, apart from the principal peak, is not greater than the area of the principal peak in the chromatogram obtained with reference solution (c) (0.3 per cent). Disregard any peak with an area less than 0.025 times that of the peak in the chromatogram obtained with reference solution (c).

Heavy metals (*2.4.8*). Dissolve 2.0 g in *water R* and dilute to 20.0 ml with the same solvent. 12 ml of the solution complies with limit test A for heavy metals (10 ppm). Prepare the standard using *lead standard solution (1 ppm Pb) R*.

Loss on drying (*2.2.32*). Not more than 0.5 per cent, determined on 1.000 g by drying in an oven at 100-105 °C for 2 h.

Sulphated ash (*2.4.14*). Not more than 0.1 per cent, determined on 1.0 g.

ASSAY

Dissolve 0.400 g in a mixture of 2 ml of *anhydrous formic acid R* and 60 ml of *acetic anhydride R* and titrate with *0.1 M perchloric acid*, determining the end-point potentiometrically (*2.2.20*).

1 ml of *0.1 M perchloric acid* is equivalent to 45.1 mg of $C_{22}H_{27}ClN_2O_4S$.

Monographs D-E

STORAGE

Store in an airtight container, protected from light.

IMPURITIES

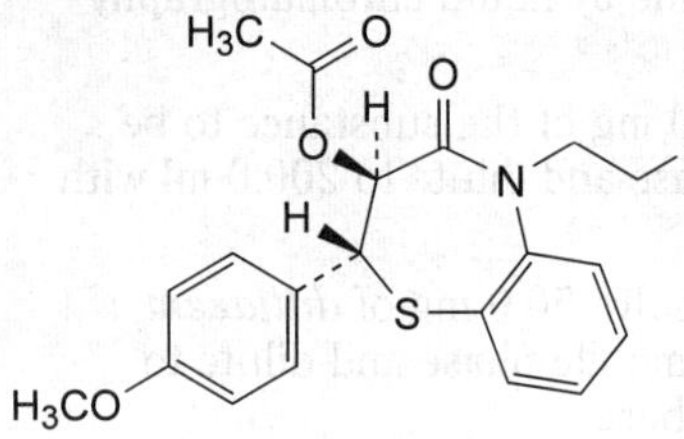

A. (2*R*,3*S*)-5-[2-(dimethylamino)ethyl]-2-(4-methoxyphenyl)-4-oxo-2,3,4,5-tetrahydro-1,5-benzothiazepin-3-yl acetate,

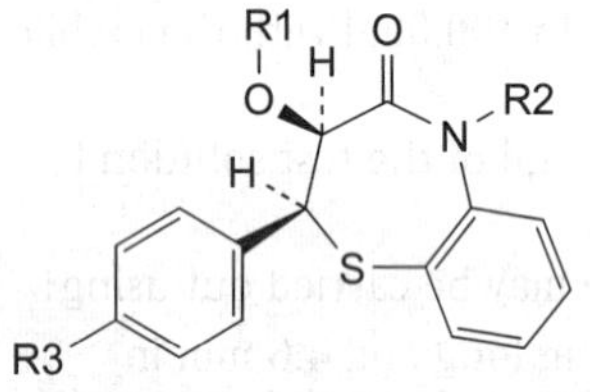

B. R1 = CO-CH_3, R2 = H, R3 = OCH_3: (2*S*,3*S*)-2-(4-methoxyphenyl)-4-oxo-2,3,4,5-tetrahydro-1,5-benzothiazepin-3-yl acetate,

C. R1 = CO-CH_3, R2 = CH_2-CH_2-N$(CH_3)_2$, R3 = OH: (2*S*,3*S*)-5-[2-(dimethylamino)ethyl]-2-(4-hydroxyphenyl)-4-oxo-2,3,4,5-tetrahydro-1,5-benzothiazepin-3-yl acetate,

D. R1 = CO-CH_3, R2 = CH_2-CH_2-NH-CH_3, R3 = OCH_3: (2*S*,3*S*)-2-(4-methoxyphenyl)-5-[2-(methylamino)ethyl]-4-oxo-2,3,4,5-tetrahydro-1,5-benzothiazepin-3-yl acetate,

E. R1 = R2 = H, R3 = OCH_3: (2*S*,3*S*)-3-hydroxy-2-(4-methoxyphenyl)-2,3-dihydro-1,5-benzothiazepin-4(5*H*)-one,

F. R1 = H, R2 = CH_2-CH_2-N$(CH_3)_2$, R3 = OCH_3: (2*S*,3*S*)-5-[2-(dimethylamino)ethyl]-3-hydroxy-2-(4-methoxyphenyl)-2,3-dihydro-1,5-benzothiazepin-4(5*H*)-one.

01/2005:0601

DIMENHYDRINATE

Dimenhydrinatum

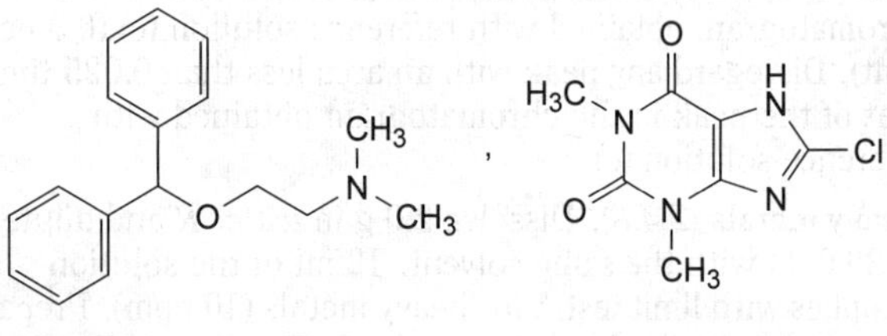

$C_{24}H_{28}ClN_5O_3$ M_r 470.0

DEFINITION

Dimenhydrinate contains not less than 53.0 per cent and not more than 55.5 per cent of diphenhydramine [2-(diphenylmethoxy)-*N*,*N*-dimethylethylamine, $C_{17}H_{21}NO$, M_r 255.4] and not less than 44.0 per cent and not more than 46.5 per cent of 8-chlorotheophylline (8-chloro-3,7-dihydro-1,3-dimethyl-1*H*-purine-2,6-dione, $C_7H_7ClN_4O_2$, M_r 214.6), both calculated with reference to the dried substance.

CHARACTERS

A white, crystalline powder or colourless crystals, slightly soluble in water, freely soluble in alcohol.

IDENTIFICATION

First identification: C.

Second identification: A, B, D.

A. Melting point (*2.2.14*): 102 °C to 106 °C.

B. Dissolve 0.1 g in a mixture of 3 ml of *water R* and 3 ml of *alcohol R*, add 6 ml of *water R* and 1 ml of *dilute hydrochloric acid R* and cool in iced water for 30 min, scratching the wall of the tube with a glass rod if necessary to initiate crystallisation. Dissolve about 10 mg of the precipitate obtained in 1 ml of *hydrochloric acid R*, add 0.1 g of *potassium chlorate R* and evaporate to dryness in a porcelain dish. A reddish residue is obtained which becomes violet-red when exposed to ammonia vapour.

C. Examine by infrared absorption spectrophotometry (*2.2.24*), comparing with the spectrum obtained with *dimenhydrinate CRS*.

D. Dissolve 0.2 g in 10 ml of *alcohol R*. Add 10 ml of *picric acid solution R* and initiate crystallisation by scratching the wall of the tube with a glass rod. The precipitate, washed with *water R* and dried at 100 °C to 105 °C, melts (*2.2.14*) at 130 °C to 134 °C.

TESTS

Appearance of solution. Dissolve 1.0 g in *alcohol R* and dilute to 20 ml with the same solvent. The solution is clear (*2.2.1*) and colourless (*2.2.2, Method II*).

pH (*2.2.3*). To 0.4 g add 20 ml of *carbon dioxide-free water R*, shake for 2 min and filter. The pH of the filtrate is 7.1 to 7.6.

Theophylline and substances related to diphenhydramine. Examine by thin-layer chromatography (*2.2.27*), using *silica gel GF_{254} R* as the coating substance.

Test solution. Dissolve 0.40 g of the substance to be examined in *methylene chloride R* and dilute to 10 ml with the same solvent.

Reference solution (a). Dissolve 20 mg of *theophylline R* in *methylene chloride R* and dilute to 100 ml with the same solvent.

Reference solution (b). Dilute 5 ml of the test solution to 100 ml with *methylene chloride R*. Dilute 10 ml of this solution to 100 ml with *methylene chloride R*.

Apply separately to the plate 5 µl of each solution. Develop over a path of 15 cm using a mixture of 1 volume of *concentrated ammonia R*, 9 volumes of *methanol R* and 90 volumes of *methylene chloride R*. Dry the plate in a current of cold air and examine in ultraviolet light at 254 nm. Any spot corresponding to theophylline in the chromatogram obtained with the test solution is not more intense than the spot in the chromatogram obtained with reference solution (a) (0.5 per cent). Spray with *potassium iodobismuthate solution R*. Allow the plate to dry in air and spray with *dilute hydrogen peroxide solution R*. Any spot in the chromatogram obtained with the test solution, apart from the principal spot, is not more intense than the spot in the chromatogram obtained with reference solution (b) (0.5 per cent). Disregard any spot extending from the starting point to an R_f of about 0.1.

Heavy metals (*2.4.8*). Dissolve 2.5 g in a mixture of 15 volumes of *water R* and 85 volumes of *acetone R* and dilute to 25 ml with the same mixture of solvents. The solution complies with limit test B for heavy metals (20 ppm). Prepare the standard using lead standard solution (2 ppm Pb) prepared by diluting *lead standard solution (100 ppm Pb) R* with a mixture of 15 volumes of *water R* and 85 volumes of *acetone R*.

Loss on drying (*2.2.32*). Not more than 0.5 per cent, determined on 1.000 g by drying *in vacuo*.

Sulphated ash (*2.4.14*). Not more than 0.2 per cent, determined on 1.0 g.

ASSAY

Diphenhydramine. Dissolve 0.200 g in 60 ml of *anhydrous acetic acid R*. Titrate with *0.1 M perchloric acid*, determining the end-point potentiometrically (*2.2.20*).

1 ml of *0.1 M perchloric acid* is equivalent to 25.54 mg of $C_{17}H_{21}NO$.

8-Chlorotheophylline. To 0.800 g add 50 ml of *water R*, 3 ml of *dilute ammonia R1* and 0.6 g of *ammonium nitrate R* and heat on a water-bath for 5 min. Add 25.0 ml of *0.1 M silver nitrate* and continue heating on a water-bath for 15 min with frequent swirling. Cool, add 25 ml of *dilute nitric acid R* and dilute to 250.0 ml with *water R*. Filter and discard the first 25 ml of the filtrate. Using 5 ml of *ferric ammonium sulphate solution R2* as indicator, titrate 100.0 ml of the filtrate with *0.1 M ammonium thiocyanate* until a yellowish-brown colour is obtained.

1 ml of *0.1 M silver nitrate* is equivalent to 21.46 mg of $C_7H_7ClN_4O_2$.

01/2005:0389

DIMERCAPROL

Dimercaprolum

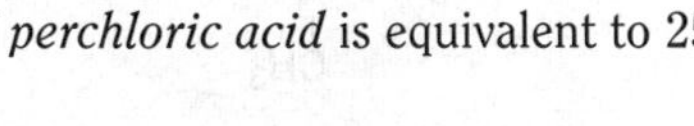

$C_3H_8OS_2$ M_r 124.2

DEFINITION

Dimercaprol contains not less than 98.5 per cent and not more than the equivalent of 101.5 per cent of (2*RS*)-2,3-disulfanylpropan-1-ol.

CHARACTERS

A clear, colourless or slightly yellow liquid, soluble in water and in arachis oil, miscible with alcohol and with benzyl benzoate.

IDENTIFICATION

A. Dissolve 0.05 ml in 2 ml of *water R*. Add 1 ml of *0.05 M iodine*. The colour of the iodine is discharged immediately.

B. Dissolve 0.1 ml in 5 ml of *water R* and add 2 ml of *copper sulphate solution R*. A bluish-black precipitate is formed which quickly becomes dark grey.

C. In a ground-glass-stoppered tube, suspend 0.6 g of *sodium bismuthate R*, previously heated to 200 °C for 2 h, in a mixture of 2.8 ml of *dilute phosphoric acid R* and 6 ml of *water R*. Add 0.2 ml of the substance to be examined, mix and allow to stand for 10 min with frequent shaking. To 1 ml of the supernatant liquid add 5 ml of a 4 g/l solution of *chromotropic acid, sodium salt R* in *sulphuric acid R* and mix. Heat for 15 min in a water-bath. A violet-red colour develops.

TESTS

Appearance. It is clear (*2.2.1*) and not more intensely coloured than reference solution B_6 or BY_6 (*2.2.2, Method II*).

Acidity or alkalinity. Dissolve 0.2 g in *carbon dioxide-free water R* and dilute to 10 ml with the same solvent. Add 0.25 ml of *bromocresol green solution R* and 0.3 ml of *0.01 M hydrochloric acid*. The solution is yellow. Not more than 0.5 ml of *0.01 M sodium hydroxide* is required to change the colour of the indicator to blue.

Refractive index (*2.2.6*): 1.568 to 1.574.

Halides. To 2.0 g add 25 ml of *alcoholic potassium hydroxide solution R* and boil under a reflux condenser for 2 h. Eliminate the alcohol by evaporation in a stream of hot air, add 20 ml of *water R* and cool. Add 40 ml of *water R* and 10 ml of *strong hydrogen peroxide solution R*, boil gently for 10 min, cool and filter rapidly. Add 10 ml of *dilute nitric acid R* and 5.0 ml of *0.1 M silver nitrate*. Using 2 ml of *ferric ammonium sulphate solution R2* as indicator, titrate with *0.1 M ammonium thiocyanate* until a reddish-yellow colour is obtained. Carry out a blank titration. The difference between the titration volumes is not greater than 1.0 ml.

ASSAY

Dissolve 0.100 g in 40 ml of *methanol R*. Add 20 ml of *0.1 M hydrochloric acid* and 50.0 ml of *0.05 M iodine*. Allow to stand for 10 min and titrate with *0.1 M sodium thiosulphate*. Carry out a blank titration.

1 ml of *0.05 M iodine* is equivalent to 6.21 mg of $C_3H_8OS_2$.

STORAGE

Store in a well-filled, airtight container, protected from light, at a temperature of 2 °C to 8 °C.

01/2005:0763

DIMETHYL SULFOXIDE

Dimethylis sulfoxidum

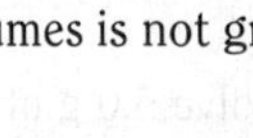

C_2H_6OS M_r 78.1

DEFINITION

Dimethyl sulfoxide is sulphinylbismethane.

CHARACTERS

A colourless liquid or colourless crystals, hygroscopic, miscible with water and with alcohol.

IDENTIFICATION

First identification: C.

Second identification: A, B, D.

A. It complies with the test for relative density (see Tests).

B. It complies with the test for refractive index (see Tests).

C. Examine by infrared absorption spectrophotometry (*2.2.24*), comparing with the spectrum obtained with *dimethyl sulfoxide CRS*.

D. Dissolve 50 mg of *nickel chloride R* in 5 ml of the substance to be examined. The solution is greenish-yellow. Heat in a water-bath at 50 °C. The colour changes to green or bluish-green. Cool. The colour changes to greenish-yellow.

TESTS

Acidity. Dissolve 50.0 g in 100 ml of *carbon dioxide-free water R*. Add 0.1 ml of *phenolphthalein solution R1*. Not more than 5.0 ml of *0.01 M sodium hydroxide* is required to produce a pink colour.

Relative density (*2.2.5*): 1.100 to 1.104.

Refractive index (*2.2.6*): 1.478 to 1.479.

Freezing point (*2.2.18*). Not less than 18.3 °C.

Absorbance (*2.2.25*). Purge with *nitrogen R* for 15 min. The absorbance, measured using *water R* as the compensation liquid, is not more than 0.30 at 275 nm and not more than 0.20 at both 285 nm and 295 nm. Examined between 270 nm and 350 nm, the substance to be examined shows no absorption maximum.

Related substances. Examine by gas chromatography (*2.2.28*), using *bibenzyl R* as the internal standard.

Internal standard solution. Dissolve 0.125 g of *bibenzyl R* in *acetone R* and dilute to 50 ml with the same solvent.

Test solution (a). Dissolve 5.0 g of the substance to be examined in *acetone R* and dilute to 10.0 ml with the same solvent.

Test solution (b). Dissolve 5.0 g of the substance to be examined in *acetone R*, add 1.0 ml of the internal standard solution and dilute to 10.0 ml with *acetone R*.

Reference solution. Dissolve 50.0 mg of the substance to be examined and 50 mg of *dimethyl sulphone R* in *acetone R*, add 10.0 ml of the internal standard solution and dilute to 100.0 ml with *acetone R*.

The chromatographic procedure may be carried out using:

– a glass column 1.5 m long and 4 mm in internal diameter, packed with *diatomaceous earth for gas chromatography R* (125 μm to 180 μm) impregnated with 10 per cent *m/m* of *polyethyleneglycol adipate R*,

– *nitrogen for chromatography R* as the carrier gas at a flow rate of 30 ml/min,

– a flame-ionisation detector,

maintaining the temperature of the column at 165 °C and that of the injection port and of the detector at 190 °C.

Inject 1 μl of the reference solution and adjust the sensitivity of the system so that the heights of the three peaks, apart from the solvent peak, are not less than 70 per cent of the full scale of the recorder. The substances elute in the following order: dimethyl sulfoxide, dimethyl sulphone, bibenzyl. The test is not valid unless, in the chromatogram obtained with the reference solution, the resolution between the peaks due to dimethyl sulfoxide and dimethyl sulphone is at least 3.

Inject 1 μl of test solution (a). In the chromatogram obtained, verify that there is no peak with the same retention time as the internal standard.

Inject 1 μl of test solution (b) and 1 μl of the reference solution. Continue the chromatography for four times the retention time of dimethyl sulfoxide, which is about 5 min. From the chromatogram obtained with the reference solution, calculate the ratio (*R*) of the area of the peak due to dimethyl sulfoxide to the area of the peak due to the internal standard. From the chromatogram obtained with test solution (b), calculate the ratio of the sum of the areas of any peaks, apart from the principal peak, the peak due to the internal standard and the peak due to the solvent, to the area of the peak due to the internal standard; this ratio is not greater than *R* (0.1 per cent).

Water (*2.5.12*). Not more than 0.2 per cent, determined on 10.0 g by the semi-micro determination of water.

STORAGE

Store in an airtight, glass container, protected from light.

01/2005:1667

DIMETHYLACETAMIDE

Dimethylacetamidum

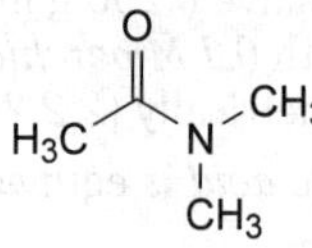

C_4H_9NO M_r 87.1

DEFINITION

N,N-Dimethylacetamide.

CHARACTERS

Appearance: clear, colourless, slightly hygroscopic liquid.

Solubility: miscible with water, with alcohol, and with most common organic solvents.

bp: about 165 °C.

IDENTIFICATION

First identification: C.

Second identification: A, B, D.

A. Relative density (*2.2.5*): 0.941 to 0.944.

B. Refractive index (*2.2.6*): 1.435 to 1.439.

C. Infrared absorption spectrophotometry (*2.2.24*).
Preparation: films.
Comparison: *dimethylacetamide CRS*.

D. Dilute 50 mg with 1 ml of *methanol R*. Add 1 ml of a 15 g/l solution of *hydroxylamine hydrochloride R* and mix. Add 1 ml of *dilute sodium hydroxide solution R*, mix and allow to stand for 30 min. Add 1 ml of *dilute hydrochloric acid R* and add 1 ml of a 100 g/l solution of *ferric chloride R* in *0.1 M hydrochloric acid*. A reddish-brown colour develops, reaching a maximum intensity after about 5 min.

TESTS

Appearance. The substance to be examined is clear (*2.2.1*) and not more intensely coloured than reference solution Y_7 (*2.2.2, Method II*).

Acidity. Dilute 50 ml with 50 ml of *water R* previously adjusted with *0.02 M potassium hydroxide* or *0.02 M hydrochloric acid* to a bluish-green colour, using 0.5 ml of *bromothymol blue solution R1* as indicator. Not more than 5.0 ml of *0.02 M potassium hydroxide* is required to restore the initial (bluish-green) colour.

Alkalinity. To 50 ml add 50 ml of *water R* previously adjusted with *0.02 M potassium hydroxide* or *0.02 M hydrochloric acid* to a yellow colour, using 0.5 ml of *bromothymol blue solution R1* as indicator. Titrate with *0.02 M hydrochloric acid*. Not more than 0.5 ml of *0.02 M hydrochloric acid* is required to restore the initial (yellow) colour.

Related substances. Gas chromatography (*2.2.28*): use the normalisation procedure.

Test solution. The substance to be examined.

Reference solution (a). Dilute a mixture of 1 ml of the substance to be examined and 1 ml of *dimethylformamide R* to 20 ml with *methylene chloride R*.

Reference solution (b). Dilute 1 ml of the substance to be examined to 20.0 ml with *methylene chloride R*. Dilute 0.1 ml of the solution to 10.0 ml with *methylene chloride R*.

Column:

- *material*: fused silica,
- *size*: l = 30 m, Ø = 0.32 mm,
- *stationary phase*: *macrogol 20 000 R* (film thickness 1 µm).

Carrier gas: *nitrogen for chromatography R*.

Linear velocity: 30 cm/s.

Split ratio: 1:20.

Temperature:

	Time (min)	Temperature (°C)
Column	0 - 15	80 → 200
Injection port		250
Detector		250

Detection: flame ionisation.

Injection: 0.5 µl.

System suitability:

- *resolution*: minimum 5.0 between the peaks due to dimethylacetamide and dimethylformamide in the chromatogram obtained with reference solution (a),
- *signal-to-noise ratio*: minimum 10 for the principal peak in the chromatogram obtained with reference solution (b).

Limits:

- *any impurity*: maximum 0.1 per cent,
- *total*: maximum 0.3 per cent,
- *disregard limit*: area of the peak in the chromatogram obtained with reference solution (b) (0.05 per cent).

Heavy metals (*2.4.8*): maximum 10 ppm.

Dilute 4.0 g to 20.0 ml with *water R*. 12 ml of the solution complies with limit test A. Prepare the standard using *lead standard solution (2 ppm Pb) R*.

Non-volatile matter: maximum 20 ppm.

Evaporate 50 g to dryness using a rotary evaporator at a pressure not exceeding 1 kPa and on a water-bath. Dry the residue in an oven at 170-175 °C. The residue weighs not more than 1 mg.

Water (*2.5.32*): maximum 0.1 per cent, determined on 0.100 g.

STORAGE

In an airtight container, protected from light.

IMPURITIES

A. acetic acid,

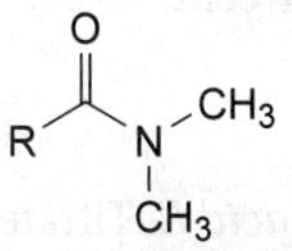

B. R = H: *N,N*-dimethylformamide,

C. R = C_2H_5: *N,N*-dimethylpropanamide,

D. R = CH_2-CH_2-CH_3: *N,N*-dimethylbutanamide.

01/2005:0138

DIMETICONE

Dimeticonum

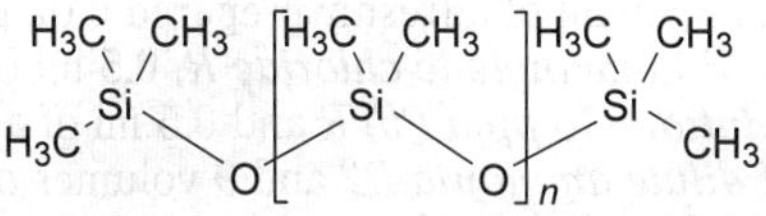

DEFINITION

Dimeticone is a poly(dimethylsiloxane) obtained by hydrolysis and polycondensation of dichlorodimethylsilane and chlorotrimethylsilane. Different grades exist which are distinguished by a number indicating the nominal viscosity placed after the name.

Their degree of polymerisation (n = 20 to 400) is such that their kinematic viscosities are nominally between 20 $mm^2 \cdot s^{-1}$ and 1300 $mm^2 \cdot s^{-1}$.

Dimeticones with a nominal viscosity of 50 $mm^2 \cdot s^{-1}$ or lower are intended for external use only.

CHARACTERS

Clear, colourless liquids of various viscosities, practically insoluble in water, very slightly soluble to practically insoluble in ethanol, miscible with ethyl acetate, with methyl ethyl ketone and with toluene.

IDENTIFICATION

A. It is identified by its kinematic viscosity at 25 °C (see Tests).

B. Examine by infrared absorption spectrophotometry (*2.2.24*) comparing with the spectrum obtained with *dimeticone CRS*. The region of the spectrum from 850 cm^{-1} to 750 cm^{-1} is not taken into account.

C. Heat 0.5 g in a test-tube over a small flame until white fumes begin to appear. Invert the tube over a 2nd tube containing 1 ml of a 1 g/l solution of *chromotropic acid, sodium salt R* in *sulphuric acid R* so that the fumes reach the solution. Shake the 2nd tube for about 10 s and heat on a water-bath for 5 min. The solution is violet.

D. In a platinum crucible, prepare the sulphated ash (*2.4.14*) using 50 mg. The residue is a white powder that gives the reaction of silicates (*2.3.1*).

TESTS

Acidity. To 2.0 g add 25 ml of a mixture of equal volumes of *ethanol R* and *ether R*, previously neutralised to 0.2 ml of *bromothymol blue solution R1* and shake. Not more than 0.15 ml of *0.01 M sodium hydroxide* is required to change the colour of the solution to blue.

Viscosity (*2.2.9*). Determine the kinematic viscosity at 25 °C. For dimeticones, the kinematic viscosity is not less than 90 per cent and not more than 110 per cent of the nominal viscosity stated on the label.

Mineral oils. Place 2 g in a test-tube and examine in ultraviolet light at 365 nm. The fluorescence is not more intense than that of a solution containing 0.1 ppm of *quinine sulphate R* in *0.005 M sulphuric acid* examined in the same conditions.

Phenylated compounds. Dissolve 5.0 g with shaking in 10 ml of *cyclohexane R*. At wavelengths from 250 nm to 270 nm, the absorbance (*2.2.25*) of the solution is not greater than 0.2.

Heavy metals. Mix 1.0 g with *methylene chloride R* and dilute to 20 ml with the same solvent. Add 1.0 ml of a freshly prepared 0.02 g/l solution of *dithizone R* in *methylene chloride R*, 0.5 ml of *water R* and 0.5 ml of a mixture of 1 volume of *dilute ammonia R2* and 9 volumes of a 2 g/l solution of *hydroxylamine hydrochloride R*. At the same time, prepare a standard as follows: to 20 ml of *methylene chloride R* add 1.0 ml of a freshly prepared 0.02 g/l solution of *dithizone R* in *methylene chloride R*, 0.5 ml of *lead standard solution (10 ppm Pb) R* and 0.5 ml of a mixture of 1 volume of *dilute ammonia R2* and 9 volumes of a 2 g/l solution of *hydroxylamine hydrochloride R*. Immediately shake each solution vigorously for 1 min. Any red colour in the test solution is not more intense than that in the standard (5 ppm).

Volatile matter. For dimeticones with a nominal viscosity greater than 50 $mm^2 \cdot s^{-1}$, not more than 0.3 per cent, determined on 1.00 g by heating in an oven at 150 °C for 2 h. Carry out the test using a dish 60 mm in diameter and 10 mm deep.

LABELLING

The label states:

- the nominal viscosity by a number placed after the name of the product,
- where applicable, that the product is intended for external use.

Monographs D-E

01/2005:1417

DIMETINDENE MALEATE

Dimetindeni maleas

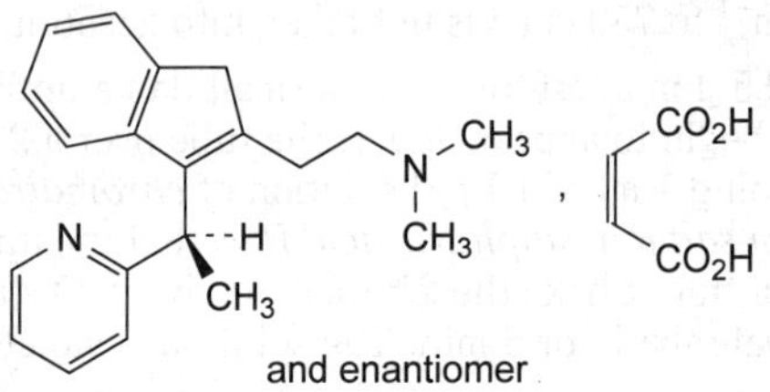

$C_{24}H_{28}N_2O_4$ M_r 408.5

DEFINITION

Dimetindene maleate contains not less than 99.0 per cent and not more than the equivalent of 101.0 per cent of *N,N*-dimethyl-2-[3-[(*RS*)-1-(pyridin-2-yl)ethyl]-1*H*-inden-2-yl]ethanamine (*Z*)-butenedioate, calculated with reference to the dried substance.

CHARACTERS

A white to almost white, crystalline powder, slightly soluble in water, soluble in methanol.

IDENTIFICATION

Examine by infrared absorption spectrophotometry (*2.2.24*), comparing with the spectrum obtained with *dimetindene maleate CRS*. Examine the substance prepared as discs.

TESTS

Solution S. Dissolve 0.20 g in *methanol R* and dilute to 20.0 ml with the same solvent.

Appearance of solution. Solution S is clear (*2.2.1*) and not more intensely coloured than Y_6 (*2.2.2, Method II*).

Optical rotation (*2.2.7*). Determined on solution S, the angle of optical rotation is − 0.10° to + 0.10°.

Related substances. Examine by gas chromatography (*2.2.28*).

Test solution. Dissolve 50.0 mg of the substance to be examined in a mixture of equal volumes of *acetone R* and *methylene chloride R* and dilute to 5.0 ml with the same mixture of solvents.

Reference solution (a). Dilute 1 ml of the test solution to 100.0 ml with a mixture of equal volumes of *acetone R* and *methylene chloride R*.

Reference solution (b). Dissolve 5.0 mg of *2-ethylpyridine R* in a mixture of equal volumes of *acetone R* and *methylene chloride R* and dilute to 50.0 ml with the same mixture of solvents. Dilute 10.0 ml of this solution to 100.0 ml with the same mixture of solvents.

The chromatographic procedure may be carried out using:

- a fused-silica column 30 m long and 0.32 mm in internal diameter coated with *polymethylphenylsiloxane R* (film thickness 0.25 μm),
- *helium for chromatography R* as the carrier gas at a linear velocity of about 30 cm/s,
- a flame-ionisation detector,

maintaining the temperature of the column at 60 °C for 1 min, then raising the temperature at a rate of 6 °C/min to 260 °C and maintaining at 260 °C for 12 min. Maintain the temperature of the injection port at 240 °C and that of the detector at 260 °C.

Inject via a split injector with a split flow of 30 ml/min for 1.3 times the retention time of the principal peak.

Inject 2 μl of reference solution (a). The symmetry factor of the principal peak in the chromatogram obtained is not greater than 1.3.

Inject 2 μl of the test solution and 2 μl of reference solution (b). In the chromatogram obtained with the test solution the area of the peak corresponding to 2-ethylpyridine is not greater than the area of the peak in the chromatogram obtained with reference solution (b) (0.1 per cent).

In the chromatogram obtained with the test solution the area of any peak, apart from the principal peak and any peak appearing during the first 8 min (2-ethylpyridine, the solvent mixture and maleic acid), is not greater than 0.2 times the area of the peak in the chromatogram with reference solution (a) (0.2 per cent) and the sum of the areas of all peaks is not greater than 0.5 times the area of the peak in the chromatogram obtained with reference solution (a) (0.5 per cent). Disregard any peak with an areas less than 0.05 times the area of the principal peak in the chromatogram obtained with the reference solution (a).

Loss on drying (*2.2.32*). Not more than 0.1 per cent, determined on 1.000 g by drying in an oven at 100 °C to 105 °C for 2 h.

Sulphated ash (*2.4.14*). Not more than 0.1 per cent, determined on 1.0 g.

ASSAY

Dissolve 0.150 g in 80 ml of *anhydrous acetic acid R*. Titrate with *0.1 M perchloric acid*, determining the end-point potentiometrically (*2.2.20*).

1 ml of *0.1 M perchloric acid* is equivalent to 20.43 mg of $C_{24}H_{28}N_2O_4$.

STORAGE

Store protected from light.

IMPURITIES

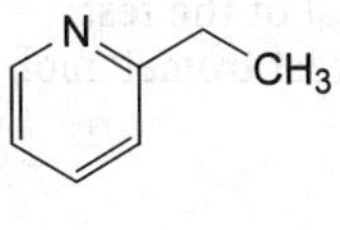

A. 2-ethylpyridine,

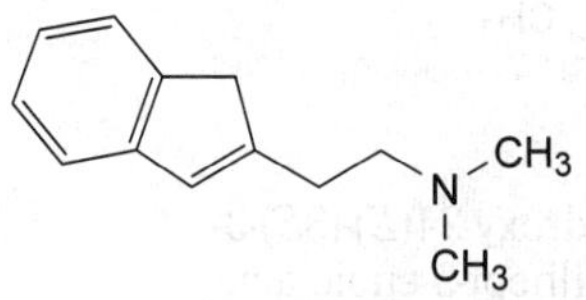

B. 2-(1*H*-inden-2-yl)-*N*,*N*-dimethylethanamine,

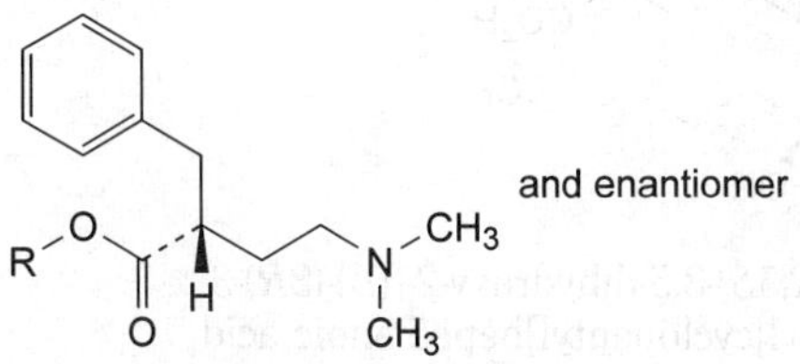

C. R = C_2H_5: ethyl (2*RS*)-2-benzyl-4-(dimethylamino)butanoate,

D. R = H: (2*RS*)-2-benzyl-4-(dimethylamino)butanoic acid,

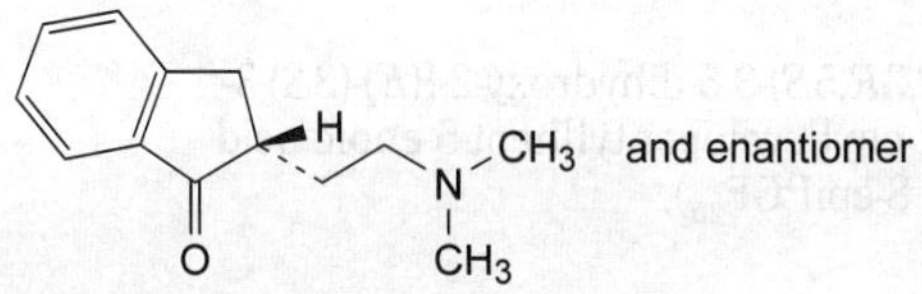

E. (2*RS*)-2-[2-(dimethylamino)ethyl]indan-1-one,

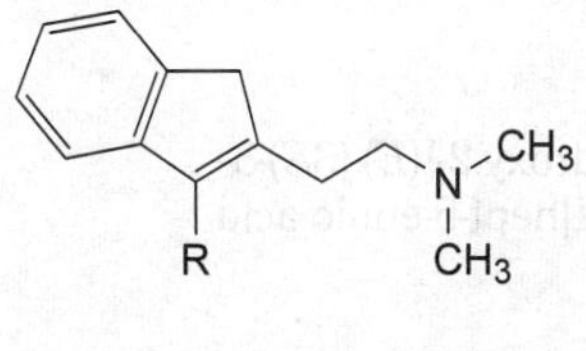

F. R = $[CH_2]_3$-CH_3: 2-(3-butyl-1*H*-inden-2-yl)-*N*,*N*-dimethylethanamine,

G. R = C_6H_5: *N*,*N*-dimethyl-2-(3-phenyl-1*H*-inden-2-yl)ethanamine,

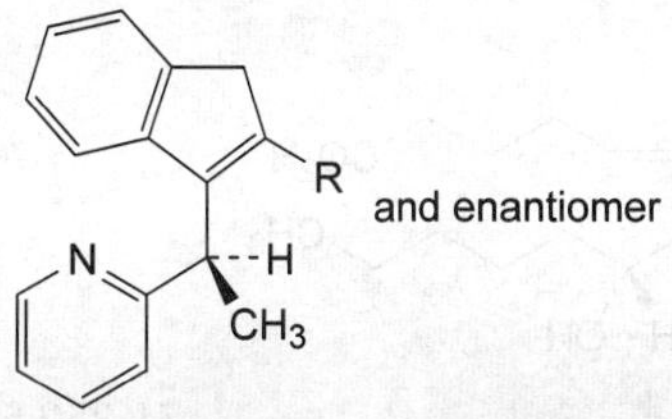

H. R = CH = CH_2: 2-[(1*RS*)-1-(2-ethenyl-1*H*-inden-3-yl)ethyl]pyridine,

I. R = CH_2-CH_2-NH-CH_3: *N*-methyl-2-[3-[(1*RS*)-1-(pyridin-2-yl)ethyl]-1*H*-inden-2-yl]ethanamine.

01/2005:1312

DINOPROST TROMETAMOL

Dinoprostum trometamolum

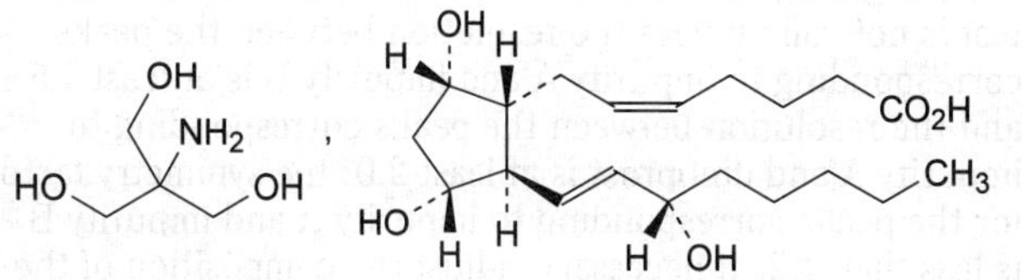

$C_{24}H_{45}NO_8$ M_r 475.6

DEFINITION

Dinoprost trometamol contains not less than 96.0 per cent and not more than the equivalent of 102.0 per cent of trometamol (*Z*)-7-[(1*R*,2*R*,3*R*,5*S*)-3,5-dihydroxy-2-[(*E*)-(3*S*)-3-hydroxyoct-1-enyl]cyclopentyl]hept-5-enoate ($PGF_{2\alpha}$), calculated with reference to the anhydrous substance.

CHARACTERS

A white or almost white powder, very soluble in water, freely soluble in alcohol, practically insoluble in acetonitrile.

IDENTIFICATION

A. Dissolve 0.100 g in *alcohol R* and dilute to 10.0 ml with the same solvent. The specific optical rotation (*2.2.7*) is + 19 to + 26, calculated with reference to the anhydrous substance.

B. Examine by infrared absorption spectrophotometry (*2.2.24*), comparing with the spectrum obtained with *dinoprost trometamol CRS*.

TESTS

Related substances. Examine by liquid chromatography (*2.2.29*).

Test solution. Dissolve 10.0 mg of the substance to be examined in a mixture of 23 volumes of *acetonitrile R* and 77 volumes of *water R* and dilute to 10.0 ml with the same mixture of solvents.

Reference solution (a). Degradation of dinoprost trometamol to impurity B. Dissolve 1 mg of the substance to be examined in 1 ml of the mobile phase and heat the solution on a water-bath at 85 °C for 5 min and cool.

Reference solution (b). Dilute 2.0 ml of the test solution to 20.0 ml with a mixture of 23 volumes of *acetonitrile R* and 77 volumes of *water R*. Dilute 2.0 ml of the solution to 20.0 ml with a mixture of 23 volumes of *acetonitrile R* and 77 volumes of *water R*.

The chromatographic procedure may be carried out using:

- a stainless steel column 0.15 m long and 3.9 mm in internal diameter packed with *octadecylsilyl silica gel for chromatography R1* (5 µm) with a pore size of 10 nm and a carbon loading of 19 per cent,
- as mobile phase at a flow rate of 1 ml/min a mixture prepared as follows: dissolve 2.44 g of *sodium dihydrogen phosphate R* in *water R* and dilute to 1000 ml with *water R*; adjust the pH to 2.5 with *phosphoric acid R* (about 0.6 ml); mix 770 ml of the buffer solution with 230 ml of *acetonitrile R1*,
- as detector a spectrophotometer set at 200 nm.

Adjust the sensitivity of the system so that the height of the principal peak in the chromatogram obtained with 20 µl of reference solution (b) is 25 per cent to 50 per cent of the full scale of the recorder.

Inject 20 µl of reference solution (a). When the chromatograms are recorded in the prescribed conditions, the retention times are: (15*R*)-PGF$_{2\alpha}$ (impurity B) about 55 min; 5,6-*trans*-PGF$_{2\alpha}$ (impurity A) about 60 min and dinoprost about 66 min. Continue the chromatography for 2.5 times the retention time of the principal peak (to elute degradation products formed during heating). The test is not valid unless the resolution between the peaks corresponding to impurity A and impurity B is at least 1.5 and the resolution between the peaks corresponding to impurity A and dinoprost is at least 2.0; the symmetry factor for the peaks corresponding to impurity A and impurity B is less than 1.2. If necessary, adjust the composition of the mobile phase by increasing the concentration of acetonitrile to decrease the retention times.

Inject separately 20 µl of the test solution and 20 µl of reference solution (b). Continue the chromatography of the test solution for 10 min after the elution of the principal peak. In the chromatogram obtained with the test solution the area of any peak corresponding to impurity A is not greater than twice the area of the principal peak obtained with reference solution (b) (2 per cent); the area of any other peak, apart from the principal peak and any peak corresponding to impurity A, is not greater than 1.5 times the area of the principal peak obtained with reference solution (b) (1.5 per cent) and not more than one such peak has an area greater than half the area of the principal peak obtained with reference solution (b) (0.5 per cent). The sum of the areas of all the peaks, apart from the principal peak and the peak corresponding to impurity A, is not greater than twice the area of the principal peak obtained with reference solution (b) (2 per cent). Disregard any peak due to the mobile phase and any peak due to trometamol (retention time about 1.5 min) and also any peak with an area of less than 0.05 times the area of the principal peak obtained with reference solution (b).

Water (*2.5.12*). Not more than 1.0 per cent, determined on 0.500 g by the semi-micro determination of water.

ASSAY

Examine by liquid chromatography (*2.2.29*).

Test solution. Dissolve 10.0 mg of the substance to be examined in a mixture of 23 volumes of *acetonitrile R* and 77 volumes of *water R* and dilute to 10.0 ml with the same mixture.

Reference solution. Dissolve 10.0 mg of *dinoprost trometamol CRS* in a mixture of 23 volumes of *acetonitrile R* and 77 volumes of *water R* and dilute to 10.0 ml with the same mixture.

The chromatographic procedure may be carried out using:

– a stainless steel column 0.15 m long and 3.9 mm in internal diameter packed with *octadecylsilyl silica gel for chromatography R1* (5 µm) with a pore size of 10 nm and a carbon loading of 19 per cent,

– as mobile phase at a flow rate of 1 ml/min a mixture prepared as follows: dissolve 2.44 g of *sodium dihydrogen phosphate R* in *water R* and dilute to 1000 ml with *water R*; adjust the pH to 2.5 with *phosphoric acid R* (about 0.6 ml); mix 730 ml of the buffer solution with 270 ml of *acetonitrile R1*,

– as detector a spectrophotometer set at 200 nm.

Adjust the sensitivity of the system so that the height of the principal peak in the chromatogram obtained with 20 µl of the reference solution is 70 per cent to 90 per cent of the full scale of the recorder. When the chromatogram is recorded under the conditions described above, the retention time is about 23 min for dinoprost.

Inject the reference solution six times. The test is not valid unless the relative standard deviation of the peak area for dinoprost is at most 2.0 per cent. Inject 20 µl of the test solution. Calculate the percentage of dinoprost trometamol.

IMPURITIES

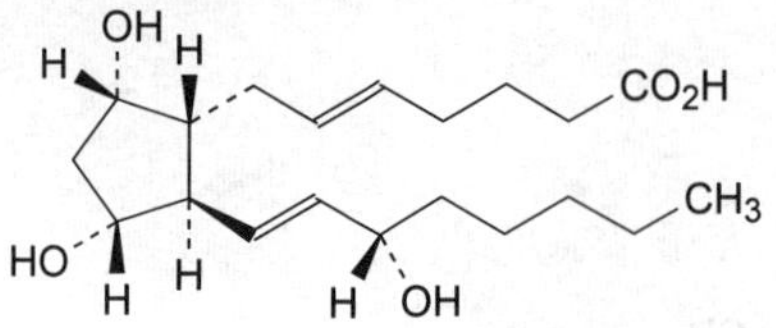

A. (*E*)-7-[(1*R*,2*R*,3*R*,5*S*)-3,5-dihydroxy-2-[(*E*)-(3*S*)-3-hydroxyoct-1-enyl]cyclopentyl]hept-5-enoic acid ((5*E*)-PGF$_{2\alpha}$; 5,6-*trans*-PGF$_{2\alpha}$),

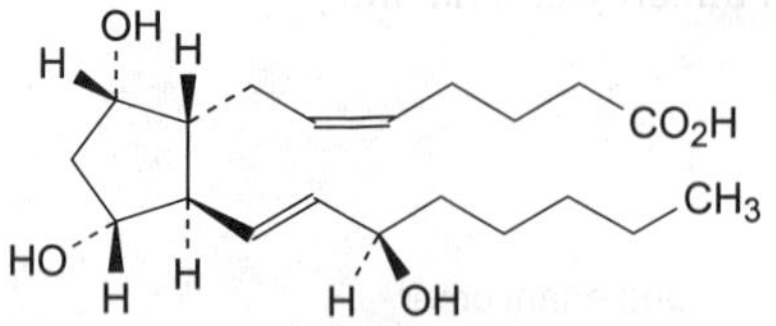

B. (*Z*)-7-[(1*R*,2*R*,3*R*,5*S*)-3,5-dihydroxy-2-[(*E*)-(3*R*)-3-hydroxyoct-1-enyl]cyclopentyl]hept-5-enoic acid ((15*R*)-PGF$_{2\alpha}$;15-epiPGF$_{2\alpha}$),

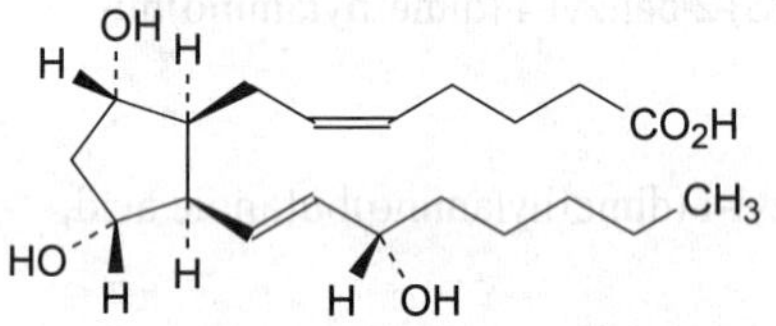

C. (*Z*)-7-[(1*S*,2*R*,3*R*,5*S*)-3,5-dihydroxy-2-[(*E*)-(3*S*)-3-hydroxyoct-1-enyl]cyclopentyl]hept-5-enoic acid ((8*S*)-PGF$_{2\alpha}$; 8-epiPGF$_{2\alpha}$),

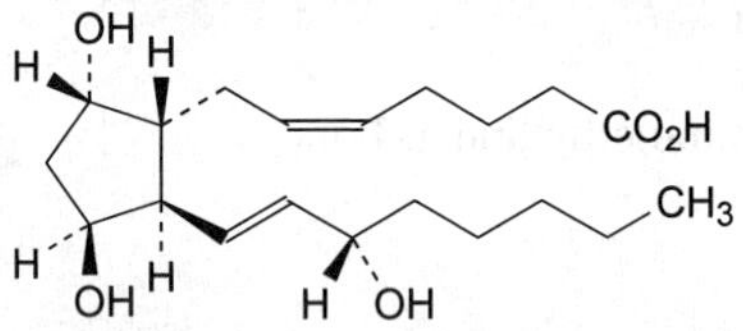

D. (*Z*)-7-[(1*R*,2*R*,3*S*,5*S*)-3,5-dihydroxy-2-[(*E*)-(3*S*)-3-hydroxyoct-1-enyl]cyclopentyl]hept-5-enoic acid (11β-PGF$_{2\alpha}$; 11-epiPGF$_{2\alpha}$).

01/2005:1311

DINOPROSTONE

Dinoprostonum

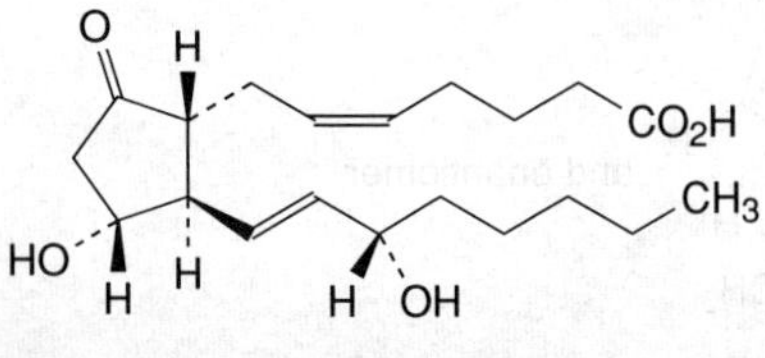

$C_{20}H_{32}O_5$ M_r 352.5

DEFINITION

(*Z*)-7-[(1*R*,2*R*,3*R*)-3-hydroxy-2-[(*E*)-(3*S*)-3-hydroxyoct-1-enyl]-5-oxocyclopentyl]hept-5-enoic acid (PGE$_2$).

Content: 95.0 per cent to 102.0 per cent (anhydrous substance).

CHARACTERS

Appearance: white or almost white, crystalline powder or colourless crystals.

Solubility: practically insoluble in water, very soluble in methanol, freely soluble in alcohol.

The substance degrades at room temperature.

IDENTIFICATION

A. Specific optical rotation (*2.2.7*): − 82 to − 90 (anhydrous substance).

Immediately before use, dissolve 50.0 mg in *alcohol R* and dilute to 10.0 ml with the same solvent.

B. Infrared absorption spectrophotometry (*2.2.24*).

Comparison: *dinoprostone CRS*.

TESTS

Prepare the solutions immediately before use.

Related substances. Liquid chromatography (*2.2.29*).

Test solution (a). Dissolve 10.0 mg of the substance to be examined in a 58 per cent *V/V* solution of *methanol R2* and dilute to 2.0 ml with the same solvent.

Test solution (b). Dissolve 20.0 mg of the substance to be examined in a 58 per cent *V/V* solution of *methanol R2* and dilute to 20.0 ml with the same solvent.

Reference solution (a). Dissolve 1 mg of *dinoprostone CRS* and 1 mg of *dinoprostone impurity C CRS* in a 58 per cent *V/V* solution of *methanol R2* and dilute to 10.0 ml with the same solvent. Dilute 4.0 ml of the solution to 10.0 ml with a 58 per cent *V/V* solution of *methanol R2*.

Reference solution (b). Dilute 0.5 ml of test solution (a) to 10.0 ml with a 58 per cent *V/V* solution of *methanol R2*. Dilute 1.0 ml of the solution to 10.0 ml with a 58 per cent *V/V* solution of *methanol R2*.

Reference solution (c). In order to prepare *in situ* the degradation compounds (impurity D and impurity E), dissolve 1 mg of the substance to be examined in 100 µl of *1 M sodium hydroxide* (the solution becomes brownish-red), wait 4 min, add 150 µl of *1 M acetic acid* (yellowish-white opalescent solution) and dilute to 5.0 ml with a 58 per cent *V/V* solution of *methanol R2*.

Reference solution (d). Dissolve 20 mg of *dinoprostone CRS* in a 58 per cent *V/V* solution of *methanol R2* and dilute to 20.0 ml with the same solvent.

Column:

- *size*: l = 0.25 m, Ø = 4.6 mm,
- *stationary phase*: *end-capped octadecylsilyl silica gel for chromatography R*,
- *temperature*: 30 °C.

Mobile phase: mix 42 volumes of a 0.2 per cent *V/V* solution of *acetic acid R* and 58 volumes of *methanol R2*.

Flow rate: 1.0 ml/min.

Detection: spectrophotometer at 210 nm.

Injection: 20 µl; inject test solution (a) and reference solutions (a), (b) and (c).

Relative retention with reference to dinoprostone (retention time = about 18 min): impurity C = about 1.2; impurity D = about 1.8; impurity E = about 2.0.

System suitability: reference solution (a):

- *resolution*: minimum of 3.8 between the peaks due to dinoprostone and to impurity C. If necessary adjust the concentration of the acetic acid solution and/or methanol (increase the concentration of the acetic acid solution to increase the retention time for dinoprostone and impurity C and increase the concentration of methanol to decrease the retention time for both compounds).

Limits:

- *correction factors*: for the calculation of contents, multiply the peak areas of the following impurities by the corresponding correction factor: impurity D = 0.2; impurity E = 0.7,
- *impurity C*: not more than 3 times the area of the principal peak in the chromatogram obtained with reference solution (b) (1.5 per cent),
- *impurity D*: not more than twice the area of the principal peak in the chromatogram obtained with reference solution (b) (1 per cent),
- *impurity E*: not more than the area of the principal peak in the chromatogram obtained with reference solution (b) (0.5 per cent),
- *any other impurity*: not more than the area of the principal peak in the chromatogram obtained with reference solution (b) (0.5 per cent),
- *total of other impurities*: not more than twice the area of the principal peak in the chromatogram obtained with reference solution (b) (1 per cent),
- *disregard limit*: 0.1 times the area of the principal peak in the chromatogram obtained with reference solution (b) (0.05 per cent).

If any peak with a relative retention to dinoprostone of about 0.8 is greater than 0.5 per cent or if the total of other impurities is greater than 1.0 per cent, record the chromatogram of test solution (a) with a detector set at 230 nm. If the area of the peak at 230 nm is twice the area of the peak at 210 nm, multiply the area at 210 nm by 0.2 (correction factor for impurity F).

Water (*2.5.12*): maximum 0.5 per cent, determined on 0.50 g.

ASSAY

Prepare the solutions immediately before use.

Liquid chromatography (*2.2.29*) as described in the test for related substances.

Injection: test solution (b) and reference solution (d).

Calculate the percentage content of $C_{20}H_{32}O_5$.

STORAGE

At a temperature not exceeding - 15 °C.

IMPURITIES

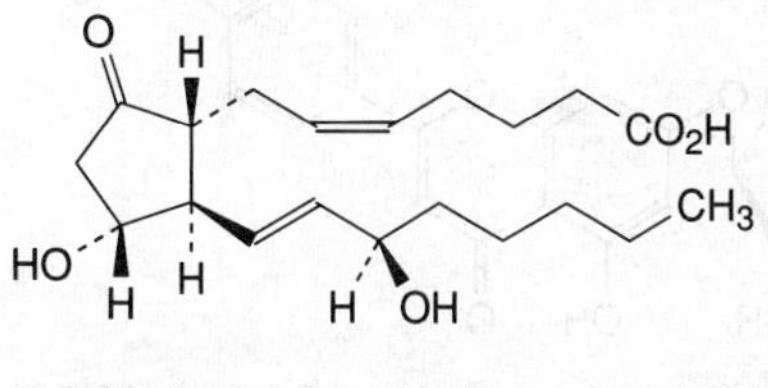

A. (*Z*)-7-[(1*R*,2*R*,3*R*)-3-hydroxy-2-[(*E*)-(3*R*)-3-hydroxyoct-1-enyl]-5-oxocyclopentyl]hept-5-enoic acid (15-epiPGE$_2$; (15*R*)-PGE$_2$),

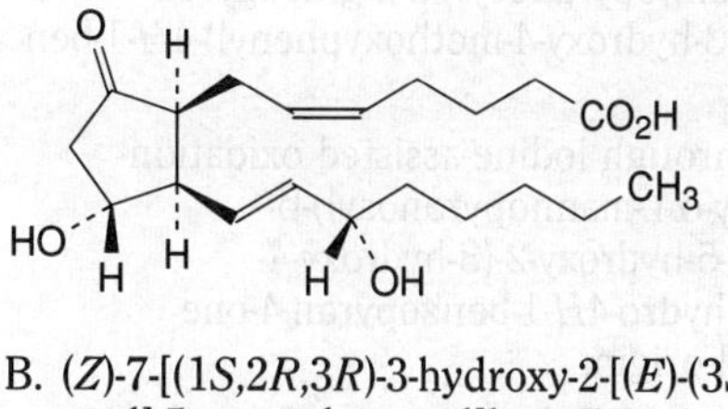

B. (*Z*)-7-[(1*S*,2*R*,3*R*)-3-hydroxy-2-[(*E*)-(3*S*)-3-hydroxyoct-1-enyl]-5-oxocyclopentyl]hept-5-enoic acid (8-epiPGE$_2$; (8*S*)-PGE$_2$),

Monographs D-E

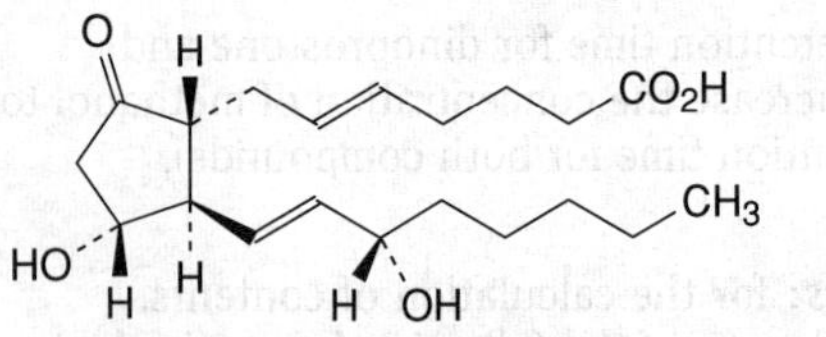

C. (*E*)-7-[(1*R*,2*R*,3*R*)-3-hydroxy-2-[(*E*)-(3*S*)-3-hydroxyoct-1-enyl]-5-oxocyclopentyl]hept-5-enoic acid (5-*trans*-PGE_2; (5*E*)-PGE_2),

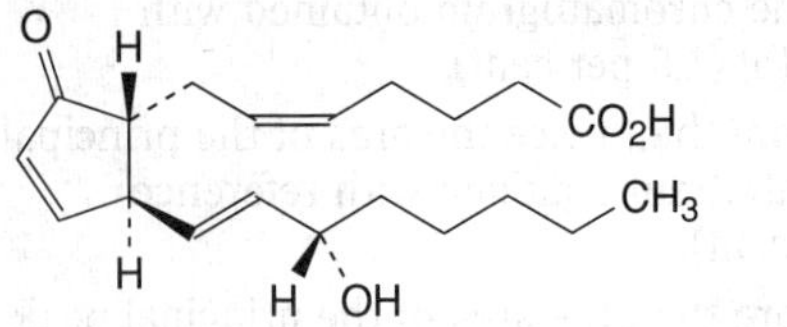

D. (*Z*)-7-[(1*R*,2*S*)-2-[(*E*)-(3*S*)-3-hydroxyoct-1-enyl]-5-oxocyclopent-3-enyl]hept-5-enoic acid (PGA_2),

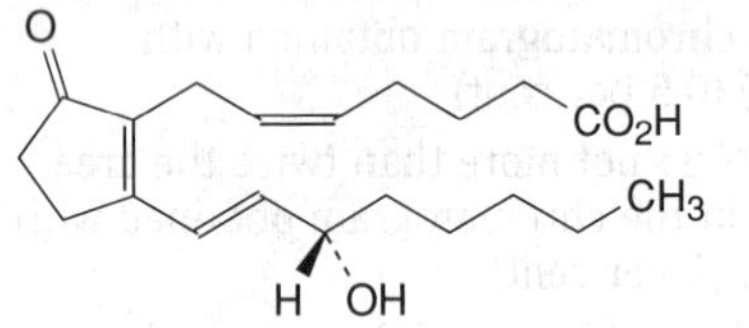

E. (*Z*)-7-[2-[(*E*)-(3*S*)-3-hydroxyoct-1-enyl]-5-oxocyclopent-1-enyl]hept-5-enoic acid (PGB_2),

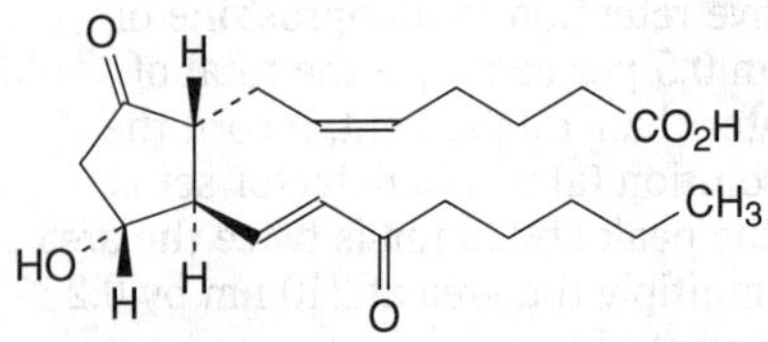

F. (*Z*)-7-[(1*R*,2*R*,3*R*)-3-hydroxy-2-[(*E*)-3-oxo-oct-1-enyl]-5-oxocyclopentyl]hept-5-enoic acid (15-oxo-PGE_2; 15-keto-PGE_2).

Monographs D-E

01/2005:1611

DIOSMIN

Diosminum

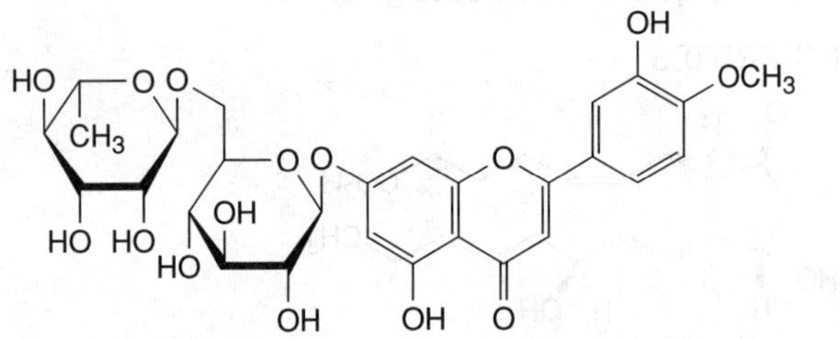

$C_{28}H_{32}O_{15}$ M_r 609

DEFINITION

7-[[6-*O*-(6-Deoxy-α-L-mannopyranosyl)-β-D-glucopyranosyl]oxy]-5-hydroxy-2-(3-hydroxy-4-methoxyphenyl)-4*H*-1-benzopyran-4-one.

Substance obtained through iodine-assisted oxidation of (2*S*)-7-[[6-*O*-(6-deoxy-α-L-mannopyranosyl)-β-D-glucopyranosyl]oxy]-5-hydroxy-2-(3-hydroxy-4-methoxyphenyl)-2,3-dihydro-4*H*-1-benzopyran-4-one (hesperidin) of natural origin.

Content: 90.0 per cent to 102.0 per cent (anhydrous substance).

CHARACTERS

Appearance: greyish-yellow or light yellow hygroscopic powder.

Solubility: practically insoluble in water, soluble in dimethyl sulphoxide, practically insoluble in alcohol. It dissolves in dilute solutions of alkali hydroxides.

IDENTIFICATION

A. Infrared absorption spectrophotometry (*2.2.24*).
Comparison: *diosmin CRS*.

B. Examine the chromatograms obtained in the assay.
Results: the principal peak in the chromatogram obtained with the test solution is similar in retention time and size to the principal peak in the chromatogram obtained with reference solution (a).

TESTS

Iodine: maximum 0.1 per cent.

Determine the total content of iodine by potentiometry, using an iodide-selective electrode (*2.2.36*), after oxygen combustion (*2.5.10*).

Test solution. Wrap 0.100 g of the substance to be examined in a piece of filter paper and place it in a sample carrier. Introduce into the flask 50 ml of a 0.2 g/l solution of *hydrazine R*. Flush the flask with oxygen for 10 min. Ignite the filter paper. Stir the contents of the flask immediately after the end of the combustion to dissolve completely the combustion products. Continue stirring for 1 h.

Reference solution. Dilute 2.0 ml of a 16.6 g/l solution of *potassium iodide R* to 100.0 ml with *water R*. Dilute 10.0 ml of the solution to 100.0 ml with *water R*.

Introduce into a beaker 30 ml of a 200 g/l solution of *potassium nitrate R* in *0.1 M nitric acid*. Immerse the electrodes and stir for 10 min. The potential of the solution (nT_1) must remain stable. Add 1 ml of the test solution and measure the potential (nT_2).

Introduce into a beaker 30 ml of a 200 g/l solution of *potassium nitrate R* in *0.1 M nitric acid*. Immerse the electrodes and stir for 10 min. The potential of the solution must remain stable (nR_1). Add 80 µl of the reference solution and measure the potential (nR_2).

The absolute value $|nT_2 - nT_1|$ is not higher than the absolute value $|nR_2 - nR_1|$.

Related substances. Liquid chromatography (*2.2.29*).

Test solution. Dissolve 25.0 mg of the substance to be examined in *dimethyl sulphoxide R* and dilute to 25.0 ml with the same solvent.

Reference solution (a). Dissolve 25.0 mg of *diosmin CRS* in *dimethyl sulphoxide R* and dilute to 25.0 ml with the same solvent.

Reference solution (b). Dilute 5.0 ml of reference solution (a) to 100.0 ml with *dimethyl sulphoxide R*.

Reference solution (c). Dissolve 5.0 mg of *diosmin for system suitability CRS* in *dimethyl sulphoxide R* and dilute to 5.0 ml with the same solvent.

Column:

- *size*: l = 0.10 m, Ø = 4.6 mm,
- *stationary phase*: *octadecylsilyl silica gel for chromatography R* (3 µm),
- *temperature*: 40 °C.

Mobile phase: *acetonitrile R, glacial acetic acid R, methanol R, water R (2:6:28:66 V/V/V/V).*

Flow rate: 1.5 ml/min.

Detection: spectrophotometer at 275 nm.

Injection: 10 µl loop injector; inject the test solution and reference solutions (b) and (c).

Run time: 6 times the retention time of diosmin.

Relative retention with reference to diosmin (retention time = about 4.6 min): impurity A = about 0.5, impurity B = about 0.6, impurity C = about 0.8, impurity D = about 2.2, impurity E = about 2.6, impurity F = about 4.5.

System suitability: reference solution (c):

– *resolution*: minimum of 2.5 between the peaks due to impurities B and C.

Limits:

– *correction factors*: for the calculation of contents, multiply the peak areas of the following impurities by the corresponding correction factor: impurity A = 0.38; impurity F = 0.61,
– *impurity A*: not more than 0.2 times the area of the principal peak in the chromatogram obtained with reference solution (b) (1 per cent),
– *impurity B*: not more than the area of the principal peak in the chromatogram obtained with reference solution (b) (5 per cent),
– *impurity C*: not more than 0.6 times the area of the principal peak in the chromatogram obtained with reference solution (b) (3 per cent),
– *impurity E*: not more than 0.6 times the area of the principal peak in the chromatogram obtained with reference solution (b) (3 per cent),
– *impurity F*: not more than 0.6 times the area of the principal peak in the chromatogram obtained with reference solution (b) (3 per cent),
– *any other impurity*: not more than 0.2 times the area of the principal peak in the chromatogram obtained with reference solution (b) (1 per cent),
– *total of other impurities and impurity A*: not more than 0.2 times the area of the principal peak in the chromatogram obtained with reference solution (b) (1 per cent),
– *total*: not more than twice the area of the principal peak in the chromatogram obtained with reference solution (b) (10 per cent),
– *disregard limit*: 0.02 times the area of the principal peak in the chromatogram obtained with reference solution (b) (0.1 per cent).

Heavy metals (*2.4.8*): maximum 20 ppm.

2.0 g complies with limit test C. Prepare the standard using 4.0 ml of *lead standard solution (10 ppm Pb) R*.

Water (*2.5.12*): maximum 6.0 per cent, determined on 0.300 g.

Sulphated ash (*2.4.14*): maximum 0.2 per cent, determined on 1.0 g.

ASSAY

Liquid chromatography (*2.2.29*), as described in the test for related substances.

Injection: test solution and reference solution (a).

STORAGE

In an airtight container.

IMPURITIES

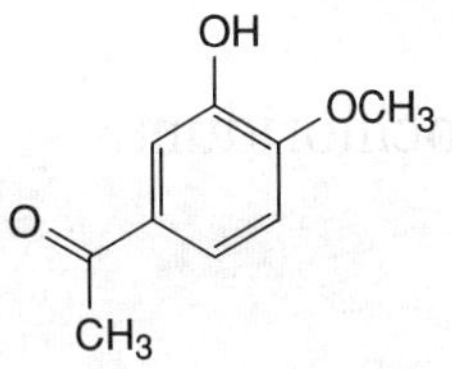

A. 1-(3-hydroxy-4-methoxyphenyl)ethanone (acetoisovanillone),

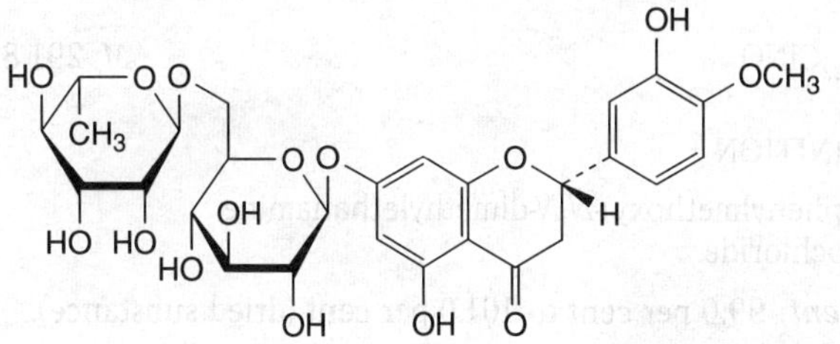

B. (2*S*)-7-[[6-*O*-(6-deoxy-α-L-mannopyranosyl)-β-D-glucopyranosyl]oxy]-5-hydroxy-2-(3-hydroxy-4-methoxyphenyl)-2,3-dihydro-4*H*-1-benzopyran-4-one (hesperidin),

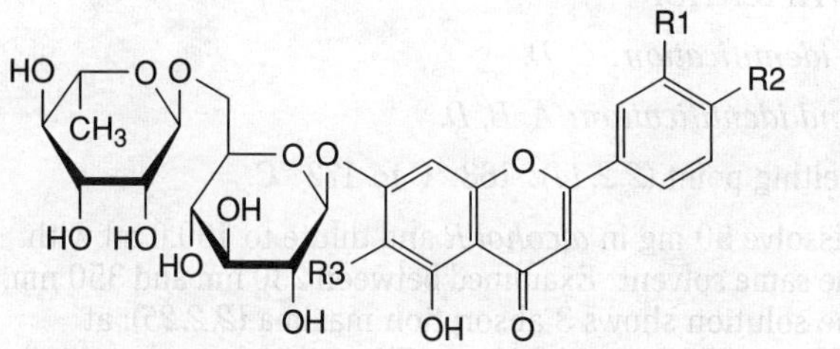

C. R1 = R3 = H, R2 = OH: 7-[[6-*O*-(6-deoxy-α-L-mannopyranosyl)-β-D-glucopyranosyl]oxy]-5-hydroxy-2-(4-hydroxyphenyl)-4*H*-1-benzopyran-4-one (isorhoifin),

D. R1 = OH, R2 = OCH_3, R3 = I: 7-[[6-*O*-(6-deoxy-α-L-mannopyranosyl)-β-D-glucopyranosyl]oxy]-5-hydroxy-2-(3-hydroxy-4-methoxyphenyl)-6-iodo-4*H*-1-benzopyran-4-one (6-iododiosmin),

E. R1 = R3 = H, R2 = OCH_3: 7-[[6-*O*-(6-deoxy-α-L-mannopyranosyl)-β-D-glucopyranosyl]oxy]-5-hydroxy-2-(4-methoxyphenyl)-4*H*-1-benzopyran-4-one (linarin),

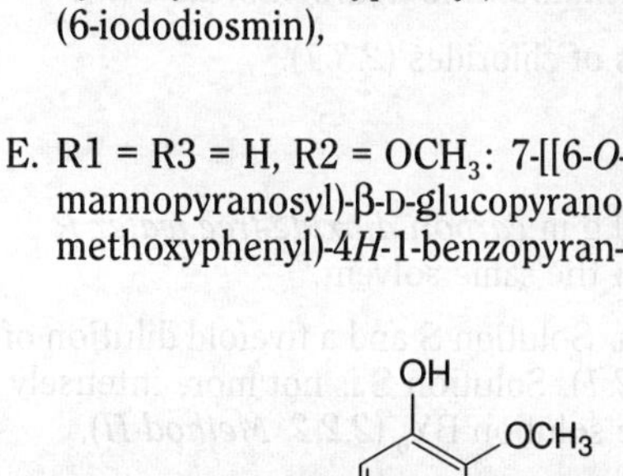

F. 5,7-dihydroxy-2-(3-hydroxy-4-methoxyphenyl)-4*H*-1-benzopyran-4-one (diosmetin).

01/2005:0023
corrected

DIPHENHYDRAMINE HYDROCHLORIDE

Diphenhydramini hydrochloridum

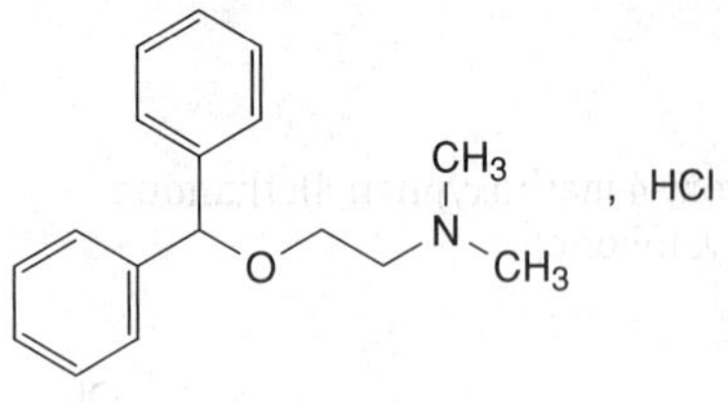

$C_{17}H_{22}ClNO$ M_r 291.8

DEFINITION

2-(Diphenylmethoxy)-*N*,*N*-dimethylethanamine hydrochloride.

Content: 99.0 per cent to 101.0 per cent (dried substance).

CHARACTERS

Appearance: white or almost white, crystalline powder.

Solubility: very soluble in water, freely soluble in alcohol.

IDENTIFICATION

First identification: C, D.

Second identification: A, B, D.

A. Melting point (*2.2.14*): 168 °C to 172 °C.

B. Dissolve 50 mg in *alcohol R* and dilute to 100.0 ml with the same solvent. Examined between 230 nm and 350 nm, the solution shows 3 absorption maxima (*2.2.25*), at 253 nm, 258 nm and 264 nm. The ratio of the absorbance measured at the maximum at 258 nm to that measured at the maximum at 253 nm is 1.1 to 1.3. The ratio of the absorbance measured at the maximum at 258 nm to that measured at the maximum at 264 nm is 1.2 to 1.4.

C. Infrared absorption spectrophotometry (*2.2.24*).

Preparation: discs.

Comparison: *diphenhydramine hydrochloride CRS*.

D. It gives the reactions of chlorides (*2.3.1*).

TESTS

Solution S. Dissolve 1.0 g in *carbon dioxide-free water R* and dilute to 20 ml with the same solvent.

Appearance of solution. Solution S and a fivefold dilution of solution S are clear (*2.2.1*). Solution S is not more intensely coloured than reference solution BY_6 (*2.2.2, Method II*).

Acidity or alkalinity. To 10 ml of solution S add 0.15 ml of *methyl red solution R* and 0.25 ml of *0.01 M hydrochloric acid*. The solution is pink. Not more than 0.5 ml of *0.01 M sodium hydroxide* is required to change the colour of the indicator to yellow.

Related substances. Liquid chromatography (*2.2.29*).

Test solution. Dissolve 70 mg of the substance to be examined in the mobile phase and dilute to 20.0 ml with the mobile phase. Dilute 2.0 ml of the solution to 10.0 ml with the mobile phase.

Reference solution (a). Dilute 1.0 ml of the test solution to 10.0 ml with the mobile phase. Dilute 1.0 ml of this solution to 20.0 ml with the mobile phase.

Reference solution (b). Dissolve 5 mg of *diphenhydramine impurity A CRS* and 5 mg of *diphenylmethanol R* in the mobile phase and dilute to 10.0 ml with the mobile phase. To 2.0 ml of this solution add 1.5 ml of the test solution and dilute to 10.0 ml with the mobile phase.

Column:

- *size*: l = 0.25 m, Ø = 4.6 mm,
- *stationary phase*: *base-deactivated octylsilyl silica gel for chromatography R* (5 µm).

Mobile phase: mix 35 volumes of *acetonitrile R* and 65 volumes of a 5.4 g/l solution of *potassium dihydrogen phosphate R* adjusted to pH 3.0 using *phosphoric acid R*.

Flow rate: 1.2 ml/min.

Detection: spectrophotometer at 220 nm.

Injection: 10 µl.

Run time: 7 times the retention time of diphenhydramine.

Relative retention with reference to diphenhydramine (retention time = about 6 min): impurity A = about 0.9; impurity B = about 1.5; impurity C = about 1.8; impurity D = about 2.6; impurity E = about 5.1.

System suitability: reference solution (b):

- *resolution*: minimum 2.0 between the peaks due to diphenhydramine and to impurity A.

Limits:

- *correction factor*: for the calculation of content, multiply the peak area of impurity D by 0.7,
- *impurity A*: not more than the area of the principal peak in the chromatogram obtained with reference solution (a) (0.5 per cent),
- *any other impurity*: not more than 0.6 times the area of the principal peak in the chromatogram obtained with reference solution (a) (0.3 per cent),
- *total*: not more than twice the area of the principal peak in the chromatogram obtained with reference solution (a) (1.0 per cent),
- *disregard limit*: 0.1 times the area of the principal peak in the chromatogram obtained with reference solution (a) (0.05 per cent).

Loss on drying (*2.2.32*): maximum 0.5 per cent, determined on 1.000 g by drying in an oven at 100-105 °C.

Sulphated ash (*2.4.14*): maximum 0.1 per cent, determined on 1.0 g.

ASSAY

Dissolve 0.250 g in 50 ml of *alcohol R* and add 5.0 ml of *0.01 M hydrochloric acid*. Carry out a potentiometric titration (*2.2.20*), using *0.1 M sodium hydroxide*. Read the volume added between the 2 points of inflexion.

1 ml of *0.1 M sodium hydroxide* is equivalent to 29.18 mg of $C_{17}H_{22}ClNO$.

STORAGE

Protected from light.

IMPURITIES

Specified impurities: A, B, C, D, E.

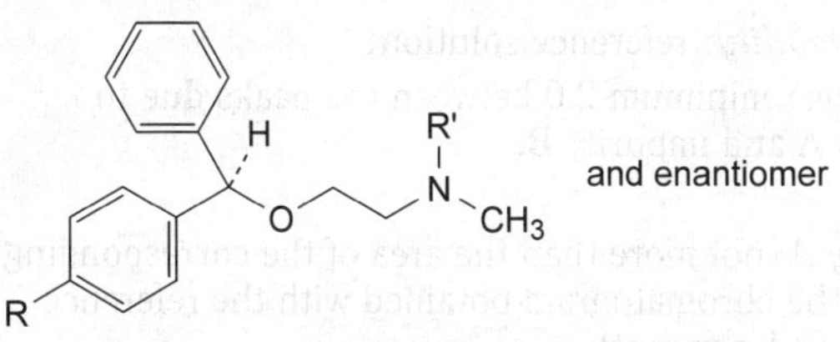

A. R = R′ = H: 2-(diphenylmethoxy)-*N*-methylethanamine,

B. R = R′ = CH_3: 2-[(*RS*)-(4-methylphenyl)phenylmethoxy]-*N,N*-dimethylethanamine,

C. R = Br, R′ = CH_3: 2-[(*RS*)-(4-bromophenyl)phenylmethoxy]-*N,N*-dimethylethanamine,

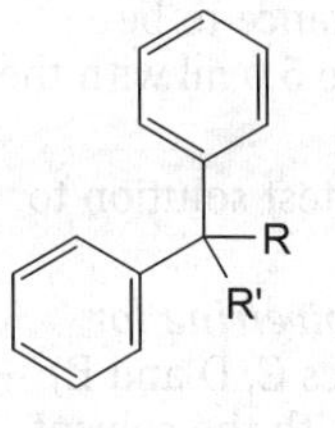

D. R = OH, R′ = H: diphenylmethanol (benzhydrol),

E. R + R′ = O: diphenylmethanone (benzophenone).

01/2005:0819

DIPHENOXYLATE HYDROCHLORIDE

Diphenoxylati hydrochloridum

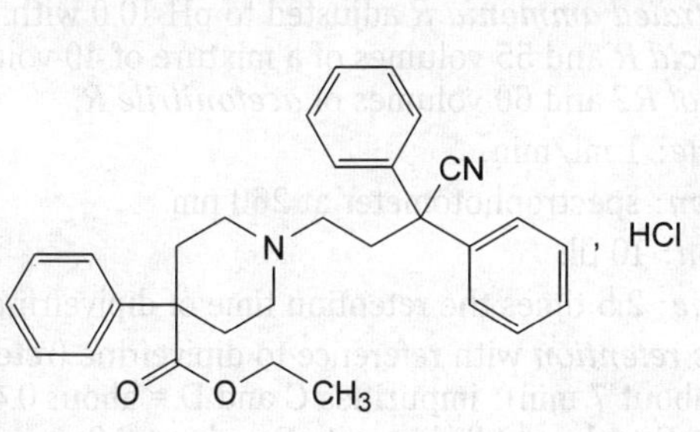

$C_{30}H_{33}ClN_2O_2$ M_r 489.1

DEFINITION

Diphenoxylate hydrochloride contains not less than 98.0 per cent and not more than the equivalent of 102.0 per cent of ethyl 1-(3-cyano-3,3-diphenylpropyl)-4-phenylpiperidine-4-carboxylate hydrochloride, calculated with reference to the dried substance.

CHARACTERS

A white or almost white, crystalline powder, very slightly soluble in water, freely soluble in methylene chloride, sparingly soluble in alcohol.

It melts at about 220 °C, with decomposition.

IDENTIFICATION

A. Examine by infrared absorption spectrophotometry (*2.2.24*), comparing with the *Ph. Eur. reference spectrum of diphenoxylate hydrochloride.*

B. Dissolve about 30 mg in 5 ml of *methanol R*. Add 0.25 ml of *nitric acid R* and 0.4 ml of *silver nitrate solution R1*. Shake and allow to stand. A curdled precipitate is formed. Centrifuge and rinse the precipitate with three quantities, each of 2 ml, of *methanol R*. Carry out this operation rapidly and protected from bright light. Suspend the precipitate in 2 ml of *water R* and add 1.5 ml of *ammonia R*. The precipitate dissolves easily.

TESTS

Appearance of solution. Dissolve 1.0 g in *methylene chloride R* and dilute to 10 ml with the same solvent. The solution is clear (*2.2.1*) and not more intensely coloured than reference solution Y_6 (*2.2.2, Method II*).

Related substances. Examine by thin-layer chromatography (*2.2.27*), using a plate coated with a suitable octadecylsilyl silica gel (5 µm) with a fluorescent indicator having an optimal intensity at 254 nm.

Test solution. Dissolve 1.0 g in a mixture of 1 volume of *methanol R* and 2 volumes of *methylene chloride R* and dilute to 20 ml with the same mixture of solvents.

Reference solution (a). Dilute 0.5 ml of the test solution to 100 ml with a mixture of 1 volume of *methanol R* and 2 volumes of *methylene chloride R*.

Reference solution (b). Dissolve 0.50 g of the substance to be examined in 25 ml of a 15 g/l solution of *potassium hydroxide R* in *methanol R* and add 1 ml of *water R*. Heat on a water-bath under a reflux condenser for 4 h. Cool and add 25 ml of *0.5 M hydrochloric acid*. Shake with 100 ml of *methylene chloride R*. Evaporate the lower layer to dryness on a water-bath. Dissolve the residue in 10 ml of a mixture of 1 volume of *methanol R* and 2 volumes of *methylene chloride R*, add 10 ml of the test solution and dilute to 25 ml with a mixture of 1 volume of *methanol R* and 2 volumes of *methylene chloride R*.

Apply separately to a plate (100 mm square) 1 µl of each solution. Develop in an unsaturated tank over a path of 7 cm using a mixture of 10 volumes of *methanol R*, 30 volumes of a 59 g/l solution of *sodium chloride R* and 60 volumes of *dioxan R*. Allow the plate to dry in an oven at 160 °C for 15 min and place the hot plate in a closed tank containing about 20 ml of *fuming nitric acid R* for 30 min. Remove the plate and heat it again at 160 °C for 15 min. Allow to cool and examine immediately in ultraviolet light at 254 nm. Any spot in the chromatogram obtained with the test solution, apart from the principal spot, is not more intense than the spot in the chromatogram obtained with reference solution (a) (0.5 per cent). The test is not valid unless the chromatogram obtained with reference solution (b) shows two clearly separated principal spots.

Loss on drying (*2.2.32*). Not more than 0.5 per cent, determined on 1.000 g by drying in an oven at 100 °C to 105 °C.

Sulphated ash (*2.4.14*). Not more than 0.1 per cent, determined on 1.0 g.

ASSAY

Dissolve 0.400 g in 40 ml of *alcohol R* and add 5.0 ml of *0.01 M hydrochloric acid*. Carry out a potentiometric titration (*2.2.20*), using *0.1 M ethanolic sodium hydroxide*. Read the volume added between the two points of inflexion.

1 ml of *0.1 M ethanolic sodium hydroxide* is equivalent to 48.91 mg of $C_{30}H_{33}ClN_2O_2$.

STORAGE

Store protected from light.

01/2005:1719

DIPIVEFRINE HYDROCHLORIDE

Dipivefrini hydrochloridum

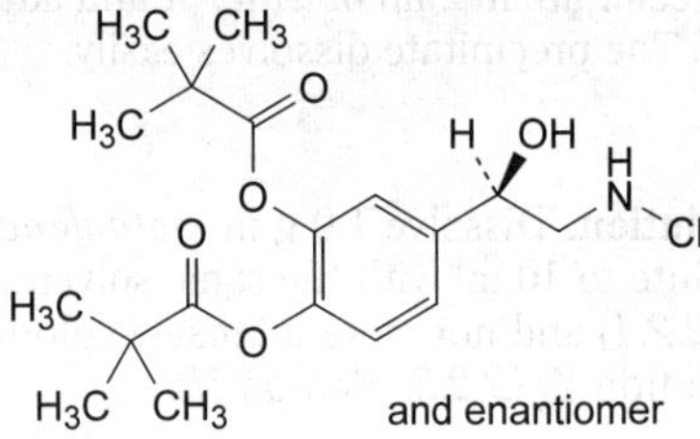

$C_{19}H_{30}ClNO_5$ M_r 387.9

DEFINITION

Hydrochloride of 4-[(1*RS*)-1-hydroxy-2-(methylamino)ethyl]-1,2-phenylene bis(2,2-dimethylpropanoate).

Content: 97.5 per cent to 102.0 per cent (dried substance).

CHARACTERS

Appearance: white or almost white, crystalline powder.

Solubility: freely soluble in water, very soluble in methanol, freely soluble in ethanol (96 per cent) and in methylene chloride.

mp: about 160 °C.

IDENTIFICATION

A. Infrared absorption spectrophotometry (*2.2.24*).
Preparation: discs.
Comparison: *dipivefrine hydrochloride CRS*.

B. It gives reaction (a) of chlorides (*2.3.1*).

TESTS

Impurities A and B. Liquid chromatography (*2.2.29*).

Test solution. Dissolve 0.100 g of the substance to be examined in *0.01 M hydrochloric acid* and dilute to 10.0 ml with the same acid.

Reference solution. Dissolve 10.0 mg of *adrenaline R* and 10.0 mg of *adrenalone hydrochloride R* in *0.01 M hydrochloric acid* and dilute to 100.0 ml with the same acid. Dilute 1.0 ml of this solution to 10.0 ml with *0.01 M hydrochloric acid. Protect this solution from light.*

Column:
- *size*: *l* = 0.15 m, Ø = 4.6 mm,
- *stationary phase*: *end-capped polar-embedded octadecylsilyl amorphous organosilica polymer R* (5 µm).

Mobile phase:
- *mobile phase A*: 0.1 per cent *V/V* solution of *anhydrous formic acid R*,
- *mobile phase B*: *methanol R2*, *acetonitrile R* (40:60 *V/V*),

Time (min)	Mobile phase A (per cent *V/V*)	Mobile phase B (per cent *V/V*)
0 - 3	100	0
3 - 5	100 → 40	0 → 60
5 - 10	40	60
10 - 11	40 → 100	60 → 0
11 - 25	100	0

Flow rate: 1 ml/min.

Detection: spectrophotometer at 260 nm.

Injection: 10 µl.

Retention times: impurity A = about 2.2 min; impurity B = about 3.2 min.

System suitability: reference solution:
- *resolution*: minimum 2.0 between the peaks due to impurity A and impurity B.

Limits:
- *impurity A*: not more than the area of the corresponding peak in the chromatogram obtained with the reference solution (0.1 per cent),
- *impurity B*: not more than the area of the corresponding peak in the chromatogram obtained with the reference solution (0.1 per cent).

Related substances. Liquid chromatography (*2.2.29*).

Solvent mixture. Mix 40 volumes of *methanol R2* and 60 volumes of *acetonitrile R*. Mix 55 volumes of this mixture and 45 volumes of *0.01 M hydrochloric acid*.

Test solution. Dissolve 50.0 mg of the substance to be examined in the solvent mixture and dilute to 5.0 ml with the solvent mixture.

Reference solution (a). Dilute 1.0 ml of the test solution to 100.0 ml with the solvent mixture.

Reference solution (b). Dissolve 5 mg of *dipivefrine for system suitability CRS* (containing impurities C, D and E) in the solvent mixture and dilute to 2.0 ml with the solvent mixture.

Reference solution (c). Dissolve 5.0 mg of *dipivefrine hydrochloride CRS* in the solvent mixture and dilute to 2.0 ml with the solvent mixture. Dilute 1.0 ml of the solution to 25.0 ml with the solvent mixture.

Column:
- *size*: *l* = 0.15 m, Ø = 4.6 mm,
- *stationary phase*: *end-capped polar-embedded octadecylsilyl amorphous organosilica polymer R* (5 µm).

Mobile phase: mix 45 volumes of a 0.7 g/l solution of *concentrated ammonia R* adjusted to pH 10.0 with *dilute acetic acid R* and 55 volumes of a mixture of 40 volumes of *methanol R2* and 60 volumes of *acetonitrile R*.

Flow rate: 1 ml/min.

Detection: spectrophotometer at 260 nm.

Injection: 10 µl.

Run time: 2.5 times the retention time of dipivefrine.

Relative retention with reference to dipivefrine (retention time = about 7 min): impurities C and D = about 0.4; impurity E = about 1.3; impurity F = about 2.0.

System suitability: reference solution (b):
- *resolution*: minimum 3.0 between the peaks due to dipivefrine and impurity E.

Limits:
- *correction factors*: for the calculation of contents, multiply the peak areas of the following impurities by the corresponding correction factor: impurities C and D = 0.5; impurity E = 0.06;
- *sum of impurities C and D*: not more than 0.3 times the area of the principal peak in the chromatogram obtained with reference solution (a) (0.3 per cent);
- *impurities E, F*: for each impurity, not more than 0.1 times the area of the principal peak in the chromatogram obtained with reference solution (a) (0.1 per cent);
- *any other impurity*: for each impurity, not more than 0.1 times the area of the principal peak in the chromatogram obtained with reference solution (a) (0.1 per cent);

– *total*: not more than 0.5 times the area of the principal peak in the chromatogram obtained with reference solution (a) (0.5 per cent);
– *disregard limit*: 0.05 times the area of the principal peak in the chromatogram obtained with reference solution (a) (0.05 per cent), disregard any peak with a mass distribution ratio of less than 0.5.

Loss on drying (*2.2.32*): maximum 1.0 per cent, determined on 1.000 g by drying *in vacuo* at 60 °C for 6 h.

Sulphated ash (*2.4.14*): maximum 0.1 per cent, determined on 1.0 g.

ASSAY

Liquid chromatography (*2.2.29*) as described in the test for related substances with the following modification.

Injection: 20 µl of reference solutions (a) and (c).

Calculate the percentage content of $C_{19}H_{30}ClNO_5$ using the chromatograms obtained with reference solutions (a) and (c) and the declared content of *dipivefrine hydrochloride CRS*.

IMPURITIES

Specified impurities: A, B, C, D, E, F.

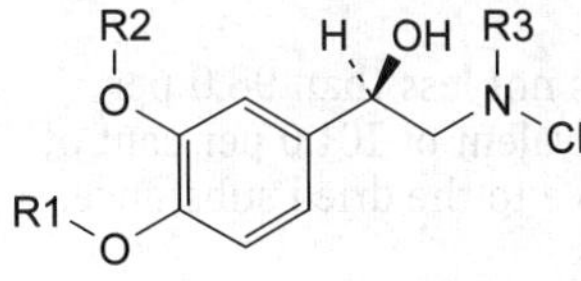

and enantiomer

A. R1 = R2 = R3 = H: 4-[(1*RS*)-1-hydroxy-2-(methylamino)ethyl]benzene-1,2-diol ((±)-adrenaline),

C. R1 = R3 = H, R2 = CO-C(CH_3)$_3$: 2-hydroxy-5-[(1*RS*)-1-hydroxy-2-(methylamino)ethyl]phenyl 2,2-dimethylpropanoate,

D. R1 = CO-C(CH_3)$_3$, R2 = R3 = H: 2-hydroxy-4-[(1*RS*)-1-hydroxy-2-(methylamino)ethyl]phenyl 2,2-dimethylpropanoate,

F. R1 = R2 = CO-C(CH_3)$_3$, R3 = C_2H_5: 4-[(1*RS*)-2-(ethylmethylamino)-1-hydroxyethyl]-1,2-phenylene bis(2,2-dimethylpropanoate),

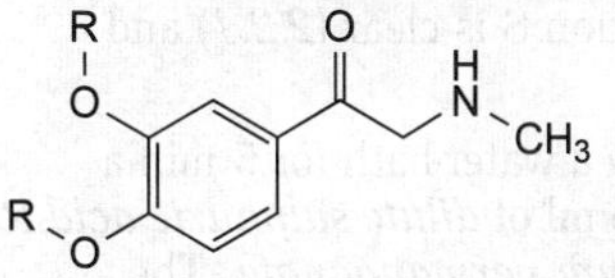

B. R = H: 1-(3,4-dihydroxyphenyl)-2-(methylamino)ethanone (adrenalone),

E. R = CO-C(CH_3)$_3$: 4-[(methylamino)acetyl]-1,2-phenylene bis(2,2-dimethylpropanoate) (adrenalone dipivalate ester).

01/2005:0898

DIPOTASSIUM CLORAZEPATE

Dikalii clorazepas

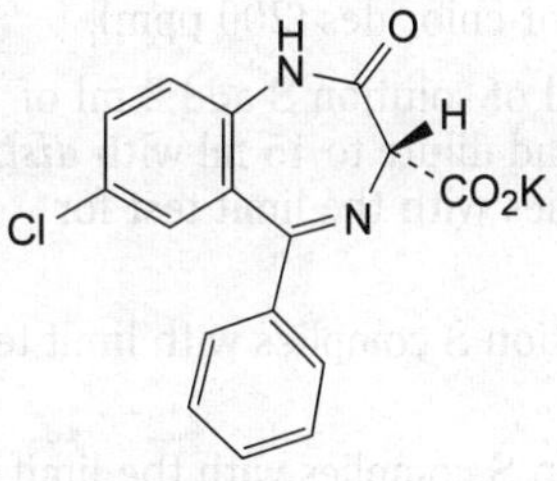

and enantiomer , KOH

$C_{16}H_{11}ClK_2N_2O_4$ M_r 408.9

DEFINITION

Potassium (3*RS*)-7-chloro-2-oxo-5-phenyl-2,3-dihydro-1*H*-1,4-benzodiazepine-3-carboxylate compound with potassium hydroxide (1:1).

Content: 99.0 per cent to 101.0 per cent (dried substance).

CHARACTERS

Appearance: white or light yellow, crystalline powder.

Solubility: freely soluble to very soluble in water, very slightly soluble in alcohol, practically insoluble in methylene chloride.

Solutions in water and in alcohol are unstable and are to be used immediately.

IDENTIFICATION

First identification: B, E.

Second identification: A, C, D, E.

A. Dissolve 10.0 mg in a 0.3 g/l solution of *potassium carbonate R* and dilute to 100.0 ml with the same solution (solution A). Dilute 10.0 ml of solution A to 100.0 ml with a 0.3 g/l solution of *potassium carbonate R* (solution B). Examined between 280 nm and 350 nm (*2.2.25*), solution A shows a broad absorption maximum at about 315 nm. The specific absorbance at the absorption maximum at 315 nm is 49 to 56. Examined between 220 nm and 280 nm (*2.2.25*), solution B shows an absorption maximum at 230 nm. The specific absorbance at the absorption maximum at 230 nm is 800 to 870.

B. Infrared absorption spectrophotometry (*2.2.24*).

Preparation: discs.

Comparison: *Ph. Eur. reference spectrum of dipotassium clorazepate.*

C. Dissolve about 20 mg in 2 ml of *sulphuric acid R*. Observed in ultraviolet light at 365 nm, the solution shows yellow fluorescence.

D. Dissolve 0.5 g in 5 ml of *water R*. Add 0.1 ml of *thymol blue solution R*. The solution is violet-blue.

E. Place 1.0 g in a crucible and add 2 ml of *dilute sulphuric acid R*. Heat at first on a water-bath, then ignite until all black particles have disappeared. Allow to cool. Take up the residue with *water R* and dilute to 20 ml with the same solvent. The solution gives reaction (b) of potassium (*2.3.1*).

TESTS

Appearance of solution. The solution is clear (*2.2.1*) and not more intensely coloured than reference solution GY_5 (*2.2.2, Method II*).

Rapidly dissolve 2.0 g with shaking in *water R* and dilute to 20.0 ml with the same solvent. Observe immediately.

Related substances. Thin-layer chromatography (*2.2.27*). *Prepare the solutions immediately before use and carry out the test protected from light.*

Test solution. Dissolve 0.20 g of the substance to be examined in *water R* and dilute to 5.0 ml with the same solvent. Shake immediately with 2 quantities, each of 5.0 ml, of *methylene chloride R*. Combine the organic layers and dilute to 10.0 ml with *methylene chloride R*.

Reference solution (a). Dissolve 10 mg of *aminochlorobenzophenone R* in *methylene chloride R* and dilute to 100.0 ml with the same solvent. Dilute 5.0 ml of the solution to 25.0 ml with *methylene chloride R*.

Reference solution (b). Dissolve 5 mg of *nordazepam CRS* in *methylene chloride R* and dilute to 25.0 ml with the same solvent. Dilute 5.0 ml of the solution to 25.0 ml with *methylene chloride R*.

Reference solution (c). Dilute 10.0 ml of reference solution (b) to 20.0 ml with *methylene chloride R*.

Reference solution (d). Dissolve 5 mg of *nordazepam CRS* and 5 mg of *nitrazepam CRS* in *methylene chloride R* and dilute to 25 ml with the same solvent.

Plate: *TLC silica gel F_{254} plate R.*

Mobile phase: *acetone R, methylene chloride R* (15:85 *V/V*).

Application: 5 µl.

Development: over 2/3 of the plate.

Drying: in air.

Detection A: examine in ultraviolet light at 254 nm.

System suitability: the chromatogram obtained with reference solution (d) shows 2 clearly separated spots.

Limits A:

– *impurity B*: any spot due to impurity B is not more intense than the spot in the chromatogram obtained with reference solution (b) (0.2 per cent),
– *any other impurity*: any spot, apart from any spot due to impurity B, is not more intense than the spot in the chromatogram obtained with reference solution (c) (0.1 per cent).

Detection B: spray with a freshly prepared 10 g/l solution of *sodium nitrite R* in *dilute hydrochloric acid R*. Dry in a current of warm air and spray with a 4 g/l solution of *naphthylethylenediamine dihydrochloride R* in *alcohol R*.

Limits B:

– *impurity A*: any spot due to impurity A is not more intense than the spot in the chromatogram obtained with reference solution (a) (0.1 per cent).

Loss on drying (*2.2.32*): maximum 0.5 per cent, determined on 1.000 g by drying *in vacuo* at 60 °C for 4 h.

ASSAY

Dissolve 0.130 g in 10 ml of *anhydrous acetic acid R*. Add 30 ml of *methylene chloride R*. Titrate with *0.1 M perchloric acid*, determining the 2 points of inflexion by potentiometry (*2.2.20*).

At the 2nd point of inflexion, 1 ml of *0.1 M perchloric acid* is equivalent to 13.63 mg of $C_{16}H_{11}ClK_2N_2O_4$.

STORAGE

In an airtight container, protected from light.

IMPURITIES

Specified impurities: *A, B.*

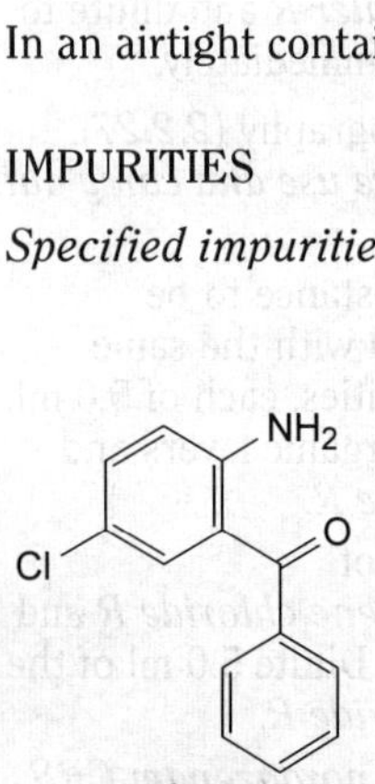

A. (2-amino-5-chlorophenyl)phenylmethanone (aminochlorobenzophenone),

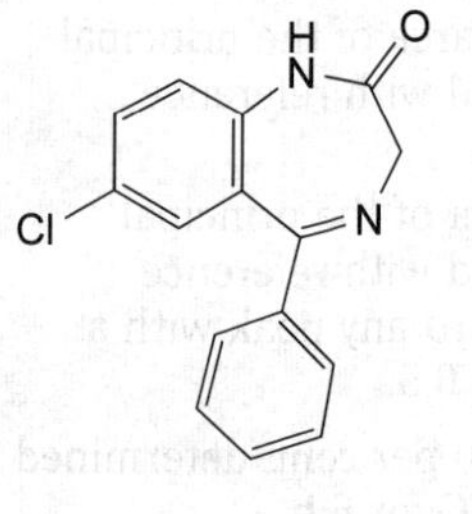

B. 7-chloro-5-phenyl-1,3-dihydro-2*H*-1,4-benzodiazepin-2-one (nordazepam).

01/2005:1003

DIPOTASSIUM PHOSPHATE

Dikalii phosphas

K_2HPO_4 M_r 174.2

DEFINITION

Dipotassium phosphate contains not less than 98.0 per cent and not more than the equivalent of 101.0 per cent of K_2HPO_4, calculated with reference to the dried substance.

CHARACTERS

A white powder or colourless crystals, very hygroscopic, very soluble in water, very slightly soluble in alcohol.

IDENTIFICATION

A. Solution S (see Tests) is slightly alkaline (*2.2.4*).

B. Solution S gives reaction (b) of phosphates (*2.3.1*).

C. Solution S gives reaction (a) of potassium (*2.3.1*).

TESTS

Solution S. Dissolve 5.0 g in *distilled water R* and dilute to 50 ml with the same solvent.

Appearance of solution. Solution S is clear (*2.2.1*) and colourless (*2.2.2, Method II*).

Reducing substances. Heat on a water-bath for 5 min a mixture of 5 ml of solution S, 5 ml of *dilute sulphuric acid R* and 0.25 ml of *0.02 M potassium permanganate*. The solution remains faintly pink.

Monopotassium phosphate. Calculated from the number of millilitres of *1 M hydrochloric acid* (10.0 ml) and of *1 M sodium hydroxide* (n_1 ml and n_2 ml) used in the assay, the ratio:

$$\frac{n_2 - 10}{10 - n_1}$$

does not exceed 0.025 (2.5 per cent).

Chlorides (*2.4.4*). To 2.5 ml of solution S add 10 ml of *dilute nitric acid R* and dilute to 15 ml with *water R*. The solution complies with the limit test for chlorides (200 ppm).

Sulphates (*2.4.13*). To 1.5 ml of solution S add 2 ml of *dilute hydrochloric acid R* and dilute to 15 ml with *distilled water R*. The solution complies with the limit test for sulphates (0.1 per cent).

Arsenic (*2.4.2*). 5 ml of solution S complies with limit test A for arsenic (2 ppm).

Iron (*2.4.9*). 10 ml of solution S complies with the limit test for iron (10 ppm).

Heavy metals (*2.4.8*). Dissolve 2.0 g in 8 ml of *water R*. Acidify with about 6 ml of *dilute hydrochloric acid R* (pH 3 to 4) and dilute to 20 ml with *water R*. 12 ml of the solution complies with limit test A for heavy metals (10 ppm). Prepare the standard using *lead standard solution (1 ppm Pb) R*.

Sodium. If intended for use in the manufacture of parenteral dosage forms, it contains not more than 0.1 per cent of Na, determined by atomic emission spectrometry (*2.2.22, Method I*).

Test solution. Dissolve 1.00 g of the substance to be examined in *water R* and dilute to 100.0 ml with the same solvent.

Reference solutions. Prepare the reference solutions using *sodium standard solution (200 ppm Na) R*, diluted as necessary with *water R*.

Measure the emission intensity at 589 nm.

Loss on drying (*2.2.32*). Not more than 2.0 per cent, determined on 1.000 g by drying in an oven at 125 °C to 130 °C.

Bacterial endotoxins (*2.6.14*): less than 1.1 IU/mg, if intended for use in the manufacture of parenteral dosage forms without a further appropriate procedure for the removal of bacterial endotoxins.

ASSAY

Dissolve 0.800 g (*m*) in 40 ml of *carbon dioxide-free water R* and add 10.0 ml of *1 M hydrochloric acid*. Using *1 M sodium hydroxide*, titrate potentiometrically (*2.2.20*) to the first inflexion point of the pH curve (n_1 ml). Continue the titration to the second inflexion point of the curve (total volume of *1 M sodium hydroxide* required, n_2 ml).

Calculate the percentage content of K_2HPO_4 from the expression:

$$\frac{1742\,(10 - n_1)}{m\,(100 - d)}$$

d = percentage loss on drying.

STORAGE

Store in an airtight container.

LABELLING

The label states:

- where applicable, that the substance is suitable for use in the manufacture of parenteral dosage forms,
- where applicable, that the substance is free from bacterial endotoxins.

01/2005:0486

DIPROPHYLLINE

Diprophyllinum

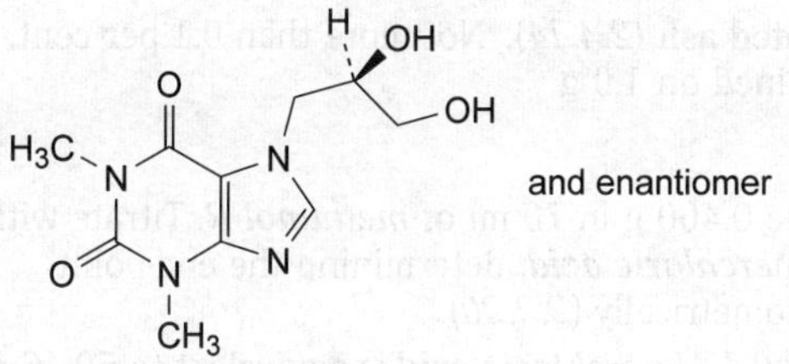

$C_{10}H_{14}N_4O_4$ M_r 254.2

DEFINITION

Diprophylline contains not less than 98.5 per cent and not more than the equivalent of 101.0 per cent of 7-[(2*RS*)-2,3-dihydroxypropyl]-1,3-dimethyl-3,7-dihydro-1*H*-purine-2,6-dione, calculated with reference to the dried substance.

CHARACTERS

A white, crystalline powder, freely soluble in water, slightly soluble in alcohol.

IDENTIFICATION

First identification: B, C.

Second identification: A, C, D.

A. Melting point (*2.2.14*): 160 °C to 165 °C.

B. Examine by infrared absorption spectrophotometry (*2.2.24*), comparing with the spectrum obtained with *diprophylline CRS*. Examine the substances as discs prepared using 0.5 mg to 1 mg of the substance to be examined in 0.3 g of *potassium bromide R*.

C. Dissolve 1 g in 5 ml of *acetic anhydride R* and boil under a reflux condenser for 15 min. Allow to cool and add 100 ml of a mixture of 20 volumes of *ether R* and 80 volumes of *light petroleum R*. Cool in iced water for at least 20 min, shaking from time to time. Filter, wash the precipitate with a mixture of 20 volumes of *ether R* and 80 volumes of *light petroleum R*, recrystallise from *alcohol R* and dry *in vacuo*. The crystals melt (*2.2.14*) at 142 °C to 148 °C.

D. It gives the reaction of xanthines (*2.3.1*).

TESTS

Solution S. Dissolve 2.5 g in *carbon dioxide-free water R* and dilute to 50 ml with the same solvent.

Appearance of solution. Solution S is clear (*2.2.1*) and colourless (*2.2.2, Method II*).

Acidity or alkalinity. To 10 ml of solution S add 0.25 ml of *bromothymol blue solution R1*. The solution is yellow or green. Not more than 0.4 ml of *0.01 M sodium hydroxide* is required to change the colour of the indicator to blue.

Related substances. Examine by thin-layer chromatography (*2.2.27*), using *silica gel HF_{254} R* as the coating substance.

Test solution. Dissolve 0.3 g of the substance to be examined in a mixture of 20 volumes of *water R* and 30 volumes of *methanol R* and dilute to 10 ml with the same mixture of solvents. *Prepare immediately before use.*

Reference solution (a). Dilute 1 ml of the test solution to 100 ml with *methanol R*.

Reference solution (b). Dilute 0.2 ml of the test solution to 100 ml with *methanol R*.

Reference solution (c). Dissolve 10 mg of *theophylline R* in *methanol R*, add 0.3 ml of the test solution and dilute to 10 ml with *methanol R*.

Apply to the plate 10 µl of each solution. Develop over a path of 15 cm using a mixture of 1 volume of *concentrated ammonia R*, 10 volumes of *ethanol R* and 90 volumes of *chloroform R*. Allow the plate to dry in air and examine in ultraviolet light at 254 nm. Any spot in the chromatogram obtained with the test solution, apart from the principal spot, is not more intense than the spot in the chromatogram obtained with reference solution (a) (1 per cent) and at most one such spot is more intense than the spot in the chromatogram obtained with reference solution (b) (0.2 per cent). The test is not valid unless the chromatogram obtained with reference solution (c) shows two clearly separated spots.

Monographs D-E

Chlorides (*2.4.4*). Dilute 2.5 ml of solution S to 15 ml with *water R*. The solution complies with the limit test for chlorides (400 ppm).

Heavy metals (*2.4.8*). 12 ml of solution S complies with limit test A for heavy metals (20 ppm). Prepare the standard using *lead standard solution (1 ppm Pb) R*.

Loss on drying (*2.2.32*). Not more than 0.5 per cent, determined on 1.000 g by drying in an oven at 100 °C to 105 °C.

Sulphated ash (*2.4.14*). Not more than 0.1 per cent, determined on 1.0 g.

ASSAY

In order to avoid overheating in the reaction medium, mix thoroughly throughout and stop the titration immediately after the end-point has been reached.

Dissolve 0.200 g in 3.0 ml of *anhydrous formic acid R* and add 50.0 ml of *acetic anhydride R*. Titrate with *0.1 M perchloric acid*, determining the end-point potentiometrically (*2.2.20*).

1 ml of *0.1 M perchloric acid* is equivalent to 25.42 mg of $C_{10}H_{14}N_4O_4$.

STORAGE

Store protected from light.

01/2005:1199

DIPYRIDAMOLE

Dipyridamolum

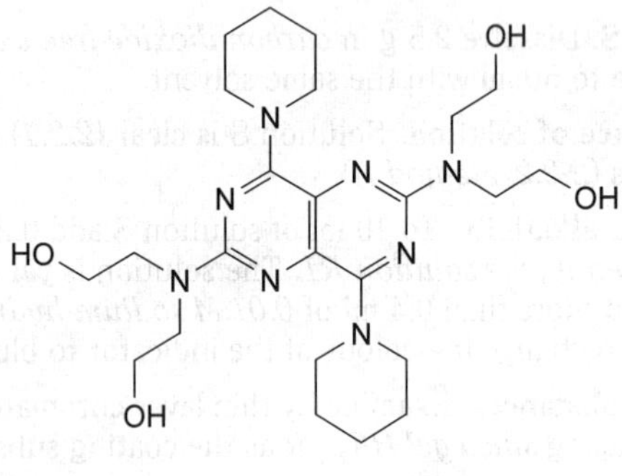

$C_{24}H_{40}N_8O_4$ M_r 504.6

DEFINITION

Dipyridamole contains not less than 98.5 per cent and not more than the equivalent of 101.5 per cent of 2,2′,2″,2‴-[[4,8-di(piperidin-1-yl)pyrimido[5,4-*d*]pyrimidine-2,6-diyl]dinitrilo]tetraethanol, calculated with reference to the dried substance.

CHARACTERS

A bright yellow, crystalline powder, practically insoluble in water, freely soluble in acetone, soluble in ethanol. It dissolves in dilute solutions of mineral acids.

IDENTIFICATION

First identification: C.

Second identification: A, B, D.

A. Melting point (*2.2.14*): 162 °C to 168 °C.

B. Dissolve 10 mg in a mixture of 1 volume of *0.1 M hydrochloric acid* and 9 volumes of *methanol R* and dilute to 50.0 ml with the same mixture of solvents. Dilute 5.0 ml of this solution to 100.0 ml with a mixture of 1 volume of *0.1 M hydrochloric acid* and 9 volumes of *methanol R*. Examined between 220 nm and 350 nm (*2.2.25*), the solution shows two absorption maxima at 232 nm and 284 nm. The ratio of the absorbance measured at the maximum at 284 nm to that measured at the maximum at 232 nm is 1.25 to 1.45.

C. Examine by infrared absorption spectrophotometry (*2.2.24*), comparing with the spectrum obtained with *dipyridamole CRS*. Examine the substances as discs prepared using *potassium bromide R*.

D. Dissolve about 5 mg in a mixture of 0.1 ml of *nitric acid R* and 2 ml of *sulphuric acid R*. An intense violet colour is produced.

TESTS

Related substances. Examine by liquid chromatography (*2.2.29*).

Test solution. Dissolve 10.0 mg in the mobile phase and dilute to 20.0 ml with the mobile phase.

Reference solution (a). Dilute 1.0 ml of the test solution to 20.0 ml with the mobile phase. Dilute 5.0 ml of this solution to 50.0 ml with the mobile phase.

Reference solution (b). Dissolve 10.0 mg of *diltiazem hydrochloride CRS* in the mobile phase and dilute to 10.0 ml with the mobile phase. Dilute 1.0 ml of this solution to 20.0 ml with reference solution (a).

The chromatographic procedure may be carried out using:

– a stainless steel column 0.25 m long and 4.6 mm in internal diameter packed with *octylsilyl silica gel for chromatography R* (5 µm),
– as mobile phase at a flow rate of 1.3 ml/min a mixture prepared as follows: dissolve 0.504 g of *potassium dihydrogen phosphate R* in 370 ml of *water R* and adjust to pH 3.0 with *phosphoric acid R*; add 80 ml of *acetonitrile R* and 550 ml of *methanol R*,
– as detector a spectrophotometer set at 290 nm,

maintaining the temperature of the column at 30 °C.

Inject 20 µl of each solution and continue the chromatography of the test solution for nine times the retention time of dipyridamole. The test is not valid unless, in the chromatogram obtained with reference solution (b), the resolution between the peaks corresponding respectively to diltiazem and dipyridamole is at least 2.0. In the chromatogram obtained with the test solution: the area of any peak, apart from the principal peak is not greater than the area of the peak in the chromatogram obtained with reference solution (a) (0.5 per cent); and the sum of the areas of all the peaks, apart from the principal peak, is not greater than twice the area of the peak in the chromatogram obtained with reference solution (a) (1 per cent). Disregard any peak with an area less than 0.1 times that of the peak in the chromatogram obtained with reference solution (a).

Chlorides (*2.4.4*). To 0.250 g add 10 ml of *water R* and strongly shake. Filter, rinse the filter with 5 ml of *water R* and dilute to 15 ml with *water R*. The combined filtrates comply with the limit test for chlorides (200 ppm).

Loss on drying (*2.2.32*). Not more than 0.5 per cent, determined on 1.000 g by drying in an oven at 100 °C to 105 °C.

Sulphated ash (*2.4.14*). Not more than 0.1 per cent, determined on 1.0 g.

ASSAY

Dissolve 0.400 g in 70 ml of *methanol R*. Titrate with *0.1 M perchloric acid*, determining the end-point potentiometrically (*2.2.20*).

1 ml of *0.1 M perchloric acid* is equivalent to 50.46 mg of $C_{24}H_{40}N_8O_4$.

STORAGE

Store protected from light.

IMPURITIES

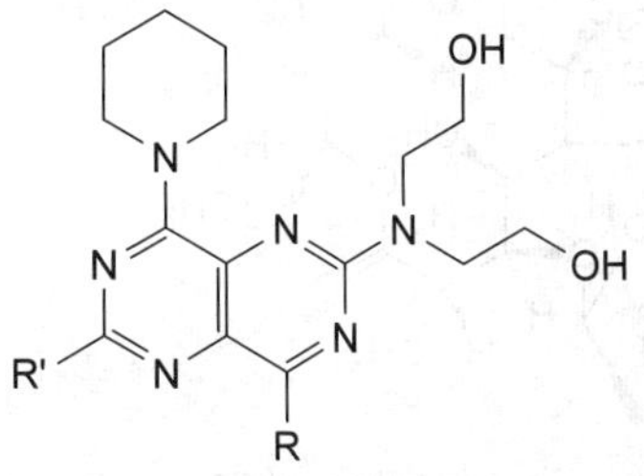

A. R = R′ = NC_5H_{10}: 2,2′-[[4,6,8-tri(piperidin-1-yl)pyrimido[5,4-*d*]pyrimidin-2-yl]nitrilo]diethanol,

B. R = R′ = $N(CH_2-CH_2OH)_2$: 2,2′,2″,2‴,2⁗,2‴″-[[8-(piperidin-1-yl)pyrimido[5,4-*d*]pyrimidine-2,4,6-triyl]trinitrilo]hexaethanol,

C. R = NC_5H_{10}, R′ = Cl: 2,2′-[[2-chloro-4,8-di(piperidin-1-yl)pyrimido[5,4-*d*]pyrimidin-6-yl]nitrilo]diethanol.

01/2005:1313

DIRITHROMYCIN

Dirithromycinum

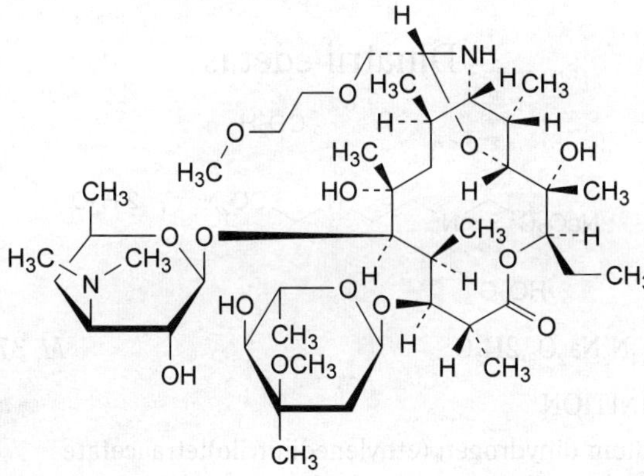

$C_{42}H_{78}N_2O_{14}$ M_r 835

DEFINITION

Dirithromycin is (1*R*,2*S*,3*R*,6*R*,7*S*,8*S*,9*R*,10*R*,12*R*,13*S*,15*R*,17*S*)-9-[[3-(dimethylamino)-3,4,6-trideoxy-β-D-*xylo*-hexopyranosyl]oxy]-3-ethyl-2,10-dihydroxy-15-[(2-methoxyethoxy)methyl]-2,6,8,10,12,17-hexamethyl-7-[(3-*C*-methyl-3-*O*-methyl-2,6-dideoxy-α-L-*ribo*-hexopyranosyl)oxy]-4,16-dioxa-14-azabicyclo[11.3.1]heptadecan-5-one (or (9*S*)-9,11-[imino[(1*R*)-2-(2-methoxyethoxy)ethylidene]oxy]-9-deoxo-11-deoxyerythromycin). The sum of the percentage contents of $C_{42}H_{78}N_2O_{14}$ and dirithromycin 15*S*-epimer is not less than 96.0 per cent and not more than the equivalent of 102.0 per cent, calculated with reference to the anhydrous substance.

CHARACTERS

A white or almost white powder, very slightly soluble in water, very soluble in methanol and in methylene chloride.

It shows polymorphism.

IDENTIFICATION

A. Examine by infrared absorption spectrophotometry (*2.2.24*), comparing with the spectrum obtained with *dirithromycin CRS*. Examine the substance prepared as discs.

B. Examine the chromatograms obtained in the assay. The retention time and size of the principal peak in the chromatogram obtained with test solution (a) are similar to those of the principal peak in the chromatogram obtained with reference solution (a).

TESTS

Related substances. Examine by liquid chromatography (*2.2.29*), as described under Assay. Inject 10 µl of reference solution (b). Adjust the sensitivity of the system so that the height of the principal peak is at least 50 per cent of the full scale of the recorder. Inject 10 µl of test solution (b) and continue the chromatography for three times the retention time of the principal peak. In the chromatogram obtained with test solution (b): the area of any peak corresponding to impurity A is not greater than 0.75 times the area of the principal peak in the chromatogram obtained with reference solution (b) (1.5 per cent); the area of any peak, apart from the principal peak and any peak corresponding to impurity A and any peak corresponding to 15*S*-epimer, is not greater than half the area of the principal peak in the chromatogram obtained with reference solution (b) (1 per cent).

Dirithromycin 15*S*-epimer. Not more than 1.5 per cent, determined by liquid chromatography (*2.2.29*), as described under Assay. Inject 10 µl of reference solution (b). Adjust the sensitivity of the system so that the height of the principal peak is at least 50 per cent of the full scale of the recorder. Inject reference solution (b) six times. The test is not valid unless the relative standard deviation of the peak area for dirithromycin is at most 5.0 per cent. Inject alternately test solution (b) and reference solution (b). Calculate the percentage content of dirithromycin 15*S*-epimer using the chromatogram obtained with reference solution (b).

Acetonitrile (*2.4.24, System A*). Not more than 0.1 per cent. Prepare the solutions using *dimethylformamide R* instead of *water R*.

Sample solution. Dissolve 0.200 g of the substance to be examined in *dimethylformamide R* and dilute to 20.0 ml with the same solvent.

The following static head-space injection conditions may be used:

- equilibration temperature: 120 °C,
- equilibration time: 60 min,
- transfer-line temperature: 125 °C.

Heavy metals (*2.4.8*). Dissolve 1.0 g in 20 ml of a mixture of equal volumes of *methanol R* and *water R*. 12 ml of the solution complies with limit test B for heavy metals (20 ppm). Prepare the standard using lead standard solution (1 ppm Pb) obtained by diluting *lead standard solution (100 ppm Pb) R* with a mixture of equal volumes of *methanol R* and *water R*.

Water (*2.5.12*). Not more than 1.0 per cent, determined on 1.00 g by the semi-micro determination of water.

Sulphated ash (*2.4.14*). Not more than 0.1 per cent, determined on 1.0 g.

ASSAY

Examine by liquid chromatography (*2.2.29*).

Solvent mixture. Mix 30 volumes of *methanol R* and 70 volumes of *acetonitrile R*.

Test solution (a). Dissolve 20.0 mg of the substance to be examined in the solvent mixture and dilute to 10.0 ml with the solvent mixture.

Test solution (b). Dissolve 0.10 g of the substance to be examined in the solvent mixture and dilute to 10.0 ml with the solvent mixture.

Reference solution (a). Dissolve 20.0 mg of *dirithromycin CRS* in the solvent mixture and dilute to 10.0 ml with the solvent mixture.

Reference solution (b). Dilute 5.0 ml of reference solution (a) to 50.0 ml with the solvent mixture.

Reference solution (c). Dissolve 20 mg of *dirithromycin CRS* in the mobile phase and dilute to 10 ml with the mobile phase. Allow to stand for 24 h before use.

The chromatographic procedure may be carried out using:

- a stainless steel column 0.25 m long and 4.6 mm in internal diameter packed with *octadecylsilyl silica gel for chromatography R* (5 µm),
- as mobile phase at a flow rate of 2.0 ml/min a mixture of: 9 volumes of *water R*; 19 volumes of *methanol R*; 28 volumes of a solution containing 1.9 g/l of *potassium dihydrogen phosphate R* and 9.1 g/l of *dipotassium hydrogen phosphate R* adjusted to pH 7.5 if necessary with a 100 g/l solution of *potassium hydroxide R*; 44 volumes of *acetonitrile R,*
- as detector a spectrophotometer set at 205 nm,

maintaining the temperature of the column at 40 °C. Inject 10 µl of reference solution (a). Adjust the sensitivity of the system so that the height of the principal peak in the chromatogram obtained is at least 50 per cent of the full scale of the recorder. Inject 10 µl of reference solution (c). When the chromatogram is recorded in the prescribed conditions, the retention times relative to dirithromycin are: impurity A about 0.7 and 15*S*-epimer about 1.1. The test is not valid unless, in the chromatogram obtained with reference solution (c), the resolution between the peaks corresponding to dirithromycin and its 15*S*-epimer is at least 2.0 (if necessary adjust the concentration of the organic modifiers in the mobile phase). Inject reference solution (a) six times. The test is not valid unless the relative standard deviation of the peak area for dirithromycin is at most 1.0 per cent. Inject alternately test solution (a) and reference solution (a).

IMPURITIES

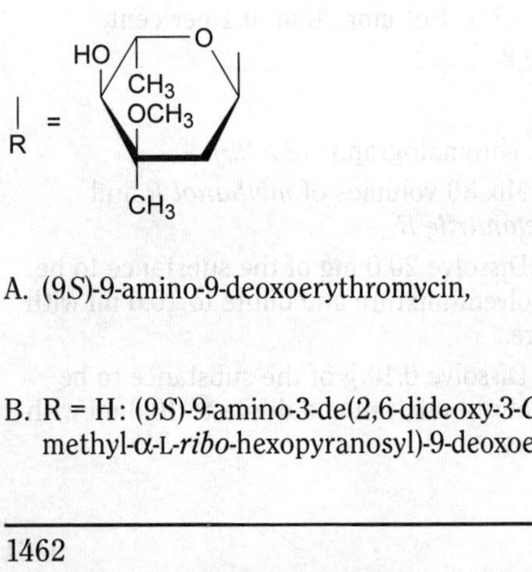

A. (9*S*)-9-amino-9-deoxoerythromycin,

B. R = H: (9*S*)-9-amino-3-de(2,6-dideoxy-3-*C*-methyl-3-*O*-methyl-α-L-*ribo*-hexopyranosyl)-9-deoxoerythromycin,

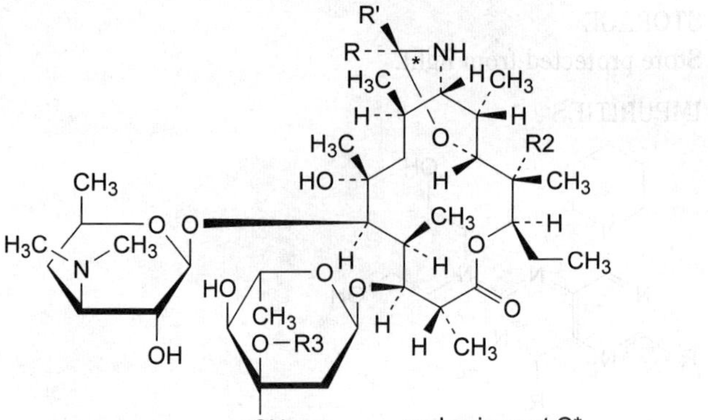

and epimer at C*

C. R = CH_2-O-CH_2-CH_2-O-CH_3, R′ = H, R2 = H, R3 = CH_3: (9*S*)-9,11-[imino[(1*RS*)-2-(2-methoxyethoxy)ethylidene]oxy]-9-deoxo-11,12-dideoxyerythromycin (dirithromycin B),

D. R = CH_2-O-CH_2-CH_2-O-CH_3, R′ = H, R2 = OH, R3 = H: (9*S*)-9,11-[imino[(1*RS*)-2-(2-methoxyethoxy)ethylidene]oxy]-3′-*O*-demethyl-9-deoxo-11-deoxyerythromycin (dirithromycin C),

E. R = CH_3, R′ = CH_3, R2 = OH, R3 = CH_3: 9,11-[imino(1-methylethylidene)oxy]-9-deoxo-11-deoxyerythromycin.

01/2005:0232

DISODIUM EDETATE

Dinatrii edetas

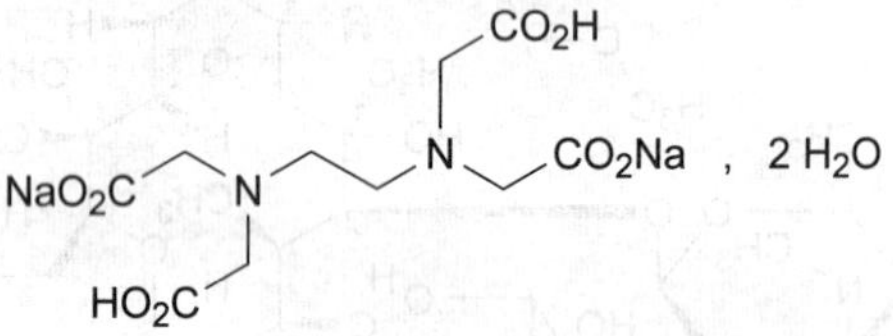

$C_{10}H_{14}N_2Na_2O_8,2H_2O$ M_r 372.2

DEFINITION

Disodium dihydrogen (ethylenedinitrilo)tetraacetate dihydrate.

Content: 98.5 per cent to 101.0 per cent.

CHARACTERS

Appearance: white, crystalline powder.

Solubility: soluble in water, practically insoluble in alcohol.

IDENTIFICATION

First identification: *A, B, D.*

Second identification: *B, C, D.*

A. Infrared absorption spectrophotometry (*2.2.24*).

Preparation: discs.

Comparison: *disodium edetate CRS.*

B. Dissolve 2 g in 25 ml of *water R*, add 6 ml of *lead nitrate solution R*, shake and add 3 ml of *potassium iodide solution R*. No yellow precipitate is formed. Make alkaline to *red litmus paper R* by the addition of *dilute ammonia R2*. Add 3 ml of *ammonium oxalate solution R*. No precipitate is formed.

C. Dissolve 0.5 g in 10 ml of *water R* and add 0.5 ml of *calcium chloride solution R*. Make alkaline to *red litmus paper R* by the addition of *dilute ammonia R2* and add 3 ml of *ammonium oxalate solution R*. No precipitate is formed.

D. It gives the reactions of sodium (*2.3.1*).

TESTS

Solution S. Dissolve 5.0 g in *carbon dioxide-free water R* and dilute to 100 ml with the same solvent.

Appearance of solution. Solution S is clear (*2.2.1*) and colourless (*2.2.2, Method II*).

pH (*2.2.3*): 4.0 to 5.5 for solution S.

Impurity A. Liquid chromatography (*2.2.29*). *Carry out the test protected from light.*

Solvent mixture. Dissolve 10.0 g of *ferric sulphate pentahydrate R* in 20 ml of *0.5 M sulphuric acid* and add 780 ml of *water R*. Adjust to pH 2.0 with *1 M sodium hydroxide* and dilute to 1000 ml with *water R*.

Test solution. Dissolve 0.100 g of the substance to be examined in the solvent mixture and dilute to 25.0 ml with the solvent mixture.

Reference solution. Dissolve 40.0 mg of *nitrilotriacetic acid R* in the solvent mixture and dilute to 100.0 ml with the solvent mixture. To 1.0 ml of the solution add 0.1 ml of the test solution and dilute to 100.0 ml with the solvent mixture.

Column:
- *size*: l = 0.10 m, Ø = 4.6 mm,
- *stationary phase*: spherical *graphitised carbon for chromatography R1* (5 µm) with a specific surface area of 120 m^2/g and a pore size of 25 nm.

Mobile phase: dissolve 50.0 mg of *ferric sulphate pentahydrate R* in 50 ml of *0.5 M sulphuric acid* and add 750 ml of *water R*. Adjust to pH 1.5 with *0.5 M sulphuric acid* or *1 M sodium hydroxide*, add 20 ml of *ethylene glycol R* and dilute to 1000 ml with *water R*.

Flow rate: 1 ml/min.

Detection: spectrophotometer at 273 nm.

Injection: 20 µl; filter the solutions and inject immediately.

Run time: 4 times the retention time of the iron complex of impurity A.

Retention times: iron complex of impurity A = about 5 min; iron complex of edetic acid = about 10 min.

System suitability: reference solution:
- *resolution*: minimum 7 between the peaks due to the iron complex of impurity A and the iron complex of edetic acid,
- *signal-to-noise ratio*: minimum 50 for the peak due to impurity A.

Limit:
- *impurity A*: not more than the area of the corresponding peak in the chromatogram obtained with the reference solution (0.1 per cent).

Iron (*2.4.9*): maximum 80 ppm.

Dilute 2.5 ml of solution S to 10 ml with *water R*. Add 0.25 g of *calcium chloride R* to the test solution and the standard before the addition of the *thioglycollic acid R*.

Heavy metals (*2.4.8*): maximum 20 ppm.

1.0 g complies with limit test D. Prepare the standard using 2 ml of *lead standard solution (10 ppm Pb) R*.

ASSAY

Dissolve 0.300 g in *water R* and dilute to 300 ml with the same solvent. Add 2 g of *hexamethylenetetramine R* and 2 ml of *dilute hydrochloric acid R*. Titrate with *0.1 M lead nitrate*, using about 50 mg of *xylenol orange triturate R* as indicator.

1 ml of *0.1 M lead nitrate* is equivalent to 37.22 mg of $C_{10}H_{14}N_2Na_2O_8,2H_2O$.

STORAGE

Protected from light.

IMPURITIES

Specified impurities: A.

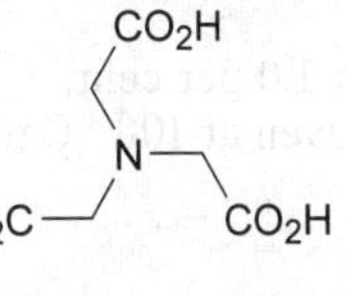

A. nitrilotriacetic acid.

01/2005:1509
corrected

DISODIUM PHOSPHATE, ANHYDROUS

Dinatrii phosphas anhydricus

Na_2HPO_4 M_r 142.0

DEFINITION

Anhydrous disodium phosphate contains not less than 98.0 per cent and not more than the equivalent of 101.0 per cent of Na_2HPO_4, calculated with reference to the dried substance.

CHARACTERS

A white powder, hygroscopic, soluble in water, practically insoluble in alcohol.

IDENTIFICATION

A. Solution S (see Tests) is slightly alkaline (*2.2.4*).

B. It complies with the test for loss on drying (see Tests).

C. Solution S (see Tests) gives reaction (b) of phosphates (*2.3.1*).

D. Solution S (see Tests) gives reaction (a) of sodium (*2.3.1*).

TESTS

Solution S. Dissolve 5.0 g in *distilled water R* and dilute to 100.0 ml with the same solvent.

Appearance of solution. Solution S is clear (*2.2.1*) and colourless (*2.2.2, Method II*).

Reducing substances. To 10 ml of solution S add 5 ml of *dilute sulphuric acid R* and 0.25 ml of *0.02 M potassium permanganate* and heat on a water-bath for 5 min. The solution retains a slight red colour.

Monosodium phosphate. Calculated from the number of millilitres of *1 M hydrochloric acid* (25 ml) and of *1 M sodium hydroxide* (n_1 ml and n_2 ml) used in the assay, the ratio:

$$\frac{n_2 - 25}{25 - n_1}$$

does not exceed 0.025.

Chlorides (*2.4.4*). 5 ml of solution S diluted to 15 ml with *dilute nitric acid R* complies with the limit test for chlorides (200 ppm).

Sulphates (*2.4.13*). To 6 ml of solution S add 2 ml of *dilute hydrochloric acid R* and dilute to 15 ml with *distilled water R*. The solution complies with the limit test for sulphates (500 ppm).

Arsenic (*2.4.2*). 10 ml of solution S complies with limit test A for arsenic (2 ppm).

Iron (*2.4.9*). 10 ml of solution S complies with the limit test for iron (20 ppm).

Heavy metals (*2.4.8*). 12 ml of solution S complies with limit test A for heavy metals (10 ppm). Prepare the standard using 5 ml of *lead standard solution (1 ppm Pb) R* and 5 ml of *water R*.

Loss on drying (*2.2.32*). Not more than 1.0 per cent, determined on 1.000 g by drying in an oven at 100 °C to 105 °C for 4 h.

ASSAY

Dissolve 1.600 g (m) in 25.0 ml of *carbon dioxide-free water R* and add 25.0 ml of *1 M hydrochloric acid*. Using *1 M sodium hydroxide*, titrate potentiometrically (*2.2.20*) to the first inflexion point (n_1 ml). Continue the titration to the second inflexion point (total volume of *1 M sodium hydroxide* required, n_2 ml).

Calculate the percentage content of Na_2HPO_4 from the expression:

$$\frac{1420\,(25 - n_1)}{m\,(100 - d)}$$

d = percentage loss on drying.

STORAGE

Store in an airtight container.

Monographs D-E

01/2005:0602

DISODIUM PHOSPHATE DIHYDRATE

Dinatrii phosphas dihydricus

$Na_2HPO_4,2H_2O$ M_r 178.0

DEFINITION

Disodium phosphate dihydrate contains not less than 98.0 per cent and not more than the equivalent of 101.0 per cent of Na_2HPO_4, calculated with reference to the dried substance.

CHARACTERS

A white or almost white powder or colourless crystals, soluble in water, practically insoluble in alcohol.

IDENTIFICATION

A. Solution S (see Tests) is slightly alkaline (*2.2.4*).

B. It complies with the test for loss on drying (see Tests).

C. Solution S gives reaction (b) of phosphates (*2.3.1*).

D. Solution S gives reaction (a) of sodium (*2.3.1*).

TESTS

Solution S. Dissolve 5.0 g in *distilled water R* and dilute to 100 ml with the same solvent.

Appearance of solution. Solution S is clear (*2.2.1*) and colourless (*2.2.2, Method II*).

Reducing substances. To 5 ml of solution S add 5 ml of *dilute sulphuric acid R* and 0.25 ml of *0.02 M potassium permanganate* and heat on a water-bath for 5 min. The solution retains a slight red colour.

Monosodium phosphate. Calculated from the number of millilitres of *1 M hydrochloric acid* (25 ml) and of *1 M sodium hydroxide* (n_1 ml and n_2 ml) used in the assay, the ratio:

$$\frac{n_2 - 25}{25 - n_1}$$

does not exceed 0.025.

Chlorides (*2.4.4*). To 2.5 ml of solution S add 10 ml of *dilute nitric acid R* and dilute to 15 ml with *water R*. The solution complies with the limit test for chlorides (400 ppm).

Sulphates (*2.4.13*). To 3 ml of solution S add 2 ml of *dilute hydrochloric acid R* and dilute to 15 ml with *distilled water R*. The solution complies with the limit test for sulphates (0.1 per cent).

Arsenic (*2.4.2*). 5 ml of solution S complies with limit test A for arsenic (4 ppm).

Iron (*2.4.9*). 5 ml of solution S diluted to 10 ml with *water R* complies with the limit test for iron (40 ppm).

Heavy metals (*2.4.8*). 12 ml of solution S complies with limit test A for heavy metals (20 ppm). Prepare the standard using *lead standard solution (1 ppm Pb) R*.

Loss on drying (*2.2.32*): 19.5 per cent to 21.0 per cent, determined on 1.000 g by drying in an oven at 130 °C.

ASSAY

Dissolve 2.000 g (m g) in 50 ml of *water R* and add 25.0 ml of *1 M hydrochloric acid*. Using *1 M sodium hydroxide*, titrate potentiometrically (*2.2.20*) to the first inflexion point of the pH curve (n_1 ml). Continue the titration to the second inflexion point of the curve (total volume of *1 M sodium hydroxide* required, n_2 ml).

Calculate the percentage content of Na_2HPO_4 from the expression:

$$\frac{1420\,(25 - n_1)}{m\,(100 - d)}$$

d = percentage loss on drying.

01/2005:0118

DISODIUM PHOSPHATE DODECAHYDRATE

Dinatrii phosphas dodecahydricus

$Na_2HPO_4,12H_2O$ M_r 358.1

DEFINITION

Disodium phosphate dodecahydrate contains not less than 98.0 per cent and not more than the equivalent of 101.0 per cent of Na_2HPO_4, calculated with reference to the anhydrous substance.

CHARACTERS

Colourless, transparent crystals, very efflorescent, very soluble in water, practically insoluble in alcohol.

IDENTIFICATION

A. Solution S (see Tests) gives the reactions of phosphates (*2.3.1*).

B. Solution S gives the reactions of sodium (*2.3.1*).

TESTS

Solution S. Dissolve 5.0 g in *distilled water R* and dilute to 50 ml with the same solvent.

Appearance of solution. Solution S is clear (*2.2.1*) and colourless (*2.2.2, Method II*).

Reducing substances. To 5 ml of solution S add 5 ml of *dilute sulphuric acid R* and 0.25 ml of *0.02 M potassium permanganate* and heat on a water-bath for 5 min. The solution retains a slight red colour.

Monosodium phosphate. Calculated from the number of millilitres of *1 M hydrochloric acid* (25 ml) and of *1 M sodium hydroxide* (n_1 ml and n_2 ml) used in the assay, the ratio:

$$\frac{n_2 - 25}{25 - n_1}$$

does not exceed 0.025.

Chlorides (*2.4.4*). To 2.5 ml of solution S add 10 ml of *dilute nitric acid R* and dilute to 15 ml with *water R*. The solution complies with the limit test for chlorides (200 ppm).

Sulphates (*2.4.13*). To 3 ml of solution S add 2 ml of *dilute hydrochloric acid R* and dilute to 15 ml with *distilled water R*. The solution complies with the limit test for sulphates (500 ppm).

Arsenic (*2.4.2*). 5 ml of solution S complies with limit test A for arsenic (2 ppm).

Iron (*2.4.9*). 5 ml of solution S diluted to 10 ml with *water R* complies with the limit test for iron (20 ppm).

Heavy metals (*2.4.8*). 12 ml of solution S complies with limit test A for heavy metals (10 ppm). Prepare the standard using *lead standard solution (1 ppm Pb) R*.

Water (*2.5.12*). 57.0 per cent to 61.0 per cent, determined on 50.0 mg by the semi-micro determination of water. Use a mixture of 10 volumes of *anhydrous methanol R* and 40 volumes of *formamide R* as solvent.

ASSAY

Dissolve 4.00 g (*m* g) in 25 ml of *water R* and add 25.0 ml of *1 M hydrochloric acid*. Using *1 M sodium hydroxide*, titrate potentiometrically (*2.2.20*) to the first inflexion point of the pH curve (n_1 ml). Continue the titration to the second inflexion point of the curve (total volume of *1 M sodium hydroxide* required, n_2 ml).

Calculate the percentage content of Na_2HPO_4 from the expression:

$$\frac{1420\,(25 - n_1)}{m\,(100 - d)}$$

d = percentage water content.

01/2005:1006

DISOPYRAMIDE

Disopyramidum

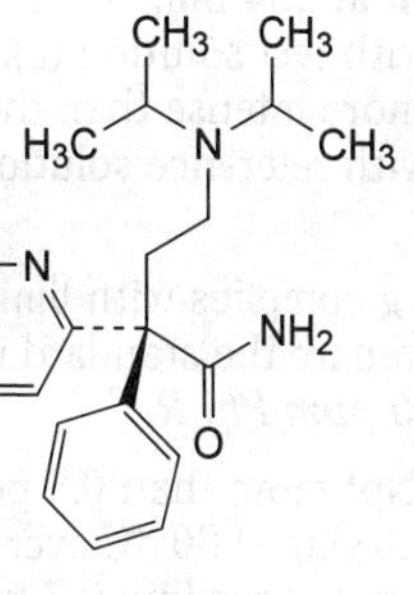

$C_{21}H_{29}N_3O$ M_r 339.5

DEFINITION

Disopyramide contains not less than 98.5 per cent and not more than the equivalent of 101.5 per cent of (2*RS*)-4-[bis(1-methylethyl)amino]-2-phenyl-2-(pyridin-2-yl)butanamide, calculated with reference to the dried substance.

CHARACTERS

A white or almost white powder, slightly soluble in water, freely soluble in methylene chloride, soluble in alcohol.

IDENTIFICATION

First identification: B.

Second identification: A, C.

A. Dissolve 40.0 mg in a 5 g/l solution of *sulphuric acid R* in *methanol R* and dilute to 100.0 ml with the same solution. Dilute 5.0 ml of this solution to 50.0 ml with a 5 g/l solution of *sulphuric acid R* in *methanol R*. Examined between 240 nm and 350 nm (*2.2.25*), the solution shows an absorption maximum at 269 nm and a shoulder at 263 nm. The specific absorbance at the maximum is 190 to 210.

B. Examine by infrared absorption spectrophotometry (*2.2.24*), comparing with the spectrum obtained with *disopyramide CRS*. Examine the substances as discs prepared by placing 50 µl of a 50 g/l solution in *methylene chloride R* on a disc of *potassium bromide R*. Dry the discs at 60 °C for 1 h before use.

C. Examine the chromatograms obtained in the test for related substances in ultraviolet light at 254 nm. The principal spot in the chromatogram obtained with test solution (b) is similar in position and size to the principal spot in the chromatogram obtained with reference solution (a). Spray with *dilute potassium iodobismuthate solution R*. Examine in daylight. The principal spot in the chromatogram obtained with test solution (b) is similar in position, colour and size to the principal spot in the chromatogram obtained with reference solution (a).

TESTS

Related substances. Examine by thin-layer chromatography (*2.2.27*), using *silica gel* GF_{254} *R* as the coating substance.

Test solution (a). Dissolve 0.20 g of the substance to be examined in *methanol R* and dilute to 10 ml with the same solvent.

Test solution (b). Dilute 1 ml of test solution (a) to 10 ml with *methanol R*.

Reference solution (a). Dissolve 20 mg of *disopyramide CRS* in *methanol R* and dilute to 10 ml with the same solvent.

Monographs D-E

Reference solution (b). Dilute 0.5 ml of test solution (b) to 20 ml with *methanol R.*

Apply to the plate 10 µl of each solution. Develop over a path of 15 cm using a mixture of 1 volume of *concentrated ammonia R*, 30 volumes of *acetone R* and 30 volumes of *cyclohexane R*. Dry the plate in a current of warm air and examine in ultraviolet light at 254 nm. Any spot in the chromatogram obtained with test solution (a), apart from the principal spot, is not more intense than the spot in the chromatogram obtained with reference solution (b) (0.25 per cent).

Heavy metals (*2.4.8*). 2.0 g complies with limit test C for heavy metals (10 ppm). Prepare the standard using 2 ml of *lead standard solution (10 ppm Pb) R.*

Loss on drying (*2.2.32*). Not more than 0.5 per cent, determined on 1.000 g by drying at 80 °C over *diphosphorus pentoxide R* at a pressure not exceeding 0.7 kPa for 2 h.

Sulphated ash (*2.4.14*). Not more than 0.2 per cent, determined on 1.0 g.

ASSAY

Dissolve 0.130 g in 30 ml of *anhydrous acetic acid R.* Add 0.2 ml of *naphtholbenzein solution R.* Titrate with *0.1 M perchloric acid* until the colour changes from yellow to green.

1 ml of *0.1 M perchloric acid* is equivalent to 16.97 mg of $C_{21}H_{29}N_3O$.

STORAGE

Store protected from light.

IMPURITIES

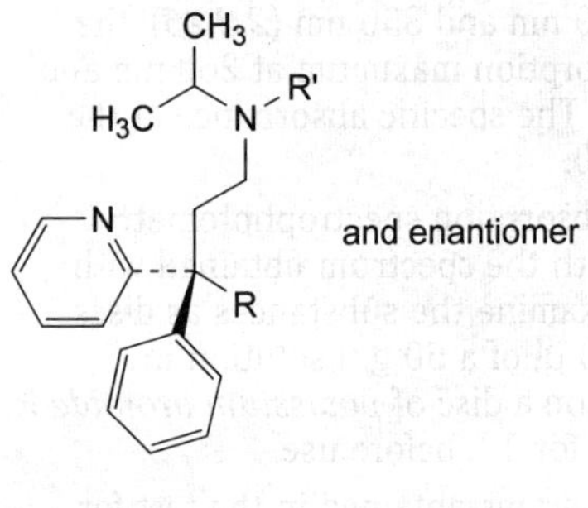

A. R = CN, R′ = $CH(CH_3)_2$: (2*RS*)-4-[bis(1-methylethyl)amino]-2-phenyl-2-(pyridin-2-yl)butanenitrile (di-isopyronitrile),

B. R = H, R′ = $CH(CH_3)_2$: (3*RS*)-*N*,*N*-bis(1-methylethyl)-3-phenyl-3-(pyridin-2-yl)propan-1-amine,

C. R = CO-NH_2, R′ = H: (2*RS*)-4-[(1-methylethyl)amino]-2-phenyl-2-(pyridin-2-yl)butanamide,

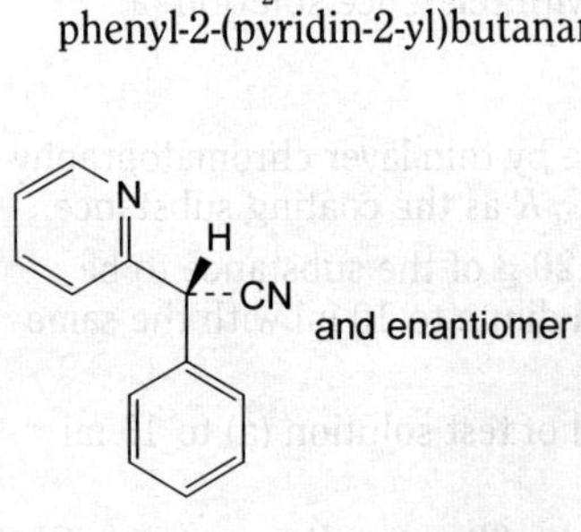

D. (*RS*)-phenyl(pyridin-2-yl)acetonitrile (pyronitrile).

01/2005:1005

DISOPYRAMIDE PHOSPHATE

Disopyramidi phosphas

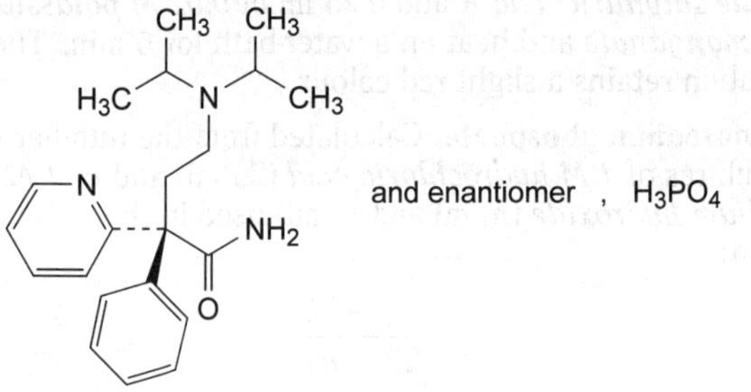

$C_{21}H_{32}N_3O_5P$ M_r 437.5

DEFINITION

Disopyramide phosphate contains not less than 98.0 per cent and not more than the equivalent of 102.0 per cent of (2*RS*)-4-[bis(1-methylethyl)amino]-2-phenyl-2-(pyridin-2-yl)butanamide dihydrogen phosphate, calculated with reference to the dried substance.

CHARACTERS

A white or almost white powder, soluble in water, sparingly soluble in alcohol, practically insoluble in methylene chloride.

IDENTIFICATION

First identification: B.

Second identification: A, C, D.

A. Dissolve 50.0 mg in a 5 g/l solution of *sulphuric acid R* in *methanol R* and dilute to 100.0 ml with the same solution. Dilute 5.0 ml of this solution to 50.0 ml with a 5 g/l solution of *sulphuric acid R* in *methanol R.* Examined between 240 nm and 350 nm (*2.2.25*), the solution shows an absorption maximum at 269 nm and a shoulder at 263 nm. The specific absorbance at the maximum is 147 to 163.

B. Examine by infrared absorption spectrophotometry (*2.2.24*), comparing with the spectrum obtained with *disopyramide phosphate CRS*. Examine the substances prepared as discs.

C. Examine the chromatograms obtained in the test for related substances in ultraviolet light at 254 nm. The principal spot in the chromatogram obtained with test solution (b) is similar in position and size to the principal spot in the chromatogram obtained with reference solution (a). Spray with *dilute potassium iodobismuthate solution R.* Examine in daylight. The principal spot in the chromatogram obtained with test solution (b) is similar in position, colour and size to the principal spot in the chromatogram obtained with reference solution (a).

D. Solution S (see Tests) gives reaction (a) of phosphates (*2.3.1*).

TESTS

Solution S. Dissolve 1.0 g in *carbon dioxide-free water R* and dilute to 20 ml with the same solvent.

Appearance of solution. Solution S is clear (*2.2.1*) and colourless (*2.2.2, Method II*).

pH (*2.2.3*). The pH of solution S is 4.0 to 5.0.

Related substances. Examine by thin-layer chromatography (*2.2.27*), using *silica gel* GF_{254} *R* as the coating substance.

Test solution (a). Dissolve 0.25 g of the substance to be examined in *methanol R* and dilute to 10 ml with the same solvent.

Test solution (b). Dilute 1 ml of test solution (a) to 10 ml with *methanol R*.

Reference solution (a). Dissolve 25 mg of *disopyramide phosphate CRS* in *methanol R* and dilute to 10 ml with the same solvent.

Reference solution (b). Dilute 1 ml of test solution (b) to 20 ml with *methanol R*.

Apply to the plate 10 µl of each solution. Develop over a path of 15 cm using a mixture of 1 volume of *concentrated ammonia R*, 30 volumes of *acetone R* and 30 volumes of *cyclohexane R*. Dry the plate in a current of warm air and examine in ultraviolet light at 254 nm. Any spot in the chromatogram obtained with test solution (a), apart from the principal spot, is not more intense than the spot in the chromatogram obtained with reference solution (b) (0.5 per cent).

Heavy metals (*2.4.8*). 2.0 g complies with limit test C for heavy metals (10 ppm). Prepare the standard using 2 ml of *lead standard solution (10 ppm Pb) R*.

Loss on drying (*2.2.32*). Not more than 0.5 per cent, determined on 1.000 g by drying in an oven at 100-105 °C.

ASSAY

Dissolve 0.180 g in 30 ml of *anhydrous acetic acid R*. Add 0.2 ml of *naphtholbenzein solution R*. Titrate with *0.1 M perchloric acid* until the colour changes from yellow to green.

1 ml of *0.1 M perchloric acid* is equivalent to 21.88 mg of $C_{21}H_{32}N_3O_5P$.

STORAGE

Store protected from light.

IMPURITIES

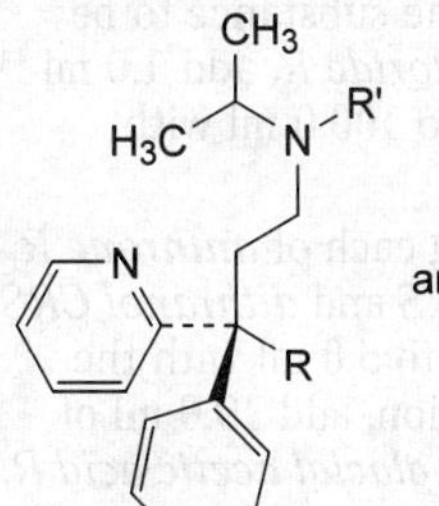

A. R = CN, R' = $CH(CH_3)_2$: (2*RS*)-4-[bis(1-methylethyl)amino]-2-phenyl-2-(pyridin-2-yl)butanenitrile (di-isopyronitrile),

B. R = H, R' = $CH(CH_3)_2$: (3*RS*)-*N*,*N*-bis(1-methylethyl)-3-phenyl-3-(pyridin-2-yl)propan-1-amine,

C. R = CO-NH_2, R' = H: (2*RS*)-4-[(1-methylethyl)amino]-2-phenyl-2-(pyridin-2-yl)butanamide,

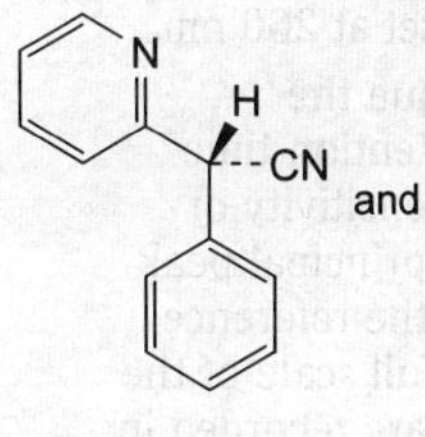

D. (*RS*)-phenyl(pyridin-2-yl)acetonitrile (pyronitrile).

01/2005:0603

DISULFIRAM

Disulfiramum

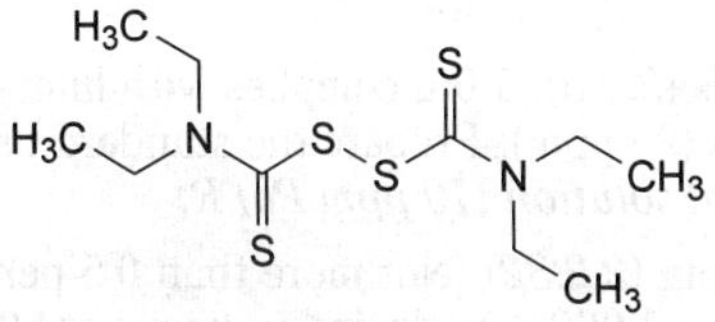

$C_{10}H_{20}N_2S_4$ M_r 296.5

DEFINITION

Disulfiram contains not less than 98.5 per cent and not more than the equivalent of 101.0 per cent of tetraethyldisulfanedicarbothioamide, calculated with reference to the dried substance.

CHARACTERS

A white or almost white, crystalline powder, practically insoluble in water, freely soluble in methylene chloride, sparingly soluble in alcohol.

IDENTIFICATION

First identification: A, B.

Second identification: A, C, D.

A. Melting point (*2.2.14*): 70 °C to 73 °C.

B. Examine by infrared absorption spectrophotometry (*2.2.24*), comparing with the spectrum obtained with *disulfiram CRS*. Examine the substances prepared as discs.

C. Examine the chromatograms obtained in the test for related substances. The principal spot in the chromatogram obtained with test solution (b) is similar in position and size to the principal spot in the chromatogram obtained with reference solution (a).

D. Dissolve about 10 mg in 10 ml of *methanol R*. Add 2 ml of a 0.5 g/l solution of *cupric chloride R* in *methanol R*. A yellow colour develops which becomes greenish-yellow.

TESTS

Related substances. Examine by thin-layer chromatography (*2.2.27*), using as the coating substance a suitable silica gel with a fluorescent indicator having an optimal intensity at 254 nm.

Test solution (a). Dissolve 0.20 g of the substance to be examined in *ethyl acetate R* and dilute to 10 ml with the same solvent.

Test solution (b). Dilute 1 ml of test solution (a) to 10 ml with *ethyl acetate R*.

Reference solution (a). Dissolve 10 mg of *disulfiram CRS* in *ethyl acetate R* and dilute to 5 ml with the same solvent.

Reference solution (b). Dilute 1 ml of test solution (b) to 20 ml with *ethyl acetate R*.

Apply to the plate 10 µl of each solution. Develop over a path of 15 cm using a mixture of 30 volumes of *butyl acetate R* and 70 volumes of *hexane R*. Allow the plate to dry in air and examine in ultraviolet light at 254 nm. Any spot in the chromatogram obtained with test solution (a), apart from the principal spot, is not more intense than the spot in the chromatogram obtained with reference solution (b) (0.5 per cent).

Diethyldithiocarbamate. Dissolve 0.20 g in 10 ml of *peroxide-free ether R*, add 5 ml of *buffer solution pH 8.0 R* and shake vigorously. Discard the upper layer and wash the lower layer with 10 ml of *peroxide-free ether R*. Add to the lower layer 0.2 ml of a 4 g/l solution of *copper sulphate R* and 5 ml of *cyclohexane R*. Shake. Any yellow colour in the upper layer is not more intense than that of a standard prepared at the same time using 0.2 ml of a freshly prepared 0.15 g/l solution of *sodium diethyldithiocarbamate R* (150 ppm).

Heavy metals (*2.4.8*). 1.0 g complies with limit test C for heavy metals (20 ppm). Prepare the standard using 2 ml of *lead standard solution (10 ppm Pb) R*.

Loss on drying (*2.2.32*). Not more than 0.5 per cent, determined on 1.000 g by drying *in vacuo* at 50 °C.

Sulphated ash (*2.4.14*). Not more than 0.1 per cent, determined on 1.0 g.

ASSAY

Dissolve 0.450 g in 80 ml of *acetone R* and add 20 ml of a 20 g/l solution of *potassium nitrate R*. Titrate with *0.1 M silver nitrate*. Determine the end-point potentiometrically (*2.2.20*), using a silver electrode and a silver-silver chloride double-junction electrode saturated with potassium nitrate.

1 ml of *0.1 M silver nitrate* is equivalent to 59.30 mg of $C_{10}H_{20}N_2S_4$.

STORAGE

Store protected from light.

IMPURITIES

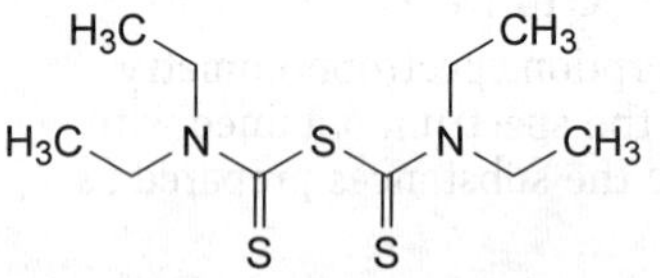

A. diethylthiocarbamic thioanhydride (sulfiram),

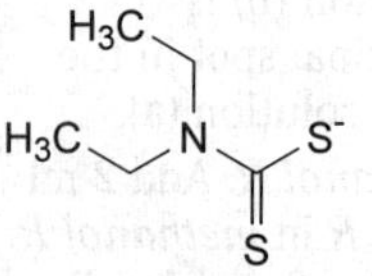

B. diethyldithiocarbamate.

01/2005:1007

DITHRANOL

Dithranolum

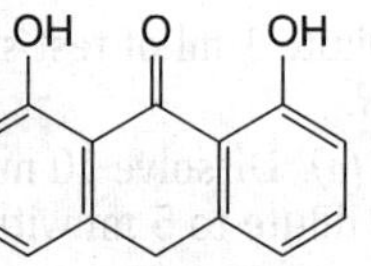

$C_{14}H_{10}O_3$ M_r 226.2

DEFINITION

Dithranol contains not less than 98.5 per cent and not more than the equivalent of 101.0 per cent of 1,8-dihydroxyanthracen-9(10*H*)-one, calculated with reference to the dried substance.

CHARACTERS

A yellow or brownish-yellow, crystalline powder, practically insoluble in water, soluble in methylene chloride, sparingly soluble in acetone, slightly soluble in alcohol. It dissolves in dilute solutions of alkali hydroxides.

Carry out all tests protected from bright light and use freshly prepared solutions.

IDENTIFICATION

First identification: A, B.

Second identification: A, C, D.

A. It melts (*2.2.14*) at 178 °C to 182 °C.

B. Examine by infrared absorption spectrophotometry (*2.2.24*), comparing with the spectrum obtained with *dithranol CRS*.

C. Examine by thin-layer chromatography (*2.2.27*), using *silica gel H R* as the coating substance.

Test solution. Dissolve 10 mg of the substance to be examined in *methylene chloride R* and dilute to 10 ml with the same solvent.

Reference solution (a). Dissolve 10 mg of *dithranol CRS* in *methylene chloride R* and dilute to 10 ml with the same solvent.

Reference solution (b). Dissolve about 5 mg of *dantron R* in 5 ml of reference solution (a).

Apply to the plate 10 µl of each solution. Develop over a path of 12 cm using a mixture of equal volumes of *hexane R* and *methylene chloride R*. Allow the plate to dry in air. Place the plate in a tank saturated with ammonia vapour until the spots appear. Examine in daylight. The principal spot in the chromatogram obtained with the test solution is similar in position, colour and size to the principal spot in the chromatogram obtained with reference solution (a). The test is not valid unless the chromatogram obtained with reference solution (b) shows 2 clearly separated spots.

D. To 5 mg add 0.1 g of *anhydrous sodium acetate R* and 1 ml of *acetic anhydride R*. Boil for 30 s. Add 20 ml of *alcohol R*. Examined in ultraviolet light at 365 nm, the solution shows a blue fluorescence.

TESTS

Related substances

A. Examine by liquid chromatography (*2.2.29*).

Test solution. Dissolve 0.200 g of the substance to be examined in 20 ml of *methylene chloride R*, add 1.0 ml of *glacial acetic acid R* and dilute to 100.0 ml with *hexane R*.

Reference solution. Dissolve 5.0 mg each of *anthrone R*, *dantron R*, *dithranol impurity C CRS* and *dithranol CRS* in *methylene chloride R* and dilute to 5.0 ml with the same solvent. To 1.0 ml of the solution, add 19.0 ml of *methylene chloride R* and 1.0 ml of *glacial acetic acid R*, and dilute to 50.0 ml with *hexane R*.

The chromatographic procedure may be carried out using:

- a stainless steel column 0.25 m long and 4.6 mm in internal diameter packed with *silica gel for chromatography R* (5 µm),
- as mobile phase at a flow rate of 2 ml/min a mixture of 1 volume of *glacial acetic acid R*, 5 volumes of *methylene chloride R* and 82 volumes of *hexane R*,
- as detector a spectrophotometer set at 260 nm.

Inject 20 µl of each solution. Continue the chromatography for 1.5 times the retention time of dithranol impurity C. Adjust the sensitivity of the system so that the height of the principal peak in the chromatogram obtained with the reference solution is about 70 per cent of the full scale of the recorder. When the chromatograms are recorded in the prescribed conditions, the substances are eluted in the following sequence: dithranol, dantron, anthrone, dithranol impurity C. The test is not valid unless, in the chromatogram obtained with the reference solution, the resolution between the peaks due to dithranol and dantron is greater than 2.0. In the chromatogram obtained with the test solution: the area of any peak corresponding to anthrone, dantron or dithranol impurity C is not greater than that of the corresponding peak in the chromatogram obtained with the reference solution (1 per cent); the area of any peak apart from the principal peak and any peaks due to anthrone, dantron and dithranol impurity C is not greater than that of the peak due to dithranol in the chromatogram obtained with the reference solution (1 per cent).

B. Examine by liquid chromatography (*2.2.29*).

Test solution. Dissolve 25.0 mg of the substance to be examined in 5 ml of *tetrahydrofuran R* and dilute to 25.0 ml with the mobile phase.

Reference solution. Dissolve 5.0 mg of *dithranol impurity D CRS* and 5.0 mg of *dithranol CRS* in 5 ml of *tetrahydrofuran R* and dilute to 10.0 ml with the mobile phase. Dilute 1.0 ml of the solution to 20.0 ml with the mobile phase.

The chromatographic procedure may be carried out using:

- a stainless steel column 0.20 m long and 4.6 mm in internal diameter packed with *octadecylsilyl silica gel for chromatography R* (5 µm),
- as mobile phase at a flow rate of 0.9 ml/min a mixture of 2.5 volumes of *glacial acetic acid R*, 40 volumes of *tetrahydrofuran R* and 60 volumes of *water R*,
- as detector a spectrophotometer set at 254 nm.

Inject 20 µl of each solution. Continue the chromatography for 3 times the retention time of the peak due to dithranol. Adjust the sensitivity of the system so that the height of the principal peak in the chromatogram obtained with the reference solution is about 50 per cent of the full scale of the recorder. The test is not valid unless, in the chromatogram obtained with the reference solution, the resolution between the peaks due to dithranol impurity D and dithranol is greater than 2.5. In the chromatogram obtained with the test solution, the area of any peak corresponding to dithranol impurity Dis not greater than that of the corresponding peak in the chromatogram obtained with the reference solution (2.5 per cent).

The total content of related substances as determined in tests A and B is not more than 3.0 per cent.

Chlorides (*2.4.4*). Shake 1.0 g with 20 ml of *water R* for 1 min and filter. Dilute 10 ml of the filtrate to 15 ml with *water R*. The solution complies with the limit test for chlorides (100 ppm).

Loss on drying (*2.2.32*). Not more than 0.5 per cent, determined on 1.000 g by drying in an oven at 100-105 °C

Sulphated ash (*2.4.14*). Not more than 0.1 per cent, determined on 1.0 g.

ASSAY

Dissolve 0.200 g in 50 ml of *anhydrous pyridine R*. Titrate with *0.1 M tetrabutylammonium hydroxide* under *nitrogen R*. Determine the end-point potentiometrically (*2.2.20*), using a glass indicator electrode and a calomel reference electrode containing, as the electrolyte, a saturated solution of *potassium chloride R* in *methanol R*.

1 ml of *0.1 M tetrabutylammonium hydroxide* is equivalent to 22.62 mg of $C_{14}H_{10}O_3$.

STORAGE

Store protected from light.

IMPURITIES

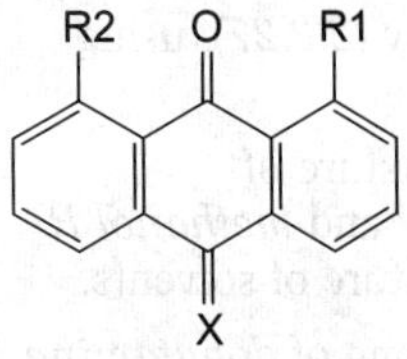

A. R1 = R2 = H, X = H_2: anthracen-9(10*H*)-one (anthrone),

B. R1 = R2 = OH, X = O: 1,8-dihydroxyanthracene-9,10-dione (danthron),

D. R1 = OH, R2 = H, X = H_2: 1-hydroxyanthracen-9(10*H*)-one,

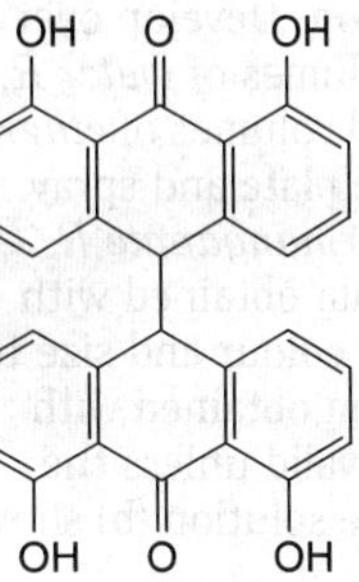

C. C. 4,4′,5,5′-tetrahydroxy-9,9′-bianthracenyl-10,10′(9*H*, 9′*H*)-dione.

01/2005:1200

DOBUTAMINE HYDROCHLORIDE

Dobutamini hydrochloridum

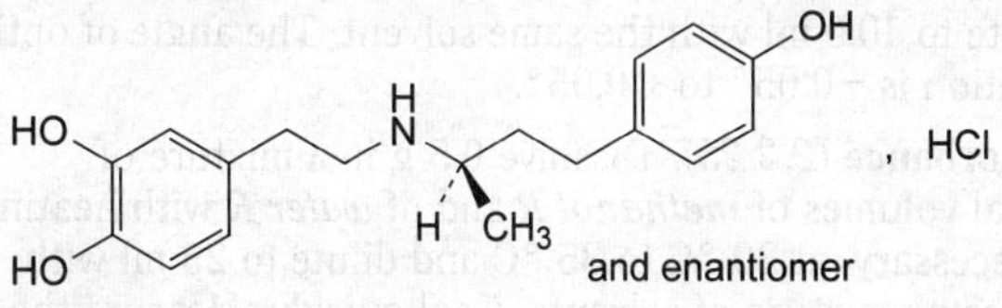

$C_{18}H_{24}ClNO_3$ M_r 337.9

DEFINITION

Dobutamine hydrochloride contains not less than 98.5 per cent and not more than the equivalent of 101.0 per cent of (*RS*)-4-[2-[[3-(4-hydroxyphenyl)-1-methylpropyl]amino]ethyl]benzene-1,2-diol hydrochloride, calculated with reference to the dried substance.

CHARACTERS

A white or almost white, crystalline powder, sparingly soluble in water, soluble in methanol, sparingly soluble in alcohol.

IDENTIFICATION

First identification: C, E.

Second identification: A, B, D, E.

A. Melting point (*2.2.14*): 189 °C to 192 °C.

B. Dissolve 20.0 mg in *methanol R* and dilute to 100.0 ml with the same solvent. Dilute 10.0 ml of the solution to 100.0 ml with *methanol R*. Examined between 220 nm and 300 nm (*2.2.25*), the solution shows two absorption maxima, at 223 nm and 281 nm. The ratio of the absorbance measured at the maximum at 281 nm to that measured at the maximum at 223 nm is 0.34 to 0.36.

C. Examine by infrared absorption spectrophotometry (*2.2.24*), comparing with the spectrum obtained with *dobutamine hydrochloride CRS*. Examine the substances prepared as discs.

D. Examine by thin-layer chromatography (*2.2.27*), using *silica gel G R* as the coating substance.

Test solution. Dissolve 10 mg in a mixture of equal volumes of *glacial acetic acid R* and *methanol R* and dilute to 10 ml with the same mixture of solvents.

Reference solution (a). Dissolve 10.0 mg of *dobutamine hydrochloride CRS* in a mixture of equal volumes of *glacial acetic acid R* and *methanol R* and dilute to 10 ml with the same mixture of solvents.

Reference solution (b). Dissolve 5.0 mg of *dopamine hydrochloride CRS* in 5 ml of the test solution.

Apply to the plate 10 µl of each solution. Develop over a path of 15 cm using a mixture of 5 volumes of *water R*, 15 volumes of *glacial acetic acid R*, 30 volumes of *ether R* and 45 volumes of *butanol R*. Dry the plate and spray with a 1 g/l solution of *potassium permanganate R*. The principal spot in the chromatogram obtained with the test solution is similar in position, colour and size to the principal spot in the chromatogram obtained with reference solution (a). The test is not valid unless the chromatogram obtained with reference solution (b) shows two clearly separated spots.

E. It gives reaction (a) of chlorides (*2.3.1*) using a mixture of equal volumes of *methanol R* and *water R*.

TESTS

Acidity or alkalinity. Dissolve 0.1 g in *water R* with gentle heating and dilute to 10 ml with the same solvent. Add 0.1 ml of *methyl red solution R* and 0.2 ml of *0.01 M sodium hydroxide*. The solution is yellow. Add 0.4 ml of *0.01 M hydrochloric acid*. The solution is red.

Optical rotation (*2.2.7*). Dissolve 0.50 g in *methanol R* and dilute to 10.0 ml with the same solvent. The angle of optical rotation is − 0.05° to + 0.05°.

Absorbance (*2.2.25*). Dissolve 0.5 g in a mixture of equal volumes of *methanol R* and of *water R* with heating, if necessary, at 30 °C to 35 °C and dilute to 25 ml with the same mixture of solvents. Cool quickly. Measure the absorbance immediately at 480 nm. The absorbance is not greater than 0.04.

Related substances. Examine by liquid chromatography (*2.2.29*).

Test solution. Dissolve 0.10 g in a mixture of 35 volumes of mobile phase B and 65 volumes of mobile phase A and dilute to 20.0 ml with the same mixture of mobile phases.

Reference solution (a). Dilute 4.0 ml of the test solution to 100.0 ml with a 0.05 g/l solution of *anisaldehyde R* in a mixture of 35 volumes of mobile phase B and 65 volumes of mobile phase A. Dilute 1.0 ml of the solution to 10.0 ml with a mixture of 35 volumes of mobile phase B and 65 volumes of mobile phase A.

Reference solution (b). Dilute 5.0 ml of the test solution to 100.0 ml with a mixture of 35 volumes of mobile phase B and 65 volumes of mobile phase A. Dilute 1.0 ml of the solution to 10.0 ml with a mixture of 35 volumes of mobile phase B and 65 volumes of mobile phase A.

The chromatographic procedure may be carried out using:

– a stainless steel column 0.15 m long and 4.6 mm in internal diameter packed with *octadecylsilyl silica gel for chromatography R* (5 µm),

– as mobile phase at a flow rate of 1 ml/min:

Mobile phase A. Dissolve 2.60 g of *sodium octanesulphonate R* in 1000 ml of *water R* and add 3 ml of *triethylamine R*; adjust to pH 2.5 with *phosphoric acid R*,

Mobile phase B. A mixture of 18 volumes of *acetonitrile R* and 82 volumes of *methanol R*,

Time (min)	Mobile phase A (per cent *V/V*)	Mobile phase B (per cent *V/V*)
0 - 5	65	35
5 - 20	65 → 20	35 → 80
20 - 25	20	80

– as detector a spectrophotometer set at 280 nm.

Inject 20 µl of reference solution (a). The test is not valid unless the resolution between the peaks corresponding to dobutamine hydrochloride and anisaldehyde is at least 4.0. Inject 20 µl of the test solution and 20 µl of reference solution (b). In the chromatogram obtained with the test solution: any peak apart from the principal peak is not greater than the principal peak in the chromatogram obtained with reference solution (b) (0.5 per cent); and the sum of the areas of all the peaks apart from the principal peak is not greater than twice the area of the principal peak in the chromatogram obtained with the reference solution (b) (1 per cent). Disregard any peak due to the solvent and any peak with an area less than 0.1 times the area of the principal peak in the chromatogram obtained with reference solution (b).

Heavy metals (*2.4.8*). 2.0 g complies with limit test C for heavy metals (10 ppm). Prepare the standard using 2 ml of *lead standard solution (10 ppm Pb) R*.

Loss on drying (*2.2.32*). Not more than 0.5 per cent, determined on 1.000 g by drying in an oven at 100 °C to 105 °C.

Sulphated ash (*2.4.14*). Not more than 0.1 per cent, determined on 1.0 g.

ASSAY

In order to avoid overheating in the reaction medium, mix thoroughly throughout and stop the titration immediately after the end-point has been reached.

Dissolve 0.250 g in 10 ml of *anhydrous formic acid R*. Add 50 ml of *acetic anhydride R*. Titrate with *0.1 M perchloric acid*, determining the end-point potentiometrically (*2.2.20*).

1 ml of *0.1 M perchloric acid* is equivalent to 33.79 mg of $C_{18}H_{24}ClNO_3$.

STORAGE

Store protected from light.

IMPURITIES

A. dopamine,

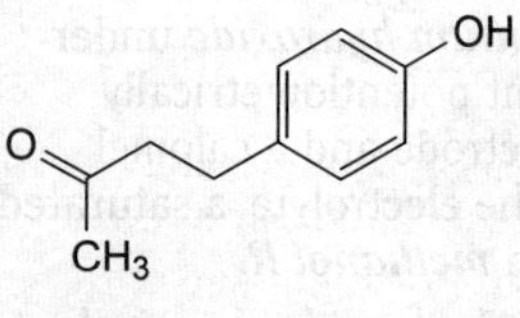

B. 4-(4-hydroxyphenyl)butan-2-one,

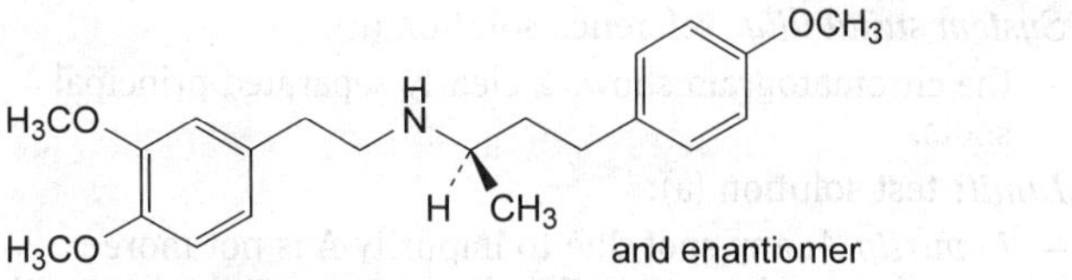

C. (2*RS*)-*N*-[2-(3,4-dimethoxyphenyl)ethyl]-4-(4-methoxyphenyl)butan-2-amine.

01/2005:1418

DOCUSATE SODIUM

Natrii docusas

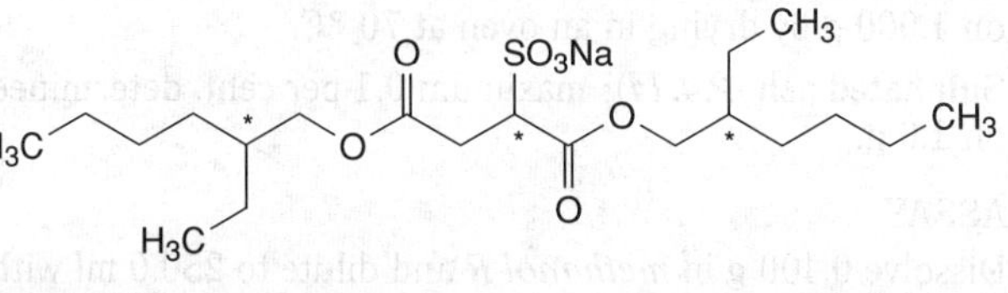

$C_{20}H_{37}NaO_7S$ M_r 444.6

DEFINITION

Sodium 1,4-bis[(2-ethylhexyl)oxy]-1,4-dioxobutane-2-sulphonate.

Content: 98.0 to 101.0 per cent (anhydrous substance).

CHARACTERS

Appearance: white or almost white, waxy masses or flakes, hygroscopic.

Solubility: sparingly soluble in water, freely soluble in alcohol and in methylene chloride.

IDENTIFICATION

A. Infrared absorption spectrophotometry (*2.2.24*).

Preparation: place about 3 mg of the substance to be examined on a sodium chloride plate, add 0.05 ml of *acetone R* and immediately cover with another sodium chloride plate. Rub the plates together to dissolve the substance to be examined, slide the plates apart and allow the acetone to evaporate.

Comparison: *Ph. Eur. reference spectrum of docusate sodium.*

B. In a crucible, ignite 0.75 g in the presence of *dilute sulphuric acid R*, until an almost white residue is obtained. Allow to cool and take up the residue with 5 ml of *water R*. Filter. 2 ml of the filtrate gives reaction (a) of sodium (*2.3.1*).

TESTS

Alkalinity. Dissolve 1.0 g in 100 ml of a mixture of equal volumes of *methanol R* and *water R*, previously neutralised to *methyl red solution R*. Add 0.1 ml of *methyl red solution R*. Not more than 0.2 ml of *0.1 M hydrochloric acid* is required to change the colour of the indicator to red.

Related non-ionic substances. Gas chromatography (*2.2.28*).

Internal standard solution. Dissolve 10 mg of *methyl behenate R* in *hexane R* and dilute to 50 ml with the same solvent.

Test solution (a). Dissolve 0.10 g of the substance to be examined in 2.0 ml of the internal standard solution and dilute to 5.0 ml with *hexane R*. Pass the solution, at a rate of about 1.5 ml/min, through a column 10 mm in internal diameter, packed with 5 g of *basic aluminium oxide R* and previously washed with 25 ml of *hexane R*. Elute with 5 ml of *hexane R* and discard the eluate. Elute with 20 ml of a mixture of equal volumes of *ether R* and *hexane R*. Evaporate the eluate to dryness and dissolve the residue in 2.0 ml of *hexane R*.

Test solution (b). Prepare as described for test solution (a) but dissolving 0.10 g of the substance to be examined in *hexane R*, diluting to 5.0 ml with the same solvent, and using a new column.

Reference solution. Dilute 2.0 ml of the internal standard solution to 5.0 ml with *hexane R*.

Column:
- *material*: glass,
- *size*: l = 2 m, Ø = 2 mm,
- *stationary phase*: *silanised diatomaceous earth for gas chromatography R* impregnated with 3 per cent *m/m* of *polymethylphenylsiloxane R*.

Carrier gas: *nitrogen for chromatography R*.

Flow rate: 30 ml/min.

Temperature:
- *column*: 230 °C,
- *injection port and detector*: 280 °C.

Detection: flame ionisation.

Injection: 1 µl.

Run time: 2.5 times the retention time of the internal standard.

System suitability: there is no peak with the same retention time as the internal standard in the chromatogram obtained with test solution (b).

Limits: test solution (a):
- *any impurity*: for each impurity, not more than the area of the peak due to the internal standard (0.4 per cent).

Chlorides: maximum 350 ppm.

Dissolve 5.0 g in 50 ml of *alcohol (50 per cent V/V) R* and add 0.1 ml of *potassium dichromate solution R*. Not more than 0.5 ml of *0.1 M silver nitrate* is required to change the colour of the indicator from yellow to orange.

Sodium sulphate: maximum 2 per cent.

Dissolve 0.25 g in 40 ml of a mixture of 20 volumes of *water R* and 80 volumes of *2-propanol R*. Adjust to pH between 2.5 and 4.0 using *perchloric acid solution R*. Add 0.4 ml of *naphtharson solution R* and 0.1 ml of a 0.125 g/l solution of *methylene blue R*. Not more than 1.5 ml of *0.025 M barium perchlorate* is required to change the colour of the indicator from yellowish-green to yellowish-pink.

Heavy metals (*2.4.8*): maximum 10 ppm.

Dissolve 4.0 g in *alcohol (80 per cent V/V) R* and dilute to 20 ml with the same solvent. 12 ml of the solution complies with limit test B. Prepare the standard using lead standard solution (2 ppm Pb) obtained by diluting *lead standard solution (100 ppm Pb) R* with *alcohol (80 per cent V/V) R*.

Water (*2.5.12*): maximum 3.0 per cent, determined on 0.250 g.

ASSAY

To 1.000 g in a 250 ml conical flask fitted with a reflux condenser add 25.0 ml of *0.5 M alcoholic potassium hydroxide* and heat on a water-bath under reflux for 45 min. Allow to cool. Add 0.25 ml of *phenolphthalein solution R1* and titrate with *0.5 M hydrochloric acid* until the red colour disappears. Carry out a blank titration.

1 ml of *0.5 M hydrochloric acid* is equivalent to 0.1112 g of $C_{20}H_{37}NaO_7S$.

STORAGE

In an airtight container.

01/2005:2078

DODECYL GALLATE

Dodecylis gallas

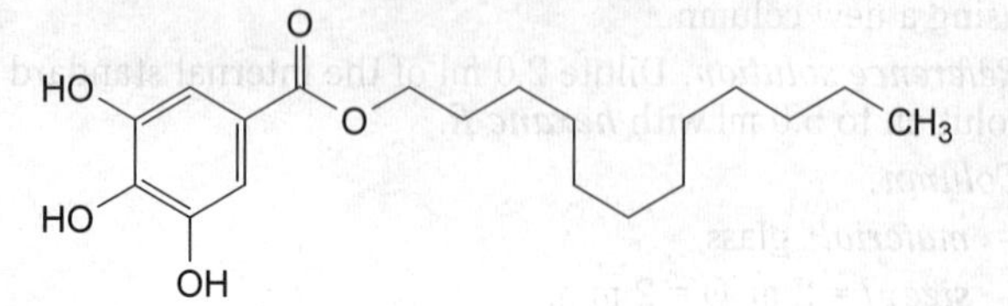

$C_{19}H_{30}O_5$ M_r 338.4

DEFINITION

Dodecyl 3,4,5-trihydroxybenzoate.

Content: 97.0 per cent to 103.0 per cent (dried substance).

CHARACTERS

Appearance: white or almost white, crystalline powder.

Solubility: very slightly soluble or practically insoluble in water, freely soluble in ethanol (96 per cent), slightly soluble in methylene chloride.

IDENTIFICATION

A. Melting point (*2.2.14*).
Determine the melting point of the substance to be examined. Mix equal parts of the substance to be examined and *dodecyl gallate CRS* and determine the melting point of the mixture. The difference between the melting points (which are about 96 °C) is not greater than 2 °C.

B. Examine the chromatograms obtained in the test for impurity A.
Results: the principal spot in the chromatogram obtained with test solution (b) is similar in position, colour and size to the principal spot in the chromatogram obtained with reference solution (a).

TESTS

Impurity A. Thin-layer chromatography (*2.2.27*).

Test solution (a). Dissolve 0.20 g of the substance to be examined in *acetone R* and dilute to 10 ml with the same solvent.

Test solution (b). Dilute 1.0 ml of test solution (a) to 20 ml with *acetone R*.

Reference solution (a). Dissolve 10 mg of *dodecyl gallate CRS* in *acetone R* and dilute to 10 ml with the same solvent.

Reference solution (b). Dissolve 20 mg of *gallic acid R* in *acetone R* and dilute to 20 ml with the same solvent.

Reference solution (c). Dilute 1.0 ml of reference solution (b) to 10 ml with *acetone R*.

Reference solution (d). Dilute 1.0 ml of reference solution (b) to 5 ml with test solution (a).

Plate: *TLC silica gel plate R*.

Mobile phase: *anhydrous formic acid R, ethyl formate R, toluene R* (10:40:50 *V/V/V*).

Application: 5 µl of test solutions (a) and (b) and reference solutions (a), (c) and (d).

Development: over 2/3 of the plate.

Drying: in air for 10 min.

Detection: spray with a mixture of 1 volume of *ferric chloride solution R1* and 9 volumes of *ethanol (96 per cent) R*.

System suitability: reference solution (d):
– the chromatogram shows 2 clearly separated principal spots.

Limit: test solution (a):
– *impurity A*: any spot due to impurity A is not more intense than the spot in the chromatogram obtained with reference solution (c) (0.5 per cent).

Chlorides (*2.4.4*): maximum 100 ppm.

To 1.65 g add 50 ml of *water R*. Shake for 5 min. Filter. 15 ml of the filtrate complies with the test.

Heavy metals (*2.4.8*): maximum 10 ppm.

2.0 g complies with limit test C. Prepare the reference solution using 2 ml of *lead standard solution (10 ppm Pb) R*.

Loss on drying (*2.2.32*): maximum 0.5 per cent, determined on 1.000 g by drying in an oven at 70 °C.

Sulphated ash (*2.4.14*): maximum 0.1 per cent, determined on 1.0 g.

ASSAY

Dissolve 0.100 g in *methanol R* and dilute to 250.0 ml with the same solvent. Dilute 5.0 ml of the solution to 200.0 ml with *methanol R*. Measure the absorbance (*2.2.25*) at the absorption maximum at 275 nm.

Calculate the content of $C_{19}H_{30}O_5$ taking the specific absorbance to be 321.

STORAGE

In a non-metallic container, protected from light.

IMPURITIES

Specified impurities: A.

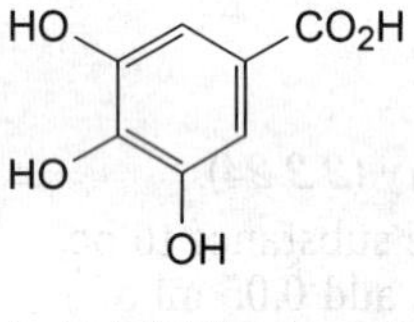

A. 3,4,5-trihydroxybenzoic acid (gallic acid).

01/2005:1510

DOG ROSE

Rosae pseudo-fructus

DEFINITION

Dog rose consists of the rose hips made up by the receptacle and the remains of the dried sepals of *Rosa canina* L., *R. pendulina* L. and other *Rosa* species, with the achenes removed. It contains not less than 0.3 per cent of ascorbic acid ($C_6H_8O_6$; M_r 176.1), calculated with reference to the dried drug.

CHARACTERS

It has the macroscopic and microscopic characters described under identification tests A and B.

IDENTIFICATION

A. It consists of fragments of the fleshy, hollow, urceolate receptacle, bearing the remains of the reduced sepals, light pink to orange-pink, the convex outer surface shiny and strongly wrinkled; bearing on its lighter inner surface abundant bristle-like hairs.

B. Reduce to a powder (355). The powder is orange-yellow. Examine under a microscope using *chloral hydrate solution R*. The powder shows numerous fragments of receptacle, the outer epidermis with orange-yellow contents and a thick cuticle, the inner epidermis composed of thin-walled cells containing cluster crystals and occasional prisms of calcium oxalate; scattered lignified cells, isodiametric, with thickened and pitted walls forming the trichome bases; abundant long, unicellar trichomes, up to 2 mm long and 30 µm to 45 µm thick, tapering towards each end, walls heavily thickened and with a waxy cuticle which may show fissures in a spiral arrangement; numerous oily orange-yellow globules.

C. Examine by thin-layer chromatography (*2.2.27*), using a *TLC silica gel F_{254} plate R*.

Test solution. To 5 g of the powdered drug (355) add 25 ml of *alcohol R*. Shake for 30 min and filter.

Reference solution. Dissolve 10 mg of *ascorbic acid R* in 5.0 ml of *alcohol (60 per cent V/V) R*.

Apply to the plate 20 µl of the test solution and 2 µl of the reference solution. Develop over a path of 15 cm using a mixture of 5 volumes of *acetic acid R*, 5 volumes of *acetone R*, 20 volumes of *methanol R* and 70 volumes of *toluene R*. Allow the plate to dry in air and examine in ultraviolet light at 254 nm. The chromatogram obtained with the test solution shows a quenching zone similar in position to the principal zone in the chromatogram obtained with the reference solution. Spray with a 0.2 g/l solution of *dichlorophenolindophenol, sodium salt R* in *alcohol R*. Examine in daylight. The chromatogram obtained with the test solution shows a white zone on a pink background similar in position and colour to the principal zone in the chromatogram obtained with the reference solution. The chromatogram also shows an intense orange-yellow zone near the solvent front and a yellow zone in the upper third (carotenoids).

TESTS

Foreign matter (*2.8.2*). Not more than 1 per cent.

Loss on drying (*2.2.32*). Not more than 10.0 per cent, determined on 1.000 g of the powdered drug (355) by drying in an oven at 100-105 °C.

Total ash (*2.4.16*). Not more than 7.0 per cent.

ASSAY

Test solution. In a round-bottomed flask, weigh 0.500 g of the freshly powdered drug (710). Add a solution of 1.0 g of *oxalic acid R* in 50.0 ml of *methanol R*. Boil under a reflux condenser for 10 min, and cool in iced water until the temperature reaches 15 °C to 20 °C. Filter. Transfer 2.0 ml of the filtrate to a 50 ml conical flask. Add successively, with gentle shaking after each addition, 2.0 ml of *dichlorophenolindophenol standard solution R* and then, exactly 60 s later, 0.5 ml of a 100 g/l solution of *thiourea R* in *alcohol (50 per cent V/V) R* and 0.7 ml of *dinitrophenylhydrazine-sulphuric acid solution R*. Heat under a reflux condenser at 50 °C for 75 min, and place immediately in iced water for 5 min. Add dropwise 5.0 ml of a mixture of 12 ml of *water R* and 50 ml of *sulphuric acid R*, taking care to carry out the addition over a period of not less than 90 s and not more than 120 s while maintaining vigorous stirring in iced water. Allow to stand for 30 min at room temperature and measure the absorbance (*2.2.25*) at 520 nm using solution A as compensation liquid.

Solution A. Treat 2.0 ml of the filtrate obtained during the preparation of the test solution as described but adding the *dinitrophenylhydrazine-sulphuric acid solution R* just before the absorbance is measured.

Reference solution. Dissolve 40.0 mg of *ascorbic acid R* in a freshly prepared 20 g/l solution of *oxalic acid R* in *methanol R* and dilute to 100.0 ml with the same solvent. Dilute 5.0 ml of the solution to 100.0 ml with the methanolic solution of oxalic acid. Treat 2.0 ml of the solution as described above for the filtrate obtained during the preparation of the test solution. Measure the absorbance (*2.2.25*) at 520 nm using solution B as compensation liquid.

Solution B. Treat 2.0 ml of the reference solution as described above for solution A.

Calculate the percentage content of ascorbic acid from the expression:

$$\frac{2.5 \times A_1 \times m_2}{A_2 \times m_1}$$

A_1 = absorbance of the test solution,

A_2 = absorbance of the reference solution,

m_1 = mass of the substance to be examined, in grams,

m_2 = mass of ascorbic acid used, in grams.

01/2005:1009

DOMPERIDONE

Domperidonum

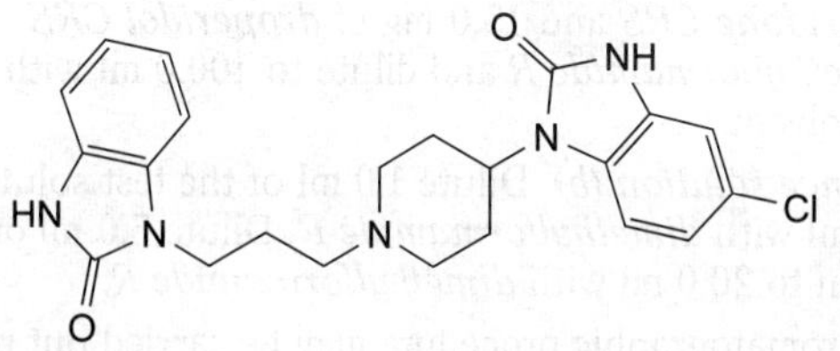

$C_{22}H_{24}ClN_5O_2$ M_r 425.9

DEFINITION

Domperidone contains not less than 99.0 per cent and not more than the equivalent of 101.0 per cent of 5-chloro-1-[1-[3-(2-oxo-2,3-dihydro-1*H*-benzimidazol-1-yl)propyl]piperidin-4-yl]-1,3-dihydro-2*H*-benzimidazol-2-one, calculated with reference to the dried substance.

CHARACTERS

A white or almost white powder, practically insoluble in water, soluble in dimethylformamide, slightly soluble in alcohol and in methanol.

IDENTIFICATION

First identification: A, B.

Second identification: A, C, D.

A. Melting point (*2.2.14*): 244 °C to 248 °C.

B. Examine by infrared absorption spectrophotometry (*2.2.24*), comparing with the spectrum obtained with *domperidone CRS*. Examine the substances prepared as discs.

C. Examine by thin-layer chromatography (*2.2.27*), using a suitable octadecylsilyl silica gel as the coating substance.

Test solution. Dissolve 20 mg of the substance to be examined in *methanol R* and dilute to 10 ml with the same solvent.

Reference solution (a). Dissolve 20 mg of *domperidone CRS* in *methanol R* and dilute to 10 ml with the same solvent.

Reference solution (b). Dissolve 20 mg of *domperidone CRS* and 20 mg of *droperidol CRS* in *methanol R* and dilute to 10 ml with the same solvent.

Apply separately to the plate 5 µl of each solution. Develop over a path of 15 cm using a mixture of 20 volumes of *ammonium acetate solution R*, 40 volumes of *dioxan R* and 40 volumes of *methanol R*. Dry the plate in a current of warm air for 15 min and expose it to iodine vapour until the spots appear. Examine in daylight. The principal spot in the chromatogram obtained with the test solution is similar in position and size to the principal spot in the chromatogram obtained with reference solution (a). The test is not valid unless the chromatogram obtained with reference solution (b) shows two clearly separated spots.

D. It gives the reaction of non-nitrogen substituted barbiturates (*2.3.1*).

TESTS

Appearance of solution. Dissolve 0.20 g in *dimethylformamide R* and dilute to 20.0 ml with the same solvent. The solution is clear (*2.2.1*) and not more intensely coloured than reference solution Y_6 (*2.2.2, Method II*).

Related substances. Examine by liquid chromatography (*2.2.29*). *Prepare the solutions immediately before use.*

Test solution. Dissolve 0.10 g of the substance to be examined in *dimethylformamide R* and dilute to 10.0 ml with the same solvent.

Reference solution (a). Dissolve 10.0 mg of *domperidone CRS* and 15.0 mg of *droperidol CRS* in *dimethylformamide R* and dilute to 100.0 ml with the same solvent.

Reference solution (b). Dilute 1.0 ml of the test solution to 100.0 ml with *dimethylformamide R*. Dilute 5.0 ml of this solution to 20.0 ml with *dimethylformamide R*.

The chromatographic procedure may be carried out using:

- a stainless steel column 0.1 m long and 4.6 mm in internal diameter packed with *base-deactivated octadecylsilyl silica gel for chromatography R* (3 µm),
- as mobile phase at a flow rate of 1.5 ml/min a mixture of 3 volumes *methanol R* and 7 volumes of a 5 g/l solution of *ammonium acetate R*, changing by linear gradient to *methanol R* over 10 min, followed by elution with *methanol R* for 2 min,
- as detector a spectrophotometer set at 280 nm.

Equilibrate the column for at least 30 min with *methanol R* and then equilibrate at the initial mobile phase composition for at least 5 min.

Adjust the sensitivity of the system so that the height of the principal peak in the chromatogram obtained with 10 µl of reference solution (b) is at least 50 per cent of the full scale of the recorder.

Inject 10 µl of reference solution (a). When the chromatogram is recorded in the prescribed conditions, the retention times are: domperidone about 6.5 min; droperidol about 7 min. The test is not valid unless the resolution between the peaks due to domperidone and droperidol is at least 2.0. If necessary, adjust the concentration of methanol in the mobile phase or adjust the time programme for the linear gradient.

Inject separately 10 µl of *dimethylformamide R* as a blank, 10 µl of the test solution and 10 µl of reference solution (b). In the chromatogram obtained with the test solution: the area of any peak, apart from the principal peak, is not greater than the area of the principal peak in the chromatogram obtained with reference solution (b) (0.25 per cent); the sum of the areas of all peaks, apart from the principal peak, is not greater than twice the area of the principal peak in the chromatogram obtained with reference solution (b) (0.5 per cent). Disregard any peak in the chromatogram obtained with the blank run and any peak with an area less than 0.2 times the area of the principal peak in the chromatogram obtained with reference solution (b).

Heavy metals (*2.4.8*). 1.0 g complies with limit test D for heavy metals (20 ppm). Prepare the standard using 2 ml of *lead standard solution (10 ppm Pb) R*.

Loss on drying (*2.2.32*). Not more than 0.5 per cent, determined on 1.000 g by drying in an oven at 100 °C to 105 °C.

Sulphated ash (*2.4.14*). Not more than 0.1 per cent, determined on 1.0 g.

ASSAY

Dissolve 0.300 g in 50 ml of a mixture of 1 volume of *anhydrous acetic acid R* and 7 volumes of *methyl ethyl ketone R*. Titrate with *0.1 M perchloric acid* until the colour changes from orange-yellow to green using 0.2 ml of *naphtholbenzein solution R* as indicator.

1 ml of *0.1 M perchloric acid* is equivalent to 42.59 mg of $C_{22}H_{24}ClN_5O_2$.

STORAGE

Store protected from light.

IMPURITIES

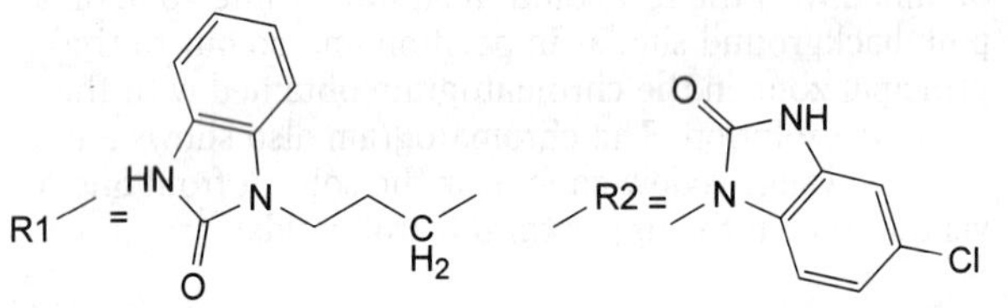

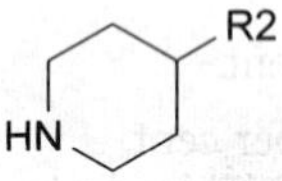

A. 5-chloro-1-(piperidin-4-yl)-1,3-dihydro-2*H*-benzimidazol-2-one,

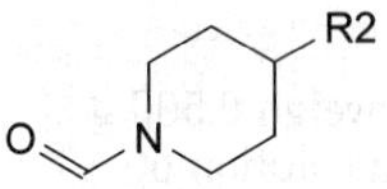

B. 4-(5-chloro-2-oxo-2,3-dihydro-1*H*-benzimidazol-1-yl)-1-formylpiperidine,

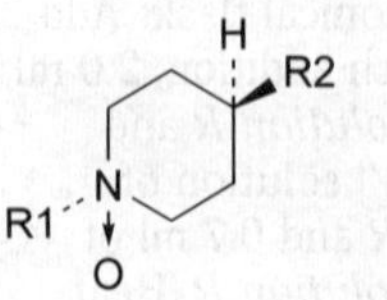

C. *cis*-4-(5-chloro-2-oxo-2,3-dihydro-1*H*-benzimidazol-1-yl)-1-[3-(2-oxo-2,3-dihydro-1*H*-benzimidazol-1-yl)propyl]piperidine 1-oxide,

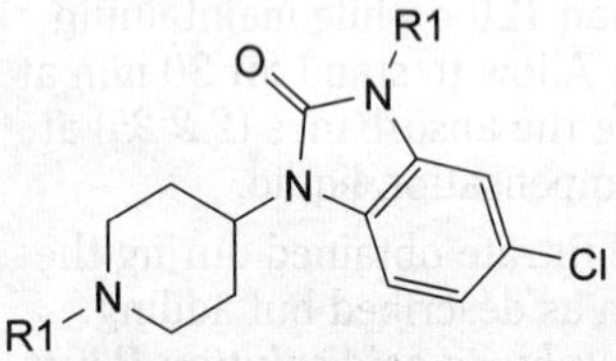

D. 5-chloro-3-[3-(2-oxo-2,3-dihydro-1*H*-benzimidazol-1-yl)propyl]-1-[1-[3-(2-oxo-2,3-dihydro-1*H*-benzimidazol-1-yl)propyl]piperidin-4-yl]-1,3-dihydro-2*H*-benzimidazol-2-one,

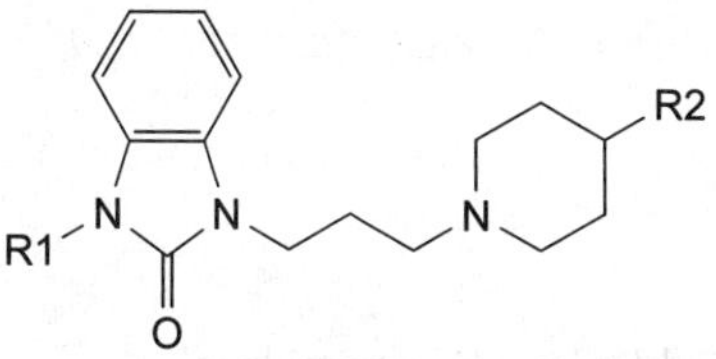

E. 1-[3-[4-(5-chloro-2-oxo-2,3-dihydro-1*H*-benzimidazol-1-yl)piperidin-1-yl]propyl]-3-[3-(2-oxo-2,3-dihydro-1*H*-benzimidazol-1-yl)propyl]-1,3-dihydro-2*H*-benzimidazol-2-one,

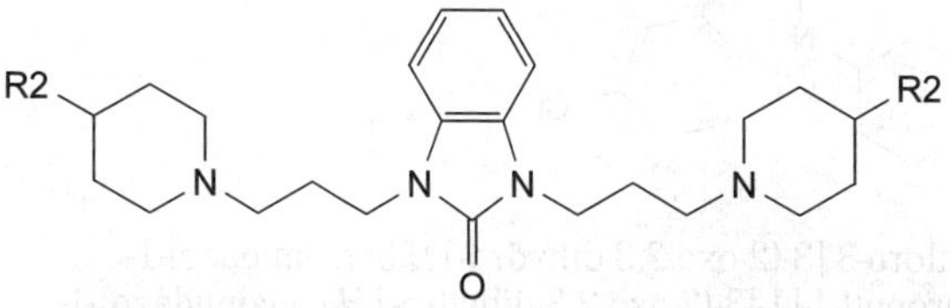

F. 1,3-bis[3-[4-(5-chloro-2-oxo-2,3-dihydro-1*H*-benzimidazol-1-yl)piperidin-1-yl]propyl]-1,3-dihydro-2*H*-benzimidazol-2-one.

01/2005:1008
corrected

DOMPERIDONE MALEATE

Domperidoni maleas

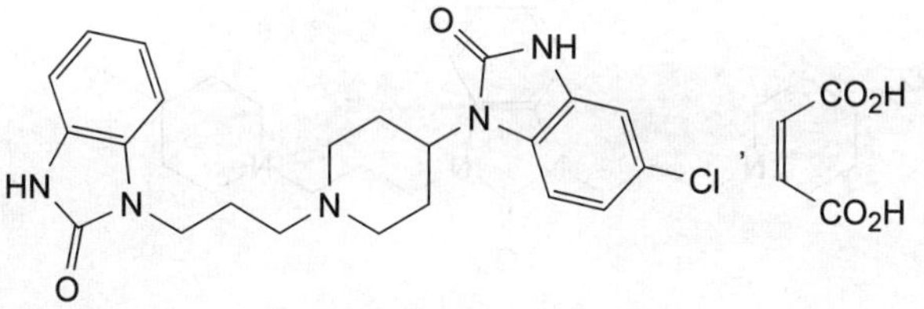

$C_{26}H_{28}ClN_5O_6$ M_r 542.0

DEFINITION

Domperidone maleate contains not less than 99.0 per cent and not more than the equivalent of 101.0 per cent of 5-chloro-1-[1-[3-(2-oxo-2,3-dihydro-1*H*-benzimidazol-1-yl)propyl]piperidin-4-yl]-1,3-dihydro-2*H*-benzimidazol-2-one hydrogen (*Z*)-butenedioate, calculated with reference to the dried substance.

CHARACTERS

A white or almost white powder, very slightly soluble in water, sparingly soluble in dimethylformamide, slightly soluble in methanol, very slightly soluble in alcohol.

It shows polymorphism.

IDENTIFICATION

First identification: A.

Second identification: B, C.

A. Examine by infrared absorption spectrophotometry (*2.2.24*), comparing with the spectrum obtained with *domperidone maleate CRS.* Examine the substances prepared as discs. If the spectra obtained show differences, dissolve the substance to be examined and the reference substance separately in the minimum volume of *2-propanol R*, evaporate to dryness on a water-bath and record new spectra using the residues.

B. Examine by thin-layer chromatography (*2.2.27*), using a suitable octadecylsilyl silica gel as the coating substance.

Test solution. Dissolve 20 mg of the substance to be examined in *methanol R* and dilute to 10 ml with the same solvent.

Reference solution (a). Dissolve 20 mg of *domperidone maleate CRS* in *methanol R* and dilute to 10 ml with the same solvent.

Reference solution (b). Dissolve 20 mg of *domperidone maleate CRS* and 20 mg of *droperidol CRS* in *methanol R* and dilute to 10 ml with the same solvent.

Apply to the plate 5 µl of each solution. Develop over a path of 15 cm using a mixture of 20 volumes of *ammonium acetate solution R*, 40 volumes of *dioxan R* and 40 volumes of *methanol R*. Dry the plate in a current of warm air for 15 min and expose it to iodine vapour until the spots appear. Examine in daylight. The principal spot in the chromatogram obtained with the test solution is similar in position and size to the principal spot in the chromatogram obtained with reference solution (a). The test is not valid unless the chromatogram obtained with reference solution (b) shows two clearly separated spots.

C. Triturate 0.1 g with a mixture of 1 ml of *strong sodium hydroxide solution R* and 3 ml of *water R*. Shake with three quantities, each of 5 ml, of *ether R*. To 0.1 ml of the aqueous layer add a solution of 10 mg of *resorcinol R* in 3 ml of *sulphuric acid R*. Heat on a water-bath for 15 min. No colour develops. To the remainder of the aqueous layer add 2 ml of *bromine solution R*. Heat on a water-bath for 15 min and then heat to boiling. Cool. To 0.1 ml of the solution add a solution of 10 mg of *resorcinol R* in in 3 ml of *sulphuric acid R*. Heat on a water-bath for 15 min. A violet colour develops.

TESTS

Appearance of solution. Dissolve 0.20 g in *dimethylformamide R* and dilute to 20.0 ml with the same solvent. The solution is clear (*2.2.1*) and not more intensely coloured than reference solution Y_6 (*2.2.2, Method II*).

Related substances. Examine by liquid chromatography (*2.2.29*). *Prepare the solutions immediately before use.*

Test solution. Dissolve 0.10 g of the substance to be examined in *dimethylformamide R* and dilute to 10.0 ml with the same solvent.

Reference solution (a). Dissolve 10.0 mg of *domperidone maleate CRS* and 15.0 mg of *droperidol CRS* in *dimethylformamide R* and dilute to 100.0 ml with the same solvent.

Reference solution (b). Dilute 1.0 ml of the test solution to 100.0 ml with *dimethylformamide R*. Dilute 5.0 ml of this solution to 20.0 ml with *dimethylformamide R.*

The chromatographic procedure may be carried out using:

– a stainless steel column 0.1 m long and 4.6 mm in internal diameter packed with *base-deactivated octadecylsilyl silica gel for chromatography R* (3 µm),

– as mobile phase at a flow rate of 1.5 ml per minute of a mixture of 3 volumes of *methanol R* and 7 volumes of a 5 g/l solution of *ammonium acetate R*, changing by linear gradient to *methanol R* over 10 min, followed by elution with *methanol R* for 2 min,

– as detector a spectrophotometer set at 280 nm.

Equilibrate the column for at least 30 min with *methanol R* and then equilibrate at the initial mobile phase composition for at least 5 min.

Adjust the sensitivity of the system so that the height of the principal peak in the chromatogram obtained with 10 µl of reference solution (b) is at least 50 per cent of the full scale of the recorder.

Inject 10 µl of reference solution (a). When the chromatogram is recorded in the prescribed conditions, the retention times are: domperidone maleate, about 6.5 min and droperidol, about 7 min. The test is not valid unless the resolution between the peaks due to domperidone maleate and droperidol is at least 2.0. If necessary, adjust the concentration of methanol in the mobile phase or adjust the time programme for the linear gradient.

Inject 10 µl of *dimethylformamide R* as a blank, 10 µl of the test solution and 10 µl of reference solution (b). In the chromatogram obtained with the test solution: the area of any peak, apart from the principal peak, is not greater than the area of the principal peak in the chromatogram obtained with reference solution (b) (0.25 per cent); the sum of the areas of all peaks, apart from the principal peak, is not greater than twice the area of the principal peak in the chromatogram obtained with reference solution (b) (0.5 per cent). Disregard any peak in the chromatogram obtained with the blank run, any peak due to maleic acid at the beginning of the chromatogram and any peak with an area less than 0.2 times that of the principal peak in the chromatogram obtained with reference solution (b).

Heavy metals (*2.4.8*). 1.0 g complies with limit test D for heavy metals (20 ppm). Prepare the standard using 2 ml of *lead standard solution (10 ppm Pb) R*.

Loss on drying (*2.2.32*). Not more than 0.5 per cent, determined on 1.000 g by drying in an oven at 100 °C to 105 °C.

Sulphated ash (*2.4.14*). Not more than 0.1 per cent, determined on 1.0 g.

ASSAY

Dissolve 0.400 g in 50 ml of *anhydrous acetic acid R*. Using 0.2 ml of *naphtholbenzein solution R* as indicator, titrate with *0.1 M perchloric acid* until the colour changes from orange-yellow to green.

1 ml of *0.1 M perchloric acid* is equivalent to 54.20 mg of $C_{26}H_{28}ClN_5O_6$.

STORAGE

Store protected from light.

IMPURITIES

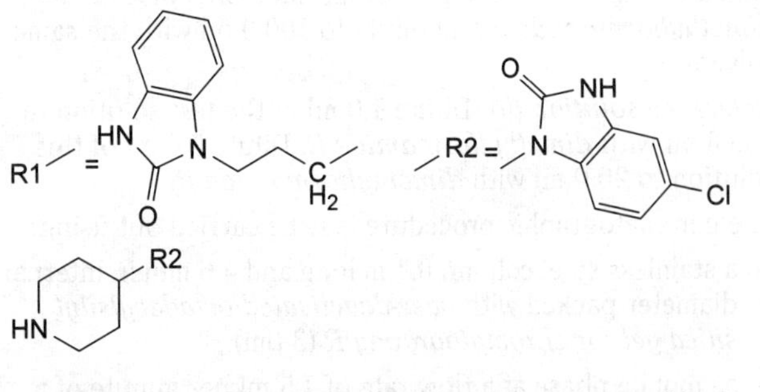

A. 5-chloro-1-(piperidin-4-yl)-1,3-dihydro-2*H*-benzimidazol-2-one,

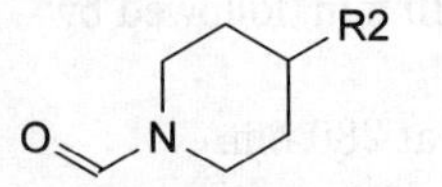

B. 4-(5-chloro-2-oxo-2,3-dihydro-1*H*-benzimidazol-1-yl)-1-formylpiperidine,

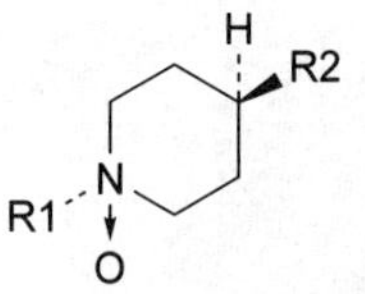

C. *cis*-4-(5-chloro-2-oxo-2,3-dihydro-1*H*-benzimidazol-1-yl)-1-[3-(2-oxo-2,3-dihydro-1*H*-benzimidazol-1-yl)propyl]piperidine 1-oxide,

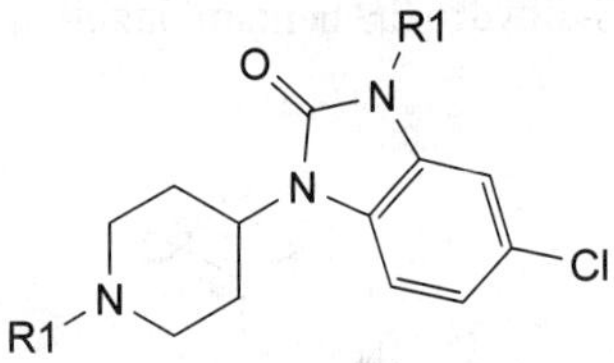

D. 5-chloro-3-[3-(2-oxo-2,3-dihydro-1*H*-benzimidazol-1-yl)propyl]-1-[1-[3-(2-oxo-2,3-dihydro-1*H*-benzimidazol-1-yl)propyl]piperidin-4-yl]-1,3-dihydro-2*H*-benzimidazol-2-one,

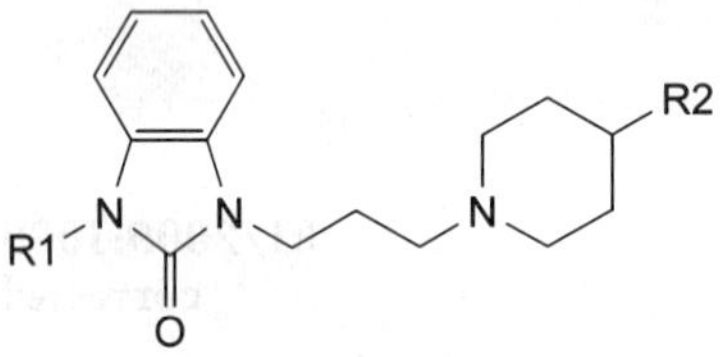

E. 1-[3-[4-(5-chloro-2-oxo-2,3-dihydro-1*H*-benzimidazol-1-yl)piperidin-1-yl]propyl]-3-[3-(2-oxo-2,3-dihydro-1*H*-benzimidazol-1-yl)propyl]-1,3-dihydro-2*H*-benzimidazol-2-one,

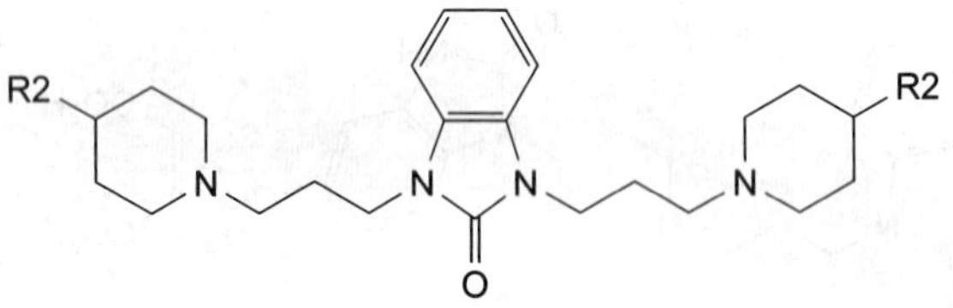

F. 1,3-bis[3-[4-(5-chloro-2-oxo-2,3-dihydro-1*H*-benzimidazol-1-yl)piperidin-1-yl]propyl]-1,3-dihydro-2*H*-benzimidazol-2-one.

01/2005:0664

DOPAMINE HYDROCHLORIDE

Dopamini hydrochloridum

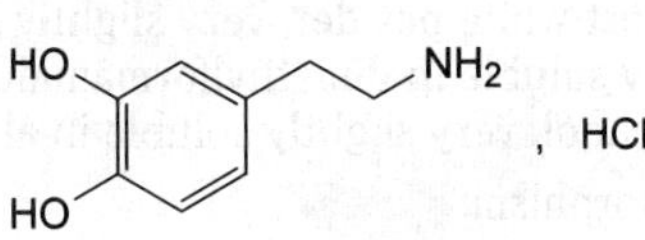

$C_8H_{12}ClNO_2$ M_r 189.6

DEFINITION

Dopamine hydrochloride contains not less than 98.0 per cent and not more than the equivalent of 102.0 per cent of 4-(2-aminoethyl)benzene-1,2-diol hydrochloride, calculated with reference to the dried substance.

CHARACTERS

A white or almost white, crystalline powder, freely soluble in water, soluble in alcohol, sparingly soluble in acetone and in methylene chloride.

IDENTIFICATION

First identification: B, E.

Second identification: A, C, D, E.

A. Dissolve 40.0 mg in *0.1 M hydrochloric acid* and dilute to 100.0 ml with the same acid. Dilute 10.0 ml of the solution to 100.0 ml with *0.1 M hydrochloric acid.* Examined between 230 nm and 350 nm (*2.2.25*), the solution shows an absorption maximum at 280 nm. The specific absorbance at the maximum is 136 to 150.

B. Examine by infrared absorption spectrophotometry (*2.2.24*), comparing with the spectrum obtained with *dopamine hydrochloride CRS*. Examine the substances as discs prepared using *potassium chloride R*.

C. Dissolve about 5 mg in a mixture of 5 ml of *1 M hydrochloric acid* and 5 ml of *water R*. Add 0.1 ml of *sodium nitrite solution R* containing 100 g/l of *ammonium molybdate R*. A yellow colour develops which becomes red on the addition of *strong sodium hydroxide solution R*.

D. Dissolve about 2 mg in 2 ml of *water R* and add 0.2 ml of *ferric chloride solution R2*. A green colour develops which changes to bluish-violet on the addition of 0.1 g of *hexamethylenetetramine R*.

E. It gives reaction (a) of chlorides (*2.3.1*).

TESTS

Appearance of solution. Dissolve 0.4 g in *water R* and dilute to 10 ml with the same solvent. The solution is clear (*2.2.1*) and not more intensely coloured than reference solution B_6 or Y_6 (*2.2.2, Method II*).

Acidity or alkalinity. Dissolve 0.5 g in *carbon dioxide-free water R* and dilute to 10 ml with the same solvent. Add 0.1 ml of *methyl red solution R* and 0.75 ml of *0.01 M sodium hydroxide*. The solution is yellow. Add 1.5 ml of *0.01 M hydrochloric acid*. The solution is red.

Related substances. Examine by thin-layer chromatography (*2.2.27*), using *silica gel G R* as the coating substance.

Test solution. Dissolve 0.15 g of the substance to be examined in *methanol R* and dilute to 5 ml with the same solvent.

Reference solution (a). Dissolve 7.5 mg of *4-O-methyldopamine hydrochloride R* in *methanol R* and dilute to 100 ml with the same solvent.

Reference solution (b). Dissolve 7.5 mg each of *3-O-methyldopamine hydrochloride R* and *4-O-methyldopamine hydrochloride R* in *methanol R* and dilute to 100 ml with the same solvent.

Apply to the plate 10 µl of each solution. Develop over a path of 15 cm using a mixture of 2 volumes of *anhydrous formic acid R*, 7 volumes of *water R*, 36 volumes of *methanol R* and 52 volumes of *chloroform R*. Allow the plate to dry in air for 15 min. Spray evenly and abundantly with a mixture of equal volumes of *potassium ferricyanide solution R* and *ferric chloride solution R1*, prepared immediately before use. Any spot in the chromatogram obtained with the test solution with an R_f value higher than that of the principal spot is not more intense than the spot in the chromatogram obtained with reference solution (a) (0.25 per cent). The test is not valid unless the chromatogram obtained with reference solution (b) shows two clearly separated spots.

Heavy metals (*2.4.8*). 1.0 g complies with limit test C for heavy metals (20 ppm). Prepare the standard using 2 ml of *lead standard solution (10 ppm Pb) R*.

Loss on drying (*2.2.32*). Not more than 0.5 per cent, determined on 1.000 g by drying in an oven at 100 °C to 105 °C for 2 h.

Sulphated ash (*2.4.14*). Not more than 0.1 per cent, determined on 1.0 g.

ASSAY

In order to avoid overheating in the reaction medium, mix thoroughly throughout and stop the titration immediately after the end-point has been reached.

Dissolve 0.1500 g in 10 ml of *anhydrous formic acid R*. Add 50 ml of *acetic anhydride R*. Titrate with *0.1 M perchloric acid*, determining the end-point potentiometrically (*2.2.20*).

1 ml of *0.1 M perchloric acid* is equivalent to 18.96 mg of $C_8H_{12}ClNO_2$.

STORAGE

Store in an airtight container, protected from light.

IMPURITIES

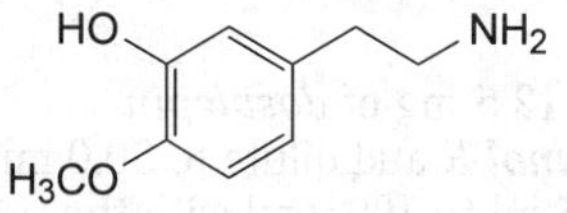

A. 5-(2-aminoethyl)-2-methoxyphenol (4-*O*-methyldopamine).

Monographs D-E

01/2005:1314

DOSULEPIN HYDROCHLORIDE

Dosulepini hydrochloridum

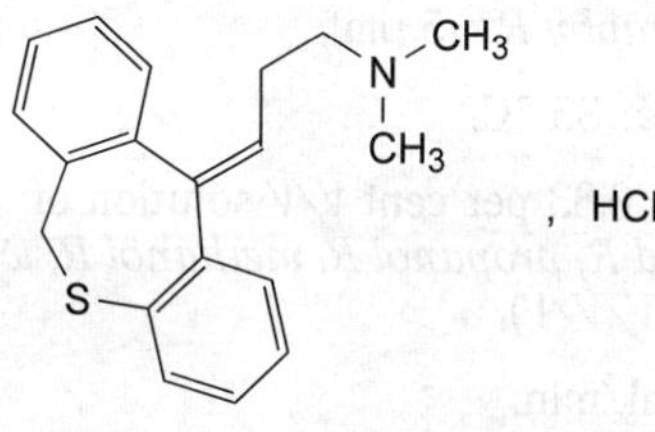

$C_{19}H_{22}ClNS$ M_r 331.9

DEFINITION

(*E*)-3-(Dibenzo[*b*,*e*]thiepin-11(6*H*)-ylidene)-*N*,*N*-dimethylpropan-1-amine hydrochloride.

Content: 98.0 per cent to 101.0 per cent (dried substance).

CHARACTERS

Appearance: white or faintly yellow, crystalline powder.

Solubility: freely soluble in water, in alcohol and in methylene chloride.

IDENTIFICATION

First identification: B, D.

Second identification: A, C, D.

A. Dissolve 25.0 mg in a 1 g/l solution of *hydrochloric acid R* in *methanol R* and dilute to 100.0 ml with the same solution. Dilute 2.0 ml to 50.0 ml with a 1 g/l solution of *hydrochloric acid R* in *methanol R*. Examined between 220 nm and 350 nm (*2.2.25*), the solution shows 2 absorption maxima at 231 nm and 306 nm and a shoulder at about 260 nm. The specific absorbance at the maximum at 231 nm is 660 to 730.

B. Infrared absorption spectrophotometry (*2.2.24*).

Preparation: discs.

Comparison: *dosulepin hydrochloride CRS*.

C. Dissolve about 1 mg in 5 ml of *sulphuric acid R*. A dark red colour is produced.

D. It gives reaction (b) of chlorides (*2.3.1*).

TESTS

Appearance of solution. The solution is clear (*2.2.1*) and not more intensely coloured than reference solution Y_5 (*2.2.2, Method II*).

Dissolve 1 g in *water R* and dilute to 20 ml with the same solvent.

pH (*2.2.3*): 4.2 to 5.2.

Dissolve 1 g in *carbon dioxide-free water R* and dilute to 10 ml with the same solvent.

Impurity E and related substances. Liquid chromatography (*2.2.29*). *Prepare the solutions immediately before use and protect from light.*

Test solution. Dissolve 50.0 mg of the substance to be examined in 5 ml of *methanol R* and dilute to 100.0 ml with the mobile phase.

Reference solution (a). Dissolve 12.5 mg of *dosulepin impurity A CRS* in 5 ml of *methanol R* and dilute to 50.0 ml with the mobile phase. Dilute 0.5 ml to 100.0 ml with the mobile phase.

Reference solution (b). Dissolve 10.0 mg of *dosulepin hydrochloride CRS* in 5 ml of *methanol R* and dilute to 20.0 ml with the mobile phase.

Column:

- *size*: *l* = 0.25 m, Ø = 4.6 mm,
- *stationary phase*: *nitrile silica gel for chromatography R1* (5 µm),
- *temperature*: 35 °C.

Mobile phase: 0.83 per cent *V/V* solution of *perchloric acid R, propanol R, methanol R, water R* (1:10:30:60 *V/V/V/V*).

Flow rate: 1 ml/min.

Detection: spectrophotometer at 229 nm.

Injection: 5 µl.

Run time: 2.5 times the retention time of dosulepin (*E*-isomer).

Relative retention with reference to dosulepin (*E*-isomer; retention time = about 25 min): impurity E = about 0.9.

System suitability: reference solution (b):

- *peak-to-valley ratio*: minimum 4, where H_p = height above the baseline of the peak due to impurity E and H_v = height above the baseline of the lowest point of the curve separating this peak from the peak due to dosulepin (*E*-isomer).

Limits:

- *impurity E*: not more than 5 per cent of the sum of the areas of the peak due to impurity E and the principal peak in the chromatogram obtained with the test solution,
- *impurity A*: not more than the area of the principal peak in the chromatogram obtained with reference solution (a) (0.25 per cent),
- *any other impurity*: not more than 0.4 times the area of the principal peak in the chromatogram obtained with reference solution (a) (0.1 per cent),
- *total of other impurities and impurity A*: not more than twice the area of the principal peak in the chromatogram obtained with reference solution (a) (0.5 per cent),
- *disregard limit*: 0.2 times the area of the principal peak in the chromatogram obtained with reference solution (a) (0.05 per cent).

Heavy metals (*2.4.8*): maximum 20 ppm.

1.0 g complies with limit test C. Prepare the standard using 2 ml of *lead standard solution (10 ppm Pb) R*.

Loss on drying (*2.2.32*): maximum 0.5 per cent, determined on 1.000 g by drying in an oven at 100-105 °C.

Sulphated ash (*2.4.14*): maximum 0.1 per cent, determined on 1.0 g.

ASSAY

Dissolve 0.250 g in a mixture of 5 ml of *anhydrous acetic acid R* and 35 ml of *acetic anhydride R*. Titrate with *0.1 M perchloric acid*, determining the end-point potentiometrically (*2.2.20*).

1 ml of *0.1 M perchloric acid* is equivalent to 33.19 mg of $C_{19}H_{22}ClNS$.

STORAGE

Protected from light.

IMPURITIES

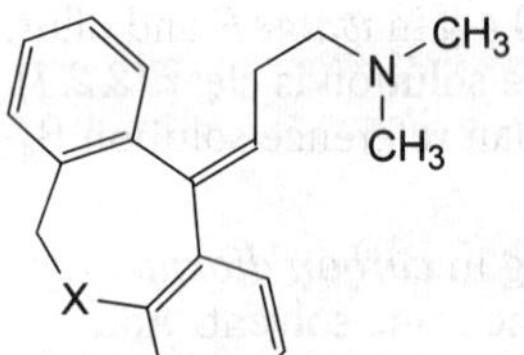

A. X = SO: (*E*)-3-(5-oxo-5λ⁴-dibenzo[*b,e*]thiepin-11(6*H*)-ylidene)-*N,N*-dimethylpropan-1-amine,

D. X = SO_2: (*E*)-3-(5,5-dioxo-5λ⁶-dibenzo[*b,e*]thiepin-11(6*H*)-ylidene)-*N,N*-dimethylpropan-1-amine,

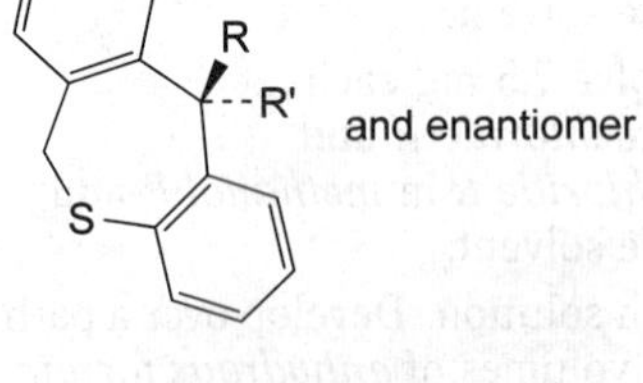

B. R + R′ = O: dibenzo[*b,e*]thiepin-11(6*H*)-one,

C. R = OH, R′ = $[CH_2]_3$-$N(CH_3)_2$: (11*RS*)-11-[3-(dimethylamino)propyl]-6,11-dihydrodibenzo[*b,e*]thiepin-11-ol,

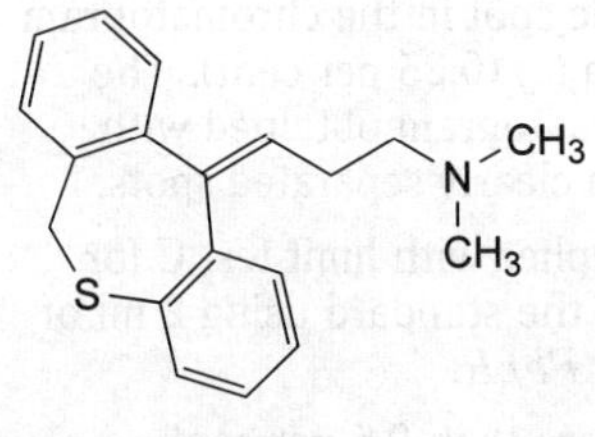

E. (*Z*)-3-(dibenzo[*b,e*]thiepin-11(6*H*)-ylidene)-*N,N*-dimethylpropan-1-amine.

01/2005:1201

DOXAPRAM HYDROCHLORIDE

Doxaprami hydrochloridum

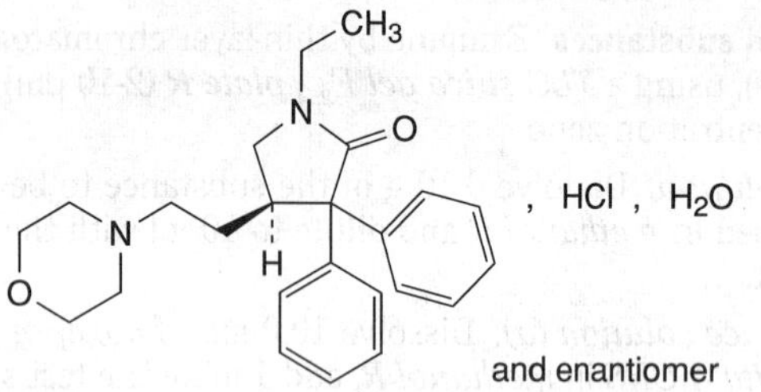

$C_{24}H_{31}ClN_2O_2,H_2O$ M_r 433.0

DEFINITION

(4*RS*)-1-Ethyl-4-[2-(morpholin-4-yl)ethyl]-3,3-diphenylpyrrolidin-2-one hydrochloride.

Content: 98.0 per cent to 100.5 per cent (dried substance).

CHARACTERS

Appearance: white or almost white, crystalline powder.

Solubility: soluble in water, in alcohol and in methylene chloride.

IDENTIFICATION

First identification: A, C.

Second identification: B, C.

A. Infrared absorption spectrophotometry (*2.2.24*).
Preparation: discs.
Comparison: *doxapram hydrochloride CRS.*

B. Thin-layer chromatography (*2.2.27*).
Test solution. Dissolve 10 mg of the substance to be examined in *methanol R* and dilute to 10 ml with the same solvent.
Reference solution. Dissolve 10 mg of *doxapram hydrochloride CRS* in *methanol R* and dilute to 10 ml with the same solvent.
Plate: *TLC silica gel plate R.*
Mobile phase: solution of *ammonia R* containing 17 g/l of NH_3, *2-propanol R, 2-methylpropanol R* (10:10:80 *V/V/V*).
Application: 10 µl.
Development: over a path of 15 cm.
Drying: in air.
Detection: spray with *dilute potassium iodobismuthate solution R* and examine immediately.
Results: the principal spot in the chromatogram obtained with the test solution is similar in position, colour and size to the principal spot in the chromatogram obtained with the reference solution.

C. It gives reaction (a) of chlorides (*2.3.1*).

TESTS

Solution S. Dissolve 2.500 g in *carbon dioxide-free water R* and dilute to 50.0 ml with the same solvent.

Appearance of solution. The solution is clear (*2.2.1*) and colourless (*2.2.2, Method II*).

Dilute 10 ml of solution S to 25 ml with *water R.*

pH (*2.2.3*): 3.5 to 5.0.

Dilute 5 ml of solution S to 25 ml with *carbon dioxide-free water R.*

Optical rotation (*2.2.7*): − 0.10° to + 0.10°, determined on solution S.

Related substances. Liquid chromatography (*2.2.29*). *Prepare the solutions immediately before use.*

Test solution. Dissolve 10.0 mg of the substance to be examined in the mobile phase and dilute to 10.0 ml with the mobile phase.

Reference solution (a). Dilute 1.0 ml of the test solution to 100.0 ml with the mobile phase.

Reference solution (b). Dilute 1.0 ml of reference solution (a) to 5.0 ml with the mobile phase.

Reference solution (c). Dissolve 5 mg of *doxapram impurity B CRS* in the mobile phase and dilute to 5.0 ml with the mobile phase. To 1.0 ml of the solution, add 1.0 ml of the test solution and dilute to 100.0 ml with the mobile phase.

Column:

- *size*: *l* = 0.25 m, Ø = 4.6 mm,
- *stationary phase*: spherical *end-capped octadecylsilyl silica gel for chromatography R* (5 µm) with a carbon loading of 14 per cent, a specific surface area of 350 m^2/g and a pore size of 10 nm.

Mobile phase: mix 50 volumes of *acetonitrile R* and 50 volumes of a 0.82 g/l solution of *sodium acetate R* adjusted to pH 4.5 with *glacial acetic acid R.*

Flow rate: 1.5 ml/min.

Detection: spectrophotometer at 214 nm.

Injection: 20 µl.

Run time: 4 times the retention time of doxapram.

Retention time: doxapram = about 6 min.

System suitability: reference solution (c):

- *resolution*: minimum of 3.0 between the peaks corresponding to doxapram and to impurity B.

Limits:

- *any impurity*: not more than the area of the principal peak in the chromatogram obtained with reference solution (b) (0.2 per cent),
- *total*: not more than the area of the principal peak in the chromatogram obtained with reference solution (a) (1.0 per cent),
- *disregard limit*: 0.05 times the area of the principal peak in the chromatogram obtained with reference solution (a) (0.05 per cent).

Heavy metals (*2.4.8*): maximum 20 ppm.

Dissolve 2.0 g in a mixture of 15 volumes of *water R* and 85 volumes of *methanol R* and dilute to 20 ml with the same mixture of solvents. 12 ml of the solution complies with limit test B. Prepare the standard using lead standard solution (2 ppm Pb) obtained by diluting *lead standard solution (100 ppm Pb) R* with a mixture of 15 volumes of *water R* and 85 volumes of *methanol R.*

Loss on drying (*2.2.32*): 3.0 per cent to 4.5 per cent, determined on 1.000 g by drying in an oven at 100-105 °C.

Sulphated ash (*2.4.14*): maximum 0.1 per cent, determined on 1.0 g.

ASSAY

Dissolve 0.300 g in a mixture of 10 ml of *0.01 M hydrochloric acid* and 50 ml of *alcohol R.* Carry out a potentiometric titration (*2.2.20*) using *0.1 M sodium hydroxide.* Read the volume added between the 2 points of inflexion.

1 ml of *0.1 M sodium hydroxide* is equivalent to 41.50 mg of $C_{24}H_{31}ClN_2O_2$.

IMPURITIES

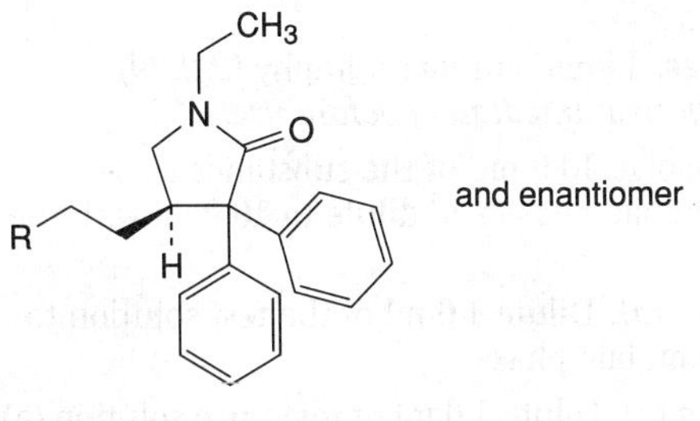

A. R = Cl: (4*RS*)-4-(2-chloroethyl)-1-ethyl-3,3-diphenylpyrrolidin-2-one,

B. R = NH-CH_2-CH_2-OH: (4*RS*)-1-ethyl-4-[2-[(2-hydroxyethyl)amino]ethyl]-3,3-diphenylpyrrolidin-2-one.

01/2005:1096
corrected

DOXEPIN HYDROCHLORIDE

Doxepini hydrochloridum

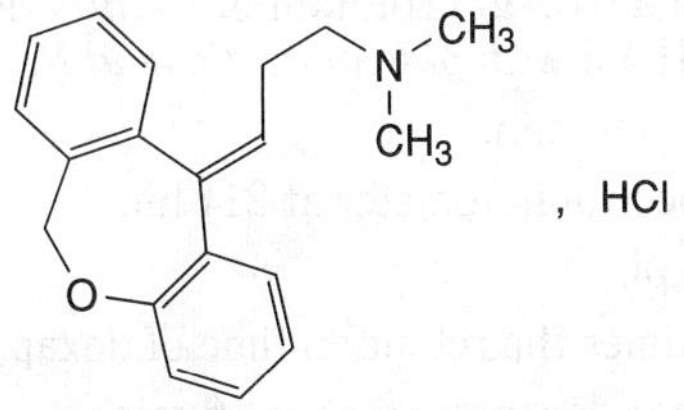

$C_{19}H_{22}ClNO$ M_r 315.8

DEFINITION

Doxepin hydrochloride is (*E*)-3-(dibenzo[*b,e*]oxepin-11(6*H*)-ylidene)-*N,N*-dimethylpropan-1-amine hydrochloride. It contains not less than 98.0 per cent and not more than the equivalent of 101.0 per cent of $C_{19}H_{22}ClNO$, calculated with reference to the dried substance.

CHARACTERS

A white or almost white, crystalline powder, freely soluble in water, in alcohol and in methylene chloride.

IDENTIFICATION

First identification: C, E.

Second identification: A, B, D, E.

A. Melting point (*2.2.14*): 185 °C to 191 °C.

B. Dissolve 50.0 mg in a 1 g/l solution of *hydrochloric acid R* in *methanol R* and dilute to 100.0 ml with the same acid solution. Dilute 5.0 ml to 50.0 ml with a 1 g/l solution of *hydrochloric acid R* in *methanol R*. Examined between 230 nm and 350 nm (*2.2.25*), the solution shows an absorption maximum at 297 nm. The specific absorbance at the maximum is 128 to 142.

C. Examine by infrared absorption spectrophotometry (*2.2.24*), comparing with the *Ph. Eur. reference spectrum of doxepin hydrochloride.*

D. Dissolve about 5 mg in 2 ml of *sulphuric acid R*. A dark red colour is produced.

E. Solution S (see Tests) gives reaction (a) of chlorides (*2.3.1*).

TESTS

Solution S. Dissolve 1.5 g in *carbon dioxide-free water R* and dilute to 30 ml with the same solvent.

Appearance of solution. Dilute 10 ml of solution S to 25 ml with *water R*. The solution is clear (*2.2.1*) and colourless (*2.2.2, Method II*).

Acidity. To 10 ml of solution S add 0.1 ml of *methyl red solution R*. Not more than 0.1 ml of *0.1 M sodium hydroxide* is required to change the colour of the indicator to yellow.

Related substances. Examine by thin-layer chromatography (*2.2.27*), using a *TLC silica gel F_{254} plate R* (2-10 μm) with a concentration zone.

Test solution. Dissolve 0.10 g of the substance to be examined in *methanol R* and dilute to 10 ml with the same solvent.

Reference solution (a). Dissolve 10.0 mg of *doxepin impurity A CRS* in *methanol R*, add 1 ml of the test solution and dilute to 10 ml with *methanol R*. Dilute 1.0 ml of this solution to 50 ml with *methanol R*.

Reference solution (b). Dissolve 10.0 mg of *doxepin impurity B CRS* in *methanol R*, add 1 ml of the test solution and dilute to 10 ml with *methanol R*. Dilute 1.0 ml of this solution to 50 ml with *methanol R*.

Reference solution (c). Dissolve 10.0 mg of *doxepin impurity B CRS* in *methanol R* and dilute to 200 ml with the same solvent.

Apply to one plate (plate A) 2 μl of the test solution and 2 μl of reference solution (a). Develop over a path of 5 cm using a mixture of 30 volumes of *methyl ethyl ketone R* and 60 volumes of *heptane R*. Doxepin remains on the starting line.

Apply to another plate (plate B) 2 μl of the test solution and 2 μl of reference solutions (b) and (c). Develop over a path of 5 cm using a mixture of 10 volumes of *methanol R* and 90 volumes of *methylene chloride R*.

Allow the plates to dry in a current of air. Spray with a solution prepared as follows: dissolve 20 g of *zinc chloride R* in 30 ml of *glacial acetic acid R*, add 3 ml of *phosphoric acid R* and 0.80 ml of *strong hydrogen peroxide solution R* and dilute to 60 ml with *water R*. Heat the plates at 120 °C for 15 min and examine immediately in ultraviolet light at 365 nm.

Plate A. In the chromatogram obtained with the test solution: any spot corresponding to impurity A is not more intense than the corresponding spot in the chromatogram obtained with reference solution (a) (0.2 per cent); any spot, apart from the principal spot and the spot corresponding to impurity A, is not more intense than the spots in the chromatogram obtained with reference solution (a) (0.2 per cent).

Plate B. In the chromatogram obtained with the test solution: any spot corresponding to impurity C (R_f about 0.12) is not more intense than the spot in the chromatogram obtained with reference solution (c) (0.5 per cent); any spot corresponding to impurity B is not more intense than the corresponding spot in the chromatogram obtained with reference solution (b) (0.2 per cent); any spot, apart from the principal spot, the spot corresponding to impurity B or the spot corresponding to impurity C, is not more intense than the spots in the chromatogram obtained with reference solution (b) (0.2 per cent).

The test is not valid unless the chromatograms obtained with reference solutions (a) and (b) show clearly visible and separated principal spots.

***Z*-Isomer.** 13.0 per cent to 18.5 per cent of the *Z*-isomer, determined by liquid chromatography (*2.2.29*).

Test solution. Dissolve 20.0 mg of the substance to be examined in the mobile phase and dilute to 20.0 ml with the

mobile phase. Dilute 1.0 ml of this solution to 10.0 ml with the mobile phase.

The chromatographic procedure may be carried out using:

- a stainless steel column 0.12 m long and 4 mm in internal diameter packed with spherical *octylsilyl silica gel for chromatography R* (5 µm) with a specific surface area of 220 m^2/g and a pore size of 80 nm,
- as mobile phase at a flow rate of 1 ml/min a mixture of 30 volumes of *methanol R* and 70 volumes of a 30 g/l solution of *sodium dihydrogen phosphate R*, previously adjusted to pH 2.5 with *phosphoric acid R*,
- as detector a spectrophotometer set at 254 nm,

maintaining the temperature of the column at 50 °C.

Inject 20 µl of the test solution. Adjust the sensitivity of the system so that the height of the principal peak is at least 50 per cent of the full scale of the recorder. The test is not valid unless the resolution between the first peak (*E*-isomer) and the second peak (*Z*-isomer) is at least 1.5.

The ratio of the area of the peak due to the *E*-isomer to the area of the peak due to the *Z*-isomer is 4.4 to 6.7.

Heavy metals (*2.4.8*). 1.0 g complies with limit test D (20 ppm). Prepare the standard using 2 ml of *lead standard solution (10 ppm Pb) R*.

Loss on drying (*2.2.32*). Not more than 0.5 per cent, determined on 1.000 g by drying in an oven at 100-105 °C.

Sulphated ash (*2.4.14*). Not more than 0.1 per cent, determined on 1.0 g.

ASSAY

Dissolve 0.250 g in a mixture of 5 ml of *anhydrous acetic acid R* and 35 ml of *acetic anhydride R*. Titrate with *0.1 M perchloric acid* until the colour changes from blue to green, using 0.2 ml of *crystal violet solution R* as indicator.

1 ml of *0.1 M perchloric acid* is equivalent to 31.58 mg of $C_{19}H_{22}ClNO$.

STORAGE

Protected from light.

IMPURITIES

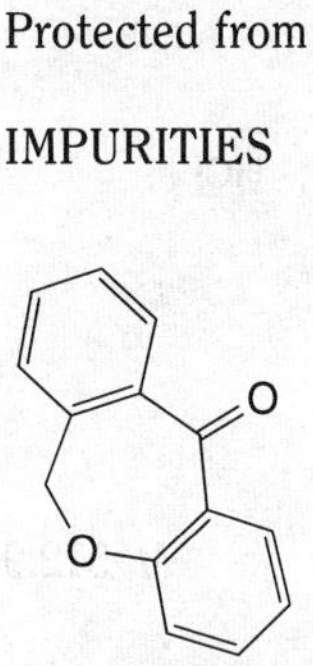

A. dibenzo[*b,e*]oxepin-11(6*H*)-one,

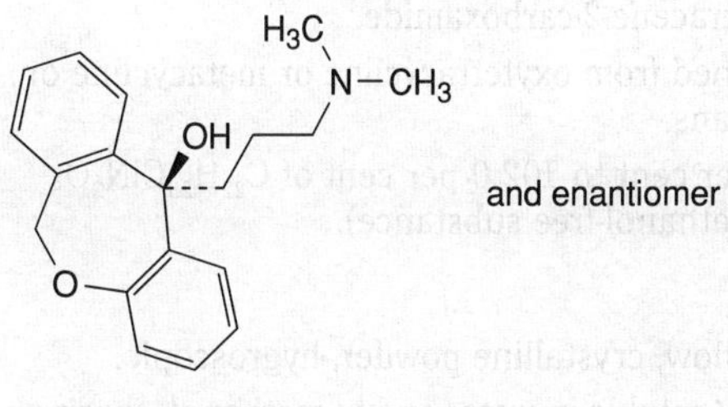

B. (11*RS*)-11-[3-(dimethylamino)propyl]-6,11-dihydrodibenzo[*b,e*]oxepin-11-ol,

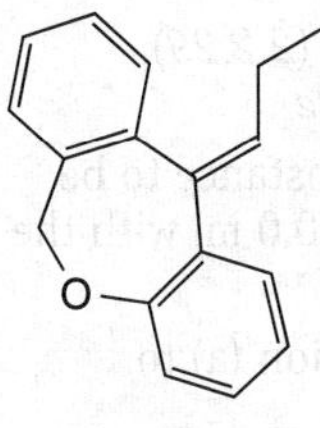

C. (*E*)-3-(dibenzo[*b,e*]oxepin-11(6*H*)-ylidene)-*N*-methylpropan-1-amine,

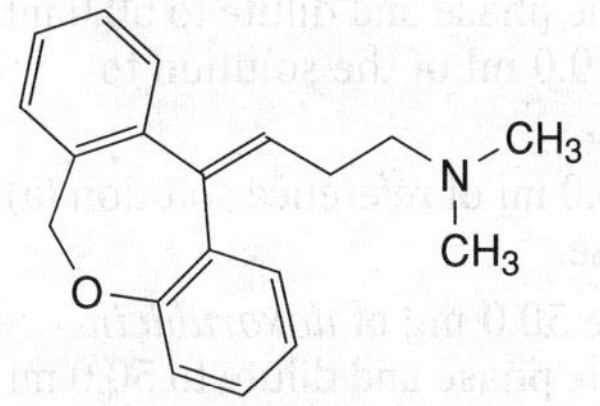

D. (*Z*)-3-(dibenzo[*b,e*]oxepin-11(6*H*)-ylidene)-*N,N*-dimethylpropan-1-amine.

01/2005:0714

DOXORUBICIN HYDROCHLORIDE

Doxorubicini hydrochloridum

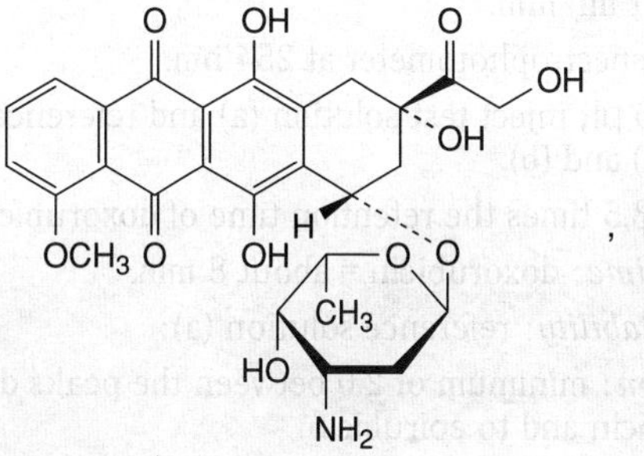

$C_{27}H_{30}ClNO_{11}$ M_r 580.0

DEFINITION

(8*S*,10*S*)-10-[(3-Amino-2,3,6-trideoxy-α-L-*lyxo*-hexopyranosyl)oxy]-6,8,11-trihydroxy-8-(hydroxyacetyl)-1-methoxy-7,8,9,10-tetrahydrotetracene-5,12-dione hydrochloride.

Substance produced by certain strains of *Streptomyces coeruleorubidus* or *Streptomyces peucetiusor* obtained by any other means.

Content: 98.0 per cent to 102.0 per cent (anhydrous, solvent-free substance).

CHARACTERS

Appearance: orange-red, crystalline powder, hygroscopic.

Solubility: soluble in water, slightly soluble in methanol.

IDENTIFICATION

A. Infrared absorption spectrophotometry (*2.2.24*).

Comparison: *doxorubicin hydrochloride CRS*.

B. Dissolve about 10 mg in 0.5 ml of *nitric acid R*, add 0.5 ml of *water R* and heat over a flame for 2 min. Allow to cool and add 0.5 ml of *silver nitrate solution R1*. A white precipitate is formed.

TESTS

pH (*2.2.3*): 4.0 to 5.5.

Dissolve 50 mg in *carbon dioxide-free water R* and dilute to 10 ml with the same solvent.

Related substances. Liquid chromatography (*2.2.29*). *Prepare the solutions immediately before use.*

Test solution (a). Dissolve 50.0 mg of the substance to be examined in the mobile phase and dilute to 50.0 ml with the mobile phase.

Test solution (b). Dilute 10.0 ml of test solution (a) to 100.0 ml with the mobile phase.

Reference solution (a). Dissolve 10.0 mg of *doxorubicin hydrochloride CRS* and 10 mg of *epirubicin hydrochloride CRS* in the mobile phase and dilute to 50.0 ml with the mobile phase. Dilute 10.0 ml of the solution to 100.0 ml with the mobile phase.

Reference solution (b). Dilute 5.0 ml of reference solution (a) to 20.0 ml with the mobile phase.

Reference solution (c). Dissolve 50.0 mg of *doxorubicin hydrochloride CRS* in the mobile phase and dilute to 50.0 ml with the mobile phase. Dilute 10.0 ml of the solution to 100.0 ml with the mobile phase.

Column:

- *size*: *l* = 0.25 m, Ø = 4.0 mm,
- *stationary phase*: *end-capped octadecylsilyl silica gel for chromatography R* (5 µm).

Mobile phase: mix equal volumes of *acetonitrile R* and a solution containing 2.88 g/l of *sodium laurilsulfate R* and 2.25 g/l of *phosphoric acid R.*

Flow rate: 1 ml/min.

Detection: spectrophotometer at 254 nm.

Injection: 5 µl; inject test solution (a) and reference solutions (a) and (b).

Run time: 3.5 times the retention time of doxorubicin.

Retention time: doxorubicin = about 8 min.

System suitability: reference solution (a):

- *resolution*: minimum of 2.0 between the peaks due to doxorubicin and to epirubicin.

Limits:

- *any impurity*: not more than the area of the peak corresponding to doxorubicin in the chromatogram obtained with reference solution (b) (0.5 per cent),
- *disregard limit*: 0.1 times the area of the peak corresponding to doxorubicin in the chromatogram obtained with reference solution (b) (0.05 per cent).

Ethanol (*2.4.24, System B*): maximum 1.0 per cent.

Water (*2.5.12*): maximum 4.0 per cent, determined on 0.100 g.

Bacterial endotoxins (*2.6.14*): less than 2.2 IU/mg, if intended for use in the manufacture of parenteral dosage forms without a further appropriate procedure for the removal of bacterial endotoxins.

ASSAY

Liquid chromatography (*2.2.29*) as described in the test for related substances.

Injection: test solution (b) and reference solution (c).

Calculate the percentage content of $C_{27}H_{30}ClNO_{11}$.

STORAGE

In an airtight container. If the substance is sterile, store in a sterile, airtight, tamper-proof container.

LABELLING

The label states, where applicable, that the substance is free from bacterial endotoxins.

IMPURITIES

A. daunorubicin,

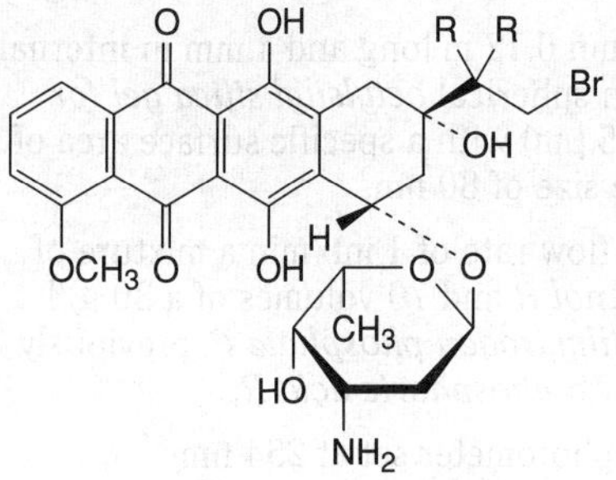

B. R = OCH_3: (8*S*,10*S*)-10[(3-amino-2,3,6-trideoxy-α-L-*lyxo*-hexopyranosyl)oxy]-8-(2-bromo-1,1-dimethoxyethyl)-6,8,11-trihydroxy-1-methoxy-7,8,9,10-tetrahydrotetracene-5,12-dione,

C. R + R = O: (8*S*,10*S*)-10[(3-amino-2,3,6-trideoxy-α-L-*lyxo*-hexopyranosyl)oxy]-8-(bromoacetyl)-6,8,11-trihydroxy-1-methoxy-7,8,9,10-tetrahydrotetracene-5,12-dione,

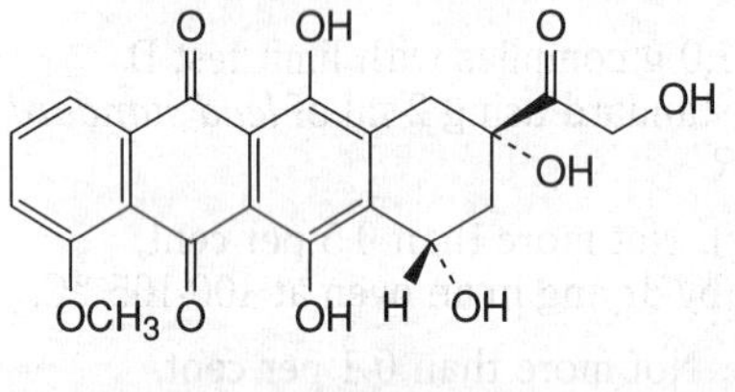

D. (8*S*,10*S*)-6,8,10,11-tetrahydroxy-8-(hydroxyacetyl)-1-methoxy-7,8,9,10-tetrahydrotetracene-5,12-dione (doxorubicin aglycone, doxorubicinone).

01/2005:0272

DOXYCYCLINE HYCLATE

Doxycyclini hyclas

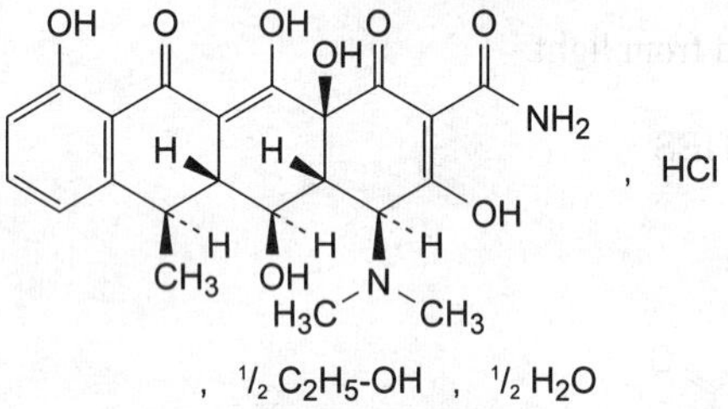

$(C_{22}H_{25}ClN_2O_8)_2,{}^1/_2C_2H_6O,{}^1/_2H_2O$ M_r 512.9

DEFINITION

Hydrochloride hemiethanol hemihydrate of (4*S*,4a*R*,5*S*,5a*R*,6*R*,12a*S*)-4-(dimethylamino)-3,5,10,12,12a-pentahydroxy-6-methyl-1,11-dioxo-1,4,4a,5,5a,6,11,12a-octahydrotetracene-2-carboxamide.

Substance obtained from oxytetracycline or metacycline or by any other means.

Content: 95.0 per cent to 102.0 per cent of $C_{22}H_{25}ClN_2O_8$ (anhydrous and ethanol-free substance).

CHARACTERS

Appearance: yellow, crystalline powder, hygroscopic.

Solubility: freely soluble in water and in methanol, sparingly soluble in ethanol (96 per cent). It dissolves in solutions of alkali hydroxides and carbonates.

IDENTIFICATION

A. Examine the chromatograms obtained in the assay.
Results: the principal peak in the chromatogram obtained with the test solution is similar in retention time and size to the principal peak in the chromatogram obtained with reference solution (a).

B. To about 2 mg add 5 ml of *sulphuric acid R*. A yellow colour develops.

C. It gives reaction (a) of chlorides (*2.3.1*).

TESTS

pH (*2.2.3*): 2.0 to 3.0.

Dissolve 0.1 g in *carbon dioxide-free water R* and dilute to 10 ml with the same solvent.

Specific optical rotation (*2.2.7*): − 105 to − 120 (anhydrous and ethanol-free substance).

Dissolve 0.250 g in a mixture of 1 volume of *1 M hydrochloric acid* and 99 volumes of *methanol R* and dilute to 25.0 ml with the same mixture of solvents. Carry out the measurement within 5 min of preparing the solution.

Specific absorbance (*2.2.25*): 300 to 335, determined at the absorption maximum at 349 nm (anhydrous and ethanol-free substance).

Dissolve 25.0 mg in a mixture of 1 volume of *1 M hydrochloric acid* and 99 volumes of *methanol R* and dilute to 25.0 ml with the same mixture of solvents. Dilute 1.0 ml of the solution to 100.0 ml with a mixture of 1 volume of *1 M hydrochloric acid* and 99 volumes of *methanol R*. Carry out the measurement within 1 h of preparing the solution.

Light-absorbing impurities. The absorbance (*2.2.25*), determined at 490 nm is maximum 0.07 (anhydrous and ethanol-free substance).

Dissolve 0.10 g in a mixture of 1 volume of *1 M hydrochloric acid* and 99 volumes of *methanol R* and dilute to 10.0 ml with the same mixture of solvents. Carry out the measurement within 1 h of preparing the solution.

Related substances. Liquid chromatography (*2.2.29*). *Prepare the solutions immediately before use.*

Test solution. Dissolve 20.0 mg of the substance to be examined in *0.01 M hydrochloric acid* and dilute to 25.0 ml with the same acid.

Reference solution (a). Dissolve 20.0 mg of *doxycycline hyclate CRS* in *0.01 M hydrochloric acid* and dilute to 25.0 ml with the same acid.

Reference solution (b). Dissolve 20.0 mg of *6-epidoxycycline hydrochloride CRS* in *0.01 M hydrochloric acid* and dilute to 25.0 ml with the same acid.

Reference solution (c). Dissolve 20.0 mg of *metacycline hydrochloride CRS* in *0.01 M hydrochloric acid* and dilute to 25.0 ml with the same acid.

Reference solution (d). Mix 4.0 ml of reference solution (a), 1.5 ml of reference solution (b) and 1.0 ml of reference solution (c) and dilute to 25.0 ml with *0.01 M hydrochloric acid.*

Reference solution (e). Mix 2.0 ml of reference solution (b) and 2.0 ml of reference solution (c) and dilute to 100.0 ml with *0.01 M hydrochloric acid.*

Column:

- *size*: *l* = 0.25 m, Ø = 4.6 mm,
- *stationary phase*: *styrene-divinylbenzene copolymer R* (8 μm),
- *temperature*: 60 °C.

Mobile phase: weigh 60.0 g of *2-methyl-2-propanol R* and transfer to a 1000 ml volumetric flask with the aid of 200 ml of *water R*; add 400 ml of *buffer solution pH 8.0 R*, 50 ml of a 10 g/l solution of *tetrabutylammonium hydrogen sulphate R* adjusted to pH 8.0 with *dilute sodium hydroxide solution R* and 10 ml of a 40 g/l solution of *sodium edetate R* adjusted to pH 8.0 with *dilute sodium hydroxide solution R*; dilute to 1000.0 ml with *water R*.

Flow rate: 1.0 ml/min.

Detection: spectrophotometer at 254 nm.

Injection: 20 μl of the test solution and reference solutions (d) and (e).

Relative retention with reference to doxycycline: impurity E = about 0.2; impurity D = about 0.3; impurity C = about 0.5; impurity F = about 1.2.

System suitability: reference solution (d):

- *resolution*: minimum 1.25 between the peaks due to impurity B (1st peak) and impurity A (2nd peak) and minimum 2.0 between the peaks due to impurity A and doxycycline (3rd peak); if necessary, adjust the 2-methyl-2-propanol content in the mobile phase;
- *symmetry factor*: maximum 1.25 for the peak due to doxycycline.

Limits:

- *impurity A*: not more than the area of the corresponding peak in the chromatogram obtained with reference solution (e) (2.0 per cent),
- *impurity B*: not more than the area of the corresponding peak in the chromatogram obtained with reference solution (e) (2.0 per cent),
- *impurities C, D, E, F*: for each impurity, not more than 0.25 times the area of the peak due to impurity A in the chromatogram obtained with reference solution (e) (0.5 per cent),
- *any other impurity*: for each impurity, not more than 0.25 times the area of the peak due to impurity A in the chromatogram obtained with reference solution (e) (0.5 per cent),
- *disregard limit*: 0.05 times the area of the peak due to impurity A in the chromatogram obtained with reference solution (e) (0.1 per cent).

Ethanol. Gas chromatography (*2.2.28*).

Internal standard solution. Dilute 0.50 ml of *propanol R* to 1000.0 ml with *water R.*

Test solution (a). Dissolve 0.10 g of the substance to be examined in *water R* and dilute to 10.0 ml with the same solvent.

Test solution (b). Dissolve 0.10 g of the substance to be examined in the internal standard solution and dilute to 10.0 ml with the same solution.

Reference solution. Dilute 0.50 ml of *ethanol R* to 100.0 ml with the internal standard solution. Dilute 1.0 ml of this solution to 10.0 ml with the internal standard solution.

Column:

- *size*: *l* = 1.5 m, Ø = 4.0 mm,
- *stationary phase*: *ethylvinylbenzene-divinylbenzene copolymer R* (150-180 μm).

Carrier gas: *nitrogen for chromatography R.*

Temperature:

- *column*: 135 °C,
- *injection port and detector*: 150 °C.

Detection: flame ionisation.

Calculate the content of ethanol taking the density (*2.2.5*) at 20 °C to be 0.790 g/ml.

Limit:

– *ethanol*: 4.3 per cent to 6.0 per cent.

Heavy metals (*2.4.8*): maximum 50 ppm.

0.5 g complies with limit test C. Prepare the reference solution using 2.5 ml of *lead standard solution (10 ppm Pb) R*.

Water (*2.5.12*): 1.4 per cent to 2.8 per cent, determined on 1.20 g.

Sulphated ash (*2.4.14*): maximum 0.4 per cent, determined on 1.0 g.

Bacterial endotoxins (*2.6.14*): less than 1.14 IU/mg, if intended for use in the manufacture of parenteral dosage forms without a further appropriate procedure for the removal of bacterial endotoxins.

ASSAY

Liquid chromatography (*2.2.29*) as described in the test for related substances with the following modification.

Injection: test solution and reference solution (a).

Calculate the percentage content of $C_{22}H_{25}ClN_2O_8$ (M_r = 480.9).

STORAGE

In an airtight container, protected from light. If the substance is sterile, store in a sterile, airtight, tamper-proof container.

LABELLING

The label states, where applicable, that the substance is free from bacterial endotoxins.

IMPURITIES

Specified impurities: A, B, C, D, E, F.

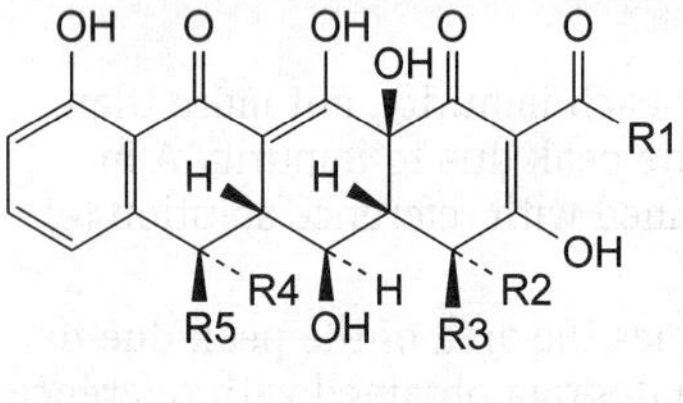

A. R1 = NH_2, R2 = R5 = H, R3 = $N(CH_3)_2$, R4 = CH_3: (4*S*,4a*R*,5*S*,5a*R*,6*S*,12a*S*)-4-(dimethylamino)-3,5,10,12,12a-pentahydroxy-6-methyl-1,11-dioxo-1,4,4a,5,5a,6,11,12a-octahydrotetracene-2-carboxamide (6-epidoxycycline),

B. R1 = NH_2, R2 = H, R3 = $N(CH_3)_2$, R4 + R5 = CH_2: (4*S*,4a*R*,5*S*,5a*R*,12a*S*)-4-(dimethylamino)-3,5,10,12,12a-pentahydroxy-6-methylene-1,11-dioxo-1,4,4a,5,5a,6,11,12a-octahydrotetracene-2-carboxamide (metacycline),

C. R1 = NH_2, R2 = $N(CH_3)_2$, R3 = R4 = H, R5 = CH_3: (4*R*,4a*R*,5*S*,5a*R*,6*R*,12a*S*)-4-(dimethylamino)-3,5,10,12,12a-pentahydroxy-6-methyl-1,11-dioxo-1,4,4a,5,5a,6,11,12a-octahydrotetracene-2-carboxamide (4-epidoxycycline),

D. R1 = NH_2, R2 = $N(CH_3)_2$, R3 = R5 = H, R4 = CH_3: (4*R*,4a*R*,5*S*,5a*R*,6*S*,12a*S*)-4-(dimethylamino)-3,5,10,12,12a-pentahydroxy-6-methyl-1,11-dioxo-1,4,4a,5,5a,6,11,12a-octahydrotetracene-2-carboxamide (4-epi-6-epidoxycycline),

E. R1 = NH_2, R2 = H, R3 = $N(CH_3)_2$, R4 = OH, R5 = CH_3: oxytetracycline,

F. R1 = CH_3, R2 = R4 = H, R3 = $N(CH_3)_2$, R5 = CH_3: (4*S*,4a*R*,5*S*,5a*R*,6*R*,12a*S*)-2-acetyl-4-(dimethylamino)-3,5,10,12,12a-pentahydroxy-6-methyl-4a,5a,6,12a-tetrahydrotetracene-1,11(4*H*,5*H*)-dione (2-acetyl-2-decarbamoyldoxycycline).

01/2005:0820

DOXYCYCLINE MONOHYDRATE

Doxycyclinum monohydricum

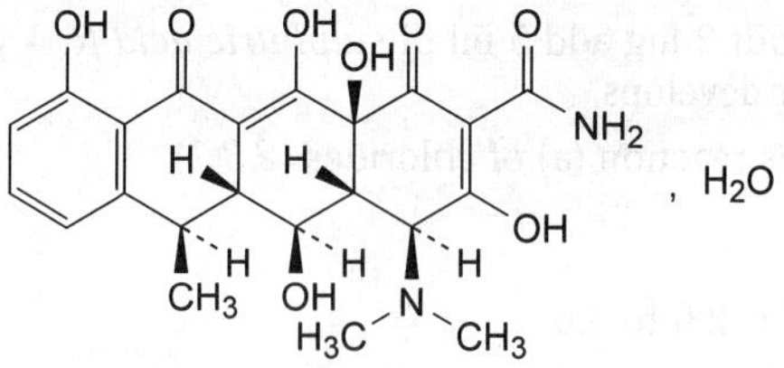

$C_{22}H_{24}N_2O_8,H_2O$ M_r 462.5

DEFINITION

(4*S*,4a*R*,5*S*,5a*R*,6*R*,12a*S*)-4-(Dimethylamino)-3,5,10,12,12a-pentahydroxy-6-methyl-1,11-dioxo-1,4,4a,5,5a,6,11,12a-octahydrotetracene-2-carboxamide monohydrate.

Substance obtained from oxytetracycline or metacycline or by any other means.

Content: 95.0 per cent to 102.0 per cent (anhydrous substance).

CHARACTERS

Appearance: yellow, crystalline powder.

Solubility: very slightly soluble in water and in alcohol. It dissolves in dilute solutions of mineral acids and in solutions of alkali hydroxides and carbonates.

IDENTIFICATION

A. Examine the chromatograms obtained in the assay.
Results: the principal peak in the chromatogram obtained with the test solution is similar in retention time and size to the principal peak in the chromatogram obtained with reference solution (a).

B. To about 2 mg add 5 ml of *sulphuric acid R*. A yellow colour develops.

C. Dissolve 25 mg in a mixture of 0.2 ml of *dilute nitric acid R* and 1.8 ml of *water R*. The solution does not give reaction (a) of chlorides (*2.3.1*).

TESTS

pH (*2.2.3*): 5.0 to 6.5.

Suspend 0.1 g in *carbon dioxide-free water R* and dilute to 10 ml with the same solvent.

Specific optical rotation (*2.2.7*): − 113 to − 130 (anhydrous substance).

Dissolve 0.250 g in a mixture of 0.5 volumes of *hydrochloric acid R* and 99.5 volumes of *methanol R* and dilute to 25.0 ml with the same mixture of solvents. Carry out the measurement within 5 min of preparing the solution.

Specific absorbance (*2.2.25*): 325 to 363 determined at the maximum at 349 nm (anhydrous substance).

Dissolve 25.0 mg in a mixture of 0.5 volumes of *hydrochloric acid R* and 99.5 volumes of *methanol R* and dilute to 50.0 ml with the same mixture of solvents. Dilute 2.0 ml of the solution to 100.0 ml with a mixture of 0.5 volumes of *1 M hydrochloric acid* and 99.5 volumes of *methanol R*. Carry out the measurement within 1 h of preparing the solution.

Light-absorbing impurities. The absorbance (*2.2.25*) determined at 490 nm has a maximum of 0.07 (anhydrous substance).

Dissolve 0.10 g in a mixture of 0.5 volumes of *hydrochloric acid R* and 99.5 volumes of *methanol R* and dilute to

10.0 ml with the same mixture of solvents. Carry out the measurement within 1 h of preparing the solution.

Related substances. Liquid chromatography (*2.2.29*). *Prepare the solutions immediately before use.*

Test solution. Dissolve 20.0 mg of the substance to be examined in *0.01 M hydrochloric acid* and dilute to 25.0 ml with the same acid.

Reference solution (a). Dissolve 20.0 mg of *doxycycline hyclate CRS* in *0.01 M hydrochloric acid* and dilute to 25.0 ml with the same acid.

Reference solution (b). Dissolve 20.0 mg of *6-epidoxycycline hydrochloride CRS* in *0.01 M hydrochloric acid* and dilute to 25.0 ml with the same acid.

Reference solution (c). Dissolve 20.0 mg of *metacycline hydrochloride CRS* in *0.01 M hydrochloric acid* and dilute to 25.0 ml with the same acid.

Reference solution (d). Mix 4.0 ml of reference solution (a), 1.5 ml of reference solution (b) and 1.0 ml of reference solution (c) and dilute to 25.0 ml with *0.01 M hydrochloric acid*.

Reference solution (e). Mix 2.0 ml of reference solution (b) and 2.0 ml of reference solution (c) and dilute to 100.0 ml with *0.01 M hydrochloric acid*.

Column:

- *size*: *l* = 0.25 m, Ø = 4.6 mm,
- *stationary phase*: *styrene-divinylbenzene copolymer R* (8 µm),
- *temperature*: 60 °C.

Mobile phase: weigh 60.0 g of *2-methyl-2-propanol R* and transfer into a 1000 ml volumetric flask with the aid of 200 ml of *water R*; add 400 ml of *buffer solution pH 8.0 R*, 50 ml of a 10 g/l solution of *tetrabutylammonium hydrogen sulphate R* adjusted to pH 8.0 with *dilute sodium hydroxide solution R* and 10 ml of a 40 g/l solution of *sodium edetate R* adjusted to pH 8.0 with *dilute sodium hydroxide solution R*; dilute to 1000.0 ml with *water R*.

Flow rate: 1.0 ml/min.

Detection: spectrophotometer at 254 nm.

Injection: 20 µl; inject the test solution and reference solutions (d) and (e).

Relative retention with reference to doxycycline: impurity E = about 0.2; impurity D = about 0.3; impurity C = about 0.5; impurity F = about 1.2.

System suitability: reference solution (d):

- *resolution*: minimum 1.25 between the peaks due to impurity B (1st peak) and impurity A (2nd peak) and minimum 2.0 between the peaks due to impurity A and doxycycline (3rd peak); if necessary, adjust the 2-methyl-2-propanol content in the mobile phase,
- *symmetry factor*: maximum 1.25 for the peak due to doxycycline.

Limits:

- *impurity A*: not more than the area of the corresponding peak in the chromatogram obtained with reference solution (e) (2.0 per cent),
- *impurity B*: not more than the area of the corresponding peak in the chromatogram obtained with reference solution (e) (2.0 per cent),
- *any other impurity*: not more than 0.25 times the area of the peak due to impurity A in the chromatogram obtained with reference solution (e) (0.5 per cent),
- *disregard limit*: 0.05 times the area of the peak due to impurity A in the chromatogram obtained with reference solution (e) (0.1 per cent).

Heavy metals (*2.4.8*): maximum 50 ppm.

0.5 g complies with limit test C. Prepare the standard using 2.5 ml of *lead standard solution (10 ppm Pb) R*.

Water (*2.5.12*): 3.6 per cent to 4.6 per cent, determined on 0.200 g.

Sulphated ash (*2.4.14*): maximum 0.4 per cent, determined on 1.0 g.

ASSAY

Liquid chromatography (*2.2.29*) as described in the test for related substances with the following modification.

Injection: test solution and reference solution (a).

Calculate the percentage content of $C_{22}H_{24}N_2O_8$.

STORAGE

Protected from light.

IMPURITIES

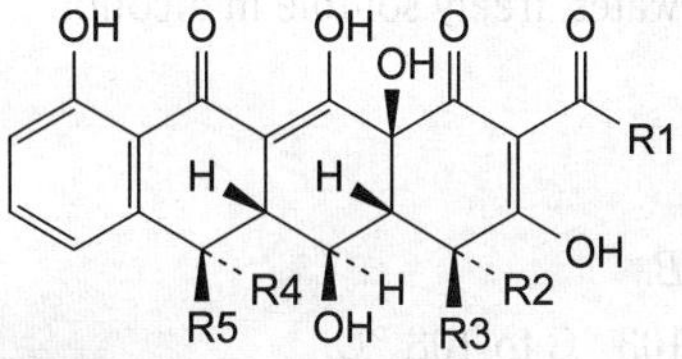

A. R1 = NH_2, R2 = R5 = H, R3 = $N(CH_3)_2$, R4 = CH_3: (4*S*,4a*R*,5*S*,5a*R*,6*S*,12a*S*)-4-(dimethylamino)-3,5,10,12,12a-pentahydroxy-6-methyl-1,11-dioxo-1,4,4a,5,5a,6,11,12a-octahydrotetracene-2-carboxamide (6-epidoxycycline),

B. R1 = NH_2, R2 = H, R3 = $N(CH_3)_2$, R4 + R5 = CH_2: (4*S*,4a*R*,5*S*,5a*R*,12a*S*)-4-(dimethylamino)-3,5,10,12,12a-pentahydroxy-6-methylene-1,11-dioxo-1,4,4a,5,5a,6,11,12a-octahydrotetracene-2-carboxamide (metacycline),

C. R1 = NH_2, R2 = $N(CH_3)_2$, R3 = R4 = H, R5 = CH_3: (4*R*,4a*R*,5*S*,5a*R*,6*R*,12a*S*)-4-(dimethylamino)-3,5,10,12,12a-pentahydroxy-6-methyl-1,11-dioxo-1,4,4a,5,5a,6,11,12a-octahydrotetracene-2-carboxamide (4-epidoxycycline),

D. R1 = NH_2, R2 = $N(CH_3)_2$, R3 = R5 = H, R4 = CH_3: (4*R*,4a*R*,5*S*,5a*R*,6*S*,12a*S*)-4-(dimethylamino)-3,5,10,12,12a-pentahydroxy-6-methyl-1,11-dioxo-1,4,4a,5,5a,6,11,12a-octahydrotetracene-2-carboxamide (4-epi-6-epidoxycycline),

E. R1 = NH_2, R2 = H, R3 = $N(CH_3)_2$, R4 = OH, R5 = CH_3: oxytetracycline,

F. R1 = CH_3, R2 = R4 = H, R3 = $N(CH_3)_2$, R5 = CH_3: (4*S*,4a*R*,5*S*,5a*R*,6*R*,12a*S*)-2-acetyl-4-(dimethylamino)-3,5,10,12,12a-pentahydroxy-6-methyl-4a,5a,6,12a-tetrahydrotetracene-1,11(4*H*,5*H*)-dione (2-acetyl-2-decarbamoyldoxycycline).

Monographs D-E

01/2005:1589

DOXYLAMINE HYDROGEN SUCCINATE

Doxylamini hydrogenosuccinas

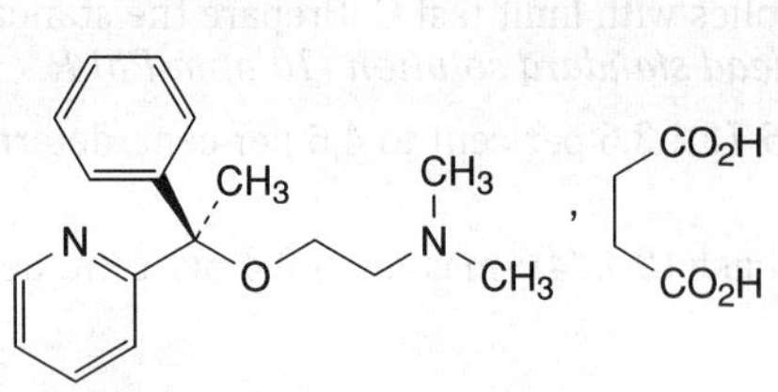

and enantiomer

$C_{21}H_{28}N_2O_5$ M_r 388.5

DEFINITION

N,N-dimethyl-2-[(1*RS*)-1-phenyl-1-(pyridin-2-yl)ethoxy(ethanamine hydrogen butanedioate.

Content: 99.0 per cent to 101.0 per cent (anhydrous substance).

CHARACTERS

Appearance: a white or almost white powder.

Solubility: very soluble in water, freely soluble in alcohol.

IDENTIFICATION

First identification: C.

Second identification: A, B.

A. Melting point (*2.2.14*): 103 °C to 108 °C.

B. Dissolve 0.200 g in *0.1 M hydrochloric acid* and dilute to 100.0 ml with the same solvent. Dilute 1.0 ml of the solution to 100.0 ml with *0.1 M hydrochloric acid*. Examined between 230 nm and 350 nm (*2.2.25*), the solution shows an absorption maximum at 262 nm. The specific absorbance at the maximum is 229 to 243 (anhydrous substance).

C. Infrared absorption spectrophotometry (*2.2.24*).
Comparison: *Ph. Eur. reference spectrum of doxylamine hydrogen succinate.*

TESTS

Appearance of solution. The solution is clear (*2.2.1*) and colourless (*2.2.2, Method II*).

Dissolve 0.4 g of the substance to be examined in *water R* and dilute to 20 ml with the same solvent.

Optical rotation (*2.2.7*): - 0.10° to + 0.10°.

Dissolve 2.50 g of the substance to be examined in *water R* and dilute to 25.0 ml with the same solvent.

Related substances. Gas chromatography (*2.2.28*).

Test solution. Dissolve 0.650 g of the substance to be examined in 20 ml of *0.1 M hydrochloric acid.* Add 3 ml of a 100 g/l solution of *sodium hydroxide R* and extract 3 times with 25 ml of *methylene chloride R*. Combine the methylene chloride extracts and filter using hydrophobic phase-separation filter paper. Rinse the filter with 10 ml of *methylene chloride R* and combine the rinsings with the methylene chloride extracts. Evaporate the solvent under reduced pressure at a temperature not exceeding 40 °C. Dissolve the residue in 20.0 ml of *ethanol R*.

Reference solution (a). Dilute 1.0 ml of the test solution to 200.0 ml with *ethanol R*.

Reference solution (b). Dissolve 40 mg of *doxylamine impurity A CRS* and 40 mg of *2-benzoylpyridine R* in *ethanol R* and dilute to 20 ml with the same solvent. Dilute 1 ml of this solution to 20 ml with *ethanol R*.

Column:

- *material*: fused silica,
- *size*: *l* = 30 m, Ø = 0.53 mm,
- *stationary phase*: *poly(dimethyl)(diphenyl)siloxane R* (film thickness 1.5 µm).

Carrier gas: *helium for chromatography R.*

Flow rate: 7 ml/min.

Temperature:

	Time (min)	Temperature (°C)
Column	0 - 12	160 → 220
	12 - 27	220
Injection port		250
Detector		250

Detection: flame ionisation.

Injection: 1 µl.

System suitability: reference solution (b):

- *resolution*: minimum 1.5 between the peaks due to impurity A and impurity D.

Limits:

- *any impurity*: not more than the area of the principal peak in the chromatogram obtained with reference solution (a) (0.5 per cent),
- *total*: not more than twice the area of the principal peak in the chromatogram obtained with reference solution (a) (1 per cent),
- *disregard limit*: 0.1 times the area of the principal peak in the chromatogram obtained with reference solution (a) (0.05 per cent).

Water (*2.5.12*): maximum 0.5 per cent, determined on 2.00 g.

Sulphated ash (*2.4.14*): maximum 0.1 per cent, determined on 1.0 g.

ASSAY

Dissolve 0.150 g in 50 ml of *anhydrous acetic acid R*. Titrate with *0.1 M perchloric acid*, determining the end-point potentiometrically (*2.2.20*).

1 ml of *0.1 M perchloric acid* is equivalent to 19.43 mg of $C_{21}H_{28}N_2O_5$.

IMPURITIES

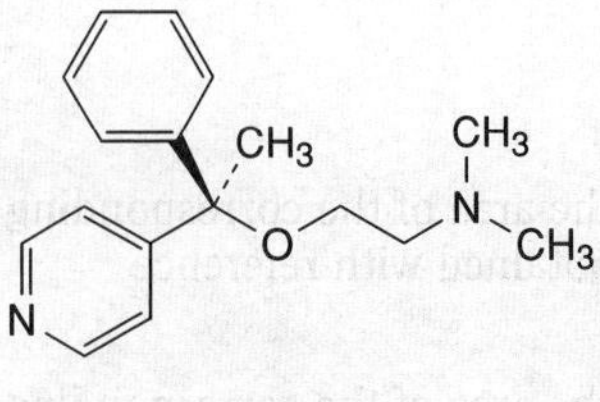

and enantiomer

A. *N,N*-dimethyl-2-[1(*RS*)-1-phenyl-1-(pyridin-4-yl)ethoxy]ethanamine,

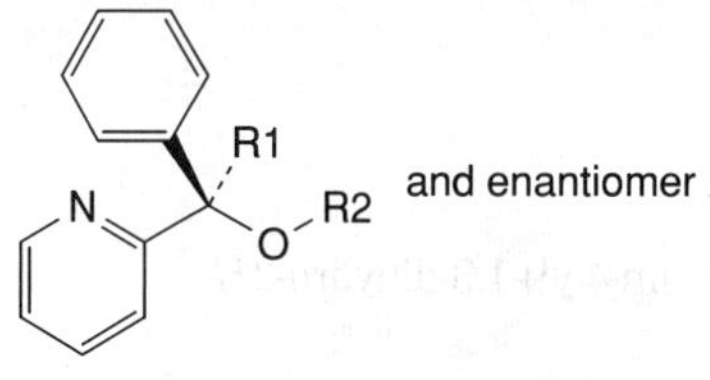

B. R1 = CH_3, R2 = H: (1*RS*)-1-phenyl-1-(pyridin-2-yl)ethanol,

C. R1 = H, R2 = CH_2-CH_2-N(CH_3)$_2$: *N,N*-dimethyl-2-[(*RS*)-1-phenyl(pyridin-2-yl)methoxy]ethanamine,

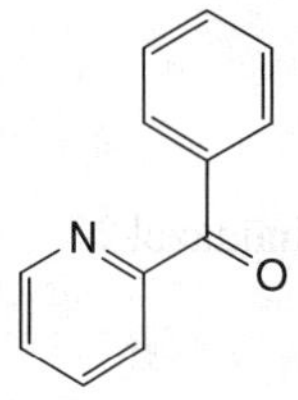

D. phenyl(pyridin-2-yl)methanone (2-benzoylpyridine).

01/2005:1010

DROPERIDOL

Droperidolum

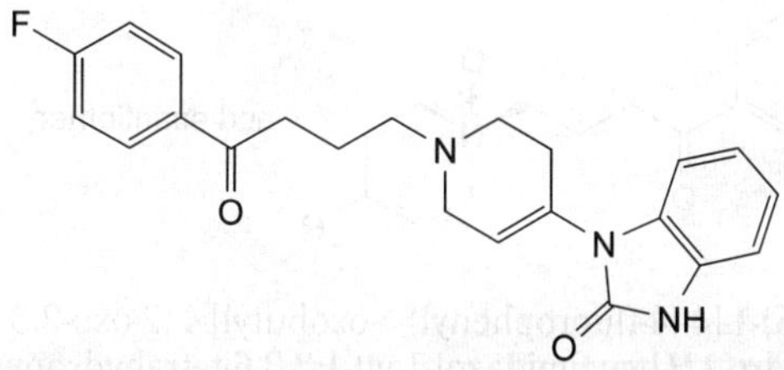

$C_{22}H_{22}FN_3O_2$ M_r 379.4

DEFINITION

Droperidol contains not less than 99.0 per cent and not more than the equivalent of 101.0 per cent of 1-[1-[4-(4-fluorophenyl)-4-oxobutyl]-1,2,3,6-tetrahydropyridin-4-yl]-1,3-dihydro-2*H*-benzimidazol-2-one, calculated with reference to the dried substance.

CHARACTERS

A white or almost white powder, practically insoluble in water, freely soluble in dimethylformamide and in methylene chloride, sparingly soluble in alcohol.

It shows polymorphism.

IDENTIFICATION

First identification: A.

Second identification: B, C, D.

A. Examine by infrared absorption spectrophotometry (*2.2.24*), comparing with the spectrum obtained with *droperidol CRS*. Examine the substances prepared as discs. If the spectra obtained show differences, dissolve the substance to be examined and the reference substance separately in the minimum volume of *acetone R*, evaporate to dryness on a water-bath and record new spectra using the residues.

B. Examine by thin-layer chromatography (*2.2.27*), using *silica gel GF_{254} R* as the coating substance.

Test solution. Dissolve 30 mg of the substance to be examined in a mixture of 1 volume of *acetone R* and 9 volumes of *methanol R* and dilute to 10 ml with the same mixture of solvents.

Reference solution (a). Dissolve 30 mg of *droperidol CRS* in a mixture of 1 volume of *acetone R* and 9 volumes of *methanol R* and dilute to 10 ml with the same mixture of solvents.

Reference solution (b). Dissolve 30 mg of *droperidol CRS* and 30 mg of *benperidol CRS* in a mixture of 1 volume of *acetone R* and 9 volumes of *methanol R* and dilute to 10 ml with the same mixture of solvents.

Apply to the plate 10 µl of each solution. Develop over a path of 15 cm using a mixture of 1 volume of *acetone R* and 9 volumes of *methanol R*. Allow the plate to dry in air and examine in ultraviolet light at 254 nm. The principal spot in the chromatogram obtained with the test solution is similar in position and size to the principal spot in the chromatogram obtained with reference solution (a). The test is not valid unless the chromatogram obtained with reference solution (b) shows 2 clearly separated spots.

C. Dissolve about 10 mg in 5 ml of *ethanol R*. Add 0.5 ml of *dinitrobenzene solution R* and 0.5 ml of *2 M alcoholic potassium hydroxide R*. A violet colour is produced and becomes brownish-red after 20 min.

D. Mix about 5 mg with 45 mg of *heavy magnesium oxide R* and ignite in a crucible until an almost white residue is obtained (usually less than 5 min). Allow to cool, add 1 ml of *water R*, 0.05 ml of *phenolphthalein solution R1* and about 1 ml of *dilute hydrochloric acid R* to render the solution colourless. Filter. To a freshly prepared mixture of 0.1 ml of *alizarin S solution R* and 0.1 ml of *zirconyl nitrate solution R*, add 1.0 ml of the filtrate. Mix, allow to stand for 5 min and compare the colour of the solution with that of a blank prepared in the same manner. The test solution is yellow and the blank is red.

TESTS

Appearance of solution. Dissolve 0.20 g in *methylene chloride R* and dilute to 20.0 ml with the same solvent. The solution is clear (*2.2.1*) and not more intensely coloured than reference solution BY_5 (*2.2.2, Method II*).

Related substances. Examine by liquid chromatography (*2.2.29*). *Prepare the solutions immediately before use.*

Test solution. Dissolve 0.10 g of the substance to be examined in *dimethylformamide R* and dilute to 10.0 ml with the same solvent.

Reference solution (a). Dissolve 2.5 mg of *droperidol CRS* and 2.5 mg of *benperidol CRS* in *dimethylformamide R* and dilute to 100.0 ml with the same solvent.

Reference solution (b). Dilute 1.0 ml of the test solution to 100.0 ml with *dimethylformamide R*. Dilute 5.0 ml of this solution to 20.0 ml with *dimethylformamide R*.

The chromatographic procedure may be carried out using:

- a stainless steel column 0.10 m long and 4.6 mm in internal diameter packed with *base-deactivated octadecylsilyl silica gel for chromatography R* (3 µm),
- as mobile phase at a flow rate of 1.5 ml/min:

  mobile phase A: *acetonitrile R*,

  mobile phase B: 10 g/l solution of *tetrabutylammonium hydrogen sulphate R1*,

Time (min)	Mobile phase A (per cent *V/V*)	Mobile phase B (per cent *V/V*)
0 - 15	0 → 40	100 → 60
15 - 20	40	60
20 - 25	40 → 0	60 → 100

- as detector a spectrophotometer set at 275 nm.

Adjust the sensitivity of the system so that the height of the principal peak in the chromatogram obtained with 10 µl of reference solution (b) is at least 50 per cent of the full scale of the recorder.

Inject 10 µl of reference solution (a). When the chromatogram is recorded in the prescribed conditions, the retention times are: benperidol about 6.5 min and droperidol about 7 min. The test is not valid unless the resolution between the peaks due to droperidol and benperidol is at least 2.0. If necessary, adjust the final concentration of acetonitrile in the mobile phase or adjust the time programme for the linear gradient.

Inject 10 µl of *dimethylformamide R* as a blank, 10 µl of the test solution and 10 µl of reference solution (b). In the chromatogram obtained with the test solution: the area of any peak, apart from the principal peak, is not greater than the area of the principal peak in the chromatogram obtained with reference solution (b) (0.25 per cent); the sum of the areas of all the peaks, apart from the principal peak, is not greater than twice the area of the principal peak in the chromatogram obtained with reference solution (b) (0.5 per cent). Disregard any peak obtained with the blank and any peak with an area less than 0.2 times the area of the principal peak in the chromatogram obtained with reference solution (b).

Heavy metals (*2.4.8*). 1.0 g complies with limit test D for heavy metals (20 ppm). Prepare the standard using 2 ml of *lead standard solution (10 ppm Pb) R*.

Loss on drying (*2.2.32*). Not more than 0.5 per cent, determined on 1.000 g by drying in an oven at 100-105 °C.

Sulphated ash (*2.4.14*). Not more than 0.1 per cent, determined on 1.0 g.

ASSAY

Dissolve 0.300 g in 50 ml of a mixture of 1 volume of *anhydrous acetic acid R* and 7 volumes of *methyl ethyl ketone R*. Using 0.2 ml of *naphtholbenzein solution R*, titrate with *0.1 M perchloric acid* until the colour changes from orange-yellow to green.

1 ml of *0.1 M perchloric acid* is equivalent to 37.94 mg of $C_{22}H_{22}FN_3O_2$.

STORAGE

Store protected from light.

IMPURITIES

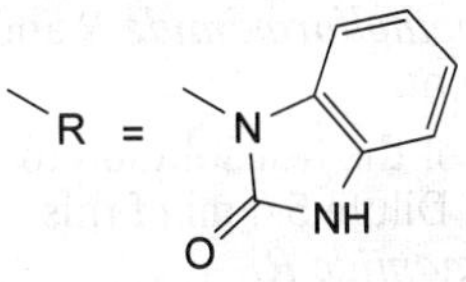

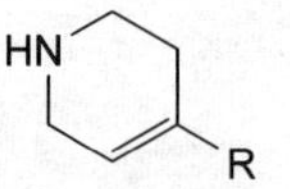

A. 1-(1,2,3,6-tetrahydropyridin-4-yl)-1,3-dihydro-2*H*-benzimidazol-2-one,

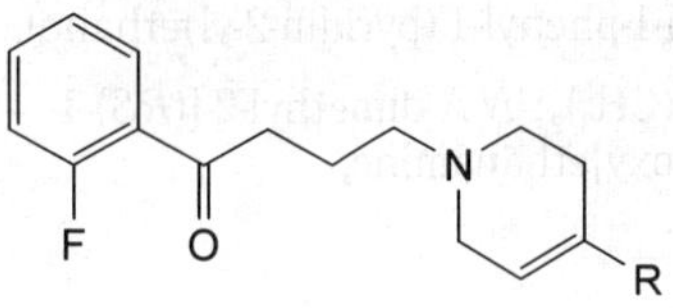

B. 1-[1-[4-(2-fluorophenyl)-4-oxobutyl]-1,2,3,6-tetrahydropyridin-4-yl]-1,3-dihydro-2*H*-benzimidazol-2-one,

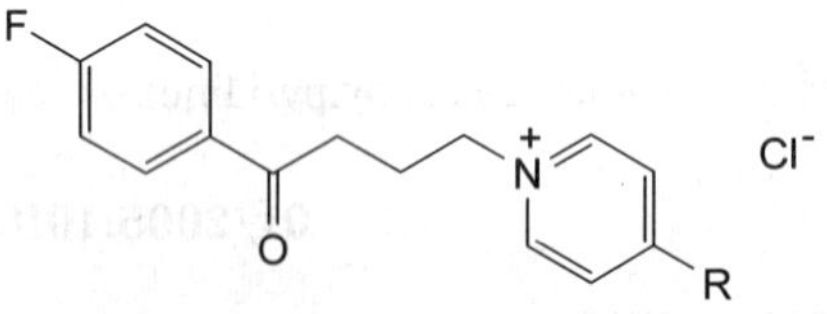

C. 1-[4-(4-fluorophenyl)-4-oxobutyl]-4-(2-oxo-2,3-dihydro-1*H*-benzimidazol-1-yl)pyridinium chloride,

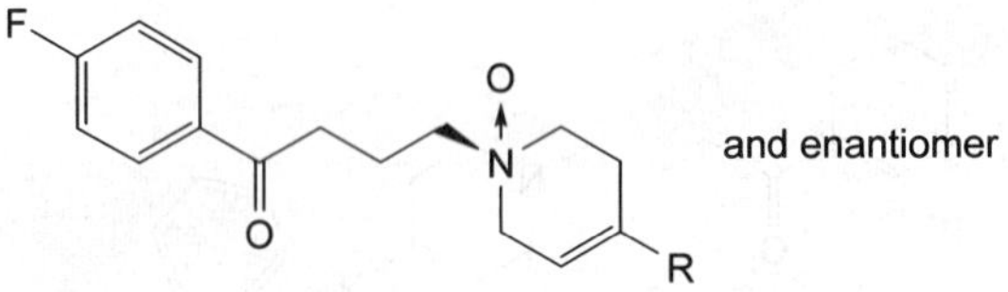

D. (1*RS*)-1-[4-(4-fluorophenyl)-4-oxobutyl]-4-(2-oxo-2,3-dihydro-1*H*-benzimidazol-1-yl)-1,2,3,6-tetrahydropyridine 1-oxide,

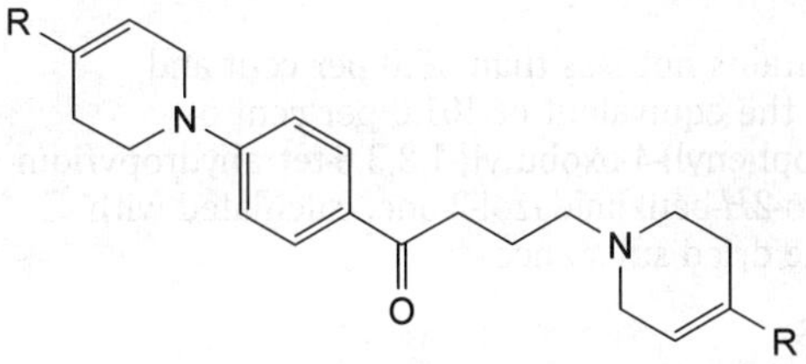

E. 1-[1-[4-[4-[4-(2-oxo-2,3-dihydro-1*H*-benzimidazol-1-yl)-3,6-dihydropyridin-1(2*H*)-yl]-1-oxobutyl]phenyl]-1,2,3,6-tetrahydropyridin-4-yl]-1,3-dihydro-2*H*-benzimidazol-2-one.

E

01/2005:2015
corrected

EBASTINE

Ebastinum

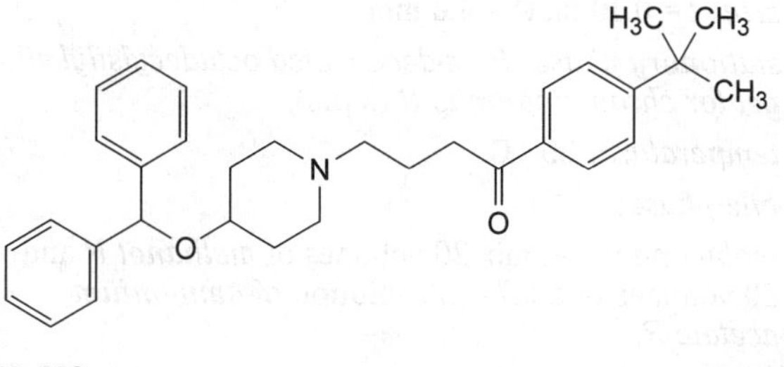

$C_{32}H_{39}NO_2$ M_r 469.7

DEFINITION

1-[4-(1,1-Dimethylethyl)phenyl]-4-[4-(diphenylmethoxy)piperidin-1-yl]butan-1-one.

Content: 99.0 per cent to 101.0 per cent (anhydrous substance).

CHARACTERS

Appearance: white or almost white, crystalline powder.

Solubility: practically insoluble in water, very soluble in methylene chloride, sparingly soluble in methanol.

mp: about 86 °C.

IDENTIFICATION

Infrared absorption spectrophotometry (*2.2.24*).

Comparison: *Ph. Eur. reference spectrum of ebastine.*

TESTS

Related substances. Liquid chromatography (*2.2.29*). *Keep the solutions protected from light.*

Solution A. Mix 65 volumes of *acetonitrile R* and 35 volumes of a 1.1 g/l solution of *phosphoric acid R* adjusted to pH 5.0 with a 40 g/l solution of *sodium hydroxide R.*

Test solution. Dissolve 0.125 g of the substance to be examined in solution A and dilute to 50.0 ml with the same solution.

Reference solution (a). Dissolve 5.0 mg of *ebastine impurity C CRS* and 5.0 mg of *ebastine impurity D CRS* in solution A and dilute to 20.0 ml with the same solution. Dilute 1.0 ml of the solution to 100.0 ml with solution A.

Reference solution (b). Dilute 1.0 ml of the test solution to 100.0 ml with solution A. Dilute 1.0 ml of this solution to 10.0 ml with solution A.

Column:

- *size*: l = 0.25 m, Ø = 4.6 mm,
- *stationary phase*: *nitrile silica gel for chromatography R* (5 µm).

Mobile phase: mix 35 volumes of *acetonitrile R* and 65 volumes of a 1.1 g/l solution of *phosphoric acid R* adjusted to pH 5.0 with a 40 g/l solution of *sodium hydroxide R.* Adjust the percentage of acetonitrile to between 30 per cent *V/V* and 40 per cent *V/V* so that the retention time of ebastine is about 110 min.

Flow rate: 1 ml/min.

Detection: spectrophotometer at 210 nm.

Injection: 10 µl.

Run time: 1.4 times the retention time of ebastine.

Relative retention with reference to ebastine: impurity A = about 0.04; impurity B = about 0.05; impurity D = about 0.20; impurity C = about 0.22; impurity F = about 0.42; impurity G = about 0.57; impurity E = about 1.14.

System suitability: reference solution (a):

- *resolution*: minimum 2.0 between the peaks due to impurity D and impurity C.

Limits:

- *impurities A, B, C, D, E, F, G*: for each impurity, not more than the area of the principal peak in the chromatogram obtained with reference solution (b) (0.1 per cent),
- *any other impurity*: for each impurity, not more than the area of the principal peak in the chromatogram obtained with reference solution (b) (0.1 per cent),
- *total*: not more than 4 times the area of the principal peak in the chromatogram obtained with reference solution (b) (0.4 per cent),
- *disregard limit*: 0.5 times the area of the principal peak in the chromatogram obtained with reference solution (b) (0.05 per cent).

Sulphates (*2.4.13*): maximum 100 ppm.

Suspend 2.5 g in 25 ml of *dilute nitric acid R.* Boil under a reflux condenser for 10 min. Cool and filter. 15 ml of the filtrate complies with the limit test for sulphates.

Water (*2.5.12*): maximum 0.5 per cent, determined on 0.500 g.

Sulphated ash (*2.4.14*): maximum 0.1 per cent, determined on 1.0 g.

ASSAY

Dissolve 0.350 g in 50 ml of *anhydrous acetic acid R.* Titrate with *0.1 M perchloric acid,* determining the end-point potentiometrically (*2.2.20*).

1 ml of *0.1 M perchloric acid* is equivalent to 46.97 mg of $C_{32}H_{39}NO_2$.

STORAGE

Protected from light.

IMPURITIES

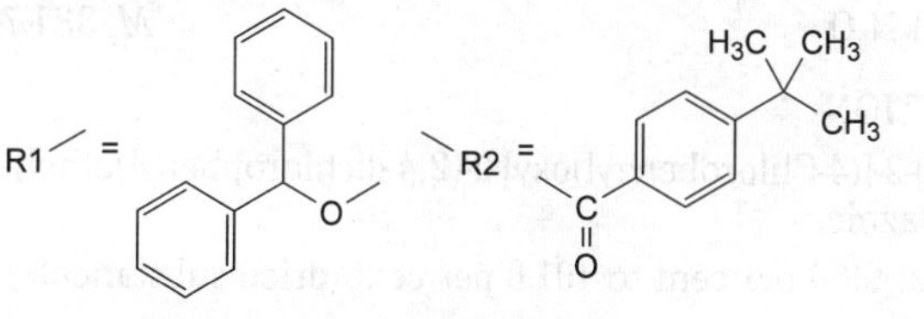

A. R1–H: diphenylmethanol (benzhydrol),

B. R2–CH_3: 1-[4-(1,1-dimethylethyl)phenyl]ethanone,

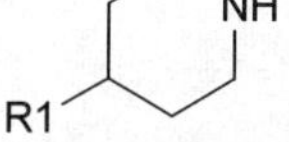

C. 4-(diphenylmethoxy)piperidine,

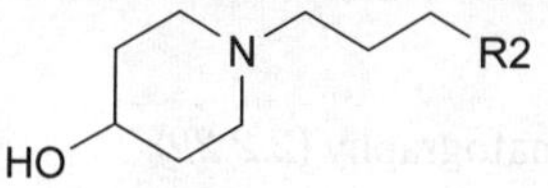

D. 1-[4-(1,1-dimethylethyl)phenyl]-4-(4-hydroxypiperidin-1-yl)butan-1-one,

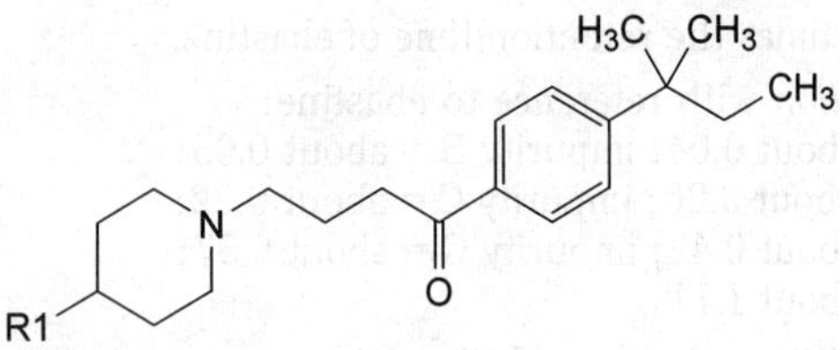

E. 1-[4-(1,1-dimethylpropyl)phenyl]-4-[4-(diphenylmethoxy)piperidin-1-yl]butan-1-one,

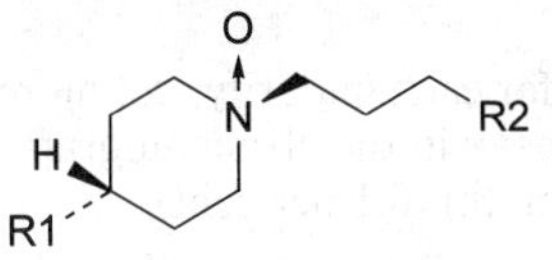

F. 1-[4-(1,1-dimethylethyl)phenyl]-4-[*cis*-4-(diphenylmethoxy)-1-oxidopiperidin-1-yl]butan-1-one,

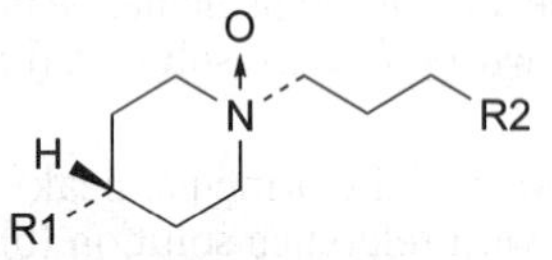

G. 1-[4-(1,1-dimethylethyl)phenyl]-4-[*trans*-4-(diphenylmethoxy)-1-oxidopiperidin-1-yl]butan-1-one.

01/2005:2049 corrected

ECONAZOLE

Econazolum

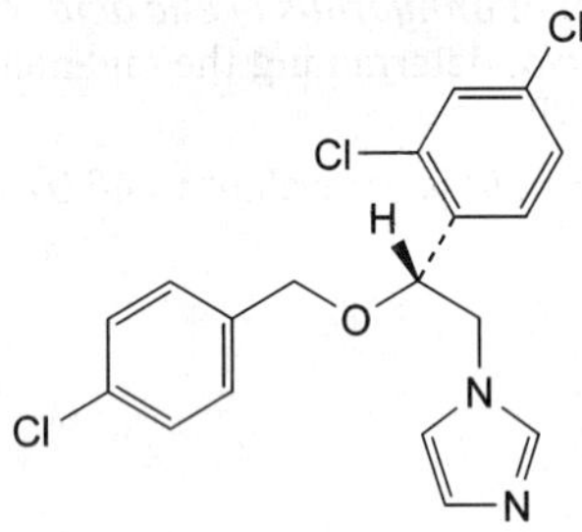

and enantiomer

$C_{18}H_{15}Cl_3N_2O$ M_r 381.7

DEFINITION

1-[(2*RS*)-2-[(4-Chlorobenzyl)oxy]-2-(2,4-dichlorophenyl)ethyl]-1*H*-imidazole.

Content: 99.0 per cent to 101.0 per cent (dried substance).

CHARACTERS

Appearance: white or almost white powder.

Solubility: practically insoluble in water, very soluble in alcohol and in methylene chloride.

IDENTIFICATION

A. Melting point (*2.2.14*): 88 °C to 92 °C.

B. Infrared absorption spectrophotometry (*2.2.24*).

Comparison: *Ph. Eur. reference spectrum of econazole.*

TESTS

Related substances. Liquid chromatography (*2.2.29*).

Test solution. Dissolve 0.100 g of the substance to be examined in *methanol R* and dilute to 10.0 ml with the same solvent.

Reference solution (a). Dissolve 10 mg of *econazole for system suitability CRS* in *methanol R* and dilute to 1.0 ml with the same solvent.

Reference solution (b). Dilute 1.0 ml of the test solution to 20.0 ml with *methanol R*. Dilute 1.0 ml of this solution to 25.0 ml with *methanol R*.

Column:

- *size*: l = 0.10 m, Ø = 4.6 mm,
- *stationary phase*: *base-deactivated octadecylsilyl silica gel for chromatography R* (3 µm),
- *temperature*: 35 °C.

Mobile phase:

- *mobile phase A*: mix 20 volumes of *methanol R* and 80 volumes of a 0.77 g/l solution of *ammonium acetate R*,
- *mobile phase B*: *methanol R*, *acetonitrile R* (40:60 *V/V*),

Time (min)	Mobile phase A (per cent *V/V*)	Mobile phase B (per cent *V/V*)
0 - 25	60 → 10	40 → 90
25 - 27	10	90
27 - 28	10 → 60	90 → 40
28 - 33	60	40

Flow rate: 1.5 ml/min.

Detection: spectrophotometer at 225 nm.

Injection: 10 µl.

Relative retention with reference to econazole (retention time = about 15 min): impurity A = about 0.2; impurity B = about 0.6; impurity C = about 1.1.

System suitability: reference solution (a):

- *peak-to-valley ratio*: minimum 1.5, where H_p = height above the baseline of the peak due to impurity C and H_v = height above the baseline of the lowest point of the curve separating this peak from the peak due to econazole.

Limits:

- *correction factor*: for the calculation of content, multiply the peak area of impurity A by 1.4,
- *impurities A, B, C*: for each impurity, not more than the area of the principal peak in the chromatogram obtained with reference solution (b) (0.2 per cent),
- *total*: not more than 1.5 times the area of the principal peak in the chromatogram obtained with reference solution (b) (0.3 per cent),
- *disregard limit*: 0.25 times the area of the principal peak in the chromatogram obtained with reference solution (b) (0.05 per cent).

Loss on drying (*2.2.32*): maximum 0.5 per cent, determined on 1.000 g by drying *in vacuo* at 60 °C for 4 h.

Sulphated ash (*2.4.14*): maximum 0.1 per cent, determined on 1.0 g.

ASSAY

Dissolve 0.300 g in 75 ml of *anhydrous acetic acid R*. Titrate with *0.1 M perchloric acid*, determining the end-point potentiometrically (*2.2.20*). Carry out a blank titration.

1 ml of *0.1 M perchloric acid* is equivalent to 38.17 mg of $C_{18}H_{15}Cl_3N_2O$.

STORAGE

Protected from light.

IMPURITIES

Specified impurities: A, B, C.

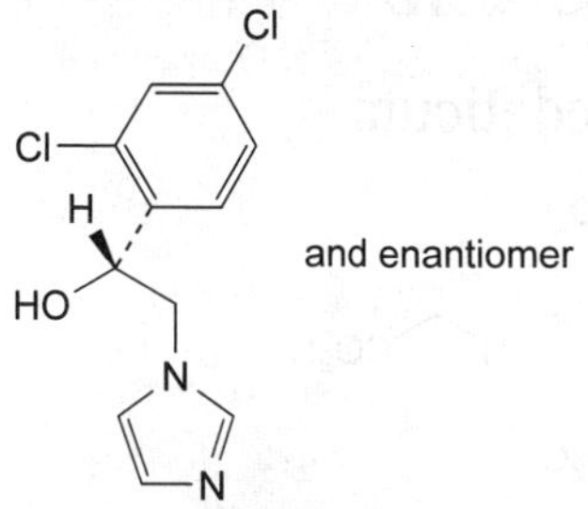

A. (1*RS*)-1-(2,4-dichlorophenyl)-2-(1*H*-imidazol-1-yl)ethanol,

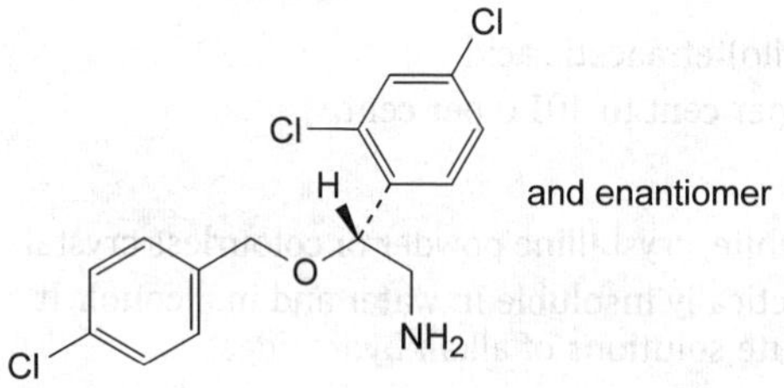

B. (2*RS*)-2-[(4-chlorobenzyl)oxy]-2-(2,4-dichlorophenyl)ethanamine,

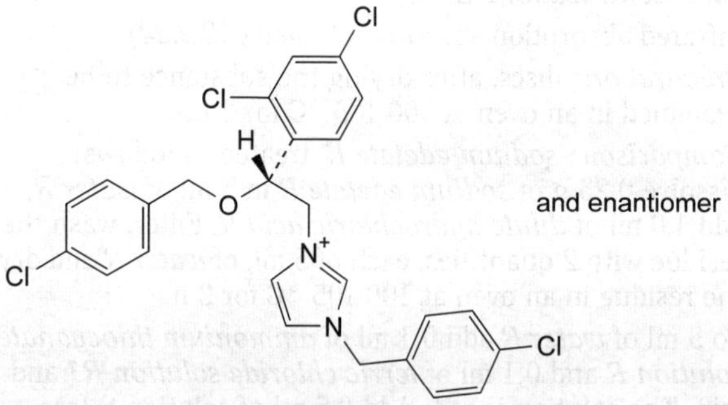

C. 1-(4-chlorobenzyl)-3-[(2*RS*)-2-[(4-chlorobenzyl)oxy]-2-(2,4-dichlorophenyl)ethyl]imidazolium.

01/2005:0665
corrected

ECONAZOLE NITRATE

Econazoli nitras

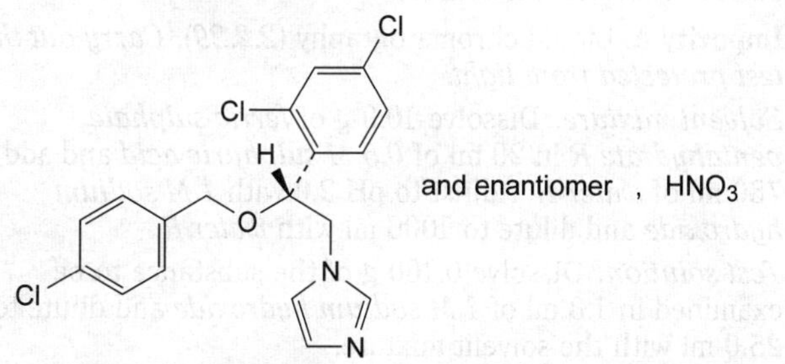

$C_{18}H_{16}Cl_3N_3O_4$ M_r 444.7

DEFINITION

1-[(2*RS*)-2-[(4-Chlorobenzyl)oxy]-2-(2,4-dichlorophenyl)ethyl]-1*H*-imidazole nitrate.

Content: 99.0 per cent to 101.0 per cent (dried substance).

CHARACTERS

Appearance: white or almost white crystalline powder.

Solubility: very slightly soluble in water, soluble in methanol, sparingly soluble in methylene chloride, slightly soluble in alcohol.

mp: about 165 °C, with decomposition.

IDENTIFICATION

Infrared absorption spectrophotometry (*2.2.24*).

Comparison: *Ph. Eur. reference spectrum of econazole nitrate.*

TESTS

Related substances. Liquid chromatography (*2.2.29*).

Test solution. Dissolve 0.100 g of the substance to be examined in *methanol R* and dilute to 10.0 ml with the same solvent.

Reference solution (a). Dissolve 10 mg of *econazole for system suitability CRS* in *methanol R* and dilute to 1.0 ml with the same solvent.

Reference solution (b). Dilute 1.0 ml of the test solution to 20.0 ml with *methanol R*. Dilute 1.0 ml of the solution to 25.0 ml with *methanol R*.

Column:

- *size*: l = 0.10 m, Ø = 4.6 mm,
- *stationary phase*: *base-deactivated octadecylsilyl silica gel for chromatography R* (3 µm),
- *temperature*: 35 °C.

Mobile phase:

- *mobile phase A*: mix 20 volumes of *methanol R* and 80 volumes of a 0.77 g/l solution of *ammonium acetate R*,
- *mobile phase B*: *methanol R*, *acetonitrile R* (40:60 *V/V*),

Time (min)	Mobile phase A (per cent *V/V*)	Mobile phase B (per cent *V/V*)
0 - 25	60 → 10	40 → 90
25 - 27	10	90
27 - 28	10 → 60	90 → 40
28 - 33	60	40

Flow rate: 1.5 ml/min.

Detection: spectrophotometer at 225 nm.

Injection: 10 µl.

Relative retention with reference to econazole (retention time = about 15 min): impurity A = about 0.2; impurity B = about 0.6; impurity C = about 1.1.

System suitability: reference solution (a):

- *peak-to-valley ratio*: minimum of 1.5, where H_p = height above the baseline of the peak due to impurity C, and H_v = height above the baseline of the lowest point of the curve separating this peak from the peak due to econazole.

Limits:

- *correction factor*: for the calculation of content, multiply the peak area of impurity A by 1.4,
- *impurities A, B, C*: for each impurity, not more than the area of the principal peak in the chromatogram obtained with reference solution (b) (0.2 per cent),
- *total*: not more than 1.5 times the area of the principal peak in the chromatogram obtained with reference solution (b) (0.3 per cent),
- *disregard limit*: 0.25 times the area of the principal peak in the chromatogram obtained with reference solution (b) (0.05 per cent); disregard the peak due to the nitrate ion at the beginning of the chromatogram.

Loss on drying (*2.2.32*): maximum 0.5 per cent, determined on 1.000 g by drying in an oven at 100-105 °C for 4 h.

Sulphated ash (*2.4.14*): maximum 0.1 per cent, determined on 1.0 g.

ASSAY

Dissolve 0.400 g in 50 ml of *anhydrous acetic acid R*. Titrate with *0.1 M perchloric acid*, determining the end-point potentiometrically (*2.2.20*). Carry out a blank titration.

1 ml of *0.1 M perchloric acid* is equivalent to 44.47 mg of $C_{18}H_{16}Cl_3N_3O_4$.

STORAGE

Protected from light.

IMPURITIES

Specified impurities: A, B, C.

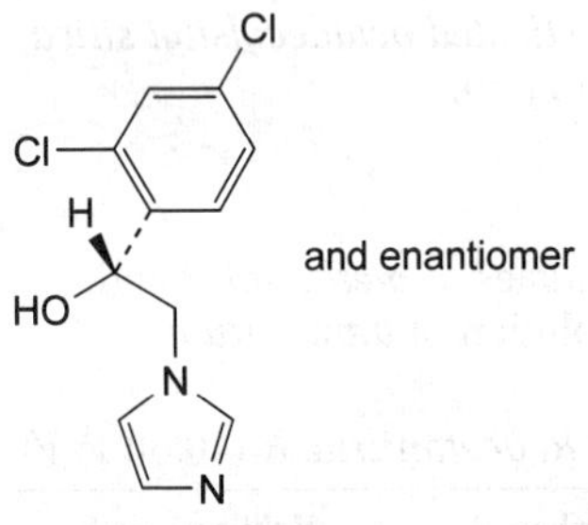

A. (1*RS*)-1-(2,4-dichlorophenyl)-2-(1*H*-imidazol-1-yl)ethanol,

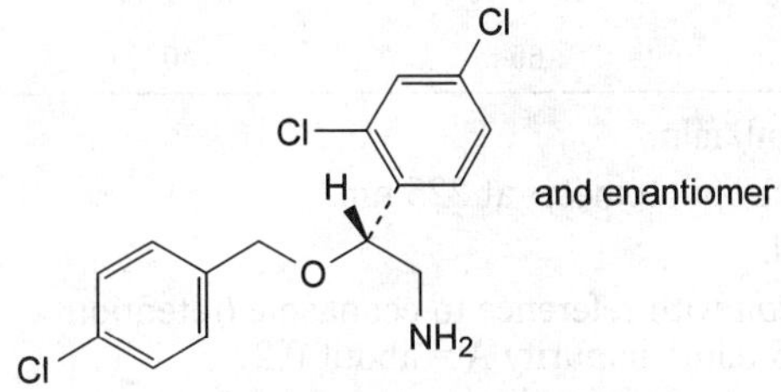

B. (2*RS*)-2-[(4-chlorobenzyl)oxy]-2-(2,4-dichlorophenyl)ethanamine,

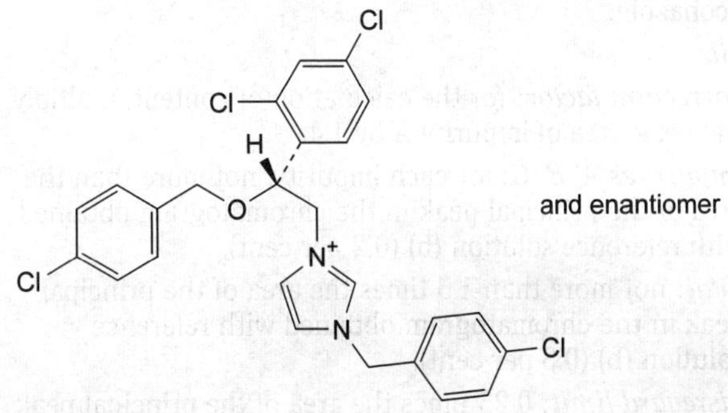

C. 1-(4-chlorobenzyl)-3-[(2*RS*)-2-[(4-chlorobenzyl)oxy]-2-(2,4-dichlorophenyl)ethyl]imidazolium.

01/2005:1612

EDETIC ACID

Acidum edeticum

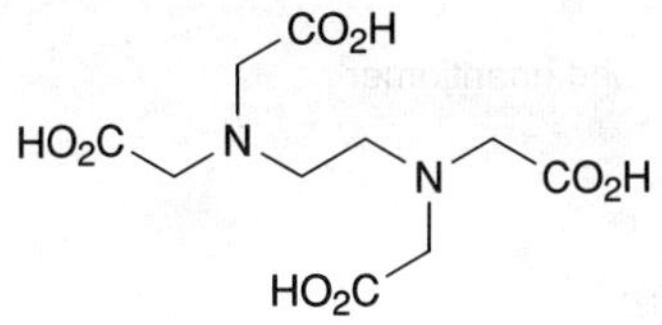

$C_{10}H_{16}N_2O_8$ M_r 292.2

DEFINITION

(Ethylenedinitrilo)tetraacetic acid.

Content: 98.0 per cent to 101.0 per cent.

CHARACTERS

Appearance: white, crystalline powder or colourless crystals.

Solubility: practically insoluble in water and in alcohol. It dissolves in dilute solutions of alkali hydroxides.

IDENTIFICATION

First identification: A.

Second identification: B, C.

A. Infrared absorption spectrophotometry (*2.2.24*).

Preparation: discs, after drying the substance to be examined in an oven at 100-105 °C for 2 h.

Comparison: *sodium edetate R*, treated as follows: dissolve 0.25 g of *sodium edetate R* in 5 ml of *water R*, add 1.0 ml of *dilute hydrochloric acid R*. Filter, wash the residue with 2 quantities, each of 5 ml, of *water R* and dry the residue in an oven at 100-105 °C for 2 h.

B. To 5 ml of *water R* add 0.1 ml of *ammonium thiocyanate solution R* and 0.1 ml of *ferric chloride solution R1* and mix. The solution is red. Add 0.5 ml of solution S (see Tests). The solution becomes yellowish.

C. To 10 ml of solution S add 0.5 ml of *calcium chloride solution R*. Make alkaline to *red litmus paper R* by the addition of *dilute ammonia R2* and add 3 ml of *ammonium oxalate solution R*. No precipitate is formed.

TESTS

Solution S. Dissolve 5.0 g in 20 ml of *dilute sodium hydroxide solution R* and dilute to 100 ml with *water R*.

Appearance of solution. Solution S is clear (*2.2.1*) and colourless (*2.2.2, Method II*).

Impurity A. Liquid chromatography (*2.2.29*). *Carry out the test protected from light.*

Solvent mixture. Dissolve 10.0 g of *ferric sulphate pentahydrate R* in 20 ml of *0.5 M sulphuric acid* and add 780 ml of *water R*. Adjust to pH 2.0 with *1 M sodium hydroxide* and dilute to 1000 ml with *water R*.

Test solution. Dissolve 0.100 g of the substance to be examined in 1.0 ml of *1 M sodium hydroxide* and dilute to 25.0 ml with the solvent mixture.

Reference solution. Dissolve 40.0 mg of *nitrilotriacetic acid R* in the solvent mixture and dilute to 100.0 ml with the solvent mixture. To 1.0 ml of the solution add 0.1 ml of the test solution and dilute to 100.0 ml with the solvent mixture.

Column:

- *size*: l = 0.10 m, Ø = 4.6 mm,
- *stationary phase*: spherical *graphitised carbon for chromatography R1* (5 μm) with a specific surface area of 120 m^2/g and a pore size of 25 nm.

Mobile phase: dissolve 50.0 mg of *ferric sulphate pentahydrate R* in 50 ml of *0.5 M sulphuric acid* and add 750 ml of *water R*. Adjust to pH 1.5 with *0.5 M sulphuric acid* or *1 M sodium hydroxide,* add 20 ml of *ethylene glycol R* and dilute to 1000 ml with *water R*.

Flow rate: 1 ml/min.

Detection: spectrophotometer at 273 nm.

Injection: 20 µl; filter the solutions and inject immediately.

Run time: 4 times the retention time of the iron complex of impurity A.

Retention time: iron complex of impurity A = about 5 min; iron complex of edetic acid = about 10 min.

System suitability: reference solution:

- *resolution*: minimum 7 between the peaks due to the iron complex of impurity A and the iron complex of edetic acid,
- *signal-to-noise ratio*: minimum 50 for the peak due to impurity A.

Limit:

- *impurity A*: not more than the area of the corresponding peak in the chromatogram obtained with the reference solution (0.1 per cent).

Chlorides (*2.4.4*): maximum 200 ppm.

To 10 ml of solution S add 8 ml of *nitric acid R* and stir for 10 min. A precipitate is formed. Filter and wash the filter with *water R*. Collect the filtrate and the washings and dilute to 20 ml with *water R*. Dilute 10 ml of this solution to 15 ml with *water R*.

Iron (*2.4.9*): maximum 80 ppm.

Dilute 2.5 ml of solution S to 10 ml with *water R* and add 0.25 g of *calcium chloride R* before adding the *thioglycollic acid R*. Allow to stand for 5 min. Also add 0.25 g of *calcium chloride R* to the standard.

Heavy metals (*2.4.8*): maximum 20 ppm.

1.0 g complies with limit test D. Use a fused-silica crucible. If necessary moisten the residue on ignition with *nitric acid R* and ignite until a white residue is obtained. Prepare the standard using 2 ml of *lead standard solution (10 ppm Pb) R*.

Sulphated ash (*2.4.14*): maximum 0.2 per cent, determined on 1.0 g.

ASSAY

Dissolve 0.250 g in 2.0 ml of *dilute sodium hydroxide solution R* and dilute to 300 ml with *water R*. Add 2 g of *hexamethylenetetramine R* and 2 ml of *dilute hydrochloric acid R*. Titrate with *0.1 M zinc sulphate* using about 50 mg of *xylenol orange triturate R* as indicator.

1 ml of *0.1 M zinc sulphate* corresponds to 29.22 mg of $C_{10}H_{16}N_2O_8$.

STORAGE

Protected from light.

IMPURITIES

Specified impurities: A.

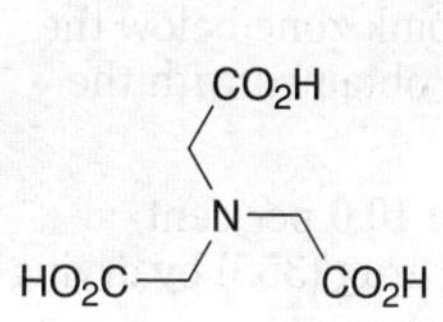

A. nitrilotriacetic acid.

01/2005:2106

EDROPHONIUM CHLORIDE

Edrophonii chloridum

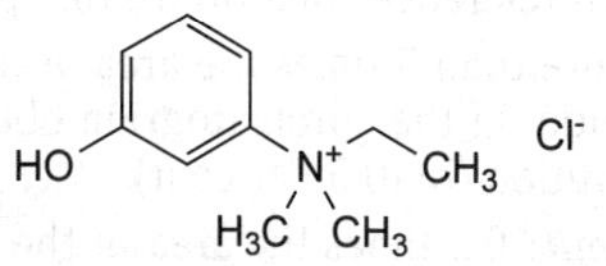

$C_{10}H_{16}ClNO$ M_r 201.7

DEFINITION

N-Ethyl-3-hydroxy-*N*,*N*-dimethylanilinium chloride.

Content: 99.0 per cent to 101.0 per cent (dried substance).

CHARACTERS

Appearance: white or almost white, crystalline powder.

Solubility: very soluble in water, freely soluble in ethanol (96 per cent), practically insoluble in methylene chloride.

IDENTIFICATION

A. Infrared absorption spectrophotometry (*2.2.24*).

Comparison: *edrophonium chloride CRS.*

B. It gives reaction (a) of chlorides (*2.3.1*).

TESTS

Appearance of solution. The solution is clear (*2.2.1*) and colourless (*2.2.2, Method II*).

Dissolve 0.5 g in *water R* and dilute to 25 ml with the same solvent.

pH (*2.2.3*): 4.0 to 5.0.

Dissolve 1.0 g in *carbon dioxide-free water R* and dilute to 10.0 ml with the same solvent.

Related substances. Liquid chromatography (*2.2.29*).

Test solution. Dissolve 50.0 mg in *water R* and dilute to 50.0 ml with the same solvent.

Reference solution (a). Dissolve 10.0 mg of *3-dimethylaminophenol R* in *acetonitrile R* and dilute to 10.0 ml with the same solvent.

Reference solution (b). Mix 1.0 ml of the test solution and 1.0 ml of reference solution (a) and dilute to 100.0 ml with *water R*. Dilute 10.0 ml of this solution to 100.0 ml with *water R*.

Column:

- *size*: *l* = 0.25 m, Ø = 4.6 mm,
- *stationary phase*: *styrene-divinylbenzene copolymer R* (8-10 µm).

Mobile phase: mix 10 volumes of *acetonitrile R* and 90 volumes of a 7.7 g/l solution of *tetramethylammonium bromide R* previously adjusted to pH 3.0 with *phosphoric acid R*.

Flow rate: 1 ml/min.

Detection: spectrophotometer at 281 nm.

Injection: 20 µl.

Run time: twice the retention time of edrophonium.

Relative retention with reference to edrophonium (retention time = about 3.8 min): impurity A = about 1.3.

System suitability: reference solution (b):

- *resolution*: minimum 2.0 between the peaks due to edrophonium and impurity A.

Limits:
- *impurity A*: not more than the area of the corresponding peak in the chromatogram obtained with reference solution (b) (0.1 per cent),
- *any other impurity*: for each impurity, not more than the area of the peak due to edrophonium in the chromatogram obtained with reference solution (b) (0.1 per cent),
- *total*: not more than 5 times the area of the peak due to edrophonium in the chromatogram obtained with reference solution (b) (0.5 per cent),
- *disregard limit*: 0.5 times the area of the peak due to edrophonium in the chromatogram obtained with reference solution (b) (0.05 per cent).

Loss on drying (*2.2.32*): maximum 0.5 per cent, determined on 1.000 g by drying in a desiccator over *diphosphorus pentoxide R* at a pressure not exceeding 0.7 kPa for 24 h.

Sulphated ash (*2.4.14*): maximum 0.1 per cent, determined on 1.0 g.

Bacterial endotoxins (*2.6.14*): less than 8.3 IU/mg.

ASSAY

Dissolve 0.150 g in 60 ml of a mixture of equal volumes of *acetic anhydride R* and *anhydrous acetic acid R*. Titrate with *0.1 M perchloric acid*, determining the end-point potentiometrically (*2.2.20*).

1 ml of *0.1 M perchloric acid* is equivalent to 20.17 mg of $C_{10}H_{16}ClNO$.

STORAGE

Protected from light.

IMPURITIES

Specified impurities: A.

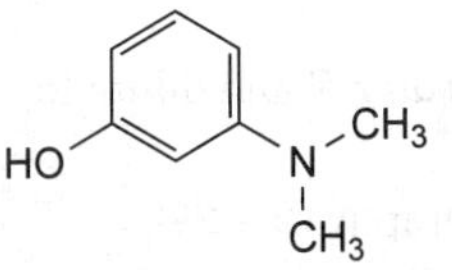

A. 3-(dimethylamino)phenol.

01/2005:1217

ELDER FLOWER

Sambuci flos

DEFINITION

Elder flower consists of the dried flowers of *Sambucus nigra* L. It contains not less than 0.80 per cent of flavonoids, calculated as isoquercitroside ($C_{21}H_{20}O_{12}$; M_r 464.4) with reference to the dried drug.

CHARACTERS

It has the macroscopic and microscopic characters described under identification tests A and B.

IDENTIFICATION

A. The flower, about 5 mm in diameter, has three small bracts (hand lens) and may have a peduncle. The five-toothed calyx is small; the corolla is light yellow, with five broadly oval petals fused at their bases into a tube. The filaments of the five yellow stamens alternate with the petals. The corolla is often isolated or attached to the stamens, to which it is fused at the base. The ovary is inferior with three locules and it bears a short style with three obtuse stigmata.

B. Reduce to a powder (355). The powder is greenish-yellow. Examine under a microscope using *chloral hydrate solution R*. The powder shows numerous spherical, sometimes ellipsoidal, pollen grains about 30 µm in diameter, with three germinal pores and very finely pitted exine; calyx epidermal cells with a striated cuticle and occasional unicellular marginal teeth from the basal region; corolla fragments with numerous small globules of volatile oil, those of the upper epidermis with slightly thickened and beaded walls and a striated cuticle; mesophyll cells of petals and sepals with idioblasts containing numerous sandy crystals of calcium oxalate.

C. Examine in ultraviolet light at 365 nm the chromatograms obtained in the test for *Sambucus ebulus*. The chromatogram obtained with the test solution shows an intense zone of light blue fluorescence due to chlorogenic acid, a zone of orange fluorescence due to rutin as well as a zone of orange fluorescence due to isoquercitrin, which appears slightly above the zone due to hyperoside in the chromatogram obtained with the reference solution. A zone of greenish-blue fluorescence appears in the chromatogram obtained with the test solution a little below the caffeic acid zone in the chromatogram obtained with the reference solution. Additional faint fluorescent zones may be present. In daylight, only the orange fluorescent zones due to rutin and isoquercitroside in the chromatogram obtained with the test solution are clearly visible.

TESTS

Foreign matter (*2.8.2*). Determined on 10 g, not more than 8 per cent of fragments of coarse pedicels and other foreign matter; not more than 15 per cent of discoloured, brown flowers.

Sambucus ebulus L. Examine by thin-layer chromatography (*2.2.27*), using a suitable silica gel as the coating substance.

Test solution. To 0.5 g of the powdered drug (355) add 10 ml of *methanol R* and heat in a water bath at 65 °C for 5 min, shaking frequently. Allow to cool and filter. Dilute the filtrate to 10 ml with *methanol R*.

Reference solution. Dissolve 1 mg of *caffeic acid R*, 1 mg of *chlorogenic acid R*, 2.5 mg of *hyperoside R* and 2.5 mg of *rutin R* in 10 ml of *methanol R*.

Apply separately to the plate, as bands, 10 µl of each solution. Develop over a path of 15 cm using a mixture of 10 volumes of *anhydrous formic acid R*, 10 volumes of *water R*, 30 volumes of *methyl ethyl ketone R* and 50 volumes of *ethyl acetate R*. Dry the plate at 100-105 °C and spray it while still warm with a 10 g/l solution of *diphenylboric acid aminoethyl ester R* in *methanol R*. Subsequently spray the plate with a 50 g/l solution of *macrogol 400 R* in *methanol R*. Allow the plate to dry in air for 30 min and examine in ultraviolet light at 365 nm. The chromatogram obtained with the reference solution shows in the lower half, with increasing R_f values, the zone of orange fluorescence due to rutin, the zone of light blue fluorescence due to chlorogenic acid and the zone of orange-yellow to orange-brown fluorescence due to hyperoside. The upper third presents a zone of greenish-blue fluorescence due to caffeic acid. The chromatogram obtained with the test solution does not show a pink zone below the zone due to rutin in the chromatogram obtained with the reference solution.

Loss on drying (*2.2.32*). Not more than 10.0 per cent, determined on 1.000 g of the powdered drug (355) by drying in an oven at 100-105 °C for 2 h.

Total ash (*2.4.16*). Not more than 10.0 per cent.

ASSAY

Stock solution. In a 100 ml round-bottomed flask, introduce 0.600 g of the powdered drug (355), add 1 ml of a 5 g/l solution of *hexamethylenetetramine R*, 20 ml of *acetone R* and 2 ml of *hydrochloric acid R1*. Boil the mixture under a reflux condenser for 30 min. Filter the liquid through a plug of absorbent cotton into a flask. Add the absorbent cotton to the residue in the round-bottomed flask and extract with two quantities, each of 20 ml, of *acetone R*, each time boiling under a reflux condenser for 10 min. Allow to cool, filter each extract through the plug of absorbent cotton into the flask. After cooling, filter the combined acetone extracts through a paper-filter into a volumetric flask, dilute to 100.0 ml with *acetone R* by rinsing the flask and the paper-filter. Introduce 20.0 ml of the solution into a separating funnel, add 20 ml of *water R* and shake the mixture with one quantity of 15 ml and then three quantities, each of 10 ml, of *ethyl acetate R*. Combine the ethyl acetate extracts in a separating funnel, wash with two quantities, each of 50 ml, of *water R*, and filter the extracts over 10 g of *anhydrous sodium sulphate R* into a volumetric flask and dilute to 50.0 ml with *ethyl acetate R*.

Test solution. To 10.0 ml of the stock solution add 1 ml of *aluminium chloride reagent R* and dilute to 25.0 ml with a 5 per cent *V/V* solution of *glacial acetic acid R* in *methanol R*.

Compensation solution. Dilute 10.0 ml of the stock solution to 25.0 ml with a 5 per cent *V/V* solution of *glacial acetic acid R* in *methanol R*.

Measure the absorbance (*2.2.25*) of the test solution after 30 min, by comparison with the compensation solution at 425 nm. Calculate the percentage content of flavonoids, calculated as isoquercitroside, from the expression:

$$\frac{A \times 1.25}{m}$$

i.e. taking the specific absorbance of isoquercitroside to be 500.

A = absorbance at 425 nm,

m = mass of the substance to be examined, in grams.

STORAGE

Store protected from light.

01/2005:1419
corrected

ELEUTHEROCOCCUS

Eleutherococci radix

DEFINITION

Dried, whole or cut underground organs of *Eleutherococcus senticosus* (Rupr. et Maxim.) Maxim.

Content: minimum 0.08 per cent for the sum of eleutheroside B (M_r 372.4) and eleutheroside E (M_r 742.7).

CHARACTERS

Macroscopic and microscopic characters described under identification tests A and B.

IDENTIFICATION

A. The rhizome is knotty, of irregular cylindrical shape, 1.5 cm to 4.0 cm in diameter; the surface is rugged, longitudinally wrinkled and greyish-brown to blackish-brown; the bark, about 2 mm thick, closely adheres to the xylem; the heartwood is light brown and the sapwood is pale yellow; the fracture shows short thin fibres in the bark and is coarsely fibrous, especially in the internal part of the xylem. The lower surface bears numerous cylindrical and knotty roots, 3.5 cm to 15 cm long and 0.3 cm to 1.5 cm in diameter; with a smooth, greyish-brown to blackish-brown surface; the bark is about 0.5 mm thick, closely adhering to the pale yellow xylem; the fracture is slightly fibrous; in places where the outer layer has been removed, the outer surface is yellowish-brown.

B. Reduce to a powder (355). The powder is yellowish-brown. Examine under a microscope, using *chloral hydrate solution R*. The powder shows numerous groups of thick-walled, lignified fibres; fragments of reticulate and bordered pitted vessels with a wide lumen; groups of secretory canals, up to 20 µm in diameter with brown contents; parenchymatous cells containing cluster crystals of calcium oxalate 10 µm to 50 µm in diameter. Examine under a microscope, using a 50 per cent *V/V* solution of *glycerol R*. The powder shows small starch granules, rounded to slightly angular in outline, single compounds or with 2 or 3 components.

C. Thin-layer chromatography (*2.2.27*).

Test solution. To 1.0 g of the powdered drug (355) add 10 ml of *alcohol (50 per cent V/V) R* and boil under reflux for 1 h. Cool and filter. Evaporate the filtrate to dryness on a water-bath. Dissolve the residue in 2.5 ml of a mixture of 5 volumes of *water R* and 20 volumes of *alcohol (50 per cent V/V) R* and filter.

Reference solution. Dissolve 2.0 mg of *esculin R* and 2.0 mg of *catalpol R* in 20 ml of a mixture of 2 volumes of *water R* and 8 volumes of *alcohol (50 per cent V/V) R*.

Plate: *TLC silica gel plate R.*

Mobile phase: *water R, methanol R, methylene chloride R* (4:30:70 *V/V/V*).

Application: 20 µl, as bands.

Development: over a path of 10 cm.

Drying: in air.

Detection A: examine in ultraviolet light at 365 nm.

Results A: the chromatogram obtained with the reference solution shows in the upper half a blue fluorescent zone (esculin).

Detection B: spray with *anisaldehyde solution R* and examine in daylight while heating at 100-105 °C for 5-10 min.

Results B: see below the sequence of the zones present in the chromatograms obtained with the reference solution and the test solution. Furthermore, other faint zones are present in the chromatogram obtained with the test solution.

Top of the plate	
	A brown zone (eleutheroside B)
Esculin: a blue fluorescent zone (marked at 365 nm)	
	A reddish-brown zone (eleutheroside E)
	_______
Catalpol: a violet-brown zone	
_______	_______
	2 brown zones
Reference solution	**Test solution**

TESTS

Foreign matter (*2.8.2*): maximum 3 per cent.

Loss on drying (*2.2.32*): maximum 10.0 per cent, determined on 1.000 g of the powdered drug (355) by drying in an oven at 100-105 °C for 2 h.

Total ash (*2.4.16*): maximum 8.0 per cent.

ASSAY

Liquid chromatography (*2.2.29*).

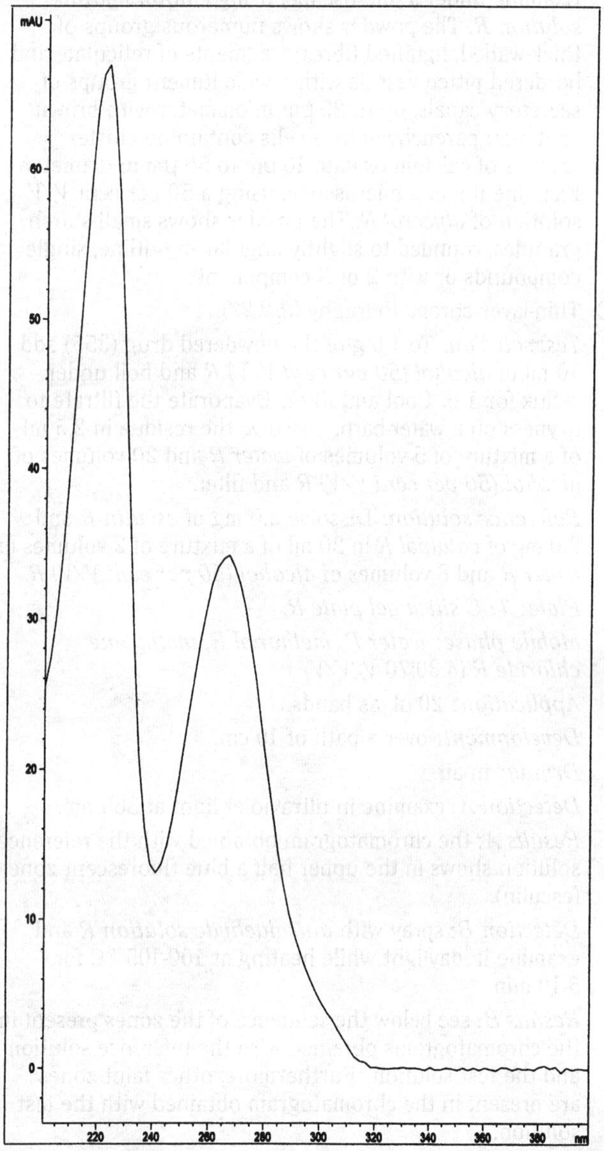

Figure 1419.-1. – *UV spectrum of eleutheroside B for the assay of eleutherococcus*

Test solution. To 0.500 g of the powdered drug (355) in a 100 ml round-bottomed flask, add 30 ml of a mixture of equal volumes of *alcohol R* and *water R*. Heat in a water-bath at 60 °C for 30 min. Allow to cool and filter through a sintered-glass filter. Collect the liquid in a 250 ml round-bottomed flask. Repeat this operation twice, using the residue obtained in the filtration step instead of the powdered drug. Add both fractions of supernatant liquid to the 250 ml round-bottomed flask. Evaporate under reduced pressure until about 10 ml of supernatant liquid is left in the flask. Transfer the supernatant liquid quantitatively to a 20.0 ml volumetric flask and dilute to 20.0 ml with a mixture of equal volumes of *alcohol R* and *water R*. Filter through a nylon filter (pore size 0.45 μm).

Reference solution (a). Dissolve 10 mg of *ferulic acid R* in a mixture of equal volumes of *methanol R* and *water R* and dilute to 20.0 ml with the same mixture of solvents.

Reference solution (b). Dissolve 10 mg of *caffeic acid R* in a mixture of equal volumes of *methanol R* and *water R* and dilute to 20.0 ml with the same mixture of solvents.

Reference solution (c). Transfer 1 ml of reference solution (a) to a 25 ml volumetric flask and dilute to 25.0 ml with a mixture of equal volumes of *methanol R* and *water R*. Filter through a nylon filter (pore size 0.45 μm).

Reference solution (d). Transfer 1 ml of reference solution (a) and 1 ml of reference solution (b) in a mixture of equal volumes of *methanol R* and *water R* and dilute to 25.0 ml with the same mixture of solvents. Filter through a nylon filter (pore size 0.45 μm).

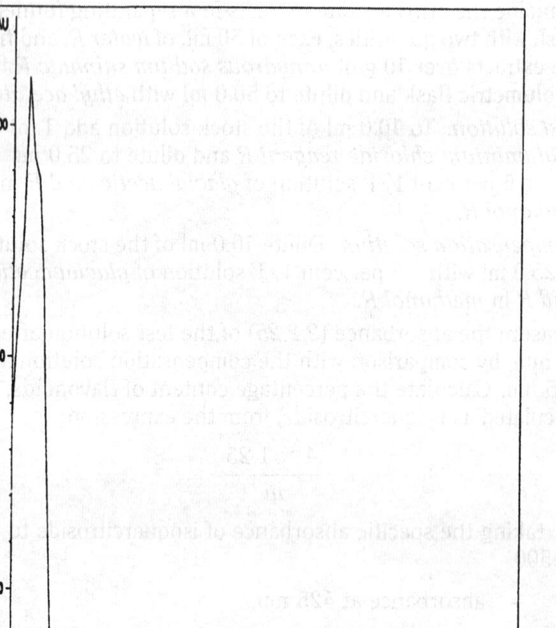

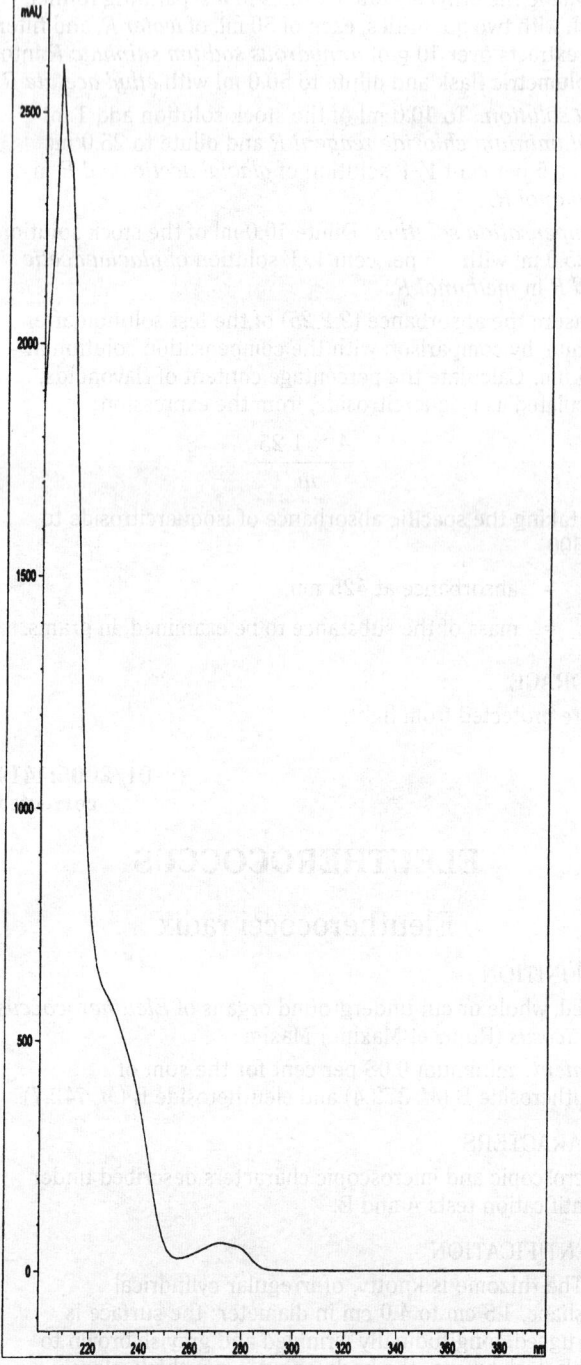

Figure 1419.-2. – *UV spectrum of eleutheroside E for the assay of eleutherococcus*

Precolumn:

- *size*: l = 0.04 m, Ø = 4.6 mm,
- *stationary phase*: *octadecylsilyl silica gel for chromatography R* (5 µm).

Column:

- *size*: l = 0.25 m, Ø = 4.6 mm,
- *stationary phase*: *octadecylsilyl silica gel for chromatography R* (5 µm).

Mobile phase:

- *mobile phase A*: *phosphoric acid R, water R* (0.5:99.5 *V/V*),
- *mobile phase B*: *acetonitrile for chromatography R*,

Time (min)	Mobile phase A (per cent *V/V*)	Mobile phase B (per cent *V/V*)
0 - 5	90	10
5 - 27	90 → 80	10 → 20
27 - 30	80 → 50	20 → 50
30 - 35	50	50
35 - 40	50 → 90	50 → 10

Flow rate: 1.0 ml/min.

Detection: spectrophotometer at 220 nm.

Injection: 20 µl of the test solution and reference solutions (c) and (d).

Retention time: eleutheroside B = about 10 min; eleutheroside E = about 22 min.

Locate the peaks due to eleutheroside B and eleutheroside E using the UV spectra shown in Figures 1419.-1 and 1419.-2.

System suitability: reference solution (d):

- *resolution*: minimum 15 between the peaks due to caffeic acid and ferulic acid.

Calculate the total percentage content of eleutheroside B and eleutheroside E from the expression:

$$\frac{(A_B \times C \times 0.73 \times 2)}{(A_R \times m)} + \frac{(A_E \times C \times 1.90 \times 2)}{(A_R \times m)}$$

A_B = area of the peak due to eleutheroside B in the chromatogram obtained with the test solution,

A_E = area of the peak due to eleutheroside E in the chromatogram obtained with the test solution,

A_R = area of the peak due to ferulic acid in the chromatogram obtained with reference solution (c),

C = concentration of ferulic acid in reference solution (c), in micrograms per millilitre,

m = mass of the drug to be examined, in milligrams.

01/2005:0080

EMETINE HYDROCHLORIDE HEPTAHYDRATE

Emetini hydrochloridum heptahydricum

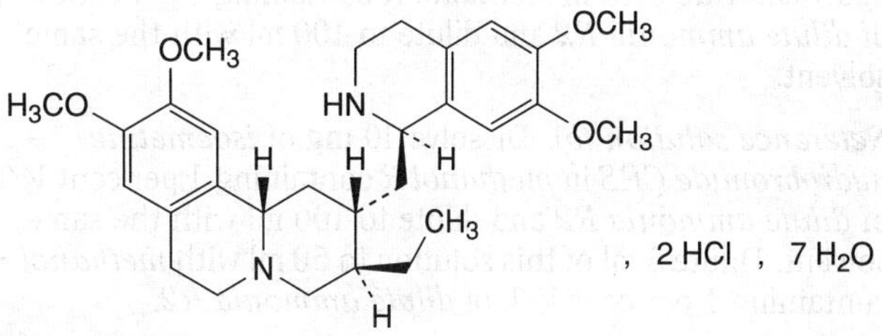

$C_{29}H_{42}Cl_2N_2O_4,7H_2O$ M_r 680

DEFINITION

Emetine hydrochloride heptahydrate contains not less than 98.0 per cent and not more than the equivalent of 102.0 per cent of (2*S*,3*R*,11b*S*)-2-[[(1*R*)-6,7-dimethoxy-1,2,3,4-tetrahydroisoquinolin-1-yl]methyl]-3-ethyl-9,10-dimethoxy-1,3,4,6,7,11b-hexahydro-2*H*-benzo[*a*]quinolizine dihydrochloride, calculated with reference to the dried substance.

CHARACTERS

A white or slightly yellowish, crystalline powder, freely soluble in water and in alcohol.

IDENTIFICATION

First identification: *A, E.*

Second identification: *B, C, D, E.*

A. Examine by infrared absorption spectrophotometry (*2.2.24*), comparing with the spectrum obtained with *emetine hydrochloride CRS*.

B. Examine the chromatograms obtained in the test for related substances in ultraviolet light at 365 nm. The principal spot in the chromatogram obtained with the test solution is similar in position, fluorescence and size to the spot in the chromatogram obtained with reference solution (a).

C. Dissolve about 10 mg in 2 ml of *dilute hydrogen peroxide solution R*, add 1 ml of *hydrochloric acid R* and heat. An orange colour develops.

D. Sprinkle about 5 mg on the surface of 1 ml of *sulphomolybdic reagent R2*. A bright-green colour develops.

E. It gives reaction (a) of chlorides (*2.3.1*).

TESTS

Solution S. Dissolve 1.25 g in *carbon dioxide-free water R* and dilute to 25 ml with the same solvent.

Appearance of solution. Solution S is clear (*2.2.1*) and not more intensely coloured than reference solution Y_5 or BY_5 (*2.2.2, Method II*).

pH (*2.2.3*). Dilute 4 ml of solution S to 10 ml with *carbon dioxide-free water R*. The pH of the solution is 4.0 to 6.0.

Specific optical rotation (*2.2.7*). Dissolve in *water R* a quantity of the substance to be examined corresponding to 1.250 g of dried substance and dilute to 25.0 ml with the same solvent. The specific optical rotation is + 16 to + 19, calculated with reference to the dried substance.

Monographs D-E

Related substances. Examine by thin-layer chromatography (*2.2.27*), using a *TLC silica gel G plate R. Prepare the solutions immediately before use.*

Test solution. Dissolve 50 mg of the substance to be examined in *methanol R* containing 1 per cent *V/V* of *dilute ammonia R2* and dilute to 100 ml with the same solvent.

Reference solution (a). Dissolve 50 mg of *emetine hydrochloride CRS* in *methanol R* containing 1 per cent *V/V* of *dilute ammonia R2* and dilute to 100 ml with the same solvent.

Reference solution (b). Dissolve 10 mg of *isoemetine hydrobromide CRS* in *methanol R* containing 1 per cent *V/V* of *dilute ammonia R2* and dilute to 100 ml with the same solvent. Dilute 5 ml of this solution to 50 ml with *methanol R* containing 1 per cent *V/V* of *dilute ammonia R2.*

Reference solution (c). Dissolve 10 mg of *cephaëline hydrochloride CRS* in *methanol R* containing 1 per cent *V/V* of *dilute ammonia R2* and dilute to 100 ml with the same solvent. Dilute 5 ml of this solution to 50 ml with *methanol R* containing 1 per cent *V/V* of *dilute ammonia R2.*

Reference solution (d). Dilute 1 ml of reference solution (a) to 100 ml with *methanol R* containing 1 per cent *V/V* of *dilute ammonia R2.*

Reference solution (e). To 1 ml of reference solution (a) add 1 ml of reference solution (b) and 1 ml of reference solution (c).

Apply to the plate 10 µl of the test solution and each of reference solutions (a), (b), (c) and (d) and 30 µl of reference solution (e). Develop over a path of 15 cm using a mixture of 0.5 volumes of *diethylamine R*, 2 volumes of *water R*, 5 volumes of *methanol R*, 20 volumes of *ethylene glycol monomethyl ether R* and 100 volumes of *chloroform R*. Allow the plate to dry in air until the solvent has evaporated. Spray in a well ventilated fume-cupboard with *chloroformic solution of iodine R* and heat at 60 °C for 15 min. Examine in ultraviolet light at 365 nm. In the chromatogram obtained with the test solution, any spots corresponding to isoemetine and cephaëline are not more intense than the spots in the chromatograms obtained with reference solutions (b) and (c) respectively (2.0 per cent); any spot, apart from the principal spot and the spots corresponding to isoemetine and cephaëline, is not more intense than the spot in the chromatogram obtained with reference solution (d) (1.0 per cent). The test is not valid unless the chromatogram obtained with reference solution (e) shows three clearly separated spots.

Loss on drying (*2.2.32*). 15.0 per cent to 19.0 per cent, determined on 1.00 g by drying in an oven at 100 °C to 105 °C for 3 h.

Sulphated ash (*2.4.14*). Not more than 0.1 per cent, determined on 1.0 g.

ASSAY

Dissolve 0.200 g in a mixture of 5.0 ml of *0.01 M hydrochloric acid* and 50 ml of *alcohol R*. Carry out a potentiometric titration (*2.2.20*), using *0.1 M sodium hydroxide*. Read the volume added between the 2 points of inflexion.

1 ml of *0.1 M sodium hydroxide* is equivalent to 27.68 mg of $C_{29}H_{42}Cl_2N_2O_4$.

STORAGE

Store protected from light.

01/2005:0081

EMETINE HYDROCHLORIDE PENTAHYDRATE

Emetini hydrochloridum pentahydricum

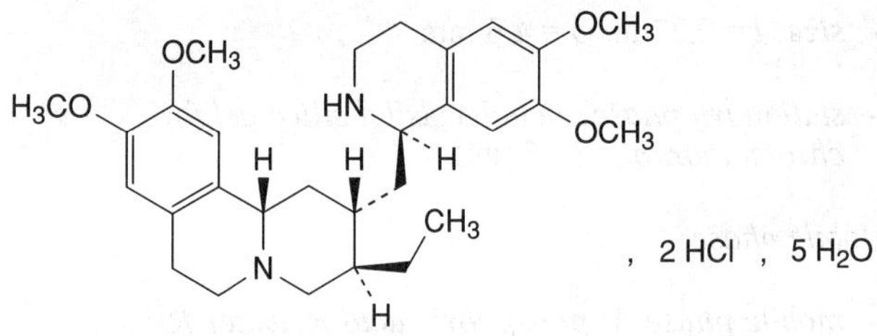

$C_{29}H_{42}Cl_2N_2O_4,5H_2O$ M_r 644

DEFINITION

Emetine hydrochloride pentahydrate contains not less than 98.0 per cent and not more than the equivalent of 102.0 per cent of (2*S*,3*R*,11b*S*)-2-[[(1*R*)-6,7-dimethoxy-1,2,3,4-tetrahydroisoquinolin-1-yl]methyl]-3-ethyl-9,10-dimethoxy-1,3,4,6,7,11b-hexahydro-2*H*-benzo[*a*]quinolizine dihydrochloride, calculated with reference to the dried substance.

CHARACTERS

A white or slightly yellowish, crystalline powder, freely soluble in water and in alcohol.

IDENTIFICATION

First identification: A, E.

Second identification: B, C, D, E.

A. Examine by infrared absorption spectrophotometry (*2.2.24*), comparing with the spectrum obtained with *emetine hydrochloride CRS.*

B. Examine the chromatograms obtained in the test for related substances in ultraviolet light at 365 nm. The principal spot in the chromatogram obtained with the test solution is similar in position, fluorescence and size to the spot in the chromatogram obtained with reference solution (a).

C. Dissolve about 10 mg in 2 ml of *dilute hydrogen peroxide solution R*, add 1 ml of *hydrochloric acid R* and heat. An orange colour develops.

D. Sprinkle about 5 mg on the surface of 1 ml of *sulphomolybdic reagent R2.* A bright-green colour develops.

E. It gives reaction (a) of chlorides (*2.3.1*).

TESTS

Solution S. Dissolve 1.25 g in *carbon dioxide-free water R* and dilute to 25 ml with the same solvent.

Appearance of solution. Solution S is clear (*2.2.1*) and not more intensely coloured than reference solution Y_5 or BY_5 (*2.2.2, Method II*).

pH (*2.2.3*). Dilute 4 ml of solution S to 10 ml with *carbon dioxide-free water R*. The pH of the solution is 4.0 to 6.0.

Specific optical rotation (*2.2.7*). Dissolve in *water R* a quantity of the substance to be examined corresponding to 1.250 g of dried substance and dilute to 25.0 ml with the same solvent. The specific optical rotation is + 16 to + 19, calculated with reference to the dried substance.

Related substances. Examine by thin-layer chromatography (*2.2.27*), using a *TLC silica gel G plate R. Prepare the solutions immediately before use.*

Test solution. Dissolve 50 mg of the substance to be examined in *methanol R* containing 1 per cent *V/V* of *dilute ammonia R2* and dilute to 100 ml with the same solvent.

Reference solution (a). Dissolve 50 mg of *emetine hydrochloride CRS* in *methanol R* containing 1 per cent *V/V* of *dilute ammonia R2* and dilute to 100 ml with the same solvent.

Reference solution (b). Dissolve 10 mg of *isoemetine hydrobromide CRS* in *methanol R* containing 1 per cent *V/V* of *dilute ammonia R2* and dilute to 100 ml with the same solvent. Dilute 5 ml of this solution to 50 ml with *methanol R* containing 1 per cent *V/V* of *dilute ammonia R2.*

Reference solution (c). Dissolve 10 mg of *cephaëline hydrochloride CRS* in *methanol R* containing 1 per cent *V/V* of *dilute ammonia R2* and dilute to 100 ml with the same solvent. Dilute 5 ml of this solution to 50 ml with *methanol R* containing 1 per cent *V/V* of *dilute ammonia R2.*

Reference solution (d). Dilute 1 ml of reference solution (a) to 100 ml with *methanol R* containing 1 per cent *V/V* of *dilute ammonia R2.*

Reference solution (e). To 1 ml of reference solution (a) add 1 ml of reference solution (b) and 1 ml of reference solution (c).

Apply to the plate 10 µl of the test solution and each of reference solutions (a), (b), (c) and (d) and 30 µl of reference solution (e). Develop over a path of 15 cm using a mixture of 0.5 volumes of *diethylamine R,* 2 volumes of *water R,* 5 volumes of *methanol R,* 20 volumes of *ethylene glycol monomethyl ether R* and 100 volumes of *chloroform R.* Allow the plate to dry in air until the solvent has evaporated. Spray in a well ventilated fume-cupboard with *chloroformic solution of iodine R* and heat at 60 °C for 15 min. Examine in ultraviolet light at 365 nm. In the chromatogram obtained with the test solution, any spots corresponding to isoemetine and cephaëline are not more intense than the spots in the chromatograms obtained with reference solutions (b) and (c) respectively (2.0 per cent); any spot, apart from the principal spot and the spots corresponding to isoemetine and cephaëline, is not more intense than the spot in the chromatogram obtained with reference solution (d) (1.0 per cent). The test is not valid unless the chromatogram obtained with reference solution (e) shows three clearly separated spots.

Loss on drying (*2.2.32*). 11.0 per cent to 15.0 per cent, determined on 1.00 g by drying in an oven at 100 °C to 105 °C for 3 h.

Sulphated ash (*2.4.14*). Not more than 0.1 per cent, determined on 1.0 g.

ASSAY

Dissolve 0.200 g in a mixture of 5.0 ml of *0.01 M hydrochloric acid* and 50 ml of *alcohol R.* Carry out a potentiometric titration (*2.2.20*), using *0.1 M sodium hydroxide.* Read the volume added between the two points of inflexion.

1 ml of *0.1 M sodium hydroxide* is equivalent to 27.68 mg of $C_{29}H_{42}Cl_2N_2O_4$.

STORAGE

Store protected from light.

01/2005:1420

ENALAPRIL MALEATE

Enalaprili maleas

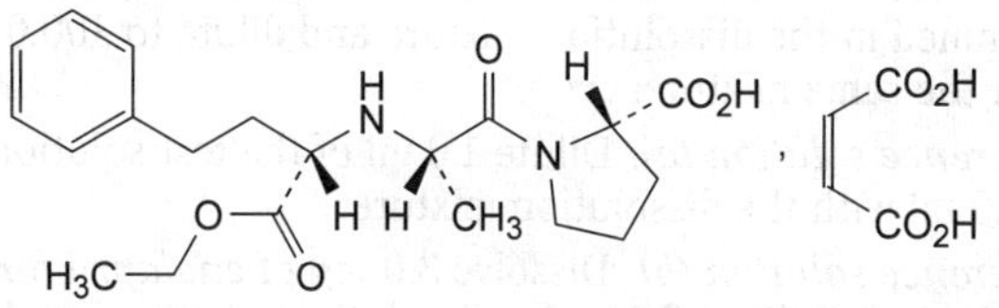

$C_{24}H_{32}N_2O_9$ M_r 492.5

DEFINITION

Enalapril maleate contains not less than 98.5 per cent and not more than the equivalent of 101.5 per cent of (2*S*)-1-[(2*S*)-2-[[(1*S*)-1-(ethoxycarbonyl)-3-phenylpropyl]amino]propanoyl]pyrrolidine-2-carboxylic acid (*Z*)-butenedioate, calculated with reference to the dried substance.

CHARACTERS

A white or almost white crystalline powder, sparingly soluble in water, freely soluble in methanol, practically insoluble in methylene chloride. It dissolves in dilute solutions of alkali hydroxides.

IDENTIFICATION

First identification: B.

Second identification: A, C, D.

A. Melting point (*2.2.14*): 143 °C to 145 °C.

B. Examine by infrared absorption spectrophotometry (*2.2.24*), comparing with the spectrum obtained with *enalapril maleate CRS.*

C. Dissolve about 30 mg in 3 ml of *water R.* Add 1 ml of *bromine water R* and heat on a water bath until bromine has disappeared completely and cool. To 0.2 ml of this solution, add 3 ml of a 3 g/l solution of *resorcinol R* in *sulphuric acid R* and heat on a water bath for 15 min. A reddish-brown colour develops.

D. To about 30 mg, add 0.5 ml of a 100 g/l solution of *hydroxylamine hydrochloride R* in *methanol R* and 1.0 ml of a 100 g/l solution of *potassium hydroxide R* in *alcohol R.* Heat to boiling, allow to cool and acidify with *dilute hydrochloric acid R.* Add 0.2 ml of *ferric chloride solution R1* diluted 1 to 10; a reddish-brown colour appears.

TESTS

Solution S. Dissolve 0.25 g in *carbon dioxide-free water R* and dilute to 25.0 ml with the same solvent.

Appearance of solution. Solution S is clear (*2.2.1*) and colourless (*2.2.2, Method II*).

pH (*2.2.3*). The pH of solution S is 2.4 to 2.9.

Specific optical rotation (*2.2.7*): − 48 to − 51, determined on solution S and calculated with reference to the dried substance.

Related substances. Examine by liquid chromatography (*2.2.29*).

Buffer solution A. Dissolve 2.8 g of *sodium dihydrogen phosphate monohydrate R* in 950 ml of *water R.* Adjust to pH 2.5 with *phosphoric acid R* and dilute to 1000 ml with *water R.*

Buffer solution B. Dissolve 2.8 g of *sodium dihydrogen phosphate monohydrate R* in 950 ml of *water R*. Adjust to pH 6.8 with *strong sodium hydroxide solution R* and dilute to 1000 ml with *water R*.

Dissolution mixture. Mix 50 ml of *acetonitrile R1* and 950 ml of buffer solution A.

Test solution. Dissolve 30.0 mg of the substance to be examined in the dissolution mixture and dilute to 100.0 ml with the same mixture.

Reference solution (a). Dilute 1.0 ml of the test solution to 100.0 ml with the dissolution mixture.

Reference solution (b). Dissolve 3.0 mg of *enalapril for system suitability CRS* in the dissolution mixture and dilute to 10.0 ml with the same mixture.

The chromatographic procedure may be carried out using:

- a stainless steel column 0.15 m long and 4.1 mm in internal diameter packed with *styrene-divinylbenzene copolymer R* (5 µm),
- as mobile phase at a flow rate of 1.4 ml/min,

  Mobile phase A. Mix 50 ml of *acetonitrile R1* and 950 ml of buffer solution B,

  Mobile phase B. Mix 340 ml of buffer solution B and 660 ml of *acetonitrile R1*,

Time (min)	Mobile phase A (per cent *V/V*)	Mobile phase B (per cent *V/V*)
0 - 20	95 → 40	5 → 60
20 - 25	40	60
25 - 26	40 → 95	60 → 5
26 - 30	95	5

- as detector a spectrophotometer set at 215 nm,

maintaining the temperature of the column at 70 °C.

Inject 50 µl of reference solution (b). When the chromatogram is recorded in the prescribed conditions, the retention times are: enalapril about 11 min and impurity A about 12 min. The test is not valid unless the resolution between the peaks corresponding to enalapril and impurity A is at least 1.5. Inject 50 µl of the test solution and 50 µl of reference solution (a). In the chromatogram obtained with the test solution: the area of any peak corresponding to impurity A is not greater than that of the principal peak in the chromatogram obtained with reference solution (a) (1.0 per cent); the area of any peak apart from the principal peak and any peak corresponding to impurity A, is not greater than 0.3 times the area of the principal peak in the chromatogram obtained with reference solution (a) (0.3 per cent) and the sum of the areas of any such peaks is not greater than the area of the principal peak in the chromatogram obtained with reference solution (a) (1.0 per cent). Disregard any peak with an area less than 0.05 times that of the principal peak in the chromatogram obtained with reference solution (a).

Heavy metals (*2.4.8*). 2.0 g complies with limit test C (10 ppm). Use 2 ml of *lead standard solution (10 ppm Pb) R*.

Loss on drying (*2.2.32*). Not more than 1.0 per cent determined on 1.000 g by heating in an oven at 100-105 °C for 3 h.

Sulphated ash (*2.4.14*). Not more than 0.1 per cent, determined on 1.0 g.

ASSAY

Dissolve 0.100 g in *carbon dioxide-free water R* and dilute to 30 ml with the same solvent. Titrate with *0.1 M sodium hydroxide* determining the end point potentiometrically (*2.2.20*). Titrate to the second point of inflexion.

1 ml of *0.1 M sodium hydroxide* is equivalent to 16.42 mg of $C_{24}H_{32}N_2O_9$.

STORAGE

Store protected from light.

IMPURITIES

Specified impurities: A, B, C, D, E, H.

Other detectable impurities: F, G, I.

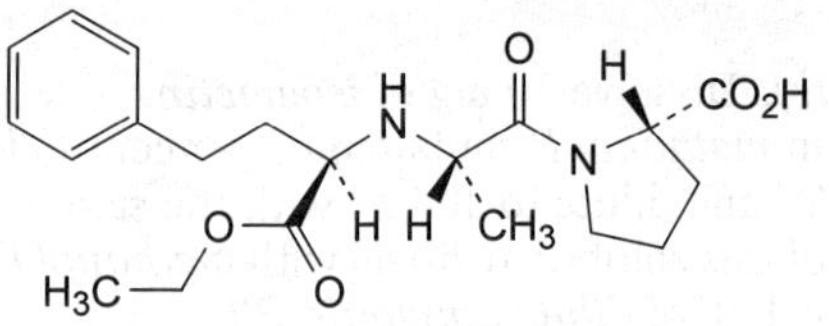

A. (2*S*)-1-[(2*S*)-2-[[(1*R*)-1-(ethoxycarbonyl)-3-phenylpropyl]amino]propanoyl]pyrrolidine-2-carboxylic acid,

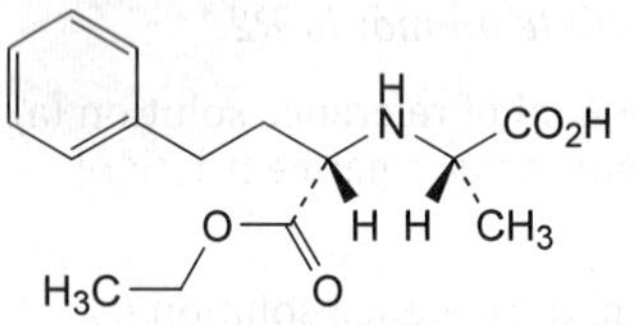

B. (2*S*)-2-[[(1*S*)-1-(ethoxycarbonyl)-3-phenylpropyl]amino]propanoic acid,

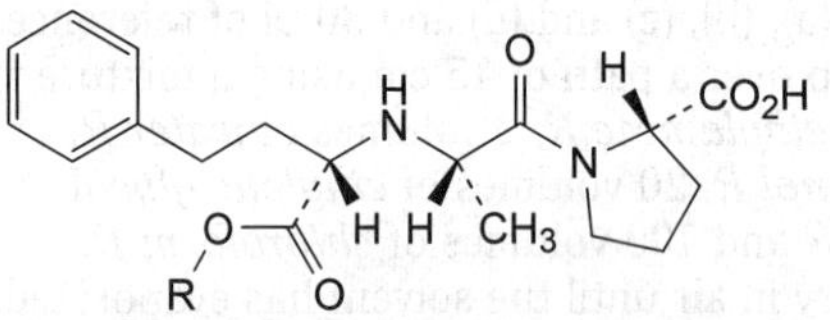

C. R = H: (2*S*)-1-[(2*S*)-2-[[(1*S*)-1-carboxy-3-phenylpropyl]amino]propanoyl]pyrrolidine-2-carboxylic acid,

E. R = CH_2-CH_2-C_6H_5: (2*S*)-1-[(2*S*)-2-[[(1*S*)-3-phenyl-1-[(2-phenylethoxy)carbonyl]propyl]amino]propanoyl]pyrrolidine-2-carboxylic acid,

F. R = C_4H_9: (2*S*)-1-[(2*S*)-2-[[(1*S*)-1-(butoxycarbonyl)-3-phenylpropyl]amino]propanoyl]pyrrolidine-2-carboxylic acid,

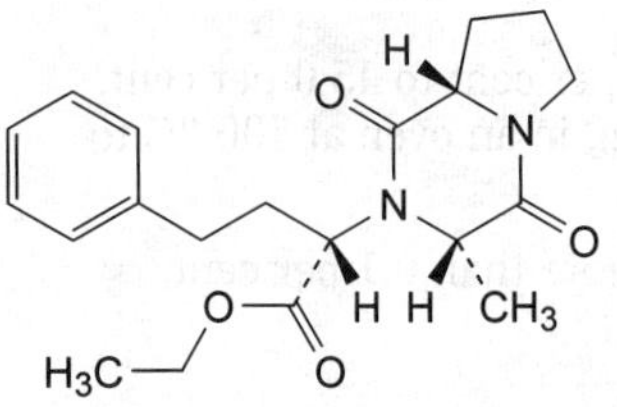

D. ethyl (2*S*)-2-[(3*S*,8a*S*)-3-methyl-1,4-dioxo-octahydropyrrolo[1,2-*a*]pyrazin-2-yl]-4-phenylbutanoate,

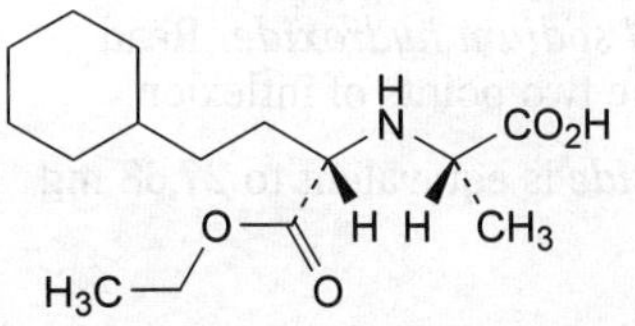

G. (2*S*)-2-[[(1*S*)-3-cyclohexyl-1-(ethoxycarbonyl)propyl]amino]propanoic acid,

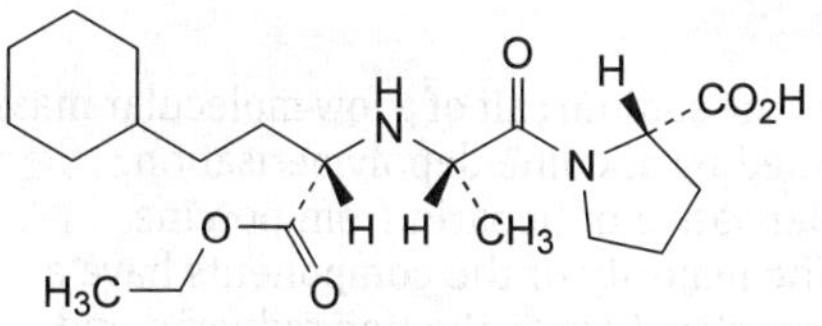

H. (2*S*)-1-[(2*S*)-2-[[(1*S*)-3-cyclohexyl-1-(ethoxycarbonyl)propyl]amino]propanoyl]pyrrolidine-2-carboxylic acid,

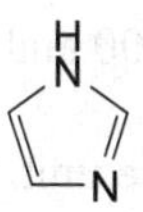

I. 1*H*-imidazole.

01/2005:1720

ENILCONAZOLE FOR VETERINARY USE

Enilconazolum ad usum veterinarium

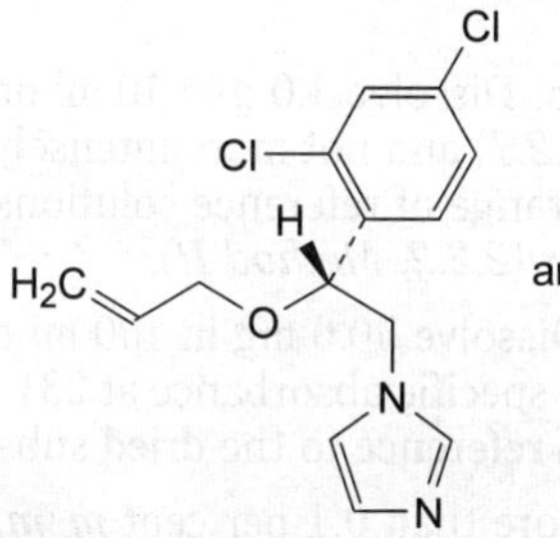

and enantiomer

$C_{14}H_{14}Cl_2N_2O$ M_r 297.2

DEFINITION

1-[(2*RS*)-2-(2,4-Dichlorophenyl)-2-(prop-2-enyloxy)ethyl]-1*H*-imidazole.

Content: 98.5 per cent to 101.5 per cent (dried substance).

CHARACTERS

Appearance: clear, yellowish, oily liquid or solid mass.

Solubility: very slightly soluble in water, freely soluble in alcohol, in methanol and in toluene.

IDENTIFICATION

Infrared absorption spectrophotometry (*2.2.24*).

Comparison: *enilconazole CRS*.

TESTS

Optical rotation (*2.2.7*): − 0.10° to + 0.10°.

Dissolve 0.1 g in *methanol R* and dilute to 10 ml with the same solvent.

Related substances. Gas chromatography (*2.2.28*). *Prepare the solutions immediately before use and protect from light.*

Test solution. Dissolve 0.100 g of the substance to be examined in *toluene R* and dilute to 100.0 ml with the same solvent.

Reference solution (a). Dissolve 10.0 mg of *enilconazole CRS* and 10.0 mg of *enilconazole impurity E CRS* in *toluene R* and dilute to 100.0 ml with the same solvent.

Reference solution (b). Dilute 5.0 ml of the test solution to 100.0 ml with *toluene R*. Dilute 1.0 ml of this solution to 10.0 ml with *toluene R*.

Column:

- *material*: fused silica,
- *size*: *l* = 25 m, Ø = 0.32 mm,
- *stationary phase*: chemically bonded *poly(dimethyl)(diphenyl)siloxane R* (film thickness 0.52 µm).

Carrier gas: *helium for chromatography R*.

Flow rate: 1.3 ml/min.

Split ratio: 1:38.

Temperature:

	Time (min)	**Temperature (°C)**
Column	0 - 6.4	100 → 260
	6.4 - 14	260
Injection port	-	250
Detector	-	300

Detection: flame ionisation.

Injection: 2 µl.

Relative retentions with reference to enilconazole (retention time = about 10 min): impurity A = about 0.6; impurity B = about 0.7; impurity C = about 0.8; impurity D = about 0.9; impurity F = about 1.1.

System suitability: reference solution (a):

- *resolution*: minimum 2.5 between the peaks due to enilconazole and impurity E.

Limits:

- *any impurity*: not more than twice the area of the principal peak in the chromatogram obtained with reference solution (b) (1.0 per cent), and not more than one such peak has an area greater than the area of the principal peak in the chromatogram obtained with reference solution (b) (0.5 per cent),
- *total*: not more than 4 times the area of the principal peak in the chromatogram obtained with reference solution (b) (2.0 per cent),
- *disregard limit*: 0.1 times the area of the principal peak in the chromatogram obtained with reference solution (b) (0.05 per cent).

Loss on drying (*2.2.32*): maximum 0.5 per cent, determined on 1.000 g by drying *in vacuo* at 40 °C for 4 h.

Sulphated ash (*2.4.14*): maximum 0.1 per cent, determined on 1.0 g.

ASSAY

Dissolve 0.230 g in 50 ml of a mixture of 1 volume of *anhydrous acetic acid R* and 7 volumes of *methyl ethyl ketone R*. Titrate with *0.1 M perchloric acid* using 0.2 ml of *naphtholbenzein solution R* as indicator.

1 ml of *0.1 M perchloric acid* is equivalent to 29.72 mg of $C_{14}H_{14}Cl_2N_2O$.

STORAGE

In an airtight container, protected from light.

IMPURITIES

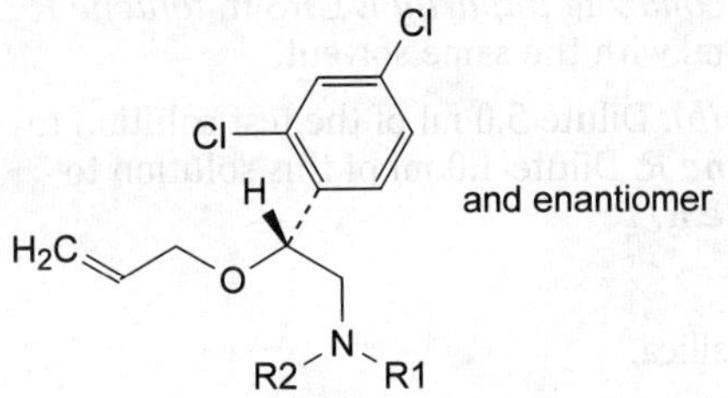

A. R1 = R2 = H: (2*RS*)-2-(2,4-dichlorophenyl)-2-(prop-2-enyloxy)ethanamine,

B. R1 = H, R2 = CH_2-CH=CH_2: *N*-[(2*RS*)-2-(2,4-dichlorophenyl)-2-(prop-2-enyloxy)ethyl]prop-2-en-1-amine,

C. R1 = CHO, R2 = H: *N*-[(2*RS*)-2-(2,4-dichlorophenyl)-2-(prop-2-enyloxy)ethyl]formamide,

D. R1 = CHO, R2 = CH_2-CH=CH_2: *N*-[(2*RS*)-2-(2,4-dichlorophenyl)-2-(prop-2-enyloxy)ethyl]-*N*-(prop-2-enyl)formamide,

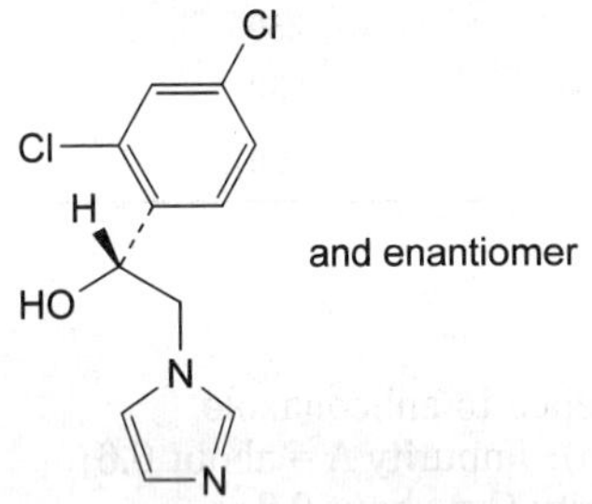

E. (1*RS*)-1-(2,4-dichlorophenyl)-2-(-1*H*-imidazol-1-yl)ethanol,

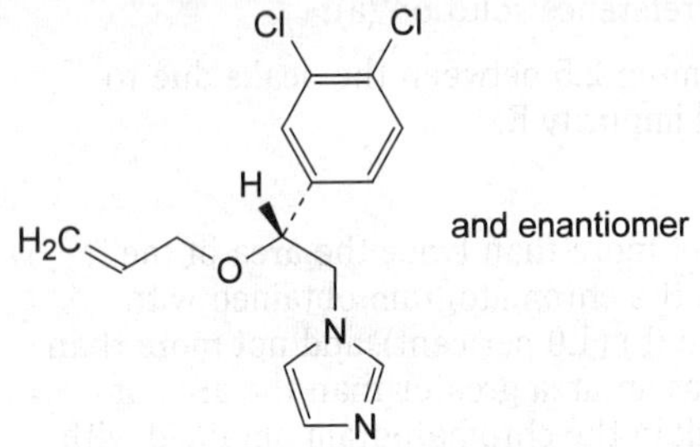

F. 1-[(2*RS*)-2-(3,4-dichlorophenyl)-2-(prop-2-enyloxy)ethyl]-1*H*-imidazole.

01/2005:1097

ENOXAPARIN SODIUM

Enoxaparinum natricum

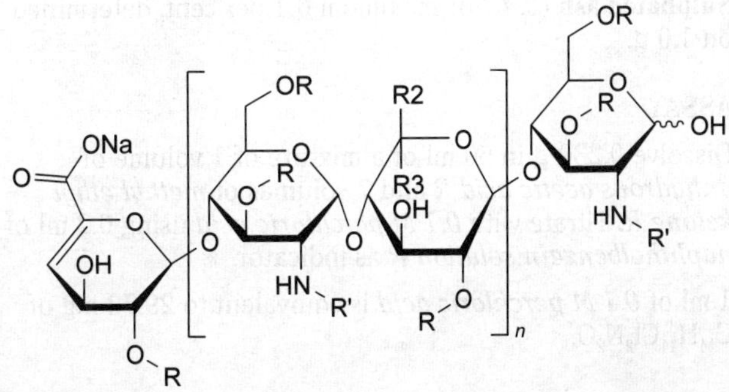

n = 1 to 21 , R = H or SO_3Na , R' = H or SO_3Na or CO-CH_3
R2 = H and R3 = CO_2Na or R2 = CO_2Na and R3 = H

DEFINITION

Enoxaparin sodium is the sodium salt of a low-molecular-mass heparin that is obtained by alkaline depolymerisation of the benzyl ester derivative of heparin from porcine intestinal mucosa. The majority of the components have a 4-enopyranose uronate structure at the non-reducing end of their chain.

Enoxaparin sodium complies with the monograph on Heparins, low-molecular-mass (0828) with the modifications and additional requirements below.

The mass-average molecular mass ranges between 3500 and 5500 with a characteristic value of about 4500.

The degree of sulphatation is about 2 per disaccharide unit.

The potency is not less than 90 IU and not more than 125 IU of anti-factor Xa activity per milligram, calculated with reference to the dried substance. The ratio of anti-factor Xa activity to anti-factor IIa activity is between 3.3 and 5.3.

IDENTIFICATION

Carry out identification test C as described in the monograph on *Heparins, low-molecular-mass (0828)*. The following requirements apply.

The mass-average molecular mass ranges between 3500 and 5500. The mass percentage of chains lower than 2000 ranges between 12.0 per cent and 20.0 per cent. The mass percentage of chains between 2000 and 8000 ranges between 68.0 per cent and 88.0 per cent.

TESTS

Appearance of solution. Dissolve 1.0 g in 10 ml of *water R*. The solution is clear (*2.2.1*) and not more intensely coloured than intensity 5 of the range of reference solutions of the most appropriate colour (*2.2.2, Method II*).

Absorbance (*2.2.25*). Dissolve 50.0 mg in 100 ml of *0.01 M hydrochloric acid*. The specific absorbance at 231 nm is 14.0 to 20.0, calculated with reference to the dried substance.

Benzyl alcohol. Not more than 0.1 per cent *m/m*, determined by liquid chromatography (*2.2.29*).

Internal standard solution. Prepare a 1 g/l solution of *3,4-dimethylphenol R* in *methanol R*.

Test solution. Dissolve about 0.500 g of the substance to be examined in 5.0 ml of *1 M sodium hydroxide*. Allow to stand for 1 h. Add 1.0 ml of *glacial acetic acid R* and 1.0 ml of the internal standard solution and dilute to 10.0 ml with *water R*.

Reference solution. Prepare a 0.25 g/l solution of *benzyl alcohol R* in *water R*. Mix 0.50 ml of this solution with 1.0 ml of the internal standard solution and dilute to 10.0 ml with *water R*.

The chromatographic procedure may be carried out using:

– a stainless steel column 0.15 m long and4.6 mm in internal diameter packed with *octylsilyl silica gel for chromatography R* (5 µm) equipped with a guard column 20 mm long and 4.6 mm in internal diameter, packed with the same material,

– as mobile phase at a flow rate of 1 ml/min a mixture of 5 volumes of *methanol R*, 15 volumes of *acetonitrile R* and 80 volumes of *water R*,

– as detector a spectrophotometer set at 256 nm.

From the chromatogram obtained with the reference solution, calculate the ratio (R_1) of the height of the peak due to benzyl alcohol to the height of the peak due to the internal standard. From the chromatogram obtained with the test solution, calculate the ratio (R_2) of the height of the peak due to benzyl alcohol to the height of the peak due to the internal standard.

Calculate the content (*m/m*) of benzyl alcohol from the following expression:

$$\frac{0.0125 \times R_2}{m \times R_1}$$

m = mass of the substance to be examined in grams.

Sodium. 11.3 to 13.5 per cent of Na calculated with reference to the dried substance and determined by atomic absorption spectrometry (*2.2.23, Method I*).

01/2005:1511

ENOXOLONE

Enoxolonum

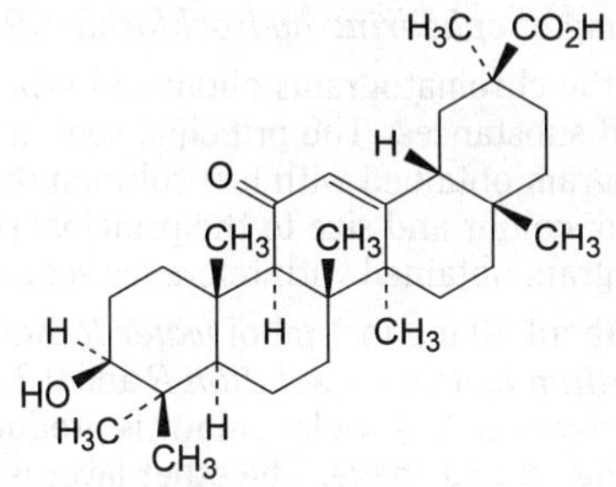

$C_{30}H_{46}O_4$ M_r 470.7

DEFINITION

(20β)-3β-Hydroxy-11-oxo-olean-12-en-29-oic acid.

Content: 98.0 per cent to 101.0 per cent (dried substance).

CHARACTERS

Appearance: white or almost white crystalline powder.

Solubility: practically insoluble in water, soluble in ethanol, sparingly soluble in methylene chloride.

It shows polymorphism.

IDENTIFICATION

First identification: A.

Second identification: B, C.

A. Examine by infrared absorption spectrophotometry (*2.2.24*).

Comparison: *enoxolone CRS.*

If the spectra obtained in the solid state show differences, dissolve 0.2 g of the substance to be examined and 0.2 g of the reference substance separately in 6 ml of *ethanol R.* Boil under a reflux condenser for 1 h and add 6 ml of *water R.* A precipitate is formed. Cool to about 10 °C and filter with the aid of vacuum. Wash the precipitate with 10 ml of *alcohol R,* dry in an oven at 80 °C and record new spectra.

B. Thin-layer chromatography (*2.2.27*).

Test solution. Dissolve 10 mg of the substance to be examined in *methylene chloride R* and dilute to 10 ml with the same solvent.

Reference solution. Dissolve 10 mg of *enoxolone CRS* in *methylene chloride R* and dilute to 10 ml with the same solvent.

Plate: *TLC silica gel plate R.*

Mobile phase: *glacial acetic acid R, acetone R, methylene chloride R (5:10:90 V/V/V).*

Application: 5 µl.

Development: over 2/3 of the plate.

Drying: in air for 5 min.

Detection: spray with *anisaldehyde solution R* and heat at 100-105 °C for 10 min.

Results: the principal spot in the chromatogram obtained with the test solution is similar in position, colour and size to the principal spot in the chromatogram obtained with the reference solution.

C. Dissolve 50 mg in 10 ml of *methylene chloride R.* To 2 ml of this solution, add 1 ml of *acetic anhydride R* and 0.3 ml of *sulphuric acid R.* A pink colour is produced.

TESTS

Appearance of solution. The solution is clear (*2.2.1*) and not more intensely coloured than reference solution Y_6 (*2.2.2, Method II*).

Dissolve 0.1 g in *ethanol R* and dilute to 10 ml with the same solvent.

Specific optical rotation (*2.2.7*): + 145 to + 154 (dried substance).

Dissolve 0.50 g in *dioxan R* and dilute to 50.0 ml with the same solvent.

Related substances. Liquid chromatography (*2.2.29*).

Test solution. Dissolve 0.10 g of the substance to be examined in the mobile phaseand dilute to 100.0 ml with the mobile phase.

Reference solution (a). Dilute 2.0 ml of the test solution to 100.0 ml with the mobile phase.

Reference solution (b). Dilute 5.0 ml of reference solution (a) to 100.0 ml with the mobile phase.

Reference solution (c). Dissolve 0.1 g of *18α-glycyrrhetinic acid R* in *tetrahydrofuran R* and dilute to 100.0 ml with the same solvent. To 2.0 ml of the solution, add 2.0 ml of the test solution and dilute to 100.0 ml with the mobile phase.

Column:

- *size*: *l* = 0.25 m, Ø = 4.6 mm,
- *stationary phase*: *octadecylsilyl silica gel for chromatography R* (5 µm),
- *temperature*: 30 °C.

Mobile phase: mix 430 volumes of *tetrahydrofuran R* and 570 volumes of a 1.36 g/l solution of *sodium acetate R* adjusted to pH 4.8 with *glacial acetic acid R.*

Flow rate: 0.8 ml/min.

Detection: spectrophotometer at 250 nm.

Injection: 20 µl loop injector; inject the test solution and the reference solutions.

Run time: 4 times the retention time of enoxolone.

System suitability:

- *resolution*: minimum of 2.0 between the peaks due to enoxolone and to 18α-glycyrrhetinic acid in the chromatogram obtained with reference solution (c).

Limits:

- *any impurity*: not more than 7 times the area of the principal peak in the chromatogram obtained with reference solution (b) (0.7 per cent),
- *total*: not more than the area of the principal peak in the chromatogram obtained with reference solution (a) (2.0 per cent),
- *disregard limit*: 0.5 times the area of the principal peak in the chromatogram obtained with reference solution (b) (0.05 per cent).

Heavy metals (*2.4.8*): maximum 20 ppm.

1.0 g complies with limit test F. Prepare the standard using 2 ml of *lead standard solution (10 ppm Pb) R.*

Monographs D-E

Loss on drying (*2.2.32*): maximum 0.5 per cent, determined on 1.000 g by drying in an oven at 100-105 °C for 4 h.

Sulphated ash (*2.4.14*): maximum 0.2 per cent, determined on 1.0 g.

ASSAY

Dissolve 0.330 g in 40 ml of *dimethylformamide R*. Titrate with *0.1 M tetrabutylammonium hydroxide*, determining the end-point potentiometrically (*2.2.20*). Carry out a blank titration.

1 ml of *0.1 M tetrabutylammonium hydroxide* is equivalent to 47.07 mg of $C_{30}H_{46}O_4$.

STORAGE

Protected from light.

IMPURITIES

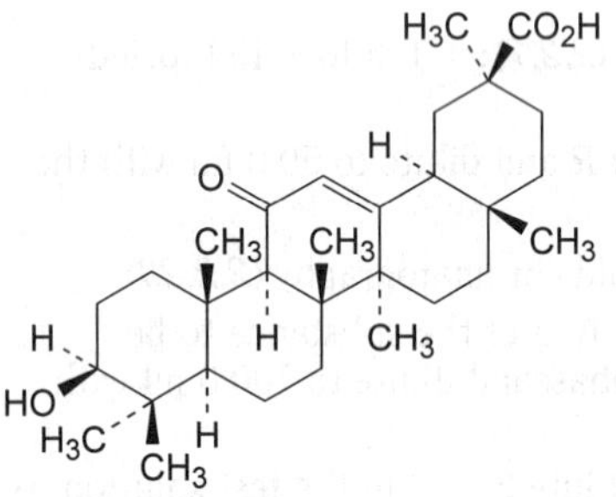

A. (20β)-3β-hydroxy-11-oxo-18α-olean-12-en-29-oic acid,

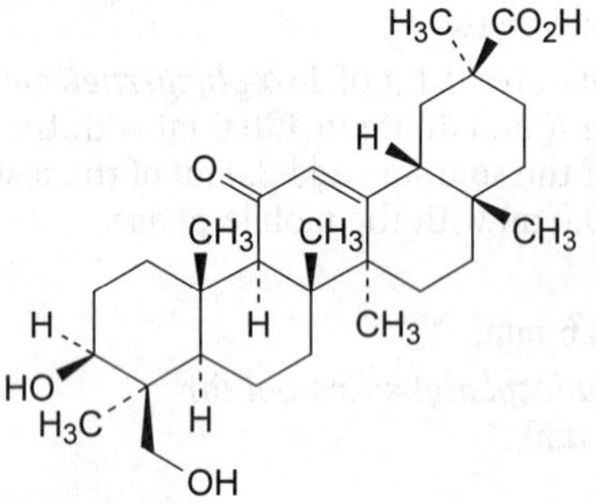

B. (4β,20β)-3β,23-dihydroxy-11-oxo-olean-12-en-29-oic acid.

01/2005:0488

EPHEDRINE, ANHYDROUS

Ephedrinum anhydricum

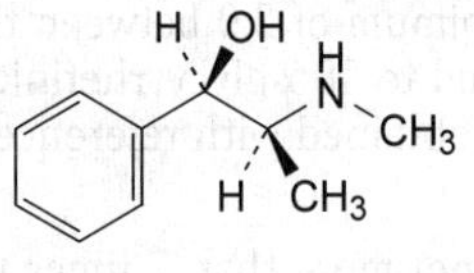

$C_{10}H_{15}NO$ M_r 165.2

DEFINITION

Anhydrous ephedrine contains not less than 99.0 per cent and not more than the equivalent of 101.0 per cent of (1*R*,2*S*)-2-methylamino-1-phenylpropan-1-ol, calculated with reference to the anhydrous substance.

CHARACTERS

A white, crystalline powder or colourless crystals, soluble in water, very soluble in alcohol.

It melts at about 36 °C.

IDENTIFICATION

First identification: B, D.

Second identification: A, C, D, E.

A. It complies with the test for specific optical rotation (see Tests).

B. Examine by infrared absorption spectrophotometry (*2.2.24*), comparing with the spectrum obtained with the base isolated from *ephedrine hydrochloride CRS*. Examine the substances in discs prepared as follows: dissolve 40 mg of the substance to be examined in 1 ml of *water R*, add 1 ml of *dilute sodium hydroxide solution R* and 4 ml of *chloroform R* and shake; dry the organic layer over 0.2 g of *anhydrous sodium sulphate R*; prepare a blank disc using about 0.3 g of *potassium bromide R*; apply dropwise to the disc 0.1 ml of the organic layer, allowing the solvent to evaporate between applications; dry the disc at 50 °C for 2 min. Repeat the operations using 50 mg of *ephedrine hydrochloride CRS*.

C. Examine the chromatograms obtained in the test for related substances. The principal spot in the chromatogram obtained with test solution (b) is similar in position, colour and size to the principal spot in the chromatogram obtained with reference solution (a).

D. Dissolve about 10 mg in 1 ml of *water R*. Add 0.2 ml of *strong sodium hydroxide solution R* and 0.2 ml of *copper sulphate solution R*. A violet colour is produced. Add 2 ml of *ether R* and shake. The ether layer is purple and the aqueous layer blue.

E. It complies with the test for water (see Tests).

TESTS

Appearance of solution. Dissolve 0.25 g in *water R* and dilute to 10 ml with the same solvent. The solution is clear (*2.2.1*) and colourless (*2.2.2, Method II*).

Specific optical rotation (*2.2.7*). Dissolve 2.25 g in 15 ml of *dilute hydrochloric acid R* and dilute to 50.0 ml with *water R*. The specific optical rotation is − 41 to − 43, calculated with reference to the anhydrous substance.

Related substances. Examine by thin-layer chromatography (*2.2.27*), using *silica gel G R* as the coating substance.

Test solution (a). Dissolve 0.2 g of the substance to be examined in *methanol R* and dilute to 10 ml with the same solvent.

Test solution (b). Dilute 1 ml of test solution (a) to 10 ml with *methanol R*.

Reference solution (a). Dissolve 25 mg of *ephedrine hydrochloride CRS* in *methanol R* and dilute to 10 ml with the same solvent.

Reference solution (b). Dilute 1.0 ml of test solution (a) to 200 ml with *methanol R*.

Apply separately to the plate 10 µl of each solution. Develop over a path of 15 cm using a mixture of 5 volumes of *chloroform R*, 15 volumes of *concentrated ammonia R* and 80 volumes of *2-propanol R*. Allow the plate to dry in air and spray with *ninhydrin solution R*. Heat at 110 °C for 5 min. Any spot in the chromatogram obtained with test solution (a), apart from the principal spot, is not more intense than the spot in the chromatogram obtained with reference solution (b) (0.5 per cent). Disregard any spot of lighter colour than the background.

Chlorides. Dissolve 0.17 g in 10 ml of *water R*. Add 5 ml of *dilute nitric acid R* and 0.5 ml of *silver nitrate solution R1*. Allow to stand for 2 min, protected from bright light. Any opalescence in the solution is not more intense than that in a standard prepared at the same time and in the same manner using 10 ml of *chloride standard solution (5 ppm Cl) R*, 5 ml of *dilute nitric acid R* and 0.5 ml of *silver nitrate solution R1* (290 ppm).

Water (*2.5.12*). Not more than 0.5 per cent, determined on 2.000 g by the semi-micro determination of water.

Sulphated ash (*2.4.14*). Not more than 0.1 per cent, determined on 1.0 g.

ASSAY

Dissolve 0.200 g in 5 ml of *alcohol R* and add 20.0 ml of *0.1 M hydrochloric acid*. Using 0.05 ml of *methyl red solution R* as indicator, titrate with *0.1 M sodium hydroxide* until a yellow colour is obtained.

1 ml of *0.1 M hydrochloric acid* is equivalent to 16.52 mg of $C_{10}H_{15}NO$.

STORAGE

Store protected from light.

01/2005:0489

EPHEDRINE HEMIHYDRATE

Ephedrinum hemihydricum

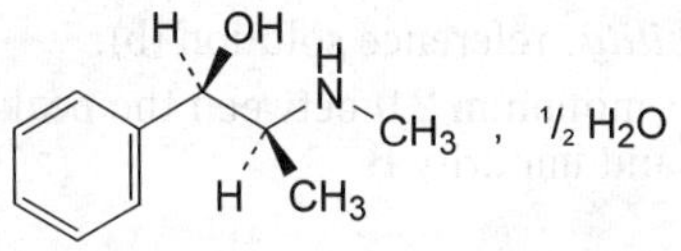

$C_{10}H_{15}NO,{}^1/_2H_2O$ M_r 174.2

DEFINITION

Ephedrine hemihydrate contains not less than 99.0 per cent and not more than the equivalent of 101.0 per cent of (1*R*,2*S*)-2-(methylamino)-1-phenylpropan-1-ol, calculated with reference to the anhydrous substance.

CHARACTERS

A white, crystalline powder or colourless crystals, soluble in water, very soluble in alcohol.

It melts at about 42 °C, determined without previous drying.

IDENTIFICATION

First identification: B, D.

Second identification: A, C, D, E.

A. It complies with the test for specific optical rotation (see Tests).

B. Examine by infrared absorption spectrophotometry (*2.2.24*), comparing with the spectrum obtained with the base isolated from *ephedrine hydrochloride CRS*. Examine the substances in discs prepared as follows: dissolve 40 mg of the substance to be examined in 1 ml of *water R*, add 1 ml of *dilute sodium hydroxide solution R* and 4 ml of *chloroform R* and shake; dry the organic layer over 0.2 g of *anhydrous sodium sulphate R*; prepare a blank disc using about 0.3 g of *potassium bromide R*; apply dropwise to the disc 0.1 ml of the organic layer, allowing the solvent to evaporate between applications; dry the disc at 50 °C for 2 min. Repeat the operations using 50 mg of *ephedrine hydrochloride CRS*.

C. Examine the chromatograms obtained in the test for related substances. The principal spot in the chromatogram obtained with test solution (b) is similar in position, colour and size to the principal spot in the chromatogram obtained with reference solution (a).

D. Dissolve about 10 mg in 1 ml of *water R*. Add 0.2 ml of *strong sodium hydroxide solution R* and 0.2 ml of *copper sulphate solution R*. A violet colour is produced. Add 2 ml of *ether R* and shake. The ether layer is purple and the aqueous layer blue.

E. It complies with the test for water (see Tests).

TESTS

Appearance of solution. Dissolve 0.25 g in *water R* and dilute to 10 ml with the same solvent. The solution is clear (*2.2.1*) and colourless (*2.2.2, Method II*).

Specific optical rotation (*2.2.7*). Dissolve 2.25 g in 15 ml of *dilute hydrochloric acid R* and dilute to 50.0 ml with *water R*. The specific optical rotation is − 41 to − 43, calculated with reference to the anhydrous substance.

Related substances. Examine by thin-layer chromatography (*2.2.27*), using *silica gel G R* as the coating substance.

Test solution (a). Dissolve 0.2 g of the substance to be examined in *methanol R* and dilute to 10 ml with the same solvent.

Test solution (b). Dilute 1 ml of test solution (a) to 10 ml with *methanol R*.

Reference solution (a). Dissolve 25 mg of *ephedrine hydrochloride CRS* in *methanol R* and dilute to 10 ml with the same solvent.

Reference solution (b). Dilute 1.0 ml of test solution (a) to 200 ml with *methanol R*.

Apply separately to the plate 10 µl of each solution. Develop over a path of 15 cm using a mixture of 5 volumes of *chloroform R*, 15 volumes of *concentrated ammonia R* and 80 volumes of *2-propanol R*. Allow the plate to dry in air and spray with *ninhydrin solution R*. Heat at 110 °C for 5 min. Any spot in the chromatogram obtained with test solution (a), apart from the principal spot, is not more intense than the spot in the chromatogram obtained with reference solution (b) (0.5 per cent). Disregard any spot of lighter colour than the background.

Chlorides. Dissolve 0.18 g in 10 ml of *water R*. Add 5 ml of *dilute nitric acid R* and 0.5 ml of *silver nitrate solution R1*. Allow to stand for 2 min, protected from bright light. Any opalescence in the solution is not more intense than that in a standard prepared at the same time and in the same manner using 10 ml of *chloride standard solution (5 ppm Cl) R*, 5 ml of *dilute nitric acid R* and 0.5 ml of *silver nitrate solution R1* (280 ppm).

Water (*2.5.12*): 4.5 per cent to 5.5 per cent, determined on 0.300 g by the semi-micro determination of water.

Sulphated ash (*2.4.14*). Not more than 0.1 per cent, determined on 1.0 g.

ASSAY

Dissolve 0.200 g in 5 ml of *alcohol R* and add 20.0 ml of *0.1 M hydrochloric acid*. Using 0.05 ml of *methyl red solution R* as indicator, titrate with *0.1 M sodium hydroxide* until a yellow colour is obtained.

1 ml of *0.1 M hydrochloric acid* is equivalent to 16.52 mg of $C_{10}H_{15}NO$.

STORAGE

Store protected from light.

01/2005:0487

EPHEDRINE HYDROCHLORIDE

Ephedrini hydrochloridum

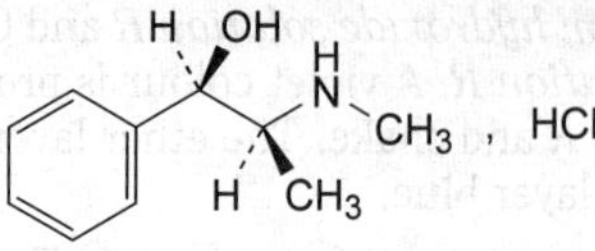

$C_{10}H_{16}ClNO$ M_r 201.7

DEFINITION

(1*R*,2*S*)-2-(Methylamino)-1-phenylpropan-1-ol hydrochloride.

Content: 99.0 per cent to 101.0 per cent (dried substance).

CHARACTERS

Appearance: white, crystalline powder or colourless crystals.

Solubility: freely soluble in water, soluble in alcohol.

mp: about 219 °C.

IDENTIFICATION

First identification: B, E.

Second identification: A, C, D, E.

A. Specific optical rotation (see Tests).

B. Infrared absorption spectrophotometry (*2.2.24*).
Comparison: *ephedrine hydrochloride CRS*.

C. Thin-layer chromatography (*2.2.27*).
Test solution. Dissolve 20 mg of the substance to be examined in *methanol R* and dilute to 10 ml with the same solvent.
Reference solution. Dissolve 10 mg of *ephedrine hydrochloride CRS* in *methanol R* and dilute to 5 ml with the same solvent.
Plate: *TLC silica gel plate R*.
Mobile phase: *methylene chloride R, concentrated ammonia R, 2-propanol R (5:15:80 V/V/V)*.
Application: 10 µl.
Development: over 2/3 of the plate.
Drying: in air.
Detection: spray with *ninhydrin solution R*; heat at 110 °C for 5 min.
Results: the principal spot in the chromatogram obtained with the test solution is similar in position, colour and size to the principal spot in the chromatogram obtained with the reference solution.

D. To 0.1 ml of solution S (see Tests) add 1 ml of *water R*, 0.2 ml of *copper sulphate solution R* and 1 ml of *strong sodium hydroxide solution R*. A violet colour is produced. Add 2 ml of *methylene chloride R* and shake. The lower (organic) layer is dark grey and the upper (aqueous) layer is blue.

E. To 5 ml of solution S (see Tests) add 5 ml of *water R*. The solution gives reaction (a) of chlorides (*2.3.1*).

TESTS

Solution S. Dissolve 5.00 g in *distilled water R* and dilute to 50.0 ml with the same solvent.

Appearance of solution. Solution S is clear (*2.2.1*) and colourless (*2.2.2, Method II*).

Acidity or alkalinity. To 10 ml of solution S add 0.1 ml of *methyl red solution R* and 0.2 ml of *0.01 M sodium hydroxide*. The solution is yellow. Add 0.4 ml of *0.01 M hydrochloric acid*. The solution is red.

Specific optical rotation (*2.2.7*): − 33.5 to − 35.5 (dried substance).

Dilute 12.5 ml of solution S to 25.0 ml with *water R*.

Related substances. Liquid chromatography (*2.2.29*).

Test solution. Dissolve 75 mg of the substance to be examined in the mobile phase and dilute to 10 ml with the mobile phase.

Reference solution (a). Dilute 2.0 ml of the test solution to 100.0 ml with the mobile phase. Dilute 1.0 ml of this solution to 10.0 ml with the mobile phase.

Reference solution (b). Dissolve 5 mg of the substance to be examined and 5 mg of *pseudoephedrine hydrochloride CRS* in the mobile phase and dilute to 50 ml with the mobile phase.

Column:
- *size*: l = 0.25 m, Ø = 4.6 mm,
- *stationary phase*: spherical *phenylsilyl silica gel for chromatography R* (5 µm).

Mobile phase: mix 6 volumes of *methanol R* and 94 volumes of a 11.6 g/l solution of *ammonium acetate R* adjusted to pH 4.0 with *glacial acetic acid R*.

Flow rate: 1.0 ml/min.

Detection: spectrophotometer at 257 nm.

Injection: 20 µl.

Run time: 2.5 times the retention time of ephedrine.

Relative retention with reference to ephedrine (retention time = about 8 min): impurity B = about 1.1; impurity A = about 1.4.

System suitability: reference solution (b):
- *resolution*: minimum 2.0 between the peaks due to ephedrine and impurity B.

Limits:
- *correction factor*: for the calculation of content, multiply the peak area of impurity A by 0.4,
- *impurity A*: not more than the area of the principal peak in the chromatogram obtained with reference solution (a) (0.2 per cent),
- *any other impurity*: for each impurity, not more than 0.5 times the area of the principal peak in the chromatogram obtained with reference solution (a) (0.1 per cent),
- *total of impurities other than A*: not more than 2.5 times the area of the principal peak in the chromatogram obtained with reference solution (a) (0.5 per cent),
- *disregard limit*: 0.25 times the area of the principal peak in the chromatogram obtained with reference solution (a) (0.05 per cent).

Sulphates (*2.4.13*): maximum 100 ppm, determined on 15 ml of solution S.

Loss on drying (*2.2.32*): maximum 0.5 per cent, determined on 1.000 g by drying in an oven at 100-105 °C.

Sulphated ash (*2.4.14*): maximum 0.1 per cent, determined on 1.0 g.

ASSAY

Dissolve 0.150 g in 50 ml of *alcohol R* and add 5.0 ml of *0.01 M hydrochloric acid*. Carry out a potentiometric titration (*2.2.20*), using *0.1 M sodium hydroxide*. Read the volume added between the 2 points of inflexion.

1 ml of *0.1 M sodium hydroxide* is equivalent to 20.17 mg of $C_{10}H_{16}ClNO$.

STORAGE

Protected from light.

IMPURITIES

Specified impurities: A.

Other detectable impurities: B.

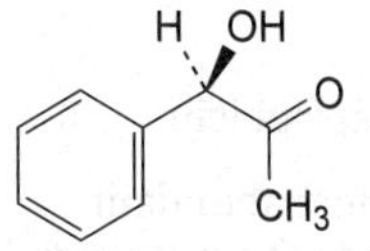

A. (−)-(1*R*)-1-hydroxy-1-phenylpropan-2-one,

B. pseudoephedrine.

01/2005:0715

EPHEDRINE HYDROCHLORIDE, RACEMIC

Ephedrini racemici hydrochloridum

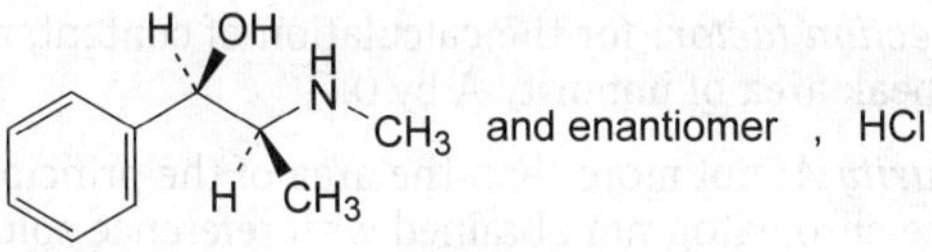

$C_{10}H_{16}ClNO$ M_r 201.7

DEFINITION

Racemic ephedrine hydrochloride contains not less than 99.0 per cent and not more than the equivalent of 101.0 per cent of (1*RS*,2*SR*)-2-(methylamino)-1-phenylpropan-1-ol hydrochloride, calculated with reference to the dried substance.

CHARACTERS

A white, crystalline powder or colourless crystals, freely soluble in water, soluble in alcohol.

It melts at about 188 °C.

IDENTIFICATION

First identification: B, E.

Second identification: A, C, D, E.

A. It complies with the test for angle of optical rotation (see Tests).

B. Examine by infrared absorption spectrophotometry (*2.2.24*), comparing with the spectrum obtained with *racemic ephedrine hydrochloride CRS.* Examine the substances prepared as discs.

C. Examine the chromatograms obtained in the test for related substances. The principal spot in the chromatogram obtained with test solution (b) is similar in position, colour and size to the principal spot in the chromatogram obtained with reference solution (a).

D. To 0.1 ml of solution S (see Tests) add 1 ml of *water R*, 0.2 ml of *copper sulphate solution R* and 1 ml of *strong sodium hydroxide solution R*. A violet colour is produced. Add 2 ml of *ether R* and shake. The ether layer is purple and the aqueous layer is blue.

E. To 5 ml of solution S add 5 ml of *water R*. The solution gives reaction (a) of chlorides (*2.3.1*).

TESTS

Solution S. Dissolve 5.00 g in *distilled water R* and dilute to 50.0 ml with the same solvent.

Appearance of solution. Solution S is clear (*2.2.1*) and colourless (*2.2.2, Method II*).

Acidity or alkalinity. To 10 ml of solution S add 0.1 ml of *methyl red solution R* and 0.1 ml of *0.01 M sodium hydroxide*; the solution is yellow. Add 0.2 ml of *0.01 M hydrochloric acid*; the solution is red.

Angle of optical rotation (*2.2.7*): + 0.2° to − 0.2°, determined on solution S.

Related substances. Examine by thin-layer chromatography (*2.2.27*), using *silica gel G R* as the coating substance.

Test solution (a). Dissolve 0.20 g of the substance to be examined in *methanol R* and dilute to 10 ml with the same solvent.

Test solution (b). Dilute 1 ml of test solution (a) to 10 ml with *methanol R.*

Reference solution (a). Dissolve 20 mg of *racemic ephedrine hydrochloride CRS* in *methanol R* and dilute to 10 ml with the same solvent.

Reference solution (b). Dilute 1 ml of test solution (a) to 200 ml with *methanol R.*

Apply separately to the plate 10 µl of each solution. Develop over a path of 15 cm using a mixture of 5 volumes of *chloroform R*, 15 volumes of *concentrated ammonia R* and 80 volumes of *2-propanol R*. Allow the plate to dry in air. Spray with *ninhydrin solution R* and heat at 110 °C for 5 min. Any spot in the chromatogram obtained with test solution (a), apart from the principal spot, is not more intense than the spot in the chromatogram obtained with reference solution (b) (0.5 per cent). Disregard any spot of lighter colour than the background.

Sulphates (*2.4.13*). 15 ml of solution S complies with the limit test for sulphates (100 ppm).

Loss on drying (*2.2.32*). Not more than 0.5 per cent, determined on 1.000 g by drying in an oven at 100 °C to 105 °C.

Sulphated ash (*2.4.14*). Not more than 0.1 per cent, determined on 1.0 g.

ASSAY

Dissolve 0.170 g in 30 ml of *alcohol R*. Add 5.0 ml of *0.01 M hydrochloric acid.* Carry out a potentiometric titration (*2.2.20*), using *0.1 M sodium hydroxide*. Read the volume added between the two points of inflexion.

1 ml of *0.1 M sodium hydroxide* corresponds to 20.17 mg of $C_{10}H_{16}ClNO$.

STORAGE

Store protected from light.

01/2005:1590

EPIRUBICIN HYDROCHLORIDE

Epirubicini hydrochloridum

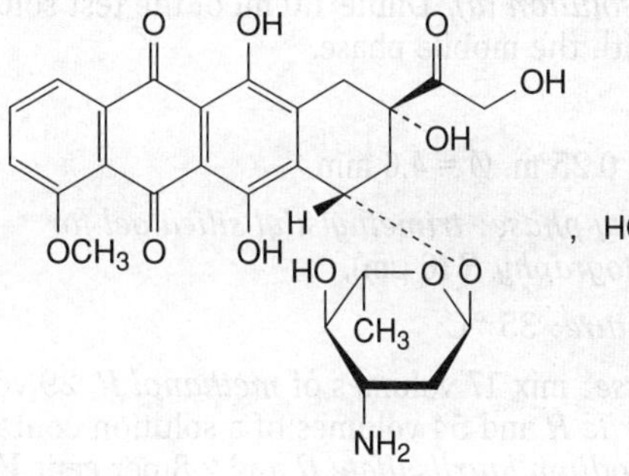

$C_{27}H_{30}ClNO_{11}$ M_r 580.0

DEFINITION

(8*S*,10*S*)-10-[(3-Amino-2,3,6-trideoxy-α-L-*arabino*-hexopyranosyl)oxy]-6,8,11-trihydroxy-8-(hydroxyacetyl)-1-methoxy-7,8,9,10-tetrahydrotetracene-5,12-dione hydrochloride.

Substance obtained by chemical transformation of a substance produced by certain strains of *Streptomyces peucetius*.

Content: 97.0 per cent to 102.0 per cent (anhydrous and acetone-free substance).

CHARACTERS

Appearance: orange-red powder.

Solubility: soluble in water and in methanol, slightly soluble in anhydrous ethanol, practically insoluble in acetone.

IDENTIFICATION

A. Infrared absorption spectrophotometry (*2.2.24*).

Comparison: *epirubicin hydrochloride CRS.*

B. Examine the chromatograms obtained in the assay.

Results: the principal peak in the chromatogram obtained with the test solution is similar in retention time to the principal peak in the chromatogram obtained with reference solution (a).

C. Dissolve about 10 mg in 0.5 ml of *nitric acid R*, add 0.5 ml of *water R* and heat over a flame for 2 min. Allow to cool and add 0.5 ml of *silver nitrate solution R1.* A white precipitate is formed.

TESTS

pH (*2.2.3*): 4.0 to 5.5.

Dissolve 50 mg in *carbon dioxide-free water R* and dilute to 10 ml with the same solvent.

Related substances. Liquid chromatography (*2.2.29*).

Test solution. Dissolve 25.0 mg of the substance to be examined in the mobile phase and dilute to 25.0 ml with the mobile phase.

Reference solution (a). Dissolve 25.0 mg of *epirubicin hydrochloride CRS* in the mobile phase and dilute to 25.0 ml with the mobile phase.

Reference solution (b). Dissolve 10 mg of *epirubicin hydrochloride CRS* and 10 mg of *doxorubicin hydrochloride CRS* in the mobile phase and dilute to 100 ml with the mobile phase.

Reference solution (c). Dissolve 10 mg of *doxorubicin hydrochloride CRS* in a mixture of 5 ml of *water R* and 5 ml of *phosphoric acid R.* Allow to stand for 30 min. Adjust to pH 2.6 with an 80 g/l solution of *sodium hydroxide R.* Add 15 ml of *acetonitrile R* and 10 ml of *methanol R.* Mix.

Reference solution (d). Dilute 1.0 ml of the test solution to 100.0 ml with the mobile phase.

Column:

- *size*: *l* = 0.25 m, Ø = 4.6 mm,
- *stationary phase*: *trimethylsilyl silica gel for chromatography R* (6 μm),
- *temperature*: 35 °C.

Mobile phase: mix 17 volumes of *methanol R*, 29 volumes of *acetonitrile R* and 54 volumes of a solution containing 3.7 g/l of *sodium laurilsulfate R* and 2.8 per cent *V/V* of *dilute phosphoric acid R.*

Flow rate: 2.5 ml/min.

Detection: spectrophotometer at 254 nm.

Injection: 10 μl of the test solution and reference solutions (b), (c) and (d).

Run time: 3.5 times the retention time of epirubicin.

Identification of impurities: use the 2nd most abundant peak present in the chromatogram obtained with reference solution (c) to identify impurity A.

Relative retention with reference to epirubicin (retention time = about 9.5 min): impurity A = about 0.3; impurity B = about 0.4; impurity C = about 0.8; impurity E = about 1.1; impurity D = about 1.5; impurity F = about 1.7; impurity G = about 2.1.

System suitability: reference solution (b):

- *resolution*: minimum 2.0 between the peaks due to impurity C and epirubicin.

Limits:

- *correction factor*: for the calculation of content, multiply the peak area of impurity A by 0.7,
- *impurity A*: not more than the area of the principal peak in the chromatogram obtained with reference solution (d) (1.0 per cent),
- *impurity C*: not more than the area of the principal peak in the chromatogram obtained with reference solution (d) (1.0 per cent),
- *any other impurity*: for each impurity, not more than 0.5 times the area of the principal peak in the chromatogram obtained with reference solution (d) (0.5 per cent),
- *total*: not more than twice the area of the principal peak in the chromatogram obtained with reference solution (d) (2.0 per cent),
- *disregard limit*: 0.05 times the area of the principal peak in the chromatogram obtained with reference solution (d) (0.05 per cent).

Acetone (*2.4.24*): maximum 1.5 per cent.

Water (*2.5.12*): maximum 4.0 per cent, determined on 0.100 g.

Bacterial endotoxins (*2.6.14*): less than 1.1 IU/mg, if intended for use in the manufacture of parenteral dosage forms without a further appropriate procedure for removal of bacterial endotoxins.

ASSAY

Liquid chromatography (*2.2.29*) as described in the test for related substances with the following modification.

Injection: test solution and reference solution (a).

Calculate the percentage content of $C_{27}H_{30}ClNO_{11}$.

STORAGE

In an airtight container, protected from light, at a temperature of 2 °C to 8 °C. If the substance is sterile, store in a sterile, airtight, tamper-proof container.

LABELLING

The label states, where applicable, that the substance is free from bacterial endotoxins.

IMPURITIES

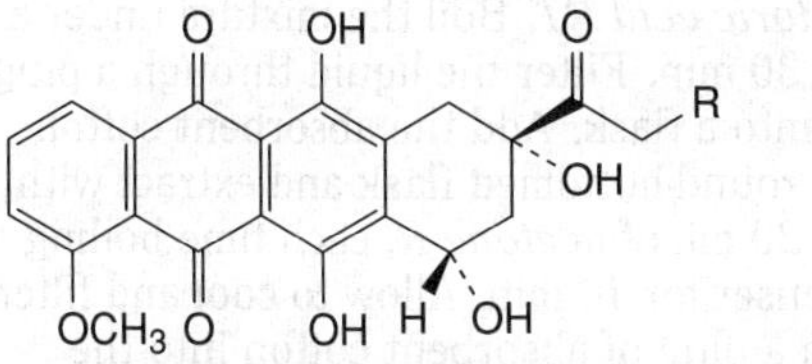

A. R = OH: (8*S*,10*S*)-6,8,10,11-tetrahydroxy-8-(hydroxyacetyl)-1-methoxy-7,8,9,10-tetrahydrotetracene-5,12-dione (doxorubicinone),

B. R = H: (8*S*,10*S*)-8-acetyl-6,8,10,11-tetrahydroxy-1-methoxy-7,8,9,10-tetrahydrotetracene-5,12-dione (daunorubicinone),

C. doxorubicin,

D. daunorubicin,

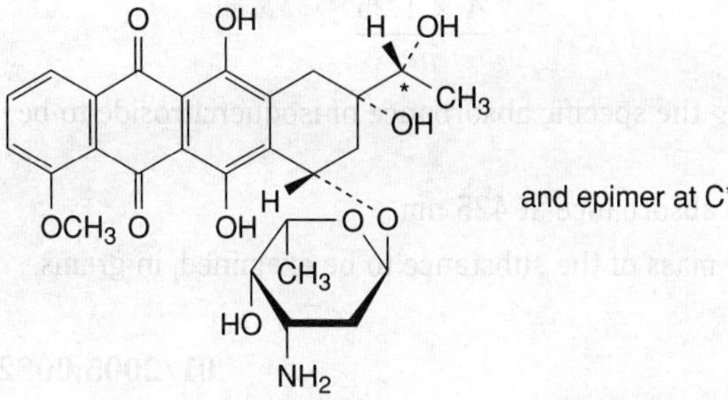

E. (8*S*,10*S*)-10-[(3-amino-2,3,6-trideoxy-α-L-*lyxo*-hexopyranosyl)oxy]-6,8,11-trihydroxy-8-[(1*RS*)-1-hydroxyethyl]-1-methoxy-7,8,9,10-tetrahydrotetracene-5,12-dione (dihydrodaunorubicin),

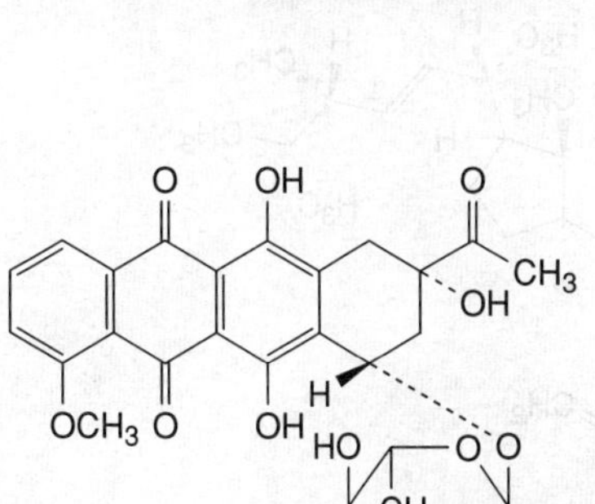

F. (8*S*,10*S*)-8-acetyl-10-[(3-amino-2,3,6-trideoxy-α-L-*arabino*-hexopyranosyl)oxy]-6,8,11-trihydroxy-1-methoxy-7,8,9,10-tetrahydrotetracene-5,12-dione (*epi*-daunorubicin),

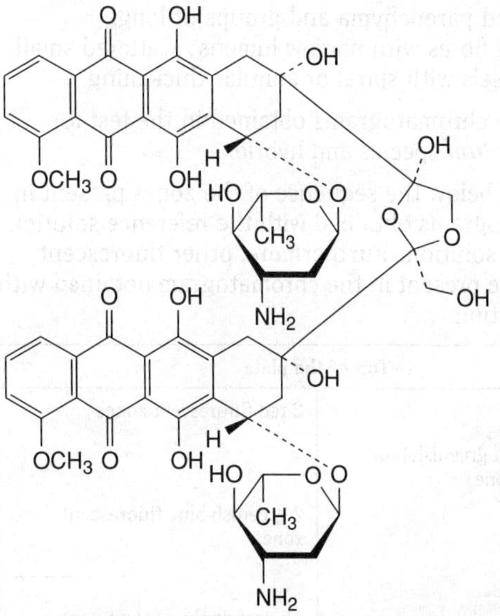

G. 8,8′-[(2*R*,4*R*)-4-hydroxy-2-(hydroxymethyl)-1,3-dioxolan-2,4-diyl]bis[(8*S*,10*S*)-10-[(3-amino-2,3,6-trideoxy-α-L-*arabino*-hexopyranosyl)oxy]-6,8,11-trihydroxy-1-methoxy-7,8,9,10-tetrahydrotetracene-5,12-dione] (epirubicin dimer).

01/2005:1825

EQUISETUM STEM

Equiseti herba

DEFINITION

Whole or cut, dried sterile aerial parts of *Equisetum arvense* L.

Content: minimum 0.3 per cent of total flavonoids expressed as isoquercitroside ($C_{21}H_{20}O_{12}$; M_r 464.4) (dried drug).

CHARACTERS

Macroscopic and microscopic characters described under identification tests A and B.

IDENTIFICATION

A. It consists of fragments of grooved stems and linear leaves, light green to greenish-grey. They are rough to the touch, brittle and crunchy when crushed. The main stems are about 0.8 mm to 4.5 mm in diameter, hollow, jointed at the nodes which occur at intervals of about 1.5 cm to 4.5 cm; distinct vertical grooves are present on the internodes, ranging in number from 4 to 14 or more. Verticils of widely spaced and erect branches, usually simple, each about 1 mm thick with 2 to 4 longitudinal grooves, occur at the nodes. The leaves are small, linear, verticillate at each node, concrescent at the base, they form a toothed sheath around the stem; with the number of teeth corresponding to the number of grooves on the stem. Each tooth, often brown, is lanceolate-triangular. The lowest internode of each branch is longer than the sheath of the stem it belongs to.

B. Reduce to a powder (355). The powder is greenish-grey. Examine under a microscope using *chloral hydrate solution R*. The powder shows the following diagnostic characters: fragments of the epidermis in surface view, composed of rectangular cells with wavy walls and paracytic stomata (*2.8.3*) with the 2 subsidiary cells covering the guard cells and having conspicuous radial ridges; in transverse sectional view the epidermis is crenate, with the protuberances formed from the contiguous walls of 2 adjacent, U-shaped cells. Fragments

Monographs D-E

of large-celled parenchyma and groups of long, non-lignified fibres with narrow lumens; scattered small, lignified vessels with spiral or annular thickening.

C. Examine the chromatograms obtained in the test for other *Equisetum* species and hybrids.

Results: see below the sequence of the zones present in the chromatograms obtained with the reference solution and the test solution. Furthermore, other fluorescent zones may be present in the chromatogram obtained with the test solution.

Top of the plate	
	2 red fluorescent zones
Caffeic acid: a greenish-blue fluorescent zone	
	2 greenish-blue fluorescent zones
_______	_______
	An orange fluorescent zone
Hyperoside: an orange fluorescent zone	
	2 greenish-blue fluorescent zones
_______	_______
Rutin: an orange fluorescent zone	
Reference solution	**Test solution**

TESTS

Foreign matter (*2.8.2*): maximum 5 per cent of stems from other *Equisetum* species and hybrids and maximum 2 per cent of other foreign matter.

Other *Equisetum* species and hybrids. Thin-layer chromatography (*2.2.27*).

Test solution. To 1.0 g of the powdered drug (355) add 10 ml of *methanol R*. Heat in a water-bath at 60 °C for 10 min with occasional shaking. Allow to cool. Filter.

Reference solution. Dissolve 1.0 mg of *caffeic acid R*, 2.5 mg of *hyperoside R* and 2.5 mg of *rutin R* in 10 ml of *methanol R*.

Plate: *TLC silica gel plate R*.

Mobile phase: *anhydrous formic acid R, glacial acetic acid R, water R, ethyl acetate R* (7.5:7.5:18:67 *V/V/V/V*).

Application: 10 µl, as bands.

Development: over a path of 10 cm.

Drying: at 100-105 °C.

Detection: spray the warm plate with a 10 g/l solution of *diphenylboric acid aminoethyl ester R* in *methanol R*. Then spray with a 50 g/l solution of *macrogol 400 R* in *methanol R*. Allow the plate to dry in air for 30 min. Examine in ultraviolet light at 365 nm.

Results: the chromatogram obtained with the test solution shows no yellow or greenish-yellow fluorescent zone shortly above the starting line.

Loss on drying (*2.2.32*): maximum 10 per cent, determined on 1.000 g of the powdered drug (355) by drying in an oven at 100-105 °C for 2 h.

Ash insoluble in hydrochloric acid (*2.8.1*): minimum 3.0 per cent and maximum 15.0 per cent.

Total ash (*2.4.16*): minimum 12.0 per cent and maximum 27.0 per cent.

ASSAY

Stock solution. In a 100 ml round-bottomed flask, introduce 0.800 g of the powdered drug (355), add 1 ml of a 5 g/l solution of *hexamethylenetetramine R*, 20 ml of *acetone R* and 2 ml of *hydrochloric acid R1*. Boil the mixture under a reflux condenser for 30 min. Filter the liquid through a plug of absorbent cotton into a flask. Add the absorbent cotton to the residue in the round-bottomed flask and extract with 2 quantities, each of 20 ml, of *acetone R*, each time boiling under a reflux condenser for 10 min. Allow to cool and filter each extract through a plug of absorbent cotton into the flask. After cooling, filter the combined acetone extracts through a filter paper into a volumetric flask and dilute to 100.0 ml with *acetone R* by rinsing the flask and the filter paper. Introduce 20.0 ml of the solution into a separating funnel, add 20 ml of *water R* and shake the mixture with 1 quantity of 15 ml and then 3 quantities, each of 10 ml, of *ethyl acetate R*. Combine the ethyl acetate extracts in a separating funnel, wash with 2 quantities, each of 50 ml, of *water R*, and filter the extracts over 10 g of *anhydrous sodium sulphate R* into a volumetric flask. Dilute to 50.0 ml with *ethyl acetate R*.

Test solution. To 10.0 ml of the stock solution add 1 ml of *aluminium chloride reagent R* and dilute to 25.0 ml with a 5 per cent *V/V* solution of *glacial acetic acid R* in *methanol R*.

Compensation solution. Dilute 10.0 ml of the stock solution to 25.0 ml with a 5 per cent *V/V* solution of *glacial acetic acid R* in *methanol R*.

Measure the absorbance (*2.2.25*) of the test solution after 30 min, by comparison with the compensation solution at 425 nm. Calculate the percentage content of flavonoids, calculated as isoquercitroside, from the expression:

$$\frac{A \times 1.25}{m}$$

i.e. taking the specific absorbance of isoquercitroside to be 500,

A = absorbance at 425 nm,

m = mass of the substance to be examined, in grams.

01/2005:0082

ERGOCALCIFEROL

Ergocalciferolum

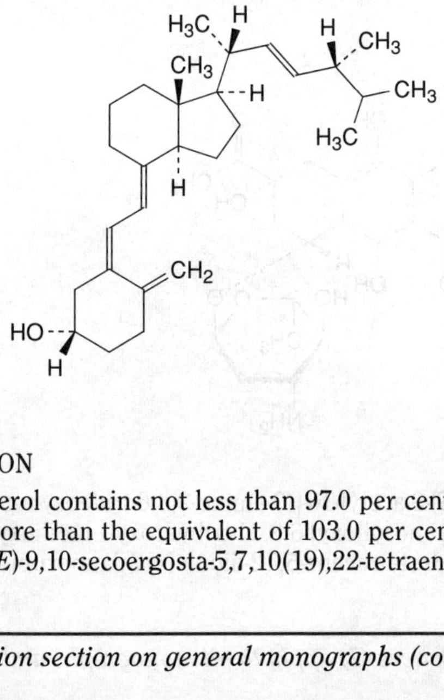

$C_{28}H_{44}O$ M_r 396.7

DEFINITION

Ergocalciferol contains not less than 97.0 per cent and not more than the equivalent of 103.0 per cent of (5*Z*,7*E*,22*E*)-9,10-secoergosta-5,7,10(19),22-tetraen-3β-ol.

1 mg of ergocalciferol is equivalent to 40 000 IU of antirachitic activity (vitamin D) in rats.

CHARACTERS

A white or slightly yellowish, crystalline powder or white or almost white crystals, practically insoluble in water, freely soluble in alcohol, soluble in fatty oils. It is sensitive to air, heat and light. Solutions in volatile solvents are unstable and are to be used immediately.

A reversible isomerisation to pre-ergocalciferol takes place in solution, depending on temperature and time. The activity is due to both compounds.

IDENTIFICATION

Examine by infrared absorption spectrophotometry (*2.2.24*), comparing with the spectrum obtained with *ergocalciferol CRS*. Examine the substances prepared as discs.

TESTS

Specific optical rotation (*2.2.7*). Dissolve 0.200 g rapidly and without heating in *aldehyde-free alcohol R* and dilute to 25.0 ml with the same solvent. The specific optical rotation, determined within 30 min of preparing the solution, is + 103 to + 107.

Reducing substances. Dissolve 0.1 g in *aldehyde-free alcohol R* and dilute to 10.0 ml with the same solvent. Add 0.5 ml of a 5 g/l solution of *tetrazolium blue R* in *aldehyde-free alcohol R* and 0.5 ml of *dilute tetramethylammonium hydroxide solution R*. Allow to stand for exactly 5 min and add 1.0 ml of *glacial acetic acid R*. Prepare a reference solution at the same time and in the same manner using 10.0 ml of a solution containing 0.2 µg/ml of *hydroquinone R* in *aldehyde-free alcohol R*. Measure the absorbance (*2.2.25*) of the two solutions at 525 nm using as the compensation liquid 10.0 ml of *aldehyde-free alcohol R* treated in the same manner. The absorbance of the test solution is not greater than that of the reference solution (20 ppm).

Ergosterol. Examine by thin-layer chromatography (*2.2.27*), using a *TLC silica gel G plate R*.

Test solution. Dissolve 0.25 g of the substance to be examined in *ethylene chloride R* containing 10 g/l of *squalane R* and 0.1 g/l of *butylhydroxytoluene R* and dilute to 5 ml with the same solvent. Prepare immediately before use.

Reference solution (a). Dissolve 0.10 g of *ergocalciferol CRS* in *ethylene chloride R* containing 10 g/l of *squalane R* and 0.1 g/l of *butylhydroxytoluene R* and dilute to 2 ml with the same solvent. Prepare immediately before use.

Reference solution (b). Dissolve 5 mg of *ergosterol CRS* in *ethylene chloride R* containing 10 g/l of *squalane R* and 0.1 g/l of *butylhydroxytoluene R* and dilute to 50 ml with the same solvent. Prepare immediately before use.

Reference solution (c). Mix equal volumes of reference solution (a) and reference solution (b). Prepare immediately before use.

Apply to the plate 10 µl of the test solution, 10 µl of reference solution (a), 10 µl of reference solution (b) and 20 µl of reference solution (c). Develop immediately, protected from light, over a path of 15 cm using a mixture of equal volumes of *cyclohexane R* and *peroxide-free ether R*, the mixture containing 0.1 g/l of *butylhydroxytoluene R*. Allow the plate to dry in air and spray three times with *antimony trichloride solution R1*. Examine the chromatograms for 3 min to 4 min after spraying. The principal spot in the chromatogram obtained with the test solution is initially orange-yellow and then becomes brown. In the chromatogram obtained with the test solution, any slowly appearing violet spot (corresponding to ergosterol) immediately below the principal spot is not more intense than the spot in the chromatogram obtained with reference solution (b) (0.2 per cent). There is no spot in the chromatogram obtained with the test solution that does not correspond to one of the spots in the chromatograms obtained with reference solutions (a) and (b). The test is not valid unless the chromatogram obtained with reference solution (c) shows two clearly separated spots.

ASSAY

Carry out the operations as rapidly as possible, avoiding exposure to actinic light and air.

Examine by liquid chromatography (*2.2.29*).

Test solution. Dissolve 10.0 mg of the substance to be examined without heating in 10.0 ml of *toluene R* and dilute to 100.0 ml with the mobile phase.

Reference solution (a). Dissolve 10.0 mg of *ergocalciferol CRS* without heating in 10.0 ml of *toluene R* and dilute to 100.0 ml with the mobile phase.

Reference solution (b). Dilute 1.0 ml of *cholecalciferol for performance test CRS* to 5.0 ml with the mobile phase. Heat in a water-bath at 90 °C under a reflux condenser for 45 min and cool.

The chromatographic procedure may be carried out using:

- a stainless steel column 0.25 m long and 4.6 mm in internal diameter packed with a suitable silica gel (5 µm),
- as mobile phase at a flow rate of 2 ml/min a mixture of 3 volumes of *pentanol R* and 997 volumes of *hexane R*,
- as detector a spectrophotometer set at 254 nm.

An automatic injection device or a sample loop is recommended. Inject a suitable volume of reference solution (b). Adjust the sensitivity of the system so that the height of the principal peak is at least 50 per cent of the full scale of the recorder. Inject reference solution (b) 6 times. When the chromatograms are recorded in the prescribed conditions, the approximate relative retention times with reference to cholecalciferol are 0.4 for pre-cholecalciferol and 0.5 for *trans*-cholecalciferol. The relative standard deviation of the response for cholecalciferol is not greater than 1 per cent and the resolution between the peaks corresponding to pre-cholecalciferol and *trans*-cholecalciferol is not less than 1.0. If necessary adjust the proportions of the constituents and the flow rate of the mobile phase to obtain this resolution.

Inject a suitable volume of reference solution (a). Adjust the sensitivity of the system so that the height of the principal peak is at least 50 per cent of the full scale of the recorder. Inject the same volume of the test solution and record the chromatogram in the same manner.

Calculate the percentage content of ergocalciferol from the expression:

$$\frac{m'}{m} \times \frac{S_D}{S'_D} \times 100$$

m = mass of the substance to be examined in the test solution, in milligrams,

m' = mass of *ergocalciferol CRS* in reference solution (a), in milligrams,

S_D = area (or height) of the peak due to ergocalciferol in the chromatogram obtained with the test solution,

S'_D = area (or height) of the peak due to ergocalciferol in the chromatogram obtained with reference solution (a).

STORAGE

Store in an airtight container, under nitrogen, protected from light, at a temperature between 2 °C and 8 °C.

The contents of an opened container are to be used immediately.

IMPURITIES

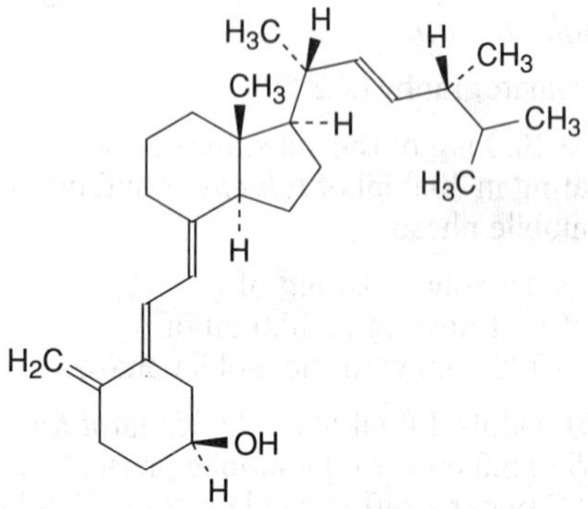

A. (5*E*,7*E*,22*E*)-9,10-secoergosta-5,7,10(19),22-tetraen-3β-ol (*trans*-vitamin D_2),

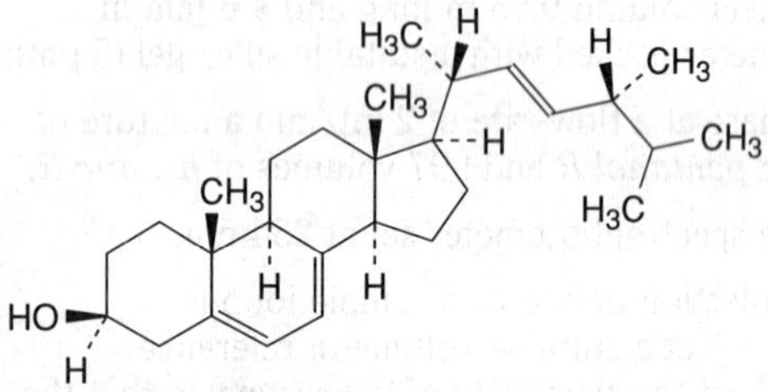

B. (22*E*)-ergosta-5,7,22-trien-3β-ol (ergosterol),

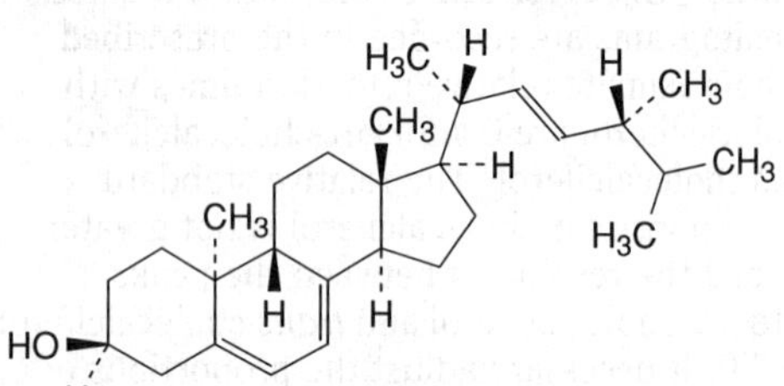

C. (9β,10α,22*E*)-ergosta-5,7,22-trien-3β-ol (lumisterol$_2$),

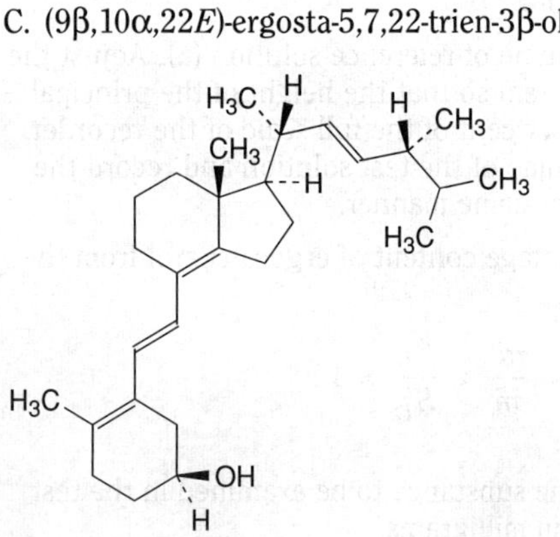

D. (6*E*,22*E*)-9,10-secoergosta-5(10),6,8(14),22-tetraen-3β-ol (iso-tachysterol$_2$),

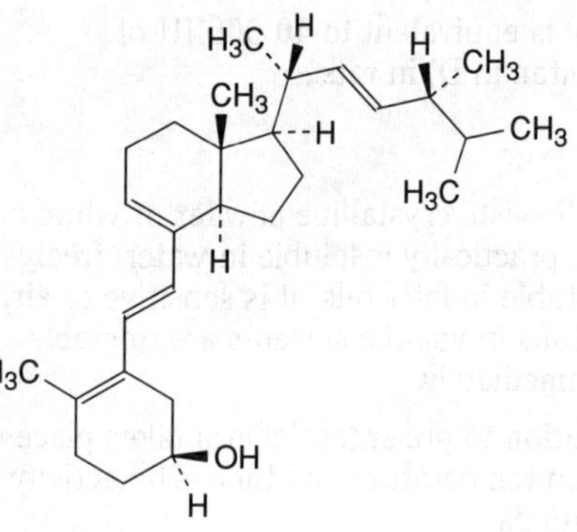

E. (6*E*,22*E*)-9,10-secoergosta-5(10),6,8,22-tetraen-3β-ol (tachysterol$_2$).

01/2005:0223

ERGOMETRINE MALEATE

Ergometrini maleas

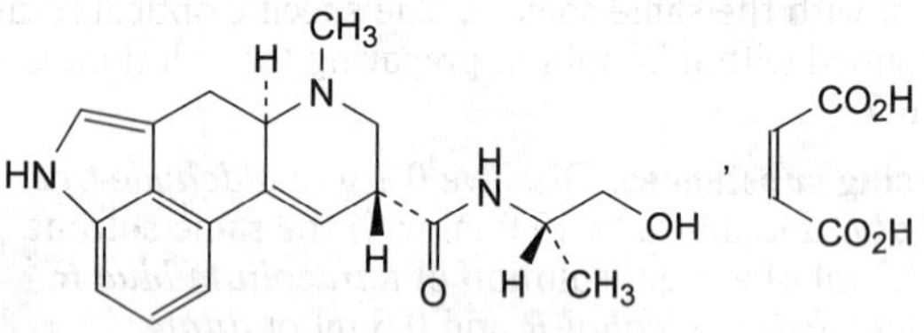

$C_{23}H_{27}N_3O_6$ M_r 441.5

DEFINITION

Ergometrine maleate contains not less than 98.0 per cent and not more than the equivalent of 101.0 per cent of (6a*R*,9*R*)-*N*-[(*S*)-2-hydroxy-1-methylethyl]-7-methyl-4,6,6a,7,8,9-hexahydro-indolo[4,3-*fg*]quinoline-9-carboxamide maleate, calculated with reference to the dried substance.

CHARACTERS

A white or slightly coloured, crystalline powder, sparingly soluble in water, slightly soluble in alcohol.

IDENTIFICATION

First identification: B, C.

Second identification: A, C, D, E.

A. Dissolve 30 mg in *0.01 M hydrochloric acid* and dilute to 100.0 ml with the same acid. Dilute 10.0 ml of the solution to 100.0 ml with *0.01 M hydrochloric acid.* Examined between 250 nm and 360 nm (*2.2.25*), the solution shows an absorption maximum at 311 nm and a minimum at 265 nm to 272 nm. The specific absorbance at the maximum is 175 to 195.

B. Examine by infrared absorption spectrophotometry (*2.2.24*), comparing with the spectrum obtained with *ergometrine maleate CRS*. Examine the substances prepared as discs.

C. Examine the chromatograms obtained in the test for related substances. The principal spot in the chromatogram obtained with test solution (b) is similar in position, colour and size to the principal spot in the chromatogram obtained with reference solution (a).

D. To 0.1 ml of solution S (see Tests) add 1 ml of *glacial acetic acid R*, 0.05 ml of *ferric chloride solution R1* and 1 ml of *phosphoric acid R* and heat in a water-bath at 80 °C. After about 10 min, a blue or violet colour develops which becomes more intense on standing.

E. Dissolve 0.1 g in a mixture of 0.5 ml of *dilute sulphuric acid R* and 2.5 ml of *water R*. Add 5 ml of *ether R* and 1 ml of *strong sodium hydroxide solution R* and shake. Separate the aqueous layer and shake with two quantities, each of 5 ml, of *ether R*. To 0.1 ml of the aqueous layer add a solution of 10 mg of *resorcinol R* in 3 ml of *sulphuric acid R*. Heat on a water-bath for 15 min. No colour develops. To the rest of the aqueous layer add 1 ml of *bromine water R*. Heat on a water-bath for 10 min, then heat to boiling and cool. To 0.2 ml of this solution add a solution of 10 mg of *resorcinol R* in 3 ml of *sulphuric acid R*. Heat on a water-bath for 15 min. A pinkish-violet colour develops.

TESTS

Solution S. Dissolve 0.100 g, without heating and protected from light, in 9 ml of *carbon dioxide-free water R* and dilute to 10.0 ml with the same solvent.

Appearance of solution. Solution S is clear (*2.2.1*) and not more intensely coloured than reference solution Y_5 or BY_5 (*2.2.2, Method II*).

pH (*2.2.3*). The pH of solution S is 3.6 to 4.4.

Specific optical rotation (*2.2.7*): + 50 to + 56, determined on solution S and calculated with reference to the dried substance.

Related substances. Examine by thin-layer chromatography (*2.2.27*), using *silica gel G R* as the coating substance. *Carry out all operations as rapidly as possible, protected from light. Prepare the test and reference solutions immediately before use.*

Test solution (a). Dissolve 50 mg of the substance to be examined in a mixture of 1 volume of *concentrated ammonia R* and 9 volumes of *alcohol (80 per cent V/V) R* and dilute to 5.0 ml with the same mixture of solvents.

Test solution (b). Dilute 1.0 ml of test solution (a) to 10.0 ml with a mixture of 1 volume of *concentrated ammonia R* and 9 volumes of *alcohol (80 per cent V/V) R.*

Reference solution (a). Dissolve 10 mg of *ergometrine maleate CRS* in a mixture of 1 volume of *concentrated ammonia R* and 9 volumes of *alcohol (80 per cent V/V) R* and dilute to 10.0 ml with the same mixture of solvents.

Reference solution (b). Dilute 5.0 ml of reference solution (a) to 50.0 ml with a mixture of 1 volume of *concentrated ammonia R* and 9 volumes of *alcohol (80 per cent V/V) R.*

Reference solution (c). To 2.0 ml of reference solution (b) add 2.0 ml of a mixture of 1 volume of *concentrated ammonia R* and 9 volumes of *alcohol (80 per cent V/V) R.*

Apply separately to the plate 5 µl of each solution. Develop immediately over a path of 14 cm using a mixture of 3 volumes of *water R*, 25 volumes of *methanol R* and 75 volumes of *chloroform R*. Dry the plate in a current of cold air and spray with *dimethylaminobenzaldehyde solution R7*. Dry the plate in a current of warm air for about 2 min. Any spot in the chromatogram obtained with test solution (a), apart from the principal spot, is not more intense than the principal spot in the chromatogram obtained with reference solution (b) (1.0 per cent) and at most one such spot is more intense than the principal spot in the chromatogram obtained with reference solution (c) (0.5 per cent).

Loss on drying (*2.2.32*). Not more than 2.0 per cent, determined on 0.20 g by drying over *diphosphorus pentoxide R* at 80 °C at a pressure not exceeding 2.7 kPa for 2 h.

ASSAY

Dissolve 0.150 g in 40 ml of *anhydrous acetic acid R*. Titrate with *0.05 M perchloric acid*, determining the end-point potentiometrically (*2.2.20*).

1 ml of *0.05 M perchloric acid* is equivalent to 22.07 mg of $C_{23}H_{27}N_3O_6$.

STORAGE

Store in an airtight, glass container, protected from light, at a temperature of 2 °C to 8 °C.

01/2005:0224

ERGOTAMINE TARTRATE

Ergotamini tartras

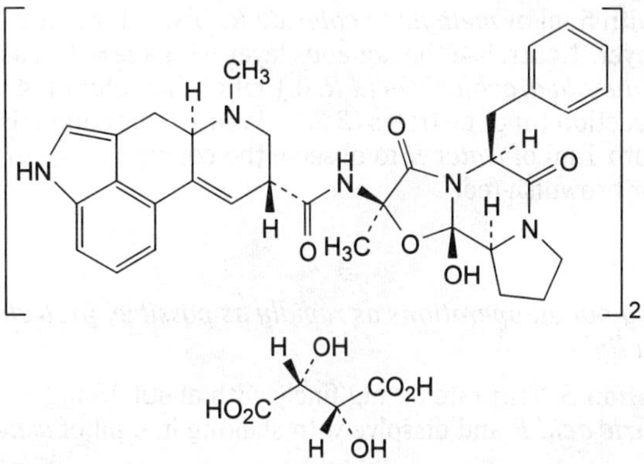

$C_{70}H_{76}N_{10}O_{16}$ M_r 1313

DEFINITION

Ergotamine tartrate contains not less than 98.0 per cent and not more than the equivalent of 101.0 per cent of bis[(6a*R*,9*R*)-*N*-[(2*R*,5*S*,10a*S*,10b*S*)-5-benzyl-10b-hydroxy-2-methyl-3,6-dioxo-octahydro-8*H*-oxazolo[3,2-*a*]pyrrolo[2,1-*c*]pyrazin-2-yl]-7-methyl-4,6,6a,7,8,9-hexahydroindolo[4,3-*fg*]quinoline-9-carboxamide] tartrate, calculated with reference to the dried substance. It may contain two molecules of methanol of crystallisation.

CHARACTERS

A white or almost white, crystalline powder or colourless crystals, slightly hygroscopic, slightly soluble in alcohol. Aqueous solutions slowly become cloudy owing to hydrolysis; this may be prevented by the addition of tartaric acid.

IDENTIFICATION

First identification: B, C.

Second identification: A, C, D, E.

A. Dissolve 50 mg in *0.01 M hydrochloric acid* and dilute to 100.0 ml with the same acid. Dilute 10.0 ml of the solution to 100.0 ml with *0.01 M hydrochloric acid.* Examined between 250 nm and 360 nm (*2.2.25*), the solution shows an absorption maximum at 311 nm to 321 nm and a minimum at 265 nm to 275 nm. The specific absorbance at the maximum is 118 to 128, calculated with reference to the dried substance.

B. Examine by infrared absorption spectrophotometry (*2.2.24*), comparing with the spectrum obtained with *ergotamine tartrate CRS*. Examine the substances as discs prepared as follows: triturate the substance to be examined and the reference substance separately with 0.2 ml of *methanol R* and then with *potassium bromide R* as prescribed in the general method.

Monographs D-E

C. Examine for not more than 1 min in ultraviolet light at 365 nm the chromatograms obtained in the test for related substances. The principal spot in the chromatogram obtained with test solution (b) is similar in position and fluorescence to the principal spot in the chromatogram obtained with reference solution (a). After spraying with *dimethylaminobenzaldehyde solution R7*, examine in daylight. The principal spot in the chromatogram obtained with test solution (b) is similar in position, colour and size to the principal spot in the chromatogram obtained with reference solution (a).

D. To 0.1 ml of solution S (see Tests) add 1 ml of *glacial acetic acid R*, 0.05 ml of *ferric chloride solution R1* and 1 ml of *phosphoric acid R* and heat in a water-bath at 80 °C. After about 10 min, a blue or violet colour develops which becomes more intense on standing.

E. Dissolve about 10 mg in 1.0 ml of *0.1 M sodium hydroxide*. Transfer to a separating funnel and shake with 5 ml of *methylene chloride R*. Discard the organic layer. Neutralise the aqueous layer with a few drops of *dilute hydrochloric acid R*. 0.1 ml of this solution gives reaction (b) of tartrates (*2.3.1*). Pour the reaction mixture into 1 ml of *water R* to observe the colour change to red or brownish-red.

TESTS

Carry out all operations as rapidly as possible, protected from light.

Solution S. Triturate 30 mg finely with about 15 mg of *tartaric acid R* and dissolve with shaking in 6 ml of *water R*.

Appearance of solution. Solution S is clear (*2.2.1*) and not more intensely coloured than reference solution Y_6 (*2.2.2, Method II*).

pH (*2.2.3*). Shake 10 mg, finely powdered, with 4 ml of *carbon dioxide-free water R*. The pH of the suspension is 4.0 to 5.5.

Specific optical rotation (*2.2.7*). Dissolve 0.40 g in 40 ml of a 10 g/l solution of *tartaric acid R*. Add 0.5 g of *sodium hydrogen carbonate R* cautiously in several portions and mix thoroughly. Shake with four quantities, each of 10 ml, of *chloroform R* previously washed with five quantities of *water R*, each of 50 ml per 100 ml of *chloroform R*. Combine the organic layers. Filter through a small filter moistened with *chloroform R* previously washed as described above. Dilute the filtrate to 50.0 ml with *chloroform R* previously washed as described above. Measure the angle of rotation.

Determine the amount of ergotamine base in the chloroformic solution as follows: to 25.0 ml of the solution add 50 ml of *anhydrous acetic acid R* and titrate with *0.05 M perchloric acid*, determining the end-point potentiometrically (*2.2.20*).

1 ml of *0.05 M perchloric acid* is equivalent to 29.08 mg of $C_{33}H_{35}N_5O_5$.

The specific optical rotation is − 154 to − 165, calculated from the angle of rotation and the concentration of ergotamine base.

Related substances. Examine by thin-layer chromatography (*2.2.27*), using a *TLC silica gel G plate R. Prepare the reference solutions and the test solutions immediately before use and in the order indicated below.*

Reference solution (a). Dissolve 10 mg of *ergotamine tartrate CRS* in a mixture of 1 volume of *methanol R* and 9 volumes of *methylene chloride R* and dilute to 10.0 ml with the same mixture of solvents.

Reference solution (b). Dilute 7.5 ml of reference solution (a) to 50.0 ml with a mixture of 1 volume of *methanol R* and 9 volumes of *methylene chloride R*.

Reference solution (c). To 2.0 ml of reference solution (b) add 4.0 ml of a mixture of 1 volume of *methanol R* and 9 volumes of *methylene chloride R*.

Test solution (a). Dissolve 50 mg of the substance to be examined in a mixture of 1 volume of *methanol R* and 9 volumes of *methylene chloride R* and dilute to 5.0 ml with the same mixture of solvents.

Test solution (b). Dilute 1.0 ml of test solution (a) to 10.0 ml with a mixture of 1 volume of *methanol R* and 9 volumes of *methylene chloride R*.

Apply immediately to the plate 5 µl of each reference solution and then 5 µl of each test solution. Expose the starting points immediately to ammonia vapour and for exactly 20 s by moving the starting line from side to side above a beaker 55 mm high and 45 mm in diameter containing about 20 ml of *concentrated ammonia R*. Dry the starting line in a current of cold air for exactly 20 s. Develop immediately over a path of 17 cm using a mixture of 5 volumes of *ethanol R*, 10 volumes of *methylene chloride R*, 15 volumes of *dimethylformamide R* and 70 volumes of *ether R*. Dry the plate in a current of cold air for about 2 min. Examine for not more than 1 min in ultraviolet light at 365 nm for the identification. Spray the plate abundantly with *dimethylaminobenzaldehyde solution R7* and dry in a current of warm air for about 2 min. Any spot in the chromatogram obtained with test solution (a), apart from the principal spot, is not more intense than the principal spot in the chromatogram obtained with reference solution (b) (1.5 per cent) and at most one such spot is more intense than the principal spot in the chromatogram obtained with reference solution (c) (0.5 per cent).

Loss on drying (*2.2.32*). Not more than 6.0 per cent, determined on 0.100 g by drying *in vacuo* at 95 °C for 6 h.

ASSAY

Dissolve 0.200 g in 40 ml of *anhydrous acetic acid R*. Titrate with *0.05 M perchloric acid*, determining the end-point potentiometrically (*2.2.20*).

1 ml of *0.05 M perchloric acid* is equivalent to 32.84 mg of $C_{70}H_{76}N_{10}O_{16}$.

STORAGE

Store in an airtight, glass container, protected from light, at a temperature of 2 °C to 8 °C.

01/2005:1803

ERYTHRITOL

Erythritolum

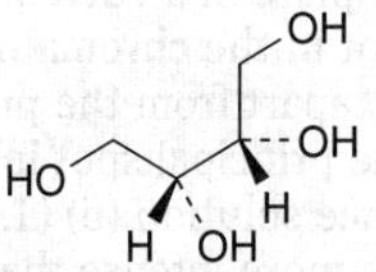

$C_4H_{10}O_4$ M_r 122.1

DEFINITION

(2*R*,3*S*)-Butane1,2,3,4-tetrol (*meso*-erythritol).

Content: 96.0 per cent to 102.0 per cent (anhydrous substance).

CHARACTERS

Appearance: white or almost white, crystalline powder or free-flowing granules.

Solubility: freely soluble in water, very slightly soluble in alcohol.

IDENTIFICATION

A. Melting point (*2.2.14*): 119 °C to 122 °C.

B. Infrared absorption spectrophotometry (*2.2.24*).

Comparison: *erythritol CRS*.

TESTS

Appearance of solution. The solution is clear (*2.2.1*) and colourless (*2.2.2, Method II*).

Dissolve 5.0 g in *water R* and dilute to 50 ml with the same solvent.

Conductivity (*2.2.38*): maximum 20 μS·cm^{-1}.

Dissolve 20.0 g in *carbon dioxide-free water R* prepared from *distilled water R* and dilute to 100.0 ml with the same solvent. Measure the conductivity of the solution, while gently stirring with a magnetic stirrer.

Related substances. Liquid chromatography (*2.2.29*).

Test solution. Dissolve 0.50 g of the substance to be examined in *water R* and dilute to 10.0 ml with the same solvent.

Reference solution (a). Dissolve 0.50 g of *erythritol CRS* in *water R* and dilute to 10.0 ml with the same solvent.

Reference solution (b). Dilute 2.0 ml of the test solution to 100.0 ml with *water R*.

Reference solution (c). Dilute 5.0 ml of reference solution (b) to 100.0 ml with *water R*.

Reference solution (d). Dissolve 1.0 g of *erythritol R* and 1.0 g of *glycerol R* in *water R* and dilute to 20.0 ml with the same solvent.

Column:

- *size*: l = 0.3 m, Ø = 7.8 mm,
- *stationary phase*: *cation-exchange resin R* (9 μm),
- *temperature*: 70 °C.

Mobile phase: 0.01 per cent *V/V* solution of *sulphuric acid R*.

Flow rate: 0.8 ml/min.

Detection: refractometer maintained at a constant temperature.

Injection: 20 μl; inject the test solution and reference solutions (b), (c) and (d).

Run time: 3 times the retention time of erythritol.

Relative retention with reference to erythritol (retention time = about 11 min): impurity A = about 0.77; impurity B = about 0.90; impurity C = about 0.94; impurity D = about 1.10.

System suitability: reference solution (d):

- *resolution*: minimum 2 between the peaks due to erythritol and impurity D.

Limits:

- *any impurity*: not more than the area of the principal peak in the chromatogram obtained with reference solution (b) (2.0 per cent),
- *total*: not more than the area of the principal peak in the chromatogram obtained with reference solution (b) (2.0 per cent),
- *disregard limit*: area of the principal peak in the chromatogram obtained with reference solution (c) (0.1 per cent).

Lead (*2.4.10*): maximum 0.5 ppm.

Water (*2.5.12*): maximum 0.5 per cent, determined on 1.00 g.

Microbial contamination. Total viable aerobic count (*2.6.12*) not more than 10^3 bacteria and 10^2 fungi per gram, determined by plate count. It complies with the tests for *Escherichia coli* and *Salmonella* (*2.6.13*). If intended for use in the manufacture of parenteral dosage forms, the total viable aerobic count (*2.6.12*) is not more than 10^2 bacteria and 10^2 fungi per gram, determined by plate count.

Bacterial endotoxins (*2.6.14*). If intended for use in the manufacture of parenteral dosage forms without a further appropriate procedure for the removal of bacterial endotoxins:

- less than 4 IU/g for parenteral dosage forms having a concentration of 100 g/l or less of erythritol,
- less than 2.5 IU/g for parenteral dosage forms having a concentration of more than 100 g/l of erythritol.

ASSAY

Liquid chromatography (*2.2.29*) as described in the test for related substances with the following modification.

Injection: test solution and reference solution (a).

Calculate the percentage content of erythritol using the chromatogram obtained with reference solution (a) and the declared content of *erythritol CRS*.

LABELLING

The label states where applicable, that the substance is suitable for use in the manufacture of parenteral dosage forms.

IMPURITIES

A. maltitol,

B. sorbitol,

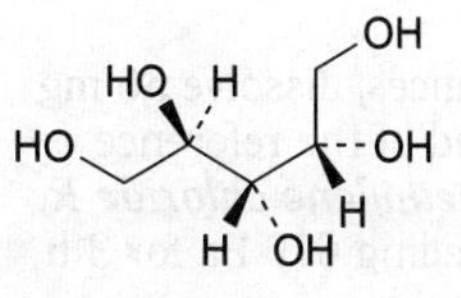

C. (2*R*,3*s*,4*S*)-pentane-1,2,3,4,5-pentol (*meso*-ribitol),

D. glycerol.

01/2005:0179

ERYTHROMYCIN

Erythromycinum

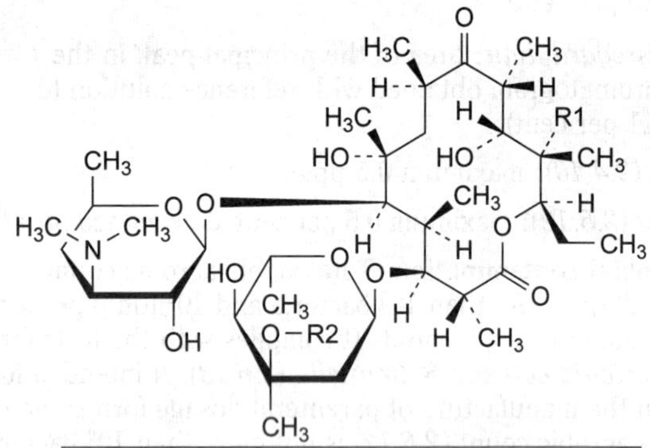

Erythromycin	Mol. Formula	M_r	R1	R2
A	$C_{37}H_{67}NO_{13}$	734	OH	CH_3
B	$C_{37}H_{67}NO_{12}$	718	H	CH_3
C	$C_{36}H_{65}NO_{13}$	720	OH	H

DEFINITION

Mixture of macrolide antibiotics produced by a strain of *Streptomyces erythreus,* the main component being (3*R*,4*S*,5*S*,6*R*,7*R*,9*R*,11*R*,12*R*,13*S*,14*R*)-4-[(2,6-dideoxy-3-*C*-methyl-3-*O*-methyl-α-L-*ribo*-hexopyranosyl)oxy]-14-ethyl-7,12,13-trihydroxy-3,5,7,9,11,13-hexamethyl-6-[(3,4,6-trideoxy-3-dimethylamino-β-D-*xylo*-hexopyranosyl)-oxy]oxacyclotetradecane-2,10-dione (erythromycin A).

Content:

- sum of the contents of erythromycin A, erythromycin B and erythromycin C: 93.0 per cent to 102.0 per cent (anhydrous substance),
- erythromycin B: maximum 5.0 per cent,
- erythromycin C: maximum 5.0 per cent.

CHARACTERS

Appearance: white or slightly yellow powder or colourless or slightly yellow crystals, slightly hygroscopic.

Solubility: slightly soluble in water (the solubility decreases as the temperature rises), freely soluble in alcohol, soluble in methanol.

IDENTIFICATION

First identification: A.

Second identification: B, C, D.

A. Infrared absorption spectrophotometry (*2.2.24*).

Comparison: *erythromycin CRS.*

Disregard any band in the region from 1980 cm^{-1} to 2050 cm^{-1}.

If the spectra obtained show differences, dissolve 50 mg of the substance to be examined and of the reference substance separately in 1.0 ml of *methylene chloride R*, dry at 60 °C at a pressure not exceeding 670 Pa for 3 h and record new spectra using the residues.

B. Thin-layer chromatography (*2.2.27*).

Test solution. Dissolve 10 mg of the substance to be examined in *methanol R* and dilute to 10 ml with the same solvent.

Reference solution (a). Dissolve 10 mg of *erythromycin A CRS* in *methanol R* and dilute to 10 ml with the same solvent.

Reference solution (b). Dissolve 20 mg of *spiramycin CRS* in *methanol R* and dilute to 10 ml with the same solvent.

Plate: *TLC silica gel G plate R.*

Mobile phase: mix 4 volumes of *2-propanol R*, 8 volumes of a 150 g/l solution of *ammonium acetate R* previously adjusted to pH 9.6 with *ammonia R* and 9 volumes of *ethyl acetate R*. Allow to settle and use the upper layer.

Application: 10 μl.

Development: over 2/3 of the plate.

Drying: in air.

Detection: spray with *anisaldehyde solution R1* and heat at 110 °C for 5 min.

Results: the principal spot in the chromatogram obtained with the test solution is similar in position, colour and size to the principal spot in the chromatogram obtained with reference solution (a) and its position and colour are different from those of the spots in the chromatogram obtained with reference solution (b).

C. To about 5 mg add 5 ml of a 0.2 g/l solution of *xanthydrol R* in a mixture of 1 volume of *hydrochloric acid R* and 99 volumes of *acetic acid R* and heat on a water-bath. A red colour develops.

D. Dissolve about 10 mg in 5 ml of *hydrochloric acid R1* and allow to stand for 10-20 min. A yellow colour develops.

TESTS

Specific optical rotation (*2.2.7*): − 71 to − 78 (anhydrous substance).

Dissolve 1.00 g in *ethanol R* and dilute to 50.0 ml with the same solvent. The specific optical rotation is determined at least 30 min after preparing the solution.

Related substances. Liquid chromatography (*2.2.29*).

Test solution. Dissolve 40.0 mg of the substance to be examined in a mixture of 1 volume of *methanol R* and 3 volumes of *phosphate buffer solution pH 7.0 R1* and dilute to 10.0 ml with the same mixture of solvents.

Reference solution (a). Dissolve 40.0 mg of *erythromycin A CRS* in a mixture of 1 volume of *methanol R* and 3 volumes of *phosphate buffer solution pH 7.0 R1* and dilute to 10.0 ml with the same mixture of solvents.

Reference solution (b). Dissolve 10.0 mg of *erythromycin B CRS* and 10.0 mg of *erythromycin C CRS* in a mixture of 1 volume of *methanol R* and 3 volumes of *phosphate buffer solution pH 7.0 R1* and dilute to 50.0 ml with the same mixture of solvents.

Reference solution (c). Dissolve 5 mg of *N-demethyl-erythromycin A CRS* in reference solution (b). Add 1.0 ml of reference solution (a) and dilute to 25 ml with reference solution (b).

Reference solution (d). Dilute 3.0 ml of reference solution (a) to 100.0 ml with a mixture of 1 volume of *methanol R* and 3 volumes of *phosphate buffer solution pH 7.0 R1.*

Reference solution (e). Transfer 40 mg of *erythromycin A CRS* to a glass vial and spread evenly such that it forms a layer not more than about 1 mm thick. Heat at 130 °C for 4 h. Allow to cool and dissolve in a mixture of 1 volume of *methanol R* and 3 volumes of *phosphate buffer solution pH 7.0 R1* and dilute to 10 ml with the same mixture of solvents.

Column:

- *size*: l = 0.25 m, Ø = 4.6 mm,
- *stationary phase*: *styrene-divinylbenzene copolymer R* (8 μm) with a pore size of 100 nm,
- *temperature*: 70 °C using a water-bath for the column and at least one-third of the tubing preceding the column.

Mobile phase: to 50 ml of a 35 g/l solution of *dipotassium hydrogen phosphate R* adjusted to pH 9.0 ± 0.05 with *dilute phosphoric acid R*, add 400 ml of *water R*, 165 ml of *2-methyl-2-propanol R* and 30 ml of *acetonitrile R*, and dilute to 1000 ml with *water R*.

Flow rate: 2.0 ml/min.

Detection: spectrophotometer at 215 nm.

Injection: 100 μl; inject the test solution and reference solutions (c), (d) and (e).

Run time: 5 times the retention time of erythromycin A.

Relative retention with reference to erythromycin A (retention time = about 15 min): impurity A = about 0.3; impurity B = about 0.45; erythromycin C = about 0.5; impurity C = about 0.9; impurity D = about 1.4; impurity F = about 1.5; erythromycin B = about 1.8; impurity E = about 4.3.

System suitability: reference solution (c):

- *resolution*: minimum 0.8 between the peaks due to impurity B and erythromycin C and minimum 5.5 between the peaks due to impurity B and erythromycin A. If necessary, adjust the concentration of 2-methyl-2-propanol in the mobile phase or reduce the flow rate to 1.5 ml or 1.0 ml/min.

Limits:

- *correction factors*: for the calculation of contents, multiply the peak areas of the following impurities (use the chromatogram obtained with reference solution (e) to identify them) by the corresponding correction factor: impurity E = 0.09; impurity F = 0.15,
- *any impurity*: not more than the area of the principal peak in the chromatogram obtained with reference solution (d) (3.0 per cent),
- *total*: not more than 2.3 times the area of the principal peak in the chromatogram obtained with reference solution (d) (7.0 per cent),
- *disregard limit*: 0.02 times the area of the principal peak in the chromatogram obtained with reference solution (d) (0.06 per cent); disregard the peaks due to erythromycin B and erythromycin C.

Thiocyanate: maximum 0.3 per cent.

Prepare the solutions immediately before use and protect from actinic light.

Compensation liquid. Dilute 1.0 ml of a 90 g/l solution of *ferric chloride R* to 50.0 ml with *methanol R*.

Test solution. Dissolve 0.100 g (m g) of the substance to be examined in 20 ml of *methanol R*, add 1.0 ml of a 90 g/l solution of *ferric chloride R* and dilute to 50.0 ml with *methanol R*.

Prepare 2 independent reference solutions.

Reference solution. Dissolve 0.100 g of *potassium thiocyanate R*, previously dried at 105 °C for 1 h, in *methanol R* and dilute to 50.0 ml with the same solvent. Dilute 5.0 ml to 50.0 ml with *methanol R*. To 5.0 ml of this solution, add 1.0 ml of a 90 g/l solution of *ferric chloride R* and dilute to 50.0 ml with *methanol R*.

Measure the absorbances (*2.2.25*) of each reference solution (A_1, A_2) and of the test solution (A) at the maximum (about 492 nm).

Suitability value:

$$S = \frac{m_2 \times A_1}{m_1 \times A_2}$$

m_1, m_2 = mass of the potassium thiocyanate used to prepare the respective reference solutions, in grams.

The test is not valid unless S is not less than 0.985 and not more than 1.015.

Calculate the percentage content of thiocyanate from the expression:

$$\frac{A \times 58.08 \times 0.5}{m \times 97.18} \times \left(\frac{m_1}{A_1} + \frac{m_2}{A_2}\right)$$

58.08 = relative molecular mass of the thiocyanate moiety,

97.18 = relative molecular mass of potassium thiocyanate.

Water (*2.5.12*): maximum 6.5 per cent, determined on 0.200 g.

Use a 100 g/l solution of *imidazole R* in *anhydrous methanol R* as the solvent.

Sulphated ash (*2.4.14*): maximum 0.2 per cent, determined on 1.0 g.

ASSAY

Liquid chromatography (*2.2.29*) as described in the test for related substances with the following modifications.

Injection: test solution and reference solutions (a) and (b).

System suitability: reference solution (a):

- *repeatability*: maximum relative standard deviation of 1.2 per cent for 6 replicate injections.

Calculate the percentage content of erythromycin A using the chromatogram obtained with reference solution (a). Calculate the percentage contents of erythromycin B and erythromycin C using the chromatogram obtained with reference solution (b).

STORAGE

Protected from light.

IMPURITIES

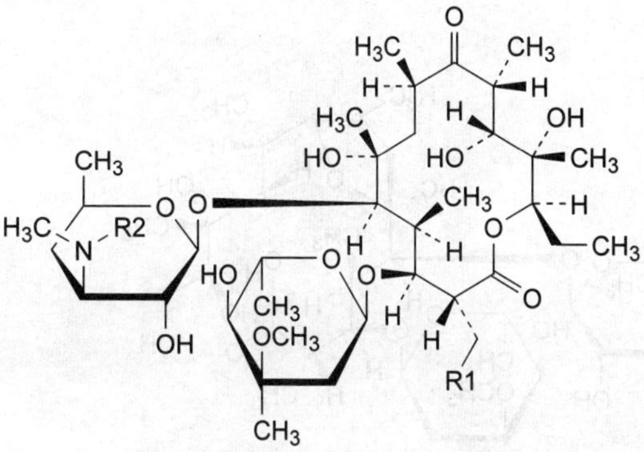

A. R1 = OH, R2 = CH_3: erythromycin F,

B. R1 = R2 = H: *N*-demethylerythromycin A,

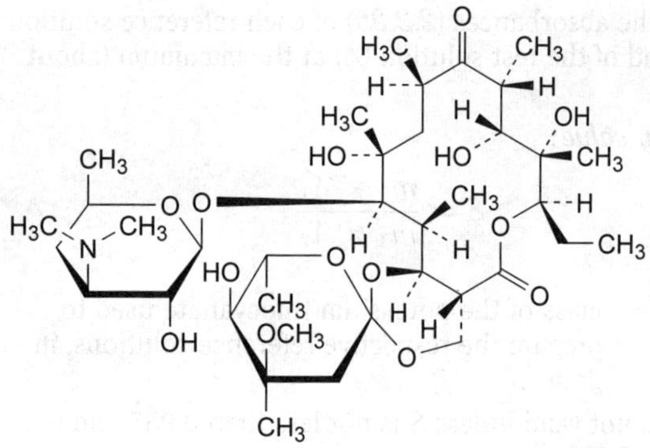

C. erythromycin E,

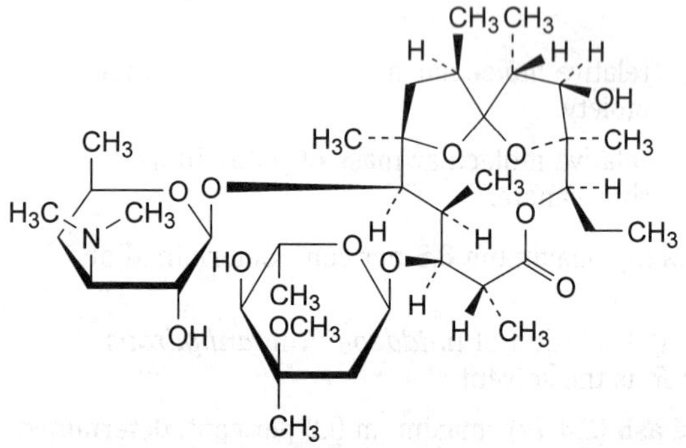

D. anhydroerythromycin A,

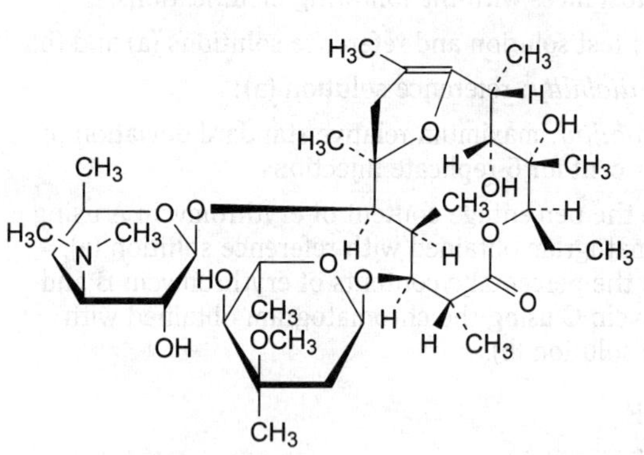

E. erythromycin A enol ether,

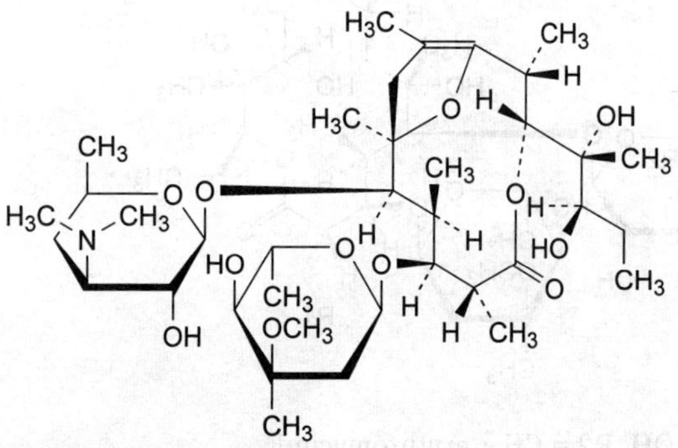

F. pseudoerythromycin A enol ether.

01/2005:0552

ERYTHROMYCIN ESTOLATE

Erythromycini estolas

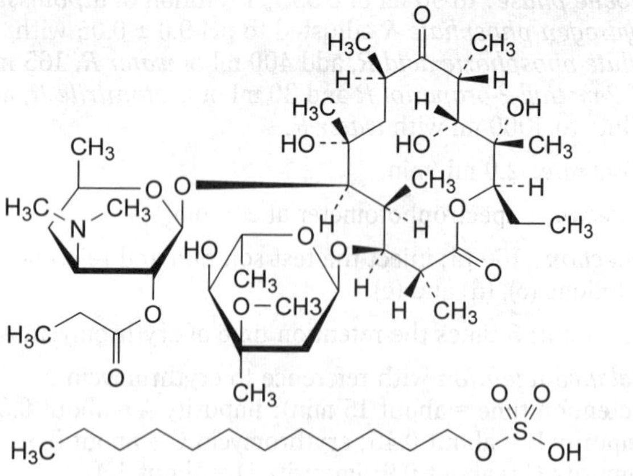

$C_{52}H_{97}NO_{18}S$ M_r 1056

DEFINITION

Erythromycin estolate (or erythromycin 2′-propionate dodecyl sulphate) is (3*R*,4*S*,5*S*,6*R*,7*R*,9*R*,11*R*,12*R*,13*S*,14*R*)-4-[(2,6-dideoxy-3-*C*-methyl-3-*O*-methyl-α-L-*ribo*-hexopyranosyl)oxy]-14-ethyl-7,12,13-trihydroxy-3,5,7,9,11,13-hexamethyl-6-[[3,4,6-trideoxy-3-(dimethylamino)-2-*O*-propionyl-β-D-*xylo*-hexopyranosyl]oxy]oxacyclotetradecane-2,10-dione dodecyl sulphate. The potency is not less than 610 IU/mg, calculated with reference to the anhydrous substance.

CHARACTERS

A white, crystalline powder, practically insoluble in water, freely soluble in alcohol, soluble in acetone. It is practically insoluble in dilute hydrochloric acid.

IDENTIFICATION

First identification: A, D.

Second identification: B, C, D.

A. Examine by infrared absorption spectrophotometry (*2.2.24*), comparing with the spectrum obtained with *erythromycin estolate CRS*.

B. Examine the chromatograms obtained in the test for related substances. The principal spot in the chromatogram obtained with test solution (b) is similar in position and colour to the principal spot in the chromatogram obtained with reference solution (a). The test is not valid unless the chromatogram obtained with reference solution (b) shows two clearly separated spots.

C. Suspend about 3 mg in 2 ml of *dilute sulphuric acid R*. Add 0.1 ml of a 0.1 g/l solution of *methylene blue R* and 2 ml of *chloroform R* and shake. The chloroform layer is blue.

D. Dissolve about 10 mg in 5 ml of *hydrochloric acid R1* and allow to stand for 10 min to 20 min. A yellow colour develops.

TESTS

pH (*2.2.3*). Suspend 0.4 g in 10 ml of *carbon dioxide-free water R*. Shake for 5 min and allow to stand. The pH of the clear supernatant liquid is 5.5 to 7.0.

Related substances. Examine by thin-layer chromatography (*2.2.27*), using *silica gel G R* as the coating substance.

Test solution (a). Dissolve 40 mg of the substance to be examined in *acetone R* and dilute to 10 ml with the same solvent.

Test solution (b). Dilute 2.5 ml of test solution (a) to 10 ml with *acetone R*.

Reference solution (a). Dissolve 10 mg of *erythromycin estolate CRS* in *acetone R* and dilute to 10 ml with the same solvent.

Reference solution (b). Dissolve 10 mg of *erythromycin estolate CRS* and 10 mg of *erythromycin ethylsuccinate CRS* in *acetone R* and dilute to 10 ml with the same solvent.

Reference solution (c). Dissolve 8 mg of *erythromycin CRS* in *acetone R* and dilute to 100 ml with the same solvent.

Apply separately to the plate 10 µl of each solution. Develop over a path of 15 cm using a mixture of 1 volume of a 150 g/l solution of *ammonium acetate R* previously adjusted to pH 7.0, 15 volumes of *alcohol R* and 85 volumes of *chloroform R*. Allow the plate to dry in air and spray with *anisaldehyde solution R*. Heat at 110 °C for 5 min and allow to cool. Any spot in the chromatogram obtained with test solution (a), apart from the principal spot, is not more intense than the spot in the chromatogram obtained with reference solution (c) (2.0 per cent).

Dodecyl sulphate. 23.0 per cent to 25.5 per cent of $C_{12}H_{26}O_4S$, calculated with reference to the anhydrous substance. Dissolve 0.500 g of the substance to be examined in 25 ml of *dimethylformamide R*. Titrate with *0.1 M sodium methoxide* using 0.05 ml of a 3 g/l solution of *thymol blue R* in *methanol R* as indicator.

1 ml of *0.1 M sodium methoxide* is equivalent to 26.64 mg of $C_{12}H_{26}O_4S$.

Water (*2.5.12*). Not more than 4.0 per cent, determined on 0.300 g by the semi-micro determination of water. Use a 100 g/l solution of *imidazole R* in *anhydrous methanol R* as the solvent.

Sulphated ash (*2.4.14*). Not more than 0.5 per cent, determined on 0.5 g.

ASSAY

Dissolve 40.0 mg in 40 ml of *methanol R*, add 20 ml of *phosphate buffer solution pH 7.0 R* and dilute to 100.0 ml with *water R*. Maintain at 60 °C for 3 h and allow to cool. Carry out the microbiological assay of antibiotics (*2.7.2*). Use *erythromycin CRS* as the reference substance.

STORAGE

Store in an airtight container, protected from light, at a temperature below 30 °C.

01/2005:0274

ERYTHROMYCIN ETHYLSUCCINATE

Erythromycini ethylsuccinas

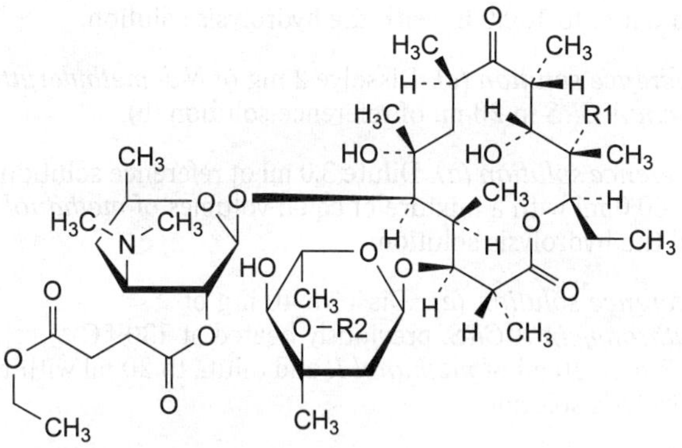

Ethylsuccinate compound	Mol. Formula	M_r	R1	R2
Erythromycin A	$C_{43}H_{75}NO_{16}$	862	OH	CH_3
Erythromycin B	$C_{43}H_{75}NO_{15}$	846	H	CH_3
Erythromycin C	$C_{42}H_{73}NO_{16}$	848	OH	H

DEFINITION

Main component: (3*R*,4*S*,5*S*,6*R*,7*R*,9*R*,11*R*,12*R*,13*S*,14*R*)-4-[(2,6-dideoxy-3-*C*-methyl-3-*O*-methyl-α-L-*ribo*-hexopyranosyl)oxy]-14-ethyl-7,12,13-trihydroxy-3,5,7,9,11,13-hexamethyl-6-[[3,4,6-trideoxy-3-(dimethylamino)-2-*O*-(4-ethoxy-4-oxobutanoyl)-β-D-*xylo*-hexopyranosyl]oxy]oxacyclotetradecane-2,10-dione (erythromycin A ethylsuccinate).

Content:

- sum of erythromycin A, erythromycin B and erythromycin C: minimum 78.0 per cent (anhydrous substance),
- erythromycin B: maximum 5.0 per cent (anhydrous substance),
- erythromycin C: maximum 5.0 per cent (anhydrous substance).

CHARACTERS

Appearance: white, crystalline powder, hygroscopic.

Solubility: practically insoluble in water, freely soluble in acetone, in ethanol and in methanol.

IDENTIFICATION

Infrared absorption spectrophotometry (*2.2.24*).

Comparison: *erythromycin ethylsuccinate CRS*.

TESTS

Specific optical rotation (*2.2.7*): − 70 to − 82 (anhydrous substance).

Dissolve 0.100 g in *acetone R* and dilute to 10.0 ml with the same solvent. Measure the angle of rotation at least 30 min after preparing the solution.

Related substances. Liquid chromatography (*2.2.29*).

Hydrolysis solution. A 20 g/l solution of *dipotassium hydrogen phosphate R* adjusted to pH 8.0 with *phosphoric acid R.*

Test solution. Dissolve 0.115 g of the substance to be examined in 25 ml of *methanol R*. Add 20 ml of the hydrolysis solution, mix and allow to stand at room temperature for at least 12 h. Dilute to 50.0 ml with the hydrolysis solution.

Reference solution (a). Dissolve 40.0 mg of *erythromycin A CRS* in 10 ml of *methanol R* and dilute to 20.0 ml with the hydrolysis solution.

Reference solution (b). Dissolve 10.0 mg of *erythromycin B CRS* and 10.0 mg of *erythromycin C CRS* in 50 ml of *methanol R*. Add 5.0 ml of reference solution (a) and dilute to 100.0 ml with the hydrolysis solution.

Reference solution (c). Dissolve 2 mg of *N-demethylerythromycin A CRS* in 20 ml of reference solution (b).

Reference solution (d). Dilute 3.0 ml of reference solution (a) to 100.0 ml with a mixture of equal volumes of *methanol R* and the hydrolysis solution.

Reference solution (e). Dissolve 40 mg of *erythromycin A CRS*, previously heated at 130 °C for 3 h, in 10 ml of *methanol R* and dilute to 20 ml with the hydrolysis solution.

Column:

- *size*: *l* = 0.25 m, Ø = 4.6 mm,
- *stationary phase*: *styrene-divinylbenzene copolymer R* (8 µm) with a pore size of 100 nm,
- *temperature*: 70 °C using a water-bath for the column and at least one third of the tubing preceding the column.

Mobile phase: to 50 ml of a 35 g/l solution of *dipotassium hydrogen phosphate R* adjusted to pH 8.0 with *dilute phosphoric acid R*, add 400 ml of *water R*, 165 ml of *2-methyl-2-propanol R* and 30 ml of *acetonitrile R*, and dilute to 1000 ml with *water R*.

Flow rate: 2.0 ml/min.

Detection: spectrophotometer at 215 nm.

Injection: 200 µl; inject the test solution and reference solutions (a), (c), (d) and (e).

Run time: 5 times the retention time of erythromycin A; begin integration after the hydrolysis peak.

Relative retention with reference to erythromycin A (retention time = about 15 min): hydrolysis peak = less than 0.3; impurity B = about 0.45; erythromycin C = about 0.5; impurity C = about 0.9; impurity G = about 1.3; impurity D = about 1,4; impurity F = about 1.5; erythromycin B = about 1.8; impurity E = about 4.3.

System suitability: reference solution (c):

- *resolution*: minimum 0.8 between the peaks due to impurity B and to erythromycin C and minimum 5.5 between the peaks due to impurity B and to erythromycin A.

Limits:

- *correction factors*: for the calculation of contents, multiply the peak areas of the following impurities by the corresponding correction factor: impurity E = 0.09; impurity F = 0.15; impurity G = 0.14; use the chromatogram obtained with reference solution (e) to identify the peaks due to impurities E and F.
- *any impurity*: not more than the area of the principal peak in the chromatogram obtained with reference solution (d) (3.0 per cent).
- *total*: not more than 1.67 times the area of the principal peak in the chromatogram obtained with reference solution (d) (5.0 per cent).
- *disregard limit*: 0.02 times the area of the principal peak in the chromatogram obtained with reference solution (d) (0.06 per cent).

Free erythromycin. Liquid chromatography (*2.2.29*).

Test solution. Dissolve 0.250 g of the substance to be examined in *acetonitrile R* and dilute to 50.0 ml with the same solvent.

Reference solution. Dissolve 75.0 mg of *erythromycin A CRS* in *acetonitrile R* and dilute to 50.0 ml with the same solvent. Dilute 5.0 ml of the solution to 25.0 ml with *acetonitrile R*.

Column:

- *size*: *l* = 0.25 m, Ø = 4.6 mm,
- *stationary phase*: *octylsilyl silica gel for chromatography R* (5 µm).

Mobile phase: mix 35 volumes of *acetonitrile R* and 65 volumes of a solution containing 3.4 g/l of *potassium dihydrogen phosphate R* and 2.0 g/l of *triethylamine R*, adjusted to pH 3.0 with *dilute phosphoric acid R*.

Flow rate: 1 ml/min.

Detection: spectrophotometer at 195 nm.

Injection: 20 µl.

Run time: twice the retention time of erythromycin A (retention time = about 8 min) for the reference solution and twice the retention time of erythromycin ethylsuccinate (retention time = about 24 min) for the test solution.

Limit:

- *free erythromycin*: not more than the area of the principal peak in the chromatogram obtained with the reference solution (6.0 per cent).

Water (*2.5.12*): maximum 3.0 per cent, determined on 0.30 g.

Use a 100 g/l solution of *imidazole R* in *anhydrous methanol R* as the solvent.

Sulphated ash (*2.4.14*): maximum 0.3 per cent, determined on 1.0 g.

ASSAY

Liquid chromatography (*2.2.29*) as described in the test for related substances.

Injection: inject the test solution and reference solutions (a) and (b).

System suitability: reference solution (a):

- *relative standard deviation*: maximum 1.2 per cent for 6 replicate injections.

Calculate the percentage content of erythromycin A using the chromatogram obtained with reference solution (a). Calculate the percentage contents of erythromycin B and erythromycin C using the chromatogram obtained with reference solution (b).

STORAGE

In an airtight container, protected from light.

IMPURITIES

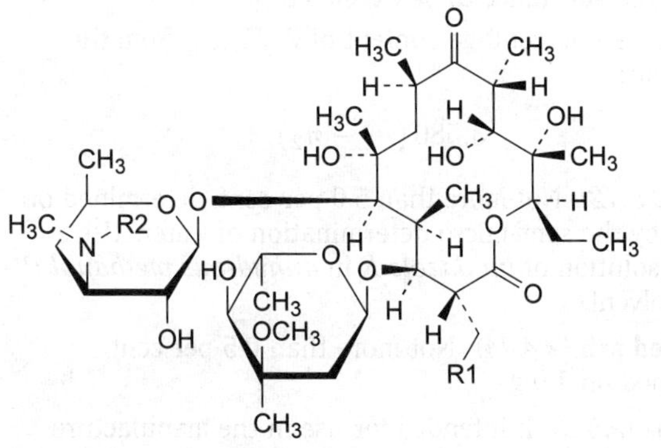

A. R1 = OH, R2 = CH_3: erythromycin F,

B. R1 = R2 = H: *N*-demethylerythromycin A,

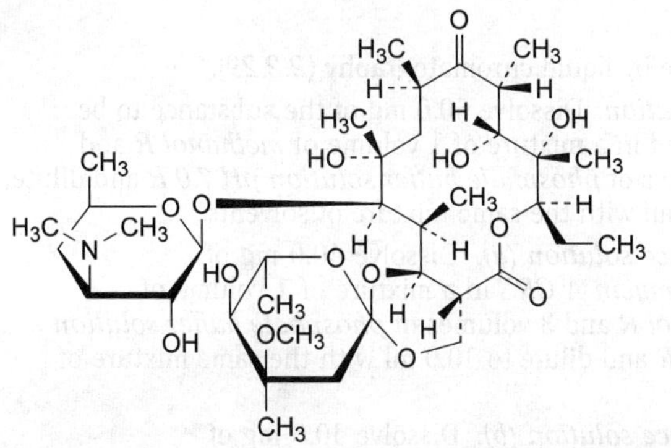

C. erythromycin E,

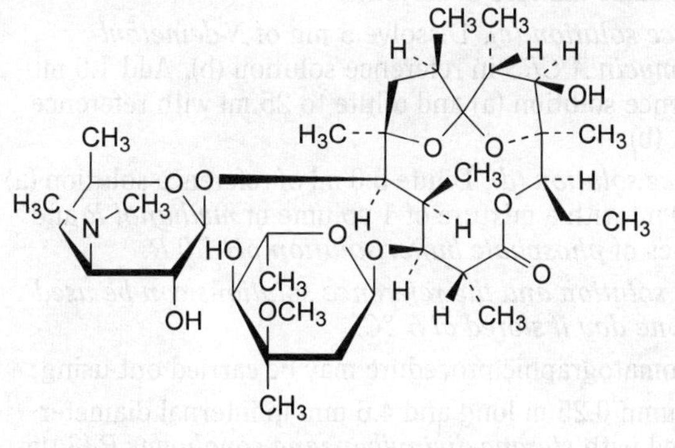

D. anhydroerythomycin A,

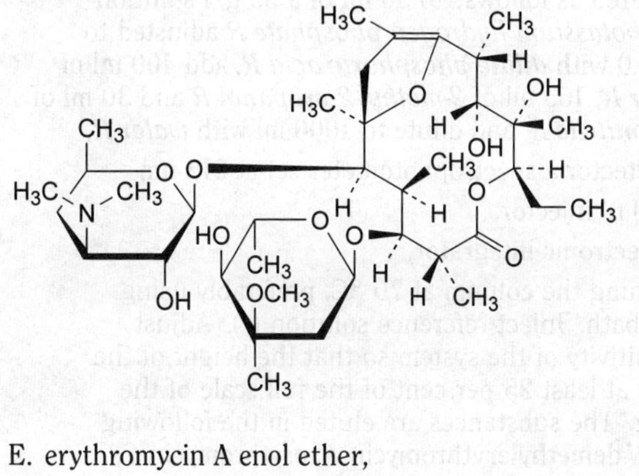

E. erythromycin A enol ether,

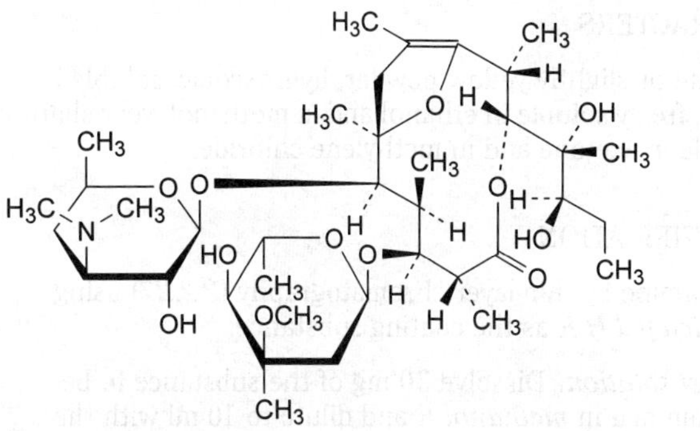

F. pseudoerythromycin A enol ether,

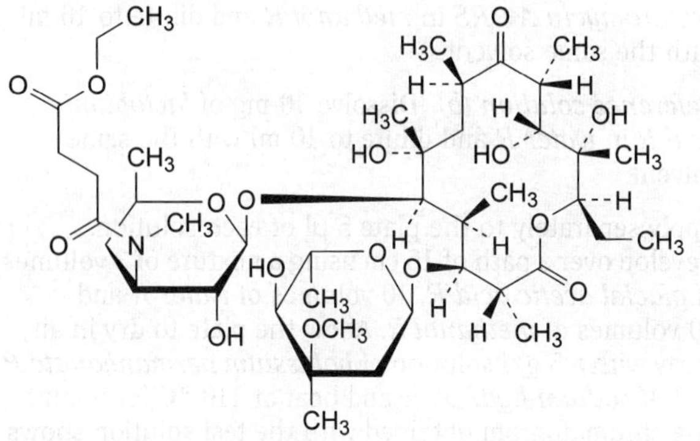

G. erythromycin *N*-ethylsuccinate.

01/2005:1098

ERYTHROMYCIN LACTOBIONATE

Erythromycini lactobionas

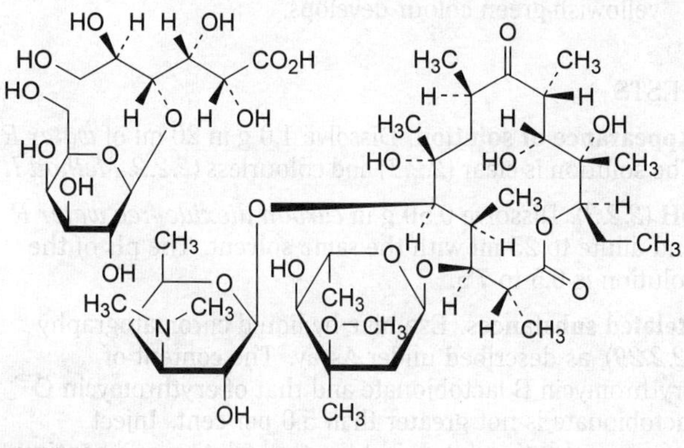

$C_{49}H_{89}NO_{25}$ M_r 1092

DEFINITION

Erythromycin lactobionate is a mixture of lactobionates of macrolide antibiotics. The main component is (3*R*,4*S*,5*S*,6*R*,7*R*,9*R*,11*R*,12*R*,13*S*,14*R*)-4-[(2,6-dideoxy-3-*C*-methyl-3-*O*-methyl-α-L-*ribo*-hexopyranosyl)oxy]-14-ethyl-7,12,13-trihydroxy-3,5,7,9,11,13-hexamethyl-6-[[3,4,6-trideoxy-3-(dimethylamino)-β-D-*xylo*-hexopyranosyl]oxy]oxacyclotetradecane-2,10-dione 4-*O*-β-D-galactopyranosyl-D-gluconate. The sum of the content of erythromycin A lactobionate, of erythromycin B lactobionate and of erythromycin C lactobionate is not less than 93.0 per cent and not more than the equivalent of 100.5 per cent, calculated with reference to the anhydrous substance.

CHARACTERS

A white or slightly yellow powder, hygroscopic, soluble in water, freely soluble in ethanol and in methanol, very slightly soluble in acetone and in methylene chloride.

IDENTIFICATION

A. Examine by thin-layer chromatography (*2.2.27*) using *silica gel H R* as the coating substance.

Test solution. Dissolve 30 mg of the substance to be examined in *methanol R* and dilute to 10 ml with the same solvent.

Reference solution (a). Dissolve 20 mg of *erythromycin A CRS* in *methanol R* and dilute to 10 ml with the same solvent.

Reference solution (b). Dissolve 10 mg of *lactobionic acid R* in *water R* and dilute to 10 ml with the same solvent.

Apply separately to the plate 5 µl of each solution. Develop over a path of 15 cm using a mixture of 3 volumes of *glacial acetic acid R*, 10 volumes of *water R* and 90 volumes of *methanol R*. Allow the plate to dry in air, spray with a 5 g/l solution of *potassium permanganate R* in *1 M sodium hydroxide* and heat at 110 °C for 5 min. The chromatogram obtained with the test solution shows two spots, one of which corresponds in position, colour and size to the principal spot in the chromatogram obtained with reference solution (a) and the other to the principal spot in the chromatogram obtained with reference solution (b).

B. To about 5 mg add 5 ml of a 0.2 g/l solution of *xanthydrol R* in a mixture of 1 volume of *hydrochloric acid R* and 99 volumes of *acetic acid R*. A red colour develops.

C. Dissolve about 10 mg in 5 ml of *hydrochloric acid R1*. A yellowish-green colour develops.

TESTS

Appearance of solution. Dissolve 1.0 g in 20 ml of *water R*. The solution is clear (*2.2.1*) and colourless (*2.2.2, Method II*).

pH (*2.2.3*). Dissolve 0.50 g in *carbon dioxide-free water R* and dilute to 25 ml with the same solvent. The pH of the solution is 6.5 to 7.5.

Related substances. Examine by liquid chromatography (*2.2.29*), as described under Assay. The content of erythromycin B lactobionate and that of erythromycin C lactobionate is not greater than 5.0 per cent. Inject reference solution (d). Inject the test solution and continue the chromatography for five times the retention time of erythromycin A. In the chromatogram obtained with the test solution, the area of any peak, apart from the peaks corresponding to erythromycin A, erythromycin B or erythromycin C, is not greater than the area of the principal peak in the chromatogram obtained with reference solution (d) (3.0 per cent).

Free lactobionic acid. Not more than 1.0 per cent of $C_{12}H_{22}O_{12}$, calculated with reference to the anhydrous substance. Dissolve 0.400 g in 50 ml of *water R*. Titrate with *0.1 M sodium hydroxide*, determining the end-point potentiometrically (*2.2.20*). Calculate the volume of *0.1 M sodium hydroxide* required per gram of the substance to be examined (n_1 ml). Dissolve 0.500 g in 40 ml of *anhydrous acetic acid R* and titrate with *0.1 M perchloric acid*, determining the end-point potentiometrically (*2.2.20*). Calculate the volume of *0.1 M perchloric acid* required per gram of the substance to be examined (n_2 ml).

Calculate the percentage content of $C_{12}H_{22}O_{12}$ from the expression:

$$3.580\,(n_1 - n_2)$$

Water (*2.5.12*). Not more than 5.0 per cent, determined on 0.200 g by the semi-micro determination of water. Use a 100 g/l solution of *imidazole R* in *anhydrous methanol R* as the solvent.

Sulphated ash (*2.4.14*). Not more than 0.5 per cent, determined on 1.0 g.

Pyrogens (*2.6.8*). If intended for use in the manufacture of parenteral dosage forms without a further appropriate procedure for the removal of pyrogens, it complies with the test for pyrogens. Inject per kilogram of the rabbit's mass 1 ml of a solution in *water for injections R* containing 7.4 mg of the substance to be examined per millilitre (equivalent to 5 mg of erythromycin).

ASSAY

Examine by liquid chromatography (*2.2.29*).

Test solution. Dissolve 60.0 mg of the substance to be examined in a mixture of 1 volume of *methanol R* and 3 volumes of *phosphate buffer solution pH 7.0 R* and dilute to 10.0 ml with the same mixture of solvents.

Reference solution (a). Dissolve 40.0 mg of *erythromycin A CRS* in a mixture of 1 volume of *methanol R* and 3 volumes of *phosphate buffer solution pH 7.0 R* and dilute to 10.0 ml with the same mixture of solvents.

Reference solution (b). Dissolve 10.0 mg of *erythromycin B CRS* and 10.0 mg of *erythromycin C CRS* in a mixture of 1 volume of *methanol R* and 3 volumes of *phosphate buffer solution pH 7.0 R* and dilute to 50.0 ml with the same mixture of solvents.

Reference solution (c). Dissolve 5 mg of *N-demethylerythromycin A CRS* in reference solution (b). Add 1.0 ml of reference solution (a) and dilute to 25 ml with reference solution (b).

Reference solution (d). Dilute 3.0 ml of reference solution (a) to 100.0 ml with a mixture of 1 volume of *methanol R* and 3 volumes of *phosphate buffer solution pH 7.0 R*.

The test solution and the reference solutions can be used within one day if stored at 5 °C.

The chromatographic procedure may be carried out using:

- a column 0.25 m long and 4.6 mm in internal diameter packed with *styrene-divinylbenzene copolymer R* (8 µm to 10 µm) with a pore size of 100 nm,
- as mobile phase at a flow rate of 2.0 ml/min a solution prepared as follows: to 50 ml of a 35 g/l solution of *dipotassium hydrogen phosphate R* adjusted to pH 9.0 with *dilute phosphoric acid R*, add 400 ml of *water R*, 165 ml of *2-methyl-2-propanol R* and 30 ml of *acetonitrile R*, and dilute to 1000 ml with *water R*,
- as detector a spectrophotometer set at 215 nm,
- a 100 µl injector,
- an electronic integrator,

maintaining the column at 70 °C, preferably using a water-bath. Inject reference solution (c). Adjust the sensitivity of the system so that the height of the peaks is at least 25 per cent of the full scale of the recorder. The substances are eluted in the following order: *N*-demethylerythromycin A, erythromycin C, erythromycin A and erythromycin B. The assay is not valid unless the resolution between the peaks corresponding to *N*-demethylerythromycin A and erythromycin C is at least 0.8 and the resolution between the peaks corresponding to *N*-demethylerythromycin A and erythromycin A is at least 5.5. If necessary, adjust the concentration of 2-methyl-2-propanol in the mobile phase or reduce the flow rate to 1.5 ml/min or 1.0 ml/min. Inject reference solution (a) six times. The assay is not valid unless the relative standard deviation of the area of the peak due to erythromycin A is at most 2.0 per cent. Inject alternately the test solution and reference solutions (a) and (b).

Calculate the percentage content of erythromycin A using the chromatogram obtained with reference solution (a). Express the result as erythromycin A lactobionate by multiplying the percentage content of erythromycin A by 1.4877. Calculate the percentage contents of erythromycin B and erythromycin C using the chromatogram obtained with reference solution (b). Express the result as erythromycin B lactobionate and as erythromycin C lactobionate by multiplying by 1.4877.

STORAGE

Store in an airtight container at a temperature not exceeding 25 °C. If the substance is sterile, store in a sterile, airtight, tamper-proof container.

LABELLING

The label states, where applicable, that the substance is free from pyrogens.

IMPURITIES

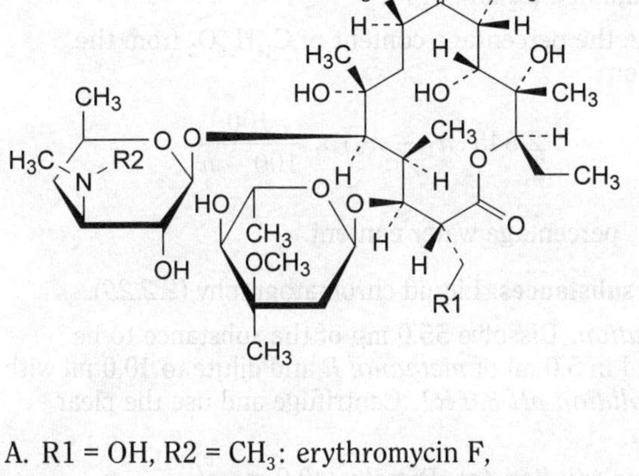

A. R1 = OH, R2 = CH_3: erythromycin F,

B. R1 = R2 = H: *N*-demethylerythromycin A,

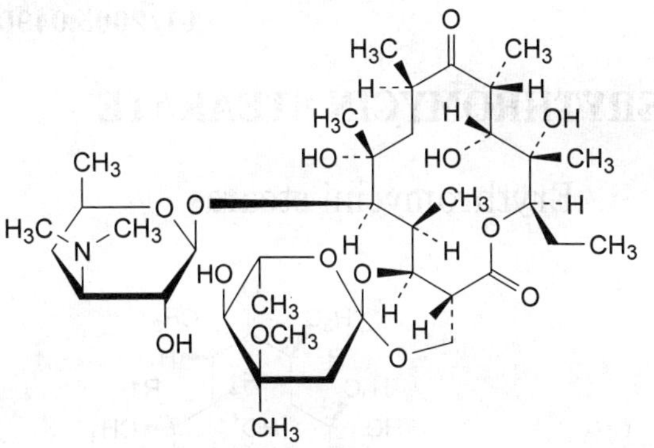

C. erythromycin E,

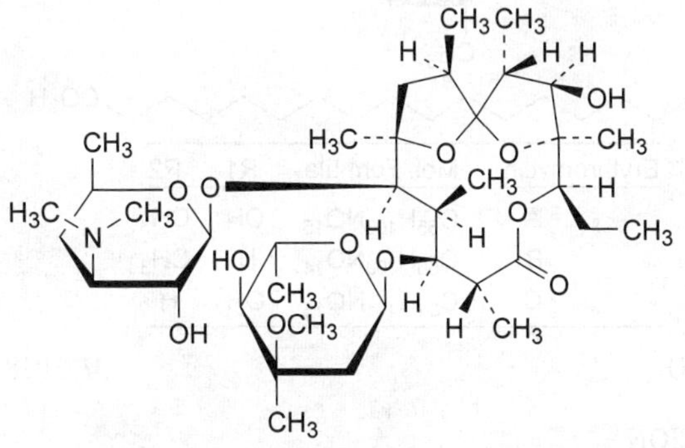

D. anhydroerythromycin A,

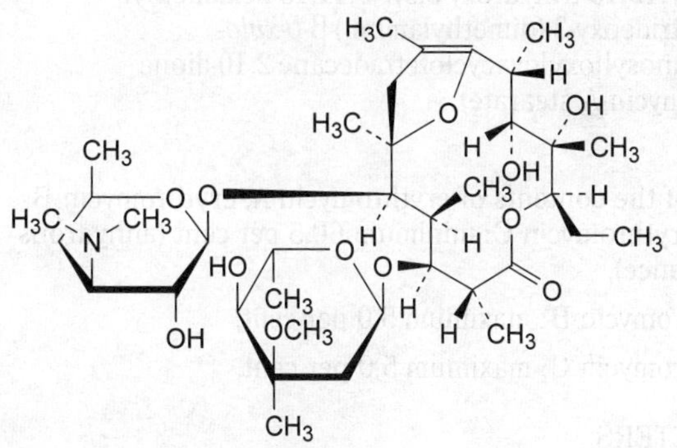

E. erythromycin A enol ether,

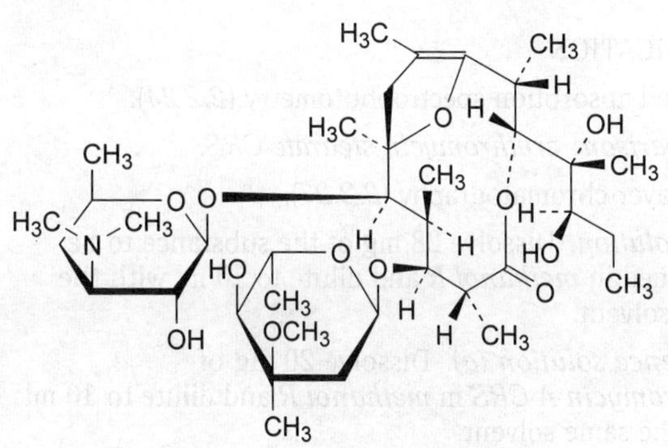

F. pseudoerythromycin A enol ether.

Monographs D-E

01/2005:0490

ERYTHROMYCIN STEARATE

Erythromycini stearas

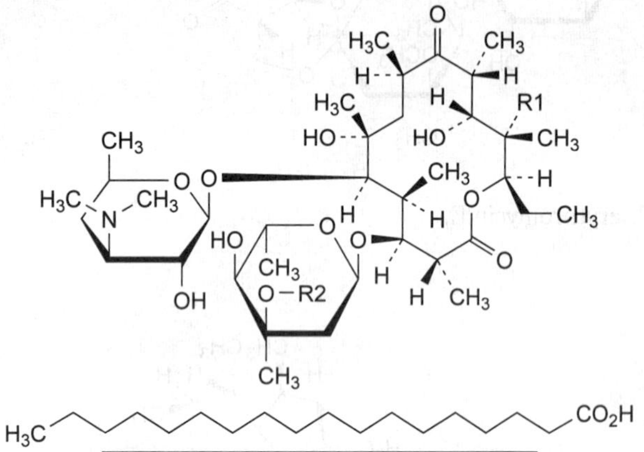

Erythromycin	Mol. Formula	R1	R2
A	$C_{55}H_{103}NO_{15}$	OH	CH_3
B	$C_{55}H_{103}NO_{14}$	H	CH_3
C	$C_{54}H_{101}NO_{15}$	OH	H

$C_{55}H_{103}NO_{15}$ M_r 1018

DEFINITION

A mixture of the stearates of erythromycin and stearic acid. The main component is the octadecanoate of (3*R*,4*S*,5*S*,6*R*,7*R*,9*R*,11*R*,12*R*,13*S*,14*R*)-4-[(2,6-dideoxy-3-*C*-methyl-3-*O*-methyl-α-L-*ribo*-hexopyranosyl)oxy]-14-ethyl-7,12,13-trihydroxy-3,5,7,9,11,13-hexamethyl-6-[[3,4,6-trideoxy-3-(dimethylamino)-β-D-*xylo*-hexopyranosyl]oxy]oxacyclotetradecane-2,10-dione (erythromycin A stearate).

Content:

- sum of the contents of erythromycin A, erythromycin B and erythromycin C: minimum 60.5 per cent (anhydrous substance),
- erythromycin B: maximum 5.0 per cent,
- erythromycin C: maximum 5.0 per cent.

CHARACTERS

Appearance: white, crystalline powder.

Solubility: practically insoluble in water, soluble in acetone and in methanol.

Solutions may be opalescent.

IDENTIFICATION

A. Infrared absorption spectrophotometry (*2.2.24*).

Comparison: *erythromycin stearate CRS*.

B. Thin-layer chromatography (*2.2.27*).

Test solution. Dissolve 28 mg of the substance to be examined in *methanol R* and dilute to 10 ml with the same solvent.

Reference solution (a). Dissolve 20 mg of *erythromycin A CRS* in *methanol R* and dilute to 10 ml with the same solvent.

Reference solution (b). Dissolve 10 mg of *stearic acid R* in *methanol R* and dilute to 10 ml with the same solvent.

Plate: *TLC silica gel G plate R*.

Mobile phase: mix 4 volumes of *2-propanol R*, 8 volumes of a 150 g/l solution of *ammonium acetate R* previously adjusted to pH 9.6 with *ammonia R* and 9 volumes of *ethyl acetate R*. Allow to settle and use the upper layer.

Application: 5 μl.

Development: over 2/3 of the plate.

Drying: in air.

Detection A: spray with a solution containing 0.2 g/l of *dichlorofluorescein R* and 0.1 g/l of *rhodamine B R* in *alcohol R*. Maintain the plate for a few seconds in the vapour above a water-bath. Examine in ultraviolet light at 365 nm.

Results A: the chromatogram obtained with the test solution shows 2 spots, one of which corresponds in position to the principal spot in the chromatogram obtained with reference solution (a) and the other to the principal spot in the chromatogram obtained with reference solution (b).

Detection B: spray the plate with *anisaldehyde solution R1*. Heat at 110 °C for 5 min and examine in daylight.

Results B: the spot in the chromatogram obtained with the test solution corresponds in position, colour and size to the principal spot in the chromatogram obtained with reference solution (a).

TESTS

Free stearic acid: maximum 14.0 per cent (anhydrous substance) of $C_{18}H_{36}O_2$.

Dissolve 0.400 g in 50 ml of *methanol R*. Titrate with *0.1 M sodium hydroxide*, determining the end-point potentiometrically (*2.2.20*). Calculate the volume of *0.1 M sodium hydroxide* required per gram of the substance to be examined (n_1 ml). Dissolve 0.500 g in 30 ml of *methylene chloride R*. If the solution is opalescent, filter and shake the residue with 3 quantities, each of 25 ml, of *methylene chloride R*. Filter, if necessary, and rinse the filter with *methylene chloride R*. Reduce the volume of the combined filtrate and rinsings to 30 ml by evaporation on a water-bath. Add 50 ml of *glacial acetic acid R* and titrate with *0.1 M perchloric acid*, determining the end-point potentiometrically (*2.2.20*). Calculate the volume of *0.1 M perchloric acid* required per gram of the substance to be examined (n_2 ml).

Calculate the percentage content of $C_{18}H_{36}O_2$ from the expression:

$$2.845\,(n_1 - n_2) \times \frac{100}{100 - h}$$

h = percentage water content.

Related substances. Liquid chromatography (*2.2.29*).

Test solution. Dissolve 55.0 mg of the substance to be examined in 5.0 ml of *methanol R* and dilute to 10.0 ml with *buffer solution pH 8.0 R1*. Centrifuge and use the clear solution.

Reference solution (a). Dissolve 40.0 mg of *erythromycin A CRS* in 5.0 ml of *methanol R* and dilute to 10.0 ml with *buffer solution pH 8.0 R1*.

Reference solution (b). Dissolve 10.0 mg of *erythromycin B CRS* and 10.0 mg of *erythromycin C CRS* in 25.0 ml of *methanol R* and dilute to 50.0 ml with *buffer solution pH 8.0 R1*.

Reference solution (c). Dissolve 5 mg of *N-demethylerythromycin A CRS* in reference solution (b). Add 1.0 ml of reference solution (a) and dilute to 25 ml with reference solution (b).

Reference solution (d). Dilute 3.0 ml of reference solution (a) to 100.0 ml with a mixture of equal volumes of *methanol R* and *buffer solution pH 8.0 R1*.

Reference solution (e). Transfer 40 mg of *erythromycin A CRS* to a glass vial and spread evenly such that it forms a layer not more than about 1 mm thick. Heat at 130 °C for 4 h. Allow to cool and dissolve in a mixture of 1 volume of *methanol R* and 3 volumes of *buffer solution pH 8.0 R1* and dilute to 10 ml with the same mixture of solvents.

Column:

- *size*: *l* = 0.25 m, Ø = 4.6 mm,
- *stationary phase*: *styrene-divinylbenzene copolymer R* (8 µm) with a pore size of 100 nm,
- *temperature*: 70 °C using a water-bath for the column and at least one third of the tubing preceding the column.

Mobile phase: to 50 ml of a 35 g/l solution of *dipotassium hydrogen phosphate R* adjusted to pH 9.0 ± 0.05 with *dilute phosphoric acid R*, add 400 ml of *water R*, 165 ml of *2-methyl-2-propanol R* and 30 ml of *acetonitrile R*, and dilute to 1000 ml with *water R*.

Flow rate: 2.0 ml/min.

Detection: spectrophotometer at 215 nm.

Injection: 100 µl; inject the test solution and reference solutions (c), (d) and (e).

Run time: 5 times the retention time of erythromycin A.

Relative retention with reference to erythromycin A (retention time = about 15 min): impurity A = about 0.3; impurity B = about 0.45; erythromycin C = about 0.5; impurity C = about 0.9; impurity D = about 1.4; impurity F = about 1.5; erythromycin B = about 1.8; impurity E = about 4.3.

System suitability: reference solution (c):

- *resolution*: minimum 0.8 between the peaks due to impurity B and to erythromycin C and minimum 5.5 between the peaks due to impurity B and to erythromycin A. If necessary, adjust the concentration of 2-methyl-2-propanol in the mobile phase or reduce the flow rate to 1.5 ml/min or 1.0 ml/min.

Limits:

- *correction factors*: for the calculation of contents, multiply the peak areas of the following impurities (use the chromatogram obtained with reference solution (e) to identify them) by the corresponding correction factor: impurity E = 0.09; impurity F = 0.15,
- *any impurity*: not more than the area of the principal peak in the chromatogram obtained with reference solution (d) (3 per cent),
- *total*: not more than twice the area of the principal peak in the chromatogram obtained with reference solution (d) (6 per cent),
- *disregard limit*: 0.02 times the area of the principal peak in the chromatogram obtained with reference solution (d) (0.06 per cent); disregard the peaks due to erythromycin B and to erythromycin C.

Water (*2.5.12*): maximum 4.0 per cent, determined on 0.300 g.

Use a 100 g/l solution of *imidazole R* in *anhydrous methanol R* as the solvent.

Sulphated ash (*2.4.14*): maximum 0.5 per cent, determined on 1.0 g.

ASSAY

Liquid chromatography (*2.2.29*) as described in the test for related substances with the following modifications.

Injection: test solution and reference solutions (a) and (b).

System suitability: reference solution (a):

- *repeatability*: maximum relative standard deviation of 1.2 per cent for 6 replicate injections.

Calculate the percentage content of erythromycin A using the chromatogram obtained with reference solution (a). Calculate the percentage contents of erythromycin B and erythromycin C using the chromatogram obtained with reference solution (b).

IMPURITIES

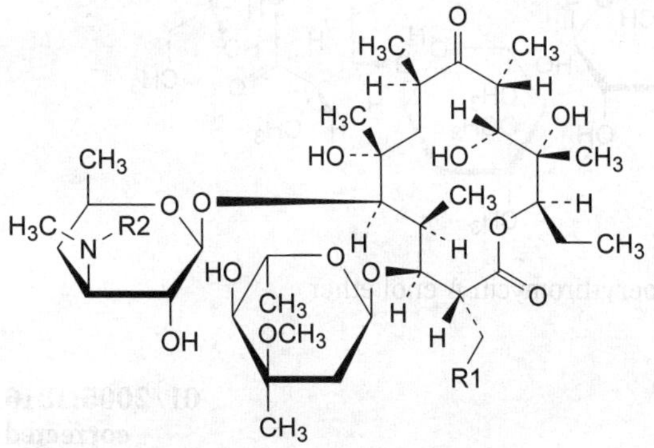

A. R1 = OH, R2 = CH_3: erythromycin F,

B. R1 = R2 = H: *N*-demethylerythromycin A,

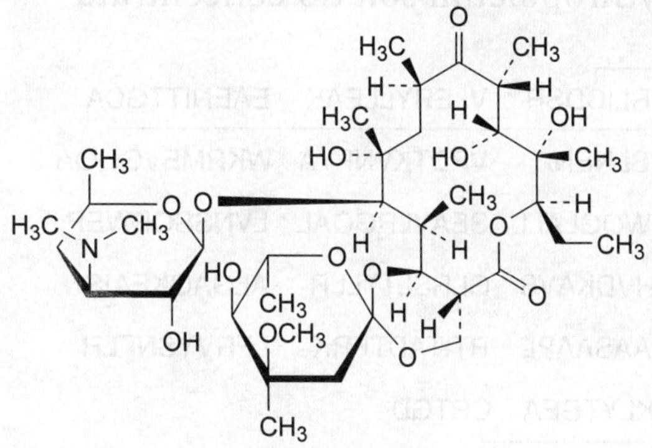

C. erythromycin E,

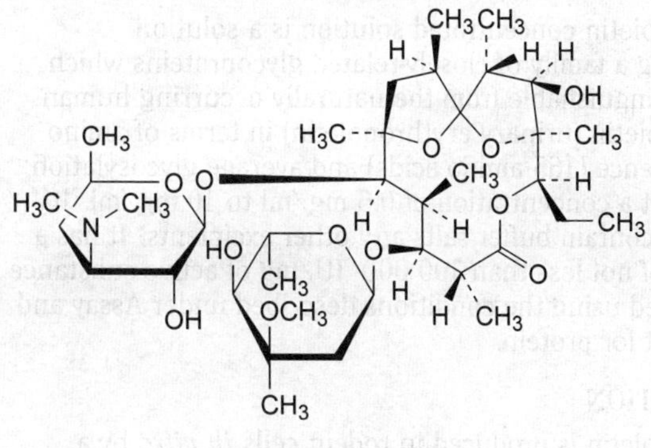

D. anhydroerythromycin A,

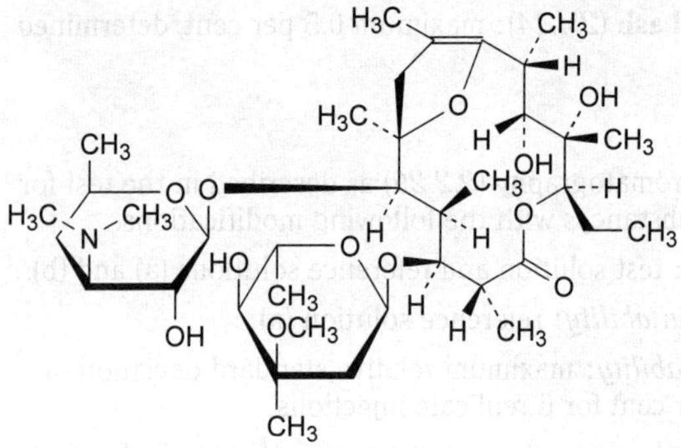

E. erythromycin A enol ether,

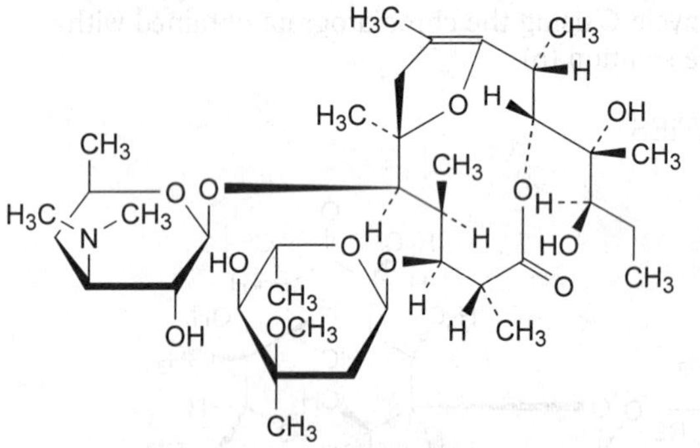

F. pseudoerythromycin A enol ether.

01/2005:1316
corrected

ERYTHROPOIETIN CONCENTRATED SOLUTION

Erythropoietini solutio concentrata

APPRLICDSR	VLERYLLEAK	EAENITTGCA
EHCSLNENIT	VPDTKVNFYA	WKRMEVGQQA
VEVWQGLALL	SEAVLRGQAL	LVNSSQPWEP
LQLHVDKAVS	GLRSLTTLLR	ALGAQKEAIS
PPDAASAAPL	RTITADTFRK	LFRVYSNFLR
GKLKLYTGEA	CRTGD	

M_r approx. 30 600

DEFINITION

Erythropoietin concentrated solution is a solution containing a family of closely-related glycoproteins which are indistinguishable from the naturally occurring human erythropoietin (urinary erythropoietin) in terms of amino acid sequence (165 amino acids) and average glycosylation pattern, at a concentration of 0.5 mg/ml to 10 mg/ml. It may also contain buffer salts and other excipients. It has a potency of not less than 100 000 IU/mg of active substance determined using the conditions described under Assay and in the test for protein.

PRODUCTION

Erythropoietin is produced in rodent cells *in vitro* by a method based on recombinant DNA technology.

Prior to batch release, the following tests are carried out on each batch of the final product, unless exemption has been granted by the competent authority.

Host cell-derived proteins: the limit is approved by the competent authority.

Host cell- and vector-derived DNA: the limit is approved by the competent authority.

CHARACTERS

Appearance: clear or slightly turbid colourless solution.

IDENTIFICATION

A. It gives the appropriate response when examined using the conditions described under Assay.

B. Capillary zone electrophoresis (*2.2.47*)

Test solution. Dilute the substance to be examined with *water R* to obtain a concentration of 1 mg/ml. Desalt 0.25 ml of the solution by passage through a micro-concentrator cartridge provided with a membrane with a molecular mass cut-off of not more than 10 000. Add 0.2 ml of *water R* to the sample and desalt again. Repeat the desalting procedure once more. Dilute the sample with *water R*, determine its protein concentration as described under Tests and adjust to a concentration of approximately 1 mg/ml with *water R*.

Reference solution. Dissolve the contents of a vial of *erythropoietin BRP* in 0.25 ml of *water R*. Proceed with desalting as described for the test solution.

Capillary:
- *material*: uncoated fused silica,
- *size*: effective length = about 100 cm, Ø = 50 µm,

Temperature: 35 °C.

CZE buffer concentrate (0.1 M sodium chloride, 0.1 M tricine, 0.1 M sodium acetate). Dissolve 0.584 g of *sodium chloride R*, 1.792 g of *tricine R* and 0.820 g of *anhydrous sodium acetate R* in *water R* and dilute to 100.0 ml with the same solvent.

1 M putrescine solution. Dissolve 0.882 g of *putrescine R* in 10 ml of *water R*. Distribute in 0.5 ml aliquots.

CZE buffer (0.01 M tricine, 0.01 M sodium chloride, 0.01 M sodium acetate, 7 M urea, 2.5 mM putrescine). Dissolve 21.0 g of *urea R* in 25 ml of *water R* by warming in a water-bath at 30 °C. Add 5.0 ml of CZE buffer concentrate and 125 µl of 1 M putrescine solution. Dilute to 50.0 ml with *water R*. Using *dilute acetic acid R*, adjust to pH 5.55 at 30 °C and filter through a 0.45 µm membrane filter.

Detection: spectrophotometer at 214 nm.

Set the autosampler to store the samples at 4 °C during analysis.

Preconditioning of the capillary: rinse the capillary for 60 min with *0.1 M sodium hydroxide* filtered through a 0.45 µm membrane filter and for 60 min with CZE buffer. Apply voltage for 12 h (20 kV).

Between-run rinsing: rinse the capillary for 10 min with *water R*, for 5 min with *0.1 M sodium hydroxide* filtered through a 0.45 µm membrane filter and for 10 min with CZE buffer.

Injection: under pressure or vacuum.

Migration: apply a field strength of 143 V/cm (15.4 kV for capillaries of 107 cm total length) for 80 min, using CZE buffer as the electrolyte in both buffer reservoirs.

System suitability: in the electropherogram obtained with the reference solution, a pattern of well separated peaks corresponding to the peaks in the *Ph. Eur. reference electropherogram of erythropoietin* (Figure 1316.-1) is seen, and the largest peak is at least 50 times greater than the baseline noise. If necessary, adjust the sample load to give peaks of sufficient height. Identify the peaks corresponding to isoforms 1 to 8. The peak corresponding to isoform 1 is detected; the resolution between the peaks corresponding to isoforms 5 and 6 is not less than 1. Repeat the separation at least 3 times. The baseline is stable, showing little drift, and the distribution of peaks is qualitatively and quantitatively similar to the distribution of peaks in the *Ph. Eur. reference electropherogram of erythropoietin*. The relative standard deviation of the migration time of the peak corresponding to isoform 2 is less than 2 per cent.

Limits: identify the peaks corresponding to isoforms 1 to 8 in the electropherogram obtained with the test solution by comparison with the electropherogram obtained with the reference solution. Calculate the percentage content of each isoform from the corresponding peak area. The percentages are within the following ranges:

Isoform number	Content (per cent)
1	0 - 15
2	0 - 15
3	5 - 20
4	10 - 35
5	15 - 40
6	10 - 35
7	0 - 20
8	0 - 15

C. Polyacrylamide gel electrophoresis and immunoblotting

(a) Polyacrylamide gel electrophoresis (*2.2.31*)

Gel dimensions: 0.75 mm thick, about 16 cm square.

Resolving gel: 12 per cent acrylamide.

Sample buffer. SDS-PAGE sample buffer (concentrated) R.

Test solution (a). Dilute the preparation to be examined in *water R* to obtain a concentration of 1.0 mg/ml. To 1 volume of this solution add 1 volume of sample buffer.

Test solution (b). Dilute the preparation to be examined in *water R* to obtain a concentration of 0.1 mg/ml. To 1 volume of this solution add 1 volume of sample buffer.

Reference solution (a). Dissolve the contents of a vial of *erythropoietin BRP* in 0.25 ml of *water R*. To 1 volume of this solution add 1 volume of sample buffer.

Reference solution (b). Dissolve the contents of a vial of *erythropoietin BRP* in *water R* and dilute with the same solvent to obtain a concentration of 0.1 mg/ml. To 1 volume of this solution add 1 volume of sample buffer.

Reference solution (c). A solution of molecular mass markers suitable for calibrating SDS-polyacrylamide gels in the range of 10-70 kDa.

Reference solution (d). A solution of pre-stained molecular mass markers suitable for calibrating SDS-polyacrylamide gels in the range of 10-70 kDa and suitable for the electrotransfer to an appropriate membrane.

Sample treatment: boil for 2 min.

Application: 20 µl, in the following order: reference solution (c), reference solution (a), test solution (a), empty well, reference solution (b), test solution (b), reference solution (d).

At the end of the separation, remove the gel-cassette from the apparatus, and cut the gel into 2 parts: the first part containing reference solution (c), reference solution (a) and test solution (a); the second part containing reference solution (b), test solution (b) and reference solution (d).

Detection: Coomassie staining on the first part of the gel.

System suitability: reference solution (c).

Validation criteria are met.

Results: the electropherogram obtained with test solution (a) shows a single diffuse band corresponding in position and intensity to the single band seen in the electropherogram obtained with reference solution (a).

(b) Immunoblotting

Transfer the second part of the gel onto a membrane suitable for the immobilisation of proteins, using commercially available electrotransfer equipment and following the manufacturer's instructions. After electrotransfer, incubate the membrane in a neutral isotonic buffer containing a suitable blocking agent (for example, 50 g/l of dried milk or 10 per cent *V/V* foetal calf serum), for 1-2 h, followed by incubation for 1-14 h in the same blocking solution with a suitable dilution of either a polyclonal or monoclonal anti-erythropoietin antibody. Detect erythropoietin-bound antibody using a suitable enzyme- or radiolabelled antibody (for example, an alkaline phosphatase-conjugated second antibody). The precise details of blocking agents, concentrations and incubation times should be optimised using the principles set out in *Immunochemical methods* (*2.7.1*).

System suitability: in the electropherogram obtained with reference solution (d), the molecular mass markers are resolved on the membrane into discrete bands, with a linear relationship between distance migrated and $logarithm_{10}$ of the molecular mass.

Results: the electropherogram obtained with test solution (b) shows a single broad band corresponding in position and intensity to the single band seen in the electropherogram obtained with reference solution (b).

D. Peptide mapping

Test solution. Dilute the preparation to be examined in *tris-acetate buffer solution pH 8.5 R* to a concentration of 1.0 mg/ml. Equilibrate the solution in *tris-acetate buffer solution pH 8.5 R* using a suitable procedure (dialysis against *tris-acetate buffer solution pH 8.5 R*, or membrane filtration using the procedure described under Identification B, but reconstituting the desalted sample with *tris-acetate buffer solution pH 8.5 R*, are suitable). Transfer the dialysed solution to a polypropylene centrifuge tube. Freshly prepare a solution of *trypsin for peptide mapping R* at a concentration of 1 mg/ml in *water R*, and add 5 µl to 0.25 ml of the dialysed solution. Cap the tube and place in a water-bath at 37 °C for 18 h. Remove the sample from the water-bath and stop the reaction immediately by freezing.

Reference solution. Dissolve the contents of a vial of *erythropoietin BRP* in 0.25 ml of *water R*. Prepare as for the test solution, ensuring that all procedures are carried out simultaneously, and under identical conditions.

Examine the 2 tryptic digests by liquid chromatography (*2.2.29*).

Monographs D-E

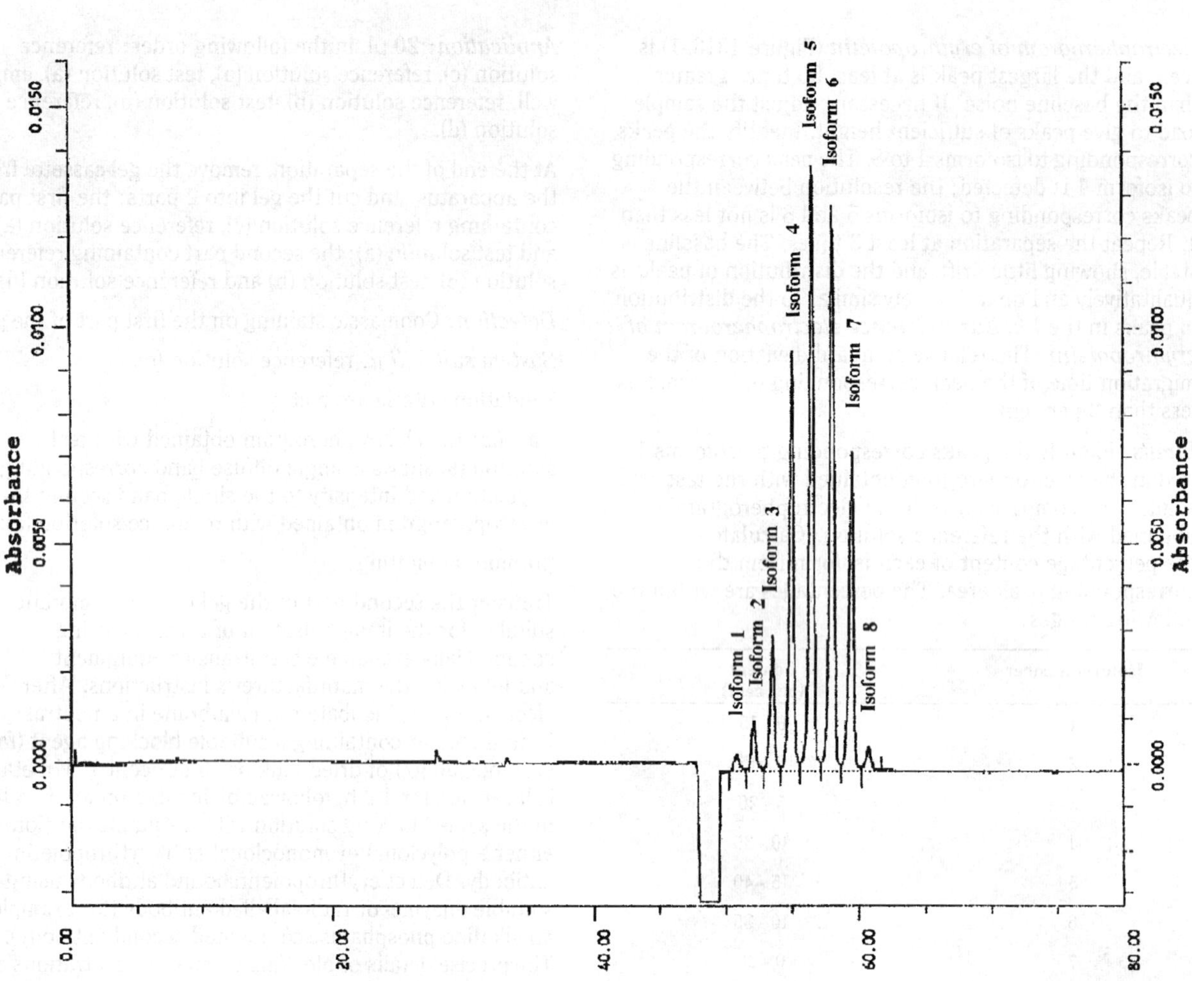

Figure 1316.-1. – *Ph. Eur. reference electropherogram of erythropoietin*

Column:
– *size*: l = 0.25 m, Ø = 4.6 mm,
– *stationary phase*: *butylsilyl silica gel R* (5-10 µm).

Mobile phase:
– *mobile phase A*: 0.06 per cent *V/V* solution of *trifluoroacetic acid R*,
– *mobile phase B*: to 100 ml of *water R* add 0.6 ml of *trifluoroacetic acid R* and dilute to 1000 ml with of *acetonitrile for chromatography R*,

Time (min)	Flow rate (ml/min)	Mobile phase A (per cent *V/V*)	Mobile phase B (per cent *V/V*)
0 - 10	0.75	100	0
10 - 125	0.75	100 → 39	0 → 61
125 - 135	1.25	39 → 17	61 → 83
135 - 145	1.25	17 → 0	83 → 100
145 - 150	1.25	100	0

Detection: spectrophotometer at 214 nm.

Equilibration: at initial conditions for at least 15 min. Carry out a blank run using the above-mentioned gradient.

Injection: 50 µl.

System suitability: the chromatogram obtained with each solution is qualitatively similar to the chromatogram of erythropoietin digest supplied with *erythropoietin BRP*.

Results: the profile of the chromatogram obtained with the test solution corresponds to that of the chromatogram obtained with the reference solution.

E. *N*-terminal sequence analysis

The first 15 amino acids are: Alanine - Proline - Proline - Arginine - Leucine - Isoleucine - (no recovered peak) - Aspartic acid - Serine - Arginine - Valine - Leucine - Glutamic acid - Arginine - Tyrosine.

Perform the Edman degradation using an automated solid-phase sequencer, operated in accordance with the manufacturer's instructions.

Desalt the equivalent of 50 µg of erythropoietin. For example, dilute a volume of the substance to be examined equivalent to 50 µg of the active substance in 1 ml of a 0.1 per cent *V/V* solution of *trifluoroacetic acid R*. Pre-wash a C18 reverse-phase sample preparation cartridge according to the instructions supplied and equilibrate the cartridge in a 0.1 per cent *V/V* solution of *trifluoroacetic acid R*. Apply the sample to the cartridge, and wash successively with a 0.1 per cent *V/V* solution of *trifluoroacetic acid R* containing 0 per cent, 10 per cent and 50 per cent *V/V* of *acetonitrile R* according to the manufacturer's instructions. Lyophilise the 50 per cent *V/V acetonitrile R* eluate.

Redissolve the desalted sample in 50 µl of a 0.1 per cent *V/V* solution of *trifluoroacetic acid R* and couple to a sequencing cartridge using the protocol provided by the manufacturer. Run 15 sequencing cycles, using the reaction conditions for proline when running the second and third cycles.

Identify the phenylthiohydantoin (PTH)-amino acids released at each sequencing cycle by reverse-phase liquid chromatography. The procedure may be carried out using the column and reagents recommended by the manufacturer of the sequencing equipment for the separation of PTH-amino-acids.

The separation procedure is calibrated using:

- the mixture of PTH-amino acids provided by the manufacturer of the sequencer, with the gradient conditions adjusted as indicated to achieve optimum resolution of all amino acids,
- a sample obtained from a blank sequencing cycle obtained as recommended by the equipment manufacturer.

TESTS

Protein (*2.5.33, Method I*): 80 per cent to 120 per cent of the stated concentration.

Test solution. Dilute the preparation to be examined in a 4 g/l solution of *ammonium hydrogen carbonate R*.

Record the absorbance spectrum between 250 nm and 400 nm. Measure the value at the absorbance maximum (276-280 nm), after correction for any light scattering, measured up to 400 nm. Calculate the concentration of erythropoietin using a specific absorbance value of 7.43.

Dimers and related substances of higher molecular mass. Size-exclusion chromatography (*2.2.30*).

Test solution. Dilute the preparation to be examined in the mobile phase to obtain a concentration of 0.2 mg/ml.

Reference solution. To 0.02 ml of the test solution add 0.98 ml of the mobile phase.

Column:

- *size*: l = 0.6 m, Ø = 7.5 mm,
- *stationary phase*: *hydrophilic silica gel for chromatography R*, of a grade suitable for fractionation of globular proteins in the molecular mass range of 20 000 to 200 000.

Mobile phase: dissolve 1.15 g of *anhydrous disodium hydrogen phosphate R*, 0.2 g of *potassium dihydrogen phosphate R* and 23.4 g of *sodium chloride R* in 1 litre of *water R* (1.5 mM potassium dihydrogen phosphate, 8.1 mM disodium hydrogen phosphate, 0.4 M sodium chloride, pH 7.4); adjust the pH to 7.4 if necessary.

Flow rate: 0.5 ml/min.

Detection: spectrophotometer at 214 nm.

Injection: 100 µl.

Run time: minimum 1 h.

System suitability: the area of the principal peak in the chromatogram obtained with the reference solution is 1.5 to 2.5 per cent of the area of the principal peak in the chromatogram obtained with the test solution.

Limit:

- *total of any peaks eluted before the principal peak*: not more than the area of the principal peak in the chromatogram obtained with the reference solution (2 per cent).

Sialic acids: minimum 10 mol of sialic acids (calculated as *N*-acetylneuraminic acid) per mole of erythropoietin.

Test solution (a). Dilute the preparation to be examined in the mobile phase used in the test for dimers and related substances of higher molecular mass to obtain a concentration of 0.3 mg/ml.

Test solution (b). To 0.5 ml of test solution (a) add 0.5 ml of the mobile phase used in the test for dimers and related substances of higher molecular mass.

Reference solution (a). Dissolve a suitable amount of *N-acetylneuraminic acid R* in *water R* to obtain a concentration of 0.1 mg/ml.

Reference solution (b). To 0.8 ml of reference solution (a) add 0.2 ml of *water R*.

Reference solution (c). To 0.6 ml of reference solution (a) add 0.4 ml of *water R*.

Reference solution (d). To 0.4 ml of reference solution (a) add 0.6 ml of *water R*.

Reference solution (e). To 0.2 ml of reference solution (a) add 0.8 ml of *water R*.

Reference solution (f). Use *water R*.

Carry out the test in triplicate. Transfer 100 µl of each of the test and reference solutions to 10 ml glass test tubes. To each tube add 1.0 ml of *resorcinol reagent R*. Stopper the tubes and incubate at 100 °C for 30 min. Cool on ice. To each tube, add 2.0 ml of a mixture of 12 volumes of *butanol R* and 48 volumes of *butyl acetate R*. Mix vigorously, and allow the 2 phases to separate. Ensuring that the upper phase is completely clear, remove the upper phase, taking care to exclude completely any of the lower phase. Measure the absorbance (*2.2.25*) of all samples at 580 nm. Using the calibration curve generated by the reference solutions, determine the content of sialic acids in each of the 2 test solutions and calculate the mean. Calculate the number of moles of sialic acids per mole of erythropoietin assuming that the relative molecular mass of erythropoietin is 30 600 and that the relative molecular mass of *N*-acetylneuraminic acid is 309.

System suitability:

- the individual replicates agree to within ± 10 per cent of each other,
- the value obtained from reference solution (a) is between 1.5 and 2.5 times that obtained with test solution (a).

Bacterial endotoxins (*2.6.14*): less than 20 IU in the volume that contains 100 000 IU of erythropoietin.

ASSAY

The activity of the preparation is compared with that of *erythropoietin BRP* and expressed in International Units (IU).

The estimated potency is not less than 80 per cent and not more than 125 per cent of the stated potency. The confidence limits of the estimated potency (P = 0.95) are not less than 64 per cent and not more than 156 per cent of the stated potency.

Carry out the determination of potency by Method A or B.

A. In polycythaemic mice

The activity of the preparation is estimated by examining, under given conditions, its effect in stimulating the incorporation of ^{59}Fe into circulating red blood cells of mice made polycythaemic by exposure to reduced atmospheric pressure.

The following schedule, using treatment in a hypobaric chamber, has been found to be suitable.

Induce polycythaemia in female mice of the same strain, weighing 16 g to 18 g. Place the mice in a hypoxic chamber and reduce the pressure to 0.6 atmospheres. After 3 days at 0.6 atmospheres, further reduce the pressure to 0.4-0.5 atmospheres and maintain the animals at this pressure for a further 11 days (the partial vacuum is interrupted daily for a maximum of 1 h at about 11:00 a.m., in order to clean the cages and feed the animals). At the end of the specified period, return the mice to normal atmospheric conditions. Randomly distribute the mice into cages, each containing 6 animals, and mark them.

Test solution (a). Dilute the substance to be examined in *phosphate-albumin buffered saline pH 7.2 R1* to obtain a concentration of 0.2 IU/ml.

Test solution (b). Mix equal volumes of test solution (a) and *phosphate-albumin buffered saline pH 7.2 R1*.

Monographs D-E

Test solution (c). Mix equal volumes of test solution (b) and *phosphate-albumin buffered saline pH 7.2 R1.*

Reference solution (a). Dissolve *erythropoietin BRP* in *phosphate-albumin buffered saline pH 7.2 R1* to obtain a concentration of 0.2 IU/ml.

Reference solution (b). Mix equal volumes of reference solution (a) and *phosphate-albumin buffered saline pH 7.2 R1.*

Reference solution (c). Mix equal volumes of reference solution (b) and *phosphate-albumin buffered saline pH 7.2 R1.*

Radiolabelled ferric [^{59}Fe] chloride solution, concentrated. Use a commercially available solution of [^{59}Fe]ferric chloride (approximate specific activity: 100-1000 MBq/mg of Fe).

Radiolabelled [^{59}Fe]ferric chloride solution. Dilute the concentrated radiolabelled [^{59}Fe]ferric chloride solution in *sodium citrate buffer solution pH 7.8 R* to obtain a solution with an activity of 3.7 × 10^4 Bq/ml.

The concentrations of the test solutions and reference solutions may need to be modified, based on the response range of the animals used.

3 days after returning the animals to atmospheric pressure, inject each animal subcutaneously with 0.2 ml of one of the solutions. The 6 animals in each cage must each receive one of the 6 different treatments (3 test solutions and 3 reference solutions), and the order of injection must be separately randomised for each cage. A minimum of 8 cages is recommended. 2 days after injection of the test or reference solution, inject each animal intraperitoneally with 0.2 ml of radiolabelled [^{59}Fe]ferric chloride solution. The order of the injections must be the same as that of the erythropoietin injections, and the time interval between administration of the erythropoietin and the radiolabelled ferric chloride solution must be the same for each animal. After a further 48 h, anaesthetise each animal by injection of a suitable anaesthetic, record body weights and withdraw blood samples (0.65 ml) into haematocrit capillaries from the bifurcation of the aorta. After determining the packed cell volume for each sample, measure the radioactivity.

Calculate the response (percentage of iron-59 in total circulating blood) for each mouse using the expression:

$$\frac{A_s \times M \times 7.5}{A_t \times V_s}$$

A_s = radioactivity in the sample,

A_t = total radioactivity injected,

7.5 = total blood volume as per cent body weight,

M = body weight, in grams,

V_s = sample volume.

Calculate the potency by the usual statistical methods for a parallel line assay. Eliminate from the calculation any animal where the packed cell volume is less than 54 per cent, or where the body weight is more than 24 g.

B. In normocythaemic mice

The assay is based on the measurement of stimulation of reticulocyte production in normocythaemic mice.

The assay may be carried out using the following procedure:

Test solution (a). Dilute the substance to be examined in *phosphate-albumin buffered saline pH 7.2 R1* to obtain a concentration of 80 IU/ml.

Test solution (b). Mix equal volumes of test solution (a) and *phosphate-albumin buffered saline pH 7.2 R1.*

Test solution (c). Mix equal volumes of test solution (b) and *phosphate-albumin buffered saline pH 7.2 R1.*

Reference solution (a). Dissolve *erythropoietin BRP* in *phosphate-albumin buffered saline pH 7.2 R1* to obtain a concentration of 80 IU/ml.

Reference solution (b). Mix equal volumes of reference solution (a) and *phosphate-albumin buffered saline pH 7.2 R1.*

Reference solution (c). Mix equal volumes of reference solution (b) and *phosphate-albumin buffered saline pH 7.2 R1.*

The exact concentrations of the test solutions and reference solutions may need to be modified, based on the response range of the animals used.

At the beginning of the assay procedure, randomly distribute mice of a suitable age and strain (8-week old B6D2F1 mice are suitable) into 6 cages. A minimum of 8 mice per cage is recommended. Inject each animal subcutaneously with 0.5 ml of the appropriate treatment (one solution per cage) and put the animal in a new cage. Combine the mice in such a way that each cage housing the treated mice contains one mouse out of the 6 different treatments (3 test solutions and 3 reference solutions, 6 mice per cage). 4 days after the injections, collect blood samples from the animals and determine the number of reticulocytes using a suitable procedure.

The following method may be employed:

The volume of blood, dilution procedure and fluorescent reagent may need to be modified to ensure maximum development and stability of fluorescence.

Colorant solution, concentrated. Use a solution of thiazole orange suitable for the determination of reticulocytes. Prepare at a concentration twice that necessary for the analysis.

Proceed with the following dilution steps. Dilute whole blood 500-fold in the buffer used to prepare the colorant solution. Dilute this solution 2-fold in the concentrated colorant solution. After staining for 3-10 min, determine the reticulocyte count microfluorometrically in a flow cytometer. The percentage of reticulocytes is determined using a biparametric histogram: number of cells/red fluorescence (620 nm).

Calculate the potency by the usual statistical methods for a parallel line assay.

STORAGE

In an airtight container at a temperature below −20 °C. Avoid repeated freezing and thawing.

LABELLING

The label states:

– the erythropoietin content in milligrams per millilitre,

– the activity in International Units per millilitre,

– the name and the concentration of any other excipients.

01/2005:1742

ESKETAMINE HYDROCHLORIDE

Esketamini hydrochloridum

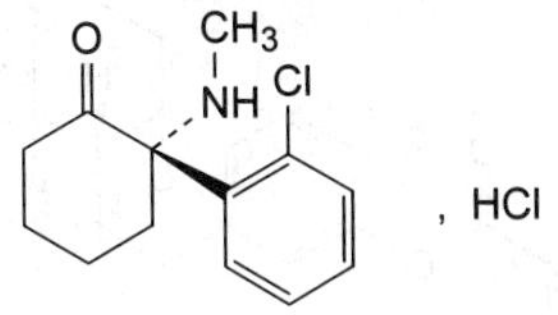

$C_{13}H_{17}Cl_2NO$ M_r 274.2

DEFINITION

(2*S*)-2-(2-Chlorophenyl)-2-(methylamino)cyclohexanone hydrochloride.

Content: 99.0 per cent to 101.0 per cent.

CHARACTERS

Appearance: white, crystalline powder.

Solubility: freely soluble in water and in methanol, soluble in alcohol.

IDENTIFICATION

A. Specific optical rotation (*2.2.7*): + 85.0 to + 95.0.

Dilute 12.5 ml of solution S (see Tests) to 40.0 ml with *water R*.

B. Infrared absorption spectrophotometry (*2.2.24*).

Comparison: *Ph. Eur. reference spectrum of esketamine hydrochloride*.

C. It gives reaction (a) of chlorides (*2.3.1*).

TESTS

Solution S. Dissolve 8.0 g in *carbon dioxide-free water R* and dilute to 50.0 ml with the same solvent.

Appearance of solution. Solution S is clear (*2.2.1*) and colourless (*2.2.2, Method II*).

pH (*2.2.3*): 3.5 to 4.5.

Dilute 12.5 ml of solution S to 20 ml with *carbon dioxide-free water R*.

Impurity D. Liquid chromatography (*2.2.29*).

Test solution. Dissolve 25.0 mg of the substance to be examined in *water R* and dilute to 100.0 ml with the same solvent.

Reference solution (a). Dissolve 5 mg of *esketamine impurity D CRS* in *water R*, add 20 ml of the test solution and dilute to 50 ml with *water R*. Dilute 10 ml of this solution to 100 ml with *water R*.

Reference solution (b). Dilute 5.0 ml of the test solution to 25.0 ml with *water R*. Dilute 5.0 ml of this solution to 50.0 ml with *water R*.

Reference solution (c). Dilute 2.5 ml of reference solution (b) to 10.0 ml with *water R*. Dilute 1.0 ml of this solution to 10.0 ml with *water R*.

Precolumn:

- *size*: *l* = 0.01 m, Ø = 3.0 mm,
- *stationary phase*: *silica gel AGP for chiral chromatography R* (5 µm),
- *temperature*: 30 °C.

Column:

- *size*: *l* = 0.125 m, Ø = 4.6 mm,
- *stationary phase*: *silica gel AGP for chiral chromatography R* (5 µm),
- *temperature*: 30 °C.

Mobile phase: mix 16 volumes of *methanol R* and 84 volumes of a 6.8 g/l solution of *potassium dihydrogen phosphate R* previously adjusted to pH 7.0 with *potassium hydroxide R*.

Flow rate: 0.8 ml/min.

Detection: spectrophotometer at 215 nm.

Injection: 20 µl.

Run time: 20 min.

Relative retention with reference to esketamine (retention time = about 10 min): impurity D = about 1.3.

System suitability:

- *resolution*: minimum 2.0 between the peaks due to esketamine and impurity D in the chromatogram obtained with reference solution (a),
- *signal-to-noise ratio*: minimum 3 for the principal peak in the chromatogram obtained with reference solution (c).

Limit:

- *impurity D*: not more than the area of the principal peak in the chromatogram obtained with reference solution (b) (2.0 per cent).

Related substances. Liquid chromatography (*2.2.29*).

Test solution. Dissolve 50.0 mg of the substance to be examined in the mobile phase and dilute to 50.0 ml with the mobile phase.

Reference solution (a). Dissolve 5 mg of *ketamine impurity A CRS* in the mobile phase (using ultrasound, if necessary) and dilute to 10 ml with the mobile phase. To 1 ml of the solution add 0.5 ml of the test solution and dilute to 100 ml with the mobile phase. Prepare immediately before use.

Reference solution (b). Dilute 1.0 ml of the test solution to 10.0 ml with the mobile phase. Dilute 1.0 ml of this solution to 20.0 ml with the mobile phase.

Column:

- *size*: *l* = 0.125 m, Ø = 4.0 mm,
- *stationary phase*: spherical *octadecylsilyl silica gel for chromatography R* (5 µm).

Mobile phase: dissolve 0.95 g of *sodium hexanesulphonate R* in 1000 ml of a mixture of 25 volumes of *acetonitrile R* and 75 volumes of *water R* and add 4 ml of *acetic acid R*.

Flow rate: 1.0 ml/min.

Detection: spectrophotometer at 215 nm.

Injection: 20 µl.

Run time: 10 times the retention time of esketamine.

Relative retention with reference to esketamine: impurity A = about 1.6; impurity B = about 3.3; impurity C = about 4.6.

System suitability: reference solution (a):

- *retention time*: esketamine = 3.0 min to 4.5 min,
- *resolution*: minimum 1.5 between the peaks due to impurity A and esketamine.

Limits:

- *impurities A, B, C*: for each impurity, not more than 0.4 times the area of the principal peak in the chromatogram obtained with reference solution (b) (0.2 per cent),

- *any other impurity*: for each impurity, not more than 0.2 times the area of the principal peak in the chromatogram obtained with reference solution (b) (0.1 per cent),
- *total*: not more than the area of the principal peak in the chromatogram obtained with reference solution (b) (0.5 per cent),
- *disregard limit*: 0.2 times the area of the principal peak in the chromatogram obtained with reference solution (b) (0.1 per cent).

Heavy metals (*2.4.8*): maximum 20 ppm.

Dilute 12.5 ml of solution S to 20 ml with *water R*. 12 ml of the solution complies with limit test A. Prepare the standard using *lead standard solution (2 ppm Pb) R*.

Sulphated ash (*2.4.14*): maximum 0.1 per cent, determined on 1.0 g.

ASSAY

Dissolve 0.200 g in 50 ml of *methanol R* and add 1.0 ml of *0.1 M hydrochloric acid*. Carry out a potentiometric titration (*2.2.20*), using *0.1 M sodium hydroxide*. Read the volume added between the 2 points of inflexion.

1 ml of *0.1 M sodium hydroxide* is equivalent to 27.42 mg of $C_{13}H_{17}Cl_2NO$.

STORAGE

Protected from light.

IMPURITIES

Specified impurities: A, B, C, D.

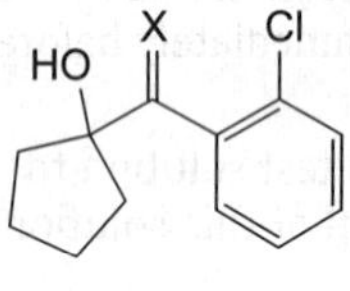

A. X = N-CH_3: 1-[(2-chlorophenyl)(methylimino)methyl]cyclopentanol,

C. X = O: (2-chlorophenyl)(1-hydroxycyclopentyl)methanone,

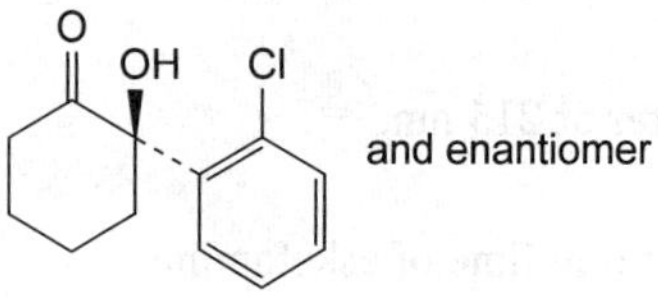

B. (2*RS*)-2-(2-chlorophenyl)-2-hydroxycyclohexanone,

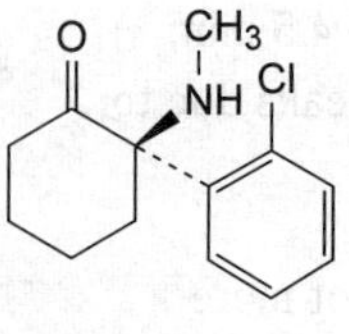

D. (2*R*)-2-(2-chlorophenyl)-2-(methylamino)cyclohexanone ((*R*)-ketamine).

01/2005:0139

ESTRADIOL BENZOATE

Estradioli benzoas

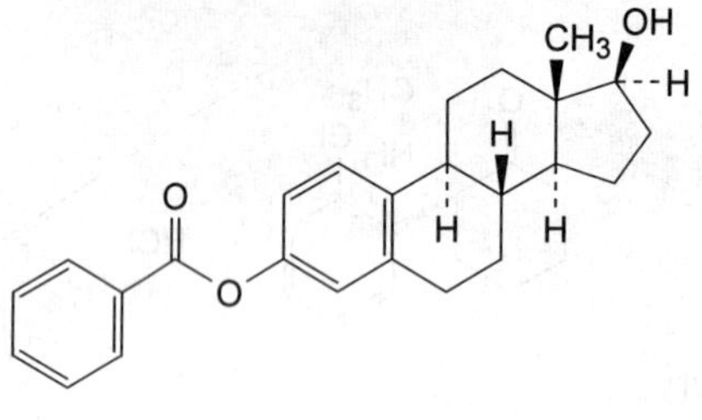

$C_{25}H_{28}O_3$ M_r 376.5

DEFINITION

17β-Hydroxyestra-1,3,5(10)-trien-3-yl benzoate.

Content: 97.0 per cent to 103.0 per cent (dried substance).

CHARACTERS

Appearance: almost white, crystalline powder or colourless crystals.

Solubility: practically insoluble in water, freely soluble in methylene chloride, sparingly soluble in acetone, slightly soluble in methanol.

It shows polymorphism.

IDENTIFICATION

Infrared absorption spectrophotometry (*2.2.24*).

Comparison: *estradiol benzoate CRS*.

If the spectra obtained in the solid state show differences, dissolve the substance to be examined and the reference substance separately in *acetone R*, evaporate to dryness and record new spectra using the residues.

TESTS

Specific optical rotation (*2.2.7*): + 55.0 to + 59.0 (dried substance).

Dissolve 0.250 g in *acetone R* and dilute to 25.0 ml with the same solvent.

Related substances. Liquid chromatography (*2.2.29*).

Test solution. Dissolve 20 mg of the substance to be examined in *acetonitrile R* and dilute to 10.0 ml with the same solvent.

Reference solution (a). Dissolve 5 mg of *estradiol benzoate impurity E CRS* in 5 ml of *acetonitrile R*, add 2.5 ml of the test solution and dilute to 10 ml with *acetonitrile R*.

Reference solution (b). Dilute 1.0 ml of the test solution to 100.0 ml with *acetonitrile R*.

Column:
- *size*: l = 0.25 m, Ø = 4.6 mm,
- *stationary phase*: *octylsilyl silica gel for chromatography R* (5 μm).

Mobile phase:
- *mobile phase A*: *water R*, *acetonitrile R* (40:60 *V/V*),
- *mobile phase B*: *acetonitrile R*,

Time (min)	Mobile phase A (per cent *V/V*)	Mobile phase B (per cent *V/V*)
0 - t_R	100	0
t_R - (t_R + 1)	100 → 10	0 → 90
(t_R + 1) - (t_R + 10)	10	90

t_R = retention time of impurity E

Flow rate: 1.0 ml/min.
Detection: spectrophotometer at 230 nm.
Injection: 10 μl.
Elution order: impurity A, impurity F, estradiol benzoate, impurity E, impurity B, impurity D, impurity C.
Relative retention with reference to estradiol benzoate: impurity C = about 1.5.
System suitability: reference solution (a):
- *resolution*: minimum 2.0 between the peaks due to estradiol benzoate and impurity E.

Limits:
- *correction factor*: for the calculation of content, multiply the peak area of impurity C by 0.7,
- *any impurity*: for each impurity, not more than 0.5 times the area of the principal peak in the chromatogram obtained with reference solution (b) (0.5 per cent),
- *total*: not more than 1.5 times the area of the principal peak in the chromatogram obtained with reference solution (b) (1.5 per cent),
- *disregard limit*: 0.05 times the area of the principal peak in the chromatogram obtained with reference solution (b) (0.05 per cent).

Loss on drying (*2.2.32*): maximum 0.5 per cent, determined on 0.5 g by drying in an oven at 100-105 °C for 3 h.

ASSAY

Dissolve 25.0 mg in *anhydrous ethanol R* and dilute to 250.0 ml with the same solvent. Dilute 10.0 ml of the solution to 100.0 ml with *anhydrous ethanol R*. Measure the absorbance (*2.2.25*) at the absorption maximum at 231 nm.
Calculate the content of $C_{25}H_{28}O_3$ taking the specific absorbance to be 500.

IMPURITIES

Specified impurities: A, B, C, D, E, F.

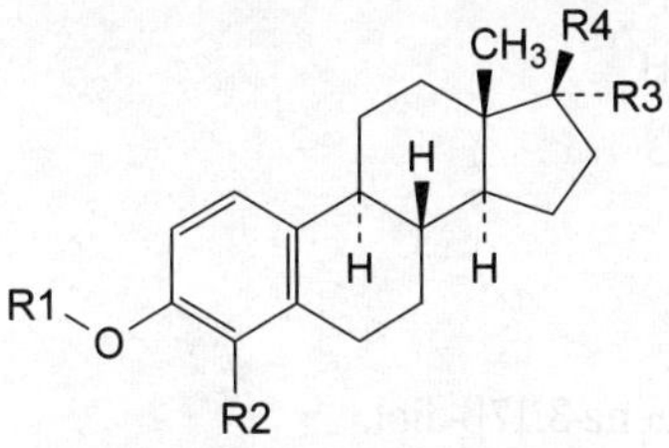

A. R1 = R2 = R3 = H, R4 = OH: estradiol,

B. R1 = CO-C_6H_5, R2 = CH_3, R3 = H, R4 = OH: 17β-hydroxy-4-methylestra-1,3,5(10)-trien-3-yl benzoate,

C. R1 = CO-C_6H_5, R2 = R3 = H, R4 = O-CO-C_6H_5: estra-1,3,5(10)-triene-3,17β-diyl dibenzoate,

D. R1 = R2 = R3 = H, R4 = O-CO-C_6H_5: 3-hydroxyestra-1,3, 5(10)-trien-17β-yl benzoate,

E. R1 = CO-C_6H_5, R2 = R4 = H, R3 = OH: 17α-hydroxyestra-1,3,5(10)-trien-3-yl benzoate,

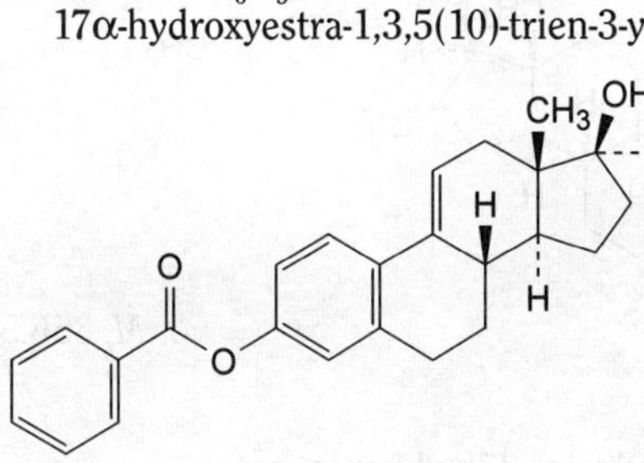

F. 17β-hydroxyestra-1,3,5(10),9(11)-tetraen-3-yl benzoate.

01/2005:0821

ESTRADIOL HEMIHYDRATE

Estradiolum hemihydricum

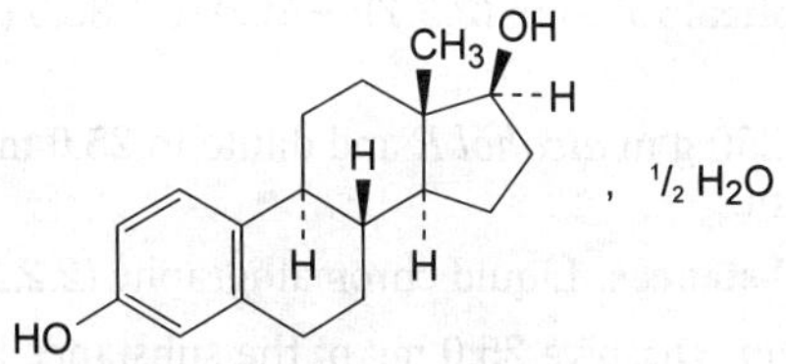

$C_{18}H_{24}O_2,{}^1/_2H_2O$ M_r 281.4

DEFINITION

Estra-1,3,5(10)-triene-3,17β-diol hemihydrate.

Content: 97.0 per cent to 103.0 per cent (anhydrous substance).

CHARACTERS

Appearance: white or almost white, crystalline powder or colourless crystals.

Solubility: practically insoluble in water, soluble in acetone, sparingly soluble in alcohol, slightly soluble in methylene chloride.

IDENTIFICATION

First identification: B.

Second identification: A, C, D, E.

A. Melting point (*2.2.14*): 175 °C to 180 °C.

B. Infrared absorption spectrophotometry (*2.2.24*).
Comparison: *estradiol hemihydrate CRS.*

C. Thin-layer chromatography (*2.2.27*).
Test solution. Dissolve 50 mg of the substance to be examined in *methanol R* and dilute to 50 ml with the same solvent.
Reference solution (a). Dissolve 50 mg of *estradiol hemihydrate CRS* in *methanol R* and dilute to 50 ml with the same solvent.
Reference solution (b). Dissolve 25 mg of *ethinylestradiol CRS* in reference solution (a) and dilute to 25 ml with reference solution (a).
Plate: *TLC silica gel plate R.*
Mobile phase: *alcohol R, toluene R (20:80 V/V).*
Application: 5 μl.
Development: over 3/4 of the plate.
Drying: in air until the solvent has evaporated.
Detection: heat at 110 °C for 10 min. Spray the hot plate with *alcoholic solution of sulphuric acid R*. Heat again at 110 °C for 10 min. Allow to cool. Examine in daylight and in ultraviolet light at 365 nm.
System suitability: the chromatogram obtained with reference solution (b) shows 2 spots which may however not be completely separated.
Results: the principal spot in the chromatogram obtained with the test solution is similar in position, colour in daylight, fluorescence in ultraviolet light at 365 nm and size to the principal spot in the chromatogram obtained with reference solution (a).

D. To about 1 mg add 0.5 ml of freshly prepared *sulphomolybdic reagent R2*. A blue colour develops which in ultraviolet light at 365 nm has an intense green fluorescence. Add 1 ml of *sulphuric acid R* and 9 ml of *water R*. The colour becomes pink with a yellowish fluorescence.

E. It complies with the test for water (see Tests).

TESTS

Specific optical rotation (*2.2.7*): + 76.0 to + 83.0 (anhydrous substance).

Dissolve 0.250 g in *alcohol R* and dilute to 25.0 ml with the same solvent.

Related substances. Liquid chromatography (*2.2.29*).

Test solution. Dissolve 25.0 mg of the substance to be examined in 10 ml of *acetonitrile R* and dilute to 25.0 ml with *methanol R2*.

Reference solution (a). Dilute 1.0 ml of the test solution to 100.0 ml with the mobile phase. Dilute 2.0 ml of the solution to 10.0 ml with the mobile phase.

Reference solution (b). Dissolve 2 mg of *17α-estradiol R* in 5.0 ml of *acetonitrile R*. Mix 2.0 ml of this solution with 1.0 ml of the test solution and dilute to 5.0 ml with the mobile phase.

Reference solution (c). Mix equal volumes of a 1 mg/ml solution of the substance to be examined in *methanol R2* and of a 1 mg/ml solution of *2,3-dichloro-5,6-dicyanobenzoquinone R* in *methanol R2*. Allow to stand for 30 min before injection.

Reference solution (d). Dissolve 5 mg of *estradiol for peak identification CRS* (estradiol hemihydrate spiked with impurities A, B and C at about 0.5 per cent) in 2 ml of *acetonitrile R* and dilute to 5 ml with *methanol R2*.

Column:

- size: *l* = 0.25 m, Ø = 4.6 mm,
- *stationary phase*: *end-capped octadecylsilyl silica gel for chromatography R* (5 µm).

Mobile phase: to 400 ml of *acetonitrile R* add 50 ml of *methanol R2* and 400 ml of *water R*; allow to stand for 10 min, dilute to 1000 ml with *water R* and mix again.

Flow rate: 1 ml/min.

Detection: spectrophotometer at 280 nm.

Equilibration: about 60 min.

Injection: 20 µl.

Run time: twice the retention time of the principal peak.

Relative retention with reference to estradiol (retention time = about 13 min): impurity D = about 0.9; impurity B = about 1.1; impurity A = about 1.4; impurity C = about 1.9.

System suitability: reference solution (b):

- *resolution*: minimum 2.5 between the peaks due to estradiol and impurity B.

Limits:

- *correction factor*: for the calculation of content, multiply the peak area of impurity D by 0.4 (use the chromatogram obtained with reference solution (c) to identify this peak),
- *impurities A, B, C, D*: for each impurity, not more than 1.5 times the area of the principal peak obtained with reference solution (a) (0.3 per cent),
- *any other impurity*: for each impurity, not more than 0.5 times the area of the principal peak obtained with reference solution (a) (0.1 per cent),
- *total*: not more than 2.5 times the area of the principal peak in the chromatogram obtained with reference solution (a) (0.5 per cent),
- *disregard limit*: 0.25 times the area of the principal peak in the chromatogram obtained with reference solution (a) (0.05 per cent).

Water (*2.5.12*): 2.9 per cent to 3.5 per cent, determined on 0.500 g.

ASSAY

Dissolve 20.0 mg in *alcohol R* and dilute to 100.0 ml with the same solvent. Dilute 5.0 ml of the solution to 50.0 ml with *0.1 M sodium hydroxide*. Allow to cool to room temperature. Measure the absorbance (*2.2.25*) of the solution at the maximum at 238 nm.

Calculate the content of $C_{18}H_{24}O_2$ taking the specific absorbance to be 335.

IMPURITIES

Specified impurities: A, B, C, D.

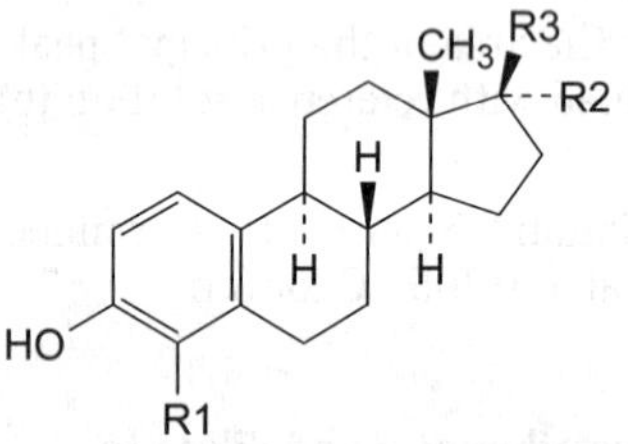

A. R1 = H, R2 + R3 = O: 3-hydroxyestra-1,3,5(10)-trien-17-one (estrone),

B. R1 = R3 = H, R2 = OH: estra-1,3,5(10)-triene-3,17α-diol (17α-estradiol),

C. R1 = CH_3, R2 = H, R3 = OH: 4-methylestra-1,3,5(10)-triene-3,17β-diol,

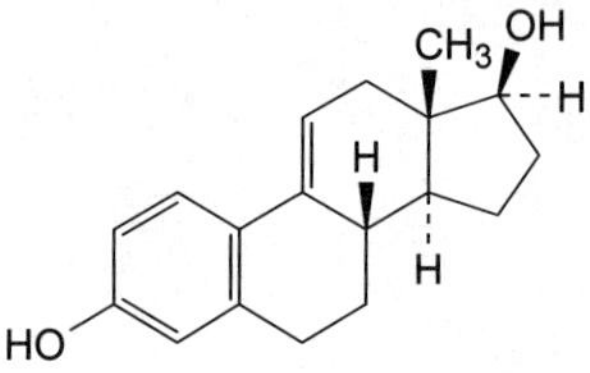

D. estra-1,3,5(10),9(11)-tetraene-3,17β-diol.

01/2005:1614

ESTRADIOL VALERATE

Estradioli valeras

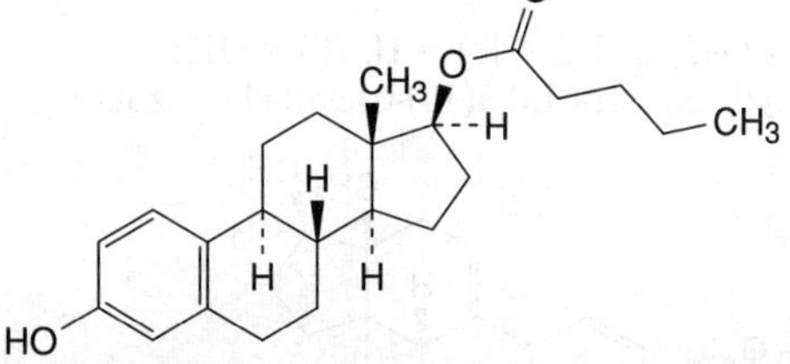

$C_{23}H_{32}O_3$ M_r 356.5

DEFINITION

3-Hydroxyestra-1,3,5(10)-trien-17β-yl pentanoate.

Content: 97.0 per cent to 103.0 per cent (dried substance).

CHARACTERS

Appearance: white or almost white, crystalline powder or colourless crystals.

Solubility: practically insoluble in water, soluble in alcohol.

mp: about 145 °C.

IDENTIFICATION

Infrared absorption spectrophotometry (*2.2.24*).

Comparison: *estradiol valerate CRS*.

TESTS

Solution S. Dissolve 0.500 g in *methanol R* and dilute to 20.0 ml with the same solvent.

Appearance of solution. Solution S is clear (*2.2.1*) and colourless (*2.2.2, Method II*).

Specific optical rotation (*2.2.7*): + 41 to + 47 (dried substance), determined on solution S.

Related substances. Liquid chromatography (*2.2.29*).

Solvent mixture. Mix 15 volumes of *water R* and 135 volumes of *acetonitrile R*.

Test solution. Dissolve 0.100 g of the substance to be examined in the solvent mixture and dilute to 10.0 ml with the solvent mixture.

Reference solution (a). Dissolve 2 mg of *estradiol valerate CRS* and 2 mg of *estradiol butyrate CRS* in the solvent mixture and dilute to 10 ml with the solvent mixture.

Reference solution (b). Dilute 0.5 ml of the test solution to 100.0 ml with the solvent mixture.

Column:
- *size*: *l* = 0.25 m, Ø = 4.6 mm,
- *stationary phase*: *octadecylsilyl silica gel for chromatography R* (5 µm),
- *temperature*: 40 °C.

Mobile phase:
- *mobile phase A*: *water R*,
- *mobile phase B*: *acetonitrile R*,

Time (min)	**Mobile phase A (per cent *V/V*)**	**Mobile phase B (per cent *V/V*)**
0 - 15	40 → 0	60 → 100
15 - 25	0	100
25 - 30	40	60
30 = 0	40	60

Flow rate: 1.0 ml/min.

Detection: spectrophotometer at 220 nm.

Injection: 10 µl.

Relative retention with reference to estradiol valerate (retention time = about 12 min): impurity F = about 0.9.

System suitability: reference solution (a):
- *resolution*: minimum of 5.0 between the peaks due to impurity F and to estradiol valerate.

Limits:
- *any impurity*: not more than the area of the principal peak in the chromatogram obtained with reference solution (b) (0.5 per cent),
- *total*: not more than twice the area of the principal peak in the chromatogram obtained with reference solution (b) (1.0 per cent),
- *disregard limit*: 0.1 times the area of the principal peak in the chromatogram obtained with reference solution (b) (0.05 per cent).

Loss on drying (*2.2.32*): maximum 1.0 per cent, determined on 0.500 g by drying in an oven at 100-105 °C for 3 h.

ASSAY

Dissolve 25.0 mg in *alcohol R* and dilute to 250.0 ml with the same solvent. Measure the absorbance (*2.2.25*) at the maximum at 280 nm.

Calculate the content of $C_{23}H_{32}O_3$ taking the specific absorbance to be 58.0.

STORAGE

Protected from light.

IMPURITIES

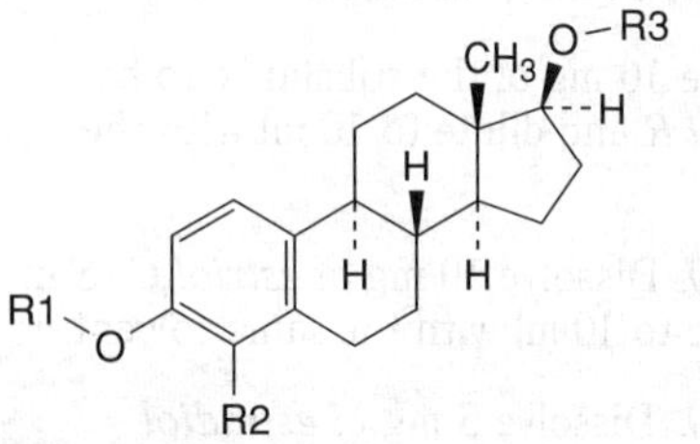

A. R1 = R2 = R3 = H: estradiol,

B. R1 = CO-$[CH_2]_3$-CH_3, R2 = R3 = H: 17β-hydroxyestra-1,3,5(10)-trien-3-yl pentanoate,

D. R1 = H,R2 = CH_3,R3 = CO-$[CH_2]_3$-CH_3: 3-hydroxy-4-methylestra-1,3,5(10)-trien-17β-yl pentanoate,

E. R1 = R3 = CO-$[CH_2]_3$-CH_3,R2 = H: estra-1,3,5(10)-trien-3,17β-diyl dipentanoate,

F. R1 = R2 = H,R3 = CO-$[CH_2]_2$-CH_3: 3-hydroxyestra-1,3,5(10)-trien-17β-yl butanoate (estradiol butyrate),

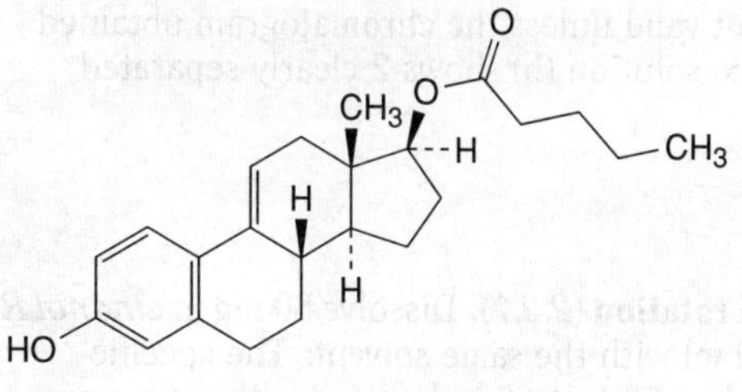

C. 3-hydroxyestra-1,3,5(10),9(11)-tetraen-17β-yl pentanoate.

01/2005:1203

ESTRIOL

Estriolum

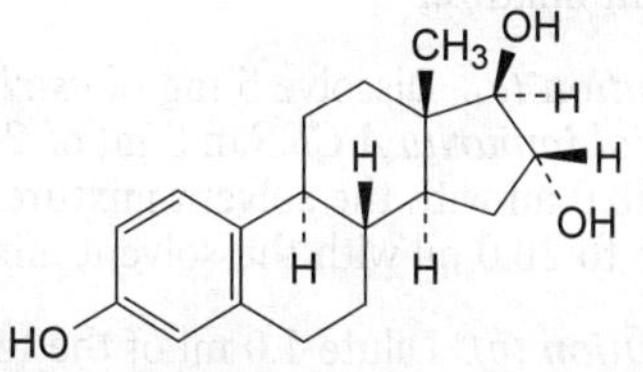

$C_{18}H_{24}O_3$ M_r 288.4

DEFINITION

Estriol contains not less than 97.0 per cent and not more than the equivalent of 103.0 per cent of estra-1,3,5(10)-triene-3,16α,17β-triol, calculated with reference to the dried substance.

Monographs D-E

CHARACTERS

A white or almost white, crystalline powder, practically insoluble in water, sparingly soluble in alcohol.

It melts about 282 °C.

IDENTIFICATION

A. Examine by infrared absorption spectrophotometry (*2.2.24*), comparing with the spectrum obtained with *estriol CRS*.

B. Examine by thin-layer chromatography (*2.2.27*), using a suitable silica gel as the coating substance.

Test solution. Dissolve 10 mg of the substance to be examined in *methanol R* and dilute to 10 ml with the same solvent.

Reference solution (a). Dissolve 10 mg of *estriol CRS* in *methanol R* and dilute to 10 ml with the same solvent.

Reference solution (b). Dissolve 5 mg of *estradiol hemihydrate CRS* in reference solution (a) and dilute to 5 ml with the same solvent.

Apply to the plate 5 µl of each solution. Develop over a path of 15 cm using a mixture of 20 volumes of *alcohol R* and 80 volumes of *toluene R*. Allow the plate to dry in air. Spray the plate with *alcoholic solution of sulphuric acid R*. Heat the plate at 100 °C for 10 min or until the spots appear. Allow to cool. Examine in daylight and ultraviolet light at 365 nm. The principal spot in the chromatogram obtained with the test solution is similar in position, colour in daylight, fluorescence in ultraviolet light at 365 nm and size to the principal spot in the chromatogram obtained with the reference solution (a). The test is not valid unless the chromatogram obtained with reference solution (b) shows 2 clearly separated spots.

TESTS

Specific optical rotation (*2.2.7*). Dissolve 80 mg in *ethanol R* and dilute to 10 ml with the same solvent. The specific optical rotation is + 60 to + 65, calculated with reference to the dried substance.

Related substances. Examine by liquid chromatography (*2.2.29*).

Solvent mixture. A mixture of 20 volumes of *2-propanol R1* and 80 volumes of *heptane R*.

Test solution. Dissolve 20.0 mg of the substance to be examined in 5 ml of *2-propanol R1* and dilute to 20.0 ml with the solvent mixture.

Reference solution (a). Dissolve 5 mg of *estriol CRS* and 2.0 mg of *estriol impurity A CRS* in 5 ml of *2-propanol R1* and dilute to 10.0 ml with the solvent mixture. Dilute 1.0 ml of the solution to 20.0 ml with the solvent mixture.

Reference solution (b). Dilute 1.0 ml of the test solution to 10.0 ml with the solvent mixture. Dilute 1.0 ml of the solution to 10.0 ml with the same solvent mixture.

The chromatographic procedure may be carried out using:

- a stainless steel column 0.15 m long and 4.0 mm in internal diameter packed with *diol silica gel for chromatography R* (5 µm),
- as mobile phase at a flow rate of 1.2 ml/min a linear gradient programme using the following conditions:

Mobile phase A. Heptane R,

Mobile phase B. 2-Propanol R1,

Time (min)	Mobile phase A (per cent V/V)	Mobile phase B (per cent V/V)	Comment
0 - 10	95 → 88	5 → 12	linear gradient
10 - 20	88	12	isocratic
20 - 30	88 → 95	12 → 5	switch to initial eluent composition
30 - 35	95	5	equilibration
35 = 0	95	5	restart gradient

- as detector a spectrophotometer set at 280 nm,

maintaining the temperature of the column at 40 °C. Equilibrate the column with a mixture of 20 per cent *V/V* of *2-propanol R1* in *heptane R* until a stable baseline is obtained.

Adjust the sensitivity of the system so that the height of the principal peak in the chromatogram obtained with 20 µl of reference solution (b) is about 25 per cent of the full scale of the recorder.

Inject 20 µl of reference solution (a). When the chromatograms are recorded in the prescribed conditions, the retention times are: estriol about 19 min and estriol impurity A about 21 min. The test is not valid unless the resolution between the peaks corresponding to estriol and estriol impurity A is at least 2.2. If the retention times increase or the resolution decreases, wash the column first with *acetone R* and then with *heptane R*.

Inject separately 20 µl of the solvent mixture as a blank, 20 µl of the test solution and 20 µl of each of the reference solutions (a) and (b). In the chromatogram obtained with the test solution: the area of any peak corresponding to estriol impurity A is not greater than half the area of the peak corresponding to estriol impurity A in the chromatogram obtained with reference solution (a) (0.5 per cent) and any other peak, apart from the principal peak, is not greater than half the area of the principal peak in the chromatogram obtained with reference solution (b) (0.5 per cent); the sum of the areas of all the peaks, apart from the principal peak and the peak corresponding to estriol impurity A, is not greater than the area of the peak in the chromatogram obtained with reference solution (b) (1 per cent). Disregard any peak due to the blank and any peak with an area less than 0.05 times the area of the principal peak in the chromatogram obtained with reference solution (b).

Loss on drying (*2.2.32*). Not more than 0.5 per cent, determined on 1.000 g by drying in an oven at 100-105 °C for 3 h.

ASSAY

Dissolve 25.0 mg in *alcohol R* and dilute to 50.0 ml with the same solvent. Dilute 10.0 ml of this solution to 50.0 ml with the same solvent. Measure the absorbance (*2.2.25*) at the maximum at 281 nm.

Calculate the content of $C_{18}H_{24}O_3$ taking the specific absorbance to be 72.5.

IMPURITIES

Specified impurities: A, B, C, D, E, F, G.

Other detectable impurities: H, I.

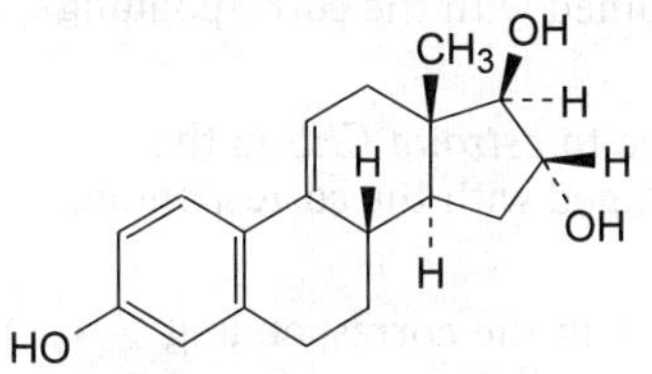

A. estra-1,3,5(10),9(11)-tetraene-3,16α,17β-triol (9,11-didehydroestriol),

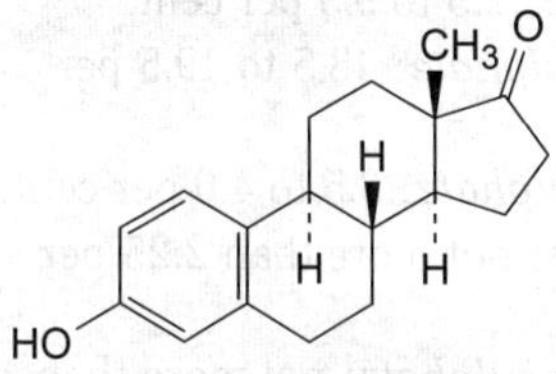

B. 3-hydroxyestra-1,3,5(10)-trien-17-one (estrone),

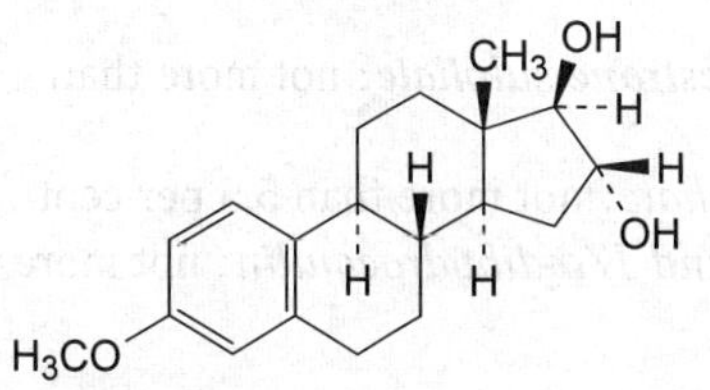

C. 3-methoxyestra-1,3,5(10)-triene-16α,17β-diol (estriol 3-methyl ether),

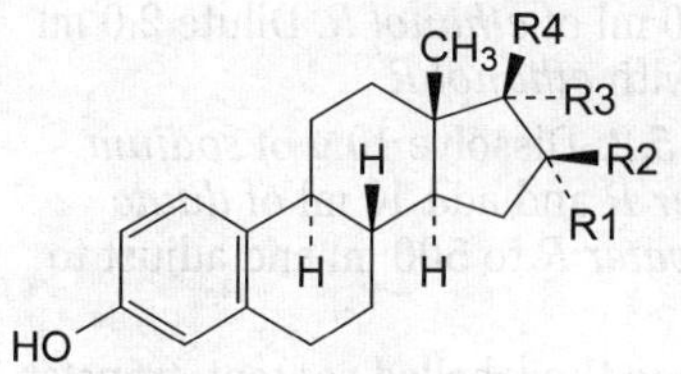

D. R1 = R2 = R3 = H, R4 = OH: estradiol,

E. R1 = R3 = OH, R2 = R4 = H: estra-1,3,5(10)-triene-3,16α, 17α-triol (17-epi-estriol),

F. R1 = R3 = H, R2 = R4 = OH: estra-1,3,5(10)-triene-3,16β, 17β-triol (16-epi-estriol),

G. R1 = R4 = H, R2 = R3 = OH: estra-1,3,5(10)-triene-3,16β, 17α-triol (16,17-epi-estriol),

H. R1 = OH, R2 = H, R3 + R4 = O: 3,16α-dihydroxyestra-1, 3,5(10)-trien-17-one,

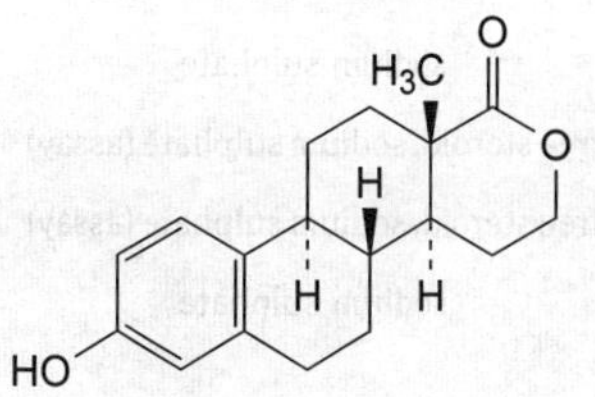

I. 3-hydroxy-17-oxa-*D*-homoestra-1,3,5(10)-trien-17a-one.

01/2005:1512

ESTROGENS, CONJUGATED

Estrogeni coniuncti

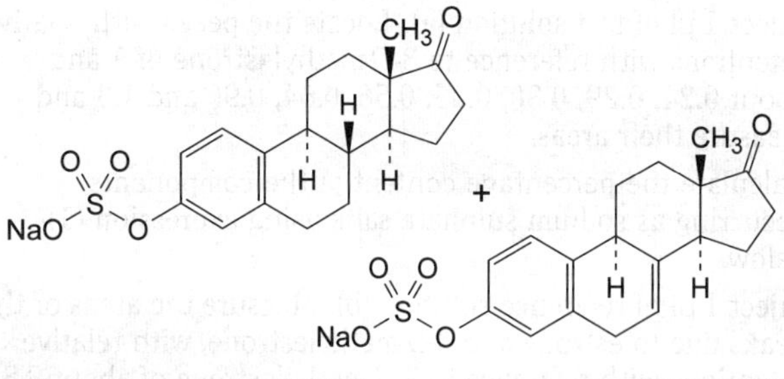

$C_{18}H_{21}O_5NaS + C_{18}H_{19}O_5NaS$ M_r 372.4 + 370.4

DEFINITION

Conjugated estrogens are a mixture of various conjugated forms of estrogens obtained from the urine of pregnant mares or by synthesis, dispersed in a suitable powdered diluent.

The two principal components are 17-oxoestra-1,3,5(10)-trien-3-yl sodium sulphate (sodium estrone sulphate) and 17-oxoestra-1,3,5(10),7-tetraen-3-yl sodium sulphate (sodium equilin sulphate). Concomitants are sodium 17α-estradiol sulphate, sodium 17α-dihydroequilin sulphate and sodium 17β-dihydroequilin sulphate.

Conjugated estrogens contain not less than 52.5 per cent and not more than 61.5 per cent of sodium estrone sulphate, not less than 22.5 per cent and not more than 30.5 per cent of sodium equilin sulphate, not less than 2.5 per cent and not more than 9.5 per cent of sodium 17α-estradiol sulphate, not less than 13.5 per cent and not more than 19.5 per cent of sodium 17α-dihydroequilin sulphate, not less than 0.5 per cent and not more than 4.0 per cent of sodium 17β-dihydroequilin sulphate. The total of sodium estrone sulphate and sodium equilin sulphate is not less than 79.5 per cent and not more than 88.0 per cent.

All percentages are related to the labelled content.

CHARACTERS

An almost white or brownish, amorphous powder.

IDENTIFICATION

A. Examine the chromatograms obtained in the assay. The retention times and sizes of the 2 principal peaks corresponding to estrone and equilin in the chromatogram obtained with test solution (a) are approximately the same as those of the 2 principal peaks in the chromatogram obtained with reference solution (a).

B. Examine the chromatogram obtained with test solution (b) in the chromatographic profile. The chromatogram exhibits additional peaks corresponding to 17α-estradiol, 17α-dihydroequilin and 17β-dihydroequilin, at relative retentions with reference to 3-*O*-methylestrone (internal standard) of about 0.24, 0.30 and 0.35 respectively.

TESTS

Chromatographic profile. Carry out the test as prescribed in the assay with the following additional information.

Test solution (b). Prepare the test solution as described in the assay, do not add the sulphatase and use 6.0 ml of the upper layer instead of 3.0 ml. Prepare a blank in the same manner.

Reference solution (b). Prepare the reference solution as described in the assay. Dilute tenfold with *ethanol R* before adding the internal standard.

Inject 1 μl of reference solution (a). Measure the areas of the peaks due to 17α-dihydroequilin, estrone and 3-*O*-methylestrone, with relative retentions with reference to 3-*O*-methylestrone of about 0.30, 0.80 and 1 respectively.

Inject 1 μl of test solution (a). Locate the peaks with relative retentions with reference to 3-*O*-methylestrone of 1 and about 0.24, 0.29, 0.30, 0.35, 0.56, 0.64, 0.90 and 1.3 and measure their areas.

Calculate the percentage content of the components occurring as sodium sulphate salts using expression (1) below.

Inject 1 μl of reference solution (b). Measure the areas of the peaks due to estrone and 3-*O*-methylestrone, with relative retentions with reference to 3-*O*-methylestrone of about 0.80 and 1 respectively.

Inject 1 μl of test solution (b). Locate the peaks with relative retentions with reference to 3-*O*-methylestrone of about 0.30, 0.80 and 0.87 and measure the sum of the areas.

Calculate the percentage content of 17α-dihydroequilin, estrone and equilin occurring as free steroids using expression (2):

$$\frac{S'_A \times S_I \times m_R \times 137.8 \times 1000}{S_R \times S'_I \times m \times LC} \quad (1)$$

$$\frac{S'_{FS} \times S_I \times m_E \times 100 \times 1000}{S_E \times S'_I \times m \times LC} \quad (2)$$

S_I = area of the peak due to the internal standard in the chromatogram obtained with the corresponding reference solution,

S'_I = area of the peak due to the internal standard in the chromatogram obtained with the corresponding test solution,

S_R = area of the peak due to the reference substance (Table 1512.-1) in the chromatogram obtained with the corresponding reference solution,

S'_A = area of the peak due to the analyte in the chromatogram obtained with the corresponding test solution,

m_R = mass of the reference substance (Table 1512.-1) in the corresponding reference solution, in milligrams,

m = mass of the substance to be examined in the corresponding test solution, in milligrams,

S'_{FS} = sum of the areas of the peaks due to 17α-dihydroequilin, estrone and equilin in the chromatogram obtained with the corresponding test solution,

S_E = area of the peak due to *estrone CRS* in the chromatogram obtained with the corresponding reference solution,

m_E = mass of *estrone CRS* in the corresponding reference solution, in milligrams,

LC = labelled content, in milligrams per gram.

The percentages are within the following ranges:

- *sodium 17α-estradiol sulphate*: 2.5 to 9.5 per cent,
- *sodium 17α-dihydroequilin sulphate*: 13.5 to 19.5 per cent,
- *sodium 17β-dihydroequilin sulphate*: 0.5 to 4.0 per cent,
- *sodium 17β-estradiol sulphate*: not more than 2.25 per cent,
- *sodium 17α-dihydroequilenin sulphate*: not more than 3.25 per cent,
- *sodium 17β-dihydroequilenin sulphate*: not more than 2.75 per cent,
- *sodium 8,9-didehydroestrone sulphate*: not more than 6.25 per cent,
- *sodium equilenin sulphate*: not more than 5.5 per cent,
- *total estrone, equilin and 17α-dihydroequilin*: not more than 1.3 per cent.

ASSAY

Examine by gas chromatography (*2.2.28*), using *3-O-methylestrone R* as the internal standard.

Internal standard solution. Dissolve 8 mg of *3-O-methylestrone R* in 10.0 ml of *ethanol R*. Dilute 2.0 ml of this solution to 10.0 ml with *ethanol R*.

Acetate buffer solution pH 5.2. Dissolve 10 g of *sodium acetate R* in 100 ml of *water R* and add 10 ml of *dilute acetic acid R*. Dilute with *water R* to 500 ml and adjust to pH 5.2 ± 0.1.

Test solution (a). Considering the labelled content, transfer an accurately weighed quantity corresponding to about 2 mg of conjugated estrogens to a 50 ml centrifuge tube containing 15 ml of acetate buffer solution pH 5.2 and 1 g of *barium chloride R*. Cap the tube tightly and shake for 30 min. If necessary, adjust the pH of the solution to

Table 1512.-1

Relative retention (to 3-*O*-methylestrone)	Analyte	Quantified with reference to CRS	Present as
0.24	17α-estradiol	*17α-dihydroequilin CRS*	sodium sulphate
0.29	17β-estradiol	*estrone CRS*	sodium sulphate
0.30	17α-dihydroequilin	*17α-dihydroequilin CRS*	free steroid, sodium sulphate (assay)
0.35	17β-dihydroequilin	*17α-dihydroequilin CRS*	sodium sulphate
0.56	17α-dihydroequilenin	*estrone CRS*	sodium sulphate
0.64	17β-dihydroequilenin	*estrone CRS*	sodium sulphate
0.80	estrone	*estrone CRS*	free steroid, sodium sulphate (assay)
0.87	equilin	*equilin CRS*	free steroid, sodium sulphate (assay)
0.90	8,9-didehydroestrone	*estrone CRS*	sodium sulphate
1	3-*O*-methylestrone	(internal standard)	
1.3	equilenin	*estrone CRS*	sodium sulphate

5.0 ± 0.5 with *acetic acid R* or a 120 g/l solution of *sodium acetate R*. Sonicate for 30 s, then shake for 30 min. Add a suitable sulphatase preparation equivalent to 2500 units and shake mechanically for 10 min in a water-bath at 50 ± 1 °C. Swirl the tube by hand, then shake mechanically for 10 min in the water-bath. Allow to cool. Add 15.0 ml of *ethylene chloride R* to the mixture, immediately cap the tube tightly and shake for 15 min. Centrifuge for 10 min or until the lower layer is clear. Draw out the organic layer to a screw cap tube and add 5 g of *anhydrous sodium sulphate R* and shake. Allow the solution to stand until clear. Protect the solution from any loss due to evaporation. Transfer 3.0 ml of the clear solution to a suitable centrifuge tube fitted with a screw cap. Add 1.0 ml of the internal standard solution. Evaporate the mixture to dryness with the aid of a stream of *nitrogen R* maintaining the temperature below 50 °C. To the dry residue add 15 μl of *anhydrous pyridine R* and 65 μl of *N,O-bis(trimethylsilyl)trifluoroacetamide R* containing 1 per cent *chlorotrimethylsilane R*. Immediately cap the tube tightly, mix thoroughly and allow to stand for 15 min. Add 0.5 ml of *toluene R* and mix mechanically.

Reference solution (a). Dissolve separately 8 mg of *estrone CRS*, 7 mg of *equilin CRS* and 5 mg of *17α-dihydroequilin CRS* in 10.0 ml of *ethanol R*. Dilute together 2.0 ml, 1.0 ml and 1.0 ml respectively of these solutions to 10.0 ml with *ethanol R*. Transfer 1.0 ml of this solution and 1.0 ml of the internal standard solution to a centrifuge tube fitted with a screw-cap. Evaporate the mixture to dryness with the aid of a stream of *nitrogen R*, maintaining the temperature below 50 °C. To the dry residue add 15 μl of *anhydrous pyridine R* and 65 μl of *N,O-bis(trimethylsilyl)trifluoroacetamide R* containing 1 per cent *chlorotrimethylsilane R*. Immediately cap the tube tightly, mix and allow to stand for 15 min. Add 0.5 ml of *toluene R*.

The chromatographic procedure may be carried out using:

- a fused-silica column 15 m long and 0.25 mm in internal diameter coated with *poly[(cyanopropyl)(methyl)][(phenyl)(methyl)]siloxane R* (film thickness 0.25 μm),
- *hydrogen for chromatography R* as the carrier gas at a flow rate of 2 ml/min,
- a flame-ionisation detector,
- a split ratio of 1:20 to 1:30,

maintaining the temperature of the column at 220 °C and that of the injection port and of the detector at 260 °C. Set the temperature and the flow rate of the carrier gas in such a manner that the required resolution is achieved.

Inject 1 μl of reference solution (a). The relative retentions with reference to 3-*O*-methylestrone are about 0.30, 0.80, 0.87, and 1 for 17α-dihydroequilin, estrone, equilin and 3-*O*-methylestrone, respectively.

The test is not valid unless the resolution between estrone and equilin is at least 1.2. The relative standard deviation of the ratio of the peak area due to estrone to that of the internal standard, obtained from at least 6 injections, is not more than 2.0 per cent.

Inject 1 μl of reference solution (a). Measure the areas of the peaks due to estrone or equilin and *O*-methylestrone. Inject 1 μl of test solution (a). Measure the areas of the peaks due to estrone, equilin and 3-*O*-methylestrone.

Calculate the percentage content of sodium estrone sulphate and sodium equilin sulphate using expression (1).

LABELLING

The label states:

- the name of the substance,
- the content of the substance,
- the nature of the diluent.

IMPURITIES AND CONCOMITANTS

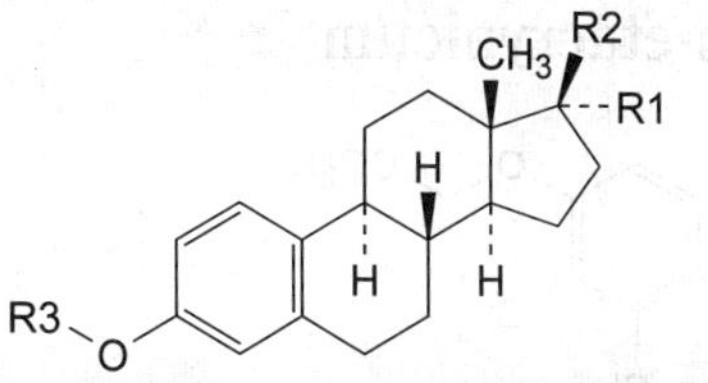

A. R1 = OH, R2 = H, R3 = SO_3Na: 17α-hydroxyestra-1,3,5(10)-trien-3-yl sodium sulphate (sodium 17α-estradiol sulphate),

D. R1 = H, R2 = OH, R3 = SO_3Na: 17β-hydroxyestra-1,3,5(10)-trien-3-yl sodium sulphate (sodium 17β-estradiol sulphate),

I. R1 + R2 = O, R3 = H: 3-hydroxyestra-1,3,5(10)-trien-17-one (estrone),

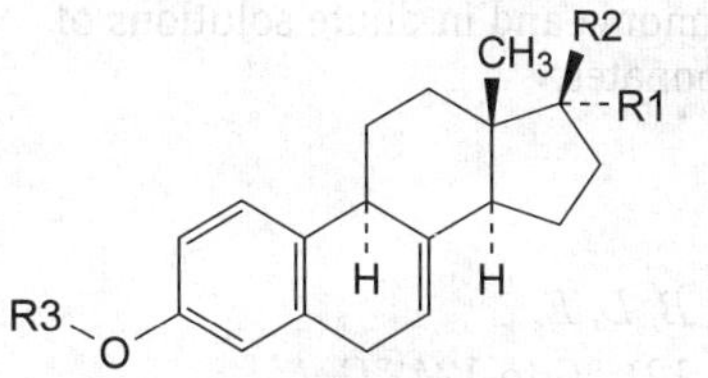

B. R1 = OH, R2 = H, R3 = SO_3Na: 17α-hydroxyestra-1,3,5(10),7-tetraen-3-yl sodium sulphate (sodium 17α-dihydroequilin sulphate),

C. R1 = H, R2 = OH, R3 = SO_3Na: 17β-hydroxyestra-1,3,5(10),7-tetraen-3-yl sodium sulphate (sodium 17β-dihydroequilin sulphate),

J. R1 + R2 = O, R3 = H: 3-hydroxyestra-1,3,5(10),7-tetraen-17-one (equilin),

K. R1 = OH, R2 = R3 = H: estra-1,3,5(10),7-tetraene-3,17α-diol (17α-dihydroequilin),

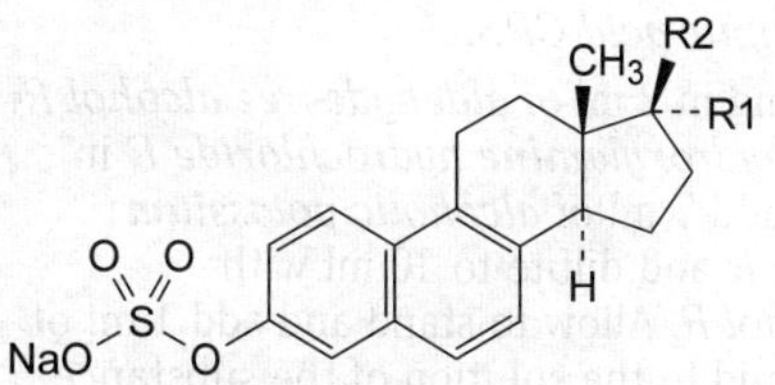

E. R1 = OH, R2 = H: 17α-hydroxyestra-1,3,5(10),6,8-pentaen-3-yl sodium sulphate (sodium 17α-dihydroequilenin sulphate),

F. R1 = H, R2 = OH: 17β-hydroxyestra-1,3,5(10),6,8-pentaen-3-yl sodium sulphate (sodium 17β-dihydroequilenin sulphate),

H. R1 + R2 = O: 17-oxoestra-1,3,5(10),6,8-pentaen-3-yl sodium sulphate (sodium equilenin sulphate),

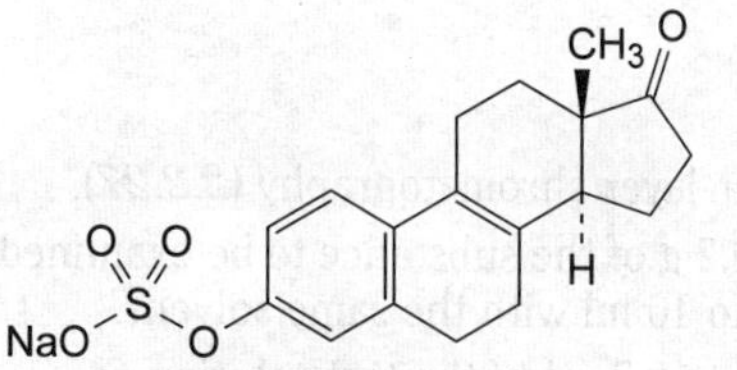

G. 17-oxoestra-1,3,5(10),8-tetraen-3-yl sodium sulphate (sodium 8,9-didehydroestrone sulphate).

01/2005:0457

ETACRYNIC ACID

Acidum etacrynicum

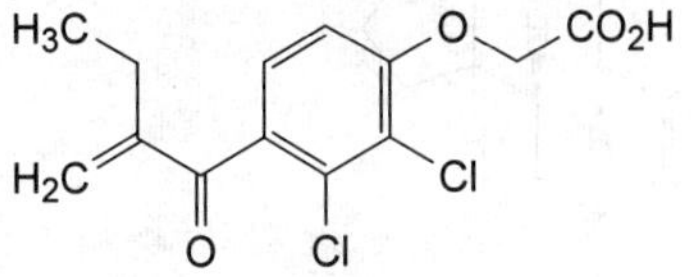

$C_{13}H_{12}Cl_2O_4$ M_r 303.1

DEFINITION

[2,3-Dichloro-4-(2-ethylpropenoyl)phenoxy]acetic acid.

Content: 98.0 per cent to 102.0 per cent (dried substance).

CHARACTERS

Appearance: white or almost white, crystalline powder.

Solubility: very slightly soluble in water, freely soluble in alcohol. It dissolves in ammonia and in dilute solutions of alkali hydroxides and carbonates.

IDENTIFICATION

First identification: C.

Second identification: A, B, D, E.

A. Melting point (*2.2.14*): 121 °C to 124 °C.

B. Dissolve 50.0 mg in a mixture of 1 volume of a 103 g/l solution of *hydrochloric acid R* and 99 volumes of *methanol R* and dilute to 100.0 ml with the same mixture of solvents. Dilute 10.0 ml of this solution to 100.0 ml with a mixture of 1 volume of a 103 g/l solution of *hydrochloric acid R* and 99 volumes of *methanol R*. Examined between 230 nm and 350 nm (*2.2.25*), the solution shows an absorption maximum at 270 nm and a shoulder at about 285 nm. The specific absorbance at the maximum at 270 nm is 110 to 120.

C. Infrared absorption spectrophotometry (*2.2.24*).
Preparation: discs.
Comparison: *etacrynic acid CRS*.

D. Dissolve about 30 mg in 2 ml of *aldehyde-free alcohol R*. Dissolve 70 mg of *hydroxylamine hydrochloride R* in 0.1 ml of *water R*, add 7 ml of *alcoholic potassium hydroxide solution R* and dilute to 10 ml with *aldehyde-free alcohol R*. Allow to stand and add 1 ml of the supernatant liquid to the solution of the substance to be examined. Heat the mixture on a water-bath for 3 min. After cooling, add 3 ml of *water R* and 0.15 ml of *hydrochloric acid R*. Examined in ultraviolet light at 254 nm, the mixture shows an intense blue fluorescence.

E. Dissolve about 25 mg in 2 ml of a 42 g/l solution of *sodium hydroxide R* and heat in a water-bath for 5 min. Cool and add 0.25 ml of a mixture of equal volumes of *water R* and *sulphuric acid R*. Add 0.5 ml of a 100 g/l solution of *chromotropic acid, sodium salt R* and, carefully, 2 ml of *sulphuric acid R*. An intense violet colour is produced.

TESTS

Related substances. Thin-layer chromatography (*2.2.27*).

Test solution. Dissolve 0.2 g of the substance to be examined in *alcohol R* and dilute to 10 ml with the same solvent.

Reference solution. Dilute 0.3 ml of the test solution to 100 ml with *alcohol R*.

Plate: *TLC silica gel F_{254} plate R.*

Mobile phase: *glacial acetic acid R, ethyl acetate R, methylene chloride R* (20:50:60 *V/V/V*).

Application: 10 µl.

Development: over 2/3 of the plate.

Drying: in air.

Detection: examine in ultraviolet light at 254 nm.

Limits:

– *any impurity*: any spots, apart from the principal spot, are not more intense than the spot in the chromatogram obtained with the reference solution (0.3 per cent).

Heavy metals (*2.4.8*): maximum 20 ppm.

1.0 g complies with limit test F. Prepare the standard using 2 ml of *lead standard solution (10 ppm Pb) R*.

Loss on drying (*2.2.32*): maximum 0.5 per cent, determined on 2.000 g by drying at 60 °C over *diphosphorus pentoxide R* at a pressure of 0.1-0.5 kPa.

Sulphated ash (*2.4.14*): maximum 0.1 per cent, determined on 1.0 g.

ASSAY

Dissolve 0.250 g in 100 ml of *methanol R* and add 5 ml of *water R*. Titrate with *0.1 M sodium hydroxide*, determining the end-point potentiometrically (*2.2.20*).

1 ml of *0.1 M sodium hydroxide* is equivalent to 30.31 mg of $C_{13}H_{12}Cl_2O_4$.

01/2005:1204

ETAMSYLATE

Etamsylatum

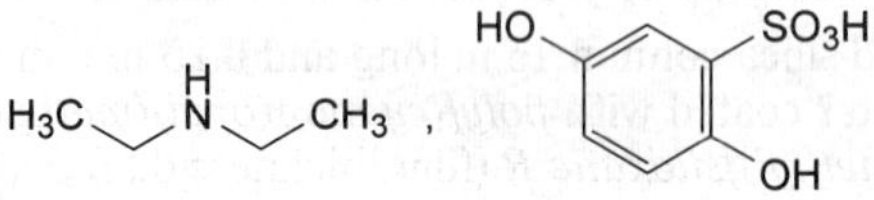

$C_{10}H_{17}NO_5S$ M_r 263.3

DEFINITION

Etamsylate contains not less than 99.0 per cent and not more than the equivalent of 101.0 per cent of *N*-ethylethanamine 2,5-dihydroxybenzenesulphonate, calculated with reference to the dried substance.

CHARACTERS

A white or almost white, crystalline powder, very soluble in water, freely soluble in methanol, soluble in ethanol, practically insoluble in methylene chloride.

It shows polymorphism.

IDENTIFICATION

First identification: B.

Second identification: A, C, D.

A. Melting point (*2.2.14*): 127 °C to 134 °C.

B. Examine by infrared absorption spectrophotometry (*2.2.24*), comparing with the spectrum obtained with *etamsylate CRS*. Examine the substances prepared as discs.

C. Dissolve 0.100 g in *water R* and dilute to 200.0 ml with the same solvent. Dilute 5.0 ml of the solution to 100.0 ml with *water R*. Examined immediately between 210 nm and 350 nm (*2.2.25*), the solution shows two absorption, maxima at 221 nm and 301 nm. The specific absorbance at the maximum at 301 nm is 145 to 151.

D. In a test-tube, introduce 2 ml of freshly prepared solution S (see Tests) and 0.5 g of *sodium hydroxide R*. Warm the mixture and place near the open end of the tube a wet strip of *red litmus paper R*. The colour of the paper becomes blue.

TESTS

Solution S. Dissolve 10.0 g in *carbon dioxide-free water R* and dilute to 100 ml with the same solvent.

Appearance of solution. Solution S, when freshly prepared,is clear (*2.2.1*) and colourless (*2.2.2, Method II*).

pH (*2.2.3*). The pH of solution S is 4.5 to 5.6.

Hydroquinone. Examine by thin-layer chromatography (*2.2.27*), using as the coating substance a suitable silica gel with a fluorescent indicator having an optimal intensity at 254 nm.

Test solution. Dissolve 2.0 g of the substance to be examined in *water R* and dilute to 10 ml with the same solvent.

Reference solution. Dissolve 10 mg of *hydroquinone R* in *water R* and dilute to 50 ml with the same solvent.

Apply to the plate 10 µl of each solution and dry the starting points in a current of cool air. Develop over a path of 15 cm using a mixture of 20 volumes of *methylene chloride R*, 30 volumes of *methyl acetate R* and 50 volumes of *ethyl acetate R*. Dry the plate in a current of hot air and examine in ultraviolet light at 254 nm. Any spot corresponding to hydroquinone in the chromatogram obtained with the test solution is not more intense than the principal spot in the chromatogram obtained with the reference solution (0.1 per cent).

Heavy metals (*2.4.8*). 1.0 g complies with limit test C for heavy metals (15 ppm). Prepare the standard using 1.5 ml of *lead standard solution (10 ppm Pb) R*.

Iron (*2.4.9*). 10 ml of solution S complies with the limit test for iron (10 ppm).

Loss on drying (*2.2.32*). Not more than 0.5 per cent, determined on 1.000 g by drying in an oven *in vacuo* at 60 °C.

Sulphated ash (*2.4.14*). Not more than 0.1 per cent, determined on 1.0 g.

ASSAY

Dissolve 0.200 g in a mixture of 10 ml of *water R* and 40 ml of *dilute sulphuric acid R*. Titrate with *0.1 M cerium sulphate*, determining the end-point potentiometrically (*2.2.20*).

1 ml of *0.1 M cerium sulphate* is equivalent to 13.16 mg of $C_{10}H_{17}NO_5S$.

STORAGE

Store in an airtight container, protected from light.

IMPURITIES

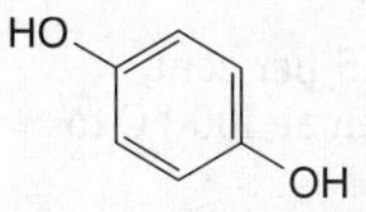

A. benzene-1,4-diol (hydroquinone).

01/2005:1591

ETHACRIDINE LACTATE MONOHYDRATE

Ethacridini lactas monohydricus

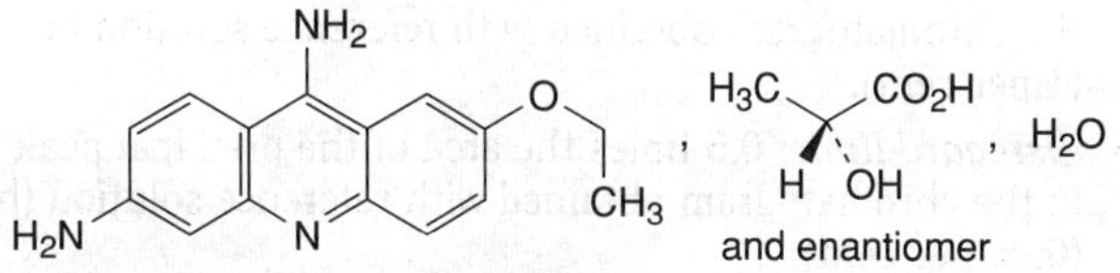

$C_{18}H_{21}N_3O_4,H_2O$ M_r 361.4

DEFINITION

7-Ethoxyacridine-3,9-diamine (2*RS*)-2-hydroxypropanoate.

Content: 99.0 per cent to 101.0 per cent (dried substance).

CHARACTERS

Appearance: yellow crystalline powder.

Solubility: sparingly soluble in water, very slightly soluble in alcohol, practically insoluble in methylene chloride.

IDENTIFICATION

First identification: A.

Second identification: B, C, D.

A. Infrared absorption spectrophotometry (*2.2.24*).
Comparison: *ethacridine lactate monohydrate CRS.*

B. Mix 0.1 ml of solution S (see Tests) and 100 ml of *water R*. The solution is greenish-yellow and shows a strong green fluorescence in ultraviolet light at 365 nm. Add 5 ml of *1 M hydrochloric acid*. The fluorescence remains.

C. To 0.5 ml of solution S add 1.0 ml of *water R*, 0.1 ml of a 10 g/l solution of *cobalt chloride R* and 0.1 ml of a 50 g/l solution of *potassium ferrocyanide R*. The solution is green.

D. To 50 ml of solution S add 10 ml of *dilute sodium hydroxide solution R*. Filter. To 5 ml of the filtrate, add 1 ml of *dilute sulphuric acid R*. 5 ml of the solution obtained gives the reaction of lactates (*2.3.1*).

TESTS

Solution S. Dissolve 2.0 g in *carbon dioxide-free water R* and dilute to 100.0 ml with the same solvent.

pH (*2.2.3*): 5.5 to 7.0 for solution S.

Related substances. Liquid chromatography (*2.2.29*).

Test solution. Dissolve 10.0 mg of the substance to be examined in the mobile phase and dilute to 25.0 ml with the mobile phase.

Reference solution (a). Dilute 1.0 ml of test solution to 100.0 ml with the mobile phase.

Reference solution (b). Dilute 1.0 ml of reference solution (a) to 10.0 ml with the mobile phase.

Column:

– *size*: *l* = 0.25 m, Ø = 4.6 mm,

– *stationary phase*: *octadecylsilyl silica gel for chromatography R* (5 µm).

Mobile phase: dissolve 1.0 g of *sodium octanesulphonate R* in a mixture of 300 ml of *acetonitrile R* and 700 ml of *phosphate buffer solution pH 2.8 R*.

Flow rate: 1 ml/min.

Detection: spectrophotometer at 268 nm.

Injection: 10 µl.

Run time: 3 times the retention time of ethacridine.

Retention time: ethacridine = about 15 min.

Limits:

- *any impurity*: not more than 3 times the area of the principal peak in the chromatogram obtained with reference solution (b) (0.3 per cent),
- *total*: not more than the area of the principal peak in the chromatogram obtained with reference solution (a) (1 per cent),
- *disregard limit*: 0.5 times the area of the principal peak in the chromatogram obtained with reference solution (b) (0.05 per cent).

Heavy metals (*2.4.8*): maximum 50 ppm.

1.0 g complies with limit test F. Prepare the standard using 5.0 ml of *lead standard solution (10 ppm Pb) R*.

Loss on drying (*2.2.32*): 4.5 per cent to 5.5 per cent, determined on 1.000 g by drying in an oven *in vacuo* at 100-105 °C.

Sulphated ash (*2.4.14*): maximum 0.1 per cent, determined on 1.0 g.

ASSAY

Dissolve 0.270 g in 5.0 ml of *anhydrous formic acid R*. Add 60.0 ml of *acetic anhydride R* and titrate with *0.1 M perchloric acid*, determining the end-point potentiometrically (*2.2.20*).

1 ml of *0.1 M perchloric acid* is equivalent to 34.34 mg of $C_{18}H_{21}N_3O_4$.

STORAGE

Protected from light.

IMPURITIES

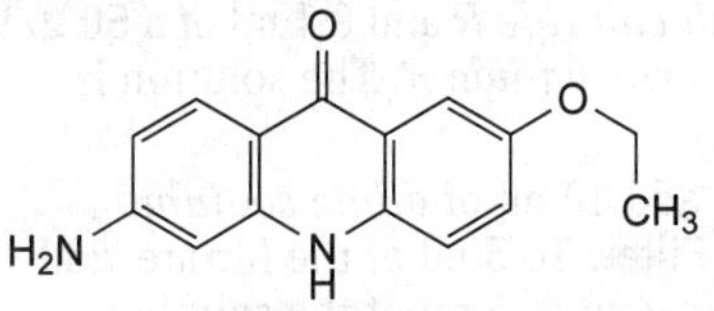

A. 6-amino-2-ethoxyacridin-9(10*H*)-one,

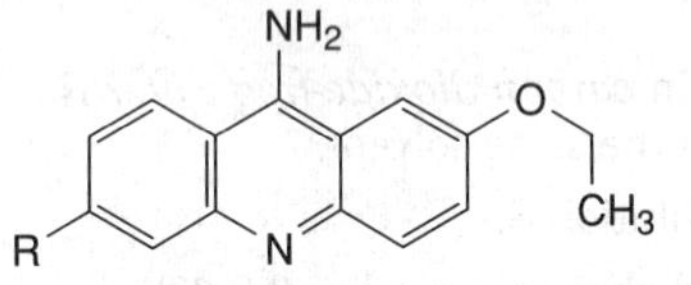

B. R = Cl: 6-chloro-2-ethoxyacridin-9-amine,

C. R = $O-CH_2-CH_2-OH$: 2-[(9-amino-7-ethoxyacridin-3-yl)oxy]ethanol.

01/2005:0553

ETHAMBUTOL HYDROCHLORIDE

Ethambutoli hydrochloridum

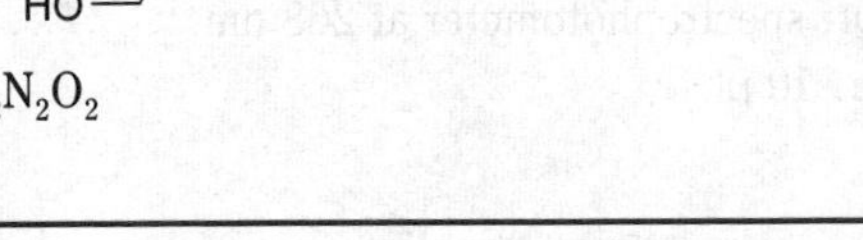

$C_{10}H_{26}Cl_2N_2O_2$ M_r 277.2

DEFINITION

Ethambutol hydrochloride contains not less than 97.0 per cent and not more than the equivalent of 101.0 per cent of 2,2′-(ethylenediimino)bis[(2*S*)-butan-1-ol] dihydrochloride, calculated with reference to the dried substance.

CHARACTERS

A white, crystalline powder, freely soluble in water, soluble in alcohol.

It melts at about 202 °C.

IDENTIFICATION

First identification: A, D.

Second identification: B, C, D.

A. Examine by infrared absorption spectrophotometry (*2.2.24*), comparing with the spectrum obtained with *ethambutol hydrochloride CRS*. Examine the substances prepared as discs.

B. Examine the chromatograms obtained in the test for 2-aminobutanol. The principal spot in the chromatogram obtained with test solution (b) is similar in position, colour and size to the principal spot in the chromatogram obtained with reference solution (b).

C. Dissolve 0.1 g in 10 ml of *water R* and add 0.2 ml of *copper sulphate solution R*. Add 0.5 ml of *dilute sodium hydroxide solution R*. A blue colour is produced.

D. It gives reaction (a) of chlorides (*2.3.1*).

TESTS

pH (*2.2.3*). Dissolve 0.2 g in 10 ml of *carbon dioxide-free water R*. The pH of the solution is 3.7 to 4.0.

2-Aminobutanol. Examine by thin-layer chromatography (*2.2.27*), using *silica gel G R* as the coating substance.

Test solution (a). Dissolve 0.50 g of the substance to be examined in *methanol R* and dilute to 10 ml with the same solvent.

Test solution (b). Dilute 1 ml of test solution (a) to 10 ml with *methanol R*.

Reference solution (a). Dissolve 50 mg of *2-aminobutanol R* in *methanol R* and dilute to 10 ml with the same solvent. Dilute 1 ml of this solution to 10 ml with *methanol R*.

Reference solution (b). Dissolve 50 mg of *ethambutol hydrochloride CRS* in *methanol R* and dilute to 10 ml with the same solvent.

Apply separately to the plate 2 µl of each solution. Develop over a path of 15 cm using a mixture of 10 volumes of *concentrated ammonia R*, 15 volumes of *water R* and 75 volumes of *methanol R*. Allow the plate to dry in air, heat at 110 °C for 10 min, cool and spray with *ninhydrin solution R1*. Heat the plate at 110 °C for 5 min. Any spot corresponding to 2-aminobutanol in the chromatogram obtained with test solution (a) is not more intense than the spot in the chromatogram obtained with reference solution (a) (1.0 per cent).

Heavy metals (*2.4.8*). 2.0 g complies with limit test C for heavy metals (10 ppm). Prepare the standard using 2 ml of *lead standard solution (10 ppm Pb) R*.

Loss on drying (*2.2.32*). Not more than 0.5 per cent, determined on 0.500 g by drying in an oven at 100 °C to 105 °C for 3 h.

Sulphated ash (*2.4.14*). Not more than 0.1 per cent, determined on 1.0 g.

ASSAY

To 70 ml of *dilute ammonia R2* add 4.0 ml of *copper sulphate solution R*, mix, add 5.0 ml of *dilute sodium hydroxide solution R* and dilute to 100 ml with *water R*. Dissolve 0.100 g of the substance to be examined in 20 ml of this solution and dilute to 25.0 ml with the same solution. Prepare a reference solution in the same manner using 0.100 g of *ethambutol hydrochloride CRS*. Measure the angle of optical rotation (*2.2.7*) of the solutions at 436 nm.

Calculate the content of $C_{10}H_{26}Cl_2N_2O_2$ from the angles of optical rotation measured and the concentrations of the solutions.

STORAGE

Store in an airtight container.

01/2005:1317

ETHANOL (96 PER CENT)

Ethanolum (96 per centum)

DEFINITION

Content:

– ethanol (C_2H_6O; M_r 46.07): 95.1 per cent *V/V* (92.6 per cent *m/m*) to 96.9 per cent *V/V* (95.2 per cent *m/m*) at 20 °C, calculated from the relative density using the alcoholimetric tables (*5.5*),

– water.

CHARACTERS

Appearance: colourless, clear, volatile, flammable liquid, hygroscopic.

Solubility: miscible with water and with methylene chloride.

It burns with a blue, smokeless flame.

bp: about 78 °C.

IDENTIFICATION

First identification: A, B.

Second identification: A, C, D.

A. It complies with the test for relative density (see Tests).

B. Infrared absorption spectrophotometry (*2.2.24*).
Comparison: *Ph. Eur. reference spectrum ethanol (96 per cent)*.

C. Mix 0.1 ml with 1 ml of a 10 g/l solution of *potassium permanganate R* and 0.2 ml of *dilute sulphuric acid R* in a test-tube. Cover immediately with a filter paper moistened with a freshly prepared solution containing 0.1 g of *sodium nitroprusside R* and 0.5 g of *piperazine hydrate R* in 5 ml of *water R*. After a few minutes, an intense blue colour appears on the paper and becomes paler after 10-15 min.

D. To 0.5 ml add 5 ml of *water R*, 2 ml of *dilute sodium hydroxide solution R*, then slowly add 2 ml of *0.05 M iodine*. A yellow precipitate is formed within 30 min.

TESTS

Appearance. It is clear (*2.2.1*) and colourless (*2.2.2, Method II*) when compared with *water R*. Dilute 1.0 ml to 20 ml with *water R*. After standing for 5 min, the dilution remains clear (*2.2.1*) when compared with *water R*.

Acidity or alkalinity. To 20 ml add 20 ml of *carbon dioxide-free water R* and 0.1 ml of *phenolphthalein solution R*. The solution is colourless. Add 1.0 ml of *0.01 M sodium hydroxide*. The solution is pink (30 ppm, expressed as acetic acid).

Relative density (*2.2.5*): 0.805 to 0.812.

Absorbance (*2.2.25*): maximum 0.40 at 240 nm, 0.30 between 250 nm and 260 nm and 0.10 between 270 nm and 340 nm.

Examine between 235 nm and 340 nm, in a 5 cm cell using *water R* as the compensation liquid. The absorption curve is smooth.

Volatile impurities. Gas chromatography (*2.2.28*).

Test solution (a). The substance to be examined.

Test solution (b). Add 150 µl of *4-methylpentan-2-ol R* to 500.0 ml of the substance to be examined.

Reference solution (a). Dilute 100 µl of *anhydrous methanol R* to 50.0 ml with the substance to be examined. Dilute 5.0 ml of the solution to 50.0 ml with the substance to be examined.

Reference solution (b). Dilute 50 µl of *anhydrous methanol R* and 50 µl of *acetaldehyde R* to 50.0 ml with the substance to be examined. Dilute 100 µl of the solution to 10.0 ml with the substance to be examined.

Reference solution (c). Dilute 150 µl of *acetal R* to 50.0 ml with the substance to be examined. Dilute 100 µl of the solution to 10.0 ml with the substance to be examined.

Reference solution (d). Dilute 100 µl of *benzene R* to 100.0 ml with the substance to be examined. Dilute 100 µl of the solution to 50.0 ml with the substance to be examined.

Column:

– *material*: fused silica,
– *size*: *l* = 30 m, Ø = 0.32 mm,
– *stationary phase*: *poly[(cyanopropyl)(phenyl)][dimethyl]siloxane R* (film thickness 1.8 µm).

Carrier gas: *helium for chromatography R*.

Linear velocity: 35 cm/s.

Split ratio: 1:20.

Temperature:

	Time (min)	Temperature (°C)
Column	0 - 12	40
	12 - 32	40 → 240
	32 - 42	240
Injection port		200
Detector		280

Detection: flame ionisation.

Injection: 1 µl.

System suitability: reference solution (b):

– *resolution*: minimum 1.5 between the first peak (acetaldehyde) and the second peak (methanol).

Limits:

– *methanol* in the chromatogram obtained with test solution (a): not more than half the area of the corresponding peak in the chromatogram obtained with reference solution (a) (200 ppm *V/V*),

– *acetaldehyde + acetal*: maximum 10 ppm *V/V*, expressed as acetaldehyde.

Monographs D-E

Calculate the sum of the contents of acetaldehyde and acetal in parts per million (*V/V*) using the following expression:

$$\frac{10 \times A_E}{A_T - A_E} + \frac{30 \times C_E}{C_T - C_E}$$

A_E = area of the acetaldehyde peak in the chromatogram obtained with test solution (a),

A_T = area of the acetaldehyde peak in the chromatogram obtained with reference solution (b),

C_E = area of the acetal peak in the chromatogram obtained with test solution (a),

C_T = area of the acetal peak in the chromatogram obtained with reference solution (c).

– *benzene*: maximum 2 ppm *V/V*.

Calculate the content of benzene in parts per million (*V/V*) using the following expression:

$$\frac{2B_E}{B_T - B_E}$$

B_E = area of the benzene peak in the chromatogram obtained with the test solution (a),

B_T = area of the benzene peak in the chromatogram obtained with reference solution (d).

If necessary, the identity of benzene can be confirmed using another suitable chromatographic system (stationary phase with a different polarity).

– *total of other impurities* in the chromatogram obtained with test solution (b): not more than the area of the peak due to 4-methylpentan-2-ol in the chromatogram obtained with test solution (b) (300 ppm),

– *disregard limit*: 0.03 times the area of the peak corresponding to 4-methylpentan-2-ol in the chromatogram obtained with test solution (b) (9 ppm).

Residue on evaporation: maximum 25 ppm *m/V*.

Evaporate 100 ml to dryness on a water-bath and dry at 100-105 °C for 1 h. The residue weighs a maximum of 2.5 mg.

STORAGE

Protected from light.

IMPURITIES

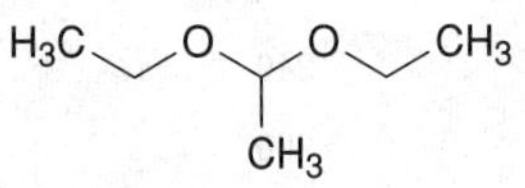

A. 1,1-diethoxyethane (acetal),

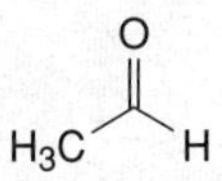

B. acetaldehyde,

C. acetone,

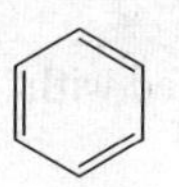

D. benzene,

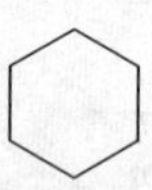

E. cyclohexane,

F. CH_3-OH: methanol,

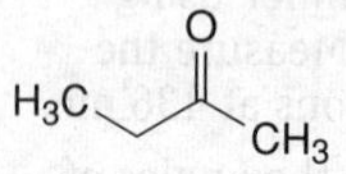

G. butan-2-one (methyl ethyl ketone),

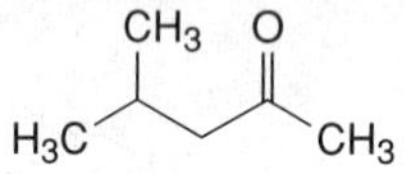

H. 4-methylpentan-2-one (methyl isobutyl ketone),

I. CH_3-$(CH_2)_2$-OH: propanol,

J. propan-2-ol (isopropyl alcohol),

K. CH_3-$(CH_2)_3$-OH: butanol,

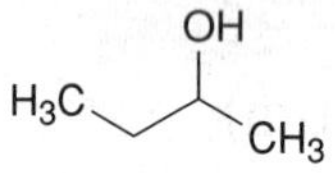

L. butan-2-ol,

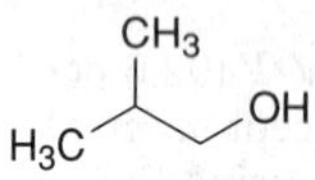

M. 2-methylpropanol (isobutanol),

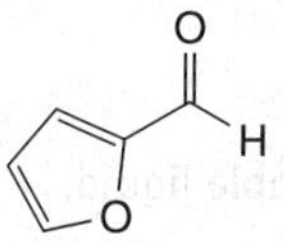

N. furane-2-carbaldehyde (furfural),

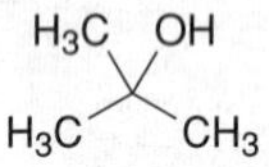

O. 2-methylpropan-2-ol (1,1-dimethylethyl alcohol),

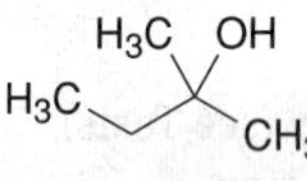

P. 2-methylbutan-2-ol,

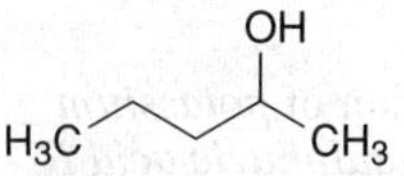

Q. pentan-2-ol,

R. CH_3-$(CH_2)_4$-OH: pentanol,

S. CH_3-$(CH_2)_5$-OH: hexanol,

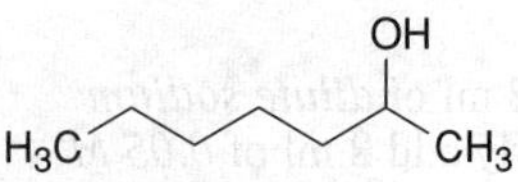

T. heptan-2-ol,

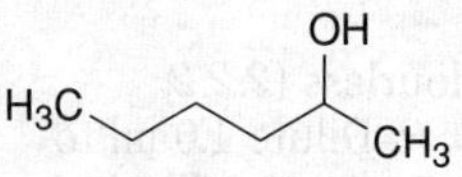

U. hexan-2-ol,

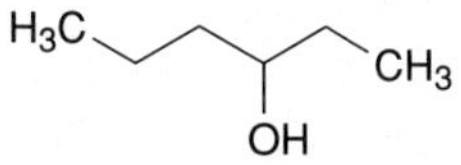

V. hexan-3-ol.

01/2005:1318

ETHANOL, ANHYDROUS

Ethanolum anhydricum

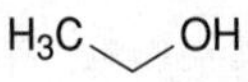

C_2H_6O M_r 46.07

DEFINITION

Content: not less than 99.5 per cent *V/V* of C_2H_6O (99.2 per cent *m/m*), at 20 °C, calculated from the relative density using the alcoholimetric tables (*5.5*).

CHARACTERS

Appearance: colourless, clear, volatile, flammable liquid, hygroscopic.

Solubility: miscible with water and with methylene chloride.

It burns with a blue, smokeless flame.

bp: about 78 °C.

IDENTIFICATION

First identification: A, B.

Second identification: A, C, D.

A. It complies with the test for relative density (see Tests).

B. Infrared absorption spectrophotometry (*2.2.24*).
Comparison: *Ph. Eur. reference spectrum of anhydrous ethanol.*

C. Mix 0.1 ml with 1 ml of a 10 g/l solution of *potassium permanganate R* and 0.2 ml of *dilute sulphuric acid R* in a test-tube. Cover immediately with a filter paper moistened with a freshly prepared solution containing 0.1 g of *sodium nitroprusside R* and 0.5 g of *piperazine hydrate R* in 5 ml of *water R*. After a few minutes, an intense blue colour appears on the paper and becomes paler after 10-15 min.

D. To 0.5 ml add 5 ml of *water R*, 2 ml of *dilute sodium hydroxide solution R*, then slowly add 2 ml of *0.05 M iodine*. A yellow precipitate is formed within 30 min.

TESTS

Appearance. It is clear (*2.2.1*) and colourless (*2.2.2, Method II*) when compared with *water R*. Dilute 1.0 ml to 20 ml with *water R*. After standing for 5 min, the dilution remains clear (*2.2.1*) when compared with *water R*.

Acidity or alkalinity. To 20 ml add 20 ml of *carbon dioxide-free water R* and 0.1 ml of *phenolphthalein solution R*. The solution is colourless. Add 1.0 ml of *0.01 M sodium hydroxide*. The solution is pink (30 ppm, expressed as acetic acid).

Relative density (*2.2.5*): 0.790 to 0.793.

Absorbance (*2.2.25*): maximum 0.40 at 240 nm, 0.30 between 250 nm and 260 nm, and 0.10 between 270 nm and 340 nm.

Examined between 235 nm and 340 nm in a 5 cm cell using *water R* as the compensation liquid. The absorption curve is smooth.

Volatile impurities. Gas chromatography (*2.2.28*).

Test solution (a). The substance to be examined.

Test solution (b). Add 150 µl of *4-methylpentan-2-ol R* to 500.0 ml of the substance to be examined.

Reference solution (a). Dilute 100 µl of *anhydrous methanol R* to 50.0 ml with the substance to be examined. Dilute 5.0 ml of the solution to 50.0 ml with the substance to be examined.

Reference solution (b). Dilute 50 µl of *anhydrous methanol R* and 50 µl of *acetaldehyde R* to 50.0 ml with the substance to be examined. Dilute 100 µl of the solution to 10.0 ml with the substance to be examined.

Reference solution (c). Dilute 150 µl of *acetal R* to 50.0 ml with the substance to be examined. Dilute 100 µl of the solution to 10.0 ml with the substance to be examined.

Reference solution (d). Dilute 100 µl of *benzene R* to 100.0 ml with the substance to be examined. Dilute 100 µl of the solution to 50.0 ml with the substance to be examined.

Column:
- *material*: fused silica,
- *size*: *l* = 30 m, Ø = 0.32 mm,
- *stationary phase*: *poly[(cyanopropyl)(phenyl)][dimethyl]siloxane R* (film thickness 1.8 µm).

Carrier gas: *helium for chromatography R.*

Linear velocity: 35 cm/s.

Split ratio: 1:20.

Temperature:

	Time (min)	**Temperature (°C)**
Column	0 - 12	40
	12 - 32	40 → 240
	32 - 42	240
Injection port		200
Detector		280

Detection: flame ionisation.

Injection: 1 µl.

System suitability: reference solution (b):
- *resolution*: minimum 1.5 between the first peak (acetaldehyde) and the second peak (methanol).

Limits:
- *methanol*: in the chromatogram obtained with test solution (a): not more than half the area of the corresponding peak in the chromatogram obtained with reference solution (a) (200 ppm *V/V*) .
- *acetaldehyde + acetal*: maximum of 10 ppm *V/V*, expressed as acetaldehyde.

Calculate the sum of the contents of acetaldehyde and acetal in parts per million (*V/V*) using the following expression:

$$\frac{10 \times A_E}{A_T - A_E} + \frac{30 \times C_E}{C_T - C_E}$$

A_E = area of the acetaldehyde peak in the chromatogram obtained with test solution (a),

A_T = area of the acetaldehyde peak in the chromatogram obtained with reference solution (b),

C_E = area of the acetal peak in the chromatogram obtained with test solution (a),

C_T = area of the acetal peak in the chromatogram obtained with reference solution (c).

- *benzene*: maximum 2 ppm *V/V*.
  Calculate the content of benzene in parts per million (*V/V*) using the following expression:

$$\frac{2B_E}{B_T - B_E}$$

B_E = area of the benzene peak in the chromatogram obtained with the test solution (a),

B_T = area of the benzene peak in the chromatogram obtained with reference solution (d).

If necessary, the identity of benzene can be confirmed using another suitable chromatographic system (stationary phase with a different polarity).

- *total of other impurities* in the chromatogram obtained with test solution (b): not more than the area of the peak due to 4-methylpentan-2-ol in the chromatogram obtained with test solution (b) (300 ppm),
- *disregard limit*: 0.03 times the area of the peak corresponding to 4-methylpentan-2-ol in the chromatogram obtained with test solution (b) (9 ppm).

Residue on evaporation: maximum 25 ppm *m/V*.

Evaporate 100 ml to dryness on a water-bath and dry at 100-105 °C for 1 h. The residue weighs a maximum of 2.5 mg.

STORAGE

Protected from light.

IMPURITIES

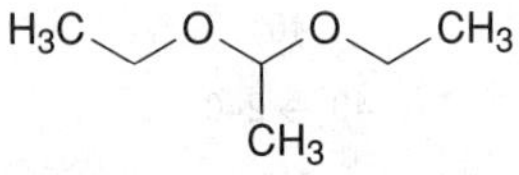

A. 1,1-diethoxyethane (acetal),

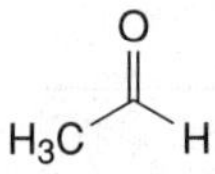

B. acetaldehyde,

C. acetone,

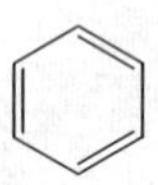

D. benzene,

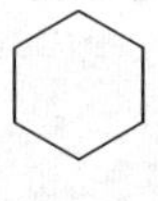

E. cyclohexane,

F. CH_3-OH: methanol,

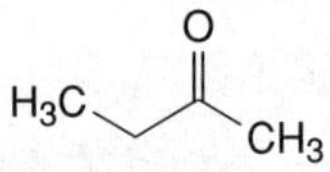

G. butan-2-one (methyl ethyl ketone),

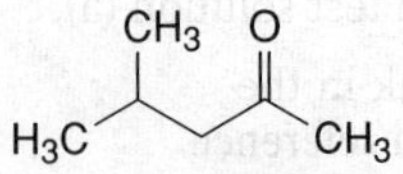

H. 4-methylpentan-2-one (methyl isobutyl ketone),

I. CH_3-$(CH_2)_2$-OH: propanol,

J. propan-2-ol (isopropyl alcohol),

K. CH_3-$(CH_2)_3$-OH: butanol,

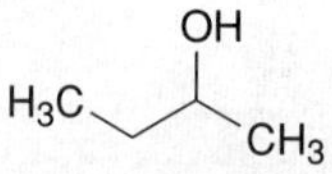

L. butan-2-ol,

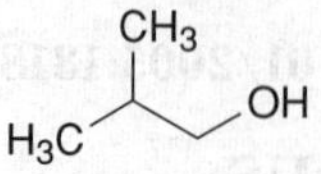

M. 2-methylpropanol (isobutanol),

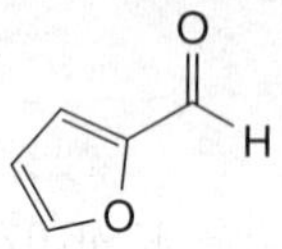

N. furane-2-carbaldehyde (furfural),

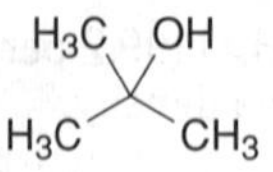

O. 2-methylpropan-2-ol (1,1-dimethylethyl alcohol),

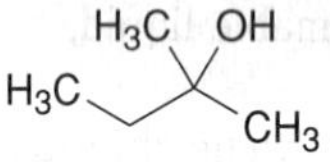

P. 2-methylbutan-2-ol,

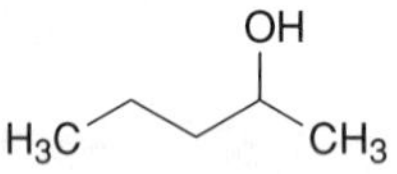

Q. pentan-2-ol,

R. CH_3-$(CH_2)_4$-OH: pentanol,

S. CH_3-$(CH_2)_5$-OH: hexanol,

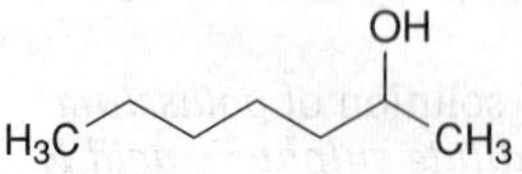

T. heptan-2-ol,

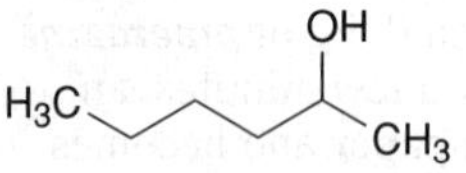

U. hexan-2-ol,

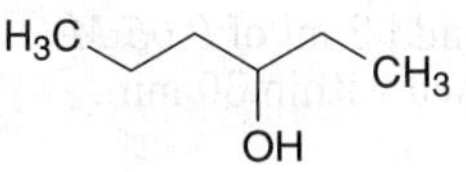

V. hexan-3-ol.

01/2005:0650

ETHER

Aether

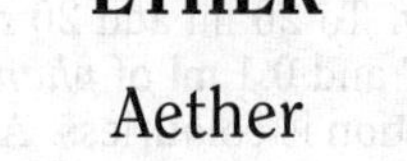

$C_4H_{10}O$ M_r 74.1

DEFINITION

Ether is diethyl ether which may contain a suitable non-volatile antioxidant at a suitable concentration.

CHARACTERS

A clear, colourless liquid, volatile, highly flammable, soluble in water, miscible with alcohol, with methylene chloride and with fatty oils.

IDENTIFICATION

A. It complies with the test for relative density (see Tests).

B. It complies with the test for distillation range (see Tests).

TESTS

Acidity. To 20 ml of *alcohol R* add 0.25 ml of *bromothymol blue solution R1* and, dropwise, *0.02 M sodium hydroxide* until a blue colour persists for 30 s. Add 25 ml of the substance to be examined, shake and add, dropwise, *0.02 M sodium hydroxide* until the blue colour reappears and persists for 30 s. Not more than 0.4 ml of *0.02 M sodium hydroxide* is required.

Relative density (*2.2.5*): 0.714 to 0.716.

Distillation range (*2.2.11*). *Do not distil if the substance to be examined does not comply with the test for peroxides.* It distils completely between 34.0 °C and 35.0 °C. Carry out the test using a suitable heating device and taking care to avoid directly heating the flask above the level of the liquid.

Non-volatile matter. *After ensuring that the substance to be examined complies with the test for peroxides,* evaporate 50 ml to dryness on a water-bath and dry the residue in an oven at 100 °C to 105 °C. The residue weighs not more than 1 mg (20 mg/l).

Substances with a foreign odour. Moisten a disc of filter paper 80 mm in diameter with 5 ml of the substance to be examined and allow to evaporate. No foreign odour is perceptible immediately after the evaporation.

Aldehydes. To 10.0 ml in a ground-glass-stoppered cylinder add 1 ml of *alkaline potassium tetraiodomercurate solution R* and shake for 10 s. Allow to stand for 5 min, protected from light. The lower layer may show yellow or reddish-brown opalescence but not grey or black opalescence.

Peroxides. Place 8 ml of *potassium iodide and starch solution R* in a 12 ml ground-glass-stoppered cylinder about 15 mm in diameter. Fill completely with the substance to be examined, mix and allow to stand protected from light for 5 min. No colour develops.

Water (*2.5.12*). Not more than 2 g/l, determined on 20 ml by the semi-micro determination of water.

STORAGE

Store in an airtight container, protected from light, at a temperature of 8 °C to 15 °C.

LABELLING

The label states, where appropriate, the name and concentration of any added non-volatile antioxidant.

01/2005:0367

ETHER, ANAESTHETIC

Aether anaestheticus

$C_4H_{10}O$ M_r 74.1

DEFINITION

Anaesthetic ether is diethyl ether which may contain a suitable non-volatile antioxidant at an appropriate concentration.

CHARACTERS

A clear, colourless liquid, volatile, very mobile, highly flammable, soluble in 15 parts of water, miscible with alcohol and with fatty oils.

IDENTIFICATION

A. It complies with the test for relative density (see Tests).

B. It complies with the test for distillation range (see Tests).

TESTS

Relative density (*2.2.5*): 0.714 to 0.716.

Distillation range (*2.2.11*). *Do not distil if the substance to be examined does not comply with the test for peroxides.* It distils completely between 34.0 °C and 35.0 °C. Carry out the test using a suitable heating device and taking care to avoid directly heating the flask above the level of the liquid.

Acids. To 20 ml of *alcohol R* add 0.25 ml of *bromothymol blue solution R1* and, dropwise, *0.02 M sodium hydroxide* until a blue colour persists for 30 s. Add 25 ml of the substance to be examined, shake and add, dropwise, *0.02 M sodium hydroxide* until the blue colour reappears and persists for 30 s. Not more than 0.4 ml of *0.02 M sodium hydroxide* is required.

Acetone and aldehydes. To 10.0 ml in a ground-glass-stoppered cylinder add 1 ml of *alkaline potassium tetra-iodomercurate solution R* and shake for 10 s. Allow to stand for 5 min, protected from light. The lower layer shows only a slight opalescence.

If the substance to be examined does not comply with the test, distil 40 ml, *after ensuring that the substance to be examined complies with the test for peroxides,* until only 5 ml remains. Collect the distillate in a receiver cooled by placing in a bath of iced water and repeat the test described above using 10.0 ml of the distillate.

Peroxides. Place 8 ml of *potassium iodide and starch solution R* in a 12 ml ground-glass-stoppered cylinder about 15 mm in diameter. Fill completely with the substance to be examined, shake vigorously and allow to stand protected from light for 30 min. No colour is produced.

Non-volatile matter. *After ensuring that the substance to be examined complies with the test for peroxides,* evaporate 50 ml to dryness on a water-bath and dry the residue at 100 °C to 105 °C. The residue weighs not more than 1 mg (20 mg/l).

Substances with a foreign odour. Moisten a disc of filter paper 80 mm in diameter with 5 ml of the substance to be examined and allow to evaporate. No foreign odour is perceptible immediately after the evaporation.

Water (*2.5.12*). Not more than 2 g/l, determined on 20 ml by the semi-micro determination of water.

STORAGE

Store in an airtight container, protected from light, at a temperature of 8 °C to 15 °C. The contents of a partly filled container may deteriorate rapidly.

LABELLING

The label states, where appropriate, the name and concentration of any added non-volatile antioxidant.

01/2005:0140

ETHINYLESTRADIOL

Ethinylestradiolum

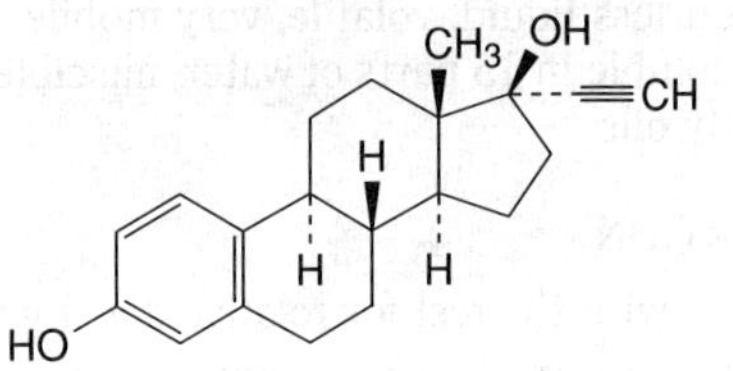

$C_{20}H_{24}O_2$ M_r 296.4

DEFINITION

19-Nor-17α-pregna-1,3,5(10)-trien-20-yne-3,17-diol.

Content: 97.0 per cent to 102.0 per cent (dried substance).

CHARACTERS

Appearance: white or slightly yellowish-white, crystalline powder.

Solubility: practically insoluble in water, freely soluble in alcohol. It dissolves in dilute alkaline solutions.

IDENTIFICATION

A. Infrared absorption spectrophotometry (*2.2.24*).

Comparison: *ethinylestradiol CRS*.

If the spectra obtained in the solid state show differences, dissolve the substance to be examined and the reference substance in *methanol R*, evaporate to dryness and record new spectra using the residues.

B. Thin-layer chromatography (*2.2.27*).

Test solution. Dissolve 25 mg of the substance to be examined in a mixture of 1 volume of *methanol R* and 9 volumes of *methylene chloride R* and dilute to 25 ml with the same mixture of solvents.

Reference solution. Dissolve 25 mg of *ethinylestradiol CRS* in a mixture of 1 volume of *methanol R* and 9 volumes of *methylene chloride R* and dilute to 25 ml with the same mixture of solvents.

Plate: *TLC silica gel G plate R*.

Mobile phase: *alcohol R, toluene R* (10:90 *V/V*).

Application: 5 µl.

Development: over a path of 15 cm.

Drying: in air until the solvent has evaporated.

Detection: heat at 110 °C for 10 min, spray the hot plate with *alcoholic solution of sulphuric acid R* and heat again at 110 °C for 10 min. Examine in daylight and in ultraviolet light at 365 nm.

Results: the principal spot in the chromatogram obtained with the test solution is similar in position, colour, fluorescence and size to the principal spot in the chromatogram obtained with the reference solution.

TESTS

Specific optical rotation (*2.2.7*): − 27 to − 30 (dried substance).

Dissolve 1.25 g in *pyridine R* and dilute to 25.0 ml with the same solvent.

Related substances. Liquid chromatography (*2.2.29*).

Test solution. Dissolve 0.10 g of the substance to be examined in the mobile phase and dilute to 100.0 ml with the mobile phase.

Reference solution (a). Dissolve 10 mg of *estradiol R* in the mobile phase, add 10.0 ml of the test solution and dilute to 50.0 ml with the mobile phase. Dilute 1.0 ml of this solution to 10.0 ml with the mobile phase.

Reference solution (b). Dilute 10.0 ml of the test solution to 50.0 ml with the mobile phase. Dilute 1.0 ml of this solution to 20.0 ml with the mobile phase.

Column:

– *size*: *l* = 0.15 m, Ø = 4.6 mm,
– *stationary phase*: *octadecylsilyl silica gel for chromatography R* (5 µm).

Mobile phase: *acetonitrile R, water R* (45:55 *V/V*).

Flow rate: 1 ml/min.

Detection: spectrophotometer at 280 nm.

Injection: 20 µl.

Run time: 2.5 times the retention time of ethinylestradiol.

Relative retention with reference to ethinylestradiol (retention time = about 4.6 min): impurity D = about 0.76, impurity B = about 0.94.

System suitability: reference solution (a):

– *resolution*: minimum 3.5 between the peaks due to impurity D and ethinylestradiol.

Limits:

– *impurity B*: not more than the area of the principal peak in the chromatogram obtained with reference solution (b) (1.0 per cent),
– *any other impurity*: not more than 0.25 times the area of the principal peak in the chromatogram obtained with reference solution (b) (0.25 per cent),
– *total of other impurities*: not more than half the area of the principal peak in the chromatogram obtained with reference solution (b) (0.5 per cent)
– *disregard limit*: 0.05 times the area of the principal peak in the chromatogram obtained with reference solution (b) (0.05 per cent)

Loss on drying (*2.2.32*): maximum 1.0 per cent, determined on 0.500 g by drying in an oven at 100-105 °C for 3 h.

ASSAY

Dissolve 0.200 g in 40 ml of *tetrahydrofuran R* and add 5 ml of a 100 g/l solution of *silver nitrate R*. Titrate with *0.1 M sodium hydroxide*, determining the end-point potentiometrically (*2.2.20*). Carry out a blank titration.

1 ml of *0.1 M sodium hydroxide* is equivalent to 29.64 mg of $C_{20}H_{24}O_2$.

STORAGE

Protected from light.

IMPURITIES

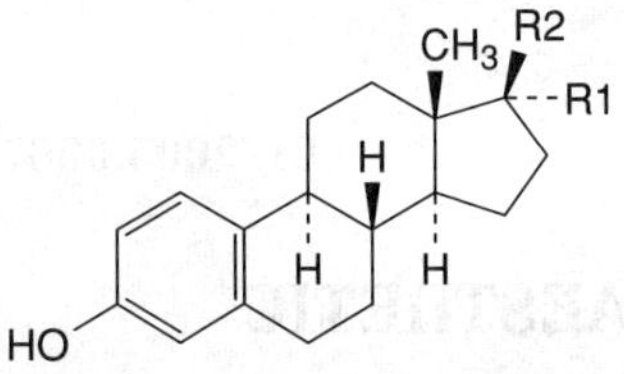

A. R1 = OH, R2 = C≡CH: 19-norpregna-1,3,5(10)-trien-20-yne-3,17-diol (17β-ethinylestradiol),

C. R1 + R2 = O: 3-hydroxyestra-1,3,5(10)-trien-17-one (estrone),

D. R1 = H, R2 = OH: estradiol,

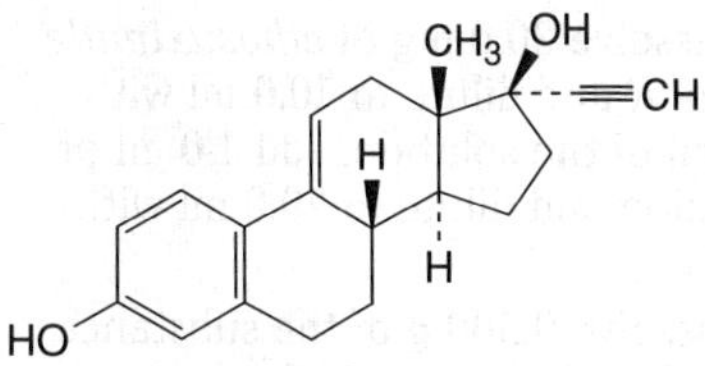

B. 19-nor-17α-pregna-1,3,5(10),9(11)-tetraen-20-yne-3,17-diol.

01/2005:0141

ETHIONAMIDE

Ethionamidum

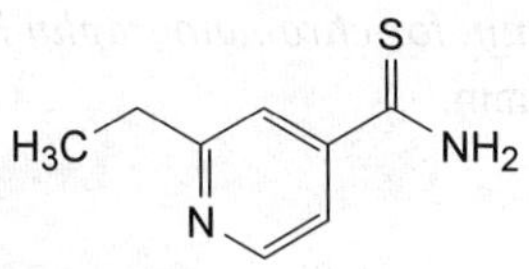

$C_8H_{10}N_2S$ M_r 166.2

DEFINITION

Ethionamide contains not less than 98.5 per cent and not more than the equivalent of 101.0 per cent of 2-ethylpyridine-4-carbothioamide, calculated with reference to the dried substance.

CHARACTERS

A yellow, crystalline powder or small, yellow crystals, practically insoluble in water, soluble in methanol, sparingly soluble in alcohol.

IDENTIFICATION

First identification: A, C.

Second identification: A, B, D.

A. Melting point (*2.2.14*): 158 °C to 164 °C.

B. Dissolve 10.0 mg in *methanol R* and dilute to 100.0 ml with the same solvent. Dilute 10.0 ml of the solution to 100.0 ml with *methanol R*. Examined between 230 nm and 350 nm (*2.2.25*), the solution shows an absorption maximum at 290 nm. The specific absorbance at the maximum is 380 to 440.

C. Examine by infrared absorption spectrophotometry (*2.2.24*), comparing with the spectrum obtained with *ethionamide CRS*.

D. Dissolve about 10 mg in 5 ml of *methanol R*. Add 5 ml of *silver nitrate solution R2*. A dark-brown precipitate is formed.

TESTS

Appearance of solution. Dissolve 0.5 g in 10 ml of *methanol R*, heating to about 50 °C. Allow to cool to room temperature. The solution is not more opalescent than reference suspension II (*2.2.1*).

Acidity. Dissolve 2.0 g in 20 ml of *methanol R*, heating to about 50 °C, and add 20 ml of *water R*. Cool slightly while shaking until crystallisation begins and then allow to cool to room temperature. Add 60 ml of *water R* and 0.2 ml of *cresol red solution R*. Not more than 0.2 ml of *0.1 M sodium hydroxide* is required to change the colour of the indicator to red.

Related substances. Examine by thin-layer chromatography (*2.2.27*), using *silica gel GF_{254} R* as the coating substance.

Test solution. Dissolve 0.2 g of the substance to be examined in *acetone R* and dilute to 10 ml with the same solvent.

Reference solution (a). Dilute 0.5 ml of the test solution to 100 ml with *acetone R*.

Reference solution (b). Dilute 0.2 ml of the test solution to 100 ml with *acetone R*.

Apply separately to the plate 10 µl of each solution. Develop over a path of 15 cm using a mixture of 10 volumes of *methanol R* and 90 volumes of *chloroform R*. Allow the plate to dry in air. Examine in ultraviolet light at 254 nm. Any spot in the chromatogram obtained with the test solution, apart from the principal spot, is not more intense than the spot in the chromatogram obtained with reference solution (a) (0.5 per cent) and at most 1 such spot is more intense than the spot in the chromatogram obtained with reference solution (b) (0.2 per cent).

Heavy metals (*2.4.8*). 1.0 g complies with limit test D for heavy metals (20 ppm). Prepare the standard using 2 ml of *lead standard solution (10 ppm Pb) R*.

Loss on drying (*2.2.32*). Not more than 0.5 per cent, determined on 1.00 g by drying in an oven at 100 °C to 105 °C for 3 h.

Sulphated ash (*2.4.14*). Not more than 0.1 per cent, determined on 1.0 g.

ASSAY

Dissolve 0.150 g in 50 ml of *anhydrous acetic acid R*. Titrate with *0.1 M perchloric acid*, determining the end-point potentiometrically (*2.2.20*).

1 ml of *0.1 M perchloric acid* is equivalent to 16.62 mg of $C_8H_{10}N_2S$.

01/2005:0764

ETHOSUXIMIDE

Ethosuximidum

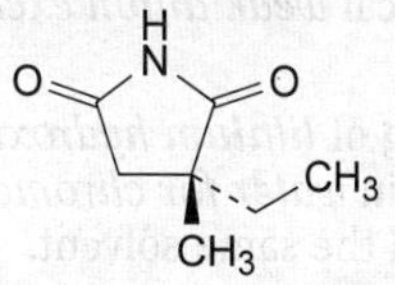

and enantiomer

$C_7H_{11}NO_2$ M_r 141.2

DEFINITION

(*RS*)-3-Ethyl-3-methylpyrrolidine-2,5-dione.

Content: 99.0 per cent to 101.0 per cent (anhydrous substance).

CHARACTERS

Appearance: white or almost white powder or waxy solid.

Solubility: freely soluble in water, very soluble in alcohol and in methylene chloride.

It shows polymorphism.

IDENTIFICATION

First identification: A, C.

Second identification: A, B, D, E.

A. Melting point (*2.2.14*): 45 °C to 50 °C.

B. Dissolve 50.0 mg in *alcohol R* and dilute to 50.0 ml with the same solvent. Examined between 230 nm and 300 nm (*2.2.25*), the solution shows an absorption maximum at 248 nm. The specific absorbance at the maximum is 8 to 9.

C. Infrared absorption spectrophotometry (*2.2.24*).

Preparation: discs of *potassium bromide R*.

Comparison: *ethosuximide CRS.*

If the spectra obtained in the solid state show differences, dissolve the substance to be examined and the reference substance separately in *methylene chloride R*, evaporate to dryness and record new spectra using the residues.

D. Dissolve 0.1 g in 3 ml of *methanol R*. Add 0.05 ml of a 100 g/l solution of *cobalt chloride R* and 0.05 ml of a 100 g/l solution of *calcium chloride R* and add 0.1 ml of *dilute sodium hydroxide solution R*. A purple colour develops and no precipitate is formed.

E. To about 10 mg add 10 mg of *resorcinol R* and 0.2 ml of *sulphuric acid R*. Heat at 140 °C for 5 min and cool. Add 5 ml of *water R* and 2 ml of *concentrated ammonia R1*. A brown colour is produced. Add about 100 ml of *water R*. A green fluorescence is produced.

TESTS

Solution S. Dissolve 2.5 g in *water R* and dilute to 25 ml with the same solvent.

Appearance of solution. Solution S is clear (*2.2.1*) and colourless (*2.2.2, Method II*).

Cyanide. Liquid chromatography (*2.2.29*).

Test solution. Dissolve 0.50 g of the substance to be examined in *water R* and dilute to 10.0 ml with the same solvent.

Reference solution (a). Dissolve 0.125 g of *potassium cyanide R* in *water R* and dilute to 50.0 ml with the same solvent. Dilute 1.0 ml to 100.0 ml with *water R*. Dilute 0.5 ml of this solution to 10.0 ml with *water R*.

Reference solution (b). Dissolve 0.50 g of the substance to be examined in *water R*, add 0.5 ml of reference solution (a) and dilute to 10.0 ml with *water R*.

Column:

- *size*: l = 0.075 m, Ø = 7.5 mm,
- *stationary phase*: spherical *weak anion exchange resin* (10 μm).

Mobile phase: dissolve 2.1 g of *lithium hydroxide R* and 85 mg of *sodium edetate R* in *water for chromatography R* and dilute to 1000.0 ml with the same solvent.

Flow rate: 2.0 ml/min.

Detection: electrochemical detector (direct amperometry) with a silver working electrode, a silver-silver chloride reference electrode, held at + 0.05 V oxidation potential, and a detector sensitivity of 20 nA full scale.

Injection: 20 μl; inject the test solution and reference solution (b).

System suitability: reference solution (b):

- *peak-to-valley ratio*: minimum 3, where H_p = height above the baseline of the peak due to cyanide and H_v = height above the baseline of the lowest point of the curve separating this peak from the peak due to ethosuximide.

Limit:

- *cyanide*: not more than half the height of the corresponding peak in the chromatogram obtained with reference solution (b) (0.5 ppm).

Related substances. Gas chromatography (*2.2.28*).

Internal standard solution. Dissolve 20 mg of *myristyl alcohol R* in *ethanol R* and dilute to 10.0 ml with the same solvent.

Test solution. Dissolve 1.00 g of the substance to be examined in *ethanol R*, add 1.0 ml of the internal standard solution and dilute to 20.0 ml with *ethanol R*.

Reference solution (a). Dissolve 20.0 mg of *ethosuximide impurity A CRS* in *ethanol R* and dilute to 10.0 ml with the same solvent. To 0.5 ml of the solution, add 1.0 ml of the internal standard solution and dilute to 20.0 ml with *ethanol R*.

Reference solution (b). Dissolve 0.500 g of the substance to be examined in *ethanol R* and dilute to 10.0 ml with the same solvent. Dilute 1.0 ml to 50.0 ml with *ethanol R*. To 2.0 ml of this solution, add 1.0 ml of the internal standard solution and dilute to 20.0 ml with *ethanol R*.

Column:

- *material*: fused silica,
- *size*: l = 30 m, Ø = 0.25 mm,
- *stationary phase*: *poly(cyanopropyl)(phenylmethyl) siloxane R* (film thickness 0.25 μm).

Carrier gas: *helium for chromatography R*.

Flow rate: 1 ml/min.

Split ratio: 1:67.

Temperature:

- *column*: 175 °C,
- *injection port and detector*: 240 °C.

Detection: flame ionisation.

Injection: 1 μl.

Run time: 1.5 times the retention time of ethosuximide.

Relative retentions with reference to the internal standard (retention time = about 8 min): impurity A = about 0.7; ethosuximide = about 1.1.

System suitability: reference solution (b):

- *resolution*: minimum 5 between the peaks due to the internal standard and to ethosuximide.

Limits:

- *impurity A*: calculate the ratio (R) of the area of the peak due to impurity A to the area of the peak due to the internal standard from the chromatogram obtained with reference solution (a); from the chromatogram obtained with the test solution, calculate the ratio of the area of any peak due to impurity A to the area of the peak due to the internal standard: this ratio is not greater than R (0.1 per cent),
- *any other impurity*: calculate the ratio (R) of half the area of the peak due to ethosuximide to the area of the peak due to the internal standard from the chromatogram obtained with reference solution (b); from the chromatogram obtained with the test solution, calculate the ratio of the area of any peak, apart from the principal peak and the peaks due to impurity A and to the internal standard, to the area of the peak due to the internal standard: this ratio is not greater than R (0.1 per cent),
- *total*: calculate the ratio (R) of the area of the peak due to ethosuximide to the area of the peak due to the internal standard from the chromatogram obtained with reference solution (b); from the chromatogram obtained with the test solution, calculate the ratio of the sum of the areas of any peaks, apart from the principal peak and the peak due to the internal standard, to the area of the peak due to the internal standard: this ratio is not greater than R (0.2 per cent),
- *disregard limit*: calculate the ratio (R) of 0.25 times the area of the peak due to impurity A to the area of the peak due to the internal standard from the chromatogram obtained with reference solution (a); from the chromatogram obtained with the test solution, calculate the ratio of the area of any peak, apart from the principal peak and the peak due to the internal

standard, to the area of the peak due to the internal standard: disregard any peak which has a ratio less than *R* (0.025 per cent).

Heavy metals (*2.4.8*): maximum 10 ppm.

12 ml of solution S complies with limit test A. Prepare the standard using *lead standard solution (1 ppm Pb) R*.

Water (*2.5.12*): maximum 0.5 per cent, determined on 1.00 g.

Sulphated ash (*2.4.14*): maximum 0.1 per cent, determined on 1.0 g.

ASSAY

Dissolve 0.120 g in 20 ml of *dimethylformamide R* and carry out a potentiometric titration (*2.2.20*) using *0.1 M tetrabutylammonium hydroxide*. Protect the solution from atmospheric carbon dioxide throughout the titration. Carry out a blank titration.

1 ml of *0.1 M tetrabutylammonium hydroxide* is equivalent to 14.12 mg of $C_7H_{11}NO_2$.

STORAGE

Protected from light.

IMPURITIES

Specified impurities: A.

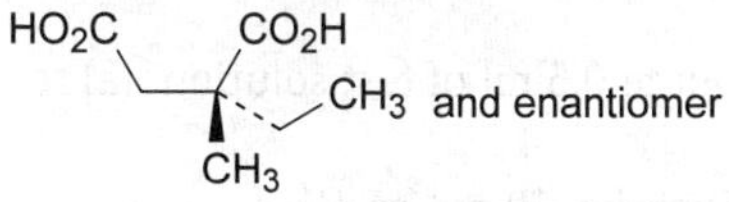

A. (2*RS*)-2-ethyl-2-methylbutanedioic acid.

01/2005:0899

ETHYL ACETATE

Ethylis acetas

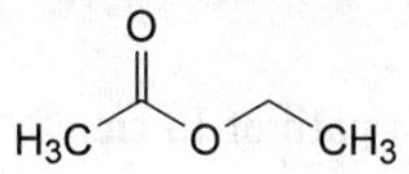

$C_4H_8O_2$ M_r 88.1

DEFINITION

Ethyl acetate is ethyl ethanoate.

CHARACTERS

A clear, colourless liquid, volatile, soluble in water, miscible with acetone, with alcohol and with methylene chloride.

IDENTIFICATION

First identification: B.

Second identification: A, C, D.

A. Boiling point (*2.2.12*): 76 °C to 78 °C.

B. Examine by infrared absorption spectrophotometry (*2.2.24*), comparing with the *Ph. Eur. reference spectrum of ethyl acetate*.

C. It gives the reaction of acetyl (*2.3.1*).

D. It gives the reaction of esters (*2.3.1*).

TESTS

Appearance of solution. A mixture of 1 ml of the substance to be examined and 15 ml of *water R* is clear (*2.2.1*) and colourless (*2.2.2, Method II*).

Acidity. To 10 ml of *alcohol R* add 0.1 ml of *phenolphthalein solution R* and *0.01 M sodium hydroxide* until the colour changes to pink. Add 5.5 ml of the substance to be examined and 0.25 ml of *0.02 M sodium hydroxide*. The solution remains pink for not less than 15 s.

Relative density (*2.2.5*): 0.898 to 0.902.

Refractive index (*2.2.6*): 1.370 to 1.373.

Reaction with sulphuric acid. Carefully add 2 ml to 10 ml of *sulphuric acid R*. After 15 min, the interface between the two liquids is not coloured.

Related substances. Examine by gas chromatography (*2.2.28*).

Test solution. The substance to be examined.

The chromatographic procedure may be carried out using:

- a glass column 2 m long and 2 mm in internal diameter, packed with *ethylvinylbenzene-divinylbenzene copolymer R* (136 µm to 173 µm),
- *nitrogen for chromatography R* as the carrier gas at a flow rate of 30 ml/min,
- a flame-ionisation detector,

raising the temperature at a rate of 8 °C/min from 90 °C to 240 °C and maintaining at 240 °C for 8 min and maintaining the temperature of the injection port and that of the detector at 240 °C.

Inject 1 µl of the test solution. In the chromatogram obtained with the test solution, the sum of the areas of any peaks apart from the principal peak is not greater than 0.2 per cent of the area of the principal peak.

Residue on evaporation. Evaporate 100.0 g to dryness on a water-bath and dry in an oven at 100 °C to 105 °C. The residue weighs not more than 3 mg (30 ppm).

Water (*2.5.12*). Not more than 0.1 per cent, determined on 10.0 ml by the semi-micro determination of water.

STORAGE

Store protected from light, at a temperature not exceeding 30 °C.

IMPURITIES

A. methyl acetate,

B. ethanol,

C. methanol.

01/2005:1319

ETHYL OLEATE

Ethylis oleas

DEFINITION

Ethyl oleate is a mixture consisting of the ethyl esters of fatty acids, mainly oleic acid. A suitable antioxidant may be added.

CHARACTERS

A clear, pale yellow or colourless liquid, practically insoluble in water, miscible with alcohol, with methylene chloride and with light petroleum (40 °C to 60 °C).

IDENTIFICATION

A. It complies with the test for relative density (see Tests).

B. It complies with the test for saponification value (see Tests).

C. It complies with the test of oleic acid (see Tests).

TESTS

Relative density (*2.2.5*): 0.866 to 0.874.

Acid value (*2.5.1*). Not more than 0.5, determined on 10.0 g.

Iodine value (*2.5.4*): 75 to 90.

Peroxide value (*2.5.5*). Not more than 10.0.

Saponification value (*2.5.6*): 177 to 188, determined on 2.0 g.

Oleic acid (*2.4.22, Method A*). The fatty acid fraction of the substance contains at least 60.0 per cent of oleic acid.

Water (*2.5.12*). Not more than 1.0 per cent, determined on 1.00 g by the semi-micro determination of water.

Total ash (*2.4.16*). Not more than 0.1 per cent, determined on 2.0 g.

STORAGE

Store protected from light.

LABELLING

The label states, where applicable, the name and concentration of any added antioxidant.

01/2005:0900

ETHYL PARAHYDROXYBENZOATE

Ethylis parahydroxybenzoas

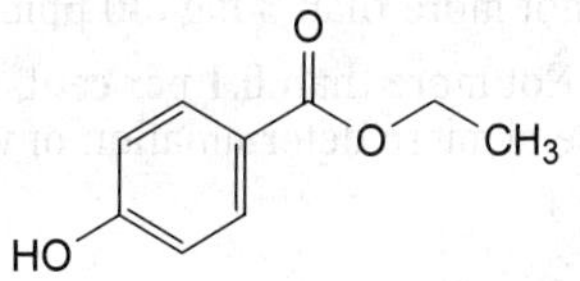

$C_9H_{10}O_3$ M_r 166.2

DEFINITION

Ethyl 4-hydroxybenzoate.

Content: 98.0 per cent to 102.0 per cent.

CHARACTERS

Appearance: white or almost white, crystalline powder or colourless crystals.

Solubility: very slightly soluble in water, freely soluble in alcohol and in methanol.

IDENTIFICATION

First identification: A, B.

Second identification: A, C, D.

A. Melting point (*2.2.14*): 115 °C to 118 °C.

B. Infrared absorption spectrophotometry (*2.2.24*).

Comparison: *ethyl parahydroxybenzoate CRS.*

C. Examine the chromatograms obtained in the test for related substances.

Results: the principal spot in the chromatogram obtained with test solution (b) is similar in position and size to the principal spot in the chromatogram obtained with reference solution (b).

D. To about 10 mg in a test-tube add 1 ml of *sodium carbonate solution R*, boil for 30 s and cool (solution A). To a further 10 mg in a similar test-tube add 1 ml of *sodium carbonate solution R*; the substance partly dissolves (solution B). Add at the same time to solution A and solution B 5 ml of *aminopyrazolone solution R* and 1 ml of *potassium ferricyanide solution R* and mix. Solution B is yellow to orange-brown. Solution A is orange to red, the colour being clearly more intense than any similar colour which may be obtained with solution B.

TESTS

Solution S. Dissolve 1.0 g in *alcohol R* and dilute to 10 ml with the same solvent.

Appearance of solution. Solution S is clear (*2.2.1*) and not more intensely coloured than reference solution BY_6 (*2.2.2, Method II*).

Acidity. To 2 ml of solution S add 3 ml of *alcohol R*, 5 ml of *carbon dioxide-free water R* and 0.1 ml of *bromocresol green solution R*. Not more than 0.1 ml of *0.1 M sodium hydroxide* is required to change the colour of the indicator to blue.

Related substances. Thin-layer chromatography (*2.2.27*).

Test solution (a). Dissolve 0.10 g of the substance to be examined in *acetone R* and dilute to 10 ml with the same solvent.

Test solution (b). Dilute 1 ml of test solution (a) to 10 ml with *acetone R*.

Reference solution (a). Dilute 0.5 ml of test solution (a) to 100 ml with *acetone R*.

Reference solution (b). Dissolve 10 mg of *ethyl parahydroxybenzoate CRS* in *acetone R* and dilute to 10 ml with the same solvent.

Reference solution (c). Dissolve 10 mg of *methyl parahydroxybenzoate R* in 1 ml of test solution (a) and dilute to 10 ml with *acetone R*.

Plate: suitable octadecylsilyl silica gel with a fluorescent indicator having an optimal intensity at 254 nm as the coating substance.

Mobile phase: *glacial acetic acid R, water R, methanol R* (1:30:70 *V/V/V*).

Application: 2 µl.

Development: over a path of 15 cm.

Drying: in air.

Detection: examine in ultraviolet light at 254 nm.

System suitability: the chromatogram obtained with reference solution (c) shows 2 clearly separated principal spots.

Limits:

- *any impurity*: any spot in the chromatogram obtained with test solution (a), apart from the principal spot, is not more intense than the spot in the chromatogram obtained with reference solution (a) (0.5 per cent).

Sulphated ash (*2.4.14*): maximum 0.1 per cent, determined on 1.0 g.

ASSAY

To 1.000 g add 20.0 ml of *1 M sodium hydroxide*. Heat at about 70 °C for 1 h. Cool rapidly in an ice bath. Prepare a blank in the same manner. Carry out the titration on the solutions at room temperature. Titrate the excess sodium hydroxide with *0.5 M sulphuric acid*, continuing the titration until the second point of inflexion and determining the end-point potentiometrically (*2.2.20*).

1 ml of *1 M sodium hydroxide* is equivalent to 166.2 mg of $C_9H_{10}O_3$.

IMPURITIES

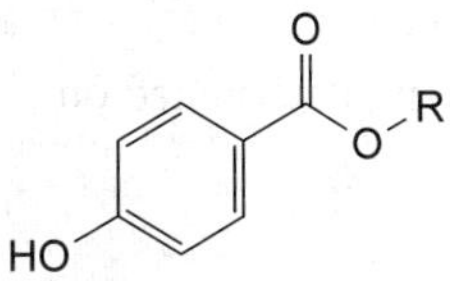

A. R = H: 4-hydroxybenzoic acid,

B. R = CH_3: methyl 4-hydroxybenzoate,

C. R = CH_2-CH_2-CH_3: propyl 4-hydroxybenzoate,

D. R = CH_2-CH_2-CH_2-CH_3: butyl 4-hydroxybenzoate.

01/2005:0822

ETHYLCELLULOSE

Ethylcellulosum

DEFINITION

Partly *O*-ethylated cellulose.

Content: 44.0 per cent to 51.0 per cent of ethoxy (-OC_2H_5) groups (dried substance).

CHARACTERS

Appearance: white or yellowish-white powder or granular powder, odourless or almost odourless.

Solubility: practically insoluble in water, soluble in methylene chloride and in a mixture of 20 g of alcohol and 80 g of toluene, slightly soluble in ethyl acetate and in methanol, practically insoluble in glycerol (85 per cent) and in propylene glycol. The solutions may show a slight opalescence.

IDENTIFICATION

A. Infrared absorption spectrophotometry (*2.2.24*).

Comparison: *Ph. Eur. reference spectrum of ethylcellulose.*

B. It complies with the limits of the assay.

TESTS

Acidity or alkalinity. To 0.5 g add 25 ml of *carbon dioxide-free water R* and shake for 15 min. Filter through a sintered-glass filter (40). To 10 ml add 0.1 ml of *phenolphthalein solution R* and 0.5 ml of *0.01 M sodium hydroxide*. The solution is pink. To 10 ml add 0.1 ml of *methyl red solution R* and 0.5 ml of *0.01 M hydrochloric acid*. The solution is red.

Viscosity (*2.2.9*). The viscosity, determined at 25 °C and expressed in mPa·s, is not less than 80.0 per cent and not more than 120.0 per cent of that stated on the label for a nominal viscosity greater than 6 mPa·s; and not less than 75.0 per cent and not more than 140.0 per cent of that stated on the label for a nominal viscosity not greater than 6 mPa·s.

Shake a quantity of the substance to be examined equivalent to 5.00 g of the dried substance with 95 g of a mixture of 20 g of *alcohol R* and 80 g of *toluene R* until the substance is dissolved. Determine the viscosity using a capillary viscometer.

Acetaldehyde: maximum 100 ppm.

Introduce 3.0 g into a 250 ml conical flask with a ground-glass stopper, add 10 ml of *water R* and stir mechanically for 1 h. Allow to stand for 24 h, filter and dilute the filtrate to 100.0 ml with *water R*. Transfer 5.0 ml to a 25 ml volumetric flask, add 5 ml of a 0.5 g/l solution of *methylbenzothiazolone hydrazone hydrochloride R* and heat in a water-bath at 60 °C for 5 min. Add 2 ml of *ferric chloride-sulphamic acid reagent R* and heat again at 60 °C for 5 min. Cool and dilute to 25.0 ml with *water R*. The solution is not more intensely coloured than a standard prepared at the same time and in the same manner using instead of the 5.0 ml of filtrate, 5.0 ml of a reference solution prepared by diluting 3.0 ml of *acetaldehyde standard solution (100 ppm C_2H_4O) R1* to 100.0 ml with *water R*.

Chlorides (*2.4.4*): maximum 0.1 per cent.

Disperse 0.250 g in 50 ml of *water R*, heat to boiling and allow to cool, shaking occasionally. Filter and discard the first 10 ml of the filtrate. Dilute 10 ml of the filtrate to 15 ml with *water R*. The solution complies with the limit test for chlorides.

Heavy metals (*2.4.8*): maximum 20 ppm.

1.0 g complies with limit test C. Prepare the standard using 2 ml of *lead standard solution (10 ppm Pb) R*.

Loss on drying (*2.2.32*): maximum 3.0 per cent, determined on 1.000 g by drying in an oven at 100-105 °C for 2 h.

Sulphated ash (*2.4.14*): maximum 0.5 per cent, determined on 1.0 g.

ASSAY

Gas chromatography (*2.2.28*).

CAUTION: hydriodic acid and its reaction by-products are highly toxic. Perform all steps for preparation of the test and reference solutions in a properly functioning hood.

Internal standard solution. Dilute 120 µl of *toluene R* to 10 ml with *o-xylene R*.

Test solution. Transfer 50.0 mg of the substance to be examined, 50.0 mg of *adipic acid R* and 2.0 ml of the internal standard solution into a suitable 5 ml thick-walled reaction vial with a pressure-tight septum-type closure. Cautiously add 2.0 ml of *hydriodic acid R*, immediately close the vial tightly and weigh the contents and the vial accurately. Shake the vial for 30 s, heat to 125 °C for 10 min, allow to cool for 2 min, shake again for 30 s and heat to 125 °C for 10 min. Afterwards allow to cool for 2 min and repeat shaking and heating for a third time. Allow the vial to cool for 45 min and reweigh. If the loss is greater than 10 mg, discard the mixture and prepare another. Use the upper layer.

Reference solution. Transfer 100.0 mg of *adipic acid R*, 4.0 ml of the internal standard solution and 4.0 ml of *hydriodic acid R* into a suitable 10 ml thick-walled reaction vial with a pressure-tight septum-type closure. Close the vial tightly and weigh the vial and contents accurately. Afterwards inject 50 µl of *iodoethane R* through the septum with a syringe, weigh the vial again and calculate the mass of iodoethane added, by difference. Shake well and allow the layers to separate.

Column:
- *material*: stainless steel,
- *size*: l = 5.0 m, Ø = 2 mm,
- *stationary phase*: *diatomaceous earth for gas chromatography R* (150-180 µm) impregnated with 3 per cent *m/m* of *poly(dimethyl)siloxane R.*

Carrier gas: *nitrogen for chromatography R.*

Flow rate: 15 ml/min.

Temperature:
- *column*: 80 °C,
- *injection port and detector*: 200 °C.

Detection: flame ionisation.

Injection: 1 µl of the upper layer of the test solution and 1 µl of the upper layer of the reference solution.

Relative retention with reference to toluene: iodoethane = about 0.6; *o*-xylene = about 2.3.

System suitability: reference solution:

– *resolution*: minimum 2.0 between the peaks due to iodoethane and toluene.

Calculate the percentage content of ethoxy groups from the following expression:

$$\frac{Q_1 \times m_2 \times 45.1 \times 100 \times 100}{2 \times Q_2 \times m_1 \times 156.0 \times (100 - d)}$$

Q_1 = ratio of iodoethane peak area to toluene peak area in the chromatogram obtained with the test solution,

Q_2 = ratio of iodoethane peak area to toluene peak area in the chromatogram obtained with the reference solution,

m_1 = mass of the substance to be examined used in the test solution, in milligrams,

m_2 = mass of iodoethane used in the reference solution, in milligrams,

d = percentage loss on drying.

LABELLING

The label states the nominal viscosity in millipascal seconds for a 5 per cent *m/m* solution.

01/2005:1421

ETHYLENE GLYCOL MONOPALMITOSTEARATE

Ethylenglycoli monopalmitostearas

DEFINITION

Mixture of ethylene glycol mono- and diesters of stearic and palmitic acids, produced from the condensation of ethylene glycol and stearic acid 50 of vegetable or animal origin (see *Stearic acid (1474)*).

Content: minimum of 50.0 per cent of monoesters.

CHARACTERS

Appearance: white or almost white, waxy solid.

Solubility: practically insoluble in water, soluble in acetone and in hot alcohol.

IDENTIFICATION

A. It complies with the test for melting point (see Tests).

B. It complies with the test for composition of fatty acids (see Tests).

C. It complies with the assay (monoesters content).

TESTS

Melting point (*2.2.15*): 54 °C to 60 °C.

Acid value (*2.5.1*): maximum 3.0, determined on 10.0 g.

Iodine value (*2.5.4*): maximum 3.0.

Saponification value (*2.5.6*): 170 to 195, determined on 2.0 g.

Composition of fatty acids (*2.4.22, Method A*). The fatty acid fraction has the following composition:

– *stearic acid*: 40.0 per cent to 60.0 per cent,

– *sum of contents of palmitic acid and stearic acid*: minimum 90.0 per cent.

Free ethylene glycol: maximum 5.0 per cent, determined as prescribed under Assay.

Total ash (*2.4.16*): maximum 0.1 per cent, determined on 1.0 g.

ASSAY

Size-exclusion chromatography (*2.2.30*).

Test solution. Into a 15 ml flask, weigh about 0.2 g (*m*), to the nearest 0.1 mg. Add 5.0 ml of *tetrahydrofuran R* and shake to dissolve. Heat gently, if necessary. Reweigh the flask and calculate the total mass of solvent and substance (*M*).

Reference solutions. Into four 15 ml flasks, weigh, to the nearest 0.1 mg, about 2.5 mg, 5.0 mg, 10.0 mg and 20.0 mg of *ethylene glycol R*. Add 5.0 ml of *tetrahydrofuran R* and shake to dissolve. Weigh the flasks again and calculate the concentration of ethylene glycol in milligrams per gram for each reference solution.

Column:

– *size*: l = 0.6 m, Ø = 7 mm,

– *stationary phase*: *styrene-divinylbenzene copolymer R* (particle diameter 5 µm and pore size 10 nm).

Mobile phase: *tetrahydrofuran R*.

Flow rate: 1 ml/min.

Detection: differential refractometer.

Injection: 40 µl.

Relative retention with reference to ethylene glycol: diesters = about 0.76, monoesters = about 0.83.

Limits:

– *free ethylene glycol*: from the calibration curve obtained with the reference solutions, determine the concentration (*C*) in milligrams per gram in the test solution and calculate the percentage content in the substance to be examined using the following expression:

$$\frac{C \times M}{m \times 10}$$

– *monoesters*: calculate the percentage content of monoesters using the following expression:

$$\frac{A}{A+B} \times (100 - D)$$

A = area of the peak due to the monoesters,

B = area of the peak due to the diesters,

D = percentage content of free ethylene glycol + percentage content of free fatty acids which may be determined using the following expression: $\frac{I_A \times 270}{561.1}$

I_A = acid value.

STORAGE

Protected from light.

01/2005:0716

ETHYLENEDIAMINE

Ethylendiaminum

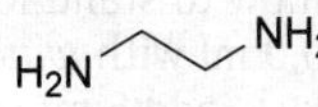

$C_2H_8N_2$ M_r 60.1

DEFINITION

Ethylenediamine contains not less than 98.0 per cent and not more than the equivalent of 101.0 per cent of ethane-1,2-diamine.

CHARACTERS

A clear, colourless or slightly yellow liquid, hygroscopic, miscible with water and with ethanol. On exposure to air, white fumes are evolved. On heating, it evaporates completely.

IDENTIFICATION

A. Relative density (*2.2.5*): 0.895 to 0.905.

B. Boiling point (*2.2.12*): 116 °C to 118 °C.

C. To 0.2 ml add 0.5 ml of *acetic anhydride R*. Boil. A crystalline mass forms after cooling, which dissolves in 5 ml of *2-propanol R* with heating. Cool the solution and add 5 ml of *ether R*. If necessary, initiate crystallisation by scratching the walls of the test-tube with a glass rod. Filter through a sintered-glass filter, wash with several portions of *ether R* and dry at 100 °C to 105 °C. The residue melts (*2.2.14*) at 173 °C to 177 °C.

TESTS

Solution S. Mix 10 g with *carbon dioxide-free water R* and dilute to 100 ml with the same solvent.

Appearance of solution. Solution S is clear (*2.2.1*) and not more intensely coloured than the reference solution BY_6 (*2.2.2, Method II*).

Carbonate. A mixture of 4 ml of solution S and 6 ml of *calcium hydroxide solution R* is not more opalescent than reference suspension II (*2.2.1*).

Chlorides (*2.4.4*). To 5 ml of solution S add 5 ml of *dilute nitric acid R* and dilute to 15 ml with *water R*. This solution complies with the limit test for chlorides (100 ppm).

Ammonia and other bases. Dissolve 1.2 g in 20 ml of *alcohol R* and add, dropwise with stirring, 4.5 ml of *hydrochloric acid R*. Evaporate to dryness on a water-bath, breaking up any resulting cake with a glass rod, and dry at 100 °C to 105 °C for 1 h.

1 g of the residue is equivalent to 0.4518 g of $C_2H_8N_2$. The percentage content of $C_2H_8N_2$ found in this test does not vary by more than 0.5 from the percentage content determined in the assay.

Iron (*2.4.9*). 10 ml of solution S complies with the limit test for iron (10 ppm).

Heavy metals (*2.4.8*). 12 ml of solution S complies with limit test A for heavy metals (10 ppm). Prepare the standard using *lead standard solution (1 ppm Pb) R*.

Residue on evaporation. Evaporate 5.00 g to dryness on a water-bath and dry at 100 °C to 105 °C for 1 h. The residue weighs not more than 15 mg (0.3 per cent).

ASSAY

Place 25.0 ml of *1 M hydrochloric acid* and 0.2 ml of *methyl red mixed solution R* in a flask. Add 0.600 g of the substance to be examined. Titrate with *1 M sodium hydroxide* until the colour changes from violet-red to green.

1 ml of *1 M hydrochloric acid* is equivalent to 30.05 mg of $C_2H_8N_2$.

STORAGE

Store in an airtight container, protected from light.

01/2005:0491

ETHYLMORPHINE HYDROCHLORIDE

Ethylmorphini hydrochloridum

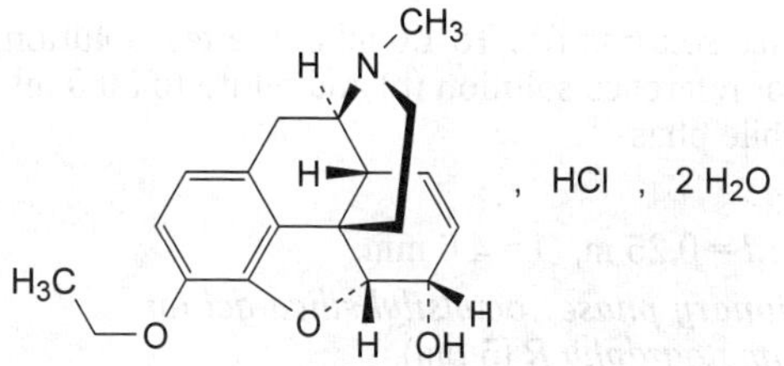

$C_{19}H_{24}ClNO_3,2H_2O$ M_r 385.9

DEFINITION

7,8-Didehydro-4,5α-epoxy-3-ethoxy-17-methylmorphinan-6α-ol hydrochloride dihydrate.

Content: 99.0 per cent to 101.0 per cent (anhydrous substance).

CHARACTERS

Appearance: white or almost white, crystalline powder.

Solubility: soluble in water and in alcohol, insoluble in cyclohexane.

IDENTIFICATION

First identification: A, D.

Second identification: B, C, D.

A. Infrared absorption spectrophotometry (*2.2.24*).
Comparison: *Ph. Eur. reference spectrum of ethylmorphine hydrochloride.*

B. In a test-tube, dissolve 0.5 g in 6 ml of *water R* and add 15 ml of *0.1 M sodium hydroxide*. Scratch the wall of the tube with a glass rod. A white, crystalline precipitate is formed. Collect the precipitate, wash and dissolve in 20 ml of *water R* heated to 80 °C. Filter and cool in iced water. The crystals, after drying *in vacuo* for 12 h, melt (*2.2.14*) at 85 °C to 89 °C.

C. To about 10 mg add 1 ml of *sulphuric acid R* and 0.05 ml of *ferric chloride solution R2*. Heat on a water-bath. A blue colour develops. Add 0.05 ml of *nitric acid R*. The colour becomes red.

D. Solution S (see Tests) gives reaction (a) of chlorides (*2.3.1*).

TESTS

Solution S. Dissolve 0.500 g in *carbon dioxide-free water R* and dilute to 25.0 ml with the same solvent.

Appearance of solution. Solution S is clear (*2.2.1*) and not more intensely coloured than reference solution BY_6 (*2.2.2, Method II*).

Acidity or alkalinity. To 10 ml of solution S add 0.05 ml of *methyl red solution R* and 0.2 ml of *0.02 M hydrochloric acid*, the solution is red. Add 0.4 ml of *0.02 M sodium hydroxide*, the solution becomes yellow.

Specific optical rotation (*2.2.7*): − 102 to − 105 (anhydrous substance), determined on solution S.

Related substances. Liquid chromatography (*2.2.29*).

Test solution. Dissolve 50.0 mg of the substance to be examined in the mobile phase and dilute to 20.0 ml with the mobile phase.

Monographs D-E

Reference solution (a). Dilute 1.0 ml of the test solution to 25.0 ml with the mobile phase. Dilute 1.0 ml of this solution to 20.0 ml with the mobile phase.

Reference solution (b). Dissolve 12.5 mg of *codeine R* in the mobile phase and dilute to 5.0 ml with the mobile phase.

Reference solution (c). Dilute 0.5 ml of reference solution (b) to 100.0 ml with the mobile phase.

Reference solution (d). To 1.0 ml of the test solution, add 1.0 ml of reference solution (b) and dilute to 50.0 ml with the mobile phase.

Column:

- *size*: l = 0.25 m, Ø = 4.6 mm,
- *stationary phase*: *octylsilyl silica gel for chromatography R* (5 µm),
- *temperature*: 30 °C.

Mobile phase: add 1.25 g of *sodium heptanesulphonate R* to a mixture of 12.5 ml of *glacial acetic acid R* and 5 ml of a 20 per cent *V/V* solution of *triethylamine R* in a mixture of equal volumes of *methanol R* and *water R*. Dilute to 1000 ml with *water R*. To 550 ml of this solution add 450 ml of *methanol R*.

Flow rate: 1 ml/min.

Detection: spectrophotometer at 230 nm.

Injection: 10 µl.

Run time: 4 times the retention time of ethylmorphine.

Relative retention with reference to ethylmorphine (retention time = about 6.2 min): impurity B = about 0.7; impurity C = about 0.8; impurity D = about 1.3; impurity A = about 2.5.

System suitability: reference solution (d):

- *resolution*: minimum 5 between the peaks due to ethylmorphine and impurity C.

Limits:

- *correction factor*: for the calculation of content, multiply the peak area of impurity D by 0.4,
- *impurities A, B, D*: for each impurity, not more than the area of the principal peak in the chromatogram obtained with reference solution (a) (0.2 per cent),
- *impurity C*: not more than the area of the principal peak in the chromatogram obtained with reference solution (c) (0.5 per cent),
- *any other impurity*: for each impurity, not more than 0.5 times the area of the principal peak in the chromatogram obtained with reference solution (a) (0.1 per cent),
- *total of impurities other than C*: not more than 2.5 times the area of the principal peak in the chromatogram obtained with reference solution (a) (0.5 per cent),
- *disregard limit*: 0.25 times the area of the principal peak in the chromatogram obtained with reference solution (a) (0.05 per cent).

Water (*2.5.12*): 8.0 per cent to 10.0 per cent, determined on 0.250 g.

Sulphated ash (*2.4.14*): maximum 0.1 per cent, determined on 1.0 g.

ASSAY

Dissolve 0.300 g in a mixture of 5 ml of *0.01 M hydrochloric acid* and 30 ml of *alcohol R*. Carry out a potentiometric titration (*2.2.20*), using *0.1 M sodium hydroxide*. Read the volume added between the 2 points of inflexion.

1 ml of *0.1 M sodium hydroxide* is equivalent to 34.99 mg of $C_{19}H_{24}ClNO_3$.

STORAGE

Protected from light.

IMPURITIES

Specified impurities: A, B, C, D.

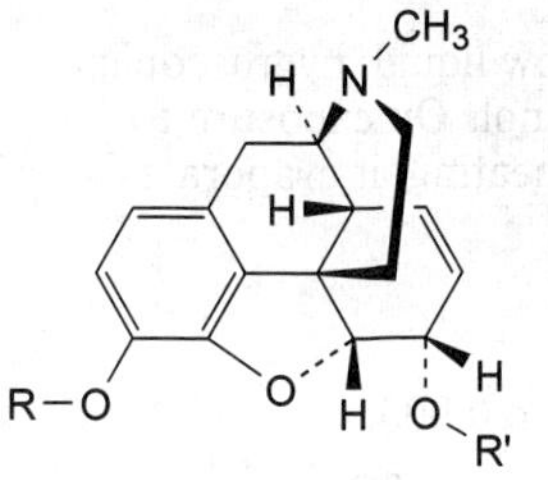

A. R = R′ = C_2H_5: 7,8-didehydro-4,5α-epoxy-3,6α-diethoxy-17-methylmorphinan,

B. R = R′ = H: morphine,

C. R = CH_3, R′ = H: codeine,

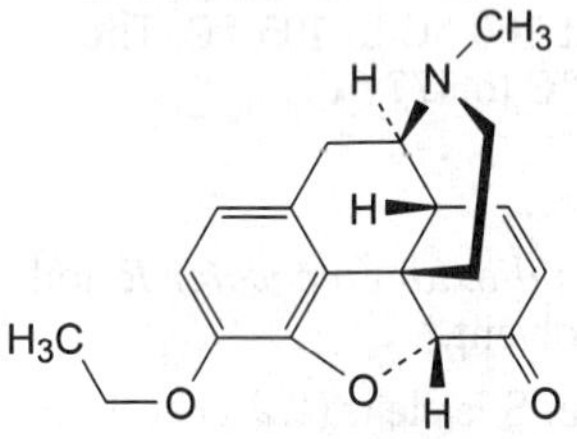

D. 7,8-didehydro-4,5α-epoxy-3-ethoxy-17-methylmorphinan-6-one (ethylmorphinone).

01/2005:1205

ETILEFRINE HYDROCHLORIDE

Etilefrini hydrochloridum

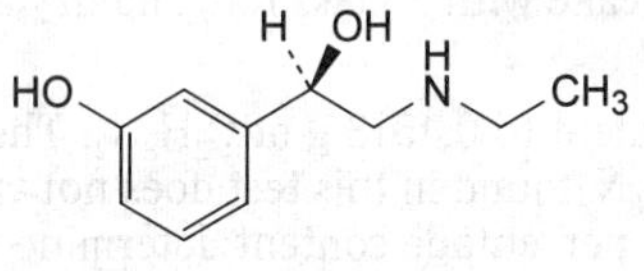

$C_{10}H_{16}ClNO_2$ M_r 217.7

DEFINITION

(1*RS*)-2-(Ethylamino)-1-(3-hydroxyphenyl)ethanol hydrochloride.

Content: 98.0 per cent to 101.0 per cent (dried substance).

CHARACTERS

Appearance: white or almost white, crystalline powder or colourless crystals.

Solubility: freely soluble in water, soluble in ethanol (96 per cent), practically insoluble in methylene chloride.

IDENTIFICATION

First identification: B, E.

Second identification: A, C, D, E.

A. Melting point (*2.2.14*): 118 °C to 122 °C.

B. Infrared absorption spectrophotometry (*2.2.24*).

Preparation: discs of *potassium chloride R*.

Comparison: *etilefrine hydrochloride CRS*.

C. Thin-layer chromatography (*2.2.27*).

Prepare the solutions protected from bright light and develop the chromatograms protected from light.

Test solution. Dissolve 25 mg of the substance to be examined in *methanol R* and dilute to 5 ml with the same solvent.

Reference solution (a). Dissolve 25 mg of *etilefrine hydrochloride CRS* in *methanol R* and dilute to 5 ml with the same solvent.

Reference solution (b). Dissolve 10 mg of *phenylephrine hydrochloride CRS* in 2 ml of reference solution (a) and dilute to 10 ml with *methanol R*.

Plate: *TLC silica gel plate R*.

Mobile phase: *concentrated ammonia R, methanol R, methylene chloride R* (5:25:70 *V/V/V*).

Application: 5 µl.

Development: over a path of 15 cm.

Drying: in a current of warm air.

Detection: spray with a 10 g/l solution of *potassium permanganate R*; examine in daylight after 15 min.

System suitability: reference solution (b):

– the chromatogram shows 2 clearly separated spots.

Results: the principal spot in the chromatogram obtained with the test solution is similar in position, colour and size to the principal spot in the chromatogram obtained with reference solution (a).

D. To 0.2 ml of solution S (see Tests), add 1 ml of *water R*, 0.1 ml of *copper sulphate solution R* and 1 ml of *strong sodium hydroxide solution R*. A blue colour is produced. Add 2 ml of *ether R* and shake. The upper layer is colourless.

E. Dilute 1 ml of solution S to 10 ml with *water R*. The solution gives reaction (a) of chlorides (*2.3.1*).

TESTS

Solution S. Dissolve 2.50 g in *carbon dioxide-free water R* prepared from *distilled water R* and dilute to 50.0 ml with the same solvent.

Appearance of solution. Solution S is clear (*2.2.1*) and colourless (*2.2.2, Method II*).

Acidity or alkalinity. Dilute 4 ml of solution S to 10 ml with *carbon dioxide-free water R*. Add 0.1 ml of *methyl red solution R* and 0.2 ml of *0.01 M sodium hydroxide*. The solution is yellow. Not more than 0.4 ml of *0.01 M hydrochloric acid* is required to change the colour of the indicator to red.

Optical rotation (*2.2.7*): − 0.10° to + 0.10°, determined on solution S.

Related substances. Liquid chromatography (*2.2.29*).

Prepare the solutions immediately before use.

Test solution. Dissolve 50.0 mg of the substance to be examined in *water R* and dilute to 50.0 ml with the same solvent.

Reference solution (a). Dilute 1.0 ml of the test solution to 10.0 ml with *water R*. Dilute 1.0 ml of this solution to 50.0 ml with *water R*.

Reference solution (b). Dissolve 10.0 mg of *etilefrine impurity A CRS* in *water R* and dilute to 50.0 ml with the same solvent. Dilute 1.0 ml of the solution to 50.0 ml with *water R*.

Reference solution (c). To 10.0 ml of reference solution (a) add 5.0 ml of reference solution (b) and dilute to 20.0 ml with *water R*.

Column:

– *size*: *l* = 0.25 m, Ø = 4.6 mm,

– *stationary phase*: *octylsilyl silica gel for chromatography R* (5 µm).

Mobile phase: mix 35 volumes of *acetonitrile R* and 65 volumes of a 1.1 g/l solution of *sodium laurilsulfate R* adjusted to pH 2.3 with *phosphoric acid R*.

Flow rate: 1 ml/min.

Detection: spectrophotometer at 220 nm.

Injection: 20 µl.

Run time: 5 times the retention time of etilefrine.

Relative retention with reference to etilefrine (retention time = about 9 min): impurity E = about 0.5; impurity C = about 0.8; impurity B = about 0.9; impurity A = about 1.2; impurity F = about 1.7; impurity D = about 4.5.

System suitability: reference solution (c):

– *resolution*: minimum 2.5 between the peaks due to etilefrine and impurity A.

Limits:

– *impurity A*: not more than the area of the principal peak in the chromatogram obtained with reference solution (b) (0.4 per cent),

– *impurities B, C, D, E*: for each impurity, not more than the area of the principal peak in the chromatogram obtained with reference solution (a) (0.2 per cent),

– *any other impurity*: for each impurity, not more than 0.5 times the area of the principal peak in the chromatogram obtained with reference solution (a) (0.1 per cent),

– *sum of impurities other than A*: not more than 5 times the area of the principal peak in the chromatogram obtained with reference solution (a) (1 per cent),

– *disregard limit*: 0.1 times the area of the principal peak in the chromatogram obtained with reference solution (a) (0.02 per cent); disregard any peak due to the solvent.

Sulphates (*2.4.13*): maximum 200 ppm, determined on 15 ml of solution S.

Heavy metals (*2.4.8*): maximum 20 ppm.

Dissolve 2.0 g in 20 ml of *water R*. 12 ml of the solution complies with limit test A. Prepare the reference solution using *lead standard solution (2 ppm Pb) R*.

Loss on drying (*2.2.32*): maximum 0.5 per cent, determined on 1.000 g by drying in an oven at 100-105 °C.

Sulphated ash (*2.4.14*): maximum 0.1 per cent, determined on 1.0 g.

ASSAY

Dissolve 0.150 g in a mixture of 20 ml of *anhydrous acetic acid R* and 50 ml of *acetic anhydride R*. Titrate with *0.1 M perchloric acid*, determining the end-point potentiometrically (*2.2.20*).

1 ml of *0.1 M perchloric acid* is equivalent to 21.77 mg of $C_{10}H_{16}ClNO_2$.

STORAGE

In an airtight container, protected from light.

Monographs D-E

IMPURITIES

Specified impurities: A, B, C, D, E.

Other detectable impurities: F.

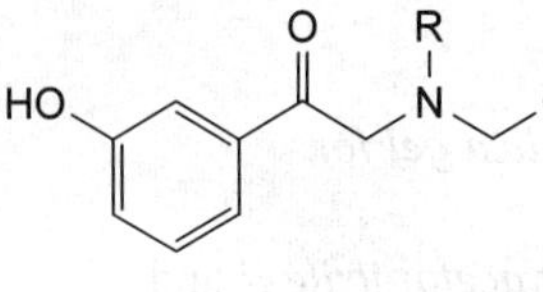

A. R = H: 2-(ethylamino)-1-(3-hydroxyphenyl)ethanone (etilefrone),

D. R = CH_2-C_6H_5: 2-(benzylethylamino)-1-(3-hydroxyphenyl)ethanone (benzyletilefrone),

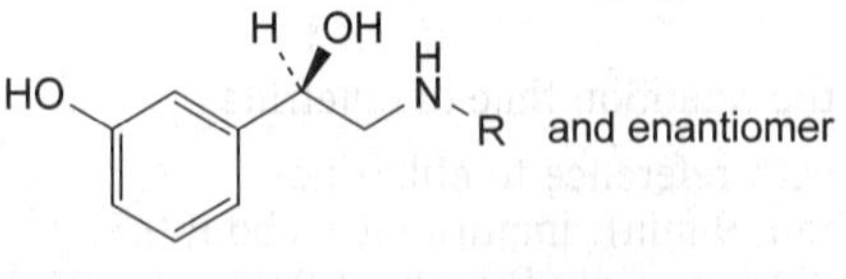

B. R = CH_3: (1*RS*)-1-(3-hydroxyphenyl)-2-(methylamino)ethanol (phenylephrine),

C. R = H: (1*RS*)-2-amino-1-(3-hydroxyphenyl)ethanol (norfenefrine),

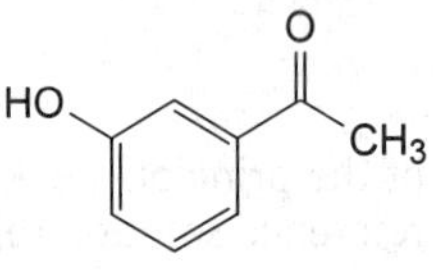

E. 1-(3-hydroxyphenyl)ethanone (3-hydroxyacetophenone),

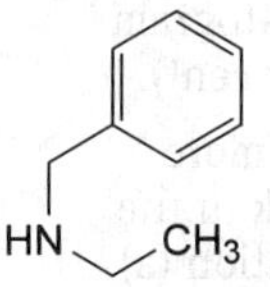

F. *N*-benzylethanamine (benzylethylamine).

01/2005:1422

ETODOLAC

Etodolacum

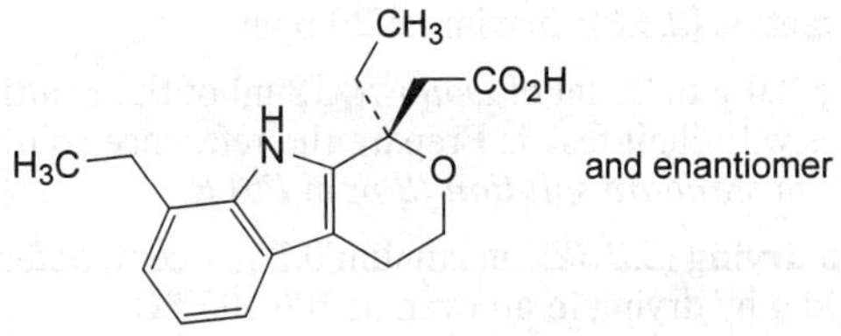

$C_{17}H_{21}NO_3$ M_r 287.4

DEFINITION

Etodolac contains not less than 98.0 per cent and not more than the equivalent of 102.0 per cent of 2-[(1*RS*)-1,8-diethyl-1,3,4,9-tetrahydropyrano[3,4-*b*]indol-1-yl]acetic acid, calculated with reference to the anhydrous substance.

CHARACTERS

A white or almost white, crystalline powder, practically insoluble in water, freely soluble in acetone and in ethanol.

IDENTIFICATION

First identification: B.

Second identification: A, C.

A. Melting point (*2.2.14*): 144 °C to 150 °C.

B. Examine by infrared absorption spectrophotometry (*2.2.24*), comparing with the spectrum obtained with *etodolac CRS*.

C. Examine by thin-layer chromatography (*2.2.27*), using a *TLC silica gel GF_{254} plate R* previously activated by heating at 105 °C for 1 h.
Test solution. Dissolve 10 mg of the substance to be examined in *acetone R* and dilute to 10 ml with the same solvent.
Reference solution. Dissolve 10 mg of *etodolac CRS* in *acetone R* and dilute to 10 ml with the same solvent.
Place the plate in an unsaturated chamber containing a mixture of 20 volumes of a 25 g/l solution of *ascorbic acid R* and 80 volumes of *methanol R*. Allow the solution to ascend 1 cm above the line of application on the plate, remove the plate and allow it to dry for at least 30 min.
Apply separately to the plate 10 µl of each solution. Develop over a path of 15 cm using a mixture of 0.5 volumes of *glacial acetic acid R*, 30 volumes of *ethanol R* and 70 volumes of *toluene R*. Allow the plate to dry in air and examine in ultraviolet light at 254 nm. The principal spot in the chromatogram obtained with the test solution is similar in position and size to the principal spot in the chromatogram obtained with the reference solution.

TESTS

Optical rotation (*2.2.7*). Dissolve 2.50 g in *methanol R* and dilute to 25.0 ml with the same solvent. The angle of optical rotation is − 0.10° to + 0.10°.

Related substances. Examine by liquid chromatography (*2.2.29*).

Test solution. Dissolve 50.0 mg of the substance to be examined in *methanol R* and dilute to 50.0 ml with the same solvent.

Reference solution (a). Dilute 5.0 ml of the test solution to 50.0 ml with *methanol R*. Dilute 5.0 ml of this solution to 100.0 ml with *methanol R*.

Reference solution (b). Dissolve 1.0 mg of *etodolac impurity H CRS* and 1.0 mg of *etodolac CRS* in *methanol R* and dilute to 50 ml with the same solvent.

The chromatographic procedure may be carried out using:

– a stainless steel column 0.15 m long and 4.6 mm in internal diameter, packed with *octadecylsilyl silica gel for chromatography R* (5 µm),

– as mobile phase at a flow rate of 1.5 ml/min:
Mobile phase A. A mixture of 312 volumes of *methanol R* and 688 volumes of a solution prepared as follows: dissolve 13.6 g of *potassium dihydrogen phosphate R* in 900 ml of *water R*, adjust the pH to 7.0 with a 300 g/l solution of *potassium hydroxide R* and dilute to 1000 ml with *water R*,
Mobile phase B. Acetonitrile R,

Time (min)	Mobile phase A (per cent *V/V*)	Mobile phase B (per cent *V/V*)	Comment
0 - 20	90 → 80	10 → 20	linear gradient
20 - 40	80 → 50	20 → 50	linear gradient
40 - 45	90	10	switch to initial conditions
45 - 55	90	10	re–equilibration

-as detector a spectrophotometer set at 225 nm, maintaining the temperature of the column at 40 °C.

Inject 10 µl of reference solution (a). Adjust the sensitivity of the system so that the height of the principal peak in the chromatogram obtained is at least 50 per cent of the full scale of the recorder. Inject 10 µl of reference solution (b). When the chromatogram is recorded in the prescribed conditions, the retention times are: impurity H about 8 min and etodolac about 9 min. The test is not valid unless the resolution between the peaks due to impurity H and etodolac is at least 5.0.

Inject separately 10 µl of the test solution and 10 µl of reference solution (a). In the chromatogram obtained with the test solution the area of any peak, apart from the principal peak, is not greater than the area of the principal peak in the chromatogram obtained with reference solution (a) (0.5 per cent); the sum of the areas of all of the peaks apart from the principal peak is not greater than twice the area of the principal peak in the chromatogram obtained with reference solution (a) (1 per cent). Disregard any peak with an area less than 0.1 times the area of the principal peak in the chromatogram obtained with reference solution (a).

Chlorides. Not more than 300 ppm. Dissolve 1.0 g of the substance to be examined in 60 ml of *methanol R*, add 10 ml of *water R* and 20 ml of *dilute nitric acid R*. Titrate with *0.01 M silver nitrate*, determining the end-point potentiometrically (*2.2.20*).

1 ml of *0.01 M silver nitrate* is equivalent to 0.3545 mg Cl.

Heavy metals (*2.4.8*). 2.0 g complies with limit test C for heavy metals (10 ppm). Prepare the standard using 2 ml of *lead standard solution (10 ppm Pb) R*.

Water (*2.5.12*). Not more than 0.5 per cent, determined on 1.000 g by the semi-micro determination of water.

Sulphated ash (*2.4.14*). Not more than 0.1 per cent, determined on 1.0 g.

ASSAY

Dissolve 0.250 g in 60 ml of *methanol R*. Titrate with *0.1 M tetrabutylammonium hydroxide* determining the end-point potentiometrically (*2.2.20*). Carry out a blank titration.

1 ml of *0.1 M tetrabutylammonium hydroxide* is equivalent to 28.74 mg of $C_{17}H_{21}NO_3$.

IMPURITIES

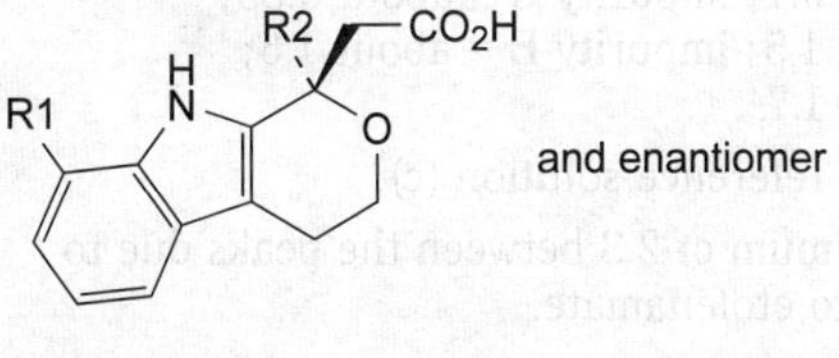

A. R1 = H, R2 = CH_2-CH_3: 2-[(1*RS*)-1-ethyl-1,3,4,9-tetrahydropyrano[3,4-*b*]indol-1-yl]acetic acid (8-desethyl etodolac),

B. R1 = CH_3, R2 = CH_2-CH_3: 2-[(1*RS*)-1-ethyl-8-methyl-1,3,4,9-tetrahydropyrano[3,4-*b*]indol-1-yl]acetic acid (8-methyl etodolac),

C. R1 = CH_2-CH_3, R2 = CH_3: 2-[(1*RS*)-8-ethyl-1-methyl-1,3,4,9-tetrahydropyrano[3,4-*b*]indol-1-yl]acetic acid (1-methyl etodolac),

D. R1 = $CH(CH_3)_2$, R2 = CH_2-CH_3: 2-[(1*RS*)-1-ethyl-8-(1-methylethyl)-1,3,4,9-tetrahydropyrano[3,4-*b*]indol-1-yl]acetic acid (8-isopropyl etodolac),

E. R1 = CH_2-CH_2-CH_3, R2 = CH_2-CH_3: 2-[(1*RS*)-1-ethyl-8-propyl-1,3,4,9-tetrahydropyrano[3,4-*b*]indol-1-yl]acetic acid (8-propyl etodolac),

F. R1 = CH_2-CH_3, R2 = $CH(CH_3)_2$: 2-[(1*RS*)-8-ethyl-1-(1-methylethyl)-1,3,4,9-tetrahydropyrano[3,4-*b*]indol-1-yl]acetic acid (1-isopropyl etodolac),

G. R1 = CH_2-CH_3, R2 = CH_2-CH_2-CH_3: 2-[(1*RS*)-8-ethyl-1-propyl-1,3,4,9-tetrahydropyrano[3,4-*b*]indol-1-yl]acetic acid (1-propyl etodolac),

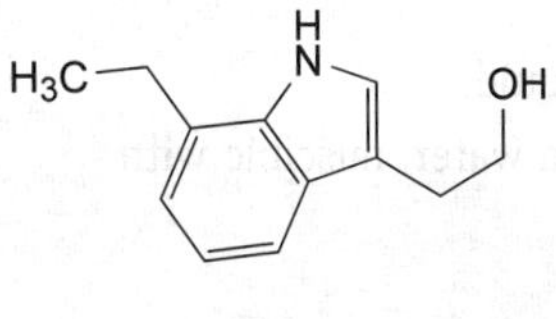

H. 2-(7-ethylindol-3-yl)ethanol,

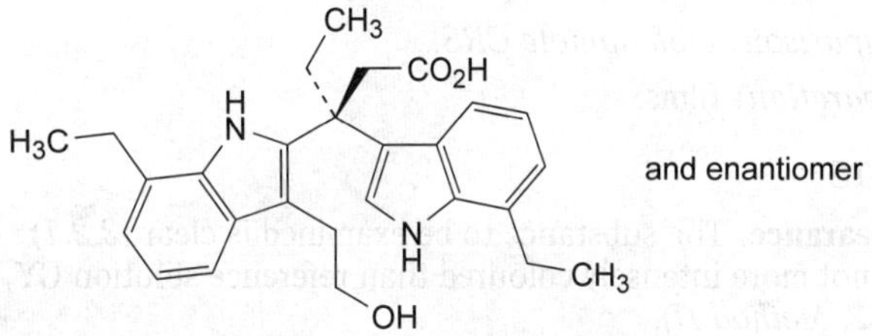

I. (3*RS*)-3-[7-ethyl-3-(2-hydroxyethyl)indol-2-yl]-3-(7-ethylindol-3-yl)pentanoic acid (etodolac dimer),

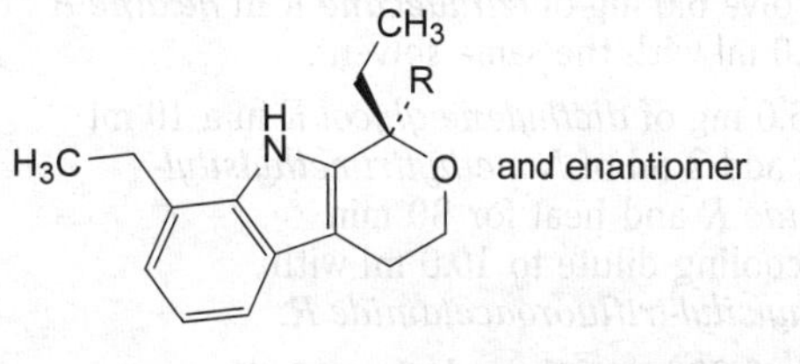

J. R = CH_3: (1*RS*)-1,8-diethyl-1-methyl-1,3,4,9-tetrahydropyrano[3,4-*b*]indole (decarboxy etodolac),

K. K. R = CH_2-CO-O-CH_3: methyl 2-[(1*RS*)-1,8-diethyl-1,3,4,9-tetrahydropyrano[3,4-*b*]indol-1-yl]acetate (etodolac methyl ester),

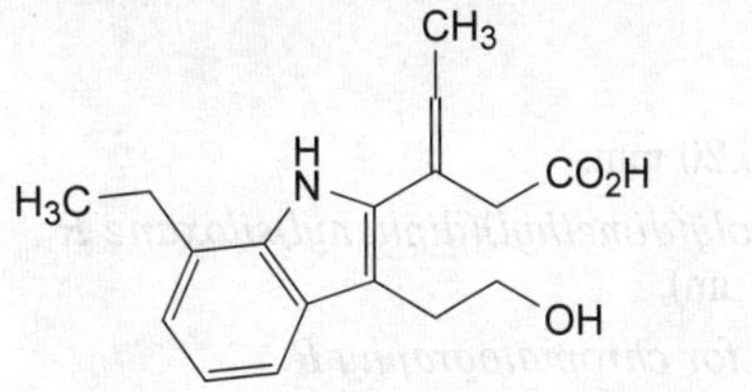

L. (*EZ*)-3-[7-ethyl-3-(2-hydroxyethyl)-1*H*-indol-2-yl]pent-3-enoic acid.

01/2005:1513

ETOFENAMATE

Etofenamatum

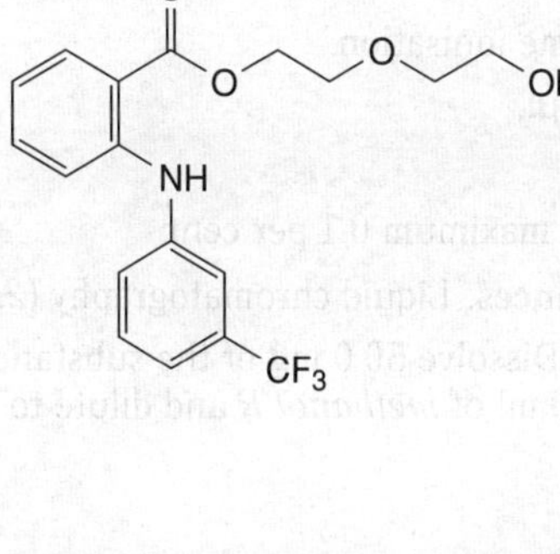

$C_{18}H_{18}F_3NO_4$ M_r 369.4

DEFINITION

2-(2-Hydroxyethoxy)ethyl 2-[[3-(trifluoromethyl)phenyl]amino]benzoate.

Content: 98.5 per cent to 101.5 per cent (anhydrous substance).

CHARACTERS

Appearance: yellowish viscous liquid.

Solubility: practically insoluble in water, miscible with alcohol and with ethyl acetate.

IDENTIFICATION

Infrared absorption spectrophotometry (*2.2.24*).

Comparison: *etofenamate CRS*.

Preparation: films.

TESTS

Appearance. The substance to be examined is clear (*2.2.1*) and not more intensely coloured than reference solution GY_1 (*2.2.2, Method II*).

Impurity F. Gas chromatography (*2.2.28*).

Internal standard: *tetradecane R*.

Solution A. Dissolve 6.0 mg of *tetradecane R* in *hexane R* and dilute to 10.0 ml with the same solvent.

Solution B. To 6.0 mg of *diethylene glycol R* in a 10 ml volumetric flask add 3 ml of *N-methyltrimethylsilyl-trifluoroacetamide R* and heat for 30 min at 50 °C. After cooling dilute to 10.0 ml with *N-methyltrimethylsilyl-trifluoroacetamide R*.

Test solution. To 0.200 g of the substance to be examined add 10 µl of solution A. Add 2 ml of *N-methyltrimethylsilyl-trifluoroacetamide R* and heat for 30 min at 50 °C.

Reference solution. To 2.0 ml of *N-methyltrimethylsilyl-trifluoroacetamide R* add 10 µl of solution A and 10 µl of solution B.

Column:

- *size*: *l* = 25 m, Ø = 0.20 mm,
- *stationary phase*: *poly(dimethyl)(diphenyl)siloxane R* (film thickness 0.33 µm).

Carrier gas: *hydrogen for chromatography R*.

Flow rate: 0.9 ml/min.

Temperature:

	Time (min)	Temperature (°C)	Rate (°C/min)
Column	0 - 13	60 → 150	7
	13 - 19	150 → 300	25
	19 - 34	300	
Injection port		150	
Detector		300	

Detection: flame ionisation.

Injection: 0.2 µl.

Limit:

- *impurity F*: maximum 0.1 per cent.

Related substances. Liquid chromatography (*2.2.29*).

Test solution. Dissolve 50.0 mg of the substance to be examined in 30 ml of *methanol R* and dilute to 50.0 ml with *water R*.

Reference solution (a). Dissolve 10.0 mg of *etofenamate impurity G CRS* in *methanol R* and dilute to 20.0 ml with the same solvent. Dilute 0.2 ml of the solution to 50.0 ml with a mixture of 40 volumes of *water R* and 60 volumes of *methanol R*.

Reference solution (b). Dilute 0.2 ml of the test solution to 100.0 ml with a mixture of 40 volumes of *water R* and 60 volumes of *methanol R*.

Reference solution (c). To 5.0 ml of reference solution (a), add 5.0 ml of reference solution (b).

Reference solution (d). Dissolve 10.0 mg of *etofenamate for peak identification CRS* (contains etofenamate spiked with about 1 per cent of impurities A, B, C, D and E) in 6.0 ml of *methanol R* and dilute to 10.0 ml with *water R*.

Column:

- *size*: *l* = 0.10 m, Ø = 4.0 mm,
- *stationary phase*: *octadecylsilyl silica gel for chromatography R* (3 µm),
- *temperature*: 40 °C.

Mobile phase:

- *mobile phase A*: dissolve 1.3 g of *ammonium phosphate R* and 4.0 g of *tetrabutylammonium hydroxide R* in 900 ml of *water R*. Adjust the pH to 8.0 with *dilute phosphoric acid R* and dilute to 1000 ml with *water R*,
- *mobile phase B*: *methanol R*,

Time	Mobile phase A (per cent *V/V*)	Mobile phase B (per cent *V/V*)
0 - 13	40	60
13 - 20	40 → 10	60 → 90
20 - 25	10	90
25 - 26	10 → 40	90 → 60
26 - 31	40	60

Flow rate: 1.2 ml/min.

Detection: spectrophotometer at 286 nm.

Injection: 20 µl.

Relative retention with reference to etofenamate (retention time = about 13 min): impurity A = about 0.2; impurity C = about 0.7; impurity G = about 0.85; impurity E = about 1.5; impurity B = about 1.6; impurity D = about 1.7.

System suitability: reference solution (c):

- *resolution*: minimum of 2.3 between the peaks due to impurity G and to etofenamate.

Limits:

- *correction factors*: for the calculation of contents, multiply the peak areas of the following impurities by the corresponding correction factor: impurity A = 0.62; impurity C = 0.45; impurity D = 0.77,
- *impurity A*: not more than 1.25 times the area of the principal peak in the chromatogram obtained with reference solution (b) (0.25 per cent),
- *impurity B*: not more than the area of the principal peak in the chromatogram obtained with reference solution (b) (0.2 per cent),
- *impurity C*: not more than the area of the principal peak in the chromatogram obtained with reference solution (b) (0.2 per cent),
- *impurity D*: not more than 2.5 times the area of the principal peak in the chromatogram obtained with reference solution (b) (0.5 per cent),

- *impurity E*: not more than the area of the principal peak in the chromatogram obtained with reference solution (b) (0.2 per cent),
- *impurity G*: not more than the area of the principal peak in the chromatogram obtained with reference solution (a) (0.2 per cent),
- *any other impurity*: not more than half the area of the principal peak in the chromatogram obtained with reference solution (b) (0.1 per cent),
- *total*: not more than 6 times the area of the principal peak in the chromatogram obtained with reference solution (b) (1.2 per cent),
- *disregard limit*: 0.25 times the area of the principal peak in the chromatogram obtained with reference solution (b) (0.05 per cent).

Heavy metals (*2.4.8*): maximum 10 ppm.

2.0 g complies with limit test C. Prepare the standard using 2 ml of *lead standard solution (10 ppm Pb) R*.

Water (*2.5.12*): maximum 0.5 per cent, determined on 1.00 g.

Sulphated ash (*2.4.14*): maximum 0.1 per cent, determined on 1.0 g.

ASSAY

To 3.000 g add 20 ml of *2-propanol R* and 20.0 ml of *1 M sodium hydroxide* and heat under reflux for 2 h. Add 0.1 ml of *bromothymol blue solution R1*. Titrate after cooling with *1 M hydrochloric acid* until the colour disappears. Carry out a blank titration.

1 ml of *1 M sodium hydroxide* is equivalent to 0.3694 g of $C_{18}H_{18}F_3NO_4$.

IMPURITIES

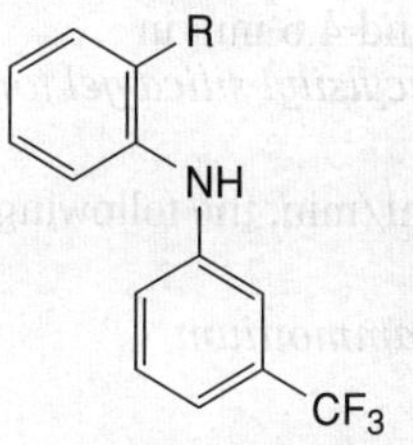

A. R = CO_2H: 2-[[3-(trifluoromethyl)phenyl]amino]benzoic acid (flufenamic acid),

B. R = $CO-O-C_4H_9$: butyl 2-[[3-(trifluoromethyl)phenyl]amino]benzoate (butyl flufenamate),

C. R = H: *N*-phenyl-3-(trifluoromethyl)aniline,

E. R = $CO-[O-CH_2-CH_2]_3-CH_2-CH_3$: 2-(2-butoxyethoxy)ethyl 2-[[3-(trifluoromethyl)phenyl]amino]benzoate,

G. R = $CO-O-CH_2-CH_2-OH$: 2-hydroxyethyl 2-[[3-(trifluoromethyl)phenyl]amino]benzoate,

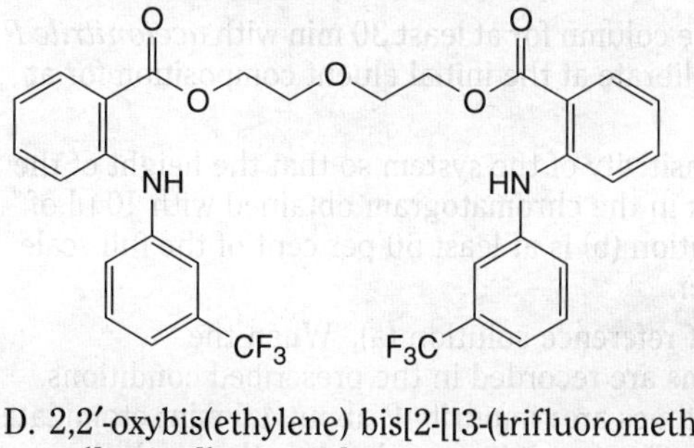

D. 2,2′-oxybis(ethylene) bis[2-[[3-(trifluoromethyl)phenyl]amino]benzoate],

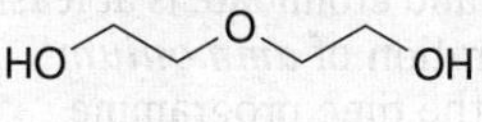

F. 2,2′-oxydiethanol.

01/2005:0492

ETOFYLLINE

Etofyllinum

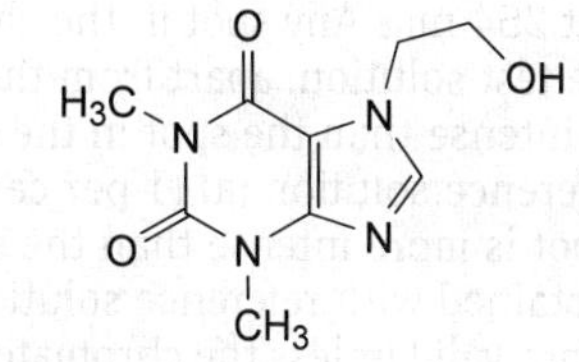

$C_9H_{12}N_4O_3$ M_r 224.2

DEFINITION

Etofylline contains not less than 98.5 per cent and not more than the equivalent of 101.0 per cent of 7-(2-hydroxyethyl)-1,3-dimethyl-3,7-dihydro-1*H*-purine-2,6-dione, calculated with reference to the dried substance.

CHARACTERS

A white, crystalline powder, soluble in water, slightly soluble in alcohol.

IDENTIFICATION

First identification: B, C.

Second identification: A, C, D.

A. Melting point (*2.2.14*): 161 °C to 166 °C.

B. Examine by infrared absorption spectrophotometry (*2.2.24*), comparing with the spectrum obtained with *etofylline CRS*. Examine the substances as discs prepared using 0.5 mg to 1 mg of the substance to be examined in 0.3 g of *potassium bromide R*.

C. Dissolve 1 g in 5 ml of *acetic anhydride R* and boil under a reflux condenser for 15 min. Allow to cool and add 100 ml of a mixture of 20 volumes of *ether R* and 80 volumes of *light petroleum R*. Cool in iced water for at least 20 min, shaking from time to time. Filter, wash the precipitate with a mixture of 20 volumes of *ether R* and 80 volumes of *light petroleum R*, recrystallise from *alcohol R* and dry *in vacuo*. The crystals melt (*2.2.14*) at 101 °C to 105 °C.

D. It gives the reaction of xanthines (*2.3.1*).

TESTS

Solution S. Dissolve 2.5 g in *carbon dioxide-free water R* and dilute to 50 ml with the same solvent.

Appearance of solution. Solution S is clear (*2.2.1*) and colourless (*2.2.2, Method II*).

Acidity or alkalinity. To 10 ml of solution S add 0.25 ml of *bromothymol blue solution R1*. The solution is yellow or green. Not more than 0.4 ml of *0.01 M sodium hydroxide* is required to change the colour of the indicator to blue.

Related substances. Examine by thin-layer chromatography (*2.2.27*), using *silica gel* HF_{254} *R* as the coating substance.

Test solution. Dissolve 0.3 g of the substance to be examined in a mixture of 20 volumes of *water R* and 30 volumes of *methanol R* and dilute to 10 ml with the same mixture of solvents. Prepare immediately before use.

Reference solution (a). Dilute 1 ml of the test solution to 100 ml with *methanol R*.

Reference solution (b). Dilute 0.2 ml of the test solution to 100 ml with *methanol R*.

Reference solution (c). Dissolve 10 mg of *theophylline R* in *methanol R,* add 0.3 ml of the test solution and dilute to 10 ml with *methanol R.*

Apply to the plate 10 µl of each solution. Develop over a path of 15 cm using a mixture of 1 volume of *concentrated ammonia R,* 10 volumes of *ethanol R* and 90 volumes of *chloroform R.* Allow the plate to dry in air and examine in ultraviolet light at 254 nm. Any spot in the chromatogram obtained with the test solution, apart from the principal spot, is not more intense than the spot in the chromatogram obtained with reference solution (a) (1 per cent) and at most one such spot is more intense than the spot in the chromatogram obtained with reference solution (b) (0.2 per cent). The test is not valid unless the chromatogram obtained with reference solution (c) shows two clearly separated spots.

Chlorides (*2.4.4*). Dilute 2.5 ml of solution S to 15 ml with *water R.* The solution complies with the limit test for chlorides (400 ppm).

Heavy metals (*2.4.8*). 12 ml of solution S complies with limit test A for heavy metals (20 ppm). Prepare the standard using *lead standard solution (1 ppm Pb) R.*

Loss on drying (*2.2.32*). Not more than 0.5 per cent, determined on 1.000 g by drying in an oven at 100 °C to 105 °C.

Sulphated ash (*2.4.14*). Not more than 0.1 per cent, determined on 1.0 g.

ASSAY

In order to avoid overheating in the reaction medium, mix thoroughly throughout and stop the titration immediately after the end-point has been reached.

Dissolve 0.200 g in 3.0 ml of *anhydrous formic acid R* and add 50.0 ml of *acetic anhydride R.* Titrate with *0.1 M perchloric acid,* determining the end-point potentiometrically (*2.2.20*).

1 ml of *0.1 M perchloric acid* is equivalent to 22.42 mg of $C_9H_{12}N_4O_3$.

STORAGE

Store protected from light.

01/2005:1514

ETOMIDATE

Etomidatum

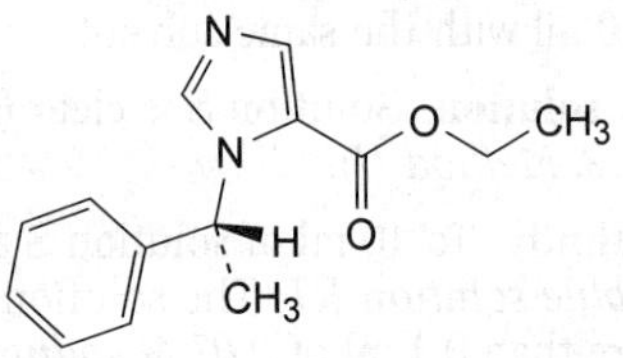

$C_{14}H_{16}N_2O_2$ M_r 244.3

DEFINITION

Etomidate contains not less than 99.0 per cent and not more than the equivalent of 101.0 per cent of ethyl 1-[(1*R*)-1-phenylethyl]-1*H*-imidazole-5-carboxylate, calculated with reference to the dried substance.

CHARACTERS

A white or almost white powder, very slightly soluble in water, freely soluble in alcohol and in methylene chloride.

It melts at about 68 °C.

IDENTIFICATION

A. Examine by infrared absorption spectrophotometry (*2.2.24*), comparing with the spectrum obtained with *etomidate CRS.*

B. It complies with the test for specific optical rotation (see Tests).

TESTS

Solution S. Dissolve 0.25 g in *ethanol R* and dilute to 25.0 ml with the same solvent.

Appearance of solution. Solution S is clear (*2.2.1*) and colourless (*2.2.2, Method II*).

Specific optical rotation (*2.2.7*): + 67 to + 70, determined on solution S and calculated with reference to the dried substance.

Related substances. Examine by liquid chromatography (*2.2.29*).

Test solution. Dissolve 0.100 g of the substance to be examined in a mixture of 50 volumes of *ethanol R* and 50 volumes of *water R* and dilute to 10.0 ml with the same mixture of solvents.

Reference solution (a). Dissolve 5.0 mg of *etomidate CRS* and 5.0 mg of *etomidate impurity B CRS* in a mixture of 50 volumes of *ethanol R* and 50 volumes of *water R* and dilute to 250.0 ml with the same mixture of solvents.

Reference solution (b). Dilute 1.0 ml of the test solution to 100.0 ml with a mixture of 50 volumes of *ethanol R* and 50 volumes of *water R.* Dilute 5.0 ml of the solution to 25.0 ml with a mixture of 50 volumes of *ethanol R* and 50 volumes of *water R.*

The chromatographic procedure may be carried out using:

– a stainless steel column 0.1 m long and 4.6 mm in internal diameter packed with *octadecylsilyl silica gel for chromatography R* (3 µm),

– as mobile phase at a flow rate of 2.0 ml/min, the following linear gradient programme:

Mobile phase A. A 5 g/l solution of *ammonium carbonate R,*

Mobile phase B. Acetonitrile R,

Time (min)	Mobile phase A (per cent *V/V*)	Mobile phase B (per cent *V/V*)	Comment
0 - 5	90 → 30	10 → 70	linear gradient
5 - 6	30 → 10	70 → 90	linear gradient
6 - 10	10	90	isocratic
10 - 11	10 → 90	90 → 10	linear gradient
11 - 15	90	10	re-equilibration

– as detector a spectrophotometer set at 235 nm.

Equilibrate the column for at least 30 min with *acetonitrile R* and then equilibrate at the initial eluent composition for at least 5 min.

Adjust the sensitivity of the system so that the height of the principal peak in the chromatogram obtained with 10 µl of reference solution (b) is at least 50 per cent of the full scale of the recorder.

Inject 10 µl of reference solution (a). When the chromatograms are recorded in the prescribed conditions, the retention times are: impurity B about 4.5 min; etomidate about 5.0 min. The test is not valid unless the resolution between the peaks due to impurity B and etomidate is at least 5.0. If necessary, adjust the concentration of *ammonium carbonate R* in the mobile phase or the time programme of the linear gradient.

Inject 10 µl of the test solution and 10 µl of reference solution (b). In the chromatogram obtained with the test solution: the area of any peak, apart from the principal peak, is not greater than the area of the principal peak in the chromatogram obtained with reference solution (b) (0.2 per cent) and the sum of the areas of any such peaks is not greater than 1.5 times the area of the principal peak in the chromatogram obtained with reference solution (b) (0.3 per cent). Disregard any peak with an area less than 0.25 times the area of the principal peak in the chromatogram obtained with reference solution (b).

Loss on drying (*2.2.32*). Not more than 0.5 per cent, determined on 1.000 g by drying *in vacuo* at 40 °C for 4 h.

Sulphated ash (*2.4.14*). Not more than 0.1 per cent, determined on 1.0 g.

ASSAY

Dissolve 0.200 g in 50 ml of a mixture of 1 volume of *anhydrous acetic acid R* and 7 volumes of *methyl ethyl ketone R* and titrate with *0.1 M perchloric acid* using 0.2 ml of *naphtholbenzein solution R* as indicator.

1 ml of *0.1 M perchloric acid* is equivalent to 24.43 mg of $C_{14}H_{16}N_2O_2$.

STORAGE

Protected from light.

IMPURITIES

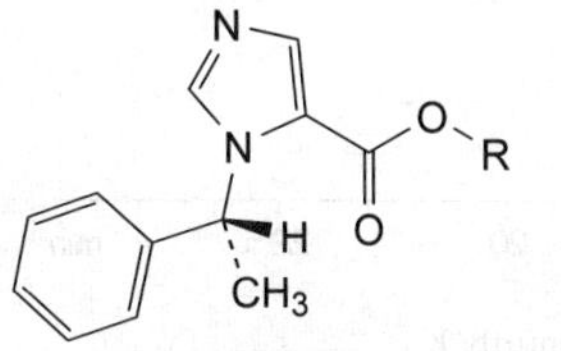

A. R = H: 1-[(1*RS*)-1-phenylethyl]-1*H*-imidazole-5-carboxylic acid,

B. R = CH_3: methyl 1-[(1*RS*)-1-phenylethyl]-1*H*-imidazole-5-carboxylate (metomidate),

C. R = $CH(CH_3)_2$: 1-methylethyl 1-[(1*RS*)-1-phenylethyl]-1*H*-imidazole-5-carboxylate.

01/2005:0823

ETOPOSIDE

Etoposidum

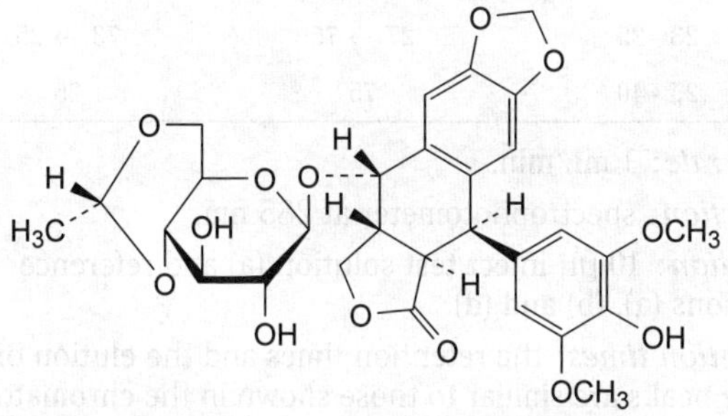

$C_{29}H_{32}O_{13}$ M_r 588.6

DEFINITION

(5*R*,5a*R*,8a*R*,9*S*)-9-[[4,6-*O*-[(*R*)-Ethylidene]-β-D-glucopyranosyl]oxy]-5-(4-hydroxy-3,5-dimethoxyphenyl)-5,8,8a,9-tetrahydroisobenzofuro[5,6-*f*][1,3]benzodioxol-6(5a*H*)-one.

Content: 98.0 per cent to 101.0 per cent (anhydrous substance).

CHARACTERS

Appearance: white or almost white crystalline powder.

Solubility: practically insoluble in water, sparingly soluble in methanol, slightly soluble in alcohol and in methylene chloride.

IDENTIFICATION

First identification: A, B.

Second identification: C, D.

A. Specific optical rotation (see Tests).

B. Infrared absorption spectrophotometry (*2.2.24*).

Comparison: *etoposide CRS.*

C. Thin-layer chromatography (*2.2.27*).

Test solution. Dissolve 10 mg of the substance to be examined in a mixture of 1 volume of *methanol R* and 9 volumes of *methylene chloride R* and dilute to 2 ml with the same mixture of solvents.

Reference solution. Dissolve 10 mg of *etoposide CRS* in a mixture of 1 volume of *methanol R* and 9 volumes of *methylene chloride R* and dilute to 2 ml with the same mixture of solvents.

Plate: plate with *silica gel H R* as coating substance.

Mobile phase: *water R, glacial acetic acid R, acetone R, methylene chloride R* (1.5:8:20:100 *V/V/V/V*).

Application: 5 µl as 10 mm bands.

Development: immediately, over a path of 17 cm.

Drying: in a current of warm air for 5 min.

Detection: spray with a mixture of 1 volume of *sulphuric acid R* and 9 volumes of *alcohol R* and heat at 140 °C for 15 min. Cover the plate immediately with a glass plate of the same size. Examine in daylight.

Results: the principal band in the chromatogram obtained with the test solution is similar in position, colour and size to the principal band in the chromatogram obtained with the reference solution.

D. In a test-tube dissolve about 5 mg in 5 ml of *glacial acetic acid R* and add 0.05 ml of *ferric chloride solution R1*. Mix and cautiously add 2 ml of *sulphuric acid R*. Avoid mixing the 2 layers. Allow to stand for about 30 min; a pink to reddish-brown ring develops at the interface and the upper layer is yellow.

TESTS

Appearance of solution. The solution is clear (*2.2.1*) and not more intensely coloured than reference solution Y_6 or BY_6 (*2.2.2, Method II*).

Dissolve 0.6 g in a mixture of 1 volume of *methanol R* and 9 volumes of *methylene chloride R* and dilute to 20 ml with the same mixture of solvents.

Specific optical rotation (*2.2.7*): − 106 to − 114 (anhydrous substance).

Dissolve 50 mg in a mixture of 1 volume of *methanol R* and 9 volumes of *methylene chloride R* and dilute to 10.0 ml with the same mixture of solvents.

Related substances. Liquid chromatography (*2.2.29*).

Test solution (a). Dissolve 40 mg of the substance to be examined in a mixture of equal volumes of mobile phase A and mobile phase B and dilute to 10.0 ml with the same mixture of mobile phases.

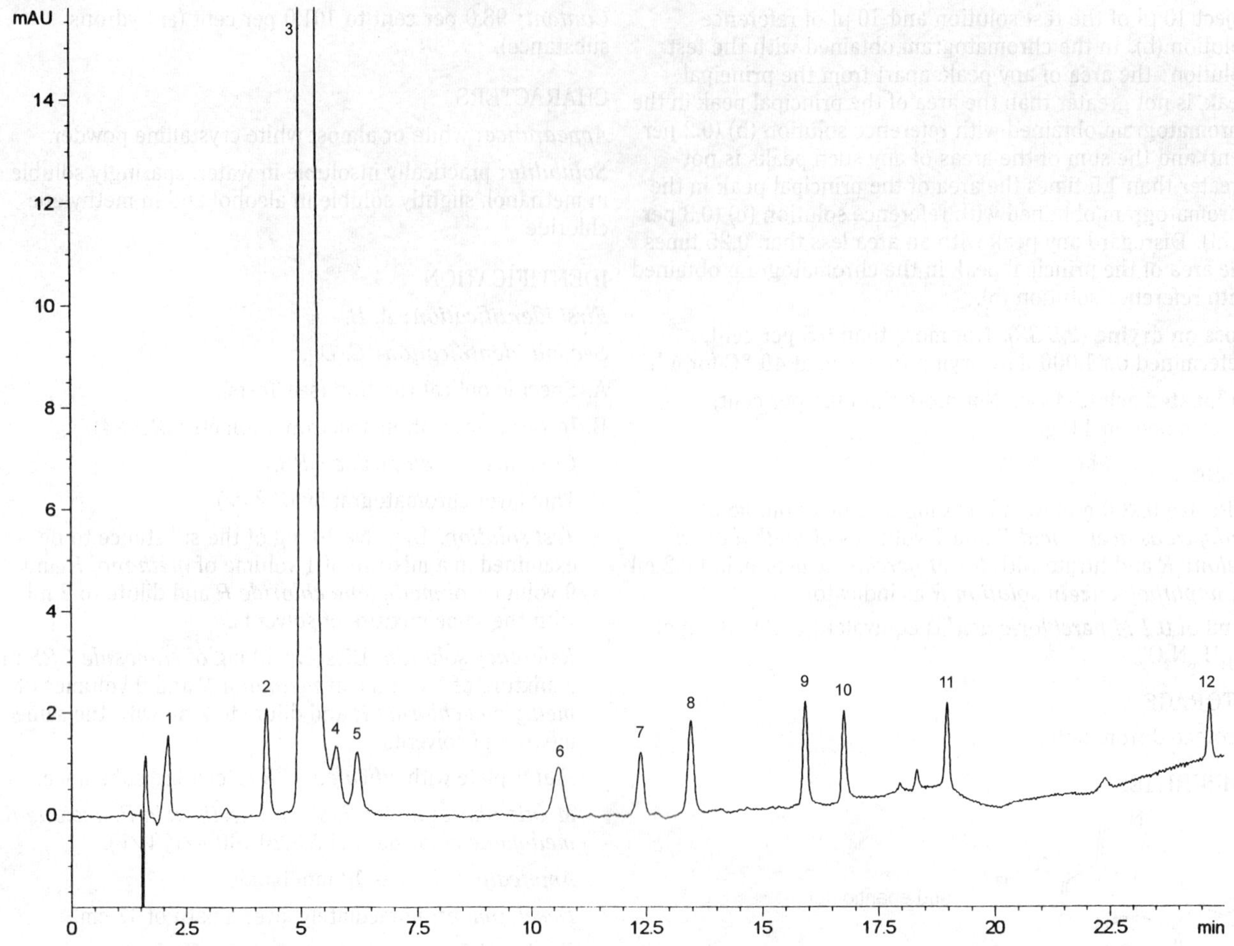

1. impurity D
2. impurity E
3. etoposide
4. impurity C
5. impurity B
6. impurity M
7. impurity I
8. impurity J
9. impurity H
10. impurity K
11. impurity A
12. impurity G

Figure 0823.-1. – *Chromatogram for the test for related substances of etoposide*

Test solution (b). Dissolve 50.0 mg of the substance to be examined in a mixture of equal volumes of mobile phase A and mobile phase B and dilute to 50.0 ml with the same mixture of mobile phases.

Reference solution (a). Dilute 1.0 ml of test solution (a) to 10.0 ml with a mixture of equal volumes of mobile phase A and mobile phase B. Dilute 1.0 ml of this solution to 20.0 ml with a mixture of equal volumes of mobile phase A and mobile phase B.

Reference solution (b). Dilute 4.0 ml of reference solution (a) to 10.0 ml with a mixture of equal volumes of mobile phase A and mobile phase B.

Reference solution (c). Dissolve 50.0 mg of *etoposide CRS* in a mixture of equal volumes of mobile phase A and mobile phase B and dilute to 50.0 ml with the same mixture of mobile phases.

Reference solution (d). To 10 ml of test solution (b), add 0.1 ml of a 4 per cent *V/V* solution of *glacial acetic acid R* and 0.1 ml of *phenolphthalein solution R*. Add *1 M sodium hydroxide* until the solution becomes faintly pink (about 0.15 ml). After 15 min, add 0.1 ml of a 4 per cent *V/V* solution of *glacial acetic acid R*.

Column:
- *size*: *l* = 0.125 m, Ø = 4.6 mm,
- *stationary phase*: *octadecylsilyl silica gel for chromatography R* (5 µm),
- *temperature*: 40 °C.

Mobile phase:
- *mobile phase A*: *triethylamine R, anhydrous formic acid R, water R* (1:1:998 *V/V/V*),
- *mobile phase B*: *triethylamine R, anhydrous formic acid R, acetonitrile R* (1:1:998 *V/V/V*),

Time (min)	Mobile phase A (per cent *V/V*)	Mobile phase B (per cent *V/V*)
0 - 7	75	25
7 - 23	75 → 27	25 → 73
23 - 25	27 → 75	73 → 25
25 - 40	75	25

Flow rate: 1 ml/min.

Detection: spectrophotometer at 285 nm.

Injection: 10 µl; inject test solution (a) and reference solutions (a), (b) and (d).

Retention times: the retention times and the elution order of the peaks are similar to those shown in the chromatogram (Figure 0823.-1).

System suitability: reference solution (d): continue the chromatography until the peak due to phenolphtalein is eluted.
- the chromatogram shows 2 principal peaks corresponding to etoposide and to impurity B. Disregard any peak due to phenolphthalein.

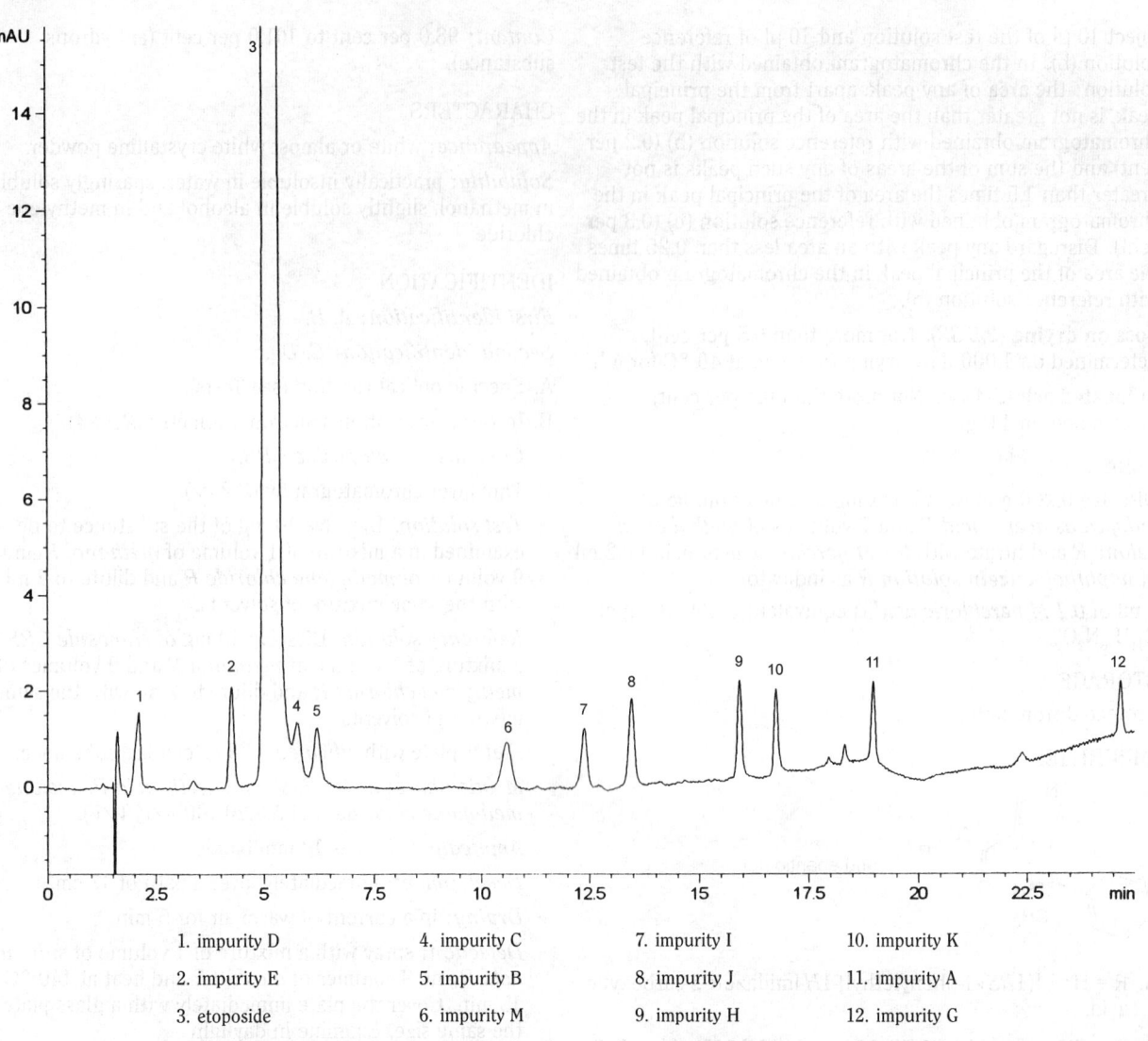

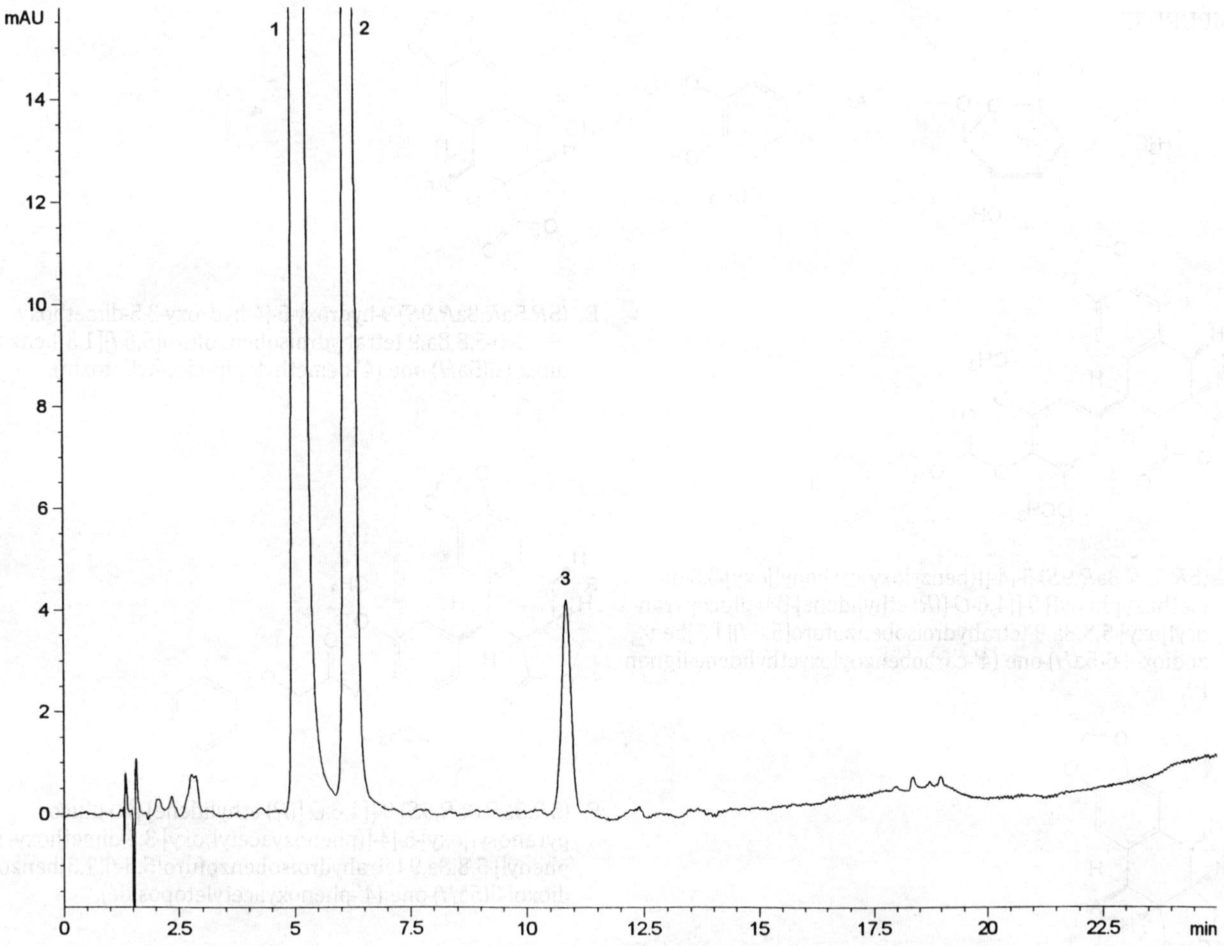

1. etoposide 2. impurity B 3. phenophthalein

Figure 0823.-2. – *Chromatogram for the test for related substances of etoposide: reference solution (d)*

– *resolution*: minimum 3.0 between the peaks due to etoposide and to impurity B.

If necessary, increase slightly the proportion of mobile phase A during the isocratic phase of the gradient. When the chromatograms are recorded under the prescribed conditions, the retention times of the peaks in the chromatogram obtained with reference solution (d) are similar to those shown in the chromatogram (Figure 0823.-2).

Limits:

– *any impurity*: not more than the area of the principal peak in the chromatogram obtained with reference solution (a) (0.5 per cent) and not more than 2 such peaks have an area greater than the area of the principal peak in the chromatogram obtained with reference solution (b) (0.2 per cent),

– *total*: not more than twice the area of the principal peak in the chromatogram obtained with reference solution (a) (1 per cent),

– *disregard limit*: 0.1 times the area of the principal peak in the chromatogram obtained with reference solution (a). Disregard any peak due to the solvent.

Heavy metals (*2.4.8*): maximum 20 ppm.

1.0 g complies with limit test C. Prepare the reference solution using 2 ml of *lead standard solution (10 ppm Pb) R.*

Water (*2.5.12*): maximum 6.0 per cent, determined on 0.250 g.

Sulphated ash (*2.4.14*): maximum 0.1 per cent, determined on 1.0 g.

ASSAY

Liquid chromatography (*2.2.29*) as described in the test for related substances with the following modifications.

Injection: test solution (b) and reference solution (c).

System suitability:

– *repeatability*: maximum relative standard deviation of 1.0 per cent after 6 injections of reference solution (c).

Calculate the percentage content of $C_{29}H_{32}O_{13}$ from the areas of the peaks and the declared content of *etoposide CRS*.

STORAGE

In an airtight container.

IMPURITIES

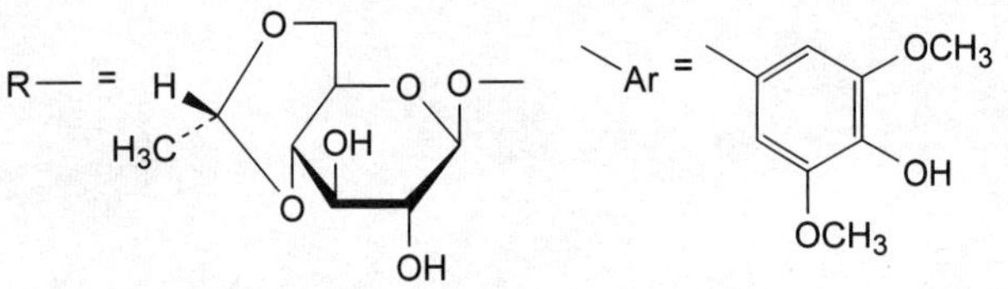

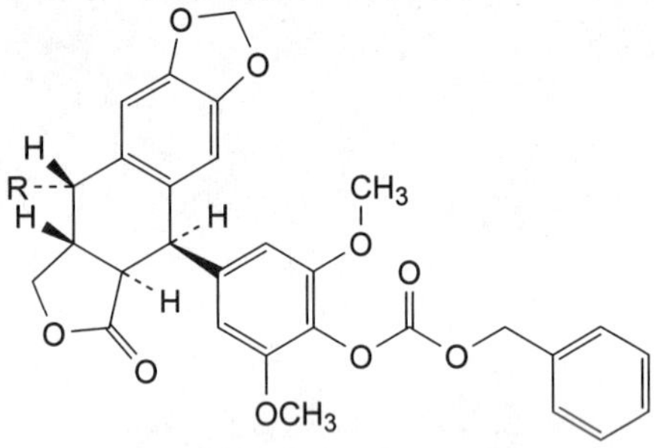

A. (5*R*,5a*R*,8a*R*,9*S*)-5-[4-[[(benzyloxy)carbonyl]oxy]-3,5-dimethoxyphenyl]-9-[[4,6-*O*-[(*R*)-ethylidene]-β-D-glucopyranosyl]oxy]-5,8,8a,9-tetrahydroisobenzofuro[5,6-*f*][1,3]benzodioxol-6(5a*H*)-one (4′-carbobenzoyloxyethylidene-lignan P),

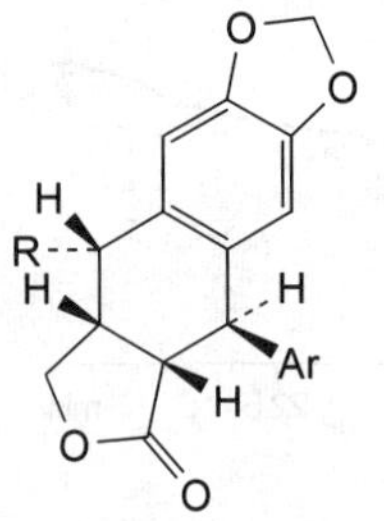

B. (5*R*,5a*S*,8a*R*,9*S*)-9-[[4,6-*O*-[(*R*)-ethylidene]-β-D-glucopyranosyl]oxy]-5-(4-hydroxy-3,5-dimethoxyphenyl)-5,8,8a,9-tetrahydroisobenzofuro[5,6-*f*][1,3]benzodioxol-6(5a*H*)-one (picroethylidene-lignan P; *cis*-etoposide),

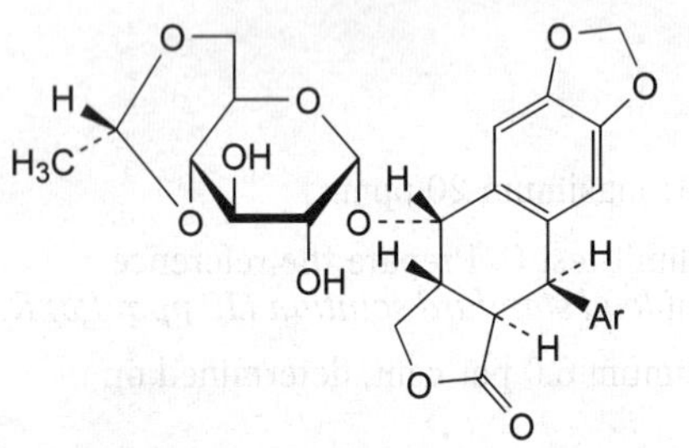

C. (5*R*,5a*R*,8a*R*,9*S*)-9-[[4,6-*O*-[(*R*)-ethylidene]-α-D-glucopyranosyl]oxy]-5-(4-hydroxy-3,5-dimethoxyphenyl)-5,8,8a,9-tetrahydroisobenzofuro[5,6-*f*][1,3]benzodioxol-6(5a*H*)-one (α-etoposide),

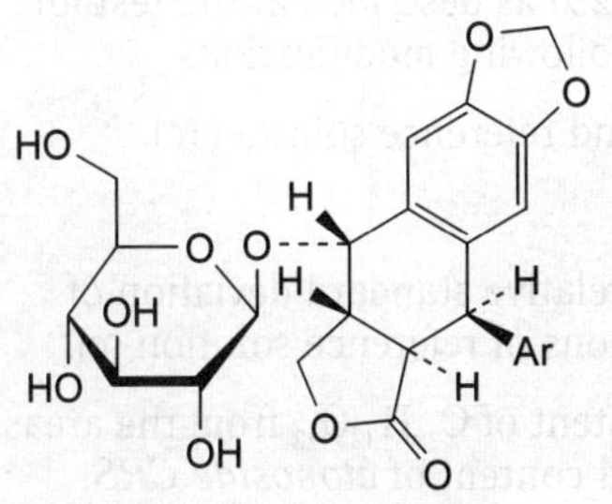

D. (5*R*,5a*R*,8a*R*,9*S*)-9-(β-D-glucopyranosyloxy)-5-(4-hydroxy-3,5-dimethoxyphenyl)-5,8,8a,9-tetrahydroisobenzofuro[5,6-*f*][1,3]benzodioxol-6(5a*H*)-one (lignan P),

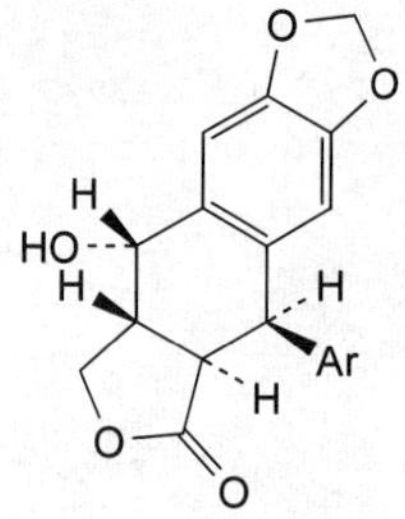

E. (5*R*,5a*R*,8a*R*,9*S*)-9-hydroxy-5-(4-hydroxy-3,5-dimethoxyphenyl)-5,8,8a,9-tetrahydroisobenzofuro[5,6-*f*][1,3]benzodioxol-6(5a*H*)-one (4′-demethylepipodophyllotoxin),

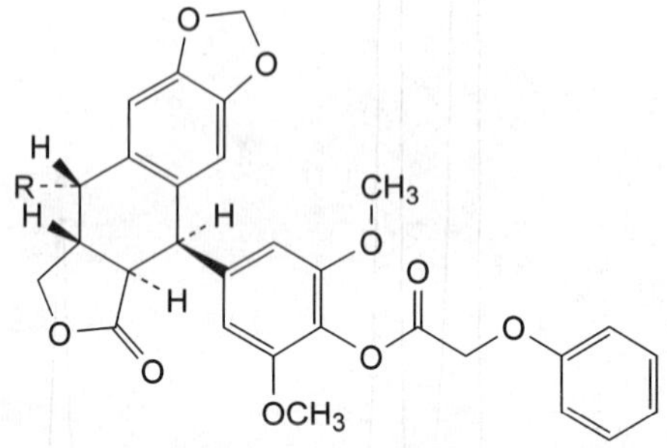

F. (5*R*,5a*R*,8a*R*,9*S*)-9-[[4,6-*O*-[(*R*)-ethylidene]-β-D-glucopyranosyl]oxy]-5-[4-[(phenoxyacetyl)oxy]-3,5-dimethoxyphenyl]-5,8,8a,9-tetrahydroisobenzofuro[5,6-*f*][1,3]benzodioxol-6(5a*H*)-one (4′-phenoxyacetyletoposide),

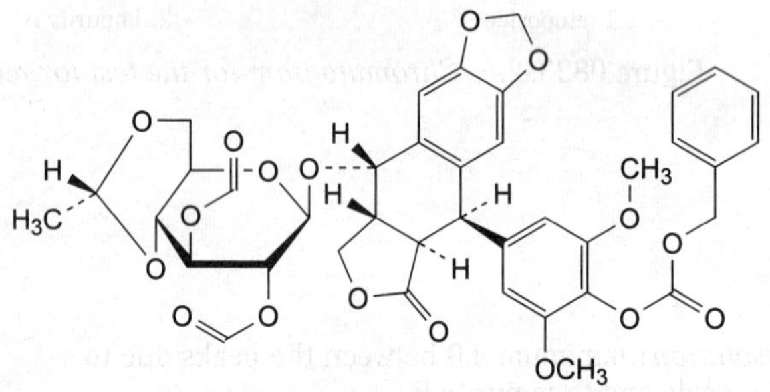

G. (5*R*,5a*R*,8a*R*,9*S*)-5-[4-[[(benzyloxy)carbonyl]oxy]-3,5-dimethoxyphenyl]-9-[[4,6-*O*-[(*R*)-ethylidene]-2,3-di-*O*-formyl-β-D-glucopyranosyl]oxy]-5,8,8a,9-tetrahydroisobenzofuro[5,6-*f*][1,3]benzodioxol-6(5a*H*)-one (4′-carbobenzoyloxydiformylethylidene-lignan P),

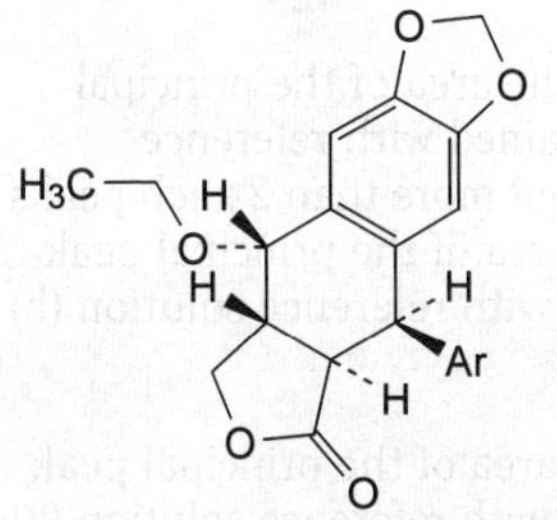

H. (5*R*,5a*R*,8a*R*,9*S*)-9-ethoxy-5-(4-hydroxy-3,5-dimethoxyphenyl)-5,8,8a,9-tetrahydroisobenzofuro[5,6-*f*][1,3]benzodioxol-6(5a*H*)-one (4′-*O*-demethyl-1-*O*-ethylepipodophyllotoxin),

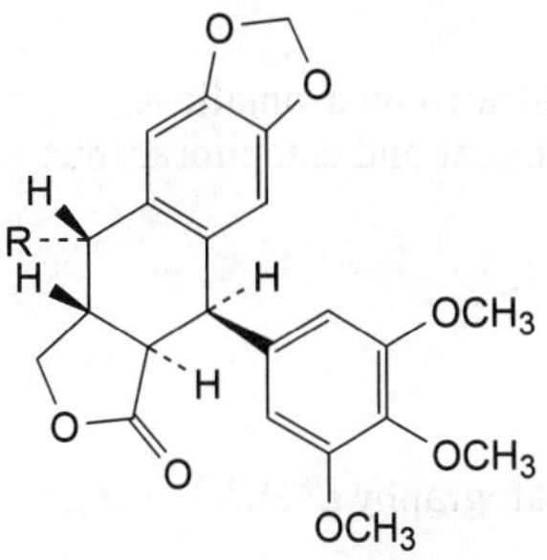

I. (5*R*,5a*R*,8a*R*,9S)-9-[[4,6-*O*-[(*R*)-ethylidene]-β-D-glucopyranosyl]oxy]-5-(3,4,5-trimethoxyphenyl)-5,8,8a,9-tetrahydroisobenzofuro[5,6-*f*][1,3]benzodioxol-6(5a*H*)-one (4-*O*-methylethylidene-lignan P),

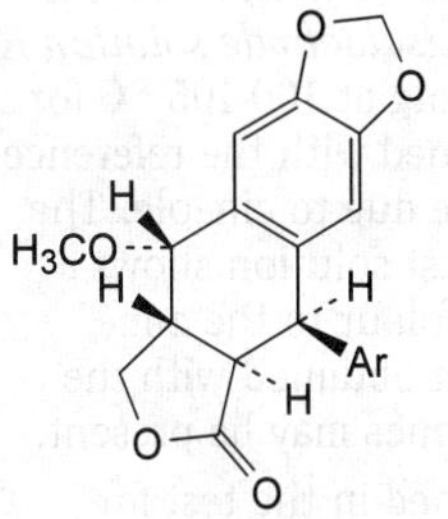

J. (5*R*,5a*R*,8a*R*,9*S*)-5-(4-hydroxy-3,5-dimethoxyphenyl)-9-methoxy-5,8,8a,9-tetrahydroisobenzofuro[5,6-*f*][1,3]benzodioxol-6(5a*H*)-one (4′-*O*-demethyl-1-*O*-methylepipodophyllotoxin),

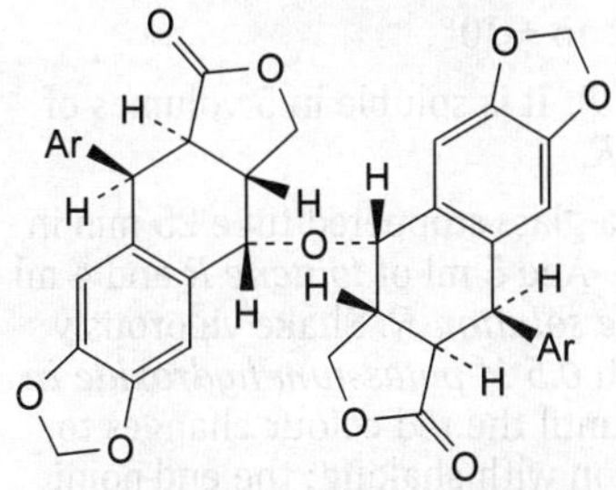

K. 9,9′-oxybis[(5*R*,5a*R*,8a*R*,9*S*)-5-(4-hydroxy-3,5-dimethoxyphenyl)-5,8,8a,9-tetrahydroisobenzofuro[5,6-*f*][1,3]benzodioxol-6(5a*H*)-one] (di-4′-*O*-demethylepipodophyllotoxin),

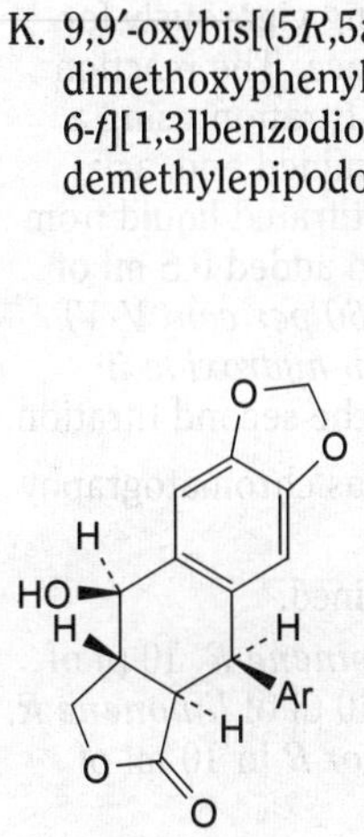

L. (5*R*,5a*R*,8a*R*,9*R*)-9-hydroxy-5-(4-hydroxy-3,5-dimethoxyphenyl)-5,8,8a,9-tetrahydroisobenzofuro[5,6-*f*][1,3]benzodioxol-6(5a*H*)-one (4′-*O*-demethylpodophyllotoxin),

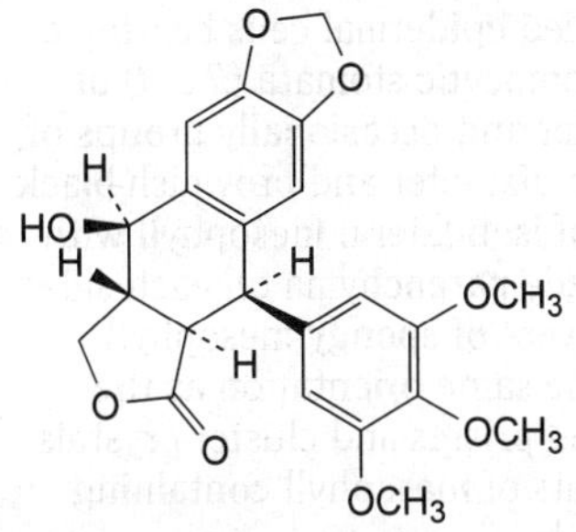

M. (5*R*,5a*R*,8a*R*,9*R*)-9-hydroxy-5-(3,4,5-trimethoxyphenyl)-5,8,8a,9-tetrahydroisobenzofuro[5,6-*f*][1,3]benzodioxol-6(5a*H*)-one (podophyllotoxin),

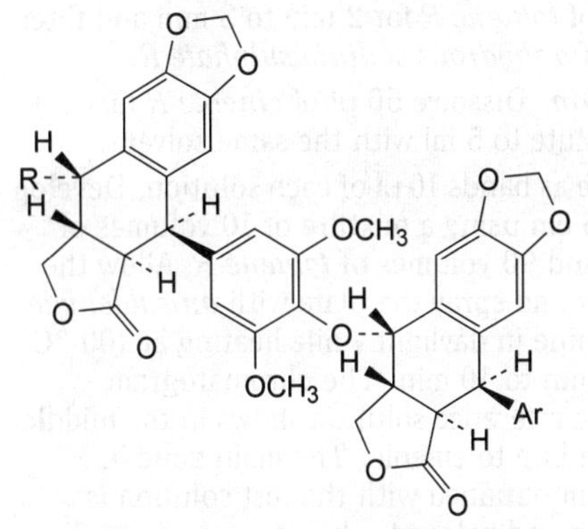

N. (5*R*,5a*R*,8a*R*,9*S*)-9-[[4,6-*O*-[(*R*)-ethylidene]-β-D-glucopyranosyl]oxy]-5-[4-[[(5*R*,5a*R*,8a*R*,9*S*)-5-(4-hydroxy-3,5-dimethoxyphenyl)-6-oxo-5,5a,6,8,8a,9-hexahydroisobenzofuro[5,6-*f*][1,3]benzodioxol-9-yl]oxy]-3,5-dimethoxyphenyl]-5,8,8a,9-tetrahydroisobenzofuro[5,6-*f*][1,3]benzodioxol-6(5a*H*)-one.

01/2005:1320

EUCALYPTUS LEAF

Eucalypti folium

DEFINITION

Eucalyptus leaf consists of the whole or cut dried leaves of older branches of *Eucalyptus globulus* Labill. The whole drug contains not less than 20 ml/kg of essential oil and the cut drug not less than 15 ml/kg of essential oil, both calculated with reference to the anhydrous drug.

CHARACTERS

The drug has an aromatic odour of cineole.

It has the macroscopic and microscopic characters described under identification tests A and B.

IDENTIFICATION

A. The leaves which are mainly greyish-green and relatively thick are elongated, elliptical and slightly sickle-shaped and usually up to 25 cm in length, and up to 5 cm in width. The petiole is twisted, strongly wrinkled and is 2 cm to 3 cm, rarely 5 cm, in length. The coriaceous, stiff leaves are entire and glabrous and have a yellowish-green mid-rib. Lateral veins anastomose near the margin to a continuous line. The margin is even and somewhat thickened. On both surfaces are minute, irregularly distributed, warty dark brown spots. Small oil glands may be seen in transmitted light.

B. Reduce to a powder (355). The powder is greyish-green. Examine under a microscope, using *chloral hydrate solution R*. The powder shows fragments of glabrous

Monographs D-E

lamina with small thick-walled epidermal cells bearing a thick cuticle, numerous anomocytic stomata (*2.8.3*) of more than 80 µm in diameter and occasionally groups of brown cork cells, 300 µm in diameter and brownish-black in their centre; fragments of isobilateral mesophyll with two or three layers of palisade parenchyma on each side and in the centre several layers of spongy mesophyll with elongated cells with the same orientation as the palisade cells and containing prisms and cluster crystals of calcium oxalate; fragments of mesophyll containing large schizogenous oil glands.

C. Examine by thin-layer chromatography (*2.2.27*), using a suitable silica gel as the coating substance.

Test solution. Shake 0.5 g of the freshly powdered drug (355) with 5 ml of *toluene R* for 2 min to 3 min and filter over about 2 g of *anhydrous sodium sulphate R.*

Reference solution. Dissolve 50 µl of *cineole R* in *toluene R* and dilute to 5 ml with the same solvent.

Apply to the plate as bands 10 µl of each solution. Develop over a path of 15 cm using a mixture of 10 volumes of *ethyl acetate R* and 90 volumes of *toluene R.* Allow the plate to dry in air and spray the plate with *anisaldehyde solution R.* Examine in daylight while heating at 100 °C to 105 °C for 5 min to 10 min. The chromatogram obtained with the reference solution shows in the middle a zone corresponding to cineole. The main zone in the chromatogram obtained with the test solution is similar in position and colour to the zone corresponding to cineole in the chromatogram obtained with the reference solution, it also shows an intense violet zone (hydrocarbons) near the solvent front and there may also be other fainter zones.

TESTS

Foreign matter (*2.8.2*). Not more than 3 per cent of dark and brown leaves, not more than 5 per cent of stems and not more than 2 per cent of other foreign matter. Cordate or ovate sessile leaves of young branches, with numerous glands on both sides, visible as points in transmitted light, are not present. Determine by using 30 g of the drug.

Water (*2.2.13*). Not more than 100 ml/kg, determined on 20.0 g of powdered drug (355) by distillation.

Total ash (*2.4.16*). Not more than 6.0 per cent.

ASSAY

Carry out the determination of essential oil in vegetable drugs (*2.8.12*). Use 10.0 g of the cut drug immediately before determination, a 500 ml round-bottomed flask, 200 ml of *water R* and 100 ml of *glycerol R* as the distillation liquid and 0.5 ml of *xylene R* in the graduated tube. Distil at a rate of 2 ml/min to 3 ml/min for 2 h.

STORAGE

Store protected from light.

01/2005:0390

EUCALYPTUS OIL

Eucalypti aetheroleum

DEFINITION

Eucalyptus oil is obtained by steam distillation and rectification from the fresh leaves or the fresh terminal branchlets of various species of *Eucalyptus* rich in 1,8-cineole. The species mainly used are *Eucalyptus globulus* Labill., *Eucalyptus polybractea* R.T. Baker and *Eucalyptus smithii* R.T. Baker.

CHARACTERS

A colourless or pale yellow liquid with an aromatic and camphoraceous odour and a pungent and camphoraceous taste.

IDENTIFICATION

First identification: B.

Second identification: A.

A. Examine by thin-layer chromatography (*2.2.27*), using a *TLC silica gel plate R.*

Test solution. Dissolve 0.1 g of the substance to be examined in *toluene R* and dilute to 10 ml with the same solvent.

Reference solution. Dissolve 50 µl of *cineole R* in *toluene R* and dilute to 5 ml with the same solvent.

Apply to the plate as bands 10 µl of each solution. Develop over a path of 15 cm using a mixture of 10 volumes of *ethyl acetate R* and 90 volumes of *toluene R.* Allow the plate to dry in air and spray with *anisaldehyde solution R* and examine in daylight while heating at 100-105 °C for 5-10 min. The chromatogram obtained with the reference solution shows in the middle a zone due to cineole. The chromatogram obtained with the test solution shows a main zone similar in position and colour to the zone due to cineole in the chromatogram obtained with the reference solution. Other weaker zones may be present.

B. Examine the chromatograms obtained in the test for chromatographic profile. The chromatogram obtained with the test solution shows 5 peaks similar in retention time to the 5 peaks in the chromatogram obtained with the reference solution.

TESTS

Relative density (*2.2.5*): 0.906 to 0.927.

Refractive index (*2.2.6*): 1.458 to 1.470.

Optical rotation (*2.2.7*): 0° to + 10°.

Solubility in alcohol (*2.8.10*). It is soluble in 5 volumes of *ethanol (70 per cent V/V) R.*

Aldehydes. Place 10 ml in a glass-stoppered tube 25 mm in diameter and 150 mm long. Add 5 ml of *toluene R* and 4 ml of *alcoholic hydroxylamine solution R.* Shake vigorously and titrate immediately with *0.5 M potassium hydroxide in alcohol (60 per cent V/V)* until the red colour changes to yellow. Continue the titration with shaking; the end-point is reached when the pure yellow colour of the indicator is permanent in the lower layer after shaking vigorously for 2 min and allowing separation to take place. The reaction is complete in about 15 min. Repeat the titration using a further 10 ml of the substance to be examined and, as a reference solution for the end-point, the titrated liquid from the first determination to which has been added 0.5 ml of *0.5 M potassium hydroxide in alcohol (60 per cent V/V).* Not more than 2.0 ml of *0.5 M potassium hydroxide in alcohol (60 per cent V/V)* is required in the second titration.

Chromatographic profile. Examine by gas chromatography (*2.2.28*).

Test solution. The substance to be examined.

Reference solution. Dissolve 80 µl of *α-pinene R,* 10 µl of *β-pinene R,* 10 µl of *α-phellandrene R,* 10 µl of *limonene R,* 0.8 ml of *cineole R* and 10 mg of *camphor R* in 10 ml of *acetone R.*

The chromatographic procedure may be carried out using:

– a fused-silica column 60 m long and about 0.25 mm in internal diameter coated with *macrogol 20 000 R* as the bonded phase,

- *helium for chromatography R* as the carrier gas at a flow rate of 1.5 ml/min,
- a flame-ionisation detector,
- a split ratio of 1:100,

maintaining the temperature of the column at 60 °C for 5 min, then raising the temperature at a rate of 5 °C/min to 200 °C and maintaining at 200 °C for 5 min; maintaining the temperature of the injection port and that of the detector at 220 °C.

Inject about 0.5 µl of the reference solution. When the chromatogram is recorded in the prescribed conditions the components elute in the order indicated in the composition of the reference solution. Record the retention times of these substances.

The assay is not valid unless: the number of theoretical plates calculated for the peak due to limonene at 110 °C is at least 30 000; the resolution between the peaks corresponding to limonene and cineole is at least 1.5.

Inject about 0.5 µl of the test solution. Using the retention times determined from the chromatogram obtained with the reference solution, locate the components of the reference solution on the chromatogram obtained with the test solution.

Determine the percentage content of these components by the normalisation procedure.

The percentages are within the following ranges:

- *α-pinene*: traces to 9.0 per cent,
- *β-pinene*: less than 1.5 per cent,
- *α-phellandrene*: less than 1.5 per cent,
- *limonene*: traces to 12.0 per cent,
- *1,8-cineole*: minimum 70.0 per cent,
- *camphor*: less than 0.1 per cent.

STORAGE

In a well-filled, airtight container, protected from light and at a temperature not exceeding 25 °C.

01/2005:1100

EUGENOL

Eugenolum

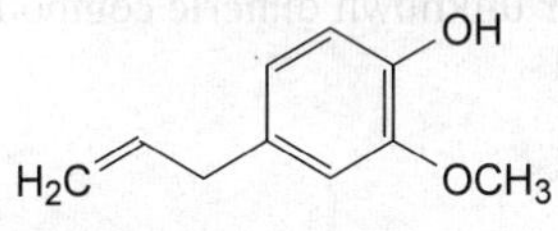

$C_{10}H_{12}O_2$ M_r 164.2

DEFINITION

Eugenol is 2-methoxy-4-(prop-2-enyl)phenol.

CHARACTERS

A colourless or pale yellow, clear liquid, darkening on exposure to air, with a strong odour of clove, practically insoluble in water, freely soluble in alcohol (70 per cent *V/V*), practically insoluble in glycerol, miscible with glacial acetic acid, with alcohol, with fatty oils and with methylene chloride.

IDENTIFICATION

First identification: B.

Second identification: A, C, D.

A. It complies with the test for refractive index (see Tests).

B. Examine by infrared absorption spectrophotometry (*2.2.24*), comparing with the spectrum obtained with *eugenol CRS*.

C. Examine by thin-layer chromatography (*2.2.27*), using a *TLC silica gel F_{254} plate R*.
Test solution. Dissolve 50 µl of the substance to be examined in *alcohol R* and dilute to 25 ml with the same solvent.
Reference solution. Dissolve 50 µl of *eugenol CRS* in *alcohol R* and dilute to 25 ml with the same solvent.
Apply to the plate 5 µl of each solution. Develop over a path of 15 cm using a mixture of 10 volumes of *ethyl acetate R* and 90 volumes of *toluene R*. Dry the plate in a current of cold air and examine in ultraviolet light at 254 nm. The principal spot in the chromatogram obtained with the test solution is similar in position and size to the principal spot in the chromatogram obtained with the reference solution. Spray with *anisaldehyde solution R*. Heat at 100-105 °C for 10 min. The principal spot in the chromatogram obtained with the test solution is similar in position, colour and size to the principal spot in the chromatogram obtained with the reference solution.

D. Dissolve 0.05 ml in 2 ml of *alcohol R* and add 0.1 ml of *ferric chloride solution R1*. A dark green colour is produced which changes to yellowish-green within 10 min.

TESTS

Relative density (*2.2.5*): 1.066 to 1.070.

Refractive index (*2.2.6*): 1.540 to 1.542.

Dimeric and oligomeric compounds. Dissolve 0.150 g of the substance to be examined in *ethanol R* and dilute to 100.0 ml with the same solvent. The absorbance of the solution (*2.2.25*) at 330 nm is not greater than 0.25.

Related substances. Examine by gas chromatography (*2.2.28*).

Test solution. Dissolve 1.00 g of the substance to be examined in *ethanol R* and dilute to 5.0 ml with the same solvent.

Reference solution (a). Dilute 1.0 ml of the test solution to 100.0 ml with *ethanol R*.

Reference solution (b). Dissolve 50 mg of *vanillin R* in 1 ml of the test solution and dilute to 5 ml with *ethanol R*.

The chromatographic procedure may be carried out using:

- a fused-silica capillary column 30 m long and 0.25 mm in internal diameter coated with a film of *polymethylphenylsiloxane R* (film thickness 0.25 µm),
- *helium for chromatography R* as the carrier gas at a flow rate of 1 ml/min,
- a flame-ionisation detector,
- a split ratio of 1:40,

	Time (min)	Temperature (°C)	Rate (°C/min)	Comment
Column	0 - 2	80		isothermal
	2 - 27	80 → 280	8	linear gradient
	27 - 47	280		isothermal
Injection port		250		
Detector		280		

Inject 1 µl of the test solution and 1 µl each of reference solutions (a) and (b). The test is not valid unless in the chromatogram obtained with reference solution (b), the relative retention time of the peak due to vanillin is at least 1.1 with respect to the peak due to eugenol. Calculate the percentage content of related substances from the areas

of the peaks in the chromatogram obtained with the test solution by the normalisation procedure; disregard the solvent peak and any peak with an area less than 0.05 times that of the principal peak in the chromatogram obtained with reference solution (a). The content of related substances with a relative retention time greater than 2.0 in respect to the main peak is not greater than 1.0 per cent; the content of any related substances is not greater than 0.5 per cent; the total content of related substances is not greater than 3.0 per cent.

Hydrocarbons. Dissolve 1 ml in 5 ml of *dilute sodium hydroxide solution R* and add 30 ml of *water R* in a stoppered test-tube. Examined immediately, the solution is yellow and clear (*2.2.1*).

Sulphated ash (*2.4.14*). Not more than 0.1 per cent, determined on 1.0 g.

STORAGE

Store in a well-filled container, protected from light.

IMPURITIES

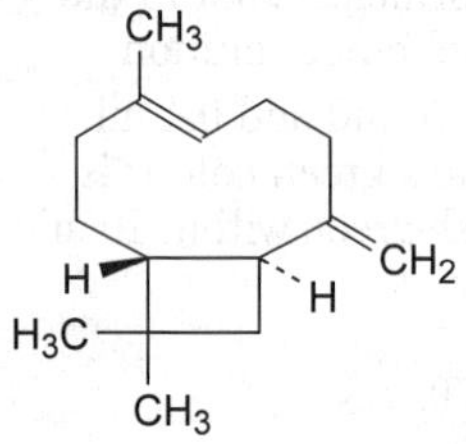

A. (1*R*,4*E*,9*S*)-4,11,11-trimethyl-8-methylenebicyclo[7.2.0]undec-4-ene (β-caryophyllene),

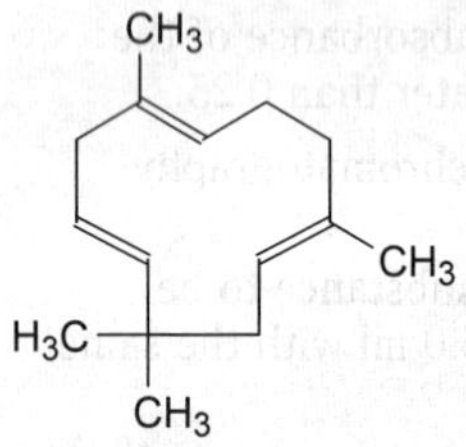

B. (1*E*,4*E*,8*E*)-2,6,6,9-tetramethylcycloundeca-1,4,8-triene (α-humulene, α-caryophyllene),

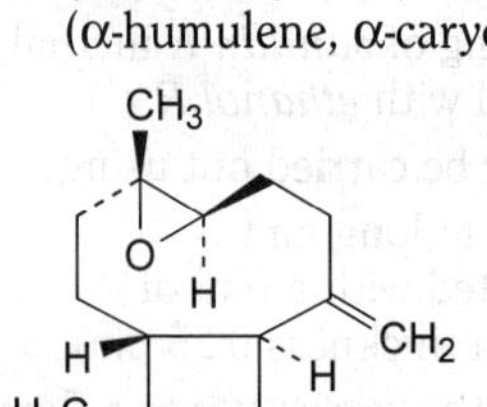

C. (1*R*,4*R*,6*R*,10*S*)-4,12,12-trimethyl-9-methylene-5-oxatricyclo[8.2.0.0^{4,6}]dodecane (β-caryophyllene oxide),

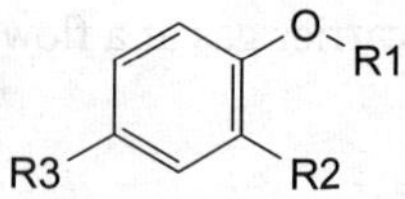

D. R1 = H, R2 = H, R3 = CH_2-CH=CH_2: 4-(prop-2-enyl)phenol,

E. R1 = CH_3, R2 = OCH_3, R3 = CH_2-CH=CH_2: 1,2-dimethoxy-4-(prop-2-enyl)benzene (eugenol methyl ether),

F. R1 = H, R2 = OCH_3, R3 = CH=CH-CH_3 (*cis*): 2-methoxy-4-[(Z)-prop-1-enyl]phenol (*cis*-isoeugenol),

G. R1 = H, R2 = OCH_3, R3 = CH=CH-CH_3 (*trans*): 2-methoxy-4-[(E)-prop-1-enyl]phenol (*trans*-isoeugenol),

H. R1 = H, R2 = OCH_3, R3 = CHO: 4-hydroxy-3-methoxybenzaldehyde (vanillin),

I. R1 = CO-CH_3, R2 = OCH_3, R3 = CH_2-CH=CH_2: 2-methoxy-4-(prop-2-enyl)phenyl acetate (acetyleugenol),

J. R1 = H, R2 = OCH_3, R3 = CO-CH=CH_2: 1-(4-hydroxy-3-methoxyphenyl)prop-2-enone,

K. R1 = H, R2 = OCH_3, R3 = CH=CH-CHO: (*E*)-3-(4-hydroxy-3-methoxyphenyl)prop-2-enal (*trans*-coniferyl aldehyde),

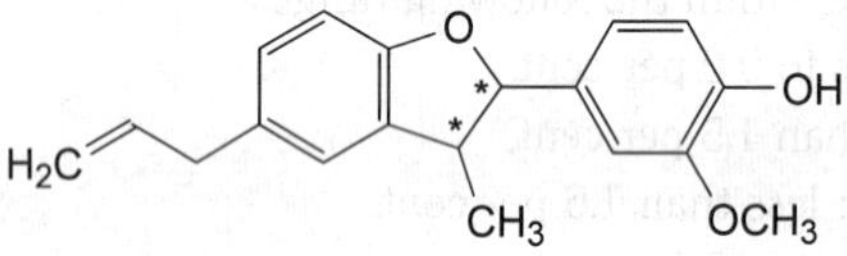

L. 2-methoxy-4-[3-methyl-5-(prop-2-enyl)-2,3-dihydrobenzofuran-2-yl]phenol (dehydrodi-isoeugenol),

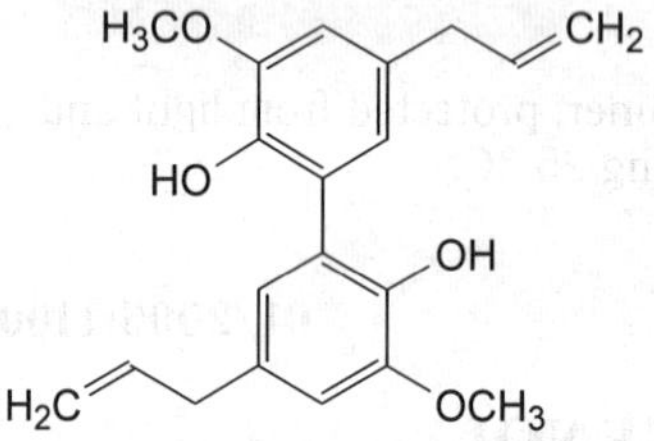

M. 3,3′-dimethoxy-5,5′-bis(prop-2-enyl)biphenyl-2,2′-diol (dehydrodieugenol),

N. O. two further unknown dimeric compounds,

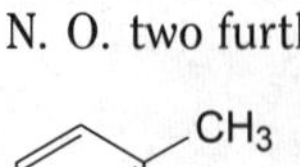

P. toluene.

F

01/2005:1012

FAMOTIDINE

Famotidinum

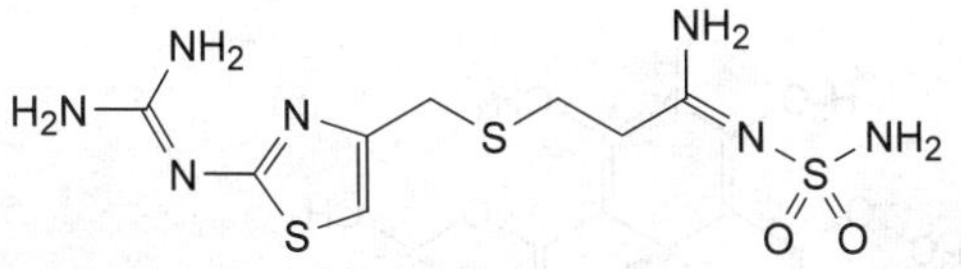

$C_8H_{15}N_7O_2S_3$ M_r 337.5

DEFINITION

3-[[[2-[(Diaminomethylene)amino]thiazol-4-yl]methyl]sulphanyl]-*N'*-sulphamoylpropanimidamide.

Content: 98.5 per cent to 101.5 per cent (dried substance).

CHARACTERS

Appearance: white or yellowish-white, crystalline powder or crystals.

Solubility: very slightly soluble in water, freely soluble in glacial acetic acid, very slightly soluble in anhydrous ethanol, practically insoluble in ethyl acetate. It dissolves in dilute mineral acids.

It shows polymorphism.

IDENTIFICATION

Infrared absorption spectrophotometry (*2.2.24*).

Preparation: discs.

Comparison: *famotidine CRS.*

If the spectra obtained show differences, suspend 0.10 g of the substance to be examined and 0.10 g of the reference substance separately in 5 ml of *water R*. Heat to boiling and allow to cool, scratching the wall of the tube with a glass rod to initiate crystallisation. Filter, wash the crystals with 2 ml of iced *water R* and dry in an oven at 80 °C at a pressure not exceeding 670 Pa for 1 h. Record new spectra using the residues.

TESTS

Appearance of solution. Dissolve 0.20 g in a 50 g/l solution of *hydrochloric acid R*, heating to 40 °C if necessary, and dilute to 20 ml with the same acid. The solution is clear (*2.2.1*) and not more intensely coloured than reference solution BY_7 (*2.2.2, Method II*).

Related substances. Liquid chromatography (*2.2.29*).

Test solution. Dissolve 12.5 mg of the substance to be examined in mobile phase A and dilute to 25.0 ml with mobile phase A.

Reference solution (a). Dilute 1.0 ml of the test solution to 10.0 ml with mobile phase A. Dilute 1.0 ml of this solution to 100.0 ml with mobile phase A.

Reference solution (b). Dissolve 2.5 mg of *famotidine impurity D CRS* in *methanol R* and dilute to 10.0 ml with the same solvent. To 1.0 ml of the solution add 0.50 ml of the test solution and dilute to 100.0 ml with mobile phase A.

Reference solution (c). Dissolve 5.0 mg of *famotidine for system suitability CRS* (famotidine containing impurities A, B, C, D, E, F, G) in mobile phase A and dilute to 10.0 ml with mobile phase A.

Column:

– *size*: *l* = 0.25 m, Ø = 4.6 mm,
– *stationary phase*: *end-capped octadecylsilyl silica gel for chromatography R* (5 µm),
– *temperature*: 50 °C.

Mobile phase:

– *mobile phase A*: mix 6 volumes of *methanol R*, 94 volumes of *acetonitrile R* and 900 volumes of a 1.882 g/l solution of *sodium hexanesulphonate R* previously adjusted to pH 3.5 with *acetic acid R*,
– *mobile phase B*: *acetonitrile R*,

Time (min)	Mobile phase A (per cent *V/V*)	Mobile phase B (per cent *V/V*)	Flow rate (ml/min)
0 - 23	100 → 96	0 → 4	1
23 - 27	96	4	1 → 2
27 - 47	96 → 78	4 → 22	2
47 - 48	78 → 100	22 → 0	2
48 - 54	100	0	2 → 1

Detection: spectrophotometer at 265 nm.

Injection: 20 µl.

Relative retention with reference to famotidine (retention time = about 21 min): impurity D = about 1.1; impurity C = about 1.2; impurity G = about 1.4; impurity F = about 1.5; impurity A = about 1.6; impurity B = about 2.0; impurity E = about 2.1.

System suitability:

– the chromatogram obtained with reference solution (c) is similar to the chromatogram supplied with *famotidine for system suitability CRS*;
– *retention time*: famotidine = 19-23 min in all the chromatograms; impurity E = maximum 48 min in the chromatogram obtained with reference solution (c);
– *resolution*: minimum 3.5 between the peaks due to famotidine and impurity D in the chromatogram obtained with reference solution (b).

Limits:

– *correction factors*: for the calculation of contents, multiply the peak areas of the following impurities by the corresponding correction factor: impurity A = 1.9; impurity B = 2.5; impurity C = 1.9; impurity F = 1.7; impurity G = 1.4;
– *impurities A, G*: for each impurity, not more than twice the area of the principal peak in the chromatogram obtained with reference solution (a) (0.2 per cent);
– *impurities B, C, D, E*: for each impurity, not more than 3 times the area of the principal peak in the chromatogram obtained with reference solution (a) (0.3 per cent), and not more than 3 such peaks have an area greater than the area of the principal peak in the chromatogram obtained with reference solution (a) (0.1 per cent);
– *impurity F*: not more than the area of the principal peak in the chromatogram obtained with reference solution (a) (0.1 per cent);
– *any other impurity*: for each impurity, not more than the area of the principal peak in the chromatogram obtained with reference solution (a) for the peaks eluting by 25 min, and not more than 0.5 times the area of the principal peak in the chromatogram obtained with reference solution (a) for the peaks eluting after 25 min (0.1 per cent);
– *total*: not more than 10 times the area of the principal peak in the chromatogram obtained with reference solution (a) (1.0 per cent);
– *disregard limit*: 0.2 times the area of the principal peak in the chromatogram obtained with reference solution (a).

Heavy metals (*2.4.8*): maximum 10 ppm.

2.0 g complies with limit test D. Prepare the reference solution using 2 ml of *lead standard solution (10 ppm Pb) R*.

Loss on drying (*2.2.32*): maximum 0.5 per cent, determined on 1.000 g by drying in an oven at 80 °C at a pressure not exceeding 670 Pa for 5 h.

Sulphated ash (*2.4.14*): maximum 0.1 per cent, determined on 1.0 g.

ASSAY

Dissolve 0.120 g in 60 ml of *anhydrous acetic acid R*. Titrate with *0.1 M perchloric acid*, determining the end-point potentiometrically (*2.2.20*).

1 ml of *0.1 M perchloric acid* is equivalent to 16.87 mg of $C_8H_{15}N_7O_2S_3$.

STORAGE

Protected from light.

IMPURITIES

Specified impurities: A, B, C, D, E, F, G.

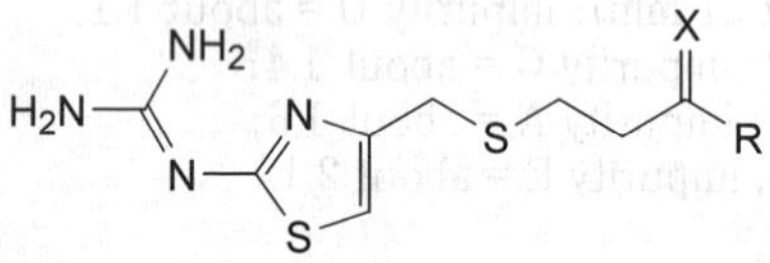

A. R = NH_2, X = NH: 3-[[[2-[(diaminomethylene)amino]thiazol-4-yl]methyl]sulphanyl]propanimidamide,

C. R = NH-SO_2-NH_2, X = O: 3-[[[2-[(diaminomethylene)amino]thiazol-4-yl]methyl]sulphanyl]-*N*-sulphamoylpropanamide,

D. R = NH_2, X = O: 3-[[[2-[(diaminomethylene)amino]thiazol-4-yl]methyl]sulphanyl]propanamide,

F. R = OH, X = O: 3-[[[2-[(diaminomethylene)amino]thiazol-4-yl]methyl]sulphanyl]propanoic acid,

G. R = NH-CN, X = NH: *N*-cyano-3-[[[2-[(diaminomethylene)amino]thiazol-4-yl]methyl]sulphanyl]propanimidamide,

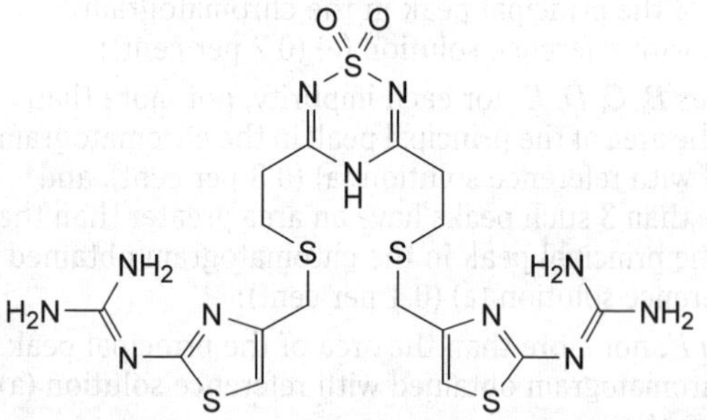

B. 3,5-bis[2-[[[2-[(diaminomethylene)amino]thiazol-4-yl]methyl]sulphanyl]ethyl]-4*H*-1,2,4,6-thiatriazine 1,1-dioxide,

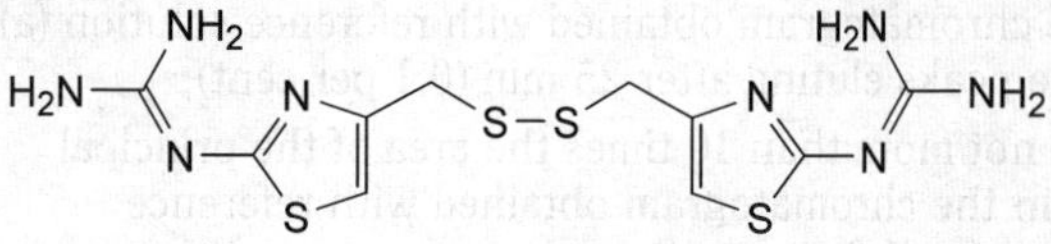

E. 2,2′-[disulphanediylbis(methylenethiazole-4,2-diyl)]diguanidine.

01/2005:1013

FELODIPINE

Felodipinum

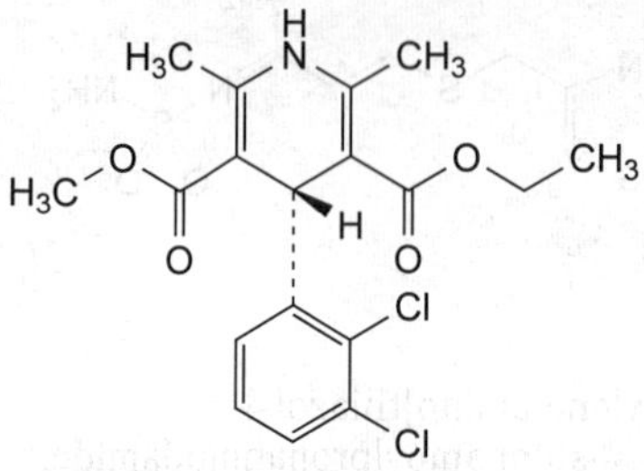

and enantiomer

$C_{18}H_{19}Cl_2NO_4$ M_r 384.3

DEFINITION

Felodipine contains not less than 99.0 per cent and not more than the equivalent of 101.0 per cent of ethyl methyl (4*RS*)-4-(2,3-dichlorophenyl)-2,6-dimethyl-1,4-dihydropyridine-3,5-dicarboxylate, calculated with reference to the dried substance.

CHARACTERS

A white or light yellow, crystalline powder, practically insoluble in water, freely soluble in acetone, in ethanol, in methanol and in methylene chloride.

IDENTIFICATION

First identification: B.

Second identification: A, C, D.

A. Dissolve 50 mg in *methanol R* and dilute to 100 ml with the same solvent. Dilute 3 ml to 100 ml with *methanol R*. Examined between 220 nm and 400 nm (*2.2.25*), the solution shows two absorption maxima, at 238 nm and 361 nm. The ratio of the absorbance measured at the maximum at 361 nm to that measured at the maximum at 238 nm is 0.34 to 0.36.

B. Examine by infrared absorption spectrophotometry (*2.2.24*), comparing with the spectrum obtained with *felodipine CRS*. Examine the substances prepared as discs.

C. Examine by thin-layer chromatography (*2.2.27*), using as the coating substance a suitable silica gel with a fluorescent indicator having an optimal intensity at 254 nm.

Test solution. Dissolve 10 mg of the substance to be examined in *methanol R* and dilute to 10 ml with the same solvent.

Reference solution (a). Dissolve 10 mg of *felodipine CRS* in *methanol R* and dilute to 10 ml with the same solvent.

Reference solution (b). Dissolve 5 mg of *nifedipine CRS* in reference solution (a) and dilute to 5 ml with the same solution.

Apply separately to the plate 5 µl of each solution. Develop over a path of 15 cm using a mixture of 40 volumes of *ethyl acetate R* and 60 volumes of *cyclohexane R*. Allow the plate to dry in air and examine in ultraviolet light at 254 nm. The principal spot in the chromatogram obtained with the test solution is similar in position, fluorescence and size to the spot in the chromatogram obtained with reference solution (a). The test is not valid unless the chromatogram obtained with reference solution (b) shows two clearly separated spots.

D. Dissolve 150 mg in a mixture of 25 ml of *2-methyl-2-propanol R* and 25 ml of *perchloric acid solution R*. Add 10 ml of *0.1 M cerium sulphate*, allow to stand for 15 min, add 3.5 ml of *strong sodium hydroxide solution R* and neutralise with *dilute sodium hydroxide solution R*. Shake with 25 ml of *methylene chloride R*. Evaporate the lower layer to dryness on a water-bath under nitrogen (the residue is also used in the test for related substances). Dissolve about 20 mg of the residue in *methanol R* and dilute to 50 ml with the same solvent. Dilute 2 ml to 50 ml with *methanol R*. Examined between 220 nm and 400 nm (*2.2.25*), the solution shows an absorption maximum at 273 nm.

TESTS

Solution S. Dissolve 1.00 g in *methanol R* and dilute to 20.0 ml with the same solvent.

Appearance of solution. Solution S is clear (*2.2.1*).

Absorbance (*2.2.25*). The absorbance of solution S at 440 nm is not greater than 0.10.

Related substances. Examine by liquid chromatography (*2.2.29*).

Test solution. Dissolve 25.0 mg of the substance to be examined in the mobile phase and dilute to 50.0 ml with the mobile phase.

Reference solution (a). Dilute 1.0 ml of the test solution to 100.0 ml with the mobile phase.

Reference solution (b). Dilute 1.0 ml of reference solution (a) to 10.0 ml with the mobile phase.

Reference solution (c). Dissolve 50.0 mg of the residue obtained in identification test D (impurity A) and 25.0 mg of *felodipine CRS* in the mobile phase and dilute to 50.0 ml with the mobile phase. Dilute 1.0 ml to 100.0 ml with the mobile phase. Dilute 1.0 ml of this solution to 10.0 ml with the mobile phase.

The chromatographic procedure may be carried out using:

– a stainless steel column 0.125 m to 0.15 m long and 4 mm in internal diameter packed with *octadecylsilyl silica gel for chromatography R* (5 µm),

– as mobile phase at a flow rate of 1 ml/min a mixture of 20 volumes of *methanol R*, 40 volumes of *acetonitrile R* and 40 volumes of a phosphate buffer solution pH 3.0, containing 0.8 g/l of *phosphoric acid R* and 8 g/l of *sodium dihydrogen phosphate R*,

– as detector a spectrophotometer set at 254 nm.

Inject 20 µl of reference solution (c). Adjust the sensitivity of the system so that the heights of the two peaks are not less than 20 per cent of the full scale of the recorder. The test is not valid unless the resolution between the first peak (impurity A) and the second peak (felodipine) is at least 2.5. Two other peaks may be observed corresponding to impurity B and impurity C. The substances elute in the following order: impurity B, impurity A, felodipine and impurity C.

Inject 20 µl of the test solution, 20 µl of reference solution (a) and 20 µl of reference solution (b). Continue the chromatography for twice the retention time of felodipine, which is about 12 min. In the chromatogram obtained with the test solution: the sum of the areas of any peaks corresponding to impurity B and impurity C is not greater than the area of the principal peak in the chromatogram obtained with reference solution (a) (1.0 per cent); the area of any peak apart from the principal peak and any peaks corresponding to impurity B and impurity C is not greater than the area of the principal peak in the chromatogram obtained with reference solution (b) (0.1 per cent) and the sum of the areas of such peaks is not greater than three times the area of the principal peak in the chromatogram obtained with reference solution (b) (0.3 per cent). Disregard any peak with an area less than 0.2 times that of the principal peak in the chromatogram obtained with reference solution (b).

Loss on drying (*2.2.32*). Not more than 0.5 per cent, determined on 1.000 g by drying in an oven at 100 °C to 105 °C for 3 h.

Sulphated ash (*2.4.14*). Not more than 0.1 per cent, determined on 1.0 g.

ASSAY

Dissolve 0.160 g in a mixture of 25 ml of *2-methyl-2-propanol R* and 25 ml of *perchloric acid solution R*. Add 0.05 ml of *ferroin R*. Titrate with *0.1 M cerium sulphate* until the pink colour disappears. Titrate slowly towards the end of the titration.

1 ml of *0.1 M cerium sulphate* is equivalent to 19.21 mg of $C_{18}H_{19}Cl_2NO_4$.

STORAGE

Store protected from light.

IMPURITIES

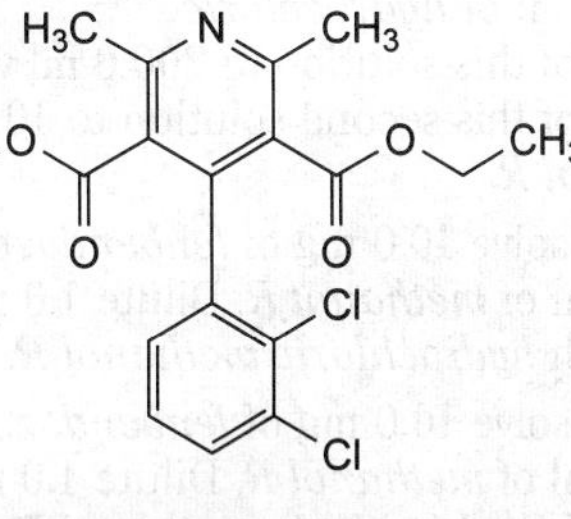

A. ethyl methyl 4-(2,3-dichlorophenyl)-2,6-dimethylpyridine-3,5-dicarboxylate,

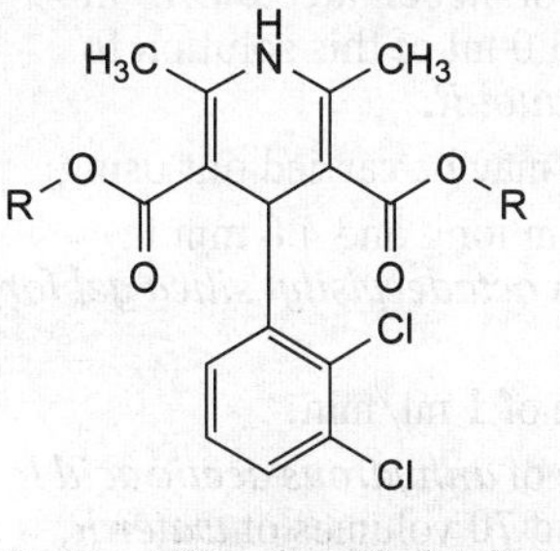

B. R = CH_3: dimethyl 4-(2,3-dichlorophenyl)-2,6-dimethyl-1,4-dihydropyridine-3,5-dicarboxylate,

C. R = C_2H_5: diethyl 4-(2,3-dichlorophenyl)-2,6-dimethyl-1,4-dihydropyridine-3,5-dicarboxylate.

01/2005:1208

FENBENDAZOLE FOR VETERINARY USE

Fenbendazolum ad usum veterinarium

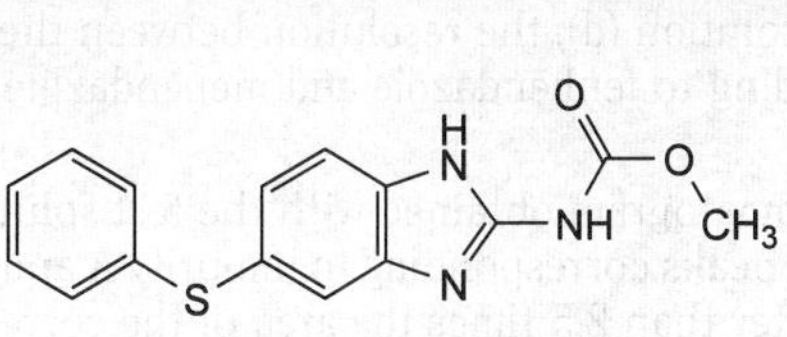

$C_{15}H_{13}N_3O_2S$ M_r 299.4

DEFINITION

Fenbendazole for veterinary use contains not less than 98.0 per cent and not more than the equivalent of 101.0 per cent of methyl [5-(phenylsulphanyl)-1*H*-benzimidazol-2-yl]carbamate, calculated with reference to the dried substance.

CHARACTERS

A white or almost white powder, practically insoluble in water, sparingly soluble in dimethylformamide, very slightly soluble in methanol.

IDENTIFICATION

Examine by infrared absorption spectrophotometry (*2.2.24*), comparing with the spectrum obtained with *fenbendazole CRS*. Examine the substances prepared as discs.

TESTS

Related substances. Examine by liquid chromatography (*2.2.29*).

Test solution. Dissolve 50.0 mg of the substance to be examined in 10.0 ml of *hydrochloric methanol R*.

Reference solution (a). Dissolve 50.0 mg of *fenbendazole CRS* in 10.0 ml of *hydrochloric methanol R*. Dilute 1.0 ml of this solution to 200.0 ml with *methanol R*. Dilute 5.0 ml of this second solution to 10.0 ml with *hydrochloric methanol R*.

Reference solution (b). Dissolve 10.0 mg of *fenbendazole impurity A CRS* in 100.0 ml of *methanol R*. Dilute 1.0 ml of this solution to 10.0 ml with *hydrochloric methanol R*.

Reference solution (c). Dissolve 10.0 mg of *fenbendazole impurity B CRS* in 100.0 ml of *methanol R*. Dilute 1.0 ml of this solution to 10.0 ml with *hydrochloric methanol R*.

Reference solution (d). Dissolve 10.0 mg of *fenbendazole CRS* and 10.0 mg of *mebendazole CRS* in 100.0 ml of *methanol R*. Dilute 1.0 ml of this solution to 10.0 ml with *hydrochloric methanol R*.

The chromatographic procedure may be carried out using:

- a stainless steel column 0.25 m long and 4.6 mm in internal diameter packed with *octadecylsilyl silica gel for chromatography R* (5 µm),
- as mobile phase at a flow rate of 1 ml/min:

  Mobile phase A. Mix 1 volume of *anhydrous acetic acid R*, 30 volumes of *methanol R* and 70 volumes of *water R*,

  Mobile phase B. Mix 1 volume of *anhydrous acetic acid R*, 30 volumes of *water R* and 70 volumes of *methanol R*,

Time (min)	Mobile phase A (per cent *V/V*)	Mobile phase B (per cent *V/V*)	Comment
0 - 10	100 → 0	0 → 100	linear gradient
10 - 40	0	100	isocratic
40 - 50	0 → 100	100 → 0	re-equilibration

- as detector a spectrophotometer set at 280 nm.

When the chromatograms are recorded in the prescribed conditions, the retention time for fenbendazole is about 19 min. Inject separately 10 µl of each solution. The test is not valid unless, in the chromatogram obtained with reference solution (d), the resolution between the peaks corresponding to fenbendazole and mebendazole is at least 1.5.

In the chromatogram obtained with the test solution: the area of the peaks corresponding to impurity A and impurity B is not greater than 2.5 times the area of the corresponding peak in the chromatograms obtained with reference solution (b) and reference solution (c) (0.5 per cent); the area of any peak, apart from the principal peak and the peaks corresponding to impurity A and impurity B respectively, is not greater than twice the area of the principal peak in the chromatogram obtained with reference solution (a) (0.5 per cent); the sum of the areas of all the peaks, apart from the principal peak, is not greater than 4 times the area of the principal peak in the chromatogram obtained with reference solution (a) (1 per cent). Disregard any peak with an area less than 0.2 times that of the principal peak in the chromatogram obtained with reference solution (a).

Heavy metals (*2.4.8*). 1.0 g complies with limit test C for heavy metals (20 ppm). Prepare the standard using 2 ml of *lead standard solution (10 ppm Pb) R*.

Loss on drying (*2.2.32*). Not more than 1.0 per cent, determined on 1.000 g by drying in an oven at 100-105 °C for 3 h.

Sulphated ash (*2.4.14*). Not more than 0.3 per cent, determined on 1.0 g.

ASSAY

Dissolve 0.200 g in 30 ml of *anhydrous acetic acid R*, warming gently if necessary. Cool and titrate with *0.1 M perchloric acid*, determining the end-point potentiometrically (*2.2.20*).

1 ml of *0.1 M perchloric acid* is equivalent to 29.94 mg of $C_{15}H_{13}N_3O_2S$.

STORAGE

Protected from light.

IMPURITIES

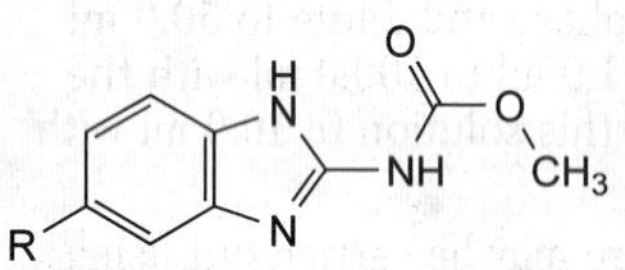

A. R = H: methyl (1*H*-benzimidazol-2-yl)carbamate,

B. R = Cl: methyl (5-chloro-1*H*-benzimidazol-2-yl)carbamate.

01/2005:1209

FENBUFEN

Fenbufenum

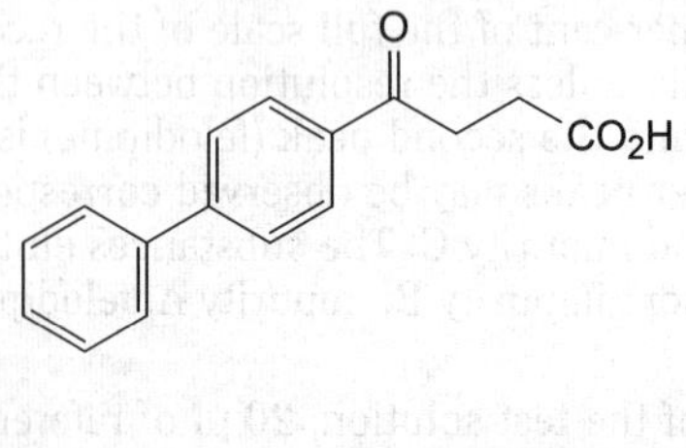

$C_{16}H_{14}O_3$ M_r 254.3

DEFINITION

Fenbufen contains not less than 98.5 per cent and not more than the equivalent of 101.0 per cent of 4-(biphenyl-4-yl)-4-oxobutanoic acid, calculated with reference to the dried substance.

CHARACTERS

A white, fine, crystalline powder, very slightly soluble in water, slightly soluble in acetone, in alcohol and in methylene chloride.

IDENTIFICATION

First identification: B.

Second identification: A, C.

A. Melting point (*2.2.14*): 186 °C to 189 °C.

B. Examine by infrared absorption spectrophotometry (*2.2.24*), comparing with the spectrum obtained with *fenbufen CRS*.

C. Examine by thin-layer chromatography (*2.2.27*), using as the coating substance a suitable silica gel with a fluorescent indicator having an optimal intensity at 254 nm.

Test solution. Dissolve 10 mg of the substance to be examined in *methylene chloride R* and dilute to 10 ml with the same solvent.

Reference solution (a). Dissolve 10 mg of *fenbufen CRS* in *methylene chloride R* and dilute to 10 ml with the same solvent.

Reference solution (b). Dissolve 10 mg of *ketoprofen CRS* in *methylene chloride R* and dilute to 10 ml with the same solvent. To 5 ml of the solution, add 5 ml of reference solution (a).

Apply to the plate 10 µl of each solution. Develop over a path of 15 cm using a mixture of 5 volumes of *anhydrous acetic acid R*, 25 volumes of *ethyl acetate R* and 75 volumes of *hexane R*. Allow the plate to dry in air and examine in ultraviolet light at 254 nm. The principal spot in the chromatogram obtained with the test solution is similar in position and size to the principal spot in the chromatogram obtained with reference solution (a). The test is not valid unless the chromatogram obtained with reference solution (b) shows two clearly separated spots.

TESTS

Related substances. Examine by liquid chromatography (*2.2.29*).

Test solution. Dissolve 50.0 mg of the substance to be examined in a mixture of 40 volumes of *dimethylformamide R* and 60 volumes of mobile phase A and dilute to 10.0 ml with the same mixture of solvents.

Reference solution (a). Dilute 0.5 ml of the test solution to 50.0 ml with a mixture of 40 volumes of *dimethylformamide R* and 60 volumes of mobile phase A. Dilute 1.0 ml of the solution to 10.0 ml with a mixture of 40 volumes of *dimethylformamide R* and 60 volumes of mobile phase A.

Reference solution (b). Dissolve 25 mg of *fenbufen CRS* and 6 mg of *ketoprofen CRS* in a mixture of 40 volumes of *dimethylformamide R* and 60 volumes of mobile phase A and dilute to 10 ml with the same mixture of solvents. Dilute 1 ml of the solution to 100 ml with a mixture of 40 volumes of *dimethylformamide R* and 60 volumes of mobile phase A.

The chromatographic procedure may be carried out using:

– a stainless steel column 0.125 m long and 4.0 mm in internal diameter packed with *octadecylsilyl silica gel for chromatography R* (5 µm),

– as mobile phase at a flow rate of 2 ml/min the following solutions:

Mobile phase A. 32 volumes of*acetonitrile R* and 68 volumes of a mixture of 1 volume of *glacial acetic acid R* and 55 volumes of *water R*,

Mobile phase B. 45 volumes of *acetonitrile R* and 55 volumes of a mixture of 1 volume of *glacial acetic acid R* and 55 volumes of *water R*,

Time (min)	Mobile phase A (per cent *V/V*)	Mobile phase B (per cent *V/V*)	Comment
0 – 15	100	0	isocratic
15 – 20	100 → 0	0 → 100	linear gradient
20 – 35	0	100	isocratic
35 – 40	0 → 100	100 → 0	linear gradient
40 – 45	100	0	re-equilibration

– as detector a spectrophotometer set at 254 nm.

Inject 20 µl of reference solution (a) and 20 µl of reference solution (b). Adjust the sensitivity of the system so that the height of the principal peak in the chromatogram obtained with reference solution (a) is at least 50 per cent of the full scale of the recorder. The test is not valid unless, in the chromatogram obtained with reference solution (b), the resolution between the peaks corresponding to ketoprofenand to fenbufen is at least 5.0.

Inject 20 µl of the test solution. In the chromatogram obtained with the test solution: the area of any peak, apart from the principal peak, is not greater than the area of the principal peak in the chromatogram obtained with reference solution (a) (0.1 per cent); the sum of the areas of any peaks, apart from the principal peak, is not greater than five times the area of the principal peak in the chromatogram obtained with reference solution (a) (0.5 per cent). Disregard any peak due to the solvent and any peak with an area less than 0.2 times that of the principal peak in the chromatogram obtained with reference solution (a).

Heavy metals (*2.4.8*). 1.0 g complies with limit test C for heavy metals (20 ppm). Prepare the standard using 2 ml of *lead standard solution (10 ppm Pb) R*.

Loss on drying (*2.2.32*). Not more than 0.5 per cent, determined on 1.000 g by drying in an oven at 100-105 °C for 3 h.

Sulphated ash (*2.4.14*). Not more than 0.1 per cent, determined on 1.0 g.

ASSAY

Dissolve 0.200 g in 75 ml of *acetone R* previously neutralised with *phenolphthalein solution R1* and add 50 ml of *water R*. Add 0.2 ml of *phenolphthalein solution R1* and titrate with *0.1 M sodium hydroxide*. Carry out a blank titration.

1 ml of *0.1 M sodium hydroxide* is equivalent to 25.43 mg of $C_{16}H_{14}O_3$.

IMPURITIES

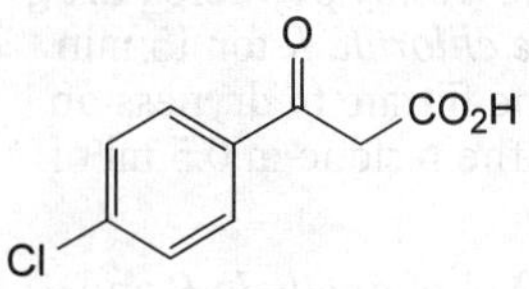

A. 3-(4-chlorophenyl)-3-oxopropanoic acid,

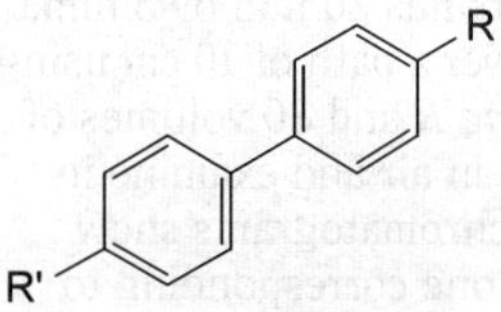

B. R = CO-CH=CH-CO_2H, R′ = H: 4-(biphenyl-4-yl)-4-oxobut-2-enoic acid,

C. R = R′ = H: biphenyl,

D. R = CO-CH_2-CH_2-CO_2H, R′ = OH: 4-(4′-hydroxybiphenyl-4-yl)-4-oxobutanoic acid.

01/2005:0824

FENNEL, BITTER

Foeniculi amari fructus

DEFINITION

Bitter fennel consists of the dry, cremocarps and mericarps of *Foeniculum vulgare* Miller sp. *vulgare* var. *vulgare*. It contains not less than 40 ml/kg of essential oil, calculated with reference to the anhydrous drug. The oil contains not less than 60.0 per cent of anethole and not less than 15.0 per cent of fenchone.

CHARACTERS

Bitter fennel is greenish-brown, brown or green.

It has the macroscopic and microscopic characters described under identification tests A and B.

IDENTIFICATION

A. The fruit of bitter fennel is a cremocarp, of almost cylindrical shape with a rounded base and a narrower summit crowned with a large stylopod. It is generally 3 mm to 12 mm long and 3 mm to 4 mm wide. The mericarps, usually free, are glabrous. Each bears five prominent slightly carenated ridges. When cut transversely, four vittae on the dorsal surface and two on the commissural surface may be seen with a lens.

B. Reduce to a powder (355). The powder is greyish-brown to greyish-yellow. Examine under a microscope using *chloral hydrate solution R*. The powder shows the following diagnostic characters: yellow fragments of wide secretory canals, often made up of yellowish-brown-walled polygonal secretory cells, frequently associated with a layer of thin-walled transversely elongated cells 2 µm to 9 µm wide, having a parquetry arrangement; reticulate parenchyma of the mesocarp; numerous fibre bundles from the ridges, often accompanied by narrow spiral vessels; very numerous endosperm fragments containing aleurone grains and very small calcium oxalate microrosette crystals, as well as some fibre bundles from the carpophore.

C. Examine by thin-layer chromatography (*2.2.27*), using *silica gel GF_{254} R* as the coating substance.

Test solution. Shake 0.3 g of the freshly powdered drug (1400) with 5.0 ml of *methylene chloride R* for 15 min. Filter and carefully evaporate the filtrate to dryness on a water-bath at 60 °C. Dissolve the residue in 0.5 ml of *toluene R*.

Reference solution. Dissolve 50 µl of *anethole R* and 10 µl of *fenchone R* in 5.0 ml of *hexane R*.

Apply separately to the plate, as bands 20 mm by 3 mm, 10 µl of each solution. Develop over a path of 10 cm using a mixture of 20 volumes of *hexane R* and 80 volumes of *toluene R*. Allow the plate to dry in air and examine in ultraviolet light at 254 nm. The chromatograms show in the central part a quenching zone corresponding to anethole. Spray the plate with *sulphuric acid R* and heat at 140 °C for 5 min to 10 min until a yellow zone corresponding to fenchone appears in the lower third of the chromatograms. Anethole appears as a violet band in the central part. The chromatogram obtained with the test solution also shows a reddish-brown zone in its upper third (terpenes).

TESTS

Estragole. The essential oil obtained in the assay contains not more than 5.0 per cent of estragole.

Operate as described in the assay for anethole and fenchone, using the following reference solution.

Reference solution. Dissolve 5 mg of *estragole R* in 0.5 ml of *xylene R*.

Determine the content of estragole by normalisation.

Foreign matter (*2.8.2*). Not more than 1.5 per cent of peduncles and not more than 1.5 per cent of other foreign matter.

Water (*2.2.13*). Not more than 80 ml/kg, determined by distillation on 20.0 g of the powdered drug (710).

Total ash (*2.4.16*). Not more than 10.0 per cent.

ASSAY

Essential oil. Carry out the determination of essential oils in vegetable drugs (*2.8.12*). Use a 500 ml round-bottomed flask and 200 ml of *water R* as the distillation liquid. Reduce the drug to a coarse powder (1400) and immediately use 5.0 g for the determination. Introduce 0.50 ml of *xylene R* in the graduated tube. Distil at a rate of 2 ml/min to 3 ml/min for 2 h.

Anethole and fenchone. Examine by gas chromatography (*2.2.28*).

Test solution. Dilute the mixture of essential oil and *xylene R* obtained in the determination of essential oil to 5.0 ml with *xylene R* and by rinsing the apparatus.

Reference solution. Dissolve 5 mg of *fenchone R* and 5 mg of *anethole R* in 0.5 ml of *xylene R*.

The chromatographic procedure may be carried out using:

– a capillary column 30 m to 60 m long and 0.3 mm in internal diameter coated with *macrogol 20 000 R*,
– *nitrogen for chromatography R* as the carrier gas at a flow rate of 0.40 ml/min and split at a ratio of 1 to 200,
– a flame-ionisation detector,

maintaining the temperature of the column at 60 °C for 4 min, then raising the temperature linearly at a rate of 5 °C per minute to 170 °C and maintaining at 170 °C for 15 min and maintaining the temperature of the injection port at 220 °C and that of the detector at 270 °C.

Inject 1 µl of the reference solution. Identify and record the retention times of the components, which are eluted in the order indicated in the composition of the reference solution.

Inject 1 µl of the test solution. Determine the contents of anethole and fenchone by normalisation.

STORAGE

Store protected from light and moisture.

01/2005:0825

FENNEL, SWEET

Foeniculi dulcis fructus

DEFINITION

Sweet fennel consists of the dry, cremocarps and mericarps of *Foeniculum vulgare* Miller sp. *vulgare* var. *dulce* (Miller) Thellung. It contains not less than 20 ml/kg of essential oil, calculated with reference to the anhydrous drug. The oil contains not less than 80.0 per cent of anethole.

CHARACTERS

Sweet fennel is pale green or pale yellowish-brown.

It has the macroscopic and microscopic characters described under identification tests A and B.

IDENTIFICATION

A. The fruit of sweet fennel is a cremocarp of almost cylindrical shape with a rounded base and a narrowed summit crowned with a large stylopod. It is generally 3 mm to 12 mm long and 3 mm to 4 mm wide. The mericarps, usually free, are glabrous. Each bears five prominent slightly carenated ridges. When cut transversely, four vittae on the dorsal surface and two on the commissural surface may be seen with a lens.

B. Reduce to a powder (355). The powder is greyish-brown to greyish-yellow. Examine under a microscope using *chloral hydrate solution R*. The powder shows the following diagnostic characters: yellow fragments of wide secretory canals, often made up of yellowish-brown-walled polygonal secretory cells, frequently associated with a layer of thin-walled transversely elongated cells 2 µm to 9 µm wide, having a parquetry arrangement; reticulate parenchyma of the mesocarp; numerous fibre bundles from the ridges, often accompanied by narrow spiral vessels; very numerous endosperm fragments containing aleurone grains and very small calcium oxalate microrosette crystals, as well as some fibre bundles from the carpophore.

C. Examine by thin-layer chromatography (*2.2.27*), using *silica gel GF_{254} R* as the coating substance.

Test solution. Shake 0.3 g of the freshly powdered drug (1400) with 5.0 ml of *methylene chloride R* for 15 min. Filter and carefully evaporate the filtrate to dryness on a water-bath at 60 °C. Dissolve the residue in 0.5 ml of *toluene R*.

Reference solution. Dissolve 60 µl of *anethole R* in 5.0 ml of *hexane R*.

Apply separately to the plate, as bands 20 mm by 3 mm, 10 µl of each solution. Develop over a path of 10 cm using a mixture of 20 volumes of *hexane R* and 80 volumes of *toluene R*. Allow the plate to dry in air and examine in ultraviolet light at 254 nm. The chromatograms show in the central part a quenching zone corresponding to anethole. Spray the plate with *sulphuric acid R* and heat at 140 °C for 5 min. Examine in daylight. The chromatograms show in the central part a violet band corresponding to anethole. The chromatogram obtained with the test solution also shows a reddish-brown zone in its upper third (terpenes).

TESTS

Estragole and fenchone. The essential oil obtained in the assay contains not more than 10.0 per cent of estragole and not more than 7.5 per cent of fenchone.

Proceed as described in the assay for anethole, using the following reference solution.

Reference solution. Dissolve 5 mg of *estragole R* and 5 mg of *fenchone R* in 0.5 ml of *xylene R*.

Determine the contents of estragole and fenchone by normalisation.

Foreign matter (*2.8.2*). Not more than 1.5 per cent of peduncles and not more than 1.5 per cent of other foreign matter.

Water (*2.2.13*). Not more than 80 ml/kg, determined by distillation on 20.0 g of the powdered drug (710).

Total ash (*2.4.16*). Not more than 10.0 per cent.

ASSAY

Essential oil. Carry out the determination of essential oils in vegetable drugs (*2.8.12*). Use a 500 ml round-bottomed flask and 200 ml of *water R* as the distillation liquid. Reduce the drug to a coarse powder (1400) and immediately use 10.0 g for the determination. Introduce 0.50 ml of *xylene R* in the graduated tube. Distil at a rate of 2 ml/min to 3 ml/min for 2 h.

Anethole. Examine by gas chromatography (*2.2.28*).

Test solution. Dilute the mixture of essential oil and *xylene R* obtained in the determination of the essential oil to 5.0 ml with *xylene R* and by rinsing the apparatus.

Reference solution. Dissolve 5 mg of *anethole R* in 0.5 ml of *xylene R*.

The chromatographic procedure may be carried out using:

- a capillary column 30 m to 60 m long and 0.3 mm in internal diameter coated with *macrogol 20 000 R*,
- *nitrogen for chromatography R* as the carrier gas at a flow rate of 0.40 ml/min and split at a ratio of 1 to 200,
- a flame-ionisation detector,

maintaining the temperature of the column at 60 °C for 4 min, then raising the temperature linearly at a rate of 5 °C per minute to 170 °C and maintaining at 170 °C for 15 min and maintaining the temperature of the injection port at 220 °C and that of the detector at 270 °C.

Inject 1 µl of each solution. Determine the content of anethole by normalisation.

STORAGE

Store protected from light and moisture.

Monographs F-H

01/2005:1322

FENOFIBRATE

Fenofibratum

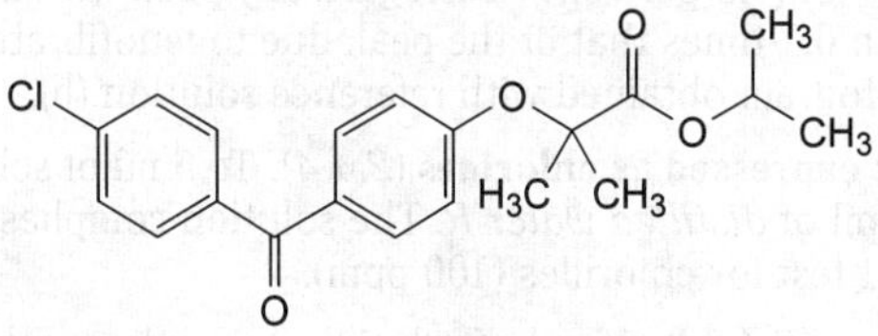

$C_{20}H_{21}ClO_4$ M_r 360.8

DEFINITION

Fenofibrate contains not less than 98.5 per cent and not more than the equivalent of 101.0 per cent of 1-methylethyl 2-[4-(4-chlorobenzoyl)phenoxy]-2-methylpropanoate, calculated with reference to the dried substance.

CHARACTERS

A white or almost white, crystalline powder, practically insoluble in water, very soluble in methylene chloride, slightly soluble in alcohol.

IDENTIFICATION

A. Melting point (*2.2.14*): 79 °C to 82 °C.

B. Examine by infrared absorption spectrophotometry (*2.2.24*), comparing with the spectrum obtained with *fenofibrate CRS*. Examine the substances prepared as discs.

TESTS

Solution S. To 5.0 g, add 25 ml of *distilled water R* and heat at 50 °C for 10 min. Cool and dilute to 50.0 ml with the same solvent. Filter. Use the filtrate as solution S.

Appearance of solution. Dissolve 0.50 g in *acetone R* and dilute to 10.0 ml with the same solvent. The solution is clear (*2.2.1*) and not more intensely coloured than reference solution BY_6 (*2.2.2, Method II*).

Acidity. Dissolve 1.0 g in 50 ml of *alcohol R* previously neutralised using 0.2 ml of *phenolphthalein solution R1*. Not more than 0.2 ml of *0.1 M sodium hydroxide* is required to change the colour of the indicator to pink.

Related substances. Examine by liquid chromatography (*2.2.29*) as described under Assay.

Inject 20 µl of reference solution (b). Adjust the sensitivity of the system so that the height of the peaks in the chromatogram obtained is at least 20 per cent of the full scale of the recorder. When the chromatograms are recorded in the prescribed conditions, the relative retention times are: impurity A about 0.34, impurity B about 0.36, impurity C about 0.50, impurity D about 0.65, impurity E about 0.80, impurity F about 0.85 and impurity G about 1.35. The test is not valid unless the resolution between the peaks corresponding to impurity A and impurity B is at least 1.5.

Inject 20 µl of reference solution (b) and 20 µl of the test solution. Continue the chromatography of the test solution for twice the retention time of fenofibrate. In the chromatogram obtained with the test solution, the area of any peak corresponding to impurity A, impurity B or impurity G is not greater than that of the corresponding peak in the chromatogram obtained with reference solution (b) (0.1 per cent for impurities A and B and 0.2 per cent for impurity G); the area of any peak, apart from the principal peak and any peaks corresponding to impurities A, B and G, is not greater than the area of the peak corresponding to fenofibrate in the chromatogram obtained with reference solution (b) (0.1 per cent); the sum of the areas of all the peaks, apart from the principal peak, is not greater than five times the area of the peak corresponding to fenofibrate in the chromatogram obtained with reference solution (b) (0.5 per cent). Disregard any peak with an area less than 0.1 times that of the peak due to fenofibrate in the chromatogram obtained with reference solution (b).

Halides expressed as chlorides (*2.4.4*). To 5 ml of solution S add 10 ml of *distilled water R*. The solution complies with the limit test for chlorides (100 ppm).

Sulphates (*2.4.13*). 15 ml of solution S complies with the limit test for sulphates (100 ppm).

Heavy metals (*2.4.8*). 1.0 g complies with limit test C for heavy metals (20 ppm). Prepare the standard using 2 ml of *lead standard solution (10 ppm Pb) R*.

Loss on drying (*2.2.32*). Not more than 0.5 per cent, determined on 1.000 g by drying *in vacuo* at 60 °C.

Sulphated ash (*2.4.14*). Not more than 0.1 per cent, determined on 1.0 g.

ASSAY

Examine by liquid chromatography (*2.2.29*).

Test solution. Dissolve 0.100 g of the substance to be examined in the mobile phase and dilute to 100.0 ml with the mobile phase.

Reference solution (a). Dissolve 25.0 mg of *fenofibrate CRS* in the mobile phase and dilute to 25.0 ml with the mobile phase.

Reference solution (b). Dissolve 10.0 mg of *fenofibrate CRS*, 10.0 mg of *fenofibrate impurity A CRS*, 10.0 mg of *fenofibrate impurity B CRS* and 20.0 mg of *fenofibrate impurity G CRS* in the mobile phase and dilute to 100.0 ml with the mobile phase. Dilute 1.0 ml of this solution to 100.0 ml with the mobile phase.

The chromatographic procedure may be carried out using:

- a stainless steel column 0.25 m long and 4.0 mm in internal diameter packed with *octadecylsilyl silica gel for chromatography R* (5 µm),
- as mobile phase at a flow rate of 1 ml/min a mixture of 30 volumes of *water R* acidified to pH 2.5 with *phosphoric acid R* and 70 volumes of *acetonitrile R*,
- as detector a spectrophotometer set at 286 nm.

Inject 5 µl of reference solution (b). Adjust the sensitivity of the system so that the height of the peaks in the chromatogram is at least 50 per cent of the full scale of the recorder. Inject 5 µl of reference solution (a) six times. The assay is not valid unless the relative standard deviation of the peak area for fenofibrate is at most 1.0 per cent. Inject 5 µl of the test solution and 5 µl of reference solution (a).

STORAGE

Store protected from light.

IMPURITIES

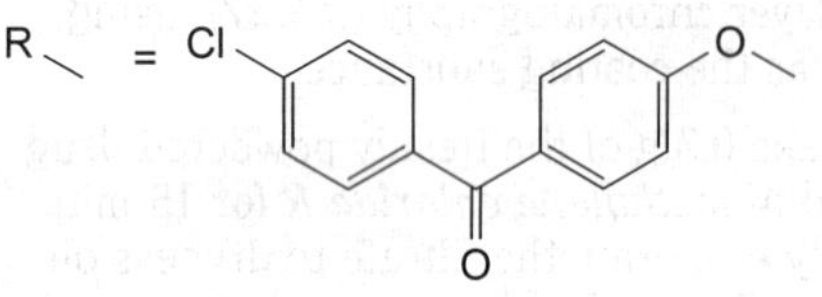

A. R-H: (4-chlorophenyl)(4-hydroxyphenyl)methanone,

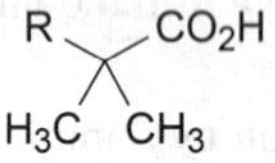

B. 2-[4-(4-chlorobenzoyl)phenoxy]-2-methylpropanoic acid (fenofibric acid),

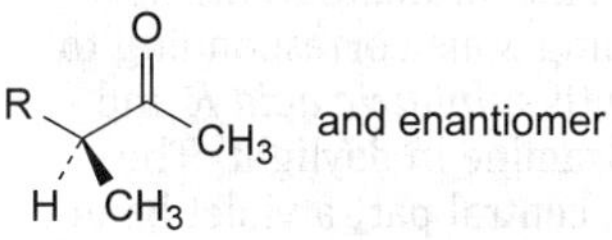

C. (3*RS*)-3-[4-(4-chlorobenzoyl)phenoxy]butan-2-one,

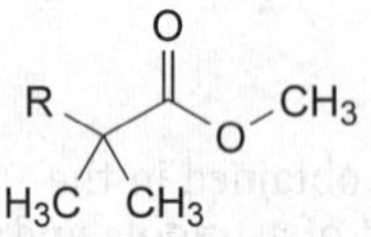

D. methyl 2-[4-(4-chlorobenzoyl)phenoxy]-2-methylpropanoate,

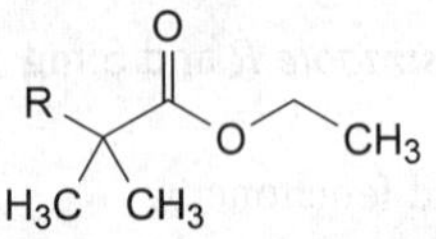

E. ethyl 2-[4-(4-chlorobenzoyl)phenoxy]-2-methylpropanoate,

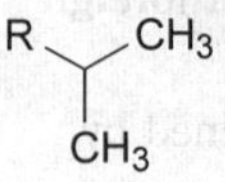

F. (4-chlorophenyl)[4-(1-methylethoxy)phenyl]methanone,

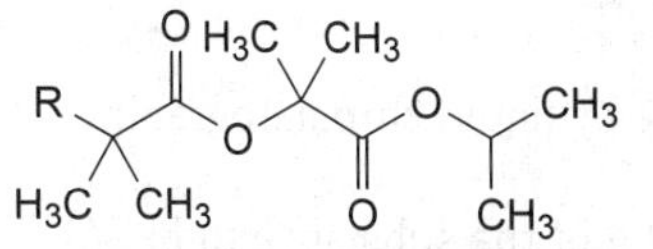

G. 1-methylethyl 2-[[2-[4-(4-chlorobenzoyl)phenoxy]-2-methylpropanoyl]oxy]-2-methylpropanoate.

01/2005:0901

FENOTEROL HYDROBROMIDE

Fenoteroli hydrobromidum

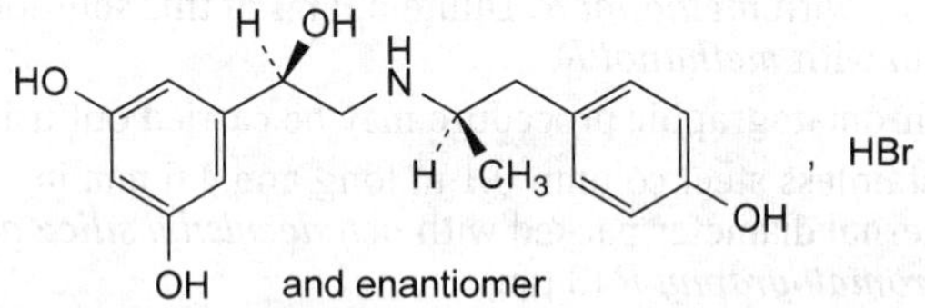

and enantiomer

$C_{17}H_{22}BrNO_4$ M_r 384.3

DEFINITION

(1*RS*)-1-(3,5-dihydoxyphenyl)-2-[[(1*RS*)-2-(4-hydroxyphenyl)-1-methylethyl]amino]ethanol hydrobromide.

Content: 99.0 per cent to 101.0 per cent (dried substance).

CHARACTERS

Appearance: white, crystalline powder.

Solubility: soluble in water and in alcohol.

IDENTIFICATION

First identification: B, E.

Second identification: A, C, D, E.

A. Dissolve 50.0 mg in *dilute hydrochloric acid R1* and dilute to 50.0 ml with the same acid. Dilute 5.0 ml to 50.0 ml with *dilute hydrochloric acid R1*. Examined between 230 nm and 350 nm (*2.2.25*), the solution shows an absorption maximum at 275 nm and a shoulder at about 280 nm. The specific absorbance at the maximum is 80 to 86.

B. Infrared absorption spectrophotometry (*2.2.24*).

Preparation: discs.

Comparison: *Ph. Eur. reference spectrum of fenoterol hydrobromide.*

C. Thin-layer chromatography (*2.2.27*).

Test solution. Dissolve 10 mg of the substance to be examined in *alcohol R* and dilute to 10 ml with the same solvent.

Reference solution. Dissolve 10 mg of *fenoterol hydrobromide CRS* in *alcohol R* and dilute to 10 ml with the same solvent.

Plate: *TLC silica gel G plate R.*

Mobile phase: *concentrated ammonia R, water R, aldehyde-free methanol R* (1.5:10:90 *V/V/V*).

Application: 2 µl.

Development: over a path of 15 cm.

Drying: in air.

Detection: spray with a 10 g/l solution of *potassium permanganate R.*

Results: the principal spot in the chromatogram obtained with the test solution is similar in position, colour and size to the principal spot in the chromatogram obtained with the reference solution.

D. Dissolve about 10 mg in a 20 g/l solution of *disodium tetraborate R* and dilute to 50 ml with the same solution. Add 1 ml of a 10 g/l solution of *aminopyrazolone R,* 10 ml of a 2 g/l solution of *potassium ferricyanide R* and 10 ml of *methylene chloride R*. Shake and allow to separate. A reddish-brown colour develops in the lower layer.

E. It gives reaction (a) of bromides (*2.3.1*).

TESTS

Solution S. Dissolve 2.00 g in *carbon dioxide-free water R* and dilute to 50.0 ml with the same solvent.

Appearance of solution. Solution S is clear (*2.2.1*) and not more intensely coloured than reference solution Y_7 (*2.2.2, Method II*).

pH (*2.2.3*): 4.2 to 5.2 for solution S.

Phenone: maximum 0.2 per cent. The absorbance (*2.2.25*) of solution S at 330 nm has a maximum of 0.42.

Diastereoisomers. Liquid chromatography (*2.2.29*). *Prepare the solutions immediately before use.*

Test solution. Dissolve 25.0 mg of the substance to be examined in *water R* and dilute to 10.0 ml with the same solvent.

Reference solution. Dissolve 25.0 mg of *fenoterol hydrobromide CRS* in *water R* and dilute to 10.0 ml with the same solvent.

Column:

– *size*: *l* = 0.25 m, Ø = 4.6 mm,

– *stationary phase*: *octadecylsilyl silica gel for chromatography R* (5 µm to 10 µm).

Mobile phase: to a mixture of 1 volume of a 9 g/l solution of *potassium dihydrogen phosphate R* and 69 volumes of a 24 g/l solution of *disodium hydrogen phosphate R,* adjusted to pH 8.5 using *phosphoric acid R,* add 30 volumes of *methanol R.*

Flow rate: 1 ml/min.

Detection: spectrophotometer at 280 nm.

Injection: 20 µl loop injector.

Sensitivity: the height of the peak due to the diastereoisomers eluting immediately after the principal peak is not less than 10 per cent of the full scale of the recorder.

System suitability: reference solution:

– the height of the trough separating the peak due to the diastereoisomers from the principal peak is less than 4 per cent of the full scale of the recorder,

– the retention time of the principal peak is less than 20 min.

Limits:

Calculate the content of diastereoisomers by determining the height of a perpendicular dropped from the apex of the peak to a line drawn from the trough between the 2 peaks to the baseline, and taking into account the declared content of diastereoisomers in *fenoterol hydrobromide CRS* (4.0 per cent).

Iron (*2.4.9*): maximum 5 ppm.

Dissolve the residue from the test for sulphated ash in 2.5 ml of *dilute hydrochloric acid R* and dilute to 10 ml with *water R*. The solution complies with the limit test for iron.

Loss on drying (*2.2.32*): maximum 0.5 per cent, determined on 1.000 g by drying in an oven at 100-105 °C.

Sulphated ash (*2.4.14*): maximum 0.1 per cent, determined on 1.0 g.

ASSAY

Dissolve 0.600 g in 50 ml of *water R* and add 5 ml of *dilute nitric acid R*, 25.0 ml of *0.1 M silver nitrate* and 2 ml of *ferric ammonium sulphate solution R2*. Shake and titrate with *0.1 M ammonium thiocyanate* until an orange colour is obtained. Carry out a blank titration.

1 ml of *0.1 M silver nitrate* is equivalent to 38.43 mg of $C_{17}H_{22}BrNO_4$.

STORAGE

Protected from light.

IMPURITIES

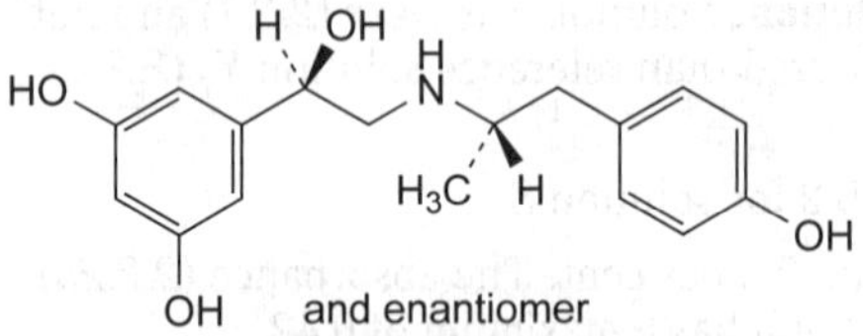

and enantiomer

A. (1*RS*)-1-(3,5-dihydoxyphenyl)-2-[[(1*SR*)-2-(4-hydroxyphenyl)-1-methylethyl]amino]ethanol,

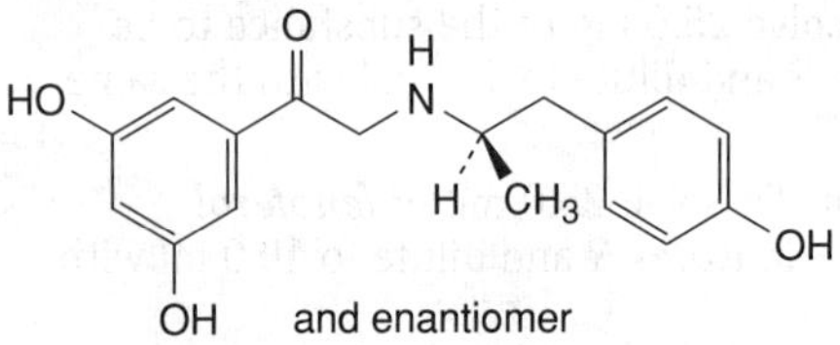

and enantiomer

B. 1-(3,5-dihydoxyphenyl)-2-[[(1*RS*)-2-(4-hydroxyphenyl)-1-methylethyl]amino]ethanone (phenone).

01/2005:1210

FENTANYL

Fentanylum

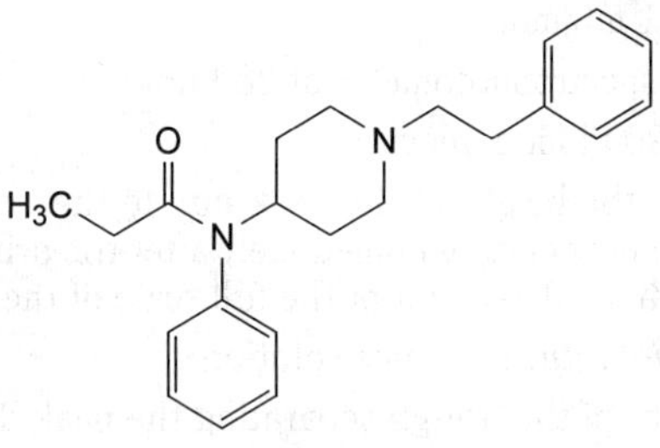

$C_{22}H_{28}N_2O$ M_r 336.5

DEFINITION

Fentanyl contains not less than 99.0 per cent and not more than the equivalent of 101.0 per cent of *N*-phenyl-*N*-[1-(2-phenylethyl)piperidin-4-yl]propanamide, calculated with reference to the dried substance.

CHARACTERS

A white or almost white powder, practically insoluble in water, freely soluble in alcohol and in methanol.

It shows polymorphism.

IDENTIFICATION

Examine by infrared absorption spectrophotometry (*2.2.24*), comparing with the *Ph. Eur. reference spectrum of fentanyl*. If the spectrum obtained in the solid state shows differences, dissolve the substance to be examined in the minimum volume of *ethanol R*, evaporate to dryness at room temperature under an air-stream and record the spectrum again using the residue.

TESTS

Related substances. Examine by liquid chromatography (*2.2.29*).

Test solution. Dissolve 0.100 g of the substance to be examined in *methanol R* and dilute to 10.0 ml with the same solvent.

Reference solution (a). In order to prepare the *in situ* degradation compound (fentanyl impurity D), dissolve 10 mg of the substance to be examined in 10.0 ml of *dilute hydrochloric acid R*. Heat on a water-bath under a reflux condenser for 4 h. Neutralise with 10.0 ml of *dilute sodium hydroxide solution R*. Evaporate to dryness on a water-bath. Cool and take up the residue in 10 ml of *methanol R*. Filter.

Reference solution (b). Dilute 1.0 ml of the test solution to 100.0 ml with *methanol R*. Dilute 5.0 ml of this solution to 20.0 ml with *methanol R*.

The chromatographic procedure may be carried out using:

- a stainless steel column 0.1 m long and 4.6 mm in internal diameter packed with *octadecylsilyl silica gel for chromatography R* (3 μm),
- as mobile phase at a flow rate of 1.5 ml/min the following mixtures:

  Mobile phase A. A 5 g/l solution of *ammonium carbonate R* in a mixture of 10 volumes of *tetrahydrofuran R* and 90 volumes of *water R*,

  Mobile phase B. *Acetonitrile R*,

Time (min)	Mobile phase A (per cent *V/V*)	Mobile phase B (per cent *V/V*)	Comment
0 - 15	90 → 40	10 → 60	linear gradient
15 - 20	40	60	isocratic elution
20 - 25	90	10	switch to initial eluent composition
20 = 0	90	10	restart gradient

- as detector a spectrophotometer set at 220 nm.

Equilibrate the column for at least 30 min with *acetonitrile R* and then equilibrate at the initial eluent composition for at least 5 min.

Adjust the sensitivity of the system so that the height of the principal peak in the chromatogram obtained with 10 μl of reference solution (b) is at least 50 per cent of the full scale of the recorder.

Inject 10 μl of reference solution (a). When the chromatograms are recorded in the prescribed conditions, the retention times are: fentanyl about 10 min and fentanyl impurity D about 12 min. The test is not valid unless the resolution between the peaks corresponding to fentanyl and fentanyl impurity D is at least 8.0. If necessary, adjust the concentration of acetonitrile in the mobile phase or adjust the time programme for the linear gradient elution.

Inject separately 10 μl of *methanol R* as a blank, 10 μl of the test solution and 10 μl of reference solution (b). In the chromatogram obtained with the test solution: the area of any peak, apart from the principal peak, is not greater than the area of the principal peak in the chromatogram obtained with reference solution (b) (0.25 per cent); the sum of the areas of all peaks, apart from the principal peak, is not greater than twice the area of the principal peak in the chromatogram obtained with reference solution (b) (0.5 per cent). Disregard any peak obtained with the blank run and any peak with an area less than 0.2 times the area of the principal peak in the chromatogram obtained with reference solution (b).

Loss on drying (*2.2.32*). Not more than 0.5 per cent, determined on 1.000 g by drying *in vacuo* at 50 °C.

ASSAY

Dissolve 0.200 g in 50 ml of a mixture of 1 volume of *anhydrous acetic acid R* and 7 volumes of *methyl ethyl ketone R* and titrate with *0.1 M perchloric acid*, using 0.2 ml of *naphtholbenzein solution R* as indicator.

1 ml of *0.1 M perchloric acid* is equivalent to 33.65 mg of $C_{22}H_{28}N_2O$.

STORAGE

Store protected from light.

IMPURITIES

Specified impurities: A, B, C, D.

Other detectable impurities: E, F, G.

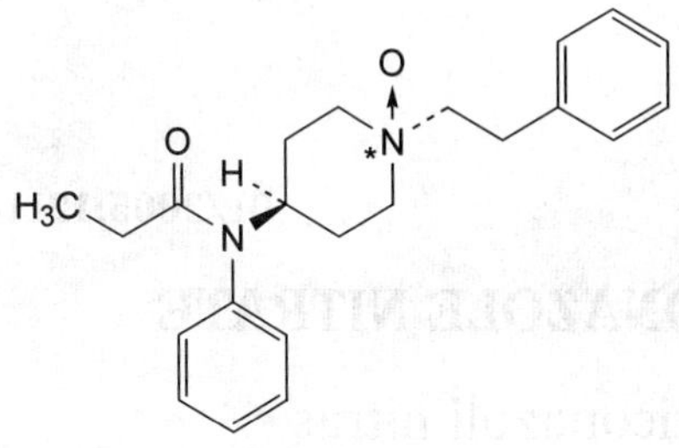

A. *N*-phenyl-*N*-[*cis,trans*-1-oxido-1-(2-phenylethyl)piperidin-4-yl]propanamide,

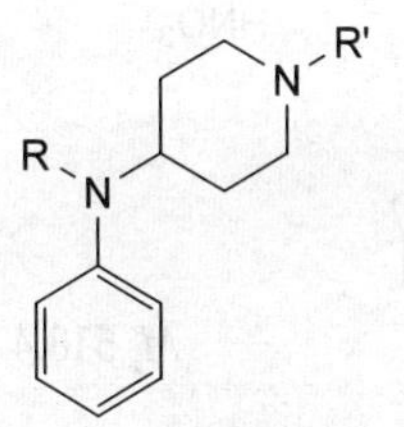

B. R = CO-C_2H_5, R′ = H: *N*-phenyl-*N*-(piperidin-4-yl)propanamide,

C. R = CO-CH_3, R′ = CH_2-CH_2-C_6H_5: *N*-phenyl-*N*-[1-(2-phenylethyl)piperidin-4-yl]acetamide,

D. R = H, R′ = CH_2-CH_2-C_6H_5: *N*-phenyl-1-(2-phenylethyl)piperidin-4-amine,

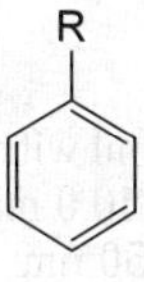

E. R = CHO: benzaldehyde,

F. R = NH_2: aniline (phenylamine),

G. R = NH-CO-C_2H_5: *N*-phenylpropanamide.

01/2005:1103

FENTANYL CITRATE

Fentanyli citras

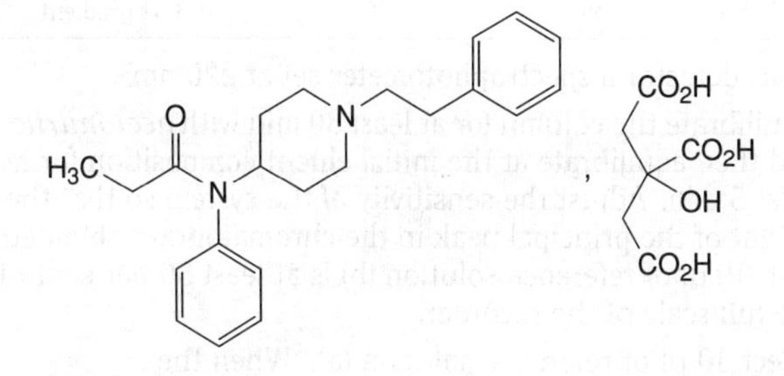

$C_{28}H_{36}N_2O_8$ M_r 528.6

DEFINITION

Fentanyl citrate contains not less than 99.0 per cent and not more than the equivalent of 101.0 per cent of *N*-phenyl-*N*-[1-(2-phenylethyl)piperidin-4-yl]propanamide dihydrogen 2-hydroxypropane-1,2,3-tricarboxylate, calculated with reference to the dried substance.

CHARACTERS

A white or almost white powder, soluble in water, freely soluble in methanol, sparingly soluble in alcohol.

It melts at about 152 °C with decomposition.

IDENTIFICATION

Examine by infrared absorption spectrophotometry (*2.2.24*), comparing with the *Ph. Eur. reference spectrum of fentanyl citrate*.

TESTS

Appearance of solution. Dissolve 0.2 g of the substance to be examined in *water R* and dilute to 20 ml with the same solvent. The solution is clear (*2.2.1*) and colourless (*2.2.2, Method II*).

Related substances. Examine by liquid chromatography (*2.2.29*).

Test solution. Dissolve 0.100 g of the substance to be examined in *methanol R* and dilute to 10.0 ml with the same solvent.

Reference solution (a). In order to prepare the *in situ* degradation compound (impurity D), dissolve 10 mg of the substance to be examined in 10.0 ml of *dilute hydrochloric acid R*. Heat on a water-bath under a reflux condenser for 4 h. Neutralise with 10.0 ml of *dilute sodium hydroxide solution R*. Evaporate to dryness on a water-bath. Cool and take up the residue in 10 ml of *methanol R*. Filter.

Reference solution (b). Dilute 1.0 ml of the test solution to 100.0 ml with *methanol R*. Dilute 5.0 ml of the solution to 20.0 ml with *methanol R*.

The chromatographic procedure may be carried out using:

- a stainless steel column 0.1 m long and 4.6 mm in internal diameter packed with *octadecylsilyl silica gel for chromatography R* (3 µm),
- as mobile phase at a flow rate of 1.5 ml/min a gradient programme using the following conditions:

Mobile phase A. A 5 g/l solution of *ammonium carbonate R* in a mixture of 10 volumes of *tetrahydrofuran R* and 90 volumes of *water R*,

Mobile phase B. Acetonitrile R,

Time (min)	Mobile phase A (per cent *V/V*)	Mobile phase B (per cent *V/V*)	Comment
0 - 15	$90 \rightarrow 40$	$10 \rightarrow 60$	linear gradient
15 - 20	40	60	isocratic elution
20 - 25	90	10	switch to initial eluent composition
25 = 0	90	10	restart gradient

– as detector a spectrophotometer set at 220 nm.

Equilibrate the column for at least 30 min with *acetonitrile R* and then equilibrate at the initial eluent composition for at least 5 min. Adjust the sensitivity of the system so that the height of the principal peak in the chromatogram obtained with 10 µl of reference solution (b) is at least 50 per cent of the full scale of the recorder.

Inject 10 µl of reference solution (a). When the chromatograms are recorded in the prescribed conditions, the retention times are: fentanyl about 10 min; impurity D about 12 min. The test is not valid unless the resolution between the peaks corresponding to fentanyl and impurity D is at least 8.0. If necessary, adjust the concentration of acetonitrile in the mobile phase or adjust the time programme for the linear gradient elution.

Inject separately 10 µl of *methanol R* as a blank, 10 µl of the test solution and 10 µl of reference solution (b). In the chromatogram obtained with the test solution: the area of any peak, apart from the principal peak, is not greater than the area of the principal peak in the chromatogram obtained with reference solution (b) (0.25 per cent); the sum of the areas of all peaks, apart from the principal peak, is not greater than twice the area of the principal peak in the chromatogram obtained with reference solution (b) (0.5 per cent). Disregard any peak obtained with the blank run and any peak with a retention time relative to the principal peak of 0.05 or less and any peak with an area less than 0.2 times the area of the principal peak in the chromatogram obtained with reference solution (b).

Loss on drying (*2.2.32*). Not more than 0.5 per cent, determined on 1.000 g by drying *in vacuo* at 60 °C.

ASSAY

Dissolve 0.300 g in 50 ml of a mixture of 1 volume of *anhydrous acetic acid R* and 7 volumes of *methyl ethyl ketone R*. Titrate with *0.1 M perchloric acid* using 0.2 ml of *naphtholbenzein solution R* as indicator.

1 ml of *0.1 M perchloric acid* is equivalent to 52.86 mg of $C_{28}H_{36}N_2O_8$.

STORAGE

Store protected from light.

IMPURITIES

Specified impurities: A, B, C, D.

Other detectable impurities: E.

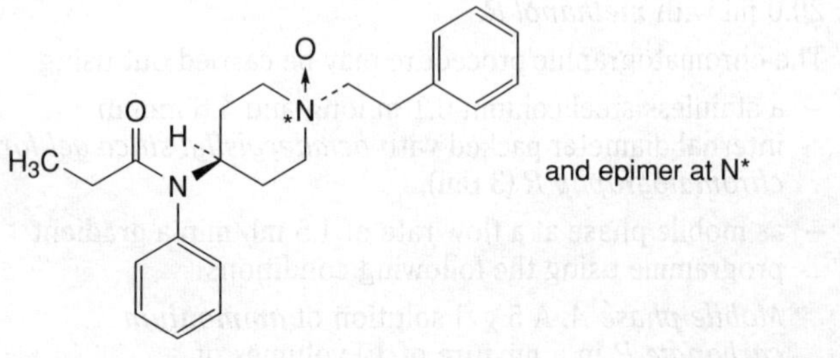

A. *N*-phenyl-*N*-[*cis,trans*-1-oxido-1-(2-phenylethyl)piperidin-4-yl]propanamide,

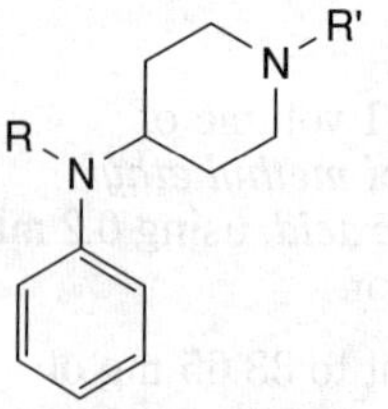

B. R = CO-C_2H_5, R′ = H: *N*-phenyl-*N*-(piperidin-4-yl)propanamide,

C. R = CO-CH_3, R′ = CH_2-CH_2-C_6H_5: *N*-phenyl-*N*-[1-(2-phenylethyl)piperidin-4-yl]acetamide,

D. R = H, R′ = CH_2-CH_2-C_6H_5: *N*-phenyl-1-(2-phenylethyl)piperidin-4-amine,

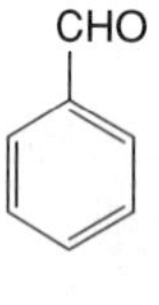

E. benzaldehyde.

01/2005:1211

FENTICONAZOLE NITRATE

Fenticonazoli nitras

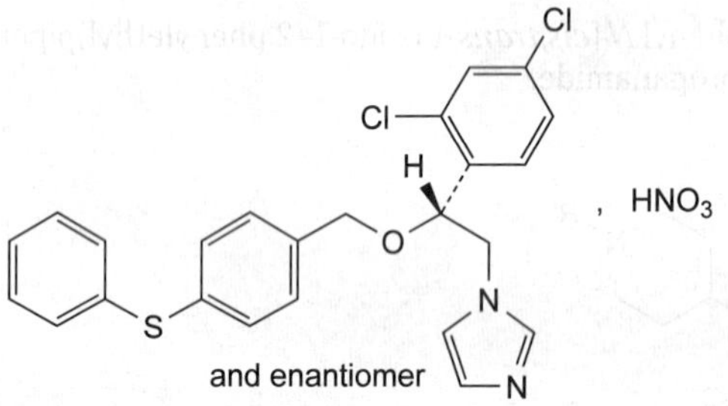

$C_{24}H_{21}Cl_2N_3O_4S$ M_r 518.4

DEFINITION

Fenticonazole nitrate contains not less than 99.0 per cent and not more than the equivalent of 101.0 per cent of 1-[(2*RS*)-2-(2,4-dichlorophenyl)-2-[[4-(phenylsulphanyl)benzyl]oxy]ethyl]-1*H*-imidazole nitrate, calculated with reference to the dried substance.

CHARACTERS

A white or almost white, crystalline powder, practically insoluble in water, freely soluble in methanol and in dimethylformamide, sparingly soluble in ethanol.

IDENTIFICATION

First identification: C, D.

Second identification: A, B, D.

A. Melting point (*2.2.14*): 134 °C to 137 °C.

B. Dissolve 20.0 mg in *ethanol R* and dilute to 100.0 ml with the same solvent. Dilute 1.0 ml of this solution to 10.0 ml with *ethanol R*. Examined between 230 nm and 350 nm (*2.2.25*), the solution shows an absorption maximum at 252 nm, a shoulder at about 270 nm and an absorption minimum at 236 nm. The specific absorption at the maximum is 260 to 280.

C. Examine by infrared absorption spectrophotometry (*2.2.24*), comparing with the spectrum obtained with *fenticonazole nitrate CRS*.

D. It gives the reaction of nitrates (*2.3.1*).

TESTS

Optical rotation (*2.2.7*). Dissolve 0.10 g in *methanol R* and dilute to 10.0 ml with the same solvent. The angle of optical rotation is − 0.10° to + 0.10°.

Related substances. Examine by liquid chromatography (*2.2.29*).

Test solution. Dissolve 25.0 mg of the substance to be examined in the mobile phase and dilute to 25.0 ml with the mobile phase.

Reference solution (a). Dilute 1.0 ml of the test solution to 200.0 ml with the mobile phase.

Reference solution (b). Dilute 10.0 ml of reference solution (a) to 25.0 ml with the mobile phase.

Reference solution (c). Dilute 1.0 ml of reference solution (a) to 10.0 ml with the mobile phase.

Reference solution (d). To 5 ml of the test solution add 5.0 mg of *fenticonazole impurity D CRS*, dissolve in the mobile phase and dilute to 100.0 ml with the mobile phase. Dilute 2.0 ml of this solution to 10.0 ml with the mobile phase.

The chromatographic procedure may be carried out using:

- a stainless steel column 0.25 m long and 4 mm in internal diameter packed with *octadecylsilyl silica gel for chromatography R* (5 µm to 10 µm),
- as mobile phase at a flow rate of 1.0 ml/min a mixture of 70 volumes of *acetonitrile R* and 30 volumes of a phosphate buffer solution prepared by dissolving 3.4 g of *potassium dihydrogen phosphate R* in 900 ml of *water R*, adjusting to pH 3.0 with *phosphoric acid R* and diluting to 1000 ml with *water R*,
- as detector a spectrophotometer set at 229 nm.

Inject 10 µl of reference solution (b). Adjust the sensitivity of the system so that the height of the peak due to fenticonazole is at least 10 per cent of the full scale of the recorder.

Inject separately 10 µl of reference solution (c) and 10 µl of reference solution (d). The test is not valid unless in the chromatogram obtained with reference solution (d), the resolution between the peak due to fenticonazole impurity D and fenticonazole is at least 2.0. The test is not valid unless in the chromatogram obtained with reference solution (c) the signal-to-noise ratio is at least five.

Inject separately 10 µl of the test solution and 10 µl of reference solution (a). Record the chromatogram obtained with the test solution for 5.5 times the retention time of the principal peak. In the chromatogram obtained with the test solution: the area of any peak apart from the principal peak and the nitric ion peak (which corresponds to the dead volume of the column), is not greater than the area of the principal peak in the chromatogram obtained with reference solution (b) (0.2 per cent) and the sum of the areas of such peaks is not greater than the area of the principal peak in the chromatogram obtained with reference solution (a) (0.5 per cent). Disregard any peak with an area less than that of the principal peak in the chromatogram obtained with reference solution (c).

Toluene. Not more than 100 ppm, determined by head-space gas chromatography (*2.2.28*), using the standard additions method.

Test solution. Disperse 0.2 g of the substance to be examined in a 10 ml vial with 5 ml of *water R*.

Reference solution. Mix 4 mg of *toluene R* with *water R* and dilute to 1000 ml. Place 5 ml of this solution in a 10 ml vial.

The chromatographic procedure may be carried out using:

- a column 25 m long and 0.32 mm in internal diameter coated with *poly(cyanopropyl)(7)phenyl(7)methyl(86)siloxane R* (film thickness 1.2 µm),
- *helium for chromatography R* as the carrier gas, split ratio 1:25, column head pressure 40 kPa,
- a flame-ionisation detector,

maintaining the temperature of the column at 80 °C, that of the injection port at 180 °C and that of the detector at 220 °C. Maintain each solution at 90 °C for 1 h, and transfer onto the column 1 ml of the vapour phase.

Loss on drying (*2.2.32*). Not more than 0.5 per cent, determined on 1.000 g by drying *in vacuo* at 60 °C.

Sulphated ash (*2.4.14*). Not more than 0.1 per cent, determined on 1.0 g.

ASSAY

Dissolve 0.450 g in 50 ml of a mixture of equal volumes of *anhydrous acetic acid R* and *methyl ethyl ketone R*. Titrate with *0.1 M perchloric acid*, determining the end-point potentiometrically (*2.2.20*).

1 ml of *0.1 M perchloric acid* is equivalent to 51.84 mg of $C_{24}H_{21}Cl_2N_3O_4S$.

STORAGE

Store protected from light.

IMPURITIES

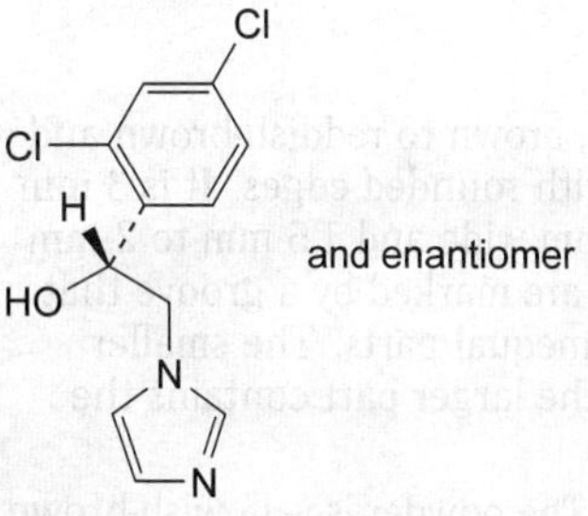

A. (*RS*)-1-(2,4-dichlorophenyl)-2-(1*H*-imidazol-1-yl)ethanol,

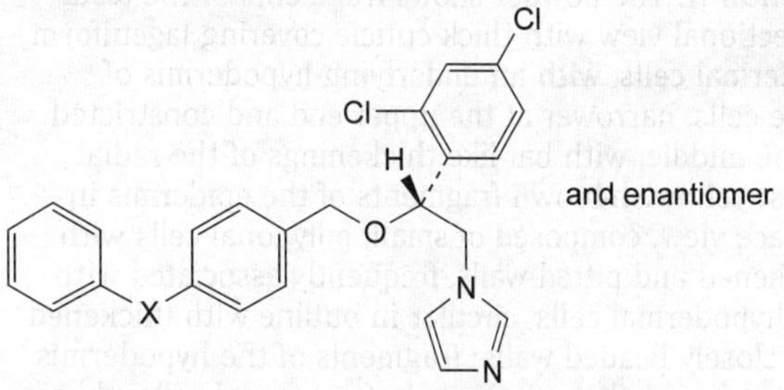

B. X = SO: 1-[(2*RS*)-2-(2,4-dichlorophenyl)-2-[[4-(phenylsulphinyl)benzyl]oxy]ethyl]-1*H*-imidazole,

C. X = SO_2: 1-[(2*RS*)-2-(2,4-dichlorophenyl)-2-[[4-(phenylsulphonyl)benzyl]oxy]ethyl]-1*H*-imidazole,

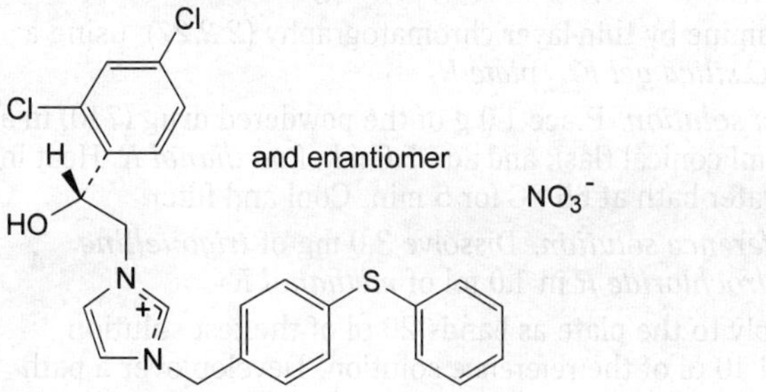

D. (*RS*)-1-[2-(2,4-dichlorophenyl)-2-hydroxyethyl]-3-[4-(phenylsulphanyl)benzyl]imidazolium nitrate,

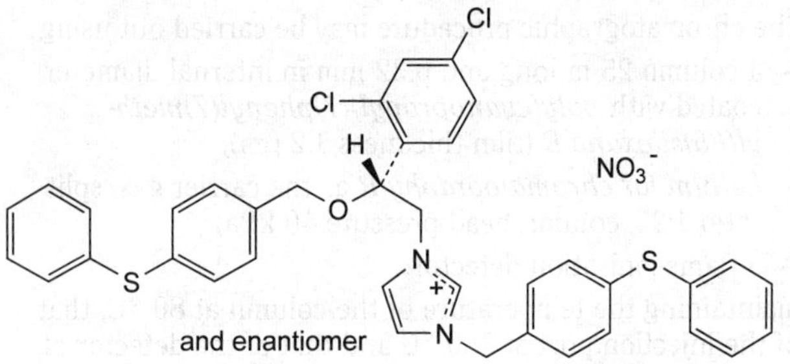

E. (RS)-1-[2-(2,4-dichlorophenyl)-2-[4-(phenylsulphanyl)benzyloxy]ethyl]-3-[4-(phenylsulphanyl)benzyl]imidazolium nitrate.

01/2005:1323

FENUGREEK

Trigonellae foenugraeci semen

DEFINITION

Fenugreek consists of the dried, ripe seeds of *Trigonella foenum-graecum* L.

CHARACTERS

Fenugreek has a strong characteristic aromatic odour.

It has the macroscopic and microscopic characters described under identification tests A and B.

IDENTIFICATION

A. The seed is hard, flattened, brown to reddish-brown and more or less rhomboidal with rounded edges. It is 3 mm to 5 mm long, 2 mm to 3 mm wide and 1.5 mm to 2 mm thick. The widest surfaces are marked by a groove that divides the seed into two unequal parts. The smaller part contains the radicle; the larger part contains the cotyledons.

B. Reduce to a powder (355). The powder is yellowish-brown. Examine under a microscope using *chloral hydrate solution R*. The powder shows fragments of the testa in sectional view with thick cuticle covering lageniform epidermal cells, with an underlying hypodermis of large cells, narrower at the upper end and constricted in the middle, with bar-like thickenings of the radial walls; yellowish-brown fragments of the epidermis in surface view, composed of small, polygonal cells with thickened and pitted walls, frequently associated with the hypodermal cells, circular in outline with thickened and closely beaded walls; fragments of the hypodermis viewed from below, composed of polygonal cells whose bar-like thickenings extend to the upper and lower walls; parenchyma of the testa with elongated, rectangular cells with slightly thickened and beaded walls; fragments of endosperm with irregularly thickened, sometimes elongated cells, containing mucilage.

C. Examine by thin-layer chromatography (*2.2.27*), using a *TLC silica gel F_{254} plate R*.

Test solution. Place 1.0 g of the powdered drug (710) in a 25 ml conical flask and add 5.0 ml of *methanol R*. Heat in a water-bath at 65 °C for 5 min. Cool and filter.

Reference solution. Dissolve 3.0 mg of *trigonelline hydrochloride R* in 1.0 ml of *methanol R*.

Apply to the plate as bands 20 µl of the test solution and 10 µl of the reference solution. Develop over a path of 10 cm using a mixture of 30 volumes of *water R* and 70 volumes of *methanol R*. Allow the plate to dry in air and examine in ultraviolet light at 254 nm. The chromatogram obtained with the test solution shows in its lower half a quenching zone similar in position and fluorescence to the zone in the chromatogram obtained with the reference solution. Spray with *potassium iodobismuthate solution R2*. The chromatogram obtained with the test solution shows an intense orange-red zone similar in position and colour to the zone in the chromatogram obtained with the reference solution. It also shows in its upper half a broad, light brownish-yellow zone (triglycerides).

TESTS

Foreign matter (*2.8.2*). It complies with the test for foreign matter.

Swelling index (*2.8.4*). Not less than 6, determined on the powdered drug (710).

Loss on drying (*2.2.32*). Not more than 12.0 per cent, determined on 1.000 g of the powdered drug by drying in an oven at 100 °C to 105 °C for 2 h.

Total ash (*2.4.16*). Not more than 5.0 per cent.

STORAGE

Store protected from light.

01/2005:1515

FERRIC CHLORIDE HEXAHYDRATE

Ferri chloridum hexahydricum

$FeCl_3,6H_2O$ M_r 270.3

DEFINITION

Ferric chloride hexahydrate contains not less than 98.0 per cent and not more than 102.0 per cent of $FeCl_3,6H_2O$.

CHARACTERS

Crystalline mass or orange-yellow to brownish-yellow crystals, very hygroscopic, very soluble in water and in alcohol, freely soluble in glycerol.

IDENTIFICATION

A. It gives reaction (a) of chlorides (*2.3.1*).

B. It gives reaction (c) of iron (*2.3.1*).

TESTS

Solution S. Dissolve 10 g in *distilled water R* and dilute to 100 ml with the same solvent.

Acidity. In a suitable polyethylene container, dissolve 3.0 g of *potassium fluoride R* in 15 ml of *water R*. Titrate with *0.1 M sodium hydroxide* using 0.1 ml of *phenolphthalein solution R* as indicator until a pink colour is obtained. Add 10 ml of solution S and allow to stand for 3 h. Filter and use 12.5 ml of the filtrate. Not more than 0.30 ml of *0.1 M sodium hydroxide* is required to change the colour of the indicator to pink.

Free chlorine. Heat 5 ml of solution S. The vapour does not turn *starch iodide paper R* blue.

Sulphates (*2.4.13*). Heat 15 ml of solution S on a water-bath and add 5 ml of *strong sodium hydroxide solution R*. Allow to cool and filter. Neutralise the filtrate to *blue litmus paper R* using *hydrochloric acid R1* and evaporate to 15 ml. The solution complies with the limit test for sulphates (100 ppm).

Ferrous ions. To 10 ml of solution S, add 1 ml of *water R*, 0.05 ml of *potassium ferricyanide solution R* followed by 4 ml of *phosphoric acid R*. After 10 min, any blue colour in the solution is not more intense than that in a standard prepared at the same time and in the same manner using 10 ml of *water R* and 1 ml of a freshly prepared 0.250 g/l solution of *ferrous sulphate R* (50 ppm Fe).

Heavy metals (*2.4.8*). Dissolve 1.0 g in 10 ml of *hydrochloric acid R1*. Add 2 ml of *strong hydrogen peroxide solution R*, then evaporate to 5 ml. Allow to cool and dilute to 20 ml with *hydrochloric acid R1* and transfer the solution to a separating funnel. Shake three times, for 3 min each time, with 20 ml of *methyl isobutyl ketone R1*. Separate the lower phase, reduce to half its volume by evaporation and dilute to 25 ml with *water R*. Neutralise 10 ml of the solution with *dilute ammonia R1* to *red litmus paper R* and dilute to 20 ml with *water R*. 12 ml of the solution complies with limit test A for heavy metals (50 ppm). Prepare the standard using *lead standard solution (1 ppm Pb) R*.

ASSAY

In a conical flask with a ground-glass stopper, dissolve 0.200 g in 20 ml of *water R*. Add 10 ml of *dilute hydrochloric acid R* and 2 g of *potassium iodide R*. Allow the stoppered flask to stand for 1 h protected from light. Titrate with *0.1 M sodium thiosulphate*, using 5 ml of *starch solution R* as indicator, added towards the end of the titration.

1 ml of *0.1 M sodium thiosulphate* is equivalent to 27.03 mg of $FeCl_3,6H_2O$.

STORAGE

Store in an airtight container, protected from light.

01/2005:0902

FERROUS FUMARATE

Ferrosi fumaras

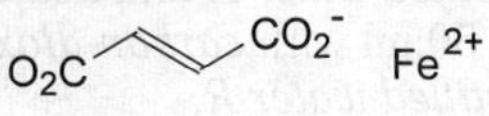

$C_4H_2FeO_4$ M_r 169.9

DEFINITION

Ferrous fumarate contains not less than 93.0 per cent and not more than the equivalent of 101.0 per cent of iron(II) (*E*)-butenedioate, calculated with reference to the dried substance.

CHARACTERS

A fine, reddish-orange or reddish-brown powder, slightly soluble in water, very slightly soluble in alcohol.

IDENTIFICATION

A. Examine by thin-layer chromatography (*2.2.27*), using a *TLC silica gel F_{254} plate R*.

Test solution. To 1.0 g add 25 ml of a mixture of equal volumes of *hydrochloric acid R* and *water R* and heat on a water-bath for 15 min. Cool and filter. Use the filtrate for identification test C. Wash the residue with 50 ml of a mixture of 1 volume of *dilute hydrochloric acid R* and 9 volumes of *water R* and discard the washings. Dry the residue at 100-105 °C. Dissolve 20 mg of the residue in *acetone R* and dilute to 10 ml with the same solvent.

Reference solution. Dissolve 20 mg of *fumaric acid CRS* in *acetone R* and dilute to 10 ml with the same solvent.

Apply to the plate 5 µl of each solution. Develop in an unsaturated tank over a path of 10 cm using a mixture of 12 volumes of *anhydrous formic acid R*, 16 volumes of *methylene chloride R*, 32 volumes of *butanol R* and 44 volumes of *heptane R*. Dry the plate at 105 °C for 15 min and examine in ultraviolet light at 254 nm. The principal spot in the chromatogram obtained with the test solution is similar in position and size to the principal spot in the chromatogram obtained with the reference solution.

B. Mix 0.5 g with 1 g of *resorcinol R*. To 0.5 g of the mixture in a crucible add 0.15 ml of *sulphuric acid R* and heat gently. A dark red semi-solid mass is formed. Add the mass, with care, to 100 ml of *water R*. An orange-yellow colour develops and the solution shows no fluorescence.

C. The filtrate obtained for the test solution in identification test A gives reaction (a) of iron (*2.3.1*).

TESTS

Solution S. Dissolve 2.0 g of the substance to be examined in a mixture of 10 ml of *lead-free hydrochloric acid R* and 80 ml of *water R*, heating slightly if necessary. Allow to cool, filter if necessary and dilute to 100 ml with *water R*.

Sulphates (*2.4.13*). Heat 0.15 g with 8 ml of *dilute hydrochloric acid R* and 20 ml of *distilled water R*. Cool in iced water, filter and dilute to 30 ml with *distilled water R*. 15 ml of this solution complies with the limit test for sulphates (0.2 per cent).

Arsenic (*2.4.2*). Mix 1.0 g with 15 ml of *water R* and 15 ml of *sulphuric acid R*. Warm to precipitate the fumaric acid completely. Cool and add 30 ml of *water R*. Filter. Wash the precipitate with *water R*. Dilute the combined filtrate and washings to 125 ml with *water R*. 25 ml of the solution complies with limit test A for arsenic (5 ppm).

Ferric ion. Not more than 2.0 per cent of ferric ion.

In a flask with a ground-glass stopper, dissolve 3.0 g in a mixture of 10 ml of *hydrochloric acid R* and 100 ml of *water R* by heating rapidly to boiling. Boil for 15 s. Cool rapidly, add 3 g of *potassium iodide R*, stopper the flask and allow to stand protected from light for 15 min. Add 2 ml of *starch solution R* as indicator. Titrate the liberated iodine with *0.1 M sodium thiosulphate*. Carry out a blank test. The difference between the volumes used in the two titrations corresponds to the amount of iodine liberated by ferric ion.

1 ml of *0.1 M sodium thiosulphate* is equivalent to 5.585 mg of ferric ion.

Cadmium. Not more than 10 ppm of Cd, determined by atomic absorption spectrometry (*2.2.23, Method I*).

Test solution. Use solution S.

Reference solutions. Prepare the solutions using *cadmium standard solution (0.1 per cent Cd) R* and diluting with a 10 per cent *V/V* solution of *lead-free hydrochloric acid R*.

Measure the absorbance at 228.8 nm using a cadmium hollow-cathode lamp as source of radiation and an air-acetylene flame.

Chromium. Not more than 200 ppm of Cr, determined by atomic absorption spectrometry (*2.2.23, Method I*).

Test solution. Use solution S.

Reference solutions. Prepare the solutions using *chromium standard solution (0.1 per cent Cr) R* and diluting with a 10 per cent *V/V* solution of *lead-free hydrochloric acid R*.

Measure the absorbance at 357.9 nm using a chromium hollow-cathode lamp as source of radiation and an air-acetylene flame.

Lead. Not more than 20 ppm of Pb, determined by atomic absorption spectrometry (*2.2.23, Method I*).

Test solution. Use solution S.

Reference solutions. Prepare the solutions using *lead standard solution (10 ppm Pb) R* and diluting with a 10 per cent *V/V* solution of *lead-free hydrochloric acid R*.

Measure the absorbance at 283.3 nm using a lead hollow-cathode lamp as the source of radiation and an air-acetylene flame.

Mercury. Not more than 1 ppm of Hg, determined by atomic absorption spectrometry (*2.2.23, Method I*).

Test solution. Use solution S.

Reference solutions. Prepare the solutions using *mercury standard solution (10 ppm Hg) R* and diluting with a 25 per cent *V/V* solution of *lead-free hydrochloric acid R*.

Following the recommendations of the manufacturer, introduce 5 ml of solution S or 5 ml of the reference solutions into the reaction vessel of the cold-vapour mercury assay accessory, add 10 ml of *water R* and 1 ml of *stannous chloride solution R1*.

Measure the absorbance at 253.7 nm using a mercury hollow-cathode lamp as the source of radiation.

Nickel. Not more than 200 ppm of Ni, determined by atomic absorption spectrometry (*2.2.23, Method I*).

Test solution. Use solution S.

Reference solutions. Prepare the solutions using *nickel standard solution (10 ppm Ni) R* and diluting with a 10 per cent *V/V* solution of *lead-free hydrochloric acid R*.

Measure the absorbance at 232 nm using a nickel hollow-cathode lamp as source of radiation and an air-acetylene flame.

Zinc. Not more than 500 ppm of Zn, determined by atomic absorption spectrometry (*2.2.23, Method I*).

Test solution. Use solution S diluted ten times.

Reference solutions. Prepare the solutions using *zinc standard solution (10 ppm Zn) R* and diluting with a 1 per cent *V/V* solution of *lead-free hydrochloric acid R*.

Measure the absorbance at 213.9 nm using a zinc hollow-cathode lamp as source of radiation and an air-acetylene flame.

Loss on drying (*2.2.32*). Not more than 1.0 per cent, determined on 1.000 g by drying in an oven at 100-105 °C.

ASSAY

Dissolve with slight heating 0.150 g in 7.5 ml of *dilute sulphuric acid R*. Cool and add 25 ml of *water R*. Add 0.1 ml of *ferroin R*. Titrate immediately with *0.1 M cerium sulphate* until the colour changes from orange to light bluish-green.

1 ml of *0.1 M cerium sulphate* is equivalent to 16.99 mg of $C_4H_2FeO_4$.

STORAGE

Store in an airtight container, protected from light.

01/2005:0493

FERROUS GLUCONATE

Ferrosi gluconas

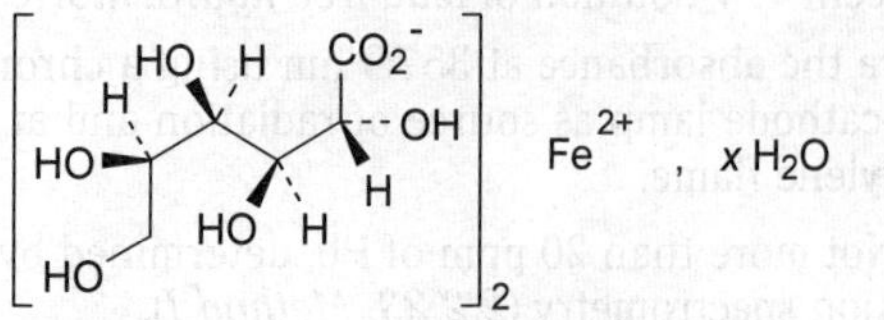

$C_{12}H_{22}FeO_{14},xH_2O$ M_r 446.1 (anhydrous substance)

DEFINITION

Ferrous gluconate is iron(II) di(D-gluconate). It contains not less than 11.8 per cent and not more than 12.5 per cent of iron(II), calculated with reference to the dried substance.

CHARACTERS

A greenish-yellow to grey powder or granules, freely but slowly soluble in water giving a greenish-brown solution, more readily soluble in hot water, practically insoluble in alcohol.

IDENTIFICATION

A. Examine by thin-layer chromatography (*2.2.27*), using a *TLC silica gel G plate R*.

Test solution. Dissolve 20 mg of the substance to be examined in 2 ml of *water R*, heating if necessary in a water-bath at 60 °C.

Reference solution. Dissolve 20 mg of *ferrous gluconate CRS* in 2 ml of *water R*, heating if necessary in a water-bath at 60 °C.

Apply separately to the plate 5 µl of each solution. Develop over a path of 10 cm using a mixture of 10 volumes of *ethyl acetate R*, 10 volumes of *concentrated ammonia R*, 30 volumes of *water R* and 50 volumes of *alcohol R*. Dry the plate at 100 °C to 105 °C for 20 min, allow to cool and spray with a 50 g/l solution of *potassium dichromate R* in a 40 per cent *m/m* solution of *sulphuric acid R*. After 5 min, the principal spot in the chromatogram obtained with the test solution is similar in position, colour and size to the principal spot in the chromatogram obtained with the reference solution.

B. 1 ml of solution S (see Tests) gives reaction (a) of iron (*2.3.1*).

TESTS

Solution S. Dissolve 5.0 g in *carbon dioxide-free water R* prepared from *distilled water R* and heated to about 60 °C, cool and dilute to 50 ml with *carbon dioxide-free water R* prepared from *distilled water R*.

Appearance of solution. Dilute 2 ml of solution S to 10 ml with *water R*. Examined against the light, the solution is clear (*2.2.1*).

pH (*2.2.3*). The pH of solution S, measured 3 h to 4 h after preparation, is 4.0 to 5.5.

Sucrose and reducing sugars. Dissolve 0.5 g in 10 ml of warm *water R* and add 1 ml of *dilute ammonia R1*. Pass *hydrogen sulphide R* through the solution and allow to stand for 30 min. Filter and wash the precipitate with two quantities, each of 5 ml, of *water R*. Acidify the combined filtrate and washings to *blue litmus paper R* with *dilute hydrochloric acid R* and add 2 ml in excess. Boil until the vapour no longer darkens *lead acetate paper R* and continue boiling, if necessary, until the volume is reduced to about 10 ml. Cool, add 15 ml of *sodium carbonate solution R*, allow to stand for 5 min and filter. Dilute the filtrate to 100 ml with *water R*. To 5 ml of this solution add 2 ml of *cupri-tartaric solution R* and boil for 1 min. Allow to stand for 1 min. No red precipitate is formed.

Chlorides (*2.4.4*). 0.8 ml of solution S diluted to 15 ml with *water R* complies with the limit test for chlorides (0.06 per cent).

Oxalates. Dissolve 5.0 g in a mixture of 10 ml of *dilute sulphuric acid R* and 40 ml of *water R*. Shake the solution with 50 ml of *ether R* for 5 min. Separate the aqueous layer and shake it with 20 ml of *ether R* for 5 min. Combine the ether layers, evaporate to dryness and dissolve the residue in 15 ml of *water R*. Filter, boil the filtrate until the volume

Monographs F-H

is reduced to 5 ml and add 1 ml of *dilute acetic acid R* and 1.5 ml of *calcium chloride solution R*. Allow to stand for 30 min. No precipitate is formed.

Sulphates (*2.4.13*). To 3.0 ml of solution S add 3 ml of *acetic acid R* and dilute to 15 ml with *distilled water R*. The solution complies with the limit test for sulphates (500 ppm). Examine the solutions against the light.

Arsenic (*2.4.2*). 0.5 g complies with limit test A for arsenic (2 ppm).

Barium. Dilute 10 ml of solution S to 50 ml with *distilled water R* and add 5 ml of *dilute sulphuric acid R*. Allow to stand for 5 min. Any opalescence in the solution is not more intense than that in a mixture of 10 ml of solution S and 45 ml of *distilled water R*.

Ferric ion. In a ground-glass-stoppered flask, dissolve 5.00 g in a mixture of 10 ml of *hydrochloric acid R* and 100 ml of *carbon dioxide-free water R*. Add 3 g of *potassium iodide R*, close the flask and allow to stand protected from light for 5 min. Titrate with *0.1 M sodium thiosulphate*, using 0.5 ml of *starch solution R*, added towards the end of the titration, as indicator. Carry out a blank titration. Not more than 9.0 ml of *0.1 M sodium thiosulphate* is used in the test (1.0 per cent).

Heavy metals (*2.4.8*). Thoroughly mix 2.5 g with 0.5 g of *magnesium oxide R1* in a silica crucible. Ignite to dull redness until a homogeneous mass is obtained. Heat at 800 °C for about 1 h, allow to cool and take up the residue in 20 ml of hot *hydrochloric acid R*. Allow to cool. Transfer the liquid to a separating funnel and shake for 3 min with three quantities, each of 20 ml, of methyl isobutyl ketone saturated with hydrochloric acid (prepared by shaking 100 ml of freshly distilled *methyl isobutyl ketone R* with 1 ml of *hydrochloric acid R*). Allow to stand, separate the aqueous layer, reduce to half its volume by boiling, allow to cool and dilute to 25 ml with *water R*. Neutralise 10 ml of this solution to *red litmus paper R* using *dilute ammonia R1* and dilute to 20 ml with *water R*. 12 ml of the solution complies with limit test A for heavy metals (20 ppm). Prepare the standard using *lead standard solution (1 ppm Pb) R*.

Loss on drying (*2.2.32*): 5.0 per cent to 10.5 per cent, determined on 0.500 g by drying in an oven at 100 °C to 105 °C for 5 h.

Microbial contamination. Total viable aerobic count (*2.6.12*) not more than 10^3 micro-organisms per gram, determined by plate count.

ASSAY

Dissolve 0.5 g of *sodium hydrogen carbonate R* in a mixture of 30 ml of *dilute sulphuric acid R* and 70 ml of *water R*. When the effervescence stops, dissolve in the solution 1.00 g of the substance to be examined with gentle shaking. Using 0.1 ml of *ferroin R* as indicator, titrate with *0.1 M ammonium and cerium nitrate* until the red colour disappears.

1 ml of *0.1 M ammonium and cerium nitrate* is equivalent to 5.585 mg of iron(II).

STORAGE

Store protected from light.

01/2005:0083

FERROUS SULPHATE HEPTAHYDRATE

Ferrosi sulfas heptahydricus

$FeSO_4,7H_2O$ M_r 278.0

DEFINITION

Content: 98.0 per cent to 105.0 per cent.

CHARACTERS

Appearance: light green, crystalline powder or bluish-green crystals, efflorescent in air.

Solubility: freely soluble in water, very soluble in boiling water, practically insoluble in alcohol.

Ferrous sulphate is oxidised in moist air, becoming brown.

IDENTIFICATION

A. It gives the reaction of sulphates (*2.3.1*).

B. It gives reaction (a) of iron (*2.3.1*).

C. It complies with the limits of the assay.

TESTS

Solution S. Dissolve 2.5 g in *carbon dioxide-free water R*, add 0.5 ml of *dilute sulphuric acid R* and dilute to 50 ml with *water R*.

Appearance of solution. Solution S is not more opalescent than reference suspension II (*2.2.1*).

pH (*2.2.3*): 3.0 to 4.0.

Dissolve 0.5 g in *carbon dioxide-free water R* and dilute to 10 ml with the same solvent.

Chlorides (*2.4.4*): maximum 300 ppm.

Dilute 3.3 ml of solution S to 10 ml with *water R* and add 5 ml of *dilute nitric acid R*. The solution complies with the limit test for chlorides. Prepare the standard using a mixture of 10 ml of *chloride standard solution (5 ppm Cl) R* and 5 ml of *dilute nitric acid R*. Use 0.15 ml of *silver nitrate solution R2* in this test.

Ferric ions: maximum 0.5 per cent.

In a ground-glass-stoppered flask, dissolve 5.00 g in a mixture of 10 ml of *hydrochloric acid R* and 100 ml of *carbon dioxide-free water R*. Add 3 g of *potassium iodide R*, close the flask and allow to stand in the dark for 5 min. Titrate the liberated iodine with *0.1 M sodium thiosulphate*, using 0.5 ml of *starch solution R*, added towards the end of the titration, as indicator. Carry out a blank test in the same conditions. Not more than 4.5 ml of *0.1 M sodium thiosulphate* is used, taking into account the blank titration.

Manganese: maximum 0.1 per cent.

Dissolve 1.0 g in 40 ml of *water R*, add 10 ml of *nitric acid R* and boil until red fumes are evolved. Add 0.5 g of *ammonium persulphate R* and boil for 10 min. Discharge any pink colour by adding dropwise a 50 g/l solution of *sodium sulphite R* and boil until any odour of sulphur dioxide is eliminated. Add 10 ml of *water R*, 5 ml of *phosphoric acid R* and 0.5 g of *sodium periodate R*, boil for 1 min and allow to cool. The solution is not more intensely coloured than a standard prepared at the same time in the same manner using 1.0 ml of *0.02 M potassium permanganate* and adding the same volumes of the same reagents.

Zinc: maximum 500 ppm.

To 5 ml of solution A obtained in the test for heavy metals add 1 ml of *potassium ferrocyanide solution R* and dilute

Monographs F-H

to 13 ml with *water R*. After 5 min, any turbidity produced is not more intense than that of a standard prepared at the same time by mixing 10 ml of *zinc standard solution (10 ppm Zn) R*, 2 ml of *hydrochloric acid R1* and 1 ml of *potassium ferrocyanide solution R*.

Heavy metals (*2.4.8*): maximum 50 ppm.

Dissolve 1.0 g in 10 ml of *hydrochloric acid R1*, add 2 ml of *strong hydrogen peroxide solution R* and boil until the volume is reduced to 5 ml. Allow to cool, dilute to 20 ml with *hydrochloric acid R1*, transfer the solution to a separating funnel and shake for 3 min with 3 quantities, each of 20 ml, of methyl isobutyl ketone saturated with hydrochloric acid (prepared by shaking 100 ml of freshly distilled *methyl isobutyl ketone R* with 1 ml of *hydrochloric acid R1*). Allow to stand, separate the aqueous layer and reduce to half its volume by boiling, allow to cool and dilute to 25 ml with *water R* (solution A). Neutralise 10 ml of solution A to *litmus paper R* using *dilute ammonia R1* and dilute to 20 ml with *water R*. 12 ml of the solution complies with limit test A. Prepare the standard using *lead standard solution (1 ppm Pb) R*.

ASSAY

Dissolve 2.5 g of *sodium hydrogen carbonate R* in a mixture of 150 ml of *water R* and 10 ml of *sulphuric acid R*. When the effervescence ceases add to the solution 0.500 g of the substance to be examined and dissolve with gentle shaking. Add 0.1 ml of *ferroin R* and titrate with *0.1 M ammonium and cerium nitrate* until the red colour disappears.

1 ml of *0.1 M ammonium and cerium nitrate* is equivalent to 27.80 mg of $FeSO_4,7H_2O$.

STORAGE

In an airtight container.

Monographs F-H

01/2005:1516

FEVERFEW

Tanaceti parthenii herba

DEFINITION

Feverfew consists of the dried, whole or fragmented aerial parts of *Tanacetum parthenium* (L.) Schultz Bip. It contains not less than 0.20 per cent of parthenolide ($C_{15}H_{20}O_3$; M_r 248.3), calculated with reference to the dried drug.

CHARACTERS

Fewerfew has a camphoraceous odour.

It has the macroscopic and microscopic characters described under identification tests A and B.

IDENTIFICATION

A. The leafy, more or less branched stem has a diameter of up to 5 mm; it is almost quadrangular, channelled longitudinally and slightly pubescent. The leaves are ovate, 2 cm to 5 cm long, sometimes up to 10 cm, yellowish-green, petiolate and alternate. They are pinnate or bipinnate, deeply divided into five to nine segments, each with a coarsely crenate margin and an obtuse apex. Both surfaces are somewhat pubescent and the midrib is prominent on the lower surface. When present, the flowering heads are 12 mm to 22 mm in diameter with long pedicels; they are clustered into broad corymbs consisting of five to thirty flower-heads. The hemispherical involucre is 6 mm to 8 mm wide and consists of many overlapping bracts, which are rather narrow, are obtuse and scarious and have membranous margins. The central flowers are yellow, hermaphrodite, tube-shaped with five teeth and have five stamens inserted in the corolla; the filaments of the stamens are separate from each other but the anthers are fused into a tube through which passes the style, bearing two stigmatic branches. The peripheral flowers are female and have a white three-toothed ligule, 2 mm to 7 mm long. The fruit is an achene, 1.2 mm to 1.5 mm long, brown when ripe, with five to ten white longitudinal ribs. It is glandular and bears a short, crenate, membranous crown.

B. Reduce to a powder (355). The powder is yellowish-green. Examine under a microscope using *chloral hydrate solution R*. The powder shows numerous large, multicellular, uniseriate covering trichomes consisting of a rhomboidal basal cell, three to five smaller, thick-walled rectangular cells and a very long, flat, slender terminal cell, often curved at a right angle to the axis of the basal cell; glandular trichomes with a short, biseriate, two to four celled stalk and a biseriate head of four cells around which the cuticle forms a bladder-like covering; epidermal cells with a very sinuous anticlinal walls, a striated cuticle and anomocytic stomata; numerous spirally and annularly thickened vessels; stratified parenchyma and collenchyma. Fragments of disc florets containing pale yellow amorphous masses and small rosette crystals of calcium oxalate may be present; spherical pollen grains about 25 µm in diameter, with three pores and a spiny exine may be present.

C. Examine by thin-layer chromatography (*2.2.27*), using a *TLC silica gel plate R*.

Test solution. To 1 g of the powdered drug (355) add 20 ml of *methanol R*. Heat in a water-bath at 60 °C for 15 min. Allow to cool and filter. Evaporate to dryness under reduced pressure and dissolve the residue in 2 ml of *methanol R*.

Reference solution. Dissolve 5 mg of *parthenolide R* in *methanol R* and dilute to 5 ml with the same solvent.

Apply to the plates as bands 20 µl of each solution. Develop over a path of 10 cm using a mixture of 15 volumes of *acetone R* and 85 volumes of *toluene R*. Allow the plate to dry in air. Spray with a 5 g/l solution of *vanillin R* in a mixture of 20 volumes of *ethanol R* and 80 volumes of *sulphuric acid R*. After 5 min examine in daylight. The chromatogram obtained with the test solution shows in its central part a blue principal zone that is similar in position, colour and size to the principal zone in the chromatogram obtained with the reference solution, and somewhat below the principal zone it may show a second blue zone. It also shows, one or two blue zones in its lower third. Other violet zones may be present.

TESTS

Foreign matter (*2.8.2*). Not more than 10.0 per cent of stem having a diameter exceeding 5 mm, and not more than 2.0 per cent of other foreign matter.

Loss on drying (*2.2.32*). Not more than 10.0 per cent, determined on 1.000 g of the powdered drug (355) by drying in an oven at 100 °C to 105 °C for 2 h.

Total ash (*2.4.16*). Not more than 12.0 per cent.

ASSAY

Examine by liquid chromatography (*2.2.29*).

Test solution. Completely reduce about 50 g to a powder (355). After homogenisation, introduce 1.00 g of the powdered drug into a flask and add 40 ml of *methanol R*. Heat in a water-bath at 60 °C for 10 min. Allow to cool and filter. Rinse the filter with 15 ml of *methanol R*. Take up the residue with 40 ml of *methanol R*. Repeat the operation. Collect the filtrates and rinsings and evaporate to dryness under reduced pressure. Take up the residue with *methanol R* and dilute to 20.0 ml with the same solvent. Dilute 10.0 ml of this solution to 50.0 ml with the mobile phase. Filter (0.45 µm).

Reference solution. Dissolve 5.0 mg of *parthenolide R* in *methanol R* and dilute to 10.0 ml with the same solvent. Dilute 2.0 ml of the solution to 50.0 ml with the mobile phase.

The chromatographic procedure may be carried out using:

– a stainless steel column 0.25 m long and 4.6 mm in internal diameter packed with *octadecylsilyl silica gel for chromatography R* (5 µm),
– as mobile phase at a flow rate of 1 ml/min a mixture of 40 volumes of *acetonitrile R* and 60 volumes of *water R*,
– as detector a spectrophotometer set at 220 nm,

Inject 20 µl of each solution. The retention time of parthenolide is about 11.5 min.

Calculate the percentage content of parthenolide from the expression:

$$\frac{A_1 \times m_2 \times 40}{A_2 \times m_1}$$

A_1 = area corresponding to the principal compound in the chromatogram obtained with the test solution,

A_2 = area corresponding to the principal compound in the chromatogram obtained with the reference solution,

m_1 = mass of the drug used in the test solution, in grams,

m_2 = mass of parthenolide in the reference solution, in grams.

STORAGE

Store protected from light.

01/2005:0903
corrected

FIBRIN SEALANT KIT

Fibrini glutinum

DEFINITION

Fibrin sealant kit is essentially composed of 2 components, namely fibrinogen concentrate (component 1), a protein fraction containing human fibrinogen and a preparation containing human thrombin (component 2). A fibrin clot is rapidly formed when the 2 thawed or reconstituted components are mixed. Other ingredients (for example, human coagulation factor XIII, a fibrinolysis inhibitor or calcium ions) and stabilisers (for example, *Human albumin solution (0255)*) may be added. No antimicrobial preservative is added.

Human constituents are obtained from plasma that complies with the requirements of the monograph on *Human plasma for fractionation (0853)*. No antibiotic is added to the plasma used.

When thawed or reconstituted as stated on the label, component 1 contains not less than 40 g/l of clottable protein; the thrombin activity of component 2 varies over a wide range (approximately 4-1000 IU/ml).

PRODUCTION

The method of preparation includes a step or steps that have been shown to remove or to inactivate known agents of infection; if substances are used for inactivation of viruses during production, the subsequent purification procedure must be validated to demonstrate that the concentration of these substances is reduced to a suitable level and any residues are such as not to compromise the safety of the preparation for patients.

Constituents or mixtures of constituents are passed through a bacteria-retentive filter and distributed aseptically into sterile containers. Containers of freeze-dried constituents are closed under vacuum or filled with oxygen-free nitrogen or other suitable inert gas before being closed. In either case, they are closed so as to exclude micro-organisms.

If the human coagulation factor XIII content in component 1 is greater than 10 units/ml, the assay of factor XIII is carried out.

CHARACTERS

Freeze-dried constituents are hygroscopic, white or pale yellow powders or friable solids. Frozen constituents are colourless or pale yellow, opaque solids. Liquid constituents are colourless or pale yellow.

For the freeze-dried or frozen constituents, reconstitute or thaw as stated on the label immediately before carrying out the identification and the tests, except those for solubility and water.

Component 1 (fibrinogen concentrate)

IDENTIFICATION

A. It complies with the limits of the assay of fibrinogen.

B. It complies with the limits of the assay of factor XIII (where applicable).

TESTS

pH (*2.2.3*): 6.5 to 8.0.

Solubility. Freeze-dried concentrates dissolve within 20 min in the volume of solvent for reconstitution and at the temperature stated on the label, forming an almost colourless, clear or slightly turbid solution.

Stability of solution. No gel formation appears at room temperature during 120 min following thawing or reconstitution.

Water. Determined by a suitable method, such as the semi-microdetermination (*2.5.12*), loss on drying (*2.2.32*) or near infrared spectrophotometry (*2.2.40*), the water content is within the limits approved by the competent authority.

Sterility (*2.6.1*). It complies with the test for sterility.

ASSAY

Fibrinogen (clottable protein). The estimated content in milligrams of clottable protein is not less than 70 per cent and not more than 130 per cent of the content stated on the label.

Mix 0.2 ml of the reconstituted preparation with 2 ml of a suitable buffer solution (pH 6.6-7.4) containing sufficient *human thrombin R* (approximately 3 IU/ml) and calcium (0.05 mol/l). Maintain at 37 °C for 20 min, separate the precipitate by centrifugation (5000 *g*, 20 min), wash thoroughly with a 9 g/l solution of *sodium chloride R* and determine the protein as nitrogen by sulphuric acid digestion (*2.5.9*). Calculate the protein content by multiplying the result by 6.0. If for a particular preparation this method cannot be applied, use another validated method for determination of fibrinogen.

Monographs F-H

Factor XIII. Where the label indicates that the human coagulation factor XIII activity is greater than 10 units/ml, the estimated activity is not less than 80 per cent and not more than 120 per cent of the activity stated on the label.

Make at least 3 suitable dilutions of thawed or reconstituted component 1 and of human normal plasma (reference preparation) using as diluent coagulation factor XIII deficient plasma or another suitable diluent. Add to each dilution suitable amounts of the following reagents:

- activator reagent, containing bovine or human thrombin, a suitable buffer, calcium chloride and a suitable inhibitor such as Gly-Pro-Arg-Pro-Ala-NH_2 which inhibits clotting of the sample but does not prevent coagulation factor XIII activation by thrombin,
- detection reagent, containing a suitable factor XIIIa-specific peptide substrate, such as Leu-Gly-Pro-Gly-Glu-Ser-Lys-Val-Ile-Gly-NH_2 and glycine ethyl ester as 2nd substrate in a suitable buffer solution,
- NADH reagent, containing glutamate dehydrogenase, α-ketoglutarate and NADH in a suitable buffer solution.

After mixing, the absorbance changes (ΔA/min) are measured at a wavelength of 340 nm, after the linear phase of the reaction is reached.

1 unit of factor XIII is equal to the activity of 1 ml of human normal plasma.

Calculate the activity of the test preparation by the usual statistical methods (*5.3*, for example). The confidence limits (P = 0.95) are not less than 80 per cent and not more than 125 per cent of the estimated activity.

Component 2 (thrombin preparation)

IDENTIFICATION

It complies with the limits of the assay of thrombin.

TESTS

pH (*2.2.3*): 5.0 to 8.0.

Solubility. Freeze-dried preparations dissolve within 5 min in the volume of solvent for reconstitution stated on the label, forming a colourless, clear or slightly turbid solution.

Water. Determined by a suitable method, such as the semi-microdetermination (*2.5.12*), loss on drying (*2.2.32*) or near infrared spectrophotometry (*2.2.40*), the water content is within the limits approved by the competent authority.

Sterility (*2.6.1*). It complies with the test for sterility.

ASSAY

Thrombin. The estimated activity is not less than 80 per cent and not more than 125 per cent of the activity stated on the label.

If necessary, dilute the reconstituted preparation to be examined to approximately 2-20 IU of thrombin per millilitre using as diluent a suitable buffer pH 7.3-7.5, such as *imidazole buffer solution pH 7.3 R* containing 10 g/l of *human albumin R* or *bovine albumin R*. To a suitable volume of the dilution, add a suitable volume of fibrinogen solution (1 g/l of clottable protein) warmed to 37 °C and start measurement of the clotting time immediately. Repeat the procedure with each of at least 3 dilutions, in the range stated above, of a reference preparation of thrombin, calibrated in International Units. Calculate the activity of the test preparation by the usual statistical methods (*5.3*, for example). The confidence limits (P = 0.95) are not less than 80 per cent and not more than 125 per cent of the estimated activity.

STORAGE

Protected from light and, for freeze-dried components, in an airtight container.

LABELLING

The label states:

- the amount of fibrinogen (milligrams of clottable protein), thrombin (International Units) per container, and coagulation factor XIII, if this is greater than 10 units/ml,
- where applicable, the name and volume of solvent to be used to reconstitute the components.

01/2005:1615

FINASTERIDE

Finasteridum

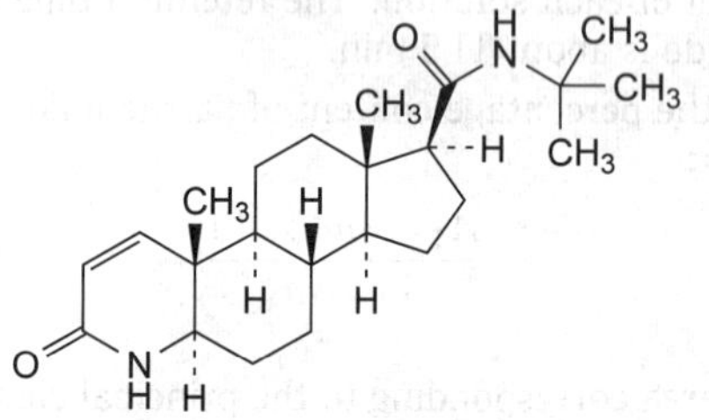

$C_{23}H_{36}N_2O_2$ M_r 372.6

DEFINITION

N-(1,1-Dimethylethyl)-3-oxo-4-aza-5α-androst-1-ene-17β-carboxamide.

Content: 98.0 per cent to 102.0 per cent (dried substance).

CHARACTERS

Appearance: white or almost white, crystalline powder.

Solubility: practically insoluble in water, freely soluble in ethanol and in methylene chloride.

It shows polymorphism.

IDENTIFICATION

Infrared absorption spectrophotometry (*2.2.24*).

Comparison: *finasteride CRS*.

If the spectra obtained in the solid state show differences, dissolve the substance to be examined and the reference substance separately in *methanol R*, evaporate to dryness and record new spectra using the residues.

TESTS

Specific optical rotation (*2.2.7*): + 12.0 to + 14.0 (dried substance).

Dissolve 0.250 g in *methanol R* and dilute to 25.0 ml with the same solvent.

Related substances. Liquid chromatography (*2.2.29*).

Test solution (a). Dissolve 25.0 mg of the substance to be examined in a mixture of equal volumes of *acetonitrile R* and *water R* and dilute to 50.0 ml with the same mixture of solvents.

Test solution (b). Dissolve 0.100 g of the substance to be examined in a mixture of equal volumes of *acetonitrile R* and *water R* and dilute to 10.0 ml with the same mixture of solvents.

Reference solution (a). Dissolve 25.0 mg of *finasteride CRS* in a mixture of equal volumes of *acetonitrile R* and *water R* and dilute to 50.0 ml with the same mixture of solvents.

Reference solution (b). Dissolve 50.0 mg of *finasteride for system suitability CRS* in a mixture of equal volumes of *acetonitrile R* and *water R* and dilute to 5.0 ml with the same mixture of solvents.

Reference solution (c). Dilute 2.0 ml of test solution (b) to 100.0 ml in a mixture of equal volumes of *acetonitrile R* and *water R*. Dilute 1.0 ml of this solution to 10.0 ml with a mixture of equal volumes of *acetonitrile R* and *water R*.

Column:

- *size*: l = 0.25 m, Ø = 4.0 mm,
- *stationary phase*: *end-capped octadecylsilyl silica gel for chromatography R* (5 µm) with a ratio of specific surface area (m^2g^{-1})/carbon-percentage less than 20,
- *temperature*: 60 °C.

Mobile phase: *acetonitrile R, tetrahydrofuran R, water R* (10:10:80 *V/V/V*).

Flow rate: 1.5 ml/min.

Detection: spectrophotometer at 210 nm.

Injection: 15 µl; inject test solution (b) and reference solutions (b) and (c).

Run time: twice the retention time of finasteride.

Relative retention with reference to finasteride (retention time = about 28 min): impurity A = about 0.94; impurity B = about 1.22; impurity C = about 1.36.

System suitability: reference solution (b):

- *peak-to-valley ratio*: minimum 2.5, where H_p = height above the baseline of the peak due to impurity A, and H_v = height above the baseline of the lowest point of the curve separating this peak from the peak due to finasteride.

Limits:

- *impurity A*: maximum 0.3 per cent, calculated from the area of the corresponding peak in the chromatogram obtained with reference solution (b) and taking into account the assigned value of impurity A in *finasteride for system suitability CRS*,
- *impurity B*: not more than 1.5 times the area of the principal peak in the chromatogram obtained with reference solution (c) (0.3 per cent),
- *impurity C*: not more than 1.5 times the area of the principal peak in the chromatogram obtained with reference solution (c) (0.3 per cent),
- *any other impurity*: not more than half the area of the principal peak in the chromatogram obtained with reference solution (c) (0.1 per cent),
- *total*: not more than 3 times the area of the principal peak in the chromatogram obtained with reference solution (c) (0.6 per cent),
- *disregard limit*: 0.25 times the area of the principal peak in the chromatogram obtained with reference solution (c) (0.05 per cent).

Loss on drying (*2.2.32*): maximum 0.5 per cent, determined on 1.000 g by drying in an oven at 100-105 °C.

ASSAY

Liquid chromatography (*2.2.29*) as described in the test for related substances.

Injection: test solution (a) and reference solution (a).

Calculate the percentage content of $C_{23}H_{36}N_2O_2$.

STORAGE

Protected from light.

IMPURITIES

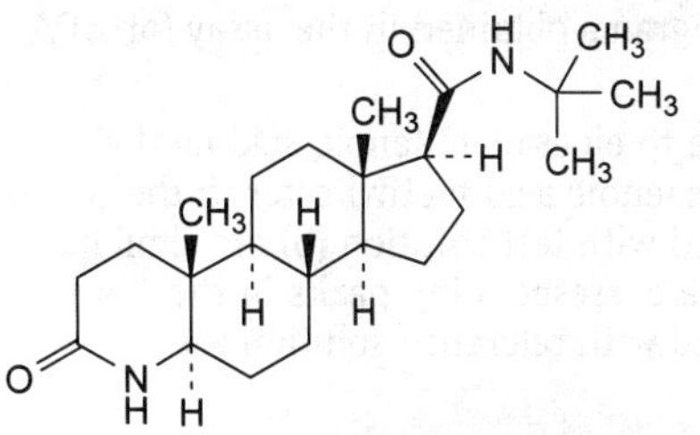

A. *N*-(1,1-dimethylethyl)-3-oxo-4-aza-5α-androstane-17β-carboxamide (dihydrofinasteride),

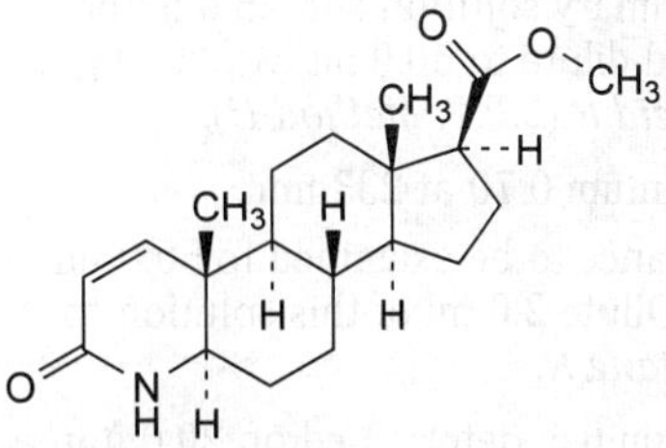

B. methyl 3-oxo-4-aza-5α-androst-1-ene-17β-carboxylate (Δ-1-aza ester),

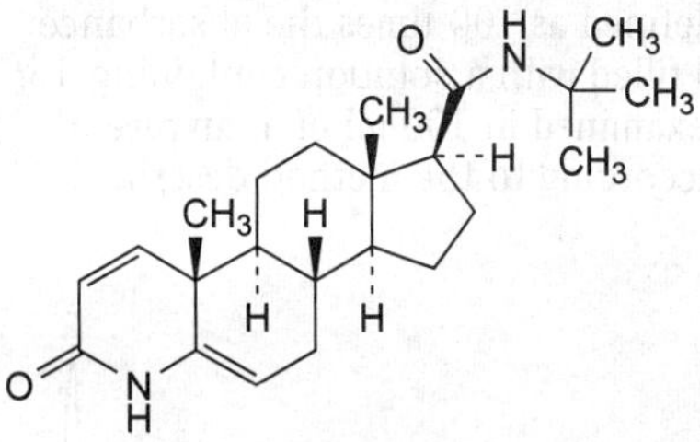

C. *N*-(1,1-dimethylethyl)-3-oxo-4-azaandrosta-1,5-diene-17β-carboxamide (Δ-1,5-aza amide).

01/2005:1912
corrected

FISH OIL, RICH IN OMEGA-3-ACIDS

Piscis oleum omega-3 acidis abundans

DEFINITION

Purified, winterised and deodorised fatty oil obtained from fish of the families *Engraulidae, Carangidae, Clupeidae, Osmeridae, Scombridae* and *Ammodytidae*. The omega-3 acids are defined as the following acids: *alpha*-linolenic acid (C18:3 n-3), moroctic acid (C18:4 n-3), eicosatetraenoic acid (C20:4 n-3), timnodonic (eicosapentaenoic) acid (C20:5 n-3; EPA), heneicosapentaenoic acid (C21:5 n-3), clupanodonic acid (C22:5 n-3) and cervonic (docosahexaenoic) acid (C22:6 n-3; DHA).

Content:

- EPA, expressed as triglycerides: minimum 13.0 per cent,
- DHA, expressed as triglycerides: minimum 9.0 per cent,
- total omega-3-acids, expressed as triglycerides: minimum 28.0 per cent.

Authorised antioxidants in concentrations not exceeding the levels specified by the competent authorities may be added.

CHARACTERS

Appearance: pale yellow liquid.

Solubility: practically insoluble in water, very soluble in acetone and in heptane, slightly soluble in ethanol.

IDENTIFICATION

Examine the chromatograms obtained in the assay for EPA and DHA.

Results: the peaks due to eicosapentaenoic acid methyl ester and to docosahexaenoic acid methyl ester in the chromatogram obtained with test solution (b) are similar in retention time to the corresponding peaks in the chromatogram obtained with reference solution (a).

TESTS

Appearance. The substance to be examined is not more intensely coloured than a reference solution prepared as follows: to 3.0 ml of red primary solution add 25.0 ml of yellow primary solution and dilute to 50.0 ml with a 10 g/l solution of *hydrochloric acid R* (*2.2.2, Method II*).

Absorbance (*2.2.25*): maximum 0.70 at 233 nm.

Dilute 0.300 g of the substance to be examined to 50.0 ml with *trimethylpentane R*. Dilute 2.0 ml of this solution to 50.0 ml with *trimethylpentane R*.

Acid value (*2.5.1*): maximum 0.5, determined on 20.0 g in 50 ml of the prescribed mixture of solvents.

Anisidine value: maximum 30.0.

The anisidine value is defined as 100 times the absorbance measured in a 1 cm cell filled with a solution containing 1 g of the substance to be examined in 100 ml of a mixture of solvents and reagents according to the method described below.

Monographs F-H

Carry out the operations as rapidly as possible, avoiding exposure to actinic light.

Test solution (a). Dilute 0.500 g of the substance to be examined to 25.0 ml with *trimethylpentane R*.

Test solution (b). To 5.0 ml of test solution (a) add 1.0 ml of a 2.5 g/l solution of *p-anisidine R* in *glacial acetic acid R*, shake and store protected from light.

Reference solution. To 5.0 ml of *trimethylpentane R* add 1.0 ml of a 2.5 g/l solution of *p-anisidine R* in *glacial acetic acid R*, shake and store protected from light.

Measure the absorbance (*2.2.25*) of test solution (a) at 350 nm using *trimethylpentane R* as the compensation liquid. Measure the absorbance of test solution (b) at 350 nm exactly 10 min after its preparation, using the reference solution as the compensation liquid.

Calculate the anisidine value from the expression:

$$\frac{25 \times (1.2\,A_s - A_b)}{m}$$

A_s = absorbance of test solution (b),

A_b = absorbance of test solution (a),

m = mass of the substance to be examined in test solution (a), in grams.

Peroxide value (*2.5.5, Method A*): maximum 10.0.

Unsaponifiable matter (*2.5.7*): maximum 1.5 per cent, determined on 5.0 g.

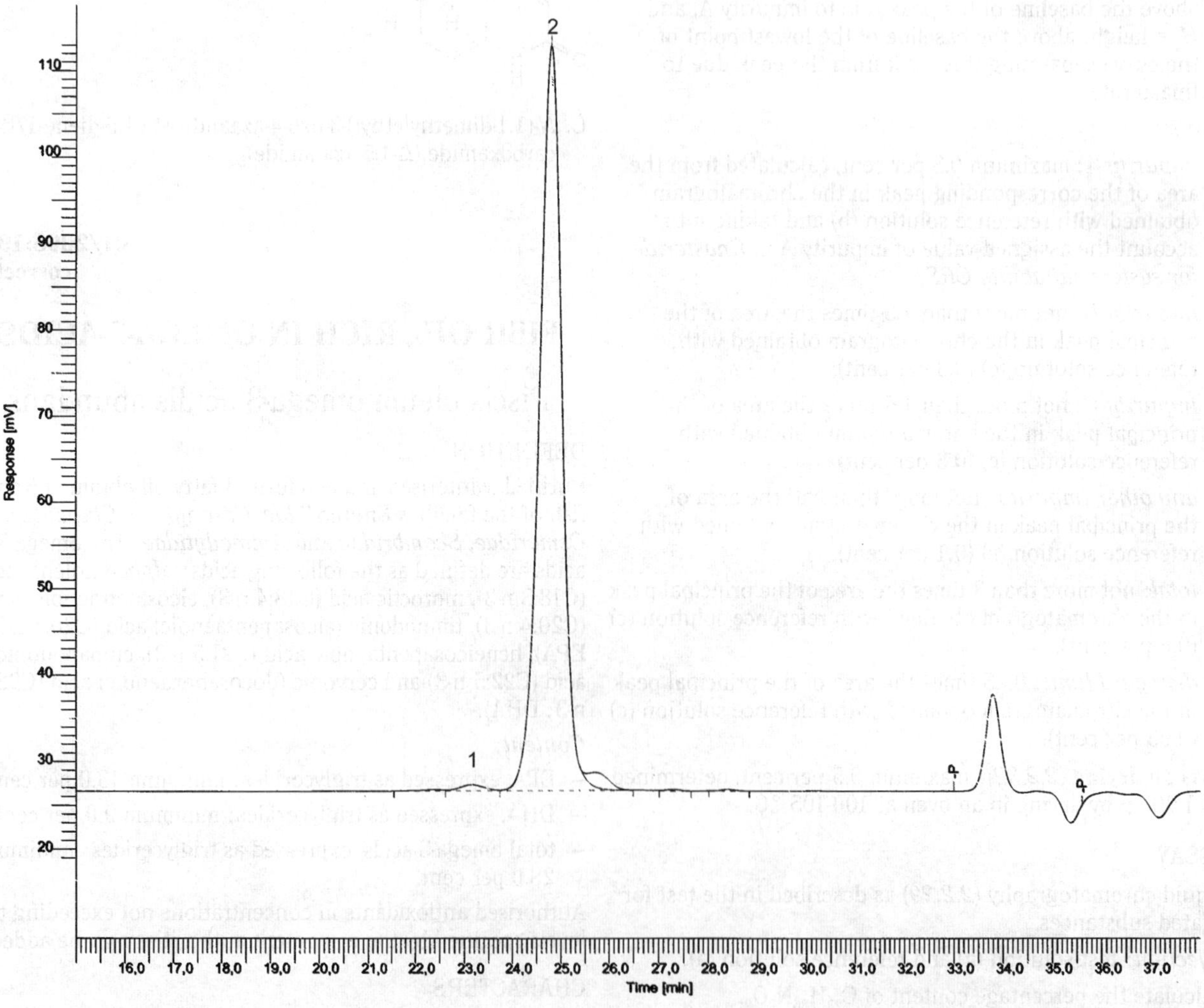

1. oligomers 2. triglycerides

Figure 1912.-1. – *Chromatogram of the test for oligomers in fish oil rich in omega-3 acids*

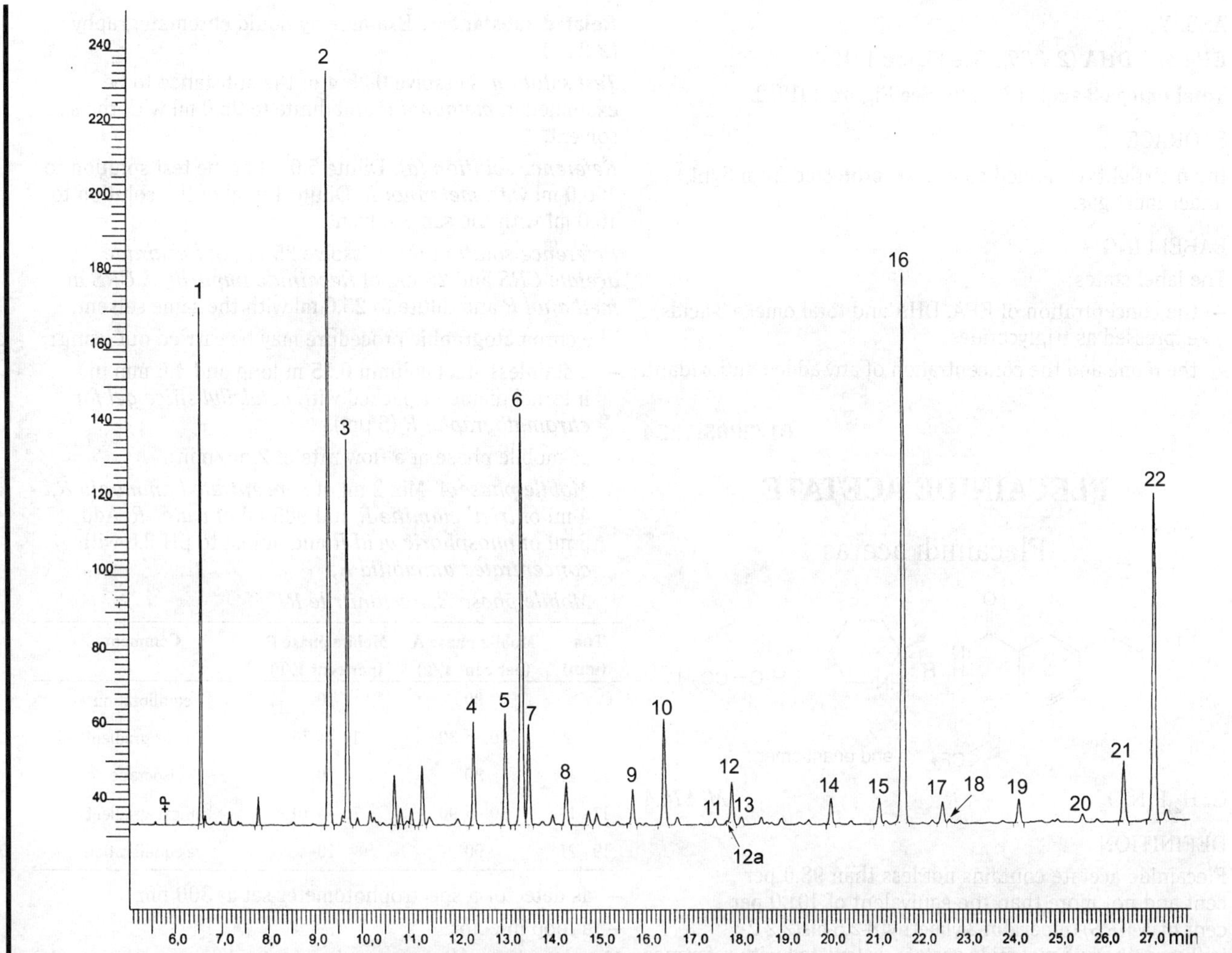

1. C14:0	6. C18:1 n-9	11. C20:0	15. C20:4 n-3	20. C22:5 n-6
2. C16:0	7. C18:1 n-7	12. C20:1 n-9	16. C20:5 n-3	21. C22:5 n-3
3. C16:1 n-7	8. C18:2 n-6	12a. C20:1 n-11	17. C22:1 n-11	22. C22:6 n-3
4. C16:4 n-1	9. C18:3 n-3	13. C20:1 n-7	18. C22:1 n-9	
5. C18:0	10. C18:4 n-3	14. C20:4 n-6	19. C21:5 n-3	

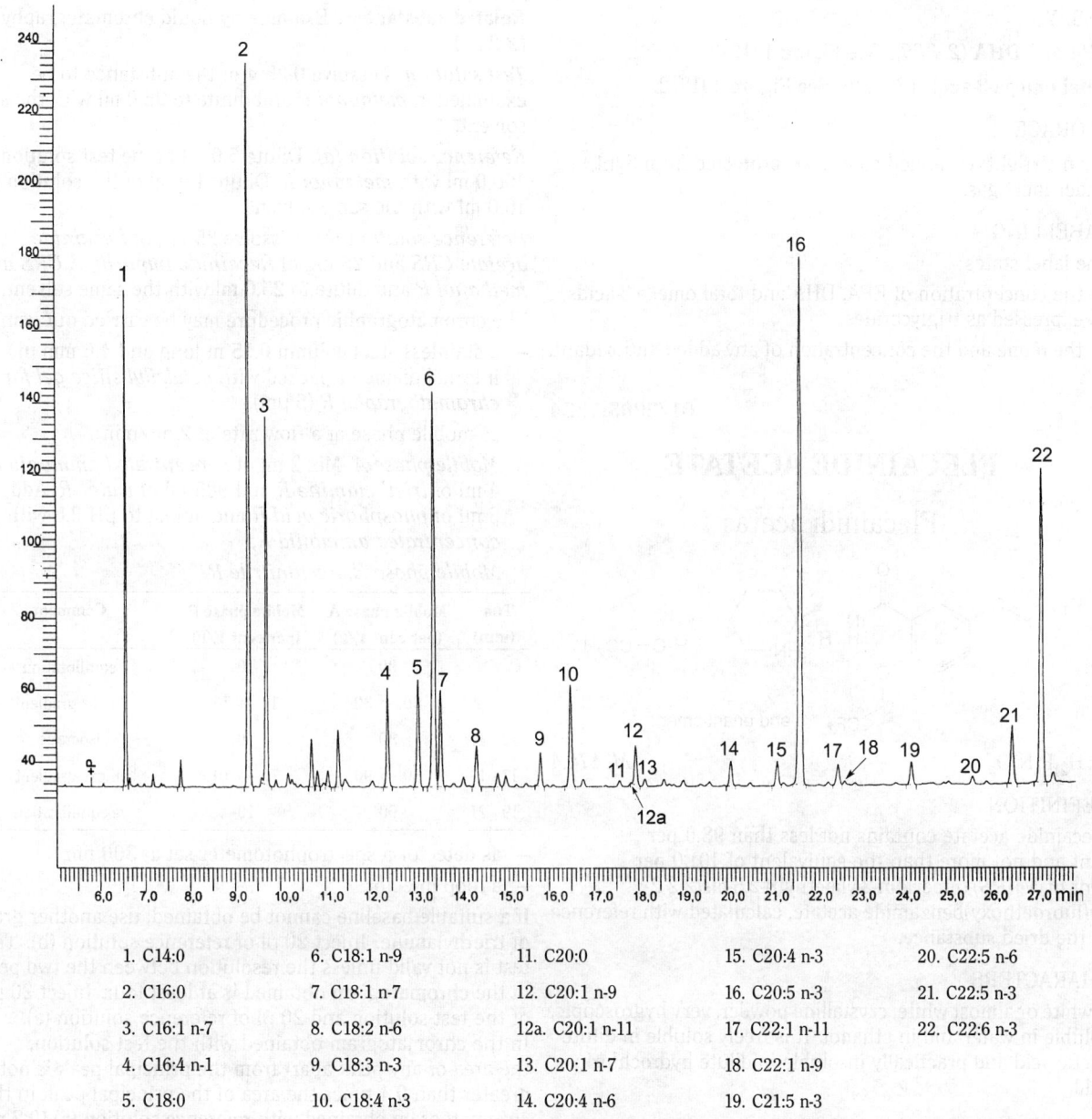

Figure 1912.-2. – *Chromatogram for the assay of total omega-3 acids in fish oil rich in omega-3 acids*

Stearin. 100 ml remains clear after cooling at 0 °C for 3 h.

Oligomers. Size-exclusion chromatography (*2.2.30*).

Test solution. Dilute 10.0 mg of the substance to be examined to 10.0 ml with *tetrahydrofuran R*.

Reference solution. In a 100 ml volumetric flask dissolve 50 mg of *monodocosahexaenoin R*, 30 mg of *didocosahexaenoin R* and 20 mg of *tridocosahexaenoin R* in *tetrahydrofuran R* and dilute to 100.0 ml with the same solvent.

Column 1:
– *size*: *l* = 0.3 m, Ø = 7.8 mm,
– *stationary phase*: *styrene-divinylbenzene copolymer R* (7 µm) with a pore size of 10 nm.

Columns 2 and 3, placed closest to the injector:
– *size*: *l* = 0.3 m, Ø = 7.8 mm,
– *stationary phase*: *styrene-divinylbenzene copolymer R* (7 µm) with a pore size of 50 nm.

Mobile phase: *tetrahydrofuran R*.

Flow rate: 0.8 ml/min.

Detection: differential refractometer.

Injection: 40 µl.

System suitability: reference solution:
– *elution order*: tridocosahexaenoin, didocosahexaenoin, monodocosahexaenoin.
– *resolution*: minimum of 2.0 between the peaks due to monodocosahexaenoin and to didocosahexaenoin and minimum of 1.0 between the peaks due to didocosahexaenoin and to tridocosahexaenoin.

Identify the peaks from the chromatogram (Figure 1912.-1). Calculate the percentage content of oligomers using the following expression:

$$\frac{B}{A} \times 100$$

A = sum of the areas of all the peaks in the chromatogram,

B = area of the peak with a retention time less than the retention time of the triglyceride peak.

Limit:
– *oligomers*: maximum 1.5 per cent.

Monographs F-H

ASSAY

EPA and DHA (*2.4.29*). See Figure 1912.-2.

Total omega-3-acids (*2.4.29*). See Figure 1912.-2.

STORAGE

In an airtight, well-filled container, protected from light, under inert gas.

LABELLING

The label states:

– the concentration of EPA, DHA and total omega-3-acids, expressed as triglycerides,

– the name and the concentration of any added antioxidant.

01/2005:1324

FLECAINIDE ACETATE

Flecainidi acetas

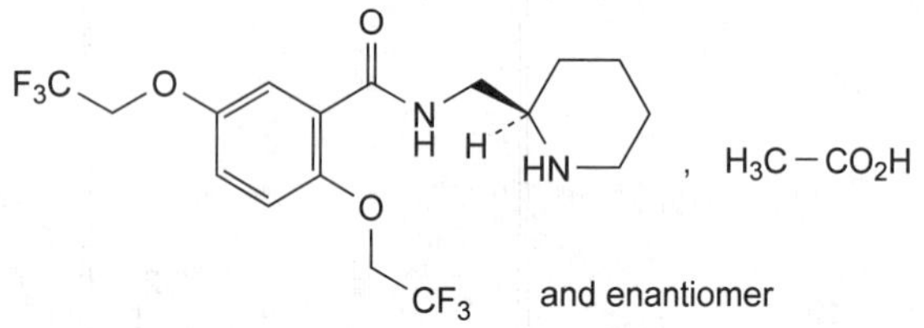

$C_{19}H_{24}F_6N_2O_5$ M_r 474.4

DEFINITION

Flecainide acetate contains not less than 98.0 per cent and not more than the equivalent of 101.0 per cent of *N*-[(*RS*)-(piperidin-2-ylmethyl)]-2,5-bis(2,2,2-trifluoroethoxy)benzamide acetate, calculated with reference to the dried substance.

CHARACTERS

A white or almost white, crystalline powder, very hygroscopic, soluble in water and in ethanol. It is freely soluble in dilute acetic acid and practically insoluble in dilute hydrochloric acid.

IDENTIFICATION

First identification: A, C.

Second identification: A, B, D.

A. Melting point (*2.2.14*): 146 °C to 152 °C. The melting range is not greater than 3 °C.

B. Dissolve 50 mg in *alcohol R* and dilute to 50.0 ml with the same solvent. Dilute 5.0 ml of the solution to 50.0 ml with the same solvent. Examined between 230 nm and 350 nm (*2.2.25*), the solution shows an absorption maximum at 298 nm. The specific absorbance at the maximum is 61 to 65.

C. Examine by infrared absorption spectrophotometry (*2.2.24*), comparing with the spectrum obtained with *flecainide acetate CRS.*

D. It gives reaction (b) of acetates (*2.3.1*).

TESTS

Appearance of solution. Dissolve 0.25 g in *water R,* add 0.05 ml of *glacial acetic acid R* and dilute to 10 ml with *water R*. The solution is clear (*2.2.1*) and colourless (*2.2.2, Method II*).

pH (*2.2.3*). Dissolve 0.25 g in *carbon dioxide-free water R* and dilute to 10 ml with the same solvent. The pH of the solution is 6.7 to 7.1.

Related substances. Examine by liquid chromatography (*2.2.29*).

Test solution. Dissolve 0.25 g of the substance to be examined in *methanol R* and dilute to 25.0 ml with the same solvent.

Reference solution (a). Dilute 5.0 ml of the test solution to 100.0 ml with *methanol R*. Dilute 1.0 ml of the solution to 10.0 ml with the same solvent.

Reference solution (b). Dissolve 25 mg of *flecainide acetate CRS* and 25 mg of *flecainide impurity A CRS* in *methanol R* and dilute to 25.0 ml with the same solvent.

The chromatographic procedure may be carried out using:

– a stainless steel column 0.15 m long and 4.6 mm in internal diameter packed with *octylsilyl silica gel for chromatography R* (5 µm),

– as mobile phase at a flow rate of 2 ml/min:

Mobile phase A. Mix 2 ml of *concentrated ammonia R,* 4 ml of *triethylamine R* and 985 ml of *water R*. Add 6 ml of *phosphoric acid R* and adjust to pH 2.8 with *concentrated ammonia R,*

Mobile phase B. Acetonitrile R,

Time (min)	Mobile phase A (per cent *V/V*)	Mobile phase B (per cent *V/V*)	Comment
	90	10	equilibration
0 - 12	90 → 30	10 → 70	linear gradient
12 - 17	30	70	isocratic
17 - 19	30 → 90	70 → 10	linear gradient
19 - 21	90	10	re-equilibration

– as detector a spectrophotometer set at 300 nm,

– a loop injector.

If a suitable baseline cannot be obtained, use another grade of triethylamine. Inject 20 µl of reference solution (b). The test is not valid unless the resolution between the two peaks in the chromatogram obtained is at least four. Inject 20 µl of the test solution and 20 µl of reference solution (a).

In the chromatogram obtained with the test solution, the area of any peak apart from the principal peak is not greater than 0.4 times the area of the principal peak in the chromatogram obtained with reference solution (a) (0.2 per cent) and the sum of the areas of all the peaks apart from the principal peak is not greater than the area of the peak in the chromatogram obtained with reference solution (a) (0.5 per cent). Disregard any peak with an area less than 0.02 times that of the principal peak in the chromatogram obtained with reference solution (a).

Impurity B. Examine by thin-layer chromatography (*2.2.27*), using a *TLC silica gel F_{254} plate R.*

Test solution. Dissolve 0.10 g of the substance to be examined in *methanol R* and dilute to 2 ml with the same solvent.

Reference solution. Dissolve 10 mg of *flecainide impurity B CRS* in *methanol R* and dilute to 100 ml with the same solvent (solution A). Dissolve 0.10 g of *flecainide acetate CRS* in solution A and dilute to 2 ml with the same solution.

Apply separately to the plate 5 µl of each solution. Develop over a path of 10 cm using a freshly prepared mixture of 5 volumes of *concentrated ammonia R* and 95 volumes of *acetone R*. Dry the plate at 100 °C to 105 °C until the ammonia has evaporated and examine in ultraviolet light at 254 nm to establish the position of the flecainide spot. Then spray with a freshly prepared 2 g/l solution of *ninhydrin R* in *methanol R* and heat at 100 °C to 110 °C for 2 min to 5 min and examine in daylight. In the chromatogram obtained with the test solution, any spot corresponding to impurity B is not more intense than the spot corresponding to impurity B in the chromatogram obtained with the reference solution (0.2 per cent). The test is not valid unless the chromatogram obtained with the reference solution shows two clearly separated spots.

Heavy metals (*2.4.8*). 1.0 g complies with limit test C for heavy metals (20 ppm). Prepare the standard using 2 ml of *lead standard solution (10 ppm Pb) R*.

Loss on drying (*2.2.32*). Not more than 0.5 per cent determined on 1.000 g by drying in an oven at 60 °C under a pressure not exceeding 0.6 kPa for 2 h.

Sulphated ash (*2.4.14*). Not more than 0.1 per cent, determined on 1.0 g in a platinum crucible.

ASSAY

Dissolve 0.400 g in 25 ml of *anhydrous acetic acid R*. Titrate with *0.1 M perchloric acid*, determining the end-point potentiometrically (*2.2.20*).

1 ml of *0.1 M perchloric acid* is equivalent to 47.44 mg of $C_{19}H_{24}F_6N_2O_5$.

STORAGE

Store protected from light.

IMPURITIES

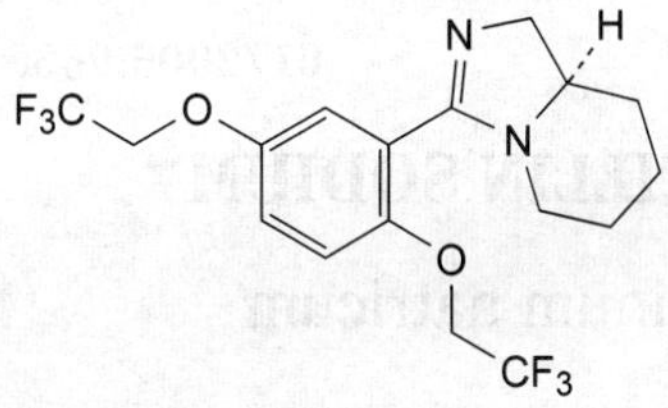

and enantiomer

A. (8a*RS*)-3-[2,5-bis(2,2,2-trifluoroethoxy)phenyl]-1,5,6,7,8,8a-hexahydroimidazo[1,5-*a*]pyridine,

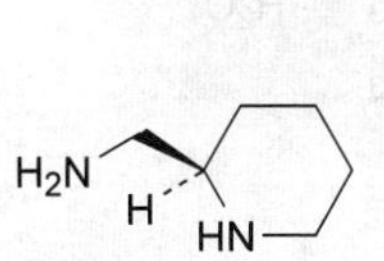

and enantiomer

B. (*RS*)-(piperidin-2-yl)methanamine,

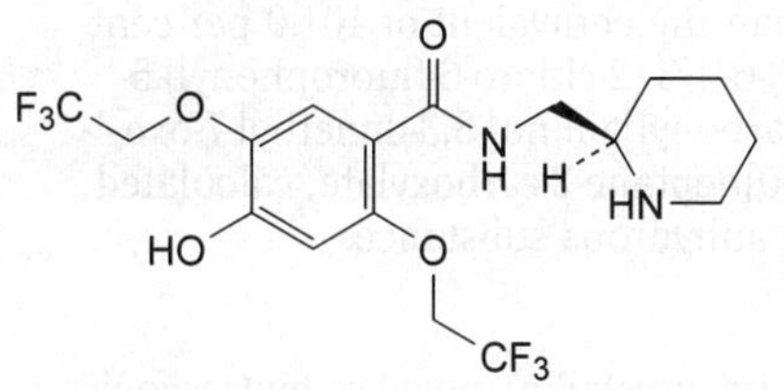

and enantiomer

C. (*RS*)-4-hydroxy-*N*-(piperidin-2-ylmethyl)-2,5-bis(2,2,2-trifluoroethoxy)benzamide,

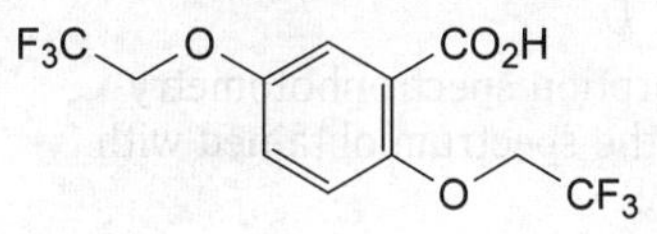

D. 2,5-bis(2,2,2-trifluoroethoxy)benzoic acid,

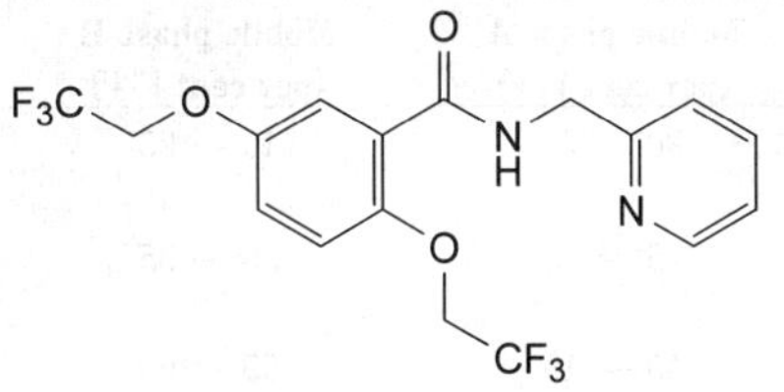

E. *N*-(pyridin-2-ylmethyl)-2,5-bis(2,2,2-trifluoroethoxy)benzamide.

01/2005:1721

FLUBENDAZOLE

Flubendazolum

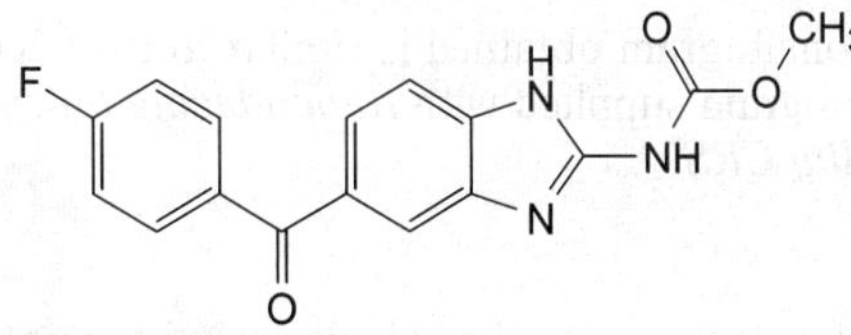

$C_{16}H_{12}FN_3O_3$ M_r 313.3

DEFINITION

Methyl [5-(4-fluorobenzoyl)-1*H*-benzimidazol-2-yl]carbamate

Content: 99.0 per cent to 101.0 per cent (dried substance).

CHARACTERS

Appearance: white or almost white powder.

Solubility: practically insoluble in water, in alcohol and in methylene chloride.

It shows polymorphism.

IDENTIFICATION

Infrared absorption spectrophotometry (*2.2.24*), without recrystallisation.

Comparison: *flubendazole CRS*.

TESTS

Related substances. Liquid chromatography (*2.2.29*).

Test solution. Dissolve 0.100 g of the substance to be examined in *dimethylformamide R* and dilute to 100.0 ml with the same solvent.

Reference solution (a). Dissolve 5 mg of *flubendazole for system suitability CRS* in *dimethylformamide R* and dilute to 5.0 ml with the same solvent.

Reference solution (b). Dilute 1.0 ml of the test solution to 100.0 ml with *dimethylformamide R*. Dilute 5.0 ml of this solution to 20.0 ml with *dimethylformamide R*.

Column:

- *size*: *l* = 0.10 m, Ø = 4.6 mm,
- *stationary phase*: *base-deactivated octadecylsilyl silica gel for chromatography R* (3 µm),
- *temperature*: 40 °C.

Mobile phase:

- *mobile phase A*: 7.5 g/l solution of *ammonium acetate R*,
- *mobile phase B*: *acetonitrile R*,

Time (min)	Mobile phase A (per cent V/V)	Mobile phase B (per cent V/V)
0 - 15	90 → 75	10 → 25
15 - 30	75 → 45	25 → 55
30 - 32	45 → 10	55 → 90
32 - 37	10	90
37 - 38	10 → 90	90 → 10
38 - 42	90	10

Flow rate: 1.2 ml/min.

Detection: spectrophotometer at 250 nm.

Injection: 10 μl.

System suitability: reference solution (a):

– the chromatogram obtained is similar to the chromatogram supplied with *flubendazole for system suitability CRS*.

Limits:

– *correction factors*: for the calculation of contents, multiply the peak areas of the following impurities by the corresponding correction factor: impurity A = 1.4; impurity C = 1.3; impurity D = 1.3; impurity G = 1.4,

– *impurities A, B, C, D, E, G*: for each impurity, not more than the area of the principal peak in the chromatogram obtained with reference solution (b) (0.25 per cent),

– *impurity F*: not more than twice the area of the principal peak in the chromatogram obtained with reference solution (b) (0.5 per cent),

– *any other impurity with a relative retention between 1.2 and 1.3*: not more than the area of the principal peak in the chromatogram obtained with reference solution (b) (0.25 per cent),

– *total*: not more than 6 times the area of the principal peak in the chromatogram obtained with reference solution (b) (1.5 per cent),

– *disregard limit*: 0.2 times the area of the principal peak in the chromatogram obtained with reference solution (b) (0.05 per cent).

Loss on drying (*2.2.32*): maximum 0.5 per cent, determined on 1.000 g by drying in an oven at 100-105 °C, for 4 h.

Sulphated ash (*2.4.14*): maximum 0.1 per cent, determined on 1.0 g.

ASSAY

Dissolve 0.250 g in 3 ml of *anhydrous formic acid R* and add 50 ml of a mixture of 1 volume of *anhydrous acetic acid R* and 7 volumes of *methyl ethyl ketone R*. Titrate with *0.1 M perchloric acid*, determining the end-point potentiometrically (*2.2.20*).

1 ml of *0.1 M perchloric acid* is equivalent to 31.33 mg of $C_{16}H_{12}FN_3O_3$.

STORAGE

Protected from light.

IMPURITIES

Specified impurities: A, B, C, D, E, F, G.

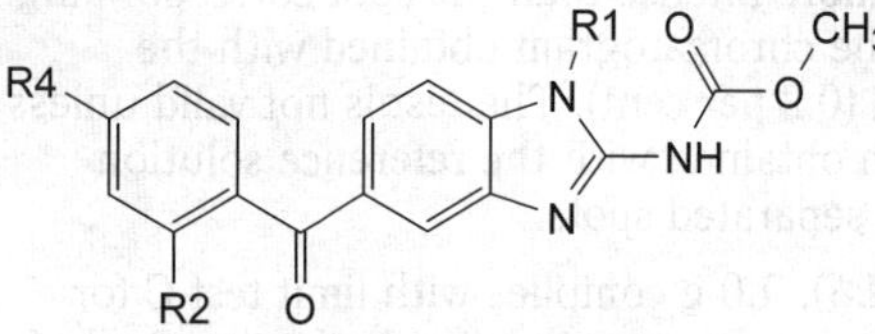

A. R1 = R2 = H, R4 = NH-CHO: methyl [5-[4-(formylamino)benzoyl]-1*H*-benzimidazol-2-yl]carbamate,

E. R1 = R4 = H, R2 = F: methyl [5-(2-fluorobenzoyl)-1*H*-benzimidazol-2-yl]carbamate,

F. R1 = CH_3, R2 = H, R4 = F: methyl [5-(4-fluorobenzoyl)-1-methyl-1*H*-benzimidazol-2-yl]carbamate,

G. R1 = R2 = H, R4 = O-CH$(CH_3)_2$: methyl [5-[4-(1-methylethoxy)benzoyl]-1*H*-benzimidazol-2-yl]carbamate,

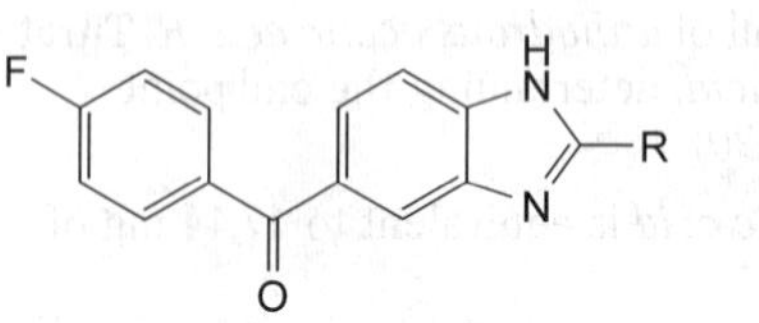

B. R = NH_2: (2-amino-1*H*-benzimidazol-5-yl)(4-fluorophenyl)methanone,

C. R = OH: (4-fluorophenyl)(2-hydroxy-1*H*-benzimidazol-5-yl)methanone,

D. R = H: (1*H*-benzimidazol-5-yl)(4-fluorophenyl)methanone.

01/2005:0668

FLUCLOXACILLIN SODIUM

Flucloxacillinum natricum

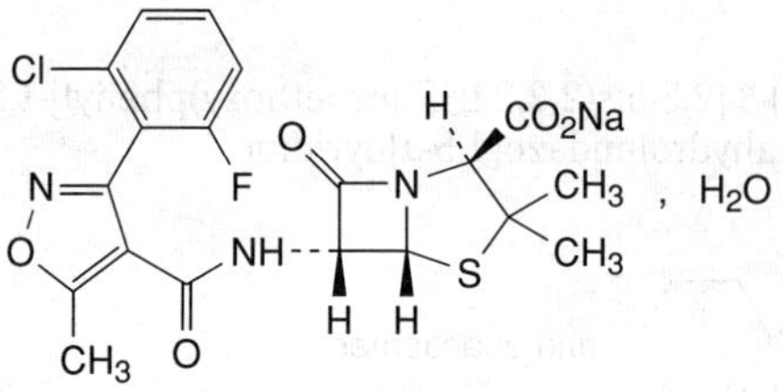

$C_{19}H_{16}ClFN_3NaO_5S,H_2O$ M_r 493.9

DEFINITION

Flucloxacillin sodium contains not less than 95.0 per cent and not more than the equivalent of 101.0 per cent of sodium (2*S*,5*R*,6*R*)-6-[[[3-(2-chloro-6-fluorophenyl)-5-methylisoxazol-4-yl]carbonyl]amino]-3,3-dimethyl-7-oxo-4-thia-1-azabicyclo[3.2.0]heptane-2-carboxylate, calculated with reference to the anhydrous substance.

CHARACTERS

A white or almost white, crystalline powder, hygroscopic, freely soluble in water and in methanol, soluble in alcohol.

IDENTIFICATION

First identification: A, D.

Second identification: B, C, D.

A. Examine by infrared absorption spectrophotometry (*2.2.24*), comparing with the spectrum obtained with *flucloxacillin sodium CRS*.

B. Examine by thin-layer chromatography (*2.2.27*), using *silanised silica gel H R* as the coating substance.

Test solution. Dissolve 25 mg of the substance to be examined in 5 ml of *water R*.

Reference solution (a). Dissolve 25 mg of *flucloxacillin sodium CRS* in 5 ml of *water R*.

Reference solution (b). Dissolve 25 mg of *cloxacillin sodium CRS*, 25 mg of *dicloxacillin sodium CRS* and 25 mg of *flucloxacillin sodium CRS* in 5 ml of *water R*.

Apply separately to the plate 1 µl of each solution. Develop over a path of 15 cm using a mixture of 30 volumes of *acetone R* and 70 volumes of a 154 g/l solution of *ammonium acetate R* adjusted to pH 5.0 with *glacial acetic acid R*. Allow the plate to dry in air and expose it to iodine vapour until the spots appear. Examine in daylight. The principal spot in the chromatogram obtained with the test solution is similar in position, colour and size to the principal spot in the chromatogram obtained with reference solution (a). The test is not valid unless the chromatogram obtained with reference solution (b) shows three clearly separated spots.

C. Place about 2 mg in a test-tube about 150 mm long and 15 mm in diameter. Moisten with 0.05 ml of *water R* and add 2 ml of *sulphuric acid-formaldehyde reagent R*. Mix the contents of the tube by swirling; the colour of the solution is slightly greenish-yellow. Place the test-tube in a water-bath for 1 min; the solution becomes yellow.

D. It gives reaction (a) of sodium (*2.3.1*).

TESTS

Solution S. Dissolve 2.50 g in *carbon dioxide-free water R* and dilute to 25.0 ml with the same solvent.

Appearance of solution. Solution S is clear (*2.2.1*). The absorbance (*2.2.25*) of solution S measured at 430 nm is not greater than 0.04.

pH (*2.2.3*). The pH of solution S is 5.0 to 7.0.

Specific optical rotation (*2.2.7*). Dissolve 0.250 g in *water R* and dilute to 25.0 ml with the same solvent. The specific optical rotation is + 158 to + 168, calculated with reference to the anhydrous substance.

Related substances. Examine by liquid chromatography (*2.2.29*) as prescribed under Assay. Inject test solution (a) and continue the chromatography for five times the retention time of the principal peak. Inject reference solution (b). In the chromatogram obtained with test solution (a): the area of any peak, apart from the principal peak, is not greater than the area of the principal peak in the chromatogram obtained with reference solution (b) (1 per cent); the sum of the areas of all peaks, apart from the principal peak, is not greater than five times the area of the principal peak in the chromatogram obtained with reference solution (b) (5 per cent). Disregard any peak with an area less than 0.05 times the area of the principal peak in the chromatogram obtained with reference solution (b).

***N,N*-Dimethylaniline** (*2.4.26, Method B*). Not more than 20 ppm.

2-Ethylhexanoic acid (*2.4.28*). Not more than 0.8 per cent *m/m*.

Water (*2.5.12*): 3.0 per cent to 4.5 per cent, determined on 0.300 g by the semi-micro determination of water.

Pyrogens (*2.6.8*). If intended for use in the manufacture of parenteral dosage forms without a further appropriate procedure for the removal of pyrogens, it complies with the test for pyrogens. Inject per kilogram of the rabbit's mass 1 ml of a solution in *water for injections R* containing 20 mg of the substance to be examined per millilitre.

ASSAY

Examine by liquid chromatography (*2.2.29*).

Test solution (a). Dissolve 50.0 mg of the substance to be examined in the mobile phase and dilute to 50.0 ml with the mobile phase.

Test solution (b). Dilute 5.0 ml of test solution (a) to 50.0 ml with the mobile phase.

Reference solution (a). Dissolve 50.0 mg of *flucloxacillin sodium CRS* in the mobile phase and dilute to 50.0 ml with the mobile phase. Dilute 5.0 ml of the solution to 50.0 ml with the mobile phase.

Reference solution (b). Dilute 5.0 ml of reference solution (a) to 50.0 ml with the mobile phase.

Reference solution (c). Dissolve 5 mg of *flucloxacillin sodium CRS* and 5 mg of *cloxacillin sodium CRS* in the mobile phase and dilute to 50.0 ml with the mobile phase.

The chromatographic procedure may be carried out using:

– a stainless steel column 0.25 m long and 4 mm in internal diameter packed with *octadecylsilyl silica gel for chromatography R* (5 µm),
– as mobile phase at a flow rate of 1 ml/min a mixture of 25 volumes of *acetonitrile R* and 75 volumes of a 2.7 g/l solution of *potassium dihydrogen phosphate R*; adjust to pH 5.0 with *dilute sodium hydroxide solution R*,
– as detector a spectrophotometer set at 225 nm,
– a 20 µl loop injector.

Inject reference solution (c). Adjust the sensitivity of the system so that the heights of the principal peaks in the chromatogram obtained are at least 50 per cent of the full scale of the recorder. The test is not valid unless the resolution between the first peak (cloxacillin) and the second peak (flucloxacillin) is at least 2.5. Inject reference solution (a) six times. The test is not valid unless the relative standard deviation of the peak area for flucloxacillin is at most 1.0 per cent. Inject alternately test solution (b) and reference solution (a).

STORAGE

Store in an airtight container, at a temperature not exceeding 25 °C. If the substance is sterile, store in a sterile, airtight, tamper-proof container.

LABELLING

The label states, where applicable, that the substance is apyrogenic.

IMPURITIES

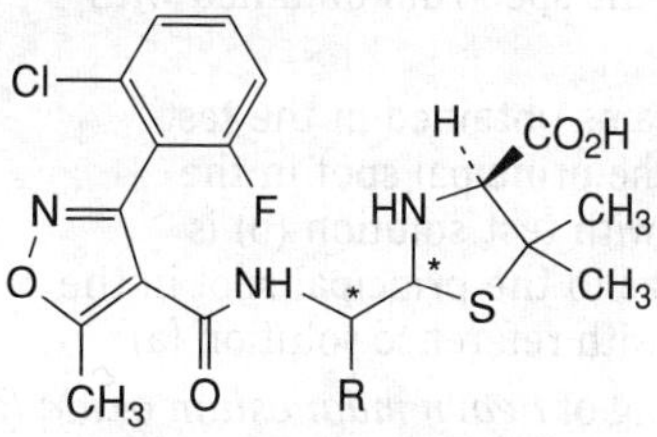

A. R = CO_2H: (4*S*)-2-[carboxy[[[3-(2-chloro-6-fluorophenyl)-5-methylisoxazol-4-yl]carbonyl]amino]methyl]-5,5-dimethylthiazolidine-4-carboxylic acid (penicilloic acids of flucloxacillin),

B. R = H: (2*RS*,4*S*)-2-[[[[3-(2-chloro-6-fluorophenyl)-5-methylisoxazol-4-yl]carbonyl]amino]methyl]-5,5-dimethylthiazolidine-4-carboxylic acid (penilloic acids of flucloxacillin),

Monographs F-H

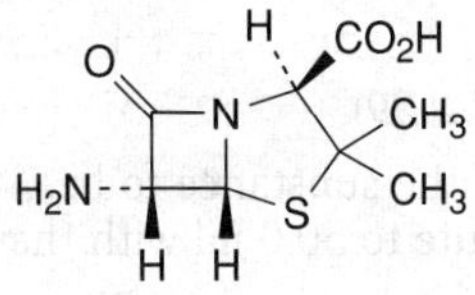

C. (2*S*,5*R*,6*R*)-6-amino-3,3-dimethyl-7-oxo-4-thia-1-azabicyclo[3.2.0]heptane-2-carboxylic acid (6-aminopenicillanic acid),

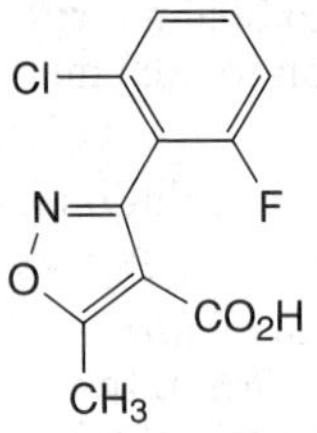

D. 3-(2-chloro-6-fluorophenyl)-5-methylisoxazole-4-carboxylic acid.

01/2005:0766

FLUCYTOSINE

Flucytosinum

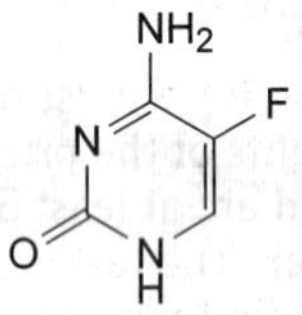

$C_4H_4FN_3O$ M_r 129.1

DEFINITION

Flucytosine contains not less than 98.5 per cent and not more than the equivalent of 101.0 per cent of 4-amino-5-fluoropyrimidin-2(1*H*)-one, calculated with reference to the dried substance.

CHARACTERS

A white or almost white, crystalline powder, sparingly soluble in water, slightly soluble in ethanol.

IDENTIFICATION

First identification: A.

Second identification: B, C, D.

A. Examine by infrared absorption spectrophotometry (*2.2.24*), comparing with the spectrum obtained with *flucytosine CRS*.

B. Examine the chromatograms obtained in the test for related substances. The principal spot in the chromatogram obtained with test solution (b) is similar in position and size to the principal spot in the chromatogram obtained with reference solution (a).

C. Mix about 5 mg with 45 mg of *heavy magnesium oxide R* and ignite in a crucible until an almost white residue is obtained (usually less than 5 min). Allow to cool, add 1 ml of *water R*, 0.05 ml of *phenolphthalein solution R1* and about 1 ml of *dilute hydrochloric acid R* to render the solution colourless. Filter and add to the filtrate a freshly prepared mixture of 0.1 ml of *alizarin S solution R* and 0.1 ml of *zirconyl nitrate solution R*. Mix, allow to stand for 5 min and compare the colour of the solution with that of a blank prepared in the same manner. The colour of the solution changes from red to yellow.

D. To 5 ml of solution S (see Tests) add 0.15 ml of *bromine water R* and shake. The colour of the solution is discharged.

TESTS

Solution S. Dissolve 0.5 g in *carbon dioxide-free water R* and dilute to 50 ml with the same solvent.

Appearance of solution. Solution S is clear (*2.2.1*) and not more intensely coloured than reference solution BY_7 or Y_7 (*2.2.2, Method II*).

Related substances. Examine by thin-layer chromatography (*2.2.27*), using a suitable silica gel as the coating substance.

Test solution (a). Dissolve 50 mg of the substance to be examined in a mixture of 10 volumes of *water R* and 15 volumes of *methanol R* and dilute to 5 ml with the same mixture of solvents.

Test solution (b). Dilute 1 ml of test solution (a) to 10 ml with a mixture of 10 volumes of *water R* and 15 volumes of *methanol R*.

Reference solution (a). Dissolve 10 mg of *flucytosine CRS* in a mixture of 10 volumes of *water R* and 15 volumes of *methanol R* and dilute to 10 ml with the same mixture of solvents.

Reference solution (b). Dilute 1 ml of test solution (b) to 100 ml with a mixture of 10 volumes of *water R* and 15 volumes of *methanol R*.

Reference solution (c). Dissolve 5 mg of *fluorouracil CRS* in 5 ml of reference solution (a).

Apply separately to the plate 10 µl of each solution. Develop over a path of 12 cm in an unsaturated tank using a mixture of 1 volume of *anhydrous formic acid R*, 15 volumes of *water R*, 25 volumes of *methanol R* and 60 volumes of *ethyl acetate R*. Allow the solvents to evaporate. At the bottom of a chromatography tank place an evaporating dish containing a mixture of 2 volumes of a 15 g/l solution of *potassium permanganate R*, 1 volume of *hydrochloric acid R1* and 1 volume of *water R*, close the tank and allow to stand for 15 min. Place the dried plate in the tank and close the tank. Leave the plate in contact with the chlorine vapour for 5 min. Withdraw the plate and place it in a current of cold air until the excess of chlorine is removed and an area of the coating below the points of application does not give a blue colour with a drop of *potassium iodide and starch solution R*. Spray with *potassium iodide and starch solution R*. Examine the plate in daylight. Any spot in the chromatogram obtained with test solution (a), apart from the principal spot, is not more intense than the spot in the chromatogram obtained with reference solution (b) (0.1 per cent). The test is not valid unless the chromatogram obtained with reference solution (c) shows two clearly separated spots.

Fluoride. Not more than 200 ppm. Carry out a potentiometric determination of fluoride ion, using a fluoride-selective indicator electrode and a silver-silver chloride reference electrode.

Prepare and store all solutions in plastic containers.

Buffer solution. Dissolve 58 g of *sodium chloride R* in 500 ml of *water R*. Add 57 ml of *glacial acetic acid R* and 200 ml of a 100 g/l solution of *cyclohexylenedinitrilotetra-acetic acid R* in *1 M sodium hydroxide*. Adjust the pH to 5.0 to 5.5 with a 200 g/l solution of *sodium hydroxide R* and dilute to 1000.0 ml with *water R*.

Test solution. Dissolve 1.00 g of the substance to be examined in *water R* and dilute to 100.0 ml with the same solvent.

Reference solutions. Dissolve 4.42 g of *sodium fluoride R,* previously dried at 120 °C for 2 h, in 300 ml of *water R* and dilute to 1000.0 ml with the same solvent (solution (a): 1.9 g/l of fluoride). Prepare three reference solutions by dilution of solution (a) 1 in 100, 1 in 1000 and 1 in 10 000.

To 20.0 ml of each reference solution, add 10.0 ml of the buffer solution and stir with a magnetic stirrer. Introduce the electrodes into the solution and allow to stand for 5 min with constant stirring. Determine the potential difference between the electrodes. Plot on semi-logarithmic graph paper the potential difference obtained for each solution as a function of concentration of fluoride. Using exactly the same conditions, determine the potential difference obtained with the test solution and calculate the content of fluoride.

Heavy metals (*2.4.8*). 1.0 g complies with limit test C for heavy metals (20 ppm). *Use aplatinum crucible.* Prepare the standard using 2 ml of *lead standard solution (10 ppm Pb) R.*

Loss on drying (*2.2.32*). Not more than 1.0 per cent, determined on 1.000 g by drying in an oven at 100 °C to 105 °C.

Sulphated ash (*2.4.14*). Not more than 0.1 per cent, determined on 1.0 g in a platinum crucible.

ASSAY

Dissolve 0.100 g in 40 ml of *anhydrous acetic acid R* and add 100 ml of *acetic anhydride R.* Titrate with *0.1 M perchloric acid* determining the end-point potentiometrically (*2.2.20*).

1 ml of *0.1 M perchloric acid* is equivalent to 12.91 mg of $C_4H_4FN_3O$.

STORAGE

Store protected from light.

01/2005:0767

FLUDROCORTISONE ACETATE

Fludrocortisoni acetas

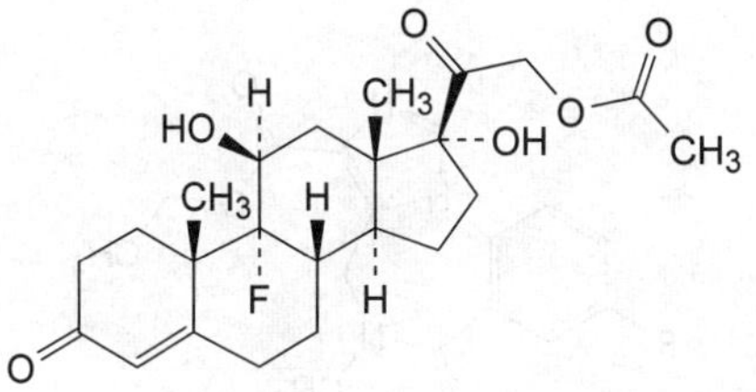

$C_{23}H_{31}FO_6$ M_r 422.5

DEFINITION

Fludrocortisone acetate contains not less than 97.0 per cent and not more than the equivalent of 103.0 per cent of 9-fluoro-11β,17-dihydroxy-3,20-dioxopregn-4-en-21-yl acetate, calculated with reference to the dried substance.

CHARACTERS

A white or almost white, crystalline powder, practically insoluble in water, sparingly soluble in ethanol.

IDENTIFICATION

First identification: A, B.

Second identification: C, D, E.

A. Examine by infrared absorption spectrophotometry (*2.2.24*), comparing with the spectrum obtained with *fludrocortisone acetate CRS.* If the spectra obtained in the solid state show differences, dissolve the substance to be examined and the reference substance separately in the minimum volume of *acetone R,* evaporate to dryness and record the spectra again using the residues.

B. Examine by thin-layer chromatography (*2.2.27*), using as the coating substance a suitable silica gel with a fluorescent indicator having an optimal intensity at 254 nm.

Test solution. Dissolve 10 mg of the substance to be examined in a mixture of 1 volume of *methanol R* and 9 volumes of *methylene chloride R* and dilute to 10 ml with the same mixture of solvents.

Reference solution (a). Dissolve 10 mg of *fludrocortisone acetate CRS* in a mixture of 1 volume of *methanol R* and 9 volumes of *methylene chloride R* and dilute to 10 ml with the same mixture of solvents.

Reference solution (b). Dissolve 5 mg of *cortisone acetate CRS* in 5 ml of reference solution (a).

Apply separately to the plate 5 µl of each solution. Prepare the mobile phase by adding a mixture of 1.2 volumes of *water R* and 8 volumes of *methanol R* to a mixture of 15 volumes of *ether R* and 77 volumes of *methylene chloride R.* Develop over a path of 15 cm. Allow the plate to dry in air and examine in ultraviolet light at 254 nm. The principal spot in the chromatogram obtained with the test solution is similar in position and size to the principal spot in the chromatogram obtained with reference solution (a). Spray the plate with *alcoholic solution of sulphuric acid R.* Heat at 120 °C for 10 min or until the spots appear. Allow to cool. Examine in daylight and in ultraviolet light at 365 nm. The principal spot in the chromatogram obtained with the test solution is similar in position, colour in daylight, fluorescence in ultraviolet light at 365 nm and size to the principal spot in the chromatogram obtained with reference solution (a). The test is not valid unless the chromatogram obtained with reference solution (b) shows two clearly separated spots.

C. Examine by thin-layer chromatography (*2.2.27*), using as the coating substance a suitable silica gel with a fluorescent indicator having an optimal intensity at 254 nm.

Test solution (a). Dissolve 25 mg of the substance to be examined in *methanol R* and dilute to 5 ml with the same solvent. (This solution is also used to prepare test solution (b)). Dilute 2 ml of the solution to 10 ml with *methylene chloride R.*

Test solution (b). Transfer 2 ml of the solution obtained during preparation of test solution (a) to a 15 ml glass tube with a ground-glass stopper or a polytetrafluoroethylene cap. Add 10 ml of *saturated methanolic potassium hydrogen carbonate solution R* and immediately pass a stream of *nitrogen R* through the solution for 5 min. Stopper the tube. Heat on a water-bath at 45 °C protected from light for 2 h 30 min. Allow to cool.

Reference solution (a). Dissolve 25 mg of *fludrocortisone acetate CRS* in *methanol R* and dilute to 5 ml with the same solvent. (This solution is also used to prepare reference solution (b)). Dilute 2 ml of the solution to 10 ml with *methylene chloride R.*

Reference solution (b). Transfer 2 ml of the solution obtained during preparation of reference solution (a) to a 15 ml glass tube with a ground-glass stopper or a polytetrafluoroethylene cap. Add 10 ml of *saturated methanolic potassium hydrogen carbonate solution R* and immediately pass a stream of *nitrogen R* through the solution for 5 min. Stopper the tube. Heat on a water bath at 45 °C protected from light for 2 h 30 min. Allow to cool.

Monographs F-H

Apply separately to the plate 5 µl of each solution. Prepare the mobile phase by adding a mixture of 1.2 volumes of *water R* and 8 volumes of *methanol R* to a mixture of 15 volumes of *ether R* and 77 volumes of *methylene chloride R*. Develop over a path of 15 cm. Allow the plate to dry in air and examine in ultraviolet light at 254 nm. The principal spot in each of the chromatograms obtained with the test solutions is similar in position and size to the principal spot in the chromatogram obtained with the corresponding reference solution. Spray with *alcoholic solution of sulphuric acid R*. Heat at 120 °C for 10 min or until the spots appear. Allow to cool. Examine in daylight and in ultraviolet light at 365 nm. The principal spot in each of the chromatograms obtained with the test solutions is similar in position, colour in daylight, fluorescence in ultraviolet light at 365 nm and size to the principal spot in the chromatogram obtained with the corresponding reference solution. The principal spots in the chromatograms obtained with test solution (b) and reference solution (b) have R_f values distinctly lower than those of the principal spots in the chromatograms obtained with test solution (a) and reference solution (a).

D. Mix about 5 mg with 45 mg of *heavy magnesium oxide R* and ignite in a crucible until an almost white residue is obtained (usually less than 5 min). Allow to cool, add 1 ml of *water R*, 0.05 ml of *phenolphthalein solution R1* and about 1 ml of *dilute hydrochloric acid R* to render the solution colourless. Filter and add to the filtrate a freshly prepared mixture of 0.1 ml of *alizarin S solution R* and 0.1 ml of *zirconyl nitrate solution R*. Mix, allow to stand for 5 min and compare the colour of the solution with that of a blank prepared in the same manner. The colour of the solution changes from red to yellow.

E. About 10 mg gives the reaction of acetyl (*2.3.1*).

TESTS

Specific optical rotation (*2.2.7*). Dissolve 0.250 g in *dioxan R* and dilute to 25.0 ml with the same solvent. The specific optical rotation is + 148 to + 156, calculated with reference to the dried substance.

Related substances. Examine by liquid chromatography (*2.2.29*).

Test solution. Dissolve 20.0 mg of the substance to be examined in the mobile phase and dilute to 10.0 ml with the mobile phase.

Reference solution (a). Dissolve 2.0 mg of *fludrocortisone acetate CRS* and 2.0 mg of *hydrocortisone acetate CRS* in the mobile phase and dilute to 50.0 ml with the mobile phase.

Reference solution (b). Dilute 1.0 ml of the test solution to 50.0 ml with the mobile phase.

The chromatographic procedure may be carried out using:

– a stainless steel column 0.2 m long and 4.6 mm in internal diameter packed with *octadecylsilyl silica gel for chromatography R*,
– as mobile phase at a flow rate of 1 ml/min a mixture of 35 volumes of *tetrahydrofuran R* and 65 volumes of *water R*,
– as detector a spectrophotometer set at 254 nm.

Adjust the sensitivity so that the height of the principal peak in the chromatogram obtained with reference solution (b) is 70 per cent to 90 per cent of the full scale of the recorder. Equilibrate the column with the mobile phase at a flow rate of 1 ml/min for about 30 min.

Inject 20 µl of reference solution (a). When the chromatograms are recorded in the conditions described above the retention times are: hydrocortisone acetate about 8.5 min and fludrocortisone acetate about 10 min. The test is not valid unless the resolution between the peaks corresponding to hydrocortisone acetate and fludrocortisone acetate is at least 1.0; if this resolution is not achieved, adjust slightly the concentration of tetrahydrofuran in the mobile phase. Increasing the concentration of tetrahydrofuran reduces the retention times.

Inject separately 20 µl of the test solution and 20 µl of reference solution (b). Continue the chromatography for twice the retention time of the principal peak. In the chromatogram obtained with the test solution: the area of any peak, apart from the principal peak, is not greater than half the area of the principal peak in the chromatogram obtained with reference solution (b) (1.0 per cent) and the sum of the areas of all such peaks, is not greater than 0.75 times the area of the principal peak in the chromatogram obtained with reference solution (b) (1.5 per cent). Disregard any peak due to the solvent and any peak with an area less than 0.025 times the area of the principal peak in the chromatogram obtained with reference solution (b).

Loss on drying (*2.2.32*). Not more than 1.0 per cent, determined on 0.500 g by drying in an oven at 100 °C to 105 °C.

ASSAY

Dissolve 10.0 mg of the substance to be examined in *alcohol R* and dilute to 100.0 ml with the same solvent. Dilute 5.0 ml of this solution to 50.0 ml with *alcohol R*. Measure the absorbance (*2.2.25*) at the maximum at 238 nm.

Calculate the content of $C_{23}H_{31}FO_6$ taking the specific absorbance to be 405.

01/2005:1326

FLUMAZENIL

Flumazenilum

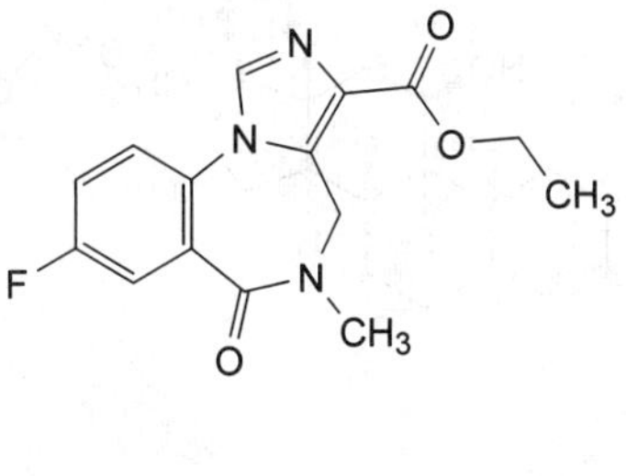

$C_{15}H_{14}FN_3O_3$ M_r 303.3

DEFINITION

Ethyl 8-fluoro-5-methyl-6-oxo-5,6-dihydro-4*H*-imidazo[1,5-*a*][1,4]benzodiazepine-3-carboxylate.

Content: 99.0 per cent to 101.0 per cent (dried substance).

CHARACTERS

Appearance: white or almost white, crystalline powder.

Solubility: very slightly soluble in water, freely soluble in methylene chloride, sparingly soluble in methanol.

mp: 198 °C to 202 °C.

IDENTIFICATION

Infrared absorption spectrophotometry (*2.2.24*).

Comparison: *Ph. Eur. reference spectrum of flumazenil*.

TESTS

Appearance of solution. The solution is clear (*2.2.1*) and is not more intensely coloured than reference solution BY_7 (*2.2.2, Method II*).

Dissolve 0.10 g in *methanol R* and dilute to 10 ml with the same solvent.

Impurity C: maximum 1 per cent.

Dissolve 0.10 g in 0.5 ml of *methylene chloride R* and dilute to 10 ml with *butanol R*. To 5.0 ml of this solution add 2.0 ml of *ninhydrin solution R* and heat in a water-bath at 95 °C for 15 min. Any blue-purple colour in the solution is not more intense than that in a standard prepared at the same time and in the same manner using 5.0 ml of a 0.1 g/l solution of *dimethylformamide diethylacetal R* in *butanol R*.

Related substances. Liquid chromatography (*2.2.29*).

Test solution. Dissolve 50.0 mg of the substance to be examined in 5 ml of *methanol R* and dilute to 25.0 ml with the mobile phase.

Reference solution (a). Dissolve 2.0 mg of *flumazenil impurity B CRS* and 2.0 mg of the substance to be examined in the mobile phase and dilute to 25.0 ml with the mobile phase. Dilute 2.0 ml of this solution to 25.0 ml with the mobile phase.

Reference solution (b). Dilute 10.0 ml of the test solution to 100.0 ml with the mobile phase. Dilute 1.0 ml of this solution to 100.0 ml with the mobile phase.

Column:

- *size*: *l* = 0.25 m, Ø = 4.6 mm,
- *stationary phase*: *end-capped octadecylsilyl silica gel for chromatography R* (5 µm).

Mobile phase: to 800 ml of *water R* adjusted to pH 2.0 with *phosphoric acid R*, add 130 ml of *methanol R* and 70 ml of *tetrahydrofuran R* and mix.

Flow rate: 1 ml/min.

Detection: spectrophotometer at 230 nm.

Injection: 20 µl.

Run time: 3 times the retention time of flumazenil.

Relative retention with reference to flumazenil (retention time = about 14 min): impurity A = about 0.4; impurity D = about 0.5; impurity E = about 0.6; impurity B = about 0.7; impurity F = about 2.4.

System suitability: reference solution (a):

- *resolution*: minimum 3.0 between the peaks due to impurity B and flumazenil.

Limits:

- *impurity B*: not more than twice the area of the principal peak in the chromatogram obtained with reference solution (b) (0.2 per cent),
- *any other impurity*: for each impurity, not more than the area of the principal peak in the chromatogram obtained with reference solution (b) (0.1 per cent),
- *total*: not more than twice the area of the principal peak in the chromatogram obtained with reference solution (b) (0.2 per cent),
- *disregard limit*: 0.5 times the area of the principal peak in the chromatogram obtained with reference solution (b) (0.05 per cent).

Loss on drying (*2.2.32*): maximum 0.5 per cent, determined on 1.000 g by drying in an oven at 100-105 °C.

Sulphated ash (*2.4.14*): maximum 0.1 per cent, determined on 1.0 g in a platinum crucible.

ASSAY

Dissolve 0.250 g in 50 ml of a mixture of 2 volumes of *acetic anhydride R* and 3 volumes of *anhydrous acetic acid R*. Titrate with *0.1 M perchloric acid*, determining the end-point potentiometrically (*2.2.20*).

1 ml of *0.1 M perchloric acid* is equivalent to 30.33 mg of $C_{15}H_{14}FN_3O_3$.

IMPURITIES

Specified impurities: B, C.

Other detectable impurities: A, D, E, F.

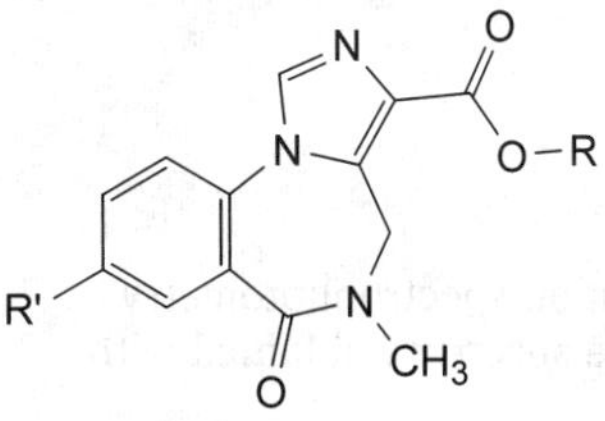

A. R = H, R′ = F: 8-fluoro-5-methyl-6-oxo-5,6-dihydro-4*H*-imidazo[1,5-*a*][1,4]benzodiazepine-3-carboxylic acid,

B. R = C_2H_5, R′ = OH: ethyl 8-hydroxy-5-methyl-6-oxo-5,6-dihydro-4*H*-imidazo[1,5-*a*][1,4]benzodiazepine-3-carboxylate,

E. R = C_2H_5, R′ = H: ethyl 5-methyl-6-oxo-5,6-dihydro-4*H*-imidazo[1,5-*a*][1,4]benzodiazepine-3-carboxylate,

F. R = C_2H_5, R′ = Cl: ethyl 8-chloro-5-methyl-6-oxo-5,6-dihydro-4*H*-imidazo[1,5-*a*][1,4]benzodiazepine-3-carboxylate,

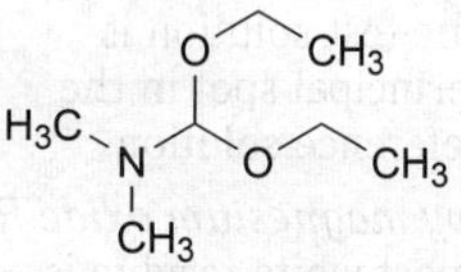

C. diethoxy-*N*,*N*-dimethylmethanamine,

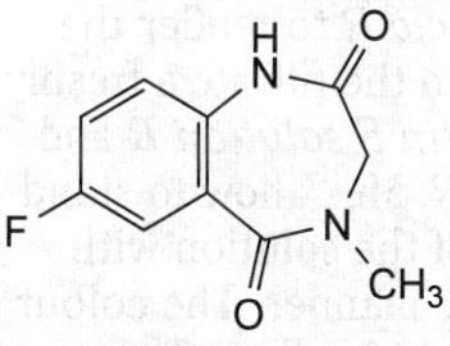

D. 7-fluoro-4-methyl-3,4-dihydro-1*H*-1,4-benzodiazepine-2,5-dione.

01/2005:1517

FLUMEQUINE

Flumequinum

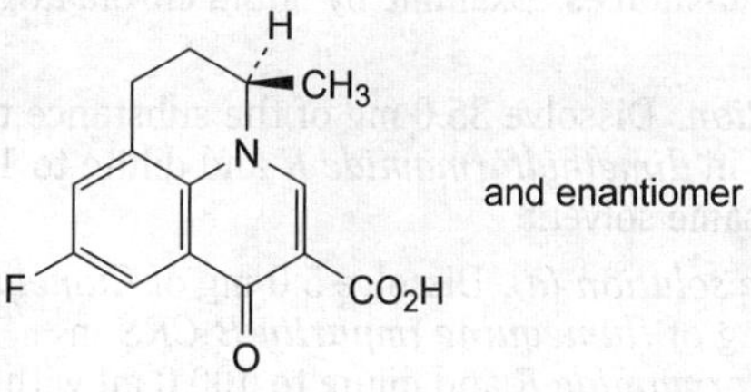

$C_{14}H_{12}FNO_3$ M_r 261.3

DEFINITION

Flumequine contains not less than 99.0 per cent and not more than the equivalent of 101.0 per cent of (*RS*)-9-fluoro-5-methyl-1-oxo-6,7-dihydro-1*H*,5*H*-benzo[*i*,*j*]quinolizine-2-carboxylic acid, calculated with reference to the dried substance.

CHARACTERS

A microcrystalline white powder, practically insoluble in water, freely soluble indilute solutions of alkali hydroxides, sparingly soluble in methylene chloride, very slightly soluble in methanol.

IDENTIFICATION

First identification: A, B.

Second identification: B, C, D.

A. Examine by infrared absorption spectrophotometry (*2.2.24*), comparing with the spectrum obtained with *flumequine CRS*.

B. It complies with the test for optical rotation (see Tests).

C. Examine by thin-layer chromatography (*2.2.27*), using a *TLC silica gel F_{254} plate R*.

Test solution. Dissolve 5 mg of the substance to be examined in 10 ml of *methylene chloride R*.

Reference solution. Dissolve 5 mg of *flumequine CRS* in 10 ml of *methylene chloride R*.

Apply to the plate 5 µl of each solution. Develop over a path of 15 cm using a mixture of 10 volumes of *ammonia R*, 10 volumes of *water R* and 90 volumes of *alcohol R*. Allow the plate to dry in air. Examine in ultraviolet light at 254 nm. The principal spot in the chromatogram obtained with the test solution is similar in position and size to the principal spot in the chromatogram obtained with the reference solution.

D. Mix about 5 mg with 45 mg of *heavy magnesium oxide R* and ignite in a crucible until an almost white residue is obtained (usually less than 5 min). Allow to cool, add 1 ml of *water R*, 0.05 ml of *phenolphthalein solution R1* and about 2 ml of *dilute hydrochloric acid R* to render the solution colourless. Filter and add to the filtrate a freshly prepared mixture of 0.1 ml of *alizarin S solution R* and 0.1 ml of *zirconyl nitrate solution R*. Mix, allow to stand for 5 min and compare the colour of the solution with that of a blank prepared in the same manner. The colour of the test solution changes from red to yellow. The colour of the blank solution remains red.

TESTS

Solution S. Dissolve 5.00 g in *0.5 M sodium hydroxide* and dilute to 50.0 ml with the same solvent.

Appearance of solution. Solution S is clear (*2.2.1*) and not more intensely coloured than reference solution BY_5 (*2.2.2, Method II*).

Optical rotation (*2.2.7*). The angle of optical rotation, determined on solution S, is − 0.10° to + 0.10°.

Related substances. Examine by liquid chromatography (*2.2.29*).

Test solution. Dissolve 35.0 mg of the substance to be examined in *dimethylformamide R* and dilute to 100.0 ml with the same solvent.

Reference solution (a). Dissolve 5.0 mg of *flumequine CRS* and 5.0 mg of *flumequine impurity B CRS* in *dimethylformamide R* and dilute to 100.0 ml with the same solvent.

Reference solution (b). Dilute 1.0 ml of the test solution to 200.0 ml with *dimethylformamide R*.

The chromatographic procedure may be carried out using:

- a stainless steel column 0.15 m long and 4.6 mm in internal diameter packed with *octadecylsilyl silica gel for chromatography R* (5 µm),
- as mobile phase at a flow rate of 0.8 ml/min a mixture of 49 volumes of *methanol R* and 51 volumes of a 1.36 g/l solution of *potassium dihydrogen phosphate R*,
- as detector a spectrophotometer set at 313 nm,
- a 10 µl loop injector.

Inject reference solution (a). When the chromatograms are recorded in the prescribed conditions, the retention times are: impurity B, about 11 min and flumequine, about 13 min. The test is not valid unless the resolution between the peaks corresponding to flumequine and impurity B is at least 2.0.

Inject separately *dimethylformamide R* as a blank, the test solution and reference solution (b). Continue the chromatography of the test solution for three times the retention time of flumequine. When the chromatograms are recorded in the prescribed conditions, the relative retention time for impurity A is about 0.67 with respect to the flumequine peak. In the chromatogram obtained with the test solution: the area of any peak, apart from the principal peak, is not greater than the area of the principal peak in the chromatogram obtained with reference solution (b) (0.5 per cent); the sum of the areas of all the peaks, apart from the principal peak, is not greater than twice the area of the principal peak in the chromatogram obtained with reference solution (b) (1 per cent). Disregard any peak obtained with dimethylformamide and any peak with an area less than 0.1 times the area of the principal peak in the chromatogram obtained with reference solution (b).

Heavy metals (*2.4.8*). 2.0 g complies with limit test C for heavy metals (10 ppm). Prepare the standard using 2 ml of *lead standard solution (10 ppm Pb) R*.

Loss on drying (*2.2.32*). Not more than 0.5 per cent, determined on 1.000 g by drying in an oven at 100 °C to 105 °C for 3 h.

Sulphated ash (*2.4.14*). Not more than 0.1 per cent, determined on 1.0 g in a platinum crucible.

ASSAY

Dissolve 0.500 g in 50 ml of *dimethylformamide R*. Titrate with *0.1 M tetrabutylammonium hydroxide*, determining the end-point potentiometrically (*2.2.20*).

1 ml of *0.1 M tetrabutylammonium hydroxide* is equivalent to 26.13 mg of $C_{14}H_{12}FNO_3$.

IMPURITIES

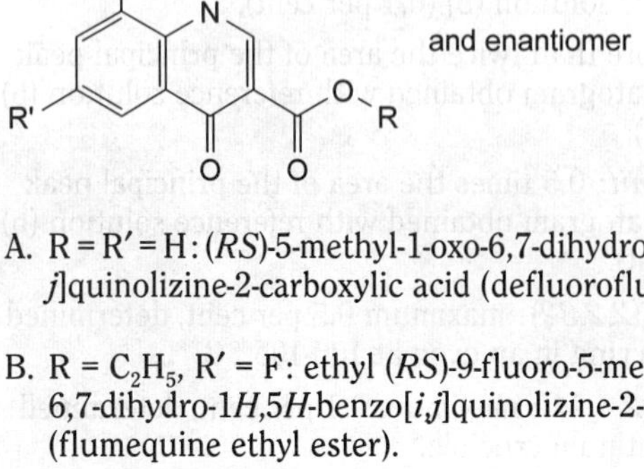

A. R = R′ = H: (*RS*)-5-methyl-1-oxo-6,7-dihydro-1*H*,5*H*-benzo[*i*,*j*]quinolizine-2-carboxylic acid (defluoroflumequine),

B. R = C_2H_5, R′ = F: ethyl (*RS*)-9-fluoro-5-methyl-1-oxo-6,7-dihydro-1*H*,5*H*-benzo[*i*,*j*]quinolizine-2-carboxylate (flumequine ethyl ester).

01/2005:1327

FLUMETASONE PIVALATE

Flumetasoni pivalas

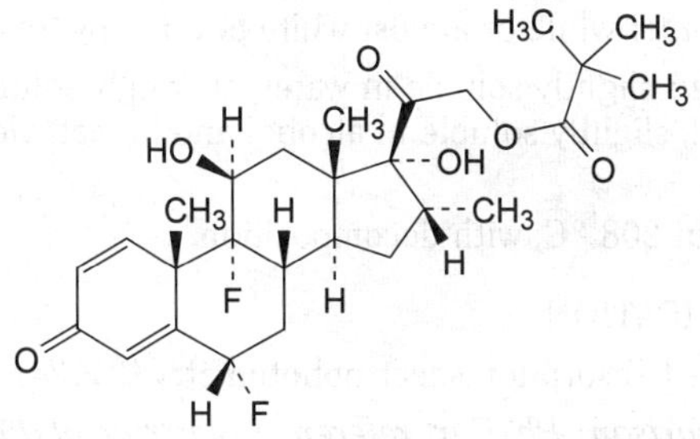

$C_{27}H_{36}F_2O_6$ M_r 494.6

DEFINITION

Flumetasone pivalate contains not less than 97.0 per cent and not more than the equivalent of 103.0 per cent of 6α,9-difluoro-11β,17-dihydroxy-16α-methyl-3,20-dioxopregna-1,4-dien-21-yl 2,2-dimethylpropanoate, calculated with reference to the dried substance.

CHARACTERS

A white or almost white, crystalline powder, practically insoluble in water, sparingly soluble in acetone, slightly soluble in alcohol and in methylene chloride.

It shows polymorphism.

IDENTIFICATION

First identification: A, B.

Second identification: B, C, D.

A. Examine by infrared absorption spectrophotometry (*2.2.24*),comparing with the spectrum obtained with *flumetasone pivalate CRS*. If the spectra obtained in the solid state show differences, dissolve the substance to be examined and the reference substance separately in *acetone R*, evaporate to dryness on a water-bath and record new spectra using the residues.

B. Examine by thin-layer chromatography (*2.2.27*), using a *TLC silica gel F_{254} plate R*.

Test solution. Dissolve 10 mg of the substance to be examined in *acetone R* and dilute to 10 ml with the same solvent.

Reference solution (a). Dissolve 10 mg of *flumetasone pivalate CRS* in *acetone R* and dilute to 10 ml with the same solvent.

Reference solution (b). Dissolve 10 mg of *desoxycortone acetate CRS* in *acetone R* and dilute to 10 ml with the same solvent. Dilute 5 ml of the solution to 10 ml with reference solution (a).

Apply to the plate 5 µl of each solution. Prepare the mobile phase by adding a mixture of 1.2 volumes of *water R* and 8 volumes of *methanol R* to a mixture of 15 volumes of *ether R* and 77 volumes of *methylene chloride R*. Develop over a path of 15 cm. Allow the plate to dry in air and examine in ultraviolet light at 254 nm. The principal spot in the chromatogram obtained with the test solution is similar in position and size to the principal spot in the chromatogram obtained with reference solution (a). Spray the plate with *alcoholic solution of sulphuric acid R*. Heat at 120 °C for 10 min or until the spots appear. Allow to cool. Examine in daylight and in ultraviolet light at 365 nm. The principal spot in the chromatogram obtained with the test solution is similar in position, colour in daylight, fluorescence in ultraviolet light at 365 nm and size to the principal spot in the chromatogram obtained with reference solution (a). The test is not valid unless the chromatogram obtained with reference solution (b) shows two clearly separated spots.

C. Add about 2 mg to 2 ml of a mixture of 0.5 ml of *water R* and 1.5 ml of *sulphuric acid R* and shake to dissolve. Within 5 min, a pink colour develops. Add the solution to 10 ml of *water R* and mix. The colour fades and a clear solution remains.

D. Mix about 5 mg with 45 mg of *heavy magnesium oxide R* and ignite in a crucible until an almost white residue is obtained (usually less than 5 min). Allow to cool, add 1 ml of *water R*, 0.05 ml of *phenolphthalein solution R1* and about 1 ml of *dilute hydrochloric acid R* to render the solution colourless. Filter. To a freshly prepared mixture of 0.1 ml of *alizarin S solution R* and 0.1 ml of *zirconyl nitrate solution R* add 1.0 ml of the filtrate. Mix, allow to stand for 5 min and compare the colour of the solution with that of a blank prepared in the same manner. The test solution is yellow and the blank is red.

TESTS

Solution S. Dissolve 0.50 g in *acetone R* and dilute to 25.0 ml with the same solvent.

Appearance of solution. Solution S is clear (*2.2.1*) and not more intensely coloured than reference solution BY_6 (*2.2.2, Method II*).

Specific optical rotation (*2.2.7*): + 69 to + 77, determined on solution S and calculated with reference to the dried substance.

Related substances. Examine by liquid chromatography (*2.2.29*).

Test solution. Dissolve 25.0 mg of the substance to be examined in the mobile phaseand dilute to 25.0 ml with the mobile phase. Dilute 5.0 ml of the solution to 50.0 ml with the mobile phase.

Reference solution (a). Dissolve 10 mg of *dexamethasone pivalate CRS* in the mobile phase and dilute to 100.0 ml with the mobile phase. Take 5.0 ml of the solution, add 5.0 ml of the test solution, mix and dilute to 50.0 ml with the mobile phase.

Reference solution (b). Dilute 2.0 ml of the test solution to 100.0 ml with the mobile phase.

The chromatographic procedure may be carried out using:

- a stainless steel column 0.25 m long and 4.6 mm in internal diameter packed with *octadecylsilyl silica gel for chromatography R* (5 µm),
- as mobile phase at a flow rate of 0.6 ml/min a mixture of 5 volumes of *tetrahydrofuran R*, 30 volumes of *acetonitrile R*, 30 volumes of *water R* and 35 volumes of *methanol R*,
- as detector a spectrophotometer set at 254 nm.

Inject 20 µl of reference solution (b). Adjust the sensitivity of the system so that the height of the principal peak in the chromatogram obtained with reference solution (b) is at least 50 per cent of the full scale of the recorder.

Inject 20 µl of reference solution (a). When the chromatograms are recorded in the prescribed conditions, the relative retention time of dexamethasone pivalate, relative to flumetasone pivalate, is about 1.1. The test is not valid unless in the chromatogram obtained with reference solution (a) the resolution between the peaks corresponding to dexamethasone pivalate and flumetasone pivalate is at least 2.8. If necessary adjust the concentration of tetrahydrofuran in the mobile phase.

Monographs F-H

Inject 20 µl of the test solution. Continue the chromatography for 1.5 times the retention time of the principal peak. In the chromatogram obtained with the test solution, the area of any peak, apart from the principal peak, is not greater than 0.75 times the area of the principal peak in the chromatogram obtained with reference solution (b) (1.5 per cent); the sum of the areas of any peaks, apart from the principal peak, is not greater than the area of the principal peak in the chromatogram obtained with reference solution (b) (2 per cent). Disregard any peak with an area less than 0.025 times the area of the principal peak in the chromatogram obtained with reference solution (b).

Loss on drying (*2.2.32*). Not more than 1.0 per cent, determined on 0.500 g by drying in an oven at 100 °C to 105 °C for 4 h.

ASSAY

Dissolve 50.0 mg in *alcohol R* and dilute to 100.0 ml with the same solvent. Dilute 2.0 ml of the solution to 100.0 ml with *alcohol R*. Measure the absorbance (*2.2.25*) at the maximum at 239 nm.

Calculate the content of $C_{27}H_{36}F_2O_6$ taking the specific absorbance to be 336.

STORAGE

Store protected from light.

IMPURITIES

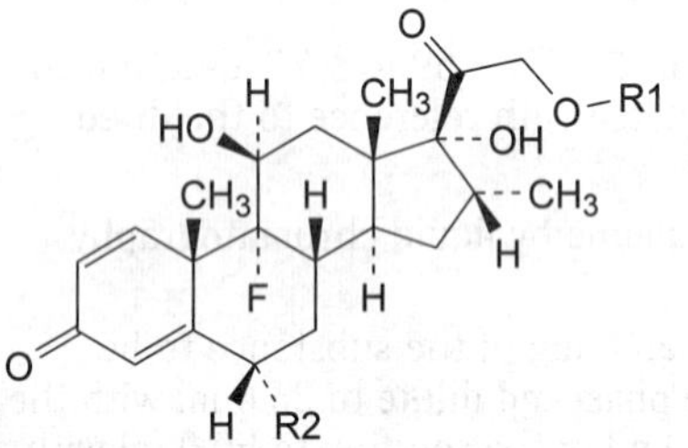

A. R1 = H, R2 = F: 6α,9-difluoro-11β,17,21-trihydroxy-16α-methylpregna-1,4-diene-3,20-dione (flumetasone),

B. R1 = CO-CH_3, R2 = F: 6α,9-difluoro-11β,17-dihydroxy-16α-methyl-3,20-dioxopregna-1,4-dien-21-yl acetate (flumetasone acetate),

C. R1 = CO-C$(CH_3)_3$, R2 = H: 9-fluoro-11β,17-dihydroxy-16α-methyl-3,20-dioxopregna-1,4-dien-21-yl 2,2-dimethylpropanoate (dexamethasone pivalate),

D. R1 = CO-C$(CH_3)_3$, R2 = Cl: 6α-chloro-9-fluoro-11β,17-dihydroxy-16α-methyl-3,20-dioxopregna-1,4-dien-21-yl 2,2-dimethylpropanoate (chlordexamethasone pivalate).

01/2005:1722

FLUNARIZINE DIHYDROCHLORIDE

Flunarizini dihydrochloridum

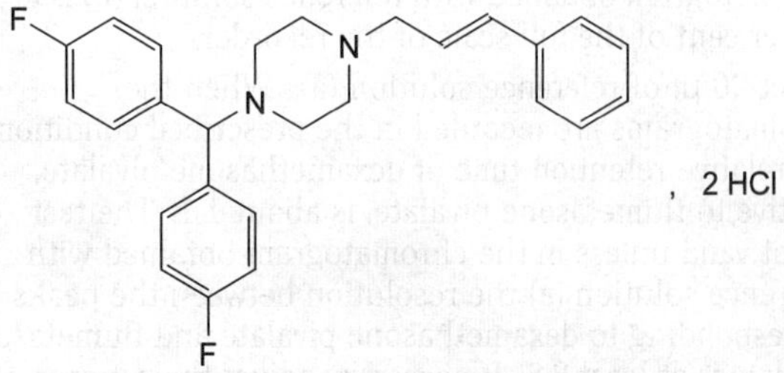

$C_{26}H_{28}Cl_2F_2N_2$ M_r 477.4

DEFINITION

1-[Bis(4-fluorophenyl)methyl]-4-[(2*E*)-3-phenylprop-2-enyl]piperazine dihydrochloride.

Content: 99.0 per cent to 101.5 per cent (dried substance).

CHARACTERS

Appearance: white or almost white powder, hygroscopic.

Solubility: slightly soluble in water, sparingly soluble in methanol, slightly soluble in alcohol and in methylene chloride.

mp: about 208 °C, with decomposition.

IDENTIFICATION

A. Infrared absorption spectrophotometry (*2.2.24*).

Comparison: *Ph. Eur. reference spectrum of flunarizine dihydrochloride.*

B. Dissolve 25 mg in 2 ml of *methanol R* and add 0.5 ml of *water R*. The solution gives reaction (a) of chlorides (*2.3.1*).

TESTS

Related substances. Liquid chromatography (*2.2.29*). *Prepare the solutions immediately before use and protect from light.*

Test solution. Dissolve 0.100 g of the substance to be examined in *methanol R* and dilute to 10.0 ml with the same solvent.

Reference solution (a). Dissolve 10 mg of *flunarizine dihydrochloride for system suitability CRS* in *methanol R* and dilute to 1.0 ml with the same solvent.

Reference solution (b). Dilute 1.0 ml of the test solution to 100.0 ml with *methanol R*. Dilute 5.0 ml of this solution to 20.0 ml with *methanol R*.

Column:

– *size*: *l* = 0.10 m, Ø = 4.6 mm,
– *stationary phase*: *base-deactivated octadecylsilyl silica gel for chromatography R* (3 µm).

Mobile phase:

– *mobile phase A*: solution containing 23.8 g/l of *tetrabutylammonium hydrogen sulphate R* and 7 g/l of *ammonium acetate R*,
– *mobile phase B*: *acetonitrile R*,

Time (min)	Mobile phase A (per cent *V/V*)	Mobile phase B (per cent *V/V*)
0 - 12	80 → 40	20 → 60
12 - 15	40	60
15 - 16	40 → 80	60 → 20
16 - 20	80	20

Flow rate: 1.5 ml/min.

Detection: spectrophotometer at 230 nm.

Injection: 10 µl.

System suitability: reference solution (a):

– *peak-to-valley ratio*: minimum 1.5, where H_p = height above the baseline of the peak due to impurity C and H_v = height above the baseline of the lowest point of the curve separating this peak from the peak due to flunarizine,
– the chromatogram obtained is concordant with the chromatogram supplied with *flunarizine dihydrochloride for system suitability CRS.*

Limits:
- *correction factor*: for the calculation of content, multiply the peak area of impurity A by 1.5,
- *impurities A, D*: for each impurity, not more than 0.4 times the area of the principal peak in the chromatogram obtained with reference solution (b) (0.1 per cent),
- *impurity B*: not more than twice the area of the principal peak in the chromatogram obtained with reference solution (b) (0.5 per cent),
- *impurity C*: not more than the area of the principal peak in the chromatogram obtained with reference solution (b) (0.25 per cent),
- *any other impurity*: for each impurity, not more than 0.4 times the area of the principal peak in the chromatogram obtained with reference solution (b) (0.1 per cent),
- *total*: not more than 4 times the area of the principal peak in the chromatogram obtained with reference solution (b) (1.0 per cent),
- *disregard limit*: 0.2 times the area of the principal peak in the chromatogram obtained with reference solution (b) (0.05 per cent).

Loss on drying (*2.2.32*): maximum 5.0 per cent, determined on 1.000 g by drying in an oven at 100-105 °C for 4 h.

Sulphated ash (*2.4.14*): maximum 0.1 per cent, determined on 1.0 g in a platinum crucible.

ASSAY

Dissolve 0.200 g in 70 ml of *alcohol R*. Carry out a potentiometric titration (*2.2.20*), using *0.1 M sodium hydroxide*. Read the volume added at the second point of inflexion. Carry out a blank titration.

1 ml of *0.1 M sodium hydroxide* is equivalent to 23.87 mg of $C_{26}H_{28}Cl_2F_2N_2$.

STORAGE

In an airtight container, protected from light.

IMPURITIES

Specified impurities: A, B, C, D.

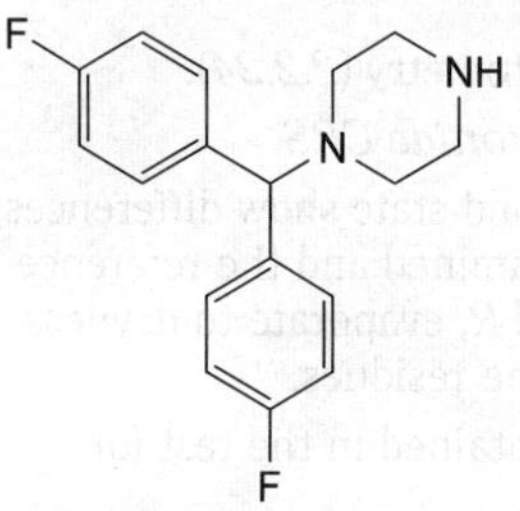

A. 1-[bis(4-fluorophenyl)methyl]piperazine,

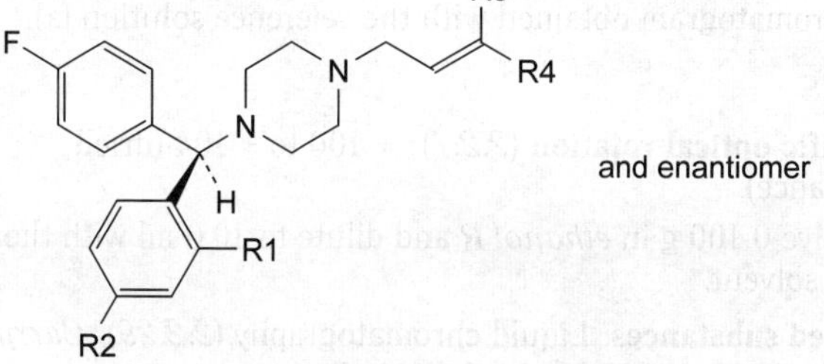

B. R1 = R2 = R3 = H, R4 = C_6H_5: 1-[(*RS*)-(4-fluorophenyl)phenylmethyl]-4-[(2*E*)-3-phenylprop-2-enyl]piperazine,

C. R1 = F, R2 = R3 = H, R4 = C_6H_5: 1-[(*RS*)-(2-fluorophenyl)(4-fluorophenyl)methyl]-4-[(2*E*)-3-phenylprop-2-enyl]piperazine,

D. R1 = R4 = H, R2 = F, R3 = C_6H_5: 1-[bis(4-fluorophenyl)methyl]-4-[(2*Z*)-3-phenylprop-2-enyl]piperazine.

01/2005:0717

FLUNITRAZEPAM

Flunitrazepamum

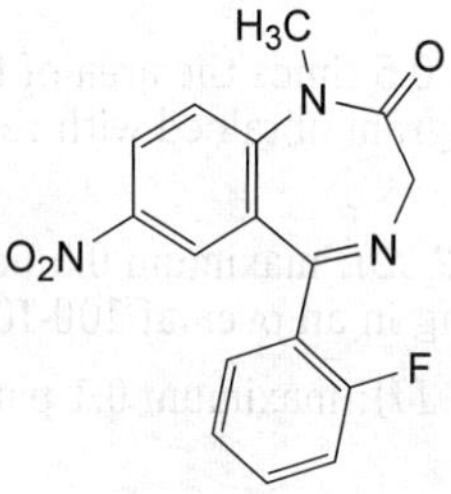

$C_{16}H_{12}FN_3O_3$ M_r 313.3

DEFINITION

5-(2-Fluorophenyl)-1-methyl-7-nitro-1,3-dihydro-2*H*-1,4-benzodiazepin-2-one.

Content: 99.0 per cent to 101.0 per cent (dried substance).

CHARACTERS

Appearance: white or yellowish, crystalline powder.

Solubility: practically insoluble in water, soluble in acetone, slightly soluble in alcohol.

IDENTIFICATION

Infrared absorption spectrophotometry (*2.2.24*).

Comparison: *Ph. Eur. reference spectrum of flunitrazepam.*

TESTS

Related substances. Liquid chromatography (*2.2.29*). *Prepare the solutions immediately before use.*

Test solution. Dissolve 100.0 mg of the substance to be examined in 10 ml of *acetonitrile R* and dilute to 50.0 ml with the mobile phase.

Reference solution (a). Dilute 1.0 ml of the test solution to 100.0 ml with the mobile phase. Dilute 5.0 ml of this solution to 50.0 ml with the mobile phase.

Reference solution (b). Dissolve 4 mg of the substance to be examined and 4 mg of *nitrazepam R* in 5 ml of *acetonitrile R* and dilute to 20.0 ml with the mobile phase. Dilute 1.0 ml of the solution to 20.0 ml with the mobile phase.

Column:
- *size*: *l* = 0.15 m, Ø = 4.6 mm,
- *stationary phase*: *octadecylsilyl silica gel for chromatography R* (5 µm).

Mobile phase: *methanol R, acetonitrile R, water R* (50:305:645 *V/V/V*).

Flow rate: 1.0 ml/min.

Detection: spectrophotometer at 254 nm.

Injection: 20 µl.

Run time: 6 times the retention time of flunitrazepam.

Relative retention with reference to flunitrazepam (retention time = about 11 min): impurity A = about 0.2; impurity B = about 0.6; impurity C = about 2.3; impurity D = about 4.0.

System suitability: reference solution (b):

– *resolution*: minimum 4.0 between the peaks due to nitrazepam and flunitrazepam.

Limits:

– *correction factor*: for the calculation of content, multiply the peak area of impurity C by 2.44,
– *any impurity*: not more than the area of the principal peak in the chromatogram obtained with reference solution (a) (0.1 per cent),
– *total*: not more than 3 times the area of the principal peak in the chromatogram obtained with reference solution (a) (0.3 per cent),
– *disregard limit*: 0.5 times the area of the principal peak in the chromatogram obtained with reference solution (a) (0.05 per cent).

Loss on drying (*2.2.32*): maximum 0.5 per cent, determined on 1.000 g by drying in an oven at 100-105 °C.

Sulphated ash (*2.4.14*): maximum 0.1 per cent, determined on 1.0 g.

ASSAY

Dissolve 0.250 g in 20 ml of *anhydrous acetic acid R* and add 50 ml of *acetic anhydride R*. Titrate with *0.1 M perchloric acid*, determining the end-point potentiometrically (*2.2.20*).

1 ml of *0.1 M perchloric acid* is equivalent to 31.33 mg of $C_{16}H_{12}FN_3O_3$.

STORAGE

Protected from light.

IMPURITIES

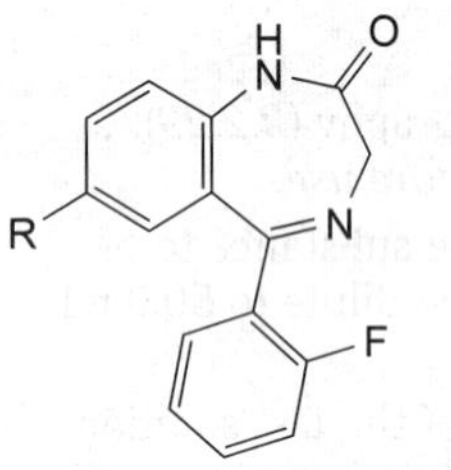

A. R = NH_2: 7-amino-5-(2-fluorophenyl)-1,3-dihydro-2*H*-1,4-benzodiazepin-2-one (7-aminodemethylflunitrazepam),

B. R = NO_2: 5-(2-fluorophenyl)-7-nitro-1,3-dihydro-2*H*-1,4-benzodiazepin-2-one (demethylflunitrazepam),

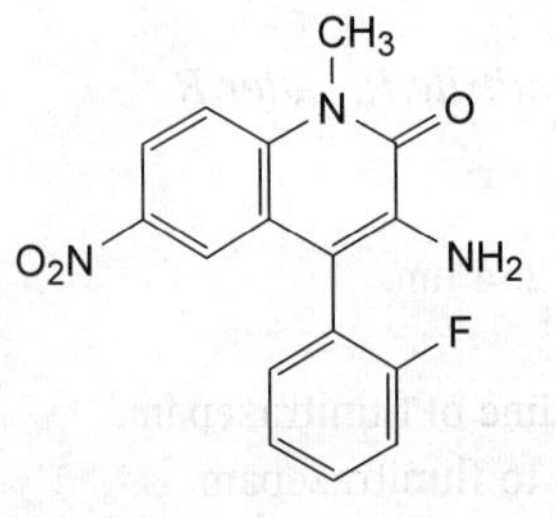

C. 3-amino-4-(2-fluorophenyl)-1-methyl-6-nitroquinolin-2(1*H*)-one,

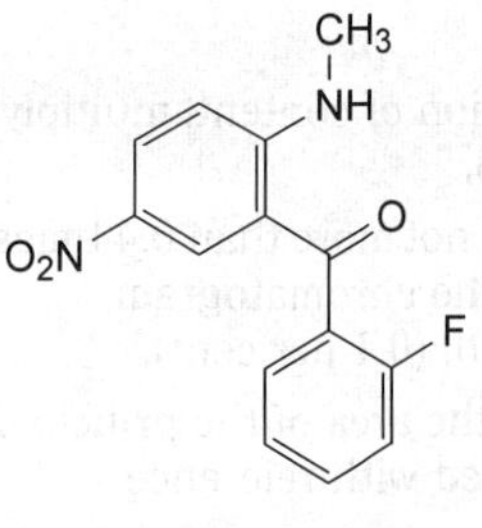

D. (2-fluorophenyl)[2-(methylamino)-5-nitrophenyl]methanone.

01/2005:0494

FLUOCINOLONE ACETONIDE

Fluocinoloni acetonidum

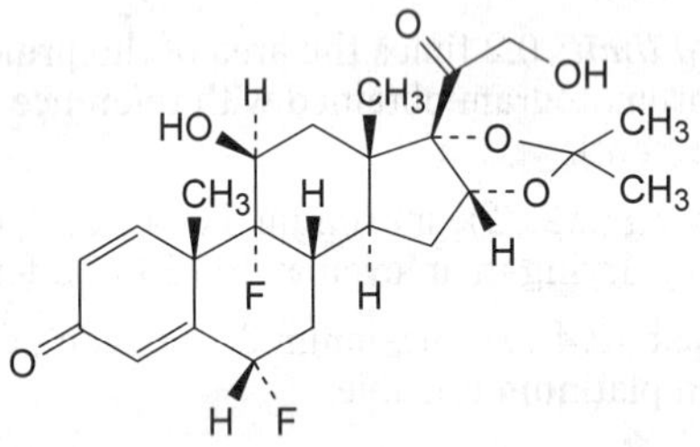

$C_{24}H_{30}F_2O_6$ M_r 452.5

DEFINITION

6α,9-Difluoro-11β,21-dihydroxy-16α,17-(1-methylethylidenedioxy)pregna-1,4-diene-3,20-dione.

Content: 97.0 per cent to 103.0 per cent (dried substance).

CHARACTERS

Appearance: white or almost white, crystalline powder.

Solubility: practically insoluble in water, soluble in acetone and in ethanol.

It shows polymorphism.

IDENTIFICATION

A. Infrared absorption spectrophotometry (*2.2.24*).

Comparison: *fluocinolone acetonide CRS.*

If the spectra obtained in the solid state show differences, dissolve the substance to be examined and the reference substance separately in *ethanol R*, evaporate to dryness and record new spectra using the residues.

B. Examine the chromatograms obtained in the test for related substances.

Results: the principal peak in the chromatogram obtained with the reference solution (b) is similar in retention time to the peak due to *fluocinolone acetonide CRS* in the chromatogram obtained with the reference solution (a).

TESTS

Specific optical rotation (*2.2.7*): + 100 to + 104 (dried substance).

Dissolve 0.100 g in *ethanol R* and dilute to 10.0 ml with the same solvent.

Related substances. Liquid chromatography (*2.2.29*). *Carry out the test protected from light.*

Test solution. Dissolve 25.0 mg of the substance to be examined in *acetonitrile R* and dilute to 10.0 ml with the same solvent.

Reference solution (a). Dissolve 2.5 mg of *fluocinolone acetonide CRS* and 2.5 mg of *triamcinolone acetonide R* in 45 ml of *acetonitrile R* and dilute to 100.0 ml with *water R.*

Reference solution (b). Dilute 1.0 ml of the test solution to 100.0 ml with *acetonitrile R.*

Column:

- *size*: *l* = 0.25 m, Ø = 4.6 mm,
- *stationary phase*: *base-deactivated end-capped octadecylsilyl silica gel for chromatography R* (5 µm).

Mobile phase: mix 450 ml of *acetonitrile R* with 500 ml of *water R* and allow to equilibrate; adjust the volume to 1000.0 ml with *water R* and mix again.

Flow rate: 1 ml/min.

Detection: spectrophotometer at 238 nm.

Injection: 20 µl.

Run time: 4 times the retention time of fluocinolone acetonide.

Retention times: triamcinolone acetonide = about 8.5 min; fluocinolone acetonide = about 10 min.

System suitability:

- *resolution*: minimum of 3.0 between the peaks due to triamcinolone acetonide and fluocinolone acetonide in the chromatogram obtained with reference solution (a).

Limits:

- *any impurity*: not more than the area of the principal peak in the chromatogram obtained with reference solution (b) (1 per cent) and not more than 1 such peak has an area greater than half the area of the principal peak in the chromatogram obtained with reference solution (b) (0.5 per cent),
- *total*: not more than 2.5 times the area of the principal peak in the chromatogram obtained with reference solution (b) (2.5 per cent),
- *disregard limit*: 0.05 times the area of the principal peak in the chromatogram obtained with reference solution (b) (0.05 per cent).

Loss on drying (*2.2.32*): maximum 1.0 per cent, determined on 1.000 g by drying in an oven at 100-105 °C for 3 h.

ASSAY

Protect the solutions from light throughout the assay.

Dissolve 50.0 mg in *alcohol R* and dilute to 50.0 ml with the same solvent. Dilute 2.0 ml of this solution to 100.0 ml with *alcohol R.* Measure the absorbance (*2.2.25*) at the maximum at 238 nm.

Calculate the content of $C_{24}H_{30}F_2O_6$ taking the specific absorbance to be 355.

STORAGE

Protected from light.

IMPURITIES

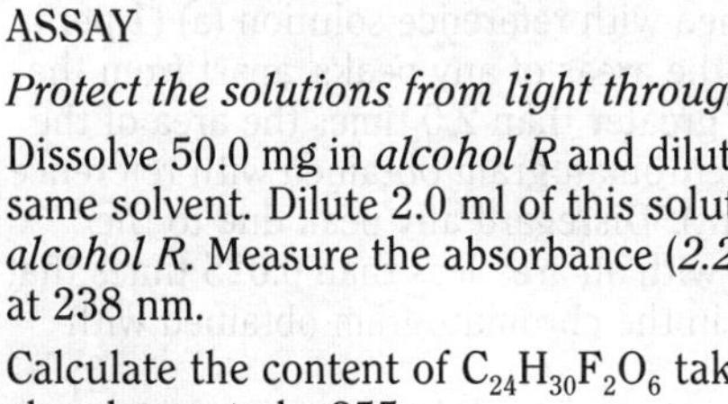

A. R = $CO\text{-}CO_2H$: 6α,9-difluoro-11β-hydroxy-16α,17-(1-methylethylidenedioxy)-3,20-dioxopregna-1,4-dien-21-oic acid,

B. R = CO_2H: 6α,9-difluoro-11β-hydroxy-16α,17-(1-methylethylidenedioxy)-3-oxoandrosta-1,4-diene-17β-carboxylic acid,

D. R = CO-CH=O: 6α,9-difluoro-11β-hydroxy-16α,17-(1-methylethylidenedioxy)-3,20-dioxopregna-1,4-dien-21-al,

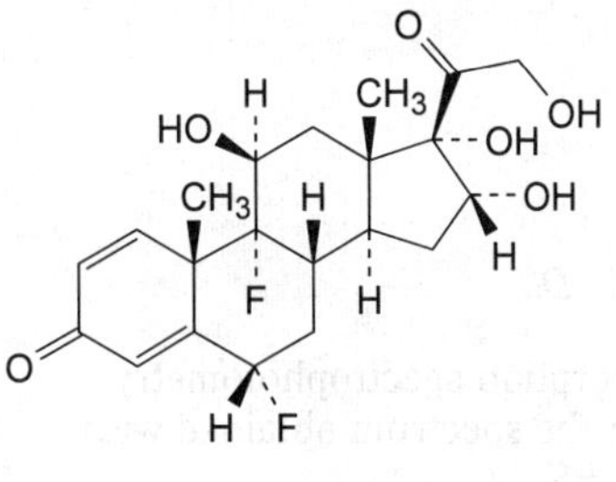

C. 6α,9-difluoro-11β,16α,17,21-tetrahydroxypregna-1,4-diene-3,20-dione (fluocinolone),

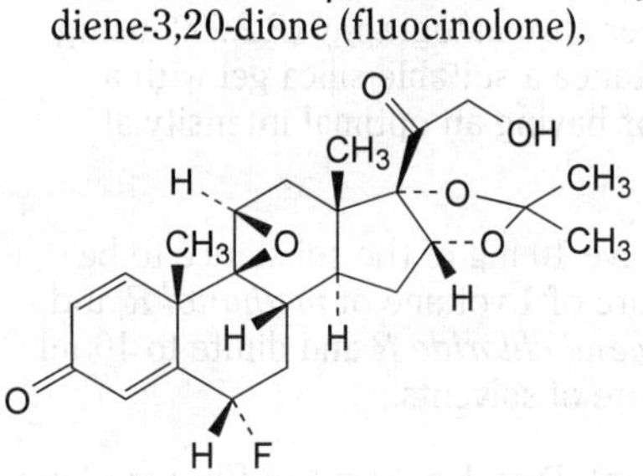

E. 9,11β-epoxy-6α-fluoro-21-hydroxy-16α,17-(1-methylethylidenedioxy)-9β-pregna-1,4-diene-3,20-dione,

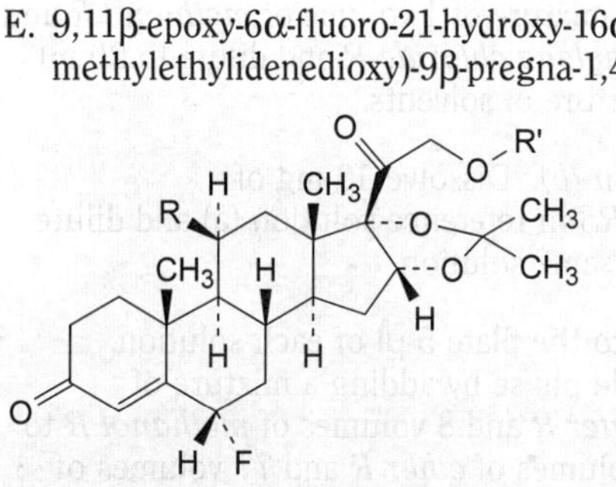

F. R = R′ = H: 6α-fluoro-21-hydroxy-16α,17-(1-methylethylidenedioxy)pregn-4-ene-3,20-dione,

G. R = OH, R′ = $CO\text{-}CH_3$: 6α-fluoro-11β-hydroxy-16α,17-(1-methylethylidenedioxy)-3,20-dioxopregn-4-en-21-yl acetate.

01/2005:1212

FLUOCORTOLONE PIVALATE

Fluocortoloni pivalas

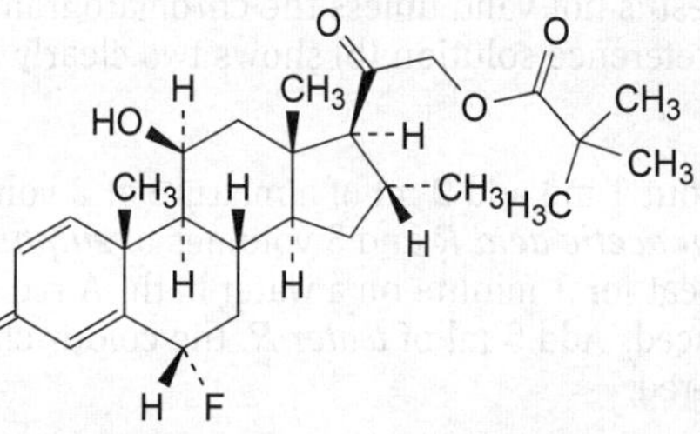

$C_{27}H_{37}FO_5$ M_r 460.6

DEFINITION

Fluocortolone pivalate contains not less than 97.0 per cent and not more than the equivalent of 103.0 per cent of 6α-fluoro-11β-hydroxy-16α-methyl-3,20-dioxopregna-1,4-dien-21-yl 2,2-dimethylpropanoate calculated with reference to the dried substance.

CHARACTERS

A white or almost white, crystalline powder, practically insoluble in water, freely soluble in methylene chloride and in dioxan, sparingly soluble in alcohol.

IDENTIFICATION

First identification: A, B.

Second identification: B, C, D.

A. Examine by infrared absorption spectrophotometry (*2.2.24*), comparing with the spectrum obtained with *fluocortolone pivalate CRS*.

B. Examine by thin-layer chromatography (*2.2.27*), using as the coating substance a suitable silica gel with a fluorescent indicator having an optimal intensity at 254 nm.

Test solution. Dissolve 10 mg of the substance to be examined in a mixture of 1 volume of *methanol R* and 9 volumes of *methylene chloride R* and dilute to 10 ml with the same mixture of solvents.

Reference solution (a). Dissolve 20 mg of *fluocortolone pivalate CRS* in a mixture of 1 volume of *methanol R* and 9 volumes of *methylene chloride R* and dilute to 20 ml with the same mixture of solvents.

Reference solution (b). Dissolve 10 mg of *norethisterone CRS* in reference solution (a) and dilute to 10 ml with the same solution.

Apply separately to the plate 5 µl of each solution. Prepare the mobile phase by adding a mixture of 1.2 volumes of *water R* and 8 volumes of *methanol R* to a mixture of 15 volumes of *ether R* and 77 volumes of *methylene chloride R*. Develop over a path of 15 cm. Allow the plate to dry in air and examine in ultraviolet light at 254 nm. The principal spot in the chromatogram obtained with the test solution is similar in position and size to the principal spot in the chromatogram obtained with reference solution (a). Spray with *alcoholic solution of sulphuric acid R*. Heat at 120 °C for 10 min or until the spots appear. Allow to cool. Examine the plate in daylight and in ultraviolet light at 365 nm. The principal spot in the chromatogram obtained with the test solution is similar in position, colour in daylight, fluorescence in ultraviolet light at 365 nm and size to the principal spot in the chromatogram obtained with reference solution (a). The test is not valid unless the chromatogram obtained with reference solution (b) shows two clearly separated spots.

C. To about 1 mg add 2 ml of a mixture of 2 volumes of *glacial acetic acid R* and 3 volumes of *sulphuric acid R* and heat for 1 minute on a water-bath. A red colour is produced. Add 5 ml of *water R*, the colour changes to violet-red.

D. Mix about 5 mg with 45 mg of *heavy magnesium oxide R* and ignite in a crucible until an almost white residue is obtained (usually less than 5 min). Allow to cool, add 1 ml of *water R*, 0.05 ml of *phenolphthalein solution R1* and about 1 ml of *dilute hydrochloric acid R* to render the solution colourless. Filter and add to the filtrate a freshly prepared mixture of 0.1 ml of *alizarin S solution R* and 0.1 ml of *zirconyl nitrate solution R*. Mix, allow to stand for 5 min and compare the colour of the solution with that of a blank prepared in the same manner. The test solution is yellow and the blank is red.

TESTS

Specific optical rotation (*2.2.7*). Dissolve 0.25 g in *dioxan R* and dilute to 25.0 ml with the same solvent. The specific optical rotation is + 100 to + 105, calculated with reference to the dried substance.

Related substances. Examine by liquid chromatography(*2.2.29*).

Test solution. Dissolve 10.0 mg of the substance to be examined in *acetonitrile R* and dilute to 10.0 ml with the same solvent.

Reference solution (a). Dilute 1.0 ml of the test solution to 100.0 ml with *acetonitrile R*.

Reference solution (b). Dissolve 2 mg of *fluocortolone pivalate CRS* and 2 mg of *prednisolone hexanoate CRS* in *acetonitrile R* and dilute to 100 ml with the same solvent.

The chromatographic procedure may be carried out using:

– a stainless steel column 0.25 m long and 4.6 mm in internal diameter packed with *octadecylsilyl silica gel for chromatography R* (5 µm),

– as mobile phase at a flow rate of 1.5 ml/min a mixture of 25 volumes of *methanol R*, 30 volumes of *acetonitrile R* and 32 volumes of *water R*,

– as detector a spectrophotometer set at 243 nm.

Inject 20 µl of reference solution (a). Adjust the sensitivity of the system so that the height of the principal peak in the chromatogram obtained is at least 50 per cent of the full scale of the recorder. Inject 20 µl of reference solution (b). The test is not valid unless, in the chromatogram obtained, the resolution between the two principal peaks is at least 5.0. Inject 20 µl of the test solution. Continue the chromatography for twice the retention time of fluocortolone pivalate. In the chromatogram obtained with the test solution: the area of any peak, apart from the principal peak, is not greater than the area of the principal peak in the chromatogram obtained with reference solution (a) (1 per cent) and the sum of the areas of any peaks, apart from the principal peak, is not greater than 2.0 times the area of the principal peak in the chromatogram obtained with reference solution (a) (2 per cent). Disregard any peak due to the solvent and any peak with an area less than 0.025 times that of the principal peak in the chromatogram obtained with reference solution (a).

Loss on drying (*2.2.32*). Not more than 1.0 per cent, determined on 1.000 g by drying in an oven at 100-105 °C.

Sulphated ash (*2.4.14*). Not more than 0.1 per cent, determined on 1.0 g.

ASSAY

Dissolve 30.0 mg in *ethanol R* and dilute to 100.0 ml with the same solvent. Dilute 5.0 ml of the solution to 100.0 ml with *ethanol R*. Measure the absorbance (*2.2.25*) at the maximum at 242 nm.

Calculate the content of $C_{27}H_{37}FO_5$ taking the specific absorbance to be 350.

STORAGE

Store protected from light.

IMPURITIES

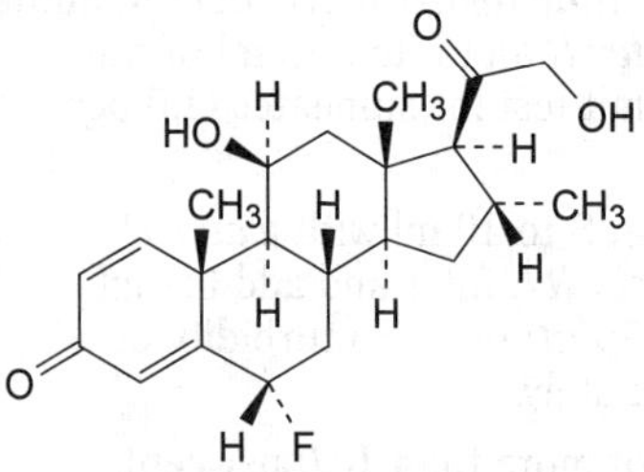

A. 6α-fluoro-11β,21-dihydroxy-16α-methylpregna-1,4-diene-3,20-dione (fluocortolone),

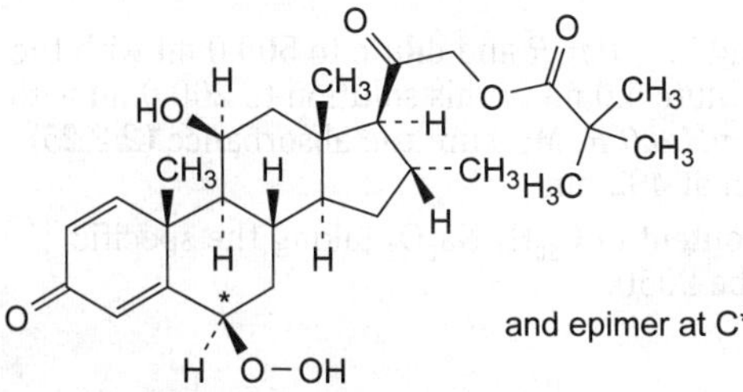

B. 6-hydroperoxy-11β-hydroxy-16α-methyl-3,20-dioxopregna-1,4-dien-21-yl 2,2-dimethylpropanoate,

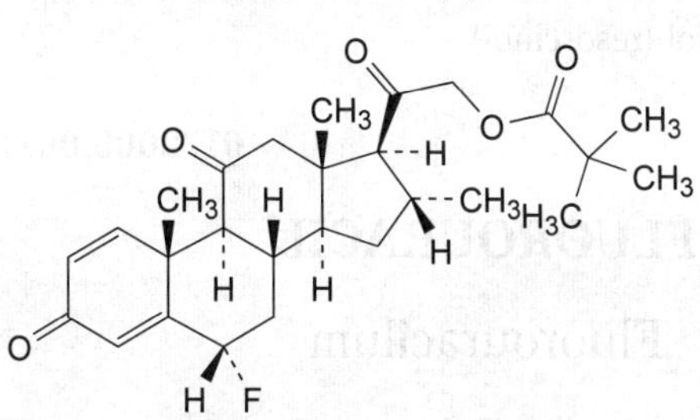

C. 6α-fluoro-16α-methyl-3,11,20-trioxopregna-1,4-dien-21-yl 2,2-dimethylpropanoate,

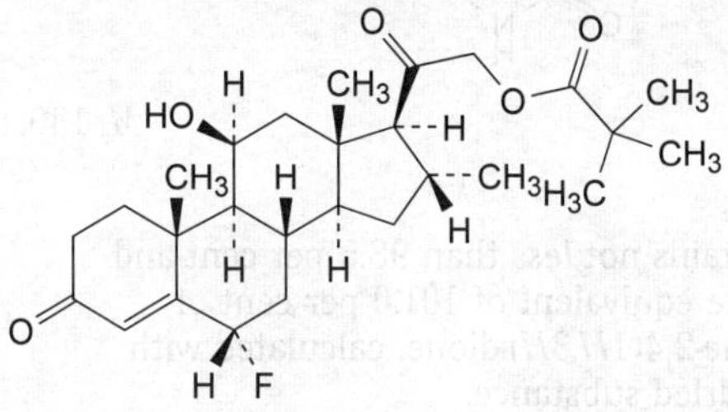

D. 6α-fluoro-11β-hydroxy-16α-methyl-3,20-dioxopregna-4-en-21-yl 2,2-dimethylpropanoate.

01/2005:1213

FLUORESCEIN SODIUM

Fluoresceinum natricum

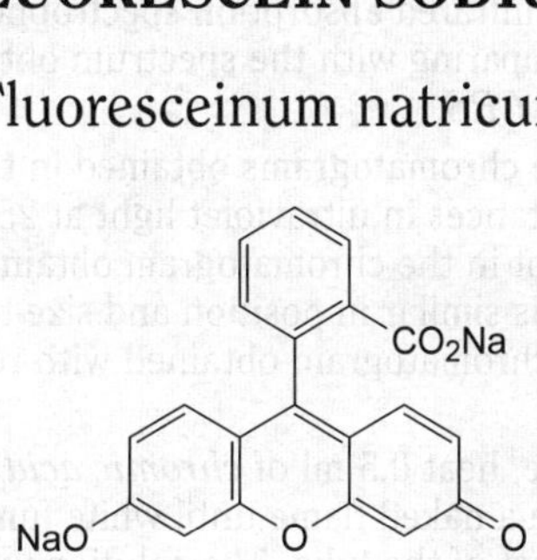

$C_{20}H_{10}Na_2O_5$ M_r 376.3

DEFINITION

Fluorescein sodium contains not less than 95.0 per cent and not more than the equivalent of 103.0 per cent of disodium 2-(3-oxo-6-oxido-3*H*-xanthen-9-yl)benzoate, calculated with reference to the dried substance.

CHARACTERS

An orange-red, fine powder, hygroscopic, freely soluble in water, soluble in alcohol, practically insoluble in hexane and in methylene chloride.

IDENTIFICATION

First identification: B, D.

Second identification: A, C, D.

A. Dilute 0.1 ml of solution S (see Tests) to 10 ml with *water R*. The solution shows yellowish-green fluorescence. The fluorescence disappears on addition of 0.1 ml of *dilute hydrochloric acid R* and reappears on addition of 0.2 ml of *dilute sodium hydroxide solution R*.

B. Examine by infrared absorption spectrophotometry (*2.2.24*), comparing with the *Ph. Eur. reference spectrum of fluorescein sodium*. Examine the substance prepared as a disc.

C. The absorption by a piece of filter paper of 0.05 ml of the solution prepared for identification A (before the addition of *dilute hydrochloric acid R*) colours the paper yellow. On exposing the moist paper to bromine vapour for 1 min and then to ammonia vapour the colour becomes deep pink.

D. Ignite 0.1 g in a porcelain crucible. Dissolve the residue in 5 ml of *water R* and filter. 2 ml of the filtrate gives reaction (a) of sodium (*2.3.1*).

TESTS

Solution S. Dissolve 1.0 g in *carbon dioxide-free water R* prepared from *distilled water R* and dilute to 50 ml with the same solvent.

Appearance of solution. Solution S is clear (*2.2.1*) and orange-yellow with yellowish-green fluorescence.

pH (*2.2.3*). The pH of solution S is 7.0 to 9.0.

Related substances and resorcinol. Examine by thin-layer chromatography (*2.2.27*), using as the coating substance a suitable silica gel.

Test solution (a). Dissolve 0.10 g of the substance to be examined in a 10 g/l solution of *hydrochloric acid R* in *methanol R* and dilute to 10 ml with the same acidic solution.

Test solution (b). Dissolve 0.250 g of the substance to be examined in 5 ml of *water R*. Transfer to a separating funnel and wash with 3 ml of *water R*. Add 2 ml of *buffer solution pH 8.0 R* and 2.5 g of *sodium chloride R*. Shake until the sodium chloride dissolves. Shake the solution obtained with two quantities, each of 25 ml, of *peroxide-free ether R*. Dry the ether layers over *anhydrous sodium sulphate R* and evaporate to dryness using a rotary evaporator. Dissolve the residue in 10 ml of a 10 g/l solution of *hydrochloric acid R* in *methanol R*.

Reference solution (a). Dilute 0.5 ml of test solution (a) to 100 ml with a 10 g/l solution of *hydrochloric acid R* in *methanol R*.

Reference solution (b). Dilute 1 ml of test solution (a) to 50 ml with a 10 g/l solution of *hydrochloric acid R* in *methanol R*. Dilute 1 ml of the solution to 10 ml with a 10 g/l solution of *hydrochloric acid R* in *methanol R*.

Reference solution (c). Dissolve 25 mg of *resorcinol R* in *methanol R* and dilute to 100 ml with the same solvent.

Reference solution (d). Dilute 10 ml of reference solution (c) to 20 ml with *water R.*

Reference solution (e). To 5 ml of reference solution (c) add 1 ml of test solution (a) and dilute to 10 ml with *methanol R.*

Apply separately to the plate 5 µl of test solutions (a) and (b) and 5 µl of reference solutions (a), (b), (d) and (e). Develop over a path of 15 cm using a mixture of 10 volumes of *methanol R* and 90 volumes of *methylene chloride R*. Allow the plate to dry in air. Examine in ultraviolet light at 365 nm. Expose the plate to iodine vapour for 30 min and examine in daylight. In the chromatogram obtained with test solution (a): any spot, apart from the principal spot, is not more intense than the principal spot in the chromatogram obtained with reference solution (a) (0.5 per cent) and not more than one such spot is more intense than the principal spot in the chromatogram obtained with reference solution (b) (0.2 per cent). In the chromatogram obtained with test solution (b) any spot corresponding to resorcinol is not more intense than the principal spot in the chromatogram obtained with reference solution (d) (0.5 per cent). The test is not valid unless the chromatogram obtained with reference solution (e) shows two clearly separated spots. The spots corresponding to resorcinol are visible only after exposing the plate to iodine vapour.

Dimethylformamide. Examine by gas chromatography (*2.2.28*) using *dimethylacetamide R* as the internal standard.

Internal standard solution. Dilute 20 µl of *dimethylacetamide R* to 100 ml with *water R.*

Test solution (a). Dissolve 1.0 g of the substance to be examined in 10 ml of *water R.* Add, with gently stirring, 10 ml of a 60 g/l solution of *hydrochloric acid R.* Allow to stand for 15 min and centrifuge. Dissolve 0.10 g of *trisodium phosphate dodecahydrate R* in 5 ml of the supernatant.

Test solution (b). Dissolve 1.0 g of the substance to be examined in 10 ml of the internal standard solution. Add, with gentle stirring, 10 ml of a 60 g/l solution of *hydrochloric acid R.* Allow to stand for 15 min and centrifuge. Dissolve 0.10 g of *trisodium phosphate dodecahydrate R* in 5 ml of the supernatant.

Reference solution. Dilute 20 µl of *dimethylformamide R* to 10 ml with *water R.* Dilute 1 ml of the solution to 10 ml with *water R.* Add 10 ml of the internal standard solution and mix.

The chromatographic procedure may be carried out using:

- a glass column 1.5 m long and 4 mm in internal diameter packed with *silanised diatomaceous earth for gas chromatography R* (135 µm to 175 µm) impregnated with 10 per cent *m/m* of *macrogol 1000 R,*
- *nitrogen for chromatography R* as the carrier gas at a flow rate of 40 ml/min,
- a flame-ionisation detector,

maintaining the temperature of the column at 120 °C and that of the injection port and of the detector at 170 °C.

Inject 2 µl of each solution. In the chromatogram obtained with test solution (b), the ratio of the area of any peak corresponding to dimethylformamide to the area of the peak due to the internal standard is not greater than the corresponding ratio in the chromatogram obtained with the reference solution (0.2 per cent).

Chlorides (*2.4.4*). To 10 ml of solution S add 90 ml of *water R* and 1 ml of *dilute nitric acid R*, wait for at least 10 min and filter. 10 ml of the filtrate diluted to 15 ml with *water R* complies with the limit test for chlorides (0.25 per cent).

Sulphates (*2.4.13*). To 5 ml of solution S add 90 ml of *distilled water R*, 2.5 ml of *dilute hydrochloric acid R*, dilute to 100 ml with *distilled water R* and filter. 15 ml of the filtrate complies with the limit test for sulphates (1.0 per cent).

Zinc. Dilute 5 ml of solution S to 10 ml with *water R.* Add 2 ml of*hydrochloric acid R1*, filter and add 0.1 ml of *potassium ferrocyanide solution R.* No turbidity or precipitate is formed immediately.

Loss on drying (*2.2.32*). Not more than 10.0 per cent, determined on 1.000 g by drying in an oven at 100 °C to 105 °C.

ASSAY

Dissolve 50.0 mg in *water R* and dilute to 500.0 ml with the same solvent. Dilute 5.0 ml of this solution to 200.0 ml with *buffer solution pH 8.0 R.* Measure the absorbance (*2.2.25*) at the maximum at 492 nm.

Calculate the content of $C_{20}H_{10}Na_2O_5$ taking the specific absorbance to be 2050.

STORAGE

Store in an airtight container, protected from light.

IMPURITIES

A. benzene-1,3-diol (resorcinol).

01/2005:0611

FLUOROURACIL

Fluorouracilum

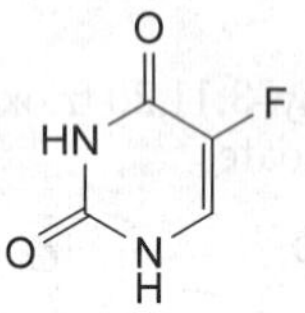

$C_4H_3FN_2O_2$ M_r 130.1

DEFINITION

Fluorouracil contains not less than 98.5 per cent and not more than the equivalent of 101.0 per cent of 5-fluoropyrimidine-2,4(1*H*,3*H*)-dione, calculated with reference to the dried substance.

CHARACTERS

A white or almost white, crystalline powder, sparingly soluble in water, slightly soluble in alcohol.

IDENTIFICATION

First identification: A.

Second identification: B, C.

A. Examine by infrared absorption spectrophotometry (*2.2.24*), comparing with the spectrum obtained with *fluorouracil CRS.*

B. Examine the chromatograms obtained in the test for related substances in ultraviolet light at 254 nm. The principal spot in the chromatogram obtained with test solution (b) is similar in position and size to the principal spot in the chromatogram obtained with reference solution (a).

C. In a test-tube, heat 0.5 ml of *chromic acid cleansing mixture R* in a naked flame until white fumes appear in the upper part of the tube. The solution wets the side of the tube and there is no appearance of greasiness. Add

Monographs F-H

about 2 mg of the substance to be examined and heat again in a naked flame until white fumes appear. The solution does not wet the sides of the tube.

TESTS

Solution S. Dissolve 0.5 g in *carbon dioxide-free water R* and dilute to 50 ml with the same solvent.

Appearance of solution. Solution S is clear (*2.2.1*) and not more intensely coloured than reference solution BY_7 or Y_7 (*2.2.2, Method II*).

pH (*2.2.3*). The pH of solution S is 4.5 to 5.0.

Related substances. Examine by thin-layer chromatography (*2.2.27*), using *silica gel GF_{254} R* as the coating substance.

Test solution (a). Dissolve 0.10 g of the substance to be examined in a mixture of equal volumes of *methanol R* and *water R* and dilute to 10.0 ml with the same mixture of solvents.

Test solution (b). Dilute 2 ml of test solution (a) to 10 ml with a mixture of equal volumes of *methanol R* and *water R*.

Reference solution (a). Dissolve 20 mg of *fluorouracil CRS* in a mixture of equal volumes of *methanol R* and *water R* and dilute to 10 ml with the same mixture of solvents.

Reference solution (b). Dilute 2.5 ml of reference solution (a) to 200 ml with a mixture of equal volumes of *methanol R* and *water R*.

Reference solution (c). Dissolve 5 mg of *5-hydroxyuracil R* in a mixture of equal volumes of *methanol R* and *water R* and dilute to 200 ml with the same mixture of solvents.

Apply to the plate 10 µl of each solution. Develop over a path of 12 cm using a mixture of 15 volumes of *methanol R*, 15 volumes of *water R* and 70 volumes of *ethyl acetate R*. Allow the plate to dry in air and examine in ultraviolet light at 254 nm. Any spot in the chromatogram obtained with test solution (a), apart from the principal spot, is not more intense than the spot in the chromatogram obtained with reference solution (b) (0.25 per cent). Spray with a freshly prepared 5 g/l solution of *fast blue B salt R* and subsequently with *0.1 M sodium hydroxide*. Any spot corresponding to 5-hydroxyuracil in the chromatogram obtained with test solution (a) is not more intense than the spot in the chromatogram obtained with reference solution (c) (0.25 per cent).

Heavy metals (*2.4.8*). *Use a platinum crucible.* 1.0 g complies with limit test C for heavy metals (20 ppm). Prepare the standard using 2 ml of *lead standard solution (10 ppm Pb) R*.

Loss on drying (*2.2.32*). Not more than 0.5 per cent, determined on 1.000 g by drying *in vacuo* at 80 °C for 4 h.

Sulphated ash (*2.4.14*). *Use a platinum crucible.* Not more than 0.1 per cent, determined on 1.0 g.

ASSAY

Dissolve 0.1000 g in 80 ml of *dimethylformamide R*, warming gently. Cool and titrate with *0.1 M tetrabutylammonium hydroxide*, using 0.25 ml of a 10 g/l solution of *thymol blue R* in *dimethylformamide R* as indicator. Carry out a blank titration.

1 ml of *0.1 M tetrabutylammonium hydroxide* is equivalent to 13.01 mg of $C_4H_3FN_2O_2$.

STORAGE

Store protected from light.

01/2005:1104

FLUOXETINE HYDROCHLORIDE

Fluoxetini hydrochloridum

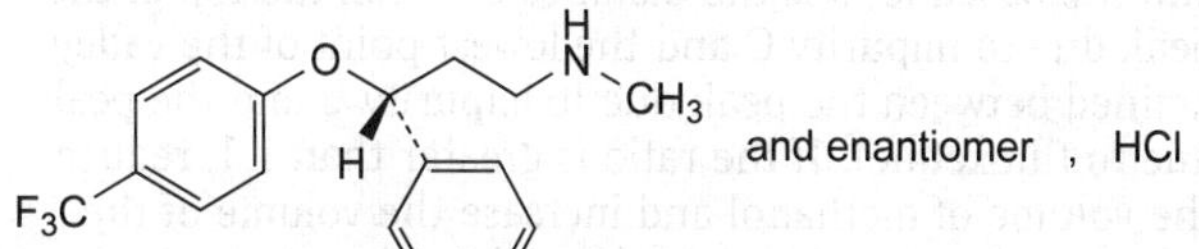

$C_{17}H_{19}ClF_3NO$ M_r 345.8

DEFINITION

Fluoxetine hydrochloride contains not less than 98.0 per cent and not more than the equivalent of 102.0 per cent of (3*RS*)-*N*-methyl-3-phenyl-3-[4-(trifluoromethyl)phenoxy]propan-1-amine hydrochloride, calculated with reference to the anhydrous, acetonitrile-free substance.

CHARACTERS

A white or almost white, crystalline powder, sparingly soluble in water, freely soluble in methanol, sparingly soluble in methylene chloride.

IDENTIFICATION

A. Examine by infrared absorption spectrophotometry (*2.2.24*), comparing with the spectrum obtained with *fluoxetine hydrochloride CRS*. Examine the substances prepared as discs.

B. It gives reaction (a) of chlorides (*2.3.1*).

TESTS

Solution S. Dissolve 2.0 g in a mixture of 15 volumes of *water R* and 85 volumes of *methanol R* and dilute to 100 ml with the same mixture of solvents.

Appearance of solution. Solution S is clear (*2.2.1*) and colourless (*2.2.2, Method II*).

pH (*2.2.3*). Dissolve 0.20 g in *carbon dioxide-free water R* and dilute to 20 ml with the same solvent. The pH of the solution is 4.5 to 6.5.

Optical rotation (*2.2.7*): −0.05° to + 0.05°, determined on solution S.

Related substances. Examine by liquid chromatography (*2.2.29*) as prescribed under Assay, setting the spectrophotometer at 215 nm.

Test solution (a). Dissolve 55.0 mg of the substance to be examined in the mobile phase and dilute to 10.0 ml with the mobile phase.

Test solution (b). Dilute 2.0 ml of test solution (a) to 10.0 ml with the mobile phase.

Reference solution. Dissolve 22.0 mg of *fluoxetine hydrochloride CRS* in 10.0 ml of *0.5 M sulphuric acid*. Heat at about 85 °C for 3 h. Allow to cool. The resulting solution contains considerable quantities of impurity A and 4-trifluoromethylphenol. To 0.4 ml of the solution, add 28.0 mg of *fluoxetine hydrochloride CRS* and about 1 mg of *fluoxetine impurity B CRS* and of *fluoxetine impurity C CRS* and dilute to 25.0 ml with the mobile phase. When the chromatograms are recorded in the prescribed conditions, the retention times relative to fluoxetine are: impurity A about 0.24, impurity B about 0.27 and impurity C about 0.94.

Inject 10 µl of the reference solution.

The test is not valid unless: in the chromatogram obtained with the reference solution, the retention time of the peak due to fluoxetine is 10 min to 18 min; the retention time of the peak due to 4-trifluoromethylphenol is not greater than 35 min; the *h/v* ratio is not greater than 1.1 (*h* is the distance between the top of the peak due to impurity C and the baseline; *v* is the distance between the top of the peak due to impurity C and the lowest point of the valley defined between the peak due to impurity C and the peak due to fluoxetine). If the ratio is greater than 1.1, reduce the volume of methanol and increase the volume of the solution of triethylamine in the mobile phase.

Inject 10 µl of test solution (a) and 10 µl of test solution (b). Continue the chromatography for 3 times the retention time of fluoxetine.

In the chromatogram obtained with test solution (b), the area of any peak due to impurity C is not greater than 0.0015 times the area of the principal peak (0.15 per cent).

In the chromatogram obtained with test solution (a): the areas of any peaks due to impurity A and impurity B are not greater than 0.0125 times the area of the principal peak in the chromatogram obtained with test solution (b) (0.25 per cent); none of the peaks, except the principal peak and the peaks due to impurity A and impurity B, has an area greater than 0.005 times the area of the principal peak in the chromatogram obtained with test solution (b) (0.1 per cent); the sum of the areas of all the peaks, apart from the principal peak, is not greater than 0.025 times the area of the principal peak in the chromatogram obtained with test solution (b) (0.5 per cent).

Disregard any peak with an area less than 0.0025 times that of the principal peak in the chromatogram obtained with test solution (b).

Acetonitrile. Not more than 0.1 per cent, determined by gas chromatography (*2.2.28*).

Test solution. Dissolve 50 mg of the substance to be examined in *dimethylformamide R* and dilute to 5.0 ml with the same solvent.

Reference solution. To 1.0 g of *acetonitrile R*, add *dimethylformamide R*, mix and dilute to 100.0 ml with the same solvent. Dilute 1.0 ml of the solution to 1000.0 ml with *dimethylformamide R*.

The chromatographic procedure may be carried out using:

- a fused-silica capillary column 30 m long and about 0.53 mm in internal diameter coated with *macrogol 20 000 R* (1 µm thick),
- *helium for chromatography R* as the carrier gas at a flow rate of 10 ml/min,
- a flame-ionisation detector,

maintaining the temperature of the column at 35 °C for 2 min then raising the temperature at a rate of 15 °C/min to 220 °C and maintaining at 220 °C for 10 min and maintaining the temperature of the injection port and that of the detector at 250 °C.

Inject 1 µl of the test solution, 1 µl of the reference solution and 1 µl of the dissolution solvent. In the chromatogram obtained with the reference solution, note the retention time of acetonitrile.

In the chromatogram obtained with the dissolution solvent, verify that there is no peak with the same retention time as acetonitrile.

The area of the peak due to acetonitrile in the chromatogram obtained with the test solution is not greater than that of the corresponding peak in the chromatogram obtained with the reference solution.

Heavy metals (*2.4.8*). 1.0 g complies with limit test C (20 ppm). Prepare the standard using 2 ml of *lead standard solution (10 ppm Pb) R*.

Water (*2.5.12*). Not more than 0.5 per cent, determined on 1.00 g by the semi-micro determination of water.

Sulphated ash (*2.4.14*). Not more than 0.1 per cent, determined on 1.0 g.

ASSAY

Examine by liquid chromatography (*2.2.29*).

Test solution. Dissolve 55.0 mg of the substance to be examined in the mobile phase and dilute to 50.0 ml with the mobile phase. Dilute 10.0 ml of the solution to 100.0 ml with the mobile phase.

Reference solution. Dissolve 55.0 mg of *fluoxetine hydrochloride CRS* in the mobile phase and dilute to 50.0 ml with the mobile phase. Dilute 10.0 ml of the solution to 100.0 ml with the mobile phase.

The chromatographic procedure may be carried out using:

- a stainless steel column 0.25 m long and 4.6 mm in internal diameter packed with *octylsilyl silica gel for chromatography R* (5 µm),
- as mobile phase at a flow rate of 1 ml/min a mixture of 8 volumes of *methanol R*, 30 volumes of *tetrahydrofuran R* and 62 volumes of a solution of *triethylamine R* prepared as follows: to 10 ml of *triethylamine R*, add 980 ml of *water R*, mix and adjust to pH 6.0 with *phosphoric acid R* (about 4.5 ml) and dilute to 1000 ml with *water R*,
- as detector a spectrophotometer set at 227 nm.

When using a recorder, adjust the sensitivity of the system so that the height of the principal peak in the chromatogram obtained with the reference solution is at least 50 per cent of the full scale of the recorder.

Adjust the volumes of methanol and the solution of triethylamine in the mobile phase so that the retention time of fluoxetine is between 10 min and 18 min.

The assay is not valid unless the symmetry factor calculated at 10 per cent of the height of the peak due to fluoxetine is at most 2.0.

Inject 10 µl of the test solution and 10 µl of the reference solution.

Calculate the content of fluoxetine hydrochloride ($C_{17}H_{19}ClF_3NO$) from the area of the peaks in the chromatograms obtained with the test solution and the reference solution using the stated content of $C_{17}H_{19}ClF_3NO$ in *fluoxetine hydrochloride CRS* and correcting for the content of water and of acetonitrile in the substance to be examined.

IMPURITIES

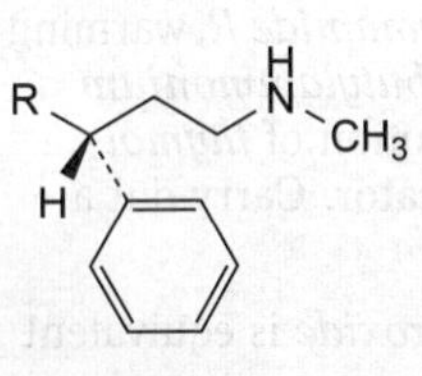

and enantiomer

A. R = OH: (1*RS*)-3-(methylamino)-1-phenylpropan-1-ol,

B. R = H: *N*-methyl-3-phenylpropan-1-amine,

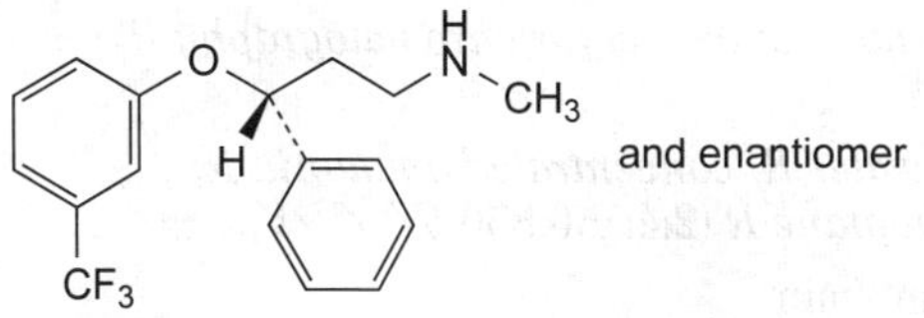

C. (3*RS*)-*N*-methyl-3-phenyl-3-[3-(trifluoromethyl)phenoxy]propan-1-amine.

01/2005:1693

FLUPENTIXOL DIHYDROCHLORIDE

Flupentixoli dihydrochloridum

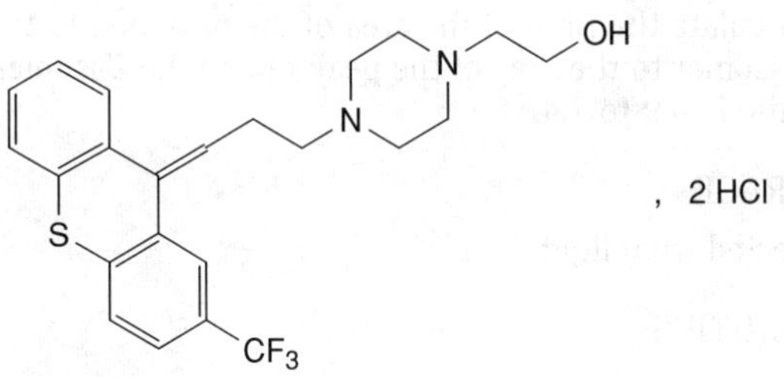

$C_{23}H_{27}Cl_2F_3N_2OS$ M_r 507.4

DEFINITION

2-[4-[3-[(*EZ*)-2-(trifluoromethyl)-9*H*-thioxanthen-9-ylidene]propyl]piperazin-1-yl]ethanol dihydrochloride.

Content:

- flupentixol dihydrochloride: 98.0 per cent to 101.5 per cent (dried substance),
- *Z*-isomer: 42.0 per cent to 52.0 per cent.

CHARACTERS

Appearance: white or almost white powder.

Solubility: very soluble in water, soluble in alcohol, practically insoluble in methylene chloride.

IDENTIFICATION

First identification: A, D.

Second identification: B, C, D.

A. Infrared absorption spectrophotometry (*2.2.24*).

Comparison: *flupentixol dihydrochloride CRS.*

B. Thin-layer chromatography (*2.2.27*).

Test solution. Dissolve 20 mg of the substance to be examined in *methanol R* and dilute to 10 ml with the same solvent.

Reference solution. Dissolve 20 mg of *flupentixol dihydrochloride CRS* in *methanol R* and dilute to 10 ml with the same solvent.

Plate: *TLC silica gel F_{254} plate R.*

Mobile phase: *water R, diethylamine R, methyl ethyl ketone R* (1:4:95 *V/V/V*).

Application: 2 μl.

Development: twice over a path of 15 cm.

Drying: in air.

Detection A: examine in ultraviolet light at 254 nm.

Results A: the principal spot in the chromatogram obtained with the test solution is similar in position and size to the principal spot in the chromatogram obtained with the reference solution. Doubling of the spot may be observed in both chromatograms.

Detection B: spray with *alcoholic solution of sulphuric acid R*; heat at 110 °C for 5 min and allow to cool; examine in ultraviolet light at 365 nm.

Results B: the principal spot in the chromatogram obtained with the test solution is similar in position and size to the principal spot in the chromatogram obtained with the reference solution. Doubling of the spot may be observed in both chromatograms.

C. Mix about 5 mg with 45 mg of *heavy magnesium oxide R* and ignite in a crucible until an almost white residue is obtained (usually less than 5 min). Allow to cool, add 1 ml of *water R*, 0.05 ml of *phenolphthalein solution R1* and about 1 ml of *dilute hydrochloric acid R* to render the solution colourless. Filter and add to the filtrate a freshly prepared mixture of 0.1 ml of *alizarin S solution R* and 0.1 ml of *zirconyl nitrate solution R*. Mix, allow to stand for 5 min and compare the colour of the solution with that of a blank prepared in the same manner. The test solution is yellow. The blank is red.

D. It gives reaction (a) of chlorides (*2.3.1*).

TESTS

Appearance of solution. The solution is clear (*2.2.1*) and not more intensely coloured than reference solution GY_6 (*2.2.2, Method II*).

Dissolve 2.0 g of the substance to be examined in *water R* and dilute to 20 ml with the same solvent.

pH (*2.2.3*): 2.0 to 3.0.

Dissolve 0.5 g in *carbon dioxide-free water R* and dilute to 50 ml with the same solvent.

Related substances. Thin-layer chromatography (*2.2.27*). *Carry out the test protected from light and prepare the solutions immediately before use.*

Test solution (a). Dissolve 0.40 g of the substance to be examined in *alcohol R* and dilute to 20 ml with the same solvent.

Test solution (b). Dilute 2.0 ml of test solution (a) to 20.0 ml with *alcohol R*.

Reference solution (a). Dilute 1.0 ml of test solution (b) to 50.0 ml with *alcohol R*.

Reference solution (b). Dilute 2.0 ml of reference solution (a) to 20.0 ml with *alcohol R*.

Reference solution (c). Dissolve 10 mg of *flupentixol impurity D CRS* in *alcohol R*, add 0.5 ml of test solution (a) and dilute to 20.0 ml with *alcohol R*.

Plate: *TLC silica gel F_{254} plate R.*

Mobile phase: *diethylamine R, toluene R, ethyl acetate R* (10:20:70 *V/V/V*).

Application: 5 μl.

Development: in an unsaturated tank over a path of 10 cm.

Drying: in air.

Detection: spray with *alcoholic solution of sulphuric acid R*, heat at 110 °C for 5 min and allow to cool; examine in ultraviolet light at 365 nm. Doubling of the spot due to flupentixol may be observed.

System suitability: the chromatogram obtained with reference solution (c) shows 2 clearly separated spots.

Limits:

- in the chromatogram obtained with test solution (a): any spots, apart from the principal spot, are not more intense than the spot, or spots in the chromatogram obtained with reference solution (a) (0.2 per cent),

– in the chromatogram obtained with test solution (b): any spots, apart from the principal spot, are not more intense than the spot or spots in the chromatogram obtained with reference solution (b) (0.2 per cent).

Impurity F. Liquid chromatography (*2.2.29*). *Carry out the test protected from light and prepare the solutions immediately before use.*

Test solution. Dissolve 20.0 mg of the substance to be examined in the mobile phase and dilute to 20.0 ml with the mobile phase.

Reference solution. Dissolve 10.0 mg of *flupentixol dihydrochloride CRS* and 10.0 mg of *flupentixol impurity F CRS* in the mobile phase and dilute to 100.0 ml with the mobile phase. Dilute 1.0 ml of the solution to 20.0 ml with the mobile phase.

Column:

- *size*: l = 0.125 m, Ø = 4.6 mm,
- *stationary phase*: *octylsilyl silica gel for chromatography R* (3 µm)

Mobile phase: mix 10 volumes of *acetonitrile R*, 55 volumes of *methanol R* and 35 volumes of a solution containing 8.72 g/l of *potassium dihydrogen phosphate R*, 0.37 g/l of *anhydrous disodium hydrogen phosphate R* and 0.77 g/l of *dodecyltrimethylammonium bromide R*.

Flow rate: 1.0 ml/min.

Detection: spectrophotometer at 270 nm.

Injection: 20 µl.

System suitability: reference solution:

- *resolution*: minimum 2.0 between the 2nd of the peaks due to impurity F and the 1st of the peaks due to flupentixol. Peak splitting may not always occur.

Limit:

- *impurity F*: not more than the area of the corresponding peak or peaks in the chromatogram obtained with the reference solution (0.5 per cent).

Heavy metals (*2.4.8*): maximum 20 ppm.

1.0 g complies with limit test C. Prepare the standard using 2 ml of *lead standard solution (10 ppm Pb) R*.

Loss on drying (*2.2.32*): maximum 2.0 per cent, determined on 1.000 g by drying in an oven at 100-105 °C.

Sulphated ash (*2.4.14*): maximum 0.1 per cent, determined on 1.0 g in a platinum crucible.

ASSAY

Flupentixol dihydrochloride. Dissolve 0.200 g in 30 ml of *alcohol R*. Carry out a potentiometric titration (*2.2.20*), using *0.1 M sodium hydroxide*. Read the volume added between the 2 points of inflexion.

1 ml of *0.1 M sodium hydroxide* is equivalent to 50.74 mg of $C_{23}H_{27}Cl_2F_3N_2OS$.

***Z*-Isomer.** Liquid chromatography (*2.2.29*).

Test solution. Dissolve 20.0 mg of the substance to be examined in the mobile phase and dilute to 50.0 ml with the mobile phase.

Reference solution. Dissolve 20.0 mg of *flupentixol dihydrochloride CRS* in the mobile phase and dilute to 50.0 ml with the mobile phase.

Column:

- *size*: l = 0.25 m, Ø = 4.0 mm,
- *stationary phase*: *silica gel for chromatography R* (5 µm).

Mobile phase: *water R, concentrated ammonia R, 2-propanol R, heptane R* (2:4:150:850 *V/V/V/V*).

Flow rate: 1.5 ml/min.

Detection: spectrophotometer at 254 nm.

Injection: 20 µl.

System suitability: reference solution:

- *resolution*: minimum 3.0 between the peaks due to *Z*-isomer (1st peak) and to *E*-isomer (2nd peak).

Results:

- calculate the percentage content of *Z*-isomer taking into account the assigned content of *Z*-isomer in *flupentixol dihydrochloride CRS*,
- calculate the ratio of the area of the peak due to the *E*-isomer to the area of the peak due to the *Z*-isomer: this ratio is 0.9 to 1.4.

STORAGE

Protected from light.

IMPURITIES

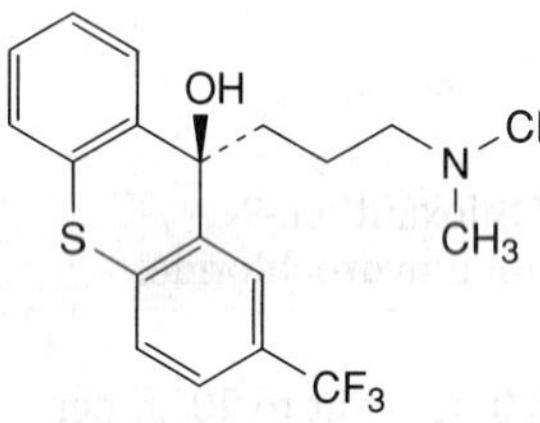

A. (9*RS*)-9-[3-(dimethylamino)propyl]-2-(trifluoromethyl)-9*H*-thioxanthen-9-ol,

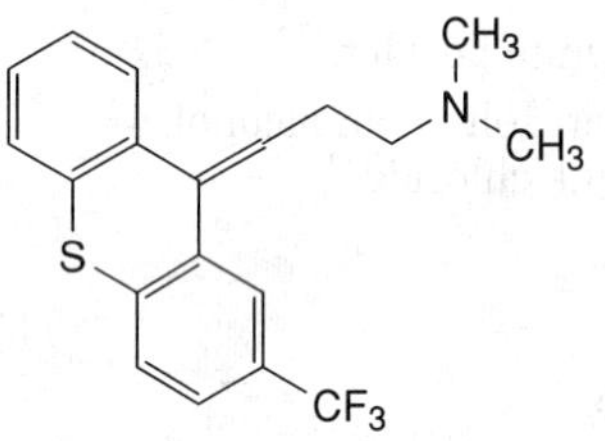

B. *N,N*-dimethyl-3-[(*EZ*)-2-(trifluoromethyl)-9*H*-thioxanthen-9-ylidene]propan-1-amine,

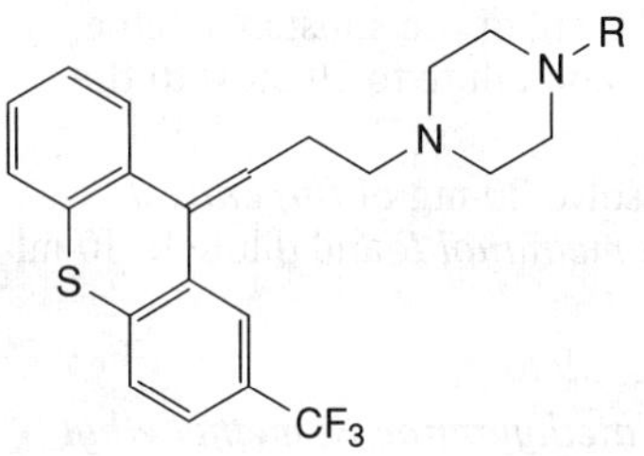

C. R = H: 1-[3-[(*EZ*)-2-(trifluoromethyl)-9*H*-thioxanthen-9-ylidene]propyl]piperazine,

D. R = CH_2-CH_2-O-CH_2-CH_2-OH: 2-[2-[4-[3-[(*EZ*)-2-(trifluoromethyl)-9*H*-thioxanthen-9-ylidene]propyl]piperazin-1-yl]ethoxy]ethanol,

E. R = CH_2-CH_2-O-CO-CH_3: 2-[4-[3-[(*EZ*)-2-(trifluoromethyl)-9*H*-thioxanthen-9-ylidene]propyl]piperazin-1-yl]ethyl acetate,

Monographs F-H

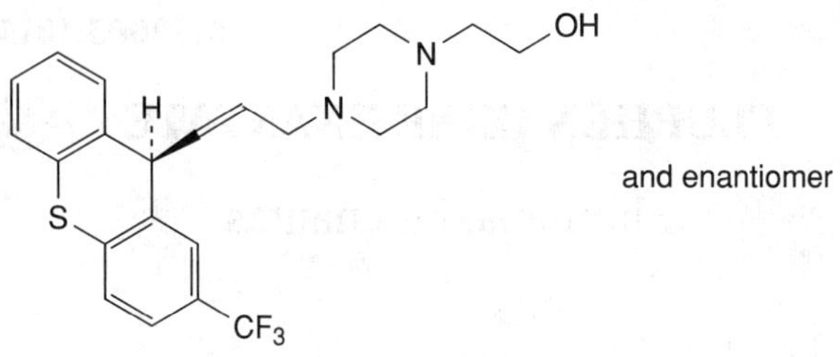

F. 2-[4-[(*EZ*)-3-[(9*RS*)-2-(trifluoromethyl)-9*H*-thioxanthen-9-yl]prop-2-enyl]piperazin-1-yl]ethanol,

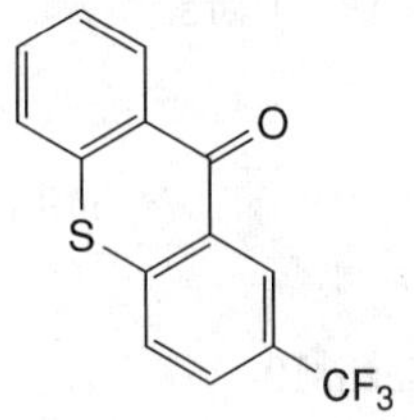

G. 2-(trifluoromethyl)-9*H*-thioxanthen-9-one.

01/2005:1014

FLUPHENAZINE DECANOATE

Fluphenazini decanoas

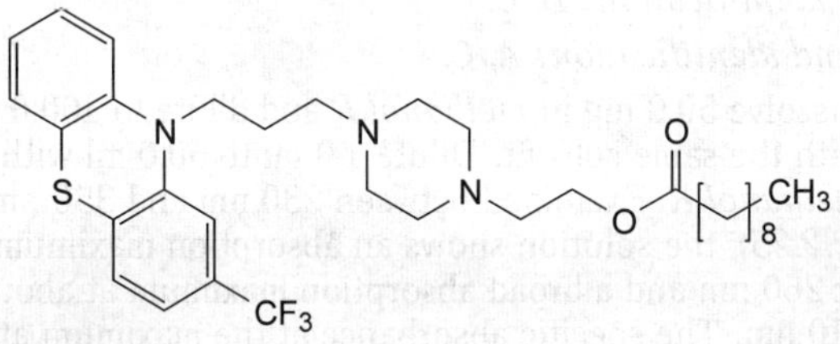

$C_{32}H_{44}F_3N_3O_2S$ M_r 591.8

DEFINITION

2-[4-[3-[2-(Trifluoromethyl)-10*H*-phenothiazin-10-yl]propyl]piperazin-1-yl]ethyl decanoate.

Content: 98.5 per cent to 101.5 per cent (dried substance).

CHARACTERS

Appearance: pale yellow, viscous liquid or yellow solid.

Solubility: practically insoluble in water, very soluble in ethanol and in methylene chloride, freely soluble in methanol.

IDENTIFICATION

First identification: B, C.

Second identification: A, C.

A. Dissolve 50.0 mg in *methanol R* and dilute to 100.0 ml with the same solvent. Dilute 1.0 ml to 50.0 ml with *methanol R*. Examined between 230 nm and 350 nm (*2.2.25*), the solution shows an absorption maximum at 260 nm and a broad absorption maximum at about 310 nm. The specific absorbance at the maximum at 260 nm is 570 to 630.

B. Infrared absorption spectrophotometry (*2.2.24*).
Preparation: apply 50 μl of a 25 g/l solution in *methylene chloride R* to a disc of *potassium bromide R*. Dry the discs at 60 °C for 1 h before use.
Comparison: *fluphenazine decanoate CRS.*

C. Thin-layer chromatography (*2.2.27*).
Test solution. Dissolve 10 mg of the substance to be examined in *methanol R* and dilute to 10 ml with the same solvent.
Reference solution (a). Dissolve 10 mg of *fluphenazine decanoate CRS* in *methanol R* and dilute to 10 ml with the same solvent.
Reference solution (b). Dissolve 5 mg of *fluphenazine enantate CRS* in reference solution (a) and dilute to 5 ml with the same solution.
Plate: *TLC octadecylsilyl silica gel F_{254} plate R.*
Mobile phase: *concentrated ammonia R1, water R, methanol R* (1:4:95 *V/V/V*).
Application: 2 μl.
Development: over a path of 8 cm.
Detection: examine in ultraviolet light at 254 nm.
System suitability: the chromatogram obtained with reference solution (b) shows 2 clearly separated spots.
Results: the principal spot in the chromatogram obtained with the test solution is similar in position and size to the principal spot in the chromatogram obtained with reference solution (a).

TESTS

Related substances. Liquid chromatography (*2.2.29*). *Carry out the test protected from light and prepare the solutions immediately before use.*

Test solution. Dissolve 10.0 mg of the substance to be examined in *acetonitrile R* and dilute to 50.0 ml with the same solvent.

Reference solution (a). Dissolve 5 mg of *fluphenazine octanoate CRS* and 5 mg of *fluphenazine enantate CRS* in *acetonitrile R* and dilute to 50 ml with the same solvent.

Reference solution (b). Dilute 5.0 ml of the test solution to 100.0 ml with a mixture of 5 volumes of mobile phase A and 95 volumes of mobile phase B. Dilute 1.0 ml of this solution to 10.0 ml with a mixture of 5 volumes of mobile phase A and 95 volumes of mobile phase B.

Reference solution (c). Dissolve 11.7 mg of *fluphenazine dihydrochloride CRS* and 5.0 mg of *fluphenazine sulphoxide CRS* in a mixture of 5 volumes of *water R* and 95 volumes of *acetonitrile R* and dilute to 100.0 ml with the same mixture of solvents. Dilute 1.0 ml to 50.0 ml with a mixture of 5 volumes of *water R* and 95 volumes of *acetonitrile R*.

Column:
- *size*: *l* = 0.25 m, Ø = 4.6 mm,
- *stationary phase*: spherical *octadecylsilyl silica gel for chromatography R* (5 μm).

Mobile phase:
- *mobile phase A*: 10 g/l solution of *ammonium carbonate R* adjusted to pH 7.5 with *dilute hydrochloric acid R,*
- *mobile phase B*: mobile phase A, *acetonitrile R, methanol R* (7.5:45:45 *V/V/V*),

Time (min)	Mobile phase A (per cent *V/V*)	Mobile phase B (per cent *V/V*)
0 - 7	20	80
7 - 17	20 → 0	80 → 100
17 - 80	0	100
80 - 81	0 → 20	100 → 80

Flow rate: 1.0 ml/min.

Detection: spectrophotometer at 260 nm.

Equilibration: at least 30 min with the mobile phase at the initial composition.

Injection: 10 µl.

Relative retention with reference to fluphenazine decanoate (retention time = about 34 min): impurity A = about 0.13; impurity B = about 0.33; impurity C = about 0.76; impurity D = about 0.82.

System suitability: reference solution (a):

- *resolution*: minimum 6 between the peaks due to impurity C and impurity D.

Limits:

- *impurity A*: not more than the area of the corresponding peak in the chromatogram obtained with reference solution (c) (0.5 per cent),
- *impurity B*: not more than the area of the corresponding peak in the chromatogram obtained with reference solution (c) (1.0 per cent),
- *any other impurity*: not more than the area of the principal peak in the chromatogram obtained with reference solution (b) (0.5 per cent),
- *total*: not more than 2.0 per cent,
- *disregard limit for any other impurity*: 0.1 times the area of the principal peak in the chromatogram obtained with reference solution (b) (0.05 per cent).

Heavy metals (*2.4.8*): maximum 20 ppm.

1.0 g complies with limit test C. Prepare the standard using 2 ml of *lead standard solution (10 ppm Pb) R*.

Loss on drying (*2.2.32*): maximum 1.0 per cent, determined on 1.000 g by drying in an oven at 60 °C at a pressure not exceeding 0.7 kPa for 3 h.

Sulphated ash (*2.4.14*): maximum 0.1 per cent, determined on 1.0 g in a platinum crucible.

ASSAY

Dissolve 0.250 g in 30 ml of *glacial acetic acid R*. Using 0.05 ml of *crystal violet solution R* as indicator, titrate with *0.1 M perchloric acid* until the colour changes from violet to green.

1 ml of *0.1 M perchloric acid* is equivalent to 29.59 mg of $C_{32}H_{44}F_3N_3O_2S$.

STORAGE

Protected from light.

IMPURITIES

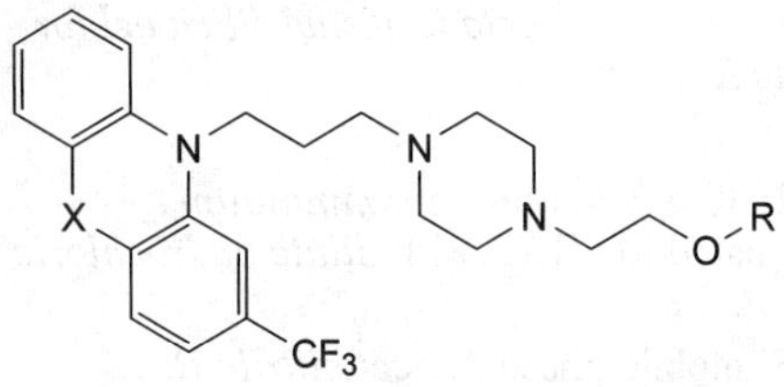

A. X = SO, R = H: fluphenazine *S*-oxide,

B. X = S, R = H: fluphenazine,

C. X = S, R = CO-$[CH_2]_5$-CH_3: fluphenazine enantate,

D. X = S, R = CO-$[CH_2]_6$-CH_3: fluphenazine octanoate,

E. X = S, R = CO-$[CH_2]_7$-CH_3: fluphenazine nonanoate,

F. X = S, R = CO-$[CH_2]_9$-CH_3: fluphenazine undecanoate,

G. X = S, R = CO-$[CH_2]_{10}$-CH_3: fluphenazine dodecanoate.

01/2005:1015

FLUPHENAZINE ENANTATE

Fluphenazini enantas

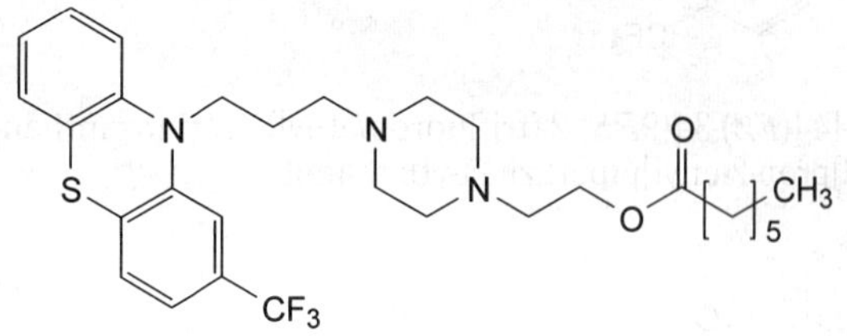

$C_{29}H_{38}F_3N_3O_2S$ M_r 549.7

DEFINITION

2-[4-[3-[2-(Trifluoromethyl)-10*H*-phenothiazin-10-yl]propyl]piperazin-1-yl]ethyl heptanoate.

Content: 98.5 per cent to 101.5 per cent (dried substance).

CHARACTERS

Appearance: pale yellow, viscous liquid or yellow solid.

Solubility: practically insoluble in water, very soluble in ethanol and in methylene chloride, freely soluble in methanol.

IDENTIFICATION

First identification: B, C.

Second identification: A, C.

A. Dissolve 50.0 mg in *methanol R* and dilute to 100.0 ml with the same solvent. Dilute 1.0 ml to 50.0 ml with *methanol R*. Examined between 230 nm and 350 nm (*2.2.25*), the solution shows an absorption maximum at 260 nm and a broad absorption maximum at about 310 nm. The specific absorbance at the maximum at 260 nm is 610 to 670.

B. Infrared absorption spectrophotometry (*2.2.24*).

Preparation: apply 50 µl of a 25 g/l solution in *methylene chloride R* to a disc of *potassium bromide R*. Dry the discs at 60 °C for 1 h before use.

Comparison: *fluphenazine enantate CRS*.

C. Thin-layer chromatography (*2.2.27*).

Test solution. Dissolve 10 mg of the substance to be examined in *methanol R* and dilute to 10 ml with the same solvent.

Reference solution (a). Dissolve 10 mg of *fluphenazine enantate CRS* in *methanol R* and dilute to 10 ml with the same solvent.

Reference solution (b). Dissolve 5 mg of *fluphenazine decanoate CRS* in reference solution (a) and dilute to 5 ml with the same solution.

Plate: *TLC octadecylsilyl silica gel F_{254} plate R*.

Mobile phase: *concentrated ammonia R1, water R, methanol R* (1:4:95 *V/V/V*).

Application: 2 µl.

Development: over a path of 8 cm.

Detection: examine in ultraviolet light at 254 nm.

System suitability: the chromatogram obtained with reference solution (b) shows 2 clearly separated spots.

Results: the principal spot in the chromatogram obtained with the test solution is similar in position and size to the principal spot in the chromatogram obtained with reference solution (a).

TESTS

Related substances. Liquid chromatography (*2.2.29*). *Carry out the test protected from light and prepare the solutions immediately before use.*

Test solution. Dissolve 10.0 mg of the substance to be examined in *acetonitrile R* and dilute to 50.0 ml with the same solvent.

Reference solution (a). Dissolve 5 mg of *fluphenazine octanoate CRS* and 5 mg of *fluphenazine enantate CRS* in *acetonitrile R* and dilute to 50 ml with the same solvent.

Reference solution (b). Dilute 5.0 ml of the test solution to 100.0 ml with a mixture of 5 volumes of mobile phase A and 95 volumes of mobile phase B. Dilute 1.0 ml of this solution to 10.0 ml with a mixture of 5 volumes of mobile phase A and 95 volumes of mobile phase B.

Reference solution (c). Dissolve 5.0 mg of *fluphenazine sulphoxide CRS* in *acetonitrile R* and dilute to 100.0 ml with the same solvent. Dilute 1.0 ml to 50.0 ml with *acetonitrile R.*

Column:
- *size*: *l* = 0.25 m, Ø = 4.6 mm,
- *stationary phase*: spherical *octadecylsilyl silica gel for chromatography R* (5 µm).

Mobile phase:
- *mobile phase A*: 10 g/l solution of *ammonium carbonate R* adjusted to pH 7.5 with *dilute hydrochloric acid R,*
- *mobile phase B*: mobile phase A, *acetonitrile R, methanol R* (7.5:45:45 *V/V/V*),

Time (min)	Mobile phase A (per cent *V/V*)	Mobile phase B (per cent *V/V*)
0 - 7	20	80
7 - 17	20 → 0	80 → 100
17 - 80	0	100
80 - 81	0 → 20	100 → 80

Flow rate: 1.0 ml/min.

Detection: spectrophotometer at 260 nm.

Equilibration: at least 30 min with the mobile phase at the initial composition.

Injection: 10 µl.

Relative retention with reference to fluphenazine enantate (retention time = about 25 min): impurity A = about 0.2; impurity D = about 1.1.

System suitability: reference solution (a):
- *resolution*: minimum 6 between the peaks due to fluphenazine enantate and impurity D.

Limits:
- *impurity A*: not more than the area of the principal peak in the chromatogram obtained with reference solution (c) (0.5 per cent),
- *any other impurity*: not more than the area of the principal peak in the chromatogram obtained with reference solution (b) (0.5 per cent),
- *total*: not more than 1.6 per cent,
- *disregard limit for any other impurity*: 0.1 times the area of the principal peak in the chromatogram obtained with reference solution (b) (0.05 per cent).

Heavy metals (*2.4.8*): maximum 20 ppm.

1.0 g complies with limit test C. Prepare the standard using 2 ml of *lead standard solution (10 ppm Pb) R.*

Loss on drying (*2.2.32*): maximum 1.0 per cent, determined on 1.000 g by drying in an oven at 60 °C at a pressure not exceeding 0.7 kPa for 3 h.

Sulphated ash (*2.4.14*): maximum 0.1 per cent, determined on 1.0 g in a platinum crucible.

ASSAY

Dissolve 0.250 g in 30 ml of *glacial acetic acid R*. Using 0.05 ml of *crystal violet solution R* as indicator titrate with *0.1 M perchloric acid* until the colour changes from violet to green.

1 ml of *0.1 M perchloric acid* is equivalent to 27.49 mg of $C_{29}H_{38}F_3N_3O_2S$.

STORAGE

Protected from light.

IMPURITIES

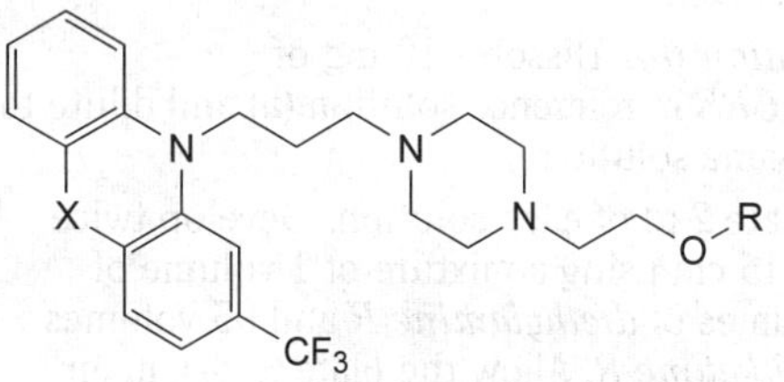

A. X = SO, R = H: fluphenazine *S*-oxide,

B. X = S, R = H: fluphenazine,

C. X = S, R = CO-$[CH_2]_8$-CH_3: fluphenazine decanoate,

D. X = S, R = CO-$[CH_2]_6$-CH_3: fluphenazine octanoate,

E. X = S, R = CO-$[CH_2]_7$-CH_3: fluphenazine nonanoate,

F. X = S, R = CO-$[CH_2]_9$-CH_3: fluphenazine undecanoate,

G. X = S, R = CO-$[CH_2]_{10}$-CH_3: fluphenazine dodecanoate.

01/2005:0904

FLUPHENAZINE HYDROCHLORIDE

Fluphenazini hydrochloridum

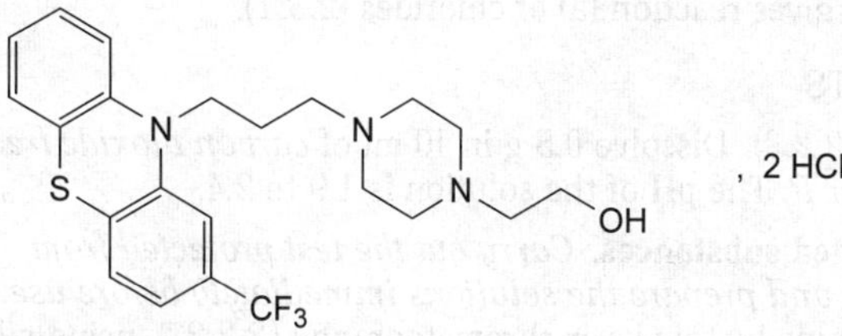

$C_{22}H_{28}Cl_2F_3N_3OS$ M_r 510.5

DEFINITION

Fluphenazine hydrochloride contains not less than 98.5 per cent and not more than the equivalent of 101.0 per cent of 2-[4-[3-[2-(trifluoromethyl)-10*H*-phenothiazin-10-yl]propyl]piperazin-1-yl]ethanol dihydrochloride, calculated with reference to the dried substance.

CHARACTERS

A white or almost white, crystalline powder, freely soluble in water, slightly soluble in alcohol and in methylene chloride.

IDENTIFICATION

First identification: *B, E.*

Second identification: *A, C, D, E.*

A. Dissolve 50.0 mg in *methanol R* and dilute to 100.0 ml with the same solvent. Dilute 2.0 ml to 100.0 ml with *methanol R*. Examined between 230 nm and 350 nm (*2.2.25*), the solution shows an absorption maximum at 260 nm and a broad absorption maximum at about 310 nm. The specific absorbance at the maximum at 260 nm is 630 to 700.

B. Examine by infrared absorption spectrophotometry (*2.2.24*), comparing with the spectrum obtained with *fluphenazine hydrochloride CRS*.

C. Examine by thin-layer chromatography (*2.2.27*), using *silica gel GF_{254} R* as the coating substance.

Test solution. Dissolve 20 mg of the substance to be examined in *methanol R* and dilute to 10 ml with the same solvent.

Reference solution (a). Dissolve 20 mg of *fluphenazine hydrochloride CRS* in *methanol R* and dilute to 10 ml with the same solvent.

Reference solution (b). Dissolve 10 mg of *perphenazine CRS* in reference solution (a) and dilute to 5 ml with the same solution.

Apply to the plate 2 µl of each solution. Develop twice over a path of 15 cm using a mixture of 1 volume of *water R*, 4 volumes of *diethylamine R* and 95 volumes of *methyl ethyl ketone R*. Allow the plate to dry in air and examine in ultraviolet light at 254 nm. The principal spot in the chromatogram obtained with the test solution is similar in position and size to the principal spot in the chromatogram obtained with reference solution (a). The test is not valid unless the chromatogram obtained with reference solution (b) shows two clearly separated principal spots.

D. Mix about 5 mg with 45 mg of *heavy magnesium oxide R* and ignite in a crucible until an almost white residue is obtained (usually less than 5 min). Allow to cool, add 1 ml of *water R*, 0.05 ml of *phenolphthalein solution R1* and about 1 ml of *dilute hydrochloric acid R* to render the solution colourless. Filter. Add 1.0 ml of the filtrate to a freshly prepared mixture of 0.1 ml of *alizarin S solution R* and 0.1 ml of *zirconyl nitrate solution R*. Mix, allow to stand for 5 min and compare the colour of the solution with that of a blank prepared in the same manner. The test solution is yellow and the blank is red.

E. It gives reaction (a) of chlorides (*2.3.1*).

TESTS

pH (*2.2.3*). Dissolve 0.5 g in 10 ml of *carbon dioxide-free water R*. The pH of the solution is 1.9 to 2.4.

Related substances. *Carry out the test protected from light and prepare the solutions immediately before use.* Examine by thin-layer chromatography (*2.2.27*), using *silica gel GF_{254} R* as the coating substance.

Test solution. Dissolve 0.20 g of the substance to be examined in a mixture of 5 volumes of *diethylamine R* and 95 volumes of *methanol R* and dilute to 10 ml with the same mixture of solvents.

Reference solution (a). Dilute 1 ml of the test solution to 100 ml with a mixture of 5 volumes of *diethylamine R* and 95 volumes of *methanol R*.

Reference solution (b). Dilute 5 ml of reference solution (a) to 10 ml with a mixture of 5 volumes of *diethylamine R* and 95 volumes of *methanol R*.

Apply to the plate 10 µl of each solution. Develop over a path of 12 cm using a mixture of 10 volumes of *acetone R*, 10 volumes of *diethylamine R* and 80 volumes of *cyclohexane R*. Allow the plate to dry in air and examine in ultraviolet light at 254 nm. Any spot in the chromatogram obtained with the test solution, apart from the principal spot, is not more intense than the spot in the chromatogram obtained with reference solution (a) (1.0 per cent) and at most one such spot is more intense than the spot in the chromatogram obtained with reference solution (b) (0.5 per cent).

Heavy metals (*2.4.8*). 1.0 g complies with limit test C for heavy metals (20 ppm). Prepare the standard using 2 ml of *lead standard solution (10 ppm Pb) R*.

Loss on drying (*2.2.32*). Not more than 1.0 per cent, determined on 0.500 g by drying in an oven at 65 °C for 3 h.

Sulphated ash (*2.4.14*). Not more than 0.1 per cent, determined on 1.0 g.

ASSAY

Dissolve 0.220 g in a mixture of 10 ml of *anhydrous formic acid R* and 40 ml of *acetic anhydride R*. Titrate with *0.1 M perchloric acid*, determining the end-point potentiometrically (*2.2.20*).

1 ml of *0.1 M perchloric acid* is equivalent to 25.52 mg of $C_{22}H_{28}Cl_2F_3N_3OS$.

STORAGE

Store protected from light.

IMPURITIES

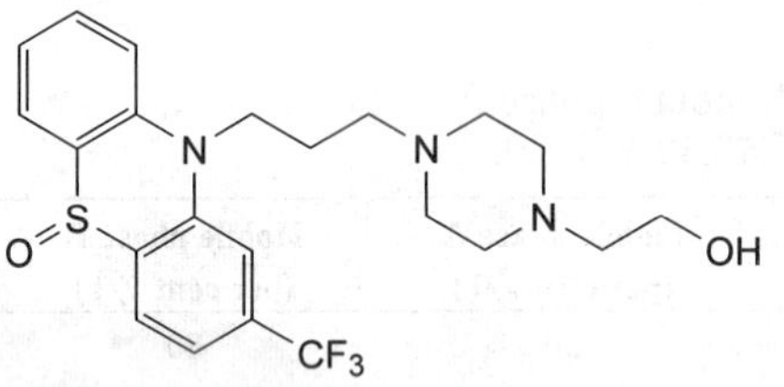

A. fluphenazine *S*-oxide.

01/2005:0905

FLURAZEPAM MONOHYDROCHLORIDE

Flurazepami monohydrochloridum

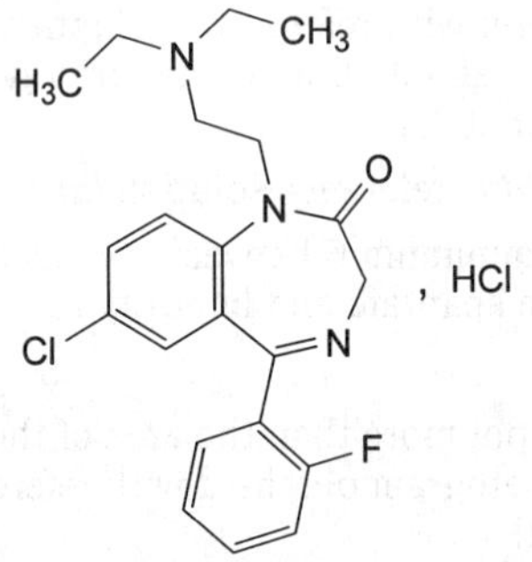

$C_{21}H_{24}Cl_2FN_3O$ M_r 424.3

DEFINITION

7-Chloro-1-[2-(diethylamino)ethyl]-5-(2-fluorophenyl)-1,3-dihydro-2*H*-1,4-benzodiazepin-2-one monohydrochloride.

Content: 99.0 per cent to 101.0 per cent (dried substance).

CHARACTERS

Appearance: white or almost white, crystalline powder.

Solubility: very soluble in water, freely soluble in alcohol.

IDENTIFICATION

A. Infrared absorption spectrophotometry (*2.2.24*).

Comparison: *Ph. Eur. reference spectrum of flurazepam monohydrochloride.*

B. It gives reaction (a) of chlorides (*2.3.1*).

TESTS

pH (*2.2.3*): 5.0 to 6.0.

Dissolve 0.50 g in *carbon dioxide-free water R* and dilute to 10 ml with the same solvent.

Related substances. Liquid chromatography (*2.2.29*). *Prepare the solutions immediately before use.*

Test solution. Dissolve 50.0 mg of the substance to be examined in the mobile phase and dilute to 50.0 ml with the mobile phase.

Reference solution (a). Dilute 1.0 ml of the test solution to 100.0 ml with the mobile phase. Dilute 5.0 ml of this solution to 50.0 ml with the mobile phase.

Reference solution (b). Dissolve 5 mg of the substance to be examined and 5 mg of *oxazepam R* in 10 ml of *acetonitrile R* and dilute to 50.0 ml with the mobile phase.

Column:

- *size*: l = 0.15 m, Ø = 4.6 mm,
- *stationary phase*: *base-deactivated octylsilyl silica gel for chromatography R* (5 μm).

Mobile phase: mix 350 volumes of *acetonitrile R* and 650 volumes of a 10.5 g/l solution of *potassium dihydrogen phosphate R* and ajust to pH 6.1 with a 40 g/l solution of *sodium hydroxide R*.

Flow rate: 1.0 ml/min.

Detection: spectrophotometer at 239 nm.

Injection: 20 μl.

Run time: 6 times the retention time of flurazepam.

Relative retention with reference to flurazepam (retention time = about 7 min): impurity C = about 1.5; impurity B = about 1.9; impurity A = about 2.4.

System suitability: reference solution (b):

- *resolution*: minimum of 4.5 between the peaks due to flurazepam and to oxazepam.

Limits:

- *correction factors*: for the calculation of contents, multiply the peak areas of the following impurities by the corresponding correction factor: impurity B = 0.61; impurity C = 0.65,
- *any impurity*: not more than the area of the principal peak in the chromatogram obtained with reference solution (a) (0.1 per cent),
- *total*: not more than 3 times the area of the principal peak in the chromatogram obtained with reference solution (a) (0.3 per cent),
- *disregard limit*: 0.5 times the area of the principal peak in the chromatogram obtained with reference solution (a) (0.05 per cent).

Fluorides (*2.4.5*): maximum 500 ppm.

0.10 g complies with the limit test for fluorides.

Loss on drying (*2.2.32*): maximum 0.5 per cent, determined on 1.000 g by drying in an oven at 100-105 °C for 4 h.

Sulphated ash (*2.4.14*): maximum 0.1 per cent, determined on 1.0 g.

ASSAY

Dissolve 0.350 g in a mixture of 1.0 ml of *0.1 M hydrochloric acid* and 50 ml of *alcohol R*. Carry out a potentiometric titration (*2.2.20*), using *0.1 M sodium hydroxide*. Read the volume added between the 2 points of inflexion.

1 ml of *0.1 M sodium hydroxide* is equivalent to 42.43 mg of $C_{21}H_{24}Cl_2FN_3O$.

STORAGE

Protected from light.

IMPURITIES

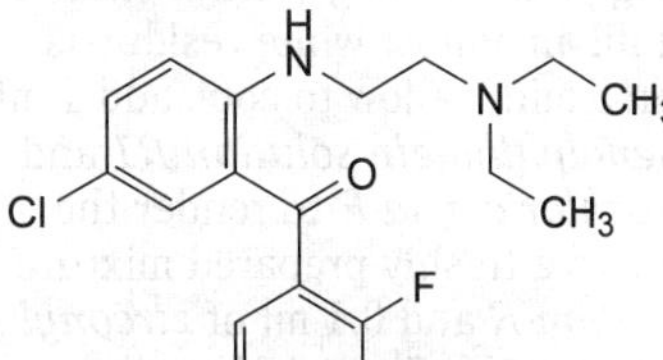

A. [5-chloro-2-[[2-(diethylamino)ethyl]amino]phenyl](2-fluorophenyl)methanone,

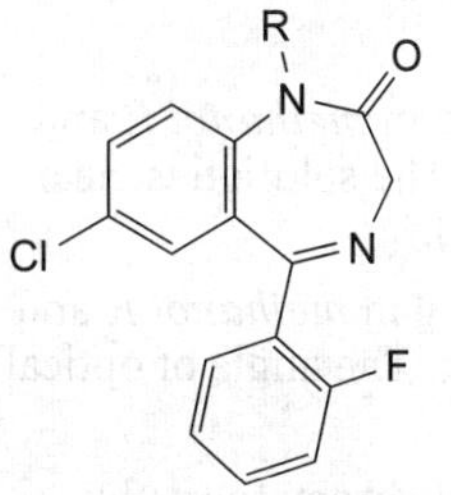

B. R = H: 7-chloro-5-(2-fluorophenyl)-1,3-dihydro-2*H*-1,4-benzodiazepin-2-one,

C. R = CHOH-CH_3: 7-chloro-5-(2-fluorophenyl)-1-[(1*RS*)-1-hydroxyethyl]-1,3-dihydro-2*H*-1,4-benzodiazepin-2-one.

01/2005:1519

FLURBIPROFEN

Flurbiprofenum

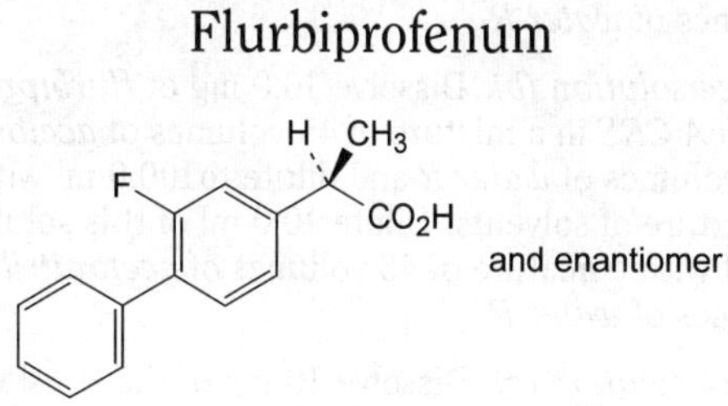

$C_{15}H_{13}FO_2$ M_r 244.3

DEFINITION

Flurbiprofen contains not less than 99.0 per cent and not more than the equivalent of 101.0 per cent of (2*RS*)-2-(2-fluorobiphenyl-4-yl)propanoic acid, calculated with reference to the dried substance.

CHARACTERS

A white or almost white, crystalline powder, practically insoluble in water, freely soluble in alcohol and in methylene chloride. It dissolves in aqueous solutions of alkali hydroxides and carbonates.

IDENTIFICATION

First identification: C, D.

Second identification: A, B, D.

A. Melting point (*2.2.14*): 114 °C to 117 °C.

B. Dissolve 0.10 g in *0.1 M sodium hydroxide* and dilute to 100.0 ml with the same alkaline solution. Dilute 1.0 ml of the solution to 100.0 ml with *0.1 M sodium hydroxide.* Examined between 230 nm and 350 nm (*2.2.25*), the solution shows an absorption maximum at 247 nm. The specific absorbance at the maximum is 780 to 820.

C. Examine by infrared absorption spectrophotometry (*2.2.24*), comparing with the spectrum obtained with *flurbiprofen CRS.*

D. Mix about 5 mg with 45 mg of *heavy magnesium oxide R* and ignite in a crucible until an almost white residue is obtained (usually less than 5 min). Allow to cool, add 1 ml of *water R,* 0.05 ml of *phenolphthalein solution R1* and about 1 ml of *dilute hydrochloric acid R* to render the solution colourless. Filter. To a freshly prepared mixture of 0.1 ml of *alizarin S solution R* and 0.1 ml of *zirconyl nitrate solution R* add 1.0 ml of the filtrate. Mix, allow to stand for 5 min and compare the colour of the solution with that of a blank prepared in the same manner. The test solution is yellow and the blank is red.

TESTS

Appearance of solution. Dissolve 1.0 g in *methanol R* and dilute to 10 ml with the same solvent. The solution is clear (*2.2.1*) and colourless (*2.2.2, Method I*).

Optical rotation (*2.2.7*). Dissolve 0.50 g in *methanol R* and dilute to 20.0 ml with the same solvent. The angle of optical rotation is − 0.1° to + 0.1°.

Related substances. Examine by liquid chromatography (*2.2.29*).

Test solution. Dissolve 0.20 g of the substance to be examined in a mixture of 45 volumes of *acetonitrile R* and 55 volumes of *water R* and dilute to 100.0 ml with the same mixture of solvents.

Reference solution (a). Dilute 1.0 ml of the test solution to 50.0 ml with a mixture of 45 volumes of *acetonitrile R* and 55 volumes of *water R.* Dilute 1.0 ml of the solution to 10.0 ml with a mixture of 45 volumes of *acetonitrile R* and 55 volumes of *water R.*

Reference solution (b). Dissolve 10.0 mg of *flurbiprofen impurity A CRS* in a mixture of 45 volumes of *acetonitrile R* and 55 volumes of *water R* and dilute to100.0 ml with the same mixture of solvents. Dilute 10.0 ml of this solution to 100.0 ml with a mixture of 45 volumes of *acetonitrile R* and 55 volumes of *water R.*

Reference solution (c). Dissolve 10 mg of the substance to be examined in a mixture of 45 volumes of *acetonitrile R* and 55 volumes of *water R* and dilute to 100.0 ml with the same mixture of solvents. Dilute 1.0 ml of the solution to 10.0 ml with reference solution (b).

The chromatographic procedure may be carried out using:

- a stainless steel column 0.15 m long and 3.9 mm in internal diameter packed with *octadecylsilyl silica gel for chromatography R* (5 µm),
- as mobile phase at a flow rate of 1 ml/min a mixture of 5 volumes of *glacial acetic acid R,* 35 volumes of *acetonitrile R* and 60 volumes of *water R,*
- as detector a spectrophotometer set at 254 nm.

Inject 10 µl of reference solution (c). Adjust the sensitivity of the system so that the heights of the two principal peaks in the chromatogram obtained are at least 40 per cent of the full scale of the recorder. The test is not valid unless the resolution between the peak corresponding to impurity A and the peak corresponding to flurbiprofen is at least 1.5. Inject 10 µl of the test solution and of reference solutions (a) and (b). Continue the chromatography for twice the retention time of flurbiprofen. In the chromatogram obtained with the test solution the area of any peak corresponding to impurity A is not greater than the area of the peak in the chromatogram obtained with reference solution (b) (0.5 per cent); the area of any peak, apart from the principal peak and the peak due to impurity A, is not greater than the area of the principal peak in the chromatogram obtained with reference solution (a) (0.2 per cent) and the sum of the areas of any such peaks is not greater than five times the area of the principal peak in the chromatogram obtained with reference solution (a) (1.0 per cent). Disregard any peak with an area less than 0.1 times that of the principal peak in the chromatogram obtained with reference solution (a) (0.02 per cent).

Heavy metals (*2.4.8*). Dissolve 2.0 g in a mixture of 10 volumes of *water R* and 90 volumes of *methanol R* and dilute to 20 ml with the same mixture of solvents. 12 ml of the solution complies with limit test B for heavy metals (10 ppm). Prepare the standard using *lead standard solution (1 ppm Pb)* obtained by diluting *lead standard solution (100 ppm Pb) R* with a mixture of 10 volumes of *water R* and 90 volumes of *methanol R.*

Loss on drying (*2.2.32*). Not more than 0.5 per cent, determined on 1.000 g by drying at 60 °C at a pressure not exceeding 0.7 kPa for 3 h.

Sulphated ash (*2.4.14*). Not more than 0.1 per cent, determined on 1.0 g in a platinum crucible.

ASSAY

Dissolve 0.200 g in 50 ml of *alcohol R.* Titrate with *0.1 M sodium hydroxide,* determining the end-point potentiometrically (*2.2.20*).

1 ml of *0.1 M sodium hydroxide* is equivalent to 24.43 mg of $C_{15}H_{13}FO_2$.

IMPURITIES

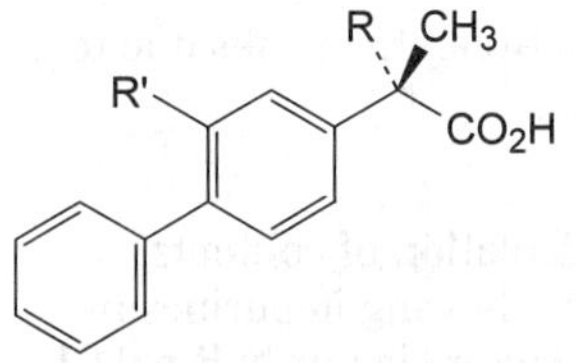

and enantiomer

A. R = R′ = H: (*2RS*)-2-(biphenyl-4-yl)propanoic acid,

B. R = $CH(CH_3)$-CO_2H: 2-(2-fluorobiphenyl-4-yl)-2,3-dimethylbutanedioic acid,

C. C. R = OH, R′ = F: (*2RS*)-2-(2-fluorobiphenyl-4-yl)-2-hydroxypropanoic acid,

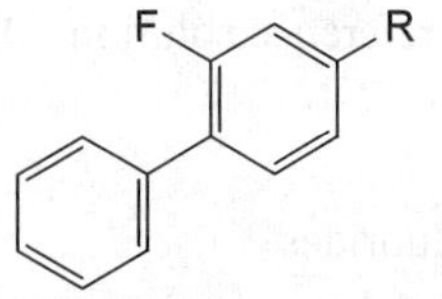

D. R = CO-CH_3: 1-(2-fluorobiphenyl-4-yl)ethanone,

E. R = CO_2H: 2-fluorobiphenyl-4-carboxylic acid.

01/2005:1723

FLUSPIRILENE

Fluspirilenum

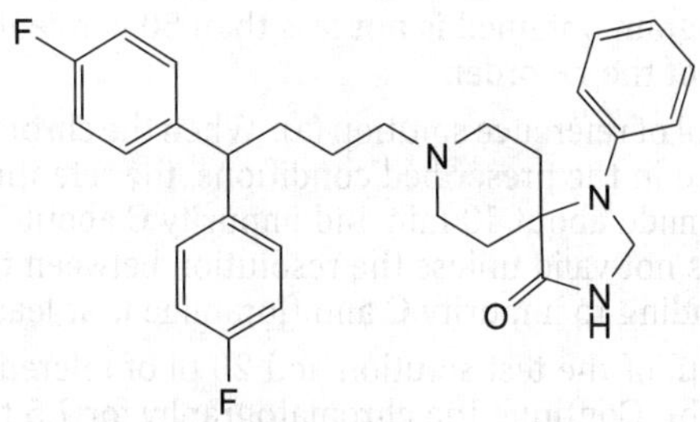

$C_{29}H_{31}F_2N_3O$ M_r 475.6

DEFINITION

8-[4,4-bis(4-Fluorophenyl)butyl]-1-phenyl-1,3,8-triazaspiro[4.5]decan-4-one.

Content: 99.0 per cent to 101.0 per cent (dried substance).

CHARACTERS

Appearance: white or almost white powder.

Solubility: practically insoluble in water, soluble in methylene chloride, slightly soluble in alcohol.

It shows polymorphism.

IDENTIFICATION

Infrared absorption spectrophotometry (*2.2.24*).

Preparation: discs.

Comparison: *fluspirilene CRS.*

If the spectra obtained show differences, dissolve the substance to be examined and the reference substance separately in *methylene chloride R*, gently evaporate to dryness and record new spectra using the residues.

TESTS

Appearance of solution. The solution is clear (*2.2.1*) and colourless (*2.2.2, Method II*).

Dissolve 0.25 g in 25 ml of *methylene chloride R*.

Related substances. Liquid chromatography (*2.2.29*).

Test solution. Dissolve 0.100 g of the substance to be examined in *dimethylformamide R* and dilute to 10.0 ml with the same solvent.

Reference solution (a). Dissolve 5.0 mg of *fluspirilene impurity C CRS* in *dimethylformamide R*, add 0.5 ml of the test solution and dilute to 100.0 ml with *dimethylformamide R.*

Reference solution (b). Dilute 1.0 ml of the test solution to 20.0 ml with *dimethylformamide R.* Dilute 1.0 ml of this solution to 25.0 ml with *dimethylformamide R.*

Column:

- *size*: *l* = 0.15 m, Ø = 4.6 mm,
- *stationary phase*: *octadecylsilyl silica gel for chromatography R* (3 µm).

Mobile phase:

- *mobile phase A*: 13.6 g/l solution of *tetrabutylammonium hydrogen sulphate R,*
- *mobile phase B*: *acetonitrile R,*

Time (min)	Mobile phase A (per cent *V/V*)	Mobile phase B (per cent *V/V*)
0 - 15	75 → 70	25 → 30
15 - 20	70	30
20 - 22	70 → 0	30 → 100
22 - 30	0	100
30 - 31	0 → 75	100 → 25
31 - 40	75	25

Flow rate: 1.2 ml/min.

Detection: spectrophotometer at 250 nm.

Injection: 10 µl.

Relative retention with reference to fluspirilene (retention time = about 15 min): impurity A = about 0.8; impurity B = about 0.93; impurity C = 0.97.

System suitability: reference solution (a):

- *resolution*: minimum 2.2 between the peaks due to impurity C and fluspirilene.

Limits:

- *impurities A, B, C*: for each impurity, not more than 1.5 times the area of the principal peak in the chromatogram obtained with reference solution (b) (0.3 per cent),
- *any other impurity*: not more than 0.5 times the area of the principal peak in the chromatogram obtained with reference solution (b) (0.1 per cent),
- *total*: not more than 3 times the area of the principal peak in the chromatogram obtained with reference solution (b) (0.6 per cent),
- *disregard limit*: 0.25 times the area of the principal peak in the chromatogram obtained with reference solution (b) (0.05 per cent).

Loss on drying (*2.2.32*): maximum 0.5 per cent, determined on 1.000 g by drying in an oven at 100-105 °C for 4 h.

Sulphated ash (*2.4.14*): maximum 0.1 per cent, determined on 1.0 g in a platinum crucible.

ASSAY

Dissolve 0.350 g in 50 ml of a mixture of 1 volume of *anhydrous acetic acid R* and 7 volumes of *methyl ethyl ketone R.* Titrate with *0.1 M perchloric acid,* determining the end-point potentiometrically (*2.2.20*). Carry out a blank titration.

1 ml of *0.1 M perchloric acid* is equivalent to 47.56 mg of $C_{29}H_{31}F_2N_3O$.

STORAGE

Protected from light.

Monographs F-H

IMPURITIES

Specified impurities: A, B, C.

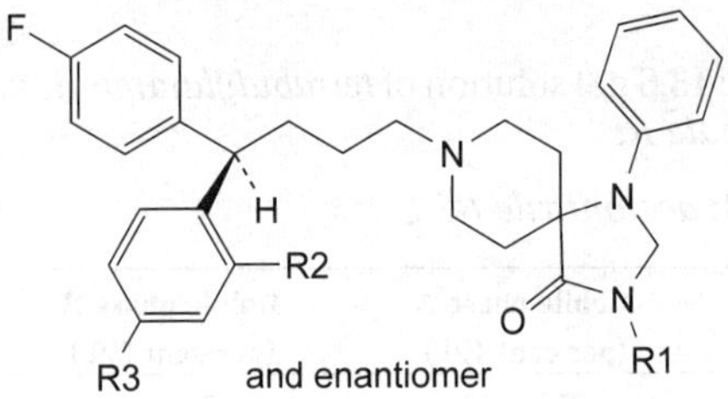

A. R1 = R2 = R3 = H: 8-[(4*RS*)-4-(4-fluorophenyl)-4-phenylbutyl]-1-phenyl-1,3,8-triazaspiro[4.5]decan-4-one,

B. R1 = R3 = H, R2 = F: 8-[(4*RS*)-4-(2-fluorophenyl)-4-(4-fluorophenyl)butyl]-1-phenyl-1,3,8-triazaspiro[4.5]decan-4-one,

C. R1 = CH_2OH, R2 = H, R3 = F: 8-[4,4-bis(4-fluorophenyl)butyl]-3-(hydroxymethyl)-1-phenyl-1,3,8-triazaspiro[4.5]decan-4-one.

01/2005:1423

FLUTAMIDE

Flutamidum

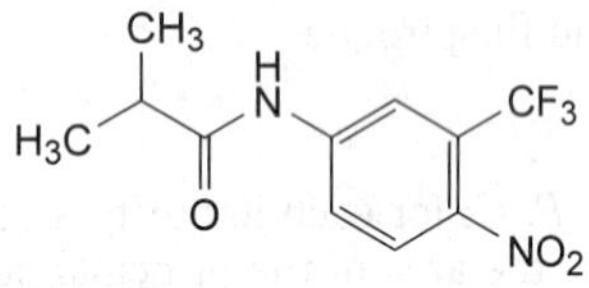

$C_{11}H_{11}F_3N_2O_3$ M_r 276.2

DEFINITION

Flutamide contains not less than 97.0 per cent and not more than the equivalent of 103.0 per cent of 2-methyl-*N*-[4-nitro-3-(trifluoromethyl)phenyl]propanamide, calculated with reference to the dried substance.

CHARACTERS

A pale yellow, crystalline powder, practically insoluble in water, freely soluble in acetone and in alcohol.

It melts at about 112 °C.

IDENTIFICATION

Examine by infrared absorption spectrophotometry (*2.2.24*), comparing with the spectrum obtained with *flutamide CRS*.

TESTS

Related substances. Examine by liquid chromatography (*2.2.29*).

Test solution. Dissolve 20.0 mg of the substance to be examined in the mobile phase and dilute to 20.0 ml with the mobile phase.

Reference solution (a). Dissolve 2 mg of *flutamide CRS* and 2 mg of *flutamide impurity C CRS* in the mobile phase and dilute to 50.0 ml with the mobile phase. Dilute 1.0 ml of this solution to 20.0 ml with the mobile phase.

Reference solution (b). Dilute 1.0 ml of the test solution to 50.0 ml with the mobile phase. Dilute 2.0 ml of this solution to 20.0 ml with the mobile phase.

The chromatographic procedure may be carried out using:

- a stainless steel column 0.25 m long and 4.0 mm in internal diameter packed with *octadecylsilyl silica gel for chromatography R* (5 µm),
- as mobile phase at a flow rate of 0.5 ml/min a mixture of equal volumes of *acetonitrile R* and *water R*,
- as detector a spectrophotometer set at 240 nm.

Inject 20 µl of reference solution (b). Adjust the sensitivity of the system so that the height of the principal peak in the chromatogram obtained is not less than 50 per cent of the full scale of the recorder.

Inject 20 µl of reference solution (a). When the chromatogram is recorded in the prescribed conditions, the retention times are: flutamide about 19 min and impurity C about 14 min. The test is not valid unless the resolution between the peaks corresponding to impurity C and flutamide is at least 10.5.

Inject 20 µl of the test solution and 20 µl of reference solution (b). Continue the chromatography for 1.5 times the retention time of the principal peak. In the chromatogram obtained with the test solution: the area of the peak corresponding to impurity C, with a retention time of about 0.72 relative to flutamide, is not greater than 1.5 times the area of the principal peak in the chromatogram obtained with reference solution (b) (0.3 per cent); the area of any other peak apart from the principal peak and the peak corresponding to impurity C is not greater than the area of the principal peak in the chromatogram obtained with reference solution (b) (0.2 per cent); the sum of the areas of the peaks apart from the principal peak is not greater than 2.5 times the area of the principal peak in the chromatogram obtained with reference solution (b) (0.5 per cent). Disregard any peak with an area less than 0.25 times the area of the principal peak in the chromatogram obtained with reference solution (b).

Heavy metals (*2.4.8*). 1.0 g complies with limit test C for heavy metals (20 ppm). Prepare the standard using 2 ml of *lead standard solution (10 ppm Pb) R*.

Loss on drying (*2.2.32*). Not more than 0.5 per cent, determined on 1.000 g by drying *in vacuo* at 60 °C for 3 h.

Sulphated ash (*2.4.14*). Not more than 0.1 per cent, determined on 1.0 g.

ASSAY

Dissolve 25.0 mg in *methanol R* and dilute to 25.0 ml with the same solvent. Dilute 2.0 ml of this solution to 100.0 ml with *methanol R*. Measure the absorbance (*2.2.25*) at the maximum at 295 nm.

Calculate the content of $C_{11}H_{11}F_3N_2O_3$ taking the specific absorbance to be 295.

STORAGE

Store protected from light.

IMPURITIES

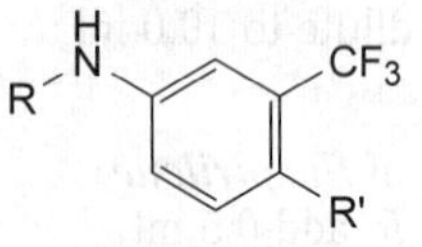

A. R = H, R′ = NO_2: 4-nitro-3-(trifluoromethyl)aniline,

B. R = CO-CH_3, R′ = NO_2: *N*-[4-nitro-3-(trifluoromethyl)phenyl]acetamide,

C. R = CO-CH_2-CH_3, R′ = NO_2: *N*-[4-nitro-3-(trifluoromethyl)phenyl]propanamide,

D. R = R′ = H: 3-(trifluoromethyl)aniline,

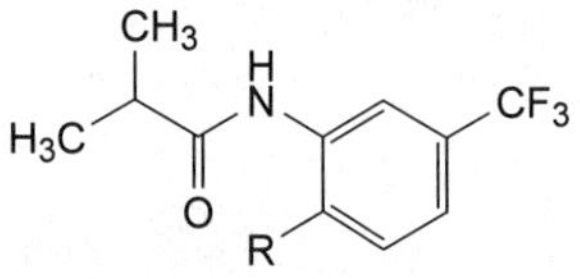

E. R = H: 2-methyl-*N*-[3-(trifluoromethyl)phenyl]propanamide,

F. R = NO_2: 2-methyl-*N*-[2-nitro-5-(trifluoromethyl)phenyl]propanamide.

01/2005:1750

FLUTICASONE PROPIONATE

Fluticasoni propionas

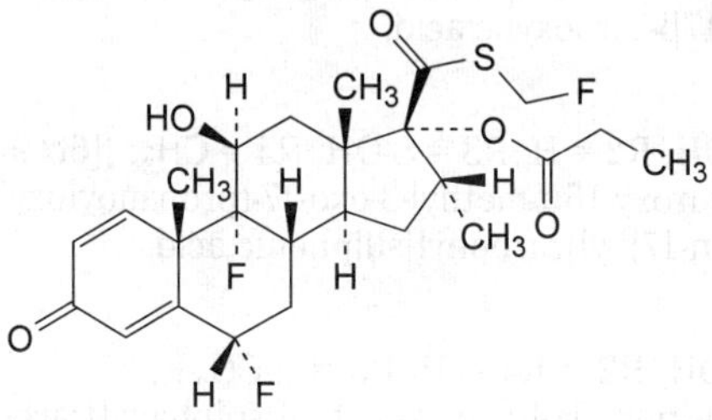

$C_{25}H_{31}F_3O_5S$ M_r 500.6

DEFINITION

6α,9-Difluoro-17-[[(fluoromethyl)sulphanyl]carbonyl]-11β-hydroxy-16α-methyl-3-oxoandrosta-1,4-dien-17α-yl propanoate.

Content: 97.0 per cent to 102.0 per cent (anhydrous and solvent-free substance).

CHARACTERS

Appearance: white or almost white powder.

Solubility: practically insoluble in water, sparingly soluble in methylene chloride, slightly soluble in alcohol.

IDENTIFICATION

A. Infrared absorption spectrophotometry (*2.2.24*).

Comparison: *fluticasone propionate CRS.*

B. Examine the chromatograms obtained in the assay.

Results: the principal peak in the chromatogram obtained with the test solution is similar in retention time to the principal peak in the chromatogram obtained with reference solution (b).

TESTS

Specific optical rotation (*2.2.7*): + 32 to + 36 (anhydrous and solvent-free substance).

Dissolve 0.25 g in *methylene chloride R* and dilute to 50.0 ml with the same solvent.

Related substances. Liquid chromatography (*2.2.29*): use the normalisation procedure.

Test solution. Dissolve 20 mg of the substance to be examined in a mixture of equal volumes of mobile phase A and mobile phase B and dilute to 100.0 ml with the same mixture of mobile phases.

Reference solution (a). Dissolve 4 mg of *fluticasone impurity D CRS* in a mixture of equal volumes of mobile phase A and mobile phase B and dilute to 100.0 ml with the same mixture of mobile phases.

Reference solution (b). Dissolve 20 mg of *fluticasone propionate CRS* in a mixture of equal volumes of mobile phase A and mobile phase B, add 1.0 ml of reference solution (a) and dilute to 100.0 ml with a mixture of equal volumes of mobile phase A and mobile phase B.

Column:

– *size*: *l* = 0.25 m, Ø = 4.6 mm,
– *stationary phase*: *octadecylsilyl silica gel for chromatography R* (5 µm),
– *temperature*: 40 °C.

Mobile phase:

– *mobile phase A*: a solution containing 0.05 per cent *V/V* of *phosphoric acid R* and 3.0 per cent *V/V* of *methanol R* in *acetonitrile R*,
– *mobile phase B*: a solution containing 0.05 per cent *V/V* of *phosphoric acid R* and 3.0 per cent *V/V* of *methanol R* in *water R*,

Time (min)	Mobile phase A (per cent *V/V*)	Mobile phase B (per cent *V/V*)
0 - 40	43 → 55	57 → 45
40 - 60	55 → 90	45 → 10
60 - 70	90	10
70 - 75	90 → 43	10 → 57

Flow rate: 1 ml/min.

Detection: spectrophotometer at 239 nm.

Injection: 50 µl; inject the test solution and reference solution (b).

Relative retention with reference to fluticasone propionate (retention time = about 30 min): impurity A = about 0.38; impurity B = about 0.46; impurity C = about 0.76; impurity D = about 0.95; impurity E = about 1.12; impurity F = about 1.18; impurity G = about 1.33; impurity H = about 1.93; impurity I = about 2.01.

System suitability: reference solution (b):

– *resolution*: minimum 1.5 between the peaks due to impurity D and to fluticasone propionate.

Limits:

– *impurities D, G*: for each impurity, maximum 0.3 per cent,
– *impurities A, B, C, E, F, H, I*: for each impurity, maximum 0.2 per cent,
– *impurity with relative retention at about 1.23*: maximum 0.2 per cent,
– *any other impurity*: maximum 0.1 per cent,
– *total*: maximum 1.2 per cent,
– *disregard limit*: 0.05 per cent.

Acetone. Gas chromatography (*2.2.28*).

Internal standard solution. Dilute 0.5 ml of *tetrahydrofuran R* to 1000 ml with *dimethylformamide R.*

Test solution. Dissolve 0.50 g of the substance to be examined in the internal standard solution and dilute to 10.0 ml with the same solution.

Reference solution. Dilute 0.40 g of *acetone R* to 100.0 ml with the internal standard solution. Dilute 1.0 ml to 10.0 ml with the internal standard solution.

Column:

– *material*: fused silica,
– *size*: *l* = 25 m, Ø = 0.53 mm,
– *stationary phase*: cross-linked *macrogol 20 000 R* (film thickness 2 µm).

Carrier gas: *nitrogen for chromatography R.*

Flow rate: 5.5 ml/min.

Monographs F-H

Temperature:

	Time (min)	Temperature (°C)
Column	0 - 3.5	60
	3.5 - 7.5	60 → 180
	7.5 - 10.5	180
Injection port		150
Detector		250

Detection: flame ionisation.

Injection: 0.1 µl.

Limit:

– *acetone*: maximum 1.0 per cent *m/m*.

Water (*2.5.12*): maximum 0.5 per cent determined on 0.250 g.

Use as solvent a mixture of equal volumes of *chloroform R* and *methanol R*.

ASSAY

Liquid chromatography (*2.2.29*).

Test solution. Dissolve 20.0 mg of the substance to be examined in the mobile phase and dilute to 50.0 ml with the mobile phase. Dilute 1.0 ml to 10.0 ml with the mobile phase.

Reference solution (a). Dissolve 20.0 mg of *fluticasone propionate CRS* in the mobile phase and dilute to 50.0 ml with the mobile phase.

Reference solution (b). Dilute 1.0 ml of reference solution (a) to 10.0 ml with the mobile phase.

Reference solution (c). Dissolve 4.0 mg of *fluticasone impurity D CRS* in the mobile phase and dilute to 50.0 ml with the mobile phase. To 1.0 ml of this solution, add 1.0 ml of reference solution (a) and dilute to 10.0 ml with the mobile phase.

Column:

– *size*: *l* = 0.25 m, Ø = 4.6 mm,

– *stationary phase*: *octadecylsilyl silica gel for chromatography R* (5 µm),

– *temperature*: 40 °C.

Mobile phase: mix 15 volumes of *acetonitrile R*, 35 volumes of a 1.15 g/l solution of *ammonium dihydrogen phosphate R* adjusted to pH 3.5 and 50 volumes of *methanol R*.

Flow rate: 1.5 ml/min.

Detection: spectrophotometer at 239 nm.

Injection: 20 µl; inject the test solution and reference solutions (b) and (c).

System suitability: reference solution (c):

– *resolution*: minimum 1.5 between the peaks due to impurity D and to fluticasone propionate.

If necessary, adjust the ratio of acetonitrile to methanol in the mobile phase.

Calculate the percentage content of $C_{25}H_{31}F_3O_5S$ using the chromatograms obtained with the test solution and reference solution (b), and the declared content of *fluticasone propionate CRS*.

STORAGE

Protected from light.

IMPURITIES

Specified impurities: A, B, C, D, E, F, G, H, I.

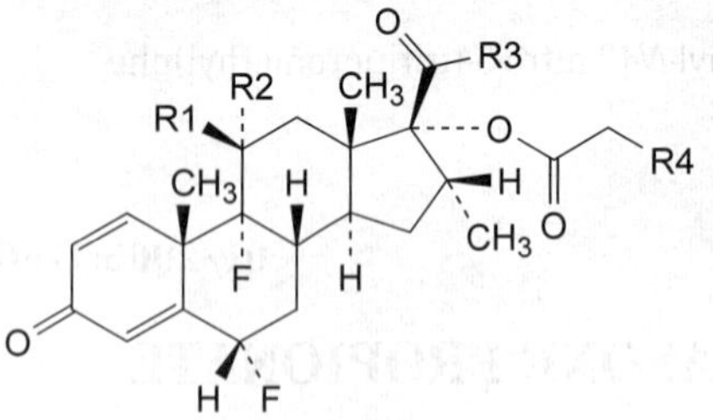

A. R1 = R3 = OH, R2 = H, R4 = CH_3: 6α,9-difluoro-11β-hydroxy-16α-methyl-3-oxo-17-(propanoyloxy)androsta-1,4-diene-17β-carboxylic acid,

B. R1 = OH, R2 = H, R3 = S-OH, R4 = CH_3: [[6α,9-difluoro-11β-hydroxy-16α-methyl-3-oxo-17-(propanoyloxy)androsta-1,4-dien-17β-yl]carbonyl]sulphenic acid,

C. R1 = OH, R2 = R4 = H, R3 = S-CH_2-F: 6α,9-difluoro-17-[[(fluoromethyl)sulphanyl]carbonyl]-11β-hydroxy-16α-methyl-3-oxoandrosta-1,4-dien-17α-yl acetate,

D. R1 = OH, R2 = H, R3 = S-CH_3, R4 = CH_3: 6α,9-difluoro-17-[(methylsulphanyl)carbonyl]-11β-hydroxy-16α-methyl-3-oxoandrosta-1,4-dien-17α-yl propanoate,

F. R1 + R2 = O, R3 = S-CH_2-F, R4 = CH_3: 6α,9-difluoro-17-[[(fluoromethyl)sulphanyl]carbonyl]-16α-methyl-3,11-dioxoandrosta-1,4-dien-17α-yl propanoate,

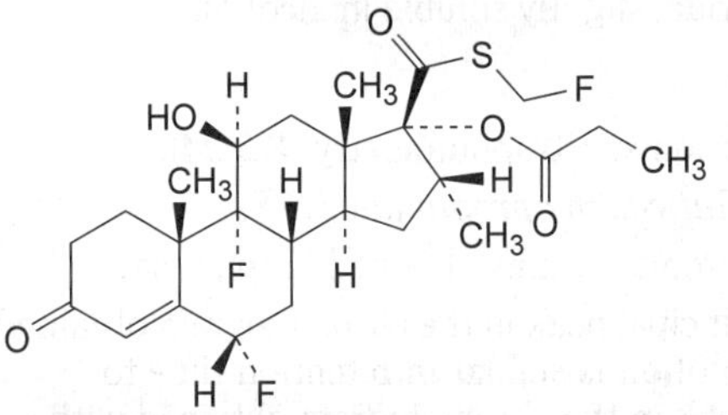

E. 6α,9-difluoro-17-[[(fluoromethyl)sulphanyl]carbonyl]-11β-hydroxy-16α-methyl-3-oxoandrost-4-en-17α-yl propanoate,

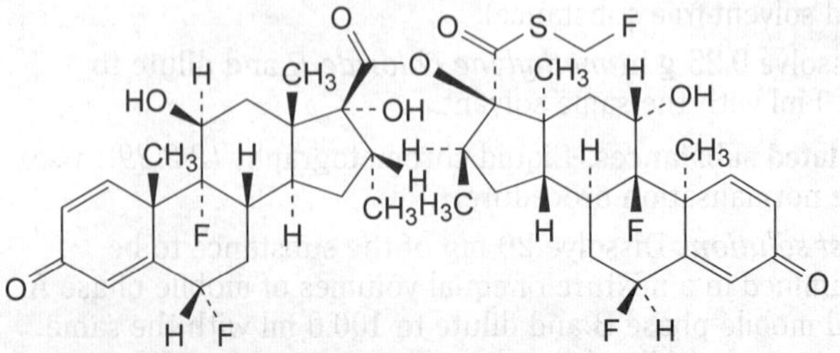

G. 6α,9-difluoro-17-[[(fluoromethyl)sulphanyl]carbonyl]-11β-hydroxy-16α-methyl-3-oxoandrosta-1,4-dien-17α-yl 6α,9-difluoro-11β,17-dihydroxy-16α-methyl-3-oxoandrosta-1,4-diene-17β-carboxylate,

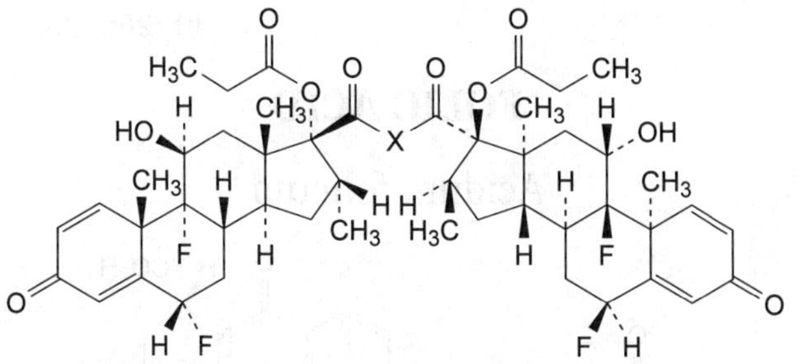

H. X = S-S: 17,17′-(disulphanediyldicarbonyl)bis(6α,9-difluoro-11β-hydroxy-16α-methyl-3-oxoandrosta-1,4-dien-17α-yl) dipropanoate,

I. X = S-S-S: 17,17′-(trisulphanediyldicarbonyl)bis(6α,9-difluoro-11β-hydroxy-16α-methyl-3-oxoandrosta-1,4-dien-17α-yl) dipropanoate.

01/2005:1424

FLUTRIMAZOLE

Flutrimazolum

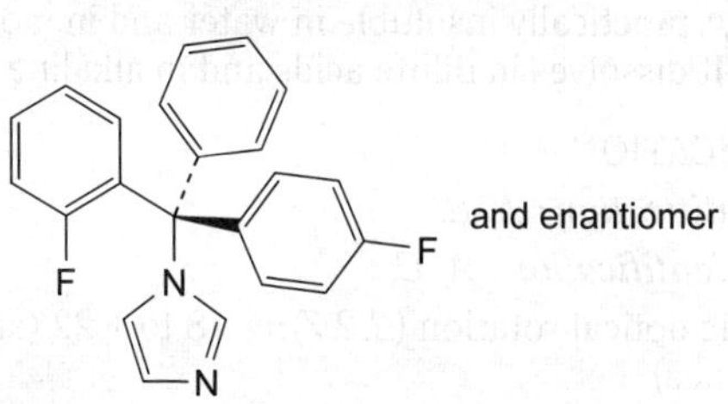

$C_{22}H_{16}F_2N_2$ M_r 346.4

DEFINITION

Flutrimazole contains not less than 99.0 per cent and not more than the equivalent of 101.0 per cent of (*RS*)-1-[(2-fluorophenyl)(4-fluorophenyl)phenylmethyl]-1*H*-imidazole, calculated with reference to the dried substance.

CHARACTERS

A white or almost white powder, practically insoluble in water, freely soluble in tetrahydrofuran and soluble in methanol.

IDENTIFICATION

First identification: B.

Second identification: A, C, D.

A. Melting point (*2.2.14*): 161 °C to 166 °C.

B. Examine by infrared absorption spectrophotometry (*2.2.24*), comparing with the spectrum obtained with *flutrimazole CRS*. Examine the substances prepared as discs.

C. Examine by thin-layer chromatography (*2.2.27*), using a *TLC silica gel F_{254} plate R*. Heat the plate at 110 °C for 1 h.

Test solution. Dissolve 20 mg of the substance to be examined in *acetone R* and dilute to 10 ml with the same solvent.

Reference solution (a). Dissolve 20 mg of *flutrimazole CRS* in *acetone R* and dilute to 10 ml with the same solvent.

Reference solution (b). Dissolve 20 mg of *flutrimazole CRS* and 10 mg of *metronidazole benzoate CRS* in *acetone R* and dilute to 10 ml with the same solvent.

Apply separately to the plate 10 µl of each solution. Develop over a path corresponding to two-thirds of the height of the plate using a mixture of 10 volumes of *2-propanol R* and90 volumes of *ethyl acetate R*. Allow the plate to dry in air and examine in ultraviolet light at 254 nm. The principal spot in the chromatogram obtained with the test solution is similar in position and size to the principal spot in the chromatogram obtained with reference solution (a). The test is not valid unless the chromatogram obtained with reference solution (b) shows two clearly separated spots.

D. Mix about 5 mg with 45 mg of *heavy magnesium oxide R* and ignite in a crucible until an almost white residue is obtained (usually less than 5 min). Allow to cool, add 1 ml of *water R*, 0.05 ml of *phenolphthalein solution R1* and about 1 ml of *dilute hydrochloric acid R* to render the solution colourless. Filter. Add 1.0 ml of the filtrate to a freshly prepared mixture of 0.1 ml of *alizarin S solution R* and 0.1 ml of *zirconyl nitrate solution R*. Mix, allow to stand for 5 min and compare the colour of the solution with that of a blank prepared in the same manner. The test solution is yellow and the blank is red.

TESTS

Solution S. Dissolve 1.00 g in *methanol R* and dilute to 50.0 ml with the same solvent.

Appearance of solution. Solution S is not more opalescent than reference suspension II (*2.2.1*) and not more intensely coloured than reference solution Y_7 (*2.2.2, Method II*).

Optical rotation (*2.2.7*). The angle of optical rotation, determined on solution S, is − 0.05° to + 0.05°.

Related substances. Examine by liquid chromatography (*2.2.29*).

Test solution. Dissolve 40.0 mg of the substance to be examined in the mobile phase and dilute to 50.0 ml with the mobile phase.

Reference solution (a). Dissolve 25.0 mg of *imidazole CRS* in the mobile phase and dilute to 50.0 ml with the mobile phase. Dilute 10.0 ml of this solution to 50.0 ml with the mobile phase.

Reference solution (b). Dissolve 30.0 mg of *flutrimazole impurity B CRS* in the mobile phase and dilute to 100.0 ml with the mobile phase.

Reference solution (c). Mix 2.0 ml of reference solution (a) and 2.0 ml of reference solution (b) and dilute to 50.0 ml with the mobile phase.

Reference solution (d). Dilute 10.0 ml of reference solution (c) to 50.0 ml with the mobile phase.

Reference solution (e). Mix 2.0 ml of the test solution and 10.0 ml of reference solution (c) and dilute to 50.0 ml with the mobile phase.

Reference solution (f). Dilute 1.0 ml of the test solution to 100.0 ml with the mobile phase. Dilute 1.0 ml of this solution to 10.0 ml with the mobile phase.

The chromatographic procedure may be carried out using:

– a stainless steel column 0.2 m long and 4.6 mm in internal diameter packed with *octylsilyl silica gel for chromatography R* (5 µm),

– as mobile phase at a flow rate of 1.3 ml/min a mixture of 40 volumes of *0.03 M phosphate buffer solution pH 7.0 R* and 60 volumes of *acetonitrile R*,

– as detector a spectrophotometer set at 220 nm.

Inject 20 µl of reference solution (e). The test is not valid unless the resolution between the first peak (imidazole) and the second peak (impurity B) is at least 2.0 and the resolution between the second peak and the third peak (flutrimazole) is at least 1.5. The symmetry factor of the first peak and the second peak is not greater than 2.0.

Inject separately 20 µl of the test solution, 20 µl of reference solution (d) and 20 µl of reference solution (f). Continue the chromatography for 2.5 times the retention time of the principal peak.

In the chromatogram obtained with the test solution:

- the area of the peak due to imidazole is not greater than the corresponding area in the chromatogram obtained with reference solution (d) (0.1 per cent);
- the area of the peak due to impurity B is not greater than the corresponding area in the chromatogram obtained with reference solution (d) (0.3 per cent);
- the area of any peak, apart from the principal peak and any peak corresponding to impurity B, is not greater than the area of the principal peak in the chromatogram obtained with reference solution (f) (0.1 per cent); the sum of the areas of any such peaks is not greater than three times the area of the principal peak in the chromatogram obtained with reference solution (f) (0.3 per cent). Disregard any peak with an area less than half the area of the principal peak in the chromatogram obtained with reference solution (f).

Heavy metals (*2.4.8*). 2.0 g complies with limit test F for heavy metals (10 ppm). Use a platinum crucible. Prepare the standard using 2 ml of *lead standard solution (10 ppm Pb) R*.

Loss on drying (*2.2.32*). Not more than 0.5 per cent, determined on 1.000 g by drying in an oven at 100 °C to 105 °C.

Sulphated ash (*2.4.14*). Not more than 0.1 per cent, determined on 1.0 g in a platinum crucible.

ASSAY

Dissolve 0.300 g in 50 ml of *anhydrous acetic acid R*. Titrate with *0.1 M perchloric acid* determining the end-point potentiometrically (*2.2.20*).

1 ml of *0.1 M perchloric acid* is equivalent to 34.64 mg of $C_{22}H_{16}F_2N_2$.

STORAGE

Store protected from light.

IMPURITIES

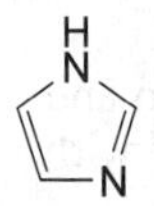

A. imidazole,

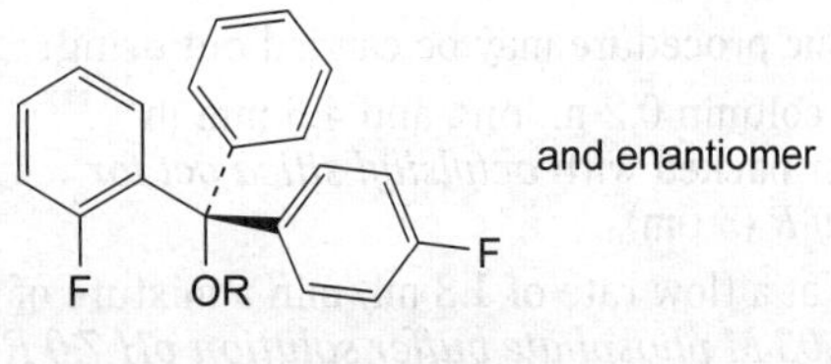

B. R = H: (*RS*)-(2-fluorophenyl)(4-fluorophenyl)phenylmethanol,

C. R = CH_3: (*RS*)-(2-fluorophenyl)(4-fluorophenyl)methoxyphenylmethane.

01/2005:0067

FOLIC ACID

Acidum folicum

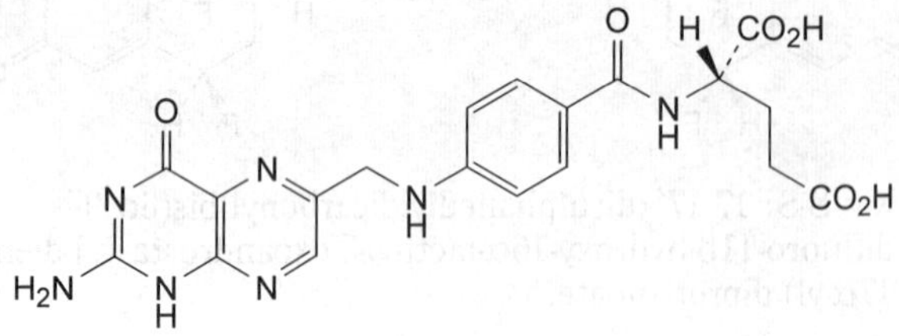

$C_{19}H_{19}N_7O_6$ M_r 441.4

DEFINITION

(2*S*)-2-[[4-[[(2-amino-4-oxo-1,4-dihydropteridin-6-yl)methyl]amino]benzoyl]amino]pentanedioic acid.

Content: 96.0 per cent to 102.0 per cent (anhydrous substance).

CHARACTERS

Appearance: yellowish or orange, crystalline powder.

Solubility: practically insoluble in water and in most organic solvents. It dissolves in dilute acids and in alkaline solutions.

IDENTIFICATION

First identification: A, B.

Second identification: A, C.

A. Specific optical rotation (*2.2.7*): + 18 to + 22 (anhydrous substance).

   Dissolve 0.25 g in *0.1 M sodium hydroxide* and dilute to 25.0 ml with the same solvent.

B. Examine the chromatograms obtained in the assay.

   Results: the principal peak in the chromatogram obtained with the test solution is similar in retention time to the principal peak in the chromatogram obtained with reference solution (a).

C. Thin-layer chromatography (*2.2.27*).

   Test solution. Dissolve 50 mg of the substance to be examined in a mixture of 2 volumes of *concentrated ammonia R* and 9 volumes of *methanol R* and dilute to 100 ml with the same mixture of solvents.

   Reference solution. Dissolve 50 mg of *folic acid CRS* in a mixture of 2 volumes of *concentrated ammonia R* and 9 volumes of *methanol R* and dilute to 100 ml with the same mixture of solvents.

   Plate: *TLC silica gel G plate R*.

   Mobile phase: *concentrated ammonia R, propanol R, alcohol R (20:20:60 V/V/V)*.

   Application: 2 µl.

   Development: over 3/4 of the plate.

   Drying: in air.

   Detection: ultraviolet light at 365 nm.

   Results: the principal spot in the chromatogram obtained with the test solution is similar in position, fluorescence and size to the principal spot in the chromatogram obtained with the reference solution.

TESTS

Related substances. Liquid chromatography (*2.2.29*).

Test solution. Dissolve 0.100 g of the substance to be examined in 5 ml of a 28.6 g/l solution of *sodium carbonate R* and dilute to 100.0 ml with the mobile phase.

Dilute 2.0 ml of this solution to 10.0 ml with the mobile phase.

Reference solution (a). Dissolve 0.100 g of *folic acid CRS* in 5 ml of a 28.6 g/l solution of *sodium carbonate R* and dilute to 100.0 ml with the mobile phase. Dilute 2.0 ml of this solution to 10.0 ml with the mobile phase.

Reference solution (b). Dissolve 20 mg of *pteroic acid R* in 5 ml of a 28.6 g/l solution of *sodium carbonate R* and dilute to 100.0 ml with the mobile phase. Mix 1.0 ml of this solution with 1.0 ml of reference solution (a) and dilute to 100.0 ml with the mobile phase.

Reference solution (c). Dilute 2.0 ml of the test solution to 20.0 ml with the mobile phase. Dilute 1.0 ml of this solution to 20.0 ml with the mobile phase.

Reference solution (d). Dissolve 10.0 mg of *N-(4-aminobenzoyl)-L-glutamic acid R* in 1 ml of a 28.6 g/l solution of *sodium carbonate R* and dilute to 100.0 ml with the mobile phase. Dilute 1.0 ml of this solution to 100.0 ml with the mobile phase.

Reference solution (e). Dissolve 12.0 mg of *pteroic acid R* in 1 ml of a 28.6 g/l solution of *sodium carbonate R* and dilute to 100.0 ml with the mobile phase. Dilute 1.0 ml of this solution to 100.0 ml with the mobile phase.

Column:

- *size*: *l* = 0.25 m, Ø = 4.0 mm,
- *stationary phase*: spherical *octylsilyl silica gel for chromatography R* (5 µm) with a carbon loading of 12.5 per cent, a specific surface of 350 m^2/g and a pore size of 10 nm.

Mobile phase: mix 12 volumes of *methanol R* and 88 volumes of a solution containing 11.16 g/l *potassium dihydrogen phosphate R* and 5.50 g/l of *dipotassium hydrogen phosphate R* solution.

Flow rate: 0.6 ml/min.

Detection: spectrophotometer at 280 nm.

Injection: 5 µl; inject the test solution and reference solutions (b), (c) (d) and (e).

Run time: 3 times the retention time of folic acid.

Relative retention with reference to folic acid (retention time = about 8.5 min): impurity A = about 0.5; impurity B = about 0.6; impurity C = about 0.9; impurity E = about 1.27; impurity D = about 1.33; impurity F = about 2.2.

System suitability: reference solution (b):

- *resolution*: minimum 4.0 between the peaks due to folic acid and to impurity D.

Limits:

- *impurity A*: not more than the area of the principal peak in the chromatogram obtained with reference solution (d) (0.5 per cent),
- *impurity D*: not more than the area of the principal peak in the chromatogram obtained with reference solution (e) (0.6 per cent),
- *any other impurity*: not more than the area of the principal peak in the chromatogram obtained with reference solution (c) (0.5 per cent),
- *total of other impurities*: not more than 2 times the area of the principal peak in the chromatogram obtained with reference solution (c) (1.0 per cent),
- *disregard limit*: 0.1 times the area of the principal peak in the chromatogram obtained with reference solution (c) (0.05 per cent).

Water (*2.5.12*): 5.0 per cent to 8.5 per cent, determined on 0.150 g.

Sulphated ash (*2.4.14*): maximum 0.2 per cent, determined on 1.0 g.

ASSAY

Liquid chromatography (*2.2.29*) as described in the test for related substances with the following modification.

Injection: test solution and reference solution (a).

STORAGE

Protected from light.

IMPURITIES

Specified impurities: A, B, C, D, E, F.

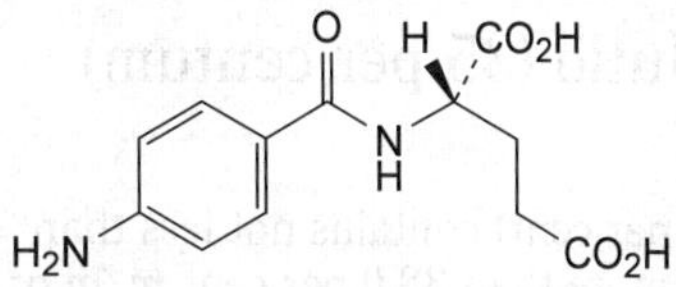

A. (2*S*)-2-[(4-aminobenzoyl)amino]pentanedioic acid (*N*-(4-aminobenzoyl)-L-glutamic acid),

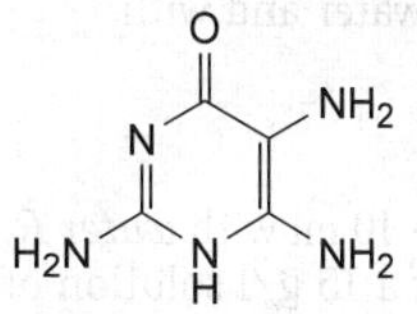

B. 2,5,6-triaminopyrimidin-4(1*H*)-one,

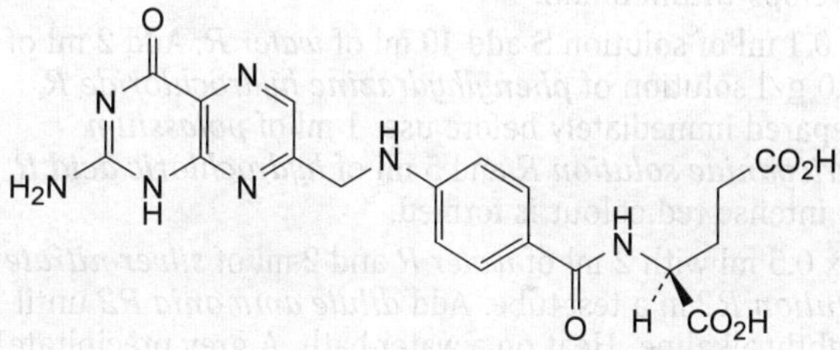

C. (2*S*)-2-[[4-[[(2-amino-4-oxo-1,4-dihydropteridin-7-yl)methyl]amino]benzoyl]amino]pentanedioic acid (isofolic acid),

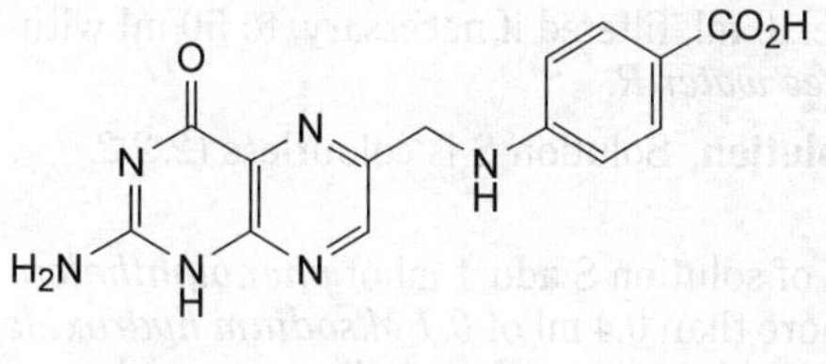

D. 4-[[(2-amino-4-oxo-1,4-dihydropteridin-6-yl)methyl]amino]benzoic acid (pteroic acid),

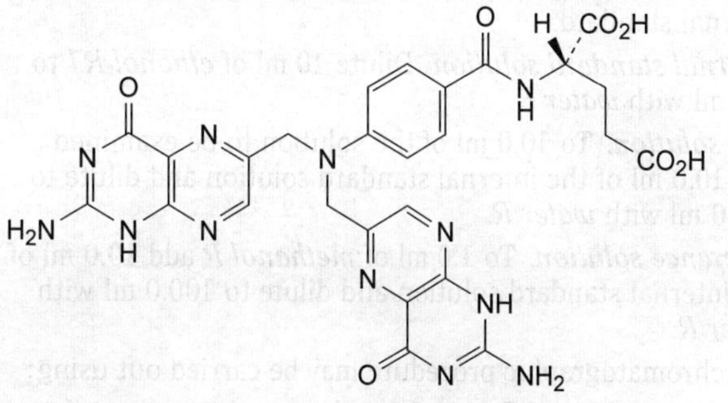

E. (2*S*)-2-[[4-[bis[(2-amino-4-oxo-1,4-dihydropteridin-6-yl)methyl]amino]benzoyl]amino]pentanedioic acid (6-pterinylfolic acid),

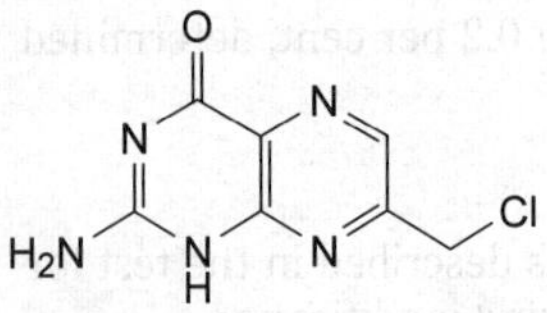

F. 2-amino-7-(chloromethyl)pteridin-4(1*H*)-one.

01/2005:0826

FORMALDEHYDE SOLUTION (35 PER CENT)

Formaldehydi solutio (35 per centum)

DEFINITION

Formaldehyde solution (35 per cent) contains not less than 34.5 per cent *m/m* and not more than 38.0 per cent *m/m* of formaldehyde (CH_2O; M_r 30.03) with methanol as stabiliser.

CHARACTERS

A clear, colourless liquid, miscible with water and with alcohol. It may be cloudy after storage.

IDENTIFICATION

A. Dilute 1 ml of solution S (see Tests) to 10 ml with *water R*. To 0.05 ml of the solution add 1 ml of a 15 g/l solution of *chromotropic acid, sodium salt R*, 2 ml of *water R* and 8 ml of *sulphuric acid R*. A violet-blue or violet-red colour develops within 5 min.

B. To 0.1 ml of solution S add 10 ml of *water R*. Add 2 ml of a 10 g/l solution of *phenylhydrazine hydrochloride R*, prepared immediately before use, 1 ml of *potassium ferricyanide solution R* and 5 ml of *hydrochloric acid R*. An intense red colour is formed.

C. Mix 0.5 ml with 2 ml of *water R* and 2 ml of *silver nitrate solution R2* in a test-tube. Add *dilute ammonia R2* until slightly alkaline. Heat on a water-bath. A grey precipitate or a silver mirror is formed.

D. It complies with the limits of the assay.

TESTS

Solution S. Dilute 10 ml, filtered if necessary, to 50 ml with *carbon dioxide-free water R*.

Appearance of solution. Solution S is colourless (*2.2.2, Method II*).

Acidity. To 10 ml of solution S add 1 ml of *phenolphthalein solution R*. Not more than 0.4 ml of *0.1 M sodium hydroxide* is required to change the colour of the indicator to red.

Methanol: 9.0 per cent *V/V* to 15.0 per cent *V/V*, determined by gas chromatography (*2.2.28*), using *ethanol R1* as the internal standard.

Internal standard solution. Dilute 10 ml of *ethanol R1* to 100 ml with *water R*.

Test solution. To 10.0 ml of the solution to be examined add 10.0 ml of the internal standard solution and dilute to 100.0 ml with *water R*.

Reference solution. To 1.0 ml of *methanol R* add 10.0 ml of the internal standard solution and dilute to 100.0 ml with *water R*.

The chromatographic procedure may be carried out using:

– a glass column 1.5 m to 2.0 m long and 2 mm to 4 mm in internal diameter packed with *ethylvinylbenzene-divinylbenzene copolymer R* (150 µm to 180 µm),
– *nitrogen for chromatography R* as the carrier gas at a flow rate of 30 ml/min to 40 ml/min,
– a flame-ionisation detector,

maintaining the temperature of the column at 120 °C and that of the injection port and of the detector at 150 °C. Inject 1 µl of the reference solution. Adjust the sensitivity of the detector so that the heights of the peaks in the chromatogram obtained are at least 50 per cent of the full scale of the recorder. The test is not valid unless the resolution between the peaks corresponding to methanol and ethanol is at least 2.0. Inject separately 1 µl of the test solution and 1 µl of the reference solution. Calculate the percentage content of methanol.

Sulphated ash (*2.4.14*). Not more than 0.1 per cent, determined on 1.0 g.

ASSAY

Into a 100 ml volumetric flask containing 2.5 ml of *water R* and 1 ml of *dilute sodium hydroxide solution R*, introduce 1.000 g of the solution to be examined, shake and dilute to 100.0 ml with *water R*. To 10.0 ml of the solution add 30.0 ml of *0.05 M iodine*. Mix and add 10 ml of *dilute sodium hydroxide solution R*. After 15 min, add 25 ml of *dilute sulphuric acid R* and 2 ml of *starch solution R*. Titrate with *0.1 M sodium thiosulphate*.

1 ml of *0.05 M iodine* is equivalent to 1.501 mg of CH_2O.

STORAGE

Store protected from light, at a temperature of 15 °C to 25 °C.

01/2005:1724

FORMOTEROL FUMARATE DIHYDRATE

Formoteroli fumaras dihydricus

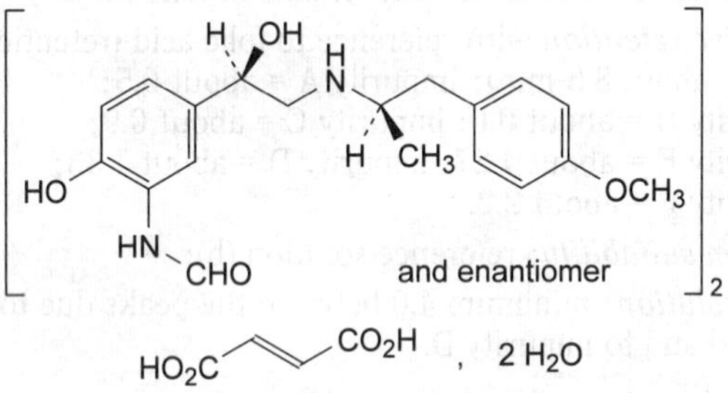

$C_{42}H_{52}N_4O_{12},2H_2O$ M_r 841

DEFINITION

N-[2-Hydroxy-5-[(1*RS*)-1-hydroxy-2-[[(1*RS*)-2-(4-methoxyphenyl)-1-methylethyl]amino]ethyl]phenyl]formamide (*E*)-butenedioate dihydrate.

Content: 98.5 per cent to 101.5 per cent (anhydrous substance).

CHARACTERS

Appearance: white or almost white or slightly yellow powder.

Solubility: slightly soluble in water, soluble in methanol, slightly soluble in 2-propanol, practically insoluble in acetonitrile.

IDENTIFICATION

Infrared absorption spectrophotometry (*2.2.24*).

Comparison: *formoterol fumarate dihydrate CRS*.

TESTS

pH (*2.2.3*): 5.5 to 6.5.

Dissolve 20 mg in *carbon dioxide-free water R* while heating to about 40 °C, allow to cool and dilute to 20 ml with the same solvent.

Optical rotation (*2.2.7*): − 0.10° to + 0.10°.

Dissolve 0.25 g in *methanol R* and dilute to 25.0 ml with the same solvent.

Related substances. Liquid chromatography (*2.2.29*).

Solution A. Dissolve 6.10 g of *sodium dihydrogen phosphate monohydrate R* and 1.03 g of *disodium hydrogen phosphate dihydrate R* in *water R* and dilute to 1000 ml with the same solvent. The pH is 6.0 ± 0.1.

Solvent mixture: *acetonitrile R*, solution A (16:84 *V/V*).

Test solution. Dissolve 20.0 mg of the substance to be examined in the solvent mixture and dilute to 100.0 ml with the solvent mixture. *Inject within 4 h of preparation, or within 24 h if stored protected from light at 4 °C.*

Reference solution (a). Dissolve 5 mg of *formoterol fumarate for system suitability CRS* (containing impurities A, B, C, D, E, F, G) in the solvent mixture and dilute to 25.0 ml with the solvent mixture.

Reference solution (b). Dilute 1.0 ml of the test solution to 25.0 ml with the solvent mixture. Dilute 1.0 ml of this solution to 20.0 ml with the solvent mixture.

Column:

- *size*: *l* = 0.15 m, Ø = 4.6 mm,
- *stationary phase*: spherical *octylsilyl silica gel for chromatography R3* (5 µm) with a pore size of 8 nm.

Mobile phase:

- *mobile phase A*: *acetonitrile R1*;
- *mobile phase B*: dissolve 3.73 g of *sodium dihydrogen phosphate monohydrate R* and 0.35 g of *phosphoric acid R* in *water R* and dilute to 1000 ml with the same solvent; the pH is 3.1 ± 0.1;

Time (min)	Mobile phase A (per cent *V/V*)	Mobile phase B (per cent *V/V*)
0 - 10	16	84
10 - 37	16 → 70	84 → 30
37 - 40	70 → 16	30 → 84
40 - 55	16	84

Flow rate: 1.0 ml/min.

Detection: spectrophotometer at 214 nm.

Injection: 20 µl, inject the solvent mixture until a repeatable profile is obtained.

Identification of impurities: use the chromatogram obtained with reference solution (a) and the chromatogram supplied with *formoterol for system suitability CRS* to identify the peaks.

Relative retention with reference to formoterol (retention time = about 12 min): impurity G = about 0.4; impurity A = about 0.5; impurity B = about 0.7; impurity C = about 1.2; impurity D = about 1.3; impurity E = about 1.8; impurity F = about 2.0; impurity H = about 2.2.

System suitability: reference solution (a):

- *resolution*: minimum 1.5 between the peaks due to impurity G and impurity A.
- *peak-to-valley ratio*: minimum 2.5, where H_p = height above the baseline of the peak due to impurity C and H_v = height above the baseline of the lowest point of the curve separating this peak from the peak due to formoterol.

Limits:

- *correction factor*: for the calculation of content, multiply the peak area of impurity A by 1.75,
- *impurity A*: not more than 1.5 times the area of the principal peak in the chromatogram obtained with reference solution (b) (0.3 per cent),
- *impurities B, C, D, F*: for each impurity, not more than the area of the principal peak in the chromatogram obtained with reference solution (b) (0.2 per cent),
- *impurity E*: not more than 0.5 times the area of the principal peak in the chromatogram obtained with reference solution (b) (0.1 per cent),
- *any other impurity*: for each impurity, not more than 0.5 times the area of the principal peak in the chromatogram obtained with reference solution (b) (0.1 per cent),
- *total*: not more than 2.5 times the area of the principal peak in the chromatogram obtained with reference solution (b) (0.5 per cent),
- *disregard limit*: 0.25 times the area of the principal peak in the chromatogram obtained with reference solution (b) (0.05 per cent).

Impurity I. Liquid chromatography (*2.2.29*).

Test solution. Dissolve 5.0 mg of the substance to be examined in *water R* and dilute to 50.0 ml with the same solvent. Sonicate if necessary.

Reference solution (a). Dissolve 5.0 mg of *formoterol for impurity I identification CRS* in *water R* and dilute to 50.0 ml with the same solvent. Sonicate if necessary.

Reference solution (b). Dilute 1.0 ml of the test solution to 20.0 ml with *water R*. Dilute 1.0 ml of this solution to 25.0 ml with *water R*.

Column:

- *size*: *l* = 0.15 m, Ø = 4.6 mm,
- *stationary phase*: *octadecyl vinyl polymer for chromatography R*.

Mobile phase: mix 12 volumes of *acetonitrile R1* with 88 volumes of a 5.3 g/l solution of *tripotassium phosphate trihydrate R* previously adjusted to pH 12.0 ± 0.1 with a 280 g/l solution of *potassium hydroxide R* or *phosphoric acid R*.

Flow rate: 0.5 ml/min.

Detection: spectrophotometer at 225 nm.

Injection: 20 µl.

Elution order: formoterol, impurity I.

System suitability: reference solution (a):

- *peak-to-valley ratio*: minimum 3.5, where H_p = height above the baseline of the peak due to impurity I and H_v = height above the baseline of the lowest point of the curve separating this peak from the peak due to formoterol.

Limit:

- *impurity I*: not more than 1.5 times the area of the principal peak in the chromatogram obtained with reference solution (b) (0.3 per cent),

Water (*2.5.12*): 4.0 per cent to 5.0 per cent, determined on 0.100 g.

ASSAY

Dissolve 0.350 g in 50 ml of *anhydrous acetic acid R*. Titrate with *0.1 M perchloric acid*, determining the end-point potentiometrically (*2.2.20*).

1 ml of *0.1 M perchloric acid* is equivalent to 40.24 mg of $C_{42}H_{52}N_4O_{12}$.

STORAGE

Protected from light.

IMPURITIES

Specified impurities: A, B, C, D, E, F, I.

Other detectable impurities: G, H.

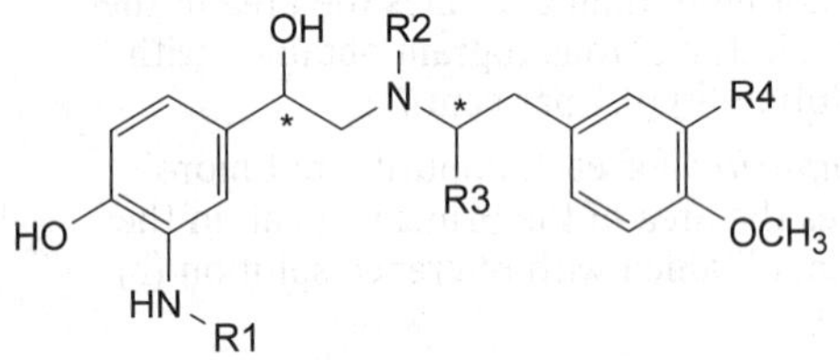

A. R1 = R2 = R4 = H, R3 = CH_3: 1-(3-amino-4-hydroxyphenyl)-2-[[2-(4-methoxyphenyl)-1-methylethyl]amino]ethanol,

B. R1 = CHO, R2 = R3 = R4 = H: *N*-[2-hydroxy-5-[(1*RS*)-1-hydroxy-2-[[2-(4-methoxyphenyl)ethyl]amino]ethyl]phenyl]formamide,

C. R1 = CO-CH_3, R2 = R4 = H, R3 = CH_3: *N*-[2-hydroxy-5-[1-hydroxy-2-[[2-(4-methoxyphenyl)-1-methylethyl]amino]ethyl]phenyl]acetamide,

D. R1 = CHO, R2 = R3 = CH_3, R4 = H: *N*-[2-hydroxy-5-[1-hydroxy-2-[methyl[2-(4-methoxyphenyl)-1-methylethyl]amino]ethyl]phenyl]formamide,

E. R1 = CHO, R2 = H, R3 = R4 = CH_3: *N*-[2-hydroxy-5-[1-hydroxy-2-[[2-(4-methoxy-3-methylphenyl)-1-methylethyl]amino]ethyl]phenyl]formamide,

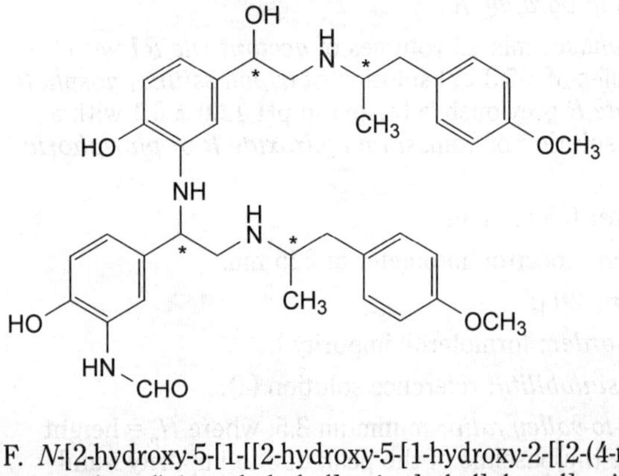

F. *N*-[2-hydroxy-5-[1-[[2-hydroxy-5-[1-hydroxy-2-[[2-(4-methoxyphenyl)-1-methylethyl]amino]ethyl]phenyl]amino]-2-[[2-(4-methoxyphenyl)-1-methylethyl]amino]ethyl]phenyl]formamide,

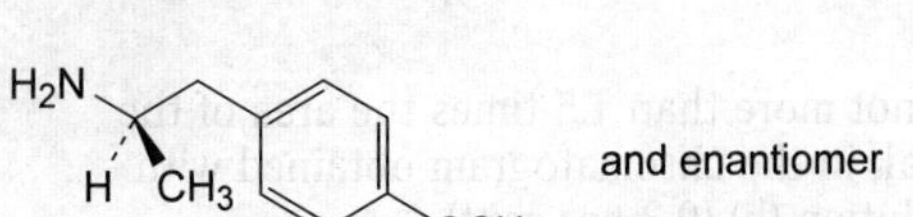

G. (2*RS*)-1-(4-methoxyphenyl)propan-2-amine,

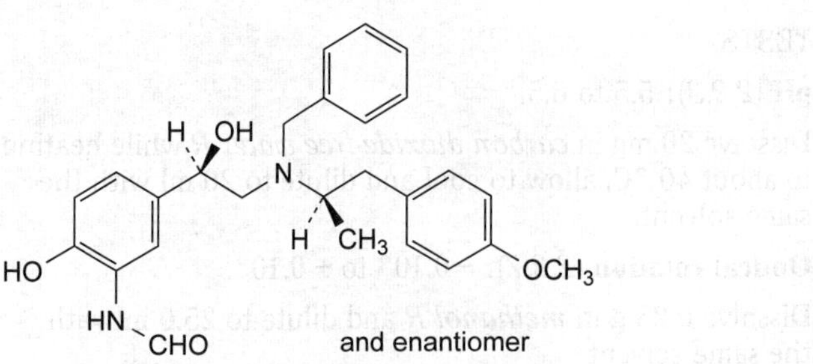

H. *N*-[5-[(1*RS*)-2-[benzyl[(1*RS*)-2-(4-methoxyphenyl)-1-methylethyl]amino]-1-hydroxyethyl]-2-hydroxyphenyl]formamide (monobenzyl analogue),

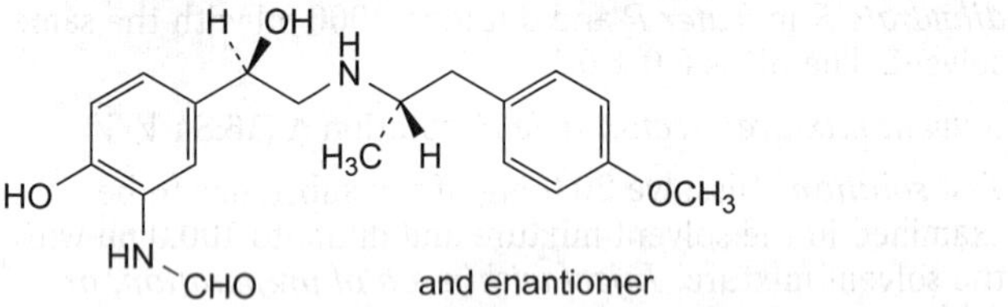

I. *N*-[2-hydroxy-5-[(1*RS*)-1-hydroxy-2-[[(1*SR*)-2-(4-methoxyphenyl)-1-methylethyl]amino]ethyl]phenyl]formamide (diastereoisomer).

01/2005:1520
corrected

FOSCARNET SODIUM HEXAHYDRATE

Foscarnetum natricum hexahydricum

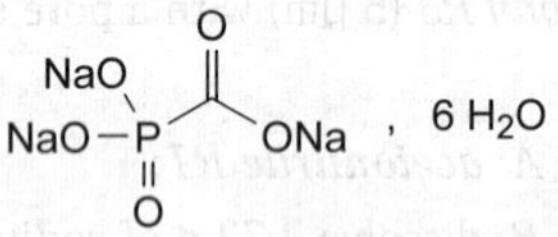

$CNa_3O_5P,6H_2O$ M_r 300.0

DEFINITION

Foscarnet sodium hexahydrate contains not less than 98.5 per cent and not more than the equivalent of 101.0 per cent of trisodium phosphonatoformate, calculated with reference to the dried substance.

CHARACTERS

A white or almost white, crystalline powder, soluble in water, practically insoluble in alcohol.

IDENTIFICATION

A. Examine by infrared absorption spectrophotometry (*2.2.24*), comparing with the spectrum obtained with *foscarnet sodium hexahydrate CRS*.

B. It gives reaction (a) of sodium (*2.3.1*).

TESTS

Solution S. Dissolve 0.5 g in *carbon dioxide-free water R* and dilute to 25 ml with the same solvent.

Appearance of solution. Solution S is not more opalescent than reference suspension I (*2.2.1*) and is colourless (*2.2.2, Method II*).

pH (*2.2.3*). The pH of solution S is 9.0 to 11.0.

Related substances. Examine by liquid chromatography (*2.2.29*).

Test solution. Dissolve 25 mg of the substance to be examined in the mobile phase and dilute to 10.0 ml with the mobile phase.

Reference solution (a). Dilute 1.0 ml of the test solution to 50.0 ml with mobile phase. Dilute 1.0 ml of this solution to 10.0 ml with the mobile phase.

Reference solution (b). Dissolve 5.0 mg of *foscarnet impurity B CRS* in the mobile phase, add 2.0 ml of the test solution and dilute to 50.0 ml with the mobile phase.

The chromatographic procedure may be carried out using:

– a stainless steel column 0.10 m long and 4.6 mm in internal diameter packed with *octadecylsilyl silica gel for chromatography R* (3 µm),

– as mobile phase at a flow rate of 1.0 ml/min a solution prepared as follows: dissolve 3.22 g of *sodium sulphate decahydrate R* in *water R*, add 3 ml of *glacial acetic acid R*, 6 ml of a 44.61 g/l solution of *sodium pyrophosphate R* and dilute to 1000 ml with *water R* (solution A); dissolve 3.22 g of *sodium sulphate decahydrate R* in *water R*, add 6.8 g of *sodium acetate R* and 6 ml of a 44.61 g/l solution of *sodium pyrophosphate R* and dilute to 1000 ml with *water R* (solution B). Mix about 700 ml of solution A and about 300 ml of solution B to obtain a solution of pH 4.4. To 1000 ml of this solution, add 0.25 g of *tetrahexylammonium hydrogen sulphate R* and 100 ml of *methanol R*.

– as detector a spectrophotometer set at 230 nm.

Inject 20 µl of reference solution (b). Continue the chromatography for 2.5 times the retention time of foscarnet. The test is not valid unless the resolution between the peaks due to foscarnet and impurity B is at least 7.

Inject 20 µl of the test solution and 20 µl of reference solution (a). In the chromatogram obtained with the test solution: the area of any peak, apart from the principal peak, is not greater than the area of the principal peak in the chromatogram obtained with reference solution (a) (0.2 per cent); the sum of the areas of all the peaks, apart from the principal peak, is not greater than twice the area of the principal peak in the chromatogram obtained with reference solution (a) (0.4 per cent). Disregard any peak with a relative retention time less than 0.6 and any peak with an area less than 0.2 times that of the peak in the chromatogram obtained with reference solution (a).

Impurity D. Examine by gas chromatography (*2.2.28*).

Test solution. Dissolve 0.25 g of the substance to be examined in 9.0 ml of *0.1 M acetic acid* using a magnetic stirrer. Add 1.0 ml of *ethanol R* and mix.

Reference solution. Dissolve 25 mg of *triethyl phosphonoformate R* in *ethanol R* and dilute to 100 ml with the same solvent. Dilute 1 ml of the solution to 10 ml with *ethanol R*.

The chromatographic procedure may be carried out using:

– a fused-silica column 25 m long and 0.31 mm in internal diameter coated with *poly(dimethyl)(diphenyl)(divinyl)siloxane R* (film thickness 0.5 µm),

– *helium for chromatography R* as the carrier gas,

– a flame-ionisation detector,

– a split mode injector of 1:20,

raising the temperature of the column from 100 °C to 180 °C at a rate of 10 °C per minute and maintaining the temperature of the injection port at 200 °C and that of the detector at 250 °C.

Inject 3 µl of each solution.

In the chromatogram obtained with the test solution the area of any peak due to impurity D is not greater than the area of the peak in the chromatogram obtained with reference solution (0.1 per cent).

Phosphate and phosphite. Examine by liquid chromatography (*2.2.29*).

Test solution. Dissolve 60.0 mg of the substance to be examined in *water R* and dilute to 25.0 ml with the same solvent.

Reference solution (a). Dissolve 28 mg of *sodium dihydrogen phosphate monohydrate R* in *water R* and dilute to 100 ml with the same solvent.

Reference solution (b). Dissolve 43 mg of *sodium phosphite pentahydrate R* in *water R* and dilute to 100 ml with the same solvent.

Reference solution (c). Dilute 1.0 ml of reference solution (a) and 1.0 ml of reference solution (b) to 25 ml with *water R*.

Reference solution (d). Dilute 3 ml of reference solution (a) and 3 ml of reference solution (b) to 25 ml with *water R*.

The chromatographic procedure may be carried out using:

– a stainless steel column 0.05 m long and 4.6 mm in internal diameter packed with an *anion exchange resin R*,

– as mobile phase at a flow rate of 1.4 ml/min a solution prepared as follows: dissolve 0.102 g of *potassium hydrogen phthalate R* in *water R*, add 2.5 ml of *1 M nitric acid* and dilute to 1000 ml with *water R*,

– as detector a spectrophotometer set at 290 nm (indirect detection).

Inject 20 µl of reference solution (d). The test is not valid unless: the resolution between the peaks due to phosphate (first peak) and phosphite is at least 2.0; the principal peak has a signal-to-noise ratio of at least ten.

Inject 20 µl of the test solution and 20 µl of reference solution (c). In the chromatogram obtained with the test solution: the area of any peak due to phosphate and phosphite is not greater than the area of the corresponding peaks in the chromatogram obtained with reference solution (c) (0.3 per cent of phosphate and 0.3 per cent of phosphite).

Heavy metals. Dissolve 1.25 g in 12.5 ml of *1 M hydrochloric acid*. Warm on a water-bath for 3 min and cool to room temperature. Transfer to a beaker and adjust the pH to about 3.5 with *dilute ammonia R1* and dilute to 25 ml with *water R* (solution A). To 12 ml of solution A, add 2.0 ml of *buffer solution pH 3.5 R*. Rapidly pour the mixture into a test tube containing one drop of *sodium sulphide solution R*. The solution is not more intensely coloured than a standard prepared simultaneously and in the same manner pouring a mixture of 5.0 ml of *lead standard solution (1 ppm Pb) R*, 5.0 ml of *water R*, 2.0 ml of solution A and 2.0 ml of *buffer solution pH 3.5 R* into a test tube containing one drop of *sodium sulphide solution R* (10 ppm).

Loss on drying (*2.2.32*): 35.0 per cent to 37.0 per cent, determined on 1.000 g by drying in an oven at 150 °C.

Bacterial endotoxins (*2.6.14*): less than 83.3 IU/g, if intended for use in the manufacture of parenteral dosage forms without a further appropriate procedure for the removal of bacterial endotoxins.

ASSAY

Dissolve 0.200 g in 50 ml of *water R*. Titrate with *0.05 M sulphuric acid*, determining the end-point potentiometrically (*2.2.20*) at the first inflexion point.

1 ml of *0.05 M sulphuric acid* is equivalent to 19.20 mg of CNa_3O_5P.

STORAGE

Store protected from light.

IMPURITIES

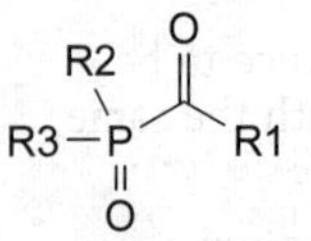

A. R1 = OC_2H_5, R2 = R3 = ONa: disodium (ethoxycarbonyl)phosphonate,

B. R1 = R2 = ONa, R3 = OC_2H_5: disodium (ethoxyoxydophosphanyl)formate,

C. R1 = R2 = OC_2H_5, R3 = ONa: ethyl sodium (ethoxycarbonyl)phosphonate,

D. R1 = R2 = R3 = OC_2H_5: methyl (diethoxyphosphoryl)formate.

01/2005:1328

FOSFOMYCIN CALCIUM

Fosfomycinum calcicum

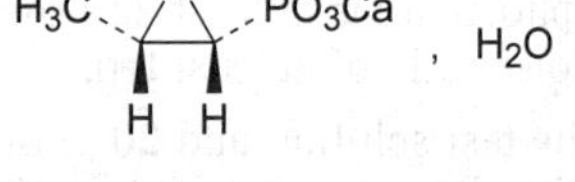

$C_3H_5CaO_4P,H_2O$ M_r 194.1

DEFINITION

Calcium fosfomycin contains not less than 95.0 per cent and not more than the equivalent of 101.0 per cent of calcium (2*R*,3*S*)-(3-methyloxiran-2-yl)phosphonate, calculated with reference to the anhydrous substance.

CHARACTERS

A white or almost white powder, slightly soluble in water, practically insoluble in acetone, in methanol and in methylene chloride.

IDENTIFICATION

First identification: A, D.

Second identification: B, C, D.

A. Examine by infrared absorption spectrophotometry (*2.2.24*), comparing with the *Ph. Eur. reference spectrum of fosfomycin calcium*. Examine the substance as discs prepared using *potassium bromide R*.

B. Dissolve about 0.1 g in 3 ml of a 25 per cent *V/V* solution of *perchloric acid R*. Add 1 ml of *0.1 M sodium periodate* and heat on a water-bath for 30 min. Allow to cool and add 50 ml of *water R*. Neutralise with a saturated solution of *sodium hydrogen carbonate R* and add 1 ml of a freshly prepared 400 g/l solution of *potassium iodide R*. Prepare a blank at the same time and in the same manner. The test solution remains colourless and the blank is orange.

C. To about 8 mg of the substance to be examined, add 2 ml of *water R*, 1 ml of *perchloric acid R* and 2 ml of *0.1 M sodium periodate*. Heat on a water-bath for 10 min and add, without cooling, 1 ml of *ammonium molybdate solution R5* and 1 ml of *aminohydroxynaphthalenesulphonic acid solution R*. Allow to stand for 30 min. A blue colour develops.

D. It gives reaction (a) of calcium (*2.3.1*).

TESTS

pH (*2.2.3*). Dissolve 20 mg in *carbon dioxide-free water R* and dilute to 20.0 ml with the same solvent. The pH of the solution is 8.1 to 9.6.

Specific optical rotation (*2.2.7*). Dissolve 2.5 g in a 125 g/l solution of *sodium edetate R* previously adjusted to pH 8.5 with *strong sodium hydroxide solution R*, and dilute to 50.0 ml with the same solution. Measured at 405 nm using a mercury lamp, the specific optical rotation is − 11.0 to − 13.0, calculated with reference to the anhydrous substance.

Calcium 1,2-(dihydroxypropyl)phosphonate. Not more than 1.5 per cent. Into a glass-stoppered flask, dissolve 0.200 g of the substance to be examined in 100.0 ml of *water R*. Add 50 ml of *0.5 M phthalate buffer solution pH 6.4 R* and 5.0 ml of *0.005 M sodium periodate*, close and shake. Allow to stand protected from light for 90 min. Add 10 ml of a freshly prepared 400 g/l solution of *potassium iodide R*, close and shake for 2 min. Titrate with *0.0025 M sodium arsenite* until the yellow colour almost disappears. Add 2 ml of *starch solution R* and titrate slowly until the colour is completely discharged. Carry out a blank test under the same conditions. Calculate the percentage content of $C_3H_7CaO_5P$ from the expression:

$$\frac{(n_1 - n_2) \times c \times 97}{m\,(100 - H)} \times 100$$

m = quantity of the substance to be examined, in milligrams,

n_1 = volume of *0.0025 M sodium arsenite* used in the blank titration,

n_2 = volume of *0.0025 M sodium arsenite* used in the titration of the test solution,

c = molarity of the sodium arsenite solution,

H = percentage content of water.

Chlorides (*2.4.4*). Dissolve 0.500 g in *water R*, add 2 ml of *nitric acid R* and dilute to 50 ml with the same acid. To 2.5 ml of the solution add 12.5 ml of *water R*. The solution complies with the limit test for chlorides (0.2 per cent).

Heavy metals (*2.4.8*). Dissolve 2.5 g of the substance to be examined in 6 ml of *glacial acetic acid R* and dilute to 25.0 ml with *water R*. 12 ml of the solution complies with limit test A for heavy metals (20 ppm). Prepare the standard using *lead standard solution (2 ppm Pb) R*.

Water (*2.5.12*): 8.5 per cent to 11.5 per cent, determined on 0.250 g by the semi-micro determination of water. Use as the solvent a mixture of 1 volume of *pyridine R* and 3 volumes of *ethylene glycol R*.

ASSAY

Into a glass-stoppered flask, dissolve 0.120 g of the substance to be examined in 20.0 ml of *0.1 M sodium periodate*. Add 5 ml of a 50 per cent *V/V* solution of *perchloric acid R* and shake. Heat in a water-bath at 37 °C for 105 min. Add 50 ml of *water R* and immediately adjust to pH 6.4 with a saturated solution of *sodium hydrogen carbonate R*. Add 10 ml of a freshly prepared 400 g/l solution of *potassium iodide R*, close and allow to stand for 2 min. Titrate with *0.1 M sodium arsenite* until the yellow colour almost disappears. Add 2 ml of *starch solution R* and titrate slowly until the colour is completely discharged. Carry out a blank test under the same conditions.

Calculate the percentage content of $C_3H_5CaO_4P$ from the expression:

$$\frac{(n_1 - n_2) \times c \times 88 \times 100}{m\,(100 - H)} \times 100 - G$$

m = quantity of the substance to be examined, in milligrams,

n_1 = volume of *0.1 M sodium arsenite* used in the blank titration,

n_2 = volume of *0.1 M sodium arsenite* used in the titration of the test solution,

c = molarity of the sodium arsenite solution,

G = percentage content of calcium 1,2-(dihydroxypropyl)phosphonate,

H = percentage content of water.

STORAGE

Store in an airtight container, protected from light.

IMPURITIES

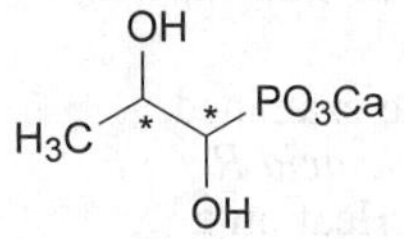

A. calcium (1,2-dihydroxypropyl)phosphonate.

01/2005:1329

FOSFOMYCIN SODIUM

Fosfomycinum natricum

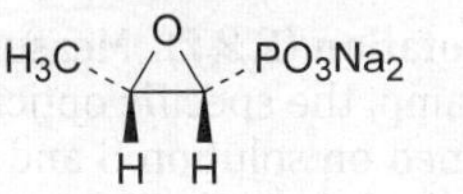

$C_3H_5Na_2O_4P$ M_r 182.0

DEFINITION

Fosfomycin sodium contains not less than 95.0 per cent and not more than the equivalent of 101.0 per cent of disodium (2*R*,3*S*)-(3-methyloxiran-2-yl)phosphonate, calculated with reference to the anhydrous substance.

CHARACTERS

A white or almost white, very hygroscopic powder, very soluble in water, sparingly soluble in methanol, practically insoluble in ethanol and in methylene chloride.

IDENTIFICATION

First identification: A, D.

Second identification: B, C, D.

A. Examine by infrared absorption spectrophotometry (*2.2.24*), comparing with the *Ph. Eur. reference spectrum of fosfomycin sodium.* Examine the substance as discs prepared using *potassium bromide R.*

B. Dissolve about 0.1 g in 3 ml of a 25 per cent *V/V* solution of *perchloric acid R.* Add 1 ml of *0.1 M sodium periodate* and heat on a water-bath for 30 min. Allow to cool and add 50 ml of *water R.* Neutralise with a saturated solution of *sodium hydrogen carbonate R* and add 1 ml of a freshly prepared 400 g/l solution of *potassium iodide R.* Prepare a blank at the same time and in the same manner. The test solution remains colourless and the blank is orange.

C. To about 8 mg of the substance to be examined, add 2 ml of *water R,* 1 ml of *perchloric acid R* and 2 ml of *0.1 M sodium periodate.* Heat on a water-bath for 10 min and add, without cooling, 1 ml of *ammonium molybdate solution R5* and 1 ml of *aminohydroxynaphthalenesulphonic acid solution R.* Allow to stand for 30 min. A blue colour develops.

D. It gives reaction (a) of sodium (*2.3.1*).

TESTS

Solution S. Dissolve 5.0 g in *carbon dioxide-free water R* and dilute to 50.0 ml with the same solvent.

Appearance of solution. Solution S is clear (*2.2.1*) and not more intensely coloured than reference solution B_9 (*2.2.2, Method II*).

pH (*2.2.3*). Dilute 10 ml of solution S to 20 ml with *carbon dioxide-free water R.* The pH of the solution is 9.0 to 10.5.

Specific optical rotation (*2.2.7*). Dissolve 2.5 g in *water R* and dilute to 50.0 ml with the same solvent. Measured at 405 nm using a mercury lamp, the specific optical rotation is − 13.0 to − 15.0, calculated with reference to the anhydrous substance.

Disodium 1,2-(dihydroxypropyl)phosphonate. Not more than 1.0 per cent. Into a glass-stoppered flask, dissolve 0.200 g of the substance to be examined in 100.0 ml of *water R.* Add 50 ml of *0.5 M phthalate buffer solution pH 6.4 R* and 5.0 ml of *0.005 M sodium periodate,* close and shake. Allow to stand protected from light for 90 min. Add 10 ml of a freshly prepared 400 g/l solution of *potassium iodide R,* close and shake for 2 min. Titrate with *0.0025 M sodium arsenite* until the yellow colour almost disappears. Add 2 ml of *starch solution R* and titrate slowly until the colour is completely discharged. Carry out a blank test under the same conditions. Calculate the percentage content of $C_3H_7Na_2O_5P$ from the expression:

$$\frac{(n_1 - n_2) \times c \times 100}{m\,(100 - H)} \times 100$$

m = quantity of the substance to be examined, in milligrams,

n_1 = volume of *0.0025 M sodium arsenite* used in the blank titration,

n_2 = volume of *0.0025 M sodium arsenite* used in the titration of the test solution,

c = molarity of the sodium arsenite solution,

H = percentage content of water.

Heavy metals (*2.4.8*). 12 ml of solution S complies with limit test A for heavy metals (20 ppm). Prepare the standard using *lead standard solution (2 ppm Pb) R.*

Water (*2.5.12*). Not more than 1.0 per cent, determined on 0.50 g by the semi-micro determination of water. Use as the solvent a mixture of 1 volume of *pyridine R* and 3 volumes of *ethylene glycol R.*

Bacterial endotoxins (*2.6.14*): less than 0.083 IU/mg, if intended for use in the manufacture of parenteral dosage forms without a further appropriate procedure for removal of bacterial endotoxins.

ASSAY

Into a glass-stoppered flask, dissolve 0.120 g of the substance to be examined in 20.0 ml of *0.1 M sodium periodate.* Add 5 ml of a 50 per cent *V/V* solution of *perchloric acid R* and shake. Heat on a water-bath at 37 °C for 105 min. Add 50 ml of *water R* and immediately adjust to pH 6.4 with a saturated solution of *sodium hydrogen carbonate R*. Add 10 ml of a freshly prepared 400 g/l solution of *potassium iodide R*, close and allow to stand for 2 min. Titrate with *0.1 M sodium arsenite* until the yellow colour almost disappears. Add 2 ml of *starch solution R* and titrate slowly until the colour is completely discharged. Carry out a blank test under the same conditions.

Calculate the percentage content of $C_3H_5Na_2O_4P$ from the expression:

$$\frac{(n_1 - n_2) \times c \times 91 \times 100}{m\,(100 - H)} \times 100 - G$$

m = quantity of the substance to be examined, in milligrams,

n_1 = volume of *0.1 M sodium arsenite* used in the blank titration,

n_2 = volume of *0.1 M sodium arsenite* used in the titration of the test solution,

c = molarity of the sodium arsenite solution,

G = percentage content of disodium 1,2-(dihydroxypropyl)phosphonate,

H = percentage content of water.

STORAGE

Store in an airtight container, protected from light. If the substance is sterile, store in a sterile, airtight, tamper-proof container.

LABELLING

The label states, where applicable, that the substance is free from bacterial endotoxins.

IMPURITIES

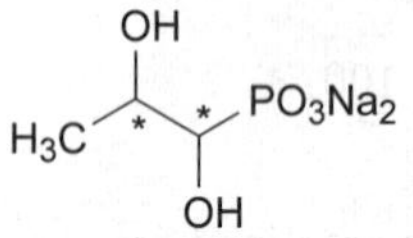

A. disodium (1,2-dihydroxypropyl)phosphonate.

01/2005:1425

FOSFOMYCIN TROMETAMOL

Fosfomycinum trometamolum

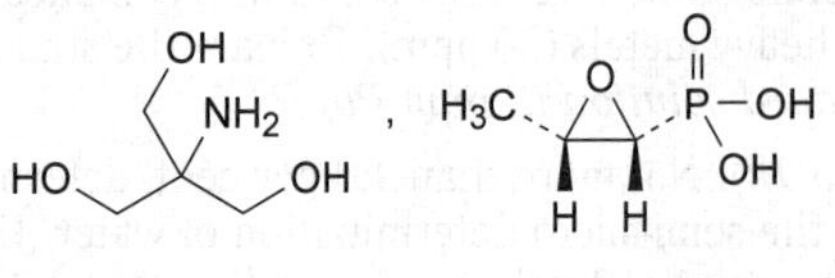

$C_7H_{18}NO_7P$ M_r 259.2

DEFINITION

Fosfomycin trometamol contains not less than 98.0 per cent and not more than the equivalent of 102.0 per cent of 1,3-dihydroxy-2-(hydroxymethyl)propan-2-aminium (2*R*,3*S*)-(3-methyloxiran-2-yl)phosphonate, calculated with reference to the anhydrous substance.

CHARACTERS

A white or almost white powder, hygroscopic, very soluble in water, slightly soluble in alcohol and in methanol, practically insoluble in acetone.

IDENTIFICATION

First identification: A.

Second identification: B, C.

A. Examine by infrared absorption spectrophotometry (*2.2.24*), comparing with the spectrum obtained with *fosfomycin trometamol CRS*.

B. Examine by thin-layer chromatography (*2.2.27*), using *cellulose for chromatography R* as the coating substance.

Test solution. Dissolve 50 mg of the substance to be examined in *water R* and dilute to 10 ml with the same solvent.

Reference solution. Dissolve 50 mg of *fosfomycin trometamol CRS* in *water R* and dilute to 10 ml with the same solvent.

Apply to the plate 10 µl of each solution. Develop over a path of 15 cm using a mixture of 10 volumes of *concentrated ammonia R*, 20 volumes of *water R* and 70 volumes of *2-propanol R*. Dry the plate in a current of warm air and expose it to iodine vapour until the spots appear. The principal spot in the chromatogram obtained with the test solution is similar in position, colour and size to the principal spot in the chromatogram obtained with the reference solution.

C. To about 15 mg of the substance to be examined, add 2 ml of *water R*, 1 ml of *perchloric acid R* and 2 ml of *0.1 M sodium periodate*. Heat on a water-bath for 10 min and add, without cooling, 1 ml of *ammonium molybdate solution R5* and 1 ml of *aminohydroxynaphthalenesulphonic acid solution R*. Allow to stand for 30 min. A blue colour develops.

TESTS

Solution S. Dissolve 1.00 g in *carbon dioxide-free water R* and dilute to 20.0 ml with the same solvent.

pH (*2.2.3*). The pH of solution S is 3.5 to 5.5.

Specific optical rotation (*2.2.7*). Measured at 365 nm using a mercury lamp, the specific optical rotation is − 13.5 to − 12.5, determined on solution S and calculated with reference to the anhydrous substance.

Related substances. Examine by liquid chromatography (*2.2.29*) as prescribed under Assay.

Inject 5 µl of the test solution, 5 µl of reference solution (b) and 5 µl of the blank solution. Continue the chromatography for twice the retention time of the peak due to fosfomycin. In the chromatogram obtained with the test solution: the area of any peak corresponding to impurity A is not greater than the area of the corresponding peak in the chromatogram obtained with reference solution (b) (0.5 per cent, calculated as trometamol salts); the area of any peak, apart from the principal peak, two peaks corresponding to trometamol and any peak corresponding to impurity A, is not greater than the area of the principal peak in the chromatogram obtained with reference solution (b) (0.5 per cent, calculated as trometamol salts). The sum of the areas of all the peaks, apart from the principal peak and the two peaks corresponding to trometamol, is not greater than twice the area of the principal peak in the chromatogram obtained with reference solution (b) (1 per cent, calculated as trometamol salts). Disregard any peak due to the blank and any peak with an area less than 0.1 times the area of the principal peak in the chromatogram obtained with reference solution (b).

Phosphates. Dissolve 0.1 g in 3 ml of *dilute nitric acid R* and dilute to 10 ml with *water R*. To 5 ml of this test solution add 5 ml of *water R* and 5 ml of *molybdovanadic reagent R*. Shake vigorously. After 5 min, any colour in the test solution is not more intense that that in a standard prepared at the same time in the same manner, using 5 ml of *phosphate standard solution (5 ppm PO_4) R* (500 ppm).

Heavy metals (*2.4.8*). Dissolve 2.0 g in *water R* and dilute to 20 ml with the same solvent. 12 ml of the solution complies with limit test A for heavy metals (10 ppm). Prepare the standard using *lead standard solution (1 ppm Pb) R.*

Water (*2.5.12*). Not more than 0.5 per cent, determined on 0.500 g by the semi-micro determination of water.

ASSAY

Examine the substance by liquid chromatography (*2.2.29*). *Prepare the solutions immediately before use.*

Test solution. Dissolve 0.60 g of the substance to be examined in the mobile phase and dilute to 5.0 ml with the mobile phase.

Reference solution (a). Dissolve 0.60 g of *fosfomycin trometamol CRS* in the mobile phase and dilute to 5.0 ml with the mobile phase.

Reference solution (b). Dissolve 8.7 mg of *fosfomycin trometamol impurity A CRS* (disodium salt) in the mobile phase and dilute to 20.0 ml with the mobile phase.

Reference solution (c). Dissolve 5 mg of *fosfomycin trometamol impurity A CRS* (disodium salt) and 10 mg of *fosfomycin trometamol CRS* in the mobile phase and dilute to 5 ml with the mobile phase.

Blank solution. A 0.3 g/l solution of *anhydrous disodium hydrogen phosphate R* in the mobile phase.

The chromatographic procedure may be carried out using:

– a stainless steel column 0.25 m long and 4.6 mm in internal diameter packed with *aminopropylsilyl silica gel for chromatography R* (5 µm),
– as mobile phase at a flow rate of 1 ml/min a 10.89 g/l solution of *potassium dihydrogen phosphate R,*
– as detector a differential refractometer maintaining the temperature at 35 °C.

When the chromatograms are recorded in the prescribed conditions, the relative retention times (to fosfomycin) are about 0.3 for the two peaks corresponding to trometamol and 0.8 for impurity A.

Inject 5 µl of reference solution (c). The test is not valid unless the resolution between the peaks corresponding to fosfomycin and impurity A is at least 1.5. Inject reference solution (a) six times. The test is not valid unless the relative standard deviation of the peak area for fosfomycin is at most 1.0 per cent. Inject alternately the test solution and reference solution (a).

Calculate the percentage content of fosfomycin trometamol.

STORAGE

Store in an airtight container.

IMPURITIES

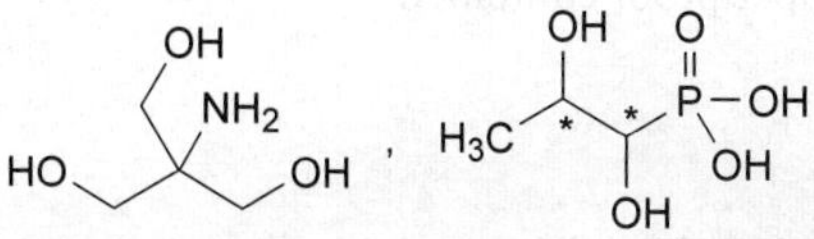

A. 1,3-dihydroxy-2-(hydroxymethyl)propan-2-aminium (1,2-dihydroxypropyl)phosphonate,

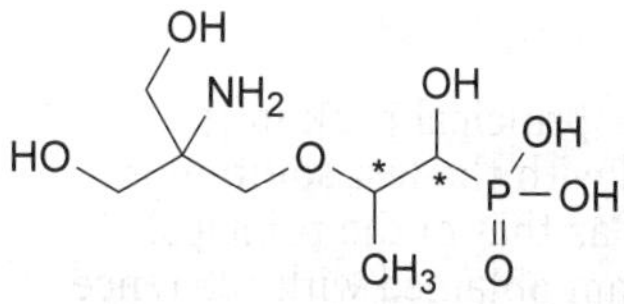

B. [2-[2-amino-3-hydroxy-2-(hydroxymethyl)propoxy]-1-hydroxypropyl]phosphonic acid,

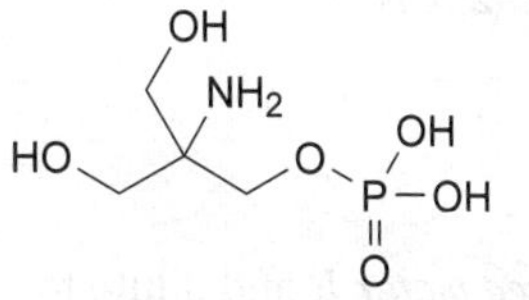

C. 2-amino-3-hydroxy-2-(hydroxymethyl)propyl dihydrogenphosphate (trometamol phosphoric ester),

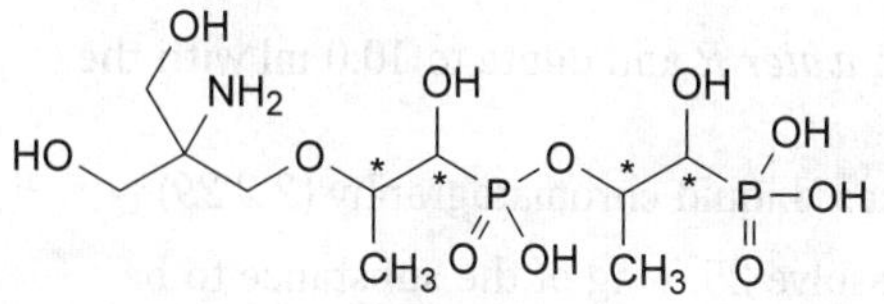

D. [2-[[[2-[2-amino-3-hydroxy-2-(hydroxymethyl)propoxy]-1-hydroxypropyl]hydroxyphosphoryl]oxy]-1-hydroxypropyl]phosphonic acid (trometamoyloxy fosfomycin dimer).

01/2005:0180 corrected

FRAMYCETIN SULPHATE

Framycetini sulfas

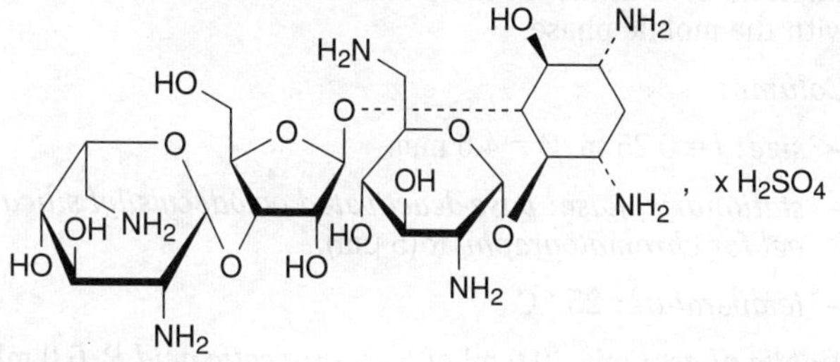

$C_{23}H_{46}N_6O_{13},xH_2SO_4$ M_r 615 (base)

DEFINITION

Sulphate of 2-deoxy-4-*O*-(2,6-diamino-2,6-dideoxy-α-D-glucopyranosyl)-5-*O*-[3-*O*-(2,6-diamino-2,6-dideoxy-β-L-idopyranosyl)-β-D-ribofuranosyl]-D-streptamine (neomycin B), a substance produced by the growth of selected strains of *Streptomyces fradiae* or *Streptomyces decaris* or obtained by any other means.

Content: minimum of 630 IU/mg (dried substance).

CHARACTERS

Appearance: white or yellowish-white powder, hygroscopic.

Solubility: freely soluble in water, very slightly soluble in alcohol, practically insoluble in acetone.

IDENTIFICATION

A. Examine the chromatograms obtained in the test for related substances.

Results:

- the retention time of the principal peak in the chromatogram obtained with the test solution is approximately the same as that of the principal peak in the chromatogram obtained with reference solution (a),
- it complies with the limit given for impurity C.

B. It gives reaction (a) of sulphates (*2.3.1*).

TESTS

pH (*2.2.3*): 6.0 to 7.0.

Dissolve 0.1 g in *carbon dioxide-free water R* and dilute to 10 ml with the same solvent.

Specific optical rotation (*2.2.7*): + 52.5 to + 55.5 (dried substance).

Dissolve 1.00 g in *water R* and dilute to 10.0 ml with the same solvent

Related substances. Liquid chromatography (*2.2.29*).

Test solution. Dissolve 25.0 mg of the substance to be examined in the mobile phase and dilute to 50.0 ml with the mobile phase.

Reference solution (a). Dissolve the contents of a vial of *framycetin sulphate CRS* in the mobile phase and dilute with the mobile phase to obtain a solution containing 0.5 mg/ml.

Reference solution (b). Dilute 3.0 ml of reference solution (a) to 100.0 ml with the mobile phase.

Reference solution (c). Dilute 1.0 ml of reference solution (a) to 100.0 ml with the mobile phase.

Reference solution (d). Dissolve the contents of a vial of *neamine CRS* (corresponding to 0.5 mg) in the mobile phase and dilute to 100.0 ml with the mobile phase.

Reference solution (e). Dissolve 10 mg of *neomycin sulphate CRS* in the mobile phase and dilute to 100.0 ml with the mobile phase.

Column:

- *size*: l = 0.25 m, Ø = 4.6 mm,
- *stationary phase*: *base-deactivated octadecylsilyl silica gel for chromatography R* (5 µm),
- *temperature*: 25 °C.

Mobile phase: mix 20.0 ml of *trifluoroacetic acid R*, 6.0 ml of *carbonate-free sodium hydroxide solution R* and 500 ml of *water R*, allow to equilibrate, dilute to 1000 ml with *water R* and degas.

Flow rate: 0.7 ml/min.

Post-column solution: *carbonate-free sodium hydroxide solution R* diluted 1 in 25 previously degassed, which is added pulse-less to the column effluent using a 375 µl polymeric mixing coil.

Flow rate: 0.5 ml/min.

Detection: pulsed amperometric detector with a gold working electrode, a silver-silver chloride reference electrode and a stainless steel auxiliary electrode which is the cell body, held at respectively 0.00 V detection, + 0.80 V oxidation and − 0.60 V reduction potentials, with pulse durations according to the instrument used.

Injection: 10 µl.

Run time: 1.5 times the retention time of neomycin B.

Relative retention with reference to neomycin B (retention time = about 10 min): impurity A = about 0.65; impurity C = about 0.9; impurity G = about 1.1.

System suitability:

- *resolution*: minimum 2.0 between the peaks due to impurity C and to neomycin B in the chromatogram obtained with reference solution (e); if necessary, adjust the volume of the carbonate-free sodium hydroxide solution in the mobile phase,
- *signal-to-noise ratio*: minimum 10 for the principal peak in the chromatogram obtained with reference solution (c).

Limits:

- *impurity A*: not more than the area of the principal peak in the chromatogram obtained with reference solution (d) and taking into account the declared content of *neamine CRS* (1.0 per cent),
- *impurity C*: not more than the area of the principal peak in the chromatogram obtained with reference solution (b) (3.0 per cent),
- *total of other impurities*: not more than the area of the principal peak in the chromatogram obtained with reference solution (b) (3.0 per cent),
- *disregard limit*: area of the principal peak in the chromatogram obtained with reference solution (c) (1.0 per cent).

Sulphate: 27.0 per cent to 31.0 per cent (dried substance).

Dissolve 0.250 g in 100 ml of *water R* and adjust the solution to pH 11 using *concentrated ammonia R*. Add 10.0 ml of *0.1 M barium chloride* and about 0.5 mg of *phthalein purple R*. Titrate with *0.1 M sodium edetate* adding 50 ml of *alcohol R* when the colour of the solution begins to change and continuing the titration until the violet-blue colour disappears.

1 ml of *0.1 M barium chloride* is equivalent to 9.606 mg of SO_4.

Loss on drying (*2.2.32*): maximum 8.0 per cent, determined on 1.000 g by drying at 60 °C over *diphosphorus pentoxide R* at a pressure not exceeding 0.7 kPa for 3 h.

Sulphated ash (*2.4.14*): maximum 1.0 per cent, determined on 1.0 g.

Sterility (*2.6.1*). If intended for introduction into body cavities without a further appropriate sterilisation procedure, it complies with the test for sterility.

Bacterial endotoxins (*2.6.14, Method D*): less than 1.3 IU/mg if intended for introduction into body cavities without a further appropriate procedure for the removal of bacterial endotoxins.

ASSAY

Carry out the microbiological assay of antibiotics (*2.7.2*). Use *framycetin sulphate CRS* as the reference substance.

STORAGE

In an airtight container, protected from light. If the substance is intended for introduction into body cavities, store in a sterile, tamper-proof container.

LABELLING

The label states:

- where applicable, that the substance is sterile,
- where applicable, that the substance is free from bacterial endotoxins.

IMPURITIES

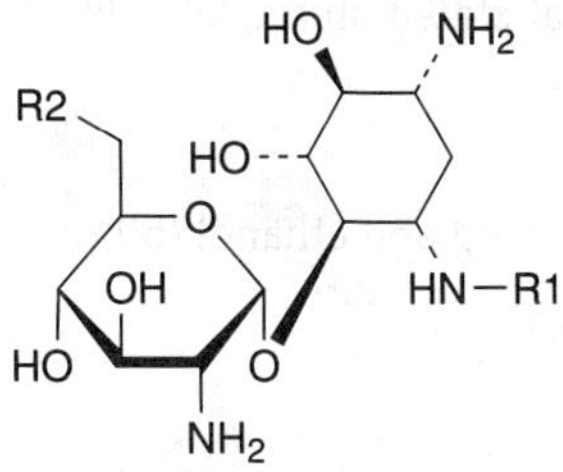

A. R1 = H, R2 = NH_2: 2-deoxy-4-*O*-(2,6-diamino-2,6-dideoxy-α-D-glucopyranosyl)-D-streptamine (neamine or neomycin A-LP),

B. R1 = CO-CH_3, R2 = NH_2: 3-*N*-acetyl-2-deoxy-4-*O*-(2,6-diamino-2,6-dideoxy-α-D-glucopyranosyl)-D-streptamine (3-acetylneamine),

D. R1 = H, R2 = OH: 4-*O*-(2-amino-2-deoxy-α-D-glucopyranosyl)-2-deoxy-D-streptamine (paromamine or neomycin D),

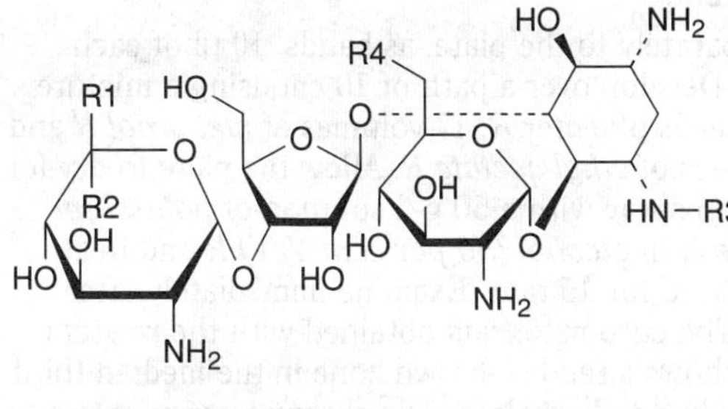

C. R1 = CH_2-NH_2, R2 = R3 = H, R4 = NH_2: 2-deoxy-4-*O*-(2,6-diamino-2,6-dideoxy-α-D-glucopyranosyl)-5-*O*-[3-*O*-(2,6-diamino-2,6-dideoxy-α-D-glucopyranosyl)-β-D-ribofuranosyl]-D-streptamine (neomycin C),

E. R1 = R3 = H, R2 = CH_2-NH_2, R4 = OH: 4-*O*-(2-amino-2-deoxy-α-D-glucopyranosyl)-2-deoxy-5-*O*-[3-*O*-(2,6-diamino-2,6-dideoxy-β-L-idopyranosyl)-β-D-ribofuranosyl]-D-streptamine (paromomycin I or neomycin E),

F. R1 = CH_2-NH_2, R2 = R3 = H, R4 = OH: 4-*O*-(2-amino-2-deoxy-α-D-glucopyranosyl)-2-deoxy-5-*O*-[3-*O*-(2,6-diamino-2,6-dideoxy-α D-glucopyranosyl)-β-D-ribofuranosyl]-D-streptamine (paromomycin II or neomycin F),

G. R1 = H, R2 = CH_2-NH_2, R3 = CO-CH_3, R4 = NH_2: 3-*N*-acetyl-2-deoxy-4-*O*-(2,6-diamino-2,6-dideoxy-α-D-glucopyranosyl)-5-*O*-[3-*O*-(2,6-diamino-2,6-dideoxy-β-L-idopyranosyl)-β-D-ribofuranosyl]-D-streptamine (neomycin B-LP).

01/2005:0025

FRANGULA BARK

Frangulae cortex

DEFINITION

Frangula bark consists of the dried, whole or fragmented bark of the stems and branches of *Rhamnus frangula* L. (*Frangula alnus* Miller). It contains not less than 7.0 per cent of glucofrangulins, expressed as glucofrangulin A ($C_{27}H_{30}O_{14}$; M_r 578.5) and calculated with reference to the dried drug.

CHARACTERS

It has the macroscopic and microscopic characters described under Identification tests A and B.

IDENTIFICATION

A. The bark occurs in curved, almost flat or rolled fragments or in single or double quilled pieces usually 0.5 mm to 2 mm thick and variable in length and width. The greyish-brown or dark brown outer surface is wrinkled longitudinally and covered with numerous greyish, transversely elongated lenticels; when the outer layers are removed, a dark red layer is exposed. The orange-brown to reddish-brown inner surface is smooth and bears fine longitudinal striations; it becomes red when treated with alkali. The fracture is short, fibrous in the inner part.

B. Reduce to a powder (355). The powder is yellowish or reddish-brown. Examine under a microscope using *chloral hydrate solution R*. The powdered drug shows: numerous phloem fibres, partially lignified, in groups with crystal sheaths containing calcium oxalate prisms; reddish-brown fragments of cork; fragments of parenchyma containing calcium oxalate cluster crystals. Sclereids are absent.

C. Examine the chromatogram obtained in the test for "Other species of *Rhamnus*; anthrones" in daylight. The chromatogram obtained with the test solution shows two orange brown zones (glucofrangulins) in the lower third and two to four red zones (frangulins, not always clearly separated, and above them frangula-emodin) in the upper third.

D. To about 50 mg of the powdered drug (180) add 25 ml of *dilute hydrochloric acid R* and heat the mixture on a water-bath for 15 min. Allow to cool, shake with 20 ml of *ether R* and discard the aqueous layer. Shake the ether layer with 10 ml of *dilute ammonia R1*. The aqueous layer becomes reddish-violet.

TESTS

Other species of *Rhamnus*; anthrones. Examine by thin-layer chromatography (*2.2.27*), using a suitable silica gel as the coating substance.

Test solution. To 0.5 g of the powdered drug (180) add 5 ml of *alcohol (70 per cent V/V) R* and heat to boiling. Cool and centrifuge. Decant the supernatant solution immediately and use within 30 min.

Reference solution. Dissolve 20 mg of *barbaloin R* in *alcohol (70 per cent V/V) R* and dilute to 10 ml with the same solvent.

Apply separately to the plate, as bands, 10 µl of each solution. Develop over a path of 10 cm using a mixture of 13 volumes of *water R*, 17 volumes of *methanol R* and 100 volumes of *ethyl acetate R*. Allow the plate to dry for 5 min, spray with a 50 g/l solution of *potassium hydroxide R* in *alcohol (50 per cent V/V) R*, and heat at 100-105 °C for 15 min. Examine in ultraviolet light at 365 nm. The chromatogram obtained with the reference solution shows a brownish-yellow zone corresponding to barbaloin in the central part. The chromatogram obtained with the test solution shows no zones of intense yellow fluorescence and no zone of orange to reddish fluorescence similar in position to the zone of barbaloin in the chromatogram obtained with the reference solution.

Apply to another plate, as a band, 10 µl of the test solution and develop as described above. Allow the plate to dry for not longer than 5 min and spray immediately with a 5 g/l solution of *nitrotetrazolium blue R* in *methanol R*. Examine the chromatogram immediately. No violet or greyish-blue zones appear.

Foreign matter (*2.8.2*). Not more than 1 per cent.

Loss on drying (*2.2.32*). Not more than 10.0 per cent, determined on 1.000 g of the powdered drug (355) by drying in an oven at 100-105 °C for 2 h.

Total ash (*2.4.16*). Not more than 6.0 per cent.

ASSAY

Carry out the assay protected from bright light.

In a tared, round-bottomed flask with a ground-glass neck, weigh 0.250 g of powdered drug (180). Add 25.0 ml of a 70 per cent *V/V* solution of *methanol R*; mix and weigh again. Heat in a water-bath under a reflux condenser for 15 min. Allow to cool, weigh and adjust to the original mass with a 70 per cent *V/V* solution of *methanol R*. Filter and transfer 5.0 ml of the filtrate to a separating funnel. Add 50 ml of *water R* and 0.1 ml of *hydrochloric acid R*. Shake with five quantities, each of 20 ml, of *light petroleum R*. Allow the layers to separate and transfer the aqueous layer to a 100 ml volumetric flask. Combine the light petroleum layers and wash with two quantities, each of 15 ml, of *water R*. Use this water for washing the separating funnel and add it to the aqueous solution in the volumetric flask. Add 5 ml of a 50 g/l solution of *sodium carbonate R* and dilute to 100.0 ml with *water R*. Discard the light petroleum layer. Transfer 40.0 ml of the aqueous solution to a 200 ml round-bottomed flask with a ground-glass neck. Add 20 ml of a 200 g/l solution of *ferric chloride R* and heat under a reflux condenser for 20 min in a water-bath with the water level above that of the liquid in the flask. Add 2 ml of *hydrochloric acid R* and continue heating for 20 min, shaking frequently, until the precipitate is dissolved. Allow to cool, transfer the mixture to a separating funnel and shake with three quantities, each of 25 ml, of *ether R*, previously used to rinse the flask. Combine the ether extracts and wash with two quantities, each of 15 ml, of *water R*. Transfer the ether layer to a volumetric flask and dilute to 100.0 ml with *ether R*. Evaporate 20.0 ml carefully to dryness and dissolve the residue in 10.0 ml of a 5 g/l solution of *magnesium acetate R* in *methanol R*. Measure the absorbance (*2.2.25*) at 515 nm using *methanol R* as the compensation liquid.

Calculate the percentage of glucofrangulins, expressed as glucofrangulin A, from the expression:

$$\frac{A \times 3.06}{m}$$

i.e. taking the specific absorbance of glucofrangulin A to be 204.

A = absorbance at 515 nm,

m = mass of the sample, in grams.

STORAGE

Store protected from light.

01/2005:1214

FRANGULA BARK DRY EXTRACT, STANDARDISED

Frangulae corticis extractum siccum normatum

DEFINITION

Standardised frangula bark dry extract is produced from *Frangula bark (0025)*. It contains not less than 15.0 per cent and not more than 30.0 per cent of glucofrangulins, expressed as glucofrangulin A ($C_{27}H_{30}O_{14}$; M_r 578.5) and calculated with reference to the dried extract. The measured content does not deviate from that stated on the label by more than ± 10 per cent.

PRODUCTION

The extract is produced from the drug and ethanol (50 to 80 per cent *V/V*) by an appropriate procedure.

CHARACTERS

A yellowish-brown, fine powder.

IDENTIFICATION

A. Examine by thin-layer chromatography (*2.2.27*), using a suitable silica gel as the coating substance.

Test solution. To 0.05 g add 5 ml of *alcohol (70 per cent V/V) R* and heat to boiling. Cool and centrifuge. Decant the supernatant solution immediately and use within 30 min.

Reference solution. Dissolve 20 mg of *barbaloin R* in *alcohol (70 per cent V/V) R* and dilute to 10 ml with the same solvent.

Apply separately to the plate, as bands, 10 µl of each solution. Develop over a path of 10 cm using a mixture of 13 volumes of *water R*, 17 volumes of *methanol R* and 100 volumes of *ethyl acetate R*. Allow the plate to dry for 5 min, then spray with a 50 g/l solution of *potassium hydroxide R* in *alcohol (50 per cent V/V) R* and heat at 100-105 °C for 15 min. Examine immediately after heating. The chromatogram obtained with the reference solution shows a reddish-brown zone in the median third corresponding to barbaloin. The chromatogram obtained with the test solution shows two orange-brown zones (glucofrangulins) in the lower third and two to four red zones (frangulins, not always clearly separated, and above them frangula-emodin) in the upper third.

B. To about 25 mg add 25 ml of *dilute hydrochloric acid R* and heat the mixture on a water-bath for 15 min. Allow to cool, shake with 20 ml of *ether R* and discard the aqueous layer. Shake the ether layer with 10 ml of *dilute ammonia R1*. The aqueous layer becomes reddish-violet.

TESTS

Loss on drying (*2.8.17*): maximum 5.0 per cent.

Microbial contamination. Total viable aerobic count (*2.6.12*) not more than 10^4 per gram of which not more than 10^2 fungi per gram, determined by plate count. It complies with the test for *Escherichia coli* and *Salmonella* (*2.6.13*).

ASSAY

Carry out the assay protected from bright light.

In a tared round-bottomed flask with a ground-glass neck, weigh 0.100 g of the preparation to be examined. Add 25.0 ml of a 70 per cent *V/V* solution of *methanol R*, mix and weigh again. Heat the flask in a water-bath under a reflux condenser at 70 °C for 15 min. Allow to cool, weigh and adjust to the original mass with a 70 per cent *V/V* solution of *methanol R*. Filter and transfer 5.0 ml of the filtrate to a separating funnel. Add 50 ml of *water R* and 0.1 ml of *hydrochloric acid R*. Shake with five quantities, each of 20 ml, of *light petroleum R1*. Allow the layers to separate and transfer the aqueous layer to a 100 ml volumetric flask. Combine the light petroleum layers and wash with two quantities, each of 15 ml, of *water R*. Use this water for washing the separating funnel and add it to the aqueous solution in the volumetric flask. Add 5 ml of a 50 g/l solution of *sodium carbonate R* and dilute to 100.0 ml with *water R*. Discard the light petroleum layer. Transfer 40.0 ml of the aqueous solution to a 200 ml round-bottomed flask with a ground-glass neck. Add 20 ml of a 200 g/l solution of *ferric chloride R* and heat under a reflux condenser for 20 min in a water-bath with the water level above that of the liquid in the flask. Add 2 ml of *hydrochloric acid R* and continue heating for 20 min, shaking frequently, until the precipitate is dissolved. Allow to cool, transfer the mixture to a separating funnel and shake with three quantities, each of 25 ml, of *ether R*, previously used to rinse the flask. Combine the ether extracts and wash with two quantities, each of 15 ml, of *water R*. Transfer the ether layer to a volumetric flask and dilute to 100.0 ml with *ether R*. Evaporate 20.0 ml carefully to dryness and dissolve the residue in 10.0 ml of a 5 g/l solution of *magnesium acetate R* in *methanol R*. Measure the absorbance (*2.2.25*) at 515 nm using *methanol R* as the compensation liquid.

Calculate the percentage of glucofrangulins, expressed as glucofrangulin A from the expression:

$$\frac{A \times 3.06}{m}$$

i.e. taking the specific absorbance of glucofrangulin A to be 204, calculated on the basis of the specific absorbance of barbaloin,

A = absorbance at 515 nm,

m = mass of the preparation to be examined, in grams.

STORAGE

Store in an airtight container, protected from light.

LABELLING

The label states the content of glucofrangulins.

01/2005:0188

FRUCTOSE

Fructosum

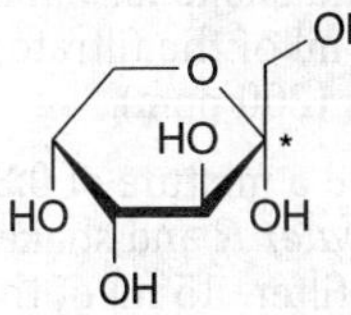

and epimer at C*

$C_6H_{12}O_6$ M_r 180.2

DEFINITION

Fructose is (-)-D-*arabino*-hex-2-ulopyranose. The substance described in this monograph is not necessarily suitable for parenteral use.

CHARACTERS

A white, crystalline powder, with a very sweet taste, very soluble in water, soluble in alcohol.

IDENTIFICATION

A. Examine by thin-layer chromatography (*2.2.27*), using *silica gel G R* as the coating substance.

Test solution. Dissolve 10 mg of the substance to be examined in a mixture of 2 volumes of *water R* and 3 volumes of *methanol R* and dilute to 20 ml with the same mixture of solvents.

Reference solution (a). Dissolve 10 mg of *fructose CRS* in a mixture of 2 volumes of *water R* and 3 volumes of *methanol R* and dilute to 20 ml with the same mixture of solvents.

Reference solution (b). Dissolve 10 mg each of *fructose CRS, glucose CRS, lactose CRS* and *sucrose CRS* in a mixture of 2 volumes of *water R* and 3 volumes of *methanol R* and dilute to 20 ml with the same mixture of solvents.

Apply separately to the plate 2 µl of each solution and thoroughly dry the starting points. Develop over a path of 15 cm using a mixture of 10 volumes of *water R*, 15 volumes of *methanol R*, 25 volumes of *anhydrous acetic acid R* and 50 volumes of *ethylene chloride R*. The solvents should be measured accurately since a slight excess of water produces cloudiness. Dry the plate in a current of warm air. Repeat the development immediately, after renewing the mobile phase. Dry the plate in a current of warm air and spray evenly with a solution of 0.5 g of *thymol R* in a mixture of 5 ml of *sulphuric acid R* and 95 ml of *alcohol R*. Heat at 130 °C for 10 min. The principal spot in the chromatogram obtained with the test solution is similar in position, colour and size to the principal spot in the chromatogram obtained with reference solution (a). The test is not valid unless the chromatogram obtained with reference solution (b) shows four clearly separated spots.

B. Dissolve 0.1 g in 10 ml of *water R*. Add 3 ml of *cupri-tartaric solution R* and heat. A red precipitate is formed.

C. To 1 ml of solution S (see Tests) add 9 ml of *water R*. To 1 ml of the solution add 5 ml of *hydrochloric acid R* and heat to 70 °C. A brown colour develops.

D. Dissolve 5 g in *water R* and dilute to 10 ml with the same solvent. To 0.5 ml of the solution add 0.2 g of *resorcinol R* and 9 ml of *dilute hydrochloric acid R* and heat on a water-bath for 2 min. A red colour develops.

TESTS

Solution S. Dissolve 10.0 g in *distilled water R* and dilute to 100 ml with the same solvent.

Appearance of solution. Dissolve 5.0 g in *water R* and dilute to 10 ml with the same solvent. The solution is clear (*2.2.1*). Add 10 ml of *water R*. The solution is colourless (*2.2.2, Method II*).

Acidity or alkalinity. Dissolve 6.0 g in 25 ml of *carbon dioxide-free water R* and add 0.3 ml of *phenolphthalein solution R*. The solution is colourless. Not more than 0.15 ml of *0.1 M sodium hydroxide* is required to change the colour of the indicator to pink.

Specific optical rotation (*2.2.7*). Dissolve 10.0 g in 80 ml of *water R*, add 0.2 ml of *dilute ammonia R1*, allow to stand for 30 min and dilute to 100.0 ml with *water R*. The specific optical rotation is − 91.0 to − 93.5, calculated with reference to the anhydrous substance.

Foreign sugars. Dissolve 5.0 g in *water R* and dilute to 10 ml with the same solvent. To 1 ml of the solution add 9 ml of *alcohol R*. Any opalescence in the solution is not more intense than that in a mixture of 1 ml of the initial solution and 9 ml of *water R*.

5-Hydroxymethylfurfural and related compounds. To 5 ml of solution S add 5 ml of *water R*. The absorbance (*2.2.25*) measured at 284 nm is not greater than 0.32.

Barium. To 10 ml of solution S add 1 ml of *dilute sulphuric acid R*. When examined immediately and after 1 h, any opalescence in the solution is not more intense than that in a mixture of 1 ml of *distilled water R* and 10 ml of solution S.

Lead in sugars (*2.4.10*). It complies with the limit test for lead in sugars (0.5 ppm).

Water (*2.5.12*). Not more than 0.5 per cent, determined on 1.00 g by the semi-micro determination of water.

Sulphated ash (*2.4.14*). Not more than 0.1 per cent. Dissolve 5.0 g in 10 ml of *water R*, add 2 ml of *sulphuric acid R*, evaporate to dryness on a water-bath and ignite to constant mass.

01/2005:0391

FUROSEMIDE

Furosemidum

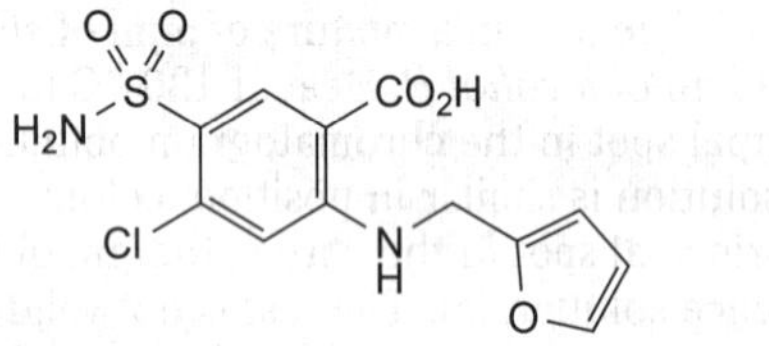

$C_{12}H_{11}ClN_2O_5S$ M_r 330.7

DEFINITION

Furosemide contains not less than 98.5 per cent and not more than the equivalent of 101.0 per cent of 4-chloro-2-[(furan-2-ylmethyl)amino]-5-sulphamoylbenzoic acid, calculated with reference to the dried substance.

CHARACTERS

A white or almost white, crystalline powder, practically insoluble in water, soluble in acetone, sparingly soluble in alcohol, practically insoluble in methylene chloride. It dissolves in dilute solutions of alkali hydroxides.

It melts at about 210 °C, with decomposition.

IDENTIFICATION

First identification: B.

Second identification: A, C.

A. Dissolve 50 mg in a 4 g/l solution of *sodium hydroxide R* and dilute to 100 ml with the same alkaline solution. Dilute 1 ml of the solution to 100 ml with a 4 g/l solution of *sodium hydroxide R*. Examined between 220 nm and 350 nm (*2.2.25*), the solution shows three absorption maxima, at 228 nm, 270 nm and 333 nm. The ratio of the absorbance measured at the maximum at 270 nm to that measured at the maximum at 228 nm is 0.52 to 0.57.

B. Examine by infrared absorption spectrophotometry (*2.2.24*), comparing with the spectrum obtained with *furosemide CRS*.

C. Dissolve about 25 mg in 10 ml of *alcohol R*. To 5 ml add 10 ml of *water R*. To 0.2 ml of this solution add 10 ml of *dilute hydrochloric acid R* and heat under a reflux condenser for 15 min. Allow to cool and add 18 ml of *1 M sodium hydroxide* and 1 ml of a 5 g/l solution of *sodium nitrite R*. Allow to stand for 3 min, add 2 ml of a 25 g/l solution of *sulphamic acid R* and mix. Add 1 ml of a 5 g/l solution of *naphthylethylenediamine dihydrochloride R*. A violet-red colour develops.

TESTS

Related substances. Examine by liquid chromatography (*2.2.29*). *Prepare the solutions immediately before use and protect from light.*

Test solution. Dissolve 50.0 mg of the substance to be examined in the mobile phase and dilute to 50.0 ml with the mobile phase.

Reference solution (a). Dissolve 20.0 mg of *furosemide impurity A CRS* in the mobile phase and dilute to 20.0 ml with the mobile phase.

Reference solution (b). Dilute a mixture of 1.0 ml of the test solution and 1.0 ml of reference solution (a) to 20.0 ml with the mobile phase. Dilute 1.0 ml of this solution to 20.0 ml with the mobile phase.

The chromatographic procedure may be carried out using:

- a stainless steel column 0.25 m long and 4.6 mm in internal diameter packed with *octylsilyl silica gel for chromatography R* (5 μm),
- as mobile phase at a flow rate of 1 ml per minute a mixture prepared as follows: dissolve 0.2 g of *potassium dihydrogen phosphate R* and 0.25 g of *cetrimide R* in 70 ml of *water R*; adjust to pH 7.0 with *ammonia R* and add 30 ml of *propanol R*,
- as detector a spectrophotometer set at 238 nm.

Inject 20 μl of reference solution (b). Adjust the sensitivity of the system so that the heights of the two peaks in the chromatogram obtained are not less than 20 per cent of the full scale of the recorder. The test is not valid unless the resolution between the first peak (furosemide impurity A) and the second peak (furosemide) is at least 4.

Inject 20 μl of the test solution. Continue the chromatography for three times the retention time of the principal peak. In the chromatogram obtained with the test solution: the area of any peak, apart from the principal peak, is not greater than the area of the first peak in the chromatogram obtained with reference solution (b) (0.25 per cent); the sum of the areas of all the peaks, apart from the principal peak, is not greater than twice the area of the first peak in the chromatogram obtained with reference solution (b) (0.5 per cent). Disregard any peak with an area less than 0.1 times the area of the first peak in the chromatogram obtained with reference solution (b).

Chlorides (*2.4.4*). To 0.5 g add a mixture of 0.2 ml of *nitric acid R* and 30 ml of *water R* and shake for 5 min. Allow to stand for 15 min and filter. 15 ml of the filtrate complies with the limit test for chlorides (200 ppm).

Sulphates (*2.4.13*). To 1.0 g add a mixture of 0.2 ml of *acetic acid R* and 30 ml of *distilled water R* and shake for 5 min. Allow to stand for 15 min and filter. 15 ml of the filtrate complies with the limit test for sulphates (300 ppm).

Heavy metals (*2.4.8*). 1.0 g complies with limit test C for heavy metals (20 ppm). Prepare the standard using 2 ml of *lead standard solution (10 ppm Pb) R*.

Loss on drying (*2.2.32*). Not more than 0.5 per cent, determined on 1.000 g by drying in an oven at 100 °C to 105 °C.

Sulphated ash (*2.4.14*). Not more than 0.1 per cent, determined on 1.0 g.

ASSAY

Dissolve 0.250 g in 20 ml of *dimethylformamide R*. Titrate with *0.1 M sodium hydroxide* using 0.2 ml of *bromothymol blue solution R2*. Carry out a blank titration.

1 ml of *0.1 M sodium hydroxide* is equivalent to 33.07 mg of $C_{12}H_{11}ClN_2O_5S$.

STORAGE

Store protected from light.

IMPURITIES

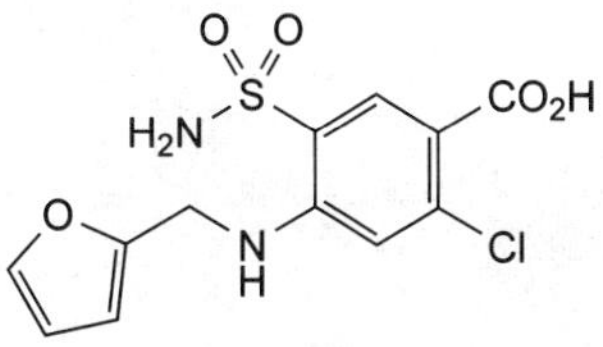

A. 2-chloro-4-[(furan-2-ylmethyl)amino]-5-sulphamoylbenzoic acid,

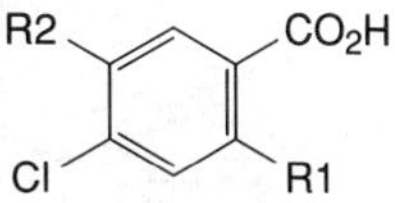

B. R1 = Cl, R2 = SO_2-NH_2: 2,4-dichloro-5-sulphamoylbenzoic acid,

C. R1 = NH_2, R2 = SO_2-NH_2: 2-amino-4-chloro-5-sulphamoylbenzoic acid,

E. R1 = Cl, R2 = H: 2,4-dichlorobenzoic acid,

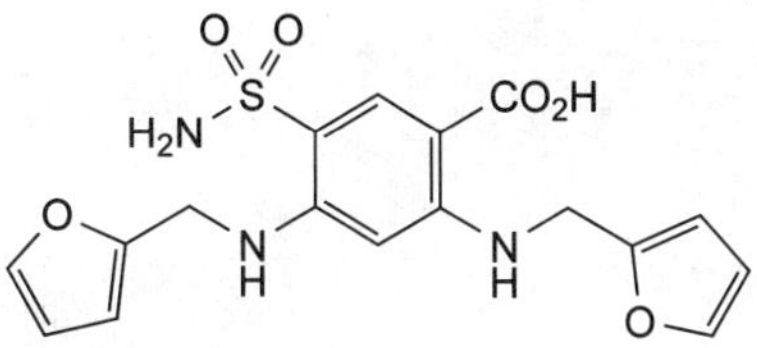

D. 2,4-bis[(furan-2-ylmethyl)amino]-5-sulphamoylbenzoic acid.

01/2005:0798

FUSIDIC ACID

Acidum fusidicum

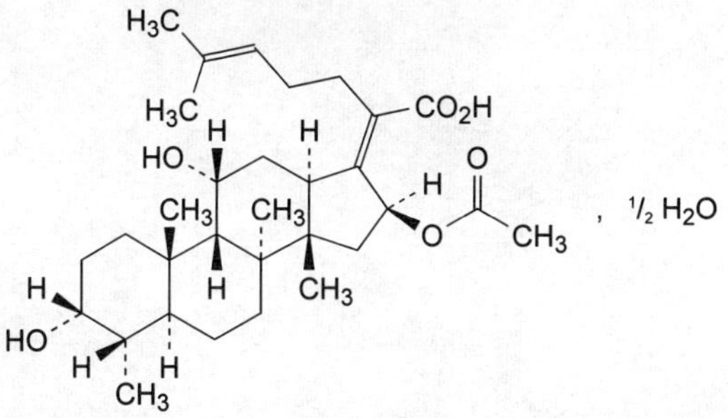

$C_{31}H_{48}O_6, {}^1/_2H_2O$ M_r 525.7

DEFINITION

Fusidic acid is *ent*-(17*Z*)-16α-(acetyloxy)-3β,11β-dihydroxy-4β,8,14-trimethyl-18-nor-5β,10α-cholesta-17(20),24-dien-21-oic acid, an antimicrobial substance produced by the growth of certain strains of *Fusidium coccineum* or by any other means. It contains not less than 97.5 per cent and not more than the equivalent of 101.0 per cent of $C_{31}H_{48}O_6$, calculated with reference to the anhydrous substance.

CHARACTERS

A white or almost white, crystalline powder, practically insoluble in water, freely soluble in alcohol.

IDENTIFICATION

A. Examine by infrared absorption spectrophotometry (*2.2.24*), comparing with the spectrum obtained with the *Ph. Eur. reference spectrum of fusidic acid.*

B. Examine by thin-layer chromatography (*2.2.27*), using *silica gel HF_{254} R* as the coating substance.

Test solution. Dissolve 20 mg of the substance to be examined in *methanol R* and dilute to 10 ml with the same solvent.

Reference solution. Dissolve 24 mg of *diethanolamine fusidate CRS* in *methanol R* and dilute to 10 ml with the same solvent.

Apply to the plate 10 μl of each solution. Develop over a path of 15 cm using a mixture of 2.5 volumes of *methanol R*, 10 volumes of *glacial acetic acid R*, 10 volumes of *cyclohexane R* and 80 volumes of *chloroform R*. Dry the plate in a current of hot air. Examine in ultraviolet light at 254 nm. The principal spot in the chromatogram obtained with the test solution is similar in position and size to the principal spot in the chromatogram obtained with the reference solution.

TESTS

Related substances. Examine by liquid chromatography (*2.2.29*).

Test solution. Dissolve 50 mg of the substance to be examined in the mobile phase and dilute to 10.0 ml with the mobile phase.

Reference solution (a). Dissolve 5 mg of *3-ketofusidic acid CRS* in 5 ml of the mobile phase. To 1.0 ml of this solution add 0.20 ml of the test solution and dilute to 20.0 ml with the mobile phase.

Reference solution (b). Dilute 20 μl of the test solution to 100.0 ml with the mobile phase.

The chromatographic procedure may be carried out using:

– a steel column 0.125 m to 0.15 m long and 4 mm to 5 mm in internal diameter packed with *octadecylsilyl silica gel for chromatography R* (5 μm),
– as mobile phase at a flow rate of 2 ml/min a mixture of 10 volumes of *methanol R*, 20 volumes of a 10 g/l solution of *phosphoric acid R*, 20 volumes of *water R* and 50 volumes of *acetonitrile R*,
– as detector a spectrophotometer set at 235 nm,
– a 20 μl loop injector.

Continue the chromatography for at least 3.5 times the retention time of the principal peak. In the chromatogram obtained with the test solution, the sum of the areas of the peaks, apart from the principal peak and the solvent peak, is not greater than twice the area of the peak corresponding to fusidic acid in the chromatogram obtained with reference solution (a) (2.0 per cent). Disregard any peak with an area less than that of the principal peak in the chromatogram obtained with reference solution (b). The test is not valid unless: the resolution between the peaks corresponding to 3-ketofusidic acid and fusidic acid in the chromatogram obtained with reference solution (a) is at least 2.5; the principal peak in the chromatogram obtained with reference solution (b) has a signal-to-noise ratio of at least 3.

Water (*2.5.12*): 1.4 per cent to 2.0 per cent, determined on 0.50 g by the semi-micro determination of water.

Sulphated ash (*2.4.14*). Not more than 0.2 per cent, determined on 1.0 g.

ASSAY

Dissolve 0.500 g in 10 ml of *alcohol R*. Add 0.5 ml of *phenolphthalein solution R*. Titrate with *0.1 M sodium hydroxide* until a pink colour is obtained.

1 ml of *0.1 M sodium hydroxide* is equivalent to 51.67 mg of $C_{31}H_{48}O_6$.

STORAGE

Store protected from light, at a temperature of 2 °C to 8 °C.

G

01/2005:1215

GALACTOSE

Galactosum

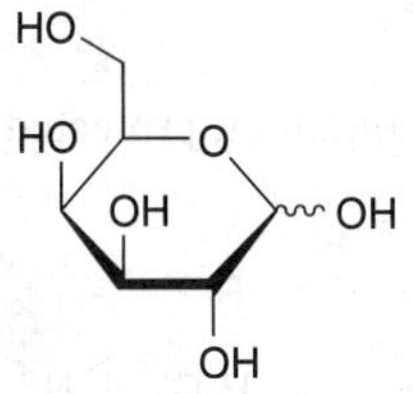

$C_6H_{12}O_6$ M_r 180.2

DEFINITION

Galactose is D-galactopyranose.

CHARACTERS

A white, crystalline or finely granulated powder, freely soluble or soluble in water, very slightly soluble in alcohol.

IDENTIFICATION

First identification: A.

Second identification: B, C.

A. Examine by infrared absorption spectrophotometry (*2.2.24*), comparing with the spectrum obtained with *galactose CRS*. Examine the substances prepared as discs.

B. Examine by thin-layer chromatography (*2.2.27*), using a suitable silica gel as the coating substance.

Test solution. Dissolve 10 mg of the substance to be examined in a mixture of 2 volumes of *water R* and 3 volumes of *methanol R* and dilute to 20 ml with the same mixture of solvents.

Reference solution (a). Dissolve 10 mg of *galactose CRS* in a mixture of 2 volumes of *water R* and 3 volumes of *methanol R* and dilute to 20 ml with the same mixture of solvents.

Reference solution (b). Dissolve 10 mg of *galactose CRS*, 10 mg of *glucose CRS* and 10 mg of *lactose CRS* in a mixture of 2 volumes of *water R* and 3 volumes of *methanol R* and dilute to 20 ml with the same mixture of solvents.

Apply to the plate 2 µl of each solution and thoroughly dry the starting points. Develop in an unsaturated tank over a path of 15 cm using a mixture of 15 volumes of *water R* and 85 volumes of *propanol R*. Dry the plate in a current of warm air. Spray uniformly with a solution of 0.5 g of *thymol R* in a mixture of 5 ml of *sulphuric acid R* and 95 ml of *alcohol R*. Heat in an oven at 130 °C for 10 min. The principal spot in the chromatogram obtained with the test solution is similar in position, colour and size to the principal spot in the chromatogram obtained with reference solution (a). The test is not valid unless the chromatogram obtained with reference solution (b) shows three clearly separated spots.

C. Dissolve 0.1 g in 10 ml of *water R*. Add 3 ml of *cupri-tartaric solution R* and heat. An orange to red precipitate is formed.

TESTS

Solution S. Dissolve, with heating in a water-bath at 50 °C, 10.0 g in *carbon dioxide-free water R* prepared from *distilled water R* and dilute to 50 ml with the same solvent.

Appearance of solution. Solution S is clear (*2.2.1*) and not more intensely coloured than reference solution B_8 (*2.2.2, Method II*).

Acidity or alkalinity. To 30 ml of solution S add 0.3 ml of *phenolphthalein solution R*. The solution is colourless. Not more than 1.5 ml of *0.01 M sodium hydroxide* is required to change the colour of the indicator to pink.

Specific optical rotation (*2.2.7*). Dissolve 10.00 g in 80 ml of *water R* and add 0.2 ml of *dilute ammonia R1*. Allow to stand for 30 min and dilute to 100.0 ml with *water R*. The specific optical rotation is + 78.0 to + 81.5, calculated with reference to the anhydrous substance.

Barium. Dilute 5 ml of solution S to 10 ml with *distilled water R*. Add 1 ml of *dilute sulphuric acid R*. When examined immediately and after 1 h, any opalescence in the solution is not more intense than that in a mixture of 5 ml of solution S and 6 ml of *distilled water R*.

Lead (*2.4.10*). It complies with the limit test for lead in sugars (0.5 ppm).

Water (*2.5.12*). Not more than 1.0 per cent, determined on 1.00 g by the semi-micro determination of water.

Sulphated ash. To 5 ml of solution S add 2 ml of *sulphuric acid R*, evaporate to dryness on a water-bath and ignite to constant mass. The residue weighs not more than 1 mg (0.1 per cent).

Microbial contamination. Total viable aerobic count (*2.6.12*) not more than 10^2 micro-organisms per gram.

01/2005:0181

GALLAMINE TRIETHIODIDE

Gallamini triethiodidum

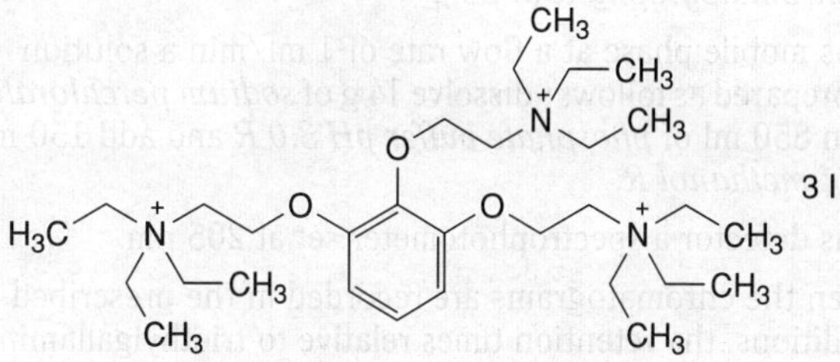

$C_{30}H_{60}I_3N_3O_3$ M_r 892

DEFINITION

Gallamine triethiodide contains not less than 98.0 per cent and not more than the equivalent of 101.0 per cent of 2,2′,2″-[benzene-1,2,3-triyltris(oxy)]tris(*N,N,N*-triethylethanaminium) triiodide, calculated with reference to the dried substance.

CHARACTERS

A white or almost white powder, hygroscopic, very soluble in water, slightly soluble in alcohol, practically insoluble in methylene chloride.

IDENTIFICATION

First identification: B, D.

Second identification: A, C, D.

A. Dissolve 50 mg in *0.01 M hydrochloric acid* and dilute to 50.0 ml with the same solvent. Dilute 1.0 ml of the solution to 100.0 ml with *0.01 M hydrochloric acid.* Examined between 220 nm and 350 nm (*2.2.25*), the solution shows an absorption maximum at 225 nm. The specific absorbance at the maximum is 500 to 550.

B. Examine by infrared absorption spectrophotometry (*2.2.24*), comparing with the spectrum obtained with *gallamine triethiodide CRS*.

Monographs F-H

C. To 5 ml of solution S (see Tests) add 1 ml of *potassium tetraiodomercurate solution R*. A yellow precipitate is formed.

D. Dilute 0.5 ml of solution S to 2 ml with *water R*. Add 0.2 ml of *dilute nitric acid R*. The solution gives reaction (a) of iodides (*2.3.1*).

TESTS

Solution S. Dissolve 0.6 g in *water R* and dilute to 30 ml with the same solvent.

Appearance of solution. Solution S is clear (*2.2.1*) and immediately after preparation is not more intensely coloured than reference solution Y_7 (*2.2.2, Method II*).

Acidity or alkalinity. To 50 ml of *water R* add 0.2 ml of *methyl red solution R*. Add either *0.01 M sulphuric acid* or *0.02 M sodium hydroxide* until an orange-yellow colour is obtained. Add 1.0 g of the substance to be examined and dissolve by shaking. Not more than 0.2 ml of *0.01 M sulphuric acid* or *0.02 M sodium hydroxide* is required to restore the orange-yellow colour.

Related substances. Examine by liquid chromatography (*2.2.29*).

Test solution. Dissolve 30.0 mg of the substance to be examined in the mobile phase and dilute to 50.0 ml with the mobile phase.

Reference solution. Dilute 1.0 ml of the test solution to 100.0 ml with the mobile phase.

The chromatographic procedure may be carried out using:

– a stainless steel column 0.25 m long and 4.6 mm in internal diameter packed with *octadecylsilyl silica gel for chromatography R* (5 µm),

– as mobile phase at a flow rate of 1 ml/min a solution prepared as follows: dissolve 14 g of *sodium perchlorate R* in 850 ml of *phosphate buffer pH 3.0 R* and add 150 ml of *methanol R*,

– as detector a spectrophotometer set at 205 nm.

When the chromatograms are recorded in the prescribed conditions, the retention times relative to triethylgallamine as perchlorate (about 40 min) are: impurity A about 0.45, impurity B about 0.50, impurity C about 0.65, impurity D about 0.75, impurity E about 0.85 and impurity F about 0.90.

Inject separately 20 µl of the test solution and 20 µl of the reference solution. Continue the chromatography for 1.5 times the retention time of triethylgallamine as perchlorate.

In the chromatogram obtained with the test solution: the area of any peak, apart from the principal peak, is not greater than the area of the principal peak in the chromatogram obtained with the reference solution (1 per cent) and the sum of the areas of such peaks is not greater than twice the area of the principal peak in the chromatogram obtained with the reference solution (2 per cent). Disregard the peak due to iodide with a retention time of zero.

Loss on drying (*2.2.32*). Not more than 1.5 per cent, determined on 1.000 g by drying in an oven at 100 °C to 105 °C.

Sulphated ash (*2.4.14*). Not more than 0.1 per cent, determined on 1.0 g.

ASSAY

In order to avoid overheating in the reaction medium, mix thoroughly throughout and stop the titration immediately after the end-point has been reached.

Dissolve 0.270 g in a mixture of 5.0 ml of *anhydrous formic acid R* and 50.0 ml of *acetic anhydride R*. Titrate with *0.1 M perchloric acid*, determining the end-point potentiometrically (*2.2.20*).

1 ml of *0.1 M perchloric acid* is equivalent to 29.72 mg of $C_{30}H_{60}I_3N_3O_3$.

STORAGE

Store in an airtight container, protected from light.

IMPURITIES

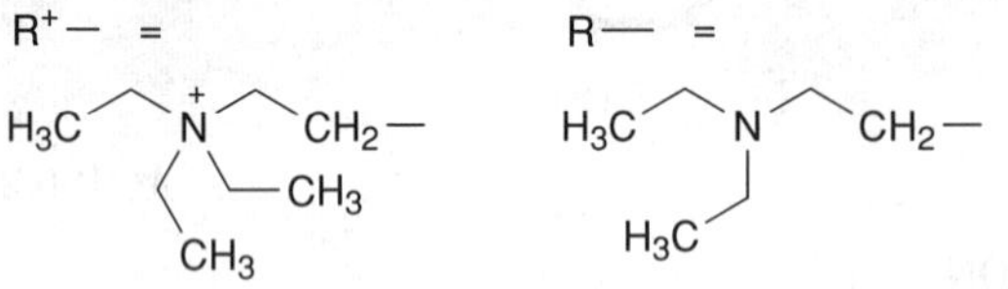

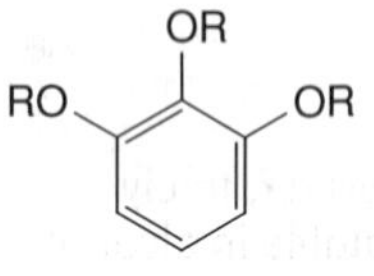

A. 2,2′,2″-[benzene-1,2,3-triyltris(oxy)]tris(*N,N*-diethylethanamine),

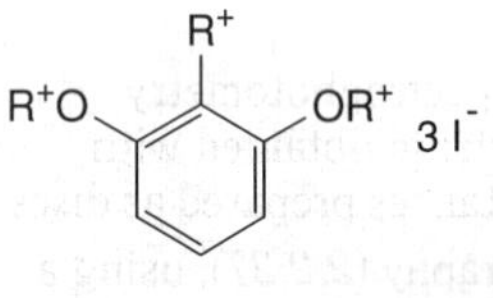

B. 2,2′-[2-[2-(triethylammonio)ethyl]-1,3-phenylene-bis(oxy)]bis(*N,N,N*-triethylethanaminium) triiodide,

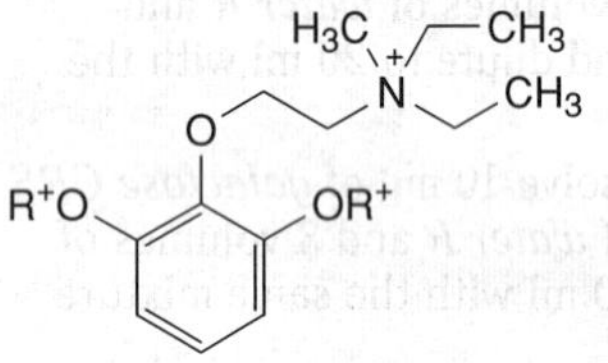

C. 2,2′-[2-[2-(diethylmethylammonio)ethoxy]-1,3-phenylenebis(oxy)]bis(*N,N,N*-triethylethanaminium) triiodide,

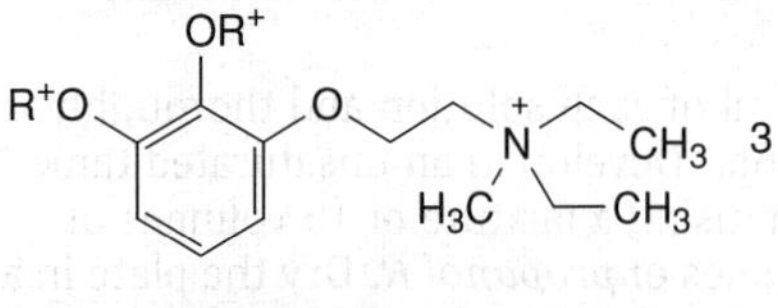

D. 2,2′-[3-[2-(diethylmethylammonio)ethoxy]-1,2-phenylenebis(oxy)]bis(*N,N,N*-triethylethanaminium) triiodide,

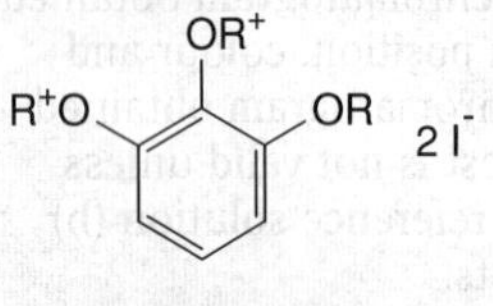

E. 2,2′-[3-[2-(diethylamino)ethoxy]-1,2-phenylene-bis(oxy)]bis(*N,N,N*-triethylethanaminium) diiodide,

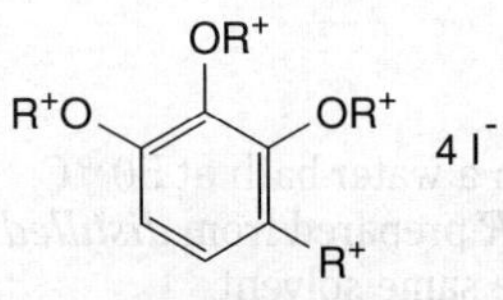

F. 2,2′,2″-[4-[2-(triethylammonio)ethyl]benzene-1,2,3triyltris(oxy)]tris(*N,N,N*-triethylethanaminium) tetraiodide.

01/2005:1216

GARLIC POWDER

Allii sativi bulbi pulvis

DEFINITION

Garlic powder is produced from the bulbs of *Allium sativum* L., cut, freeze-dried or dried at a temperature not exceeding 65 °C and powdered. It contains not less than 0.45 per cent of allicin ($C_6H_{10}OS_2$; M_r 162.3), calculated with reference to the dried drug.

CHARACTERS

A light yellowish powder.

It shows the microscopic characters described under Identification test A.

IDENTIFICATION

A. Examine under a microscope using *chloral hydrate solution R*. The powder shows numerous fragments of parenchyma and groups of spiral or annular vessels accompanied by thin-walled parenchyma.

B. Examine by thin-layer chromatography (*2.2.27*), using a suitable silica gel as the coating substance.

Test solution. To 1.0 g of garlic powder add 5.0 ml of *methanol R*, shake for 60 s and filter.

Reference solution. Dissolve 5 mg of *alanine R* in 10 ml of *water R* and dilute to 20 ml with *methanol R*.

Apply separately to the plate, as bands, 20 µl of the test solution and 10 µl of the reference solution. Develop over a path of 10 cm using a mixture of 20 volumes of *glacial acetic acid R*, 20 volumes of *propanol R*, 20 volumes of *water R* and 40 volumes of *ethanol R*. Allow the plate to dry in air. Spray with a 2 g/l solution of *ninhydrin R* in a mixture of 5 volumes of *glacial acetic acid R* and 95 volumes of *butanol R* and heat at 105 °C to 110 °C for 5 min to 10 min. Examine in daylight. The chromatogram obtained with the reference solution shows a violet zone (alanine) in its central third. The chromatogram obtained with the test solution shows a violet or brownish-red zone similar in position to that in the chromatogram obtained with the reference solution and corresponding to alliin; above and below this zone are other, generally fainter, violet zones.

TESTS

Starch. Examine the powdered drug under a microscope using *water R*. Add *iodine solution R1*. No blue colour develops.

Loss on drying (*2.2.32*). Not more than 7.0 per cent, determined on 1.000 g of the powdered drug by drying in an oven at 100-105 °C.

Total ash (*2.4.16*). Not more than 5.0 per cent.

ASSAY

Examine by liquid chromatography (*2.2.29*), using *butyl parahydroxybenzoate R* as the internal standard. *Carry out the assay as quickly as possible.*

Internal standard solution. Dissolve 20.0 mg of *butyl parahydroxybenzoate R* in 100.0 ml of a mixture of equal volumes of *methanol R* and *water R*.

Test solution. To 0.800 g of garlic powder add 20.0 ml of *water R* and homogenise the mixture in an ultrasonic bath at 4 °C for 5 min. Allow to stand at room temperature for 30 min. Then centrifuge for 30 min. Dilute 10.0 ml of the supernatant to 25.0 ml with a mixture of 40 volumes of a 1 per cent *V/V* solution of *anhydrous formic acid R* and 60 volumes of *methanol R* (stock solution). Shake and centrifuge for 5 min. Place 0.50 ml of the internal standard solution in a volumetric flask and dilute to 10.0 ml with the stock solution.

The chromatographic procedure may be carried out using:

- a stainless steel column 0.25 m long and 4 mm in internal diameter packed with silanised *octadecylsilyl silica gel for chromatography R* (5 µm) combined with a stainless steel precolumn 20 mm long and 4 mm in internal diameter packed with silanised *octadecylsilyl silica gel for chromatography R* (5 µm),
- as mobile phase at a flow rate of 0.8 ml/min a mixture of 40 volumes of a 1 per cent *V/V* solution of *anhydrous formic acid R* and 60 volumes of *methanol R*,
- a loop injector,
- as detector a spectrophotometer set at 254 nm.

Inject 1 µl of the internal standard solution. Inject 10 µl of the test solution. Adjust the sensitivity of the system so that the height of the peak due to butyl parahydroxybenzoate in the chromatogram obtained with the test solution is about 50 per cent of the full scale of the recorder.

Calculate the percentage of allicin from the expression:

$$\frac{S_1 \times m_2 \times 22.75}{S_2 \times m_1}$$

S_1 = area of the peak corresponding to allicin (most prominent peak),

S_2 = area of the peak corresponding to butyl parahydroxybenzoate in the chromatogram obtained with the test solution,

m_1 = mass of the drug, in grams,

m_2 = mass of butyl parahydroxybenzoate in grams in 100.0 ml of the internal standard solution. 1 mg of butylparahydroxybenzoate corresponds to 8.65 mg of allicin.

STORAGE

Store protected from light.

01/2005:0330

GELATIN

Gelatina

DEFINITION

Purified protein obtained either by partial acid hydrolysis (type A), partial alkaline hydrolysis (type B) or enzymatic hydrolysis of collagen from animals (including fish and poultry); it may also be a mixture of different types.

The hydrolysis leads to gelling or non-gelling product grades. Both product grades are covered by this monograph.

Gelatin described in this monograph is not suitable for parenteral use or for other special purposes.

CHARACTERS

Appearance: faintly yellow or light yellowish-brown, solid, usually occurring as translucent sheets, shreds, granules or powder.

Solubility: practically insoluble in common organic solvents; gelling grades swell in cold water and give on heating a colloidal solution which on cooling forms a more or less firm gel.

Monographs F-H

The isoelectric point is a relevant quality parameter for use of gelatin in different applications: for type A gelatin it is typically between pH 6.0 and pH 9.5 and for type B gelatin is typically between pH 4.7 and pH 5.6. These ranges cover a variety of different gelatins and for specific applications a narrower tolerance is usually applied.

Different gelatins form aqueous solutions that vary in clarity and colour. For a particular application, a suitable specification for clarity and colour is usually applied.

IDENTIFICATION

A. To 2 ml of solution S (see Tests) add 0.05 ml of *copper sulphate solution R*. Mix and add 0.5 ml of *dilute sodium hydroxide solution R*. A violet colour is produced.

B. To 0.5 g in a test-tube add 10 ml of *water R*. Allow to stand for 10 min, heat at 60 °C for 15 min and keep the tube upright at 0 °C for 6 h. Invert the tube; the contents immediately flow out for non-gelling grades and do not flow out immediately for gelling grades.

Monographs F-H

TESTS

Solution S. Dissolve 1.00 g in *carbon dioxide-free water R* at about 55 °C, dilute to 100 ml with the same solvent and keep the solution at this temperature to carry out the tests.

pH (*2.2.3*): 3.8 to 7.6 for solution S.

Conductivity (*2.2.38*): maximum 1 mS·cm^{-1}, determined on a 1.0 per cent solution at 30 ± 1.0 °C.

Sulphur dioxide (*2.5.29*): maximum 50 ppm.

Peroxides: maximum 10 ppm, determined using *peroxide test strips R*.

Peroxidase transfers oxygen from peroxides to an organic redox indicator which is converted to a blue oxidation product. The intensity of the colour obtained is proportional to the quantity of peroxide and can be compared with a colour scale provided with the test strips, to determine the peroxide concentration.

Suitability test. Dip a test strip for 1 s into *hydrogen peroxide standard solution (10 ppm H_2O_2) R*, such that the reaction zone is properly wetted. Remove the test strip, shake off excess liquid and compare the reaction zone after 15 s with the colour scale provided with the test strips used. The colour must match that of the 10 ppm concentration, otherwise the test is invalid.

Test. Weigh 20.0 ± 0.1 g of the substance to be tested in a beaker and add 80.0 ± 0.2 ml of *water R*. Stir to moisten all gelatin and allow the sample to stand at room temperature for 1-3 h. Cover the beaker with a watch-glass. Place the beaker for 20 ± 5 min in a water bath at 65 ± 2 °C to dissolve the sample. Stir the contents of the beaker with a glass rod to achieve a homogeneous solution. Dip a test strip for 1 s into the test solution, such that the reaction zone is properly wetted. Remove the test strip, shake off excess liquid and compare the reaction zone after 15 s with the colour scale provided with the test strips used. Multiply the concentration read from the colour scale by a factor of 5 to calculate the concentration in parts per million of peroxide in the test substance.

Gel strength (Bloom value): 80 to 120 per cent of the labelled nominal value.

The gel strength is expressed as the mass in grams necessary to produce the force which, applied to a plunger 12.7 mm in diameter, makes a depression 4 mm deep in a gel having a concentration of 6.67 per cent *m/m* and matured at 10 °C.

Apparatus. Texture analyser or gelometer with:

- a cylindrical piston 12.7 ± 0.1 mm in diameter with a plane pressure surface with a sharp bottom edge,
- a bottle 59 ± 1 mm in internal diameter and 85 mm high.

Adjust the apparatus according to the manufacturer's manual. Settings are: distance 4 mm, test speed 0.5 mm/s.

Method. Perform the test in duplicate. Place 7.5 g of the substance to be tested in each bottle. Add 105 ml of *water R*, place a watch-glass over each bottle and allow to stand for 1-4 h. Heat in a water-bath at 65 ± 2 °C for 15 min. While heating, gently stir with a glass rod. Ensure that the solution is uniform and that any condensed water on the inner walls of the bottle is incorporated. Allow to cool at room temperature for 15 min and transfer the bottles to a thermostatically controlled bath at 10.0 ± 0.1 °C, and fitted with a device to ensure that the platform on which the bottles stand is perfectly horizontal. Close the bottles with a rubber stopper and allow to stand for 17 ± 1 h. Remove the sample bottles from the bath and quickly wipe the water from the exterior of the bottle. Centre consecutively the 2 bottles on the platform of the apparatus so that the plunger contacts the sample as nearly at its midpoint as possible and start the measurement. Report the result as the average of the 2 measurements.

Iron: maximum 30 ppm.

Atomic absorption spectrometry (*2.2.23, Method I*).

Test solution. To 5.00 g of the substance to be examined, in a conical flask, add 10 ml of *hydrochloric acid R*. Close the flask and place in a water-bath at 75-80 °C for 2 h. Allow to cool and adjust the content of the flask to 100.0 g with *water R*.

Reference solutions. Prepare the reference solutions using *iron standard solution (8 ppm Fe) R*, diluted as necessary with *water R*.

Wavelength: 248.3 nm.

Chromium: maximum 10 ppm.

Atomic absorption spectrometry (*2.2.23, Method I*).

Test solution. Test solution described in the test for iron.

Reference solutions. Prepare the reference solutions using *chromium standard solution (100 ppm Cr) R*, diluted if necessary with *water R*.

Wavelength: 357.9 nm.

Zinc: maximum 30 ppm.

Atomic absorption spectrometry (*2.2.23, Method I*).

Test solution. Test solution described in the test for iron.

Reference solutions. Prepare the reference solutions using *zinc standard solution (10 ppm Zn) R*, diluted if necessary with *water R*.

Wavelength: 213.9 nm.

Loss on drying (*2.2.32*): maximum 15.0 per cent, determined on 1.000 g, by drying in an oven at 100-105 °C.

Microbial contamination. Total viable aerobic count (*2.6.12*) not more than 10^3 micro-organisms per gram, determined by plate count. It complies with the tests for *Escherichia coli* and *Salmonella* (*2.6.13*).

STORAGE

Protect from heat and moisture.

LABELLING

The label states the gel strength (Bloom value) or that it is a non-gelling grade.

01/2005:0331
corrected

GENTAMICIN SULPHATE

Gentamicini sulfas

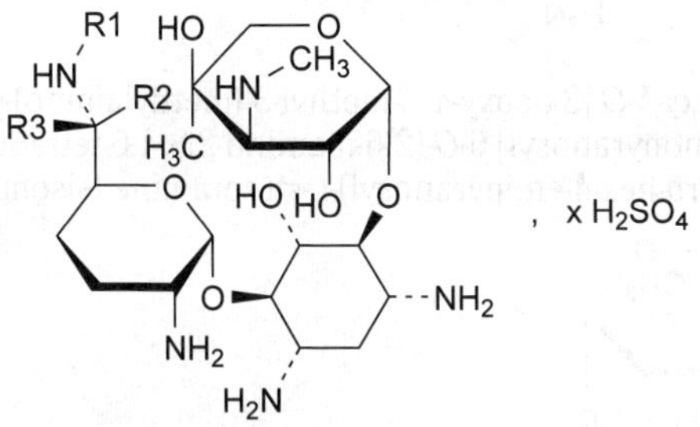

Gentamicin	Mol. Formula	R1	R2	R3
C1	$C_{21}H_{43}N_5O_7$	CH_3	CH_3	H
C1a	$C_{19}H_{39}N_5O_7$	H	H	H
C2	$C_{20}H_{41}N_5O_7$	H	CH_3	H
C2a	$C_{20}H_{41}N_5O_7$	H	H	CH_3
C2b	$C_{20}H_{41}N_5O_7$	CH_3	H	H

DEFINITION

Mixture of the sulphates of antimicrobial substances produced by *Micromonospora purpurea*, the main components being gentamicins C1, C1a, C2, C2a and C2b.

Content: minimum 590 IU/mg (anhydrous substance).

CHARACTERS

Appearance: white or almost white, hygroscopic powder.

Solubility: freely soluble in water, practically insoluble in alcohol.

IDENTIFICATION

First identification: C, D.

Second identification: A, B, D.

A. Dissolve about 10 mg in 1 ml of *water R* and add 5 ml of a 400 g/l solution of *sulphuric acid R*. Heat on a water-bath for 100 min, cool and dilute to 25 ml with *water R*. Examined between 240 nm and 330 nm (*2.2.25*), the solution shows no absorption maximum.

B. Thin-layer chromatography (*2.2.27*).

Test solution. Dissolve 25 mg of the substance to be examined in *water R* and dilute to 5 ml with the same solvent.

Reference solution. Dissolve 25 mg of *gentamicin sulphate CRS* in *water R* and dilute to 5 ml with the same solvent.

Plate: *TLC silica gel plate R.*

Mobile phase: the lower layer of a mixture of equal volumes of *concentrated ammonia R, methanol R* and *methylene chloride R.*

Application: 10 µl.

Development: over 2/3 of the plate.

Drying: in air.

Detection: spray with *ninhydrin solution R1* and heat at 110 °C for 5 min.

Results: the 3 principal spots in the chromatogram obtained with the test solution are similar in position, colour and size to the 3 principal spots in the chromatogram obtained with the reference solution.

C. Examine the chromatograms obtained in the test for composition.

Results: the chromatogram obtained with the test solution shows 5 principal peaks having the same retention times as the 5 principal peaks in the chromatogram obtained with reference solution (a).

D. It gives reaction (a) of sulphates (*2.3.1*).

TESTS

Solution S. Dissolve 0.8 g in *carbon dioxide-free water R* and dilute to 20 ml with the same solvent.

Appearance of solution. Solution S is clear (*2.2.1*) and not more intensely coloured than intensity 6 of the range of reference solutions of the most appropriate colour (*2.2.2, Method II*).

pH (*2.2.3*): 3.5 to 5.5 for solution S.

Specific optical rotation (*2.2.7*): + 107 to + 121 (anhydrous substance).

Dissolve 2.5 g in *water R* and dilute to 25.0 ml with the same solvent.

Composition. Liquid chromatography (*2.2.29*): use the normalisation procedure taking into account only the peaks due to gentamicins C1, C1a, C2, C2a and C2b; use the chromatogram supplied with *gentamicin sulphate CRS* to identify the corresponding peaks.

Test solution. Dissolve 50 mg of the substance to be examined in the mobile phase and dilute to 100.0 ml with the mobile phase.

Reference solution (a). Dissolve the content of a vial of *gentamicin sulphate CRS* in the mobile phase and dilute with the mobile phase to obtain a solution containing 0.5 mg/ml.

Reference solution (b). Dilute 5.0 ml of reference solution (a) to 100.0 ml with the mobile phase.

Column:
- *size*: l = 0.25 m, Ø = 4.6 mm,
- *stationary phase*: *styrene-divinylbenzene copolymer R* (8 µm) with a pore size of 100 nm,
- *temperature*: 55 °C.

Mobile phase: a mixture prepared with *carbon dioxide-free water R* containing 60 g/l of *anhydrous sodium sulphate R*, 1.75 g/l of *sodium octanesulphonate R*, 8 ml/l of *tetrahydrofuran R*, 50 ml/l of *0.2 M potassium dihydrogen phosphate R* previously adjusted to pH 3.0 with *dilute phosphoric acid R* and degassed.

Flow rate: 1.0 ml/min.

Post-column solution: a *carbonate-free sodium hydroxide solution R* diluted 1 to 25, previously degassed, which is added pulse-less to the column effluent using a 375 µl polymeric mixing coil.

Flow rate: 0.3 ml/min.

Detection: pulsed amperometric detector or equivalent with a gold indicator electrode, a silver-silver chloride reference electrode, and a stainless steel auxiliary electrode which is the cell body, held at respectively + 0.05 V detection, + 0.75 V oxidation and − 0.15 V reduction potentials, with pulse durations according to the instrument used.

Injection: 20 µl.

Run time: 1.2 times the retention time of gentamicin C1.

Monographs F-H

System suitability: reference solution (a):

- *peak-to-valley ratio*: minimum 2.0 where H_p = height above the baseline of the peak due to gentamicin C2a, and H_v = height above the baseline of the lowest point of the curve separating this peak from the peak due to gentamicin C2.

Limits:

- *gentamicin C1*: 20.0 per cent to 40.0 per cent,
- *gentamicin C1a*: 10.0 per cent to 30.0 per cent,
- *sum of gentamicins C2, C2a, and C2b*: 40.0 per cent to 60.0 per cent,
- *disregard limit*: the area of the peak due to gentamicin C1a in the chromatogram obtained with reference solution (b).

Related substances. Liquid chromatography (*2.2.29*) as described in the test for composition.

Limits (for related substances eluting before gentamicin C1a):

- *any impurity*: maximum 3.0 per cent,
- *total*: maximum 10.0 per cent.

Methanol (*2.4.24, System B*): maximum 1.0 per cent.

Sulphate: 32.0 per cent to 35.0 per cent (anhydrous substance).

Dissolve 0.250 g in 100 ml of *distilled water R* and adjust the solution to pH 11 using *concentrated ammonia R*. Add 10.0 ml of *0.1 M barium chloride* and about 0.5 mg of *phthalein purple R*. Titrate with *0.1 M sodium edetate*, adding 50 ml of *alcohol R* when the colour of the solution begins to change and continue the titration until the violet-blue colour disappears.

1 ml of *0.1 M barium chloride* is equivalent to 9.606 mg of SO_4.

Water (*2.5.12*): maximum 15.0 per cent, determined on 0.300 g.

Sulphated ash (*2.4.14*): maximum 1.0 per cent, determined on 0.50 g.

Bacterial endotoxins (*2.6.14*): less than 0.71 IU/mg, if intended for use in the manufacture of parenteral dosage forms without a further appropriate procedure for the removal of bacterial endotoxins.

ASSAY

Carry out the microbiological assay of antibiotics (*2.7.2*).

STORAGE

In an airtight container. If the substance is sterile, store in a sterile, airtight, tamper-proof container.

LABELLING

The label states, where applicable, that the substance is free from bacterial endotoxins.

IMPURITIES

Specified impurities: A, B, C.

Other detectable impurities: D, E.

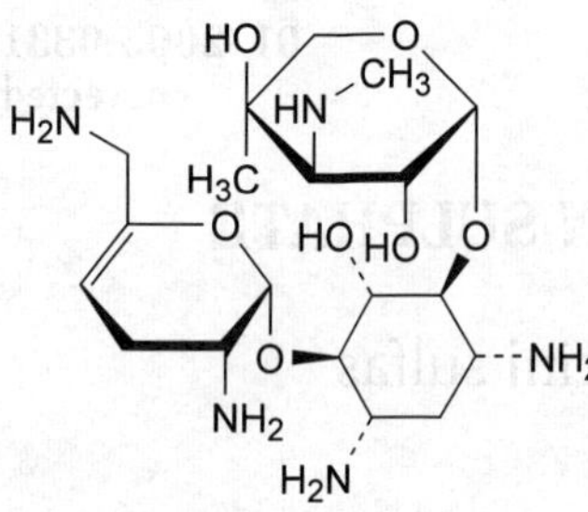

A. 2-deoxy-4-*O*-[3-deoxy-4-*C*-methyl-3-(methylamino)-β-L-arabinopyranosyl]-6-*O*-(2,6-diamino-2,3,4,6-tetradeoxy-α-D-*glycero*-hex-4-enopyranosyl)-L-streptamine (sisomicin),

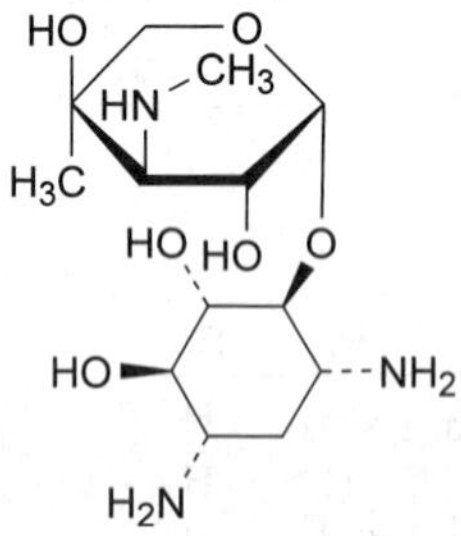

B. 2-deoxy-4-*O*-[3-deoxy-4-*C*-methyl-3-(methylamino)-β-L-arabinopyranosyl]-L-streptamine (garamine),

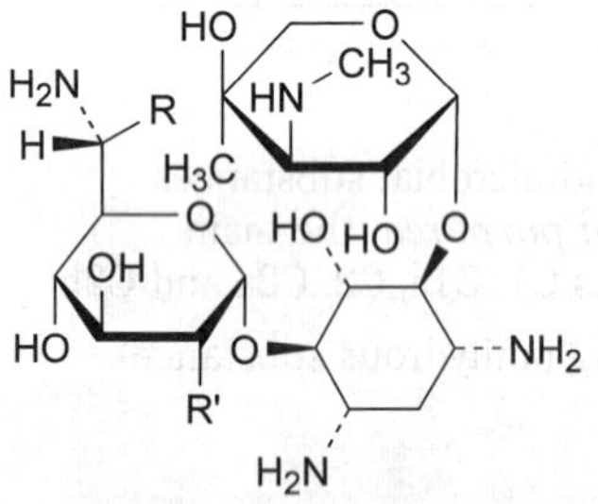

C. R = CH_3, R′ = OH: 4-*O*-(6-amino-6,7-dideoxy-D-*glycero*-α-D-*gluco*-heptopyranosyl)-2-deoxy-6-*O*-[3-deoxy-4-*C*-methyl-3-(methylamino)-β-L-arabinopyranosyl]-D-streptamine (gentamicin B_1),

D. R = H, R′ = NH_2: 2-deoxy-4-*O*-[3-deoxy-4-*C*-methyl-3-(methylamino)-β-L-arabinopyranosyl]-6-*O*-(2,6-diamino-2,6-dideoxy-α-D-*gluco*-hexopyranosyl)-L-streptamine,

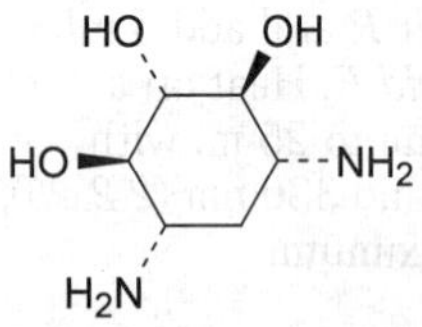

E. 2-deoxystreptamine.

01/2005:0392

GENTIAN ROOT

Gentianae radix

DEFINITION

Dried, fragmented underground organs of *Gentiana lutea* L.

CHARACTERS

Gentian root occurs as single or branched subcylindrical pieces of various lengths and usually 10 mm to 40 mm thick but occasionally up to 80 mm thick at the crown.

Macroscopic and microscopic characters described under identification tests A and B.

Characteristic odour and strong and persistent bitter taste.

IDENTIFICATION

A. The surface is brownish-grey, and the colour of a transverse section is yellowish to reddish-yellow, but not reddish-brown. The root is longitudinally wrinkled and bears occasional rootlet scars. The branches of the rhizome frequently bear a terminal bud and are always encircled by closely arranged leaf scars. The rhizome and root are brittle when dry and break with a short fracture but they absorb moisture readily to become flexible. The smoothed, transversely cut surface shows a bark, occupying about one-third of the radius, separated by the well-marked cambium from an indistinctly radiate and mainly parenchymatous xylem.

B. Reduce to a powder (355). The powder is light brown or yellowish-brown. Examine under a microscope using *chloral hydrate solution R*. The powder shows the following diagnostic characters: fragments of the subero-phellodermic layer, consisting of thin-walled yellowish-brown cork cells and thick-walled collenchyma (phello-derm); fragments of cortical and ligneous parenchymatous cells with moderately thickened walls containing droplets of oil and small prisms and minute needles of calcium oxalate; fragments of lignified vessels with spiral or reticulate thickening.

C. Thin-layer chromatography (*2.2.27*).

Test solution. To 1.0 g of the powdered drug (355) add 25 ml of *methanol R*, shake for 15 min and filter. Evaporate the filtrate to dryness under reduced pressure, at a temperature not exceeding 50 °C. Take up the residue with small quantities of *methanol R* so as to obtain 5 ml of a solution, which may contain a sediment.

Reference solution. Dissolve 5 mg of *phenazone R* and 5 mg of *hyperoside R* in 10 ml of *methanol R*.

Plate: *TLC silica gel F_{254} plate R*.

Mobile phase: *water R, anhydrous formic acid R, ethyl formate R (4:8:88 V/V/V)*.

Application: 20 µl, as bands.

Development: over a path of 8 cm, in an unsaturated tank.

Drying: in air.

Detection A: examine in ultraviolet light at 254 nm.

Results A: see below the sequence of the zones present in the chromatograms obtained with the reference solution and the test solution. Furthermore, other zones may be present in the chromatogram obtained with the test solution.

Top of the plate	
	A prominent quenching zone
Phenazone: a quenching zone	
	A weak quenching zone (amarogentin)
_______	_______
	_______
Hyperoside: a quenching zone	A prominent quenching zone (gentiopicroside)
Reference solution	**Test solution**

Detection B: spray with a 10 per cent *V/V* solution of *potassium hydroxide R* in *methanol R* and then with a freshly prepared 2 g/l solution of *fast blue B salt R* in a mixture of *ethanol R* and *water R* (50:50 *V/V*). Examine in daylight.

Results B: see below the sequence of the zones present in the chromatograms obtained with the reference solution and the test solution. Furthermore, other zones may be present in the chromatogram obtained with the test solution.

Top of the plate	
	A prominent dark violet zone
	A violet-red zone (amarogentin)
_______	_______
_______	_______
Hyperoside: a brownish-red zone	A weak light brown zone (gentiopicroside)
Reference solution	**Test solution**

TESTS

Chromatography. Examine the chromatograms obtained in identification test C, detection B.

Results: the chromatogram obtained with the test solution does not show violet zones immediately above the zone due to amarogentine (other species of *Gentiana*).

Bitterness value (*2.8.15*): minimum 10 000.

Water-soluble extractive: minimum 33 per cent.

To 5.0 g of powdered drug (710) add 200 ml of boiling *water R*. Allow to stand for 10 min, shaking occasionally. Allow to cool, dilute to 200.0 ml with *water R* and filter. Evaporate 20.0 ml of the filtrate to dryness on a water-bath. Dry the residue in an oven at 100-105 °C. The residue weighs a minimum of 0.165 g.

Total ash (*2.4.16*): maximum 6.0 per cent.

01/2005:1870

GENTIAN TINCTURE

Gentianae tinctura

DEFINITION

Tincture produced from *Gentian root (0392)*.

PRODUCTION

The tincture is produced from 1 part of the comminuted drug and 5 parts of ethanol (70 per cent *V/V*) by a suitable procedure.

CHARACTERS

Appearance: yellowish-brown or reddish-brown liquid.

It has a strong bitter taste.

IDENTIFICATION

Thin-layer chromatography (*2.2.27*).

Test solution. The tincture to be examined.

Reference solution. Dissolve 5 mg of *phenazone R* and 5 mg of *hyperoside R* in 10 ml of *methanol R*.

Plate: *TLC silica gel F_{254} plate R* .

Mobile phase: *water R, anhydrous formic acid R, ethyl formate R (4:8:88 V/V/V)*.

Application: 20 µl, as bands.

Development: over a path of 8 cm, in an unsaturated tank.

Drying: in air.

Detection A: examine in ultraviolet light at 254 nm.

Monographs F-H

Results A: see below the sequence of the zones present in the chromatograms obtained with the reference solution and the test solution. Furthermore, other zones may be present in the chromatogram obtained with the test solution.

Top of the plate	
	A prominent quenching zone
Phenazone: a quenching zone	
	A weak quenching zone (amarogentin)
_______	_______
_______	_______
Hyperoside: a quenching zone	A prominent quenching zone (gentiopicroside)
Reference solution	**Test solution**

Detection B: spray with a 10 per cent *V/V* solution of *potassium hydroxide R* in *methanol R* and then with a freshly prepared 2 g/l solution of *fast blue B salt R* in a mixture of *ethanol R* and *water R* (50:50 *V/V*). Examine in daylight.

Results B: see below the sequence of the zones present in the chromatograms obtained with the reference solution and the test solution. Furthermore, other zones may be present in the chromatogram obtained with the test solution.

Top of the plate	
	A prominent dark violet zone
	A violet-red zone (amarogentin)
_______	_______
_______	_______
Hyperoside: a brownish-red zone	A weak light brown zone (gentiopicroside)
Reference solution	**Test solution**

TESTS

Ethanol content (*2.9.10*): 62 per cent *V/V* to 67 per cent *V/V*.

Bitterness value (*2.8.15*): minimum 1000.

Dry residue (*2.8.16*): minimum 5.0 per cent *m/m*, determined on 3.00 g.

01/2005:1522

GINGER

Zingiberis rhizoma

DEFINITION

Ginger consists of the dried, whole or cut rhizome of *Zingiber officinale* Roscoe, with the cork removed, either completely or from the wide flat surfaces only. Whole or cut, it contains not less than 15 ml/kg of essential oil, calculated with reference to the anhydrous drug.

CHARACTERS

Ginger has a characteristic aromatic odour and a spicy and burning taste.

It has the macroscopic and microscopic characters described under identification tests A and B.

IDENTIFICATION

A. The rhizome is laterally compressed, bearing short, flattened, obovate oblique branches on the upper side, each sometimes having a depressed scar at the apex; the whole rhizomes are about 5 cm to 10 cm long, 1.5 cm to 3 cm or 4 cm wide and 1 cm to 1.5 cm thick, sometimes split longitudinally. The scraped rhizome with a light-brown external surface shows longitudinal striations and occasional loose fibres; the outer surface of the unscraped rhizome varies from pale to dark brown and is more or less covered with cork which shows conspicuous, narrow, longitudinal and transverse ridges; the cork readily exfoliates from the lateral surfaces but persists between the branches. The fracture is short and starchy with projecting fibres. The smoothed transversely cut surface exhibits a narrow cortex separated by an endodermis from a much wider stele; it shows numerous, scattered, fibrovascular bundles and abundant scattered oleoresin cells with yellow contents. The unscraped rhizome shows, in addition, an outer layer of dark brown cork.

B. Reduce to a powder (355). The powder is pale yellow to brownish. Examine under a microscope using *chloral hydrate solution R*. The powder shows groups of large, thin-walled, septate fibres, with one wall frequently dentate; fairly large vessels with reticulate thickening and often accompanied by narrow, thin-walled cells containing brown pigment; abundant thin-walled parenchyma of the ground tissue, some cells containing brown oleoresin; fragments of brown cork, usually seen in surface view. Examine under a microscope using a 50 per cent *V/V* solution of *glycerol R*. The powder shows abundant starch granules, simple, flattened, oblong to oval or irregular, up to about 50 µm long and 25 µm wide, with a small point hilum situated at the narrower end; occasional granules show faint, transverse striations.

C. Examine by thin-layer chromatography (*2.2.27*), using a *TLC silica gel plate R*.

Test solution. To 1.0 g of the powdered drug (710) add 5 ml of *methanol R*. Shake for 15 min and filter.

Reference solution. Dissolve 10 µl of *citral R* and 10 mg of *resorcinol R* in 10 ml of *methanol R*. Prepare the solution immediately before use.

Apply to the plate as bands, 20 µl of each solution. Develop over a path of 15 cm in an unsaturated chromatographic tank using a mixture of 40 volumes of *hexane R* and 60 volumes of *ether R*. Allow the plate to dry in air. Spray the plate with a 10 g/l solution of *vanillin R* in *sulphuric acid R* and examine in daylight while heating at 100 °C to 105 °C for 10 min. The chromatogram obtained with the reference solution shows in the lower half an intense red zone (resorcinol) and in the upper half two violet zones (citral). The chromatogram obtained with the test solution shows below the resorcinol zone in the chromatogram obtained with the reference solution two intense violet zones (gingerols) and in the middle, between the resorcinol and citral zones in the chromatogram obtained with the reference solution, two other less intense violet zones (shogaols). Other zones may be present.

TESTS

Foreign matter (*2.8.2*). It complies with the test for foreign matter.

Water (*2.2.13*). Not more than 100 ml/kg, determined by distillation on 20.0 g of the powdered drug (710).

Total ash (*2.4.16*). Not more than 6.0 per cent.

ASSAY

Carry out the determination of essential oils in vegetable drugs (*2.8.12*). Use 20.0 g of the freshly, coarsely powdered drug, a 1000 ml round-bottomed flask, 10 drops of *liquid paraffin R* or other antifoam, 500 ml of *water R* as distillation liquid and 0.5 ml of *xylene R* in the graduated tube. Distil at a rate of 2 ml/min to 3 ml/min for 4 h.

STORAGE

Store protected from light.

01/2005:1828

GINKGO LEAF

Ginkgo folium

DEFINITION

Whole or fragmented, dried leaf of *Ginkgo biloba* L.

Content: not less than 0.5 per cent of flavonoids, calculated as flavone glycosides (M_r 757) (dried drug).

CHARACTERS

Ginkgo leaf is greyish or yellowish-green or yellowish-brown.

Macroscopic and microscopic characters described under identification tests A and B.

IDENTIFICATION

A. The upper surface of ginkgo leaf is slightly darker than the lower surface. The petioles of the leaf are about 4 cm to 9 cm long. The lamina is about 4 cm to 10 cm wide, fan-shaped, usually bilobate or sometimes undivided. Both surfaces are smooth, and the venation dichotomous, the veins appearing to radiate from the base; they are equally prominent on both surfaces. The distal margin is incised, irregularly and to different degrees, and irregularly lobate or emarginate. The lateral margins are entire and taper towards the base.

B. Reduce to a powder (355). The powder is greyish or yellowish-green or yellowish-brown. Examine under a microscope using *chloral hydrate solution R*. The powder shows irregularly-shaped fragments of the lamina in surface view, the upper epidermis consisting of elongated cells with irregularly sinuous walls, the lower epidermal cells smaller, with a finely striated cuticle and each cell shortly papillose; stomata about 60 µm, large, deeply sunken with 6 to 8 subsidiary cells, are more numerous in the lower epidermis; abundant large cluster crystals of calcium oxalate of various sizes in the mesophyll; fragments of fibro-vascular tissue from the petiole and veins.

C. Thin-layer chromatography (*2.2.27*).

Test solution. To 2.0 g of the powdered drug (710) add 10 ml of *methanol R*. Heat in a water-bath at 65 °C for 10 min. Shake frequently. Allow to cool to room temperature and filter.

Reference solution. Dissolve 1.0 mg of *chlorogenic acid R* and 3.0 mg of *rutin R* in 20 ml of *methanol R*.

Plate: *TLC silica gel plate R*.

Mobile phase: *anhydrous formic acid R, glacial acetic acid R, water R, ethyl acetate R* (7.5:7.5:17.5:67.5 *V/V/V/V*).

Application: 20 µl, as bands.

Development: over a path of 17 cm.

Drying: at 100-105 °C.

Detection: spray the warm plate with a 10 g/l solution of *diphenylboric acid aminoethyl ester R* in *methanol R*. Subsequently spray with the same volume of a 50 g/l solution of *macrogol 400 R* in *methanol R*. Allow the plate to dry in air for about 30 min. Examine in ultraviolet light at 365 nm.

Results: see below the sequence of the zones present in the chromatograms obtained with the reference and test solutions. Furthermore, other weaker fluorescent zones may be present in the chromatogram obtained with the test solution.

Top of the plate	
	A yellowish-brown fluorescent zone
	A green fluorescent zone
	2 yellowish-brown fluorescent zones
	An intense light blue fluorescent zone sometimes overlapped by a greenish-brown fluorescent zone
Chlorogenic acid: a light blue fluorescent zone	
	A green fluorescent zone
Rutin: a yellowish-brown fluorescent zone	2 yellowish-brown fluorescent zones
	A green fluorescent zone
	A yellowish-brown fluorescent zone
Reference solution	**Test solution**

TESTS

Foreign matter (*2.8.2*): maximum 5 per cent of stems and 2 per cent of other foreign matter.

Loss on drying (*2.2.32*): maximum 11.0 per cent, determined on 1.000 g of the powdered drug (355) by drying in an oven at 100-105 °C for 2 h.

Total ash (*2.4.16*): maximum 11.0 per cent.

ASSAY

Flavonoids. Liquid chromatography (*2.2.29*).

Test solution. Heat 2.500 g of the powdered drug (710) in 50 ml of a 60 per cent *V/V* solution of *acetone R* under a reflux condenser for 30 min. Filter and collect the filtrate. Extract the drug residue a second time in the same manner, using 40 ml of a 60 per cent *V/V* solution of *acetone R* and filter. Collect the filtrates and dilute to 100.0 ml with a 60 per cent *V/V* solution of *acetone R*. Evaporate 50.0 ml of the solution to eliminate the acetone and transfer to a 50.0 ml vial, rinsing with 30 ml of *methanol R*. Add 4.4 ml of *hydrochloric acid R1*, dilute to 50.0 ml with *water R* and centrifuge. Place 10 ml of the supernatant liquid in a 10 ml brown-glass vial. Close with a rubber seal and an aluminium cap and heat on a water-bath for 25 min. Allow to cool to room temperature.

Reference solution. Dissolve 10.0 mg of *quercetin dihydrate R* in 20 ml of *methanol R*. Add 15.0 ml of *dilute hydrochloric acid R* and 5 ml of *water R* and dilute to 50.0 ml with *methanol R*.

Column:

- *stationary phase*: *octadecylsilyl silica gel for chromatography R* (5 µm),
- *size*: l = 0.125 m, Ø = 4 mm,
- *temperature*: 25 °C.

Mobile phase:

- *mobile phase A*: 0.3 g/l solution of *phosphoric acid R* adjusted to pH 2.0,
- *mobile phase B*: *methanol R*,

Time (min)	Mobile phase A (per cent V/V)	Mobile phase B (per cent V/V)
0 - 1	60	40
1 - 20	60 → 45	40 → 55
20 - 21	45 → 0	55 → 100
21 - 25	0	100

Flow rate: 1.0 ml/min.

Detector: spectrophotometer at 370 nm.

Injection: 10 μl.

Relative retention with reference to quercetin (retention time = about 12.5 min): kaempferol = about 1.4; isorhamnetin= about 1.5.

System suitability:

– *resolution*: minimum 1.5 between the peaks due to kaempferol and to isorhamnetin.

Do not take into account peaks eluting before the quercetin peak or after the isorhamnetin peak in the chromatogram obtained with the test solution.

Calculate the percentage content of flavonoids, expressed as flavone glycosides, from the expression:

$$2 \times \frac{F_1 \times m_1 \times 2.514 \times p}{F_2 \times m_2}$$

F_1 = sum of the areas of all the considered peaks in the chromatogram obtained with the test solution,

F_2 = area of the peak corresponding to quercetin in the chromatogram obtained with the reference solution,

m_1 = mass of quercetin used to prepare the reference solution, in grams,

m_2 = mass of the drug to be examined used to prepare the test solution, in grams,

p = percentage content of anhydrous quercetin in *quercetin dihydrate R*.

01/2005:1523

GINSENG

Ginseng radix

DEFINITION

Ginseng consists of the whole or cut dried root of *Panax ginseng* C. A. Meyer. It contains not less than 0.40 per cent of combined ginsenosides Rg1($C_{42}H_{72}O_{14}$,$2H_2O$; M_r 837) and Rb1 ($C_{54}H_{92}O_{23}$,$3H_2O$; M_r 1163), calculated with reference to the dried drug.

CHARACTERS

It has the macroscopic and microscopic characters described under identification tests A and B.

IDENTIFICATION

A. The principal root is fusiform or cylindrical, sometimes branched, up to about 20 cm long and 2.5 cm in diameter, and may be curved or markedly re-curved. The surface is pale yellow to cream and shows longitudinal ridges; stem scars may be seen at the crown. The fracture is short. The transversely-cut surface shows a wide outer zone with scattered orange-red resin canals and a finely radiate inner region. The rootlets, numerous in the lower part, are fine with a small diameter.

B. Reduce to a powder (355). Examine under a microscope using *chloral hydrate solution R*. The light yellow powder shows abundant fragments of thin-walled parenchymatous cells and fragments of large secretory canals containing yellowish-brown resin. The powder occasionally shows non-lignified tracheids and partially-lignified vessels with spiral or reticulate thickening, occurring singly or in small groups, and scattered cluster crystals of calcium oxalate. Examine under a microscope using a mixture of equal volumes of *glycerol R* and *water R*. The starch granules are very abundant, simple or two or three compound, and range from 1 μm to 10 μm in diameter.

C. Examine by thin-layer chromatography (*2.2.27*), using a *TLC silica gel plate R*.

Test solution. Boil 1.0 g of the powdered drug (355) under a reflux condenser with 10 ml of a 70 per cent *V/V* solution of *methanol R* for 15 min. Filter after cooling and dilute to 10.0 ml with *methanol R*.

Reference solution. Dissolve 5.0 mg of *aescin R* and 5.0 mg of *arbutin R* in 1 ml of *methanol R*.

Apply to the plate as bands 20 μl of each solution. Develop over a path of 10 cm, in an unsaturated tank, using the upper layer of a mixture of 25 ml of *ethyl acetate R*, 50 ml of *water R* and 100 ml of *butanol R*, which has been allowed to separate for 10 min. Allow the plate to dry in air. Spray with *anisaldehyde solution R* and heat at 105 °C to 110 °C for 5 min to 10 min. Examine in daylight. The chromatogram obtained with the reference solution shows in the upper third a brown zone corresponding to arbutin, and in the lower third a grey zone corresponding to aescin. Between these two zones, a little below the zone corresponding to arbutin in the chromatogram obtained with the reference solution, the chromatogram obtained with the test solution shows two violet-grey zones due to ginsenoside Rg1 (upper zone) and to ginsenoside Re (lower zone). The violet-grey zone due to ginsenoside Rb1 is similar in position to the grey zone due to aescin in the chromatogram obtained with the reference solution. Between the zones corresponding to ginsenoside Rb1 and Re other, less intense, bands are present; the zone closest to the starting point corresponds to ginsenoside Rc. Other zones are visible in the lower third of the chromatogram.

TESTS

Foreign matter (*2.8.2*). It complies with the test for foreign matter.

Panax quinquefolium. Examine the chromatograms obtained in the assay. The chromatogram obtained with the test solution shows the peak corresponding to ginsenoside Rf. In the case of a substitution by *Panax quinquefolium* no peak corresponding to ginsenoside Rf is present.

Loss on drying (*2.2.32*). Not more than 10.0 per cent, determined on 1.000 g of the powdered drug (355) by drying in an oven at 100 °C to 105 °C.

Total ash (*2.4.16*). Not more than 7.0 per cent.

Ash insoluble in hydrochloric acid (*2.8.1*). Not more than 1.0 per cent.

ASSAY

Examine by liquid chromatography (*2.2.29*).

Test solution. Reduce about 50 g to a powder (355). Place 1.00 g of the powdered drug and 70 ml of a 50 per cent *V/V* solution of *methanol R* in a 250 ml round-bottomed flask. After adding a few grains of pumice, boil on a water-bath under a reflux condenser for 1 h. After cooling, centrifuge and collect the supernatant liquid. Treat the residue as described above. Mix the collected liquids and evaporate to dryness under reduced pressure at a temperature not exceeding 60 °C. Take up the residue with 10 ml of a buffer solution containing 3.5 g of *sodium dihydrogen phosphate R* and 7.2 g of *potassium dihydrogen phosphate R* in 1000 ml of *water R* (solution A).

Wash a cartridge containing about 360 mg of a suitable *octadecylsilyl silica gel for chromatography R* with 5 ml of *methanol R* followed by 20 ml of *water R*. Apply 5 ml of solution A to the cartridge. Elute with 20 ml of *water R*, followed by 15 ml of a 30 per cent *V/V* solution of *methanol R*. Discard the eluates. Elute with 20 ml of *methanol R*. Evaporate the eluate to dryness and take up the residue with 2 ml of *methanol R*. Discard the eluates after checking that no ginsenosides are present, otherwise repeat the assay with a cartridge from a different manufacturer.

Reference solution. Dissolve 3.0 mg of *ginsenoside Rb1 R*, 3.0 mg of *ginsenoside Rg1 R* and 3.0 mg of *ginsenoside Rf R*, accurately weighed, in *methanol R* and dilute to 10 ml with the same solvent.

The chromatographic procedure may be carried out using:
- a stainless steel column 0.10 m long and 4.6 mm in internal diameter packed with *aminopropylsilyl silica gel for chromatography R*,
- as mobile phase at a flow rate of 2 ml/min:
  Mobile phase A. Acetonitrile R,
  Mobile phase B. Water R,

Time (min)	Mobile phase A (per cent *V/V*)	Mobile phase B (per cent *V/V*)
0 - 14	90	10
14 - 18	90 → 80	10 → 20
18 - 55	80	20
55 - 60	90	10

- a 20 µl loop injector,
- as detector a spectrophotometer set at 203 nm.

Inject the reference solution and adjust the sensitivity of the system so that the heights of the peaks due to ginsenosides are about 50 per cent of the full scale of the recorder. The test is not valid unless the resolution between the peaks corresponding to ginsenoside Rf and ginsenoside Rg1 is at least 1.0.

Inject the test solution.

Calculate the percentage content of ginsenosides Rb1 and Rg1 from the expression:

$$\frac{A_1 \times m_2 \times 40}{m_1 \times A_{\mathrm{Rb1}}} + \frac{A_2 \times m_3 \times 40}{m_1 \times A_{\mathrm{Rg1}}}$$

A_1 = area of the peak due to ginsenoside Rb1 in the chromatogram obtained with the test solution,

A_2 = area of the peak due to ginsenoside Rg1 in the chromatogram obtained with the test solution,

A_{Rb1} = area of the peak due to ginsenoside Rb1 in the chromatogram obtained with the reference solution,

A_{Rg1} = area of the peak due to ginsenoside Rg1 in the chromatogram obtained with the reference solution,

m_1 = mass of the drug to be examined, in grams,

m_2 = mass of ginsenoside Rb1, in grams,

m_3 = mass of ginsenoside Rg1, in grams.

STORAGE

Store protected from light.

01/2005:0718

GLIBENCLAMIDE

Glibenclamidum

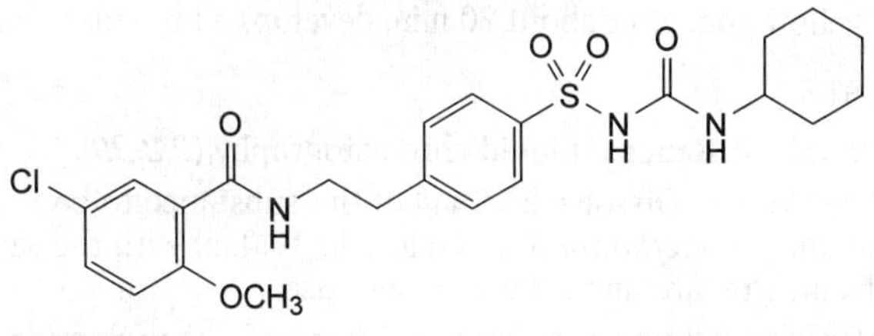

$C_{23}H_{28}ClN_3O_5S$ M_r 494.0

DEFINITION

1-[[4-[2-[(5-Chloro-2-methoxybenzoyl)amino]ethyl]phenyl]sulphonyl]-3-cyclohexylurea.

Content: 99.0 per cent to 101.0 per cent (dried substance).

CHARACTERS

Appearance: white or almost white, crystalline powder.

Solubility: practically insoluble in water, sparingly soluble in methylene chloride, slightly soluble in alcohol and in methanol.

IDENTIFICATION

First identification: A, C.

Second identification: A, B, D, E.

A. Melting point (*2.2.14*): 169 °C to 174 °C.

B. Dissolve 50.0 mg in *methanol R*, with the aid of ultrasound if necessary, and dilute to 50.0 ml with the same solvent. To 10.0 ml of the solution add 1.0 ml of a 103 g/l solution of *hydrochloric acid R* and dilute to 100.0 ml with *methanol R*. Examined between 230 nm and 350 nm (*2.2.25*), the solution shows an absorption maximum at 300 nm and a less intense maximum at 275 nm. The specific absorbances at the maxima are 61 to 65 and 27 to 32, respectively.

C. Infrared absorption spectrophotometry (*2.2.24*).
Preparation: discs of *potassium bromide R*.
Comparison: *glibenclamide CRS*.
If the spectra obtained show differences, moisten separately the substance to be examined and the reference substance with *methanol R*, triturate, dry at 100-105 °C and record the spectra again.

D. Thin-layer chromatography (*2.2.27*).
Test solution. Dissolve 10 mg of the substance to be examined in a mixture of equal volumes of *methanol R* and *methylene chloride R* and dilute to 10 ml with the same mixture of solvents.
Reference solution. Dissolve 10 mg of *glibenclamide CRS* in a mixture of equal volumes of *methanol R* and *methylene chloride R* and dilute to 10 ml with the same mixture of solvents.
Plate: *TLC silica gel GF_{254} plate R.*
Mobile phase: *alcohol R, glacial acetic acid R, cyclohexane R, methylene chloride R* (5:5:45:45 *V/V/V/V*).
Application: 10 µl.
Development: over a path of 10 cm.
Drying: in air.

Monographs F-H

Detection: examine in ultraviolet light at 254 nm.

Results: the principal spot in the chromatogram obtained with the test solution is similar in position and size to the principal spot in the chromatogram obtained with the reference solution.

E. Dissolve 20 mg in 2 ml of *sulphuric acid R*. The solution is colourless and shows blue fluorescence in ultraviolet light at 365 nm. Dissolve 0.1 g of *chloral hydrate R* in the solution. Within about 5 min, the colour changes to deep yellow and, after about 20 min, develops a brownish tinge.

TESTS

Related substances. Liquid chromatography (*2.2.29*).

Test solution. Dissolve 25.0 mg of the substance to be examined in *methanol R* and dilute to 10.0 ml with the same solvent. Prepare immediately before use.

Reference solution (a). Dissolve 5.0 mg of *glibenclamide impurity A CRS* and 5.0 mg of *glibenclamide impurity B CRS* in *methanol R* and dilute to 100.0 ml with the same solvent. Dilute 5.0 ml of the solution to 20.0 ml with *methanol R*.

Reference solution (b). Dilute 2.0 ml of the test solution to 100.0 ml with *methanol R*. Dilute 5.0 ml of this solution to 50.0 ml with *methanol R*.

Reference solution (c). Dissolve 5 mg of *gliclazide CRS* in *methanol R*, add 2 ml of the test solution and dilute to 100 ml with *methanol R*. Dilute 1 ml of this solution to 10 ml with *methanol R*.

Column:
- *size*: *l* = 0.10 m, Ø = 4.6 mm,
- *stationary phase*: spherical *base-deactivated end-capped octadecylsilyl silica gel for chromatography R* (3 μm),
- *temperature*: 35 °C.

Mobile phase:
- *mobile phase A*: mix 20 ml of a 101.8 g/l solution of freshly distilled *triethylamine R* adjusted to pH 3.0 using *phosphoric acid R*, and 50 ml of *acetonitrile R*; dilute to 1000 ml with *water R*,
- *mobile phase B*: mobile phase A, *water R*, *acetonitrile R* (20:65:915 *V/V/V*),

Time (min)	Mobile phase A (per cent *V/V*)	Mobile phase B (per cent *V/V*)
0 - 15	45	55
15 - 30	45 → 5	55 → 95
30 - 40	5	95
40 - 41	5 → 45	95 → 55
41 - 55	45	55

Flow rate: 0.8 ml/min.

Detection: spectrophotometer at 230 nm.

Injection: 10 μl.

Relative retention with reference to glibenclamide (retention time = about 5 min): impurity A = about 0.5; impurity B = about 0.6.

System suitability: reference solution (c):
- *resolution*: minimum 5.0 between the peaks due to glibenclamide and gliclazide.

Limits:
- *impurity A*: not more than the area of the corresponding peak in the chromatogram obtained with reference solution (a) (0.5 per cent),
- *impurity B*: not more than the area of the corresponding peak in the chromatogram obtained with reference solution (a) (0.5 per cent),
- *any other impurity*: not more than the area of the principal peak in the chromatogram obtained with reference solution (b) (0.2 per cent), and not more than 2 such peaks have an area greater than half the area of the principal peak in the chromatogram obtained with reference solution (b) (0.1 per cent),
- *total of other impurities*: not more than 2.5 times the area of the principal peak in the chromatogram obtained with reference solution (b) (0.5 per cent),
- *disregard limit*: 0.25 times the area of the principal peak in the chromatogram obtained with reference solution (b) (0.05 per cent).

Heavy metals (*2.4.8*): maximum 20 ppm.

1.0 g complies with limit test D. Prepare the standard using 2 ml of *lead standard solution (10 ppm Pb) R*.

Loss on drying (*2.2.32*): maximum 1.0 per cent, determined on 1.000 g by drying in an oven at 100-105 °C.

Sulphated ash (*2.4.14*): maximum 0.1 per cent, determined on 1.0 g.

ASSAY

Dissolve 0.400 g with heating in 100 ml of *alcohol R*. Titrate with *0.1 M sodium hydroxide*, using 1.0 ml of *phenolphthalein solution R* as indicator, until a pink colour is obtained.

1 ml of *0.1 M sodium hydroxide* is equivalent to 49.40 mg of $C_{23}H_{28}ClN_3O_5S$.

IMPURITIES

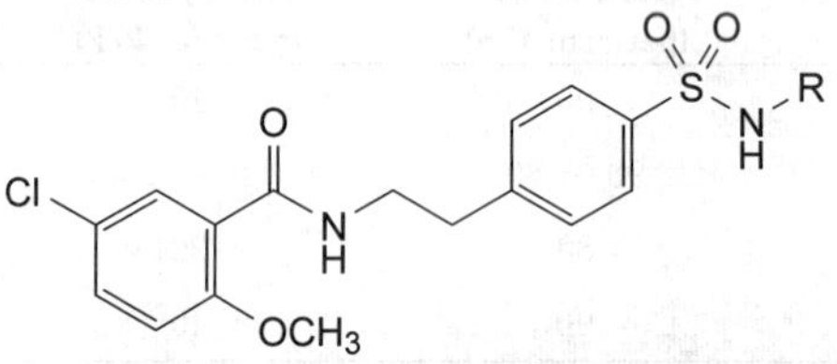

A. R = H: 5-chloro-2-methoxy-*N*-[2-(4-sulphamoylphenyl)ethyl]benzamide,

B. R = CO-OCH$_3$: methyl [[4-[2-[(5-chloro-2-methoxybenzoyl)amino]ethyl]phenyl]sulphonyl]carbamate.

01/2005:1524

GLICLAZIDE

Gliclazidum

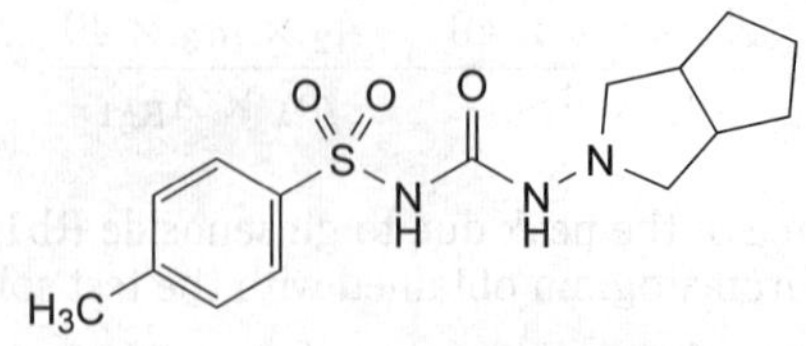

$C_{15}H_{21}N_3O_3S$ M_r 323.4

DEFINITION

Gliclazide contains not less than 99.0 per cent and not more than the equivalent of 101.0 per cent of 1-(hexahydrocyclopenta[*c*]pyrrol-2(1*H*)-yl)-3-[(4-methylphenyl)sulphonyl]urea, calculated with reference to the dried substance.

CHARACTERS

A white or almost white powder, practically insoluble in water, freely soluble in methylene chloride, sparingly soluble in acetone, slightly soluble in alcohol.

IDENTIFICATION

Examine by infrared absorption spectrophotometry (*2.2.24*), comparing with the spectrum obtained with *gliclazide CRS*. Examine the substances prepared as discs.

TESTS

Related substances. Examine by liquid chromatography (*2.2.29*). *Prepare the solutions immediately before use.*

Test solution. Dissolve 50.0 mg of the substance to be examined in 23 ml of *acetonitrile R* and dilute to 50.0 ml with *water R*.

Reference solution (a). Dilute 1.0 ml of the test solution to 100.0 ml with a mixture of 45 volumes of *acetonitrile R* and 55 volumes of *water R*. Dilute 10.0 ml of the solution to 100.0 ml with a mixture of 45 volumes of *acetonitrile R* and 55 volumes of *water R*.

Reference solution (b). Dissolve 5 mg of the substance to be examined and 15 mg of *gliclazide impurity F CRS* in 23 ml of *acetonitrile R* and dilute to 50 ml with *water R*. Dilute 1 ml of the solution to 20 ml with a mixture of 45 volumes of *acetonitrile R* and 55 volumes of *water R*.

Reference solution (c). Dissolve 10.0 mg of *gliclazide impurity F CRS* in 45 ml of *acetonitrile R* and dilute to 100.0 ml with *water R*. Dilute 1.0 ml of the solution to 100.0 ml with a mixture of 45 volumes of *acetonitrile R* and 55 volumes of *water R*.

The chromatographic procedure may be carried out using:

- a stainless steel column 0.25 m long and 4 mm in internal diameter packed with *octylsilyl silica gel for chromatography R* (5 µm),
- as mobile phase at a flow rate of 0.9 ml/min a mixture of 0.1 volumes of *triethylamine R*, 0.1 volumes of *trifluoroacetic acid R*, 45 volumes of *acetonitrile R* and 55 volumes of *water R*,
- as detector a spectrophotometer set at 235 nm.

Inject 20 µl of reference solution (b). Adjust the sensitivity of the system so that the heights of the 2 principal peaks in the chromatogram obtained with reference solution (b) are at least 50 per cent of the full scale of the recorder. The test is not valid unless in the chromatogram obtained the resolution between the two principal peaks is at least 1.8.

Inject 20 µl of the test solution and 20 µl each of reference solutions (a) and (c). Continue the chromatography of the test solution for twice the retention time of gliclazide. In the chromatogram obtained with the test solution: the area of any peak corresponding to impurity F is not greater than the area of the corresponding peak in the chromatogram obtained with reference solution (c) (0.1 per cent); the area of any peaks, apart from the principal peak and the peak due to impurity F, is not greater than the area of the principal peak in the chromatogram obtained with reference solution (a) (0.1 per cent); the sum of the areas of any such peaks is not greater than twice the area of the principal peak in the chromatogram obtained with reference solution (a) (0.2 per cent). Disregard any peak with an area less than 0.2 times that of the principal peak in the chromatogram obtained with reference solution (a).

Impurity B. Examine by liquid chromatography (*2.2.29*) as described in the test for related substances.

Test solution. Dissolve 0.400 g in 2.5 ml of *dimethyl sulphoxide R* and dilute to 10.0 ml with *water R*. Stir for 10 min, store at 4 °C for 30 min and filter.

Reference solution (a). Dissolve 20.0 mg of *gliclazide impurity B CRS* in *dimethyl sulphoxide R* and dilute to 100.0 ml with the same solvent. To 1.0 ml of the solution, add 12 ml of *dimethyl sulphoxide R* and dilute to 50.0 ml with *water R*.

Reference solution (b). To 1.0 ml of reference solution (a), add 12 ml of *dimethyl sulphoxide R* and dilute to 50.0 ml with *water R*.

Inject 50 µl of the test solution and 50 µl of reference solution (b). In the chromatogram obtained with the test solution, the area of any peak corresponding to impurity B is not greater than the area of the corresponding peak in the chromatogram obtained with reference solution (b) (2 ppm).

Heavy metals (*2.4.8*). 1.5 g complies with limit test F for heavy metals (10 ppm). Prepare the standard using 1.5 ml of *lead standard solution (10 ppm Pb) R*.

Loss on drying (*2.2.32*). Not more than 0.25 per cent, determined on 1.000 g by drying in an oven at 100 °C to 105 °C for 2 h.

Sulphated ash (*2.4.14*). Not more than 0.1 per cent, determined on 1.0 g.

ASSAY

Dissolve 0.250 g in 50 ml of *anhydrous acetic acid R*. Titrate with *0.1 M perchloric acid*, determining the end-point potentiometrically (*2.2.20*).

1 ml of *0.1 M perchloric acid* is equivalent to 32.34 mg of $C_{15}H_{21}N_3O_3S$.

IMPURITIES

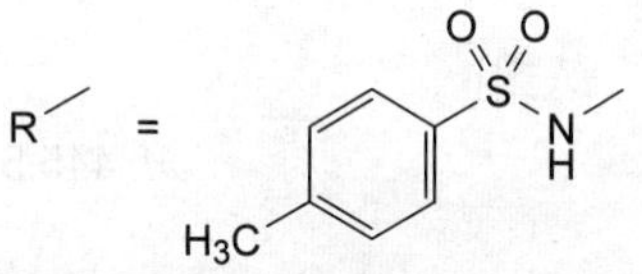

A. R-H: 4-methylbenzenesulphonamide,

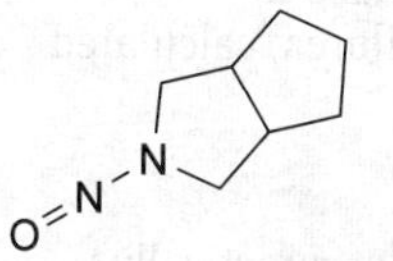

B. 2-nitroso-octahydrocyclopenta[*c*]pyrrole,

C. R-CO-O-C_2H_5: ethyl [(4-methylphenyl)sulphonyl]carbamate,

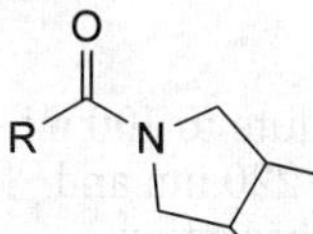

D. *N*-[(4-methylphenyl)sulphonyl]hexahydrocyclopenta[*c*]pyrrol-2(1*H*)-carboxamide,

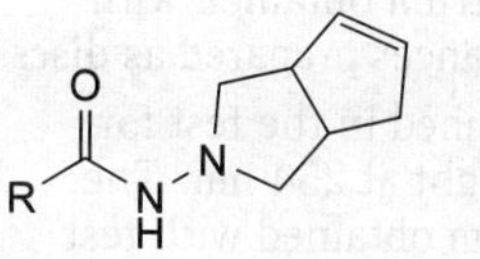

E. 1-[(4-methylphenyl)sulphonyl]-3-(3,3a,4,6a-tetrahydrocyclopenta[*c*]pyrrol-2(1*H*)-yl)urea,

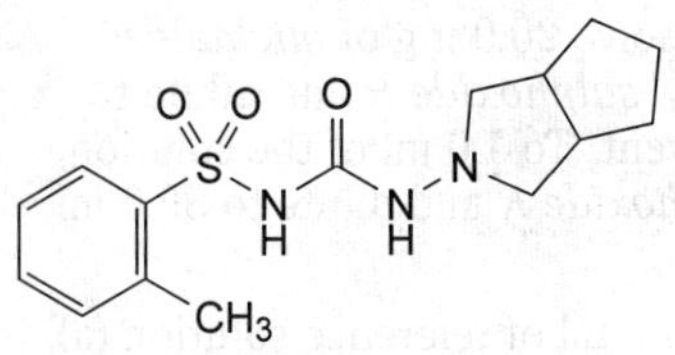

F. 1-(hexahydrocyclopenta[*c*]pyrrol-2(1*H*)-yl)-3-[(2-methylphenyl)sulphonyl]urea,

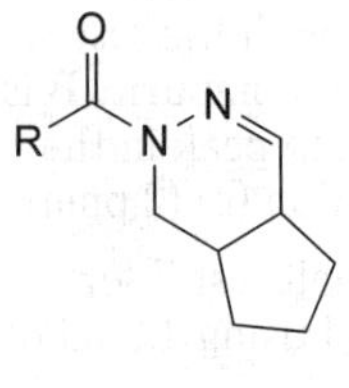

G. *N*-[(4-methylphenyl)sulphonyl]-1,4a,5,6,7,7a-hexahydro-2*H*-cyclopenta[*d*]pyridazine-2-carboxamide.

01/2005:0906

GLIPIZIDE

Glipizidum

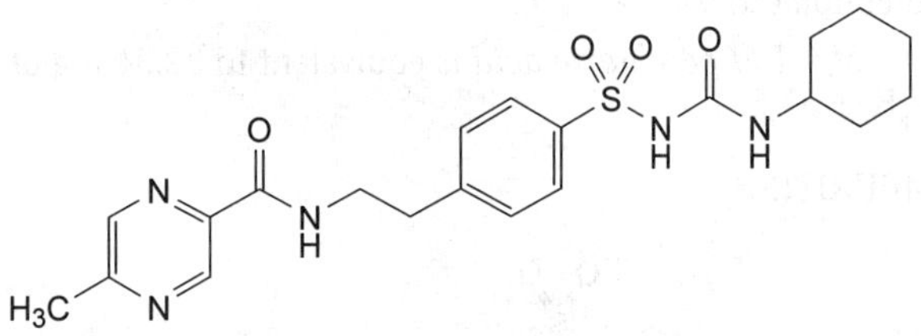

$C_{21}H_{27}N_5O_4S$ M_r 445.5

DEFINITION

Glipizide contains not less than 98.0 per cent and not more than the equivalent of 102.0 per cent of 1-cyclohexyl-3-[[4-[2-[[(5-methylpyrazin-2-yl)carbonyl]amino]ethyl]phenyl]sulphonyl]urea, calculated with reference to the dried substance.

CHARACTERS

A white or almost white, crystalline powder, practically insoluble in water, soluble in methylene chloride, sparingly soluble in acetone, practically insoluble in alcohol. It dissolves in dilute solutions of alkali hydroxides.

IDENTIFICATION

First identification: B.

Second identification: A, C, D.

A. Dissolve about 2 mg in *methanol R* and dilute to 100 ml with the same solvent. Examined between 220 nm and 350 nm (*2.2.25*), the solution shows two absorption maxima, at 226 nm and 274 nm. The ratio of the absorbance measured at the maximum of 226 nm to that measured at the maximum at 274 nm is 2.0 to 2.4.

B. Examine by infrared absorption spectrophotometry (*2.2.24*), comparing with the spectrum obtained with *glipizide CRS*. Examine the substances prepared as discs.

C. Examine the chromatograms obtained in the test for related substances in ultraviolet light at 254 nm. The principal spot in the chromatogram obtained with test solution (b) is similar in position and size to the principal spot in the chromatogram obtained with reference solution (a).

D. Dissolve 50 mg in 5 ml of *dioxan R*. Add 1 ml of a 5 g/l solution of *fluorodinitrobenzene R* in *dioxan R* and boil for 2-3 min. A yellow colour is produced.

TESTS

Related substances. Examine by thin-layer chromatography (*2.2.27*), using *silica gel* GF_{254} *R* as the coating substance.

Test solution (a). Dissolve 0.20 g of the substance to be examined in a mixture of equal volumes of *methanol R* and of *methylene chloride R* and dilute to 10 ml with the same mixture of solvents.

Test solution (b). Dilute 1 ml of test solution (a) to 20 ml with a mixture of equal volumes of *methanol R* and *methylene chloride R*.

Reference solution (a). Dissolve 10 mg of *glipizide CRS* in a mixture of equal volumes of *methanol R* and *methylene chloride R* and dilute to 10 ml with the same mixture of solvents.

Reference solution (b). Dissolve 5 mg of *glipizide impurity A CRS* in a mixture of equal volumes of *methanol R* and *methylene chloride R* and dilute to 50 ml with the same mixture of solvents.

Reference solution (c). Dilute 0.5 ml of test solution (a) to 100 ml with a mixture of equal volumes of *methanol R* and *methylene chloride R*.

Reference solution (d). Dilute 4 ml of reference solution (c) to 10 ml with a mixture of equal volumes of *methanol R* and *methylene chloride R*.

Reference solution (e). Dilute 5 ml of test solution (a) to 10 ml with reference solution (b).

Apply to the plate 10 µl of each solution. Develop over a path of 15 cm using a mixture of 25 volumes of *anhydrous formic acid R*, 25 volumes of *ethyl acetate R* and 50 volumes of *methylene chloride R*. Allow the plate to dry in air and examine in ultraviolet light at 254 nm. In the chromatogram obtained with test solution (a): any spot corresponding to glipizide impurity A is not more intense than the spot in the chromatogram obtained with reference solution (b) (0.5 per cent); any spot apart from the principal spot and the spot corresponding to glipizide impurity A is not more intense than the spot in the chromatogram obtained with reference solution (c) (0.5 per cent) and not more than two such spots are more intense than the spot in the chromatogram obtained with reference solution (d) (0.2 per cent). The test is not valid unless the chromatogram obtained with reference solution (e) shows two clearly separated spots.

Cyclohexylamine. Not more than 100 ppm, determined by gas chromatography (*2.2.28*), using *decane R* as internal standard.

Internal standard solution. Dissolve 25 mg of *decane R* in *hexane R* and dilute to 100 ml with the same solvent. Dilute 5 ml of this solution to 50 ml with *hexane R*.

Test solution (a). Dissolve 3.0 g of the substance to be examined in 50 ml of a 12 g/l solution of *sodium hydroxide R* and shake with two quantities, each of 5.0 ml, of *hexane R*. Use the combined upper layers.

Test solution (b). Dissolve 3.0 g of the substance to be examined in 50 ml of a 12 g/l solution of *sodium hydroxide R* and shake with two quantities, each of 5.0 ml, of the internal standard solution. Use the combined upper layers.

Reference solution. Dissolve 30.0 mg of *cyclohexylamine R* in a 17.5 g/l solution of *hydrochloric acid R* and dilute to 100.0 ml with the same acid. To 1.0 ml of this solution add 50 ml of a 12 g/l solution of *sodium hydroxide R* and shake with two quantities, each of 5.0 ml, of the internal standard solution. Use the combined upper layers.

Monographs F-H

The chromatographic procedure may be carried out using:

- a glass column 1.5 m long and 4 mm in internal diameter packed with *silanised diatomaceous earth for gas chromatography R* impregnated with 10 per cent *m/m* of *macrogol 20 000 R* and 4 per cent *m/m* of *potassium hydroxide R,*
- *nitrogen for chromatography R* as the carrier gas at a flow rate of 30 ml/min,
- a flame-ionisation detector,

maintaining the temperature of the column at 80 °C and that of the injection port and of the detector at 120 °C.

Inject 1 µl of the reference solution and adjust the sensitivity of the detector so that the heights of the first peak (decane) and the second peak (cyclohexylamine) are not less than 50 per cent of the full scale of the recorder. The test is not valid unless the resolution between these two peaks is at least 2. Inject 1 µl of test solution (a). In the chromatogram obtained, verify that there is no peak with the same retention time as that of the internal standard. Inject separately 1 µl of test solution (b) and 1 µl of the reference solution. From the chromatogram obtained with the reference solution, calculate the ratio (*R*) of the area of the peak due to cyclohexylamine to the area of the peak due to the internal standard. From the chromatogram obtained with test solution (b), calculate the ratio of the area of any peak corresponding to cyclohexylamine to the area of the peak due to the internal standard: this ratio is not greater than *R*.

Heavy metals (*2.4.8*). 2.0 g complies with limit test C for heavy metals (20 ppm). Prepare the standard using 4 ml of *lead standard solution (10 ppm Pb) R.*

Loss on drying (*2.2.32*). Not more than 0.5 per cent, determined on 1.000 g by drying in an oven at 100-105 °C.

Sulphated ash (*2.4.14*). Not more than 0.2 per cent, determined on 1.0 g.

ASSAY

Dissolve 0.400 g in 50 ml of *dimethylformamide R.* Titrate with *0.1 M lithium methoxide* using 0.2 ml of *quinaldine red solution R* as indicator until the colour changes from red to colourless.

1 ml of *0.1 M lithium methoxide* is equivalent to 44.55 mg of $C_{21}H_{27}N_5O_4S$.

IMPURITIES

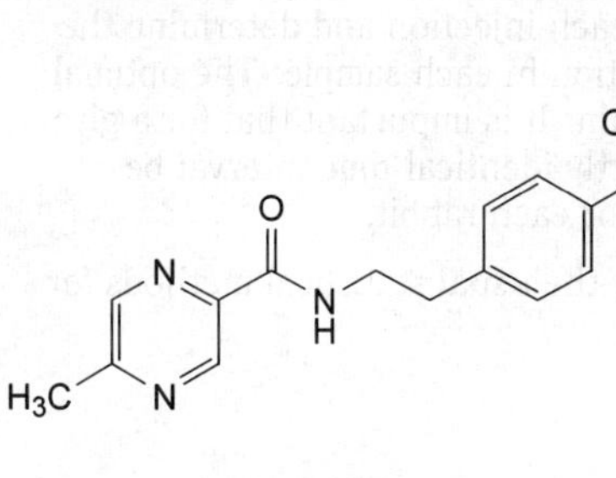

A. 5-methyl-*N*-[2-(4-sulphamoylphenyl)ethyl]pyrazine-2-carboxamide,

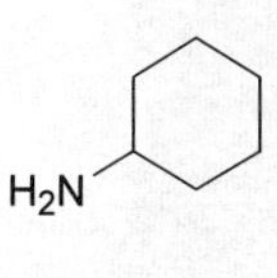

B. cyclohexanamine.

01/2005:0612

GLUCAGON

Glucagonum

H-His–Ser–Gln–Gly–Thr–Phe–Thr–Ser–Asp–Tyr–(10)
Ser–Lys–Tyr–Leu–Asp–Ser–Arg–Arg–Ala–Gln–(20)
Asp–Phe–Val–Gln–Trp–Leu–Met–Asn–Thr–OH

$C_{153}H_{225}N_{43}O_{49}S$ M_r 3482

DEFINITION

Glucagon is a polypeptide hormone obtained from beef or pork pancreas and which increases the blood-glucose concentration by promoting rapid breakdown of liver glycogen. The potency is not less than 1 IU/mg, calculated with reference to the dried substance. Glucagon is prepared in conditions designed to minimise microbial contamination.

CHARACTERS

A white or almost white powder, practically insoluble in water and in most organic solvents. It dissolves in dilute mineral acids and in dilute solutions of the alkali hydroxides.

IDENTIFICATION

A. It causes a rise of blood-glucose concentration in the test animals when injected as prescribed in the assay.

B. Examine the electropherograms obtained in the test for related substances. The principal band in the electropherogram obtained with test solution (a) corresponds in position to the principal band in the electropherogram obtained with reference solution (a).

TESTS

Absorbance. Dissolve 2.5 mg in *0.01 M hydrochloric acid* and dilute to 10.0 ml with the same acid. The specific absorbance (*2.2.25*) determined at the maximum at 276 nm is 21 to 25, calculated with reference to the dried substance.

Related substances. Examine by polyacrylamide gel electrophoresis (*2.2.31*), using rod gels 75 mm long and 5 mm in diameter and, as buffer, *tris-glycine buffer solution pH 8.3 R.* The electrode in the upper reservoir is the cathode and that in the lower reservoir the anode.

Use the following gel mixture: mix 1 volume of a solution containing in 100 ml 36.6 mg of *tris(hydroxymethyl)aminomethane R,* 0.23 ml of *tetramethylethylenediamine R* and 48.0 ml of *1 M hydrochloric acid* and 2 volumes of a solution containing in 100 ml 0.735 g of *methylene-bisacrylamide R* and 30.0 g of *acrylamide R.* Add sufficient *urea R* to give a concentration of 480 g/l in the final solution and dilute to 7 volumes with *water R.* If necessary, heat to not more than 40 °C to dissolve the urea. Degas the solution and add 1 volume of a 5.6 g/l solution of *ammonium persulphate R.*

Test solution (a). Dissolve 10 mg of the substance to be examined in 0.5 ml of *0.01 M sodium hydroxide.*

Test solution (b). Dilute 0.25 ml of test solution (a) to 5 ml with *0.01 M sodium hydroxide.*

Reference solution (a). Dissolve a quantity of *glucagon CRS* equivalent to 5 IU in *0.01 M sodium hydroxide* and dilute to 25 ml with the same solvent.

Reference solution (b). Dilute 8 ml of reference solution (a) to 10 ml with *0.01 M sodium hydroxide.*

Reference solution (c). Dilute 6 ml of reference solution (a) to 10 ml with *0.01 M sodium hydroxide.*

Reference solution (d). Dilute 4 ml of reference solution (a) to 10 ml with *0.01 M sodium hydroxide.*

Reference solution (e). Dilute 2 ml of reference solution (a) to 10 ml with *0.01 M sodium hydroxide.*

Apply 100 µl of each solution to the surface of a gel. After the addition of the buffer, add 0.2 ml of *bromophenol blue solution R*. Allow electrophoresis to take place with a constant current of 1 mA per tube for 30 min and then increase the current to 3 mA per tube. Immerse the gels in a 125 g/l solution of *trichloroacetic acid R* for at least 1 h. For each 10 ml of trichloroacetic acid solution used add 0.5 ml of a 2.5 g/l solution of *acid blue 90 R* and allow to stand for 12 h. Remove the staining solution and wash twice with a mixture of 1 volume of *acetic acid R* and 4 volumes of *water R*, discard the washings and store the gels in a similar mixture of *acetic acid R* and *water R*. Examine the electropherograms using a cold-light illuminator. In the electropherograms obtained with test solution (a), any band, other than the bromophenol blue band, that migrates between two and three times the distance of the principal band is not more intense than the principal band in the electropherogram obtained with reference solution (e). In the electropherogram obtained with test solution (b), any band that migrates immediately in front of the principal band is not more intense than the principal band in the electropherogram obtained with reference solution (a). The test is not valid unless a band is seen in the electropherogram obtained with reference solution (e) and a gradation of intensity of staining is seen in the electropherograms obtained with reference solutions (a) to (e).

Monographs F-H

Nitrogen: 16.0 per cent to 18.5 per cent, determined by the method of sulphuric acid digestion (*2.5.9*) and calculated with reference to the dried substance.

Zinc. Not more than 0.15 per cent of Zn, determined by atomic absorption spectrometry (*2.2.23, Method I*).

Test solution. Dissolve 50.0 mg of the substance to be examined in *0.01 M hydrochloric acid* and dilute to 25.0 ml with the same acid. Dilute if necessary with *0.01 M hydrochloric acid* to obtain a zinc concentration of 0.4 µg/ml to 1.6 µg/ml.

Reference solutions. Use solutions containing 0.10 µg, 0.40 µg, 0.80 µg, 1.00 µg, 1.20 µg and 1.60 µg of Zn per millilitre, freshly prepared by diluting *zinc standard solution (5 mg/ml Zn) R* with *0.01 M hydrochloric acid.*

Measure the absorbance at 213.9 nm using a zinc hollow-cathode lamp as the source of radiation and an air-acetylene flame of suitable composition (for example, 2 litres of acetylene and 11 litres of air per minute).

Loss on drying (*2.2.32*). Not more than 10.0 per cent, determined on 50.0 mg by drying at 105 °C for 24 h.

ASSAY

The potency of glucagon is determined by comparing, in given conditions, the hyperglycaemic effect it produces with that produced by the International Standard or by a reference preparation calibrated in International Units.

The International Unit is the specific hyperglycaemic activity contained in a stated amount of the International Standard which consists of a quantity of freeze-dried glucagon to which lactose and sodium chloride have been added. The equivalence in International units of the International Standard is stated by the World Health Organisation.

The estimated potency is not less than 80 per cent and not more than 125 per cent of the stated potency. The confidence limits ($P = 0.95$) of the estimated potency are not less than 64 per cent and not more than 156 per cent of the stated potency.

Reference solution. Dissolve the entire contents of an ampoule of the reference preparation in 2 ml of a 9 g/l solution of *sodium chloride R* adjusted to pH 3.0 with *hydrochloric acid R* and dilute with the same solvent to obtain a solution containing, for example, 0.1 IU/ml. Store the solution at 2 °C to 8 °C and use within 2 days.

Use in the test healthy rabbits, the difference in mass between the heaviest and the lightest being not greater than 1.2 kg (for example, rabbits with body masses in the range 1.8 kg to 2.8 kg). Keep the rabbits in the laboratory under uniform conditions on a uniform diet for a least 1 week before use in the assay. Handle the rabbits with care to avoid undue excitement.

Inject intramuscularly into each rabbit 48 h before the test 1 ml of a 25 g/l solution of cortisone acetate and withhold all food but not water from 16 h before each test day until after the withdrawal of the last blood sample on that day. Distribute the rabbits at random into four equal groups of not fewer than four rabbits.

Prepare two dilutions of the reference solution with a concentration ratio of 1 to 4, for example 0.006 IU/ml (reference dilution 1) and 0.024 IU/ml (reference dilution 2). Use as diluent a 9 g/l solution of *sodium chloride R* adjusted to pH 3.0 with *hydrochloric acid R*. Use the same diluent to dissolve the substance to be examined and to prepare two dilutions, one of which (test dilution 1) is presumed, on the basis of the stated potency to contain the same number of units per millilitre as reference dilution 1 and the other (test dilution 2) the same number of units per millilitre as reference dilution 2. Inject 1.0 ml of each dilution subcutaneously giving the doses in the order indicated in the following table, the second injection being made approximately 24 h after the first injection.

Group of rabbits	First injection	Second injection
1	reference dilution 1	test dilution 2
2	reference dilution 2	test dilution 1
3	test dilution 1	reference dilution 2
4	test dilution 2	reference dilution 1

Take a suitable blood sample from the marginal ear vein of each rabbit 1 h after each injection and determine the blood-glucose concentration in each sample. The optimal time depends on the strain. It is important that for a given assay a definite and exactly identical time interval be scrupulously respected for each rabbit.

Calculate the potency by the usual statistical methods for the twin cross-over assay.

STORAGE

Store in an airtight container, at a temperature below 8 °C and preferably at −20 °C.

LABELLING

The label states:

- the number of units per container,
- the number of units per milligram,
- the storage conditions.

01/2005:1635

GLUCAGON, HUMAN

Glucagonum humanum

H-His-Ser-Gln-Gly-Thr-Phe-Thr-Ser-Asp-Tyr-
10
Ser-Lys-Tyr-Leu-Asp-Ser-Arg-Arg-Ala-Gln-
20
Asp-Phe-Val-Gln-Trp-Leu-Met-Asn-Thr-OH

$C_{153}H_{225}N_{43}O_{49}S$ M_r 3483

DEFINITION

Polypeptide having the same structure (29 amino-acids) as the hormone produced by the α-cells of the human pancreas which increases the blood-glucose concentration by promoting rapid breakdown of liver glycogen.

Content: 92.5 per cent to 105.0 per cent (anhydrous substance).

PRODUCTION

Human glucagon is produced by a method based on recombinant DNA (rDNA) technology. During the course of product development it must be demonstrated that the manufacturing process produces a product having a biological activity of not less than 1 IU/mg using a suitable validated bioassay, based on hyperglycaemia measurement.

Host-cell-derived proteins: the limit is approved by the competent authority.

Host-cell- and vector-derived DNA: the limit is approved by the competent authority.

CHARACTERS

Appearance: white or almost white powder.

Solubility: practically insoluble in water and in most organic solvents, soluble in dilute mineral acids and in dilute solutions of alkali hydroxides.

IDENTIFICATION

A. Peptide mapping. Liquid chromatography (*2.2.29*).

Test solution. Prepare a 10 mg/ml solution of the substance to be examined in *0.01 M hydrochloric acid.* Mix 200 µl of the solution with 800 µl of *0.1 M ammonium carbonate buffer solution pH 10.3 R* (diluted stock solution). Freshly prepare a 2.0 mg/ml solution of *α-chymotrypsin for peptide mapping R* in *0.1 M ammonium carbonate buffer solution pH 10.3 R* and add 25 µl to the diluted stock solution of the substance to be examined. Place the test solution in a closed vial at 37 °C for 2 h. Remove the vial and stop the reaction immediately by the addition of 120 µl of *glacial acetic acid R.*

Reference solution. Prepare at the same time and in the same manner as for the test solution but using *human glucagon CRS* instead of the substance to be examined.

Column:
- *size*: *l* = 0.05 m, Ø = 4 mm,
- *stationary phase*: *octadecylsilyl silica gel for chromatography R* (5 µm).

Mobile phase:
- *mobile phase A*: mix 500 µl of *trifluoroacetic acid R* and 1000 ml of *water R,*
- *mobile phase B*: mix 500 µl of *trifluoroacetic acid R* with 600 ml of *ethanol R* and add 400 ml of *water R,*

Time (min)	Mobile phase A (per cent *V/V*)	Mobile phase B (per cent *V/V*)
0 - 35	100 → 53	0 → 47
35 - 45	53 → 0	47 → 100
45 - 46	0 → 100	100 → 0
46 - 75	100	0

Flow rate: 1.0 ml/min.

Detection: spectrophotometer at 215 nm.

Equilibration: mobile phase A for at least 15 min.

Injection: 10 µl.

Results: the profile of the chromatogram obtained with the test solution corresponds to that of the chromatogram obtained with the reference solution.

B. Examine the chromatograms obtained in the assay. The principal peak in the chromatogram obtained with the test solution is similar in retention time to the principal peak in the chromatogram obtained with the reference solution.

TESTS

Specific absorbance (*2.2.25*): 21 to 25, determined at the maximum at 276 nm (anhydrous substance).

Dissolve 2.5 mg in *0.01 M hydrochloric acid* and dilute to 10.0 ml with the same solvent.

Deamidated glucagon. Liquid chromatography (*2.2.29*): use the normalisation procedure.

Test solution. Dissolve the substance to be examined in *0.01 M hydrochloric acid* to obtain a concentration of 1.0 mg/ml.

Resolution solution. Dissolve the substance to be examined in *0.1 M hydrochloric acid* to obtain a concentration of 1.0 mg/ml. Incubate in an oven at 60 °C for 2 h. Immediately after degradation, adjust to pH 2.5 with *1 M sodium hydroxide.*

Column:
- *material*: glass,
- *size*: *l* = 0.05 m, Ø = 5 mm,
- *stationary phase*: *anion exchange resin R2.*

Mobile phase:
- *mobile phase A*: mix 1000 ml of *tris-hydrochloride buffer solution pH 8.3 R* and 1000 ml of *ethanol R,*
- *mobile phase B*: dissolve 29.2 g of *sodium chloride R* in 1000 ml of *tris-hydrochloride buffer solution pH 8.3 R;* add 1000 ml of *ethanol R,*

Time (min)	Mobile phase A (per cent *V/V*)	Mobile phase B (per cent *V/V*)
0 - 4	100	0
4 - 30	100 → 78	0 → 22
30 - 34	78 → 45	22 → 55
34 - 38	45 → 20	55 → 80
38 - 40	20 → 100	80 → 0
40 - 60	100	0

Flow rate: 0.6 ml/min.

Detection: spectrophotometer at 230 nm.

Equilibration: mobile phase A for at least 15 min.

Injection: 60 µl.

System suitability: resolution solution:
- *retention time*: glucagon = about 10 min; 4 deamidated forms: between 15 min and 40 min,

- *resolution*: baseline separation of the 4 deamidated forms and glucagon.

Limit:

- *total of the 4 deamidated forms*: maximum 0.5 per cent, calculated from the peaks eluting between 10 min and 40 min.

Related proteins. Liquid chromatography (*2.2.29*): use the normalisation procedure.

2.8 M urea solution. Dissolve 16.8 g of *urea R* in *0.01 M hydrochloric acid* and dilute to 100 ml with the same solvent.

Test solution. Dissolve the substance to be examined in *0.01 M hydrochloric acid* to obtain a concentration of 1.0 mg/ml. *Maintain the solution at 2-8 °C and use within 24 h.*

Reference solution. Dissolve the contents of a vial of *human glucagon CRS* in *0.01 M hydrochloric acid* to obtain a concentration of 1.0 mg/ml. *Maintain the solution at 2-8 °C and use within 24 h.*

Resolution solution. Dissolve 10 mg of the substance to be examined in 10 ml of 2.8 M urea solution. Adjust to pH 7 with *1 M sodium hydroxide* and place the sealed vial at about 50 °C for about 2 h. Cool and adjust to pH 2.5 with *1 M hydrochloric acid. Maintain the solution at 2-8 °C and use within 2 h.*

Column:

- *size*: l = 0.25 m, Ø = 4.6 mm,
- *stationary phase*: *octadecylsilyl silica gel for chromatography R* (5 µm) with a pore size of 30 nm,
- *temperature*: 45 °C.

Mobile phase:

- *mobile phase A*: dissolve 14.2 g of *anhydrous sodium sulphate R* in 400 ml of *water R*; add 1.35 ml of *phosphoric acid R* and adjust to pH 2.5 (*2.2.3*) with *ethanolamine R*; add 100 ml of *acetonitrile for chromatography R*,
- *mobile phase B*: *acetonitrile for chromatography R*, *water R* (40:60 *V/V*),

Time (min)	Mobile phase A (per cent *V/V*)	Mobile phase B (per cent *V/V*)
0 - 23	57	43
23 - 29	57 → 10	43 → 90
29 - 30	10	90
30 - 31	10 → 57	90 → 43
31 - 75	57	43

Flow rate: 1.0 ml/min.

Detection: spectrophotometer at 214 nm.

Injection: 25 µl; inject the test solution and the resolution solution.

System suitability: resolution solution:

- *retention time*: glucagon = about 20 min; carbamoylglucagon = about 22 min,
- *resolution*: minimum 1.3 between the peaks due to glucagon and carbamoylglucagon,
- *symmetry factor*: 0.6 to 1 for the peak due to glucagon.

Limit:

- *total of all impurities*: maximum 2.5 per cent.

Water (*2.5.12*): maximum 10 per cent, determined on 20.0 mg.

Bacterial endotoxins (*2.6.14*): less than 10 IU/mg.

ASSAY

Liquid chromatography (*2.2.29*) as described in the test for related proteins with the following modifications.

Injection: test solution and reference solution.

Calculate the content of human glucagon ($C_{153}H_{225}N_{43}O_{49}S$) from the declared content of $C_{153}H_{225}N_{43}O_{49}S$ in *human glucagon CRS.*

STORAGE

In an airtight container, protected from light, at a temperature lower than − 15 °C.

01/2005:0177

GLUCOSE, ANHYDROUS

Glucosum anhydricum

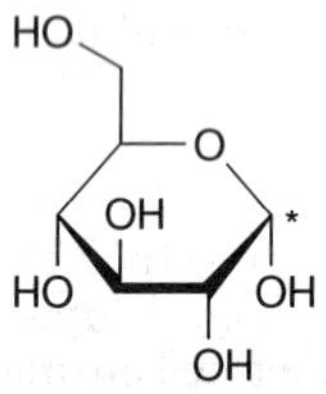

$C_6H_{12}O_6$ M_r 180.2

DEFINITION

Anhydrous glucose is (+)-D-glucopyranose.

CHARACTERS

A white, crystalline powder, with a sweet taste, freely soluble in water, sparingly soluble in alcohol.

IDENTIFICATION

A. Specific optical rotation (see Tests): + 52.5 to + 53.3.

B. Examine by thin-layer chromatography (*2.2.27*), using *silica gel G R* as the coating substance.

Test solution. Dissolve 10 mg of the substance to be examined in a mixture of 2 volumes of *water R* and 3 volumes of *methanol R* and dilute to 20 ml with the same mixture of solvents.

Reference solution (a). Dissolve 10 mg of *glucose CRS* in a mixture of 2 volumes of *water R* and 3 volumes of *methanol R* and dilute to 20 ml with the same mixture of solvents.

Reference solution (b). Dissolve 10 mg each of *fructose CRS, glucose CRS, lactose CRS* and *sucrose CRS* in a mixture of 2 volumes of water R and 3 volumes of *methanol R* and dilute to 20 ml with the same mixture of solvents.

Apply separately to the plate 2 µl of each solution and thoroughly dry the starting points. Develop over a path of 15 cm using a mixture of 10 volumes of *water R*, 15 volumes of *methanol R*, 25 volumes of *anhydrous acetic acid R* and 50 volumes of *ethylene chloride R*. The solvents should be measured accurately since a slight excess of water produces cloudiness. Dry the plate in a current of warm air. Repeat the development immediately, after renewing the mobile phase. Dry the plate in a current of warm air and spray evenly with a solution of 0.5 g of *thymol R* in a mixture of 5 ml of *sulphuric acid R* and 95 ml of *alcohol R*. Heat at 130 °C for 10 min. The principal spot in the chromatogram obtained with the test solution is similar in position, colour and size to the principal spot in the chromatogram obtained with

Monographs F-H

reference solution (a). The test is not valid unless the chromatogram obtained with reference solution (b) shows four clearly separated spots.

C. Dissolve 0.1 g in 10 ml of *water R*. Add 3 ml of *cupri-tartaric solution R* and heat. A red precipitate is formed.

TESTS

Solution S. Dissolve 10.0 g in *distilled water R* and dilute to 100 ml with the same solvent.

Appearance of solution. Dissolve 10.0 g in 15 ml of *water R*. The solution is clear (*2.2.1*), odourless, and not more intensely coloured than reference solution BY_7 (*2.2.2, Method II*).

Acidity or alkalinity. Dissolve 6.0 g in 25 ml of *carbon dioxide-free water R* and add 0.3 ml of *phenolphthalein solution R*. The solution is colourless. Not more than 0.15 ml of *0.1 M sodium hydroxide* is required to change the colour of the indicator to pink.

Specific optical rotation (*2.2.7*). Dissolve 10.0 g in 80 ml of *water R*, add 0.2 ml of *dilute ammonia R1*, allow to stand for 30 min and dilute to 100.0 ml with *water R*. The specific optical rotation is + 52.5 to + 53.3, calculated with reference to the anhydrous substance.

Foreign sugars, soluble starch, dextrins. Dissolve 1.0 g by boiling in 30 ml of *alcohol (90 per cent V/V) R*. Cool; the appearance of the solution shows no change.

Sulphites. Dissolve 5.0 g in 40 ml of *water R*, add 2.0 ml of *0.1 M sodium hydroxide* and dilute to 50.0 ml with *water R*. To 10.0 ml of the solution, add 1 ml of a 310 g/l solution of *hydrochloric acid R*, 2.0 ml of *decolorised fuchsin solution R1* and 2.0 ml of a 0.5 per cent *V/V* solution of *formaldehyde R*. Allow to stand for 30 min and measure the absorbance (*2.2.25*) at the maximum at 583 nm. Prepare a standard as follows. Dissolve 76 mg of *sodium metabisulphite R* in *water R* and dilute to 50.0 ml with the same solvent. Dilute 5.0 ml of this solution to 100.0 ml with *water R*. To 3.0 ml of this solution add 4.0 ml of *0.1 M sodium hydroxide* and dilute to 100.0 ml with *water R*. Immediately add to 10.0 ml of this solution 1 ml of a 310 g/l solution of *hydrochloric acid R*, 2.0 ml of *decolorised fuchsin solution R1* and 2.0 ml of a 0.5 per cent *V/V* solution of *formaldehyde R*. Allow to stand for 30 min and measure the absorbance at the maximum at 583 nm. Use as compensation liquid for both measurements a solution prepared in the same manner using 10.0 ml of *water R*. The absorbance of the test solution is not greater than that of the standard (15 ppm of SO_2)

Chlorides (*2.4.4*). 4 ml of solution S diluted to 15 ml with *water R* complies with the limit test for chlorides (125 ppm).

Sulphates (*2.4.13*). 7.5 ml of solution S diluted to 15 ml with *distilled water R* complies with the limit test for sulphates (200 ppm).

Arsenic (*2.4.2*). 1.0 g complies with limit test A for arsenic (1 ppm).

Barium. To 10 ml of solution S add 1 ml of *dilute sulphuric acid R*. When examined immediately and after 1 h, any opalescence in the solution is not more intense than that in a mixture of 1 ml of *distilled water R* and 10 ml of solution S.

Calcium (*2.4.3*). 5 ml of solution S diluted to 15 ml with *distilled water R* complies with the limit test for calcium (200 ppm).

Lead in sugars (*2.4.10*). It complies with the limit test for lead in sugars (0.5 ppm).

Water (*2.5.12*). Not more than 1.0 per cent, determined on 0.50 g by the semi-micro determination of water.

Sulphated ash (*2.4.14*). Not more than 0.1 per cent. Dissolve 5.0 g in 5 ml of *water R*, add 2 ml of *sulphuric acid R*, evaporate to dryness on a water-bath and ignite to constant mass. If necessary, repeat the heating with *sulphuric acid R*.

Pyrogens (*2.6.8*). If intended for use in large-volume preparations for parenteral use, the competent authority may require that it comply with the test for pyrogens carried out as follows. Inject per kilogram of the rabbit's mass 10 ml of a solution containing 50 mg per millilitre of the substance to be examined in *water for injections R*.

LABELLING

The label states where applicable, that the substance is apyrogenic.

01/2005:1330

GLUCOSE, LIQUID

Glucosum liquidum

DEFINITION

Liquid glucose is an aqueous solution containing a mixture of glucose, oligosaccharides and polysaccharides obtained by hydrolysis of starch. It contains not less than 70.0 per cent of dry matter. The degree of hydrolysis expressed as dextrose equivalent (DE) is not less than 20 (nominal value).

CHARACTERS

A clear, colourless or brown, viscous liquid, miscible with water. The substance may partly or totally solidify at room temperature and liquefies again when heated to 50 °C.

IDENTIFICATION

A. Dissolve 0.1 g in 2.5 ml of *water R* and heat with 2.5 ml of *cupri-tartaric solution R*. A red precipitate is formed.

B. Dip, for 1 s, a suitable stick with a reactive pad containing glucose-oxidase, peroxidase and a hydrogen-donating substance, such as tetramethylbenzidine, in a 5 g/l solution of the substance to be examined. Observe the colour of the reactive pad; within 60 s the colour changes from yellow to green or blue.

C. It is a clear, colourless or brown, viscous liquid, miscible with water. The substance may partly or totally solidify at room temperature and liquefies again when heated to 50 °C.

D. It complies with the test for dextrose equivalent (see Tests).

TESTS

Solution S. Dissolve 25.0 g in *carbon dioxide-free water R* and dilute to 50.0 ml with the same solvent.

pH (*2.2.3*). The pH of a mixture of 1 ml of a 223.6 g/l solution of *potassium chloride R* and 30 ml of solution S is 4.0 to 6.0.

Sulphur dioxide (*2.5.29*). Not more than 20 ppm. Not more than 400 ppm if intended for the production of lozenges or pastilles obtained by high boiling techniques, provided that the final product does not contain more than 50 ppm of sulphur dioxide.

Heavy metals (*2.4.8*). Dilute 2 ml of solution S to 30 ml with *water R*. The solution complies with limit test E for heavy metals (10 ppm). Prepare the standard using 10 ml of *lead standard solution (1 ppm Pb) R*.

Monographs F-H

Loss on drying (*2.2.32*). Not more than 30.0 per cent, determined on 1.000 g. Triturate the sample with 3.000 g of *kieselguhr G R*, previously dried at 80 °C under reduced pressure for 2 h, and dry at 80 °C under reduced pressure for 2 h.

Sulphated ash (*2.4.14*). Not more than 0.5 per cent, determined on 1.0 g.

Dextrose equivalent. Weigh an amount of the substance to be examined equivalent to 2.85-3.15 g of reducing carbohydrates, calculated as dextrose equivalent, into a 500 ml volumetric flask. Dissolve in *water R* and dilute to 500.0 ml with the same solvent. Transfer the solution to a 50 ml burette.

Pipette 25.0 ml of *cupri-tartaric solution R* into a 250 ml flask and add 18.5 ml of the test solution from the burette, mix and add boiling chips. Place the flask on a hot plate, previously adjusted so that the solution begins to boil after 2 min ± 15 s. Leave to boil for exactly 120 s, add 1 ml of a 1 g/l solution of *methylene blue R* and titrate with the test solution (V_1) until the blue colour disappears. Maintain the solution at boiling throughout the titration.

Standardise the cupri-tartaric solution using a 6.00 g/l solution of *glucose R* (V_0).

Calculate the dextrose equivalent (DE) from the equation:

$$\mathrm{DE} = \frac{300 \times V_0 \times 100}{V_1 \times M \times D}$$

V_0 = total volume of glucose standard solution, in millilitres,

V_1 = total volume of test solution, in millilitres,

M = mass of the sample, in grams,

D = percentage content of dry matter in the substance.

The dextrose equivalent (DE) is within 10 per cent of the nominal value.

LABELLING

The label states the dextrose equivalent (DE) (= nominal value).

01/2005:1525

GLUCOSE, LIQUID, SPRAY-DRIED

Glucosum liquidum dispersione desiccatum

DEFINITION

Spray-dried liquid glucose is a mixture of glucose, oligosaccharides and polysaccharides, obtained by the partial hydrolysis of starch. The degree of hydrolysis, expressed as dextrose equivalent (DE), is not less than 20 (nominal value).

CHARACTERS

A white or almost white, slightly hygroscopic powder or granules, freely soluble in water.

IDENTIFICATION

A. Dissolve 0.1 g in 2.5 ml of *water R* and heat with 2.5 ml of *cupri-tartaric solution R*. A red precipitate is formed.

B. Dip, for 1 s, a suitable stick with a reactive pad containing glucose-oxidase, peroxidase and a hydrogen-donating substance, such as tetramethylbenzidine, in a 5 g/l solution of the substance to be examined. Observe the colour of the reactive pad; within 60 s the colour changes from yellow to green or blue.

C. It is a powder or granules.

D. It complies with the test for dextrose equivalent (see Tests).

TESTS

Solution S. Dissolve 12.5 g in *carbon dioxide-free water R* and dilute to 50.0 ml with the same solvent.

pH (*2.2.3*). The pH of a mixture of 1 ml of a 223.6 g/l solution of *potassium chloride R* and 30 ml of solution S is 4.0 to 7.0.

Sulphur dioxide (*2.5.29*). Not more than 20 ppm.

Heavy metals (*2.4.8*). Dilute 4 ml of solution S to 30 ml with *water R*. The solution complies with limit test E (10 ppm). Prepare the standard using 10 ml of *lead standard solution (1 ppm Pb) R*.

Loss on drying (*2.2.32*). Not more than 6.0 per cent, determined on 10.00 g by drying in an oven at 100-105 °C.

Sulphated ash (*2.4.14*). Not more than 0.5 per cent, determined on 1.0 g.

Dextrose equivalent. Weigh an amount of the substance to be examined equivalent to 2.85-3.15 g of reducing carbohydrates, calculated as dextrose equivalent, into a 500 ml volumetric flask. Dissolve in *water R* and dilute to 500.0 ml with the same solvent. Transfer the solution to a 50 ml burette.

Pipette 25.0 ml of *cupri-tartaric solution R* into a 250 ml flask and add 18.5 ml of the test solution from the burette, mix and add boiling chips. Place the flask on a hot plate, previously adjusted so that the solution begins to boil after 2 min ± 15 s. Allow to boil for exactly 120 s, add 1 ml of a 1 g/l solution of *methylene blue R* and titrate with the test solution (V_1) until the blue colour disappears. Maintain the solution at boiling throughout the titration.

Standardise the cupri-tartaric solution using a 6.00 g/l solution of *glucose R* (V_0).

Calculate the dextrose equivalent (DE) from the equation:

$$\mathrm{DE} = \frac{300 \times V_0 \times 100}{V_1 \times M \times D}$$

V_0 = total volume of glucose standard solution, in millilitres,

V_1 = total volume of test solution, in millilitres,

M = mass of the sample, in grams,

D = percentage content of dry matter in the substance.

The dextrose equivalent (DE) is within 10 per cent of the nominal value.

Microbial contamination. Total viable aerobic count (*2.6.12*) not more than 10^3 bacteria and 10^2 fungi per gram, determined by plate count. It complies with the tests for *Escherichia coli* and *Salmonella* (*2.6.13*).

LABELLING

The label states the dextrose equivalent (DE) (= nominal value).

01/2005:0178

GLUCOSE MONOHYDRATE

Glucosum monohydricum

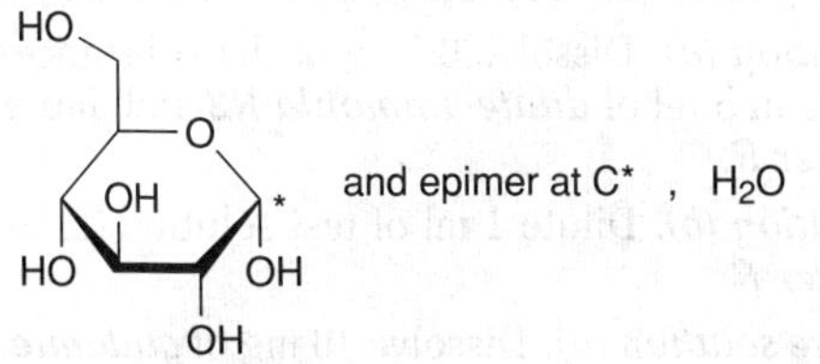

$C_6H_{12}O_6,H_2O$ M_r 198.2

DEFINITION

Glucose monohydrate is the monohydrate of (+)-D-glucopyranose.

CHARACTERS

A white, crystalline powder, with a sweet taste, freely soluble in water, sparingly soluble in alcohol.

IDENTIFICATION

A. Specific optical rotation (see Tests): + 52.5 to + 53.3.

B. Examine by thin-layer chromatography (*2.2.27*), using *silica gel G R* as the coating substance.

Test solution. Dissolve 10 mg of the substance to be examined in a mixture of 2 volumes of *water R* and 3 volumes of *methanol R* and dilute to 20 ml with the same mixture of solvents.

Reference solution (a). Dissolve 10 mg of *glucose CRS* in a mixture of 2 volumes of *water R* and 3 volumes of *methanol R* and dilute to 20 ml with the same mixture of solvents.

Reference solution (b). Dissolve 10 mg each of *fructose CRS, glucose CRS, lactose CRS* and *sucrose CRS* in a mixture of 2 volumes of *water R* and 3 volumes of *methanol R* and dilute to 20 ml with the same mixture of solvents.

Apply separately to the plate 2 µl of each solution and thoroughly dry the starting points. Develop over a path of 15 cm using a mixture of 10 volumes of *water R*, 15 volumes of *methanol R*, 25 volumes of *anhydrous acetic acid R* and 50 volumes of *ethylene chloride R*. The solvents should be measured accurately since a slight excess of water produces cloudiness. Dry the plate in a current of warm air. Repeat the development immediately, after renewing the mobile phase. Dry the plate in a current of warm air and spray evenly with a solution of 0.5 g of *thymol R* in a mixture of 5 ml of *sulphuric acid R* and 95 ml of *alcohol R*. Heat at 130 °C for 10 min. The principal spot in the chromatogram obtained with the test solution is similar in position, colour and size to the principal spot in the chromatogram obtained with reference solution (a). The test is not valid unless the chromatogram obtained with reference solution (b) shows 4 clearly separated spots.

C. Dissolve 0.1 g in 10 ml of *water R*. Add 3 ml of *cupri-tartaric solution R* and heat. A red precipitate is formed.

TESTS

Solution S. Dissolve 10.0 g in *distilled water R* and dilute to 100 ml with the same solvent.

Appearance of solution. Dissolve 10.0 g in 15 ml of *water R*. The solution is clear (*2.2.1*), odourless, and not more intensely coloured than reference solution BY_7 (*2.2.2, Method II*).

Acidity or alkalinity. Dissolve 6.0 g in 25 ml of *carbon dioxide-free water R* and add 0.3 ml of *phenolphthalein solution R*. The solution is colourless. Not more than 0.15 ml of *0.1 M sodium hydroxide* is required to change the colour of the indicator to pink.

Specific optical rotation (*2.2.7*). Dissolve 10.0 g in 80 ml of *water R*, add 0.2 ml of *dilute ammonia R1*, allow to stand for 30 min and dilute to 100.0 ml with *water R*. The specific optical rotation is + 52.5 to + 53.3, calculated with reference to the anhydrous substance.

Foreign sugars, soluble starch, dextrins. Dissolve 1.0 g by boiling in 30 ml of *alcohol (90 per cent V/V) R*. Cool; the appearance of the solution shows no change.

Sulphites. Dissolve 5.0 g in 40 ml of *water R*, add 2.0 ml of *0.1 M sodium hydroxide* and dilute to 50.0 ml with *water R*. To 10.0 ml of the solution, add 1 ml of a 310 g/l solution of *hydrochloric acid R*, 2.0 ml of *decolorised fuchsin solution R1* and 2.0 ml of a 0.5 per cent *V/V* solution of *formaldehyde R*. Allow to stand for 30 min and measure the absorbance (*2.2.25*) at the maximum at 583 nm. Prepare a standard as follows. Dissolve 76 mg of *sodium metabisulphite R* in *water R* and dilute to 50.0 ml with the same solvent. Dilute 5.0 ml of this solution to 100.0 ml with *water R*. To 3.0 ml of this solution add 4.0 ml of *0.1 M sodium hydroxide* and dilute to 100.0 ml with *water R*. Immediately add to 10.0 ml of this solution 1 ml of a 310 g/l solution of *hydrochloric acid R*, 2.0 ml of *decolorised fuchsin solution R1* and 2.0 ml of a 0.5 per cent *V/V* solution of *formaldehyde R*. Allow to stand for 30 min and measure the absorbance at the maximum at 583 nm. Use as compensation liquid for both measurements a solution prepared in the same manner using 10.0 ml of *water R*. The absorbance of the test solution is not greater than that of the standard (15 ppm of SO_2).

Chlorides (*2.4.4*). 4 ml of solution S diluted to 15 ml with *water R* complies with the limit test for chlorides (125 ppm).

Sulphates (*2.4.13*). 7.5 ml of solution S diluted to 15 ml with *distilled water R* complies with the limit test for sulphates (200 ppm).

Arsenic (*2.4.2*). 1.0 g complies with limit test A for arsenic (1 ppm).

Barium. To 10 ml of solution S add 1 ml of *dilute sulphuric acid R*. When examined immediately and after 1 h, any opalescence in the solution is not more intense than that in a mixture of 1 ml of *distilled water R* and 10 ml of solution S.

Calcium (*2.4.3*). 5 ml of solution S diluted to 15 ml with *distilled water R* complies with the limit test for calcium (200 ppm).

Lead in sugars (*2.4.10*). It complies with the limit test for lead in sugars (0.5 ppm).

Water (*2.5.12*). 7.0 per cent to 9.5 per cent, determined on 0.50 g by the semi-micro determination of water.

Sulphated ash (*2.4.14*). Not more than 0.1 per cent. Dissolve 5.0 g in 5 ml of *water R*, add 2 ml of *sulphuric acid R*, evaporate to dryness on a water-bath and ignite to constant mass. If necessary, repeat the heating with *sulphuric acid R*.

Pyrogens (*2.6.8*). If intended for use in large-volume preparations for parenteral use, the competent authority may require that it comply with the test for pyrogens carried

Monographs F-H

out as follows. Inject per kilogram of the rabbit's mass 10 ml of a solution containing 55 mg per millilitre of the substance to be examined in *water for injections R*.

LABELLING

The label states where applicable, that the substance is apyrogenic.

01/2005:0750

GLUTAMIC ACID

Acidum glutamicum

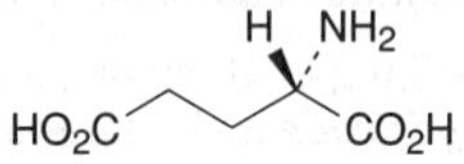

$C_5H_9NO_4$ M_r 147.1

DEFINITION

Glutamic acid contains not less than 98.5 per cent and not more than the equivalent of 100.5 per cent of (2*S*)-2-aminopentanedioic acid, calculated with reference to the dried substance.

CHARACTERS

A white, crystalline powder or colourless crystals, freely soluble in boiling water, slightly soluble in cold water, practically insoluble in acetic acid, in acetone and in alcohol.

IDENTIFICATION

First identification: A, B.

Second identification: A, C, D.

A. It complies with the test for specific optical rotation (see Tests).

B. Examine by infrared absorption spectrophotometry (*2.2.24*), comparing with the spectrum obtained with *glutamic acid CRS*. Examine the substances prepared as discs. If the spectra obtained show differences, dissolve the substance to be examined and the reference substance separately in the minimum quantity of *water R*, evaporate to dryness at 60 °C and record new spectra using the residues.

C. Examine the chromatograms obtained in the test for ninhydrin-positive substances. The principal spot in the chromatogram obtained with test solution (b) is similar in position, colour and size to the principal spot in the chromatogram obtained with reference solution (a).

D. To 2.0 ml of solution S (see Tests) add 0.1 ml of *phenolphthalein solution R* and 3.0 ml to 3.5 ml of *1 M sodium hydroxide* to change the colour of the indicator to red. Add a mixture of 3 ml of *formaldehyde solution R*, 3 ml of *carbon dioxide-free water R* and 0.1 ml of *phenolphthalein solution R*, to which sufficient *1 M sodium hydroxide* has been added to produce a pink colour. The solution is decolourised. Add *1 M sodium hydroxide* until a red colour is produced. The total volume of *1 M sodium hydroxide* used is 4.0 ml to 4.7 ml.

TESTS

Solution S. Dissolve 5.00 g in *1 M hydrochloric acid* with gentle heating, and dilute to 50.0 ml with the same acid.

Appearance of solution. Solution S is clear (*2.2.1*) and colourless (*Method II, 2.2.2*).

Specific optical rotation (*2.2.7*): + 30.5 to + 32.5, determined on solution S and calculated with reference to the dried substance.

Ninhydrin-positive substances. Examine by thin-layer chromatography (*2.2.27*), using a *TLC silica gel plate R*.

Test solution (a). Dissolve 0.10 g of the substance to be examined in 5 ml of *dilute ammonia R2* and dilute to 10 ml with *water R*.

Test solution (b). Dilute 1 ml of test solution (a) to 50 ml with *water R*.

Reference solution (a). Dissolve 10 mg of *glutamic acid CRS* in *water R* and dilute to 50 ml with the same solvent.

Reference solution (b). Dilute 5 ml of test solution (b) to 20 ml with *water R*.

Reference solution (c). Dissolve 10 mg of *glutamic acid CRS* and 10 mg of *aspartic acid CRS* in *water R* and dilute to 25 ml with the same solvent.

Apply to the plate 5 µl of each solution. Dry the plate in a current of air for 15 min. Develop over a path of 15 cm using a mixture of 20 volumes of *glacial acetic acid R*, 20 volumes of *water R* and 60 volumes of *butanol R*. Allow the plate to dry in air, spray with *ninhydrin solution R* and heat at 100-105 °C for 15 min. Any spot in the chromatogram obtained with test solution (a), apart from the principal spot, is not more intense than the spot in the chromatogram obtained with reference solution (b) (0.5 per cent). The test is not valid unless the chromatogram obtained with reference solution (c) shows 2 clearly separated spots.

Chlorides (*2.4.4*). Dissolve 0.25 g in 3 ml of *dilute nitric acid R* and dilute to 15 ml with *water R*. The solution, to which 1 ml of *water R* is added instead of *dilute nitric acid R*, complies with the limit test for chlorides (200 ppm).

Sulphates (*2.4.13*). Dilute 5 ml of solution S to 15 ml with *distilled water R*. The solution complies with the limit test for sulphates (300 ppm).

Ammonium (*2.4.1*). 50 mg complies with limit test B for ammonium (200 ppm). Prepare the standard using 0.1 ml of *ammonium standard solution (100 ppm NH_4) R*.

Iron (*2.4.9*). In a separating funnel, dissolve 1.0 g in 10 ml of *dilute hydrochloric acid R*. Shake with 3 quantities, each of 10 ml, of *methyl isobutyl ketone R1*, shaking for 3 min each time. To the combined organic layers add 10 ml of *water R* and shake for 3 min. The aqueous layer complies with the limit test for iron (10 ppm).

Heavy metals (*2.4.8*). 2.0 g complies with limit test D for heavy metals (10 ppm). Prepare the standard using 2 ml of *lead standard solution (10 ppm Pb) R*.

Loss on drying (*2.2.32*). Not more than 0.5 per cent, determined on 1.000 g by drying in an oven at 100-105 °C.

Sulphated ash (*2.4.14*). Not more than 0.1 per cent, determined on 1.0 g.

ASSAY

Dissolve 0.130 g in 50 ml of *carbon dioxide-free water R* with gentle heating. Cool. Using 0.1 ml of *bromothymol blue solution R1* as indicator, titrate with *0.1 M sodium hydroxide* until the colour changes from yellow to blue.

1 ml of *0.1 M sodium hydroxide* is equivalent to 14.71 mg of $C_5H_9NO_4$.

STORAGE

Protected from light.

01/2005:0496
corrected

GLYCEROL

Glycerolum

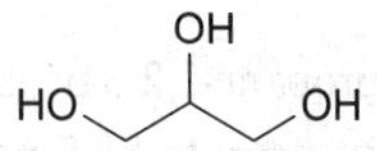

$C_3H_8O_3$ M_r 92.1

DEFINITION

Propane-1,2,3-triol.

Content: 98.0 per cent *m/m* to 101.0 per cent *m/m* (anhydrous substance).

CHARACTERS

Aspect: syrupy liquid, unctuous to the touch, colourless or almost colourless, clear, very hygroscopic.

Solubility: miscible with water and with alcohol, slightly soluble in acetone, practically insoluble in fatty oils and in essential oils.

IDENTIFICATION

First identification: A, B.

Second identification: A, C, D.

A. It complies with the test for refractive index (see Tests).

B. Infrared absorption spectrophotometry (*2.2.24*).

Preparation: to 5 ml add 1 ml of *water R* and mix carefully.

Comparison: *Ph. Eur. reference spectrum of glycerol (85 per cent).*

C. Mix 1 ml with 0.5 ml of *nitric acid R*. Superimpose 0.5 ml of *potassium dichromate solution R*. A blue ring develops at the interface of the liquids. Within 10 min, the blue colour does not diffuse into the lower layer.

D. Heat 1 ml with 2 g of *potassium hydrogen sulphate R* in an evaporating dish. Vapours (acrolein) are evolved which blacken filter paper impregnated with *alkaline potassium tetraiodomercurate solution R*.

TESTS

Solution S. Dilute 100.0 g to 200.0 ml with *carbon dioxide-free water R*.

Appearance of solution. Solution S is clear (*2.2.1*). Dilute 10 ml of solution S to 25 ml with *water R*. The solution is colourless (*2.2.2, Method II*).

Acidity or alkalinity. To 50 ml of solution S add 0.5 ml of *phenolphthalein solution R*. The solution is colourless. Not more than 0.2 ml of *0.1 M sodium hydroxide* is required to change the colour of the indicator to pink.

Refractive index (*2.2.6*): 1.470 to 1.475.

Aldehydes: maximum 10 ppm.

Place 7.5 ml of solution S in a ground-glass-stoppered flask and add 7.5 ml of *water R* and 1.0 ml of *decolorised pararosaniline solution R*. Close the flask and allow to stand for 1 h at a temperature of 25 ± 1 °C. The absorbance (*2.2.25*) of the solution measured at 552 nm is not greater than that of a standard prepared at the same time and in the same manner using 7.5 ml of *formaldehyde standard solution (5 ppm CH_2O) R* and 7.5 ml of *water R*. The test is not valid unless the standard is pink.

Esters. Add 10.0 ml of *0.1 M sodium hydroxide* to the final solution obtained in the test for acidity or alkalinity. Boil under a reflux condenser for 5 min. Cool. Add 0.5 ml of *phenolphthalein solution R* and titrate with *0.1 M hydrochloric acid*. Not less than 8.0 ml of *0.1 M hydrochloric acid* is required to change the colour of the indicator.

Impurity A and related substances. Gas chromatography (*2.2.28*).

Test solution. Dilute 10.0 ml of solution S to 100.0 ml with *water R*.

Reference solution (a). Dilute 10.0 g of *glycerol R1* to 20.0 ml with *water R*. Dilute 10.0 ml of the solution to 100.0 ml with *water R*.

Reference solution (b). Dissolve 1.000 g of *diethylene glycol R* in *water R* and dilute to 100.0 ml with the same solvent.

Reference solution (c). Dilute 1.0 ml of reference solution (b) to 10.0 ml with reference solution (a). Dilute 1.0 ml of this solution to 20.0 ml with reference solution (a).

Reference solution (d). Mix 1.0 ml of the test solution and 5.0 ml of reference solution (b) and dilute to 100.0 ml with *water R*. Dilute 1.0 ml of this solution to 10.0 ml with *water R*.

Reference solution (e). Dilute 5.0 ml of reference solution (b) to 100.0 ml with *water R*.

Column:

– *size*: *l* = 30 m, Ø = 0.53 mm,

– *stationary phase*: 6 per cent polycyanopropylphenyl siloxane and 94 per cent of polydimethylsiloxane.

Carrier gas: *helium for chromatography R.*

Split ratio: 1:10.

Linear velocity: 38 cm/s.

Temperature:

	Time (min)	Temperature (°C)
Column	0	100
	0 - 16	100 → 220
	16 - 20	220
Injection port		220
Detector		250

Detection: flame ionisation.

Injection: 0.5 µl.

Elution order: impurity A, glycerol.

System suitability: reference solution (d):

– *resolution*: minimum 7.0 between the peaks due to impurity A and glycerol.

Limits:

– *impurity A*: not more than the area of the corresponding peak in the chromatogram obtained with reference solution (c) (0.1 per cent),

– *any other impurity with a retention time less than the retention time of glycerol*: not more than the area of the peak due to impurity A in the chromatogram obtained with reference solution (c) (0.1 per cent),

– *total of all impurities with retention times greater than the retention time of glycerol*: not more than 5 times the area of the peak due to impurity A in the chromatogram obtained with reference solution (c) (0.5 per cent),

– *disregard limit*: 0.05 times the area of the peak due to impurity A in the chromatogram obtained with reference solution (e) (0.05 per cent).

Halogenated compounds: maximum 35 ppm.

To 10 ml of solution S add 1 ml of *dilute sodium hydroxide solution R*, 5 ml of *water R* and 50 mg of *halogen-free nickel-aluminium alloy R*. Heat on a water-bath for 10 min, allow to cool and filter. Rinse the flask and the filter with *water R* until 25 ml of filtrate is obtained. To 5 ml of the filtrate add 4 ml of *alcohol R*, 2.5 ml of *water R*, 0.5 ml of *nitric acid R* and 0.05 ml of *silver nitrate solution R2* and mix. Allow to stand for 2 min. Any opalescence in the solution is not more intense than that in a standard prepared at the same time by mixing 7.0 ml of *chloride standard solution (5 ppm Cl) R*, 4 ml of *alcohol R*, 0.5 ml of *water R*, 0.5 ml of *nitric acid R* and 0.05 ml of *silver nitrate solution R2*.

Sugars. To 10 ml of solution S add 1 ml of *dilute sulphuric acid R* and heat on a water-bath for 5 min. Add 3 ml of carbonate-free *dilute sodium hydroxide solution R* (prepared by the method described for carbonate-free *1 M sodium hydroxide* (*4.2.2*)), mix and add dropwise 1 ml of freshly prepared *copper sulphate solution R*. The solution is clear and blue. Continue heating on the water-bath for 5 min. The solution remains blue and no precipitate is formed.

Chlorides (*2.4.4*): maximum 10 ppm.

1 ml of solution S diluted to 15 ml with *water R* complies with the limit test for chlorides. Prepare the standard using 1 ml of *chloride standard solution (5 ppm Cl) R* diluted to 15 ml with *water R*.

Heavy metals (*2.4.8*): maximum 5 ppm.

Dilute 8 ml of solution S to 20 ml with *water R*. 12 ml of the solution complies with limit test A. Prepare the standard using *lead standard solution (1 ppm Pb) R*.

Water (*2.5.12*): maximum 2.0 per cent, determined on 1.000 g.

Sulphated ash (*2.4.14*): maximum 0.01 per cent, determined on 5.0 g after heating to boiling and ignition.

ASSAY

Thoroughly mix 0.075 g with 45 ml of *water R*. Add 25.0 ml of a mixture of 1 volume of *0.1 M sulphuric acid* and 20 volumes of *0.1 M sodium periodate*. Allow to stand protected from light for 15 min. Add 5.0 ml of a 500 g/l solution of *ethylene glycol R* and allow to stand protected from light for 20 min. Using 0.5 ml of *phenolphthalein solution R* as indicator, titrate with *0.1 M sodium hydroxide*. Carry out a blank titration.

1 ml of *0.1 M sodium hydroxide* is equivalent to 9.21 mg of $C_3H_8O_3$.

STORAGE

In an airtight container.

IMPURITIES

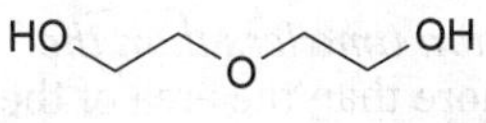

A. 2,2'-oxydiethanol (diethylene glycol),

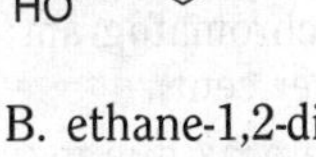

B. ethane-1,2-diol (ethylene glycol),

C. propylene glycol.

01/2005:0497
corrected

GLYCEROL (85 PER CENT)

Glycerolum (85 per centum)

DEFINITION

Aqueous solution of propane-1,2,3-triol.

Content: 83.5 per cent *m/m* to 88.5 per cent *m/m* of propane-1,2,3-triol ($C_3H_8O_3$; M_r 92.1).

CHARACTERS

Aspect: syrupy liquid, unctuous to the touch, colourless or almost colourless, clear, very hygroscopic.

Solubility: miscible with water and with alcohol, slightly soluble in acetone, practically insoluble in fatty oils and in essential oils.

IDENTIFICATION

First identification: A, B.

Second identification: A, C, D.

A. It complies with the test for refractive index (see Tests).

B. Infrared absorption spectrophotometry (*2.2.24*).

Comparison: *Ph. Eur. reference spectrum of glycerol (85 per cent).*

C. Mix 1 ml with 0.5 ml of *nitric acid R*. Superimpose 0.5 ml of *potassium dichromate solution R*. A blue ring develops at the interface of the liquids. Within 10 min, the blue colour does not diffuse into the lower layer.

D. Heat 1 ml with 2 g of *potassium hydrogen sulphate R* in an evaporating dish. Vapours (acrolein) are evolved which blacken filter paper impregnated with *alkaline potassium tetraiodomercurate solution R*.

TESTS

Solution S. Dilute 117.6 g to 200.0 ml with *carbon dioxide-free water R*.

Appearance of solution. Solution S is clear (*2.2.1*). Dilute 10 ml of solution S to 25 ml with *water R*. The solution is colourless (*2.2.2, Method II*).

Acidity or alkalinity. To 50 ml of solution S add 0.5 ml of *phenolphthalein solution R*. The solution is colourless. Not more than 0.2 ml of *0.1 M sodium hydroxide* is required to change the colour of the indicator to pink.

Refractive index (*2.2.6*): 1.449 to 1.455.

Aldehydes: maximum 10 ppm.

Place 7.5 ml of solution S in a ground-glass-stoppered flask and add 7.5 ml of *water R* and 1.0 ml of *decolorised pararosaniline solution R*. Close the flask and allow to stand for 1 h at a temperature of 25 ± 1 °C. The absorbance (*2.2.25*) of the solution measured at 552 nm is not greater than that of a standard prepared at the same time and in the same manner using 7.5 ml of *formaldehyde standard solution (5 ppm CH_2O) R* and 7.5 ml of *water R*. The test is not valid unless the standard is pink.

Esters. Add 10.0 ml of *0.1 M sodium hydroxide* to the final solution obtained in the test for acidity or alkalinity. Boil under a reflux condenser for 5 min. Cool. Add 0.5 ml of *phenolphthalein solution R* and titrate with *0.1 M hydrochloric acid*. Not less than 8.0 ml of *0.1 M hydrochloric acid* is required to change the colour of the indicator.

Impurity A and related substances. Gas chromatography (*2.2.28*).

Test solution. Dilute 10.0 ml of solution S to 100.0 ml with *water R*.

Reference solution (a). Dilute 11.8 g of *glycerol (85 per cent) R1* to 20.0 ml with *water R*. Dilute 10.0 ml of the solution to 100.0 ml with *water R*.

Reference solution (b). Dissolve 1.000 g of *diethylene glycol R* in *water R* and dilute to 100.0 ml with the same solvent.

Reference solution (c). Dilute 1.0 ml of reference solution (b) to 10.0 ml with reference solution (a). Dilute 1.0 ml of this solution to 20.0 ml with reference solution (a).

Reference solution (d). Mix 1.0 ml of the test solution and 5.0 ml of reference solution (b) and dilute to 100.0 ml with *water R*. Dilute 1.0 ml of this solution to 10.0 ml with *water R*.

Reference solution (e). Dilute 5.0 ml of reference solution (b) to 100.0 ml with *water R*.

Column:
- *size*: *l* = 30 m, Ø = 0.53 mm,
- *stationary phase*: 6 per cent polycyanolpropylphenyl siloxane and 94 per cent of polydimethylsiloxane.

Carrier gas: *helium for chromatography R*.

Split ratio: 1:10.

Linear velocity: 38 cm/s.

Temperature:

	Time (min)	Temperature (°C)
Column	0	100
	0 - 16	100 → 220
	16 - 20	220
Injection port		220
Detector		250

Detection: flame ionisation.

Injection: 0.5 μl.

Elution order: impurity A, glycerol.

System suitability: reference solution (d):
- *resolution*: minimum 7.0 between the peaks due to impurity A and glycerol.

Limits:
- *impurity A*: not more than the area of the corresponding peak in the chromatogram obtained with reference solution (c) (0.1 per cent),
- *any other impurity with a retention time less than the retention time of glycerol*: not more than the area of the peak due to impurity A in the chromatogram obtained with reference solution (c) (0.1 per cent),
- *total of all impurities with retention times greater than the retention time of glycerol*: not more than 5 times the area of the peak due to impurity A in the chromatogram obtained with reference solution (c) (0.5 per cent),
- *disregard limit*: 0.05 times the area of the peak due to impurity A in the chromatogram obtained with reference solution (e) (0.05 per cent).

Halogenated compounds: maximum 30 ppm.

To 10 ml of solution S add 1 ml of *dilute sodium hydroxide solution R*, 5 ml of *water R* and 50 mg of *halogen-free nickel-aluminium alloy R*. Heat on a water-bath for 10 min, allow to cool and filter. Rinse the flask and the filter with *water R* until 25 ml of filtrate is obtained. To 5 ml of the filtrate add 4 ml of *alcohol R*, 2.5 ml of *water R*, 0.5 ml of *nitric acid R* and 0.05 ml of *silver nitrate solution R2* and mix. Allow to stand for 2 min. Any opalescence in the solution is not more intense than that in a standard prepared at the same time by mixing 7.0 ml of *chloride standard solution (5 ppm Cl) R*, 4 ml of *alcohol R*, 0.5 ml of *water R*, 0.5 ml of *nitric acid R* and 0.05 ml of *silver nitrate solution R2*.

Sugars. To 10 ml of solution S add 1 ml of *dilute sulphuric acid R* and heat on a water-bath for 5 min. Add 3 ml of carbonate-free *dilute sodium hydroxide solution R* (prepared by the method described for carbonate-free *1 M sodium hydroxide (4.2.2)*), mix and add dropwise 1 ml of freshly prepared *copper sulphate solution R*. The solution is clear and blue. Continue heating on the water-bath for 5 min. The solution remains blue and no precipitate is formed.

Chlorides (*2.4.4*): maximum 10 ppm.

1 ml of solution S diluted to 15 ml with *water R* complies with the limit test for chlorides. Prepare the standard using 1 ml of *chloride standard solution (5 ppm Cl) R* diluted to 15 ml with *water R*.

Heavy metals (*2.4.8*): maximum 5 ppm.

Dilute 8 ml of solution S to 20 ml with *water R*. 12 ml of the solution complies with limit test A. Prepare the standard using *lead standard solution (1 ppm Pb) R*.

Water (*2.5.12*): 12.0 per cent to 16.0 per cent, determined on 0.200 g.

Sulphated ash (*2.4.14*): maximum 0.01 per cent, determined on 5.0 g after heating to boiling and ignition.

ASSAY

Thoroughly mix 0.075 g with 45 ml of *water R*. Add 25.0 ml of a mixture of 1 volume of *0.1 M sulphuric acid* and 20 volumes of *0.1 M sodium periodate*. Allow to stand protected from light for 15 min. Add 5.0 ml of a 500 g/l solution of *ethylene glycol R* and allow to stand protected from light for 20 min. Using 0.5 ml of *phenolphthalein solution R* as indicator, titrate with *0.1 M sodium hydroxide*. Carry out a blank titration.

1 ml of *0.1 M sodium hydroxide* is equivalent to 9.21 mg of $C_3H_8O_3$.

STORAGE

In an airtight container.

IMPURITIES

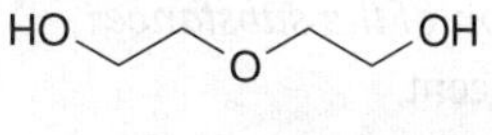

A. 2,2′-oxydiethanol (diethylene glycol),

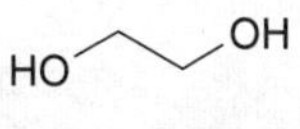

B. ethane-1,2-diol (ethylene glycol),

C. propylene glycol.

01/2005:1427

GLYCEROL DIBEHENATE

Glyceroli dibehenas

DEFINITION

Mixture of diacylglycerols, mainly dibehenylglycerol, together with variable quantities of mono- and triacylglycerols, obtained by esterification of glycerol with behenic acid.

Content:
- monoacylglycerols: 13.0 per cent to 21.0 per cent,

– diacylglycerols: 40.0 per cent to 60.0 per cent,
– triacylglycerols: 21.0 per cent to 35.0 per cent.

CHARACTERS

Appearance: hard, waxy mass or powder or white or almost white, unctuous flakes.

Solubility: practically insoluble in water, soluble in methylene chloride and partly soluble in hot alcohol.

IDENTIFICATION

A. Melting point (*2.2.14*): 65 °C to 77 °C.

B. Thin-layer chromatography (*2.2.27*).

Test solution. Dissolve 1.0 g of the substance to be examined in *toluene R*, with gentle heating and dilute to 20 ml with the same solvent.

Reference solution. Dissolve 1.0 g of *glycerol dibehenate CRS* in *toluene R*, with gentle heating and dilute to 20 ml with the same solvent.

Plate: *TLC silica gel plate R.*

Mobile phase: *hexane R, ether R* (30:70 *V/V*).

Application: 10 µl.

Development: over a path of 15 cm.

Drying: in air.

Detection: spray with a 0.1 g/l solution of *rhodamine B R* in *alcohol R*. Examine in ultraviolet light at 365 nm.

Results: the spots in the chromatogram obtained with the test solution are similar in position to those in the chromatogram obtained with the reference solution.

C. It complies with the test for composition of fatty acids (see Tests).

TESTS

Acid value (*2.5.1*): maximum 4.0, determined on 1.0 g, using a mixture of equal volumes of *alcohol R* and *toluene R* as solvent and with gentle heating.

Iodine value (*2.5.4*): maximum 3.0.

Saponification value (*2.5.6*): 145 to 165.

Carry out the titration with heating.

Free glycerol: maximum 1.0 per cent, determined as described under Assay.

Composition of fatty acids. Gas chromatography (*2.4.22, Method C*), raising the temperature of the column to 240 °C.

Composition of the fatty acid fraction of the substance:

– *palmitic acid*: maximum 3.0 per cent,
– *stearic acid*: maximum 5.0 per cent,
– *arachidic acid*: maximum 10.0 per cent,
– *behenic acid*: minimum 83.0 per cent,
– *lignoceric acid*: maximum 3.0 per cent,
– *erucic acid*: maximum 3.0 per cent.

Nickel (*2.4.27*): maximum 1 ppm.

Water (*2.5.12*): maximum 1.0 per cent, determined on 1.00 g. Use *pyridine R* as the solvent.

Total ash (*2.4.16*): maximum 0.1 per cent, determined on 1.00 g.

ASSAY

Size-exclusion chromatography (*2.2.30*).

Test solution. Into a 15 ml flask, weigh about 0.2 g (*m*), to the nearest 0.1 mg. Add 5 ml of *tetrahydrofuran R*, warm the flask slightly (about 35 °C) and shake until dissolution is obtained. Reweigh the flask and calculate the total mass of solvent and substance (*M*).

Reference solutions. In four 15 ml flasks, weigh to the nearest 0.1 mg about 2 mg, 5 mg, 10 mg and 20 mg respectively of *glycerol R*. Add 5 ml of *tetrahydrofuran R* and shake until well mixed. Weigh the flasks again and calculate the concentration of glycerol in milligrams per gram for each reference solution.

Column:

– *size*: l = 0.6 m, Ø = 7 mm,
– *stationary phase*: *styrene-divinylbenzene copolymer R* (5 µm) with a pore size of 10 nm.

Mobile phase: *tetrahydrofuran R.*

Flow rate: 1 ml/min.

Detection: differential refractive index.

Injection: 40 µl; when injecting the test solution, maintain the flask at about 35 °C in order to avoid precipitation.

Relative retentions with reference to glycerol: monoacylglycerols = about 0.82; diacylglycerols = about 0.76; triacylglycerols = about 0.73.

From the calibration curve obtained with the reference solutions determine the concentration (*C*) in milligrams per gram of glycerol in the test solution.

Calculate the percentage content of free glycerol in the substance to be examined using the following expression:

$$\frac{C \times M}{m \times 10}$$

Calculate the percentage content of mono-, di- and triacylglycerols in the substance to be examined by the normalisation procedure.

01/2005:1428

GLYCEROL DISTEARATE

Glyceroli distearas

DEFINITION

Glycerol distearate is a mixture of diacylglycerols, mainly distearoylglycerol, together with variable quantities of mono- and triacylglycerols. It contains 8.0 per cent to 22.0 per cent of monoacylglycerols, 40.0 per cent to 60.0 per cent of diacylglycerols and 25.0 per cent to 35.0 per cent of triacylglycerols, obtained by partial glycerolysis of vegetable oils containing triacylglycerols of palmitic or stearic acid or by esterification of glycerol with stearic acid 50 (type I), stearic acid 70 (type II) or stearic acid 95 (type III) (see *Stearic acid (1474)*). The fatty acids may be of vegetable or animal origin.

CHARACTERS

A hard, waxy mass or powder or white or almost white, unctuous flakes, insoluble in water, soluble in methylene chloride, partly soluble in hot alcohol.

IDENTIFICATION

A. Melting point (*2.2.14*): 50 °C to 60 °C (type I and II), 50 °C to 70 °C (type III).

B. Examine by thin-layer chromatography (*2.2.27*), using a *TLC silica gel plate R.*

Test solution. Dissolve 1.0 g of the substance to be examined in *methylene chloride R*, with gentle heating and dilute to 20 ml with the same solvent.

Reference solution. Dissolve 1.0 g of *glycerol distearate CRS* in *methylene chloride R*, with gentle heating and dilute to 20 ml with the same solvent.

Apply to the plate 10 µl of each solution. Develop over a path of 15 cm using a mixture of 30 volumes of *hexane R* and 70 volumes of *ether R*. Allow the plate to dry in air. Spray with a 0.1 g/l solution of *rhodamine B R* in *alcohol R* and examine in ultraviolet light at 365 nm. The spots in the chromatogram obtained with the test solution are similar in position to those in the chromatogram obtained with the reference solution.

C. It complies with the test for composition of fatty acids according to the type stated on the label (see Tests).

D. It complies with the limits of the assay (diacylglycerol content).

TESTS

Acid value (*2.5.1*). Not more than 6.0, determined on 1.0 g, using a mixture of equal volumes of *alcohol R* and *toluene R* as solvent and with gentle heating.

Iodine value (*2.5.4*). Not more than 3.0.

Saponification value (*2.5.6*): 165 to 195, determined on 2.0 g. Carry out the titration with heating.

Free glycerol. Not more than 1.0 per cent, determined as described under Assay.

Composition of fatty acids (*2.4.22, Method C*). The fatty-acid fraction of the substance to be examined has the following composition:

	Fatty acid used for production by esterification	Composition of fatty acids
Glycerol distearate type I	Stearic acid 50	Stearic acid: 40.0 per cent to 60.0 per cent Sum of the contents of palmitic and stearic acids: not less than 90.0 per cent
Glycerol distearate type II	Stearic acid 70	Stearic acid: 60.0 per cent to 80.0 per cent Sum of palmitic and stearic acids: not less than 90.0 per cent
Glycerol distearate type III	Stearic acid 95	Stearic acid: 90.0 per cent to 99.0 per cent Sum of the contents of palmitic and stearic acids: not less than 96.0 per cent

Nickel (*2.4.27*). Not more than 1 ppm of Ni.

Water (*2.5.12*). Not more than 1.0 per cent, determined on 1.00 g by the semi-micro determination of water. Use *pyridine R* as the solvent.

Total ash (*2.4.16*). Not more than 0.1 per cent, determined on 1.00 g.

ASSAY

Determine the free glycerol content and the mono-, di- and triacylglycerol contents by size-exclusion chromatography (*2.2.30*).

Test solution. Into a 15 ml flask, weigh about 0.2 g (*m*), to the nearest 0.1 mg. Add 5 ml of *tetrahydrofuran R* and shake to dissolve. Reweigh the flask and calculate the total mass of solvent and substance (*M*).

Reference solutions. Into four 15 ml flasks, respectively weigh, to the nearest 0.1 mg, about 2 mg, 5 mg, 10 mg and 20 mg of *glycerol R*. Add 5 ml of *tetrahydrofuran R* and shake until well mixed. Weigh the flasks again and calculate the concentration of glycerol in milligrams per gram for each reference solution.

The chromatographic procedure may be carried out using:

- a gel-permeation column 0.6 m long and 7 mm in internal diameter packed with *styrene-divinylbenzene copolymer R* (particle diameter 5 µm and porosity 10 nm),
- as mobile phase at a flow rate of 1 ml/min *tetrahydrofuran R*,
- a differential refractive index detector.

Inject 40 µl of each solution. When the chromatograms are recorded in the prescribed conditions, the retention times relative to glycerol are 0.84 for the monoacylglycerols, 0.78 for the diacylglycerols and 0.75 for the triacylglycerols. From the calibration curve obtained with the reference solutions determine the concentration (*C*) in milligrams per gram of glycerol in the test solution.

Calculate the percentage content of free glycerol in the substance to be examined using the following expression:

$$\frac{C \times M}{m \times 10}$$

Calculate the percentage content of mono-, di- and triacylglycerols in the substance to be examined by the normalisation procedure.

LABELLING

The label states the type of glycerol distearate.

01/2005:1429

GLYCEROL MONOLINOLEATE

Glyceroli monolinoleas

DEFINITION

Glycerol monolinoleate is a mixture of monoacylglycerols, mainly mono-oleoyl- and monolinoleoylglycerol, together with variable quantities of di- and triacylglycerols. It contains 32.0 per cent to 52.0 per cent of monoacylglycerols, 40.0 per cent to 55.0 per cent of diacylglycerols and 5.0 per cent to 20.0 per cent of triacylglycerols, obtained by partial glycerolysis of vegetable oils mainly containing triacylglycerols of linoleic acid. A suitable antioxidant may be added.

CHARACTERS

Amber, oily liquids which may be partially solidified at room temperature, practically insoluble in water, freely soluble in methylene chloride.

IDENTIFICATION

A. It complies with the test for iodine value (see Tests).

B. Examine by thin-layer chromatography (*2.2.27*), using a *TLC silica gel plate R*.

Test solution. Dissolve 1.0 g of the substance to be examined in *methylene chloride R* and dilute to 20 ml with the same solvent.

Reference solution. Dissolve 1.0 g of *glycerol monolinoleate CRS* in *methylene chloride R* and dilute to 20 ml with the same solvent.

Apply to the plate 10 µl of each solution. Develop over a path of 15 cm using a mixture of 30 volumes of *hexane R* and 70 volumes of *ether R*. Allow the plate to dry in air. Spray with a 0.1 g/l solution of *rhodamine B R* in *alcohol R* and examine in ultraviolet light at 365 nm. The spots in the chromatogram obtained with the test solution are similar in position to those in the chromatogram obtained with the reference solution.

C. It complies with the test for composition of fatty acids (see Tests).

TESTS

Acid value (*2.5.1*). Not more than 6.0, determined on 1.0 g.

Iodine value (*2.5.4*): 100 to 140.

Peroxide value (*2.5.5, Method A*). Not more than 12.0, determined on 2.0 g.

Saponification value (*2.5.6*): 160 to 180, determined on 2.0 g.

Free glycerol. Not more than 6.0 per cent, determined as described under Assay.

Composition of fatty acids (*2.4.22, Method C*). The fatty-acid fraction of the substance has the following composition:

- *palmitic acid*: 4.0 per cent to 20.0 per cent,
- *stearic acid*: not more than 6.0 per cent,
- *oleic acid*: 10.0 per cent to 35.0 per cent,
- *linoleic acid*: not less than 50.0 per cent,
- *linolenic acid*: not more than 2.0 per cent,
- *arachidic acid*: not more than 1.0 per cent,
- *eicosenoic acid*: not more than 1.0 per cent.

Water (*2.5.12*). Not more than 1.0 per cent, determined on 1.00 g by the semi-micro determination of water. Use as the solvent a mixture of equal volumes of *anhydrous methanol R* and *methylene chloride R*.

Total ash (*2.4.16*). Not more than 0.1 per cent, determined on 1.00 g.

ASSAY

Determine the free glycerol content and the mono-, di- and triacylglycerol contents by size-exclusion chromatography (*2.2.30*).

Test solution. Into a 15 ml flask, weigh about 0.2 g (*m*), to the nearest 0.1 mg. Add 5 ml of *tetrahydrofuran R* and shake to dissolve. Reweigh the flask and calculate the total mass of solvent and substance (*M*).

Reference solutions. Into four 15 ml flasks, respectively weigh, to the nearest 0.1 mg, about 2.5 mg, 5 mg, 10 mg and 20 mg of *glycerol R*. Add 5 ml of *tetrahydrofuran R* and shake until well mixed. Weigh the flasks again and calculate the concentration of glycerol in milligrams per gram for each reference solution.

The chromatographic procedure may be carried out using:

- a gel-permeation column 0.6 m long and 7 mm in internal diameter packed with *styrene-divinylbenzene copolymer R* (particle diameter 5 µm and porosity 10 nm),
- as mobile phase at a flow rate of 1 ml/min *tetrahydrofuran R*,
- a differential refractive index detector.

Inject 40 µl of each solution. When the chromatograms are recorded in the prescribed conditions, the retention times relative to glycerol are about 0.86 for the monoacylglycerols, about 0.80 for the diacylglycerols and about 0.76 for the triacylglycerols. From the calibration curve obtained with the reference solutions determine the concentration (*C*) in milligrams per gram of glycerol in the test solution.

Calculate the percentage content of free glycerol in the substance to be examined using the following expression:

$$\frac{C \times M}{m \times 10}$$

Calculate the percentage content of mono-, di- and triacylglycerols in the substance to be examined by the normalisation procedure.

STORAGE

Store in an airtight container, protected from light.

LABELLING

The label states the name and concentration of any added antioxidant.

01/2005:1430

GLYCEROL MONO-OLEATES

Glyceroli mono-oleates

DEFINITION

Glycerol mono-oleates are mixtures of monoacylglycerols, mainly mono-oleoylglycerol, together with variable quantities of di- and triacylglycerols. They are defined by the nominal content of monoacylglycerols and obtained by partial glycerolysis of vegetable oils mainly containing triacylglycerols of oleic acid or by esterification of glycerol by oleic acid, this fatty acid being of vegetable or animal origin.

	Nominal content of acylglycerol (per cent)		
	40	60	90
Monoacylglycerols	32.0 - 52.0	55.0 - 65.0	90.0 - 101.0
Diacylglycerols	30.0 - 50.0	15.0 - 35.0	< 10.0
Triacylglycerols	5.0 - 20.0	2.0 - 10.0	< 2.0

A suitable antioxidant may be added.

CHARACTERS

Amber, oily liquids which may be partially solidified at room temperature, practically insoluble in water, freely soluble in methylene chloride.

IDENTIFICATION

A. It complies with the test for iodine value (see Tests).

B. Examine by thin-layer chromatography (*2.2.27*), using a *TLC silica gel plate R*.

Test solution. Dissolve 1.0 g of the substance to be examined in *methylene chloride R* and dilute to 20 ml with the same solvent.

Reference solution. Dissolve 1.0 g of *glycerol mono-oleate CRS* in *methylene chloride R* and dilute to 20 ml with the same solvent.

Apply to the plate 10 µl of each solution. Develop over a path of 15 cm using a mixture of 30 volumes of *hexane R* and 70 volumes of *ether R*. Allow the plate to dry in air. Spray with a 0.1 g/l solution of *rhodamine B R* in *alcohol R* and examine in ultraviolet light at 365 nm. The spots in the chromatogram obtained with the test solution are similar in position to those in the chromatogram obtained with the reference solution.

C. It complies with the limits of the assay (monoacylglycerol content).

TESTS

Acid value (*2.5.1*). Not more than 6.0, determined on 1.0 g.

Iodine value (*2.5.4*): 65.0 to 95.0.

Peroxide value (*2.5.5*). Not more than 12.0, determined on 2.0 g.

Saponification value (*2.5.6*): 150 to 170, determined on 2.0 g.

Free glycerol. Not more than 6.0 per cent, determined as described under Assay.

Composition of fatty acids (*2.4.22, Method C*). The fatty-acid fraction of the substance has the following composition:

- *palmitic acid*: not more than 12.0 per cent,
- *stearic acid*: not more than 6.0 per cent,
- *oleic acid*: not less than 60.0 per cent,
- *linoleic acid*: not more than 35.0 per cent,
- *linolenic acid*: not more than 2.0 per cent,
- *arachidic acid*: not more than 2.0 per cent,
- *eicosenoic acid*: not more than 2.0 per cent.

Water (*2.5.12*). Not more than 1.0 per cent, determined on 1.00 g by the semi-micro determination of water. Use as the solvent a mixture of equal volumes of *anhydrous methanol R* and *methylene chloride R*.

Total ash (*2.4.16*). Not more than 0.1 per cent, determined on 1.00 g.

ASSAY

Determine the free glycerol content and the mono-, di- and triacylglycerol contents by size-exclusion chromatography (*2.2.30*).

Test solution. Into a 15 ml flask, weigh about 0.2 g (*m*), to the nearest 0.1 mg. Add 5 ml of *tetrahydrofuran R* and shake to dissolve. Reweigh the flask and calculate the total mass of solvent and substance (*M*).

Reference solutions. Into four 15 ml flasks, respectively weigh, to the nearest 0.1 mg, about 2.5 mg, 5 mg, 10 mg and 20 mg of *glycerol R*. Add 5 ml of *tetrahydrofuran R* and shake until well mixed. Weigh the flasks again and calculate the concentration of glycerol in milligrams per gram for each reference solution.

The chromatographic procedure may be carried out using:

- a gel-permeation column 0.6 m long and 7 mm in internal diameter packed with *styrene-divinylbenzene copolymer R* (particle diameter 5 µm and porosity 10 nm),
- as mobile phase at a flow rate of 1 ml/min *tetrahydrofuran R*,
- a differential refractive index detector.

Inject 40 µl of each solution. When the chromatograms are recorded in the prescribed conditions, the retention times relative to glycerol are about 0.85 for the monoacylglycerols, about 0.79 for the diacylglycerols and about 0.76 for the triacylglycerols. From the calibration curve obtained with the reference solutions determine the concentration (*C*) in milligrams per gram of glycerol in the test solution.

Calculate the percentage content of free glycerol in the substance to be examined using the following expression:

$$\frac{C \times M}{m \times 10}$$

Calculate the percentage content of mono-, di- and triacylglycerols in the substance to be examined by the normalisation procedure.

STORAGE

Store in an airtight container, protected from light.

LABELLING

The label states:

- the nominal content of monoacylglycerol,
- the name and concentration of any added antioxidant.

01/2005:0495

GLYCEROL MONOSTEARATE 40-55

Glyceroli monostearas 40-55

DEFINITION

Glycerol monostearate 40-55 is a mixture of monoacylglycerols, mainly monostearoylglycerol, together with variable quantities of di- and triacylglycerols. It contains 40.0 per cent to 55.0 per cent of monoacylglycerols, 30.0 per cent to 45.0 per cent of diacylglycerols and 5.0 per cent to 15.0 per cent of triacylglycerols, obtained by partial glycerolysis of vegetable oils mainly containing triacylglycerols of palmitic or stearic acid or by esterification of glycerol with stearic acid 50 (type I), stearic acid 70 (type II) or stearic acid 95 (type III) (see *Stearic acid (1474)*). The fatty acids may be of vegetable or animal origin.

CHARACTERS

A hard, waxy mass or unctuous powder or flakes, white or almost white, practically insoluble in water, soluble in alcohol at 60 °C.

IDENTIFICATION

A. Melting point (*2.2.15*): 54 °C to 64 °C. Introduce the melted substance into the capillary tubes and allow to stand for 24 h in a well-closed container.

B. Examine by thin-layer chromatography (*2.2.27*), using a *TLC silica gel plate R*.

Test solution. Dissolve 1.0 g of the substance to be examined in *methylene chloride R*, with gentle heating, and dilute to 20 ml with the same solvent.

Reference solution. Dissolve 1.0 g of *glycerol monostearate 40-55 CRS* in *methylene chloride R*, with gentle heating, and dilute to 20 ml with the same solvent.

Apply to the plate 10 µl of each solution. Develop over a path of 15 cm using a mixture of 30 volumes of *hexane R* and 70 volumes of *ether R*. Allow the plate to dry in air. Spray with a 0.1 g/l solution of *rhodamine B R* in *alcohol R* and examine in ultraviolet light at 365 nm. The spots in the chromatogram obtained with the test solution are similar in position to those in the chromatogram obtained with the reference solution.

C. It complies with the test for composition of fatty acids according to the type stated on the label (see Tests).

D. It complies with the limits of the assay (monoacylglycerol content).

TESTS

Acid value (*2.5.1*). Not more than 3.0, determined on 1.0 g, using a mixture of equal volumes of *alcohol R* and *toluene R* as solvent and heating gently.

Iodine value (*2.5.4*). Not more than 3.0.

Saponification value (*2.5.6*): 158 to 177, determined on 2.0 g. Carry out the titration with heating.

Free glycerol. Not more than 6.0 per cent, determined as described under Assay.

Monographs F-H

Composition of fatty acids (*2.4.22, Method C*). The fatty acid fraction of the substance to be examined has the following composition:

	Fatty acid used for production by esterification	Composition of fatty acids
Glycerol monostearate 40-55 type I	Stearic acid 50	*Stearic acid*: 40.0 per cent to 60.0 per cent *Sum of the contents of palmitic and stearic acids*: not less than 90.0 per cent
Glycerol monostearate 40-55 type II	Stearic acid 70	*Stearic acid*: 60.0 per cent to 80.0 per cent *Sum of palmitic and stearic acids*: not less than 90.0 per cent
Glycerol monostearate 40-55 type III	Stearic acid 95	*Stearic acid*: 90.0 per cent to 99.0 per cent *Sum of the contents of palmitic and stearic acids*: not less than 96.0 per cent

Nickel (*2.4.27*). Not more than 1 ppm of Ni.

Water (*2.5.12*). Not more than 1.0 per cent, determined on 1.00 g by the semi-micro determination of water. Use *pyridine R* as the solvent and heat gently.

Total ash (*2.4.16*). Not more than 0.1 per cent, determined on 1.00 g.

ASSAY

Determine the free glycerol content and the mono-, di- and triacylglycerol contents by size-exclusion chromatography (*2.2.30*).

Test solution. Into a 15 ml flask, weigh about 0.2 g (*m*), to the nearest 0.1 mg. Add 5 ml of *tetrahydrofuran R* and shake to dissolve. Reweigh the flask and calculate the total mass of solvent and substance (*M*).

Reference solutions. Into four 15 ml flasks, respectively weigh, to the nearest 0.1 mg, about 2.5 mg, 5 mg, 10 mg and 20 mg of *glycerol R*. Add 5 ml of *tetrahydrofuran R* and shake until well mixed. Weigh the flasks again and calculate the concentration of glycerol in milligrams per gram for each reference solution.

The chromatographic procedure may be carried out using:

– a gel-permeation column 0.6 m long and 7 mm in internal diameter packed with *styrene-divinylbenzene copolymer R* (particle diameter 5 µm and porosity 10 nm),

– as mobile phase at a flow rate of 1 ml/min *tetrahydrofuran R*,

– a differential refractive index detector.

Inject 40 µl of each solution. When the chromatograms are recorded in the prescribed conditions, the retention times relative to glycerol are about 0.86 for the monoacylglycerols, about 0.81 for the diacylglycerols and about 0.77 for the triacylglycerols. From the calibration curve obtained with the reference solutions determine the concentration (*C*) in milligrams per gram of glycerol in the test solution.

Calculate the percentage content of free glycerol in the substance to be examined using the following expression:

$$\frac{C \times M}{m \times 10}$$

Calculate the percentage content of mono-, di- and triacylglycerols in the substance to be examined by the normalisation procedure.

LABELLING

The label states the type of glycerol monostearate 40-55.

01/2005:1331

GLYCERYL TRINITRATE SOLUTION

Glyceroli trinitratis solutio

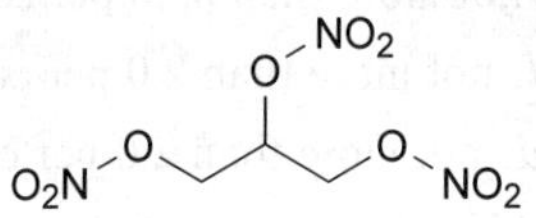

$C_3H_5N_3O_9$ M_r 227.1

DEFINITION

Ethanolic solution of glyceryl trinitrate.

Content: 1 per cent *m/m* to 10 per cent *m/m* of propane-1,2,3-triyl trinitrate and 96.5 per cent to 102.5 per cent of the declared content of glyceryl trinitrate stated on the label.

CHARACTERS

Appearance: clear, colourless or slightly yellow solution.

Solubility: miscible with acetone and with ethanol.

Solubility of pure glyceryl trinitrate: practically insoluble in water, freely soluble in ethanol, miscible with acetone.

IDENTIFICATION

First identification: A, C.

Second identification: B, C.

Upon diluting glyceryl trinitrate solution, care must be taken to always use anhydrous ethanol, otherwise droplets of pure glyceryl trinitrate may precipitate from the solution.

After examination, the residues and the solutions obtained in both the identification and the test sections must be heated on a water-bath for 5 min with dilute sodium hydroxide solution R.

A. Infrared absorption spectrophotometry (*2.2.24*).

Preparation: place 50 µl of a solution diluted, if necessary, with *ethanol R*, to contain 10 g/l of glyceryl trinitrate, on a disc of *potassium bromide R* and evaporate the solvent *in vacuo*.

Comparison: *Ph. Eur. reference spectrum of glyceryl trinitrate.*

B. Thin-layer chromatography (*2.2.27*).

Test solution. Dilute a quantity of the substance to be examined corresponding to 50 mg of glyceryl trinitrate to 100 ml with *acetone R*.

Reference solution. Dilute 0.05 ml of *glyceryl trinitrate solution CRS* to 1 ml with *acetone R*.

Plate: *TLC silica gel G plate R.*

Mobile phase: *ethyl acetate R, toluene R* (20:80 *V/V*).

Application: 5 µl.

Development: over 2/3 of the plate.

Drying: in air.

Detection: spray with freshly prepared *potassium iodide and starch solution R*. Expose the plate to ultraviolet light at 254 nm for 15 min. Examine in daylight.

Results: the principal spot in the chromatogram obtained with the test solution is similar in position, colour and size to the principal spot in the chromatogram obtained with the reference solution.

C. It complies with the limits of the assay.

TESTS

Upon diluting glyceryl trinitrate solution, care must be taken always to use anhydrous ethanol, otherwise droplets of pure glyceryl trinitrate may precipitate from the solution.

After examination, the residues and the solutions obtained in both the identification and the test sections must be heated on a water-bath for 5 min with dilute sodium hydroxide solution R.

Appearance of solution. If necessary dilute the solution to be examined to a concentration of 10 g/l with *ethanol R*. The solution is not more intensely coloured than reference solution Y_7 (*2.2.2, Method II*).

Inorganic nitrates. Thin-layer chromatography (*2.2.27*).

Test solution. If necessary dilute the solution to be examined to a concentration of 10 g/l with *ethanol R*.

Reference solution. Dissolve 5 mg of *potassium nitrate R* in 1 ml of *water R* and dilute to 100 ml with *alcohol R*.

Plate: *TLC silica gel plate R*.

Mobile phase: *glacial acetic acid R, acetone R, toluene R* (15:30:60 *V/V/V*).

Application: 10 µl.

Development: over 2/3 of the plate.

Drying: in a current of air until the acetic acid is completely removed.

Detection: spray intensively with freshly prepared *potassium iodide and starch solution R*. Expose the plate to ultraviolet light at 254 nm for 15 min. Examine in daylight.

Limit:

- *nitrate ion*: any spot corresponding to the nitrate ion in the chromatogram obtained with the test solution is not more intense than the spot in the chromatogram obtained with the reference solution (0.5 per cent of the content of glyceryl trinitrate calculated as potassium nitrate).

Related substances. Liquid chromatography (*2.2.29*).

Test solution. Dissolve a quantity of the substance to be examined corresponding to 2 mg of glyceryl trinitrate in the mobile phase and dilute to 20.0 ml with the mobile phase.

Reference solution (a). Dissolve 0.10 g of *glyceryl trinitrate solution CRS* and a quantity of *diluted pentaerythrityl tetranitrate CRS* equivalent to 1.0 mg of pentaerythrityl tetranitrate in the mobile phase and dilute to 100.0 ml with the mobile phase. Sonicate and filter if necessary.

Reference solution (b). Dilute 1.0 ml of the test solution to 100.0 ml with the mobile phase.

Column:

- *size*: *l* = 0.25 m, Ø = 4.6 mm,
- *stationary phase*: *octadecylsilyl silica gel for chromatography R* (5 µm).

Mobile phase: *acetonitrile R, water R* (50:50 *V/V*).

Flow rate: 1 ml/min.

Detection: spectrophotometer at 210 nm.

Injection: 20 µl.

Run time: 3 times the retention time of the principal peak.

System suitability: reference solution (a):

- *resolution*: minimum 2.0 between the peaks due to glyceryl trinitrate and to pentaerythrityl tetranitrate.

Limits:

- *any impurity*: not more than the area of the principal peak in the chromatogram obtained with reference solution (b) (1 per cent, calculated as glyceryl trinitrate),
- *total*: not more than 3 times the area of the principal peak in the chromatogram obtained with reference solution (b) (3 per cent, calculated as glyceryl trinitrate),
- *disregard limit*: 0.1 times the area of the principal peak in the chromatogram obtained with reference solution (b) (0.1 per cent).

ASSAY

Test solution. Prepare a solution containing 1.0 mg of glyceryl trinitrate in 250.0 ml of *methanol R*.

Reference solution. Dissolve 70.0 mg of *sodium nitrite R* in *methanol R* and dilute to 250.0 ml with the same solvent. Dilute 5.0 ml of the solution to 500.0 ml with *methanol R*.

Into three 50 ml volumetric flasks introduce 10.0 ml of the test solution, 10.0 ml of the reference solution and 10 ml of *methanol R* as a blank. To each flask add 5 ml of *dilute sodium hydroxide solution R*, close the flask, mix and allow to stand at room temperature for 30 min. Add 10 ml of *sulphanilic acid solution R* and 10 ml of *dilute hydrochloric acid R* and mix. After exactly 4 min, add 10 ml of *naphthylethylenediamine dihydrochloride solution R*, dilute to volume with *water R* and mix. After 10 min read the absorbance (*2.2.25*) of the test solution and the reference solution at 540 nm using the blank solution as the compensation liquid.

Calculate the amount of glyceryl trinitrate in milligrams in the test solution from the following expression:

$$\frac{A_T \times m_S \times C}{A_R \times m_T \times 60.8 \times 100}$$

A_T = absorption of the test solution,

m_T = mass of the substance to be examined, in milligrams,

C = percentage content of sodium nitrite used as reference,

A_R = absorption of the reference solution,

m_S = mass of sodium nitrite, in milligrams.

STORAGE

Store diluted solutions (10 g/l) protected from light, at a temperature of 2 °C to 15 °C. Store more concentrated solutions protected from light, at a temperature of 15 °C to 20 °C.

LABELLING

The label states the declared content of glyceryl trinitrate.

IMPURITIES

A. inorganic nitrates,

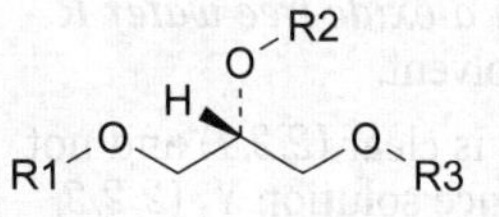

and enantiomer

B. R1 = NO_2, R2 = R3 = H: (2*RS*)-2,3-dihydroxypropyl nitrate,

C. R1 = R3 = H, R2 = NO_2: 2-hydroxy-1-(hydroxymethyl)ethyl nitrate,

D. R1 = R2 = NO_2, R3 = H: (2*RS*)-3-hydroxypropane-1,2-diyl dinitrate,

E. R1 = R3 = NO_2, R2 = H: 2-hydroxypropane-1,3-diyl dinitrate.

01/2005:0614
corrected

GLYCINE

Glycinum

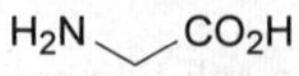

$C_2H_5NO_2$ M_r 75.1

DEFINITION

2-Aminoacetic acid.

Content: 98.5 per cent to 101.0 per cent (dried substance).

CHARACTERS

Appearance: white or almost white, crystalline powder.

Solubility: freely soluble in water, very slightly soluble in alcohol.

It shows polymorphism.

IDENTIFICATION

First identification: A.

Second identification: B, C.

A. Infrared absorption spectrophotometry (*2.2.24*).

Preparation: discs. Use about 1 mg for 0.4 g of *potassium bromide R*.

Comparison: *glycine CRS*.

If the spectra obtained in the solid state show differences, dissolve the substance to be examined and the reference substance separately in the smallest necessary quantity of *alcohol (60 per cent V/V) R*, evaporate to dryness and record the spectra again.

B. Examine the chromatograms obtained in the test for ninhydrin-positive substances.

Results: the principal spot in the chromatogram obtained with test solution (b) is similar in position, colour and size to the principal spot in the chromatogram obtained with reference solution (a).

C. Dissolve 50 mg in 5 ml of *water R*, add 1 ml of *strong sodium hypochlorite solution R* and boil for 2 min. Add 1 ml of *hydrochloric acid R* and boil for 4-5 min. Add 2 ml of *hydrochloric acid R* and 1 ml of a 20 g/l solution of *resorcinol R*, boil for 1 min and cool. Add 10 ml of *water R* and mix. To 5 ml of the solution add 6 ml of *dilute sodium hydroxide solution R*. The solution is violet with greenish-yellow fluorescence. After a few minutes, the colour becomes orange and then yellow and an intense fluorescence remains.

TESTS

Solution S. Dissolve 5.0 g in *carbon dioxide-free water R* and dilute to 50 ml with the same solvent.

Appearance of solution. Solution S is clear (*2.2.1*) and not more intensely coloured than reference solution Y_7 (*2.2.2, Method II*).

pH (*2.2.3*): 5.9 to 6.4.

Dilute 10 ml of solution S to 20 ml with *carbon dioxide-free water R*.

Ninhydrin-positive substances. Thin-layer chromatography (*2.2.27*).

Test solution (a). Dissolve 0.10 g of the substance to be examined in *water R* and dilute to 10.0 ml with the same solvent.

Test solution (b). Dilute 1.0 ml of test solution (a) to 10.0 ml with *water R*.

Reference solution (a). Dissolve 10 mg of *glycine CRS* in *water R* and dilute to 10.0 ml with the same solvent.

Reference solution (b). Dilute 1.0 ml of test solution (a) to 200 ml with *water R*.

Reference solution (c). Dissolve 10 mg of *glycine CRS* and 10 mg of *alanine CRS* in *water R* and dilute to 25 ml with the same solvent.

Plate: *cellulose for chromatography R* as the coating substance.

Mobile phase: *glacial acetic acid R, water R, butanol R* (20:20:60 *V/V/V*).

Application: 5 µl.

Development: over 2/3 of the plate.

Drying: at 80 °C for 30 min.

Detection: spray with *ninhydrin solution R* and dry at 100-105 °C for 15 min.

System suitability: the chromatogram obtained with reference solution (c) shows 2 clearly separated spots.

Limits: in the chromatogram obtained with test solution (a):

– *any impurity*: any spots, apart from the principal spot, are not more intense than the principal spot in the chromatogram obtained with reference solution (b) (0.5 per cent).

Chlorides (*2.4.4*): maximum 75 ppm.

Dissolve 0.67 g in *water R* and dilute to 15 ml with the same solvent. The solution complies with the limit test for chlorides.

Heavy metals (*2.4.8*): maximum 10 ppm.

12 ml of solution S complies with limit test A. Prepare the standard using *lead standard solution (1 ppm Pb) R*.

Loss on drying (*2.2.32*): maximum 0.5 per cent, determined on 1.000 g by drying in an oven at 100-105 °C for 2 h.

Sulphated ash (*2.4.14*): maximum 0.1 per cent, determined on 1.0 g.

ASSAY

Dissolve 70.0 mg in 3 ml of *anhydrous formic acid R* and add 30 ml of *anhydrous acetic acid R*. Immediately after dissolution, titrate with *0.1 M perchloric acid*, determining the end-point potentiometrically (*2.2.20*).

1 ml of *0.1 M perchloric acid* is equivalent to 7.51 mg of $C_2H_5NO_2$.

01/2005:1892
corrected

GOLDENROD

Solidaginis herba

DEFINITION

Whole or cut, dried, flowering aerial parts of *Solidago gigantea* Ait or *S. canadensis* L., their varieties or hybrids and/or mixtures of these.

Content: minimum 2.5 per cent of flavonoids, expressed as hyperoside ($C_{21}H_{20}O_{12}$; M_r 464.4) (dried drug).

CHARACTERS

Macroscopic and microscopic characters described under identification tests A and B.

IDENTIFICATION

A. The stems are greenish-yellow or greenish-brown, partly tinted reddish, roundish, more or less conspicuously grooved, glabrous and smooth in the lower part, slightly or densely pubescent in the upper part. They are solid with a whitish pith.

The leaves are green, sessile, lanceolate, with a serrate margin, 8 cm to 12 cm long and about 1 cm to 3 cm wide, the upper surface is green and more or less glabrous, the lower surface is greyish-green and pubescent, especially on the veins. The inflorescence consists of a number of unilateral, curved racemes which together form a pyramidal panicle at the end of the stems.

Each capitulum has an involucre composed of linear-lanceolate, imbricated yellowish-green bracts, surrounding a single row of yellow ligulate florets about the same length as the involucre; yellow, radially arranged tubular florets, as long as, or longer, than the ligulate florets; a brownish inferior ovary surmounted by a white pappus of silky hairs.

B. Reduce to a powder (355). The powder is greyish-green. Examine under a microscope using *chloral hydrate solution R*. The powder shows pappus bristles and their fragments, consisting of multiseriate trichomes composed of elongated cells with the tips free from the surface and forming pointed projections over the entire length; fragments of the leaf mesophyll with vascular bundles accompanied by secretory cells; fragments of the leaf epidermis with sinuous to wavy-walled cells and stomata of the anomocytic type (*2.8.3*); uniseriate covering trichomes with up to 5 or 6 cells, some whip-like with a thicker-walled terminal cell; fragments of the style with long, slender papillae; fragments of the stem with reticulate and spiral vessels; pollen grains, with 3 germinal pores and a spiny exine; numerous whisk-shaped hairs, a few isolated twin-hairs from the ovary, absence of multicellular trichomes with a terminal cell bent at a right angle.

C. Thin-layer chromatography (*2.2.27*), as described in the test for *Solidago virgaurea* with the following modifications.

Detection: spray with a 10 g/l solution of *diphenylboric acid aminoethyl ester R* in *methanol R* and then with a 50 g/l solution of *macrogol 400 R* in *methanol R*. Allow to stand for 30 min. Examine in ultraviolet light at 365 nm.

Results: see below the sequence of the zones present in the chromatograms obtained with the reference solution and the test solution. Furthermore, other zones may be present in the chromatogram obtained with the test solution.

Top of the plate	
Caffeic acid: a light blue fluorescent zone.	
	A bluish-green fluorescent zone.
Quercitrin: a yellowish-brown fluorescent zone.	A faint to intense yellowish-brown fluorescent zone.
	A more or less intense yellowish brown zone.
Chlorogenic acid: a light blue fluorescent zone.	A light blue zone and/or a yellow fluorescent zone.
Rutin: an orange fluorescent zone.	A faint to intense yellowish-brown fluorescent zone.
Reference solution	**Test solution**

TESTS

Foreign matter (*2.8.2*): maximum 5 per cent of brownish parts and maximum 2 per cent of other foreign matter.

Solidago virgaurea. Thin-layer chromatography (*2.2.27*).

Test solution. To 0.75 g of the powdered drug (355) add 5 ml of *methanol R* and boil in a water-bath under a reflux condenser for 10 min. Cool and filter.

Reference solution. Dissolve 1.0 mg of *chlorogenic acid R*, 1.0 mg of *caffeic acid R*, 2.5 mg of *quercitrin R* and 2.5 mg of *rutin R* in 10 ml of *methanol R*.

Plate: *TLC silica gel plate R*.

Mobile phase: *anhydrous formic acid R, water R, methyl ethyl ketone R, ethyl acetate R* (6:6:18:30 *V/V/V/V*).

Application: 20 µl of the test solution and 10 µl of the reference solution, as bands.

Development: over a path of 10 cm.

Drying: at 100-105 °C.

Detection: spray with *anisaldehyde solution R* and heat at 100-105 °C for 10 min. Examine in ultraviolet light at 365 nm.

Results: the chromatograms obtained with the reference solution and the test solution show a greyish-green fluorescent zone in the lower third (rutin). The chromatogram obtained with the test solution does not show a dark grey or dark brown zone (leiocarposide) below the zone due to rutin.

Loss on drying (*2.2.32*): maximum 10 per cent, determined on 0.500 g of the powdered drug (355) by drying in an oven at 100-105 °C for 2 h.

Total ash (*2.4.16*): maximum 7.0 per cent.

Ash insoluble in hydrochloric acid (*2.8.1*): maximum 1.0 per cent.

ASSAY

Stock solution. In a 100 ml round-bottomed flask, introduce 0.200 g of the powdered drug (250), add 1 ml of a 5 g/l solution of *hexamethylenetetramine R*, 20 ml of *acetone R* and 2 ml of *hydrochloric acid R1*. Boil the mixture under a reflux condenser for 30 min. Filter the liquid through a small plug of absorbent cotton into a 100 ml flask. Add the absorbent cotton to the residue in the round-bottomed flask, extract with 2 quantities, each of 20 ml of *acetone R*, each time boiling under a reflux condenser for 10 min. Allow to cool. Filter the combined acetone extracts through a filter paper into a volumetric flask. Rinse the flask and the filter paper and dilute to 100.0 ml with *acetone R*. Introduce 20.0 ml of the solution into a suitable separating funnel, add 20 ml of *water R* and shake the mixture with 1 quantity of 15 ml and then 3 quantities, each of 10 ml, of *ethyl acetate R*. Combine the ethyl acetate extracts in a separating funnel, wash twice with 50 ml of *water R* and filter the extracts over 10 g of *anhydrous sodium sulphate R* into a volumetric flask. Dilute to 50.0 ml with *ethyl acetate R*, rinsing the separating funnel and the sodium sulphate.

Test solution. To 10.0 ml of the stock solution add 1.0 ml of *aluminium chloride reagent R* and dilute to 25.0 ml with a 5 per cent *V/V* solution of *glacial acetic acid R* in *methanol R*.

Compensation solution. Dilute 10.0 ml of the stock solution to 25.0 ml with a 5 per cent *V/V* solution of *glacial acetic acid R* in *methanol R*.

Measure the absorbance of the test solution (*2.2.25*) at 425 nm after 30 min by comparison with the compensation solution.

Calculate the percentage content of flavonoids, expressed as hyperoside, from the expression:

$$\frac{A \times 1.25}{m}$$

i.e. taking the value of the specific absorbance of hyperoside to be 500.

A = absorbance measured at 425 nm,

m = mass of the drug to be examined, in grams.

01/2005:1893 corrected

GOLDENROD, EUROPEAN

Solidaginis virgaureae herba

DEFINITION

Whole or cut, dried, flowering aerial parts of *Solidago virgaurea* L.

Content: minimum 1.0 per cent of flavonoids, expressed as hyperoside ($C_{21}H_{20}O_{12}$; M_r 464.4) (dried drug).

CHARACTERS

Macroscopic and microscopic characters described under identification tests A and B.

IDENTIFICATION

A. The stem is cylindrical, striated, the lower part often reddish-violet, sometimes entirely glabrous or pubescent with short, bent, apically directed hairs. The basal leaves are obovate to oblanceolate, with a serrate margin, and taper at the base into a long, winged petiole; the cauline leaves are alternate, smaller than the basal leaves and more elliptical in outline, with an entire or slightly toothed margin; they are sessile or with only a short petiole. Both surfaces of the leaves are glabrous or only slightly pubescent with a prominent reticulate venation on the lower surface. The capitula form a tightly packed panicle. At the base of the pedicels there are 2, small, linear bracts with scarious margins. The involucre consists of 2 to 4 rows of loosely-arranged, imbricate bracts, each bract greenish-yellow with a smooth and shiny inner surface, the outer surface hairy or glabrous, with a scarious margin. Each capitulum contains from 6 to 12 widely separated female ray florets, about twice as long as the bracts, and about 10 to 30 hermaphrodite, tubular florets. All florets are yellow. The brown, inferior ovary tapers towards the base and has a ribbed surface, covered with scattered hairs; it is surmounted by a whitish pappus composed of smooth or rough, bristly hairs.

B. Reduce to a powder (355). The powder is light green. Examine under a microscope using *chloral hydrate solution R*. The powder shows fragments of the leaf in surface view, those of the upper epidermis composed of polygonal cells with straight, beaded walls and distinct cuticular striations, those of the lower epidermis more sinuous with fewer striations and numerous anomocytic stomata (*2.8.3*); occasional leaf fragments showing cells containing small, isolated cluster crystals of calcium oxalate; uniseriate, conical covering trichomes from the leaves and the bracts with up to about 10 cells, some of the shorter trichomes showing a terminal cell extended and pennant-like; occasional glandular trichomes with a 1 or 2 celled stalk and a unicellular, elongated head; rare paired, covering trichomes from the ovary with a distinctly pitted central wall and a bifid apex; abundant pappus hairs and their fragments, multiseriate with the marginal cells overlapping outwards; groups of fibres and vascular tissue from the stems; fragments of the epidermis of the petals with striated cuticle and occasional long, biseriate glandular trichomes; pollen grains spherical, with 3 pores and a spiny exine.

C. Thin-layer chromatography (*2.2.27*) as described in the test for *Solidago gigantea* and *Solidago canadensis*.

Detection: spray 1 of the 2 plates with *anisaldehyde solution R* and heat at 105-110 °C for 10 min. Examine the plate in daylight.

Results: see below the sequence of the zones present in the chromatograms obtained with the reference solution and the test solution. Furthermore, other fluorescent zones may be present in the chromatogram obtained with the test solution.

Top of the plate	
	A violet zone
Quercitrin: a yellow zone	
_______	_______
	A faint yellow zone (nicotiflorin)
Rutin: a yellow zone	A yellow zone (rutin)
Leiocarposide: a brownish zone	A brownish zone (leiocarposide)
_______	_______
	A greenish zone
Reference solution	**Test solution**

TESTS

Foreign matter (*2.8.2*): maximum 5 per cent of brown coloured matter and maximum 2 per cent of other foreign matter.

Solidago gigantea* and *Solidago canadensis. Thin-layer chromatography (*2.2.27*).

Test solution. To 0.75 g of the powdered drug (355) add 5 ml of *methanol R* and heat on a water-bath under a reflux condenser for 10 min. Cool and filter.

Reference solution. Dissolve 1.0 mg of *chlorogenic acid R*, 2.5 mg of *quercitrin R*, 2.5 mg of *rutin R* and 5 mg of *leiocarposide R* in 10 ml of *methanol R*.

Plate: *TLC silica gel plate R* (2 plates).

Mobile phase: *anhydrous formic acid R, water R, methyl ethyl ketone R, ethyl acetate R* (6:6:18:30 *V/V/V/V*).

Application: 20 µl, as bands.

Development: over a path of 10 cm.

Drying: in air.

Detection: spray 1 of the 2 plates with a 10 g/l solution of *diphenylboric acid aminoethyl ester R* in *methanol R* and then with a 50 g/l solution of *macrogol 400 R* in *methanol R*. Examine in ultraviolet light at 365 nm after 30 min.

Results: see below the sequence of zones present in the chromatograms obtained with the reference solution and the test solution. Furthermore, other fluorescent zones may be present in the chromatogram obtained with the test solution. The chromatogram obtained with the test solution shows no strong orange fluorescent zone similar in position to the zone of quercitrin in the chromatogram obtained with the reference solution.

Top of the plate	
	A light blue fluorescent zone
Quercitrin: an orange fluorescent zone	
_______	_______
Chlorogenic acid: a light blue fluorescent zone	A light blue fluorescent zone (chlorogenic acid)
Rutin: an orange fluorescent zone	An orange fluorescent zone (rutin)
_______	_______
Reference solution	**Test solution**

Loss on drying (*2.2.32*): maximum 12 per cent, determined on 1.000 g of the powdered drug (355) by drying in an oven at 100-105 °C for 2 h.

Total ash (*2.4.16*): maximum 8.0 per cent.

ASSAY

Stock solution. In a 100 ml round-bottomed flask, place 0.200 g of the powdered drug (355), add 1 ml of a 5 g/l solution of *hexamethylenetetramine R*, 20 ml of *acetone R* and 2 ml of *hydrochloric acid R1*. Boil the mixture in a water-bath under a reflux condenser for 30 min. Filter the liquid through a small plug of absorbent cotton into a 100 ml flask. Add the absorbent cotton to the residue in the round-bottomed flask and extract with 2 quantities, each of 20 ml, of *acetone R*, each time boiling under a reflux condenser for 10 min. Allow to cool. Filter the combined acetone extracts through filter paper, dilute to 100.0 ml with *acetone R*, rinsing the volumetric flask and the filter paper with acetone. Introduce 20.0 ml of the solution into a suitable separating funnel, add 20 ml of *water R* and shake the mixture with 1 quantity of 15 ml and then with 3 quantities, each of 10 ml, of *ethyl acetate R*. Combine the ethyl acetate extracts in a separating funnel, wash twice with 50 ml of *water R* and filter the extracts over 10 g of *anhydrous sodium sulphate R* into a volumetric flask. Dilute to 50.0 ml with *ethyl acetate R*, rinsing the separating funnel and the sodium sulphate.

Test solution. To 10.0 ml of the stock solution add 1.0 ml of *aluminium chloride reagent R* and dilute to 25.0 ml with a 5 per cent *V/V* solution of *glacial acetic acid R* in *methanol R*.

Compensation liquid. Dilute 10.0 ml of the stock solution to 25.0 ml with a 5 per cent *V/V* solution of *glacial acetic acid R* in *methanol R*.

After 30 min, measure the absorbance (*2.2.25*) of the test solution at 425 nm by comparison with the compensation liquid.

Calculate the percentage content of flavonoids, expressed as hyperoside, from the expression:

$$\frac{A \times 1.25}{m}$$

i.e. taking the specific absorbance of hyperoside to be 500.

A = measured absorbance at 425 nm,

m = mass of the drug to be examined, in grams.

01/2005:1831

GOLDENSEAL RHIZOME

Hydrastis rhizoma

DEFINITION

Whole or cut, dried rhizome and root of *Hydrastis canadensis* L.

Content:

– hydrastine ($C_{21}H_{21}NO_6$; M_r 383.4): minimum 2.5 per cent (dried drug),

– berberine ($C_{20}H_{19}NO_5$; M_r 353.4): minimum 3.0 per cent (dried drug).

CHARACTERS

Macroscopic and microscopic characters described under identification tests A and B.

IDENTIFICATION

A. The rhizome is tortuous and knotty, about 5 cm long and 5 mm to 10 mm thick. The surface is yellowish to brownish-grey and irregularly wrinkled, and bears the remains of numerous slender, wiry roots; stem bases and scale leaves occur on the upper surface. The fracture is short and resinous. The transversely-cut surface is yellowish-brown and shows a fairly wide bark, a ring of from about 12 to 20 widely separated xylem bundles and a large, central pith.

B. Reduce to a powder (180). The powder is greenish-yellow. Examine under a microscope using *chloral hydrate solution R*. The powder shows the following diagnostic characters: abundant thin-walled parenchyma; occasional fragments of yellowish-brown cork from the rhizome and roots; groups of small vessels with conspicuous perforations in the oblique end walls and with simple or bordered, slit-shaped pits; infrequent groups of thin-walled, pitted fibres, usually found associated with the vessels; numerous ovoid or spherical, orange-brown granular masses. Examine under a microscope using a 50 per cent *V/V* solution of *glycerol R*. The powder shows abundant starch granules, mostly simple but sometimes compound with up to 4 components; the granules are small, spherical to ovoid, up to about 10 µm in diameter, occasionally with a small, rounded or slit-shaped hilum.

C. Thin-layer chromatography (*2.2.27*).

Test solution. Sonicate for 10 min 250 mg of powdered drug (180) in 4 ml of a mixture of 20 ml of *water R* and 80 ml of *methanol R* and filter. Wash the residue twice with 2 ml of *methanol R*. Combine the solutions and dilute to 20 ml with *methanol R*.

Reference solution. Dissolve 5 mg of *hydrastine hydrochloride R* and 5 mg of *berberine chloride R* in 20 ml of *methanol R*.

Plate: *TLC silica gel plate R*.

Mobile phase: *anhydrous formic acid R, water R, ethyl acetate R* (10:10:80 *V/V/V*).

Application: 20 µl as bands.

Development: over a path of 15 cm.

Drying: in air.

Detection: examine in ultraviolet light at 365 nm.

Results: see below the sequence of the zones present in the chromatograms obtained with the reference solution and the test solution. Furthermore other fluorescent zones may be present in the chromatogram obtained with the test solution.

Monographs F-H

Top of the plate	
———	———
Berberine: a bright yellow fluorescent zone	A bright yellow fluorescent zone (berberine)
Hydrastine: a deep blue fluorescent zone	A deep blue fluorescent zone (hydrastine)
———	———
	A bright light blue fluorescent zone (hydrastinine)
	A deep blue fluorescent zone
Reference solution	**Test solution**

TESTS

Foreign matter (*2.8.2*): maximum 2 per cent *m/m*.

Loss on drying (*2.2.32*): maximum 10.0 per cent, determined on 1.000 g of the powdered drug (180) by drying in an oven at 100-105 °C for 2 h.

Total ash (*2.4.16*): maximum 8.0 per cent.

Ash insoluble in hydrochloric acid (*2.8.1*): maximum 4.0 per cent.

ASSAY

Liquid chromatography (*2.2.29*).

Test solution. To 1.000 g of the powdered drug (355) in a 100 ml round-bottomed flask, add 50 ml of a 10 ml/l solution of *concentrated ammonia R* in *alcohol R* and boil the mixture under a reflux condenser for 30 min. Allow to cool to room temperature and filter the liquid through a plug of absorbent cotton into a flask. Add the absorbent cotton to the residue in the round-bottomed flask and repeat the extraction with a further 2 quantities, each of 30 ml of a 10 ml/l solution of *concentrated ammonia R* in *alcohol R*, each time boiling under a reflux condenser for 10 min and filtering through a plug of absorbent cotton in the same flask as previously. Filter the combined filtrates through a filter-paper into a 250 ml round-bottomed flask, and rinse flask and filter with 20 ml of a 10 ml/l solution of *concentrated ammonia R* in *alcohol R*. Evaporate the filtrate to dryness *in vacuo* in a water-bath at 55 °C. Dissolve the residue in 50.0 ml of the mobile phase. Dilute 10.0 ml of this solution to 250.0 ml with the mobile phase.

Reference solution. Dissolve 10 mg of *hydrastine hydrochloride R* and 10 mg of *berberine chloride R* in *methanol R* and dilute to 100.0 ml with the same solvent.

Column:

- *size*: l = 0.125 m, Ø = 4 mm,
- *stationary phase*: *end-capped octadecylsilyl silica gel for chromatography R* (5 μm).

Mobile phase: dissolve 9.93 g of *potassium dihydrogen phosphate R* in 730 ml of *water R*, add 270 ml of *acetonitrile R* and mix.

Flow rate: 1.2 ml/min.

Detection: spectrophotometer at 235 nm.

Injection: 10 μl.

System suitability: reference solution:

- *elution order*: when the chromatograms are recorded in the prescribed conditions, the components elute in the order indicated in the composition of the reference solution; record the retention times of these substances;
- *resolution*: minimum 1.5 between the peaks due to hydrastine and berberine.

Using the retention times determined from the chromatogram obtained with the reference solution, locate the components of the reference solution on the chromatogram obtained with the test solution.

Calculate the percentage content of each alkaloid (hydrastine and berberine) from the following expression:

$$\frac{A_1 \times m_2 \times p}{A_2 \times m_1} \times 12.5$$

A_1 = area of the peak due to hydrastine or berberine in the chromatogram obtained with the test solution,

A_2 = area of the peak due to hydrastine or berberine in the chromatogram obtained with the reference solution,

m_1 = mass of the drug to be examined, in grams,

m_2 = mass of hydrastine hydrochloride or berberine chloride in the reference solution, in grams,

p = percentage content of hydrastine in *hydrastine hydrochloride R* or berberine in *berberine chloride R*.

01/2005:0827
corrected

GONADORELIN ACETATE

Gonadorelini acetas

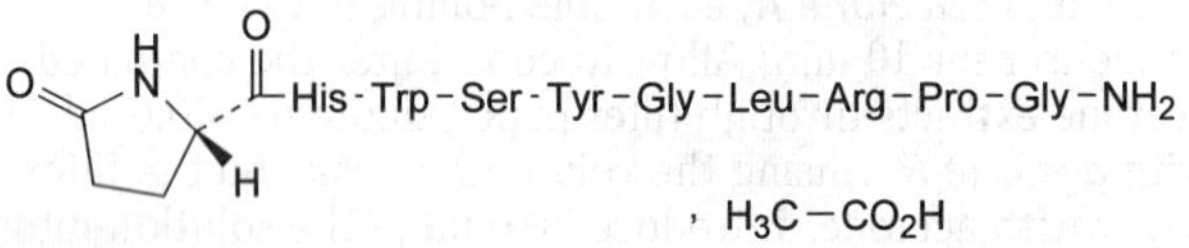

$C_{57}H_{79}N_{17}O_{15}$ M_r 1242

DEFINITION

Gonadorelin acetate is the acetate form of a hypothalamic peptide that stimulates the release of follicle-stimulating hormone and luteinising hormone from the pituitary gland. It contains not less than 95.0 per cent and not more than the equivalent of 102.0 per cent of the peptide $C_{55}H_{75}N_{17}O_{13}$, calculated with reference to the anhydrous, acetic acid-free substance. It is obtained by chemical synthesis.

CHARACTERS

A white or slightly yellowish powder, soluble in water and in a 1 per cent *V/V* solution of glacial acetic acid, sparingly soluble in methanol.

IDENTIFICATION

A. Examine the chromatograms obtained in the assay. The retention time and size of the principal peak in the chromatogram obtained with the test solution are approximately the same as those of the principal peak in the chromatogram obtained with reference solution (a).

B. Examine by thin-layer chromatography (*2.2.27*), using a *TLC silica gel G plate R*.
Use the test solution and reference solution (a) prepared under Assay.
Apply to the plate 10 μl of each solution. Develop over a path of 15 cm using a mixture of 6 volumes of *glacial acetic acid R*, 14 volumes of *water R*, 45 volumes of *methanol R* and 60 volumes of *methylene chloride R*. Allow the plate to dry in air for 5 min. At the bottom of a chromatography tank, place an evaporating dish containing a mixture of 10 ml of a 50 g/l solution of

potassium permanganate R and 3 ml of *hydrochloric acid R*, close the tank and allow to stand. Place the dried plate in the tank and close the tank. Leave the plate in contact with the chlorine vapour for 2 min. Withdraw the plate and place it in a current of cold air until the excess of chlorine is removed and an area of coating below the points of application no longer gives a blue colour with 0.05 ml of *potassium iodide and starch solution R*. Spray with *potassium iodide and starch solution R*. The principal spot in the chromatogram obtained with the test solution corresponds in position and size to the principal spot in the chromatogram obtained with reference solution (a).

TESTS

Appearance of solution. A 10 g/l solution is clear (*2.2.1*) and not more intensely coloured than reference solution Y_5 (*2.2.2, Method II*).

Specific optical rotation (*2.2.7*). Dissolve 10.0 mg in 1.0 ml of a 1 per cent *V/V* solution of *glacial acetic acid R*. The specific optical rotation is − 54 to − 66, calculated on the basis of the peptide content as determined in the assay.

Absorbance (*2.2.25*). Dissolve 10.0 mg in *water R* and dilute to 100.0 ml with the same solvent. The absorbance, determined at the maximum at 278 nm, corrected to a 10 mg/100 ml solution on the basis of the peptide content determined in the assay, is 0.55 to 0.61.

Amino acids. Examine by means of an amino-acid analyser. Standardise the apparatus with a mixture containing equimolar amounts of ammonia, glycine and the L-form of the following amino acids:

lysine	threonine	alanine	leucine
histidine	serine	valine	tyrosine
arginine	glutamic acid	methionine	phenylalanine
aspartic acid	proline	isoleucine	

together with half the equimolar amount of L-cystine. For the validation of the method, an appropriate internal standard, such as *DL-norleucine R*, is used.

Test solution. Place 1.0 mg of the substance to be examined in a rigorously cleaned hard-glass tube 100 mm long and 6 mm in internal diameter. Add a suitable amount of a 50 per cent *V/V* solution of *hydrochloric acid R*. Immerse the tube in a freezing mixture at − 5 °C, reduce the pressure to below 133 Pa and seal. Heat at 110 °C to 115 °C for 16 h. Cool, open the tube, transfer the contents to a 10 ml flask with the aid of five quantities, each of 0.2 ml, of *water R* and evaporate to dryness over *potassium hydroxide R* under reduced pressure. Take up the residue in *water R* and evaporate to dryness over *potassium hydroxide R* under reduced pressure; repeat these operations once. Take up the residue in a buffer solution suitable for the amino-acid analyser used and dilute to a suitable volume with the same buffer solution. Apply a suitable volume to the amino-acid analyser.

Express the content of each amino acid in moles. Calculate the relative proportions of the amino acids, taking one-eighth of the sum of the number of moles of histidine, glutamic acid, leucine, proline, glycine, tyrosine and arginine as equal to one. The values fall within the following limits: serine 0.7 to 1.05; glutamic acid 0.95 to 1.05; proline 0.95 to 1.05; glycine 1.9 to 2.1; leucine 0.9 to 1.1; tyrosine 0.7 to 1.05; histidine 0.95 to 1.05 and arginine 0.95 to 1.05. Lysine and isoleucine are absent; not more than traces of other amino acids are present, with the exception of tryptophan.

Related substances. Examine by liquid chromatography (*2.2.29*) as described under Assay.

Inject 20 µl of reference solution (b). Adjust the sensitivity of the system so that the height of the principal peak in the chromatogram obtained is at least 50 per cent of the full scale of the recorder.

Inject 20 µl of the test solution. Continue the chromatography for twice the retention time of gonadorelin. In the chromatogram obtained with the test solution: the area of any peak apart from the principal peak, is not greater than twice the area of the principal peak in the chromatogram obtained with reference solution (b) (2 per cent); the sum of the areas of the peaks, apart from the principal peak, is not greater than 5 times the area of the principal peak in the chromatogram obtained with reference solution (b) (5 per cent). Disregard any peak with an area less than 0.05 times that of the principal peak in the chromatogram obtained with reference solution (b) (0.05 per cent).

Acetic acid (*2.5.34*): 4.0 per cent to 7.5 per cent.

Test solution. Dissolve 10.0 mg of the substance to be examined in a mixture of 5 volumes of mobile phase B and 95 volumes of mobile phase A and dilute to 10.0 ml with the same mixture of solvents.

Water (*2.5.12*). Not more than 7.0 per cent, determined on 0.200 g by the semi-micro determination of water.

Bacterial endotoxins (*2.6.14*): less than 70 IU/mg, if intended for use in the manufacture of parenteral dosage forms without a further appropriate procedure for the removal of bacterial endotoxins.

ASSAY

Examine by liquid chromatography (*2.2.29*).

Test solution. Dissolve 5.0 mg of the substance to be examined in *water R* and dilute to 10.0 ml with the same solvent.

Reference solution (a). Dissolve the contents of a vial of *gonadorelin CRS* in *water R* to obtain a concentration of 0.5 mg/ml.

Reference solution (b). Dilute 1.0 ml of the test solution to 100.0 ml with *water R*.

Reference solution (c). Dissolve 2.5 mg of the substance to be examined in 1 ml of *0.1 M hydrochloric acid* and heat in a water-bath at 65 °C for 4 h. Add 1 ml of *0.1 M sodium hydroxide* and dilute to 5.0 ml with *water R*.

The chromatographic procedure may be carried out using:

– a stainless steel column 0.12 m long and 4.0 mm in internal diameter packed with *octadecylsilyl silica gel for chromatography R* (5 µm),

– as mobile phase at a flow rate of 1.5 ml/min a mixture of 13 volumes of *acetonitrile R* and 87 volumes of a 1.18 per cent *V/V* solution of *phosphoric acid R* (adjusted to pH 2.3 with *triethylamine R*),

– as detector a spectrophotometer set at 215 nm.

Inject 20 µl of reference solution (c). The test is not valid unless the resolution between the first and second peaks is at least 2.0.

Inject 20 µl of the test solution and 20 µl of reference solution (a).

Calculate the content of gonadorelin ($C_{55}H_{75}N_{17}O_{13}$) from the peak areas in the chromatograms obtained with the test solution and reference solution (a) and the declared content of $C_{55}H_{75}N_{17}O_{13}$ in *gonadorelin CRS*.

STORAGE

Store in an airtight container, protected from light at a temperature of 2 °C to 8 °C. If the substance is sterile, store in a sterile, airtight, tamper-proof container.

LABELLING

The label states:

– the mass of peptide in the container,
– where applicable, that the substance is free from bacterial endotoxins.

01/2005:0498

GONADOTROPHIN, CHORIONIC

Gonadotropinum chorionicum

DEFINITION

Chorionic gonadotrophin is a dry preparation of placental glycoproteins which have luteinising activity. The potency is not less than 2500 IU/mg.

PRODUCTION

Chorionic gonadotrophin is extracted from the urine of pregnant women using a suitable fractionation procedure. It is either dried under reduced pressure or freeze-dried. It is prepared in conditions designed to minimise or eliminate microbial and viral contamination. The manufacturing process must have been shown to reduce any viral contamination such as hepatitis virus or HIV by appropriate validated methods.

CHARACTERS

Appearance: white to yellowish-white, amorphous powder.

Solubility: soluble in water.

IDENTIFICATION

When administered to immature rats as prescribed in the assay, it causes an increase in the mass of the seminal vesicles and of the prostate gland.

TESTS

Water (*2.5.32*): maximum 5.0 per cent.

Bacterial endotoxins (*2.6.14*): less than 0.02 IU per IU of chorionic gonadotrophin, if intended for use in the manufacture of parenteral dosage forms without a further appropriate procedure for the removal of bacterial endotoxins.

ASSAY

The potency of chorionic gonadotrophin is estimated by comparing under given conditions its effect of increasing the mass of the seminal vesicles (or the prostate gland) of immature rats with the same effect of the International Standard of chorionic gonadotrophin or of a reference preparation calibrated in International Units.

The International Unit is the activity contained in a stated amount of the International Standard, which consists of a mixture of a freeze-dried extract of chorionic gonadotrophin from the urine of pregnant women with lactose. The equivalence in International Units of the International Standard is stated by the World Health Organisation.

Use immature male rats of the same strain, 19 to 28 days old, differing in age by not more than 3 days and having body masses such that the difference between the heaviest and the lightest rat is not more than 10 g. Assign the rats at random to 6 equal groups of at least 5 animals. If sets of 6 litter mates are available, assign one litter mate from each set to each group and mark according to litter.

Choose 3 doses of the reference preparation and 3 doses of the preparation to be examined such that the smallest dose is sufficient to produce a positive response in some of the rats and the largest dose does not produce a maximal response in all the rats. Use doses in geometric progression and as an initial approximation total doses of 4 IU, 8 IU and 16 IU may be tried although the dose will depend on the sensitivity of the animals used, which may vary widely.

Dissolve separately the total quantities of the preparation to be examined and of the reference preparation corresponding to the daily doses to be used in sufficient *phosphate-albumin buffered saline pH 7.2 R* such that the daily dose is administered in a volume of about 0.5 ml. Add a suitable antimicrobial preservative such as 4 g/l of phenol or 0.02 g/l of thiomersal. Store the solutions at 5 ± 3 °C.

Inject subcutaneously into each rat the daily dose allocated to its group, on 4 consecutive days at the same time each day. On the fifth day, about 24 h after the last injection, kill the rats and remove the seminal vesicles. Remove any extraneous fluid and tissue and weigh the vesicles immediately. Calculate the results by the usual statistical methods, using the mass of the vesicles as the response. (The precision of the assay may be improved by a suitable correction of the organ mass with reference to the body mass of the animal from which it was taken; an analysis of covariance may be used).

The estimated potency is not less than 80 per cent and not more than 125 per cent of the stated potency. The confidence limits ($P = 0.95$) of the estimated potency are not less than 64 per cent and not more than 156 per cent of the stated potency.

STORAGE

In an airtight, tamper-proof container, protected from light at a temperature of 2 °C to 8 °C. If the substance is sterile, store in a sterile, airtight, tamper-proof container.

LABELLING

The label states:

– the number of International Units per container,
– the potency in International Units per milligram,
– where applicable, that the substance is free from bacterial endotoxins.

01/2005:0719

GONADOTROPHIN, EQUINE SERUM, FOR VETERINARY USE

Gonadotropinum sericum equinum ad usum veterinarium

DEFINITION

Equine serum gonadotrophin for veterinary use is a dry preparation of a glycoprotein fraction obtained from the serum or plasma of pregnant mares. It has follicle-stimulating and luteinising activities. The potency is not less than 1000 IU of gonadotrophin activity per milligram, calculated with reference to the anhydrous substance.

PRODUCTION

Equine serum gonadotrophin may be prepared by precipitation with alcohol (70 per cent *V/V*) and further purification by a suitable form of chromatography. It is prepared in conditions designed to minimise microbial contamination.

CHARACTERS

Appearance: white or pale grey, amorphous powder.

Solubility: soluble in water.

IDENTIFICATION

When administered as prescribed in the assay it causes an increase in the mass of the ovaries of immature female rats.

TESTS

Water (*2.5.12*): maximum 10.0 per cent, determined on 80 mg.

Bacterial endotoxins (*2.6.14, method C*): less than 0.035 IU per IU of equine serum gonadotrophin, if intended for use in the manufacture of parenteral dosage forms without a further appropriate procedure for the removal of bacterial endotoxins.

ASSAY

The potency of equine serum gonadotrophin is estimated by comparing under given conditions its effect of increasing the mass of the ovaries of immature female rats with the same effect of the International Standard of equine serum gonadotrophin or of a reference preparation calibrated in International Units.

The International Unit is the activity contained in a stated amount of the International Standard, which consists of a mixture of a freeze-dried extract of equine serum gonadotrophin from the serum of pregnant mares with lactose. The equivalence in International Units of the International Standard is stated by the World Health Organisation.

Use immature female rats of the same strain, 21 to 28 days old, differing in age by not more than 3 days and having masses such that the difference between the heaviest and the lightest rat is not more than 10 g. Assign the rats at random to 6 equal groups of not fewer than 5 animals. If sets of 6 litter mates are available, assign one litter mate from each set to each group and mark according to litter.

Choose 3 doses of the reference preparation and 3 doses of the preparation to be examined such that the smallest dose is sufficient to produce a positive response in some of the rats and the largest dose does not produce a maximal response in all the rats. Use doses in geometric progression: as an initial approximation total doses of 8 IU, 12 IU and 18 IU may be tried, although the dose will depend on the sensitivity of the animals used and may vary widely.

Dissolve separately the total quantities of the preparation to be examined and of the reference preparation corresponding to the doses to be used in sufficient of a sterile 9 g/l solution of *sodium chloride R* containing 1 mg/ml of *bovine albumin R* such that each single dose is administered in a volume of about 0.2 ml. Store the solutions at 5 ± 3 °C.

Inject subcutaneously into each rat the dose allocated to its group. Repeat the injections 18 h, 21 h, 24 h, 42 h and 48 h after the first injection. Not less than 40 h and not more than 72 h after the last injection, kill the rats and remove the ovaries. Remove any extraneous fluid and tissue and weigh the 2 ovaries immediately. Calculate the results by the usual statistical methods, using the combined mass of the 2 ovaries of each animal as the response.

The estimated potency is not less than 80 per cent and not more than 125 per cent of the stated potency. The confidence limits ($P = 0.95$) of the estimated potency are not less than 64 per cent and not more than 156 per cent of the stated potency.

STORAGE

In an airtight container, protected from light, at a temperature not exceeding 8 °C. If the substance is sterile, store in a sterile, airtight, tamper-proof container.

LABELLING

The label states:

- the potency in International Units per milligram,
- where applicable, that the substance is free from bacterial endotoxins.

01/2005:1636

GOSERELIN

Goserelinum

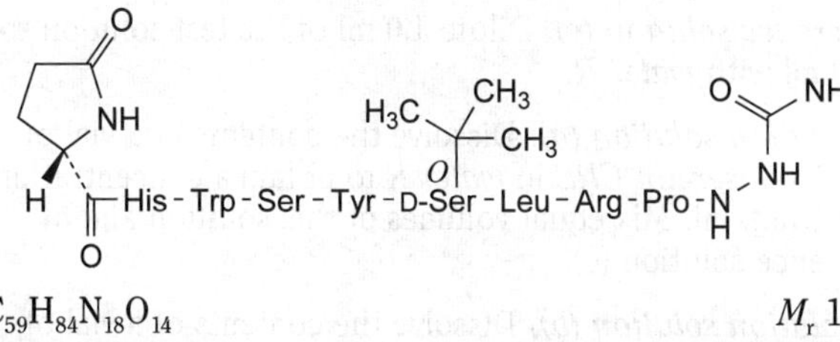

$C_{59}H_{84}N_{18}O_{14}$ M_r 1269

DEFINITION

1-Carbamoyl-2-[5-oxo-L-prolyl-L-histidyl-L-tryptophyl-L-seryl-L-tyrosyl-*O*-(1,1-dimethylethyl)-D-seryl-L-leucyl-L-arginyl-L-prolyl]diazane.

Synthetic nonapeptide analogue of the hypothalamic decapeptide, gonadorelin. It is obtained by chemical synthesis and is available as an acetate.

Content: 94.5 per cent to 103.0 per cent of the peptide $C_{59}H_{84}N_{18}O_{14}$ (anhydrous and acetic-acid free substance).

CHARACTERS

Appearance: white or almost white powder.

Solubility: soluble in water, freely soluble in glacial acetic acid. It dissolves in dilute solutions of mineral acids and alkali hydroxides.

IDENTIFICATION

A. Nuclear magnetic resonance spectrometry (*2.2.33*).

Preparation: 40 mg/ml solution of the substance to be examined in *deuterium oxide R* adjusted to pH 4.0 with *deuterated acetic acid R*.

Results: the ^{13}C, proton decoupled NMR spectrum obtained is qualitatively similar to the *Ph. Eur. reference spectrum of goserelin*.

B. Examine the chromatograms obtained in the assay.

Results: the principal peak in the chromatogram obtained with the test solution is similar in retention time and size to the principal peak in the chromatogram obtained with reference solution (a).

C. Amino acid analysis (*2.2.56*). For protein hydrolysis use Method 1 and for analysis use Method 1.

Express the content of each amino acid in moles. Calculate the relative proportions of the amino acids taking one sixth of the sum of the number of moles of glutamic acid, histidine, tyrosine, leucine, arginine, proline as equal to 1. The values fall within the following limits: glutamic acid, histidine, tyrosine, leucine, arginine and proline 0.9 to 1.1; serine 1.6 to 2.2. Not more than traces of other amino acids are present, with the exception of tryptophan.

TESTS

Specific optical rotation (*2.2.7*): −52 to −56 (anhydrous and acetic-acid free substance).

Dissolve the substance to be examined in *water R* to obtain a concentration of 2 mg/ml.

Related substances. Liquid chromatography (*2.2.29*).

Test solution. Dissolve the substance to be examined in *water R* to obtain a concentration of 1.0 mg/ml.

Reference solution (a). Dissolve the contents of a vial of *goserelin CRS* in *water R* to obtain a concentration of 1.0 mg/ml.

Reference solution (b). Dilute 1.0 ml of the test solution to 100 ml with *water R*.

Reference solution (c). Dilute 1.0 ml of the test solution to 10.0 ml with *water R*.

Resolution solution (a). Dissolve the contents of a vial of *4-D-Ser-goserelin CRS* in *water R* to obtain a concentration of 0.1 mg/ml. Mix equal volumes of this solution and of reference solution (c).

Resolution solution (b). Dissolve the contents of a vial of *goserelin validation mixture CRS* with 1.0 ml of *water R*.

Column:

- *size*: *l* = 0.15 m, Ø = 4.6 mm,
- *stationary phase*: *octadecylsilyl amorphous organosilica polymer R* (3.5 μm) with a pore size of 12.5 nm,
- *temperature*: 50-55 °C.

Mobile phase: *trifluoroacetic acid R, acetonitrile for chromatography R, water R* (0.5:200:800 *V/V/V*).

Flow rate: 0.7-1.2 ml/min.

Detection: spectrophotometer at 220 nm.

Injection: 10 μl of the test solution, reference solution (b) and the resolution solutions.

Run time: 90 min.

Relative retention with reference to goserelin: impurity A = about 0.67; impurity C = about 0.78; impurity B = about 0.79; impurity D = about 0.85; impurity E = about 0.89; impurity F = about 0.92; impurity G = about 0.94; impurity H = about 0.98; impurity I = about 1.43; impurity J = about 1.53; impurity K = about 1.67; impurity L = about 1.77.

System suitability:

- *retention time*: goserelin = 40 min to 50 min in the chromatogram obtained with resolution solution (b); adjust the flow rate of the mobile phase if necessary; if adjusting the flow rate does not result in a correct retention time of the principal peak, change the composition of acetonitrile in the mobile phase to obtain the requested retention time for goserelin;
- *resolution*: minimum 7.0 between the peaks due to impurity A and goserelin in the chromatogram obtained with resolution solution (a);
- *symmetry factor*: 0.8 to 2.5 for the peaks due to impurity A and goserelin in the chromatogram obtained with resolution solution (a);
- the chromatogram obtained with resolution solution (b) is similar to the chromatogram supplied with *goserelin validation mixture CRS*. 2 peaks eluting prior to the principal peak and corresponding to impurity E and impurity G, are clearly visible. 3 peaks eluting after the principal peak are clearly visible.

Limits:

- *impurity E*: not more than the area of the principal peak in the chromatogram obtained with reference solution (b) (1.0 per cent),
- *any other impurity*: for each impurity, not more than 0.5 times the area of the principal peak in the chromatogram obtained with reference solution (b) (0.5 per cent),
- *total*: not more than 2.5 times the area of the principal peak in the chromatogram obtained with reference solution (b) (2.5 per cent),
- *disregard limit*: 0.05 times the area of the principal peak in the chromatogram obtained with reference solution (b) (0.05 per cent).

Acetic acid (*2.5.34*): 4.5 per cent to 15.0 per cent.

Test solution. Dissolve 10.0 mg of the substance to be examined in a mixture of 5 volumes of mobile phase B and 95 volumes of mobile phase A and dilute to 10.0 ml with the same mixture of mobile phases.

Water (*2.5.32*): maximum 10.0 per cent.

Bacterial endotoxins (*2.6.14*): less than 16 IU/mg, if intended for use in the manufacture of parenteral dosage forms without a further appropriate procedure for the removal of bacterial endotoxins.

ASSAY

Liquid chromatography (*2.2.29*) as described in the test for related substances with the following modifications.

Injection: test solution and reference solution (a).

Run time: 60 min.

Calculate the content of goserelin ($C_{59}H_{84}N_{18}O_{14}$) using the chromatograms obtained with the test solution and reference solution (a) and the declared content of $C_{59}H_{84}N_{18}O_{14}$ in *goserelin CRS*.

STORAGE

In an airtight container, protected from light, at a temperature of 2 °C to 8 °C.

LABELLING

The label states:

- the mass of peptide in the container,
- where applicable, that the substance is free from bacterial endotoxins.

IMPURITIES

Specified impurities: A, B, C, D, E, F, G, H, I, J, K, L.

Monographs F-H

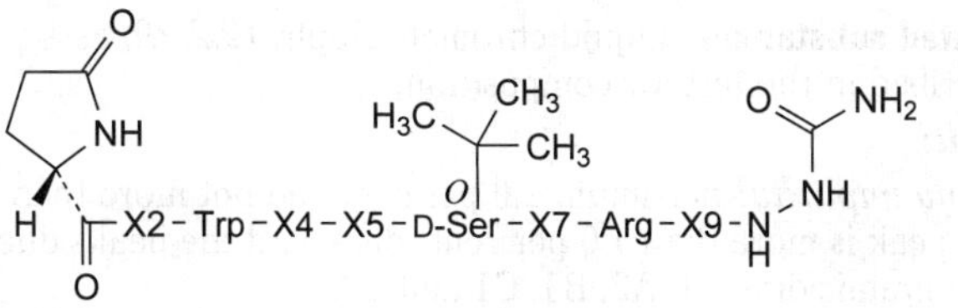

A. X2 = L-His, X4 = D-Ser, X5 = L-Tyr, X7 = L-Leu, X9 = L-Pro: [4-D-serine]goserelin,

C. X2 = L-His, X4 = L-Ser, X5 = L-Tyr, X7 = L-Leu, X9 = D-Pro: [9-D-proline]goserelin,

F. X2 = L-His, X4 = L-Ser, X5 = D-Tyr, X7 = L-Leu, X9 = L-Pro: [5-D-tyrosine]goserelin,

G. X2 = D-His, X4 = L-Ser, X5 = L-Tyr, X7 = L-Leu, X9 = L-Pro: [2-D-histidine]goserelin,

L. X2 = L-His, X4 = L-Ser, X5 = L-Tyr, X7 = D-Leu, X9 = L-Pro: [7-D-leucine]goserelin,

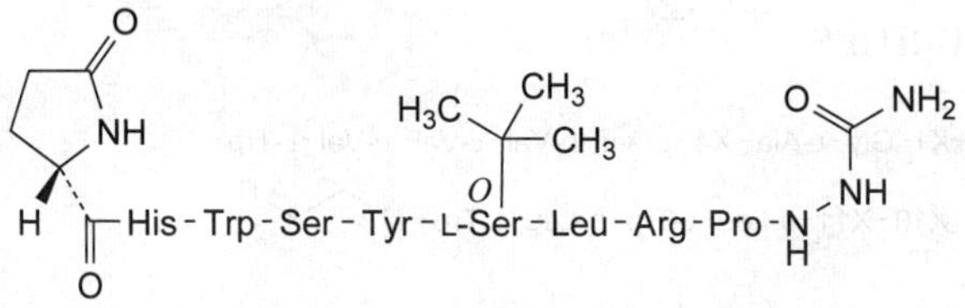

B. [6-[*O*-(1,1-dimethylethyl)-L-serine]]goserelin,

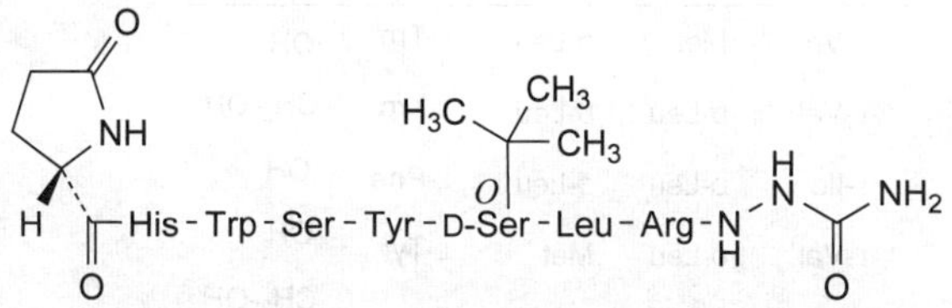

D. 1-carbamoylyl-2-[5-oxo-L-prolyl-L-histidyl-L-tryptophyl-L-seryl-L-tyrosyl-*O*-(1,1-dimethylethyl)-D-seryl-L-leucyl-L-arginyl]diazane,

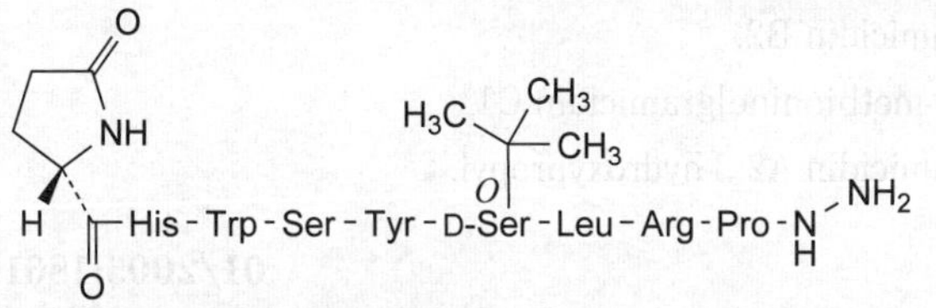

E. 5-oxo-L-prolyl-L-histidyl-L-tryptophyl-L-seryl-L-tyrosyl-*O*-(1,1-dimethylethyl)-D-seryl-L-leucyl-L-arginyl-L-prolinohydrazide,

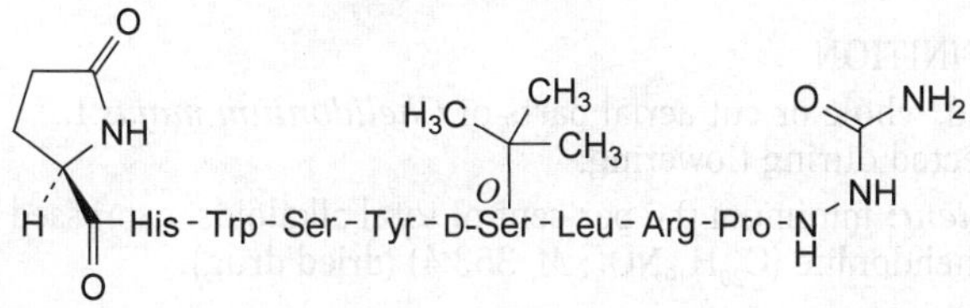

H. [1-(5-oxo-D-proline)]goserelin,

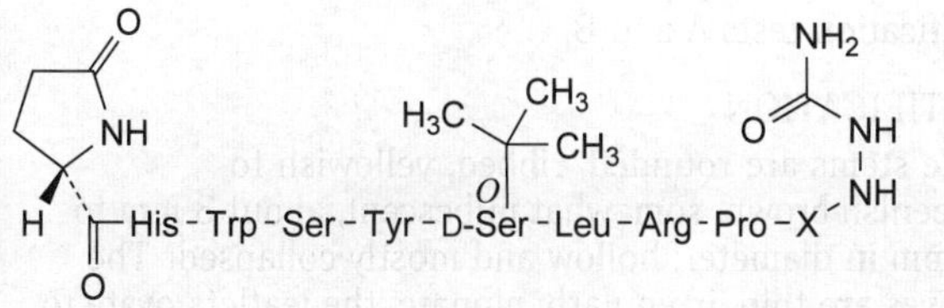

I. X = Pro-Pro: endo-8a,8b-di-L-proline-goserelin,

J. X = Pro: endo-8a-L-proline-goserelin,

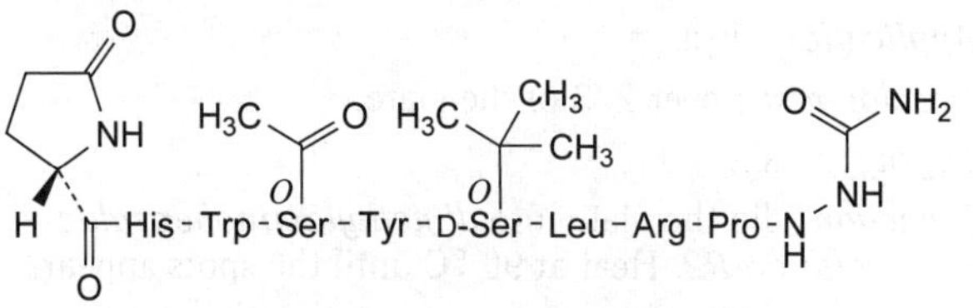

K. O^4-acetylgoserelin.

01/2005:0907

GRAMICIDIN

Gramicidinum

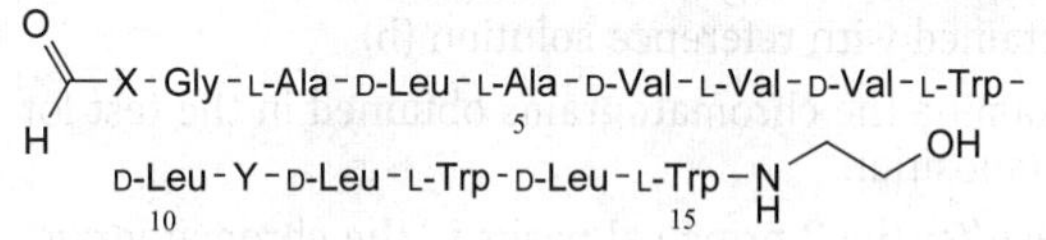

Gramicidin	X	Y	Mol. formula	M_r
A1	L-Val	L-Trp	$C_{99}H_{140}N_{20}O_{17}$	1882
A2	L-Ile	L-Trp	$C_{100}H_{142}N_{20}O_{17}$	1896
B1	L-Val	L-Phe	$C_{97}H_{139}N_{19}O_{17}$	1843
C1	L-Val	L-Tyr	$C_{97}H_{139}N_{19}O_{18}$	1859
C2	L-Ile	L-Tyr	$C_{98}H_{141}N_{19}O_{18}$	1873

DEFINITION

Gramicidin consists of a family of antimicrobial linear polypeptides, usually obtained by extraction from tyrothricin, the complex isolated from the fermentation broth of *Brevibacillus brevis* Dubos. The main component is gramicidin A1, together with gramicidins A2, B1, C1 and C2 in particular.

Content: minimum 900 IU/mg (dried substance).

CHARACTERS

Appearance: white or almost white, crystalline powder, slightly hygroscopic.

Solubility: practically insoluble in water, soluble in methanol, sparingly soluble in alcohol.

mp: about 230 °C.

IDENTIFICATION

First identification: A, C.

Second identification: A, B.

A. Dissolve 0.100 g in *alcohol R* and dilute to 100.0 ml with the same solvent. Dilute 5.0 ml of this solution to 100.0 ml with *alcohol R*. Examined between 240 nm and 320 nm (*2.2.25*), the solution shows 2 absorption maxima, at 282 nm and 290 nm, a shoulder at about 275 nm and an absorption minimum at 247 nm. The specific absorbance at the maximum at 282 nm is 105 to 125.

B. Thin-layer chromatography (*2.2.27*).

Test solution. Dissolve 5 mg of the substance to be examined in 6.0 ml of *alcohol R*.

Reference solution (a). Dissolve 5 mg of *gramicidin CRS* in 6.0 ml of *alcohol R*.

Reference solution (b). Dissolve 5 mg of *tyrothricin CRS* in 6.0 ml of *alcohol R*.

Plate: *TLC silica gel plate R.*

Mobile phase: *methanol R, butanol R, water R, glacial acetic acid R, butyl acetate R* (3:9:15:24:49 *V/V/V/V/V*).

Application: 1 µl.

Development: over 2/3 of the plate.

Drying: in air.

Detection: dip the plate into *dimethylaminobenzaldehyde solution R2*. Heat at 90 °C until the spots appear.

System suitability: the chromatogram obtained with reference solution (b) shows 2 clearly separated spots or 2 clearly separated groups of spots.

Results: the principal spot or group of principal spots in the chromatogram obtained with the test solution is similar in position, colour and size to the principal spot or group of principal spots in the chromatogram obtained with reference solution (a) and to the spot or group of spots with the highest R_f value in the chromatogram obtained with reference solution (b).

C. Examine the chromatograms obtained in the test for composition.

Results: the 3 principal peaks in the chromatogram obtained with the test solution are similar in retention time to the 3 principal peaks in the chromatogram obtained with reference solution (a).

TESTS

Composition. Liquid chromatography (*2.2.29*): use the normalisation procedure.

Test solution. Dissolve 25 mg of the substance to be examined in 10 ml of *methanol R* and dilute to 25 ml with the mobile phase.

Reference solution (a). Dissolve 25 mg of *gramicidin CRS* in 10 ml of *methanol R* and dilute to 25 ml with the mobile phase.

Reference solution (b). Dilute 1.0 ml of reference solution (a) to 50.0 ml with the mobile phase. Dilute 1.0 ml of this solution to 10.0 ml with the mobile phase.

Column:

- *size*: *l* = 0.25 m, Ø = 4.6 mm,
- *stationary phase*: *base-deactivated end-capped octadecylsilyl silica gel for chromatography R* (5 µm),
- *temperature*: 50 °C.

Mobile phase: *water R, methanol R* (29:71 *V/V*).

Flow rate: 1.0 ml/min.

Detection: spectrophotometer at 282 nm.

Injection: 20 µl.

Run time: 2.5 times the retention time of gramicidin A1.

Relative retention with reference to gramicidin A1 (retention time = about 22 min): gramicidin C1 = about 0.7; gramicidin C2 = about 0.8; gramicidin A2 = about 1.2; gramicidin B1 = about 1.9.

System suitability: reference solution (a):

- *resolution*: minimum 1.5 between the peaks due to gramicidin A1 and gramicidin A2,
- the chromatogram obtained is concordant with the chromatogram supplied with *gramicidin CRS*.

Composition:

- *sum of the contents of gramicidins A1, A2, B1, C1 and C2*: minimum 95.0 per cent,
- *ratio of the content of gramicidin A1 to the sum of the contents of gramicidins A1, A2, B1, C1 and C2*: minimum 60.0 per cent,
- *disregard limit*: the area of the peak due to gramicidin A1 in the chromatogram obtained with reference solution (b).

Related substances. Liquid chromatography (*2.2.29*) as described in the test for composition.

Limit:

- *any impurity*: maximum 2.0 per cent and not more than 1 peak is more than 1.0 per cent; disregard the peaks due to gramicidins A1, A2, B1, C1 and C2.

Loss on drying (*2.2.32*): maximum 3.0 per cent, determined on 1.000 g by drying over *diphosphorus pentoxide R* at 60 °C at a pressure not exceeding 0.1 kPa for 3 h.

Sulphated ash (*2.4.14*): maximum 1.0 per cent, determined on 1.0 g.

ASSAY

Carry out the microbiological assay of antibiotics (*2.7.2*), using the turbidimetric method. Use *gramicidin CRS* as the reference substance.

STORAGE

In an airtight container, protected from light.

IMPURITIES

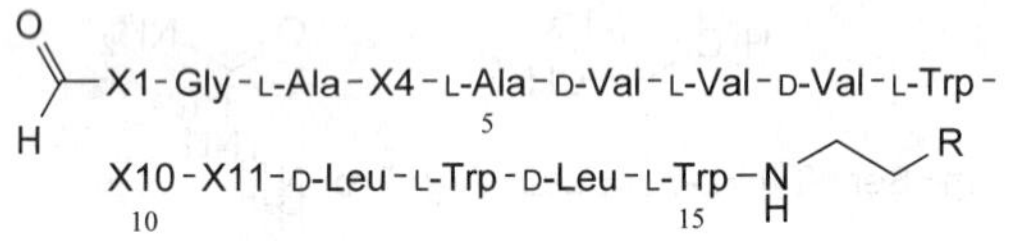

Impurity	X1	X4	X10	X11	R
A	L-Val	Met	D-Leu	L-Trp	OH
B	L-Val	D-Leu	D-Leu	L-Trp	CH_2-OH
C	L-Ile	D-Leu	D-Leu	L-Phe	OH
D	L-Val	D-Leu	Met	L-Tyr	OH
E	L-Ile	D-Leu	D-Leu	L-Trp	CH_2-OH

A. [4-methionine]gramicidin A1,

B. gramicidin A1 3-hydroxypropyl,

C. gramicidin B2,

D. [10-methionine]gramicidin C1,

E. gramicidin A2 3-hydroxypropyl.

01/2005:1861

GREATER CELANDINE

Chelidonii herba

DEFINITION

Dried, whole or cut aerial parts of *Chelidonium majus* L. collected during flowering.

Content: minimum 0.6 per cent of total alkaloids, expressed as chelidonine ($C_{20}H_{19}NO_5$; M_r 353.4) (dried drug).

CHARACTERS

Macroscopic and microscopic characters described under identification tests A and B.

IDENTIFICATION

A. The stems are rounded, ribbed, yellowish to greenish-brown, somewhat pubescent, about 3 mm to 7 mm in diameter, hollow and mostly collapsed. The leaves are thin, irregularly pinnate, the leaflets ovate to oblong with coarsely dentate margins, the terminal leaflet often three-lobed; the adaxial surface is bluish-green and glabrous, the abaxial surface paler and pubescent, especially on the veins. The flowers have 2 deeply concavo-convex sepals, readily removed, and 4 yellow, broadly ovate, spreading petals about 8 mm to 10 mm long; the stamens are numerous, yellow, and a short style arises from a superior ovary; long, capsular, immature fruits are rarely present.

B. Reduce to a powder (355). The powder is dark greyish-green to brownish-green. Examine under a microscope using *chloral hydrate solution R*. The powder shows the following diagnostic characters: numerous fragments of leaves in surface view, the epidermal cells with sinuous walls; anomocytic stomata (*2.8.3*) occur on the abaxial surface only; covering trichomes long, uniseriate, with thin walls and usually fragmented; vascular tissue from the leaves and stems with groups of fibres, pitted and spirally thickened vessels and associated latex tubes with yellowish-brown contents; occasional fragments of the corolla with thin-walled, partly papillose cells containing numerous pale yellow droplets of oil; spherical pollen grains about 30 µm to 40 µm in diameter with 3 pores and a finely pitted exine.

C. Thin-layer chromatography (*2.2.27*).

Test solution. To 0.4 g of the powdered drug (710) add 50 ml of *dilute acetic acid R*. Boil the mixture under a reflux condenser in a water-bath for 30 min. Cool and filter. To the filtrate add *concentrated ammonia R* until a strong alkaline reaction is produced. Shake with 30 ml of *methylene chloride R*. Dry the organic layer over *anhydrous sodium sulphate R*, filter and evaporate *in vacuo* to dryness. Dissolve the residue in 1.0 ml of *methanol R*.

Reference solution. Dissolve 2 mg of *papaverine hydrochloride R* and 2 mg of *methyl red R* in 10 ml of *alcohol R*.

Plate: *TLC silica gel plate R*.

Mobile phase: *anhydrous formic acid R, water R, propanol R* (1:9:90 *V/V/V*).

Application: 10 µl as bands.

Development: over a path of 10 cm.

Drying: in air.

Detection: spray with *potassium iodobismuthate solution R* and dry the plate in air; spray with *sodium nitrite solution R* and allow the plate to dry in air; examine in daylight.

Results: see below the sequence of the zones present in the chromatograms obtained with the reference solution and the test solution. Furthermore, other weaker zones may be present in the chromatogram obtained with the test solution.

Top of the plate	
——	——
Methyl red: a red zone	A brown zone
	A brown zone
Papaverine: a greyish-brown zone	A greyish-brown zone
——	——
	A brown zone
	A brown zone
Reference solution	**Test solution**

TESTS

Foreign matter (*2.8.2*): maximum 10 per cent.

Loss on drying (*2.2.32*): maximum 10.0 per cent, determined on 1.000 g of the powdered drug (355) by drying in an oven at 100-105 °C for 2 h.

Total ash (*2.4.16*): maximum 13.0 per cent.

ASSAY

Test solution. To 0.750 g of the powdered drug (710), add 200 ml of *dilute acetic acid R* and heat on a water-bath for 30 min, shaking frequently. Cool and dilute to 250.0 ml with *dilute acetic acid R*. Filter. Discard the first 20 ml of the filtrate. To 30.0 ml of the filtrate add 6.0 ml of *concentrated ammonia R* and 100.0 ml of *methylene chloride R*. Shake for 30 min. Separate the organic layer, place 50.0 ml in a 100 ml round-bottomed flask and evaporate to dryness *in vacuo* at a temperature not exceeding 40 °C. Dissolve the residue in about 2-3 ml of *alcohol R*, warming slightly. Transfer the solution to a 25 ml volumetric flask by rinsing the round-bottomed flask with *dilute sulphuric acid R* and dilute to 25.0 ml with the same solvent. To 5.0 ml of the solution, add 5.0 ml of a 10 g/l solution of *chromotropic acid, sodium salt R* in *sulphuric acid R* in a 25 ml volumetric flask, stopper the flask and mix carefully. Dilute to 25.0 ml with *sulphuric acid R* and stopper the flask.

Compensation solution. At the same time and in the same manner, place in a 25 ml volumetric flask 5.0 ml of *dilute sulphuric acid R* and 5.0 ml of a 10 g/l solution of *chromotropic acid, sodium salt R* in *sulphuric acid R*, stopper the flask and mix carefully. Dilute to 25.0 ml with *sulphuric acid R* and stopper the flask.

Place both solutions on a water-bath for 10 min. Cool to about 20 °C and dilute if necessary to 25.0 ml with *sulphuric acid R*. Measure the absorbance (*2.2.25*) of the test solution at 570 nm.

Calculate the percentage content of total alkaloids, expressed as chelidonine, from the expression:

$$\frac{A \times 2.23}{m}$$

i.e. taking the specific absorbance of chelidonine to be 933.

A = absorbance at 570 nm,

m = mass of the substance to be examined, in grams.

01/2005:0182

GRISEOFULVIN

Griseofulvinum

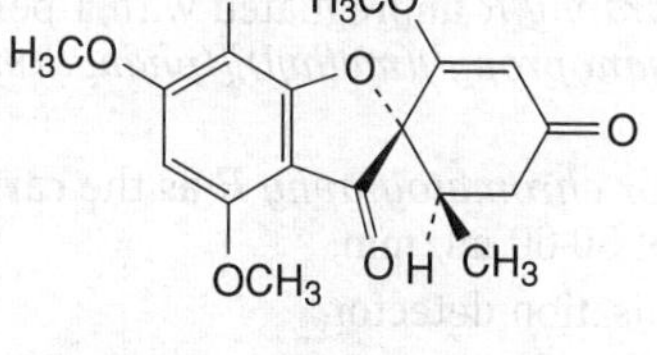

$C_{17}H_{17}ClO_6$ M_r 352.8

DEFINITION

Griseofulvin is (1′*S*,3-6′*R*)-7-chloro-2′,4,6-trimethoxy-6′-methylspiro[benzofuran-2(3*H*),1′-[2]cyclohexene]-3,4′-dione, a substance produced by the growth of certain strains of *Penicillium griseofulvum* or obtained by any other means. It contains not less than 97.0 per cent and not more than the equivalent of 102.0 per cent of $C_{17}H_{17}ClO_6$, calculated with reference to the dried substance.

CHARACTERS

A white or yellowish-white, microfine powder, the particles of which are generally up to 5 µm in maximum dimension although larger particles which may occasionally exceed 30 µm may be present, tasteless, practically insoluble in water, freely soluble in dimethylformamide and in tetrachloroethane, slightly soluble in ethanol and in methanol.

It melts at about 220 °C.

IDENTIFICATION

A. Examine by infrared absorption spectrophotometry (*2.2.24*), comparing with the spectrum obtained with *griseofulvin CRS*.

B. Dissolve about 5 mg in 1 ml of *sulphuric acid R* and add about 5 mg of powdered *potassium dichromate R*. A wine-red colour develops.

TESTS

Appearance of solution. Dissolve 0.75 g in *dimethylformamide R* and dilute to 10 ml with the same solvent. The solution is clear (*2.2.1*) and not more intensely coloured than reference solution Y_4 (*2.2.2, Method II*).

Acidity. Suspend 0.25 g in 20 ml of *alcohol R* and add 0.1 ml of *phenolphthalein solution R*. Not more than 1.0 ml of *0.02 M sodium hydroxide* is required to change the colour of the indicator.

Specific optical rotation (*2.2.7*). Dissolve 0.250 g in *dimethylformamide R* and dilute to 25.0 ml with the same solvent. The specific optical rotation is + 354 to + 364, calculated with reference to the dried substance.

Related substances. Examine by gas chromatography (*2.2.28*), using *diphenylanthracene R* as the internal standard.

Internal standard solution. Dissolve 0.2 g of *diphenylanthracene R* in *acetone R* and dilute to 100.0 ml with the same solvent.

Test solution (a). Dissolve 0.10 g of the substance to be examined in *acetone R* and dilute to 10.0 ml with the same solvent.

Test solution (b). Dissolve 0.10 g of the substance to be examined in *acetone R*, add 1.0 ml of the internal standard solution and dilute to 10.0 ml with *acetone R*.

Reference solution. Dissolve 5.0 mg of *griseofulvin CRS* in *acetone R*, add 1.0 ml of the internal standard solution and dilute to 10.0 ml with *acetone R*.

The chromatographic procedure may be carried out using:

- a glass column 1 m long and 4 mm in internal diameter packed with *diatomaceous earth for gas chromatography R* impregnated with 1 per cent *m/m* of *poly[(cyanopropyl)(methyl)][(phenyl)(methyl)]siloxane R*,
- *nitrogen for chromatography R* as the carrier gas at a flow rate of 50-60 ml/min,
- a flame-ionisation detector.

Maintain the temperature of the column at 250 °C, that of the injection port at 270 °C and that of the detector at 300 °C. Continue the chromatography for three times the period of time required for the appearance of the peak corresponding to griseofulvin which is about 11 min. For the chromatogram obtained with the reference solution, determine the ratio of the area of the peak corresponding to griseofulvin to the area of the peak corresponding to the internal standard. For the chromatogram obtained with test solution (b), determine the ratio of the area of the peak corresponding to dechloro-griseofulvin (distance t_R about 0.6 times that of griseofulvin) to the area of the peak corresponding to the internal standard, determine also the ratio of the area of the peak corresponding to dehydrogriseofulvin (distance t_R about 1.4 times that of griseofulvin) to the area of the peak corresponding to the internal standard.

The ratios calculated from the chromatogram obtained with test solution (b) divided by the ratio calculated from the chromatogram obtained with the reference solution are less than 0.6 for dechlorogriseofulvin and less than 0.15 for dehydrogriseofulvin.

Substances soluble in light petroleum. Shake 1.0 g with 20 ml of *light petroleum R*. Boil under a reflux condenser for 10 min. Cool, filter and wash with three quantities, each of 15 ml, of *light petroleum R*. Combine the filtrate and washings, evaporate to dryness on a water-bath and dry at 100 °C to 105 °C for 1 h. The residue weighs not more than 2 mg (0.2 per cent).

Loss on drying (*2.2.32*). Not more than 1.0 per cent, determined on 1.00 g by drying in an oven at 100 °C to 105 °C.

Sulphated ash (*2.4.14*). Not more than 0.2 per cent, determined on 1.0 g.

Abnormal toxicity. To each of five healthy mice, each weighing 17 g to 22 g, administer orally a suspension of 0.1 g of the substance to be examined in 0.5 ml to 1 ml of *water R*. None of the mice dies within 48 h.

ASSAY

Dissolve 80.0 mg in *ethanol R* and dilute to 200.0 ml with the same solvent. Dilute 2.0 ml of the solution to 100.0 ml with *ethanol R*. Measure the absorbance (*2.2.25*) at the maximum at 291 nm. Calculate the content of $C_{17}H_{17}ClO_6$, taking the specific absorbance to be 686.

01/2005:0615
corrected

GUAIFENESIN

Guaifenesinum

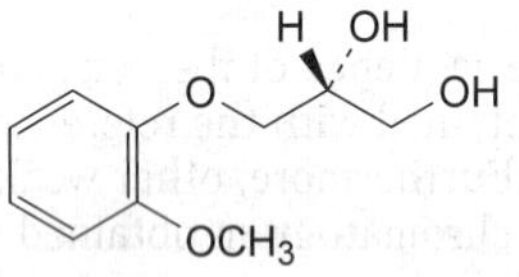

and enantiomer

$C_{10}H_{14}O_4$ M_r 198.2

DEFINITION

(2*RS*)-3-(2-Methoxyphenoxy)propane-1,2-diol.

Content: 98.0 per cent to 102.0 per cent (dried substance).

CHARACTERS

Appearance: white or almost white, crystalline powder.

Solubility: sparingly soluble in water, soluble in alcohol.

IDENTIFICATION

First identification: B.

Second identification: A, C.

A. Melting point (*2.2.14*): 79 °C to 83 °C.

B. Infrared absorption spectrophotometry (*2.2.24*).

Comparison: *guaifenesin CRS*.

C. Thin-layer chromatography (*2.2.27*).

Test solution. Dissolve 30 mg of the substance to be examined in *methanol R* and dilute to 10 ml with the same solvent.

Reference solution. Dissolve 30 mg of *guaifenesin CRS* in *methanol R* and dilute to 10 ml with the same solvent.

Plate: *TLC silica gel G plate R*.

Mobile phase: *methylene chloride R, propanol R* (20:80 *V/V*).

Application: 5 µl.

Development: over 2/3 of the plate.

Drying: in air.

Detection: spray with a mixture of equal volumes of a 10 g/l solution of *potassium ferricyanide R*, a 200 g/l solution of *ferric chloride R* and *alcohol R*.

Results: the principal spot in the chromatogram obtained with the test solution is similar in position, colour and size to the principal spot in the chromatogram obtained with the reference solution.

TESTS

Solution S. Dissolve 1.0 g in *carbon dioxide-free water R*, heating gently if necessary, and dilute to 50 ml with the same solvent.

Appearance of solution. Solution S is clear (*2.2.1*) and colourless (*2.2.2, Method II*).

Acidity or alkalinity. To 10 ml of solution S add 0.05 ml of *phenolphthalein solution R1*. Not more than 0.1 ml of *0.01 M sodium hydroxide* is required to change the colour of the indicator. To 10 ml of solution S add 0.15 ml of *methyl red solution R*. Not more than 0.1 ml of *0.01 M hydrochloric acid* is required to change the colour of the indicator to red.

Related substances. Liquid chromatography (*2.2.29*).

Test solution. Dissolve 0.100 g of the substance to be examined in *acetonitrile R* and dilute to 50.0 ml with the same solvent.

Reference solution (a). Dilute 1.0 ml of the test solution to 20.0 ml with *acetonitrile R*. Dilute 1.0 ml of this solution to 10.0 ml with *acetonitrile R*.

Reference solution (b). Dissolve 10.0 mg of *guaiacol R* in *acetonitrile R* and dilute to 50.0 ml with the same solvent. Dilute 0.5 ml of this solution to 50.0 ml with *acetonitrile R*.

Reference solution (c). Dissolve 50.0 mg of *guaiacol R* in *acetonitrile R* and dilute to 50.0 ml with the same solvent. Dilute 5.0 ml of this solution to 10.0 ml with the test solution.

Column:

- *size*: l = 0.25 m, Ø = 4.6 mm,
- *stationary phase*: *octadecylsilyl silica gel for chromatography R* (5 µm).

Mobile phase:

- *mobile phase A*: *glacial acetic acid R, water R* (10:990 *V/V*),
- *mobile phase B*: *acetonitrile R*,

Time (min)	Mobile phase A (per cent *V/V*)	Mobile phase B (per cent *V/V*)
0 - 32	80 → 50	20 → 50
32 - 33	50 → 80	50 → 20
33 - 40	80	20

Flow rate: 1 ml/min.

Detection: spectrophotometer at 276 nm.

Injection: 10 µl.

Relative retention with reference to guaifenesin (retention time = about 8 min): impurity B = about 0.9; impurity A = about 1.4; impurity C = about 3.1; impurity D = about 3.7.

System suitability: reference solution (c):

- *resolution*: minimum 3.0 between the peaks due to guaifenesin and impurity A.

Limits:

- *impurity A*: not more than the area of the principal peak in the chromatogram obtained with reference solution (b) (0.1 per cent),
- *impurity B*: not more than twice the area of the principal peak in the chromatogram obtained with reference solution (a) (1.0 per cent),
- *any other impurity*: not more than the area of the principal peak in the chromatogram obtained with reference solution (a) (0.5 per cent),
- *total (excluding impurity B)*: not more than twice the area of the principal peak in the chromatogram obtained with reference solution (a) (1.0 per cent),
- *disregard level*: 0.1 times the area of the principal peak in the chromatogram obtained with reference solution (a) (0.05 per cent).

Chlorides and monochlorhydrins: maximum of 250 ppm.

To 10 ml of solution S add 2 ml of *dilute sodium hydroxide solution R* and heat on a water-bath for 5 min. Cool and add 3 ml of *dilute nitric acid R*. The resulting solution complies with the limit test for chlorides (*2.4.4*).

Heavy metals (*2.4.8*): maximum of 25 ppm.

Dissolve 2.0 g in a mixture of 1 volume of *water R* and 9 volumes of *alcohol R* and dilute to 25 ml with the same mixture of solvents. 12 ml of the solution complies with limit test B. Prepare the standard using lead standard solution (2 ppm Pb) prepared by diluting *lead standard solution (100 ppm Pb) R* with a mixture of 1 volume of *water R* and 9 volumes of *alcohol R*.

Loss on drying (*2.2.32*): maximum 0.5 per cent, determined on 1.000 g by drying *in vacuo* at 60 °C for 3 h.

Sulphated ash (*2.4.14*): maximum 0.1 per cent, determined on 1.0 g.

ASSAY

To 0.500 g (m g) add 10.0 ml of a freshly prepared mixture of 1 volume of *acetic anhydride R* and 7 volumes of *pyridine R*. Boil under a reflux condenser for 45 min. Cool and add 25 ml of *water R*. Using 0.25 ml of *phenolphthalein solution R* as indicator, titrate with *1 M sodium hydroxide* (n_1 ml). Carry out a blank titration (n_2 ml).

Calculate the percentage content of $C_{10}H_{14}O_4$ from the expression:

$$\frac{19.82\,(n_2 - n_1)}{2m}$$

IMPURITIES

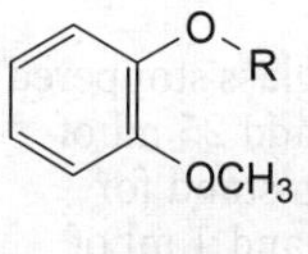

A. R = H: 2-methoxyphenol (guaiacol),

B. R = $CH(CH_2OH)_2$: 2-(2-methoxyphenoxy)propane-1,3-diol (B-isomer),

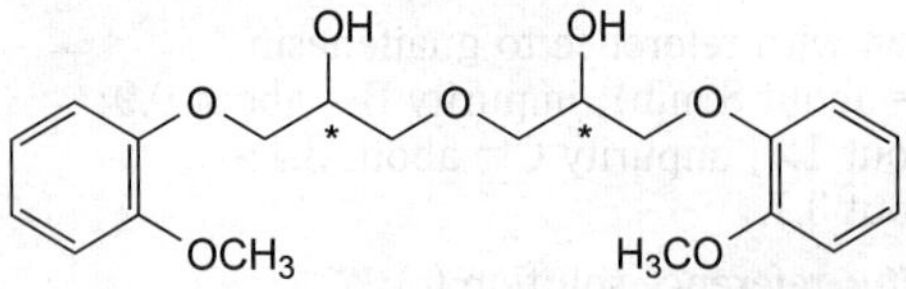

C. 1,1′-oxybis[3-(2-methoxyphenoxy)propan-2-ol] (bisether),

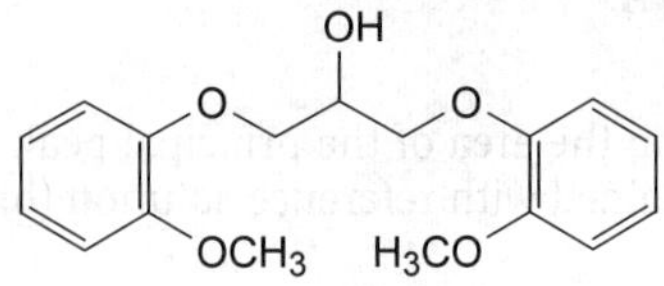

D. 1,3-bis(2-methoxyphenoxy)propan-2-ol.

01/2005:0027

GUANETHIDINE MONOSULPHATE

Guanethidini monosulfas

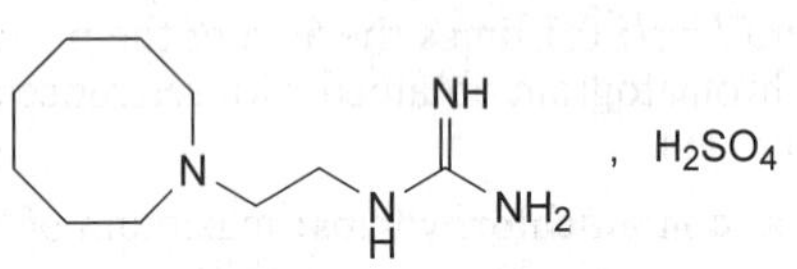

$C_{10}H_{24}N_4O_4S$ M_r 296.4

DEFINITION

Guanethidine monosulphate contains not less than 99.0 per cent and not more than the equivalent of 101.0 per cent of 1-[2-(hexahydroazocin-1(2*H*)-yl)ethyl]guanidine monosulphate, calculated with reference to the dried substance.

CHARACTERS

A colourless, crystalline powder, freely soluble in water, practically insoluble in alcohol.

It melts at about 250 °C, with decomposition.

IDENTIFICATION

A. Dissolve about 25 mg in 25 ml of *water R*, add 20 ml of *picric acid solution R* and filter. The precipitate, washed with *water R* and dried at 100 °C to 105 °C, melts (*2.2.14*) at about 154 °C.

B. Dissolve about 25 mg in 5 ml of *water R*. Add 1 ml of *strong sodium hydroxide solution R*, 1 ml of *α-naphthol solution R* and, dropwise with shaking, 0.5 ml of *strong sodium hypochlorite solution R*. A bright pink precipitate is formed and becomes violet-red on standing.

C. It gives the reactions of sulphates (*2.3.1*).

TESTS

Solution S. Dissolve 0.4 g in *carbon dioxide-free water R* and dilute to 20 ml with the same solvent.

Appearance of solution. Solution S is not more intensely coloured than reference solution GY_6 (*2.2.2, Method II*).

pH (*2.2.3*). The pH of solution S is 4.7 to 5.5.

Oxidisable substances. In a conical, ground-glass-stoppered flask, dissolve 1.0 g in 25 ml of *water R* and add 25 ml of *dilute sodium hydroxide solution R*. Allow to stand for 10 min and add 1 g of *potassium bromide R* and 1 ml of *0.0083 M potassium bromate*. Acidify with 30 ml of *dilute hydrochloric acid R*. Mix and allow to stand in the dark for 5 min. Add 2 g of *potassium iodide R* and shake. Allow to stand for 2 min and titrate the liberated iodine with *0.05 M sodium thiosulphate*, using *starch solution R* as indicator. Not less than 0.3 ml of *0.05 M sodium thiosulphate* is required to decolorise the solution.

Heavy metals (*2.4.8*). 2.0 g complies with limit test C (10 ppm). Prepare the standard using 2 ml of *lead standard solution (10 ppm Pb) R*.

Loss on drying (*2.2.32*). Not more than 0.5 per cent, determined on 1.00 g by drying in an oven at 100 °C to 105 °C.

Sulphated ash (*2.4.14*). Not more than 0.1 per cent, determined on 1.0 g.

ASSAY

Dissolve 0.250 g, warming if necessary, in 30 ml of *anhydrous acetic acid R* and add 15 ml of *acetic anhydride R*. Titrate with *0.1 M perchloric acid*, determining the end-point potentiometrically (*2.2.20*).

1 ml of *0.1 M perchloric acid* is equivalent to 29.64 mg of $C_{10}H_{24}N_4O_4S$.

STORAGE

Protected from light.

01/2005:1218

GUAR

Cyamopsidis seminis pulvis

DEFINITION

Guar is obtained by grinding the endosperms of seeds of *Cyamopsis tetragonolobus* (L.) Taub. It consists mainly of guar galactomannan.

CHARACTERS

A white or almost white powder, yielding a mucilage of variable viscosity when dissolved in water, practically insoluble in alcohol.

It has the microscopic characters described under Identification test A.

IDENTIFICATION

A. Examined under a microscope in *glycerol R*, the substance to be examined (125) shows pyriform to ovoid cells, usually isolated, having very thick walls around a central somewhat elongated lumen with granular contents, and smaller polyhedral cells, isolated or in clusters, with thinner walls.

B. In a conical flask place 2 g, add rapidly 45 ml of *water R* and stir vigorously for 30 s. After 5-10 min a stiff gel forms which does not flow when the flask is inverted.

C. Mix a suspension of 0.1 g in 10 ml of *water R* with 1 ml of a 10 g/l solution of *disodium tetraborate R*; the mixture soon gels.

D. Examine by thin-layer chromatography (*2.2.27*), using a suitable silica gel as the coating substance.

Test solution. To 10 mg in a thick-walled, centrifuge test tube add 2 ml of a 100 g/l solution of *trifluoroacetic acid R*, shake vigorously to dissolve the forming gel, stopper the test tube and heat the mixture at 120 °C for 1 h. Centrifuge the hydrolysate, transfer the clear supernatant liquid carefully into a 50 ml flask, add 10 ml of *water R* and evaporate the solution to dryness under reduced pressure. To the resulting clear film add 0.1 ml of *water R* and 0.9 ml of *methanol R*. Centrifuge to separate the amorphous precipitate. Dilute the supernatant liquid, if necessary, to 1 ml with *methanol R*.

Reference solution. Dissolve 10 mg of *galactose R*, 10 mg of *mannose R* in 2 ml of *water R* and dilute to 20 ml with *methanol R*.

Apply separately to the plate as bands 5 µl of each solution. Develop over a path of 15 cm using a mixture of 15 volumes of *water R* and 85 volumes of *acetonitrile R*. Spray with *aminohippuric acid reagent R* and dry the plate at 120 °C for 5 min. The chromatogram obtained with the reference solution shows in the lower part, two clearly separated brownish zones (galactose and mannose in order of increasing R_f value). The chromatogram obtained with the test solution shows two zones corresponding to galactose and mannose.

TESTS

Tragacanth, sterculia gum, agar, alginates, carrageenan. To a small amount of the substance to be examined add 0.2 ml of freshly prepared *ruthenium red solution R*. Examined under a microscope the cell walls do not stain red.

Protein. Not more than 8.0 per cent. Carry out the determination of nitrogen by the method of sulphuric acid digestion (*2.5.9*) using 0.170 g. Multiply the result by 6.25.

Apparent viscosity. Moisten 1.00 g calculated with reference to the dried substance with 2.5 ml of *2-propanol R*. While stirring, dilute to 100.0 ml with *water R*. After 1 h, determine the viscosity (*2.2.10*) using a rotating viscometer at 20 °C and a shear rate of 100 s^{-1}. The apparent viscosity is not less than 85 per cent and not more than 115 per cent of the value stated on the label.

Loss on drying (*2.2.32*). Not more than 15.0 per cent, determined on 1.000 g by drying in an oven at 100-105 °C for 5 h.

Total ash (*2.4.16*). Not more than 1.8 per cent.

Microbial contamination. Total viable aerobic count (*2.6.12*) not more than 10^4 micro-organisms per gram, determined by plate count. It complies with the tests for *Escherichia coli* and for *Salmonella* (*2.6.13*).

LABELLING

The label states the apparent viscosity in millipascal seconds for a 10 g/l solution.

01/2005:0908

GUAR GALACTOMANNAN

Guar galactomannanum

DEFINITION

Guar galactomannan is obtained from the seeds of *Cyamopsis tetragonolobus* (L.) Taub. by grinding of the endosperms and subsequent partial hydrolysis. The main components are polysaccharides composed of D-galactose and D-mannose at molecular ratios of 1:1.4 to 1:2. The molecules consist of a linear main chain of β-(1→4)-glycosidically linked mannopyranoses and single α-(1→6)-glycosidically linked galactopyranoses.

CHARACTERS

A yellowish-white powder, soluble in cold water and in hot water, practically insoluble in organic solvents.

IDENTIFICATION

A. Mix 5 g of solution S (see Tests) with 0.5 ml of a 10 g/l solution of *disodium tetraborate R*. A gel forms within a short time.

B. Heat 20 g of solution S in a water-bath for 10 min. Allow to cool and adjust to the original mass with *water R*. The solution does not gel.

C. Examine by thin-layer chromatography (*2.2.27*), using *silica gel G R* as the coating substance.

Test solution. To 10 mg of the substance to be examined in a thick-walled centrifuge tube add 2 ml of a 230 g/l solution of *trifluoroacetic acid R*, shake vigorously to dissolve the forming gel, stopper the test tube and heat the mixture at 120 °C for 1 h. Centrifuge the hydrolysate, transfer the clear supernatant liquid carefully into a 50 ml flask, add 10 ml of *water R* and evaporate the solution to dryness under reduced pressure. Take up the residue in 10 ml of *water R* and evaporate again to dryness under reduced pressure. To the resulting clear film, which has no odour of acetic acid, add 0.1 ml of *water R* and 1 ml of *methanol R*. Centrifuge to separate the amorphous precipitate. Dilute the supernatant liquid, if necessary, to 1 ml with *methanol R*.

Reference solution. Dissolve 10 mg of *galactose R* and 10 mg of *mannose R* in 2 ml of *water R* and dilute to 10 ml with *methanol R*.

Apply separately to the plate, as bands 20 mm by 3 mm, 5 µl of each solution. Develop over a path of 15 cm using a mixture of 15 volumes of *water R* and 85 volumes of *acetonitrile R*. Spray with *aminohippuric acid reagent R* and heat at 120 °C for 5 min. The chromatogram obtained with the reference solution shows in the lower part two clearly separated brownish zones (galactose and mannose in order of increasing R_f value). The chromatogram obtained with the test solution shows two zones corresponding to galactose and mannose.

TESTS

Solution S. Moisten 1.0 g with 2 ml of *2-propanol R*. While stirring, dilute with *water R* to 100 g and stir until the substance is uniformly dispersed. Allow to stand for at least 1 h. If the apparent viscosity is below 200 mPa·s, use 3.0 g of substance instead of 1.0 g.

pH (*2.2.3*). The pH of solution S is 5.5 to 7.5.

Apparent viscosity. Moisten a quantity of the substance to be examined equivalent to 2.00 g of the dried substance with 2.5 ml of *2-propanol R* and, while stirring, dilute to 100.0 ml with *water R*. After 1 h, determine the viscosity (*2.2.10*) using a rotating viscometer at 20 °C and a shear rate of 100 s^{-1}. The apparent viscosity is not less than 75 per cent and not more than 140 per cent of the value stated on the label.

Insoluble matter. In a 250 ml flask disperse, while stirring, 1.50 g in a mixture of 1.6 ml of *sulphuric acid R* and 150 ml of *water R* and weigh. Immerse the flask in a water-bath and heat under a reflux condenser for 6 h. Adjust to the original mass with *water R*. Filter the hot solution through a tared, sintered-glass filter (160). Rinse the filter with hot *water R* and dry at 100 °C to 105 °C. The residue weighs not more than 105 mg (7.0 per cent).

Protein. Not more than 5.0 per cent. Carry out the determination of nitrogen by sulphuric acid digestion (*2.5.9*), using 0.400 g of substance. Multiply the result by 6.25.

Tragacanth, sterculia gum, agar, alginates and carrageenan. To a small amount of the substance to be examined, add 0.2 ml of freshly prepared *ruthenium red solution R*. Examined under a microscope, none of the structures are stained red.

Loss on drying (*2.2.32*). Not more than 15.0 per cent, determined on 1.000 g by drying in an oven at 100 °C to 105 °C for 5 h.

Monographs F-H

Total ash (*2.4.16*). Not more than 1.8 per cent, determined on 1.00 g after wetting with 10 ml of *water R*.

Microbial contamination. Total viable aerobic count (*2.6.12*) not more than 10^3 micro-organisms per gram, determined by plate-count. It complies with the tests for *Escherichia coli* and for *Salmonella* (*2.6.13*).

LABELLING

The label states the apparent viscosity in millipascal seconds for a 20 g/l solution.

H

01/2005:1167

HAEMODIALYSIS SOLUTIONS, CONCENTRATED, WATER FOR DILUTING

Aqua ad dilutionem solutionium concentratarum ad haemodialysim

The following monograph is given for information.

The analytical methods described and the limits proposed are intended to be used for validating the procedure for obtaining the water.

DEFINITION

Water for diluting concentrated haemodialysis solutions is obtained from potable water by distillation, by reverse osmosis, by ion exchange or by any other suitable method. The conditions of preparation, transfer and storage are designed to minimise the risk of chemical and microbial contamination.

When water obtained by one of the methods described above is not available, potable water may be used for home dialysis. Because the chemical composition of potable water varies considerably from one locality to another, consideration must be given to its chemical composition to enable adjustments to be made to the content of ions so that the concentrations in the diluted solution correspond to the intended use.

Attention has also to be paid to the possible presence of residues from water treatment (for example, chloramines) and volatile halogenated hydrocarbons.

For the surveillance of the quality of water for diluting concentrated haemodialysis solutions, the following methods may be used to determine the chemical composition and/or to detect the presence of possible contaminants together with suggested limits to be obtained.

CHARACTERS

Clear, colourless, tasteless liquid.

TESTS

Acidity or alkalinity. To 10 ml of the water to be examined, freshly boiled and cooled in a borosilicate glass flask, add 0.05 ml of *methyl red solution R*. The solution is not red. To 10 ml of the water to be examined add 0.1 ml of *bromothymol blue solution R1*. The solution is not blue.

Oxidisable substances. To 100 ml of the water to be examined add 10 ml of *dilute sulphuric acid R* and 0.1 ml of *0.02 M potassium permanganate* and boil for 5 min. The solution remains faintly pink.

Total available chlorine: maximum 0.1 ppm.

In a 125 ml test-tube (A), place successively 5 ml of *buffer solution pH 6.5 R*, 5 ml of *diethylphenylenediamine sulphate solution R* and 1 g of *potassium iodide R*. In a second 125 ml test-tube (B), place successively 5 ml of *buffer solution pH 6.5 R* and 5 ml of *diethylphenylenediamine sulphate solution R*. Add as simultaneously as possible to tube A 100 ml of the water to be examined and to tube B a reference solution prepared as follows: to 1 ml of a 10 mg/l solution of *potassium iodate R*, add 1 g of *potassium iodide R* and 1 ml of *dilute sulphuric acid R*; allow to stand for 1 min, add 1 ml of *dilute sodium hydroxide solution R* and dilute to 100 ml with *water R*. Any colour in the mixture obtained with the water to be examined is not more intense than that in the mixture obtained with the reference solution.

Chlorides (*2.4.4*): maximum 50 ppm.

Dilute 1 ml of the water to be examined to 15 ml with *water R*. The solution complies with the limit test for chlorides.

Fluorides: maximum 0.2 ppm.

Potentiometry (*2.2.36, Method I*): use as indicator electrode a fluoride-selective solid-membrane electrode and as reference electrode a silver-silver chloride electrode.

Test solution. The water to be examined.

Reference solutions. Dilute 2.0 ml, 4.0 ml and 10.0 ml of *fluoride standard solution (1 ppm F) R* respectively to 20.0 ml with *total-ionic-strength-adjustment buffer R1*.

Carry out the measurement of each solution.

Nitrates: maximum 2 ppm.

Dilute 2 ml of the water to be examined to 100 ml with *nitrate-free water R*. Place 5 ml of the dilution in a test-tube immersed in iced water, add 0.4 ml of a 100 g/l solution of *potassium chloride R* and 0.1 ml of *diphenylamine solution R* and then, dropwise and with shaking, 5 ml of *sulphuric acid R*. Transfer the tube to a water-bath at 50 °C. Allow to stand for 15 min. Any blue colour in the solution is not more intense than that in a standard prepared at the same time and in the same manner using a mixture of 0.1 ml of *nitrate standard solution (2 ppm NO_3) R* and 4.9 ml of *nitrate-free water R*.

Sulphates (*2.4.13*): maximum 50 ppm.

Dilute 3 ml of the water to be examined to 15 ml with *distilled water R*. The solution complies with the limit test for sulphates.

Aluminium (*2.4.17*): maximum 10 µg/l.

Prescribed solution. To 400 ml of the water to be examined add 10 ml of *acetate buffer solution pH 6.0 R* and 100 ml of *water R*.

Reference solution. Mix 2 ml of *aluminium standard solution (2 ppm Al) R*, 10 ml of *acetate buffer solution pH 6.0 R* and 98 ml of *water R*.

Blank solution. Mix 10 ml of *acetate buffer solution pH 6.0 R* and 100 ml of *water R*.

Ammonium: maximum 0.2 ppm.

To 20 ml of the water to be examined in a flat-bottomed and transparent tube, add 1 ml of *alkaline potassium tetraiodomercurate solution R*. Allow to stand for 5 min. The solution is not more intensely coloured than a standard prepared at the same time and in the same manner using a mixture of 4 ml of *ammonium standard solution (1 ppm NH_4) R* and 16 ml of *ammonium-free water R*. Examine the solutions along the vertical axis of the tube.

Calcium: maximum 2 ppm.

Atomic absorption spectrometry (*2.2.23, Method I*).

Test solution. The water to be examined.

Reference solutions. Prepare reference solutions (1 ppm to 5 ppm) using *calcium standard solution (400 ppm Ca) R*.

Source: calcium hollow-cathode lamp.

Wavelength: 422.7 nm.

Atomisation device: oxidising air-acetylene flame.

Magnesium: maximum 2 ppm.

Atomic absorption spectrometry (*2.2.23, Method I*).

Test solution. Dilute 10 ml of the water to be examined to 100 ml with *distilled water R*.

Reference solutions. Prepare reference solutions (0.1 ppm to 0.5 ppm) using *magnesium standard solution (100 ppm Mg) R*.

Source: magnesium hollow-cathode lamp.

Monographs F-H

Wavelength: 285.2 nm.

Atomisation device: oxidising air-acetylene flame.

Mercury: maximum 0.001 ppm.

Atomic absorption spectrometry (*2.2.23, Method I*).

Test solution. Add 5 ml of *nitric acid R* per litre of the water to be examined. In a 50 ml borosilicate glass flask with a ground-glass-stopper, place 20 ml of the water to be examined and add 1 ml of *dilute nitric acid R* and shake. Add 0.3 ml of *bromine water R1*. Stopper the flask, shake and heat the stoppered flask at 45 °C for 4 h. Allow to cool. If the solution does not become yellow, add 0.3 ml of *bromine water R1* and re-heat at 45 °C for 4 h. Add 0.5 ml of a freshly prepared 10 g/l solution of *hydroxylamine hydrochloride R*. Shake. Allow to stand for 20 min.

Reference solutions. Use freshly prepared reference solutions (0.0005 ppm to 0.002 ppm) obtained by diluting *mercury standard solution (1000 ppm Hg) R* with a 5 per cent *V/V* solution of *dilute nitric acid R* and treat as described for the test solution.

To a volume of solution suitable for the instrument to be used, add *stannous chloride solution R2* equal to 1/5 of this volume. Fit immediately the device for the entrainment of the mercury vapour. Wait 20 s and pass through the device a stream of *nitrogen R* as the carrier gas.

Source: mercury hollow-cathode tube or a discharge lamp.

Wavelength: 253.7 nm.

Atomisation device: flameless system whereby the mercury can be entrained in the form of cold vapour.

Potassium: maximum 2 ppm.

Atomic emission spectrometry (*2.2.22, Method I*).

Test solution (a). Dilute 50.0 ml of the water to be examined to 100 ml with *distilled water R*. Carry out a determination using this solution. If the potassium content is more than 0.75 mg/l, further dilute the water to be examined with *distilled water R*.

Test solution (b). Take 50.0 ml of the water to be examined or, if necessary, the water to be examined diluted as described in the preparation of test solution (a). Add 1.25 ml of *potassium standard solution (20 ppm K) R* and dilute to 100.0 ml with *distilled water R*.

Reference solutions. Prepare reference solutions (0 ppm; 0.25 ppm; 0.50 ppm; 0.75 ppm; 1 ppm) using *potassium standard solution (20 ppm K) R*.

Wavelength: 766.5 nm.

Calculate the potassium content of the water to be examined in parts per million from the expression:

$$\frac{p \times n_1 \times 0.5}{n_2 - n_1}$$

p = dilution factor used for the preparation of test solution (a),

n_1 = measured value of test solution (a),

n_2 = measured value of test solution (b).

Sodium: maximum 50 ppm.

Atomic emission spectrometry (*2.2.22, Method I*).

Test solution. The water to be examined. If the sodium content is more than 10 mg/l, dilute with *distilled water R* to obtain a concentration suitable for the apparatus used.

Reference solutions. Prepare reference solutions (0 ppm; 2.5 ppm; 5.0 ppm; 7.5 ppm; 10 ppm) using *sodium standard solution (200 ppm Na) R*.

Wavelength: 589 nm.

Zinc: maximum 0.1 ppm.

Atomic absorption spectrometry (*2.2.23, Method I*): use sampling and analytical equipment free from zinc or not liable to yield zinc under the conditions of use.

Test solution. The water to be examined.

Reference solutions. Prepare reference solutions (0.05 ppm to 0.15 ppm) using *zinc standard solution (100 ppm Zn) R*.

Source: zinc hollow-cathode lamp.

Wavelength: 213.9 nm.

Atomisation device: oxidising air-acetylene flame.

Heavy metals (*2.4.8*): maximum 0.1 ppm.

Heat 200 ml of the water to be examined in a glass evaporating dish on a water-bath until the volume is reduced to 20 ml. 12 ml of the solution complies with limit test A. Prepare the standard using *lead standard solution (1 ppm Pb) R*.

Microbial contamination. Total viable aerobic count (*2.6.12*) not more than 10^2 micro-organisms per millilitre, determined by plate count.

Bacterial endotoxins (*2.6.14*): less than 0.25 IU/ml.

01/2005:0128

HAEMODIALYSIS, SOLUTIONS FOR

Solutiones ad haemodialysim

DEFINITION

Solutions for haemodialysis are solutions of electrolytes with a concentration close to the electrolytic composition of plasma. Glucose may be included in the formulation.

Because of the large volumes used, haemodialysis solutions are usually prepared by diluting a concentrated solution with water of suitable quality (see the monograph on *Haemodialysis solutions concentrated, water for diluting (1167)*), using for example an automatic dosing device.

Concentrated solutions for haemodialysis

Concentrated haemodialysis solutions are prepared and stored using materials and methods designed to produce solutions having as low a degree of microbial contamination as possible. In certain circumstances, it may be necessary to use sterile solutions.

During dilution and use, precautions are taken to avoid microbial contamination. Diluted solutions are to be used immediately after preparation.

Concentrated solutions for haemodialysis are supplied in:

- rigid, semi-rigid or flexible plastic containers,
- glass containers.

Three types of concentrated solutions are used:

1. Concentrated solutions with acetate or lactate

Several formulations of concentrated solutions are used. The concentrations of the components in the solutions are such that after dilution to the stated volume the concentrations of the components per litre are usually in the following ranges:

Table 0128.-1.

	Expression in mmol	Expression in mEq
Sodium	130 - 145	130 - 145
Potassium	0 - 3.0	0 - 3.0
Calcium	0 - 2.0	0 - 4.0
Magnesium	0 - 1.2	0 - 2.4
Acetate or lactate	32 - 45	32 - 45
Chloride	90 - 120	90 - 120
Glucose	0 - 12.0	

Concentrated solutions with acetate or lactate are diluted before use.

2. Concentrated acidic solutions

Several formulations of concentrated solutions are used. The concentrations of the components in the solutions are such that after dilution to the stated volume and before neutralisation with sodium hydrogen carbonate the concentrations of the components per litre are usually in the following ranges:

Table 0128.-2.

	Expression in mmol	Expression in mEq
Sodium	80 - 110	80 - 110
Potassium	0 - 3.0	0 - 3.0
Calcium	0 - 2.0	0 - 4.0
Magnesium	0 - 1.2	0 - 2.4
Acetic acid	2.5 - 10	2.5 - 10
Chloride	90 - 120	90 - 120
Glucose	0 - 12.0	

Sodium hydrogen carbonate must be added immediately before use to a final concentration of not more than 45 mmol/l. The concentrated solution of sodium hydrogen carbonate is supplied in a separate container. The concentrated acidic solutions and the concentrated solutions of sodium hydrogen carbonate are diluted and mixed immediately before use using a suitable device. Alternatively, solid sodium hydrogen carbonate may be used to prepare the solution.

3. Concentrated solutions without buffer

Several formulations of concentrated solutions without buffer are used. The concentrations of the components in the solutions are such that after dilution to the stated volume, the concentrations of the components per litre are usually in the following ranges:

Table 0128.-3.

	Expression in mmol	Expression in mEq
Sodium	130 - 145	130 - 145
Potassium	0 - 3.0	0 - 3.0
Calcium	0 - 2.0	0 - 4.0
Magnesium	0 - 1.2	0 - 2.4
Chloride	130 - 155	130 - 155
Glucose	0 - 12.0	

Concentrated solutions without buffer are used together with parenteral administration of suitable hydrogen carbonate solutions.

IDENTIFICATION

According to the stated composition, the solution to be examined gives the following identification reactions (*2.3.1*):

- potassium: reaction (b);
- calcium: reaction (a);
- sodium: reaction (b);
- chlorides: reaction (a);
- lactates;
- carbonates and hydrogen carbonates;
- acetates:
  - if the solution is free from glucose, use reaction (b),
  - if the solution contains glucose, use the following method: to 5 ml of the solution to be examined add 1 ml of *hydrochloric acid R* in a test tube fitted with a stopper and a bent tube, heat and collect a few millilitres of distillate; carry out reaction (b) of acetates on the distillate;
- magnesium: to 0.1 ml of *titan yellow solution R* add 10 ml of *water R*, 2 ml of the solution to be examined and 1 ml of a 4.2 g/l solution of *sodium hydroxide R*; a pink colour is produced;
- glucose: to 5 ml of the solution to be examined, add 2 ml of *dilute sodium hydroxide solution R* and 0.05 ml of *copper sulphate solution R*; the solution is blue and clear; heat to boiling; an abundant red precipitate is formed.

TESTS

Appearance of solution. The solution to be examined is clear (*2.2.1*). If it does not contain glucose, it is colourless (*2.2.2, Method I*). If it contains glucose, it is not more intensely coloured than reference solution Y_7 (*2.2.2, Method I*).

Aluminium (*2.4.17*): maximum 0.1 mg/l.

Prescribed solution. Take 20 ml of the solution to be examined, adjust to pH 6.0 and add 10 ml of *acetate buffer solution pH 6.0 R*.

Reference solution. Mix 1 ml of *aluminium standard solution (2 ppm Al) R*, 10 ml of *acetate buffer solution pH 6.0 R* and 9 ml of *water R*.

Blank solution. Mix 10 ml of *acetate buffer solution pH 6.0 R* and 10 ml of *water R*.

Extractable volume (*2.9.17*). The volume measured is not less than the nominal volume stated on the label.

Sterility (*2.6.1*). If the label states that the concentrated haemodialysis solution is sterile, it complies with the test for sterility.

Bacterial endotoxins (*2.6.14*): less than 0.5 IU/ml in the solution diluted for use.

Pyrogens (*2.6.8*). Solutions for which a validated test for bacterial endotoxins cannot be carried out comply with the test for pyrogens. Dilute the solution to be examined with *water for injections R* to the concentration prescribed for use. Inject 10 ml of the solution per kilogram of the rabbit's mass.

ASSAY

Determine the density (2.2.5) of the concentrated solution and calculate the content in grams per litre and in millimoles per litre.

Sodium: 97.5 per cent to 102.5 per cent of the content of sodium (Na) stated on the label.

Atomic emission spectrometry (*2.2.22, Method I*).

Monographs F-H

Test solution. Dilute 5.0 ml of the solution to be examined to 100.0 ml with *water R*. Dilute 2.0 ml of this solution to 50.0 ml with *water R*. To 1.0 ml of this solution add 10 ml of *lanthanum chloride solution R* and dilute to 100.0 ml with *water R*.

Reference solutions. Into 4 identical volumetric flasks each containing 10 ml of *lanthanum chloride solution R*, introduce respectively 1.0 ml, 2.0 ml, 4.0 ml and 5.0 ml of *sodium standard solution (10 ppm Na) R* and dilute to 100.0 ml with *water R*.

Wavelength: 589.0 nm.

Potassium: 95.0 per cent to 105.0 per cent of the content of potassium (K) stated on the label.

Atomic absorption spectrometry (*2.2.23, Method I*).

Test solution. Dilute with *water R* an accurately weighed quantity of the solution to be examined to a concentration suitable for the instrument to be used. To 100 ml of this solution add 10 ml of a 22 g/l solution of *sodium chloride R*.

Reference solutions. Prepare the reference solutions using *potassium standard solution (100 ppm K) R*. To 100 ml of each reference solution add 10 ml of a 22 g/l solution of *sodium chloride R*.

Source: potassium hollow-cathode lamp.

Wavelength: 766.5 nm.

Atomisation device: air-acetylene flame.

Calcium: 95.0 per cent to 105.0 per cent of the content of calcium (Ca) stated on the label.

Atomic absorption spectrometry (*2.2.23, Method I*).

Test solution. Dilute 5.0 ml of the solution to be examined to 100.0 ml with *water R*. To 3.0 ml of this solution add 5 ml of *lanthanum chloride solution R* and dilute to 50.0 ml with *water R*.

Reference solutions. Into 4 keep volumetric flasks each containing 5 ml of *lanthanum chloride solution R*, introduce respectively 2.5 ml, 5.0 ml, 7.0 ml and 10.0 ml of *calcium standard solution (10 ppm Ca) R* and dilute to 50.0 ml with *water R*.

Source: calcium hollow-cathode lamp.

Wavelength: 422.7 nm.

Atomisation device: air-acetylene flame.

Magnesium: 95.0 per cent to 105.0 per cent of the content of magnesium (Mg) stated on the label.

Atomic absorption spectrometry (*2.2.23, Method I*).

Test solution. Dilute 5.0 ml of the solution to be examined to 100.0 ml with *water R*. To 2.0 ml of this solution add 5 ml of *lanthanum chloride solution R* and dilute to 50.0 ml with *water R*.

Reference solutions. Into 4 identical volumetric flasks each containing 5 ml of *lanthanum chloride solution R*, introduce respectively 1.0 ml, 2.0 ml, 3.0 ml and 4.0 ml of *magnesium standard solution (10 ppm Mg) R* and dilute to 50.0 ml with *water R*.

Source: magnesium hollow-cathode lamp.

Wavelength: 285.2 nm.

Atomisation device: air-acetylene flame.

Total chloride: 95.0 per cent to 105.0 per cent of the content of chloride (Cl) stated on the label.

Dilute to 50 ml with *water R* an accurately measured volume of the solution to be examined containing the equivalent of about 60 mg of chloride. Add 5 ml of *dilute nitric acid R*, 25.0 ml of *0.1 M silver nitrate* and 2 ml of *dibutyl phthalate R*. Shake. Using 2 ml of *ferric ammonium sulphate solution R2* as indicator, titrate with *0.1 M ammonium thiocyanate* until a reddish-yellow colour is obtained.

1 ml of *0.1 M silver nitrate* is equivalent to 3.545 mg of Cl.

Acetate: 95.0 per cent to 105.0 per cent of the content of acetate stated on the label.

To a volume of the solution to be examined, corresponding to about 0.7 mmol of acetate, add 10.0 ml of *0.1 M hydrochloric acid*. Carry out a potentiometric titration (*2.2.20*), using *0.1 M sodium hydroxide*. Read the volume added between the 2 points of inflexion.

1 ml of *0.1 M sodium hydroxide* is equivalent to 0.1 mmol of acetate.

Lactate: 95.0 per cent to 105.0 per cent of the content of lactate stated on the label.

To a volume of the solution to be examined, corresponding to about 0.7 mmol of lactate, add 10.0 ml of *0.1 M hydrochloric acid*. Then add 50 ml of *acetonitrile R*. Carry out a potentiometric titration (*2.2.20*), using *0.1 M sodium hydroxide*. Read the volume added between the 2 points of inflexion.

1 ml of *0.1 M sodium hydroxide* is equivalent to 0.1 mmol of lactate.

Sodium hydrogen carbonate: 95.0 per cent to 105.0 per cent of the content of sodium hydrogen carbonate stated on the label.

Titrate with *0.1 M hydrochloric acid* a volume of the solution to be examined corresponding to about 0.1 g of sodium hydrogen carbonate, determining the end-point potentiometrically (*2.2.20*).

1 ml of *0.1 M hydrochloric acid* is equivalent to 8.40 mg of $NaHCO_3$.

Reducing sugars (expressed as anhydrous glucose): 95.0 per cent to 105.0 per cent of the content of glucose stated on the label.

Transfer a volume of the solution to be examined containing the equivalent of 25 mg of glucose to a 250 ml conical flask with a ground-glass neck and add 25.0 ml of *cupri-citric solution R*. Add a few grains of pumice, fit a reflux condenser, heat so that boiling occurs within 2 min and maintain boiling for exactly 10 min. Cool and add 3 g of *potassium iodide R* dissolved in 3 ml of *water R*. Carefully add, in small amounts, 25 ml of a 25 per cent *m/m* solution of *sulphuric acid R*. Titrate with *0.1 M sodium thiosulphate* using *starch solution R*, added towards the end of the titration, as indicator. Carry out a blank titration using 25.0 ml of *water R*.

Calculate the content of reducing sugars, expressed as anhydrous glucose ($C_6H_{12}O_6$), using Table 0128.-4:

Table 0128.-4.

Volume of *0.1 M sodium thiosulphate* (ml)	Anhydrous glucose (mg)
8	19.8
9	22.4
10	25.0
11	27.6
12	30.3
13	33.0
14	35.7
15	38.5
16	41.3

STORAGE

Store at a temperature not below 4 °C.

LABELLING

The label states:

- the formula of the concentrated solution for haemodialysis expressed in grams per litre and in millimoles per litre,
- the nominal volume of the solution in the container,
- where applicable, that the concentrated solution is sterile,
- the storage conditions,
- that the concentrated solution is to be diluted immediately before use,
- the dilution to be made,
- that the volume taken for use is to be measured accurately,
- the ionic formula for the diluted solution ready for use in millimoles per litre,
- that any unused portion of solution is to be discarded,
- where applicable, that sodium hydrogen carbonate is to be added before use.

01/2005:0861

HAEMOFILTRATION AND FOR HAEMODIAFILTRATION, SOLUTIONS FOR

Solutiones ad haemocolaturam haemodiacolaturamque

DEFINITION

Solutions for haemofiltration and for haemodiafiltration are preparations for parenteral use containing electrolytes with a concentration close to the electrolytic composition of plasma. Glucose may be included in the formulation.

Solutions for haemofiltration and for haemodiafiltration are supplied in:

- rigid or semi-rigid plastic containers,
- flexible plastic containers inside closed protective envelopes,
- glass containers.

The containers and closures comply with the requirements for containers for preparations for parenteral use (*3.2. Containers*).

In haemofiltration and haemodiafiltration, the following formulations are used. The concentrations of the components per litre of solution are usually in the following range:

Table 0861.-1.

	Expression in mmol	**Expression in mEq**
Sodium	125 - 150	125 - 150
Potassium	0 - 4.5	0 - 4.5
Calcium	1.0 - 2.5	2.0 - 5.0
Magnesium	0.25 - 1.5	0.50 - 3.0
Acetate and/or lactate and/or hydrogen carbonate	30 - 60	30 - 60
Chloride	90 - 120	90 - 120
Glucose	0 - 25	

When hydrogen carbonate is present, the solution of sodium hydrogen carbonate is supplied in a container or a separate compartment and is added to the electrolyte solution immediately before use.

In haemofiltration and in haemodiafiltration, the following formulations may also be used:

Table 0861.-2.

	Expression in mmol	**Expression in mEq**
Sodium	130 - 167	130 - 167
Potassium	0 - 4.0	0 - 4.0
Hydrogen carbonate	20 - 167	20 - 167
Chloride	0 - 147	0 - 147

Antioxidants such as metabisulphite salts are not added to the solutions.

IDENTIFICATION

According to the stated composition, the solution to be examined gives the following identification reactions (*2.3.1*):

- potassium: reaction (b);
- calcium: reaction (a);
- sodium: reaction (b);
- chlorides: reaction (a);
- acetates:

  if the solution is free from glucose, use reaction (b),

  if the solution contains glucose, use the following method: to 5 ml of the solution to be examined add 1 ml of *hydrochloric acid R* in a test-tube fitted with a stopper and a bent tube, heat and collect a few millilitres of distillate; carry out reaction (b) of acetates on the distillate;
- lactates;
- carbonates and hydrogen carbonates;
- magnesium: to 0.1 ml of *titan yellow solution R* add 10 ml of *water R*, 2 ml of the solution to be examined and 1 ml of *1 M sodium hydroxide*; a pink colour is produced;
- glucose: to 5 ml of the solution to be examined, add 2 ml of *dilute sodium hydroxide solution R* and 0.05 ml of *copper sulphate solution R*; the solution is blue and clear; heat to boiling; an abundant red precipitate is formed.

TESTS

Appearance of solution. The solution is clear (*2.2.1*). If it does not contain glucose, it is colourless (*2.2.2, Method I*). If it contains glucose, it is not more intensely coloured than reference solution Y_7 (*2.2.2, Method I*).

pH (*2.2.3*). The pH of the solution is 5.0 to 7.5. If the solution contains glucose, the pH is 4.5 to 6.5. If the solution contains hydrogen carbonate, the pH is 7.0 to 8.5.

Hydroxymethylfurfural. To a volume of the solution containing the equivalent of 25 mg of glucose, add 5.0 ml of a 100 g/l solution of *p-toluidine R* in *2-propanol R* containing 10 per cent *V/V* of *glacial acetic acid R* and 1.0 ml of a 5 g/l solution of *barbituric acid R*. The absorbance (*2.2.25*), determined at 550 nm after allowing the mixture to stand for 2 min to 3 min, is not greater than that of a standard prepared at the same time in the same manner using a solution containing 10 µg of *hydroxymethylfurfural R* in the same volume as the solution to be examined. If the solution contains hydrogen carbonate, use as the standard a solution containing 20 µg of *hydroxymethylfurfural R*.

Aluminium (*2.4.17*). Take 200 ml, adjust to pH 6.0 and add 10 ml of *acetate buffer solution pH 6.0 R*. The solution complies with the limit test for aluminium (10 µg/l). Use as the reference solution a mixture of 1 ml of *aluminium standard solution (2 ppm Al) R*, 10 ml of *acetate*

Monographs F-H

buffer solution pH 6.0 R and 9 ml of *water R*. To prepare the blank use a mixture of 10 ml of *acetate buffer solution pH 6.0 R* and 10 ml of *water R*.

Particulate contamination. Carry out the test for sub-visible particles (*2.9.19*) using 50 ml of solution.

Table 0861.-3.

Particles larger than	10 μm	25 μm
Maximum number of particles per millilitre	25	3

Extractable volume (*2.9.17*). The solution complies with the test prescribed for parenteral infusions.

Sterility (*2.6.1*). The solution complies with the test for sterility.

Bacterial endotoxins (*2.6.14*): less than 0.25 IU/ml.

Pyrogens (*2.6.8*). Solutions for which a validated test for bacterial endotoxins cannot be carried out comply with the test for pyrogens. Inject per kilogram of the rabbit's mass 10 ml of the solution.

ASSAY

Sodium: 97.5 per cent to 102.5 per cent of the content of sodium (Na) stated on the label, determined by atomic absorption spectrometry (*2.2.23, Method II*).

Test solution. If necessary, dilute the solution to be examined with *water R* to a concentration suitable for the instrument to be used.

Reference solutions. Prepare the reference solutions using *sodium standard solution (200 ppm Na) R*.

Measure the absorbance at 589.0 nm using a sodium hollow-cathode lamp as source of radiation and an air-propane or an air-acetylene flame.

Potassium. 95.0 per cent to 105.0 per cent of the content of potassium (K) stated on the label, determined by atomic absorption spectrometry (*2.2.23, Method I*).

Test solution. If necessary, dilute the solution to be examined with *water R* to a concentration suitable for the instrument to be used. To 100 ml of the solution add 10 ml of a 22 g/l solution of *sodium chloride R*.

Reference solutions. Prepare the reference solutions using *potassium standard solution (100 ppm K) R*. To 100 ml of each reference solution add 10 ml of a 22 g/l solution of *sodium chloride R*.

Measure the absorbance at 766.5 nm using a potassium hollow-cathode lamp as source of radiation and an air-propane or an air-acetylene flame.

Calcium. 95.0 per cent to 105.0 per cent of the content of calcium (Ca) stated on the label, determined by atomic absorption spectrometry (*2.2.23, Method I*).

Test solution. If necessary, dilute the solution to be examined with *water R* to a concentration suitable for the instrument to be used.

Reference solutions. Prepare the reference solutions using *calcium standard solution (400 ppm Ca) R*.

Measure the absorbance at 422.7 nm using a calcium hollow-cathode lamp as source of radiation and an air-propane or an air-acetylene flame.

Magnesium. 95.0 per cent to 105.0 per cent of the content of magnesium (Mg) stated on the label, determined by atomic absorption spectrometry (*2.2.23, Method I*).

Test solution. If necessary, dilute the solution to be examined with *water R* to a concentration suitable for the instrument to be used.

Reference solutions. Prepare the reference solutions using *magnesium standard solution (100 ppm Mg) R*.

Measure the absorbance at 285.2 nm using a magnesium hollow-cathode lamp as source of radiation and an air-propane or an air-acetylene flame.

Total chloride: 95.0 per cent to 105.0 per cent of the content of chloride (Cl) stated on the label. Dilute to 50 ml with *water R* an accurately measured volume of the solution to be examined containing the equivalent of about 60 mg of chloride. Add 5 ml of *dilute nitric acid R*, 25.0 ml of *0.1 M silver nitrate* and 2 ml of *dibutyl phthalate R*. Shake. Using 2 ml of *ferric ammonium sulphate solution R2* as indicator, titrate with *0.1 M ammonium thiocyanate* until a reddish-yellow colour is obtained.

1 ml of *0.1 M silver nitrate* is equivalent to 3.545 mg of Cl.

Acetate: 95.0 per cent to 105.0 per cent of the content of acetate stated on the label. To a volume of the solution to be examined, corresponding to about 0.7 mmol of acetate, add 10.0 ml of *0.1 M hydrochloric acid*. Carry out a potentiometric titration (*2.2.20*), using *0.1 M sodium hydroxide*. Read the volume added between the two points of inflexion.

1 ml of *0.1 M sodium hydroxide* is equivalent to 0.1 mmol of acetate.

Lactate: 95.0 per cent to 105.0 per cent of the content of lactate stated on the label. To a volume of the solution to be examined, corresponding to about 0.7 mmol of lactate, add 10.0 ml of *0.1 M hydrochloric acid*. Add 50 ml of *acetonitrile R*. Carry out a potentiometric titration (*2.2.20*), using *0.1 M sodium hydroxide*. Read the volume added between the two points of inflexion.

1 ml of *0.1 M sodium hydroxide* is equivalent to 0.1 mmol of lactate.

Sodium hydrogen carbonate: 95.0 per cent to 105.0 per cent of the content of sodium hydrogen carbonate stated on the label. Titrate with *0.1 M hydrochloric acid*, a volume of the solution to be examined corresponding to about 0.1 g of sodium hydrogen carbonate, determining the end-point potentiometrically (*2.2.20*).

1 ml of *0.1 M hydrochloric acid* is equivalent to 8.40 mg of $NaHCO_3$.

Lactate and hydrogen carbonate: 95.0 per cent to 105.0 per cent of the content of lactates and/or hydrogen carbonates stated on the label. Examine by liquid chromatography (*2.2.29*).

Test solution. Solution to be examined.

Reference solution. Dissolve in 100 ml of *water for chromatography R* quantities of lactates and bicarbonates, accurately weighed, in order to obtain solutions having concentrations representing about 90 per cent, 100 per cent and 110 per cent of the concentrations indicated on the label.

The chromatographic procedure may be carried out using:

- a column 0.30 m long and 7.8 mm in internal diameter packed with *cation exchange resin R* (9 μm),
- as mobile phase at a flow rate of 0.6 ml/min *0.005 M sulphuric acid* previously degassed with *helium R*,
- a differential refractometer detector,

maintaining the temperature of the column at 85 °C.

Inject in duplicate 20 μl of test solution and 20 μl of each reference solution. When the chromatograms are recorded in the prescribed conditions, the peaks elute in the following order: lactates then hydrogen carbonates.

Determine the concentration of lactates and hydrogen carbonates in the test solution by interpolating the peak area for lactate and the peak height for hydrogen carbonate from the linear regression curve obtained with the reference solutions.

Reducing sugars (expressed as anhydrous glucose). 95.0 per cent to 105.0 per cent of the content of glucose stated on the label. Transfer a volume of the solution to be examined containing the equivalent of 25 mg of glucose to a 250 ml conical flask with a ground-glass neck and add 25.0 ml of *cupri-citric solution R*. Add a few grains of pumice, fit a reflux condenser, heat so that boiling occurs within 2 min and boil for exactly 10 min. Cool and add 3 g of *potassium iodide R* dissolved in 3 ml of *water R*. Carefully add, in small amounts, 25 ml of a 25 per cent *m/m* solution of *sulphuric acid R*. Titrate with *0.1 M sodium thiosulphate* using *starch solution R*, added towards the end of titration, as indicator. Carry out a blank titration using 25.0 ml of *water R*.

Calculate the content of reducing sugars expressed as anhydrous glucose ($C_6H_{12}O_6$), using Table 0861.-4:

Table 0861.-4.

Volume of 0.1 M sodium thiosulphate (ml)	Anhydrous glucose (mg)
8	19.8
9	22.4
10	25.0
11	27.6
12	30.3
13	33.0
14	35.7
15	38.5
16	41.3

STORAGE

Store at a temperature not lower than 4 °C.

LABELLING

The label states:

– the formula of the solution for haemofiltration or haemodiafiltration, expressed in grams per litre and in millimoles per litre,

– the calculated osmolarity, expressed in milliosmoles per litre,

– the nominal volume of the solution for haemofiltration or haemodiafiltration in the container,

– that the solution is free from bacterial endotoxins, or where applicable, that it is apyrogenic,

– the storage conditions,

– that any unused portion of solution is to be discarded.

01/2005:1979 corrected

HALOFANTRINE HYDROCHLORIDE

Halofantrini hydrochloridum

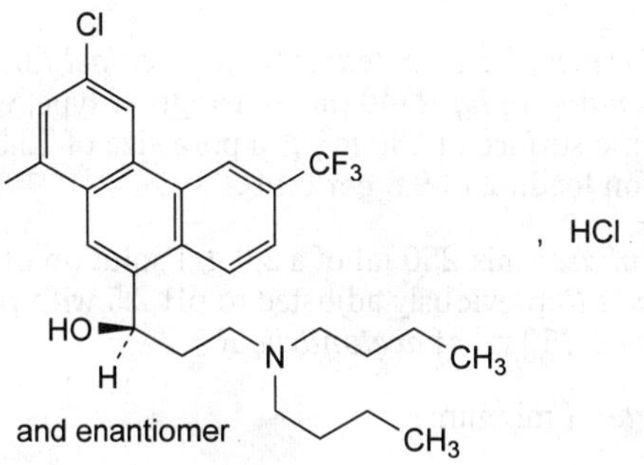

$C_{26}H_{31}Cl_3F_3NO$ M_r 536.9

DEFINITION

(1*RS*)-3-(Dibutylamino)-1-[1,3-dichloro-6-(trifluoromethyl)phenanthren-9-yl]propan-1-ol hydrochloride.

Content: 97.5 per cent to 102.0 per cent (dried substance).

CHARACTERS

Appearance: white or almost white powder.

Solubility: practically insoluble in water, freely soluble in methanol, sparingly soluble in alcohol.

It shows polymorphism.

IDENTIFICATION

A. Infrared absorption spectrophotometry (*2.2.24*).

Comparison: *halofantrine hydrochloride CRS*.

If the spectra obtained in the solid state show differences, dissolve the substance to be examined and the reference substance separately in *methyl ethyl ketone R*, evaporate to dryness and record new spectra using the residues.

B. It gives reaction (b) of chlorides (*2.3.1*).

TESTS

Optical rotation (*2.2.7*): − 0.10° to + 0.10°.

Dissolve 1.00 g in *alcohol R* and dilute to 100.0 ml with the same solvent.

Absorbance (*2.2.25*): maximum 0.085 at 450 nm.

Dissolve 0.200 g in *methanol R* and dilute to 10.0 ml with the same solvent.

Related substances. Liquid chromatography (*2.2.29*).

Test solution (a). Dissolve 40.0 mg of the substance to be examined in the mobile phase and dilute to 100.0 ml with the mobile phase.

Test solution (b). Dilute 5.0 ml of test solution (a) to 50.0 ml with the mobile phase.

Reference solution (a). Dissolve 40.0 mg of *halofantrine hydrochloride CRS* in the mobile phase and dilute to 100.0 ml with the mobile phase.

Reference solution (b). Dilute 5.0 ml of reference solution (a) to 50.0 ml with the mobile phase.

Reference solution (c). Dilute 1.0 ml of test solution (a) to 100.0 ml with the mobile phase. Dilute 5.0 ml of the solution to 50.0 ml with the mobile phase.

Monographs F-H

Reference solution (d). Dissolve 10.0 mg of *halofantrine impurity C CRS* in the mobile phase and dilute to 25 ml with the mobile phase. To 5.0 ml of the solution, add 5.0 ml of reference solution (a) and dilute to 50.0 ml with the mobile phase.

Column:

- *size*: l = 0.30 m, Ø = 3.9 mm,
- *stationary phase*: *octadecylsilyl silica gel for chromatography R* (10 µm) of irregular type, with a specific surface of 330 m²/g, a pore size of 12.5 nm and a carbon loading of 9.8 per cent .

Mobile phase: mix 250 ml of a 2.0 g/l solution of *sodium hydroxide R*, previously adjusted to pH 2.5 with *perchloric acid R* and 750 ml of *acetonitrile R*.

Flow rate: 1 ml/min.

Detection: spectrophotometer at 260 nm.

Injection: 20 µl; inject the test solution (a) and reference solutions (c) and (d).

Run time: 5 times the retention time of halofantrine which is about 6 min.

System suitability:

- *resolution*: minimum 3.3 between the peaks due to halofantrine and impurity C in the chromatogram obtained with reference solution (d).

Limits:

- *any impurity*: not more than twice the area of the principal peak in the chromatogram obtained with reference solution (c) (0.2 per cent),
- *total*: not more than 5 times the area of the principal peak in the chromatogram obtained with reference solution (c) (0.5 per cent),
- *disregard limit*: 0.5 times the area of the principal peak in the chromatogram obtained with reference solution (c) (0.05 per cent).

Heavy metals (*2.4.8*): maximum 20 ppm.

1.0 g complies with limit test C. Prepare the standard using 2 ml of *lead standard solution (10 ppm Pb) R*.

Loss on drying (*2.2.32*): maximum 0.5 per cent, determined on 1.000 g by drying in an oven at 100-105 °C for 4 h.

Sulphated ash (*2.4.14*): maximum 0.1 per cent, determined on 1.0 g.

ASSAY

Liquid chromatography (*2.2.29*) as described in the test for related substances.

Injection: test solution (b) and reference solution (b).

Calculate the percentage content of halofantrine hydrochloride.

STORAGE

Protected from light.

IMPURITIES

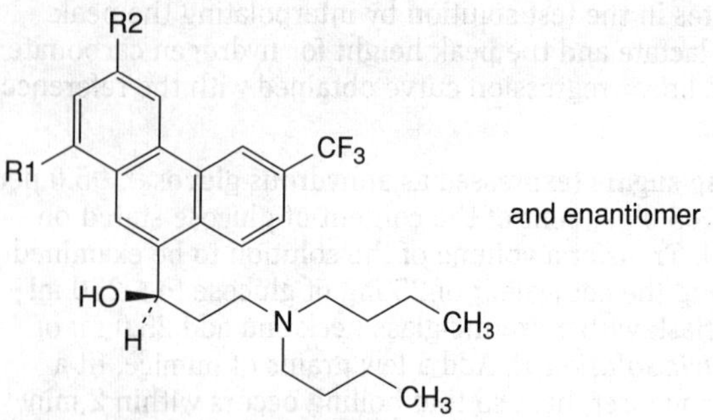

A. R1 = H, R2 = Cl: (1*RS*)-1-[3-chloro-6-(trifluoromethyl)phenanthren-9-yl]-3-(dibutylamino)propan-1-ol (1-dechlorohalofantrine),

B. R1 = Cl, R2 = H: (1*RS*)-1-[1-chloro-6-(trifluoromethyl)phenanthren-9-yl]-3-(dibutylamino)propan-1-ol (3-dechlorohalofantrine),

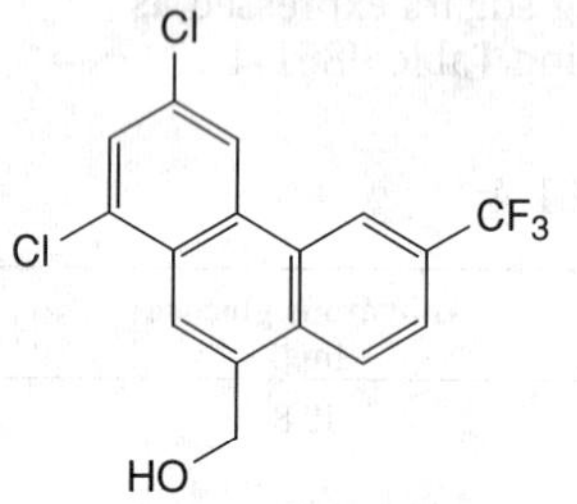

C. [1,3-dichloro-6-(trifluoromethyl)phenanthren-9-yl]methanol.

01/2005:0616

HALOPERIDOL

Haloperidolum

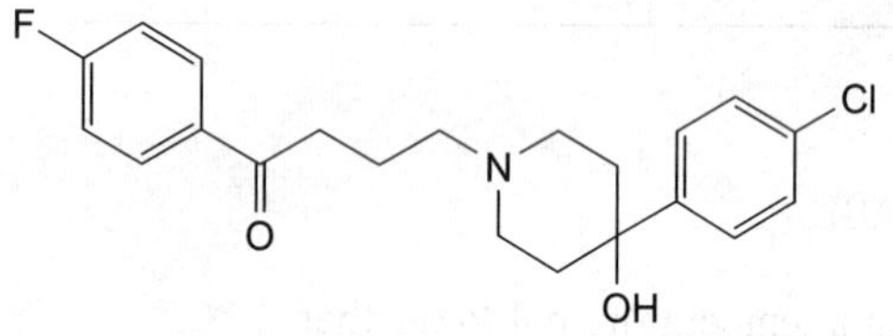

$C_{21}H_{23}ClFNO_2$ M_r 375.9

DEFINITION

Haloperidol contains not less than 99.0 per cent and not more than the equivalent of 101.0 per cent of 4-[4-(4-chlorophenyl)-4-hydroxypiperidin-1-yl]-1-(4-fluorophenyl)butan-1-one, calculated with reference to the dried substance.

CHARACTERS

A white or almost white powder, practically insoluble in water, slightly soluble in alcohol, in methanol and in methylene chloride.

IDENTIFICATION

First identification: B, E.

Second identification: A, C, D, E.

A. Melting point (*2.2.14*): 150 °C to 153 °C.

B. Examine by infrared absorption spectrophotometry (*2.2.24*), comparing with the spectrum obtained with *haloperidol CRS*. Examine the substances prepared as discs.

C. Examine by thin-layer chromatography (*2.2.27*), using a suitable octadecylsilyl silica gel as the coating substance.

Test solution. Dissolve 10 mg of the substance to be examined in *methanol R* and dilute to 10 ml with the same solvent.

Reference solution (a). Dissolve 10 mg of *haloperidol CRS* in *methanol R* and dilute to 10 ml with the same solvent.

Reference solution (b). Dissolve 10 mg of *haloperidol CRS* and 10 mg of *bromperidol CRS* in *methanol R* and dilute to 10 ml with the same solvent.

Apply to the plate 1 µl of each solution. Develop in an unsaturated tank over a path of 15 cm using a mixture of 10 volumes of *tetrahydrofuran R*, 45 volumes of *methanol R* and 45 volumes of a 58 g/l solution of *sodium chloride R*. Allow the plate to dry in air and examine in ultraviolet light at 254 nm. The principal spot in the chromatogram obtained with the test solution is similar in position and size to the principal spot in the chromatogram obtained with reference solution (a). The test is not valid unless the chromatogram obtained with reference solution (b) shows 2 spots which may, however, not be completely separated.

D. Dissolve about 10 mg in 5 ml of *ethanol R*. Add 0.5 ml of *dinitrobenzene solution R* and 0.5 ml of *2 M alcoholic potassium hydroxide R*. A violet colour is produced and becomes brownish-red after 20 min.

E. To 0.1 g in a porcelain crucible add 0.5 g of *anhydrous sodium carbonate R*. Heat over an open flame for 10 min. Allow to cool. Take up the residue with 5 ml of *dilute nitric acid R* and filter. To 1 ml of the filtrate add 1 ml of *water R*. The solution gives reaction (a) of chlorides (*2.3.1*).

TESTS

Appearance of solution. Dissolve 0.2 g in 20 ml of a 1 per cent *V/V* solution of *lactic acid R*. The solution is clear (*2.2.1*) and not more intensely coloured than reference solution Y_7 (*2.2.2, Method II*).

Related substances. Examine by liquid chromatography (*2.2.29*). *Prepare the solutions immediately before use and protect from light.*

Test solution. Dissolve 0.100 g of the substance to be examined in *methanol R* and dilute to 10.0 ml with the same solvent.

Reference solution (a). Dissolve 5.0 mg of *haloperidol CRS* and 2.5 mg of *bromperidol CRS* in *methanol R* and dilute to 50.0 ml with the same solvent.

Reference solution (b). Dilute 5.0 ml of the test solution to 100.0 ml with *methanol R*. Dilute 1.0 ml of this solution to 10.0 ml with *methanol R*.

The chromatographic procedure may be carried out using:

– a stainless steel column 0.1 m long and 4.6 mm in internal diameter packed with *base-deactivated octadecylsilyl silica gel for chromatography R* (3 µm),

– as mobile phase at a flow rate of 1.5 ml/min:

Mobile phase A. A 17 g/l solution of *tetrabutylammonium hydrogen sulphate R1*,

Mobile phase B. Acetonitrile R,

Time (min)	Mobile phase A (per cent *V/V*)	Mobile phase B (per cent *V/V*)	Comment
0 - 15	90 → 50	10 → 50	linear gradient
15 - 20	50	50	isocratic elution
20 - 25	90	10	switch to initial eluent composition
25 = 0	90	10	restart gradient

– as detector a spectrophotometer set at 230 nm.

Adjust the sensitivity of the system so that the height of the principal peak in the chromatogram obtained with 10 µl of reference solution (b) is at least 50 per cent of the full scale of the recorder.

Inject 10 µl of reference solution (a). When the chromatogram is recorded in the prescribed conditions, the retention times are: haloperidol about 5.5 min and bromperidol about 6 min. The test is not valid unless the resolution between the peaks due to haloperidol and bromperidol is at least 3.0. If necessary, adjust the concentration of acetonitrile in the mobile phase or adjust the time programme for the linear-gradient elution.

Inject separately 10 µl of *methanol R* as a blank, 10 µl of the test solution and 10 µl of reference solution (b). In the chromatogram obtained with the test solution: the area of any peak, apart from the principal peak, is not greater than the area of the principal peak in the chromatogram obtained with reference solution (b) (0.5 per cent); the sum of the areas of all peaks, apart from the principal peak, is not greater than twice the area of the principal peak in the chromatogram obtained with reference solution (b) (1 per cent). Disregard any peak obtained with the blank and any peak with an area less than 0.1 times the area of the principal peak in the chromatogram obtained with reference solution (b).

Loss on drying (*2.2.32*). Not more than 0.5 per cent, determined on 1.000 g by drying in an oven at 100-105 °C.

Sulphated ash (*2.4.14*). Not more than 0.1 per cent, determined on 1.0 g using a platinum crucible.

ASSAY

Dissolve 0.300 g in 50 ml of a mixture of 1 volume of *anhydrous acetic acid R* and 7 volumes of *methyl ethyl ketone R*. Titrate with *0.1 M perchloric acid*, using 0.2 ml of *naphtholbenzein solution R* as indicator.

1 ml of *0.1 M perchloric acid* is equivalent to 37.59 mg of $C_{21}H_{23}ClFNO_2$.

STORAGE

Store protected from light.

IMPURITIES

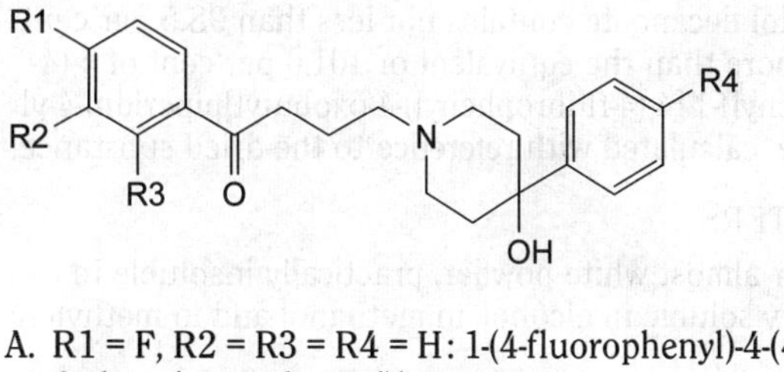

A. R1 = F, R2 = R3 = R4 = H: 1-(4-fluorophenyl)-4-(4-hydroxy-4-phenylpiperidin-1-yl)butan-1-one,

B. R1 = R2 = H, R3 = F, R4 = Cl: 4-[4-(4-chlorophenyl)-4-hydroxypiperidin-1-yl]-1-(2-fluorophenyl)butan-1-one,

C. R1 = F, R2 = C_2H_5, R3 = H, R4 = Cl: 4-[4-(4-chlorophenyl)-4-hydroxypiperidin-1-yl]-1-(3-ethyl-4-fluorophenyl)butan-1-one,

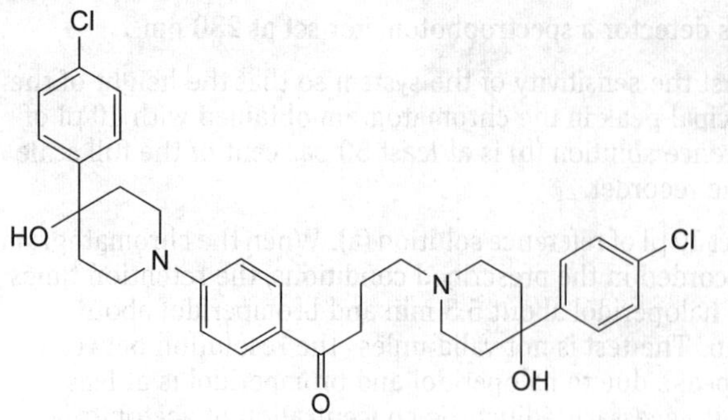

D. 4-[4-(4-chlorophenyl)-4-hydroxypiperidin-1-yl]-1-[4-[4-(4-chlorophenyl)-4-hydroxypiperidin-1-yl]phenyl]butan-1-one,

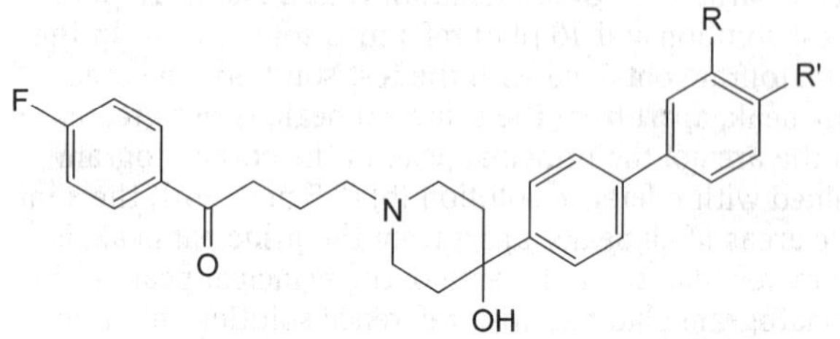

E. R = H, R′ = Cl: 4-[4-(4′-chlorobiphenyl-4-yl)-4-hydroxypiperidin-1-yl]-1-(4-fluorophenyl)butan-1-one,

F. R = Cl, R′ = H: 4-[4-(3′-chlorobiphenyl-4-yl)-4-hydroxypiperidin-1-yl]-1-(4-fluorophenyl)butan-1-one.

01/2005:1431

HALOPERIDOL DECANOATE

Haloperidoli decanoas

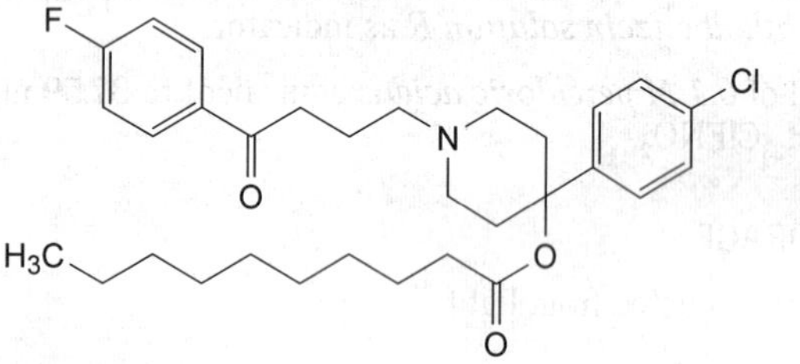

$C_{31}H_{41}ClFNO_3$ M_r 530.1

DEFINITION

Haloperidol decanoate contains not less than 98.5 per cent and not more than the equivalent of 101.0 per cent of 4-(4-chlorophenyl)-1-[4-(4-fluorophenyl)-4-oxobutyl]piperidin-4-yl decanoate, calculated with reference to the dried substance.

CHARACTERS

A white or almost white powder, practically insoluble in water, very soluble in alcohol, in methanol and in methylene chloride.

It melts at about 42 °C.

IDENTIFICATION

A. Examine by infrared absorption spectrophotometry (*2.2.24*), comparing with the spectrum obtained with *haloperidol decanoate CRS*. Examine the substances prepared as mulls in *liquid paraffin R*.

B. To 0.1 g in a porcelain crucible add 0.5 g of *anhydrous sodium carbonate R*. Heat over an open flame for 10 min. Allow to cool. Take up the residue with 5 ml of *dilute nitric acid R* and filter. To 1 ml of the filtrate add 1 ml of *water R*. The solution gives reaction (a) of chlorides (*2.3.1*).

TESTS

Appearance of solution. Dissolve 2.0 g in *methylene chloride R* and dilute to 20 ml with the same solvent. The solution is clear (*2.2.1*) and not more intensely coloured than reference solution B_5 (*2.2.2, Method II*).

Related substances. Examine by liquid chromatography (*2.2.29*). *Prepare the solutions immediately before use and protect from light.*

Test solution. Dissolve 0.100 g of the substance to be examined in *methanol R* and dilute to 10.0 ml with the same solvent.

Reference solution (a). Dissolve 2.5 mg of *bromperidol decanoate CRS* and 2.5 mg of *haloperidol decanoate CRS* in *methanol R* and dilute to 50.0 ml with the same solvent.

Reference solution (b). Dilute 5.0 ml of the test solution to 100.0 ml with *methanol R*. Dilute 1.0 ml of this solution to 10.0 ml with *methanol R*.

The chromatographic procedure may be carried out using:

– a stainless steel column 0.1 m long and 4.0 mm in internal diameter packed with *base-deactivated octadecylsilyl silica gel for chromatography R* (3 µm),

– as mobile phase at a flow rate of 1.5 ml/min the following linear gradient programme:

Mobile phase A. A 27 g/l solution of *tetrabutylammonium hydrogen sulphate R*,

Mobile phase B. Acetonitrile R,

Time (min)	Mobile phase A (per cent *V/V*)	Mobile phase B (per cent *V/V*)	Comment
0 - 30	80 → 40	20 → 60	linear gradient
30 - 35	40	60	isocratic elution
35 - 40	40 → 80	60 → 20	switch to initial eluent composition
40 = 0	80	20	restart gradient

– as detector a spectrophotometer set at 230 nm.

Equilibrate the column for at least 30 min with *acetonitrile R* and then equilibrate at the initial eluent composition for at least 5 min.

Adjust the sensitivity of the system so that the height of the principal peak in the chromatogram obtained with 10 µl of reference solution (b) is at least 50 per cent of the full scale of the recorder.

Inject 10 µl of reference solution (a). When the chromatogram is recorded in the prescribed conditions the retention times are: haloperidol decanoate about 24 min and bromperidol decanoate about 24.5 min. The test is not valid unless the resolution between the peaks due to haloperidol decanoate and bromperidol decanoate is at least 1.5. If necessary, adjust the gradient or the time programme for the linear gradient elution.

Inject 10 µl of *methanol R* as a blank, 10 µl of the test solution and 10 µl of reference solution (b). In the chromatogram obtained with the test solution: the area of any peak apart from the principal peak, is not greater than the area of the principal peak in the chromatogram obtained with reference solution (b) (0.5 per cent); the sum of the areas of all the peaks apart from the principal peak, is not greater than three times the area of the principal peak in the chromatogram obtained with the reference solution (b) (1.5 per cent). Disregard any peak due to the blank and any peak with an area less than 0.1 times the area of the principal peak in the chromatogram obtained with reference solution (b).

Loss on drying (*2.2.32*). Not more than 0.5 per cent, determined on 1.000 g by drying *in vacuo* at 30 °C.

Sulphated ash (*2.4.14*). Not more than 0.1 per cent, determined on 1.0 g in a platinum crucible.

ASSAY

Dissolve 0.425 g in 50 ml of a mixture of 1 volume of *anhydrous acetic acid R* and 7 volumes of *methyl ethyl ketone R*. Titrate with *0.1 M perchloric acid* using 0.2 ml of *naphtholbenzein solution R* as indicator.

1 ml of *0.1 M perchloric acid* is equivalent to 53.01 mg of $C_{31}H_{41}ClFNO_3$.

STORAGE

Store at room temperature below 25 °C, protected from light.

IMPURITIES

Specified impurities: A, B, C, D, E, F, G, H, I, J, K.

Other detectable impurities: L.

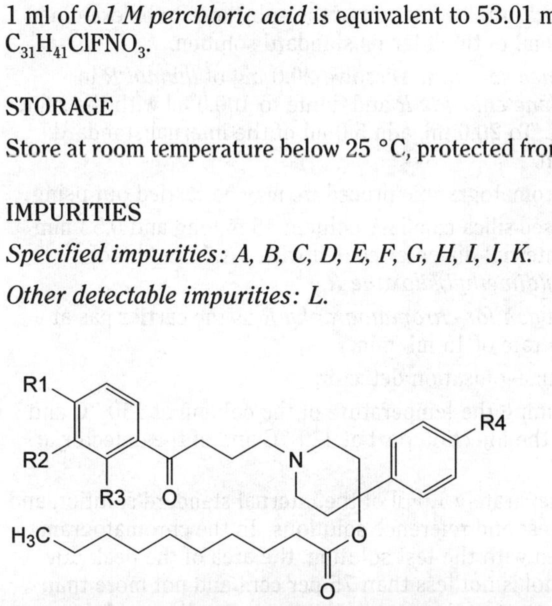

A. R1 = F, R2 = R3 = R4 = H: 1-[4-(4-fluorophenyl)-4-oxobutyl]-4-phenylpiperidin-4-yl decanoate,

B. R1 = R2 = H, R3 = F, R4 = Cl: 4-(4-chlorophenyl)-1-[4-(2-fluorophenyl)-4-oxobutyl]piperidin-4-yl decanoate,

C. R1 = F, R2 = C_2H_5, R3 = H, R4 = Cl: 4-(4-chlorophenyl)-1-[4-(3-ethyl-4-fluorophenyl)-4-oxobutyl]piperidin-4-yl decanoate,

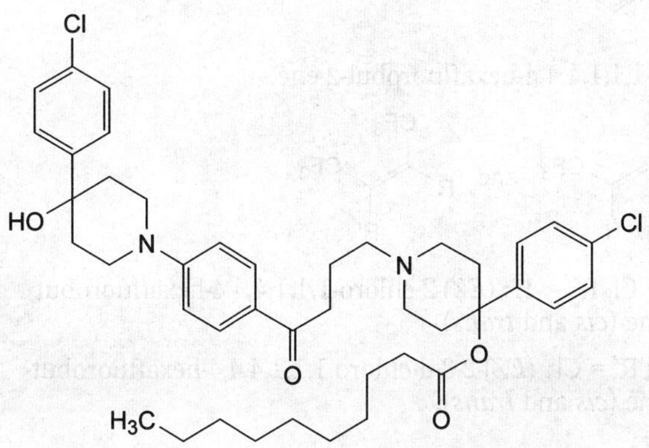

D. 4-(4-chlorophenyl)-1-[4-[4-[4-(4-chlorophenyl)-4-hydroxypiperidin-1-yl]phenyl]-4-oxobutyl]piperidin-4-yl decanoate,

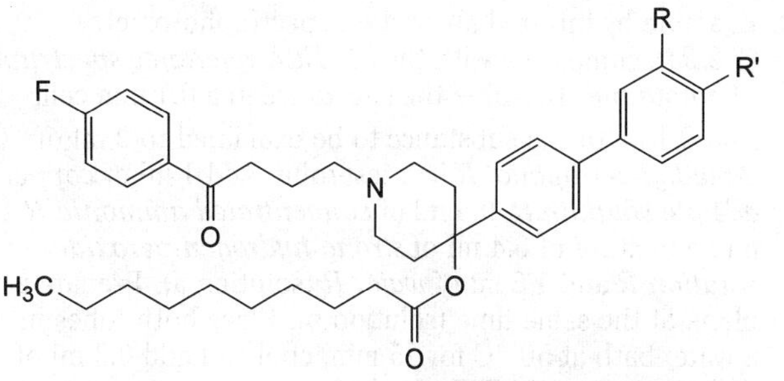

E. R = H, R′ = Cl: 4-(4′-chlorobiphenyl-4-yl)-1-[4-(4-fluorophenyl)-4-oxobutyl]piperidin-4-yl decanoate,

F. R = Cl, R′ = H: 4-(3′-chlorobiphenyl-4-yl)-1-[4-(4-fluorophenyl)-4-oxobutyl]piperidin-4-yl decanoate,

G. haloperidol,

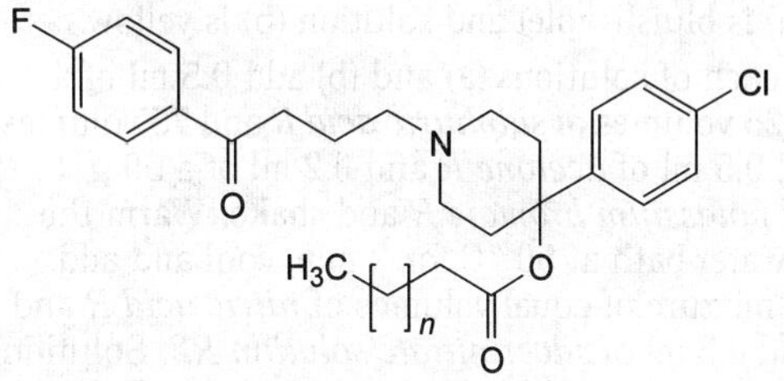

H. *n* = 5: 4-(4-chlorophenyl)-1-[4-(4-fluorophenyl)-4-oxobutyl]piperidin-4-yl octanoate,

I. *n* = 6: 4-(4-chlorophenyl)-1-[4-(4-fluorophenyl)-4-oxobutyl]piperidin-4-yl nonanoate,

J. *n* = 8: 4-(4-chlorophenyl)-1-[4-(4-fluorophenyl)-4-oxobutyl]piperidin-4-yl undecanoate,

K. *n* = 9: 4-(4-chlorophenyl)-1-[4-(4-fluorophenyl)-4-oxobutyl]piperidin-4-yl dodecanoate,

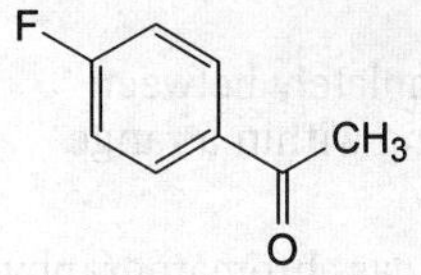

L. 1-(4-fluorophenyl)ethanone.

01/2005:0393

HALOTHANE

Halothanum

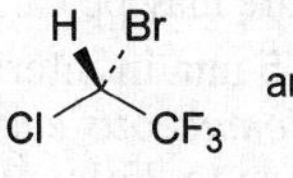

$C_2HBrClF_3$ M_r 197.4

DEFINITION

Halothane is (*RS*)-2-bromo-2-chloro-1,1,1-trifluoroethane to which 0.01 per cent *m/m* of thymol has been added.

CHARACTERS

A clear, colourless, mobile, heavy, non-flammable liquid, slightly soluble in water, miscible with ethanol and with trichloroethylene.

IDENTIFICATION

First identification: B.

Second identification: A, C.

A. It complies with the test for distillation range (see Tests).

B. Examine by infrared absorption spectrophotometry (*2.2.24*), comparing with the *Ph. Eur. reference spectrum of halothane*. Examine the substance in a 0.1 mm cell.

C. Add 0.1 ml of the substance to be examined to 2 ml of *2-methyl-2-propanol R* in a test-tube. Add 1 ml of *copper edetate solution R*, 0.5 ml of *concentrated ammonia R* and a mixture of 0.4 ml of *strong hydrogen peroxide solution R* and 1.6 ml of *water R* (solution a). Prepare a blank at the same time (solution b). Place both tubes in a water-bath at 50 °C for 15 min, cool and add 0.3 ml of *glacial acetic acid R*. To 1 ml of each of solutions (a) and (b) add 0.5 ml of a mixture of equal volumes of freshly prepared *alizarin S solution R* and *zirconyl nitrate solution R*. Solution (a) is yellow and solution (b) is red.

To 1 ml of each of solutions (a) and (b) add 1 ml of *buffer solution pH 5.2 R*, 1 ml of *phenol red solution R* diluted 1 in 10 with *water R* and 0.1 ml of *chloramine solution R*. Solution (a) is bluish-violet and solution (b) is yellow.

To 2 ml of each of solutions (a) and (b) add 0.5 ml of a mixture of 25 volumes of *sulphuric acid R* and 75 volumes of *water R*, 0.5 ml of *acetone R* and 0.2 ml of a 50 g/l solution of *potassium bromate R* and shake. Warm the tubes in a water-bath at 50 °C for 2 min, cool and add 0.5 ml of a mixture of equal volumes of *nitric acid R* and *water R* and 0.5 ml of *silver nitrate solution R2*. Solution (a) is opalescent and a white precipitate is formed after a few minutes; solution (b) remains clear.

TESTS

Acidity or alkalinity. To 20 ml add 20 ml of *carbon dioxide-free water R*, shake for 3 min and allow to stand. Separate the aqueous layer and add 0.2 ml of *bromocresol purple solution R*. Not more than 0.1 ml of *0.01 M sodium hydroxide* or 0.6 ml of *0.01 M hydrochloric acid* is required to change the colour of the indicator.

Relative density (*2.2.5*): 1.872 to 1.877.

Distillation range (*2.2.11*). It distils completely between 49.0 °C and 51.0 °C, 95 per cent distilling within a range of 1.0 °C.

Volatile related substances. Examine by gas chromatography (*2.2.28*), using *trichlorotrifluoroethane CRS* as the internal standard.

Test solution (a). Use the substance to be examined.

Test solution (b). Dilute 5.0 ml of *trichlorotrifluoroethane CRS* to 100.0 ml with the substance to be examined. Dilute 1.0 ml of the solution to 100.0 ml with the substance to be examined. Dilute 1.0 ml of this solution to 10.0 ml with the substance to be examined.

The chromatographic procedure may be carried out using:

- a column 2.75 m long and 5 mm in internal diameter packed with *silanised diatomaceous earth for gas chromatography R1* (180 µm to 250 µm), the first 1.8 m being impregnated with 30 per cent *m/m* of *macrogol 400 R* and the remainder with 30 per cent *m/m* of *dinonyl phthalate R*,
- *nitrogen for chromatography R* as the carrier gas at a flow rate of 30 ml/min,
- a flame-ionisation detector,

maintaining the temperature of the column at 50 °C. Inject 5 µl of test solutions (a) and (b).

In the chromatogram obtained with test solution (b), the sum of the areas of the peaks, apart from the principal peak and the peak due to the internal standard, is not greater than the area of the peak due to the internal standard, corrected if necessary for any impurity with the same retention time as the internal standard (0.005 per cent).

Bromides and chlorides. To 10 ml add 20 ml of *water R* and shake for 3 min. To 5 ml of the aqueous layer add 5 ml of *water R*, 0.05 ml of *nitric acid R* and 0.2 ml of *silver nitrate solution R1*. The solution is not more opalescent than a mixture of 5 ml of the aqueous layer and 5 ml of *water R*.

Bromine and chlorine. To 10 ml of the aqueous layer obtained in the test for bromides and chlorides add 1 ml of *potassium iodide and starch solution R*. No blue colour is produced.

Thymol. Examine by gas chromatography (*2.2.28*), using *menthol R* as the internal standard.

Internal standard solution. Dissolve 0.10 g of *menthol R* in *methylene chloride R* and dilute to 100.0 ml with the same solvent.

Test solution. To 20.0 ml of the substance to be examined add 5.0 ml of the internal standard solution.

Reference solution. Dissolve 20.0 mg of *thymol R* in *methylene chloride R* and dilute to 100.0 ml with the same solvent. To 20.0 ml, add 5.0 ml of the internal standard solution.

The chromatographic procedure may be carried out using:

- a fused-silica capillary column 15 m long and 0.53 mm in internal diameter coated with a 1.5 µm film of *poly(dimethyl)siloxane R*,
- *nitrogen for chromatography R* as the carrier gas at a flow rate of 15 ml/min,
- a flame-ionisation detector,

maintaining the temperature of the column at 150 °C and that of the injection port at 170 °C and of the detector at 200 °C.

Inject separately 1.0 µl of the internal standard solution and of the test and reference solutions. In the chromatogram obtained with the test solution, the area of the peak due to thymol is not less than 75 per cent and not more than 115 per cent of the area of the corresponding peak in the chromatogram obtained with the reference solution (0.008 per cent *m/m* to 0.012 per cent *m/m*).

Non-volatile matter. Evaporate 50 ml to dryness on a water-bath and dry the residue in an oven at 100 °C to 105 °C for 2 h. The residue weighs not more than 1 mg (20 mg/l).

STORAGE

Store in an airtight container, protected from light, at a temperature not exceeding 25 °C. The choice of material for the container is made taking into account the particular reactivity of halothane with certain metals.

IMPURITIES

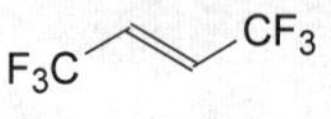

A. (*E*)-1,1,1,4,4,4-hexafluorobut-2-ene,

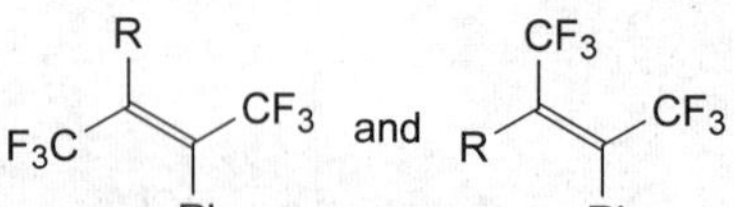

B. R = Cl, R′ = H: (*EZ*)-2-chloro-1,1,1,4,4,4-hexafluorobut-2-ene (*cis* and *trans*),

C. R = R′ = Cl: (*EZ*)-2,3-dichloro-1,1,1,4,4,4-hexafluorobut-2-ene (*cis* and *trans*),

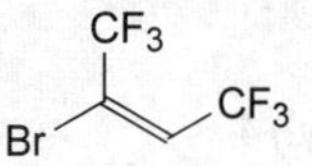

D. (*E*)-2-bromo-1,1,1,4,4,4-hexafluorobut-2-ene,

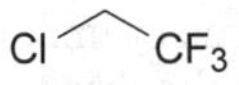

E. 2-chloro-1,1,1-trifluoroethane,

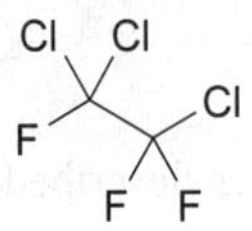

F. 1,1,2-trichloro-1,2,2-trifluoroethane,

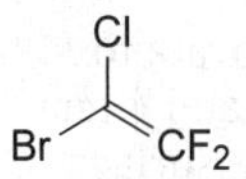

G. 1-bromo-1-chloro-2,2-difluoroethene,

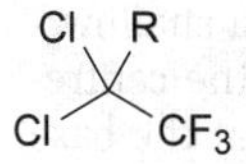

H. R = H: 2,2-dichloro-1,1,1-trifluoroethane,

I. R = Br: 1-bromo-1,1-dichloro-2,2,2-trifluoroethane,

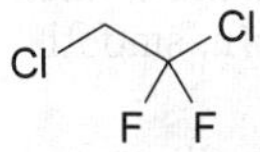

J. 1,2-dichloro-1,1-difluoroethane.

01/2005:0909

HAMAMELIS LEAF

Hamamelidis folium

DEFINITION

Hamamelis leaf consists of the whole or cut, dried leaf of *Hamamelis virginiana* L. It contains not less than 3 per cent of tannins, expressed as pyrogallol ($C_6H_6O_3$; M_r 126.1), calculated with reference to the dried drug.

CHARACTERS

It has the macroscopic and microscopic characters described under identification tests A and B.

IDENTIFICATION

A. The leaf is green or greenish-brown, often broken, crumpled and compressed into more or less compact masses. The lamina is broadly ovate to obovate; the base is oblique and asymmetric and the apex is acute or, rarely, obtuse. The margins of the lamina are roughly crenate or dentate. The venation is pinnate and prominent on the abaxial surface. Usually, four to six pairs of secondary veins are attached to the main vein, emerging at an acute angle and curving gently to the marginal points where there are fine veins often at right angles to the secondary veins.

B. Reduce to a powder (355). The powder is brownish-green. Examine under a microscope using *chloral hydrate solution R*. The powder shows fragments of adaxial epidermis with wavy anticlinal walls; abaxial epidermis with stomata mainly paracytic (*2.8.3*); star-shaped covering trichomes, either entire or broken, composed of four to twelve unicellular branches which are united by their bases, elongated, conical and curved, usually up to 250 µm long, thick-walled and with a clearly visible lumen with contents often brown in colour; fibres are lignified and thick-walled, isolated or in groups, and they are accompanied by a sheath of prismatic calcium oxalate crystals; small, cylindrical parenchymatous cells of palisade; irregular-shaped cells of spongy mesophyll; sclereids, frequently enlarged at one or both ends, 150 µm to 180 µm long, whole or fragmented; fragments of annular or spiral vessels; isolated prisms of calcium oxalate.

C. Examine by thin-layer chromatography (*2.2.27*), using a *TLC silica gel G plate R*.

Test solution. To 1.0 g of the powdered drug (355) add 10 ml of *alcohol (60 per cent V/V) R*, shake for 15 min and filter.

Reference solution (a). Dissolve 30 mg of *tannic acid R* in 5 ml of *alcohol (60 per cent V/V) R*.

Reference solution (b). Dissolve 5 mg of *gallic acid R* in 5 ml of *alcohol (60 per cent V/V) R*.

Apply to the plate as bands 10 µl of each solution. Develop over a path of 10 cm using a mixture of 10 volumes of *anhydrous formic acid R*, 10 volumes of *water R* and 80 volumes of *ethyl formate R*. Dry the plate at 100 °C to 105 °C for 10 min and allow to cool. Spray with *ferric chloride solution R2* until bluish-grey zones (phenolic compounds) appear. The chromatogram obtained with the test solution shows in its lower third a principal zone similar in position to the principal zone in the chromatogram obtained with reference solution (a) and, in its upper part, a narrow zone similar in position to the principal zone in the chromatogram obtained with reference solution (b). The chromatogram obtained with the test solution shows in addition several slightly coloured zones in the central part.

TESTS

Foreign matter (*2.8.2*). Not more than 7 per cent of stem and not more than 2 per cent of other foreign matter, determined on 50 g.

Loss on drying (*2.2.32*). Not more than 10.0 per cent, determined on 2.000 g of powdered drug (355) by drying in an oven at 100 °C to 105 °C for 4 h.

Total ash (*2.4.16*). Not more than 7.0 per cent.

Ash insoluble in hydrochloric acid (*2.8.1*). Not more than 2.0 per cent.

ASSAY

Carry out the determination of tannins in herbal drugs (*2.8.14*). Use 0.750 g of the powdered drug (180).

STORAGE

Store protected from light.

01/2005:0462

HARD FAT

Adeps solidus

DEFINITION

Hard fat consists of a mixture of triglycerides, diglycerides and monoglycerides, which may be obtained either by esterification of fatty acids of natural origin with glycerol or by transesterification of natural fats. Each type of hard fat is characterised by its melting point, its hydroxyl value and its saponification value. It contains no additives.

CHARACTERS

A white or almost white, waxy, brittle mass, practically insoluble in water, slightly soluble in ethanol. When heated to 50 °C, it melts giving a colourless or slightly yellowish liquid.

IDENTIFICATION

Examine by thin-layer chromatography (*2.2.27*), using *silica gel G R* as the coating substance.

Test solution. Dissolve 1.0 g of the substance to be examined in *ethylene chloride R* and dilute to 10 ml with the same solvent.

Apply to the plate 2 µl of the test solution. Develop over a path of 12 cm with a mixture of 10 volumes of *ether R* and 90 volumes of *ethylene chloride R*. Allow the plate to dry in air and expose to iodine vapour until the spots appear. Examine in daylight. The chromatogram shows a spot with an R_f value of about 0.6, corresponding to triglycerides (R_{st} 1) and spots corresponding to 1,3-diglycerides (R_{st} 0.5) and to 1,2-di-glycerides (R_{st} 0.3). A spot corresponding to 1-monoglycerides may also be visible (R_{st} 0.05).

TESTS

Alkaline impurities. Dissolve 2.00 g in a mixture of 1.5 ml of *alcohol R* and 3.0 ml of *ether R*. Add 0.05 ml of *bromophenol blue solution R*. Not more than 0.15 ml of *0.01 M hydrochloric acid* is required to change the colour of the indicator to yellow.

Melting point (*2.2.15*): 30 °C to 45 °C; the melting point does not differ by more than 2 °C from the nominal value. Introduce the melted substance into the capillary tube and allow to stand at a temperature below 10 °C for 24 h.

Acid value (*2.5.1*). Not more than 0.5. Dissolve 5.0 g in 50 ml of the prescribed mixture of solvents.

Hydroxyl value (*2.5.3, Method A*). The hydroxyl value is not more than 50 and does not differ by more than 5 units from the nominal value. If the nominal value is less than 5, the hydroxyl value is not more than 5.

Iodine value (*2.5.4*). Not more than 3.

Peroxide value (*2.5.5*). Not more than 3.

Saponification value (*2.5.6*): 210 to 260, determined on 2.0 g. The saponification value does not differ by more than 5 per cent from the nominal value.

Unsaponifiable matter (*2.5.7*). Not more than 0.6 per cent, determined on 5.0 g.

Heavy metals (*2.4.8*). 2.0 g complies with limit test D for heavy metals (10 ppm). Prepare the standard using 2 ml of *lead standard solution (10 ppm Pb) R*.

Total ash (*2.4.16*). Not more than 0.05 per cent, determined on 2.00 g.

STORAGE

Store protected from light and heat.

LABELLING

The label states:

- the nominal melting point,
- the nominal hydroxyl value,
- the nominal saponification value.

01/2005:1220

HAWTHORN BERRIES

Crataegi fructus

DEFINITION

Hawthorn berries consist of the dried false fruits of *Crataegus monogyna* Jacq. (Lindm.), or *Crataegus laevigata* (Poir.) D.C. (synonym: *Crataegus oxyacantha* L.) or their hybrids or a mixture of these false fruits. They contain not less than 1.0 per cent of procyanidins, calculated as cyanidin chloride ($C_{15}H_{11}ClO_6$; M_r 322.7) with reference to the dried drug.

CHARACTERS

The false fruit has a sweet mucilaginous taste.

It has the macroscopic and microscopic characters described under identification tests A and B.

IDENTIFICATION

A. The false fruit of *Crataegus monogyna* is obovate to globular. It is generally 6 mm to 10 mm long and 4 mm to 8 mm wide, reddish-brown to dark red. The surface is pitted or, more rarely, reticulated. The upper end of the fruit is crowned by the remains of five reflexed sepals surrounding a small sunken disc with a shallow, raised rim. The remains of the style occur in the centre of the disc with tufts of stiff, colourless hairs at the base. At the lower end of the fruit a short length of pedicel or, more frequently, a small pale circular scar where the pedicel was attached. The receptacle is fleshy and encloses a yellowish-brown, ovoid fruit with a hard, thick wall containing a single, elongated, pale brown, smooth and shiny seed.

The false fruit of *Crataegus laevigata* is up to 13 mm long. It contains two to three stony fruits, ventrally flattened, with short hairs at the top. Frequently, in the centre of the disc of the false fruit occur the remains of the two styles.

B. Reduce to a powder (355). The powder is greyish-red. Examine under a microscope using *chloral hydrate solution R*. The powder shows covering trichomes from inside the disc which are long, unicellular, frequently bent, tapering to a point, with smooth, much thickened and lignified walls, parenchymatous receptacle fragments the outer layer with red colouring matter, some cells of the inner layers containing small cluster crystals of calcium oxalate; occasional fragments including groups of sclereids and vascular strands with associated files of cells containing prisms of calcium oxalate; pericarp fragments consisting of large thick-walled sclereids with numerous pits, some of which are conspicuously branched; a few fragments of the testa having an epidermal layer composed of hexagonal, mucilaginous cells beneath which is a yellowish-brown pigment layer containing numerous elongated prisms of calcium oxalate; thin-walled parenchyma of the endosperm and cotyledons containing aleurone grains and globules of fixed oil.

C. Examine by thin-layer chromatography (*2.2.27*), using a suitable silica gel as the coating substance.

Test solution. To 1.0 g of the powdered drug (355) add 10 ml of *methanol R* and heat in a water bath at 65 °C for 5 min. Shake frequently. Allow to cool to room temperature and filter. Dilute the filtrate to 10 ml with *methanol R*.

Reference solution. Dissolve 2 mg of *chlorogenic acid R*, 2 mg of *caffeic acid R*, 5 mg of *hyperoside R* and 5 mg of *rutin R* in 20 ml of *methanol R*.

Apply separately to the plate, as bands, 30 µl of the test solution and 10 µl of the reference solution. Develop over a path of 15 cm using as the mobile phase a mixture of 10 volumes of *anhydrous formic acid R*, 10 volumes of *water R*, 30 volumes of *methyl ethyl ketone R* and 50 volumes of *ethyl acetate R*. Dry the plate at 100-105 °C and spray whilst hot with a 10 g/l solution of *diphenylboric acid aminoethyl ester R* in *methanol R*. Subsequently spray the plate with a 50 g/l solution of *macrogol 400 R* in *methanol R*. Allow the plate to dry in air for 30 min and examine in ultraviolet light at 365 nm. The chromatogram obtained with the reference solution shows in the lower half, in order of increasing R_f values, the yellowish-brown fluorescent zone of rutin, the light blue fluorescent zone of chlorogenic acid and the yellowish-brown fluorescent zone of hyperoside; in the upper third appears the light blue fluorescent zone of caffeic acid. The chromatogram obtained with the test solution shows three zones similar in position and fluorescence to the zones due to chlorogenic acid, hyperoside and caffeic acid in the chromatogram obtained with the reference solution and three weak reddish fluorescent zones, one corresponding to the rutin zone in the chromatogram obtained with the reference solution and both of the others located above the hyperoside zone. Below and above the caffeic acid zone some light blue zones appear.

TESTS

Foreign matter (*2.8.2*). Not more than 2 per cent. Not more than 5 per cent of deteriorated false fruit. It does not contain fruits of other *Crataegus* species (*C. nigra* Waldst. et Kit., *C. pentagyna* Waldst. et Kit. ex Willd. and *C. azarolus* L.) which are characterised by the presence of more than three hard stones.

Loss on drying (*2.2.32*). Not more than 12.0 per cent, determined on 1.000 g of the powdered drug (355) by drying in an oven at 100-105 °C for 2 h.

Total ash (*2.4.16*). Not more than 5.0 per cent.

ASSAY

To 2.50 g of the powdered drug (355) add 30 ml of *alcohol (70 per cent V/V) R*. Heat under a reflux condenser for 30 min and filter. Wash the residue with 10.0 ml of *alcohol (70 per cent V/V) R*. Add to the filtrate 15.0 ml of *hydrochloric acid R1* and 10.0 ml of *water R*. Heat under a reflux condenser for 80 min. Allow to cool, filter and wash the residue with *alcohol (70 per cent V/V) R* until the filtrate is colourless. Dilute the filtrate to 250.0 ml with *alcohol (70 per cent V/V) R*. Evaporate 50.0 ml of this solution in a round-bottomed flask to about 3 ml and transfer it to a separating funnel. Rinse the round-bottomed flask sequentially with 10 ml and 5 ml of *water R* and transfer to the separating funnel. Shake the combined solution with three quantities, each of 15 ml, of *butanol R*. Combine the organic layers and dilute to 100.0 ml with *butanol R*. Measure the absorbance (*2.2.25*) of the solution at 545 nm.

Calculate the percentage content of procyanidins, as cyanidin chloride, from the expression:

$$\frac{A \times 500}{75 \times m}$$

i.e. taking the specific absorbance of cyanidin chloride to be 75.

A = absorbance at 545 nm,

m = mass of the substance to be examined, in grams.

STORAGE

Store protected from light.

01/2005:1432

HAWTHORN LEAF AND FLOWER

Crataegi folium cum flore

DEFINITION

Whole or cut, dried flower bearing branches of *Crataegus monogyna* Jacq. (Lindm.), *C. laevigata* (Poiret) D.C. (*C. oxyacanthoides* Thuill.) or their hybrids or, more rarely, other European *Crataegus* species including *C. pentagyna* Waldst. et Kit. ex Willd., *C. nigra* Waldst. et Kit., *C. azarolus* L.

Content: minimum 1.5 per cent of flavonoids expressed as hyperoside ($C_{21}H_{20}O_{12}$; M_r 464.4) (dried drug).

CHARACTERS

Macroscopic and microscopic characters described under identification tests A and B.

IDENTIFICATION

A. The stems are dark brown, woody, 1-2.5 mm in diameter, bearing alternate, petiolate leaves with small, often deciduous stipules and corymbs of numerous small white flowers. The leaves are more or less deeply lobed with slightly serrate or almost entire margins; those of *C. laevigata* are pinnately lobed or pinnatifid with 3, 5 or 7 obtuse lobes, those of *C. monogyna* pinnatisect with 3 or 5 acute lobes; the adaxial surface is dark green to brownish-green, the abaxial surface is lighter greyish-green and shows a prominent, dense, reticulate venation. The leaves of *C. laevigata, C. monogyna* and *C. pentagyna* are glabrous or bear only isolated trichomes, those of *C. azarolus* and *C. nigra* are densely pubescent. The flowers have a brownish-green tubular calyx composed of 5 free, reflexed sepals, a corolla composed of 5 free, yellowish-white to brownish, rounded or broadly ovate and shortly unguiculate petals and numerous stamens. The ovary is fused to the calyx and consists of 1 to 5 carpels, each with a long style and containing a single ovule; in *C. monogyna* there is 1 carpel, in *C. laevigata* 2 or 3, in *C. azarolus* 2 or 3, or sometimes only 1, in *C. pentagyna* 5 or, rarely, 4.

B. Reduce to a powder (355). The powder is yellowish-green. Examine under a microscope using *chloral hydrate solution R*. The powder shows unicellular covering trichomes, usually with a thick wall and wide lumen, almost straight to slightly curved, pitted at the base; fragments of leaf epidermis with cells which have sinuous to polygonal anticlinal walls and with large anomocytic stomata (*2.8.3*) surrounded by 4 to 7 subsidiary cells; parenchymatous cells of the mesophyll containing calcium oxalate clusters, usually measuring 10-20 µm, those associated with the veins containing groups of small prism crystals; fragments of petals showing rounded polygonal epidermal cells, strongly papillose, with thick walls, the cuticle of which clearly shows wavy striations; fragments of anthers showing endothecium with an arched and regularly thickened margin; fragments of stems containing collenchymatous cells, bordered pitted vessels and groups of lignified sclerenchymatous fibres with narrow lumina; numerous spherical to elliptical or triangular pollen grains up to 45 µm in diameter, with 3 germinal pores and a faintly granular exine.

C. Thin-layer chromatography (*2.2.27*).

Test solution. To 1.0 g of the powdered drug (355) add 10 ml of *methanol R* and heat in a water-bath at 65 °C under a reflux condenser for 5 min. Cool and filter.

Monographs F-H

Reference solution. Dissolve 1.0 mg of *chlorogenic acid R* and 2.5 mg of *hyperoside R* in 10 ml of *methanol R*.

Plate: *TLC silica gel plate R.*

Mobile phase: *anhydrous formic acid R, water R, methyl ethyl ketone R, ethyl acetate R* (10:10:30:50 *V/V/V/V*).

Application: 20 µl as bands.

Development: over a path of 15 cm.

Drying: at 100-105 °C.

Detection: spray with a 10 g/l solution of *diphenylboric acid aminoethyl ester R* in *methanol R*. Subsequently spray with a 50 g/l solution of *macrogol 400 R* in *methanol R*. Allow the plate to dry in air for about 30 min. Examine in ultraviolet light at 365 nm.

Results: see below the sequence of the zones present in the chromatograms obtained with the reference solution and the test solution. Furthermore, other fluorescent zones may be present in the chromatogram obtained with the test solution.

Top of the plate	
—	—
	A yellowish-green fluorescent zone (vitexin)
Hyperoside: a yellowish-orange fluorescent zone	A yellowish-orange fluorescent zone (hyperoside)
Chlorogenic acid: a light blue fluorescent zone	A light blue fluorescent zone (chlorogenic acid)
	A yellowish-green fluorescent zone (vitexin-2″-rhamnoside)
—	—
Reference solution	**Test solution**

TESTS

Foreign matter (*2.8.2*): maximum 8 per cent of lignified branches with a diameter greater than 2.5 mm and maximum 2 per cent of other foreign matter.

Loss on drying (*2.2.32*): maximum 10.0 per cent, determined on 1.000 g of powdered drug (355) by drying in an oven at 100-105 °C for 2 h.

Total ash (*2.4.16*): maximum 10.0 per cent.

ASSAY

Stock solution. In a 200 ml flask introduce 0.400 g of the powdered drug (250) and 40 ml of *alcohol (60 per cent V/V) R*. Heat in a water-bath at 60 °C for 10 min, shaking frequently. Allow to cool and filter through a plug of absorbent cotton into a 100 ml volumetric flask. Transfer the absorbent cotton with the drug residue back into the 200 ml flask, add 40 ml of *alcohol (60 per cent V/V) R* and heat again in a water-bath at 60 °C for 10 min, shaking frequently. Allow to cool and filter into the same 100 ml volumetric flask as previously. Rinse the 200 ml flask and filter with a further quantity of *alcohol (60 per cent V/V) R* and transfer to the same 100 ml volumetric flask. Dilute to volume with *alcohol (60 per cent V/V) R* and filter.

Test solution. Introduce 5.0 ml of the stock solution into a round-bottomed flask and evaporate to dryness under reduced pressure. Take up the residue with 8 ml of a mixture of 10 volumes of *methanol R* and 100 volumes of *glacial acetic acid R* and transfer into a 25 ml volumetric flask. Rinse the round-bottomed flask with 3 ml of a mixture of 10 volumes of *methanol R* and 100 volumes of *glacial acetic acid R* and transfer into the same 25 ml volumetric flask as previously. Add 10.0 ml of a solution containing 25.0 g/l of *boric acid R* and 20.0 g/l of *oxalic acid R* in *anhydrous formic acid R* and dilute to 25.0 ml with *anhydrous acetic acid R*.

Compensation liquid. Introduce 5.0 ml of the stock solution into a round-bottomed flask and evaporate to dryness under reduced pressure. Take up the residue with 8 ml of a mixture of 10 volumes of *methanol R* and 100 volumes of *glacial acetic acid R* and transfer it into a 25 ml volumetric flask. Rinse the round-bottomed flask with 3 ml of a mixture of 10 volumes of *methanol R* and 100 volumes of *glacial acetic acid R* and transfer into the same 25 ml volumetric flask as previously. Add 10.0 ml of *anhydrous formic acid R* and dilute to 25.0 ml with *anhydrous acetic acid R*.

Measure the absorbance (*2.2.25*) of the test solution at 410 nm after 30 min.

Calculate the percentage content of total flavonoids expressed as hyperoside from the expression:

$$\frac{A \times 1.235}{m}$$

i.e. taking the value of the specific absorbance of hyperoside at 410 nm to be 405.

A = absorbance of the test solution at 410 nm,

m = mass of the drug to be examined, in grams.

01/2005:1865

HAWTHORN LEAF AND FLOWER DRY EXTRACT

Crataegi folii cum flore extractum siccum

DEFINITION

Extract produced from *Hawthorn leaf and flower (1432)*.

Content:

- for aqueous extracts: minimum 2.5 per cent of flavonoids, expressed as hyperoside ($C_{21}H_{20}O_{12}$; M_r 464.4) (dried extract);
- for hydroalcoholic extracts: minimum 6.0 per cent of flavonoids, expressed as hyperoside ($C_{21}H_{20}O_{12}$; M_r 464.4) (dried extract).

PRODUCTION

The extract is produced from the drug by a suitable procedure using either water or a hydroalcoholic solvent equivalent in strength to a minimum of 45 per cent *V/V* ethanol.

CHARACTERS

Appearance: light brown or greenish-brown powder.

IDENTIFICATION

Thin-layer chromatography (*2.2.27*).

Test solution. Suspend 0.2 g of the extract to be examined in 20 ml of *alcohol (70 per cent V/V) R* and filter.

Reference solution. Dissolve 1 mg of *chlorogenic acid R*, 2.5 mg of *hyperoside R* and 2.5 mg of *rutin R* in 10 ml of *methanol R*.

Plate: *TLC silica gel plate R.*

Mobile phase: *anhydrous formic acid R, water R, methyl ethyl ketone R, ethyl acetate R* (10:10:30:50 *V/V/V/V*).

Application: 20 µl of the test solution and 10 µl of the reference solution, as bands.

Development: over a path of 15 cm.

Drying: at 100-105 °C.

Detection: spray the plate whilst hot with a 10 g/l solution of *diphenylboric acid aminoethyl ester R* in *methanol R*; subsequently spray the plate with a 50 g/l solution of *macrogol 400 R* in *methanol R*; allow the plate to dry in air for 30 min and examine in ultraviolet light at 365 nm.

Results: see below the sequence of the zones present in the chromatograms obtained with the reference solution and the test solution. Furthermore, other fluorescent zones may be present in the chromatogram obtained with the test solution.

Top of the plate	
	A light yellow fluorescent zone
Hyperoside: a yellowish-orange fluorescent zone	A yellowish-orange fluorescent zone (hyperoside)
Chlorogenic acid: a light blue fluorescent zone	A light blue fluorescent zone (chlorogenic acid)
	A yellowish-green fluorescent zone (vitexin 2″-rhamnoside)
Rutin: a yellowish-orange fluorescent zone	A yellowish-orange fluorescent zone (rutin)
Reference solution	**Test solution**

TESTS

Methanol (*2.9.11*): maximum 0.05 per cent *V/V*.

Loss on drying (*2.2.32*): maximum 6.0 per cent, determined on 0.500 g of the extract to be examined by drying in an oven at 100-105 °C for 2 h.

ASSAY

Stock solution. Dissolve 0.100 g of the extract to be examined in *alcohol (60 per cent V/V) R* and dilute to 100.0 ml with the same solvent.

Test solution. Introduce 5.0 ml of the stock solution into a round-bottomed flask and evaporate to dryness under reduced pressure. Dissolve the residue in 8 ml of a mixture of 10 volumes of *methanol R* and 100 volumes of *glacial acetic acid R* and transfer into a 25 ml volumetric flask. Rinse the round-bottomed flask with 3 ml of a mixture of 10 volumes of *methanol R* and 100 volumes of *glacial acetic acid R* and transfer into the 25 ml volumetric flask. Add 10.0 ml of a solution containing 25.0 g/l of *boric acid R* and 20.0 g/l of *oxalic acid R* in *anhydrous formic acid R* and dilute to 25.0 ml with *anhydrous acetic acid R*.

Compensation liquid. Introduce 5.0 ml of the stock solution into a round-bottomed flask and evaporate to dryness under reduced pressure. Dissolve the residue in 8 ml of a mixture of 10 volumes of *methanol R* and 100 volumes of *glacial acetic acid R* and transfer into a 25 ml volumetric flask. Rinse the round-bottomed flask with 3 ml of a mixture of 10 volumes of *methanol R* and 100 volumes of *glacial acetic acid R* and transfer into the 25 ml volumetric flask. Add 10.0 ml of *anhydrous formic acid R* and dilute to 25.0 ml with *anhydrous acetic acid R*.

After 30 min measure the absorbance (*2.2.25*) of the test solution at 410 nm by comparison with the compensation liquid.

Calculate the percentage content of total flavonoids, calculated as hyperoside, from the expression:

$$\frac{A \times 1.235}{m}$$

i.e. taking the specific absorbance to be 405.

A = absorbance at 410 nm,

m = mass of the extract to be examined, in grams.

01/2005:0332

HEPARIN CALCIUM

Heparinum calcicum

DEFINITION

Heparin calcium is a preparation containing the calcium salt of a sulphated glucosaminoglycan present in mammalian tissues. On complete hydrolysis, it liberates D-glucosamine, D-glucuronic acid, L-iduronic acid, acetic acid and sulphuric acid. It has the characteristic property of delaying the clotting of freshly shed blood. The potency of heparin calcium intended for parenteral administration is not less than 150 IU/mg, calculated with reference to the dried substance. The potency of heparin calcium not intended for parenteral administration is not less than 120 IU/mg, calculated with reference to the dried substance.

PRODUCTION

It is prepared from the lungs of oxen or from the intestinal mucosae of oxen, pigs or sheep.

It is produced by methods of manufacturing designed to minimise or eliminate microbial contamination and substances lowering blood pressure.

CHARACTERS

A white or almost white powder, moderately hygroscopic, freely soluble in water.

IDENTIFICATION

A. It delays the clotting of recalcified citrated sheep plasma (see Assay).

B. Dissolve 0.40 g in *water R* and dilute to 10.0 ml with the same solvent. The specific optical rotation (*2.2.7*) is not less than + 35.

C. Examine by zone electrophoresis (*2.2.31*) using *agarose for electrophoresis R* as the supporting medium. To equilibrate the agarose and as electrolyte solution use a mixture of 50 ml of *glacial acetic acid R* and 800 ml of *water R* adjusted to pH 3 by addition of *lithium hydroxide R* and diluted to 1000.0 ml with *water R*.

Test solution. Dissolve 25 mg of the substance to be examined in *water R* and dilute to 10 ml with the same solvent.

Reference solution. Dilute *heparin sodium BRP* with an equal volume of *water R*.

Apply separately to the strip 2 µl to 3 µl of each solution. Pass a current of 1 mA to 2 mA per centimetre of strip width at a potential difference of 300 V for about 10 min. Stain the strips using a 1 g/l solution of *toluidine blue R* and remove the excess by washing. The ratio of the mobility of the principal band or bands in the electropherogram obtained with the test solution to the mobility of the band in the electropherogram obtained with the reference solution is 0.9 to 1.1.

D. It gives the reactions of calcium (*2.3.1*).

TESTS

Appearance of solution. Dissolve a quantity equivalent to 50 000 IU in *water R* and dilute to 10 ml with the same solvent. The solution is clear (*2.2.1*) and not more intensely coloured than degree 5 of the range of reference solutions of the most appropriate colour (*2.2.2, Method II*).

Monographs F-H

pH (*2.2.3*). Dissolve 0.1 g in *carbon dioxide-free water R* and dilute to 10 ml with the same solvent. The pH of the solution is 5.5 to 8.0.

Protein and nucleotidic impurities. Dissolve 40 mg in 10 ml of *water R*. The absorbance (*2.2.25*) measured at 260 nm is not greater than 0.20 and that measured at 280 nm is not greater than 0.15.

Nitrogen. Not more than 2.5 per cent, calculated with reference to the dried substance. Carry out the determination of nitrogen by sulphuric acid digestion (*2.5.9*), using 0.100 g.

Calcium: 9.5 per cent to 11.5 per cent of Ca, calculated with reference to the dried substance. Determine the calcium by complexometric titration (*2.5.11*), using 0.200 g.

Heavy metals (*2.4.8*). 0.5 g complies with limit test C for heavy metals (30 ppm). Prepare the standard using 1.5 ml of *lead standard solution (10 ppm Pb) R*.

Loss on drying (*2.2.32*). Not more than 8.0 per cent, determined on 1.000 g by drying at 60 °C over *diphosphorus pentoxide R* at a pressure not exceeding 670 Pa for 3 h.

Sulphated ash (*2.4.14*): 32 per cent to 40 per cent, determined on 0.20 g and calculated with reference to the dried substance.

Bacterial endotoxins (*2.6.14*): less than 0.01 IU per IU of heparin, if intended for use in the manufacture of parenteral dosage forms without a further appropriate procedure for removal of bacterial endotoxins. The addition of divalent cations may be necessary in order to fulfil the validation criteria.

ASSAY

Carry out the assay of heparin (*2.7.5*). The estimated potency is not less than 90 per cent and not more than 111 per cent of the stated potency. The confidence limits of the estimated potency ($P = 0.95$) are not less than 80 per cent and not more than 125 per cent of the stated potency.

STORAGE

Store in an airtight container. If the substance is sterile, store in a sterile, airtight, tamper-proof container.

LABELLING

The label states:

– the number of International Units per milligram,
– the name and quantity of any added substance,
– where applicable, that the substance is free from bacterial endotoxins.

01/2005:0333

HEPARIN SODIUM

Heparinum natricum

DEFINITION

Heparin sodium is a preparation containing the sodium salt of a sulphated glucosaminoglycan present in mammalian tissues. On complete hydrolysis, it liberates D-glucosamine, D-glucuronic acid, L-iduronic acid, acetic acid and sulphuric acid. It has the characteristic property of delaying the clotting of freshly shed blood. The potency of heparin sodium intended for parenteral administration is not less than 150 IU/mg, calculated with reference to the dried substance. The potency of heparin sodium not intended for parenteral administration is not less than 120 IU/mg, calculated with reference to the dried substance.

PRODUCTION

It is prepared from the lungs of oxen or from the intestinal mucosae of oxen, pigs or sheep.
It is produced by methods of manufacturing designed to minimise or eliminate microbial contamination and substances lowering blood pressure.

CHARACTERS

A white or almost white powder, moderately hygroscopic, freely soluble in water.

IDENTIFICATION

A. It delays the clotting of recalcified citrated sheep plasma (see Assay).

B. Dissolve 0.40 g in *water R* and dilute to 10.0 ml with the same solvent. The specific optical rotation (*2.2.7*) is not less than + 35.

C. Examine by zone electrophoresis (*2.2.31*) using *agarose for electrophoresis R* as the supporting medium. To equilibrate the agarose and as electrolyte solution use a mixture of 50 ml of *glacial acetic acid R* and 800 ml of *water R* adjusted to pH 3 by addition of *lithium hydroxide R* and diluted to 1000.0 ml with *water R*.

Test solution. Dissolve 25 mg of the substance to be examined in *water R* and dilute to 10 ml with the same solvent.

Reference solution. Dilute *heparin sodium BRP* with an equal volume of *water R*.

Apply separately to the strip 2 µl to 3 µl of each solution. Pass a current of 1 mA to 2 mA per centimetre of strip width at a potential difference of 300 V for about 10 min. Stain the strips using a 1 g/l solution of *toluidine blue R* and remove the excess by washing. The ratio of the mobility of the principal band or bands in the electropherogram obtained with the test solution to the mobility of the band in the electropherogram obtained with the reference solution is 0.9 to 1.1.

D. The residue obtained in the test for sulphated ash (see Tests) gives reaction (a) of sodium (*2.3.1*).

TESTS

Appearance of solution. Dissolve a quantity equivalent to 50 000 IU in *water R* and dilute to 10 ml with the same solvent. The solution is clear (*2.2.1*) and not more intensely coloured than intensity 5 of the range of reference solutions of the most appropriate colour (*2.2.2, Method II*).

pH (*2.2.3*). Dissolve 0.1 g in *carbon dioxide-free water R* and dilute to 10 ml with the same solvent. The pH of the solution is 5.5 to 8.0.

Protein and nucleotidic impurities. Dissolve 40 mg in 10 ml of *water R*. The absorbance (*2.2.25*) measured at 260 nm is not greater than 0.20 and that measured at 280 nm is not greater than 0.15.

Nitrogen. Not more than 2.5 per cent, calculated with reference to the dried substance. Carry out the determination of nitrogen by sulphuric acid digestion (*2.5.9*), using 0.100 g.

Sodium: 9.5 per cent to 12.5 per cent of Na, calculated with reference to the dried substance and determined by atomic absorption spectrometry (*2.2.23, Method I*).

Test solution. Dissolve 50 mg of the substance to be examined in *0.1 M hydrochloric acid* containing 1.27 mg of *caesium chloride R* per millilitre and dilute to 100.0 ml with the same solvent.

Reference solutions. Prepare reference solutions containing 25 ppm, 50 ppm and 75 ppm of Na, using *sodium standard solution (200 ppm Na) R* diluted with *0.1 M hydrochloric acid* containing 1.27 mg of *caesium chloride R* per millilitre.

Measure the absorbance at 330.3 nm using a sodium hollow-cathode lamp as the source of radiation and a flame of suitable composition (for example 11 litres of air and 2 litres of acetylene per minute).

Heavy metals (*2.4.8*). 0.5 g complies with limit test C for heavy metals (30 ppm). Prepare the standard using 1.5 ml of *lead standard solution (10 ppm Pb) R*.

Loss on drying (*2.2.32*). Not more than 8.0 per cent, determined on 1.000 g by drying at 60 °C over *diphosphorus pentoxide R* at a pressure not exceeding 670 Pa for 3 h.

Sulphated ash (*2.4.14*): 30 per cent to 43 per cent, determined on 0.20 g and calculated with reference to the dried substance.

Bacterial endotoxins (*2.6.14*): less than 0.01 IU per IU of heparin, if intended for use in the manufacture of parenteral dosage forms without a further appropriate procedure for removal of bacterial endotoxins.

ASSAY

Carry out the assay of heparin (*2.7.5*). The estimated potency is not less than 90 per cent and not more than 111 per cent of the stated potency. The confidence limits of the estimated potency (P = 0.95) are not less than 80 per cent and not more than 125 per cent of the stated potency.

STORAGE

Store in an airtight container. If the substance is sterile, store in a sterile, airtight, tamper-proof container.

LABELLING

The label states:

- the number of International Units per milligram,
- the name and quantity of any added substance,
- where applicable, that the substance is free from bacterial endotoxins.

01/2005:0828
corrected

HEPARINS, LOW-MOLECULAR-MASS

Heparina massae molecularis minoris

DEFINITION

Salts of sulphated glucosaminoglycans having a mass-average molecular mass less than 8000 and for which at least 60 per cent of the total mass has a molecular mass less than 8000. Low-molecular-mass heparins display different chemical structures at the reducing, or the non-reducing end of the polysaccharide chains.

The potency is not less than 70 IU of anti-factor Xa activity per milligram, calculated with reference to the dried substance. The ratio of anti-factor Xa activity to anti-factor IIa activity, determined as described under Assay, is not less than 1.5.

PRODUCTION

Low-molecular-mass heparins are produced in conditions designed to minimise microbial contamination.

Low-molecular-mass heparins are obtained by fractionation or depolymerisation of heparin of natural origin that complies with the monograph on *Heparin sodium (0333)* or *Heparin calcium (0332)*, whichever is appropriate, for parenteral use, unless otherwise justified and authorised. For each type of low-molecular-mass heparin the batch-to-batch consistency is ensured by demonstrating, for example, that the mass-average molecular mass and the mass percentage within defined molecular-mass ranges lower than 8000 are not less than 75 per cent and not more than 125 per cent of the mean value stated as type specification. The same limits apply also to the ratio of anti-factor Xa activity to anti-factor IIa activity.

Nucleotide and protein impurities of the source material. Dissolve 40 mg of the source material before fractionation in 10 ml of *water R*. The absorbance (*2.2.25*) measured at 260 nm and 280 nm is not greater than 0.20 and 0.15, respectively.

CHARACTERS

Appearance: white or almost white powder, hygroscopic.

Solubility: freely soluble in water.

IDENTIFICATION

A. Nuclear magnetic resonance spectrometry (*2.2.33*) using a pulsed (Fourier transform) spectrometer operating at 75 MHz for ^{13}C.

Test solution. Dissolve 0.200 g of the substance to be examined in a mixture of 0.2 ml of *deuterium oxide R* and 0.8 ml of *water R*.

Reference solution. Dissolve 0.200 g of the appropriate specific low-molecular-mass heparin CRS in a mixture of 0.2 ml of *deuterium oxide R* and 0.8 ml of *water R*.

Record the spectra at 40 °C, using cells 5 mm in diameter. Use *deuterated methanol R* as internal reference at δ = 50.0 ppm.

Results: the spectrum obtained with the test solution is similar to that obtained with the reference solution containing the appropriate specific low-molecular-mass heparin CRS.

B. The ratio of anti-factor Xa activity to anti-factor IIa activity, determined as described under Assay, is not less than 1.5.

C. Size-exclusion chromatography (*2.2.30*).

Test solution. Dissolve 20 mg of the substance to be examined in 2 ml of the mobile phase.

Reference solution. Dissolve 20 mg of *low-molecular-mass heparin for calibration CRS* in 2 ml of the mobile phase.

Column:

- *size*: l = 0.30 m, Ø = 7.5 mm,
- *stationary phase*: appropriate porous silica beads (5 µm) with a fractionation range for proteins of approximately 15 000 to 100 000,
- *number of theoretical plates*: minimum of 20 000 per metre.

Mobile phase: 28.4 g/l solution of *anhydrous sodium sulphate R* adjusted to pH 5.0 using *dilute sulphuric acid R*.

Flow rate: 0.5 ml/min.

Detection: differential refractometer.

Injection: 25 µl.

Calibration. For detection, use a differential refractometer (RI) detector connected in series to a ultraviolet spectrophotometer set (UV) at 234 nm such that the UV monitor is connected to the column outlet, and the RI detector to the UV-monitor outlet.

Monographs F-H

It is necessary to measure the time lapse between the 2 detectors accurately, so that chromatograms from them can be aligned correctly. The retention times used in the calibration must be those from the RI detector.

The normalisation factor used to calculate the molecular weight from the RI/UV ratio is obtained as follows: calculate the total area under the UV_{234} (ΣUV_{234}) and the RI (ΣRI) curves by numerical integration over the range of interest (i.e. excluding salt and solvent peaks at the end of the chromatogram). Calculate the ratio *r* using the following expression:

$$\frac{\sum \mathrm{RI}}{\sum \mathrm{UV}_{234}}$$

Calculate the factor *f* using the following expression:

$$\frac{M_{na}}{r}$$

M_{na} = the known number-average molecular mass of the *low-molecular-mass heparin for calibration CRS* found in the leaflet supplied with the CRS.

Provided the UV_{234} and the RI responses are aligned, the molecular mass *M* at any point is calculated from:

$$f\frac{\mathrm{RI}}{\mathrm{UV}_{234}}$$

The resulting table of retention times and molecular masses may be used to derive a calibration for the chromatographic system by fitting a suitable mathematical relationship to the data. A polynomial of the third degree is recommended. *It must be stressed that the extrapolation of this fitted calibration curve to higher molecular masses is not valid.*

Inject 25 µl of the test solution and record the chromatogram for a period of time, ensuring complete elution of sample and solvent peaks.

The mass-average molecular mass is defined by the expression:

$$\frac{\sum (\mathrm{RI}_i M_i)}{\sum \mathrm{RI}_i}$$

RI_i = mass of substance eluting in the fraction *i*

M_i = molecular mass corresponding to fraction *i*.

The value for the mass-average molecular mass is not greater than 8000 and at least 60 per cent of the total mass has a molecular mass lower than 8000. In addition, the molecular mass parameters of a given substance do not differ by more than 25 per cent from those of the corresponding reference substance.

D. It gives reaction (a) of sodium or the reactions of calcium (as appropriate) (*2.3.1*).

TESTS

pH (*2.2.3*): 5.5 to 8.0.

Dissolve 0.1 g in *carbon dioxide-free water R* and dilute to 10 ml with the same solvent.

Nitrogen (*2.5.9*): 1.5 per cent to 2.5 per cent (dried substance).

Calcium (*2.5.11*): 9.5 per cent to 11.5 per cent (dried substance), if prepared from heparin complying with the monograph on *Heparin calcium (0332)*. Use 0.200 g.

Sodium (*2.2.23, Method I*): 9.5 per cent to 12.5 per cent (dried substance), if prepared from heparin complying with the monograph on *Heparin sodium (0333)*.

Atomic absorption spectrometry.

Test solution. Dissolve 50 mg of the substance to be examined in *0.1 M hydrochloric acid* containing 1.27 mg of *caesium chloride R* per millilitre and dilute to 100.0 ml with the same solvent.

Reference solutions. Prepare reference solutions (25 ppm, 50 ppm and 75 ppm) using *sodium standard solution (200 ppm Na) R* diluted with *0.1 M hydrochloric acid* containing 1.27 mg of *caesium chloride R* per millilitre.

Source: sodium hollow-cathode lamp.

Wavelength: 330.3 nm.

Atomisation device: flame of suitable composition (for example, 11 litres of air and 2 litres of acetylene per minute).

Molar ratio of sulphate ions to carboxylate ions (*2.2.38*): minimum 1.8.

The sample of heparin used in this titration must be free from ionisable impurities, particularly salts.

Weigh 0.100 g of the substance to be examined taking the necessary measures to avoid the problems linked to hygroscopicity.

Take up into about 20 ml of double-glass-distilled *water R*. Cool to 4 °C and apply 2.0 ml of this solution to a pre-cooled column (approximately 10 × 1 cm), packed with a suitable *cation exchange resin R*. Wash through with double-glass-distilled *water R* into the titration vessel up to a final volume of about 10-15 ml (*the titration vessel must be just large enough to hold the electrodes from the conductivity meter, a small stirrer bar and a fine flexible tube from the outlet of a 2 ml burette*). Stir magnetically. When the conductivity reading is constant, note it and titrate with *0.05 M sodium hydroxide* added in approximately 50 µl portions. Record the burette level and the conductivity meter reading a few seconds after each addition until the end-point is reached.

For each measured figure, calculate the number of milliequivalents of sodium hydroxide added from the volume and the known concentration of the sodium hydroxide solution. Plot on a graph the figures for conductivity (as *y*-axis) against the figures of milliequivalent of sodium hydroxide (as *x*-axis). The graph will have 3, approximately linear sections: an initial steep downward slope, a middle slight rise and a final steep rise. Estimate the best straight lines through these 3 parts of the graph. At the points where the first and second lines intersect, and where the second and third lines intersect, draw perpendiculars to the *x*-axis to estimate the milliequivalents of sodium hydroxide taken up by the sample at those points. The point where the first and second lines intersect will give the number of milliequivalents of sodium hydroxide taken up by the sulphate groups, and the point where the second and third lines intersect will give the number of milliequivalents taken up by the sulphate and carboxylate groups together. The difference between the 2 will therefore give the number of milliequivalents taken up by the carboxylate groups.

Heavy metals (*2.4.8*): maximum 30 ppm.

0.5 g complies with limit test C. Prepare the standard using 1.5 ml of *lead standard solution (10 ppm Pb) R*.

Loss on drying (*2.2.32*): maximum 10.0 per cent, determined on 1.000 g by drying at 60 °C over *diphosphorus pentoxide R* at a pressure not exceeding 670 Pa for 3 h.

Bacterial endotoxins (*2.6.14*): less than 0.01 IU per International Unit of anti-Xa activity, if intended for use in the manufacture of parenteral dosage forms without a further appropriate procedure for the removal of bacterial endotoxins. The addition of divalent cations may be necessary to fulfil the validation criteria.

ASSAY

The anticoagulant activity of low-molecular-mass heparins is determined *in vitro* by 2 assays which determine its ability to accelerate the inhibition of factor Xa (anti-Xa assay) and thrombin, factor IIa (anti-IIa assay), by antithrombin III.

The International Units for anti-Xa and anti-IIa activity are the activities contained in a stated amount of the International Standard for low-molecular-mass heparin.

Low-molecular-mass heparin for assay BRP, calibrated in International Units by comparison with the International Standard using the 2 assays given below, is used as reference preparation.

ANTI-FACTOR Xa ACTIVITY

Reference and test solutions

Prepare 4 independent series of 4 dilutions each, of the substance to be examined and of the reference preparation of low-molecular-mass heparin in *tris(hydroxymethyl)aminomethane sodium chloride buffer solution pH 7.4 R*; the concentration range should be within 0.025 IU to 0.2 IU of anti-factor Xa activity per millilitre and the dilutions chosen should give a linear response when results are plotted as absorbance against log concentration.

Procedure

Label 16 tubes in duplicate: T_1, T_2, T_3, T_4 for the dilutions of the substance to be examined and S_1, S_2, S_3, S_4 for the dilutions of the reference preparation. To each tube add 50 µl of *antithrombin III solution R1* and 50 µl of the appropriate dilution of the substance to be examined, or the reference preparation. After each addition, mix but do not allow bubbles to form. Treating the tubes in the order S_1, S_2, S_3, S_4, T_1, T_2, T_3, T_4, T_1, T_2, T_3, T_4, S_1, S_2, S_3, S_4, allow to equilibrate at 37 °C (water-bath or heating block) for 1 min and add to each tube 100 µl of *bovine factor Xa solution R*. Incubate for exactly 1 min and add 250 µl of *chromophore substrate R1*. Stop the reaction after exactly 4 min by adding 375 µl of *acetic acid R*. Transfer the mixtures to semi-micro cuvettes and measure the absorbance (*2.2.25*) at 405 nm using a suitable reading device. Determine the blank amidolytic activity at the beginning and at the end of the procedure in a similar manner, using *tris(hydroxymethyl)aminomethane sodium chloride buffer solution pH 7.4 R* instead of the reference and test solutions; the 2 blank values do not differ significantly. Calculate the regression of the absorbance on log concentrations of the solutions of the substance to be examined and of the reference preparation of low-molecular-mass heparins and calculate the potency of the substance to be examined in International Units of anti-factor Xa activity per millilitre using the usual statistical methods for parallel-line assays.

ANTI-FACTOR IIa ACTIVITY

Reference and test solutions

Prepare 4 independent series of 4 dilutions each, of the substance to be examined and of the reference preparation of low molecular-mass heparin in *tris(hydroxymethyl)aminomethane sodium chloride buffer solution pH 7.4 R*; the concentration range should be within 0.015 IU to 0.075 IU of anti-factor IIa activity per millilitre and the dilutions chosen should give a linear response when results are plotted as absorbance against log concentration.

Procedure

Label 16 tubes in duplicate: T_1, T_2, T_3, T_4 for the dilutions of the substance to be examined and S_1, S_2, S_3, S_4 for the dilutions of the reference preparation. To each tube add 50 µl of *antithrombin III solution R2* and 50 µl of the appropriate dilution of the substance to be examined or the reference preparation. After each addition, mix but do not allow bubbles to form. Treating the tubes in the order S_1, S_2, S_3, S_4, T_1, T_2, T_3, T_4, T_1, T_2, T_3, T_4, S_1, S_2, S_3, S_4, allow to equilibrate at 37 °C (water-bath or heating block) for 1 min and add to each tube 100 µl of *human thrombin solution R*. Incubate for exactly 1 min and add 250 µl of *chromophore substrate R2*. Stop the reaction after exactly 4 min by adding 375 µl of *acetic acid R*. Transfer the mixtures to semi-micro cuvettes and measure the absorbance (*2.2.25*) at 405 nm using a suitable reading device. Determine the blank amidolytic activity at the beginning and at the end of the procedure in a similar manner, using *tris(hydroxymethyl)aminomethane sodium chloride buffer solution pH 7.4 R* instead of the reference and test solutions; the 2 blank values do not differ significantly. Calculate the regression of the absorbance on log concentrations of the solutions of the substance to be examined and of the reference preparation of low-molecular-mass heparins, and calculate the potency of the substance to be examined in International Units of anti-factor IIa activity per millilitre using the usual statistical methods for parallel-line assays.

LABELLING

The label states:

- the number of International Units of anti-factor Xa activity per milligram,
- the number of International Units of anti-factor IIa activity per milligram,
- the mass-average molecular mass and the percentage of molecules within defined molecular mass ranges,
- where applicable, that the substance is free from bacterial endotoxins,
- where applicable, that the contents are the sodium salt,
- where applicable, that the contents are the calcium salt.

STORAGE

In an airtight tamper-proof container. If the product is sterile and free of bacterial endotoxins, store in a sterile and apyrogenic container.

01/2005:1980
corrected

HEPTAMINOL HYDROCHLORIDE

Heptaminoli hydrochloridum

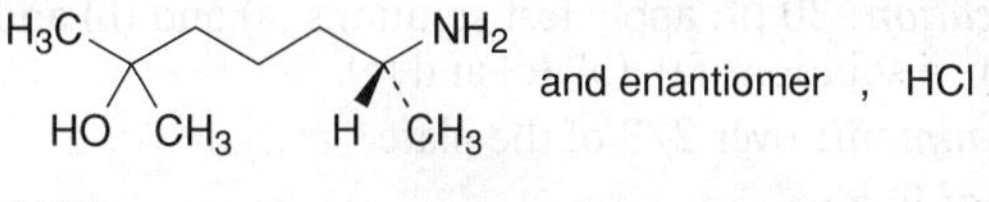

$C_8H_{20}ClNO$ M_r 181.7

DEFINITION

(6*RS*)-6-Amino-2-methylheptan-2-ol hydrochloride.

Content: 99.0 per cent to 101.0 per cent (dried substance).

CHARACTERS

Appearance: white or almost white, crystalline powder.

Solubility: freely soluble in water, soluble in alcohol, practically insoluble in methylene chloride.

IDENTIFICATION

First identification: B, D.

Second identification: A, C, D.

A. To 1 ml of solution S (see Tests) add 4 ml of *water R* and 2 ml of a 200 g/l solution of *ammonium and cerium nitrate R* in *4 M nitric acid*. An orange-brown colour develops.

B. Infrared absorption spectrophotometry (*2.2.24*).

Comparison: *heptaminol hydrochloride CRS*.

C. Examine the chromatograms obtained in the test for related substances.

Detection: examine in daylight.

Results: the principal spot in the chromatogram obtained with test solution (b) is similar in position, colour and size to the principal spot in the chromatogram obtained with reference solution (b).

D. It gives reaction (a) of chlorides (*2.3.1*).

TESTS

Solution S. Dissolve 5.0 g in *carbon dioxide-free water R* and dilute to 50 ml with the same solvent.

Appearance of solution. Solution S is clear (*2.2.1*) and not more intensely coloured than reference solution BY_6 (*2.2.2, Method II*).

Acidity or alkalinity. To 10 ml of solution S add 0.1 ml of *methyl red solution R* and 0.3 ml of *0.01 M hydrochloric acid*. The solution is red. Add 0.6 ml of *0.01 M sodium hydroxide*. The solution is yellow.

Related substances. Thin-layer chromatography (*2.2.27*).

Test solution (a). Dissolve 0.50 g of the substance to be examined in *methanol R* and dilute to 5.0 ml with the same solvent.

Test solution (b). Dilute 1.0 ml of test solution (a) to 10 ml with *methanol R*.

Reference solution (a). Dilute 3.0 ml of test solution (a) to 10.0 ml with *methanol R*. Dilute 1.0 ml of this solution to 50.0 ml with *methanol R*.

Reference solution (b). Dissolve 0.10 g of *heptaminol hydrochloride CRS* in *methanol R* and dilute to 10 ml with the same solvent.

Reference solution (c). Dissolve 10.0 mg of *heptaminol impurity A CRS* in *methanol R* and dilute to 5.0 ml with the same solvent.

Reference solution (d). Dilute 1.0 ml of reference solution (c) to 10.0 ml with *methanol R*.

Reference solution (e). To 2.5 ml of reference solution (c) add 0.5 ml of test solution (b) and dilute to 5 ml with *methanol R*.

Plate: *TLC silica gel G plate R*.

Mobile phase: *concentrated ammonia R, dioxan R, 2-propanol R* (10:50:50 *V/V/V*).

Application: 10 µl; apply test solutions (a) and (b) and reference solutions (a), (b), (d) and (e).

Development: over 2/3 of the plate.

Drying: in air.

Detection: expose the plate to iodine vapour for at least 15 h.

System suitability: the chromatogram obtained with reference solution (e) shows 2 clearly separated principal spots and the chromatogram obtained with reference solution (a) shows a single principal spot.

Limits: in the chromatogram obtained with test solution (a):

- *impurity A*: any spot corresponding to impurity A is not more intense than the spot in the chromatogram obtained with reference solution (d) (0.2 per cent),
- *any other impurity*: any spot, apart from the principal spot and any spot corresponding to impurity A is not more intense than the spot in the chromatogram obtained with reference solution (a) (0.6 per cent).

Heavy metals (*2.4.8*): maximum 10 ppm.

12 ml of solution S complies with limit test A. Prepare the standard using *lead standard solution (1 ppm Pb) R*.

Loss on drying (*2.2.32*): maximum 0.5 per cent, determined on 1.000 g by drying in an oven at 100-105 °C for 4 h.

Sulphated ash (*2.4.14*): maximum 0.1 per cent, determined on 1.0 g.

ASSAY

Dissolve 0.140 g in 50 ml of *alcohol R* and add 5.0 ml of *0.01 M hydrochloric acid*. Carry out a potentiometric titration (*2.2.20*), using *0.1 M sodium hydroxide*. Read the volume added between the 2 points of inflexion.

1 ml of *0.1 M sodium hydroxide* is equivalent to 18.17 mg of $C_8H_{20}ClNO$.

IMPURITIES

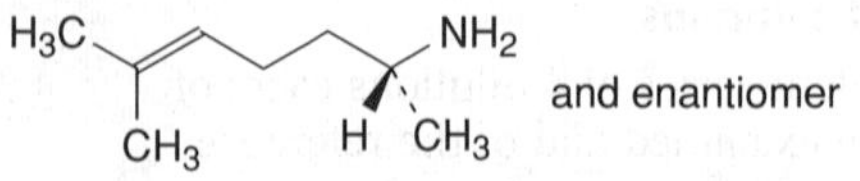

A. (2*RS*)-6-methylhept-5-en-2-amine.

01/2005:1436

HEXAMIDINE DIISETIONATE

Hexamidini diisetionas

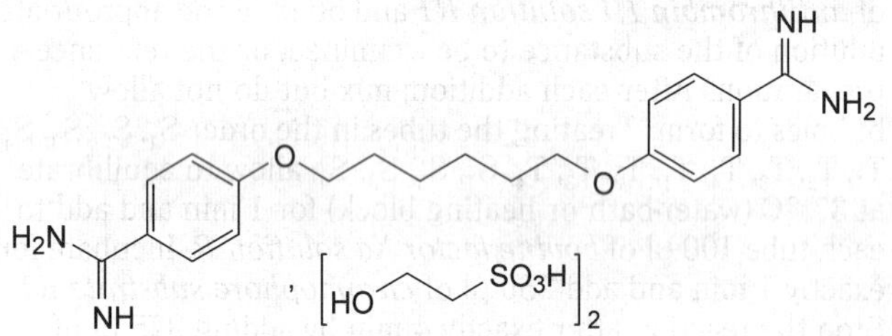

$C_{24}H_{38}N_4O_{10}S_2$ M_r 607

DEFINITION

Hexamidine diisetionate contains not less than 98.5 per cent and not more than the equivalent of 101.5 per cent of 4,4′-(hexane-1,6-diyldioxy)dibenzimidamide bis(2-hydroxyethanesulphonate), calculated with reference to the dried substance.

CHARACTERS

A white or slightly yellow powder, hygroscopic, sparingly soluble in water, slightly soluble in alcohol, practically insoluble in methylene chloride.

IDENTIFICATION

A. Examine by infrared absorption spectrophotometry (*2.2.24*), comparing with the spectrum obtained with *hexamidine diisetionate CRS*.

B. Dissolve about 40 mg in 5 ml of *water R* and add dropwise with shaking, 1 ml of a 100 g/l solution of *sodium chloride R*. Allow to stand for 5 min. An abundant shimmering white precipitate forms slowly.

TESTS

Appearance of solution. Dissolve 0.5 g in *carbon dioxide-free water R* heating at about 70 °C and dilute to 10 ml with the same solvent. Allow to cool to room temperature for 10 min to 15 min. The solution is not more opalescent than reference suspension II (*2.2.1*) and not more intensely coloured than intensity 6 of the range of reference solutions of the most appropriate colour (*2.2.2, Method II*).

Acidity or alkalinity. Dissolve 2.0 g in *water R* heating at about 50 °C and dilute to 20 ml with *water R* heating at about 50 °C. Allow to cool to about 35 °C, add 0.1 ml of *methyl red solution R*. Not more than 0.25 ml of *0.05 M hydrochloric acid* or *0.05 M sodium hydroxide* is required to change the colour of the indicator.

Related substances. Examine by liquid chromatography (*2.2.29*).

Test solution. Dissolve 20.0 mg of the substance to be examined in mobile phase A and dilute to 100.0 ml with mobile phase A.

Reference solution (a). Dilute 1.0 ml of the test solution to 100.0 ml with the mobile phase A.

Reference solution (b). Dissolve 5 mg of the substance to be examined and 5 mg of *pentamidine diisetionate CRS* in mobile phase A and dilute to 100 ml with mobile phase A. Dilute 2 ml of the solution to 5 ml with mobile phase A.

The chromatographic procedure may be carried out using:

- a stainless steel column 0.25 m long and 4.6 mm in internal diameter, packed with *styrene-divinylbenzene copolymer R* (8 μm),
- as mobile phase at a flow rate of 1 ml/min:

  Mobile phase A. Mix 20 volumes of *acetonitrile R* and 80 volumes of a 6.8 g/l solution of *potassium dihydrogen phosphate R* adjusted to pH 3 using *phosphoric acid R*,

  Mobile phase B. Mix equal volumes of *acetonitrile R* and of a 6.8 g/l solution of *potassium dihydrogen phosphate R* adjusted to pH 3 using *phosphoric acid R*,

Time (min)	Mobile phase A (per cent *V/V*)	Mobile phase B (per cent *V/V*)	Comment
0 - 30	100 → 0	0 → 100	linear gradient
30 - 35	0	100	isocratic
35 - 40	0 → 100	100 → 0	re-equilibration

- as detector a spectrophotometer set at 263 nm.

Inject 20 μl of reference solution (a) and 20 μl of reference solution (b). Adjust the sensitivity of the system so that the height of the principal peak in the chromatogram obtained with reference solution (a) is at least 50 per cent of the full scale of the recorder. The test is not valid unless, in the chromatogram obtained with reference solution (b), the resolution between the peak corresponding respectively to hexamidine diisetionate and pentamidine diisetionate is at least 5.

Inject 20 μl of the test solution. In the chromatogram obtained, the area of any peak, apart from the principal peak, is not greater than the area of the principal peak in the chromatogram obtained with reference solution (a) (1 per cent) and not more than one such peak has an area greater than half the area of the principal peak in the chromatogram obtained with reference solution (a) (0.5 per cent); the sum of the areas of all the peaks, apart from the principal peak, is not greater than 1.5 times the area of the principal peak in the chromatogram obtained with reference solution (a) (1.5 per cent). Disregard any peak with an area less than 0.05 times that of the principal peak in the chromatogram obtained with reference solution (a).

Loss on drying (*2.2.32*). Not more than 0.5 per cent, determined on 1.000 g by drying in an oven at 100 °C to 105 °C.

Sulphated ash (*2.4.14*). Not more than 0.1 per cent, determined on 1.0 g.

ASSAY

Dissolve 0.250 g in 50 ml of *dimethylformamide R*. Titrate with *0.1 M tetrabutylammonium hydroxide* under a current of *nitrogen R*, determining the end-point potentiometrically (*2.2.20*).

1 ml of *0.1 M tetrabutylammonium hydroxide* is equivalent to 30.35 mg of $C_{24}H_{38}N_4O_{10}S_2$.

STORAGE

Store in an airtight container.

IMPURITIES

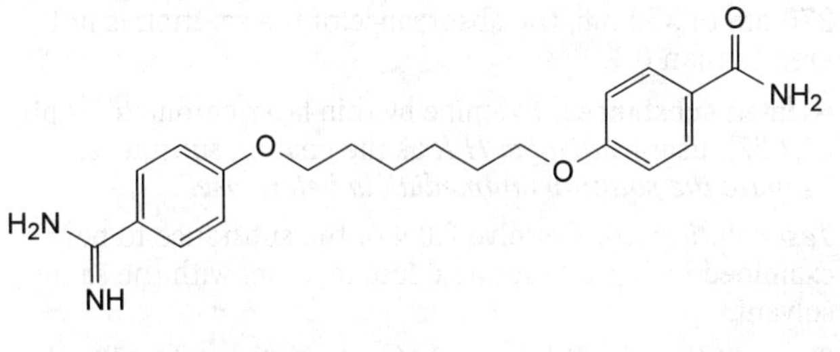

A. 4-[[6-(4-carbamimidoylphenoxy)hexyl]oxy]benzamide.

01/2005:1221

HEXETIDINE

Hexetidinum

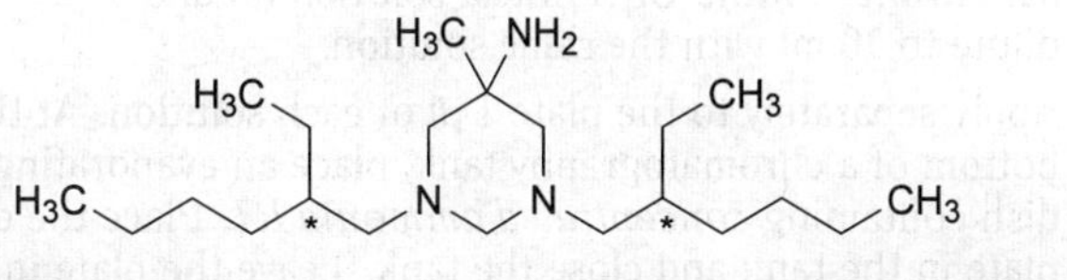

$C_{21}H_{45}N_3$ M_r 339.6

DEFINITION

Hexetidine contains not less than 98.0 per cent and not more than the equivalent of 102.0 per cent of 1,3-bis(2-ethylhexyl)]-5-methylhexahydropyrimidin-5-amine.

CHARACTERS

An oily liquid, colourless or slightly yellow, very slightly soluble in water, very soluble in acetone, in alcohol and in methylene chloride. It dissolves in dilute mineral acids.

IDENTIFICATION

First identification: A.

Second identification: B, C, D.

A. Examine by infrared absorption spectrophotometry (*2.2.24*), comparing with the spectrum obtained with *hexetidine CRS*.

B. Examine the chromatograms obtained in the test for related substances. The principal spot in the chromatogram obtained with test solution (b) is similar in position, colour and size to the principal spot in the chromatogram obtained with reference solution (a).

C. To 0.2 ml add 2 ml of *sulphuric acid R* and 2 mg of *chromotropic acid, sodium salt R*. Heat in a water-bath at 60 °C. A violet colour develops.

D. Dissolve 0.2 ml in 1 ml of *methylene chloride R*. Add 0.5 ml of *copper sulphate solution R*, 0.05 ml of *0.25 M alcoholic sulphuric acid R* and 5 ml of *water R*. Shake, then allow to stand. The lower layer becomes deep blue.

TESTS

Appearance. The substance to be examined is clear (*2.2.1*)and not more intensely coloured than reference solution Y_5 or reference solution GY_5 (*2.2.2, Method II*).

Relative density (*2.2.5*): 0.864 to 0.870.

Refractive index (*2.2.6*): 1.461 to 1.467.

Optical rotation (*2.2.7*). Dissolve 1.0 g in *ethanol R* and dilute to 10.0 ml with the same solvent. The angle of optical rotation is − 0.10° to + 0.10°.

Absorbance (*2.2.25*). Dissolve 0.50 g in *heptane R* and dilute to 50.0 ml with the same solvent. At wavelengths from 270 nm to 350 nm, the absorbance of the solution is not greater than 0.1.

Related substances. Examine by thin-layer chromatography (*2.2.27*), using *silica gel H R* as the coating substance. *Prepare the solutions immediately before use.*

Test solution (a). Dissolve 2.0 g of the substance to be examined in *heptane R* and dilute to 20 ml with the same solvent.

Test solution (b). Dilute 1 ml of test solution (a) to 10 ml with *heptane R*.

Reference solution (a). Dissolve 20 mg of *hexetidine CRS* in *heptane R* and dilute to 2 ml with the same solvent.

Reference solution (b). Dilute 1 ml of test solution (a) to 100 ml with *heptane R*.

Reference solution (c). Dilute 5 ml of reference solution (b) to 10 ml with *heptane R*.

Reference solution (d). Dissolve 10 mg of *dehydrohexetidine CRS* in test solution (a) and dilute to 10 ml with the same solution.

Apply separately to the plate 1 µl of each solution. At the bottom of a chromatography tank, place an evaporating dish containing *concentrated ammonia R1*. Place the dried plate in the tank and close the tank. Leave the plate in contact with the ammonia vapour for 15 min. Withdraw the plate and place it in a current of air to remove the ammonia vapour. Develop over a path of 15 cm using a mixture of 20 volumes of *methanol R* and 80 volumes of *toluene R*. Allow the plate to dry in air. Expose the plate to iodine vapour for 30 min. Any spot in the chromatogram obtained with test solution (a), apart from the principal spot, is not more intense than the spot in the chromatogram obtained with reference solution (b) (1 per cent) and at most two such spots are more intense than the spot in the chromatogram obtained with reference solution (c) (0.5 per cent). The test is not valid unless the chromatogram obtained with reference solution (d) shows two clearly separated spots.

Heavy metals (*2.4.8*). Dissolve 2.0 g in a mixture of 15 volumes of *water R* and 85 volumes of *acetone R* and dilute to 20 ml with the same mixture of solvents. 12 ml of the solution complies with limit test B for heavy metals (10 ppm). Prepare the standard using lead standard solution (1 ppm Pb) obtained by diluting *lead standard solution (100 ppm Pb) R* with a mixture of 15 volumes of *water R* and 85 volumes of *acetone R*.

Sulphated ash (*2.4.14*). Not more than 0.1 per cent, determined on 1.0 g.

ASSAY

Dissolve 0.150 g in 80 ml of *anhydrous acetic acid R*. Titrate with *0.1 M perchloric acid*, determining the end-point potentiometrically (*2.2.20*).

1 ml of *0.1 M perchloric acid* is equivalent to 16.98 mg of $C_{21}H_{45}N_3$.

STORAGE

Store protected from light.

IMPURITIES

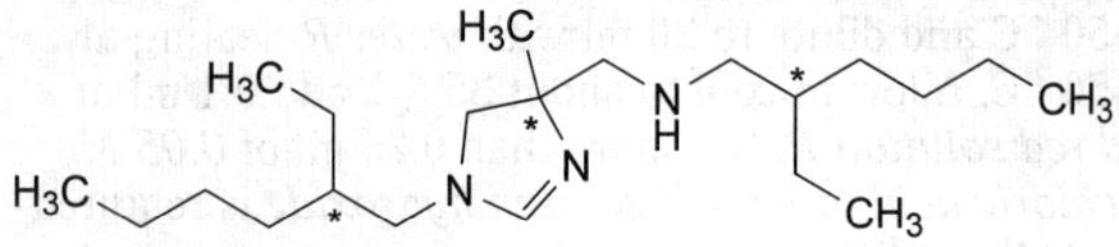

A. 2-ethyl-*N*-[[1-(2-ethylhexyl)-4-methyl-4,5-dihydro-1*H*-imidazol-4-yl]methyl]hexan-1-amine (dehydrohexetidine),

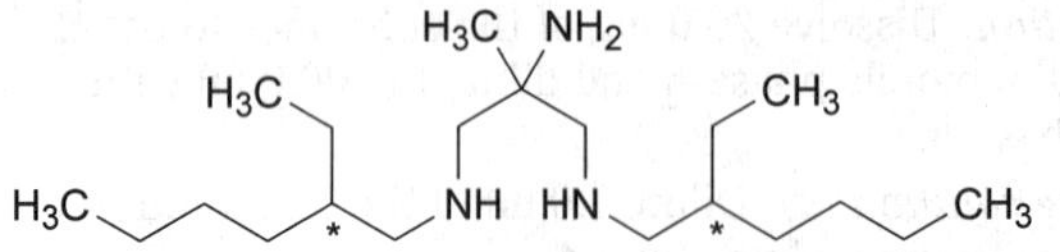

B. N^1,N^3-bis(2-ethylhexyl)-2-methylpropane-1,2,3-triamine (triamine),

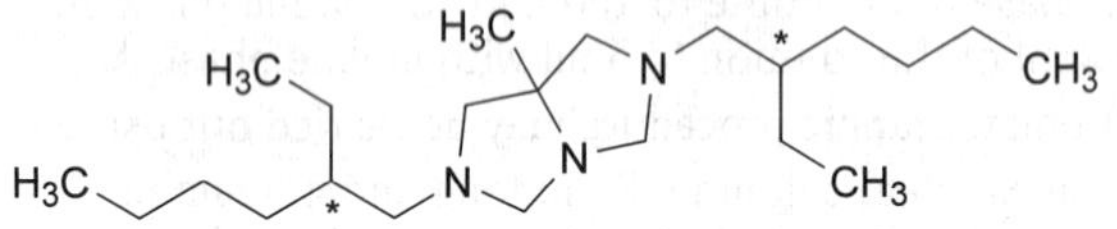

C. 2,6-bis(2-ethylhexyl)-7a-methylhexahydro-1*H*-imidazo[1,5-*c*]imidazole (hexedine),

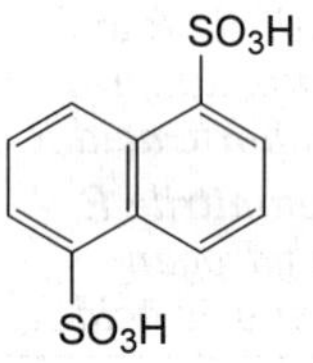

D. naphthalene-1,5-disulphonic acid.

01/2005:0183

HEXOBARBITAL

Hexobarbitalum

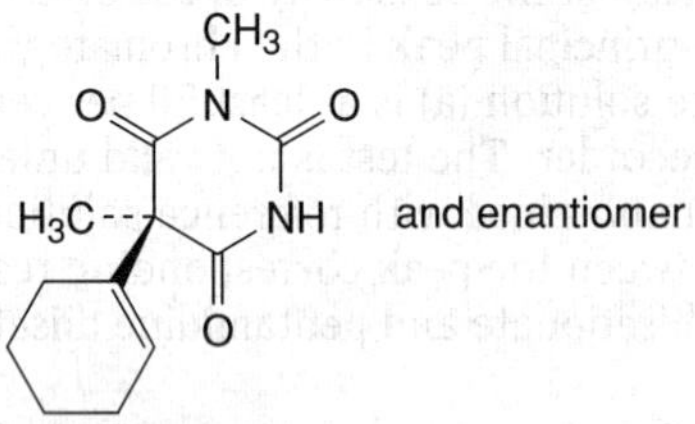

$C_{12}H_{16}N_2O_3$ M_r 236.3

DEFINITION

Hexobarbital contains not less than 99.0 per cent and not more than the equivalent of 101.0 per cent of (5*RS*)-5-(cyclohex-1-enyl)-1,5-dimethylpyrimidine-2,4,6(1*H*,3*H*,5*H*)-trione, calculated with reference to the dried substance.

CHARACTERS

A white, crystalline powder, very slightly soluble in water, sparingly soluble in alcohol. It forms water-soluble compounds with alkali hydroxides and carbonates and with ammonia.

IDENTIFICATION

First identification: A, B.

Second identification: A, C, D.

A. Determine the melting point (*2.2.14*) of the substance to be examined. Mix equal parts of the substance to be examined and *hexobarbital CRS* and determine the melting point of the mixture. The difference between the melting points (which are about 146 °C) is not greater than 2 °C.

B. Examine by infrared absorption spectrophotometry (*2.2.24*), comparing with the spectrum obtained with *hexobarbital CRS*.

C. Examine by thin-layer chromatography (*2.2.27*), using *silica gel GF_{254} R* as the coating substance.

Test solution. Dissolve 0.1 g of the substance to be examined in *chloroform R* and dilute to 100 ml with the same solvent.

Reference solution. Dissolve 0.1 g of *hexobarbital CRS* in *chloroform R* and dilute to 100 ml with the same solvent.

Apply separately to the plate 10 µl of each solution. Develop over a path of 18 cm using the lower layer of a mixture of 5 volumes of *concentrated ammonia R*, 15 volumes of *alcohol R* and 80 volumes of *chloroform R*. Examine immediately in ultraviolet light at 254 nm. The principal spot in the chromatogram obtained with the test solution is similar in position and size to the principal spot in the chromatogram obtained with the reference solution.

D. To about 10 mg add 1.0 ml of a 10 g/l solution of *vanillin R* in *alcohol R* and 2 ml of a cooled mixture of 1 volume of *water R* and 2 volumes of *sulphuric acid R*. Shake and allow to stand for 5 min. A greenish-yellow colour develops. Heat on a water-bath for 10 min. The colour becomes dark red.

TESTS

Appearance of solution. Dissolve 1.0 g in a mixture of 4 ml of *dilute sodium hydroxide solution R* and 6 ml of *water R*. The solution is clear (*2.2.1*) and not more intensely coloured than reference solution Y_6 (*2.2.2, Method II*).

Acidity. Boil 1.0 g with 50 ml of *water R* for 2 min, allow to cool and filter. To 10 ml of the filtrate add 0.15 ml of *methyl red solution R*. The solution is orange-yellow. Not more than 0.1 ml of *0.1 M sodium hydroxide* is required to produce a pure yellow colour.

Related substances. Examine by thin-layer chromatography (*2.2.27*), using *silica gel GF_{254} R* as the coating substance.

Test solution. Dissolve 1.0 g of the substance to be examined in *chloroform R* and dilute to 100 ml with the same solvent.

Reference solution. Dilute 0.5 ml of the test solution to 100 ml with *chloroform R*.

Apply separately to the plate 20 µl of each solution. Develop over a path of 15 cm using the lower layer of a mixture of 5 volumes of *concentrated ammonia R*, 15 volumes of *alcohol R* and 80 volumes of *chloroform R*. Examine immediately in ultraviolet light at 254 nm. Any spot in the chromatogram obtained with the test solution, apart from the principal spot, is not more intense than the spot in the chromatogram obtained with the reference solution (0.5 per cent).

Loss on drying (*2.2.32*). Not more than 0.5 per cent, determined on 1.00 g by drying in an oven at 100 °C to 105 °C.

Sulphated ash (*2.4.14*). Not more than 0.1 per cent, determined on 1.0 g.

ASSAY

Dissolve 0.200 g in 5 ml of *pyridine R*. Add 0.5 ml of *thymolphthalein solution R* and 10 ml of *silver nitrate solution in pyridine R*. Titrate with *0.1 M ethanolic sodium hydroxide* until a pure blue colour is obtained. Carry out a blank titration.

1 ml of *0.1 M ethanolic sodium hydroxide* is equivalent to 23.63 mg of $C_{12}H_{16}N_2O_3$.

01/2005:1437

HEXYLRESORCINOL

Hexylresorcinolum

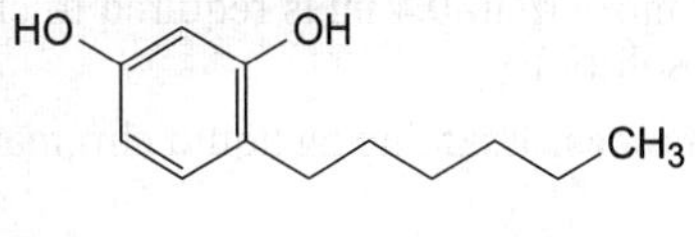

$C_{12}H_{18}O_2$ M_r 194.3

DEFINITION

Hexylresorcinol contains not less than 98.0 per cent and not more than the equivalent of 101.0 per cent of 4-hexylbenzene-1,3-diol calculated with reference to the anhydrous substance.

CHARACTERS

A colourless, yellowish or reddish, crystalline powder or needles, turning brownish-pink on exposure to light or air, very slightly soluble in water, freely soluble in alcohol and in methylene chloride.

It shows polymorphism.

IDENTIFICATION

First identification: B.

Second identification: A, C, D.

A. Melting point (*2.2.14*): 66 °C to 68 °C. Melting may occur at about 60 °C, followed by solidification and a second melting between 66 °C and 68 °C.

B. Examine by infrared absorption spectrophotometry (*2.2.24*), comparing with the spectrum obtained with *hexylresorcinol CRS*. If the spectra obtained in the solid state show differences, dissolve the substance to be examined and the reference substance separately in *methanol R*, evaporate to dryness and record new spectra using the residues.

C. Examine by thin-layer chromatography (*2.2.27*), using a *TLC silica gel G plate R*.

Test solution. Dilute 0.1 ml of solution S (see Tests) to 10 ml with *alcohol R*.

Reference solution (a). Dissolve 10 mg of *hexylresorcinol CRS* in *alcohol R* and dilute to 10 ml with the same solvent.

Reference solution (b). Dissolve 10 mg of *hexylresorcinol CRS* and 10 mg of *resorcinol R* in *alcohol R* and dilute to 10 ml with the same solvent.

Apply to the plate 10 µl of each solution. Develop over a path corresponding to two thirds of the plate height with a mixture of equal volumes of *methyl ethyl ketone R* and *pentane R*. Allow the plate to dry in air for 5 min. Spray the plate with 3 ml of *anisaldehyde solution R* and heat at 100 °C to 105 °C for 5 min. The principal spot in the chromatogram obtained with the test solution is similar in position, colour and size to the principal spot in the chromatogram obtained with reference solution (a).

The test is not valid unless the chromatogram obtained with reference solution (b) shows two clearly separated principal spots.

D. Dissolve 0.1 g in 1 ml of *alcohol R*. Add one drop of *ferric chloride solution R1*. A green colour is produced. Add *dilute ammonia R1*. The solution becomes brown.

TESTS

Solution S. Dissolve 1.0 g in *alcohol R* and dilute to 10.0 ml with the same solvent.

Appearance of solution. Solution S is clear (*2.2.1*).

Acidity. Dissolve 0.5 g in a mixture of 25 ml of *carbon dioxide-free water R* and 25 ml of *ether R* previously neutralised to *phenolphthalein solution R1* and titrate with *0.1 M sodium hydroxide*, shaking vigorously after each addition. Not more than 0.4 ml is required to change the colour of the solution.

Related substances. Examine by liquid chromatography (*2.2.29*).

Test solution. Dissolve 0.1 g of the substance to be examined in the mobile phase and dilute to 10.0 ml with the mobile phase.

Reference solution (a). Dilute 1.0 ml of the test solution to 200.0 ml with the mobile phase.

Reference solution (b). Dissolve 20.0 mg of *phenol R* in the mobile phase and dilute to 100.0 ml with the mobile phase.

Reference solution (c). Dissolve 20.0 mg of *resorcinol R* in the mobile phase and dilute to 100.0 ml with the mobile phase.

Reference solution (d). To 8.0 ml of reference solution (a) add 2.0 ml of reference solution (b), 2.0 ml of reference solution (c) and dilute to 20.0 ml with the mobile phase.

The chromatographic procedure may be carried out using:

- a stainless steel column 0.25 m long and 4.6 mm in internal diameter packed with *octadecylsilyl silica gel for chromatography R* (5 µm),
- as mobile phase at a flow rate of 1 ml/min a mixture of 25 volumes of a 3.0 g/l solution of *glacial acetic acid R*, adjusted to pH 5.9 with *dilute ammonia R1* and 75 volumes of *methanol R*,
- as detector a spectrophotometer set at 281 nm,
- a loop injector.

Inject 20 µl of reference solution (d). Adjust the sensitivity of the system so that the heights of the three principal peaks in the chromatogram obtained are at least 20 per cent of the full scale of the recorder. The test is not valid unless the resolution between the second peak (phenol) and the third peak (hexylresorcinol) is at least 5.0.

Inject 20 µl of the test solution and 20 µl of reference solution (a). Continue the chromatography of the test solution for twice the retention time of hexylresorcinol. In the chromatogram obtained with the test solution: the areas corresponding to phenol and resorcinol are not greater than the areas of the corresponding peaks in the chromatograms obtained with reference solution (d) (0.2 per cent); the area of any peak, apart from the principal peak and the peaks corresponding to phenol and resorcinol is not greater than the area of the principal peak in the chromatogram obtained with reference solution (a) (0.5 per cent); the sum of the areas of such peaks is not greater than twice the area of the principal peak obtained with reference solution (a) (1 per cent). Disregard any peak with an area less than 0.1 times the area of the principal peak in the chromatogram obtained with reference solution (a).

Water (*2.5.12*). Not more than 0.5 per cent determined on 1.000 g by the semi-micro determination of water.

Sulphated ash (*2.4.14*). Not more than 0.1 per cent, determined on 1.0 g.

ASSAY

Dissolve 0.100 g in 10 ml of *methanol R* in a ground-glass-stoppered flask, add 30.0 ml of *0.0167 M potassium bromate* and 2 g of *potassium bromide R*. Shake to dissolve the substance and add 15 ml of *dilute sulphuric acid R*. Stopper the flask, shake and allow to stand in the dark for 15 min, stirring continuously. Add 5 ml of *methylene chloride R* and a solution of 1 g of *potassium iodide R* in 10 ml of *water R*, allow to stand in the dark for 15 min, stirring continuously. Titrate with *0.1 M sodium thiosulphate*, using 1 ml of *starch solution R*, shaking thoroughly. Carry out a blank titration under the same conditions.

1 ml of *0.0167 M potassium bromate* is equivalent to 4.857 mg of $C_{12}H_{18}O_2$.

STORAGE

Store in an airtight container, protected from light.

IMPURITIES

A. phenol,

B. resorcinol.

01/2005:0143

HISTAMINE DIHYDROCHLORIDE

Histamini dihydrochloridum

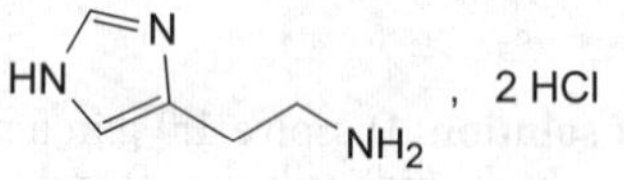

$C_5H_{11}Cl_2N_3$ M_r 184.1

DEFINITION

Histamine dihydrochloride contains not less than 98.5 per cent and not more than the equivalent of 101.0 per cent of 2-(1*H*-imidazol-4-yl)ethanamine dihydrochloride, calculated with reference to the dried substance.

CHARACTERS

A white, crystalline powder or colourless crystals, hygroscopic, very soluble in water, soluble in alcohol.

IDENTIFICATION

First identification: A, D.

Second identification: B, C, D.

A. Examine by infrared absorption spectrophotometry (*2.2.24*), comparing with the spectrum obtained with *histamine dihydrochloride CRS*. Examine as discs prepared using 1 mg of substance.

B. Examine the chromatograms obtained in the test for histidine. The principal spot in the chromatogram obtained with test solution (b) is similar in position, colour and size to the principal spot in the chromatogram obtained with reference solution (a).

C. Dissolve 0.1 g in 7 ml of *water R* and add 3 ml of a 200 g/l solution of *sodium hydroxide R*. Dissolve 50 mg of *sulphanilic acid R* in a mixture of 0.1 ml of *hydrochloric acid R* and 10 ml of *water R* and add 0.1 ml of *sodium nitrite solution R*. Add the second solution to the first and mix. A red colour is produced.

D. It gives reaction (a) of chlorides (*2.3.1*).

TESTS

Solution S. Dissolve 0.5 g in *carbon dioxide-free water R* prepared from *distilled water R* and dilute to 10 ml with the same solvent.

Appearance of solution. Solution S is clear (*2.2.1*) and not more intensely coloured than reference solution Y_7 (*2.2.2, Method II*).

pH (*2.2.3*). The pH of solution S is 2.85 to 3.60.

Histidine. Examine by thin-layer chromatography (*2.2.27*), using a *TLC silica gel G plate R*.

Test solution (a). Dissolve 0.5 g of the substance to be examined in *water R* and dilute to 10 ml with the same solvent.

Test solution (b). Dilute 2 ml of test solution (a) to 10 ml with *water R*.

Reference solution (a). Dissolve 0.1 g of *histamine dihydrochloride CRS* in *water R* and dilute to 10 ml with the same solvent.

Reference solution (b). Dissolve 50 mg of *histidine monohydrochloride R* in *water R* and dilute to 100 ml with the same solvent.

Reference solution (c). Mix 1 ml of test solution (a) and 1 ml of reference solution (b).

Apply to the plate 1 µl of test solution (a), 1 µl of test solution (b), 1 µl of reference solution (a), 1 µl of reference solution (b) and 2 µl of reference solution (c). Develop over a path of 15 cm using a mixture of 5 volumes of *concentrated ammonia R*, 20 volumes of *water R* and 75 volumes of *acetonitrile R*. Dry the plate in a current of air. Repeat the development in the same direction, dry the plate in a current of air and spray with *ninhydrin solution R1*. Heat the plate at 110 °C for 10 min. Any spot corresponding to histidine in the chromatogram obtained with test solution (a) is not more intense than the spot in the chromatogram obtained with reference solution (b) (1 per cent). The test is not valid unless the chromatogram obtained with reference solution (c) shows 2 clearly separated spots.

Sulphates (*2.4.13*). 3 ml of solution S diluted to 15 ml with *distilled water R* complies with the limit test for sulphates (0.1 per cent).

Loss on drying (*2.2.32*). Not more than 0.5 per cent, determined on 0.20 g by drying in an oven at 100-105 °C.

Sulphated ash (*2.4.14*). Not more than 0.1 per cent, determined on 0.5 g.

ASSAY

Dissolve 0.080 g in a mixture of 5.0 ml of *0.01 M hydrochloric acid* and 50 ml of *alcohol R*. Carry out a potentiometric titration (*2.2.20*), using *0.1 M sodium hydroxide*. Read the volume added between the first and third points of inflexion.

1 ml of *0.1 M sodium hydroxide* is equivalent to 9.203 mg of $C_5H_{11}Cl_2N_3$.

STORAGE

Store in an airtight container, protected from light.

01/2005:0144

HISTAMINE PHOSPHATE

Histamini phosphas

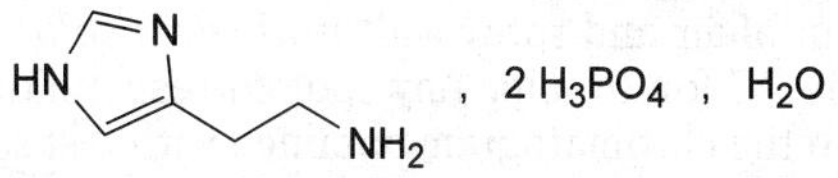

$C_5H_{15}N_3O_8P_2,H_2O$ M_r 325.2

DEFINITION

Histamine phosphate contains not less than 98.0 per cent and not more than the equivalent of 101.0 per cent of 2-(1*H*-imidazol-4-yl)ethanamine diphosphate, calculated with reference to the anhydrous substance.

CHARACTERS

Colourless, long prismatic crystals, freely soluble in water, slightly soluble in alcohol.

IDENTIFICATION

First identification: A, D.

Second identification: B, C, D.

A. Examine by infrared absorption spectrophotometry (*2.2.24*), comparing with the spectrum obtained with *histamine phosphate CRS*. Examine as discs prepared using 1 mg of substance.

B. Examine the chromatograms obtained in the test for histidine. The principal spot in the chromatogram obtained with test solution (b) is similar in position, colour and size to the principal spot in the chromatogram obtained with reference solution (a).

C. Dissolve 0.1 g in 7 ml of *water R* and add 3 ml of a 200 g/l solution of *sodium hydroxide R*. Dissolve 50 mg of *sulphanilic acid R* in a mixture of 0.1 ml of *hydrochloric acid R* and 10 ml of *water R* and add 0.1 ml of *sodium nitrite solution R*. Add the second solution to the first and mix. A red colour is produced.

D. It gives reaction (a) of phosphates (*2.3.1*).

TESTS

Solution S. Dissolve 0.5 g in *carbon dioxide-free water R* prepared from *distilled water R* and dilute to 10 ml with the same solvent.

Appearance of solution. Solution S is clear (*2.2.1*) and not more intensely coloured than reference solution BY_7 (*2.2.2, Method II*).

pH (*2.2.3*). The pH of solution S is 3.75 to 3.95.

Histidine. Examine by thin-layer chromatography (*2.2.27*), using *silica gel G R* as the coating substance.

Test solution (a). Dissolve 0.5 g of the substance to be examined in *water R* and dilute to 10 ml with the same solvent.

Test solution (b). Dilute 2 ml of test solution (a) to 10 ml with *water R*.

Reference solution (a). Dissolve 0.1 g of *histamine phosphate CRS* in *water R* and dilute to 10 ml with the same solvent.

Reference solution (b). Dissolve 50 mg of *histidine monohydrochloride R* in *water R* and dilute to 100 ml with the same solvent.

Reference solution (c). Mix 1 ml of test solution (a) and 1 ml of reference solution (b).

Apply separately to the plate 1 µl of test solution (a), 1 µl of test solution (b), 1 µl of reference solution (a), 1 µl of reference solution (b) and 2 µl of reference solution (c). Develop over a path of 15 cm using a mixture of 5 volumes of *concentrated ammonia R*, 20 volumes of *water R* and 75 volumes of *acetonitrile R*. Dry the plate in a current of air. Repeat the development in the same direction, dry the plate in a current of air and spray with *ninhydrin solution R1*. Heat at 110 °C for 10 min. Any spot corresponding to histidine in the chromatogram obtained with test solution (a) is not more intense than the spot in the chromatogram obtained with reference solution (b) (1 per cent). The test is not valid unless the chromatogram obtained with reference solution (c) shows 2 clearly separated spots.

Sulphates (*2.4.13*). 3 ml of solution S diluted to 15 ml with *distilled water R* complies with the limit test for sulphates (0.1 per cent).

Water (*2.5.12*). 5.0 per cent to 6.2 per cent, determined on 0.30 g by the semi-micro determination of water.

ASSAY

Dissolve 0.140 g in 5 ml of *anhydrous formic acid R* and add 20 ml of *anhydrous acetic acid R*. Titrate with *0.1 M perchloric acid,* determining the end-point potentiometrically (*2.2.20*). Carry out a blank titration.

1 ml of *0.1 M perchloric acid* is equivalent to 15.36 mg of $C_5H_{15}N_3O_8P_2$.

STORAGE

Store protected from light.

Monographs F-H

01/2005:0911

HISTIDINE

Histidinum

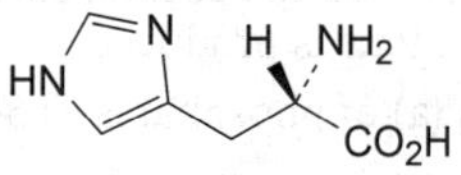

$C_6H_9N_3O_2$ M_r 155.2

DEFINITION

(*S*)-2-Amino-3-(imidazol-4-yl)propanoic acid.

Content: 98.5 per cent to 101.0 per cent (dried substance).

CHARACTERS

Appearance: white, crystalline powder or colourless crystals.

Solubility: soluble in water, very slightly soluble in alcohol.

IDENTIFICATION

First identification: A, B.

Second identification: A, C, D.

A. It complies with the test for specific optical rotation (see Tests).

B. Infrared absorption spectrophotometry (*2.2.24*).

Preparation: discs.

Comparison: *histidine CRS.*

If the spectra obtained show differences, dissolve the substance to be examined and the reference substance separately in the minimum volume of *water R*, evaporate to dryness at 60 °C and record new spectra using the residues.

C. Examine the chromatograms obtained in the test for ninhydrin-positive substances. The principal spot in the chromatogram obtained with test solution (b) is similar in position, colour and size to the principal spot in the chromatogram obtained with reference solution (a).

D. Dissolve 0.1 g in 7 ml of *water R* and add 3 ml of a 200 g/l solution of *sodium hydroxide R*. Dissolve 50 mg of *sulphanilic acid R* in a mixture of 0.1 ml of *hydrochloric acid R* and 10 ml of *water R* and add 0.1 ml of *sodium nitrite solution R*. Add the second solution to the first and mix. An orange-red colour develops.

TESTS

Solution S. Dissolve 2.5 g in *distilled water R*, heating in a water-bath and dilute to 50 ml with the same solvent.

Appearance of solution. Solution S is clear (*2.2.1*) and not more intensely coloured than reference solution BY_7 (*2.2.2, Method II*).

Specific optical rotation (*2.2.7*): + 11.4 to + 12.4 (dried substance).

Dissolve 2.75 g in 12.0 ml of *hydrochloric acid R1* and dilute to 25.0 ml with *water R*.

Ninhydrin-positive substances. Thin-layer chromatography (*2.2.27*).

Test solution (a). Dissolve 0.10 g of the substance to be examined in *water R* and dilute to 10 ml with the same solvent.

Test solution (b). Dilute 1 ml of test solution (a) to 50 ml with *water R*.

Reference solution (a). Dissolve 10 mg of *histidine CRS* in *water R* and dilute to 50 ml with the same solvent.

Reference solution (b). Dilute 5 ml of test solution (b) to 20 ml with *water R*.

Reference solution (c). Dissolve 10 mg of *histidine CRS* and 10 mg of *proline CRS* in *water R* and dilute to 25 ml with the same solvent.

Plate: *TLC silica gel plate R.*

Mobile phase: *glacial acetic acid R, water R, butanol R* (20:20:60 *V/V/V*).

Application: 5 µl.

Development: over 2/3 of the plate.

Drying: in air.

Detection: spray with *ninhydrin solution R* and heat at 100-105 °C for 15 min.

System suitability: the chromatogram obtained with reference solution (c) shows 2 clearly separated spots.

Limits:

– *any impurity*: any spots in the chromatogram obtained with test solution (a), apart from the principal spot, are not more intense than the spot in the chromatogram obtained with reference solution (b) (0.5 per cent).

Chlorides (*2.4.4*): maximum 200 ppm.

Dilute 5 ml of solution S to 15 ml with *water R*.

Sulphates (*2.4.13*): maximum 300 ppm.

Dilute 10 ml of solution S to 15 ml with *distilled water R*.

Ammonium (*2.4.1*): maximum 200 ppm, determined on 50 mg.

Prepare the standard using 0.1 ml of *ammonium standard solution (100 ppm NH_4) R*.

Iron (*2.4.9*): maximum 10 ppm.

In a separating funnel, dissolve 1.0 g in 10 ml of *dilute hydrochloric acid R*. Shake with 3 quantities, each of 10 ml, of *methyl isobutyl ketone R1*, shaking for 3 min each time.

To the combined organic layers add 10 ml of *water R* and shake for 3 min. The aqueous layer complies with the limit test for iron.

Heavy metals (*2.4.8*): maximum 10 ppm.

Dissolve 2.0 g in a mixture of 3 ml of *dilute hydrochloric acid R* and 15 ml of *water R*, with gentle warming if necessary, and dilute to 20 ml with *water R*. 12 ml of the solution complies with limit test A. Prepare the standard using *lead standard solution (1 ppm Pb) R*.

Loss on drying (*2.2.32*): maximum 0.5 per cent, determined on 1.000 g by drying in an oven at 100-105 °C.

Sulphated ash (*2.4.14*): maximum 0.1 per cent, determined on 1.0 g.

ASSAY

Dissolve 0.130 g in 50 ml of *water R*. Titrate with *0.1 M hydrochloric acid*, determining the end-point potentiometrically (*2.2.20*).

1 ml of *0.1 M hydrochloric acid* is equivalent to 15.52 mg of $C_6H_9N_3O_2$.

STORAGE

Protected from light.

01/2005:0910

HISTIDINE HYDROCHLORIDE MONOHYDRATE

Histidini hydrochloridum monohydricum

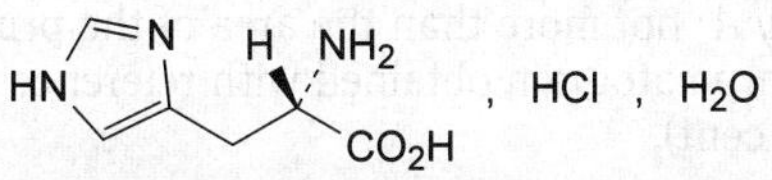

$C_6H_{10}ClN_3O_2,H_2O$ M_r 209.6

DEFINITION

Histidine hydrochloride monohydrate contains not less than 98.5 per cent and not more than the equivalent of 101.0 per cent of the hydrochloride of (*S*)-2-amino-3-(imidazol-4-yl)propanoic acid, calculated with reference to the dried substance.

CHARACTERS

A white, crystalline powder or colourless crystals, freely soluble in water, slightly soluble in alcohol.

IDENTIFICATION

First identification: A, B, C, F.

Second identification: A, B, D, E, F.

A. It complies with the test for specific optical rotation (see Tests).

B. It complies with the test for the pH (see Tests).

C. Examine by infrared absorption spectrophotometry (*2.2.24*), comparing with the spectrum obtained with *histidine hydrochloride monohydrate CRS*. Examine the substances prepared as discs.

D. Examine the chromatograms obtained in the test for ninhydrin-positive substances. The principal spot in the chromatogram obtained with test solution (b) is similar in position, colour and size to the principal spot in the chromatogram obtained with reference solution (a).

E. Dissolve 0.1 g in 7 ml of *water R* and add 3 ml of a 200 g/l solution of *sodium hydroxide R*. Dissolve 50 mg of *sulphanilic acid R* in a mixture of 0.1 ml of *hydrochloric acid R* and 10 ml of *water R* and add 0.1 ml of *sodium nitrite solution R*. Add the second solution to the first and mix. An orange-red colour develops.

F. About 20 mg gives reaction (a) of chlorides (*2.3.1*).

TESTS

Solution S. Dissolve 2.5 g in *carbon dioxide-free water R* prepared from *distilled water R* and dilute to 50 ml with the same solvent.

Appearance of solution. Solution S is clear (*2.2.1*) and not more intensely coloured than reference solution BY_6 (*2.2.2, Method II*).

pH (*2.2.3*). The pH of solution S is 3.0 to 5.0.

Specific optical rotation (*2.2.7*). Dissolve 2.75 g in 12.0 ml of *hydrochloric acid R1* and dilute to 25.0 ml with *water R*. The specific optical rotation is + 9.2 to + 10.6, calculated with reference to the dried substance.

Ninhydrin-positive substances. Examine by thin-layer chromatography (*2.2.27*), using a *TLC silica gel plate R*.

Test solution (a). Dissolve 0.10 g of the substance to be examined in *water R* and dilute to 10 ml with the same solvent.

Test solution (b). Dilute 1 ml of test solution (a) to 50 ml with *water R*.

Reference solution (a). Dissolve 10 mg of *histidine hydrochloride monohydrate CRS* in *water R* and dilute to 50 ml with the same solvent.

Reference solution (b). Dilute 5 ml of test solution (b) to 20 ml with *water R*.

Reference solution (c). Dissolve 10 mg of *histidine hydrochloride monohydrate CRS* and 10 mg of *proline CRS* in *water R* and dilute to 25 ml with the same solvent.

Apply separately to the plate 5 µl of each solution. Dry the plate in a current of air. Develop over a path of 15 cm using a mixture of 20 volumes of *glacial acetic acid R*, 20 volumes of *water R* and 60 volumes of *butanol R*. Allow the plate to dry in air. Spray with *ninhydrin solution R* and heat at 100 °C to 105 °C for 15 min. Any spot in the chromatogram obtained with test solution (a), apart from the principal spot, is not more intense than the spot in the chromatogram obtained with reference solution (b) (0.5 per cent). The test is not valid unless the chromatogram obtained with reference solution (c) shows two clearly separated principal spots.

Sulphates (*2.4.13*). Dilute 10 ml of solution S to 15 ml with *distilled water R*. The solution complies with the limit test for sulphates (300 ppm).

Ammonium (*2.4.1*). 50 mg complies with limit test B for ammonium (200 ppm). Prepare the standard using 0.1 ml of *ammonium standard solution (100 ppm NH_4) R*.

Iron (*2.4.9*). In a separating funnel, dissolve 1.0 g in 10 ml of *dilute hydrochloric acid R*. Shake with three quantities, each of 10 ml, of *methyl isobutyl ketone R1*, shaking for 3 min each time. To the combined organic layers add 10 ml of *water R* and shake for 3 min. The aqueous layer complies with the limit test for iron (10 ppm).

Heavy metals (*2.4.8*). Dissolve 2.0 g in *water R* and dilute to 20 ml with the same solvent. 12 ml of the solution complies with limit test A for heavy metals (10 ppm). Prepare the standard using *lead standard solution (1 ppm Pb) R*.

Loss on drying (*2.2.32*): 7.0 per cent to 10.0 per cent, determined on 1.000 g by drying in an oven at 145 °C to 150 °C.

Sulphated ash (*2.4.14*). Not more than 0.1 per cent, determined on 1.0 g.

ASSAY

Dissolve 0.160 g in 50 ml of *carbon dioxide-free water R*. Titrate with *0.1 M sodium hydroxide*, determining the end-point potentiometrically (*2.2.20*).

1 ml of *0.1 M sodium hydroxide* is equivalent to 19.16 mg of $C_6H_{10}ClN_3O_2$.

STORAGE

Store protected from light.

01/2005:0500

HOMATROPINE HYDROBROMIDE

Homatropini hydrobromidum

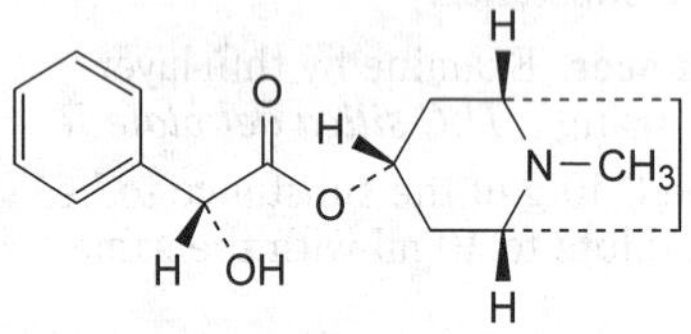

$C_{16}H_{22}BrNO_3$ M_r 356.3

DEFINITION

(1*R*,3*r*,5*S*)-8-Methyl-8-azabicyclo[3.2.1]oct-3-yl (2*RS*)-2-hydroxy-2-phenylacetate hydrobromide.

Content: 99.0 per cent to 101.0 per cent (dried substance).

CHARACTERS

Appearance: white, crystalline powder or colourless crystals.

Solubility: freely soluble in water, sparingly soluble in alcohol.

mp: about 215 °C, with decomposition.

IDENTIFICATION

First identification: A, C.

Second identification: B, C.

A. Infrared absorption spectrophotometry (*2.2.24*).
   Comparison: *homatropine hydrobromide CRS*.

B. Dissolve 50 mg in 1 ml of *water R* and add 2 ml of *dilute acetic acid R*. Heat and add 4 ml of *picric acid solution R*. Allow to cool, shaking occasionally. Collect the crystals, wash with 2 quantities, each of 3 ml, of iced *water R* and dry at 100-105 °C. The crystals melt (*2.2.14*) at 182 °C to 186 °C.

C. It gives reaction (a) of bromides (*2.3.1*).

TESTS

Solution S. Dissolve 1.25 g in *carbon dioxide-free water R* and dilute to 25 ml with the same solvent.

Appearance of solution. Solution S is clear (*2.2.1*) and colourless (*2.2.2, Method II*).

pH (*2.2.3*): 5.0 to 6.5 for solution S.

Related substances. Liquid chromatography (*2.2.29*).

Test solution. Dissolve 50.0 mg of the substance to be examined in the mobile phase and dilute to 25.0 ml with the mobile phase.

Reference solution (a). Dilute 5.0 ml of the test solution to 100.0 ml with the mobile phase. Dilute 5.0 ml of this solution to 50.0 ml with the mobile phase.

Reference solution (b). Dilute 5.0 ml of reference solution (a) to 25.0 ml with the mobile phase.

Reference solution (c). Dissolve 5.0 mg of *hyoscine hydrobromide CRS* in the mobile phase and dilute to 50.0 ml with the mobile phase. To 10.0 ml of this solution add 0.5 ml of the test solution and dilute to 100.0 ml with the mobile phase.

Column:
- *size*: l = 0.1 m, Ø = 4.6 mm,
- *stationary phase*: *octadecylsilyl silica gel for chromatography R* (3 µm),
- *temperature*: 40 °C.

Mobile phase: mix 33 volumes of *methanol R2* and 67 volumes of a solution prepared as follows: dissolve 6.8 g of *potassium dihydrogen phosphate R* and 7.0 g of *sodium heptanesulphonate monohydrate R* in 1000 ml of *water R* and adjust to pH 2.7 with a 330 g/l solution of *phosphoric acid R*.

Flow rate: 1.5 ml/min.

Detection: spectrophotometer at 210 nm.

Injection: 10 µl.

Run time: 3 times the retention time of homatropine.

Relative retention with reference to homatropine (retention time = about 6.8 min): impurity C = about 0.2; impurity A = about 0.9; impurity B = about 1.1; impurity D = about 1.9.

System suitability: reference solution (c):
- *resolution*: minimum 1.5 between the peaks due to homatropine and impurity B,
- *symmetry factor*: maximum 2.5 for the peak due to homatropine.

Limits:
- *impurity A*: not more than the area of the principal peak in the chromatogram obtained with reference solution (a) (0.5 per cent),
- *impurities B, C, D*: for each impurity, not more than the area of the principal peak in the chromatogram obtained with reference solution (b) (0.1 per cent),
- *any other impurity*: for each impurity, not more than the area of the principal peak in the chromatogram obtained with reference solution (b) (0.1 per cent),
- *total*: not more than twice the area of the principal peak in the chromatogram obtained with reference solution (a) (1.0 per cent); disregard the peak due to the bromide ion which appears close to the peak due to the solvent,
- *disregard limit*: 0.5 times the area of the principal peak in the chromatogram obtained with reference solution (b) (0.05 per cent).

Loss on drying (*2.2.32*): maximum 0.5 per cent, determined on 1.000 g by drying in an oven at 100-105 °C.

Sulphated ash (*2.4.14*): maximum 0.1 per cent, determined on 1.0 g.

ASSAY

Dissolve 0.300 g in a mixture of 5.0 ml of *0.01 M hydrochloric acid* and 50 ml of *alcohol R*. Carry out a potentiometric titration (*2.2.20*), using *0.1 M sodium hydroxide*. Read the volume added between the 2 points of inflexion.

1 ml of *0.1 M sodium hydroxide* is equivalent to 35.63 mg of $C_{16}H_{22}BrNO_3$.

STORAGE

Protected from light.

IMPURITIES

Specified impurities: A, B, C, D.

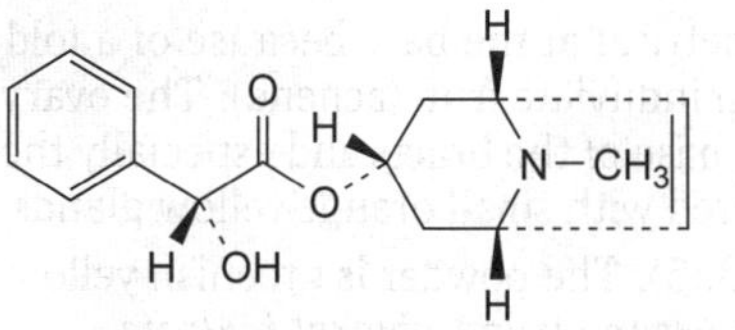

A. (1*R*,3*s*,5*S*)-8-methyl-8-azabicyclo[3.2.1]oct-6-en-3-yl (2*RS*)-2-hydroxy-2-phenylacetate (dehydrohomatropine),

B. hyoscine,

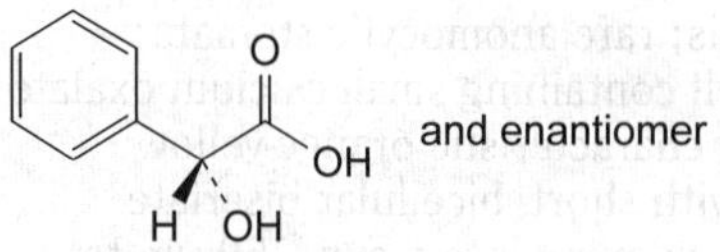

C. (2*RS*)-2-hydroxy-2-phenylacetic acid (mandelic acid),

D. atropine.

01/2005:0720

HOMATROPINE METHYLBROMIDE

Homatropini methylbromidum

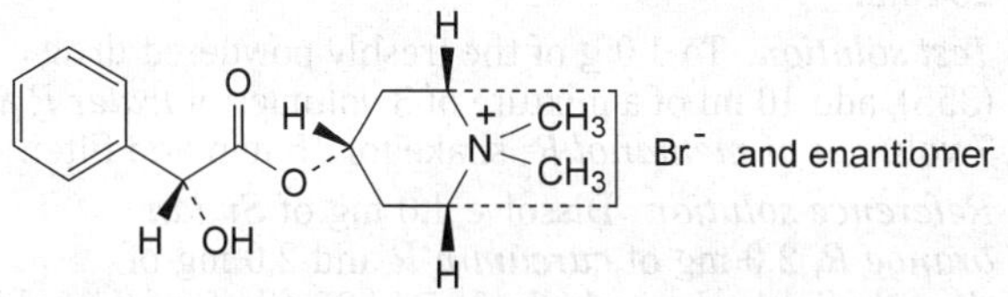

$C_{17}H_{24}BrNO_3$ M_r 370.3

DEFINITION

(1*R*,3*r*,5*S*)-3-[[(2*RS*)-2-hydroxy-2-phenylacetyl]oxy]-8,8-dimethyl-8-azoniabicyclo[3.2.1]octane bromide.

Content: 98.5 per cent to 101.0 per cent (dried substance).

CHARACTERS

Appearance: white, crystalline powder or colourless crystals.

Solubility: freely soluble in water, soluble in alcohol.

mp: about 190 °C.

IDENTIFICATION

First identification: A, C.

Second identification: B, C.

A. Infrared absorption spectrophotometry (*2.2.24*).
Comparison: *homatropine methylbromide CRS*.

B. Dissolve 50 mg in 1 ml of *water R* and add 2 ml of *dilute acetic acid R*. Heat and add 4 ml of *picric acid solution R*. Allow to cool, shaking occasionally. The crystals, washed with 2 quantities, each of 3 ml, of iced *water R* and dried at 100-105 °C melt (*2.2.14*) at 132 °C to 138 °C.

C. It gives reaction (a) of bromides (*2.3.1*).

TESTS

Solution S. Dissolve 1.25 g in *carbon dioxide-free water R* and dilute to 25 ml with the same solvent.

Appearance of solution. Solution S is clear (*2.2.1*) and colourless (*2.2.2, Method II*).

pH (*2.2.3*): 4.5 to 6.5 for solution S.

Related substances. Liquid chromatography (*2.2.29*).

Solvent mixture: *acetonitrile R*, mobile phase A (9:41 *V/V*).

Test solution. Dissolve 50.0 mg of the substance to be examined in the solvent mixture and dilute to 25.0 ml with the solvent mixture.

Reference solution (a). Dilute 5.0 ml of the test solution to 100.0 ml with the solvent mixture. Dilute 5.0 ml of the solution to 50.0 ml with the solvent mixture.

Reference solution (b). Dilute 5.0 ml of reference solution (a) to 25.0 ml with the solvent mixture.

Reference solution (c). Dissolve 5.0 mg of *homatropine hydrobromide CRS* in the solvent mixture and dilute to 50.0 ml with the solvent mixture. To 10.0 ml of the solution add 0.5 ml of the test solution and dilute to 100.0 ml with the solvent mixture.

Column:

- *size*: *l* = 0.15 m, Ø = 4.6 mm,
- *stationary phase*: *octadecylsilyl silica gel for chromatography R* (3 µm),
- *temperature*: 25 °C.

Mobile phase:

- *mobile phase A*: dissolve 3.4 g of *potassium dihydrogen phosphate R* and 5.0 g of *sodium heptanesulphonate monohydrate R* in 1000 ml of *water R*, and adjust to pH 3.0 with a 330 g/l solution of *phosphoric acid R*,
- *mobile phase B*: mix 400 ml of mobile phase A and 600 ml of *acetonitrile R*,

Time (min)	Mobile phase A (per cent *V/V*)	Mobile phase B (per cent *V/V*)
0 - 2	70	30
2 - 15	70 → 30	30 → 70
15 - 20	30 → 70	70 → 30

Flow rate: 1.4 ml/min.

Detection: spectrophotometer at 210 nm.

Injection: 10 µl.

Relative retention with reference to homatropine methylbromide (retention time = about 4.8 min): impurity C = about 0.7; impurity A = about 0.9; impurity B = about 1.2; impurity D = about 1.3; impurity E = about 1.4; impurity F = about 1.7.

System suitability: reference solution (c):

- *resolution*: minimum 2.5 between the peaks due to homatropine methylbromide and impurity B,
- *symmetry factor*: maximum 2.5 for the peak due to homatropine methylbromide.

Limits:

- *impurities A, B*: for each impurity, not more than the area of the principal peak in the chromatogram obtained with reference solution (a) (0.5 per cent),
- *impurities C, D, E, F*: for each impurity, not more than the area of the principal peak in the chromatogram obtained with reference solution (b) (0.1 per cent),
- *any other impurity*: for each impurity, not more than the area of the principal peak in the chromatogram obtained with reference solution (b) (0.1 per cent),
- *total*: not more than twice the area of the principal peak in the chromatogram obtained with reference solution (a) (1.0 per cent); disregard the peak due to the bromide ion which appears close to the peak due to the solvent,
- *disregard limit*: 0.5 times the area of the principal peak in the chromatogram obtained with reference solution (b) (0.05 per cent).

Loss on drying (*2.2.32*): maximum 0.5 per cent, determined on 1.000 g by drying in an oven at 100-105 °C.

Sulphated ash (*2.4.14*): maximum 0.1 per cent, determined on 1.0 g.

ASSAY

Dissolve 0.300 g in 10 ml of *water R*. Titrate with *0.1 M silver nitrate*. Determine the end-point potentiometrically (*2.2.20*), using a silver indicator electrode and a silver-silver chloride reference electrode.

1 ml of *0.1 M silver nitrate* is equivalent to 37.03 mg of $C_{17}H_{24}BrNO_3$.

STORAGE

Protected from light.

IMPURITIES

Specified impurities: A, B, C, D, E, F.

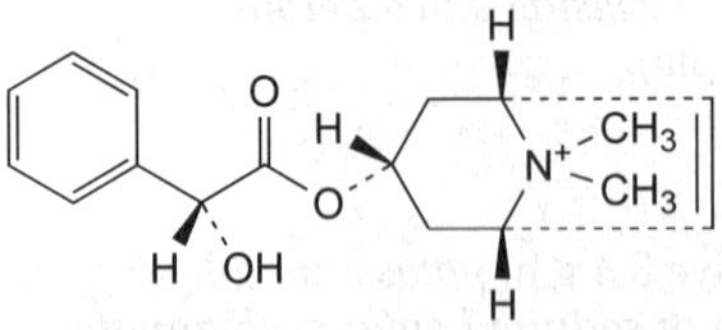

A. (1*R*,3*s*,5*S*)-3-[[(2*RS*)-2-hydroxy-2-phenylacetyl]oxy]-8,8-dimethyl-8-azoniabicyclo[3.2.1]oct-6-ene (methyldehydrohomatropine),

B. homatropine,

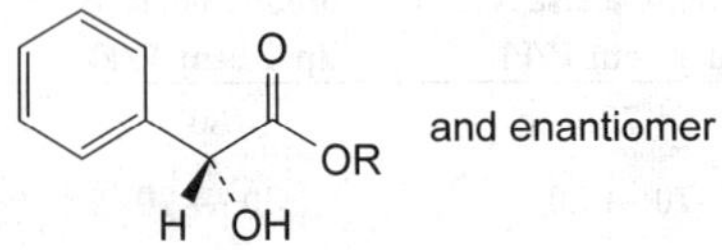

C. R = H: (2*RS*)-2-hydroxy-2-phenylacetic acid (mandelic acid),

F. R = CH_3: methyl (2*RS*)-2-hydroxy-2-phenylacetate (methyl mandelate),

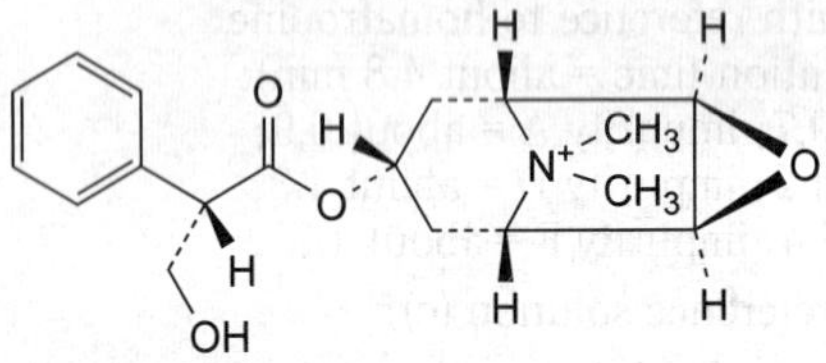

D. (1*R*,2*R*,4*S*,5*S*,7*s*)-7-[[(2*S*)-3-hydroxy-2-phenylpropanoyl]oxy]-9,9-dimethyl-3-oxa-9-azoniatricyclo[3.3.1.0^{2,4}]nonane (methylhyoscine),

E. methylatropine.

01/2005:1222

HOP STROBILE

Lupuli flos

DEFINITION

Hop strobile consists of the dried, generally whole, female inflorescences of *Humulus lupulus* L.

CHARACTERS

It has a characteristic, aromatic odour.

It has the macroscopic and microscopic characters described in identification tests A and B.

IDENTIFICATION

A. Hop strobiles are generally isolated and 2 cm to 5 cm long, petiolate, ovoid, made up of many oval, greenish-yellow, sessile, membranous, overlapping bracts. The external bracts are flattened and symmetrical. The internal bracts are longer and asymmetrical at the base because of a fold generally encircling an induviate fruit (achene). The ovary or rarely the fruit, the base of the bracts and especially the induvial fold, are covered with small orange-yellow glands.

B. Reduce to a powder (355). The powder is greenish-yellow. Examine under a microscope using *chloral hydrate solution R*. The powder shows the following diagnostic characters: fragments of bracts and bracteoles covered by polygonal, irregular epidermal cells with wavy walls; unicellular, conical, straight or curved covering trichomes with thin, smooth walls; rare anomocytic stomata; fragments of mesophyll containing small calcium oxalate cluster crystals; many characteristic orange-yellow glandular trichomes with short, bicellular biseriate stalks, bearing a part widening into a cup, 150 µm to 250 µm in diameter, made up of a hemispherical layer of secretory cells with a cuticle that has been detached and distended by the accumulation of oleoresinous secretions; fragments of elongated sclerenchymatous cells of the testa with thick walls showing striations and numerous pits.

C. Examine by thin-layer chromatography (*2.2.27*), using as the coating substance a suitable silica gel with a fluorescent indicator having an optimal intensity at 254 nm.

Test solution. To 1.0 g of the freshly powdered drug (355), add 10 ml of a mixture of 3 volumes of *water R* and 7 volumes of *methanol R*; shake for 15 min and filter.

Reference solution. Dissolve 1.0 mg of *Sudan orange R*, 2.0 mg of *curcumin R* and 2.0 mg of *dimethylaminobenzaldehyde R* in 20 ml of *methanol R*.

Apply to the plate as bands, 20 µl of each solution. Develop over a path of 15 cm using a mixture of 2 volumes of *anhydrous acetic acid R*, 38 volumes of *ethyl acetate R* and 60 volumes of *cyclohexane R*. Allow the plate to dry in air and examine in ultraviolet light at 254 nm. The chromatogram obtained with the reference solution shows three quenching bands; in the lower quarter is the faint curcumin band, somewhat below the middle is the dimethylaminobenzaldehyde band and above the band due to Sudan orange. The chromatogram obtained with the test solution shows a number of quenching bands similar in position to the bands in the chromatogram obtained with the reference solution; at about the level of curcumin is a faint band due to xanthohumol, near the level of dimethylaminobenzaldehyde are bands due to humulones, and near the level of Sudan orange are bands due to lupulones. Examine in ultraviolet light at 365 nm. In the chromatogram obtained with the test solution the bands due to lupulones show blue fluorescence, the bands due to humulones brown fluorescence and the band due to xanthohumol dark brown fluorescence. Spray with *dilute phosphomolybdotungstic reagent R*. Expose the plate to ammonia vapour. Examine in daylight. In the chromatogram obtained with the test solution, the bands due to humulones and to lupulones are bluish-grey and the band due to xanthohumol is greenish-grey. In the chromatogram obtained with the reference solution, the bands are bluish-grey to brownish-grey.

TESTS

Foreign matter (*2.8.2*). It complies with the test for foreign matter.

Matter extractable by alcohol (70 per cent *V/V*). To 10.0 g of the powdered drug (355) add 300 ml of *alcohol (70 per cent V/V) R* and heat for 10 min on a water bath under a reflux condenser. Allow to cool, filter and discard the first 10 ml of the filtrate. Evaporate 30.0 ml of the filtrate to dryness on a water-bath and dry in an oven at 100 °C to 105 °C for 2 h. The mass of the residue is not less than 0.250 g (25.0 per cent).

Loss on drying (*2.2.32*). Not more than 10.0 per cent, determined on 1.000 g of the powdered drug (355) by drying in an oven at 100 °C to 105 °C for 2 h.

Total ash (*2.4.16*). Not more than 12.0 per cent.

STORAGE

Store protected from light.

01/2005:0255

HUMAN ALBUMIN SOLUTION

Albumini humani solutio

DEFINITION

Human albumin solution is an aqueous solution of protein obtained from plasma that complies with the requirements of the monograph on *Plasma for fractionation, human (0853)*.

PRODUCTION

Separation of the albumin is carried out under controlled conditions, particularly of pH, ionic strength and temperature so that in the final product not less than 95 per cent of the total protein is albumin. Human albumin solution is prepared as a concentrated solution containing 150 g/l to 250 g/l of total protein or as an isotonic solution containing 35 g/l to 50 g/l of total protein. A suitable stabiliser against the effects of heat, such as sodium caprylate (sodium octanoate) or *N*-acetyltryptophan or a combination of these two, at a suitable concentration, may be added but no antimicrobial preservative is added at any stage during preparation. The solution is passed through a bacteria-retentive filter and distributed aseptically into sterile containers which are then closed so as to prevent contamination. The solution in its final container is heated to 60 ± 1.0 °C and maintained at this temperature for not less than 10 h. The containers are then incubated at 30-32 °C for not less than 14 days or at 20-25 °C for not less than 4 weeks and examined visually for evidence of microbial contamination.

CHARACTERS

A clear, slightly viscous liquid; it is almost colourless, yellow, amber or green.

IDENTIFICATION

Examine by a suitable immunoelectrophoresis technique. Using antiserum to normal human serum, compare normal human serum and the preparation to be examined, both diluted to contain 10 g/l of protein. The main component of the preparation to be examined corresponds to the main component of normal human serum. The preparation may show the presence of small quantities of other plasma proteins.

TESTS

pH (*2.2.3*): 6.7 to 7.3.

Dilute the preparation to be examined with a 9 g/l solution of *sodium chloride R* to obtain a solution containing 10 g/l of protein.

Total protein. Dilute the preparation to be examined with a 9 g/l solution of *sodium chloride R* to obtain a solution containing about 15 mg of protein in 2 ml. To 2.0 ml of this solution in a round-bottomed centrifuge tube add 2 ml of a 75 g/l solution of *sodium molybdate R* and 2 ml of a mixture of 1 volume of *nitrogen-free sulphuric acid R* and 30 volumes of *water R*. Shake, centrifuge for 5 min, decant the supernatant liquid and allow the inverted tube to drain on filter paper. Determine the nitrogen in the residue by the method of sulphuric acid digestion (*2.5.9*) and calculate the quantity of protein by multiplying by 6.25. The preparation contains not less than 95 per cent and not more than 105 per cent of the quantity of protein stated on the label.

Protein composition. Zone electrophoresis (*2.2.31*).

Use strips of suitable cellulose acetate gel as the supporting medium and *barbital buffer solution pH 8.6 R1* as the electrolyte solution.

Test solution. Dilute the preparation to be examined with a 9 g/l solution of *sodium chloride R* to a protein concentration of 20 g/l.

Reference solution. Dilute *human albumin for electrophoresis BRP* with a 9 g/l solution of *sodium chloride R* to a protein concentration of 20 g/l.

To a strip apply 2.5 µl of the test solution as a 10 mm band or apply 0.25 µl per millimetre if a narrower strip is used. To another strip, apply in the same manner the same volume of the reference solution. Apply a suitable electric field such that the most rapid band migrates at least 30 mm. Treat the strips with *amido black 10B solution R* for 5 min. Decolorise with a mixture of 10 volumes of *glacial acetic acid R* and 90 volumes of *methanol R* until the background is just free of colour. Develop the transparency of the strips with a mixture of 19 volumes of *glacial acetic acid R* and 81 volumes of *methanol R*. Measure the absorbance of the bands at 600 nm in an instrument having a linear response over the range of measurement. Calculate the result as the mean of 3 measurements of each strip. In the electropherogram obtained with the test solution, not more than 5 per cent of the protein has a mobility different from that of the principal band. The test is not valid unless, in the electropherogram obtained with the reference preparation, the proportion of protein in the principal band is within the limits stated in the leaflet accompanying the reference preparation.

Molecular size distribution. Liquid chromatography (*2.2.29*).

Test solution. Dilute the preparation to be examined with a 9 g/l solution of *sodium chloride R* to a concentration suitable for the chromatographic system used. A concentration in the range 4 g/l to 12 g/l and injection of 50 µg to 600 µg of protein are usually suitable.

Column:

- *size*: l = 0.6 m, Ø = 7.5 mm,
- *stationary phase*: *hydrophilic silica gel for chromatography R*, of a grade suitable for fractionation of globular proteins with relative molecular masses in the range 10 000 to 500 000.

Mobile phase: dissolve 4.873 g of *disodium hydrogen phosphate dihydrate R*, 1.741 g of *sodium dihydrogen phosphate monohydrate R*, 11.688 g of *sodium chloride R* and 50 mg of *sodium azide R* in 1 litre of *water R*.

Flow rate: 0.5 ml/min.

Detection: spectrophotometer at 280 nm.

The peak due to polymers and aggregates is located in the part of the chromatogram representing the void volume. Disregard the peak due to the stabiliser. The area of the peak due to polymers and aggregates is not greater than 10 per cent of the total area of the chromatogram (corresponding to about 5 per cent of polymers and aggregates).

Monographs F-H

Haem. Dilute the preparation to be examined using a 9 g/l solution of *sodium chloride R* to obtain a solution containing 10 g/l of protein. The absorbance (*2.2.25*) of the solution measured at 403 nm using *water R* as the compensation liquid is not greater than 0.15.

Prekallikrein activator (*2.6.15*): maximum 35 IU/ml.

Aluminium: maximum 200 µg of Al per litre.

Atomic absorption spectrometry (*2.2.23, Method I*). Use a furnace as atomic generator. *Use plastic containers for preparation of the solutions. Wash equipment in nitric acid (200 g/l* HNO_3*) before use.*

Test solution. Use the preparation to be examined.

Validation solution. Use *human albumin for aluminium validation BRP*.

Reference solutions. Prepare a suitable range of reference solutions by adding suitable volumes of *aluminium standard solution (10 ppm Al) R* to known volumes of *water R*. Dilute the solutions as necessary using nitric acid (10 g/l HNO_3) containing 1.7 g/l of *magnesium nitrate R* and 0.05 per cent *V/V* of *octoxinol 10 R*. Measure the absorbance at 309.3 nm. The test is not valid unless the aluminium content determined for *human albumin for aluminium validation BRP* is within 20 per cent of the value stated in the leaflet accompanying the reference preparation.

Potassium: maximum 0.05 mmol of K per gram of protein. Atomic emission spectrometry (*2.2.22, Method I*).

Wavelength: 766.5 nm.

Sodium: maximum 160 mmol of Na per litre and not less than 95 per cent and not more than 105 per cent of the content of Na stated on the label. Atomic emission spectrometry (*2.2.22, Method I*).

Wavelength: 589 nm.

Sterility (*2.6.1*). It complies with the test for sterility.

Pyrogens (*2.6.8*). It complies with the test for pyrogens. For a solution containing 35 g/l to 50 g/l of protein, inject per kilogram of the rabbit's mass 10 ml of the preparation to be examined. For a solution containing 150 g/l to 250 g/l of protein, inject per kilogram of the rabbit's mass 5 ml of the preparation to be examined.

STORAGE

Protected from light.

LABELLING

The label states:

- the name of the preparation,
- the volume of the preparation,
- the content of protein expressed in grams per litre,
- the content of sodium expressed in millimoles per litre,
- that the product is not to be used if it is cloudy or if a deposit has formed,
- the name and concentration of any added substance (for example stabiliser).

Monographs F-H

01/2005:0557

HUMAN ANTI-D IMMUNOGLOBULIN

Immunoglobulinum humanum anti-D

DEFINITION

Human anti-D immunoglobulin is a liquid or freeze-dried preparation containing immunoglobulins, mainly immunoglobulin G. The preparation is intended for intramuscular administration. It contains specific antibodies against erythrocyte D-antigen and may also contain small quantities of other blood-group antibodies. *Human normal immunoglobulin (0338)* may be added.

It complies with the monograph on *Human normal immunoglobulin (0338)*, except for the minimum number of donors and the minimum total protein content. For products prepared by a method that eliminates immunoglobulins with specificities other than anti-D, where authorised, the test for antibodies to hepatitis B surface antigen is not required.

PRODUCTION

Human anti-D immunoglobulin is preferably obtained from the plasma of donors with a sufficient titre of previously acquired anti-D antibodies. Where necessary, in order to ensure an adequate supply of human anti-D immunoglobulin, it is obtained from plasma derived from donors immunised with D-positive erythrocytes that are compatible in relevant blood group systems in order to avoid formation of undesirable antibodies.

ERYTHROCYTE DONORS

Erythrocyte donors complies with the requirements for donors prescribed in the monograph *Human plasma for fractionation (0853)*.

IMMUNISATION

Immunisation of the plasma donor is carried out under proper medical supervision. Recommendations concerning donor immunisation, including testing of erythrocyte donors, have been formulated by the World Health Organisation (*Requirements for the collection, processing and quality control of blood, blood components and plasma derivatives*, WHO Technical Report Series, No. 840, 1994 or subsequent revision).

POOLED PLASMA

To limit the potential B19 virus burden in plasma pools used for the manufacture of anti-D immunoglobulin, the plasma pool is tested for B19 virus using validated nucleic acid amplification techniques (*2.6.21*).

B19 virus DNA: maximum 10^4 IU/ml.

A positive control with 10^4 IU of B19 virus DNA per millilitre and, to test for inhibitors, an internal control prepared by addition of a suitable marker to a sample of the plasma pool are included in the test. The test is invalid if the positive control is non-reactive or if the result obtained with the internal control indicates the presence of inhibitors.

B19 virus DNA for NAT testing BRP is suitable for use as a positive control.

If *Human normal immunoglobulin (0338)* is added to the preparation, the plasma pool from which it is derived complies with the above requirement for B19 virus DNA.

POTENCY

Carry out the assay of human anti-D immunoglobulin (*2.7.13, Method A*). The estimated potency is not less than 90 per cent of the stated potency. The confidence limits ($P = 0.95$) are not less than 80 per cent and not more than 120 per cent of the estimated potency.

Method B or C (*2.7.13*) may be used for potency determination if a satisfactory correlation with the results obtained by Method A has been established for the particular product.

STORAGE

See *Human normal immunoglobulin (0338)*.

LABELLING

See *Human normal immunoglobulin (0338)*.

The label states the number of International Units per container.

01/2005:1527
corrected

HUMAN ANTI-D IMMUNOGLOBULIN FOR INTRAVENOUS ADMINISTRATION

Immunoglobulinum humanum anti-D ad usum intravenosum

DEFINITION

Human anti-D immunoglobulin for intravenous administration is a liquid or freeze-dried preparation containing immunoglobulins, mainly immunoglobulin G. It contains specific antibodies against erythrocyte D-antigen and may also contain small quantities of other blood-group antibodies. *Human normal immunoglobulin for intravenous administration (0918)* may be added.

It complies with the monograph on *Human normal immunoglobulin for intravenous administration (0918)*, except for the minimum number of donors, the minimum total protein content, the limit for osmolality and the limit for prekallikrein activator. For products prepared by a method that eliminates immunoglobulins with specificities other than anti-D: where authorised, the test for antibodies to hepatitis B surface antigen is not required; a suitable test for Fc function is carried out instead of that described in chapter *2.7.9*, which is not applicable to such a product.

PRODUCTION

Human anti-D immunoglobulin is preferably obtained from the plasma of donors with a sufficient titre of previously acquired anti-D antibodies. Where necessary, in order to ensure an adequate supply of human anti-D immunoglobulin, it is obtained from plasma derived from donors immunised with D-positive erythrocytes that are compatible in relevant blood group systems in order to avoid formation of undesirable antibodies.

ERYTHROCYTE DONORS

Erythrocyte donors comply with the requirements for donors prescribed in the monograph *Human plasma for fractionation (0853)*.

IMMUNISATION

Immunisation of the plasma donor is carried out under proper medical supervision. Recommendations concerning donor immunisation, including testing of erythrocyte donors, have been formulated by the World Health Organisation (***Requirements for the collection, processing and quality control of blood, blood components and plasma derivatives,*** WHO Technical Report Series, No. 840, 1994 or subsequent revision).

POOLED PLASMA

To limit the potential B19 virus burden in plasma pools used for the manufacture of anti-D immunoglobulin, the plasma pool is tested for B19 virus using validated nucleic acid amplification techniques (*2.6.21*).

B19 virus DNA: maximum 10^4 IU/ml.

A positive control with 10^4 IU of B19 virus DNA per millilitre and, to test for inhibitors, an internal control prepared by addition of a suitable marker to a sample of the plasma pool are included in the test. The test is invalid if the positive control is non-reactive or if the result obtained with the internal control indicates the presence of inhibitors.

B19 virus DNA for NAT testing BRP is suitable for use as a positive control.

If *Human normal immunoglobulin for intravenous administration (0918)* is added to the preparation, the plasma pool from which it is derived complies with the above requirement for B19 virus DNA.

POTENCY

Carry out the assay of human anti-D immunoglobulin (*2.7.13, Method A*). The estimated potency is not less than 90 per cent of the stated potency. The confidence limits (P = 0.95) are not less than 80 per cent and not more than 120 per cent of the estimated potency.

Method B or C (*2.7.13*) may be used for potency determination if a satisfactory correlation with the results obtained by Method A has been established for the particular product.

STORAGE

See *Human normal immunoglobulin for intravenous administration (0918)*.

LABELLING

See *Human normal immunoglobulin for intravenous administration (0918)*.

The label states the number of International Units per container.

01/2005:0878

HUMAN ANTITHROMBIN III CONCENTRATE

Antithrombinum III humanum densatum

DEFINITION

Human antithrombin III concentrate is a preparation of a glycoprotein fraction obtained from human plasma that inactivates thrombin in the presence of an excess of heparin. It is obtained from plasma that complies with the requirements of the monograph on *Human plasma for fractionation (0853)*.

When reconstituted in the volume of solvent stated on the label, the potency is not less than 25 IU of antithrombin III per millilitre.

PRODUCTION

The method of preparation includes a step or steps that have been shown to remove or to inactivate known agents of infection; if substances are used for inactivation of viruses during production, the subsequent purification procedure must be validated to demonstrate that the concentration of these substances is reduced to a suitable level and any residues are such as not to compromise the safety of the preparation for patients.

The antithrombin III is purified and concentrated and a suitable stabiliser may be added. The specific activity is not less than 3 IU of antithrombin III per milligram of total protein, excluding albumin. The antithrombin III concentrate is passed through a bacteria-retentive filter, distributed aseptically into its final, sterile containers and immediately frozen. It is then freeze-dried and the containers are closed under vacuum or in an atmosphere of inert gas. No antimicrobial preservative is added at any stage of production.

Monographs F-H

VALIDATION TEST

It shall be demonstrated that the manufacturing process yields a product that consistently complies with the following test.

Heparin-binding fraction. Examine by agarose gel electrophoresis (*2.2.31*). Prepare a 10 g/l solution of *agarose for electrophoresis R* containing 15 IU of *heparin R* per millilitre in *barbital buffer solution pH 8.4 R*. Pour 5 ml of this solution onto a glass plate 5 cm square. Cool at 4 °C for 30 min. Cut 2 wells 2 mm in diameter 1 cm and 4 cm from the side of the plate and 1 cm from the cathode. Introduce into one well 5 µl of the preparation to be examined, diluted to an activity of about 1 IU of antithrombin III per millilitre. Introduce into the other well 5 µl of a solution of a marker dye such as *bromophenol blue R*. Allow the electrophoresis to proceed at 4 °C, using a constant electric field of 7 V/cm, until the dye reaches the anode.

Cut across the agarose gel 1.5 cm from that side of the plate on which the preparation to be examined was applied and remove the larger portion of the gel leaving a band 1.5 cm wide containing the material to be examined. Replace the removed portion with an even layer consisting of 3.5 ml of a 10 g/l solution of *agarose for electrophoresis R* in *barbital buffer solution pH 8.4 R*, containing a rabbit anti-human antithrombin III antiserum at a suitable concentration, previously determined, to give adequate peak heights of at least 1.5 cm. Place the plate with the original gel at the cathode so that a second electrophoretic migration can occur at right angles to the first. Allow this second electrophoresis to proceed using a constant electric field of 2 V/cm for 16 h. Cover the plates with filter paper and several layers of thick lint soaked in a 9 g/l solution of *sodium chloride R* and compress for 2 h, renewing the saline several times. Rinse with *water R*, dry the plates and stain with *acid blue 92 solution R*.

Calculate the fraction of antithrombin III bound to heparin, which is the peak closest to the anode, with respect to the total amount of antithrombin III, by measuring the area defined by the 2 precipitation peaks.

The fraction of antithrombin III able to bind to heparin is not less than 60 per cent.

CHARACTERS

A white, hygroscopic, friable solid or a powder.

Reconstitute the preparation to be examined as stated on the label immediately before carrying out the identification, the tests (except those for solubility, total protein and water), and the assay.

IDENTIFICATION

It complies with the limits of the assay.

TESTS

pH (*2.2.3*): 6.0 to 7.5.

Solubility. It dissolves completely under gentle swirling within 10 min in the volume of the solvent stated on the label, forming a clear or slightly turbid, colourless solution.

Osmolality (*2.2.35*): minimum 240 mosmol/kg.

Total protein. If necessary, dilute an accurately measured volume of the preparation to be examined with *water R* to obtain a solution containing about 15 mg of protein in 2 ml. To 2.0 ml of the solution in a round-bottomed centrifuge tube add 2 ml of a 75 g/l solution of *sodium molybdate R* and 2 ml of a mixture of 1 volume of *nitrogen-free sulphuric acid R* and 30 volumes of *water R*. Shake, centrifuge for 5 min, decant the supernatant liquid and allow the inverted tube to drain on filter paper. Determine the nitrogen in the residue by the method of sulphuric acid digestion (*2.5.9*) and calculate the amount of protein by multiplying the result by 6.25.

Heparin (*2.7.5*): maximum 0.1 IU of heparin activity per International Unit of antithrombin III activity. It is necessary to validate the method for assay of heparin for each specific preparation to be examined to allow for interference by antithrombin III.

Water. Determined by a suitable method, such as the semi-micro determination of water (*2.5.12*), loss on drying (*2.2.32*) or near infrared spectrophotometry (*2.2.40*), the water content is within the limits approved by the competent authority.

Sterility (*2.6.1*). It complies with the test for sterility.

Pyrogens (*2.6.8*). It complies with the test for pyrogens. Inject per kilogram of the rabbit's mass a volume of the preparation to be examined equivalent to 50 IU of antithrombin III, calculated from the activity stated on the label.

ASSAY

Assay of human antithrombin III (*2.7.17*).

The estimated potency is not less than 80 per cent and not more than 120 per cent of the potency stated on the label. The confidence limits ($P = 0.95$) are not less than 90 per cent and not more than 110 per cent of the estimated potency.

STORAGE

Protected from light, in an airtight container.

LABELLING

The label states:

- the content of antithrombin III expressed in International Units per container.
- the name and volume of solvent to be used to reconstitute the preparation,
- where applicable, the amount of albumin present as a stabiliser.

01/2005:1224

HUMAN COAGULATION FACTOR VII

Factor VII coagulationis humanus

DEFINITION

Human coagulation factor VII is a plasma protein fraction that contains the single-chain glycoprotein factor VII and may also contain small amounts of the activated form, the two-chain derivative factor VIIa. It may also contain coagulation factors II, IX and X and protein C and protein S. It is obtained from human plasma that complies with the monograph on *Human plasma for fractionation (0853)*.

The potency of the preparation, reconstituted as stated on the label, is not less than 15 IU of factor VII per millilitre.

PRODUCTION

The method of preparation is designed to minimise activation of any coagulation factor (to minimise potential thrombogenicity) and includes a step or steps that have been shown to remove or to inactivate known agents of infection; if substances are used for inactivation of viruses during production, the subsequent purification procedure must be validated to demonstrate that the concentration of these substances is reduced to a suitable level and that any residues are such as not to compromise the safety of the preparation for patients.

Monographs F-H

The specific activity is not less than 2 IU of factor VII per milligram of total protein, before the addition of any protein stabiliser.

The factor VII fraction is dissolved in a suitable liquid. Heparin, antithrombin and other auxiliary substances such as a stabiliser may be added. No antimicrobial preservative is added. The solution is passed through a bacteria-retentive filter, distributed aseptically into the final containers and immediately frozen. It is subsequently freeze-dried and the containers are closed under vacuum or under an inert gas.

CONSISTENCY OF THE METHOD OF PRODUCTION

The consistency of the method of production with respect to the activities of factors II, IX and X of the preparation, expressed in International Units relative to the activity of factor VII, shall be demonstrated.

The consistency of the method of production with respect to the activity of factor VIIa of the preparation shall be demonstrated. The activity of factor VIIa may be determined, for example, using a recombinant soluble tissue factor that does not activate factor VII but possesses a cofactor function specific for factor VIIa; after incubation of a mixture of the recombinant soluble tissue factor with phospholipids reagent and the dilution of the test sample in factor VII-deficient plasma, calcium chloride is added and the clotting time determined; the clotting time is inversely related to the factor VIIa activity of the test sample.

CHARACTERS

A hygroscopic powder or friable solid that may be white, pale yellow, green or blue.

Reconstitute the preparation to be examined as stated on the label immediately before carrying out the identification, tests (except those for solubility and water) and assay.

IDENTIFICATION

It complies with the limits of the assay.

TESTS

Solubility. To a container of the preparation to be examined add the volume of liquid stated on the label at the recommended temperature. The preparation dissolves completely with gentle swirling within 10 min, giving a clear or slightly opalescent solution that may be coloured.

pH (*2.2.3*): 6.5 to 7.5.

Osmolality (*2.2.35*): minimum 240 mosmol/kg.

Total protein. If necessary, dilute an accurately measured volume of the reconstituted preparation with a 9 g/l solution of *sodium chloride R* to obtain a solution expected to contain about 15 mg of protein in 2 ml. To 2.0 ml of the solution in a round-bottomed centrifuge tube add 2 ml of a 75 g/l solution of *sodium molybdate R* and 2 ml of a mixture of 1 volume of *nitrogen-free sulphuric acid R* and 30 volumes of *water R*. Shake, centrifuge for 5 min, decant the supernatant liquid and allow the inverted tube to drain on filter paper. Determine the nitrogen in the residue by the method of sulphuric acid digestion (*2.5.9*) and calculate the amount of protein by multiplying the result by 6.25.

Activated coagulation factors (*2.6.22*). For each of the dilutions, the coagulation time is not less than 150 s.

Heparin. If heparin has been added during preparation, determine the amount present by the assay of heparin in coagulation factor concentrates (*2.7.12*). The preparation to be examined contains not more than the amount of heparin stated on the label and in any case not more than 0.5 IU of heparin per International Unit of factor VII.

Thrombin. If the preparation to be examined contains heparin, determine the amount present as described in the test for heparin and neutralise the heparin by addition of *protamine sulphate R* (10 µg of protamine sulphate neutralises 1 IU of heparin). In each of 2 test-tubes, mix equal volumes of the reconstituted preparation and a 3 g/l solution of *fibrinogen R*. Keep one of the tubes at 37 °C for 6 h and the other at room temperature for 24 h. In a third tube, mix a volume of the fibrinogen solution with an equal volume of a solution of *human thrombin R* (1 IU/ml) and place the tube in a water-bath at 37 °C. No coagulation occurs in the tubes containing the preparation to be examined. Coagulation occurs within 30 s in the tube containing thrombin.

Factor II. Carry out the assay of human coagulation factor II (*2.7.18*).

The estimated content is not more than 125 per cent of the stated content. The confidence limits ($P = 0.95$) are not less than 90 per cent and not more than 111 per cent of the estimated potency.

Factor IX. Carry out the assay of human coagulation factor IX (*2.7.11*).

The estimated content is not more than 125 per cent of the stated content. The confidence limits ($P = 0.95$) are not less than 80 per cent and not more than 125 per cent of the estimated potency.

Factor X. Carry out the assay of human coagulation factor X (*2.7.19*).

The estimated content is not more than 125 per cent of the stated content. The confidence limits ($P = 0.95$) are not less than 90 per cent and not more than 111 per cent of the estimated potency.

Water. Determined by a suitable method, such as the semi-micro determination of water (*2.5.12*), loss on drying (*2.2.32*) or near-infrared spectrometry (*2.2.40*), the water content is within the limits approved by the competent authority.

Sterility (*2.6.1*). It complies with the test for sterility.

Pyrogens (*2.6.8*). It complies with the test for pyrogens. Inject per kilogram of the rabbit's mass a volume equivalent to not less than 30 IU of factor VII.

ASSAY

Assay of human coagulation factor VII (*2.7.10*).

The estimated potency is not less than 80 per cent and not more than 125 per cent of the stated potency. The confidence limits ($P = 0.95$) are not less than 80 per cent and not more than 125 per cent of the estimated potency.

STORAGE

In an airtight container, protected from light.

LABELLING

The label states:

- the number of International Units of factor VII per container,
- the maximum content of International Units of factor II, factor IX and factor X per container,
- the amount of protein per container,
- the name and quantity of any added substances, including where applicable, heparin,
- the name and volume of the liquid to be used for reconstitution,
- that the transmission of infectious agents cannot be totally excluded when medicinal products prepared from human blood or plasma are administered.

Monographs F-H

01/2005:0275

HUMAN COAGULATION FACTOR VIII

Factor VIII coagulationis humanus

DEFINITION

Human coagulation factor VIII is a plasma protein fraction that contains the glycoprotein coagulation factor VIII together with varying amounts of von Willebrand factor, depending on the method of preparation. It is prepared from human plasma that complies with the monograph on *Human plasma for fractionation (0853)*.

The potency of the preparation, reconstituted as stated on the label, is not less than 20 IU of factor VIII:C per millilitre.

PRODUCTION

The method of preparation includes a step or steps that have been shown to remove or to inactivate known agents of infection; if substances are used for the inactivation of viruses during production, the subsequent purification procedure must be validated to demonstrate that the concentration of these substances is reduced to a suitable level and that any residues are such as not to compromise the safety of the preparation for patients.

The specific activity is not less than 1 IU of factor VIII:C per milligram of total protein before the addition of any protein stabiliser.

The factor VIII fraction is dissolved in a suitable liquid. Auxiliary substances such as a stabiliser may be added. No antimicrobial preservative is added. The solution is passed through a bacteria-retentive filter, distributed aseptically into the final containers and immediately frozen. It is subsequently freeze-dried and the containers are closed under vacuum or under an inert gas.

Validation test applied to products stated to have von Willebrand factor activity. For products intended for treatment of von Willebrand's disease it shall be demonstrated that the manufacturing process yields a product with a consistent composition with respect to von Willebrand factor. This composition may be characterised in a number of ways. For example, the number and the relative amount of the different multimers may be determined by sodium dodecyl sulphate (SDS) agarose gel electrophoresis (about 1 per cent agarose) with or without Western blot analysis on nitrocellulose, using a normal human plasma pool as reference; visualisation of the multimeric pattern may be performed using an immunoenzymatic technique and quantitative evaluation may be carried out by densitometric analysis or by other suitable methods.

von Willebrand factor activity. For products intended for treatment of von Willebrand's disease the von Willebrand factor activity is determined by a suitable method using a reference preparation of the same type as the preparation to be examined, calibrated against the International Standard for von Willebrand factor in plasma. Suitable methods include determination of ristocetin cofactor activity and determination of collagen-binding activity. The following method for determination of ristocetin cofactor activity is given as an example of a suitable method.

Ristocetin cofactor activity. Carry out appropriate dilutions of the preparation to be examined and of the reference preparation using as diluent a solution containing 9 g/l of *sodium chloride R* and 50 g/l of human albumin. Add to each dilution suitable amounts of a von Willebrand reagent containing stabilised human platelets and ristocetin A. Mix on a glass plate by moving it gently in circles for 1 min. Allow to stand for a further 1 min and read the result against a dark background with side lighting. The last dilution which shows clearly visible agglutination indicates the ristocetin cofactor titre of the sample. Use diluent as a negative control.

The estimated potency is not less than 60 per cent and not more than 140 per cent of the potency approved for the particular product.

CHARACTERS

A white or pale yellow, hygroscopic powder or friable solid.

Reconstitute the preparation to be examined as stated on the label immediately before carrying out the identification, tests (except those for solubility and water) and assay.

IDENTIFICATION

It complies with the limits of the assay.

TESTS

pH (*2.2.3*): 6.5 to 7.5.

Solubility. To a container of the preparation to be examined add the volume of the solvent stated on the label at the recommended temperature. The preparation dissolves completely with gentle swirling within 10 min, giving a clear or slightly opalescent, colourless or slightly yellow solution.

Osmolality (*2.2.35*): minimum 240 mosmol/kg.

Total protein. If necessary, dilute an accurately measured volume of the preparation to be examined with a 9 g/l solution of *sodium chloride R* to obtain a solution containing about 15 mg of protein in 2 ml. To 2.0 ml of the solution in a round-bottomed centrifuge tube add 2 ml of a 75 g/l solution of *sodium molybdate R* and 2 ml of a mixture of 1 volume of *nitrogen-free sulphuric acid R* and 30 volumes of *water R*. Shake, centrifuge for 5 min, decant the supernatant liquid and allow the inverted tube to drain on filter paper. Determine the nitrogen in the residue by the method of sulphuric acid digestion (*2.5.9*) and calculate the amount of protein by multiplying the result by 6.25.

For some products, especially those without a protein stabiliser such as albumin, this method may not be applicable and another validated method for protein determination must therefore be performed.

Haemagglutinins anti-A and anti-B. Dilute the preparation with a 9 g/l solution of *sodium chloride R* to contain 3 IU of factor VIII:C per millilitre. Carry out the indirect determination of haemagglutinins A and B (*2.6.20*). The 1 to 64 dilutions do not show agglutination.

Hepatitis B surface antigen. Examine the reconstituted preparation by a suitably sensitive method such as enzyme immunoassay (*2.7.1*). Hepatitis B surface antigen is not detected.

Water. Determined by a suitable method, such as the semi-micro determination of water (*2.5.12*), loss on drying (*2.2.32*) or near infrared spectrophotometry (*2.2.40*), the water content is within the limits approved by the competent authority.

Sterility (*2.6.1*). It complies with the test for sterility.

Pyrogens (*2.6.8*). It complies with the test for pyrogens. Inject per kilogram of the rabbit's mass a volume of the preparation to be examined equivalent to not less than 50 IU of factor VIII:C.

ASSAY

Assay of human coagulation factor VIII (*2.7.4*).

Monographs F-H

The estimated potency is not less than 80 per cent and not more than 120 per cent of the stated potency. The confidence limits ($P = 0.95$) are not less than 80 per cent and not more than 120 per cent of the estimated potency.

STORAGE

In an airtight container, protected from light.

LABELLING

The label states:

- the number of International Units of factor VIII:C and, where applicable, of von Willebrand factor in the container,
- the amount of protein in the container,
- the name and quantity of any added substance,
- the name and volume of the liquid to be used for reconstitution,
- that the transmission of infectious agents cannot be totally excluded when medicinal products prepared from human blood or plasma are administered.

01/2005:1643

HUMAN COAGULATION FACTOR VIII (rDNA)

Factor VIII coagulationis humanus (ADNr)

DEFINITION

Human coagulation factor VIII (rDNA) is a freeze-dried preparation of glycoproteins having the same activity as coagulation factor VIII in human plasma. It acts as a cofactor of the activation of factor X in the presence of factor IXa, phospholipids and calcium ions.

Human coagulation factor VIII circulates in plasma mainly as a two-chain glycosylated protein with 1 heavy (relative molecular mass of about 200 000) and 1 light (relative molecular mass 80 000) chain held together by divalent metal ions. Human coagulation factor VIII (rDNA) is prepared as full-length factor VIII (octocog alfa), or as a shortened two-chain structure (relative molecular mass 90 000 and 80 000), in which the B-domain has been deleted from the heavy chain (moroctocog alfa).

Full-length human rDNA coagulation factor VIII contains 25 potential *N*-glycosylation sites, 19 in the B domain of the heavy chain, 3 in the remaining part of the heavy chain (relative molecular mass 90 000) and 3 in the light chain (relative molecular mass 80 000). The different products are characterised by their molecular size and post-translational modification and/or other modifications.

PRODUCTION

Human coagulation factor VIII (rDNA) is produced by recombinant DNA technology in mammalian cell culture. It is produced under conditions designed to minimise microbial contamination.

Purified bulk factor VIII (rDNA) may contain added human albumin and/or other stabilising agents, as well as other auxiliary substances to provide, for example, correct pH and osmolality.

The specific activity is not less than 2000 IU of factor VIII:C per milligram of total protein before the addition of any protein stabiliser, and varies depending on purity and the type of modification of molecular structure of factor VIII.

The quality of the bulk preparation is controlled using one or more manufacturer's reference preparations as reference.

MANUFACTURER'S REFERENCE PREPARATIONS

During development, reference preparations are established for subsequent verification of batch consistency during production, and for control of bulk and final preparation. They are derived from representative batches of purified bulk factor VIII (rDNA) that are extensively characterised by tests including those described below and whose procoagulant and other relevant functional properties have been ascertained and compared, wherever possible, with the International Standard for factor VIII concentrate. The reference preparations are suitably characterised for their intended purpose and are stored in suitably sized aliquots under conditions ensuring their stability.

PURIFIED BULK FACTOR VIII (rDNA)

The purified bulk complies with a suitable combination of the following tests for characterisation of integrity of the factor VIII (rDNA). Where any substance added during preparation of the purified bulk interferes with a test, the test is carried out before addition of that substance. Where applicable, the characterisation tests may alternatively be carried out on the finished product.

Specific biological activity or ratio of factor VIII activity to factor VIII antigen. Carry out the assay of human coagulation factor VIII (*2.7.4*). The protein content, or where a protein stabiliser is present, the factor VIII antigen content, is determined by a suitable method and the specific biological activity or the ratio of factor VIII activity to factor VIII antigen is calculated.

Protein composition. The protein composition is determined by a selection of appropriate characterisation techniques which may include peptide mapping, Western blots, HPLC, gel electrophoresis, capillary electrophoresis, mass spectrometry or other techniques to monitor integrity and purity. The protein composition is comparable to that of the manufacturer's reference preparation.

Molecular size distribution. Using size-exclusion chromatography (*2.2.30*), the molecular size distribution is comparable to that of the manufacturer's reference preparation.

Peptide mapping (*2.2.55*). There is no significant difference between the test protein and the manufacturer's reference preparation.

Carbohydrates/sialic acid. To monitor batch-to-batch consistency, the monosaccharide content and the degree of sialylation or the oligosaccharide profile are monitored and correspond to those of the manufacturer's reference preparation.

FINAL LOT

It complies with the requirements under Identification, Tests and Assay.

Excipients: 80 per cent to 120 per cent of the stated content, determined by a suitable method, where applicable.

CHARACTERS

Appearance: white or slightly yellow powder or friable mass.

IDENTIFICATION

A. It complies with the limits of the assay.

B. The distribution of characteristic peptide bands corresponds with that of the manufacturer's reference preparation (SDS-PAGE or Western blot).

TESTS

Reconstitute the preparation as stated on the label immediately before carrying out the tests (except those for solubility and water) and assay.

Solubility. It dissolves within 5 min at 20-25 °C, giving a clear or slightly opalescent solution.

pH (*2.2.3*): 6.5 to 7.5.

Osmolality (*2.2.35*): minimum 240 mosmol/kg.

Water. Determined by a suitable method, such as the semi-micro determination of water (*2.5.12*), loss on drying (*2.2.32*) or near infrared spectrophotometry (*2.2.40*), the water content is within the limits approved by the competent authority.

Sterility (*2.6.1*). It complies with the test for sterility.

Bacterial endotoxins (*2.6.14*): less than 3 IU in the volume that contains 100 IU of factor VIII activity.

ASSAY

Carry out the assay of human coagulation factor VIII (*2.7.4*).

The estimated potency is not less than 80 per cent and not more than 125 per cent of the stated potency. The confidence limits ($P = 0.95$) are not less than 80 per cent and not more than 120 per cent of the estimated potency.

STORAGE

Protected from light.

LABELLING

The label states:

- the factor VIII content in International Units,
- the name and amount of any excipient,
- the composition and volume of the liquid to be used for reconstitution.

01/2005:1223

HUMAN COAGULATION FACTOR IX

Factor IX coagulationis humanus

DEFINITION

Human coagulation factor IX is a plasma protein fraction containing coagulation factor IX, prepared by a method that effectively separates factor IX from other prothrombin complex factors (factors II, VII and X). It is obtained from human plasma that complies with the monograph on *Human plasma for fractionation (0853)*.

The potency of the preparation, reconstituted as stated on the label, is not less than 20 IU of factor IX per millilitre.

PRODUCTION

The method of preparation is designed to maintain functional integrity of factor IX, to minimise activation of any coagulation factor (to minimise potential thrombogenicity) and includes a step or steps that have been shown to remove or to inactivate known agents of infection; if substances are used for inactivation of viruses during production, the subsequent purification procedure must be validated to demonstrate that the concentration of these substances is reduced to a suitable level and that any residues are such as not to compromise the safety of the preparation for patients.

The specific activity is not less than 50 IU of factor IX per milligram of total protein, before the addition of any protein stabiliser.

The factor IX fraction is dissolved in a suitable liquid. Heparin, antithrombin and other auxiliary substances such as a stabiliser may be included. No antimicrobial preservative is added. The solution is passed through a bacteria-retentive filter, distributed aseptically into the final containers and immediately frozen. It is subsequently freeze-dried and the containers are closed under vacuum or under an inert gas.

CONSISTENCY OF THE METHOD OF PRODUCTION

The consistency of the method of production is evaluated by suitable analytical procedures that are determined during process development and which normally include:

- assay of factor IX,
- determination of activated coagulation factors,
- determination of activities of factors II, VII and X which shall be shown to be not more than 5 per cent of the activity of factor IX.

CHARACTERS

A white or pale yellow, hygroscopic powder or friable solid.

Reconstitute the preparation to be examined as stated on the label, immediately before carrying out the identification, tests (except those for solubility and water) and assay.

IDENTIFICATION

It complies with the limits of the assay.

TESTS

pH (*2.2.3*): 6.5 to 7.5.

Solubility. To a container of the preparation to be examined add the volume of the liquid stated on the label at the recommended temperature. The preparation dissolves completely with gentle swirling within 10 min, giving a clear or slightly opalescent, colourless solution.

Osmolality (*2.2.35*): minimum 240 mosmol/kg.

Total protein. If necessary, dilute an accurately measured volume of the preparation to be examined with a 9 g/l solution of *sodium chloride R*, to obtain a solution which may be expected to contain about 15 mg of protein in 2 ml. To 2.0 ml of that solution, in a round-bottomed centrifuge tube, add 2 ml of a 75 g/l solution of *sodium molybdate R* and 2 ml of a mixture of 1 volume of *nitrogen-free sulphuric acid R* and 30 volumes of *water R*. Shake, centrifuge for 5 min, decant the supernatant liquid and allow the inverted tube to drain on filter paper. Determine the nitrogen in the residue by the method of sulphuric acid digestion (*2.5.9*) and calculate the amount of protein by multiplying the result by 6.25.

For some products, especially those without a protein stabiliser such as albumin, this method may not be applicable. Another validated method for protein determination must therefore be performed.

Activated coagulation factors (*2.6.22*). If necessary, dilute the preparation to be examined to contain 20 IU of factor IX per millilitre. For each of the dilutions the coagulation time is not less than 150 s.

Heparin. If heparin has been added during preparation, determine the amount by the assay of heparin in coagulation factor concentrates (*2.7.12*). The preparation to be examined contains not more than the amount of heparin stated on the label and in any case not more than 0.5 IU of heparin per International Unit of factor IX.

Water. Determined by a suitable method, such as the semi-micro determination of water (*2.5.12*), loss on drying (*2.2.32*) or near infrared spectrophotometry (*2.2.40*), the water content is within the limits approved by the competent authority.

Sterility (*2.6.1*). It complies with the test for sterility.

Pyrogens (*2.6.8*). It complies with the test for pyrogens. Inject per kilogram of the rabbit's mass a volume equivalent to not less than 50 IU of factor IX.

ASSAY

Assay of human blood coagulation factor IX (*2.7.11*).

The estimated potency is not less than 80 per cent and not more than 125 per cent of the stated potency. The confidence limits ($P = 0.95$) are not less than 80 per cent and not more than 125 per cent of the estimated potency.

STORAGE

In an airtight container, protected from light.

LABELLING

The label states:

- the number of International Units of factor IX per container,
- the amount of protein per container,
- the name and quantity of any added substances including, where applicable, heparin,
- the name and volume of the liquid to be used for reconstitution,
- that the transmission of infectious agents cannot be totally excluded when medicinal products prepared from human blood or plasma are administered.

01/2005:1644

HUMAN COAGULATION FACTOR XI

Factor XI coagulationis humanus

DEFINITION

Human coagulation factor XI is a plasma protein fraction containing coagulation factor XI. It is obtained from *Human plasma for fractionation (0853)*.

When reconstituted as stated on the label, the potency is not less than 50 units of factor XI per millilitre.

PRODUCTION

The method of preparation includes a step or steps that have been shown to remove or to inactivate known agents of infection; if substances are used for inactivation of viruses during production, the subsequent purification procedure must be validated to demonstrate that the concentration of these substances is reduced to a suitable level and any residues are such as not to compromise the safety of the preparation for patients.

After preparation, the factor XI fraction is dissolved in a suitable liquid. Heparin, C_1-esterase inhibitor and antithrombin III may be added. The solution is distributed into the final containers and immediately frozen. It is subsequently freeze-dried and the containers are closed under vacuum or under nitrogen. No antimicrobial preservative is added.

CHARACTERS

A white powder or friable solid.

Reconstitute the preparation to be examined as stated on the label immediately before carrying out the identification, tests (except those for solubility and water) and assay.

IDENTIFICATION

The assay of factor XI serves also to identify the preparation.

TESTS

Solubility. To a container of the preparation to be examined, add the volume of liquid stated on the label at room temperature. The preparation dissolves completely with gentle swirling within 10 min.

pH (*2.2.3*): 6.8 to 7.4.

Osmolality (*2.2.35*): minimum 240 mosmol/kg.

Total protein (*2.5.33*). The preparation to be examined contains not more than the amount of protein stated on the label.

Activated coagulation factors (*2.6.22*). For each of the dilutions, the coagulation time is not less than 150 s.

Heparin (*2.7.12*). If heparin has been added, the preparation to be examined contains not more than the amount of heparin stated on the label and in any case not more than 0.5 IU of heparin per unit of factor XI.

Antithrombin III (*2.7.17*). If antithrombin III has been added, the preparation to be examined contains not more than the amount of antithrombin III stated on the label.

C_1-esterase inhibitor. If C_1-esterase inhibitor has been added, the preparation to be examined contains not more than the amount of C_1-esterase inhibitor stated on the label.

The C_1-esterase inhibitor content of the preparation to be examined is determined by comparing its ability to inhibit C_1-esterase with the same ability of a reference preparation consisting of human normal plasma. 1 unit of C_1-esterase is equal to the activity of 1 ml of human normal plasma. Varying quantities of the preparation to be examined are mixed with an excess of C_1-esterase and the remaining C_1-esterase activity is determined using a suitable chromogenic substrate.

Method. Reconstitute the preparation as stated on the label. Prepare an appropriate series of 3 or 4 independent dilutions from 1 unit/ml of factor XI, for both the preparation to be examined and the reference preparation, using a solution containing 9 g/l of *sodium chloride R* and either 10 g/l of *human albumin R* or 10 g/l of *bovine albumin R*. Warm all solutions to 37 °C in a water bath for 1-2 min before use. Place a suitable amount of C_1-esterase solution in tubes or in microtitre plate wells and incubate at 37 °C. Add a suitable amount of one of the dilutions of the reference preparation or of the preparation to be examined and incubate at 37 °C for 5 min. Add a suitable amount of a suitable chromogenic substrate such as methoxycarbonyl-L-lysyl(ε-benzyloxycarbonyl)-glycyl-L-arginine 4-nitroanilide. Read the rate of increase of absorbance (ΔA/min) at 405 nm. Carry out a blank test using *tris(hydroxymethyl)aminomethane sodium chloride buffer solution pH 7.4 R* instead of the C_1-esterase and the substrate.

Calculate the C_1-esterase inhibitor content using the usual statistical methods (for example, *5.3.*).

Anti-A and anti-B haemagglutinins (*2.6.20*). The 1 to 64 dilutions do not show agglutination.

Water. Determined by a suitable method, such as the semi-micro determination of water (*2.5.12*), loss on drying (*2.2.32*) or near infrared spectrophotometry (*2.2.40*), the water content is within the limits approved by the competent authority.

Sterility (*2.6.1*). The reconstituted preparation complies with the test for sterility.

Monographs F-H

Pyrogens (*2.6.8*). The reconstituted preparation complies with the test for pyrogens. Inject per kilogram of the rabbit's mass a volume of the reconstituted preparation equivalent to 100 units of factor XI, calculated from the activity stated on the label.

ASSAY

Carry out the assay of human coagulation factor XI (*2.7.22*).

The estimated potency is not less than 80 per cent and not more than 120 per cent of the stated potency. The confidence limits ($P = 0.95$) are not less than 80 per cent and not more than 125 per cent of the estimated potency.

STORAGE

Protected from light, at a temperature of 2 °C to 8 °C.

LABELLING

The label states:

– the number of units per container,

– the maximum amount of protein per container,

– where applicable, the amount of heparin per container,

– where applicable, the amount of antithrombin III per container,

– where applicable, the amount of C_1-esterase inhibitor per container,

– the name and volume of the liquid to be used for reconstitution.

Monographs F-H

01/2005:0024

HUMAN FIBRINOGEN

Fibrinogenum humanum

DEFINITION

Human fibrinogen contains the soluble constituent of human plasma that is transformed to fibrin on the addition of thrombin. It is obtained from *Human plasma for fractionation (0853)*. The preparation may contain auxiliary substances such as salts, buffers and stabilisers.

When dissolved in the volume of the solvent stated on the label, the solution contains not less than 10 g/l of fibrinogen.

PRODUCTION

The method of preparation includes a step or steps that have been shown to remove or to inactivate known agents of infection; if substances are used for inactivation of viruses during production, the subsequent purification procedure must be validated to demonstrate that the concentration of these substances is reduced to a suitable level and any residues are such as not to compromise the safety of the preparation for patients.

No antibiotic is added to the plasma used and no antimicrobial preservative is included in the preparation. The preparation is freeze-dried.

The method of preparation is such as to obtain fibrinogen with a specific activity (fibrinogen content with respect to total protein content) not less than 80 per cent. The fibrinogen content is determined by a suitable method such as that described under Assay and the total protein content is determined by a suitable method such as that described under Total protein in *Human albumin solution (0255)*. If a protein stabiliser (for example, human albumin) is added to the preparation, the requirement for specific activity applies to the fibrinogen before addition of the stabiliser. Albumin may also be obtained with fibrinogen during fractionation and a specific determination of albumin is then carried out by a suitable immunochemical method (*2.7.1*) and the quantity of albumin determined is subtracted from the total protein content for the calculation of the specific activity.

CHARACTERS

A white or pale yellow, hygroscopic powder or friable solid.

IDENTIFICATION

It complies with the limits of the assay.

TESTS

pH (*2.2.3*): 6.5 to 7.5.

Osmolality (*2.2.35*): minimum 240 mosmol/kg.

Solubility. Add the volume of solvent stated on the label to the contents of a container. The preparation dissolves within 30 min at 20-25 °C, forming an almost colourless, slightly opalescent solution.

Stability of solution. Allow the reconstituted solution to stand at 20-25 °C. No gel formation appears within 60 min of reconstitution.

Hepatitis B surface antigen. Examine the reconstituted preparation by an immunochemical method (*2.7.1*) of suitable sensitivity, such as radio-immunoassay. Hepatitis B surface antigen is not detected.

Water. Determined by a suitable method, such as the semi-micro determination of water (*2.5.12*), loss on drying (*2.2.32*) or near infrared spectrophotometry (*2.2.40*), the water content is within the limits approved by the competent authority.

Sterility (*2.6.1*). The reconstituted preparation complies with the test for sterility.

Pyrogens (*2.6.8*). The reconstituted preparation complies with the test for pyrogens. Inject per kilogram of the rabbit's mass a volume of the reconstituted preparation equivalent to not less than 30 mg of fibrinogen, calculated from the quantity stated on the label.

ASSAY

Mix 0.2 ml of the reconstituted preparation with 2 ml of a suitable buffer solution (pH 6.6-6.8) containing sufficient thrombin (approximately 3 IU/ml) and calcium (0.05 mol/l). Maintain at 37 °C for 20 min, separate the precipitate by centrifugation (5000 *g*, 20 min), wash thoroughly with a 9 g/l solution of *sodium chloride R*. Determine the nitrogen content by sulphuric acid digestion (*2.5.9*) and calculate the fibrinogen (clottable protein) content by multiplying the result by 6.0. The content is not less than 70 per cent and not more than 130 per cent of the amount of fibrinogen stated on the label.

STORAGE

In an airtight container, protected from light.

LABELLING

The label states:

– the amount of fibrinogen in the container,

– the name and volume of the solvent to be used to reconstitute the preparation,

– where applicable, the name and quantity of protein stabiliser in the preparation.

01/2005:0769

HUMAN HEPATITIS A IMMUNOGLOBULIN

Immunoglobulinum humanum hepatitidis A

DEFINITION

Human hepatitis A immunoglobulin is a liquid or freeze-dried preparation containing immunoglobulins, mainly immunoglobulin G. The preparation is intended for intramuscular administration. It is obtained from plasma from selected donors having antibodies against hepatitis A virus. *Human normal immunoglobulin (0338)* may be added.

It complies with the monograph on *Human normal immunoglobulin (0338)*, except for the minimum number of donors and the minimum total protein content.

POTENCY

The potency is determined by comparing the antibody titre of the immunoglobulin to be examined with that of a reference preparation calibrated in International Units, using an immunoassay of suitable sensitivity and specificity (*2.7.1*).

The International Unit is the activity contained in a stated amount of the International Standard for anti-hepatitis A immunoglobulin. The equivalence in International Units of the International Standard is stated by the World Health Organisation.

Human hepatitis A immunoglobulin BRP is calibrated in International Units by comparison with the International Standard.

The stated potency is not less than 600 IU/ml. The estimated potency is not less than the stated potency. The confidence limits (P = 0.95) of the estimated potency are not less than 80 per cent and not more than 125 per cent.

STORAGE

See *Human normal immunoglobulin (0338)*.

LABELLING

See *Human normal immunoglobulin (0338)*.

The label states the number of International Units per container.

01/2005:0722

HUMAN HEPATITIS B IMMUNOGLOBULIN

Immunoglobulinum humanum hepatitidis B

DEFINITION

Human hepatitis B immunoglobulin is a liquid or freeze-dried preparation containing immunoglobulins, mainly immunoglobulin G. The preparation is intended for intramuscular administration. It is obtained from plasma from selected and/or immunised donors having antibodies against hepatitis B surface antigen. *Human normal immunoglobulin (0338)* may be added.

It complies with the monograph on *Human normal immunoglobulin (0338)*, except for the minimum number of donors and the minimum total protein content.

POTENCY

The potency is determined by comparing the antibody titre of the immunoglobulin to be examined with that of a reference preparation calibrated in International Units, using an immunoassay of suitable sensitivity and specificity (*2.7.1*).

The International Unit is the activity contained in a stated amount of the International Reference Preparation of hepatitis B immunoglobulin. The equivalence in International Units of the International Reference Preparation is stated by the World Health Organisation.

The stated potency is not less than 100 IU/ml. The estimated potency is not less than the stated potency. The confidence limits (P = 0.95) of the estimated potency are not less than 80 per cent and not more than 125 per cent.

STORAGE

See *Human normal immunoglobulin (0338)*.

LABELLING

See *Human normal immunoglobulin (0338)*.

The label states the number of International Units per container.

01/2005:1016

HUMAN HEPATITIS B IMMUNOGLOBULIN FOR INTRAVENOUS ADMINISTRATION

Immunoglobulinum humanum hepatitidis B ad usum intravenosum

DEFINITION

Human hepatitis B immunoglobulin for intravenous administration is a liquid or freeze-dried preparation containing immunoglobulins, mainly immunoglobulin G. It is obtained from plasma from selected and/or immunised donors having antibodies against hepatitis B surface antigen. *Human normal immunoglobulin for intravenous administration (0918)* may be added.

It complies with the monograph on *Human normal immunoglobulinum for intravenous administration (0918)*, except for the minimum number of donors, the minimum total protein content and the limit for osmolality.

POTENCY

The potency is determined by comparing the antibody titre of the immunoglobulin to be examined with that of a reference preparation calibrated in International Units, using an immunoassay (*2.7.1*) of suitable sensitivity and specificity.

The International Unit is the activity contained in a stated amount of the International Reference Preparation of hepatitis B immunoglobulin. The equivalence in International Units of the International Reference Preparation is stated by the World Health Organisation.

The stated potency is not less than 50 IU/ml. The estimated potency is not less than the stated potency. The confidence limits (P = 0.95) are not less than 80 per cent and not more than 120 per cent of the estimated potency.

STORAGE

See *Human normal immunoglobulin for intravenous administration (0918)*.

LABELLING

See *Human normal immunoglobulin for intravenous administration (0918)*.

Monographs F-H

The label states the minimum number of International Units of hepatitis B immunoglobulin per container.

01/2005:0397

HUMAN MEASLES IMMUNOGLOBULIN

Immunoglobulinum humanum morbillicum

DEFINITION

Human measles immunoglobulin is a liquid or freeze-dried preparation containing immunoglobulins, mainly immunoglobulin G. The preparation is intended for intramuscular administration. It is obtained from plasma containing specific antibodies against the measles virus. *Human normal immunoglobulin (0338)* may be added.

It complies with the monograph on *Human normal immunoglobulin (0338)*, except for the minimum number of donors and the minimum total protein content.

POTENCY

The potency of the liquid preparation and of the freeze-dried preparation after reconstitution as stated on the label is not less than 50 IU per millilitre of neutralising antibody against measles virus.

The potency is determined by comparing the antibody titres of the immunoglobulin to be examined and of a reference preparation calibrated in International Units, using a challenge dose of measles virus in a suitable cell culture system. A method of equal sensitivity and precision may be used providing that the competent authority is satisfied that it correlates with neutralising activity for the measles virus by comparison with the reference preparation.

The International Unit is the specific neutralising activity for measles virus contained in a stated amount of the International Standard for human anti-measles serum. The equivalence in International Units of the International Reference Preparation is stated by the World Health Organisation.

Prepare serial two-fold dilutions of the immunoglobulin to be examined and of the reference preparation. Mix each dilution with an equal volume of a suspension of measles virus containing about 100 $CCID_{50}$ in 0.1 ml and incubate protected from light at 37 °C for 2 h. Using not fewer than six cell cultures per mixture, inoculate 0.2 ml of each mixture into each of the cell cultures allocated to that mixture and incubate for not less than 10 days. Examine the cultures for viral activity and compare the dilution containing the smallest quantity of the immunoglobulin which neutralises the virus with that of the corresponding dilution of the reference preparation.

Calculate the potency of the immunoglobulin to be examined in International Units per millilitre of neutralising antibody against measles virus.

STORAGE

See *Human normal immunoglobulin (0338)*.

LABELLING

See *Human normal immunoglobulin (0338)*.

The label states the number of International Units per container.

01/2005:0338

HUMAN NORMAL IMMUNOGLOBULIN

Immunoglobulinum humanum normale

DEFINITION

Human normal immunoglobulin is a liquid or freeze-dried preparation containing immunoglobulins, mainly immunoglobulin G (IgG). Other proteins may be present. Human normal immunoglobulin contains the IgG antibodies of normal subjects. It is intended for intramuscular injection.

Human normal immunoglobulin is obtained from plasma that complies with the requirements of the monograph on *Human plasma for fractionation (0853)*. No antibiotic is added to the plasma used.

PRODUCTION

The method of preparation includes a step or steps that have been shown to remove or to inactivate known agents of infection; if substances are used for inactivation of viruses, it shall have been shown that any residues present in the final product have no adverse effects on the patients treated with the immunoglobulin.

The product shall have been shown, by suitable tests in animals and evaluation during clinical trials, to be well tolerated when administered intramuscularly.

Human normal immunoglobulin is prepared from pooled material from at least 1000 donors by a method that has been shown to yield a product that:

- does not transmit infection;
- at a protein concentration of 160 g/l, contains antibodies for at least 2 of which (one viral and one bacterial) an International Standard or Reference Preparation is available, the concentration of such antibodies being at least 10 times that in the initial pooled material.

Human normal immunoglobulin is prepared as a stabilised solution, for example in a 9 g/l solution of sodium chloride, a 22.5 g/l solution of glycine or, if the preparation is to be freeze-dried, a 60 g/l solution of glycine. Multidose preparations contain an antimicrobial preservative. Single-dose preparations do not contain an antimicrobial preservative. Any antimicrobial preservative or stabilising agent used shall have been shown to have no deleterious effect on the final product in the amount present. The solution is passed through a bacteria-retentive filter. The preparation may subsequently be freeze-dried and the containers closed under vacuum or under an inert gas.

The stability of the preparation is demonstrated by suitable tests carried out during development studies.

CHARACTERS

The liquid preparation is clear and pale-yellow to light-brown; during storage it may show formation of slight turbidity or a small amount of particulate matter. The freeze-dried preparation is a hygroscopic, white or slightly yellow powder or solid, friable mass.

For the freeze-dried preparation, reconstitute as stated on the label immediately before carrying out the identification and the tests, except those for solubility and water.

IDENTIFICATION

Examine by a suitable immunoelectrophoresis technique. Using antiserum to normal human serum, compare normal human serum and the preparation to be examined, both diluted to contain 10 g/l of protein. The main component of the preparation to be examined corresponds to the IgG component of normal human serum. The solution may show the presence of small quantities of other plasma proteins.

TESTS

Solubility. For the freeze-dried preparation, add the volume of the liquid stated on the label. The preparation dissolves completely within 20 min at 20-25 °C.

pH (*2.2.3*): 5.0 to 7.2.

Dilute the preparation to be examined with a 9 g/l solution of *sodium chloride R* to obtain a solution containing 10 g/l of protein.

Total protein. Dilute the preparation to be examined with a 9 g/l solution of *sodium chloride R* to obtain a solution containing about 15 mg of protein in 2 ml. To 2.0 ml of this solution in a round-bottomed centrifuge tube add 2 ml of a 75 g/l solution of *sodium molybdate R* and 2 ml of a mixture of 1 volume of *nitrogen-free sulphuric acid R* and 30 volumes of *water R*. Shake, centrifuge for 5 min, decant the supernatant liquid and allow the inverted tube to drain on filter paper. Determine the nitrogen in the residue by the method of sulphuric acid digestion (*2.5.9*) and calculate the content of protein by multiplying the result by 6.25. The preparation contains not less than 100 g/l and not more than 180 g/l of protein and not less than 90 per cent and not more than 110 per cent of the quantity of protein stated on the label.

Protein composition. Examine by zone electrophoresis (*2.2.31*), using strips of suitable cellulose acetate gel as the supporting medium and *barbital buffer solution pH 8.6 R1* as the electrolyte solution.

Test solution. Dilute the preparation to be examined with a 9 g/l solution of *sodium chloride R* to a protein concentration of 50 g/l.

Reference solution. Reconstitute *human immunoglobulin for electrophoresis BRP* and dilute with a 9 g/l solution of *sodium chloride R* to a protein concentration of 50 g/l.

To a strip apply 2.5 µl of the test solution as a 10 mm band or apply 0.25 µl per millimetre if a narrower strip is used. To another strip apply in the same manner the same volume of the reference solution. Apply a suitable electric field such that the albumin band of normal human serum applied on a control strip migrates at least 30 mm. Stain the strip with *amido black 10B solution R* for 5 min. Decolourise with a mixture of 10 volumes of *glacial acetic acid R* and 90 volumes of *methanol R* so that the background is just free of colour. Develop the transparency of the strips with a mixture of 19 volumes of *glacial acetic acid R* and 81 volumes of *methanol R*. Measure the absorbance of the bands at 600 nm in an instrument having a linear response over the range of measurement. Calculate the result as the mean of 3 measurements of each strip. In the electropherogram obtained with the test solution, not more than 10 per cent of the protein has a mobility different from that of the principal band. The test is not valid unless, in the electropherogram obtained with the reference preparation, the proportion of protein in the principal band is within the limits stated in the leaflet accompanying the reference preparation.

Distribution of molecular size. Liquid chromatography (*2.2.29*).

Test solution. Dilute the preparation to be examined with a 9 g/l solution of *sodium chloride R* to a concentration suitable for the chromatographic system used. A concentration in the range 4 g/l to 12 g/l and injection of 50 µg to 600 µg of protein are usually suitable.

Reference solution. Dilute *human immunoglobulin BRP* with a 9 g/l solution of *sodium chloride R* to the same protein concentration as the test solution.

Column:

- *size*: l = 0.6 m, Ø = 7.5 mm,
- *stationary phase*: *hydrophilic silica gel for chromatography R*, of a grade suitable for fractionation of globular proteins with relative molecular masses in the range 10 000 to 500 000.

Mobile phase: dissolve 4.873 g of *disodium hydrogen phosphate dihydrate R*, 1.741 g of *sodium dihydrogen phosphate monohydrate R*, 11.688 g of *sodium chloride R* and 50 mg of *sodium azide R* in 1 litre of *water R*.

Flow rate: 0.5 ml/min.

Detection: spectrophotometer at 280 nm.

In the chromatogram obtained with the reference solution, the principal peak corresponds to IgG monomer and there is a peak corresponding to dimer with a relative retention to the principal peak of about 0.85. Identify the peaks in the chromatogram obtained with the test solution by comparison with the chromatogram obtained with the reference solution; any peak with a retention time shorter than that of dimer corresponds to polymers and aggregates. The preparation to be examined complies with the test if, in the chromatogram obtained with the test solution:

- *relative retention*: for monomer and dimer, the relative retention to the corresponding peak in the chromatogram obtained with the reference solution is 1 ± 0.02;
- *peak area*: the sum of the peak areas of monomer and dimer represent not less than 85 per cent of the total area of the chromatogram and the sum of the peak area of polymers and aggregates represents not more than 10 per cent of the total area of the chromatogram.

Water. Determined by a suitable method, such as the semi-micro determination of water (*2.5.12*), loss on drying (*2.2.32*) or near infrared spectrophotometry (*2.2.40*), the water content is within the limits approved by the competent authority.

Sterility (*2.6.1*). It complies with the test for sterility.

Pyrogens (*2.6.8*). It complies with the test for pyrogens. Inject 1 ml per kilogram of the rabbit's mass.

Antibody to hepatitis B surface antigen. Not less than 0.5 IU/g of immunoglobulin, determined by a suitable immunochemical method (*2.7.1*).

Antibody to hepatitis A virus. If intended for use in the prophylaxis of hepatitis A, it complies with the following additional requirement. Determine the antibody content by comparison with a reference preparation calibrated in International Units, using an immunoassay of suitable sensitivity and specificity (*2.7.1*).

The International Unit is the activity contained in a stated amount of the International Standard for anti-hepatitis A immunoglobulin. The equivalence in International Units of the International Standard is stated by the World Health Organisation.

Human hepatitis A immunoglobulin BRP is calibrated in International Units by comparison with the International Standard.

The stated potency is not less than 100 IU/ml. The estimated potency is not less than the stated potency. The confidence limits (P = 0.95) of the estimated potency are not less than 80 per cent and not more than 125 per cent.

STORAGE

For the liquid preparation, store in a colourless glass container, protected from light. For the freeze-dried preparation, store in an airtight colourless glass container, protected from light.

LABELLING

The label states:

- for liquid preparations, the volume of the preparation in the container and the protein content expressed in grams per litre,
- for freeze-dried preparations, the quantity of protein in the container,
- the route of administration,
- for freeze-dried preparations, the name or composition and the volume of the reconstituting liquid to be added,
- where applicable, that the preparation is suitable for use in the prophylaxis of hepatitis A infection,
- where applicable, the anti-hepatitis A virus activity in International Units per millilitre,
- where applicable, the name and amount of antimicrobial preservative in the preparation.

01/2005:0918

HUMAN NORMAL IMMUNOGLOBULIN FOR INTRAVENOUS ADMINISTRATION

Immunoglobulinum humanum normale ad usum intravenosum

DEFINITION

Human normal immunoglobulin for intravenous administration is a liquid or freeze-dried preparation containing immunoglobulins, mainly immunoglobulin G (IgG). Other proteins may be present. Human normal immunoglobulin for intravenous administration contains the IgG antibodies of normal subjects. This monograph does not apply to products intentionally prepared to contain fragments or chemically modified IgG.

Human normal immunoglobulin for intravenous administration is obtained from plasma that complies with the requirements of the monograph on *Human plasma for fractionation (0853)*. No antibiotic is added to the plasma used.

PRODUCTION

The method of preparation includes a step or steps that have been shown to remove or to inactivate known agents of infection; if substances are used for inactivation of viruses, it shall have been shown that any residues present in the final product have no adverse effects on the patients treated with the immunoglobulin.

The product shall have been shown, by suitable tests in animals and evaluation during clinical trials, to be well tolerated when administered intravenously.

Human normal immunoglobulin is prepared from pooled material from not fewer than 1000 donors by a method that has been shown to yield a product that:

- does not transmit infection,
- at an immunoglobulin concentration of 50 g/l, contains antibodies for at least 2 of which (one viral and one bacterial) an International Standard or Reference Preparation is available, the concentration of such antibodies being at least 3 times that in the initial pooled material,
- has a defined distribution of immunoglobulin G subclasses,
- complies with the test for Fc function of immunoglobulin (*2.7.9*).

Human normal immunoglobulin for intravenous administration is prepared as a stabilised solution or as a freeze-dried preparation. A stabiliser may be added. In both cases the preparation is passed through a bacteria-retentive filter. The preparation may subsequently be freeze-dried and the containers closed under vacuum or under an inert gas. No antimicrobial preservative is added either during fractionation or at the stage of the final bulk solution.

The stability of the preparation is demonstrated by suitable tests carried out during development studies.

CHARACTERS

The liquid preparation is clear or slightly opalescent and colourless or pale yellow. The freeze-dried preparation is a hygroscopic, white or slightly yellow powder or solid friable mass.

For the freeze-dried preparation, reconstitute as stated on the label immediately before carrying out the identification and the tests, except those for solubility and water.

IDENTIFICATION

Examine by a suitable immunoelectrophoresis technique. Using antiserum to normal human serum, compare normal human serum and the preparation to be examined, both diluted to contain 10 g/l of protein. The main component of the preparation to be examined corresponds to the IgG component of normal human serum. The preparation to be examined may show the presence of small quantities of other plasma proteins; if human albumin has been added as a stabiliser, it may be seen as a major component.

TESTS

Solubility. For the freeze-dried preparation, add the volume of the liquid stated on the label. The preparation dissolves completely within 30 min at 20-25 °C.

pH (*2.2.3*): 4.0 to 7.4.

Dilute the preparation to be examined with a 9 g/l solution of *sodium chloride R* to obtain a solution containing 10 g/l of protein.

Osmolality (*2.2.35*): minimum 240 mosmol/kg.

Total protein. Dilute the preparation to be examined with a 9 g/l solution of *sodium chloride R* to obtain a solution containing about 15 mg of protein in 2 ml. To 2.0 ml of this solution in a round-bottomed centrifuge tube add 2 ml of a 75 g/l solution of *sodium molybdate R* and 2 ml of a mixture of 1 volume of *nitrogen-free sulphuric acid R* and 30 volumes of *water R*. Shake, centrifuge for 5 min, decant the supernatant liquid and allow the inverted tube to drain on filter paper. Determine the nitrogen in the centrifugation residue by the method of sulphuric acid digestion (*2.5.9*) and calculate the content of protein by multiplying the result by 6.25. The preparation contains not less than 30 g/l of protein and not less than 90 per cent and not more than 110 per cent of the quantity of protein stated on the label.

Protein composition. Examine by zone electrophoresis (*2.2.31*), using strips of suitable cellulose acetate gel as the supporting medium and *barbital buffer solution pH 8.6 R1* as the electrolyte solution.

Test solution. Dilute the preparation to be examined with a 9 g/l solution of *sodium chloride R* to an immunoglobulin concentration of 30 g/l.

Reference solution. Reconstitute *human immunoglobulin for electrophoresis BRP* and dilute with a 9 g/l solution of *sodium chloride R* to a protein concentration of 30 g/l.

To a strip apply 4.0 µl of the test solution as a 10 mm band or apply 0.4 µl per millimetre if a narrower strip is used. To another strip apply in the same manner the same volume of the reference solution. Apply a suitable electric field such that the albumin band of normal human serum applied on a control strip migrates at least 30 mm. Stain the strips with *amido black 10B solution R* for 5 min. Decolourise with a mixture of 10 volumes of *glacial acetic acid R* and 90 volumes of *methanol R* so that the background is just free of colour. Develop the transparency of the strips with a mixture of 19 volumes of *glacial acetic acid R* and 81 volumes of *methanol R*. Measure the absorbance of the bands at 600 nm in an instrument having a linear response over the range of measurement. Calculate the result as the mean of 3 measurements of each strip. In the electropherogram obtained with the test solution, not more than 5 per cent of protein has a mobility different from that of the principal band. This limit is not applicable if albumin has been added to the preparation as a stabiliser; for such preparations, a test for protein composition is carried out during manufacture before addition of the stabiliser. The test is not valid unless, in the electropherogram obtained with the reference preparation, the proportion of protein in the principal band is within the limits stated in the leaflet accompanying the reference preparation.

Distribution of molecular size. Liquid chromatography (*2.2.29*).

Test solution. Dilute the preparation to be examined with a 9 g/l solution of *sodium chloride R* to a concentration suitable for the chromatographic system used. A concentration in the range 4 g/l to 12 g/l and injection of 50 µg to 600 µg of protein are usually suitable.

Reference solution. Dilute *human immunoglobulin BRP* with a 9 g/l solution of *sodium chloride R* to the same protein concentration as the test solution.

Column:

- *size*: l = 0.6 m, Ø = 7.5 mm,
- *stationary phase*: *hydrophilic silica gel for chromatography R* of a grade suitable for fractionation of globular proteins with relative molecular masses in the range 10 000 to 500 000.

Mobile phase: dissolve 4.873 g of *disodium hydrogen phosphate dihydrate R*, 1.741 g of *sodium dihydrogen phosphate monohydrate R*, 11.688 g of *sodium chloride R* and 50 mg of *sodium azide R* in 1 litre of *water R*.

Flow rate: 0.5 ml/min.

Detection: spectrophotometer at 280 nm.

In the chromatogram obtained with the reference solution, the principal peak corresponds to IgG monomer and there is a peak corresponding to dimer with a relative retention to the principal peak of about 0.85. Identify the peaks in the chromatogram obtained with the test solution by comparison with the chromatogram obtained with the reference solution; any peak with a retention time shorter than that of dimer corresponds to polymers and aggregates. The preparation to be examined complies with the test if, in the chromatogram obtained with the test solution:

- *relative retention*: for monomer and dimer, the relative retention to the corresponding peak in the chromatogram obtained with the reference solution is 1 ± 0.02;
- *peak area*: the sum of the peak areas of monomer and dimer represent not less than 90 per cent of the total area of the chromatogram and the sum of the peak area of polymers and aggregates represents not more than 3 per cent of the total area of the chromatogram. This requirement does not apply to products where albumin has been added as a stabiliser; for products stabilised with albumin, a test for distribution of molecular size is carried out during manufacture before addition of the stabiliser.

Anticomplementary activity (*2.6.17*). The consumption of complement is not greater than 50 per cent (1 CH_{50} per milligram of immunoglobulin).

Prekallikrein activator (*2.6.15*): maximum 35 IU/ml, calculated with reference to a dilution of the preparation to be examined containing 30 g/l of immunoglobulin.

Anti-A and anti-B haemagglutinins (*2.6.20*). Carry out the tests for anti-A and anti-B haemagglutinins. If the preparation to be examined contains more than 30 g/l of immunoglobulin, dilute to this concentration before preparing the dilutions to be used in the test. The 1:64 dilutions do not show agglutination.

Water. Determined by a suitable method, such as the semi-micro determination of water (*2.5.12*), loss on drying (*2.2.32*) or near infrared spectrophotometry (*2.2.40*), the water content is within the limits approved by the competent authority.

Sterility (*2.6.1*). It complies with the test for sterility.

Pyrogens (*2.6.8*). It complies with the test for pyrogens. Inject per kilogram of the rabbit's mass a volume equivalent to 0.5 g of immunoglobulin but not more than 10 ml per kilogram of body mass.

Antibody to hepatitis B surface antigen: minimum 0.5 IU/g of immunoglobulin, determined by a suitable immunochemical method (*2.7.1*).

STORAGE

For the liquid preparation, store in a colourless glass container, protected from light, at the temperature stated on the label. For the freeze-dried preparation, store in an airtight colourless glass container, protected from light, at a temperature not exceeding 25 °C.

LABELLING

The label states:

- for liquid preparations, the volume of the preparation in the container and the protein content expressed in grams per litre,
- for freeze-dried preparations, the quantity of protein in the container,
- the amount of immunoglobulin in the container,
- the route of administration,
- for freeze-dried preparations, the name or composition and the volume of the reconstituting liquid to be added,
- the distribution of subclasses of immunoglobulin G present in the preparation,
- where applicable, the amount of albumin added as a stabiliser,
- the maximum content of immunoglobulin A.

01/2005:0853
corrected

HUMAN PLASMA FOR FRACTIONATION

Plasma humanum ad separationem

DEFINITION

Human plasma for fractionation is the liquid part of human blood remaining after separation of the cellular elements from blood collected in a receptacle containing an anticoagulant, or separated by continuous filtration or centrifugation of anticoagulated blood in an apheresis procedure; it is intended for the manufacture of plasma-derived products.

PRODUCTION

DONORS

Only a carefully selected, healthy donor who, as far as can be ascertained after medical examination, laboratory blood tests and a study of the donor's medical history, is free from detectable agents of infection transmissible by plasma-derived products may be used. Recommendations in this field are made by the Council of Europe [*Recommendation No. R (95) 15 on the preparation, use and quality assurance of blood components,* or subsequent revision] and the European Union [*Council Recommendation of 29 June 1998 on the suitability of blood and plasma donors and the screening of donated blood in the European Community* (98/463/EC)].

Immunisation of donors. Immunisation of donors to obtain immunoglobulins with specified activities may be carried out when sufficient supplies of material of suitable quality cannot be obtained from naturally immunised donors. Recommendations for such immunisation are formulated by the World Health Organisation (*Requirements for the collection, processing and quality control of blood, blood components and plasma derivatives,* WHO Technical Report Series, No. 840, 1994 or subsequent revision).

Records. Records of donors and donations made are kept in such a way that, while maintaining the required degree of confidentiality concerning the donor's identity, the origin of each donation in a plasma pool and the results of the corresponding acceptance procedures and laboratory tests can be traced.

Laboratory tests. Laboratory tests are carried out for each donation to detect the following viral markers:

1. antibodies against human immunodeficiency virus 1 (anti-HIV-1),
2. antibodies against human immunodeficiency virus 2 (anti-HIV-2),
3. hepatitis B surface antigen (HBsAg),
4. antibodies against hepatitis C virus (anti-HCV).

Pending complete harmonisation of the laboratory tests to be carried out, the competent authority may require that a test for alanine aminotransferase (ALT) also be carried out.

The test methods used are of suitable sensitivity and specificity and comply with the regulations in force. If a repeat-reactive result is found in any of these tests, the donation is not accepted.

INDIVIDUAL PLASMA UNITS

The plasma is prepared by a method that removes cells and cell debris as completely as possible. Whether prepared from whole blood or by plasmapheresis, the plasma is separated from the cells by a method designed to prevent the introduction of micro-organisms. No antibacterial or antifungal agent is added to the plasma. The containers comply with the requirements for glass containers (*3.2.1*) or for plastic containers for blood and blood components (*3.2.3*). The containers are closed so as to prevent contamination.

If 2 or more units are pooled prior to freezing, the operations are carried out using sterile connecting devices or under aseptic conditions and using containers that have not previously been used.

When obtained by plasmapheresis, plasma intended for the recovery of proteins that are labile in plasma is frozen by cooling rapidly at − 30 °C or below as soon as possible and at the latest within 24 h of collection.

When obtained from whole blood, plasma intended for the recovery of proteins that are labile in plasma is separated from cellular elements and is frozen by cooling rapidly at − 30 °C or below as soon as possible and at the latest within 24 h of collection.

When obtained from whole blood, plasma intended solely for the recovery of proteins that are not labile in plasma is separated from cellular elements and frozen at − 20 °C or below as soon as possible and at the latest within 72 h of collection.

It is not intended that the determination of total protein and factor VIII shown below be carried out on each unit of plasma. They are rather given as guidelines for good manufacturing practice, the test for factor VIII being relevant for plasma intended for use in the preparation of concentrates of labile proteins.

The total protein content of a unit of plasma depends on the serum protein content of the donor and the degree of dilution inherent in the donation procedure. When plasma is obtained from a suitable donor and using the intended proportion of anticoagulant solution, a total protein content complying with the limit of 50 g/l is obtained. If a volume of blood or plasma smaller than intended is collected into the anticoagulant solution, the resulting plasma is not necessarily unsuitable for pooling for fractionation. The aim of good manufacturing practice must be to achieve the prescribed limit for all normal donations.

Preservation of factor VIII in the donation depends on the collection procedure and the subsequent handling of the blood and plasma. With good practice, 0.7 IU/ml can usually be achieved, but units of plasma with a lower activity may still be suitable for use in the production of coagulation factor concentrates. The aim of good manufacturing practice is to conserve labile proteins as much as possible.

Total protein. Carry out the test using a pool of not fewer than 10 units. Dilute the pool with a 9 g/l solution of *sodium chloride R* to obtain a solution containing about 15 mg of protein in 2 ml. To 2.0 ml of this solution in a round-bottomed centrifuge tube add 2 ml of a 75 g/l solution of *sodium molybdate R* and 2 ml of a mixture of 1 volume of *nitrogen-free sulphuric acid R* and 30 volumes of *water R*. Shake, centrifuge for 5 min, decant the supernatant liquid and allow the inverted tube to drain on filter paper. Determine the nitrogen in the residue by the method of sulphuric acid digestion (*2.5.9*) and calculate the protein content by multiplying the quantity of nitrogen by 6.25. The total protein content is not less than 50 g/l.

Factor VIII. Carry out the test using a pool of not fewer than 10 units. Thaw the samples to be examined, if necessary, at 37 °C. Carry out the assay of factor VIII (*2.7.4*), using a reference plasma calibrated against the International Standard for blood coagulation factor VIII in plasma. The activity is not less than 0.7 IU/ml.

Monographs F-H

POOLED PLASMA

During the manufacture of plasma products, the first homogeneous pool of plasma (for example, after removal of cryoprecipitate) is tested for HBsAg, for hepatitis C virus antibodies and for HIV antibodies using test methods of suitable sensitivity and specificity; the pool must give negative results in these tests.

The plasma pool is also tested for hepatitis C virus RNA using a validated nucleic acid amplification technique (*2.6.21*). A positive control with 100 IU/ml of hepatitis C virus RNA and, to test for inhibitors, an internal control prepared by addition of a suitable marker to a sample of the plasma pool are included in the test. The test is invalid if the positive control is non-reactive or if the result obtained with the internal control indicates the presence of inhibitors. The plasma pool complies with the test if it is found non-reactive for hepatitis C virus RNA.

Hepatitis C virus RNA for NAT testing BRP is suitable for use as a positive control.

CHARACTERS

Before freezing, a clear to slightly turbid liquid without visible signs of haemolysis; it may vary in colour from light yellow to green.

STORAGE

Store and transport frozen plasma at or below − 20 °C; the plasma may still be used for fractionation if the temperature is between − 20 °C and − 15 °C for not more than a total of 72 h without exceeding − 15 °C on more than one occasion as long as the temperature is at all times − 5 °C or lower.

LABELLING

The label enables each individual unit to be traced to a specific donor.

01/2005:1646
corrected

HUMAN PLASMA (POOLED AND TREATED FOR VIRUS INACTIVATION)

Plasma humanum collectum deinde conditum ad viros exstinguendos

DEFINITION

Human plasma pooled and treated for virus inactivation is a frozen or freeze-dried, sterile, non-pyrogenic preparation obtained from human plasma derived from donors belonging to the same ABO blood group. The preparation is thawed or reconstituted before use to give a solution for infusion.

The human plasma used complies with the monograph on *Human plasma for fractionation (0853)*.

PRODUCTION

The units of plasma to be used are cooled to − 30 °C or lower within 6 h of separation of cells and in any case within 24 h of collection.

The pool is prepared by mixing units of plasma belonging to the same ABO blood group.

The pool of plasma is tested for hepatitis B surface antigen (HBsAg), for hepatitis C virus antibodies and for HIV antibodies using test methods of suitable sensitivity and specificity; the pool must give negative results in these tests.

The plasma pool is also tested for hepatitis C virus RNA using a validated nucleic acid amplification technique (*2.6.21*). A positive control with 100 IU of hepatitis C virus RNA per millilitre and, to test for inhibitors, an internal control prepared by addition of a suitable marker to a sample of the plasma pool are included in the test. The test is invalid if the positive control is non-reactive or if the result obtained with the internal control indicates the presence of inhibitors. The pool complies with the test if it is found non-reactive for hepatitis C virus RNA.

Hepatitis C virus RNA for NAT testing BRP is suitable for use as a positive control.

To limit the potential burden of B19 virus in plasma pools, the plasma pool is also tested for B19 virus using a validated nucleic acid amplification technique (*2.6.21*).

A positive control with 10^4 IU of B19 virus DNA per millilitre and, to test for inhibitors, an internal control prepared by addition of a suitable marker to a sample of the plasma pool are included in the test. The test is invalid if the positive control is non-reactive or if the result obtained with the internal control indicates the presence of inhibitors. The plasma pool contains not more than 10^4 IU of B19 virus DNA per millilitre.

B19 virus DNA for NAT testing BRP is suitable for use as a positive control.

The method of preparation is designed to minimise activation of any coagulation factor (to minimise potential thrombogenicity) and includes a step, or steps that have been shown to inactivate known agents of infection; if substances are used for the inactivation of viruses during production, the subsequent purification procedure must be validated to demonstrate that the concentration of these substances is reduced to a suitable level and that any residues are such as not to compromise the safety of the preparation for patients.

A typical method to inactivate enveloped viruses is the solvent-detergent process which uses treatment with a combination of tributyl phosphate and octoxinol 10; these reagents are subsequently removed by oil extraction or by solid phase extraction so that the amount in the final product is less than 2 μg/ml for tributyl phosphate and less than 5 μg/ml for octoxinol 10.

No antimicrobial preservative is added.

The solution is passed through a bacteria-retentive filter, distributed aseptically into the final containers and immediately frozen; it may subsequently be freeze-dried.

Plastic containers comply with the requirements for sterile plastic containers for human blood and blood components (*3.2.3*).

Glass containers comply with the requirements for glass containers for pharmaceutical use (*3.2.1*).

CHARACTERS

The frozen preparation, after thawing, is a clear or slightly opalescent liquid free from solid and gelatinous particles. The freeze-dried preparation is an almost white or slightly yellow powder or friable solid.

Thaw or reconstitute the preparation to be examined as stated on the label immediately before carrying out the identification, tests and assay.

IDENTIFICATION

A. Examine by electrophoresis (*2.2.31*) comparing with normal human plasma. The electropherograms show the same bands.

B. It complies with the test for anti-A and anti-B haemagglutinins (see Tests).

TESTS

pH (*2.2.3*): 6.5 to 7.6.

Monographs F-H

Osmolality (*2.2.35*): minimum 240 mosmol/kg.

Total protein: minimum 45 g/l.

Dilute with a 9 g/l solution of *sodium chloride R* to obtain a solution containing about 15 mg of protein in 2 ml. To 2.0 ml of this solution in a round-bottomed centrifuge tube add 2 ml of a 75 g/l solution of *sodium molybdate R* and 2 ml of a mixture of 1 volume of *nitrogen-free sulphuric acid R* and 30 volumes of *water R*. Shake, centrifuge for 5 min, decant the supernatant liquid and allow the inverted tube to drain on filter paper. Determine the nitrogen in the residue by the method of sulphuric acid digestion (*2.5.9*) and calculate the quantity of protein by multiplying the result by 6.25.

Activated coagulation factors (*2.6.22*). It complies with the test for activated coagulation factors. Carry out the test with 0.1 ml of the preparation to be examined instead of 1 to 10 and 1 to 100 dilutions. The coagulation time for the tube containing the preparation to be examined is not less than 150 s.

Anti-A and anti-B haemagglutinins (*2.6.20*). The presence of haemagglutinin (anti-A or anti-B) corresponds to the blood group stated on the label.

Hepatitis A virus antibodies: minimum 2 IU/ml, determined by a suitable immunochemical method (*2.7.1*).

Human hepatitis A immunoglobulin BRP is suitable for use as a reference preparation.

Irregular erythrocyte antibodies. The preparation to be examined does not show the presence of irregular erythrocyte antibodies when examined without dilution by an indirect antiglobulin test.

Citrate. Liquid chromatography (*2.2.29*).

Test solution. Dilute the preparation to be examined with an equal volume of a 9 g/l solution of *sodium chloride R*. Filter the solution using a filter with 0.45 µm pores.

Reference solution. Dissolve 0.300 g of *sodium citrate R* in *water R* and dilute to 100.0 ml with the same solvent.

Column:

– *size*: l = 0.3 m, Ø = 7.8 mm,

– *stationary phase*: *cation exchange resin R* (9 µm).

Mobile phase: 0.51 g/l solution of *sulphuric acid R*.

Flow rate: 0.5 ml/min.

Detection: spectrophotometer at 215 nm.

Equilibration: 15 min.

Injection: 10 µl.

Retention time: citrate = about 10 min.

Limit:

– *citrate*: maximum 25 mmol/l.

Calcium: maximum 5.0 mmol/l.

Atomic absorption spectrometry (*2.2.23, Method I*).

Source: calcium hollow-cathode lamp using a transmission band preferably of 0.5 nm.

Wavelength: 622 nm.

Atomisation device: air-acetylene or acetylene-propane flame.

Potassium: maximum 5.0 mmol/l.

Atomic emission spectrometry (*2.2.22, Method I*).

Wavelength: 766.5 nm.

Sodium: maximum 200 mmol/l.

Atomic emission spectrometry (*2.2.22, Method I*).

Wavelength: 589 nm.

Water: for the freeze-dried product: determined by a suitable method, such as the semi-micro determination of water (*2.5.12*), loss on drying (*2.2.32*) or near-infrared spectrometry (*2.2.40*), the water content is within the limits approved by the competent authority.

Sterility (*2.6.1*). It complies with the test for sterility.

Pyrogens (*2.6.8*). It complies with the test for pyrogens. Inject 3 ml per kilogram of the rabbit's mass.

ASSAY

Factor VIII. Carry out the assay of coagulation factor VIII (*2.7.4*) using a reference plasma calibrated against the International Standard for blood coagulation factor VIII in plasma.

The estimated potency is not less than 0.5 IU/ml. The confidence limits (P = 0.95) are not less than 80 per cent and not more than 120 per cent of the estimated potency.

Factor V. Using *imidazole buffer solution pH 7.3 R*, prepare 3 twofold dilutions of the preparation to be examined, preferably in duplicate, from 1 in 10 to 1 in 40. Test each dilution as follows: mix 0.1 ml of *plasma substrate deficient in factor V R*, 0.1 ml of the dilution to be examined, 0.1 ml of *thromboplastin R* and 0.1 ml of a 3.5 g/l solution of *calcium chloride R*; measure the coagulation times, i.e. the interval between the moment at which the calcium chloride solution is added and the first indication of the formation of fibrin, which may be observed visually or by means of a suitable apparatus.

In the same manner, determine the coagulation time of 4 twofold dilutions (1 in 10 to 1 in 80) of human normal plasma in *imidazole buffer solution pH 7.3 R*. 1 unit of factor V is equal to the activity of 1 ml of human normal plasma. Human normal plasma is prepared by pooling plasma units from not fewer than 30 donors and stored at −30 °C or lower.

Check the validity of the assay and calculate the potency of the test preparation by the usual statistical methods for a parallel-line assay (for example, *5.3*).

The estimated potency is not less than 0.5 IU/ml. The confidence limits (P = 0.95) are not less than 80 per cent and not more than 120 per cent of the estimated potency.

Factor XI. Carry out the assay of human coagulation factor XI (*2.7.22*) using as reference human normal plasma (see above under Factor V).

The estimated potency is not less than 0.5 IU/ml. The confidence limits (P = 0.95) are not less than 80 per cent and not more than 125 per cent of the estimated potency.

LABELLING

The label states:

– the ABO blood group,

– the method used for virus inactivation.

01/2005:0554

HUMAN PROTHROMBIN COMPLEX

Prothrombinum multiplex humanum

DEFINITION

Human prothrombin complex is a plasma protein fraction containing blood coagulation factor IX together with variable amounts of coagulation factors II, VII and X; the presence and proportion of these additional factors depends on the method of fractionation. It is obtained from human plasma that complies with the monograph on *Human plasma for fractionation (0853)*.

The potency of the preparation, reconstituted as stated on the label, is not less than 20 IU of factor IX per millilitre.

PRODUCTION

The method of preparation is designed to minimise activation of any coagulation factor (to minimise potential thrombogenicity) and includes a step or steps that have been shown to remove or to inactivate known agents of infection; if substances are used for inactivation of viruses during production, the subsequent purification procedure must be validated to demonstrate that the concentration of these substances is reduced to a suitable level and that any residues are such as not to compromise the safety of the preparation for patients.

The specific activity is not less than 0.6 IU of factor IX per milligram of total protein, before the addition of any protein stabiliser.

The prothrombin complex fraction is dissolved in a suitable liquid. Heparin, antithrombin and other auxiliary substances such as a stabiliser may be added. No antimicrobial preservative is added. The solution is passed through a bacteria-retentive filter, distributed aseptically into the final containers and immediately frozen. It is subsequently freeze-dried and the containers are closed under vacuum or under an inert gas.

CHARACTERS

A white or slightly coloured powder or friable solid, very hygroscopic.

Reconstitute the preparation to be examined as stated on the label immediately before carrying out the identification, tests (except those for solubility and water) and assay.

IDENTIFICATION

It complies with the limits of the assay for coagulation factor IX activity and, where applicable, those for factors II, VII and X.

TESTS

Solubility. To a container of the preparation to be examined add the volume of the liquid stated on the label at the recommended temperature. The preparation dissolves completely with gentle swirling within 10 min, giving a clear solution that may be coloured.

pH (*2.2.3*): 6.5 to 7.5.

Osmolality (*2.2.35*): minimum 240 mosmol/kg.

Total protein. If necessary, dilute an accurately measured volume of the reconstituted preparation with a 9 g/l solution of *sodium chloride R* to obtain a solution expected to contain about 15 mg of protein in 2 ml. To 2.0 ml of the solution in a round-bottomed centrifuge tube add 2 ml of a 75 g/l solution of *sodium molybdate R* and 2 ml of a mixture of 1 volume of *nitrogen-free sulphuric acid R* and 30 volumes of *water R*. Shake, centrifuge for 5 min, decant the supernatant liquid and allow the inverted tube to drain on filter paper. Determine the nitrogen in the residue by the method of sulphuric acid digestion (*2.5.9*) and calculate the amount of protein by multiplying the result by 6.25.

Activated coagulation factors (*2.6.22*). If necessary, dilute the preparation to be examined to contain 20 IU of factor IX per millilitre. For each of the dilutions, the coagulation time is not less than 150 s.

Heparin. If heparin has been added during preparation, determine the amount present by the assay of heparin in coagulation factor concentrates (*2.7.12*). The preparation to be examined contains not more than the amount of heparin stated on the label and in any case not more than 0.5 IU of heparin per International Unit of factor IX.

Thrombin. If the preparation to be examined contains heparin, determine the amount present as described in the test for heparin and neutralise it by addition of *protamine sulphate R* (10 µg of protamine sulphate neutralises 1 IU of heparin). In each of 2 test-tubes, mix equal volumes of the reconstituted preparation and a 3 g/l solution of *fibrinogen R*. Keep one of the tubes at 37 °C for 6 h and the other at room temperature for 24 h. In a third tube, mix a volume of the fibrinogen solution with an equal volume of a solution of *human thrombin R* (1 IU/ml) and place the tube in a water-bath at 37 °C. No coagulation occurs in the tubes containing the preparation to be examined. Coagulation occurs within 30 s in the tube containing thrombin.

Water. Determined by a suitable method, such as the semi-micro determination of water (*2.5.12*), loss on drying (*2.2.32*) or near-infrared spectrometry (*2.2.40*), the water content is within the limits approved by the competent authority.

Sterility (*2.6.1*). It complies with the test for sterility.

Pyrogens (*2.6.8*). It complies with the test for pyrogens. Inject per kilogram of the rabbit's mass a volume of the reconstituted preparation equivalent to not less than 30 IU of factor IX.

ASSAY

Factor IX. Carry out the assay of human coagulation factor IX (*2.7.11*).

The estimated potency is not less than 80 per cent and not more than 125 per cent of the stated potency. The confidence interval ($P = 0.95$) of the estimated potency is not greater than 80 per cent to 125 per cent.

Factor II. Carry out the assay of human coagulation factor II (*2.7.18*).

The estimated potency is not less than 80 per cent and not more than 125 per cent of the stated potency. The confidence interval ($P = 0.95$) of the estimated potency is not greater than 90 per cent to 111 per cent.

Factor VII. If the label states that the preparation contains factor VII, carry out the assay of human coagulation factor VII (*2.7.10*).

The estimated potency is not less than 80 per cent and not more than 125 per cent of the stated potency. The confidence interval ($P = 0.95$) of the estimated potency is not greater than 80 per cent to 125 per cent.

Factor X. Carry out the assay of human coagulation factor X (*2.7.19*).

The estimated potency is not less than 80 per cent and not more than 125 per cent of the stated potency. The confidence interval ($P = 0.95$) of the estimated potency is not greater than 90 per cent to 111 per cent.

STORAGE

In an airtight container, protected from light.

LABELLING

The label states:

- the number of International Units of factor IX, factor II and factor X per container,
- where applicable, the number of International Units of factor VII per container,

Monographs F-H

- where applicable, that the preparation contains protein C and/or protein S,
- the amount of protein per container,
- the name and quantity of any added substances, including where applicable, heparin,
- the name and quantity of the liquid to be used for reconstitution,
- that the transmission of infectious agents cannot be totally excluded when medicinal products prepared from human blood or plasma are administered.

01/2005:0723

HUMAN RABIES IMMUNOGLOBULIN

Immunoglobulinum humanum rabicum

DEFINITION

Human rabies immunoglobulin is a liquid or freeze-dried preparation containing immunoglobulins, mainly immunoglobulin G. The preparation is intended for intramuscular administration. It is obtained from plasma from donors immunised against rabies. It contains specific antibodies neutralising the rabies virus. *Human normal immunoglobulin (0338)* may be added.

It complies with the monograph on *Human normal immunoglobulin (0338)*, except for the minimum number of donors and the minimum total protein content.

POTENCY

The potency is determined by comparing the dose of immunoglobulin required to neutralise the infectivity of a rabies virus suspension with the dose of a reference preparation, calibrated in International Units, required to produce the same degree of neutralisation (*2.7.1*). The test is performed in sensitive cell cultures and the presence of unneutralised virus is revealed by immunofluorescence.

The International Unit is the specific neutralising activity for rabies virus in a stated amount of the International Standard for anti-rabies immunoglobulin. The equivalence in International Units of the International Standard is stated by the World Health Organisation.

Human rabies immunoglobulin BRP is calibrated in International Units by comparison with the International Standard.

Carry out the test in suitable sensitive cells. It is usual to use the BHK 21 cell line, grown in the medium described below, between the 18th and 30th passage levels counted from the ATCC seed lot. Harvest the cells after 2 to 4 days of growth, treat with trypsin and prepare a suspension containing 500 000 cells per millilitre (cell suspension). 10 min before using this suspension add 10 μg of *diethylamino-ethyldextran R* per millilitre, if necessary, to increase the sensitivity of the cells.

Use a fixed virus strain grown in sensitive cells, such as the CVS strain of rabies virus adapted to growth in the BHK 21 cell line (seed virus suspension). Estimate the titre of the seed virus suspension as follows.

Prepare a series of dilutions of the viral suspension. In the chambers of cell-culture slides (8 chambers per slide), place 0.1 ml of each dilution and 0.1 ml of medium and add 0.2 ml of the cell suspension. Incubate in an atmosphere of carbon dioxide at 37 °C for 24 h. Carry out fixation, immunofluorescence staining and evaluation as described below. Determine the end-point titre of the seed virus suspension and prepare the working virus dilution corresponding to 100 $CCID_{50}$ per 0.1 ml.

For each assay, check the amount of virus used by performing a control titration: from the dilution corresponding to 100 $CCID_{50}$ per 0.1 ml, make three tenfold dilutions. Add 0.1 ml of each dilution to four chambers containing 0.1 ml of medium and add 0.2 ml of the cell suspension. The test is not valid unless the titre lies between 30 $CCID_{50}$ and 300 $CCID_{50}$.

Dilute the reference preparation to a concentration of 2 IU/ml using non-supplemented culture medium (stock reference dilution, stored below − 80 °C). Prepare two suitable predilutions (1:8 and 1:10) of the stock reference dilution so that the dilution of the reference preparation that reduces the number of fluorescent fields by 50 per cent lies within the four dilutions of the cell-culture slide. Add 0.1 ml of the medium to each chamber, except the first in each of two rows, to which add respectively 0.2 ml of the two predilutions of the stock reference dilution transferring successively 0.1 ml to the other chambers.

Dilute the preparation to be examined 1 in 100 using non-supplemented medium (stock immunoglobulin dilution) - to reduce to a minimum errors due to viscosity of the undiluted preparation - and make three suitable predilutions so that the dilution of the preparation to be examined that reduces the number of fluorescent fields by 50 per cent lies within the four dilutions of the cell-culture slide. Add 0.1 ml of the medium to all the chambers except the first in each of three rows, to which add respectively 0.2 ml of the three predilutions of the stock immunoglobulin dilution. Prepare a series of twofold dilutions transferring successively 0.1 ml to the other chambers.

To all the chambers containing the dilutions of the reference preparation and the dilutions of the preparation to be examined, add 0.1 ml of the virus suspension corresponding to 100 $CCID_{50}$ per 0.1 ml (working virus dilution), shake manually, allow to stand in an atmosphere of carbon dioxide at 37 °C for 90 min, add 0.2 ml of the cell suspension, shake manually and allow to stand in an atmosphere of carbon dioxide at 37 °C for 24 h.

After 24 h, discard the medium and remove the plastic walls. Wash the cell monolayer with *phosphate buffered saline pH 7.4 R* and then with a mixture of 20 volumes of *water R* and 80 volumes of *acetone R* and fix in a mixture of 20 volumes of *water R* and 80 volumes of *acetone R* at − 20 °C for 3 min. Spread on the slides *fluorescein-conjugated rabies antiserum R* ready for use. Allow to stand in an atmosphere with a high level of moisture at 37 °C for 30 min. Wash with *phosphate buffered saline pH 7.4 R* and dry. Examine twenty fields in each chamber at a magnification of 250 ×, using a microscope equipped for fluorescence readings. Note the number of fields with at least one fluorescent cell. Check the test dose used in the virus titration slide and determine the dilution of the reference preparation and the dilution of the preparation to be examined that reduce the number of fluorescent fields by 50 per cent, calculating the two or three dilutions together using probit analysis. The test is not valid unless the statistical analysis shows a significant slope of the dose-response curve and no evidence of deviation from linearity or parallelism.

The stated potency is not less than 150 IU/ml. The estimated potency is not less than the stated potency and is not greater than twice the stated potency. The confidence limits (P = 0.95) of the estimated potency are not less than 80 per cent and not more than 125 per cent.

CULTURE MEDIUM FOR GROWTH OF BHK 21 CELLS

Commercially available media that have a slightly different composition from that shown below may also be used.

Sodium chloride	6.4 g
Potassium chloride	0.40 g
Calcium chloride, anhydrous	0.20 g
Magnesium sulphate, heptahydrate	0.20 g
Sodium dihydrogen phosphate, monohydrate	0.124 g
Glucose monohydrate	4.5 g
Ferric nitrate, nonahydrate	0.10 mg
L-Arginine hydrochloride	42.0 mg
L-Cystine	24.0 mg
L-Histidine	16.0 mg
L-Isoleucine	52.0 mg
L-Leucine	52.0 mg
L-Lysine hydrochloride	74.0 mg
L-Phenylalanine	33.0 mg
L-Threonine	48.0 mg
L-Tryptophan	8.0 mg
L-Tyrosine	36.0 mg
L-Valine	47.0 mg
L-Methionine	15.0 mg
L-Glutamine	0.292 g
i-Inositol	3.60 mg
Choline chloride	2.0 mg
Folic acid	2.0 mg
Nicotinamide	2.0 mg
Calcium pantothenate	2.0 mg
Pyridoxal hydrochloride	2.0 mg
Thiamine hydrochloride	2.0 mg
Riboflavine	0.2 mg
Phenol red	15.0 mg
Sodium hydrogen carbonate	2.75 g
Water to	1000 ml

The medium is supplemented with:

Foetal calf serum (heated at 56 °C for 30 min)	10 per cent
Tryptose phosphate broth	10 per cent
Benzylpenicillin sodium	60 mg/l
Streptomycin	0.1 g/l

STORAGE

See *Human normal immunoglobulin (0338)*.

LABELLING

See *Human normal immunoglobulin (0338)*.

The label states the number of International Units per container.

01/2005:0617

HUMAN RUBELLA IMMUNOGLOBULIN

Immunoglobulinum humanum rubellae

DEFINITION

Human rubella immunoglobulin is a liquid or freeze-dried preparation containing immunoglobulins, mainly immunoglobulin G. The preparation is intended for intramuscular administration. It is obtained from plasma containing specific antibodies against rubella virus. *Human normal immunoglobulin (0338)* may be added.

It complies with the monograph on *Human normal immunoglobulin (0338)*, except for the minimum number of donors and the minimum total protein content.

POTENCY

The potency is determined by comparing the activity of the preparation to be examined in a suitable haemagglutination-inhibition test with that of a reference preparation calibrated in International Units.

The International Unit is the activity contained in a stated amount of the International Standard for anti-rubella immunoglobulin. The equivalence in International Units of the International Reference Preparation is stated by the World Health Organisation.

The estimated potency is not less than 4500 IU/ml. The confidence limits ($P = 0.95$) of the estimate of potency are not less than 50 per cent and not more than 200 per cent of the stated potency.

STORAGE

See *Human normal immunoglobulin (0338)*.

LABELLING

See *Human normal immunoglobulin (0338)*.

The label states the number of International Units per millilitre.

01/2005:0398

HUMAN TETANUS IMMUNOGLOBULIN

Immunoglobulinum humanum tetanicum

DEFINITION

Human tetanus immunoglobulin is a liquid or freeze-dried preparation containing immunoglobulins, mainly immunoglobulin G. The preparation is intended for intramuscular administration. It is obtained from plasma containing specific antibodies against the toxin of *Clostridium tetani*. *Human normal immunoglobulin (0338)* may be added.

It complies with the monograph on *Human normal immunoglobulin (0338)*, except for the minimum number of donors and the minimum total protein content.

PRODUCTION

During development, a satisfactory relationship shall be established between the potency determined by immunoassay as described under Potency and that determined by means of the following test for toxin-neutralising capacity in mice.

Toxin-neutralising capacity in mice. The potency is determined by comparing the quantity necessary to protect mice against the paralytic effects of a fixed quantity of

Monographs F-H

tetanus toxin with the quantity of a reference preparation of human tetanus immunoglobulin, calibrated in International Units, necessary to give the same protection.

The International Unit of antitoxin is the specific neutralising activity for tetanus toxin contained in a stated amount of the International Standard, which consists of freeze-dried human immunoglobulin. The equivalence in International Units of the International Standard is stated by the World Health Organisation.

Human tetanus immunoglobulin BRP is calibrated in International Units by comparison with the International Standard.

Selection of animals. Use mice weighing 16 g to 20 g.

Preparation of the test toxin. Prepare the test toxin by a suitable method from the sterile filtrate of a culture in liquid medium of *C. tetani.* The two methods shown below are given as examples and any other suitable method may be used.

(1) To the filtrate of an approximately 9-day culture add 1 to 2 volumes of *glycerol R* and store the mixture in the liquid state at a temperature slightly below 0 °C.

(2) Precipitate the toxin by addition to the filtrate of *ammonium sulphate R,* dry the precipitate *in vacuo* over *diphosphorus pentoxide R,* reduce to a powder and store dry, either in sealed ampoules or *in vacuo* over *diphosphorus pentoxide R.*

Determination of test dose of toxin (Lp/10 dose). Prepare a solution of the reference preparation in a suitable liquid such that it contains 0.5 IU of antitoxin per millilitre. If the test toxin is stored dry, reconstitute it using a suitable liquid. Prepare mixtures of the solution of the reference preparation and the test toxin such that each contains 2.0 ml of the solution of the reference preparation, one of a graded series of volumes of the test toxin and sufficient of a suitable liquid to bring the volume to 5.0 ml. Allow the mixtures to stand, protected from light, for 60 min. Using six mice for each mixture, inject a dose of 0.5 ml subcutaneously into each mouse. Observe the mice for 96 h. Mice that become paralysed may be killed. The test dose of toxin is the quantity in 0.5 ml of the mixture made with the smallest amount of toxin capable of causing, despite partial neutralisation by the reference preparation, paralysis in all six mice injected with the mixture, within the observation period.

Determination of potency of the immunoglobulin. Prepare a solution of the reference preparation in a suitable liquid such that it contains 0.5 IU of antitoxin per millilitre. Prepare a solution of the test toxin in a suitable liquid such that it contains five test doses per millilitre. Prepare mixtures of the solution of the test toxin and the immunoglobulin to be examined such that each contains 2.0 ml of the solution of the test toxin, one of a graded series of volumes of the immunoglobulin to be examined and sufficient of a suitable liquid to bring the total volume to 5.0 ml. Also prepare mixtures of the solution of the test toxin and the solution of the reference preparation such that each contains 2.0 ml of the solution of the test toxin, one of a graded series of volumes of the solution of the reference preparation centred on that volume (2.0 ml) that contains 1 IU and sufficient of a suitable liquid to bring the total volume to 5.0 ml. Allow the mixtures to stand, protected from light, for 60 min. Using six mice for each mixture, inject subcutaneously a dose of 0.5 ml into each mouse. Observe the mice for 96 h. Mice that become paralysed may be killed. The mixture that contains the largest volume of immunoglobulin that fails to protect the mice from paralysis contains 1 IU. This quantity is used to calculate the potency of the immunoglobulin in International Units per millilitre.

The test is not valid unless all the mice injected with mixtures containing 2.0 ml or less of the solution of the reference preparation show paralysis and all those injected with mixtures containing more do not.

POTENCY

The potency is determined by comparing the antibody titre of the immunoglobulin to be examined with that of a reference preparation calibrated in International Units, using an immunoassay of suitable sensitivity and specificity (*2.7.1*).

The International Unit is the activity contained in a stated amount of the International Standard for anti-tetanus immunoglobulin. The equivalence in International Units of the International Standard is stated by the World Health Organisation.

Human tetanus immunoglobulin BRP is calibrated in International Units by comparison with the International Standard.

The stated potency is not less than 100 IU of tetanus antitoxin per millilitre. The estimated potency is not less than the stated potency. The confidence limits (P = 0.95) of the estimated potency are not less than 80 per cent and not more than 125 per cent.

STORAGE

See *Human normal immunoglobulin (0338).*

LABELLING

See *Human normal immunoglobulin (0338).*

The label states the number of International Units per container.

01/2005:0724

HUMAN VARICELLA IMMUNOGLOBULIN

Immunoglobulinum humanum varicellae

DEFINITION

Human varicella immunoglobulin is a liquid or freeze-dried preparation containing immunoglobulins, mainly immunoglobulin G. The preparation is intended for intramuscular administration. It is obtained from plasma from selected donors having antibodies against *Herpesvirus varicellae. Human normal immunoglobulin (0338)* may be added.

It complies with the monograph on *Human normal immunoglobulin (0338)* except for the minimum number of donors, the minimum total protein content and, where authorised, the test for antibody to hepatitis B surface antigen.

POTENCY

The potency is determined by comparing the antibody titre of the immunoglobulin to be examined with that of a reference preparation calibrated in International Units, using an immunoassay of suitable sensitivity and specificity (*2.7.1*).

The International Unit is the activity contained in a stated amount of the International Standard for anti varicella-zoster. The equivalence in International Units of the International Standard is stated by the World Health Organisation.

The stated potency is not less than 100 IU/ml. The estimated potency is not less than the stated potency. The confidence limits (P = 0.95) of the estimated potency are not less than 80 per cent and not more than 125 per cent.

Monographs F-H

STORAGE

See *Human normal immunoglobulin (0338)*.

LABELLING

See *Human normal immunoglobulin (0338)*.

The label states the number of International Units per container.

01/2005:1528

HUMAN VARICELLA IMMUNOGLOBULIN FOR INTRAVENOUS ADMINISTRATION

Immunoglobulinum humanum varicellae ad usum intravenosum

DEFINITION

Human varicella immunoglobulin for intravenous administration is a liquid or freeze-dried preparation containing immunoglobulins, mainly immunoglobulin G. It is obtained from plasma from selected donors having antibodies against human herpesvirus 3 (varicella-zoster virus 1). *Human normal immunoglobulin for intravenous administration (0918)* may be added.

It complies with the monograph on *Human normal immunoglobulin for intravenous administration (0918)*, except for the minimum number of donors, the minimum total protein content and the limit for osmolality.

POTENCY

The potency is determined by comparing the antibody titre of the immunoglobulin to be examined with that of a reference preparation calibrated in International Units, using an immunoassay of suitable sensitivity and specificity (*2.7.1*).

The International Unit is the activity contained in a stated amount of the International Standard for anti varicella-zoster immunoglobulin. The equivalence in International Units of the International Standard is stated by the World Health Organisation.

The stated potency is not less than 25 IU/ml. The estimated potency is not less than the stated potency. The confidence limits (P = 0.95) of the estimated potency are not less than 80 per cent and not more than 125 per cent.

STORAGE

See *Human normal immunoglobulin for intravenous administration (0918)*.

LABELLING

See *Human normal immunoglobulin for intravenous administration (0918)*.

The label states the number of International Units per container.

01/2005:0912
corrected

HYALURONIDASE

Hyaluronidasum

DEFINITION

Hyaluronidase is an enzyme extracted from mammalian testes (for example bovine testes) and capable of hydrolysing mucopolysaccharides of the hyaluronic acid type. It contains not less than 300 IU of hyaluronidase activity per milligram, calculated with reference to the dried substance. It may contain a suitable stabiliser.

PRODUCTION

The animals from which hyaluronidase is derived must fulfil the requirements for the health of animals suitable for human consumption to the satisfaction of the competent authority.

Hyaluronidase is produced using a validated method of extraction and purification in conditions designed to minimise the degree of microbial contamination; the method of preparation must have been shown to reduce any contamination by viruses or other known infectious agents to acceptable limits.

CHARACTERS

A white or yellowish-white, amorphous powder, soluble in water, practically insoluble in acetone and in ethanol.

IDENTIFICATION

A solution containing the equivalent of 100 IU of hyaluronidase in 1 ml of a 9 g/l solution of *sodium chloride R* depolymerises an equal volume of a 10 g/l solution of *sodium hyaluronate BRP* in 1 min at 20 °C as shown by a pronounced decrease in viscosity. This action is destroyed by heating the hyaluronidase at 100 °C for 30 min.

TESTS

Appearance of solution. Dissolve 0.10 g of the substance to be examined in *water R* and dilute to 10 ml. The solution is clear (*2.2.1*).

pH (*2.2.3*). Dissolve 30 mg in 10 ml of *carbon dioxide-free water R*. The pH of the solution is 4.5 to 7.5.

Loss on drying (*2.2.32*). Not more than 5.0 per cent, determined on 0.500 g by drying at 60 °C at a pressure not exceeding 670 Pa for 2 h.

Bacterial endotoxins (*2.6.14*): less than 0.2 IU per IU of hyaluronidase.

ASSAY

The activity of hyaluronidase is determined by comparing the rate at which it hydrolyses *sodium hyaluronate BRP* with the rate obtained with the International Standard, or a reference preparation calibrated in International Units, using a slope-ratio assay.

Substrate solution. To 0.10 g of *sodium hyaluronate BRP* in a 25 ml conical flask add slowly 20.0 ml of *water R* at 4 °C. The rate of addition must be slow enough to allow the substrate particles to swell (about 5 min). Maintain at 4 °C and stir for at least 12 h. Store at 4 °C and use within 4 days.

For the test solution and the reference solution, prepare the solution and carry out the dilution at 0 °C to 4 °C.

Test solution. Dissolve a suitable amount of the substance to be examined in *hyaluronidase diluent R* so as to obtain a solution containing 0.6 ± 0.3 IU of hyaluronidase per millilitre.

Reference solution. Dissolve a suitable amount of *hyaluronidase BRP* in *hyaluronidase diluent R* so as to obtain a solution containing 0.6 IU of hyaluronidase per millilitre.

In a reaction vessel, mix 1.50 ml of *phosphate buffer solution pH 6.4 R* and 1.0 ml of the substrate solution and equilibrate at 37 ± 0.1 °C. At time t_1 = 0 (first chronometer) add 0.50 ml of the test solution containing E_t mg of the enzyme to be examined, mix, measure the viscosity of the solution using a suitable viscometer maintained at 37 ± 0.1 °C and record the outflow time t_2 using a second chronometer (graduated in 0.1 second intervals), several times during about 20 min (read on the first chronometer). The following viscometer has been found suitable: Ubbelohde microviscometer (DIN 51 562, Part 2), capillary type MII, viscometer constant about 0.1 mm²/s².

Repeat the procedure using 0.50 ml of the reference solution containing E_r mg of *hyaluronidase BRP*.

Calculate the viscosity ratio from the expression:

$$\eta_r = \frac{k \times t_2}{0.6915}$$

k = the viscometer constant in mm²/s² (indicated on the viscometer),

t_2 = the outflow time (in seconds) of the solution.

0.6915 = the kinematic viscosity in mm²/s of the buffer solution at 37 °C.

Since the enzymatic reaction continues during the outflow time measurements, the real reaction time equals $t_1 + t_2/2$, half of the outflow time ($t_2/2$) for which a certain measurement is valid being added to the time t_1 at which the measurement is started. Plot $(\ln \eta_r)^{-1}$ as a function of the reaction time ($t_1 + t_2/2$) in seconds. A linear relationship is obtained. Calculate the slope for the substance to be examined (b_t) and the reference preparation (b_r).

Calculate the specific activity in International Units per milligram from the expression:

$$\frac{b_t}{b_r} \times \frac{E_r}{E_t} \times A$$

A = the specific activity of *hyaluronidase BRP* in International Units per milligram.

Carry out the complete procedure at least three times and calculate the average activity of the substance to be examined.

STORAGE

Store in an airtight container at a temperature of 2 °C to 8 °C. If the substance is sterile, store in a sterile, tamper-proof container.

LABELLING

The label states the activity in International Units per milligram.

01/2005:0829

HYDRALAZINE HYDROCHLORIDE

Hydralazini hydrochloridum

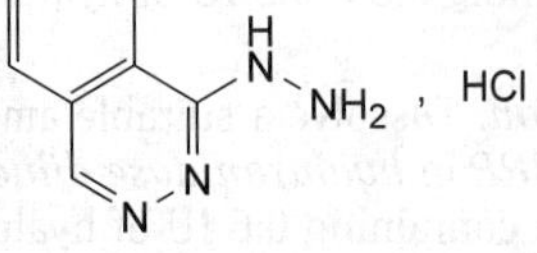

$C_8H_9ClN_4$ M_r 196.6

DEFINITION

Hydralazine hydrochloride contains not less than 98.5 per cent and not more than the equivalent of 101.0 per cent of 1-hydrazinophthalazine hydrochloride, calculated with reference to the dried substance.

CHARACTERS

A white or almost white, crystalline powder, soluble in water, slightly soluble in alcohol, very slightly soluble in methylene chloride.

It melts at about 275 °C, with decomposition.

IDENTIFICATION

First identification: B, E.

Second identification: A, C, D, E.

A. Dissolve 50 mg in *water R* and dilute to 100 ml with the same solvent. Dilute 2 ml of the solution to 100 ml with *water R*. Examined between 220 nm and 350 nm (*2.2.25*), the solution shows four absorption maxima, at 240 nm, 260 nm, 303 nm and 315 nm. The ratio of the absorbance measured at the maximum at 240 nm to that measured at the maximum at 303 nm is 2.0 to 2.2.

B. Examine by infrared spectrophotometry (*2.2.24*), comparing with the spectrum obtained with *hydralazine hydrochloride CRS*. Examine the substances prepared as discs.

C. Dissolve 0.5 g in a mixture of 8 ml of *dilute hydrochloric acid R* and 100 ml of *water R*. Add 2 ml of *sodium nitrite solution R*, allow to stand for 10 min and filter. The precipitate, washed with *water R* and dried at 100 °C to 105 °C, melts (*2.2.14*) at 209 °C to 212 °C.

D. Dissolve about 10 mg in 2 ml of *water R*. Add 2 ml of a 20 g/l solution of *nitrobenzaldehyde R* in *alcohol R*. An orange precipitate is formed.

E. It gives reaction (a) of chlorides (*2.3.1*).

TESTS

Solution S. Dissolve 0.5 g in *carbon dioxide-free water R* and dilute to 25 ml with the same solvent.

Appearance of solution. Dilute 4 ml of solution S to 20 ml with *water R*. The solution is clear (*2.2.1*) and not more intensely coloured than reference solution GY_6 (*2.2.2, Method II*).

pH (*2.2.3*). The pH of solution S is 3.5 to 4.2.

Related substances. Examine by liquid chromatography (*2.2.29*).

Test solution. Dissolve 25.0 mg of the substance to be examined in the mobile phase and dilute to 50.0 ml with the mobile phase.

Reference solution (a). Dilute 1.0 ml of the test solution to 100.0 ml with the mobile phase.

Reference solution (b). Dilute 10.0 ml of reference solution (a) to 50.0 ml with the mobile phase.

Reference solution (c). Dissolve 25.0 mg of *phthalazine R* in the mobile phase and dilute to 50.0 ml with the mobile phase. Dilute 4.0 ml of this solution to 100.0 ml with the mobile phase.

Reference solution (d). Dilute a mixture of 4.0 ml of the test solution and 10.0 ml of reference solution (c) to 100.0 ml with the mobile phase.

The solutions must be analysed within one working day.

The chromatographic procedure may be carried out using:

– a stainless steel column 0.25 m long and 4.6 mm in internal diameter packed with *nitrile silica gel for chromatography R1* (10 µm),

– as mobile phase at a flow rate of 1 ml/min a solution prepared as follows: to 22 volumes of *acetonitrile R* add 78 volumes of a solution containing 1.44 g of *sodium laurilsulfate R* and 0.75 g of *tetrabutylammonium bromide R* per litre and adjust the mixture to pH 3.0 with *0.05 M sulphuric acid*,

– as detector a spectrophotometer set at 230 nm.

Inject 20 µl of reference solution (a) and adjust the sensitivity of the detector so that the height of the principal peak in the chromatogram is not less than 70 per cent of the full scale of the recorder. When the chromatograms are recorded in the prescribed conditions, the retention time of hydralazine is about 10 min to 12 min. If necessary, adjust the concentration of acetonitrile in the mobile phase. Inject 20 µl of the test solution and continue the chromatography for three times the retention time of hydralazine. Inject 20 µl of reference solution (b). The area of any peak in the chromatogram obtained with the test solution, apart from the peaks due to the solvent and to hydralazine, is not greater than the area of the peak in the chromatogram obtained with reference solution (b) (0.2 per cent).

The test is not valid unless: the chromatogram obtained with reference solution (d) shows two principal peaks and the resolution between the peaks is at least 2.5; the principal peak in the chromatogram obtained with reference solution (b) has a signal-to-noise ratio of at least 3.

Hydrazine. Examine by thin-layer chromatography (*2.2.27*), using *silica gel G R* as the coating substance.

Test solution. Dissolve 0.12 g of the substance to be examined in 4 ml of *water R* and add 4 ml of a 150 g/l solution of *salicylaldehyde R* in *methanol R* and 0.2 ml of *hydrochloric acid R*. Mix and keep at a temperature not exceeding 25 °C for 2 h to 4 h, until the precipitate formed has sedimented. Add 4 ml of *toluene R*, shake vigorously and centrifuge. Transfer the clear supernatant liquid to a 100 ml separating funnel, separate the toluene layer and shake vigorously, each time for 3 min, with two quantities, each of 20 ml, of a 200 g/l solution of *sodium metabisulphite R* and with two quantities, each of 50 ml, of *water R*. Separate the toluene layer which is the test solution.

Reference solution (a). Dissolve 12 mg of *hydrazine sulphate R* in *dilute hydrochloric acid R* and dilute to 100.0 ml with the same acid. Dilute 1.0 ml of this solution to 100.0 ml with *dilute hydrochloric acid R*.

Reference solution (b). Prepare the solution at the same time and in the same manner as described for the test solution, using 1.0 ml of reference solution (a) and 3 ml of *water R*.

Apply to the plate 20 µl of the test solution and 20 µl of reference solution (b). Develop over a path of 10 cm using a mixture of 10 volumes of *alcohol R* and 90 volumes of *toluene R*. Allow the plate to dry in air and examine in ultraviolet light at 365 nm. Any spot showing yellow fluorescence in the chromatogram obtained with the test solution is not more intense than the corresponding spot in the chromatogram obtained with reference solution (b) (10 ppm of hydrazine).

Heavy metals (*2.4.8*). 1.0 g complies with limit test C for heavy metals (20 ppm). Prepare the standard using 2 ml of *lead standard solution (10 ppm Pb) R*.

Loss on drying (*2.2.32*). Not more than 0.5 per cent, determined on 1.000 g by drying *in vacuo*.

Sulphated ash (*2.4.14*). Not more than 0.1 per cent, determined on 1.0 g.

ASSAY

Dissolve 80.0 mg in 25 ml of *water R*. Add 35 ml of *hydrochloric acid R* and titrate with *0.05 M potassium iodate*, determining the end-point potentiometrically (*2.2.20*), using a calomel reference electrode and a platinum indicator electrode.

1 ml of *0.05 M potassium iodate* is equivalent to 9.832 mg of $C_8H_9ClN_4$.

STORAGE

Store protected from light.

01/2005:0002

HYDROCHLORIC ACID, CONCENTRATED

Acidum hydrochloridum concentratum

HCl M_r 36.46

DEFINITION

Concentrated hydrochloric acid contains not less than 35.0 per cent *m/m* and not more than 39.0 per cent *m/m* of HCl.

CHARACTERS

A clear, colourless, fuming liquid, miscible with water.

It has a relative density of about 1.18.

IDENTIFICATION

A. Dilute with *water R*. The solution is strongly acid (*2.2.4*).

B. It gives the reactions of chlorides (*2.3.1*).

C. It complies with the limits of the assay.

TESTS

Appearance of solution. To 2 ml add 8 ml of *water R*. The solution is clear (*2.2.1*) and colourless (*2.2.2, Method II*).

Free chlorine. To 15 ml add 100 ml of *carbon dioxide-free water R*, 1 ml of a 100 g/l solution of *potassium iodide R* and 0.5 ml of *iodide-free starch solution R*. Allow to stand in the dark for 2 min. Any blue colour disappears on the addition of 0.2 ml of *0.01 M sodium thiosulphate* (4 ppm).

Sulphates (*2.4.13*). To 6.4 ml add 10 mg of *sodium hydrogen carbonate R* and evaporate to dryness on a water-bath. Dissolve the residue in 15 ml of *distilled water R*. The solution complies with the limit test for sulphates (20 ppm).

Heavy metals (*2.4.8*). Dissolve the residue obtained in the test for residue on evaporation in 1 ml of *dilute hydrochloric acid R* and dilute to 25 ml with *water R*. Dilute 5 ml of this solution to 20 ml with *water R*. 12 ml of the solution complies with limit test A for heavy metals (2 ppm). Prepare the standard using *lead standard solution (2 ppm Pb) R*.

Residue on evaporation. Evaporate 100.0 g to dryness on a water-bath and dry at 100 °C to 105 °C. The residue weighs not more than 10 mg (0.01 per cent).

ASSAY

Weigh accurately a ground-glass-stoppered flask containing 30 ml of *water R*. Introduce 1.5 ml of the acid and weigh again. Titrate with *1 M sodium hydroxide*, using *methyl red solution R* as indicator.

1 ml of *1 M sodium hydroxide* is equivalent to 36.46 mg of HCl.

STORAGE

Store in a stoppered container made of glass or another inert material, at a temperature below 30 °C.

01/2005:0003

HYDROCHLORIC ACID, DILUTE

Acidum hydrochloridum dilutum

DEFINITION

Dilute hydrochloric acid contains 9.5 per cent *m/m* to 10.5 per cent *m/m* of HCl (M_r 36.46).

PREPARATION

To 274 g of concentrated hydrochloric acid add 726 g of *water R* and mix.

IDENTIFICATION

A. It is strongly acid (*2.2.4*).

B. It gives the reactions of chlorides (*2.3.1*).

C. It complies with the limits of the assay.

TESTS

Appearance. It is clear (*2.2.1*) and colourless (*2.2.2, Method II*).

Free chlorine. To 60 ml add 50 ml of *carbon dioxide-free water R*, 1 ml of a 100 g/l solution of *potassium iodide R* and 0.5 ml of *iodide-free starch solution R*. Allow to stand in the dark for 2 min. Any blue colour disappears on the addition of 0.2 ml of *0.01 M sodium thiosulphate* (1 ppm).

Sulphates (*2.4.13*). To 26 ml add 10 mg of *sodium hydrogen carbonate R* and evaporate to dryness on a water-bath. Dissolve the residue in 15 ml of *distilled water R*. The solution complies with the limit test for sulphates (5 ppm).

Heavy metals (*2.4.8*). Dissolve the residue obtained in the test for residue on evaporation in 1 ml of *dilute hydrochloric acid R* and dilute to 25 ml with *water R*. Dilute 5 ml of this solution to 20 ml with *water R*. 12 ml of the solution complies with limit test A for heavy metals (2 ppm). Prepare the standard using *lead standard solution (2 ppm Pb) R*.

Residue on evaporation. Evaporate 100.0 g to dryness on a water-bath and dry at 100 °C to 105 °C. The residue weighs not more than 10 mg (0.01 per cent).

ASSAY

To 6.00 g add 30 ml of *water R*. Titrate with *1 M sodium hydroxide*, using *methyl red solution R* as indicator.

1 ml of *1 M sodium hydroxide* is equivalent to 36.46 mg of HCl.

01/2005:0394

HYDROCHLOROTHIAZIDE

Hydrochlorothiazidum

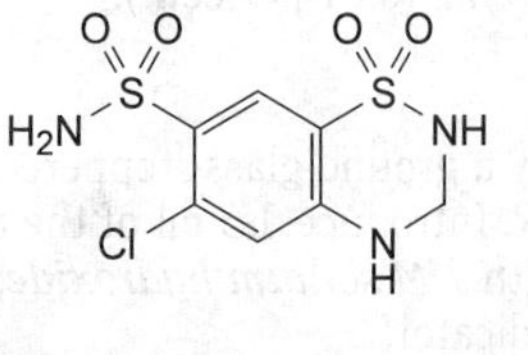

$C_7H_8ClN_3O_4S_2$ M_r 297.7

DEFINITION

Hydrochlorothiazide contains not less than 98.0 per cent and not more than the equivalent of 102.0 per cent of 6-chloro-3,4-dihydro-2*H*-1,2,4-benzothiadiazine-7-sulphonamide 1,1-dioxide, calculated with reference to the dried substance.

CHARACTERS

A white or almost white, crystalline powder, very slightly soluble in water, soluble in acetone, sparingly soluble in alcohol. It dissolves in dilute solutions of alkali hydroxides.

IDENTIFICATION

First identification: B.

Second identification: A, C, D.

A. Dissolve 50.0 mg in 10 ml of *0.1 M sodium hydroxide* and dilute to 100.0 ml with *water R*. Dilute 2.0 ml of this solution to 100.0 ml with *0.01 M sodium hydroxide*. Examined between 250 nm and 350 nm (*2.2.25*), the solution shows absorption maxima at 273 nm and at 323 nm. The ratio of the absorbance measured at the maximum at 273 nm to that measured at 323 nm is 5.4 to 5.7.

B. Examine by infrared absorption spectrophotometry (*2.2.24*), comparing with the spectrum obtained with *hydrochlorothiazide CRS*.

C. Examine by thin-layer chromatography (*2.2.27*), using as the coating substance a suitable silica gel with a fluorescent indicator having an optimal intensity at 254 nm.

Test solution. Dissolve 50 mg in *acetone R* and dilute to 10 ml with the same solvent.

Reference solution (a). Dissolve 50 mg of *hydrochlorothiazide CRS* in *acetone R* and dilute to 10 ml with the same solvent.

Reference solution (b). Dissolve 25 mg of *chlorothiazide R* in reference solution (a) and dilute to 5 ml with the same reference solution.

Apply separately to the plate 2 µl of each solution. Develop over a path of 10 cm using *ethyl acetate R*. Dry the plate in a current of air and examine in ultraviolet light at 254 nm. The principal spot in the chromatogram obtained with the test solution is similar in position and size to the principal spot in the chromatogram obtained with reference solution (a). The test is not valid unless the chromatogram obtained with reference solution (b) shows two clearly separated spots.

D. Gently heat about 1 mg with 2 ml of a freshly prepared 0.5 g/l solution of *chromotropic acid, sodium salt R* in a cooled mixture of 35 volumes of *water R* and 65 volumes of *sulphuric acid R*. A violet colour develops.

TESTS

Acidity or alkalinity. Shake 0.5 g of the powdered substance to be examined with 25 ml of *water R* for 2 min and filter. To 10 ml of the filtrate, add 0.2 ml of *0.01 M sodium hydroxide* and 0.15 ml of *methyl red solution R*. The solution is yellow. Not more than 0.4 ml of *0.01 M hydrochloric acid* is required to change the colour of the indicator to red.

Related substances. Examine by liquid chromatography (*2.2.29*).

Solvent solution. Dilute 50.0 ml of a mixture of equal volumes of *acetonitrile R* and *methanol R* to 200.0 ml with *phosphate buffer solution pH 3.2 R1*.

Test solution. Dissolve 30.0 mg of the substance to be examined in 5 ml of a mixture of equal volumes of *acetonitrile R* and *methanol R*, using sonication if necessary, and dilute to 20.0 ml with *phosphate buffer solution pH 3.2 R1*.

Reference solution (a). Dissolve 15.0 mg of *hydrochlorothiazide CRS* and 15.0 mg of *chlorothiazide CRS* in 25.0 ml of a mixture of equal volumes of *acetonitrile R* and *methanol R*, using sonication if necessary, and dilute to 100.0 ml with *phosphate buffer solution pH 3.2 R1*. Dilute 5.0 ml to 100.0 ml with the solvent solution.

Reference solution (b). Dilute 1.0 ml of the test solution to 50.0 ml with the solvent solution. Dilute 5.0 ml of this solution to 20.0 ml with the solvent solution.

The chromatographic procedure may be carried out using:

- a stainless steel column 0.1 m long and 4.6 mm in internal diameter packed with *octadecylsilyl silica gel for chromatography R* (3 µm),
- as mobile phase at a flow rate of 0.8 ml/min:
  Mobile phase A. To 940 ml of *phosphate buffer solution pH 3.2 R1* add 60.0 ml of *methanol R* and 10.0 ml of *tetrahydrofuran R* and mix,
  Mobile phase B. To a mixture of 500 ml of *methanol R* and 500 ml of *phosphate buffer solution pH 3.2 R1* add 50.0 ml of *tetrahydrofuran R* and mix,

Time (min)	Mobile phase A (per cent *V/V*)	Mobile phase B (per cent *V/V*)	Comment
0 - 17	100 → 55	0 → 45	linear gradient
17 - 30	55	45	isocratic
30 - 35	55 → 100	45 → 0	linear gradient
35 - 50	100	0	isocratic
50 = 0	100	0	return to initial eluent composition

- as detector a spectrophotometer set at 224 nm.

Equilibrate the column for at least 20 min with mobile phase A. Adjust the sensitivity of the system so that the height of the principal peak in the chromatogram obtained with 10 µl of reference solution (b) is at least 50 per cent of the full scale of the recorder.

Inject 10 µl of reference solution (a). When the chromatogram is recorded in the prescribed conditions, the retention times are: chlorothiazide about 7 min and hydrochlorothiazide about 8 min. The test is not valid unless the resolution between the peaks corresponding to chlorothiazide and hydrochlorothiazide is at least 2.5. If necessary, adjust slightly the composition of the mobile phase or the time programme of the linear gradient.

Inject separately 10 µl of the solvent solution as a blank, 10 µl of the test solution and 10 µl of reference solution (b). In the chromatogram obtained with the test solution: the area of any peak, apart from the principal peak, is not greater than the area of the principal peak in the chromatogram obtained with reference solution (b) (0.5 per cent); the sum of the areas of all peaks, apart from the principal peak, is not greater than twice the area of the principal peak in the chromatogram obtained with reference solution (b) (1 per cent). Disregard any peak due to the solvent solution and any peak with an area less than 0.1 times the area of the principal peak in the chromatogram obtained with reference solution (b).

Chlorides (*2.4.4*). Dissolve 1.0 g in 25 ml of *acetone R* and dilute to 30 ml with *water R*. 15 ml complies with the limit test for chlorides (100 ppm). Prepare the standard using 5 ml of *acetone R* containing 15 per cent *V/V* of *water R* and 10 ml of *chloride standard solution (5 ppm Cl) R*.

Loss on drying (*2.2.32*). Not more than 0.5 per cent, determined on 1.000 g by drying in an oven at 100 °C to 105 °C.

Sulphated ash (*2.4.14*). Not more than 0.1 per cent, determined on 1.0 g.

ASSAY

Dissolve 0.120 g in 50 ml of *dimethyl sulphoxide R*. Titrate with *0.1 M tetrabutylammonium hydroxide in 2-propanol*, determining the end-point potentiometrically (*2.2.20*) at the second point of inflexion. Carry out a blank titration.

1 ml of *0.1 M tetrabutylammonium hydroxide in 2-propanol* is equivalent to 14.88 mg of $C_7H_8ClN_3O_4S_2$.

IMPURITIES

A. chlorothiazide,

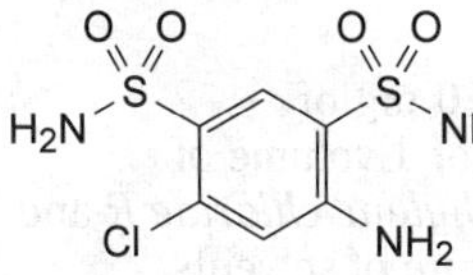

B. 4-amino-6-chlorobenzene-1,3-disulphonamide (salamide),

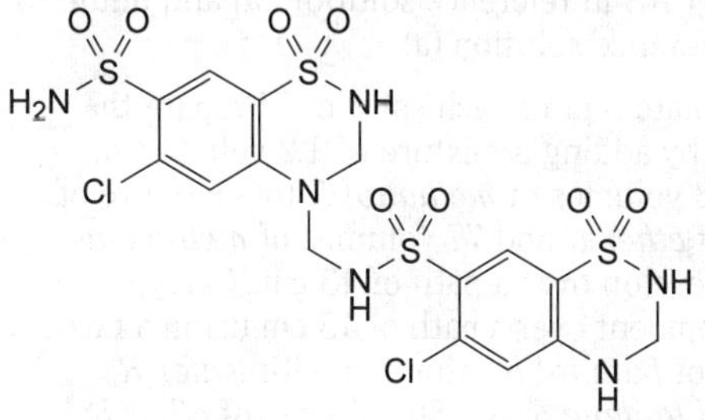

C. 6-chloro-*N*-[(6-chloro-7-sulphamoyl-2,3-dihydro-4*H*-1,2,4-benzothiadiazin-4-yl 1,1-dioxide)methyl]-3,4-dihydro-2*H*-1,2,4-benzothiadiazine-7-sulphonamide 1,1-dioxide.

01/2005:0335

HYDROCORTISONE

Hydrocortisonum

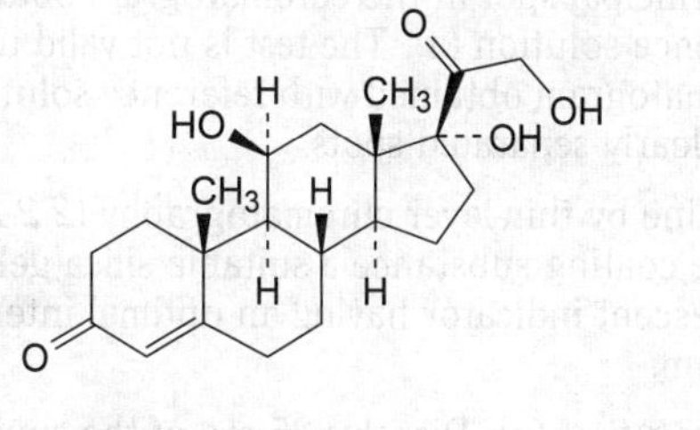

$C_{21}H_{30}O_5$ M_r 362.5

DEFINITION

Hydrocortisone contains not less than 97.0 per cent and not more than the equivalent of 103.0 per cent of 11β,17,21-trihydroxypregn-4-ene-3,20-dione, calculated with reference to the dried substance.

CHARACTERS

A white or almost white, crystalline powder, practically insoluble in water, sparingly soluble in acetone and in alcohol, slightly soluble in methylene chloride.

It shows polymorphism.

IDENTIFICATION

First identification: A, B.

Second identification: C, D.

A. Examine by infrared absorption spectrophotometry (*2.2.24*), comparing with the spectrum obtained with *hydrocortisone CRS*. If the spectra obtained in the solid state show differences, dissolve the substance to be examined and the reference substance separately in the minimum volume of *acetone R*, evaporate to dryness on a water-bath and record new spectra using the residues.

B. Examine by thin-layer chromatography (*2.2.27*), using as the coating substance a suitable silica gel with a fluorescent indicator having an optimal intensity at 254 nm.

Test solution. Dissolve 10 mg of the substance to be examined in a mixture of 1 volume of *methanol R* and 9 volumes of *methylene chloride R* and dilute to 10 ml with the same mixture of solvents.

Reference solution (a). Dissolve 20 mg of *hydrocortisone CRS* in a mixture of 1 volume of *methanol R* and 9 volumes of *methylene chloride R* and dilute to 20 ml with the same mixture of solvents.

Reference solution (b). Dissolve 10 mg of *prednisolone CRS* in reference solution (a) and dilute to 10 ml with reference solution (a).

Apply to the plate 5 µl of each solution. Prepare the mobile phase by adding a mixture of 1.2 volumes of *water R* and 8 volumes of *methanol R* to a mixture of 15 volumes of *ether R* and 77 volumes of *methylene chloride R*. Develop over a path of 15 cm. Carry out a second development over a path of 15 cm using a mixture of 5 volumes of *butanol R* saturated with *water R*, 15 volumes of *toluene R* and 80 volumes of *ether R*. Allow the plate to dry in air. Examine in ultraviolet light at 254 nm. The principal spot in the chromatogram obtained with the test solution is similar in position and size to the principal spot in the chromatogram obtained with reference solution (a). Spray with *alcoholic solution of sulphuric acid R*. Heat at 120 °C for 10 min or until the spots appear. Allow to cool. Examine the chromatograms in daylight and in ultraviolet light at 365 nm. The principal spot in the chromatogram obtained with the test solution is similar in position, colour in daylight, fluorescence in ultraviolet light at 365 nm and size to the principal spot in the chromatogram obtained with reference solution (a). The test is not valid unless the chromatogram obtained with reference solution (b) shows two clearly separated spots.

C. Examine by thin-layer chromatography (*2.2.27*), using as the coating substance a suitable silica gel with a fluorescent indicator having an optimal intensity at 254 nm.

Test solution (a). Dissolve 25 mg of the substance to be examined in *methanol R* and dilute to 5 ml with the same solvent. This solution is also used to prepare test solution (b). Dilute 2 ml of the solution to 10 ml with *methylene chloride R*.

Test solution (b). Transfer 0.4 ml of the solution obtained during preparation of test solution (a) to a glass tube 100 mm long and 20 mm in diameter and fitted with a ground-glass stopper or a polytetrafluoroethylene cap and evaporate the solvent with gentle heating under a stream of *nitrogen R*. Add 2 ml of a 15 per cent *V/V* solution of *glacial acetic acid R* and 50 mg of *sodium bismuthate R*. Stopper the tube and shake the suspension for 1 h in a mechanical shaker, protected from light. Add 2 ml of a 15 per cent *V/V* solution of *glacial acetic acid R* and filter into a 50 ml separating funnel, washing the filter with two quantities, each of 5 ml, of *water R*. Shake the clear filtrate with 10 ml of *methylene chloride R*. Wash the organic layer with 5 ml of *1 M sodium hydroxide* and two quantities, each of 5 ml, of *water R*. Dry over *anhydrous sodium sulphate R*.

Reference solution (a). Dissolve 25 mg of *hydrocortisone CRS* in *methanol R* and dilute to 5 ml with the same solvent. This solution is also used to prepare reference solution (b). Dilute 2 ml of the solution to 10 ml with *methylene chloride R*.

Reference solution (b). Transfer 0.4 ml of the solution obtained during preparation of reference solution (a) to a glass tube 100 mm long and 20 mm in diameter and fitted with a ground-glass stopper or a polytetrafluoroethylene cap and evaporate the solvent with gentle heating under a stream of *nitrogen R*. Add 2 ml of a 15 per cent *V/V* solution of *glacial acetic acid R* and 50 mg of *sodium bismuthate R*. Stopper the tube and shake the suspension for 1 h in a mechanical shaker protected from light. Add 2 ml of a 15 per cent *V/V* solution of *glacial acetic acid R* and filter into a 50 ml separating funnel, washing the filter with two quantities, each of 5 ml, of *water R*. Shake the clear filtrate with 10 ml of *methylene chloride R*. Wash the organic layer with 5 ml of *1 M sodium hydroxide* and two quantities, each of 5 ml, of *water R*. Dry over *anhydrous sodium sulphate R*.

Apply to the plate 5 µl of test solution (a), 5 µl of reference solution (a), 25 µl of test solution (b) and 25 µl of reference solution (b), applying the latter two in small quantities to obtain small spots. Prepare the mobile phase by adding a mixture of 1.2 volumes of *water R* and 8 volumes of *methanol R* to a mixture of 15 volumes of *ether R* and 77 volumes of *methylene chloride R*. Develop over a path of 15 cm. Carry out a second development over a path of 15 cm using a mixture of 5 volumes of *butanol R* saturated with *water R*, 15 volumes of *toluene R* and 80 volumes of *ether R*. Allow the plate to dry in air and examine in ultraviolet light at 254 nm. The principal spot in each of the chromatograms obtained with the test solutions is similar in position and size to the principal spot in the chromatogram obtained with the corresponding reference solution. Spray with *alcoholic solution of sulphuric acid R* and heat at 120 °C for 10 min or until the spots appear. Allow to cool. Examine the plate in daylight and in ultraviolet light at 365 nm. The principal spot in each of the chromatograms obtained with the test solutions is similar in position, colour in daylight, fluorescence in ultraviolet light at 365 nm and size to the principal spot in the chromatogram obtained with the corresponding reference solution. The principal spots in the chromatograms obtained with test solution (b) and reference solution (b) have an R_f value distinctly higher than that of the principal spots in the chromatograms obtained with test solution (a) and reference solution (a).

D. Add about 2 mg to 2 ml of *sulphuric acid R* and shake to dissolve. Within 5 min, an intense brownish-red colour develops with a green fluorescence which is particularly intense when examined in ultraviolet light at 365 nm. Add the solution to 10 ml of *water R* and mix. The colour fades and a clear solution remains. The fluorescence in ultraviolet light does not disappear.

TESTS

Specific optical rotation (*2.2.7*). Dissolve 0.250 g in *dioxan R* and dilute to 25.0 ml with the same solvent. The specific optical rotation is + 150 to + 156, calculated with reference to the dried substance.

Related substances. Examine by liquid chromatography (*2.2.29*). *Prepare the solutions immediately before use.*

Test solution. Dissolve 25.0 mg of the substance to be examined in 2 ml of *tetrahydrofuran R* and dilute to 10.0 ml with *water R*.

Reference solution (a). Dissolve 2 mg of *hydrocortisone CRS* and 2 mg of *prednisolone CRS* in the mobile phase and dilute to 100.0 ml with the mobile phase.

Reference solution (b). Dilute 1.0 ml of the test solution to 100.0 ml with the mobile phase.

The chromatographic procedure may be carried out using:

- a stainless steel column 0.25 m long and 4.6 mm in internal diameter packed with *base-deactivated end-capped octadecylsilyl silica gel for chromatography R* (5 μm),
- as mobile phase at a flow rate of 1 ml/min a mixture prepared as follows: in a 1000 ml volumetric flask mix 220 ml of *tetrahydrofuran R* with 700 ml of *water R* and allow to equilibrate; dilute to 1000 ml with *water R* and mix again,
- as detector a spectrophotometer set at 254 nm,

maintaining the temperature of the column at 45 °C.

Equilibrate the column with the mobile phase at a flow rate of 1 ml/min for about 30 min.

Adjust the sensitivity of the system so that the height of the principal peak in the chromatogram obtained with 20 μl of reference solution (b) is at least 50 per cent of the full scale of the recorder.

Inject 20 μl of reference solution (a). When the chromatograms are recorded in the prescribed conditions, the retention times are: prednisolone about 14 min and hydrocortisone about 15.5 min. The test is not valid unless the resolution between the peaks due to prednisolone and hydrocortisone is at least 2.2. If necessary, adjust the concentration of *tetrahydrofuran R* in the mobile phase.

Inject separately 20 μl of the solvent mixture of the test solution as a blank, 20 μl of the test solution and 20 μl of reference solution (b). Continue the chromatography of the test solution for four times the retention time of the principal peak. In the chromatogram obtained with the test solution: the area of any peak, apart from the principal peak, is not greater than half the area of the principal peak in the chromatogram obtained with reference solution (b) (0.5 per cent): the sum of the areas of all the peaks, apart from the principal peak, is not greater than 1.5 times the area of the principal peak in the chromatogram obtained with reference solution (b) (1.5 per cent). Disregard any peak obtained with the blank run and any peak with an area less than 0.05 times the area of the principal peak in the chromatogram obtained with reference solution (b).

Loss on drying (*2.2.32*). Not more than 1.0 per cent, determined on 0.500 g by drying in an oven at 100 °C to 105 °C.

ASSAY

Dissolve 0.100 g in *alcohol R* and dilute to 100.0 ml with the same solvent. Dilute 2.0 ml of the solution to 100.0 ml with *alcohol R*. Measure the absorbance (*2.2.25*) at the maximum at 241.5 nm.

Calculate the content of $C_{21}H_{30}O_5$ taking the specific absorbance to be 440.

STORAGE

Store protected from light.

IMPURITIES

A. prednisolone,

B. cortisone,

C. hydrocortisone acetate,

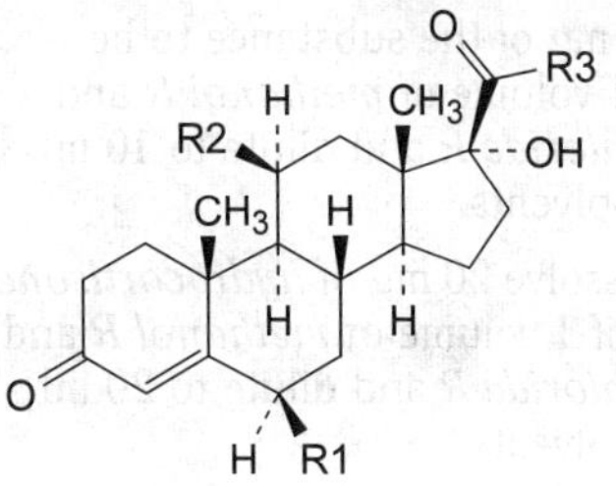

D. R1 = R2 = OH, R3 = CH_2OH: 6β,11β,17,21-tetrahydroxypregn-4-ene-3,20-dione (6β-hydroxyhydrocortisone),

F. R1 = R2 = H, R3 = CH_2OH: 17,21-dihydroxypregn-4-ene-3,20-dione (Reichstein's substance),

G. R1 = H, R2 = OH, R3 = CHO: 11β,17-dihydroxy-3,20-dioxopregn-4-en-21-al,

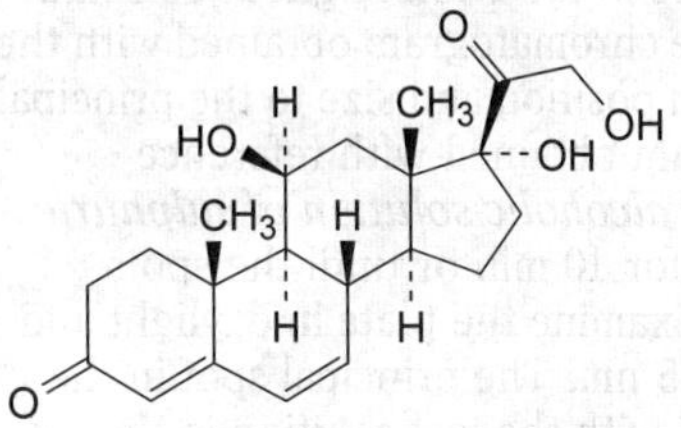

E. 11β,17,21-trihydroxypregna-4,6-diene-3,20-dione (Δ6-hydrocortisone).

01/2005:0334

HYDROCORTISONE ACETATE

Hydrocortisoni acetas

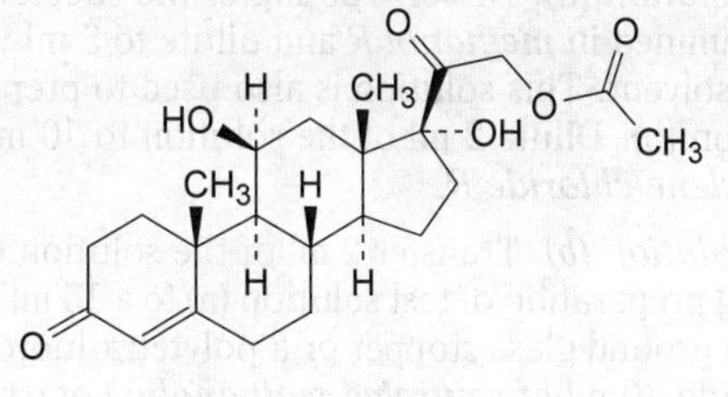

$C_{23}H_{32}O_6$ M_r 404.5

DEFINITION

Hydrocortisone acetate contains not less than 97.0 per cent and not more than the equivalent of 103.0 per cent of 11β,17-dihydroxy-3,20-dioxopregn-4-en-21-yl acetate, calculated with reference to the dried substance.

CHARACTERS

A white or almost white, crystalline powder, practically insoluble in water, slightly soluble in ethanol and in methylene chloride.

It melts at about 220 °C, with decomposition.

IDENTIFICATION

First identification: A, B.

Second identification: C, D, E.

A. Examine by infrared absorption spectrophotometry (*2.2.24*), comparing with the spectrum obtained with *hydrocortisone acetate CRS*.

B. Examine by thin-layer chromatography (*2.2.27*), using as the coating substance a suitable silica gel with a fluorescent indicator having an optimal intensity at 254 nm.

Test solution. Dissolve 10 mg of the substance to be examined in a mixture of 1 volume of *methanol R* and 9 volumes of *methylene chloride R* and dilute to 10 ml with the same mixture of solvents.

Reference solution (a). Dissolve 20 mg of *hydrocortisone acetate CRS* in a mixture of 1 volume of *methanol R* and 9 volumes of *methylene chloride R* and dilute to 20 ml with the same mixture of solvents.

Reference solution (b). Dissolve 10 mg of *cortisone acetate R* in reference solution (a) and dilute to 10 ml with reference solution (a).

Apply to the plate 5 µl of each solution. Prepare the mobile phase by adding a mixture of 1.2 volumes of *water R* and 8 volumes of *methanol R* to a mixture of 15 volumes of *ether R* and 77 volumes of *methylene chloride R*. Develop over a path of 15 cm. Allow the plate to dry in air and examine in ultraviolet light at 254 nm. The principal spot in the chromatogram obtained with the test solution is similar in position and size to the principal spot in the chromatogram obtained with reference solution (a). Spray with *alcoholic solution of sulphuric acid R*. Heat at 120 °C for 10 min or until the spots appear. Allow to cool. Examine the plate in daylight and in ultraviolet light at 365 nm. The principal spot in the chromatogram obtained with the test solution is similar in position, colour in daylight, fluorescence in ultraviolet light at 365 nm and size to the principal spot in the chromatogram obtained with reference solution (a). The test is not valid unless the chromatogram obtained with reference solution (b) shows two clearly separated spots.

C. Examine by thin-layer chromatography (*2.2.27*), using as the coating substance a suitable silica gel with a fluorescent indicator having an optimal intensity at 254 nm.

Test solution (a). Dissolve 25 mg of the substance to be examined in *methanol R* and dilute to 5 ml with the same solvent. This solution is also used to prepare test solution (b). Dilute 2 ml of the solution to 10 ml with *methylene chloride R*.

Test solution (b). Transfer 2 ml of the solution obtained during preparation of test solution (a) to a 15 ml glass tube with a ground-glass stopper or a polytetrafluoroethylene cap. Add 10 ml of *saturated methanolic potassium hydrogen carbonate solution R* and immediately pass a stream of *nitrogen R* briskly through the solution for 5 min. Stopper the tube. Heat in a water-bath at 45 °C protected from light for 2 h 30 min. Allow to cool.

Reference solution (a). Dissolve 25 mg of *hydrocortisone acetate CRS* in *methanol R* and dilute to 5 ml with the same solvent. This solution is also used to prepare reference solution (b). Dilute 2 ml of the solution to 10 ml with *methylene chloride R*.

Reference solution (b). Transfer 2 ml of the solution obtained during preparation of reference solution (a) to a 15 ml glass tube with a ground-glass stopper or a polytetrafluoroethylene cap. Add 10 ml of *saturated methanolic potassium hydrogen carbonate solution R* and immediately pass a stream of *nitrogen R* briskly through the solution for 5 min. Stopper the tube. Heat in a water-bath at 45 °C protected from light for 2 h 30 min. Allow to cool.

Apply to the plate 5 µl of each solution. Prepare the mobile phase by adding a mixture of 1.2 volumes of *water R* and 8 volumes of *methanol R* to a mixture of 15 volumes of *ether R* and 77 volumes of *methylene chloride R*. Develop over a path of 15 cm. Allow the plate to dry in air and examine in ultraviolet light at 254 nm. The principal spot in each of the chromatograms obtained with the test solutions is similar in position and size to the principal spot in the chromatogram obtained with the corresponding reference solution. Spray with *alcoholic solution of sulphuric acid R* and heat at 120 °C for 10 min or until the spots appear. Allow to cool. Examine in daylight and in ultraviolet light at 365 nm. The principal spot in each of the chromatograms obtained with the test solutions is similar in position, colour in daylight, fluorescence in ultraviolet light at 365 nm and size to the principal spot in the chromatogram obtained with the corresponding reference solution. The principal spots in the chromatograms obtained with test solution (b) and reference solution (b) have an R_f value distinctly lower than that of the principal spots in the chromatograms obtained with test solution (a) and reference solution (a).

D. Add about 2 mg to 2 ml of *sulphuric acid R* and shake to dissolve. Within 5 min an intense brownish-red colour develops with a green fluorescence which is particularly intense when viewed in ultraviolet light at 365 nm. Add the solution to 10 ml of *water R* and mix. The colour fades and the fluorescence in ultraviolet light does not disappear.

E. About 10 mg gives the reaction of acetyl (*2.3.1*).

TESTS

Specific optical rotation (*2.2.7*). Dissolve 0.250 g in *dioxan R* and dilute to 25.0 ml with the same solvent. The specific optical rotation is + 158 to + 167, calculated with reference to the dried substance.

Related substances. Examine by liquid chromatography (*2.2.29*).

Test solution. Dissolve 25.0 mg of the substance to be examined in *methanol R* and dilute to 10.0 ml with the same solvent.

Reference solution (a). Dissolve 2 mg of *hydrocortisone acetate CRS* and 2 mg of *cortisone acetate R* in the mobile phase and dilute to 100.0 ml with the mobile phase.

Reference solution (b). Dilute 1.0 ml of the test solution to 100.0 ml with the mobile phase.

The chromatographic procedure may be carried out using:

– a stainless steel column 0.25 m long and 4.6 mm in internal diameter packed with *octadecylsilyl silica gel for chromatography R* (5 µm),
– as mobile phase at a flow rate of 1 ml/min a mixture prepared as follows: in a 1000 ml volumetric flask mix 400 ml of *acetonitrile R* with 550 ml of *water R* and allow to equilibrate; adjust the volume to 1000 ml with *water R* and mix again,
– as detector a spectrophotometer set at 254 nm.

Equilibrate the column with the mobile phase at a flow rate of 1 ml/min for about 30 min.

Adjust the sensitivity of the system so that the height of the principal peak in the chromatogram obtained with 20 µl of reference solution (b) is not less than 50 per cent of the full scale of the recorder.

Inject 20 µl of reference solution (a). When the chromatograms are recorded in the prescribed conditions the retention times are: hydrocortisone acetate, about 10 min and cortisone acetate, about 12 min. The test is not valid unless the resolution between the peaks due to hydrocortisone acetate and cortisone acetate is at least 4.2; if necessary, adjust the concentration of acetonitrile in the mobile phase.

Inject separately 20 µl of the test solution and 20 µl of reference solution (b). Continue the chromatography for 2.5 times the retention time of the principal peak. In the chromatogram obtained with the test solution: the area of any peak, apart from the principal peak, is not greater than the area of the principal peak in the chromatogram obtained with reference solution (b) (1.0 per cent) and not more than one such peak has an area greater than half the area of the principal peak in the chromatogram obtained with reference solution (b) (0.5 per cent); the sum of the areas of all the peaks, apart from the principal peak, is not greater than 1.5 times the area of the principal peak in the chromatogram obtained with reference solution (b) (1.5 per cent). Disregard any peak due to the solvent and any peak with an area less than 0.05 times the area of the principal peak in the chromatogram obtained with reference solution (b).

Loss on drying (*2.2.32*). Not more than 0.5 per cent, determined on 0.500 g by drying in an oven at 100 °C to 105 °C.

ASSAY

Dissolve 0.100 g in *alcohol R* and dilute to 100.0 ml with the same solvent. Dilute 2.0 ml of the solution to 100.0 ml with *alcohol R*. Measure the absorbance (*2.2.25*) at the maximum of 241.5 nm.

Calculate the content of $C_{23}H_{32}O_6$ taking the specific absorbance to be 395.

STORAGE

Store protected from light.

01/2005:0768

HYDROCORTISONE HYDROGEN SUCCINATE

Hydrocortisoni hydrogenosuccinas

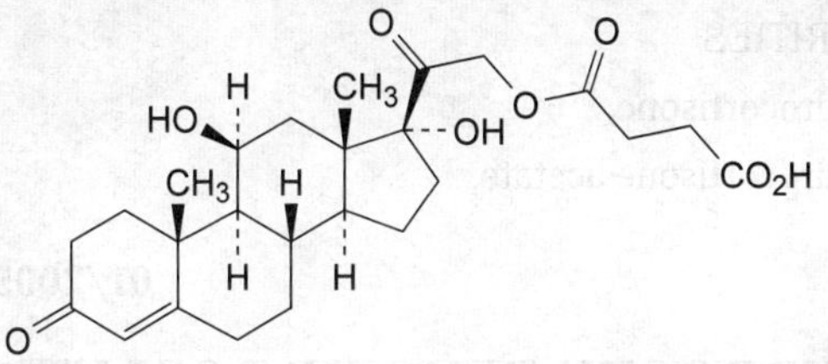

$C_{25}H_{34}O_8$ M_r 462.5

DEFINITION

Hydrocortisone hydrogen succinate contains not less than 97.0 per cent and not more than the equivalent of 103.0 per cent of 11β,17-dihydroxy-3,20-dioxopregn-4-en-21-yl hydrogen butanedioate, calculated with reference to the dried substance.

CHARACTERS

A white or almost white powder, hygroscopic, practically insoluble in water, freely soluble in acetone and in ethanol. It dissolves in dilute solutions of alkali carbonates and alkali hydroxides.

IDENTIFICATION

First identification: A, B.

Second identification: C, D.

A. Examine by infrared absorption spectrophotometry (*2.2.24*), comparing with the spectrum obtained with *hydrocortisone hydrogen succinate CRS*. Dry the substances before use at 100 °C to 105 °C for 3 h.

B. Examine by thin-layer chromatography (*2.2.27*), using as the coating substance a suitable silica gel with a fluorescent indicator having an optimal intensity at 254 nm.

Test solution. Dissolve 10 mg of the substance to be examined in a mixture of 1 volume of *methanol R* and 9 volumes of *methylene chloride R* and dilute to 10 ml with the same mixture of solvents.

Reference solution (a). Dissolve 20 mg of *hydrocortisone hydrogen succinate CRS* in a mixture of 1 volume of *methanol R* and 9 volumes of *methylene chloride R* and dilute to 20 ml with the same mixture of solvents.

Reference solution (b). Dissolve 10 mg of *methylprednisolone hydrogen succinate CRS* in reference solution (a) and dilute to 10 ml with reference solution (a).

Apply separately to the plate 5 µl of each solution. Develop over a path of 15 cm using a mixture of 0.1 volumes of *anhydrous formic acid R*, 1 volume of *ethanol R* and 15 volumes of *methylene chloride R*. Allow the plate to dry in air and examine in ultraviolet light at 254 nm. The principal spot in the chromatogram obtained with the test solution is similar in position and size to the principal spot in the chromatogram obtained with reference solution (a). Spray the plate with *alcoholic solution of sulphuric acid R*. Heat at 120 °C for 10 min or until the spots appear. Allow to cool. Examine in daylight and in ultraviolet light at 365 nm. The principal spot in the chromatogram obtained with the test solution is similar in position, colour in daylight, fluorescence in ultraviolet light at 365 nm and size to the principal spot in the chromatogram obtained with reference solution (a). The test is not valid unless the chromatogram obtained with reference solution (b) shows two spots which may however not be completely separated.

C. Examine by thin-layer chromatography (*2.2.27*), using as the coating substance a suitable silica gel with a fluorescent indicator having an optimal intensity at 254 nm.

Test solution (a). Dissolve 25 mg of the substance to be examined in *methanol R* with gentle heating and dilute to 5 ml with the same solvent. (This solution is also used to prepare test solution (b)). Dilute 2 ml of the solution to 10 ml with *methylene chloride R*.

Test solution (b). Transfer 2 ml of the solution obtained during preparation of test solution (a) to a 15 ml glass tube with a ground-glass stopper or a polytetrafluoroeth-ylene cap. Add 10 ml of a 0.8 g/l solution of *sodium hydroxide R* in *methanol R* and immediately pass a stream of *nitrogen R* briskly through the solution for 5 min. Stopper the tube. Heat in a water-bath at 45 °C, protected from light, for 30 min. Allow to cool.

Reference solution (a). Dissolve 25 mg of *hydrocortisone hydrogen succinate CRS* in *methanol R* with gentle heating and dilute to 5 ml with the same solvent. (This solution is also used to prepare reference solution (b)). Dilute 2 ml of the solution to 10 ml with *methylene chloride R*.

Reference solution (b). Transfer 2 ml of the solution obtained during preparation of reference solution (a) to a 15 ml glass tube with a ground-glass stopper or a polytetra-fluoroethylene cap. Add 10 ml of a 0.8 g/l solution of *sodium hydroxide R* in *methanol R* and immediately pass a stream of *nitrogen R* briskly through the solution for 5 min. Stopper the tube. Heat in a water-bath at 45 °C, protected from light, for 30 min. Allow to cool.

Apply separately to the plate 5 μl of each solution. Prepare the mobile phase by adding a mixture of 1.2 volumes of *water R* and 8 volumes of *methanol R* to a mixture of 15 volumes of *ether R* and 77 volumes of *methylene chloride R*. Develop over a path of 15 cm. Allow the plate to dry in air and examine in ultraviolet light at 254 nm. The principal spot in each of the chromatograms obtained with the test solutions is similar in position and size to the principal spot in the chromatogram obtained with the corresponding reference solution. Spray the plate with *alcoholic solution of sulphuric acid R*. Heat at 120 °C for 10 min or until the spots appear. Allow to cool. Examine in daylight and in ultraviolet light at 365 nm. The principal spot in the chromatograms obtained with the test solutions is similar in position, colour in daylight, fluorescence in ultraviolet light at 365 nm and size to the principal spot in the chromatogram obtained with the corresponding reference solution. The principal spot in each of the chromatograms obtained with test solution (b) and reference solution (b) has an R_f value distinctly higher than that of the principal spots in each of the chromatograms obtained with test solution (a) and reference solution (a).

D. Add about 2 mg to 2 ml of *sulphuric acid R* and shake to dissolve. Within 5 min, an intense brownish-red colour develops with a green fluorescence which is particularly intense when viewed in ultraviolet light at 365 nm. Add the solution to 10 ml of *water R* and mix. The colour fades and a clear solution remains. The fluorescence in ultraviolet light does not disappear.

TESTS

Appearance of solution. Dissolve 0.10 g in 5 ml of *sodium hydrogen carbonate solution R*. The solution is clear (*2.2.1*).

Specific optical rotation (*2.2.7*). Dissolve 0.250 g in *ethanol R* and dilute to 25.0 ml with the same solvent. The specific optical rotation is + 147 to + 153, calculated with reference to the dried substance.

Related substances. Examine by liquid chromatography (*2.2.29*).

Test solution. Dissolve 25.0 mg of the substance to be examined in a mixture of equal volumes of *acetonitrile R* and *water R* and dilute to 10.0 ml with the same solvent.

Reference solution (a). Dissolve 2 mg of *hydrocortisone hydrogen succinate CRS* and 2 mg of *dexamethasone CRS* in 50 ml of *acetonitrile R* and dilute to 100.0 ml with *water R*.

Reference solution (b). Dilute 1.0 ml of the test solution to 100.0 ml with a mixture of equal volumes of *acetonitrile R* and *water R*.

The chromatographic procedure may be carried out using:

- a stainless steel column 0.25 m long and 4.6 mm in internal diameter packed with *octadecylsilyl silica gel for chromatography R* (5 μm),
- as mobile phase at a flow rate of 1 ml/min a mixture prepared as follows: in a 1000 ml volumetric flask mix 330 ml of *acetonitrile R* with 600 ml of *water R* and 1.0 ml of *phosphoric acid R* and allow to equilibrate; dilute to 1000 ml with *water R* and mix again,
- as detector a spectrophotometer set at 254 nm.

Equilibrate the column with the mobile phase at a flow rate of 1 ml/min for about 30 min.

Adjust the sensitivity of the system so that the height of the principal peak in the chromatogram obtained with 20 μl of reference solution (b) is not less than 50 per cent of the full scale of the recorder.

Inject 20 μl of reference solution (a). When the chromatograms are recorded in the conditions described above the retention times are: dexamethasone, about 12.5 min and hydrocortisone hydrogen succinate, about 15 min. The test is not valid unless the resolution between the peaks corresponding to dexamethasone and hydrocortisone hydrogen succinate is a least 5.0; if necessary, adjust the concentration of acetonitrile in the mobile phase.

Inject separately 20 μl of the test solution and 20 μl of reference solution (b). Continue the chromatography for twice the retention time of the principal peak. In the chromatogram obtained with the test solution: the area of any peak, apart from the principal peak, is not greater than half the area of the principal peak in the chromatogram obtained with reference solution (b) (0.5 per cent); the sum of the areas of all the peaks, apart from the principal peak, is not greater than 0.75 times the area of the principal peak in the chromatogram obtained with reference solution (b) (0.75 per cent). Disregard any peak due to the solvent and any peak with an area less than 0.05 times the area of the principal peak in the chromatogram obtained with reference solution (b).

Loss on drying (*2.2.32*). Not more than 4.0 per cent, determined on 1.000 g by drying in an oven at 100 °C to 105 °C.

Sulphated ash (*2.4.14*). Not more than 0.1 per cent, determined on 1.0 g.

ASSAY

Dissolve 0.100 g in *alcohol R* and dilute to 100.0 ml with the same solvent. Dilute 2.0 ml to 100.0 ml with *alcohol R*. Measure the absorbance (*2.2.25*) at the maximum at 241.5 nm.

Calculate the content of $C_{25}H_{34}O_8$ taking the specific absorbance to be 353.

STORAGE

Store in an airtight container, protected from light.

IMPURITIES

A. hydrocortisone,

B. hydrocortisone acetate.

01/2005:0395

HYDROGEN PEROXIDE SOLUTION (3 PER CENT)

Hydrogenii peroxidum 3 per centum

DEFINITION

Hydrogen peroxide solution (3 per cent) contains not less than 2.5 per cent *m/m* and not more than 3.5 per cent *m/m* of H_2O_2 (M_r 34.01). One volume of this solution corresponds to about ten times its volume of oxygen. A suitable stabiliser may be added.

CHARACTERS

A colourless, clear liquid.

IDENTIFICATION

A. To 2 ml add 0.2 ml of *dilute sulphuric acid R* and 0.2 ml of *0.02 M potassium permanganate*. The solution becomes colourless or slightly pink within 2 min.

B. To 0.5 ml add 1 ml of *dilute sulphuric acid R*, 2 ml of *ether R* and 0.1 ml of *potassium chromate solution R* and shake. The ether layer is blue.

C. It complies with the requirement for the content of H_2O_2.

TESTS

Acidity. To 10 ml add 20 ml of *water R* and 0.25 ml of *methyl red solution R*. Not less than 0.05 ml and not more than 1.0 ml of *0.1 M sodium hydroxide* is required to change the colour of the indicator.

Organic stabilisers. Shake 20 ml with 10 ml of *chloroform R* and then with two quantities, each of 5 ml, of *chloroform R*. Evaporate the combined chloroform layers under reduced pressure at a temperature not exceeding 25 °C and dry the residue in a desiccator. The residue weighs not more than 5 mg (250 ppm).

Non-volatile residue. Allow 10 ml to stand in a platinum dish until all effervescence has ceased. Evaporate the solution to dryness on a water-bath and dry the residue at 100 °C to 105 °C. The residue weighs not more than 20 mg (2 g/l).

ASSAY

Dilute 10.0 g to 100.0 ml with *water R*. To 10.0 ml of this solution add 20 ml of *dilute sulphuric acid R*. Titrate with *0.02 M potassium permanganate* until a pink colour is obtained.

1 ml of *0.02 M potassium permanganate* is equivalent to 1.701 mg of H_2O_2 or 0.56 ml of oxygen.

STORAGE

Store protected from light; if the solution does not contain a stabiliser, store at a temperature below 15 °C.

LABELLING

If the solution contains a stabiliser, the label states that the contents are stabilised. The competent authority may require that the name of the stabiliser be stated on the label.

CAUTION

It decomposes in contact with oxidisable organic matter and with certain metals and if allowed to become alkaline.

01/2005:0396

HYDROGEN PEROXIDE SOLUTION (30 PER CENT)

Hydrogenii peroxidum 30 per centum

DEFINITION

Hydrogen peroxide solution (30 per cent) contains not less than 29.0 per cent *m/m* and not more than 31.0 per cent *m/m* of H_2O_2 (M_r 34.01). One volume of this solution corresponds to about 110 times its volume of oxygen. A suitable stabiliser may be added.

CHARACTERS

A colourless, clear liquid.

IDENTIFICATION

A. To 1 ml add 0.2 ml of *dilute sulphuric acid R* and 0.25 ml of *0.02 M potassium permanganate*. The solution becomes colourless with evolution of gas.

B. To 0.05 ml add 2 ml of *dilute sulphuric acid R*, 2 ml of *ether R* and 0.05 ml of *potassium chromate solution R* and shake. The ether layer is blue.

C. It complies with the requirement for the content of H_2O_2.

TESTS

Acidity. To 10 ml add 100 ml of *water R* and 0.25 ml of *methyl red solution R*. Not less than 0.05 ml and not more than 0.5 ml of *0.1 M sodium hydroxide* is required to change the colour of the indicator.

Organic stabilisers. Shake 20 ml with 10 ml of *chloroform R* and then with two quantities, each 5 ml, of *chloroform R*. Evaporate the combined chloroform layers under reduced pressure at a temperature not exceeding 25 °C and dry the residue in a desiccator. The residue weighs not more than 10 mg (500 ppm).

Non-volatile residue. Allow 10 ml to stand in a platinum dish until all effervescence has ceased, cooling if necessary. Evaporate the solution to dryness on a water-bath and dry the residue at 100 °C to 105 °C. The residue weighs not more than 20 mg (2 g/l).

ASSAY

Dilute 1.00 g to 100.0 ml with *water R*. To 10.0 ml of this solution add 20 ml of *dilute sulphuric acid R*. Titrate with *0.02 M potassium permanganate* until a pink colour is obtained.

1 ml of *0.02 M potassium permanganate* is equivalent to 1.701 mg of H_2O_2 or 0.56 ml of oxygen.

STORAGE

Store protected from light; if the solution does not contain a stabiliser, store at a temperature below 15 °C.

LABELLING

If the solution contains a stabiliser, the label states that the contents are stabilised. The competent authority may require that the name of the stabiliser be stated on the label.

CAUTION

It decomposes vigorously in contact with oxidisable organic matter and with certain metals and if allowed to become alkaline.

01/2005:2099

HYDROMORPHONE HYDROCHLORIDE

Hydromorphoni hydrochloridum

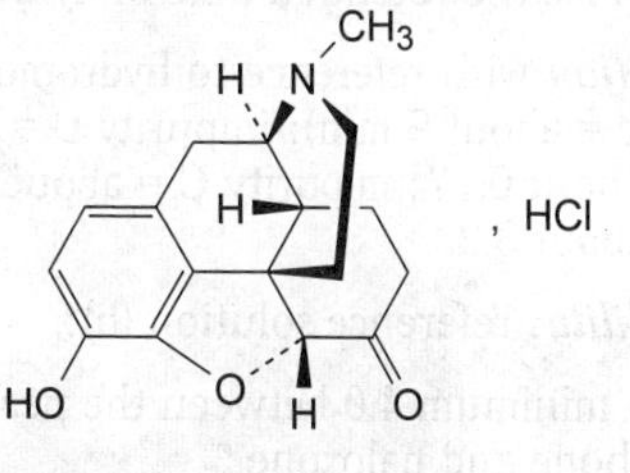

$C_{17}H_{20}ClNO_3$ M_r 321.8

DEFINITION

4,5α-Epoxy-3-hydroxy-17-methylmorphinan-6-one hydrochloride.

Content: 99.0 per cent to 101.0 per cent (dried substance).

CHARACTERS

Appearance: white or almost white, crystalline powder.

Solubility: freely soluble in water, very slightly soluble in ethanol (96 per cent), practically insoluble in methylene chloride.

IDENTIFICATION

A. Infrared absorption spectrophotometry (*2.2.24*).

Comparison: *hydromorphone hydrochloride CRS*.

B. It gives reaction (a) of chlorides (*2.3.1*).

TESTS

Solution S. Dissolve 1.250 g in *carbon dioxide-free water R* and dilute to 25.0 ml with the same solvent.

Appearance of solution. Solution S is clear (*2.2.1*) and not more intensely coloured than reference solution BY_5 (*2.2.2, Method II*).

Acidity or alkalinity. To 2 ml of solution S add 0.1 ml of *methyl red solution R*. The solution is not yellow. To 2 ml of solution S add 0.05 ml of *bromocresol green solution R*. The solution is not yellow.

Specific optical rotation (*2.2.7*): − 136 to − 140 (dried substance), determined on solution S.

Related substances. Liquid chromatography (*2.2.29*).

Test solution. Dissolve 0.100 g of the substance to be examined in *water R*, sonicating if necessary and dilute to 100.0 ml with the same solvent.

Reference solution (a). Dilute 1.0 ml of the test solution to 100.0 ml with *water R*. Dilute 1.0 ml of this solution to 10.0 ml with *water R*.

Reference solution (b). To 5 ml of the test solution add 5 mg of *naloxone hydrochloride dihydrate CRS* and dilute to 50 ml with *water R*.

Column:

- *size*: *l* = 0.25 m, Ø = 4.6 mm,
- *stationary phase*: *base-deactivated end-capped octadecylsilyl silica gel for chromatography R* (5 µm).

Mobile phase: dissolve 18.29 g of *diethylamine R* and 2.88 g of *sodium laurilsulfate R* in *water R* and dilute to 1000 ml with the same solvent. Adjust 800 ml of this solution to pH 3.0 with *phosphoric acid R*. Add 100 ml of *acetonitrile R* and 100 ml of *methanol R*.

Flow rate: 1 ml/min.

Detection: spectrophotometer at 284 nm.

Injection: 20 µl.

Run time: 4 times the retention time of hydromorphone.

Relative retention with reference to hydromorphone (retention time = about 9 min): impurity D = about 0.72; impurity B = about 0.77; impurity C = about 0.82; impurity A = about 3.2.

System suitability: reference solution (b):

- *resolution*: minimum 4.0 between the peaks due to hydromorphone and naloxone.

Limits:

- *impurity A*: not more than 3 times the area of the principal peak in the chromatogram obtained with reference solution (a) (0.3 per cent),
- *impurities B, C, D*: for each impurity, not more than twice the area of the principal peak in the chromatogram obtained with reference solution (a) (0.2 per cent),
- *any other impurity*: for each impurity, not more than the area of the principal peak in the chromatogram obtained with reference solution (a) (0.1 per cent),
- *total*: not more than 5 times the area of the principal peak in the chromatogram obtained with reference solution (a) (0.5 per cent),
- *disregard limit*: 0.5 times the area of the principal peak in the chromatogram obtained with reference solution (a) (0.05 per cent).

Loss on drying (*2.2.32*): maximum 0.5 per cent, determined on 1.000 g by drying in an oven at 100-105 °C.

Sulphated ash (*2.4.14*): maximum 0.1 per cent, determined on the residue obtained in the test for loss on drying.

ASSAY

Dissolve 0.250 g in 50 ml of *ethanol (96 per cent) R* and add 5.0 ml of *0.01 M hydrochloric acid*. Carry out a potentiometric titration (*2.2.20*), using *0.1 M sodium hydroxide*. Read the volume added between the 2 points of inflexion.

1 ml of *0.1 M sodium hydroxide* is equivalent to 32.18 mg of $C_{17}H_{20}ClNO_3$.

STORAGE

Protected from light.

IMPURITIES

Specified impurities: *A, B, C, D*.

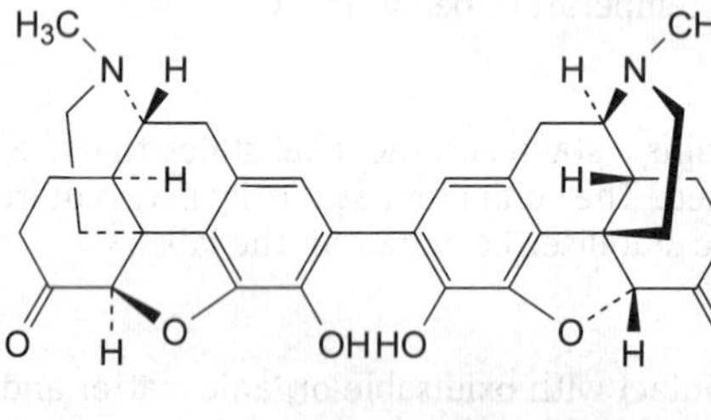

A. 4,5α:4′,5′α-diepoxy-3,3′-dihydroxy-17,17′-dimethyl-2,2′-bimorphinanyl-6,6′-dione (pseudohydromorphone),

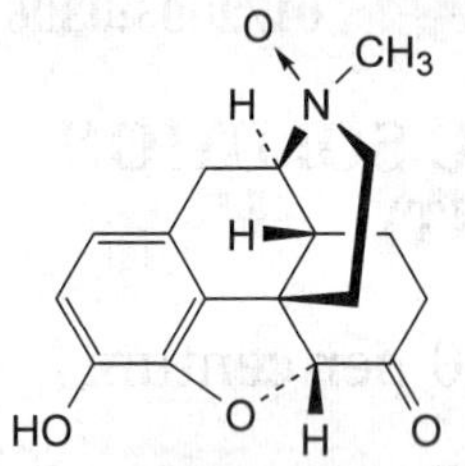

B. 4,5α-epoxy-3-hydroxy-17-methylmorphinan-6-one 17-oxide (hydromorphone *N*-oxide),

C. morphine,

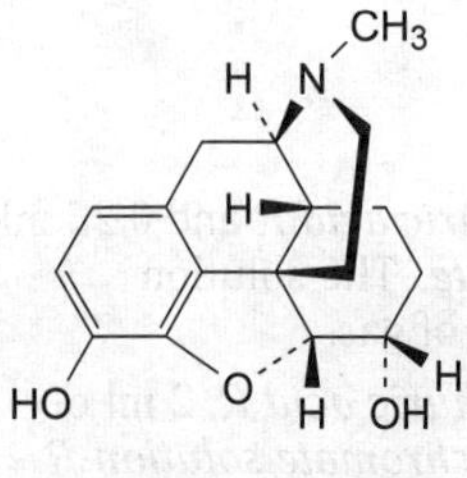

D. 4,5α-epoxy-17-methylmorphinan-3,6α-diol (dihydromorphine).

01/2005:0913

HYDROXOCOBALAMIN ACETATE

Hydroxocobalamini acetas

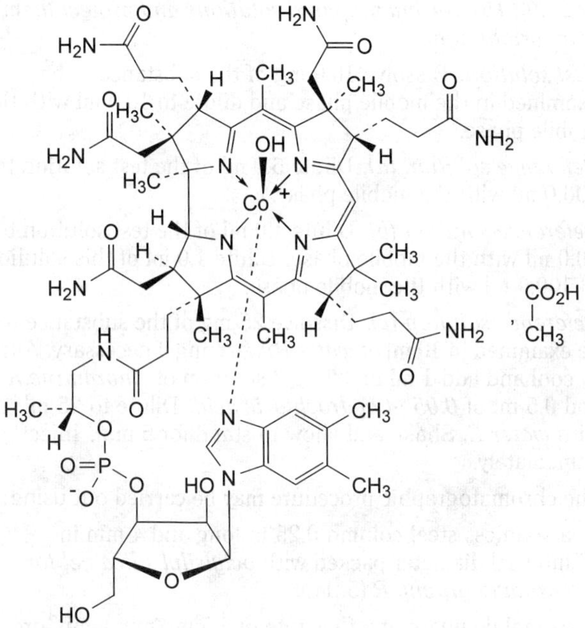

$C_{64}H_{93}CoN_{13}O_{17}P$ M_r 1406

DEFINITION

Hydroxocobalamin acetate contains not less than 96.0 per cent and not more than the equivalent of 102.0 per cent of Coα-[α-(5,6-dimethylbenzimidazolyl)]-Coβ-hydroxocobamide acetate, calculated with reference to the dried substance.

CHARACTERS

A dark red, crystalline powder or dark red crystals, soluble in water, very hygroscopic. Some decomposition may occur on drying.

IDENTIFICATION

A. Dissolve 2.5 mg in a solution containing 0.8 per cent *V/V* of *glacial acetic acid R* and 10.9 g/l of *sodium acetate R* and dilute to 100 ml with the same solution. Examined between 260 nm and 610 nm (*2.2.25*), the solution shows three absorption maxima, at 274 nm, 351 nm and 525 nm. The ratio of the absorbance at the maximum at 274 nm to that at the maximum at 351 nm is 0.75 to 0.83. The ratio of the absorbance at the maximum at 525 nm to that at the maximum at 351 nm is 0.31 to 0.35.

B. Examine by thin-layer chromatography (*2.2.27*), using *silica gel G R* as the coating substance. *Carry out the test protected from light.*

Test solution. Dissolve 2 mg of the substance to be examined in 1 ml of a mixture of equal volumes of *alcohol R* and *water R*.

Reference solution. Dissolve 2 mg of *hydroxocobalamin CRS* in 1 ml of a mixture of equal volumes of *alcohol R* and *water R*.

Apply to the plate 10 µl of each solution. Develop in an unlined tank over a path of 12 cm using a mixture of 25 volumes of *dilute ammonia R1* and 75 volumes of *methanol R*. Allow the plate to dry in air. Examine in daylight. The principal spot in the chromatogram obtained with the test solution is similar in position, colour and size to the principal spot in the chromatogram obtained with the reference solution.

C. It gives reaction (a) of acetates (*2.3.1*).

TESTS

Related substances. Examine by liquid chromatography (*2.2.29*). *Use freshly prepared solutions and protect them from bright light.*

Test solution. Dissolve 10.0 mg of the substance to be examined in the mobile phase and dilute to 10.0 ml with the mobile phase.

Reference solution (a). Dilute 5.0 ml of the test solution to 100.0 ml with the mobile phase.

Reference solution (b). Dilute 1.0 ml of the test solution to 10.0 ml with the mobile phase. Dilute 1.0 ml of this solution to 100.0 ml with the mobile phase.

Reference solution (c). Dissolve 25 mg of the substance to be examined in 10 ml of *water R*, warming if necessary. Allow to cool and add 1 ml of a 20 g/l solution of *chloramine R* and 0.5 ml of *0.05 M hydrochloric acid.* Dilute to 25 ml with *water R*. Shake and allow to stand for 5 min. Inject immediately.

The chromatographic procedure may be carried out using:

- a stainless steel column 0.25 m long and 4 mm in internal diameter packed with *octylsilyl silica gel for chromatography R* (5 µm),
- as mobile phase at a flow rate of 1.5 ml/min a mixture prepared as follows: mix 19.5 volumes of *methanol R* and 80.5 volumes of a solution containing 15 g/l of *citric acid R* and 8.1 g/l of *disodium hydrogen phosphate R*,
- as detector a spectrophotometer set at 351 nm,
- a loop injector,

Inject separately 20 µl of each solution and continue the chromatography for four times the retention time of the principal peak in the chromatogram obtained with reference solution (a). In the chromatogram obtained with the test solution, the sum of the areas of any peaks apart from the principal peak is not greater than the area of the principal peak in the chromatogram obtained with reference solution (a) (5 per cent). Disregard any peak whose area is less than that of the principal peak in the chromatogram obtained with reference solution (b). The test is not valid unless: the chromatogram obtained with reference solution (c) shows three principal peaks and the resolution between each pair of adjacent peaks is at least 3.0; the chromatogram obtained with reference solution (b) shows one principal peak with a signal-to-noise ratio of at least 5.

Loss on drying (*2.2.32*): 8.0 per cent to 12.0 per cent, determined on 0.400 g by drying at 100-105 °C at a pressure not exceeding 0.7 kPa.

ASSAY

Protect the solutions from light throughout the assay. Dissolve 25.0 mg in a solution containing 0.8 per cent *V/V* of *glacial acetic acid R* and 10.9 g/l of *sodium acetate R* and dilute to 1000.0 ml with the same solvent. Measure the absorbance of the resulting solution at the maximum at 351 nm (*2.2.25*).

Calculate the content of $C_{64}H_{93}CoN_{13}O_{17}P$ taking the specific absorbance to be 187.

STORAGE

Store in an airtight container, protected from light, at a temperature of 2 °C to 8 °C.

01/2005:0914

HYDROXOCOBALAMIN CHLORIDE

Hydroxocobalamini chloridum

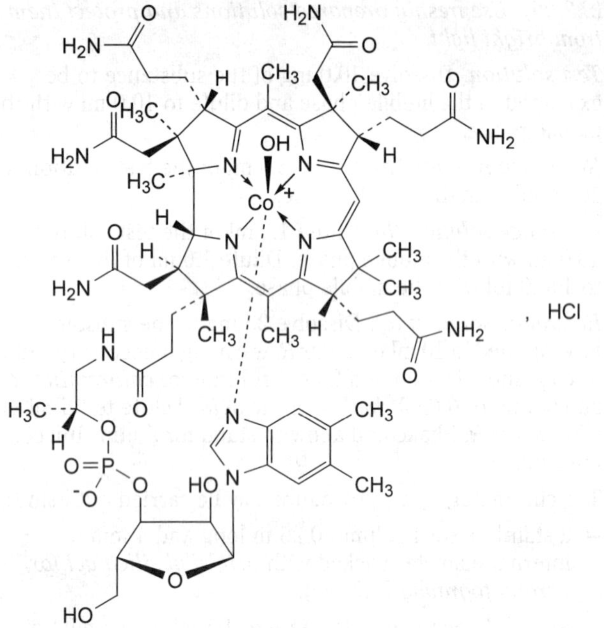

$C_{62}H_{90}ClCoN_{13}O_{15}P$ M_r 1383

DEFINITION

Hydroxocobalamin chloride contains not less than 96.0 per cent and not more than the equivalent of 102.0 per cent of Coα-[α-(5,6-dimethylbenzimidazolyl)]-Coβ-hydroxocobamide chloride, calculated with reference to the dried substance.

CHARACTERS

A dark red, crystalline powder or dark red crystals, soluble in water, very hygroscopic. Some decomposition may occur on drying.

IDENTIFICATION

A. Dissolve 2.5 mg in a solution containing 0.8 per cent *V/V* of *glacial acetic acid R* and 10.9 g/l of *sodium acetate R* and dilute to 100 ml with the same solution. Examined between 260 nm and 610 nm (*2.2.25*), the solution shows three absorption maxima, at 274 nm, 351 nm and 525 nm. The ratio of the absorbance at the maximum at 274 nm to that at the maximum at 351 nm is 0.75 to 0.83. The ratio of the absorbance at the maximum at 525 nm to that at the maximum at 351 nm is 0.31 to 0.35.

B. Examine by thin-layer chromatography (*2.2.27*), using *silica gel G R* as the coating substance. *Carry out the test protected from light.*

Test solution. Dissolve 2 mg of the substance to be examined in 1 ml of a mixture of equal volumes of *alcohol R* and *water R.*

Reference solution. Dissolve 2 mg of *hydroxocobalamin CRS* in 1 ml of a mixture of equal volumes of *alcohol R* and *water R.*

Apply to the plate 10 µl of each solution. Develop in an unlined tank over a path of 12 cm using a mixture of 25 volumes of *dilute ammonia R1* and 75 volumes of *methanol R*. Allow the plate to dry in air. Examine in daylight. The principal spot in the chromatogram obtained with the test solution is similar in position, colour and size to the principal spot in the chromatogram obtained with the reference solution.

C. It gives reaction (a) of chlorides (*2.3.1*).

TESTS

Related substances. Examine by liquid chromatography (*2.2.29*). *Use freshly prepared solutions and protect them from bright light.*

Test solution. Dissolve 10.0 mg of the substance to be examined in the mobile phase and dilute to 10.0 ml with the mobile phase.

Reference solution (a). Dilute 5.0 ml of the test solution to 100.0 ml with the mobile phase.

Reference solution (b). Dilute 1.0 ml of the test solution to 10.0 ml with the mobile phase. Dilute 1.0 ml of this solution to 100.0 ml with the mobile phase.

Reference solution (c). Dissolve 25 mg of the substance to be examined in 10 ml of *water R*, warming if necessary. Allow to cool and add 1 ml of a 20 g/l solution of *chloramine R* and 0.5 ml of *0.05 M hydrochloric acid*. Dilute to 25 ml with *water R*. Shake and allow to stand for 5 min. Inject immediately.

The chromatographic procedure may be carried out using:

- a stainless steel column 0.25 m long and 4 mm in internal diameter packed with *octylsilyl silica gel for chromatography R* (5 µm),
- as mobile phase at a flow rate of 1.5 ml/min a mixture prepared as follows: mix 19.5 volumes of *methanol R* and 80.5 volumes of a solution containing 15 g/l of *citric acid R* and 8.1 g/l of *disodium hydrogen phosphate R*,
- as detector a spectrophotometer set at 351 nm,
- a loop injector.

Inject separately 20 µl of each solution and continue the chromatography for four times the retention time of the principal peak in the chromatogram obtained with reference solution (a). In the chromatogram obtained with the test solution, the sum of the areas of any peaks apart from the principal peak is not greater than the area of the principal peak in the chromatogram obtained with reference solution (a) (5 per cent). Disregard any peak whose area is less than that of the principal peak in the chromatogram obtained with reference solution (b). The test is not valid unless: the chromatogram obtained with reference solution (c) shows three principal peaks and the resolution between each pair of adjacent peaks is at least 3.0; the chromatogram obtained with reference solution (b) shows one principal peak with a signal-to-noise ratio of at least 5.

Loss on drying (*2.2.32*): 8.0 per cent to 12.0 per cent, determined on 0.400 g by drying at 100-105 °C at a pressure not exceeding 0.7 kPa.

ASSAY

Protect the solutions from light throughout the assay. Dissolve 25.0 mg in a solution containing 0.8 per cent *V/V* of *glacial acetic acid R* and 10.9 g/l of *sodium acetate R* and dilute to 1000.0 ml with the same solvent. Measure the absorbance of the resulting solution at the maximum at 351 nm (*2.2.25*).

Calculate the content of $C_{62}H_{90}ClCoN_{13}O_{15}P$ taking the specific absorbance to be 190.

STORAGE

Store in an airtight container protected from light, at a temperature of 2 °C to 8 °C.

01/2005:0915

HYDROXOCOBALAMIN SULPHATE

Hydroxocobalamini sulfas

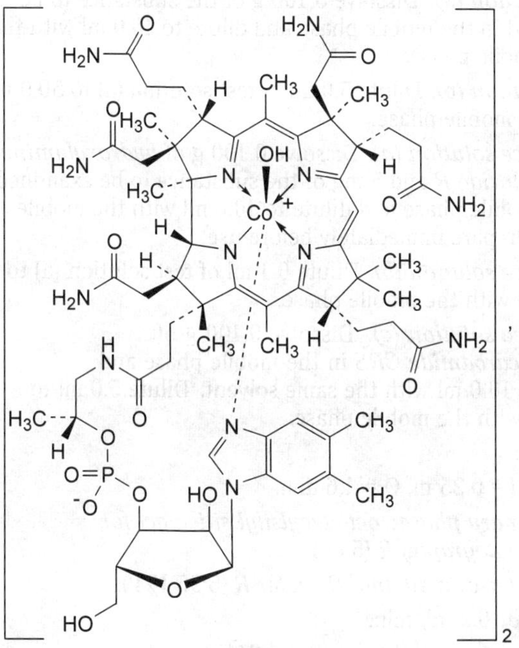

$C_{124}H_{180}Co_2N_{26}O_{34}P_2S$ M_r 2791

DEFINITION

Hydroxocobalamin sulphate contains not less than 96.0 per cent and not more than the equivalent of 102.0 per cent of di-(Coα-[α-(5,6-dimethylbenzimidazolyl)]-Coβ-hydroxocobamide) sulphate, calculated with reference to the dried substance.

CHARACTERS

A dark red, crystalline powder or dark red crystals, soluble in water, very hygroscopic. Some decomposition may occur on drying.

IDENTIFICATION

A. Dissolve 2.5 mg in a solution containing 0.8 per cent *V/V* of *glacial acetic acid R* and 10.9 g/l of *sodium acetate R* and dilute to 100 ml with the same solution. Examined between 260 nm and 610 nm (*2.2.25*), the solution shows three absorption maxima, at 274 nm, 351 nm and 525 nm. The ratio of the absorbance at the maximum at 274 nm to that at the maximum at 351 nm is 0.75 to 0.83. The ratio of the absorbance at the maximum at 525 nm to that at the maximum at 351 nm is 0.31 to 0.35.

B. Examine by thin-layer chromatography (*2.2.27*), using *silica gel G R* as the coating substance. *Carry out the test protected from light.*

Test solution. Dissolve 2 mg of the substance to be examined in 1 ml of a mixture of equal volumes of *alcohol R* and *water R*.

Reference solution. Dissolve 2 mg of *hydroxocobalamin CRS* in 1 ml of a mixture of equal volumes of *alcohol R* and *water R*.

Apply separately to the plate 10 µl of each solution. Develop in an unlined tank over a path of 12 cm using a mixture of 25 volumes of *dilute ammonia R1* and 75 volumes of *methanol R*. Allow the plate to dry in air. Examine in daylight. The principal spot in the chromatogram obtained with the test solution is similar in position, colour and size to the principal spot in the chromatogram obtained with the reference solution.

C. It gives reaction (a) of sulphates (*2.3.1*).

TESTS

Related substances. Examine by liquid chromatography (*2.2.29*). *Use freshly prepared solutions and protect them from bright light.*

Test solution. Dissolve 10.0 mg of the substance to be examined in the mobile phase and dilute to 10.0 ml with the mobile phase.

Reference solution (a). Dilute 5.0 ml of the test solution to 100.0 ml with the mobile phase.

Reference solution (b). Dilute 1.0 ml of the test solution to 10.0 ml with the mobile phase. Dilute 1.0 ml of this solution to 100.0 ml with the mobile phase.

Reference solution (c). Dissolve 25 mg of the substance to be examined in 10 ml of *water R*, warming if necessary. Allow to cool and add 1 ml of a 20 g/l solution of *chloramine R* and 0.5 ml of *0.05 M hydrochloric acid*. Dilute to 25 ml with *water R*. Shake and allow to stand for 5 min. Inject immediately.

The chromatographic procedure may be carried out using:

- a stainless steel column 0.25 m long and 4 mm in internal diameter packed with *octylsilyl silica gel for chromatography R* (5 µm),
- as mobile phase at a flow rate of 1.5 ml/min a mixture prepared as follows: mix 19.5 volumes of *methanol R* and 80.5 volumes of a solution containing 15 g/l of *citric acid R* and 8.1 g/l of *disodium hydrogen phosphate R*,
- as detector a spectrophotometer set at 351 nm,
- a loop injector.

Inject separately 20 µl of each solution and continue the chromatography for four times the retention time of the principal peak in the chromatogram obtained with reference solution (a). In the chromatogram obtained with the test solution, the sum of the areas of any peaks apart from the principal peak is not greater than the area of the principal peak in the chromatogram obtained with reference solution (a) (5 per cent). Disregard any peak whose area is less than that of the principal peak in the chromatogram obtained with reference solution (b). The test is not valid unless: the chromatogram obtained with reference solution (c) shows three principal peaks and the resolution between each pair of adjacent peaks is at least 3.0; the chromatogram obtained with reference solution (b) shows one principal peak with a signal-to-noise ratio of at least 5.

Loss on drying (*2.2.32*): 8.0 per cent to 16.0 per cent, determined on 0.400 g by drying at 100 °C to 105 °C at a pressure not exceeding 0.7 kPa.

ASSAY

Protect the solutions from light throughout the assay. Dissolve 25.0 mg in a solution containing 0.8 per cent *V/V* of *glacial acetic acid R* and 10.9 g/l of *sodium acetate R* and dilute to 1000.0 ml with the same solvent. Measure the absorbance of the resulting solution at the maximum at 351 nm (*2.2.25*).

Calculate the content of $C_{124}H_{180}Co_2N_{26}O_{34}P_2S$ taking the specific absorbance to be 188.

STORAGE

Store in an airtight container protected from light, at a temperature of 2 °C to 8 °C.

Monographs F-H

01/2005:1616
corrected

HYDROXYCARBAMIDE

Hydroxycarbamidum

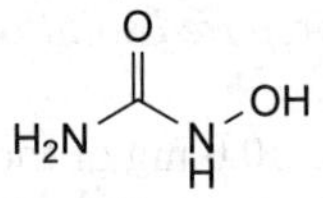

$CH_4N_2O_2$ M_r 76.1

DEFINITION

N-Hydroxyurea.

Content: 97.5 per cent to 102.0 per cent (anhydrous substance).

CHARACTERS

Appearance: white or almost white, crystalline powder, hygroscopic.

Solubility: freely soluble in water, practically insoluble in alcohol.

It shows polymorphism.

IDENTIFICATION

A. Infrared absorption spectrophotometry (*2.2.24*).

Comparison: *hydroxycarbamide CRS*.

If the spectra obtained in the solid state show differences dissolve the substance to be examined and the reference substance separately in *alcohol R*, evaporate to dryness and record new spectra using the residues.

B. Examine the chromatograms obtained in the test for urea.

Results: the principal spot in the chromatogram obtained with the test solution is similar in position and size to the principal spot in the chromatogram obtained with reference solution (c).

TESTS

Urea. Thin-layer chromatography (*2.2.27*).

Test solution. Dissolve 50 mg of the substance to be examined in *water R* and dilute to 1.0 ml with the same solvent.

Reference solution (a). Dissolve 12.5 mg of *urea R* in *water R* and dilute to 50 ml with the same solvent.

Reference solution (b). Dissolve 5 mg of the substance to be examined and 5 mg of *urea R* in *water R* and dilute to 20 ml with the same solvent.

Reference solution (c). Dissolve 50 mg of *hydroxycarbamide CRS* in *water R* and dilute to 1 ml with the same solvent.

Plate: *TLC silica gel plate R*.

Mobile phase: *pyridine R, water R, ethyl acetate R* (2:2:10 *V/V/V*).

Application: 10 µl.

Development: over 2/3 of the plate.

Drying: in air.

Detection: spray with a 10 g/l solution of *dimethylaminobenzaldehyde R* in *1 M hydrochloric acid*.

System suitability: the test is not valid unless the chromatogram obtained with reference solution (b) shows 2 clearly separated spots.

Limit:

- *urea*: any spot corresponding to urea in the chromatogram obtained with the test solution is not more intense than the spot in the chromatogram obtained with the reference solution (a) (0.5 per cent).

Related substances. Liquid chromatography (*2.2.29*).

Test solution (a). Dissolve 0.100 g of the substance to be examined in the mobile phase and dilute to 10.0 ml with the same mobile phase.

Test solution (b). Dilute 5.0 ml of test solution (a) to 50.0 ml with the mobile phase.

Reference solution (a). Dissolve 0.100 g of *hydroxylamine hydrochloride R* and 5 mg of the substance to be examined in the mobile phase and dilute to 10.0 ml with the mobile phase. Prepare immediately before use.

Reference solution (b). Dilute 0.1 ml of test solution (a) to 100.0 ml with the mobile phase.

Reference solution (c). Dissolve 0.100 g of *hydroxycarbamide CRS* in the mobile phase and dilute to 10.0 ml with the same solvent. Dilute 5.0 ml to 50.0 ml with the mobile phase.

Column:

- *size*: l = 0.25 m, Ø = 4.6 mm,
- *stationary phase*: *octadecylsilyl silica gel for chromatography R* (5 µm).

Mobile phase: *methanol R, water R* (5:95 *V/V*).

Flow rate: 0.5 ml/min.

Detection: spectrophotometer at 214 nm.

Injection: 20 µl; inject test solution (a) and reference solutions (a) and (b).

Run time: 3 times the retention time of hydroxycarbamide which is about 5 min.

System suitability: reference solution (a):

- *resolution*: minimum of 1.0 between the peaks due to impurity A and to hydroxycarbamide.

Limits:

- *any impurity*: not more than the area of the principal peak in the chromatogram obtained with reference solution (b) (0.1 per cent),
- *total*: not more than 2 times the area of the principal peak in the chromatogram obtained with reference solution (b) (0.2 per cent),
- *disregard limit*: 0.2 times the area of the principal peak in the chromatogram obtained with reference solution (b) (0.02 per cent).

Chlorides (*2.4.4*): maximum 50 ppm.

Dissolve 1.0 g in *water R* and dilute to 15 ml with the same solvent. The solution complies with the limit test for chlorides.

Heavy metals (*2.4.8*): maximum 10 ppm.

Dissolve 2.0 g in *water R* and dilute to 20 ml with the same solvent. 12 ml of the solution complies with limit test A. Prepare the standard using *lead standard solution (1 ppm Pb) R*.

Water (*2.5.12*): maximum 0.5 per cent, determined on 2.00 g.

Sulphated ash (*2.4.14*): maximum 0.1 per cent, determined on 1.0 g.

ASSAY

Liquid chromatography (*2.2.29*) as described in the test for related substances.

Injection: test solution (b) and reference solution (c).

STORAGE

In an airtight container, protected from light.

IMPURITIES

A. H_2N-OH: hydroxylamine.

01/2005:1225

HYDROXYETHYL SALICYLATE

Hydroxyethylis salicylas

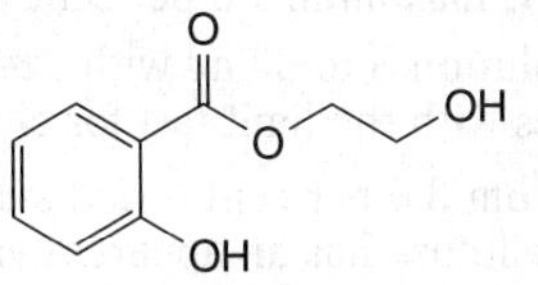

$C_9H_{10}O_4$ M_r 182.2

DEFINITION

2-Hydroxyethyl 2-hydroxybenzoate.

Content: 98.0 per cent to 102.0 per cent.

CHARACTERS

Appearance: oily, colourless or almost colourless liquid, or colourless crystals.

Solubility: sparingly soluble in water, very soluble in acetone and in methylene chloride, freely soluble in alcohol.

Mp: about 21 °C.

IDENTIFICATION

First identification: A, B.

Second identification: A, C, D, E.

A. It complies with the test for refractive index (see Tests).

B. Infrared absorption spectrophotometry (*2.2.24*).

Preparation: thin films.

Comparison: *hydroxyethyl salicylate CRS*.

C. Examine the chromatograms obtained in the test for related substances.

Results: the principal spot in the chromatogram obtained with test solution (b) is similar in position and size to the principal spot in the chromatogram obtained with reference solution (a).

D. To 1 ml of solution S (see Tests), add 1 ml of *water R* and 0.2 ml of *ferric chloride solution R2*. A violet-red colour appears which disappears immediately after the addition of 2 ml of *dilute acetic acid R*. A very faint violet colour may remain.

E. In a test tube 160 mm long, mix 1.0 g with 2.0 g of finely powdered *manganese sulphate R*. Insert 2 cm into the test-tube a strip of filter paper impregnated with a freshly prepared mixture of 1 volume of a 20 per cent *V/V* solution of *diethanolamine R* and 11 volumes of a 50 g/l solution of *sodium nitroprusside R* adjusted to pH 9.8 with *1 M hydrochloric acid*. Heat the test-tube over a naked flame for 1-2 min. The filter paper becomes blue.

TESTS

Solution S. Dissolve 2.5 g in 40 ml of *alcohol R* and dilute to 50 ml with *distilled water R*.

Appearance of solution. Solution S is clear (*2.2.1*) and colourless (*2.2.2, Method II*).

Acidity or alkalinity. To 2 ml of solution S add 0.1 ml of *methyl red solution R* and 0.2 ml of *0.01 M sodium hydroxide*. The solution is yellow. Add 0.3 ml of *0.01 M hydrochloric acid*. The solution is red.

Relative density (*2.2.5*): 1.252 to 1.257.

Refractive index (*2.2.6*): 1.548 to 1.551.

Related substances. Thin-layer chromatography (*2.2.27*).

Test solution (a). Dissolve 0.50 g of the substance to be examined in *methanol R* and dilute to 10 ml with the same solvent.

Test solution (b). Dilute 2 ml of test solution (a) to 50 ml with *methanol R*.

Reference solution (a). Dissolve 50.0 mg of *hydroxyethyl salicylate CRS* in *methanol R* and dilute to 25 ml with the same solvent.

Reference solution (b). Dilute 2.5 ml of test solution (b) to 10 ml with *methanol R*.

Reference solution (c). Dissolve 0.10 g of *ethylene glycol R* in *methanol R* and dilute to 50 ml with the same solvent. Dilute 1.25 ml of the solution to 10 ml with *methanol R*.

Plate: *TLC silica gel F_{254} plate R*.

Mobile phase: *ethyl acetate R, glacial acetic acid R, cyclohexane R* (20:20:60 *V/V/V*).

Application: 10 µl.

Development: over a path of 15 cm.

Drying: in a current of cold air.

Detection A: in ultraviolet light at 254 nm.

Limits A:

– *any impurity*: any spot in the chromatogram obtained with test solution (a), apart from the principal spot, is not more intense than the spot in the chromatogram obtained with reference solution (b) (1 per cent).

Detection B: spray the plate with *ammonium vanadate solution R* and heat at 100 °C for 10 min. Allow to cool for 10 min and examine in daylight.

Limits B: in the chromatogram obtained with test solution (a):

– *impurity B*: any spot corresponding to impurity B is not more intense than the spot in the chromatogram obtained with reference solution (c) (0.5 per cent),

– *any other impurity*: any spot, apart from the principal spot and any spot corresponding to impurity B is not more intense than the spot in the chromatogram obtained with reference solution (b) (1 per cent).

System suitability: the chromatogram obtained with reference solution (c) shows a clearly visible spot.

Chlorides (*2.4.4*): maximum 100 ppm.

Dilute 10 ml of solution S to 15 ml with *water R*. The solution complies with the limit test for chlorides.

Sulphates (*2.4.13*): maximum 250 ppm.

Dilute 12 ml of solution S to 15 ml with *distilled water R*. The solution complies with the limit test for sulphates.

Sulphated ash (*2.4.14*): maximum 0.1 per cent, determined on 1.0 g.

ASSAY

In a flask with a ground-glass stopper, dissolve 0.125 g in 30 ml of *glacial acetic acid R*. Add 10 ml of *dilute sulphuric acid R*, 1.5 g of *potassium bromide R* and 50.0 ml of *0.0167 M potassium bromate*. Immediately close the flask and allow to stand protected from light for 15 min. Add 1.5 g of *potassium iodide R* immediately after removing the stopper and titrate with *0.1 M sodium thiosulphate*, adding 1 ml of *starch solution R* towards the end of the titration. Carry out a blank titration.

1 ml of *0.0167 M potassium bromate* is equivalent to 4.555 mg of $C_9H_{10}O_4$.

STORAGE

Protected from light.

IMPURITIES

A. salicylic acid,

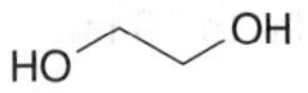

B. ethane-1,2-diol (ethylene glycol).

01/2005:0336

HYDROXYETHYLCELLULOSE

Hydroxyethylcellulosum

DEFINITION

Partly *O*-(2-hydroxyethylated) cellulose.

CHARACTERS

Appearance: white, yellowish-white or greyish-white powder or granules.

Solubility: soluble in hot and cold water giving a colloidal solution, practically insoluble in acetone, in alcohol and in toluene.

IDENTIFICATION

A. Heat 10 ml of solution S (see Tests) to boiling. The solution remains clear.

B. To 10 ml of solution S add 0.3 ml of *dilute acetic acid R* and 2.5 ml of a 100 g/l solution of *tannic acid R*. A yellowish-white, flocculent precipitate is formed which dissolves in *dilute ammonia R1*.

C. In a test-tube about 160 mm in length, thoroughly mix 1 g with 2 g of finely powdered *manganese sulphate R*. Introduce to a depth of 2 cm into the upper part of the tube a strip of filter paper impregnated with a freshly prepared mixture of 1 volume of a 200 g/l solution of *diethanolamine R* and 11 volumes of a 50 g/l solution of *sodium nitroprusside R*, adjusted to about pH 9.8 with *1 M hydrochloric acid*. Insert the tube 8 cm into a silicone-oil bath and heat at 190-200 °C. The filter paper becomes blue within 10 min. Carry out a blank test.

D. Dissolve 0.2 g completely, without heating, in 15 ml of a 700 g/l solution of *sulphuric acid R*. Pour the solution with stirring into 100 ml of iced *water R* and dilute to 250 ml with iced *water R*. In a test-tube, mix thoroughly while cooling in iced water 1 ml of the solution with 8 ml of *sulphuric acid R*, added dropwise. Heat on a water-bath for exactly 3 min and immediately cool in iced water. While the mixture is cold, carefully add 0.6 ml of *ninhydrin solution R2* and mix well. Allow to stand at 25 °C. A pink colour is produced immediately and does not become violet within 100 min.

TESTS

Solution S. Disperse a quantity of the substance to be examined equivalent to 1.0 g of the dried substance in 50 ml of *carbon dioxide-free water R*. After 10 min, dilute to 100 ml with *carbon dioxide-free water R* and stir until dissolution is complete.

pH (*2.2.3*): 5.5 to 8.5 for solution S.

Apparent viscosity (*2.2.10*): 75 per cent to 140 per cent of the value stated on the label.

While stirring, introduce a quantity of the substance to be examined equivalent to 2.00 g of the dried substance into 50 g of *water R*. Dilute to 100.0 g with *water R* and stir until dissolution is complete. Determine the viscosity using a rotating viscometer at 25 °C and at a shear rate of 100 s^{-1} for substances with an expected viscosity up to 100 mPa·s, at a shear rate of 10 s^{-1} for substances with an expected viscosity between 100 mPa·s and 20 000 mPa·s and at a shear rate of 1 s^{-1} for substances with an expected viscosity above 20 000 mPa·s. If it is impossible to obtain a shear rate of exactly 1 s^{-1}, 10 s^{-1} or 100 s^{-1} respectively, use a rate slightly higher and a rate slightly lower and interpolate.

Chlorides (*2.4.4*): maximum 1.0 per cent.

Dilute 1 ml of solution S to 30 ml with *water R*. 15 ml of the solution complies with the limit test for chlorides.

Nitrates: maximum 3.0 per cent (dried substance), if hydroxyethylcellulose has an apparent viscosity of 1000 mPa·s or less and maximum 0.2 per cent (dried substance), if hydroxyethylcellulose has an apparent viscosity of more than 1000 mPa·s.

Determine potentiometrically (*2.2.36, Method I*) using as indicator a nitrate selective electrode and a silver-silver chloride electrode with *0.1 M ammonium sulphate* as reference electrolyte.

Prepare the solutions immediately before use.

Buffer solution. To a mixture of 50 ml of *1 M sulphuric acid* and 800 ml of *water R*, add 135 g of *potassium dihydrogen phosphate R* and dilute to 1000 ml with *water R*.

Buffered water. Dilute 80 ml of buffer solution to 2000 ml with *water R*.

Nitrate standard solution (500 ppm NO_3). Dissolve 0.8154 g of *potassium nitrate R* in 500 ml of buffered water and dilute to 1000.0 ml with the same solvent.

Test solution. Dissolve 0.50 g of the substance to be examined in buffered water and dilute to 100.0 ml with the same solvent.

Reference solutions. If hydroxyethylcellulose has an apparent viscosity of 1000 mPa·s or less, dilute 10.0 ml, 20.0 ml and 40.0 ml of nitrate standard solution (500 ppm NO_3) to 100.0 ml with buffered water and mix.

If hydroxyethylcellulose has an apparent viscosity of more than 1000 mPa·s, dilute 1.0 ml, 2.0 ml and 4.0 ml of nitrate standard solution (500 ppm NO_3) to 100.0 ml with buffered water and mix.

Carry out the measurements for each solution. Calculate the concentration of nitrates using the calibration curve.

Glyoxal: maximum 20 ppm.

Introduce 1.0 g into a test tube with a ground-glass stopper and add 10.0 ml of *ethanol R*. Stopper the tube and stir mechanically for 30 min. Centrifuge. To 2.0 ml of the supernatant liquid add 5.0 ml of a 4 g/l solution of *methylbenzothiazolone hydrazone hydrochloride R* in an 80 per cent *V/V* solution of *glacial acetic acid R* in *water R*. Shake to homogenise. After 2 h, the solution is not more intensely coloured than a standard prepared at the same time and in the same manner using 2.0 ml of *glyoxal standard solution (2 ppm $C_2H_2O_2$) R* instead of the 2.0 ml of supernatant liquid.

Ethylene oxide. Head-space gas chromatography (*2.4.25*).

Test preparation. Place 1.00 g of the substance to be examined in a 5 ml vial (other sizes may be used depending on the operating conditions) and add 1 ml of *water R*. It swells in water but does not dissolve.

Reference preparation (a). Place 1.00 g of the substance to be examined into an identical 5 ml vial. Add 0.2 ml of cooled *ethylene oxide solution R2* and 0.8 ml of *water R*. It swells in water but does not dissolve.

Reference preparation (b). To 0.1 ml of *ethylene oxide solution R2* in a 5 ml vial add 0.1 ml of a freshly prepared 10 mg/l solution of *acetaldehyde R*.

Close the vials immediately with a butyl rubber membrane stopper, coated with aluminium or polytetrafluoroethylene and secured with an aluminium crimped cap.

Limit:

– *ethylene oxide*: maximum 1 ppm.

2-Chloroethanol. Head-space gas chromatography (*2.2.28*).

Test preparation. To 50 mg of the substance to be examined in a 10 ml vial (other size may be used depending on the operating conditions), add 2 μl of *2-propanol R*. Seal the flask and mix.

Reference preparation (a). Dissolve 0.125 g of *2-chloroethanol R* and dilute to 50.0 ml with *2-propanol R*. Dilute 1.0 ml of the solution to 10.0 ml with *2-propanol R*.

Reference preparation (b). To 50 mg of the substance to be examined into an identical 10 ml vial, add 2 μl of reference solution (a). Seal the flask and mix.

Close the vials immediately with a butyl rubber membrane stopper, coated with aluminium or polytetrafluoroethylene and secured with an aluminium crimped cap.

Column:

– *size*: l = 50 m, Ø = 0.32 mm,

– *stationary phase*: *poly(dimethyl)siloxane R* (1.2 μm).

Carrier gas: *helium for chromatography R.*

Flow rate: 25-35 cm/s.

Split ratio: 1:10.

Static head-space conditions which may be used:

– *equilibration temperature*: 110 °C,

– *equilibration time*: 20 min,

– *temperature of injection system*: 115 °C.

Temperature:

	Time (min)	Temperature (°C)
Column	0 - 6	60
	6 - 16	60 → 110
	16 - 31	110 → 230
	31 - 36	230
Injection port		150
Detector		250

Detection: flame ionisation.

Injection: 2 ml.

Retention time: 2-chloroethanol = about 7.8 min.

Limit:

– *2-chloroethanol*: not more than 0.5 times the area of the peak due to 2-chloroethanol in reference solution (b) (10 ppm).

Heavy metals (*2.4.8*): maximum 20 ppm.

1.0 g complies with limit test C. Prepare the standard using 2 ml of *lead standard solution (10 ppm Pb) R.*

Loss on drying (*2.2.32*): maximum 10.0 per cent, determined on 1.000 g by drying in an oven at 100-105 °C for 3 h.

Sulphated ash (*2.4.14*): maximum 4.0 per cent, determined on 1.0 g.

LABELLING

The label states the apparent viscosity, in millipascal seconds for a 2 per cent *m/m* solution.

01/2005:1804

HYDROXYPROPYLBETADEX

Hydroxypropylbetadexum

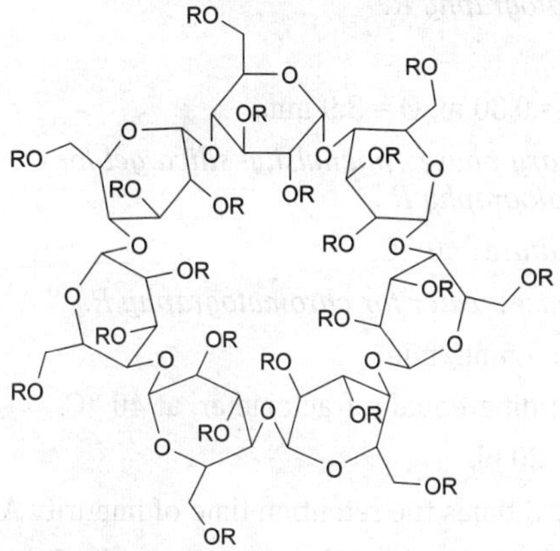

R = -[CH₂-CH(CH₃)-O]ₙ-H   *n* = 0, 1, 2...

$C_{42}H_{70}O_{35}(C_3H_6O)_x$ with x = 7 *MS*

DEFINITION

Hydroxypropylbetadex (β-cyclodextrin, 2-hydroxypropyl ether) is a partially substituted poly(hydroxypropyl) ether of betadex. The number of hydroxypropyl groups per anhydroglucose unit, expressed as Molar Substitution (*MS*), is not less than 0.40 and not more than 1.50 and is within 10 per cent of the value stated on the label.

CHARACTERS

Appearance: white or almost white, amorphous or crystalline powder.

Solubility: freely soluble in water and in propylene glycol.

IDENTIFICATION

A. Infrared absorption spectrophotometry (*2.2.24*).

Comparison: *hydroxypropylbetadex CRS.*

Results: the spectrum obtained with the substance to be examined shows the same absorption bands as the spectrum obtained with *hydroxypropylbetadex CRS*. Due to the difference in the substitution of the substance, the intensity of some absorption bands can vary.

B. It complies with the test for appearance of solution (see Tests).

TESTS

Solution S. Dissolve 5.0 g in *carbon dioxide-free water R* prepared from *distilled water R* and dilute to 50.0 ml with the same solvent.

Appearance of solution. The solution is clear (*2.2.1*) and colourless (*2.2.2, Method II*) and remains so after cooling at room temperature.

Dissolve 1.0 g in 2.0 ml of *water R*, with heating.

Conductivity (*2.2.38*): maximum 200 μS·cm^{-1}.

Measure the conductivity of solution S, while gently stirring with a magnetic stirrer.

Monographs F-H

Related substances. Liquid chromatography (*2.2.29*).

Test solution. Dissolve 2.50 g of the substance to be examined in *water R* with heating, cool and dilute to 25.0 ml with the same solvent.

Reference solution (a). Dissolve 0.15 g of *betadex CRS* and 0.25 g of *propylene glycol R* in *water R* and dilute to 10.0 ml with the same solvent.

Reference solution (b). Dilute 5.0 ml of reference solution (a) to 50.0 ml with *water R*.

Precolumn:

- *stationary phase*: *phenylsilyl silica gel for chromatography R*.

Column:

- *size*: l = 0.30 m, Ø = 3.9 mm,
- *stationary phase*: *phenylsilyl silica gel for chromatography R* ,
- *temperature*: 40 °C.

Mobile phase: *water for chromatography R*.

Flow rate: 1.5 ml/min.

Detection: differential refractometer, at 40 °C.

Injection: 20 µl.

Run time: 3 times the retention time of impurity A.

Relative retention with reference to impurity B (retention time = about 2.5 min): impurity A = about 4.2; hydroxypropylbetadex = about 6 for the beginning of the elution.

Hydroxypropylbetadex elutes as a very wide peak or several peaks.

System suitability: reference solution (a):

- *resolution*: minimum 4 between the peaks due to impurity A and impurity B.

Limits:

- *impurity A*: not more than the area of the corresponding peak in the chromatogram obtained with reference solution (b) (1.5 per cent),
- *impurity B*: not more than the area of the corresponding peak in the chromatogram obtained with reference solution (b) (2.5 per cent),
- *any other impurity*: not more than 0.04 times the area of the peak due to impurity B in the chromatogram obtained with reference solution (b) (0.1 per cent),
- *total of other impurities*: not more than 0.4 times the area of the peak due to impurity B in the chromatogram obtained with reference solution (b) (1.0 per cent),
- *disregard limit*: 0.02 times the area of the peak due to impurity B in the chromatogram obtained with reference solution (b) (0.05 per cent); disregard any peak eluting before impurity B and after impurity A.

Heavy metals (*2.4.8*): maximum 20 ppm.

12 ml of solution S complies with limit test A. Prepare the standard using *lead standard solution (2 ppm Pb) R*.

Loss on drying (*2.2.32*): maximum 10.0 per cent, determined on 1.000 g by drying in an oven at 120 °C for 2 h.

Molar substitution. Nuclear magnetic resonance spectrometry (*2.2.33*).

The Molar Substitution (*MS*) is calculated from the ratio between the signal from the 3 protons of the methyl group, which is part of the hydroxypropyl group and the signal from the proton attached to the carbon C_1 (glycosidic proton) of the anhydroglucose units.

Use a Fourier transform nuclear magnetic resonance spectrometer of minimum frequency 250 MHz, suited to perform a proton spectrum and to carry out quantitative analysis, at a temperature of at least 25 °C.

Introduce not less than the equivalent of 10.0 mg of the substance to be examined (dried substance) into a 5 mm NMR tube, equipped with a spinner in order to record the spectrum in rotation. Add approximately 0.75 ml of *deuterium oxide R1*. Cap the tube, mix thoroughly and adapt the spinner.

Make the appropriate instrument settings (frequency, gain, digital resolution, sample rotation, shims, probe tuning, resolution/data point, receiver gain etc.) so as to obtain a suitable spectrum for quantitative analysis (good FID (Free Induction Decay), no distortion of the spectrum after Fourier transform and phase corrections). The relaxation delay must be adapted to the pulse angle in order to have sufficient relaxation of the protons concerned between 2 pulses (for example: 10 s for a 90° pulse).

Record the FID, with at least 8 scans, so as to obtain a spectral window comprised, at least, between 0 ppm and 6.2 ppm, referring to the signal of exchangeable protons (solvent) at 4.8 ppm (25 °C).

Make a zero filling of at least 3-fold in size relative to the acquisition data file and transform the FID to the spectrum without any correction of Gaussian broadening factor (GB = 0) and with a line broadening factor up to maximum 0.2 (LB ≤ 0.2). Call the integration sub-routine after phase corrections and baseline correction between 0.5 ppm and 6.2 ppm.

Measure the peak areas of the doublet from the methyl groups at 1.2 ppm (A_1), and of the signals of the glycosidic protons between 5 ppm and 5.4 ppm (A_2).

The molar substitution is obtained using the formula:

$$MS = \frac{A_1}{(3 \times A_2)}$$

A_1 = area of the signal due to the 3 protons of the methyl groups, which are part of the hydroxypropyl groups,

A_2 = area of the signals due to the glycosidic protons.

The degree of substitution is the number of hydroxypropyl groups per molecule of β-cyclodextrin and is obtained by multiplying the *MS* by 7.

Microbial contamination. Total viable aerobic count (*2.6.12*) not more than 10^3 bacteria and 10^2 fungi per gram, determined by plate count. If intended for use in the manufacture of parenteral dosage forms, the total viable aerobic count is not more than 10^2 bacteria and 10^2 fungi per gram. It complies with the tests for *Escherichia coli* and *Salmonella* (*2.6.13*).

Bacterial endotoxins (*2.6.14*): less than 10 IU/g, if intended for use in the manufacture of parenteral dosage forms without a further appropriate procedure for the removal of bacterial endotoxins.

LABELLING

The label states:

- the molar substitution (*MS*),
- where applicable, that the substance is suitable for use in the manufacture of parenteral dosage forms.

IMPURITIES

A. betadex,

B. propylene glycol.

01/2005:0337

HYDROXYPROPYLCELLULOSE

Hydroxypropylcellulosum

DEFINITION

Hydroxypropylcellulose is a partly *O*-(2-hydroxypropylated) cellulose. It may contain not more than 0.6 per cent of silica (SiO_2).

CHARACTERS

A white or yellowish-white powder or granules, hygroscopic after drying, soluble in cold water, in glacial acetic acid, in ethanol, in methanol and in propylene glycol and in a mixture of 10 parts of methanol and 90 parts of methylene chloride giving colloidal solutions, sparingly soluble or slightly soluble in acetone depending on the degree of substitution, practically insoluble in hot water, in ethylene glycol and in toluene.

IDENTIFICATION

A. Heat 10 ml of solution S (see Tests) in a water-bath while stirring. At a temperature above 40 °C the solution becomes cloudy or a flocculent precipitate is formed. The solution becomes clear again on cooling.

B. To 10 ml of solution S add 0.3 ml of *dilute acetic acid R* and 2.5 ml of a 100 g/l solution of *tannic acid R*. A yellowish-white, flocculent precipitate is formed which dissolves in *dilute ammonia R1*.

C. In a test-tube about 160 mm long, thoroughly mix 1 g with 2 g of finely powdered *manganese sulphate R*. Introduce to a depth of 2 cm into the upper part of the tube a strip of filter paper impregnated with a freshly prepared mixture of 1 volume of a 20 per cent *V/V* solution of *diethanolamine R* and 11 volumes of a 50 g/l solution of *sodium nitroprusside R*, adjusted to about pH 9.8 with *1 M hydrochloric acid*. Insert the tube 8 cm into a silicone-oil bath at 190 °C to 200 °C. The filter paper becomes blue within 10 min. Carry out a blank test.

D. Dissolve 0.2 g completely, without heating, in 15 ml of a 70 per cent *m/m* solution of *sulphuric acid R*. Pour the solution with stirring into 100 ml of iced *water R* and dilute to 250 ml with iced *water R*. In a test-tube, mix thoroughly while cooling in iced water 1 ml of the solution with 8 ml of *sulphuric acid R*, added dropwise. Heat in a water-bath for exactly 3 min and immediately cool in iced water. While the mixture is cold, carefully add 0.6 ml of *ninhydrin solution R2* and mix well. Allow to stand at 25 °C. A pink colour is produced immediately and becomes violet within 100 min.

E. Place 1 ml of solution S on a glass plate. After evaporation of the water a thin film is formed.

F. 0.2 g does not dissolve in 10 ml of *toluene R* but dissolves completely in 10 ml of *ethanol R*.

TESTS

Solution S. While stirring, introduce a quantity of the substance to be examined equivalent to 1.0 g of the dried substance into 50 g of *carbon dioxide-free water R* heated to 90 °C. Allow to cool, adjust the mass of the solution to 100 g with *carbon dioxide-free water R* and stir until dissolution is complete.

Appearance of solution. Solution S is not more opalescent than reference suspension III (*2.2.1*) and not more intensely coloured than reference solution Y_6 (*2.2.2, Method II*).

pH (*2.2.3*). The pH of solution S is 5.0 to 8.5.

Apparent viscosity. While stirring, introduce a quantity of the substance to be examined equivalent to 6.00 g of the dried substance into 150 g of *water R* heated to 90 °C. Stir with a propeller-type stirrer for 10 min, place the flask in a bath of iced water, continue the stirring and allow to remain in the bath of iced water for 40 min to ensure that dissolution is complete. Adjust the mass of the solution to 300 g and centrifuge the solution to expel any entrapped air. Adjust the temperature of the solution to 20 ± 0.1 °C. Determine the viscosity (*2.2.10*) with a rotating viscometer at 20 °C and a shear rate of 10 s^{-1}. The apparent viscosity is not less than 75 per cent and not more than 140 per cent of the value stated on the label.

For a product of low viscosity, use a quantity of the substance to be examined sufficient to prepare a solution of the concentration stated on the label.

Silica. Not more than 0.6 per cent. To the residue obtained in the test for sulphated ash add sufficient *alcohol R* to moisten the residue completely. Add 6 ml of *hydrofluoric acid R* in small portions. Evaporate to dryness at 95 °C to 105 °C, taking care to avoid loss from sputtering. Cool and rinse the wall of the platinum crucible with 6 ml of *hydrofluoric acid R*. Add 0.5 ml of *sulphuric acid R* and evaporate to dryness. Progressively increase the temperature, ignite at 900 °C, allow to cool in a desiccator and weigh. The difference between the mass of the residue obtained in the test for sulphated ash and the mass of the final residue is equal to the amount of silica in the substance to be examined.

Chlorides (*2.4.4*). 1 ml of solution S diluted to 15 ml with *water R* complies with the limit test for chlorides (0.5 per cent).

Heavy metals (*2.4.8*). 1.0 g complies with limit test C for heavy metals (20 ppm). Prepare the standard using 2 ml of *lead standard solution (10 ppm Pb) R*.

Loss on drying (*2.2.32*). Not more than 7.0 per cent, determined on 1.000 g by drying in an oven at 100-105 °C.

Sulphated ash (*2.4.14*). Not more than 1.6 per cent, determined on 1.0 g using a platinum crucible.

LABELLING

The label states:

- the apparent viscosity in millipascal seconds for a 2 per cent *m/m* solution,
- for a product of low viscosity, the concentration of the solution to be used and the apparent viscosity in millipascal seconds.
- where applicable, that the substance contains silica.

Monographs F-H

01/2005:0916

HYDROXYZINE HYDROCHLORIDE

Hydroxyzini hydrochloridum

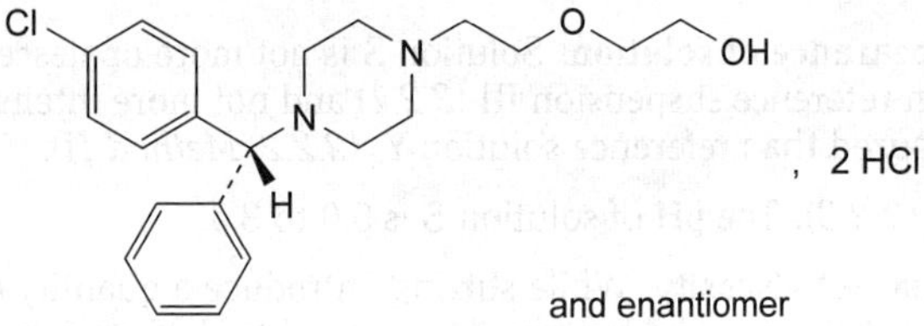

$C_{21}H_{29}Cl_3N_2O_2$ M_r 447.8

DEFINITION

Hydroxyzine hydrochloride contains not less than 99.0 per cent and not more than the equivalent of 101.0 per cent of (*RS*)-2-[2-[4-[(4-chlorophenyl)phenylmethyl]piperazin-1-yl]ethoxy]ethanol dihydrochloride, calculated with reference to the dried substance.

CHARACTERS

A white or almost white, crystalline powder, hygroscopic, freely soluble in water and in alcohol, very slightly soluble in acetone.

It melts at about 200 °C, with decomposition.

IDENTIFICATION

First identification: A, D.

Second identification: B, C, D.

A. Examine by infrared absorption spectrophotometry (*2.2.24*), comparing with the spectrum obtained with *hydroxyzine hydrochloride CRS*. Examine the substances prepared as discs.

B. Examine by thin-layer chromatography (*2.2.27*), using a *TLC silica gel G plate R*.

Test solution. Dissolve 0.50 g of the substance to be examined in a mixture of equal volumes of *methanol R* and *methylene chloride R* and dilute to 10 ml with the same mixture of solvents.

Reference solution (a). Dissolve 0.50 g of *hydroxyzine hydrochloride CRS* in a mixture of equal volumes of *methanol R* and *methylene chloride R* and dilute to 10 ml with the same mixture of solvents.

Reference solution (b). Dissolve 0.50 g of *meclozine hydrochloride R* in a mixture of equal volumes of *methanol R* and *methylene chloride R* and dilute to 10 ml with the same mixture of solvents. Dilute 1 ml to 2 ml with reference solution (a).

Apply to the plate 2 µl of each solution. Develop over a path of 15 cm using a mixture of 1 volume of *concentrated ammonia R*, 24 volumes of *alcohol R* and 75 volumes of *toluene R*. Allow the plate to dry in air. Spray with *potassium iodobismuthate solution R2*. The principal spot in the chromatogram obtained with the test solution is similar in position, colour and size to the principal spot in the chromatogram obtained with reference solution (a). The test is not valid unless the chromatogram obtained with reference solution (b) shows two clearly separated principal spots.

C. Dissolve 0.1 g in *alcohol R* and dilute to 15 ml with the same solvent. Add 15 ml of a saturated solution of *picric acid R* in *alcohol R*. Allow to stand for 15 min. A precipitate is formed. Filter. Recrystallise from *alcohol R*. Initiate crystallisation, if necessary, by scratching the wall of the tube with a glass rod. The crystals melt (*2.2.14*) at 189 °C to 192 °C.

D. It gives reaction (a) of chlorides (*2.3.1*).

TESTS

Solution S. Dissolve 2.0 g in *water R* and dilute to 20.0 ml with the same solvent.

Appearance of solution. Solution S is clear (*2.2.1*) and not more intensely coloured than reference solution Y_7 (*2.2.2, Method II*).

Optical rotation (*2.2.7*): − 0.10° to + 0.10°, determined on solution S.

Related substances. Examine by liquid chromatography (*2.2.29*).

Test solution. Dissolve 10.0 mg of the substance to be examined in the mobile phase and dilute to 10.0 ml with the mobile phase.

Reference solution (a). Dissolve 10.0 mg of *hydroxyzine hydrochloride CRS* in the mobile phase and dilute to 10.0 ml with the mobile phase.

Reference solution (b). Dilute 3.0 ml of the test solution to 200.0 ml with the mobile phase. Dilute 5.0 ml to 25.0 ml with the mobile phase.

The chromatographic procedure may be carried out using:

- a stainless steel column 0.15 m long and 4.6 mm in internal diameter packed with *base-deactivated octadecylsilyl silica gel for chromatography R* (3 µm),
- as mobile phase at a flow rate of 1 ml/min a mixture prepared as follows: dissolve 0.5 g of *sodium methanesulphonate R* in a mixture of 14 volumes of *triethylamine R*, 300 volumes of *acetonitrile R* and 686 volumes of *water R*; adjust to pH 2.7 with *sulphuric acid R*,
- as detector a spectrophotometer set at 230 nm.

Inject 20 µl of reference solution (a) and 20 µl of reference solution (b). Adjust the sensitivity of the system so that the height of the principal peak in the chromatogram obtained with reference solution (b) is at least 50 per cent of the full scale of the recorder.

In the chromatogram obtained with reference solution (a), measure the height (*A*) above the baseline of the peak immediately before the principal peak and the height (*B*) above the baseline of the lowest point of the curve (*B*) separating this peak from the peak due to hydroxyzine. The test is not valid unless *A* is greater than ten times *B*.

Inject 20 µl of the test solution and 20 µl of reference solution (b). Continue the chromatography for 2.5 times the retention time of the principal peak. In the chromatogram obtained with the test solution: the area of any peak, apart from the principal peak, is not greater than one third of the area of the principal peak in the chromatogram obtained with reference solution (b) (0.1 per cent); the sum of the areas of all the peaks, apart from the principal peak, is not greater than the area of the principal peak in the chromatogram obtained with reference solution (b) (0.3 per cent). Disregard any peak with an area less than 0.1 times that of the principal peak in the chromatogram obtained with reference solution (b).

Heavy metals (*2.4.8*). 12 ml of solution S complies with limit test A for heavy metals (10 ppm). Prepare the standard using *lead standard solution (1 ppm Pb) R*.

Loss on drying (*2.2.32*). Not more than 5.0 per cent, determined on 1.000 g by drying in an oven at 100-105 °C.

Sulphated ash (*2.4.14*). Not more than 0.1 per cent, determined on 1.0 g.

ASSAY

Dissolve 0.200 g in 10 ml of *anhydrous acetic acid R*. Add 40 ml of *acetic anhydride R*. Titrate with *0.1 M perchloric acid*, determining the end-point potentiometrically (*2.2.20*).

1 ml of *0.1 M perchloric acid* is equivalent to 22.39 mg of $C_{21}H_{29}Cl_3N_2O_2$.

STORAGE

Store in an airtight container, protected from light.

IMPURITIES

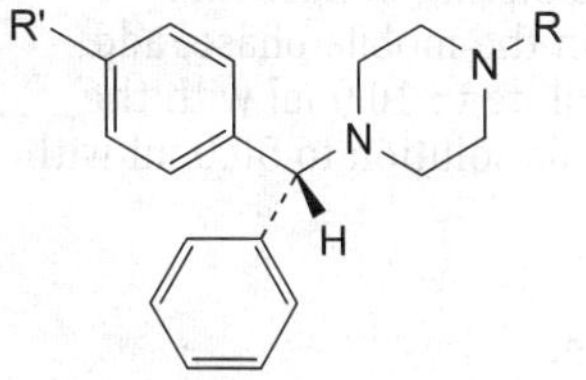

A. R = H, R′ = Cl: (*RS*)-1-[(4-chlorophenyl)phenylmethyl]piperazine,

B. R = CH_2-CH_2-O-CH_2-CH_2-OH, R′ = H: 2-[2-[4-(diphenylmethyl)piperazin-1-yl]ethoxy]ethanol (decloxizine).

01/2005:1786

HYMECROMONE

Hymecromonum

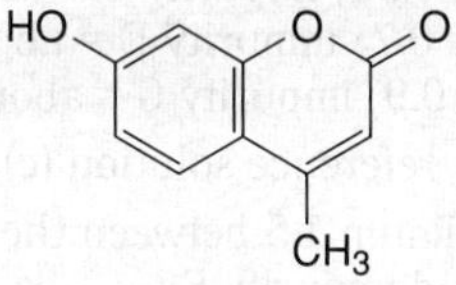

$C_{10}H_8O_3$ M_r 176.2

DEFINITION

7-Hydroxy-4-methyl-2*H*-1-benzopyran-2-one.

Content: 99.0 per cent to 101.0 per cent (dried substance).

CHARACTERS

Appearance: almost white crystalline powder.

Solubility: very slightly soluble in water, sparingly soluble in methanol, slightly soluble in methylene chloride. It dissolves in dilute solutions of ammonia.

IDENTIFICATION

Infrared absorption spectrophotometry (*2.2.24*).

Comparison: *hymecromone CRS*.

TESTS

Absorbance (*2.2.25*). Dissolve 50 mg in 10 ml of *ammonium chloride buffer solution pH 10.4 R* and dilute to 100.0 ml with *water R*. To 1.0 ml of the solution, add 10 ml of *ammonium chloride buffer solution pH 10.4 R* and dilute to 100.0 ml with *water R*. Examined between 200 nm and 400 nm, the solution shows 2 absorption maxima, at 229 nm and 360 nm, and an absorption minimum at 276 nm. The specific absorbance at the maximum at 360 nm is 1020 to 1120.

Related substances. Liquid chromatography (*2.2.29*).

Buffer solution. To 280 ml of a 1.56 g/l solution of *sodium dihydrogen phosphate R*, add 720 ml of a 3.58 g/l solution of *disodium hydrogen phosphate R*. Adjust to pH 7 with a 100 g/l solution of *phosphoric acid R*.

Test solution. Dissolve 10 mg of the substance to be examined in the mobile phase and dilute to 10.0 ml with the mobile phase.

Reference solution (a). Dissolve 20 mg of *hymecromone CRS*, 10 mg of *hymecromone impurity A CRS* and 10 mg of *hymecromone impurity B CRS* in the mobile phase and dilute to 100.0 ml with the mobile phase.

Reference solution (b). Dilute 1.0 ml of reference solution (a) to 200.0 ml with the mobile phase.

Column:

- *size*: l = 0.25 m, Ø = 4 mm,
- *stationary phase*: spherical *octadecylsilyl silica gel for chromatography R* (10 µm).

Mobile phase: *methanol R*, buffer solution (465:535 *V/V*).

Flow rate: 1.0 ml/min.

Detection: spectrophotometer at 270 nm.

Injection: 20 µl.

Run time: 1.5 times the retention time of hymecromone.

Relative retention with reference to hymecromone (retention time = about 6 min): impurity A = about 0.5; impurity B = about 0.7.

System suitability: reference solution (a):

- *resolution*: minimum of 2 between the peaks due to impurity A and to impurity B and minimum of 3 between the peaks due to impurity B and to hymecromone.

Limits:

- *impurity A*: not more than the area of the corresponding peak in the chromatogram obtained with reference solution (b) (0.05 per cent),
- *impurity B*: not more than the area of the corresponding peak in the chromatogram obtained with reference solution (b) (0.05 per cent),
- *any other impurity*: not more than the area of the peak due to hymecromone in the chromatogram obtained with reference solution (b) (0.1 per cent),
- *total*: not more than twice the area of the peak due to hymecromone in the chromatogram obtained with reference solution (b) (0.2 per cent),
- *disregard limit*: 0.1 times the area of the peak due to hymecromone in the chromatogram obtained with reference solution (b) (0.01 per cent).

Heavy metals (*2.4.8*): maximum 10 ppm.

Dissolve 1.5 g in a mixture of 15 volumes of *water R* and 85 volumes of *dimethylformamide R* and dilute to 18 ml with the same mixture of solvents. The solution complies with limit test B. Prepare the standard using a lead standard solution (1 ppm Pb) obtained by diluting *lead standard solution (100 ppm Pb) R* with a mixture of 15 volumes of *water R* and 85 volumes of *dimethylformamide R*.

Loss on drying (*2.2.32*): maximum 0.5 per cent, determined on 1.000 g by drying in an oven at 100-105 °C for 4 h.

Sulphated ash (*2.4.14*): maximum 0.1 per cent, determined on 1.0 g.

ASSAY

Dissolve 0.100 g in 80 ml of *2-propanol R*. Titrate with *0.1 M tetrabutylammonium hydroxide in 2-propanol* determining the end-point potentiometrically (*2.2.20*). Carry out a blank titration.

Monographs F-H

1 ml of *0.1 M tetrabutylammonium hydroxide in 2-propanol* is equivalent to 17.62 mg of $C_{10}H_8O_3$.

STORAGE

Protected from light.

IMPURITIES

A. resorcinol,

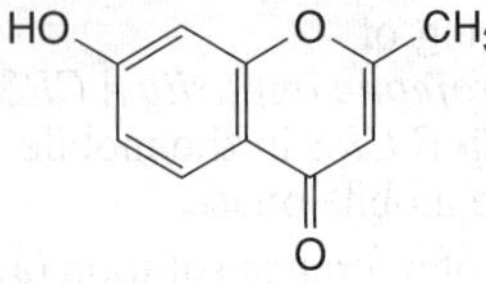

B. 7-hydroxy-2-methyl-4*H*-1-benzopyran-4-one.

01/2005:0737

HYOSCINE BUTYLBROMIDE

Hyoscini butylbromidum
Scopolamini butylbromidum

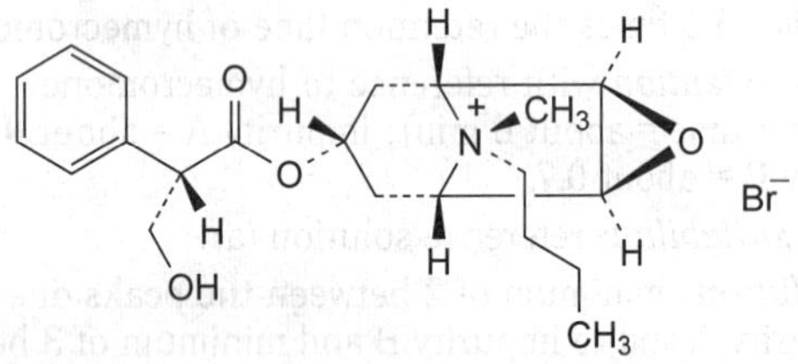

$C_{21}H_{30}BrNO_4$ M_r 440.4

DEFINITION

(1*R*,2*R*,4*S*,5*S*,7*s*,9*r*)-9-Butyl-7-[[(2*S*)-3-hydroxy-2-phenylpropanoyl]oxy]-9-methyl-3-oxa-9-azoniatricyclo[3.3.1.0^{2,4}]nonane bromide.

Content: 98.0 per cent to 101.0 per cent (dried substance).

CHARACTERS

Appearance: white or almost white, crystalline powder.

Solubility: freely soluble in water and in methylene chloride, sparingly soluble in anhydrous ethanol.

IDENTIFICATION

First identification: A, C, F.

Second identification: A, B, D, E, F.

A. It complies with the test for specific optical rotation (see Tests).

B. Melting point (*2.2.14*): 139 °C to 141 °C.

C. Infrared absorption spectrophotometry (*2.2.24*).

Comparison: *hyoscine butylbromide CRS.*

D. To about 1 mg add 0.2 ml of *nitric acid R* and evaporate to dryness on a water-bath. Dissolve the residue in 2 ml of *acetone R* and add 0.1 ml of a 30 g/l solution of *potassium hydroxide R* in *methanol R*. A violet colour develops.

E. To 5 ml of solution S (see Tests) add 2 ml of *dilute sodium hydroxide solution R*. No precipitate is formed.

F. It gives reaction (a) of bromides (*2.3.1*).

TESTS

Solution S. Dissolve 1.25 g in *carbon dioxide-free water R* and dilute to 25.0 ml with the same solvent.

Appearance of solution. Solution S is clear (*2.2.1*) and colourless (*2.2.2, Method II*).

pH (*2.2.3*): 5.5 to 6.5 for solution S.

Specific optical rotation (*2.2.7*): − 18 to − 20 (dried substance), determined on solution S.

Related substances. Liquid chromatography (*2.2.29*).

Test solution. Dissolve 50.0 mg of the substance to be examined in the mobile phase and dilute to 10.0 ml with the mobile phase.

Reference solution (a). Dilute 1.0 ml of the test solution to 50.0 ml with the mobile phase. Dilute 5.0 ml of this solution to 50.0 ml with the mobile phase.

Reference solution (b). Dilute 10.0 ml of reference solution (a) to 20.0 ml with the mobile phase.

Reference solution (c). Dissolve 5.0 mg of *hyoscine butylbromide impurity E CRS* in the mobile phase, add 1.0 ml of the test solution and dilute to 10.0 ml with the mobile phase. Dilute 5.0 ml of this solution to 50.0 ml with the mobile phase.

Column:

- *size*: *l* = 0.125 m, Ø = 4.0 mm,
- *stationary phase*: *octylsilyl silica gel for chromatography R* (4 µm),
- *temperature*: 25 ± 1 °C.

Mobile phase: dissolve 5.8 g of *sodium dodecyl sulphate R* in a mixture of 410 ml of *acetonitrile R* and 605 ml of a 7.0 g/l solution of *potassium dihydrogen phosphate R* previously adjusted to pH 3.3 with *0.05 M phosphoric acid.*

Flow rate: 2.0 ml/min.

Detection: spectrophotometer at 210 nm.

Injection: 10 µl.

Run time: 3.5 times the retention time of butylhyoscine.

Relative retention with reference to butylhyoscine (retention time = about 7.0 min): impurity B = about 0.1; impurity A = about 0.36; impurity C = about 0.40; impurity D = about 0.7; impurity E = about 0.8; impurity F = about 0.9; impurity G = about 3.0.

System suitability: reference solution (c):

- *resolution*: minimum 1.5 between the peaks due to butylhyoscine and impurity E,
- *symmetry factor*: maximum 2.5 for the peak due to butylhyoscine.

Limits:

- *correction factors*: for the calculation of contents, multiply the peak areas of the following impurities by the corresponding correction factor: impurity B = 0.3; impurity G = 0.6;
- *impurity A*: not more than the area of the principal peak in the chromatogram obtained with reference solution (b) (0.1 per cent);
- *impurities B, C, D, E, F, G*: for each impurity, not more than the area of the principal peak in the chromatogram obtained with reference solution (a) (0.2 per cent);
- *any other impurity*: for each impurity, not more than the area of the principal peak in the chromatogram obtained with reference solution (b) (0.1 per cent);
- *total*: not more than twice the area of the principal peak in the chromatogram obtained with reference solution (a) (0.4 per cent); disregard any peak due to the bromide ion which appears close to the solvent peak;
- *disregard limit*: 0.5 times the area of the principal peak in the chromatogram obtained with reference solution (b) (0.05 per cent).

Loss on drying (*2.2.32*): maximum 2.5 per cent, determined on 0.500 g by drying in an oven at 100-105 °C.

Sulphated ash (*2.4.14*): maximum 0.1 per cent, determined on 0.5 g.

ASSAY

Dissolve 0.400 g in 50 ml of *water R*. Titrate with *0.1 M silver nitrate*, determining the end-point potentiometrically (*2.2.20*) using a silver indicator electrode and a silver-silver chloride reference electrode.

1 ml of *0.1 M silver nitrate* is equivalent to 44.04 mg of $C_{21}H_{30}BrNO_4$.

IMPURITIES

Specified impurities: A, B, C, D, E, F, G.

A. hyoscine,

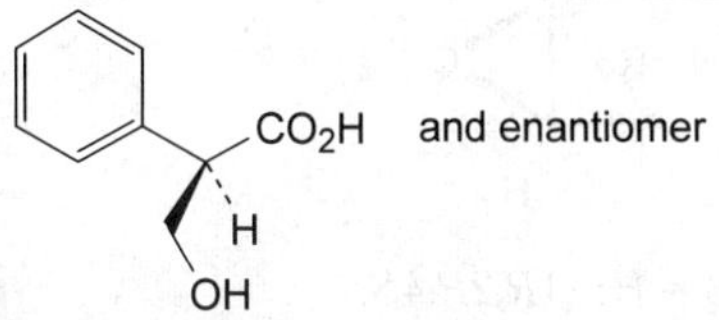

B. (2*RS*)-3-hydroxy-2-phenylpropanoic acid (DL-tropic acid),

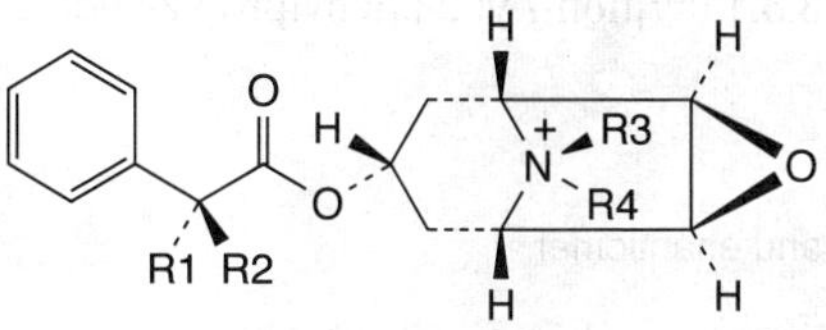

C. R1 = CH_2OH, R2 = H, R3 = R4 = CH_3: (1*R*,2*R*,4*S*,5*S*,7*s*)-7-[[(2*S*)-3-hydroxy-2-phenylpropanoyl]oxy]-9,9-dimethyl-3-oxa-9-azoniatricyclo[3.3.1.0^{2,4}]nonane (methylhyoscine),

D. R1 = CH_2OH, R2 = H, R3 = CH_3, R4 = CH_2-CH_2-CH_3: (1*R*,2*R*,4*S*,5*S*,7*s*,9*r*)-7-[[(2*S*)-3-hydroxy-2-phenylpropanoyl]oxy]-9-methyl-9-propyl-3-oxa-9-azoniatricyclo[3.3.1.0^{2,4}]nonane (propylhyoscine),

F. R1 = CH_2OH, R2 = H, R3 = CH_2-CH_2-CH_2-CH_3, R4 = CH_3: (1*R*,2*R*,4*S*,5*S*,7*s*,9*s*)-9-butyl-7-[[(2*S*)-3-hydroxy-2-phenylpropanoyl]oxy]-9-methyl-3-oxa-9-azoniatricyclo[3.3.1.0^{2,4}]nonane (pseudo-isomer),

G. R1 + R2 = CH_2 , R3 = CH_3, R4 = CH_2-CH_2-CH_2-CH_3: (1*R*,2*R*,4*S*,5*S*,7*s*,9*r*)-9-butyl-9-methyl-7-[(2-phenylprop-2-enoyl)oxy]-3-oxa-9-azoniatricyclo[3.3.1.0^{2,4}]nonane (apo-*N*-butylhyoscine);

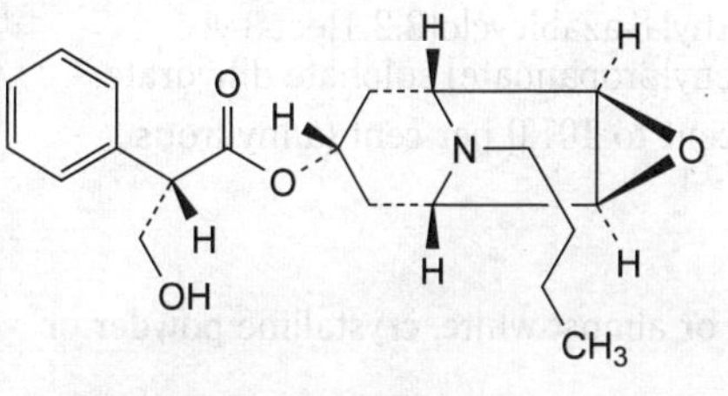

E. (1*R*,2*R*,4*S*,5*S*,7*s*)-9-butyl-3-oxa-9-azatricyclo[3.3.1.0^{2,4}]nonan-7-yl (2*S*)-3-hydroxy-2-phenylpropanoate (*N*-butylhyoscine).

01/2005:0106

HYOSCINE HYDROBROMIDE

Hyoscini hydrobromidum
Scopolamini hydrobromidum

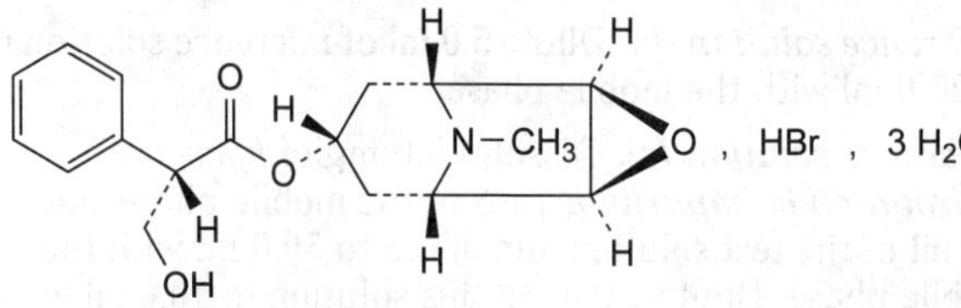

$C_{17}H_{22}BrNO_4,3H_2O$ — M_r 438.3

DEFINITION

(1*R*,2*R*,4*S*,5*S*,7*s*)-9-Methyl-3-oxa-9-azatricyclo[3.3.1.0^{2,4}]non-7-yl (2*S*)-3-hydroxy-2-phenylpropanoate hydrobromide trihydrate.

Content: 99.0 per cent to 101.0 per cent (anhydrous substance).

CHARACTERS

Appearance: white or almost white, crystalline powder or colourless crystals, efflorescent.

Solubility: freely soluble in water, soluble in ethanol (96 per cent).

IDENTIFICATION

First identification: B, E.

Second identification: A, C, D, E.

A. It complies with the test for specific optical rotation (see Tests).

B. Infrared absorption spectrophotometry (*2.2.24*).

Comparison: *hyoscine hydrobromide CRS.*

If the spectra obtained in the solid state show differences, proceed as follows: dissolve 3 mg of the substance to be examined in 1 ml of *ethanol (96 per cent) R* and evaporate to dryness on a water-bath; dissolve the residue in 0.5 ml of *methylene chloride R* and add 0.2 g of *potassium bromide R* and 15 ml of *ether R*; allow to stand for 5 min shaking frequently; decant; dry the residue on a water-bath until the solvents have evaporated; using the residue prepare a disc and dry at 100-105 °C for 3 h. Repeat the procedure with *hyoscine hydrobromide CRS* and record the spectra.

C. Dissolve about 50 mg in 5 ml of *water R* and add 5 ml of *picric acid solution R* dropwise and with shaking. The precipitate, washed with *water R* and dried at 100-105 °C for 2 h, melts (*2.2.14*) at 188 °C to 193 °C.

D. To about 1 mg add 0.2 ml of *fuming nitric acid R* and evaporate to dryness on a water-bath. Dissolve the residue in 2 ml of *acetone R* and add 0.1 ml of a 30 g/l solution of *potassium hydroxide R* in *methanol R*. A violet colour develops.

E. It gives reaction (a) of bromides (*2.3.1*).

TESTS

Solution S. Dissolve 2.50 g in *carbon dioxide-free water R* and dilute to 50.0 ml with the same solvent.

pH (*2.2.3*): 4.0 to 5.5 for solution S.

Specific optical rotation (*2.2.7*): − 24 to − 27 (anhydrous substance), determined on solution S.

Related substances. Liquid chromatography (*2.2.29*).

Test solution. Dissolve 70.0 mg of the substance to be examined in the mobile phase and dilute to 50.0 ml with the mobile phase.

Reference solution (a). Dilute 2.0 ml of the test solution to 100.0 ml with the mobile phase. Dilute 5.0 ml of this solution to 20.0 ml with the mobile phase.

Reference solution (b). Dilute 5.0 ml of reference solution (a) to 25.0 ml with the mobile phase.

Reference solution (c). Dissolve 5.0 mg of *hyoscine hydrobromide impurity B CRS* in the mobile phase, add 5.0 ml of the test solution and dilute to 50.0 ml with the mobile phase. Dilute 1.0 ml of this solution to 10.0 ml with the mobile phase.

Column:

- *size*: l = 0.125 m, Ø = 4.0 mm,
- *stationary phase*: *octylsilyl silica gel for chromatography R* (3 µm),
- *temperature*: 25 ± 1 °C.

Mobile phase: mix 330 ml of *acetonitrile R* with 670 ml of a 2.5 g/l solution of *sodium dodecyl sulphate R* previously adjusted to pH 2.5 with *3 M phosphoric acid.*

Flow rate: 1.5 ml/min.

Detection: spectrophotometer at 210 nm.

Injection: 5 µl.

Run time: 3 times the retention time of hyoscine.

Relative retention with reference to hyoscine (retention time = about 5.0 min): impurity D = about 0.2; impurity B = about 0.9; impurity A = about 1.3; impurity C = about 2.4.

System suitability: reference solution (c):

- *resolution*: minimum 1.5 between the peaks due to impurity B and hyoscine,
- *symmetry factor*: maximum 2.5 for the peak due to hyoscine.

Limits:

- *correction factors*: for the calculation of contents, multiply the peak areas of the following impurities by the corresponding correction factor: impurity D = 0.3; impurity C = 0.6;
- *impurity B*: not more than the area of the principal peak in the chromatogram obtained with reference solution (a) (0.5 per cent);
- *impurities A, C, D*: for each impurity, not more than the area of the principal peak in the chromatogram obtained with reference solution (b) (0.1 per cent);
- *any other impurity*: for each impurity, not more than the area of the principal peak in the chromatogram obtained with reference solution (b) (0.1 per cent);
- *total*: not more than 1.4 times the area of the principal peak in the chromatogram obtained with reference solution (a) (0.7 per cent); disregard any peak due to the bromide ion which appears close to the solvent peak;
- *disregard limit*: 0.5 times the area of the principal peak in the chromatogram obtained with reference solution (b) (0.05 per cent).

Water (*2.5.12*): 10.0 per cent to 13.0 per cent, determined on 0.20 g.

Sulphated ash (*2.4.14*): maximum 0.1 per cent, determined on 1.0 g.

Monographs F-H

ASSAY

Dissolve 0.300 g in a mixture of 5.0 ml of *0.01 M hydrochloric acid* and 50 ml of *ethanol (96 per cent) R*. Carry out a potentiometric titration (*2.2.20*), using *0.1 M sodium hydroxide* free from carbonate. Read the volume added between the 2 points of inflexion.

1 ml of *0.1 M sodium hydroxide* is equivalent to 38.43 mg of $C_{17}H_{22}BrNO_4$.

STORAGE

In a well-filled, airtight container of small capacity, protected from light.

IMPURITIES

Specified impurities: A, B, C, D.

A. hyoscyamine,

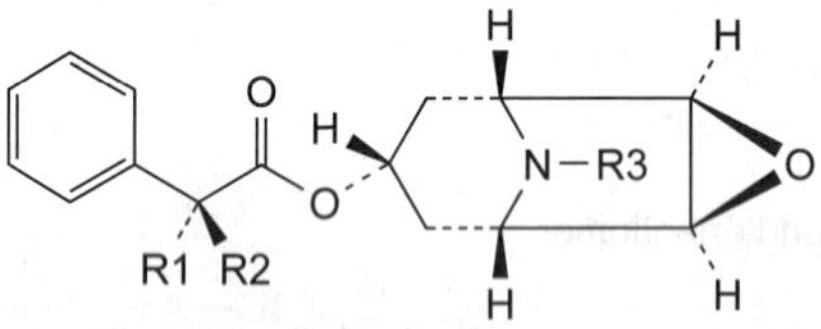

B. R1 = CH_2OH, R2 = R3 = H: (1*R*,2*R*,4*S*,5*S*,7*s*)-3-oxa-9-azatricyclo[3.3.1.0[2,4]]non-7-yl (2*S*)-3-hydroxy-2-phenylpropanoate (norhyoscine),

C. R1 + R2 = CH_2, R3 = CH_3: (1*R*,2*R*,4*S*,5*S*,7*s*)-9-methyl-3-oxa-9-azatricyclo[3.3.1.0[2,4]]non-7-yl 2-phenylprop-2-enoate (apohyoscine),

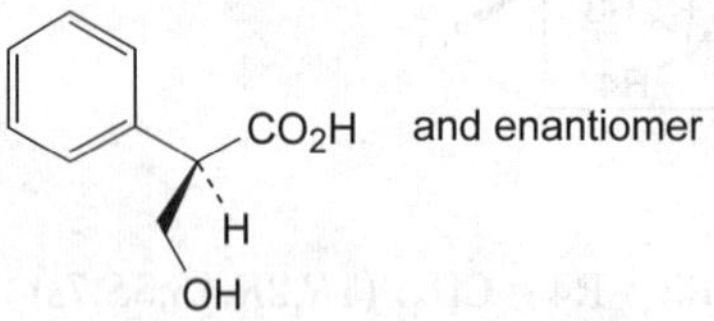

D. (2*RS*)-3-hydroxy-2-phenylpropanoic acid (DL-tropic acid).

01/2005:0501

HYOSCYAMINE SULPHATE

Hyoscyamini sulfas

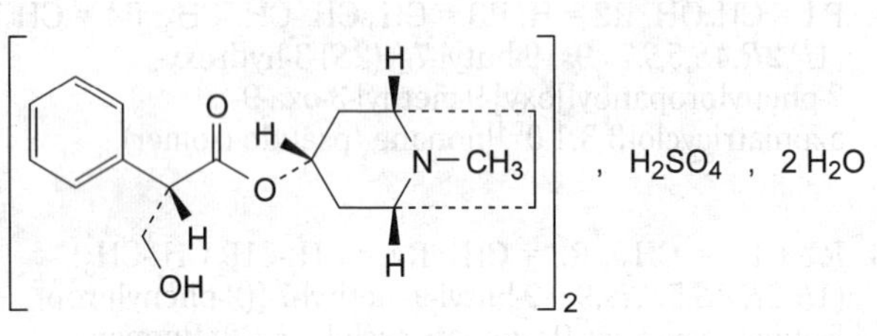

$C_{34}H_{48}N_2O_{10}S,2H_2O$ M_r 713

DEFINITION

Bis[(1*R*,3*r*,5*S*)-8-methyl-8-azabicyclo[3.2.1]oct-3-yl (2*S*)-3-hydroxy-2-phenylpropanoate] sulphate dihydrate.

Content: 98.0 per cent to 101.0 per cent (anhydrous substance).

CHARACTERS

Appearance: white or almost white, crystalline powder or colourless needles.

Solubility: very soluble in water, sparingly soluble or soluble in ethanol (96 per cent).

IDENTIFICATION

First identification: A, B, E.

Second identification: C, D, E.

A. It complies with the test for specific optical rotation (see Tests).

B. Infrared absorption spectrophotometry (*2.2.24*).

Comparison: *hyoscyamine sulphate CRS.*

C. To 0.5 ml of solution S (see Tests) add 2 ml of *dilute acetic acid R* and heat. To the hot solution add 4 ml of *picric acid solution R.* Allow to cool, shaking occasionally. Collect the crystals, wash with 2 quantities, each of 3 ml, of iced *water R* and dry at 100-105 °C. The crystals melt (*2.2.14*) at 164 °C to 168 °C.

D. To about 1 mg add 0.2 ml of *fuming nitric acid R* and evaporate to dryness on a water-bath. Dissolve the residue in 2 ml of *acetone R* and add 0.2 ml of a 30 g/l solution of *potassium hydroxide R* in *methanol R.* A violet colour develops.

E. It gives reaction (a) of sulphates (*2.3.1*).

TESTS

Solution S. Dissolve 2.50 g in *water R* and dilute to 50.0 ml with the same solvent.

Appearance of solution. Solution S is not more intensely coloured than reference solution BY_6 (*2.2.2, Method II*).

pH (*2.2.3*): 4.5 to 6.2.

Dissolve 0.5 g in *carbon dioxide-free water R* and dilute to 25 ml with the same solvent.

Specific optical rotation (*2.2.7*): − 24 to − 29 (anhydrous substance), determined on solution S.

Related substances. Liquid chromatography (*2.2.29*).

Test solution. Dissolve 60.0 mg of the substance to be examined in mobile phase A and dilute to 50.0 ml with mobile phase A. Dilute 10.0 ml of the solution to 50.0 ml with mobile phase A.

Reference solution (a). Dilute 5.0 ml of the test solution to 100.0 ml with mobile phase A. Dilute 5.0 ml of this solution to 50.0 ml with mobile phase A.

Reference solution (b). Dilute 5.0 ml of reference solution (a) to 25.0 ml with mobile phase A.

Reference solution (c). Dissolve 5.0 mg of *hyoscyamine impurity E CRS* in mobile phase A, add 1.0 ml of the test solution and dilute to 20.0 ml with mobile phase A. Dilute 5.0 ml of this solution to 25.0 ml with mobile phase A.

Column:

- *size*: *l* = 0.10 m, Ø = 4.6 mm,
- *stationary phase*: *octadecylsilyl silica gel for chromatography R* (3 µm),
- *temperature*: 25 ± 1 °C.

Mobile phase:

- *mobile phase A*: dissolve 3.5 g of *sodium dodecyl sulphate R* in 606 ml of a 7.0 g/l solution of *potassium dihydrogen phosphate R* previously adjusted to pH 3.3 with *0.05 M phosphoric acid* and mix with 320 ml of *acetonitrile R*,
- *mobile phase B*: *acetonitrile R*,

Time (min)	Mobile phase A (per cent *V/V*)	Mobile phase B (per cent *V/V*)
0 - 2.0	95	5
2.0 - 20.0	95 → 70	5 → 30
20.0 - 20.1	70 → 95	30 → 5
20.1 - 25.0	95	5

Flow rate: 1.0 ml/min.

Detection: spectrophotometer at 210 nm.

Injection: 10 µl.

Relative retention with reference to hyoscyamine (retention time = about 10.5 min): impurity A = about 0.2; impurity B = about 0.67; impurity C = about 0.72; impurity D = about 0.8; impurity E = about 0.9; impurity F = about 1.1; impurity G = about 1.8.

System suitability: reference solution (c):

- *resolution*: minimum 2.5 between the peaks due to hyoscyamine and impurity E,
- *symmetry factor*: maximum 2.5 for the peak due to hyoscyamine.

Limits:

- *correction factors*: for the calculation of contents, multiply the peak areas of the following impurities by the corresponding correction factor: impurity A = 0.3; impurity G = 0.6;
- *impurity E*: not more than 3 times the area of the principal peak in the chromatogram obtained with reference solution (b) (0.3 per cent);
- *impurities A, B, C, D, F, G*: for each impurity, not more than twice the area of the principal peak in the chromatogram obtained with reference solution (b) (0.2 per cent);
- *any other impurity*: for each impurity, not more than the area of the principal peak in the chromatogram obtained with reference solution (b) (0.1 per cent);
- *total*: not more than the area of the principal peak in the chromatogram obtained with reference solution (a) (0.5 per cent);
- *disregard limit*: 0.1 times the area of the principal peak in the chromatogram obtained with reference solution (a) (0.05 per cent).

Water (*2.5.12*): 2.0 per cent to 5.5 per cent, determined on 0.500 g.

Sulphated ash (*2.4.14*): maximum 0.1 per cent, determined on 1.0 g.

ASSAY

Dissolve 0.500 g in 25 ml of *anhydrous acetic acid R.* Titrate with *0.1 M perchloric acid,* determining the end-point potentiometrically (*2.2.20*).

1 ml of *0.1 M perchloric acid* is equivalent to 67.7 mg of $C_{34}H_{48}N_2O_{10}S$.

STORAGE

In an airtight container, protected from light.

IMPURITIES

Specified impurities: A, B, C, D, E, F, G.

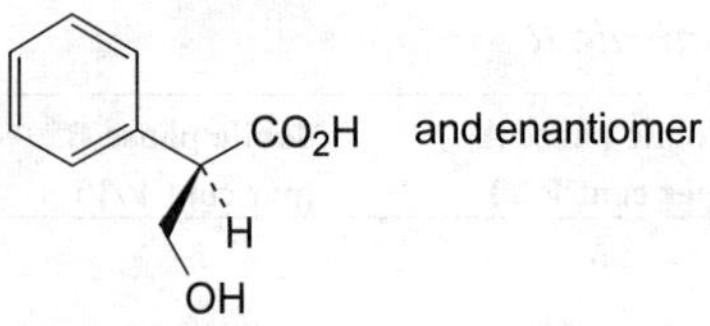

A. (2*RS*)-3-hydroxy-2-phenylpropanoic acid (DL-tropic acid),

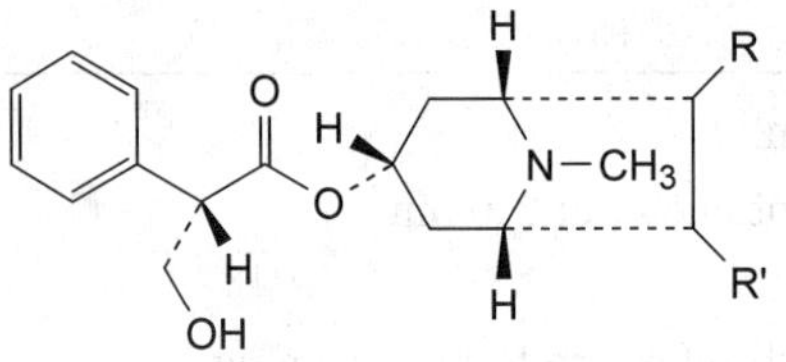

B. R = OH, R′ = H: (1*R*,3*S*,5*R*,6*RS*)-6-hydroxy-8-methyl-8-azabicyclo[3.2.1]oct-3-yl (2*S*)-3-hydroxy-2-phenylpropanoate (7-hydroxyhyoscyamine),

C. R = H, R′ = OH: (1*S*,3*R*,5*S*,6*RS*)-6-hydroxy-8-methyl-8-azabicyclo[3.2.1]oct-3-yl (2*S*)-3-hydroxy-2-phenylpropanoate (6-hydroxyhyoscyamine),

D. hyoscine,

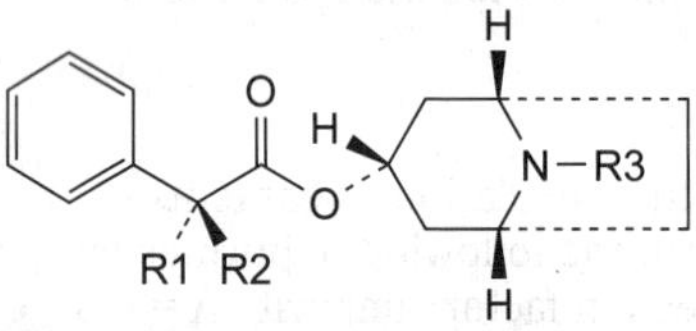

E. R1 = CH_2OH, R2 = R3 = H: (1*R*,3*r*,5*S*)-8-azabicyclo[3.2.1]oct-3-yl (2*S*)-3-hydroxy-2-phenylpropanoate (norhyoscyamine),

G. R1 + R2 = CH_2, R3 = CH_3: (1*R*,3*r*,5*S*)-8-methyl-8-azabicyclo[3.2.1]oct-3-yl 2-phenylprop-2-enoate (apoatropine),

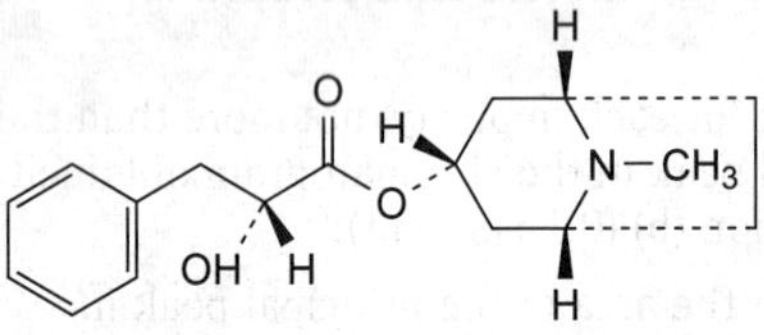

F. (1*R*,3*r*,5*S*)-8-methyl-8-azabicyclo[3.2.1]oct-3-yl (2*R*)-2-hydroxy-3-phenylpropanoate (littorine).

01/2005:0348

HYPROMELLOSE

Hypromellosum

DEFINITION

Hypromellose (hydroxypropylmethylcellulose) is a partly *O*-methylated and *O*-(2-hydroxypropylated) cellulose.

CHARACTERS

A white, yellowish-white or greyish-white powder or granules, hygroscopic after drying, practically insoluble in hot water, in acetone, in ethanol and in toluene. It dissolves in cold water giving a colloidal solution.

IDENTIFICATION

A. Heat 10 ml of solution S (see Tests) in a water-bath while stirring. At a temperature above 50 °C the solution becomes cloudy or a flocculent precipitate is formed. The solution becomes clear again on cooling.

B. To 10 ml of solution S add 0.3 ml of *dilute acetic acid R* and 2.5 ml of a 100 g/l solution of *tannic acid R*. A yellowish-white, flocculent precipitate is formed which dissolves in *dilute ammonia R1*.

C. In a test-tube about 160 mm long, thoroughly mix 1 g with 2 g of finely powdered *manganese sulphate R*. Introduce to a depth of 2 cm into the upper part of the tube a strip of filter paper impregnated with a freshly prepared mixture of 1 volume of a 20 per cent *V/V* solution of *diethanolamine R* and 11 volumes of a 50 g/l solution of *sodium nitroprusside R*, adjusted to about pH 9.8 with *1 M hydrochloric acid*. Insert the tube 8 cm into a silicone-oil bath at 190 °C to 200 °C. The filter paper becomes blue within 10 min. Carry out a blank test.

D. Dissolve 0.2 g completely, without heating, in 15 ml of a 70 per cent *m/m* solution of *sulphuric acid R*. Pour the solution with stirring into 100 ml of iced *water R* and dilute to 250 ml with iced *water R*. In a test-tube, mix thoroughly while cooling in iced water 1 ml of the solution with 8 ml of *sulphuric acid R*, added dropwise. Heat in a water-bath for exactly 3 min and immediately cool in iced water. While the mixture is cold, carefully add 0.6 ml of *ninhydrin solution R2* and mix well. Allow to stand at 25 °C. A pink colour is produced immediately and becomes violet within 100 min.

E. Place 1 ml of solution S on a glass plate. After evaporation of the water a thin film is formed.

F. 0.2 g does not dissolve in 10 ml of *toluene R* nor in 10 ml of *ethanol R*.

TESTS

Solution S. While stirring, introduce a quantity of the substance to be examined equivalent to 1.0 g of the dried substance into 50 g of *carbon dioxide-free water R* heated to 90 °C. Allow to cool, adjust the mass of the solution to 100 g with *carbon dioxide-free water R* and stir until dissolution is complete.

Appearance of solution. Solution S is not more opalescent than reference suspension III (*2.2.1*) and not more intensely coloured than reference solution Y_6 (*2.2.2, Method II*).

pH (*2.2.3*). The pH of solution S is 5.5 to 8.0.

Apparent viscosity. While stirring, introduce a quantity of the substance to be examined equivalent to 6.00 g of the dried substance into 150 g of *water R* heated to 90 °C. Stir with a propeller-type stirrer for 10 min, place the flask in a bath of iced water, continue the stirring and allow to remain in the bath of iced water for 40 min to ensure that dissolution is complete. Adjust the mass of the solution to 300 g, and centrifuge the solution to expel any entrapped air. Adjust the temperature of the solution to 20 ± 0.1 °C. Determine the viscosity (*2.2.10*) with a rotating viscometer at 20 °C and a shear rate of 10 s^{-1}. The apparent viscosity is not less than 75 per cent and not more than 140 per cent of the value stated on the label.

Chlorides (*2.4.4*). 1 ml of solution S diluted to 15 ml with *water R* complies with the limit test for chlorides (0.5 per cent).

Heavy metals (*2.4.8*). 1.0 g complies with limit test C for heavy metals (20 ppm). Prepare the standard using 2 ml of *lead standard solution (10 ppm Pb) R*.

Loss on drying (*2.2.32*). Not more than 10.0 per cent, determined on 1.000 g by drying in an oven at 100 °C to 105 °C.

Sulphated ash (*2.4.14*). Not more than 1.0 per cent, determined on 1.0 g.

LABELLING

The label states the apparent viscosity in millipascal seconds for a 2 per cent *m/m* solution.

01/2005:0347

HYPROMELLOSE PHTHALATE

Hypromellosi phthalas

DEFINITION

Hypromellose phthalate (hydroxypropylmethylcellulose phthalate) is a monophthalic acid ester of hypromellose. It contains methoxy (-OCH_3) and 2-hydroxypropoxy (-$OCH_2CHOHCH_3$) groups and not less than 21.0 per cent and not more than 35.0 per cent of phthaloyl (*o*-carboxybenzoyl $C_8H_5O_3$) groups, calculated with reference to the anhydrous substance.

CHARACTERS

White or slightly off-white, free-flowing flakes or a granular powder, practically insoluble in water, soluble in a mixture of equal volumes of acetone and methanol and in a mixture of equal volumes of methanol and methylene chloride, very slightly soluble in acetone and in toluene, practically insoluble in ethanol.

IDENTIFICATION

A. Examine by infrared absorption spectrophotometry (*2.2.24*), comparing with the *Ph. Eur. reference spectrum of hypromellose phthalate.*

B. Dissolve about 40 mg in 1 ml of a mixture of equal volumes of *acetone R* and of *methanol R*. Allow the solution to flow over a glass plate and dry. A colourless, transparent film is formed.

TESTS

Free phthalic acid. Examine by liquid chromatography (*2.2.29*).

Test solution. Dissolve 0.20 g of the substance to be examined in about 50 ml of *acetonitrile R* with the aid of ultrasound. Add 10 ml of *water R*, cool to room temperature and dilute to 100.0 ml with *acetonitrile R*.

Reference solution. Dissolve 5.0 mg of *phthalic acid R* in 125 ml of *acetonitrile R*. Add 25 ml of *water R* and dilute to 250.0 ml with *acetonitrile R*.

The chromatographic procedure may be carried out using:

- a column 0.25 m long and 4.6 mm in internal diameter packed with octadecylsilane chemically bound to porous silica or ceramic micro-particles (5 µm to 10 µm),
- as mobile phase at a flow rate of 2 ml/min a mixture of 15 volumes of *acetonitrile R* and 85 volumes of an 8.5 g/l solution of *cyanoacetic acid R*,
- as detector a spectrophotometer set at 235 nm.

Inject 20 µl of the reference solution. Adjust the sensitivity of the system so that the height of the principal peak, apart from the peaks due to the solvent, is at least 50 per cent of the full scale of the recorder.

Inject 20 µl of the test solution. In the chromatogram obtained with the test solution, the area of any peak corresponding to phthalic acid is not greater than the area of the principal peak in the chromatogram obtained with the reference solution (1 per cent).

Chlorides. Dissolve 1.0 g in 40.0 ml of *0.2 M sodium hydroxide*, add 0.05 ml of *phenolphthalein solution R* and *dilute nitric acid R* dropwise and with stirring until the red colour disappears. Add an additional 20.0 ml of *dilute nitric acid R* with stirring. Heat on a water-bath with stirring until the gel-like precipitate formed becomes granular. Cool and centrifuge. Separate the liquid phase and wash the residue with three quantities, each of 20 ml, of *water R*, separating the washings by centrifugation. Combine the liquid phases, filter, add 5.0 ml of *0.1 M silver nitrate*, dilute to 200.0 ml with *water R* and mix. 50.0 ml of the solution is not more opalescent than a standard prepared by treating 0.5 ml of *0.01 M hydrochloric acid* with 10.0 ml of *0.2 M sodium hydroxide*, adding 7 ml of *dilute nitric acid R*, 5.0 ml of *0.1 M silver nitrate* and diluting to 50.0 ml with *water R* (0.07 per cent).

Heavy metals (*2.4.8*). 2.0 g complies with limit test C for heavy metals (10 ppm). Prepare the standard using 2 ml of *lead standard solution (10 ppm Pb) R*.

Sulphated ash (*2.4.14*). Not more than 0.2 per cent, determined on 1.0 g.

Water (*2.5.12*). Not more than 5.0 per cent, determined on 0.500 g by the semi-micro determination of water using 50 ml of *anhydrous methanol R* as the solvent.

ASSAY

Dissolve 1.000 g in 50 ml of a mixture of 1 volume of *water R*, 2 volumes of *acetone R* and 2 volumes of *alcohol R*. Add 0.1 ml of *phenolphthalein solution R* and titrate with *0.1 M sodium hydroxide* until a faint pink colour is obtained. Carry out a blank titration.

Calculate the percentage content of phthaloyl groups from the expression:

$$\frac{149n}{(100-a)\,m} - 1.795S$$

a = percentage content of water,

m = mass of the substance to be examined, in grams,

n = number of millilitres of *0.1 M sodium hydroxide* used,

S = percentage content of free phthalic acid (see Tests).

STORAGE

Store in an airtight container.

Monographs F-H

I

01/2005:0721

IBUPROFEN

Ibuprofenum

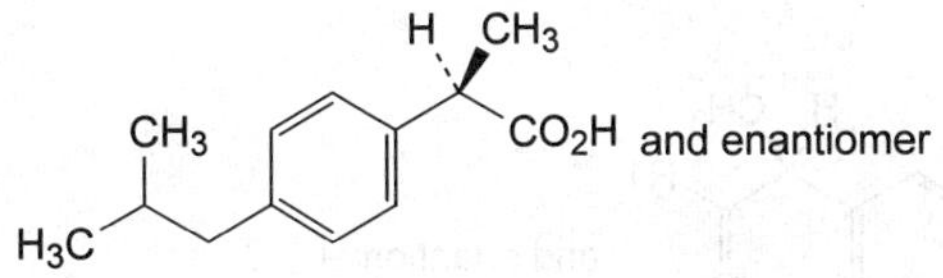

$C_{13}H_{18}O_2$ M_r 206.3

DEFINITION

(2*RS*)-2-[4-(2-Methylpropyl)phenyl]propanoic acid.

Content: 98.5 per cent to 101.0 per cent (dried substance).

CHARACTERS

Appearance: white, crystalline powder or colourless crystals.

Solubility: practically insoluble in water, freely soluble in acetone, in methanol and in methylene chloride. It dissolves in dilute solutions of alkali hydroxides and carbonates.

IDENTIFICATION

First identification: *A, C.*

Second identification: *A, B, D.*

A. Melting point (*2.2.14*): 75 °C to 78 °C.

B. Dissolve 50.0 mg in a 4 g/l solution of *sodium hydroxide R* and dilute to 100.0 ml with the same alkaline solution. Examined between 240 nm and 300 nm (*2.2.25*), using a spectrophotometer with a band width of 1.0 nm and a scan speed of not more than 50 nm/min, the solution shows a shoulder at 258 nm and 2 absorption maxima, at 264 nm and 272 nm. The ratio of the absorbance measured at the maximum at 264 nm to that measured at the shoulder at 258 nm is 1.20 to 1.30. The ratio of the absorbance measured at the maximum at 272 nm to that measured at the shoulder at 258 nm is 1.00 to 1.10.

C. Infrared absorption spectrophotometry (*2.2.24*).

Preparation: discs.

Comparison: *ibuprofen CRS.*

D. Thin-layer chromatography (*2.2.27*).

Test solution. Dissolve 50 mg of the substance to be examined in *methylene chloride R* and dilute to 10 ml with the same solvent.

Reference solution. Dissolve 50 mg of *ibuprofen CRS* in *methylene chloride R* and dilute to 10 ml with the same solvent.

Plate: *TLC silica gel plate R.*

Mobile phase: *anhydrous acetic acid R, ethyl acetate R, hexane R* (5:24:71 *V/V/V*).

Application: 5 µl.

Development: over a path of 10 cm.

Drying: at 120 °C for 30 min.

Detection: lightly spray with a 10 g/l solution of *potassium permanganate R* in *dilute sulphuric acid R* and heat at 120 °C for 20 min. Examine in ultraviolet light at 365 nm.

Results: the principal spot in the chromatogram obtained with the test solution is similar in position, colour and size to the principal spot in the chromatogram obtained with the reference solution.

TESTS

Solution S. Dissolve 2.0 g in *methanol R* and dilute to 20 ml with the same solvent.

Appearance of solution. Solution S is clear (*2.2.1*) and colourless (*2.2.2, Method II*).

Angle of optical rotation (*2.2.7*): − 0.05° to + 0.05°.

Dissolve 0.50 g in *methanol R* and dilute to 20.0 ml with the same solvent.

Related substances. Liquid chromatography (*2.2.29*).

Test solution. Dissolve 20 mg of the substance to be examined in 2 ml of *acetonitrile R* and dilute to 10.0 ml with mobile phase A.

Reference solution (a). Dilute 1.0 ml of the test solution to 100.0 ml with mobile phase A.

Reference solution (b). Dissolve 20 mg of *ibuprofen CRS* in 2 ml of *acetonitrile R*, add 1.0 ml of a 0.06 g/l solution of *ibuprofen impurity B CRS* in *acetonitrile R* and dilute to 10.0 ml with mobile phase A.

Column:

– *size*: *l* = 0.15 m, Ø = 4.6 mm,

– *stationary phase*: *octadecylsilyl silica gel for chromatography R* (5 µm).

Mobile phase:

– *mobile phase A*: mix 0.5 volumes of *phosphoric acid R*, 340 volumes of *acetonitrile R* and 600 volumes of *water R*; allow to equilibrate and dilute to 1000 volumes with *water R*,

– *mobile phase B*: *acetonitrile R*,

Time (min)	Mobile phase A (per cent *V/V*)	Mobile phase B (per cent *V/V*)
0 - 25	100	0
25 - 55	100 → 15	0 → 85
55 - 70	15	85
70 - 75	15 → 100	85 → 0

Flow rate: 2 ml/min.

Detection: spectrophotometer at 214 nm.

Equilibration: for about 45 min with mobile phase A.

Injection: 20 µl.

System suitability: reference solution (b):

– *peak-to-valley ratio*: minimum of 1.5, where H_p = height above the baseline of the peak due to impurity B, and H_v = height above the baseline of the lowest point of the curve separating this peak from the peak due to ibuprofen. If necessary, adjust the concentration of acetonitrile in mobile phase A.

Limits:

– *impurity B*: not more than the area of the corresponding peak in the chromatogram obtained with reference solution (b) (0.3 per cent),

– *any other impurity*: not more than 0.3 times the area of the principal peak in the chromatogram obtained with reference solution (a) (0.3 per cent),

– *total of all impurities apart from impurity B*: not more than 0.7 times the area of the principal peak in the chromatogram obtained with reference solution (a) (0.7 per cent),

– *disregard limit*: 0.05 times the area of the principal peak in the chromatogram obtained with reference solution (a) (0.05 per cent).

Monographs I-L

Impurity F. Gas chromatography (*2.2.28*): use the normalisation procedure.

Methylating solution. Dilute 1 ml of *N,N-dimethylformamide dimethyl acetal R* and 1 ml of *pyridine R* to 10 ml with *ethyl acetate R*.

Test solution. Weigh about 50.0 mg of the substance to be examined into a sealable vial, dissolve in 1.0 ml of *ethyl acetate R*, add 1 ml of methylating solution, seal and heat at 100 °C in a block heater for 20 min. Allow to cool. Remove the reagents under a stream of nitrogen at room temperature. Dissolve the residue in 5 ml of *ethyl acetate R*.

Reference solution (a). Dissolve 0.5 mg of *ibuprofen impurity F CRS* in *ethyl acetate R* and dilute to 10.0 ml with the same solvent.

Reference solution (b). Weigh about 50.0 mg of *ibuprofen CRS* into a sealable vial, dissolve in 1.0 ml of reference solution (a), add 1 ml of methylating solution, seal and heat at 100 °C in a block heater for 20 min. Allow to cool. Remove the reagents under a stream of nitrogen at room temperature. Dissolve the residue in 5 ml of *ethyl acetate R*.

Column:

- *material*: fused-silica,
- *size*: *l* = 25 m, Ø = 0.53 mm,
- *stationary phase*: *macrogol 20 000 R* (film thickness 2 µm).

Carrier gas: *helium for chromatography R.*

Flow rate: 5.0 ml/min.

Temperature:

- *column*: 150 °C,
- *injection port*: 200 °C,
- *detector*: 250 °C.

Detection: flame-ionisation.

Injection: 1 µl; inject the test solution and reference solution (b).

Run time: twice the retention time of ibuprofen.

System suitability:

- *relative retention* with reference to ibuprofen (retention time = about 17 min): impurity F = about 1.5.

Limit:

- *impurity F*: maximum 0.1 per cent.

Heavy metals (*2.4.8*): maximum 10 ppm.

12 ml of solution S complies with limit test B. Prepare the standard using lead standard solution (1 ppm Pb) prepared by diluting *lead standard solution (100 ppm Pb) R* with *methanol R.*

Loss on drying (*2.2.32*): maximum 0.5 per cent, determined on 1.000 g by drying *in vacuo* over *diphosphorus pentoxide R.*

Sulphated ash (*2.4.14*): maximum 0.1 per cent, determined on 1.0 g.

ASSAY

Dissolve 0.450 g in 50 ml of *methanol R*. Add 0.4 ml of *phenolphthalein solution R1*. Titrate with *0.1 M sodium hydroxide* until a red colour is obtained. Carry out a blank titration.

1 ml of *0.1 M sodium hydroxide* is equivalent to 20.63 mg of $C_{13}H_{18}O_2$.

IMPURITIES

Specified impurities: A, B, C, D, E.

Other detectable impurities: F, G, H, I, J, K, L, M, N, O, P, Q, R.

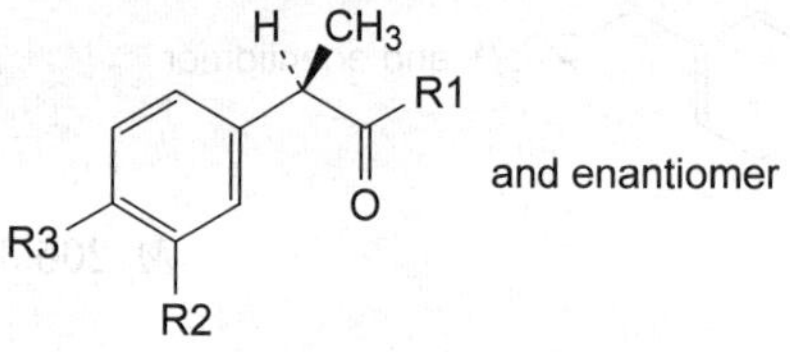

A. R1 = OH, R2 = CH_2-$CH(CH_3)_2$, R3 = H: (2*RS*)-2-[3-(2-methylpropyl)phenyl]propanoic acid,

B. R1 = OH, R2 = H, R3 = $[CH_2]_3$-CH_3: (2*RS*)-2-(4-butylphenyl)propanoic acid,

C. R1 = NH_2, R2 = H, R3 = CH_2-$CH(CH_3)_2$: (2*RS*)-2-[4-(2-methylpropyl)phenyl]propanamide,

D. R1 = OH, R2 = H, R3 = CH_3: (2*RS*)-2-(4-methylphenyl)propanoic acid,

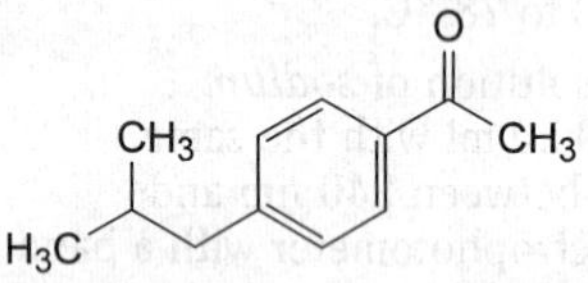

E. 1-[4-(2-methylpropyl)phenyl]ethanone,

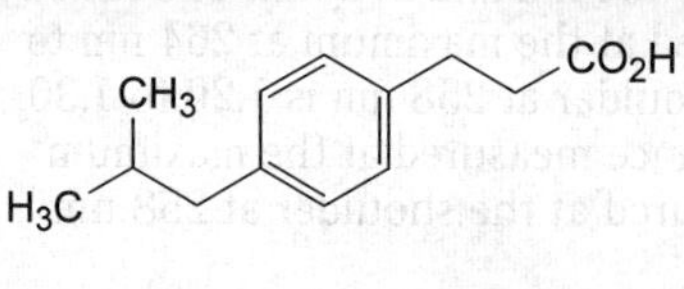

F. 3-[4-(2-methylpropyl)phenyl]propanoic acid,

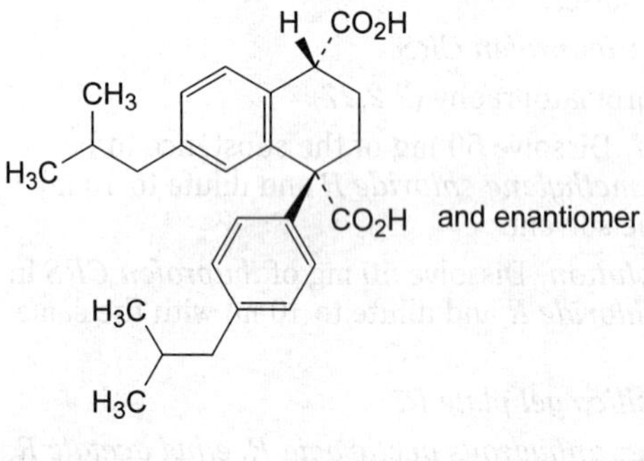

G. *cis*-7-(2-methylpropyl)-1-[4-(2-methylpropyl)phenyl]-1,2,3,4-tetrahydronaphthalene-1,4-dicarboxylic acid,

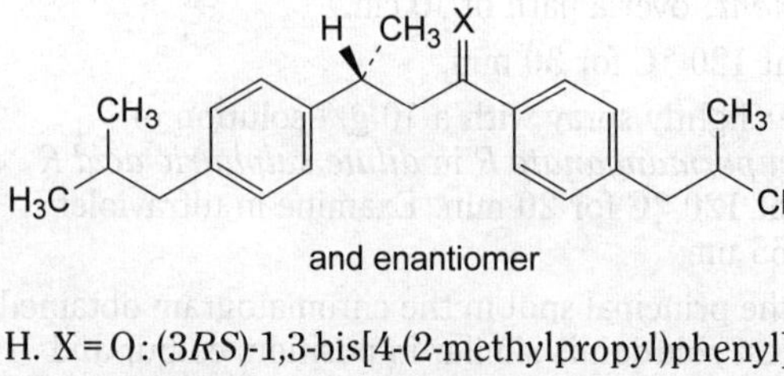

H. X = O: (3*RS*)-1,3-bis[4-(2-methylpropyl)phenyl]butan-1-one,

I. X = H_2: (3*RS*)-1,3-bis[4-(2-methylpropyl)phenyl]butane,

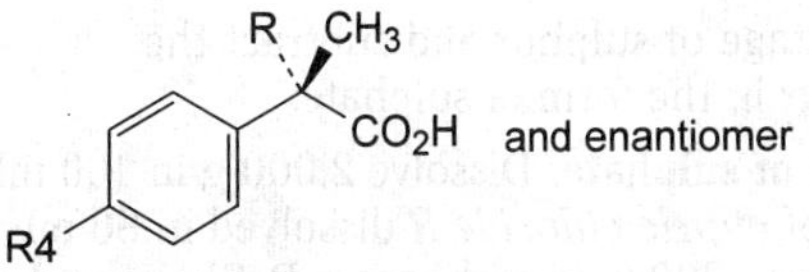

J. R = H, R4 = CO-$CH(CH_3)_2$: (2*RS*)-2-[4-(2-methylpropanoyl)phenyl]propanoic acid,

K. R = H, R4 = CHO: (2*RS*)-2-(4-formylphenyl)propanoic acid,

L. R = H, R4 = CHOH-$CH(CH_3)_2$: 2-[4-(1-hydroxy-2-methylpropyl)phenyl]propanoic acid,

M. R = OH, R4 = CH_2-$CH(CH_3)_2$: (2*RS*)-2-hydroxy-2-[4-(2-methylpropyl)phenyl]propanoic acid,

N. R = H, R4 = C_2H_5: (2*RS*)-2-(4-ethylphenyl)propanoic acid,

O. R = H, R4 = $CH(CH_3)$-C_2H_5: 2-[4-(1-methylpropyl)phenyl]propanoic acid,

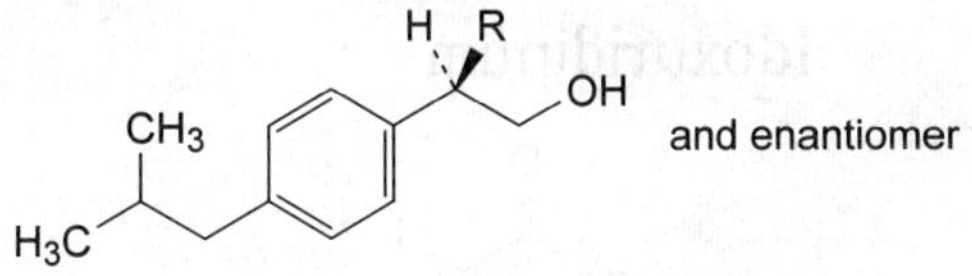

P. R = CH_3: (2*RS*)-2-[4-(2-methylpropyl)phenyl]propan-1-ol,

Q. R = H: 2-[4-(2-methylpropyl)phenyl]ethanol,

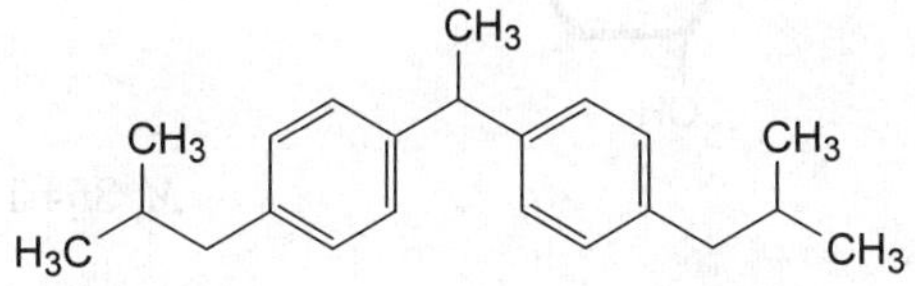

R. 1,1-bis[4-(2-methylpropyl)phenyl]ethane.

01/2005:1439

ICELAND MOSS

Lichen islandicus

DEFINITION

Iceland moss consists of the whole or cut dried thallus of *Cetraria islandica* (L.) Acharius s.l.

CHARACTERS

Iceland moss has a bitter, mucilaginous taste.

It has the macroscopic and microscopic characters described under identification tests A and B.

IDENTIFICATION

A. The thallus, up to 15 cm long, is irregularly dichotomous and consists of glabrous, groove-shaped or almost flat, stiff, brittle bands, 0.3 cm to 1.5 cm wide and about 0.5 mm thick, sometimes serrated with the margin appearing ciliated (pycnidia). The upper surface is greenish to greenish-brown, the lower surface is greyish-white to light brownish and shows whitish, depressed spots (so-called respiratory cavities). On the apexes of the terminal lobes, very rarely, there are brown, discoid apothecia.

B. Reduce to a powder (355). The powder is greyish-brown. Examine under a microscope, using *chloral hydrate solution R*. The powder shows numerous fragments of the pseudoparenchyma consisting of narrow-lumened, thick-walled hyphae from the marginal layer and wide-lumened hyphae from the adjacent layer consisting of loosely entwined hyphae, in which, in the medullary zone, greenish to brownish algae cells up to 15 µm in diameter, are embedded; occasionally marginal fragments of the thallus with tube-like or cylindrical spermogonia, up to about 160 µm wide and up to about 400 µm long.

C. To 1.0 g of the powdered drug (355) add 10 ml of *water R* and boil for 2 min to 3 min. The greyish-brown solution forms a gel after cooling.

D. Examine the chromatograms obtained in the test for other lichen species. The chromatogram obtained with the test solution shows the violet to grey zone of fumaroprotocetraric acid located slightly below the zone of caffeic acid in the chromatogram obtained with the reference solution. Other fainter zones are present.

TESTS

Foreign matter (*2.8.2*). Not more than 5 per cent.

Other lichen species. Examine by thin-layer chromatography (*2.2.27*), using a *TLC silica gel plate R*.

Test solution. To 1.0 g of the powdered drug (355) add 5 ml of *acetone R* and heat in a water-bath under a reflux condenser for 2 min to 3 min. Cool and filter.

Reference solution. Dissolve 5 mg of *anethole R* and 5 mg of *caffeic acid R* in 2 ml of *acetone R*.

Apply to the plate as bands 20 µl of the test solution and 10 µl of the reference solution. Develop over a path of 10 cm, using a mixture of 5 volumes of *acetone R*, 5 volumes of *methanol R*, 10 volumes of *glacial acetic acid R* and 80 volumes of *toluene R*. Allow the plate to dry in air and spray the plate with *anisaldehyde solution R*. Examine in daylight while heating at 100 °C to 105 °C for 5 min to 10 min. The chromatogram obtained with the reference solution shows in the lower half a greyish-blue to violet-blue zone (caffeic acid) and in the upper half a blue to blue-violet zone (anethole). The chromatogram obtained with the test solution shows no red-violet zone a little below the zone of anethole in the chromatogram obtained with the reference solution.

Loss on drying (*2.2.32*). Not more than 12.0 per cent, determined on 1.000 g of powdered drug (355) by drying in an oven at 100 °C to 105 °C for 2 h.

Total ash (*2.4.16*). Not more than 3.0 per cent.

Swelling value (*2.8.4*). Not less than 4.5, determined on the powdered drug (355).

STORAGE

Store in an airtight container, protected from light.

01/2005:0917

ICHTHAMMOL

Ichthammolum

DEFINITION

Ichthammol is obtained by distillation from certain bituminous schists, sulphonation of the distillate and neutralisation of the product with ammonia. It contains not less than 50.0 per cent *m/m* and not more than 56.0 per cent *m/m* of dry matter, not less than 4.5 per cent *m/m* and not more than 7.0 per cent *m/m* of total ammonia (NH_3; M_r 17.03) and not less than 10.5 per cent *m/m* of organically combined sulphur, calculated with reference to the dried substance; not more than 20.0 per cent *m/m* of the total sulphur is in the form of sulphate.

CHARACTERS

A dense, blackish-brown liquid, miscible with water and with glycerol, slightly soluble in alcohol, in fatty oils and in liquid paraffin. It forms homogeneous mixtures with wool fat and soft paraffin.

IDENTIFICATION

A. Dissolve 1.5 g in 15 ml of *water R* (solution A). To 2 ml of solution A add 2 ml of *hydrochloric acid R*. A resinous precipitate is formed. Decant the supernatant liquid. The precipitate is partly soluble in *ether R*.

B. 2 ml of solution A, obtained in identification test A, gives the reaction of ammonium salts and salts of volatile bases (*2.3.1*).

C. Evaporate and ignite the mixture of solution A and *dilute sodium hydroxide solution R* obtained in identification test B. Take up the residue with 5 ml of *dilute hydrochloric acid R*. Gas is evolved which turns *lead acetate paper R* brown or black. Filter the solution. The filtrate gives reaction (a) of sulphates (*2.3.1*).

TESTS

Acidity or alkalinity. To 10.0 ml of the clear filtrate obtained in the assay of total ammonia add 0.05 ml of *methyl red solution R*. Not more than 0.2 ml of *0.02 M hydrochloric acid* or *0.02 M sodium hydroxide* is required to change the colour of the indicator.

Relative density (*2.2.5*): 1.040 to 1.085, determined on a mixture of equal volumes of the substance to be examined and *water R*.

Sulphated ash (*2.4.14*). Not more than 0.3 per cent, determined on 1.00 g.

ASSAY

Dry matter. Weigh 1.000 g in a tared flask containing 2 g of *sand R*, previously dried to constant mass, and a small glass rod. Heat on a water-bath for 2 h with frequent stirring and dry in an oven at 100 °C to 105 °C until two consecutive weighings do not differ by more than 2.0 mg; the second weighing is carried out after drying again for 1 h.

Total ammonia. Dissolve 2.50 g in 25 ml of warm *water R*. Rinse the solution into a 250 ml volumetric flask, add 200 ml of *sodium chloride solution R* and dilute to 250.0 ml with *water R*. Filter the solution, discarding the first 20 ml of filtrate. To 100.0 ml of the clear filtrate add 25 ml of *formaldehyde solution R*, neutralised to *phenolphthalein solution R1*. Titrate with *0.1 M sodium hydroxide* until a faint pink colour is obtained.

1 ml of *0.1 M sodium hydroxide* is equivalent to 1.703 mg of NH_3.

Organically combined sulphur. Mix 0.500 g with 4 g of *anhydrous sodium carbonate R* and 3 ml of *methylene chloride R* in a porcelain crucible of about 50 ml capacity, warm and stir until all the methylene chloride has evaporated. Add 10 g of coarsely powdered *copper nitrate R*, mix thoroughly and heat the mixture very gently using a small flame. When the initial reaction has subsided, increase the temperature slightly until most of the material has blackened. Cool, place the crucible in a large beaker, add 20 ml of *hydrochloric acid R* and, when the reaction has ceased, add 100 ml of *water R* and boil until all the copper oxide has dissolved. Filter the solution, add 400 ml of *water R*, heat to boiling and add 20 ml of *barium chloride solution R1*. Allow to stand for 2 h, filter, wash with *water R*, dry and ignite at about 600 °C until two successive weighings do not differ by more than 0.2 per cent of the mass of the residue.

1 g of residue is equivalent to 0.1374 g of total sulphur.

Calculate the percentage of sulphur and subtract the percentage of sulphur in the form of sulphate.

Sulphur in the form of sulphate. Dissolve 2.000 g in 100 ml of *water R*, add 2 g of *cupric chloride R* dissolved in 80 ml of *water R* and dilute to 200.0 ml with *water R*. Shake and filter. Heat 100.0 ml of the filtrate almost to boiling, add 1 ml of *hydrochloric acid R* and 5 ml of *barium chloride solution R1* dropwise and heat on a water-bath. Filter, wash the precipitate with *water R*, dry and ignite at about 600 °C until two successive weighings do not differ by more than 0.2 per cent of the mass of the residue.

1 g of residue is equivalent to 0.1374 g of sulphur present in the form of sulphate.

Calculate the percentage of sulphur in the form of sulphate.

01/2005:0669

IDOXURIDINE

Idoxuridinum

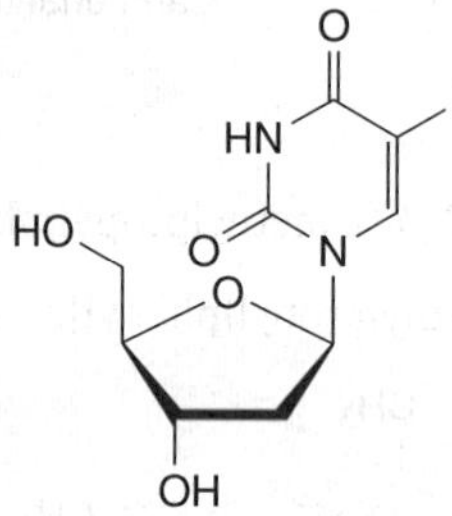

$C_9H_{11}IN_2O_5$ M_r 354.1

DEFINITION

Idoxuridine contains not less than 98.0 per cent and not more than the equivalent of 101.0 per cent of 5-iodo-1-(2-deoxy-β-D-*erythro*-pentofuranosyl)pyrimidine-2,4(1*H*,3*H*)-dione, calculated with reference to the dried substance.

CHARACTERS

A white or almost white, crystalline powder, slightly soluble in water and in alcohol. It dissolves in dilute solutions of alkali hydroxides.

It melts at about 180 °C, with decomposition.

IDENTIFICATION

First identification: A.

Second identification: B, C, D.

A. Examine by infrared absorption spectrophotometry (*2.2.24*), comparing with the spectrum obtained with *idoxuridine CRS*. Examine the substances as discs prepared using 1 mg of the substance to be examined and of the reference substance each in 0.3 g of *potassium bromide R*.

B. Examine the chromatograms obtained in the test for related substances. The principal spot in the chromatogram obtained with test solution (b) is similar in position and size to the principal spot in the chromatogram obtained with reference solution (c).

C. Heat about 5 mg in a test-tube over a naked flame. Violet vapour is evolved.

D. Disperse about 2 mg in 1 ml of *water R* and add 2 ml of *diphenylamine solution R2*. Heat in a water-bath for 10 min. A persistent light-blue colour develops.

TESTS

Solution S. Dissolve 0.500 g in *1 M sodium hydroxide* and dilute to 50.0 ml with the same solvent.

Appearance of solution. Solution S is clear (*2.2.1*) and colourless (*2.2.2, Method II*).

pH (*2.2.3*). Dissolve 0.10 g in *carbon dioxide-free water R* and dilute to 100 ml with the same solvent. The pH of the solution is 5.5 to 6.5.

Specific optical rotation (*2.2.7*): + 28 to + 32, determined on solution S and calculated with reference to the dried substance.

Related substances. Examine by thin-layer chromatography (*2.2.27*), using as coating substance a suitable silica gel with a fluorescent indicator having an optimal intensity at 254 nm.

Test solution (a). Dissolve 0.20 g of the substance to be examined in a mixture of 1 volume of *concentrated ammonia R* and 5 volumes of *methanol R* and dilute to 5 ml with the same mixture of solvents.

Test solution (b). Dilute 1 ml of test solution (a) to 10 ml with a mixture of 1 volume of *concentrated ammonia R* and 5 volumes of *methanol R*.

Reference solution (a). Dissolve 20 mg of *5-iodouracil R*, 20 mg of *2′-deoxyuridine R* and 20 mg of *5-bromo-2′-deoxyuridine R* in a mixture of 1 volume of *concentrated ammonia R* and 5 volumes of *methanol R* and dilute to 100 ml with the same mixture of solvents.

Reference solution (b). Dissolve 0.20 g of the substance to be examined in 5 ml of reference solution (a).

Reference solution (c). Dissolve 20 mg of *idoxuridine CRS* in a mixture of 1 volume of *concentrated ammonia R* and 5 volumes of *methanol R* and dilute to 5 ml with the same mixture of solvents.

Reference solution (d). Dilute 1 ml of test solution (b) to 20 ml with a mixture of 1 volume of *concentrated ammonia R* and 5 volumes of *methanol R*.

Apply separately to the plate 5 µl of each solution. Develop twice over a path of 15 cm using a mixture of 10 volumes of *concentrated ammonia R*, 40 volumes of *chloroform R* and 50 volumes of *2-propanol R*, drying the plate in a current of cold air after each development. Examine in ultraviolet light at 254 nm. In the chromatogram obtained with test solution (a): any spots corresponding to 5-iodouracil, 2′-deoxyuridine and 5-bromo-2′-deoxyuridine are not more intense than the corresponding spots in the chromatogram obtained with reference solution (a) (0.5 per cent); any spot, apart from the principal spot and the spots corresponding to 5-iodouracil, 2′-deoxyuridine and 5-bromo-2′-deoxyuridine, is not more intense than the spot in the chromatogram obtained with reference solution (d) (0.5 per cent). The test is not valid unless the chromatogram obtained with reference solution (b) shows four clearly separated spots.

Iodide. Dissolve 0.25 g in 25 ml of *0.1 M sodium hydroxide*, add 5 ml of *dilute hydrochloric acid R* and dilute to 50 ml with *water R*. Allow to stand for 10 min and filter. To 25 ml of the filtrate add 5 ml of *dilute hydrogen peroxide solution R* and 10 ml of *chloroform R* and shake. Any pink colour in the organic layer is not more intense than that in a standard prepared at the same time in the same manner using 1 ml of a 0.33 g/l solution of *potassium iodide R* instead of the substance to be examined (0.1 per cent).

Loss on drying (*2.2.32*). Not more than 1.0 per cent, determined on 1.000 g by drying *in vacuo* at 60 °C.

Sulphated ash (*2.4.14*). Not more than 0.1 per cent, determined on 1.0 g.

ASSAY

Dissolve 0.3000 g in 20 ml of *dimethylformamide R*. Titrate with *0.1 M tetrabutylammonium hydroxide*, determining the end-point potentiometrically (*2.2.20*).

1 ml of *0.1 M tetrabutylammonium hydroxide* is equivalent to 35.41 mg of $C_9H_{11}IN_2O_5$.

STORAGE

Store protected from light.

01/2005:1529
corrected

IFOSFAMIDE

Ifosfamidum

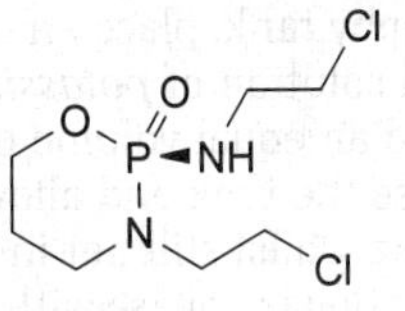

and enantiomer

$C_7H_{15}Cl_2N_2O_2P$ M_r 261.1

DEFINITION

Ifosfamide contains not less than 98.0 per cent and not more than the equivalent of 102.0 per cent of (*RS*)-*N*,3-bis(2-chloroethyl)-1,3,2-oxazaphosphinan-2-amine 2-oxide, calculated with reference to the anhydrous substance.

CHARACTERS

A white or almost white, fine, crystalline powder, hygroscopic, soluble in water, freely soluble in methylene chloride.

IDENTIFICATION

Examine by infrared absorption spectrophotometry (*2.2.24*), comparing with the *Ph. Eur. reference spectrum of ifosfamide*. Examine the substance prepared as a disc.

TESTS

Solution S. Dissolve 5.0 g in *carbon dioxide-free water R* and dilute to 50.0 ml with the same solvent.

Appearance of solution. Solution S is clear (*2.2.1*) and not more intensely coloured than reference solution Y_7 (*2.2.2, Method II*).

Acidity or alkalinity. Dilute 5 ml of solution S to 50 ml with *carbon dioxide-free water R*. To 10 ml of this solution add 0.1 ml of *methyl red solution R*. Not more than 0.1 ml of *0.01 M hydrochloric acid* is required to change the colour of the indicator to red. To another 10 ml of the solution add 0.1 ml of *phenolphthalein solution R*. Not more than 0.3 ml of *0.01 M sodium hydroxide* is required to change the colour of the indicator to pink.

Optical rotation (*2.2.7*). The angle of optical rotation, determined on solution S, is − 0.10° to + 0.10°.

Related substances

A. Examine by thin-layer chromatography (*2.2.27*), using a *TLC silica gel plate R*.

Test solution. Dissolve 1.00 g of the substance to be examined in a mixture of equal volumes of *methanol R* and *water R* and dilute to 10 ml with the same mixture of solvents.

Reference solution (a). Dissolve 25 mg of *ifosfamide impurity A CRS* and 25 mg of *chloroethylamine hydrochloride R* (impurity C) ina mixture of equal volumes of *methanol R* and *water R* and dilute to 100 ml with the same mixture of solvents.

Monographs I-L

Reference solution (b). Dissolve 15 mg of *ifosfamide impurity B CRS* ina mixture of equal volumes of *methanol R* and *water R* and dilute to 100 ml with the same mixture of solvents.

Reference solution (c). Dissolve 5 mg of *ethanolamine R* (impurity D), 20 mg of *ifosfamide impurity A CRS* and 80 mg of *chloroethylamine hydrochloride R* (impurity C) in a mixture of equal volumes of *methanol R* and *water R* and dilute to 100 ml with the same mixture of solvents.

Apply to the plate 10 µl of each solution. Develop over a path of 15 cm using a mixture of 10 volumes of *water R*, 15 volumes of *methanol R*, 25 volumes of *anhydrous acetic acid R* and 50 volumes of *methylene chloride R*. Dry the plate at 115 °C for 45 min. At the bottom of a chromatography tank, place an evaporating dish containing a 3.2 g/l solution of *potassium permanganate R* and add an equal volume of *dilute hydrochloric acid R*, close the tank and allow to stand for 10 min. Place the plate whilst still hot in the tank, avoiding contact of the stationary phase with the solution, and close the tank. Leave the plate in contact with the chlorine vapour for 20 min. Withdraw the plate and place it in a current of cold air until the excess of chlorine is removed (about 20 min) and an area of coating below the points of application does not give a blue colour with a drop of *potassium iodide and starch solution R*. Avoid prolonged exposure to cold air. Immerse the plate in a 1 g/l solution of *tetramethylbenzidine R* in *alcohol R* for 5 s. Allow the plate to dry and examine. In the chromatogram obtained with the test solution: any spot corresponding to impurity A or impurity C is not more intense than the corresponding spot in the chromatogram obtained with reference solution (a) (0.25 per cent); any spot corresponding to impurity B is not more intense than the corresponding spot in the chromatogram obtained with reference solution (b) (0.15 per cent); any other spot is not more intense than the principal spot in the chromatogram obtained with reference solution (b) (0.15 per cent). The test is not valid unless the chromatogram obtained with reference solution (c) shows 3 clearly separated spots.

B. Examine by thin-layer chromatography (*2.2.27*), using a *TLC silica gel plate R*.

Test solution. Dissolve 0.200 g of the substance to be examined in a mixture of equal volumes of *methanol R* and *methylene chloride R* and dilute to 10 ml with the same mixture of solvents.

Reference solution (a). Dissolve 5 mg of *ifosfamide impurity E CRS* and 5 mg of *ifosfamide impurity F CRS* in a mixture of equal volumes of *methanol R* and *methylene chloride R* and dilute to 100 ml with the same mixture of solvents.

Reference solution (b). Dissolve 10 mg of *ifosfamide impurity E CRS* and 10 mg of *ifosfamide CRS* in a mixture of equal volumes of *methanol R* and *methylene chloride R* and dilute to 100 ml with the same mixture of solvents.

Apply to the plate 5 µl of each solution. Develop over a path of 15 cm using a mixture of 1 volume of *methylene chloride R* and 10 volumes of *acetone R*. Dry the plate at 115 °C for 45 min. Proceed as described in Related substances test A. Any spot corresponding to impurity E or impurity F in the chromatogram obtained with the test solution is not more intense than the corresponding spot in the chromatogram obtained with reference solution (a) (0.25 per cent). The test is not valid unless the chromatogram obtained with reference solution (b) shows 2 clearly separated spots.

Chlorides (*2.4.4*). Dilute 5 ml of solution S to 15 ml with *water R*. The freshly prepared solution complies with the limit test for chlorides (100 ppm).

Heavy metals (*2.4.8*). 12 ml of solution S complies with limit test A for heavy metals (10 ppm). Prepare the standard using *lead standard solution (1 ppm Pb) R*.

Water (*2.5.12*). Not more than 0.5 per cent, determined on 1.00 g by the semi-micro determination of water.

ASSAY

Examine by liquid chromatography (*2.2.29*). *Use the solutions within 24 h.*

Solution A. Dissolve 50.0 mg of *ethyl parahydroxybenzoate R* in 25 ml of *alcohol R*, dilute to 100.0 ml with *water R* and mix.

Test solution. To 0.150 g of the substance to be examined add 10.0 ml of solution A and dilute to 250.0 ml with *water R*.

Reference solution. To 15.0 mg of *ifosfamide CRS* add 1.0 ml of solution A and dilute to 25.0 ml with *water R*.

The chromatography may be carried out using:

– a stainless steel column 0.25 m long and 4.6 mm in internal diameter packed with *octadecylsilyl silica gel for chromatography R* (5 µm),
– as mobile phase at a flow rate of 1.5 ml/min a mixture of 30 volumes of *acetonitrile R* and 70 volumes of *water R*,
– as detector a spectrophotometer set at 195 nm.

Inject 1 µl of the reference solution six times. The assay is not valid unless the resolution between the peaks due to ifosfamide and to ethyl parahydroxybenzoate is not less than 6.0 and the relative standard deviation of the peak area for ifosfamide is at most 2.0 per cent.

Inject 1 µl of the test solution. Calculate the percentage content of $C_7H_{15}Cl_2N_2O_2P$ from the area of the corresponding peak in the chromatogram obtained and the declared content of *ifosfamide CRS*.

STORAGE

Store in an airtight container.

IMPURITIES

Specified impurities: *A, B, C, E, F.*

Other detectable impurities: *D.*

Related substances test A

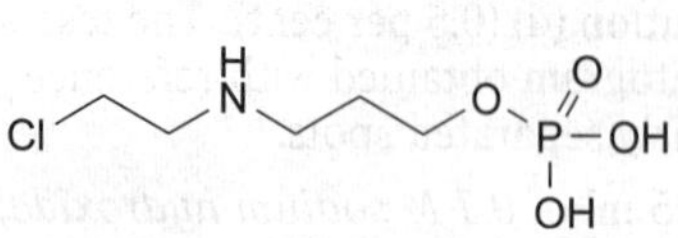

A. 3-[(2-chloroethyl)amino]propyl dihydrogen phosphate,

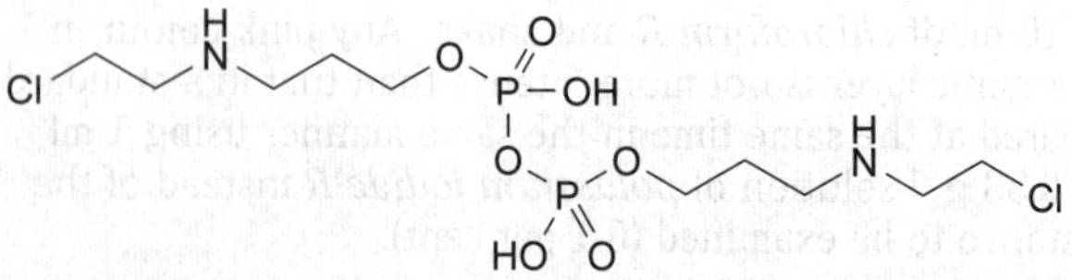

B. bis[3-[(2-chloroethyl)amino]propyl] dihydrogen diphosphate,

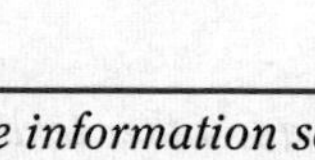

C. R = Cl: 2-chloroethanamine,

D. R = OH: 2-aminoethanol.

Related substances test B

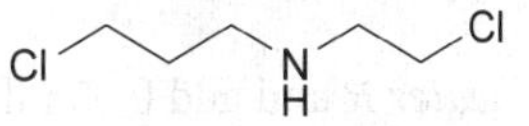

E. 3-chloro-*N*-(2-chloroethyl)propan-1-amine,

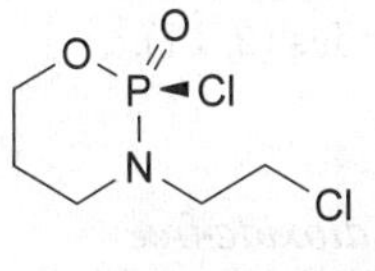

F. (*RS*)-2-chloro-3-(2-chloroethyl)-1,3,2-oxazaphosphinane 2-oxide.

01/2005:1226

IMIPENEM

Imipenemum

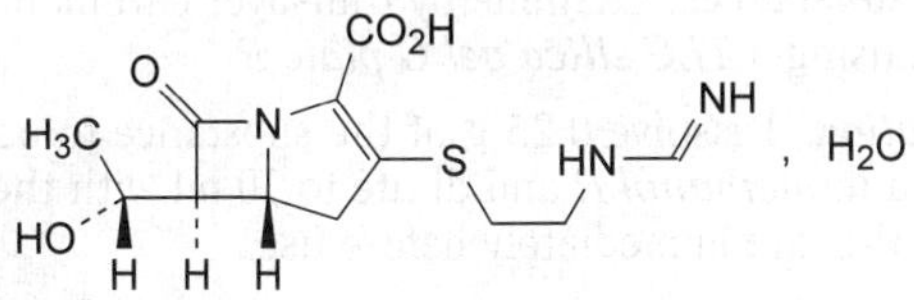

$C_{12}H_{17}N_3O_4S,H_2O$ M_r 317.4

DEFINITION

Imipenem contains not less than 98.0 per cent and not more than the equivalent of 101.0 per cent of (5*R*,6*S*)-6-[(*R*)-1-hydroxyethyl]-3-[[2-[(iminomethyl)amino]ethyl]sulphanyl]-7-oxo-1-azabicyclo[3.2.0]hept-2-ene-2-carboxylic acid, calculated with reference to the anhydrous substance.

CHARACTERS

A white to almost white or pale yellow powder, sparingly soluble in water, slightly soluble in methanol.

IDENTIFICATION

Examine by infrared absorption spectroscopy (*2.2.24*), comparing with the spectrum obtained with *imipenem CRS*.

TESTS

Appearance of solution. Dissolve 0.500 g in *phosphate buffer solution pH 7.0 R3* and dilute to 50 ml with the same solution. The solution is not more opalescent than reference suspension II (*2.2.1*) and not more intensely coloured than intensity 6 of the range of the reference solutions of the most appropriate colour (*2.2.2, Method II*).

pH (*2.2.3*). Dissolve 0.500 g in *carbon dioxide-free water R* and dilute to 100.0 ml with the same solvent. The pH of the solution is 4.5 to 7.0.

Specific optical rotation (*2.2.7*). Dissolve 0.125 g in *phosphate buffer solution pH 7.0 R3* and dilute to 25.0 ml with the same solution. The specific optical rotation measured at 25 °C is + 84 to + 89, calculated with reference to the anhydrous substance.

Related substances. Examine by liquid chromatography (*2.2.29*), as described under Assay. Inject 20 µl of reference solution (b). Adjust the sensitivity of the system so that the height of the principal peak in the chromatogram obtained is at least 50 per cent of the full scale of the recorder. Inject 20 µl of the test solution and continue the chromatography for twice the retention time of the principal peak. In the chromatogram obtained with the test solution: the area of any peak corresponding to thienamycin is not greater than that of the principal peak in the chromatogram obtained with reference solution (b) (1 per cent); the area of any peak, apart from the principal peak and any peak corresponding to thienamycin, is not greater than 0.3 times the area of the principal peak in the chromatogram obtained with reference solution (b) (0.3 per cent); the sum of the areas of all the peaks, apart from the principal peak and any peak corresponding to thienamycin, is not greater than the area of the principal peak in the chromatogram obtained with reference solution (b) (1 per cent). Disregard any peak with an area less than 0.1 times the area of the principal peak in the chromatogram obtained with reference solution (b).

Water (*2.5.12*): 5.0 per cent to 8.0 per cent, determined on 0.200 g by the semi-micro determination of water. Use an iodosulphurous reagent containing imidazole instead of pyridine and a clean container for each determination.

Sulphated ash (*2.4.14*). Not more than 0.2 per cent, determined on 1.0 g.

Bacterial endotoxins (*2.6.14*): less than 0.17 IU/mg, if intended for use in the manufacture of parenteral dosage forms without a further appropriate procedure for removal of bacterial endotoxins.

ASSAY

Examine by liquid chromatography (*2.2.29*).

Keep the solutions in an ice-bath and use within 8 h of preparation.

Test solution. Dissolve 40.0 mg of the substance to be examined in a mixture of 0.7 volumes of *acetonitrile R* and 99.3 volumes of a 0.135 g/l solution of *dipotassium hydrogen phosphate R* adjusted to pH 6.8 with *dilute phosphoric acid R* and dilute to 100.0 ml with the same mixture of solvents.

Reference solution (a). Dissolve 40.0 mg of *imipenem CRS* in a mixture of 0.7 volumes of *acetonitrile R* and 99.3 volumes of a 0.135 g/l solution of *dipotassium hydrogen phosphate R* adjusted to pH 6.8 with *dilute phosphoric acid R* and dilute to 100.0 ml with the same mixture of solvents.

Reference solution (b). Dilute 1.0 ml of the test solution to 100.0 ml with a mixture of 0.7 volumes of *acetonitrile R* and 99.3 volumes of a 0.135 g/l solution of *dipotassium hydrogen phosphate R* adjusted to pH 6.8 with *dilute phosphoric acid R.*

Reference solution (c). Heat at 80 °C for 5 min 20 ml of the test solution previously adjusted to pH 10 with *sodium hydroxide solution R.*

The chromatographic procedure may be carried out using:

– a stainless steel column 0.25 m long and 4.6 mm in internal diameter packed with *octadecylsilyl silica gel for chromatography R* (5 µm),
– as mobile phase at a flow rate of 1.0 ml/min a mixture of 0.7 volumes of *acetonitrile R* and 99.3 volumes of a 8.7 g/l solution of *dipotassium hydrogen phosphate R* adjusted to pH 7.3 with *dilute phosphoric acid R*,
– as detector a spectrophotometer set at 254 nm.

Inject 20 µl of reference solution (a). Adjust the sensitivity of the system so that the height of the principal peak in the chromatogram obtained is at least 50 per cent of the full scale of the recorder. Inject 20 µl of reference solution (c). When the chromatograms are recorded in the prescribed conditions, the retention time of imipenem is about 9 min and the relative retention time of thienamycin relative to imipenem is about 0.8. The assay is not valid unless the resolution between the peaks corresponding to imipenem and thienamycin is at least 3.5. Inject 20 µl of reference solution (a) six times. The test is not valid unless the relative standard deviation of the peak area for imipenem is at most 1.0 per cent. Inject alternately the test solution and reference solution (a).

STORAGE

Store in an airtight container, at a temperature of 2 °C to 8 °C. If the substance is sterile, store in a sterile, airtight, tamper-proof container.

LABELLING

The label states, where applicable, that the substance is free from bacterial endotoxins.

IMPURITIES

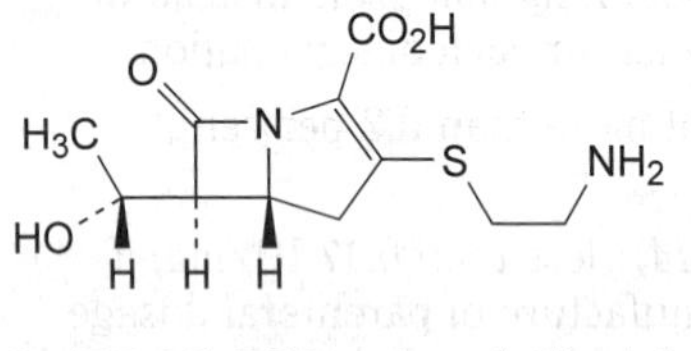

A. (5*R*,6*S*)-3-[(2-aminoethyl)sulphanyl]-6-[(*R*)-1-hydroxyethyl]-7-oxo-1-azabicyclo[3.2.0]hept-2-ene-2-carboxylic acid (thienamycin).

01/2005:0029
corrected

IMIPRAMINE HYDROCHLORIDE

Imipramini hydrochloridum

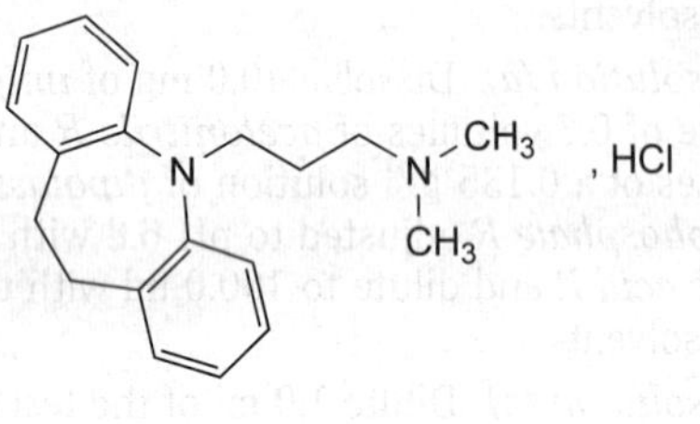

$C_{19}H_{25}ClN_2$ M_r 316.9

DEFINITION

Imipramine hydrochloride contains not less than 98.5 per cent and not more than the equivalent of 101.0 per cent of 3-(10,11-dihydro-5*H*-dibenzo[*b,f*]azepin-5-yl)-*N,N*-dimethylpropan-1-amine hydrochloride, calculated with reference to the dried substance.

CHARACTERS

A white or slightly yellow, crystalline powder, freely soluble in water and in alcohol.

IDENTIFICATION

First identification: A, C, F.

Second identification: A, B, D, E, F.

A. Melting point (*2.2.14*): 170 °C to 174 °C.

B. Dissolve 20 mg in *0.01 M hydrochloric acid* and dilute to 100.0 ml with the same acid. Dilute 1.0 ml of the solution to 10.0 ml with *0.01 M hydrochloric acid.* Examined between 230 nm and 350 nm, the solution shows a single absorption maximum (*2.2.25*), at 251 nm, and a shoulder at 270 nm. The specific absorbance at the maximum is about 260.

C. Examine by infrared absorption spectrophotometry (*2.2.24*), comparing with the spectrum obtained with *imipramine hydrochloride CRS*. Examine the substances prepared as discs.

D. Dissolve about 5 mg in 2 ml of *nitric acid R*. An intense blue colour develops.

E. Dissolve about 50 mg in 3 ml of *water R* and add 0.05 ml of a 25 g/l solution of *quinhydrone R* in *methanol R*. No red colour develops within 15 min.

F. About 20 mg gives reaction (a) of chlorides (*2.3.1*).

TESTS

Solution S. To 3.0 g add 20 ml of *carbon dioxide-free water R,* dissolve rapidly by shaking and triturating with a glass rod and dilute to 30 ml with the same solvent.

Appearance of solution. Solution S is clear (*2.2.1*). Immediately after preparation, dilute solution S with an equal volume of *water R*. This solution is not more intensely coloured than reference solution BY_6 (*2.2.2, Method II*).

pH (*2.2.3*). The pH of solution S, measured immediately after preparation, is 3.6 to 5.0.

Related substances. Examine by thin-layer chromatography (*2.2.27*), using a *TLC silica gel G plate R*.

Test solution. Dissolve 0.25 g of the substance to be examined in *methanol R* and dilute to 10 ml with the same solvent. Prepare immediately before use.

Reference solution (a). Dilute 1 ml of the test solution to 10 ml with *methanol R*. Dilute 1 ml of this solution to 50 ml with *methanol R*.

Reference solution (b). Dissolve 5 mg of *iminodibenzyl R* in *methanol R* and dilute to 100 ml with the same solvent. Prepare immediately before use.

Apply to the plate 10 µl of each solution. Develop over a path of 12 cm using a mixture of 5 volumes of *hydrochloric acid R*, 5 volumes of *water R*, 35 volumes of *glacial acetic acid R* and 55 volumes of *ethyl acetate R*. Allow the plate to dry in air for 5 min and spray with a 5 g/l solution of *potassium dichromate R* in a mixture of 1 volume of *sulphuric acid R* and 4 volumes of *water R*. Examine the plate immediately. The chromatogram obtained with the test solution shows a blue principal spot. In the chromatogram obtained with the test solution: any spot corresponding to iminodibenzyl is not more intense than the spot in the chromatogram obtained with reference solution (b) (0.2 per cent); any spot apart from the principal spot and any spot corresponding to iminodibenzyl, is not more intense than the spot in the chromatogram obtained with reference solution (a) (0.2 per cent).

Heavy metals (*2.4.8*). 2.0 g complies with limit test C for heavy metals (20 ppm). Prepare the standard using 4 ml of *lead standard solution (10 ppm Pb) R*.

Loss on drying (*2.2.32*). Not more than 0.5 per cent, determined on 1.00 g by drying in an oven at 100 °C to 105 °C.

Sulphated ash (*2.4.14*). Not more than 0.1 per cent, determined on 1.0 g.

ASSAY

Dissolve 0.250 g in 50 ml of *alcohol R* and add 5.0 ml of *0.01 M hydrochloric acid.* Carry out a potentiometric titration (*2.2.20*), using *0.1 M sodium hydroxide*. Read the volume added between the 2 points of inflexion.

1 ml of *0.1 M sodium hydroxide* is equivalent to 31.69 mg of $C_{19}H_{25}ClN_2$.

STORAGE

Store protected from light.

01/2005:1108

INDAPAMIDE

Indapamidum

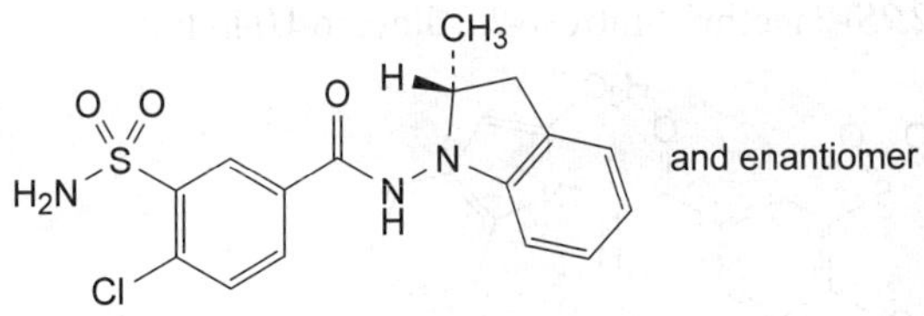

$C_{16}H_{16}ClN_3O_3S$ M_r 365.8

DEFINITION

Indapamide contains not less than 98.0 per cent and not more than the equivalent of 102.0 per cent of 4-chloro-*N*-[(2*RS*)-2-methyl-2,3-dihydro-1*H*-indol-1-yl]-3-sulphamoylbenzamide, calculated with reference to the anhydrous substance.

CHARACTERS

A white or almost white powder, practically insoluble in water, soluble in alcohol.

IDENTIFICATION

First identification: B.

Second identification: A, C.

A. Dissolve 50.0 mg in *alcohol R* and dilute to 100.0 ml with the same solvent. Dilute 2.0 ml of the solution to 100.0 ml with *alcohol R*. Examined between 220 nm and 350 nm (*2.2.25*), the solution shows an absorption maximum at 242 nm and two shoulders, at 279 nm and 287 nm. The specific absorbance at the maximum is 590 to 630.

B. Examine by infrared absorption spectrophotometry (*2.2.24*), comparing with the spectrum obtained with *indapamide CRS*. Examine the substances prepared as discs using *potassium bromide R*.

C. Examine by thin-layer chromatography (*2.2.27*), using *silica gel GF_{254} R* as the coating substance.

Test solution. Dissolve 20 mg of the substance to be examined in *alcohol R* and dilute to 10 ml with the same solvent.

Reference solution (a). Dissolve 20 mg of *indapamide CRS* in *alcohol R* and dilute to 10 ml with the same solvent.

Reference solution (b). Dissolve 10 mg of *indometacin R* in 5 ml of reference solution (a) and dilute to 10 ml with *alcohol R*.

Apply to the plate 10 µl of each solution. Develop over a path of 15 cm using a mixture of 1 volume of *glacial acetic acid R*, 20 volumes of *acetone R* and 79 volumes of *toluene R*. Allow the plate to dry in air and examine in ultraviolet light at 254 nm. The principal spot in the chromatogram obtained with the test solution is similar in position and size to the principal spot in the chromatogram obtained with reference solution (a). The test is not valid unless the chromatogram obtained with reference solution (b) shows two clearly separated spots.

TESTS

Optical rotation (*2.2.7*). Dissolve 0.250 g in *ethanol R* and dilute to 25.0 ml with the same solvent. The angle of optical rotation is − 0.02° to + 0.02°.

Related substances. Examine by liquid chromatography (*2.2.29*) as described under Assay.

Adjust the sensitivity of the system so that the height of the principal peak in the chromatogram obtained with reference solution (b) is not less than 15 per cent of the full scale of the recorder.

Inject 10 µl of each solution and continue the chromatography for 2.5 times the retention time of the principal peak. The test is not valid unless in the chromatogram obtained with reference solution (d): the resolution between the peak corresponding to indapamide and the peak corresponding to methylnitrosoindoline is at least 4.0; the principal peak in the chromatogram obtained with reference solution (b) has a signal-to-noise ratio of at least 6.

In the chromatogram obtained with the test solution: the area of any peak corresponding to indapamide impurity B is not greater than the area of the principal peak in the chromatogram obtained with reference solution (a) (0.3 per cent); the area of any peak, apart from the principal peak and any peak corresponding to indapamide impurity B, is not greater than the area of the principal peak in the chromatogram obtained with reference solution (b) (0.1 per cent); the sum of the areas of all the peaks, apart from the principal peak, is not greater than five times the area of the principal peak in the chromatogram obtained with reference solution (b) (0.5 per cent). Disregard any peak with an area less than 0.5 times the area of the principal peak in the chromatogram obtained with reference solution (b).

Methylnitrosoindoline. Not more than 5 ppm, determined by liquid chromatography (*2.2.29*). *Carry out the test protected from light.*

Test solution. Dissolve 25.0 mg of the substance to be examined in 1 ml of *acetonitrile R* and dilute to 10.0 ml with *water R*. Shake for 15 min. Allow to stand at 4 °C for 1 h and filter.

Reference solution. Dissolve 25.0 mg of the substance to be examined in 1.0 ml of a 0.125 mg/l solution of *methylnitrosoindoline CRS* in *acetonitrile R* and dilute to 10.0 ml with *water R*. Shake for 15 min. Allow to stand at 4 °C for 1 h and filter.

The chromatographic procedure may be carried out using:

– a stainless steel column 0.15 m long and 4.6 mm in internal diameter packed with *octadecylsilyl silica gel for chromatography R* (5 µm),

– as mobile phase at a flow rate of 1.4 ml/min a mixture of 7 volumes of *acetonitrile R*, 20 volumes of *tetrahydrofuran R* and 73 volumes of a 1.5 g/l solution of *triethylamine R* adjusted to pH 2.8 with *phosphoric acid R*,

– as detector a spectrophotometer set at 305 nm,

maintaining the temperature of the column at 30 °C.

Inject 0.1 ml of the solutions.

In the chromatogram obtained with the reference solution, measure from the baseline the height *A* of the peak corresponding to methylnitrosoindoline, appearing just before the principal peak, and the height *B* corresponding to the lowest point in the curve between this peak and the principal peak.

The test is not valid unless in the chromatogram obtained with the reference solution: the difference between *A* and *B* is at least 85 per cent of height *A*, the peak corresponding to methylnitrosoindoline appearing just before the principal peak has a signal-to-noise ratio of at least 3.

In the chromatogram obtained with the test solution, the area of any peak corresponding to methylnitrosoindoline is not greater than the difference between the areas of the peaks corresponding to methylnitrosoindoline in the chromatograms obtained with the reference solution and the test solution.

Heavy metals (*2.4.8*). 2.0 g complies with limit test C for heavy metals (10 ppm). Prepare the standard using 2 ml of *lead standard solution (10 ppm Pb) R*.

Water (*2.5.12*). Not more than 3.0 per cent, determined on 0.10 g by the semi-micro determination of water.

Sulphated ash (*2.4.14*). Not more than 0.1 per cent, determined on 1.0 g.

ASSAY

Examine by liquid chromatography (*2.2.29*). *Carry out the assay protected from light and prepare the solutions immediately before use or maintain them at 4 °C.*

Test solution. Dissolve 20.0 mg of the substance to be examined in 7 ml of a mixture of equal volumes of *acetonitrile R* and *methanol R* and dilute to 20.0 ml with a 0.2 g/l solution of *sodium edetate R.*

Reference solution (a). Dissolve 30.0 mg of *indapamide impurity B CRS* in 35 ml of a mixture of equal volumes of *acetonitrile R* and *methanol R* and dilute to 100.0 ml with a 0.2 g/l solution of *sodium edetate R.* To 1.0 ml of the solution, add 35 ml of a mixture of equal volumes of *acetonitrile R* and *methanol R* and dilute to 100.0 ml with a 0.2 g/l solution of *sodium edetate R.*

Reference solution (b). Dilute 1.0 ml of the test solution to 50.0 ml with a mixture of 17.5 volumes of *acetonitrile R,* 17.5 volumes of *methanol R* and 65 volumes of a 0.2 g/l solution of *sodium edetate R.* Dilute 1.0 ml of the solution to 20.0 ml with a mixture of 17.5 volumes of *acetonitrile R,* 17.5 volumes of *methanol R* and 65 volumes of a 0.2 g/l solution of *sodium edetate R.*

Reference solution (c). Dissolve 20.0 mg of *indapamide CRS* in 7 ml of a mixture of equal volumes of *acetonitrile R* and *methanol R* and dilute to 20.0 ml with a 0.2 g/l solution of *sodium edetate R.*

Reference solution (d). Dissolve 25.0 mg of *indapamide CRS* and 45.0 mg of *methylnitrosoindoline CRS* in 17.5 ml of a mixture of equal volumes of *acetonitrile R* and *methanol R* and dilute to 50.0 ml with a 0.2 g/l solution of *sodium edetate R.*

The chromatographic procedure may be carried out using:

- a stainless steel column 0.20 m long and 4.6 mm in internal diameter packed with *octadecylsilyl silica gel for chromatography R* (5 µm),
- as mobile phase at a flow rate of 2 ml/min a mixture of 0.1 volumes of *glacial acetic acid R,* 17.5 volumes of *acetonitrile R,* 17.5 volumes of *methanol R* and 65 volumes of a 0.2 g/l solution of *sodium edetate R,*
- as detector a spectrophotometer set at 254 nm,

maintaining the temperature of the column at 40 °C.

When the chromatograms are recorded at the prescribed conditions, the retention time of the principal peak in the chromatogram obtained with refererence solution (c) is about 11 min.

Inject reference solution (c) six times. The test is not valid unless the relative standard deviation of the peak area for indapamide is at most 1.0 per cent. If necessary, adjust the integrator parameters. Inject alternately the test solution and reference solution (c).

Calculate the per cent *m/m* content of anhydrous substance.

STORAGE

Store protected from light.

IMPURITIES

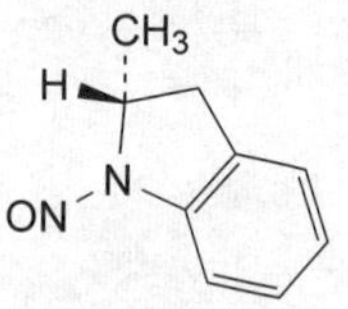

and enantiomer

A. (2*RS*)-2-methyl-1-nitroso-2,3-dihydro-1*H*-indole,

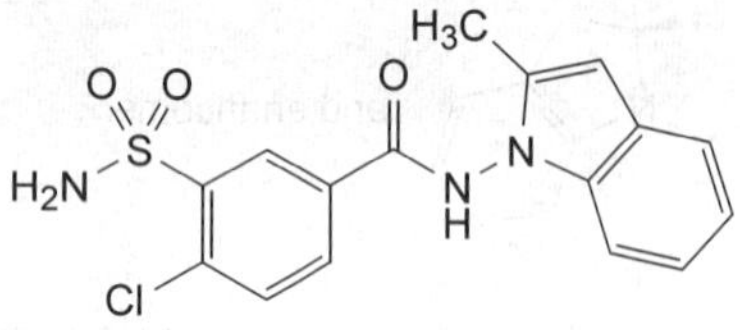

B. 4-chloro-*N*-(2-methyl-1*H*-indol-1-yl]-3-sulphamoylbenzamide.

01/2005:0092

INDOMETACIN

Indometacinum

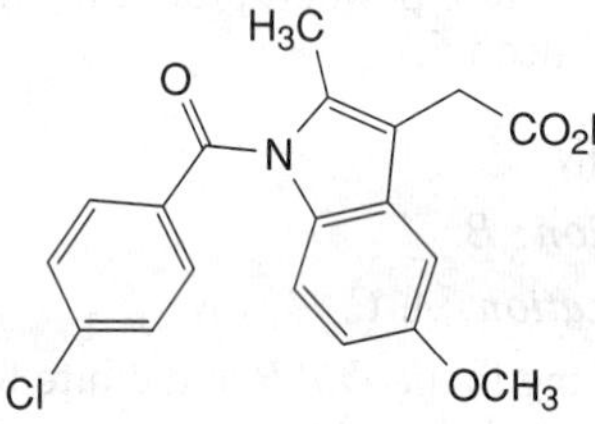

$C_{19}H_{16}ClNO_4$ M_r 357.8

DEFINITION

Indometacin contains not less than 98.5 per cent and not more than the equivalent of 100.5 per cent of [1-(4-chlorobenzoyl)-5-methoxy-2-methylindol-3-yl]acetic acid, calculated with reference to the dried substance.

CHARACTERS

A white or yellow, crystalline powder, practically insoluble in water, sparingly soluble in alcohol.

IDENTIFICATION

First identification: A, C.

Second identification: A, B, D, E.

A. Melting point (*2.2.14*): 158 °C to 162 °C.

B. Dissolve 25 mg in a mixture of 1 volume of *1 M hydrochloric acid* and 9 volumes of *methanol R* and dilute to 100.0 ml with the same mixture of solvents. Dilute 10.0 ml of the solution to 100.0 ml with a mixture of 1 volume of *1 M hydrochloric acid* and 9 volumes of *methanol R.* Examined between 300 nm and 350 nm (*2.2.25*), the solution shows an absorption maximum at 318 nm. The specific absorbance at the maximum is 170 to 190.

C. Examine by infrared absorption spectrophotometry (*2.2.24*), comparing with the spectrum obtained with *indometacin CRS.* Examine the substances in the solid state without recrystallisation.

D. Dissolve 0.1 g in 10 ml of *alcohol R,* heating slightly if necessary. To 0.1 ml of the solution add 2 ml of a freshly prepared mixture of 1 volume of a 250 g/l solution of *hydroxylamine hydrochloride R* and 3 volumes of *dilute sodium hydroxide solution R.* Add 2 ml of *dilute hydrochloric acid R* and 1 ml of *ferric chloride solution R2* and mix. A violet-pink colour develops.

E. To 0.5 ml of the solution in alcohol prepared in identification test D, add 0.5 ml of *dimethylaminobenzaldehyde solution R2*. A precipitate is formed that dissolves on shaking. Heat on a water-bath. A bluish-green colour is produced. Continue to heat for 5 min and cool in iced water for 2 min. A precipitate is formed and the colour changes to light greyish-green. Add 3 ml of *alcohol R*. The solution is clear and violet-pink in colour.

TESTS

Related substances. Examine by thin-layer chromatography (*2.2.27*), using *silica gel HF_{254} R* as the coating substance. Prepare the slurry using a 46.8 g/l solution of *sodium dihydrogen phosphate R*.

Test solution. Dissolve 0.2 g of the substance to be examined in *methanol R* and dilute to 10 ml with the same solvent. Prepare immediately before use.

Reference solution. Dilute 1 ml of the test solution to 200 ml with *methanol R*.

Apply separately to the plate 10 µl of each solution. Develop over a path of 15 cm using a mixture of 30 volumes of *light petroleum R* and 70 volumes of *ether R*. Allow the plate to dry in air and examine in ultraviolet light at 254 nm. Any spot in the chromatogram obtained with the test solution, apart from the principal spot, is not more intense than the spot in the chromatogram obtained with the reference solution (0.5 per cent).

Heavy metals (*2.4.8*). 2.0 g complies with limit test C for heavy metals (20 ppm). Prepare the standard using 4 ml of *lead standard solution (10 ppm Pb) R*.

Loss on drying (*2.2.32*). Not more than 0.5 per cent, determined on 1.000 g by drying in an oven at 100 °C to 105 °C.

Sulphated ash (*2.4.14*). Not more than 0.1 per cent, determined on 1.0 g.

ASSAY

Dissolve 0.300 g in 75 ml of *acetone R*, through which *nitrogen R*, free from carbon dioxide, has been passed for 15 min. Maintain a constant stream of nitrogen through the solution. Add 0.1 ml of *phenolphthalein solution R*. Titrate with *0.1 M sodium hydroxide*. Carry out a blank titration.

1 ml of *0.1 M sodium hydroxide* is equivalent to 35.78 mg of $C_{19}H_{16}ClNO_4$.

STORAGE

Store protected from light.

IMPURITIES

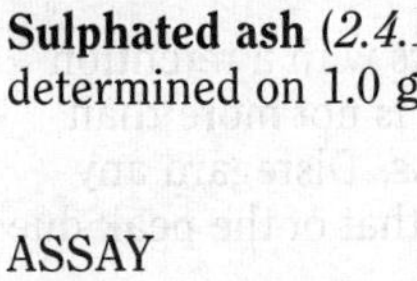

A. 4-chlorobenzoic acid.

01/2005:2084

INSULIN ASPART

Insulinum aspartum

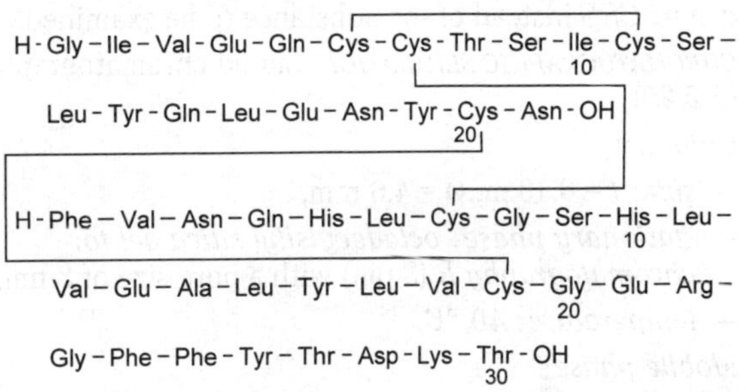

$C_{256}H_{381}N_{65}O_{79}S_6$ M_r 5826

DEFINITION

28^B-L-Aspartate insulin (human).

Insulin aspart is a 2-chain peptide containing 51 amino acids. The A-chain is composed of 21 amino acids and the B-chain is composed of 30 amino acids. It is identical in primary structure to human insulin, except that it has aspartic acid instead of proline at position 28 of the B-chain. As in human insulin, insulin aspart contains 2 interchain disulphide bonds and 1 intrachain disulphide bond.

Content: 90.0 per cent to 104.0 per cent of insulin aspart $C_{256}H_{381}N_{65}O_{79}S_6$ plus A21Asp insulin aspart, B3Asp insulin aspart, B3isoAsp insulin aspart and B28isoAsp insulin aspart (dried substance).

By convention, for the purpose of labelling insulin aspart preparations, 0.0350 mg of insulin aspart is equivalent to 1 unit.

PRODUCTION

Insulin aspart is produced by a method based on recombinant DNA (rDNA) technology under conditions designed to minimise the degree of microbial contamination.

Prior to release the following tests are carried out on each batch of the final bulk product, unless exemption has been granted by the competent authority.

Host-cell-derived proteins. The limit is approved by the competent authority.

Single-chain precursor. The limit is approved by the competent authority. Use a suitably sensitive method.

CHARACTERS

Appearance: white or almost white powder.

Solubility: practically insoluble in ethanol (96 per cent), in methanol and in aqueous solutions with a pH around 5.1. In aqueous solutions below pH 3.5 or above pH 6.5, the solubility is greater than or equal to 25 mg/ml.

IDENTIFICATION

A. Examine the chromatograms obtained in the assay.
Results: the principal peak in the chromatogram obtained with the test solution is similar in retention time to the principal peak in the chromatogram obtained with reference solution (a).

B. Peptide mapping (*2.2.55*).
SELECTIVE CLEAVAGE OF THE PEPTIDE BONDS
Test solution. Prepare a 2.0 mg/ml solution of the substance to be examined in *0.01 M hydrochloric acid* and transfer 25 µl of this solution to a clean tube. Add 100 µl of *HEPES buffer solution pH 7.5 R* and 20 µl of

a 1 mg/ml solution of *Staphylococcus aureus strain V8 protease R*. Cap the tube and incubate at 25 °C for 6 h. Stop the reaction by adding 145 µl of *sulphate buffer solution pH 2.0 R*.

Reference solution. Prepare at the same time and in the same manner as for the test solution, but using *insulin aspart CRS* instead of the substance to be examined.

CHROMATOGRAPHIC SEPARATION. Liquid chromatography (*2.2.29*).

Column:

- *size*: *l* = 0.10 m, Ø = 4.6 mm,
- *stationary phase*: *octadecylsilyl silica gel for chromatography R* (3 µm) with a pore size of 8 nm,
- *temperature*: 40 °C.

Mobile phase:

- *mobile phase A*: mix 100 ml of *acetonitrile for chromatography R*, 200 ml of *sulphate buffer solution pH 2.0 R* and 700 ml of *water R*; filter and degas;
- *mobile phase B*: mix 200 ml of *sulphate buffer solution pH 2.0 R*, 400 ml of *acetonitrile for chromatography R* and 400 ml of *water R*; filter and degas;

Time (min)	Mobile phase A (per cent *V/V*)	Mobile phase B (per cent *V/V*)
0 - 60	90 → 30	10 → 70
60 - 65	30 → 0	70 → 100
65 - 70	0	100

Flow rate: 1 ml/min.

Detection: spectrophotometer at 214 nm.

Equilibration: at initial conditions for at least 15 min. Carry out a blank run using the above-mentioned gradient.

Injection: 50 µl.

System suitability:

- the chromatograms obtained with the test solution and the reference solution are qualitatively similar to the chromatogram of insulin aspart digest supplied with *insulin aspart CRS*,
- in the chromatogram obtained with the reference solution, identify the peaks due to digest fragments I, II and III:

  symmetry factor: maximum 1.5, for the peaks due to fragments II and III,

  resolution : minimum 8.0, between the peaks due to fragments II and III.

Results: the profile of the chromatogram obtained with the test solution corresponds to that of the chromatogram obtained with the reference solution.

NOTE: the retention times of fragments I, II and IV are the same as for human insulin. The retention time of fragment III differs from human insulin due to substitution of proline by aspartic acid.

TESTS

Impurities with molecular masses greater than that of insulin aspart. Size-exclusion chromatography (*2.2.30*): use the normalisation procedure.

Test solution. Prepare a solution containing 4 mg/ml of the substance to be examined in *0.01 M hydrochloric acid*. Maintain the solution at 2-8 °C and use within 48 h.

Resolution solution. Use a solution of insulin (about 4 mg/ml), containing more than 0.4 per cent of high molecular mass proteins. An injectable insulin preparation, whether a solution or a suspension, that has been clarified with a sufficient amount of *6 M hydrochloric acid*, containing the indicated percentage of high molecular mass proteins, or a solution prepared from insulin, dissolved in *0.01 M hydrochloric acid* may be used. Insulin containing the indicated percentage of high molecular mass proteins may be prepared by allowing insulin powder to stand at room temperature for about 10 days. Maintain the solution at 2-8 °C and use within 7 days.

Column:

- *size*: *l* = 0.3 m, Ø = 7.8 mm,
- *stationary phase*: *hydrophilic silica gel for chromatography R* (5-10 µm) with a pore size of 12-12.5 nm, of a grade suitable for the separation of insulin monomer from dimer and polymers.

Mobile phase: mix 15 volumes of *glacial acetic acid R*, 20 volumes of *acetonitrile for chromatography R* and 65 volumes of a 1.0 g/l solution of *arginine R*; filter and degas.

Flow rate: 0.5 ml/min.

Detection: spectrophotometer at 276 nm.

Equilibration: at least 3 injections of the resolution solution; the column is equilibrated when repeatable results are obtained from 2 subsequent injections.

Injection: 100 µl.

Run time: about 35 min.

Retention time: insulin aspart polymers = 13-17 min; insulin aspart dimer = about 17.5 min; insulin aspart monomer = about 20 min; salts = about 22 min.

System suitability: resolution solution:

- *peak-to-valley ratio*: minimum 2.0, where H_p = height above the baseline of the peak due to the dimer and H_v = height above the baseline of the lowest point of the curve separating this peak from the peak due to the monomer.

Limits: the sum of the areas of the peaks with a retention time less than that of the principal peak is not more than 0.5 per cent of the total area of the peaks. Disregard any peak with a retention time greater than that of the peak due to insulin aspart monomer.

Related proteins. Liquid chromatography (*2.2.29*) as described under Assay: use the normalisation procedure.

Limits:

- *B28isoAsp insulin aspart*: maximum 1.0 per cent,
- *total of the peaks due to A21Asp insulin aspart, B3Asp insulin aspart and B3isoAsp insulin aspart*: maximum 2.0 per cent,
- *total of other impurities*: maximum 1.5 per cent.

Loss on drying (*2.2.32*): maximum 10.0 per cent, determined on 0.200 g by drying in an oven at 100-105 °C for 24 h.

Sulphated ash (*2.4.14*): maximum 6.0 per cent, determined on 0.200 g (dried substance).

Bacterial endotoxins (*2.6.14*): less than 10 IU/mg, if intended for use in the manufacture of parenteral dosage forms without a further appropriate procedure for the removal of bacterial endotoxins.

ASSAY

Liquid chromatography (*2.2.29*).

Test solution. Dissolve the substance to be examined in *0.01 M hydrochloric acid* to obtain a concentration of 4.0 mg/ml. Maintain the solution at 2-8 °C and use within 24 h.

Reference solution (a). Dissolve the contents of a vial of *insulin aspart CRS* in *0.01 M hydrochloric acid* to obtain a concentration of 4.0 mg/ml. Maintain the solution at 2-8 °C and use within 48 h.
Reference solution (b). Mix equal volumes of reference solution (a) and *water R*. Maintain the solution at 2-8 °C and use within 48 h.
Resolution solution. Use an appropriate solution with a content of B3Asp insulin aspart and A21Asp insulin aspart of not less than 1 per cent. This may be achieved by storing reference solution (a) at room temperature for about 1-3 days. Maintain the solution at 2-8 °C and use within 72 h.
Column:
- *size*: *l* = 0.25 m, Ø = 4 mm,
- *stationary phase*: *octadecylsilyl silica gel for chromatography R* (5 µm),
- *temperature*: 40 °C.

Mobile phase:
- *mobile phase A*: dissolve 142.0 g of *anhydrous sodium sulphate R* in *water R*; add 13.5 ml of *phosphoric acid R* and dilute to 5000 ml with *water R*; adjust to pH 3.6, if necessary, with *strong sodium hydroxide solution R*; filter and degas; mix 9 volumes of the solution with 1 volume of *acetonitrile for chromatography R*; filter and degas;
- *mobile phase B*: mix equal volumes of *water R* and *acetonitrile for chromatography R*; filter and degas;

Time (min)	Mobile phase A (per cent *V/V*)	Mobile phase B (per cent *V/V*)
0 - 35	58	42
35 - 40	58 → 20	42 → 80
40 - 45	20	80
45 - 46	20 → 58	80 → 42
46 - 60	58	42

Flow rate: 1 ml/min.
Detection: spectrophotometer at 214 nm.
Injection: 10 µl.
Relative retention with reference to insulin aspart (retention time = 20-24 min): B28isoAsp insulin aspart = about 0.9; B3Asp insulin aspart plus A21Asp insulin aspart (generally coeluted) = about 1.3; B3isoAsp insulin aspart = about 1.5.
System suitability: resolution solution:
- *resolution*: minimum 2.0 between the peak due to insulin aspart and the peak due to A21Asp insulin aspart and to B3Asp insulin aspart.

Calculate the content of insulin aspart $C_{256}H_{381}N_{65}O_{79}S_6$, plus B28isoAsp insulin aspart, A21Asp insulin aspart, B3Asp insulin aspart and B3isoAsp insulin aspart using the areas of the corresponding peaks in the chromatograms obtained with the test solution and reference solution (a) and the declared content of insulin aspart plus B28isoAsp insulin aspart, A21Asp insulin aspart, B3Asp insulin aspart and B3isoAsp insulin aspart in *insulin aspart CRS*.

STORAGE

In an airtight container, protected from light, at or below − 18 °C until released by the manufacturer. When thawed, insulin aspart is stored at 5 ± 3 °C and used for manufacturing preparations within a short period of time. To avoid absorption of humidity from the air during weighing, insulin aspart must be at room temperature before opening the container.

LABELLING

The label states, where applicable, that the substance is free from bacterial endotoxins.

01/2005:1637
corrected

INSULIN, BOVINE

Insulinum bovinum

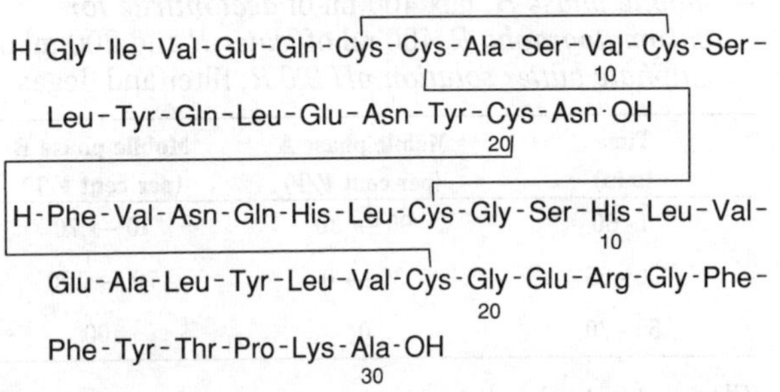

$C_{254}H_{377}N_{65}O_{75}S_6$ M_r 5734

DEFINITION

Bovine insulin is the natural antidiabetic principle obtained from beef pancreas and purified. The content of bovine insulin $C_{254}H_{377}N_{65}O_{75}S_6$ plus A21 desamido bovine insulin is not less than 93.0 per cent and not more than 105.0 per cent, calculated with reference to the dried substance.
By convention, for the purpose of labelling insulin preparations, 0.0342 mg of bovine insulin is equivalent to 1 IU of insulin.

PRODUCTION

The animals from which bovine insulin is derived must fulfil the requirements for the health of animals suitable for human consumption to the satisfaction of the competent authority.
The manufacturing process is validated to demonstrate suitable inactivation or removal of any contamination by viruses or other infectious agents.

CHARACTERS

Appearance: white or almost white powder.
Solubility: practically insoluble in water and in ethanol. It dissolves in dilute mineral acids and with decomposition in dilute solutions of alkali hydroxides.

IDENTIFICATION

A. Examine the chromatograms obtained in the assay.
Results: the retention time of the principal peak in the chromatogram obtained with the test solution corresponds to that of the principal peak in the chromatogram obtained with reference solution (c).

B. Peptide mapping.
Test solution. Prepare a 2.0 mg/ml solution of the substance to be examined in *0.01 M hydrochloric acid* and transfer 500 µl of this solution to a clean tube. Add 2.0 ml of *HEPES buffer solution pH 7.5 R* and 400 µl of a 1 mg/ml solution of *Staphylococcus aureus strain V8 protease R*. Cap the tube and incubate at 25 °C for 6 h. Stop the reaction by adding 2.9 ml of *sulphate buffer solution pH 2.0 R*.
Reference solution. Prepare at the same time and in the same manner as for the test solution but using *bovine insulin CRS* instead of the substance to be examined.
Examine the digests by liquid chromatography (*2.2.29*).

Monographs I-L

Column:

- *size*: *l* = 0.10 m, Ø = 4.6 mm,
- *stationary phase*: *octadecylsilyl silica gel for chromatography R* (3 µm),
- *temperature*: 40 °C.

Mobile phase:

- *mobile phase A*: mix 100 ml of *acetonitrile for chromatography R*, 700 ml of *water R* and 200 ml of *sulphate buffer solution pH 2.0 R*; filter and degas;
- *mobile phase B*: mix 400 ml of *acetonitrile for chromatography R*, 400 ml of *water R* and 200 ml of *sulphate buffer solution pH 2.0 R*; filter and degas;

Time (min)	Mobile phase A (per cent *V/V*)	Mobile phase B (per cent *V/V*)
0 - 60	90 → 30	10 → 70
60 - 65	30 → 0	70 → 100
65 - 70	0	100

Flow rate: 1 ml/min.

Detection: spectrophotometer at 214 nm.

Equilibration: at initial conditions for at least 15 min. Carry out a blank run using the above-mentioned gradient.

Injection: 50 µl.

System suitability: the chromatograms obtained with the test solution and the reference solution are qualitatively similar to the chromatogram of bovine insulin digest supplied with *bovine insulin CRS*. In the chromatogram obtained with the reference solution, identify the peaks due to digest fragments I, II and III. The symmetry factor of the peaks due to fragments II and III is not greater than 1.5, and the resolution between the 2 peaks is at least 1.9.

Results: the profile of the chromatogram obtained with the test solution corresponds to that of the chromatogram obtained with the reference solution.

NOTE: The retention time of fragment I is the same for porcine insulin and for human insulin. The retention times of fragments II and IV are the same for all insulins. The retention time of fragment III is the same for bovine insulin and for porcine insulin.

TESTS

Impurities with molecular masses greater than that of insulin. Size-exclusion chromatography (*2.2.30*): use the normalisation procedure.

Test solution. Dissolve 4 mg of the substance to be examined in 1.0 ml of *0.01 M hydrochloric acid*.

Resolution solution. Use a solution of insulin (approximately 4 mg/ml), containing more than 0.4 per cent of high molecular mass proteins. An injectable insulin preparation, whether a solution or a suspension, that has been clarified with a sufficient amount of *6 M hydrochloric acid*, containing the indicated percentage of high molecular mass proteins, or a solution prepared from insulin, dissolved in *0.01 M hydrochloric acid*, may be used. Insulin containing the indicated percentage of high molecular mass proteins may be prepared by allowing insulin powder to stand at room temperature for about 10 days.

Maintain the solutions at 2-10 °C and use within 7 days. If an automatic injector is used, maintain the temperature at 2-10 °C.

Column:

- *size*: *l* = 0.3 m, Ø = at least 7.5 mm,
- *stationary phase*: *hydrophilic silica gel for chromatography R* (5-10 µm), of a grade suitable for the separation of insulin monomer from dimer and polymers.

Mobile phase: mix of 15 volumes of *glacial acetic acid R*, 20 volumes of *acetonitrile R* and 65 volumes of a 1.0 g/l solution of *arginine R*; filter and degas.

Flow rate: 0.5 ml/min.

Detection: spectrophotometer at 276 nm.

Equilibration: before using a new column for chromatographic analysis, equilibrate by repeated injections of an insulin solution containing high molecular mass proteins. This can be done by at least 3 injections of the resolution solution. The column is equilibrated when repeatable results are obtained from 2 subsequent injections.

Injection: 100 µl.

Run time: about 35 min.

Retention times: polymeric insulin complexes = 13-17 min; covalent insulin dimer = about 17.5 min; insulin monomer = about 20 min; salts = about 22 min.

System suitability: resolution solution:

- *peak-to-valley ratio*: minimum 2.0, where H_p = height above the baseline of the peak due to the dimer and H_v = height above the baseline of the lowest point of the curve separating this peak from the peak due to the monomer.

Limits: the sum of the areas of any peaks with a retention time less than that of the principal peak is not greater than 1.0 per cent of the total area of the peaks. Disregard any peak with a retention time greater than that of the insulin peak.

Related proteins. Liquid chromatography (*2.2.29*) as described under Assay, following the elution conditions as described in the table below:

Time (min)	Mobile phase A (per cent *V/V*)	Mobile phase B (per cent *V/V*)
0 - 30	42	58
30 - 44	42 → 11	58 → 89
44 - 50	11	89

Maintain the solutions at 2-10 °C and use within 24 h. Perform a system suitability test (resolution, linearity) as described under Assay. If necessary, the relative proportions of the mobile phases may be adjusted to ensure complete elution of A21 desamido porcine insulin before commencement of the gradient. The profile of the gradient may also be adjusted to ensure complete elution of all insulin related impurities.

Inject 20 µl of reference solution (c) and 20 µl of the test solution. If necessary, adjust the injection volume to between 10 µl and 20 µl in accordance with the results obtained in the test for linearity as described under Assay. Record the chromatograms for approximately 50 min. In the chromatogram obtained with reference solution (c), A21 desamido bovine insulin appears as a small peak after the principal peak and has a relative retention of about 1.3 with reference to the principal peak. In the chromatogram obtained with the test solution, the area of the peak due to A21 desamido bovine insulin is not greater than 3.0 per cent of the total area of the peaks; the sum of the areas of all the peaks, apart from those due to bovine insulin and A21 desamido bovine insulin, is not greater than 3.0 per cent of the total area of the peaks.

Bovine proinsulin-like immunoreactivity (PLI): maximum 10 ppm, calculated with reference to the dried substance.

Use a suitably sensitive immunochemical method (*2.7.1*) such as radio-immunoassay, using the International Reference Reagent for bovine proinsulin to calibrate the method.

Zinc: maximum 1.0 per cent, calculated with reference to the dried substance.

Atomic absorption spectrometry (*2.2.23, Method I*).

Test solution. Dissolve 50.0 mg of the substance to be examined in *0.01 M hydrochloric acid* and dilute to 25.0 ml with the same acid. Dilute if necessary to a suitable concentration (for example, 0.4 µg to 1.6 µg of Zn per millilitre) with *0.01 M hydrochloric acid.*

Reference solutions. Use solutions containing 0.40 µg, 0.80 µg, 1.00 µg, 1.20 µg and 1.60 µg of Zn per millilitre, freshly prepared by diluting *zinc standard solution (5 mg/ml Zn) R* with *0.01 M hydrochloric acid.*

Source: zinc hollow-cathode lamp.

Wavelength: 213.9 nm.

Flame: air-acetylene flame of suitable composition (for example, 11 litres of air and 2 litres of acetylene per minute).

Loss on drying (*2.2.32*): maximum 10.0 per cent, determined on 0.200 g by drying in an oven at 100-105 °C for 24 h.

Sulphated ash (*2.4.14*): maximum 2.5 per cent, determined on 0.200 g and calculated with reference to the dried substance.

Bacterial endotoxins (*2.6.14*): less than 10 IU/mg, if intended for use in the manufacture of parenteral dosage forms without a further appropriate procedure for the removal of bacterial endotoxins.

ASSAY

Liquid chromatography (*2.2.29*).

Test solution. Dissolve 40.0 mg of the substance to be examined in *0.01 M hydrochloric acid* and dilute to 10.0 ml with the same solvent.

Reference solution (a). Dissolve the contents of a vial of *human insulin CRS* in *0.01 M hydrochloric acid* to obtain a concentration of 4.0 mg/ml.

Reference solution (b). Dissolve the contents of a vial of *porcine insulin CRS* in *0.01 M hydrochloric acid* to obtain a concentration of 4.0 mg/ml.

Reference solution (c). Dissolve 40.0 mg of *bovine insulin CRS* in 10.0 ml of *0.01 M hydrochloric acid.*

Reference solution (d). Dilute 1.0 ml of reference solution (c) to 10.0 ml with *0.01 M hydrochloric acid.*

Resolution solution. Mix 1.0 ml of reference solution (a) and 1.0 ml of reference solution (b).

Maintain the solutions at 2-10 °C and use within 48 h. If an automatic injector is used, maintain the temperature at 2-10 °C.

Column:

- *size*: l = 0.25 m, Ø = 4.6 mm,
- *stationary phase*: *octadecylsilyl silica gel for chromatography R* (5 µm),
- *temperature*: 40 °C.

Mobile phase: mix 42 volumes of mobile phase A and 58 volumes of mobile phase B, adjusting the composition of the mixture if necessary.

Prepare and maintain the following solutions at a temperature of at least 20 °C:

- *mobile phase A*: dissolve 28.4 g of *anhydrous sodium sulphate R* in *water R* and dilute to 1000 ml with the same solvent; add 2.7 ml of *phosphoric acid R*; adjust to pH 2.3, if necessary, with *ethanolamine R*; filter and degas;
- *mobile phase B*: mix 550 ml of mobile phase A with 450 ml of *acetonitrile R*. Warm the solution to a temperature of at least 20 °C in order to avoid precipitation (mixing of mobile phase A with acetonitrile is endothermic); filter and degas.

Flow rate: 1 ml/min.

Detection: spectrophotometer at 214 nm.

System suitability:

- *resolution*: inject 20 µl of the resolution solution and 20 µl of reference solution (b). Record the chromatogram of the resolution solution until the peak corresponding to the principal peak in the chromatogram obtained with reference solution (b) is clearly visible. In the chromatogram obtained with the resolution solution, identify the peaks due to porcine insulin and human insulin. The test is not valid unless the resolution between the peaks corresponding to human insulin and porcine insulin is at least 1.2. If necessary, adjust the concentration of acetonitrile in the mobile phase until this resolution is achieved.
- *linearity*: inject 20 µl each of reference solutions (c) and (d). The test is not valid unless the area of the principal peak in the chromatogram obtained with reference solution (c) is 10 ± 0.5 times the area of the principal peak in the chromatogram obtained with reference solution (d). If this test fails, adjust the injection volume to between 10 µl and 20 µl, in order that the responses are within the linearity range of the detector.

Injection: 20 µl of the test solution.

Calculate the content of bovine insulin $C_{254}H_{377}N_{65}O_{75}S_6$ plus A21 desamido bovine insulin from the area of the principal peak and the area of the peak corresponding to A21 desamido bovine insulin in the chromatograms obtained with the test solution and reference solution (c) and the declared content of bovine insulin plus A21 desamido bovine insulin in *bovine insulin CRS.*

STORAGE

In an airtight container, protected from light, at − 20 °C until released by the manufacturer. When thawed, insulin may be stored at 5 ± 3 °C and used for manufacturing preparations within a short period of time. To avoid absorption of humidity from the air during weighing, the insulin must be at room temperature.

LABELLING

The label states where applicable, that the substance is free from bacterial endotoxins.

Monographs I-J

01/2005:0838

INSULIN, HUMAN

Insulinum humanum

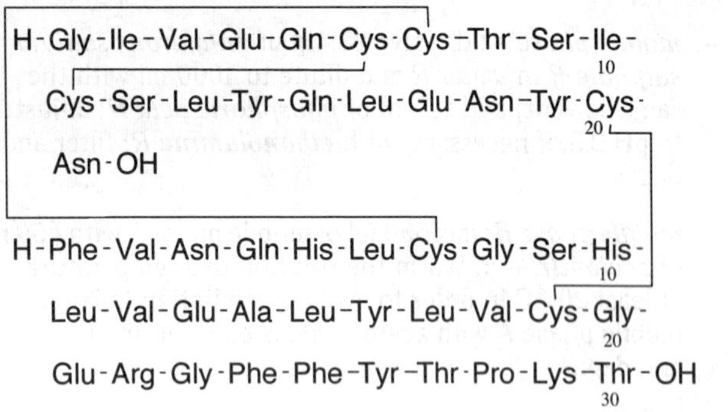

$C_{257}H_{383}N_{65}O_{77}S_6$ M_r 5808

DEFINITION

Human insulin is a 2-chain peptide having the structure of the antidiabetic hormone produced by the human pancreas.

Content: 95.0 per cent to 105.0 per cent of human insulin $C_{257}H_{383}N_{65}O_{77}S_6$ plus A21 desamido human insulin (dried substance).

By convention, for the purpose of labelling insulin preparations, 0.0347 mg of human insulin is equivalent to 1 IU of insulin.

PRODUCTION

Human insulin is produced either by enzymatic modification and suitable purification of insulin obtained from the pancreas of the pig or by a method based on recombinant DNA (rDNA) technology.

Human insulin is produced under conditions designed to minimise the degree of microbial contamination.

For human insulin produced by enzymatic modification of insulin obtained from the pancreas of the pig, the manufacturing process is validated to demonstrate removal of any residual proteolytic activity. The competent authority may require additional tests.

For human insulin produced by a method based on rDNA technology, prior to release the following tests are carried out on each batch of the final bulk product, unless exemption has been granted by the competent authority.

Host-cell-derived proteins. The limit is approved by the competent authority.

Single chain precursor. The limit is approved by the competent authority. Use a suitably sensitive method.

CHARACTERS

Appearance: white or almost white powder.

Solubility: practically insoluble in water and in ethanol (96 per cent). It dissolves in dilute mineral acids and with decomposition in dilute solutions of alkali hydroxides.

IDENTIFICATION

A. Examine the chromatograms obtained in the assay.

Results: the principal peak in the chromatogram obtained with the test solution is similar in retention time to the principal peak in the chromatogram obtained with reference solution (a).

B. Peptide mapping (*2.2.55*).

SELECTIVE CLEAVAGE OF THE PEPTIDE BONDS

Test solution. Prepare a 2.0 mg/ml solution of the substance to be examined in *0.01 M hydrochloric acid* and transfer 500 µl of this solution to a clean tube. Add 2.0 ml of *HEPES buffer solution pH 7.5 R* and 400 µl of a 1 mg/ml solution of *Staphylococcus aureus strain V8 protease R*. Cap the tube and incubate at 25 °C for 6 h. Stop the reaction by adding 2.9 ml of *sulphate buffer solution pH 2.0 R*.

Reference solution. Prepare at the same time and in the same manner as for the test solution but using *human insulin CRS* instead of the substance to be examined.

CHROMATOGRAPHIC SEPARATION. Liquid chromatography (*2.2.29*).

Column:

- *size*: l = 0.10 m, Ø = 4.6 mm,
- *stationary phase*: *octadecylsilyl silica gel for chromatography R* (3 µm) with a pore size of 8 nm,
- *temperature*: 40 °C.

Mobile phase:

- *mobile phase A*: mix 100 ml of *acetonitrile for chromatography R*, 200 ml of *sulphate buffer solution pH 2.0 R* and 700 ml of *water R*; filter and degas;
- *mobile phase B*: mix 200 ml of *sulphate buffer solution pH 2.0 R*, 400 ml of *acetonitrile for chromatography R* and 400 ml of *water R*; filter and degas;

Time (min)	Mobile phase A (per cent *V/V*)	Mobile phase B (per cent *V/V*)
0 - 60	90 → 30	10 → 70
60 - 65	30 → 0	70 → 100
65 - 70	0	100

Flow rate: 1 ml/min.

Detection: spectrophotometer at 214 nm.

Equilibration: at initial conditions for at least 15 min. Carry out a blank run using the above-mentioned gradient.

Injection: 50 µl.

System suitability:

- the chromatograms obtained with the test solution and the reference solution are qualitatively similar to the chromatogram of human insulin digest supplied with *human insulin CRS*,
- in the chromatogram obtained with the reference solution, identify the peaks due to digest fragments I, II and III:

  symmetry factor: maximum 1.5 for the peaks due to fragments II and III,

  resolution: minimum 3.4 between the peaks due to fragments II and III.

Results: the profile of the chromatogram obtained with the test solution corresponds to that of the chromatogram obtained with the reference solution.

NOTE: the retention time of fragment I is the same for porcine insulin and for human insulin. The retention times of fragments II and IV are the same for all insulins. The retention time of fragment III is the same for bovine insulin and for porcine insulin.

TESTS

Impurities with molecular masses greater than that of insulin. Size-exclusion chromatography (*2.2.30*): use the normalisation procedure.

Test solution. Prepare a solution containing 4 mg/ml of the substance to be examined in *0.01 M hydrochloric acid*.

Resolution solution. Use a solution of insulin (about 4 mg/ml), containing more than 0.4 per cent of high molecular mass proteins. An injectable insulin preparation, whether a solution or a suspension, that has been clarified with a sufficient amount of *6 M hydrochloric acid*, containing the indicated percentage of high molecular mass proteins, or a solution prepared from insulin, dissolved in *0.01 M hydrochloric acid*, may be used. Insulin containing the indicated percentage of high molecular mass proteins may be prepared by allowing insulin powder to stand at room temperature for about 10 days.

Maintain the solutions at 2-8 °C and use within 7 days. If an automatic injector is used, maintain the temperature at 2-8 °C.

Column:

- *size*: l = 0.3 m, Ø = minimum 7.5 mm,
- *stationary phase*: *hydrophilic silica gel for chromatography R* (5-10 µm) with a pore size of 12-12.5 nm, of a grade suitable for the separation of insulin monomer from dimer and polymers.

Mobile phase: mix 15 volumes of *glacial acetic acid R*, 20 volumes of *acetonitrile R* and 65 volumes of a 1.0 g/l solution of *arginine R*; filter and degas.

Flow rate: 0.5 ml/min.

Detection: spectrophotometer at 276 nm.

Equilibration: before using a new column for chromatographic analysis, equilibrate by repeated injections of an insulin solution containing high molecular mass proteins. This can be done by at least 3 injections of the resolution solution. The column is equilibrated when repeatable results are obtained from 2 subsequent injections.

Injection: 100 µl.

Run time: about 35 min.

Retention time: polymeric insulin complexes = 13-17 min; covalent insulin dimer = about 17.5 min; insulin monomer = about 20 min; salts = about 22 min.

System suitability: resolution solution:

- *peak-to-valley ratio*: minimum 2.0, where H_p = height above the baseline of the peak due to the dimer and H_v = height above the baseline of the lowest point of the curve separating this peak from the peak due to the monomer.

Limits: the sum of the areas of any peaks with a retention time less than that of the principal peak is not greater than 1.0 per cent of the total area of the peaks. Disregard any peak with a retention time greater than that of the peak due to insulin.

Related proteins. Liquid chromatography (*2.2.29*) as described under Assay, following the elution conditions as described below:

Time (min)	Mobile phase A (per cent *V/V*)	Mobile phase B (per cent *V/V*)
0 - 30	42	58
30 - 44	42 → 11	58 → 89
44 - 50	11	89

Maintain the solutions at 2-8 °C and use within 24 h. Perform a system suitability test (resolution, linearity) as described in the assay. If necessary, the relative proportions of the mobile phases may be adjusted to ensure complete elution of A21 desamido porcine insulin before commencement of the gradient. The profile of the gradient may also be adjusted to ensure complete elution of all insulin related impurities.

Inject 20 µl of reference solution (a), 20 µl of reference solution (b), 20 µl of reference solution (c) and 20 µl of the test solution. If necessary, adjust the injection volume to a volume between 10 µl and 20 µl in accordance with the results obtained in the test for linearity as described in the assay. Record the chromatograms for approximately 50 min. In the chromatogram obtained with reference solution (a), A21 desamido human insulin appears as a small peak after the principal peak and has a retention time of about 1.3 relative to the principal peak. In the chromatogram obtained with the test solution, the area of the peak due to A21 desamido human insulin is not greater than 2.0 per cent of the total area of the peaks; the sum of the areas of all peaks, apart from those due to human insulin and that due to A21 desamido human insulin, is not greater than 2.0 per cent of the total area of the peaks. For semisynthetic human insulin only: in the chromatogram obtained with the test solution, the area of any peak corresponding to the principal peak in the chromatogram obtained with reference solution (b) is not greater than the area of the corresponding peak in the chromatogram obtained with reference solution (c) (1.0 per cent of porcine insulin in human insulin).

The following test applies only to human insulin produced by enzymatic modification of porcine insulin.

Proinsulin-like immunoreactivity (PLI): maximum 10 ppm, calculated with reference to the dried substance and determined by a suitably sensitive immunochemical method (*2.7.1*) such as radio-immunoassay. Use the International Reference Reagent for porcine proinsulin to calibrate the method.

Zinc: maximum 1.0 per cent (dried substance).

Atomic absorption spectrometry (*2.2.23, Method I*).

Test solution. Dissolve 50.0 mg of the substance to be examined in *0.01 M hydrochloric acid* and dilute to 25.0 ml with the same acid. Dilute if necessary to a suitable concentration (for example, 0.4-1.6 µg of Zn per millilitre) with *0.01 M hydrochloric acid*.

Reference solutions. Use solutions containing 0.40 µg, 0.80 µg, 1.00 µg, 1.20 µg and 1.60 µg of Zn per millilitre, freshly prepared by diluting *zinc standard solution (5 mg/ml Zn) R* with *0.01 M hydrochloric acid*.

Source: zinc hollow-cathode lamp.

Wavelength: 213.9 nm.

Atomisation device: air-acetylene flame of suitable composition (for example, 11 litres of air and 2 litres of acetylene per minute).

Loss on drying (*2.2.32*): maximum 10.0 per cent, determined on 0.200 g by drying in an oven at 100-105 °C for 24 h.

Sulphated ash (*2.4.14*): maximum 2.5 per cent, determined on 0.200 g (dried substance).

Bacterial endotoxins (*2.6.14*): less than 10 IU/mg, if intended for use in the manufacture of parenteral dosage forms without a further appropriate procedure for removal of bacterial endotoxins.

ASSAY

Liquid chromatography (*2.2.29*).

Monographs I-J

Test solution. Dissolve 40.0 mg of the substance to be examined in *0.01 M hydrochloric acid* and dilute to 10.0 ml with the same solvent.

Reference solution (a). Dissolve the contents of a vial of *human insulin CRS* in *0.01 M hydrochloric acid* to obtain a concentration of 4.0 mg/ml.

Reference solution (b). Dissolve the contents of a vial of *porcine insulin CRS* in *0.01 M hydrochloric acid* to obtain a concentration of 4.0 mg/ml.

Reference solution (c). Dilute 1.0 ml of reference solution (b) to 50.0 ml with *0.01 M hydrochloric acid.* To 1.0 ml of this solution add 1.0 ml of reference solution (a).

Reference solution (d). Dilute 1.0 ml of reference solution (a) to 10.0 ml with *0.01 M hydrochloric acid.*

Resolution solution. Mix 1.0 ml of reference solution (a) and 1.0 ml of reference solution (b).

Maintain the solutions at 2-8 °C and use within 48 h. If an automatic injector is used, maintain at 2-8 °C.

Column:

- *size*: l = 0.25 , Ø = 4.6 mm,
- *stationary phase*: *octadecylsilyl silica gel for chromatography R* (5 µm),
- *temperature*: 40 °C.

Mobile phase: mix 42 volumes of mobile phase A and 58 volumes of mobile phase B, adjusting the composition of the mixture if necessary.

Prepare and maintain the following solutions at a temperature of at least 20 °C:

- *mobile phase A*: dissolve 28.4 g of *anhydrous sodium sulphate R* in *water R* and dilute to 1000 ml with the same solvent; add 2.7 ml of *phosphoric acid R*; adjust to pH 2.3, if necessary, with *ethanolamine R*; filter and degas;
- *mobile phase B*: mix 550 ml of mobile phase A with 450 ml of *acetonitrile R.* Warm the solution to a temperature of at least 20 °C in order to avoid precipitation (mixing of mobile phase A with acetonitrile is endothermic); filter and degas.

Flow rate: 1 ml/min.

Detection: spectrophotometer at 214 nm.

System suitability:

- *resolution*: inject 20 µl of the resolution solution and 20 µl of reference solution (b). Record the chromatogram of the resolution solution until the peak corresponding to the principal peak in the chromatogram obtained with reference solution (b) is clearly visible. In the chromatogram obtained with the resolution solution, identify the peaks due to porcine insulin and human insulin. The test is not valid unless the resolution between the peaks due to human insulin and porcine insulin is at least 1.2. If necessary, adjust the concentration of acetonitrile in the mobile phase until this resolution is achieved.
- *linearity*: inject 20 µl each of reference solutions (a) and (d). The test is not valid unless the area of the principal peak in the chromatogram obtained with reference solution (a) is 10 ± 0.5 times the area of the principal peak in the chromatogram obtained with reference solution (d). If this test fails, adjust the injection volume to between 10 µl and 20 µl, in order that the responses are within the linearity range of the detector.

Injection: 20 µl of the test solution and reference solution (a).

Calculate the content of human insulin $C_{257}H_{383}N_{65}O_{77}S_6$ plus A21 desamido human insulin using the areas of the corresponding peaks in the chromatograms obtained with the test solution and reference solution (a) and the declared content of human insulin plus A21 desamido human insulin in *human insulin CRS*.

STORAGE

In an airtight container, protected from light, at − 18 °C or below, until released by the manufacturer. When thawed, insulin is stored at 5 ± 3 °C and used for manufacturing preparations within a short period of time. To avoid absorption of humidity from the air during weighing, the insulin must be at room temperature.

LABELLING

The label states:

- whether the substance is produced by enzymatic modification of porcine insulin or by rDNA technology,
- where applicable, that the substance is free from bacterial endotoxins.

01/2005:0831

INSULIN INJECTION, BIPHASIC

Insulini biphasici iniectabilium

Biphasic insulin injection complies with the monograph on Insulin preparations, injectable (0854) with the amendments prescribed below.

DEFINITION

Biphasic insulin injection is a sterile suspension of crystals containing bovine insulin in a solution of porcine insulin.

CHARACTERS

A white suspension. When examined under a microscope, the majority of the particles are seen to be rhombohedral crystals, with a maximum dimension measured from corner to corner through the crystal greater than 10 µm but rarely exceeding 40 µm.

IDENTIFICATION

Examine the chromatograms obtained in the assay. The position of the peaks due to the two insulins in the chromatogram obtained with the test solution correspond to those of the principal peaks in the chromatogram obtained with the appropriate reference solution.

TESTS

pH (*2.2.3*). The pH of the suspension to be examined is 6.6 to 7.2.

Insulin in the supernatant: 22.0 per cent to 28.0 per cent of insulin in solution. Determine by the method described in the test for insulin in the supernatant in the monograph on *Insulin preparations, injectable (0854)*.

Total zinc: 26.0 µg to 37.5 µg per 100 IU of insulin. Determine by the method described in the monograph on *Insulin preparations, injectable (0854)*.

01/2005:0832

INSULIN INJECTION, BIPHASIC ISOPHANE

Insulini isophani biphasici iniectabilium

Biphasic isophane insulin injection complies with the monograph on Insulin preparations, injectable (0854) with the exception of the test for Insulin in the supernatant and with the amendments prescribed below for the other tests.

DEFINITION

Biphasic isophane insulin injection is a sterile buffered suspension of either porcine or human insulin, complexed with protamine sulphate or another suitable protamine, in a solution of insulin of the same species.

PRODUCTION

Biphasic isophane insulin injection is prepared by carrying out the procedures described in the monograph on *Insulin preparations, injectable (0854).*

Biphasic isophane insulin injection is produced by mixing, in defined ratios, soluble insulin injection and isophane insulin injection. The defined ratios shall be demonstrated by a test method which has been approved by the competent authority to comply with the label claim.

CHARACTERS

A white suspension which on standing deposits a white sediment and leaves a colourless or almost colourless supernatant liquid; the sediment is readily resuspended by gently shaking. When examined under a microscope, the particles are seen to be rod-shaped crystals, the majority with a maximum dimension greater than 1 µm but rarely exceeding 60 µm, free from large aggregates.

IDENTIFICATION

Examine the chromatograms obtained in the Assay. The position of the peak due to insulin in the chromatogram obtained with the test solution corresponds to that of the principal peak obtained with the appropriate reference solution.

TESTS

Total zinc. Not more than 40.0 µg per 100 IU of insulin, determined as described in the monograph on *Insulin preparations, injectable (0854).*

LABELLING

The label states in addition to the indications mentioned in the monograph on *Insulin preparations, injectable (0854)* the ratio of soluble insulin injection to isophane insulin injection used in the manufacturing process of biphasic isophane insulin injection.

01/2005:0833

INSULIN INJECTION, ISOPHANE

Insulini isophani iniectabilium

Isophane insulin injection complies with the monograph on Insulin preparations, injectable (0854) with the modifications prescribed below.

DEFINITION

Isophane insulin injection is a sterile suspension of bovine, porcine or human insulin, complexed with protamine sulphate or another suitable protamine.

PRODUCTION

Isophane insulin injection is prepared by carrying out the procedures described in the monograph on *Insulin preparations, injectable (0854).*

The amount of protamine is based on the known isophane ratio and is not less than the equivalent of 0.3 mg and not more than the equivalent of 0.6 mg of protamine sulphate for each 100 IU of insulin in the insulin-protamine complex.

CHARACTERS

A white suspension which on standing deposits a white sediment and leaves a colourless or almost colourless supernatant liquid; the sediment is readily resuspended by gently shaking. When examined under a microscope, the particles are seen to be rod-shaped crystals, the majority with a maximum dimension greater than 1 µm but rarely exceeding 60 µm, free from large aggregates.

IDENTIFICATION

Examine the chromatograms obtained in the Assay. The position of the peak due to insulin in the chromatogram obtained with the test solution corresponds to that of the principal peak in the chromatogram obtained with the appropriate reference solution.

TESTS

Total zinc. Not more than 40.0 µg per 100 IU of insulin, determined as described in the monograph on *Insulin preparations, injectable (0854).*

01/2005:0834

INSULIN INJECTION, SOLUBLE

Insulini solubilis iniectabilium

Soluble insulin injection complies with the monograph on Insulin preparations, injectable (0854) with the amendments prescribed below.

DEFINITION

Soluble insulin injection is a neutral, sterile solution of bovine, porcine or human insulin.

CHARACTERS

A colourless liquid, free from turbidity and foreign matter; during storage, traces of a very fine sediment may be deposited.

IDENTIFICATION

Examine the chromatograms obtained in the assay. The position of the peak due to insulin in the chromatogram obtained with the test solution corresponds to that of the principal peak obtained with the appropriate reference solution.

TESTS

Total zinc. Not more than 40.0 µg per 100 IU of insulin.

Determine by the method described in the monograph on *Insulin preparations, injectable (0854).*

Use the following test solution.

Test solution. Dilute a volume of the gently shaken preparation containing 200 IU to 25.0 ml with *water R.* Dilute if necessary to a suitable concentration (for example, 0.4 µg to 1.6 µg of Zn per millilitre) with *water R.*

Monographs I-L

01/2005:2085

INSULIN LISPRO

Insulinum lisprum

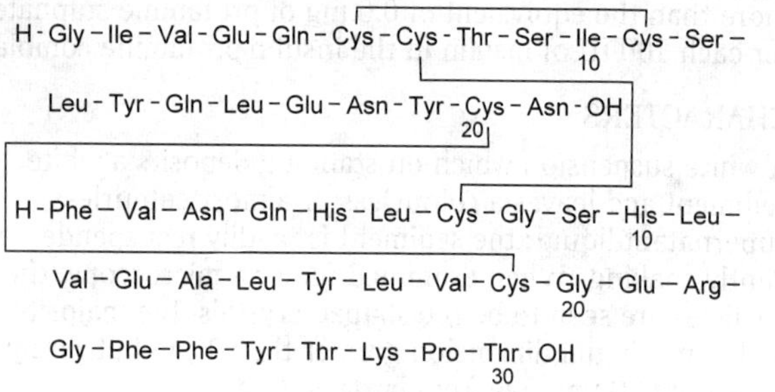

$C_{257}H_{383}N_{65}O_{77}S_6$ M_r 5808

DEFINITION

28^B-L-Lysine-29^B-L-proline insulin (human).

Insulin lispro is a 2-chain peptide containing 51 amino acids. The A-chain is composed of 21 amino acids and the B-chain is composed of 30 amino acids. It is identical in primary structure to human insulin, only differing in amino acid sequence at positions 28 and 29 of the B-chain. Human insulin is Pro(B28), Lys(B29), whereas insulin lispro is Lys(B28), Pro(B29). As in human insulin, insulin lispro contains 2 interchain disulphide bonds and 1 intrachain disulphide bond.

Content: 94.0 per cent to 104.0 per cent (dried substance).

By convention, for the purpose of labelling insulin lispro preparations, 0.0347 mg of insulin lispro is equivalent to 1 unit.

PRODUCTION

Insulin lispro is produced by a method based on recombinant DNA (rDNA) technology under conditions designed to minimise the degree of microbial contamination.

Prior to release the following tests are carried out on each batch of final bulk product, unless exemption has been granted by the competent authority.

Host-cell-derived proteins. The limit is approved by the competent authority.

Single-chain precursor. The limit is approved by the competent authority. Use a suitably sensitive method.

CHARACTERS

Appearance: white or almost white powder.

Solubility: practically insoluble in water and in ethanol (96 per cent). It dissolves in dilute mineral acids and with decomposition in dilute solutions of alkali hydroxides.

IDENTIFICATION

A. Examine the chromatograms obtained in the assay.

Results: the principal peak in the chromatogram obtained with the test solution is similar in retention time to the principal peak in the chromatogram obtained with the reference solution.

B. Peptide mapping (*2.2.55*).

SELECTIVE CLEAVAGE OF THE PEPTIDE BONDS

Test solution. Prepare a 2.0 mg/ml solution of the substance to be examined in *0.01 M hydrochloric acid* and transfer 500 µl of this solution to a clean tube. Add 2.0 ml of *HEPES buffer solution pH 7.5 R* and 400 µl of a 1 mg/ml solution of *Staphylococcus aureus strain V8 protease R*. Cap the tube and incubate at 25 °C for 6 h. Stop the reaction by adding 2.9 ml of *sulphate buffer solution pH 2.0 R*.

Reference solution. Prepare at the same time and in the same manner as for the test solution but using *insulin lispro CRS* instead of the substance to be examined.

CHROMATOGRAPHIC SEPARATION. Liquid chromatography (*2.2.29*).

Column:
- *size*: l = 0.10 m, Ø = 4.6 mm,
- *stationary phase*: *octadecylsilyl silica gel for chromatography R* (3 µm) with a pore size of 8 nm,
- *temperature*: 40 °C.

Mobile phase:
- *mobile phase A*: mix 100 ml of *acetonitrile for chromatography R*, 200 ml of *sulphate buffer solution pH 2.0 R* and 700 ml of *water R*; filter and degas;
- *mobile phase B*: mix 200 ml of *sulphate buffer solution pH 2.0 R*, 400 ml of *acetonitrile for chromatography R* and 400 ml of *water R*; filter and degas;

Time (min)	Mobile phase A (per cent *V/V*)	Mobile phase B (per cent *V/V*)
0 - 60	90 → 30	10 → 70
60 - 65	30 → 0	70 → 100
65 - 70	0	100

Flow rate: 1 ml/min.

Detection: spectrophotometer at 214 nm.

Equilibration: at initial conditions for at least 15 min. Carry out a blank run using the above-mentioned gradient.

Injection: 50 µl.

System suitability:
- the chromatograms obtained with the test solution and the reference solution are qualitatively similar to the chromatogram of insulin lispro digest supplied with *insulin lispro CRS*,
- in the chromatogram obtained with the reference solution, identify the peaks due to digest fragments I, II and III:

  symmetry factor: maximum 1.5 for the peaks due to fragments II and III,

  resolution: minimum 8.0 between the peaks due to fragments II and III.

Results: the profile of the chromatogram obtained with the test solution corresponds to that of the chromatogram obtained with the reference solution.

NOTE: the retention times of fragments I, II and IV are the same as for human insulin. The retention time of fragment III differs from human insulin due to differences in sequence at positions 28 and 29 of the B-chain.

TESTS

Impurities with molecular masses greater than that of insulin lispro. Size-exclusion chromatography (*2.2.30*): use the normalisation procedure.

Test solution. Prepare a solution containing 4 mg/ml of the substance to be examined in *0.01 M hydrochloric acid*. Maintain the solution at 2-8 °C and use within 48 h.

Resolution solution. Use a solution of insulin (about 4 mg/ml), containing more than 0.4 per cent of high molecular mass proteins. An injectable insulin preparation, whether a solution or a suspension, that has been clarified with a sufficient amount of *6 M hydrochloric acid,* containing the indicated percentage of high molecular mass proteins, or a solution prepared from insulin, dissolved in *0.01 M hydrochloric acid,* may be used. Insulin containing the indicated percentage of high molecular mass proteins may be prepared by allowing insulin powder to stand at room temperature for about 10 days. Maintain the solution at 2-8 °C and use within 8 days.

Column:

– *size*: *l* = 0.30 m, Ø = 7.8 mm,

– *stationary phase*: *hydrophilic silica gel for chromatography R* (5-10 µm) with a pore size of 12-12.5 nm, of a grade suitable for the separation of insulin monomer from dimer and polymers.

Mobile phase: mix 15 volumes of *glacial acetic acid R*, 20 volumes of *acetonitrile for chromatography R* and 65 volumes of a 1.0 g/l solution of *arginine R*; filter and degas.

Flow rate: 0.5 ml/min.

Detection: spectrophotometer at 276 nm.

Equilibration: at least 3 injections of the resolution solution; the column is equilibrated when repeatable results are obtained for 2 subsequent injections.

Injection: 100 µl.

Run time: about 35 min.

Retention time: insulin lispro polymers = 13-17 min; insulin lispro dimer = about 17.5 min; insulin lispro monomer = about 20 min; salts = about 22 min.

System suitability: resolution solution:

– *peak-to-valley ratio*: minimum 2.0, where H_p = height above the baseline of the peak due to the dimer and H_v = height above the baseline of the lowest point of the curve separating this peak from the peak due to the monomer,

– *symmetry factor*: maximum 2.0 for the peak due to insulin lispro.

Limits: the sum of the areas of the peaks with a retention time less than that of the principal peak is not more than 0.25 per cent of the total area of the peaks. Disregard any peak with a retention time greater than that of the peak due to insulin lispro monomer.

Related proteins. Liquid chromatography (*2.2.29*): use the normalisation procedure.

Test solution. Dissolve 3.5 mg of the substance to be examined in 1.0 ml of *0.01 M hydrochloric acid.* Maintain the solution at 2-8 °C and use within 56 h.

Resolution solution. Dissolve 3.5 mg of the substance to be examined in 1.0 ml of *0.01 M hydrochloric acid.* Allow to stand at room temperature to obtain a solution containing between 0.8 per cent and 11 per cent of A21 desamido insulin lispro.

Column:

– *size*: *l* = 0.25 m, Ø = 4.6 mm,

– *stationary phase*: *octadecylsilyl silica gel for chromatography R* (5 µm) with a pore size of 30 nm,

– *temperature*: 40 °C.

Mobile phase:

– *mobile phase A*: mix 82 volumes of a 28.4 g/l solution of *anhydrous sodium sulphate R* adjusted to pH 2.3 with *phosphoric acid R* and 18 volumes of *acetonitrile for chromatography R*; filter and degas;

– *mobile phase B*: mix equal volumes of a 28.4 g/l solution of *anhydrous sodium sulphate R* adjusted to pH 2.3 with *phosphoric acid R* and *acetonitrile for chromatography R*; filter and degas;

Time (min)	Mobile phase A (per cent *V/V*)	Mobile phase B (per cent *V/V*)
0 - 60	81	19
60 - 83	81 → 51	19 → 49
83 - 84	51 → 81	49 → 19
84 - 94	81	19

Flow rate: 1 ml/min.

Detection: spectrophotometer at 214 nm.

Injection: 20 µl.

Retention time: adjust the mobile phase composition to obtain a retention time of about 41 min for insulin lispro; A21 desamido insulin lispro elutes near the start of the gradient elution.

System suitability: resolution solution:

– *resolution*: minimum 1.5 between the 1st peak (insulin lispro) and the 2nd peak (A21 desamido insulin lispro),

– *symmetry factor*: maximum 2.0 for the peak due to insulin lispro.

Limits:

– *A21 desamido insulin lispro*: maximum 1.0 per cent,

– *any other impurity*: maximum 0.50 per cent,

– *total (excluding A21)*: maximum 2.0 per cent.

Zinc: maximum 1.0 per cent (dried substance).

Atomic absorption spectrometry (*2.2.23, Method I*).

Test solution. Dissolve at least 50 mg of the substance to be examined in *0.01 M hydrochloric acid* and dilute to 25 ml with the same acid. Dilute if necessary to a suitable concentration (for example 0.4-0.6 µg of Zn per millilitre) with *0.01 M hydrochloric acid.*

Reference solutions. Use solutions of concentrations which bracket the expected zinc concentration of the samples, for example, 0.2-0.8 µg of Zn per millilitre, freshly prepared by diluting *zinc standard solution (5 mg/ml Zn) R* with *0.01 M hydrochloric acid.*

Source: zinc hollow-cathode lamp.

Wavelength: 213.9 nm.

Atomisation device: air-acetylene flame of suitable composition (for example, 11 litres of air and 2 litres of acetylene per minute).

Loss on drying (*2.2.32*): maximum 10.0 per cent, determined on 0.200 g by drying in an oven at 100-105 °C for 16 h.

Sulphated ash (*2.4.14*): maximum 2.5 per cent, determined on 0.200 g (dried substance).

Bacterial endotoxins (*2.6.14, Method D*): less than 10 IU/mg, if intended for use in the manufacture of parenteral dosage forms without a further appropriate procedure for the removal of bacterial endotoxins.

ASSAY

Liquid chromatography (*2.2.29*).

Test solution. Dissolve the substance to be examined in *0.01 M hydrochloric acid* to obtain a concentration of 0.8 mg/ml. Maintain the solution at 2-8 °C and use within 48 h.

Reference solution. Dissolve the contents of a vial of *insulin lispro CRS* in *0.01 M hydrochloric acid* to obtain a concentration of 0.8 mg/ml. Maintain the solution at 2-8 °C and use within 48 h.

Resolution solution. Dissolve about 10 mg of the substance to be examined in 10 ml of *0.01 M hydrochloric acid.* Allow to stand at room temperature to obtain a solution containing between 0.8 per cent and 11 per cent of A21 desamido insulin lispro. Maintain the solution at 2-8 °C and use within 14 days.

Column:
- *size*: l = 0.10 m, Ø = 4.6 mm,
- *stationary phase*: *octadecylsilyl silica gel for chromatography R* (3 µm) with a pore size of 8 nm,
- *temperature*: 40 °C.

Mobile phase: mix 745 volumes of a 28.4 g/l solution of *anhydrous sodium sulphate R* adjusted to pH 2.3 with *phosphoric acid R* and 255 volumes of *acetonitrile for chromatography R*; filter and degas.

Flow rate: 0.8 ml/min.

Detection: spectrophotometer at 214 nm.

Injection: 20 µl.

Retention time: insulin lispro = about 24 min.

System suitability:
- *resolution*: minimum 1.8 between the 1st peak (insulin lispro) and the 2nd peak (A21 desamido insulin lispro), in the chromatogram obtained with the resolution solution,
- *repeatability*: maximum relative standard deviation of 1.1 per cent after 3 injections of the reference solution.

Calculate the content of insulin lispro $C_{257}H_{383}N_{65}O_{77}S_6$ using the chromatograms obtained with the test solution and the reference solution and the declared content of $C_{257}H_{383}N_{65}O_{77}S_6$ in *insulin lispro CRS*.

STORAGE

In an airtight container, protected from light, at or below − 18 °C. When thawed, insulin lispro is stored and weighed under conditions defined by the manufacturer to maintain the quality attributes of the drug substance and is used for manufacturing preparations within a short period of time. To avoid absorption of humidity from the air during weighing, insulin lispro must be at room temperature before opening the container.

LABELLING

The label states, where applicable, that the substance is free from bacterial endotoxins.

01/2005:1638
corrected

INSULIN, PORCINE

Insulinum porcinum

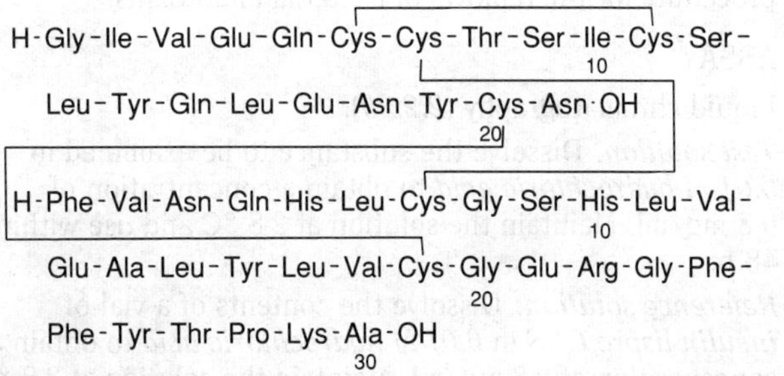

$C_{256}H_{381}N_{65}O_{76}S_6$ M_r 5778

DEFINITION

Porcine insulin is the natural antidiabetic principle obtained from pork pancreas and purified. The content of porcine insulin $C_{256}H_{381}N_{65}O_{76}S_6$ plus A21 desamido porcine insulin is not less than 95.0 per cent and not more than 105.0 per cent, calculated with reference to the dried substance.

By convention, for the purpose of labelling insulin preparations, 0.0345 mg of porcine insulin is equivalent to 1 IU of insulin.

PRODUCTION

The animals from which porcine insulin is derived must fulfil the requirements for the health of animals suitable for human consumption to the satisfaction of the competent authority.

The manufacturing process is validated to demonstrate suitable inactivation or removal of any contamination by viruses or other infectious agents.

CHARACTERS

Appearance: white or almost white powder.

Solubility: practically insoluble in water and in ethanol. It dissolves in dilute mineral acids and with decomposition in dilute solutions of alkali hydroxides.

IDENTIFICATION

A. Examine the chromatograms obtained in the assay.

Results: the retention time of the principal peak in the chromatogram obtained with the test solution corresponds to that of the principal peak in the chromatogram obtained with reference solution (b).

B. Peptide mapping.

Test solution. Prepare a 2.0 mg/ml solution of the substance to be examined in *0.01 M hydrochloric acid* and transfer 500 µl of this solution to a clean tube. Add 2.0 ml of *HEPES buffer solution pH 7.5 R* and 400 µl of a 1 mg/ml solution of *Staphylococcus aureus strain V8 protease R*. Cap the tube and incubate at 25 °C for 6 h. Stop the reaction by adding 2.9 ml of *sulphate buffer solution pH 2.0 R.*

Reference solution. Prepare at the same time and in the same manner as for the test solution but using *porcine insulin CRS* instead of the substance to be examined.

Examine the digests by liquid chromatography (*2.2.29*).

Column:
- *size*: l = 0.10 m, Ø = 4.6 mm,
- *stationary phase*: *octadecylsilyl silica gel for chromatography R* (3 µm),
- *temperature*: 40 °C.

Mobile phase:
- *mobile phase A*: mix 100 ml of *acetonitrile for chromatography R*, 700 ml of *water R* and 200 ml of *sulphate buffer solution pH 2.0 R*; filter and degas;
- *mobile phase B*: mix 400 ml of *acetonitrile for chromatography R*, 400 ml of *water R* and 200 ml of *sulphate buffer solution pH 2.0 R*; filter and degas;

Time (min)	Mobile phase A (per cent *V/V*)	Mobile phase B (per cent *V/V*)
0 - 60	90 → 30	10 → 70
60 - 65	30 → 0	70 → 100
65 - 70	0	100

Flow rate: 1 ml/min.

Detection: spectrophotometer at 214 nm.

Equilibration: at initial conditions for at least 15 min. Carry out a blank run using the above-mentioned gradient.

Injection: 50 µl.

System suitability: the chromatograms obtained with the test solution and the reference solution are qualitatively similar to the chromatogram of porcine insulin digest supplied with *porcine insulin CRS*. In the chromatogram obtained with the reference solution, identify the peaks due to digest fragments I, II and III. The symmetry factor of the peaks due to fragments II and III is not greater than 1.5, and the resolution between the 2 peaks is at least 1.9.

Results: the profile of the chromatogram obtained with the test solution corresponds to that of the chromatogram obtained with the reference solution.

NOTE: the retention time of fragment I is the same for porcine insulin and for human insulin. The retention times of fragments II and IV are the same for all insulins. The retention time of fragment III is the same for bovine insulin and for porcine insulin.

TESTS

Impurities with molecular masses greater than that of insulin. Size-exclusion chromatography (*2.2.30*): use the normalisation procedure.

Test solution. Dissolve 4 mg of the substance to be examined in 1.0 ml of *0.01 M hydrochloric acid.*

Resolution solution. Use a solution of insulin (approximately 4 mg/ml), containing more than 0.4 per cent of high molecular mass proteins. An injectable insulin preparation, whether a solution or a suspension, that has been clarified with a sufficient amount of *6 M hydrochloric acid*, containing the indicated percentage of high molecular mass proteins, or a solution prepared from insulin, dissolved in *0.01 M hydrochloric acid*, may be used. Insulin containing the indicated percentage of high molecular mass proteins may be prepared by allowing insulin powder to stand at room temperature for about 10 days.

Maintain the solutions at 2-10 °C and use within 7 days. If an automatic injector is used, maintain the temperature at 2-10 °C.

Column:

- *size*: l = 0.3 m, Ø = at least 7.5 mm,
- *stationary phase*: *hydrophilic silica gel for chromatography R* (5-10 µm), of a grade suitable for the separation of insulin monomer from dimer and polymers.

Mobile phase: mix 15 volumes of *glacial acetic acid R*, 20 volumes of *acetonitrile R* and 65 volumes of a 1.0 g/l solution of *arginine R*; filter and degas.

Flow rate: 0.5 ml/min.

Detection: spectrophotometer at 276 nm.

Equilibration: before using a new column for chromatographic analysis, equilibrate by repeated injections of an insulin solution containing high molecular mass proteins. This can be done by at least 3 injections of the resolution solution. The column is equilibrated when repeatable results are obtained from 2 subsequent injections.

Injection: 100 µl.

Run time: about 35 min.

Retention times: polymeric insulin complexes = 13-17 min; covalent insulin dimer = about 17.5 min; insulin monomer = about 20 min; salts = about 22 min.

System suitability: resolution solution:

- *peak-to-valley ratio*: minimum 2.0, where H_p = height above the baseline of the peak due to the dimer and H_v = height above the baseline of the lowest point of the curve separating this peak from the peak due to the monomer.

Limits: the sum of the areas of any peaks with a retention time less than that of the principal peak is not greater than 1.0 per cent of the total area of the peaks. Disregard any peak with a retention time greater than that of the insulin peak.

Related proteins. Liquid chromatography (*2.2.29*) as described under Assay, following the elution conditions as described in the table below:

Time (min)	Mobile phase A (per cent *V/V*)	Mobile phase B (per cent *V/V*)
0 - 30	42	58
30 - 44	42 → 11	58 → 89
44 - 50	11	89

Maintain the solutions at 2-10 °C and use within 24 h. Perform a system suitability test (resolution, linearity) as described under Assay. If necessary, the relative proportions of the mobile phases may be adjusted to ensure complete elution of A21 desamido porcine insulin before commencement of the gradient. The profile of the gradient may also be adjusted to ensure complete elution of all insulin related impurities.

Inject 20 µl of reference solution (b) and 20 µl of the test solution. If necessary, adjust the injection volume to between 10 µl and 20 µl in accordance with the results obtained in the test for linearity as described under Assay. Record the chromatograms for approximately 50 min. In the chromatogram obtained with reference solution (b), A21 desamido porcine insulin appears as a small peak after the principal peak and has a relative retention of about 1.3 with reference to the principal peak. In the chromatogram obtained with the test solution, the area of the peak due to A21 desamido porcine insulin is not greater than 2.0 per cent of the total area of the peaks; the sum of the areas of all the peaks, apart from those due to porcine insulin and A21 desamido porcine insulin, is not greater than 2.0 per cent of the total area of the peaks.

Porcine proinsulin-like immunoreactivity (PLI): maximum 10 ppm, calculated with reference to the dried substance.

Use a suitably sensitive immunochemical method (*2.7.1*) such as radio-immunoassay, using the International Reference Reagent for porcine proinsulin to calibrate the method.

Zinc: maximum 1.0 per cent, calculated with reference to the dried substance.

Atomic absorption spectrometry (*2.2.23, Method I*).

Test solution. Dissolve 50.0 mg of the substance to be examined in *0.01 M hydrochloric acid* and dilute to 25.0 ml with the same acid. Dilute if necessary to a suitable concentration (for example, 0.4 µg to 1.6 µg of Zn per millilitre) with *0.01 M hydrochloric acid.*

Reference solutions. Use solutions containing 0.40 µg, 0.80 µg, 1.00 µg, 1.20 µg and 1.60 µg of Zn per millilitre, freshly prepared by diluting *zinc standard solution (5 mg/ml Zn) R* with *0.01 M hydrochloric acid.*

Source: zinc hollow-cathode lamp.

Wavelength: 213.9 nm.

Flame: air-acetylene flame of suitable composition (for example, 11 litres of air and 2 litres of acetylene per minute).

Loss on drying (*2.2.32*): maximum 10.0 per cent, determined on 0.200 g by drying in an oven at 100-105 °C for 24 h.

Monographs I-J

Sulphated ash (*2.4.14*): maximum 2.5 per cent, determined on 0.200 g and calculated with reference to the dried substance.

Bacterial endotoxins (*2.6.14*): less than 10 IU/mg, if intended for use in the manufacture of parenteral dosage forms without a further appropriate procedure for the removal of bacterial endotoxins.

ASSAY

Liquid chromatography (*2.2.29*).

Test solution. Dissolve 40.0 mg of the substance to be examined in *0.01 M hydrochloric acid* and dilute to 10.0 ml with the same solvent.

Reference solution (a). Dissolve the contents of a vial of *human insulin CRS* in *0.01 M hydrochloric acid* to obtain a concentration of 4.0 mg/ml.

Reference solution (b). Dissolve the contents of a vial of *porcine insulin CRS* in *0.01 M hydrochloric acid* to obtain a concentration of 4.0 mg/ml.

Reference solution (c). Dilute 1.0 ml of reference solution (b) to 10.0 ml with *0.01 M hydrochloric acid.*

Resolution solution. Mix 1.0 ml of reference solution (a) and 1.0 ml of reference solution (b).

Maintain the solutions at 2-10 °C and use within 48 h. If an automatic injector is used, maintain the temperature at 2-10 °C.

Column:

- *size*: l = 0.25 , Ø = 4.6 mm,
- *stationary phase*: *octadecylsilyl silica gel for chromatography R* (5 μm),
- *temperature*: 40 °C.

Mobile phase: mix 42 volumes of mobile phase A and 58 volumes of mobile phase B, adjusting the composition of the mixture if necessary.

Prepare and maintain the following solutions at a temperature of at least 20 °C:

- *mobile phase A*: dissolve 28.4 g of *anhydrous sodium sulphate R* in *water R* and dilute to 1000 ml with the same solvent; add 2.7 ml of *phosphoric acid R*; adjust to pH 2.3, if necessary, with *ethanolamine R*; filter and degas;
- *mobile phase B*: mix 550 ml of mobile phase A with 450 ml of *acetonitrile R*. Warm the solution to a temperature of at least 20 °C in order to avoid precipitation (mixing of mobile phase A with acetonitrile is endothermic); filter and degas.

Flow rate: 1 ml/min.

Detection: spectrophotometer at 214 nm.

System suitability:

- *resolution*: inject 20 μl of the resolution solution and 20 μl of reference solution (b). Record the chromatogram of the resolution solution until the peak corresponding to the principal peak in the chromatogram obtained with reference solution (b) is clearly visible. In the chromatogram obtained with the resolution solution, identify the peaks due to porcine insulin and human insulin. The test is not valid unless the resolution between the peaks corresponding to human insulin and porcine insulin is at least 1.2. If necessary, adjust the concentration of acetonitrile in the mobile phase until this resolution is achieved.
- *linearity*: inject 20 μl each of reference solutions (b) and (c). The test is not valid unless the area of the principal peak in the chromatogram obtained with reference solution (b) is 10 ± 0.5 times the area of the principal peak in the chromatogram obtained with reference solution (c). If this test fails, adjust the injection volume to between 10 μl and 20 μl, in order that the responses are within the linearity range of the detector.

Injection: 20 μl of the test solution.

Calculate the content of porcine insulin $C_{256}H_{381}N_{65}O_{76}S_6$ plus A21 desamido porcine insulin from the area of the principal peak and the area of the peak corresponding to A21 desamido porcine insulin in the chromatograms obtained with the test solution and reference solution (b) and the declared content of porcine insulin plus A21 desamido porcine insulin in *porcine insulin CRS*.

STORAGE

In an airtight container, protected from light, at − 20 °C until released by the manufacturer. When thawed, insulin may be stored at 5 ± 3 °C and used for manufacturing preparations within a short period of time. To avoid absorption of humidity from the air during weighing, the insulin must be at room temperature.

LABELLING

The label states where applicable, that the substance is free from bacterial endotoxins.

01/2005:0854

INSULIN PREPARATIONS, INJECTABLE

Praeparationes insulini iniectabiles

Injectable insulin preparations comply with the requirements for Injections prescribed in the monograph on Parenteral preparations (0520).

DEFINITION

Injectable insulin preparations are sterile preparations of *Insulin, human (0838)*, *Insulin, bovine (1637)* or *Insulin, porcine (1638)*. They contain not less than 90.0 per cent and not more than the equivalent of 110.0 per cent of the amount of insulin stated on the label. They are either solutions or suspensions or they are prepared by combining solutions and suspensions.

PRODUCTION

The methods of preparation are designed to confer suitable properties with respect to the onset and duration of therapeutic action.

The following procedures are carried out in a suitable sequence, depending on the method of preparation:

- addition of suitable antimicrobial preservatives,
- addition of a suitable substance or substances to render the preparation isotonic with blood,
- addition of a suitable substance or substances to adjust the pH to the appropriate value,
- determination of the strength of the insulin-containing component or components followed, where necessary, by adjustment so that the final preparation contains the requisite number of International Units per millilitre,
- sterilisation by filtration of the insulin-containing component or components; once this procedure has been carried out all subsequent procedures are carried out aseptically using materials that have been sterilised by a suitable method.

In addition, where appropriate, suitable substances are added and suitable procedures carried out to confer the appropriate physical form on the insulin-containing component or components. The final preparation is distributed aseptically into sterile containers which are closed so as to exclude microbial contamination.

TESTS

pH (*2.2.3*). The pH of the solution or suspension is 6.9 to 7.8, unless otherwise prescribed in the specific monograph.

Insulin in the supernatant. For injectable insulin preparations that are suspensions, not more than 2.5 per cent of the total insulin content, unless otherwise stated. Centrifuge 10 ml of the suspension at 1500 *g* for 10 min and carefully separate the supernatant liquid and the residue. Determine the insulin content of the supernatant liquid (*S*) by a suitable method, for example using the chromatographic conditions described under Assay. Calculate the percentage of the insulin in solution from the expression:

$$\frac{100S}{T}$$

where *T* is the total insulin content determined as described under the Assay.

Impurities with molecular masses greater than that of insulin. Examine by size-exclusion chromatography (*2.2.30*).

Test solution. Add 4 µl of *6 M hydrochloric acid* per millilitre of the preparation to be examined, whether a suspension or a solution, to obtain a clear acid insulin solution. When sampling a suspension, agitate the material prior to sampling in order to obtain a homogeneous sample. If a suspension does not turn clear within 5 min of the initial addition of hydrochloric acid, add small aliquots of acid (less than 4 µl per millilitre) until a solution is obtained. Preparations with concentrations higher than 100 IU/ml need to be diluted with *0.01 M hydrochloric acid* to avoid overloading the column with insulin monomer.

Resolution solution. Use a solution of insulin (approximately 4 mg/ml), containing more than 0.4 per cent of high molecular mass proteins. An injectable insulin preparation, whether a solution or a suspension, that has been clarified with a sufficient amount of *6 M hydrochloric acid*, containing the indicated percentage of high molecular mass proteins, or a solution prepared from insulin, dissolved in *0.01 M hydrochloric acid*, may be used. Insulin containing the indicated percentage of high molecular mass proteins may be prepared by allowing insulin powder to stand at room temperature for about ten days.

Maintain the solutions at 2 °C to 10 °C and use within 30 h (soluble insulin injection) or 7 days (other insulin preparations). If an automatic injector is used, maintain the temperature at 2 °C to 10 °C.

The chromatographic procedure may be carried out using:

- a column 0.3 m long and at least 7.5 mm in internal diameter packed with *hydrophilic silica gel for chromatography R* (5 µm to 10 µm), of a grade suitable for the separation of insulin monomer from dimers and polymers,
- as mobile phase at a flow rate of 0.5 ml/min a mixture consisting of 15 volumes of *glacial acetic acid R*, 20 volumes of *acetonitrile R* and 65 volumes of a 1.0 g/l solution of *arginine R*; filter and degas,
- as detector a spectrophotometer set at 276 nm.

Equilibration of the column. Before using a new column for chromatographic analysis, equilibrate by repeated injections of an insulin solution containing high molecular mass proteins. This can be done by at least three injections of the resolution solution. The column is equilibrated when repeatable results are obtained from two subsequent injections. If protamine-containing samples are to be analysed, the equilibration of the column is performed using a solution containing protamine.

Inject 100 µl of the resolution solution. When the chromatograms are recorded under the prescribed conditions, the retention times are: polymeric insulin complexes or covalent insulin-protamine complex: about 13 min to 17 min, covalent insulin dimer: about 17.5 min, insulin monomer: about 20 min, salts: about 22 min. If the sample solution contains preservatives, for example methyl paraben, *m*-cresol or phenol, these compounds elute later. The test is not valid unless the resolution, defined by the ratio of the height of the dimer peak to the height above the baseline of the valley separating the monomer and dimer peaks, is at least 2.0.

Inject 100 µl of the test solution. Record the chromatogram for approximately 35 min. In the chromatogram obtained, the sum of the areas of any peak with a retention time less than that of the insulin peak is not greater than 3.0 per cent (protamine containing preparations) or 2.0 per cent (non-protamine containing preparations) of the total area of the peaks. Disregard any peak with a retention time greater than that of the insulin peak.

Related proteins. Examine by liquid chromatography (*2.2.29*) as described under Assay, following the elution conditions as described in the table below:

Time (min)	Mobile phase A (per cent *V/V*)	Mobile phase B (per cent *V/V*)	Comment
0 - 30	42	58	isocratic
30 - 44	42 → 11	58 → 89	linear gradient
44 - 50	11	89	isocratic

Maintain the solutions at 2 °C to 10 °C and use within 24 h. Perform a system suitability check (resolution, linearity) as described under Assay. If necessary, the relative proportions of the mobile phases may be adjusted to ensure complete elution of A21 desamido porcine insulin before commencement of the gradient. The profile of the gradient may also be adjusted to ensure complete elution of all insulin related impurities.

Inject 20 µl of the test solution and 20 µl of either reference solution (a), for insulin preparations containing 100 IU/ml, or reference solution (b), for insulin preparations containing 40 IU/ml. If necessary, adjust the injection volume to a volume between 10 µl and 20 µl in accordance with the results obtained in the test for linearity as described under Assay. Record the chromatograms for approximately 50 min. If necessary, make further adjustments to the mobile phase in order to ensure that the antimicrobial preservatives present in the test solution are well separated from the insulin and show a shorter retention time. A small reduction in the concentration of acetonitrile increases the retention time of the insulin peaks relatively more than those of the preservatives. In the chromatogram obtained with either reference solution (a), or reference solution (b), as appropriate, A21 desamido insulin appears as a small peak after the principal peak and has a retention time of about 1.3 relative to the principal peak, due to insulin. In the chromatogram obtained with the test solution the area of the peak due to A21 desamido insulin is not greater than 5.0 per cent of the total area of the peaks; the sum of the areas of any other peaks, apart from those due to insulin and A21 desamido insulin is not greater than 6.0 per cent of the total area of the peaks. Disregard the peaks due to the preservatives and protamine (early eluting peaks).

Total zinc. Not more than the amount stated in the individual monograph, determined by atomic absorption spectrometry (*2.2.23, Method I*).

Use the following method, unless otherwise prescribed in the specific monograph.

Test solution. Shake the preparation gently and dilute a volume containing 200 IU of insulin to 25.0 ml with *0.01 M hydrochloric acid*. Dilute if necessary to a suitable concentration of zinc (for example 0.4 µg to 1.6 µg of Zn per millilitre) with *0.01 M hydrochloric acid*.

Reference solutions. Use solutions containing 0.40 µg, 0.80 µg, 1.00 µg, 1.20 µg and 1.60 µg of Zn per millilitre, freshly prepared by diluting *zinc standard solution (5 mg/ml Zn) R* with *0.01 M hydrochloric acid*.

Measure the absorbance at 213.9 nm using a zinc hollow-cathode lamp as source of radiation and an air-acetylene flame of suitable composition (for example 11 litres of air and 2 litres of acetylene per minute).

Zinc in solution. Where applicable, not more than the amount stated in the individual monograph, determined by atomic absorption spectrometry (*2.2.23, Method I*).

Test solution. Centrifuge the preparation to be examined and dilute 1 ml of the clear supernatant liquid obtained to 25.0 ml with *water R*. Dilute if necessary to a suitable concentration of zinc (for example 0.4 µg to 1.6 µg of Zn per millilitre) with *water R*.

Reference solutions. Use solutions containing 0.40 µg, 0.80 µg, 1.00 µg, 1.20 µg and 1.60 µg of Zn per millilitre, freshly prepared by diluting *zinc standard solution (5 mg/ml Zn) R* with *0.01 M hydrochloric acid*.

Measure the absorbance at 213.9 nm using a zinc hollow-cathode lamp as source of radiation and an air-acetylene flame of suitable composition (for example 11 litres of air and 2 litres of acetylene per minute).

Bacterial endotoxins (*2.6.14*): less than 80 IU per 100 IU of insulin.

ASSAY

Examine by liquid chromatography (*2.2.29*).

Test solution. Add 4 µl of *6 M hydrochloric acid* per millilitre of the preparation to be examined, whether a suspension or a solution, to obtain a clear solution. When sampling a suspension, shake the material prior to sampling in order to obtain a homogeneous sample. If a suspension does not turn clear within 5 min of the initial addition of acid, add small aliquots of acid (less than 4 µl per millilitre) until a solution is obtained. For a preparation containing more than 100 IU ml, an additional dilution with *0.01 M hydrochloric acid* is necessary to avoid overloading the column.

Reference solution (a). For a preparation containing a single species of insulin, dissolve in *0.01 M hydrochloric acid*, as appropriate, the contents of a vial of *human insulin CRS* or *porcine insulin CRS*, or a defined quantity of *bovine insulin CRS* to obtain a concentration of 4.0 mg/ml. For a preparation containing both bovine and porcine insulins, mix 1.0 ml of a solution containing 4.0 mg of *bovine insulin CRS* per millilitre of *0.01 M hydrochloric acid* and 1.0 ml of a solution containing 4.0 mg of *porcine insulin CRS* per millilitre of *0.01 M hydrochloric acid. Reference solution (a) is used for the assay of insulin preparations containing 100 IU/ml.*

Reference solution (b). Dilute 4.0 ml of reference solution (a) to 10.0 ml with *0.01 M hydrochloric acid. Reference solution (b) is used for the assay of insulin preparations containing 40 IU/ml.*

Reference solution (c). Dissolve the contents of a vial of *human insulin CRS* in *0.01 M hydrochloric acid* to obtain a concentration of 4.0 mg/ml.

Reference solution (d). Dissolve the contents of a vial of *porcine insulin CRS* in *0.01 M hydrochloric acid* to obtain a concentration of 4.0 mg/ml.

Reference solution (e). Dilute 1.0 ml of reference solution (a) to 10.0 ml with *0.01 M hydrochloric acid*.

Reference solution (f). Dilute 1.0 ml of reference solution (b) to 10.0 ml with *0.01 M hydrochloric acid*.

Resolution solution. Mix 1.0 ml of reference solution (c) and 1.0 ml of reference solution (d).

Maintain the solutions at 2 °C to 10 °C and use within 48 h. If an automatic injector is used, maintain the temperature at 2 °C to 10 °C.

The chromatographic procedure may be carried out using:

– a stainless steel column 0.25 m long and 4.6 mm in internal diameter packed with *octadecylsilyl silica gel for chromatography R* (5 µm),

– as mobile phase at a flow rate of 1 ml/min the following solutions prepared and maintained at a temperature not lower than 20 °C:

  Mobile phase A. Dissolve 28.4 g of *anhydrous sodium sulphate R* in *water R* and dilute to 1000 ml with the same solvent; add 2.7 ml of *phosphoric acid R*; adjust the pH to 2.3, if necessary, with *ethanolamine R*; filter and degas,

  Mobile phase B. Mix 550 ml of mobile phase A with 450 ml of *acetonitrile R*. Warm the solution to a temperature not lower than 20 °C in order to avoid precipitation (mixing of mobile phase A with acetonitrile is endothermic); filter and degas,

– as detector a spectrophotometer set at 214 nm,

maintaining the temperature of the column at 40 °C.

Elute with a mixture of 42 volumes of mobile phase A and 58 volumes of mobile phase B, adjusted if necessary.

Inject 20 µl of the resolution solution and 20 µl of reference solution (d). Record the chromatogram of the resolution solution until the peak corresponding to the principal peak in the chromatogram obtained with reference solution (d) is clearly visible. In the chromatogram obtained with the resolution solution, identify the peaks due to porcine insulin and human insulin. The test is not valid unless the resolution between the peaks due to human insulin and porcine insulin is at least 1.2. If necessary, adjust the concentration of acetonitrile in the mobile phase until this resolution is achieved.

Inject 20 µl of the test solution and 20 µl of either reference solutions (a) and (e), for insulin preparations containing 100 IU/ml, or 20 µl of reference solutions (b) and (f), for insulin preparations containing 40 IU/ml. If necessary, make further adjustments of the mobile phase in order to ensure that the antimicrobial preservatives present in the test solution are well separated from the insulin and show shorter retention times. A small reduction in the concentration of acetonitrile increases the retention time of the insulin peaks relatively more than those of the preservatives. If necessary, after having carried out the chromatography of a solution wash the column with a mixture of equal volumes of *acetonitrile R* and *water R* for a sufficient time to ensure elution of any interfering substances before injecting the next solution. The test is not valid unless the area of the principal peak in the chromatogram obtained with reference solution (a) or (b) is 10 ± 0.5 times the area of the principal peak in the chromatogram obtained with reference solution (e) or (f). If this test fails, adjust the injection volume between 10 µl and 20 µl, in order to be in the linearity range of the detector.

Calculate the content of insulin plus A21 desamido insulin from the area of the peak due to the bovine, porcine or human insulin and that of any peak due to the A21 desamido insulin, using the declared content of insulin plus A21 desamido insulin in *bovine insulin CRS, porcine insulin CRS* or *human insulin CRS*, as appropriate. For preparations containing both bovine and porcine insulin use the sum of the areas of both the bovine and porcine insulin peaks and of the peaks due to the A21 desamido insulin(1) derivatives.

STORAGE

Unless otherwise prescribed, store in a sterile, airtight, tamper-proof container, protected from light, at a temperature of 2 °C to 8 °C. Insulin preparations are not to be frozen.

LABELLING

The label states:

- the potency in International Units per millilitre,
- the concentration in terms of the number of milligrams of insulin per millilitre (for preparations containing both bovine insulin and porcine insulin the concentration is stated as the combined amount of both insulins),
- where applicable, that the substance is produced by enzymatic modification of porcine insulin,
- where applicable, that the substance is produced by recombinant DNA technology,
- where applicable, the animal species of origin,
- that the preparation must not be frozen,
- where applicable, that the preparation must be resuspended before use.

01/2005:0837

INSULIN ZINC INJECTABLE SUSPENSION

Insulini zinci suspensio iniectabilis

Insulin zinc injectable suspension complies with the monograph on Insulin preparations, injectable (0854) with the amendments prescribed below.

DEFINITION

Insulin zinc injectable suspension is a sterile neutral suspension of bovine insulin and/or porcine insulin or of human insulin with a suitable zinc salt; the insulin is in a form which is practically insoluble in water.

PRODUCTION

Insulin zinc injectable suspension is prepared by carrying out the procedures described in the monograph on *Insulin preparations, injectable (0854)*.

Insulin zinc injectable suspension is produced by mixing insulin zinc injectable suspension (crystalline) and insulin zinc injectable suspension (amorphous) in a ratio of 7 to 3.

CHARACTERS

A white suspension which on standing deposits a white sediment and leaves a colourless or almost colourless supernatant liquid; the sediment is readily resuspended by gently shaking. When examined under a microscope, the majority of the particles are seen to be rhombohedral crystals with a maximum dimension when measured from corner to corner through the crystal greater than 10 µm but rarely exceeding 40 µm; a considerable proportion of the particles are seen to have no uniform shape and a maximum dimension rarely exceeding 2 µm.

IDENTIFICATION

Examine the chromatograms obtained in the Assay.

For preparations made from a single species of insulin (bovine, porcine or human), the position of the peak due to insulin in the chromatogram obtained with the test solution corresponds to that of the principal peak in the chromatogram obtained with the appropriate reference solution. For preparations made from a mixture of bovine and porcine insulin, the positions of the peaks due to the two insulins in the chromatogram obtained with the test solution correspond to those of the principal peaks in the chromatogram obtained with the appropriate reference solution.

TESTS

Insulin not extractable with buffered acetone solution: 63 per cent to 77 per cent of the total insulin content. Centrifuge a volume of the substance to be examined containing 200 IU of insulin and discard the supernatant liquid. Suspend the residue in 1.65 ml of *water R*, add 3.3 ml of *buffered acetone solution R*, stir for 3 min, again centrifuge, discard the supernatant liquid and repeat all the operations with the residue. Dissolve the residue using a suitable procedure, for example dissolve in *0.1 M hydrochloric acid* to give a final volume of 2.0 ml. Determine the insulin content of the residue (*R*) and determine the total insulin content (*T*) of an equal volume of the suspension by a suitable method. Calculate the percentage of insulin not extractable with buffered acetone solution from the expression:

$$\frac{100R}{T}$$

Total zinc: 0.12 mg to 0.25 mg per 100 IU of insulin, determined as described in the monograph on *Insulin preparations, injectable (0854)*.

Zinc in solution: 20 per cent to 65 per cent of the total zinc is in the form of zinc in solution. Determine by the method described in the monograph on *Insulin preparations, injectable (0854)*.

01/2005:0835

INSULIN ZINC INJECTABLE SUSPENSION (AMORPHOUS)

Insulini zinci amorphi suspensio iniectabilis

Insulin zinc injectable suspension (amorphous) complies with the monograph on Insulin preparations, injectable (0854) with the amendments prescribed below.

DEFINITION

Insulin zinc injectable suspension (amorphous) is a sterile neutral suspension of bovine, porcine or human insulin complexed with a suitable zinc salt; the insulin is in a form which is practically insoluble in water.

(1) 100 IU are equivalent to 3.47 mg of human insulin, to 3.45 mg of porcine insulin and to 3.42 mg of bovine insulin.

CHARACTERS

A white suspension which on standing deposits a white sediment and leaves a colourless or almost colourless supernatant liquid; the sediment is readily resuspended by gently shaking. When examined under a microscope, the particles are seen to have no uniform shape and a maximum dimension rarely exceeding 2 µm.

IDENTIFICATION

Examine the chromatograms obtained in the Assay. The position of the peak due to insulin in the chromatogram obtained with the test solution corresponds to that of the principal peak in the chromatogram obtained with the appropriate reference solution.

TESTS

Total zinc. 0.12 mg to 0.25 mg per 100 IU of insulin, determined as described in the monograph on *Insulin preparations, injectable (0854)*.

Zinc in solution. 20 per cent to 65 per cent of the total zinc is in the form of zinc in solution. Determine by the method described in the monograph on *Insulin preparations, injectable (0854)*.

01/2005:0836

INSULIN ZINC INJECTABLE SUSPENSION (CRYSTALLINE)

Insulini zinci cristallini suspensio iniectabilis

Insulin zinc injectable suspension (crystalline) complies with the monograph on Insulin preparations, injectable (0854) with the amendments prescribed below.

DEFINITION

Insulin zinc injectable suspension (crystalline) is a sterile neutral suspension of bovine, porcine or human insulin, complexed with a suitable zinc salt; the insulin is in a form which is practically insoluble in water.

CHARACTERS

A white suspension which on standing deposits a white sediment and leaves a colourless or almost colourless supernatant liquid; the sediment is readily resuspended by gently shaking. When examined under a microscope, the particles are seen to be rhombohedral crystals, the majority having a maximum dimension when measured from corner to corner through the crystal greater than 10 µm but rarely exceeding 40 µm.

IDENTIFICATION

Examine the chromatograms obtained in the Assay. The position of the peak due to insulin in the chromatogram obtained with the test solution corresponds to that of the principal peak in the chromatogram obtained with the appropriate reference solution.

TESTS

Insulin not extractable with buffered acetone solution. Not less than 90 per cent of the total insulin content. Centrifuge a volume of the substance to be examined containing 200 IU of insulin and discard the supernatant liquid. Suspend the residue in 1.65 ml of *water R*, add 3.3 ml of *buffered acetone solution R*, stir for 3 min, again centrifuge, discard the supernatant liquid and repeat all the operations with the residue. Dissolve the residue using a suitable procedure, for example dissolve in *0.1 M hydrochloric acid* to give a final volume of 2.0 ml. Determine the insulin content of the residue (*R*) and determine the total insulin content (*T*) of an equal volume of the suspension by a suitable method. Calculate the percentage of insulin not extractable with buffered acetone solution from the expression:

$$\frac{100R}{T}$$

Total zinc: 0.12 mg to 0.25 mg per 100 IU of insulin, determined as described in the monograph on *Insulin preparations, injectable (0854)*.

Zinc in solution: 20 per cent to 65 per cent of the total zinc is in the form of zinc in solution. Determine by the method described in the monograph on *Insulin preparations, injectable (0854)*.

01/2005:1110
corrected

INTERFERON ALFA-2 CONCENTRATED SOLUTION

Interferoni alfa-2 solutio concentrata

```
CDLPQTHSLG  SRRTLMLLAQ  MRX1ISLFSCL  KDRHDFGFPQ
EEFGNQFQKA  ETIPVLHEMI  QQIFNLFSTK   DSSAAWDETL
LDKFYTELYQ  QLNDLEACVI  QGVGVTETPL   MKEDSILAVR
KYFQRITLYL  KEKKYSPCAW  EVVRAEIMRS   FSLTSNLQES
LRSKE
```

DEFINITION

Interferon alfa-2 concentrated solution is a solution of a protein that is produced according to the information coded by the alfa-2 sub-species of interferon alfa gene and that exerts non-specific antiviral activity, at least in homologous cells, through cellular metabolic processes involving synthesis of both ribonucleic acid and protein. Interferon alfa-2 concentrated solution also exerts antiproliferative activity. Different types of alfa-2 interferon, varying in the amino acid residue at position 23, are designated by a letter in lower case.

Designation	**Residue at position 23 (X_1)**
alfa-2a	Lys
alfa-2b	Arg

This monograph applies to interferon alfa-2a and -2b concentrated solutions.

The potency of interferon alfa-2 concentrated solution is not less than 1.4×10^8 IU per milligram of protein. Interferon alfa-2 concentrated solution contains not less than 2×10^8 IU of interferon alfa-2 per millilitre.

PRODUCTION

Interferon alfa-2 concentrated solution is produced by a method based on recombinant DNA (rDNA) technology using bacteria as host cells. It is produced under conditions designed to minimise microbial contamination of the product.

Interferon alfa-2 concentrated solution complies with the following additional requirements.

Host-cell-derived proteins. The limit is approved by the competent authority.

Host-cell- or vector-derived DNA. The limit is approved by the competent authority.

CHARACTERS

A clear, colourless or slightly yellowish liquid.

IDENTIFICATION

A. It shows the expected biological activity (see Assay).

B. Examine by isoelectric focusing.

Test solution. Dilute the preparation to be examined with *water R* to a protein concentration of 1 mg/ml.

Reference solution. Prepare a 1 mg/ml solution of the appropriate *interferon alfa-2 CRS* in *water R.*

Isoelectric point calibration solution pI range 3.0 to 10.0. Prepare and use according to the manufacturer's instructions.

Use a suitable apparatus connected with a recirculating temperature controlled water-bath set at 10 °C and gels for isoelectric focusing with a pH gradient from 3.5 to 9.5. Operate the apparatus in accordance with the manufacturer's instructions. Use as the anode solution *phosphoric acid R* (98 g/l H_3PO_4)and as the cathode solution *1 M sodium hydroxide.* Samples are applied to the gel by filter papers. Place sample application filters on the gel close to the cathode.

Apply 15 µl of the test solution and 15 µl of the reference solution. Start the isoelectric focusing at 1500 V and 50 mA. Turn off the power after 30 min, remove the application filters and reconnect the power supply for 1 h. Keep the power constant during the focusing process. After focusing, immerse the gel in a suitable volume of a solution containing115 g/l of *trichloroacetic acid R* and 34.5 g/l of *sulphosalicylic acid R* in *water R* and agitate the container gently for 60 min. Transfer the gel to a mixture of 32 volumes of *glacial acetic acid R,* 100 volumes of *ethanol R* and 268 volumes of *water R,* and soak for 5 min. Immerse the gel for 10 min in a staining solution prewarmed to 60 °C in which 1.2 g/l of *acid blue 83 R* has been added to the previous mixture of glacial acetic acid, ethanol and water. Wash the gel in several containers with the previous mixture of glacial acetic acid, ethanol and water and keep the gel in this mixture until the background is clear (12 h to 24 h). After adequate destaining, soak the gel for 1 h in a 10 per cent *V/V* solution of *glycerol R* in the previous mixture of glacial acetic acid, ethanol and water.

The principal bands of the electropherogram obtained with the test solution correspond in position to the principal bands of the electropherogram obtained with the reference solution. Plot the migration distances of the isoelectric point markers versus their isoelectric points and determine the isoelectric points of the principal components of the test solution and the reference solution. They do not differ by more than 0.2 pI unit. The test is not valid unless the isoelectric point markers are distributed along the entire length of the gel and the isoelectric points of the principal bands in the electropherogram obtained with the reference solution are between 5.8 and 6.3.

C. Examine the electropherograms obtained under reducing conditions in the test for impurities of molecular masses differing from that of interferon alfa-2. The principal band in the electropherogram obtained with test solution (a) corresponds in position to the principal band in the electropherogram obtained with reference solution (a).

D. Examine by peptide mapping.

Test solution. Dilute the preparation to be examined in *water R* to a protein concentration of 1.5 mg/ml. Transfer 25 µl to a polypropylene or glass tube of 1.5 ml capacity. Add 1.6 µl of *1 M phosphate buffer solution pH 8.0 R,* 2.8 µl of a freshly prepared 1.0 mg/ml solution of *trypsin for peptide mapping R* in *water R* and 3.6 µl of *water R* and mix vigorously. Cap the tube and place it in a water-bath at 37 °C for 18 h, then add 100 µl of a 573 g/l solution of *guanidine hydrochloride R* and mix well. Add 7 µl of 154.2 g/l solution of *dithiothreitol R* and mix well. Place the capped tube in boiling water for 1 min. Cool to room temperature.

Reference solution. Prepare at the same time and in the same manner as for the test solution but use a 1.5 mg ml solution of the appropriate *interferon alfa-2 CRS* in *water R.*

Examine by liquid chromatography (*2.2.29*).

The chromatographic procedure may be carried out using:

– a stainless steel column 0.10 m long and 4.6 mm in internal diameter packed with *octadecylsilyl silica gel for chromatography R* (5 µm) with a pore size of 30 nm,

– as mobile phase at a flow rate of 1.0 ml/min:

Mobile phase A. Dilute 1 ml of *trifluoroacetic acid R* to 1000 ml with *water R,*

Mobile phase B. To 100 ml of *water R* add 1 ml of *trifluoroacetic acid R* and dilute to 1000 ml with *acetonitrile for chromatography R,*

Time (min)	Mobile phase A (per cent *V/V*)	Mobile phase B (per cent *V/V*)	Comment
0 - 8	100	0	isocratic
8 - 68	100 → 40	0 → 60	linear gradient
68 - 72	40	60	isocratic
72 - 75	40 → 100	60 → 0	linear gradient
75 - 80	100	0	re-equilibration

– as detector a spectrophotometer set at 214 nm,

maintaining the temperature of the column at 30 °C.

Equilibrate the column with mobile phase A for at least 15 min.

Inject 100 µl of the test solution and 100 µl of the reference solution. The test is not valid unless the chromatogram obtained with each solution is qualitatively similar to the chromatogram of interferon alfa-2 digest supplied with the appropriate *interferon alfa-2 CRS.* The profile of the chromatogram obtained with the test solution corresponds to that of the chromatogram obtained with the reference solution.

TESTS

Impurities of molecular masses differing from that of interferon alfa-2. Examine by SDS polyacrylamide gel electrophoresis (*2.2.31*). The test is performed under both reducing and non-reducing conditions, using resolving gels of 14 per cent acrylamide and silver staining as the detection method.

Sample buffer (non-reducing conditions). Mix equal volumes of *water R* and *concentrated SDS PAGE sample buffer R.*

Sample buffer (reducing conditions). Mix equal volumes of *water R* and *concentrated SDS PAGE sample buffer for reducing conditions R* containing 2-mercaptoethanol as the reducing agent.

Test solution (a). Dilute the preparation to be examined in sample buffer to a protein concentration of 0.5 mg/ml.

Test solution (b). Dilute 0.20 ml of test solution (a) to 1 ml with sample buffer.

Reference solution (a). Prepare a 0.625 mg/ml solution of the appropriate *interferon alfa-2 CRS* in sample buffer.

Reference solution (b). Dilute 0.20 ml of reference solution (a) to 1 ml with sample buffer.

Reference solution (c). Dilute 0.20 ml of reference solution (b) to 1 ml with sample buffer.

Reference solution (d). Dilute 0.20 ml of reference solution (c) to 1 ml with sample buffer.

Reference solution (e). Dilute 0.20 ml of reference solution (d) to 1 ml with sample buffer.

Reference solution (f). Use a solution of molecular mass standards suitable for calibrating SDS-PAGE gels in the range 15 kDa to 67 kDa.

Place test and reference solutions, contained in covered test-tubes, on a water-bath for 2 min.

Apply 10 µl of reference solution (f) and 50 µl of each of the other solutions to the stacking gel wells. Perform the electrophoresis under the conditions recommended by the manufacturer of the equipment. Detect proteins in the gel by silver staining.

The test is not valid unless: the validation criteria are met (*2.2.31*); a band is seen in the electropherogram obtained with reference solution (e); and a gradation of intensity of staining is seen in the electropherograms obtained, respectively, with test solution (a) and test solution (b) and with reference solutions (a) to (e).

The electropherogram obtained with test solution (a) under reducing conditions may show, in addition to the principal band, less intense bands with molecular masses lower than the principal band. No such band is more intense than the principal band in the electropherogram obtained with reference solution (d) (1.0 per cent) and not more than three such bands are more intense than the principal band in the electropherogram obtained with reference solution (e) (0.2 per cent).

The electropherogram obtained with test solution (a) under non-reducing conditions may show, in addition to the principal band, less intense bands with molecular masses higher than the principal band. No such band is more intense than the principal band in the electropherogram obtained with reference solution (d) (1.0 per cent) and not more than three such bands are more intense than the principal band in the electropherogram obtained with reference solution (e) (0.2 per cent).

Related proteins. Examine by liquid chromatography (*2.2.29*).

Test solution. Dilute the preparation to be examined with *water R* to a protein concentration of 1 mg/ml.

0.25 per cent m/m hydrogen peroxide solution. Dilute *dilute hydrogen peroxide solution R* in *water R* in order to obtain a 0.25 per cent *m/m* solution.

Reference solution. To a volume of the test solution, add a suitable volume of 0.25 per cent *m/m* hydrogen peroxide solution to give a final hydrogen peroxide concentration of 0.005 per cent *m/m*, and allow to stand at room temperature for 1 h, or for the length of time that will generate about 5 per cent oxidised interferon. Add 12.5 mg of *L-methionine R* per millilitre of solution. Allow to stand at room temperature for 1 h. Store the solutions for not longer than 24 h at a temperature of 2 °C to 8 °C.

The chromatographic procedure may be carried out using:

– a stainless steel column 0.25 m long and 4.6 mm in internal diameter packed with *octadecylsilyl silica gel for chromatography R* (5 µm) with a pore size of 30 nm,

– as mobile phase at a flow rate of 1.0 ml/min:

Mobile phase A. To 700 ml of *water R* add 2 ml of *trifluoroacetic acid R* and 300 ml of *acetonitrile for chromatography R*,

Mobile phase B. To 200 ml of *water R* add 2 ml of *trifluoroacetic acid R* and 800 ml of *acetonitrile for chromatography R*,

Time (min)	Mobile phase A (per cent *V/V*)	Mobile phase B (per cent *V/V*)	Comment
0 - 1	72	28	isocratic
1 - 5	72 → 67	28 → 33	linear gradient
5 - 20	67 → 63	33 → 37	linear gradient
20 - 30	63 → 57	37 → 43	linear gradient
30 - 40	57 → 40	43 → 60	linear gradient
40 - 42	40	60	isocratic
42 - 50	40 → 72	60 → 28	linear gradient
50 - 60	72	28	re-equilibration

– as detector a spectrophotometer set at 210 nm.

Equilibrate the column with the mobile phases in the initial gradient ratio for at least 15 min. Inject 50 µl of each solution.

In the chromatograms obtained, interferon alfa-2 elutes at a retention time of about 20 min. In the chromatogram obtained with the reference solution a peak related to oxidised interferon appears at a retention time of about 0.9 relative to the principal peak. The test is not valid unless the resolution between the peaks corresponding to oxidised interferon and interferon is at least 1.0. Consider only the peaks whose retention time is 0.7 to 1.4 relative to that of the principal peak. In the chromatogram obtained with the test solution, the area of any peak, apart from the principal peak, is not greater than 3.0 per cent of the total area of all of the peaks. The sum of the areas of any peaks other than the principal peak is not greater than 5.0 per cent of the total area of all of the peaks.

Bacterial endotoxins (*2.6.14*): less than 100 IU in the volume that contains 1.0 mg of protein.

ASSAY

Protein

Test solution. Dilute the preparation to be examined with *water R* to obtain a concentration of about 0.5 mg/ml of interferon alfa-2.

Reference solutions. Prepare a stock solution of 0.5 mg/ml of *bovine albumin R*. Prepare eight dilutions of the stock solution containing between 3 µg/ml and 30 µg/ml of *bovine albumin R*.

Prepare 30-fold and 50-fold dilutions of the test solution. Add 1.25 ml of a mixture prepared the same day by combining 2.0 ml of a 20 g/l solution of *copper sulphate R* in *water R*, 2.0 ml of a 40 g/l solution of *sodium tartrate R* in *water R* and 96.0 ml of a 40 g/l solution of *sodium carbonate R* in *0.2 M sodium hydroxide* to test-tubes containing 1.5 ml of *water R* (blank), 1.5 ml of the different dilutions of the test solution or 1.5 ml of the reference solutions. Mix after each addition. After approximately 10 min, add to each test-tube 0.25 ml of a mixture of equal volumes of *water R* and *phosphomolybdotungstic reagent R*. Mix after each addition. After approximately 30 min, measure the absorbance (*2.2.25*) of each solution at 750 nm using the blank as the compensation liquid. Draw a calibration curve from the absorbances of the eight reference solutions and the corresponding protein contents and read from the curve the content of protein in the test solution.

Potency

The potency of interferon alfa-2 is estimated by comparing its effect to protect cells against a viral cytopathic effect with the same effect of the appropriate International Standard of human recombinant interferon alfa-2 or of a reference preparation calibrated in International Units.

The International Unit is the activity contained in a stated amount of the appropriate International Standard. The equivalence in International Units of the International Standard is stated by the World Health Organisation.

Carry out the assay by a suitable method, based on the following design.

Use, in standard culture conditions, an established cell line sensitive to the cytopathic effect of a suitable virus (a human diploid fibroblast cell line, free of microbial contamination, responsive to interferon and sensitive to encephalomyocarditis virus, is suitable).

The following cell cultures and virus have shown to be suitable: MDBK cells (ATCC No. CCL22), or Mouse L cells (NCTC clone 929; ATCC No. CCL 1) as the cell culture and vesicular stomatitis virus VSV, Indiana strain (ATCC No. VR-158) as the infective agent; or human diploid fibroblast FS-71 cells responsive to interferon as the cell culture, and encephalomyocarditis virus (ATCC No. VR-129B) as the infective agent.

Incubate in at least four series, cells with three or more different concentrations of the preparation to be examined and the reference preparation in a microtitre plate and include in each series appropriate controls of untreated cells. Choose the concentrations of the preparations such that the lowest concentration produces some protection and the largest concentration produces less than maximal protection against the viral cytopathic effect. Add at a suitable time the cytopathic virus to all wells with the exception of a sufficient number of wells in all series, which are left with uninfected control cells. Determine the cytopathic effect of virus quantitatively with a suitable method. Calculate the potency of the preparation to be examined by the usual statistical methods for a parallel line assay.

The estimated potency is not less than 80 per cent and not more than 125 per cent of the stated potency. The confidence limits of the estimated potency ($P = 0.95$) are not less than 64 per cent and not more than 156 per cent of the stated potency.

STORAGE

Store in an airtight container, protected from light, at or below − 20 °C.

LABELLING

The label states:

- the type of interferon (alfa-2a or alfa-2b),
- the type of production.

01/2005:1440
corrected

INTERFERON GAMMA-1b CONCENTRATED SOLUTION

Interferoni gamma-1b solutio concentrata

$C_{734}H_{1166}N_{204}O_{216}S_5$ M_r 16 465

DEFINITION

Interferon gamma-1b concentrated solution is a solution of the *N*-terminal methionyl form of interferon gamma, a protein which is produced and secreted by human antigen-stimulated T lymphocytes in response to viral infections and various other inducers. It has specific immunomodulatory properties, such as potent phagocyte-activating effects. The protein consists of non-covalent dimers of two identical monomers. The formula of the monomer is as follows:

```
                                             M
QDPYVKEAEN  LKKYFNAGHS  DVADNGTLFL  GILKNWKEES
DRKIMQSQIV  SFYFKLFKNF  KDDQSIQKSV  ETIKEDMNVK
FFNSNKKKRD  DFEKLTNYSV  TDLNVQRKAI  HELIQVMAEL
SPAAKTGKRK  RSQMLFRGR
```

The potency of interferon gamma-1b is not less than 20×10^6 IU per milligram of protein. Interferon gamma-1b concentrated solution contains not less than 30×10^6 IU of interferon gamma-1b per millilitre.

PRODUCTION

Interferon gamma-1b concentrated solution is produced by a method based on recombinant DNA technology, using bacteria as host-cells. It is produced under conditions designed to minimise microbial contamination.

Interferon gamma-1b concentrated solution complies with the following additional requirements.

Host-cell derived proteins. The limit is approved by the competent authority.

Host-cell- and vector-derived DNA. The limit is approved by the competent authority.

CHARACTERS

A clear, colourless or slightly yellowish liquid.

IDENTIFICATION

A. It shows the expected biological activity when tested as prescribed in the assay.

B. Examine the electropherograms obtained in the test for impurities of molecular masses differing from that of interferon gamma-1b. The principal bands in the electropherogram obtained with the test solution correspond in position to the principal bands in the electropherogram obtained with reference solution (a).

C. Examine by peptide mapping.

Solution A. Prepare a solution containing 1.2 g/l of *tris(hydroxymethyl)aminomethane R*, 8.2 g/l of *anhydrous sodium acetate R*, 0.02 g/l of *calcium chloride R* and adjust to pH 8.3 (*2.2.3*) with *dilute acetic acid R*. Add *polysorbate 20 R* to a concentration of 0.1 per cent *V/V*.

Test solution. Desalt a volume of the preparation to be examined containing 1 mg of protein by a suitable procedure. For example, filter in a microcentrifuge tube and reconstitute with 500 µl of solution A. Add 10 µl of a freshly prepared 1 mg/ml solution of *trypsin for peptide mapping R* in *water R* and mix gently by inversion. Incubate at 30 °C to 37 °C for 24 h, add 100 µl of *phosphoric acid R* per millilitre of digested sample and mix by inversion.

Reference solution. Dilute *interferon gamma-1b CRS* in *water R* to obtain a concentration of 1 mg/ml. Prepare as for the test solution, ensuring that all procedures are carried out simultaneously and under identical conditions.

Examine by liquid chromatography (*2.2.29*).

The chromatographic procedure may be carried out using:

– a stainless steel column, 0.15 m long and 4.6 mm in internal diameter packed with *octadecylsilyl silica gel for chromatography R* (10 µm),

– as mobile phase at a flow rate of 1.0 ml/min:

Mobile phase A (0.05 M sodium phosphate buffer solution pH 3.3). Solution I: dissolve 7.80 g of *sodium dihydrogen phosphate R* in *water R* and dilute to 1000.0 ml with the same solvent. Solution II: dilute 0.33 ml of *phosphoric acid R* to 100.0 ml with *water R*. Mix 920 ml of solution I and 80 ml of solution II. Adjust the pH (*2.2.3*) if necessary,

Mobile phase B. Acetonitrile for chromatography R,

with the following elution conditions (if necessary, the gradient may be modified to improve the separation of the digest):

Time (min)	Mobile phase A (per cent *V/V*)	Mobile phase B (per cent *V/V*)
0 - 30	100 → 80	0 → 20
30 - 50	80 → 60	20 → 40
50 - 51	60 → 30	40 → 70
51 - 59	30	70
59 - 60	30 → 100	70 → 0

– as detector a spectrophotometer set at 214 nm,

maintaining the temperature of the column at 40 °C.

Equilibrate the column for at least 15 min at the initial elution composition. Carry out a blank run using the above-mentioned gradient.

Inject 100 µl of the test solution and 100 µl of the reference solution. The test is not valid unless the chromatogram obtained with each solution is qualitatively similar to the chromatogram of interferon gamma-1b digest supplied with *interferon gamma-1b CRS*. The profile of the chromatogram obtained with the test solution corresponds to that of the chromatogram obtained with the reference solution.

D. Examine by *N*-terminal sequence analysis.

Use an automated solid-phase sequencer, operated in accordance with the manufacturer's instructions.

Equilibrate by a suitable procedure the equivalent of 100 µg of interferon gamma-1b in a 10 g/l solution of *ammonium hydrogen carbonate R*, pH 9.0.

Identify the phenylthiohydantoin (PTH)-amino acids released at each sequencing cycle by reverse-phase liquid chromatography. The procedure may be carried out using the column and reagents recommended by the manufacturer of the sequencing equipment for the separation of PTH-amino acids.

The separation procedure is calibrated using:

– the mixture of PTH-amino acids provided by the manufacturer, with the gradient conditions adjusted as indicated to achieve optimum resolution of all amino acids,

– a sample from a blank sequencing cycle, obtained as recommended by the equipment manufacturer.

The first fifteen amino acids are:

Met-Gln-Asp-Pro-Tyr-Val-Lys-Glu-Ala-Glu-Asn-Leu-Lys-Lys-Tyr.

TESTS

Appearance. The preparation to be examined is clear (*2.2.1*) and not more intensely coloured than reference solution Y_7 (*2.2.2, Method II*).

pH (*2.2.3*). The pH of the preparation to be examined is 4.5 to 5.5.

Covalent dimers and oligomers. Not greater than 2 per cent, determined by size-exclusion chromatography (*2.2.30*).

Test solution. Dilute the preparation to be examined with the mobile phase to a protein concentration of 0.1 mg/ml.

Reference solution (a). Dilute *interferon gamma-1b CRS* with the mobile phase to a protein concentration of 0.1 mg/ml.

Reference solution (b). Prepare a mixture of the following molecular mass standards: bovine albumin, ovalbumin, trypsinogen, lysozyme, at a concentration of 0.1 mg/ml to 0.2 mg/ml for each standard.

The chromatographic procedure may be carried out using:

– a stainless steel column 0.3 m long and 7.8 mm in internal diameter packed with *hydrophilic silica gel for chromatography R*, of a grade suitable for fractionation of globular proteins in the molecular weight range of 10 000 to 500 000 (5 µm),

– as mobile phase at a flow rate of 1.0 ml/min a mixture prepared as follows (0.2 M sodium phosphate buffer solution pH 6.8). Solution I: dissolve 31.2 g of *sodium dihydrogen phosphate R* and 1.0 g of *sodium dodecyl sulphate R* in *water R* and dilute to 1000.0 ml with the same solvent. Solution II: dissolve 28.4 g of *anhydrous disodium hydrogen phosphate R* and 1.0 g of *sodium dodecyl sulphate R* in *water R* and dilute to 1000.0 ml with the same solvent. Mix 450 ml of solution I and 550 ml of solution II. Adjust the pH (*2.2.3*) if necessary,

– as detector a spectrophotometer set at 210 nm to 214 nm.

Inject 200 µl of each solution. The test is not valid unless: the molecular mass standards in reference solution (b) are well separated; the retention time of the principal peak in the chromatogram obtained with reference solution (a) is between the retention time of trypsinogen and lysozyme in the chromatogram obtained with reference solution (b).

Compare the chromatograms obtained with the test solution and with reference solution (a). There are no additional shoulders or peaks in the chromatogram obtained with the test solution compared with the chromatogram obtained with reference solution (a).

Calculate the percentage content of covalent dimers and oligomers.

Monomer and aggregates. Examine by size-exclusion chromatography (*2.2.30*). The content of monomer and aggregates is not greater than 2 per cent.

Solution A. Prepare a solution of the following composition: 0.59 g/l of *succinic acid R* and 40 g/l of *mannitol R*, adjusted to pH 5.0 (*2.2.3*) with *sodium hydroxide solution R.*

Test solution. Dilute the preparation to be examined with solution A to a protein concentration of 1 mg/ml.

Reference solution. Dilute *interferon gamma-1b CRS* with solution A to a protein concentration of 1 mg/ml.

Resolution solution. Prepare 500 µl of a mixture consisting of 0.04 mg/ml of *bovine albumin R* and 0.2 mg/ml of *interferon gamma-1b CRS* in solution A. Use this solution within 24 h of preparation.

The chromatographic procedure may be carried out using:

– a stainless steel column 0.3 m long and 7.8 mm in internal diameter packed with *hydrophilic silica gel for chromatography R*, of a grade suitable for fractionation of globular proteins in the molecular weight range of 10 000 - 300 000 (5 µm),

– as mobile phase at a flow rate of 0.8 ml/min a 89.5 g/l solution of *potassium chloride R* (1.2 M),

– as detector a spectrophotometer set at 214 nm.

Inject 20 µl of the resolution solution. In the chromatogram obtained, the retention time of the principal peak, corresponding to the native interferon gamma-1b dimer, is about 10 min. bovine albumin elutes at a relative retention time of about 0.85, relative to the main peak. The test is not valid unless the resolution between the peaks corresponding to bovine albumin and interferon gamma-1b is at least 1.5.

Inject 20 µl of the test solution and 20 µl of the reference solution. The chromatograms obtained show principal peaks with identical retention times. Calculate the percentage content of monomer and aggregates from the peak area of the monomer peak and of peaks which elute prior to the native interferon gamma-1b peak in the chromatogram obtained with the test solution, by the normalisation procedure, disregarding any peak due to the solvent.

Deamidated and oxidised forms and heterodimers. Examine by liquid chromatography (*2.2.29*). The content of deamidated and oxidised forms is not greater than 10 per cent. The content of heterodimers is not greater than 3 per cent.

Test solution. Dilute the preparation to be examined with *water R* to a protein concentration of 1 mg/ml.

Reference solution. Dilute *interferon gamma-1b CRS* with *water R* to a protein concentration of 1 mg/ml.

Resolution solution. Use *interferon gamma-1b validation solution CRS.*

The chromatographic procedure may be carried out using:

– a stainless steel column 0.075 m long and 7.5 mm in internal diameter packed with an appropriate hydrophilic polymethacrylate, strong cation exchange gel (10 µm, 100 nm),

– as mobile phase at a flow rate of 1.2 ml/min:

Mobile phase A (0.05 M ammonium acetate buffer pH 6.5). A 3.86 g/l solution of *ammonium acetate R*, adjusted to pH 6.5 with *dilute acetic acid R*,

Mobile phase B (1.2 M ammonium acetate buffer pH 6.5). A 92.5 g/l solution of *ammonium acetate R*, adjusted to pH 6.5 with *dilute acetic acid R*,

with the following elution conditions (if necessary, the slope of the gradient may be modified to improve the separation).

Time (min)	Mobile phase A (per cent *V/V*)	Mobile phase B (per cent *V/V*)
0 - 1	100	0
2 - 30	100 → 0	0 → 100
31 - 35	0	100
36 - 37	0 → 100	100 → 0
38 - 47	100	0

– as detector a spectrophotometer set at 280 nm,

maintaining the temperature of the column at 35 °C.

Inject 25 µl of the resolution solution. In the chromatogram obtained, the retention time of the principal peak is about 26 min. Deamidated and oxidised forms co-elute at a relative retention time of about 0.95, relative to the principal peak. The test is not valid unless the resolution, defined by the ratio of the height of the peak corresponding to the deamidated and oxidised forms to the height above the baseline of the valley separating the two peaks, is at least 1.2.

Inject 25 µl of the test solution and 25 µl of the reference solution. The chromatograms obtained show principal peaks with identical retention times. Calculate the percentage content of deamidated and oxidised interferon gamma-1b as a percentage of the area of the main peak. Heterodimers have relative retention times of 0.7 and 0.85 relative to the main peak. Calculate the percentage of heterodimers as a percentage of the sum of the areas of all peaks.

Impurities of molecular masses differing from that of interferon gamma-1b. Examine by polyacrylamide gel electrophoresis (*2.2.31*). The test is performed under both reducing and non-reducing conditions, using resolving gels of 15 per cent acrylamide and silver staining as the detection method.

Sample buffer (non-reducing conditions). Dissolve 3.78 g of *tris(hydroxymethyl)aminomethane R*, 10.0 g of *sodium dodecyl sulphate R* and 0.100 g of *bromophenol blue R* in *water R*. Add 50.0 ml of *glycerol R* and dilute to 80 ml with *water R*. Adjust the pH (*2.2.3*) to 6.8 with *hydrochloric acid R* and dilute to 100 ml with *water R*.

Sample buffer (reducing conditions). Dissolve 3.78 g of *tris(hydroxymethyl)aminomethane R*, 10.0 g of *sodium dodecyl sulphate R* and 0.100 g of *bromophenol blue R* in *water R*. Add 50.0 ml of *glycerol R* and dilute to 80 ml with *water R*. Adjust the pH (*2.2.3*) to 6.8 with *hydrochloric acid R* and dilute to 100 ml with *water R*. Immediately before use, add *dithiothreitol R* to a final concentration of 250 mM.

Test solution. Dilute the preparation to be examined in *water R* to a protein concentration of 1 mg/ml. Dilute 150 µl of the solution with 38 µl of sample buffer.

Reference solution (a). Prepare in the same manner as for the test solution, but using *interferon gamma-1b CRS* instead of the preparation to be examined.

Reference solution (b) (5 ng control). Mix 50 µl of a 0.01 mg/ml solution of *bovine albumin R* with 2000 µl of *water R* and 450 µl of sample buffer.

Reference solution (c) (2 ng control). Mix 20 µl of a 0.01 mg/ml solution of *bovine albumin R* with 2000 µl of *water R* and 450 µl of sample buffer.

Reference solution (d). Use a solution of molecular mass standards suitable for calibrating SDS-polyacrylamide gels in the range of 10 kDa to 70 kDa.

Leave each solution, contained in a test tube, at ambient temperature for 15 min, then store on ice.

Apply 25 µl of each solution to the stacking gel wells. Perform the electrophoresis under the conditions recommended by the manufacturer of the equipment. Detect proteins in the gel by silver staining.

The test is not valid unless: the validation criteria are met (*2.2.31*); a band is seen in the electropherograms obtained with reference solutions (b) and (c).

The principal band in the electropherogram obtained with the test solution is similar in intensity to the principal band in the electropherogram obtained with reference solution (a). In the electropherogram obtained with the test solution, no significant bands are observed that are not present in the electropherogram obtained with reference solution (a) (0.01 per cent). A significant band is defined as any band whose intensity is greater than or equal to that of the band in the electropherogram obtained with reference solution (c).

Norleucine. Not more than 0.2 mole of norleucine per mole of interferon gamma-1b, determined by amino acid analysis.

Test solution. Add 2.5 ml of the preparation to be examined onto a column suitable for the desalting of proteins previously equilibrated with 25 ml of a 10 per cent *V/V* solution of *acetic acid R*. Elute the sample with another 2.5 ml of a 10 per cent *V/V* solution of *acetic acid R*. Determine the protein content by measuring the absorbance of this solution as described under Protein, in the Assay section. Pipette a volume containing the equivalent of 100 µg of interferon gamma-1b into each of three reaction vials. Evaporate to dryness under reduced pressure.

Perform the hydrolysis of the three samples as follows. Add to each reaction vial 200 µl of a 50 per cent *V/V* solution of *hydrochloric acid R* containing 1 per cent *V/V* of *phenol R*, evacuate the samples, purge with nitrogen and hydrolyse in the gas phase. Heat the reaction vials at 110 °C for 22 h. After hydrolysis evaporate to dryness under reduced pressure.

Perform the derivatisation of the samples as follows. Prepare immediately before use a mixture consisting of two volumes of *ethanol R*, one volume of *water R* and one volume of *triethylamine R*. Add 50 µl of this solution to each reaction vial and shake lightly. Evaporate to dryness under reduced pressure. Add to each vial 50 µl of a mixture consisting of 7 volumes of *ethanol R*, one volume of *water R*, one volume of *triethylamine R* and one volume of *phenyl isothiocyanate R*. Shake lightly and allow to stand at room temperature for about 15 min. Evaporate to dryness under reduced pressure. Reconstitute the samples in 250 µl of mobile phase A.

Norleucine stock solution. Prepare a 250 nmol/ml solution of *DL-norleucine R* in *0.01 M hydrochloric acid. This solution may be kept for two months at 4 °C.*

Leucine stock solution. Prepare a 250 nmol/ml solution of *leucine R* in *0.01 M hydrochloric acid. This solution may be kept at 4 °C for two months.*

Reference solution. Mix 10 µl of norleucine stock solution with 100 µl of leucine stock solution in each of the three reaction vials. Evaporate to dryness under reduced pressure. Perform the derivatisation of the samples as described for the preparation of the test solution.

Examine by liquid chromatography (*2.2.29*).

The chromatographic procedure may be carried out using:

– a stainless steel column 0.15 m long and 3.9 mm in diameter packed with *octadecylsilyl silica gel for chromatography R* (4 µm),

– as mobile phase at a flow rate of 1.0 ml/min:

Mobile phase A. Mix 70 volumes of a 19 g/l solution of *sodium acetate R* containing 0.05 per cent *V/V* of *triethylamine R* and adjusted to pH 6.4 with *dilute acetic acid R* and 30 volumes of mobile phase B,

Mobile phase B. Mix 40 volumes of *water R* and 60 volumes of *acetonitrile R*,

Time (min)	Mobile phase A (per cent *V/V*)	Mobile phase B (per cent *V/V*)	Comment
0 - 7	100	0	isocratic
7 - 7.1	100 → 0	0 → 100	linear gradient
7.1 - 10	0	100	washing step
10 - 10.1	0 → 100	100 → 0	linear gradient
10.1 - 15	100	0	re-equilibration

– as detector a spectrophotometer set at 254 nm, maintaining the temperature of the column at 43 °C.

Inject 50 µl of each solution.

In the chromatograms obtained with the test solution, identify the peaks corresponding to leucine and norleucine. The retention time of norleucine is 6.2 min to 7 min.

Calculate the content of norleucine (in moles of norleucine per mole of interferon gamma-1b) from the peak areas of leucine and norleucine in the chromatograms obtained with the reference and test solutions, considering that there are 10 moles of leucine per mole of interferon gamma-1b.

Bacterial endotoxins (*2.6.14*): less than 5 IU in the volume that contains 20 × 10^6 IU of interferon gamma-1b.

ASSAY

Protein (*2.2.25*). Dilute the substance to be examined in *water R* to obtain a concentration of 1 mg/ml. Record the absorbance spectrum between 220 nm and 340 nm. Measure the value at the absorbance maximum of 280 nm, after correction for any light scattering due to turbidity measured at 316 nm. Calculate the concentration of interferon gamma-1b using a specific absorbance value of 7.5.

Potency. The potency of interferon gamma-1b is estimated by evaluating the increase of the expression of human-leukocyte-antigen-DR (HLA-DR) due to the interferon gamma-1b present in test solutions during cultivation of the cells, and comparing this increase with the same effect of the appropriate International Standard of human recombinant interferon gamma or of a reference preparation calibrated in International Units.

The International Unit is the activity contained in a stated amount of the appropriate International Standard. The equivalence in International Units of the International Standard is stated by the World Health Organisation.

Carry out the assay by a suitable method, based on the following design.

Use COLO 205 cells under standard culture conditions. Trypsinise a 3- to 5-day-old flask of COLO 205 cells and prepare a cell suspension at a concentration of 1.0 × 10^6 cells/ml.

Add 100 µl of the dilution medium to all wells of a 96-well microtitre plate. Add an additional 100 µl of this solution to the wells designed for the blanks. Add 100 µl of each solution to be tested onto the plate and carry out a series of twofold dilution steps in order to obtain a standard curve. Then add 100 µl of the cell suspension to all wells and incubate the plate under appropriate conditions for cell cultivation.

After cultivation remove the growth medium and wash and fix cells to the plate. Add an antibody able to detect HLA-DR expressed due to the presence of interferon gamma-1b and incubate under appropriate conditions. After washing the plate, incubate with an antibody conjugated to a marker enzyme which is able to detect the anti-HLA-DR antibody. After this incubation step, wash the plate and add an appropriate substrate solution. Stop the reaction. Measure the absorbance of the solution and calculate the potency of the preparation to be examined by the usual statistical methods.

The estimated specific activity is not less than 80 per cent and not more than 125 per cent of the stated potency. The confidence limits (P = 0.95) are not less than 70 per cent and not more than 140 per cent of the estimated potency.

STORAGE

Store in an airtight container, protected from light and at a temperature of − 70 °C.

01/2005:0031

IODINE

Iodum

I_2 M_r 253.8

DEFINITION

Iodine contains not less than 99.5 per cent and not more than the equivalent of 100.5 per cent of I.

CHARACTERS

Greyish-violet, brittle plates or fine crystals with a metallic sheen, very slightly soluble in water, soluble in alcohol, slightly soluble in glycerol, very soluble in concentrated solutions of iodides. Iodine volatilises slowly at room temperature.

IDENTIFICATION

A. Heat a few fragments in a test-tube. Violet vapour is evolved and a bluish-black crystalline sublimate is formed.

B. To a saturated solution add *starch solution R*. A blue colour is produced. Heat until decolourised. On cooling, the colour reappears.

TESTS

Solution S. Triturate 3.0 g with 20 ml of *water R*, filter, wash the filter with *water R* and dilute the filtrate to 30 ml with the same solvent. To the solution add 1 g of *zinc powder R*. When the solution is decolourised, filter, wash the filter with *water R* and dilute to 40 ml with the same solvent.

Bromides and chlorides. To 10 ml of solution S add 3 ml of *ammonia R* and 6 ml of *silver nitrate solution R2*. Filter, wash the filter with *water R* and dilute the filtrate to 20 ml with the same solvent. To 10 ml of the solution add 1.5 ml of *nitric acid R*. After 1 min, any opalescence in the solution is not more intense than that in a standard prepared at the same time by mixing 10.75 ml of *water R*, 0.25 ml of *0.01 M hydrochloric acid*, 0.2 ml of *dilute nitric acid R* and 0.3 ml of *silver nitrate solution R2* (250 ppm).

Non-volatile substances. Heat 1.00 g in a porcelain dish on a water-bath until the iodine has volatilised. Dry the residue at 100 °C to 105 °C. The residue weighs not more than 1 mg (0.1 per cent).

ASSAY

Introduce 0.200 g into a flask containing 1 g of *potassium iodide R* and 2 ml of *water R* and add 1 ml of *dilute acetic acid R*. When dissolution is complete, add 50 ml of *water R* and titrate with *0.1 M sodium thiosulphate*, using *starch solution R* as indicator.

1 ml of *0.1 M sodium thiosulphate* is equivalent to 12.69 mg of I.

01/2005:1114

IOHEXOL

Iohexolum

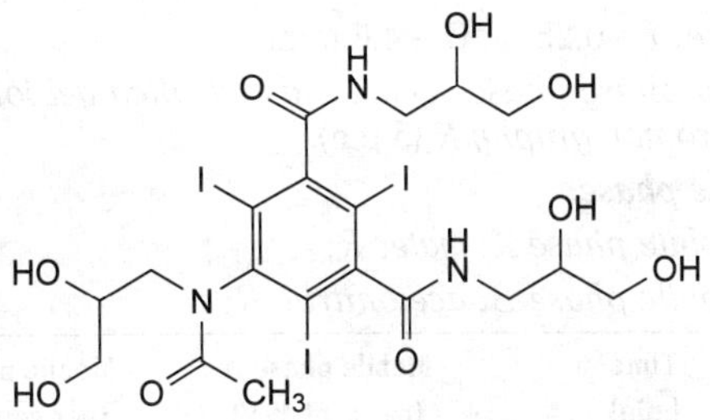

$C_{19}H_{26}I_3N_3O_9$ M_r 821

DEFINITION

5-[Acetyl(2,3-dihydroxypropyl)amino]-*N*,*N'*-bis(2,3-dihydroxypropyl)-2,4,6-triiodobenzene-1,3-dicarboxamide.

The substance is a mixture of diastereoisomers and atropisomers.

Content: 98.0 per cent to 101.0 per cent (anhydrous substance).

CHARACTERS

Appearance: white or greyish-white, hygroscopic powder.

Solubility: very soluble in water, freely soluble in methanol, practically insoluble in methylene chloride.

IDENTIFICATION

A. Infrared absorption spectrophotometry (*2.2.24*).

Comparison: *iohexol CRS*.

B. Examine the chromatograms obtained in test A for related substances (see Tests).

Results: the principal peaks in the chromatogram obtained with reference solution (b) are similar in retention time and size to the peaks due to iohexol in the chromatogram obtained with reference solution (a).

TESTS

Solution S. Dissolve 5.0 g in *water R* and dilute to 50.0 ml with the same solvent.

Appearance of solution. Solution S is clear (*2.2.1*) and not more intensely coloured than reference solution Y_7 (*2.2.2, Method II*).

Related substances

A. Liquid chromatography (*2.2.29*).

NOTE: iohexol gives rise to 2 non-resolved peaks in the chromatogram due to endo-exo isomerism. In addition, a small peak (also due to iohexol) usually appears at the leading edge of the 1st principal peak. This small peak has a retention time about 1.2 min less than the 1st principal peak.

Test solution. Dissolve 0.150 g of the substance to be examined in *water R* and dilute to 100.0 ml with the same solvent.

Reference solution (a). Dissolve 15.0 mg of *iohexol CRS* and 15.0 mg of *iohexol impurity A CRS* in a mixture of 1-2 drops of *dilute sodium hydroxide solution R* and 10 ml of *water R* and dilute to 100.0 ml with *water R*. Dilute 1.0 ml of this solution to 10.0 ml with *water R*.

Reference solution (b). Dilute 1.0 ml of the test solution to 100.0 ml with *water R*.

Reference solution (c). Dissolve 5.0 mg of *iohexol for peak identification CRS* (containing impurities B, C, D and E) in *water R* and dilute to 5.0 ml with the same solvent.

Blank solution: *water R.*

Column:

- *size*: *l* = 0.25 m, Ø = 4.6 mm,
- *stationary phase*: *octadecylsilyl silica gel for chromatography R* (5 µm).

Mobile phase:

- *mobile phase A*: *water R;*
- *mobile phase B*: *acetonitrile R;*

Time (min)	Mobile phase A (per cent *V/V*)	Mobile phase B (per cent *V/V*)
0 - 60	99 → 87	1 → 13
60 - 65	87 → 99	13 → 1

Flow rate: 1 ml/min.

Detection: spectrophotometer at 254 nm.

Equilibration: at the initial eluent composition for at least 10 min.

Injection: 10 µl.

Retention times: impurity A and impurity H = about 17 min; iohexol (peaks corresponding to *endo-exo* isomerism) = about 20 min.

System suitability: reference solution (a):

- *resolution*: minimum 5.0 between the peak due to impurity A and the 2nd and greater peak due to iohexol.

Limits:

- *sum of impurities B, C, D and E* (relative retention with reference to the 2nd and greater peak due to iohexol between 1.1 and 1.4): not more than 0.6 times the total area of the principal peaks in the chromatogram obtained with reference solution (b) (0.6 per cent); use the chromatogram obtained with reference solution (c) to identify the corresponding peaks;
- *sum of impurities A and H*: not more than 0.5 times the total area of the principal peaks in the chromatogram obtained with reference solution (b) (0.5 per cent);
- *impurities M, N, O, P, Q*: for each impurity, not more than 0.1 times the total area of the principal peaks in the chromatogram obtained with reference solution (b) (0.1 per cent);
- *any other impurity*: for each impurity, not more than 0.1 times the total area of the principal peaks in the chromatogram obtained with reference solution (b) (0.1 per cent);
- *total*: not more than 1.5 times the total area of the principal peaks in the chromatogram obtained with reference solution (b) (1.5 per cent);
- *disregard limit*: 0.03 times the total area of the principal peaks in the chromatogram obtained with reference solution (b) (0.03 per cent); disregard any peak observed with the blank.

B. Thin-layer chromatography (*2.2.27*).

Test solution. Dissolve 1.0 g of the substance to be examined in *water R* and dilute to 10.0 ml with the same solvent.

Reference solution (a). Dissolve 50 mg of *iohexol impurity J CRS* and 50 mg of *iohexol CRS* in *water R* and dilute to 10.0 ml with the same solvent.

Reference solution (b). Dilute 1.0 ml of the test solution to 10.0 ml with *water R.* Dilute 1.0 ml of this solution to 50.0 ml with *water R.*

Plate: *TLC silica gel F_{254} plate R.*

Preconditioning: wash the plate with the mobile phase, dry at room temperature for 30 min, then at 90 °C for 1 h.

Mobile phase: *concentrated ammonia R, methanol R, 2-propanol R, acetone R* (16:16:28:40 *V/V/V/V*).

Application: 10 µl.

Development: over half of the plate.

Drying: in air.

Detection: examine in ultraviolet light at 254 nm.

System suitability: reference solution (a):

- the chromatogram shows 2 clearly separated spots.

Limits:

- *any impurity*: any spot in the chromatogram obtained with the test solution, apart from the principal spot, is not more intense than the spot in the chromatogram obtained with reference solution (b) (0.2 per cent).

3-Chloropropane-1,2-diol. Gas chromatography (*2.2.28*).

Test solution. Dissolve 1.0 g of the substance to be examined in 1.0 ml of *water R.* Shake with 4 quantities, each of 2 ml, of *methyl acetate R.* Dry the combined upper layers over *anhydrous sodium sulphate R.* Filter and concentrate to about 0.7 ml using a warm water bath at 60 °C and a stream of nitrogen and dilute to 1.0 ml with *methyl acetate R.*

Reference solution. Dissolve 0.25 g of *3-chloropropane-1,2-diol R* in 100.0 ml of *methyl acetate R.* Dilute 1.0 ml of this solution with 100.0 ml of *methyl acetate R.*

Column:

- *material*: fused silica,
- *size*: *l* = 25 m, Ø = 0.33 mm,
- *stationary phase*: *polymethylphenylsiloxane R* (film thickness 1 µm).

Carrier gas: *helium for chromatography R.*

Flow rate: 1 ml/min.

Temperature:

	Time (min)	Temperature (°C)
Column	0 - 2	80
	2 - 8	80 → 170
	8 - 10	170
Injection port		230
Detector		250

Detection: flame ionisation.

Injection: 2 µl (splitless for 30 s).

System suitability: reference solution:

- *retention time*: 3-chloropropane-1,2-diol = about 8 min.

Limit:

- *3-chloropropane-1,2-diol*: not more than the area of the principal peak in the chromatogram obtained with the reference solution (25 ppm).

Free aromatic amine: maximum 500 ppm.

Test solution. Transfer 0.200 g of the substance to be examined to a 25 ml volumetric flask and dissolve in 15.0 ml of *water R.*

Reference solution. Dissolve 5.0 mg of *iohexol impurity J CRS* in *water R* and dilute to 5.0 ml with *water R.* Dilute 1.0 ml of this solution to 100.0 ml with *water R.* Mix 10.0 ml of this solution with 5.0 ml of *water R* in a 25 ml volumetric flask.

Blank solution. Transfer 15.0 ml of *water R* to a 25 ml volumetric flask.

In conducting the following steps, keep the flasks in iced water and protected as much as possible from light until all of the reagents have been added.

Place the 3 flasks containing respectively the test solution, the reference solution and the blank solution in iced water, protected from light, for 5 min. Add 1.5 ml of *hydrochloric acid R1* and mix by swirling. Add 1.0 ml of a 20 g/l solution of *sodium nitrite R*, mix and allow to stand for 4 min. Add 1.0 ml of a 40 g/l solution of *sulphamic acid R*, swirl gently until gas liberation has ceased and allow to stand for 1 min. *(CAUTION: considerable pressure is produced).* Add 1.0 ml of a freshly prepared 3 g/l solution of *naphthylethylenediamine dihydrochloride R* in a mixture of 30 volumes of *water R* and 70 volumes of *propylene glycol R* and mix. Remove the flasks from the iced water, dilute to 25.0 ml with *water R*, mix and allow to stand for 5 min. Simultaneously determine the absorbance (*2.2.25*) at 495 nm of the solutions obtained from the test solution and the reference solution in 5 cm cells, using the blank as the compensation liquid. The absorbance of the test solution is not greater than that of the reference solution.

Iodide: maximum 10 ppm.

Dissolve 6.000 g in *water R* and dilute to 20 ml with the same solvent. Add 2.0 ml of *0.001 M potassium iodide.* Titrate with *0.001 M silver nitrate.* Determine the end-point potentiometrically (*2.2.20*), using a silver indicator electrode and an appropriate reference electrode. Subtract the volume of titrant corresponding to the 2.0 ml of *0.001 M potassium iodide,* determined by titrating a blank to which is added 2.0 ml of *0.001 M potassium iodide* and use the residual value to calculate the iodide content.

1 ml of *0.001 M silver nitrate* is equivalent to 126.9 µg of I^-.

Ionic compounds (*2.2.38*): maximum 0.01 per cent *m/m* calculated as sodium chloride.

Rinse all glassware with distilled water R 5 times before use.

Test solution. Dissolve 1.0 g of the substance to be examined in *water R* and dilute to 50.0 ml with the same solvent.

Reference solution. Dissolve 20.0 mg of *sodium chloride R* in *water R* and dilute to 100.0 ml with the same solvent. Dilute 1.0 ml of this solution to 100.0 ml with *water R.*

Measure the conductivity of the test solution and the reference solution using a suitable conductivity meter. The conductivity of the test solution is not greater than that of the reference solution.

Heavy metals (*2.4.8*): maximum 10 ppm.

12 ml of solution S complies with limit test A. Prepare the reference solution using *lead standard solution (1 ppm Pb) R.*

Water (*2.5.12*): maximum 4.0 per cent, determined on 1.00 g.

ASSAY

To 0.500 g in a 125 ml round-bottomed flask add 25 ml of a 50 g/l solution of *sodium hydroxide R,* 0.5 g of *zinc powder R* and a few glass beads. Boil under a reflux condenser for 30 min. Allow to cool and rinse the condenser with 20 ml of *water R,* adding the rinsings to the flask. Filter through a sintered-glass filter and wash the filter with several quantities of *water R.* Collect the filtrate and washings. Add 5 ml of *glacial acetic acid R* and titrate immediately with *0.1 M silver nitrate.* Determine the end-point potentiometrically (*2.2.20*).

1 ml of *0.1 M silver nitrate* is equivalent to 27.37 mg of $C_{19}H_{26}I_3N_3O_9$.

STORAGE

In an airtight container, protected from light and moisture.

IMPURITIES

Specified impurities: A, B, C, D, E, F, G, H, I, J, K, L, M, N, O, P, Q.

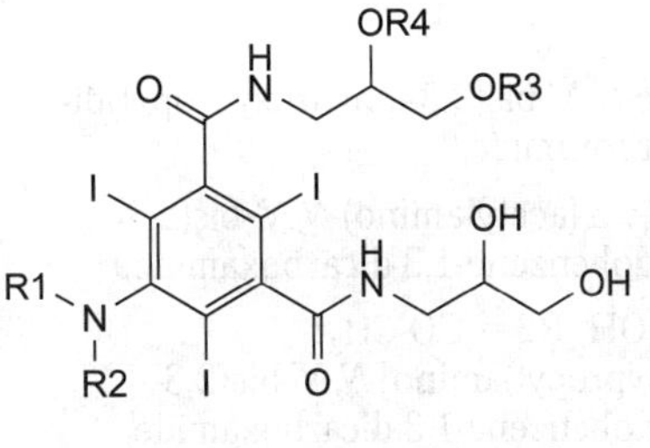

A. R1 = $CO\text{-}CH_3$, R2 = R3 = R4 = H: 5-(acetylamino)-*N*,*N'*-bis(2,3-dihydroxypropyl)-2,4,6-triiodobenzene-1,3-dicarboxamide,

J. R1 = R2 = R3 = R4 = H: 5-amino-*N*,*N'*-bis(2,3-dihydroxypropyl)-2,4,6-triiodobenzene-1,3-dicarboxamide,

P. R1 = R2 = $CO\text{-}CH_3$, R3 = $CH_2\text{-}CHOH\text{-}CH_2OH$, R4 = H: 5-(diacetylamino)-*N*-[3-(2,3-dihydroxypropoxy)-2-hydroxypropyl]-*N'*-(2,3-dihydroxypropyl)-2,4,6-triiodobenzene-1,3-dicarboxamide,

Q. R1 = R2 = $CO\text{-}CH_3$, R3 = H, R4 = $CH_2\text{-}CHOH\text{-}CH_2OH$: 5-(diacetylamino)-*N*-[2-(2,3-dihydroxypropoxy)-3-hydroxypropyl]-*N'*-(2,3-dihydroxypropyl)-2,4,6-triiodobenzene-1,3-dicarboxamide,

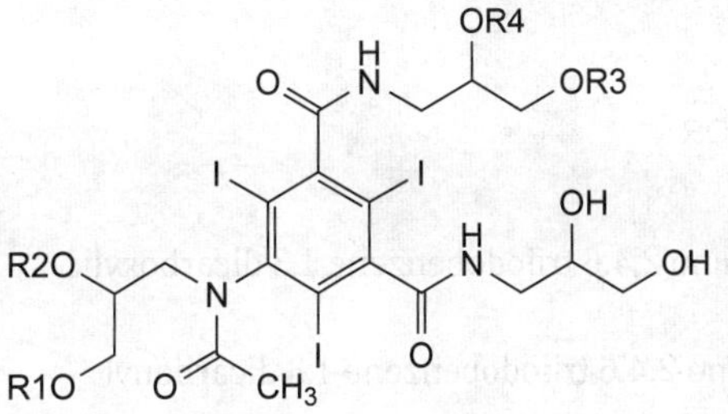

B. R1 = $CH_2\text{-}CHOH\text{-}CH_2OH$, R2 = R3 = R4 = H: 5-[acetyl[3-(2,3-dihydroxypropoxy)-2-hydroxypropyl]amino]-*N*,*N'*-bis(2,3-dihydroxypropyl)-2,4,6-triiodobenzene-1,3-dicarboxamide,

C. R2 = $CH_2\text{-}CHOH\text{-}CH_2OH$, R1 = R3 = R4 = H: 5-[acetyl[2-(2,3-dihydroxypropoxy)-3-hydroxypropyl]amino]-*N*,*N'*-bis(2,3-dihydroxypropyl)-2,4,6-triiodobenzene-1,3-dicarboxamide,

D. R3 = $CH_2\text{-}CHOH\text{-}CH_2OH$, R1 = R2 = R4 = H: 5-[acetyl(2,3-dihydroxypropyl)amino]-*N*-[3-(2,3-dihydroxypropoxy)-2-hydroxypropyl]-*N'*-(2,3-dihydroxypropyl)-2,4,6-triiodobenzene-1,3-dicarboxamide,

E. R4 = $CH_2\text{-}CHOH\text{-}CH_2OH$, R1 = R2 = R3 = H: 5-[acetyl(2,3-dihydroxypropyl)amino]-*N*-[2-(2,3-dihydroxypropoxy)-3-hydroxypropyl]-*N'*-(2,3-dihydroxypropyl)-2,4,6-triiodobenzene-1,3-dicarboxamide,

N. R4 = $CO\text{-}CH_3$, R1 = R2 = R3 = H: 5-[acetyl(2,3-dihydroxypropyl)amino]-*N*-[2-(acetyloxy)-3-hydroxypropyl]-*N'*-(2,3-dihydroxypropyl)-2,4,6-triiodobenzene-1,3-dicarboxamide,

O. R3 = $CO\text{-}CH_3$, R1 = R2 = R4 = H: 5-[acetyl(2,3-dihydroxypropyl)amino]-*N*-[3-(acetyloxy)-2-hydroxypropyl]-*N'*-(2,3-dihydroxypropyl)-2,4,6-triiodobenzene-1,3-dicarboxamide,

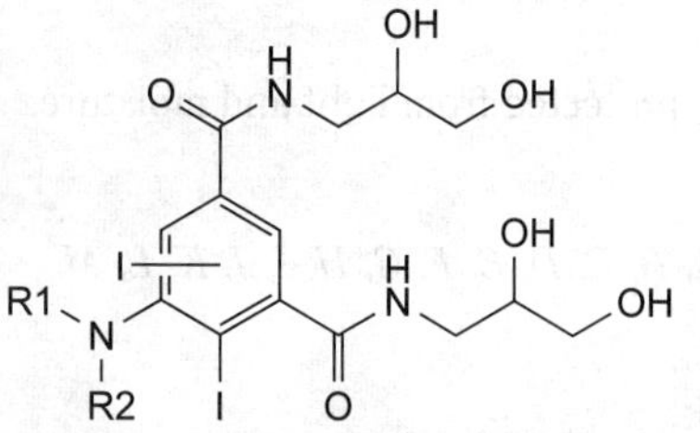

F. R1 = R2 = H: 5-amino-*N,N'*-bis(2,3-dihydroxypropyl)diiodobenzene-1,3-dicarboxamide,

G. R1 = H, R2 = CO-CH_3: 5-(acetylamino)-*N,N'*-bis(2,3-dihydroxypropyl)diiodobenzene-1,3-dicarboxamide,

H. R1 = CH_2-CHOH-CH_2OH, R2 = CO-CH_3: 5-[acetyl(2,3-dihydroxypropyl)amino]-*N,N'*-bis(2,3-dihydroxypropyl)diiodobenzene-1,3-dicarboxamide,

M. R1 = CH_2-CHOH-CH_2OH, R2 = H: *N,N'*-bis(2,3-dihydroxypropyl)-5-[(2,3-dihydroxypropyl)amino]diiodobenzene-1,3-dicarboxamide,

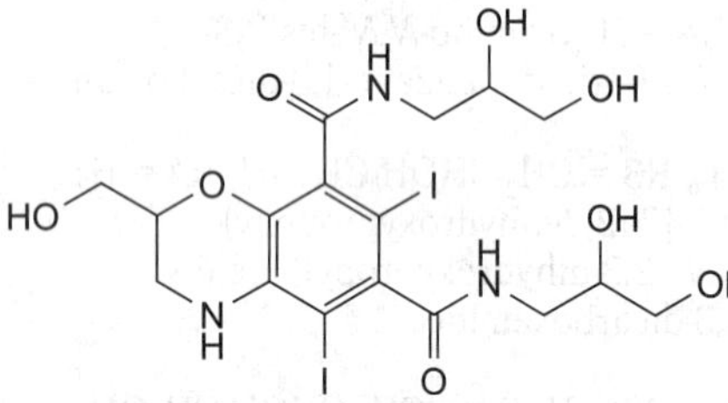

I. *N,N'*-bis(2,3-dihydroxypropyl)-2-(hydroxymethyl)-5,7-diiodo-3,4-dihydro-2*H*-1,4-benzoxazine-6,8-dicarboxamide,

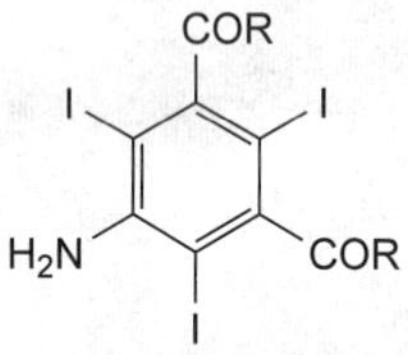

K. R = OH: 5-amino-2,4,6-triiodobenzene-1,3-dicarboxylic acid,

L. R = Cl: 5-amino-2,4,6-triiodobenzene-1,3-dicarbonyl dichloride.

01/2005:1115

IOPAMIDOL

Iopamidolum

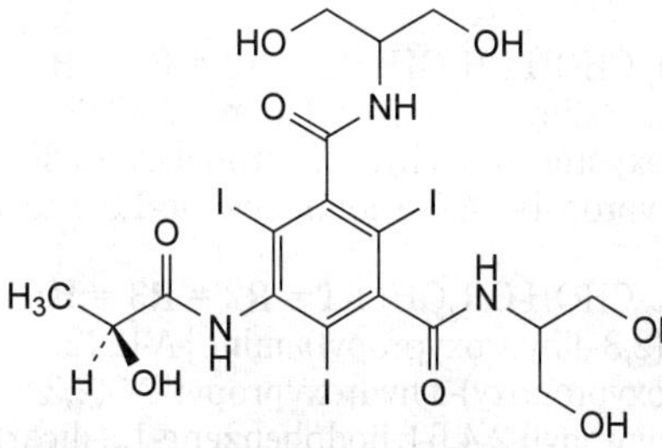

$C_{17}H_{22}I_3N_3O_8$ M_r 777

DEFINITION

N,N'-Bis[2-hydroxy-1-(hydroxymethyl)ethyl]-5-[[(2*S*)-2-hydroxypropanoyl]amino]-2,4,6-triiodobenzene-1,3-dicarboxamide.

Content: 98.5 per cent to 101.0 per cent (dried substance).

CHARACTERS

Appearance: white or almost white powder.

Solubility: freely soluble in water, very slightly soluble in methanol, practically insoluble in ethanol (96 per cent) and in methylene chloride.

IDENTIFICATION

A. Infrared absorption spectrophotometry (*2.2.24*).
Comparison: *iopamidol CRS*.

B. It complies with the test for loss on drying (see Tests).

C. It complies with the test for specific optical rotation (see Tests).

TESTS

Appearance of solution. The solution is clear (*2.2.1*) and colourless (*2.2.2, Method II*).

Dissolve 1 g in *water R* and dilute to 50 ml with the same solvent.

Acidity or alkalinity. Dissolve 10.0 g in *carbon dioxide-free water R* and dilute to 100 ml with the same solvent. Not more than 0.75 ml of *0.01 M hydrochloric acid* or 1.4 ml of *0.01 M sodium hydroxide* is required to adjust to pH 7.0 (*2.2.3*).

Specific optical rotation (*2.2.7*): − 4.6 to − 5.2 (dried substance), determined at 436 nm.

Dissolve 10.0 g, with heating if necessary, in *water R* and dilute to 25.0 ml with the same solvent.

Related substances. Liquid chromatography (*2.2.29*).

Test solution. Dissolve 0.50 g of the substance to be examined in *water R* and dilute to 50.0 ml with the same solvent.

Reference solution (a). Dissolve 5.0 mg of *iopamidol impurity H CRS* in *water R* and dilute to 100.0 ml with the same solvent.

Reference solution (b). Dilute 2.0 ml of the test solution to 20.0 ml with *water R*. Dilute 1.0 ml of this solution to 50.0 ml with *water R*.

Reference solution (c). Add 0.1 ml of the test solution to 20 ml of reference solution (a) and dilute to 50 ml with *water R*.

Column: 2 columns coupled in series,
- *size*: *l* = 0.25 m, Ø = 4.6 mm,
- *stationary phase*: *phenylsilyl silica gel for chromatography R* (5 µm),
- *temperature*: 60 °C.

Mobile phase:
- *mobile phase A*: *water R*,
- *mobile phase B*: *acetonitrile R, water R* (50:50 *V/V*),

Time (min)	Mobile phase A (per cent *V/V*)	Mobile phase B (per cent *V/V*)
0 - 18	100	0
18 - 40	100 - 62	0 - 38
40 - 45	62 - 50	38 - 50
45 - 50	50 - 100	50 - 0
50 - 60	100	0

Flow rate: 2.0 ml/min.

Detection: spectrophotometer at 240 nm.

Injection: 20 µl.

Relative retention with reference to iopamidol (retention time = about 14.6 min): impurity D = about 0.1; impurity B = about 0.6; impurities I and H = about 0.9; impurity G = about 1.1; impurity K = about 1.2; impurity C = about 1.3; impurity J = about 1.5; impurity A = about 1.8; impurity E = about 2.2; impurity F = about 2.3.

System suitability: reference solution (c):

- *resolution*: minimum 2.0 between the peaks due to impurity H and iopamidol.

Limits:

- *sum of impurities H and I*: not more than the area of the principal peak in the chromatogram obtained with reference solution (a) (0.5 per cent),
- *impurities A, B, C, D, E, F, G, J, K*: for each impurity, not more than 0.5 times the area of the principal peak in the chromatogram obtained with reference solution (b) (0.1 per cent),
- *any other impurity*: for each impurity, not more than 0.5 times the area of the principal peak in the chromatogram obtained with reference solution (b) (0.1 per cent),
- *total of other impurities*: not more than the area of the principal peak in the chromatogram obtained with reference solution (b) (0.2 per cent),
- *disregard limit*: 0.05 times the area of the principal peak in the chromatogram obtained with reference solution (b) (0.01 per cent).

Free aromatic amines: maximum 200 ppm.

Keep the solutions and reagents in iced water, protected from bright light.

Test solution. In a 25 ml volumetric flask, dissolve 0.500 g of the substance to be examined in 20.0 ml of *water R*.

Reference solution. In a 25 ml volumetric flask, mix 4.0 ml of a 25.0 mg/l solution of *iopamidol impurity A CRS* with 16.0 ml of *water R*.

Blank solution. Place 20.0 ml of *water R* in a 25 ml volumetric flask.

Place the flasks in iced water, protected from light, for 5 min. Add 1.0 ml of *hydrochloric acid R* to each flask, mix and allow to stand for 5 min. Add 1.0 ml of a 20 g/l solution of *sodium nitrite R* prepared immediately before use, mix and allow to stand for 5 min. Add 1.0 ml of a 120 g/l solution of *ammonium sulphamate R*, swirl gently until gas liberation has ceased, and allow to stand for 5 min. *(CAUTION: considerable pressure is produced).* Add 1.0 ml of a freshly prepared 1 g/l solution of *naphthylethylenediamine dihydrochloride R* and mix. Remove the flasks from the iced water and allow to stand for 10 min. Dilute to 25.0 ml with *water R* and mix. Measure immediately the absorbance (*2.2.25*) at 500 nm of the solutions obtained from the test solution and the reference solution using, as the compensation liquid, the solution obtained from the blank solution.

The absorbance of the test solution is not greater than that of the reference solution.

Free iodine: maximum 10 ppm.

Dissolve 2.0 g in 25 ml of *water R* in a ground-glass stoppered centrifuge tube. Add 5 ml of *toluene R* and 5 ml of *diluted sulphuric acid R*. Shake and centrifuge. Any red colour of the upper layer is not more intense than that of the upper phase obtained in the same way from 22 ml of *water R*, 2 ml of *iodide standard solution (10 ppm I) R*, 5 ml of *dilute sulphuric acid R*, 1 ml of *concentrated hydrogen peroxide solution R* and 5 ml of *toluene R*.

Iodide: maximum 10 ppm.

Dissolve 6.000 g in *water R* and dilute to 20 ml with the same solvent. Add 2.0 ml of *0.001 M potassium iodide*. Carry out a potentiometric titration (*2.2.20*) with *0.001 M silver nitrate* using a silver indicator electrode and an appropriate reference electrode. Subtract the volume of titrant corresponding to the 2.0 ml of *0.001 M potassium iodide*, determined by titrating a blank to which is added 2.0 ml of *0.001 M potassium iodide* and use the residual value to calculate the iodide content.

1 ml of *0.001 M silver nitrate* is equivalent to 126.9 μg of iodide.

Heavy metals (*2.4.8*): maximum 10 ppm.

2.0 g complies with limit test C. Prepare the reference solution using 2 ml of *lead standard solution (10 ppm Pb) R*.

Loss on drying (*2.2.32*): maximum 0.5 per cent, determined on 1.000 g by drying in an oven at 100-105 °C.

Sulphated ash (*2.4.14*): maximum 0.1 per cent, determined on 1.0 g.

Bacterial endotoxins (*2.6.14*): less than 1.4 IU/g, if intended for use in the manufacture of parenteral dosage forms without a further appropriate procedure for the removal of bacterial endotoxins.

ASSAY

To 0.300 g in a 250 ml round-bottomed flask add 5 ml of *strong sodium hydroxide solution R*, 20 ml of *water R*, 1 g of *zinc powder R* and a few glass beads. Boil under a reflux condenser for 30 min. Allow to cool and rinse the condenser with 20 ml of *water R*, adding the rinsings to the flask. Filter through a sintered-glass filter and wash the filter with several quantities of *water R*. Collect the filtrate and washings. Add 5 ml of *glacial acetic acid R* and titrate immediately with *0.1 M silver nitrate*. Determine the end-point potentiometrically (*2.2.20*) using a suitable electrode system such as silver-silver chloride.

1 ml of *0.1 M silver nitrate* is equivalent to 25.90 mg of $C_{17}H_{22}I_3N_3O_8$.

STORAGE

Protected from light. If the substance is sterile, store in a sterile, airtight, tamper-proof container.

LABELLING

The label states, where applicable, that the substance is free from bacterial endotoxins.

IMPURITIES

Specified impurities: A, B, C, D, E, F, G, H, I, J, K.

Monographs I-L

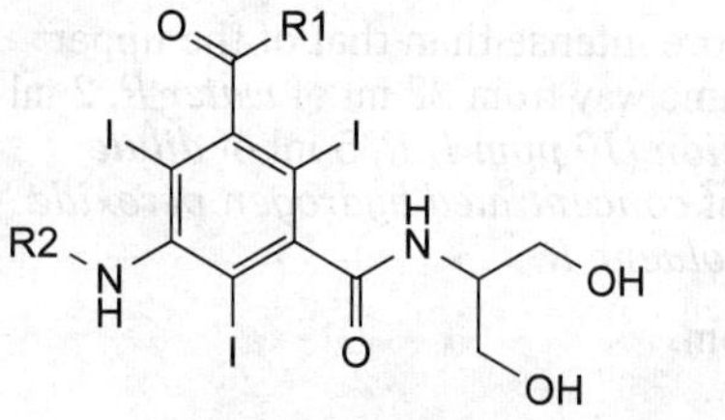

A. R1 = NH-CH(CH_2OH)$_2$, R2 = H: 5-amino-*N,N'*-bis[2-hydroxy-1-(hydroxymethyl)ethyl]-2,4,6-triiodobenzene-1,3-dicarboxamide,

B. R1 = NH-CH(CH_2OH)$_2$, R2 = CO-CH_2OH: 5-[(hydroxyacetyl)amino]-*N,N'*-bis[2-hydroxy-1-(hydroxymethyl)ethyl]-2,4,6-triiodobenzene-1,3-dicarboxamide,

C. R1 = NH-CH(CH_2OH)$_2$, R2 = CO-CH_3: 5-(acetylamino)-*N,N'*-bis[2-hydroxy-1-(hydroxymethyl)ethyl]-2,4,6-triiodobenzene-1,3-dicarboxamide,

D. R1 = H, R2 = CO-CHOH-CH_3: 3-[[2-hydroxy-1-(hydroxymethyl)ethyl]carbamoyl]-5-[[(2*S*)-2-hydroxypropanoyl]amino]-2,4,6-triiodobenzoic acid,

E. R1 = NH-CH(CH_2OH)$_2$, R2 = CO-CH(CH_3)-O-CO-CH_3: (1*S*)-2-[[3,5-bis[[2-hydroxy-1-(hydroxymethyl)ethyl]carbamoyl]-2,4,6-triiodophenyl]amino]-1-methyl-2-oxoethyl acetate,

F. R1 = N(CH_3)$_2$, R2 = CO-CHOH-CH_3: *N'*-[2-hydroxy-1-(hydroxymethyl)ethyl]-5-[[(2*S*)-2-hydroxypropanoyl]amino]-2,4,6-triiodo-*N,N*-dimethylbenzene-1,3-dicarboxamide,

G. R1 = NH-CH_2-CHOH-CH_2OH, R2 = CO-CHOH-CH_3: *N*-(2,3-dihydroxypropyl)-*N'*-[2-hydroxy-1-(hydroxymethyl)ethyl]-5-[[(2*S*)-2-hydroxypropanoyl]amino]-2,4,6-triiodobenzene-1,3-dicarboxamide,

J. R1 = NH-CH_2-CH_2OH, R2 = CO-CHOH-CH_3: *N*-(2-hydroxyethyl)-*N'*-[2-hydroxy-1-(hydroxymethyl)ethyl]-5-[[(2*S*)-2-hydroxypropanoyl]amino]-2,4,6-triiodobenzene-1,3-dicarboxamide,

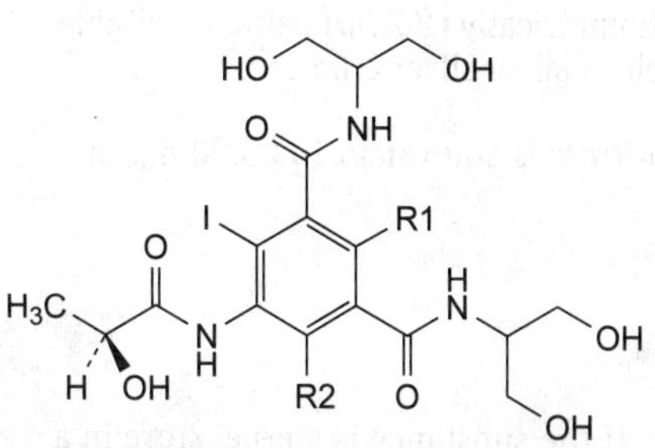

H. R1 = I, R2 = Cl: 4-chloro-*N,N'*-bis[2-hydroxy-1-(hydroxymethyl)ethyl]-5-[[(2*S*)-2-hydroxypropanoyl]amino]-2,6-diiodobenzene-1,3-dicarboxamide,

I. R1 = Cl, R2 = I: 2-chloro-*N,N'*-bis[2-hydroxy-1-(hydroxymethyl)ethyl]-5-[[(2*S*)-2-hydroxypropanoyl]amino]-4,6-diiodobenzene-1,3-dicarboxamide,

K. R1 = I, R2 = H: *N,N'*-bis[2-hydroxy-1-(hydroxymethyl)ethyl]-5-[[(2*S*)-2-hydroxypropanoyl]amino]-2,4-diiodobenzene-1,3-dicarboxamide.

01/2005:0700

IOPANOIC ACID

Acidum iopanoicum

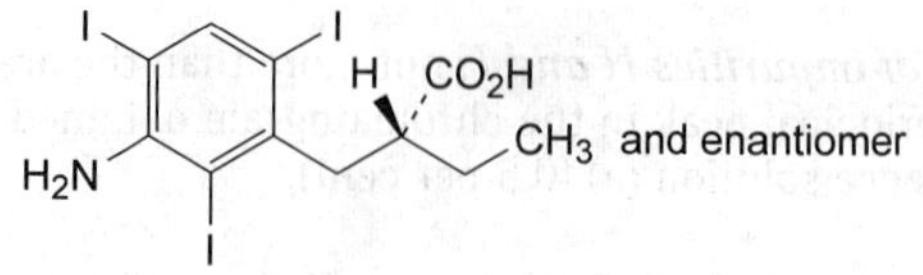

$C_{11}H_{12}I_3NO_2$ M_r 571

DEFINITION

Iopanoic acid contains not less than 98.5 per cent and not more than the equivalent of 101.0 per cent of (*RS*)-2-(3-amino-2,4,6-tri-iodobenzyl)butanoic acid, calculated with reference to the dried substance.

CHARACTERS

A white or yellowish-white powder, practically insoluble in water, soluble in ethanol and in methanol. It dissolves in dilute solutions of alkali hydroxides.

IDENTIFICATION

First identification: B.

Second identification: A, C, D.

A. Melting point (*2.2.14*): about 155 °C, with decomposition.

B. Examine by infrared absorption spectrophotometry (*2.2.24*), comparing with the spectrum obtained with *iopanoic acid CRS.*

C. Examine the chromatograms obtained in the test for related substances (see Tests). Spray the plate with a 1 g/l solution of *4-dimethylaminocinnamaldehyde R* in a mixture of 1 volume of *hydrochloric acid R* and 99 volumes of *alcohol R*. The principal spot in the chromatogram obtained with test solution (b) is similar in position, colour and size to the principal spot in the chromatogram obtained with reference solution (a).

D. Heat 50 mg carefully in a small porcelain dish over a flame. Violet vapour is evolved.

TESTS

Appearance of solution. Dissolve 1.0 g in *1 M sodium hydroxide* and dilute to 20 ml with the same solvent. The solution is clear (*2.2.1*) and not more intensely coloured than reference solution Y_3 (*2.2.2, Method II*).

Related substances. Examine by thin-layer chromatography (*2.2.27*), using *silica gel GF_{254} R* as the coating substance.

Test solution (a). Dissolve 1.0 g of the substance to be examined in a mixture of 3 volumes of *ammonia R* and 97 volumes of *methanol R* and dilute to 10 ml with the same mixture of solvents.

Test solution (b). Dilute 1 ml of test solution (a) to 10 ml with a mixture of 3 volumes of *ammonia R* and 97 volumes of *methanol R.*

Reference solution (a). Dissolve 50 mg of *iopanoic acid CRS* in a mixture of 3 volumes of *ammonia R* and 97 volumes of *methanol R* and dilute to 5 ml with the same mixture of solvents.

Reference solution (b). Dilute 1 ml of test solution (b) to 50 ml with a mixture of 3 volumes of *ammonia R* and 97 volumes of *methanol R.*

Apply separately to the plate 5 µl of each solution. Develop over a path of 10 cm using a mixture of 10 volumes of *concentrated ammonia R,* 20 volumes of *methanol R,*

20 volumes of *toluene R* and 50 volumes of *dioxan R*. Examine in ultraviolet light at 254 nm. Any spot in the chromatogram obtained with test solution (a), apart from the principal spot, is not more intense than the spot in the chromatogram obtained with reference solution (b) (0.2 per cent).

Halides. To 0.46 g add 10 ml of *nitric acid R* and 15 ml of *water R*. Shake for 5 min and filter. 15 ml of the filtrate complies with the limit test for chlorides (*2.4.4*) (180 ppm, expressed as chloride).

Loss on drying (*2.2.32*). Not more than 0.5 per cent, determined on 1.000 g by drying in an oven at 100 °C to 105 °C for 1 h.

Sulphated ash (*2.4.14*). Not more than 0.1 per cent, determined on 1.0 g.

ASSAY

To 0.150 g in a 250 ml round-bottomed flask add 5 ml of *strong sodium hydroxide solution R*, 20 ml of *water R*, 1 g of *zinc powder R* and a few glass beads. Boil under a reflux condenser for 60 min. Allow to cool and rinse the condenser with 20 ml of *water R*, adding the rinsings to the flask. Filter through a sintered-glass filter and wash the filter with several quantities of *water R*. Collect the filtrate and washings. Add 40 ml of *dilute sulphuric acid R* and titrate immediately with *0.1 M silver nitrate*. Determine the end-point potentiometrically (*2.2.20*), using a suitable electrode system such as silver-mercurous sulphate.

1 ml of *0.1 M silver nitrate* is equivalent to 19.03 mg of $C_{11}H_{12}I_3NO_2$.

STORAGE

Store protected from light.

01/2005:0751

IOTALAMIC ACID

Acidum iotalamicum

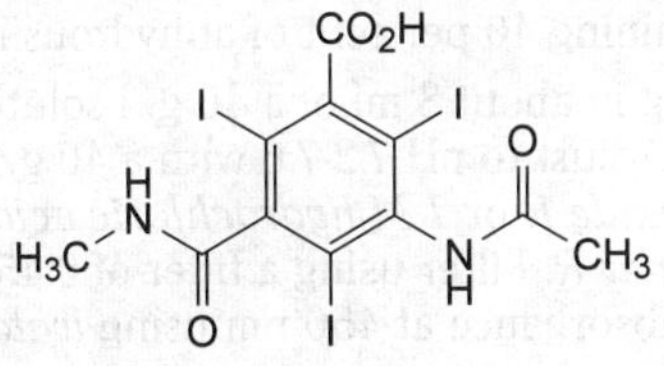

$C_{11}H_9I_3N_2O_4$ M_r 614

DEFINITION

Iotalamic acid contains not less than 98.5 per cent and not more than the equivalent of 101.0 per cent of 3-(acetylamino)-2,4,6-tri-iodo-5-(methylcarbamoyl)benzoic acid, calculated with reference to the dried substance.

CHARACTERS

A white or almost white powder, slightly soluble in water and in alcohol. It dissolves in dilute solutions of alkali hydroxides.

IDENTIFICATION

First identification: A.

Second identification: B, C.

A. Examine by infrared absorption spectrophotometry (*2.2.24*), comparing with the spectrum obtained with *iotalamic acid CRS*.

B. Examine by thin-layer chromatography (*2.2.27*), using a *TLC silica gel GF_{254} plate R*.

Test solution. Dissolve 50 mg of the substance to be examined in *methanol R* containing 3 per cent *V/V* of *ammonia R* and dilute to 5 ml with the same solvent.

Reference solution. Dissolve 50 mg of *iotalamic acid CRS* in *methanol R* containing 3 per cent *V/V* of *ammonia R* and dilute to 5 ml with the same solvent.

Apply separately to the plate 5 µl of each solution. Develop over a path of 15 cm using a mixture of 20 volumes of *anhydrous formic acid R*, 25 volumes of *methyl ethyl ketone R* and 60 volumes of *toluene R*. Allow the plate to dry until the solvents have evaporated and examine in ultraviolet light at 254 nm. The principal spot in the chromatogram obtained with the test solution is similar in position and size to the principal spot in the chromatogram obtained with the reference solution.

C. Heat 50 mg gently in a small porcelain dish over a flame. Violet vapour is evolved.

TESTS

Appearance of solution. Dissolve 1.0 g in *1 M sodium hydroxide* and dilute to 20 ml with the same solvent. The solution is clear (*2.2.1*) and colourless (*2.2.2, Method II*).

Related substances. Examine by thin-layer chromatography (*2.2.27*), using a *TLC silica gel GF_{254} plate R*.

Test solution. Dissolve 1.0 g of the substance to be examined in *methanol R* containing 3 per cent *V/V* of *ammonia R* and dilute to 10 ml with the same solvent.

Reference solution (a). Dilute 1 ml of the test solution to 50 ml with *water R*. Dilute 1 ml of the solution to 10 ml with *water R*.

Reference solution (b). Dissolve 1 mg of *iotalamic acid impurity A CRS* in 5 ml of reference solution (a).

Apply to the plate 5 µl of each solution. Develop over a path of 10 cm using a mixture of 1 volume of *glacial acetic acid R*, 1 volume of *anhydrous formic acid R*, 1 volume of *methanol R*, 5 volumes of *ether R* and 10 volumes of *methylene chloride R*. Allow the plate to dry until the solvents have evaporated. Examine in ultraviolet light at 254 nm. Any spot in the chromatogram obtained with the test solution, apart from the principal spot, is not more intense than the spot in the chromatogram obtained with reference solution (a) (0.2 per cent). The test is not valid unless the chromatogram obtained with reference solution (b) shows two clearly separated principal spots.

Halides. Dissolve 0.55 g in a mixture of 4 ml of *dilute sodium hydroxide solution R* and 15 ml of *water R*. Add 6 ml of *dilute nitric acid R* and filter. 15 ml of the filtrate complies with the limit test for chlorides (*2.4.4*) (150 ppm, expressed as chloride).

Impurity A. Not more than 0.05 per cent *m/m* determined by absorption spectrophotometry (*2.2.25*).

Test solution. Transfer 0.500 g of the substance to be examined to a 50 ml volumetric flask, add 14 ml of *water R*, shake and add 1 ml of *dilute sodium hydroxide solution R*.

Reference solution. Prepare the reference solution by mixing 10.0 ml of a 8.5 g/l solution of *sodium hydroxide R* containing 25 µg/ml of *iotalamic acid impurity A CRS* with 5 ml of *water R* in a 50 ml volumetric flask.

Blank solution. Transfer 14 ml of *water R* and 1 ml of *dilute sodium hydroxide solution R* to a 50 ml volumetric flask.

In conducting the following steps, keep the flasks in iced water and protected as far as possible from light until all of the reagents have been added.

Place all three of the flasks containing the test solution, the reference solution and the blank solution in iced water, protected from light. Add 5 ml of a 5 g/l solution of *sodium*

Monographs I-L

nitrite R and 12 ml of *dilute hydrochloric acid R*. Shake gently and allow to stand for exactly 2 min after adding the hydrochloric acid. Add 10 ml of a 20 g/l solution of *ammonium sulphamate R*. Allow to stand for 5 min shaking frequently (*CAUTION: considerable pressure is produced*), and add 0.15 ml of a 100 g/l solution of *α-naphthol R* in *alcohol R*. Shake and allow to stand for 5 min. Add 3.5 ml of *buffer solution pH 10.9 R*, mix and dilute to 50.0 ml with *water R*. Concomitantly and within 20 min determine the absorbance at 485 nm of the solutions obtained from the test solution and the reference solution in 5 cm cells, using the blank as the compensation liquid.

Calculate the content of impurity A.

Iodide. Not more than 20 ppm, determined by potentiometric titration (*2.2.20*). Dissolve 6.000 g in 20 ml of *1 M sodium hydroxide*, add 10 ml of *water R* and adjust to pH 4.5 to 5.5 with *acetic acid R*. Add 2.0 ml of *0.001 M potassium iodide*. Titrate with *0.001 M silver nitrate* using a silver indicator electrode and an appropriate reference electrode. Subtract the volume of titrant corresponding to the 2.0 ml of *0.001 M potassium iodide*, determined by titrating a blank to which is added 2.0 ml of *0.001 M potassium iodide* and use the residual value to calculate the iodide content.

1 ml of *0.001 M silver nitrate* is equivalent to 126.9 μg of iodide.

Heavy metals (*2.4.8*). Dissolve 2.0 g in 4 ml of *dilute sodium hydroxide solution R* and dilute to 20 ml with *water R*. 12 ml of this solution complies with limit test A for heavy metals (20 ppm). Prepare the standard using *lead standard solution (2 ppm Pb) R*.

Loss on drying (*2.2.32*). Not more than 0.5 per cent, determined on 0.300 g by drying in an oven at 100 °C to 105 °C.

Sulphated ash (*2.4.14*). Not more than 0.1 per cent, determined on 1.0 g.

ASSAY

To 0.150 g in a 250 ml round-bottomed flask add 5 ml of *strong sodium hydroxide solution R*, 20 ml of *water R*, 1 g of *zinc powder R* and a few glass beads. Boil under a reflux condenser for 30 min. Allow to cool and rinse the condenser with 20 ml of *water R*, adding the rinsings to the flask. Filter through a sintered-glass filter and wash the filter with several quantities of *water R*. Collect the filtrate and washings. Add 40 ml of *dilute sulphuric acid R* and titrate immediately with *0.1 M silver nitrate*. Determine the end-point potentiometrically (*2.2.20*), using a suitable electrode system such as silver-mercurous sulphate.

1 ml of *0.1 M silver nitrate* is equivalent to 20.47 mg of $C_{11}H_9I_3N_2O_4$.

STORAGE

Store protected from light.

IMPURITIES

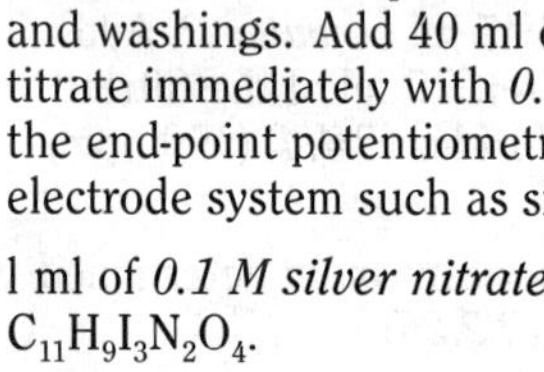

A. 3-amino-2,4,6-triiodo-5-(methylcarbamoyl)benzoic acid.

01/2005:2009
corrected

IOXAGLIC ACID

Acidum ioxaglicum

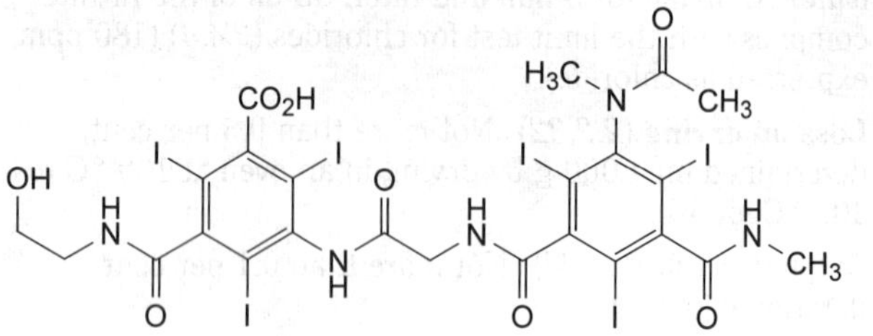

$C_{24}H_{21}I_6N_5O_8$ M_r 1269

DEFINITION

3-[[[[3-(Acetylmethylamino)-2,4,6-triiodo-5-(methylcarbamoyl)benzoyl]amino]acetyl]amino]-5-[(2-hydroxyethyl)carbamoyl]-2,4,6-triiodobenzoic acid.

Content: 98.5 per cent to 101.5 per cent (anhydrous substance).

CHARACTERS

Appearance: white or almost white powder, hygroscopic.

Solubility: very slightly soluble in water, slightly soluble in alcohol, very slightly soluble in methylene chloride. It dissolves in dilute solutions of alkali hydroxides.

IDENTIFICATION

Infrared absorption spectrophotometry (*2.2.24*).

Comparison: *ioxaglic acid CRS*.

TESTS

Appearance of solution. The solution is clear (*2.2.1*).

Dissolve 1.0 g in a 40 g/l solution of *sodium hydroxide R* and dilute to 20 ml with the same solution.

Absorbance (*2.2.25*): maximum 0.18, calculated for a solution containing 40 per cent of anhydrous ioxaglic acid.

Dissolve 10.0 g in about 8 ml of a 40 g/l solution of *sodium hydroxide R*. Adjust to pH 7.2-7.6 with a 40 g/l solution of *sodium hydroxide R* or *1 M hydrochloric acid*. Dilute to 25 ml with *water R*. Filter using a filter of 0.45 μm pore size. Measure the absorbance at 450 nm using *water R* as the compensation liquid.

Related substances. Liquid chromatography (*2.2.29*): use the normalisation procedure.

Test solution. Dissolve 0.10 g of the substance to be examined in about 40 ml of a mixture of 5 volumes of *acetonitrile R* and 95 volumes of *water R*. Add 0.5 ml ± 0.1 ml of a 4 g/l solution of *sodium hydroxide R* and dilute to 50.0 ml with a mixture of 5 volumes of *acetonitrile R* and 95 volumes of *water R*. Shake until dissolution is complete (using ultrasound, if necessary).

Reference solution (a). Dissolve 0.10 g of *ioxaglic acid CRS* in about 40 ml of a mixture of 5 volumes of *acetonitrile R* and 95 volumes of *water R*. Add 0.5 ml ± 0.1 ml of a 4 g/l solution of *sodium hydroxide R* and dilute to 50.0 ml with a mixture of 5 volumes of *acetonitrile R* and 95 volumes of *water R*. Shake until dissolution is complete (using ultrasound, if necessary).

Reference solution (b). Dissolve 5 mg of *ioxaglic acid impurity A CRS* in a mixture of 5 volumes of *acetonitrile R* and 95 volumes of *water R* and dilute to 50.0 ml with the same mixture of solvents. Dilute 1.0 ml of the solution to 50.0 ml with a mixture of 5 volumes of *acetonitrile R* and 95 volumes of *water R*.

Column:

– *size*: l = 0.25 m, Ø = 4.6 mm,

– *stationary phase*: spherical end-capped *octylsilyl silica gel for chromatography R* (5 µm) with a specific surface area of not less than 335 m^2/g, a pore size of 10 nm and a carbon loading of not less than 12 per cent,

– *temperature*: 25 °C.

Mobile phase:

– *mobile phase A*: 136 mg/l solution of *potassium dihydrogen phosphate R* adjusted to pH 3.0 with *phosphoric acid R*,

– *mobile phase B*: *acetonitrile R*,

Time (min)	Mobile phase A (per cent *V/V*)	Mobile phase B (per cent *V/V*)
0 - 5	95 → 90	5 → 10
5 - 40	90	10
40 - 85	90 → 70	10 → 30
85 - 115	70	30
115 - 120	70 → 50	30 → 50
120 - 125	50	50
125 - 130	50 → 95	50 → 5
130 - 140	95	5

Flow rate: 0.8 ml/min.

Detection: spectrophotometer at 242 nm.

Injection: 10 µl.

System suitability:

– *retention time*: ioxaglic acid = about 65 min (reference solution (a)), impurity A = about 22 min (reference solution (b)),

– the chromatogram obtained with reference solution (a) is similar to the chromatogram provided with *ioxaglic acid CRS*,

– *peak-to-valley ratio*: minimum 1.3, where H_p = height above the baseline of the peak due to impurity C and H_v = height above the baseline of the lowest point of the curve separating this peak from the peak due to ioxaglic acid in the chromatogram obtained with reference solution (a).

Limit: locate the impurities by comparison with the chromatogram provided with *ioxaglic acid CRS*.

– *impurity A*: not more than 0.1 per cent,

– *impurity B*: not more than 0.3 per cent,

– *impurity C*: not more than 0.3 per cent,

– *impurity E*: not more than 0.7 per cent,

– *impurity F*: not more than 0.4 per cent,

– *impurity D (sum of the peaks D1, D2, D3 and D4)*: not more than 0.7 per cent,

– *any other impurity*: not more than 0.2 per cent,

– *total*: not more than 2 per cent,

– *disregard limit*: 0.05 per cent; disregard any peak appearing at a retention time greater than 125 min.

Iodides: maximum 50 ppm.

Disperse 10.0 g in 50 ml of *water R*. Add 8 ml of *1 M sodium hydroxide*. After dissolution and homogenisation, add 1.0 ml of *glacial acetic acid R*. Immediately titrate with *0.001 M silver nitrate*, determining the end-point potentiometrically (*2.2.20*), using a silver indicator electrode and a suitable reference electrode.

1 ml of *0.001 M silver nitrate* is equivalent to 0.1269 mg of iodides.

Heavy metals (*2.4.8*): maximum 10 ppm.

Dissolve 2.0 g in 4 ml of a 40 g/l solution of *sodium hydroxide R* and dilute to 20 ml with *water R*. 12 ml of the solution complies with limit test A. Prepare the standard using 1 ml of *lead standard solution (10 ppm Pb) R*.

Water (*2.5.12*): maximum 5.0 per cent, determined on 0.100 g.

Sulphated ash (*2.4.14*): maximum 0.1 per cent, determined on 1.0 g. Use *sulphuric acid R* instead of *dilute sulphuric acid R*.

ASSAY

In a round-bottomed flask, place 0.100 g of the substance to be examined, add 5 ml of *strong sodium hydroxide solution R*, 20 ml of *water R*, 1 g of *zinc powder R* and a few glass beads. Fit the flask with a reflux condenser and boil for 30 min. Cool and rinse the condenser with 20 ml of *water R*. Add the rinsing liquid to the contents of the flask. Filter through a sintered-glass filter, wash the filter 3 times with 15 ml of *water R* and add the washings to the filtrate. Add 40 ml of *dilute sulphuric acid R* and titrate immediately with *0.05 M silver nitrate*. Determine the end-point potentiometrically (*2.2.20*), using a suitable electrode combination such as the silver/mercurous sulphate system.

1 ml of *0.05 M silver nitrate* is equivalent to 10.58 mg of $C_{24}H_{21}I_6N_5O_8$.

STORAGE

In an airtight container, protected from light.

IMPURITIES

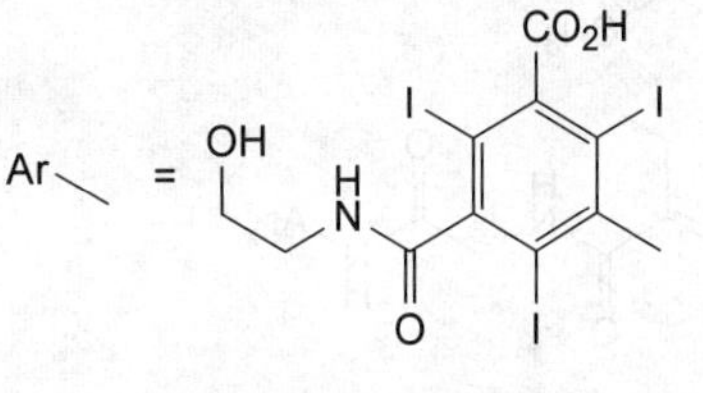

A. Ar-NH_2: 3-amino-5-[(2-hydroxyethyl)carbamoyl]-2,4,6-triiodobenzoic acid,

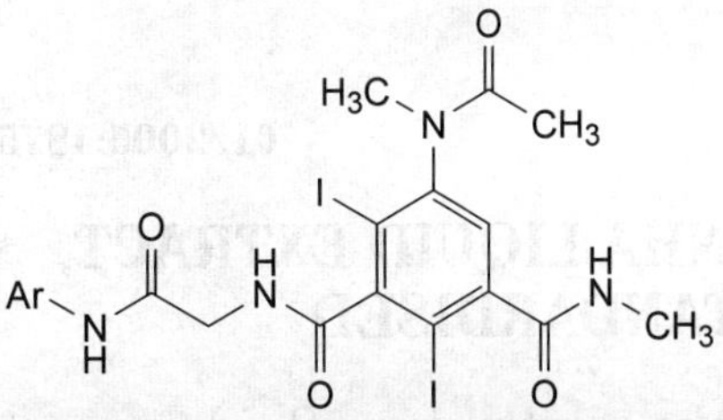

B. 3-[[[[3-(acetylmethylamino)-2,6-diiodo-5-(methylcarbamoyl)benzoyl]amino]acetyl]amino]-5-[(2-hydroxyethyl)carbamoyl]-2,4,6-triiodobenzoic acid,

C. specified impurity whose structure is unknown,

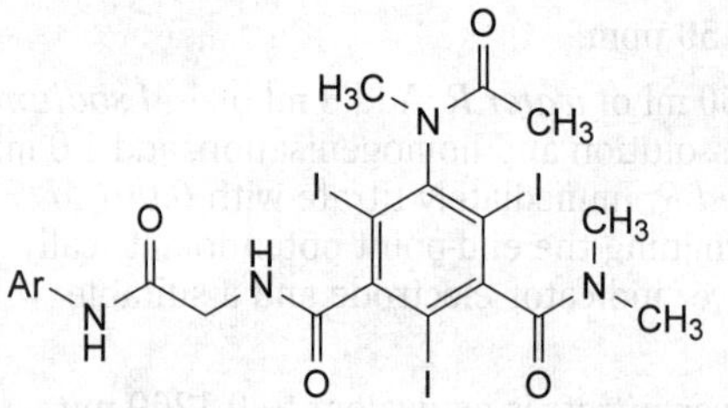

D. D1, D2, D3 and D4: 3-[[[[3-(acetylmethylamino)-5-(dimethylcarbamoyl)-2,4,6-triiodobenzoyl]amino]acetyl]amino]-5-[(2-hydroxyethyl)carbamoyl]-2,4,6-triiodobenzoic acid,

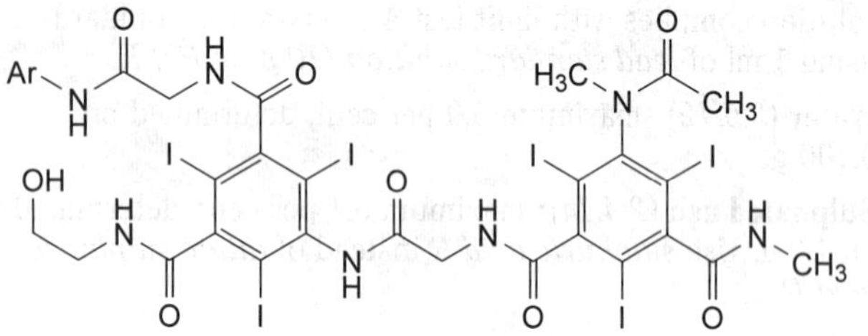

E. 3-[[[[3-[[[[3-(acetylmethylamino)-2,4,6-triiodo-5-(methylcarbamoyl)benzoyl]amino]acetyl]amino]-5-[(2-hydroxyethyl)carbamoyl]-2,4,6-triiodobenzoyl]amino]acetyl]amino]-5-[(2-hydroxyethyl)carbamoyl]-2,4,6-triiodobenzoic acid,

F. specified impurity whose structure is unknown,

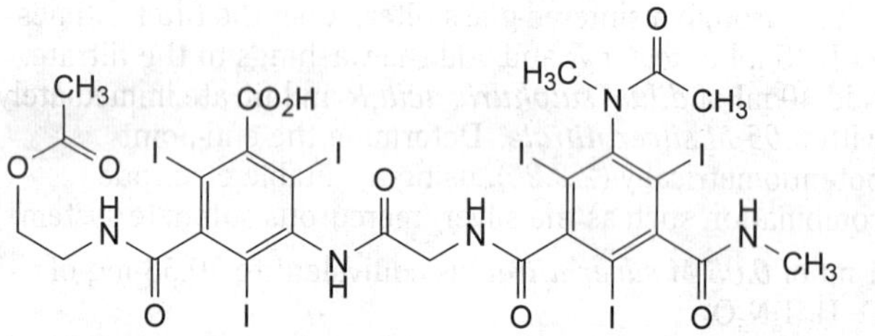

G. 3-[[[[3-(acetylmethylamino)-2,4,6-triiodo-5-(methylcarbamoyl)benzoyl]amino]acetyl]amino]-5-[[2-(acetyloxy)ethyl]carbamoyl]-2,4,6-triiodobenzoic acid,

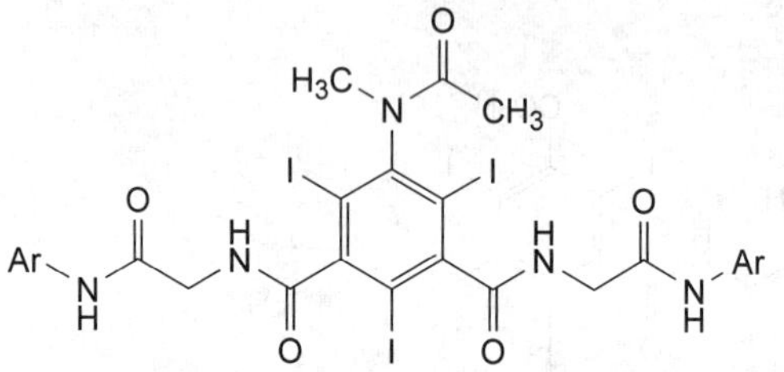

H. 3,3′-[[5-(acetylmethylamino)-2,4,6-triiodo-1,3-phenylene]bis(carbonyliminomethylenecarbonylimino)]bis[5-[(2-hydroxyethyl)carbamoyl]-2,4,6-triiodobenzoic] acid.

01/2005:1875

IPECACUANHA LIQUID EXTRACT, STANDARDISED

Ipecacuanhae extractum fluidum normatum

DEFINITION

Standardised liquid extract produced from *Ipecacuanha root (0094).*

Content: minimum 1.80 per cent and maximum 2.20 per cent of total alkaloids, calculated as emetine ($C_{29}H_{40}N_2O_4$; M_r 480.7).

PRODUCTION

The extract is produced from the herbal drug and solvent of suitable strength by an appropriate procedure.

CHARACTERS

Appearance: dark-brown liquid.

IDENTIFICATION

Thin-layer chromatography (*2.2.27*).

Test solution. Dilute 5.0 ml of the extract to be examined to 50 ml with *alcohol (70 per cent V/V) R*. To 2.0 ml of this solution add 2 ml of *water R* and 0.1 ml of *concentrated ammonia R*. Add 10 ml of *ether R* and shake. Separate the upper layer, dry it over about 2 g of *anhydrous sodium sulphate R* and filter.

Reference solution. Dissolve 2.5 mg of *emetine hydrochloride CRS* and 3 mg of *cephaëline hydrochloride CRS* in *methanol R* and dilute to 10 ml with the same solvent.

Plate: *TLC silica gel plate R.*

Mobile phase: *concentrated ammonia R, methanol R, ethyl acetate R, toluene R* (2:15:18:65 *V/V/V/V*).

Application: 10 µl, as bands.

Development: over a path of 10 cm.

Drying: in air.

Detection A: spray with a 5 g/l solution of *iodine R* in *alcohol R*. Heat at 60 °C for 10 min and allow to cool for 30 min. Examine in daylight.

Results A: see below the sequence of the zones present in the chromatograms obtained with the reference solution and the test solution. Furthermore, other zones may be present in the chromatogram obtained with the test solution.

Top of the plate	
_______	_______
_______	_______
Emetine: a yellow zone	A yellow zone (emetine)
Cephaëline: a light brown zone	A light brown zone (cephaëline)
Reference solution	**Test solution**

Detection B: examine in ultraviolet light at 365 nm.

Results B: see below the sequence of the zones present in the chromatograms obtained with the reference solution and the test solution. Furthermore, other faint fluorescent zones are present in the chromatogram obtained with the test solution.

Top of the plate	
_______	_______
	_______
Emetine: an intense yellow fluorescent zone	An intense yellow fluorescent zone (emetine)
Cephaëline: a light blue or orange-yellow fluorescent zone	A light blue or orange-yellow fluorescent zone (cephaëline)
Reference solution	**Test solution**

With a liquid extract from *Cephaelis acuminata* root, the zones of emetine and cephaëline in the chromatogram obtained with the test solution are of similar size.

With a liquid extract from *Cephaelis ipecacuanha* root, the zone of emetine is much larger than the zone of cephaëline in the chromatogram obtained with the test solution.

TESTS

Ethanol (*2.9.10*): minimum 95 per cent and maximum 105 per cent of the quantity stated on the label.

ASSAY

Dilute 1.00 g of the extract to be examined to 10 ml with *alcohol (70 per cent V/V) R* and transfer to a chromatography column about 0.2 m long and about 15 mm in internal diameter, containing 8 g of *basic aluminium oxide R*, using a glass rod. After infiltration into the aluminium oxide layer, rinse the flask, glass rod and internal wall of the column with 3 quantities, each of 2 ml, of *alcohol (70 per cent V/V) R*. Elute in portions with 40 ml of *alcohol (70 per cent V/V) R*. Avoid disturbance or drying of the surface of the aluminium oxide layer. Collect the eluate in a 100 ml flask. Evaporate the eluate on a water-bath to about 10 ml. Allow to cool. Add 10.0 ml of *0.02 M hydrochloric acid* and 20 ml of *carbon dioxide-free water R*. Titrate the excess acid with *0.02 M sodium hydroxide* using 0.15 ml of *methyl red mixed solution R* as indicator.

Perform a blank assay by repeating the assay but replacing the extract to be examined with 10.0 ml of alcohol of the strength stated on the label.

1 ml of *0.02 M hydrochloric acid* is equivalent to 4.807 mg of total alkaloids, calculated as emetine.

01/2005:0093

IPECACUANHA, PREPARED

Ipecacuanhae pulvis normatus

DEFINITION

Prepared ipecacuanha is ipecacuanha root powder (180) adjusted, if necessary, by the addition of powdered lactose or ipecacuanha root powder with a lower alkaloidal content to contain 1.9 per cent to 2.1 per cent of total alkaloids, calculated as emetine ($C_{29}H_{40}N_2O_4$; M_r 480.7) with reference to the dried drug.

CHARACTERS

Light grey to yellowish-brown powder with a slight odour.

IDENTIFICATION

A. Examine under a microscope, using *chloral hydrate solution R*. The powder shows the following diagnostic characters: parenchymatous cells, raphides of calcium oxalate up to 80 µm in length either in bundles or scattered throughout the powder; fragments of tracheids and vessels usually 10 µm to 20 µm in diameter, with bordered pits; larger vessels and sclereids from the rhizome. Examine under a microscope using a 50 per cent *V/V* solution of *glycerol R*. The powder shows simple or two- to eight-compound starch granules contained in parenchymatous cells, the simple granules being up to 15 µm in diameter in *C. ipecacuanha* and up to 22 µm in diameter in *C. acuminata*. Examined in *glycerol (85 per cent) R*, it may be seen to contain lactose crystals.

B. Examine by thin-layer chromatography (*2.2.27*), using a suitable silica gel as the coating substance.

Test solution. To 0.1 g in a test-tube add 0.05 ml of *concentrated ammonia R* and 5 ml of *ether R* and stir the mixture vigorously with a glass rod. Allow to stand for 30 min and filter.

Reference solution. Dissolve 2.5 mg of *emetine hydrochloride CRS* and 3 mg of *cephaëline hydrochloride CRS* in *methanol R* and dilute to 20 ml with the same solvent.

Apply separately to the plate as bands 10 µl of each solution. Develop over a path of 10 cm using a mixture of 2 volumes of *concentrated ammonia R*, 15 volumes of *methanol R*, 18 volumes of *ethyl acetate R* and 65 volumes of *toluene R*. Allow the plate to dry in air. Spray with a 5 g/l solution of *iodine R* in *alcohol R* and heat at 60 °C for 10 min. Examine in daylight. The chromatograms obtained with the test solution and with the reference solution show in the lower part a yellow zone corresponding to emetine and below it a light brown zone corresponding to cephaëline. Examine in ultraviolet light at 365 nm. The zone corresponding to emetine shows an intense yellow fluorescence and that corresponding to cephaëline a light blue fluorescence. The chromatogram obtained with the test solution shows also faint fluorescent zones.

With *C. acuminata* the principal zones in the chromatogram obtained with the test solution are similar in position, fluorescence and size to the zones in the chromatogram obtained with the reference solution.

With *C. ipecacuanha* the only difference is that the zone corresponding to cephaëline in the chromatogram obtained with the test solution is much smaller than the corresponding zone in the chromatogram obtained with the reference solution.

TESTS

Loss on drying (*2.2.32*). Not more than 5.0 per cent, determined on 1.000 g by drying in an oven at 100 °C to 105 °C.

Total ash (*2.4.16*). Not more than 5.0 per cent.

Ash insoluble in hydrochloric acid (*2.8.1*). Not more than 3.0 per cent.

ASSAY

To 7.5 g in a dry flask, add 100 ml of *ether R* and shake for 5 min. Add 5 ml of *dilute ammonia R1*, shake for 1 h, add 5 ml of *water R* and shake vigorously. Decant the ether layer into a flask through a plug of cotton. Wash the residue in the flask with two quantities, each of 25 ml, of *ether R*, decanting each portion through the same plug of cotton. Combine the ether solutions and eliminate the ether by distillation. Dissolve the residue in 2 ml of *alcohol (90 per cent V/V) R*, evaporate the alcohol to dryness and heat at 100 °C for 5 min. Dissolve the residue in 5 ml of previously neutralised *alcohol (90 per cent V/V) R*, warming on a water-bath, add 15.0 ml of *0.1 M hydrochloric acid* and titrate the excess acid with *0.1 M sodium hydroxide* using 0.5 ml of *methyl red mixed solution R* as indicator.

1 ml of *0.1 M hydrochloric acid* is equivalent to 24.03 mg of total alkaloids, calculated as emetine.

STORAGE

Store in an airtight container, protected from light.

01/2005:0094

IPECACUANHA ROOT

Ipecacuanhae radix

DEFINITION

Ipecacuanha root consists of the fragmented and dried underground organs of *Cephaelis ipecacuanha* (Brot.) A. Rich., known as Matto Grosso ipecacuanha, or of *Cephaelis acuminata* Karsten, known as Costa Rica ipecacuanha, or of a mixture of both species. It contains not less than 2.0 per cent of total alkaloids, calculated as emetine ($C_{29}H_{40}N_2O_4$; M_r 480.7) with reference to the dried drug. The principal alkaloids are emetine and cephaëline.

CHARACTERS

Ipecacuanha root has a slight odour.

It has the macroscopic and microscopic characters described under identification tests A and B.

IDENTIFICATION

A. *C. ipecacuanha.* The root occurs as somewhat tortuous pieces, from dark reddish-brown to very dark brown, seldom more than 15 cm long or 6 mm thick, closely annulated externally, having rounded ridges completely encircling the root; the fracture is short in the bark and splintery in the wood. The transversely cut surface shows a wide greyish bark and a small uniformly dense wood. The rhizome occurs as short lengths usually attached to roots, cylindrical, up to 2 mm in diameter, finely wrinkled longitudinally and with pith occupying approximately one-sixth of the whole diameter.

C. acuminata. The root in general resembles the root of *C. ipecacuanha*, but differs in the following particulars: it is often up to 9 mm thick; the external surface is greyish-brown or reddish-brown with transverse ridges at intervals of usually 1 mm to 3 mm, the ridges being about 0.5 mm to 1 mm wide, extending about half-way round the circumference and fading at the extremities into the general surface level.

B. Reduce to a powder (355). The powder is light grey to yellowish-brown. Examine under a microscope, using *chloral hydrate solution R*. The powder shows the following diagnostic characters: parenchymatous cells, raphides of calcium oxalate up to 80 µm in length either in bundles or scattered throughout the powder; fragments of tracheids and vessels usually 10 µm to 20 µm in diameter, with bordered pits; larger vessels and sclereids from the rhizome. Examine under a microscope using a 50 per cent *V/V* solution of *glycerol R*. The powder shows simple or two- to eight-compound starch granules contained in parenchymatous cells, the simple granules being up to 15 µm in diameter in *C. ipecacuanha* and up to 22 µm in diameter in *C. acuminata.*

C. Examine by thin-layer chromatography (*2.2.27*), using a suitable silica gel as the coating substance.

Test solution. To 0.1 g of the powdered drug (180) in a test-tube add 0.05 ml of *concentrated ammonia R* and 5 ml of *ether R* and stir the mixture vigorously with a glass rod. Allow to stand for 30 min and filter.

Reference solution. Dissolve 2.5 mg of *emetine hydrochloride CRS* and 3 mg of *cephaëline hydrochloride CRS* in *methanol R* and dilute to 20 ml with the same solvent.

Apply separately to the plate as bands 10 µl of each solution. Develop over a path of 10 cm using a mixture of 2 volumes of *concentrated ammonia R*, 15 volumes of *methanol R*, 18 volumes of *ethyl acetate R* and 65 volumes of *toluene R*. Allow the plate to dry in air. Spray with a 5 g/l solution of *iodine R* in *alcohol R* and heat at 60 °C for 10 min. Examine in daylight. The chromatograms obtained with the test solution and with the reference solution show in the lower part a yellow zone corresponding to emetine and below it a light brown zone corresponding to cephaëline. Examine in ultraviolet light at 365 nm. The zone corresponding to emetine shows an intense yellow fluorescence and that corresponding to cephaëline a light blue fluorescence. The chromatogram obtained with the test solution shows also faint fluorescent zones.

With *C. acuminata* the principal zones in the chromatogram obtained with the test solution are similar in position, fluorescence and size to the zones in the chromatogram obtained with the reference solution.

With *C. ipecacuanha* the only difference is that the zone corresponding to cephaëline in the chromatogram obtained with the test solution is much smaller than the corresponding zone in the chromatogram obtained with the reference solution.

TESTS

Foreign matter (*2.8.2*). It complies with the test for foreign matter.

Loss on drying (*2.2.32*). Not more than 10.0 per cent, determined on 1.000 g of powdered drug (180) by drying in an oven at 100-105 °C.

Total ash (*2.4.16*). Not more than 5.0 per cent.

Ash insoluble in hydrochloric acid (*2.8.1*). Not more than 3.0 per cent.

ASSAY

To 7.5 g of the powdered drug (180) in a dry flask, add 100 ml of *ether R* and shake for 5 min. Add 5 ml of *dilute ammonia R1*, shake for 1 h, add 5 ml of *water R* and shake vigorously. Decant the ether layer into a flask through a plug of cotton. Wash the residue in the flask with 2 quantities, each of 25 ml, of *ether R*, decanting each portion through the same plug of cotton. Combine the ether solutions and eliminate the ether by distillation. Dissolve the residue in 2 ml of *alcohol (90 per cent V/V) R*, evaporate the alcohol to dryness and heat at 100 °C for 5 min. Dissolve the residue in 5 ml of previously neutralised *alcohol (90 per cent V/V) R*, warming on a water-bath, add 15.0 ml of *0.1 M hydrochloric acid* and titrate the excess acid with *0.1 M sodium hydroxide* using 0.5 ml of *methyl red mixed solution R* as indicator.

1 ml of *0.1 M hydrochloric acid* is equivalent to 24.03 mg of total alkaloids, calculated as emetine.

STORAGE

Store protected from light and moisture.

01/2005:1530

IPECACUANHA TINCTURE, STANDARDISED

Ipecacuanhae tinctura normata

DEFINITION

Tincture produced from *Ipecacuanha root (0094)*.

Content: 0.18 per cent (*m/m*) to 0.22 per cent (*m/m*) of total alkaloids, calculated as emetine ($C_{29}H_{40}N_2O_4$; M_r 480.7).

PRODUCTION

The tincture is produced by a suitable procedure from the herbal drug and ethanol of suitable strength.

CHARACTERS

Appearance: yellowish-brown liquid.

IDENTIFICATION

Thin-layer chromatography (*2.2.27*).

Test solution. To 2.0 ml of the tincture to be examined add 2 ml of *water R* and 0.1 ml of *concentrated ammonia R*. Add 10 ml of *ether R* and shake. Separate the ether layer, dry it over about 2 g of *anhydrous sodium sulphate R* and filter.

Reference solution. Dissolve 2.5 mg of *emetine hydrochloride CRS* and 3 mg of *cephaëline hydrochloride CRS* in *methanol R* and dilute to 10 ml with the same solvent.

Plate: *TLC silica gel plate R.*

Mobile phase: *concentrated ammonia R, methanol R, ethyl acetate R, toluene R* (2:15:18:65 *V/V/V/V*).

Application: 10 µl, as bands.

Development: over a path of 10 cm.

Drying: in air.

Detection A: spray the plate with a 5 g/l solution of *iodine R* in *alcohol R* and heat at 60 °C for 10 min. Examine in daylight.

Results A: see below the sequence of the zones present in the chromatograms obtained with the reference solution and the test solution.

Top of the plate	
_______	_______
_______	_______
Emetine: a yellow zone	A yellow zone (emetine)
Cephaëline: a light brown zone	A light brown zone (cephaëline)
Reference solution	**Test solution**

Detection B: examine the plate in ultraviolet light at 365 nm.

Results B: see below the sequence of the zones present in the chromatograms obtained with the reference solution and the test solution. Furthermore, other faint fluorescent zones are present in the chromatogram obtained with the test solution.

Top of the plate	
_______	_______
_______	_______
Emetine: an intense yellow fluorescent zone	An intense yellow fluorescent zone (emetine)
Cephaëline: a light blue or orange-yellow fluorescent zone	A light blue or orange-yellow fluorescent zone (cephaëline)
Reference solution	**Test solution**

With a tincture from *Cephaelis acuminata* root the zones of emetine and cephaëline in the chromatogram obtained with the test solution are similar in size.

With a tincture from *Cephaelis ipecacuanha* root the zone of emetine is much larger than the zone of cephaëline in the chromatogram obtained with the test solution.

TESTS

Ethanol (*2.9.10*): 95 per cent to 105 per cent of the quantity stated on the label.

ASSAY

Transfer 10.00 g of the tincture to be examined to a chromatography column about 0.2 m long and about 15 mm in internal diameter, filled with 8 g of *basic aluminium oxide R*. After infiltration into the aluminium oxide layer rinse the internal wall of the column with 3 quantities, each of 2 ml, of *alcohol (70 per cent V/V) R*. Elute in portions, with 40 ml of *alcohol (70 per cent V/V) R*. Avoid whirling or drying of the surface of the aluminium oxide layer. Collect the eluate in a 100 ml flask. Evaporate the eluate on a water-bath to about 10 ml. Allow to cool. Add 10.0 ml of *0.02 M hydrochloric acid* and 20 ml of *carbon dioxide-free water R*. Titrate the excess acid with *0.02 M sodium hydroxide* using 0.15 ml of *methyl red mixed solution R* as indicator.

Perform a blank assay replacing the tincture to be examined with 10.0 ml of alcohol of the strength stated on the label.

1 ml of *0.02 M hydrochloric acid* is equivalent to 4.807 mg of total alkaloids, calculated as emetine.

01/2005:0919

IPRATROPIUM BROMIDE

Ipratropii bromidum

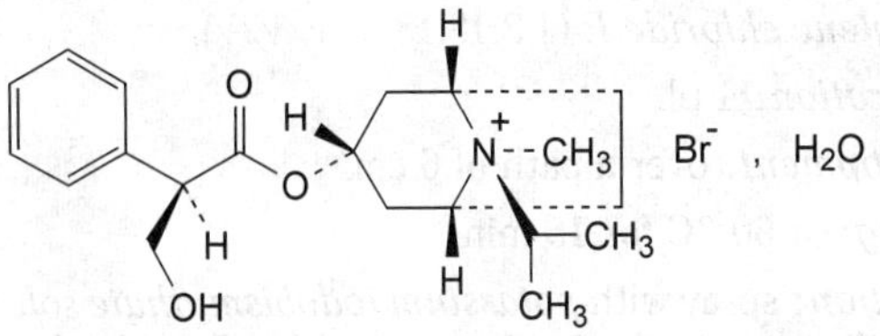

and enantiomer

$C_{20}H_{30}BrNO_3,H_2O$ M_r 430.4

DEFINITION

(1*R*,3*r*,5*S*,8*r*)-3-[[(2*RS*)-3-Hydroxy-2-phenylpropanoyl]oxy]-8-methyl-8-(1-methylethyl)-8-azoniabicyclo[3.2.1]octane bromide monohydrate.

Content: 99.0 per cent to 100.5 per cent (anhydrous substance).

CHARACTERS

Appearance: white or almost white, crystalline powder.

Solubility: soluble in water, freely soluble in methanol, slightly soluble in alcohol.

mp: about 230 °C, with decomposition.

IDENTIFICATION

First identification: A, E.

Second identification: B, C, D, E.

A. Infrared absorption spectrophotometry (*2.2.24*).
Comparison: *ipratropium bromide CRS.*

B. Examine the chromatograms obtained in the test for impurity A.
Results: the principal spot in the chromatogram obtained with the test solution is similar in position, colour and size to the principal spot in the chromatogram obtained with reference solution (a).

C. To 5 ml of solution S (see Tests), add 2 ml of *dilute sodium hydroxide solution R*. No precipitate is formed.

D. To about 1 mg add 0.2 ml of *nitric acid R* and evaporate to dryness on a water-bath. Dissolve the residue in 2 ml of *acetone R* and add 0.1 ml of a 30 g/l solution of *potassium hydroxide R* in *methanol R*. A violet colour develops.

E. It gives reaction (a) of bromides (*2.3.1*).

TESTS

Solution S. Dissolve 0.50 g in *carbon dioxide-free water R* and dilute to 50.0 ml with the same solvent.

Appearance of solution. Solution S is clear (*2.2.1*) and not more intensely coloured than reference solution GY_7 (*2.2.2, Method II*).

pH (*2.2.3*): 5.0 to 7.5 for solution S.

Monographs I-L

Impurity A. Thin-layer chromatography (*2.2.27*).

Test solution. Dissolve 20 mg of the substance to be examined in *methanol R* and dilute to 1.0 ml with the same solvent.

Reference solution (a). Dissolve 20 mg of *ipratropium bromide CRS* in *methanol R* and dilute to 1.0 ml with the same solvent.

Reference solution (b). Dissolve 20 mg of *methylatropine bromide CRS* in 1.0 ml of reference solution (a).

Reference solution (c). Dissolve 5 mg of *ipratropium impurity A CRS* in 100.0 ml of *methanol R*. Dilute 2.0 ml of the solution to 5.0 ml with *methanol R*.

Plate: *TLC silica gel plate R* (2-10 µm).

Mobile phase: *anhydrous formic acid R, water R, alcohol R, methylene chloride R* (1:3:18:18 *V/V/V/V*).

Application: 1 µl.

Development: over a path of 6 cm.

Drying: at 60 °C for 15 min.

Detection: spray with *potassium iodobismuthate solution R*, allow the plate to dry in air, spray with a 50 g/l solution of *sodium nitrite R* and protect immediately with a sheet of glass.

System suitability: the chromatogram obtained with reference solution (b) shows 2 clearly separated principal spots.

Limits:

– *impurity A*: any spot due to impurity A is not more intense than the principal spot in the chromatogram obtained with reference solution (c) (0.1 per cent).

Related substances. Liquid chromatography (*2.2.29*).

Test solution. Dissolve 0.200 g of the substance to be examined in the mobile phase and dilute to 20.0 ml with the mobile phase.

Reference solution (a). Dissolve 10.0 mg of *ipratropium bromide CRS* in the mobile phase and dilute to 20.0 ml with the mobile phase. Dilute 1.0 ml of the solution to 50.0 ml with the mobile phase.

Reference solution (b). Dissolve 5 mg of *ipratropium bromide CRS* and 5 mg of *ipratropium impurity B CRS* in 1 ml of *methanol R* and dilute to 25.0 ml with the mobile phase. Dilute 1.0 ml of the solution to 20.0 ml with the mobile phase.

Column:

– *size*: *l* = 0.15 m, Ø = 3.9 mm,

– *stationary phase*: *octadecylsilyl silica gel for chromatography R* (5 µm),

– *temperature*: 30 °C.

Mobile phase: dissolve 12.4 g of *sodium dihydrogen phosphate R* and 1.7 g of *tetrapropylammonium chloride R* in 870 ml of *water R*; adjust to pH 5.5 with a 180 g/l solution of *disodium hydrogen phosphate R* and add 130 ml of *methanol R*.

Flow rate: 1.5 ml/min.

Detection: spectrophotometer at 220 nm.

Injection: 5 µl.

Run time: 6 times the retention time of ipratropium.

Relative retention with reference to ipratropium (retention time = about 4.9 min): impurity C = about 0.7; impurity B = about 1.2; impurity D = about 1.8; impurity E = about 2.3; impurity F = about 5.1.

System suitability: reference solution (b):

– *resolution*: minimum 3.0 between the peaks due to impurity B and ipratropium,

– *symmetry factor*: maximum 2.5 for the principal peak.

Limits:

– *correction factors*: for the calculation of contents, multiply the peak areas of the following impurities by the corresponding correction factor: impurity C = 0.3; impurity D = 0.2; impurity F = 0.5;

– *impurity D*: not more than 0.5 times the area of the principal peak in the chromatogram obtained with reference solution (a) (0.05 per cent);

– *any other impurity*: not more than the area of the principal peak in the chromatogram obtained with reference solution (a) (0.1 per cent);

– *total*: not more than 2.5 times the area of the principal peak in the chromatogram obtained with reference solution (a) (0.25 per cent);

– *disregard limit*: one-third of the area of the principal peak in the chromatogram obtained with reference solution (a) (0.03 per cent).

Water (*2.5.12*): 3.9 per cent to 4.4 per cent, determined on 0.50 g.

Sulphated ash (*2.4.14*): maximum 0.1 per cent, determined on 1.0 g.

ASSAY

Dissolve 0.350 g in 50 ml of *water R* and add 3 ml of *dilute nitric acid R*. Titrate with *0.1 M silver nitrate*, determining the end-point potentiometrically (*2.2.20*).

1 ml of *0.1 M silver nitrate* is equivalent to 41.24 mg of $C_{20}H_{30}BrNO_3$.

IMPURITIES

Specified impurities: A, B, C, D.

Other detectable impurities: E, F.

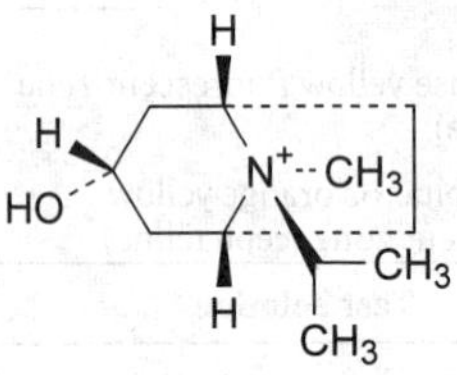

A. (1*R*,3*r*,5*S*,8*r*)-3-hydroxy-8-methyl-8-(1-methylethyl)-8-azoniabicyclo[3.2.1]octane,

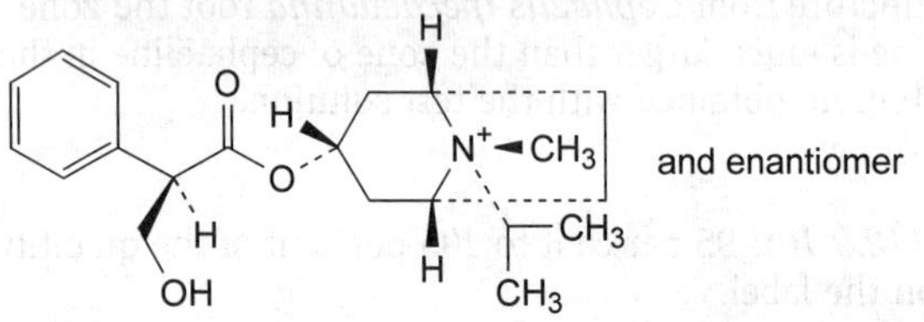

B. (1*R*,3*r*,5*S*,8*s*)-3-[[(2*RS*)-3-hydroxy-2-phenylpropanoyl]oxy]-8-methyl-8-(1-methylethyl)-8-azoniabicyclo[3.2.1]octane,

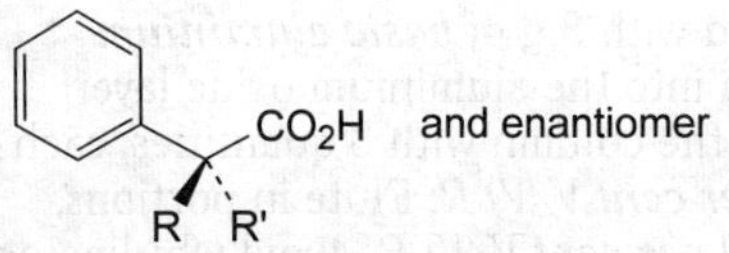

C. R = CH_2-OH, R′ = H: (2*RS*)-3-hydroxy-2-phenylpropanoic acid (DL-tropic acid),

D. R + R′ = CH_2: 2-phenylpropenoic acid (atropic acid),

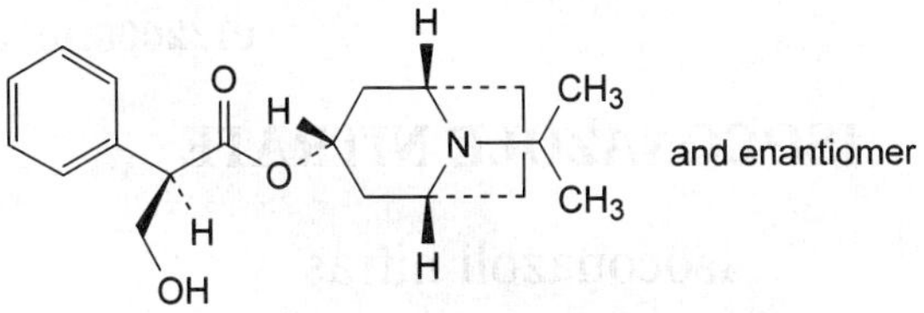

E. (1*R*,3*r*,5*S*)-8-(1-methylethyl)-8-azabicyclo[3.2.1]oct-3-yl (2*RS*)-3-hydroxy-2-phenylpropanoate,

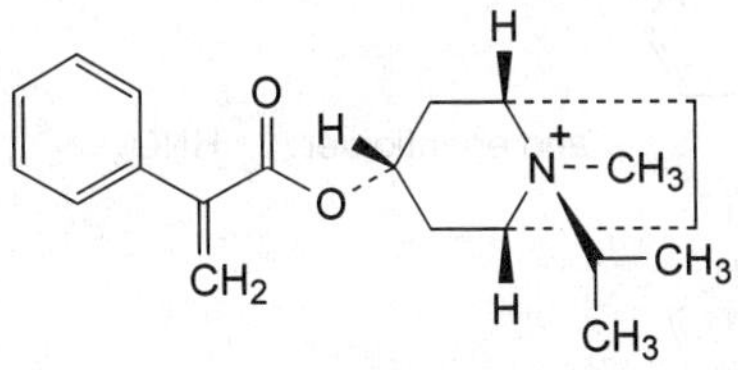

F. (1*R*,3*r*,5*S*,8*r*)-8-methyl-8-(1-methylethyl)-3-[(2-phenylpropenoyl)oxy]-8-azoniabicyclo[3.2.1]octane.

01/2005:1018

ISOCONAZOLE

Isoconazolum

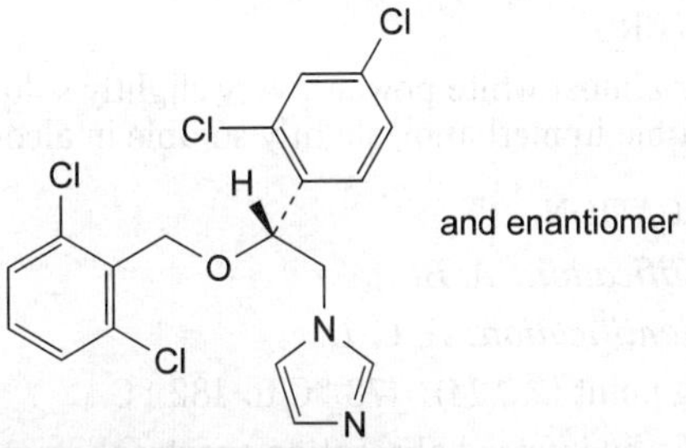

$C_{18}H_{14}Cl_4N_2O$ M_r 416.1

DEFINITION

Isoconazole contains not less than 99.0 per cent and not more than the equivalent of 101.0 per cent of 1-[(2*RS*)-2-[(2,6-dichlorobenzyl)oxy]-2-(2,4-dichlorophenyl)ethyl]-1*H*-imidazole, calculated with reference to the dried substance.

CHARACTERS

A white or almost white powder, practically insoluble in water, very soluble in methanol, freely soluble in alcohol.

IDENTIFICATION

First identification: A, B.

Second identification: A, C, D.

A. Melting point (*2.2.14*): 111 °C to 115 °C.

B. Examine by infrared absorption spectrophotometry (*2.2.24*), comparing with the spectrum obtained with *isoconazole CRS*. Examine the substances prepared as discs.

C. Examine by thin-layer chromatography (*2.2.27*), using a suitable octadecylsilyl silica gel as the coating substance.

Test solution. Dissolve 30 mg of the substance to be examined in *methanol R* and dilute to 5 ml with the same solvent.

Reference solution (a). Dissolve 30 mg of *isoconazole CRS* in *methanol R* and dilute to 5 ml with the same solvent.

Reference solution (b). Dissolve 30 mg of *isoconazole CRS* and 30 mg of *econazole nitrate CRS* in *methanol R* and dilute to 5 ml with the same solvent.

Apply separately to the plate 5 µl of each solution. Develop over a path of 15 cm using a mixture of 20 volumes of *ammonium acetate solution R*, 40 volumes of *dioxan R* and 40 volumes of *methanol R*. Dry the plate in a current of warm air for 15 min and expose it to iodine vapour until the spots appear. Examine in daylight. The principal spot in the chromatogram obtained with the test solution is similar in position, colour and size to the principal spot in the chromatogram obtained with reference solution (a). The test is not valid unless the chromatogram obtained with reference solution (b) shows 2 clearly separated spots.

D. To about 30 mg in a porcelain crucible add 0.3 g of *anhydrous sodium carbonate R*. Heat over an open flame for 10 min. Allow to cool. Take up the residue with 5 ml of *dilute nitric acid R* and filter. To 1 ml of the filtrate add 1 ml of *water R*. The solution gives reaction (a) of chlorides (*2.3.1*).

TESTS

Solution S. Dissolve 0.20 g in *methanol R* and dilute to 20.0 ml with the same solvent.

Appearance of solution. Solution S is clear (*2.2.1*) and is not more intensely coloured than reference solution Y_6 (*2.2.2, Method II*).

Optical rotation (*2.2.7*). The angle of optical rotation, determined on solution S, is − 0.10° to + 0.10°.

Related substances. Examine by liquid chromatography (*2.2.29*).

Test solution. Dissolve 0.100 g of the substance to be examined in 3.2 ml of *methanol R*. Add 3.0 ml of *acetonitrile R* and dilute to 10.0 ml with a solution of *ammonium acetate R* (6.0 g in 380 ml of *water R*).

Reference solution (a). Dissolve 2.5 mg of *isoconazole CRS* and 2.5 mg of *econazole nitrate CRS* in the mobile phase and dilute to 100.0 ml with the mobile phase.

Reference solution (b). Dilute 1.0 ml of the test solution to 100.0 ml with the mobile phase. Dilute 5.0 ml of this solution to 20.0 ml with the mobile phase.

The chromatographic procedure may be carried out using:

- a stainless steel column 0.1 m long and 4.6 mm in internal diameter packed with *octadecylsilyl silica gel for chromatography R* (3 µm),
- as mobile phase at a flow rate of 2 ml/min a solution of 6.0 g of *ammonium acetate R* in a mixture of 300 ml of *acetonitrile R*, 320 ml of *methanol R* and 380 ml of *water R*,
- as detector a spectrophotometer set at 235 nm.

Equilibrate the column with the mobile phase at a flow rate of 2 ml/min for about 30 min.

Adjust the sensitivity of the system so that the height of the principal peak in the chromatogram obtained with 10 µl of reference solution (b) is not less than 50 per cent of the full scale of the recorder.

Inject 10 µl of reference solution (a). When the chromatogram is recorded in the prescribed conditions, the retention times are: econazole, about 10 min; isoconazole, about 14 min. The test is not valid unless the resolution between the peaks corresponding to econazole and isoconazole is at least 5.0. If necessary, adjust the composition of the mobile phase.

Inject separately 10 µl of the test solution and 10 µl of reference solution (b). Continue the chromatography for 1.5 times the retention time of the principal peak. In the chromatogram obtained with the test solution: the area of any peak, apart from the principal peak, is not greater than the area of the principal peak in the chromatogram obtained with reference solution (b) (0.25 per cent); the sum of the areas of all the peaks, apart from the principal peak, is not greater than twice the area of the principal peak in the chromatogram obtained with reference solution (b) (0.5 per cent). Disregard any peaks due to the solvent and any peak with an area less than 0.2 times that of the principal peak in the chromatogram obtained with reference solution (b).

Loss on drying (*2.2.32*). Not more than 0.5 per cent, determined on 1.000 g by drying in an oven at 100 °C to 105 °C for 2 h.

Sulphated ash (*2.4.14*). Not more than 0.1 per cent, determined on 1.0 g.

ASSAY

Dissolve 0.300 g in 50 ml of a mixture of 1 volume of *anhydrous acetic acid R* and 7 volumes of *methyl ethyl ketone R*. Using 0.2 ml of *naphtholbenzein solution R* as indicator, titrate with *0.1 M perchloric acid* until the colour changes from orange-yellow to green.

1 ml of *0.1 M perchloric acid* is equivalent to 41.61 mg of $C_{18}H_{14}Cl_4N_2O$.

STORAGE

Store protected from light.

IMPURITIES

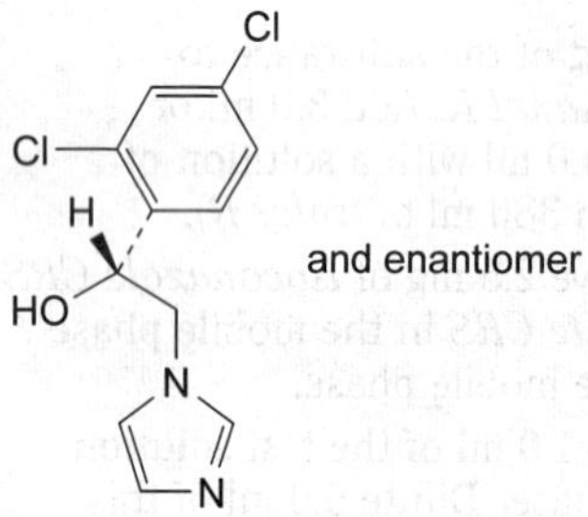

B. (1*RS*)-1-(2,4-dichlorophenyl)-2-(1*H*-imidazol-1-yl)ethanol,

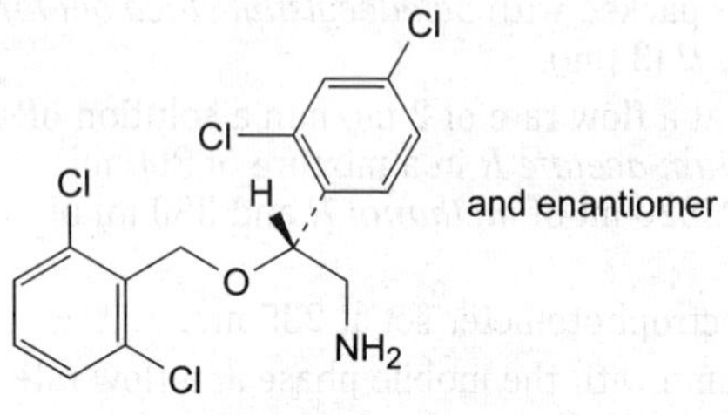

C. (2*RS*)-2-[(2,6-dichlorobenzyl)oxy]-2-(2,4-dichlorophenyl)ethanamine,

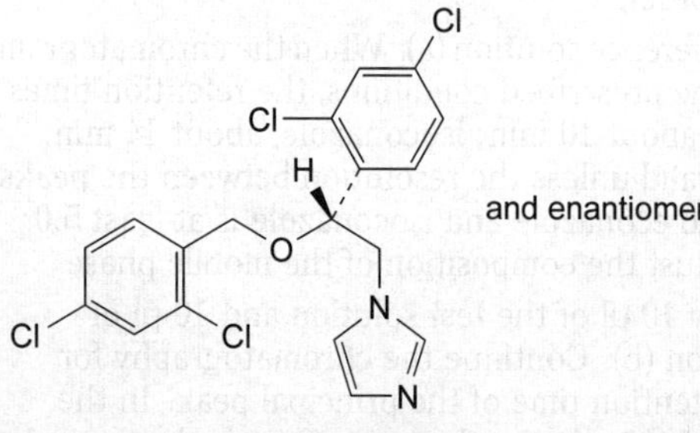

D. 1-[(2*RS*)-2-[(2,4-dichlorobenzyl)oxy]-2-(2,4-dichlorophenyl)ethyl]-1*H*-imidazole.

01/2005:1017

ISOCONAZOLE NITRATE

Isoconazoli nitras

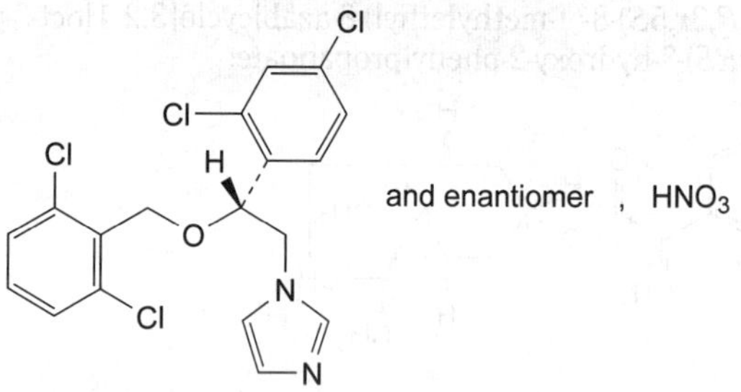

$C_{18}H_{15}Cl_4N_3O_4$ M_r 479.1

DEFINITION

Isoconazole nitrate contains not less than 99.0 per cent and not more than the equivalent of 101.0 per cent of 1-[(2*RS*)-2-[(2,6-dichlorobenzyl)oxy]-2-(2,4-dichlorophenyl)ethyl]-1*H*-imidazole, calculated with reference to the dried substance.

CHARACTERS

A white or almost white powder, very slightly soluble in water, soluble in methanol, slightly soluble in alcohol.

IDENTIFICATION

First identification: A, B.

Second identification: A, C, D.

A. Melting point (*2.2.14*): 178 °C to 182 °C.

B. Examine by infrared absorption spectrophotometry (*2.2.24*), comparing with the spectrum obtained with *isoconazole nitrate CRS*. Examine the substances prepared as discs.

C. Examine by thin-layer chromatography (*2.2.27*), using a suitable octadecylsilyl silica gel as the coating substance.

Test solution. Dissolve 30 mg of the substance to be examined in *methanol R* and dilute to 5 ml with the same solvent.

Reference solution (a). Dissolve 30 mg of *isoconazole nitrate CRS* in *methanol R* and dilute to 5 ml with the same solvent.

Reference solution (b). Dissolve 30 mg of *isoconazole nitrate CRS* and 30 mg of *econazole nitrate CRS* in *methanol R* and dilute to 5 ml with the same solvent.

Apply separately to the plate 5 µl of each solution. Develop over a path of 15 cm using a mixture of 20 volumes of *ammonium acetate solution R*, 40 volumes of *dioxan R* and 40 volumes of *methanol R*. Dry the plate in a current of warm air for 15 min and expose it to iodine vapour until the spots appear. Examine in daylight. The principal spot in the chromatogram obtained with the test solution is similar in position, colour and size to the principal spot in the chromatogram obtained with reference solution (a). The test is not valid unless the chromatogram obtained with reference solution (b) shows two clearly separated spots.

D. It gives the reaction of nitrates (*2.3.1*).

TESTS

Solution S. Dissolve 0.20 g in *methanol R* and dilute to 20.0 ml with the same solvent.

Appearance of solution. Solution S is clear (*2.2.1*) and is not more intensely coloured than reference solution Y_7 (*2.2.2, Method II*).

Optical rotation (*2.2.7*). The angle of optical rotation, determined on solution S, is − 0.10° to + 0.10°.

Related substances. Examine by liquid chromatography (*2.2.29*).

Test solution. Dissolve 0.100 g of the substance to be examined in the mobile phase and dilute to 10.0 ml with the mobile phase.

Reference solution (a). Dissolve 2.5 mg of *isoconazole nitrate CRS* and 2.5 mg of *econazole nitrate CRS* in the mobile phase and dilute to 100.0 ml with the mobile phase.

Reference solution (b). Dilute 1.0 ml of the test solution to 100.0 ml with the mobile phase. Dilute 5.0 ml of this solution to 20.0 ml with the mobile phase.

The chromatographic procedure may be carried out using:

– a stainless steel column 0.1 m long and 4.6 mm in internal diameter packed with *octadecylsilyl silica gel for chromatography R* (3 μm),
– as mobile phase at a flow rate of 2 ml/min a solution of 6.0 g of *ammonium acetate R* in a mixture of 300 ml of *acetonitrile R*, 320 ml of *methanol R* and 380 ml of *water R*,
– as detector a spectrophotometer set at 235 nm.

Equilibrate the column with the mobile phase at a flow rate of 2 ml/min for about 30 min.

Adjust the sensitivity of the system so that the height of the principal peak in the chromatogram obtained with 10 μl of reference solution (b) is at least 50 per cent of the full scale of the recorder.

Inject 10 μl of reference solution (a). When the chromatogram is recorded in the prescribed conditions, the retention times are: econazole, about 10 min and isoconazole, about 14 min. The test is not valid unless the resolution between the peaks due to econazole and isoconazole is not less than 5.0. If necessary, adjust the composition of the mobile phase.

Inject separately 10 μl of the test solution and 10 μl of reference solution (b). Continue the chromatography for 1.5 times the retention time of the principal peak. In the chromatogram obtained with the test solution: the area of any peak, apart from the principal peak, is not greater than the area of the principal peak in the chromatogram obtained with reference solution (b) (0.25 per cent); the sum of the areas of all the peaks, apart from the principal peak, is not greater than twice the area of the principal peak in the chromatogram obtained with reference solution (b) (0.5 per cent). Disregard any peaks due to the solvent and to nitrate ion and any peak with an area less than 0.2 times that of the principal peak in the chromatogram obtained with reference solution (b).

Loss on drying (*2.2.32*). Not more than 0.5 per cent, determined on 1.000 g by drying in an oven at 100 °C to 105 °C for 2 h.

Sulphated ash (*2.4.14*). Not more than 0.1 per cent, determined on 1.0 g.

ASSAY

Dissolve 0.350 g in 75 ml of a mixture of 1 volume of *anhydrous acetic acid R* and 7 volumes of *methyl ethyl ketone R* and titrate with *0.1 M perchloric acid*. Determine the end-point potentiometrically (*2.2.20*).

1 ml of *0.1 M perchloric acid* is equivalent to 47.91 mg of $C_{18}H_{15}Cl_4N_3O_4$.

STORAGE

Store protected from light.

IMPURITIES

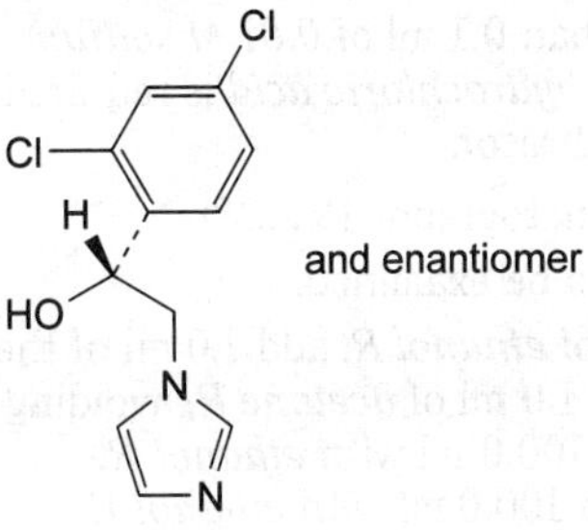

A. (1*RS*)-1-(2,4-dichlorophenyl)-2-(1*H*-imidazol-1-yl)ethanol,

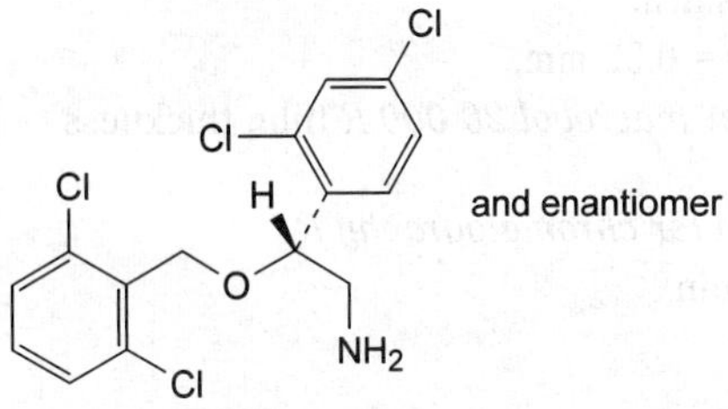

B. (2*RS*)-2-[(2,6-dichlorobenzyl)oxy]-2-(2,4-dichlorophenyl)ethanamine,

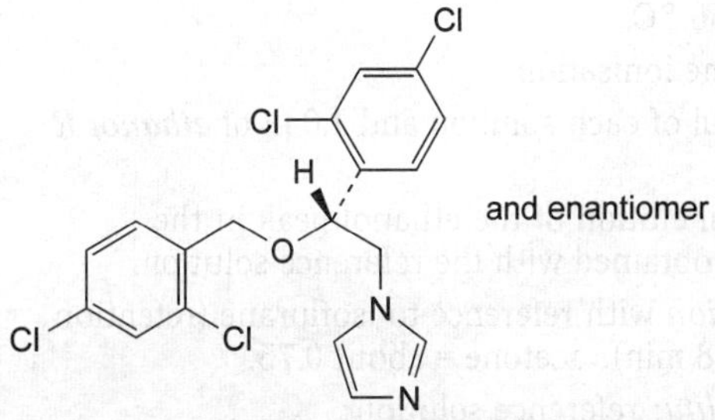

C. 1-[(2*RS*)-2-[(2,4-dichlorobenzyl)oxy]-2-(2,4-dichlorophenyl)ethyl]-1*H*-imidazole.

01/2005:1673
corrected

ISOFLURANE

Isofluranum

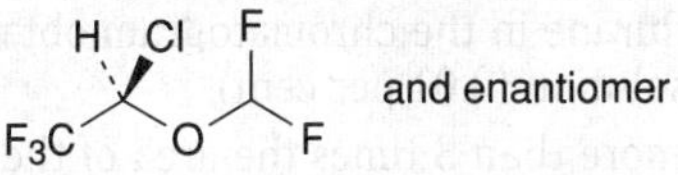

$C_3H_2ClF_5O$ M_r 184.5

DEFINITION

(2*RS*)-2-Chloro-2-(difluoromethoxy)-1,1,1-trifluoroethane.

CHARACTERS

Appearance: clear, colourless, mobile, heavy liquid.

Solubility: practically insoluble in water, miscible with ethanol and trichloroethylene.

bp: about 48 °C.

It is non-flammable.

IDENTIFICATION

Infrared absorption spectrophotometry (*2.2.24*).

Preparation: examine the substance in the gaseous state.

Comparison: *Ph. Eur. reference spectrum of isoflurane*.

TESTS

Acidity or alkalinity. To 20 ml add 20 ml of *carbon dioxide-free water R*, shake for 3 min and allow to stand. Collect the upper layer and add 0.2 ml of *bromocresol purple solution R*. Not more than 0.1 ml of *0.01 M sodium hydroxide* or 0.6 ml of *0.01 M hydrochloric acid* is required to change the colour of the indicator.

Related substances. Gas chromatography (*2.2.28*).

Test solution. The substance to be examined.

Reference solution. To 80 ml of *ethanol R*, add 1.0 ml of the substance to be examined and 1.0 ml of *acetone R*, avoiding loss by evaporation. Dilute to 100.0 ml with *ethanol R*. Dilute 1.0 ml of the solution to 100.0 ml with *ethanol R*.

Column:
- *material*: fused silica,
- *size*: l = 30 m, Ø = 0.32 mm,
- *stationary phase*: *macrogol 20 000 R* (film thickness 0.25 μm).

Carrier gas: *helium for chromatography R*.

Flow rate: 1.0 ml/min.

Split ratio: 1:25.

Temperature:
- *column*: 35 °C,
- *injection port*: 150 °C,
- *detector*: 250 °C.

Detection: flame ionisation.

Injection: 1.0 μl of each solution and 1.0 μl of *ethanol R* as a blank.

Run time: until elution of the ethanol peak in the chromatogram obtained with the reference solution.

Relative retention with reference to isoflurane (retention time = about 3.8 min): acetone = about 0.75.

System suitability: reference solution:
- *resolution*: minimum of 5 between the peaks due to acetone and to isoflurane,
- *repeatability*: maximum relative standard deviation 15.0 per cent for the peak due to isoflurane after 3 injections.

Limits:
- *acetone*: not more than the area of the corresponding peak in the chromatogram obtained with the reference solution (0.01 per cent),
- *any other impurity*: not more than the area of the peak due to isoflurane in the chromatogram obtained with the reference solution (0.01 per cent),
- *total*: not more than 3 times the area of the peak due to isoflurane in the chromatogram obtained with the reference solution (0.03 per cent),
- *disregard limit*: 0.1 times the area of the peak due to isoflurane in the chromatogram obtained with the reference solution (0.001 per cent).

Chlorides (*2.4.4*): maximum 10 ppm.

To 10 ml add 10 ml of *0.01 M sodium hydroxide* and shake for 3 min. To 5 ml of the upper layer add 10 ml of *water R*. The solution complies with the limit test for chlorides.

Fluorides: maximum 10 ppm.

Determine by potentiometry (*2.2.36, Method I*) using a fluoride-selective indicator-electrode and a silver-silver chloride reference electrode.

Test solution. To 10.0 ml in a separating funnel, add 10 ml of a mixture of 30.0 ml of *dilute ammonia R2* and 70.0 ml of *distilled water R*. Shake for 1 min and collect the upper layer. Repeat this extraction procedure twice collecting the upper layer each time. Adjust the combined upper layers to pH 5.2 using *dilute hydrochloric acid R*. Add 5.0 ml of *fluoride standard solution (1 ppm F) R* and dilute to 50.0 ml with *distilled water R*. To 20.0 ml of the solution add 20.0 ml of *total-ionic-strength-adjustment buffer R* and dilute to 50.0 ml with *distilled water R*.

Reference solutions. To each of 5.0 ml, 4.0 ml, 3.0 ml, 2.0 ml and 1.0 ml of *fluoride standard solution (10 ppm F) R* add 20.0 ml of *total-ionic-strength-adjustment buffer R* and dilute to 50.0 ml with *distilled water R*.

Carry out the measurements on 20 ml of each solution. Calculate the concentration of fluorides using the calibration curve, taking into account the addition of fluoride to the test solution.

Non-volatile matter: maximum 200 mg/l.

Evaporate 10.0 ml to dryness with the aid of a stream of cold air and dry the residue at 50 °C for 2 h. The residue weighs a maximum of 2.0 mg.

Water (*2.5.12*): maximum 1.0 mg/ml, determined on 10.0 ml.

STORAGE

In an airtight container, protected from light.

IMPURITIES

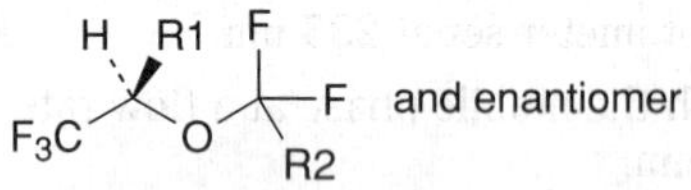

A. R1 = H, R2 = Cl: 2-(chlorodifluoromethoxy)-1,1,1-trifluoroethane,

B. R1 = R2 = H: 2-(difluoromethoxy)-1,1,1-trifluoroethane,

C. R1 = R2 = Cl: (2*RS*)-2-chloro-2-(chlorodifluoromethoxy)-1,1,1-trifluoroethane,

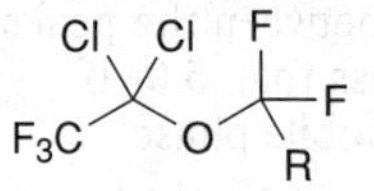

D. R = H: 1,1-dichloro-1-(difluoromethoxy)-2,2,2-trifluoroethane,

E. R = Cl: 1,1-dichloro-1-(chlorodifluoromethoxy)-2,2,2-trifluoroethane,

F. acetone.

01/2005:0770

ISOLEUCINE

Isoleucinum

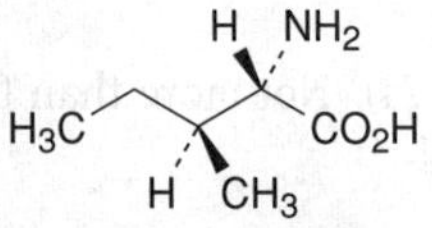

$C_6H_{13}NO_2$ M_r 131.2

DEFINITION

Isoleucine contains not less than 98.5 per cent and not more than the equivalent of 101.0 per cent of (2*S*,3*S*)-2-amino-3-methylpentanoic acid, calculated with reference to the dried substance.

CHARACTERS

White or almost white, crystalline powder or flakes, sparingly soluble in water, slightly soluble in alcohol. It dissolves in dilute mineral acids and in dilute solutions of alkali hydroxides.

IDENTIFICATION

First identification: A, C.

Second identification: A, B, D.

A. It complies with the test for specific optical rotation (see Tests).

B. Dissolve 0.5 g in *water R* and dilute to 25 ml with the same solvent. The solution is dextrorotatory.

C. Examine by infrared absorption spectrophotometry (*2.2.24*), comparing with the spectrum obtained with *isoleucine CRS*. Examine the substances prepared as discs.

D. Examine the chromatograms obtained in the test for ninhydrin-positive substances. The principal spot in the chromatogram obtained with test solution (b) is similar in position, colour and size to the principal spot in the chromatogram obtained with reference solution (a).

TESTS

Appearance of solution. Dissolve 0.5 g in *1 M hydrochloric acid* and dilute to 10 ml with the same acid. The solution is clear (*2.2.1*) and not more intensely coloured than reference solution BY_6 (*2.2.2, Method II*).

Specific optical rotation (*2.2.7*). Dissolve 1.00 g in *hydrochloric acid R1* and dilute to 25.0 ml with the same acid. The specific optical rotation is + 40.0 to + 43.0, calculated with reference to the dried substance.

Ninhydrin-positive substances. Examine by thin-layer chromatography (*2.2.27*), using a *TLC silica gel plate R*.

Test solution (a). Dissolve 0.10 g of the substance to be examined in *0.1 M hydrochloric acid* and dilute to 10 ml with the same acid.

Test solution (b). Dilute 1 ml of test solution (a) to 50 ml with *water R*.

Reference solution (a). Dissolve 10 mg of *isoleucine CRS* in *0.1 M hydrochloric acid* and dilute to 50 ml with the same acid.

Reference solution (b). Dilute 5 ml of test solution (b) to 20 ml with *water R*.

Reference solution (c). Dissolve 10 mg of *isoleucine CRS* and 10 mg of *valine CRS* in *0.1 M hydrochloric acid* and dilute to 25 ml with the same acid.

Apply separately to the plate 5 µl of each solution. Develop over a path of 15 cm using a mixture of 20 volumes of *glacial acetic acid R*, 20 volumes of *water R* and 60 volumes of *butanol R*. Allow the plate to dry in air, spray with *ninhydrin solution R* and heat at 100-105 °C for 15 min. Any spot in the chromatogram obtained with test solution (a), apart from the principal spot, is not more intense than the spot in the chromatogram obtained with reference solution (b) (0.5 per cent). The test is not valid unless the chromatogram obtained with reference solution (c) shows 2 clearly separated spots.

Chlorides (*2.4.4*). Dissolve 0.25 g in *water R* and dilute to 15 ml with the same solvent. The solution complies with the limit test for chlorides (200 ppm).

Sulphates (*2.4.13*). Dissolve 0.5 g in 3 ml of *dilute hydrochloric acid R* and dilute to 15 ml with *distilled water R*. The solution complies with the limit test for sulphates (300 ppm).

Ammonium (*2.4.1*). 50 mg complies with limit test B for ammonium (200 ppm). Prepare the standard using 0.1 ml of *ammonium standard solution (100 ppm NH_4) R*.

Iron (*2.4.9*). In a separating funnel, dissolve 1.0 g in 10 ml of *dilute hydrochloric acid R*. Shake with 3 quantities, each of 10 ml, of *methyl isobutyl ketone R1*, shaking for 3 min each time. To the combined organic layers add 10 ml of *water R* and shake for 3 min. The aqueous layer complies with the limit test for iron (10 ppm).

Heavy metals (*2.4.8*). 2.0 g complies with limit test D for heavy metals (10 ppm). Prepare the standard using 2 ml of *lead standard solution (10 ppm Pb) R*.

Loss on drying (*2.2.32*). Not more than 0.5 per cent, determined on 1.000 g by drying in an oven at 100-105 °C.

Sulphated ash (*2.4.14*). Not more than 0.1 per cent, determined on 1.0 g.

ASSAY

Dissolve 0.100 g in 3 ml of *anhydrous formic acid R*. Add 30 ml of *anhydrous acetic acid R*. Using 0.1 ml of *naphtholbenzein solution R* as indicator, titrate with *0.1 M perchloric acid* until the colour changes from brownish-yellow to green.

1 ml of *0.1 M perchloric acid* is equivalent to 13.12 mg of $C_6H_{13}NO_2$.

STORAGE

Store protected from light.

01/2005:1531

ISOMALT

Isomaltum

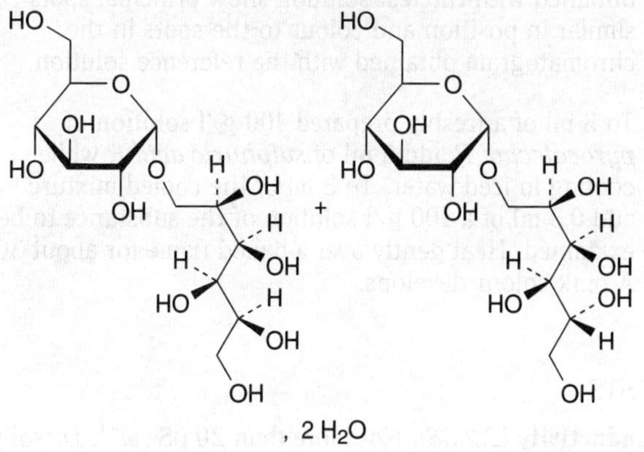

$C_{12}H_{24}O_{11}$ M_r 344.3

$C_{12}H_{24}O_{11},2H_2O$ M_r 380.3

DEFINITION

Isomalt contains not less than 98.0 per cent and not more than the equivalent of 102.0 per cent of a mixture of 6-*O*-α-D-glucopyranosyl-D-glucitol (6-*O*-α-D-glucopyranosyl-D-sorbitol; 1,6-GPS) and 1-*O*-α-D-glucopyranosyl-D-mannitol (1,1-GPM) and neither of the 2 components is less than 3.0 per cent, calculated with reference to the anhydrous substance. The percentage content of 1,6-GPS and 1,1-GPM is stated on the label.

CHARACTERS

A white or almost white powder or granules, freely soluble in water, practically insoluble in ethanol.

IDENTIFICATION

First identification: A.

Second identification: B, C.

A. Examine the chromatograms obtained in the assay. The 2 principal peaks in the chromatogram obtained with the test solution are similar in retention time to the 2 principal peaks in the chromatogram obtained with reference solution (a).

B. Examine by thin layer chromatography (*2.2.27*) using a *TLC silica gel F_{254} plate R.*

Test solution. Dissolve 50 mg of the substance to be examined in *water R* and dilute to 10 ml with the same solvent.

Reference solution. Dissolve 50 mg of *isomalt CRS* in *water R* and dilute to 10 ml with the same solvent.

Apply to the plate 1 µl of each solution and thoroughly dry the starting points in warm air. Develop over a path of 10 cm using a mixture of 5 volumes of *acetic acid R,* 5 volumes of *propionic acid R,* 10 volumes of *water R,* 50 volumes of *ethyl acetate R* and 50 volumes of *pyridine R.* Dry the plate in a current of warm air and dip for 3 s in a 1 g/l solution of *sodium periodate R.* Dry the plate in a current of hot air. Dip the plate for 3 s in a mixture of 1 volume of *acetic acid R,* 1 volume of *anisaldehyde R,* 5 volumes of *sulphuric acid R* and 90 volumes of *ethanol R.* Dry the plate in a current of hot air until coloured spots become visible. The background colour may be brightened in warm steam. Examine in daylight. The chromatogram obtained with the reference solution shows 2 blue-grey spots with R_f values of about 0.13 (1,6-GPS) and 0.16 (1,1-GPM). The chromatogram obtained with the test solution show principal spots similar in position and colour to the spots in the chromatogram obtained with the reference solution.

C. To 3 ml of a freshly prepared 100 g/l solution of *pyrocatechol R* add 6 ml of *sulphuric acid R* while cooling in iced water. To 3 ml of the cooled mixture add 0.3 ml of a 100 g/l solution of the substance to be examined. Heat gently over a naked flame for about 30 s. A pink colour develops.

TESTS

Conductivity (*2.2.38*). Not more than 20 µS·cm^{-1}. Dissolve 20.0 g in *carbon dioxide-free water R* prepared from *distilled water R* and dilute to 100.0 ml with the same solvent. Measure the conductivity of the solution while gently stirring with a magnetic stirrer.

Reducing sugars. Dissolve 3.3 g in 10 ml of *water R* with the aid of gentle heat. Cool and add 20 ml of *cupri-citric solution R* and a few glass beads. Heat so that the boiling begins after 4 min and maintain boiling for 3 min. Cool rapidly and add 100 ml of a 2.4 per cent *V/V* solution of *glacial acetic acid R* and 20.0 ml of *0.025 M iodine.* With continuous shaking, add 25 ml of a mixture of 6 volumes of *hydrochloric acid R* and 94 volumes of *water R* and, when the precipitate has dissolved, titrate the excess of iodine with *0.05 M sodium thiosulphate* using 1 ml of *starch solution R* as indicator, added towards the end of the titration. Not less than 12.8 ml of *0.05 M sodium thiosulphate* is required (0.3 per cent, calculated as glucose).

Related products. Examine the chromatograms obtained in the assay. In the chromatogram obtained with the test solution: the area of any peak corresponding to mannitol or sorbitol is not greater than the area of the corresponding peak in the chromatogram obtained with reference solution (b) (0.5 per cent); the area of any peak, apart from the 2 principal peaks corresponding to 1,1-GPM and 1,6-GPS and the peaks corresponding to mannitol and sorbitol, is not greater than the area of the peak due to sorbitol in the chromatogram obtained with reference solution (b) (0.5 per cent); the sum of the area of all the peaks apart from the peaks corresponding to 1,1-GPM and 1,6-GPS is not greater than 4 times the area of the peak due to sorbitol in the chromatogram obtained with reference solution (b) (2 per cent). Disregard any peak with an area less than 0.2 times that of the peak due to sorbitol in the chromatogram obtained with reference solution (b) (0.1 per cent).

Lead (*2.4.10*). It complies with the limit test for lead in sugars (0.5 ppm).

Nickel (*2.4.15*). It complies with the limit test for nickel in polyols (1 ppm).

Water (*2.5.12*). Not more than 7.0 per cent, determined on 0.3 g by the semi-micro determination of water. As solvent, use a mixture of 20 ml of *anhydrous methanol R* and 20 ml of *formamide R* at 50 ± 5 °C.

ASSAY

Examine by liquid chromatography (*2.2.29*).

Test solution. Dissolve 1.00 g of the substance to be examined in 20 ml of *water R* and dilute to 50.0 ml with the same solvent.

Reference solution (a). Dissolve 1.00 g of *isomalt CRS* in 20 ml of *water R* and dilute to 50.0 ml with the same solvent.

Reference solution (b). Dissolve 10.0 mg of *sorbitol CRS* and 10.0 mg of *mannitol CRS* in 20 ml of *water R* and dilute to 100.0 ml with the same solvent.

The chromatographic procedure may be carried out using:

- a stainless steel precolumn 30 mm long and 4.6 mm in internal diameter and a stainless steel column 0.3 m long and 7.8 mm in internal diameter, both packed with a *strong cation-exchange resin (calcium form) R* (9 µm) and maintained at 80 ± 1 °C,
- as mobile phase at a flow rate of 0.5 ml/min degassed *water R,*
- as detector a differential refractometer maintained at a constant temperature.

Inject 20 µl of each solution and continue the chromatography until sorbitol is completely eluted (about 25 min). When the chromatograms are recorded in the prescribed conditions, the retention time of 1,1-GPM is about 12.3 min and the relative retentions to 1,1-GPM are: 1,6-GPS about 1.2, mannitol about 1.6, sorbitol about 2.0 and isomaltulose about 0.8.

Calculate the percentage content of isomalt (1,1-GPM and 1,6-GPS) from the areas of the peaks of 1,1-GPM and 1,6-GPS and the declared content of 1,1-GPM and 1,6-GPS in *isomalt CRS.*

LABELLING

The label states the percentage content of 1,6-GPS and 1,1-GPM.

IMPURITIES

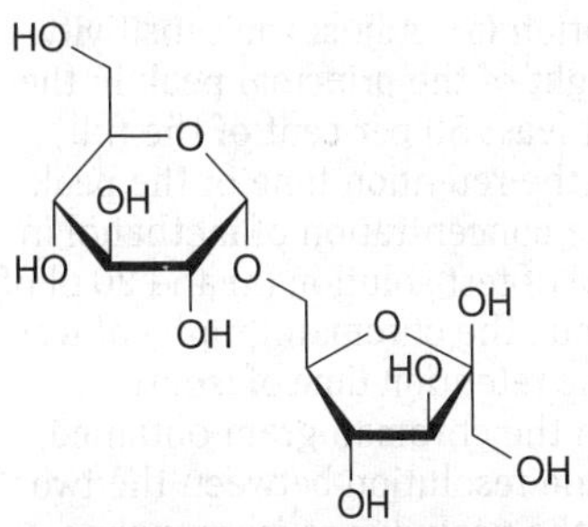

A. 6-*O*-α-D-glucopyranosyl-β-D-*arabino*-hex-2-ulofuranose (isomaltulose),

B. mannitol,

C. sorbitol,

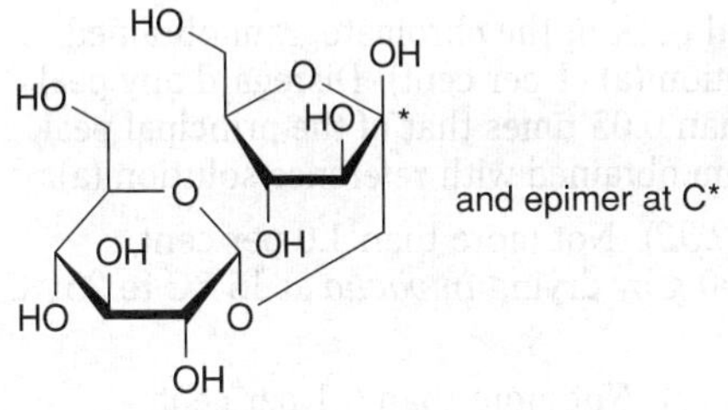

D. 1-*O*-α-D-glucopyranosyl-D-*arabino*-hex-2-ulofuranose (trehalulose).

01/2005:0146

ISONIAZID

Isoniazidum

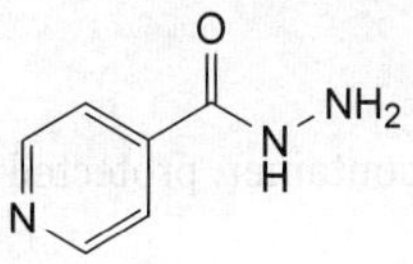

$C_6H_7N_3O$ M_r 137.1

DEFINITION

Isoniazid contains not less than 99.0 per cent and not more than the equivalent of 101.0 per cent of pyridine-4-carbohydrazide, calculated with reference to the dried substance.

CHARACTERS

A white, crystalline powder or colourless crystals, freely soluble in water, sparingly soluble in alcohol.

IDENTIFICATION

First identification: A, B.

Second identification: A, C.

A. Melting point (*2.2.14*): 170 °C to 174 °C.

B. Examine by infrared absorption spectrophotometry (*2.2.24*), comparing with the spectrum obtained with *isoniazid CRS*.

C. Dissolve 0.1 g in 2 ml of *water R* and add 10 ml of a warm 10 g/l solution of *vanillin R*. Allow to stand and scratch the wall of the test tube with a glass rod. A yellow precipitate is formed, which, after recrystallisation from 5 ml of *alcohol (70 per cent V/V) R* and drying at 100 °C to 105 °C, melts (*2.2.14*) at 226 °C to 231 °C.

TESTS

Solution S. Dissolve 2.5 g in *carbon dioxide-free water R* and dilute to 50 ml with the same solvent.

Appearance of solution. Solution S is clear (*2.2.1*) and not more intensely coloured than reference solution BY_7 (*2.2.2, Method II*).

pH (*2.2.3*). The pH of solution S is 6.0 to 8.0.

Hydrazine and related substances. Examine by thin-layer chromatography (*2.2.27*), using *silica gel GF_{254} R* as the coating substance.

Test solution. Dissolve 1.0 g of the substance to be examined in a mixture of equal volumes of *acetone R* and *water R* and dilute to 10.0 ml with the same mixture of solvents.

Reference solution. Dissolve 50.0 mg of *hydrazine sulphate R* in 50 ml of *water R* and dilute to 100.0 ml with *acetone R*. To 10.0 ml of this solution add 0.2 ml of the test solution and dilute to 100.0 ml with a mixture of equal volumes of *acetone R* and *water R*.

Apply separately to the plate 5 µl of each solution and develop over a path of 15 cm using a mixture of 10 volumes of *water R*, 20 volumes of *acetone R*, 20 volumes of *methanol R* and 50 volumes of *ethyl acetate R*. Allow the plate to dry in air and examine in ultraviolet light at 254 nm. Any spot in the chromatogram obtained with the test solution, apart from the principal spot, is not more intense than the spot in the chromatogram obtained with the reference solution (0.2 per cent). Spray the plate with *dimethylaminobenzaldehyde solution R1*. Examine in daylight. An additional spot, corresponding to hydrazine, appears in the chromatogram obtained with the reference solution. Any corresponding spot in the chromatogram obtained with the test solution is not more intense than the spot corresponding to hydrazine in the chromatogram obtained with the reference solution (0.05 per cent).

Heavy metals (*2.4.8*). 2.0 g complies with limit test C for heavy metals (10 ppm). Prepare the standard using 2 ml of *lead standard solution (10 ppm Pb) R*.

Loss on drying (*2.2.32*). Not more than 0.5 per cent, determined on 1.00 g by drying in an oven at 100 °C to 105 °C.

Sulphated ash (*2.4.14*). Not more than 0.1 per cent, determined on 1.0 g.

ASSAY

Dissolve 0.250 g in *water R* and dilute to 100.0 ml with the same solvent. To 20.0 ml of the solution add 100 ml of *water R*, 20 ml of *hydrochloric acid R*, 0.2 g of *potassium bromide R* and 0.05 ml of *methyl red solution R*. Titrate dropwise with *0.0167 M potassium bromate*, shaking continuously, until the red colour disappears.

1 ml of *0.0167 M potassium bromate* is equivalent to 3.429 mg of $C_6H_7N_3O$.

01/2005:1332

ISOPRENALINE HYDROCHLORIDE

Isoprenalini hydrochloridum

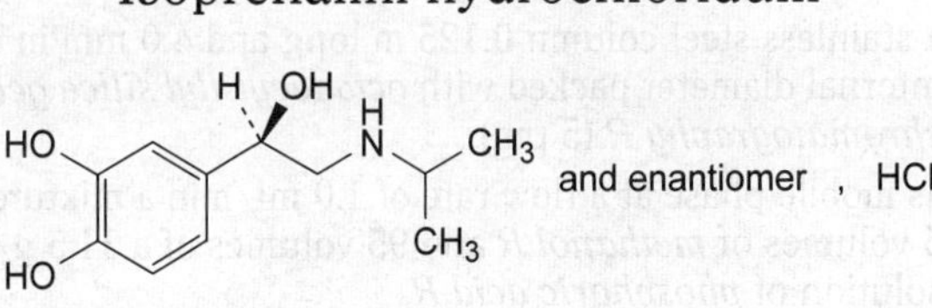

$C_{11}H_{18}ClNO_3$ M_r 247.7

DEFINITION

Isoprenaline hydrochloride contains not less than 98.0 per cent and not more than the equivalent of 101.5 per cent of (1*RS*)-1-(3,4-dihydroxyphenyl)-2-[(1-methylethyl)amino]ethanol hydrochloride, calculated with reference to the dried substance.

CHARACTERS

A white or almost white, crystalline powder, freely soluble in water, sparingly soluble in alcohol, practically insoluble in methylene chloride.

IDENTIFICATION

First identification: B, C, E.

Second identification: A, C, D, E.

A. Melting point (*2.2.14*): 165 °C to 170 °C, with decomposition.

B. Examine by infrared absorption spectrophotometry (*2.2.24*), comparing with the spectrum obtained with *isoprenaline hydrochloride CRS*. Examine the substances as discs.

C. It complies with the test for optical rotation (see Tests).

D. To 0.1 ml of solution S (see Tests) add 0.05 ml of *ferric chloride solution R1* and 0.9 ml of *water R*. A green colour is produced. Add dropwise *sodium hydrogen carbonate solution R*. The colour becomes blue then red.

E. To 0.5 ml of solution S add 1.5 ml of *water R*. The solution gives reaction (a) of chlorides (*2.3.1*).

TESTS

Prepare the solutions immediately before use.

Solution S. Dissolve 2.5 g in *carbon dioxide-free water R* and dilute to 25.0 ml with the same solvent.

Appearance of solution. Solution S is clear (*2.2.1*) and not more intensely coloured than reference solution B_7 or BY_7 (*2.2.2, Method II*).

pH (*2.2.3*). The pH of a mixture of 5 ml of solution S and 5 ml of *carbon dioxide-free water R* is 4.3 to 5.5.

Optical rotation (*2.2.7*). The angle of optical rotation, determined on solution S, is − 0.10° to + 0.10°.

Related substances. Examine by liquid chromatography (*2.2.29*).

Test solution (a). Dissolve 50.0 mg of the substance to be examined in the mobile phase and dilute to 10.0 ml with the mobile phase.

Test solution (b). Dilute 0.5 ml of test solution (a) to 100.0 ml with the mobile phase.

Reference solution (a). Dissolve 2.5 mg of *isoprenaline hydrochloride CRS* in the mobile phase and dilute to 100.0 ml with the mobile phase.

Reference solution (b). Dissolve 2.5 mg of *orciprenaline sulphate CRS* in the mobile phase and dilute to 100.0 ml with the mobile phase.

Reference solution (c). To 1.0 ml of test solution (b) add 1.0 ml of reference solution (b) and dilute to 20.0 ml with the mobile phase.

The chromatographic procedure may be carried out using:

– a stainless steel column 0.125 m long and 4.0 mm in internal diameter packed with *octadecylsilyl silica gel for chromatography R* (5 µm),
– as mobile phase at a flow rate of 1.0 ml/min a mixture of 5 volumes of *methanol R* and 95 volumes of a 11.5 g/l solution of *phosphoric acid R*,
– as detector a spectrophotometer set at 280 nm,
– a loop injector.

Inject 20 µl of reference solution (a). Adjust the sensitivity of the system so that the height of the principal peak in the chromatogram obtained is at least 50 per cent of the full scale of the recorder. Adjust the retention time of the peak to about 3 min by varying the concentration of methanol in the mobile phase. Inject 20 µl of test solution (a) and 20 µl of reference solution (c). Continue the chromatography of test solution (a) for seven times the retention time of isoprenaline. The test is not valid unless in the chromatogram obtained with reference solution (c): the resolution between the two principal peaks is at least 3; the peak due to isoprenaline has a signal-to-noise ratio of at least 3.

In the chromatogram obtained with test solution (a): the area of any peak, apart from the principal peak, is not greater than the area of the principal peak in the chromatogram obtained with reference solution (a) (0.5 per cent) and the sum of the areas of such peaks is not greater than twice the area of the principal peak in the chromatogram obtained with reference solution (a) (1 per cent). Disregard any peak with an area less than 0.05 times that of the principal peak in the chromatogram obtained with reference solution (a).

Loss on drying (*2.2.32*). Not more than 1.0 per cent, determined on 1.000 g by drying *in vacuo* at 15 °C to 25 °C for 4 h.

Sulphated ash (*2.4.14*). Not more than 0.1 per cent, determined on 1.0 g.

ASSAY

In order to avoid overheating in the reaction medium, mix thoroughly throughout and stop the titration immediately after the end-point has been reached.

Dissolve 0.150 g in 10 ml of *anhydrous formic acid R* and add 50 ml of *acetic anhydride R*. Titrate with *0.1 M perchloric acid*, determining the end-point potentiometrically (*2.2.20*).

1 ml of *0.1 M perchloric acid* is equivalent to 24.77 mg of $C_{11}H_{18}ClNO_3$.

STORAGE

Store in an airtight container, protected from light.

IMPURITIES

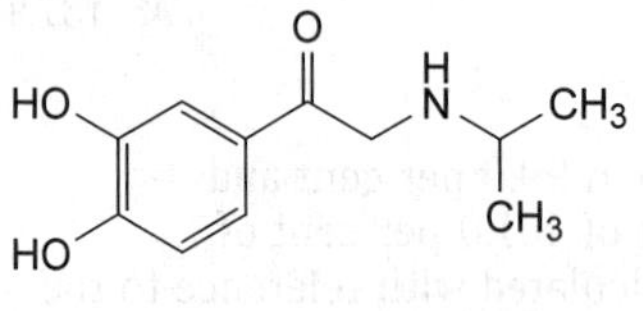

A. 1-(3,4-dihydroxyphenyl)-2-[(1-methylethyl)amino]ethanone.

01/2005:0502

ISOPRENALINE SULPHATE

Isoprenalini sulfas

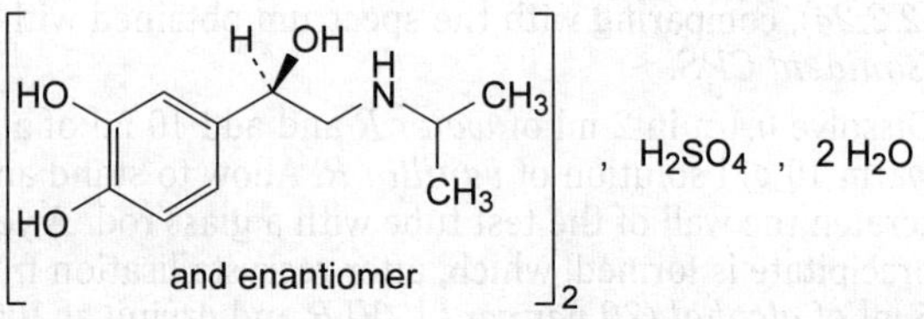

$C_{22}H_{36}N_2O_{10}S,2H_2O$ M_r 556.6

DEFINITION

Isoprenaline sulphate contains not less than 98.0 per cent and not more than the equivalent of 102.0 per cent of bis[(1*RS*)-1-(3,4-dihydroxyphenyl)-2-[(1-methylethyl)amino]ethanol] sulphate, calculated with reference to the anhydrous substance.

CHARACTERS

A white or almost white, crystalline powder, freely soluble in water, very slightly soluble in alcohol.

It melts at about 128 °C, with decomposition.

IDENTIFICATION

First identification: A, D.

Second identification: B, C, D.

A. Dissolve 0.5 g of the substance to be examined in 1.5 ml of *water R* and add 3.5 ml of *2-propanol R*. Scratch the wall of the tube with a glass rod to initiate crystallisation. Collect the crystals and dry *in vacuo* at 60 °C over *diphosphorus pentoxide R*. Repeat the operations with *isoprenaline sulphate CRS*. Examine by infrared absorption spectrophotometry (*2.2.24*), comparing with the spectrum obtained with *isoprenaline sulphate CRS*.

B. To 0.1 ml of solution S (see Tests) add 0.9 ml of *water R* and 0.05 ml of *ferric chloride solution R1*. A green colour is produced. Add dropwise *sodium hydrogen carbonate solution R*. The colour becomes blue and then red.

C. Dilute 1 ml of solution S to 10 ml with *water R* and add 0.25 ml of *silver nitrate solution R1*. A shining, grey, fine precipitate is formed within 10 min and the solution becomes pink.

D. Solution S gives reaction (a) of sulphates (*2.3.1*).

TESTS

Solution S. Dissolve 5.0 g in *carbon dioxide-free water R* and dilute to 50 ml with the same solvent. Use within 2 h of preparation.

Appearance of solution. Solution S is clear (*2.2.1*) and not more intensely coloured than reference solution Y_6 (*2.2.2, Method II*).

pH (*2.2.3*). Dilute 5 ml of solution S to 10 ml with *carbon dioxide-free water R*. The pH of the solution is 4.3 to 5.5.

Isoprenalone. Dissolve 0.20 g in *0.005 M sulphuric acid* and dilute to 100.0 ml with the same solvent. The absorbance (*2.2.25*) measured at 310 nm is not greater than 0.20.

Water (*2.5.12*): 5.0 per cent to 7.5 per cent, determined on 0.200 g by the semi-micro determination of water.

Sulphated ash (*2.4.14*). Not more than 0.1 per cent, determined on 1.0 g.

ASSAY

Dissolve 0.400 g in 20 ml of *anhydrous acetic acid R*, warming gently if necessary and add 20 ml of *methyl isobutyl ketone R*. Titrate with *0.1 M perchloric acid* determining the end-point potentiometrically (*2.2.20*).

1 ml of *0.1 M perchloric acid* is equivalent to 52.06 mg of $C_{22}H_{36}N_2O_{10}S$.

STORAGE

Store in an airtight container, protected from light.

01/2005:0970

ISOPROPYL ALCOHOL

Alcohol isopropylicus

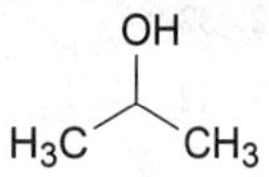

C_3H_8O M_r 60.1

DEFINITION

Propan-2-ol.

CHARACTERS

Appearance: clear, colourless liquid.

Solubility: miscible with water and with alcohol.

IDENTIFICATION

A. Relative density (*2.2.5*): 0.785 to 0.789.

B. Refractive index (*2.2.6*): 1.376 to 1.379.

C. To 1 ml add 2 ml of *potassium dichromate solution R* and 1 ml of *dilute sulphuric acid R*. Boil. Vapour is produced which changes the colour of a piece of filter paper impregnated with *nitrobenzaldehyde solution R* to green. Moisten the filter paper with *dilute hydrochloric acid R*. The colour changes to blue.

TESTS

Appearance. The substance to be examined is clear (*2.2.1*) and colourless (*2.2.2, Method II*). Dilute 1 ml to 20 ml with *water R*. After 5 min, the solution is clear (*2.2.1*).

Acidity or alkalinity. Gently boil 25 ml for 5 min. Add 25 ml of *carbon dioxide-free water R* and allow to cool protected from carbon dioxide in the air. Add 0.1 ml of *phenolphthalein solution R*. The solution is colourless. Not more than 0.6 ml of *0.01 M sodium hydroxide* is required to change the colour of the indicator to pale pink.

Absorbance (*2.2.25*): maximum 0.30 at 230 nm, 0.10 at 250 nm, 0.03 at 270 nm, 0.02 at 290 nm and 0.01 at 310 nm. The absorbance is measured between 230 nm and 310 nm using *water R* as the compensation liquid. The absorption curve is smooth.

Benzene and related substances. Gas chromatography (*2.2.28*).

Test solution (a). The substance to be examined.

Test solution (b). Dilute 1.0 ml of *2-butanol R1* to 50.0 ml with test solution (a). Dilute 5.0 ml of the solution to 100.0 ml with test solution (a).

Reference solution (a). Dilute 0.5 ml of *2-butanol R1* and 0.5 ml of *propanol R* to 50.0 ml with test solution (a). Dilute 5.0 ml of the solution to 50.0 ml with test solution (a).

Reference solution (b). Dilute 100 µl of *benzene R* to 100.0 ml with test solution (a). Dilute 0.20 ml of the solution to 100.0 ml with test solution (a).

Column:

- *material*: fused silica,
- *size*: l = 30 m, Ø = 0.32 mm,
- *stationary phase*: *poly[(cyanopropyl)(phenyl)][dimethyl]siloxane R* (film thickness 1.8 µm).

Carrier gas: *helium for chromatography R*.

Auxiliary gas: *nitrogen for chromatography R* or *helium for chromatography R*.

Linear velocity: 35 cm/s.

Monographs I-L

Split ratio: 1:5.

Temperature:

	Time (min)	Temperature (°C)
Column	0 - 12	40
	12 - 32	40 → 240
	32 - 42	240
Injection port		280
Detector		280

Detection: flame ionisation.

Injection: 1 µl.

Retention time: benzene = about 10 min.

System suitability: reference solution (a):

– *resolution*: minimum of 10 between the first peak (propanol) and the second peak (2-butanol).

Limits:

– *benzene* (test solution (a)): not more than half of the area of the corresponding peak in the chromatogram obtained with reference solution (b) (2 ppm), after the sensitivity has been adjusted so that the height of the peak due to benzene in the chromatogram obtained with reference solution (b) represents at least 10 per cent of the full scale of the recorder.

– *total of impurities apart from 2-butanol* (test solution (b)): not more than 3 times the area of the peak due to 2-butanol in the chromatogram obtained with test solution (b) (0.3 per cent), after the sensitivity has been adjusted so that the height of the 2 peaks following the principal peak in the chromatogram obtained with reference solution (a) represents at least 50 per cent of the full scale of the recorder.

Peroxides. In a 12 ml test-tube with a ground-glass stopper and a diameter of about 15 mm, introduce 8 ml of *potassium iodide and starch solution R*. Fill completely with the substance to be examined. Shake vigorously and allow to stand protected from light for 30 min. No colour develops.

Non-volatile substances: maximum 20 ppm.

Evaporate 100 g to dryness on a water-bath *after having verified that it complies with the test for peroxides* and dry in an oven at 100-105 °C. The residue weighs a maximum of 2 mg.

Water (*2.5.12*): maximum 0.5 per cent, determined on 5.0 g.

STORAGE

Protected from light.

IMPURITIES

A. acetone,

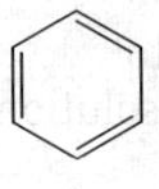

B. benzene,

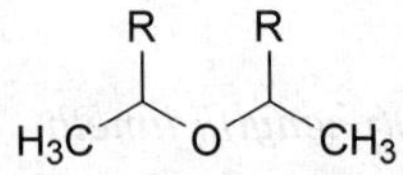

C. R = CH_3: 2-(1-methylethoxy)propane (diisopropyl ether),

D. R = H: ethoxyethane (diethyl ether),

E. CH_3-OH: methanol,

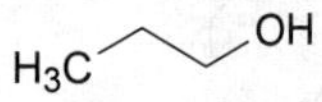

F. propan-1-ol (*n*-propanol).

01/2005:0725

ISOPROPYL MYRISTATE

Isopropylis myristas

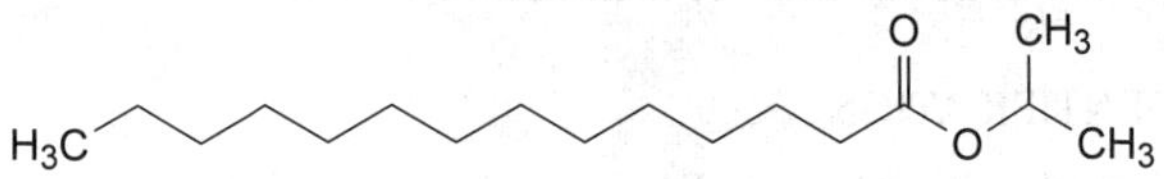

$C_{17}H_{34}O_2$ M_r 270.5

DEFINITION

1-Methylethyl tetradecanoate together with variable amounts of other fatty acid isopropyl esters.

Content: minimum 90.0 per cent of $C_{17}H_{34}O_2$.

CHARACTERS

Appearance: clear, colourless, oily liquid.

Solubility: immiscible with water, miscible with alcohol, with methylene chloride, with fatty oils and with liquid paraffin.

Relative density: about 0.853.

IDENTIFICATION

First identification: *B*.

Second identification: *A, C*.

A. It complies with the test for saponification value (see Tests).

B. Examine the chromatograms obtained in the assay.
Results: the principal peak in the chromatogram obtained with the test solution is similar in retention time to the principal peak in the chromatogram obtained with the reference solution.

C. Superpose 2 ml of a 1 g/l solution in *alcohol R* on a freshly prepared solution of 20 mg of *dimethylaminobenzaldehyde R* in 2 ml of *sulphuric acid R*. After 2 min, a yellowish-red colour appears at the junction of the 2 liquids and gradually becomes red.

TESTS

Appearance of solution. The solution is clear (*2.2.1*) and not more intensely coloured than reference solution Y_7 (*2.2.2, Method II*).

Dissolve 2.0 g in *methanol R* and dilute to 20 ml with the same solvent.

Refractive index (*2.2.6*): 1.434 to 1.437.

Viscosity (*2.2.9*): 5 mPa·s to 6 mPa·s.

Acid value (*2.5.1*): maximum 1.0.

Iodine value (*2.5.4*): maximum 1.0.

Saponification value (*2.5.6*): 202 to 212.

Water (*2.5.12*): maximum 0.1 per cent, determined on 5.0 g.

Total ash (*2.4.16*): maximum 0.1 per cent, determined on 1.0 g.

ASSAY

Gas chromatography (*2.2.28*).

Internal standard solution. Dissolve 50.0 mg of *tricosane R* in *heptane R* and dilute to 250.0 ml with the same solvent.

Test solution. Dissolve 20.0 mg of the substance to be examined in the internal standard solution and dilute to 100.0 ml with the same solution.

Reference solution. Dissolve 20.0 mg of *isopropyl tetradecanoate CRS* in the internal standard solution and dilute to 100.0 ml with the same solution.

Column:
- *material*: fused silica,
- *size*: l = 50 m, Ø = 0.2 mm,
- *stationary phase*: *poly(cyanopropyl)siloxane R* (film thickness 0.2 µm).

Carrier gas: *helium for chromatography R.*

Flow rate: 1 ml/min.

Split ratio: 1:40.

Temperature:

	Time (min)	Temperature (°C)
Column	0 - 6	125 → 185
Injection port		250
Detector		250

Detection: flame ionisation.

Injection: 2 µl.

Calculate the percentage content of $C_{17}H_{34}O_2$ in the substance to be examined.

STORAGE

Protected from light.

01/2005:0839

ISOPROPYL PALMITATE

Isopropylis palmitas

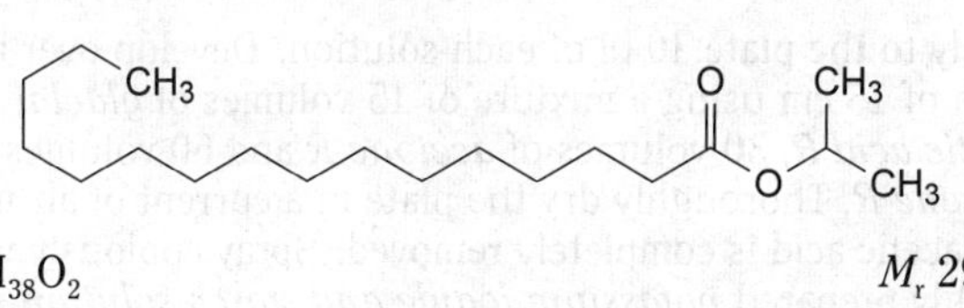

$C_{19}H_{38}O_2$ — M_r 298.5

DEFINITION

1-Methylethyl hexadecanoate together with varying amounts of other fatty acid isopropyl esters.

Content: minimum 90.0 per cent of $C_{19}H_{38}O_2$.

CHARACTERS

Appearance: clear, colourless, oily liquid.

Solubility: immiscible with water, miscible with alcohol, with methylene chloride, with fatty oils and with liquid paraffin.

Relative density: about 0.854.

IDENTIFICATION

First identification: B.

Second identification: A, C.

A. It complies with the test for saponification value (see Tests).

B. Examine the chromatograms obtained in the assay.

Results: the principal peak in the chromatogram obtained with the test solution is similar in retention time to the principal peak in the chromatogram obtained with the reference solution.

C. Superpose 2 ml of a 1 g/l solution in *alcohol R* on a freshly prepared solution of 20 mg of *dimethylaminobenzaldehyde R* in 2 ml of *sulphuric acid R*. After 2 min, a yellowish-red colour appears at the junction of the 2 liquids which gradually becomes red.

TESTS

Appearance of solution. The solution is clear (*2.2.1*) and not more intensely coloured than reference solution Y_7 (*2.2.2, Method II*).

Dissolve 2.0 g in *methanol R* and dilute to 20 ml with the same solvent.

Refractive index (*2.2.6*): 1.436 to 1.440.

Viscosity (*2.2.9*): 5 mPa·s to 10 mPa·s.

Acid value (*2.5.1*): maximum 1.0.

Iodine value (*2.5.4*): maximum 1.0.

Saponification value (*2.5.6*): 183 to 193.

Water (*2.5.12*): maximum 0.1 per cent, determined on 5.0 g.

Total ash (*2.4.16*): maximum 0.1 per cent, determined on 1.0 g.

ASSAY

Gas chromatography (*2.2.28*).

Internal standard solution. Dissolve 50.0 mg of *tricosane R* in *heptane R* and dilute to 250.0 ml with the same solvent.

Test solution. Dissolve 20.0 mg of the substance to be examined in the internal standard solution and dilute to 100.0 ml with the same solution.

Reference solution. Dissolve 20.0 mg of *isopropyl hexadecanoate CRS* in the internal standard solution and dilute to 100.0 ml with the same solution.

Column:
- *material*: fused silica,
- *size*: l = 50 m, Ø = 0.2 mm,
- *stationary phase*: *poly(cyanopropyl)siloxane R* (film thickness 0.2 µm).

Carrier gas: *helium for chromatography R.*

Flow rate: 1 ml/min.

Split ratio: 1:40.

Temperature:

	Time (min)	Temperature (°C)
Column	0 - 6	125 → 185
Injection port		250
Detector		250

Detection: flame ionisation.

Injection: 2 µl.

Calculate the percentage content of $C_{19}H_{38}O_2$ in the substance to be examined.

STORAGE

Protected from light.

Monographs I-L

01/2005:1117

ISOSORBIDE DINITRATE, DILUTED

Isosorbidi dinitras dilutus

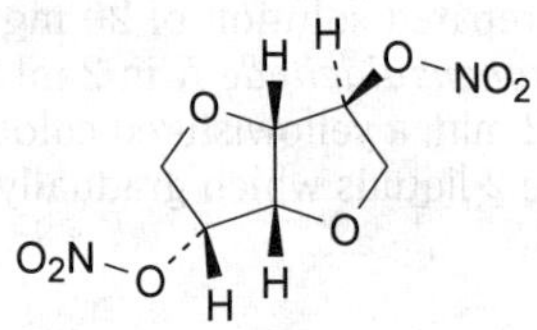

$C_6H_8N_2O_8$ M_r 236.1

DEFINITION

Diluted isosorbide dinitrate is a dry mixture of isosorbide dinitrate and *Lactose monohydrate (0187)* or *Mannitol (0559)*. It contains not less than 95.0 per cent *m/m* and not more than 105.0 per cent *m/m* of the content of 1,4:3,6-dianhydro-D-glucitol 2,5-dinitrate stated on the label.

CAUTION: Undiluted isosorbide dinitrate may explode if subjected to percussion or excessive heat. Appropriate precautions must be taken and only very small quantities should be handled.

CHARACTERS

Undiluted isosorbide dinitrate is a fine, white, crystalline powder, very slightly soluble in water, very soluble in acetone, sparingly soluble in alcohol.

The solubility of the diluted product depends on the diluent and its concentration.

IDENTIFICATION

First identification: A, C, D.

Second identification: B, C, D.

A. Examine by infrared absorption spectrophotometry (*2.2.24*) the residue obtained in identification test D, comparing with the spectrum of the residue obtained in the same way with *isosorbide dinitrate CRS*. Examine the residues prepared as discs.

B. Examine by thin-layer chromatography (*2.2.27*), using *silica gel G R* as the coating substance.

Test solution. Shake a quantity of the substance to be examined corresponding to 10 mg of isosorbide dinitrate with 10 ml of *alcohol R* for 5 min and filter.

Reference solution. Shake a quantity of *isosorbide dinitrate CRS* corresponding to 10 mg of isosorbide dinitrate with 10 ml of *alcohol R* for 5 min and filter.

Apply to the plate 10 µl of each solution. Develop over a path of 15 cm using a mixture of 5 volumes of *methanol R* and 95 volumes of *methylene chloride R*. Dry the plate in a current of air. Spray with freshly prepared *potassium iodide and starch solution R*. Expose to ultraviolet light at 254 nm for 15 min. Examine in daylight. The principal spot in the chromatogram obtained with the test solution is similar in position, colour and size to the principal spot in the chromatogram obtained with the reference solution.

C. Examine by thin-layer chromatography (*2.2.27*), using *silica gel G R* as the coating substance.

Test solution. Shake a quantity of the substance to be examined corresponding to 0.10 g of lactose or mannitol with 10 ml of *water R*. Filter if necessary.

Reference solution (a). Dissolve 0.10 g of *lactose R* in *water R* and dilute to 10 ml with the same solvent.

Reference solution (b). Dissolve 0.10 g of *mannitol R* in *water R* and dilute to 10 ml with the same solvent.

Reference solution (c). Mix equal volumes of reference solutions (a) and (b).

Apply to the plate 1 µl of each solution and thoroughly dry the starting points. Develop over a path of 15 cm using a mixture of 10 volumes of *water R*, 15 volumes of *methanol R*, 25 volumes of *anhydrous acetic acid R* and 50 volumes of *ethylene chloride R*, measured accurately since a slight excess of water produces cloudiness. Dry the plate in a current of warm air. Repeat immediately the development after renewing the mobile phase. Dry the plate in a current of warm air. Spray with *4-aminobenzoic acid solution R*. Dry the plate in a current of cold air until the acetone is removed. Heat the plate at 100 °C for 15 min. Allow to cool and spray with a 2 g/l solution of *sodium periodate R*. Dry the plate in a current of cold air. Heat the plate at 100 °C for 15 min. The principal spot in the chromatogram obtained with the test solution is similar in position, colour and size to the principal spot in the chromatogram obtained with reference solution (a) for lactose or to the principal spot in the chromatogram obtained with reference solution (b) for mannitol. The identification is not valid unless the chromatogram obtained with reference solution (c) shows two clearly separated spots.

D. Shake a quantity of the substance to be examined corresponding to 25 mg of isosorbide dinitrate with 10 ml of *acetone R*, for 5 min. Filter, evaporate to dryness at a temperature below 40 °C and dry the residue over *diphosphorus pentoxide R* at a pressure of 0.7 kPa for 16 h. The melting point (*2.2.14*) of the residue is 69 °C to 72 °C.

TESTS

Inorganic nitrates. Examine by thin-layer chromatography (*2.2.27*), using *silica gel H R* as the coating substance.

Test solution. Shake a quantity of the substance to be examined corresponding to 0.10 g of isosorbide dinitrate with 5 ml of *alcohol R* and filter.

Reference solution. Dissolve 10 mg of *potassium nitrate R* in 1 ml of *water R* and dilute to 100 ml with *alcohol R*.

Apply to the plate 10 µl of each solution. Develop over a path of 15 cm using a mixture of 15 volumes of *glacial acetic acid R*, 30 volumes of *acetone R* and 60 volumes of *toluene R*. Thoroughly dry the plate in a current of air until the acetic acid is completely removed. Spray copiously with freshly prepared *potassium iodide and starch solution R*. Expose the plate to ultraviolet light at 254 nm for 15 min. Examine in daylight. Any spot corresponding to nitrate ion in the chromatogram obtained with the test solution is not more intense than the spot in the chromatogram obtained with the reference solution (0.5 per cent, calculated as potassium nitrate).

Isosorbide 5-nitrate and isosorbide 2-nitrate. Examine by liquid chromatography (*2.2.29*) as described under Assay, changing the detection to 210-215 nm.

When the chromatograms are recorded in the prescribed conditions, the retention times are: isosorbide dinitrate, about 5 min; isosorbide 2-nitrate, about 8 min; isosorbide 5-nitrate about 11 min.

Inject 10 µl of reference solution (c). When a recorder is used, adjust the sensitivity of the system so that the height of the principal peak in the chromatogram obtained with reference solution (c) is not less than 20 per cent of the full scale of the recorder.

Monographs I-L

Inject 10 µl of reference solution (e). The test is not valid unless in the chromatogram obtained with reference solution (e), the resolution between the peaks corresponding to isosorbide dinitrate and isosorbide 2-nitrate is at least 6.0.

Inject 10 µl of test solution (a), 10 µl of reference solution (c) and 10 µl of reference solution (d). In the chromatogram obtained with test solution (a): the area of any peak corresponding to isosorbide 2-nitrate is not greater than the area of the principal peak in the chromatogram obtained with reference solution (c) (0.5 per cent); the area of any peak corresponding to isosorbide 5-nitrate is not greater than the area of the principal peak in the chromatogram obtained with reference solution (d) (0.5 per cent).

ASSAY

Examine by liquid chromatography (*2.2.29*).

Test solution (a). Sonicate a quantity of the substance to be examined corresponding to 25.0 mg of isosorbide dinitrate with 20 ml of the mobile phase for 15 min and dilute to 25.0 ml with the mobile phase. Filter the solution through a suitable membrane filter.

Test solution (b). Dilute 1.0 ml of test solution (a) to 10.0 ml with the mobile phase.

Reference solution (a). Sonicate a quantity of *isosorbide dinitrate CRS* corresponding to 25.0 mg of isosorbide dinitrate with 20 ml of the mobile phase for 15 min and dilute to 25.0 ml with the mobile phase. Filter the solution through a suitable membrane filter.

Reference solution (b). Dilute 1.0 ml of reference solution (a) to 10.0 ml with the mobile phase.

Reference solution (c). Dissolve 10.0 mg of *isosorbide 2-nitrate CRS* in the mobile phase and dilute to 10.0 ml with the mobile phase. Dilute 0.1 ml of this solution to 20.0 ml with the mobile phase.

Reference solution (d). Dissolve 10.0 mg of *isosorbide mononitrate CRS* in the mobile phase and dilute to 10.0 ml with the mobile phase. Dilute 0.1 ml of this solution to 20.0 ml with the mobile phase.

Reference solution (e). Dissolve 5 mg of *isosorbide 2-nitrate CRS* in the mobile phase and dilute to 10 ml with the mobile phase. To 1 ml of this solution, add 0.5 ml of reference solution (a) and dilute to 10 ml with the mobile phase.

The chromatographic procedure may be carried out using:
- a stainless steel column 0.25 m long and 4.6 mm in internal diameter packed with *aminopropylmethylsilyl silica gel for chromatography R* (10 µm),
- as mobile phase at a flow rate of 1 ml/min a mixture of 15 volumes of *ethanol R* and 85 volumes of *trimethylpentane R*,
- as detector a spectrophotometer set at 230 nm.

Inject 20 µl of reference solution (b). When a recorder is used, adjust the sensitivity of the system so that the height of the principal peak in the chromatogram obtained is not less than 50 per cent of the full scale of the recorder. If the areas of the peaks from two successive injections do not agree to within 1.0 per cent, then inject a further four times and calculate, for the six injections, the relative standard deviation. The assay is not valid unless the relative standard deviation for the six injections is at most 2.0 per cent. Inject test solution (b) and reference solution (b), alternately.

Calculate the content of isosorbide dinitrate as a percentage of the declared content.

STORAGE

Store protected from light.

LABELLING

The label states the percentage content of isosorbide dinitrate.

IMPURITIES

A. inorganic nitrates,

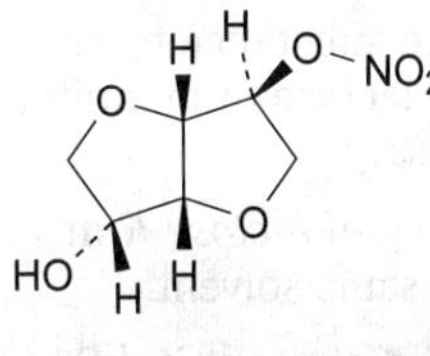

B. isosorbide 2-nitrate,

C. isosorbide mononitrate (isosorbide 5-nitrate).

01/2005:1118

ISOSORBIDE MONONITRATE, DILUTED

Isosorbidi mononitras dilutus

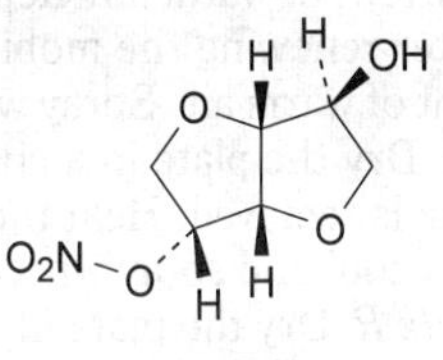

$C_6H_9NO_6$ M_r 191.1

DEFINITION

Diluted isosorbide mononitrate is a dry mixture of isosorbide mononitrate and *Lactose monohydrate (0187)* or *Mannitol (0559)*. It contains not less than 95.0 per cent *m/m* and not more than 105.0 per cent *m/m* of the content of 1,4:3,6-dianhydro-D-glucitol 5-nitrate stated on the label.

CHARACTERS

Undiluted isosorbide mononitrate is a white, crystalline powder, freely soluble in water, in acetone, in alcohol and in methylene chloride.

The solubility of the diluted product depends on the diluent and its concentration.

IDENTIFICATION

First identification: A, C, D.

Second identification: B, C, D.

A. Examine by infrared absorption spectrophotometry (*2.2.24*)the residue obtained in identification test D, comparing with the spectrum obtained with *isosorbide mononitrate CRS*. Examine the substances prepared as discs.

B. Examine by thin-layer chromatography (*2.2.27*), using *silica gel G R* as the coating substance.

Test solution. Shake a quantity of the substance to be examined corresponding to 10 mg of isosorbide mononitrate with 10 ml of *alcohol R* for 5 min and filter.

Reference solution. Dissolve 10 mg of *isosorbide mononitrate CRS* in *alcohol R* and dilute to 10 ml with the same solvent.

Apply to the plate 10 µl of each solution. Develop over a path of 15 cm using a mixture of 5 volumes of *methanol R* and 95 volumes of *methylene chloride R*. Dry the plate in a current of air. Spray with freshly prepared *potassium iodide and starch solution R*. Expose to ultraviolet light at 254 nm for 15 min. Examine in daylight. The principal spot in the chromatogram obtained with the test solution is similar in position, colour and size to the principal spot in the chromatogram obtained with the reference solution.

C. Examine by thin-layer chromatography (*2.2.27*), using *silica gel G R* as the coating substance.

Test solution. Shake a quantity of the substance to be examined corresponding to 0.10 g of lactose or mannitol with 10 ml of *water R*. Filter if necessary.

Reference solution (a). Dissolve 0.10 g of *lactose R* in *water R* and dilute to 10 ml with the same solvent.

Reference solution (b). Dissolve 0.10 g of *mannitol R* in *water R* and dilute to 10 ml with the same solvent.

Reference solution (c). Mix equal volumes of reference solutions (a) and (b).

Apply to the plate 1 µl of each solution and thoroughly dry the starting points. Develop over a path of 15 cm using a mixture of 10 volumes of *water R*, 15 volumes of *methanol R*, 25 volumes of *anhydrous acetic acid R* and 50 volumes of *ethylene chloride R*, measured accurately since a slight excess of water produces cloudiness. Dry the plate in a current of warm air. Repeat immediately the development after renewing the mobile phase. Dry the plate in a current of warm air. Spray with *4-aminobenzoic acid solution R*. Dry the plate in a current of cold air until the acetone is removed. Heat the plate at 100 °C for 15 min. Allow to cool and spray with a 2 g/l solution of *sodium periodate R*. Dry the plate in a current of cold air. Heat the plate at 100 °C for 15 min. The principal spot in the chromatogram obtained with the test solution is similar in position, colour and size to the principal spot in the chromatogram obtained with reference solution (a) for lactose or to the principal spot in the chromatogram obtained with reference solution (b) for mannitol. The identification is not valid unless the chromatogram obtained with reference solution (c) shows two clearly separated spots.

D. Shake a quantity of the substance to be examined corresponding to 25 mg of isosorbide mononitrate with 10 ml of *acetone R* for 5 min. Filter, evaporate to dryness at a temperature below 40 °C and dry the residue over *diphosphorus pentoxide R* at a pressure of 0.7 kPa for 16 h. The melting point (*2.2.14*) of the residue is 89 °C to 91 °C.

TESTS

Inorganic nitrates. Examine by thin-layer chromatography (*2.2.27*), using *silica gel H R* as the coating substance.

Test solution. Shake a quantity of the substance to be examined corresponding to 0.10 g of isosorbide mononitrate with 5 ml of *alcohol R* and filter.

Reference solution. Dissolve 10 mg of *potassium nitrate R* in 1 ml of *water R* and dilute to 100 ml with *alcohol R*.

Apply separately to the plate 10 µl of each solution. Develop over a path of 15 cm using a mixture of 15 volumes of *glacial acetic acid R*, 30 volumes of *acetone R* and 60 volumes of *toluene R*. Thoroughly dry the plate in a current of air until the acetic acid is completely removed. Spray copiously with freshly prepared *potassium iodide and starch solution R*. Expose the plate to ultraviolet light at 254 nm for 15 min. Examine in daylight. Any spot corresponding to nitrate ion in the chromatogram obtained with the test solution is not more intense than the spot in the chromatogram obtained with the reference solution (0.5 per cent, calculated as potassium nitrate).

Isosorbide dinitrate and isosorbide 2-nitrate. Examine by liquid chromatography (*2.2.29*) as described under Assay, changing the detection to 210 nm to 215 nm.

When the chromatograms are recorded in the prescribed conditions, the retention times are: isosorbide dinitrate about 5 min, isosorbide-2-nitrate about 8 min and isosorbide 5-nitrate about 11 min.

Inject 10 µl of reference solution (b). When a recorder is used, adjust the sensitivity of the system so that the height of the principal peak in the chromatogram obtained with reference solution (b) is at least 20 per cent of the full scale of the recorder.

Inject 10 µl of reference solution (d). The test is not valid unless, in the chromatogram obtained with reference solution (d), the resolution between the peaks corresponding to isosorbide 2-nitrate and isosorbide 5-nitrate is at least 4.0.

Inject 10 µl of test solution (a), 10 µl of reference solution (b) and 10 µl of reference solution (c). In the chromatogram obtained with test solution (a): the area of any peak corresponding to isosorbide 2-nitrate is not greater than the area of the principal peak in the chromatogram obtained with reference solution (b) (0.5 per cent); the area of any peak corresponding to isosorbide dinitrate is not greater than the area of the principal peak in the chromatogram obtained with reference solution (c) (0.5 per cent).

ASSAY

Examine by liquid chromatography (*2.2.29*).

Test solution (a). Sonicate a quantity of the substance to be examined corresponding to 25.0 mg of isosorbide mononitrate with 20 ml of the mobile phase for 15 min and dilute to 25.0 ml with the mobile phase. Filter the solution through a suitable membrane filter.

Test solution (b). Dilute 1.0 ml of test solution (a) to 10.0 ml with the mobile phase.

Reference solution (a). Dissolve 25.0 mg of *isosorbide mononitrate CRS* in the mobile phase and dilute to 25.0 ml with the mobile phase. Dilute 1.0 ml of the solution to 10.0 ml with the mobile phase.

Reference solution (b). Dissolve 10.0 mg of *isosorbide-2-nitrate CRS* in the mobile phase and dilute to 10.0 ml with the mobile phase. Dilute 0.1 ml of the solution to 20.0 ml with the mobile phase.

Reference solution (c). Sonicate a quantity of *isosorbide dinitrate CRS* corresponding to 10.0 mg of isosorbide dinitrate in 15 ml of the mobile phase for 15 min and dilute to 20.0 ml with the mobile phase. Filter the solution through a suitable membrane filter. Dilute 0.1 ml of the solution to 10.0 ml with the mobile phase.

Reference solution (d). Dissolve 5 mg of *isosorbide mononitrate CRS* and 5 mg of *isosorbide-2-nitrate CRS* in the mobile phase and dilute to 10 ml with the mobile phase. Dilute 1 ml of the solution to 10 ml with the mobile phase.

The chromatographic procedure may be carried out using:

– a stainless steel column 0.25 m long and4.6 mm in internal diameter packed with *aminopropylmethylsilyl silica gel for chromatography R* (10 µm),
– as mobile phase at a flow rate of 1 ml/min a mixture of 15 volumes of *ethanol R* and 85 volumes of *trimethylpentane R*,
– as detector a spectrophotometer set at 230 nm.

Inject 20 µl of reference solution (a). When a recorder is used, adjust the sensitivity of the system so that the height of the principal peak in the chromatogram obtained with reference solution (a) is at least 50 per cent of the full scale of the recorder. If the areas of the peaks from two successive

Monographs I-L

injections do not agree to within 1.0 per cent, then inject a further four times and calculate, for the six injections, the relative standard deviation. The assay is not valid unless the relative standard deviation for the six injections is at most 2.0 per cent. Inject test solution (b) and reference solution (a), alternately.

Calculate the content of isosorbide mononitrate as a percentage of the declared content.

STORAGE

Store protected from light.

LABELLING

The label states the percentage content of isosorbide mononitrate.

IMPURITIES

A. inorganic nitrates,

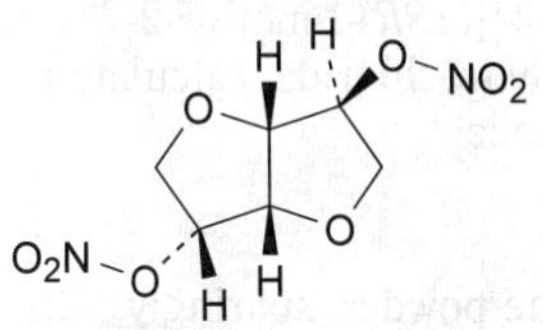

B. isosorbide dinitrate,

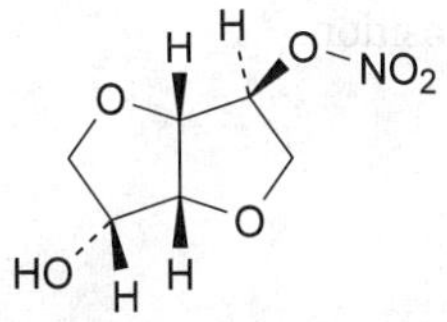

C. isosorbide 2-nitrate.

01/2005:1019

ISOTRETINOIN

Isotretinoinum

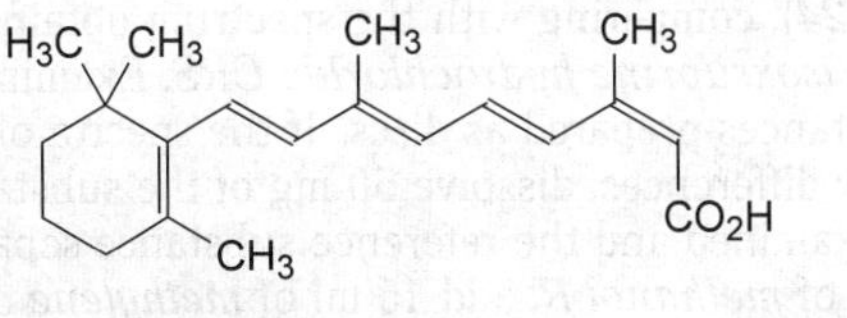

$C_{20}H_{28}O_2$ M_r 300.4

DEFINITION

Isotretinoin contains not less than 98.0 per cent and not more than the equivalent of 102.0 per cent of (2*Z*,4*E*,6*E*,8*E*)-3,7-dimethyl-9-(2,6,6-trimethylcyclohex-1-enyl)nona-2,4,6,8-tetraenoic acid, calculated with reference to the dried substance.

CHARACTERS

A yellow or light-orange, crystalline powder, practically insoluble in water, soluble in methylene chloride, slightly soluble in alcohol. It is sensitive to air, heat and light, especially in solution.

Carry out all operations as rapidly as possible and avoid exposure to actinic light; use freshly prepared solutions.

IDENTIFICATION

First identification: A, B.

Second identification: A, C, D.

A. Dissolve 75.0 mg in 5 ml of *methylene chloride R* and dilute immediately to 100.0 ml with acidified 2-propanol (prepared by diluting 1 ml of *0.01 M hydrochloric acid* to 1000 ml with *2-propanol R*). Dilute 5.0 ml of this solution to 100.0 ml with the acidified 2-propanol (solution A). Dilute 5.0 ml of solution A to 50.0 ml with the acidified 2-propanol. Examined between 300 nm and 400 nm (*2.2.25*), the solution shows an absorption maximum at 354 nm. The specific absorbance at the maximum is 1290 to 1420.

B. Examine by infrared absorption spectrophotometry (*2.2.24*), comparing with the spectrum obtained with *isotretinoin CRS*. Examine the substances prepared as discs.

C. Examine by thin-layer chromatography (*2.2.27*), using a *TLC silica gel GF_{254} plate R*.

Test solution. Dissolve 10 mg of the substance to be examined in *methylene chloride R* and dilute to 10 ml with the same solvent.

Reference solution (a). Dissolve 10 mg of *isotretinoin CRS* in *methylene chloride R* and dilute to 10 ml with the same solvent.

Reference solution (b). Dissolve 10 mg of *isotretinoin CRS* and 10 mg of *tretinoin CRS* in *methylene chloride R* and dilute to 10 ml with the same solvent.

Apply separately to the plate 5 µl of each solution. Develop over a path of 15 cm using a mixture of 2 volumes of *glacial acetic acid R*, 4 volumes of *acetone R*, 40 volumes of *peroxide-free ether R* and 54 volumes of *cyclohexane R*. Allow the plate to dry in air and examine in ultraviolet light at 254 nm. The principal spot in the chromatogram obtained with the test solution is similar in position and size to the principal spot in the chromatogram obtained with reference solution (a). The test is not valid unless the chromatogram obtained with reference solution (b) shows two clearly separated principal spots.

D. Dissolve about 5 mg in 2 ml of *antimony trichloride solution R*. An intense red colour develops and later becomes violet.

TESTS

Related substances. Examine by liquid chromatography (*2.2.29*).

Test solution. Dissolve 0.100 g of the substance to be examined in *methanol R* and dilute to 50.0 ml with the same solvent.

Reference solution (a). Dissolve 10.0 mg of *tretinoin CRS* in *methanol R* and dilute to 10.0 ml with the same solvent.

Reference solution (b). Dilute 1.0 ml of reference solution (a) to 25.0 ml with *methanol R*.

Reference solution (c). Mix 1.0 ml of reference solution (a) with 0.5 ml of the test solution and dilute to 25.0 ml with *methanol R*.

Reference solution (d). Dilute 0.5 ml of the test solution to 100.0 ml with *methanol R*.

The chromatographic procedure may be carried out using:

- a stainless steel column 0.15 m long and 4.6 mm in internal diameter packed with *octadecylsilyl silica gel for chromatography R* (3 µm),
- as mobile phase at a flow rate of 1.0 ml/min a mixture of 5 volumes of *glacial acetic acid R*, 225 volumes of *water R* and 770 volumes of *methanol R*.
- as detector a spectrophotometer set at 355 nm.

Monographs I-L

Inject separately 10 µl of each of reference solutions (b), (c) and (d) and of the test solution. Adjust the sensitivity of the detector so that the height of the principal peak in the chromatogram obtained with reference solution (b) is not less than 70 per cent of the full scale of the recorder. The test is not valid unless the resolution between the peaks due to isotretinoin and tretinoin in the chromatogram obtained with reference solution (c) is at least 2.0. In the chromatogram obtained with the test solution: the area of any peak due to tretinoin is not greater than the area of the principal peak in the chromatogram obtained with reference solution (b) (2.0 per cent); the sum of the areas of any peaks, apart from the principal peak and any peak due to tretinoin, is not greater than the area of the principal peak in the chromatogram obtained with reference solution (d) (0.5 per cent).

Heavy metals (*2.4.8*). 0.5 g complies with limit test D for heavy metals (20 ppm). Prepare the standard using 1 ml of *lead standard solution (10 ppm Pb) R*.

Loss on drying (*2.2.32*). Not more than 0.5 per cent, determined on 1.000 g by drying *in vacuo* for 16 h.

Sulphated ash (*2.4.14*). Not more than 0.1 per cent, determined on 1.0 g.

ASSAY

Dissolve 0.200 g in 70 ml of *acetone R*. Titrate with *0.1 M tetrabutylammonium hydroxide* determining the end-point potentiometrically (*2.2.20*).

1 ml of *0.1 M tetrabutylammonium hydroxide* is equivalent to 30.04 mg of $C_{20}H_{28}O_2$.

STORAGE

Store in an airtight container, protected from light, at a temperature not exceeding 25 °C.

It is recommended that the contents of an opened container be used as soon as possible and any unused part be protected by an atmosphere of an inert gas.

IMPURITIES

A. tretinoin,

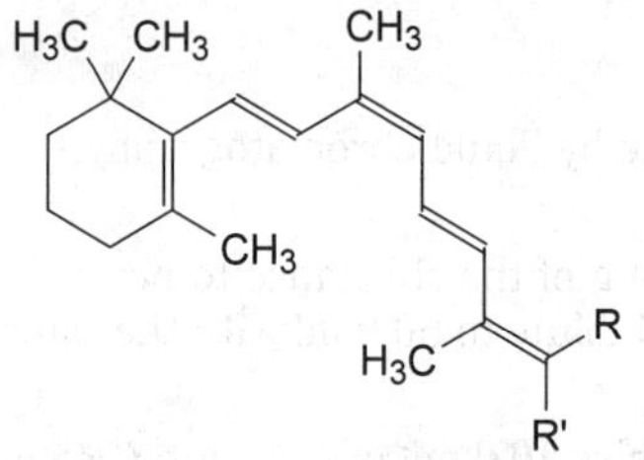

B. R = CO_2H, R′ = H: (2*Z*,4*E*,6*Z*,8*E*)-3,7-dimethyl-9-(2,6,6-trimethylcyclohex-1-enyl)nona-2,4,6,8-tetraenoic acid (9,13-di-*cis*-retinoic acid),

D. R = H, R′ = CO_2H: (2*E*,4*E*,6*Z*,8*E*)-3,7-dimethyl-9-(2,6,6-trimethylcyclohex-1-enyl)nona-2,4,6,8-tetraenoic acid (9-*cis*-retinoic acid),

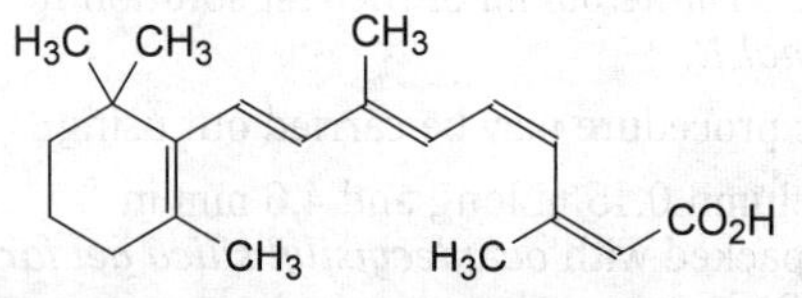

C. (2*Z*,4*Z*,6*E*,8*E*)-3,7-dimethyl-9-(2,6,6-trimethylcyclohex-1-enyl)nona-2,4,6,8-tetraenoic acid (11,13-di-*cis*-retinoic acid),

E. oxidation products of isotretinoin.

01/2005:1119

ISOXSUPRINE HYDROCHLORIDE

Isoxsuprini hydrochloridum

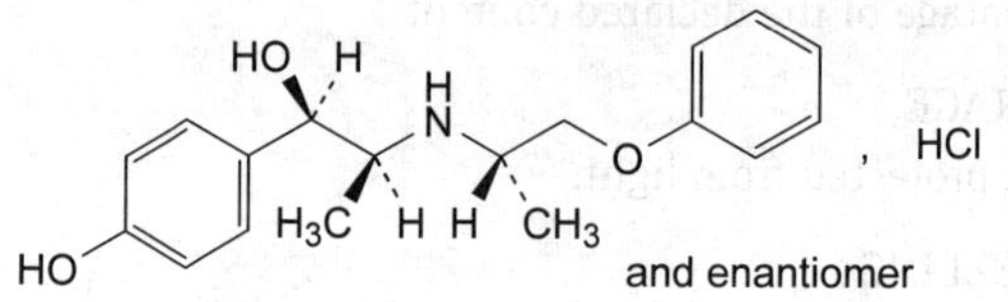

$C_{18}H_{24}ClNO_3$ M_r 337.8

DEFINITION

Isoxsuprine hydrochloride contains not less than 99.0 per cent and not more than the equivalent of 101.0 per cent of (1*RS*,2*SR*)-1-(4-hydroxyphenyl)-2-[[(1*SR*)-1-methyl-2-phenoxyethyl]amino]propan-1-ol hydrochloride, calculated with reference to the dried substance.

CHARACTERS

A white or almost white, crystalline powder, sparingly soluble in water and in alcohol, practically insoluble in methylene chloride.

It melts at about 205 °C, with decomposition.

IDENTIFICATION

First identification: B, E.

Second identification: A, C, D, E.

A. Dissolve 50.0 mg in *0.1 M hydrochloric acid* and dilute to 50.0 ml with the same acid. Dilute 10.0 ml of this solution to 100.0 ml with *0.1 M hydrochloric acid.* Examined between 230 nm and 350 nm (*2.2.25*), the solution shows two absorption maxima, at 269 nm and 275 nm. The specific absorbance at these maxima are 71 to 74 and 70 to 73, respectively. The test is not valid unless, in the test for resolution (*2.2.25*), the ratio of the absorbances is at least 1.7.

B. Examine by infrared absorption spectrophotometry (*2.2.24*), comparing with the spectrum obtained with *isoxsuprine hydrochloride CRS*. Examine the substances prepared as discs. If the spectra obtained show differences, dissolve 50 mg of the substance to be examined and the reference substance separately in 2 ml of *methanol R*, add 15 ml of *methylene chloride R*, evaporate to dryness and record new spectra using the residues.

C. Examine by thin-layer chromatography (*2.2.27*), using *silica gel G R* as the coating substance.

Test solution. Dissolve 20 mg of the substance to be examined in *methanol R* and dilute to 10 ml with the same solvent.

Reference solution. Dissolve 20 mg of *isoxsuprine hydrochloride CRS* in *methanol R* and dilute to 10 ml with the same solvent.

Apply to the plate 10 µl of each solution. Develop over a path of 12 cm using a mixture of 0.25 volumes of *concentrated ammonia R*, 15 volumes of *methanol R* and 85 volumes of *methylene chloride R*. Dry the plate in a current of warm air and spray with a 10 g/l solution of *potassium permanganate R*. The principal spot in the chromatogram obtained with the test solution is similar in position, colour and size to the principal spot in the chromatogram obtained with the reference solution.

D. To 1 ml of solution S (see Tests) add 0.05 ml of *copper sulphate solution R* and 0.5 ml of *strong sodium hydroxide solution R*. The solution becomes blue. Add 1 ml of *ether R* and shake. Allow to separate. The upper layer remains colourless.

E. 2 ml of solution S gives reaction (a) of chlorides (*2.3.1*).

TESTS

Solution S. Dissolve 0.50 g, with gentle heating if necessary, in *carbon dioxide-free water R*, cool and dilute to 50.0 ml with the same solvent.

Appearance of solution. Solution S is clear (*2.2.1*) and colourless (*2.2.2, Method II*).

pH (*2.2.3*). The pH of solution S is 4.5 to 6.0.

Optical rotation (*2.2.7*). The angle of optical rotation of solution S is − 0.05° to + 0.05°.

Phenones. Dissolve 10.0 mg in *water R* and dilute to 100.0 ml with the same solvent. The absorbance (*2.2.25*) measured at the maximum at 310 nm is not greater than 0.10 (1.0 per cent, calculated as impurity B).

Related substances. *Prepare the solutions immediately before use.* Examine by gas chromatography (*2.2.28*), using *hexacosane R* as the internal standard.

Internal standard solution (a). Dissolve 0.1 g of *hexacosane R* in *trimethylpentane R* and dilute to 20 ml with the same solvent.

Internal standard solution (b). Dilute 1 ml of internal standard solution (a) to 50 ml with *trimethylpentane R*.

Test solution. To 10.0 mg of the substance to be examined, add 0.5 ml of *N-trimethylsilylimidazole R*. Heat to 65 °C for 10 min. Allow to cool, then add 2.0 ml of the internal standard solution (b) and 2.0 ml of *water R*. Shake. Use the upper layer.

Reference solution (a). To 10.0 mg of the substance to be examined, add 0.5 ml of *N-trimethylsilylimidazole R*. Heat to 65 °C for 10 min. Allow to cool, then add 2.0 ml of the internal standard solution (a) and 2.0 ml of *water R*. Shake. Dilute 1.0 ml of the upper layer to 50.0 ml with *trimethylpentane R*.

Reference solution (b). To 10.0 mg of the substance to be examined, add 0.5 ml of *N-trimethylsilylimidazole R*. Heat to 65 °C for 10 min. Allow to cool, then add 2.0 ml of *trimethylpentane R* and 2.0 ml of *water R*. Shake. Use the upper layer.

The chromatographic procedure may be carried out using:

- a glass column 1.5 m long and 4 mm in internal diameter, packed with *silanised diatomaceous earth for gas chromatography R* (125-135 µm) impregnated with 3 per cent *m/m* of *poly(dimethyl)siloxane R*,
- *nitrogen for chromatography R* as the carrier gas at a flow rate of 30 ml/min,
- a flame-ionisation detector,

maintaining the temperature of the column at 195 °C for 25 min, then raising the temperature at a rate of 5 °C/min to 215 °C and maintaining at 215 °C for 10 min, and maintaining the temperature of the injection port and that of the detector at 225 °C.

Inject 1 µl of reference solution (a). The substances elute in the following order: isoxsuprine and hexacosane. Adjust the sensitivity of the detector so that the heights of the two principal peaks are not less than 50 per cent of the full scale of the recorder. The test is not valid unless, in the chromatogram obtained, the resolution between the peaks corresponding to isoxsuprine and hexacosane is at least 5.0.

Inject 1 µl of reference solution (b). In the chromatogram obtained, verify that there is no peak with the same retention time as the internal standard.

Inject 1 µl of the test solution and 1 µl of reference solution (a). From the chromatogram obtained with reference solution (a), calculate the ratio (*R*) of the area of the peak due to the trimethylsilyl derivative of isoxsuprine to the area of the peak due to the internal standard. From the chromatogram obtained with the test solution, calculate the ratio of the sum of the areas of any peaks, apart from the principal peak, the peak due to the internal standard and the peak due to the solvent, to the area of the peak due to the internal standard: this ratio is not greater than *R* (2.0 per cent).

Heavy metals (*2.4.8*). 1.0 g complies with limit test C for heavy metals (20 ppm). Prepare the standard using 2 ml of *lead standard solution (10 ppm Pb) R*.

Loss on drying (*2.2.32*). Not more than 0.5 per cent, determined on 1.000 g by drying in an oven at 100-105 °C.

Sulphated ash (*2.4.14*). Not more than 0.1 per cent, determined on 1.0 g.

ASSAY

Dissolve 0.250 g in 80 ml of *alcohol R* and add 1.0 ml of *0.1 M hydrochloric acid*. Carry out a potentiometric titration (*2.2.20*), using *0.1 M sodium hydroxide*. Read the volume added between the two points of inflexion.

1 ml of *0.1 M sodium hydroxide* is equivalent to 33.78 mg of $C_{18}H_{24}ClNO_3$.

STORAGE

Store protected from light.

IMPURITIES

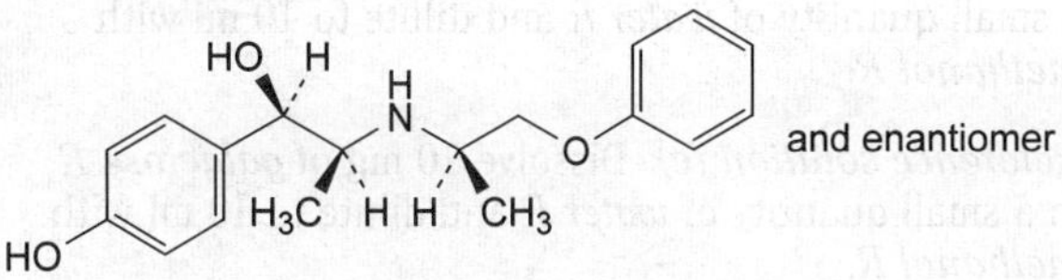

A. (1*RS*,2*SR*)-1-(4-hydroxyphenyl)-2-[[(1*RS*)-1-methyl-2-phenoxyethyl]amino]propan-1-ol,

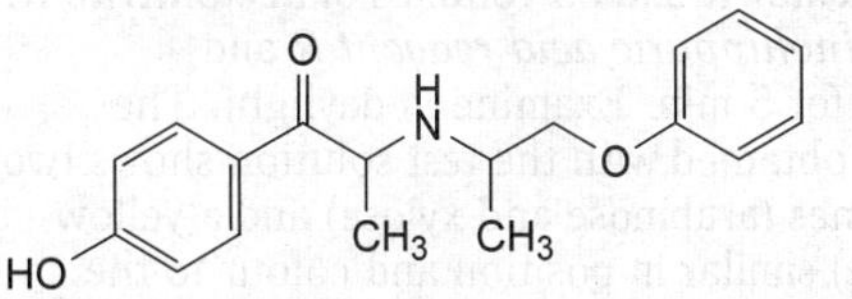

B. 1-(4-hydroxyphenyl)-2-[(1-methyl-2-phenoxyethyl)amino]propan-1-one.

01/2005:1334

ISPAGHULA HUSK

Plantaginis ovatae seminis tegumentum

DEFINITION

Ispaghula husk consists of the episperm and collapsed adjacent layers removed from the seeds of *Plantago ovata* Forssk. (*P. ispaghula* Roxb.).

CHARACTERS

It has the macroscopic and microscopic characters described under identification tests A and B.

Monographs I-L

IDENTIFICATION

A. Ispaghula husk consists of pinkish-beige fragments or flakes up to about 2 mm long and 1 mm wide, some showing a light brown spot corresponding to the location of the embryo before it was removed from the seed.

B. Reduce to a powder (355). The powder is pale yellow. Examine under a microscope using *lactic reagent R*. The powder shows mainly fragments of the episperm with polygonal cells filled with mucilage; fragments of the inner layers of the testa with brownish thin-walled cells often associated with the outer layers of the endosperm. Examine under a microscope using a 50 per cent *V/V* solution of *glycerol R*. The powder shows occasional starch granules, single or in groups of two to four, measuring 3 µm to 25 µm in diameter.

C. Examine by thin-layer chromatography (*2.2.27*), using a *TLC silica gel plate R*.

Test solution. To 10 mg of the powdered drug (355) in a thick-walled centrifuge tube add 2 ml of a 230 g/l solution of *trifluoroacetic acid R* and shake vigorously. Stopper the test tube and heat the mixture at 120 °C for 1 h. Centrifuge the hydrolysate, transfer the clear supernatant liquid into a 50 ml flask, add 10 ml of *water R* and evaporate the solution to dryness under reduced pressure. Take up the residue in 10 ml of *water R* and evaporate again to dryness under reduced pressure. Take up the residue with 2 ml of *methanol R*.

Reference solution (a). Dissolve 10 mg of *arabinose R* in a small quantity of *water R* and dilute to 10 ml with *methanol R*.

Reference solution (b). Dissolve 10 mg of *xylose R* in a small quantity of *water R* and dilute to 10 ml with *methanol R*.

Reference solution (c). Dissolve 10 mg of *galactose R* in a small quantity of *water R* and dilute to 10 ml with *methanol R*.

Apply to the plate, as bands, 10 µl of each solution. Develop over a path of 15 cm using a mixture of 15 volumes of *water R* and 85 volumes of *acetonitrile R*. Spray with *aminohippuric acid reagent R* and heat at 120 °C for 5 min. Examine in daylight. The chromatogram obtained with the test solution shows two orange-pink zones (arabinose and xylose) and a yellow zone (galactose) similar in position and colour to the zones in the chromatograms obtained with the reference solutions.

TESTS

Foreign matter (*2.8.2*). It complies with the test for foreign matter, determined on 5.0 g of the substance to be examined.

Swelling index (*2.8.4*). Not less than 40, determined on 0.1 g of the powdered drug (355).

Loss on drying (*2.2.32*). Not more than 12.0 per cent, determined on 1.000 g of the powdered drug (355) by drying in an oven at 100-105 °C for 2 h.

Total ash (*2.4.16*). Not more than 4.0 per cent.

STORAGE

Store in a well closed container, protected from light.

01/2005:1333

ISPAGHULA SEED

Plantaginis ovatae semen

DEFINITION

Dried ripe seeds of *Plantago ovata* Forssk. (*P. ispaghula* Roxb.).

CHARACTERS

Macroscopic and microscopic characters described under identification tests A and B.

IDENTIFICATION

A. Ispaghula seed is pinkish-beige, smooth, boat-shaped and curved. It is 1.5 mm to 3.5 mm long, 1.5 mm to 2 mm wide and 1 mm to 1.5 mm thick. The concave surface shows in the centre a light coloured spot corresponding to the hilum. The convex surface shows a light brown spot corresponding to the location of the embryo and takes up about one quarter of the length of the seed.

B. Reduce to a powder (355). The powder is pale brown. Examine under a microscope using *lactic reagent R*. The powder shows mainly fragments of the episperm with polygonal cells filled with mucilage; fragments of the inner layers of the testa with brownish thin-walled cells often associated with the outer layers of the endosperm; fragments of the endosperm with cells with thick cellulose walls containing aleurone grains and oil droplets; a few fragments of embryo with thin-walled cells. Examine under a microscope using a 50 per cent *V/V* solution of *glycerol R*. The powder shows starch granules, single or in groups of 2 to 4 and measuring 3 µm to 25 µm in diameter.

C. Thin-layer chromatography (*2.2.27*).

Test solution. To 50 mg of the powdered drug (355) in a thick-walled centrifuge tube add 2 ml of a 230 g/l solution of *trifluoroacetic acid R*, and shake vigorously. Stopper the test tube and heat the mixture at 120 °C for 1 h. Centrifuge the hydrolysate, transfer the clear supernatant liquid into a 50 ml flask, add 10 ml of *water R* and evaporate the solution to dryness under reduced pressure. Take up the residue in 10 ml of *water R* and evaporate again to dryness under reduced pressure. Take up the residue in 2 ml of *methanol R*.

Reference solution (a). Dissolve 10 mg of *arabinose R* in a small quantity of *water R* and dilute to 10 ml with *methanol R*.

Reference solution (b). Dissolve 10 mg of *xylose R* in a small quantity of *water R* and dilute to 10 ml with *methanol R*.

Reference solution (c). Dissolve 10 mg of *galactose R* in a small quantity of *water R* and dilute to 10 ml with *methanol R*.

Plate: *TLC silica gel plate R*.

Mobile phase: *water R, acetonitrile R* (15:85 *V/V*).

Application: 10 µl, as bands.

Development: over a path of 15 cm.

Detection: Spray with *aminohippuric acid reagent R* and heat at 120 °C for 5 min. Examine in daylight.

Results: see below the sequence of the zones present in the chromatograms obtained with the reference and the test solutions.

Top of the plate	
Xylose: an orange-pink zone	An orange-pink zone (xylose)
Arabinose: an orange-pink zone	An orange-pink zone (arabinose)
Galactose: a yellow zone	A yellow zone (galactose)
Reference solution	**Test solution**

TESTS

Foreign matter (*2.8.2*): maximum 2 per cent, determined on 10.0 g of the drug.

Swelling index (*2.8.4*): minimum 9.

Loss on drying (*2.2.32*): maximum 10.0 per cent, determined on 1.000 g of the powdered drug (355) by drying in an oven at 100-105 °C for 2 h.

Total ash (*2.4.16*): maximum 4.0 per cent.

01/2005:2110

ISRADIPINE

Isradipinum

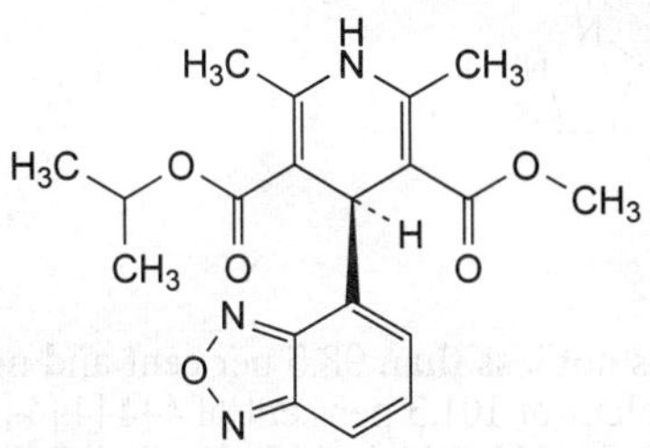

$C_{19}H_{21}N_3O_5$ M_r 371.4

DEFINITION

Methyl 1-methylethyl (4*RS*)-4-(2,1,3-benzoxadiazol-4-yl)-2,6-dimethyl-1,4-dihydropyridine-3,5-dicarboxylate.

Content: 97.0 per cent to 102.0 per cent (dried substance).

CHARACTERS

Appearance: yellow, crystalline powder.

Solubility: practically insoluble in water, freely soluble in acetone, soluble in methanol.

mp: about 168 °C.

IDENTIFICATION

Infrared absorption spectrophotometry (*2.2.24*).

Comparison: isradipine CRS.

TESTS

Related substances. Liquid chromatography (*2.2.29*).

Test solution (a). Dissolve 50.0 mg of the substance to be examined in 1 ml of *methanol R*, using an ultrasonic bath if necessary, and dilute to 25.0 ml with the mobile phase.

Test solution (b). Dissolve 50.0 mg of the substance to be examined in 2 ml of *methanol R* and dilute to 250.0 ml with the mobile phase.

Reference solution (a). Dilute 1.0 ml of test solution (a) to 100.0 ml with the mobile phase. Dilute 1.0 ml of this solution to 10.0 ml with the mobile phase.

Reference solution (b). Dissolve 2 mg of the substance to be examined and 2 mg of *isradipine impurity D CRS* in the mobile phase and dilute to 10.0 ml with the mobile phase. Dilute 1.0 ml of the solution to 10.0 ml with the mobile phase.

Reference solution (c). Dissolve 50.0 mg of *isradipine CRS* in 2 ml of *methanol R* and dilute to 250.0 ml with the mobile phase.

Column:
- *size*: l = 0.10 m, Ø = 4.6 mm,
- *stationary phase*: *octadecylsilyl silica gel for chromatography R* (5 µm).

Mobile phase: *acetonitrile R, tetrahydrofuran R, water R* (125:270:625 *V/V/V*).

Flow rate: 1.2 ml/min.

Detection: spectrophotometer at 230 nm.

Injection: 20 µl of test solution (a) and reference solutions (a) and (b).

Run time: 5 times the retention time of isradipine.

Identification of impurities: use the chromatogram supplied with *isradipine CRS* to identify the peak due to impurity B.

Relative retention with reference to isradipine (retention time = about 7 min): impurity D = about 0.9; impurity B = about 1.8.

System suitability: reference solution (b):
- *resolution*: minimum 2.0 between the peaks due to isradipine and impurity D.

Limits:
- *correction factor*: for the calculation of content, multiply the peak area of impurity D by 1.4,
- *impurity B*: not more than 8 times the area of the principal peak in the chromatogram obtained with reference solution (a) (0.8 per cent),
- *impurity D*: not more than the area of the principal peak in the chromatogram obtained with reference solution (a) (0.1 per cent),
- *any other impurity*: for each impurity, not more than the area of the principal peak in the chromatogram obtained with reference solution (a) (0.1 per cent),
- *total*: not more than 10 times the area of the principal peak in the chromatogram obtained with reference solution (a) (1.0 per cent),
- *disregard limit*: 0.5 times the area of the principal peak in the chromatogram obtained with reference solution (a) (0.05 per cent).

Loss on drying (*2.2.32*): maximum 0.2 per cent, determined on 1.000 g by drying in an oven at 100-105 °C for 4 h.

Sulphated ash (*2.4.14*): maximum 0.1 per cent, determined on 1.0 g.

ASSAY

Liquid chromatography (*2.2.29*) as described in the test for related substances with the following modifications.

Detection: spectrophotometer at 326 nm.

Injection: test solution (b) and reference solution (c).

Run time: twice the retention time of isradipine.

Calculate the percentage content of isradipine from the areas of the peaks and the declared content of *isradipine CRS*.

STORAGE

Protected from light.

IMPURITIES

Specified impurities: B, D.

Other detectable impurities: A, C, E.

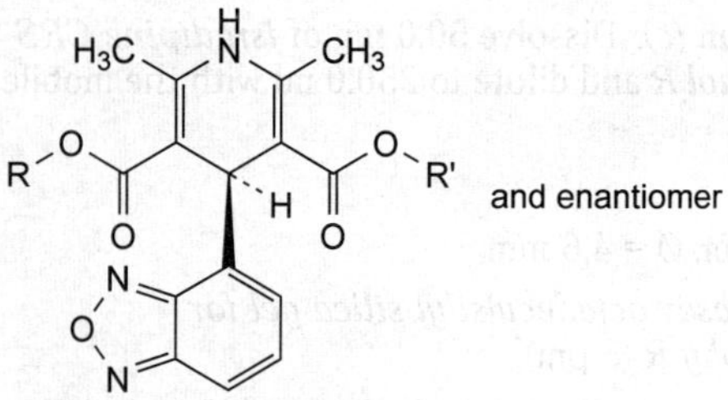

A. R = C_2H_5, R' = CH_3: ethyl methyl (4*RS*)-4-(2,1,3-benzoxadiazol-4-yl)-2,6-dimethyl-1,4-dihydropyridine-3,5-dicarboxylate,

B. R = R' = $CH(CH_3)_2$: bis(1-methylethyl) (4*RS*)-4-(2,1,3-benzoxadiazol-4-yl)-2,6-dimethyl-1,4-dihydropyridine-3,5-dicarboxylate,

C. R = R' = CH_3: dimethyl (4*RS*)-4-(2,1,3-benzoxadiazol-4-yl)-2,6-dimethyl-1,4-dihydropyridine-3,5-dicarboxylate,

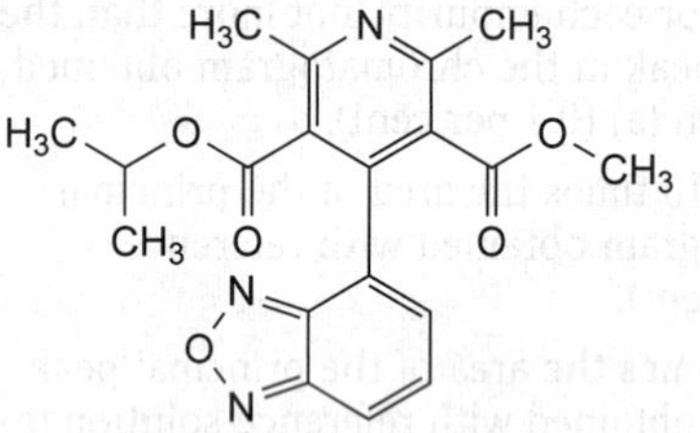

D. methyl 1-methylethyl 4-(2,1,3-benzoxadiazol-4-yl)-2,6-dimethylpyridine-3,5-dicarboxylate,

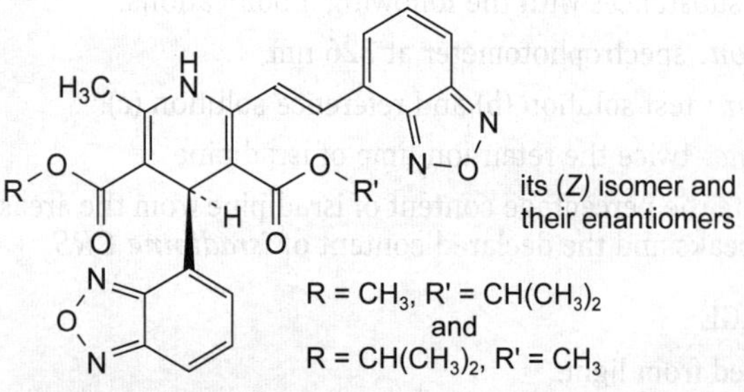

E. methyl 1-methylethyl (4*RS*)-4-(2,1,3-benzoxadiazol-4-yl)-2-[(*EZ*)-2-(2,1,3-benzoxadiazol-4-yl)ethenyl]-6-methyl-1,4-dihydropyridine-3,5-dicarboxylate.

01/2005:1335

ITRACONAZOLE

Itraconazolum

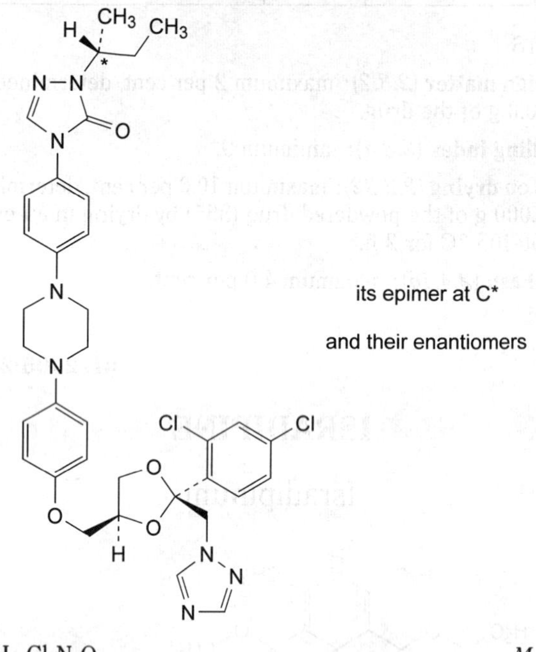

$C_{35}H_{38}Cl_2N_8O_4$ M_r 706

DEFINITION

Itraconazole contains not less than 98.5 per cent and not more than the equivalent of 101.5 per cent of 4-[4-[4-[4-[[*cis*-2-(2,4-dichlorophenyl)-2-(1*H*-1,2,4-triazol-1-ylmethyl)-1,3-dioxolan-4-yl]methoxy]phenyl]piperazin-1-yl]phenyl]-2-[(1*RS*)-1-methylpropyl]-2,4-dihydro-3*H*-1,2,4-triazol-3-one, calculated with reference to the dried substance.

CHARACTERS

A white or almost white powder, practically insoluble in water, freely soluble in methylene chloride, sparingly soluble in tetrahydrofuran, very slightly soluble in alcohol.

IDENTIFICATION

First identification: B.

Second identification: A, C, D.

A. Melting point (*2.2.14*): 166 °C to 170 °C.

B. Examine by infrared spectrophotometry (*2.2.24*), comparing with the spectrum obtained with *itraconazole CRS*. Examine the substance prepared as discs.

C. Examine by thin-layer chromatography (*2.2.27*), using a suitable octadecylsilyl silica gel as the coating substance.

Test solution. Dissolve 30 mg of the substance to be examined in a mixture of equal volumes of *methanol R* and *methylene chloride R* and dilute to 5 ml with the same mixture of solvents.

Reference solution (a). Dissolve 30 mg of *itraconazole CRS* in a mixture of equal volumes of *methanol R* and *methylene chloride R* and dilute to 5 ml with the same mixture of solvents.

Reference solution (b). Dissolve 30 mg of *itraconazole CRS* and 30 mg of *ketoconazole CRS* in a mixture of equal volumes of *methanol R* and *methylene chloride R* and dilute to 5 ml with the same mixture of solvents.

Apply to the plate 5 µl of each solution. Develop in an unsaturated tank over a path of 10 cm using a mixture of 20 volumes of *ammonium acetate solution R*, 40 volumes of *dioxan R* and 40 volumes of *methanol R*. Dry the plate in a current of warm air for 15 min and expose it to iodine vapour until the spots appear. Examine in daylight. The principal spot in the chromatogram obtained with the test solution is similar in position, colour and size to the principal spot in the chromatogram obtained with reference solution (a). The test is not valid unless the chromatogram obtained with reference solution (b) shows two clearly separated spots.

D. To 30 mg in a porcelain crucible add 0.3 g of *anhydrous sodium carbonate R*. Heat over an open flame for 10 min. Allow to cool. Take up the residue with 5 ml of *dilute nitric acid R* and filter. To 1 ml of the filtrate add 1 ml of *water R*. The solution gives reaction (a) of chlorides (*2.3.1*).

TESTS

Solution S. Dissolve 2.0 g in *methylene chloride R* and dilute to 20.0 ml with the same solvent.

Appearance of solution. Solution S is clear (*2.2.1*) and not more intensely coloured than reference solution BY_6 (*2.2.2, Method II*).

Optical rotation (*2.2.7*). The angle of optical rotation is − 0.10° to + 0.10°, determined on solution S.

Related substances. Examine by liquid chromatography (*2.2.29*).

Test solution. Dissolve 0.100 g of the substance to be examined in a mixture of equal volumes of *methanol R* and *tetrahydrofuran R* and dilute to 10.0 ml with the same mixture of solvents.

Reference solution (a). Dissolve 5.0 mg of *itraconazole CRS* and 5.0 mg of *miconazole CRS* in a mixture of equal volumes of *methanol R* and *tetrahydrofuran R* and dilute to 100.0 ml with the same mixture of solvents.

Reference solution (b). Dilute 1.0 ml of the test solution to 100.0 ml with a mixture of equal volumes of *methanol R* and *tetrahydrofuran R*. Dilute to 5.0 ml of this solution to 10.0 ml with the same mixture of solvents.

The chromatographic procedure may be carried out using:

- a stainless steel column 0.1 m long and 4.0 mm in internal diameter packed with *base-deactivated octadecylsilyl silica gel for chromatography R* (3 µm),
- as mobile phase at a flow rate of 1.5 ml/min a gradient programme using the following conditions:

  Mobile phase A. A 27.2 g/l solution of *tetrabutylammonium hydrogen sulphate R*,

  Mobile phase B. Acetonitrile R,

Time (min)	Mobile phase A (per cent *V/V*)	Mobile phase B (per cent *V/V*)	Comment
0 - 20	80 → 50	20 → 50	linear gradient
20 - 25	50	50	isocratic elution
25 - 30	80	20	switch to initial eluent composition
30 = 0	80	20	restart gradient

- as detector a spectrophotometer set at 225 nm.

Equilibrate the column for at least 30 min with *acetonitrile R* at a flow rate of 1.5 ml/min and then equilibrate at the initial eluent composition for at least 5 min.

Adjust the sensitivity of the system so that the height of the principal peak in the chromatogram obtained with 10 µl of reference solution (b) is at least 50 per cent of the full scale of the recorder.

Inject 10 µl of reference solution (a). When the chromatogram is recorded in the prescribed conditions, the retention times are: miconazole about 10.5 min and itraconazole about 11 min. The test is not valid unless the resolution between the peaks corresponding to miconazole and itraconazole is at least 2.0. If necessary, adjust the concentration of acetonitrile in the mobile phase or adjust the time programme for the linear gradient elution.

Inject separately 10 µl of the mixture of equal volumes of *methanol R* and *tetrahydrofuran R* as a blank, 10 µl of the test solution and 10 µl of reference solution (b). In the chromatogram obtained with the test solution: the area of any peak, apart from the principal peak, is not greater than that of the principal peak in the chromatogram obtained with reference solution (b) (0.5 per cent); the sum of the areas of all the peaks, apart from the principal peak, is not greater than 2.5 times the area of the principal peak in the chromatogram obtained with reference solution (b) (1.25 per cent). Disregard any peak obtained with the blank run and any peak with an area less than 0.1 times the area of the principal peak in the chromatogram obtained with reference solution (b).

Loss on drying (*2.2.32*). Not more than 0.5 per cent, determined on 1.000 g by drying in an oven at 100 °C to 105 °C for 4 h.

Sulphated ash (*2.4.14*). Not more than 0.1 per cent, determined on 1.0 g.

ASSAY

Dissolve 0.300 g in 70 ml of a mixture of 1 volume of *anhydrous acetic acid R* and 7 volumes of *methyl ethyl ketone R*. Titrate with *0.1 M perchloric acid*, determining the end-point potentiometrically at the second point of inflexion (*2.2.20*).

1 ml of *0.1 M perchloric acid* is equivalent to 35.3 mg of $C_{35}H_{38}Cl_2N_8O_4$.

STORAGE

Store protected from light.

IMPURITIES

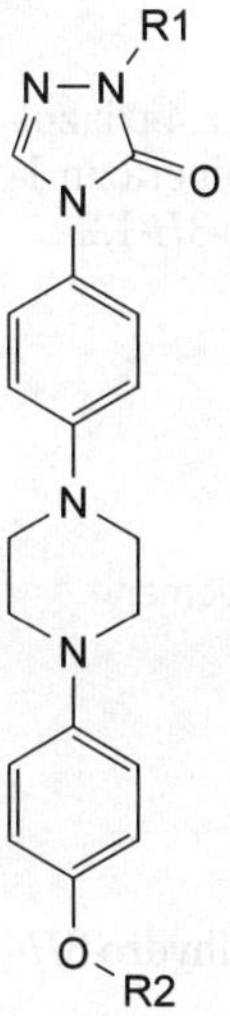

Monographs I-L

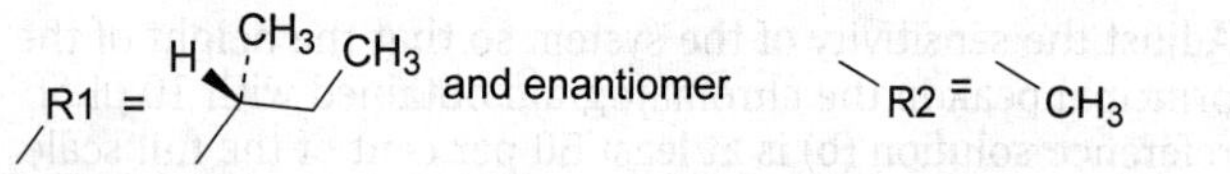

A. 4-[4-[4-(4-methoxyphenyl)piperazin-1-yl]phenyl]-2-[(1*RS*)-1-methylpropyl]-2,4-dihydro-3*H*-1,2,4-triazol-3-one,

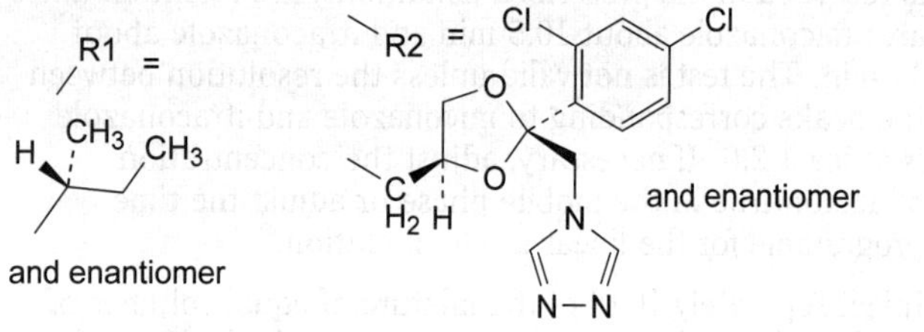

B. 4-[4-[4-[4-[[*cis*-2-(2,4-dichlorophenyl)-2-(4*H*-1,2,4-triazol-4-ylmethyl)-1,3-dioxolan-4-yl]methoxy]phenyl]piperazin-1-yl]phenyl]-2-[(1*RS*)-1-methylpropyl]-2,4-dihydro-3*H*-1,2,4-triazol-3-one,

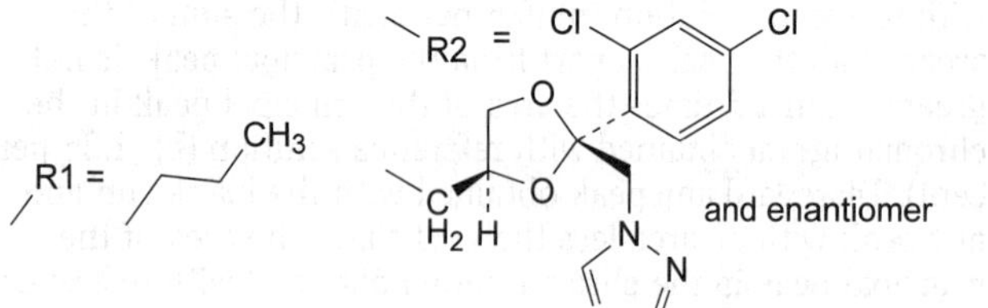

C. 4-[4-[4-[4-[[*cis*-2-(2,4-dichlorophenyl)-2-(1*H*-1,2,4-triazol-1-ylmethyl)-1,3-dioxolan-4-yl]methoxy]phenyl]piperazin-1-yl]phenyl]-2-propyl-2,4-dihydro-3*H*-1,2,4-triazol-3-one,

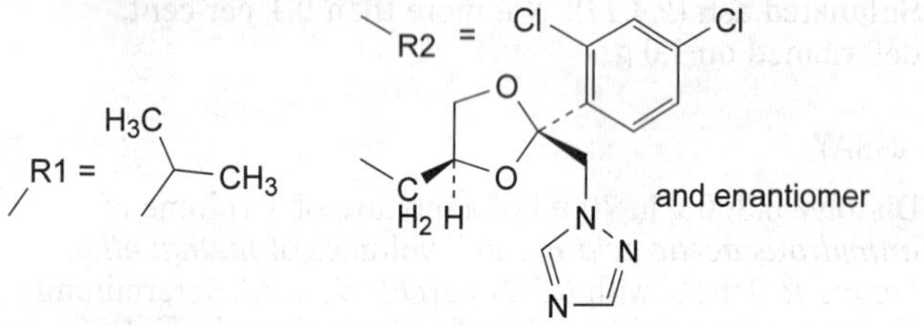

D. 4-[4-[4-[4-[[*cis*-2-(2,4-dichlorophenyl)-2-(1*H*-1,2,4-triazol-1-ylmethyl)-1,3-dioxolan-4-yl]methoxy]phenyl]piperazin-1-yl]phenyl]-2-(1-methylethyl)-2,4-dihydro-3*H*-1,2,4-triazol-3-one,

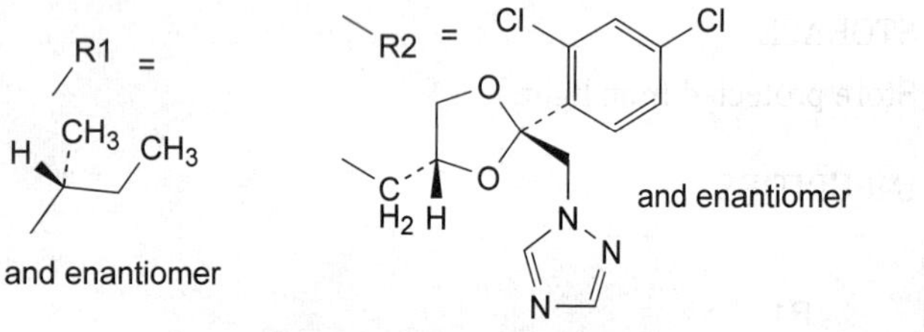

E. 4-[4-[4-[4-[[*trans*-2-(2,4-dichlorophenyl)-2-(1*H*-1,2,4-triazol-1-ylmethyl)-1,3-dioxolan-4-yl]methoxy]phenyl]piperazin-1-yl]phenyl]-2-[(1*RS*)-1-methylpropyl]-2,4-dihydro-3*H*-1,2,4-triazol- 3-one,

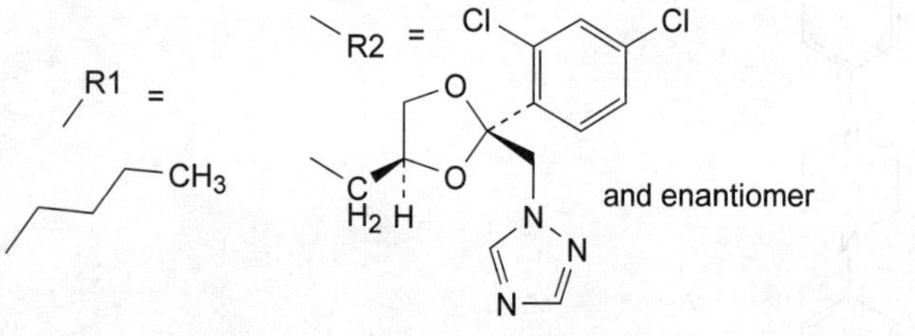

F. 2-butyl-4-[4-[4-[4-[[*cis*-2-(2,4-dichlorophenyl)-2-(1*H*-1,2,4-triazol-1-ylmethyl)-1,3-dioxolan-4-yl]methoxy]phenyl]piperazin-1-yl]phenyl]-2,4-dihydro-3*H*-1,2,4-triazol-3-one,

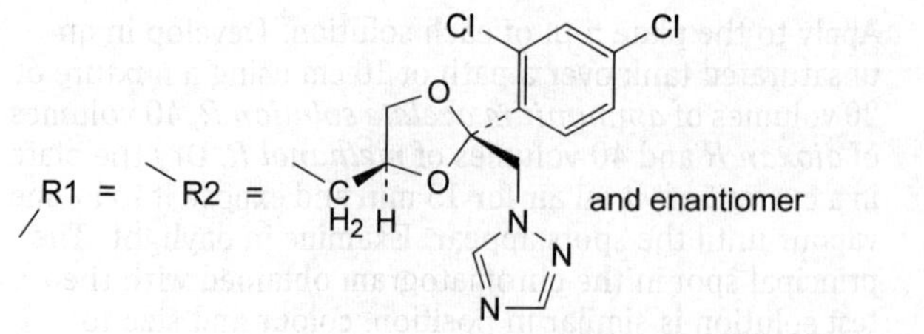

G. 4-[4-[4-[4-[[*cis*-2-(2,4-dichlorophenyl)-2-(1*H*-1,2,4-triazol-1-ylmethyl)-1,3-dioxolan-4-yl]methoxy]phenyl]piperazin-1-yl]phenyl]-2-[[*cis*-2-(2,4-dichlorophenyl)-2-(1*H*-1,2,4-triazol-1-ylmethyl)-1,3-dioxolan-4-yl]methyl]-2,4-dihydro-3*H*-1,2,4-triazol-3-one.

01/2005:1336
corrected

IVERMECTIN

Ivermectinum

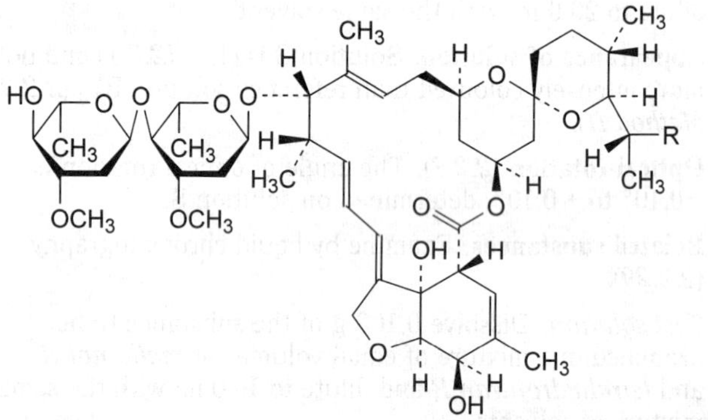

Component	R	Molecular formula	M_r
H_2B_{1a}	CH_2-CH_3	$C_{48}H_{74}O_{14}$	875
H_2B_{1b}	CH_3	$C_{47}H_{72}O_{14}$	861

DEFINITION

Mixture of (2a*E*,4*E*,5′*S*,6*S*,6′*R*,7*S*,8*E*,11*R*,13*R*,15*S*,17a*R*,20*R*,20a*R*,20b*S*)-7-[[2,6-dideoxy-4-*O*-(2,6-dideoxy-3-*O*-methyl-α-L-*arabino*-hexopyranosyl)-3-*O*-methyl-α-L-*arabino*-hexopyranosyl]oxy]-20,20b-dihydroxy-5′,6,8,19-tetramethyl-6′-[(1*S*)-1-methylpropyl]-3′,4′,5′,6,6′,7,10,11,14,15,17a,20,20a,20b-tetradecahydrospiro[11,15-methano-2*H*,13*H*,17*H*-furo[4,3,2-*pq*][2,6]benzodioxacyclooctadecene-13,2′-[2*H*]pyran]-17-one (or 5-*O*-demethyl-22,23-dihydroavermectin A_{1a}) (component H_2B_{1a}) and (2a*E*,4*E*,5′*S*,6*S*,6′*R*,7*S*,8*E*,11*R*,13*R*,15*S*,17a*R*,20*R*,20a*R*,20b*S*)-7-[[2,6-dideoxy-4-*O*-(2,6-dideoxy-3-*O*-methyl-α-L-*arabino*-hexopyranosyl)-3-*O*-methyl-α-L-*arabino*-hexopyranosyl]oxy]-20,20b-dihydroxy-5′,6,8,19-tetramethyl-6′-(1-methylethyl)-3′,4′,5′,6,6′,7,10,11,14,15,17a,20,20a,20b-tetradecahydrospiro[11,15-methano-2*H*,13*H*,17*H*-furo[4,3,2-*pq*][2,6]benzodioxacyclooctadecene-13,2′-[2*H*]pyran]-17-one (or 5-*O*-demethyl-25-de(1-methylpropyl)-25-(1-methylethyl)-22,23-dihydroavermectin A_{1a}) (component H_2B_{1b}).

Content:

– ivermectin (H_2B_{1a} + H_2B_{1b}): 95.0 per cent to 102.0 per cent (anhydrous and solvent-free substance),
– ratio H_2B_{1a}/(H_2B_{1a} + H_2B_{1b}) (areas by liquid chromatography): minimum 90.0 per cent.

CHARACTERS

Appearance: white or yellowish-white, crystalline powder, slightly hygroscopic.

Solubility: practically insoluble in water, freely soluble in methylene chloride, soluble in alcohol.

IDENTIFICATION

A. Infrared absorption spectrophotometry (*2.2.24*).

Comparison: *ivermectin CRS.*

B. Examine the chromatograms obtained in the assay.

Results: the retention times and sizes of the 2 principal peaks in the chromatogram obtained with the test solution are similar to those of the 2 principal peaks in the chromatogram obtained with reference solution (a).

TESTS

Appearance of solution. The solution is clear (*2.2.1*) and not more intensely coloured than reference solution BY_7 (*2.2.2, Method II*).

Dissolve 1.0 g in 50 ml of *toluene R*.

Specific optical rotation (*2.2.7*): − 17 to − 20 (anhydrous and solvent-free substance).

Dissolve 0.250 g in *methanol R* and dilute to 10.0 ml with the same solvent.

Related substances. Liquid chromatography (*2.2.29*).

Test solution. Dissolve 40.0 mg of the substance to be examined in *methanol R* and dilute to 50.0 ml with the same solvent.

Reference solution (a). Dissolve 40.0 mg of *ivermectin CRS* in *methanol R* and dilute to 50.0 ml with the same solvent.

Reference solution (b). Dilute 1.0 ml of reference solution (a) to 100.0 ml with *methanol R.*

Reference solution (c). Dilute 5.0 ml of reference solution (b) to 100.0 ml with *methanol R.*

Column:
- size: l = 0.25 m, Ø = 4.6 mm,
- *stationary phase*: *octadecylsilyl silica gel for chromatography R* (5 µm).

Mobile phase: *water R, methanol R, acetonitrile R* (15:34:51 *V/V/V*).

Flow rate: 1 ml/min.

Detection: spectrophotometer at 254 nm.

Injection: 20 µl.

System suitability:
- *resolution*: minimum of 3.0 between the first peak (component H_2B_{1b}) and the second peak (component H_2B_{1a}) in the chromatogram obtained with reference solution (a),
- *signal-to-noise ratio*: minimum of 10 for the principal peak in the chromatogram obtained with reference solution (c),
- *symmetry factor*: maximum of 2.5 for the principal peak in the chromatogram obtained with reference solution (a).

Limits:
- *impurity with a relative retention of 1.3 to 1.5* with reference to the principal peak: not more than 2.5 times the area of the principal peak in the chromatogram obtained with reference solution (b) (2.5 per cent),
- *any other impurity* (apart from the 2 principal peaks): not more than the area of the principal peak in the chromatogram obtained with reference solution (b) (1 per cent),
- *total*: not more than 5 times the area of the principal peak in the chromatogram obtained with reference solution (b) (5 per cent),
- *disregard limit*: area of the principal peak in the chromatogram obtained with reference solution (c) (0.05 per cent).

Ethanol and formamide. Gas chromatography (*2.2.28*).

Internal standard solution. Dilute 0.5 ml of *propanol R* to 100 ml with *water R.*

Test solution. In a centrifuge tube, dissolve 0.120 g of the substance to be examined in 2.0 ml of *m-xylene R* (if necessary heat in a water-bath at 40-50 °C). Add 2.0 ml of *water R,* mix thoroughly and centrifuge. Remove the upper layer and extract it with 2.0 ml of *water R.* Discard the upper layer and combine the aqueous layers. Add 1.0 ml of the internal standard solution. Centrifuge and discard any remaining *m*-xylene.

Reference solution (a). Dilute 3.0 g of *ethanol R* to 100.0 ml with *water R.*

Reference solution (b). Dilute 1.0 g of *formamide R* to 100.0 ml with *water R.*

Reference solution (c). Dilute 5.0 ml of reference solution (a) and 5.0 ml of reference solution (b) to 50.0 ml with *water R.* Introduce 2.0 ml of this solution into a centrifuge tube, add 2.0 ml of *m-xylene R,* mix thoroughly and centrifuge. Remove the upper layer and extract it with 2.0 ml of *water R.* Discard the upper layer and combine the aqueous layers. Add 1.0 ml of the internal standard solution. Centrifuge and discard any remaining *m*-xylene.

Reference solution (d). Dilute 10.0 ml of reference solution (a) and 10.0 ml of reference solution (b) to 50.0 ml with *water R.* Treat as prescribed for reference solution (c) (from "Introduce 2.0 ml of this solution...").

Column:
- *material*: fused silica,
- *size*: l = 30 m, Ø = 0.53 mm,
- *stationary phase*: *macrogol 20 000 R* (film thickness 1 µm).

Carrier gas: *helium for chromatography R.*

Flow rate: 7.5 ml/min.

Split ratio: 1:10.

Temperature:

	Time (min)	Temperature (°C)
Column	0 - 2	50 → 80
	2 - 8	80 → 240
Injection port		220
Detector		280

Detection: flame ionisation.

Injection: 1 µl; inject the test solution and reference solutions (c) and (d).

Limits:
- *ethanol*: maximum 5.0 per cent,
- *formamide*: maximum 3.0 per cent.

Heavy metals (*2.4.8*): maximum 20 ppm.

1.0 g complies with limit test C. Prepare the standard using 2 ml of *lead standard solution (10 ppm Pb) R.*

Water (*2.5.12*): maximum 1.0 per cent, determined on 0.50 g.

Sulphated ash (*2.4.14*): maximum 0.1 per cent, determined on 1.0 g.

ASSAY

Liquid chromatography (*2.2.29*) as described in the test for related substances.

Injection: 20 µl; inject the test solution and reference solution (a).

Calculate the percentage contents of ivermectin (H_2B_{1a} + H_2B_{1b}) and the ratio $H_2B_{1a}/(H_2B_{1a} + H_2B_{1b})$ using the declared contents of *ivermectin CRS*.

STORAGE

In an airtight container.

IMPURITIES

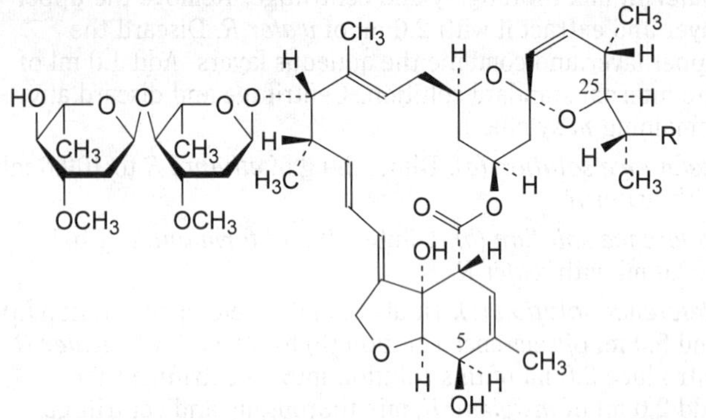

A. R = C_2H_5: 5-*O*-demethylavermectin A_{1a} (avermectin B_{1a}),

B. R = CH_3: 5-*O*-demethyl-25-de(1-methylpropyl)-25-(1-methylethyl)avermectin A_{1a} (avermectin B_{1b}),

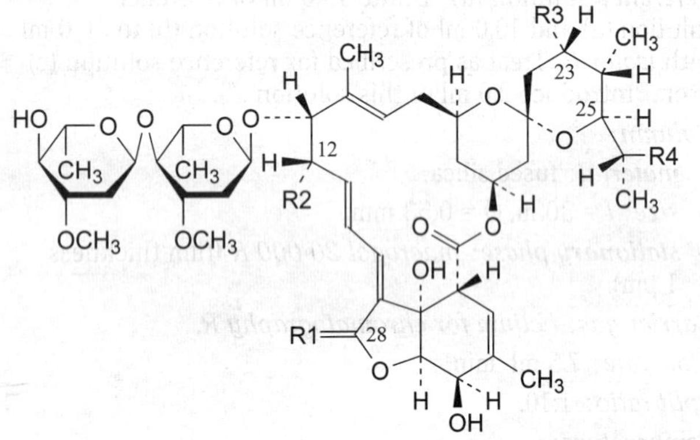

C. R1 = H_2, R2 = CH_3, R3 = OH, R4 = C_2H_5: (23*S*)-5-*O*-demethyl-23-hydroxy-22,23-dihydroavermectin A_{1a} (avermectin B_{2a}),

D. R1 = O, R2 = CH_3, R3 = H, R4 = C_2H_5: 5-*O*-demethyl-28-oxo-22,23-dihydroavermectin A_{1a} (28-oxoH_2B_{1a}),

E. R1 = H_2, R2 = C_2H_5, R3 = H, R4 = C_2H_5: 5-*O*,12-didemethyl-12-ethyl-22,23-dihydroavermectin A_{1a} (12-demethyl-12-ethyl-H_2B_{1a}),

F. R1 = H_2, R2 = C_2H_5, R3 = H, R4 = CH_3: 5-*O*,12-didemethyl-25-de(1-methylpropyl)-12-ethyl-25-(1-methylethyl)-22,23-dihydroavermectin A_{1a} (12-demethyl-12-ethyl-H_2B_{1b}),

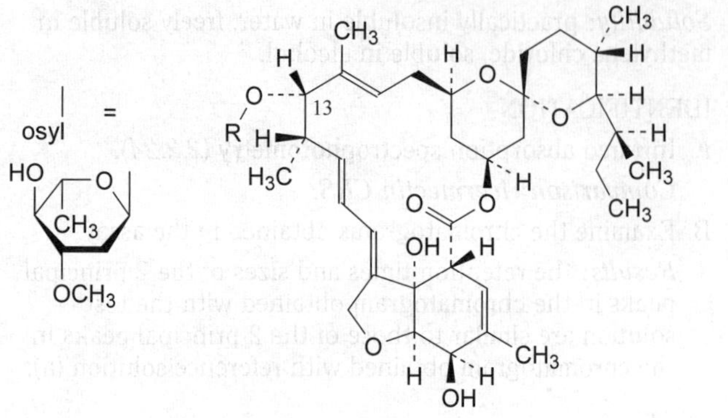

G. R = H: (6*R*,13*S*,25*R*)-5-*O*-demethyl-28-deoxy-6,28-epoxy-13-hydroxy-25-[(1*S*)-1-methylpropyl]milbemycin B (H_2B_{1a} aglycone),

H. R = osyl: 4′-*O*-de(2,6-dideoxy-3-*O*-methyl-α-L-*arabino*-hexopyranosyl)-5-*O*-demethyl-22,23-dihydroavermectin A_{1a},

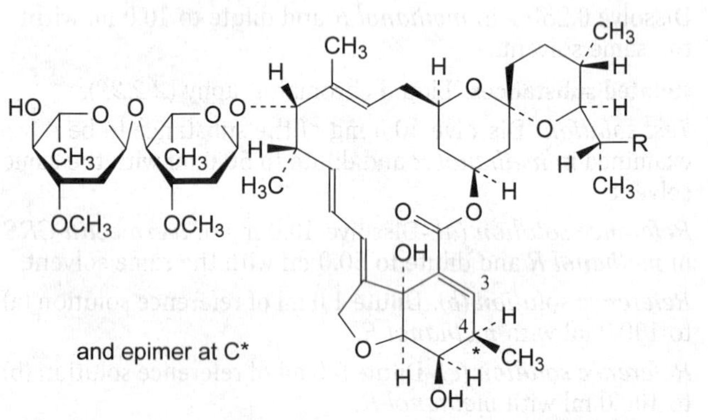

I. R = C_2H_5: 2,3-didehydro-5-*O*-demethyl-3,4,22,23-tetrahydroavermectin A_{1a} ($\Delta^{2,3}$ H_2B_{1a}),

J. R = CH_3: 2,3-didehydro-5-*O*-demethyl-25-de(1-methylpropyl)-25-(1-methylethyl)-3,4,22,23-tetrahydroavermectin A_{1a} ($\Delta^{2,3}$ H_2B_{1b}),

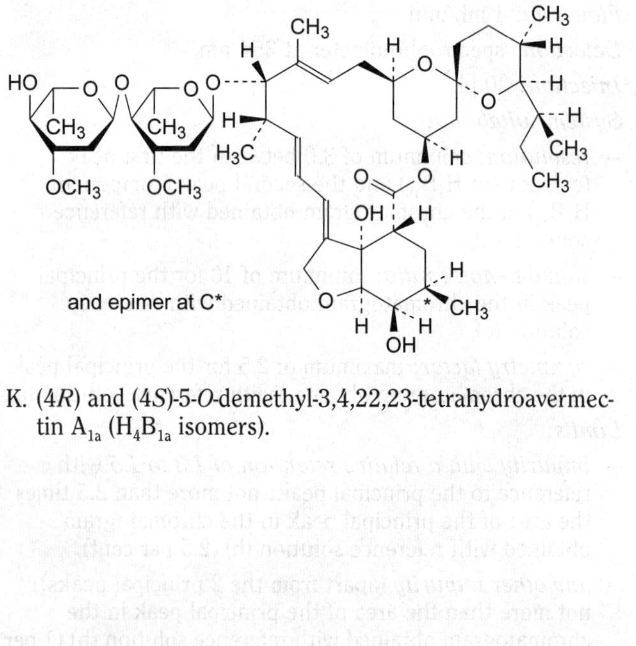

K. (4*R*) and (4*S*)-5-*O*-demethyl-3,4,22,23-tetrahydroavermectin A_{1a} (H_4B_{1a} isomers).

J

01/2005:1229

JAVA TEA

Orthosiphonis folium

DEFINITION

Fragmented, dried leaves and tops of stems of *Orthosiphon stamineus* Benth. (*O. aristatus* Miq.; *O. spicatus* Bak.).

Content: minimum 0.05 per cent of sinensetin ($C_{20}H_{20}O_7$; M_r 372.4) (dried drug).

CHARACTERS

Macroscopic and microscopic characters described under identification tests A and B.

IDENTIFICATION

A. The leaves are friable, up to 7.5 cm in length and 2.5 cm in width. The petiole is short. The lamina is oval to lanceolate, the apex acuminate and the base cuneate. The abaxial surface of the leaves is light greyish-green and the adaxial surface is dark green to brownish-green. The venation is pinnate with few secondary veins. Examined under a lens (× 10), the secondary veins, after running parallel to the midrib, diverge at an acute angle. The margin is irregularly and roughly dentate, sometimes crenate and the abaxial surface is slightly curved. The petioles are thin, quadrangular, 4 mm to 8 mm long and, like the primary venation, usually violet-coloured. Occasionally, inflorescences in clusters of bluish-white to violet flowers, not yet opened, are found.

B. Reduce to a powder (355). The powder is dark green. Examine under a microscope using *chloral hydrate solution R*. The powder shows fragments of epidermis, with cells with sinuous outlines bearing unicellular or bicellular conical covering trichomes and articulated uniseriate trichomes up to 450 µm long, consisting of 3 to 8 cells with thick pitted walls; capitate trichomes with unicellular or bicellular heads; secretory trichomes with unicellular stalks and usually tetracellular heads; diacytic stomata (*2.8.3*), which are more numerous on the lower epidermis.

C. Thin-layer chromatography (*2.2.27*).

Test solution. Shake 1 g of the powdered drug (710) for 5 min with 10 ml of *methanol R* in a water-bath at 60 °C and filter the cooled solution.

Reference solution. Dissolve 1 mg of *sinensetin R* in *methanol R* and dilute to 20 ml with the same solvent.

Plate: *TLC silica gel plate R*.

Mobile phase: *methanol R, ethyl acetate R, toluene R* (5:40:55 *V/V/V*).

Application: 10 µl, as bands.

Development: over a path of 10 cm.

Drying: in air.

Detection: examine in ultraviolet light at 365 nm.

Results: see below the sequence of the zones present in the chromatogram obtained with the reference solution and the test solution. Furthermore, red fluorescent zones are present in the lower third and near the solvent front of the chromatogram obtained with the test solution.

Top of the plate	
	1 or 2 more or less intense blue to violet-blue fluorescent zones
———	———
Sinensetin: an intense light blue fluorescent zone	A major blue fluorescent zone (sinensetin)
———	———
	2 bluish fluorescent zones
Reference solution	**Test solution**

TESTS

Foreign matter (*2.8.2*): maximum 5 per cent of stems with a diameter greater than 1 mm; maximum 2 per cent of other foreign matter.

Loss on drying (*2.2.32*): maximum 11.0 per cent, determined on 1.000 g of the powdered drug (355) by drying in an oven at 100-105 °C for 2 h.

Total ash (*2.4.16*): maximum 12.5 per cent.

ASSAY

Liquid chromatography (*2.2.29*).

Test solution. Heat 2.5 g of the powdered drug (355) and 100 ml of *methylene chloride R* on a water-bath for 30 min with stirring. Filter. Collect the filtrate and repeat the operation twice, in the same manner, on the filtration residue. Combine the filtrates. Evaporate the solvent under reduced pressure. Dissolve the residue in 25.0 ml of the mobile phase, using an ultrasonic bath if necessary. Filter the solution through a nitrocellulose filter with a pore size of 0.45 µm.

Reference solution. In a 100.0 ml graduated flask dissolve 5 mg (m_2) of *sinensetin R* in 25.0 ml of the mobile phase and dilute to 100.0 ml with the mobile phase.

Column:

– *size*: l = 0.25 m, Ø = 4.6 mm,

– *stationary phase*: *octadecylsilyl silica gel for chromatography R* (5 µm).

Mobile phase: *tetrahydrofuran R, acetic acid R, water R, methanol R* (5:8:42:45 *V/V/V/V*).

Flow rate: 0.5 ml/min.

Detection: spectrophotometer at 258 nm.

Injection: 20 µl.

Calculate the percentage content of sinensetin from the expression:

$$\frac{m_2 \times F_1 \times 25}{m_1 \times F_2}$$

F_1 = area of the peak corresponding to sinensetin in the chromatogram obtained with the test solution,

F_2 = area of the peak corresponding to sinensetin in the chromatogram obtained with the reference solution,

m_1 = mass of the drug to be examined, in grams

m_2 = mass of sinensetin in the reference solution, in grams.

01/2005:1983

JOSAMYCIN

Josamycinum

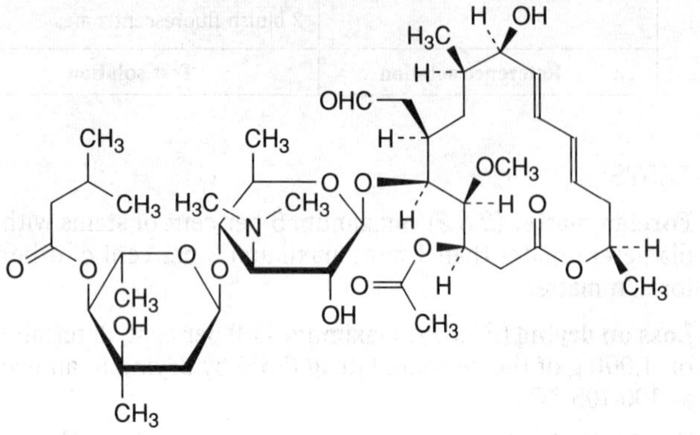

$C_{42}H_{69}NO_{15}$ M_r 828

DEFINITION

Josamycin is a macrolide antibiotic produced by certain strains of *Streptomyces narbonensis* var. *josamyceticus* var. *nova*, or obtained by any other means. The main component is (4*R*,5*S*,6*S*,7*R*,9*R*,10*R*,11*E*,13*E*,16*R*)-4-(acetyloxy)-6-[[3,6-dideoxy-4-*O*-[2,6-dideoxy-3-*C*-methyl-4-*O*-(3-methylbutanoyl)-α-L-*ribo*-hexopyranosyl]-3-(dimethylamino)-β-D-glucopyranosyl]oxy]-10-hydroxy-5-methoxy-9,16-dimethyl-7-(2-oxoethyl)oxacyclohexadeca-11,13-dien-2-one.

Content: minimum 900 Ph. Eur. U./mg (dried substance).

CHARACTERS

Appearance: white or slightly yellowish powder, slightly hygroscopic.

Solubility: very slightly soluble in water, freely soluble in methanol and in methylene chloride, soluble in acetone.

IDENTIFICATION

First identification: A, B.

Second identification: B, C.

A. Dissolve 0.10 g in *methanol R* and dilute to 100.0 ml with the same solvent. Dilute 1.0 ml of the solution to 50.0 ml with *methanol R*. Examined between 220 nm and 350 nm (*2.2.25*), the solution shows an absorption maximum at 232 nm. The specific absorbance at the maximum is 330 to 370.

B. Examine the chromatograms obtained in the test for related substances.

Results: the principal spot in the chromatogram obtained with the test solution is similar in position, colour and size to the principal spot in the chromatogram obtained with reference solution (a) and its position is different from that of the principal spot in the chromatograms obtained with reference solutions (d) and (e).

C. Dissolve about 10 mg in 5 ml of *hydrochloric acid R1* and allow to stand for 10-20 min. A pink colour develops, turning brown.

TESTS

Appearance of solution. The solution is clear (*2.2.1*) and not more intensely coloured than reference solution BY_4 (*2.2.2, Method II*).

Dissolve 1.0 g in *methanol R* and dilute to 10 ml with the same solvent.

Specific optical rotation (*2.2.7*): − 65 to − 75 (dried substance).

Dissolve 1.000 g in *methanol R* and dilute to 100.0 ml with the same solvent. Allow to stand for 30 min before measuring the angle of rotation.

Related substances. Thin-layer chromatography (*2.2.27*).

Test solution. Dissolve 0.10 g of the substance to be examined in *methanol R* and dilute to 10 ml with the same solvent.

Reference solution (a). Dissolve 0.10 g of *josamycin CRS* in *methanol R* and dilute to 10 ml with the same solvent.

Reference solution (b). Dilute 1 ml of reference solution (a) to 10 ml with *methanol R*.

Reference solution (c). Dilute 1 ml of reference solution (a) to 20 ml with *methanol R*.

Reference solution (d). Dissolve 0.10 g of *josamycin propionate CRS* in *methanol R* and dilute to 10 ml with the same solvent.

Reference solution (e). Dissolve 0.10 g of *spiramycin CRS* in *methylene chloride R* and dilute to 10 ml with the same solvent.

Reference solution (f). Dissolve 10 mg of *josamycin CRS* and 10 mg of *josamycin propionate CRS* in 1 ml of *methanol R*.

Plate: *TLC silica gel G plate R*.

Mobile phase: *methanol R, acetone R, ethyl acetate R, toluene R, hexane R* (8:10:20:25:30 *V/V/V/V/V*).

Application: 10 µl.

Development: over a path of 15 cm.

Drying: at 100 °C for 10 min.

Detection: spray with *dilute sulphuric acid R* and heat at 100 °C for 10 min.

System suitability: the chromatogram obtained with reference solution (f) shows 2 clearly separated principal spots.

Limits:

– *any impurity*: any spot, apart from the principal spot, is not more intense than the spot in the chromatogram obtained with reference solution (b) (10 per cent) and not more than 1 such spot is more intense than the spot in the chromatogram obtained with reference solution (c) (5 per cent).

Heavy metals (*2.4.8*): maximum 30 ppm.

1.0 g complies with limit test C. Prepare the standard using 3 ml of *lead standard solution (10 ppm Pb) R*.

Loss on drying (*2.2.32*): maximum 1.0 per cent, determined on 1.000 g by drying in an oven *in vacuo* at 60 °C for 3 h.

Sulphated ash (*2.4.14*): maximum 0.2 per cent, determined on 1.0 g.

ASSAY

Dissolve 30.0 mg in 5 ml of *methanol R* and dilute to 100.0 ml with *water R*.

Carry out the microbiological assay of antibiotics (*2.7.2*).

STORAGE

In an airtight container.

01/2005:1982

JOSAMYCIN PROPIONATE

Josamycini propionas

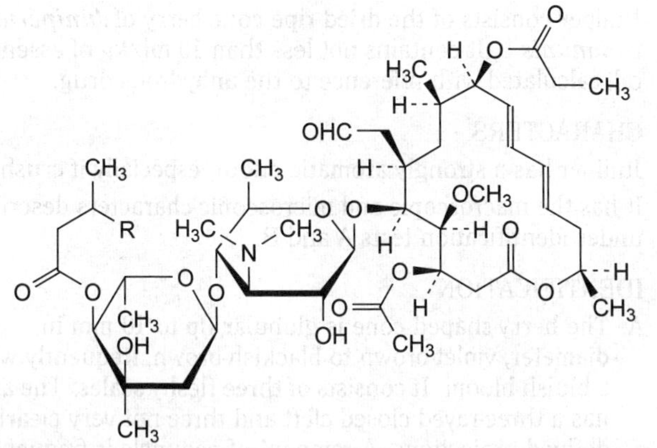

Leucomycin propionate	R	Mol. Formula	Mr
A3	CH_3	$C_{45}H_{73}NO_{16}$	884
A4	H	$C_{44}H_{71}NO_{16}$	870

DEFINITION

Propionyl ester of a macrolide antibiotic produced by certain strains of *Streptomyces narbonensis* var. *josamyceticus* var. *nova*, or obtained by any other means. The main component is (4*R*,5*S*,6*S*,7*R*,9*R*,10*R*,11*E*,13*E*,16*R*)-4-(acetyloxy)-6-[[3,6-dideoxy-4-*O*-[2,6-dideoxy-3-*C*-methyl-4-*O*-(3-methylbutanoyl)-α-L-*ribo*-hexopyranosyl]-3-(dimethylamino)-β-D-glucopyranosyl]oxy]-5-methoxy-9,16-dimethyl-7-(2-oxoethyl)-10-(propanoyloxy)oxacyclohexadeca-11,13-dien-2-one propionate (leucomycin A3 propionate).

Content:

– minimum 843 Ph. Eur. U./mg (dried substance).

CHARACTERS

Appearance: white or slightly yellowish, crystalline, slightly hygroscopic powder.

Solubility: practically insoluble in water, freely soluble in methanol and in methylene chloride, soluble in acetone.

IDENTIFICATION

First identification: A, B.

Second identification: B, C.

Prepare solutions in methanol immediately before use.

A. Dissolve 0.10 g in *methanol R* and dilute to 100.0 ml with the same solvent. Dilute 1.0 ml of the solution to 50.0 ml with *methanol R*. Examined between 220 nm and 350 nm (*2.2.25*), the solution shows an absorption maximum at 231 nm. The specific absorbance at the absorption maximum is 310 to 350.

B. Thin-layer chromatography (*2.2.27*).

Test solution. Dissolve 10 mg of the substance to be examined in *methanol R* and dilute to 1 ml with the same solvent.

Reference solution (a). Dissolve 10 mg of *josamycin propionate CRS* in *methanol R* and dilute to 1 ml with the same solvent.

Reference solution (b). Dissolve 10 mg of *josamycin CRS* in *methanol R* and dilute to 1 ml with the same solvent.

Reference solution (c). Dissolve 10 mg of *spiramycin CRS* in *methylene chloride R* and dilute to 1 ml with the same solvent.

Reference solution (d). Mix 0.5 ml of reference solution (a) with 0.5 ml of reference solution (b).

Plate: *TLC silica gel G plate R*.

Mobile phase: *methanol R, acetone R, ethyl acetate R, toluene R, hexane R* (8:10:20:25:30 *V/V/V/V/V*).

Application: 10 µl.

Development: over 2/3 of the plate.

Drying: at 100 °C for 10 min.

Detection: spray with *dilute sulphuric acid R* and heat at 100 °C for 10 min.

System suitability: the chromatogram obtained with reference solution (d) shows 2 clearly separated principal spots.

Results: the principal spot in the chromatogram obtained with the test solution is similar in position, colour and size to the principal spot in the chromatogram obtained with reference solution (a) and its position is different from that of the principal spot in the chromatograms obtained with reference solutions (b) and (c).

C. Dissolve about 10 mg in 5 ml of *hydrochloric acid R1* and allow to stand for 10-20 min. A pink colour develops, turning brown.

TESTS

Appearance of solution. The solution is clear (*2.2.1*) and not more intensely coloured than reference solution BY_4 (*2.2.2, Method II*).

Dissolve 1 g in *methanol R* and dilute to 10 ml with the same solvent.

Specific optical rotation (*2.2.7*): − 65 to − 75 (dried substance).

Dissolve 1.000 g in *methanol R* and dilute to 100.0 ml with the same solvent. Allow to stand for 30 min before measuring the angle of rotation.

Related substances. Liquid chromatography (*2.2.29*).

Test solution. Dissolve 50.0 mg of the substance to be examined in *acetonitrile for chromatography R* and dilute to 100.0 ml with the same solvent.

Reference solution (a). Dissolve 50.0 mg of *josamycin propionate CRS* in *acetonitrile for chromatography R* and dilute to 100.0 ml with the same solvent.

Reference solution (b). Dissolve 5 mg of the substance to be examined in 10 ml of *methanol R* and add 40 µl of *dilute phosphoric acid R*. Mix, allow to stand for 5 min and inject.

Reference solution (c). Dilute 2.0 ml of reference solution (a) to 100.0 ml with *acetonitrile for chromatography R*.

Column:

– *size*: *l* = 0.15 m, Ø = 3.9 mm,

– *stationary phase*: *end-capped octadecylsilyl silica gel for chromatography R* (5 µm),

– *temperature*: 30 °C.

Mobile phase: *acetonitrile R*, a 15.4 g/l solution of *ammonium acetate R* previously adjusted to pH 6.0 with *dilute phosphoric acid R* (60:40 *V/V*).

Flow rate: 1.0 ml/min.

Detection: spectrophotometer at 232 nm.

Injection: 20 µl of the test solution and reference solutions (b) and (c).

Run time: 3 times the retention time of leucomycin A3 propionate.

Relative retention with reference to leucomycin A3 propionate (retention time = about 18 min): impurity E = about 0.2; impurity A = about 0.3; impurity B = about 0.5; leucomycin A4 propionate = about 0.7; impurity C = about 1.4; impurity D = about 2.0.

System suitability: reference solution (b):

- *resolution*: minimum 2.0 between the 2 peaks eluting with a relative retention with reference to leucomycin A3 propionate of about 0.5 and 0.7 respectively.

Limits:

- *impurity D*: not more than 1.5 times the area of the principal peak in the chromatogram obtained with reference solution (c),
- *impurities A, B, C, E*: for each impurity, not more than the area of the principal peak in the chromatogram obtained with reference solution (c),
- *any other impurity*: for each impurity, not more than the area of the principal peak in the chromatogram obtained with reference solution (c),
- *total*: not more than 7 times the area of the principal peak in the chromatogram obtained with reference solution (c),
- *disregard limit*: 0.1 times the area of the principal peak in the chromatogram obtained with reference solution (c).

Loss on drying (*2.2.32*): maximum 1.0 per cent, determined on 1.000 g by drying in an oven *in vacuo* at 60 °C for 3 h.

Sulphated ash (*2.4.14*): maximum 0.2 per cent, determined on 1.0 g.

ASSAY

Dissolve 40.0 mg in 20 ml of *methanol R* and dilute to 100.0 ml with *phosphate buffer solution pH 5.6 R*.

Carry out the microbiological assay of antibiotics (*2.7.2*).

STORAGE

In an airtight container.

IMPURITIES

Specified impurities: A, B, C, D, E.

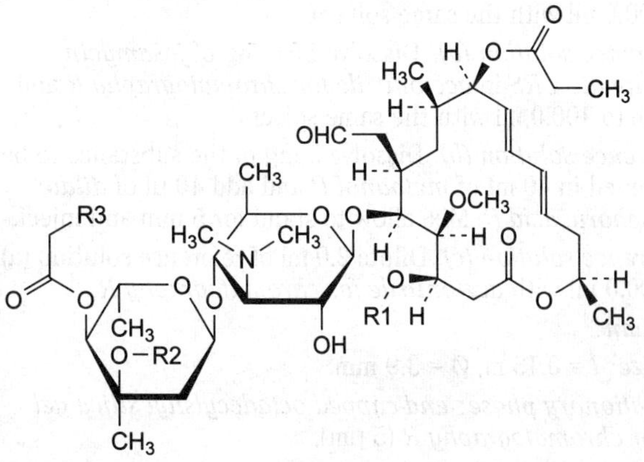

A. R1 = CO-CH_3, R2 = R3 = H: leucomycin A8 9-propionate,

B. R1 = R2 = H, R3 = C_2H_5: leucomycin A5 9-propionate,

C. R1 = CO-C_2H_5, R2 = H, R3 = $CH(CH_3)_2$: platenomycin A1 9-propionate,

D. R1 = CO-CH_3, R2 = CO-C_2H_5, R3 = $CH(CH_3)_2$: leucomycin A3 3″,9-dipropionate,

E. josamycin.

01/2005:1532

JUNIPER

Iuniperi pseudo-fructus

DEFINITION

Juniper consists of the dried ripe cone berry of *Juniperus communis* L. It contains not less than 10 ml/kg of essential oil, calculated with reference to the anhydrous drug.

CHARACTERS

Juniper has a strongly aromatic odour, especially if crushed.

It has the macroscopic and microscopic characters described under identification tests A and B.

IDENTIFICATION

A. The berry-shaped cone is globular up to 10 mm in diameter, violet-brown to blackish-brown, frequently with a bluish bloom. It consists of three fleshy scales. The apex has a three-rayed closed cleft and three not very clearly defined projections. A remnant of peduncle is frequently attached at the base. The fleshy part is crumbly and brownish. It contains three, seldom two, small, elongated, extremely hard seeds that have three sharp edges and are slightly rounded at the back, acuminate at the apex. The seeds are fused with the fleshy part of the cone berry in the lower part on the outside of their bases. Very large, oval oil glands containing sticky resin lie at the outer surface of the seeds.

B. Reduce to a powder (355). The powder is brown. Examine under a microscope, using *chloral hydrate solution R*. The powder shows fragments of epidermis of the cone berry wall containing cells with thick, pitted colourless walls and brown glandular content, occasionally with anomocytic stomata (*2.8.3*); fragments of the three-rayed apical cleft of the cone berry with spaces and epidermal cells interlocked by papillous outgrowths; fragments of the hypodermis with collenchymatous thickened cells; fragments of the mesocarp consisting of large thin-walled parenchymatous cells, usually rounded, with large intercellular spaces and irregular, large, usually scarcely pitted, yellow idioblasts (barrel cells); fragments of schizogenous oil cells; fragments of the testa with thick-walled, pitted colourless sclereids containing one or several prism crystals of calcium oxalate; fragments of the endosperm and embryonic tissue with thin-walled cells containing fatty oil and aleurone grains.

C. Examine by thin-layer chromatography (*2.2.27*), using a *TLC silica gel plate R*.

Test solution. Dilute the oil-xylene mixture obtained in the assay to 5.0 ml with *hexane R*.

Reference solution. Dissolve 4.0 mg of *guaiazulene R* and 50 µl of *cineole R* in 10 ml of *hexane R*.

Apply to the plate as bands 20 µl of the test solution and 10 µl of the reference solution. Develop over a path of 15 cm using a mixture of 5 volumes of *ethyl acetate R* and 95 volumes of *toluene R*. Allow the plate to dry in air. Spray the plate with *anisaldehyde solution R* and examine in daylight while heating at 100 °C to 105 °C for 5 min to 10 min. The chromatogram obtained with the reference solution shows a red zone (guaiazulene) in the upper half and a brownish-violet to greyish-violet zone (cineole) in the lower half. The chromatogram obtained with the test solution shows a strong violet zone (mono- and sesquiterpenes) similar in position to the zone due to guaiazulene in the chromatogram obtained with the reference solution, a reddish-violet zone a little above the zone corresponding to cineole in the chromatogram obtained with the reference solution, a greyish-violet zone (terpinen-4-ol) a little below the zone corresponding to cineole in the chromatogram obtained with the reference solution and just below it a blue zone. A faint violet zone may be present in a similar position to the zone corresponding to cineole. Further zones are present.

TESTS

Foreign matter (*2.8.2*). Not more than 5 per cent of unripe or discoloured cone berries and not more than 2 per cent of other foreign matter.

Water (*2.2.13*). Not more than 120 ml/kg, determined by distillation on 20.0 g of the crushed drug.

Total ash (*2.4.16*). Not more than 4.0 per cent.

ASSAY

Carry out the determination of essential oils in vegetable drugs (*2.8.12*). Use a 500 ml round-bottomed flask, 200 ml of *water R* as the distillation liquid and 0.5 ml of *xylene R* in the graduated tube. Crush the drug and immediately use 20.0 g for the determination. Distil at a rate of 3 ml/min to 4 ml/min for 90 min.

STORAGE

Store protected from light.

01/2005:1832

JUNIPER OIL

Iuniperi aetheroleum

DEFINITION

Essential oil obtained by steam distillation from the ripe, non-fermented berry cones of *Juniperus communis* L. A suitable antioxidant may be added.

CHARACTERS

Appearance: mobile, colourless to yellowish liquid, with a characteristic odour.

IDENTIFICATION

First identification: B.

Second identification: A.

A. Thin-layer chromatography (*2.2.27*).

Test solution. Dissolve 0.2 ml of the substance to be examined in 5 ml of *heptane R*.

Reference solution. Dissolve 20 mg of *α-terpineol R* and 20 μl of *terpinen-4-ol R* in 25 ml of *heptane R*.

Plate: *TLC silica gel plate R.*

Mobile phase: *ethyl acetate R, toluene R* (5:95 *V/V*).

Application: 20 μl, as bands.

Development: over a path of 12 cm.

Drying: in air.

Detection: spray with *anisaldehyde solution R* and heat at 100-105 °C until the zones appear. Examine immediately in daylight.

Results: see below the sequence of the zones present in the chromatograms obtained with the reference solution and the test solution.

Top of the plate	
	An intense brownish-violet zone
	A brown zone
	A violet-pink zone
Terpinen-4-ol: a brownish-violet zone	A brownish-violet zone (terpinen-4-ol)
	A violet zone
α-Terpineol: a violet or brownish-violet zone	A violet or brownish-violet zone (α-terpineol)
Reference solution	**Test solution**

B. Examine the chromatograms obtained in the test for chromatographic profile.

Results: the characteristic peaks in the chromatogram obtained with the test solution are similar in retention time to those in the chromatogram obtained with the reference solution.

TESTS

Relative density (*2.2.5*): 0.857 to 0.876.

Refractive index (*2.2.6*): 1.471 to 1.483.

Optical rotation (*2.2.7*): − 15° to − 0.5°.

Peroxide value (*2.5.5*): maximum 20.

Fatty oils and resinified essential oils (*2.8.7*). It complies with the test for fatty oils and resinified essential oils.

Chromatographic profile. Gas chromatography (*2.2.28*): use the normalisation procedure.

Test solution. Dissolve 60 mg of the substance to be examined in *trimethylpentane R* and dilute to 5.0 ml with the same solvent.

Reference solution. Mix 25 μl each of *α-pinene R, sabinene R, β-pinene R, β-myrcene R, α-phellandrene R, limonene R, terpinen-4-ol R, bornyl acetate R* and *β-caryophyllene R* and dilute to 25.0 ml with *trimethylpentane R*.

Column:

– *material*: fused silica,

– *size*: *l* = 30 m (a film thickness of 1 μm may be used) to 60 m (a film thickness of 0.2 μm may be used), Ø = 0.25-0.53 mm,

– *stationary phase*: *poly(dimethyl)(diphenyl)siloxane R.*

Carrier gas: *helium for chromatography R.*

Flow rate: 2.0 ml/min.

Split ratio: 1:50.

Temperature:

	Time (min)	Temperature (°C)
Column	0 - 1	60
	1 - 58	60→230
Injection port		250
Detector		250

Detection: flame ionisation.

Injection: 0.5 μl.

Elution order: order indicated in the composition of the reference solution. Record the retention times of these substances.

System suitability: reference solution:

– *resolution*: minimum 1.5 between the peaks due to sabinene and β-pinene.

Monographs I-L

Using the retention times determined from the chromatogram obtained with the reference solution, locate the components of the reference solution in the chromatogram obtained with the test solution.

Determine the percentage content of the components. Disregard the peak due to trimethylpentane and peaks comprising less than 0.01 per cent of the total surface area. The percentages are within the following ranges:

- *α-pinene*: 20 per cent to 50 per cent,
- *sabinene*: less than 20 per cent,
- *β-pinene*: 1.0 per cent to 12 per cent
- *β-myrcene*: 1.0 per cent to 35 per cent,
- *α-phellandrene*: less than 1.0 per cent,
- *limonene*: 2.0 per cent to 12 per cent,
- *terpinen-4-ol*: 0.5 per cent to 10 per cent,
- *bornyl acetate*: less than 2.0 per cent,
- *β-caryophyllene*: less than 7.0 per cent.

STORAGE

In a well-filled, airtight container, protected from light, at a temperature not exceeding 25 °C.

LABELLING

The label states the name and concentration of any added antioxidant.

Monographs I-L

K

01/2005:0033

KANAMYCIN ACID SULPHATE

Kanamycini sulfas acidus

DEFINITION

Kanamycin acid sulphate is a form of kanamycin sulphate prepared by adding sulphuric acid to a solution of kanamycin monosulphate and drying by a suitable method. The potency is not less than 670 IU/mg, calculated with reference to the dried substance.

PRODUCTION

It is produced by methods of manufacture designed to eliminate or minimise substances lowering blood pressure. The method of manufacture is validated to demonstrate that the product if tested would comply with the following test:

Abnormal toxicity (*2.6.9*). Inject into each mouse 0.5 ml of a solution containing 2 mg per millilitre of the substance to be examined.

CHARACTERS

A white or almost white powder, hygroscopic, soluble in about 1 part of water, practically insoluble in acetone and in alcohol.

IDENTIFICATION

A. Examine by thin-layer chromatography (*2.2.27*), using a plate coated with a 0.75 mm layer of the following mixture: mix 0.3 g of *carbomer R* with 240 ml of *water R* and allow to stand, with moderate shaking, for 1 h; adjust to pH 7 by the gradual addition, with continuous shaking, of *dilute sodium hydroxide solution R* and add 30 g of *silica gel H R*.

Heat the plate at 110 °C for 1 h, allow to cool and use immediately.

Test solution. Dissolve 10 mg of the substance to be examined in *water R* and dilute to 10 ml with the same solvent.

Reference solution (a). Dissolve 10 mg of *kanamycin monosulphate CRS* in *water R* and dilute to 10 ml with the same solvent.

Reference solution (b). Dissolve 10 mg of *kanamycin monosulphate CRS*, 10 mg of *neomycin sulphate CRS* and 10 mg of *streptomycin sulphate CRS* in *water R* and dilute to 10 ml with the same solvent.

Apply separately to the plate 10 µl of each solution. Develop over a path of 12 cm using a 70 g/l solution of *potassium dihydrogen phosphate R*. Dry the plate in a current of warm air and spray with a mixture of equal volumes of a 2 g/l solution of *dihydroxynaphthalene R* in *alcohol R* and a 460 g/l solution of *sulphuric acid R*. Heat at 150 °C for 5 min to 10 min. The principal spot in the chromatogram obtained with the test solution is similar in position, colour and size to the principal spot in the chromatogram obtained with reference solution (a). The test is not valid unless the chromatogram obtained with reference solution (b) shows 3 clearly separated spots.

B. Dissolve 0.5 g in 10 ml of *water R*. Add 10 ml of *picric acid solution R*. Initiate crystallisation if necessary by scratching the wall of the tube with a glass rod and allow to stand. Collect the crystals, wash with 20 ml of *water R* and filter. Dry at 100 °C. The crystals melt (*2.2.14*) at about 235 °C, with decomposition.

C. Dissolve about 50 mg in 2 ml of *water R*. Add 1 ml of a 10 g/l solution of *ninhydrin R* and heat for a few minutes on a water-bath. A violet colour develops.

D. It gives the reactions of sulphates (*2.3.1*).

TESTS

Solution S. Dissolve 0.20 g in *carbon dioxide-free water R* and dilute to 20.0 ml with the same solvent.

pH (*2.2.3*). The pH of solution S is 5.5 to 7.5.

Specific optical rotation (*2.2.7*). +103 to +115, determined on solution S and calculated with reference to the dried substance.

Kanamycin B. Examine by thin-layer chromatography (*2.2.27*), using a plate prepared as prescribed under identification test A.

Heat the plate at 110 °C for 1 h, allow to cool and use immediately.

Test solution. Dissolve 0.11 g of the substance to be examined in *water R* and dilute to 20 ml with the same solvent.

Reference solution. Dissolve 4 mg of *kanamycin B sulphate CRS* in *water R* and dilute to 20 ml with the same solvent.

Apply separately to the plate 4 µl of each solution. Develop over a path of 12 cm using a 70 g/l solution of *potassium dihydrogen phosphate R*. Dry the plate in a current of warm air and spray with *ninhydrin and stannous chloride reagent R*. Heat the plate at 110 °C for 15 min. Any spot corresponding to kanamycin B in the chromatogram obtained with the test solution is not more intense than the spot in the chromatogram obtained with the reference solution (4.0 per cent).

Loss on drying (*2.2.32*). Not more than 5.0 per cent, determined on 1.00 g by drying at 60 °C at a pressure not exceeding 670 Pa for 3 h.

Sulphated ash (*2.4.14*). Not more than 0.5 per cent, determined on 1.0 g.

Sulphate. 23.0 per cent to 26.0 per cent of sulphate (SO_4), calculated with reference to the dried substance. Dissolve 0.175 g in 100 ml of *water R* and adjust the solution to pH 11 using *concentrated ammonia R*. Add 10.0 ml of *0.1 M barium chloride* and about 0.5 mg of *phthalein purple R*. Titrate with *0.1 M sodium edetate* adding 50 ml of *alcohol R* when the colour of the solution begins to change and continue the titration until the violet-blue colour disappears.

1 ml of *0.1 M barium chloride* is equivalent to 9.606 mg of sulphate (SO_4).

Pyrogens (*2.6.8*). If intended for use in the manufacture of parenteral dosage forms without a further appropriate procedure for the removal of pyrogens, it complies with the test for pyrogens. Inject per kilogram of the rabbit's mass 1 ml of a solution in *water for injections R* containing 10 mg per millilitre of the substance to be examined.

ASSAY

Carry out the microbiological assay of antibiotics (*2.7.2*). Use *kanamycin monosulphate CRS* as the reference substance.

STORAGE

If the substance is sterile, store in a sterile, tamper-proof container.

LABELLING

The label states, where applicable, that the substance is apyrogenic.

Monographs I-L

01/2005:0032

KANAMYCIN MONOSULPHATE

Kanamycini monosulfas

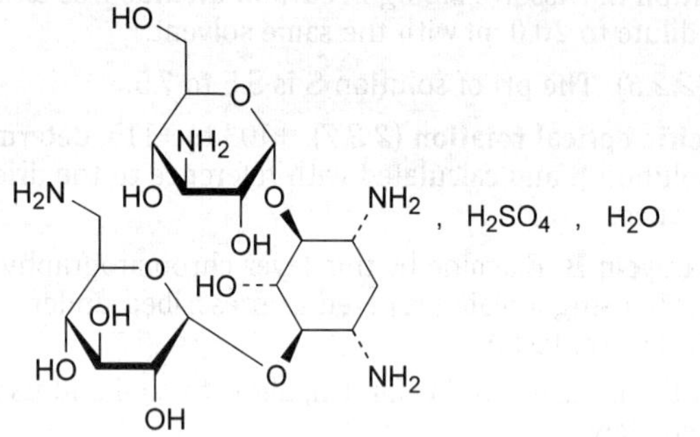

$C_{18}H_{38}N_4O_{15}S,H_2O$ M_r 601

DEFINITION

Kanamycin monosulphate is 6-*O*-(3-amino-3-deoxy-α-D-glucopyranosyl)-4-*O*-(6-amino-6-deoxy-α-D-glucopyranosyl)-2-deoxy-D-streptamine sulphate, an antimicrobial substance produced by the growth of certain strains of *Streptomyces kanamyceticus*. The potency is not less than 750 IU/mg, calculated with reference to the dried substance.

PRODUCTION

It is produced by methods of manufacture designed to eliminate or minimise substances lowering blood pressure. The method of manufacture is validated to demonstrate that the product if tested would comply with the following test:

Abnormal toxicity (*2.6.9*). Inject into each mouse 0.5 ml of a solution containing 2 mg per millilitre of the substance to be examined.

CHARACTERS

A white or almost white, crystalline powder, soluble in about 8 parts of water, practically insoluble in acetone and in alcohol.

IDENTIFICATION

A. Examine by thin-layer chromatography (*2.2.27*), using a plate coated with a 0.75 mm layer of the following mixture: mix 0.3 g of *carbomer R* with 240 ml of *water R* and allow to stand, with moderate shaking, for 1 h; adjust to pH 7 by the gradual addition, with continuous shaking, of *dilute sodium hydroxide solution R* and add 30 g of *silica gel H R*.

Heat the plate at 110 °C for 1 h, allow to cool and use immediately.

Test solution. Dissolve 10 mg of the substance to be examined in *water R* and dilute to 10 ml with the same solvent.

Reference solution (a). Dissolve 10 mg of *kanamycin monosulphate CRS* in *water R* and dilute to 10 ml with the same solvent.

Reference solution (b). Dissolve 10 mg of *kanamycin monosulphate CRS*, 10 mg of *neomycin sulphate CRS* and 10 mg of *streptomycin sulphate CRS* in *water R* and dilute to 10 ml with the same solvent.

Apply separately to the plate 10 µl of each solution. Develop over a path of 12 cm using a 70 g/l solution of *potassium dihydrogen phosphate R*. Dry the plate in a current of warm air and spray with a mixture of equal volumes of a 2 g/l solution of *dihydroxynaphthalene R* in *alcohol R* and a 460 g/l solution of *sulphuric acid R*. Heat at 150 °C for 5 min to 10 min. The principal spot in the chromatogram obtained with the test solution is similar in position, colour and size to the principal spot in the chromatogram obtained with reference solution (a). The test is not valid unless the chromatogram obtained with reference solution (b) shows three clearly separated spots.

B. Dissolve 0.5 g in 10 ml of *water R*. Add 10 ml of *picric acid solution R*. Initiate crystallisation if necessary by scratching the wall of the tube with a glass rod and allow to stand. Collect the crystals, wash with 20 ml of *water R* and filter. Dry at 100 °C. The crystals melt (*2.2.14*) at about 235 °C, with decomposition.

C. Dissolve about 50 mg in 2 ml of *water R*. Add 1 ml of a 10 g/l solution of *ninhydrin R* and heat for a few minutes on a water-bath. A violet colour develops.

D. It gives the reactions of sulphates (*2.3.1*).

TESTS

Solution S. Dissolve 0.20 g in *carbon dioxide-free water R* and dilute to 20.0 ml with the same solvent.

pH (*2.2.3*). The pH of solution S is 6.5 to 8.5.

Specific optical rotation (*2.2.7*). +112 to +123, determined on solution S and calculated with reference to the dried substance.

Kanamycin B. Examine by thin-layer chromatography (*2.2.27*), using a plate prepared as prescribed under identification test A. Heat the plate at 110 °C for 1 h, allow to cool and use immediately.

Test solution. Dissolve 0.1 g of the substance to be examined in *water R* and dilute to 20 ml with the same solvent.

Reference solution. Dissolve 4 mg of *kanamycin B sulphate CRS* in *water R* and dilute to 20 ml with the same solvent.

Apply separately to the plate 4 µl of each solution. Develop over a path of 12 cm using a 70 g/l solution of *potassium dihydrogen phosphate R*. Dry the plate in a current of warm air and spray with *ninhydrin and stannous chloride reagent R*. Heat the plate at 110 °C for 15 min. Any spot corresponding to kanamycin B in the chromatogram obtained with the test solution is not more intense than the spot in the chromatogram obtained with the reference solution.

Loss on drying (*2.2.32*). Not more than 1.5 per cent, determined on 1.00 g by drying at 60 °C at a pressure not exceeding 670 Pa for 3 h.

Sulphated ash (*2.4.14*). Not more than 0.5 per cent, determined on 1.0 g.

Sulphate. 15.0 per cent to 17.0 per cent of sulphate (SO_4), calculated with reference to the dried substance. Dissolve 0.250 g in 100 ml of *water R* and adjust the solution to pH 11 using *concentrated ammonia R*. Add 10.0 ml of *0.1 M barium chloride* and about 0.5 mg of *phthalein purple R*. Titrate with *0.1 M sodium edetate* adding 50 ml of *alcohol R* when the colour of the solution begins to change and continue the titration until the violet-blue colour disappears.

1 ml of *0.1 M barium chloride* is equivalent to 9.606 mg of sulphate (SO_4).

Pyrogens (*2.6.8*). If intended for use in the manufacture of parenteral dosage forms without a further appropriate procedure for the removal of pyrogens, it complies with the test for pyrogens. Inject per kilogram of the rabbit's mass 1 ml of a solution in *water for injections R* containing 10 mg per millilitre of the substance to be examined.

ASSAY

Carry out the microbiological assay of antibiotics (*2.7.2*).

STORAGE

If the substance is sterile, store in a sterile, tamper-proof container.

LABELLING

The label states, where applicable, that the substance is apyrogenic.

01/2005:0503

KAOLIN, HEAVY

Kaolinum ponderosum

DEFINITION

Heavy kaolin is a purified, natural, hydrated aluminium silicate of variable composition.

CHARACTERS

A fine, white or greyish-white, unctuous powder, practically insoluble in water and in organic solvents.

IDENTIFICATION

A. To 0.5 g in a metal crucible add 1 g of *potassium nitrate R* and 3 g of *sodium carbonate R* and heat until the mixture melts. Allow to cool. To the residue add 20 ml of boiling *water R*, mix and filter. Wash the residue with 50 ml of *water R*. To the residue add 1 ml of *hydrochloric acid R* and 5 ml of *water R*. Filter. To the filtrate add 1 ml of *strong sodium hydroxide solution R* and filter. To the filtrate add 3 ml of *ammonium chloride solution R*. A gelatinous white precipitate is formed.

B. Add 2.0 g in twenty portions to 100 ml of a 10 g/l solution of *sodium laurilsulfate R* in a 100 ml graduated cylinder about 30 mm in diameter. Allow 2 min between additions for each portion to settle. Allow to stand for 2 h. The apparent volume of the sediment is not greater than 5 ml.

C. 0.25 g gives the reaction of silicates (*2.3.1*).

TESTS

Solution S. To 4 g add a mixture of 6 ml of *acetic acid R* and 34 ml of *distilled water R*, shake for 1 min and filter.

Acidity or alkalinity. To 1.0 g add 20 ml of *carbon dioxide-free water R*, shake for 2 min and filter. To 10 ml of the filtrate add 0.1 ml of *phenolphthalein solution R*. The solution is colourless. Not more than 0.25 ml of *0.01 M sodium hydroxide* is required to change the colour of the indicator to pink.

Organic impurities. Heat 0.3 g to redness in a calcination tube. The residue is only slightly more coloured than the original substance.

Adsorption power. To 1.0 g in a ground-glass-stoppered test-tube add 10.0 ml of a 3.7 g/l solution of *methylene blue R* and shake for 2 min. Allow to settle. Centrifuge and dilute the solution 1 in 100 with *water R*. The solution is not more intensely coloured than a 0.03 g/l solution of *methylene blue R*.

Swelling power. Triturate 2 g with 2 ml of *water R*. The mixture does not flow.

Substances soluble in mineral acids. To 5.0 g add 7.5 ml of *dilute hydrochloric acid R* and 27.5 ml of *water R* and boil for 5 min. Filter, wash the residue on the filter with *water R* and dilute the combined filtrate and washings to 50.0 ml with *water R*. To 10.0 ml of the solution add 1.5 ml of *dilute sulphuric acid R*, evaporate to dryness on a water-bath and ignite. The residue weighs not more than 10 mg (1 per cent).

Chlorides (*2.4.4*). 2 ml of solution S diluted to 15 ml with *water R* complies with the limit test for chlorides (250 ppm).

Sulphates (*2.4.13*). 1.5 ml of solution S diluted to 15 ml with *distilled water R* complies with the limit test for sulphates (0.1 per cent).

Calcium (*2.4.3*). 4 ml of solution S diluted to 15 ml with *distilled water R* complies with the limit test for calcium (250 ppm).

Heavy metals (*2.4.8*). To 5 ml of the solution prepared for the test for substances soluble in mineral acids add 5 ml of *water R*, 10 ml of *hydrochloric acid R* and 25 ml of *methyl isobutyl ketone R*. Shake for 2 min. Separate the layers. Evaporate the aqueous layer to dryness on a water-bath. Dissolve the residue in 1 ml of *acetic acid R* and dilute to 25 ml with *water R*. Filter. 12 ml of the solution complies with limit test A for heavy metals (50 ppm) Prepare the standard using *lead standard solution (1 ppm Pb) R*.

Heavy kaolin intended for internal use complies with the requirements of the monograph modified as shown below for the test for heavy metals.

Heavy metals (*2.4.8*). To 10 ml of the solution prepared for the test for substances soluble in mineral acids add 10 ml of *water R*, 20 ml of *hydrochloric acid R* and 25 ml of *methyl isobutyl ketone R*. Shake for 2 min. Separate the layers. Evaporate the aqueous layer to dryness on a water-bath. Dissolve the residue in 1 ml of *acetic acid R* and dilute to 25 ml with *water R*. Filter. 12 ml of the solution complies with limit test A for heavy metals (25 ppm). Prepare the standard using *lead standard solution (1 ppm Pb) R*.

Microbial contamination. Total viable aerobic count (*2.6.12*) not more than 10^3 micro-organisms per gram, determined by plate-count.

LABELLING

The label states, where applicable, that the substance is suitable for internal use.

01/2005:1426

KELP

Fucus vel Ascophyllum

DEFINITION

Fragmented dried thallus of *Fucus vesiculosus* L. or *F. serratus* L. or *Ascophyllum nodosum* Le Jolis.

Content: minimum 0.03 per cent and maximum 0.2 per cent of total iodine (A_r 126.9) (dried drug).

CHARACTERS

Salty and mucilaginous taste, unpleasant marine odour.

Macroscopic and microscopic characters described under identification tests A and B.

IDENTIFICATION

A. The drug consists of fragments with a corneous consistency, blackish-brown to greenish-brown, sometimes covered with whitish efflorescence. The thallus consists of a ribbon-like blade, branching dichotomously with prominent central ribs (pseudoveins). *F. vesiculosus* typically shows a foliose blade with smooth edges and bears occasional ovoid, single or paired, air vesicles. The ends of certain branches are of ovoid shape and a little widened. They bear numerous reproductive organs (conceptacles). *F. serratus* has a foliose blade with a serrate margin and no vesicles, the branches bearing conceptacles are less swollen. The thallus of *A. nodosum* is irregularly branched, without pseudo-midrib. It shows single ovoid air vesicles; the falciform conceptacles are located at the end of small branches.

B. Reduce to a powder (355). The powder is greenish-brown. Examine under a microscope using *chloral hydrate solution R*. The powder shows fragments of surface tissue with regular isodiametric cells with brown contents, and fragments of deep tissue with colourless, elongated cells arranged in long filaments with large mucilaginous spaces between them. Thick-walled cells in files and in closely packed groups, from the pseudovein, are sometimes visible.

C. To 1 g of the powdered drug (355) add 20 ml of a 2 per cent *V/V* solution of *hydrochloric acid R*. Shake vigorously and filter. Wash the residue with 10 ml of *water R* and filter. To the residue add 10 ml of a 200 g/l solution of *sodium carbonate R*. Shake and centrifuge. Collect the supernatant liquid. Adjust to pH 1.5 using *sulphuric acid R*. A white, flocculent precipitate is slowly formed.

TESTS

Foreign matter (*2.8.2*): maximum 2 per cent *m/m*.

Arsenic (*2.4.27*) : maximum 90 ppm.

Cadmium (*2.4.27*) : maximum 4 ppm.

Lead (*2.4.27*) : maximum 5 ppm.

Mercury (*2.4.27*) : maximum 0.1 ppm.

Swelling index (*2.8.4*): minimum 6.

Loss on drying (*2.2.32*): maximum 15.0 per cent, determined on 1.000 g by drying in an oven at 100-105 °C, for 2 h.

Total ash (*2.4.16*): maximum 24 per cent.

Ash insoluble in hydrochloric acid (*2.8.1*): maximum 3.0 per cent.

ASSAY

TOTAL IODINE. To 1.000 g of the powdered drug, in a tall silica crucible, add 5 ml of *water R* and 5 g of *potassium hydroxide R*. Stir with a magnesium rod. Heat on a water bath. Add 1 g of *potassium carbonate R*. Mix, add the tip of the magnesium rod with the residues of the drug and dry, first on a water-bath then over an open flame. Incinerate raising the temperature progressively to not more than 600 °C. Allow to cool. Add 20 ml of *water R* and heat gently to boiling, stirring with a glass rod. Filter the hot mixture through an unpleated filter, into a conical flask. Rinse the residue with 4 quantities, each of 20 ml, of hot *water R*. Rinse the filter and the crucible with 50 ml of hot *water R*. Combine the solutions. Allow to cool. Neutralise with *dilute sulphuric acid R* in the presence of *methyl orange solution R*. Add 3 ml of *dilute sulphuric acid R* and 1 ml of *bromine water R*. The solution is yellow. After 5 min add 0.6 ml of a 50 g/l solution of *phenol R*. The solution is clear. Acidify with 5 ml of *phosphoric acid R* and add 0.2 g of *potassium iodide R*. Allow to stand for 5 min protected from light. Add 1 ml of *starch solution R* and titrate with *0.01 M sodium thiosulphate*.

1 ml of *0.01 M sodium thiosulphate* is equivalent to 0.2115 mg of iodine.

LABELLING

The label states the species of kelp present.

01/2005:1020

KETAMINE HYDROCHLORIDE

Ketamini hydrochloridum

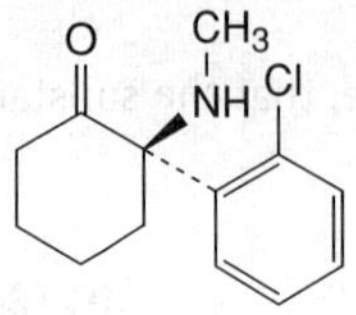

and enantiomer , HCl

$C_{13}H_{17}Cl_2NO$ M_r 274.2

DEFINITION

(*RS*)-2-(2-Chlorophenyl)-2-(methylamino)cyclohexanone hydrochloride.

Content: 99.0 per cent to 101.0 per cent.

CHARACTERS

Appearance: white, crystalline powder.

Solubility: freely soluble in water and in methanol, soluble in alcohol.

mp: about 260 °C, with decomposition.

IDENTIFICATION

A. Optical rotation (see Tests).

B. Infrared absorption spectrophotometry (*2.2.24*).

Comparison: *Ph. Eur. reference spectrum of ketamine hydrochloride*.

C. It gives reaction (a) of chlorides (*2.3.1*).

TESTS

Solution S. Dissolve 5.0 g in *carbon dioxide-free water R* and dilute to 25.0 ml with the same solvent.

Appearance of solution. Solution S is clear (*2.2.1*) and colourless (*2.2.2, Method II*).

pH (*2.2.3*): 3.5 to 4.1

Dilute 10 ml of solution S to 20 ml with *carbon dioxide-free water R*.

Optical rotation (*2.2.7*): −0.2° to + 0.2°.

Dilute 2.5 ml of solution S to 25.0 ml with *water R*.

Related substances. Liquid chromatography (*2.2.29*).

Test solution. Dissolve 50.0 mg of the substance to be examined in the mobile phase and dilute to 50.0 ml with the mobile phase.

Reference solution (a). Dissolve 25.0 mg of *ketamine impurity A CRS* in the mobile phase and dilute to 50.0 ml with the mobile phase (using ultrasound, if necessary). To 1.0 ml of the solution, add 0.5 ml of the test solution and dilute to 100.0 ml with the mobile phase. Prepare immediately before use.

Reference solution (b). Dilute 1.0 ml of the test solution to 10.0 ml with the mobile phase. Dilute 1.0 ml of the solution to 20.0 ml with the mobile phase.

Precolumn:

- *size*: *l* = 4 mm, Ø = 4.0 mm,
- *stationary phase*: spherical *octadecylsilyl silica gel for chromatography R* (5 µm).

Column:

- *size*: *l* = 0.125 m, Ø = 4.0 mm,
- *stationary phase*: spherical *octadecylsilyl silica gel for chromatography R* (5 µm).

Mobile phase: dissolve 0.95 g of *sodium hexanesulphonate R* in 1 litre of a mixture of 25 volumes of *acetonitrile R* and 75 volumes of *water R* and add 4 ml of *acetic acid R*.

Flow rate: 1.0 ml/min.

Detection: spectrophotometer at 215 nm.

Injection: 20 µl.

Run time: 10 times the retention time of ketamine.

System suitability: reference solution (a):

- *retention time*: ketamine = 3 min to 4.5 min,
- *resolution*: minimum of 1.5 between the peaks due to impurity A and to ketamine.

Limits:

- *total*: not more than the area of the principal peak in the chromatogram obtained with reference solution (b) (0.5 per cent),
- *disregard limit*: 0.2 times the area of the principal peak in the chromatogram obtained with reference solution (b) (0.1 per cent).

Heavy metals (*2.4.8*): maximum 20 ppm.

Dilute 10 ml of solution S to 20 ml with *water R*. 12 ml of the solution complies with limit test A. Prepare the standard using *lead standard solution (2 ppm Pb) R*.

Sulphated ash (*2.4.14*): maximum 0.1 per cent, determined on 1.0 g.

ASSAY

Dissolve 0.200 g in 50 ml of *methanol R* and add 1.0 ml of *0.1 M hydrochloric acid*. Carry out a potentiometric titration (*2.2.20*), using *0.1 M sodium hydroxide*. Read the volume added between the 2 points of inflexion.

1 ml of *0.1 M sodium hydroxide* is equivalent to 27.42 mg of $C_{13}H_{17}Cl_2NO$.

STORAGE

Protected from light.

IMPURITIES

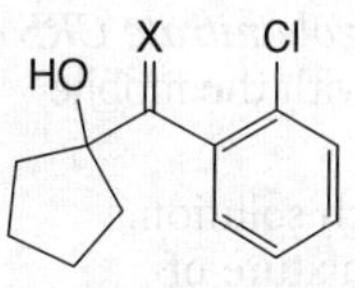

A. X = N-CH_3: 1-[(2-chlorophenyl)(methylimino)methyl]cyclopentanol,

C. X = O: (2-chlorophenyl)(1-hydroxycyclopentyl)methanone,

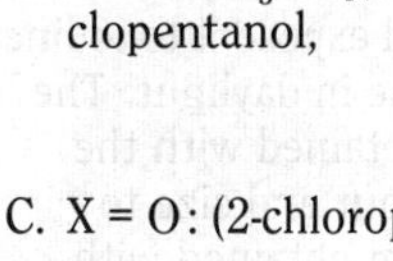

and enantiomer

B. (2*RS*)-2-(2-chlorophenyl)-2-hydroxycyclohexanone.

01/2005:1746

KETOBEMIDONE HYDROCHLORIDE

Cetobemidoni hydrochloridum

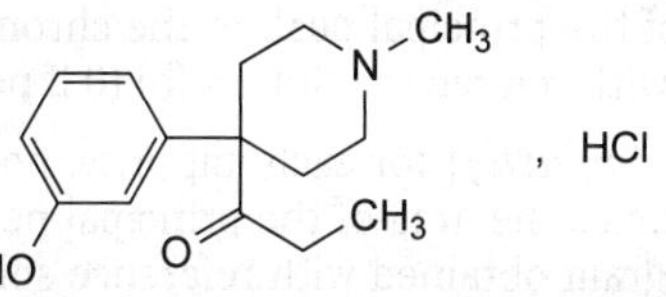

$C_{15}H_{22}ClNO_2$ M_r 283.8

DEFINITION

1-[4-(3-Hydroxyphenyl)-1-methylpiperidin-4-yl]propan-1-one hydrochloride.

Content: 99.0 per cent to 101.0 per cent (anhydrous substance).

CHARACTERS

Appearance: white or almost white, crystalline powder.

Solubility: freely soluble in water, soluble in alcohol, very slightly soluble in methylene chloride.

IDENTIFICATION

A. Infrared absorption spectrophotometry (*2.2.24*).

Comparison: *Ph. Eur. reference spectrum of ketobemidone hydrochloride*.

B. Solution S (see Tests) gives reaction (a) of chlorides (*2.3.1*).

TESTS

Solution S. Dissolve 0.250 g in *carbon dioxide-free water R* and dilute to 25.0 ml with the same solvent.

Appearance of solution. Solution S is clear (*2.2.1*) and not more intensely coloured than reference solution B_8 (*2.2.2, Method II*).

pH (*2.2.3*): 4.5 to 5.5 for solution S.

Related substances. Liquid chromatography (*2.2.29*).

Solution A: 1.54 g/l solution of *ammonium acetate R* adjusted to pH 8.0 with *dilute ammonia R1*.

Test solution. Dissolve 50.0 mg of the substance to be examined in solution A and dilute to 25.0 ml with the same solution.

Reference solution (a). Dissolve 1 mg of *ketobemidone impurity B CRS* and 1 mg of *ketobemidone impurity C CRS* in solution A and dilute to 25 ml with the same solution.

Reference solution (b). Dilute 1.0 ml of the test solution to 100.0 ml with solution A. Dilute 20.0 ml of this solution to 100.0 ml with solution A.

Column:

- *size*: *l* = 0.25 m, Ø = 4.6 mm,
- *stationary phase*: *phenylhexylsilyl silica gel for chromatography R* (5 µm),
- *temperature*: 40 °C.

Mobile phase: *acetonitrile R*, solution A (20:80 *V/V*).

Flow rate: 1.5 ml/min.

Detection: spectrophotometer at 278 nm.

Injection: 20 µl.

Run time: 4.5 times the retention time of ketobemidone.

Relative retention with reference to ketobemidone (retention time = about 10 min): impurity A = about 0.4; impurity B = about 0.6; impurity C = about 0.7; impurity D = about 3.5; impurity E = about 4.2.

System suitability: reference solution (a):

- *resolution*: minimum 4.0 between the peaks due to impurity B and impurity C.

Limits:

- *impurities A, B, C, D*: for each impurity, not more than the area of the principal peak in the chromatogram obtained with reference solution (b) (0.2 per cent),
- *any other impurity*: for each impurity, not more than 0.5 times the area of the principal peak in the chromatogram obtained with reference solution (b) (0.1 per cent),
- *total*: not more than 3.5 times the area of the principal peak in the chromatogram obtained with reference solution (b) (0.7 per cent),
- *disregard limit*: 0.25 times the area of the principal peak in the chromatogram obtained with reference solution (b) (0.05 per cent).

Water (*2.5.12*): maximum 1.0 per cent, determined on 0.50 g.

Sulphated ash (*2.4.14*): maximum 0.1 per cent, determined on 1.0 g.

ASSAY

Dissolve 0.200 g in a mixture of 5.0 ml of *0.01 M hydrochloric acid* and 50 ml of *alcohol R*. Carry out a potentiometric titration (*2.2.20*) using *0.1 M sodium hydroxide*. Read the volume added between the 2 points of inflexion.

1 ml of *0.1 M sodium hydroxide* is equivalent to 28.38 mg of $C_{15}H_{22}ClNO_2$.

IMPURITIES

Specified impurities: A, B, C, D.

Other detectable impurities: E.

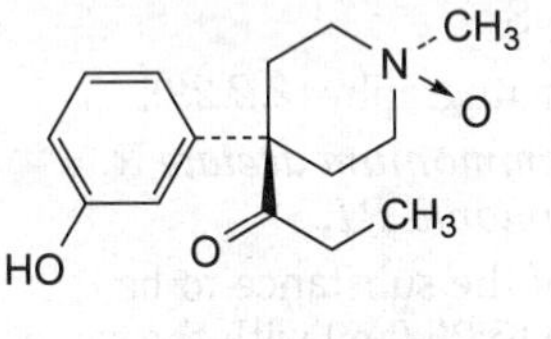

and *trans* isomer

A. 1-[4-(3-hydroxyphenyl)-1-methyl-1-oxidopiperidin-4-yl]propan-1-one (*cis* and *trans* isomers),

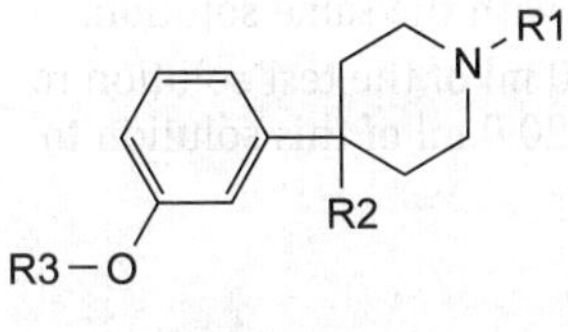

B. R1 = CH_3, R2 = CO-CH_3, R3 = H: 1-[4-(3-hydroxyphenyl)-1-methylpiperidin-4-yl]ethanone,

C. R1 = R3 = H, R2 = CO-CH_2-CH_3: 1-[4-(3-hydroxyphenyl)piperidin-4-yl]propan-1-one,

D. R1 = R3 = CH_3, R2 = CO-CH_2-CH_3: 1-[4-(3-methoxyphenyl)-1-methylpiperidin-4-yl]propan-1-one,

E. R1 = CH_3, R2 = CN, R3 = H: 4-(3-hydroxyphenyl)-1-methylpiperidine-4-carbonitrile.

01/2005:0921

KETOCONAZOLE

Ketoconazolum

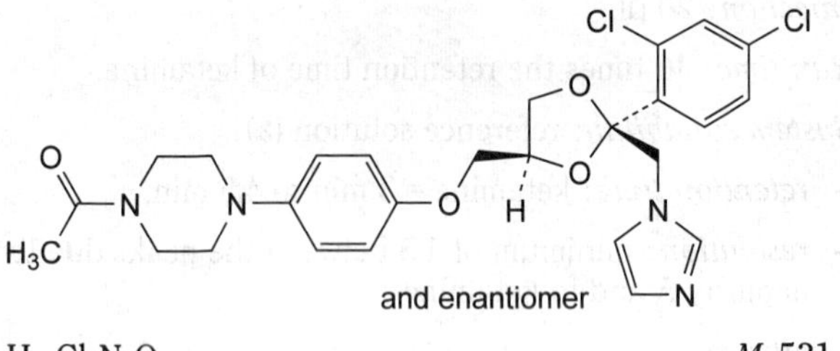

$C_{26}H_{28}Cl_2N_4O_4$ M_r 531.4

DEFINITION

Ketoconazole contains not less than 99.0 per cent and not more than the equivalent of 101.0 per cent of 1-acetyl-4-[4-[[(2*RS*,4*SR*)-2-(2,4-dichlorophenyl)-2-(1*H*-imidazol-1-ylmethyl)-1,3-dioxolan-4-yl]methoxy]phenyl]piperazine, calculated with reference to the dried substance.

CHARACTERS

A white or almost white powder, practically insoluble in water, freely soluble in methylene chloride, soluble in methanol, sparingly soluble in alcohol.

IDENTIFICATION

First identification: B.

Second identification: A, C, D.

A. Melting point (*2.2.14*): 148 °C to 152 °C.

B. Examine by infrared absorption spectrophotometry (*2.2.24*), comparing with the spectrum obtained with *ketoconazole CRS*. Examine the substances prepared as discs.

C. Examine by thin-layer chromatography (*2.2.27*), using a suitable octadecylsilyl silica gel as the coating substance.

Test solution. Dissolve 30 mg of the substance to be examined in the mobile phase and dilute to 5 ml with the mobile phase.

Reference solution (a). Dissolve 30 mg of *ketoconazole CRS* in the mobile phase and dilute to 5 ml with the mobile phase.

Reference solution (b). Dissolve 30 mg of *ketoconazole CRS* and 30 mg of *econazole nitrate CRS* in the mobile phase and dilute to 5 ml with the mobile phase.

Apply separately to the plate 5 µl of each solution. Develop over a path of 15 cm using a mixture of 20 volumes of *ammonium acetate solution R*, 40 volumes of *dioxan R* and 40 volumes of *methanol R*. Dry the plate in a current of warm air for 15 min and expose it to iodine vapour until the spots appear. Examine in daylight. The principal spot in the chromatogram obtained with the test solution is similar in position, colour and size to the principal spot in the chromatogram obtained with reference solution (a). The test is not valid unless the chromatogram obtained with reference solution (b) shows two clearly separated spots.

D. To about 30 mg in a porcelain crucible add 0.3 g of *anhydrous sodium carbonate R*. Heat over an open flame for 10 min. Allow to cool. Take up the residue with 5 ml of *dilute nitric acid R* and filter. To 1 ml of the filtrate add 1 ml of *water R*. The solution gives reaction (a) of chlorides (*2.3.1*).

TESTS

Solution S. Dissolve 1.0 g in *methylene chloride R* and dilute to 10 ml with the same solvent.

Appearance of solution. Solution S is clear (*2.2.1*) and not more intensely coloured than reference solution BY_4 (*2.2.2, Method II*).

Optical rotation (*2.2.7*). The angle of optical rotation, determined on solution S, is − 0.10° to + 0.10°.

Related substances. Examine by liquid chromatography (*2.2.29*).

Test solution. Dissolve 0.100 g of the substance to be examined in *methanol R* and dilute to 10.0 ml with the same solvent.

Reference solution (a). Dissolve 2.5 mg of *ketoconazole CRS* and 2.5 mg of *loperamide hydrochloride CRS* in *methanol R* and dilute to 50.0 ml with the same solvent.

Reference solution (b). Dilute 5.0 ml of the test solution to 100.0 ml with *methanol R*. Dilute 1.0 ml of this solution to 10.0 ml with *methanol R*.

The chromatographic procedure may be carried out using:

– a stainless steel column 0.10 m long and 4.6 mm in internal diameter packed with *octadecylsilyl silica gel for chromatography R* (3 µm),
– as mobile phase at a flow rate of 2 ml/min a mixture of 0.5 volumes of *acetonitrile R* and 9.5 volumes of a 3.4 g/l solution of *tetrabutylammonium hydrogen sulphate R* changing by linear-gradient elution to a mixture of 5 volumes of *acetonitrile R* and 5 volumes of a 3.4 g/l solution of *tetrabutylammonium hydrogen sulphate R* over 10 min, followed by the final elution mixture for 5 min,
– as detector a spectrophotometer set at 220 nm.

Equilibrate the column for at least 30 min with *acetonitrile R* and then equilibrate at the initial elution composition for at least 5 min.

Adjust the sensitivity of the system so that the height of the principal peak in the chromatogram obtained with 10 µl of reference solution (b) is at least 50 per cent of the full scale of the recorder.

Inject 10 µl of reference solution (a). When the chromatograms are recorded in the prescribed conditions, the retention times are: ketoconazole about 6 min and loperamide hydrochloride about 8 min. The test is not valid unless the resolution between the peaks corresponding to ketoconazole and loperamide hydrochloride is at least 15. If necessary, adjust the final concentration of acetonitrile in the mobile phase or adjust the time programme for the linear-gradient elution.

Inject separately 10 µl of *methanol R* as a blank, 10 µl of the test solution and 10 µl of reference solution (b). In the chromatogram obtained with the test solution, the sum of the areas of all peaks, apart from the principal peak, is not greater than the area of the principal peak in the chromatogram obtained with reference solution (b) (0.5 per cent). Disregard any peak obtained with the blank and any peak with an area less than 0.1 times that of the principal peak in the chromatogram obtained with reference solution (b).

Heavy metals (*2.4.8*). 1.0 g complies with limit test D for heavy metals (20 ppm). Prepare the standard using 2 ml of *lead standard solution (10 ppm Pb) R*.

Loss on drying (*2.2.32*). Not more than 0.5 per cent, determined on 1.000 g by drying in an oven at 100 °C to 105 °C.

Sulphated ash (*2.4.14*). Not more than 0.1 per cent, determined on 1.0 g.

ASSAY

Dissolve 0.200 g in 70 ml of a mixture of 1 volume of *anhydrous acetic acid R* and 7 volumes of *methyl ethyl ketone R*. Titrate with *0.1 M perchloric acid*, determining the end-point potentiometrically (*2.2.20*).

1 ml of *0.1 M perchloric acid* is equivalent to 26.57 mg of $C_{26}H_{28}Cl_2N_4O_4$.

STORAGE

Store protected from light.

IMPURITIES

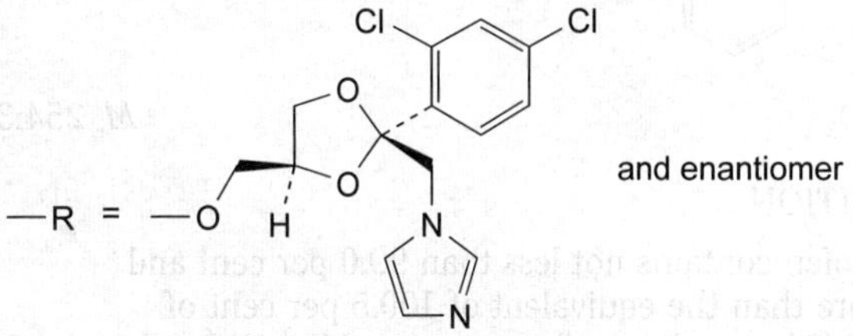

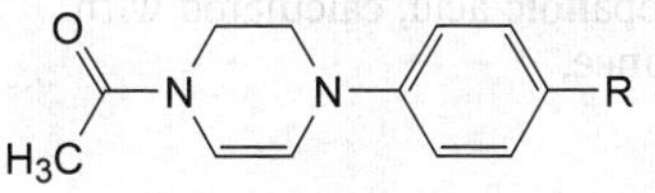

A. 1-acetyl-4-[4-[[(2*RS*,4*SR*)-2-(2,4-dichlorophenyl)-2-(1*H*-imidazol-1-ylmethyl)-1,3-dioxolan-4-yl]methoxy]phenyl]1, 2,3,4-tetrahydropyrazine,

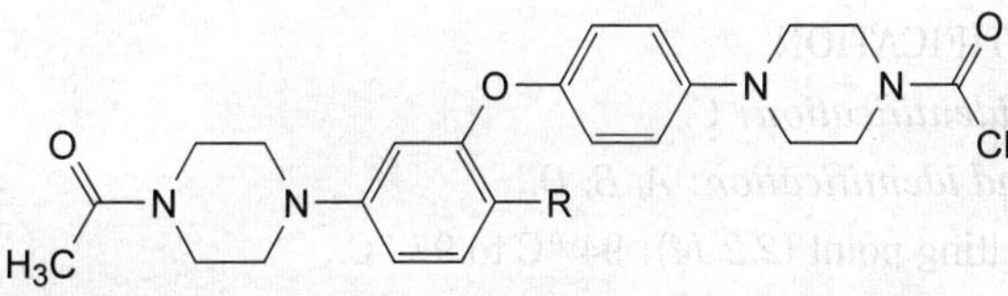

B. 1-acetyl-4-[4-[[(2*RS*,4*SR*)-2-(2,4-dichlorophenyl)-2-(1*H*-imidazol-1-ylmethyl)-1,3-dioxolan-4-yl]methoxy]-3-[4-(4-acetylpiperazin-1-yl)phenoxy]phenyl]piperazine,

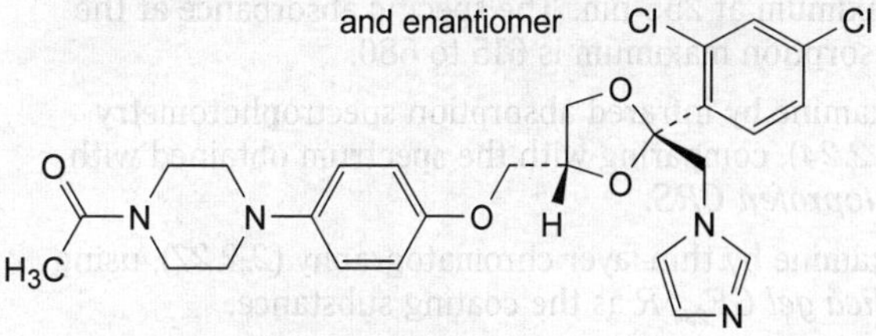

C. 1-acetyl-4-[4-[[(2*RS*,4*RS*)-2-(2,4-dichlorophenyl)-2-(1*H*-imidazol-1-ylmethyl)-1,3-dioxolan-4-yl]methoxy]phenyl]piperazine,

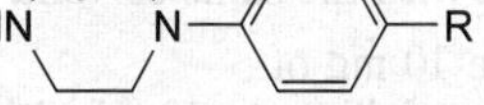

D. 1-[4-[[(2*RS*,4*SR*)-2-(2,4-dichlorophenyl)-2-(1*H*-imidazol-1-ylmethyl)-1,3-dioxolan-4-yl]methoxy]phenyl]piperazine.

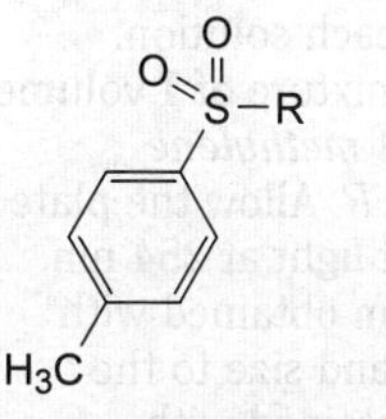

E. [(2*RS*,4*SR*)-2-(2,4-dichlorophenyl)-2-(1*H*-imidazol-1-ylmethyl)-1,3-dioxolan-4-yl]methyl 4-methylbenzenesulphonate.

01/2005:0922

KETOPROFEN

Ketoprofenum

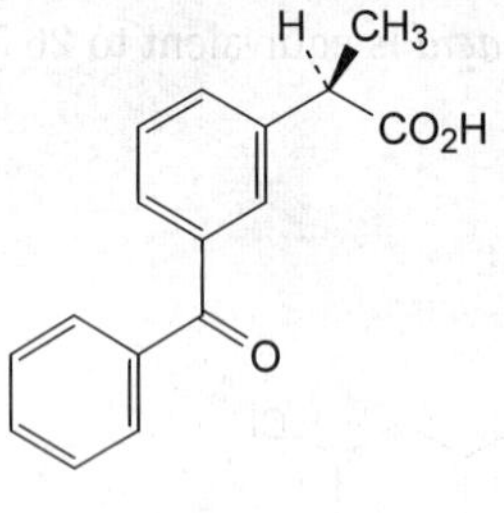

$C_{16}H_{14}O_3$ M_r 254.3

DEFINITION

Ketoprofen contains not less than 99.0 per cent and not more than the equivalent of 100.5 per cent of (2*RS*)-2-(3-benzoylphenyl)propanoic acid, calculated with reference to the dried substance.

CHARACTERS

A white or almost white, crystalline powder, practically insoluble in water, freely soluble in acetone, in ethanol (96 per cent) and in methylene chloride.

IDENTIFICATION

First identification: C.

Second identification: A, B, D.

A. Melting point (*2.2.14*): 94 °C to 97 °C.

B. Dissolve 50.0 mg in *ethanol (96 per cent) R* and dilute to 100.0 ml with the same solvent. Dilute 1.0 ml to 50.0 ml with *ethanol (96 per cent) R*. Examined between 230 nm and 350 nm (*2.2.25*), the solution shows an absorption maximum at 255 nm. The specific absorbance at the absorption maximum is 615 to 680.

C. Examine by infrared absorption spectrophotometry (*2.2.24*), comparing with the spectrum obtained with *ketoprofen CRS*.

D. Examine by thin-layer chromatography (*2.2.27*), using *silica gel* GF_{254} *R* as the coating substance.

Test solution. Dissolve 10 mg of the substance to be examined in *acetone R* and dilute to 10 ml with the same solvent.

Reference solution (a). Dissolve 10 mg of *ketoprofen CRS* in *acetone R* and dilute to 10 ml with the same solvent.

Reference solution (b). Dissolve 10 mg of *indometacin CRS* in *acetone R* and dilute to 10 ml with the same solvent. To 1 ml of the solution add 1 ml of reference solution (a).

Apply separately to the plate 10 µl of each solution. Develop over a path of 15 cm using a mixture of 1 volume of *glacial acetic acid R*, 49 volumes of *methylene chloride R* and 50 volumes of *acetone R*. Allow the plate to dry in air and examine in ultraviolet light at 254 nm. The principal spot in the chromatogram obtained with the test solution is similar in position and size to the principal spot in the chromatogram obtained with reference solution (a). The test is not valid unless the chromatogram obtained with reference solution (b) shows 2 clearly separated principal spots.

TESTS

Appearance of solution. Dissolve 1.0 g in *acetone R* and dilute to 10 ml with the same solvent. The solution is clear (*2.2.1*) and not more intensely coloured than reference solution Y_6 (*2.2.2, Method II*).

Related substances. *Prepare the solutions immediately before use.* Examine by liquid chromatography (*2.2.29*).

Test solution. Dissolve 20.0 mg of the substance to be examined in the mobile phase and dilute to 20.0 ml with the mobile phase.

Reference solution (a). Dilute 1.0 ml of the test solution to 50.0 ml with the mobile phase. Dilute 1.0 ml to 10.0 ml with the mobile phase.

Reference solution (b). Dissolve 5.0 mg of *ketoprofen impurity A CRS* in the mobile phase and dilute to 50.0 ml with the mobile phase. Dilute 1.0 ml to 50.0 ml with the mobile phase.

Reference solution (c). Dissolve 5.0 mg of *ketoprofen impurity C CRS* in the mobile phase and dilute to 50.0 ml with the mobile phase. Dilute 1.0 ml to 50.0 ml with the mobile phase.

Reference solution (d). Dilute 1.0 ml of the test solution to 100.0 ml with the mobile phase. To 1.0 ml add 1.0 ml of reference solution (b).

The chromatographic procedure may be carried out using:

- a stainless steel column 0.15 m long and 4.6 mm in internal diameter packed with a spherical *octadecylsilyl silica gel for chromatography R* (5 µm) with a specific surface area of 350 m^2/g and a pore size of 10 nm,
- as mobile phase at a flow rate of 1 ml/min a mixture of 2 volumes of *phosphate buffer solution pH 3.5 R*, freshly prepared, 43 volumes of *acetonitrile R* and 55 volumes of *water R*,
- as detector a spectrophotometer set at 233 nm,
- a loop injector.

Inject 20 µl of reference solution (d). The substances are eluted in the following order: ketoprofen and ketoprofen impurity A. Adjust the sensitivity of the detector so that the heights of the 2 principal peaks in the chromatogram obtained are not less than 50 per cent of the full scale of the recorder. The test is not valid unless the resolution between the peaks corresponding to ketoprofen and ketoprofen impurity A is at least 7.0.

Inject 20 µl of the test solution, 20 µl of reference solution (a), 20 µl of reference solution (b) and 20 µl of reference solution (c). Continue the chromatography of the test solution for 7 times the retention time of ketoprofen. The relative retentions with reference to ketoprofen (retention time = about 7 min) are as follows: impurity C = about 0.34; impurity H = about 0.39; impurity G = about 0.46; impurity E = about 0.69; impurity B = about 0.73; impurity D = about 1.35; impurity I = about 1.43; impurity A = about 1.50; impurity J = about 1.86; impurity F = about 1.95; impurity K = about 2.27; impurity L = about 2.49. In the chromatogram obtained with the test solution: the areas of any peaks corresponding to ketoprofen impurity A and ketoprofen impurity C are not greater than the areas of the principal peaks in the chromatograms obtained with reference solution (b) and reference solution (c), respectively (0.2 per cent); the area of any peak, apart from the principal peak and any peaks corresponding to ketoprofen impurity A and ketoprofen impurity C, is not greater than the area of the principal peak in the chromatogram obtained with reference solution (a) (0.2 per cent); the sum of the areas of all the peaks, apart from the principal peak and any peaks corresponding to the

2 named impurities, is not greater than twice the area of the principal peak in the chromatogram obtained with reference solution (a) (0.4 per cent). Disregard any peak with an area less than 0.1 times the area of the principal peak in the chromatogram obtained with reference solution (a).

Heavy metals (*2.4.8*). 2.0 g complies with limit test C for heavy metals (10 ppm). Prepare the reference solution using 2 ml of *lead standard solution (10 ppm Pb) R*.

Loss on drying (*2.2.32*). Not more than 0.5 per cent, determined on 1.000 g at 60 °C at a pressure not exceeding 670 Pa.

Sulphated ash (*2.4.14*). Not more than 0.1 per cent, determined on 1.0 g.

ASSAY

Dissolve 0.200 g in 25 ml of *ethanol (96 per cent) R*. Add 25 ml of *water R*. Titrate with *0.1 M sodium hydroxide*, determining the end-point potentiometrically (*2.2.20*).

1 ml of *0.1 M sodium hydroxide* is equivalent to 25.43 mg of $C_{16}H_{14}O_3$.

IMPURITIES

Specified impurities: A, B, C, D, E, F.

Other detectable impurities: G, H, I, J, K, L.

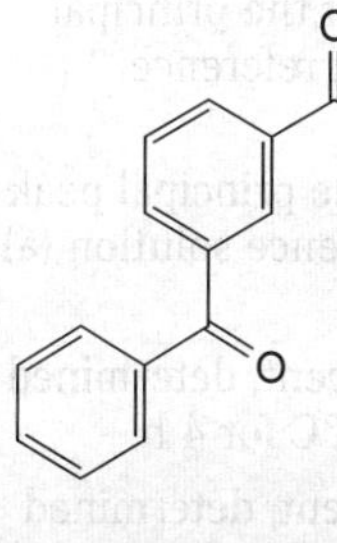

A. 1-(3-benzoylphenyl)ethanone,

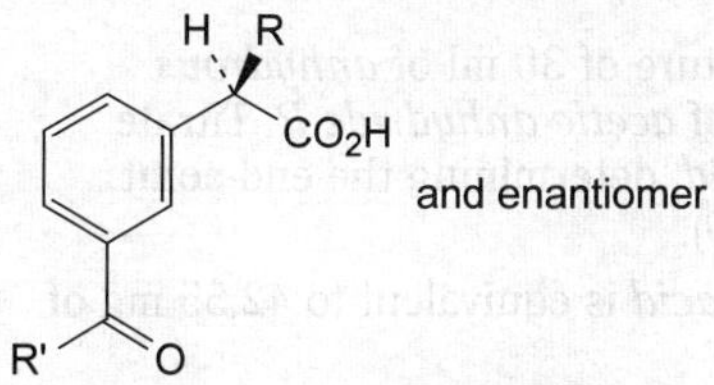

B. R = H, R′ = C_6H_5: (3-benzoylphenyl)acetic acid,

C. R = CH_3, R′ = OH: 3-[(1*RS*)-1-carboxyethyl]benzoic acid,

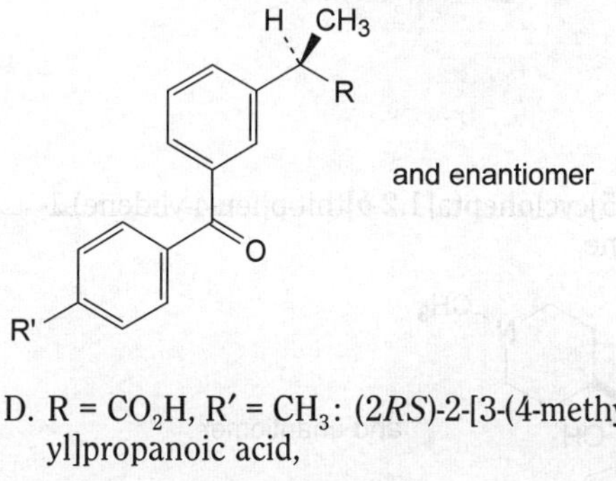

D. R = CO_2H, R′ = CH_3: (2*RS*)-2-[3-(4-methylbenzoyl)phenyl]propanoic acid,

E. R = CO-NH_2, R′ = H: (2*RS*)-2-(3-benzoylphenyl)propanamide,

F. R = CN, R′ = H: (2*RS*)-2-(3-benzoylphenyl)propanenitrile,

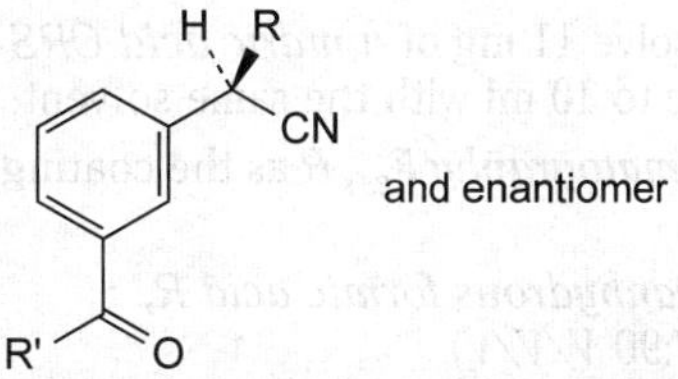

G. R = CH_3, R′ = OH: 3-[(1*RS*)-1-cyanoethyl]benzoic acid,

H. R = H, R′ = OH: 3-(cyanomethyl)benzoic acid,

I. R = H, R′ = C_6H_5: (3-benzoylphenyl)ethanenitrile,

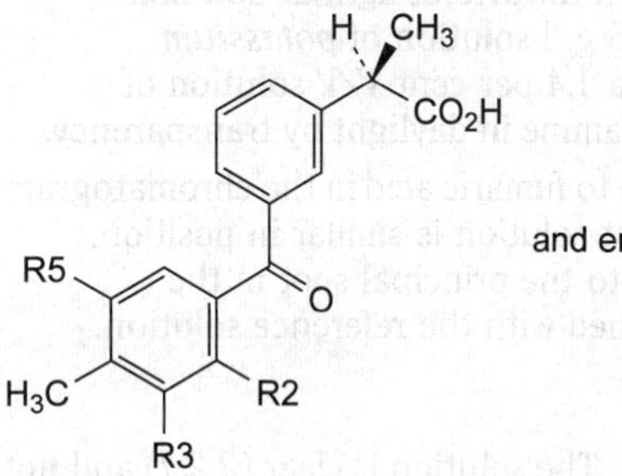

J. R2 = CH_3, R3 = R5 = H: (2*RS*)-2-[3-(2,4-dimethylbenzoyl)phenyl]propanoic acid,

K. R2 = R3 = CH_3, R5 = H + R2 = H, R3 = R5 = CH_3: mixture of (2*RS*)-2-[3-(2,3,4-trimethylbenzoyl)phenyl]propanoic acid and (2*RS*)-2-[3-(3,4,5-trimethylbenzoyl)phenyl]propanoic acid,

L. R2 = R5 = CH_3, R3 = H: (2*RS*)-2-[3-(2,4,5-trimethylbenzoyl)phenyl]propanoic acid.

01/2005:1592

KETOTIFEN HYDROGEN FUMARATE

Ketotifeni hydrogenofumaras

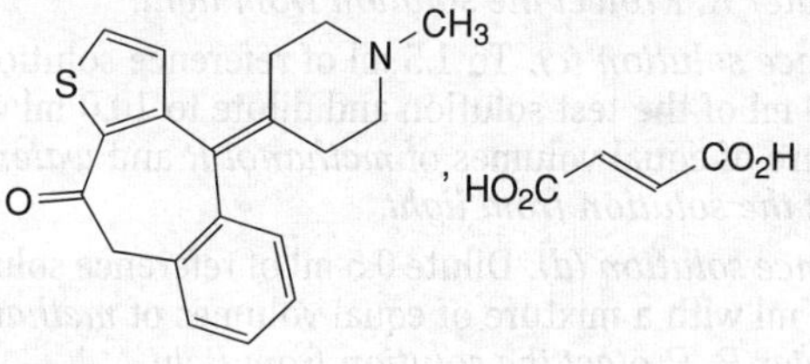

$C_{23}H_{23}NO_5S$ M_r 425.5

DEFINITION

4-(1-Methylpiperidin-4-ylidene)-4,9-dihydro-10*H*-benzo[4,5]cyclohepta[1,2-*b*]thiophen-10-one hydrogen (*E*)-butenedioate.

Content: 98.5 per cent to 101.0 per cent (dried substance).

CHARACTERS

Appearance: white to brownish-yellow, fine, crystalline powder.

Solubility: sparingly soluble in water, slightly soluble in methanol, very slightly soluble in acetonitrile.

IDENTIFICATION

A. Infrared absorption spectrophotometry (*2.2.24*).

Comparison: *Ph. Eur. reference spectrum of ketotifen hydrogen fumarate.*

B. Thin-layer chromatography (*2.2.27*).

Test solution. Dissolve 40 mg of the substance to be examined in *methanol R* and dilute to 10 ml with the same solvent.

Reference solution. Dissolve 11 mg of *fumaric acid CRS* in *methanol R* and dilute to 10 ml with the same solvent.

Plate: *cellulose for chromatography F_{254} R* as the coating substance.

Mobile phase: *water R, anhydrous formic acid R, di-isopropyl ether R* (3:7:90 *V/V/V*).

Application: 5 µl.

Development: over a path of 17 cm.

Drying: in a current of warm air.

Detection: examine in ultraviolet light at 254 nm. Spray lightly with a 5 g/l solution of *potassium permanganate R* in a 1.4 per cent *V/V* solution of *sulphuric acid R*. Examine in daylight by transparency.

Results: the spot due to fumaric acid in the chromatogram obtained with the test solution is similar in position, colour and intensity to the principal spot in the chromatogram obtained with the reference solution.

TESTS

Appearance of solution. The solution is clear (*2.2.1*) and not more intensely coloured than reference solution Y_4, BY_4 or B_4 (*2.2.2, Method II*).

Dissolve 0.2 g in *methanol R* and dilute to 10 ml with the same solvent.

Related substances. Liquid chromatography (*2.2.29*).

Test solution. Dissolve 30.0 mg of the substance to be examined in a mixture of equal volumes of *methanol R* and *water R* and dilute to 100.0 ml with the same mixture of solvents.

Reference solution (a). Dilute 1.0 ml of the test solution to 50.0 ml with a mixture of equal volumes of *methanol R* and *water R*. Dilute 1.0 ml to 10.0 ml with a mixture of equal volumes of *methanol R* and *water R*.

Reference solution (b). Dissolve 3.0 mg of *ketotifen impurity G CRS* in 10 ml of *methanol R* and dilute to 20.0 ml with *water R*. *Protect the solution from light.*

Reference solution (c). To 1.5 ml of reference solution (b) add 1.0 ml of the test solution and dilute to 10.0 ml with a mixture of equal volumes of *methanol R* and *water R*. *Protect the solution from light.*

Reference solution (d). Dilute 0.5 ml of reference solution (b) to 50.0 ml with a mixture of equal volumes of *methanol R* and *water R*. *Protect the solution from light.*

Column:

- *size*: l = 0.15 m, Ø = 4.0 mm,
- *stationary phase*: *octadecylsilyl silica gel for chromatography R* (3 µm),
- *temperature*: 40 °C.

Mobile phase:

- *mobile phase A*: mix 175 µl of *triethylamine R* and 500 ml of *water R*,
- *mobile phase B*: mix 175 µl of *triethylamine R* and 500 ml of *methanol R*,

Time (min)	Mobile phase A (per cent *V/V*)	Mobile phase B (per cent *V/V*)
0 - 12	40	60
12 - 20	40 → 10	60 → 90
20 - 25	10	90
25 - 26	10 → 40	90 → 60
26 - 31	40	60

Flow rate: 1.0 ml/min.

Detection: spectrophotometer at 297 nm.

Injection: 20 µl; inject the test solution and reference solutions (a), (c) and (d).

Relative retentions with reference to ketotifen: impurity D = about 0.31; impurity C = about 0.61; impurity G = about 0.86; impurity E = about 1.18; impurity F = about 1.36; impurity B = about 1.72; impurity A = about 2.15.

System suitability:

- *resolution*: minimum of 1.5 between the peaks due to ketotifen and to impurity G in the chromatogram obtained with reference solution (c),
- *signal-to-noise ratio*: minimum of 70 for the principal peak in the chromatogram obtained with reference solution (d).

Limits:

- *correction factor*: for the calculation of contents, multiply the area of the corresponding peak by the following correction factor: impurity G = 1.36,
- *impurity G*: not more than the area of the principal peak in the chromatogram obtained with reference solution (a) (0.2 per cent),
- *any impurity*: not more than the area of the principal peak in the chromatogram obtained with reference solution (a) (0.2 per cent),
- *total*: not more than 2.5 times the area of the principal peak in the chromatogram obtained with reference solution (a) (0.5 per cent),
- *disregard limit*: 0.25 times the area of the principal peak in the chromatogram obtained with reference solution (a) (0.05 per cent).

Loss on drying (*2.2.32*): maximum 0.5 per cent, determined on 1.000 g by drying in an oven at 100-105 °C for 4 h.

Sulphated ash (*2.4.14*): maximum 0.1 per cent, determined on 1.0 g.

ASSAY

Dissolve 0.350 g in a mixture of 30 ml of *anhydrous acetic acid R* and 30 ml of *acetic anhydride R*. Titrate with *0.1 M perchloric acid*, determining the end-point potentiometrically (*2.2.20*).

1 ml of *0.1 M perchloric acid* is equivalent to 42.55 mg of $C_{23}H_{23}NO_5S$.

IMPURITIES

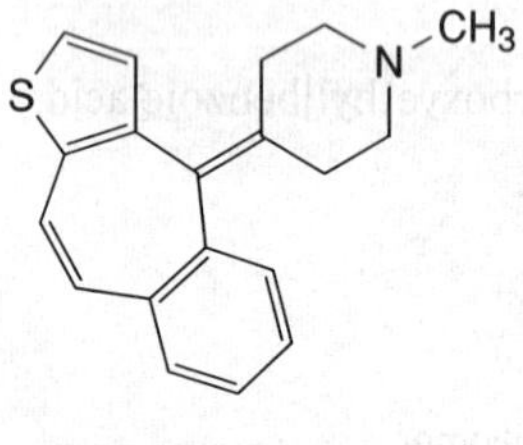

A. 4-(4*H*-benzo[4,5]cyclohepta[1,2-*b*]thiophen-4-ylidene)-1-methylpiperidine,

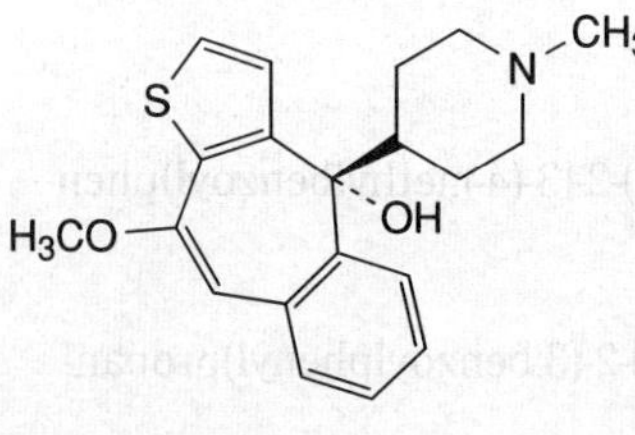

and enantiomer

B. (4*RS*)-10-methoxy-4-(1-methylpiperidin-4-yl)-4*H*-benzo[4,5]cyclohepta[1,2-*b*]thiophen-4-ol,

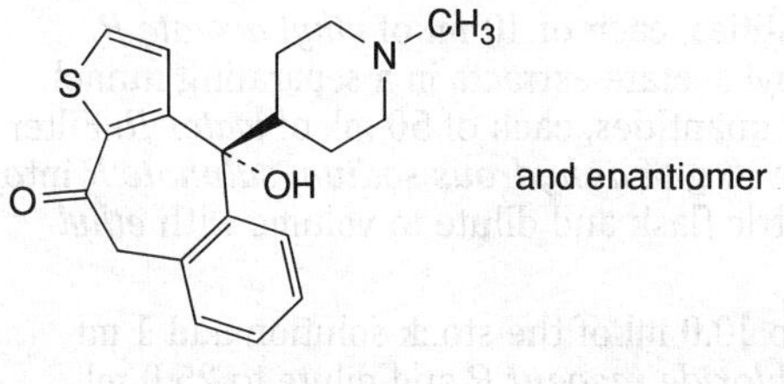

C. (4*RS*)-4-hydroxy-4-(1-methylpiperidin-4-yl)-4,9-dihydro-10*H*-benzo[4,5]cyclohepta[1,2-*b*]thiophen-10-one,

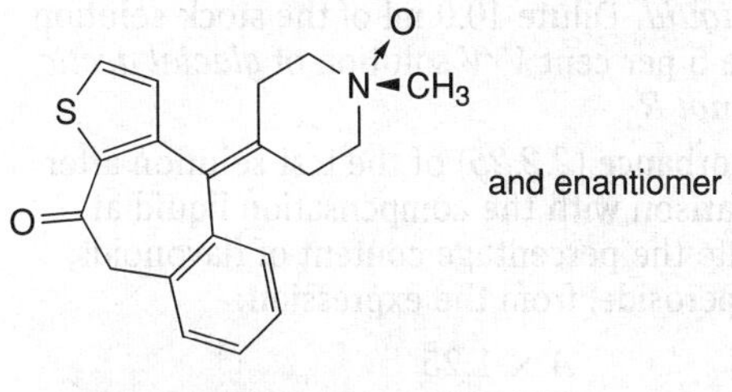

D. 4-[(*aRaS*)-1-methylpiperidin-4-ylidene]-4,9-dihydro-10*H*-benzo[4,5]cyclohepta[1,2-*b*]thiophen-10-one *N*-oxide (ketotifen *N*-oxide),

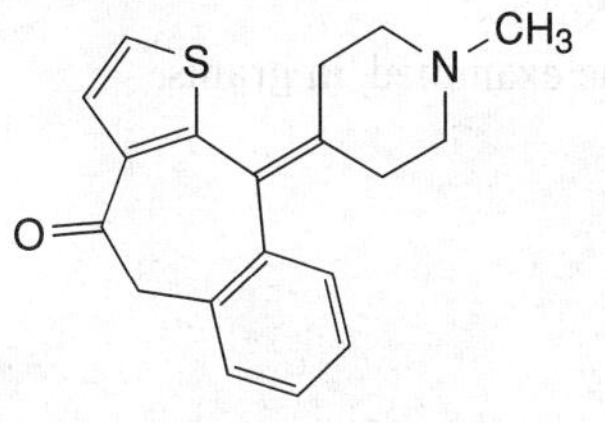

E. 10-(1-methylpiperidin-4-ylidene)-5,10-dihydro-4*H*-benzo[5,6]cyclohepta[1,2-*b*]thiophen-4-one,

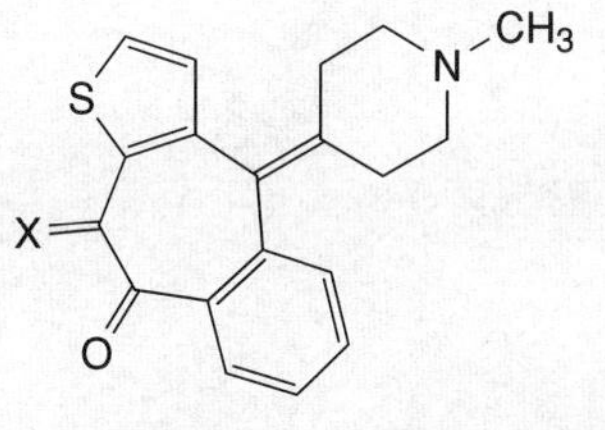

F. X = H_2: 4-(1-methylpiperidin-4-ylidene)-4,10-dihydro-9*H*-benzo[4,5]cyclohepta[1,2-*b*]thiophen-9-one,

G. X = O: 4-(1-methylpiperidin-4-ylidene)-4*H*-benzo[4,5]cyclohepta[1,2-*b*]thiophen-9,10-dione.

01/2005:1885

KNOTGRASS

Polygoni avicularis herba

DEFINITION

Whole or cut dried flowering aerial parts of *Polygonum aviculare* L. *s.l.*

Content: minimum 0.30 per cent of flavonoids, expressed as hyperoside ($C_{21}H_{20}O_{12}$; M_r 464.4) (dried drug).

CHARACTERS

Macroscopic and microscopic characters described under identification tests A and B.

IDENTIFICATION

A. The stem is 0.5 mm to 2 mm thick, branched, with nodes, cylindrical or slightly angular and longitudinally striated. It bears sessile or shortly petiolate, glabrous entire leaves, which differ widely in shape and size. The sheath-like stipules (ochrea) are lacerate and silvery. The small axillary flowers have 5 greenish-white perianth segments, the tips of which are often coloured red. The fruits are 2 mm to 4 mm, brown to black triangular nuts, usually punctate or striate.

B. Reduce to a powder (355). The powder is greenish-brown. Examine under a microscope using *chloral hydrate solution R*. The powder shows the following diagnostic characters: fragments of the leaf epidermis with polygonal to sinuous cell walls and numerous anisocytic stomata (*2.8.3*), with a striated cuticle; fragments of leaves and stems containing numerous calcium oxalate clusters, some of them very large; groups of thick-walled fibres from the hypodermis of the stem; globular pollen grains with smooth exine and 3 germinal pores; occasional brown fragments of the exocarp composed of cells with thick sinuous walls. Examine under a microscope using a 675 g/l solution of *potassium hydroxide R*. Heat gently. The epidermis of the leaves and a few cells of the mesophyll stain red to reddish-violet. Examine under a microscope using a 0.1 g/l solution of *ferric chloride R*. Leaf fragments are stained almost black.

C. Thin-layer chromatography (*2.2.27*).

Test solution. To 1.0 g of the powdered drug (355) add 10 ml of *methanol R*. Heat the mixture under a reflux condenser, in a water-bath for 10 min. Cool and filter.

Reference solution. Dissolve 1 mg of *caffeic acid R*, 2.5 mg of *hyperoside R* and 1 mg of *chlorogenic acid R* in 10 ml of *methanol R*.

Plate: *TLC silica gel plate R*.

Mobile phase: *anhydrous formic acid R, glacial acetic acid R, water R, ethyl acetate R* (7:7:14:72 *V/V/V/V*).

Application: 20 µl, as bands.

Development: over a path of 10 cm.

Drying: at 100-105 °C.

Detection: spray with a 10 g/l solution of *diphenylboric acid aminoethyl ester R* in *methanol R* subsequently spray with a 50 g/l solution of *macrogol 400 R* in *methanol R*. Allow the plate to dry in air for about 30 min. Examine in ultraviolet light at 365 nm.

Results: see below the sequence of the fluorescent zones present in the chromatograms obtained with the reference solution and the test solution. Furthermore, other fluorescent zones are present in the chromatogram obtained with the test solution.

Top of the plate	
Caffeic acid: a light blue fluorescent zone	1 or 2 blue fluorescent zones (caffeic acid)
_______	_______
	1 or 2 yellowish-green fluorescent zones
	A yellow fluorescent zone
Hyperoside: a yellowish-brown fluorescent zone	
	A yellowish-brown fluorescent zone
Chlorogenic acid: a light blue fluorescent zone	A light blue fluorescent zone (chlorogenic acid)
_______	_______
	A yellowish-brown fluorescent zone
Reference solution	**Test solution**

TESTS

Foreign matter (*2.8.2*): maximum 2 per cent of roots and maximum 2 per cent of other foreign matter.

Loss on drying (*2.2.32*): maximum 10.0 per cent, determined on 1.000 g of powdered drug (710) by drying in an oven at 100-105 °C for 2 h.

Total ash (*2.4.16*): maximum 10.0 per cent.

ASSAY

Stock solution. In a 100 ml round-bottomed flask, place 0.800 g of the powdered drug (355), add 1 ml of a 5 g/l solution of *hexamethylenetetramine R*, 20 ml of *acetone R* and 2 ml of *hydrochloric acid R1*. Boil the mixture under a reflux condenser for 30 min. Filter the liquid through a plug of absorbent cotton into a flask. Add the absorbent cotton to the residue in the round-bottomed flask and extract with 2 quantities, each of 20 ml, of *acetone R*, each time boiling under a reflux condenser for 10 min. Allow to cool, filter each extract through the plug of absorbent cotton into the flask. Filter the combined acetone extracts through a filter paper into a volumetric flask, dilute to 100.0 ml with *acetone R* rinsing the flask and the filter paper. Introduce 20.0 ml of the solution into a separating funnel, add 20 ml of *water R* and shake the mixture with 1 quantity of 15 ml and then 3 quantities, each of 10 ml of *ethyl acetate R*. Combine the ethyl acetate extracts in a separating funnel and wash with 2 quantities, each of 50 ml, of *water R*. Filter the extracts over 10 g of *anhydrous sodium sulphate R* into a 50 ml volume tric flask and dilute to volume with *ethyl acetate R*.

Test solution. To 10.0 ml of the stock solution add 1 ml of *aluminium chloride reagent R* and dilute to 25.0 ml with a 5 per cent *V/V* solution of *glacial acetic acid R* in *methanol R*.

Compensation liquid. Dilute 10.0 ml of the stock solution to 25.0 ml with a 5 per cent *V/V* solution of *glacial acetic acid R* in *methanol R*.

Measure the absorbance (*2.2.25*) of the test solution after 30 min by comparison with the compensation liquid at 425 nm. Calculate the percentage content of flavonoids, calculated as hyperoside, from the expression:

$$\frac{A \times 1.25}{m}$$

i.e. taking the specific absorbance of hyperoside to be 500.

A = absorbance at 425 nm,

m = mass of the drug to be examined, in grams.

L

01/2005:0923

LABETALOL HYDROCHLORIDE

Labetaloli hydrochloridum

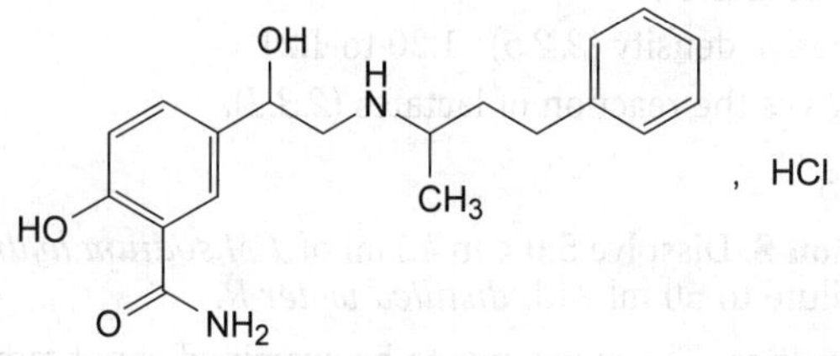

$C_{19}H_{25}ClN_2O_3$ M_r 364.9

DEFINITION

Labetalol hydrochloride contains not less than 98.5 per cent and not more than the equivalent of 101.0 per cent of 2-hydroxy-5-[1-hydroxy-2-[(1-methyl-3-phenylpropyl)amino]ethyl]benzamide hydrochloride, calculated with reference to the dried substance.

CHARACTERS

A white or almost white powder, sparingly soluble in water and in alcohol, practically insoluble in methylene chloride.

IDENTIFICATION

First identification: A, C, E.

Second identification: A, B, D, E.

A. Determined on solution S (see Tests), the angle of optical rotation (*2.2.7*) is + 0.05° to − 0.05°.

B. Dissolve 25.0 mg in *0.1 M hydrochloric acid* and dilute to 250.0 ml with the same acid. Examined between 230 nm and 350 nm (*2.2.25*), the solution shows an absorption maximum at 302 nm. The specific absorbance at the maximum is 83 to 88.

C. Examine by infrared absorption spectrophotometry (*2.2.24*), comparing with the spectrum obtained with *labetalol hydrochloride CRS*.

D. Examine by thin-layer chromatography (*2.2.27*), using as the coating substance a suitable octadecylsilyl silica gel with a fluorescent indicator having an optimal intensity at 254 nm.

Test solution. Dissolve 10 mg of the substance to be examined in 1 ml of *alcohol R*.

Reference solution (a). Dissolve 10 mg of *labetalol hydrochloride CRS* in 1 ml of *alcohol R*.

Reference solution (b). Dissolve 10 mg of *labetalol hydrochloride CRS* and 10 mg of *propranolol hydrochloride CRS* in *alcohol R* and dilute to 5 ml with the same solvent.

Apply separately to the plate 2 µl of each solution. Place the plate in a chromatographic tank immediately after the addition of the mobile phase consisting of a mixture of 0.5 volumes of *perchloric acid R*, 50 volumes of *water R* and 80 volumes of *methanol R*. Close the tank and develop over a path of 15 cm. Allow the plate to dry in air and examine in ultraviolet light at 254 nm. The principal spot in the chromatogram obtained with the test solution is similar in position and size to the principal spot in the chromatogram obtained with reference solution (a). The test is not valid unless the chromatogram obtained with reference solution (b) shows two clearly separated spots.

E. It gives reaction (a) of chlorides (*2.3.1*).

TESTS

Solution S. Dissolve 0.50 g in *carbon dioxide-free water R* and dilute to 50 ml with the same solvent. *Solution S must be freshly prepared.*

Appearance of solution. Solution S is clear (*2.2.1*) and not more intensely coloured than intensity 6 of the range of reference solutions of the most appropriate colour (*2.2.2, Method II*).

pH (*2.2.3*). The pH of solution S is 4.0 to 5.0.

Diastereoisomer ratio. Examine by gas chromatography (*2.2.28*).

Test solution. Dissolve 2.0 mg of the substance to be examined in 1.0 ml of a 12.0 g/l solution of *butylboronic acid R* in *anhydrous pyridine R* and allow to stand for 20 min.

The chromatographic procedure may be carried out using:

- a glass column 1.5 m long and 4 mm in internal diameter packed with *silanised diatomaceous earth for gas chromatography R* (125 µm to 150 µm) impregnated with 3 per cent *m/m* of *polymethylphenylsiloxane R*,
- *nitrogen for chromatography R* as the carrier gas at a flow rate of 40 ml/min,
- a flame-ionisation detector,

maintaining the temperature of the column, and that of the injection port and the detector at 300 °C.

Inject 2 µl of the test solution. Two peaks, each corresponding to a pair of diastereoisomers, appear in the chromatogram. Adjust the sensitivity of the system so that in the chromatogram obtained, the height of the taller of the diastereoisomer peaks is about 80 per cent of the full scale of the recorder. The test is not valid unless the height of the trough separating these peaks is less than 5 per cent of the full scale of the recorder. The area of each peak is not less than 45 per cent and not more than 55 per cent of the total area of the two peaks.

Related substances. Examine by liquid chromatography (*2.2.29*).

Test solution. Dissolve 50.0 mg of the substance to be examined in the mobile phase and dilute to 10.0 ml with the mobile phase.

Reference solution. Dilute 0.5 ml of the test solution to 100.0 ml with the mobile phase.

The chromatographic procedure may be carried out using:

- a stainless steel column 0.15 m long and 4.6 mm in internal diameter packed with *octadecylsilyl silica gel for chromatography R* (5 µm),
- as mobile phase at a flow rate of 1 ml/min a mixture of 150 ml of *tetrahydrofuran R*, 300 ml of *methanol R*, 550 ml of *water R*, 0.82 g of *tetrabutylammonium hydrogen sulphate R*, 1 g of *sodium octyl sulphate R* and 10 ml of a 10 per cent *V/V* solution of *sulphuric acid R*,
- as detector a spectrophotometer set at 229 nm.

Equilibrate the column with the mobile phase at a flow rate of 1 ml/min for about 30 min.

Adjust the sensitivity of the system so that the height of the principal peak in the chromatogram obtained with 20 µl of the reference solution is at least 50 per cent of the full scale of the recorder. When the chromatograms are recorded in the prescribed conditions, the retention time of the principal peak is 10 min to 15 min. If necessary, adjust the water content of the mobile phase ensuring that the 2:1 ratio of methanol to tetrahydrofuran is maintained.

Inject separately 20 µl of each solution. Continue the chromatography for three times the retention time of the principal peak. In the chromatogram obtained with the test solution: the area of any peak, apart from the principal peak, is not greater than 0.6 times that of the principal peak in the chromatogram obtained with the reference solution (0.3 per cent); the sum of the areas of any such peaks is not greater than the area of the principal peak in the chromatogram obtained with the reference solution (0.5 per cent). Disregard any peak due to the solvent and any peak with an area less than 0.1 times the area of the principal peak in the chromatogram obtained with the reference solution.

Heavy metals (*2.4.8*). 1.0 g complies with limit test C for heavy metals (20 ppm). Prepare the standard using 2 ml of *lead standard solution (10 ppm Pb) R*.

Loss on drying (*2.2.32*). Not more than 1.0 per cent, determined on 1.000 g by drying in an oven at 100 °C to 105 °C at a pressure not exceeding 0.7 kPa.

Sulphated ash (*2.4.14*). Not more than 0.1 per cent, determined on 1.0 g.

ASSAY

In order to avoid overheating in the reaction medium, mix thoroughly throughout and stop the titration immediately after the end-point has been reached.

Dissolve 0.200 g in a mixture of 10 ml of *anhydrous formic acid R* and 40 ml of *acetic anhydride R*. Titrate with *0.1 M perchloric acid*, determining the end-point potentiometrically (*2.2.20*).

1 ml of *0.1 M perchloric acid* is equivalent to 36.49 mg of $C_{19}H_{25}ClN_2O_3$.

IMPURITIES

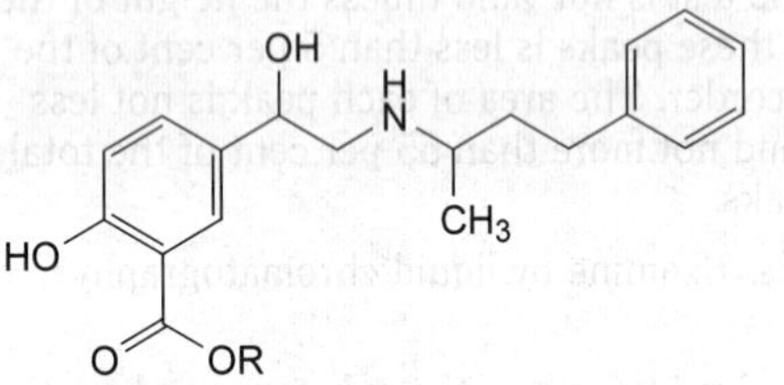

A. R = H: 2-hydroxy-5-[1-hydroxy-2-[(1-methyl-3-phenylpropyl)-amino]ethyl]benzoic acid,

B. R = CH_3: methyl 2-hydroxy-5-[1-hydroxy-2-[(1-methyl-3-phenylpropyl)amino]ethyl]benzoate.

01/2005:0458

LACTIC ACID

Acidum lacticum

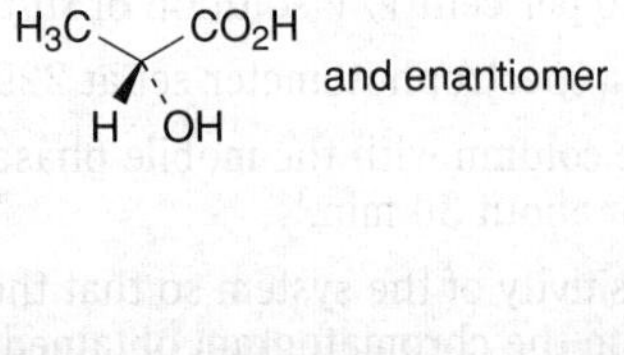

$C_3H_6O_3$ M_r 90.1

DEFINITION

Mixture of 2-hydroxypropanoic acid, its condensation products, such as lactoyl-lactic acid and polylactic acids, and water. The equilibrium between lactic acid and polylactic acids depends on the concentration and temperature. It is usually the racemate ((*RS*)-lactic acid).

Content: 88.0 per cent *m/m* to 92.0 per cent *m/m* of $C_3H_6O_3$.

CHARACTERS

Appearance: colourless or slightly yellow, syrupy liquid.

Solubility: miscible with water and with alcohol.

IDENTIFICATION

A. Dissolve 1 g in 10 ml of *water R*. The solution is strongly acidic (*2.2.4*).

B. Relative density (*2.2.5*): 1.20 to 1.21.

C. It gives the reaction of lactates (*2.3.1*).

TESTS

Solution S. Dissolve 5.0 g in 42 ml of *1 M sodium hydroxide* and dilute to 50 ml with *distilled water R*.

Appearance. The substance to be examined is not more intensely coloured than reference solution Y_6 (*2.2.2, Method II*).

Ether-insoluble substances. Dissolve 1.0 g in 25 ml of *ether R*. The solution is not more opalescent than the solvent used for the test.

Sugars and other reducing substances. To 1 ml of solution S add 1 ml of *1 M hydrochloric acid*, heat to boiling, allow to cool and add 1.5 ml of *1 M sodium hydroxide* and 2 ml of *cupri-tartaric solution R*. Heat to boiling. No red or greenish precipitate is formed.

Methanol (*2.4.24*): maximum 50 ppm, if intended for use in the manufacture of parenteral dosage forms.

Citric, oxalic and phosphoric acids. To 5 ml of solution S add *dilute ammonia R1* until slightly alkaline (*2.2.4*). Add 1 ml of *calcium chloride solution R*. Heat on a water-bath for 5 min. Both before and after heating, any opalescence in the solution is not more intense than that in a mixture of 1 ml of *water R* and 5 ml of solution S.

Sulphates (*2.4.13*): maximum 200 ppm.

7.5 ml of solution S diluted to 15 ml with *distilled water R* complies with the limit test for sulphates.

Calcium (*2.4.3*): maximum 200 ppm.

5 ml of solution S diluted to 15 ml with *distilled water R* complies with the limit test for calcium.

Heavy metals (*2.4.8*): maximum 10 ppm.

12 ml of solution S complies with limit test A. Prepare the standard using *lead standard solution (1 ppm Pb) R*.

Sulphated ash (*2.4.14*): maximum 0.1 per cent, determined on 1.0 g.

Bacterial endotoxins (*2.6.14*): less than 5 IU/g, if intended for use in the manufacture of parenteral dosage forms without a further appropriate procedure for the elimination of bacterial endotoxins.

ASSAY

Place 1.000 g in a ground-glass-stoppered flask and add 10 ml of *water R* and 20.0 ml of *1 M sodium hydroxide*. Close the flask and allow to stand for 30 min. Using 0.5 ml of *phenolphthalein solution R* as indicator, titrate with *1 M hydrochloric acid* until the pink colour is discharged.

1 ml of *1 M sodium hydroxide* is equivalent to 90.1 mg of $C_3H_6O_3$.

LABELLING

The label states:

– where applicable, that the substance is free from bacterial endotoxins,

– where applicable, that the substance is suitable for use in the manufacture of parenteral dosage forms.

01/2005:1771

(S)-LACTIC ACID

Acidum (*S*)-lacticum

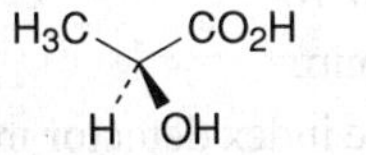

$C_3H_6O_3$ M_r 90.1

DEFINITION

Mixture of (*S*)-2-hydroxypropanoic acid, its condensation products, such as lactoyl-lactic acid and polylactic acids, and water. The equilibrium between lactic acid and polylactic acids depends on the concentration and temperature.

Content: 88.0 per cent *m/m* to 92.0 per cent *m/m* of $C_3H_6O_3$, not less than 95.0 per cent of which is the (*S*)-enantiomer.

CHARACTERS

Appearance: colourless or slightly yellow, syrupy liquid.

Solubility: miscible with water and with alcohol.

IDENTIFICATION

A. Dissolve 1 g in 10 ml of *water R*. The solution is strongly acidic (*2.2.4*).

B. Relative density (*2.2.5*): 1.20 to 1.21.

C. It gives the reaction of lactates (*2.3.1*).

D. It complies with the limits of the assay.

TESTS

Solution S. Dissolve 5.0 g in 42 ml of *1 M sodium hydroxide* and dilute to 50 ml with *distilled water R*.

Appearance. The substance to be examined is not more intensely coloured than reference solution Y_6 (*2.2.2, Method II*).

Ether-insoluble substances. Dissolve 1.0 g in 25 ml of *ether R*. The solution is not more opalescent than the solvent used for the test.

Sugars and other reducing substances. To 1 ml of solution S add 1 ml of *1 M hydrochloric acid*, heat to boiling, allow to cool and add 1.5 ml of *1 M sodium hydroxide* and 2 ml of *cupri-tartaric solution R*. Heat to boiling. No red or greenish precipitate is formed.

Methanol (*2.4.24*): maximum 50 ppm, if intended for use in the manufacture of parenteral dosage forms.

Citric, oxalic and phosphoric acids. To 5 ml of solution S add *dilute ammonia R1* until slightly alkaline (*2.2.4*). Add 1 ml of *calcium chloride solution R*. Heat on a water-bath for 5 min. Both before and after heating, any opalescence in the solution is not more intense than that in a mixture of 1 ml of *water R* and 5 ml of solution S.

Sulphates (*2.4.13*): maximum 200 ppm.

7.5 ml of solution S diluted to 15 ml with *distilled water R* complies with the limit test for sulphates.

Calcium (*2.4.3*): maximum 200 ppm.

5 ml of solution S diluted to 15 ml with *distilled water R* complies with the limit test for calcium.

Heavy metals (*2.4.8*): maximum 10 ppm.

12 ml of solution S complies with limit test A. Prepare the standard using *lead standard solution (1 ppm Pb) R*.

Sulphated ash (*2.4.14*): maximum 0.1 per cent, determined on 1.0 g.

Bacterial endotoxins (*2.6.14*): less than 5 IU/g if intended for use in the manufacture of parenteral dosage forms without a further appropriate procedure for the elimination of bacterial endotoxins.

ASSAY

Place 1.000 g in a ground-glass-stoppered flask and add 10 ml of *water R* and 20.0 ml of *1 M sodium hydroxide*. Close the flask and allow to stand for 30 min. Using 0.5 ml of *phenolphthalein solution R* as indicator, titrate with *1 M hydrochloric acid* until the pink colour is discharged.

1 ml of *1 M sodium hydroxide* is equivalent to 90.1 mg of $C_3H_6O_3$.

(S)-enantiomer

Transfer an amount of the substance to be examined equivalent to 2.00 g of lactic acid into a round-bottomed flask, add 25 ml of *1 M sodium hydroxide* and boil gently for 15 min. Cool down and adjust to pH 7.0 using *1 M hydrochloric acid*. Add 5.0 g of *ammonium molybdate R*, dissolve and dilute to 50.0 ml with *water R*. Filter and measure the angle of optical rotation (*2.2.7*). Calculate the percentage content of (*S*)-enantiomer using the expression:

$$50 + \left(24.18 \times \alpha \times \frac{2.222}{m} \times \frac{90}{c}\right)$$

α = angle of optical rotation (absolute value),

m = mass of the substance to be examined, in grams,

c = percentage content of $C_3H_6O_3$ in the substance to be examined.

The complex of (*S*)-lactic acid formed under these test conditions is laevorotatory.

LABELLING

The label states:

– where applicable, that the substance is free from bacterial endotoxins,

– where applicable, that the substance is suitable for use in the manufacture of parenteral dosage forms.

01/2005:1337

LACTITOL MONOHYDRATE

Lactitolum monohydricum

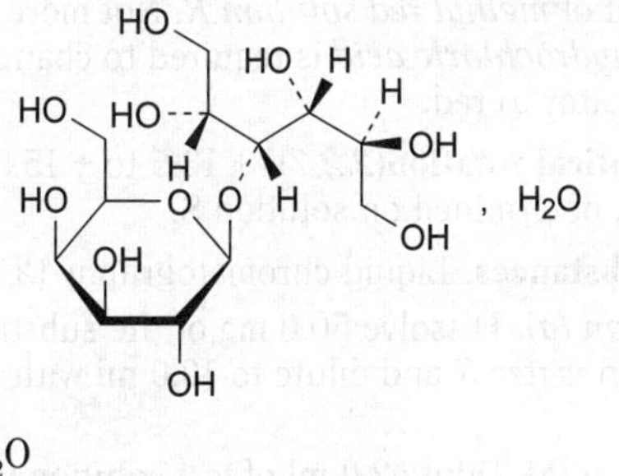

$C_{12}H_{24}O_{11},H_2O$ M_r 362.3

DEFINITION

4-*O*-(β-D-galactopyranosyl)-D-glucitol.

Content: 96.5 per cent to 102.0 per cent (anhydrous substance).

CHARACTERS

Appearance: white, crystalline powder.

Solubility: very soluble in water, slightly soluble in alcohol, practically insoluble in methylene chloride

IDENTIFICATION

First identification: B.

Second identification: A, C.

A. Specific optical rotation (see Tests).

B. Infrared absorption spectrophotometry (*2.2.24*).

Comparison: *lactitol monohydrate CRS.*

C. Thin-layer chromatography (*2.2.27*).

Test solution. Dissolve 50 mg of the substance to be examined in *methanol R* and dilute to 20 ml with the same solvent.

Reference solution (a). Dissolve 5 mg of *lactitol monohydrate CRS* in *methanol R* and dilute to 2 ml with the same solvent.

Reference solution (b). Dissolve 5 mg of *sorbitol CRS* in 2 ml of reference solution (a) and dilute to 20 ml with *methanol R.*

Plate: *TLC silica gel G plate R.*

Mobile phase: *water R, acetonitrile R* (25:75 *V/V*).

Application: 2 µl.

Development: over 2/3 of the plate.

Drying: in air.

Detection: spray with *4-aminobenzoic acid solution R.* Dry the plate in a current of cold air until the solvent is removed. Heat at 100 °C for 15 min. Allow to cool and spray with a 2 g/l solution of *sodium periodate R.* Dry the plate in a current of cold air. Heat at 100 °C for 15 min.

System suitability: the chromatogram obtained with reference solution (b) shows 2 clearly separated spots.

Results: the principal spot in the chromatogram obtained with the test solution is similar in position, colour and size to the principal spot in the chromatogram obtained with reference solution (a).

TESTS

Solution S. Dissolve 5.000 g in *carbon dioxide-free water R* and dilute to 50.0 ml with the same solvent.

Appearance of solution. Solution S is clear (*2.2.1*) and not more intensely coloured than reference solution BY_7 (*2.2.2, Method II*).

Acidity or alkalinity. To 10 ml of solution S add 10 ml of *carbon dioxide-free water R.* To 10 ml of this solution add 0.05 ml of *phenolphthalein solution R.* Not more than 0.2 ml of *0.01 M sodium hydroxide* is required to change the colour of the indicator to pink. To a further 10 ml of the solution add 0.05 ml of *methyl red solution R.* Not more than 0.3 ml of *0.01 M hydrochloric acid* is required to change the colour of the indicator to red.

Specific optical rotation(*2.2.7*): + 13.5 to + 15.5 (anhydrous substance), determined on solution S.

Related substances. Liquid chromatography (*2.2.29*).

Test solution (a). Dissolve 50.0 mg of the substance to be examined in *water R* and dilute to 10.0 ml with the same solvent.

Test solution (b). Dilute 2.0 ml of test solution (a) to 50.0 ml with *water R.*

Reference solution (a). Dissolve 5.0 mg of *lactitol monohydrate CRS* and 5 mg of *glycerol R* in *water R* and dilute to 25.0 ml with the same solvent.

Reference solution (b). Dilute 1.0 ml of test solution (a) to 100.0 ml with *water R.* Dilute 5.0 ml of this solution to 100.0 ml with *water R.*

Reference solution (c). Dilute 2.5 ml of reference solution (a) to 10.0 ml with *water R.*

Column:

- *size*: *l* = 0.30 m, Ø = 7.8 mm,
- *stationary phase*: *strong cation exchange resin (calcium form) R,*
- *temperature*: 60 °C.

Mobile phase: *water R.*

Flow rate: 0.6 ml/min.

Detection: refractive index detector maintained at a constant temperature.

Injection: 100 µl; inject test solution (a) and reference solutions (b) and (c).

Run time: 2.5 times the retention time of lactitol.

Relative retention with reference to lactitol (retention time = about 13 min): impurity A = about 0.7; impurity B = about 0.8; glycerol = about 1.3; impurity C = about 1.5; impurity D = about 1.8; impurity E = about 1.9.

System suitability: reference solution (c):

- *resolution*: minimum 5 between the peaks due to lactitol and glycerol.

Limits:

- *impurity B*: not more than the area of the peak due to lactitol in the chromatogram obtained with reference solution (c) (1.0 per cent),
- *total of other impurities*: not more than the area of the peak due to lactitol in the chromatogram obtained with reference solution (c) (1.0 per cent),
- *disregard limit*: the area of the principal peak in the chromatogram obtained with reference solution (b) (0.05 per cent); disregard any peak due to the solvent.

Reducing sugars: maximum 0.2 per cent.

Dissolve 5.0 g in 3 ml of *water R* with gentle heating. Cool and add 20 ml of *cupri-citric solution R* and a few glass beads. Heat so that boiling begins after 4 min and maintain boiling for 3 min. Cool rapidly and add 100 ml of a 2.4 per cent *V/V* solution of *glacial acetic acid R* and 20.0 ml of *0.025 M iodine.* With continuous shaking, add 25 ml of a mixture of 6 volumes of *hydrochloric acid R* and 94 volumes of *water R.* When the precipitate has dissolved, titrate the excess of iodine with *0.05 M sodium thiosulphate* using 1 ml of *starch solution R* added towards the end of the titration, as indicator. Not less than 12.8 ml of *0.05 M sodium thiosulphate* is required.

Lead (*2.4.10*): maximum 0.5 ppm.

Nickel (*2.4.15*): maximum 1 ppm.

Water (*2.5.12*): 4.5 per cent to 5.5 per cent, determined on 0.30 g.

Sulphated ash (*2.4.14*): maximum 0.1 per cent, determined on 1.0 g.

Microbial contamination. Total viable aerobic count (*2.6.12*) not more than 10^3 micro-organisms per gram. It complies with the tests for *Escherichia coli, Salmonella* and *Pseudomonas aeruginosa* (*2.6.13*).

ASSAY

Liquid chromatography (*2.2.29*) as described in the test for related substances with the following modification.

Injection: test solution (b) and reference solution (a).

Calculate the percentage content of $C_{12}H_{24}O_{11}$ using the chromatograms obtained with test solution (b) and reference solution (a) and the declared content of *lactitol monohydrate CRS.*

Monographs I-L

IMPURITIES

Specified impurities: A, B, C, D, E.

A. lactose,

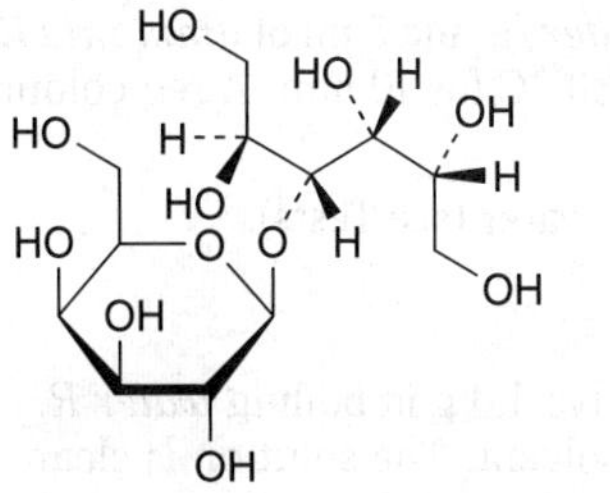

B. lactulitol,

C. mannitol,

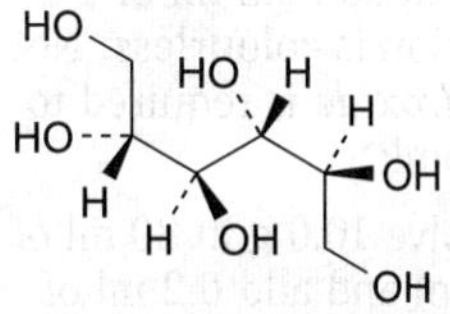

D. dulcitol (galactitol),

E. sorbitol.

01/2005:1647

LACTOBIONIC ACID

Acidum lactobionicum

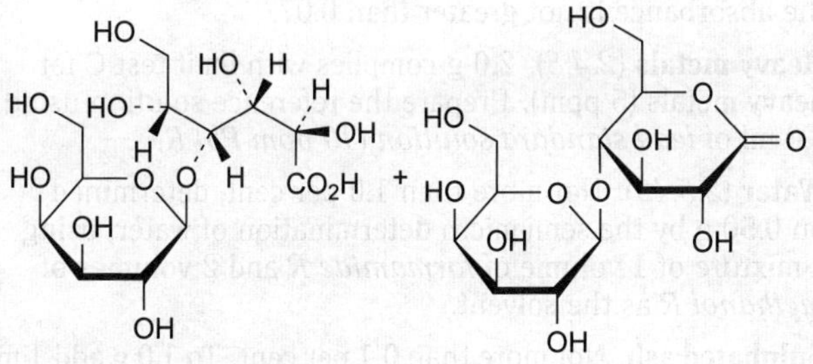

$C_{12}H_{22}O_{12}$ (acid form) M_r 358.3

$C_{12}H_{20}O_{11}$ (δ-lactone) M_r 340.3

DEFINITION

Mixture in variable proportions of 4-*O*-β-D-galactopyranosyl-D-gluconic acid and 4-*O*-β-D-galactopyranosyl-D-glucono-1,5-lactone.

Content: 98.0 per cent to 102.0 per cent (anhydrous substance).

CHARACTERS

Appearance: white or almost white powder.

Solubility: freely soluble in water, slightly soluble in glacial acetic acid, in anhydrous ethanol and in methanol.

mp: about 125 °C with decomposition.

IDENTIFICATION

A. Infrared absorption spectrophotometry (*2.2.24*).

Comparison: *lactobionic acid CRS.*

If the spectra obtained show differences, dissolve the substance to be examined and the reference substance separately in *water R*, dry at 105 °C and record new spectra using the residues.

B. Thin-layer chromatography (*2.2.27*).

Test solution. Dissolve 10 mg of the substance to be examined in *water R* and dilute to 1 ml with the same solvent.

Reference solution. Dissolve 10 mg of *lactobionic acid CRS* in *water R* and dilute to 1 ml with the same solvent.

Plate: *TLC silica gel plate R.*

Mobile phase: *concentrated ammonia R1, ethyl acetate R, water R, methanol R* (2:2:2:4 *V/V/V/V*).

Application: 5 µl.

Development: over 3/4 of the plate.

Detection: spray 3 times with *ammonium molybdate solution R6* and heat in an oven at 110 °C for 15 min.

Results: the principal spot in the chromatogram obtained with the test solution is similar in position and colour to the principal spot in the chromatogram obtained with the reference solution.

TESTS

Appearance of solution. The solution is clear (*2.2.1*) and not more intensely coloured than reference solution Y_5 (*2.2.2, Method II*).

Dissolve 3.0 g in 25 ml of *water R*.

Specific optical rotation (*2.2.7*): + 23.0 to + 29.0 (anhydrous substance).

Dissolve 1.0 g in 80 ml of *water R* and dilute to 100.0 ml with the same solvent. Allow to stand for 24 h.

Reducing sugars: maximum 0.2 per cent, calculated as glucose.

Dissolve 5.0 g in 25 ml of *water R* with the aid of gentle heat. Cool and add 20 ml of *cupri-citric solution R* and a few glass beads. Heat so that boiling begins after 4 min and maintain boiling for 3 min. Cool rapidly and add 100 ml of a 2.4 per cent *V/V* solution of *glacial acetic acid R* and 20.0 ml of *0.025 M iodine.* With continuous shaking, add 25 ml of a mixture of 6 volumes of *hydrochloric acid R* and 94 volumes of *water R* and, when the precipitate has dissolved, titrate the excess of iodine with *0.05 M sodium thiosulphate* using 1 ml of *starch solution R*, added towards the end of the titration, as indicator. Not less than 12.8 ml of *0.05 M sodium thiosulphate* is required.

Heavy metals (*2.4.8*): maximum 20 ppm.

1.0 g complies with limit test E. Prepare the reference solution using 2 ml of *lead standard solution (10 ppm Pb) R.*

Water (*2.5.12*): maximum 5.0 per cent, determined on 0.50 g. Use a mixture of 1 volume of *formamide R* and 2 volumes of *methanol R* as solvent.

Total ash (*2.4.16*): maximum 0.2 per cent.

ASSAY

Dissolve 0.350 g in 50 ml of *carbon dioxide-free water R*, previously heated to 30 °C. Immediately titrate with *0.1 M sodium hydroxide* and determine the 2 equivalence points potentiometrically (*2.2.20*).

The first equivalence point (V_1) corresponds to the acid form of lactobionic acid and the second equivalence point ($V_2 - V_1$) corresponds to the δ-lactone form.

1 ml of *0.1 M sodium hydroxide* is equivalent to 35.83 mg of $C_{12}H_{22}O_{12}$.

1 ml of *0.1 M sodium hydroxide* is equivalent to 34.03 mg of $C_{12}H_{20}O_{11}$.

The sum of the 2 results is expressed as a percentage content of lactobionic acid.

01/2005:1061

LACTOSE, ANHYDROUS

Lactosum anhydricum

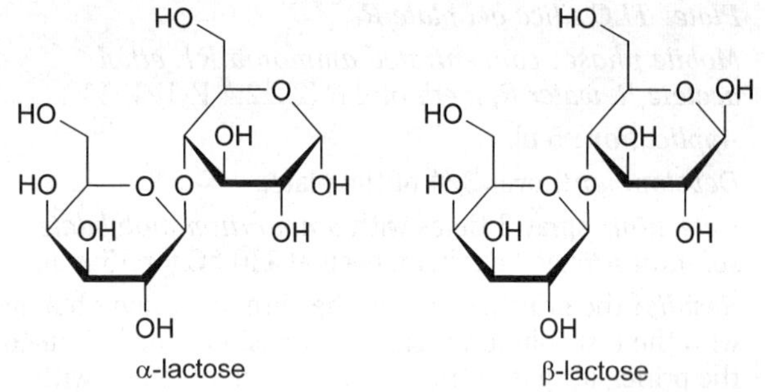

$C_{12}H_{22}O_{11}$ M_r 342.3

DEFINITION

Anhydrous lactose is *O*-β-D-galactopyranosyl-(1→4)-β-D-glucopyranose or a mixture of *O*-β-D-galactopyranosyl-(1→4)-α-D-glucopyranose and *O*-β-D-galactopyranosyl-(1→4)-β-D-glucopyranose.

CHARACTERS

A white or almost white, crystalline powder, freely but slowly soluble in water, practically insoluble in ethanol (96 per cent).

IDENTIFICATION

First identification: A, D.

Second identification: B, C, D.

A. Examine by infrared absorption spectrophotometry (*2.2.24*), comparing with the spectrum obtained with *anhydrous lactose CRS*.

B. Examine by thin-layer chromatography (*2.2.27*), using a *TLC silica gel G plate R*.

Test solution. Dissolve 10 mg of the substance to be examined in a mixture of 2 volumes of *water R* and 3 volumes of *methanol R* and dilute to 20 ml with the same mixture of solvents.

Reference solution (a). Dissolve 10 mg of *anhydrous lactose CRS* in a mixture of 2 volumes of *water R* and 3 volumes of *methanol R* and dilute to 20 ml with the same mixture of solvents.

Reference solution (b). Dissolve 10 mg each of *glucose CRS, anhydrous lactose CRS, fructose CRS* and *sucrose CRS* in a mixture of 2 volumes of *water R* and 3 volumes of *methanol R* and dilute to 20 ml with the same mixture of solvents.

Apply separately to the plate 2 µl of each solution and thoroughly dry the starting points. Develop over a path of 15 cm using a mixture of 10 volumes of *water R*, 15 volumes of *methanol R*, 25 volumes of *glacial acetic acid R* and 50 volumes of *ethylene chloride R*, measured accurately since a slight excess of water produces cloudiness. Dry the plate in a current of warm air. Repeat the development immediately, after renewing the mobile phase. Dry the plate in a current of warm air and spray evenly with a solution of 0.5 g of *thymol R* in a mixture of 5 ml of *sulphuric acid R* and 95 ml of *alcohol R*. Heat at 130 °C for 10 min. The principal spot in the chromatogram obtained with the test solution is similar in position, colour and size to the principal spot in the chromatogram obtained with reference solution (a). The test is not valid unless the chromatogram obtained with reference solution (b) shows 4 clearly separated spots.

C. Dissolve 0.25 g in 5 ml of *water R*. Add 5 ml of *ammonia R* and heat in a water-bath at 80 °C for 10 min. A red colour develops.

D. It complies with the test for water (see Tests).

TESTS

Appearance of solution. Dissolve 1.0 g in boiling *water R*, dilute to 10 ml with the same solvent. The solution is clear (*2.2.1*) and not more intensely coloured than reference solution BY_7 (*2.2.2, Method II*).

Acidity or alkalinity. Dissolve 6.0 g by heating in 25 ml of *carbon dioxide-free water R*, cool and add 0.3 ml of *phenolphthalein solution R*. The solution is colourless. Not more than 0.4 ml of *0.1 M sodium hydroxide* is required to change the colour of the indicator to pink.

Specific optical rotation (*2.2.7*). Dissolve 10.0 g in 80 ml of *water R*, heating to 50 °C. Allow to cool and add 0.2 ml of *dilute ammonia R1*. Allow to stand for 30 min and dilute to 100.0 ml with *water R*. The specific optical rotation is + 54.4 to + 55.9, calculated with reference to the anhydrous substance.

Absorbance (*2.2.25*). Dissolve 1.0 g in boiling *water R* and dilute to 10.0 ml with the same solvent (solution A). The absorbance of the solution measured at 400 nm is not greater than 0.04. Dilute 1.0 ml of solution A to 10.0 ml with *water R*. Examine the solution from 210 nm to 300 nm. At wavelengths from 210 nm to 220 nm, the absorbance is not greater than 0.25. At wavelengths from 270 nm to 300 nm, the absorbance is not greater than 0.07.

Heavy metals (*2.4.8*). 2.0 g complies with limit test C for heavy metals (5 ppm). Prepare the reference solution using 1.0 ml of *lead standard solution (10 ppm Pb) R*.

Water (*2.5.12*). Not more than 1.0 per cent, determined on 0.50 g by the semi-micro determination of water, using a mixture of 1 volume of *formamide R* and 2 volumes of *methanol R* as the solvent.

Sulphated ash. Not more than 0.1 per cent. To 1.0 g add 1 ml of *sulphuric acid R*, evaporate to dryness on a water-bath and ignite to constant mass.

Microbial contamination. Total viable aerobic count (*2.6.12*) not more than 10^2 micro-organisms per gram, determined by plate-count. It complies with the test for *Escherichia coli* (*2.6.13*)

FUNCTIONALITY-RELATED CHARACTERISTICS

The following test are not mandatory requirements but in view of their known importance for achieving consistency in manufacture, quality and performance of medicinal products, it is recommended that suppliers should verify these characteristics and provide information on the results and analytical method applied to users. The methods indicated below have been found suitable however, other methods may be used.

Anhydrous lactose is predominantly used as a filler/diluent in solid dosage forms (compressed and powder). The following characteristics are relevant for this type of application.

Particle size distribution. Determine by laser diffraction or sieve analysis.

Bulk and tapped density (*2.9.15*). Determine the bulk density and the tapped density. Calculate the Hausner index using the following expression:

$$\frac{V_0}{V_f}$$

V_0 = volume of bulk substance,

V_f = volume of tapped substance.

α-Lactose and β-lactose. Gas chromatography (*2.2.28*).

Silylation reagent. Mix 28 volumes of *N-trimethylsilylimidazole R* and 72 volumes of *pyridine R*.

Test solution. Dissolve about 1 mg of the substance to be examined in 0.45 ml of *dimethyl sulphoxide R*. Add 1.8 ml of the silylation reagent. Mix gently and allow to stand for 20 min.

Reference solution. Prepare a mixture of *α-lactose monohydrate R* and *β-lactose R* having an anomeric ratio of about 1:1 based on the labelled anomeric contents of the α-lactose monohydrate and β-lactose. Dissolve about 1 mg of this mixture in 0.45 ml of *dimethyl sulphoxide R*. Add 1.8 ml of the silylation reagent. Mix gently and allow to stand for 20 min.

Column:

- *material*: glass,
- *size*: *l* = 0.9 m, Ø = 4 mm,
- *stationary phase*: *silanised diatomaceous earth for gas chromatography R* impregnated with 3 per cent *m/m* of *poly[(cyanopropyl)(methyl)][(phenyl)(methyl)] siloxane R*.

Carrier gas: *helium for chromatography R*.

Flow rate: 40 ml/min.

Temperature:

- *column*: 215 °C,
- *injection port and detector*: 275 °C.

Detection: flame ionisation.

Injection: 2 µl.

System suitability: reference solution:

- *relative retention* with reference to β-lactose: α-lactose = about 0.7,
- *resolution*: minimum 3.0 between the peaks due to α-lactose and β-lactose.

Calculate the percentage content of α-lactose from the expression:

$$\frac{100S_a}{S_a + S_b}$$

Calculate the percentage content of β-lactose from the expression:

$$\frac{100S_b}{S_a + S_b}$$

S_a = area of the peak due to α-lactose,

S_b = area of the peak due to β-lactose.

Loss on drying (*2.2.32*). Determine on 1.000 g by drying in an oven at 80 °C for 2 h.

01/2005:0187

LACTOSE MONOHYDRATE

Lactosum monohydricum

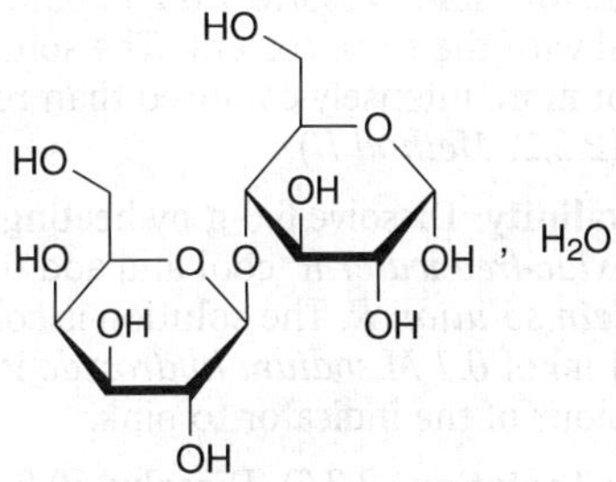

$C_{12}H_{22}O_{11},H_2O$ M_r 360.3

DEFINITION

Lactose monohydrate is the monohydrate of *O*-β-D-galactopyranosyl-(1→4)-α-D-glucopyranose.

CHARACTERS

A white or almost white, crystalline powder, freely but slowly soluble in water, practically insoluble in ethanol (96 per cent).

IDENTIFICATION

First identification: A, D.

Second identification: B, C, D.

A. Examine by infrared absorption spectrophotometry (*2.2.24*), comparing with the spectrum obtained with *lactose CRS*.

B. Examine by thin-layer chromatography (*2.2.27*), using a *TLC silica gel G plate R*.

Test solution. Dissolve 10 mg of the substance to be examined in a mixture of 2 volumes of *water R* and 3 volumes of *methanol R* and dilute to 20 ml with the same mixture of solvents.

Reference solution (a). Dissolve 10 mg of *lactose CRS* in a mixture of 2 volumes of *water R* and 3 volumes of *methanol R* and dilute to 20 ml with the same mixture of solvents.

Reference solution (b). Dissolve 10 mg each of *fructose CRS, glucose CRS, lactose CRS* and *sucrose CRS* in a mixture of 2 volumes of *water R* and 3 volumes of *methanol R* and dilute to 20 ml with the same mixture of solvents.

Apply separately to the plate 2 µl of each solution and thoroughly dry the starting points. Develop over a path of 15 cm using a mixture of 10 volumes of *water R*, 15 volumes of *methanol R*, 25 volumes of *glacial acetic acid R* and 50 volumes of *ethylene chloride R*, measured accurately since a slight excess of water produces cloudiness. Dry the plate in a current of warm air. Repeat the development immediately, after renewing the mobile phase. Dry the plate in a current of warm air and spray evenly with a solution of 0.5 g of *thymol R* in a mixture of 5 ml of *sulphuric acid R* and 95 ml of *alcohol R*. Heat at 130 °C for 10 min. The principal spot in the chromatogram obtained with the test solution is similar in position, colour and size to the principal spot in the chromatogram obtained with reference solution (a). The test is not valid unless the chromatogram obtained with reference solution (b) shows 4 clearly separated spots.

Monographs I-L

C. Dissolve 0.25 g in 5 ml of *water R*. Add 5 ml of *ammonia R* and heat in a water-bath at 80 °C for 10 min. A red colour develops.

D. It complies with the test for water (see Tests).

TESTS

Appearance of solution. Dissolve 1.0 g in boiling *water R*, dilute to 10 ml with the same solvent. The solution is clear (*2.2.1*) and not more intensely coloured than reference solution BY_7 (*2.2.2, Method II*).

Acidity or alkalinity. Dissolve 6.0 g by heating in 25 ml of *carbon dioxide-free water R*, cool and add 0.3 ml of *phenolphthalein solution R*. The solution is colourless. Not more than 0.4 ml of *0.1 M sodium hydroxide* is required to change the colour of the indicator to pink.

Specific optical rotation (*2.2.7*). Dissolve 10.0 g in 80 ml of *water R*, heating to 50 °C. Allow to cool and add 0.2 ml of *dilute ammonia R1*. Allow to stand for 30 min and dilute to 100.0 ml with *water R*. The specific optical rotation is + 54.4 to + 55.9, calculated with reference to the anhydrous substance.

Absorbance (*2.2.25*). Dissolve 1.0 g in boiling *water R* and dilute to 10.0 ml with the same solvent (solution A). The absorbance of the solution measured at 400 nm is not greater than 0.04. Dilute 1.0 ml of solution A to 10.0 ml with *water R*. Examine the solution from 210 nm to 300 nm. At wavelengths from 210 nm to 220 nm, the absorbance is not greater than 0.25. At wavelengths from 270 nm to 300 nm, the absorbance is not greater than 0.07.

Heavy metals (*2.4.8*). Dissolve 4.0 g in *water R* with warming, add 1 ml of *0.1 M hydrochloric acid* and dilute to 20 ml with *water R*. 12 ml of the solution complies with limit test A for heavy metals (5 ppm). Prepare the reference solution using *lead standard solution (1 ppm Pb) R*.

Water (*2.5.12*): 4.5 per cent to 5.5 per cent, determined on 0.50 g by the semi-micro determination of water, using a mixture of 1 volume of *formamide R* and 2 volumes of *methanol R* as the solvent.

Sulphated ash. Not more than 0.1 per cent. To 1.0 g add 1 ml of *sulphuric acid R*, evaporate to dryness on a water-bath and ignite to constant mass.

Microbial contamination. Total viable aerobic count (*2.6.12*) not more than 10^2 micro-organisms per gram, determined by plate-count. It complies with the test for *Escherichia coli* (*2.6.13*).

STORAGE

In an airtight container.

FUNCTIONALITY-RELATED CHARACTERISTICS

The following test are not mandatory requirements but in view of their known importance for achieving consistency in manufacture, quality and performance of medicinal products, it is recommended that suppliers should verify these characteristics and provide information on the results and analytical method applied to users. The methods indicated below have been found suitable however, other methods may be used.

Lactose monohydrate is predominantly used as a filler/diluent in solid dosage forms (compressed and powder). The following characteristics are relevant for this type of application.

Particle size distribution. Determine by laser diffraction or sieve analysis.

Bulk and tapped density (*2.9.15*). Determine the bulk density and the tapped density. Calculate the Hausner Index using the following expression:

$$\frac{V_0}{V_f}$$

V_0 = volume of bulk substance,

V_f = volume of tapped substance.

01/2005:1230

LACTULOSE

Lactulosum

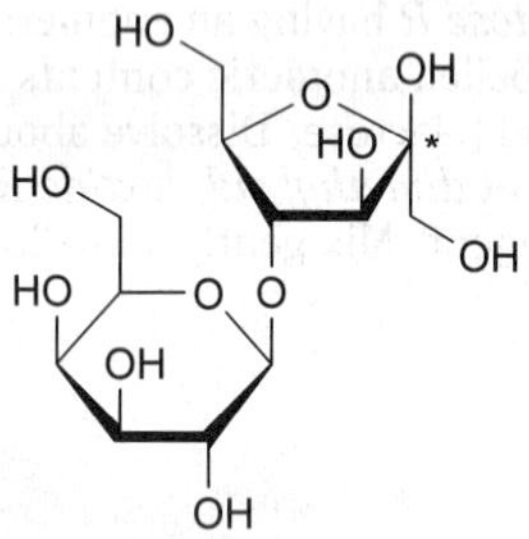

and epimer at C*

$C_{12}H_{22}O_{11}$ M_r 342.3

DEFINITION

Lactulose contains not less than 95.0 per cent and not more than the equivalent of 102.0 per cent of 4-*O*-(β-D-galactopyranosyl)-D-*arabino*-hex-2-ulofuranose, calculated with reference to the anhydrous substance.

CHARACTERS

A white or almost white, crystalline powder, freely soluble in water, sparingly soluble in methanol, practically insoluble in toluene.

It melts at about 168 °C.

IDENTIFICATION

First identification: B, C, D, E.

Second identification: A, C, D, E.

A. Examine by thin-layer chromatography (*2.2.27*), using *silica gel G R* as the coating substance.

Test solution. Dissolve 50.0 mg of the substance to be examined in *water R* and dilute to 10.0 ml with the same solvent.

Reference solution. Dissolve 50.0 mg of *lactulose CRS* in *water R* and dilute to 10.0 ml with the same solvent.

Apply separately to the plate 2 µl of each solution. Develop over a path of 15 cm using a mixture of 10 volumes of *glacial acetic acid R*, 15 volumes of a 50 g/l solution of *boric acid R*, 20 volumes of *methanol R* and 55 volumes of *ethyl acetate R*. Dry the plate at 100-105 °C for 5 min and allow to cool. Spray the plate with a 1.0 g/l solution of *1,3-dihydroxynaphthalene R* in a mixture of 10 volumes of *sulphuric acid R* and 90 volumes of *methanol R*. Heat the plate at 110 °C for 5 min. The principal spot in the chromatogram obtained with the test solution is similar in position, colour and size to the principal spot in the chromatogram obtained with the reference solution.

Monographs I-L

B. Examine the chromatograms obtained in the Assay. The principal peak in the chromatogram obtained with the test solution is similar in position and size to the principal peak in the chromatogram obtained with reference solution (b).

C. Dissolve 0.05 g in 10 ml of *water R*. Add 3 ml of *cupri-tartaric solution R* and heat. A red precipitate is formed.

D. Dissolve 0.125 g in 5 ml of *water R*. Add 5 ml of *ammonia R*. Heat on a water-bath at 80 °C for 10 min. A red colour develops.

E. It complies with the test for specific optical rotation (see Tests).

TESTS

Solution S. Dissolve 3.0 g in *carbon dioxide-free water R* and dilute to 50 ml with the same solvent.

Appearance of solution. Solution S is clear (*2.2.1*) and not more intensely coloured than reference solution BY_5 (*2.2.2, Method II*).

pH (*2.2.3*). To 10 ml of solution S add 0.1 ml of a saturated solution of *potassium chloride R*. The pH of the solution is 3.0 to 7.0.

Specific optical rotation (*2.2.7*). Dissolve 1.25 g of the substance to be examined in *water R*, add 0.2 ml of *concentrated ammonia R* and dilute to 25.0 ml with *water R*. The specific optical rotation is − 46.0 to − 50.0, calculated with reference to the anhydrous substance.

Related substances. Examine the chromatograms obtained in the Assay. In the chromatogram obtained with the test solution, the sum of the areas of any peaks corresponding to galactose, lactose, epilactose, tagatose and fructose is not greater than the area of the peak corresponding to lactulose in the chromatogram obtained with reference solution (a) (3 per cent).

Methanol. Examine by head-space gas chromatography (*2.2.28*).

Internal standard solution. Mix 0.5 ml of *propanol R* with 100.0 ml of *water R*. Dilute 1.0 ml to 100.0 ml with *water R*. Dilute 5.0 ml to 50.0 ml with *water R*.

Test solution. To 79 mg of the substance to be examined in a 20 ml vial add 1.0 ml of the internal standard solution and 5 µl of a 0.1 per cent *V/V* solution of *methanol R*.

Reference solution. To 1.0 ml of the internal standard solution in a 20 ml vial add 5 µl of a 0.1 per cent *V/V* solution of *methanol R*.

The chromatographic procedure may be carried out using:

– a column 2 m long and 2 mm in internal diameter packed with *ethylvinylbenzene-divinylbenzene copolymer R* (180 µm),
– *helium for chromatography R* as the carrier gas at a flow rate of 30 ml/min,
– a flame-ionisation detector,

maintaining the temperature of the column at 140 °C, that of the injection port at 200 °C and that of the detector at 220 °C. Maintain each solution at 60 °C for 1 h, pressurise for 1 min and transfer onto the column 1 ml of the gaseous phase.

In the chromatogram obtained with the test solution, the ratio of the area of the methanol peak to that of the internal standard peak is not greater than twice the corresponding ratio for the chromatogram obtained with the reference solution (50 ppm, calculated assuming the density (*2.2.5*) of methanol to be 0.79 g/ml at 20 °C).

Boron. *Avoid where possible the use of glassware.*

Reference solution. Dissolve 50.0 mg of *boric acid R* in *water R* and dilute to 100.0 ml with the same solvent. Dilute 5.0 ml of this solution to 100.0 ml with *water R*. *Keep in a well-closed polyethylene container.*

In 4 polyethylene 25 ml flasks, place:

– 0.50 g of the substance to be examined dissolved in 2.0 ml of *water R* (solution A),
– 0.50 g of the substance to be examined dissolved in 1.0 ml of the reference solution and 1.0 ml of *water R* (solution B),
– 1.0 ml of the reference solution and 1.0 ml of *water R* (solution C),
– 2.0 ml of *water R* (solution D).

To each flask, add 4.0 ml of *acetate-edetate buffer solution pH 5.5 R*. Mix and add 4.0 ml of freshly prepared *azomethine H solution R*. Mix and allow to stand for 1 h. Measure the absorbance (*2.2.25*) of solutions A, B and C at 420 nm, using solution D as the compensation liquid. The test is not valid unless the absorbance of solution C is at least 0.25. The absorbance of solution B is not less than twice that of solution A (9 ppm of boron).

Lead (*2.4.10*). It complies with the limit test for lead in sugars (0.5 ppm).

Water (*2.5.12*). Not more than 2.5 per cent, determined on 0.500 g by the semi-micro determination of water.

Sulphated ash (*2.4.14*). Not more than 0.1 per cent, determined on 1.0 g.

Microbial contamination. Total viable aerobic count (*2.6.12*) not more than 10^2 micro-organisms per gram, determined by plate count. It complies with the test for *Escherichia coli* (*2.6.13*).

ASSAY

Examine by liquid chromatography (*2.2.29*).

Test solution. Dissolve 1.00 g of the substance to be examined in 10 ml of *water R*. Add 12.5 ml of *acetonitrile R* with gentle heating and dilute to 25.0 ml with *water R*.

Reference solution (a). To 3 ml of the test solution add 47.5 ml of *acetonitrile R* with gentle heating and dilute to 100.0 ml with *water R*.

Reference solution (b). Dissolve 1.00 g of *lactulose CRS* in 10 ml of *water R*. Add 12.5 ml of *acetonitrile R* with gentle heating and dilute to 25.0 ml with *water R*.

Reference solution (c). Dissolve the contents of 1 vial of *lactulose for system suitability CRS* in 1 ml of a mixture of equal volumes of *acetonitrile R* and *water R*.

The chromatographic procedure may be carried out using:

– a stainless steel column 0.05 m long and 4.6 mm in internal diameter followed by a stainless steel column 0.15 m long and 4.6 mm in internal diameter, both packed with *aminopropylsilyl silica gel for chromatography R* (3 µm) and maintained at 38 ± 1 °C,
– as mobile phase at a flow rate of 1.0 ml/min a mixture prepared as follows: dissolve 0.253 g of *sodium dihydrogen phosphate R* in 220 ml of *water R* and add 780 ml of *acetonitrile R*,
– as detector a refractometer maintained at a constant temperature.

When the chromatograms are recorded in the prescribed conditions, the retention time of lactulose is about 18.3 min and relative retentions to lactulose are about 0.38 for tagatose, 0.42 for fructose, 0.57 for galactose, 0.90 for epilactose and 1.17 for lactose.

Monographs I-L

Inject 20 µl of reference solution (c). The test is not valid unless the chromatogram obtained has a similar profile to the chromatogram supplied with *lactulose for system suitability CRS* and the resolution between the peaks corresponding to lactulose and epilactose is at least 1.3. If necessary, adjust the concentration of *acetonitrile R* in the mobile phase to between 75.0 per cent *V/V* and 82.0 per cent *V/V* to achieve the prescribed resolution.

Inject separately 20 µl of the test solution and 20 µl of reference solution (b) and continue the chromatography for 2.5 times the retention time of lactulose. Calculate the percentage content of $C_{12}H_{22}O_{11}$ (lactulose) from the areas of the peaks and the declared content of *lactulose CRS*.

IMPURITIES

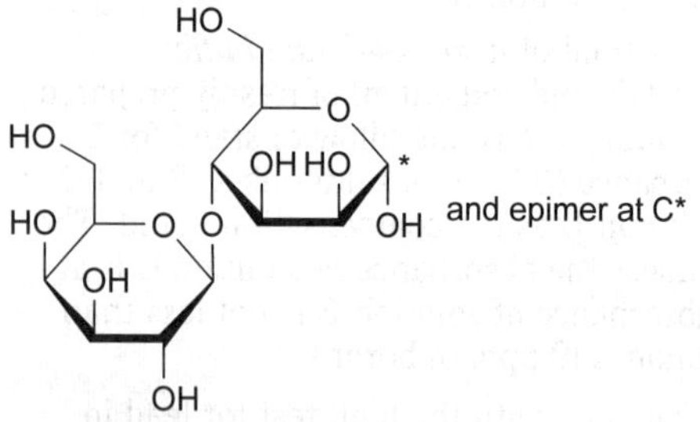

A. 4-*O*-(β-D-galactopyranosyl)-D-mannopyranose (epilactose),

B. galactose,

C. lactose,

D. fructose,

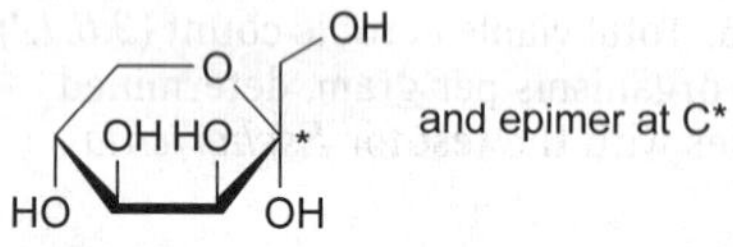

E. D-*lyxo*-hex-2-ulopyranose (tagatose).

01/2005:0924

LACTULOSE, LIQUID

Lactulosum liquidum

DEFINITION

Liquid lactulose is an aqueous solution of 4-*O*-(β-D-galactopyranosyl)-D-*arabino*-hex-2-ulofuranose normally prepared by alkaline isomerisation of lactose. It may contain lesser amounts of other sugars including lactose, epilactose, galactose, tagatose and fructose. It contains not less than 620 g/l of lactulose ($C_{12}H_{22}O_{11}$; M_r 342.3) and not less than 95.0 per cent and not more than 105.0 per cent of the declared content of lactulose. It may contain a suitable antimicrobial preservative.

CHARACTERS

A clear, viscous liquid, colourless or pale brownish-yellow, miscible with water. It may be a supersaturated solution or may contain crystals which disappear on heating.

A 10 per cent *V/V* solution is laevorotatory.

IDENTIFICATION

First identification: B, C, D.

Second identification: A, C, D.

A. Examine by thin-layer chromatography (*2.2.27*), using *silica gel G R* as the coating substance.

Test solution. Dilute 0.50 g of the substance to be examined to 50 ml with *water R*.

Reference solution. Dissolve 60 mg of *lactulose CRS* in *water R* and dilute to 10 ml with the same solvent.

Apply separately to the plate 2 µl of each solution. Develop over a path of 15 cm using a mixture of 10 volumes of *glacial acetic acid R*, 15 volumes of a 50 g/l solution of *boric acid R*, 20 volumes of *methanol R* and 55 volumes of *ethyl acetate R*. Dry the plate at 100-105 °C for 5 min and allow to cool. Spray the plate with a 1.0 g/l solution of *1,3-dihydroxynaphthalene R* in a mixture of 10 volumes of *sulphuric acid R* and 90 volumes of *methanol R*. Heat the plate at 110 °C for 5 min. The principal spot in the chromatogram obtained with the test solution is similar in position, colour and size to the principal spot in the chromatogram obtained with the reference solution.

B. Examine the chromatograms obtained in the Assay. The retention time of the principal peak in the chromatogram obtained with the test solution is approximately the same as that of the principal peak in the chromatogram obtained with reference solution (b).

C. To 0.1 g add 10 ml of *water R* and 3 ml of *cupri-tartaric solution R* and heat. A red precipitate is formed.

D. To 0.25 g add 5 ml of *water R* and 5 ml of *ammonia R*. Heat in a water-bath at 80 °C for 10 min. A red colour develops.

TESTS

Solution S. Mix 10 g with *carbon dioxide-free water R* and dilute to 100 ml with the same solvent.

Appearance of solution. Solution S is clear (*2.2.1*) and not more intensely coloured than reference solution BY_5 (*2.2.2, Method II*).

pH (*2.2.3*). To 10 ml of solution S, add 0.1 ml of a saturated solution of *potassium chloride R*. The pH of the solution is 3.0 to 7.0.

Related substances. Examine the chromatograms obtained in the Assay. In the chromatogram obtained with the test solution: the area of any peak corresponding to galactose is not greater than 3 times the area of the peak corresponding to lactulose in the chromatogram obtained with reference solution (a) (15 per cent); the area of any peak corresponding to lactose is not greater than twice the area of the peak corresponding to lactulose in the chromatogram obtained with reference solution (a) (10 per cent); the area of any peak corresponding to epilactose is not greater than twice the area of the peak corresponding to lactulose in the chromatogram obtained with reference solution (a) (10 per cent); the area of any peak corresponding to tagatose is not greater than 0.8 times the area of the peak corresponding to lactulose in the chromatogram obtained with reference solution (a) (4 per cent); the area of any peak corresponding to fructose is not greater than 0.2 times the area of the peak corresponding to lactulose in the chromatogram obtained with reference solution (a) (1 per cent).

Methanol. Examine by head-space gas chromatography (*2.2.28*).

Internal standard solution. Mix 0.5 ml of *propanol R* with 100.0 ml of *water R*. Dilute 1.0 ml to 100.0 ml with *water R*. Dilute 5.0 ml to 50.0 ml with *water R*.

Test solution. To 0.13 g of the substance to be examined in a 20 ml vial add 1.0 ml of the internal standard solution. Add 5 µl of a 0.1 per cent *V/V* solution of *methanol R*.

Reference solution. To 1.0 ml of the internal standard solution in a 20 ml vial add 5 µl of a 0.1 per cent *V/V* solution of *methanol R*.

The chromatographic procedure may be carried out using:

- a column 2 m long and 2 mm in internal diameter packed with *ethylvinylbenzene-divinylbenzene copolymer R* (180 μm),
- *helium for chromatography R* as the carrier gas at a flow rate of 30 ml/min,
- a flame-ionisation detector,

maintaining the temperature of the column at 140 °C, that of the injection port at 200 °C and that of the detector at 220 °C. Maintain each solution at 60 °C for 1 h, pressurise for 1 min and transfer onto the column 1 ml of the gaseous phase.

In the chromatogram obtained with the test solution, the ratio of the area of the methanol peak to that of the internal standard peak is not greater than twice the corresponding ratio for the chromatogram obtained with the reference solution (30 ppm calculated assuming the density (*2.2.5*) of methanol to be 0.79 g/ml at 20 °C).

Sulphites. Mix 5.0 g with 40 ml of *water R*, add 2.0 ml of *0.1 M sodium hydroxide* and dilute to 100 ml with *water R*. To 10.0 ml of the solution, add 1.0 ml of *hydrochloric acid R1*, 2.0 ml of *decolorised fuchsin solution R1* and 2.0 ml of a 0.5 per cent *V/V* solution of *formaldehyde R*. Allow to stand for 30 min and measure the absorbance (*2.2.25*) of the solution at 583 nm using as the compensation liquid a solution prepared simultaneously and in the same manner using 10.0 ml of *water R* instead of the solution of the substance to be examined. The absorbance is not greater than that of a reference solution prepared simultaneously and in the same manner, using 10.0 ml of *sulphite standard solution (1.5 ppm SO_2) R* instead of the solution of the substance to be examined (30 ppm).

Boron. *Avoid where possible the use of glassware.*

Reference solution. Dissolve 56.0 mg of *boric acid R* in *water R* and dilute to 100.0 ml with the same solvent. Dilute 5.0 ml of this solution to 100.0 ml with *water R*. *Keep in a well-closed polyethylene container.*

In 4 polyethylene 25 ml flasks, place:

- 1.00 g of the substance to be examined and 1 ml of *water R* (solution A),
- 1.00 g of the substance to be examined and 1 ml of the reference solution (solution B),
- 1 ml of the reference solution and 1 ml of *water R* (solution C),
- 2 ml of *water R* (solution D).

To each flask, add 4.0 ml of *acetate-edetate buffer solution pH 5.5 R*. Mix and add 4.0 ml of freshly prepared *azomethine H solution R*. Mix and allow to stand for 1 h. Measure the absorbance (*2.2.25*) of solutions A, B and C at 420 nm, using solution D as the compensation liquid. The test is not valid unless the absorbance of solution C is at least 0.25. The absorbance of solution B is not less than twice that of solution A (5 ppm of B).

Lead (*2.4.10*). It complies with the limit test for lead in sugars (0.5 ppm, calculated with reference to the declared content of lactulose).

Sulphated ash (*2.4.14*). Not more than 0.2 per cent, determined on 1.5 g and calculated with reference to the declared content of lactulose.

Microbial contamination. Total viable aerobic count (*2.6.12*) not more than 10^2 micro-organisms per gram, determined by plate count. It complies with the test for *Escherichia coli* (*2.6.13*).

ASSAY

Examine by liquid chromatography (*2.2.29*).

Test solution. Mix 4.00 g of the substance to be examined with 20 ml of *water R*. Add 25.0 ml of *acetonitrile R* with gentle heating and dilute to 50.0 ml with *water R*.

Reference solution (a). To 5 ml of the test solution, add 47.5 ml of *acetonitrile R* with gentle heating and dilute to 100.0 ml with *water R*.

Reference solution (b). Dissolve 2.00 g of *lactulose CRS* in 20 ml of *water R*. Add 25.0 ml of *acetonitrile R* with gentle heating and dilute to 50.0 ml with *water R*.

Reference solution (c). Dissolve the contents of 1 vial of *lactulose for system suitability CRS* in 1 ml of a mixture of equal volumes of *acetonitrile R* and *water R*.

The chromatographic procedure may be carried out using:

- a stainless steel column 0.05 m long and 4.6 mm in internal diameter followed by a stainless steel column 0.15 m long and 4.6 mm in internal diameter, both packed with *aminopropylsilyl silica gel for chromatography R* (3 μm) and maintained at 38 ± 1 °C,
- as mobile phase at a flow rate of 1.0 ml/min a mixture prepared as follows: dissolve 0.253 g of *sodium dihydrogen phosphate R* in 220 ml of *water R* and add 780 ml of *acetonitrile R*,
- as detector a refractometer maintained at a constant temperature.

When the chromatograms are recorded in the prescribed conditions, the retention time of lactulose is about 18 min and relative retentions to lactulose are about: 0.38 for tagatose, 0.42 for fructose, 0.57 for galactose, 0.90 for epilactose and 1.17 for lactose.

Inject 20 μl of reference solution (c). The test is not valid unless the chromatogram obtained has a similar profile to the chromatogram supplied with *lactulose for system suitability CRS* and the resolution between the peaks corresponding to lactulose and epilactose is at least 1.3. If necessary, adjust the concentration of *acetonitrile R* in the mobile phase to between 75.0 per cent *V/V* and 82.0 per cent *V/V* to achieve the prescribed resolution.

Inject separately 20 μl of the test solution and 20 μl of reference solution (b) and continue the chromatography for 2.5 times the retention time of lactulose. Calculate the percentage content of $C_{12}H_{22}O_{11}$ (lactulose) from the areas of the peaks and the declared content of *lactulose CRS*.

LABELLING

The label states:

- the declared content of lactulose,
- the name and concentration of any added antimicrobial preservative.

Monographs I-L

IMPURITIES

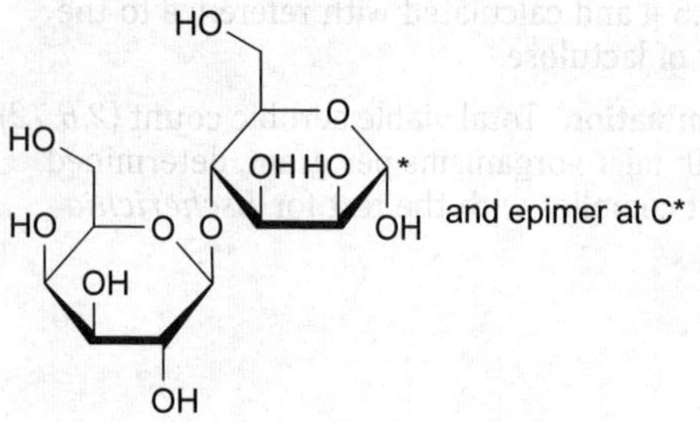

A. 4-*O*-(β-D-galactopyranosyl)-D-mannopyranose (epilactose),

B. galactose,

C. lactose,

D. fructose,

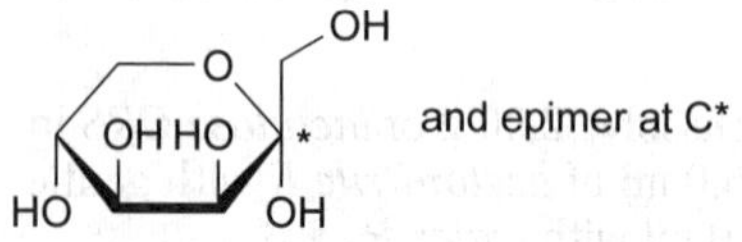

E. D-*lyxo*-hex-2-ulopyranose (tagatose).

01/2005:1231

LAUROYL MACROGOLGLYCERIDES

Macrogolglyceridorum laurates

DEFINITION

Lauroyl macrogolglycerides are mixtures of monoesters, diesters and triesters of glycerol and monoesters and diesters of macrogols with a mean relative molecular mass between 300 and 1500. They are obtained by partial alcoholysis of saturated oils mainly containing triglycerides of lauric acid using macrogol or by esterification of glycerol and macrogol with saturated fatty acids or by mixing of glycerol esters and condensates of ethylene oxide with the fatty acids of these hydrogenated oils.

CHARACTERS

Pale yellow waxy solids, dispersible in hot water, freely soluble in methylene chloride.

IDENTIFICATION

A. Examine by thin-layer chromatography (*2.2.27*), using a suitable silica gel as the coating substance.

Test solution. Dissolve 1.0 g of the substance to be examined in *methylene chloride R* and dilute to 20 ml with the same solvent.

Apply to the plate 10 μl of the test solution. Develop over a path of 15 cm using a mixture of 30 volumes of *hexane R* and 70 volumes of *ether R*. Allow the plate to dry in air. Spray with a 0.1 g/l solution of *rhodamine B R* in *alcohol R* and examine in ultraviolet light at 365 nm. The chromatogram shows a spot corresponding to triglycerides with an R_f value of about 0.9 (R_{st} 1) and spots corresponding to 1,3-diglycerides (R_{st} 0.7), to 1,2-diglycerides (R_{st} 0.6), to monoglycerides (R_{st} 0.1) and to esters of macrogol (R_{st} 0).

B. They comply with the test for hydroxyl value (see Tests).

C. They comply with the test for fatty acid composition (see Tests).

D. They comply with the test for saponification value (see Tests).

TESTS

Drop point (*2.2.17*). Introduce into the cup the substance to be examined which has been melted by heating for 1 h in an oven at 100 ± 2 °C and allow to stand for 5 h at about 5 °C. The drop point is indicated in Table 1231.-1.

Table 1231.-1

Ethylene oxide units per molecule (nominal value)	Type of macrogol	Drop point
6	300	33 to 38
8	400	36 to 41
12	600	38 to 43
32	1500	42.5 to 47.5

Acid value (*2.5.1*). Not more than 2.0, determined on 2.0 g.

Hydroxyl value (*2.5.3, Method A*). The ranges are presented in Table 1231.-2, determined on 1.0 g.

Table 1231.-2

Ethylene oxide units per molecule (nominal value)	Type of macrogol	Hydroxyl value
6	300	65 to 85
8	400	60 to 80
12	600	50 to 70
32	1500	36 to 56

Peroxide value (*2.5.5*). Not more than 6.0, determined on 2.0 g.

Saponification value (*2.5.6*). The ranges are presented in Table 1231.-3, determined on 2.0 g.

Table 1231.-3

Ethylene oxide units per molecule (nominal value)	Type of macrogol	Saponification value
6	300	190 to 204
8	400	170 to 190
12	600	150 to 170
32	1500	79 to 93

Alkaline impurities. Introduce 5.0 g into a test tube and carefully add a mixture, neutralised if necessary with *0.01 M hydrochloric acid* or with *0.01 M sodium hydroxide*, of 0.05 ml of a 0.4 g/l solution of *bromophenol blue R* in *alcohol R*, 0.3 ml of *water R* and 10 ml of *alcohol R*. Shake and allow to stand. Not more than 1.0 ml of *0.01 M hydrochloric acid* is required to change the colour of the upper layer to yellow.

Free glycerol. Not more than 3.0 per cent. Dissolve 1.20 g in 25.0 ml of *methylene chloride R*. Heat if necessary. After cooling, add 100 ml of *water R*. Shake and add 25.0 ml of a 6 g/l solution of *periodic acid R*. Shake and allow to stand for 30 min. Add 40 ml of a 75 g/l solution of *potassium iodide R*. Allow to stand for 1 min. Add 1 ml of *starch solution R*. Titrate the iodine with *0.1 M sodium thiosulphate*. Carry out a blank titration.

1 ml of *0.1 M sodium thiosulphate* is equivalent to 2.3 mg of glycerol.

Composition of fatty acids (*2.4.22, Method A*). The fatty acid fraction has the following composition:

– *caprylic acid*: not more than 15.0 per cent,
– *capric acid*: not more than 12.0 per cent,
– *lauric acid*: 30.0 per cent to 50.0 per cent,

Monographs I-L

- *myristic acid*: 5.0 per cent to 25.0 per cent,
- *palmitic acid*: 4.0 per cent to 25.0 per cent,
- *stearic acid*: 5.0 per cent to 35.0 per cent.

Ethylene oxide and dioxan (*2.4.25*). Not more than 1 ppm of ethylene oxide and not more than 10 ppm of dioxan.

Heavy metals (*2.4.8*). 2.0 g complies with limit test C for heavy metals (10 ppm). Prepare the standard using 2 ml of *lead standard solution (10 ppm Pb) R*.

Water (*2.5.12*). Not more than 1.0 per cent, determined on 1.0 g by the semi-micro determination of water using a mixture of 30 volumes of *anhydrous methanol R* and 70 volumes of *methylene chloride R* as solvent.

Total ash (*2.4.16*). Not more than 0.1 per cent, determined on 1.0 g.

LABELLING

The label states the type of macrogol used (mean relative molecular mass) or the number of units of ethylene oxide per molecule (nominal value).

01/2005:1534

LAVENDER FLOWER

Lavandulae flos

DEFINITION

Lavender flower consists of the dried flower of *Lavandula angustifolia* P. Mill. (*L. officinalis* Chaix). It contains not less than 13 ml/kg of essential oil, calculated with reference to the anhydrous drug.

CHARACTERS

Lavender flower has a strongly aromatic odour.

It has the macroscopic and microscopic characters described under identification tests A and B.

IDENTIFICATION

First identification: A, B, D.
Second identification: A, B, C.

A. The flower has a short peduncle and consists of a bluish-grey tubular calyx divided distally into four very short teeth and a small rounded lobe, a blue bilabial corolla with the upper lip bifid and the lower lip trilobate, four didynamous stamens with ovoid anthers.

B. Reduce to a powder (355). The powder is bluish-grey. Examine under a microscope using *chloral hydrate solution R*. The powder shows covering trichomes bifurcating at one or more levels; secretory trichomes with short stalks and eight-celled heads of the *Labiatae* type; secretory trichomes with unicellular or multicellular stalks and unicellular heads; secretory trichomes with long uneven stalks and unicellular heads, separated from the peduncle by an intermediary cell with a smooth cuticle; certain such trichomes show a crown of small spheroid cells just below the insertion point of the intermediary cell on the peduncle; fragments of warty epidermis from the inner surface of the petals; fragments of calyx epidermis with sinuous-walled cells and containing prismatic crystals of calcium oxalate; spherical pollen grains which have a diameter of about 45 µm and an exine with six slit-like germinal pores and six ribbon-like groins radiating from the poles.

C. Examine by thin-layer chromatography (*2.2.27*), using a *TLC silica gel plate R*.

Test solution. To 0.5 g of the powdered drug (355) add 5 ml of *hexane R*, shake for 5 min and filter.

Reference solution. Dissolve 10 µl of *linalol R* and 10 µl of *linalyl acetate R* in 5 ml of *hexane R*.

Apply to the plate as bands 10 µl of each solution. Develop over a path of 15 cm using a mixture of 5 volumes of *ethyl acetate R* and 95 volumes of *toluene R*. Allow the plate to dry in air. Spray the plate with *anisaldehyde solution R* and examine in daylight while heating at 100 °C to 105 °C for 5 min to 10 min. The chromatogram obtained with the reference solution shows in the lower third a greyish-blue zone (linalol) and in the middle third a greyish-blue zone (linalyl acetate). The chromatogram obtained with the test solution shows zones corresponding to linalol and linalyl acetate and in the middle, between these zones, a redish-violet zone (epoxydihydrocaryophyllene). Further zones are also present.

D. Examine the chromatograms obtained in the test for other species and varieties of lavender. The five principal peaks in the chromatogram obtained with the reference solution are similar in retention time to peaks in the chromatogram obtained with the test solution. Among them are mainly linalol and linalyl acetate peaks.

TESTS

Foreign matter (*2.8.2*). Not more than 3 per cent of stems and not more than 2 per cent of other foreign matter.

Other species and varieties of lavender. Examine by gas chromatography (*2.2.28*).

Test solution. Dilute 0.2 ml of the essential oil-xylene mixture obtained in the assay to 5 ml with *hexane R*, add 1 g of *anhydrous sodium sulphate R*, shake and use the supernatant liquid.

Reference solution. Dissolve 0.1 g of *limonene R*, 0.2 g of *cineole R*, 0.05 g of *camphor R*, 0.4 g of *linalol R*, 0.6 g of *linalyl acetate R* and 0.2 g of *α-terpineol R* in 100 ml of *hexane R*.

The chromatographic procedure may be carried out using:

- a fused-silica column about 60 m long and about 0.25 mm in internal diameter, coated with *macrogol 20 000 R*,
- *helium for chromatography R* as the carrier gas at a flow rate of 1.5 ml per/min,
- a flame-ionisation detector,
- a split ratio of 1:100,

with the following temperature programme:

	Time (min)	Temperature (°C)	Rate (°C/min)	Comment
Column	0 - 15	70	–	isothermal
	15 - 70	70 → 180	2	linear gradient
Injection port		220		
Detector		220		

Inject the same volume of each solution. When the chromatograms are recorded under the prescribed conditions, the components are eluted in the order indicated in the composition of the reference solution. Record the retention times of these substances.

The test is not valid unless: the number of theoretical plates calculated from the limonene peak at 110 °C is at least 30 000, and the resolution between the peak corresponding to limonene and that corresponding to cineole is at least 1.5.

Using the retention times determined from the chromatogram obtained with the reference solution, locate the six components of the reference solution in the chromatogram obtained with the test solution. Disregard the peaks due to hexane and xylene.
In the chromatogram obtained with the test solution the area of the peak due to camphor is not greater than 1 per cent of the total area of the peaks.

Water (*2.2.13*). Not more than 100 ml/kg, determined by distillation using 20.0 g of drug.

Total ash (*2.4.16*). Not more than 9.0 per cent.

ASSAY

Carry out the determination of essential oils in vegetable drugs (*2.8.12*). Use 20.0 g of the drug, a 1000 ml round-bottomed flask, 500 ml of *water R* as the distillation liquid and 0.5 ml of *xylene R* in the graduated tube. Distil at a rate of 2 ml/min to 3 ml/min for 2 h.

STORAGE

Store protected from light.

01/2005:1338

LAVENDER OIL

Lavandulae aetheroleum

DEFINITION

Essential oil obtained by steam distillation from the flowering tops of *Lavandula angustifolia* Miller (*Lavandula officinalis* Chaix).

CHARACTERS

Appearance: colourless or pale yellow, clear liquid.

It has a characteristic odour.

IDENTIFICATION

First identification: B.

Second identification: A.

A. Thin-layer chromatography (*2.2.27*).

Test solution. Dissolve 20 µl of the substance to be examined in 1 ml of *toluene R.*

Reference solution. Dissolve 10 µl of *linalol R* and 10 µl of *linalyl acetate R* in 1 ml of *toluene R.*

Plate: *TLC silica gel plate R.*

Mobile phase: *ethyl acetate R, toluene R* (5:95 *V/V*).

Application: 10 µl as bands.

Development: twice, 5 min apart, over a path of 10 cm.

Drying: in air.

Detection: spray with *anisaldehyde solution R* and heat at 100-105 °C for 5-10 min. Examine immediately in daylight.

Results: see below the sequence of zones present in the chromatograms obtained with the reference solution and the test solution. Furthermore, other violet-red or greenish-brown zones are present in the chromatogram obtained with the test solution above the zone of linalyl acetate up to the solvent front.

Top of the plate	
	Several violet-red or greenish-brown zones
———	———
Linalyl acetate: a violet to brown zone	
	A violet to brown zone (linalyl acetate)
	A violet-red zone
	Possibly a weak violet-brown zone (cineole)
———	———
Linalol: a violet to brown zone	A violet to brown zone (linalol)
	A weak brownish-green zone
	Several unresolved zones
Reference solution	**Test solution**

B. Examine the chromatograms obtained in the test for chromatographic profile.

Results: the characteristic peaks in the chromatogram obtained with the test solution are similar in retention time to those in the chromatogram obtained with reference solution (a).

TESTS

Relative density (*2.2.5*): 0.878 to 0.892.

Refractive index (*2.2.6*): 1.455 to 1.466.

Optical rotation (*2.2.7*): − 12.5° to − 7.0°.

Acid value (*2.5.1*): maximum 1.0, determined on 5.0 g of the substance to be examined dissolved in 50 ml of the prescribed mixture of solvents.

Chromatographic profile. Gas chromatography (*2.2.28*): use the normalisation procedure.

Test solution. The substance to be examined.

Reference solution (a). Dissolve 0.1 g of *limonene R*, 0.2 g of *cineole R*, 0.2 g of *3-octanone R*, 0.05 g of *camphor R*, 0.4 g of *linalol R*, 0.6 g of *linalyl acetate R*, 0.2 g of *terpinen-4-ol R*, 0.1 g of *lavandulyl acetate R*, 0.2 g of *lavandulol R* and 0.2 g of *α-terpineol R* in 5 ml of *hexane R*.

Reference solution (b). Dissolve 5 mg of *3-octanone R* in *hexane R* and dilute to 10 ml with the same solvent.

Column:

– *material*: fused silica,
– *size*: *l* = 60 m , Ø = 0.25 mm,
– *stationary phase*: *macrogol 20 000 R* (film thickness 0.25 mm).

Carrier gas: *helium for chromatography R.*

Flow rate: 1.5 ml/min.

Split ratio: 1:100.

Temperature:

	Time (min)	Temperature (°C)
Column	0 - 15	70
	15 - 70	70 → 180
Injection port		220
Detector		220

Detection: flame ionisation.

Injection: 0.2 µl.

Elution order: order indicated in the composition of reference solution (a). Record the retention times of these substances.

System suitability: reference solution (a):

– *resolution*: minimum 1.4 between the peaks due to terpinen-4-ol and lavandulyl acetate.

Using the retention times determined from the chromatogram obtained with reference solution (a), locate the components of reference solution (a) in the chromatogram obtained with the test solution.

Determine the percentage content of each of these components. The percentages are within the following ranges:

– *limonene*: less than 1.0 per cent,
– *cineole*: less than 2.5 per cent,
– *3-octanone*: 0.1 per cent to 2.5 per cent,
– *camphor*: less than 1.2 per cent,
– *linalol*: 20.0 per cent to 45.0 per cent,
– *linalyl acetate*: 25.0 per cent to 46.0 per cent,
– *terpinen-4-ol*: 0.1 per cent to 6.0 per cent,
– *lavandulyl acetate*: more than 0.2 per cent,
– *lavandulol*: more than 0.1 per cent,
– *α-terpineol*: less than 2.0 per cent.
– *disregard limit*: area of the peak in the chromatogram obtained with reference solution (b) (0.05 per cent).

Chiral purity. Gas chromatography (*2.2.28*).

Test solution. Dissolve 0.02 g of the substance to be examined in *pentane R* and dilute to 10 ml with the same solvent.

Reference solution. Dissolve 10 µl of *linalol R*, add 10 µl of *linalyl acetate R* and 5 mg of *borneol R* in *pentane R* and dilute to 10 ml with the same solvent.

Column:

– *material*: fused silica,
– *size*: l = 25 m, Ø = 0.25 mm,
– *stationary phase*: *modified β-cyclodextrin for chiral chromatography R* (film thickness 0.25 µm).

Carrier gas: *helium for chromatography R.*

Flow rate: 1.3 ml/min.

Split ratio: 1:30.

Temperature:

	Time (min)	Temperature (°C)
Column	0 - 65	50 → 180
Injection port		230
Detector		230

Detection: flame ionisation.

Injection: 1 µl.

System suitability: reference solution:

– *resolution*: minimum 5.5 between the peaks due to (*R*)-linalol (1st peak) and (*S*)-linalol (2nd peak), minimum 2.9 between the peaks due to (*S*)-linalol and borneol (3rd peak) and minimum 2.7 between the peaks due to (*R*)-linalyl acetate (4th peak) and (*S*)-linalyl acetate (5th peak).

Limits: calculate the percentage content of the specified (*S*)-enantiomers from the expression:

$$\frac{A_S}{A_S + A_R} \times 100$$

A_S = area of the peak due to the corresponding (*S*)-enantiomer,

A_R = area of the peak due to the corresponding (*R*)-enantiomer.

– *(S)-linalol*: maximum 12 per cent,
– *(S)-linalyl acetate*: maximum 1 per cent.

STORAGE

In a well-filled, airtight container, protected from light, at a temperature not exceeding 25 °C.

01/2005:0620 corrected

LEMON OIL

Limonis aetheroleum

DEFINITION

Essential oil obtained by suitable mechanical means, without the aid of heat, from the fresh peel of *Citrus limon* (L.) Burman fil.

CHARACTERS

Appearance: clear, mobile, pale yellow to greenish-yellow liquid with a characteristic odour. It may become cloudy at low temperatures.

IDENTIFICATION

First identification: B.

Second identification: A.

A. Thin-layer chromatography (*2.2.27*).

Test solution. Mix 1 ml of the substance to be examined in 1 ml of *toluene R*.

Reference solution. Dissolve 10 mg of *citropten R* and 50 µl of *citral R* in *toluene R* and dilute to 10 ml with the same solvent.

Plate: *TLC silica gel GF_{254} plate R.*

Mobile phase: *ethyl acetate R, toluene R* (15:85 *V/V*).

Application: 10 µl, as bands.

Development: over a path of 15 cm.

Drying: in air.

Detection A: examine in ultraviolet light at 254 nm.

Results A: see below the sequence of the zones present in the chromatograms obtained with the reference solution and the test solution.

Top of the plate	
	A quenching zone (bergamotin)
Citral: a quenching zone	A quenching zone (citral)
	A dark blue zone (5-geranyloxy-7-methoxycoumarin)
Citropten: a light blue fluorescent zone	A light blue fluorescent zone (citropten)
	A quenching zone (psoralen derivative)
	A quenching zone (biakangelicin)
Reference solution	**Test solution**

Monographs I-L

Detection B: examine in ultraviolet light at 365 nm.

Results B: see below the sequence of the zones present in the chromatograms obtained with the reference solution and the test solution.

Top of the plate	
	A yellow fluorescent zone (bergamotin)
Citral: a quenching zone	A quenching zone (citral)
	A bright blue fluorescent zone (5-geranyloxy-7-methoxycoumarin)
Citropten: a bright blue fluorescent zone	A bright violet-blue fluorescent zone (citropten)
	A yellow fluorescent zone (psoralen derivative)
	An orange zone (biakangelicin)
Reference solution	**Test solution**

B. Examine the chromatograms obtained in the test for chromatographic profile.

Results: the characteristic peaks in the chromatogram obtained with the test solution are similar in retention time to those in the chromatogram obtained with the reference solution.

TESTS

Relative density (*2.2.5*): 0.850 to 0.858.

Refractive index (*2.2.6*): 1.473 to 1.476.

Optical rotation (*2.2.7*): + 57° to + 70°.

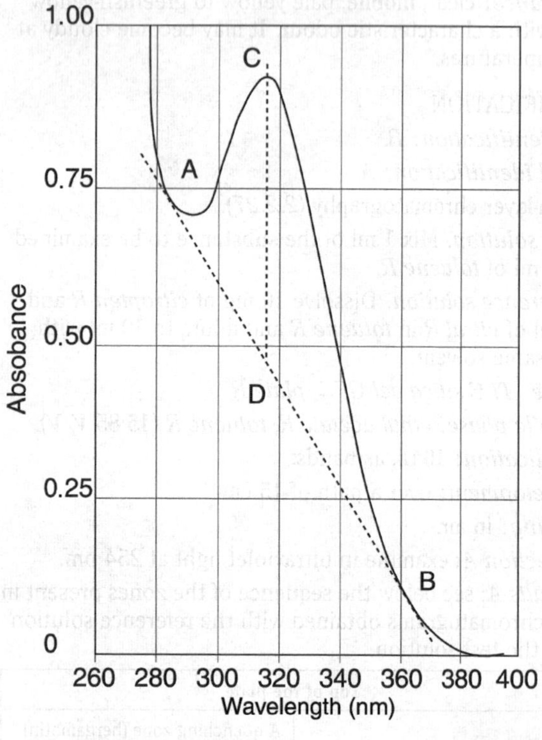

Figure 0620.-1. – *Typical spectrum of lemon oil for the test for absorbance*

Absorbance (*2.2.25*). Dissolve 0.250 g of the substance to be examined in *alcohol R*, mix and dilute to 100.0 ml with the same solvent. Measure the absorbance over the range 260 nm to 400 nm. If a manual instrument is used, measure the absorbance at 5 nm intervals from 260 nm to about 12 nm before the expected absorption maximum, then at 3 nm intervals for 3 readings and at 1 nm intervals to about 5 nm beyond the maximum and finally at 10 nm intervals to 400 nm. Plot a curve representing the absorption spectrum with the absorbances as ordinates and the wavelengths as abscissae. Draw as a baseline the tangent between *A* and *B* (Figure 0620.-1). The absorption maximum *C* is situated at 315 ± 3 nm. From *C* draw a line perpendicular to the axis of abscissae and intersecting *AB* at *D*. Deduct the absorbance corresponding to point *D* from that corresponding to point *C*. The value *C* – *D* is 0.20 to 0.96 and for Italian-type lemon oil it is not less than 0.45.

Fatty oils and resinified essential oils (*2.8.7*). It complies with the test for fatty oils and resinified essential oils.

Chromatographic profile. Gas chromatography (*2.2.28*): use the normalisation procedure.

Test solution. The substance to be examined.

Reference solution. Dissolve 20 µl of *β-pinene R*, 10 µl of *sabinene R*, 100 µl of *limonene R*, 10 µl of *γ-terpinene R*, 5 µl of *β-caryophyllene R*, 20 µl of *citral R*, 5 µl of *α-terpineol R*, 5 µl of *neryl acetate R* and 5 µl of *geranyl acetate R* in 1 ml of *acetone R*.

Column:

- *material*: fused silica,
- *size*: *l* = 30 m (a film thickness of 1 µm may be used) to 60 m (a film thickness of 0.2 µm may be used), Ø = 0.25-0.53 mm,
- *stationary phase*: *macrogol 20 000 R*.

Carrier gas: *helium for chromatography R*.

Flow rate: 1.0 ml/min.

Split ratio: 1:100.

Temperature:

	Time (min)	Temperature (°C)
Column	0 - 6	45
	6 - 21	45 → 90
	21 - 39	90 → 180
	39 - 55	180
Injection port		220
Detector		220

Detection: flame ionisation.

Injection: 0.5 µl of the reference solution and 0.2 µl of the test solution.

Elution order: order indicated in the composition of the reference solution. Record the retention times of these substances.

System suitability: reference solution:

- *resolution*: minimum 1.5 between the peaks due to β-pinene and sabinene and minimum 1.5 between the peaks due to geranial and geranyl acetate.

Using the retention times determined from the chromatogram obtained with the reference solution, locate the components of the reference solution in the chromatogram obtained with the test solution.

Determine the percentage content of these components. The percentages are within the following ranges:

- *β-pinene*: 7.0 per cent to 17.0 per cent,
- *sabinene*: 1.0 per cent to 3.0 per cent,
- *limonene*: 56.0 per cent to 78.0 per cent,
- *γ-terpinene*: 6.0 per cent to 12.0 per cent,
- *β-caryophyllene*: maximum 0.5 per cent,
- *neral*: 0.3 per cent to 1.5 per cent,
- *α-terpineol*: maximum 0.6 per cent,
- *neryl acetate*: 0.2 per cent to 0.9 per cent,
- *geranial*: 0.5 per cent to 2.3 per cent,

Monographs I-L

– *geranyl acetate*: 0.1 per cent to 0.8 per cent.

Residue on evaporation (*2.8.9*): 1.8 per cent to 3.6 per cent after heating on the water-bath for 4 h.

STORAGE

In a well-filled, airtight container, protected from light, at a temperature not exceeding 25 °C.

LABELLING

The label states, where applicable, that the contents are Italian-type lemon oil.

01/2005:0771

LEUCINE

Leucinum

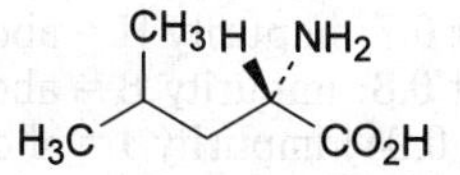

$C_6H_{13}NO_2$ M_r 131.2

DEFINITION

Leucine contains not less than 98.5 per cent and not more than the equivalent of 101.0 per cent of (*S*)-2-amino-4-methylpentanoic acid, calculated with reference to the dried substance.

CHARACTERS

White or almost white crystalline powder or shiny flakes, sparingly soluble in water, practically insoluble in alcohol. It dissolves in dilute mineral acids and in dilute solutions of alkali hydroxides.

IDENTIFICATION

First identification: A, C.

Second identification: A, B, D.

A. It complies with the test for specific optical rotation (see Tests).

B. Dissolve 0.50 g in *water R* and dilute to 25 ml with the same solvent. The solution is laevorotatory.

C. Examine by infrared absorption spectrophotometry (*2.2.24*), comparing with the spectrum obtained with *leucine CRS*. Examine the substances prepared as discs.

D. Examine the chromatograms obtained in the test for ninhydrin-positive substances. The principal spot in the chromatogram obtained with test solution (b) is similar in position, colour and size to the principal spot in the chromatogram obtained with reference solution (a).

TESTS

Appearance of solution. Dissolve 0.5 g in *1 M hydrochloric acid* and dilute to 10 ml with the same acid. The solution is clear (*2.2.1*) and not more intensely coloured than reference solution BY_6 (*2.2.2, Method II*).

Specific optical rotation (*2.2.7*). Dissolve 1.00 g in *hydrochloric acid R1* and dilute to 25.0 ml with the same acid. The specific optical rotation is + 14.5 to + 16.5, calculated with reference to the dried substance.

Ninhydrin-positive substances. Examine by thin-layer chromatography (*2.2.27*), using a *TLC silica gel plate R*.

Test solution (a). Dissolve 0.10 g of the substance to be examined in *0.1 M hydrochloric acid* and dilute to 10 ml with the same acid.

Test solution (b). Dilute 1 ml of test solution (a) to 50 ml with *water R*.

Reference solution (a). Dissolve 10 mg of *leucine CRS* in *0.1 M hydrochloric acid* and dilute to 50 ml with the same acid.

Reference solution (b). Dilute 5 ml of test solution (b) to 20 ml with *water R*.

Reference solution (c). Dissolve 10 mg of *leucine CRS* and 10 mg of *valine CRS* in *0.1 M hydrochloric acid* and dilute to 25 ml with the same acid.

Apply separately to the plate 5 µl of each solution. Allow the plate to dry in air. Develop over a path of 15 cm using a mixture of 20 volumes of *glacial acetic acid R*, 20 volumes of *water R* and 60 volumes of *butanol R*. Allow the plate to dry in air, spray with *ninhydrin solution R* and heat at 100 °C to 105 °C for 15 min. Any spot in the chromatogram obtained with test solution (a), apart from the principal spot, is not more intense than the spot in the chromatogram obtained with reference solution (b) (0.5 per cent). The test is not valid unless the chromatogram obtained with reference solution (c) shows two clearly separated spots.

Chlorides (*2.4.4*). Dissolve 0.25 g in *water R* and dilute to 15 ml with the same solvent. The solution complies with the limit test for chlorides (200 ppm).

Sulphates (*2.4.13*). Dissolve 0.5 g in 3 ml of *dilute hydrochloric acid R* and dilute to 15 ml with *distilled water R*. The solution complies with the limit test for sulphates (300 ppm).

Ammonium (*2.4.1*). 50 mg complies with limit test B for ammonium (200 ppm). Prepare the standard using 0.1 ml of *ammonium standard solution (100 ppm NH_4) R*.

Iron (*2.4.9*). In a separating funnel, dissolve 1.0 g in 10 ml of *dilute hydrochloric acid R*. Shake with three quantities, each of 10 ml, of *methyl isobutyl ketone R1*, shaking for 3 min each time. To the combined organic layers add 10 ml of *water R* and shake for 3 min. The aqueous layer complies with the limit test for iron (10 ppm).

Heavy metals (*2.4.8*). 2.0 g complies with limit test D for heavy metals (10 ppm). Prepare the standard using 2 ml of *lead standard solution (10 ppm Pb) R*.

Loss on drying (*2.2.32*). Not more than 0.5 per cent, determined on 1.000 g by drying in an oven at 100 °C to 105 °C.

Sulphated ash (*2.4.14*). Not more than 0.1 per cent, determined on 1.0 g.

ASSAY

Dissolve 0.100 g in 3 ml of *anhydrous formic acid R*. Add 30 ml of *anhydrous acetic acid R*. Titrate with *0.1 M perchloric acid* using 0.1 ml of *naphtholbenzein solution R* as indicator, until the colour changes from brownish-yellow to green.

1 ml of *0.1 M perchloric acid* is equivalent to 13.12 mg of $C_6H_{13}NO_2$.

STORAGE

Store protected from light.

01/2005:1442

LEUPRORELIN

Leuprorelinum

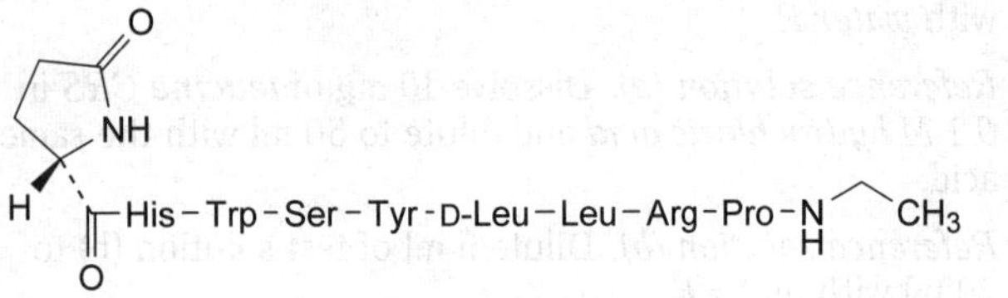

$C_{59}H_{84}N_{16}O_{12}$ M_r 1209

DEFINITION

5-Oxo-L-prolyl-L-histidyl-L-tryptophyl-L-seryl-L-tyrosyl-D-leucyl-L-leucyl-L-arginyl-*N*-ethyl-L-prolinamide.

Synthetic nonapeptide analogue of the hypothalamic peptide, gonadorelin. It is obtained by chemical synthesis and is available as an acetate.

Content: 97.0 per cent to 103.0 per cent (anhydrous and acetic acid-free substance).

CHARACTERS

Appearance: hygroscopic, white or almost white powder.

IDENTIFICATION

A. Infrared absorption spectrophotometry (*2.2.24*).
   Preparation: discs of *potassium bromide R*.
   Comparison: *Ph. Eur. reference spectrum of leuprorelin*.

B. Examine the chromatograms obtained in the assay.
   Results: the principal peak in the chromatogram obtained with test solution (b) is similar in retention time and size to the principal peak in the chromatogram obtained with reference solution (b).

C. Amino acid analysis (*2.2.56*). For hydrolysis use Method 1 and for analysis use Method 1.
   Express the content of each amino acid in moles. Calculate the relative proportions of the amino acids taking one seventh of the sum of the number of moles of histidine, glutamic acid, leucine, proline, tyrosine and arginine as equal to 1. The values fall within the following limits: serine present; glutamic acid = 0.85 to 1.1; proline = 0.85 to 1.1; leucine = 1.8 to 2.2; tyrosine = 0.85 to 1.1; histidine = 0.85 to 1.1 and arginine = 0.85 to 1.1. Not more than traces of other amino acids are present, with the exception of tryptophan.

TESTS

Specific optical rotation (*2.2.7*): − 38.0 to − 42.0 (anhydrous and acetic acid-free substance).

Dissolve the substance to be examined in a 1 per cent *V/V* solution of *glacial acetic acid R* to obtain a concentration of 10.0 mg/ml.

Related substances. Liquid chromatography (*2.2.29*): use the normalisation procedure.

Test solution (a). Dissolve the substance to be examined in the mobile phase to obtain a concentration of 1.0 mg/ml.

Test solution (b). Dilute 1.0 ml of test solution (a) to 20.0 ml with the mobile phase.

Reference solution (a). Dissolve *leuprorelin CRS* in the mobile phase to obtain a concentration of 1.0 mg/ml.

Reference solution (b). Dilute 1.0 ml of reference solution (a) to 20.0 ml with the mobile phase.

Resolution solution. Dilute 5.0 ml of reference solution (a) to 50.0 ml with *water R*. To 5 ml of the solution add 100 µl of *1 M sodium hydroxide* and shake vigorously. Heat in an oven at 100 °C for 60 min, cool immediately and add 50 µl of *dilute phosphoric acid R*. Shake vigorously.

Column:
- *size*: *l* = 0.10 m, Ø = 4.6 mm,
- *stationary phase*: *octadecylsilyl silica gel for chromatography R* (3 µm).

Mobile phase: dissolve about 15.2 g of *triethylamine R* in 800 ml of *water R*, adjust to pH 3.0 with *phosphoric acid R* and dilute to 1000 ml with *water R*. Add 850 ml of this solution to 150 ml of a mixture of 2 volumes of *propanol R* and 3 volumes of *acetonitrile R*.

Flow rate: 1.0-1.5 ml/min.

Detection: spectrophotometer at 220 nm.

Injection: 20 µl of test solution (a) and the resolution solution.

Run time: 90 min.

Relative retention with reference to leuprorelin (retention time = 41-49 min): impurity E = about 0.7; impurity F = about 0.7; impurity H = about 0.78; impurity A = about 0.8; impurity B = about 0.9; impurity I = about 0.94; impurity J = about 1.09; impurity C = about 1.2; impurity G = about 1.3; impurity K = about 1.31; impurity D = about 1.5.

System suitability: resolution solution:
- *resolution*: minimum 1.5 between the peaks due to impurity B and leuprorelin.

Limits:
- *impurity D*: maximum 1.0 per cent,
- *impurities A, B, C*: for each impurity, maximum 0.5 per cent,
- *any other impurity*: for each impurity, maximum 0.5 per cent,
- *total*: maximum 2.5 per cent,
- *disregard limit*: 0.1 per cent.

Acetic acid (*2.5.34*): 4.7 per cent to 9.0 per cent.

Test solution. Dissolve 10.0 mg of the substance to be examined in a mixture of 5 volumes of mobile phase B and 95 volumes of mobile phase A and dilute to 10.0 ml with the same mixture of mobile phases.

Water (*2.5.32*): maximum 5.0 per cent.

Sulphated ash (*2.4.14*): maximum 0.3 per cent.

Bacterial endotoxins (*2.6.14, Method D*): less than 16.7 IU/mg, if intended for use in the manufacture of parenteral dosage forms without a further appropriate procedure for removal of bacterial endotoxins.

ASSAY

Liquid chromatography (*2.2.29*) as described in the test for related substances with the following modifications.

Run time: 60 min.

Injection: 20 µl of test solution (b) and reference solution (b).

Calculate the content of leuprorelin ($C_{59}H_{84}N_{16}O_{12}$) using the areas of the peaks and the declared content of $C_{59}H_{84}N_{16}O_{12}$ in *leuprorelin CRS*.

STORAGE

In an airtight container, protected from light, at a temperature not exceeding 30 °C.

If the substance is sterile, store in a sterile, airtight, tamper-proof container.

LABELLING

The label states:

- the mass of peptide in the container,
- where applicable, that the substance is free from bacterial endotoxins.

IMPURITIES

Specified impurities: A, B, C, D.

Other detectable impurities: E, F, G, H, I, J, K.

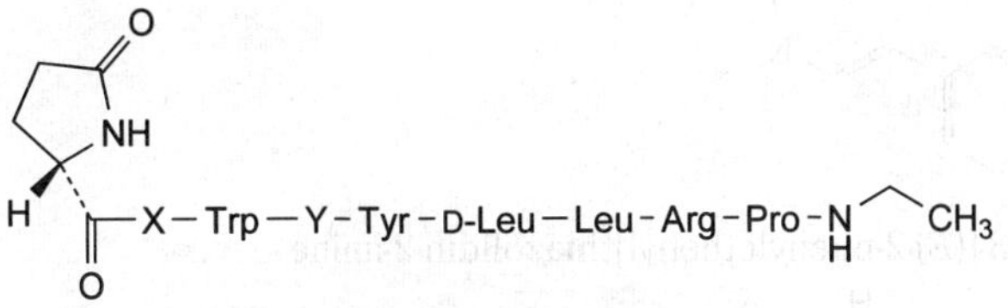

A. X = L-His, Y = D-Ser: [4-D-serine]leuprorelin,

B. X = D-His, Y = L-Ser: [2-D-histidine]leuprorelin,

F. X = D-His, Y = D-Ser: [2-D-histidine,4-D-serine]leuprorelin,

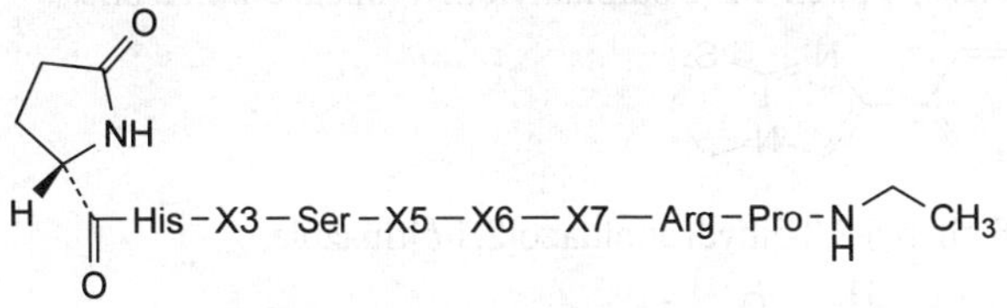

C. X3 = L-Trp, X5 = L-Tyr, X6 = X7 = L-Leu: [6-L-leucine]leuprorelin,

E. X3 = D-Trp, X5 = L-Tyr, X6 = D-Leu, X7 = L-Leu: [3-D-tryptophane]leuprorelin,

G. X3 = L-Trp, X5 = D-Tyr, X6 = D-Leu, X7 = L-Leu: [5-D-tyrosine]leuprorelin,

H. X3 = L-Trp, X5 = L-Tyr, X6 = X7 = D-Leu: [7-D-leucine]leuprorelin,

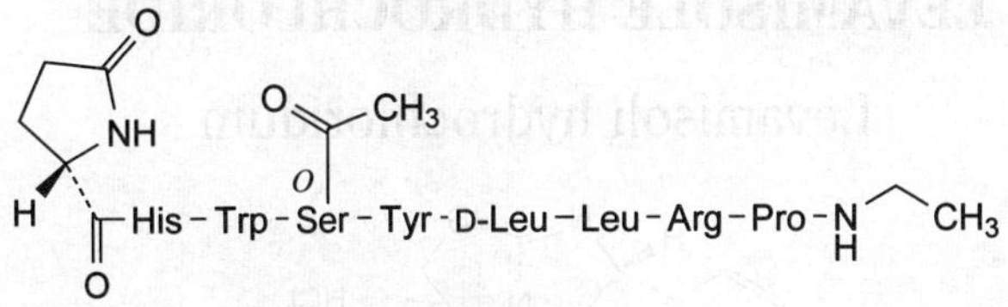

D. [4-(*O*-acetyl-L-serine)]leuprorelin,

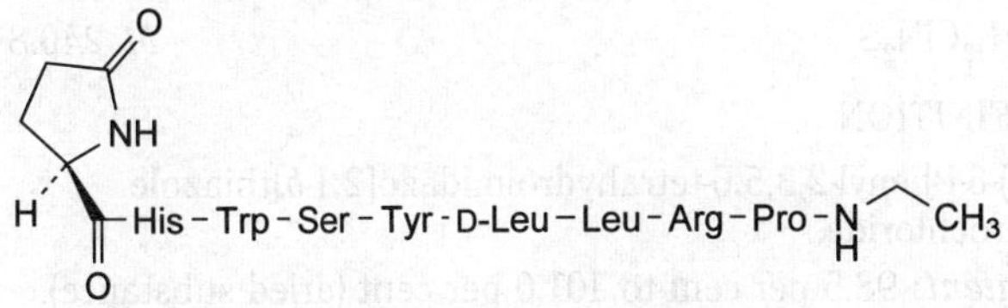

I. [1-(5-oxo-D-proline)]leuprorelin,

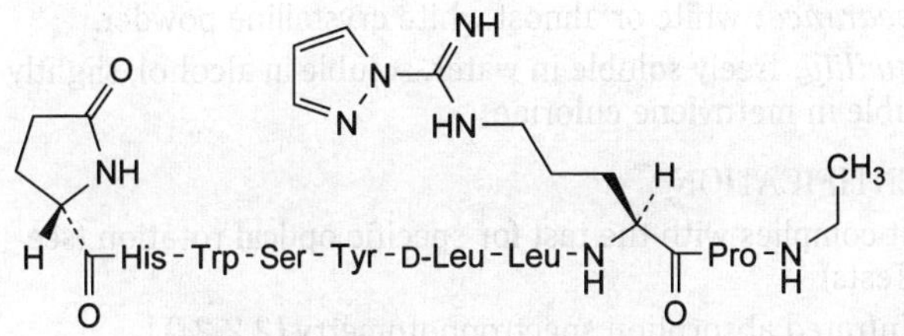

J. [8-[5-*N*-[imino(1*H*-pyrazol-1-yl)methyl]-L-ornithine]]leuprorelin,

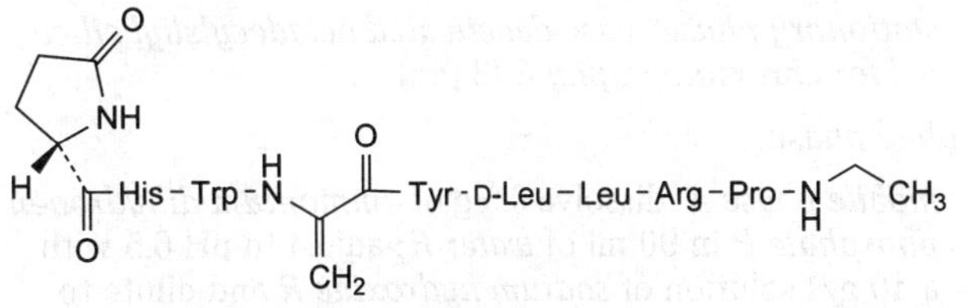

K. [4-dehydroalanine]leuprorelin.

01/2005:1728

LEVAMISOLE FOR VETERINARY USE

Levamisolum ad usum veterinarium

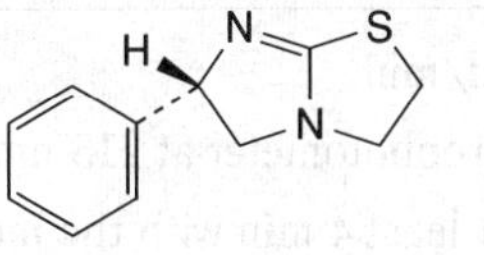

$C_{11}H_{12}N_2S$ M_r 204.3

DEFINITION

(6*S*)-6-Phenyl-2,3,5,6-tetrahydroimidazo[2,1-*b*]thiazole.

Content: 98.5 per cent to 101.5 per cent (anhydrous substance).

CHARACTERS

Appearance: white or almost white powder.

Solubility: slightly soluble in water, freely soluble in alcohol and in methanol.

It shows polymorphism.

IDENTIFICATION

A. It complies with the test for specific optical rotation (see Tests).

B. Infrared absorption spectrophotometry (*2.2.24*).

Comparison: *Ph. Eur. reference spectrum of levamisole.*

If the spectra show differences, dissolve the substance to be examined in *methylene chloride R*, evaporate to dryness and record a new spectrum using the residue.

TESTS

Solution S. Dissolve 2.50 g in *ethanol R* and dilute to 50.0 ml with the same solvent.

Appearance of solution. Solution S is clear (*2.2.1*) and not more intensely coloured than reference solution BY_6 (*2.2.2, Method II*).

Specific optical rotation (*2.2.7*): − 85 to − 89 (anhydrous substance), determined on solution S.

Related substances. Liquid chromatography (*2.2.29*). *Prepare the solutions immediately before use, protect from light and keep below 25 °C.*

Test solution. Dissolve 0.100 g of the substance to be examined in *methanol R* and dilute to 10.0 ml with the same solvent.

Reference solution (a). Dissolve 50 mg of *levamisole hydrochloride for system suitability CRS* in *methanol R*, add 0.5 ml of *concentrated ammonia R* and dilute to 5.0 ml with *methanol R*.

Reference solution (b). Dilute 1.0 ml of the test solution to 100.0 ml with *methanol R*. Dilute 5.0 ml of the solution to 25.0 ml with *methanol R*.

Column:

- *size*: *l* = 0.10 m, Ø = 4.6 mm,

- *stationary phase*: *base-deactivated octadecylsilyl silica gel for chromatography R* (3 µm).

Mobile phase:

- *mobile phase A*: dissolve 0.5 g of *ammonium dihydrogen phosphate R* in 90 ml of *water R*; adjust to pH 6.5 with a 40 g/l solution of *sodium hydroxide R* and dilute to 100 ml with *water R*,
- *mobile phase B*: *acetonitrile R*.

Time (min)	Mobile phase A (per cent *V/V*)	Mobile phase B (per cent *V/V*)
0 - 8	90 → 30	10 → 70
8 - 10	30	70
10 - 11	30 → 90	70 → 10

Flow rate: 1.5 ml/min.

Detection: spectrophotometer at 215 nm.

Equilibration: at least 4 min with the mobile phase at the initial composition.

Injection: 10 µl.

Relative retention with reference to levamisole (retention time = about 3 min): impurity A = about 0.9; impurity B = about 1.4; impurity C = about 1.5; impurity D = about 1.6; impurity E = about 2.0.

System suitability: reference solution (a):

- the chromatogram obtained is similar to the chromatogram supplied with *levamisole hydrochloride for system suitability CRS*.

Limits:

- *correction factors*: for the calculation of content, multiply the peak areas of the following impurities by the corresponding correction factor: impurity A = 2.0; impurity B = 1.7; impurity C = 2.9; impurity D = 1.3; impurity E = 2.7;
- *impurities A, B, C, D, E*: for each impurity, not more than the area of the principal peak in the chromatogram obtained with reference solution (b) (0.2 per cent);
- *any other impurity*: not more than half the area of the principal peak in the chromatogram obtained with reference solution (b) (0.1 per cent);
- *total*: not more than 1.5 times the area of the principal peak in the chromatogram obtained with reference solution (b) (0.3 per cent);
- *disregard limit*: 0.25 times the area of the principal peak in the chromatogram obtained with reference solution (b) (0.05 per cent).

Water (*2.5.12*): maximum 0.5 per cent, determined on 1.00 g.

Sulphated ash (*2.4.14*): maximum 0.1 per cent, determined on 1.0 g.

ASSAY

Dissolve 0.150 g in 50 ml of a mixture of 1 volume of *anhydrous acetic acid R* and 7 volumes of *methyl ethyl ketone R*. Titrate with *0.1 M perchloric acid*, using 0.2 ml of *naphtholbenzein solution R* as indicator.

1 ml of *0.1 M perchloric acid* is equivalent to 20.43 mg of $C_{11}H_{12}N_2S$.

STORAGE

In an airtight container, protected from light.

IMPURITIES

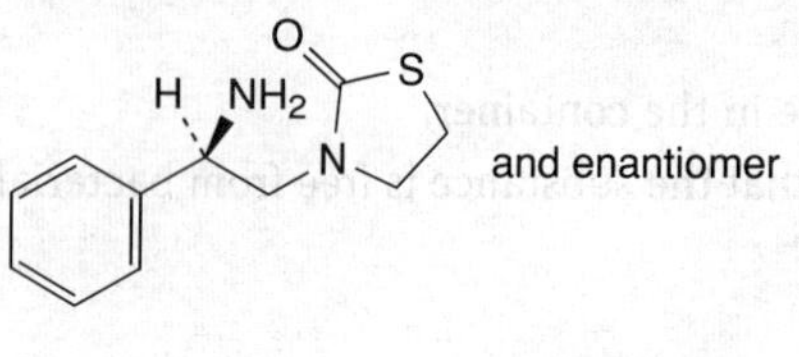

A. 3-[(2*RS*)-2-amino-2-phenylethyl]thiazolidin-2-one,

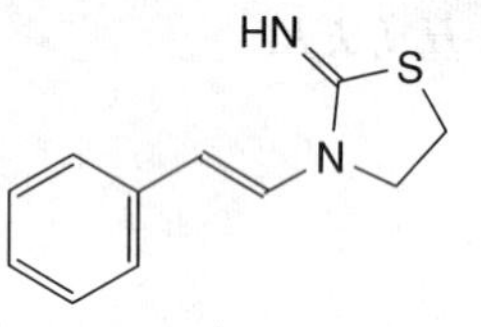

B. 3-[(*E*)-2-phenylethenyl]thiazolidin-2-imine,

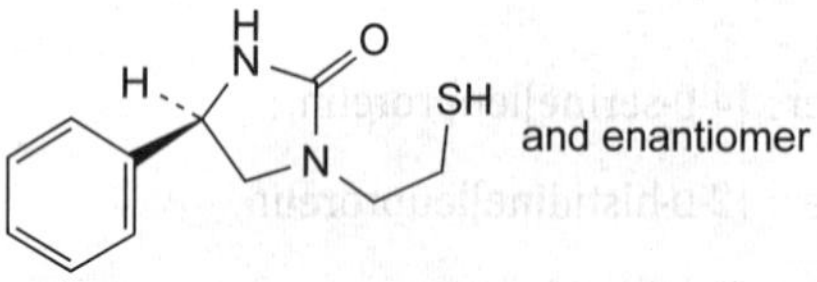

C. (4*RS*)-4-phenyl-1-(2-sulphanylethyl)imidazolidin-2-one,

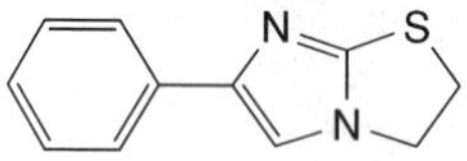

D. 6-phenyl-2,3-dihydroimidazo[2,1-*b*]thiazole,

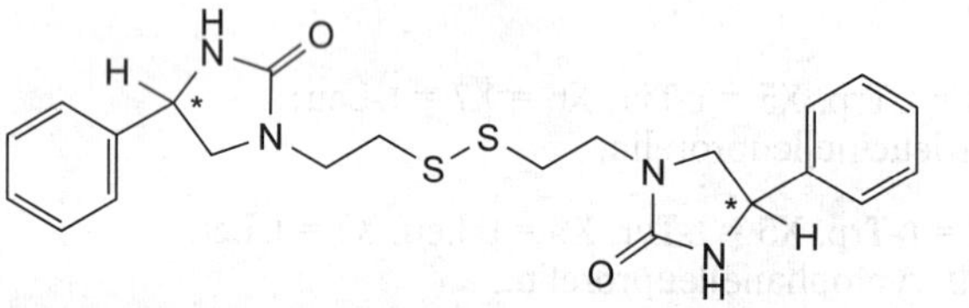

E. 1,1′-[(disulphane-1,2-diyl)bis(ethylene)]bis[(4*RS*)-4-phenylimidazolidin-2-one].

01/2005:0726

LEVAMISOLE HYDROCHLORIDE

Levamisoli hydrochloridum

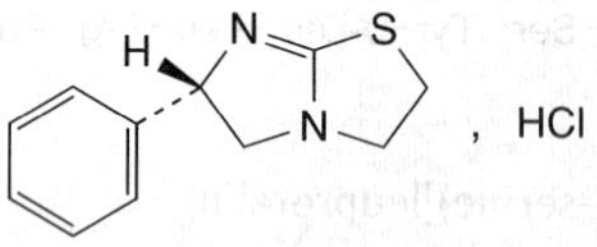

$C_{11}H_{13}ClN_2S$ M_r 240.8

DEFINITION

(6*S*)-6-Phenyl-2,3,5,6-tetrahydroimidazo[2,1-*b*]thiazole hydrochloride.

Content: 98.5 per cent to 101.0 per cent (dried substance).

CHARACTERS

Appearance: white or almost white crystalline powder.

Solubility: freely soluble in water, soluble in alcohol, slightly soluble in methylene chloride.

IDENTIFICATION

A. It complies with the test for specific optical rotation (see Tests).

B. Infrared absorption spectrophotometry (*2.2.24*).

Preparation: discs.

Comparison: *levamisole hydrochloride CRS*.

C. It gives reaction (a) of chlorides (*2.3.1*).

TESTS

Solution S. Dissolve 2.50 g in *carbon dioxide-free water R* and dilute to 50.0 ml with the same solvent.

Appearance of solution. Solution S is clear (*2.2.1*) and not more intensely coloured than reference solution Y_7 (*2.2.2, Method II*).

pH (*2.2.3*): 3.0 to 4.5 for solution S.

Specific optical rotation (*2.2.7*): − 121 to − 128(dried substance), determined on solution S.

Related substances. Liquid chromatography (*2.2.29*). *Prepare the solutions immediately before use, protect from light and keep below 25 °C.*

Test solution. Dissolve 0.100 g of the substance to be examined in *methanol R*, add 1.0 ml of *concentrated ammonia R* and dilute to 10.0 ml with *methanol R*.

Reference solution (a). Dissolve 50 mg of *levamisole hydrochloride for system suitability CRS* in *methanol R*, add 0.5 ml of *concentrated ammonia R* and dilute to 5.0 ml with *methanol R*.

Reference solution (b). Dilute 1.0 ml of the test solution to 100.0 ml with *methanol R*. Dilute 5.0 ml of the solution to 25.0 ml with *methanol R*.

Column:

- *size*: *l* = 0.10 m, Ø = 4.6 mm,
- *stationary phase*: *base-deactivated octadecylsilyl silica gel for chromatography R* (3 µm).

Mobile phase:

- *mobile phase A*: dissolve 0.5 g of *ammonium dihydrogen phosphate R* in 90 ml of *water R*; adjust to pH 6.5 with a 40 g/l solution of *sodium hydroxide R* and dilute to 100 ml with *water R*,
- *mobile phase B*: *acetonitrile R*,

Time (min)	Mobile phase A (per cent *V/V*)	Mobile phase B (per cent *V/V*)
0 - 8	90 → 30	10 → 70
8 - 10	30	70
10 - 11	30 → 90	70 → 10

Flow rate: 1.5 ml/min.

Detection: spectrophotometer at 215 nm.

Equilibration: at least 4 min with the mobile phase at the initial composition.

Injection: 10 µl.

Relative retention with reference to levamisole (retention time = about 3 min): impurity A = about 0.9; impurity B = about 1.4; impurity C = about 1.5; impurity D = about 1.6; impurity E = about 2.0.

System suitability: reference solution (a):

- the chromatogram obtained is similar to the chromatogram supplied with *levamisole hydrochloride for system suitability CRS.*

Limits:

- *correction factors*: for the calculation of contents, multiply the peak areas of the following impurities by the corresponding correction factor: impurity A = 2.0; impurity B = 1.7; impurity C = 2.9; impurity D = 1.3; impurity E = 2.7;
- *impurities A, B, C, D, E*: for each impurity, not more than the area of the principal peak in the chromatogram obtained with reference solution (b) (0.2 per cent);
- *any other impurity*: not more than half the area of the principal peak in the chromatogram obtained with reference solution (b) (0.1 per cent);
- *total*: not more than 1.5 times the area of the principal peak in the chromatogram obtained with reference solution (b) (0.3 per cent);
- *disregard limit*: 0.25 times the area of the principal peak in the chromatogram obtained with reference solution (b) (0.05 per cent).

Heavy metals (*2.4.8*): maximum 20 ppm.

12 ml of solution S complies with limit test A. Prepare the standard using *lead standard solution (1 ppm Pb) R.*

Loss on drying (*2.2.32*): maximum 0.5 per cent, determined on 1.000 g by drying in an oven at 100-105 °C for 4 h.

Sulphated ash (*2.4.14*): maximum 0.1 per cent, determined on 1.0 g.

ASSAY

Dissolve 0.200 g in 30 ml of *alcohol R* and add 5.0 ml of *0.01 M hydrochloric acid.* Carry out a potentiometric titration (*2.2.20*), using *0.1 M sodium hydroxide.* Read the volume added between the 2 points of inflexion.

1 ml of *0.1 M sodium hydroxide* is equivalent to 24.08 mg of $C_{11}H_{13}ClN_2S$.

STORAGE

Protected from light.

IMPURITIES

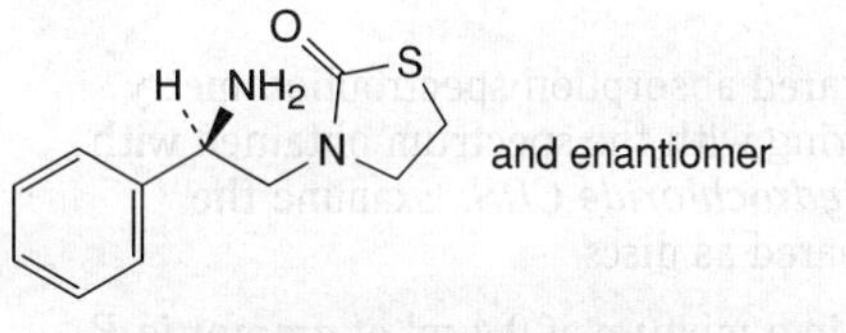

A. 3-[(2*RS*)-2-amino-2-phenylethyl]thiazolidin-2-one,

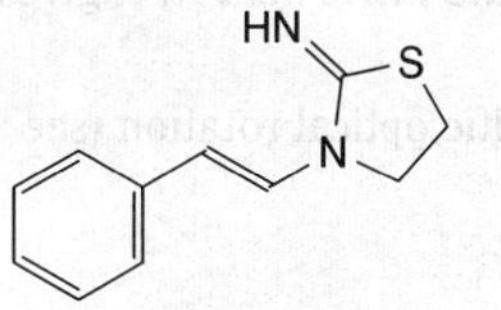

B. 3-[(*E*)-2-phenylethenyl]thiazolidin-2-imine,

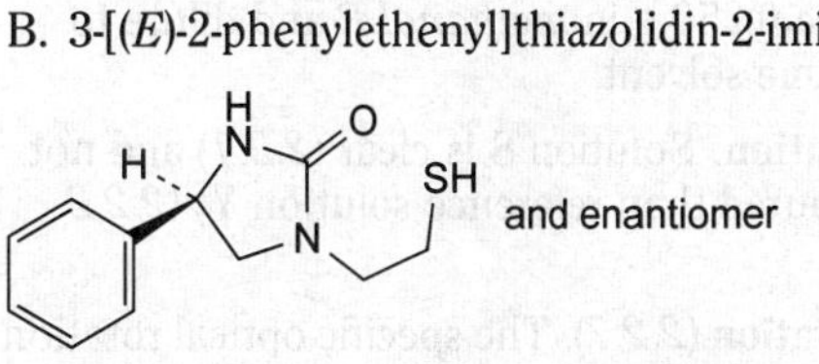

C. (4*RS*)-4-phenyl-1-(2-sulphanylethyl)imidazolidin-2-one,

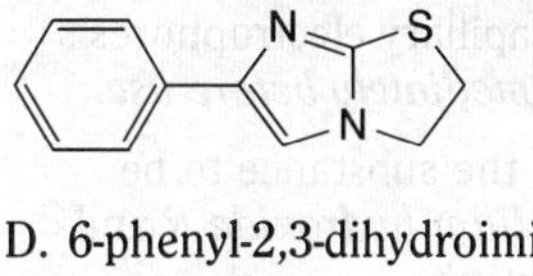

D. 6-phenyl-2,3-dihydroimidazo[2,1-*b*]thiazole,

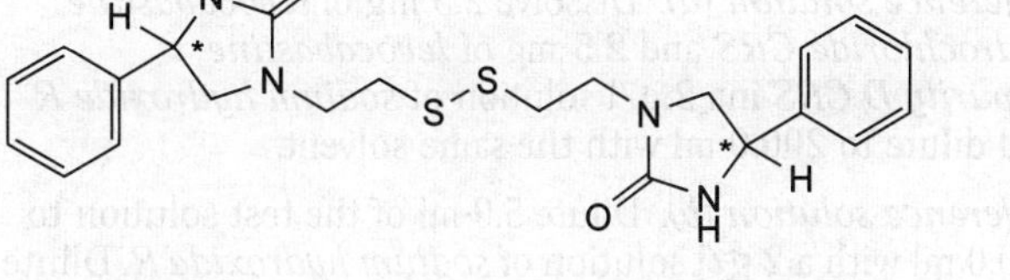

E. 1,1′-[(disulphane-1,2-diyl)bis(ethylene)]bis[(4*RS*)-4-phenylimidazolidin-2-one].

01/2005:1484

LEVOCABASTINE HYDROCHLORIDE

Levocabastini hydrochloridum

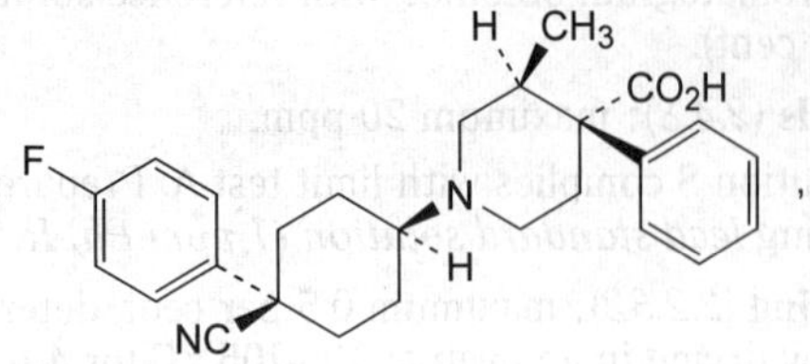

$C_{26}H_{30}ClFN_2O_2$ M_r 457.0

DEFINITION

Levocabastine hydrochloride contains not less than 98.5 per cent and not more than the equivalent of 101.5 per cent of (3*S*,4*R*)-1-[*cis*-4-cyano-4-(4-fluorophenyl)cyclohexyl]-3-methyl-4-phenylpiperidine-4-carboxylic acid monohydrochloride, calculated with reference to the dried substance.

CHARACTERS

A white or almost white powder, practically insoluble in water, sparingly soluble in methanol, slightly soluble in alcohol and in a 2 g/l solution of sodium hydroxide.

IDENTIFICATION

A. Examine by infrared absorption spectrophotometry (*2.2.24*), comparing with the spectrum obtained with *levocabastine hydrochloride CRS*. Examine the substances prepared as discs.

B. Dissolve 50 mg in a mixture of 0.4 ml of *ammonia R* and 2 ml of *water R*. Mix, allow to stand for 5 min and filter. Acidify the filtrate with *dilute nitric acid R*. It gives reaction (a) of chlorides (*2.3.1*).

C. It complies with the test for specific optical rotation (see Tests).

TESTS

Solution S. Dissolve 0.250 g in *methanol R* and dilute to 25.0 ml with the same solvent.

Appearance of solution. Solution S is clear (*2.2.1*) and not more intensely coloured than reference solution Y_7 (*2.2.2, Method II*).

Specific optical rotation (*2.2.7*). The specific optical rotation is − 102 to − 106, determined on solution S, calculated with reference to the dried substance.

Related substances. Examine by capillary electrophoresis (*2.2.47*). *Prepare the solutions immediately before use.*

Test solution. Dissolve 25.0 mg of the substance to be examined in a 2 g/l solution of *sodium hydroxide R* and dilute to 10.0 ml with the same solvent.

Reference solution (a). Dissolve 2.5 mg of *levocabastine hydrochloride CRS* and 2.5 mg of *levocabastine impurity D CRS* ina 2 g/l solution of *sodium hydroxide R* and dilute to 200.0 ml with the same solvent.

Reference solution (b). Dilute 5.0 ml of the test solution to 100.0 ml with a 2 g/l solution of *sodium hydroxide R*. Dilute 1.0 ml of the solution to 10.0 ml with a 2 g/l solution of *sodium hydroxide R*.

The micellar electrokinetic chromatographic procedure may be carried out using:

- an uncoated fused-silica capillary with the length to the detector cell of 0.5 m and 75 µm in internal diameter;
- an electrolyte solution prepared as follows: dissolve 1.08 g of *sodium dodecyl sulphate R* and 0.650 g of *hydroxypropyl-β-cyclodextrin R* in 5 ml of *2-propanol R* and dilute to 50.0 ml with buffer solution pH 9.0 prepared as follows: dissolve 1.39 g of *boric acid R* in *water R* and adjust to pH 9.0 with *1 M sodium hydroxide* (about 9 ml). Dilute to 100.0 ml with *water R*;
- as detector a spectrophotometer set at 214 nm;
- an injection of 5 s under a pressure of 3450 Pa;
- the following current gradient:

Time (min)	Current (µA)
0 - 0.17	0 → 75
0.17 - 15	75 → 130
15 - 40	130
40 – 60	130 → 200

maintaining the temperature of the capillary at 50 °C.

Equilibrate the capillary for 2 min with a 2 g/l solution of *sodium hydroxide R* and then equilibrate with the electrolyte solution for at least 5 min.

Inject reference solution (a). When the electropherogram is recorded in the prescribed conditions, the migration times are: levocabastine about 28 min and impurity D about 30 min. The test is not valid unless the resolution between the peaks due to levocabastine and impurity D is at least 4. If necessary adjust the current gradient.

Inject a 2 g/l solution of *sodium hydroxide R* as a blank, the test solution and reference solution (b). In the electropherogram obtained with the test solution: the area of any peak, apart from the principal peak, is not greater than the area of the principal peak in the electropherogram obtained with reference solution (b) (0.5 per cent); the sum of the areas of all peaks, apart from the principal peak, is not greater than twice the area of the principal peak in the electropherogram obtained with reference solution (b) (1.0 per cent). Disregard any peak obtained with the blank and any peak with an area less than 0.1 times the area of the principal peak in the electropherogram obtained with reference solution (b) (0.05 per cent).

Loss on drying (*2.2.32*). Not more than 0.5 per cent, determined on 1.000 g by drying in an oven at 100-105 °C.

Sulphated ash (*2.4.14*). Not more than 0.1 per cent, determined on 1.0 g in a platinum crucible.

ASSAY

Dissolve 0.175 g in 50 ml of *alcohol R* and add 5.0 ml of *0.01 M hydrochloric acid*. Carry out a potentiometric titration (*2.2.20*), using *0.1 M sodium hydroxide*. Read the volume added between the first and third point of inflexion.

1 ml of *0.1 M sodium hydroxide* is equivalent to 22.85 mg of $C_{26}H_{30}ClFN_2O_2$.

STORAGE

Store protected from light.

IMPURITIES

Specified impurities: A, B, C, D, E.

Other detectable impurities: F, G, H, I.

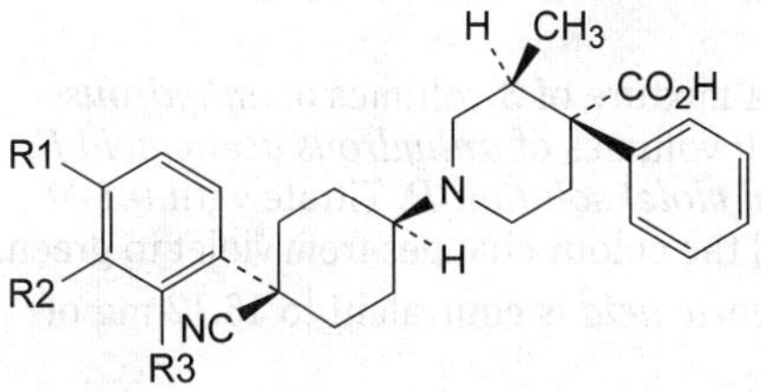

A. R1 = R2 = R3 = H: (3*S*,4*R*)-1-(*cis*-4-cyano-4-phenylcyclohexyl)-3-methyl-4-phenylpiperidine-4-carboxylic acid,

B. R1 = R2 = H, R3 = F: (3*S*,4*R*)-1-[*cis*-4-cyano-4-(2-fluorophenyl)cyclohexyl]-3-methyl-4-phenylpiperidine-4-carboxylic acid,

C. R1 = H, R2 = F, R3 = H: (3*S*,4*R*)-1-[*cis*-4-cyano-4-(3-fluorophenyl)cyclohexyl]-3-methyl-4-phenylpiperidine-4-carboxylic acid,

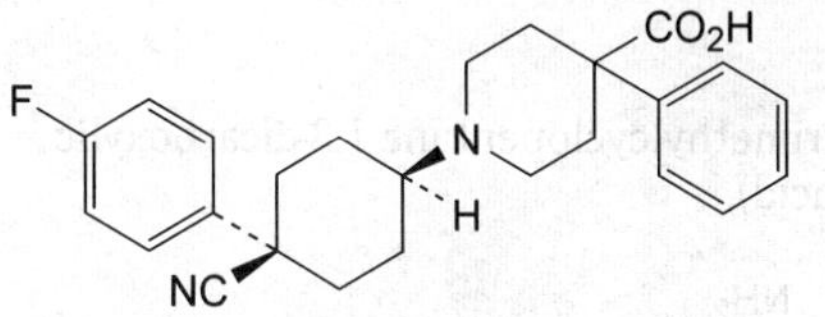

D. 1-[*cis*-4-cyano-4-(4-fluorophenyl)cyclohexyl]-4-phenylpiperidine-4-carboxylic acid,

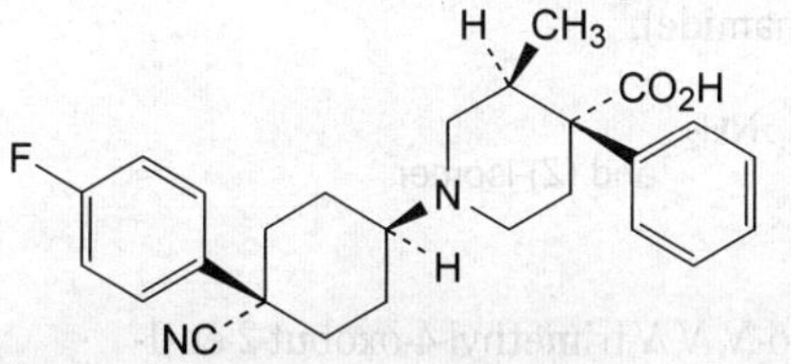

E. (3*S*,4*R*)-1-[*trans*-4-cyano-4-(4-fluorophenyl)cyclohexyl]-3-methyl-4-phenylpiperidine-4-carboxylic acid,

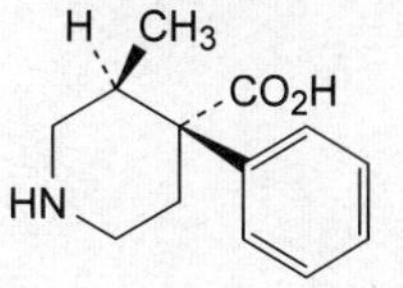

F. (3*S*,4*R*)-3-methyl-4-phenylpiperidine-4-carboxylic acid,

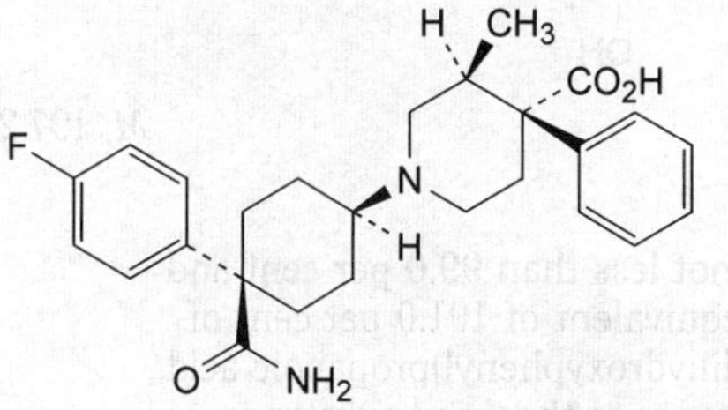

G. (3*S*,4*R*)-1-[*cis*-4-carbamoyl-4-(4-fluorophenyl)cyclohexyl]-3-methyl-4-phenylpiperidine-4-carboxylic acid,

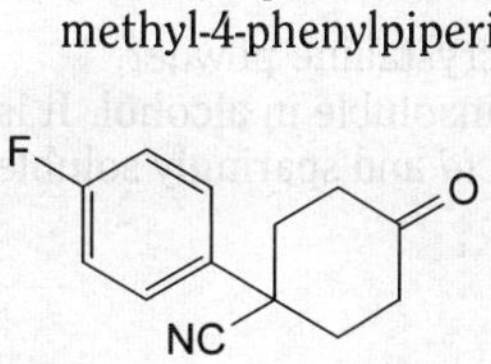

H. 1-(4-fluorophenyl)-4-oxocyclohexanecarbonitrile,

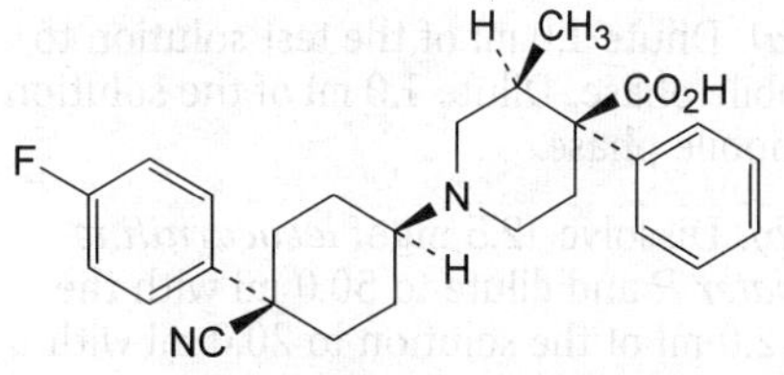

I. (3*S*,4*S*)-1-[*cis*-4-cyano-4-(4-fluorophenyl)cyclohexyl]-3-methyl-4-phenylpiperidine-4-carboxylic acid.

01/2005:1339

LEVOCARNITINE

Levocarnitinum

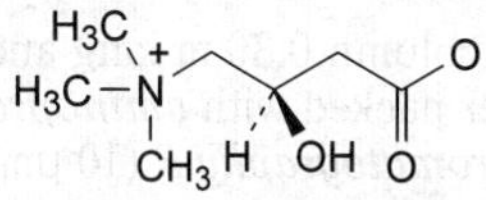

$C_7H_{15}NO_3$ M_r 161.2

DEFINITION

Levocarnitine contains not less than 98.0 per cent and not more than the equivalent of 102.0 per cent of (3*R*)-3-hydroxy-4-(trimethylammonio)butanoate, calculated with reference to the anhydrous substance.

CHARACTERS

A white, crystalline powder or colourless crystals, hygroscopic, freely soluble in water, soluble in warm alcohol, practically insoluble in acetone.

IDENTIFICATION

First identification: A, B.

Second identification: A, C.

A. It complies with the test for specific optical rotation (see Tests).

B. Examine by infrared absorption spectrophotometry (*2.2.24*), comparing with the spectrum obtained with *levocarnitine CRS*. Examine the substances, previously dried *in vacuo* at 50 °C for 5 h, prepared as discs.

C. To 1 ml of solution S (see Tests) add 9 ml of *water R*, 10 ml of *dilute sulphuric acid R* and 30 ml of *ammonium reineckate solution R*. A pink precipitate is formed. Allow to stand for 30 min. Filter and wash with *water R*, with *alcohol R* and then with *acetone R* and dry at 80 °C. The precipitate melts (*2.2.14*) at 147 °C to 150 °C.

TESTS

Solution S. Dissolve 5.00 g in *carbon dioxide-free water R* prepared from *distilled water R* and dilute to 50.0 ml with the same solvent.

Appearance of solution. Solution S is clear (*2.2.1*) and colourless (*2.2.2, Method II*).

pH (*2.2.3*). Dilute 10 ml of solution S to 20 ml with *carbon dioxide-free water R*. The pH of the solution is 6.5 to 8.5.

Specific optical rotation (*2.2.7*): − 29.0 to − 32.0, determined on solution S and calculated with reference to the anhydrous substance.

Related substances. Examine by liquid chromatography (*2.2.29*).

Test solution. Dissolve 0.10 g of the substance to be examined in the mobile phase and dilute to 20.0 ml with the mobile phase.

Reference solution (a). Dilute 1.0 ml of the test solution to 100.0 ml with the mobile phase. Dilute 1.0 ml of the solution to 10.0 ml with the mobile phase.

Reference solution (b). Dissolve 12.5 mgof *levocarnitine impurity A CRS* in *water R* and dilute to 50.0 ml with the same solvent. Dilute 2.0 ml of the solution to 20.0 ml with the mobile phase.

Reference solution (c). Dissolve 10.0 mg of *levocarnitine impurity A CRS* in *water R* and dilute to 10.0 ml with the same solvent. Dilute 2.0 ml of the solution to 20.0 ml with the mobile phase.

Reference solution (d). Dissolve 0.100 g of *levocarnitine CRS* in reference solution (c) and dilute to 10.0 ml with the same solution.

The chromatographic procedure may be carried out using:

– a stainless steel column 0.30 m long and 3.9 mm in internal diameter packed with *aminopropylmethylsilyl silica gel for chromatography R* (10 µm),

– as mobile phase at a flow rate of 1 ml/min a mixture of 35 volumes of a 6.81 g/l solution of *potassium dihydrogen phosphate R* adjusted to pH 4.7 with *dilute sodium hydroxide solution R*, and 65 volumes of *acetonitrile R*,

– as detector a spectrophotometer set at 205 nm,

maintaining the temperature of the column at 30 °C.

When the chromatograms are recorded under the prescribed conditions, the retention times are: about 9.6 min for levocarnitine and about 10.6 min for levocarnitine impurity A. Adjust the sensitivity of the system so that the height of the principal peak in the chromatogram obtained with reference solution (b) is at least 20 per cent of the full scale of the recorder.

Inject 25 µl of reference solution (d) and continue the chromatography for 15 min. The test is not valid unless, in the chromatogram obtained with reference solution (d), the resolution between the peaks corresponding to levocarnitine and to levocarnitine impurity A is at least 0.9.

Inject 25 µl of the test solution, 25 µl of reference solution (a) and 25 µl of reference solution (b). In the chromatogram obtained with the test solution: the area of any peak corresponding to levocarnitine impurity A is not greater than the area of the principal peak in the chromatogram obtained with reference solution (b) (0.5 per cent); the area of any peak, apart from the principal peak and the peak due to levocarnitine impurity A, is not greater than the area of the principal peak in the chromatogram obtained with reference solution (a) (0.1 per cent).

Chlorides (*2.4.4*). Dilute 2.5 ml of solution S to 15 ml with *water R*. The solution complies with the limit test for chlorides (200 ppm).

Sulphates (*2.4.13*). Dilute 5 ml of solution S to 15 ml with *distilled water R*. The solution complies with the limit test for sulphates (300 ppm).

Heavy metals (*2.4.8*). 12 ml of solution S complies with limit test A for heavy metals (10 ppm). Prepare the standard using *lead standard solution (1 ppm Pb) R*.

Water (*2.5.12*). Not more than 1.0 per cent, determined on 2.00 g by the semi-micro determination of water.

Sulphated ash (*2.4.14*). Not more than 0.1 per cent, determined on 1.0 g.

ASSAY

Dissolve 0.125 g in a mixture of 3 volumes of *anhydrous formic acid R* and 50 volumes of *anhydrous acetic acid R*. Add 0.2 ml of *crystal violet solution R*. Titrate with *0.1 M perchloric acid* until the colour changes from violet to green.

1 ml of *0.1 M perchloric acid* is equivalent to 16.12 mg of $C_7H_{15}NO_3$.

STORAGE

Store in an airtight container.

IMPURITIES

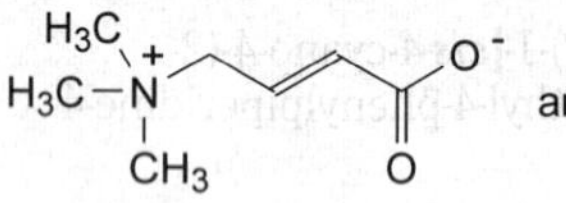

A. (*E*)- or (*Z*)-4-(trimethylammonio)but-2-enoate,

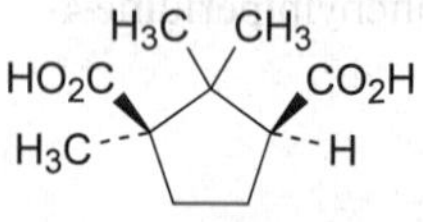

B. (1*RS*,3*SR*)-1,2,2-trimethylcyclopentane-1,3-dicarboxylic acid (camphoric acid),

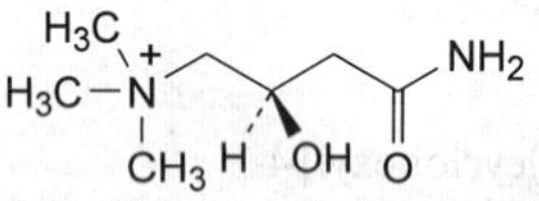

C. (2*R*)-4-amino-2-hydroxy-*N*,*N*,*N*-trimethyl-4-oxobutan-1-aminium (carnitinamide),

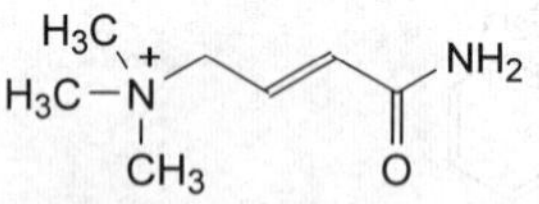

D. (*E*)- or (*Z*)-4-amino-*N*,*N*,*N*-trimethyl-4-oxobut-2-en-1-aminium.

01/2005:0038

LEVODOPA

Levodopum

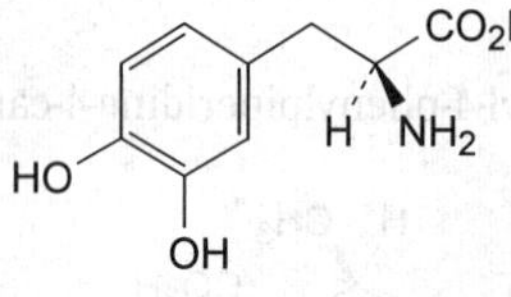

$C_9H_{11}NO_4$ M_r 197.2

DEFINITION

Levodopa contains not less than 99.0 per cent and not more than the equivalent of 101.0 per cent of (2*S*)-2-amino-3-(3,4-dihydroxyphenyl)propanoic acid, calculated with reference to the dried substance.

CHARACTERS

A white or slightly cream-coloured, crystalline powder, slightly soluble in water, practically insoluble in alcohol. It is freely soluble in *1 M hydrochloric acid* and sparingly soluble in *0.1 M hydrochloric acid*.

IDENTIFICATION

First identification: A.

Second identification: B, C, D.

A. Examine by infrared absorption spectrophotometry (*2.2.24*) comparing with the spectrum obtained with *levodopa CRS*.

B. Dissolve about 2 mg in 2 ml of *water R* and add 0.2 ml of *ferric chloride solution R2*. A green colour develops which changes to bluish-violet on the addition of 0.1 g of *hexamethylenetetramine R*.

C. Dissolve about 5 mg in a mixture of 5 ml of *1 M hydrochloric acid* and 5 ml of *water R*. Add 0.1 ml of *sodium nitrite solution R* containing 100 g/l of *ammonium molybdate R*. A yellow colour develops which changes to red on the addition of *strong sodium hydroxide solution R*.

D. To about 5 mg add 1 ml of *water R*, 1 ml of *pyridine R* and about 5 mg of *nitrobenzoyl chloride R*, mix and allow to stand for 3 min. A violet colour develops which changes to pale yellow on boiling the mixture. Add, while shaking, 0.2 ml of *sodium carbonate solution R*. The violet colour reappears.

TESTS

Appearance of solution. Dissolve 1.0 g in *1 M hydrochloric acid* and dilute to 25 ml with the same solvent. The solution is not more intensely coloured than reference solution BY_6 (*2.2.2, Method II*).

pH (*2.2.3*). Shake 0.10 g for 15 min with 10 ml of *carbon dioxide-free water R*. The pH of the suspension is 4.5 to 7.0

Optical rotation (*2.2.7*). Dissolve a quantity equivalent to 0.200 g of the dried substance and 5 g of *hexamethylenetetramine R* in 10 ml of *1 M hydrochloric acid* and dilute to 25.0 ml with the same acid. Allow the solution to stand protected from light for 3 h. The angle of optical rotation is − 1.27° to − 1.34°.

Absorbance (*2.2.25*). Dissolve 30.0 mg in *0.1 M hydrochloric acid* and dilute to 100.0 ml with the same acid. Dilute 10.0 ml of this solution to 100.0 ml with *0.1 M hydrochloric acid*. Examined between 230 nm and 350 nm, the solution shows a single absorption maximum, at 280 nm. The specific absorbance at this maximum is 137 to 147, calculated with reference to the dried substance.

Related substances. Examine by thin-layer chromatography (*2.2.27*), using *cellulose for chromatography R* as the coating substance.

Test solution. Dissolve 0.1 g of the substance to be examined in 5 ml of *anhydrous formic acid R* and dilute to 10 ml with *methanol R*. Prepare immediately before use.

Reference solution (a). Dilute 0.5 ml of the test solution to 100 ml with *methanol R*.

Reference solution (b). Dissolve 30 mg of *tyrosine R* in 1 ml of *anhydrous formic acid R* and dilute to 100 ml with *methanol R*. Mix 1 ml of this solution with 1 ml of the test solution.

Apply separately to the plate as bands 20 mm long 10 µl of the test solution, 10 µl of reference solution (a) and 20 µl of reference solution (b). Dry in a current of air. Develop over a path of 15 cm using a mixture of 25 volumes of *glacial acetic acid R*, 25 volumes of *water R* and 50 volumes of *butanol R*. Dry the plate in a current of warm air and spray with a freshly prepared mixture of equal volumes of a 100 g/l solution of *ferric chloride R* and a 50 g/l solution of *potassium ferricyanide R*. Examine the chromatograms immediately. Any spot in the chromatogram obtained with the test solution, apart from the principal spot is not more intense than the spot in the chromatogram obtained with reference solution (a) (0.5 per cent). The test is not valid unless the chromatogram obtained with reference solution (b) shows, above the principal spot, a distinct spot which is more intense than the spot in the chromatogram obtained with reference solution (a).

Heavy metals (*2.4.8*). 2.0 g complies with limit test C for heavy metals (10 ppm). Prepare the standard using 2 ml of *lead standard solution (10 ppm Pb) R*.

Loss on drying (*2.2.32*). Not more than 1.0 per cent, determined on 0.50 g by drying in an oven at 100 °C to 105 °C.

Sulphated ash (*2.4.14*). Not more than 0.1 per cent, determined on 1.0 g.

ASSAY

Dissolve 0.180 g, heating if necessary in 5 ml of *anhydrous formic acid R* and add 25 ml of *anhydrous acetic acid R* and 25 ml of *dioxan R*. Titrate with *0.1 M perchloric acid*, using 0.1 ml of *crystal violet solution R* as indicator, until a green colour is obtained.

1 ml of *0.1 M perchloric acid* is equivalent to 19.72 mg of $C_9H_{11}NO_4$.

STORAGE

Store protected from light.

01/2005:1535

LEVODROPROPIZINE

Levodropropizinum

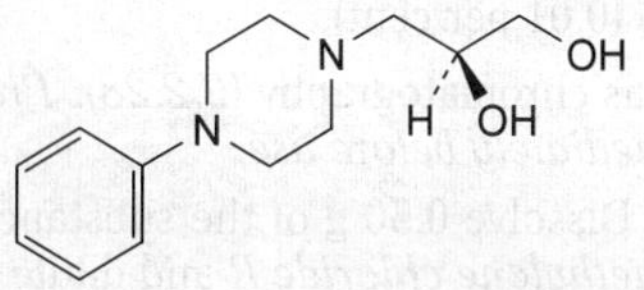

$C_{13}H_{20}N_2O_2$ M_r 236.3

DEFINITION

(2*S*)-3-(4-Phenylpiperazin-1-yl)propane-1,2-diol.

Content: 98.5 per cent to 101.0 per cent (dried substance).

CHARACTERS

Appearance: white or almost white powder.

Solubility: slightly soluble in water, freely soluble in dilute acetic acid and in methanol, slightly soluble in alcohol.

IDENTIFICATION

A. Specific optical rotation (*2.2.7*): − 30.0 to − 33.5 (dried substance).

Dissolve 1.50 g in a 21 g/l solution of *hydrochloric acid R* and dilute to 50.0 ml with the same acid.

B. Infrared absorption spectrophotometry (*2.2.24*).

Comparison: *levodropropizine CRS*.

TESTS

pH (*2.2.3*): 9.2 to 10.2.

Suspend 2.5 g in *carbon dioxide-free water R*, heat to dissolve, cool to room temperature and dilute to 100 ml with the same solvent.

Impurity B and related substances. Liquid chromatography (*2.2.29*).

Test solution. Dissolve 24.0 mg of the substance to be examined in the mobile phase and dilute to 100.0 ml with the mobile phase.

Monographs I-L

Reference solution (a). Dissolve 12.0 mg of *1-phenylpiperazine R* in *methanol R* and dilute to 100.0 ml with the same solvent. Dilute 1.0 ml to 100.0 ml with the mobile phase.

Reference solution (b). Mix 0.5 ml of the test solution with 1 ml of reference solution (a) and dilute to 100 ml with the mobile phase.

Column:

- *size*: *l* = 0.15 m, Ø = 4.6 mm,
- *stationary phase*: *base-deactivated octylsilyl silica gel for chromatography R* (5 μm).

Mobile phase: mix 12 volumes of *methanol R* and 88 volumes of a 6.81 g/l solution of *potassium dihydrogen phosphate R*, adjusted to pH 3.0 with *phosphoric acid R*.

Flow rate: 1.5 ml/min.

Detection: spectrophotometer at 254 nm.

Injection: 20 μl.

System suitability: reference solution (b):

- *resolution*: minimum 2.0 between the peaks due to levodropropizine and to impurity B.

Limits:

- *impurity B*: not more than the area of the corresponding peak in the chromatogram obtained with reference solution (a) (0.5 per cent),
- *any other impurity*: not more than 0.2 times the area of the peak due to impurity B in the chromatogram obtained with reference solution (a) (0.1 per cent),
- *disregard limit*: 0.02 times the area of the peak due to impurity B in the chromatogram obtained with reference solution (a) (0.01 per cent).

Impurity C. Gas chromatography (*2.2.28*). *Prepare the solutions immediately before use.*

Test solution. Dissolve 0.50 g of the substance to be examined in *methylene chloride R* and dilute to 2.5 ml with the same solvent.

Reference solution (a). Dissolve 0.20 g of *glycidol R* in *methylene chloride R* and dilute to 100.0 ml with the same solvent. Dilute 0.5 ml of this solution to 100.0 ml with *methylene chloride R*.

Reference solution (b). Dissolve 0.50 g of the substance to be examined in *methylene chloride R*, add 0.5 ml of reference solution (a) and dilute to 2.5 ml with *methylene chloride R*.

Column:

- *material*: fused silica,
- *size*: *l* = 30 m, Ø = 0.53 mm,
- *stationary phase*: *poly[(cyanopropyl)(phenyl)][dimethyl]siloxane R* (film thickness 3 μm).

Carrier gas: *helium for chromatography R*.

Flow rate: 2.5 ml/min.

Split ratio: 1:8.

Temperature:

- *column*: 140 °C,
- *injection port*: 170 °C,
- *detector*: 250 °C.

Detection: flame ionisation.

Injection: 1 μl; inject the test solution and reference solution (b).

Use a split-liner consisting of a column about 1 cm long packed with glass wool.

At the end of a series of tests, heat the column at 250 °C for 4-6 h.

Limit:

- *impurity C*: not more than half the area of the corresponding peak in the chromatogram obtained with reference solution (b) (10 ppm).

Enantiomeric purity. Liquid chromatography (*2.2.29*).

Test solution. Dissolve 10.0 mg of the substance to be examined in 10.0 ml of a mixture of 40 volumes of *ethanol R* and 60 volumes of *hexane R*. Dilute 1.0 ml of the solution to 50.0 ml with a mixture of 40 volumes of *ethanol R* and 60 volumes of *hexane R*.

Reference solution (a). Dissolve 10.0 mg of *levodropropizine CRS* in 10.0 ml of a mixture of 40 volumes of *ethanol R* and 60 volumes of *hexane R*. Dilute 1.0 ml of the solution to 50.0 ml with a mixture of 40 volumes of *ethanol R* and 60 volumes of *hexane R*.

Reference solution (b). Dissolve 10.0 mg of *levodropropizine impurity A CRS* in 10.0 ml of a mixture of 40 volumes of *ethanol R* and 60 volumes of *hexane R*. Dilute 1.0 ml of the solution to 50.0 ml with a mixture of 40 volumes of *ethanol R* and 60 volumes of *hexane R*.

Reference solution (c). Dilute 1.0 ml of reference solution (b) to 50.0 ml with a mixture of 40 volumes of *ethanol R* and 60 volumes of *hexane R*.

Reference solution (d). Mix 1 ml of reference solution (a) and 1 ml of reference solution (b).

Column:

- *size*: *l* = 0.25 m, Ø = 4.6 mm,
- *stationary phase*: *silica gel OD for chiral separations R*.

Mobile phase: *diethylamine R, ethanol R, hexane R* (0.2:5:95 *V/V/V*).

Flow rate: 0.8 ml/min.

Detection: spectrophotometer at 254 nm.

Injection: 20 μl; inject the test solution and reference solutions (a), (c) and (d).

Elution order: impurity A, levodropropizine.

System suitability:

- *retention times*: the retention times of the principal peaks in the chromatograms obtained with the test solution and reference solution (a) are similar,
- *resolution*: minimum 2.0 between the peaks due to impurity A and to levodropropizine in the chromatogram obtained with reference solution (d).

Limit:

- *impurity A*: not more than the area of the corresponding peak in the chromatogram obtained with reference solution (c) (2 per cent).

Loss on drying (*2.2.32*): maximum 1.0 per cent, determined on 0.500 g by drying *in vacuo* at 60 °C over *diphosphorus pentoxide R* at a pressure of 0.15 kPa to 0.25 kPa for 4 h.

Sulphated ash (*2.4.14*): maximum 0.2 per cent, determined on 1.0 g.

ASSAY

Dissolve 0.100 g in 50 ml of *anhydrous acetic acid R*. Carry out a potentiometric titration (*2.2.20*), using *0.1 M perchloric acid*. Read the volume added at the second point of inflexion.

1 ml of *0.1 M perchloric acid* is equivalent to 11.82 mg of $C_{13}H_{20}N_2O_2$.

STORAGE

Protected from light.

IMPURITIES

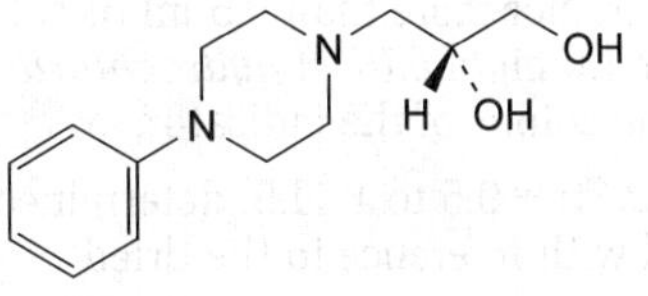

A. (2*R*)-3-(4-phenylpiperazin-1-yl)propane-1,2-diol (dextrodropropizine),

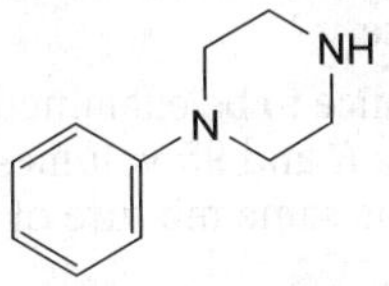

B. 1-phenylpiperazine,

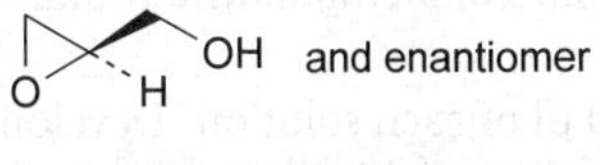

C. [(2*RS*)-oxiran-2-yl]methanol (glycidol).

01/2005:0619

LEVOMENTHOL

Levomentholum

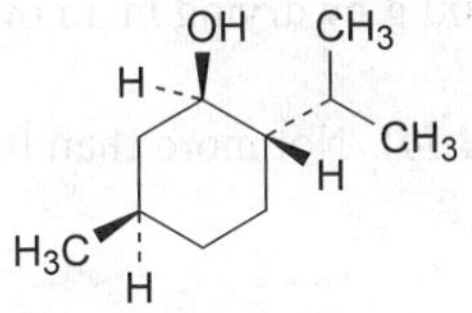

$C_{10}H_{20}O$ M_r 156.3

DEFINITION

Levomenthol is (1*R*,2*S*,5*R*)-5-methyl-2-(1-methylethyl)cyclohexanol.

CHARACTERS

Prismatic or acicular, colourless, shiny crystals, practically insoluble in water, very soluble in alcohol and in light petroleum, freely soluble in fatty oils and in liquid paraffin, very slightly soluble in glycerol.

It melts at about 43 °C.

IDENTIFICATION

First identification: A, C.

Second identification: B, D.

A. It complies with the test for specific optical rotation (see Tests).

B. Examine by thin-layer chromatography (*2.2.27*), using *silica gel G R* as the coating substance.

Test solution. Dissolve 25 mg of the substance to be examined in *methanol R* and dilute to 5 ml with the same solvent.

Reference solution. Dissolve 25 mg of *menthol CRS* in *methanol R* and dilute to 5 ml with the same solvent.

Apply separately to the plate 2 µl of each solution. Develop over a path of 15 cm using a mixture of 5 volumes of *ethyl acetate R* and 95 volumes of *toluene R*. Allow the plate to dry in air until the solvents have evaporated and spray with *anisaldehyde solution R*. Heat at 100 °C to 105 °C for 5 min to 10 min. The principal spot in the chromatogram obtained with the test solution is similar in position, colour and size to the principal spot in the chromatogram obtained with the reference solution.

C. Examine the chromatograms obtained in the test for related substances. The principal peak in the chromatogram obtained with test solution (b) is similar in position and approximate dimensions to the principal peak in the chromatogram obtained with reference solution (c).

D. Dissolve 0.20 g in 0.5 ml of *anhydrous pyridine R*. Add 3 ml of a 150 g/l solution of *dinitrobenzoyl chloride R* in *anhydrous pyridine R*. Heat on a water-bath for 10 min. Add 7.0 ml of *water R* in small quantities with stirring and allow to stand in iced water for 30 min. A precipitate is formed. Allow to stand and decant the supernatant liquid. Wash the precipitate with two quantities, each of 5 ml, of iced *water R*, recrystallise from 10 ml of *acetone R*, wash with iced *acetone R* and dry at 75 °C at a pressure not exceeding 2.7 kPa for 30 min. The crystals melt (*2.2.14*) at 154 °C to 157 °C.

TESTS

Solution S. Dissolve 2.50 g in 10 ml of *alcohol R* and dilute to 25.0 ml with the same solvent.

Appearance of solution. Solution S is clear (*2.2.1*) and colourless (*2.2.2, Method II*).

Acidity or alkalinity. Dissolve 1.0 g in *alcohol R* and dilute to 10 ml with the same solvent. Add 0.1 ml of *phenolphthalein solution R*; the solution is colourless. Not more than 0.5 ml of *0.01 M sodium hydroxide* is required to change the colour of the indicator to pink.

Specific optical rotation (*2.2.7*): − 48 to − 51, determined on solution S.

Related substances. Examine by gas chromatography (*2.2.28*).

Test solution (a). Dissolve 0.20 g of the substance to be examined in *methylene chloride R* and dilute to 50.0 ml with the same solvent.

Test solution (b). Dilute 1.0 ml of test solution (a) to 10.0 ml with *methylene chloride R*.

Reference solution (a). Dissolve 40.0 mg of the substance to be examined and 40.0 mg of *isomenthol R* in *methylene chloride R* and dilute to 100.0 ml with the same solvent.

Reference solution (b). Dilute 0.10 ml of test solution (a) to 100.0 ml with *methylene chloride R*.

Reference solution (c). Dissolve 40.0 mg of *menthol CRS* in *methylene chloride R* and dilute to 100.0 ml with the same solvent.

The chromatographic procedure may be carried out using:

- a glass column 2.0 m long and 2 mm internal diameter packed with *diatomaceous earth for gas chromatography R* impregnated with 15 per cent *m/m* of *macrogol 1500 R*,
- *nitrogen for chromatography R* as the carrier gas at a flow rate of 30 ml/min,
- a flame-ionisation detector,

maintaining the temperature of the column at 120 °C, that of the injection port at 150 °C and that of the detector at 200 °C.

Inject separately 1 µl of each solution. Record the chromatograms for twice the retention time of the peak corresponding to menthol. In the chromatogram obtained with test solution (a), the sum of the areas of the peaks, apart from the principal peak, is not greater than 1 per cent of the area of the principal peak. Disregard any peak due to the solvent and any peak whose area is less than 0.05 per cent of the area of the principal peak. The test is not valid unless: in the chromatogram obtained with reference solution (a) the resolution between the peaks corresponding to menthol and isomenthol is not less than 1.4 and the principal peak in the chromatogram obtained with reference solution (b) has a signal-to-noise ratio of not less than 5.

Residue on evaporation. Evaporate 2.00 g on a water-bath and heat in an oven at 100 °C to 105 °C for 1 h. The residue weighs not more than 1.0 mg (0.05 per cent).

01/2005:0505

LEVOMEPROMAZINE HYDROCHLORIDE

Levomepromazini hydrochloridum

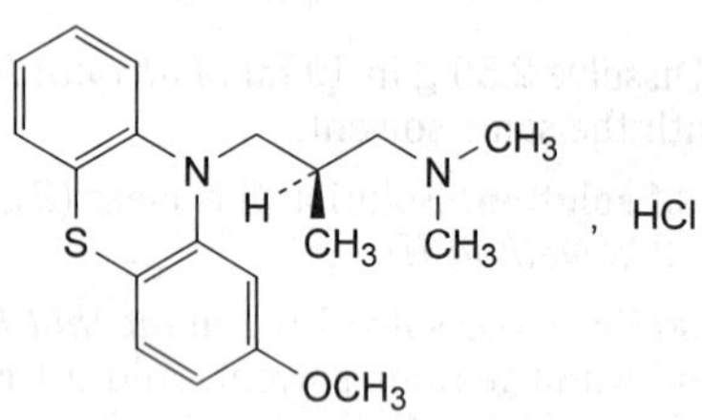

$C_{19}H_{25}ClN_2OS$ M_r 364.9

DEFINITION

Levomepromazine hydrochloride contains not less than 98.5 per cent and not more than the equivalent of 101.0 per cent of (2*R*)-3-(2-methoxy-10*H*-phenothiazin-10-yl)-*N*,*N*,2-trimethylpropan-1-amine hydrochloride, calculated with reference to the dried substance.

CHARACTERS

A white or very slightly yellow, crystalline powder, slightly hygroscopic, freely soluble in water and in alcohol. It deteriorates when exposed to air and light. It exists in two forms, one melting at about 142 °C and the other at about 162 °C.

IDENTIFICATION

A. *Prepare the solution protected from bright light and carry out the measurements immediately.* Dissolve 50.0 mg in *water R* and dilute to 500.0 ml with the same solvent. Dilute 10.0 ml of this solution to 100.0 ml with *water R*. Examined between 230 nm and 340 nm (*2.2.25*), the solution shows two absorption maxima, at 250 nm and 302 nm. The specific absorbance at the maximum at 250 nm is 640 to 700.

B. It complies with the identification test for phenothiazines by thin-layer chromatography (*2.3.3*).

C. Introduce 0.2 g into a 100 ml separating funnel. Add 5 ml of *water R* and 0.5 ml of *strong sodium hydroxide solution R*. Shake vigorously with two quantities, each of 10 ml, of *ether R*. Combine the ether layers, dry over *anhydrous sodium sulphate R* and evaporate to dryness. Keep the residue at 100 °C to 105 °C for 15 min and allow to crystallise in iced water. Initiate crystallisation if necessary by scratching the wall of the flask with a glass rod. Dry the crystals at 60 °C for 2 h. The crystals melt (*2.2.14*) at 122 °C to 128 °C.

D. It gives reaction (b) of chlorides (*2.3.1*).

TESTS

Solution S. Dissolve 2.50 g in *carbon dioxide-free water R* and dilute to 25.0 ml with the same solvent.

Acidity or alkalinity. To 10 ml of solution S add 0.1 ml of *bromocresol green solution R*. Not more than 0.5 ml of *0.01 M sodium hydroxide* or 1.0 ml of *0.01 M hydrochloric acid* is required to change the colour of the indicator.

Specific optical rotation (*2.2.7*): + 9.5 to + 11.5, determined on solution S and calculated with reference to the dried substance.

Related substances. *Carry out the test protected from bright light.* Examine by thin-layer chromatography (*2.2.27*), using *silica gel GF_{254} R* as the coating substance.

Test solution. Dissolve 0.2 g of the substance to be examined in a mixture of 5 volumes of *diethylamine R* and 95 volumes of *methanol R* and dilute to 10 ml with the same mixture of solvents. Prepare immediately before use.

Reference solution. Dilute 0.5 ml of the test solution to 100 ml with a mixture of 5 volumes of *diethylamine R* and 95 volumes of *methanol R*.

Apply separately to the plate 10 µl of each solution. Develop over a path of 15 cm using a mixture of 10 volumes of *acetone R*, 10 volumes of *diethylamine R* and 80 volumes of *cyclohexane R*. Allow the plate to dry in air and examine in ultraviolet light at 254 nm. Any spot in the chromatogram obtained with the test solution, apart from the principal spot, is not more intense than the spot in the chromatogram obtained with the reference solution (0.5 per cent).

Loss on drying (*2.2.32*). Not more than 1.0 per cent, determined on 1.000 g by drying in an oven at 100 °C to 105 °C for 3 h.

Sulphated ash (*2.4.14*). Not more than 0.1 per cent, determined on 1.0 g.

ASSAY

Dissolve 0.300 g in 5 ml of *water R* and add 50 ml of *2-propanol R*. Titrate with *0.1 M sodium hydroxide*, determining the end-point potentiometrically (*2.2.20*).

1 ml of *0.1 M sodium hydroxide* is equivalent to 36.49 mg of $C_{19}H_{25}ClN_2OS$.

STORAGE

Store in an airtight container, protected from light.

01/2005:0925

LEVOMEPROMAZINE MALEATE

Levomepromazini maleas

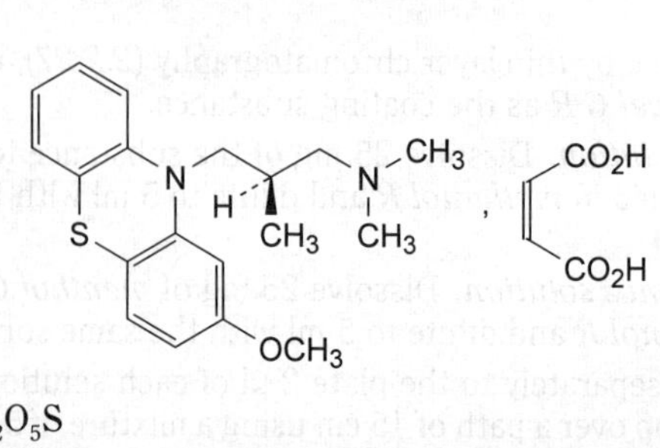

$C_{23}H_{28}N_2O_5S$ M_r 444.6

DEFINITION

Levomepromazine maleate contains not less than 98.5 per cent and not more than the equivalent of 101.0 per cent of (2*R*)-3-(2-methoxy-10*H*-phenothiazin-10-yl)-*N*,*N*,2-trimethylpropan-1-amine (*Z*)-butenedioate, calculated with reference to the dried substance.

CHARACTERS

A white or slightly yellowish, crystalline powder, slightly soluble in water, sparingly soluble in methylene chloride, slightly soluble in alcohol. It deteriorates when exposed to air and light.

It melts at about 186 °C, with decomposition.

IDENTIFICATION

First identification: A, B.

Second identification: A, C, D.

A. It complies with the test for specific optical rotation (see Tests).

B. Examine by infrared absorption spectrophotometry (*2.2.24*), comparing with the spectrum obtained with *levomepromazine maleate CRS*. Examine the substances prepared as discs.

C. It complies with the identification test for phenothiazines by thin-layer chromatography (*2.3.3*).

D. Examine by thin-layer chromatography (*2.2.27*), using *silica gel GF_{254} R* as the coating substance.

Test solution. Dissolve 0.20 g of the substance to be examined in a mixture of 10 volumes of *water R* and 90 volumes of *acetone R* and dilute to 10 ml with the same mixture of solvents.

Reference solution. Dissolve 50 mg of *maleic acid CRS* in a mixture of 10 volumes of *water R* and 90 volumes of *acetone R* and dilute to 10 ml with the same mixture of solvents.

Apply separately to the plate as bands 10 mm by 2 mm 5 µl of each solution. Develop over a path of 12 cm using a mixture of 3 volumes of *water R*, 7 volumes of *anhydrous formic acid R* and 90 volumes of *di-isopropyl ether R*. Dry the plate at 120 °C for 10 min and examine in ultraviolet light at 254 nm. The chromatogram obtained with the test solution shows a band at the starting-point and another band similar in position and size to the principal band in the chromatogram obtained with the reference solution.

TESTS

pH (*2.2.3*). *Carry out the test protected from bright light.* Introduce 0.50 g into a conical flask and add 25.0 ml of *carbon dioxide-free water R*. Shake and allow the solids to settle. The pH of the supernatant solution is 3.5 to 5.5.

Specific optical rotation (*2.2.7*). Dissolve 1.25 g in *dimethylformamide R* and dilute to 25.0 ml with the same solvent. The specific optical rotation is − 7.0 to − 8.5, calculated with reference to the dried substance.

Related substances. *Carry out the test protected from bright light and prepare the solutions immediately before use.* Examine by thin-layer chromatography (*2.2.27*), using *silica gel GF_{254} R* as the coating substance.

Test solution. Dissolve 0.20 g of the substance to be examined in a mixture of 10 volumes of *water R* and 90 volumes of *acetone R* and dilute to 10 ml with the same mixture of solvents.

Reference solution. Dilute 0.5 ml of the test solution to 100 ml with a mixture of 10 volumes of *water R* and 90 volumes of *acetone R*.

Apply separately to the plate 10 µl of each solution. Develop over a path of 15 cm using a mixture of 10 volumes of *acetone R*, 10 volumes of *diethylamine R* and 80 volumes of *cyclohexane R*. Allow the plate to dry in air and examine in ultraviolet light at 254 nm. Any spot in the chromatogram obtained with the test solution, apart from the principal spot, is not more intense than the spot in the chromatogram obtained with the reference solution (0.5 per cent).

Loss on drying (*2.2.32*). Not more than 0.5 per cent, determined on 1.000 g by drying in an oven at 100 °C to 105 °C for 3 h.

Sulphated ash (*2.4.14*). Not more than 0.1 per cent, determined on 1.0 g.

ASSAY

Dissolve 0.350 g in 50 ml of *anhydrous acetic acid R*. Titrate with *0.1 M perchloric acid*, determining the end-point potentiometrically (*2.2.20*).

1 ml of *0.1 M perchloric acid* is equivalent to 44.46 mg of $C_{23}H_{28}N_2O_5S$.

STORAGE

Store protected from light.

IMPURITIES

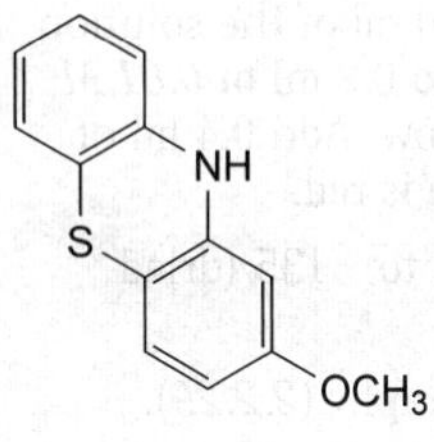

A. 2-methoxyphenothiazine,

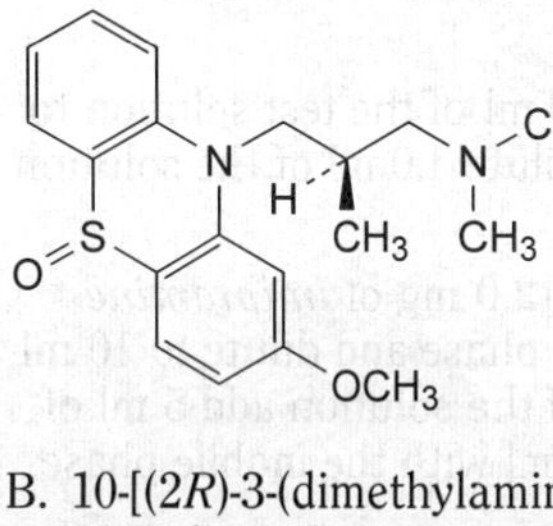

B. 10-[(2*R*)-3-(dimethylamino)-2-methylpropyl]-2-methoxy-10*H*-phenothiazine 5-oxide.

01/2005:1787

LEVOMETHADONE HYDROCHLORIDE

Levomethadoni hydrochloridum

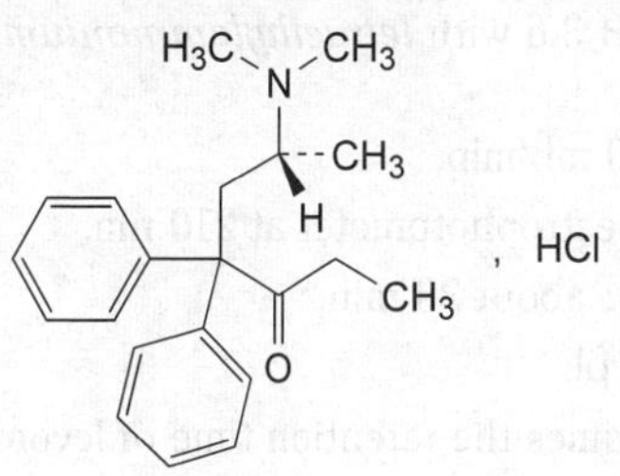

$C_{21}H_{28}ClNO$ M_r 345.9

DEFINITION

(6*R*)-6-(Dimethylamino)-4,4-diphenylheptan-3-one hydrochloride.

Content: 99.0 per cent to 101.0 per cent (dried substance).

CHARACTERS

Appearance: white, crystalline powder.

Solubility: soluble in water, freely soluble in alcohol.

IDENTIFICATION

First identification: A, C, D.

Second identification: A, B, D.

A. Specific optical rotation (see Tests).

B. Melting point (*2.2.14*): 239 °C to 242 °C.

C. Infrared absorption spectrophotometry (*2.2.24*).

Comparison: *Ph. Eur. reference spectrum of methadone hydrochloride.*

D. Dilute 1 ml of solution S (see Tests) to 5 ml with *water R* and add 1 ml of *dilute ammonia R1*. Mix, allow to stand for 5 min and filter. The filtrate gives reaction (a) of chlorides (*2.3.1*).

TESTS

Solution S. Dissolve 2.50 g in *carbon dioxide-free water R* and dilute to 50.0 ml with the same solvent.

Appearance of solution. Solution S is clear (*2.2.1*) and colourless (*2.2.2, Method II*).

Acidity or alkalinity. Dilute 10 ml of solution S to 25 ml with *carbon dioxide-free water R*. To 10 ml of the solution add 0.2 ml of *methyl red solution R* and 0.2 ml of *0.01 M sodium hydroxide*. The solution is yellow. Add 0.4 ml of *0.01 M hydrochloric acid*. The solution is red.

Specific optical rotation (*2.2.7*): − 125 to − 135 (dried substance), determined on solution S.

Related substances. Liquid chromatography (*2.2.29*).

Test solution. Dissolve 25.0 mg of the substance to be examined in the mobile phase and dilute to 100.0 ml with the mobile phase.

Reference solution (a). Dilute 1.0 ml of the test solution to 50.0 ml with the mobile phase. Dilute 1.0 ml of the solution to 10.0 ml with the mobile phase.

Reference solution (b). Dissolve 12.0 mg of *imipramine hydrochloride CRS* in the mobile phase and dilute to 10 ml with the mobile phase. To 1 ml of the solution add 5 ml of the test solution and dilute to 10 ml with the mobile phase.

Column:

- *size*: *l* = 0.125 m, Ø = 4.6 mm,
- *stationary phase*: *octadecylsilyl silica gel for chromatography R* (5 µm),
- *temperature*: 25 °C.

Mobile phase: mix 35 volumes of *acetonitrile R* and 65 volumes of an 11.5 g/l solution of *phosphoric acid R* adjusted to pH 3.6 with *tetraethylammonium hydroxide solution R*.

Flow rate: 1.0 ml/min.

Detection: spectrophotometer at 210 nm.

Equilibration: about 30 min.

Injection: 10 µl.

Run time: 7 times the retention time of levomethadone.

Retention time: levomethadone = about 5 min.

System suitability: reference solution (b):

- *resolution*: minimum 2.5 between the peaks due to imipramine and levomethadone.

Limits:

- *any impurity*: not more than half the area of the principal peak in the chromatogram obtained with reference solution (a) (0.1 per cent),
- *total*: not more than 2.5 times the area of the principal peak in the chromatogram obtained with reference solution (a) (0.5 per cent),
- *disregard limit*: 0.25 times the area of the principal peak in the chromatogram obtained with reference solution (a) (0.05 per cent).

Dextromethadone. Liquid chromatography (*2.2.29*).

Test solution. Dissolve 40.0 mg of the substance to be examined in the mobile phase and dilute to 100.0 ml with the mobile phase.

Reference solution. Dilute 1.0 ml of the test solution to 10.0 ml with the mobile phase. Dilute 1.0 ml of the solution to 20.0 ml with the mobile phase.

Column:

- *size*: *l* = 0.25 m, Ø = 4.6 mm,
- *stationary phase*: *2-hydroxypropylbetadex for chromatography R* (5 µm),
- *temperature*: 10 °C.

Mobile phase: mix 1 volume of *triethylamine R* adjusted to pH 4.0 with *phosphoric acid R*, 15 volumes of *acetonitrile R* and 85 volumes of a 13.6 g/l solution of *potassium dihydrogen phosphate R*.

Flow rate: 0.7 ml/min.

Detection: spectrophotometer at 210 nm.

Equilibration: about 30 min.

Injection: 10 µl.

Relative retention with reference to levomethadone: dextromethadone = about 1.4.

System suitability: test solution:

- *number of theoretical plates*: minimum 2000, calculated for the peak due to levomethadone,
- *tailing factor*: maximum 3 for the peak due to levomethadone.

Limit:

- *dextromethadone*: not more than the area of the principal peak in the chromatogram obtained with the reference solution (0.5 per cent).

Loss on drying (*2.2.32*): maximum 0.5 per cent, determined on 1.000 g by drying in an oven at 100-105 °C.

Sulphated ash (*2.4.14*): maximum 0.1 per cent, determined on 1.0 g.

ASSAY

Dissolve 0.300 g in a mixture of 40 ml of *water R* and 5 ml of *acetic acid R*. Titrate with *0.1 M silver nitrate*. Determine the end-point potentiometrically (*2.2.20*), using a silver electrode.

1 ml of *0.1 M silver nitrate* is equivalent to 34.59 mg of $C_{21}H_{28}ClNO$.

STORAGE

Protected from light.

IMPURITIES

Specified impurities: A, B, C, D, E, F.

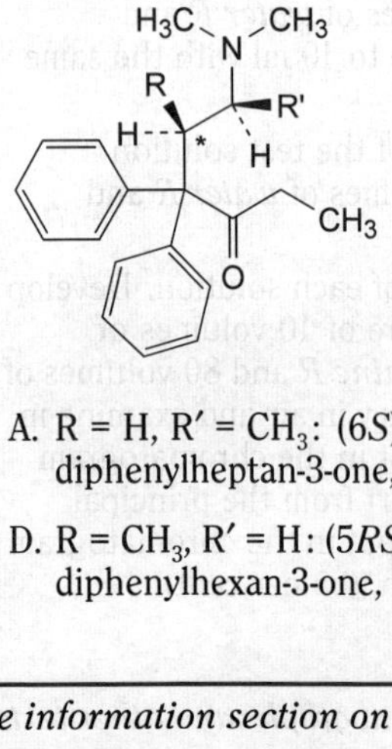

and epimer at C*

A. R = H, R′ = CH_3: (6*S*)-6-(dimethylamino)-4,4-diphenylheptan-3-one,

D. R = CH_3, R′ = H: (5*RS*)-6-(dimethylamino)-5-methyl-4,4-diphenylhexan-3-one,

Monographs I-L

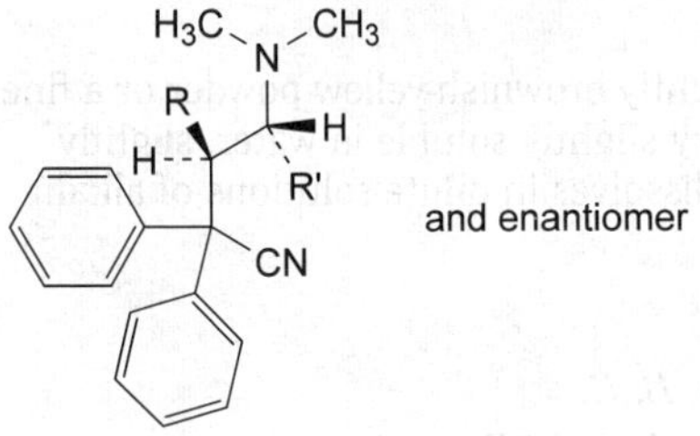

B. R = H, R′ = CH_3: (4*RS*)-4-(dimethylamino)-2,2-diphenylpentanenitrile,

C. R = CH_3,R′ = H: (3*RS*)-4-(dimethylamino)-3-methyl-2,2-diphenylbutanenitrile,

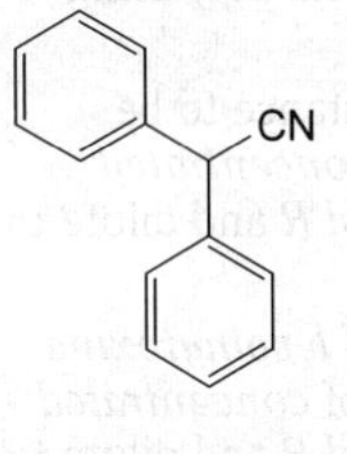

E. diphenylacetonitrile,

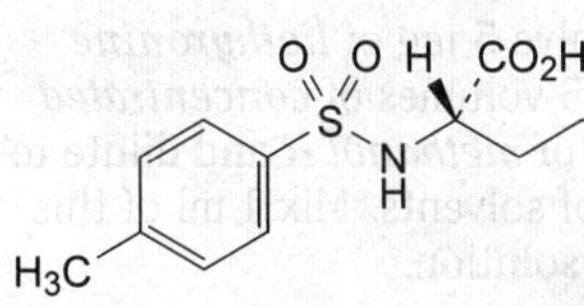

F. (2*S*)-2-[[(4-methylphenyl)sulphonyl]amino]pentanedioic acid (*N*-*p*-tosyl-L-glutamic acid).

01/2005:0926

LEVONORGESTREL

Levonorgestrelum

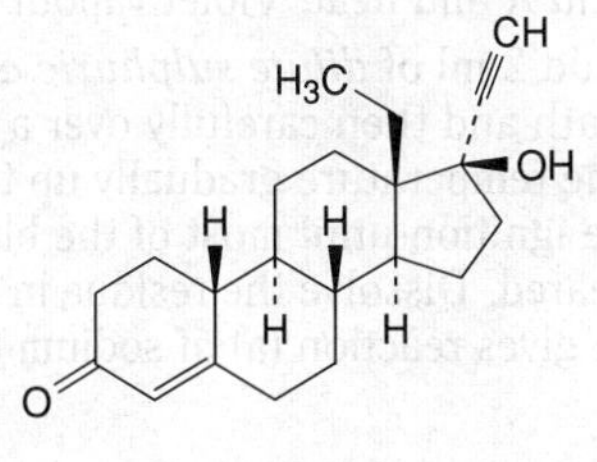

$C_{21}H_{28}O_2$ *M*r 312.5

DEFINITION

Levonorgestrel contains not less than 98.0 per cent and not more than the equivalent of 102.0 per cent of 13β-ethyl-17β-hydroxy-18,19-dinor-17α-pregn-4-en-20-yn-3-one, calculated with reference to the dried substance.

CHARACTERS

A white or almost white, crystalline powder, practically insoluble in water, sparingly soluble in methylene chloride, slightly soluble in alcohol.

IDENTIFICATION

A. It complies with the test for specific optical rotation (see Tests).

B. Examine by infrared absorption spectrophotometry (*2.2.24*), comparing with the spectrum obtained with *levonorgestrel CRS*.

TESTS

Specific optical rotation (*2.2.7*). Dissolve 0.200 g in *chloroform R* and dilute to 10.0 ml with the same solvent. The specific optical rotation is - 30 to - 35.

Related substances. Examine by thin-layer chromatography (*2.2.27*), using *silica gel G R* as the coating substance.

Test solution. Dissolve 0.2 g of the substance to be examined in *chloroform R* and dilute to 10 ml with the same solvent.

Reference solution (a). Dilute 1 ml of the test solution to 10 ml with *methylene chloride R*. Dilute 1 ml of this solution to 20 ml with *methylene chloride R*.

Reference solution (b). Dilute 4 ml of reference solution (a) to 10 ml with *methylene chloride R*.

Reference solution (c) Dissolve 5 mg of *levonorgestrel CRS* and 5 mg of *ethinylestradiol CRS* in *methylene chloride R* and dilute to 50 ml with the same solvent.

Apply separately to the plate 10 µl of each solution. Develop over a path of 15 cm using a mixture of 20 volumes of *ethyl acetate R* and 80 volumes of *methylene chloride R*. Allow the plate to dry in air, spray with a 100 g/l solution of *phosphomolybdic acid R* in *alcohol R*, heat at 100 °C to 105 °C for 15 min and examine immediately. Any spot in the chromatogram obtained with the test solution, apart from the principal spot, is not more intense than the principal spot in the chromatogram obtained with reference solution (a) (0.5 per cent) and at most two such spots are more intense than the spot in the chromatogram obtained with reference solution (b) (0.2 per cent). The test is not valid unless the chromatogram obtained with reference solution (c) shows two clearly separated spots.

Loss on drying (*2.2.32*). Not more than 0.5 per cent, determined on 1.000 g by drying in an oven at 100-105 °C.

Sulphated ash (*2.4.14*). Not more than 0.1 per cent, determined on 1.0 g.

ASSAY

Dissolve 0.200 g in 45 ml of *tetrahydrofuran R*. Add 10 ml of a 100 g/l solution of *silver nitrate R*. After 1 min, titrate with *0.1 M sodium hydroxide*, determining the end-point potentiometrically (*2.2.20*). Carry out a blank titration.

1 ml of *0.1 M sodium hydroxide* is equivalent to 31.25 mg $C_{21}H_{28}O_2$.

STORAGE

Store protected from light.

IMPURITIES

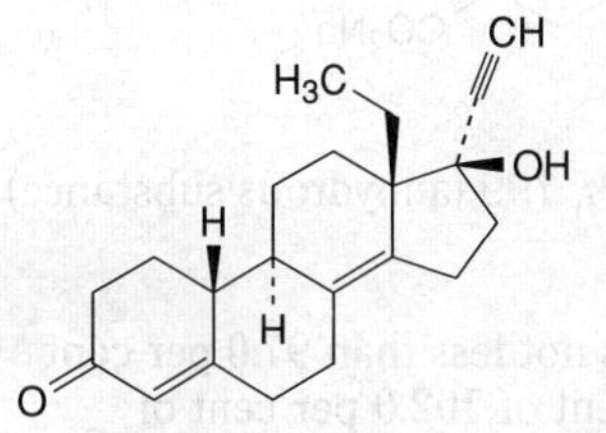

A. 13-ethyl-17-hydroxy-18,19-dinor-17α-pregna-4,8(14)-dien-20-yn-3-one,

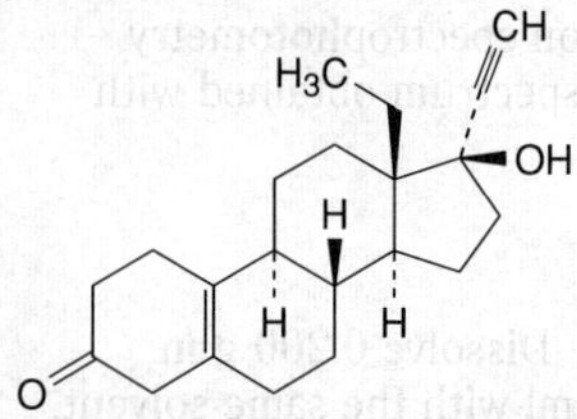

B. 13-ethyl-17-hydroxy-18,19-dinor-17α-pregn-5(10)-en-20-yn-3-one,

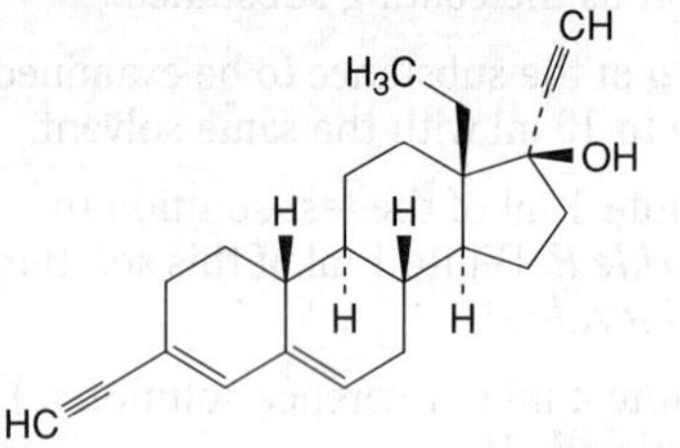

C. 13-ethyl-3-ethynyl-18,19-dinor-17α-pregna-3,5-dien-20-yn-17-ol,

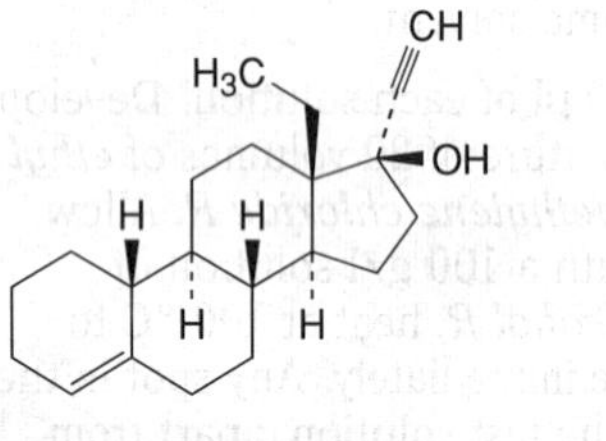

D. 13-ethyl-18,19-dinor-17α-pregn-4-en-20-yn-17-ol,

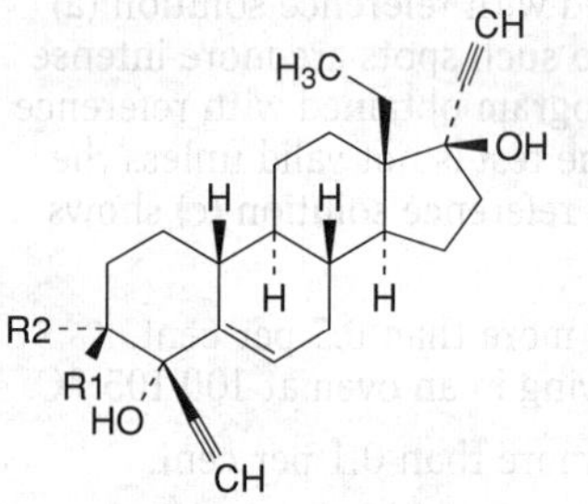

E. R1 = OH, R2 = C≡CH: 13-ethyl-3,4-diethynyl-18,19-dinor-17α-pregn-5-en-20-yn-3β,4α,17-triol,

F. R1 = C≡CH, R2 = OH: 13-ethyl-3,4-diethynyl-18,19-dinor-17α-pregn-5-en-20-yn-3α,4α,17-triol.

01/2005:0401

LEVOTHYROXINE SODIUM

Levothyroxinum natricum

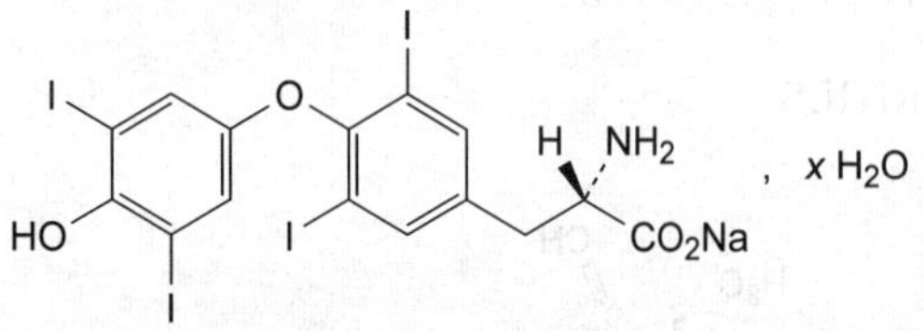

$C_{15}H_{10}I_4NNaO_4,xH_2O$ M_r 799 (anhydrous substance)

DEFINITION

Levothyroxine sodium contains not less than 97.0 per cent and not more than the equivalent of 102.0 per cent of sodium (2*S*)-2-amino-3-[4-(4-hydroxy-3,5-diiodophenoxy)-3,5-diiodophenyl]propanoate, calculated with reference to the dried substance. It contains a variable amount of water.

CHARACTERS

An almost white or slightly brownish-yellow powder or a fine, crystalline powder, very slightly soluble in water, slightly soluble in alcohol. It dissolves in dilute solutions of alkali hydroxides.

IDENTIFICATION

First identification: A, B, E.

Second identification: A, C, D, E.

A. It complies with the test for specific optical rotation (see Tests).

B. Examine by infrared absorption spectrophotometry (*2.2.24*), comparing with the spectrum obtained with *levothyroxine sodium CRS*.

C. Examine by thin-layer chromatography (*2.2.27*), using *silica gel G R* as the coating substance.

Test solution. Dissolve 5 mg of the substance to be examined in a mixture of 5 volumes of *concentrated ammonia R* and 70 volumes of *methanol R* and dilute to 5 ml with the same mixture of solvents.

Reference solution (a). Dissolve 5 mg of *levothyroxine sodium CRS* in a mixture of 5 volumes of *concentrated ammonia R* and 70 volumes of *methanol R* and dilute to 5 ml with the same mixture of solvents.

Reference solution (b). Dissolve 5 mg of *liothyronine sodium CRS* in a mixture of 5 volumes of *concentrated ammonia R* and 70 volumes of *methanol R* and dilute to 5 ml with the same mixture of solvents. Mix 1 ml of this solution and 1 ml of the test solution.

Apply separately to the plate 5 µl of each solution. Develop over a path of 15 cm using a mixture of 20 volumes of *concentrated ammonia R*, 35 volumes of *2-propanol R* and 55 volumes of *ethyl acetate R*. Allow the plate to dry in air and spray with *ninhydrin solution R*. Heat at 100 °C to 105 °C until the spots appear. Examine in daylight. The principal spot in the chromatogram obtained with the test solution is similar in position, colour and size to the principal spot in the chromatogram obtained with reference solution (a). The test is not valid unless the chromatogram obtained with reference solution (b) shows two clearly separated spots.

D. To about 50 mg in a porcelain dish add a few drops of *sulphuric acid R* and heat. Violet vapour is evolved.

E. To 200 mg add 2 ml of *dilute sulphuric acid R*. Heat on a water-bath and then carefully over a naked flame, increasing the temperature gradually up to about 600 °C. Continue the ignition until most of the black particles have disappeared. Dissolve the residue in 2 ml of *water R*. The solution gives reaction (a) of sodium (*2.3.1*).

TESTS

Solution S. Dissolve 0.500 g in 23 ml of a gently boiling mixture of 1 volume of *1 M hydrochloric acid* and 4 volumes of *alcohol R*. Cool and dilute to 25.0 ml with the same mixture of solvents.

Appearance of solution. Freshly prepared solution S is not more intensely coloured than reference solution BY_3 (*2.2.2, Method II*).

Specific optical rotation (*2.2.7*): + 16 to + 20, determined on solution S and calculated with reference to the dried substance.

Liothyronine and other related substances. Examine the chromatograms obtained in the assay. In the chromatogram obtained with test solution (a), the area of any peak corresponding to liothyronine is not greater than that of the principal peak in the chromatogram obtained with reference solution (b) (1.0 per cent) and the sum of the areas of all the peaks apart from the principal peak and any peak corresponding to liothyronine is not greater than the area of the principal peak in the chromatogram obtained with reference solution (a) (1.0 per cent). Disregard any peak with an area less than that of the peak in the chromatogram obtained with reference solution (d).

Loss on drying (*2.2.32*): 6.0 per cent to 12.0 per cent, determined on 0.100 g by drying in an oven at 100 °C to 105 °C.

ASSAY

Examine by liquid chromatography (*2.2.29*). *Protect the solutions from light throughout the assay.*

Test solution (a). Dissolve 20.0 mg of the substance to be examined in *methanolic sodium hydroxide solution R* and dilute to 100.0 ml with the same solvent.

Test solution (b). Dilute 2.0 ml of test solution (a) to 200 ml with *methanolic sodium hydroxide solution R.*

Reference solution (a). Dissolve 20.0 mg of *levothyroxine CRS* in *methanolic sodium hydroxide solution R* and dilute to 100.0 ml with the same solvent. Dilute 2.0 ml of this solution to 200 ml with *methanolic sodium hydroxide solution R.*

Reference solution (b). Dissolve 5 mg of *liothyronine sodium CRS* in *methanolic sodium hydroxide solution R* and dilute to 50.0 ml with the same solvent. Dilute 10.0 ml of this solution to 50 ml with *methanolic sodium hydroxide solution R.* Dilute 10.0 ml of this solution to 100 ml with *methanolic sodium hydroxide solution R.*

Reference solution (c). Mix equal volumes of reference solution (a) and reference solution (b).

Reference solution (d). Dilute 1 ml of reference solution (a) to 10 ml with *methanolic sodium hydroxide solution R.*

The chromatographic procedure may be carried out using:

- a column 0.25 m long and 4 mm in internal diameter packed with *nitrile silica gel for chromatography R* (5 µm to 10 µm),
- as mobile phase at a flow rate of 1 ml/min a mixture of 1 volume of *phosphoric acid R*, 300 volumes of *acetonitrile R* and 700 volumes of *water R*,
- as detector a spectrophotometer set at 225 nm,
- a loop injector.

Inject separately 50 µl of each solution. Continue the chromatography for 3.5 times the retention time of the principal peak. The assay is not valid unless the resolution between the peaks corresponding to levothyroxine and liothyronine in the chromatogram obtained with reference solution (c) is at least 4 and the principal peak in the chromatogram obtained with reference solution (d) has a signal-to-noise ratio of at least 5. Calculate the percentage of $C_{15}H_{10}I_4NNaO_4$ from the expression:

$$\frac{S_u}{0.972 S_r} \times C_r$$

S_u = area of the peak corresponding to levothyroxine in the chromatogram obtained with test solution (b);

S_r = area of the peak corresponding to levothyroxine in the chromatogram obtained with reference solution (a);

C_r = declared content of $C_{15}H_{11}I_4NO_4$ in *levothyroxine CRS.*

STORAGE

Store in an airtight container, protected from light, at 2 °C to 8 °C.

01/2005:0727

LIDOCAINE

Lidocainum

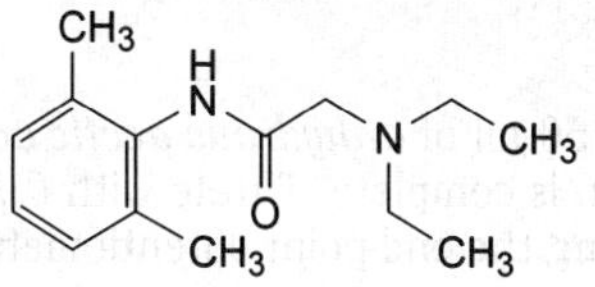

$C_{14}H_{22}N_2O$ M_r 234.3

DEFINITION

Lidocaine contains not less than 99.0 per cent and not more than the equivalent of 101.0 per cent of 2-(diethylamino)-*N*-(2,6-dimethylphenyl)acetamide, calculated with reference to the anhydrous substance.

CHARACTERS

A white or almost white, crystalline powder, practically insoluble in water, very soluble in alcohol and in methylene chloride.

IDENTIFICATION

First identification: A, B.

Second identification: A, C, D, E.

A. Melting point (*2.2.14*): 66 °C to 70 °C, determined without previous drying.

B. Examine by infrared absorption spectrophotometry (*2.2.24*), comparing with the spectrum obtained with *lidocaine CRS.*

C. Dissolve 0.20 g in a mixture of 0.5 ml of *dilute hydrochloric acid R* and 10 ml of *water R* with warming and add 10 ml of *picric acid solution R*. The precipitate, washed with *water R* and dried, melts (*2.2.14*) at about 230 °C, with decomposition.

D. To about 5 mg add 0.5 ml of *fuming nitric acid R*. Evaporate to dryness on a water-bath, cool and dissolve the residue in 5 ml of *acetone R*. Add 0.2 ml of *alcoholic potassium hydroxide solution R*. A green colour is produced.

E. Dissolve about 0.1 g in 1 ml of *alcohol R* and add 0.5 ml of a 100 g/l solution of *cobalt nitrate R*. A bluish-green precipitate is formed.

TESTS

Appearance of solution. Dissolve 1.0 g in 3 ml of *dilute hydrochloric acid R* and dilute to 10 ml with *water R*. The solution is clear (*2.2.1*) and colourless (*2.2.2, Method II*).

2,6-Dimethylaniline. Dissolve 0.25 g in *methanol R* and dilute to 10 ml with the same solvent. To 2 ml of the solution add 1 ml of a freshly prepared 10 g/l solution of *dimethylaminobenzaldehyde R* in *methanol R* and 2 ml of *glacial acetic acid R* and allow to stand for 10 min. Any yellow colour in the solution is not more intense than that in a standard prepared at the same time and in the same manner using 2 ml of a 2.5 mg/l solution of *2,6-dimethylaniline R* in *methanol R* (100 ppm).

Chlorides (*2.4.4*). Dissolve 1.4 g in a mixture of 3 ml of *dilute nitric acid R* and 12 ml of *water R*. The solution complies with the limit test for chlorides (35 ppm).

Monographs I-L

Sulphates (*2.4.13*). Dissolve 0.2 g in 5 ml of *alcohol R* and dilute to 20 ml with *distilled water R*. 15 ml of the solution complies with the limit test for sulphates (0.1 per cent).

Heavy metals (*2.4.8*). 1.0 g complies with limit test C for heavy metals (20 ppm). Prepare the standard using 2 ml of *lead standard solution (10 ppm Pb) R*.

Water (*2.5.12*). Not more than 1.0 per cent, determined on 1.000 g by the semi-micro determination of water.

Sulphated ash (*2.4.14*). Not more than 0.1 per cent, determined on 1.0 g.

ASSAY

To 0.200 g add 50 ml of *anhydrous acetic acid R* and stir until dissolution is complete. Titrate with *0.1 M perchloric acid*, determining the end-point potentiometrically (*2.2.20*).

1 ml of *0.1 M perchloric acid* is equivalent to 23.43 mg of $C_{14}H_{22}N_2O$.

01/2005:0227

LIDOCAINE HYDROCHLORIDE

Lidocaini hydrochloridum

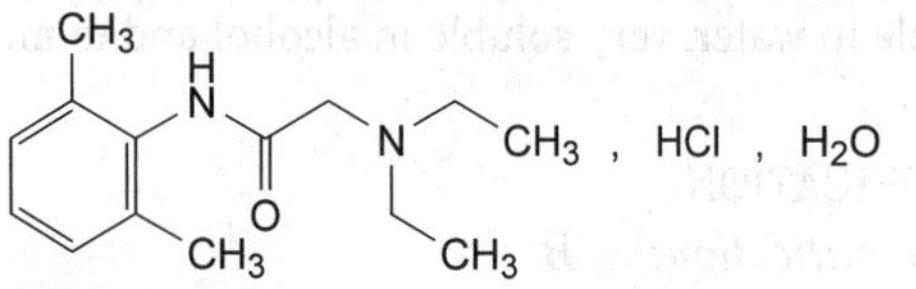

$C_{14}H_{23}ClN_2O,H_2O$ M_r 288.8

DEFINITION

Lidocaine hydrochloride contains not less than 99.0 per cent and not more than the equivalent of 101.0 per cent of 2-(diethylamino)-*N*-(2,6-dimethylphenyl)acetamide hydrochloride, calculated with reference to the anhydrous substance.

CHARACTERS

A white, crystalline powder, very soluble in water, freely soluble in alcohol.

IDENTIFICATION

First identification: A, B, F.

Second identification: A, C, D, E, F.

A. Melting point (*2.2.14*): 74 °C to 79 °C, determined without previous drying.

B. Examine by infrared absorption spectrophotometry (*2.2.24*), comparing with the spectrum obtained with *lidocaine hydrochloride CRS*.

C. Dissolve 0.2 g in 10 ml of *water R* and add 10 ml of *picric acid solution R*. The precipitate, washed with *water R* and dried, melts (*2.2.14*) at about 230 °C.

D. To about 5 mg add 0.5 ml of *fuming nitric acid R*. Evaporate to dryness on a water-bath, cool and dissolve the residue in 5 ml of *acetone R*. Add 0.2 ml of *alcoholic potassium hydroxide solution R*. A green colour is produced.

E. To 5 ml of solution S (see Tests) add 5 ml of *water R* and make alkaline with *dilute sodium hydroxide solution R*. Collect the precipitate on a filter and wash with *water R*. Dissolve half of the precipitate in 1 ml of *alcohol R* and add 0.5 ml of a 100 g/l solution of *cobalt nitrate R*. A bluish-green precipitate is formed.

F. It gives reaction (a) of chlorides (*2.3.1*).

TESTS

Solution S. Dissolve 1.0 g in *carbon dioxide-free water R* and dilute to 20 ml with the same solvent.

Appearance of solution. Solution S is clear (*2.2.1*) and colourless (*2.2.2, Method II*).

pH (*2.2.3*). Dilute 1 ml of solution S to 10 ml with *carbon dioxide-free water R*. The pH of the solution is 4.0 to 5.5.

Impurity A

Solution (a). Dissolve 0.25 g of the substance to be examined in *methanol R* and dilute to 10 ml with the same solvent. This solution is used to prepare the test solution.

Solution (b). Dissolve 50 mg of *2,6-dimethylaniline R* in *methanol R* and dilute to 100 ml with the same solvent. Dilute 1 ml of the solution to 100 ml with *methanol R*. This solution is used to prepare the standard.

Using three flat-bottomed tubes, place in the first 2 ml of solution (a), in the second 1 ml of solution (b) and 1 ml of *methanol R* and in the third 2 ml of *methanol R* (used to prepare a blank). To each tube add 1 ml of a freshly prepared 10 g/l solution of *dimethylaminobenzaldehyde R* in *methanol R* and 2 ml of *glacial acetic acid R* and allow to stand at room temperature for 10 min. The intensity of the yellow colour of the test solution is between that of the blank and that of the standard (100 ppm).

Heavy metals (*2.4.8*). Dissolve 1.0 g in *water R* and dilute to 25 ml with the same solvent. Carry out the prefiltration. 10 ml of the prefiltrate complies with limit test E for heavy metals (5 ppm). Prepare the standard using 2 ml of *lead standard solution (1 ppm Pb) R*.

Water (*2.5.12*): 5.5 per cent to 7.0 per cent, determined on 0.25 g by the semi-micro determination of water.

Sulphated ash (*2.4.14*). Not more than 0.1 per cent, determined on 1.0 g.

ASSAY

Dissolve 0.220 g in 50 ml of *alcohol R* and add 5.0 ml of *0.01 M hydrochloric acid.* Carry out a potentiometric titration (*2.2.20*), using *0.1 M sodium hydroxide*. Read the volume added between the 2 inflexion points.

1 ml of *0.1 M sodium hydroxide* is equivalent to 27.08 mg of $C_{14}H_{23}ClN_2O$.

STORAGE

Store protected from light.

IMPURITIES

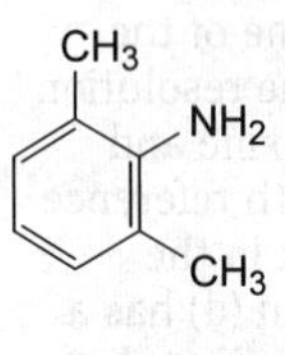

A. 2,6-dimethylaniline.

01/2005:0957

LIME FLOWER

Tiliae flos

DEFINITION

Lime flower consists of the whole, dried inflorescence of *Tilia cordata* Miller, of *Tilia platyphyllos* Scop., of *Tilia × vulgaris* Heyne or a mixture of these.

CHARACTERS

Lime flower has a faint aromatic odour and a faint, sweet and mucilaginous taste.

It has the macroscopic and microscopic characters described under identification tests A and B.

IDENTIFICATION

A. The inflorescence is yellowish-green. The main axis of the inflorescence bears a linguiform bract, membranous, yellowish-green, practically glabrous, the central vein of which is joined for up to about half of its length with the peduncle. The inflorescence usually consists of two to seven flowers, occasionally up to sixteen. The sepals are detached easily from the perianth; they are up to 6 mm long, their abaxial surface is usually glabrous, their adaxial surface and their borders are strongly pubescent. The five spatulate, thin petals are yellowish-white, up to 8 mm long. They show fine venation and their borders only are sometimes covered with isolated trichomes. The numerous stamens are free and usually constitute five groups. The superior ovary has a pistil with a somewhat 5-lobate stigma.

B. Separate the inflorescence into its different parts. Examine under a microscope using *chloral hydrate solution R*. The adaxial epidermis of the bract shows cells with straight or slightly sinuous anticlinal walls; the abaxial epidermis shows cells with wavy-sinuous anticlinal walls and anomocytic stomata (*2.8.3*). Isolated cells in the mesophyll contain small calcium oxalate cluster crystals. The parenchyma of the sepals shows, particularly near the veins, numerous mucilaginous cells and cells containing small calcium oxalate clusters. The adaxial epidermis of sepals bears bent, thick-walled covering trichomes, unicellular or stellate with up to five cells. The epidermal cells of the petals show straight anticlinal walls with a striated cuticle without stomata. The parenchyma of the petals shows small calcium oxalate clusters and especially in its acuminate part mucilaginous cells. The pollen grains have a diameter of about 30 µm to 40 µm and are oval or slightly triangular with three germinal pores and a finely granulated exine. The ovary is glabrous or densely covered with trichomes, often very twisted, unicellular or stellate with two to four branches.

C. Examine by thin-layer chromatography (*2.2.27*), using a suitable silica gel as the coating substance.

Test solution. Shake 1.0 g of the powdered drug (355) with 10 ml of *methanol R* in a water-bath at 65 °C for 5 min. Allow to cool and filter.

Reference solution. Dissolve 2.0 mg of *caffeic acid R*, 5 mg of *hyperoside R* and 5 mg of *rutin R* in 10 ml of *methanol R*.

Apply separately to the plate as bands 10 µl of each solution. Develop over a path of 15 cm using a mixture of 10 volumes of *anhydrous formic acid R*, 10 volumes of *water R*, 30 volumes of *methyl ethyl ketone R* and 50 volumes of *ethyl acetate R*. Dry the plate at 100 °C to 105 °C and spray the warm plate with a 10 g/l solution of *diphenylboric acid aminoethyl ester R* in *methanol R*. Then spray the plate with a 50 g/l solution of *macrogol 400 R* in *methanol R*. Allow the plate to dry for about 30 min and examine in ultraviolet light at 365 nm. The chromatogram obtained with the reference solution shows in order of increasing R_f value zones corresponding to rutin and hyperoside with yellowish-orange to brownish-orange fluorescence and a zone corresponding to caffeic acid with greenish-blue fluorescence. In the chromatogram obtained with the test solution, the main zone shows brownish-yellow to orange fluorescence. This zone is situated just above the zone of hyperoside in the chromatogram obtained with the reference solution. In daylight, this zone stands out from the other zones as the main zone. At the R_f level of rutin there is also a zone of brownish-yellow fluorescence. Below this zone, two zones of yellow fluorescence may be present. Between the zones of rutin and hyperoside, zones of orange and yellow fluorescence are visible. Between the zones of hyperoside and caffeic acid, up to five zones of yellow to orange fluorescence are present. Immediately below the zone of caffeic acid is a zone of a blue fluorescence.

TESTS

Foreign matter (*2.8.2*). Not more than 2 per cent, determined on 30 g. There are no inflorescences with a bract bearing at the abaxial face stellate, five- to eight-rayed trichomes and flowers having an apparent double corolla by transformation of five stamens into petal-like staminoids and having a pistil which is not lobular nor indented. 6-merous flowers occur only occasionally (*Tilia americana* L., *Tilia tomentosa* Moench).

Loss on drying (*2.2.32*). Not more than 12.0 per cent, determined on 1.000 g of the powdered drug (355) by drying in an oven at 100 °C to 105 °C for 2 h.

Total ash (*2.4.16*). Not more than 8.0 per cent.

STORAGE

Store protected from light.

01/2005:0583

LINCOMYCIN HYDROCHLORIDE

Lincomycini hydrochloridum

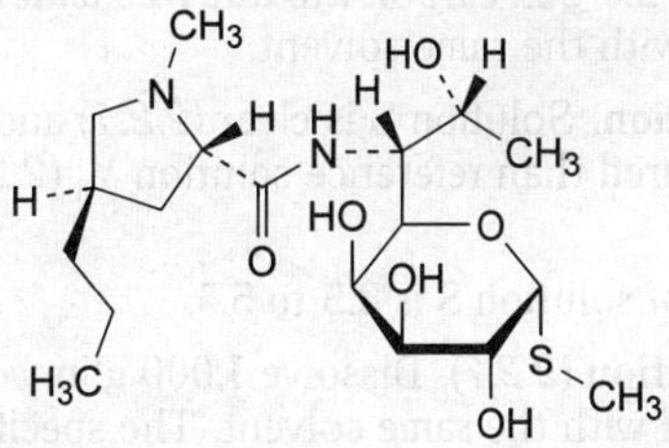

$C_{18}H_{35}ClN_2O_6S,H_2O$ M_r 461.0

DEFINITION

Lincomycin hydrochloride consists mainly of the methyl 6,8-dideoxy-6-[[[(2*S*,4*R*)-1-methyl-4-propylpyrrolidin-2-yl]carbonyl]amino]-1-thio-D-*erythro*-α-D-*galacto*-octopyranoside hydrochloride, an antimicrobial substance produced by *Streptomyces lincolnensis* var. *lincolnensis* or by any other means. It contains not less than 82.5 per cent and not more than 93.0 per cent of lincomycin ($C_{18}H_{34}N_2O_6S$), calculated with reference to the anhydrous substance.

CHARACTERS

A white or almost white, crystalline powder, very soluble in water, slightly soluble in alcohol, very slightly soluble in acetone.

IDENTIFICATION

First identification: A, D.

Second identification: B, C, D.

A. Examine by infrared absorption spectrophotometry (*2.2.24*), comparing with the spectrum obtained with *lincomycin hydrochloride CRS*.

B. Examine by thin-layer chromatography (*2.2.27*), using *silica gel G R* as the coating substance.

Test solution. Dissolve 10 mg of the substance to be examined in *methanol R* and dilute to 10 ml with the same solvent.

Reference solution (a). Dissolve 10 mg of *lincomycin hydrochloride CRS* in *methanol R* and dilute to 10 ml with the same solvent.

Reference solution (b). Dissolve 10 mg of *lincomycin hydrochloride CRS* and 10 mg of *clindamycin hydrochloride CRS* in *methanol R* and dilute to 10 ml with the same solvent.

Apply separately to the plate 5 µl of each solution. Develop over a path of 15 cm using the upper layer from a mixture of 20 volumes of *2-propanol R*, 40 volumes of a 150 g/l solution of *ammonium acetate R* previously adjusted to pH 9.6 with *ammonia R* and 45 volumes of *ethyl acetate R*. Allow the plate to dry in air and spray with a 1 g/l solution of *potassium permanganate R*. The principal spot in the chromatogram obtained with the test solution is similar in position, colour and size to the principal spot in the chromatogram obtained with reference solution (a). The test is not valid unless the chromatogram obtained with reference solution (b) shows two clearly separated spots.

C. Dissolve about 10 mg in 2 ml of *dilute hydrochloric acid R* and heat in a water-bath for 3 min. Add 3 ml of *sodium carbonate solution R* and 1 ml of a 20 g/l solution of *sodium nitroprusside R*. A violet-red colour develops.

D. Dissolve 0.1 g in *water R* and dilute to 10 ml with the same solvent. The solution gives reaction (a) of chlorides (*2.3.1*).

TESTS

Solution S. Dissolve 2.0 g in *carbon dioxide-free water R* and dilute to 20 ml with the same solvent.

Appearance of solution. Solution S is clear (*2.2.1*) and not more intensely coloured than reference solution Y_6 (*2.2.2, Method II*).

pH (*2.2.3*). The pH of solution S is 3.5 to 5.5.

Specific optical rotation (*2.2.7*). Dissolve 1.000 g in *water R* and dilute to 25.0 ml with the same solvent. The specific optical rotation is + 135 to + 150, calculated with reference to the anhydrous substance.

Lincomycin B. Examine the chromatogram obtained in the assay with test solution (a). The area of the peak due to lincomycin B, which is eluted just before lincomycin, is not more than 5 per cent of the area of the peak due to lincomycin.

Heavy metals (*2.4.8*). 2.0 g complies with limit test C for heavy metals (5 ppm). Prepare the standard using 1.0 ml of *lead standard solution (10 ppm Pb) R*.

Water (*2.5.12*). 3.1 per cent to 4.6 per cent, determined on 0.500 g by the semi-micro determination of water.

Sulphated ash (*2.4.14*). Not more than 0.5 per cent, determined on 1.0 g.

Bacterial endotoxins (*2.6.14*): less than 0.50 IU/mg, if intended for use in the manufacture of parenteral dosage forms without a further appropriate procedure for removal of bacterial endotoxins.

ASSAY

Examine by gas chromatography (*2.2.28*), using *dotriacontane R* as the internal standard.

Internal standard solution. Dissolve 0.200 g of *dotriacontane R* in *chloroform R* and dilute to 25.0 ml with the same solvent.

Test solution (a). Dissolve 0.100 g of the substance to be examined in a 20 g/l solution of *imidazole R* in *chloroform R* and dilute to 100.0 ml with the same solution. Shake until dissolution is complete. Place 4.0 ml of the solution in a ground-glass-stoppered 15 ml centrifuge tube. Add 1.0 ml of a mixture of 1 volume of *chlorotrimethylsilane R* and 99 volumes of *N,O-bis(trimethylsilyl)acetamide R* and swirl gently. Position the glass stopper loosely in the tube and heat at 65 °C for 30 min.

Test solution (b). Prepare as described for test solution (a) but add 10.0 ml of the internal standard solution before dissolution of the substance to be examined.

Reference solution. Prepare as described for test solution (a) using 0.100 g of *lincomycin hydrochloride CRS* instead of the substance to be examined and adding 10.0 ml of the internal standard solution before dissolution of the reference substance.

The chromatographic procedure may be carried out using:

- a glass column 1.5 m long and 3 mm in internal diameter packed with *silanised diatomaceous earth for gas chromatography R* impregnated with 3 per cent *m/m* of *poly(methylphenylsiloxane) R*,
- *helium for chromatography R* as the carrier gas at a flow rate of about 45 ml/min,
- a flame-ionisation detector,

maintaining the temperature of the column at 260 °C and that of the injection port and of the detector between 260 °C and 290 °C. Inject the chosen volume of the test solutions and the reference solution.

STORAGE

Store in an airtight container at a temperature not exceeding 30 °C. If the substance is sterile, store in a sterile, airtight, tamper-proof container.

LABELLING

The label states, where applicable, that the substance is free from bacterial endotoxins.

01/2005:0772

LINDANE

Lindanum

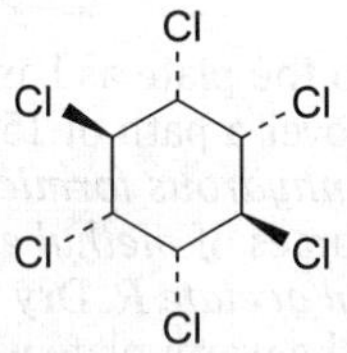

$C_6H_6Cl_6$ M_r 290.8

DEFINITION

Lindane contains not less than 99.0 per cent and not more than the equivalent of 100.5 per cent of *r*-1,*c*-2,*t*-3,*c*-4,*c*-5,*t*-6-hexachlorocyclohexane.

CHARACTERS

A white or almost white, crystalline powder, practically insoluble in water, freely soluble in acetone, soluble in ethanol.

IDENTIFICATION

First identification: A, B.

Second identification: A, C, D.

A. Melting point (*2.2.14*): 112 °C to 115 °C.

B. Examine by infrared absorption spectrophotometry (*2.2.24*), comparing with the spectrum obtained with *lindane CRS*. Examine the substances prepared as discs.

C. Examine the chromatograms obtained in the test for related substances. The principal spot in the chromatogram obtained with test solution (b) is similar in position, colour and size to the principal spot in the chromatogram obtained with reference solution (a).

D. Dissolve about 5 mg in 4 ml of *alcohol R*. Add 1 ml of *0.5 M potassium hydroxide alcoholic*. Allow to stand for 10 min. The solution gives reaction (a) of chlorides (*2.3.1*).

TESTS

Appearance of solution. Dissolve 0.50 g in *acetone R* and dilute to 10 ml with the same solvent. The solution is clear (*2.2.1*) and not more intensely coloured than reference solution B_7 (*2.2.2, Method II*).

Related substances. Examine by thin-layer chromatography (*2.2.27*), using *silica gel G R* as the coating substance.

Test solution (a). Dissolve 1.0 g of the substance to be examined in *chloroform R* and dilute to 10 ml with the same solvent.

Test solution (b). Dilute 1 ml of test solution (a) to 10 ml with *chloroform R*.

Reference solution (a). Dissolve 0.1 g of *lindane CRS* in *chloroform R* and dilute to 10 ml with the same solvent.

Reference solution (b). Dilute 1 ml of test solution (b) to 10 ml with *chloroform R*.

Reference solution (c). Dissolve 10 mg of *α-hexachlorocyclohexane CRS* in test solution (a) and dilute to 5 ml with the same solvent.

Apply separately to the plate 1 µl of each solution. Develop over a path of 12 cm using a mixture of 10 volumes of *chloroform R* and 90 volumes of *cyclohexane R*. Dry the plate in a current of air, irradiate with ultraviolet light at 254 nm for 15 min and spray with a 6 g/l solution of *dicarboxidine hydrochloride R* in *alcohol (90 per cent V/V) R*. Examine in daylight. Any spot in the chromatogram obtained with test solution (a), apart from the principal spot, is not more intense than the spot in the chromatogram obtained with reference solution (b) (1.0 per cent). The test is not valid unless the chromatogram obtained with reference solution (c) shows two clearly separated spots.

Chlorides (*2.4.4*). To 0.75 g, finely powdered, add 15 ml of *water R*. Boil for 1 min. Allow to cool, shaking frequently, and filter. To 10 ml of the filtrate add 3 ml of *water R* and 2 ml of *alcohol R*. The solution complies with the limit test for chlorides (100 ppm).

Sulphated ash (*2.4.14*). Not more than 0.1 per cent, determined on 1.0 g.

ASSAY

To 0.200 g add 10 ml of *alcohol R* and warm on a water-bath until dissolved. Cool, add 20 ml of *0.5 M alcoholic potassium hydroxide* and allow to stand for 10 min, swirling frequently. Add 50 ml of *water R*, 20 ml of *dilute nitric acid R*, 25.0 ml of *0.1 M silver nitrate* and 5 ml of *ferric ammonium sulphate solution R2*. Titrate with *0.1 M ammonium thiocyanate* until a reddish-yellow colour is obtained. Carry out a blank titration.

1 ml of *0.1 M silver nitrate* is equivalent to 9.694 mg of $C_6H_6Cl_6$.

STORAGE

Store protected from light.

01/2005:1232

LINOLEOYL MACROGOLGLYCERIDES

Macrogolglyceridorum linoleates

DEFINITION

Linoleoyl macrogolglycerides are mixtures of monoesters, diesters and triesters of glycerol and monoesters and diesters of macrogols. They are obtained by partial alcoholysis of an unsaturated oil mainly containing triglycerides of linoleic acid using macrogol with a mean relative molecular mass between 300 and 400 or by esterification of glycerol and macrogol with unsaturated fatty acids or by mixing of glycerol esters and condensates of ethylene oxide with the fatty acids of this unsaturated oil.

CHARACTERS

Amber, oily liquids which may give rise to a deposit after prolonged periods at 20 °C, practically insoluble but dispersible in water, freely soluble in methylene chloride. The viscosity at 40 °C is about 35 mPa·s, the relative density at 20 °C is about 0.95, the refractive index at 20 °C is about 1.47.

IDENTIFICATION

A. Examine by thin-layer chromatography (*2.2.27*), using a suitable silica gel as the coating substance.

Test solution. Dissolve 1.0 g of the substance to be examined in *methylene chloride R* and dilute to 20 ml with the same solvent.

Apply to the plate 10 µl of the test solution. Develop over a path of 15 cm using a mixture of 30 volumes of *hexane R* and 70 volumes of *ether R*. Allow the plate to dry in air. Spray with a 0.1 g/l solution of *rhodamine B R* in *alcohol R* and examine in ultraviolet light at 365 nm. The chromatogram shows a spot corresponding to triglycerides with an R_f value of about 0.9 (R_{st} 1) and spots corresponding to 1,3-diglycerides (R_{st} 0.7), to 1,2-diglycerides (R_{st} 0.6), to monoglycerides (R_{st} 0.1) and to esters of macrogol (R_{st} 0).

B. They comply with the test for hydroxyl value (see Tests).

C. They comply with the test for fatty acid composition (see Tests).

D. They comply with the test for saponification value (see Tests).

TESTS

Acid value (*2.5.1*). Not more than 2.0, determined on 2.0 g.

Hydroxyl value (*2.5.3, Method A*): 45 to 65, determined on 1.0 g.

Iodine value (*2.5.4*): 90 to 110.

Peroxide value (*2.5.5*). Not more than 12.0, determined on 2.0 g.

Saponification value (*2.5.6*): 150 to 170, determined on 2.0 g.

Alkaline impurities. Into a test-tube introduce 5.0 g and carefully add a mixture, neutralised if necessary with *0.01 M hydrochloric acid* or with *0.01 M sodium hydroxide*, of 0.05 ml of a 0.4 g/l solution of *bromophenol blue R* in *alcohol R*, 0.3 ml of *water R* and 10 ml of *alcohol R*.

Monographs I-L

Shake and allow to stand. Not more than 1.0 ml of *0.01 M hydrochloric acid* is required to change the colour of the upper layer to yellow.

Free glycerol. Not more than 3.0 per cent. Dissolve 1.20 g in 25.0 ml of *methylene chloride R*. Heat if necessary. After cooling, add 100 ml of *water R*. Shake and add 25.0 ml of a 6 g/l solution of *periodic acid R*. Shake and allow to stand for 30 min. Add 40 ml of a 75 g/l solution of *potassium iodide R*. Allow to stand for 1 min. Add 1 ml of *starch solution R*. Titrate the iodine with *0.1 M sodium thiosulphate*. Carry out a blank titration.

1 ml of *0.1 M sodium thiosulphate* is equivalent to 2.3 mg of glycerol.

Composition of fatty acids (*2.4.22, Method A*). The fatty acid fraction has the following composition:

- *palmitic acid*: 4.0 per cent to 20.0 per cent,
- *stearic acid*: not more than 6.0 per cent,
- *oleic acid*: 20.0 per cent to 35.0 per cent,
- *linoleic acid*: 50.0 per cent to 65.0 per cent,
- *linolenic acid*: not more than 2.0 per cent,
- *arachidic acid*: not more than 1.0 per cent,
- *eicosenoic acid*: not more than 1.0 per cent.

Ethylene oxide and dioxan (*2.4.25*). Not more than 1 ppm of ethylene oxide and not more than 10 ppm of dioxan.

Heavy metals (*2.4.8*). 2.0 g complies with limit test C for heavy metals (10 ppm). Prepare the standard using 2 ml of *lead standard solution (10 ppm Pb) R*.

Water (*2.5.12*). Not more than 1.0 per cent, determined on 1.0 g by the semi-micro determination of water, use a mixture of 30 volumes of *anhydrous methanol R* and 70 volumes of *methylene chloride R* as solvent.

Total ash (*2.4.16*). Not more than 0.1 per cent, determined on 1.0 g.

STORAGE

Store protected from light at room temperature.

LABELLING

The label states the type of macrogol used (mean relative molecular mass) or the number of units of ethylene oxide per molecule (nominal value).

01/2005:0095

LINSEED

Lini semen

DEFINITION

Linseed consists of the dried ripe seeds of *Linum usitatissimum* L.

DESCRIPTION

The seeds have a flattened, elongated ovoid shape and are 4 mm to 6 mm long, 2 mm to 3 mm wide and 1.5 mm to 2 mm thick; one end is rounded and the other end forms an oblique point near which the hilum appears as a slight depression. The testa is dark reddish-brown, smooth and glossy but when viewed with a lens the surface is seen to be minutely pitted. The interior of the testa has a narrow, whitish endosperm and an embryo composed of 2 large, flattened, yellowish and oily cotyledons; the radicle points towards the hilum.

Examined under a microscope, the testa is composed of an epidermis of isodiametric cells with mucilaginous outer walls and suberised inner walls; within this is an area of collenchymatous cells followed by a single layer of longitudinally elongated sclereids, each 120 µm to 190 µm long and 12 µm to 15 µm wide, with thickened and pitted walls; the testa has a hyaline layer composed of thin-walled parenchyma and the inner epidermis formed of a layer of flattened polygonal cells each containing a mass of orange-brown pigment. The endosperm and cotyledons are composed of polygonal parenchymatous cells with slightly thickened walls, containing aleurone grains up to 20 µm in diameter and globules of fatty oil; starch is absent.

The powder is greasy to the touch; it is yellowish-brown and has a slight characteristic odour and a mucilaginous and oily taste. It consists of: fragments of the outer epidermal cells of the testa filled with mucilage; sub-epidermal collenchymatous layer seen in surface view as round cells with distinct triangular intercellular spaces often in connection with groups of elongated sclereids with pitted walls; thin-walled pitted cells of the hyaline layer often remaining attached to the elongated sclereids and crossing them at approximately right angles; pigmented cells of the inner epidermis of the testa; parenchyma of the endosperm and cotyledons containing aleurone grains and fatty oil. Starch granules are absent.

TESTS

Odour and taste. The drug does not have a rancid odour or taste.

Foreign matter (*2.8.2*). Not more than 1.5 per cent.

Swelling index (*2.8.4*). Not less than 4 for the whole drug and not less than 4.5 for the powdered drug (710).

Sulphated ash (*2.4.14*). Not more than 6.0 per cent, determined on 1.00 g of powdered drug.

STORAGE

Store protected from light.

01/2005:1908

LINSEED OIL, VIRGIN

Lini oleum virginale

DEFINITION

Virgin oil obtained by cold expression from ripe seeds of *Linum usitatissimum* L. A suitable antioxidant may be added.

CHARACTERS

Appearance: clear, yellow or brownish-yellow liquid, on exposure to air turning dark and gradually thickening. When cooled, it becomes a soft mass at about − 20 °C.

Solubility: very slightly soluble in alcohol, miscible with light petroleum.

Relative density: about 0.931.

Refractive index: about 1.480.

IDENTIFICATION

First identification: B, C.

Second identification: A, B.

A. Identification of fatty oils by thin-layer chromatography (*2.3.2*). The chromatogram obtained is similar to the type chromatogram for linseed oil.

B. It complies with the test for iodine value (see Tests).

C. It complies with the test for composition of fatty acids (see Tests).

Monographs I-L

TESTS

Acid value (*2.5.1*): maximum 4.5.

Iodine value (*2.5.4*): 160 to 200.

Peroxide value (*2.5.5*): maximum 15.0.

Saponification value (*2.5.6*): 188 to 195. Carry out the saponification for 1 h.

Unsaponifiable matter (*2.5.7*): maximum 1.5 per cent, determined on 5.0 g.

Composition of fatty acids. Gas chromatography (*2.4.22, Method C*). Use the calibration mixture in Table 2.4.22.-3.

Composition of the fatty-acid fraction of the oil:

- *fatty acids with a chain length less than* C_{16}: maximum 1.0 per cent,
- *palmitic acid*: 3.0 per cent to 8.0 per cent,
- *palmitoleic acid* (equivalent chain length on polyethyleneglycol adipate 16.3): maximum 1.0 per cent,
- *stearic acid*: 2.0 per cent to 8.0 per cent,
- *oleic acid* (equivalent chain length on polyethyleneglycol adipate 18.3): 11.0 per cent to 35.0 per cent,
- *linoleic acid* (equivalent chain length on polyethyleneglycol adipate 18.9): 11.0 per cent to 24.0 per cent,
- *linolenic acid* (equivalent chain length on polyethyleneglycol adipate 19.7): 35.0 per cent to 65.0 per cent,
- *arachidic acid*: maximum 1.0 per cent.

Cadmium (*2.4.27*): maximum 0.5 ppm.

Water (*2.5.32*): maximum 0.1 per cent, determined on 5.00 g.

STORAGE

In an airtight container, protected from light.

LABELLING

The label states the name and concentration of any added antioxidant.

01/2005:0728

LIOTHYRONINE SODIUM

Liothyroninum natricum

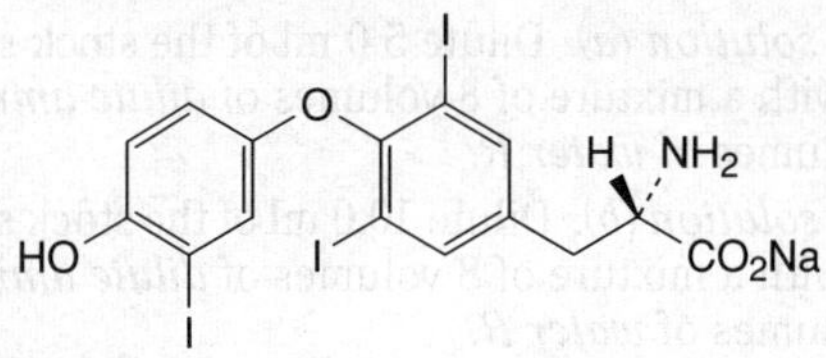

$C_{15}H_{11}I_3NNaO_4$ M_r 673

DEFINITION

Liothyronine sodium contains not less than 95.0 per cent and not more than the equivalent of 102.0 per cent of sodium (2*S*)-2-amino-3-[4-(4-hydroxy-3-iodophenoxy)-3,5-diiodophenyl]propanoate, calculated with reference to the dried substance.

CHARACTERS

A white or slightly coloured powder, practically insoluble in water, slightly soluble in alcohol. It dissolves in dilute solutions of alkali hydroxides.

IDENTIFICATION

First identification: A, C, E.

Second identification: A, B, D, E.

A. It complies with the test for specific optical rotation (see Tests).

B. Dissolve 10.0 mg in *0.1 M sodium hydroxide* and dilute to 100.0 ml with the same solvent. Examined between 230 nm and 350 nm (*2.2.25*), the solution shows an absorption maximum at 319 nm. The specific absorbance at the maximum is 63 to 69, calculated with reference to the dried substance.

C. Examine by infrared absorption spectrophotometry (*2.2.24*), comparing with the spectrum obtained with *liothyronine sodium CRS*.

D. To about 50 mg in a porcelain dish add a few drops of *sulphuric acid R* and heat. Violet vapour is evolved.

E. Dissolve the residue obtained in the test for sulphated ash in 2 ml of *water R*. The solution gives reaction (a) of sodium (*2.3.1*).

TESTS

Solution S. Dissolve 0.250 g in a mixture of 1 volume of *1 M hydrochloric acid* and 4 volumes of *alcohol R* and dilute to 25.0 ml with the same mixture of solvents.

Appearance of solution. Freshly prepared solution S is not more intensely coloured than intensity 5 of the range of reference solutions of the most appropriate colour (*2.2.2, Method II*).

Specific optical rotation (*2.2.7*). + 18.0 to + 22.0, determined on solution S and calculated with reference to the dried substance.

Levothyroxine and other related substances. Examine the chromatograms obtained in the assay. In the chromatogram obtained with test solution (a), the area of any peak corresponding to levothyroxine is not greater than that of the principal peak in the chromatogram obtained with reference solution (c) (5.0 per cent) and the sum of the areas of all the peaks apart from the principal peak and any peak corresponding to levothyroxine is not greater than half the area of the principal peak in the chromatogram obtained with reference solution (c) (2.5 per cent). Disregard any peak with an area less than that of the peak in the chromatogram obtained with reference solution (e).

Chlorides. Not more than 2.0 per cent, expressed as NaCl and calculated with reference to the dried substance. Dissolve 0.500 g in a 2 g/l solution of *sodium hydroxide R* and dilute to 100 ml with the same solvent. Add 15 ml of *dilute nitric acid R* and titrate with *0.05 M silver nitrate*, determining the end-point potentiometrically (*2.2.20*).

1 ml of *0.05 M silver nitrate* is equivalent to 2.93 mg of NaCl.

Loss on drying (*2.2.32*). Not more than 4.0 per cent, determined on 0.500 g by drying in an oven at 105 °C for 2 h.

Sulphated ash (*2.4.14*). 9.0 per cent to 12.2 per cent, determined on 0.200 g and calculated with reference to the dried substance.

ASSAY

Examine by liquid chromatography (*2.2.29*).

Test solution (a). Dissolve 20.0 mg in *methanolic sodium hydroxide solution R* and dilute to 100.0 ml with the same solvent.

Test solution (b). Dilute 5.0 ml of test solution (a) to 200 ml with *methanolic sodium hydroxide solution R*.

Reference solution (a). Dissolve 20.0 mg of *liothyronine sodium CRS* in *methanolic sodium hydroxide solution R* and dilute to 100.0 ml with the same solvent.

Reference solution (b). Dilute 5.0 ml of reference solution (a) to 200 ml with *methanolic sodium hydroxide solution R*.

Reference solution (c). Dissolve 5 mg of *levothyroxine sodium CRS* in *methanolic sodium hydroxide solution R* and dilute to 50.0 ml with same solvent. Dilute 10.0 ml of this solution to 100.0 ml with *methanolic sodium hydroxide solution R*.

Reference solution (d). Mix equal volumes of reference solution (b) and reference solution (c).

Reference solution (e). Dilute 1.0 ml of reference solution (b) to 25.0 ml with *methanolic sodium hydroxide solution R*.

The chromatographic procedure may be carried out using:

- a column 0.25 m long and 4 mm in internal diameter packed with *nitrile silica gel for chromatography R* (5-10 µm),
- as mobile phase at a flow rate of 1 ml/min a mixture of 5 volumes of *phosphoric acid R*, 300 volumes of *acetonitrile R* and 700 volumes of *water R*,
- as detector a spectrophotometer set at 225 nm,
- a loop injector.

Inject separately 50 µl of each solution. Record the chromatogram obtained with test solution (a) for 5 times the retention time of the principal peak. The test is not valid unless the resolution between the peaks corresponding to liothyronine and levothyroxine in the chromatogram obtained with reference solution (d) is at least 4 and the principal peak in the chromatogram obtained with reference solution (e) has a signal-to-noise ratio of at least 5. Calculate the content of $C_{15}H_{11}I_3NNaO_4$ from the peak areas in the chromatograms obtained with test solution (b) and reference solution (b) and the declared content of $C_{15}H_{11}I_3NNaO_4$ in *liothyronine sodium CRS*.

STORAGE

Store in an airtight container, protected from light, at a temperature between 2 °C and 8 °C.

01/2005:1536

LIQUORICE ETHANOLIC LIQUID EXTRACT, STANDARDISED

Liquiritiae extractum fluidum ethanolicum normatum

DEFINITION

Standardised liquorice ethanolic liquid extract is produced from *Liquorice root (0277)*. It contains not less than 3.0 per cent and not more than 5.0 per cent of glycyrrhizic acid ($C_{42}H_{62}O_{16}$; M_r 823).

PRODUCTION

The extract is produced from the drug and alcohol (70 per cent *V/V*), with an appropriate procedure for liquid extracts.

CHARACTERS

A dark brown, clear liquid with a faint characteristic odour and a sweet taste.

IDENTIFICATION

Examine by thin-layer chromatography (*2.2.27*), using a *TLC silica gel F_{254} plate R*.

Test solution. Place 1.0 g of the extract to be examined in a 50 ml round-bottomed flask, add 16.0 ml of *water R* and 4.0 ml of *hydrochloric acid R1* and heat on a water-bath under a reflux condenser for 30 min. Allow to cool and filter. Dry the filter and the round-bottomed flask at 105 °C for 60 min. Transfer the filter to the round-bottomed flask, add 20 ml of *ether R* and heat in a water-bath at 40 °C under a reflux condenser for 5 min. Allow to cool and filter. Evaporate the filtrate to dryness and dissolve the residue in 5.0 ml of *ether R*.

Reference solution. Dissolve 5.0 mg of *glycyrrhetic acid R* and 5.0 mg of *thymol R* in 5 ml of *ether R*.

Apply to the plate, as bands, 10 µl of each solution. Develop over a path of 15 cm using a mixture of 1 volume of *concentrated ammonia R*, 9 volumes of *water R*, 25 volumes of *alcohol R* and 65 volumes of *ethyl acetate R*. Allow the plate to dry in air for 5 min and examine in ultraviolet light at 254 nm. The chromatograms obtained with the test solution and the reference solution show in the lower half a quenching zone due to glycyrrhetic acid. Spray the plate with *anisaldehyde solution R*. Heat at 100 °C to 105 °C for 5 min to 10 min and examine in daylight. The chromatogram obtained with the reference solution shows in the lower half, a violet zone (glycyrrhetic acid) and, in the upper third, a red zone (thymol). The chromatogram obtained with the test solution shows, in the lower half, a violet zone corresponding to glycyrrhetic acid in the chromatogram obtained with the reference solution and, in the upper third, below the zone of thymol in the chromatogram obtained with the reference solution, a yellow zone due to isoliquiritigenin. Further zones are present.

TESTS

Ethanol content (*2.9.10*). 52 per cent *V/V* to 65 per cent *V/V*.

Methanol and 2-propanol (*2.9.11*): maximum 0.05 per cent *V/V* of methanol and maximum 0.05 per cent *V/V* of 2-propanol.

ASSAY

Examine by liquid chromatography (*2.2.29*).

Test solution. Dilute 1.000 g of the liquid extract to 100 ml with a mixture of 8 volumes of *dilute ammonia R1* and 92 volumes of *water R*. Centrifuge. Dilute 2.0 ml of the supernatant to 100.0 ml with a mixture of 8 volumes of *dilute ammonia R1* and 92 volumes of *water R*.

Stock solution. Dissolve 0.130 g of *monoammonium glycyrrhizate CRS* in a mixture of 8 volumes of *dilute ammonia R1* and 92 volumes of *water R* and dilute to 100.0 ml with the same mixture of solvents.

Reference solution (a). Dilute 5.0 ml of the stock solution to 100.0 ml with a mixture of 8 volumes of *dilute ammonia R1* and 92 volumes of *water R*.

Reference solution (b). Dilute 10.0 ml of the stock solution to 100.0 ml with a mixture of 8 volumes of *dilute ammonia R1* and 92 volumes of *water R*.

Reference solution (c). Dilute 15.0 ml of the stock solution to 100.0 ml with a mixture of 8 volumes of *dilute ammonia R1* and 92 volumes of *water R*.

The chromatographic procedure may be carried out using:

- a stainless steel column 0.10 m long and 4 mm in internal diameter packed with *octadecylsilyl silica gel for chromatography R* (5 µm),
- as mobile phase at a flow rate of 1.5 ml/min a mixture of 6 volumes of *glacial acetic acid R*, 30 volumes of *acetonitrile R* and 64 volumes of *water R*,
- as detector a spectrophotometer set at 254 nm.

Inject 10 µl of reference solution (c). Adjust the sensitivity of the system so that the heights of the peaks are at least 50 per cent of the full scale of the recorder. Inject each reference solution and determine the peak areas.

Establish a calibration curve with the concentrations of the reference solutions (g/100 ml) as the abscissa and the corresponding peak areas as the ordinate.

Inject 10 µl of the test solution. Using the retention times and the peak areas determined from the chromatograms obtained with the reference solutions, locate and integrate the peak due to glycyrrhizic acid in the chromatogram obtained with the test solution.

Calculate the percentage content of glycyrrhizic acid from the expression:

$$A \times \frac{5}{m} \times B \times \frac{822}{840}$$

- A = concentration of monoammonium glycyrrhizate in the test solution, determined from the calibration curve, in g/100 ml,
- B = declared percentage content of *monoammonium glycyrrhizate CRS*,
- m = mass of the liquid extract in grams,
- 822 = molecular mass of glycyrrhizic acid,
- 840 = molecular mass of monoammonium glycyrrhizate (without any water of crystallisation).

STORAGE

Store protected from light.

01/2005:0277

LIQUORICE ROOT

Liquiritiae radix

DEFINITION

Liquorice root consists of the dried unpeeled or peeled, whole or cut root and stolons of *Glycyrrhiza glabra* L.

It contains not less than 4.0 per cent of glycyrrhizic acid ($C_{42}H_{62}O_{16}$, M_r 823), calculated with reference to the dried drug.

CHARACTERS

It has the macroscopic and microscopic characters described under Identification tests A and B.

IDENTIFICATION

A. The root has few branches. Its bark is brownish-grey to brown with longitudinal striations and bears traces of lateral roots. The cylindrical stolons are 1 cm to 2 cm in diameter; their external appearance is similar to that of the root but there are occasional small buds. The fracture of the root and the stolon is granular and fibrous. The cork layer is thin; the secondary phloem region is thick and light yellow with radial striations. The yellow xylem cylinder is compact, with a radiate structure. The stolon has a central pith, which is absent from the root. The external part of the bark is absent from the peeled root.

B. Reduce to a powder (355). The powder is light yellow to faintly greyish. Examine under a microscope using *chloral hydrate solution R*. The powder shows fragments of yellow thick-walled fibres, 700 µm to 1200 µm long and 10 µm to 20 µm wide with a punctiform lumen, often accompanied by crystal sheaths containing prisms of calcium oxalate 10 µm to 35 µm long and 2 µm to 5 µm wide. The walls of the large vessels are yellow, 5 µm to 10 µm thick lignified and have numerous bordered pits with a slit-shaped aperture; fragments of cork consisting of thin-walled cells and isolated prisms of calcium oxalate occur as well as fragments of parenchymatous tissue. Fragments of cork are absent from the peeled root. Examine under a microscope using a mixture of equal volumes of *glycerol R* and *water R*. The powder shows simple, round or oval starch granules, 2 µm to 20 µm in diameter.

C. Examine by thin-layer chromatography (*2.2.27*), using as the coating substance a suitable silica gel with a fluorescent indicator having an optimal intensity at 254 nm.

Test solution. To 0.50 g of the powdered drug (180) in a 50 ml round-bottomed flask add 16.0 ml of *water R* and 4.0 ml of *hydrochloric acid R1* and heat on a water-bath under a reflux condenser for 30 min. Cool and filter. Dry the filter and the round-bottomed flask at 105 °C for 60 min. Place the filter in the round-bottomed flask, add 20.0 ml of *ether R* and heat in a water-bath at 40 °C under a reflux condenser for 5 min. Cool and filter. Evaporate the filtrate to dryness. Dissolve the residue in 5.0 ml of *ether R*.

Reference solution. Dissolve 5.0 mg of *glycyrrhetic acid R* and 5.0 mg of *thymol R* in 5.0 ml of *ether R*.

Apply separately to the plate as bands 10 µl of each solution. Develop over a path of 15 cm using a mixture of 1 volume of *concentrated ammonia R*, 9 volumes of *water R*, 25 volumes of *alcohol R* and 65 volumes of *ethyl acetate R*. Allow the plate to dry in air for 5 min and examine in ultraviolet light at 254 nm. The chromatograms obtained with the test solution and with the reference solution show in the lower half a quenching zone due to glycyrrhetic acid. Spray the plate with *anisaldehyde solution R*, and heat at 100-105 °C for 5 min to 10 min. Examine in daylight. The chromatogram obtained with the reference solution shows in the lower half the violet zone of glycyrrhetic acid and in the upper third the red zone of thymol. The chromatogram obtained with the test solution shows in the lower half of violet zone corresponding to the zone of glycyrrhetic acid in the chromatogram obtained with the reference solution and a yellow zone (isoliquiridigenine) in the upper third under the zone of thymol in the chromatogram obtained with the reference solution. Further zones may be present.

TESTS

Loss on drying (*2.2.32*). Not more than 10.0 per cent, determined on 1.000 g of powdered drug (355) by drying in an oven at 100-105 °C for 2 h.

Total ash (*2.4.16*). Not more than 10.0 per cent for the unpeeled drug and not more than 6.0 per cent for the peeled drug.

Ash insoluble in hydrochloric acid (*2.8.1*). Not more than 2.0 per cent for the unpeeled drug and not more than 0.5 per cent for the peeled drug.

ASSAY

Examine by liquid chromatography (*2.2.29*).

Test solution. Place 1.000 g of the powdered drug (180) in a 150 ml ground glass conical flask. Add 100.0 ml of an 8 g/l solution of *ammonia R* and treat in a ultrasonic bath for 30 min. Centrifuge a part of the supernatant layer and dilute 1.0 ml to 5.0 ml with an 8 g/l solution of *ammonia R*. Filter the solution through a filter (0.45 µm) and use the filtrate as the test solution.

Stock solution. Dissolve 0.130 g of *monoammonium glycyrrhizate CRS* in an 8 g/l solution of *ammonia R* and dilute to 100.0 ml with the same solvent.

Monographs I-L

Reference solution (a). Dilute 5.0 ml of the stock solution to 100.0 ml with an 8 g/l solution of *ammonia R.*

Reference solution (b). Dilute 10.0 ml of the stock solution to 100.0 ml with an 8 g/l solution of *ammonia R.*

Reference solution (c). Dilute 15.0 ml of the stock solution to 100.0 ml with an 8 g/l solution of *ammonia R.*

The chromatographic procedure may be carried out using:

– a stainless steel column 0.10 m long and 4 mm in internal diameter packed with *octadecylsilyl silica gel for chromatography R* (5 µm),
– as mobile phase at a flow rate of 1.5 ml/min a mixture of 6 volumes of *glacial acetic acid R*, 30 volumes of *acetonitrile R* and 64 volumes of *water R*,
– as detector a spectrophotometer set at 254 nm,
– a 10 µl loop injector.

Inject reference solution (c). Adjust the sensitivity of the system so that the height of the peaks are at least 50 per cent of the full scale of the recorder. Inject each reference solution and determine the peak areas.

Establish a calibration curve with the concentration of the reference solutions (g/100 ml) as the abscissa and the corresponding areas as the ordinate.

Inject the test solution. Using the retention time and the peak area determined from the chromatograms obtained with the reference solutions, locate and integrate the peak due to glycyrrhizic acid in the chromatogram obtained with the test solution.

Calculate the percentage content of glycyrrhizic acid from the expression:

$$A \times \frac{5}{m} \times B \times \frac{822}{840}$$

A = concentration of monoammonium glycyrrhizate in the test solution determined from the calibration curve, in g/100 ml,

B = declared percentage content of *monoammonium glycyrrhizate CRS*,

m = mass of the drug, in grams,

822 = molecular weight of glycyrrhizic acid,

840 = molecular weight of the monoammonium glycyrrhizate (without any water of crystallisation).

STORAGE

Store protected from light.

LABELLING

The label states whether the drug is peeled or unpeeled.

01/2005:1120
corrected

LISINOPRIL DIHYDRATE

Lisinoprilum dihydricum

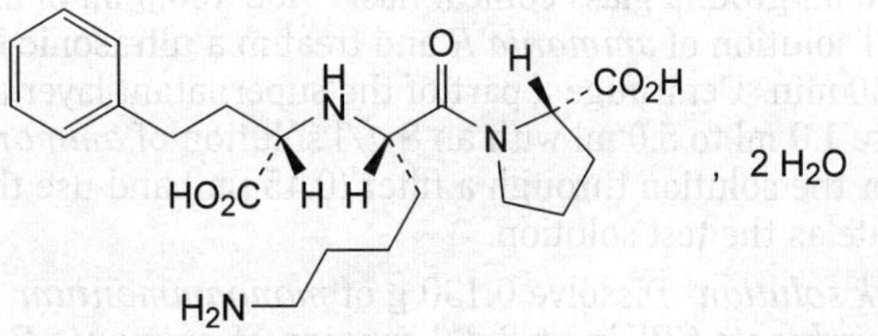

$C_{21}H_{31}N_3O_5,2H_2O$ M_r 441.5

DEFINITION

Lisinopril dihydrate contains not less than 98.5 per cent and not more than the equivalent of 101.5 per cent of (2*S*)-1-[(2*S*)-6-amino-2-[[(1*S*)-1-carboxy-3-phenylpropyl]amino]hexanoyl]pyrrole-2-carboxylic acid, calculated with reference to the anhydrous substance.

CHARACTERS

A white or almost white, crystalline powder, soluble in water, sparingly soluble in methanol, practically insoluble in acetone and in ethanol.

IDENTIFICATION

Examine by infrared absorption spectrophotometry (*2.2.24*), comparing with the spectrum obtained with *lisinopril dihydrate CRS*. Examine the substances prepared as discs.

TESTS

Specific optical rotation (*2.2.7*). Dissolve 0.5 g in *zinc acetate solution R* and dilute to 50.0 ml with the same solvent. The specific optical rotation is − 43 to − 47, calculated with reference to the anhydrous substance.

Related substances. Examine by liquid chromatography (*2.2.29*).

Test solution. Dissolve 20.0 mg of the substance to be examined in mobile phase A and dilute to 10.0 ml with the same mobile phase.

Reference solution (a). Dissolve the contents of 1 vial of *lisinopril dihydrate for performance test CRS* with 1.0 ml of mobile phase A.

Reference solution (b). Dilute 0.5 ml of the test solution to 50.0 ml with mobile phase A.

The chromatographic procedure may be carried out using:

– a stainless steel column 0.25 m long and 4.6 mm in internal diameter packed with *octylsilyl silica gel for chromatography R,*
– as mobile phase at a flow rate of 1.8 ml/min:
Mobile phase A. Prepare a mixture of 30 volumes of *acetonitrile R* and 970 volumes of a 3.12 g/l *sodium dihydrogen phosphate R* solution adjusted to pH 5.0 with a 50 g/l solution of *sodium hydroxide R,*
Mobile phase B. Prepare a mixture of 200 ml of *acetonitrile R* and 800 ml of a 3.12 g/l *sodium dihydrogen phosphate R* solution adjusted to pH 5.0 with a 50 g/l solution of *sodium hydroxide R,*

Time (min)	Mobile phase A (per cent *V/V*)	Mobile phase B (per cent *V/V*)	Comment
0 - 35	100 → 70	0 → 30	linear gradient
35 - 45	70	30	isocratic
45 - 50	70 → 100	30 → 0	switch to initial eluent composition
50 = 0	100	0	restart gradient

– as detector a spectrophotometer set at 210 nm,

maintaining the temperature of the column at 50 °C.

Equilibrate the column with mobile phase A for at least 30 min. Adjust the sensitivity of the system so that the height of the principal peak in the chromatogram obtained with 20 µl of reference solution (b) is at least 50 per cent of the full scale of the recorder.

Inject 20 µl of reference solution (a). The resulting chromatogram resembles that of the specimen chromatogram supplied with *lisinopril dihydrate for performance test CRS* in that the peaks due to impurity A and impurity E fall on either side of the peak due to lisinopril. Measure the heights *A1* and *A2* above the baseline of the peaks due to impurity A and impurity E and the heights *B1* and *B2* above the baseline of the lowest points of the curve separating these peaks from the peak due to lisinopril. The test is not valid unless *A1* is greater than nine times *B1* and *A2* is greater than nine times *B2*.

If necessary, adjust the pH of the mobile phase to 4.5 with *phosphoric acid R* and repeat the chromatography. A further adjustment to pH 4.0 may be necessary with some columns before satisfactory separation of impurity A, lisinopril and impurity E is obtained. If, after adjustment, the retention time of the peak due to impurities C and D becomes extended to the point where integration becomes difficult, increase the content of mobile phase B from 30 per cent to 40 per cent over the interval from 35 min to 45 min from the start of the chromatogram. Maintain this concentration for a further 10 min. Return the concentration of mobile phase A to 100 per cent over the next 10 min prior to the next injection.

Inject 20 µl of the test solution and 20 µl of reference solution (b). In the chromatogram obtained with the test solution: the area of any peak due to impurity E is not greater than 0.3 times the area of the principal peak in the chromatogram obtained with reference solution (b) (0.3 per cent); the area of any peak, apart from the principal peak and any peak due to impurity E, is not greater than 0.3 times the area of the principal peak in the chromatogram obtained with reference solution (b) (0.3 per cent) and the sum of the areas of all such peaks is not greater than half the area of the principal peak in the chromatogram obtained with reference solution (b) (0.5 per cent). Disregard any peak due to the solvent, any peak occurring in the first 3 minutes and any peak with an area less than 0.05 times the area of the principal peak in the chromatogram obtained with reference solution (b).

Water (*2.5.12*): 8.0 to 9.5 per cent, determined on 0.200 g by the semi-micro determination of water.

Sulphated ash (*2.4.14*). Not more than 0.1 per cent, determined on 1.0 g.

ASSAY

Dissolve 0.350 g in 50 ml of *distilled water R.* Titrate with *0.1 M sodium hydroxide,* determining the end-point potentiometrically (*2.2.20*).

1 ml of *0.1 M sodium hydroxide* is equivalent to 40.55 mg of $C_{21}H_{31}N_3O_5$.

IMPURITIES

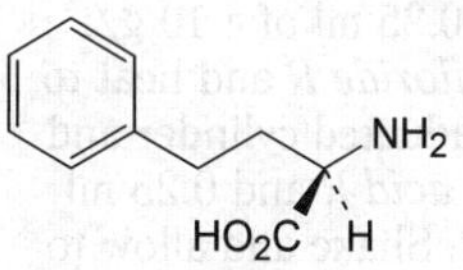
and enantiomer

A. (*2RS*)-2-amino-4-phenylbutanoic acid,

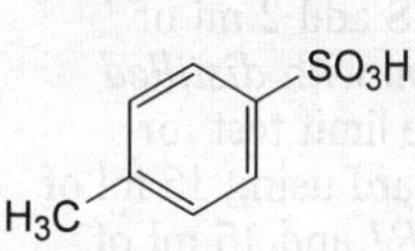

B. 4-methylbenzenesulphonic acid,

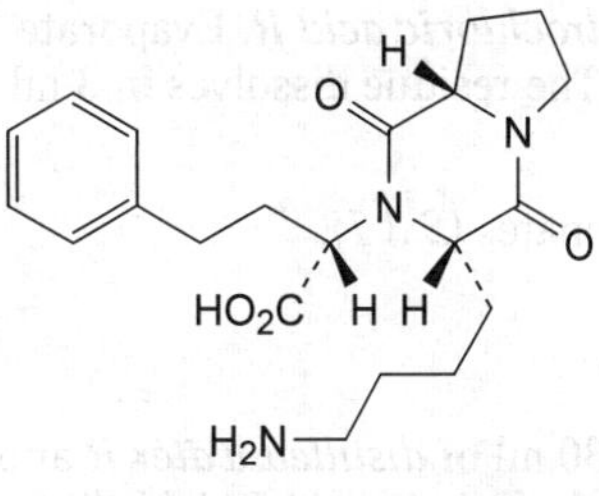

C. (2*S*)-2-[(3*S*,8a*S*)-3-(4-aminobutyl)-1,4-dioxohexahydro-pyrrolo[1,2-*a*]pyrazin-2(1*H*)-yl]-4-phenylbutanoic acid (*S,S,S*-diketopiperazine),

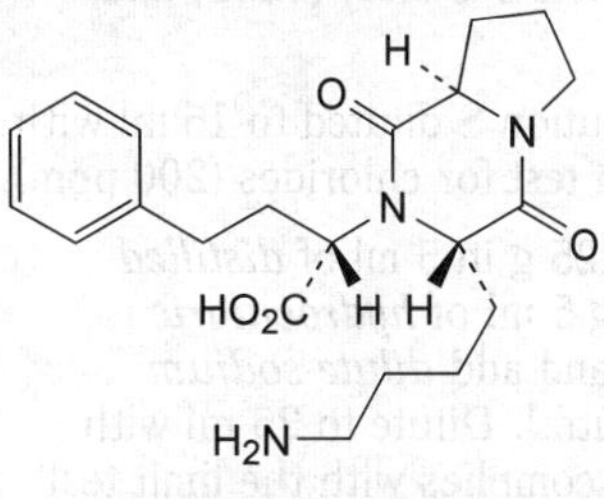

D. (2*S*)-2-[(3*S*,8a*R*)-3-(4-aminobutyl)-1,4-dioxohexahydro-pyrrolo[1,2-*a*]pyrazin-2(1*H*)-yl]-4-phenylbutanoic acid (*R,S,S*-diketopiperazine),

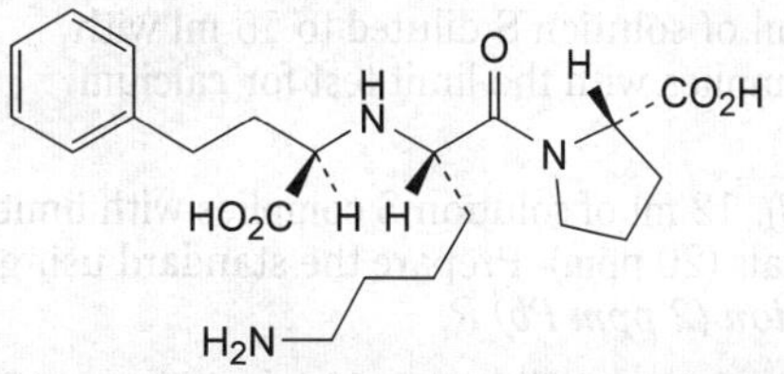

E. (2*S*)-1-[(2*S*)-6-amino-2-[[(1*R*)-1-carboxy-3-phenylpropyl]amino]hexanoyl]pyrrole-2-carboxylic acid (lisinopril *R,S,S*-isomer),

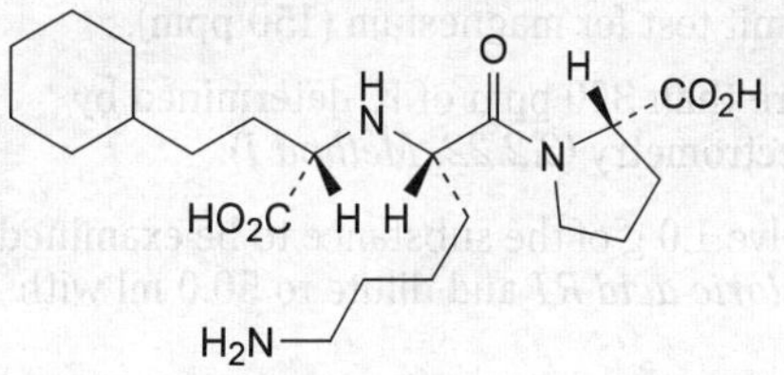

F. (2*S*)-1-[(2*S*)-6-amino-2-[[(1*S*)-1-carboxy-3-cyclohexylpropyl]amino]hexanoyl]pyrrole-2-carboxylic acid (cyclohexyl analogue).

01/2005:0228

LITHIUM CARBONATE

Lithii carbonas

Li_2CO_3 M_r 73.9

DEFINITION

Lithium carbonate contains not less than 98.5 per cent and not more than the equivalent of 100.5 per cent of Li_2CO_3.

CHARACTERS

A white powder, slightly soluble in water, practically insoluble in alcohol.

IDENTIFICATION

A. When moistened with *hydrochloric acid R*, it gives a red colour to a non-luminous flame.

B. Dissolve 0.2 g in 1 ml of *hydrochloric acid R*. Evaporate to dryness on a water-bath. The residue dissolves in 3 ml of *alcohol R*.

C. It gives the reaction of carbonates (*2.3.1*).

TESTS

Solution S. Suspend 10.0 g in 30 ml of *distilled water R* and dissolve by the addition of 22 ml of *nitric acid R*. Add *dilute sodium hydroxide solution R* until the solution is neutral and dilute to 100 ml with *distilled water R*.

Appearance of solution. Solution S is clear (*2.2.1*) and colourless (*2.2.2, Method II*).

Chlorides (*2.4.4*). 2.5 ml of solution S diluted to 15 ml with *water R* complies with the limit test for chlorides (200 ppm).

Sulphates (*2.4.13*). Disperse 1.25 g in 5 ml of *distilled water R* and dissolve by adding 5 ml of *hydrochloric acid R1*. Boil for 2 min. Cool and add *dilute sodium hydroxide solution R* until neutral. Dilute to 25 ml with *distilled water R*. The solution complies with the limit test for sulphates (200 ppm).

Arsenic (*2.4.2*). 0.5 g complies with limit test A for arsenic (2 ppm).

Calcium (*2.4.3*). 5 ml of solution S diluted to 15 ml with *distilled water R* complies with the limit test for calcium (200 ppm).

Heavy metals (*2.4.8*). 12 ml of solution S complies with limit test A for heavy metals (20 ppm). Prepare the standard using *lead standard solution (2 ppm Pb) R*.

Iron (*2.4.9*). 5 ml of solution S diluted to 10 ml with *water R* complies with the limit test for iron (20 ppm).

Magnesium (*2.4.6*). Dilute 1 ml of solution S to 10 ml with *water R*. 6.7 ml of this solution diluted to 10 ml with *water R* complies with the limit test for magnesium (150 ppm).

Potassium. Not more than 300 ppm of K, determined by atomic emission spectrometry (*2.2.22, Method I*).

Test solution. Dissolve 1.0 g of the substance to be examined in 10 ml of *hydrochloric acid R1* and dilute to 50.0 ml with *water R*.

Reference solutions. Prepare the reference solutions using a solution of *potassium chloride R* containing 500 µg of K per millilitre, diluted as required.

Measure the emission intensity at 766.5 nm.

Sodium. Not more than 300 ppm of Na, determined by atomic emission spectrometry (*2.2.22, Method I*).

Test solution. Dissolve 1.0 g of the substance to be examined in 10 ml of *hydrochloric acid R1* and dilute to 50.0 ml with *water R*.

Reference solutions. Prepare the reference solutions using a solution of *sodium chloride R* containing 500 µg of Na per millilitre, diluted as required.

Measure the emission intensity at 589 nm.

ASSAY

Dissolve 0.500 g in 25.0 ml of *1 M hydrochloric acid*. Titrate with *1 M sodium hydroxide*, using *methyl orange solution R* as indicator.

1 ml of *1 M hydrochloric acid* is equivalent to 36.95 mg of Li_2CO_3.

01/2005:0621

LITHIUM CITRATE

Lithii citras

$C_6H_5Li_3O_7,4H_2O$ M_r 282.0

DEFINITION

Lithium citrate contains not less than 98.0 per cent and not more than the equivalent of 102.0 per cent of trilithium 2-hydroxypropane-1,2,3-tricarboxylate, calculated with reference to the anhydrous substance.

CHARACTERS

A white or almost white, fine crystalline powder, freely soluble in water, slightly soluble in alcohol.

IDENTIFICATION

A. When moistened with *hydrochloric acid R*, it gives a red colour to a non-luminous flame.

B. Dilute 3 ml of solution S (see Tests) to 10 ml with *water R*. Add 3 ml of *potassium ferriperiodate solution R*. A white or yellowish-white precipitate is formed.

C. To 1 ml of solution S add 4 ml of *water R*. The solution gives the reaction of citrates (*2.3.1*).

TESTS

Solution S. Dissolve 10.0 g in *carbon dioxide-free water R* prepared from *distilled water R* and dilute to 100 ml with the same solvent.

Appearance of solution. Solution S is clear (*2.2.1*) and colourless (*2.2.2, Method II*).

Acidity or alkalinity. To 10 ml of solution S add 0.1 ml of *phenolphthalein solution R*. Not more than 0.2 ml of *0.1 M hydrochloric acid* or *0.1 M sodium hydroxide* is required to change the colour of the indicator.

Readily carbonisable substances. To 0.20 g of the powdered substance to be examined add 10 ml of *sulphuric acid R* and heat in a water-bath at 90 ± 1 °C for 60 min. Cool rapidly. The solution is not more intensely coloured than reference solution Y_2 or GY_2 (*2.2.2, Method II*).

Chlorides (*2.4.4*). Dilute 5 ml of solution S to 15 ml with *water R*. The solution complies with the limit test for chlorides (100 ppm).

Oxalates. Dissolve 0.50 g in 4 ml of *water R*, add 3 ml of *hydrochloric acid R* and 1 g of granulated *zinc R* and heat on a water-bath for 1 min. Allow to stand for 2 min, decant the liquid into a test-tube containing 0.25 ml of a 10 g/l solution of *phenylhydrazine hydrochloride R* and heat to boiling. Cool rapidly, transfer to a graduated cylinder and add an equal volume of *hydrochloric acid R* and 0.25 ml of *potassium ferricyanide solution R*. Shake and allow to stand for 30 min. Any pink colour in the solution is not more intense than that in a standard prepared at the same time and in the same manner using 4 ml of a 0.05 g/l solution of *oxalic acid R* (300 ppm, calculated as anhydrous oxalate ion).

Sulphates (*2.4.13*). To 3 ml of solution S add 2 ml of *hydrochloric acid R1* and dilute to 17 ml with *distilled water R*. The solution complies with the limit test for sulphates (500 ppm). Prepare the standard using 15 ml of a mixture of 2 ml of *hydrochloric acid R1* and 15 ml of *sulphate standard solution (10 ppm SO_4) R* and compare the opalescence after 15 min.

Monographs I-L

Heavy metals (*2.4.8*). 12 ml of solution S complies with limit test A for heavy metals (10 ppm). Prepare the standard using *lead standard solution (1 ppm Pb) R*.

Water (*2.5.12*): 24.0 per cent to 27.0 per cent, determined on 0.100 g by the semi-micro determination of water. After adding the substance to be examined, stir for 15 min before titrating. Carry out a blank titration.

ASSAY

Dissolve 80.0 mg in 50 ml of *anhydrous acetic acid R*, heating to about 50 °C. Allow to cool. Titrate with *0.1 M perchloric acid*, using 0.25 ml of *naphtholbenzein solution R* as indicator, until the colour changes from yellow to green.

1 ml of *0.1 M perchloric acid* is equivalent to 7.00 mg of $C_6H_5Li_3O_7$.

STORAGE

Store in an airtight container.

01/2005:1988
corrected

LOBELINE HYDROCHLORIDE

Lobelini hydrochloridum

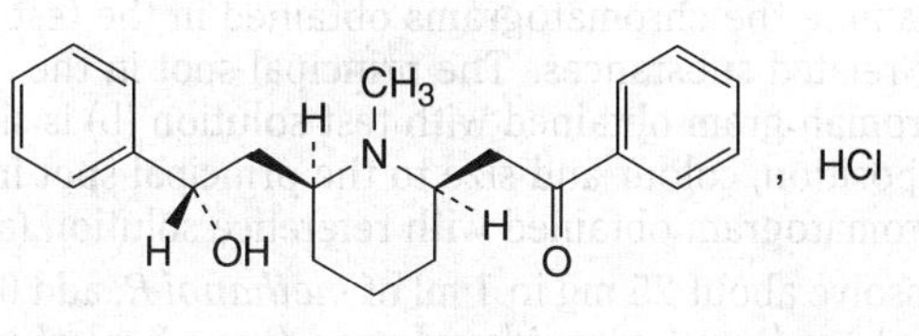

$C_{22}H_{28}ClNO_2$ M_r 373.9

DEFINITION

2-[(2*R*,6*S*)-6-[(2*S*)-2-Hydroxy-2-phenylethyl]-1-methylpiperidin-2-yl]-1-phenylethanone hydrochloride.

Content: 99.0 per cent to 101.0 per cent (dried substance).

CHARACTERS

Appearance: white or almost white, microcrystalline powder.

Solubility: sparingly soluble in water, freely soluble in alcohol, soluble in methylene chloride.

IDENTIFICATION

First identification: A, B.

Second identification: B, C.

A. Infrared absorption spectrophotometry (*2.2.24*).

Comparison: *lobeline hydrochloride CRS.*

B. Solution S (see Tests) gives reaction (a) of chlorides (*2.3.1*).

C. Examine the chromatograms obtained in the test for foreign alkaloids.

Results: the principal spot in the chromatogram obtained with test solution (b) is similar in position and size to the principal spot in the chromatogram obtained with reference solution (b).

TESTS

Solution S. Dissolve 0.250 g in *carbon dioxide-free water R* prepared from *distilled water R* and dilute to 25.0 ml with the same solvent.

Appearance of solution. Solution S is clear (*2.2.1*) and colourless (*2.2.2, Method II*).

pH (*2.2.3*): 4.6 to 6.4 for solution S.

Specific optical rotation (*2.2.7*): − 55 to − 59 (dried substance), determined on solution S.

Foreign alkaloids. Thin-layer chromatography (*2.2.27*).

Test solution (a). Dissolve 0.10 g of the substance to be examined in *methanol R* and dilute to 5.0 ml with the same solvent.

Test solution (b). Dilute 1 ml of test solution (a) to 10 ml with *methanol R.*

Reference solution (a). Dilute 0.1 ml of test solution (a) to 10 ml with *methanol R.*

Reference solution (b). Dissolve 10 mg of *lobeline hydrochloride CRS* in *methanol R* and dilute to 5 ml with the same solvent.

Plate: *TLC silica gel GF_{254} plate R.*

Mobile phase: *diethylamine R, cyclohexane R (10:90 V/V).*

Application: 10 µl.

Development: over 2/3 of the plate.

Drying: at 120 °C.

Detection: examine in ultraviolet light at 254 nm.

Limits: in the chromatogram obtained with test solution (a):

– *any impurity*: any spot, apart from the principal spot, is not more intense than the spot in the chromatogram obtained with reference solution (a) (1 per cent).

Related substances. Liquid chromatography (*2.2.29*).

Test solution. Dissolve 10.0 mg of the substance to be examined in the mobile phase and dilute to 10.0 ml with the mobile phase.

Reference solution (a). Dilute 1.0 ml of the test solution to 100.0 ml with the mobile phase. Dilute 1.0 ml of this solution to 10.0 ml with the mobile phase.

Reference solution (b). Dissolve 5 mg of *phenytoin CRS* in the mobile phase and dilute to 100.0 ml with the mobile phase. To 1 ml of the solution add 0.1 ml of the test solution and dilute to 25 ml with the mobile phase.

Column:

– *size*: *l* = 0.25 m, Ø = 4 mm,

– *stationary phase*: spherical *end-capped octylsilyl silica gel for chromatography R* (5 µm).

Mobile phase: dissolve 1.0 g of *sodium methanesulphonate R* and 2.50 g of *disodium hydrogen phosphate dihydrate R* in a mixture of 3 volumes of a 6.7 per cent *V/V* solution of *phosphoric acid R*, 29 volumes of *acetonitrile R* and 70 volumes of *water R* and dilute to 1000 ml with the same mixture of solvents.

Flow rate: 1.5 ml/min.

Detection: spectrophotometer at 210 nm.

Injection: 10 µl.

Run time: 2 times the retention time of lobeline which is about 17 min.

System suitability: reference solution (b):

– *resolution*: minimum 4.0 between the peaks due to phenytoin and to lobeline.

Limits:

– *any impurity*: not more than the area of the principal peak in the chromatogram obtained with reference solution (a) (0.1 per cent),

– *total*: maximum of 2 times the area of the principal peak in the chromatogram obtained with reference solution (a) (0.2 per cent),

– *disregard level*: 0.5 times the area of the principal peak in the chromatogram obtained with reference solution (a) (0.05 per cent).

Monographs I-L

Sulphates (*2.4.13*): maximum 0.1 per cent.

15 ml of solution S complies with the limit test for sulphates.

Loss on drying (*2.2.32*): maximum 1.0 per cent, determined on 1.000 g *in vacuo*.

Sulphated ash (*2.4.14*): maximum 0.1 per cent, determined on the residue obtained in the test for loss on drying.

ASSAY

Dissolve 0.300 g in 50 ml of *alcohol R*. Add 5 ml of *0.01 M hydrochloric acid*. Carry out a potentiometric titration (*2.2.20*), using *0.1 M sodium hydroxide*. Read the volume added between the 2 points of inflexion.

1 ml of *0.1 M sodium hydroxide* is equivalent to 37.39 mg of $C_{22}H_{28}ClNO_2$.

STORAGE

Protected from light.

IMPURITIES

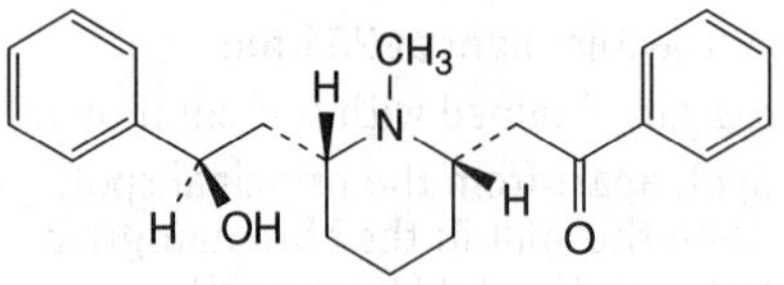

A. 2-[(2*S*,6*R*)-6-[(2*R*)-2-hydroxy-2-phenylethyl]-1-methylpiperidin-2-yl]-1-phenylethanone ((+)-lobeline),

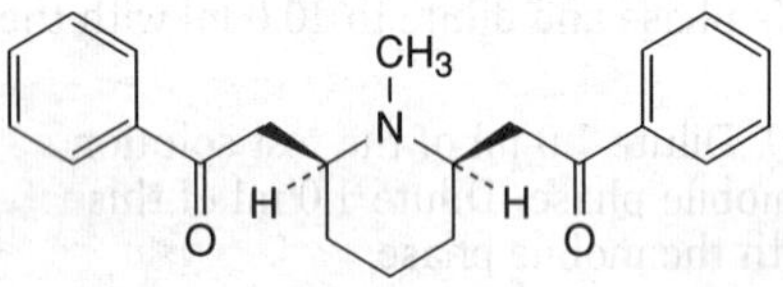

B. 2,2′-[(2*R*,6*S*)-1-methylpiperidine-2,6-diyl]bis(1-phenylethanone) (lobelanine),

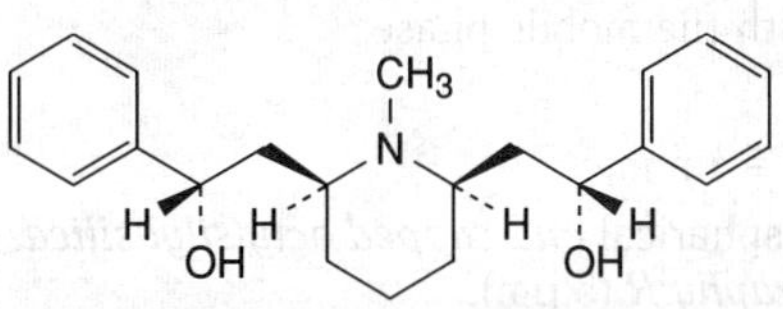

C. *meso*-(1*R*,1′*S*)-2,2′-[(2*R*,6*S*)-1-methylpiperidine-2,6-diyl]bis(1-phenylethanol) (lobelanidine),

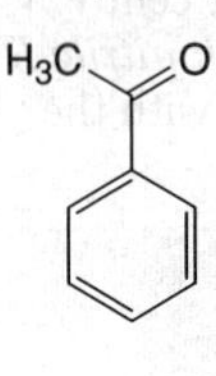

D. acetophenone.

01/2005:0928
corrected

LOMUSTINE

Lomustinum

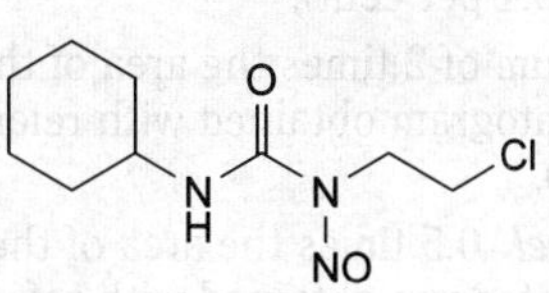

$C_9H_{16}ClN_3O_2$ M_r 233.7

DEFINITION

Lomustine contains not less than 98.5 per cent and not more than the equivalent of 100.5 per cent of 1-(2-chloroethyl)-3-cyclohexyl-1-nitrosourea, calculated with reference to the dried substance.

CHARACTERS

A yellow, crystalline powder, practically insoluble in water, freely soluble in acetone and in methylene chloride, soluble in alcohol.

Carry out the tests protected from light and prepare all the solutions immediately before use.

IDENTIFICATION

First identification: C.

Second identification: A, B, D, E.

A. Melting point (*2.2.14*): 89 °C to 91 °C.

B. Dissolve 50.0 mg in *alcohol R* and dilute to 50.0 ml with the same solvent. Dilute 2.0 ml to 100.0 ml with *alcohol R*. Examined between 220 nm and 350 nm (*2.2.25*), the solution shows an absorption maximum at 230 nm. The specific absorbance at the maximum is 250 to 270.

C. Examine by infrared absorption spectrophotometry (*2.2.24*), comparing with the spectrum obtained with *lomustine CRS*. Examine the substances prepared as discs.

D. Examine the chromatograms obtained in the test for related substances. The principal spot in the chromatogram obtained with test solution (b) is similar in position, colour and size to the principal spot in the chromatogram obtained with reference solution (a).

E. Dissolve about 25 mg in 1 ml of *methanol R*, add 0.1 ml of *dilute sodium hydroxide solution R* and 2 ml of *water R*. Acidify by adding dropwise *dilute nitric acid R*. Filter. The filtrate gives reaction (a) of chlorides (*2.3.1*).

TESTS

Related substances

A. Examine by thin-layer chromatography (*2.2.27*), using *silica gel G R* as the coating substance.

Test solution (a). Dissolve 0.25 g of the substance to be examined in *methanol R* and dilute to 10 ml with the same solvent.

Test solution (b). Dilute 1 ml of test solution (a) to 25 ml with *methanol R*.

Reference solution (a). Dissolve 10 mg of *lomustine CRS* in *methanol R* and dilute to 10 ml with the same solvent.

Reference solution (b). Dilute 1 ml of test solution (b) to 10 ml with *methanol R*.

Reference solution (c). Dilute 1 ml of test solution (b) to 20 ml with *methanol R*.

Reference solution (d). Dissolve 10 mg of *lomustine CRS* and 10 mg of *dicyclohexylurea R* in *methanol R* and dilute to 10 ml with the same solvent.

Apply separately to the plate 5 µl of each solution. Develop over a path of 15 cm using a mixture of 20 volumes of *glacial acetic acid R* and 80 volumes of *toluene R*. Dry the plate at 110 °C for 1 h. At the bottom of a chromatography tank, place an evaporating dish containing a mixture of 1 volume of *hydrochloric acid R1*, 1 volume of *water R* and 2 volumes of a 15 g/l solution of *potassium permanganate R*, close the tank and allow to stand for 15 min. Place the dried plate in the tank and close the tank. Leave the plate in contact with the chlorine vapour for 5 min. Withdraw the plate and place it in a current of cold air until the excess of chlorine is removed and an area of coating below the points of application does not give a blue colour with a drop of *potassium iodide and starch solution R*. Spray with *potassium iodide and starch solution R*. Any spot in the chromatogram obtained with test solution (a), apart from the principal spot, is not more intense than the spot in the chromatogram obtained with reference solution (b) (0.4 per cent) and at most one such spot is more intense than the spot in the chromatogram obtained with reference solution (c) (0.2 per cent). The test is not valid unless the chromatogram obtained with reference solution (d) shows two clearly separated principal spots.

B. Examine by liquid chromatography (*2.2.29*).

Test solution. Dissolve 0.25 g of the substance to be examined in *methanol R* and dilute to 10.0 ml the same solvent.

Reference solution. Dilute 1.0 ml of the test solution to 100.0 ml with *methanol R*.

The chromatographic procedure may be carried out using:

– a stainless steel column 0.25 m long and 4 mm in internal diameter packed with *octadecylsilyl silica gel for chromatography R* (5 µm to 10 µm),
– as mobile phase at a flow rate of 2 ml/min a mixture of 50 volumes of *methanol R* and 50 volumes of *water R*,
– as detector a spectrophotometer set at 230 nm,
– a loop injector.

Inject 20 µl of the reference solution. Adjust the sensitivity of the system so that the height of the principal peak in the chromatogram obtained with the reference solution is at least 50 per cent of the full scale of the recorder. Inject separately 20 µl of each solution. In the chromatogram obtained with the test solution, the sum of the areas of any peaks apart from the principal peak is not greater than the area of the principal peak in the chromatogram obtained with the reference solution (1 per cent). Disregard any peak due to the solvent and any peak with an area less than 0.05 times that of the principal peak in the chromatogram obtained with the reference solution.

Chlorides (*2.4.4*). Dissolve 0.24 g in 4 ml of *methanol R* and add 20 ml of *water R*. Allow to stand for 20 min and filter. To 10 ml of the filtrate, add 5 ml of *methanol R*. The solution complies with the limit test for chlorides (500 ppm). When preparing the standard, replace the 5 ml of *water R* with 5 ml of *methanol R*.

Loss on drying (*2.2.32*). Not more than 1.0 per cent, determined on 1.000 g by drying in a desiccator over *diphosphorus pentoxide R* at a pressure not exceeding 0.7 kPa for 24 h.

ASSAY

Dissolve 0.200 g in about 3 ml of *alcohol R* and add 20 ml of a 200 g/l solution of *potassium hydroxide R* and boil under a reflux condenser for 2 h. Add 75 ml of *water R* and 4 ml of *nitric acid R*. Cool and titrate with *0.1 M silver nitrate*, determining the end-point potentiometrically (*2.2.20*). Carry out a blank titration.

1 ml of *0.1 M silver nitrate* is equivalent to 23.37 mg of $C_9H_{16}ClN_3O_2$.

STORAGE

Store protected from light.

IMPURITIES

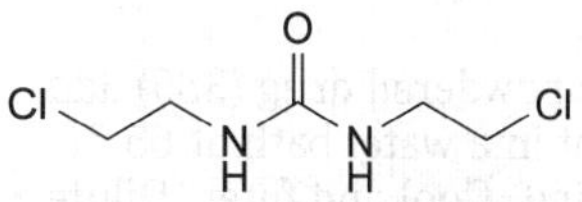

A. 1,3-bis(2-chloroethyl)urea,

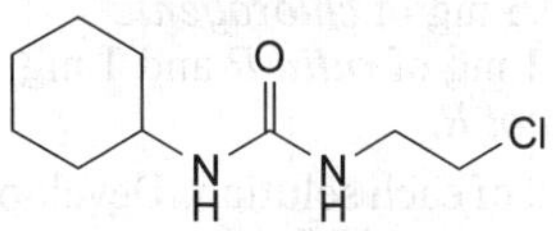

B. 1-(2-chloroethyl)-3-cyclohexylurea,

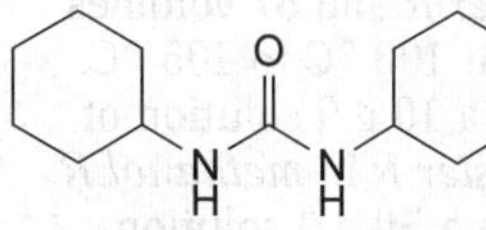

C. 1,3-dicyclohexylurea.

01/2005:1537

LOOSESTRIFE

Lythri herba

DEFINITION

Loosestrife consists of the dried flowering tops, whole or cut, of *Lythrum salicaria* L. It contains not less than 5.0 per cent of tannins, expressed as pyrogallol ($C_6H_6O_3$; M_r 126.1) and calculated with reference to the dried drug.

CHARACTERS

It has the macroscopic and microscopic characters described under identification tests A and B.

IDENTIFICATION

A. The stems are rigid, four-angled, branching at the top, brownish-green, longitudinally wrinkled and pubescent. The leaves are opposite, decussate, rarely verticillate in threes and sometimes alternate at the inflorescence which forms a long terminal spike. The leaves are sessile, lanceolate and cordate at the base, 5 cm to 15 cm long and 1 cm to 2.5 cm wide, pubescent on the lower surface; the subsidiary veins form arcs that anastomose near the leaf margin. The flowers have a pubescent, tubular, persistent gamosepalous calyx, 4 mm to 8 mm long, consisting of 6 sepals bearing 6 small, triangular teeth alternating with 6 large acute teeth at least half as long as the tube; a polypetalous corolla consisting of 6 violet-pink petals, each expanded at the top with a wavy outline and narrowing at the base. The androecium consists of 2 verticils of 6 stamens (one verticil with short, barely emerging stamens, the other with long stamens extending well out of the corolla). The fruit, if formed, is a small capsule included in the persistent calyx.

B. Reduce to a powder (355). The powder is greenish-yellow. Examine under a microscope using *chloral hydrate solution R*. The powder shows unicellular or bicellular, uniseriate, thick-walled, finely pitted covering trichomes from the lower epidermis of the stem and leaf; numerous uniseriate, unicellular or bicellular, thin-walled, finely pitted covering trichomes from the calyx; transparent violet-pink fragments from the petals; numerous cluster crystals of calcium oxalate; pollen grains with 3 pores and a thin and slightly granular exine; fragments of the upper epidermis with large polygonal cells and sinuous walls; fragments of the lower epidermis with smaller polygonal cells and anomocytic stomata (*2.8.3*).

C. Examine by thin-layer chromatography (*2.2.27*), using a *TLC silica gel plate R*.

Test solution. To 1.0 g of the powdered drug (355) add 10 ml of *methanol R* and heat in a water-bath at 65 °C for 5 min with frequent shaking. Cool and filter. Dilute the filtrate to 10 ml with *methanol R*.

Reference solution. Dissolve 0.5 mg of *chlorogenic acid R*, 1 mg of *hyperoside R*, 1 mg of *rutin R* and 1 mg of *vitexin R* in 10 ml of *methanol R*.

Apply to the plate as bands 10 µl of each solution. Develop over a path of 15 cm using a mixture of 7.5 volumes of *anhydrous acetic acid R*, 7.5 volumes of *anhydrous formic acid R*, 18 volumes of *water R* and 67 volumes of *ethyl acetate R*. Dry the plate at 100 °C to 105 °C and spray it while still warm with a 10 g/l solution of *diphenylboric acid aminoethyl ester R* in *methanol R*. Subsequently spray the plate with a 50 g/l solution of *macrogol 400 R* in *methanol R*. Allow the plate to dry in air for 30 min and examine in ultraviolet light at 365 nm. The chromatogram obtained with the reference solution shows in the lower third a yellowish-brown fluorescent zone (rutin) and in the middle third a light blue fluorescent zone (chlorogenic acid), above it a yellowish-brown fluorescent zone (hyperoside) and a green fluorescent zone (vitexin). The chromatogram obtained with the test solution shows a bright green fluorescent zone slightly above the rutin zone in the chromatogram obtained with the reference solution, a yellow fluorescent zone similar in position to the chlorogenic acid zone in the chromatogram obtained with the reference solution, a yellow fluorescent zone similar in position to the hyperoside zone in the chromatogram obtained with the reference solution and a bright green fluorescent zone corresponding to the vitexin zone in the chromatogram obtained with the reference solution.

TESTS

Foreign matter (*2.8.2*). It complies with the test for foreign matter.

Loss on drying (*2.2.32*). Not more than 12.0 per cent, determined on 1.000 g of the powdered drug (355) by drying in an oven at 100 °C to 105 °C.

Total ash (*2.4.16*). Not more than 7.0 per cent.

ASSAY

Carry out the determination of tannins in herbal drugs (*2.8.14*). Use 0.750 g of the powdered drug (180).

STORAGE

Store protected from light.

Monographs I-L

01/2005:0929

LOPERAMIDE HYDROCHLORIDE

Loperamidi hydrochloridum

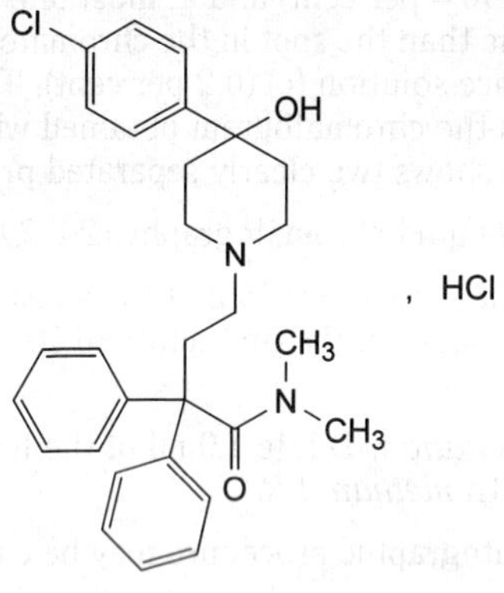

$C_{29}H_{34}Cl_2N_2O_2$ M_r 513.5

DEFINITION

4-[4-(4-Chlorophenyl)-4-hydroxypiperidin-1-yl]-*N*,*N*-dimethyl-2,2-diphenylbutanamide hydrochloride.

Content: 99.0 per cent to 101.0 per cent (dried substance).

CHARACTERS

Appearance: white or almost white powder.

Solubility: slightly soluble in water, freely soluble in alcohol and in methanol.

It shows polymorphism.

IDENTIFICATION

Infrared absorption spectrophotometry (*2.2.24*).

Comparison: *loperamide hydrochloride CRS*.

If the spectra obtained show differences, dissolve the substance to be examined and the reference substance separately in the minimum volume of *methylene chloride R*, evaporate to dryness and record new spectra using the residues.

TESTS

Related substances. Liquid chromatography (*2.2.29*).

Test solution. Dissolve 0.100 g of the substance to be examined in *methanol R* and dilute to 10.0 ml with the same solvent.

Reference solution (a). Dissolve 10.0 mg of *loperamide hydrochloride for system suitability CRS* in *methanol R* and dilute to 1.0 ml with the same solvent.

Reference solution (b). Dilute 1.0 ml of the test solution to 20.0 ml with *methanol R*. Dilute 1.0 ml of this solution to 25.0 ml with *methanol R*.

Column:

– *size*: l = 0.10 m, Ø = 4.6 mm,

– *stationary phase*: *base-deactivated octadecylsilyl silica gel for chromatography R* (3 µm),

– *temperature*: 35 °C.

Mobile phase:

– *mobile phase A*: 17.0 g/l solution of *tetrabutylammonium hydrogen sulphate R1*,

– *mobile phase B*: *acetonitrile R*,

Time (min)	Mobile phase A (per cent *V/V*)	Mobile phase B (per cent *V/V*)
0 - 15	90 → 30	10 → 70
15 - 17	30	70
17 - 19	30 → 90	70 → 10
19 - 24	90	10

Flow rate: 1.5 ml/min.

Detection: spectrophotometer at 220 nm.

Injection: 10 µl.

System suitability: reference solution (a):

- *peak-to-valley ratio*: minimum 1.5, where H_p = height above the baseline of the peak due to impurity G and H_v = height above the baseline of the lowest point of the curve separating this peak from the peak due to impurity H;
- *peak-to-valley ratio*: minimum 1.5, where H_p = height above the baseline of the peak due to impurity E and H_v = height above the baseline of the lowest point of the curve separating this peak from the peak due to impurity A;
- the chromatogram obtained is concordant with the chromatogram supplied with *loperamide hydrochloride for system suitability CRS*.

Limits:

- *correction factors*: for the calculation of contents, multiply the peak areas of the following impurities by the corresponding correction factor: impurity A = 1.3; impurity D = 1.7;
- *impurities A, B, C, D, E, F, G, H*: for each impurity, not more than the area of the principal peak in the chromatogram obtained with reference solution (b) (0.2 per cent);
- *any other impurity*: not more than 0.5 times the area of the principal peak in the chromatogram obtained with reference solution (b) (0.1 per cent);
- *total*: not more than 1.5 times the area of the principal peak in the chromatogram obtained with reference solution (b) (0.3 per cent);
- *disregard limit*: 0.25 times the area of the principal peak in the chromatogram obtained with reference solution (b) (0.05 per cent).

Loss on drying (*2.2.32*): maximum 0.5 per cent, determined on 1.000 g by drying in an oven at 100-105 °C for 4 h.

Sulphated ash (*2.4.14*): maximum 0.1 per cent, determined on 1.0 g.

ASSAY

Dissolve 0.400 g in 50 ml of *alcohol R* and add 5.0 ml of *0.01 M hydrochloric acid.* Carry out a potentiometric titration (*2.2.20*), using *0.1 M sodium hydroxide.* Read the volume added between the 2 points of inflexion.

1 ml of *0.1 M sodium hydroxide* is equivalent to 51.35 mg of $C_{29}H_{34}Cl_2N_2O_2$.

STORAGE

Protected from light.

IMPURITIES

Specified impurities: A, B, C, D, E, F, G, H.

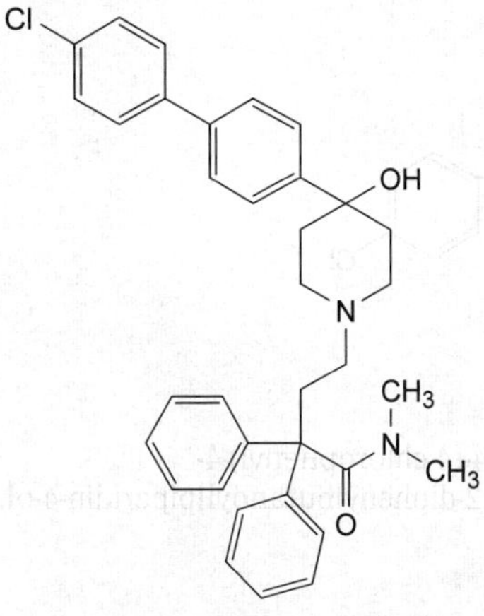

A. 4-[4-(4′-chlorobiphenyl-4-yl)-4-hydroxypiperidin-1-yl]-*N,N*-dimethyl-2,2-diphenylbutanamide,

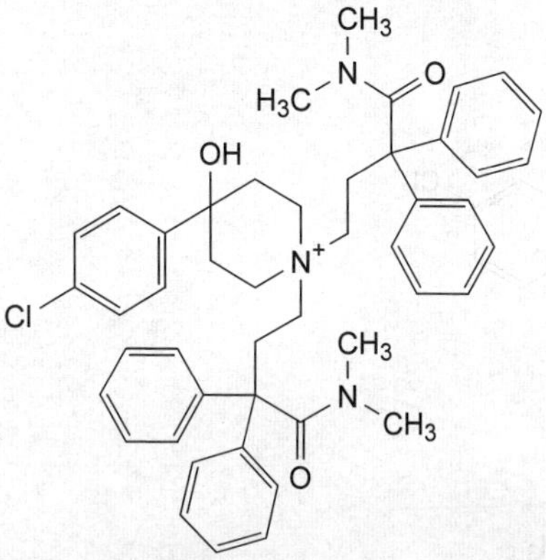

B. 4-(4-chlorophenyl)-1,1-bis[4-(dimethylamino)-4-oxo-3,3-diphenylbutyl]-4-hydroxypiperidinium,

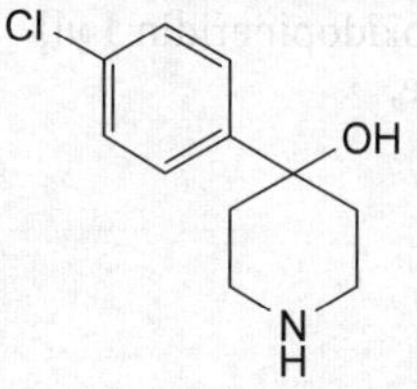

C. 4-(4-chlorophenyl)piperidin-4-ol,

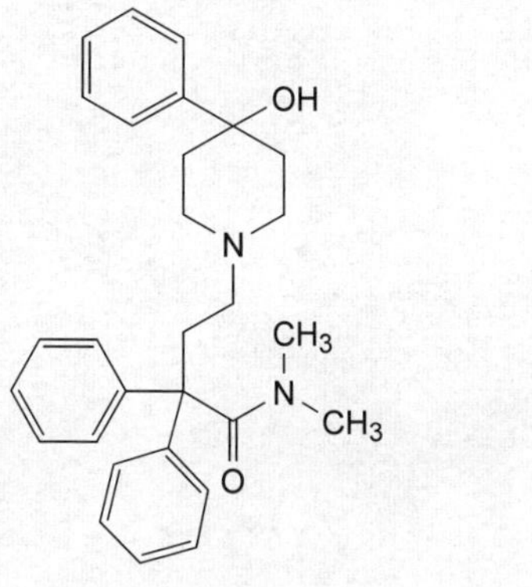

D. 4-(4-hydroxy-4-phenylpiperidin-1-yl)-*N,N*-dimethyl-2,2-diphenylbutanamide,

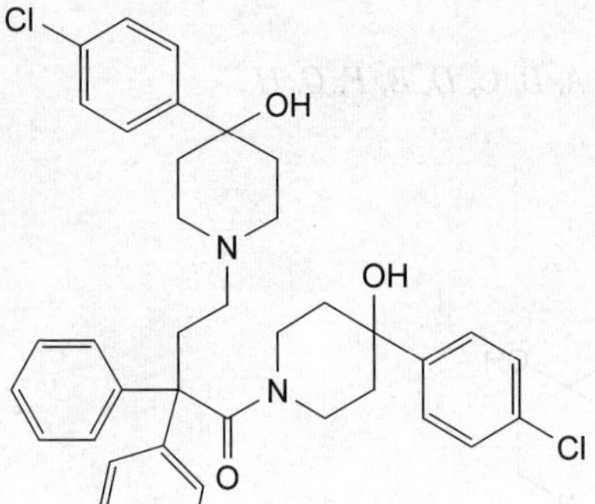

E. 4-(4-chlorophenyl)-1-[4-[4-(4-chlorophenyl)-4-hydroxypiperidin-1-yl]-2,2-diphenylbutanoyl]piperidin-4-ol,

F. loperamide oxide,

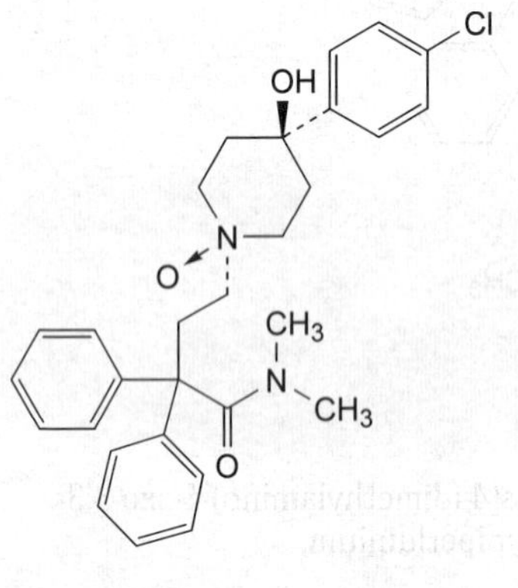

G. 4-[*cis*-4-(4-chlorophenyl)-4-hydroxy-1-oxidopiperidin-1-yl]-*N,N*-dimethyl-2,2-diphenylbutanamide,

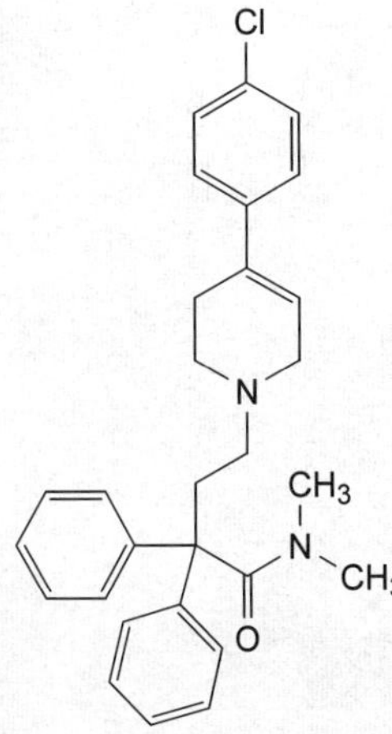

H. 4-[4-(4-chlorophenyl)-3,6-dihydropyridin-1(2*H*)-yl]-*N,N*-dimethyl-2,2-diphenylbutanamide.

01/2005:1729

LOPERAMIDE OXIDE MONOHYDRATE

Loperamidi oxidum monohydricum

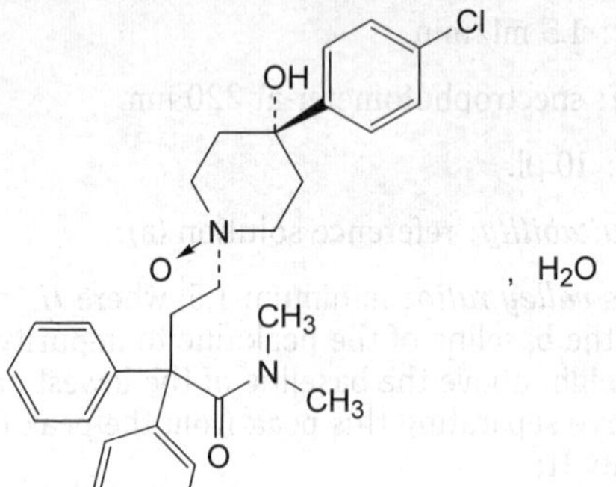

$C_{29}H_{33}ClN_2O_3,H_2O$ M_r 511.1

DEFINITION

4-[*trans*-4-(4-Chlorophenyl)-4-hydroxy-1-oxidopiperidin-1-yl]-*N,N*-dimethyl-2,2-diphenylbutanamide monohydrate.

Content: 99.0 per cent to 101.0 per cent (anhydrous substance).

CHARACTERS

Appearance: white or almost white powder, slightly hygroscopic.

Solubility: practically insoluble in water, freely soluble in alcohol and in methylene chloride.

mp: about 152 °C, with decomposition.

IDENTIFICATION

Infrared absorption spectrophotometry (*2.2.24*).

Comparison: *loperamide oxide monohydrate CRS*.

TESTS

Related substances. Liquid chromatography (*2.2.29*).

Test solution. Dissolve 0.100 g of the substance to be examined in *methanol R* and dilute to 10.0 ml with the same solvent.

Reference solution (a). Dissolve 5.0 mg of *loperamide hydrochloride CRS* in *methanol R*, add 0.5 ml of the test solution and dilute to 100.0 ml with *methanol R*.

Reference solution (b). Dilute 1.0 ml of the test solution to 20.0 ml with *methanol R*. Dilute 1.0 ml of this solution to 25.0 ml with *methanol R*.

Column:

– *size*: l = 0.10 m, Ø = 4.6 mm,
– *stationary phase*: *base-deactivated octadecylsilyl silica gel for chromatography R* (3 µm),
– *temperature*: 35 °C.

Mobile phase:

– *mobile phase A*: 17.0 g/l solution of *tetrabutylammonium hydrogen sulphate R1*,
– *mobile phase B*: *acetonitrile R*,

Time (min)	Mobile phase A (per cent *V/V*)	Mobile phase B (per cent *V/V*)
0 - 15	90 → 30	10 → 70
15 - 17	30	70
17 - 19	30 → 90	70 → 10
19 - 24	90	10

Flow rate: 1.5 ml/min.

Detection: spectrophotometer at 220 nm.

Injection: 10 µl.

Relative retention with reference to loperamide oxide (retention time = about 7 min): impurity A = about 0.9; impurity B = about 1.11; impurity C = about 1.13.

System suitability: reference solution (a):

- *resolution*: minimum 3.8 between the peaks due to loperamide oxide and impurity A.

Limits:

- *impurities A, B, C*: for each impurity, not more than the area of the principal peak in the chromatogram obtained with reference solution (b) (0.2 per cent),
- *any other impurity*: not more than 0.5 times the area of the principal peak in the chromatogram obtained with reference solution (b) (0.1 per cent),
- *total*: not more than 1.5 times the area of the principal peak in the chromatogram obtained with reference solution (b) (0.3 per cent),
- *disregard limit*: 0.25 times the area of the principal peak in the chromatogram obtained with reference solution (b) (0.05 per cent).

Water (*2.5.12*): 3.4 per cent to 4.2 per cent, determined on 0.500 g.

Sulphated ash (*2.4.14*): maximum 0.1 per cent, determined on 1.0 g.

ASSAY

Dissolve 0.350 g in 50 ml of a mixture of 1 volume of *anhydrous acetic acid R* and 7 volumes of *methyl ethyl ketone R*. Titrate with *0.1 M perchloric acid* using 0.2 ml of *naphtholbenzein solution R* as indicator.

1 ml of *0.1 M perchloric acid* is equivalent to 49.30 mg of $C_{29}H_{33}ClN_2O_3$.

STORAGE

In an airtight container, protected from light.

IMPURITIES

Specified impurities: A, B, C.

A. loperamide,

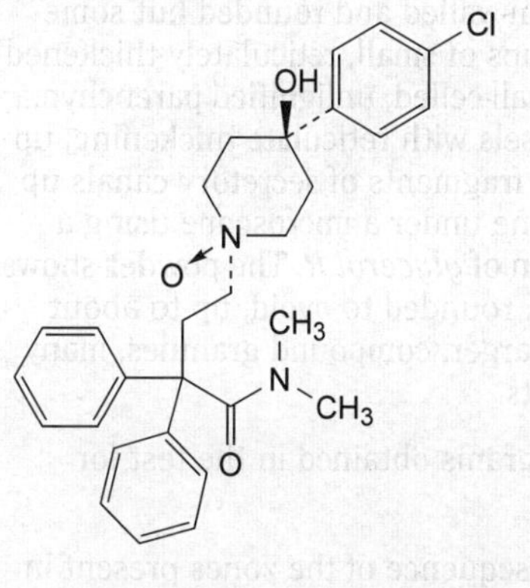

B. 4-[*cis*-4-(4-chlorophenyl)-4-hydroxy-1-oxidopiperidin-1-yl]-*N,N*-dimethyl-2,2-diphenylbutanamide,

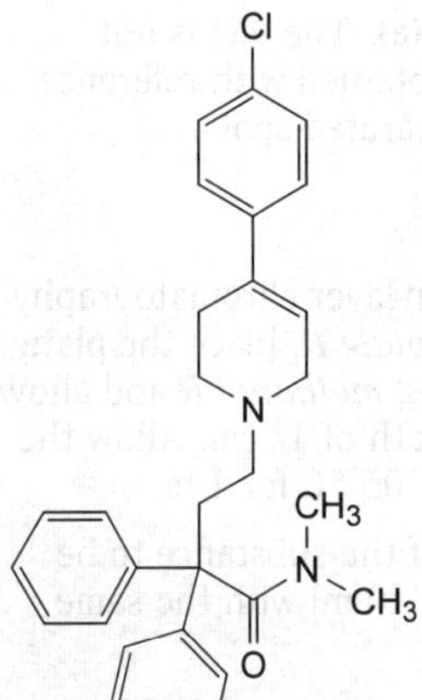

C. 4-[4-(4-chlorophenyl)-3,6-dihydropyridin-1(2*H*)-yl]-*N,N*-dimethyl-2,2-diphenylbutanamide.

01/2005:1121

LORAZEPAM

Lorazepamum

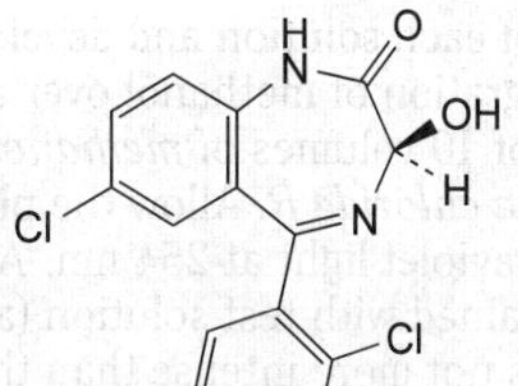

and enantiomer

$C_{15}H_{10}Cl_2N_2O_2$ M_r 321.2

DEFINITION

Lorazepam contains not less than 98.5 per cent and not more than the equivalent of 102.0 per cent of (*RS*)-7-chloro-5-(2-chlorophenyl)-3-hydroxy-1,3-dihydro-2*H*-1,4-benzodiazepin-2-one, calculated with reference to the dried substance.

CHARACTERS

A white or almost white, crystalline powder, practically insoluble in water, sparingly soluble in alcohol, sparingly soluble or slightly soluble in methylene chloride.

It shows polymorphism.

IDENTIFICATION

First identification: B.

Second identification: A, C.

A. Dissolve 10.0 mg in *alcohol R* and dilute to 100.0 ml with the same solvent. Dilute 10.0 ml of this solution to 100.0 ml with *alcohol R*. Examined between 210 nm and 280 nm (*2.2.25*), the solution shows an absorption maximum at 230 nm. The specific absorbance at the maximum is 1070 to 1170.

B. Examine by infrared absorption spectrophotometry between 600 cm^{-1} and 2000 cm^{-1} (*2.2.24*), comparing with the spectrum obtained with *lorazepam CRS*. Examine the substances as discs prepared using *potassium bromide R*.

C. Examine the chromatograms obtained in the test for related substances. The principal spot in the chromatogram obtained with test solution (b) is similar in position and size to the spot in the chromatogram obtained with reference solution (a). The test is not valid unless the chromatogram obtained with reference solution (d) shows two clearly separated spots.

TESTS

Related substances. Examine by thin-layer chromatography (*2.2.27*), using a *TLC silica gel F_{254} plate R*. Place the plate in a chromatographic tank containing *methanol R* and allow the solvent front to migrate over a path of 17 cm. Allow the plate to dry in air and heat it at 100-105 °C for 1 h.

Test solution (a). Dissolve 0.200 g of the substance to be examined in *acetone R* and dilute to 10 ml with the same solvent.

Test solution (b). Dilute 2 ml of test solution (a) to 50 ml with *acetone R*.

Reference solution (a). Dissolve 20 mg of *lorazepam CRS* in *acetone R* and dilute to 25 ml with the same solvent.

Reference solution (b). Dilute 1 ml of test solution (b) to 20 ml with *acetone R*.

Reference solution (c). Dilute 5 ml of reference solution (b) to 10 ml with *acetone R*.

Reference solution (d). Dissolve 4 mg of *nitrazepam CRS* in *acetone R*, add 5 ml of reference solution (a) and dilute to 20 ml with *acetone R*.

Apply to the plate 20 µl of each solution and develop in the direction used for the migration of methanol over a path of 12 cm with a mixture of 10 volumes of *methanol R* and 100 volumes of *methylene chloride R*. Allow the plate to dry in air and examine in ultraviolet light at 254 nm. Any spot in the chromatogram obtained with test solution (a), apart from the principal spot, is not more intense than the spot in the chromatogram obtained with reference solution (b) (0.2 per cent) and at most one such spot is more intense than the spot in the chromatogram obtained with reference solution (c) (0.1 per cent).

Loss on drying (*2.2.32*). Not more than 0.5 per cent, determined on 1.000 g under high vacuum at 100-105 °C.

Sulphated ash (*2.4.14*). Not more than 0.1 per cent, determined on 1.0 g.

ASSAY

Dissolve 0.250 g in 30 ml of *dimethylformamide R*. Titrate with *0.1 M tetrabutylammonium hydroxide*, determining the end-point potentiometrically (*2.2.20*). Protect the solution from atmospheric carbon dioxide throughout the titration.

1 ml of *0.1 M tetrabutylammonium hydroxide* is equivalent to 32.12 mg of $C_{15}H_{10}Cl_2N_2O_2$.

STORAGE

Store in an airtight container, protected from light.

IMPURITIES

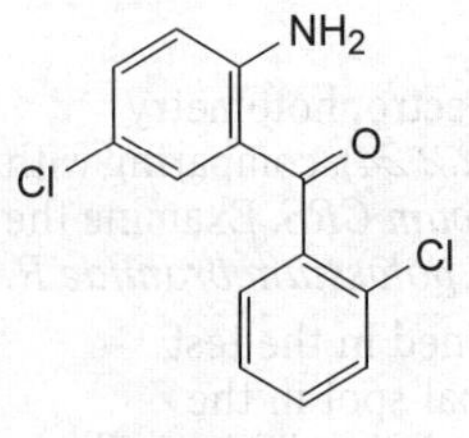

A. (2-amino-5-chlorophenyl)(2-chlorophenyl)methanone,

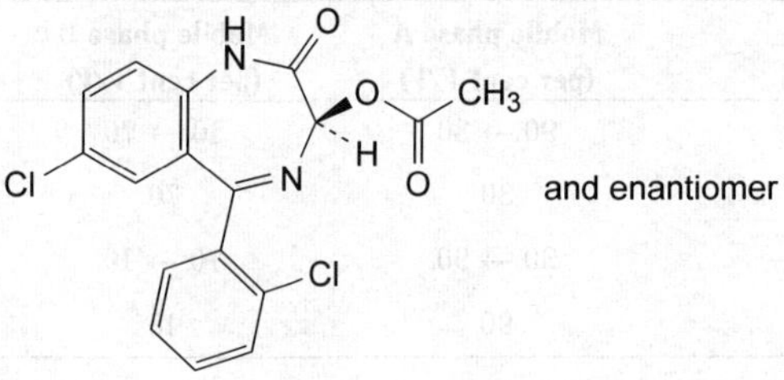

B. (3*RS*)-7-chloro-5-(2-chlorophenyl)-2-oxo-2,3-dihydro-1*H*-1,4-benzodiazepin-3-yl acetate.

01/2005:1233

LOVAGE ROOT

Levistici radix

DEFINITION

Whole or cut, dried rhizome and root of *Levisticum officinale* Koch.

Content: minimum 4.0 ml/kg of essential oil for the whole drug and minimum 3.0 ml/kg of essential oil for the cut drug (dried drug).

CHARACTERS

Macroscopic and microscopic characters described under identification tests A and B.

IDENTIFICATION

A. The rhizome and the large roots are often split longitudinally. The rhizome is short, up to 5 cm in diameter, light greyish-brown or yellowish-brown, simple or with several protuberances; the roots, showing little ramification, are the same colour as the rhizome; they are usually up to 1.5 cm thick and up to about 25 cm long; the fracture is usually smooth and shows a very wide yellowish-white bark and a narrow brownish-yellow wood.

B. Reduce to a powder (355). The powder is brownish-yellow. Examine under a microscope using *chloral hydrate solution R*. The powder shows: cork cells, polygonal or rounded in surface view, with brown contents; abundant parenchyma, mostly thin-walled and rounded but some with thicker walls; groups of small, reticulately thickened vessels embedded in small-celled, unlignified parenchyma; fragments of larger vessels with reticulate thickening, up to 125 µm in diameter; fragments of secretory canals up to 180 µm wide. Examine under a microscope using a 50 per cent *V/V* solution of *glycerol R*. The powder shows starch granules, simple, rounded to ovoid, up to about 12 µm, and numerous larger, compound granules, many with several components.

C. Examine the chromatograms obtained in the test for Angelica root.

Results: see below the sequence of the zones present in the chromatograms obtained with the reference solution and the test solution.

Top of the plate	
_______	_______
Eugenol: (marked at 254 nm)	
	An intense pale blue to white fluorescent zone
	An intense pale blue to white fluorescent zone
Coumarin: (marked at 254 nm)	
_______	_______
	1 or 2 less intense pale blue to white fluorescent zones
Reference solution	**Test solution**

TESTS

Angelica root. Thin-layer chromatography (*2.2.27*).

Test solution. To 1.0 g of the freshly powdered drug (355) add 5 ml of *methanol R* and boil for 30 s. Cool and filter.

Reference solution. Dissolve 5 mg of *coumarin R* and 25 µl of *eugenol R* in 10 ml of *methanol R*.

Plate: *TLC silica gel F_{254} plate R*.

Mobile phase: *methylene chloride R, toluene R* (50:50 *V/V*).

Application: 20 µl, as bands.

Development: twice over a path of 10 cm.

Drying: in air.

Detection: examine in ultraviolet light at 254 nm. Mark the quenching zones due to coumarin and eugenol on the chromatogram obtained with the reference solution. Examine in ultraviolet light at 365 nm.

Results: the chromatogram obtained with the test solution shows no blue or yellow fluorescent zones in the lower third.

Foreign matter (*2.8.2*): maximum 3 per cent, determined on 50 g.

Loss on drying (*2.2.32*): maximum 12.0 per cent, determined on 1.000 g of the powdered drug (355) by drying in an oven at 100-105 °C for 2 h.

Total ash (*2.4.16*): maximum 8.0 per cent.

Ash insoluble in hydrochloric acid (*2.8.1*): maximum 2.0 per cent.

ASSAY

Carry out the determination of essential oils in vegetable drugs (*2.8.12*). Use a 2 litre flask, 10 drops of *liquid paraffin R*, 500 ml of *water R* as the distillation liquid and 0.50 ml of *xylene R* in the graduated tube. Reduce the drug to a powder (500) and immediately use 40.0 g for the determination. Distil at a rate of 2-3 ml/min for 4 h.

01/2005:1538

LOVASTATIN

Lovastatinum

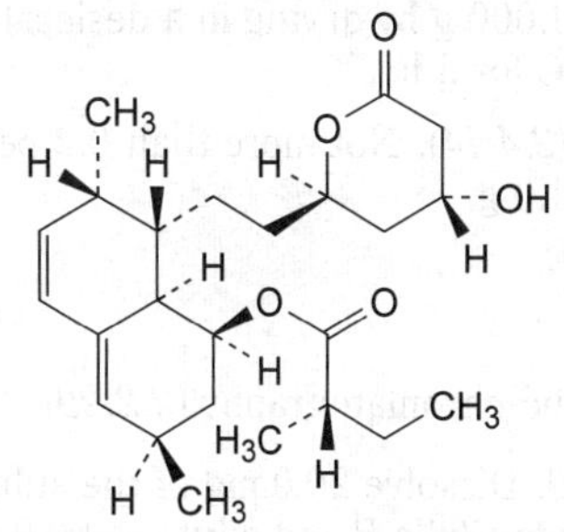

$C_{24}H_{36}O_5$ M_r 404.5

DEFINITION

Lovastatin contains not less than 97.0 per cent and not more than the equivalent of 102.0 per cent of (1*S*,3*R*,7*S*,8*S*,8a*R*)-8-[2-[(2*R*,4*R*)-4-hydroxy-6-oxotetrahydro-2*H*-pyran-2-yl]ethyl]-3,7-dimethyl-1,2,3,7,8,8a-hexahydronaphthalen-1-yl (2*S*)-2-methylbutanoate, calculated with reference to the dried substance.

CHARACTERS

A white or almost white crystalline powder, practically insoluble in water, soluble in acetone, sparingly soluble in ethanol.

IDENTIFICATION

A. It complies with the test for specific optical rotation (see Tests).

B. Examine by infrared absorption spectrophotometry (*2.2.24*), comparing with the spectrum obtained with *lovastatin CRS*. Examine the substances prepared as discs.

TESTS

Appearance of solution. Dissolve 0.200 g in *acetonitrile R* and dilute to 20.0 ml with the same solvent. The solution is clear (*2.2.1*) and not more intensely coloured than reference solution B_6 or BY_6 (*2.2.2, Method II*).

Specific optical rotation (*2.2.7*). Dissolve 0.125 g in *acetonitrile R* and dilute to 25.0 ml with the same solvent. The specific optical rotation is + 325 to + 340, calculated with reference to the dried substance.

Related substances. Examine by liquid chromatography (*2.2.29*) as described under Assay.

Inject 10 µl of reference solution (b). Adjust the sensitivity of the system so that the height of the principal peak is at least 20 per cent of the full scale of the recorder. Inject 10 µl of test solution (a). When the chromatograms are recorded under the prescribed conditions the relative retentions are: impurity A about 0.8, impurity B about 0.6, impurity C about 1.2 and impurity D about 2.3 (retention time of lovastatin: about 7 min). In the chromatogram obtained with test solution (a): the area of any peak, apart from the principal peak, is not greater than 0.6 times the area of the principal peak in the chromatogram obtained with reference solution (b) (0.3 per cent); the sum of the areas of all peaks, apart from the principal peak, is not greater than twice the area of the principal peak in the chromatogram obtained with reference solution (b) (1 per cent). Disregard any peak with an area less than 0.1 times the area of the principal peak in the chromatogram obtained with reference solution (b) (0.05 per cent).

Heavy metals (*2.4.8*). 1.0 g complies with limit test C for heavy metals (20 ppm). Prepare the standard using 2 ml of *lead standard solution (10 ppm Pb) R*.

Loss on drying (*2.2.32*). Not more than 0.5 per cent, determined on 1.000 g by drying in a desiccator under high vacuum at 60 °C for 3 h.

Sulphated ash (*2.4.14*). Not more than 0.2 per cent, determined on 1.0 g.

ASSAY

Examine by liquid chromatography (*2.2.29*).

Test solution (a). Dissolve 20.0 mg of the substance to be examined in *acetonitrile R* and dilute to 50.0 ml with the same solvent.

Test solution (b). Dilute 10.0 ml of test solution (a) to 20.0 ml with *acetonitrile R*.

Reference solution (a). Dissolve 10.0 mg of *lovastatin CRS* in *acetonitrile R* and dilute to 50.0 ml with the same solvent.

Reference solution (b). Dilute 0.5 ml of test solution (a) to 100.0 ml with *acetonitrile R*.

Reference solution (c). To 5.0 ml of reference solution (a) add 1 mg of *simvastatin CRS* and dilute to 50.0 ml with *acetonitrile R*.

The chromatographic procedure may be carried out using:

– a stainless steel column 0.25 m long and 4.6 mm in internal diameter packed with *octylsilyl silica gel for chromatography R* (5 µm),

– as mobile phase at a flow rate of 1.5 ml/min:

Mobile phase A. Acetonitrile R,

Mobile phase B. A 0.1 per cent *V/V* solution of *phosphoric acid R,*

Time (min)	Mobile phase A (per cent V/V)	Mobile phase B (per cent V/V)	Comment
0 - 5	60	40	isocratic
5 - 7	60 → 65	40 → 35	linear gradient
7 - 13	65 → 90	35 → 10	linear gradient
13 - 15	90	10	isocratic
15 - 17	90 → 60	10 → 40	linear gradient
17 - 20	60	40	re-equilibration

– as detector a spectrophotometer set at 238 nm.

Inject 10 µl of reference solution (c). The test is not valid unless, in the chromatogram obtained, the resolution between the peaks corresponding to simvastatin and lovastatin is at least 5.0. When the chromatograms are recorded in the prescribed conditions the relative retention of simvastatin is about 1.1 (retention time of lovastatin: about 7 min). Inject 10 µl of reference solution (a). Adjust the sensitivity of the system so that the height of the principal peak is at least 50 per cent of the full scale of the recorder. Inject 10 µl of test solution (b).

Calculate the content of $C_{24}H_{36}O_5$ from the peak areas in the chromatograms obtained with test solution (b) and reference solution (a), and the declared content of $C_{24}H_{36}O_5$ in *lovastatin CRS*.

STORAGE

Store under nitrogen at a temperature of 2 °C to 8 °C.

IMPURITIES

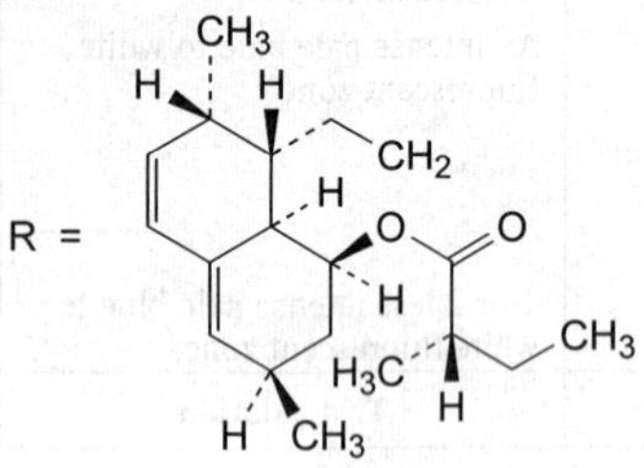

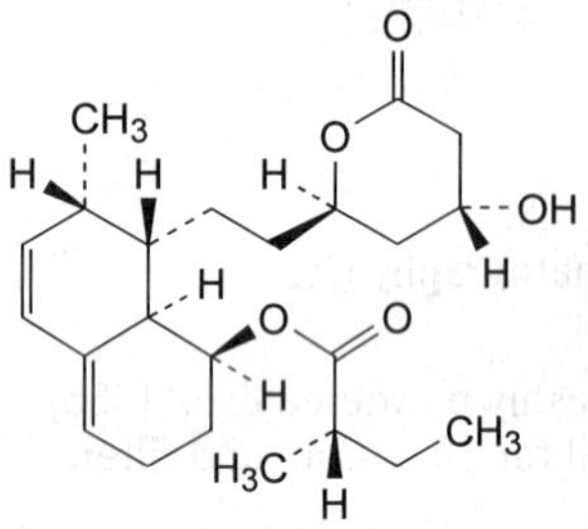

A. (1*S*,7*S*,8*S*,8a*R*)-8-[2-[(2*R*,4*R*)-4-hydroxy-6-oxotetrahydro-2*H*-pyran-2-yl]ethyl]-7-methyl-1,2,3,7,8,8a-hexahydronaphthalen-1-yl (2*S*)-2-methylbutanoate (mevastatin),

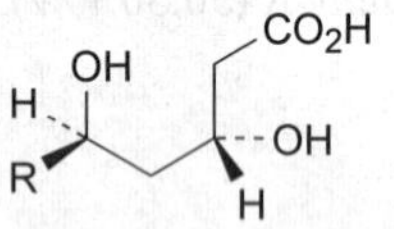

B. (3*R*,5*R*)-7-[(1*S*,2*S*,6*R*,8*S*,8a*R*)-2,6-dimethyl-8-[[(2*S*)-2-methylbutanoyl]oxy]-1,2,6,7,8,8a-hexahydronaphthalen-1-yl]-3,5-dihydroxyheptanoic acid (hydroxyacid lovastatin),

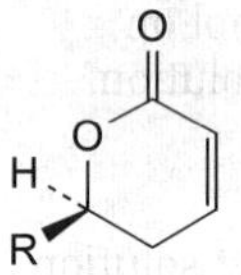

C. (1*S*,3*R*,7*S*,8*S*,8a*R*)-3,7-dimethyl-8-[2-[(2*R*)-6-oxo-3,6-dihydro-2*H*-pyran-2-yl]ethyl]-1,2,3,7,8,8a-hexahydronaphthalen-1-yl (2*S*)-2-methylbutanoate (dehydrolovastatin),

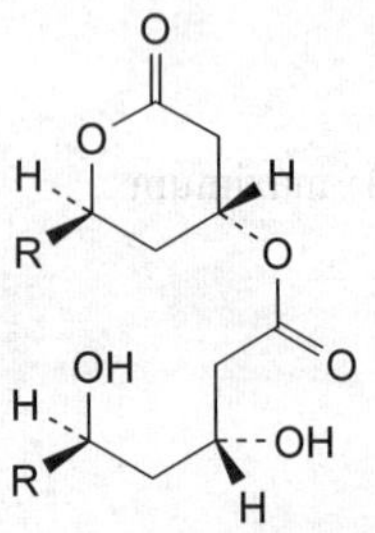

D. (2*R*,4*R*)-2-[2-[(1*S*,2*S*,6*R*,8*S*,8a*R*)-2,6-dimethyl-8-[[(2*S*)-2-methylbutanoyl]oxy]-1,2,6,7,8,8a-hexahydronaphthalen-1-yl]ethyl]-6-oxotetrahydro-2*H*-pyran-4-yl (3*R*,5*R*)-7-[(1*S*,2*S*,6*R*,8*S*,8a*R*)-2,6-dimethyl-8-[[(2*S*)-2-methylbutanoyl]oxy]-1,2,6,7,8,8a-hexahydronaphthalen-1-yl]-3,5-dihydroxyheptanoate (lovastatin dimer).

01/2005:0558

LYNESTRENOL

Lynestrenolum

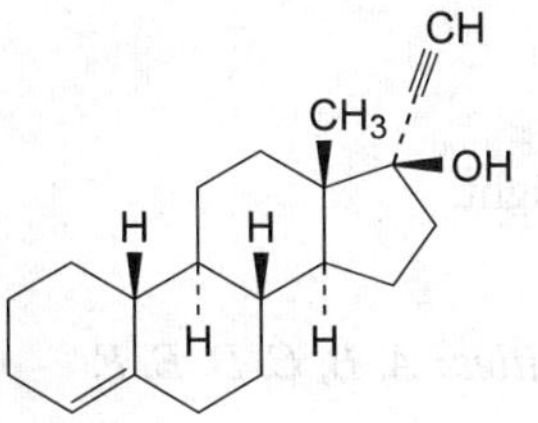

$C_{20}H_{28}O$ M_r 284.4

DEFINITION

Lynestrenol contains not less than 98.0 per cent and not more than the equivalent of 102.0 per cent of 19-nor-17α-pregn-4-en-20-yn-17-ol, calculated with reference to the dried substance.

CHARACTERS

A white or almost white, crystalline powder, practically insoluble in water, soluble in acetone and in alcohol.

IDENTIFICATION

First identification: B.

Second identification: A, C.

A. Melting point (*2.2.14*): 161 °C to 165 °C.

B. Examine by infrared absorption spectrophotometry (*2.2.24*), comparing with the spectrum obtained with *lynestrenol CRS.*

C. Examine the chromatograms obtained in the test for related substances in ultraviolet light at 365 nm. The principal spot in the chromatogram obtained with test solution (b) is similar in position, fluorescence and size to the principal spot in the chromatogram obtained with reference solution (b).

TESTS

Appearance of solution. Dissolve 0.2 g in *alcohol R* and dilute to 10 ml with the same solvent. The solution is clear (*2.2.1*) and colourless (*2.2.2, Method II*).

Specific optical rotation (*2.2.7*). Dissolve 0.900 g in *alcohol R* and dilute to 25.0 ml with the same solvent. The specific optical rotation is − 9.5 to − 11, calculated with reference to the dried substance.

Related substances. Examine by thin-layer chromatography (*2.2.27*), using *silica gel G R* as the coating substance.

Test solution (a). Dissolve 0.125 g of the substance to be examined in *chloroform R* and dilute to 25 ml with the same solvent.

Test solution (b). Dilute 5 ml of test solution (a) to 10 ml with *chloroform R.*

Reference solution (a). Dilute 1 ml of test solution (a) to 100 ml with *chloroform R.* Dilute 5 ml of the solution to 10 ml with *chloroform R.*

Reference solution (b). Dissolve 25 mg of *lynestrenol CRS* in *chloroform R* and dilute to 10 ml with the same solvent.

Apply separately to the plate 10 µl of each solution. Develop over a path of 15 cm using a mixture of 20 volumes of *acetone R* and 80 volumes of *heptane R.* Allow the plate to dry in air, spray with *0.25 M alcoholic sulphuric acid R* and heat at 105 °C for 10 min. Examine in ultraviolet light at 365 nm. Any spot in the chromatogram obtained with test solution (a), apart from the principal spot, is not more intense than the spot in the chromatogram obtained with reference solution (a) (0.5 per cent).

Loss on drying (*2.2.32*). Not more than 0.5 per cent, determined on 0.500 g by drying in an oven at 100 °C to 105 °C.

ASSAY

Dissolve 0.150 g in 40 ml of *tetrahydrofuran R* and add 5.0 ml of a 100 g/l solution of *silver nitrate R.* Titrate with *0.1 M sodium hydroxide.* Determine the end-point potentiometrically (*2.2.20*), using a glass indicator electrode and as comparison electrode a silver-silver chloride double-junction electrode with a saturated solution of *potassium nitrate R* as junction liquid. Carry out a blank titration.

1 ml of *0.1 M sodium hydroxide* is equivalent to 28.44 mg of $C_{20}H_{28}O$.

STORAGE

Store protected from light.

01/2005:2114

LYSINE ACETATE

Lysini acetas

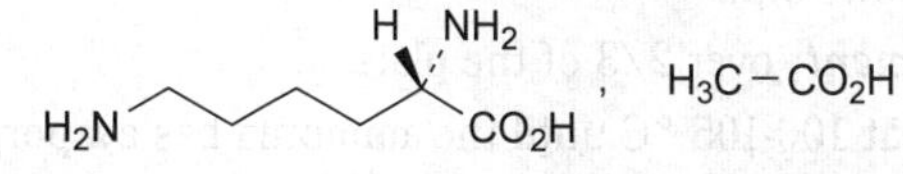

$C_8H_{18}N_2O_4$ M_r 206.2

DEFINITION

(2*S*)-2,6-Diaminohexanoic acid acetate.

Content: 98.5 per cent to 101.0 per cent (dried substance).

CHARACTERS

Appearance: white or almost white, crystalline powder or colourless crystals.

Solubility: freely soluble in water, very slightly soluble in ethanol (96 per cent).

It shows polymorphism.

IDENTIFICATION

First identification: A, B, E.

Second identification: A, C, D, E.

A. It complies with the test for specific optical rotation (see Tests).

B. Infrared absorption spectrophotometry (*2.2.24*).

Comparison: *lysine acetate CRS.*

If the spectra obtained in the solid state show differences, dissolve the substance to be examined and the reference substance separately in the minimum volume of *water R,* evaporate to dryness at 60 °C and record new spectra using the residues.

C. Examine the chromatograms obtained in the test for ninhydrin-positive substances.

Results: the principal spot in the chromatogram obtained with test solution (b) is similar in position, colour and size to the principal spot in the chromatogram obtained with reference solution (a).

D. To 0.1 ml of solution S (see Tests) add 2 ml of *water R* and 1 ml of a 50 g/l solution of *phosphomolybdic acid R.* A yellowish-white precipitate is formed.

E. It gives reaction (a) of acetates (*2.3.1*).

TESTS

Solution S. Dissolve 5.0 g in *distilled water R* and dilute to 50 ml with the same solvent.

Appearance of solution. Solution S is clear (*2.2.1*) and colourless (*2.2.2, Method II*).

Specific optical rotation (*2.2.7*): + 8.5 to + 10.0 (dried substance), determined on solution S.

Ninhydrin-positive substances. Thin-layer chromatography (*2.2.27*).

Test solution (a). Dissolve 0.10 g of the substance to be examined in *water R* and dilute to 10 ml with the same solvent.

Test solution (b). Dilute 1.0 ml of test solution (a) to 50 ml with *water R.*

Reference solution (a). Dissolve 10 mg of *lysine acetate CRS* in *water R* and dilute to 50 ml with the same solvent.

Reference solution (b). Dilute 5 ml of test solution (b) to 20 ml with *water R.*

Reference solution (c). Dissolve 10 mg of *lysine acetate CRS* and 10 mg of *arginine CRS* in *water R* and dilute to 25 ml with the same solvent.

Plate: *TLC silica gel plate R.*

Mobile phase: *concentrated ammonia R, 2-propanol R* (30:70 *V/V*).

Application: 5 µl.

Development: over 2/3 of the plate.

Drying: at 100-105 °C until the ammonia has evaporated.

Detection: spray with *ninhydrin solution R* and heat at 100-105 °C for 15 min.

System suitability: reference solution (c):

– the chromatogram shows 2 clearly separated spots.

Limits: test solution (a):

– *any impurity*: any spot, apart from the principal spot, is not more intense than the principal spot in the chromatogram obtained with reference solution (b) (0.5 per cent).

Chlorides (*2.4.4*): maximum 200 ppm.

Dilute 2.5 ml of solution S to 15 ml with *water R.*

Sulphates (*2.4.13*): maximum 300 ppm.

Dilute 5 ml of solution S to 15 ml with *distilled water R.*

Ammonium (*2.4.1, Method B*): maximum 200 ppm, determined on 50 mg.

Prepare the standard using 0.1 ml of *ammonium standard solution (100 ppm NH_4) R.*

Iron (*2.4.9*): maximum 30 ppm.

In a separating funnel, dissolve 0.33 g in 10 ml of *dilute hydrochloric acid R.* Shake with 3 quantities, each of 10 ml, of *methyl isobutyl ketone R1*, shaking for 3 min each time. To the combined organic layers add 10 ml of *water R* and shake for 3 min. The aqueous layer complies with the limit test for iron.

Heavy metals (*2.4.8*): maximum 10 ppm.

12 ml of solution S complies with limit test A. Prepare the reference solution using *lead standard solution (1 ppm Pb) R.*

Loss on drying (*2.2.32*): maximum 0.5 per cent, determined on 1.000 g by drying in an oven at 60 °C for 3 h.

Sulphated ash (*2.4.14*): maximum 0.1 per cent, determined on 1.0 g.

ASSAY

Dissolve 80 mg in 3 ml of *anhydrous formic acid R.* Add 50 ml of *anhydrous acetic acid R.* Titrate with *0.1 M perchloric acid*, determining the end-point potentiometrically (*2.2.20*). Carry out a blank titration.

1 ml of *0.1 M perchloric acid* is equivalent to 10.31 mg of $C_8H_{18}N_2O_4$.

STORAGE

Protected from light.

IMPURITIES

Specified impurities: A, B, C, D, E, F.

A. aspartic acid,

B. glutamic acid,

C. alanine,

D. valine,

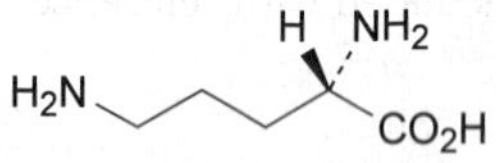

E. (2*S*)-2,5-diaminopentanoic acid (ornithine),

F. arginine.

01/2005:0930

LYSINE HYDROCHLORIDE

Lysini hydrochloridum

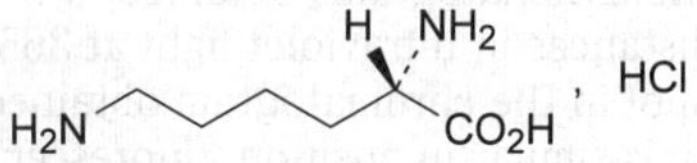

$C_6H_{15}ClN_2O_2$ $\qquad$ M_r 182.7

DEFINITION

Lysine hydrochloride contains not less than 98.5 per cent and not more than the equivalent of 101.0 per cent of (*S*)-2,6-diaminohexanoic acid hydrochloride, calculated with reference to the dried substance.

CHARACTERS

A white, crystalline powder or colourless crystals, freely soluble in water, slightly soluble in alcohol.

IDENTIFICATION

First identification: A, B, E.

Second identification: A, C, D, E.

A. It complies with the test for specific optical rotation (see Tests).

B. Examine by infrared absorption spectrophotometry (*2.2.24*), comparing with the spectrum obtained with *lysine hydrochloride CRS*. Examine the substances prepared as discs. If the spectra obtained show differences, dissolve the substance to be examined and the reference substance separately in the minimum volume of *water R*, evaporate to dryness at 60 °C, and record new spectra using the residues.

C. Examine the chromatograms obtained in the test for ninhydrin-positive substances. The principal spot in the chromatogram obtained with test solution (b) is similar in position, colour and size to the principal spot in the chromatogram obtained with reference solution (a).

D. To 0.1 ml of solution S (see Tests) add 2 ml of *water R* and 1 ml of a 50 g/l solution of *phosphomolybdic acid R*. A yellowish-white precipitate is formed.

E. To 0.1 ml of solution S add 2 ml of *water R*. The solution gives reaction (a) of chlorides (*2.3.1*).

TESTS

Solution S. Dissolve 5.0 g in *carbon dioxide-free water R* prepared from *distilled water R* and dilute to 50 ml with the same solvent.

Appearance of solution. Solution S is clear (*2.2.1*) and not more intensely coloured than reference solution B_7 or GY_7 (*2.2.2, Method II*).

Specific optical rotation (*2.2.7*). Dissolve 2.00 g in *hydrochloric acid R1* and dilute to 25.0 ml with the same acid. The specific optical rotation is + 21.0 to + 22.5, calculated with reference to the dried substance.

Ninhydrin-positive substances. Examine by thin-layer chromatography (*2.2.27*), using a *TLC silica gel plate R*.

Test solution (a). Dissolve 0.10 g of the substance to be examined in *water R* and dilute to 10 ml with the same solvent.

Test solution (b). Dilute 1 ml of test solution (a) to 50 ml with *water R*.

Reference solution (a). Dissolve 10 mg of *lysine hydrochloride CRS* in *water R* and dilute to 50 ml with the same solvent.

Reference solution (b). Dilute 5 ml of test solution (b) to 20 ml with *water R*.

Reference solution (c). Dissolve 10 mg of *lysine hydrochloride CRS* and 10 mg of *arginine CRS* in *water R* and dilute to 25 ml with the same solvent.

Apply separately to the plate 5 µl of each solution. Develop over a path of 15 cm using a mixture of 30 volumes of *concentrated ammonia R* and 70 volumes of *2-propanol R*. Dry the plate at 100 °C to 105 °C until the ammonia disappears completely. Spray with *ninhydrin solution R* and heat at 100 °C to 105 °C for 15 min. Any spot in the chromatogram obtained with test solution (a), apart from the principal spot, is not more intense than the spot in the chromatogram obtained with reference solution (b) (0.5 per cent). The test is not valid unless the chromatogram obtained with reference solution (c) shows two clearly separated principal spots.

Sulphates (*2.4.13*). Dilute 5 ml of solution S to 15 ml with *distilled water R*. The solution complies with the limit test for sulphates (300 ppm).

Ammonium (*2.4.1*). 50 mg complies with limit test B for ammonium (200 ppm). Prepare the standard using 0.1 ml of *ammonium standard solution (100 ppm NH_4) R*.

Iron (*2.4.9*). In a separating funnel, dissolve 0.33 g in 10 ml of *dilute hydrochloric acid R*. Shake with three quantities, each of 10 ml, of *methyl isobutyl ketone R1*, shaking for 3 min each time. To the combined organic layers add 10 ml of *water R* and shake for 3 min. The aqueous layer complies with the limit test for iron (30 ppm).

Heavy metals (*2.4.8*). 12 ml of solution S complies with limit test A for heavy metals (10 ppm). Prepare the standard using *lead standard solution (1 ppm Pb) R*.

Loss on drying (*2.2.32*). Not more than 0.5 per cent, determined on 1.000 g by drying in an oven at 100 °C to 105 °C.

Sulphated ash (*2.4.14*). Not more than 0.1 per cent, determined on 1.0 g.

ASSAY

Dissolve 0.150 g in 5 ml of *anhydrous formic acid R*. Add 50 ml of *anhydrous acetic acid R*. Titrate with *0.1 M perchloric acid*, determining the end-point potentiometrically (*2.2.20*).

1 ml of *0.1 M perchloric acid* is equivalent to 18.27 mg of $C_6H_{15}ClN_2O_2$.

STORAGE

Store protected from light.

M

Monographs M

01/2005:1443

MACROGOL 6 GLYCEROL CAPRYLOCAPRATE

Macrogol 6 glyceroli caprylocapras

DEFINITION

Macrogol 6 glycerol caprylocaprate is a mixture of mainly mono- and diesters of polyoxyethylene glycerol ethers mainly with caprylic (octanoic) and capric (decanoic) acids. The average content of the ethylene oxide is 6 units per molecule. Macrogol 6 glycerol caprylocaprate may be obtained by ethoxylation of glycerol and esterification with distilled coconut or palm kernel fatty acids, or by ethoxylation of mono- and diglycerides of caprylic and capric acids.

CHARACTERS

A pale yellow liquid, partly soluble in water, freely soluble in castor oil, in glycerol, in isopropanol and in propylene glycol.

It has a viscosity of about 145 mPa·s.

IDENTIFICATION

A. Dissolve 1.0 g in 99 g of a mixture of 10 volumes of *2-propanol R* and 90 volumes of *water R*. Heat the solution obtained to about 40 °C. A turbidity is produced. Allow to cool until the turbidity disappears. The cloud point is between 15 °C and 35 °C.

B. It complies with the test for saponification value (see Tests).

C. It complies with the test for composition of fatty acids (see Tests).

TESTS

Appearance. The substance to be examined is clear (*2.2.1*) and not more intensely coloured than reference solution Y_2 (*2.2.2, Method I*).

Alkalinity. Dissolve 2.0 g in a hot mixture of 10 ml of *alcohol R* and 10 ml of *water R*. Add 0.1 ml of *bromothymol blue solution R1*. Not more than 0.5 ml of *0.1 M hydrochloric acid* is required to change the colour of the indicator to yellow.

Acid value (*2.5.1*). Not more than 5.0, determined on 5.0 g.

Hydroxyl value (*2.5.3, Method A*): 165 to 225.

Saponification value (*2.5.6*): 85 to 105, determined on 2.0 g.

Composition of fatty acids (*2.4.22, Method A*). The fatty acid fraction has the following composition:

- *caproic acid*: not more than 2.0 per cent,
- *caprylic acid*: 50.0 per cent to 80.0 per cent,
- *capric acid*: 20.0 per cent to 50.0 per cent,
- *lauric acid*: not more than 3.0 per cent,
- *myristic acid*: not more than 1.0 per cent.

Ethylene oxide and dioxan (*2.4.25*). Not more than 1 ppm of ethylene oxide and not more than 10 ppm of dioxan.

Water (*2.5.12*). Not more than 1.0 per cent, determined on 1.00 g by the semi-micro determination of water.

Total ash (*2.4.16*). Not more than 0.3 per cent, determined on 1.0 g.

01/2005:2052

MACROGOL 15 HYDROXYSTEARATE

Macrogoli 15 hydroxystearas

DEFINITION

Mixture of mainly monoesters and diesters of 12-hydroxystearic acid and macrogols obtained by ethoxylation of 12-hydroxystearic acid. The number of moles of ethylene oxide reacted per mole of 12-hydroxystearic acid is 15 (nominal value). It contains free macrogols.

CHARACTERS

Appearance: yellowish, waxy mass.

Solubility: very soluble in water, soluble in alcohol, insoluble in liquid paraffin.

It solidifies at about 25 °C.

IDENTIFICATION

A. Thin-layer chromatography (*2.2.27*).

Test solution. To 1.0 g add 100 ml of a 100 g/l solution of *potassium hydroxide R* and boil under a reflux condenser for 30 min. Acidify the warm solution with 20 ml of *hydrochloric acid R* and cool to room temperature. Shake the mixture with 50 ml of *ether R* and allow to stand until a separation of the layers is visible. Separate the clear upper layer, add 5 g of *anhydrous sodium sulphate R*, wait for 30 min, filter and evaporate to dryness on a water-bath. Dissolve 50 mg of the residue in 25 ml of *ether R*.

Reference solution. Dissolve 50 mg of *12-hydroxystearic acid R* in 25 ml of *methylene chloride R*.

Plate: *octadecylsilyl silica gel for chromatography R* as the coating substance.

Mobile phase: *methylene chloride R, glacial acetic acid R, acetone R* (10:40:50 *V/V/V*).

Application: 2 µl.

Development: over 2/3 of the plate.

Drying: in a current of cold air.

Detection: spray with a 80 g/l solution of *phosphomolybdic acid R* in *2-propanol R* and heat at 120 °C for 1-2 min.

Results: the principal spot in the chromatogram obtained with the test solution is similar in position and colour to the principal spot in the chromatogram obtained with the reference solution.

B. Dissolve 15.0 g in 50 ml of *water R*. The viscosity (*2.2.9*) has a maximum of 20 mPa·s.

C. It complies with the test for free macrogols (see Tests).

TESTS

Appearance of solution. The solution is not more opalescent than reference suspension III (*2.2.1*) and not more intensely coloured than reference solution B_6 or BY_6 (*2.2.2, Method II*).

Dissolve 2.0 g in *water R* and dilute to 20 ml with the same solvent.

Acid value (*2.5.1*): maximum 1.0, determined on 2.0 g.

Hydroxyl value (*2.5.3, Method A*): 90 to 110.

Iodine value (*2.5.4*): maximum 2.0.

Peroxide value (*2.5.5, Method A*): maximum 5.0.

Saponification value (*2.5.6*): 53 to 63.

Monographs M

Free macrogols. Size-exclusion chromatography (*2.2.30*).

Test solution. Dissolve 1.20 g of the substance to be examined in the mobile phase and dilute to 250.0 ml with the mobile phase.

Reference solution (a). Dissolve about 0.4 g of *macrogol 1000 R* in the mobile phase and dilute to 250.0 ml with the mobile phase.

Reference solution (b). Dilute 50.0 ml of reference solution (a) to 100.0 ml with the mobile phase.

Precolumns (2):

– *size*: l = 0.125 m, Ø = 4 mm,

– *stationary phase*: spherical *octadecylsilyl silica gel for chromatography R* (5 μm) with a pore size of 10 nm.

Column:

– *size*: l = 0.30 m, Ø = 7.8 mm,

– *stationary phase*: *hydroxylated polymethacrylate gel R* (6 μm) with a pore size of 12 nm.

Connect both precolumns to the column using a 3-way valve and switch the mobile phase flow according to the following programme:

– 0-114 s: precolumn 1 and column,

– 115 s to the end: precolumn 2 and column,

– 115 s to 7 min: flow back of precolumn 1.

Mobile phase: *water R, methanol R* (2:8 *V/V*).

Flow rate: 1.1 ml/min.

Detection: refractometer.

Injection: 50 μl.

Calculate the percentage content of free macrogols using the following expression:

$$\frac{A_1 \times m_2 \times 200}{m_1 \times (A_2 + 2A_3)}$$

m_1 = mass of the substance to be examined in the test solution, in grams,

m_2 = mass of *macrogol 1000 R* in reference solution (a), in grams,

A_1 = area of the peak due to free macrogols in the substance to be examined in the chromatogram obtained with the test solution,

A_2 = area of the peak due to macrogol 1000 in the chromatogram obtained with reference solution (a),

A_3 = area of the peak due to macrogol 1000 in the chromatogram obtained with reference solution (b).

Limit:

– *free macrogols*: 27.0 per cent to 39.0 per cent.

Ethylene oxide and dioxan (*2.4.25*): maximum 1 ppm of ethylene oxide and maximum 50 ppm of dioxan.

Nickel (*2.4.27*): maximum 1 ppm.

Water (*2.5.12*): maximum 1.0 per cent, determined on 2.00 g.

Total ash (*2.4.16*): maximum 0.3 per cent, determined on 1.0 g.

STORAGE

In an airtight container.

01/2005:2044

MACROGOL 20 GLYCEROL MONOSTEARATE

Macrogol 20 glyceroli monostearas

DEFINITION

Macrogol 20 glycerol monostearate is obtained by ethoxylation with ethylene oxide of different types of glycerol stearates, mainly *Glycerol monostearate 40-55 (0495)*. The number of moles of ethylene oxide reacted per mole of glycerol stearate is 20 (nominal value).

CHARACTERS

Appearance: pale yellow, oily liquid or gel.

Solubility: soluble in water at 40 °C and above and in alcohol, practically insoluble in light liquid paraffin and in fatty oils.

Relative density: about 1.07.

IDENTIFICATION

A. It complies with the test for hydroxyl value (see Tests).

B. It complies with the test for saponification value (see Tests).

C. It complies with the test for composition of fatty acids (see Tests).

D. Place 1 g in a test-tube and add 0.1 ml of *sulphuric acid R*. Heat the tube until white fumes appear. The fumes turn filter paper impregnated with *alkaline potassium tetraiodomercurate solution R* black.

TESTS

Acid value (*2.5.1*): maximum 2.0, determined on 5.0 g.

Hydroxyl value (*2.5.3, Method B*): 65 to 85, determined on 0.350 g.

Iodine value (*2.5.4*): maximum 2.0.

Peroxide value (*2.5.5*): maximum 6.0.

Saponification value (*2.5.6*): 40 to 60.

Composition of fatty acids. Gas chromatography (*2.4.22, Method C*).

Composition of the fatty acid fraction of the substance:

Type of macrogol 20 glycerol monostearate	Type of glycerol stearate used	Composition of fatty acids
Type I	Type I (obtained using stearic acid 50)	*Stearic acid*: 40.0 per cent to 60.0 per cent, *Sum of the contents of palmitic and stearic acids*: minimum 90.0 per cent.
Type II	Type II (obtained using stearic acid 70)	*Stearic acid*: 60.0 per cent to 80.0 per cent, *Sum of the contents of palmitic and stearic acids*: minimum 90.0 per cent.
Type III	Type III (obtained using stearic acid 95)	*Stearic acid*: 90.0 per cent to 99.0 per cent, *Sum of the contents of palmitic and stearic acids*: minimum 96.0 per cent.

Ethylene oxide and dioxan (*2.4.25, Method A*): maximum 1 ppm of ethylene oxide and 10 ppm of dioxan.

Heavy metals (*2.4.8*): maximum 10 ppm.

2.0 g complies with limit test C. Prepare the standard using 2 ml of *lead standard solution (10 ppm Pb) R*.

Water (*2.5.12*): maximum 3.0 per cent, determined on 1.00 g.

Total ash (*2.4.16*): maximum 0.2 per cent, determined on 1.0 g.

STORAGE

Protected from light.

LABELLING

The label states the type of macrogol 20 glycerol monostearate.

01/2005:1123

MACROGOL CETOSTEARYL ETHER

Macrogoli aether cetostearylicus

DEFINITION

Macrogol cetostearyl ether is a mixture of ethers of mixed macrogols with linear fatty alcohols, mainly cetostearyl alcohol. It may contain some free macrogols and it contains various amounts of free cetostearyl alcohol. The amount of ethylene oxide reacted with cetostearyl alcohol is from 2 to 33 units per molecule (nominal value).

CHARACTERS

A waxy, white or yellowish-white, unctuous mass, pellets, microbeads or flakes.

Macrogol cetostearyl ether with low numbers of ethylene oxide units per molecule is practically insoluble in water, soluble in alcohol and in methylene chloride.

Macrogol cetostearyl ether with higher numbers of ethylene oxide units per molecule is dispersible or soluble in water, soluble in alcohol and in methylene chloride.

It solidifies at 32 °C to 52 °C.

IDENTIFICATION

A. It complies with the test for hydroxyl value (see Tests).

B. It complies with the test for iodine value (see Tests).

C. It complies with the test for saponification value (see Tests).

D. Examine by thin-layer chromatography (*2.2.27*), using a suitable silica gel as the coating substance.

Test solution. Dissolve the amount of substance to be examined (given in Table 1123.-1) in a mixture of 1 volume of *water R* and 9 volumes of *methanol R* and dilute to 75 ml with the same mixture of solvents.

Table 1123.-1

Ethylene oxide units per molecule	Amount to be dissolved
2 - 6	5.0 g
10 - 22	10.0 g
25 - 33	15.0 g

Add 60 ml of *hexane R* and shake for 3 min. The formation of foam can be reduced by the addition of some drops of *alcohol R*. Pass the hexane layer through a filter with *anhydrous sodium sulphate R*, wash the filter with 3 quantities, each of 10 ml, of *hexane R* and evaporate the combined filtrates to dryness. Dissolve 0.05 g of the residue in 10 ml of *methanol R* (sometimes the solution is opalescent).

Reference solution. Dissolve 25 mg of *stearyl alcohol CRS* in *methanol R* and dilute to 25 ml with the same solvent.

Apply separately to the plate 20 µl of each solution. Develop over a path of 15 cm using *ethyl acetate R*. Dry and spray with vanillin-sulphuric acid reagent prepared as follows: dissolve 0.50 g of *vanillin R* in 50.0 ml of *alcohol R* and dilute to 100.0 ml with *sulphuric acid R*. Allow the plate to dry in air. Heat the plate at about 130 °C for 15 min and allow to cool in air. The chromatogram obtained with the test solution shows several spots; one of these spots corresponds to the principal spot in the chromatogram obtained with the reference solution.

E. Dissolve or disperse 0.1 g in 5 ml of *alcohol R*, add 2 ml of *water R*, 10 ml of *dilute hydrochloric acid R*, 10 ml of *barium chloride solution R1* and 10 ml of a 100 g/l solution of *phosphomolybdic acid R*. A precipitate is formed.

TESTS

Appearance of solution. Dissolve 5.0 g in *alcohol R* and dilute to 50 ml with the same solvent. The solution is not more intensely coloured than reference solution BY_5 (*2.2.2, Method II*).

Alkalinity. Dissolve 2.0 g in a hot mixture of 10 ml of *water R* and 10 ml of *alcohol R*. Add 0.1 ml of *bromothymol blue solution R1*. Not more than 0.5 ml of *0.1 M hydrochloric acid* is required to change the colour of the indicator to yellow.

Acid value (*2.5.1*). Not more than 1.0, determined on 5.0 g.

Hydroxyl value (*2.5.3, Method A*).

Ethylene oxide units per molecule (nominal value)	Hydroxyl value
2	150 - 180
3	135 - 155
5 - 6	100 - 134
10	75 - 90
12	67 - 77
15	58 - 67
20 - 22	40 - 55
25	36 - 46
30 - 33	32 - 40

Iodine value (*2.5.4*). Not more than 2.0.

Saponification value (*2.5.6*). Not more than 3.0, determined on 10.0 g.

Ethylene oxide and dioxan (*2.4.25*). Not more than 1 ppm of ethylene oxide and not more than 10 ppm of dioxan.

Water (*2.5.12*). Not more than 3.0 per cent, determined on 2.00 g by the semi-micro determination of water.

Total ash (*2.4.16*). Not more than 0.2 per cent, determined on 2.0 g.

STORAGE

Store in an airtight container.

LABELLING

The label states the amount of ethylene oxide reacted with cetostearyl alcohol (nominal value).

Monographs M

01/2005:1124

MACROGOL LAURYL ETHER

Macrogoli aether laurilicum

DEFINITION

Mixture of ethers of mixed macrogols with fatty alcohols, mainly $C_{12}H_{26}O$. It contains a variable amount of free $C_{12}H_{26}O$ and it may contain free macrogols. The number of moles of ethylene oxide reacted per mole of $C_{12}H_{26}O$ is 3 to 23 (nominal value).

CHARACTERS

– Macrogol lauryl ether with 3 to 5 units of ethylene oxide per molecule.
  Appearance: colourless liquid.
  Solubility: practically insoluble in water, soluble or dispersible in alcohol, practically insoluble in light petroleum.
– Macrogol lauryl ether with 9 to 23 units of ethylene oxide per molecule.
  Appearance: white, waxy mass.
  Solubility: soluble or dispersible in water, soluble in alcohol, practically insoluble in light petroleum.

IDENTIFICATION

A. It complies with the test for hydroxyl value (see Tests).
B. It complies with the test for iodine value (see Tests).
C. It complies with the test for saponification value (see Tests).
D. Dissolve or disperse 0.1 g in 5 ml of *alcohol R*, add 10 ml of *dilute hydrochloric acid R*, 10 ml of *barium chloride solution R1* and 10 ml of a 100 g/l solution of *phosphomolybdic acid R*. A precipitate is formed.

TESTS

Appearance of solution. The solution is not more intensely coloured than reference solution BY_5 (*2.2.2, Method II*).

Dissolve 5.0 g in *alcohol R* and dilute to 50 ml with the same solvent.

Alkalinity. Dissolve 2.0 g in a hot mixture of 10 ml of *water R* and 10 ml of *alcohol R*. Add 0.1 ml of *bromothymol blue solution R1*. Not more than 0.5 ml of *0.1 M hydrochloric acid* is required to change the colour of the indicator to yellow.

Acid value (*2.5.1*): maximum 1.0, determined on 5.0 g.

Hydroxyl value (*2.5.3, Method A*).

Ethylene oxide units per molecule (nominal value)	Hydroxyl value
3	165 - 180
4	145 - 165
5	130 - 140
9	90 - 100
10	85 - 95
12	73 - 83
15	64 - 74
20 - 23	40 - 60

Iodine value (*2.5.4*): maximum 2.0.

Saponification value (*2.5.6*): maximum 3.0, determined on 10.0 g.

Ethylene oxide and dioxan (*2.4.25*): maximum 1 ppm of ethylene oxide and maximum 10 ppm of dioxan.

Water (*2.5.12*): maximum 3.0 per cent, determined on 2.00 g.

Total ash (*2.4.16*): maximum 0.2 per cent, determined on 2.0 g.

STORAGE

In an airtight container.

LABELLING

The label states the number of moles of ethylene oxide reacted per mole of $C_{12}H_{26}O$ (nominal value).

01/2005:1618

MACROGOL OLEATE

Macrogoli oleas

DEFINITION

A mixture of monoesters and diesters of mainly oleic acid and macrogols. It may be obtained by ethoxylation of *Oleic acid (0799)* or by esterification of macrogols with oleic acid of animal or vegetable origin. It may contain free macrogols. The average polymer length is equivalent to 5-6 or 10 ethylene oxide units per molecule (nominal value). A suitable antioxidant may be added.

CHARACTERS

Appearance: slightly yellowish, viscous liquid.

Solubility: dispersible in water, soluble in alcohol and in 2-propanol, dispersible in oils, miscible with fatty oils and with waxes.

Refractive index: about 1.466.

IDENTIFICATION

First identification: *A, C.*

Second identification: *A, B.*

A. It complies with the test for saponification value (see Tests).
B. Thin-layer chromatography (*2.2.27*).
   Test solution. To 20 mg add 10 ml of *methylene chloride R* and mix.
   Plate: *TLC silica gel F_{254} plate R.*
   Mobile phase: 25 per cent *V/V* solution of *concentrated ammonia R*, *2-propanol R* (20:80 *V/V*).
   Application: 10 µl.
   Development: over a path of 15 cm.
   Drying: in air.
   Detection: spray with *potassium iodobismuthate solution R4*. Examine the plate about 10 min later.
   Results: the chromatogram obtained shows 3 principal spots, corresponding, in order of increasing R_f value, to free macrogol, macrogol mono-oleate and macrogol dioleate.
C. It complies with the test for composition of fatty acids (see Tests).

TESTS

Alkalinity. Dissolve 2.0 g in *alcohol R* and dilute to 20 ml with the same solvent. To 2 ml of this solution add 0.05 ml of *phenol red solution R*. The solution is not red.

Acid value (*2.5.1*): maximum 1.0, determined on 10.0 g.

Hydroxyl value (*2.5.3, Method A*): see Table 1618.-1.

Iodine value (*2.5.4*): see Table 1618.-1.

Monographs M

Peroxide value (*2.5.5*): maximum 12.0.

Saponification value (*2.5.6*): see Table 1618.-1.

Table 1618.-1

	5-6 ethylene oxide units	10 ethylene oxide units
Hydroxyl value	50 - 70	65 - 90
Iodine value	50 - 60	27 - 34
Saponification value	105 - 120	68 - 85

Composition of fatty acids. Gas chromatography (*2.4.22, Method A*).

Composition:

- *myristic acid*: maximum 5.0 per cent,
- *stearic acid*: maximum 6.0 per cent,
- *palmitic acid*: maximum 16.0 per cent,
- *palmitoleic acid*: maximum 8.0 per cent,
- *oleic acid*: 65.0 per cent to 88.0 per cent,
- *linoleic acid*: maximum 18.0 per cent,
- *linolenic acid*: maximum 4.0 per cent,
- *fatty acids with a chain length greater than* C_{18}: maximum 4.0 per cent.

Residual ethylene oxide and dioxan (*2.4.25*): maximum 1 ppm of residual ethylene oxide and 10 ppm of residual dioxan.

Water (*2.5.12*): maximum 2.0 per cent, determined on 1.00 g using *anhydrous methanol R* as the solvent.

Total ash (*2.4.16*): maximum 0.3 per cent, determined on 1.0 g.

STORAGE

In an airtight container.

LABELLING

The label states:

- the number of ethylene oxide units per molecule (nominal value),
- the name and concentration of any added antioxidant.

01/2005:1125

MACROGOL OLEYL ETHER

Macrogoli aether oleicum

DEFINITION

Mixture of ethers of mixed macrogols with linear fatty alcohols, mainly oleyl alcohol. It contains a variable amount of free oleyl alcohol and it may contain free macrogols. The number of moles of ethylene oxide reacted per mole of oleyl alcohol is 2 to 20 (nominal value). A suitable antioxidant may be added.

CHARACTERS

- Macrogol oleyl ether with 2 to 5 units of ethylene oxide per molecule.

  Appearance: yellow liquid.

  Solubility: practically insoluble in water, soluble in alcohol, practically insoluble in light petroleum.
- Macrogol oleyl ether with 10 to 20 units of ethylene oxide per molecule.

  Appearance: yellowish-white waxy mass.

  Solubility: dispersible or soluble in water, soluble in alcohol, practically insoluble in light petroleum.

IDENTIFICATION

A. It complies with the test for hydroxyl value (see Tests).

B. It complies with the test for iodine value (see Tests).

C. It complies with the test for saponification value (see Tests).

D. Dissolve or disperse 0.1 g in 5 ml of *alcohol R*, add 2 ml of *water R*, 10 ml of *dilute hydrochloric acid R*, 10 ml of *barium chloride solution R1* and 10 ml of a 100 g/l solution of *phosphomolybdic acid R*. A precipitate is formed.

TESTS

Appearance of solution. The solution is not more intensely coloured than reference solution BY_5 (*2.2.2, Method II*).

Dissolve 5.0 g in *alcohol R* and dilute to 50 ml with the same solvent.

Alkalinity. Dissolve 2.0 g in a hot mixture of 10 ml of *water R* and 10 ml of *alcohol R*. Add 0.1 ml of *bromothymol blue solution R1*. Not more than 0.5 ml of *0.1 M hydrochloric acid* is required to change the colour of the indicator to yellow.

Acid value (*2.5.1*): maximum 1.0, determined on 5.0 g.

Hydroxyl value (*2.5.3, Method A*). See Table 1125.-1.

Iodine value (*2.5.4*). See Table 1125.-1.

Table 1125.-1

Ethylene oxide units per molecule (nominal value)	Hydroxyl value	Iodine value
2	158 - 178	48 - 74*
5	110 - 125	48 - 56
10	75 - 95	24 - 38
20	40 - 65	14 - 24

* This broad range is needed since 2 different grades of oleyl alcohol may be used for the synthesis. The iodine value does not differ by more than 5 units from the nominal iodine value and is within the limits stated in the table.

Peroxide value (*2.5.5*): maximum 10.0.

Saponification value (*2.5.6*): maximum 3.0.

Ethylene oxide and dioxan (*2.4.25*): maximum 1 ppm of ethylene oxide and 10 ppm of dioxan.

Water (*2.5.12*): maximum 3.0 per cent, determined on 2.00 g.

Total ash (*2.4.16*): maximum 0.2 per cent, determined on 2.0 g.

STORAGE

In an airtight container, protected from light.

LABELLING

The label states:

- the number of moles of ethylene oxide reacted per mole of oleyl alcohol (nominal value),
- the name and concentration of any added antioxidant,
- the nominal iodine value for the type with 2 units of ethylene oxide per molecule.

01/2005:1234

MACROGOL STEARATE

Macrogoli stearas

DEFINITION

Mixture of monoesters and diesters of mainly stearic acid and/or palmitic acid and macrogols. It may be obtained by ethoxylation or by esterification of macrogols with stearic acid 50 (type I) or stearic acid 95 (type II) (see *Stearic acid (1474)*). It may contain free macrogols. The average polymer length is equivalent to 6 to 100 ethylene oxide units per molecule (nominal value).

CHARACTERS

Appearance: white or slightly yellowish waxy mass.

Solubility: soluble in alcohol and in 2-propanol. Macrogol stearate corresponding to a product with 6 to 9 units of ethylene oxide per molecule is practically insoluble, but freely dispersible in water and miscible with fatty oils and with waxes. Macrogol stearate corresponding to a product with 20 to 100 units of ethylene oxide per molecule is soluble in water and practically insoluble in fatty oils and in waxes.

IDENTIFICATION

A. It complies with the test for saponification value (see Tests).

B. It complies with the test for composition of fatty acids (see Tests).

TESTS

Alkalinity. Dissolve 2.0 g in *alcohol R* and dilute to 20 ml with the same solvent. To 2 ml of this solution add 0.05 ml of *phenol red solution R*. The solution is not red.

Melting point (*2.2.15*). See Table 1234.-1.

Melt about 10 g at 80-90 °C. Introduce into the tube by capillary action, a sufficient amount of the substance, to form in the tube a column of the prescribed height. Allow to stand at 0 °C for 2 h.

Acid value (*2.5.1*): maximum 2.0, determined on 2.0 g.

Hydroxyl value (*2.5.3, Method A*). See Table 1234.-1.

Iodine value (*2.5.4*): maximum 2.0.

Saponification value (*2.5.6*). See Table 1234.-1.

Table 1234.-1

Ethylene oxide units per molecule (nominal value)	Melting point (°C)	Hydroxyl value	Saponification value
6		90 - 110	85 - 105
8 - 9	26 - 35	80 - 105	88 - 100
20	33 - 40	50 - 62	46 - 56
40 - 50	38 - 52	23 - 40	20 - 35
100	48 - 60	15 - 30	5 - 20

Reducing substances. Dissolve or disperse 2.0 g in *water R* and dilute to 20 ml with the same solvent. Mix 1.0 ml of the solution with 9 ml of *0.1 M sodium hydroxide* and 0.5 ml of *triphenyltetrazolium chloride solution R*. Heat in a water-bath at 70 °C. After 5 min, the solution is not more intensely coloured than a mixture of 0.15 ml of yellow primary solution, 0.9 ml of red primary solution and 8.95 ml of a 10 g/l solution of *hydrochloric acid R* (*2.2.2, Method II*).

Composition of fatty acids. Gas chromatography (*2.4.22, Method C*).

Composition of the fatty acid fraction of the substance:

	Type of fatty acid used	Composition of fatty acids
Macrogol stearate type I	Stearic acid 50	*Stearic acid*: 40.0 per cent to 60.0 per cent, *Sum of the contents of palmitic and stearic acids*: not less than 90.0 per cent.
Macrogol stearate type II	Stearic acid 95	*Stearic acid*: 90.0 per cent to 99.0 per cent, *Sum of the contents of palmitic and stearic acids*: not less than 96.0 per cent.

Ethylene oxide and dioxan (*2.4.25*): maximum 1 ppm of ethylene oxide and 10 ppm of dioxan.

Heavy metals (*2.4.8*): maximum 10 ppm.

2.0 g complies with limit test C. Prepare the standard using 2 ml of *lead standard solution (10 ppm Pb) R*.

Water (*2.5.12*): maximum 3.0 per cent, determined on 0.50 g. Use as the solvent a mixture of equal volumes of *anhydrous methanol R* and *methylene chloride R*.

Total ash (*2.4.16*): maximum 0.3 per cent, determined on 1.0 g.

STORAGE

In an airtight container.

LABELLING

The label states:

– the number of ethylene oxide units per molecule (nominal value),

– the type of macrogol stearate.

01/2005:1340

MACROGOL STEARYL ETHER

Macrogoli aether stearylicus

DEFINITION

Macrogol stearyl ether is a mixture of ethers obtained by ethoxylation of stearyl alcohol. It may contain some free macrogols and various amounts of free stearyl alcohol. The amount of ethylene oxide reacted with stearyl alcohol is 2 to 20 units per molecule (nominal value).

CHARACTERS

A white to yellowish-white, waxy, unctuous mass, pellets, microbeads or flakes.

Macrogol stearyl ether with 2 units of ethylene oxide per molecule is practically insoluble in water, soluble in alcohol with heating and in methylene chloride. Macrogol stearyl ether with 10 units of ethylene oxide per molecule is soluble in water and in alcohol. Macrogol stearyl ether with 20 units of ethylene oxide per molecule is soluble in water, in alcohol and in methylene chloride.

After melting, it solidifies at about 45 °C.

IDENTIFICATION

A. It complies with the test for hydroxyl value (see Tests).

B. It complies with the test for iodine value (see Tests).

C. It complies with the test for saponification value (see Tests).

D. Examine by thin-layer chromatography (*2.2.27*), using a *TLC silica gel plate R*.

Test solution. Dissolve 10.0 g in a mixture of 1 volume of *water R* and 9 volumes of *methanol R* and dilute to 75 ml with the same mixture of solvents. Add 60 ml of *heptane R* and shake for 3 min. The formation of foam can be reduced by the addition of a few drops of *alcohol R*. Filter the upper layer through *anhydrous sodium sulphate R*, wash the filter with 3 quantities, each of 10 ml, of *heptane R* and evaporate the combined filtrates to dryness. Dissolve 50 mg of the residue in 10 ml of *methanol R* (the solution may be opalescent).

Reference solution. Dissolve 25 mg of *stearyl alcohol CRS* in *methanol R* and dilute to 25 ml with the same solvent.

Apply to the plate 20 µl of each solution. Develop over a path of 15 cm using *ethyl acetate R*. Dry and spray with vanillin-sulphuric acid reagent prepared as follows: dissolve 0.5 g of *vanillin R* in 50 ml of *alcohol R* and dilute to 100 ml with *sulphuric acid R*. Allow the plate to dry in air. Heat the plate at about 130 °C for 15 min and allow to cool in air. The chromatogram obtained in the test solution shows several spots; one of these spots corresponds to the principal spot in the chromatogram obtained with the reference solution.

E. Dissolve or disperse 0.1 g in 5 ml of *alcohol R*, add 2 ml of *water R*, 10 ml of *dilute hydrochloric acid R*, 10 ml of *barium chloride solution R1* and 10 ml of a 100 g/l solution of *phosphomolybdic acid R*. A precipitate is formed.

TESTS

Appearance of solution. Dissolve 5.0 g in *alcohol R* and dilute to 50 ml with the same solvent. The solution is not more intensely coloured than reference solution BY_5 (*2.2.2, Method II*).

Alkalinity. Dissolve 2.0 g in a hot mixture of 10 ml of *alcohol R* and 10 ml of *water R*. Add 0.1 ml of *bromothymol blue solution R1*. Not more than 0.5 ml of *0.1 M hydrochloric acid* is required to change the colour of the indicator to yellow.

Acid value (*2.5.1*). Not more than 1.0, determined on 5.0 g.

Hydroxyl value (*2.5.3, Method A*). See Table 1340.-1.

Table 1340.-1

Ethylene oxide units per molecule (nominal value)	Hydroxyl value
2	150 to 180
10	75 to 90
20	40 to 60

Iodine value (*2.5.4*). Not more than 2.0.

Saponification value (*2.5.6*). Not more than 3.0, determined on 10.0 g.

Ethylene oxide and dioxan (*2.4.25*). Not more than 1 ppm of ethylene oxide and not more than 10 ppm of dioxan.

Water (*2.5.12*). Not more than 3.0 per cent, determined on 1.00 g by the semi-micro determination of water.

STORAGE

Store in an airtight container.

LABELLING

The label states the number of ethylene oxide units reacted with stearyl alcohol (nominal value).

01/2005:1122

MACROGOLGLYCEROL COCOATES

Macrogolglyceroli cocoates

DEFINITION

Macrogol glycerol cocoates are mixtures of mono-, di- and triesters of ethoxylated glycerol with fatty acids of vegetable origin having a composition corresponding to the fatty acid composition of the oil extracted from the hard, dried fraction of the endosperm of *Cocos nucifera* L. The average content of ethylene oxide is either 7 units per molecule or 23 units per molecule (nominal value).

CHARACTERS

A clear, yellowish, oily liquid, soluble in water and in alcohol and practically insoluble in light petroleum (50 °C to 70 °C) for macrogol 7 glycerol cocoate; soluble in water and in alcohol and practically insoluble in light petroleum (50 °C to 70 °C) for macrogol 23 glycerol cocoate. Macrogol 7 glycerol cocoate has a relative density of about 1.05 and macrogol 23 glycerol cocoate has a relative density of about 1.09.

IDENTIFICATION

A. Dissolve 1.0 g of macrogol 7 glycerol cocoate in 99 g of a mixture of 10 volumes of *2-propanol R* and 90 volumes of *water R*. Heat the solution to about 65 °C. A turbidity is produced. Allow to cool until the turbidity disappears. The cloud point is between 35 °C and 54 °C.
Heat a 10 g/l solution of macrogol 23 glycerol cocoate in a 100 g/l solution of *sodium chloride R* to about 90 °C. A turbidity is produced. Allow to cool until the turbidity disappears. The cloud point is between 65 °C and 85 °C.

B. They comply with the test for iodine value (see Tests).

C. They comply with the test for saponification value (see Tests).

TESTS

Appearance. The substance to be examined is clear (*2.2.1*) and not more intensely coloured than reference solution Y_2 (*2.2.2, Method I*).

Alkalinity. Dissolve 2.0 g in a hot mixture of 10 ml of *water R* and 10 ml of *alcohol R*. Add 0.1 ml of *bromothymol blue solution R1*. Not more than 0.5 ml of *0.1 M hydrochloric acid* is required to change the colour of the indicator to yellow.

Acid value (*2.5.1*). Not more than 5.0, determined on 5.0 g.

Hydroxyl value (*2.5.3, Method A*). See Table 1122.-1.

Saponification value (*2.5.6*). See Table 1122.-1.

Table 1122.-1

Number of units of ethylene oxide (nominal value)	Hydroxyl value	Saponification value (determined on 2.0 g)
7	170 to 210	85 to 105
23	80 to 100	40 to 50

Iodine value (*2.5.4*). Not more than 5.0.

Composition of fatty acids (*2.4.22, Method A*). The fatty acid fraction has the following composition:

- *caproic acid*: not more than 1.0 per cent,
- *caprylic acid*: 5.0 per cent to 10.0 per cent,
- *capric acid*: 4.0 per cent to 10.0 per cent,
- *lauric acid*: 40.0 per cent to 55.0 per cent,
- *myristic acid*: 14.0 per cent to 23.0 per cent,

Monographs M

- *palmitic acid*: 8.0 per cent to 12.0 per cent,
- *stearic acid*: 1.0 per cent to 5.0 per cent,
- *oleic acid*: 5.0 per cent to 10.0 per cent,
- *linoleic acid*: not more than 3.0 per cent.

Ethylene oxide and dioxan (*2.4.25*). Not more than 1 ppm of ethylene oxide and not more than 10 ppm of dioxan.

Water (*2.5.12*). Not more than 1.0 per cent, determined on 1.0 g by the semi-micro determination of water.

Total ash (*2.4.16*). Not more than 0.3 per cent, determined on 1.0 g.

LABELLING

The label states the number of ethylene oxide units per molecule (nominal value).

01/2005:1083

MACROGOLGLYCEROL HYDROXYSTEARATE

Macrogolglyceroli hydroxystearas

DEFINITION

Contains mainly trihydroxystearyl glycerol ethoxylated with 7 to 60 molecules of ethylene oxide (nominal value), with small amounts of macrogol hydroxystearate and of the corresponding free glycols. It results from the reaction of hydrogenated castor oil with ethylene oxide.

CHARACTERS

Appearance: if less than 10 units of ethylene oxide per molecule: yellowish, turbid, viscous liquid; if more than 20 units of ethylene oxide per molecule: white or yellowish semi-liquid or pasty mass.

Solubility: if less than 10 units of ethylene oxide per molecule: practically insoluble in water, soluble in acetone, dispersible in alcohol; if more than 20 units of ethylene oxide per molecule: freely soluble in water, in acetone and in alcohol, practically insoluble in light petroleum.

IDENTIFICATION

A. It complies with the test for iodine value (see Tests).

B. It complies with the test for saponification value (see Tests).

C. Thin-layer chromatography (*2.2.27*).

Test solution. To 1 g of the substance to be examined, add 100 ml of a 100 g/l solution of *potassium hydroxide R* and boil under a reflux condenser for 30 min. Allow to cool. Acidify the solution with 20 ml of *hydrochloric acid R*. Shake the mixture with 50 ml of *ether R* and allow to stand until separation of the layers is obtained. Transfer the clear upper layer to a suitable tube, add 5 g of *anhydrous sodium sulphate R*, close the tube and allow to stand for 30 min. Filter and evaporate the filtrate to dryness on a water-bath. Dissolve 50 mg of the residue in 25 ml of *ether R*.

Reference solution. Dissolve 50 mg of *12-hydroxystearic acid R* in *methylene chloride R* and dilute to 25 ml with the same solvent.

Plate: *TLC octadecylsilyl silica gel plate R*.

Mobile phase: *methylene chloride R, glacial acetic acid R, acetone R (10:40:50 V/V/V)*.

Application: 2 µl.

Development: over a path of 8 cm.

Drying: in a current of cold air.

Detection: spray with a 80 g/l solution of *phosphomolybdic acid R* in *2-propanol R* and heat at 120 °C for about 1-2 min.

Results: the principal spot in the chromatogram obtained with the test solution is similar in position and colour to the principal spot in the chromatogram obtained with the reference solution.

D. Place about 2 g in a test-tube and add 0.2 ml of *sulphuric acid R*. Close the tube using a stopper fitted with a glass tube bent twice at right angles. Heat the tube until white fumes appear. Collect the fumes in 1 ml of *mercuric chloride solution R*. A white precipitate is formed and the fumes turn a filter paper impregnated with *alkaline potassium tetraiodomercurate solution R* black.

TESTS

Solution S. Dissolve 5.0 g of macrogolglycerol hydroxystearate with less than 10 units of ethylene oxide per molecule in a mixture of 50 volumes of *acetone R* and 50 volumes of *ethanol R* and dilute to 50 ml with the same mixture of solvents.

Dissolve 5.0 g of macrogolglycerol hydroxystearate with more than 20 units of ethylene oxide per molecule in *carbon dioxide-free water R* and dilute to 50 ml with the same solvent.

Appearance of solution. Solution S is not more opalescent than reference suspension III (*2.2.1*) and not more intensely coloured than reference solution BY_6 (*2.2.2, Method II*).

Alkalinity. To 2 ml of solution S add 0.5 ml of *bromothymol blue solution R1*. The solution is not blue.

Acid value (*2.5.1*): maximum 2.0, determined on 5.0 g.

Hydroxyl value (*2.5.3, Method A*). See Table 1083.-1.

Iodine value (*2.5.4*): maximum 5.0.

Saponification value (*2.5.6*). See Table 1083.-1.

Table 1083.-1

Ethylene oxide units per molecule (nominal value)	Hydroxyl value	Saponification value
7	115 - 135	125 - 140
25	70 - 90	70 - 90
40	60 - 80	45 - 69
60	45 - 67	40 - 51

Residual ethylene oxide and dioxan (*2.4.25*): maximum 1 ppm of residual ethylene oxide and 10 ppm of residual dioxan.

Heavy metals (*2.4.8*).

Substances soluble in acetone/ethanol: maximum 10 ppm.

12 ml of solution S complies with limit test B. Prepare the standard using lead standard solution (1 ppm Pb) obtained by diluting *lead standard solution (100 ppm Pb) R* with a mixture of equal volumes of *acetone R* and *ethanol R*.

Substances soluble in water: maximum 10 ppm.

12 ml of solution S complies with limit test A. Prepare the standard using *lead standard solution (1 ppm Pb) R*.

Water (*2.5.12*): maximum 3.0 per cent, determined on 2.000 g.

Total ash (*2.4.16*): maximum 0.3 per cent, determined on 2.0 g.

LABELLING

The label states the number of ethylene oxide units per molecule (nominal value).

01/2005:1082

MACROGOLGLYCEROL RICINOLEATE

Macrogolglyceroli ricinoleas

DEFINITION

Contains mainly ricinoleyl glycerol ethoxylated with 30 to 50 molecules of ethylene oxide (nominal value), with small amounts of macrogol ricinoleate and of the corresponding free glycols. It results from the reaction of castor oil with ethylene oxide.

CHARACTERS

Appearance: clear, yellow viscous liquid or semi-solid.

Solubility: freely soluble in water, very soluble in methylene chloride, freely soluble in alcohol.

Relative density: about 1.05.

Viscosity: 500 mPa·s to 800 mPa·s at 25 °C.

IDENTIFICATION

A. It complies with the test for iodine value (see Tests).

B. It complies with the test for saponification value (see Tests).

C. Thin-layer chromatography (*2.2.27*).

Test solution. To 1 g of the substance to be examined add 100 ml of a 100 g/l solution of *potassium hydroxide R* and boil under a reflux condenser for 30 min. Allow to cool. Acidify the solution with 20 ml of *hydrochloric acid R.* Shake the mixture with 50 ml of *ether R* and allow to stand until separation of the layers is obtained. Transfer the clear upper layer to a suitable tube, add 5 g of *anhydrous sodium sulphate R,* close the tube and allow to stand for 30 min. Filter and evaporate the filtrate to dryness on a water-bath. Dissolve 50 mg of the residue in 25 ml of *ether R.*

Reference solution. Dissolve 50 mg of *ricinoleic acid R* in *methylene chloride R* and dilute to 25 ml with the same solvent.

Plate: *TLC octadecylsilyl silica gel plate R.*

Mobile phase: *methylene chloride R, glacial acetic acid R, acetone R* (10:40:50 *V/V/V*).

Application: 2 µl.

Development: over a path of 8 cm.

Drying: in a current of cold air.

Detection: spray with an 80 g/l solution of *phosphomolybdic acid R* in *2-propanol R* and heat at 120 °C for 1-2 min.

Results: the principal spot in the chromatogram obtained with the test solution is similar in position and colour to the principal spot in the chromatogram obtained with the reference solution.

D. Place about 2 g of the substance to be examined in a test-tube and add 0.2 ml of *sulphuric acid R.* Close the tube using a stopper fitted with a glass tube bent twice at right angles. Heat the tube until white fumes appear. Collect the fumes in 1 ml of *mercuric chloride solution R.* A white precipitate is formed and the fumes turn a filter paper impregnated with *alkaline potassium tetraiodomercurate solution R* black.

TESTS

Solution S. Dissolve 5.0 g in *carbon dioxide-free water R* and dilute to 50 ml with the same solvent.

Appearance of solution. Solution S is not more opalescent than reference suspension III (*2.2.1*) and not more intensely coloured than reference solution BY_6 (*2.2.2, Method II*).

Alkalinity. Dissolve 2.0 g in a hot mixture of 10 ml of *water R* and 10 ml of *alcohol R.* Add 0.1 ml of *bromothymol blue solution R1.* Not more than 0.5 ml of *0.1 M hydrochloric acid* is required to change the colour of the indicator to yellow.

Acid value (*2.5.1*): maximum 2.0, determined on 5.0 g.

Hydroxyl value (*2.5.3, Method A*). See Table 1082.-1.

Iodine value (*2.5.4*): 25 to 35.

Saponification value (*2.5.6*). See Table 1082.-1.

Table 1082.-1

Ethylene oxide units per molecule (nominal value)	Hydroxyl value	Saponification value
30 - 35	65 - 82	60 - 75
50	48 - 68	38 - 52

Residual ethylene oxide and dioxan (*2.4.25*): maximum 1 ppm of residual ethylene oxide and 10 ppm of residual dioxan.

Heavy metals (*2.4.8*): maximum 10 ppm.

12 ml of solution S, filtered if necessary, complies with limit test A. Prepare the standard using *lead standard solution (1 ppm Pb) R.*

Water (*2.5.12*): maximum 3.0 per cent, determined on 2.000 g.

Total ash (*2.4.16*): maximum 0.3 per cent, determined on 2.0 g.

STORAGE

Store protected from light.

LABELLING

The label states the amount of ethylene oxide reacted with castor oil (nominal value).

01/2005:1444

MACROGOLS

Macrogola

DEFINITION

Mixtures of polymers with the general formula $H\text{-}(OCH_2\text{-}CH_2)_n\text{-}OH$ where n represents the average number of oxyethylene groups. The type of macrogol is defined by a number that indicates the average relative molecular mass. A suitable stabiliser may be added.

CHARACTERS

Type of macrogol	Appearance	Solubility
300 400 600	clear, viscous, colourless or almost colourless hygroscopic liquid	miscible with water, very soluble in acetone, in alcohol, and in methylene chloride, practically insoluble in fatty oils and in mineral oils
1000	white or almost white, hygroscopic solid with a waxy or paraffin-like appearance	very soluble in water, freely soluble in alcohol and in methylene chloride, practically insoluble in fatty oils and in mineral oils
1500	white or almost white solid with a waxy or paraffin-like appearance	very soluble in water and in methylene chloride, freely soluble in alcohol, practically insoluble in fatty oils and in mineral oils
3000 3350	white or almost white solid with a waxy or paraffin-like appearance	very soluble in water and in methylene chloride, very slightly soluble in alcohol, practically insoluble in fatty oils and in mineral oils
4000 6000 8000	white or almost white solid with a waxy or paraffin-like appearance	very soluble in water and in methylene chloride, practically insoluble in alcohol and in fatty oils and in mineral oils
20 000 35 000	white or almost white solid with a waxy or paraffin-like appearance	very soluble in water, soluble in methylene chloride, practically insoluble in alcohol and in fatty oils and in mineral oils

IDENTIFICATION

A. It complies with the test for viscosity (see Tests).

B. To 1 g in a test-tube add 0.5 ml of *sulphuric acid R*, close the test-tube with a stopper fitted with a bent delivery tube and heat until white fumes are evolved. Collect the fumes via the delivery tube into 1 ml of *mercuric chloride solution R*. An abundant white, crystalline precipitate is formed.

C. To 0.1 g add 0.1 g of *potassium thiocyanate R* and 0.1 g of *cobalt nitrate R* and mix thoroughly with a glass rod. Add 5 ml of *methylene chloride R* and shake. The liquid phase becomes blue.

TESTS

Appearance of solution. The solution is clear (*2.2.1*) and not more intensely coloured than reference solution BY_6 (*2.2.2, Method II*).

Dissolve 12.5 g in *water R* and dilute to 50 ml with the same solvent.

Acidity or alkalinity. Dissolve 5.0 g in 50 ml of *carbon dioxide-free water R* and add 0.15 ml of *bromothymol blue solution R1*. The solution is yellow or green. Not more than 0.1 ml of *0.1 M sodium hydroxide* is required to change the colour of the indicator to blue.

Viscosity (*2.2.9*). The viscosity is calculated using a density given in Table 1444.-1.

Table 1444.-1

Type of macrogol	Kinematic viscosity ($mm^2 \cdot s^{-1}$)	Dynamic viscosity (mPa·s)	Density* (g/ml)
300	71 - 94	80 - 105	1.120
400	94 - 116	105 - 130	1.120
600	13.9 - 18.5	15 - 20	1.080
1000	20.4 - 27.7	22 - 30	1.080
1500	31 - 46	34 - 50	1.080
3000	69 - 93	75 - 100	1.080
3350	76 - 110	83 - 120	1.080
4000	102 - 158	110 - 170	1.080
6000	185 - 250	200 - 270	1.080
8000	240 - 472	260 - 510	1.080
20 000	2500 - 3200	2700 - 3500	1.080
35 000	10 000 - 13 000	11 000 - 14 000	1.080

*Density of the substance for macrogols 300 and 400. Density of the 50 per cent *m/m* solution for the other macrogols.

For macrogols having a relative molecular mass greater than 400, determine the viscosity on a 50 per cent *m/m* solution of the substance to be examined.

Freezing point (*2.2.18*). See Table 1444.-2.

Table 1444.-2

Type of macrogol	Freezing point (°C)
600	15 - 25
1000	35 - 40
1500	42 - 48
3000	50 - 56
3350	53 - 57
4000	53 - 59
6000	55 - 61
8000	55 - 62
20 000	minimum 57
35 000	minimum 57

Hydroxyl value. Introduce *m* g (see Table 1444.-3) into a dry conical flask fitted with a reflux condenser. Add 25.0 ml of *phthalic anhydride solution R*, swirl to dissolve and boil under a reflux condenser on a hot plate for 60 min. Allow to cool. Rinse the condenser first with 25 ml of *pyridine R* and then with 25 ml of *water R*, add 1.5 ml of *phenolphthalein solution R* and titrate with *1 M sodium hydroxide* until a faint pink colour is obtained (n_1 ml). Carry out a blank test (n_2 ml). Calculate the hydroxyl value using the expression:

$$\frac{56.1 \times (n_2 - n_1)}{m}$$

Table 1444.-3

Type of macrogol	Hydroxyl value	m (g)
300	340 - 394	1.5
400	264 - 300	1.9
600	178 - 197	3.5
1000	107 - 118	5.0
1500	70 - 80	7.0
3000	34 - 42	12.0
3350	30 - 38	12.0
4000	25 - 32	14.0
6000	16 - 22	18.0
8000	12 - 16	24.0
20 000	-	-
35 000	-	-

For macrogols having a relative molecular mass greater than 1000, if the water content is more than 0.5 per cent, dry a sample of suitable mass at 100-105 °C for 2 h and carry out the determination of the hydroxyl value on the dried sample.

Reducing substances. Dissolve 1 g in 1 ml of a 10 g/l solution of *resorcinol R* and warm gently if necessary. Add 2 ml of *hydrochloric acid R*. After 5 min the solution is not more intensely coloured than reference solution R_3 (*2.2.2, Method I*).

Formaldehyde: maximum 30 ppm.

Test solution. To 1.00 g add 0.25 ml of *chromotropic acid, sodium salt solution R*, cool in iced water and add 5.0 ml of *sulphuric acid R*. Allow to stand for 15 min and complete slowly to 10 ml with *water R*.

Reference solution. Dilute 0.860 g of *formaldehyde solution R* to 100 ml with *water R*. Dilute 1.0 ml of this solution to 100 ml with *water R*. In a 10 ml flask, mix 1.00 ml of this solution with 0.25 ml of *chromotropic acid, sodium salt solution R*, cool in iced water and add 5.0 ml of *sulphuric acid R*. Allow to stand for 15 min and complete slowly to 10 ml with *water R*.

Blank solution. In a 10 ml flask mix 1.00 ml of *water R* with 0.25 ml of *chromotropic acid, sodium salt solution R*, cool in iced water and add 5.0 ml of *sulphuric acid R*. Complete slowly to 10 ml with *water R*.

Determine the absorbance (*2.2.25*) of the test solution at 567 nm, against the blank solution. It is not higher than that of the reference solution.

If the use of macrogols with a higher content of formaldehyde may have adverse effects, the competent authority may impose a limit of not more than 15 ppm.

Ethylene glycol and diethylene glycol: *carry out this test only if the macrogol has a relative molecular mass below 1000.*

Gas chromatography (*2.2.28*).

Test solution. Dissolve 5.00 g of the substance to be examined in *acetone R* and dilute to 100.0 ml with the same solvent.

Reference solution. Dissolve 0.10 g of *ethylene glycol R* and 0.50 g of *diethylene glycol R* in *acetone R* and dilute to 100.0 ml with the same solvent. Dilute 1.0 ml of this solution to 10.0 ml with *acetone R*.

Column:
- *material*: glass,
- *size*: l = 1.8 m, Ø = 2 mm,
- *stationary phase*: *silanised diatomaceous earth for gas chromatography R*, impregnated with 5 per cent *m/m* of *macrogol 20 000 R*,

Carrier gas: *nitrogen for chromatography R*.

Flow rate: 30 ml/min.

Temperature:
- *column*: if necessary, precondition the column by heating at 200 °C for about 15 h; adjust the initial temperature of the column to obtain a retention time of 14-16 min for diethylene glycol; raise the temperature of the column by about 30 °C at a rate of 2 °C/min but without exceeding 170 °C;
- *injection port and detector*: 250 °C.

Detection: flame ionisation.

Injection: 2 µl.

Carry out 5 replicate injections to check the repeatability of the response.

Limit: maximum 0.4 per cent, calculated as the sum of the contents of ethylene glycol and diethylene glycol.

Ethylene oxide and dioxan (*2.4.25*): maximum 1 ppm of ethylene oxide and 10 ppm of dioxan.

Heavy metals (*2.4.8*): maximum 20 ppm.

Dissolve 2.0 g in *water R* and dilute to 20 ml with the same solvent. 12 ml of the solution complies with limit test A. Prepare the standard using *lead standard solution (2 ppm Pb) R*.

Water (*2.5.12*): maximum 2.0 per cent for macrogol with a relative molecular mass not greater than 1000 and maximum 1.0 per cent for macrogol with a relative molecular mass greater than 1000, determined on 2.00 g.

Sulphated ash (*2.4.14*): maximum 0.2 per cent, determined on 1.0 g.

STORAGE

In an airtight container.

LABELLING

The label states:
- the type of macrogol,
- the name and the concentration of any added stabiliser,
- the content of formaldehyde.

01/2005:1539
corrected

MAGALDRATE

Magaldratum

$Al_5Mg_{10}(OH)_{31}(SO_4)_2,xH_2O$ M_r 1097 (anhydrous substance)

DEFINITION

Magaldrate is composed of aluminium and magnesium hydroxides and sulphates. Its composition corresponds approximately to the formula $Al_5Mg_{10}(OH)_{31}(SO_4)_2,xH_2O$. It contains not less than 90.0 per cent and not more than the equivalent of 105.0 per cent of $Al_5Mg_{10}(OH)_{31}(SO_4)_2$, calculated with reference to the dried substance.

CHARACTERS

A white or almost white, crystalline powder, practically insoluble in water and in alcohol, soluble in dilute mineral acids.

Monographs M

IDENTIFICATION

A. Dissolve 0.6 g in 20 ml of *3 M hydrochloric acid*, add about 30 ml of *water R* and heat to boiling. Adjust to pH 6.2 with *dilute ammonia R1*, continue boiling for a further 2 min, filter and retain the precipitate and the filtrate. To 2 ml of the filtrate add 2 ml of *ammonium chloride solution R* and neutralise with a solution prepared by dissolving 2 g of *ammonium carbonate R* and 2 ml of *dilute ammonia R1* in 20 ml of *water R*; no precipitate is produced. Add *disodium hydrogen phosphate solution R*; a white, crystalline precipitate is produced which does not dissolve in *dilute ammonia R1*.

B. The precipitate retained in identification test A gives the reaction of aluminium (*2.3.1*).

C. The filtrate retained in identification test A gives reaction (a) of sulphates (*2.3.1*).

TESTS

Soluble chlorides. Disperse 1 g in 50 ml of *water R*, boil for 5 min, cool, dilute again to 50.0 ml, mix and filter. To 25.0 ml of the filtrate add 0.2 ml of *potassium chromate solution R* and titrate with *0.1 M silver nitrate* until a persistent violet-red colour is obtained. Not more than 5.0 ml of *0.1 M silver nitrate* is required (3.5 per cent).

Soluble sulphates. To 2.5 ml of the filtrate obtained in the test for soluble chlorides, add 30 ml of *water R*, neutralise to *blue litmus paper R* with *hydrochloric acid R*, add 3 ml of *1 M hydrochloric acid*, 3 ml of a 120 g/l solution of *barium chloride R* and dilute to 50 ml with *water R*. Mix and allow to stand for 10 min. Any opalescence in the test solution is not more intense than that of a standard prepared at the same time in the same manner using 1 ml of *0.01 M sulphuric acid* instead of 2.5 ml of filtrate (1.9 per cent).

Sulphates. 16.0 per cent to 21.0 per cent, calculated with reference to the dried substance. Dissolve 0.875 g in a mixture of 5 ml of *glacial acetic acid R* and 10 ml of *water R* and dilute to 25 ml with *water R*. Prepare a chromatographic column of 1 cm in internal diameter containing 15 ml of *cation exchange resin R* (150 µm to 300 µm), previously washed with 30 ml of *water R*. Transfer 5.0 ml of the solution to be examined to the column and elute with 15 ml of *water R*. To the eluate add 5 ml of a 53.6 g/l solution of *magnesium acetate R*, 32 ml of *methanol R* and 0.2 ml of *alizarin S solution R*. Add from a burette about 4.0 ml of *0.05 M barium chloride*, add a further 0.2 ml of *alizarin S solution R* and slowly complete the titration until the yellow colour disappears and a violet-red tinge is visible.

1 ml of *0.05 M barium chloride* is equivalent to 4.803 mg of SO_4.

Aluminium hydroxide: 32.1 per cent to 45.9 per cent, calculated with reference to the dried substance. Dissolve 0.800 g in 10 ml of *dilute hydrochloric acid R1*, heating on a water-bath. Cool and dilute to 50.0 ml with *water R*. To 10.0 ml of the solution, add *dilute ammonia R1* until a precipitate begins to appear. Add the smallest quantity of *dilute hydrochloric acid R* needed to dissolve the precipitate and dilute to 20 ml with *water R*. Carry out the complexometric titration of aluminium (*2.5.11*).

1 ml of *0.1 M sodium edetate* is equivalent to 7.80 mg of $Al(OH)_3$.

Magnesium hydroxide: 49.2 per cent to 66.6 per cent, calculated with reference to the dried substance. Dissolve 0.100 g in 2 ml of *dilute hydrochloric acid R* and carry out the complexometric titration of magnesium (*2.5.11*).

1 ml of *0.1 M sodium edetate* is equivalent to 5.832 mg of $Mg(OH)_2$.

Sodium. Not more than 0.10 per cent of Na, determined by atomic absorption spectrometry (*2.2.23, Method I*).

Test solution. Weigh 2.00 g of the substance to be examined into a 100 ml volumetric flask, place in an ice-bath, add 5 ml of *nitric acid R* and swirl to mix. Allow to warm to room temperature and dilute to 100 ml with *water R*. Filter, if necessary, to obtain a clear solution. Dilute 10.0 ml of the filtrate to 100.0 ml with *water R*.

Reference solutions. Prepare the reference solutions using *sodium standard solution (200 ppm Na) R*, diluted as necessary with *dilute nitric acid R*.

Measure the absorbance at 589 nm using a sodium hollow-cathode lamp as a source of radiation and an air-acetylene flame.

Heavy metals (*2.4.8*). Dissolve 2.0 g in 30 ml of *hydrochloric acid R1* and shake with 50 ml of *methyl isobutyl ketone R* for 2 min. Allow to stand, separate the aqueous layer and evaporate to dryness. Dissolve the residue in 30 ml of *water R*. 12 ml of the solution complies with limit test A for heavy metals (30 ppm). Prepare the standard using *lead standard solution (2 ppm Pb) R*.

Loss on drying (*2.2.32*): 10.0 per cent to 20.0 per cent, determined on 1.000 g by drying in an oven at 200 °C for 4 h.

ASSAY

To 1.500 g add 50.0 ml of *1 M hydrochloric acid*. Titrate the excess hydrochloric acid with *1 M sodium hydroxide* to pH 3.0, determining the end-point potentiometrically (*2.2.20*). Carry out a blank titration.

1 ml of *1 M hydrochloric acid* is equivalent to 35.40 mg of $Al_5Mg_{10}(OH)_{31}(SO_4)_2$.

01/2005:2035

MAGNESIUM ACETATE TETRAHYDRATE

Magnesii acetas tetrahydricus

$Mg(CH_3COO)_2,4H_2O$ M_r 214.5

DEFINITION

Content: 98.0 per cent to 101.0 per cent of magnesium acetate (anhydrous substance).

CHARACTERS

Appearance: colourless crystals or white, crystalline powder.

Solubility: freely soluble in water and in alcohol.

IDENTIFICATION

A. Dissolve about 100 mg in 2 ml of *water R*. Add 1 ml of *dilute ammonia R1* and heat. A white precipitate is formed that dissolves slowly on addition of 5 ml of *ammonium chloride solution R*. Add 1 ml of *disodium hydrogen phosphate solution R*. A white crystalline precipitate is formed.

B. It gives reaction (b) of acetates (*2.3.1*).

TESTS

pH (*2.2.3*): 7.5 to 8.5.

Dissolve 2.5 g in *carbon dioxide-free water R* and dilute to 50 ml with the same solvent.

Chlorides (*2.4.4*): maximum 330 ppm.

Dissolve 1.0 g in *water R* and dilute to 100 ml with the same solvent. 15 ml of the solution complies with the limit test for chlorides.

Nitrates: maximum 3 ppm.

Dissolve 1.0 g in *distilled water R* and dilute to 10 ml with the same solvent, add 5 mg of *sodium chloride R*, 0.05 ml of *indigo carmine solution R* and while stirring, 10 ml of *nitrogen-free sulphuric acid R*. A blue colour is produced which persists for at least 10 min.

Sulphates (*2.4.13*): maximum 600 ppm.

Dissolve 0.25 g in *distilled water R* and dilute to 15 ml with the same solvent.

Aluminium (*2.4.17*): maximum 1 ppm.

Prescribed solution. Dissolve 4.0 g in *water R* and dilute to 100 ml with the same solvent. Add 10 ml of *acetate buffer solution pH 6.0 R*.

Reference solution. Mix 2 ml of *aluminium standard solution (2 ppm Al) R*, 10 ml of *acetate buffer solution pH 6.0 R* and 98 ml of *water R*.

Blank solution. Mix 10 ml of *acetate buffer solution pH 6.0 R* and 100 ml of *water R*.

Calcium (*2.4.3*): maximum 100 ppm.

Dissolve 1.0 g in *distilled water R* and dilute to 15 ml with the same solvent.

Potassium: maximum 0.1 per cent.

Atomic emission spectrometry (*2.2.22, Method II*).

Test solution. Dissolve 0.5 g in *water R* and dilute to 100 ml with the same solvent.

Reference solutions. Prepare the reference solutions using *potassium standard solution (600 ppm K) R*, diluted as necessary with *water R*.

Wavelength: 766.5 nm.

Sodium: maximum 0.5 per cent.

Atomic emission spectrometry (*2.2.22, Method II*).

Test solution. Dissolve 1.0 g in *water R* and dilute to 100 ml with the same solvent.

Reference solutions. Prepare the reference solutions using *sodium standard solution (200 ppm Na) R*, diluted as necessary with *water R*.

Wavelength: 589.0 nm.

Heavy metals (*2.4.8*): maximum 40 ppm.

Dissolve 1.0 g in *water R* and dilute to 20 ml with the same solvent. 12 ml of the solution complies with limit test A. Prepare the standard using *lead standard solution (2 ppm Pb) R*.

Readily oxidisable substances. Dissolve 2.0 g in 100 ml of boiling *water R*, add 6 ml of a 150 g/l solution of *sulphuric acid R* and 0.3 ml of *0.02 M potassium permanganate*. Mix and boil gently for 5 min. The pink colour is not completely discharged.

Water (*2.5.12*): 33.0 per cent to 35.0 per cent, determined on 0.100 g.

ASSAY

Dissolve 0.150 g in 300 ml of *water R*. Carry out the complexometric titration of magnesium (*2.5.11*).

1 ml of *0.1 M sodium edetate* is equivalent to 14.24 mg of $C_4H_6MgO_4$.

01/2005:1445

MAGNESIUM ASPARTATE DIHYDRATE

Magnesii aspartas dihydricus

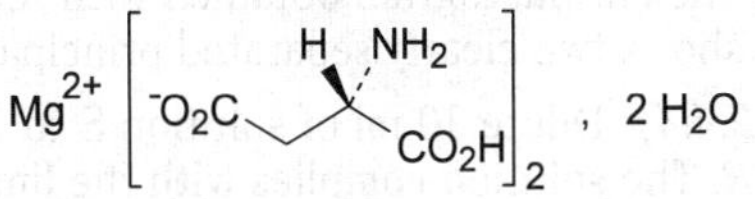

$C_8H_{12}MgN_2O_8,2H_2O$ M_r 324.5

DEFINITION

Magnesium aspartate dihydrate contains not less than 98.0 per cent and not more than the equivalent of 102.0 per cent of magnesium di[(*S*)-2-aminohydrogenobutane-1,4-dioate], calculated with reference to the anhydrous substance.

CHARACTERS

A white, crystalline powder or colourless crystals, freely soluble in water.

IDENTIFICATION

A. It complies with the test for specific optical rotation (see Tests).

B. Examine the chromatograms obtained in the test for ninhydrin-positive substances. The principal spot in the chromatogram obtained with test solution (b) is similar in position, colour and size to the principal spot in the chromatogram obtained with reference solution (a).

C. Ignite about 15 mg until a white residue is obtained. Dissolve the residue in 1 ml of *dilute hydrochloric acid R*, neutralise to *red litmus paper R* by the addition of *dilute sodium hydroxide solution R* and filter if necessary. The solution gives the reaction of magnesium (*2.3.1*).

TESTS

Solution S. Dissolve 2.5 g in *carbon dioxide-free water R* prepared from *distilled water R* and dilute to 100 ml with the same solvent.

Appearance of solution. Solution S is clear (*2.2.1*) and colourless (*2.2.2, Method II*).

pH (*2.2.3*). The pH of solution S is 6.0 to 8.0.

Specific optical rotation (*2.2.7*). Dissolve 0.50 g in a 515 g/l solution of *hydrochloric acid R* and dilute to 25.0 ml with the same acid. The specific optical rotation is + 20.5 to + 23.0, calculated with reference to the anhydrous substance.

Ninhydrin-positive substances. Examine by thin-layer chromatography (*2.2.27*), using a *TLC silica gel plate R*.

Test solution (a). Dissolve 0.10 g of the substance to be examined in *water R* and dilute to 10 ml withthe same solvent.

Test solution (b). Dilute 1 ml of test solution (a) to 50 ml with *water R*.

Reference solution (a). Dissolve 10 mg of *magnesium aspartate dihydrate CRS* in *water R* and dilute to 50 ml with the same solvent.

Reference solution (b). Dilute 5 ml of test solution (b) to 20 ml with *water R*.

Reference solution (c). Dissolve 10 mg of *magnesium aspartate dihydrate CRS* and 10 mg of *glutamic acid CRS* in 2 ml of *water R* and dilute to 25 ml with the same solvent.

Apply to the plate 5 µl of each solution. Allow the plate to dry in air. Develop over a path of 15 cm using a mixture of 20 volumes of *glacial acetic acid R*, 20 volumes of *water R* and 60 volumes of *butanol R*. Allow the plate to dry in air and spray with *ninhydrin solution R*. Heat at 100 °C to 105 °C for 15 min. Any spot in the chromatogram obtained with test solution (a), apart from the principal spot, is not more intense than the spot in the chromatogram obtained with reference solution (b) (0.5 per cent). The test is not valid unless the chromatogram obtained with reference solution (c) shows two clearly separated principal spots.

Chlorides (*2.4.4*). Dilute 10 ml of solution S to 15 ml with *water R*. The solution complies with the limit test for chlorides (200 ppm).

Sulphates (*2.4.13*). Dilute 12 ml of solution S to 15 ml with *distilled water R*. The solution complies with the limit test for sulphates (500 ppm). Carry out the evaluation of the test after 30 min.

Ammonium (*2.4.1*). 50 mg complies with limit test B for ammonium (200 ppm). Prepare the standard using 0.1 ml of *ammonium standard solution (100 ppm NH_4) R*.

Iron (*2.4.9*). In a separating funnel, dissolve 0.20 g in 10 ml of *dilute hydrochloric acid R*. Shake with three quantities, each of 10 ml, of *methyl isobutyl ketone R1*, shaking for 3 min each time. To the combined organic layers add 10 ml of *water R* and shake for 3 min. The aqueous layer complies with the limit test for iron (50 ppm).

Heavy metals (*2.4.8*). Dissolve 2.0 g with gentle heating in 20 ml of *water R*. 12 ml of the solution complies with limit test A for heavy metals (10 ppm). Prepare the standard using *lead standard solution (1 ppm Pb) R*.

Water (*2.5.12*). 10.0 per cent to 14.0 per cent, determined on 0.100 g by the semi-micro determination of water. Dissolve the substance in 10 ml of *formamide R1* at 50 °C protected from moisture, add 10 ml of *anhydrous methanol R* and allow to cool. Carry out a blank determination.

ASSAY

Dissolve 0.260 g in 10 ml of *water R* and carry out the complexometric titration of magnesium (*2.5.11*).

1 ml of *0.1 M sodium edetate* is equivalent to 28.85 mg of $C_8H_{12}MgN_2O_8$.

IMPURITIES

A. aspartic acid.

01/2005:0043

MAGNESIUM CARBONATE, HEAVY

Magnesii subcarbonas ponderosus

DEFINITION

Hydrated basic magnesium carbonate.

Content: 40.0 per cent to 45.0 per cent, calculated as MgO (M_r 40.30).

CHARACTERS

Appearance: white powder.

Solubility: practically insoluble in water. It dissolves in dilute acids with strong effervescence.

IDENTIFICATION

A. 15 g has an apparent volume (*2.9.15*) before setting about 30 ml.

B. It gives the reaction of carbonates (*2.3.1*).

C. Dissolve about 15 mg in 2 ml of *dilute nitric acid R* and neutralise with *dilute sodium hydroxide solution R*. The solution gives the reaction of magnesium (*2.3.1*).

TESTS

Solution S. Dissolve 5.0 g in 100 ml of *dilute acetic acid R*. When the effervescence has ceased, boil for 2 min, cool and dilute to 100 ml with the same acid. Filter, if necessary, through a previously ignited and tared porcelain or silica filter crucible of suitable porosity to give a clear filtrate.

Appearance of solution. Solution S is not more intensely coloured than reference solution B_4 (*2.2.2, Method II*).

Soluble substances: maximum 1.0 per cent.

Mix 2.00 g with 100 ml of *water R* and boil for 5 min. Filter whilst hot through a sintered-glass filter (40), allow to cool and dilute to 100 ml with *water R*. Evaporate 50 ml of the filtrate to dryness and dry at 100-105 °C. The residue weighs not more than 10 mg.

Substances insoluble in acetic acid: maximum 0.05 per cent.

Any residue obtained during the preparation of solution S, washed, dried, and ignited at 600 °C, weighs not more than 2.5 mg.

Chlorides (*2.4.4*): maximum 0.07 per cent.

1.5 ml of solution S diluted to 15 ml with *water R* complies with the limit test for chlorides.

Sulphates (*2.4.13*): maximum 0.6 per cent.

0.5 ml of solution S diluted to 15 ml with *distilled water R* complies with the limit test for sulphates.

Arsenic (*2.4.2*): maximum 2 ppm.

10 ml of solution S complies with limit test A.

Calcium (*2.4.3*): maximum 0.75 per cent.

Dilute 2.6 ml of solution S to 150 ml with *distilled water R*. 15 ml of the solution complies with the limit test for calcium.

Iron (*2.4.9*): maximum 400 ppm.

Dissolve 0.1 g in 3 ml of *dilute hydrochloric acid R* and dilute to 10 ml with *water R*. 2.5 ml of the solution diluted to 10 ml with *water R* complies with the limit test for iron.

Heavy metals (*2.4.8*): maximum 20 ppm.

To 20 ml of solution S add 15 ml of *hydrochloric acid R1* and shake with 25 ml of *methyl isobutyl ketone R* for 2 min. Allow to stand, separate the aqueous layer and evaporate to dryness. Dissolve the residue in 1 ml of *acetic acid R* and dilute to 20 ml with *water R*. 12 ml of the solution complies with limit test A. Prepare the standard using *lead standard solution (1 ppm Pb) R*.

ASSAY

Dissolve 0.150 g in a mixture of 20 ml of *water R* and 2 ml of *dilute hydrochloric acid R*. Carry out the complexometric titration of magnesium (*2.5.11*).

1 ml of *0.1 M sodium edetate* is equivalent to 4.030 mg of MgO.

01/2005:0042

MAGNESIUM CARBONATE, LIGHT

Magnesii subcarbonas levis

DEFINITION

Hydrated basic magnesium carbonate.

Content: 40.0 per cent to 45.0 per cent, calculated as MgO (M_r 40.30).

CHARACTERS

Appearance: white powder.

Solubility: practically insoluble in water. It dissolves in dilute acids with strong effervescence.

IDENTIFICATION

A. 15 g has an apparent volume (*2.9.15*) before settling of about 180 ml.

B. It gives the reaction of carbonates (*2.3.1*).

C. Dissolve about 15 mg in 2 ml of *dilute nitric acid R* and neutralise with *dilute sodium hydroxide solution R*. The solution gives the reaction of magnesium (*2.3.1*).

TESTS

Solution S. Dissolve 5.0 g in 100 ml of *dilute acetic acid R*. When the effervescence has ceased, boil for 2 min, cool and dilute to 100 ml with the same acid. Filter, if necessary, through a previously ignited and tared porcelain or silica filter crucible of suitable porosity to give a clear filtrate.

Appearance of solution. Solution S is not more intensely coloured than reference solution B_4 (*2.2.2, Method II*).

Soluble substances: maximum 1.0 per cent.

Mix 2.00 g with 100 ml of *water R* and boil for 5 min. Filter whilst hot through a sintered-glass filter (40), allow to cool and dilute to 100 ml with *water R*. Evaporate 50 ml of the filtrate to dryness and dry at 100-105 °C. The residue weighs not more than 10 mg.

Substances insoluble in acetic acid: maximum 0.05 per cent.

Any residue obtained during the preparation of solution S, washed, dried and ignited at 600 °C, weighs not more than 2.5 mg.

Chlorides (*2.4.4*): maximum 0.07 per cent.

1.5 ml of solution S diluted to 15 ml with *water R* complies with the limit test for chlorides.

Sulphates (*2.4.13*): maximum 0.3 per cent.

1 ml of solution S diluted to 15 ml with *distilled water R* complies with the limit test for sulphates.

Arsenic (*2.4.2*): maximum 2 ppm.

10 ml of solution S complies with limit test A.

Calcium (*2.4.3*): maximum 0.75 per cent.

Dilute 2.6 ml of solution S to 150 ml with *distilled water R*. 15 ml of the solution complies with the limit test for calcium.

Iron (*2.4.9*): maximum 400 ppm.

Dissolve 0.1 g in 3 ml of *dilute hydrochloric acid R* and dilute to 10 ml with *water R*. 2.5 ml of the solution diluted to 10 ml with *water R* complies with the limit test for iron.

Heavy metals (*2.4.8*): maximum 20 ppm.

To 20 ml of solution S add 15 ml of *hydrochloric acid R1* and shake with 25 ml of *methyl isobutyl ketone R* for 2 min. Allow to stand, separate the aqueous layer and evaporate to dryness. Dissolve the residue in 1 ml of *acetic acid R* and dilute to 20 ml with *water R*. 12 ml of the solution complies with limit test A. Prepare the standard using *lead standard solution (1 ppm Pb) R*.

ASSAY

Dissolve 0.150 g in a mixture of 20 ml of *water R* and 2 ml of *dilute hydrochloric acid R*. Carry out the complexometric titration of magnesium (*2.5.11*).

1 ml of *0.1 M sodium edetate* is equivalent to 4.030 mg of MgO.

01/2005:1341

MAGNESIUM CHLORIDE 4.5-HYDRATE

Magnesii chloridum 4.5-hydricum

$MgCl_2,xH_2O$ with x≃4. 5 M_r 95.21 (anhydrous substance)

DEFINITION

Magnesium chloride 4.5 - hydrate contains not less than 98.5 per cent and not more than the equivalent of 101.0 per cent of $MgCl_2$, calculated with reference to the anhydrous substance.

CHARACTERS

A white or almost white granular powder, hygroscopic, very soluble in water, freely soluble in alcohol.

IDENTIFICATION

A. It complies with the test for water (see Tests).

B. It gives reaction (a) of chlorides (*2.3.1*).

C. It gives the reaction of magnesium (*2.3.1*).

TESTS

Solution S. Dissolve 10.0 g in *carbon dioxide-free water R* prepared from *distilled water R* and dilute to 100.0 ml with the same solvent.

Appearance of solution. Solution S is clear (*2.2.1*) and colourless (*2.2.2, Method II*).

Acidity or alkalinity. To 5 ml of solution S add 0.05 ml of *phenol red solution R*. Not more than 0.3 ml of *0.01 M hydrochloric acid* or *0.01 M sodium hydroxide* is required to change the colour of the indicator.

Bromides. Dilute 2.0 ml of solution S to 10.0 ml with *water R*. To 1.0 ml of the solution add 4.0 ml of *water R*, 2.0 ml of *phenol red solution R3* and 1.0 ml of *chloramine solution R2* and mix immediately. After exactly 2 min add 0.30 ml of *0.1 M sodium thiosulphate*, mix and dilute to 10.0 ml with *water R*. The absorbance (*2.2.25*) of the solution measured at 590 nm, using *water R* as the compensation liquid, is not greater than that of a standard prepared at the same time and in the same manner using 5.0 ml of a 3 mg/l solution of *potassium bromide R* (500 ppm).

Sulphates (*2.4.13*). 15 ml of solution S complies with the limit test for sulphates (100 ppm).

Aluminium (*2.4.17*). If intended for use in the manufacture of peritoneal dialysis solutions, haemodialysis solutions, or haemofiltration solutions it complies with the test for aluminium. Dissolve 4 g in 100 ml of *water R* and add 10 ml of *acetate buffer solution pH 6.0 R*. The solution complies with the limit test for aluminium (1 ppm). Use as the reference solution a mixture of 2 ml of *aluminium standard solution (2 ppm Al) R*, 10 ml of *acetate buffer solution pH 6.0 R* and 98 ml of *water R*. To prepare the blank use a mixture of 10 ml of *acetate buffer solution pH 6.0 R* and 100 ml of *water R*.

Arsenic (*2.4.2*). 0.5 g complies with limit test A for arsenic (2 ppm).

Calcium (*2.4.3*). Dilute 1 ml of solution S to 15 ml with *distilled water R*. The solution complies with the limit test for calcium (0.1 per cent).

Heavy metals (*2.4.8*). 12 ml of solution S complies with limit test A for heavy metals (10 ppm). Prepare the standard using *lead standard solution (1 ppm Pb) R*.

Iron (*2.4.9*). 10 ml of solution S complies with the limit test for iron (10 ppm).

Potassium. If intended for use in the manufacture of parenteral dosage forms, not more than 500 ppm of K, determined by atomic emission spectrometry (*2.2.22, Method I*).

Test solution. Dissolve 1.00 g of the substance to be examined in *water R* and dilute to 100.0 ml with the same solvent.

Reference solution. Dissolve 1.144 g of *potassium chloride R* in *water R*, previously dried at 100 °C to 105 °C for 3 h, and dilute to 1000.0 ml with the same solvent (600 µg of K per millilitre). Dilute as required.

Measure the emission intensity at 766.5 nm.

Water (*2.5.12*): 44.0 per cent to 48.0 per cent, determined on 50.0 mg by the semi-micro determination of water.

ASSAY

Dissolve 0.250 g in 50 ml of *water R*. Carry out the complexometric titration of magnesium (*2.5.11*).

1 ml of *0.1 M sodium edetate* is equivalent to 9.521 mg of $MgCl_2$.

STORAGE

Store in an airtight container.

LABELLING

The label states:

– where applicable, that the substance is suitable for use in the manufacture of peritoneal dialysis solutions, haemodialysis solutions or haemofiltration solutions,

– where applicable, that the substance is suitable for use in the manufacture of parenteral dosage forms.

01/2005:0402

MAGNESIUM CHLORIDE HEXAHYDRATE

Magnesii chloridum hexahydricum

$MgCl_2,6H_2O$ M_r 203.3

DEFINITION

Magnesium chloride hexahydrate contains not less than 98.0 per cent and not more than the equivalent of 101.0 per cent of $MgCl_2,6H_2O$.

CHARACTERS

Colourless crystals, hygroscopic, very soluble in water, freely soluble in alcohol.

IDENTIFICATION

A. It complies with the test for water (see Tests).

B. It gives reaction (a) of chlorides (*2.3.1*).

C. It gives the reaction of magnesium (*2.3.1*).

TESTS

Solution S. Dissolve 10.0 g in *carbon dioxide-free water R* prepared from *distilled water R* and dilute to 100.0 ml with the same solvent.

Appearance of solution. Solution S is clear (*2.2.1*) and colourless (*2.2.2, Method II*).

Acidity or alkalinity. To 5 ml of solution S add 0.05 ml of *phenol red solution R*. Not more than 0.3 ml of *0.01 M hydrochloric acid* or *0.01 M sodium hydroxide* is required to change the colour of the indicator.

Bromides. Dilute 2.0 ml of solution S to 10.0 ml with *water R*. To 1.0 ml of the solution add 4.0 ml of *water R*, 2.0 ml of *phenol red solution R3* and 1.0 ml of *chloramine solution R2* and mix immediately. After exactly 2 min, add 0.30 ml of *0.1 M sodium thiosulphate*, mix and dilute to 10.0 ml with *water R*. The absorbance (*2.2.25*) of the solution measured at 590 nm, using *water R* as the compensation liquid, is not greater than that of a standard prepared at the same time and in the same manner using 5.0 ml of a 3 mg/l solution of *potassium bromide R* (500 ppm).

Sulphates (*2.4.13*). 15 ml of solution S complies with the limit test for sulphates (100 ppm).

Aluminium (*2.4.17*). If intended for use in the manufacture of peritoneal dialysis solutions, haemodialysis solutions, or haemofiltration solutions, it complies with the test for aluminium. Dissolve 4 g in 100 ml of *water R* and add 10 ml of *acetate buffer solution pH 6.0 R*. The solution complies with the limit test for aluminium (1 ppm). Use as the reference solution a mixture of 2 ml of *aluminium standard solution (2 ppm Al) R*, 10 ml of *acetate buffer solution pH 6.0 R* and 98 ml of *water R*. To prepare the blank use a mixture of 10 ml of *acetate buffer solution pH 6.0 R* and 100 ml of *water R*.

Arsenic (*2.4.2*). 0.5 g complies with limit test A for arsenic (2 ppm).

Calcium (*2.4.3*). Dilute 1 ml of solution S to 15 ml with *distilled water R*. The solution complies with the limit test for calcium (0.1 per cent).

Heavy metals (*2.4.8*). 12 ml of solution S complies with limit test A for heavy metals (10 ppm). Prepare the standard using *lead standard solution (1 ppm Pb) R*.

Iron (*2.4.9*). 10 ml of solution S complies with the limit test for iron (10 ppm).

Potassium. If intended for use in the manufacture of parenteral dosage forms, not more than 500 ppm of K, determined by atomic emission spectrometry (*2.2.22, Method I*).

Test solution. Dissolve 1.00 g of the substance to be examined in *water R* and dilute to 100.0 ml with the same solvent.

Reference solution. Dissolve 1.144 g of *potassium chloride R*, previously dried at 100 °C to 105 °C for 3 h in *water R* and dilute to 1000.0 ml with the same solvent (600 µg of K per millilitre). Dilute as required.

Measure the emission intensity at 766.5 nm.

Water (*2.5.12*). 51.0 per cent to 55.0 per cent, determined on 50.0 mg by the semi-micro determination of water.

ASSAY

Dissolve 0.300 g in 50 ml of *water R*. Carry out the complexometric titration of magnesium (*2.5.11*).

1 ml of *0.1 M sodium edetate* is equivalent to 20.33 mg of $MgCl_2,6H_2O$.

STORAGE

Store in an airtight container.

LABELLING

The label states:

– where applicable, that the substance is suitable for use in the manufacture of peritoneal dialysis solutions, haemodialysis solutions or haemofiltration solutions,

– where applicable, that the substance is suitable for use in the manufacture of parenteral dosage forms.

01/2005:1446

MAGNESIUM GLYCEROPHOSPHATE

Magnesii glycerophosphas

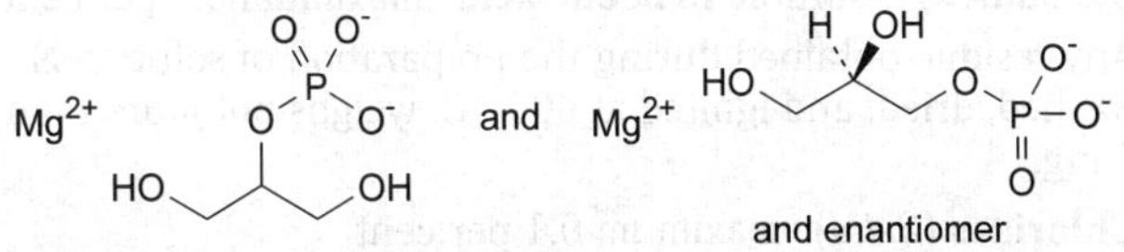

and enantiomer

$C_3H_7MgO_6P$ M_r 194.4

DEFINITION

Magnesium glycerophosphate is a mixture, in variable proportions, of magnesium (*RS*)-2,3-dihydroxypropyl phosphate, and of magnesium 2-hydroxy-1-(hydroxymethyl)ethyl phosphate, which may be hydrated. Magnesium glycerophosphate contains not less than 11.0 per cent and not more than 12.5 per cent of Mg, calculated with reference to the dried substance.

CHARACTERS

A white powder, hygroscopic, practically insoluble in alcohol. It dissolves in dilute solutions of acids.

IDENTIFICATION

A. Mix 1 g with 1 g of *potassium hydrogen sulphate R* in a test tube fitted with a glass tube. Heat strongly and direct the white vapour towards a piece of filter paper impregnated with a freshly prepared 10 g/l solution of *sodium nitroprusside R*. The filter paper develops a blue colour in contact with *piperidine R*.

B. Ignite 0.1 g in a crucible. Take up the residue with 5 ml of *nitric acid R* and heat on a water-bath for 1 min. Filter. The filtrate gives reaction (b) of phosphates (*2.3.1*).

C. It gives the reaction of magnesium (*2.3.1*).

TESTS

Solution S. Dissolve 2.5 g in *carbon dioxide-free water R* prepared from *distilled water R*, and dilute to 50 ml with the same solvent.

Appearance of solution. Solution S is not more opalescent than reference suspension III (*2.2.1*).

Acidity. Dissolve 1.0 g in 100 ml of *carbon dioxide-free water R*. Add 0.1 ml of *phenolphthalein solution R*. Not more than 1.5 ml of *0.1 M sodium hydroxide* is required to change the colour of the indicator.

Glycerol and alcohol-soluble substances. Shake 1.0 g with 25 ml of *alcohol R* for 2 min. Filter and wash the residue with 5 ml of *alcohol R*. Combine the filtrate and the washings, evaporate to dryness on a water-bath and dry the residue at 70 °C for 1 h. The residue weighs not more than 15 mg (1.5 per cent).

Chlorides (*2.4.4*). Dissolve 1.0 g in *water R* and dilute to 100 ml with the same solvent. Dilute 3.5 ml of the solution to 15 ml with *water R*. The solution complies with the limit test for chlorides (0.15 per cent).

Phosphates (*2.4.11*). Dilute 4 ml of solution S to 100 ml with *water R*. Dilute 1 ml of the solution to 100 ml with *water R*. The solution complies with the limit test for phosphates (0.5 per cent).

Sulphates (*2.4.13*). Dilute 3 ml of solution S to 15 ml with *distilled water R*. The solution complies with the limit test for sulphates (0.1 per cent).

Iron (*2.4.9*). Dissolve 67 mg in *water R* and dilute to 10 ml with the same solvent. The solution complies with the limit test for iron (150 ppm).

Heavy metals (*2.4.8*). To 20 ml of solution S add 15 ml of *hydrochloric acid R* and shake with 25 ml of *methyl isobutyl ketone R* for 2 min. Allow to stand, separate the aqueous layer and evaporate to dryness. Dissolve the residue in 2.5 ml of *acetic acid R* and dilute to 20 ml with *water R*. 12 ml of the solution complies with limit test A for heavy metals (20 ppm). Prepare the standard using *lead standard solution (1 ppm Pb) R*.

Loss on drying (*2.2.32*). Not more than 12.0 per cent, determined on 1.000 g by drying in an oven at 150 °C for 4 h.

ASSAY

Dissolve 0.200 g in 40 ml of *water R*. Carry out the complexometric titration of magnesium (*2.5.11*).

1 ml of *0.1 M sodium edetate* is equivalent to 2.431 mg of Mg.

STORAGE

Store in an airtight container.

01/2005:0039

MAGNESIUM HYDROXIDE

Magnesii hydroxidum

$Mg(OH)_2$ M_r 58.32

DEFINITION

Content: 95.0 per cent to 100.5 per cent of $Mg(OH)_2$.

CHARACTERS

Appearance: white, fine, amorphous powder.

Solubility: practically insoluble in water. It dissolves in dilute acids.

IDENTIFICATION

A. Dissolve about 15 mg in 2 ml of *dilute nitric acid R* and neutralise with *dilute sodium hydroxide solution R*. The solution gives the reaction of magnesium (*2.3.1*).

B. It complies with the test for loss on ignition (see Tests).

TESTS

Solution S. Dissolve 5.0 g in a mixture of 50 ml of *acetic acid R* and 50 ml of *distilled water R*. Not more than slight effervescence is produced. Boil for 2 min, cool and dilute to 100 ml with *dilute acetic acid R*. Filter, if necessary, through a previously ignited and tared porcelain or silica filter crucible of suitable porosity to give a clear filtrate.

Appearance of solution. Solution S is not more intensely coloured than reference solution B_3 (*2.2.2, Method II*).

Soluble substances: maximum 2.0 per cent.

Mix 2.00 g with 100 ml of *water R* and boil for 5 min. Filter whilst hot through a sintered-glass filter (40), allow to cool and dilute to 100 ml with *water R*. Evaporate 50 ml of the filtrate to dryness and dry at 100-105 °C. The residue weighs not more than 20 mg.

Substances insoluble in acetic acid: maximum 0.1 per cent.

Any residue obtained during the preparation of solution S, washed, dried, and ignited at 600 °C, weighs not more than 5 mg.

Chlorides (*2.4.4*): maximum 0.1 per cent.

1 ml of solution S diluted to 15 ml with *water R* complies with the limit test for chlorides.

Sulphates (*2.4.13*): maximum 0.5 per cent.

0.6 ml of solution S diluted to 15 ml with *distilled water R* complies with the limit test for sulphates.

Arsenic (*2.4.2*): maximum 4 ppm.

5 ml of solution S complies with limit test A.

Calcium (*2.4.3*): maximum 1.5 per cent.

Dilute 1.3 ml of solution S to 150 ml with *distilled water R*. 15 ml of the solution complies with the limit test for calcium.

Iron (*2.4.9*): maximum 0.07 per cent.

Dissolve 0.15 g in 5 ml of *dilute hydrochloric acid R* and dilute to 10 ml with *water R*. 1 ml of this solution diluted to 10 ml with *water R* complies with the limit test for iron.

Heavy metals (*2.4.8*): maximum 30 ppm.

Dissolve 2.0 g in 20 ml of *hydrochloric acid R1* and shake with 25 ml of *methyl isobutyl ketone R* for 2 min. Allow to stand, separate the aqueous layer and evaporate to dryness. Dissolve the residue in 30 ml of *water R*. 12 ml of the solution complies with limit test A. Prepare the standard using *lead standard solution (2 ppm Pb) R*.

Loss on ignition: 29.0 per cent to 32.5 per cent.

Heat 0.5 g gradually to 900 °C and ignite to constant mass.

ASSAY

Dissolve 0.100 g in a mixture of 20 ml of *water R* and 2 ml of *dilute hydrochloric acid R* and carry out the complexometric titration of magnesium (*2.5.11*).

1 ml of *0.1 M sodium edetate* is equivalent to 5.832 mg of $Mg(OH)_2$.

Monographs M

01/2005:0041

MAGNESIUM OXIDE, HEAVY

Magnesii oxidum ponderosum

MgO M_r 40.30

DEFINITION

Content: from 98.0 per cent to 100.5 per cent of MgO (ignited substance).

CHARACTERS

Appearance: fine, white powder.

Solubility: practically insoluble in water. It dissolves in dilute acids with at most slight effervescence.

IDENTIFICATION

A. 15 g has an apparent volume (*2.9.15*) before settling of about 30 ml.

B. Dissolve about 15 mg in 2 ml of *dilute nitric acid R* and neutralise with *dilute sodium hydroxide solution R*. The solution gives the reaction of magnesium (*2.3.1*).

C. It complies with the test for loss on ignition (see Tests).

TESTS

Solution S. Dissolve 5.0 g in a mixture of 30 ml of *distilled water R* and 70 ml of *acetic acid R*, boil for 2 min, cool and dilute to 100 ml with *dilute acetic acid R*. Filter, if necessary, through a previously ignited and tared porcelain or silica filter crucible of suitable porosity to give a clear solution.

Appearance of solution. Solution S is not more intensely coloured than reference solution B3 (*2.2.2, Method II*).

Soluble substances: maximum 2.0 per cent.

Mix 2.00 g with 100 ml of *water R* and boil for 5 min. Filter whilst hot through a sintered-glass filter (40), allow to cool and dilute to 100 ml with *water R*. Evaporate 50 ml of the filtrate to dryness and dry at 100-105 °C. The residue weighs not more than 20 mg.

Substances insoluble in acetic acid: maximum 0.1 per cent.

Any residue obtained during the preparation of solution S, washed, dried, and ignited at 600 °C, weighs not more than 5 mg.

Chlorides (*2.4.4*): maximum 0.1 per cent.

1 ml of solution S diluted to 15 ml with *water R* complies with the limit test for chlorides.

Sulphates (*2.4.13*): maximum 1.0 per cent.

0.3 ml of solution S diluted to 15 ml with *distilled water R* complies with the limit test for sulphates.

Arsenic (*2.4.2*): maximum 4 ppm.

5 ml of solution S complies with limit test A.

Calcium (*2.4.3*): maximum 1.5 per cent.

Dilute 1.3 ml of solution S to 150 ml with *distilled water R*. 15 ml of the solution complies with the limit test for calcium.

Iron (*2.4.9*): maximum 0.07 per cent.

Dissolve 0.15 g in 5 ml of *dilute hydrochloric acid R* and dilute to 10 ml with *water R*. 1 ml of the solution diluted to 10 ml with *water R* complies with the limit test for iron.

Heavy metals (*2.4.8*): maximum 30 ppm.

To 20 ml of solution S add 15 ml of *hydrochloric acid R1* and shake with 25 ml of *methyl isobutyl ketone R* for 2 min. Separate the layers, evaporate the aqueous layer to dryness, dissolve the residue in 1 ml of *acetic acid R* and dilute to 30 ml with *water R*. 12 ml of the solution complies with limit test A. Prepare the standard using *lead standard solution (1 ppm Pb) R*.

Loss on ignition: maximum 8.0 per cent, determined on 1.00 g at 900 °C.

ASSAY

Dissolve 0.320 g in 20 ml of *dilute hydrochloric acid R* and dilute to 100.0 ml with *water R*. Using 20.0 ml of the solution, carry out the complexometric titration of magnesium (*2.5.11*).

1 ml of *0.1 M sodium edetate* is equivalent to 4.030 mg of MgO.

01/2005:0040

MAGNESIUM OXIDE, LIGHT

Magnesii oxidum leve

MgO M_r 40.30

DEFINITION

Content: 98.0 per cent to 100.5 per cent of MgO (ignited substance).

CHARACTERS

Appearance: fine, white, amorphous powder.

Solubility: practically insoluble in water. It dissolves in dilute acids with at most slight effervescence.

IDENTIFICATION

A. 15 g has an apparent volume (*2.9.15*) before settling of about 150 ml.

B. Dissolve about 15 mg in 2 ml of *dilute nitric acid R* and neutralise with *dilute sodium hydroxide solution R*. The solution gives the reaction of magnesium (*2.3.1*).

C. It complies with the test for loss on ignition (see Tests).

TESTS

Solution S. Dissolve 5.0 g in a mixture of 30 ml of *distilled water R* and 70 ml of *acetic acid R*, boil for 2 min, cool and dilute to 100 ml with *dilute acetic acid R*. Filter if necessary through a previously ignited and tared porcelain or silica filter crucible of a suitable porosity to give a clear filtrate.

Appearance of solution. Solution S is not more intensely coloured than reference solution B_2 (*2.2.2, Method II*).

Soluble substances: maximum 2.0 per cent.

To 2.00 g add 100 ml of *water R* and heat to boiling for 5 min. Filter whilst hot through a sintered-glass filter (40), allow to cool and dilute to 100 ml with *water R*. Evaporate 50 ml of the filtrate to dryness and dry at 100-105 °C. The residue weighs not more than 20 mg.

Substances insoluble in acetic acid: maximum 0.1 per cent.

Any residue obtained during the preparation of solution S, washed, dried, and ignited at 600 °C, weighs not more than 5 mg.

Chlorides (*2.4.4*): maximum 0.15 per cent.

0.7 ml of solution S diluted to 15 ml with *water R* complies with the limit test for chlorides.

Sulphates (*2.4.13*): maximum 1.0 per cent.

0.3 ml of solution S diluted to 15 ml with *distilled water R* complies with the limit test for sulphates.

Arsenic (*2.4.2*): maximum 4 ppm.

5 ml of solution S complies with limit test A.

Calcium (*2.4.3*): maximum 1.5 per cent.

Dilute 1.3 ml of solution S to 150 ml with *distilled water R*. 15 ml of the solution complies with the limit test for calcium.

Iron (*2.4.9*): maximum 0.1 per cent.

Dissolve 50 mg in 5 ml of *dilute hydrochloric acid R* and dilute to 10 ml with *water R*. 2 ml of this solution diluted to 10 ml with *water R* complies with the limit test for iron.

Heavy metals (*2.4.8*): maximum 30 ppm.

To 20 ml of solution S add 15 ml of *hydrochloric acid R1* and shake with 25 ml of *methyl isobutyl ketone R* for 2 min. Allow to stand, separate the aqueous layer and evaporate to dryness. Dissolve the residue in 1.5 ml of *acetic acid R* and dilute to 30 ml with *water R*. 12 ml of the solution complies with limit test A. Prepare the standard using *lead standard solution (1 ppm Pb) R*.

Loss on ignition: maximum 8.0 per cent, determined on 1.00 g at 900 °C.

ASSAY

Dissolve 0.320 g in 20 ml of *dilute hydrochloric acid R* and dilute to 100.0 ml with *water R*. Using 20.0 ml of the solution, carry out the complexometric titration of magnesium (*2.5.11*).

1 ml of *0.1 M sodium edetate* is equivalent to 4.030 mg of MgO.

01/2005:1540

MAGNESIUM PEROXIDE

Magnesii peroxidum

DEFINITION

Magnesium peroxide is a mixture of magnesium peroxide and magnesium oxide. It contains not less than 22.0 per cent and not more than 28.0 per cent of MgO_2 (M_r 56.30).

CHARACTERS

A white or slightly yellow, amorphous, light powder, practically insoluble in water and in alcohol. It dissolves in dilute mineral acids.

IDENTIFICATION

A. Dissolve about 15 mg in 2 ml of *dilute nitric acid R* and neutralise with *dilute sodium hydroxide solution R*. The solution gives the reaction of magnesium (*2.3.1*).

B. Dissolve 0.1 g in 2 ml of *dilute sulphuric acid R* and dilute to 10 ml with *water R*. Shake 1 ml of the solution with 5 ml of *ether R* and 0.5 ml of *potassium dichromate solution R1*. The ether layer is blue.

TESTS

Solution S1. Dissolve cautiously 5.0 g in 40 ml of *hydrochloric acid R1*. Cautiously evaporate the solution to a volume of 10 ml and dilute to 100 ml with a mixture of equal volumes of *acetic acid R* and *distilled water R*. Filter, if necessary, through a previously ignited and tared porcelain or silica filter crucible of suitable porosity to give a clear filtrate. Keep the residue for the test for acid insoluble substances.

Solution S2. Dilute 5 ml of solution S1 to 25 ml with *distilled water R*.

Appearance of solution. Solution S1 is not more intensely coloured than reference solution B_4 (*2.2.2, Method II*).

Acid insoluble substances. Any residue obtained during the preparation of solution S1, washed, dried and ignited at 600 °C, weighs not more than 5 mg (0.1 per cent).

Acidity or alkalinity. To 2.0 g add 100 ml of *carbon dioxide-free water R* and heat to boiling for 5 min. Filter whilst hot through a sintered-glass filter (40), allow to cool and dilute to 100 ml with *carbon dioxide-free water R*. To 15 ml of the filtrate, add 0.1 ml of *phenolphthalein solution R*. The solution is red. Not more than 0.2 ml of *0.1 M hydrochloric acid* is necessary to change the colour of the indicator. Keep the filtrate for the test for soluble substances.

Soluble substances. Take 50 ml of the filtrate obtained in the test for acidity or alkalinity, evaporate to dryness and dry at 100 °C to 105 °C. The residue weighs not more than 15 mg (1.5 per cent).

Chlorides (*2.4.4*). Dissolve 50 mg in 5 ml of *dilute nitric acid R* and dilute to 15 ml with *water R*. The solution complies with the limit test for chlorides (0.1 per cent).

Sulphates (*2.4.13*). 3 ml of solution S2 diluted to 15 ml with *distilled water R* complies with the limit test for sulphates (0.5 per cent).

Arsenic (*2.4.2*). 5 ml of solution S1 complies with limit test A for arsenic (4 ppm).

Calcium (*2.4.3*). 1 ml of solution S2 diluted to 15 ml with *distilled water R* complies with the limit test for calcium (1.0 per cent).

Monographs M

Iron (*2.4.9*). 2 ml of solution S2 diluted to 10 ml with *water R* complies with the limit test for iron (500 ppm).

Heavy metals (*2.4.8*). To 20 ml of solution S1 add 15 ml of *hydrochloric acid R1* and shake with 25 ml of *methyl isobutyl ketone R* for 2 min. Allow to stand, separate the aqueous layer and evaporate to dryness. Dissolve the residue in 1.5 ml of *acetic acid R* and dilute to 30 ml with *water R*. 12 ml of the solution complies with limit test A for heavy metals (30 ppm). Prepare the standard using *lead standard solution (1 ppm Pb) R*.

ASSAY

Dissolve 80.0 mg, shaking cautiously, in a mixture, previously cooled to 20 °C, of 10 ml of *sulphuric acid R* and 90 ml of *water R*. Titrate with *0.02 M potassium permanganate* until a pink colour is obtained.

1 ml of *0.02 M potassium permanganate* is equivalent to 2.815 mg of MgO_2.

STORAGE

Store protected from light.

01/2005:1619

MAGNESIUM PIDOLATE

Magnesii pidolas

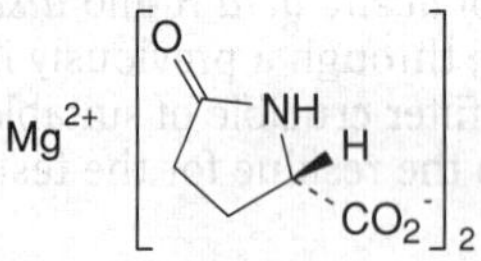

$C_{10}H_{12}N_2O_6Mg$ M_r 280.5

DEFINITION

Magnesium bis[(2*S*)-5-oxopyrrolidine-2-carboxylate].

Content: 8.49 per cent to 8.84 per cent of Mg (A_r = 24.31) (anhydrous substance).

CHARACTERS

Appearance: amorphous, white or almost white powder, hygroscopic.

Solubility: very soluble in water, soluble in methanol, practically insoluble in methylene chloride.

IDENTIFICATION

A. Thin-layer chromatography (*2.2.27*).

Test solution. Dissolve 60 mg in 2 ml of *water R* and dilute to 10 ml with *methanol R*.

Reference solution. Dissolve 55 mg of *pidolic acid CRS* in 2 ml of *water R* and dilute to 10 ml with *methanol R*.

Plate: *TLC silica gel plate R*.

Mobile phase: *methanol R, glacial acetic acid R, methylene chloride R* (15:20:65 *V/V/V*).

Application: 1 µl.

Development: over 2/3 of the plate.

Drying: at 100-105 °C for 15 min.

Detection: spray with *concentrated sodium hypochlorite solution R*. Allow to stand for 10 min and spray abundantly with *glacial acetic acid R*. Allow to stand again for 10 min and dry the plate at 100-105 °C for 2 min. Spray with *potassium iodide and starch solution R* until spots appear.

Results: the principal spot in the chromatogram obtained with the test solution is similar in position, colour and size to the principal spot in the chromatogram obtained with the reference solution. The chromatogram obtained with the test solution may show 2 faint secondary spots.

B. To 0.15 ml of solution S (see Tests) add 1.8 ml of *water R*. The solution gives the reaction of magnesium (*2.3.1*).

TESTS

Solution S. Dissolve 5.00 g in *carbon dioxide-free water R* prepared from *distilled water R* and dilute to 50.0 ml with the same solvent.

Appearance of solution. Solution S is clear (*2.2.1*) and not more intensely coloured than reference solution B_8 (*2.2.2, Method I*).

pH (*2.2.3*): 5.5 to 7.0 for solution S.

Specific optical rotation (*2.2.7*): − 23.3 to − 26.5 (anhydrous substance), determined on solution S.

Related substances. Liquid chromatography (*2.2.29*).

Test solution. Dissolve 0.500 g of the substance to be examined in the mobile phase and dilute to 100.0 ml with the mobile phase.

Reference solution (a). Dilute 1.0 ml of the test solution to 100.0 ml with the mobile phase.

Reference solution (b). Dissolve 50.0 mg *pidolate impurity B CRS* in the mobile phase and dilute to 100.0 ml with the mobile phase. Dilute 5.0 ml of the solution to 50.0 ml with the mobile phase.

Reference solution (c). Dilute 10.0 ml of reference solution (b) to 100.0 ml with the mobile phase.

Reference solution (d). Dilute 1.0 ml of *nitrate standard solution (100 ppm NO_3) R* to 100.0 ml with the mobile phase.

Reference solution (e). Dilute 6.0 ml of reference solution (a) to 10.0 ml with reference solution (b).

Column:

– *size*: *l* = 0.25 m, Ø = 4.6 mm,

– *stationary phase*: *octadecylsilyl silica gel for chromatography R* (5 µm).

Mobile phase: dissolve 1.56 g of *sodium dihydrogen phosphate R* in 1000 ml of *water R* and adjust to pH 2.5 with a 10 per cent *V/V* solution of *phosphoric acid R*.

Flow rate: 1.5 ml/min.

Detection: spectrophotometer at 210 nm.

Injection: 10 µl loop injector; inject the test solution and reference solutions (b), (c), (d) and (e).

Run time: 4 times the retention time of pidolic acid.

Retention times: pidolic acid = about 4.5 min; impurity B = about 7.5 min.

System suitability: reference solution (e):

– *resolution*: minimum 10 between the peaks due to pidolic acid and to impurity B.

Limits:

– *impurity B*: not more than the area of the principal peak in the chromatogram obtained with reference solution (b) (1.0 per cent),

– *total of other impurities*: not more than half of the area of the principal peak in the chromatogram obtained with reference solution (b) (0.5 per cent),

– *disregard limit*: not more than 0.5 times the area of the principal peak in the chromatogram obtained with reference solution (c) (0.05 per cent); disregard any peak corresponding to the nitrate ion (NO_3^-).

Impurity A. Thin-layer chromatography (*2.2.27*).

Test solution. Dissolve 0.250 g of the substance to be examined in 4 ml of *water R* and dilute to 50.0 ml with *methanol R*.

Reference solution (a). Dissolve 60.0 mg of *glutamic acid R* in 50 ml of *water R* and dilute to 100.0 ml with *methanol R*. Dilute 1.0 ml of the solution to 20.0 ml with *methanol R*.

Reference solution (b). Dissolve 10 mg of *glutamic acid R* and 10 mg of *aspartic acid R* in *water R* and dilute to 25 ml with the same solvent. Dilute 1 ml of the solution to 10 ml with *water R*.

Plate: *TLC silica gel plate R.*

Mobile phase: *glacial acetic acid R, water R, butanol R* (20:20:60 *V/V/V*).

Application: 5 µl.

Development: over 2/3 of the plate.

Drying: in air.

Detection: spray with *ninhydrin solution R* and heat at 100-105 °C for 15 min.

System suitability: the test is not valid unless the chromatogram obtained with reference solution (b) shows 2 clearly separated spots.

Limit:

- *impurity A*: any spot corresponding to impurity A in the chromatogram obtained with the test solution is not more intense that the spot in the chromatogram obtained with reference solution (a) (0.6 per cent).

Chlorides (*2.4.4*): maximum 500 ppm.

Dilute 1.0 ml of solution S to 15.0 ml of *water R*. The solution complies with the limit test for chlorides.

Nitrates. Examine the chromatogram obtained with the test solution in the test for related substances.

Limit:

- *nitrates*: not more than the area of the principal peak in the chromatogram obtained with reference solution (d) (200 ppm).

Sulphates (*2.4.13*): maximum 0.1 per cent.

Dilute 1.5 ml of solution S to 15.0 ml with *distilled water R*. The solution complies with the limit test for sulphates.

Arsenic (*2.4.2*): maximum 2 ppm.

5.0 ml of solution S complies with limit test A.

Iron (*2.4.9*): maximum 200 ppm.

Dilute 0.5 ml of solution S to 10 ml of *water R*. The solution complies with the limit test for iron.

Heavy metals (*2.4.8*): maximum 20 ppm.

12 ml of solution S complies with limit test A. Prepare the standard using *lead standard solution (2 ppm Pb) R*.

Water (*2.5.12*): maximum 8.0 per cent, determined on 0.200 g.

ASSAY

Dissolve 0.300 g in 50 ml of *water R*. Carry out the complexometric titration of magnesium (*2.5.11*).

1 ml of *0.1 M sodium edetate* is equivalent to 2.431 mg of Mg.

STORAGE

In an airtight container.

IMPURITIES

A. glutamic acid,

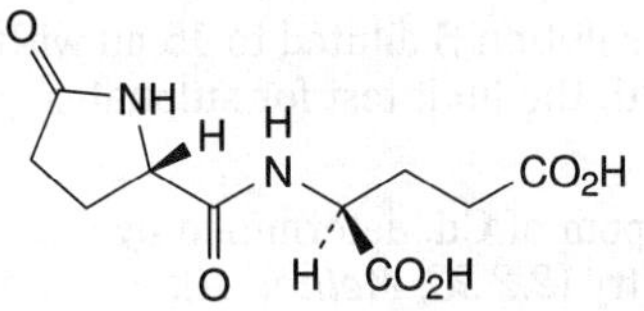

B. (2*S*)-2-[[[(2*S*)-5-oxopyrrolidin-2-yl]carbonyl]amino]pentanedioic acid.

01/2005:0229

MAGNESIUM STEARATE

Magnesii stearas

DEFINITION

Magnesium stearate is a mixture of magnesium salts of different fatty acids consisting mainly of stearic acid [$(C_{17}H_{35}COO)_2Mg$; M_r 591.3] and palmitic acid [$(C_{15}H_{31}COO)_2Mg$; M_r 535.1] with minor proportions of other fatty acids. It contains not less than 4.0 per cent and not more than 5.0 per cent of Mg (A_r 24.30), calculated with reference to the dried substance. The fatty acid fraction contains not less than 40.0 per cent of stearic acid and the sum of stearic acid and palmitic acid is not less than 90.0 per cent.

CHARACTERS

A white, very fine, light powder, greasy to the touch, practically insoluble in water and in ethanol.

IDENTIFICATION

First identification: *C, D.*

Second identification: *A, B, D.*

A. The residue obtained in the preparation of solution S (see Tests) has a freezing point (*2.2.18*) not lower than 53 °C.

B. The acid value of the fatty acids (*2.5.1*) is 195 to 210, determined on 0.200 g of the residue obtained in the preparation of solution S dissolved in 25 ml of the prescribed mixture of solvents.

C. Examine the chromatograms obtained in the test for fatty acid composition. The retention times of the principal peaks in the chromatogram obtained with the test solution are approximately the same as those of the principal peaks in the chromatogram obtained with the reference solution.

D. 1 ml of solution S gives the reaction of magnesium (*2.3.1*).

TESTS

Solution S. To 5.0 g add 50 ml of *peroxide-free ether R*, 20 ml of *dilute nitric acid R* and 20 ml of *distilled water R* and heat under a reflux condenser until dissolution is complete. Allow to cool. In a separating funnel, separate the aqueous layer and shake the ether layer with 2 quantities, each of 4 ml, of *distilled water R*. Combine the aqueous layers, wash with 15 ml of *peroxide-free ether R* and dilute to 50 ml with *distilled water R* (solution S). Evaporate the organic layer to dryness and dry the residue at 100-105 °C. Keep the residue for identification tests A and B.

Acidity or alkalinity. To 1.0 g add 20 ml of *carbon dioxide-free water R* and boil for 1 min with continuous stirring. Cool and filter. To 10 ml of the filtrate add 0.05 ml of *bromothymol blue solution R1*. Not more than 0.5 ml of *0.01 M hydrochloric acid* or *0.01 M sodium hydroxide* is required to change the colour of the indicator.

Chlorides (*2.4.4*). 0.5 ml of solution S diluted to 15 ml with *water R* complies with the limit test for chlorides (0.1 per cent).

Monographs M

Sulphates (*2.4.13*). 0.3 ml of solution S diluted to 15 ml with *distilled water R* complies with the limit test for sulphates (0.5 per cent).

Cadmium. Not more than 3 ppm of Cd, determined by atomic absorption spectrometry (*2.2.23, Method II*).

Test solution. Place 50.0 mg of the substance to be examined in a polytetrafluoroethylene digestion bomb and add 0.5 ml of a mixture of 1 volume of *hydrochloric acid R* and 5 volumes of *cadmium- and lead-free nitric acid R*. Allow to digest at 170 °C for 5 h. Allow to cool. Dissolve the residue in *water R* and dilute to 5.0 ml with the same solvent.

Reference solutions. Prepare the reference solutions using *cadmium standard solution (10 ppm Cd) R*, diluted as necessary with a 1 per cent *V/V* solution of *hydrochloric acid R*.

Measure the absorbance at 228.8 nm, using a cadmium hollow-cathode lamp as a source of radiation and a graphite furnace as atomic generator.

Lead. Not more than 10 ppm of Pb, determined by atomic absorption spectrometry (*2.2.23, Method II*).

Test solution. Use the solution described in the test for cadmium.

Reference solutions. Prepare the reference solutions using *lead standard solution (10 ppm Pb) R*, diluted as necessary with *water R*.

Measure the absorbance at 283.3 nm, using a lead hollow-cathode lamp as a source of radiation and a graphite furnace as atomic generator, depending on the apparatus the line at 217.0 nm may be used.

Nickel. Not more than 5 ppm of Ni, determined by atomic absorption spectrometry (*2.2.23, Method II*).

Test solution. Use the solution described in the test for cadmium.

Reference solutions. Prepare the reference solutions using *nickel standard solution (10 ppm Ni) R*, diluted as necessary with *water R*.

Measure the absorbance at 232.0 nm, using a nickel hollow-cathode lamp as a source of radiation and a graphite furnace as atomic generator.

Loss on drying (*2.2.32*). Not more than 6.0 per cent, determined on 1.000 g by drying in an oven at 100-105 °C.

Microbial contamination. Total viable aerobic count (*2.6.12*) not more than 10^3 micro-organisms per gram, determined by plate count. It complies with the test for *Escherichia coli* (*2.6.13*).

ASSAY

Magnesium. To 0.500 g in a 250 ml conical flask add 50 ml of a mixture of equal volumes of *butanol R* and *ethanol R*, 5 ml of *concentrated ammonia R*, 3 ml of *ammonium chloride buffer solution pH 10.0 R*, 30.0 ml of *0.1 M sodium edetate* and 15 mg of *mordant black 11 triturate R*. Heat to 45-50 °C until the solution is clear and titrate with *0.1 M zinc sulphate* until the colour changes from blue to violet. Carry out a blank titration.

1 ml of *0.1 M sodium edetate* is equivalent to 2.431 mg of Mg.

Fatty acid composition. Examine by gas chromatography (*2.2.28*).

Test solution. In a conical flask fitted with a reflux condenser, dissolve 0.10 g of the substance to be examined in 5 ml of *boron trifluoride-methanol solution R*. Boil under a reflux condenser for 10 min. Add 4 ml of *heptane R* through the condenser and boil again under a reflux condenser for 10 min. Allow to cool. Add 20 ml of a *saturated sodium chloride solution R*. Shake and allow the layers to separate. Remove about 2 ml of the organic layer and dry over 0.2 g of *anhydrous sodium sulphate R*. Dilute 1.0 ml of the solution to 10.0 ml with *heptane R*.

Reference solution. Prepare the reference solution in the same manner as the test solution using 50.0 mg of *palmitic acid CRS* and 50.0 mg of *stearic acid CRS* instead of magnesium stearate.

The chromatographic procedure may be carried out using:

- a fused-silica column 30 m long and 0.32 mm in internal diameter coated with *macrogol 20 000 R* (film thickness 0.5 µm),
- *helium for chromatography R* as the carrier gas at a flow rate of 2.4 ml/min,
- a flame-ionisation detector,

with the following temperature programme:

	Time (min)	Temperature (°C)	Rate (°C/min)	Comment
Column	0 - 2	70	–	isothermal
	2 - 36	70 → 240	5	linear gradient
	36 - 41	240	–	isothermal
Injection port		220		
Detector		260		

Inject 1 µl of the reference solution. When the chromatogram is recorded in the prescribed conditions, the relative retention of methyl palmitate to that of methyl stearate is about 0.88. The test is not valid unless, in the chromatogram obtained with the reference solution, the resolution between the peaks corresponding to methyl stearate and methyl palmitate is at least 5.0.

Inject 1 µl of the test solution. Calculate the percentage content of stearic acid and palmitic acid from the areas of the peaks in the chromatogram obtained with the test solution by the normalisation procedure, disregarding the peak due to the solvent.

FUNCTIONALITY-RELATED CHARACTERISTICS

The following test is not a mandatory requirement but in view of its known importance for achieving consistency in manufacture, quality and performance of medicinal products, it is recommended that suppliers should verify this characteristic and provide information on the result and the analytical method applied to users. The method indicated below has been found suitable but other methods may be used.

The following characteristic is relevant for magnesium stearate used as a lubricant in solid dosage forms (compressed and powder).

Specific surface area (*2.9.26, Method I*). Determine the specific surface area in the P/P_0 range of 0.05 to 0.15.

Sample outgassing: 2 h at 40 °C.

01/2005:0044

MAGNESIUM SULPHATE HEPTAHYDRATE

Magnesii sulfas heptahydricus

$MgSO_4,7H_2O$ M_r 246.5

DEFINITION

Magnesium sulphate heptahydrate contains not less than 99.0 per cent and not more than the equivalent of 100.5 per cent of $MgSO_4$, calculated with reference to the dried substance.

CHARACTERS

A white, crystalline powder or brilliant, colourless crystals, freely soluble in water, very soluble in boiling water, practically insoluble in alcohol.

IDENTIFICATION

A. It gives the reactions of sulphates (*2.3.1*).

B. It gives the reaction of magnesium (*2.3.1*).

TESTS

Solution S. Dissolve 5.0 g in *water R* and dilute to 50 ml with the same solvent.

Appearance of solution. Solution S is clear (*2.2.1*) and colourless (*2.2.2, Method II*).

Acidity or alkalinity. To 10 ml of solution S add 0.05 ml of *phenol red solution R*. Not more than 0.2 ml of *0.01 M hydrochloric acid* or *0.01 M sodium hydroxide* is required to change the colour of the indicator.

Chlorides (*2.4.4*). 1.7 ml of solution S diluted to 15 ml with *water R* complies with the limit test for chlorides (300 ppm).

Arsenic (*2.4.2*). 0.5 g complies with limit test A for arsenic (2 ppm).

Iron (*2.4.9*). 5 ml of solution S diluted to 10 ml with *water R* complies with the limit test for iron (20 ppm).

Heavy metals (*2.4.8*). 12 ml of solution S complies with limit test A for heavy metals (10 ppm). Prepare the standard using *lead standard solution (1 ppm Pb) R*.

Loss on drying (*2.2.32*). 48.0 per cent to 52.0 per cent, determined on 0.500 g by drying in an oven at 110 °C to 120 °C for 1 h and then at 400 °C to constant mass.

ASSAY

Dissolve 0.450 g in 100 ml of *water R* and carry out the complexometric titration of magnesium (*2.5.11*).

1 ml of *0.1 M sodium edetate* is equivalent to 12.04 mg of $MgSO_4$.

01/2005:0403

MAGNESIUM TRISILICATE

Magnesii trisilicas

DEFINITION

Magnesium trisilicate has a variable composition corresponding approximately to $Mg_2Si_3O_8{\cdot}xH_2O$ and contains not less than the equivalent of 29.0 per cent of magnesium oxide (MgO; M_r 40.30) and not less than the equivalent of 65.0 per cent of silicon dioxide (SiO_2; M_r 60.1), both calculated with reference to the ignited substance.

CHARACTERS

A white powder, practically insoluble in water and in alcohol.

IDENTIFICATION

A. 0.25 g gives the reaction of silicates (*2.3.1*).

B. 1 ml of solution S (see Tests) neutralised with *dilute sodium hydroxide solution R* gives the reaction of magnesium (*2.3.1*).

TESTS

Solution S. To 2.0 g add a mixture of 4 ml of *nitric acid R* and 4 ml of *distilled water R*. Heat to boiling with frequent shaking. Add 12 ml of *distilled water R* and allow to cool. Filter or centrifuge to obtain a clear solution and dilute to 20 ml with *distilled water R*.

Alkalinity. To 10.0 g in a 200 ml conical flask, add 100.0 g of *water R* and heat on a water-bath for 30 min. Allow to cool and make up to the initial mass with *water R*. Allow to stand and filter or centrifuge until a clear liquid is obtained. To 10 ml of the liquid add 0.1 ml of *phenolphthalein solution R*. Not more than 1.0 ml of *0.1 M hydrochloric acid* is required to change the colour of the indicator.

Water-soluble salts. In a platinum dish, evaporate to dryness on a water-bath 20.0 ml of the liquid obtained in the test for alkalinity. The residue, ignited to constant mass at 900 °C, weighs not more than 30 mg (1.5 per cent).

Chlorides (*2.4.4*). 0.5 ml of solution S diluted to 15 ml with *water R* complies with the limit test for chlorides (500 ppm). Prepare the standard using a mixture of 5 ml of *chloride standard solution (5 ppm Cl) R* and 10 ml of *water R*.

Sulphates (*2.4.13*). 0.3 ml of solution S diluted to 15 ml with *distilled water R* complies with the limit test for sulphates (0.5 per cent).

Arsenic (*2.4.2*). 2.5 ml of solution S complies with limit test A for arsenic (4 ppm).

Heavy metals (*2.4.8*). Neutralise 10 ml of solution S with *dilute ammonia R1*, using *metanil yellow solution R* as an external indicator. Dilute to 20 ml with *water R* and filter if necessary. 12 ml of the solution complies with limit test A for heavy metals (40 ppm). Prepare the standard using *lead standard solution (2 ppm Pb) R*.

Loss on ignition: 17 per cent to 34 per cent, determined on 0.5 g ignited to constant mass at 900 °C in a platinum crucible.

Acid-absorbing capacity. Suspend 0.25 g in *0.1 M hydrochloric acid*, dilute to 100.0 ml with the same acid and allow to stand for 2 h in a water-bath at 37 ± 0.5 °C, with frequent shaking. Allow to cool. To 20.0 ml of the supernatant solution add 0.1 ml of *bromophenol blue solution R* and titrate with *0.1 M sodium hydroxide* until a blue colour is obtained. The acid-absorbing capacity is not less than 100.0 ml of *0.1 M hydrochloric acid* per gram.

ASSAY

Magnesium oxide. To 1.000 g in a 200 ml conical flask, add 35 ml of *hydrochloric acid R* and 60 ml of *water R* and heat in a water-bath for 15 min. Allow to cool, filter, wash the conical flask and the residue with *water R* and dilute the combined filtrate and washings to 250.0 ml with *water R*. Neutralise 50.0 ml of the solution with *strong sodium hydroxide solution R* (about 8 ml). Carry out the complexometric titration of magnesium (*2.5.11*).

1 ml of *0.1 M sodium edetate* is equivalent to 4.030 mg of MgO.

Silicon dioxide. To 0.700 g add 10 ml of *dilute sulphuric acid R* and 10 ml of *water R*. Heat for 90 min on a water-bath with frequent shaking, replacing the evaporated water. Allow to cool and decant onto an ashless filter paper (diameter 7 cm). Wash the precipitate by decantation with three quantities, each of 5 ml, of hot *water R*, transfer it to the filter and wash it with hot *water R* until 1 ml of the filtrate remains clear after the addition of 0.05 ml of *dilute hydrochloric* *acid R* and 2 ml of *barium chloride solution R1*. Incinerate the filter and its contents in a platinum crucible, then ignite the residue (SiO_2) at 900 °C to constant mass.

01/2005:1342

MAIZE OIL, REFINED

Maydis oleum raffinatum

DEFINITION

Refined maize oil is the fatty oil obtained from the seeds of *Zea mays* L. by expression or by extraction, then refined.

CHARACTERS

A clear, light yellow or yellow oil, practically insoluble in water and in alcohol, miscible with light petroleum (bp: 40 °C to 60 °C) and with methylene chloride.

It has a relative density of about 0.920 and a refractive index of about 1.474.

IDENTIFICATION

A. Carry out the identification of fatty oils by thin-layer chromatography (*2.3.2*). The chromatogram obtained with the test solution is similar to that obtained with the reference solution.

B. It complies with the test for composition of fatty acids (see Tests).

TESTS

Acid value (*2.5.1*). Not more than 0.5, determined on 10.0 g. If intended for use in the manufacture of parenteral dosage forms, not more than 0.3.

Peroxide value (*2.5.5*). Not more than 10.0. If intended for use in the manufacture of parenteral dosage forms, not more than 5.0.

Unsaponifiable matter (*2.5.7*). Not more than 2.8 per cent, determined on 5.0 g.

Alkaline impurities (*2.4.19*). It complies with the test for alkaline impurities in fatty oils.

Composition of fatty acids (*2.4.22, Method A*). The fatty-acid fraction of the oil has the following composition:

- *fatty acids of chain length less than* C_{16}: not more than 0.6 per cent,
- *palmitic acid*: 8.6 per cent to 16.5 per cent,
- *stearic acid*: not more than 3.3 per cent,
- *oleic acid*: 20.0 per cent to 42.2 per cent (equivalent chain length on polyethyleneglycol adipate 18.3),
- *linoleic acid*: 39.4 per cent to 65.6 per cent (equivalent chain length on polyethyleneglycol adipate 18.9),
- *linolenic acid*: 0.5 per cent to 1.5 per cent (equivalent chain length on polyethyleneglycol adipate 19.7),
- *arachidic acid*: not more than 0.8 per cent,
- *eicosenoic acid*: not more than 0.5 per cent (equivalent chain length on polyethyleneglycol adipate 20.3),
- *behenic acid*: not more than 0.5 per cent,
- *other fatty acids*: not more than 0.5 per cent.

Sterols. Determined by gas chromatography (*2.4.23*), the sterol fraction of the oil contains not more than 0.3 per cent of brassicasterol.

Water (*2.5.32*). If intended for use in the manufacture of parenteral dosage forms, not more than 0.1 per cent, determined on 5.00 g by the micro-determination of water. Use a mixture of equal volumes of *decanol R* and *anhydrous methanol R* as the solvent.

STORAGE

Store protected from light, at a temperature not exceeding 25 °C.

LABELLING

The label states:

- where applicable, that the substance is suitable for use in the manufacture of parenteral dosage forms,
- whether the oil is obtained by mechanical expression or by extraction.

01/2005:0344

MAIZE STARCH

Maydis amylum

DEFINITION

Maize starch is obtained from the caryopsis of *Zea mays* L.

CHARACTERS

Appearance: matt, white to slightly yellowish, very fine powder which creaks when pressed between the fingers.

Solubility: practically insoluble in cold water and in alcohol.

The presence of granules with cracks or irregularities on the edge is exceptional.

It is tasteless.

IDENTIFICATION

A. Examined under a microscope, using not less than 20 × magnification and using equal volumes of *glycerol R* and *water R*, it appears as either angular polyhedral granules of irregular sizes with diameters ranging from about 2 µm to about 23 µm or as rounded or spheroidal granules of irregular sizes with diameters ranging from about 25 µm to about 35 µm. The central hilum consists of a distinct cavity or two-to five-rayed cleft and there are no concentric striations. Between crossed nicol prisms, the starch granules show a distinct black cross intersecting at the hilum.

B. Suspend 1 g in 50 ml of *water R*, boil for 1 min and cool. A thin, cloudy mucilage is formed.

C. To 10 ml of the mucilage obtained in identification test B add 0.04 ml of *iodine solution R1*. An orange-red to dark blue colour is produced which disappears on heating.

TESTS

pH (*2.2.3*): 4.0 to 7.0.

Shake 5.0 g with 25.0 ml of *carbon dioxide-free water R* for 60 s. Allow to stand for 15 min.

Foreign matter. Examined under a microscope using a mixture of equal volumes of *glycerol R* and *water R*, not more than traces of matter other than starch granules are present. No starch grains of any other origin are present.

Oxidising substances (*2.5.30*): maximum 20 ppm, calculated as H_2O_2.

Sulphur dioxide (*2.5.29*): maximum 50 ppm.

Iron (*2.4.9*): maximum 10 ppm.

Shake 1.5 g with 15 ml of *dilute hydrochloric acid R*. Filter. The filtrate complies with the limit test for iron.

Loss on drying (*2.2.32*): maximum 15.0 per cent, determined on 1.000 g by drying in an oven at 130 °C for 90 min.

Sulphated ash (*2.4.14*): maximum 0.6 per cent, determined on 1.0 g.

Microbial contamination. Total viable aerobic count (*2.6.12*) not more than 10^3 bacteria and 10^2 fungi per gram, determined by plate count. It complies with the test for *Escherichia coli* (*2.6.13*).

STORAGE

In an airtight container.

01/2005:1343

MALATHION

Malathionum

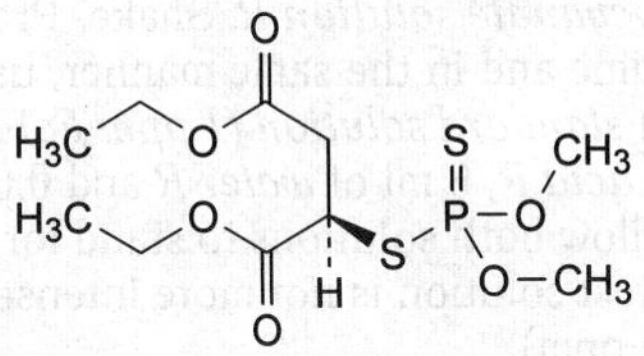

$C_{10}H_{19}O_6PS_2$ — M_r 330.4

DEFINITION

Malathion contains not less than 98.0 per cent and not more than the equivalent of 102.0 per cent of diethyl (2*RS*)-2-(dimethoxyphosphinodithioyl)butanedioate, calculated with reference to the anhydrous substance.

CHARACTERS

A clear, colourless or slightly yellowish liquid, slightly soluble in water, miscible with alcohol and with acetone, with cyclohexane and with vegetable oils.

It freezes at about 3 °C.

IDENTIFICATION

Examine by infrared absorption spectrophotometry (*2.2.24*), comparing with the spectrum obtained with *malathion CRS*.

TESTS

Relative density (*2.2.5*): 1.220 to 1.240.

Optical rotation (*2.2.7*). Dissolve 2.50 g in *alcohol R* and dilute to 25.0 ml with the same solvent. The angle of optical rotation is −0.1° to + 0.1°.

Related substances. Examine by liquid chromatography (*2.2.29*) as prescribed under Assay.

Inject 20 µl of test solution (a) and 20 µl of reference solution (d). In the chromatogram obtained with test solution (a): the area of any peak due to impurity A is not greater than three times the area of the corresponding peak in the chromatogram obtained with reference solution (d) (0.3 per cent); the area of any peak due to impurity B is not greater than the area of the corresponding peak in the chromatogram obtained with reference solution (d) (0.1 per cent); the sum of the areas of all the peaks apart from the principal peak and any peak due to impurity A or impurity B is not greater than twice the area of the principal peak in the chromatogram obtained with reference solution (b) (1 per cent). Disregard any peak with an area less than 0.1 times that of the area of the principal peak in the chromatogram obtained with reference solution (b).

Water (*2.5.12*). Not more than 0.1 per cent, determined on 2.000 g by the semi-micro determination of water.

ASSAY

Examine by liquid chromatography (*2.2.29*).

Test solution (a). Dissolve 0.10 g of the substance to be examined in a mixture of 1 volume of *water R* and 3 volumes of *acetonitrile R* and dilute to 5.0 ml with the same mixture of solvents.

Test solution (b). Take 1.0 ml of test solution (a) and dilute to 10.0 ml with a mixture of 1 volume of *water R* and 3 volumes of *acetonitrile R*.

Reference solution (a). Dissolve 0.100 g of *malathion CRS* in a mixture of 1 volume of *water R* and 3 volumes of *acetonitrile R* and dilute to 50.0 ml with the same mixture of solvents.

Reference solution (b). Take 0.5 ml of test solution (a) and dilute to 100.0 ml with a mixture of 1 volume of *water R* and 3 volumes of *acetonitrile R*.

Reference solution (c). Dissolve 5.0 mg of *malathion impurity A CRS* and 5.0 mg of *malathion impurity B CRS* in a mixture of 1 volume of *water R* and 3 volumes of *acetonitrile R* and dilute to 50.0 ml with the same mixture of solvents.

Reference solution (d). Take 2.0 ml of reference solution (c) and dilute to 10.0 ml with a mixture of 1 volume of *water R* and 3 volumes of *acetonitrile R*.

The chromatographic procedure may be carried out using:

- a stainless steel column 0.15 m long and4.6 mm in internal diameter packed with *octadecylsilyl silica gel for chromatography R* (10 µm),
- as mobile phase at a flow rate of 1 ml/min a mixture of 45 volumes of *acetonitrile R* and 55 volumes of *water R*,
- as detector a spectrophotometer set at 210 nm,

maintaining the temperature of the column at 35 °C.

Inject 20 µl of reference solution (b) and 20 µl of reference solution (c).

When the chromatograms are recorded in the prescribed conditions, the retention times are: impurity B about 3.5 min; impurity A about 5 min and malathion about 16 min. Adjust the sensitivity of the system so that the height of the principal peak in the chromatogram obtained with reference solution (b) is at least 50 per cent of the full scale of the recorder. The test is not valid unless in the chromatogram obtained with reference solution (c) the resolution between the peaks corresponding to impurity A and impurity B is at least 2.0. Inject reference solution (a) six times. The assay is not valid unless the relative standard deviation of the peak area for malathion is at most 1.0 per cent.

Inject alternately test solution (b) and reference solution (a). Calculate the percentage content of malathion.

STORAGE

Store in an airtight container, protected from light.

IMPURITIES

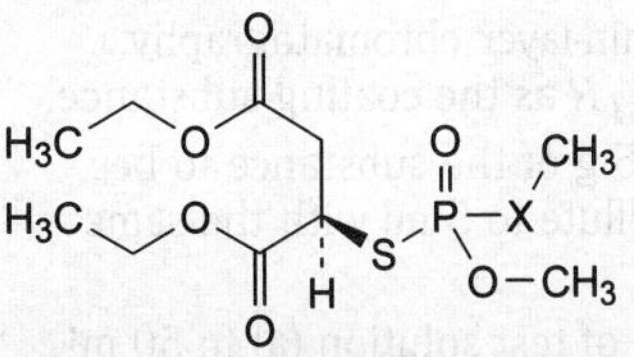

A. X = S: diethyl (2*RS*)-2-[(methoxy)(methylsulphanyl)-*S*-phosphinothioyl]butanedioate (isomalathion),

B. X = O: diethyl (2*RS*)-2-(dimethoxy-*S*-phosphinothioyl)butanedioate (maloxon),

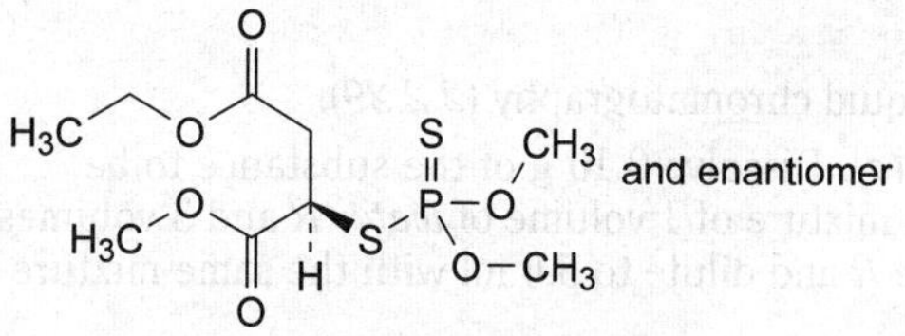

C. ethyl and methyl (2*RS*)-2-(dimethoxyphosphinodithioyl)butanedioate (methyl analogue).

01/2005:0365

MALEIC ACID

Acidum maleicum

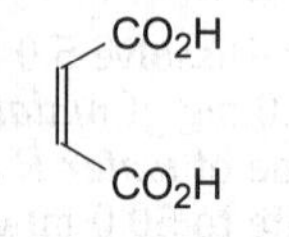

$C_4H_4O_4$ M_r 116.1

DEFINITION

Maleic acid contains not less than 99.0 per cent and not more than the equivalent of 101.0 per cent of (*Z*)-butenedioic acid, calculated with reference to the anhydrous substance.

CHARACTERS

A white, crystalline powder, freely soluble in water and in alcohol.

IDENTIFICATION

A. Dilute 5 ml of solution S (see Tests) to 10 ml with *water R*. The pH of the dilution is less than 2.

B. Examine the chromatograms obtained in the test for fumaric acid. The principal spot in the chromatogram obtained with test solution (b) is similar in position and size to the principal spot in the chromatogram obtained with reference solution (a).

C. Dissolve 0.1 g in 10 ml of *water R* (solution a). To 0.3 ml of solution (a) add a solution of 10 mg of *resorcinol R* in 3 ml of *sulphuric acid R*. Heat on a water-bath for 15 min; no colour develops. To 3 ml of solution (a) add 1 ml of *bromine water R*. Heat on a water-bath to remove the bromine (15 min), heat to boiling and cool. To 0.2 ml of this solution add a solution of 10 mg of *resorcinol R* in 3 ml of *sulphuric acid R*. Heat on a water-bath for 15 min. A violet-pink colour develops.

TESTS

Solution S. Dissolve 5.0 g in *water R* and dilute to 50 ml with the same solvent.

Appearance of solution. Solution S is clear (*2.2.1*) and not more intensely coloured than reference solution Y_7 (*2.2.2, Method II*).

Fumaric acid. Examine by thin-layer chromatography (*2.2.27*), using *silica gel GF_{254} R* as the coating substance.

Test solution (a). Dissolve 0.5 g of the substance to be examined in *acetone R* and dilute to 5 ml with the same solvent.

Test solution (b). Dilute 1 ml of test solution (a) to 50 ml with *acetone R*.

Reference solution (a). Dissolve 20 mg of *maleic acid CRS* in *acetone R* and dilute to 10 ml with the same solvent.

Reference solution (b). Dissolve 15 mg of *fumaric acid CRS* in *acetone R* and dilute to 10 ml with the same solvent.

Reference solution (c). Mix 5 ml of reference solution (a) and 5 ml of reference solution (b).

Apply separately to the plate 5 µl of test solutions (a) and (b), 5 µl of reference solutions (a) and (b) and 10 µl of reference solution (c). Develop in a non-saturated tank over a path of 10 cm using a mixture of 12 volumes of *anhydrous formic acid R*, 16 volumes of *chloroform R*, 32 volumes of *butanol R* and 44 volumes of *heptane R*. Dry the plate at 100 °C for 15 min and examine in ultraviolet light at 254 nm. Any spot corresponding to fumaric acid in the chromatogram obtained with test solution (a) is not more intense than the spot in the chromatogram obtained with reference solution (b) (1.5 per cent). The test is not valid unless the chromatogram obtained with reference solution (c) shows two clearly separated spots.

Iron. To 10 ml of solution S add 2 ml of *dilute hydrochloric acid R* and 0.05 ml of *bromine water R*. After 5 min, remove the excess of bromine by passing a current of air and add 3 ml of *potassium thiocyanate solution R*. Shake. Prepare a standard at the same time and in the same manner, using a mixture of 5 ml of *iron standard solution (1 ppm Fe) R*, 1 ml of *dilute hydrochloric acid R*, 6 ml of *water R* and 0.05 ml of *bromine water R*. Allow both solutions to stand for 5 min. Any red colour in the test solution is not more intense than that in the standard (5 ppm).

Heavy metals (*2.4.8*). 1.0 g complies with limit test D for heavy metals (10 ppm). Prepare the standard using 1 ml of *lead standard solution (10 ppm Pb) R*.

Water (*2.5.12*). Not more than 2.0 per cent, determined on 1.00 g by the semi-micro determination of water.

Sulphated ash (*2.4.14*). Not more than 0.1 per cent, determined on 1.0 g.

ASSAY

Dissolve 0.500 g in 50 ml of *water R*. Titrate with *1 M sodium hydroxide* using 0.5 ml of *phenolphthalein solution R* as indicator.

1 ml of *1 M sodium hydroxide* is equivalent to 58.04 mg of $C_4H_4O_4$.

STORAGE

Store in a glass container, protected from light.

01/2005:2080

MALIC ACID

Acidum malicum

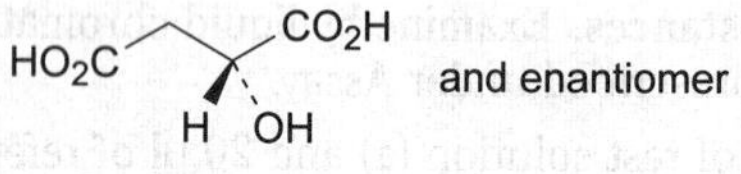

$C_4H_6O_5$ M_r 134.1

DEFINITION

(2*RS*)-2-Hydroxybutanedioic acid.

Content: 99.0 per cent to 101.0 per cent (anhydrous substance).

CHARACTERS

Appearance: white, crystalline powder.

Solubility: freely soluble in water and in alcohol, sparingly soluble in acetone.

IDENTIFICATION

A. Melting point (*2.2.14*): 128 °C to 132 °C.

B. Infrared absorption spectrophotometry (*2.2.24*).
Comparison: *Ph. Eur. reference spectrum of malic acid.*

TESTS

Solution S. Dissolve 5.00 g in *water R* and dilute to 25 ml with the same solvent.

Appearance of solution. Solution S is clear (*2.2.1*) and colourless (*2.2.2, Method II*).

Optical rotation (*2.2.7*): −0.10° to + 0.10°, determined on solution S.

Water-insoluble substances: maximum 0.1 per cent.

Dissolve 25.0 g in 100 ml of *water R*, filter the solution through a tared sintered-glass filter crucible (16), wash the filter with hot *water R* and dry at 100-105 °C to constant weight. The residue weighs a maximum of 25 mg.

Related substances. Liquid chromatography (*2.2.29*).

Test solution. Dissolve 100.0 mg of the substance to be examined in the mobile phase and dilute to 100.0 ml with the mobile phase.

Reference solution (a). Dissolve 10.0 mg of *fumaric acid R* and 4.0 mg of *maleic acid R* in 25 ml of the mobile phase and dilute to 50.0 ml with the mobile phase.

Reference solution (b). Dilute 2.5 ml of reference solution (a) to 100.0 ml with the mobile phase.

Reference solution (c). Dissolve 20.0 mg of the substance to be examined in the mobile phase, add 1.0 ml of reference solution (a) and dilute to 20.0 ml with the mobile phase.

Column:

- *size*: l = 0.30 m, Ø = 7.8 mm,
- *stationary phase*: *ion-exclusion resin for chromatography R* (9 µm),
- *temperature*: 37 °C.

Mobile phase: *0.005 M sulphuric acid*.

Flow rate: 0.6 ml/min.

Detection: spectrophotometer at 210 nm.

Injection: 20 µl.

Run time: twice the retention time of the principal peak in the chromatogram obtained with the test solution.

Relative retention with reference to malic acid (retention time = about 10 min): impurity B = about 0.8; impurity A = about 1.5.

System suitability: reference solution (c):

- *resolution*: minimum 2.5 between the peaks due to impurity B and malic acid.

Limits:

- *impurity A*: not more than twice the area of the corresponding peak in the chromatogram obtained with reference solution (b) (1.0 per cent),
- *impurity B*: not more than 0.25 times the area of the corresponding peak in the chromatogram obtained with reference solution (b) (0.05 per cent),
- *any other impurity*: for each impurity, not more than 0.5 times the area of the peak due to impurity B in the chromatogram obtained with reference solution (b) (0.1 per cent),
- *total of other impurities*: not more than 2.5 times the area of the peak due to impurity B in the chromatogram obtained with reference solution (b) (0.5 per cent),
- *disregard limit*: 0.1 times the area of the peak due to impurity B in the chromatogram obtained with reference solution (b) (0.02 per cent).

Heavy metals (*2.4.8*): maximum 20 ppm.

1.0 g complies with limit test F. Prepare the standard using 2 ml of *lead standard solution (10 ppm Pb) R*.

Water (*2.5.12*): maximum 2.0 per cent, determined on 1.00 g.

Sulphated ash (*2.4.14*): maximum 0.1 per cent, determined on 1.0 g.

ASSAY

Dissolve 0.500 g in 50 ml of *carbon dioxide-free water R*. Titrate with *1 M sodium hydroxide* determining the end-point potentiometrically (*2.2.20*).

1 ml of *1 M sodium hydroxide* is equivalent to 67.05 mg of $C_4H_6O_5$.

IMPURITIES

Specified impurities: *A, B*.

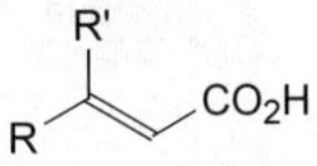

A. R = CO_2H, R′ = H: (*E*)-butenedioic acid (fumaric acid),

B. R = H, R′ = CO_2H: (*Z*)-butenedioic acid (maleic acid).

01/2005:1541

MALLOW FLOWER

Malvae sylvestris flos

DEFINITION

Mallow flower consists of the whole or fragmented dried flower of *Malva sylvestris* L. or its cultivated varieties.

CHARACTERS

It has the macroscopic and microscopic characters described under identification tests A and B.

IDENTIFICATION

A. The flower consists of an epicalyx with three oblong or elliptical-lanceolate parts that are shorter than those of the calyx and situated immediately below it; a calyx with five pubescent triangular lobes, gamosepalous at the base; a corolla three to four times longer than the calyx with five wedge-shaped, notched petals fused to the staminal tube at their base; numerous stamens, the filaments of which fuse into a staminal tube covered by small star-shaped trichomes and occasional simple trichomes visible using a lens; numerous wrinkled carpels, glabrous or sometimes pubescent, enclosed in the staminal tube and arranged into a circle around a central style ending with numerous filiform stigmas. In cultivated varieties, the epicalyx is 3 to 7 partite, the calyx 5 to 8 partite and the corolla 5 to 10 partite.

B. Reduce to a powder (355). The powder is bluish-grey. Examine under a microscope using *chloral hydrate solution R*. The powder shows unicellular, thick-walled, stiff trichomes, up to 2 mm in length; small unicellular covering trichomes, somewhat curved, either isolated or in small star-shaped groups of 2 to 6; capitate glandular trichomes with multicellular heads; mesophyll fragments with vessels accompanied by cluster crystals of calcium oxalate; spherical pollen grains, about 150 µm in diameter, with a roughly spiny exine.

When mounted with *alcohol R*, numerous elongated cells containing mucilage are seen in the petal fragments.

C. Examine by thin-layer chromatography (*2.2.27*) using a *TLC silica gel plate R*.

Test solution. To 1 g of the powdered drug (355) add 10 ml of *alcohol (60 per cent V/V) R*. Stir for 15 min and filter.

Reference solution. A 0.5 g/l solution of *quinaldine red R* in *alcohol R*.

Monographs M

Apply to the plate as bands 10 µl of the test solution and 5 µl of the reference solution.

Develop over a path of 10 cm using a mixture of 15 volumes of *acetic acid R*, 30 volumes of *water R* and 60 volumes of *butanol R*. Allow the plate to dry in air. Examine the chromatograms in daylight. The chromatogram obtained with the reference solution shows an orange-red zone in the upper part of the middle third. The chromatogram obtained with the test solution shows, below the zone in the chromatogram obtained with the reference solution, two violet zones in the middle third; the principal zone (6″-malonyl malvin) is situated just below the other violet zone (malvin).

TESTS

Foreign matter (*2.8.2*). It complies with the test for foreign matter.

Swelling index (*2.8.4*). Not less than 15, determined on 0.2 g of the powdered drug (710) humidified with 0.5 ml of *ethanol R*.

Loss on drying (*2.2.32*). Not more than 12.0 per cent, determined on 1.000 g of the powdered drug by drying in an oven at 100 °C to 105 °C.

Total ash (*2.4.16*). Not more than 14.0 per cent.

Ash insoluble in hydrochloric acid (*2.8.1*). Not more than 2.0 per cent.

STORAGE

Store protected from light.

01/2005:1235

MALTITOL

Maltitolum

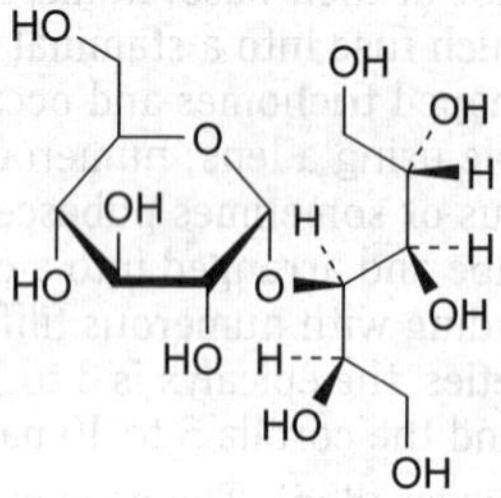

$C_{12}H_{24}O_{11}$ M_r 344.3

DEFINITION

Maltitol contains not less than 98.0 per cent and not more than the equivalent of 102.0 per cent of 4-*O*-α-D-glucopyranosyl-D-glucitol (D-maltitol), calculated with reference to the anhydrous substance.

CHARACTERS

A white, crystalline powder, very soluble in water, practically insoluble in ethanol.

IDENTIFICATION

First identification: A.

Second identification: B, C, D.

A. Examine by infrared absorption spectrophotometry (*2.2.24*), comparing with the spectrum obtained with *maltitol CRS*. Examine the substances prepared as discs.

B. Melting point (*2.2.14*): 148 °C to 151 °C.

C. Dissolve 5.00 g in *water R* and dilute to 100.0 ml with the same solvent. The specific optical rotation (*2.2.7*) is + 105.5 to + 108.5, calculated with reference to the anhydrous substance.

D. Examine by thin-layer chromatography (*2.2.27*),using a *TLC silica gel G plate R*.

Test solution. Dissolve 25 mg of the substance to be examined in *water R* and dilute to 10 ml with the same solvent.

Reference solution (a). Dissolve 25 mg of *maltitol CRS* in *water R* and dilute to 10 ml with the same solvent.

Reference solution (b). Dissolve 25 mg of *maltitol CRS* and 25 mg of *sorbitol CRS* in *water R* and dilute to 10 ml with the same solvent.

Apply to the plate 2 µl of each solution. Develop over a path of 17 cm using a mixture of 10 volumes of *water R*, 20 volumes of *ethyl acetate R* and 70 volumes of *propanol R*. Allow the plate to dry in air and spray with *4-aminobenzoic acid solution R*. Dry the plate in a current of cold air until the acetone is removed. Heat the plate at 100-105 °C for 15 min. Allow to cool and spray with a 2 g/l solution of *sodium periodate R*. Dry the plate in a current of cold air. Heat the plate at 100 °C for 15 min. The principal spot in the chromatogram obtained with the test solution is similar in position, colour and size to the principal spot in the chromatogram obtained with the reference solution (a). The test is not valid unless the chromatogram obtained with reference solution (b) shows two clearly separated spots.

TESTS

Appearance of solution. Dissolve 5.0 g in *water R* and dilute to 50 ml with the same solvent. The solution is clear (*2.2.1*) and colourless (*2.2.2, Method II*).

Conductivity (*2.2.38*). Not more than 20 µS·cm^{-1}.

Dissolve 20.0 g in *carbon dioxide-free water R* prepared from *distilled water R* and dilute to 100.0 ml with the same solvent. Measure the conductivity of the solution at a temperature of 20 °C, while gently stirring with a magnetic stirrer.

Reducing sugars. Dissolve 5.0 g in 6 ml of *water R* with the aid of gentle heat. Cool and add 20 ml of *cupri-citric solution R* and a few glass beads. Heat so that boiling begins after 4 min and maintain boiling for 3 min. Cool rapidly and add 100 ml of a 2.4 per cent *V/V* solution of *glacial acetic acid R* and 20.0 ml of *0.025 M iodine*. With continuous shaking, add 25 ml of a mixture of 6 volumes of *hydrochloric acid R* and 94 volumes of *water R* and, when the precipitate has dissolved, titrate the excess of iodine with *0.05 M sodium thiosulphate* using 1 ml of *starch solution R*, added towards the end of the titration, as indicator. Not less than 12.8 ml of *0.05 M sodium thiosulphate* is required (0.2 per cent, calculated as glucose equivalent).

Related substances. Examine by liquid chromatography (*2.2.29*) as described under Assay. Inject 20 µl of reference solution (b). Adjust the sensitivity of the system so that the height of the peak due to maltitol is at least 50 per cent of the full scale of the recorder. Inject 20 µl of the test solution and continue the chromatogram for three times the retention time of maltitol. In the chromatogram obtained with the test solution: the area of any peak, apart from the principal peak, is not greater than the area of the principal peak in the chromatogram obtained with reference solution (b) (1 per cent); the sum of the areas of all the peaks, apart from the principal peak, is not greater than twice the area of the principal peak in the chromatogram obtained with reference solution (b) (2 per cent). Disregard any peak with an area less than the area of the principal peak in the chromatogram obtained with reference solution (c) (0.1 per cent).

Lead (*2.4.10*). It complies with the limit test for lead in sugars (0.5 ppm).

Nickel (*2.4.15*). It complies with the limit test for nickel in polyols (1 ppm).

Water (*2.5.12*). Not more than 1.0 per cent, determined on 1.00 g by the semi-micro determination of water.

Microbial contamination. If intended for use in the manufacture of parenteral dosage forms the total viable aerobic count (*2.6.12*) is not more than 10^2 bacteria and 10^2 fungi per gram, determined by plate count; it complies with the tests for *Escherichia coli* and *Salmonella* (*2.6.13*).

Bacterial endotoxins (*2.6.14*): if intended for use in the manufacture of parenteral dosage forms without a further appropriate procedure for the removal of bacterial endotoxins, less than 4 IU/g for parenteral dosage forms having a concentration of less than 100 g/l of maltitol, and less than 2.5 IU/g for parenteral dosage forms having a concentration of 100 g/l or more of maltitol.

ASSAY

Examine by liquid chromatography (*2.2.29*).

Test solution. Dissolve 5.0 g of the substance to be examined in 20 ml of *water R* and dilute to 100.0 ml with the same solvent.

Reference solution (a). Dissolve 0.50 g of *maltitol CRS* in 2.0 ml of *water R* and dilute to 10.0 ml with the same solvent.

Reference solution (b). Dilute 1.0 ml of the test solution to 100.0 ml with *water R.*

Reference solution (c). Dilute 10.0 ml of reference solution (b) to 100.0 ml with *water R.*

Reference solution (d). Dissolve 0.5 g of *maltitol R* and 0.5 g of *sorbitol R* in 5 ml of *water R* and dilute to 10.0 ml with the same solvent.

The chromatography may be carried out using:

- a stainless steel column 0.3 m long and 7.8 mm in internal diameter packed with *strong cation exchange resin (calcium form) R* (9 µm) and maintained at 85 ± 1 °C,
- as mobile phase at a flow rate of 0.5 ml/min, degassed *water R,*
- as detector a refractometer maintained at a constant temperature.

Inject 20 µl of reference solution (d). Continue the chromatography for three times the retention time of maltitol.

When the chromatograms are recorded in the prescribed conditions, the retention time of maltitol is about 16 min and the relative retentions with reference to maltitol are: sorbitol about 1.8 and maltotriitol about 0.8. The test is not valid unless the resolution between the peaks due to maltitol and to sorbitol is at least 2 in the chromatogram obtained with reference solution (d).

Inject 20 µl of the test solution and 20 µl of reference solution (a). Continue the chromatography for three times the retention time of maltitol.

Calculate the percentage content of D-maltitol from the areas of the peaks and the declared content of *maltitol CRS.*

LABELLING

The label states:

- where applicable, the maximum concentration of bacterial endotoxins,
- where applicable, that the substance is suitable for use in the manufacture of parenteral dosage forms.

IMPURITIES

A. sorbitol,

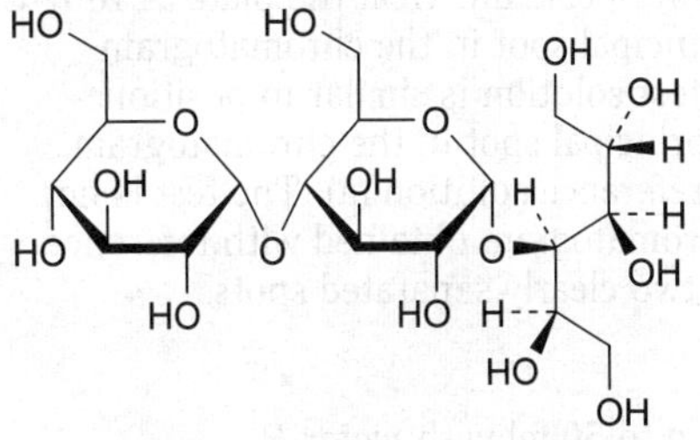

B. *O*-α-D-glucopyranosyl-(1→4)-*O*-α-D-glucopyranosyl-(1→4)-D-glucitol (maltotriitol).

01/2005:1236
corrected

MALTITOL, LIQUID

Maltitolum liquidum

DEFINITION

Liquid maltitol is an aqueous solution of a hydrogenated, partly hydrolysed starch. It contains not less than 68.0 per cent *m/m* and not more than 85.0 per cent *m/m* of anhydrous substance composed of a mixture of mainly 4-*O*-α-D-glucopyranosyl-D-glucitol (D-maltitol) with D-glucitol (D-sorbitol) and hydrogenated oligo- and polysaccharides. It contains not less than 50.0 per cent *m/m* of D-maltitol ($C_{12}H_{24}O_{11}$) and not more than 8.0 per cent *m/m* of D-sorbitol ($C_6H_{14}O_6$), both calculated with reference to the anhydrous substance. It contains not less than 95.0 per cent and not more than 105.0 per cent of the content of D-maltitol stated on the label.

CHARACTERS

A clear, colourless, syrupy liquid, miscible with water and with glycerol.

IDENTIFICATION

First identification: A.

Second identification: B, C.

A. Examine the chromatograms obtained in the assay. The principal peak in the chromatogram obtained with the test solution is similar in retention time to the principal peak in the chromatogram obtained with reference solution (a).

B. To 3 ml of a freshly prepared 100 g/l solution of *pyrocatechol R,* add 6 ml of *sulphuric acid R* while cooling in iced water. To 3 ml of the cooled mixture, add 0.3 ml of solution S (see Tests). Heat gently over a naked-flame for about 30 s. A pink colour develops.

C. Examine by thin-layer chromatography (*2.2.27*), using a *TLC silica gel G plate R.*

Test solution. Dilute 0.35 g of the substance to be examined to 100 ml with *water R.*

Reference solution (a). Dissolve 20 mg of *maltitol CRS* in *water R* and dilute to 10 ml with the same solvent.

Reference solution (b). Dissolve 20 mg of *maltitol CRS* and 20 mg of *sorbitol CRS* in *water R* and dilute to 10 ml with the same solvent.

Apply to the plate 2 µl of each solution. Develop over a path of 17 cm using a mixture of 10 volumes of *water R,* 20 volumes of *ethyl acetate R* and 70 volumes

Monographs M

of *propanol R*. Allow the plate to dry in air and spray with *4-aminobenzoic acid solution R*. Dry the plate in a current of cold air until the acetone is removed. Heat the plate at 100 °C to 105 °C for 15 min. Allow to cool and spray with a 2 g/l solution of *sodium periodate R*. Dry the plate in a current of cold air. Heat the plate at 100 °C for 15 min. The principal spot in the chromatogram obtained with the test solution is similar in position and colour to the principal spot in the chromatogram obtained with the reference solution (a). The test is not valid unless the chromatogram obtained with reference solution (b) shows two clearly separated spots.

TESTS

Solution S. Dilute 7.0 g to 50 ml with *water R*.

Appearance of solution. Solution S is clear (*2.2.1*) and colourless (*2.2.2, Method II*).

Conductivity (*2.2.38*). Not more than 10 μS·cm^{-1} measured on the undiluted liquid maltitol while gently stirring with a magnetic stirrer.

Reducing sugars. To 5.0 g add 6 ml of *water R*, 20 ml of *cupri-citric solution R* and a few glass beads. Heat so that boiling begins after 4 min and maintain boiling for 3 min. Cool rapidly and add 100 ml of a 2.4 per cent *V/V* solution of *glacial acetic acid R* and 20.0 ml of *0.025 M iodine*. With continuous shaking, add 25 ml of a mixture of 6 volumes of *hydrochloric acid R* and 94 volumes of *water R* and, when the precipitate has dissolved, titrate the excess of iodine with *0.05 M sodium thiosulphate* using 1 ml of *starch solution R*, added towards the end of the titration, as indicator. Not less than 12.8 ml of *0.05 M sodium thiosulphate* is required (0.2 per cent calculated as glucose equivalent).

Lead (*2.4.10*). It complies with the limit test for lead in sugars (0.5 ppm).

Nickel (*2.4.15*). It complies with the limit test for nickel in polyols (1 ppm).

Water (*2.5.12*). Not less than 15.0 per cent and not more than 32.0 per cent *m/m* determined on 0.100 g by the semi-micro determination of water.

ASSAY

Examine by liquid chromatography (*2.2.29*).

Test solution. Mix 1.00 g of the solution to be examined with 20 ml of *water R* and dilute to 50.0 ml with the same solvent.

Reference solution (a). Dissolve 50.0 mg of *maltitol CRS* in 2 ml of *water R* and dilute to 5.0 ml with the same solvent.

Reference solution (b). Dissolve 8.0 mg of *sorbitol CRS* in 2 ml of *water R* and dilute to 5.0 ml with the same solvent.

Reference solution (c). Dissolve 50 mg of *maltitol R* and 50 mg of *sorbitol R* in 2 ml of *water R* and dilute to 5.0 ml with the same solvent.

The chromatographic procedure may be carried out using:

- a stainless steel column 0.3 m long and 7.8 mm in internal diameter packed with a *strong cation exchange resin (calcium form) R* (9 μm) and maintained at 85 °C ± 2 °C,
- as mobile phase at a flow rate of 0.5 ml/min degassed *water R*,
- as detector a refractometer maintained at a constant temperature.

Inject 20 μl of reference solution (c). Continue the chromatography for three times the retention time of maltitol.

When the chromatogram is recorded in the prescribed conditions, the retention time of maltitol is about 16 min and the relative retention of sorbitol is about 1.8. The test is not valid unless the resolution between the peaks due to sorbitol and to maltitol is at least 2 in the chromatogram obtained with reference solution (c).

Inject 20 μl of the test solution, 20 μl of reference solution (a) and 20 μl of reference solution (b). Continue the chromatography for three times the retention time of maltitol.

Calculate the percentage contents of D-maltitol and D-sorbitol from the areas of the peaks and the declared contents of *maltitol CRS* and *sorbitol CRS*.

LABELLING

The label states the content of D-maltitol.

01/2005:1542

MALTODEXTRIN

Maltodextrinum

DEFINITION

Maltodextrin is a mixture of glucose, disaccharides and polysaccharides, obtained by the partial hydrolysis of starch. The degree of hydrolysis, expressed as dextrose equivalent (DE), is not more than 20 (nominal value).

CHARACTERS

A white or almost white, slightly hygroscopic powder or granules, freely soluble in water.

IDENTIFICATION

A. Dissolve 0.1 g in 2.5 ml of *water R* and heat with 2.5 ml of *cupri-tartaric solution R*. A red precipitate is formed.

B. Dip, for 1 s, a suitable stick with a reactive pad containing glucose-oxidase, peroxidase and a hydrogen-donating substance, such as tetramethylbenzidine, in a 100 g/l solution of the substance to be examined. Observe the colour of the reactive pad; within 60 s the colour changes from yellow to green or blue.

C. It is a powder or granules.

D. It complies with the test for dextrose equivalent (see Tests).

TESTS

Solution S. Dissolve 12.5 g in *carbon dioxide-free water R* and dilute to 50.0 ml with the same solvent.

pH (*2.2.3*). The pH of a mixture of 30 ml of solution S and 1 ml of a 223.6 g/l solution of *potassium chloride R* is 4.0 to 7.0.

Sulphur dioxide (*2.5.29*). Not more than 20 ppm.

Heavy metals (*2.4.8*). Dilute 4 ml of solution S to 30 ml with *water R*. The solution complies with limit test E for heavy metals (10 ppm). Prepare the standard using 10 ml of *lead standard solution (1 ppm Pb) R*.

Loss on drying (*2.2.32*). Not more than 6.0 per cent, determined on 10.00 g by drying in an oven at 100-105 °C.

Sulphated ash (*2.4.14*). Not more than 0.5 per cent, determined on 1.0 g.

Dextrose equivalent. Weigh an amount of the sample to be examined equivalent to 2.85-3.15 g of reducing carbohydrates, calculated as dextrose equivalent, into a 500 ml volumetric flask. Dissolve in *water R* and dilute to 500.0 ml with the same solvent. Transfer the solution to a 50 ml burette.

Pipette 25.0 ml of *cupri-tartaric solution R* into a 250 ml flask and add 18.5 ml of the sample solution from the burette, mix and add boiling chips. Place the flask on a hot plate, previously adjusted so that the solution begins to boil within 2 min ± 15 s. Allow to boil for exactly 120 s, add 1 ml of a 1 g/l solution of *methylene blue R* and titrate with the sample solution (V_1) until the blue colour disappears. Maintain the solution at boiling throughout the titration.

Standardise the cupri-tartaric solution using a 6.00 g/l solution of *glucose R* (V_0).

Calculate the dextrose equivalent (DE) from the equation:

$$DE = \frac{300 \times V_0 \times 100}{V_1 \times M \times D}$$

V_0 = total volume of glucose standard solution, in millilitres,

V_1 = total volume of sample solution, in millilitres,

M = sample weight, in grams,

D = percentage content of dry matter in the substance.

The dextrose equivalent (DE) is within 2 DE units of the nominal value.

Microbial contamination. Total viable aerobic count (*2.6.12*) not more than 10^3 bacteria and 10^2 fungi per gram, determined by plate count. It complies with the test for *Escherichia coli* and *Salmonella* (*2.6.13*).

LABELLING

The label states the dextrose equivalent (DE) (= nominal value).

01/2005:1543

MANGANESE SULPHATE MONOHYDRATE

Mangani sulfas monohydricus

$MnSO_4,H_2O$ M_r 169.0

DEFINITION

Manganese sulphate monohydrate contains not less than 99.0 per cent and not more than the equivalent of 101.0 per cent of $MnSO_4$, calculated with reference to the ignited substance.

CHARACTERS

A pale pink crystalline powder, slightly hygroscopic, freely soluble in water, practically insoluble in alcohol.

IDENTIFICATION

A. Solution S (see Tests) gives reaction (a) of sulphates (*2.3.1*).

B. Dissolve 50 mg in 5 ml of *water R*. Add 0.5 ml of *ammonium sulphide solution R*. A pale pink precipitate is formed which dissolves on the addition of 1 ml of *anhydrous acetic acid R*.

C. It complies with the test for loss on ignition (see Tests).

TESTS

Solution S. Dissolve 10.0 g in *distilled water R* and dilute to 100 ml with the same solvent.

Appearance of solution. Solution S is not more opalescent than reference suspension II (*2.2.1*).

Chlorides (*2.4.4*). Dilute 5 ml of solution S to 15 ml with *water R*. The solution complies with the limit test for chlorides (100 ppm).

Iron (*2.4.9*). 10 ml of solution S complies with the limit test for iron (10 ppm).

Zinc. To 10 ml of solution S add 1 ml of *sulphuric acid R* and 0.1 ml of *potassium ferrocyanide solution R*. After 30 s, any opalescence in the solution is not more intense than that in a mixture of 5 ml of *zinc standard solution (10 ppm Zn) R*, 5 ml of *water R*, 1 ml of *sulphuric acid R* and 0.1 ml of *potassium ferrocyanide solution R* (50 ppm).

Heavy metals (*2.4.8*). 12 ml of solution S complies with limit test A for heavy metals (20 ppm). Prepare the standard using *lead standard solution (2 ppm Pb) R*.

Loss on ignition: 10.0 per cent to 12.0 per cent, determined on 1.00 g at 500 °C.

ASSAY

Dissolve 0.150 g in 50 ml of *water R*. Add 10 mg of *ascorbic acid R*, 20 ml of *ammonium chloride buffer solution pH 10.0 R* and 0.2 ml of a 2 g/l solution of *mordant black 11 R* in *triethanolamine R*. Titrate with *0.1 M sodium edetate* until the colour changes from violet to pure blue.

1 ml of *0.1 M sodium edetate* is equivalent to 15.10 mg of $MnSO_4$.

01/2005:0559

MANNITOL

Mannitolum

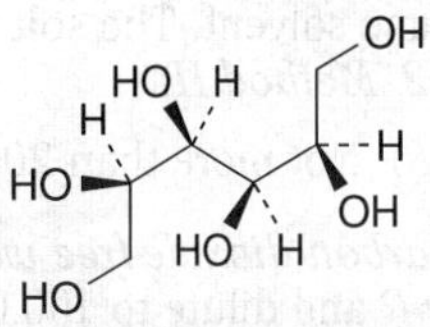

$C_6H_{14}O_6$ M_r 182.2

DEFINITION

Mannitol contains not less than 98.0 per cent and not more than the equivalent of 102.0 per cent of D-mannitol, calculated with reference to the anhydrous substance.

CHARACTERS

White or almost white, crystalline powder or free-flowing granules, freely soluble in water, very slightly soluble in alcohol.

It shows polymorphism.

IDENTIFICATION

First identification: A.

Second identification: B, C, D.

A. Examine by infrared absorption spectrophotometry (*2.2.24*), comparing with the spectrum obtained with *mannitol CRS*. Examine the substances prepared as discs. If the spectra obtained show differences, dissolve the substance to be examined and the reference substance separately in *water R*, evaporate to dryness and record new spectra using the residues.

B. Melting point (*2.2.14*): 165 °C to 170 °C.

C. Examine by thin-layer chromatography (*2.2.27*), using a *TLC silica gel G plate R*.

Test solution. Dissolve 25 mg of the substance to be examined in *water R* and dilute to 10 ml with the same solvent.

Reference solution (a). Dissolve 25 mg of *mannitol CRS* in *water R* and dilute to 10 ml with the same solvent.

Reference solution (b). Dissolve 25 mg of *mannitol CRS* and 25 mg of *sorbitol CRS* in *water R* and dilute to 10 ml with the same solvent.

Apply to the plate 2 µl of each solution. Develop over a path of 17 cm using a mixture of 10 volumes of *water R*, 20 volumes of *ethyl acetate R* and 70 volumes of *propanol R*. Allow the plate to dry in air and spray with *4-aminobenzoic acid solution R*. Dry the plate in a current of cold air until the acetone is removed. Heat the plate at 100 °C for 15 min. Allow to cool and spray with a 2 g/l solution of *sodium periodate R*. Dry the plate in a current of cold air. Heat the plate at 100 °C for 15 min. The principal spot in the chromatogram obtained with the test solution is similar in position, colour and size to the principal spot in the chromatogram obtained with reference solution (a). The test is not valid unless the chromatogram obtained with reference solution (b) shows 2 clearly separated spots.

D. Dissolve 2.00 g of the substance to be examined and 2.6 g of *disodium tetraborate R* in about 20 ml of *water R* at a temperature of 30 °C; shake continuously for 15-30 min without further heating. Dilute the resulting clear solution to 25.0 ml with *water R*. The specific optical rotation (*2.2.7*) is + 23 to + 25, calculated with reference to the anhydrous substance.

TESTS

Appearance of solution. Dissolve 5.0 g in *water R* and dilute to 50 ml with the same solvent. The solution is clear (*2.2.1*) and colourless (*2.2.2, Method II*).

Conductivity (*2.2.38*). Not more than 20 µS·cm^{-1}.

Dissolve 20.0 g in *carbon dioxide-free water R* prepared from *distilled water R* and dilute to 100.0 ml with the same solvent. Measure the conductivity of the solution while gently stirring with a magnetic stirrer.

Reducing sugars. Dissolve 5.0 g in 25 ml of *water R* with the aid of gentle heat. Cool and add 20 ml of *cupri-citric solution R* and a few glass beads. Heat so that boiling begins after 4 min and maintain boiling for 3 min. Cool rapidly and add 100 ml of a 2.4 per cent *V/V* solution of *glacial acetic acid R* and 20.0 ml of *0.025 M iodine*. With continuous shaking, add 25 ml of a mixture of 6 volumes of *hydrochloric acid R* and 94 volumes of *water R* and, when the precipitate has dissolved, titrate the excess of iodine with *0.05 M sodium thiosulphate* using 1 ml of *starch solution R*, added towards the end of the titration, as indicator. Not less than 12.8 ml of *0.05 M sodium thiosulphate* is required (0.2 per cent, calculated as glucose equivalent).

Related substances. Examine by liquid chromatography (*2.2.29*) as described under Assay. Inject 20 µl of reference solution (b). Adjust the sensitivity of the system so that the height of the peak due to mannitol is at least 50 per cent of the full scale of the recorder. Inject 20 µl of the test solution and of reference solution (c) and continue the chromatography for twice the retention time of mannitol. In the chromatogram obtained with the test solution: the area of any peak, apart from the principal peak, is not greater than the area of the principal peak in the chromatogram obtained with reference solution (b) (2 per cent); the sum of the areas of all the peaks, apart from the principal peak, is not greater than the area of the principal peak in the chromatogram obtained with reference solution (b) (2 per cent). Disregard any peak with an area less than the area of the principal peak in the chromatogram obtained with reference solution (c) (0.1 per cent).

Lead (*2.4.10*). It complies with the limit test for lead in sugars (0.5 ppm). Dissolve the substance to be examined in 150.0 ml of the prescribed mixture of solvents.

Nickel (*2.4.15*). It complies with the limit test for nickel in polyols (1 ppm). Dissolve the substance to be examined in 150.0 ml of the prescribed mixture of solvents.

Water (*2.5.12*). Not more than 0.5 per cent, determined on 1.00 g by the semi-micro determination of water.

Microbial contamination. If intended for use in the manufacture of parenteral dosage forms, the total viable aerobic count (*2.6.12*) is not more than 10^2 bacteria and 10^2 fungi per gram, determined by plate count. It complies with the tests for *Escherichia coli* and *Salmonella* (*2.6.13*).

Bacterial endotoxins (*2.6.14*): if intended for use in the manufacture of parenteral dosage forms without a further appropriate procedure for the removal of bacterial endotoxins, less than 4 IU/g for parenteral dosage forms having a concentration of 100 g/l or less of mannitol, and less than 2.5 IU/g for parenteral dosage forms having a concentration of more than 100 g/l of mannitol.

ASSAY

Examine by liquid chromatography (*2.2.29*).

Test solution. Dissolve 5.0 g of the substance to be examined in 25 ml of *water R* and dilute to 100.0 ml with the same solvent.

Reference solution (a). Dissolve 0.50 g of *mannitol CRS* in 2.5 ml of *water R* and dilute to 10.0 ml with the same solvent.

Reference solution (b). Dilute 2.0 ml of the test solution to 100.0 ml with *water R*.

Reference solution (c). Dilute 5.0 ml of reference solution (b) to 100.0 ml with *water R*.

Reference solution (d). Dissolve 0.5 g of *mannitol R* and 0.5 g of *sorbitol R* in 5 ml of *water R* and dilute to 10.0 ml with the same solvent.

The chromatography may be carried out using:

- a stainless steel column 0.3 m long and 7.8 mm in internal diameter packed with *strong cation exchange resin (calcium form) R* (9 µm) and maintained at 85 ± 1 °C,
- as mobile phase at a flow rate of 0.5 ml/min, degassed *water R*,
- as detector a refractometer maintained at a constant temperature.

Inject 20 µl of reference solution (d). Continue the chromatography for 3 times the retention time of mannitol. When the chromatograms are recorded in the prescribed conditions, the retention time of mannitol is about 22 min and the relative retention of sorbitol with reference to mannitol is about 1.25. The test is not valid unless the resolution between the peaks due to mannitol and to sorbitol is at least 2 in the chromatogram obtained with reference solution (d).

Inject 20 µl of the test solution and 20 µl of reference solution (a). Continue the chromatography for twice the retention time of mannitol.

Calculate the percentage content of D-mannitol from the areas of the peaks and the declared content of *mannitol CRS*.

LABELLING

The label states:

- where applicable, the maximum concentration of bacterial endotoxins,
- where applicable, that the substance is suitable for use in the manufacture of parenteral dosage forms.

Monographs M

IMPURITIES

A. sorbitol,

B. maltitol,

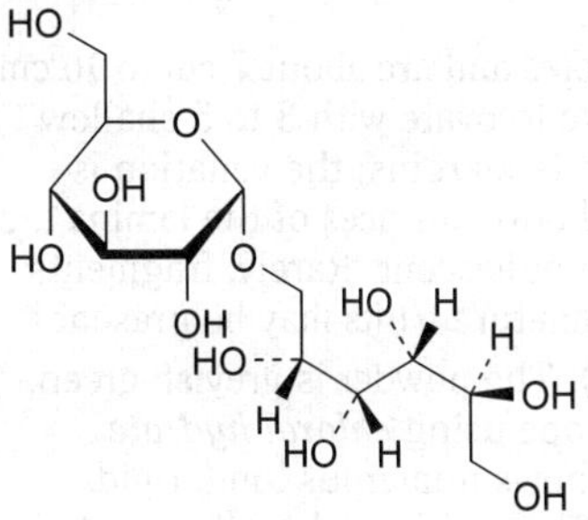

C. 6-*O*-α-D-glucopyranosyl-D-glucitol (isomaltitol).

01/2005:1237

MAPROTILINE HYDROCHLORIDE

Maprotilini hydrochloridum

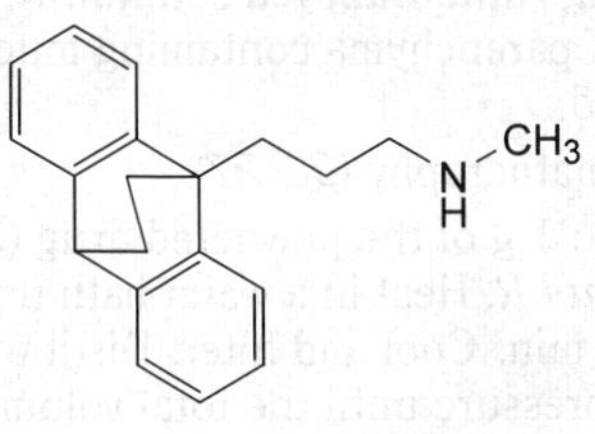

$C_{20}H_{24}ClN$ — M_r 313.9

DEFINITION

Maprotiline hydrochloride contains not less than 99.0 per cent and not more than the equivalent of 101.0 per cent of 3-(9,10-ethanoanthracen-9(10*H*)-yl)-*N*-methylpropan-1-amine hydrochloride, calculated with reference to the dried substance.

CHARACTERS

A white or almost white, crystalline powder, slightly soluble in water, freely soluble in methanol, soluble in alcohol, sparingly soluble in methylene chloride, very slightly soluble in acetone.

It shows polymorphism.

IDENTIFICATION

First identification: B, D.

Second identification: A, C, D.

A. Dissolve 10 mg in *1 M hydrochloric acid* and dilute to 100 ml with the same acid. Examined between 250 nm and 300 nm (*2.2.25*), the solution shows two absorption maxima, at 265 nm and 272 nm, and an absorption minimum at 268 nm. The ratio of the absorbance measured at the maximum at 272 nm to that measured at the maximum at 265 nm is 1.1 to 1.3.

B. Examine by infrared absorption spectrophotometry (*2.2.24*), comparing with the spectrum obtained with *maprotiline hydrochloride CRS*. Examine the substances prepared as discs. If the spectra obtained show differences, dissolve the substance to be examined and the reference substance separately in *methanol R*, evaporate to dryness and record new spectra using the residues.

C. Examine by thin-layer chromatography (*2.2.27*), using as the coating substance a suitable silica gel with a fluorescent indicator having an optimal intensity at 254 nm.

Test solution. Dissolve 25 mg of the substance to be examined in *methanol R* and dilute to 5 ml with the same solvent.

Reference solution (a). Dissolve 25 mg of *maprotiline hydrochloride CRS* in *methanol R* and dilute to 5 ml with the same solvent.

Reference solution (b). Dissolve 10 mg of *maprotiline impurity D CRS* in reference solution (a) and dilute to 2 ml with the same solution.

Apply to the plate 5 µl of each solution. Develop over a path of 10 cm using a mixture of 4 volumes of *ethyl acetate R*, 5 volumes of *dilute ammonia R1* and 14 volumes of *2-butanol R*. Dry the plate in a current of warm air and examine at 254 nm. The principal spot in the chromatogram obtained with the test solution is similar in position and size to the principal spot in the chromatogram obtained with reference solution (a). The test is not valid unless the chromatogram obtained with reference solution (b) shows two clearly separated principal spots.

D. Dilute 0.5 ml of solution S (see Tests) to 2 ml with *methanol R*. The solution gives reaction (a) of chlorides (*2.3.1*).

TESTS

Solution S. Dissolve 1.0 g in *methanol R* and dilute to 20 ml with the same solvent.

Appearance of solution. Solution S is clear (*2.2.1*) and not more intensely coloured than reference solution BY_6 (*2.2.2, Method II*).

Related substances. Examine by liquid chromatography (*2.2.29*).

Test solution. Dissolve 0.10 g of the substance to be examined in the mobile phase and dilute to 100.0 ml with the mobile phase.

Reference solution (a). Dilute 1.0 ml of the test solution to 10.0 ml with the mobile phase. Dilute 2.0 ml of the solution to 100.0 ml with the mobile phase.

Reference solution (b). Dissolve 1.0 mg of *maprotiline impurity D CRS* in the test solution and dilute to 10.0 ml with the same solution.

The chromatographic procedure may be carried out using:

– a stainless steel column 0.25 m long and 4.6 mm in internal diameter packed with *silica gel for chromatography R* (5 µm),

– as mobile phase a flow rate of 1 ml/min a mixture as prepared as follows: dissolve about 0.580 g of *ammonium acetate R* in 200 ml of *water R* and add 2 ml of a 70 g/l solution of *concentrated ammonia R*; add 150 ml of *2-propanol R* and 650 ml of *methanol R*; the resulting apparent pH value is between 8.2 and 8.4,

– as detector a spectrophotometer set at 272 nm.

When the chromatograms are recorded in the prescribed conditions, the retention time of maprotiline is about 10.3 min and retention times relative to maprotiline are: impurity A about 0.3, impurity B about 0.47, impurity C about 0.74, impurity D about 0.81, impurity E about 1.26.

Inject 20 µl of reference solution (b). Adjust the sensitivity of the system so that the height of the principal peak (maprotiline) in the chromatogram is at least 50 per cent of the full scale of the recorder. The test is not valid unless, in the chromatogram obtained, the resolution between the peaks corresponding to impurity D and maprotiline is between 1.8 and 3.2. If necessary adjust the mobile phase by adding a 50 per cent *V/V* solution of *acetic acid R* if the resolution is less than 1.8, or by adding a 70 g/l solution of *concentrated ammonia R* if the resolution is greater than 3.2, to adjust the pH in steps of 0.1 pH units. Inject 20 µl of the test solution and 20 µl of reference solution (a). Continue the chromatography of the test solution for 1.5 times the retention time of the principal peak. In the chromatogram obtained with the test solution: the area of any peak, apart from the principal peak, is not greater than the area of the principal peak in the chromatogram obtained with reference solution (a) (0.2 per cent); the sum of the areas of all the peaks, apart from the principal peak, is not greater than five times the area of the principal peak in the chromatogram obtained with reference solution (a) (1 per cent). Disregard any peak with an area less than 0.1 times that of the principal peak in the chromatogram obtained with reference solution (a).

Loss on drying (*2.2.32*). Not more than 1.0 per cent, determined on 1.000 g by drying in an oven at 80 °C at a pressure not exceeding 2.5 kPa for 6 h.

Sulphated ash (*2.4.14*). Not more than 0.1 per cent, determined on 1.0 g.

ASSAY

Dissolve 0.250 g in a mixture of 5 ml of *0.1 M hydrochloric acid* and 50 ml of *alcohol R*. Carry out a potentiometric titration (*2.2.20*), using *0.1 M sodium hydroxide*. Read the volume added between the two points of inflexion.

1 ml of *0.1 M sodium hydroxide* is equivalent to 31.39 mg of $C_{20}H_{24}ClN$.

IMPURITIES

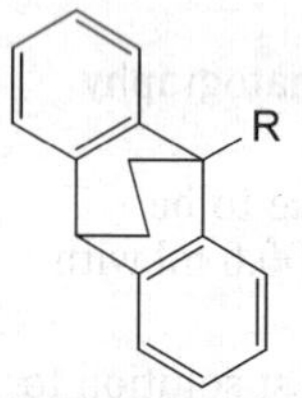

A. R = $CH=CH-CH=O$: 3-(9,10-ethanoanthracen-9(10*H*)-yl)prop-2-enal,

C. R = $CH_2-CH_2-CH_2-NH_2$: 3-(9,10-ethanoanthracen-9(10*H*)-yl)propan-1-amine,

D. R = $CH=CH-CH_2-NH-CH_3$: 3-(9,10-ethanoanthracen-9(10*H*)-yl)-*N*-methylprop-2-en-1-amine (dehydromaprotiline),

E. R = $CH_2-CH_2-CH_2-N(CH_3)_2$: 3-(9,10-ethanoanthracen-9(10*H*)-yl)-*N*,*N*-dimethylpropan-1-amine,

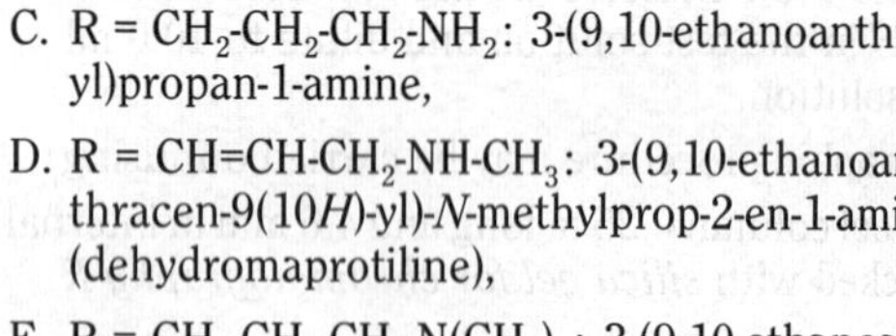

B. 3-(9,10-ethanoanthracen-9(10*H*)-yl)-*N*-[3-(9,10-ethanoanthracen-9(10*H*)-yl)propyl]-*N*-methylpropan-1-amine.

01/2005:1856

MARSHMALLOW LEAF

Althaeae folium

DEFINITION

Whole or cut dried leaf of *Althaea officinalis* L.

CHARACTERS

Macroscopic and microscopic characters described under identification tests A and B.

IDENTIFICATION

A. The leaves have long petioles and are about 7 cm to 10 cm long; the lamina is cordate to ovate with 3 to 5 shallow lobes and crenate to dentate margins; the venation is palmate. The petioles and both surfaces of the lamina are greyish-green and densely pubescent. Rarely, fragments of the inflorescence or immature fruits may be present.

B. Reduce to a powder (355). The powder is greyish-green. Examine under a microscope using *chloral hydrate solution R*. The powder shows numerous long, rigid, unicellular covering trichomes with thick walls, pointed at the apex, angular and pitted at the base where they are sometimes still united to form stellate structures with up to 8 components; few secretory trichomes with unicellular stalks and globular, multicellular heads; fragments of the leaf epidermis with anomocytic or paracytic stomata (*2.8.3*); cluster crystals of calcium oxalate, isolated or in the parenchyma of the mesophyll; fragments of veins with small, spiral or annular vessels. Examine under a microscope using *ruthenium red solution R*. The powder shows groups of parenchyma containing mucilage which stains orange-red.

C. Thin-layer chromatography (*2.2.27*).

Test solution. To 1 g of the powdered drug (355) add 10 ml of *methanol R*. Heat in a water-bath under a reflux condenser for 5 min. Cool and filter. Distil the filtrate under reduced pressure until the total volume is about 2 ml.

Reference solution. Dissolve 2.5 mg of *quercitrin R* and 2.5 mg of *chlorogenic acid R* in 10 ml of *methanol R*.

Plate: *TLC silica gel plate R.*

Mobile phase: *anhydrous formic acid R, glacial acetic acid R, water R, ethyl acetate R* (11:11:27:100 *V/V/V/V*).

Application: 10 µl, as bands.

Development: over a path of 15 cm.

Drying: at 100-105 °C.

Detection: spray with a 10 g/l solution of *diphenylboric acid aminoethyl ester R* in *methanol R*, then with a 50 g/l solution of *macrogol 400 R* in *methanol R*. Allow the plate to dry in air for 30 min. Examine in ultraviolet light at 365 nm.

Results: see below the sequence of the zones present in the chromatograms obtained with the reference solution and the test solution. Furthermore, other fluorescent zones may be present in the chromatogram obtained with the test solution.

Top of the plate	
	A blue fluorescent zone
	A yellow fluorescent zone
Quercitrin: an orange zone	
	An orange fluorescent zone
	An orange fluorescent zone
Chlorogenic acid: a blue fluorescent zone	
	A blue fluorescent zone
	An orange fluorescent zone
	An intense yellow fluorescent zone
Reference solution	**Test solution**

TESTS

Foreign matter (*2.8.2*): maximum 4 per cent of leaves infected by *Puccinia malvacearum*, showing red spots and maximum 2 per cent of other foreign matter.

Loss on drying (*2.2.32*): maximum 10.0 per cent, determined on 1.000 g of the powdered drug (355) by drying in an oven at 100-105 °C for 2 h.

Total ash (*2.4.16*): maximum 18.0 per cent.

Swelling index (*2.8.4*): minimum 12, determined on 0.2 g of the powdered drug (355).

Ash insoluble in hydrochloric acid (*2.8.1*): maximum 2.0 per cent.

01/2005:1126

MARSHMALLOW ROOT

Althaeae radix

DEFINITION

Marshmallow root consists of the peeled or unpeeled, whole or cut, dried root of *Althaea officinalis* L.

CHARACTERS

It has the macroscopic and microscopic characters described under identification tests A and B.

IDENTIFICATION

A. The unpeeled, non-fragmented drug consists of cylindrical, slightly twisted roots, up to 2 cm thick, with deep longitudinal furrows. The outer surface is greyish-brown and bears numerous rootlet scars. The fracture is fibrous externally, rugged and granular internally. The section shows a more or less thick, whitish bark with brownish periderm, separated by the well-marked, brownish cambium from a white xylem. The stratified structure of the bark and the radiate structure of xylem become more distinct when moistened.

The peeled drug has a greyish-white finely fibrous outer surface. Cork and external cortical parenchyma are absent.

B. Reduce to a powder (355). The powder is brownish-grey (unpeeled root) or whitish (peeled root). Examine under a microscope using *chloral hydrate solution R*. The powder shows the following diagnostic characters: fragments of colourless, mainly unlignified, thick-walled fibres with pointed or split ends; fragments of bordered, pitted or scalariformly thickened vessels; cluster crystals of calcium oxalate about 20 µm to 35 µm, mostly 25 µm to 30 µm in size; parenchymatous cells containing mucilage; fragments of cork with thin-walled, tabular cells in the unpeeled root. Examine under a microscope using *water R*. The powder shows numerous starch granules about 3 µm to 25 µm in size occasionally with a longitudinal hilum. The starch grains are mostly simple, a few being two to four compound.

TESTS

Foreign matter (*2.8.2*). Not more than 2 per cent of brown deteriorated drug. Not more than 2 per cent of cork in the peeled root.

Swelling index (*2.8.4*). Not less than 10, determined on the powdered drug (710).

Loss on drying (*2.2.32*). Not more than 12.0 per cent, determined on 1.000 g of powdered drug (710) by drying in an oven at 100 °C to 105 °C for 2 h.

Total ash (*2.4.16*). Not more than 6.0 per cent for peeled root and not more than 8.0 per cent for the unpeeled root.

STORAGE

Store protected from light.

01/2005:1876

MASTIC

Mastix

DEFINITION

Dried resinous exudate obtained from stems and branches of *Pistacia lentiscus* L. var. *latifolius* Coss.

Content: minimum 10 ml/kg of essential oil (anhydrous drug).

CHARACTERS

Macroscopic characters described under identification test A.

IDENTIFICATION

A. Small light yellow to greenish-yellow, non-uniform, spherical or pyriform, clear or opaque, hard glassy fragments.

B. Thin-layer chromatography (*2.2.27*).

Test solution. Dissolve 1 g of the substance to be examined in 10 ml of *methylene chloride R* and filter after 1-2 min.

Reference solution. Dissolve 25 mg of *eugenol R* and 25 mg of *borneol R* in 3 ml of *methylene chloride R*.

Plate: *TLC silica gel plate R*.

Mobile phase: *light petroleum R, toluene R* (5:95 *V/V*).

Application: 1 µl, as bands.

Development: over a path of 10 cm.

Drying: in air.

Detection: spray with *vanillin reagent R* and heat at 100-105 °C for 5 min.

Results: see below the sequence of the zones present in the chromatograms obtained with the reference solution and the test solution. Furthermore, other zones of various colours may be present in the chromatogram obtained with the test solution.

Top of the plate	
	A violet zone
_______	_______
	A pale violet zone
	A very pale violet zone
_______	_______
Eugenol: a brown zone	A blue zone
Borneol: a greenish-blue zone	A bluish-violet zone
	A dark violet zone
Reference solution	**Test solution**

TESTS

Acid value (*2.5.1*): 50 to 70, determined on 1.0 g.

Foreign matter (*2.8.2*): maximum 2 per cent *m/m*.

Water (*2.2.13*): maximum 10 ml/kg, determined on 25.0 g of the drug reduced to a coarse powder (1400).

Total ash (*2.4.16*): maximum 0.5 per cent.

ASSAY

Essential oil (*2.8.12*). Use a 500 ml round-bottomed flask and 200 ml of *water R* as the distillation liquid. Reduce the drug to a coarse powder (1400) and immediately use 20.0 g for the determination. Introduce 0.50 ml of *xylene R* in the graduated tube. Distil at a rate of 2-3 ml/min for 2 h.

STORAGE

Do not powder.

01/2005:0404

MATRICARIA FLOWER

Matricariae flos

DEFINITION

Dried capitula of *Matricaria recutita* L. (*Chamomilla recutita* (L.) Rauschert).

Content:

– blue essential oil: minimum 4 ml/kg (dried drug),

– total apigenin 7-glucoside ($C_{21}H_{20}O_{10}$): minimum 0.25 per cent (dried drug).

CHARACTERS

Macroscopic and microscopic characters described under identification tests A and B.

IDENTIFICATION

A. Capitula, when spread out, consisting of an involucre made up of many bracts arranged in 1 to 3 rows; an elongated-conical receptacle, occasionally hemispherical (young capitula); 12 to 20 marginal ligulate florets with a white ligule; several dozen yellow central tubular florets. The involucre bracts are ovate to lanceolate, with a brownish-grey scarious margin. The receptacle is hollow, without paleae. The corolla of the ligulate florets has a brownish-yellow tube at the base extending to form a white, elongated-oval ligule. The inferior ovary is dark brown, ovoid to spherical, and has a long style and bifid stigma. The tubular florets are yellow and have a five-toothed corolla tube, 5 syngenesious, epipetalous stamens and a gynoecium similar to that of the ligulate florets.

B. Separate the capitulum into its different parts. Examine under a microscope using *chloral hydrate solution R*. The bracts have a margin composed of thin-walled cells and a central region composed of elongated sclereids with occasional stomata. The inner epidermis of the corolla of the ligulate florets, in surface view, consisting of thin-walled, polygonal cells, slightly papillose, those of the outer epidermis markedly sinuous and strongly striated; corolla of the tubular florets with longitudinally elongated epidermal cells, and with small groups of papillae near the apex of the lobes. Glandular trichomes each consisting of a short stalk and a head of 2 to 3 tiers of 2 cells each occur on the outer surfaces of the bracts and on the corollas of both types of florets. The ovaries have a sclerous ring at the base and the wall is composed of vertical bands of thin-walled, longitudinally elongated cells with numerous glandular trichomes, alternating with fusiform groups of small, radially elongated cells containing mucilage. The cells at the apex of the stigmas are extended to form rounded papillae. Numerous small, cluster crystals of calcium oxalate occur in the inner tissues of the ovaries and the anther lobes. Pollen grains spherical to triangular, about 30 µm in diameter with 3 pores and a spiny exine.

C. Thin-layer chromatography (*2.2.27*).

Test solution. Dilute 50 µl of essential oil obtained in the assay of essential oil in 1 ml of *xylene R*.

Reference solution. Dissolve 2 µl of *chamazulene R*, 5 µl of *levomenol R* and 10 mg of *bornyl acetate R* in 5 ml of *toluene R*.

Plate: *TLC silica gel plate R.*

Mobile phase: *ethyl acetate R, toluene R* (5:95 *V/V*).

Application: 10 µl, as bands.

Development: over a path of 10 cm.

Drying: in air.

Detection: spray with *anisaldehyde solution R* and heat at 100-105 °C for 5-10 min. Examine immediately in daylight.

Results: see below the sequence of the zones present in the chromatograms obtained with the reference solution and the test solution. Furthermore, other zones are present in the chromatogram obtained with the test solution.

Top of the plate	
	1 or 2 blue to bluish-violet zones
Chamazulene: a red to reddish-violet zone	A red to reddish-violet zone (chamazulene)
Bornyl acetate: a yellowish-brown zone	
	A brown zone (en-yne-dicycloether)
Levomenol: a reddish-violet to bluish-violet zone	A reddish-violet to bluish-violet zone (levomenol)
Reference solution	**Test solution**

TESTS

Broken drug: maximum 25 per cent, determined on 20.0 g, passes through a sieve (710).

Foreign matter (*2.8.2*): maximum 2 per cent *m/m*.

Loss on drying (*2.2.32*): maximum 12.0 per cent, determined on 1.000 g of the powdered drug (355) by drying in an oven at 100-105 °C for 2 h.

Total ash (*2.4.16*): maximum 13.0 per cent.

ASSAY

Essential oil (*2.8.12*). Use 30 g of whole drug, a 1000 ml flask, 300 ml of *water R* as distillation liquid and 0.50 ml of *xylene R* in the graduated tube. Distil at a rate of 3-4 ml/min for 4 h. Towards the end of this period, stop the flow of water to the condenser assembly but continue distilling until the blue, steam-volatile components have reached the lower end of the condenser. Immediately re-start the flow of water to the condenser assembly to avoid warming the separation space. Stop the distillation after a further 10 min.

Total apigenin 7-glucoside. Liquid chromatography (*2.2.29*).

Test solution. Reduce 40 g of the drug to a powder (500). Place 2.00 g of the powdered drug in a 500 ml round-bottomed flask. Add 200 ml of *alcohol R*. Heat the mixture under a reflux condenser on a water-bath for 15 min. Cool and filter. Rinse the filter and the residue with a few millilitres of *alcohol R*. To the filtrate add 10 ml of freshly prepared *dilute sodium hydroxide solution R* and heat the mixture under a reflux condenser on a water-bath for about 1 h. Cool. Dilute to 250.0 ml with *alcohol R*. To 50.0 ml of the solution add 0.5 g of *citric acid R*. Shake for 5 min and filter. Dilute 5.0 ml to 10.0 ml with the mobile phase (initial mixture).

Reference solution (a). Dissolve 10.0 mg of *apigenin 7-glucoside R* in 100.0 ml of *methanol R*. Dilute 25.0 ml of this solution to 200 ml with the mobile phase (initial mixture).

Reference solution (b). Dissolve 10.0 mg of *5,7-dihydroxy-4-methylcoumarin R* in 100.0 ml of *methanol R*. Dilute 25.0 ml of this solution to 100 ml of the mobile phase (initial mixture). To 4.0 ml of this solution add 4.0 ml of reference solution (a) and dilute to 10.0 ml with the mobile phase (initial mixture).

Precolumn:

- *size*: l = 8 mm, Ø = 4.6 mm,
- *stationary phase*: *octadecylsilyl silica gel for chromatography R* (5 µm).

Column:

- *size*: l = 0.25 m, Ø = 4.6 mm,
- *stationary phase*: *octadecylsilyl silica gel for chromatography R* (5 µm).

Mobile phase:

- *mobile phase A*: *phosphoric acid R, water R* (0.5:99.5 *V/V*).
- *mobile phase B*: *phosphoric acid R, acetonitrile R* (0.5:99.5 *V/V*).

Time (min)	Mobile phase A (per cent *V/V*)	Mobile phase B (per cent *V/V*)
0 - 9	75	25
9 - 19	75 → 25	25 → 75
19 - 24	25	75
24 - 29	25 → 75	75 → 25
29 - 30	75 → 90	25 → 10

Flow rate: 1 ml/min.

Detection: spectrophotometer at 340 nm.

Injection: 20 µl.

System suitability: reference solution (b):

- *resolution*: minimum 1.8 between the peaks due to apigenin 7-glucoside and 5,7-dihydroxy-4-methylcoumarin.

Calculate the percentage content of total apigenin 7-glucoside from the expression:

$$\frac{A_1 \times m_2}{A_2 \times m_1} \times P \times 0.625$$

A_1 = area of the peak due to apigenin 7-glucoside in the chromatogram obtained with the test solution,

A_2 = area of the peak due to apigenin 7-glucoside in the chromatogram obtained with the reference solution,

m_1 = mass of the drug in the test solution, in grams,

m_2 = mass of *apigenin 7-glucoside R* in reference solution (a), in grams,

P = percentage content of apigenin 7-glucoside in the reagent.

01/2005:1544

MATRICARIA LIQUID EXTRACT

Matricariae extractum fluidum

DEFINITION

Matricaria liquid extract is produced from *Matricaria flower (0404)*. It contains not less than 0.30 per cent of blue residual oil.

PRODUCTION

The extract is produced from the drug and a mixture of 2.5 parts of a 10 per cent *m/m* solution of ammonia (NH_3), 47.5 parts of water and 50 parts of alcohol with an appropriate procedure for liquid extracts.

CHARACTERS

A brownish, clear liquid with an intense characteristic odour and characteristic bitter taste; miscible with water and with alcohol with development of turbidity, soluble in alcohol (50 per cent *V/V*).

IDENTIFICATION

A. Examine by thin-layer chromatography (*2.2.27*), using a *TLC silica gel* F_{254} *plate R*.

Test solution. Place 10 ml of the extract in a separating funnel and shake with 2 quantities, each of 10 ml, of *pentane R*. Combine the pentane layers, dry over 2 g of *anhydrous sodium sulphate R* and filter. Evaporate the filtrate to dryness on a water-bath and dissolve the residue in 0.5 ml of *toluene R*.

Reference solution. Dissolve 4 mg of *guaiazulene R*, 20 mg of *levomenol R* and 20 mg of *bornyl acetate R* in 10 ml of *toluene R*.

Apply to the plate as bands 10 µl of each solution. Develop over a path of 10 cm using a mixture of 5 volumes of *ethyl acetate R* and 95 volumes of *toluene R*. Allow the plate to dry in air and examine in ultraviolet light at 254 nm. The chromatogram obtained with the test solution shows several quenching zones, of which 2 main zones are in the middle third (en-yne-dicycloether). Examine in ultraviolet light at 365 nm. The chromatogram obtained with the test solution shows in the middle part an intense blue fluorescent zone (herniarin). Spray the plate with *anisaldehyde solution R*. Examine in daylight while heating at 100-105 °C for 5-10 min. The chromatogram obtained with the reference solution shows in the lower third a reddish-violet to bluish-violet zone (levomenol), in the middle third a yellowish-brown to greyish-green zone (bornyl acetate) and in the upper third a red to reddish-violet zone (guaiazulene). The chromatogram obtained with the test solution shows in the lower third yellowish-brown to greenish-yellow and violet zones and a reddish-violet to bluish-violet zone corresponding to levomenol in the chromatogram obtained with the reference solution; a brownish zone (en-yne-dicycloether) similar in position to bornyl acetate in the chromatogram obtained with the reference solution; a red or reddish-violet zone (chamazulene) corresponding to guaiazulene in the chromatogram obtained with the reference solution and immediately above it 1 or 2 blue to bluish-violet zones; further weak zones may be present in the chromatogram obtained with the test solution.

B. Examine by thin-layer chromatography (*2.2.27*), using a *TLC silica gel plate R*.

Test solution. Use the extract.

Monographs M

Reference solution. Dissolve 1.0 mg of *chlorogenic acid R*, 2.5 mg of *hyperoside R* and 2.5 mg of *rutin R* in 10 ml of *methanol R*.

Apply to the plate as bands 10 µl of each solution. Develop over a path of 15 cm using a mixture of 7.5 volumes of *anhydrous formic acid R*, 7.5 volumes of *glacial acetic acid R*, 18 volumes of *water R*, and 67 volumes of *ethyl acetate R*. Dry the plate at 100-105 °C and spray the warm plate with a 10 g/l solution of *diphenylboric acid aminoethyl ester R* in *methanol R*. Subsequently spray the plate with a 50 g/l solution of *macrogol 400 R* in *methanol R*. Allow the plate to dry in air for about 30 min and examine in ultraviolet light at 365 nm. The chromatogram obtained with the reference solution shows in the middle part a light blue fluorescent zone (chlorogenic acid), below it a yellowish-brown fluorescent zone (rutin) and above it a yellowish-brown fluorescent zone (hyperoside). The chromatogram obtained with the test solution shows a yellowish-brown fluorescent zone corresponding to the zone of rutin in the chromatogram obtained with the reference solution, a light blue fluorescent zone corresponding to the zone of chlorogenic acid in the chromatogram obtained with the reference solution, a yellowish-brown fluorescent zone similar in position to the zone of hyperoside in the chromatogram obtained with the reference solution; it also shows above the yellowish-brown fluorescent zone a green fluorescent zone, then several bluish or greenish fluorescent zones and near the solvent front a yellowish fluorescent zone.

TESTS

Ethanol (*2.9.10*): 38 per cent *V/V* to 53 per cent *V/V*.

Dry residue (*2.8.16*): minimum 12.0 per cent.

ASSAY

Place 20.0 g in a 1000 ml round-bottomed flask, add 300 ml of *water R* and distil until 200 ml has been collected in a flask. Transfer the distillate into a separating funnel. Dissolve 65 g of *sodium chloride R* in the distillate and shake with 3 quantities, each of 30 ml, of *pentane R* previously used to rinse the reflux condenser and the flask. Combine the pentane layers, dry over 2 g of *anhydrous sodium sulphate R* and filter into a tared 100 ml round-bottomed flask which has been dried in a desiccator for 3 h. Rinse the anhydrous sodium sulphate and the filter with 2 quantities, each of 20 ml, of *pentane R*. Evaporate the pentane in a water-bath at 45 °C. The residue of pentane is eliminated in a current of air for 3 min. Dry the flask in a desiccator for 3 h and weigh. The residual oil is blue (chamazulene).

01/2005:1836

MATRICARIA OIL

Matricariae aetheroleum

DEFINITION

Blue essential oil obtained by steam distillation from the fresh or dried flower-heads or flowering tops of *Matricaria recutita* L. (*Chamomilla recutita* L. Rauschert). There are 2 types of matricaria oil which are characterised as rich in bisabolol oxides, or rich in levomenol.

CHARACTERS

Appearance: clear, intensely blue, viscous liquid.

It has an intense characteristic odour.

IDENTIFICATION

First identification: B.

Second identification: A.

A. Thin-layer chromatography (*2.2.27*).

Test solution. Dissolve 20 µl of the substance to be examined in 1.0 ml of *toluene R*.

Reference solution. Dissolve 2 mg of *guaiazulene R*, 5 µl of *levomenol R* and 10 mg of *bornyl acetate R* in 5.0 ml of *toluene R*.

Plate: *TLC silica gel plate R.*

Mobile phase: *ethyl acetate R, toluene R* (5:95 *V/V*).

Application: 10 µl, as bands.

Development: over a path of 10 cm.

Drying: in air.

Detection A: examine in daylight.

Results A: see below for the sequence of the zones present in the chromatograms obtained with the reference solution and the test solution.

Top of the plate	
Guaiazulene: a blue zone	A blue zone (chamazulene)
_______	_______
_______	_______
Reference solution	**Test solution**

Detection B: spray with *anisaldehyde solution R* and heat at 100-105 °C for 5-10 min. Examine immediately in daylight.

Results B: see below for the sequence of the zones present in the chromatograms obtained with the reference solution and the test solution. Furthermore, yellowish-brown to greenish-yellow zones (lower third), violet zones (lower third) and further weak zones may be present in the chromatogram obtained with the test solution.

Top of the plate	
	1 or 2 blue to bluish-violet zones
Guaiazulene: a red to reddish-violet zone	A red to reddish-violet zone (chamazulene)
_______	_______
Bornyl acetate: a yellowish-brown to greyish-green zone	A brown zone (en-yne-dicycloether)
	_______
Levomenol: a reddish-violet to bluish-violet zone	A reddish-violet to bluish-violet zone (levomenol)
	A brownish zone
Reference solution	**Test solution**

B. Examine the chromatograms obtained in the test for chromatographic profile.

Results: the characteristic peaks corresponding to levomenol and to chamazulene in the chromatogram obtained with the test solution are similar in retention time to those in the chromatogram obtained with the reference solution.

TESTS

Chromatographic profile. Gas chromatography (*2.2.28*): use the normalisation procedure.

Test solution. Dissolve 20 µl of the oil to be examined in *cyclohexane R* and dilute to 5.0 ml with the same solvent.

Reference solution. Dissolve 20 µl of *levomenol R*, 5 mg of *chamazulene R* and 6 mg of *guaiazulene R* in *cyclohexane R* and dilute to 5.0 ml with the same solvent.

Column:

– *material*: fused silica,
– *size*: *l* = 30 m (a film thickness of 1 µm may be used) to 60 m (a film thickness of 0.2 µm may be used), Ø = 0.25-0.53 mm, when using a column longer than 30 m, an adjustment of the temperature programme may be necessary,
– *stationary phase*: *macrogol 20 000 R*.

Carrier gas: *helium for chromatography R*.

Flow rate: 1-2 ml/min.

Split ratio: 1:100.

Temperature:

	Time (min)	Temperature (°C)
Column	0 – 40	70 → 230
	40 – 50	230
Injection port		250
Detector		250

Detection: flame ionisation.

Injection: 1.0 µl.

Elution order: order indicated in the composition of the reference solution. Record the retention times of these substances.

Relative retention with reference to chamazulene (retention time = about 34.4 min): β-farnesene = about 0.5; bisabolol oxide B = about 0.8; bisabolone = about 0.87; levomenol = about 0.9; bisabolol oxide A = about 1.02.

System suitability: reference solution:

– *resolution*: minimum of 1.5 between the peaks due to chamazulene and to guaiazulene.

Using the retention times determined from the chromatogram obtained with the reference solution, locate levomenol and chamazulene in the chromatogram obtained with the test solution; locate bisabolol oxides (bisabolol oxide B, bisabolone and bisabolol oxide A) using Figures 1836.-1 and 1836.-2 (disregard the peak due to cyclohexane). The chromatogram obtained with the test solution does not show a peak with the retention time of guaiazulene.

Determine the percentage content of the components. The limits are within the following ranges.

	Matricaria oil rich in bisabolol oxides (per cent)	Matricaria oil rich in levomenol (per cent)
Bisabolol oxides	29 - 81	
Levomenol		10 - 65
Chamazulene	≥ 1.0	≥ 1.0
Total of bisabolol oxides and levomenol		≥ 20

STORAGE

In a well-filled, airtight container, protected from light at a temperature not exceeding 25 °C.

LABELLING

The label states the type of matricaria oil (rich in bisabolol oxides or rich in levomenol).

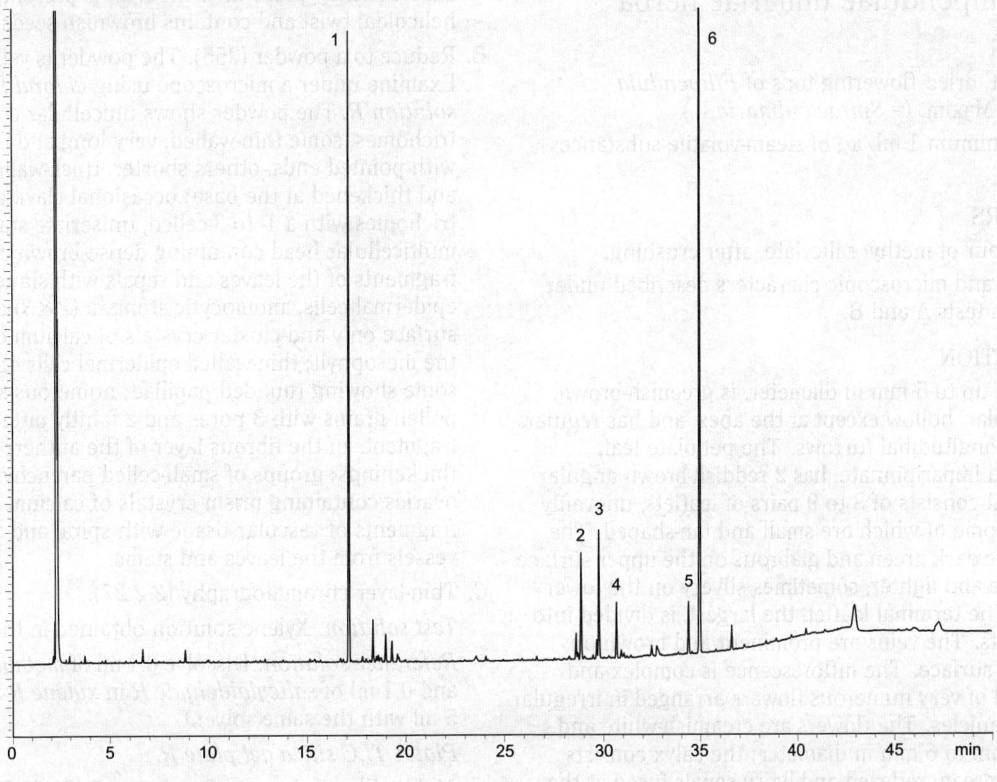

1. β-farnesene
2. bisabolol oxide B
3. bisabolone
4. levomenol
5. chamazulene
6. bisabolol oxide A

Figure 1836.-1. – *Chromatogram of matricaria oil rich in bisabolol oxides*

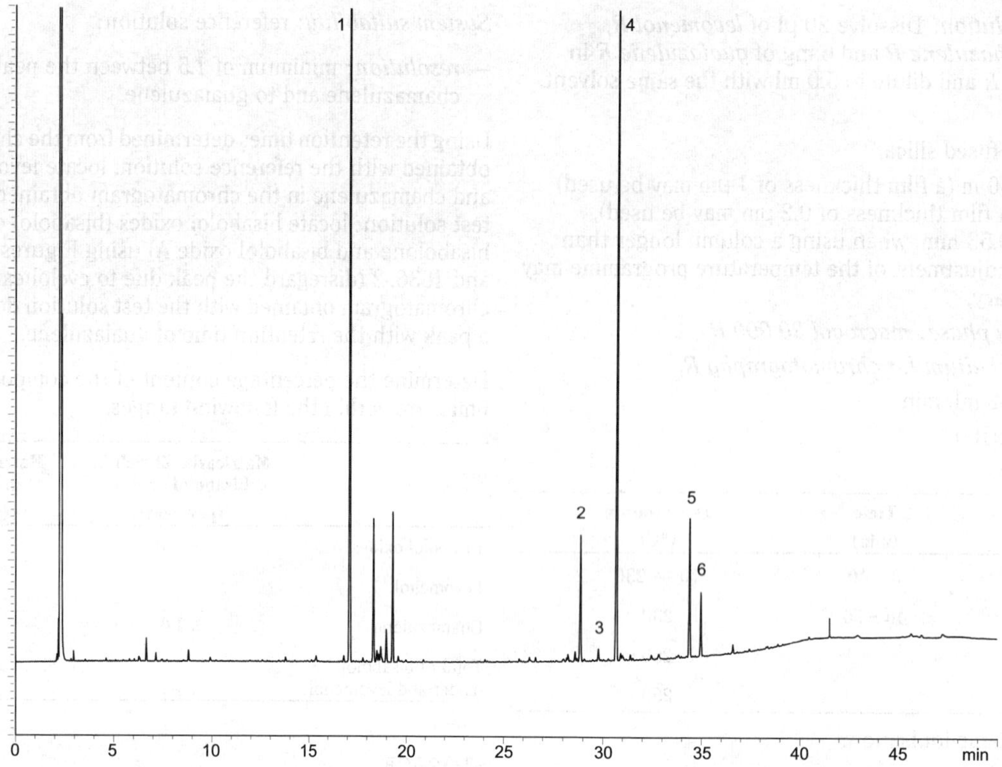

1. β-farnesene
2. bisabolol oxide B
3. bisabolone
4. levomenol
5. chamazulene
6. bisabolol oxide A

Figure 1836.-2. – *Chromatogram of matricaria oil rich in levomenol*

01/2005:1868

MEADOWSWEET

Filipendulae ulmariae herba

DEFINITION

Whole or cut, dried flowering tops of *Filipendula ulmaria* (L.) Maxim. (= *Spiraea ulmaria* L.).

Content: minimum 1 ml/kg of steam-volatile substances (dried drug).

CHARACTERS

Aromatic odour of methyl salicylate, after crushing.

Macroscopic and microscopic characters described under identification tests A and B.

IDENTIFICATION

A. The stem, up to 5 mm in diameter, is greenish-brown, stiff, angular, hollow except at the apex, and has regular, straight, longitudinal furrows. The petiolate leaf, compound imparipinnate, has 2 reddish-brown angular stipules. It consists of 3 to 9 pairs of leaflets, unevenly dentate, some of which are small and fan-shaped. The leaflets are dark green and glabrous on the upper surface, tomentose and lighter, sometimes silvery on the lower surface. The terminal leaflet, the largest, is divided into 3 segments. The veins are prominent and brown on the lower surface. The inflorescence is complex and composed of very numerous flowers arranged in irregular cymose panicles. The flowers are creamish-white and about 3 mm to 6 mm in diameter; the calyx consists of 5 dark green, reflexed and hairy sepals fused at the base to a concave receptacle; the 5 free petals, which are readily detached, are pale yellow, obovate and distinctly narrowed at the base; the stamens are numerous with rounded anthers and they extend beyond the petals; the gynoecium consists of about 4 to 6 carpels, each with a short style and a globular stigma; the carpels become twisted together spirally to form yellowish-brown fruits with a helicoidal twist. Unopened flower buds are frequently present. If the fruit is present, it has a helicoidal twist and contains brownish seeds.

B. Reduce to a powder (355). The powder is yellowish-green. Examine under a microscope using *chloral hydrate solution R*. The powder shows unicellular covering trichomes, some thin-walled, very long and flexuous, with pointed ends, others shorter, thick-walled, conical and thickened at the base; occasional clavate glandular trichomes with a 1- to 3-celled, uniseriate stalk and a multicellular head containing dense brown contents; fragments of the leaves and sepals with sinuous to wavy epidermal cells, anomocytic stomata (*2.8.3*) on the lower surface only and cluster crystals of calcium oxalate in the mesophyll; thin-walled epidermal cells of the petals, some showing rounded papillae; numerous spherical pollen grains with 3 pores and a faintly pitted exine; fragments of the fibrous layer of the anthers with stellate thickenings; groups of small-celled parenchyma from the ovaries containing prism crystals of calcium oxalate; fragments of vascular tissue with spiral and annular vessels from the leaves and stems.

C. Thin-layer chromatography (*2.2.27*).

Test solution. Xylene solution obtained in the assay.

Reference solution. Dissolve 0.1 ml of *methyl salicylate R* and 0.1 ml of *salicylaldehyde R* in *xylene R* and dilute to 5 ml with the same solvent.

Plate: *TLC silica gel plate R*.

Mobile phase: *hexane R, toluene R* (50:50 *V/V*).

Application: 10 μl, as bands.

Development: over a path of 10 cm.

Drying: in air.

Detection: spray the plate with 3 ml of *ferric chloride solution R3* and examine in daylight.

Results: see below the sequence of the zones present in the chromatograms obtained with the reference solution and the test solution. Furthermore, other zones are present in the chromatogram obtained with the test solution.

Top of the plate	
___	___
Methyl salicylate: a violet-brown zone	A violet-brown zone (methyl salicylate)
Salicylaldehyde: a violet-brown zone	A violet-brown zone (salicylaldehyde)
Reference solution	**Test solution**

TESTS

Foreign matter (*2.8.2*): maximum 5.0 per cent of stems with a diameter greater than 5 mm and maximum 2.0 per cent of foreign matter.

Loss on drying (*2.2.32*): maximum 12.0 per cent, determined on 1.000 g of the powdered drug (355) by drying in an oven at 100-105 °C for 2 h.

Total ash (*2.4.16*): maximum 7.0 per cent.

ASSAY

Examine according to the method described for the determination of essential oils in vegetable drugs (*2.8.12*). Use 50.0 g, a 1000 ml flask and 300 ml of *dilute hydrochloric acid R* as distillation liquid and 0.5 ml of *xylene R* in the graduated tube. Distil at a rate of 2-3 ml/min for 2 h.

01/2005:0845

MEBENDAZOLE

Mebendazolum

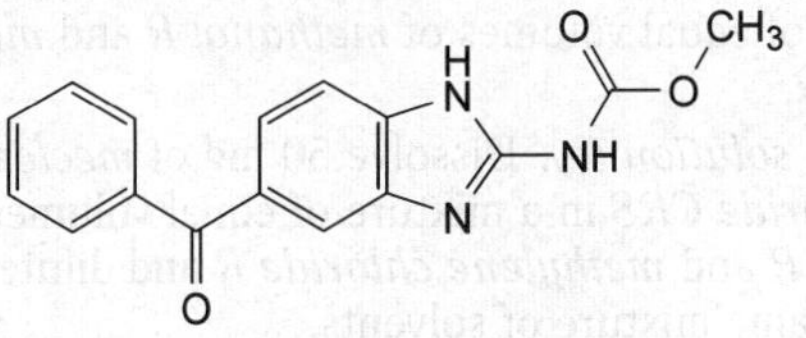

$C_{16}H_{13}N_3O_3$ M_r 295.3

DEFINITION

Methyl (5-benzoyl-1*H*-benzimidazol-2-yl)carbamate.

Content: 99.0 per cent to 101.0 per cent (dried substance).

CHARACTERS

Appearance: white or almost white powder.

Solubility: practically insoluble in water, in alcohol and in methylene chloride.

It shows polymorphism.

IDENTIFICATION

Infrared absorption spectrophotometry (*2.2.24*).

Comparison: *Ph. Eur. reference spectrum of mebendazole.*

TESTS

Related substances. Liquid chromatography (*2.2.29*).

Test solution. Dissolve 25.0 mg of the substance to be examined in *dimethylformamide R* and dilute to 25.0 ml with the same solvent.

Reference solution (a). Dissolve 5.0 mg of *mebendazole for system suitability CRS* in *dimethylformamide R* and dilute to 5.0 ml with the same solvent.

Reference solution (b). Dilute 1.0 ml of the test solution to 100.0 ml with *dimethylformamide R*. Dilute 5.0 ml of this solution to 20.0 ml with *dimethylformamide R*.

Column:

– *size*: *l* = 0.10 m, Ø = 4.6 mm,
– *stationary phase*: *base-deactivated octadecylsilyl silica gel for chromatography R* (3 µm),
– *temperature*: 40 °C.

Mobile phase:

– *mobile phase A*: 7.5 g/l solution of *ammonium acetate R*,
– *mobile phase B*: *acetonitrile R*,

Time (min)	Mobile phase A (per cent *V/V*)	Mobile phase B (per cent *V/V*)
0 - 15	80 → 70	20 → 30
15 - 20	70 → 10	30 → 90
20 - 25	10	90
25 - 26	10 → 80	90 → 20
26 - 30	80	20

Flow rate: 1.2 ml/min.

Detection: spectrophotometer at 250 nm.

Injection: 10 µl.

System suitability: reference solution (a):

– the chromatogram obtained is similar to the chromatogram supplied with *mebendazole for system suitability CRS.*

Limits:

– *correction factor*: for the calculation of content, multiply the peak area of impurity G by 1.4,
– *impurity G*: not more than twice the area of the principal peak in the chromatogram obtained with reference solution (b) (0.5 per cent),
– *any other impurity*: not more than the area of the principal peak in the chromatogram obtained with reference solution (b) (0.25 per cent),
– *total*: not more than 4 times the area of the principal peak in the chromatogram obtained with reference solution (b) (1.0 per cent),
– *disregard limit*: 0.2 times the area of the principal peak in the chromatogram obtained with reference solution (b) (0.05 per cent).

Loss on drying (*2.2.32*): maximum 0.5 per cent, determined on 1.000 g by drying in an oven at 100-105 °C for 4 h.

Sulphated ash (*2.4.14*): maximum 0.1 per cent, determined on 1.0 g.

ASSAY

Dissolve 0.250 g in 3 ml of *anhydrous formic acid R* and add 50 ml of a mixture of 1 volume of *anhydrous acetic acid R* and 7 volumes of *methyl ethyl ketone R*. Titrate with *0.1 M perchloric acid*, determining the end-point potentiometrically (*2.2.20*).

1 ml of *0.1 M perchloric acid* is equivalent to 29.53 mg of $C_{16}H_{13}N_3O_3$.

STORAGE

Protected from light.

IMPURITIES

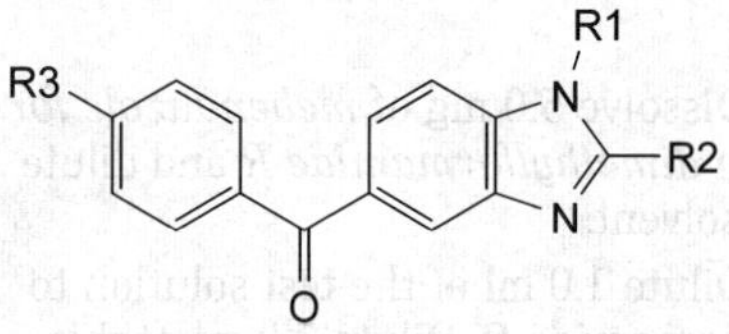

A. R1 = R3 = H, R2 = NH_2: (2-amino-1*H*-benzimidazol-5-yl)phenylmethanone,

B. R1 = R3 = H, R2 = OH: (2-hydroxy-1*H*-benzimidazol-5-yl)phenylmethanone,

C. R1 = CH_3, R2 = NH_2, R3 = H: (2-amino-1-methyl-1*H*-benzimidazol-5-yl)phenylmethanone,

D. R1 = CH_3, R2 = NH-CO-OCH_3, R3 = H: methyl (5-benzoyl-1-methyl-1*H*-benzimidazol-2-yl)carbamate,

E. R1 = R3 = H, R2 = NH-CO-OC_2H_5: ethyl (5-benzoyl-1*H*-benzimidazol-2-yl)carbamate,

F. R1 = H, R2 = NH-CO-OCH_3, R3 = CH_3: methyl [5-(4-methylbenzoyl)-1*H*-benzimidazol-2-yl]carbamate,

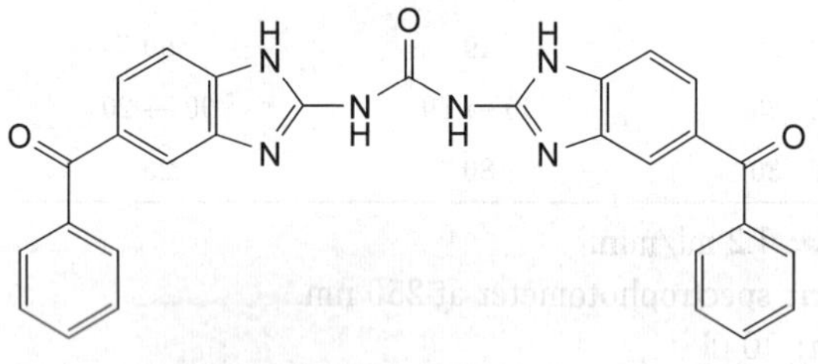

G. *N,N'*-bis(5-benzoyl-1*H*-benzimidazol-2-yl)urea.

01/2005:0622

MECLOZINE HYDROCHLORIDE

Meclozini hydrochloridum

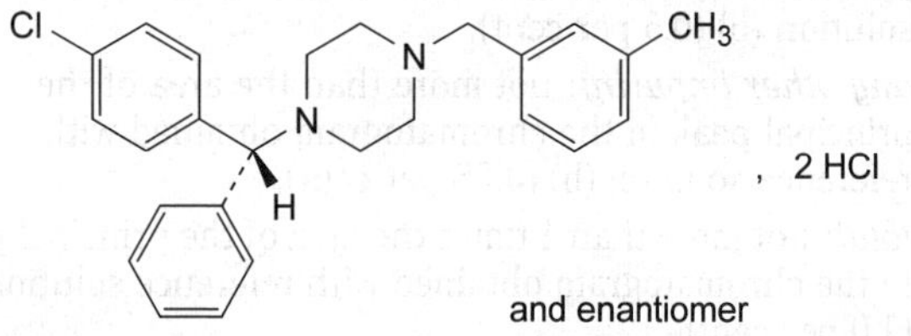

and enantiomer

$C_{25}H_{29}Cl_3N_2$ M_r 463.9

DEFINITION

Meclozine hydrochloride contains not less than 98.0 per cent and not more than the equivalent of 102.0 per cent of 1-[(*RS*)-(4-chlorophenyl)phenylmethyl]-4-(3-methylbenzyl)piperazine dihydrochloride, calculated with reference to the anhydrous substance.

CHARACTERS

A yellow or yellowish-white, crystalline powder, slightly soluble in water, soluble in alcohol and in methylene chloride.

IDENTIFICATION

First identification: B, D.

Second identification: A, C, D.

A. Dissolve 15.0 mg in *0.1 M hydrochloric acid* and dilute to 100.0 ml with the same acid. Dilute 10.0 ml of this solution to 100.0 ml with *0.1 M hydrochloric acid*. Examined between 220 nm and 350 nm (*2.2.25*), the solution shows an absorption maximum at 232 nm and weak absorbance without a defined maximum between 260 nm and 300 nm. The specific absorbance at the maximum is 345 to 380, calculated with reference to the anhydrous substance.

B. Examine by infrared absorption spectrophotometry (*2.2.24*), comparing with the spectrum obtained with *meclozine hydrochloride CRS*. Examine the substances prepared as discs using *potassium chloride R*.

C. Examine the chromatograms obtained in the test for related substances. The principal spot in the chromatogram obtained with test solution (b) is similar in position, colour and size to the principal spot in the chromatogram obtained with reference solution (a).

D. Dissolve about 15 mg in 2 ml of *alcohol R*. The solution gives reaction (a) of chlorides (*2.3.1*).

TESTS

Appearance of solution. Dissolve 0.50 g in *alcohol R* and dilute to 25 ml with the same solvent. The solution is clear (*2.2.1*) and not more intensely coloured than reference solution Y_6 (*2.2.2, Method II*).

Acidity or alkalinity. Calculate the acidity or alkalinity from the titration volumes noted in the Assay using the equation:

$$A = V_2 - 2V_1$$

V_1 = volume of *0.1 M sodium hydroxide* added at the first point of inflexion,

V_2 = volume of *0.1 M sodium hydroxide* added at the second point of inflexion.

A is − 0.3 ml to 0.3 ml for 0.3500 g of the substance to be examined.

Related substances. Examine by thin-layer chromatography (*2.2.27*), using *silica gel G R* as the coating substance.

Test solution (a). Dissolve 0.50 g of the substance to be examined in a mixture of equal volumes of *methanol R* and *methylene chloride R* and dilute to 10 ml with the same mixture of solvents.

Test solution (b). Dilute 1 ml of test solution (a) to 10 ml with a mixture of equal volumes of *methanol R* and *methylene chloride R*.

Reference solution (a). Dissolve 50 mg of *meclozine hydrochloride CRS* in a mixture of equal volumes of *methanol R* and *methylene chloride R* and dilute to 10 ml with the same mixture of solvents.

Reference solution (b). Dilute 0.5 ml of test solution (b) to 10 ml with a mixture of equal volumes of *methanol R* and *methylene chloride R*.

Apply separately to the plate 10 µl of each solution. Develop over a path of 15 cm using a mixture of 0.5 volumes of *concentrated ammonia R*, 5 volumes of *methanol R*, 30 volumes of *toluene R* and 60 volumes of *methylene chloride R*. Allow the plate to dry in air and spray with *dilute potassium iodobismuthate solution R*. Any spot in the chromatogram obtained with test solution (a), apart from the principal spot, is not more intense than the spot in the chromatogram obtained with reference solution (b) (0.5 per cent). Disregard any yellowish-white spot at the starting point.

Water (*2.5.12*). Not more than 5.0 per cent, determined on 0.200 g by the semi-micro determination of water.

Sulphated ash (*2.4.14*). Not more than 0.1 per cent, determined on 1.0 g.

ASSAY

Dissolve 0.3500 g in 50 ml of *alcohol R*. Carry out a potentiometric titration (*2.2.20*), using *0.1 M sodium hydroxide*. Read the volume added between the two points of inflexion.

1 ml of *0.1 M sodium hydroxide* is equivalent to 46.39 mg of $C_{25}H_{29}Cl_3N_2$.

STORAGE

Store in an airtight container.

01/2005:0673

MEDROXYPROGESTERONE ACETATE

Medroxyprogesteroni acetas

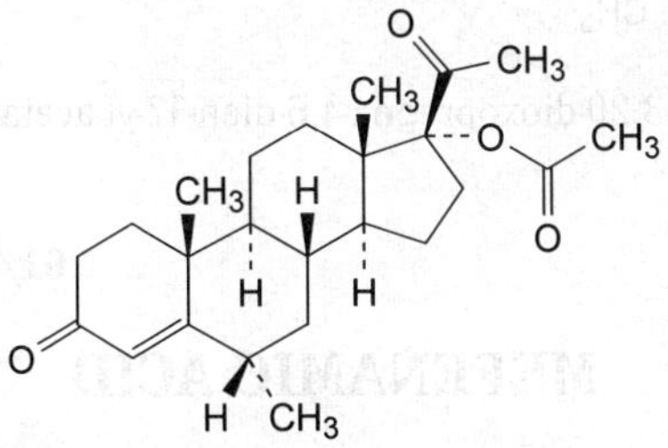

$C_{24}H_{34}O_4$ M_r 386.5

DEFINITION

Medroxyprogesterone acetate contains not less than 97.0 per cent and not more than the equivalent of 103.0 per cent of 6α-methyl-3,20-dioxopregn-4-en-17-yl acetate, calculated with reference to the dried substance.

CHARACTERS

A white or almost white, crystalline powder, practically insoluble in water, freely soluble in methylene chloride, soluble in acetone and in dioxan, sparingly soluble in alcohol.

IDENTIFICATION

First identification: A, B.

Second identification: A, C.

A. Melting point (*2.2.14*): 205 °C to 209 °C.

B. Examine by infrared absorption spectrophotometry (*2.2.24*), comparing with the spectrum obtained with *medroxyprogesterone acetate CRS*.

C. Examine the chromatogram obtained in the test for impurity F after spraying at 365 nm. The principal spot in the chromatogram obtained with test solution (b) is similar in position, fluorescence in ultraviolet light at 365 nm and size to the principal spot in the chromatogram obtained with reference solution (b).

TESTS

Specific optical rotation (*2.2.7*). Dissolve 0.250 g in *dioxan R* and dilute to 25.0 ml with the same solvent. The specific optical rotation is + 45 to + 51, calculated with reference to the dried substance.

Impurity F (6α-methyl-3,20-dioxo-5β-pregnan-17-yl acetate). Examine by thin-layer chromatography (*2.2.27*), using a *TLC silica gel plate R*.

Test solution (a). Dissolve 0.200 g of the substance to be examined in *methylene chloride R* and dilute to 10.0 ml with the same solvent.

Test solution (b). Dilute 1 ml of test solution (a) to 20 ml with *methylene chloride R*.

Reference solution (a). Add to 20.0 mg of *medroxyprogesterone acetate for performance test CRS* (containing 0.5 per cent of impurity F) 1.0 ml of *methylene chloride R* and dissolve.

Reference solution (b). Dissolve 10 mg of *medroxyprogesterone acetate CRS* in *methylene chloride R* and dilute to 10 ml with the same solvent.

Apply separately to the plate 10 µl of each solution. Develop over a path of 10 cm using a mixture of 10 volumes of *tetrahydrofuran R*, 45 volumes of *1,1-dimethylethyl methyl ether R* and 45 volumes of *hexane R*. Allow the plate to dry in air and carry out a second development in the same direction over a path of 10 cm with the same mixture. Allow the plate to dry at 120 °C for 10 min. Spray with a 200 g/l solution of *toluenesulphonic acid R* in *alcohol R*. Heat at 120 °C for 10 min. Allow to cool. Examine the chromatograms in ultraviolet light at 365 nm. In the chromatogram obtained with test solution (a) any blue fluorescent spot with an R_f value higher than the principal spot due to medroxyprogesterone acetate is not more intense than the corresponding blue fluorescent spot of impurity F in the chromatogram obtained with reference solution (a) (0.5 per cent). The test is not valid unless the chromatogram obtained with reference solution (a) shows two clearly separated spots.

Related substances. Examine by liquid chromatography (*2.2.29*).

Test solution. Dissolve 25.0 mg of the substance to be examined in 1 ml of *tetrahydrofuran R* and dilute to 10.0 ml with the mobile phase.

Reference solution (a). Dissolve 2 mg of *medroxyprogesterone acetate CRS* and 5 mg of *megestrol acetate CRS* in the mobile phase and dilute to 100.0 ml with the mobile phase.

Reference solution (b). Dilute 1.0 ml of the test solution to 100.0 ml with the mobile phase.

The chromatographic procedure may be carried out using:

– a stainless steel column 0.25 m long and 4.6 mm in internal diameter packed with *base-deactivated end-capped octadecylsilyl silica gel for chromatography R* (5 µm),

– as mobile phase at a flow rate of 2 ml/min a mixture prepared as follows: in a 1000 ml volumetric flask mix 100 ml of *tetrahydrofuran R* with 350 ml of *acetonitrile R* and 500 ml of *water R*; allow to equilibrate and adjust the volume to 1000 ml with *water R* and mix again,

– as detector a spectrophotometer set at 254 nm,

maintaining the temperature of the column at 40 °C.

Equilibrate the column with the mobile phase at a flow rate of 2 ml/min for about 30 min.

Adjust the sensitivity of the system so that the height of the principal peak in the chromatogram obtained with 20 µl of reference solution (b) is at least 50 per cent of the full scale of the recorder.

Inject 20 µl of reference solution (a). When the chromatograms are recorded in the prescribed conditions, the retention times are: megestrol acetate about 14.5 min and medroxyprogesterone acetate about 16.5 min. The test is not valid unless the resolution between the peaks corresponding to megestrol acetate and medroxyprogesterone acetate is at least 3.3. If necessary, adjust the concentration of acetonitrile and/or tetrahydrofuran in the mobile phase.

Inject 20 µl of the solvent mixture of the test solution as a blank, 20 µl of the test solution and 20 µl of reference solution (b). Continue the chromatography of the test

Monographs M

solution for 1.5 times the retention time of the principal peak. In the chromatogram obtained with the test solution: the area of any peak, apart from the principal peak, is not greater than the area of the principal peak in the chromatogram obtained with reference solution (b) (1 per cent); the sum of the areas of all the peaks, apart from the principal peak, is not greater than 1.5 times the area of the principal peak in the chromatogram obtained with reference solution (b) (1.5 per cent). Disregard any peak due to the blank and any peak with an area less than 0.05 times the area of the principal peak in the chromatogram obtained with reference solution (b).

Loss on drying (*2.2.32*). Not more than 1.0 per cent, determined on 0.500 g by drying in an oven at 100 °C to 105 °C for 3 h.

ASSAY

Dissolve 50.0 mg in *alcohol R* and dilute to 50.0 ml with the same solvent. Dilute 2.0 ml of the solution to 100.0 ml with *alcohol R*. Measure the absorbance (*2.2.25*) at the maximum at 241 nm.

Calculate the content of $C_{24}H_{34}O_4$, taking the specific absorbance to be 420.

STORAGE

Store protected from light.

IMPURITIES

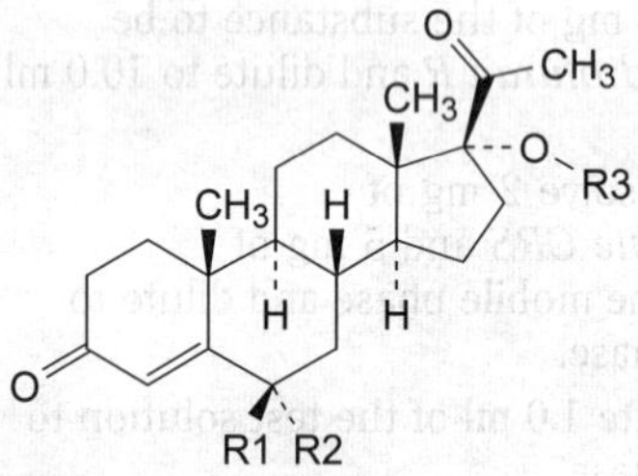

A. R1 = OH, R2 = CH_3, R3 = CO-CH_3: 6β-hydroxy-6-methyl-3,20-dioxopregn-4-en-17-yl acetate (6β-hydroxymedroxyprogesterone acetate),

B. R1 = H, R2 = CH_3, R3 = H: 17-hydroxy-6α-methylpregn-4-ene-3,20-dione (medroxyprogesterone),

D. R1 = CH_3, R2 = H, R3 = CO-CH_3: 6β-methyl-3,20-dioxopregn-4-en-17-yl acetate (6-epimedroxyprogesterone acetate),

E. R1 + R2 = CH_2, R3 = CO-CH_3: 6-methylene-3,20-dioxopregn-4-en-17-yl acetate (6-methylenehydroxyprogesterone acetate),

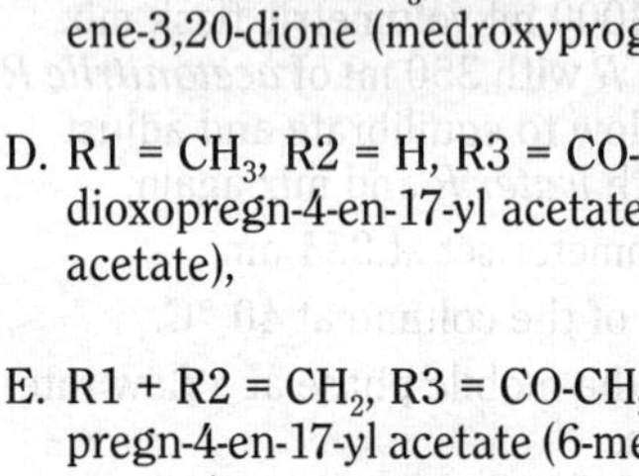

C. 6α,17a-dimethyl-3,17-dioxo-*D*-homoandrost-4-en-17aα-yl acetate,

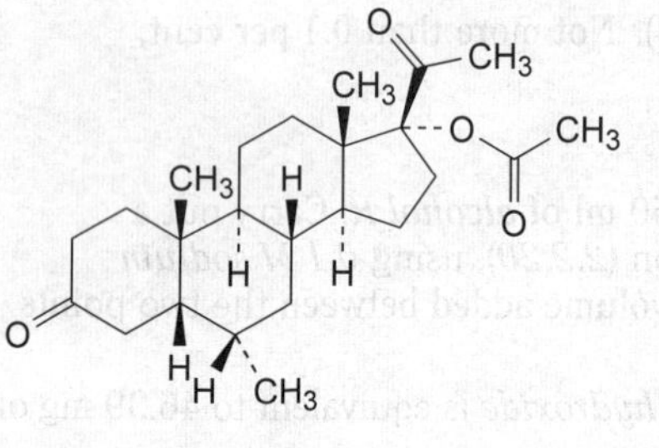

F. 6α-methyl-3,20-dioxo-5β-pregnan-17-yl acetate (4,5β-dihydromedroxyprogesterone acetate),

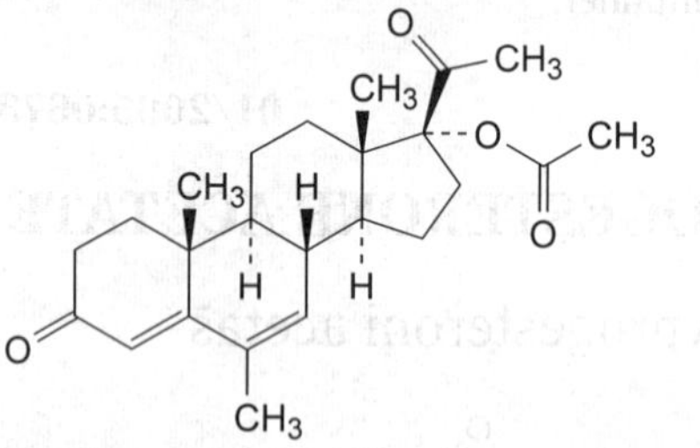

G. 6-methyl-3,20-dioxopregna-4,6-dien-17-yl acetate.

01/2005:1240

MEFENAMIC ACID

Acidum mefenamicum

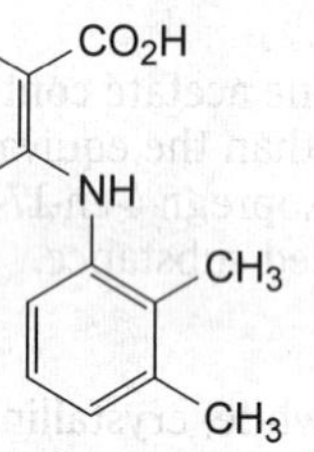

$C_{15}H_{15}NO_2$ M_r 241.3

DEFINITION

Mefenamic acid contains not less than 99.0 per cent and not more than the equivalent of 100.5 per cent of 2-[(2,3-dimethylphenyl)amino]benzoic acid, calculated with reference to the dried substance.

CHARACTERS

A white or almost white, microcrystalline powder, practically insoluble in water, slightly soluble in alcohol and in methylene chloride. It dissolves in dilute solutions of alkali hydroxides.

It shows polymorphism.

IDENTIFICATION

First identification: B.

Second identification: A, C, D.

A. Dissolve 20 mg in a mixture of 1 volume of *1 M hydrochloric acid* and 99 volumes of *methanol R* and dilute to 100 ml with the same mixture of solvents. Dilute 5 ml of the solution to 50 ml with a mixture of 1 volume of *1 M hydrochloric acid* and 99 volumes of *methanol R*. Examined between 250 nm and 380 nm (*2.2.25*), the solution shows two absorption maxima, at 279 nm and 350 nm. The ratio of the absorbance measured at the maximum at 279 nm to that measured at 350 nm is 1.1 to 1.3.

B. Examine by infrared absorption spectrophotometry (*2.2.24*), comparing with the spectrum obtained with *mefenamic acid CRS*. Examine the substances prepared as discs. If the spectra obtained show differences, dissolve the substance to be examined and the reference substance separately in *alcohol R*, evaporate to dryness and record new spectra using the residues.

C. Dissolve about 25 mg in 15 ml of *methylene chloride R* and examine in ultraviolet light at 365 nm; the solution exhibits a strong greenish-yellow fluorescence. Carefully add 0.5 ml of a saturated solution of *trichloroacetic acid R* dropwise and examine in ultraviolet light at 365 nm. The solution does not exhibit fluorescence.

D. Dissolve about 5 mg in 2 ml of *sulphuric acid R* and add 0.05 ml of *potassium dichromate solution R1*. An intense blue colour is produced, turning rapidly to brownish-green.

TESTS

Related substances. Examine by thin-layer chromatography (*2.2.27*), using a *TLC silica gel GF_{254} plate R*.

Test solution. Dissolve 0.125 g of the substance to be examined in a mixture of 1 volume of *methanol R* and 3 volumes of *methylene chloride R* and dilute to 5 ml with the same mixture of solvents.

Reference solution (a). Dilute 1 ml of the test solution to 50 ml with a mixture of 1 volume of *methanol R* and 3 volumes of *methylene chloride R*. Dilute 1 ml of the solution to 10 ml with a mixture of 1 volume of *methanol R* and 3 volumes of *methylene chloride R*.

Reference solution (b). Dissolve 5 mg of *flufenamic acid R* and 5 mg of *mefenamic acid CRS* in a mixture of 1 volume of *methanol R* and 3 volumes of *methylene chloride R* and dilute to 10 ml with the same mixture of solvents.

Apply to the plate 20 µl of each solution. Develop over a path of 15 cm using a mixture of 1 volume of *glacial acetic acid R*, 25 volumes of *dioxan R* and 90 volumes of *toluene R*. Dry the plate in a current of warm air. Expose the plate to iodine vapour for 5 min and examine in ultraviolet light at 254 nm. Any spot in the chromatogram obtained with the test solution, apart from the principal spot, is not more intense than the spot in the chromatogram obtained with reference solution (a) (0.2 per cent). The test is not valid unless the chromatogram obtained with reference solution (b) shows two clearly separated spots.

2,3-Dimethylaniline

Solution (a). Dissolve 0.250 g of the substance to be examined in a mixture of 1 volume of *methanol R* and 3 volumes of *methylene chloride R* and dilute to 10 ml with the same mixture of solvents. This solution is used to prepare the test solution.

Solution (b). Dissolve 50 mg of *2,3-dimethylaniline R* in a mixture of 1 volume of *methanol R* and 3 volumes of *methylene chloride R* and dilute to 100 ml with the same mixture of solvents. Dilute 1 ml of the solution to 100 ml with a mixture of 1 volume of *methanol R* and 3 volumes of *methylene chloride R*. This solution is used to prepare the standard.

Using three flat-bottomed tubes, place in the first 2 ml of solution (a), in the second 1 ml of solution (b) and 1 ml of a mixture of 1 volume of *methanol R* and 3 volumes of *methylene chloride R* and in the third 2 ml of a mixture of 1 volume of *methanol R* and 3 volumes of *methylene chloride R* (used to prepare a blank). To each tube add 1 ml of a freshly prepared 10 g/l solution of *dimethylaminobenzaldehyde R* in *methanol R* and 2 ml of *glacial acetic acid R* and allow to stand at room temperature for 10 min. The intensity of the yellow colour of the test solution is between that of the blank and that of the standard (100 ppm).

Copper. Not more than 10 ppm of Cu, determined by atomic absorption spectrometry (*2.2.23, Method I*).

Test solution. Place 1.00 g of the substance to be examined in a silica crucible, moisten with *sulphuric acid R*, heat cautiously on a flame for 30 min and then progressively to 650 °C. Continue ignition until all black particles have disappeared. Allow to cool, dissolve the residue in *0.1 M hydrochloric acid* and dilute to 25.0 ml with the same acid.

Reference solutions. Prepare the reference solutions using *copper standard solution (0.1 per cent Cu) R*, diluted as necessary with *0.1 M nitric acid.*

Measure the absorbance at 324.8 nm using a copper hollow-cathode lamp as a source of radiation and an air-acetylene flame.

Loss on drying (*2.2.32*). Not more than 0.5 per cent, determined on 1.000 g by drying at 100 °C to 105 °C.

Sulphated ash (*2.4.14*). Not more than 0.1 per cent, determined on 1.0 g.

ASSAY

Dissolve with the aid of ultrasound 0.200 g in 100 ml of warm *ethanol R*, previously neutralised to *phenol red solution R*. Add 0.1 ml of *phenol red solution R* and titrate with *0.1 M sodium hydroxide.*

1 ml of *0.1 M sodium hydroxide* is equivalent to 24.13 mg of $C_{15}H_{15}NO_2$.

IMPURITIES

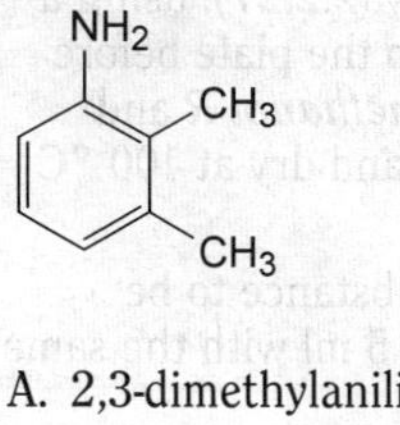

A. 2,3-dimethylaniline,

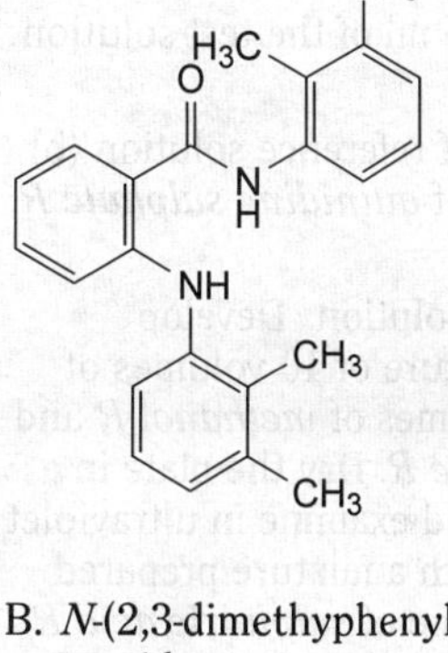

B. *N*-(2,3-dimethyphenyl)-2-[(2,3-dimethylphenyl)amino]benzamide.

01/2005:1241

MEFLOQUINE HYDROCHLORIDE

Mefloquini hydrochloridum

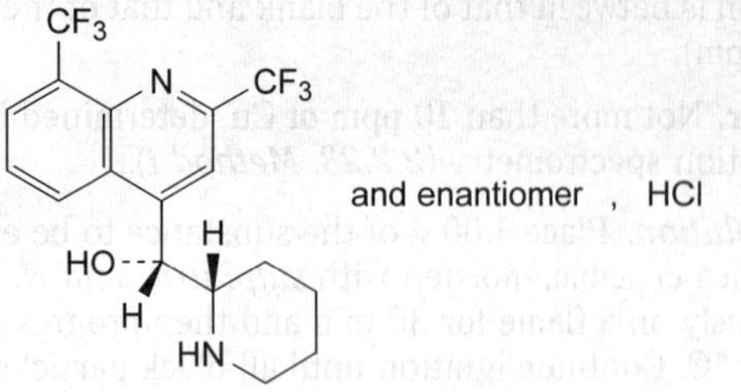

$C_{17}H_{17}ClF_6N_2O$ M_r 414.8

DEFINITION

Mefloquine hydrochloride contains not less than 99.0 per cent and not more than the equivalent of 101.0 per cent of (*RS*)-[2,8-bis(trifluoromethyl)quinolin-4-yl][(2*SR*)-piperidin-2-yl]methanol hydrochloride, calculated with reference to the anhydrous substance.

CHARACTERS

A white or slightly yellow, crystalline powder, very slightly soluble in water, freely soluble in methanol, soluble in alcohol.

It melts at about 260 °C, with decomposition.

It shows polymorphism.

IDENTIFICATION

First identification: A, E.

Second identification: B, C, D, E.

A. Examine by infrared absorption spectrophotometry (*2.2.24*), comparing with the spectrum obtained with *mefloquine hydrochloride CRS*. If the spectra obtained show differences, dissolve the substance to be examined and the reference substance separately in *methanol R*, evaporate to dryness and record new spectra using the residues.

B. Examine by thin-layer chromatography (*2.2.27*), using a *TLC silica gel* F_{254} *plate R*. Predevelop the plate before use with a mixture of 20 volumes of *methanol R* and 80 volumes of *methylene chloride R*, and dry at 100 °C to 105 °C for 15 min before use.

Test solution. Dissolve 8 mg of the substance to be examined in *methanol R* and dilute to 5 ml with the same solvent.

Reference solution (a). Dissolve 8 mg of *mefloquine hydrochloride CRS* in *methanol R* and dilute to 5 ml with the same solvent.

Reference solution (b). Dilute 2.5 ml of the test solution to 100 ml with *methanol R*.

Reference solution (c). To 1 ml of reference solution (b) add 1 ml of a 0.016 g/l solution of *quinidine sulphate R* in *methanol R*.

Apply to the plate 20 µl of each solution. Develop over a path of 10 cm using a mixture of 10 volumes of *anhydrous acetic acid R*, 10 volumes of *methanol R* and 80 volumes of *methylene chloride R*. Dry the plate in a current of warm air for 15 min and examine in ultraviolet light at 254 nm. Lightly spray with a mixture prepared immediately before use of 1 volume of *sulphuric acid R* and 40 volumes of *iodoplatinate reagent R*. Spray with *strong hydrogen peroxide solution R*. The principal spot in the chromatogram obtained with the test solution is similar in position, colour and size to the principal spot in the chromatogram obtained with reference solution (a). The test is not valid unless the chromatogram obtained with reference solution (c) shows two clearly separated spots.

C. Mix about 10 mg with 45 mg of *heavy magnesium oxide R* and ignite in a crucible until a practically white residue is obtained. Allow to cool, add 2 ml of *water R*, 0.05 ml of *phenolphthalein solution R1* and about 1 ml of *dilute hydrochloric acid R* to make the solution colourless. Filter. To the filtrate add a freshly prepared mixture of 0.1 ml of *alizarin S solution R* and 0.1 ml of *zirconyl nitrate solution R*. Mix, allow to stand for 5 min and compare the colour of the solution with a blank prepared in the same manner. The colour of the test solution is yellow and that of the blank is red.

D. To about 20 mg add 0.2 ml of *sulphuric acid R*. Blue fluorescence appears in ultraviolet light at 365 nm.

E. It gives reaction (b) of chlorides (*2.3.1*).

TESTS

Solution S. Dissolve 2.50 g in *methanol R* and dilute to 50.0 ml with the same solvent.

Appearance of solution. Solution S is clear (*2.2.1*) and not more intensely coloured than reference solution BY_7 (*2.2.2, Method I*).

Optical rotation (*2.2.7*): − 0.2° to + 0.2°, determined on solution S.

Related substances. Examine by liquid chromatography (*2.2.29*).

Test solution. Dissolve 0.10 g of the substance to be examined in the mobile phase and dilute to 25.0 ml with the mobile phase.

Reference solution (a). Dilute 1.0 ml of the test solution to 50.0 ml with the mobile phase. Dilute 1.0 ml of the solution to 20.0 ml the mobile phase.

Reference solution (b). Dissolve 8 mg of *mefloquine hydrochloride CRS* and 8 mg of *quinidine sulphate R* in the mobile phase and dilute to 50.0 ml with the mobile phase. Dilute 5.0 ml of the solution to 100.0 ml with the mobile phase.

The chromatographic procedure may be carried out using:

– a stainless steel precolumn 0.025 m long and 4 mm in internal diameter and a stainless steel column 0.25 m long and 4 mm in internal diameter, both packed with *end-capped octadecylsilyl silica gel for chromatography R* (5 µm),

– as mobile phase at a flow rate of 0.8 ml/min a mixture prepared as follows: dissolve 1 g of *tetraheptylammonium bromide R* in a mixture of 200 volumes of *methanol R*, 400 volumes of a 1.5 g/l solution of *sodium hydrogen sulphate R* and 400 volumes of *acetonitrile R*,

– as detector a spectrophotometer set at 280 nm.

Equilibrate the column with the mobile phase at a flow rate of 2 ml/min for about 30 min.

Inject 20 µl of reference solution (a). Adjust the sensitivity of the system so that the height of the principal peak is at least 50 per cent of the full scale of the recorder.

Inject 20 µl of reference solution (b).When the chromatograms are recorded in the prescribed conditions, the retention times are: quinidine about 2 min, mefloquine about 4 min, impurity B about 15 min, impurity A about 36 min.

The test is not valid unless, in the chromatogram obtained with reference solution (b), the resolution between quinidine and mefloquine is at least 8.5.

Inject 20 µl of the test solution and 20 µl of reference solution (a). Continue the chromatography for 10 times the retention time of the principal peak. In the chromatogram obtained with the test solution: the area of any peak with a relative retention with reference to mefloquine of about 0.7 is not greater than twice the area of the principal peak in the chromatogram obtained with reference solution (a) (0.2 per cent); the area of any peaks apart from the principal peak is not greater than the area of the principal peak in the chromatogram obtained with reference solution (a) (0.1 per cent) and the sum of the areas of any such peaks is not greater than five times the area of the principal peak in the chromatogram obtained with reference solution (a) (0.5 per cent). Disregard any peak with an area less than 0.2 times that of the principal peak in the chromatogram obtained with reference solution (a) (0.02 per cent).

Heavy metals (*2.4.8*). 1.0 g complies with limit test C for heavy metals (20 ppm). Prepare the standard using 2 ml of *lead standard solution (10 ppm Pb) R*.

Water (*2.5.12*). Not more than 3.0 per cent, determined on 1.000 g by the semi-micro determination of water.

Sulphated ash (*2.4.14*). Not more than 0.1 per cent, determined on 1.0 g.

ASSAY

Dissolve 0.350 g in 15 ml of *anhydrous formic acid R* and add 40 ml of *acetic anhydride R*. Titrate with *0.1 M perchloric acid,* determining the end-point potentiometrically (*2.2.20*).

1 ml of *0.1 M perchloric acid* is equivalent to 41.48 mg of $C_{17}H_{17}ClF_6N_2O$.

STORAGE

Store protected from light.

IMPURITIES

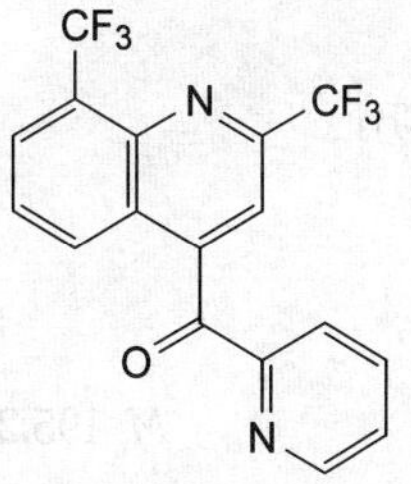

A. [2,8-bis(trifluoromethyl)quinolin-4-yl](pyridin-2-yl)methanone,

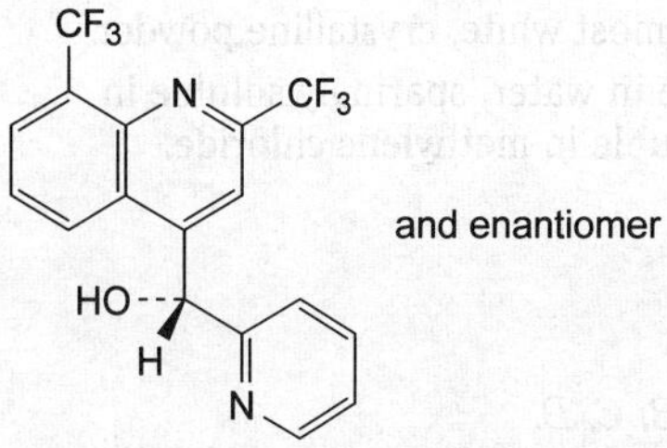

B. (*RS*)-[2,8-bis(trifluoromethyl)quinolin-4-yl](pyridin-2-yl)methanol,

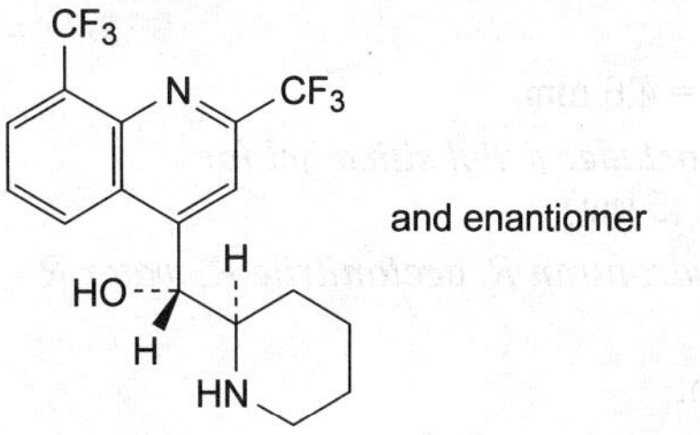

C. (*RS*)-[2,8-bis(trifluoromethyl)quinolin-4-yl][(2*RS*)-piperidin-2-yl]methanol.

01/2005:1593

MEGESTROL ACETATE

Megestroli acetas

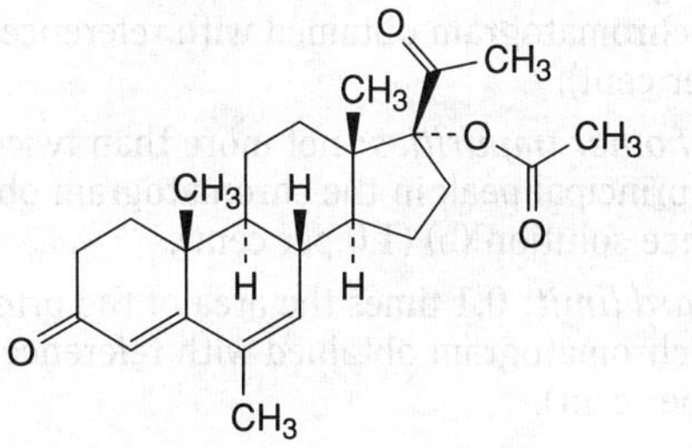

$C_{24}H_{32}O_4$ M_r 384.5

DEFINITION

6-Methyl-3,20-dioxopregna-4,6-dien-17-yl acetate.

Content: 97.0 per cent to 103.0 per cent (dried substance).

CHARACTERS

Appearance: a white or almost white, crystalline powder.

Solubility: practically insoluble in water, soluble in acetone, sparingly soluble in alcohol.

mp: about 217 °C.

IDENTIFICATION

Infrared absorption spectrophotometry (*2.2.24*).

Comparison: *Ph. Eur. reference spectrum of megestrol acetate.*

TESTS

Specific optical rotation (*2.2.7*): + 14.0 to + 17.0 (dried substance).

Dissolve 2.50 g in *methylene chloride R* and dilute to 25.0 ml with the same solvent.

Related substances. Liquid chromatography (*2.2.29*).

Test solution. Dissolve 25.0 mg of the substance to be examined in a mixture of 145 volumes of *tetrahydrofuran R* and 255 volumes of *acetonitrile R,* dilute to 20 ml with the same mixture of solvents and then dilute to 50.0 ml with *water R*.

Reference solution (a). Dissolve 25.0 mg of *medroxyprogesterone acetate CRS* in a mixture of 145 volumes of *tetrahydrofuran R* and 255 volumes of *acetonitrile R,* dilute to 20 ml with the same mixture of solvents and then dilute to 50.0 ml with *water R*.

Reference solution (b). Dilute 1.0 ml of reference solution (a) to 200.0 ml with the mobile phase.

Reference solution (c). To 3 ml of the test solution, add 1 ml of reference solution (a) and dilute to 50 ml with the mobile phase.

Column:
- *size*: *l* = 0.25 m, Ø = 4.6 mm,
- *stationary phase*: *octadecylsilyl silica gel for chromatography R* (5 µm).

Mobile phase: *tetrahydrofuran R, acetonitrile R, water R* (145:255:600 *V/V/V*).

Flow rate: 1.5 ml/min.

Detection: spectrophotometer at 254 nm.

Injection: 20 µl.

Sensitivity: reference solution (b).

Run time: 1.5 times the retention time of megestrol acetate.

System suitability: reference solution (c):
- *resolution*: minimum 4.0 between the peaks corresponding to impurity A and megestrol acetate.

Limits:
- *impurity A*: not more than the area of the principal peak in the chromatogram obtained with reference solution (b) (0.5 per cent),
- *total of other impurities*: not more than twice the area of the principal peak in the chromatogram obtained with reference solution (b) (1.0 per cent),
- *disregard limit*: 0.1 times the area of the principal peak in the chromatogram obtained with reference solution (b) (0.05 per cent).

Loss on drying (*2.2.32*): maximum 0.5 per cent, determined on 1.000 g by drying in an oven at 100-105 °C.

ASSAY

Dissolve 15.0 mg in *ethanol R* and dilute to 100.0 ml with the same solvent. Dilute 5.0 ml of the solution to 100.0 ml with *ethanol R*. Measure the absorbance (*2.2.25*) at the maximum at 287 nm.

Calculate the content of $C_{24}H_{32}O_4$ taking the specific absorbance to be 640.

STORAGE

Protected from light.

IMPURITIES

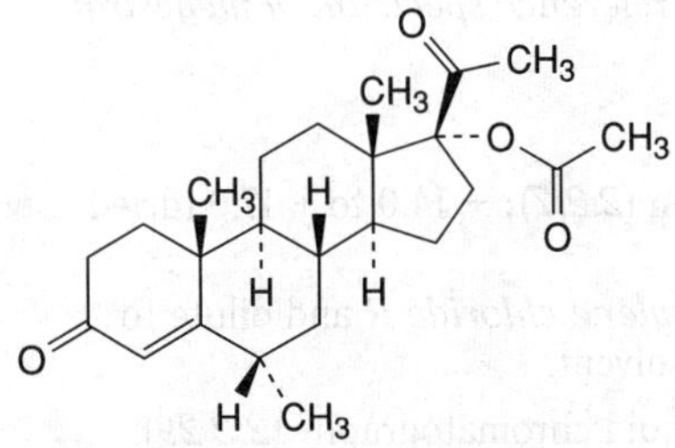

A. 6α-methyl-3,20-dioxopregn-4-en-17-yl acetate (medroxyprogesterone acetate),

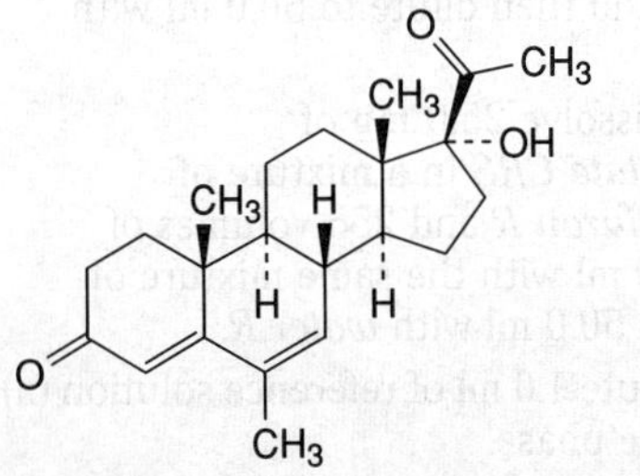

B. 6-methyl-17-hydroxypregna-4,6-diene-3,20-dione (megestrol),

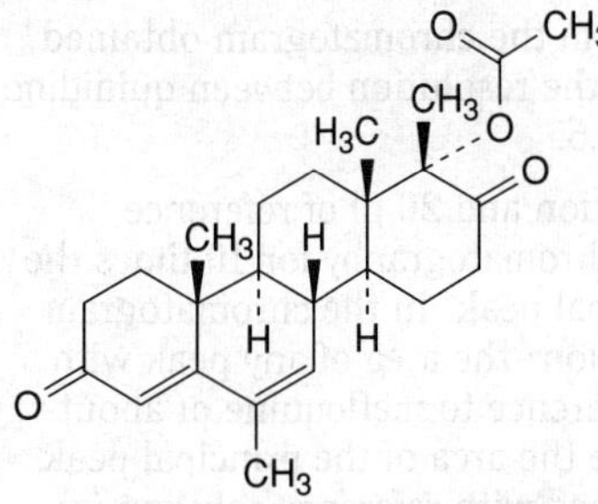

C. 6,17a-dimethyl-3,17-dioxo-*D*-homoandrosta-4,6-dien-17aα-yl acetate (*D-homo* megestrol acetate),

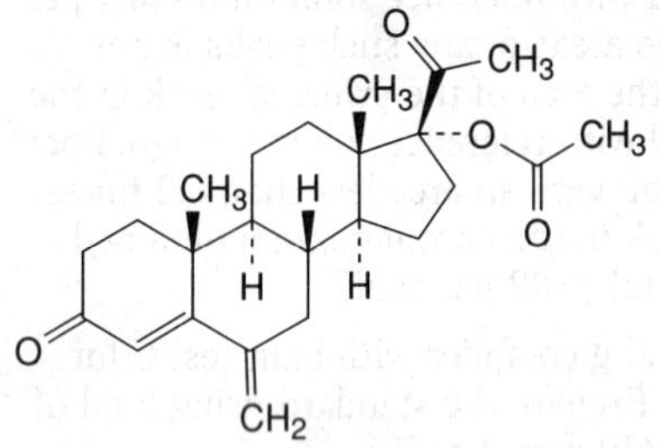

D. 6-methylene-3,20-dioxopregn-4-en-17-yl acetate (6-methylene hydroxyprogesterone acetate),

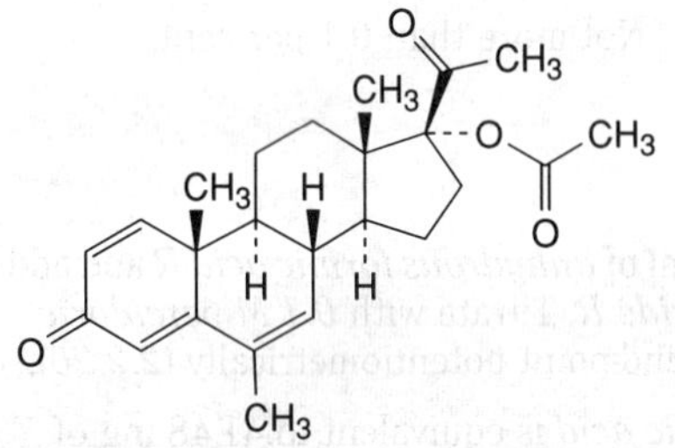

E. 6-methyl-3,20-dioxopregna-1,4,6-trien-17-yl acetate.

01/2005:2055

MEGLUMINE

Megluminum

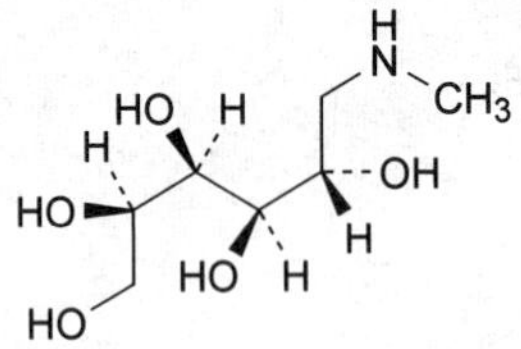

$C_7H_{17}NO_5$ M_r 195.2

DEFINITION

1-Deoxy-1-(methylamino)-D-glucitol.

Content: 99.0 per cent to 101.0 per cent (dried substance).

CHARACTERS

Appearance: white or almost white, crystalline powder.

Solubility: freely soluble in water, sparingly soluble in alcohol, practically insoluble in methylene chloride.

mp: about 128 °C.

IDENTIFICATION

First identification: A.

Second identification: B, C, D.

A. Infrared absorption spectrophotometry (*2.2.24*).

Comparison: *Ph. Eur. reference spectrum of meglumine.*

B. To 5 ml of *water R,* add 0.5 ml of *paraldehyde R* and 1 ml of *dilute sulphuric acid R.* Shake vigorously and heat on a water-bath until opalescence appears. Allow to stand for 15 min. To 1 ml of this solution add 0.2 ml of a freshly prepared 100 g/l solution of *sodium nitroprusside R,* 50 mg of the substance to be examined and 2 ml of a 50 g/l solution of *disodium tetraborate R.* A blue colour develops.

C. Dissolve 0.1 g in 2 ml of *nitric acid R.* Add 5 ml of a 6.4 g/l solution of *sodium periodate R,* then add 5 ml of *nitric acid R* and 25 ml of a 17 g/l solution of *silver nitrate R.* Allow to stand in the dark for 10 min. A white precipitate is formed.

D. It complies with the limits of the assay.

TESTS

Solution S. Dissolve 20.0 g in *distilled water R* and dilute to 100.0 ml with the same solvent.

Appearance of solution. The solution is clear (*2.2.1*) and its absorbance (*2.2.25*) at 420 nm is maximum 0.03.

Dissolve the residue obtained in the test for loss on drying in *water R* and dilute to 10 ml with the same solvent.

Specific optical rotation (*2.2.7*): − 16.0 to − 17.0 (dried substance).

Dilute 12.5 ml of solution S to 25.0 ml with *water R.*

Reducing substances: maximum 0.2 per cent, expressed as glucose.

Dilute 1.25 ml of solution S to 2.5 ml with *water R,* add 2 ml of *cupri-tartaric solution R.* Heat on a water-bath for 10 min. Cool under running water for 1 min and then sonicate the tube for 20 s. Immediately filter through a filter 25 mm in diameter and 0.5 µm in pore size. Rinse with 10 ml of *water R.* Prepare a standard in the same manner using 2.5 ml of a solution obtained by dissolving 20 mg of *glucose R* in *water R* and diluting to 100 ml with the same solvent.

Any precipitate on the membrane filter obtained with the test solution is not more intensely coloured than the precipitate obtained with the standard.

Chlorides (*2.4.4*): maximum 100 ppm.

To 2.5 ml of solution S add 12.5 ml of *water R.*

Sulphates (*2.4.13*): maximum 150 ppm.

To 5 ml of solution S add 10 ml of *distilled water R.*

Iron: maximum 10 ppm.

To 10 ml of solution S, adjusted to pH 1 by adding 0.8 ml of *hydrochloric acid R,* add 0.05 ml of *bromine water R.* Allow to stand for 5 min, evaporate the excess of bromine in a current of air and add 3 ml of *potassium thiocyanate solution R.* Prepare a reference solution at the same time and in the same manner using 10 ml of *iron standard solution (2 ppm Fe) R,* to which 2 ml of *hydrochloric acid R* has been added.

After 5 min, any red colour in the test solution is not more intense than that in the reference solution.

Heavy metals (*2.4.8*): maximum 10 ppm.

Adjust 10 ml of solution S to pH 3-4 with *dilute acetic acid R.* Dilute to 20 ml with *water R.* 12 ml of the solution complies with limit test A. Prepare the standard using *lead standard solution (1 ppm Pb) R.*

Loss on drying (*2.2.32*): maximum 0.5 per cent, determined on 1.000 g by drying in an oven at 100-105 °C for 3 h.

Sulphated ash (*2.4.14*): maximum 0.1 per cent, determined on 1.0 g.

Bacterial endotoxins (*2.6.14*): less than 1.5 IU/g.

ASSAY

Dissolve 0.180 g in 30 ml of *water R.* Titrate with *0.05 M sulphuric acid,* determining the end-point potentiometrically (*2.2.20*).

1 ml of *0.05 M sulphuric acid* is equivalent to 19.52 mg of $C_7H_{17}NO_5$.

01/2005:1447

MELISSA LEAF

Melissae folium

DEFINITION

Melissa leaf consists of the dried leaf of *Melissa officinalis* L. It contains not less than 4.0 per cent of total hydroxycinnamic derivatives expressed as rosmarinic acid ($C_{18}H_{16}O_8$; M_r 360.3), calculated with reference to the dried drug.

CHARACTERS

Melissa leaf has an odour reminiscent of lemon.

It has the macroscopic and microscopic characters described under identification tests A and B.

IDENTIFICATION

A. Melissa leaf has a petiole varying length and is oval, cordate and up to about 8 cm long and 5 cm wide. The lamina is thin and the under surface has a conspicuous, raised, reticulate venation; the margins are roughly dentate or crenate. The upper surface is bright green and the lower surface is lighter in colour.

B. Reduce to a powder (355). The powder is greenish. Examine under a microscope using *chloral hydrate solution R.* The powder shows fragments of the leaf epidermis with sinuous walls; short, straight, unicellular, conical covering trichomes with a finely striated cuticle; multicellular, uniseriate covering trichomes with pointed ends and thick, warty cuticles; eight-celled secretory trichomes of lamiaceous type; secretory trichomes with unicellular to tricellular stalks and unicellular or, more rarely bicellular, heads; diacytic stomata (*2.8.3*), on the lower surface only.

C. Examine by thin-layer chromatography (*2.2.27*), using a *TLC silica gel plate R.*

Test solution. Place 2.0 g of the powdered drug (355) in a 250 ml round-bottomed flask and add 100 ml of *water R.* Distil for 1 h using the apparatus for the determination of essential oils in vegetable drugs (*2.8.12*) and 0.5 ml of *xylene R* in the graduated tube. After distillation transfer the organic phase to a 1 ml volumetric flask rinsing the graduated tube of the apparatus with the aid of a small portion of *xylene R* and dilute to 1.0 ml with the same solvent.

Reference solution. Dissolve 1.0 µl of *citronellal R* and 10.0 µl of *citral R* in 25 ml of *xylene R.*

Apply to the plate as bands 10 µl of the reference solution and 20 µl of the test solution. Develop over a path of 15 cm using a mixture of 10 volumes of *ethyl acetate R* and 90 volumes of *hexane R.* Allow the plate to dry in air. Spray the plate with *anisaldehyde solution R.* Examine in daylight while heating at 100 °C to 105 °C for 10 min to 15 min. The chromatogram obtained with the reference solution shows in the lower third a greyish-violet to bluish-violet double zone (citral) and above it a grey to greyish-violet zone (citronellal). The chromatogram obtained with the test solution shows zones similar in position and colour to the zones in the chromatogram

Monographs M

obtained with the reference solution and between these zones a reddish-violet zone (epoxycaryophyllene). Further zones may be present.

TESTS

Foreign matter (*2.8.2*). Not more than 10 per cent of stems having a diameter greater than 1 mm and not more than 2 per cent of other foreign matters, determined on 20 g.

Loss on drying (*2.2.32*). Not more than 10.0 per cent, determined on 1.000 g of the powdered drug (355) by drying in an oven at 100 °C to 105 °C for 2 h.

Total ash (*2.4.16*). Not more than 12.0 per cent.

ASSAY

Stock solution. To 0.200 g of the powdered drug (355) add 190 ml of *alcohol (50 per cent V/V) R*. Boil in a water-bath under a reflux condenser for 30 min. Allow to cool and filter. Rinse the filter with 10 ml of *alcohol (50 per cent V/V) R*. Combine the filtrate and the rinsings in a volumetric flask and dilute to 200.0 ml with *alcohol (50 per cent V/V) R*.

Test solution. To 1.0 ml of the stock solution in a test-tube add 2 ml of *0.5 M hydrochloric acid*, 2 ml of a solution prepared by dissolving 10 g of *sodium nitrite R* and 10 g of *sodium molybdate R* in 100 ml of *water R* and then add 2 ml of *dilute sodium hydroxide solution R* and dilute to 10.0 ml with *water R* and mix.

Compensation solution. In another test-tube place 1.0 ml of the stock solution, 2 ml of *0.5 M hydrochloric acid*, 2 ml of *dilute sodium hydroxide solution R* and dilute to 10.0 ml with *water R*.

Immediately measure the absorbance (*2.2.25*) of the test solution at 505 nm by comparison with the compensation solution.

Calculate the percentage content of total hydroxycinnamic derivatives, expressed as rosmarinic acid, from the expression:

$$\frac{A \times 5}{m}$$

i.e. taking the specific absorbance to be 400 for rosmarinic acid at 505 nm.

A = absorbance of the test solution at 505 nm,

m = mass of the substance to be examined, in grams.

STORAGE

Store protected from light.

01/2005:0507

MENADIONE

Menadionum

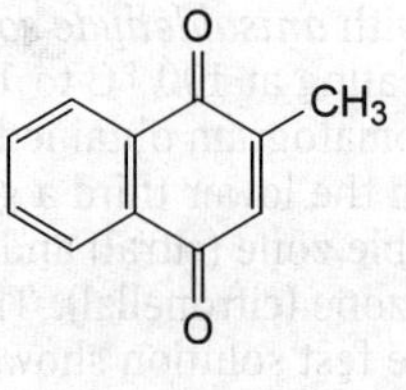

$C_{11}H_8O_2$ M_r 172.2

DEFINITION

Menadione contains not less than 98.5 per cent and not more than the equivalent of 101.0 per cent of 2-methylnaphthalene-1,4-dione, calculated with reference to the dried substance.

CHARACTERS

A pale-yellow, crystalline powder, practically insoluble in water, freely soluble in toluene, sparingly soluble in alcohol and in methanol. It is unstable in light.

IDENTIFICATION

First identification: A, B.

Second identification: A, C, D.

A. Melting point (*2.2.14*): 105 °C to 108 °C.

B. Examine by infrared absorption spectrophotometry (*2.2.24*), comparing with the spectrum obtained with *menadione CRS*.

C. Dissolve about 1 mg in 5 ml of *alcohol R*, add 2 ml of *ammonia R* and 0.2 ml of *ethyl cyanoacetate R*. An intense bluish-violet colour develops. Add 2 ml of *hydrochloric acid R*. The colour disappears.

D. Dissolve about 10 mg in 1 ml of *alcohol R*, add 1 ml of *hydrochloric acid R* and heat in a water-bath. A red colour develops.

TESTS

Related substances. *Carry out the test protected from bright light.* Examine by thin-layer chromatography (*2.2.27*), using *silica gel GF_{254} R* as the coating substance.

Test solution. Dissolve 0.2 g of the substance to be examined in *acetone R* and dilute to 10 ml with the same solvent.

Reference solution. Dilute 0.5 ml of the test solution to 100 ml with *acetone R*.

Apply separately to the plate 5 µl of each solution. Develop over a path of 15 cm using a mixture of 1 volume of *nitromethane R*, 2 volumes of *acetone R*, 5 volumes of *ethylene chloride R* and 90 volumes of *cyclohexane R*. Dry the plate in a current of hot air. Repeat the development and drying a further two times. Examine in ultraviolet light at 254 nm. Any spot in the chromatogram obtained with the test solution, apart from the principal spot, is not more intense than the spot in the chromatogram obtained with the reference solution (0.5 per cent).

Loss on drying (*2.2.32*). Not more than 0.5 per cent, determined on 1.000 g by drying over *diphosphorus pentoxide R* at a pressure of 2 kPa to 3 kPa for 4 h.

Sulphated ash (*2.4.14*). Not more than 0.1 per cent, determined on 1.0 g.

ASSAY

Dissolve 0.150 g in 15 ml of *glacial acetic acid R* in a flask with a stopper fitted with a valve. Add 15 ml of *dilute hydrochloric acid R* and 1 g of *zinc powder R*. Close the flask. Allow the mixture to stand for 60 min, protected from light, with occasional shaking. Filter the solution over a cotton wad, wash with three quantities, each of 10 ml, of *carbon dioxide-free water R*. Add 0.1 ml of *ferroin R* and immediately titrate the combined filtrate and washings with *0.1 M ammonium and cerium nitrate*.

1 ml of *0.1 M ammonium and cerium nitrate* is equivalent to 8.61 mg of $C_{11}H_8O_2$.

STORAGE

Store protected from light.

01/2005:0623

MENTHOL, RACEMIC

Mentholum racemicum

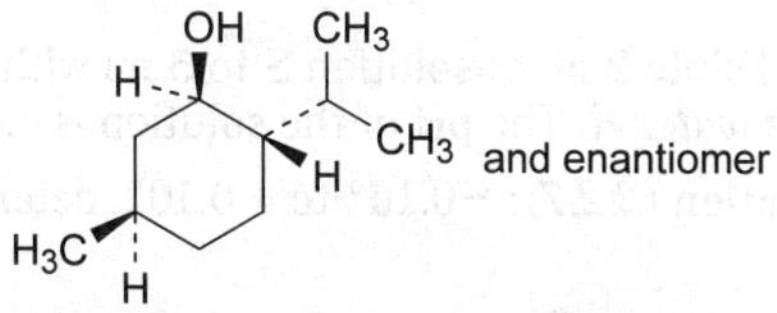

$C_{10}H_{20}O$ M_r 156.3

DEFINITION

Racemic menthol is a mixture of equal parts of (1*RS*,2*SR*,5*RS*)-5-methyl-2-(1-methylethyl)cyclohexanol.

CHARACTERS

A free-flowing or agglomerated, crystalline powder or prismatic or acicular, colourless, shiny crystals, practically insoluble in water, very soluble in alcohol and in light petroleum, freely soluble in fatty oils and in liquid paraffin, very slightly soluble in glycerol.

It melts at about 34 °C.

IDENTIFICATION

First identification: A, C.

Second identification: B, D.

A. It complies with the test for angle of optical rotation (see Tests).

B. Examine by thin-layer chromatography (*2.2.27*), using *silica gel G R* as the coating substance.

Test solution. Dissolve 25 mg of the substance to be examined in *methanol R* and dilute to 5 ml with the same solvent.

Reference solution. Dissolve 25 mg of *menthol CRS* in *methanol R* and dilute to 5 ml with the same solvent.

Apply separately to the plate 2 µl of each solution. Develop over a path of 15 cm using a mixture of 5 volumes of *ethyl acetate R* and 95 volumes of *toluene R*. Allow the plate to dry in air until the solvents have evaporated and spray with *anisaldehyde solution R*. Heat at 100 °C to 105 °C for 5 min to 10 min. The principal spot in the chromatogram obtained with the test solution is similar in position, colour and size to the principal spot in the chromatogram obtained with the reference solution.

C. Examine the chromatograms obtained in the test for related substances. The principal peak in the chromatogram obtained with test solution (b) is similar in position and approximate dimensions to the principal peak in the chromatogram obtained with reference solution (c).

D. Dissolve 0.20 g in 0.5 ml of *anhydrous pyridine R*. Add 3 ml of a 150 g/l solution of *dinitrobenzoyl chloride R* in *anhydrous pyridine R*. Heat on a water-bath for 10 min. Add 7.0 ml of *water R* in small quantities with stirring and allow to stand in iced water for 30 min. A precipitate is formed. Allow to stand and decant the supernatant liquid. Wash the precipitate with two quantities, each of 5 ml, of iced *water R*, recrystallise from 10 ml of *acetone R*, wash with iced *acetone R* and dry at 75 °C at a pressure not exceeding 2.7 kPa for 30 min. The crystals melt (*2.2.14*) at 130 °C to 131 °C.

TESTS

Solution S. Dissolve 2.50 g in 10 ml of *alcohol R* and dilute to 25.0 ml with the same solvent.

Appearance of solution. Solution S is clear (*2.2.1*) and colourless (*2.2.2, Method II*).

Acidity or alkalinity. Dissolve 1.0 g in *alcohol R* and dilute to 10 ml with the same solvent. Add 0.1 ml of *phenolphthalein solution R*; the solution is colourless. Not more than 0.5 ml of *0.01 M sodium hydroxide* is required to change the colour of the indicator to pink.

Optical rotation (*2.2.7*). The angle of optical rotation of solution S is + 0.2° to − 0.2°.

Related substances. Examine by gas chromatography (*2.2.28*).

Test solution (a). Dissolve 0.20 g of the substance to be examined in *methylene chloride R* and dilute to 50.0 ml with the same solvent.

Test solution (b). Dilute 1.0 ml of test solution (a) to 10.0 ml with *methylene chloride R*.

Reference solution (a). Dissolve 40.0 mg of the substance to be examined and 40.0 mg of *isomenthol R* in *methylene chloride R* and dilute to 100.0 ml with the same solvent.

Reference solution (b). Dilute 0.10 ml of test solution (a) to 100.0 ml with *methylene chloride R*.

Reference solution (c). Dissolve 40.0 mg of *menthol CRS* in *methylene chloride R* and dilute to 100.0 ml with the same solvent.

The chromatographic procedure may be carried out using:

- a glass column 2.0 m long and 2 mm in internal diameter packed with *diatomaceous earth for gas chromatography R* impregnated with 15 per cent *m/m* of *macrogol 1500 R*,
- *nitrogen for chromatography R* as carrier gas at a flow rate of 30 ml/min,
- a flame-ionisation detector,

maintaining the temperature of the column at 120 °C, that of the injection port at 150 °C and that of the detector at 200 °C.

Inject separately 1 µl of each solution. Record the chromatograms for twice the retention time of the peak corresponding to menthol. In the chromatogram obtained with test solution (a), the sum of the areas of the peaks, apart from the principal peak, is not greater than 1 per cent of the area of the principal peak. Disregard any peak due to the solvent and any peak whose area is less than 0.05 per cent of the area of the principal peak. The test is not valid unless: in the chromatogram obtained with reference solution (a) the resolution between the peaks corresponding to menthol and isomenthol is at least 1.4 and the principal peak in the chromatogram obtained with reference solution (b) has a signal-to-noise ratio of at least 5.

Residue on evaporation. Evaporate 2.00 g on a water-bath and heat in an oven at 100 °C to 105 °C for 1 h. The residue weighs not more than 1.0 mg (0.05 per cent).

Monographs M

01/2005:1242

MEPIVACAINE HYDROCHLORIDE

Mepivacaini hydrochloridum

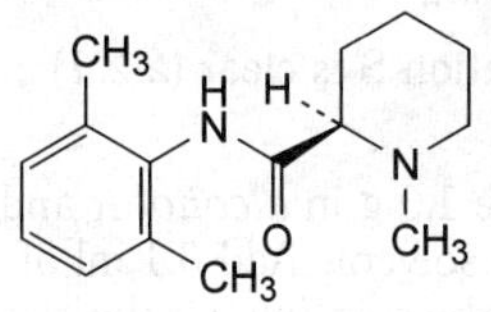

and enantiomer , HCl

$C_{15}H_{23}ClN_2O$ M_r 282.8

DEFINITION

Mepivacaine hydrochloride contains not less than 98.5 per cent and not more than the equivalent of 101.0 per cent of (*RS*)-*N*-(2,6-dimethylphenyl)-1-methylpiperidine-2-carboxamide hydrochloride, calculated with reference to the dried substance.

CHARACTERS

A white, crystalline powder, freely soluble in water and in alcohol, very slightly soluble in methylene chloride.

It melts at about 260 °C with decomposition.

IDENTIFICATION

First identification: A, B, D.

Second identification: B, C, D.

A. Examine by infrared absorption spectrophotometry (*2.2.24*), comparing with the spectrum obtained with *mepivacaine hydrochloride CRS*. Examine the substances prepared as discs.

B. Examine by thin-layer chromatography (*2.2.27*), using as the coating substance a suitable silica gel with a fluorescent indicator having an optimal intensity at 254 nm.

Test solution. Dissolve 20 mg of the substance to be examined in *alcohol R* and dilute to 5 ml with the same solvent.

Reference solution (a). Dissolve 20 mg of *mepivacaine hydrochloride CRS* in *alcohol R* and dilute to 5 ml with the same solvent.

Reference solution (b). Dissolve 20 mg of *mepivacaine hydrochloride CRS* and 20 mg of *lidocaine hydrochloride CRS* in *alcohol R* and dilute to 5 ml with the same solvent.

Apply to the plate 10 µl of each solution. Develop over a path of 12 cm using a mixture of 1 volume of *concentrated ammonia R*, 5 volumes of *methanol R* and 100 volumes of *ether R*. Allow the plate to dry in air and examine in ultraviolet light at 254 nm. The principal spot in the chromatogram obtained with the test solution is similar in position and size to the principal spot in the chromatogram obtained with reference solution (a). The test is not valid unless the chromatogram obtained with reference solution (b) shows two clearly separated principal spots.

C. To 5 ml of solution S (see Tests) add 1 ml of *dilute sodium hydroxide solution R* and shake with two quantities, each of 10 ml, of *ether R*. Dry the combined upper layers over *anhydrous sodium sulphate R*. Filter and evaporate the ether on a water-bath. Dry the residue at 100-105 °C for 2 h. The melting point (*2.2.14*) is 151 °C to 155 °C.

D. It gives reaction (a) of chlorides (*2.3.1*).

TESTS

Solution S. Dissolve 1.5 g in *carbon dioxide-free water R* and dilute to 30 ml with the same solvent.

Appearance of solution. Solution S is clear (*2.2.1*) and not more intensely coloured than reference solution B_7 (*2.2.2, Method II*).

pH (*2.2.3*). Dilute 2 ml of solution S to 5 ml with *carbon dioxide-free water R*. The pH of the solution is 4.0 to 5.0.

Optical rotation (*2.2.7*): −0.10° to + 0.10°, determined on solution S.

Related substances. Examine by liquid chromatography (*2.2.29*).

Test solution. Dissolve 20.0 mg of the substance to be examined in the mobile phase and dilute to 10.0 ml with the mobile phase.

Reference solution (a). Dissolve 20.0 mg of the substance to be examined and 30.0 mg of *mepivacaine impurity B CRS* in the mobile phase and dilute to 100.0 ml with the mobile phase. Dilute 1.0 ml of the solution to 100.0 ml with the mobile phase.

Reference solution (b). Dilute 1.0 ml of the test solution to 100.0 ml with the mobile phase. Dilute 1.0 ml of the solution to 10.0 ml with the mobile phase.

The chromatographic procedure may be carried out using:

- a stainless steel column 0.125 m long and 4.6 mm in internal diameter packed with *base-deactivated octadecylsilyl silica gel for chromatography R* (5 µm),
- as mobile phase at a flow rate of 1 ml/min a mixture of 35 volumes of *acetonitrile R* and 65 volumes of a 2.25 g/l solution of *phosphoric acid R* (adjusted to pH 7.6 with *strong sodium hydroxide solution R*),
- as detector a spectrophotometer set at 220 nm.

Inject 20 µl of reference solution (a). Adjust the sensitivity of the system so that the heights of the two principal peaks in the chromatogram obtained are at least 20 per cent of the full scale of the recorder. The test is not valid unless the resolution between the peaks corresponding to mepivacaine impurity B and mepivacaine is at least 2.5.

Inject 20 µl of the test solution and 20 µl of reference solution (b). Continue the chromatography of the test solution for three times the retention time of mepivacaine. In the chromatogram obtained with the test solution: the area of any peak, apart from the principal peak, is not greater than twice the area of the principal peak in the chromatogram obtained with reference solution (b) (0.2 per cent) and the area of not more than one of these peaks is greater than the area of the principal peak in the chromatogram obtained with reference solution (b) (0.1 per cent); the sum of the areas of all the peaks, apart from the principal peak, is not greater than five times the area of the principal peak in the chromatogram obtained with reference solution (b) (0.5 per cent). Disregard any peak with an area less than 0.2 times the area of the principal peak in the chromatogram obtained with reference solution (b).

2,6-Dimethylaniline. Dissolve 0.50 g in *methanol R* and dilute to 10 ml with the same solvent. To 2 ml of the solution add 1 ml of a freshly prepared 10 g/l solution of *dimethylaminobenzaldehyde R* in *methanol R* and 2 ml of *glacial acetic acid R* and allow to stand for 10 min. Any yellow colour in the solution is not more intense than that in a standard prepared at the same time and in the same manner using 2 ml of a 5 mg/l solution of *2,6-dimethylaniline R* in *methanol R* (100 ppm).

Heavy metals (*2.4.8*). Dissolve 1.0 g in *water R* and dilute to 25 ml with the same solvent. Carry out the prefiltration. 10 ml of the filtrate complies with limit test E for heavy metals (5 ppm). Prepare the standard using 2 ml of *lead standard solution (1 ppm Pb) R*.

Loss on drying (*2.2.32*). Not more than 1.0 per cent, determined on 1.000 g by drying in an oven at 100-105 °C.

Sulphated ash (*2.4.14*). Not more than 0.1 per cent, determined on 1.0 g.

ASSAY

Dissolve 0.250 g in a mixture of 5.0 ml of *0.01 M hydrochloric acid* and 50 ml of *alcohol R*. Carry out a potentiometric titration (*2.2.20*), using *0.1 M sodium hydroxide*. Read the volume added between the two points of inflexion.

1 ml of *0.1 M sodium hydroxide* is equivalent to 28.28 mg of $C_{15}H_{23}ClN_2O$.

IMPURITIES

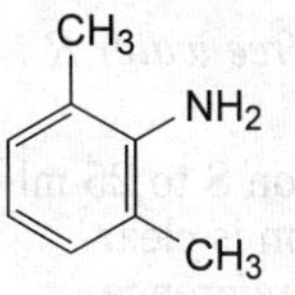

A. 2,6-dimethylaniline,

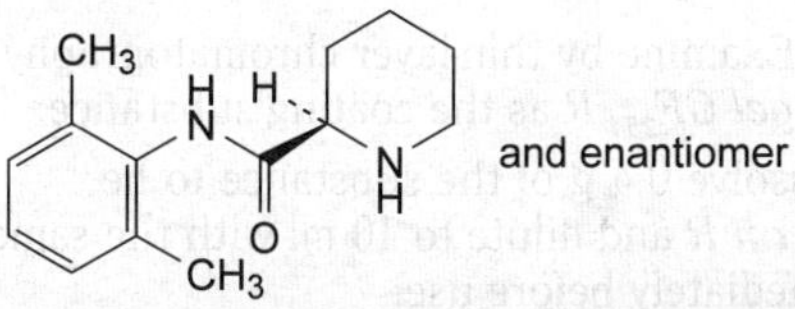

B. (*RS*)-*N*-(2,6-dimethylphenyl)piperidine-2-carboxamide,

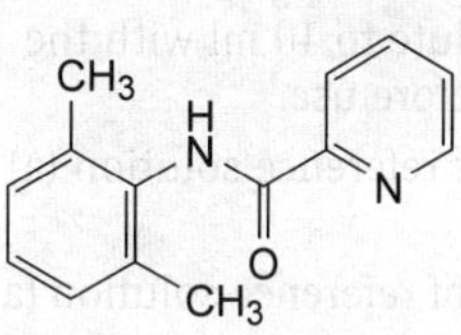

C. *N*-(2,6-dimethylphenyl)pyridine-2-carboxamide,

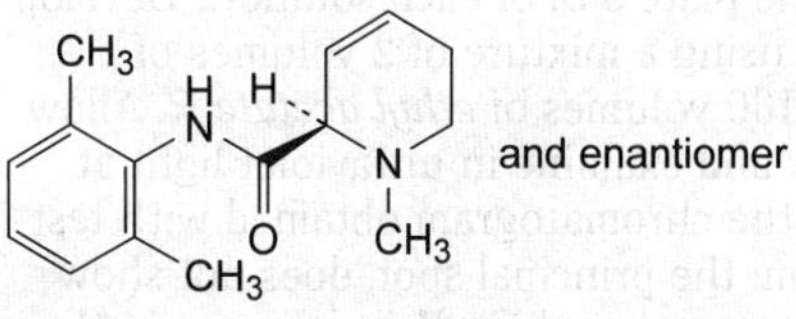

D. (*RS*)-*N*-(2,6-dimethylphenyl)-1-methyl-1,2,5,6-tetrahydropyridine-2-carboxamide,

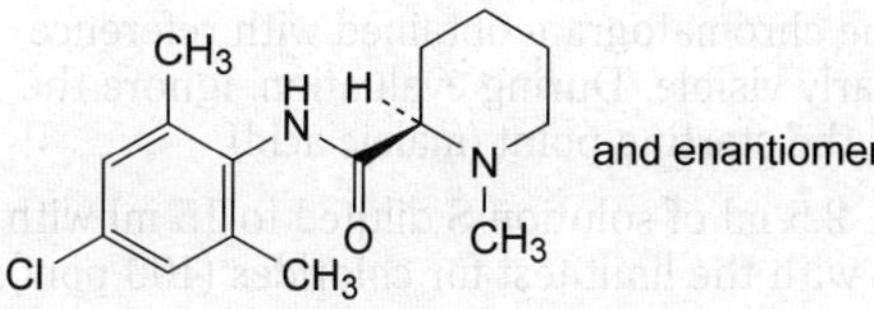

E. (*RS*)-*N*-(4-chloro-2,6-dimethylphenyl)-1-methylpiperidine-2-carboxamide.

01/2005:0407

MEPROBAMATE

Meprobamatum

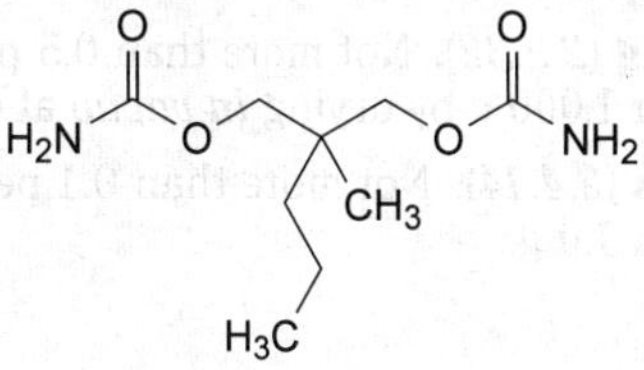

$C_9H_{18}N_2O_4$ M_r 218.3

DEFINITION

Meprobamate contains not less than 97.0 per cent and not more than the equivalent of 101.0 per cent of 2-methyl-2-propylpropane-1,3-diyl dicarbamate, calculated with reference to the dried substance.

CHARACTERS

A white or almost white, amorphous or crystalline powder, slightly soluble in water, freely soluble in alcohol.

IDENTIFICATION

First identification: A, B.

Second identification: A, C, D.

A. Melting point (*2.2.14*): 104 °C to 108 °C.

B. Examine by infrared absorption spectrophotometry (*2.2.24*), comparing with the spectrum obtained with *meprobamate CRS*.

C. To 0.5 g add 1 ml of *acetic anhydride R* and 0.05 ml of *sulphuric acid R*, mix and allow to stand for 30 min, shaking frequently. Pour the solution dropwise into 50 ml of *water R*, mix and allow to stand. Initiate crystallisation by scratching the wall of the tube with a glass rod. Collect the precipitate by filtration, wash and dry at 60 °C. The precipitate melts (*2.2.14*) at 124 °C to 128 °C.

D. Dissolve 0.2 g in 15 ml of *0.5 M alcoholic potassium hydroxide* and boil under a reflux condenser for 15 min. Add 0.5 ml of *glacial acetic acid R* and 1 ml of a 50 g/l solution of *cobalt nitrate R* in *ethanol R*. A deep-blue colour develops.

TESTS

Appearance of solution. Dissolve 1.0 g in 20 ml of *ethanol R*. The solution is clear (*2.2.1*) and colourless (*2.2.2, Method II*).

Related substances. Examine by thin-layer chromatography (*2.2.27*), using *silica gel G R* as the coating substance.

Test solution. Dissolve 0.20 g of the substance to be examined in *alcohol R* and dilute to 10 ml with the same solvent.

Reference solution. Dilute 0.1 ml of the test solution to 10 ml with *alcohol R*.

Apply separately to the plate 5 µl of each solution. Develop over a path of 15 cm using a mixture of 10 volumes of *pyridine R*, 30 volumes of *acetone R* and 70 volumes of *hexane R*. Dry the plate at 120 °C for 30 min, allow to cool and spray with a solution of 0.25 g of *vanillin R* in a cooled mixture of 10 ml of *alcohol R* and 40 ml of *sulphuric acid R* and heat at 100 °C to 105 °C for 30 min. Any spot in the chromatogram obtained with the test solution, apart from the principal spot, is not more intense than the spot in the chromatogram obtained with the reference solution (1.0 per cent).

Heavy metals (*2.4.8*). Dissolve 2.0 g in a mixture of 15 volumes of *water R* and 85 volumes of *acetone R* and dilute to 20 ml with the same mixture of solvents. 12 ml of the solution complies with limit test B for heavy metals (10 ppm). Prepare the standard using lead standard solution (1 ppm Pb) obtained by diluting *lead standard solution (100 ppm Pb) R* with the mixture of *water R* and *acetone R*.

Loss on drying (*2.2.32*). Not more than 0.5 per cent, determined on 1.000 g by drying *in vacuo* at 60 °C.

Sulphated ash (*2.4.14*). Not more than 0.1 per cent, determined on 1.0 g.

ASSAY

Dissolve 0.1000 g in 15 ml of a 25 per cent *V/V* solution of *sulphuric acid R* and boil under a reflux condenser for 3 h. Cool, dissolve by cautiously adding 30 ml of *water R*, cool again and place in a steam-distillation apparatus. Add 40 ml of *strong sodium hydroxide solution R* and distil immediately by passing steam through the mixture. Collect the distillate into 40 ml of a 40 g/l solution of *boric acid R* until the total volume in the receiver reaches about 200 ml. Add 0.25 ml of *methyl red mixed solution R*. Titrate with *0.1 M hydrochloric acid* until the colour changes from green to violet. Carry out a blank titration.

1 ml of *0.1 M hydrochloric acid* is equivalent to 10.91 mg of $C_9H_{18}N_2O_4$.

01/2005:0278

MEPYRAMINE MALEATE

Mepyramini maleas

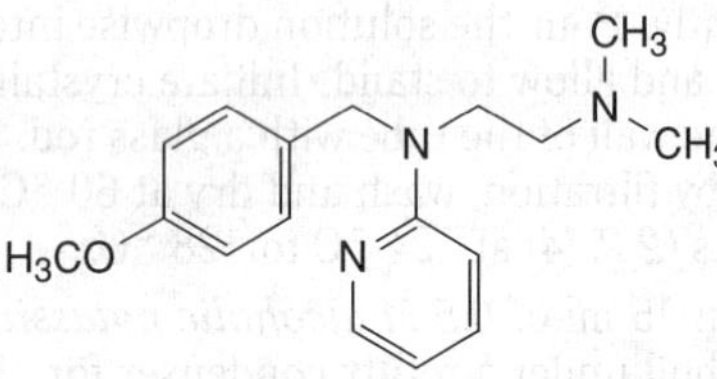

$C_{21}H_{27}N_3O_5$ M_r 401.5

DEFINITION

Mepyramine maleate contains not less than 99.0 per cent and not more than the equivalent of 101.0 per cent of *N*-(4-methoxybenzyl)-*N'*,*N'*-dimethyl-*N*-(pyridin-2-yl)ethane-1, 2-diamine (*Z*)-butenedioate, calculated with reference to the dried substance.

CHARACTERS

A white or slightly yellowish, crystalline powder, very soluble in water, freely soluble in alcohol.

IDENTIFICATION

First identification: A, B.

Second identification: A, C, D, E.

A. Melting point (*2.2.14*): 99 °C to 103 °C.

B. Examine by infrared absorption spectrophotometry (*2.2.24*), comparing with the spectrum obtained with *mepyramine maleate CRS*. Examine the substances as 50 g/l solutions in *methylene chloride R* using a 0.1 mm cell.

C. Dissolve 0.100 g in *0.01 M hydrochloric acid* and dilute to 100.0 ml with the same acid. Dilute 1.0 ml of this solution to 100.0 ml with *0.01 M hydrochloric acid*. Examined between 220 nm and 350 nm (*2.2.25*), the solution shows two absorption maxima, at 239 nm and 316 nm. The specific absorbances at the maxima are 431 to 477 and 196 to 220, respectively.

D. Examine the chromatograms obtained in the test for related substances. The principal spot in the chromatogram obtained with test solution (b) is similar in position and size to the principal spot in the chromatogram obtained with reference solution (b).

E. Triturate 0.1 g with 3 ml of *water R* and 1 ml of *strong sodium hydroxide solution R*. Shake with three quantities, each of 5 ml, of *ether R*. To 0.1 ml of the aqueous layer add a solution of 10 mg of *resorcinol R* in 3 ml of *sulphuric acid R*. Heat on a water-bath for 15 min; no colour develops. To the rest of the aqueous layer add 1 ml of *bromine water R*. Heat on a water-bath for 15 min and then heat to boiling and cool. To 0.2 ml of this solution add a solution of 10 mg of *resorcinol R* in 3 ml of *sulphuric acid R*. Heat on a water-bath for 15 min. A violet-pink colour develops.

TESTS

Solution S. Dissolve 5.0 g in *carbon dioxide-free water R* and dilute to 25 ml with the same solvent.

Appearance of solution. Dilute 5 ml of solution S to 25 ml with *carbon dioxide-free water R*. The solution is clear (*2.2.1*) and not more intensely coloured than reference solution Y_6 (*2.2.2, Method II*).

pH (*2.2.3*). Dilute 1 ml of solution S to 10 ml with *carbon dioxide-free water R*. The pH of this solution is 4.9 to 5.2.

Related substances. Examine by thin-layer chromatography (*2.2.27*), using *silica gel GF_{254} R* as the coating substance.

Test solution (a). Dissolve 0.4 g of the substance to be examined in *chloroform R* and dilute to 10 ml with the same solvent. Prepare immediately before use.

Test solution (b). Dilute 1 ml of test solution (a) to 10 ml with *chloroform R*.

Reference solution (a). Dissolve 0.4 g of *mepyramine maleate CRS* in *chloroform R* and dilute to 10 ml with the same solvent. Prepare immediately before use.

Reference solution (b). Dilute 1 ml of reference solution (a) to 10 ml with *chloroform R*.

Reference solution (c). Dilute 0.1 ml of reference solution (a) to 50 ml with *chloroform R*.

Reference solution (d). To 2 ml of reference solution (c) add 2 ml of *chloroform R*.

Apply separately to the plate 5 µl of each solution. Develop over a path of 15 cm using a mixture of 2 volumes of *diethylamine R* and 100 volumes of *ethyl acetate R*. Allow the plate to dry in air and examine in ultraviolet light at 254 nm. Any spot in the chromatogram obtained with test solution (a), apart from the principal spot, does not show more intense fluorescence quenching than the spot in the chromatogram obtained with reference solution (c) (0.2 per cent). The test is not valid unless the principal spots in the chromatograms obtained with test solution (a) and with reference solution (a) have R_f values not less than 0.2 and the spot in the chromatogram obtained with reference solution (d) is clearly visible. During evaluation, ignore the spot remaining at the starting point (maleic acid).

Chlorides (*2.4.4*). 2.5 ml of solution S diluted to 15 ml with *water R* complies with the limit test for chlorides (100 ppm).

Heavy metals (*2.4.8*). 1.0 g complies with limit test D for heavy metals (20 ppm). Prepare the standard using 2 ml of *lead standard solution (10 ppm Pb) R*.

Loss on drying (*2.2.32*). Not more than 0.25 per cent, determined on 1.00 g by drying in an oven at 80 °C.

Sulphated ash (*2.4.14*). Not more than 0.1 per cent, determined on the residue obtained in the test for loss on drying.

ASSAY

Dissolve 0.150 g in 40 ml of *anhydrous acetic acid R*. Titrate with *0.1 M perchloric acid* determining the end-point potentiometrically (*2.2.20*).

1 ml of *0.1 M perchloric acid* is equivalent to 20.07 mg of $C_{21}H_{27}N_3O_5$.

STORAGE

Store protected from light.

01/2005:0096

MERCAPTOPURINE

Mercaptopurinum

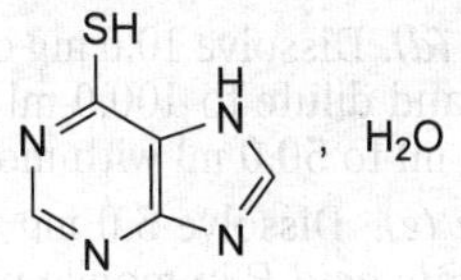

$C_5H_4N_4S,H_2O$ M_r 170.2

DEFINITION

Mercaptopurine contains not less than 98.5 per cent and not more than the equivalent of 101.0 per cent of 7*H*-purine-6-thiol, calculated with reference to the anhydrous substance.

CHARACTERS

A yellow, crystalline powder, practically insoluble in water, slightly soluble in alcohol. It dissolves in solutions of alkali hydroxides.

IDENTIFICATION

A. Dissolve 20 mg in 5 ml of *dimethyl sulphoxide R* and dilute to 100 ml with *0.1 M hydrochloric acid.* Dilute 5 ml of the solution to 200 ml with *0.1 M hydrochloric acid.* Examined between 230 nm and 350 nm (*2.2.25*), the solution shows only one absorption maximum, at 325 nm.

B. Dissolve about 20 mg in 20 ml of *alcohol R* heated to 60 °C and add 1 ml of a saturated solution of *mercuric acetate R* in *alcohol R*. A white precipitate is formed.

C. Dissolve about 20 mg in 20 ml of *alcohol R* heated to 60 °C and add 1 ml of a 10 g/l solution of *lead acetate R* in *alcohol R*. A yellow precipitate is formed.

TESTS

Hypoxanthine. Examine by thin-layer chromatography (*2.2.27*), using *silica gel GF* $_{254}$ *R* as the coating substance.

Test solution. Dissolve 50 mg of the substance to be examined in 1 ml of *dimethyl sulphoxide R* and dilute to 10 ml with *methanol R*.

Reference solution. Dissolve 10 mg of *hypoxanthine R* in 10 ml of *dimethyl sulphoxide R* and dilute to 100 ml with *methanol R*.

Apply separately to the plate 5 µl of each solution. Develop over a path of 10 cm using a mixture of 3 volumes of *concentrated ammonia R*, 7 volumes of *water R* and 90 volumes of *acetone R*. Allow the plate to dry in air and examine in ultraviolet light at 254 nm. Any spot corresponding to hypoxanthine in the chromatogram obtained with the test solution is not more intense than the spot in the chromatogram obtained with the reference solution (2.0 per cent).

Water (*2.5.12*). 10.0 per cent to 12.0 per cent, determined on 0.250 g by the semi-micro determination of water.

Sulphated ash (*2.4.14*). Not more than 0.1 per cent, determined on 1.0 g.

ASSAY

Dissolve 0.100 g in 50 ml of *dimethylformamide R*. Titrate with *0.1 M tetrabutylammonium hydroxide,* determining the end-point potentiometrically (*2.2.20*).

1 ml of *0.1 M tetrabutylammonium hydroxide* is equivalent to 15.22 mg of $C_5H_4N_4S$.

STORAGE

Store protected from light.

01/2005:0120

MERCURIC CHLORIDE

Hydrargyri dichloridum

$HgCl_2$ M_r 271.5

DEFINITION

Mercuric chloride contains not less than 99.5 per cent and not more than the equivalent of 100.5 per cent of $HgCl_2$, calculated with reference to the dried substance.

CHARACTERS

A white, crystalline powder or colourless or white crystals or heavy crystalline masses, soluble in water and in glycerol, freely soluble in alcohol.

IDENTIFICATION

A. It gives the reactions of chlorides (*2.3.1*).

B. Solution S (see Tests) gives the reactions of mercury (*2.3.1*).

TESTS

Solution S. Dissolve 1.0 g in *carbon dioxide-free water R* and dilute to 20 ml with the same solvent.

Appearance of solution. Solution S is not more opalescent than reference suspension II (*2.2.1*) and is colourless (*2.2.2, Method II*).

Acidity or alkalinity. To 10 ml of solution S add 0.1 ml of *methyl red solution R*. The solution is red. Add 0.5 g of *sodium chloride R*. The solution becomes yellow. Not more than 0.5 ml of *0.01 M hydrochloric acid* is required to change the colour to red.

Mercurous chloride. Dissolve 1.0 g in 30 ml of *ether R*. The solution shows no opalescence.

Loss on drying (*2.2.32*). Not more than 1.0 per cent, determined on 2.00 g by drying *in vacuo* for 24 h.

ASSAY

Dissolve 0.500 g in 100 ml of *water R*. Add 20.0 ml of *0.1 M sodium edetate* and 5 ml of *buffer solution pH 10.9 R*. Allow to stand for 15 min. Add 0.1 g of *mordant black 11 triturate R* and titrate with *0.1 M zinc sulphate* until the colour changes to purple. Add 3 g of *potassium iodide R*, allow to stand for 2 min, add a further 0.1 g of *mordant black 11 triturate R* and titrate with *0.1 M zinc sulphate.*

1 ml of *0.1 M zinc sulphate* used in the second titration is equivalent to 27.15 mg of $HgCl_2$.

STORAGE

Store protected from light.

01/2005:1699

MESALAZINE

Mesalazinum

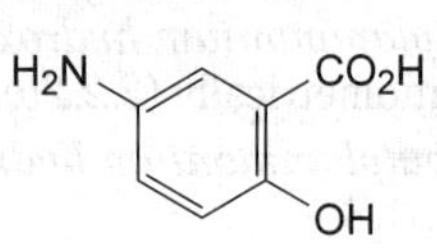

$C_7H_7NO_3$ M_r 153.1

DEFINITION

5-Amino-2-hydroxybenzoic acid.

Content: 98.5 per cent to 101.0 per cent (dried substance).

CHARACTERS

Appearance: almost white or light grey or light pink powder or crystals.

Solubility: very slightly soluble in water, practically insoluble in alcohol. It dissolves in dilute solutions of alkali hydroxides and in dilute hydrochloric acid.

IDENTIFICATION

First identification: B.

Second identification: A, C.

A. Dissolve 50.0 mg in 10 ml of a 10.3 g/l solution of *hydrochloric acid R* and dilute to 100.0 ml with the same acid. Dilute 5.0 ml to 200.0 ml with a 10.3 g/l solution of *hydrochloric acid R*. Examined between 210 nm and 250 nm (*2.2.25*), the solution shows an absorption maximum at about 230 nm. The specific absorbance at the maximum is 430 to 450.

B. Infrared absorption spectrophotometry (*2.2.24*).

Preparation: discs.

Comparison: *mesalazine CRS*.

C. Thin-layer chromatography (*2.2.27*).

Test solution. Dissolve 50 mg of the substance to be examined in 10 ml of a mixture of equal volumes of *glacial acetic acid R* and *water R* and dilute to 20.0 ml with *methanol R*.

Reference solution. Dissolve 50 mg of *mesalazine CRS* in 10 ml of a mixture of equal volumes of *glacial acetic acid R* and *water R* and dilute to 20.0 ml with *methanol R*.

Plate: a suitable silica gel as the coating substance.

Mobile phase: *glacial acetic acid R, methanol R, methyl isobutyl ketone R* (10:40:50 *V/V/V*).

Application: 5 µl.

Development: over a path of 10 cm.

Drying: in air.

Detection: examine in ultraviolet light at 365 nm.

Results: the principal spot in the chromatogram obtained with the test solution is similar in position, colour and size to the principal spot in the chromatogram obtained with the reference solution.

TESTS

Appearance of solution. *Maintain the solutions at 40 °C during preparation and measurements.* Dissolve 0.5 g in *1 M hydrochloric acid* and dilute to 20 ml with the same acid. The solution is clear (*2.2.1*). Immediately measure the absorbance (*2.2.25*) of the solution at 440 nm and 650 nm. The absorbance is not greater than 0.15 at 440 nm and 0.10 at 650 nm.

Reducing substances. Dissolve 0.10 g in *dilute hydrochloric acid R* and dilute to 25 ml with the same acid. Add 0.2 ml of *starch solution R* and 0.25 ml of *0.01 M iodine*. Allow to stand for 2 min. The solution is blue or violet-brown.

Related substances. Liquid chromatography (*2.2.29*). *Use freshly prepared solutions and mobile phases.*

Test solution. Dissolve 50.0 mg of the substance to be examined in mobile phase A and dilute to 50.0 ml with mobile phase A.

Reference solution (a). Dilute 1.0 ml of the test solution to 100.0 ml with mobile phase A.

Reference solution (b). Dissolve 5.0 mg of *3-aminobenzoic acid R* in mobile phase A and dilute to 100.0 ml with mobile phase A. Dilute 1.0 ml to 25.0 ml with the test solution.

Reference solution (c). Dissolve 5.0 mg of *3-aminobenzoic acid R* in mobile phase A and dilute to 100.0 ml with mobile phase A. Dilute 1.0 ml to 50.0 ml with mobile phase A.

Reference solution (d). Dissolve 10.0 mg of *3-aminophenol R* in mobile phase A and dilute to 100.0 ml with mobile phase A. Dilute 1.0 ml to 50.0 ml with mobile phase A.

Reference solution (e). Dissolve 5.0 mg of *2,5-dihydroxybenzoic acid R* in mobile phase A and dilute to 100.0 ml with mobile phase A. Dilute 1.0 ml to 50.0 ml with mobile phase A.

Reference solution (f). Dissolve 15.0 mg of *salicylic acid R* in mobile phase A and dilute to 100.0 ml with mobile phase A. Dilute 1.0 ml to 50.0 ml with mobile phase A.

Blank solution. Mobile phase A.

Column:

- *size*: l = 0.25 m, Ø = 4.6 mm,
- *stationary phase*: spherical *base-deactivated octylsilyl silica gel for chromatography R* (5 µm).

Mobile phase:

- *mobile phase A*: dissolve 2.2 g of *perchloric acid R* and 1.0 g of *phosphoric acid R* in *water R* and dilute to 1000.0 ml with the same solvent,
- *mobile phase B*: dissolve 1.7 g of *perchloric acid R* and 1.0 g of *phosphoric acid R* in *acetonitrile R* and dilute to 1000.0 ml with the same solvent,

Time (min)	Mobile phase A (per cent *V/V*)	Mobile phase B (per cent *V/V*)
0 - 7	100	0
7 - 25	100 → 40	0 → 60
25 - 30	40 → 100	60 → 0
30 - 40	100	0

Flow rate: 1.25 ml/min.

Detection: spectrophotometer at 220 nm.

Injection: 10 µl.

Relative retention with reference to mesalazine (retention time = about 5 min): impurity B = about 0.8; impurity D = about 1.2; impurity G = about 3.1; impurity H = about 3.9.

System suitability: reference solution (b):

- *peak-to-valley ratio*: minimum 1.5, where H_p = height above the baseline of the peak due to impurity D and H_v = height above the baseline of the lowest point of the curve separating this peak from the peak due to mesalazine.

Limits:

- *impurity B*: not more than the area of the principal peak in the chromatogram obtained with reference solution (d) (0.2 per cent),
- *impurity D*: not more than the area of the principal peak in the chromatogram obtained with reference solution (c) (0.1 per cent),
- *impurity G*: not more than the area of the principal peak in the chromatogram obtained with reference solution (e) (0.1 per cent),
- *impurity H*: not more than the area of the principal peak in the chromatogram obtained with reference solution (f) (0.3 per cent),
- *any other impurity*: not more than 0.1 times the area of the principal peak in the chromatogram obtained with reference solution (a) (0.1 per cent),
- *total*: not more than the area of the principal peak in the chromatogram obtained with reference solution (a) (1.0 per cent),
- *disregard limit*: 0.05 times the area of the principal peak in the chromatogram obtained with reference solution (a) (0.05 per cent). Disregard any peaks obtained with the blank solution.

Impurity A and impurity C. Liquid chromatography (*2.2.29*). *Use freshly prepared mobile phases.*

Test solution. Dissolve 50.0 mg of the substance to be examined in mobile phase A and dilute to 50.0 ml with mobile phase A.

Reference solution (a). Dissolve 5.0 mg of *2-aminophenol R* in mobile phase A and dilute to 100.0 ml with mobile phase A. Dilute 10.0 ml to 100.0 ml with mobile phase A.

Reference solution (b). Dissolve 5.0 mg of *4-aminophenol R* in mobile phase A and dilute to 250.0 ml with mobile phase A. To 1.0 ml of this solution, add 1.0 ml of reference solution (a) and dilute to 100.0 ml with mobile phase A.

Reference solution (c). Dilute 1.0 ml of the test solution to 200.0 ml with mobile phase A. To 5.0 ml of this solution add 5.0 ml of reference solution (a).

Column:

- *size*: *l* = 0.25 m, Ø = 4.6 mm,
- *stationary phase*: spherical *end-capped octadecylsilyl silica gel for chromatography R* (3 µm).

Mobile phase:

- *mobile phase A*: dissolve 2.2 g of *perchloric acid R* and 1.0 g of *phosphoric acid R* in *water R* and dilute to 1000.0 ml with the same solvent,
- *mobile phase B*: dissolve 1.7 g of *perchloric acid R* and 1.0 g of *phosphoric acid R* in *acetonitrile R* and dilute to 1000.0 ml with the same solvent,

Time (min)	Mobile phase A (per cent *V/V*)	Mobile phase B (per cent *V/V*)
0 - 8	100	0
8 - 25	100 → 40	0 → 60
25 - 30	40 → 100	60 → 0
30 - 40	100	0

Flow rate: 1.0 ml/min.

Detection: spectrophotometer at 220 nm.

Injection: 20 µl; inject the test solution and reference solutions (b) and (c).

Relative retention with reference to mesalazine (retention time = about 9 min): impurity A = about 0.5; impurity C = about 0.9.

System suitability: reference solution (c):

- *resolution*: minimum 3 between the peaks due to impurity C and mesalazine.

Limits:

- *impurity A*: not more than the area of the corresponding peak in the chromatogram obtained with reference solution (b) (200 ppm),
- *impurity C*: not more than 4 times the area of the corresponding peak in the chromatogram obtained with reference solution (b) (200 ppm).

Impurity K. Liquid chromatography (*2.2.29*).

Test solution. Dissolve 40.0 mg of the substance to be examined in the mobile phase and dilute to 20.0 ml with the mobile phase.

Reference solution. Dissolve 27.8 mg of *aniline hydrochloride R* in the mobile phase and dilute to 100.0 ml with the mobile phase. Dilute 0.20 ml of this solution to 20.0 ml with the mobile phase. Dilute 0.20 ml of this solution to 20.0 ml with the mobile phase.

Column:

- *size*: *l* = 0.25 m, Ø = 4 mm,
- *stationary phase*: spherical *octadecylsilyl silica gel for chromatography R* (5 µm),
- *temperature*: 40 °C.

Mobile phase: mix 15 volumes of *methanol R* and 85 volumes of a solution containing 1.41 g/l of *potassium dihydrogen phosphate R* and 0.47 g/l of *disodium hydrogen phosphate dihydrate R* previously adjusted to pH 8.0 with a 42 g/l solution of *sodium hydroxide R.*

Flow rate: 1.0 ml/min.

Detection: spectrophotometer at 205 nm.

Injection: 50 µl.

Retention time: impurity K = about 15 min.

System suitability: reference solution:

- *signal-to-noise ratio*: minimum 10 for the principal peak.

Limit:

- *impurity K*: not more than the area of the corresponding peak in the chromatogram obtained with the reference solution (10 ppm).

Chlorides: maximum 0.1 per cent.

Dissolve 1.50 g in 50 ml of *anhydrous formic acid R.* Add 100 ml of *water R* and 5 ml of *2 M nitric acid.* Titrate with *0.005 M silver nitrate* determining the end-point potentiometrically (*2.2.20*).

1 ml of *0.005 M silver nitrate* is equivalent to 0.1773 mg of Cl.

Sulphates (*2.4.13*): maximum 200 ppm.

Shake 1.0 g with 20 ml of *distilled water R* for 1 min and filter. 15 ml of the filtrate complies with the limit test for sulphates.

Heavy metals (*2.4.8*): maximum 20 ppm.

1.0 g complies with limit test F. Prepare the standard using 2 ml of *lead standard solution (10 ppm Pb) R.*

Loss on drying (*2.2.32*): maximum 0.5 per cent, determined on 1.000 g by drying in an oven at 100-105 °C.

Sulphated ash (*2.4.14*): maximum 0.2 per cent, determined on 1.0 g.

ASSAY

Dissolve 50.0 mg in 100 ml of boiling *water R.* Cool rapidly to room temperature and titrate with *0.1 M sodium hydroxide,* determining the end-point potentiometrically (*2.2.20*).

Monographs M

1 ml of *0.1 M sodium hydroxide* is equivalent to 15.31 mg of $C_7H_7NO_3$.

STORAGE

In an airtight container, protected from light.

IMPURITIES

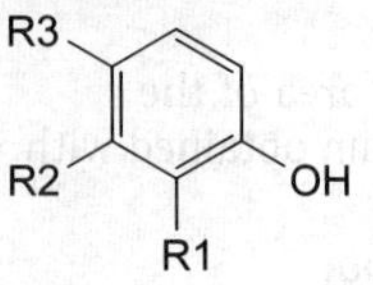

A. R1 = R2 = H, R3 = NH_2: 4-aminophenol,

B. R1 = R3 = H, R2 = NH_2: 3-aminophenol,

C. R1 = NH_2, R2 = R3 = H: 2-aminophenol,

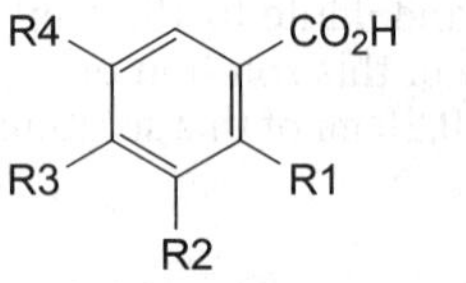

D. R1 = R3 = R4 = H, R2 = NH_2: 3-aminobenzoic acid,

E. R1 = OH, R2 = R4 = H, R3 = NH_2: 4-amino-2-hydroxybenzoic acid (4-aminosalicylic acid),

F. R1 = OH, R2 = NH_2, R3 = R4 = H: 3-amino-2-hydroxybenzoic acid (3-aminosalicylic acid),

G. R1 = R4 = OH, R2 = R3 = H: 2,5-dihydroxybenzoic acid,

H. R1 = OH, R2 = R3 = R4 = H: 2-hydroxybenzoic acid (salicylic acid),

I. R1 = OH, R2 = R3 = H, R4 = N=N-C_6H_5: 2-hydroxy-5-(phenyldiazenyl)benzoic acid (phenylazosalicylic acid),

J. R1 = OH, R2 = R4 = NH_2, R3 = H: 3,5-diamino-2-hydroxybenzoic acid (diaminosalicylic acid),

L. R1 = Cl, R2 = R3 = R4 = H: 2-chlorobenzoic acid,

M. R1 = Cl, R2 = R3 = H, R4 = NO_2: 2-chloro-5-nitrobenzoic acid,

N. R1 = OH, R2 = R3 = H, R4 = NO_2: 2-hydroxy-5-nitrobenzoic acid (5-nitrosalicylic acid),

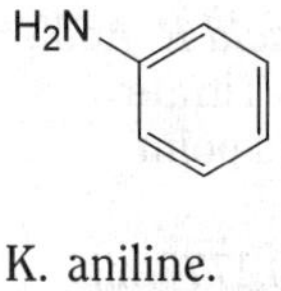

K. aniline.

01/2005:1674

MESNA

Mesnum

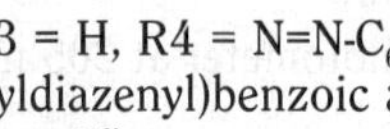

$C_2H_5NaO_3S_2$ M_r 164.2

DEFINITION

Sodium 2-sulphanylethanesulphonate.

Content: 96.0 per cent to 102.0 per cent (dried substance).

CHARACTERS

Appearance: white or slightly yellow, crystalline powder, hygroscopic.

Solubility: freely soluble in water, slightly soluble in alcohol, practically insoluble in cyclohexane.

IDENTIFICATION

A. Infrared absorption spectrophotometry (*2.2.24*).

Comparison: *Ph. Eur. reference spectrum of mesna.*

B. It gives reaction (a) of sodium (*2.3.1*).

TESTS

Solution S. Dissolve 10.0 g in *carbon dioxide-free water R* prepared from *distilled water R* and dilute to 50 ml with the same solvent.

Appearance of solution. Solution S is not more opalescent than reference suspension II (*2.2.1*) and not more intensely coloured than reference solution Y_7 (*2.2.2, Method II*).

pH (*2.2.3*): 4.5 to 6.0.

Dilute 10 ml of solution S to 20 ml with *carbon dioxide-free water R*.

Related substances. Liquid chromatography (*2.2.29*).

Test solution. Dissolve 0.10 g of the substance to be examined in the mobile phase and dilute to 25.0 ml with the mobile phase.

Reference solution (a). Dissolve 4.0 mg of *mesna impurity C CRS* in the mobile phase and dilute to 50.0 ml with the mobile phase. Dilute 2.0 ml of the solution to 20.0 ml with the mobile phase.

Reference solution (b). Dissolve 6.0 mg of *mesna impurity D CRS* in the mobile phase and dilute to 5.0 ml with the mobile phase. Dilute 1.0 ml of the solution to 10.0 ml with the mobile phase.

Reference solution (c). Dilute 3.0 ml of the test solution to 10.0 ml with the mobile phase. Dilute 1.0 ml of the solution to 100.0 ml with the mobile phase.

Reference solution (d). Dilute 6.0 ml of reference solution (c) to 20.0 ml with the mobile phase. To 10 ml of the solution, add 10 ml of reference solution (a).

Column:

- *size*: *l* = 0.25 m, Ø = 4.6 mm,
- *stationary phase*: *octadecylsilyl silica gel for chromatography R* (10 µm).

Mobile phase: dissolve 2.94 g of *potassium dihydrogen phosphate R*, 2.94 g of *dipotassium hydrogen phosphate R* and 2.6 g of *tetrabutylammonium hydrogen sulphate R* in about 600 ml of *water R*. Adjust to pH 2.3 with *phosphoric acid R*, add 335 ml of *methanol R* and dilute to 1000 ml with *water R*.

Flow rate: 1 ml/min.

Detection: spectrophotometer at 235 nm.

Injection: 20 µl.

Run time: 4 times the retention time of mesna.

Relative retention with reference to mesna (retention time = about 4.8): impurities A and B = about 0.6; impurity E = about 0.8; impurity C = about 1.4; impurity D = about 2.3.

System suitability: reference solution (d):

- *resolution*: minimum 3.0 between the peaks corresponding to mesna and to impurity C.

Limits:

- *correction factor*: for the calculation of contents, multiply the peak areas of impurities A, B and E by 0.01,
- *impurity C*: not more than the area of the corresponding peak in the chromatogram obtained with reference solution (a) (0.2 per cent),

– *impurity D*: not more than the area of the corresponding peak in the chromatogram obtained with reference solution (b) (3.0 per cent),
– *impurities A, B, E*: for each impurity, not more than the area of the principal peak in the chromatogram obtained with reference solution (c) (0.3 per cent),
– *any other impurity*: for each impurity, not more than one third the area of the principal peak in the chromatogram obtained with reference solution (c) (0.1 per cent),
– *total of other impurities*: not more than the area of the principal peak in the chromatogram obtained with reference solution (c) (0.3 per cent),
– *disregard limit*: 0.15 times the area of the principal peak in the chromatogram obtained with reference solution (c) (0.045 per cent).

Chlorides (*2.4.4*): maximum 250 ppm.

Dilute 1 ml of solution S to 15 ml with *water R*.

Sulphates (*2.4.13*): maximum 300 ppm.

Dilute 5 ml of solution S to 30 ml with *distilled water R*. 15 ml of the solution complies with the limit test for sulphates.

Disodium edetate: maximum 500 ppm.

Dissolve 4.000 g in 90 ml of *water R* and adjust to pH 4.5 using *0.1 M hydrochloric acid*. Add 10 ml of *acetate buffer solution pH 4.5 R* and 50 ml of *2-propanol R*. Add 2 ml of a 0.25 g/l solution of *dithizone R* in *2-propanol R*. Titrate with *0.01 M zinc sulphate* until the colour changes from bluish-grey to pink.

1 ml of *0.01 M zinc sulphate* is equivalent to 3.72 mg of $C_{10}H_{14}N_2Na_2O_8,2H_2O$.

Heavy metals (*2.4.8*): maximum 10 ppm.

Dilute 10 ml of solution S to 20 ml with *water R*. 12 ml of the solution complies with limit test A. Prepare the standard using *lead standard solution (1 ppm Pb) R*.

Loss on drying (*2.2.32*): maximum 1.0 per cent, determined on 1.000 g under high vacuum at 60 °C for 2 h.

ASSAY

Dissolve 0.120 g in 10 ml of *water R*. Add 10 ml of *1 M sulphuric acid* and 10.0 ml of *0.1 M iodine*. Titrate with *0.1 M sodium thiosulphate* adding 1 ml of *starch solution R* near the endpoint. Carry out a blank titration.

1 ml of *0.1 M sodium thiosulphate* is equivalent to 16.42 mg of $C_2H_5NaO_3S_2$.

STORAGE

In an airtight container.

IMPURITIES

Specified impurities: A, B, C, D, E.

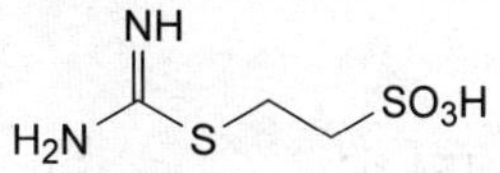

A. 2-(carbamimidoylsulphanyl)ethanesulphonic acid,

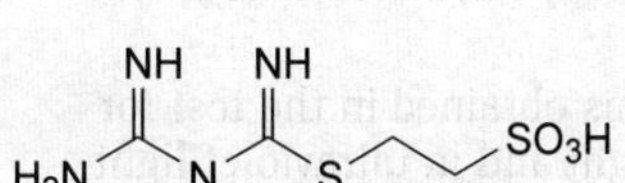

B. 2-[[(guanidino)(imino)methyl]sulphanyl]ethanesulphonic acid,

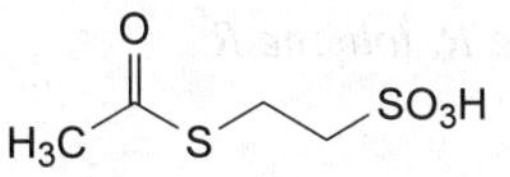

C. 2-(acetylsulphanyl)ethanesulphonic acid,

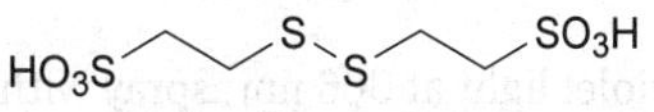

D. 2,2′-(disulphanediyl)bis(ethanesulphonic acid),

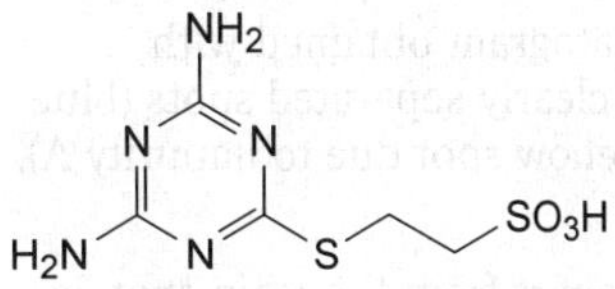

E. 2-(4,6-diamino-1,3,5-triazin-2-yl)sulphanylethanesulphonic acid.

01/2005:1730

MESTEROLONE

Mesterolonum

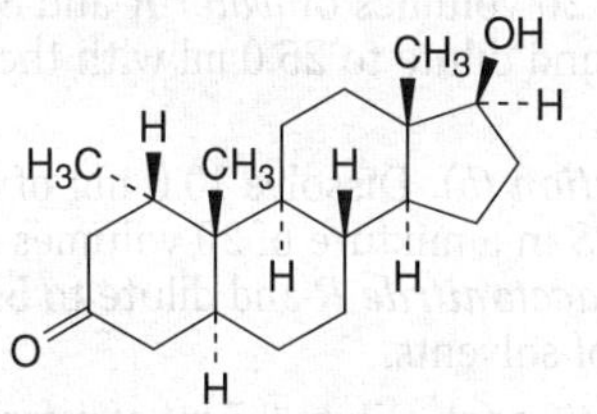

$C_{20}H_{32}O_2$ M_r 304.5

DEFINITION

17β-Hydroxy-1α-methyl-5α-androstan-3-one.

Content: 98.0 per cent to 102.0 per cent (dried substance).

CHARACTERS

Appearance: white or yellowish crystalline powder.

Solubility: practically insoluble in water, sparingly soluble in acetone, in ethyl acetate and in methanol.

IDENTIFICATION

A. Melting point (*2.2.14*): 206 °C to 211 °C.

B. Infrared absorption spectrophotometry (*2.2.24*).
Preparation: discs.
Comparison: *mesterolone CRS*.

TESTS

Specific optical rotation (*2.2.7*): + 20 to + 24 (dried substance).

Dissolve 0.200 g in *methylene chloride R* and dilute to 10.0 ml with the same solvent.

Impurity B: maximum 0.5 per cent.

Thin-layer chromatography (*2.2.27*).

Test solution. Dissolve 100.0 mg of the substance to be examined in a mixture of equal volumes of *methanol R* and *methylene chloride R* and dilute to 10.0 ml with the same mixture of solvents.

Reference solution (a). Dilute 1.0 ml of the test solution to 200.0 ml with a mixture of equal volumes of *methanol R* and *methylene chloride R*.

Reference solution (b). Dissolve 5.0 mg of *mesterolone impurity A CRS* in reference solution (a) and dilute to 100.0 ml with the same solution.

Plate: *TLC silica gel plate R*.

Mobile phase: *methanol R*, *acetone R*, *toluene R* (2:15:85 *V/V/V*).

Application: 10 µl.

Development: over 2/3 of the plate.

Drying: in air.

Detection: examine in ultraviolet light at 366 nm; spray with a 200 g/l solution of *toluenesulphonic acid R* in *alcohol R* and heat the plate for 10 min at 120 °C.

System suitability: the chromatogram obtained with reference solution (b) shows 2 clearly separated spots (blue spot due to mesterolone and yellow spot due to impurity A).

Limit:

– *impurity B*: any blue spot, apart from the main spot, is not more intense than the spot in the chromatogram obtained with reference solution (a) (0.5 per cent).

Related substances. Liquid chromatography (*2.2.29*).

Test solution. Dissolve 50.0 mg of the substance to be examined in a mixture of 20 volumes of *water R* and 80 volumes of *acetonitrile R* and dilute to 25.0 ml with the same mixture of solvents.

Reference solution (a). Dissolve 50.0 mg of *mesterolone CRS* in a mixture of 20 volumes of *water R* and 80 volumes of *acetonitrile R* and dilute to 25.0 ml with the same mixture of solvents.

Reference solution (b). Dissolve 10.0 mg of *mesterolone impurity A CRS* in a mixture of 20 volumes of *water R* and 80 volumes of *acetonitrile R* and dilute to 5.0 ml with the same mixture of solvents.

Reference solution (c). Dilute 0.5 ml of reference solution (a) and 0.5 ml of reference solution (b) to 100.0 ml with a mixture of 20 volumes of *water R* and 80 volumes of *acetonitrile R*.

Column:

– *size*: *l* = 0.25 m, Ø = 4.6 mm,
– *stationary phase*: *octadecylsilyl silica gel for chromatography R* (3 µm).

Mobile phase: *acetonitrile R*, *water R*, *methanol R* (20:40:60 *V/V/V*).

Flow rate: 0.9 ml/min.

Detection: spectrophotometer at 200 nm.

Injection: 50 µl; inject the test solution and reference solution (c).

Run time: 3 times the retention time of mesterolone.

Relative retention with reference to mesterolone (retention time = about 22 min): impurity A = about 0.7.

System suitability: reference solution (c):

– *resolution*: minimum 6.0 between the peaks due to impurity A and to mesterolone.

Limits:

– *impurity A*: not more than the area of the peak due to impurity A in the chromatogram obtained with reference solution (c) (0.5 per cent),
– *any other impurity*: not more than half the area of the peak due to mesterolone in the chromatogram obtained with reference solution (c) (0.25 per cent),
– *total*: not more than 1.5 times the area of the peak due to mesterolone in the chromatogram obtained with reference solution (c) (0.75 per cent),
– *disregard limit*: 0.1 times the area of the peak due to mesterolone in the chromatogram obtained with reference solution (c) (0.05 per cent).

Loss on drying (*2.2.32*): maximum 0.5 per cent, determined on 1.000 g by drying in an oven at 100-105 °C.

Sulphated ash (*2.4.14*): maximum 0.1 per cent, determined on 1.0 g.

ASSAY

Liquid chromatography (*2.2.29*) as described in the test for related substances.

Injection: 10 µl; inject the test solution and reference solution (a).

Calculate the percentage content of $C_{20}H_{32}O_2$.

IMPURITIES

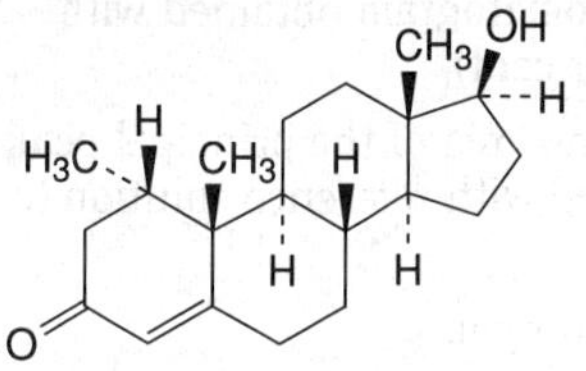

A. 17β-hydroxy-1α-methylandrost-4-en-3-one,

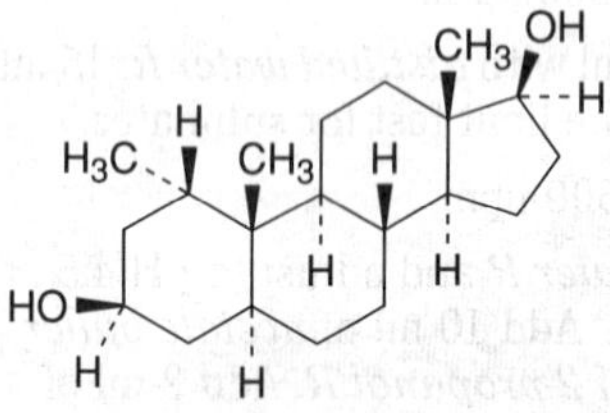

B. 1α-methyl-5α-androstane-3β,17β-diol.

01/2005:0509

MESTRANOL

Mestranolum

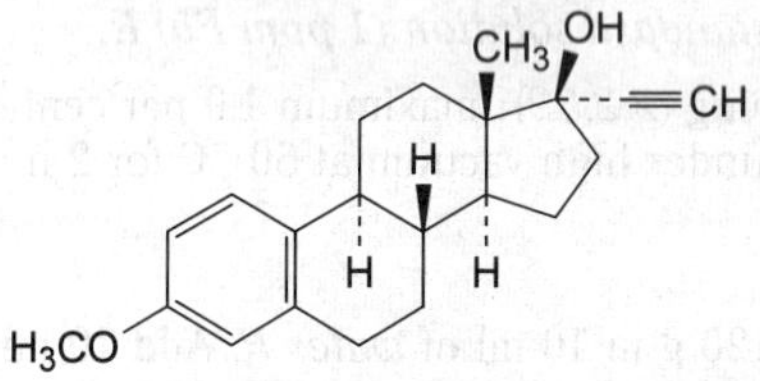

$C_{21}H_{26}O_2$ M_r 310.4

DEFINITION

Mestranol contains not less than 98.0 per cent and not more than the equivalent of 102.0 per cent of 3-methoxy-19-nor-17α-pregna-1,3,5(10)-trien-20-yn-17-ol, calculated with reference to the dried substance.

CHARACTERS

A white or almost white, crystalline powder, practically insoluble in water, sparingly soluble in alcohol.

IDENTIFICATION

First identification: B.

Second identification: A, C, D.

A. Melting point (*2.2.14*): 150 °C to 154 °C.

B. Examine by infrared absorption spectrophotometry (*2.2.24*), comparing with the spectrum obtained with *mestranol CRS*.

C. Examine the chromatograms obtained in the test for related substances in daylight and in ultraviolet light at 365 nm. The principal spot in the chromatogram obtained with test solution (b) is similar in position, colour, fluorescence and size to the principal spot in the chromatogram obtained with reference solution (a).

D. Dissolve about 5 mg in 1 ml of *sulphuric acid R*. A red colour develops with a greenish-yellow fluorescence in ultraviolet light at 365 nm. Add the solution to 10 ml of *water R* and mix. The solution becomes pink and a pink to violet precipitate is formed on standing.

TESTS

Specific optical rotation (*2.2.7*). Dissolve 0.100 g in *anhydrous pyridine R* and dilute to 10.0 ml with the same solvent. The specific optical rotation is − 20 to − 24, calculated with reference to the dried substance.

Absorbance (*2.2.25*). Dissolve 25.0 mg in *alcohol R* and dilute to 25.0 ml with the same solvent. Dilute 10.0 ml of this solution to 100.0 ml with *alcohol R*. Examined between 260 nm and 310 nm, the solution shows two absorption maxima, at 279 nm and 288 nm, and a minimum at 286 nm. The specific absorbances at the maxima are 62 to 68 and 59 to 64, respectively.

Related substances. Examine by thin-layer chromatography (*2.2.27*), using *silica gel G R* as the coating substance.

Test solution (a). Dissolve 0.10 g of the substance to be examined in *chloroform R* and dilute to 10 ml with the same solvent.

Test solution (b). Dilute 1 ml of test solution (a) to 10 ml with *chloroform R*.

Reference solution (a). Dissolve 10 mg of *mestranol CRS* in *chloroform R* and dilute to 10 ml with the same solvent.

Reference solution (b). Dilute 1 ml of test solution (b) to 10 ml with *chloroform R*.

Reference solution (c). Dilute 5 ml of reference solution (b) to 10 ml with *chloroform R*.

Apply separately to the plate 5 µl of each solution. Develop over a path of 15 cm using a mixture of 10 volumes of *alcohol R* and 90 volumes of *toluene R*. Allow the plate to dry in air until the solvent has evaporated. Heat at 110 °C for 10 min. Spray the hot plate with *alcoholic solution of sulphuric acid R*. Heat again at 110 °C for 10 min. Examine in daylight and in ultraviolet light at 365 nm. Any spot in the chromatogram obtained with test solution (a), apart from the principal spot, is not more intense than the spot in the chromatogram obtained with reference solution (b) (1.0 per cent) and at most one such spot is more intense than the spot in the chromatogram obtained with reference solution (c) (0.5 per cent).

Loss on drying (*2.2.32*). Not more than 1.0 per cent, determined on 0.500 g by drying in an oven at 100 °C to 105 °C for 3 h.

ASSAY

Dissolve 0.200 g in 40 ml of *tetrahydrofuran R* and add 5 ml of a 100 g/l solution of *silver nitrate R*. Titrate with *0.1 M sodium hydroxide,* determining the end-point potentiometrically (*2.2.20*). Carry out a blank titration.

1 ml of *0.1 M sodium hydroxide* is equivalent to 31.04 mg of $C_{21}H_{26}O_2$.

STORAGE

Store protected from light.

01/2005:2077

METACRESOL

Metacresolum

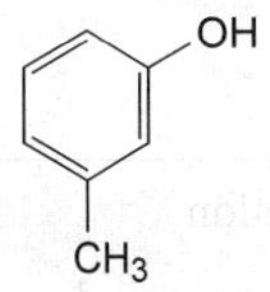

C_7H_8O M_r 108.1

DEFINITION

3-Methylphenol.

CHARACTERS

Appearance: colourless or yellowish liquid.

Solubility: sparingly soluble in water, miscible with alcohol and with methylene chloride.

Relative density: about 1.03.

mp: about 11 °C.

bp: about 202 °C.

IDENTIFICATION

Infrared absorption spectrophotometry (*2.2.24*).

Comparison: *Ph. Eur. reference spectrum of metacresol.*

TESTS

Solution S. Dissolve 1.5 g in *carbon dioxide-free water R* and dilute to 100 ml with the same solvent.

Appearance of solution. Freshly prepared solution S is not more opalescent than reference suspension III (*2.2.1*) and not more intensely coloured than reference solution BY_7 (*2.2.2, Method II*).

Acidity. To 25 ml of solution S, add 0.15 ml of *methyl red solution R*. The solution is red. Not more than 0.5 ml of *0.01 M sodium hydroxide* is required to change the colour of the indicator to yellow.

Related substances. Gas chromatography (*2.2.28*): use the normalisation procedure.

Test solution. Dissolve 0.250 g of the substance to be examined in *methanol R* and dilute to 100.0 ml with the same solvent.

Reference solution (a). Dissolve 25 mg of *cresol R*, 25 mg of *p-cresol R* and 25 mg of the substance to be examined in *methanol R* and dilute to 20 ml with the same solvent.

Reference solution (b). Dilute 1.0 ml of the test solution to 100.0 ml with *methanol R*. Dilute 1.0 ml to 20.0 ml with *methanol R*.

Column:

– *material*: fused silica,
– *size*: *l* = 25 m, Ø = 0.25 mm,
– *stationary phase*: *poly[(cyanopropyl)(methyl)][(phenyl)(methyl)]siloxane R* (0.2 µm).

Carrier gas: *helium for chromatography R*.

Flow rate: 1.5 ml/min.

Split ratio: 1:50.

Temperature:

	Time (min)	Temperature (°C)
Column	0 - 35	100
	35 - 40	100 → 150
	40 - 50	150
Injection port		200
Detector		200

Detection: flame ionisation.

Injection: 0.5 μl.

Relative retention with reference to metacresol (retention time = about 28 min): impurity B = about 0.75; impurity C = about 0.98.

System suitability: reference solution (a):

– *resolution*: minimum 1.4 between the peaks due to impurity C and metacresol.

Limits:

– *impurities B, C*: for each impurity, not more than 0.5 per cent,
– *any other impurity*: for each impurity, not more than 0.1 per cent,
– *total*: not more than 1.0 per cent.
– *disregard limit*: the area of the peak due to metacresol in the chromatogram obtained with reference solution (b) (0.05 per cent).

Residue on evaporation: maximum 0.1 per cent.

Evaporate 2.0 g to dryness on a water-bath under a fume hood and dry at 100-105 °C for 1 h. The residue weighs a maximum of 2 mg.

STORAGE

In an airtight container, protected from light.

IMPURITIES

Specified impurities: B, C.

Other detectable impurities: A, D, E, F, G, H, I, J, K, L, M.

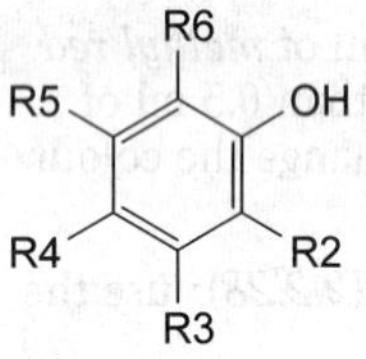

A. R2 = R3 = R4 = R5 = R6 = H: phenol,

B. R2 = CH_3, R3 = R4 = R5 = R6 = H: 2-methylphenol (*o*-cresol, cresol),

C. R2 = R3 = R5 = R6 = H, R4 = CH_3: 4-methylphenol (*p*-cresol),

D. R2 = R6 = CH_3, R3 = R4 = R5 = H: 2,6-dimethylphenol (2,6-xylenol),

E. R2 = C_2H_5, R3 = R4 = R5 = R6 = H: 2-ethylphenol (*o*-ethylphenol),

F. R2 = R4 = CH_3, R3 = R5 = R6 = H: 2,4-dimethylphenol (2,4-xylenol),

G. R2 = R5 = CH_3, R3 = R4 = R6 = H: 2,5-dimethylphenol (2,5-xylenol),

H. R2 = $CH(CH_3)_2$, R3 = R4 = R5 = R6 = H: 2-(1-methylethyl)phenol,

I. R2 = R3 = CH_3, R4 = R5 = R6 = H: 2,3-dimethylphenol (2,3-xylenol),

J. R2 = R4 = R6 = H, R3 = R5 = CH_3: 3,5-dimethylphenol (3,5-xylenol),

K. R2 = R3 = R5 = R6 = H, R4 = C_2H_5: 4-ethylphenol (*p*-ethylphenol),

L. R2 = R5 = R6 = H, R3 = R4 = CH_3: 3,4-dimethylphenol (3,4-xylenol),

M. R2 = R3 = R5 = CH_3, R4 = R6 = H: 2,3,5-trimethylphenol.

01/2005:1346

METAMIZOLE SODIUM

Metamizolum natricum

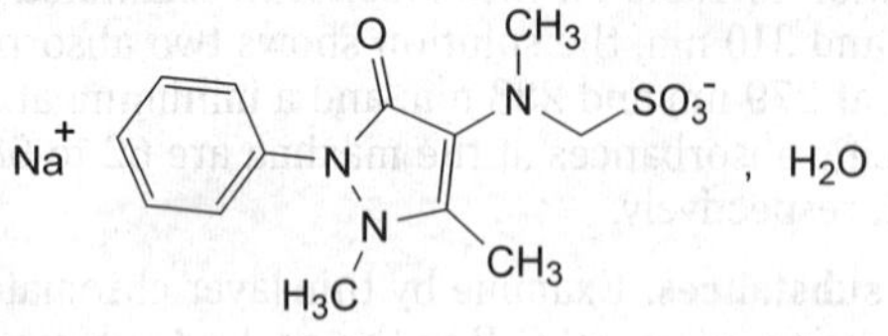

$C_{13}H_{16}N_3NaO_4S,H_2O$ M_r 351.4

DEFINITION

Metamizole sodium contains not less than 99.0 and not more than the equivalent of 100.5 per cent of sodium [(1,5-dimethyl-3-oxo-2-phenyl-2,3-dihydro-1*H*-pyrazol-4-yl)-*N*-methylamino]methanesulphonate, calculated with reference to the dried substance.

CHARACTERS

A white or almost white, crystalline powder, very soluble in water, soluble in alcohol.

IDENTIFICATION

First identification: A, D.

Second identification: B, C, D.

A. Examine by infrared absorption spectrophotometry (*2.2.24*), comparing with the spectrum obtained with *metamizole sodium CRS*.

B. Dissolve 50 mg in 1 ml of *strong hydrogen peroxide solution R*. A blue colour is produced which fades rapidly and turns to intense red in a few minutes.

C. Place 0.10 g in a test tube, add some beads of glass and dissolve the substance in 1.5 ml of *water R*. Add 1.5 ml of *dilute hydrochloric acid R* and place a filter paper wetted with a solution of 20 mg of *potassium iodate R* in 2 ml of *starch solution R* at the open end of the test tube. Heat gently, the evolving vapour of sulphur dioxide colours the filter paper blue. After heating gently for 1 min take a glass rod with a drop of a 10 g/l solution of *chromotropic acid, sodium salt R* in *sulphuric acid R* and place in the opening of the tube. Within 10 min, a blue-violet colour develops in the drop of the reagent.

D. 0.5 ml of solution S (see Tests) gives reaction (a) of sodium (*2.3.1*).

TESTS

Solution S. Dissolve 2.0 g in *carbon dioxide-free water R* and dilute to 40 ml with the same solvent.

Appearance of solution. Solution S is clear (*2.2.1*) and immediately after preparation, not more intensely coloured than reference solution BY_6 (*2.2.2, Method I*).

Acidity or alkalinity. To 5 ml of solution S, add 0.1 ml of *phenolphthalein solution R1*. The solution is colourless. Not more than 0.1 ml of *0.02 M sodium hydroxide* is required to change the colour of the indicator to pink.

Related substances. Examine by liquid chromatography (*2.2.29*).

Prepare the solutions immediately before use.

Test solution. Dissolve 50.0 mg of the substance to be examined in *methanol R* and dilute to 10.0 ml with the same solvent.

Reference solution (a). Dissolve 10.0 mg of *metamizole impurity A CRS* in *methanol R* and dilute to 20.0 ml with the same solvent.

Reference solution (b). Dilute 1.0 ml of reference solution (a) to 20.0 ml with *methanol R*.

Reference solution (c). Dissolve 40 mg of *metamizole sodium CRS* in *methanol R* and dilute to 20.0 ml with the same solvent.

Reference solution (d). Take 10 ml of reference solution (c) and boil under a reflux condenser for 10 min. Allow to cool to room temperature and dilute to 20.0 ml with *methanol R*.

Reference solution (e). To 6 ml of reference solution (a) add 1 ml of reference solution (c).

The chromatographic procedure may be carried out using:

– a stainless steel column 0.25 m long and 4.6 mm in internal diameter packed with *base-deactivated octadecylsilyl silica gel for chromatography R* (5 µm),

– as mobile phase at a flow rate of 1.0 ml/min a mixture of 28 volumes of *methanol R* and 72 volumes of a buffer solution prepared by adjusting a mixture of 1000 volumes of a 6.0 g/l solution of *sodium dihydrogen phosphate R* and 1 volume of *triethylamine R* to pH 7.0 with *strong sodium hydroxide solution R*,

– as detector a spectrophotometer set at 254 nm.

When the chromatograms are recorded in the prescribed conditions, the substances elute in the following order: impurity A, metamizole, impurity B, impurity C and impurity D. Inject 10 µl of reference solution (b). Adjust the sensitivity of the system so that the height of the principal peak in the chromatogram obtained is at least 50 per cent of the full scale of the recorder.

Inject 10 µl of reference solution (d). The chromatogram shows two principal peaks due to metamizole and impurity C.

Inject 10 µl of reference solution (e). The test is not valid unless in the chromatogram obtained the resolution between the peaks corresponding to impurity A and metamizole is at least 2.5.

Inject 10 µl of the test solution and 10 µl of reference solution (b) and continue the chromatography for 3.5 times the retention time of metamizole. In the chromatogram obtained with the test solution: the area of any peak corresponding to impurity C is not greater than the area of the principal peak in the chromatogram obtained with reference solution (b) (0.5 per cent), the area of any peaks, apart from the principal peak and the peak due to impurity C is not greater than 0.4 times the area of the principal peak in the chromatogram obtained with reference solution (b) (0.2 per cent). The sum of the areas of all the peaks, apart from the principal peak, is not greater than the area of the principal peak in the chromatogram obtained with reference solution (b) (0.5 per cent). Disregard any peak with an area less than 0.05 times that of the principal peak in the chromatogram obtained with the reference solution (b).

Sulphates (*2.4.13*). Dissolve 0.150 g in *distilled water R* and dilute to 15 ml with the same solvent. The solution complies with the limit test for sulphates (0.1 per cent).

Heavy metals (*2.4.8*). Dissolve 2.0 g in *water R* and dilute to 20 ml with the same solvent. 12 ml of the freshly prepared solution complies with limit test A for heavy metals (20 ppm). Prepare the standard using *lead standard solution (2 ppm Pb) R*.

Loss on drying (*2.2.32*): 4.9 per cent to 5.3 per cent, determined on 1.000 g by drying in an oven at 100 °C to 105 °C.

ASSAY

Dissolve 0.200 g in 10 ml of *0.01 M hydrochloric acid* previously cooled in iced water and titrate immediately, dropwise, with *0.05 M iodine*. Before each addition of *0.05 M iodine* dissolve the precipitate by swirling. At the end of the titration add 2 ml of *starch solution R* and titrate until the blue colour of the solution persists for at least 2 min. The temperature of the solution during the titration must not exceed 10 °C.

1 ml of *0.05 M iodine* is equivalent to 16.67 mg of $C_{13}H_{16}N_3NaO_4S$.

STORAGE

Store protected from light.

IMPURITIES

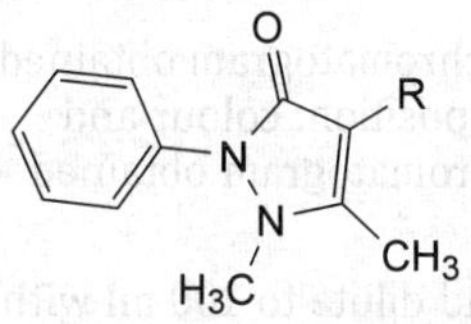

A. R = NHCHO: 4-formylamino-1,5-dimethyl-2-phenyl-1,2-dihydro-3*H*-pyrazol-3-one,

B. R = NH_2: 4-amino-1,5-dimethyl-2-phenyl-1,2-dihydro-3*H*-pyrazol-3-one,

C. R = $NHCH_3$: 4-methylamino-1,5-dimethyl-2-phenyl-1,2-dihydro-3*H*-pyrazol-3-one,

D. R = $N(CH_3)_2$: 4-dimethylamino-1,5-dimethyl-2-phenyl-1,2-dihydro-3*H*-pyrazol-3-one.

01/2005:0931

METFORMIN HYDROCHLORIDE

Metformini hydrochloridum

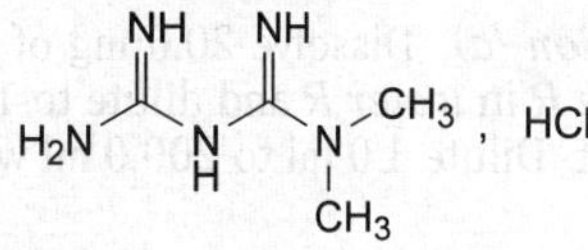

$C_4H_{12}ClN_5$ M_r 165.6

DEFINITION

1,1-Dimethylbiguanide hydrochloride.

Content: 98.5 per cent to 101.0 per cent (dried substance).

CHARACTERS

Appearance: white crystals.

Solubility: freely soluble in water, slightly soluble in alcohol, practically insoluble in acetone and in methylene chloride.

IDENTIFICATION

First identification: B, E.

Second identification: A, C, D, E.

A. Melting point (*2.2.14*): 222 °C to 226 °C.

B. Infrared absorption spectrophotometry (*2.2.24*).

Preparation: discs of *potassium chloride R*.

Comparison: *metformin hydrochloride CRS*.

C. Thin-layer chromatography (*2.2.27*).

Test solution. Dissolve 20 mg of the substance to be examined in *water R* and dilute to 5 ml with the same solvent.

Reference solution. Dissolve 20 mg of *metformin hydrochloride CRS* in *water R* and dilute to 5 ml with the same solvent.

Plate: *TLC silica gel G plate R*.

Mobile phase: upper layer of a mixture of 10 volumes of *glacial acetic acid R*, 40 volumes of *butanol R* and 50 volumes of *water R*.

Application: 5 μl.

Development: over a path of 15 cm.

Drying: at 100-105 °C for 15 min.

Detection: spray with a mixture of equal volumes of a 100 g/l solution of *sodium nitroprusside R*, a 100 g/l solution of *potassium ferricyanide R* and a 100 g/l solution of *sodium hydroxide R*, prepared 20 min before use.

Results: the principal spot in the chromatogram obtained with the test solution is similar in position, colour and size to the principal spot in the chromatogram obtained with the reference solution.

D. Dissolve about 5 mg in *water R* and dilute to 100 ml with the same solvent. To 2 ml of the solution add 0.25 ml of *strong sodium hydroxide solution R* and 0.10 ml of *α-naphthol solution R*. Mix and allow to stand in iced water for 15 min. Add 0.5 ml of *sodium hypobromite solution R* and mix. A pink colour develops.

E. It gives reaction (a) of chlorides (*2.3.1*).

TESTS

Solution S. Dissolve 2.0 g in *water R* and dilute to 20 ml with the same solvent.

Appearance of solution. Solution S is clear (*2.2.1*) and colourless (*2.2.2, Method II*).

Related substances. Liquid chromatography (*2.2.29*).

Test solution. Dissolve 0.50 g of the substance to be examined in the mobile phase and dilute to 100.0 ml with the mobile phase.

Reference solution (a). Dissolve 20.0 mg of *cyanoguanidine R* in *water R* and dilute to 100.0 ml with the same solvent. Dilute 1.0 ml to 200.0 ml with the mobile phase.

Reference solution (b). Dilute 1.0 ml of the test solution to 50.0 ml with the mobile phase. Dilute 1.0 ml of this solution to 20.0 ml with the mobile phase.

Reference solution (c). Dissolve 10.0 mg of *melamine R* in about 90 ml of *water R*. Add 5.0 ml of the test solution and dilute to 100.0 ml with *water R*. Dilute 1.0 ml of this solution to 50.0 ml with the mobile phase.

Column:

– *size*: l = 0.25 m, Ø = 4.6 mm,
– *stationary phase*: irregular, porous silica gel to which benzenesulphonic acid groups have been chemically bonded (10 μm),

or

– *size*: l = 0.11 m, Ø = 4.7 mm,
– *stationary phase*: regular, porous silica gel to which benzenesulphonic acid groups have been chemically bonded (5 μm).

Mobile phase: 17 g/l solution of *ammonium dihydrogen phosphate R* adjusted to pH 3.0 with *phosphoric acid R*.

Flow rate: 1 ml/min.

Detection: spectrophotometer at 218 nm.

Injection: 20 μl.

Run time: twice the retention time of metformin hydrochloride.

System suitability: reference solution (c):

– *resolution*: minimum of 10 between the peaks due to melamine and to metformin hydrochloride.

Limits:

– *impurity A*: not more than the area of the corresponding peak in the chromatogram obtained with reference solution (a) (0.02 per cent),
– *any other impurity*: not more than the area of the principal peak in the chromatogram obtained with reference solution (b) (0.1 per cent).

Heavy metals (*2.4.8*): maximum 10 ppm.

12 ml of solution S complies with limit test A. Prepare the standard using *lead standard solution (1 ppm Pb) R*.

Loss on drying (*2.2.32*): maximum 0.5 per cent, determined on 1.000 g by drying in an oven at 100-105 °C for 5 h.

Sulphated ash (*2.4.14*): maximum 0.1 per cent, determined on 1.0 g.

ASSAY

Dissolve 0.100 g in 4 ml of *anhydrous formic acid R*. Add 80 ml of *acetonitrile R*. Carry out the titration immediately. Titrate with *0.1 M perchloric acid*, determining the end-point potentiometrically (*2.2.20*).

1 ml of *0.1 M perchloric acid* is equivalent to 16.56 mg of $C_4H_{12}ClN_5$.

IMPURITIES

Specified impurities: A.

Other detectable impurities: B, C, D, E, F.

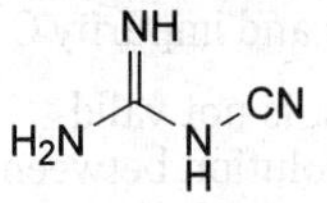

A. cyanoguanidine,

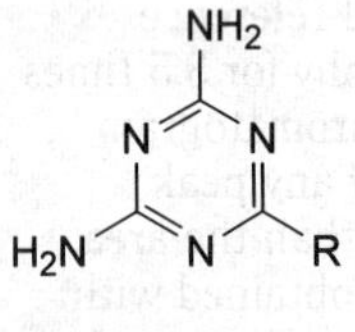

B. R = $NH-C(=NH)-NH_2$: (4,6-diamino-1,3,5-triazin-2-yl)guanidine,

C. R = $N(CH_3)_2$: *N,N*-dimethyl-1,3,5-triazine-2,4,6-triamine,

D. R = NH_2: 1,3,5-triazine-2,4,6-triamine (melamine),

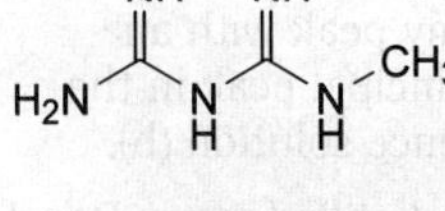

E. 1-methylbiguanide,

F. $CH_3-NH-CH_3$: *N*-methylmethanamine.

01/2005:1128

METHACRYLIC ACID - ETHYL ACRYLATE COPOLYMER (1:1)

Acidum methacrylicum et ethylis acrylas polymerisatum 1:1

DEFINITION

Methacrylic acid - ethyl acrylate copolymer (1:1) is a copolymer of methacrylic acid and ethyl acrylate having a mean relative molecular mass of about 250 000. The ratio of carboxylic groups to ester groups is about 1:1. It may contain suitable surface-active agents such as sodium dodecyl sulphate and polysorbate 80. It contains not less than 46.0 per cent *m/m* and not more than 50.6 per cent *m/m* of methacrylic acid units, calculated with reference to the dried substance.

CHARACTERS

A white, free-flowing powder, practically insoluble in water, freely soluble in ethanol and in 2-propanol, practically insoluble in ethyl acetate. It is freely soluble in a 40 g/l solution of sodium hydroxide.

IDENTIFICATION

A. Examine by infrared absorption spectrophotometry (*2.2.24*), comparing with the *Ph. Eur. reference spectrum of methacrylic acid - ethyl acrylate copolymer (1:1)*.

B. It complies with the limits of the assay.

TESTS

Apparent viscosity. Dissolve a quantity of substance to be examined corresponding to 37.5 g of the dried substance in a mixture of 7.9 g of *water R* and 254.6 g of *2-propanol R*. Determine the viscosity (*2.2.10*) using a rotating viscometer at 20 °C. At a shear rate of 10 s^{-1}, the apparent viscosity is not less than 100 mPa·s and not more than 200 mPa·s.

Appearance of a film. Place 1 ml of the solution prepared for the apparent viscosity test on a glass plate and allow to dry. A clear brittle film is formed.

Ethyl acrylate and methacrylic acid. Total content: not more than 0.1 per cent, determined by liquid chromatography (*2.2.29*).

Blank solution. To 50.0 ml of *methanol R* add 25.0 ml of mobile phase.

Test solution. Dissolve 40 mg of the substance to be examined in 50.0 ml of *methanol R* and add 25.0 ml of mobile phase.

Reference solution. Dissolve 10 mg each of *ethyl acrylate R* and *methacrylic acid R* in *methanol R* and dilute to 50.0 ml with the same solvent. Dilute 0.1 ml of this solution to 50.0 ml with *methanol R* and add 25.0 ml of mobile phase.

The chromatographic procedure may be carried out using:

– a stainless steel column 0.10 m long and 4 mm in internal diameter packed with *octadecylsilyl silica gel for chromatography R* (5 μm),

– as mobile phase at a flow rate of 2.5 ml/min a mixture of 30 volumes of *methanol R* and 70 volumes of *phosphate buffer solution pH 2.0 R*,

– as detector a spectrophotometer set at 202 nm.

Inject 50 μl of each solution. The test is not valid unless the resolution between the peaks corresponding to ethyl acrylate and methacrylic acid in the chromatogram obtained with the reference solution is at least 2.0. The test is not valid if the chromatogram obtained with the blank solution shows peaks with the same retention times as ethyl acrylate or methacrylic acid.

Calculate the percentage content of monomers from the area of the peaks in the chromatograms obtained with the test solution and the reference solution and from the content of monomers in the reference solution.

Loss on drying (*2.2.32*). Not more than 5.0 per cent, determined on 1.000 g by drying at 100 °C to 105 °C for 6 h.

Sulphated ash (*2.4.14*). Not more than 0.4 per cent, determined on 1.0 g.

ASSAY

Dissolve 1.000 g in a mixture of 40 ml of *water R* and 60 ml of *2-propanol R*. Titrate slowly while stirring with *0.5 M sodium hydroxide*, using *phenolphthalein solution R* as indicator.

1 ml of *0.5 M sodium hydroxide* is equivalent to 43.05 mg of $C_4H_6O_2$ (methacrylic acid units).

LABELLING

The label states, where applicable, the name and concentration of any surface-active agents.

01/2005:1129

METHACRYLIC ACID - ETHYL ACRYLATE COPOLYMER (1:1) DISPERSION 30 PER CENT

Acidum methacrylicum et ethylis acrylas polymerisatum 1:1 dispersio 30 per centum

DEFINITION

Methacrylic acid - ethyl acrylate copolymer (1:1) dispersion 30 per cent is a dispersion in water of a copolymer of methacrylic acid and ethyl acrylate having a mean relative molecular mass of about 250 000. The ratio of carboxylic groups to ester groups is about 1:1. It may contain suitable surface-active agents such as sodium dodecyl sulphate and polysorbate 80. It contains not less than 46.0 per cent *m/m* and not more than 50.6 per cent *m/m* of methacrylic acid units, calculated with reference to the residue on evaporation.

CHARACTERS

An opaque, white, slightly viscous liquid, miscible with water. On addition of solvents such as acetone, ethanol or 2-propanol, a precipitate is formed which dissolves on addition of excess solvent. It is miscible with a 40 g/l solution of sodium hydroxide.

It is sensitive to spoilage by microbial contaminants.

IDENTIFICATION

A. Examine by infrared absorption spectrophotometry (*2.2.24*), comparing with the *Ph. Eur. reference spectrum of methacrylic acid - ethyl acrylate copolymer (1:1) dispersion 30 per cent*.

B. It complies with the limits of the assay.

TESTS

Apparent viscosity. Determine the viscosity (*2.2.10*) using a rotating viscometer at 20 °C. At a shear rate of 50 s^{-1}, the apparent viscosity is not more than 15 mPa·s.

Appearance of a film. Place 1 ml on a glass plate and allow to dry. A clear, brittle film is formed.

Monographs M

Particulate matter. Filter 100.0 g through a tared stainless steel sieve (90). Rinse with *water R* until a clear filtrate is obtained and dry at 100 °C to 105 °C. The mass of the residue is not more than 1.00 g.

Ethyl acrylate and methacrylic acid. Total content not more than 0.1 per cent, determined by liquid chromatography (*2.2.29*) and calculated with reference to the dried substance.

Blank solution. To 50.0 ml of *methanol R* add 25.0 ml of mobile phase.

Test solution. Dissolve 40 mg of the substance to be examined in 50.0 ml of *methanol R* and add 25.0 ml of mobile phase.

Reference solution. Dissolve 10 mg each of *ethyl acrylate R* and *methacrylic acid R* in *methanol R* and dilute to 50.0 ml with the same solvent. Dilute 0.1 ml of this solution to 50.0 ml with *methanol R* and add 25.0 ml of mobile phase.

The chromatographic procedure may be carried out using:

- a stainless steel column 0.10 m long and 4 mm in internal diameter packed with *octadecylsilyl silica gel for chromatography R* (5 µm),
- as mobile phase at a flow rate of 2.5 ml/min a mixture of 30 volumes of *methanol R* and 70 volumes of *phosphate buffer solution pH 2.0 R*,

as detector a spectrophotometer set at 202 nm.

Inject 50 µl of each solution. The test is not valid unless the resolution between the peaks corresponding to ethyl acrylate and methacrylic acid in the chromatogram obtained with the reference solution is at least 2.0. The test is not valid if the chromatogram obtained with the blank solution shows peaks with the same retention times as ethyl acrylate or methacrylic acid.

Calculate the percentage content of monomers from the area of the peaks in the chromatograms obtained with the test solution and the reference solution and from the content of monomers in the reference solution.

Residue on evaporation. Dry 1.000 g at 110 °C for 5 h. The residue weighs not less than 0.285 g and not more than 0.315 g.

Sulphated ash (*2.4.14*). Not more than 0.2 per cent, determined on 1.0 g.

Microbial contamination. Total viable aerobic count (*2.6.12*) not more than 10^3 micro-organisms per gram, determined by plate count.

ASSAY

Dissolve 1.500 g in a mixture of 40 ml of *water R* and 60 ml of *2-propanol R*. Titrate slowly while stirring with *0.5 M sodium hydroxide*, using *phenolphthalein solution R* as indicator.

1 ml of *0.5 M sodium hydroxide* is equivalent to 43.05 mg of $C_4H_6O_2$ (methacrylic acid units).

STORAGE

Store protected from freezing. Handle the substance so as to minimise microbial contamination.

LABELLING

The label states, where applicable, the name and concentration of any surface-active agents.

Monographs M

01/2005:1127

METHACRYLIC ACID - METHYL METHACRYLATE COPOLYMER (1:1)

Acidum methacrylicum et methylis methacrylas polymerisatum 1:1

DEFINITION

Methacrylic acid - methyl methacrylate copolymer (1:1) is a copolymer of methacrylic acid and methyl methacrylate having a mean relative molecular mass of about 135 000. The ratio of carboxylic groups to ester groups is about 1:1. It contains not less than 46.0 per cent *m/m* and not more than 50.6 per cent of methacrylic acid units, calculated with reference to the dried substance.

CHARACTERS

A white, free-flowing powder, practically insoluble in water, freely soluble in ethanol and in 2-propanol, practically insoluble in ethyl acetate. It is freely soluble in a 40 g/l solution of sodium hydroxide.

IDENTIFICATION

A. Examine by infrared absorption spectrophotometry (*2.2.24*), comparing with the *Ph. Eur. reference spectrum of methacrylic acid - methyl methacrylate copolymer (1:1)*.

B. It complies with the limits of the assay.

TESTS

Apparent viscosity. Dissolve a quantity of substance to be examined corresponding to 37.5 g of the dried substance in a mixture of 7.9 g of *water R* and 254.6 g of *2-propanol R*. Determine the viscosity (*2.2.10*) using a rotating viscometer at 20 °C. At a shear rate of 10 s^{-1}, the apparent viscosity is not less than 50 mPa·s and not more than 200 mPa·s.

Appearance of a film. Place 1 ml of the solution prepared for the viscosity test on a glass plate and allow to dry. A clear brittle film is formed.

Methyl methacrylate and methacrylic acid. Total content: not more than 0.1 per cent, determined by liquid chromatography (*2.2.29*).

Blank solution. To 50.0 ml of *methanol R* add 25.0 ml of mobile phase.

Test solution. Dissolve 40 mg of the substance to be examined in 50.0 ml of *methanol R* and add 25.0 ml of mobile phase.

Reference solution. Dissolve 10 mg each of *methyl methacrylate R* and *methacrylic acid R* in *methanol R* and dilute to 50.0 ml with the same solvent. Dilute 0.1 ml of this solution to 50.0 ml with *methanol R* and add 25.0 ml of mobile phase.

The chromatographic procedure may be carried out using:

- a stainless steel column 0.10 m long and 4 mm in internal diameter packed with *octadecylsilyl silica gel for chromatography R* (5 µm),
- as mobile phase at a flow rate of 2.5 ml/min a mixture of 30 volumes of *methanol R* and 70 volumes of *phosphate buffer solution pH 2.0 R*,
- as detector a spectrophotometer set at 202 nm.

Inject 50 µl of each solution. The test is not valid unless the resolution between the peaks corresponding to methyl methacrylate and methacrylic acid in the chromatogram obtained with the reference solution is at least 2.0. The test is not valid if the chromatogram obtained with the blank solution shows peaks with the same retention times as methyl methacrylate or methacrylic acid.

Calculate the percentage content of monomers from the area of the peaks in the chromatograms obtained with the test solution and the reference solution and from the content of monomers in the reference solution.

Loss on drying (*2.2.32*). Not more than 5.0 per cent, determined on 1.000 g by drying at 100 °C to 105 °C for 6 h.

Sulphated ash (*2.4.14*). Not more than 0.1 per cent, determined on 1.0 g.

ASSAY

Dissolve 1.000 g in a mixture of 40 ml of *water R* and 60 ml of *2-propanol R*. Titrate slowly while stirring with *0.5 M sodium hydroxide*, using *phenolphthalein solution R* as indicator.

1 ml of *0.5 M sodium hydroxide* is equivalent to 43.05 mg of $C_4H_6O_2$ (methacrylic acid units).

01/2005:1130

METHACRYLIC ACID - METHYL METHACRYLATE COPOLYMER (1:2)

Acidum methacrylicum et methylis methacrylas polymerisatum 1:2

DEFINITION

Methacrylic acid - methyl methacrylate copolymer (1:2) is a copolymer of methacrylic acid and methyl methacrylate having a mean relative molecular mass of about 135 000. The ratio of carboxylic groups to ester groups is about 1:2. It contains not less than 27.6 per cent *m/m* and not more than 30.7 per cent *m/m* of methacrylic acid units, calculated with reference to the dried substance.

CHARACTERS

A white, free-flowing powder, practically insoluble in water, freely soluble in ethanol and in 2-propanol, practically insoluble in ethyl acetate. It is freely soluble in a 40 g/l solution of sodium hydroxide.

IDENTIFICATION

A. Examine by infrared absorption spectrophotometry (*2.2.24*), comparing with the *Ph. Eur. reference spectrum of methacrylic acid - methyl methacrylate copolymer (1:2)*.

B. It complies with the limits of the assay.

TESTS

Apparent viscosity. Dissolve a quantity of substance to be examined corresponding to 37.5 g of the dried substance in a mixture of 7.9 g of *water R* and 254.6 g of *2-propanol R*. Determine the viscosity (*2.2.10*) using a rotating viscometer at 20 °C. At a shear rate of 10 s^{-1}, the apparent viscosity is not less than 50 mPa·s and not more than 200 mPa·s.

Appearance of a film. Place 1 ml of the solution prepared for the viscosity test on a glass plate and allow to dry. A clear brittle film is formed.

Methyl methacrylate and methacrylic acid. Total content: not more than 0.1 per cent, determined by liquid chromatography (*2.2.29*).

Blank solution. To 50.0 ml of *methanol R* add 25.0 ml of mobile phase.

Test solution. Dissolve 40 mg of the substance to be examined in 50.0 ml of *methanol R* and add 25.0 ml of mobile phase.

Reference solution. Dissolve 10 mg each of *methyl methacrylate R* and *methacrylic acid R* in *methanol R* and dilute to 50.0 ml with the same solvent. Dilute 0.1 ml of this solution to 50.0 ml with *methanol R* and add 25.0 ml of mobile phase.

The chromatographic procedure may be carried out using:
- a stainless steel column 0.10 m long and 4 mm in internal diameter packed with *octadecylsilyl silica gel for chromatography R* (5 µm),
- as mobile phase at a flow rate of 2.5 ml/min a mixture of 30 volumes of *methanol R* and 70 volumes of *phosphate buffer solution pH 2.0 R*,
- as detector a spectrophotometer set at 202 nm.

Inject 50 µl of each solution. The test is not valid unless the resolution between the peaks corresponding to methyl methacrylate and methacrylic acid in the chromatogram obtained with the reference solution is at least 2.0. The test is not valid if the chromatogram obtained with the blank solution shows peaks with the same retention times as methyl methacrylate or methacrylic acid.

Calculate the percentage content of monomers from the area of the peaks in the chromatograms obtained with the test solution and the reference solution and from the content of monomers in the reference solution.

Loss on drying (*2.2.32*). Not more than 5.0 per cent, determined on 1.000 g by drying in an oven at 100 °C to 105 °C for 6 h.

Sulphated ash (*2.4.14*). Not more than 0.1 per cent, determined on 1.0 g.

ASSAY

Dissolve 1.000 g in a mixture of 40 ml of *water R* and 60 ml of *2-propanol R*.Titrate slowly while stirring with *0.5 M sodium hydroxide*, using *phenolphthalein solution R* as indicator.

1 ml of *0.5 M sodium hydroxide* is equivalent to 43.05 mg of $C_4H_6O_2$ (methacrylic acid units).

01/2005:0408

METHADONE HYDROCHLORIDE

Methadoni hydrochloridum

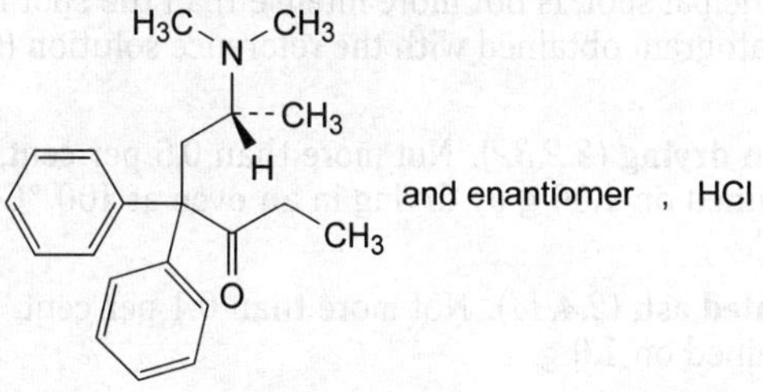

$C_{21}H_{28}ClNO$ M_r 345.9

DEFINITION

Methadone hydrochloride contains not less than 99.0 per cent and not more than the equivalent of 101.0 per cent of (6*RS*)-6-(dimethylamino)-4,4-diphenylheptan-3-one hydrochloride, calculated with reference to the dried substance.

CHARACTERS

A white, crystalline powder, soluble in water, freely soluble in alcohol.

IDENTIFICATION

First identification: A, C, E.

Second identification: A, B, D, E.

A. The optical rotation (*2.2.7*) of solution S (see Tests) measured in a 2 dm tube is − 0.05° to + 0.05°.

B. Melting point (*2.2.14*): 233 °C to 236 °C.

C. Examine by infrared absorption spectrophotometry (*2.2.24*), comparing with the *Ph. Eur. reference spectrum of methadone hydrochloride.*

D. To 2.0 ml of solution S add 1 ml of *0.1 M hydrochloric acid* and 6 ml of *ammonium thiocyanate solution R*. A white precipitate is formed which becomes crystalline on stirring for a few minutes. The crystalline precipitate, dried at 100 °C to 105 °C, melts (*2.2.14*) at 143 °C to 148 °C.

E. Dilute 1 ml of solution S to 5 ml with *water R* and add 1 ml of *dilute ammonia R1*. Mix, allow to stand for 5 min and filter. The filtrate gives reaction (a) of chlorides (*2.3.1*).

TESTS

Solution S. Dissolve 2.50 g in *carbon dioxide-free water R* and dilute to 50.0 ml with the same solvent.

Appearance of solution. Solution S is clear (*2.2.1*) and colourless (*2.2.2, Method II*).

Acidity or alkalinity. Dilute 10 ml of solution S to 25 ml with *carbon dioxide-free water R*. To 10 ml of the solution add 0.2 ml of *methyl red solution R* and 0.2 ml of *0.01 M sodium hydroxide*. The solution is yellow. Add 0.4 ml of *0.01 M hydrochloric acid*. The solution is red.

Related substances. Examine by thin-layer chromatography (*2.2.27*), using *silica gel G R* as the coating substance.

Test solution. Dissolve 0.5 g of the substance to be examined in *alcohol R* and dilute to 10 ml with the same solvent.

Reference solution. Dilute 1 ml of the test solution to 10 ml with *alcohol R*. Dilute 1 ml of this solution to 100 ml with *alcohol R*.

Apply to the plate 10 µl of each solution. Develop over a path of 15 cm using a mixture of 10 volumes of *water R*, 30 volumes of *glacial acetic acid R* and 60 volumes of *alcohol R*. Allow the plate to dry in air and spray with *dilute potassium iodobismuthate solution R*. Any spot in the chromatogram obtained with the test solution, apart from the principal spot, is not more intense than the spot in the chromatogram obtained with the reference solution (0.1 per cent).

Loss on drying (*2.2.32*). Not more than 0.5 per cent, determined on 1.00 g by drying in an oven at 100 °C to 105 °C.

Sulphated ash (*2.4.14*). Not more than 0.1 per cent, determined on 1.0 g.

ASSAY

Dissolve 0.300 g in 50 ml of *anhydrous acetic acid R*. Add 5 ml of *mercuric acetate solution R*. Using 0.1 ml of *crystal violet solution R* as indicator, titrate with *0.1 M perchloric acid* until the colour changes from violet-blue to green.

1 ml of *0.1 M perchloric acid* is equivalent to 34.59 mg of $C_{21}H_{28}ClNO$.

STORAGE

Store protected from light.

01/2005:0510

METHAQUALONE

Methaqualonum

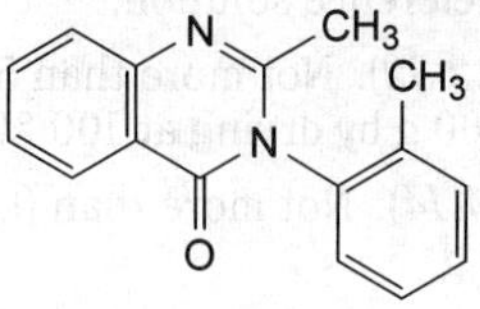

$C_{16}H_{14}N_2O$ M_r 250.3

DEFINITION

Methaqualone contains not less than 99.0 per cent and not more than the equivalent of 101.0 per cent of 2-methyl-3-(2-methylphenyl)quinazolin-4(3*H*)-one, calculated with reference to the dried substance.

CHARACTERS

A white or almost white, crystalline powder, very slightly soluble in water, soluble in alcohol. It dissolves in dilute sulphuric acid.

IDENTIFICATION

First identification: A, C.

Second identification: A, B, D.

A. Melting point (*2.2.14*): 114 °C to 117 °C.

B. Dissolve 50.0 mg in *0.1 M hydrochloric acid*, warming if necessary, and dilute to 100.0 ml with the same acid. Dilute 1.0 ml of this solution to 100.0 ml with *0.1 M hydrochloric acid*. Examined between 220 nm and 300 nm (*2.2.25*), the solution shows two absorption maxima, at 235 nm and 270 nm. The specific absorbances at the maxima are 1270 to 1390 and 315 to 345, respectively.

C. Examine by infrared absorption spectrophotometry (*2.2.24*), comparing with the *Ph. Eur. reference spectrum of methaqualone.*

D. Dissolve about 10 mg in 2 ml of *alcohol R*. Add 1 ml of *dimethylaminobenzaldehyde solution R1* and heat on a water-bath for 5 min. A reddish-orange colour develops.

TESTS

Appearance of solution. Dissolve 1.0 g in *methanol R* and dilute to 25 ml with the same solvent. The solution is clear (*2.2.1*) and not more intensely coloured than reference solution BY_7 (*2.2.2, Method II*).

Acidity. Shake 0.6 g with 30 ml of *carbon dioxide-free water R* for 5 min and filter. To 10 ml of the filtrate add 0.1 ml of *phenolphthalein solution R*. Not more than 0.2 ml of *0.01 M sodium hydroxide* is required to change the colour of the indicator.

2-Aminobenzoic acid. Dissolve 1.00 g in a mixture of 1 volume of *water R* and 3 volumes of *alcohol R* and dilute to 50.0 ml with the same mixture of solvents (test solution). Prepare a reference solution as follows: dissolve 40 mg of *2-aminobenzoic acid R* in a mixture of 1 volume of *water R* and 3 volumes of *alcohol R* and dilute to 100.0 ml with the same mixture of solvents; dilute 10.0 ml of this solution to 100.0 ml with a mixture of 1 volume of *water R* and 3 volumes of *alcohol R*; dilute 0.5 ml of this solution to 50.0 ml with a mixture of 1 volume of *water R* and 3 volumes of *alcohol R* (reference solution). To the test solution and to the reference solution add 5 ml of *dilute hydrochloric acid R* and cool in iced water for 5 min. Add 0.1 ml of *sodium nitrite solution R* and cool again in iced water for 5 min. Add 1.5 ml of a freshly prepared 10 g/l solution of *sulphamic acid R* and shake until the colour of the solution is discharged. Add 2.5 ml of a freshly prepared 2 g/l solution of *naphthylethylenediamine dihydrochloride R* and allow to stand for 2 h 30 min. Examine the solutions as described for *2.2.2, Method II*. The test solution is not more intensely coloured than the reference solution (20 ppm).

***o*-Toluidine**. Dissolve 0.50 g in *acetone R* and dilute to 10.0 ml with the same solvent (test solution). Prepare a reference solution as follows: dissolve 50 mg of freshly distilled *o-toluidine R* in 5 ml of *acetone R* and dilute to 100.0 ml with *dilute hydrochloric acid R*; dilute 10.0 ml of the solution to 100.0 ml with *dilute hydrochloric acid R*; dilute 0.1 ml of this solution to 10.0 ml with *acetone R* (reference solution). To the test solution and to the reference solution add 5 ml of *water R* and cool in iced water for 5 min. Add 0.1 ml of *sodium nitrite solution R* and cool again in iced water for 5 min. Add 10 ml of a freshly prepared 2 g/l solution of *β-naphthol R* in *dilute sodium hydroxide solution R*. Examine the solutions as described for *2.2.2, Method II*. The test solution is not more intensely coloured than the reference solution (10 ppm).

Heavy metals (*2.4.8*). 1.0 g complies with limit test C for heavy metals (20 ppm). Prepare the standard using 2 ml of *lead standard solution (10 ppm Pb) R*.

Loss on drying (*2.2.32*). Not more than 1.0 per cent, determined on 1.000 g by drying in an oven at 100 °C to 105 °C.

Sulphated ash (*2.4.14*). Not more than 0.1 per cent, determined on 1.0 g.

ASSAY

Dissolve 0.200 g in 30 ml of *anhydrous acetic acid R*. Titrate with *0.1 M perchloric acid*, determining the end-point potentiometrically (*2.2.20*).

1 ml of *0.1 M perchloric acid* is equivalent to 25.03 mg of $C_{16}H_{14}N_2O$.

STORAGE

Store protected from light.

01/2005:1545

METHENAMINE

Methenaminum

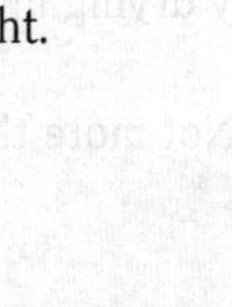

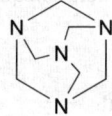

$C_6H_{12}N_4$ M_r 140.2

DEFINITION

Methenamine contains not less than 99.0 per cent and not more than the equivalent of 100.5 per cent of 1,3,5,7-tetra-azotricyclo[3.3.1.1^{3,7}]decane, calculated with reference to the dried substance.

CHARACTERS

A white, crystalline powder or colourless crystals, freely soluble in water, soluble in alcohol and in methylene chloride.

IDENTIFICATION

First identification: A.

Second identification: B, C, D.

A. Examine by infrared absorption spectrophotometry (*2.2.24*), comparing with the *Ph. Eur. reference spectrum of methenamine*.

B. To 1 ml of solution S (see Tests) add 1 ml of *sulphuric acid R* and immediately heat to boiling. Allow to cool. To 1 ml of the solution add 4 ml of *water R* and 5 ml of *acetylacetone reagent R1*. Heat on a water-bath for 5 min. An intense yellow colour develops.

C. To 1 ml of solution S add 1 ml of *dilute sulphuric acid R* and immediately heat to boiling. The solution gives the reaction of ammonium salts and salts of volatile bases (*2.3.1*).

D. Dissolve 10 mg in 5 ml of *water R* and acidify with *dilute hydrochloric acid R*. Add 1 ml of *potassium iodobismuthate solution R*. An orange precipitate is formed immediately.

TESTS

Solution S. Dissolve 10.0 g in *carbon dioxide-free water R* prepared from *distilled water R* and dilute to 100 ml with the same solvent.

Appearance of solution. Solution S is clear (*2.2.1*) and colourless (*2.2.2, Method II*).

Acidity or alkalinity. To 5 ml of solution S add 0.1 ml of *phenolphthalein solution R*. Not more than 0.2 ml of *0.1 M hydrochloric acid* or *0.1 M sodium hydroxide* is required to change the colour of the indicator.

Free formaldehyde. Dissolve 0.8 g in *water R* and dilute to 8 ml with the same solvent. Add 2 ml of *ammoniacal silver nitrate solution R*. After 5 min, any grey colour in the solution is not more intense than that in a standard prepared at the same time and in the same manner with a mixture of 8 ml of freshly prepared *formaldehyde standard solution (5 ppm CH_2O) R* and 2 ml of *ammoniacal silver nitrate solution R* (50 ppm).

Chlorides (*2.4.4*). Dilute 5 ml of solution S to 15 ml with *water R*. The solution complies with the limit test for chlorides (100 ppm).

Sulphates (*2.4.13*). 15 ml of solution S complies with the limit test for sulphates (100 ppm).

Ammonium (*2.4.1*). Dilute 2 ml of freshly prepared solution S to 13 ml with *water R*. Add 2 ml of *dilute sodium hydroxide solution R*. The solution complies with the limit test for ammonium (50 ppm).

Heavy metals (*2.4.8*). 12 ml of solution S complies with limit test A for heavy metals (20 ppm). Prepare the standard using *lead standard solution (2 ppm Pb) R*.

Loss on drying (*2.2.32*). Not more than 2.0 per cent, determined on 1.000 g by drying in a desiccator.

ASSAY

Dissolve 0.100 g in 30 ml of *methanol R*. Titrate with *0.1 M perchloric acid*, determining the end-point potentiometrically (*2.2.20*).

1 ml of *0.1 M perchloric acid* is equivalent to 14.02 mg of $C_6H_{12}N_4$.

STORAGE

Store protected from light.

01/2005:1027

METHIONINE

Methioninum

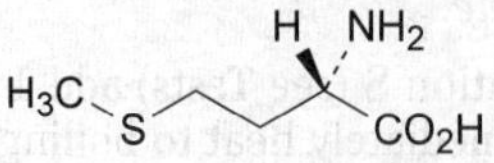

$C_5H_{11}NO_2S$ M_r 149.2

DEFINITION

Methionine contains not less than 99.0 per cent and not more than the equivalent of 101.0 per cent of (2*S*)-2-amino-4-(methylsulphanyl)butanoic acid, calculated with reference to the dried substance.

CHARACTERS

A white or almost white, crystalline powder or colourless crystals, soluble in water, very slightly soluble in alcohol.

IDENTIFICATION

First identification: A, B.

Second identification: A, C, D.

A. It complies with the test for specific optical rotation (see Tests).

B. Examine by infrared absorption spectrophotometry (*2.2.24*), comparing with the spectrum obtained with *methionine CRS*. Examine the substances prepared as discs.

C. Examine the chromatograms obtained in the test for ninhydrin-positive substances. The principal spot in the chromatogram obtained with test solution (b) is similar in position, colour and size to the principal spot in the chromatogram obtained with reference solution (a).

D. Dissolve 0.1 g of the substance to be examined and 0.1 g of *glycine R* in 4.5 ml of *dilute sodium hydroxide solution R*. Add 1 ml of a 25 g/l solution of *sodium nitroprusside R*. Heat to 40 °C for 10 min. Allow to cool and add 2 ml of a mixture of 1 volume of *phosphoric acid R* and 9 volumes of *hydrochloric acid R*. A dark red colour develops.

TESTS

Solution S. Dissolve 2.5 g in *carbon dioxide-free water R* and dilute to 100 ml with the same solvent.

Appearance of solution. Solution S is clear (*2.2.1*) and colourless (*2.2.2, Method II*).

pH (*2.2.3*). The pH of solution S is 5.5 to 6.5.

Specific optical rotation (*2.2.7*). Dissolve 1.00 g in *hydrochloric acid R1* and dilute to 50.0 ml with the same acid. The specific optical rotation is + 22.5 to + 24.0, calculated with reference to the dried substance.

Ninhydrin-positive substances. Examine by thin-layer chromatography (*2.2.27*), using a *TLC silica gel plate R*.

Test solution (a). Dissolve 0.10 g of the substance to be examined in *dilute hydrochloric acid R* and dilute to 10 ml with the same acid.

Test solution (b). Dilute 1 ml of test solution (a) to 50 ml with *water R*.

Reference solution (a). Dissolve 10 mg of *methionine CRS* in a 10 g/l solution of *hydrochloric acid R* and dilute to 50 ml with the same acid solution.

Reference solution (b). Dilute 5 ml of test solution (b) to 20 ml with *water R*.

Reference solution (c). Dissolve 10 mg of *methionine CRS* and 10 mg of *serine CRS* in a 10 g/l solution of *hydrochloric acid R* and dilute to 25 ml with the same acid solution.

Apply separately to the plate 5 µl of each solution. Develop over a path of 15 cm using a mixture of 20 volumes of *glacial acetic acid R*, 20 volumes of *water R* and 60 volumes of *butanol R*. Allow the plate to dry in air, spray with *ninhydrin solution R* and heat at 100 °C to 105 °C for 15 min. Any spot in the chromatogram obtained with test solution (a), apart from the principal spot, is not more intense than the spot in the chromatogram obtained with reference solution (b) (0.5 per cent). The test is not valid unless the chromatogram obtained with reference solution (c) shows two clearly separated spots.

Chlorides. To 10 ml of solution S add 25 ml of *water R*, 5 ml of *dilute nitric acid R* and 10 ml of *silver nitrate solution R2*. Allow to stand protected from light for 5 min. Any opalescence in the solution is not more intense than that in a standard prepared at the same time and in the same manner using 10 ml of *chloride standard solution (5 ppm Cl) R* (200 ppm). Examine the tubes laterally against a black background.

Sulphates (*2.4.13*). Dissolve 0.5 g in 3 ml of *dilute hydrochloric acid R* and dilute to 15 ml with *distilled water R*. The solution complies with the limit test for sulphates (300 ppm).

Ammonium (*2.4.1*). 0.10 g complies with limit test B for ammonium (200 ppm). Prepare the standard using 0.2 ml of *ammonium standard solution (100 ppm NH_4) R*.

Iron (*2.4.9*). In a separating funnel, dissolve 1.0 g in 10 ml of *dilute hydrochloric acid R*. Shake with three quantities, each of 10 ml, of *methyl isobutyl ketone R1*, shaking for 3 min each time. To the combined upper layers add 10 ml of *water R* and shake for 3 min. The lower layer complies with the limit test for iron (10 ppm).

Heavy metals (*2.4.8*). 2.0 g complies with limit test C for heavy metals (10 ppm). Prepare the standard using 2 ml of *lead standard solution (10 ppm Pb) R*.

Loss on drying (*2.2.32*). Not more than 0.5 per cent, determined on 1.000 g by drying in an oven at 100 °C to 105 °C.

Sulphated ash (*2.4.14*). Not more than 0.1 per cent, determined on 1.0 g.

ASSAY

Dissolve 0.125 g in 5 ml of *anhydrous formic acid R*. Add 30 ml of *anhydrous acetic acid R*. Titrate with *0.1 M perchloric acid*, determining the end-point potentiometrically (*2.2.20*).

1 ml of *0.1 M perchloric acid* is equivalent to 14.92 mg of $C_5H_{11}NO_2S$.

STORAGE

Store protected from light.

01/2005:0624

DL-METHIONINE

DL-Methioninum

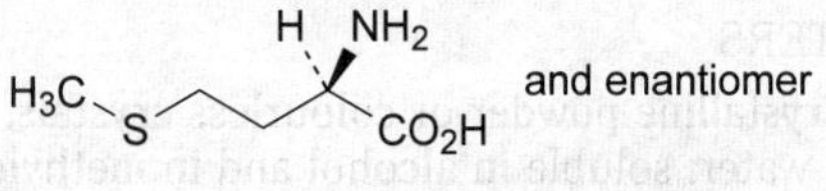

$C_5H_{11}NO_2S$ M_r 149.2

DEFINITION

DL-Methionine contains not less than 99.0 per cent and not more than the equivalent of 101.0 per cent of (2*RS*)-2-amino-4-(methylsulphanyl)butanoic acid, calculated with reference to the dried substance.

CHARACTERS

Almost white, crystalline powder or small flakes, sparingly soluble in water, very slightly soluble in alcohol. It dissolves in dilute acids and in dilute solutions of the alkali hydroxides.

It melts at about 270 °C (instantaneous method).

IDENTIFICATION

First identification: A, C.

Second identification: B, C, D.

A. Examine by infrared absorption spectrophotometry (*2.2.24*), comparing with the spectrum obtained with *DL-methionine CRS*. Dry the substances at 105 °C.

B. Examine the chromatograms obtained in the test for related substances. The principal spot in the chromatogram obtained with test solution (b) is similar in position, colour and size to the principal spot in the chromatogram obtained with reference solution (a).

C. Dissolve 2.50 g in *1 M hydrochloric acid* and dilute to 50.0 ml with the same acid. The angle of optical rotation (*2.2.7*) is − 0.05° to + 0.05°.

D. Dissolve 0.1 g of the substance to be examined and 0.1 g of *glycine R* in 4.5 ml of *dilute sodium hydroxide solution R*. Add 1 ml of a 25 g/l solution of *sodium nitroprusside R*. Heat to 40 °C for 10 min. Allow to cool and add 2 ml of a mixture of 1 volume of *phosphoric acid R* and 9 volumes of *hydrochloric acid R*. A deep-red colour develops.

TESTS

Solution S. Dissolve 1.0 g in *carbon dioxide-free water R* and dilute to 50 ml with the same solvent.

Appearance of solution. Solution S is clear (*2.2.1*) and colourless (*2.2.2, Method II*).

pH (*2.2.3*). The pH of solution S is 5.4 to 6.1.

Related substances. Examine by thin-layer chromatography (*2.2.27*), using *silica gel G R* as the coating substance.

Test solution (a). Dissolve 0.2 g in *water R* and dilute to 10 ml with the same solvent.

Test solution (b). Dilute 1 ml of test solution (a) to 50 ml with *water R*.

Reference solution (a). Dissolve 20 mg of *DL-methionine CRS* in *water R* and dilute to 50 ml with the same solvent.

Reference solution (b). Dilute 1 ml of reference solution (a) to 10 ml with *water R*.

Apply separately to the plate 5 µl of each solution. Develop over a path of 10 cm using a mixture of 20 volumes of *glacial acetic acid R*, 20 volumes of *water R* and 60 volumes of *butanol R*. Allow the plate to dry in air and spray with *ninhydrin solution R*. Heat the plate at 100 °C to 105 °C for 15 min. Any spot in the chromatogram obtained with test solution (a), apart from the principal spot, is not more intense than the spot in the chromatogram obtained with reference solution (b) (0.2 per cent).

Chlorides. Dissolve 0.25 g in 35 ml of *water R*. Add 5 ml of *dilute nitric acid R* and 10 ml of *silver nitrate solution R2*. Allow to stand protected from light for 5 min. Any opalescence in the solution is not more intense than that in a standard prepared at the same time in the same manner using a mixture of 10 ml of *chloride standard solution (5 ppm Cl) R* and 25 ml of *water R* (200 ppm). Examine the tubes laterally against a black background.

Sulphates (*2.4.13*). Dissolve 1.0 g in 20 ml of *distilled water R*, heating to 60 °C. Cool to 10 °C and filter. 15 ml of the solution complies with the limit test for sulphates (200 ppm).

Heavy metals (*2.4.8*). 1.0 g complies with limit test D for heavy metals (20 ppm). Prepare the standard using 2 ml of *lead standard solution (10 ppm Pb) R*.

Loss on drying (*2.2.32*). Not more than 0.5 per cent, determined on 1.000 g by drying in an oven at 100 °C to 105 °C.

Sulphated ash (*2.4.14*). Not more than 0.1 per cent, determined on 1.0 g.

ASSAY

Dissolve 0.140 g in 3 ml of *anhydrous formic acid R*. Add 30 ml of *anhydrous acetic acid R*. Immediately after dissolution, titrate with *0.1 M perchloric acid*, determining the end-point potentiometrically (*2.2.20*).

1 ml of *0.1 M perchloric acid* is equivalent to 14.92 mg of $C_5H_{11}NO_2S$.

STORAGE

Store protected from light.

01/2005:0560

METHOTREXATE

Methotrexatum

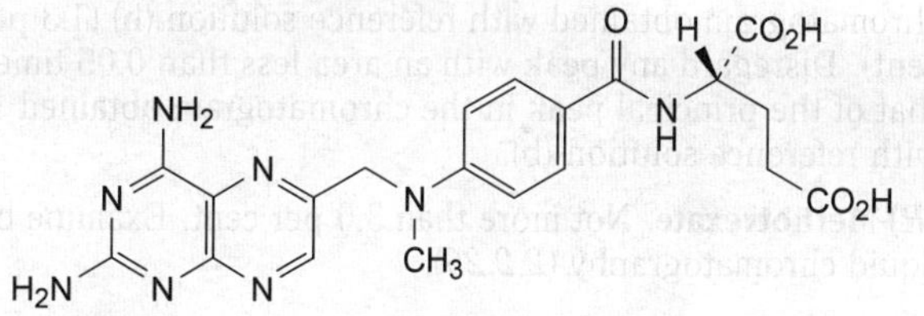

$C_{20}H_{22}N_8O_5$ M_r 454.4

DEFINITION

Methotrexate contains not less than 98.0 per cent and not more than the equivalent of 102.0 per cent of (2*S*)-2-[[4-[[(2,4-diaminopteridin-6-yl)methyl]methylamino]benzoyl]amino]pentanedioic acid, calculated with reference to the anhydrous substance.

CHARACTERS

A yellow or orange, crystalline, hygroscopic powder, practically insoluble in water, in alcohol and in methylene chloride. It dissolves in dilute solutions of mineral acids and in dilute solutions of alkali hydroxides and carbonates.

IDENTIFICATION

A. Dissolve 0.250 g in a 14 g/l solution of *sodium carbonate R* and dilute to 25.0 ml with the same solution. The specific optical rotation (*2.2.7*) is + 19 to + 24 calculated with reference to the anhydrous substance.

B. Dissolve 10 mg in a 4 g/l solution of *sodium hydroxide R* and dilute to 100 ml with the same solvent. Dilute 10 ml of this solution to 100 ml with a 4 g/l solution of *sodium hydroxide R*. Examined between 230 nm and 380 nm (*2.2.25*), the solution shows three absorption maxima, at

Monographs M

258 nm, 302 nm and 371 nm, respectively. The ratio of the absorbance measured at the maximum at 302 nm to that measured at the maximum at 371 nm is 2.8 to 3.3.

C. Examine by infrared absorption spectrophotometry (*2.2.24*), comparing with the spectrum obtained with *methotrexate CRS*.

TESTS

Related substances. Examine by liquid chromatography (*2.2.29*), as prescribed under Assay but setting the spectrophotometer at 265 nm.

Inject 20 µl of reference solution (c). The test is not valid unless in the chromatogram obtained, the resolution between the peaks corresponding to impurity D and methotrexate respectively is at least 2.0.

Inject 20 µl of the test solution and 20 µl of reference solution (b). Continue the chromatography for three times the retention time of methotrexate.

When the chromatograms are recorded in the prescribed conditions, the approximate relative retention times are the following: impurity A = 0.2; impurity B = 0.3; impurity C = 0.4; impurity D = 0.8; impurity E = 2.3.

In the chromatogram obtained with the test solution, the area of at most five peaks, apart from the principal peak, is greater than 0.2 times the area of the principal peak in the chromatogram obtained with reference solution (b) (0.1 per cent) and no such peak has an area greater than that of the principal peak in the chromatogram obtained with reference solution (b) (0.5 per cent). The sum of the areas of all the peaks, apart from the principal peak, is not greater than 2.6 times the area of the principal peak in the chromatogram obtained with reference solution (b) (1.3 per cent). Disregard any peak with an area less than 0.05 times that of the principal peak in the chromatogram obtained with reference solution (b).

(*R*)-Methotrexate. Not more than 3.0 per cent. Examine by liquid chromatography (*2.2.29*).

Test solution. Dissolve 20.0 mg of the substance to be examined in the mobile phase and dilute to 100.0 ml with the mobile phase.

Reference solution (a). Dilute 1.0 ml of the test solution to 100.0 ml with the mobile phase.

Reference solution (b). Dissolve 4.0 mg of *(RS)-methotrexate R* in the mobile phase and dilute to 100.0 ml with the mobile phase.

The chromatographic procedure may be carried out using:

- a stainless steel column 0.15 m long and 4.0 mm in internal diameter packed with *bovine albumin R* bound to *silica gel for chromatography R* (film thickness 7 µm; pore size 30 nm),
- as mobile phase at a flow rate of 1.5 ml/min a solution prepared as follows: to 500 ml of a 7.1 g/l solution of *anhydrous disodium hydrogen phosphate R* add 600 ml of a 6.9 g/l solution of *sodium dihydrogen phosphate monohydrate R* and mix. Adjust to pH 6.9 with *dilute sodium hydroxide solution R*. To 920 ml of this mixture add 80 ml of *propanol R*,
- as detector a spectrophotometer set at 302 nm.

Inject 20 µl of each solution. The test is not valid unless in the chromatogram obtained with reference solution (b); the resolution between the peaks corresponding to (*S*)-methotrexate and (*R*)-methotrexate respectively is at least 3.0.

In the chromatogram obtained with the test solution the area of any peak corresponding to (*R*)-methotrexate is not greater than three times the area of the principal peak in the chromatogram obtained with reference solution (a) (3.0 per cent).

Heavy metals (*2.4.8*). 1.0 g complies with limit test C for heavy metals (50 ppm). Prepare the standard using 5 ml of *lead standard solution (10 ppm Pb) R*.

Water (*2.5.12*). Not more than 13.0 per cent, determined on 0.10 g by the semi-micro determination of water.

Sulphated ash (*2.4.14*). Not more than 0.1 per cent, determined on 1.0 g.

ASSAY

Examine by liquid chromatography (*2.2.29*).

Test solution. Dissolve 25.0 mg of the substance to be examined in the mobile phase and dilute to 250.0 ml with the mobile phase.

Reference solution (a). Dissolve 25.0 mg of *methotrexate CRS* in the mobile phase and dilute to 250.0 ml with the mobile phase.

Reference solution (b). Dilute 0.5 ml of reference solution (a) to 100.0 ml with the mobile phase.

Reference solution (c). Dissolve 25.0 mg of the substance to be examined and 25.0 mg of *methotrexate impurity D CRS* in the mobile phase and dilute to 250.0 ml with the mobile phase.

The chromatographic procedure may be carried out using:

- a stainless steel column 0.25 m long and 4.6 mm in internal diameter packed with *base-deactivated octadecylsilyl silica gel for chromatography R* (5 µm),
- as mobile phase at a flow rate of 1.2 ml/min a mixture of 7 volumes of *acetonitrile R* and 93 volumes of a solution obtained as follows: dissolve 7.8 g of *citric acid R* and 17.9 g of *anhydrous disodium hydrogen phosphate R* in *water R* and dilute to 1000 ml with the same solvent,
- as detector a spectrophotometer set at 302 nm.

Inject reference solution (a) six times. The assay is not valid unless the relative standard deviation of the area of the methotrexate peak is not greater than 2.0 per cent. Inject 20 µl of the test solution and 20 µl of reference solution (a). Calculate the percentage content of methotrexate using the chromatograms obtained with the test solution and reference solution (a)

STORAGE

Store in an airtight container, protected from light.

IMPURITIES

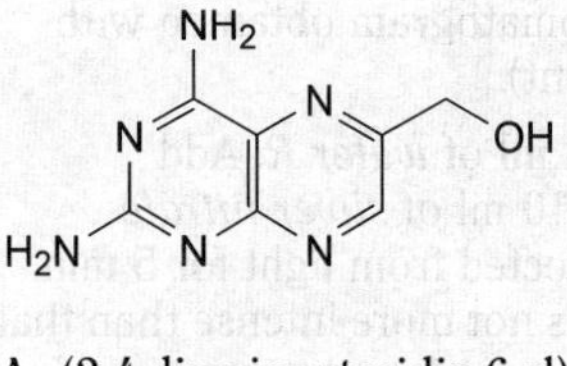

A. (2,4-diaminopteridin-6-yl)methanol,

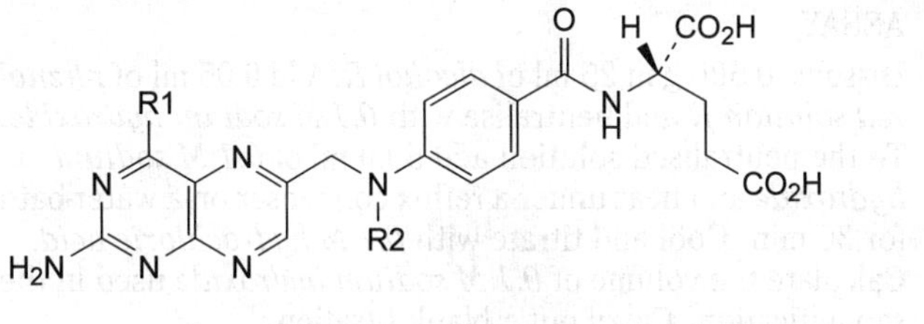

B. R1 = NH_2, R2 = H: (2*S*)-2-[[4-[[(2,4-diaminopteridin-6-yl)methyl]amino]benzoyl]amino]pentanedioic acid (4-aminofolic acid, aminopteridine),

C. R1 = OH, R2 = CH_3: (2*S*)-2-[[4-[[(2-amino-4-hydroxypteridin-6-yl)methyl]methylamino]benzoyl]amino]pentanedioic acid (*N*-methylfolic acid, methopteridine),

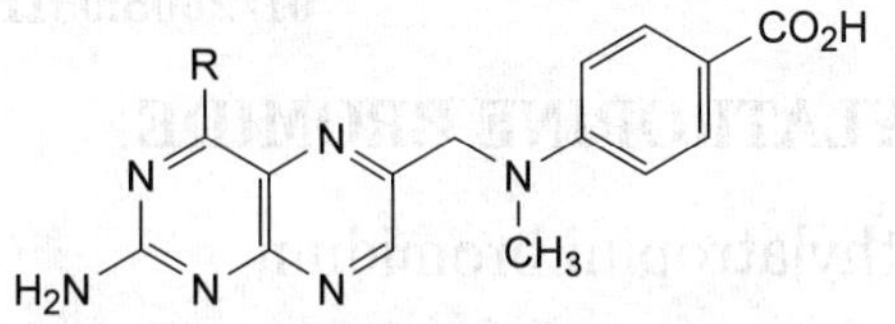

D. R = OH: 4-[[(2-amino-4-hydroxypteridin-6-yl)methyl]methylamino]benzoic acid (N^{10}-methylpteroic acid),

E. R = NH_2: 4-[[(2,4-diaminopteridin-6-yl)methyl]methylamino]benzoic acid (2,4-diamino-N^{10}-methylpterioc acid, APA),

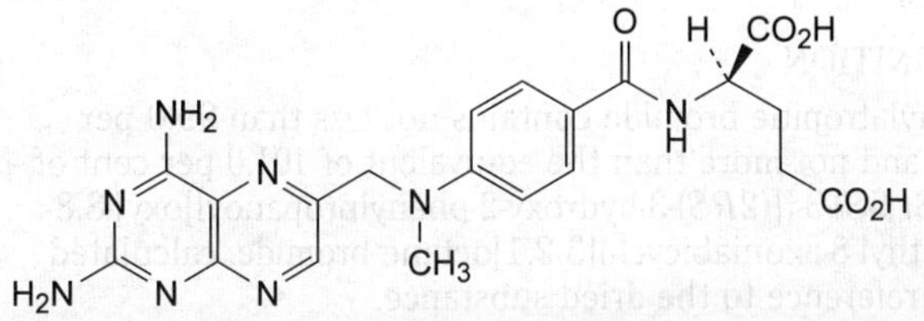

F. (2*R*)-2-[[4-[[(2,4-diaminopteridin-6-yl)methyl]methylamino]benzoyl]amino]pentanedioic acid ((*R*)-methotrexate).

01/2005:0409

METHYL PARAHYDROXYBENZOATE

Methylis parahydroxybenzoas

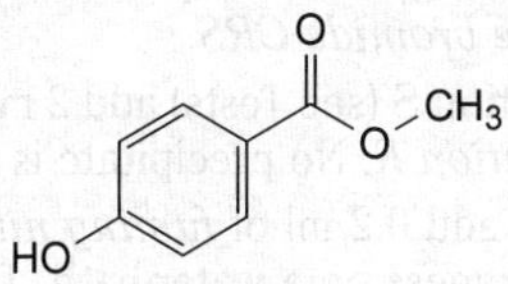

$C_8H_8O_3$ M_r 152.1

DEFINITION

Methyl 4-hydroxybenzoate.

Content: 98.0 per cent to 102.0 per cent.

CHARACTERS

Appearance: white, crystalline powder or colourless crystals.

Solubility: very slightly soluble in water, freely soluble in alcohol and in methanol.

IDENTIFICATION

First identification: A, B.

Second identification: A, C, D.

A. Melting point (*2.2.14*): 125 °C to 128 °C.

B. Infrared absorption spectrophotometry (*2.2.24*).

Comparison: *methyl parahydroxybenzoate CRS.*

C. Examine the chromatograms obtained in the test for related substances.

Results: the principal spot in the chromatogram obtained with test solution (b) is similar in position and size to the principal spot in the chromatogram obtained with reference solution (b).

D. To about 10 mg in a test-tube add 1 ml of *sodium carbonate solution R*, boil for 30 s and cool (solution A). To a further 10 mg in a similar test-tube add 1 ml of *sodium carbonate solution R*; the substance partly dissolves (solution B). Add at the same time to solution A and solution B 5 ml of *aminopyrazolone solution R* and 1 ml of *potassium ferricyanide solution R* and mix. Solution B is yellow to orange-brown. Solution A is orange to red, the colour being clearly more intense than any similar colour which may be obtained with solution B.

TESTS

Solution S. Dissolve 1.0 g in *alcohol R* and dilute to 10 ml with the same solvent.

Appearance of solution. Solution S is clear (*2.2.1*) and not more intensely coloured than reference solution BY_6 (*2.2.2, Method II*).

Acidity. To 2 ml of solution S add 3 ml of *alcohol R*, 5 ml of *carbon dioxide-free water R* and 0.1 ml of *bromocresol green solution R*. Not more than 0.1 ml of *0.1 M sodium hydroxide* is required to change the colour of the indicator to blue.

Related substances. Thin-layer chromatography (*2.2.27*).

Test solution (a). Dissolve 0.10 g of the substance to be examined in *acetone R* and dilute to 10 ml with the same solvent.

Test solution (b). Dilute 1 ml of test solution (a) to 10 ml with *acetone R*.

Reference solution (a). Dilute 0.5 ml of test solution (a) to 100 ml with *acetone R*.

Reference solution (b). Dissolve 10 mg of *methyl parahydroxybenzoate CRS* in *acetone R* and dilute to 10 ml with the same solvent.

Reference solution (c). Dissolve 10 mg of *ethyl parahydroxybenzoate CRS* in 1 ml of test solution (a) and dilute to 10 ml with *acetone R*.

Plate: suitable octadecylsilyl silica gel with a fluorescent indicator having an optimal intensity at 254 nm as the coating substance.

Mobile phase: *glacial acetic acid R, water R, methanol R* (1:30:70 *V/V/V*).

Application: 2 µl.

Development: over a path of 15 cm.

Drying: in air.

Detection: examine in ultraviolet light at 254 nm.

System suitability: the chromatogram obtained with reference solution (c) shows 2 clearly separated principal spots.

Limits:

– *any impurity*: any spot in the chromatogram obtained with test solution (a), apart from the principal spot, is not more intense than the spot in the chromatogram obtained with reference solution (a) (0.5 per cent).

Sulphated ash (*2.4.14*): maximum 0.1 per cent, determined on 1.0 g.

ASSAY

To 1.000 g add 20.0 ml of *1 M sodium hydroxide*. Heat at about 70 °C for 1 h. Cool rapidly in an ice bath. Prepare a blank in the same manner. Carry out the titration on the solutions at room temperature. Titrate the excess sodium hydroxide with *0.5 M sulphuric acid*, continuing the titration until the second point of inflexion and determining the end-point potentiometrically (*2.2.20*).

1 ml of *1 M sodium hydroxide* is equivalent to 152.1 mg of $C_8H_8O_3$.

IMPURITIES

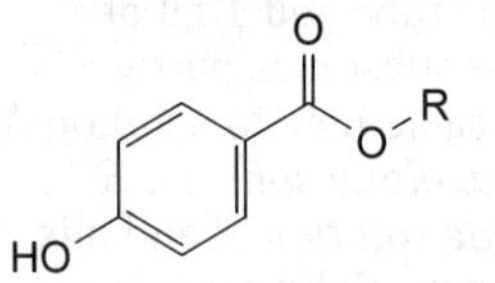

A. R = H: 4-hydroxybenzoic acid,

B. R = CH_2-CH_3: ethyl 4-hydroxybenzoate,

C. R = CH_2-CH_2-CH_3: propyl 4-hydroxybenzoate,

D. R = CH_2-CH_2-CH_2-CH_3: butyl 4-hydroxybenzoate.

01/2005:0230

METHYL SALICYLATE

Methylis salicylas

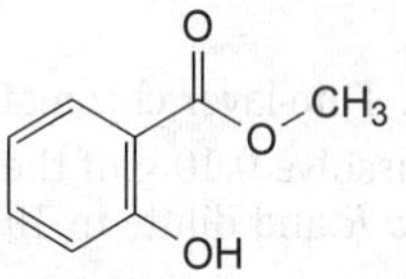

$C_8H_8O_3$ M_r 152.1

DEFINITION

Methyl salicylate contains not less than 99.0 per cent *m/m* and not more than the equivalent of 100.5 per cent *m/m* of methyl 2-hydroxybenzoate.

CHARACTERS

A colourless or slightly yellow liquid, very slightly soluble in water, miscible with alcohol and with fatty and essential oils.

IDENTIFICATION

A. Heat 0.25 ml with 2 ml of *dilute sodium hydroxide solution R* on a water-bath for 5 min. Add 3 ml of *dilute sulphuric acid R*. A crystalline precipitate is formed. Filter. The precipitate, washed with *water R* and dried at 100 °C to 105 °C, melts (*2.2.14*) at 156 °C to 161 °C.

B. To 10 ml of a saturated solution add 0.05 ml of *ferric chloride solution R1*. A violet colour develops.

TESTS

Appearance of solution. To 2 ml add 10 ml of *alcohol R*. The solution is clear (*2.2.1*) and not more intensely coloured than reference solution Y_7 (*2.2.2, Method II*).

Acidity. Dissolve 5.0 g in a mixture of 0.2 ml of *bromocresol green solution R* and 50 ml of *alcohol R* previously neutralised to a blue colour by addition of *0.1 M sodium hydroxide*. Not more than 0.4 ml of *0.1 M sodium hydroxide* is required to restore the blue colour.

Refractive index (*2.2.6*): 1.535 to 1.538.

Relative density (*2.2.5*): 1.180 to 1.186.

ASSAY

Dissolve 0.500 g in 25 ml of *alcohol R*. Add 0.05 ml of *phenol red solution R* and neutralise with *0.1 M sodium hydroxide*. To the neutralised solution add 50.0 ml of *0.1 M sodium hydroxide* and heat under a reflux condenser on a water-bath for 30 min. Cool and titrate with *0.1 M hydrochloric acid*. Calculate the volume of *0.1 M sodium hydroxide* used in the saponification. Carry out a blank titration.

1 ml of *0.1 M sodium hydroxide* is equivalent to 15.21 mg of $C_8H_8O_3$.

STORAGE

Store protected from light.

01/2005:0511

METHYLATROPINE BROMIDE

Methylatropini bromidum

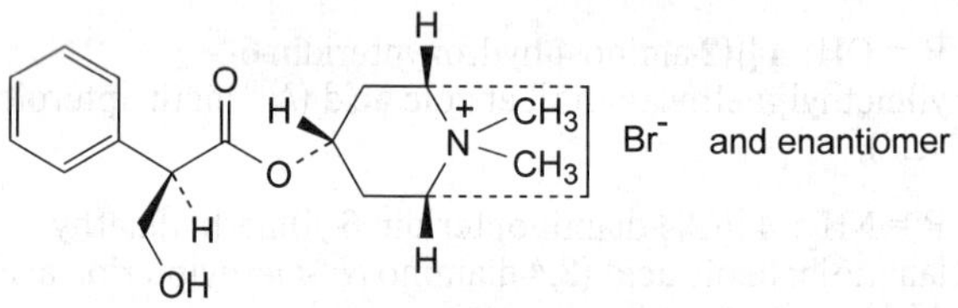

$C_{18}H_{26}BrNO_3$ M_r 384.3

DEFINITION

Methylatropine bromide contains not less than 99.0 per cent and not more than the equivalent of 101.0 per cent of (1*R*,3*r*,5*S*)-3-[[(2*RS*)-3-hydroxy-2-phenylpropanoyl]oxy]-8,8-dimethyl-8-azoniabicyclo[3.2.1]octane bromide, calculated with reference to the dried substance.

CHARACTERS

A white, crystalline powder or colourless crystals, freely soluble in water, sparingly soluble in alcohol.

It melts at about 219 °C, with decomposition.

IDENTIFICATION

First identification: B, E.

Second identification: A, C, D, E.

A. It complies with the test for optical rotation (see Tests).

B. Examine by infrared absorption spectrophotometry (*2.2.24*), comparing with the spectrum obtained with *methylatropine bromide CRS*.

C. To 5 ml of solution S (see Tests) add 2 ml of *dilute sodium hydroxide solution R*. No precipitate is formed.

D. To about 1 mg add 0.2 ml of *fuming nitric acid R* and evaporate to dryness on a water-bath. Dissolve the residue in 2 ml of *acetone R* and add 0.1 ml of a 30 g/l solution of *potassium hydroxide R* in *methanol R*. A violet colour develops.

E. It gives reaction (a) of bromides (*2.3.1*).

TESTS

Solution S. Dissolve 1.25 g in *carbon dioxide-free water R* and dilute to 25 ml with the same solvent.

Appearance of solution. Solution S is clear (*2.2.1*) and not more intensely coloured than reference solution B_9 (*2.2.2, Method II*).

Acidity or alkalinity. To 10 ml of solution S add 0.1 ml of *phenolphthalein solution R*; the solution is colourless. Add 0.5 ml of *0.01 M sodium hydroxide*; the solution is red.

Optical rotation (*2.2.7*). Dissolve 2.50 g in *water R* and dilute to 25.0 ml with the same solvent. The angle of optical rotation, measured in a 2 dm tube, is − 0.25° to + 0.05°.

Related substances. Examine by thin-layer chromatography (*2.2.27*), using a *TLC silica gel G plate R*.

Test solution. Dissolve 0.2 g of the substance to be examined in a mixture of 1 volume of *water R* and 9 volumes of *methanol R* and dilute to 5 ml with the same mixture of solvents.

Reference solution. Dilute 0.5 ml of the test solution to 100 ml with a mixture of 1 volume of *water R* and 9 volumes of *methanol R*.

Apply to the plate 5 µl of each solution. Develop over a path of 15 cm using a mixture of 10 volumes of *methanol R*, 15 volumes of *anhydrous formic acid R*, 15 volumes of *water R* and 60 volumes of *ethyl acetate R*. Dry the plate at 100 °C to 105 °C until the solvent has evaporated, allow to cool and spray with *dilute potassium iodobismuthate solution R* until the spots appear. Any spot in the chromatogram obtained with the test solution, apart from the principal spot, is not more intense than the spot in the chromatogram obtained with the reference solution (0.5 per cent).

Apomethylatropine. Dissolve 0.10 g in *0.01 M hydrochloric acid* and dilute to 100.0 ml with the same acid. Measure the absorbances (*2.2.25*) at the maxima at 252 nm and 257 nm. The ratio of the absorbance at 257 nm to that at 252 nm is at least 1.19.

Loss on drying (*2.2.32*). Not more than 0.5 per cent, determined on 0.500 g by drying in an oven at 100 °C to 105 °C.

Sulphated ash (*2.4.14*). Not more than 0.1 per cent, determined on the residue obtained in the test for loss on drying.

ASSAY

Dissolve 0.300 g in 50 ml of *anhydrous acetic acid R*, warming slightly if necessary. Titrate with *0.1 M perchloric acid*, determining the end-point potentiometrically (*2.2.20*).

1 ml of *0.1 M perchloric acid* is equivalent to 38.43 mg of $C_{18}H_{26}BrNO_3$.

STORAGE

Store protected from light.

01/2005:0512

METHYLATROPINE NITRATE

Methylatropini nitras

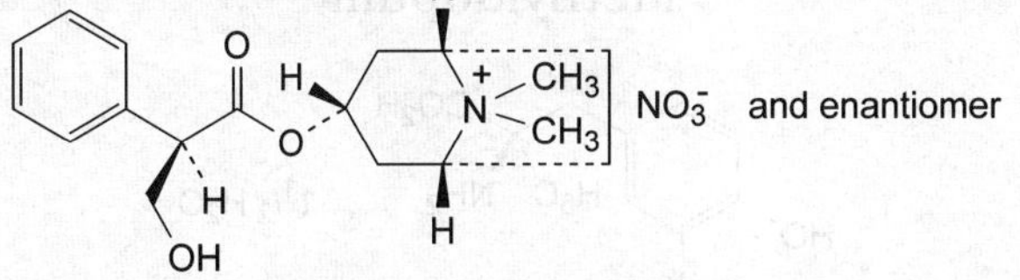

$C_{18}H_{26}N_2O_6$ M_r 366.4

DEFINITION

Methylatropine nitrate contains not less than 99.0 per cent and not more than the equivalent of 101.0 per cent of (1*R*,3*r*,5*S*)-3-[[(2*RS*)-3-hydroxy-2-phenylpropanoyl]oxy]-8,8-dimethyl-8-azoniabicyclo[3.2.1]octane nitrate, calculated with reference to the dried substance.

CHARACTERS

A white, crystalline powder or colourless crystals, freely soluble in water, soluble in alcohol.

It melts at about 167 °C.

IDENTIFICATION

First identification: B, E.

Second identification: A, C, D, E.

A. It complies with the test for optical rotation (see Tests).

B. Examine by infrared absorption spectrophotometry (*2.2.24*), comparing with the spectrum obtained with *methylatropine nitrate CRS*.

C. To a mixture of 2.5 ml of solution S (see Tests) and 2.5 ml of *water R* add 2 ml of *dilute sodium hydroxide solution R*. No precipitate is formed.

D. To about 1 mg add 0.2 ml of *fuming nitric acid R* and evaporate to dryness on a water-bath. Dissolve the residue in 2 ml of *acetone R* and add 0.25 ml of a 30 g/l solution of *potassium hydroxide R* in *methanol R*. A violet colour develops.

E. To 0.05 ml of *diphenylamine solution R* add 0.05 ml of a 1 in 10 dilution of solution S. An intense blue colour is produced.

TESTS

Solution S. Dissolve 1.25 g in *carbon dioxide-free water R* and dilute to 25 ml with the same solvent.

Appearance of solution. Solution S is clear (*2.2.1*) and not more intensely coloured than reference solution B_9 (*2.2.2, Method II*).

Acidity or alkalinity. To 10 ml of solution S add 0.1 ml of *phenolphthalein solution R*; the solution is colourless. Add 0.5 ml of *0.01 M sodium hydroxide*; the solution is red.

Optical rotation (*2.2.7*). Dissolve 2.50 g in *water R* and dilute to 25.0 ml with the same solvent. The angle of optical rotation, measured in a 2 dm tube, is − 0.25° to + 0.05°.

Related substances. Examine by thin-layer chromatography (*2.2.27*), using *silica gel G R* as the coating substance.

Test solution. Dissolve 0.2 g of the substance to be examined in a mixture of 1 volume of *water R* and 9 volumes of *methanol R* and dilute to 5 ml with the same mixture of solvents.

Reference solution. Dilute 0.5 ml of the test solution to 100 ml with a mixture of 1 volume of *water R* and 9 volumes of *methanol R*.

Apply to the plate 5 µl of each solution. Develop over a path of 15 cm using a mixture of 10 volumes of *methanol R*, 15 volumes of *anhydrous formic acid R*, 15 volumes of *water R* and 60 volumes of *ethyl acetate R*. Dry the plate at 100 °C to 105 °C until the solvent has evaporated, allow to cool and spray with *dilute potassium iodobismuthate solution R* until the spots appear. Any spot in the chromatogram obtained with the test solution, apart from the principal spot, is not more intense than the spot in the chromatogram obtained with the reference solution (0.5 per cent).

Apomethylatropine. Dissolve 0.10 g in *0.01 M hydrochloric acid* and dilute to 100.0 ml with the same acid. Measure the absorbances (*2.2.25*) at the maxima at 252 nm and 257 nm. The ratio of the absorbance at 257 nm to that at 252 nm is not less than 1.17.

Halides. 15 ml of solution S complies with the limit test for chlorides (*2.4.4*). Prepare the standard using 1.5 ml of *chloride standard solution (5 ppm Cl) R* (10 ppm).

Monographs M

Silver. Dissolve 1.0 g in 10 ml of *water R* and add 0.1 ml of *sodium sulphide solution R*. Allow to stand for 2 min. The solution is not more intensely coloured than reference solution B_8 (*2.2.2, Method II*) (10 ppm).

Loss on drying (*2.2.32*). Not more than 0.5 per cent, determined on 0.500 g by drying in an oven at 100 °C to 105 °C.

Sulphated ash (*2.4.14*). Not more than 0.1 per cent, determined on the residue obtained in the test for loss on drying.

ASSAY

Dissolve 0.300 g in 50 ml of *anhydrous acetic acid R*. Titrate with *0.1 M perchloric acid* determining the end-point potentiometrically (*2.2.20*).

1 ml of *0.1 M perchloric acid* is equivalent to 36.64 mg of $C_{18}H_{26}N_2O_6$.

STORAGE

Store protected from light.

01/2005:0345

METHYLCELLULOSE

Methylcellulosum

DEFINITION

Methylcellulose is a partly *O*-methylated cellulose.

CHARACTERS

A white, yellowish-white or greyish-white powder or granules, hygroscopic after drying, practically insoluble in hot water, in acetone, in ethanol and in toluene. It dissolves in cold water giving a colloidal solution.

IDENTIFICATION

A. Heat 10 ml of solution S (see Tests) in a water-bath while stirring. At a temperature above 50 °C the solution becomes cloudy or a flocculent precipitate is formed. The solution becomes clear again on cooling.

B. To 10 ml of solution S add 0.3 ml of *dilute acetic acid R* and 2.5 ml of a 100 g/l solution of *tannic acid R*. A yellowish-white, flocculent precipitate is formed which dissolves in *dilute ammonia R1*.

C. In a test-tube about 160 mm long, thoroughly mix 1 g with 2 g of finely powdered *manganese sulphate R*. Introduce to a depth of 2 cm into the upper part of the tube a strip of filter paper impregnated with a freshly prepared mixture of 1 volume of a 20 per cent *V/V* solution of *diethanolamine R* and 11 volumes of a 50 g/l solution of *sodium nitroprusside R*, adjusted to about pH 9.8 with *1 M hydrochloric acid*. Insert the tube 8 cm into a silicone-oil bath at 190 °C to 200 °C. The filter paper does not become blue within 10 min. Carry out a blank test.

D. Dissolve 0.2 g completely, without heating, in 15 ml of a 70 per cent *m/m* solution of *sulphuric acid R*. Pour the solution with stirring into 100 ml of iced *water R* and dilute to 250 ml with iced *water R*. In a test-tube, mix thoroughly while cooling in iced water 1 ml of the solution with 8 ml of *sulphuric acid R*, added dropwise. Heat in a water-bath for exactly 3 min and immediately cool in iced water. While the mixture is cold, carefully add 0.6 ml of *ninhydrin solution R2* and mix well. Allow to stand at 25 °C. A pink colour is produced immediately and does not become violet within 100 min.

E. Place 1 ml of solution S on a glass plate. After evaporation of the water a thin film is formed.

F. 0.2 g does not dissolve in 10 ml of *toluene R* nor in 10 ml of *ethanol R*.

TESTS

Solution S. While stirring, introduce a quantity of the substance to be examined equivalent to 1.0 g of the dried substance into 50 g of *carbon dioxide-free water R* heated to 90 °C. Allow to cool, adjust the mass of the solution to 100 g with *carbon dioxide-free water R* and stir until dissolution is complete. Allow to stand at 2 °C to 8 °C for 1 h before carrying out the test for appearance of solution.

Appearance of solution. Solution S is not more opalescent than reference suspension III (*2.2.1*) and not more intensely coloured than reference solution Y_6 (*2.2.2, Method II*).

pH (*2.2.3*). The pH of solution S is 5.5 to 8.0.

Apparent viscosity. While stirring, introduce a quantity of the substance to be examined equivalent to 6.00 g of the dried substance into 150 g of *water R* heated to 90 °C. Stir with a propeller-type stirrer for 10 min, place the flask in a bath of iced water, continue the stirring, and allow to remain in the bath of iced water for 40 min to ensure that dissolution is complete. Adjust the mass of the solution to 300 g, and centrifuge the solution to expel any entrapped air. Adjust the temperature of the solution to 20 ± 0.1 °C. Determine the viscosity (*2.2.10*) with a rotating viscometer at 20 °C and a shear rate of $10\ s^{-1}$. The apparent viscosity is not less than 75 per cent and not more than 140 per cent of the value stated on the label.

Chlorides (*2.4.4*). 1 ml of solution S diluted to 15 ml with *water R* complies with the limit test for chlorides (0.5 per cent).

Heavy metals (*2.4.8*). 1.0 g complies with limit test C for heavy metals (20 ppm). Prepare the standard using 2 ml of *lead standard solution (10 ppm Pb) R*.

Loss on drying (*2.2.32*). Not more than 10.0 per cent, determined on 1.000 g by drying in an oven at 100 °C to 105 °C.

Sulphated ash (*2.4.14*). Not more than 1.0 per cent, determined on 1.000 g.

LABELLING

The label states the apparent viscosity in millipascal seconds for a 2 per cent *m/m* solution.

01/2005:0045

METHYLDOPA

Methyldopum

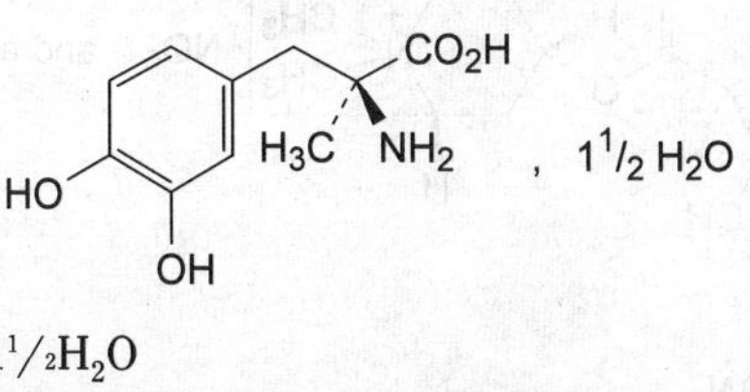

$C_{10}H_{13}NO_4,1^1/_2H_2O$ M_r 238.2

DEFINITION

Methyldopa contains not less than 98.5 per cent and not more than the equivalent of 101.0 per cent of (2*S*)-2-amino-3-(3,4-dihydroxyphenyl)-2-methylpropanoic acid, calculated with reference to the anhydrous substance.

CHARACTERS

A white or yellowish white, crystalline powder or colourless or almost colourless crystals, slightly soluble in water, very slightly soluble in alcohol. It is freely soluble in dilute mineral acids.

IDENTIFICATION

First identification: A.

Second identification: B, C, D.

A. Examine by infrared absorption spectrophotometry (*2.2.24*), comparing with the spectrum obtained with *methyldopa CRS*.

B. Dissolve about 2 mg in 2 ml of *water R* and add 0.2 ml of *ferric chloride solution R2*. A green colour develops which changes to bluish-violet on the addition of 0.1 g of *hexamethylenetetramine R*.

C. Dissolve about 5 mg in a mixture of 5 ml of *1 M hydrochloric acid* and 5 ml of *water R*. Add 0.1 ml of *sodium nitrite solution R* containing 100 g/l of *ammonium molybdate R*. A yellow colour is produced which becomes brownish-red on the addition of *strong sodium hydroxide solution R*.

D. To about 5 mg add 1 ml of *water R*, 1 ml of *pyridine R* and about 5 mg of *nitrobenzoyl chloride R* and heat to boiling. Add, while shaking, 0.2 ml of *sodium carbonate solution R*. An orange or amber colour develops.

TESTS

Appearance of solution. Dissolve 1.0 g in *1 M hydrochloric acid* and dilute to 25 ml with the same solvent. The solution is not more intensely coloured than reference solution BY_6 or B_6 (*2.2.2, Method II*).

Acidity. Dissolve 1.0 g with heating in 100 ml of *carbon dioxide-free water R*. Add 0.1 ml of *methyl red solution R*. Not more than 0.5 ml of *0.1 M sodium hydroxide* is required to produce the pure yellow colour of the indicator.

Optical rotation (*2.2.7*). Dissolve a quantity equivalent to 2.20 g of the anhydrous substance in *aluminium chloride solution R* and dilute to 50.0 ml with the same solution. The angle of optical rotation is − 1.10° to − 1.23°.

Absorbance (*2.2.25*). Dissolve 40.0 mg in *0.1 M hydrochloric acid* and dilute to 100.0 ml with the same acid. Dilute 10.0 ml of this solution to 100.0 ml with *0.1 M hydrochloric acid*. Examined between 230 nm and 350 nm, the solution shows a single absorption maximum, at 280 nm. The specific absorbance at this maximum is 122 to 137, calculated with reference to the anhydrous substance.

Methoxymethyldopa and related substances. Examine by thin-layer chromatography (*2.2.27*), using *cellulose for chromatography R* as the coating substance.

Test solution. Dissolve 0.1 g of the substance to be examined in a mixture of 0.4 ml of *hydrochloric acid R1* and 9.6 ml of *methanol R*.

Reference solution (a). Dissolve 5 mg of *3-methoxymethyldopa CRS* in 100 ml of *methanol R*.

Reference solution (b). To 1 ml of the test solution add 1 ml of reference solution (a).

Apply separately to the plate 10 µl of the test solution, 10 µl of reference solution (a) and 20 µl of reference solution (b). Develop over a path of 10 cm using a mixture of 15 volumes of *glacial acetic acid R*, 25 volumes of *water R* and 65 volumes of *butanol R*. Dry the plate immediately in a current of warm air and spray with a mixture of 5 volumes of a 50 g/l solution of *sodium nitrite R* and 45 volumes of a 3 g/l solution of *nitroaniline R* in a mixture of 20 volumes of *water R* and 80 volumes of *hydrochloric acid R*. Dry the plate immediately in a current of warm air and spray with a 200 g/l solution of *sodium carbonate R*. Examine the chromatograms immediately. Any spot in the chromatogram obtained with the test solution, apart from the principal spot, is not more intense than the spot in the chromatogram obtained with reference solution (a) (0.5 per cent). The test is not valid unless the chromatogram obtained with reference solution (b) shows 2 clearly separated spots.

Heavy metals (*2.4.8*). 1.0 g complies with limit test C for heavy metals (20 ppm). Prepare the standard using 2 ml of *lead standard solution (10 ppm Pb) R*.

Water (*2.5.12*). 10.0 per cent to 13.0 per cent, determined on 0.20 g by the semi-micro determination of water.

Sulphated ash (*2.4.14*). Not more than 0.1 per cent, determined on 1.0 g.

ASSAY

Dissolve 0.200 g in a mixture of 15 ml of *anhydrous formic acid R* 30 ml of *anhydrous acetic acid R* and 30 ml of *dioxan R*. Titrate with *0.1 M perchloric acid* until a green colour is obtained using 0.1 ml of *crystal violet solution R* as indicator.

1 ml of *0.1 M perchloric acid* is equivalent to 21.12 mg of $C_{10}H_{13}NO_4$.

STORAGE

Store protected from light.

01/2005:0932

METHYLENE CHLORIDE

Methyleni chloridum

CH_2Cl_2 M_r 84.9

DEFINITION

Methylene chloride is dichloromethane. It may contain not more than 2.0 per cent *V/V* of ethanol and/or not more than 0.03 per cent *V/V* of 2-methylbut-2-ene as stabiliser.

CHARACTERS

A clear, colourless, volatile liquid, sparingly soluble in water, miscible with alcohol.

IDENTIFICATION

First identification: B, C.

Second identification: A, D, E.

A. It complies with the test for relative density (see Tests).

B. It complies with the test for refractive index (see Tests).

C. Examine the chromatograms obtained in the test for ethanol, 2-methylbut-2-ene and other related substances. The retention time and size of the principal peak in the chromatogram obtained with test solution (b) are approximately the same as those of the principal peak in the chromatogram obtained with reference solution (a).

D. Heat 2 ml with 2 g of *potassium hydroxide R* and 20 ml of *alcohol R* under a reflux condenser for 30 min. Allow to cool. Add 15 ml of *dilute sulphuric acid R* and filter. To 1 ml of the filtrate add 1 ml of a 15 g/l solution of *chromotropic acid, sodium salt R*, 2 ml of *water R* and 8 ml of *sulphuric acid R*. A violet colour is produced.

E. 2 ml of the filtrate obtained in identification test D gives reaction (a) of chlorides (*2.3.1*).

Monographs M

TESTS

Appearance. It is clear (*2.2.1*) and colourless (*2.2.2, Method II*).

Acidity. To 50 ml of *methanol R* previously neutralised to 0.1 ml of *bromothymol blue solution R1*, add 50 g of the substance to be examined. Not more than 0.15 ml of *0.1 M sodium hydroxide* is required to change the colour of the indicator to blue.

Relative density (*2.2.5*): 1.320 to 1.332.

Refractive index (*2.2.6*): 1.423 to 1.425.

Ethanol, 2-methylbut-2-ene and other related substances. Examine by gas chromatography (*2.2.28*).

Test solution (a). The substance to be examined.

Test solution (b). Dilute 0.5 ml of test solution (a) to 100.0 ml with *water R*.

Reference solution (a). Dilute 0.5 ml of *methylene chloride CRS* to 100.0 ml with *water R*.

Reference solution (b). Dilute 2.0 ml of test solution (b) to 10.0 ml with *water R*.

Reference solution (c). To 20.0 ml of *ethanol R*, add 0.3 ml of *2-methylbut-2-ene R* and dilute to 100.0 ml with test solution (a). Dilute 1.0 ml of the solution to 10.0 ml with test solution (a).

Reference solution (d). Dilute 0.1 ml of *methanol R* and 0.1 ml of *methylene chloride CRS* to 100.0 ml with *water R*.

The chromatographic procedure may be carried out using:

- a glass column 2 m long and 2 mm in internal diameter, packed with *ethylvinylbenzene-divinylbenzene copolymer R* (136 µm to 173 µm),
- *nitrogen for chromatography R* as the carrier gas at a flow rate of 30 ml/min,
- a flame-ionisation detector,

maintaining the temperature of the column at 90 °C until injection, then raising the temperature at a rate of 4 °C per minute to 190 °C and maintaining at 190 °C for 15 min and maintaining the temperature of the injection port and the detector at 240 °C.

Inject 1 µl of reference solution (d). If a recorder is used, adjust the sensitivity of the detector such that the height of the peak due to methanol is not less than 25 per cent of the full scale of the recorder. The test is not valid unless: in the chromatogram obtained with reference solution (d), the resolution between the peaks corresponding to methanol and methylene chloride is at least 3.0.

Inject twice 2 µl of reference solution (c). If the peaks obtained show an area difference greater than 1.0 per cent, verify the repeatability by making four separate injections of reference solution (c); the test is not valid unless the relative standard deviation of the peak area is not more than 5.0 per cent.

Inject 2 µl of test solution (a), 2 µl of reference solution (b) and 2 µl of reference solution (c). In the chromatogram obtained with test solution (a): the areas of any peaks corresponding to ethanol and 2-methylbut-2-ene respectively are not greater than the difference between the areas of the peaks due to ethanol and 2-methylbut-2-ene in the chromatogram obtained with reference solution (c) and those of the peaks due to ethanol and 2-methylbut-2-ene in the chromatogram obtained with test solution (a) (2.0 per cent and 0.03 per cent, respectively).

In the chromatogram obtained with test solution (a), the sum of the areas of any peaks apart from the principal peak and any peaks due to ethanol and 2-methylbut-2-ene, is not greater than the area of the principal peak in the chromatogram obtained with reference solution (b) (0.1 per cent).

Free chlorine. Place 5 ml in a ground-glass-stoppered tube. Add 5 ml of a 100 g/l solution of *potassium iodide R* and 0.2 g of *soluble starch R*. Shake for 30 s and allow to stand for 5 min. No blue colour develops.

Heavy metals (*2.4.8*). Evaporate 25.0 g to dryness on a water-bath. Allow to cool. Add 1 ml of *hydrochloric acid R* and evaporate again. Dissolve the residue in 1 ml of *acetic acid R* and dilute to 25 ml with *water R*. 12 ml of the solution complies with limit test A for heavy metals (1 ppm). Prepare the standard using 10 ml of *lead standard solution (1 ppm Pb) R*.

Residue on evaporation. Evaporate 50.0 g to dryness on a water-bath and dry at 100 °C to 105 °C for 30 min. The residue weighs not more than 1 mg (20 ppm).

Water (*2.5.12*). Not more than 0.05 per cent *m/m*, determined on 10.00 g by the semi-micro determination of water.

STORAGE

Store in an airtight container, protected from light.

LABELLING

The label states the name and the concentration of any stabilisers.

IMPURITIES

A. carbon tetrachloride,

B. chloroform,

C. ethanol,

D. methanol,

E. 2-methylbut-2-ene.

01/2005:0346

METHYLHYDROXYETHYLCELLULOSE

Methylhydroxyethylcellulosum

DEFINITION

Methylhydroxyethylcellulose is a partly *O*-methylated and *O*-(2-hydroxyethylated) cellulose.

CHARACTERS

A white, yellowish-white or greyish-white powder or granules, hygroscopic after drying, practically insoluble in hot water, in acetone, in ethanol and in toluene. It dissolves in cold water giving a colloidal solution.

IDENTIFICATION

A. Heat 10 ml of solution S (see Tests) in a water-bath while stirring. At a temperature above 50 °C, the solution becomes cloudy or a flocculent precipitate is formed. The solution becomes clear again on cooling.

B. To 10 ml of solution S add 0.3 ml of *dilute acetic acid R* and 2.5 ml of a 100 g/l solution of *tannic acid R*. A yellowish-white, flocculent precipitate is formed which dissolves in *dilute ammonia R1*.

C. In a test-tube about 160 mm long, thoroughly mix 1 g with 2 g of finely powdered *manganese sulphate R*. Introduce to a depth of 2 cm into the upper part of the tube a strip of filter paper impregnated with a freshly prepared mixture of 1 volume of a 20 per cent *V/V* solution of *diethanolamine R* and 11 volumes of a 50 g/l solution of *sodium nitroprusside R,* adjusted to about pH 9.8 with *1 M hydrochloric acid*. Insert the tube 8 cm into a silicone-oil bath at 190 °C to 200 °C. The filter paper becomes blue within 10 min. Carry out a blank test.

D. Dissolve 0.2 g completely, without heating, in 15 ml of a 70 per cent *m/m* solution of *sulphuric acid R*. Pour the solution with stirring into 100 ml of iced *water R* and dilute to 250 ml with iced *water R*. In a test-tube, mix thoroughly, while cooling in iced water, 1 ml of the solution with 8 ml of *sulphuric acid R,* added dropwise. Heat in a water-bath for exactly 3 min and immediately cool in iced water. While the mixture is cold, carefully add 0.6 ml of *ninhydrin solution R2* and mix well. Allow to stand at 25 °C. A pink colour is produced immediately and does not become violet within 100 min.

E. Place 1 ml of solution S on a glass plate. After evaporation of the water a thin film is formed.

TESTS

Solution S. While stirring, introduce a quantity of the substance to be examined equivalent to 1.0 g of the dried substance into 50 g of *carbon dioxide-free water R* heated to 90 °C. Allow to cool, adjust the mass of the solution to 100 g with *carbon dioxide-free water R* and stir until dissolution is complete.

Appearance of solution. Solution S is not more opalescent than reference suspension III (*2.2.1*) and not more intensely coloured than reference solution Y_6 (*2.2.2, Method II*).

pH (*2.2.3*). The pH of solution S is 5.5 to 8.0.

Apparent viscosity. While stirring, introduce a quantity of the substance to be examined equivalent to 6.00 g of the dried substance into 150 g of *water R* heated to 90 °C. Stir with a propeller-type stirrer for 10 min, place the flask in a bath of iced water, continue the stirring and allow to remain in the bath of iced water for 40 min to ensure that dissolution is complete. Adjust the mass of the solution to 300 g and centrifuge the solution to expel any entrapped air. Adjust the temperature of the solution to 20 ± 0.1 °C. Determine the viscosity (*2.2.10*) with a rotating viscometer at 20 °C and a shear rate of 10 s^{-1}. The apparent viscosity is not less than 75 per cent and not more than 140 per cent of the value stated on the label.

Chlorides (*2.4.4*). 1 ml of solution S diluted to 15 ml with *water R* complies with the limit test for chlorides (0.5 per cent).

Heavy metals (*2.4.8*). 1.0 g complies with limit test C for heavy metals (20 ppm). Prepare the standard using 2 ml of *lead standard solution (10 ppm Pb) R*.

Loss on drying (*2.2.32*). Not more than 10.0 per cent, determined on 1.000 g by drying in an oven at 100 °C to 105 °C.

Sulphated ash (*2.4.14*). Not more than 1.0 per cent, determined on 1.000 g.

LABELLING

The label states the apparent viscosity in millipascal seconds for a 2 per cent *m/m* solution.

01/2005:0189

METHYLPHENOBARBITAL

Methylphenobarbitalum

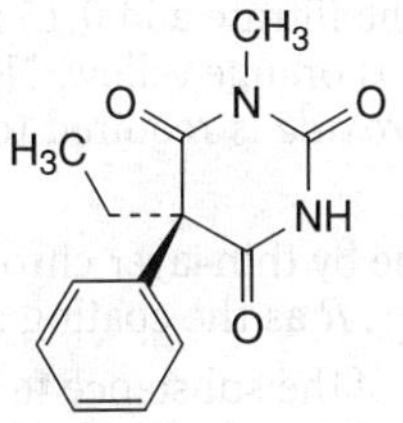

and enantiomer

$C_{13}H_{14}N_2O_3$ M_r 246.3

DEFINITION

Methylphenobarbital contains not less than 99.0 per cent and not more than the equivalent of 102.0 per cent of (5*RS*)-5-ethyl-1-methyl-5-phenylpyrimidine-2,4,6(1*H*,3*H*,5*H*)-trione, calculated with reference to the dried substance.

CHARACTERS

A white, crystalline powder or colourless crystals, practically insoluble in water, very slightly soluble in ethanol. It forms water-soluble compounds with alkali hydroxides and carbonates and with ammonia.

IDENTIFICATION

First identification: A, B.

Second identification: A, C, D.

A. Determine the melting point (*2.2.14*) of the substance to be examined. Mix equal parts of the substance to be examined and *methylphenobarbital CRS* and determine the melting point of the mixture. The difference between the two melting points (which are about 178 °C) is not greater than 2 °C.

B. Examine by infrared absorption spectrophotometry (*2.2.24*), comparing with the spectrum obtained with *methylphenobarbital CRS*.

C. Examine by thin-layer chromatography (*2.2.27*), using *silica gel GF_{254} R* as the coating substance.

Test solution. Dissolve 0.1 g of the substance to be examined in *chloroform R* and dilute to 100 ml with the same solvent.

Reference solution. Dissolve 0.1 g of *methylphenobarbital CRS* in *chloroform R* and dilute to 100 ml with the same solvent.

Apply separately to the plate 10 µl of each solution. Develop over a path of 18 cm using the lower layer of a mixture of 5 volumes of *concentrated ammonia R*, 15 volumes of *alcohol R* and 80 volumes of *chloroform R*. Examine immediately in ultraviolet light at 254 nm. The principal spot in the chromatogram obtained with the test solution is similar in position and size to the principal spot in the chromatogram obtained with the reference solution.

D. To about 10 mg add 0.2 ml of *sulphuric acid R* and 0.1 ml of *nitric acid R*. Heat on a water-bath for 10 min. Cool in iced water and add 5 ml of *water R* and 5 ml of *strong sodium hydroxide solution R*. Add 5 ml of *acetone R*, shake and allow to stand. A dark-red colour develops in the upper layer.

TESTS

Appearance of solution. Dissolve 1.0 g, with gentle heating, in a mixture of 4 ml of *dilute sodium hydroxide solution R* and 6 ml of *water R*. The solution is clear (*2.2.1*) and not more intensely coloured than reference solution Y_6 (*2.2.2, Method II*).

Acidity. Boil 1.0 g with 50 ml of *water R* for 2 min, allow to cool and filter. To 10 ml of the filtrate add 0.15 ml of *methyl red solution R*. The solution is orange-yellow. Not more than 0.1 ml of *0.1 M sodium hydroxide* is required to produce a pure yellow colour.

Related substances. Examine by thin-layer chromatography (*2.2.27*), using *silica gel GF_{254} R* as the coating substance.

Test solution. Dissolve 1.0 g of the substance to be examined in *chloroform R* and dilute to 100 ml with the same solvent.

Reference solution. Dissolve 0.1 g of *phenobarbital CRS* in *chloroform R* and dilute to 100 ml with the same solvent. Dilute 10 ml of the solution to 100 ml with *chloroform R*.

Apply separately to the plate 20 µl of each solution. Develop over a path of 15 cm using the lower layer of a mixture of 5 volumes of *concentrated ammonia R*, 15 volumes of *alcohol R* and 80 volumes of *chloroform R*. Examine immediately in ultraviolet light at 254 nm. Spray with *diphenylcarbazone mercuric reagent R*. Allow the plate to dry in air and spray with freshly prepared *alcoholic potassium hydroxide solution R* diluted 1 in 5 with *aldehyde-free alcohol R*. Heat at 100 °C to 105 °C for 5 min and examine immediately. When examined in ultraviolet light and after spraying, any spot in the chromatogram obtained with the test solution, apart from the principal spot, is not more intense than the spot in the chromatogram obtained with the reference solution (1.0 per cent).

Loss on drying (*2.2.32*). Not more than 0.5 per cent, determined on 1.00 g by drying in an oven at 100 °C to 105 °C.

Sulphated ash (*2.4.14*). Not more than 0.1 per cent, determined on 1.0 g.

ASSAY

Dissolve 0.200 g in 5 ml of *pyridine R*. Add 0.5 ml of *thymolphthalein solution R* and 10 ml of *silver nitrate solution in pyridine R*. Titrate with *0.1 M ethanolic sodium hydroxide* until a pure blue colour is obtained. Carry out a blank titration.

1 ml of *0.1 M ethanolic sodium hydroxide* is equivalent to 24.63 mg of $C_{13}H_{14}N_2O_3$.

01/2005:0561

METHYLPREDNISOLONE

Methylprednisolonum

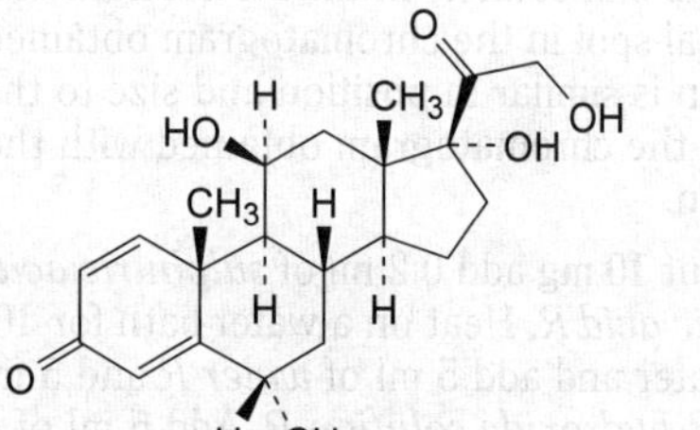

$C_{22}H_{30}O_5$ M_r 374.5

DEFINITION

Methylprednisolone contains not less than 97.0 per cent and not more than the equivalent of 103.0 per cent of 11β,17,21-trihydroxy-6α-methylpregna-1,4-diene-3,20-dione, calculated with reference to the dried substance.

CHARACTERS

A white or almost white, crystalline powder, practically insoluble in water, sparingly soluble in alcohol, slightly soluble in acetone and in methylene chloride.

It shows polymorphism.

IDENTIFICATION

First identification: A, B.

Second identification: C, D.

A. Examine by infrared absorption spectrophotometry (*2.2.24*), comparing with the spectrum obtained with *methylprednisolone CRS*. If the spectra obtained in the solid state show differences, dissolve the substance to be examined and the reference substance separately in the minimum volume of *acetone R*, evaporate to dryness on a water-bath and record new spectra using the residues.

B. Examine by thin-layer chromatography (*2.2.27*), using a *TLC silica gel F_{254} plate R*.

Test solution. Dissolve 10 mg of the substance to be examined in a mixture of 1 volume of *methanol R* and 9 volumes of *methylene chloride R* and dilute to 10 ml with the same mixture of solvents.

Reference solution (a). Dissolve 20 mg of *methylprednisolone CRS* in a mixture of 1 volume of *methanol R* and 9 volumes of *methylene chloride R* and dilute to 20 ml with the same mixture of solvents.

Reference solution (b). Dissolve 10 mg of *hydrocortisone CRS* in reference solution (a) and dilute to 10 ml with reference solution (a).

Apply to the plate 5 µl of each solution. Prepare the mobile phase by adding a mixture of 1.2 volumes of *water R* and 8 volumes of *methanol R* to a mixture of 15 volumes of *ether R* and 77 volumes of *methylene chloride R*. Develop over a path of 15 cm. Carry out a second development over a path of 15 cm using a mixture of 5 volumes of *butanol R* saturated with *water R*, 15 volumes of *toluene R* and 80 volumes of *ether R*. Allow the plate to dry in air and examine in ultraviolet light at 254 nm. The principal spot in the chromatogram obtained with the test solution is similar in position and size to the principal spot in the chromatogram obtained with reference solution (a). Spray with *alcoholic solution of sulphuric acid R*. Heat at 120 °C for 10 min or until the spots appear. Allow to cool. Examine the chromatograms in daylight and in ultraviolet light at 365 nm. The principal spot in the chromatogram obtained with the test solution is similar in position, colour in daylight, fluorescence in ultraviolet light at 365 nm and size to the principal spot in the chromatogram obtained with reference solution (a). The test is not valid unless the chromatogram obtained with reference solution (b) shows two clearly separated spots.

C. Examine by thin-layer chromatography (*2.2.27*), using a *TLC silica gel F_{254} plate R*.

Test solution (a). Dissolve 25 mg of the substance to be examined in *methanol R* and dilute to 5 ml with the same solvent. This solution is also used to prepare test solution (b). Dilute 2 ml of the solution to 10 ml with *methylene chloride R*.

Test solution (b). Transfer 0.4 ml of the solution obtained during the preparation of test solution (a) to a glass tube 100 mm long and 20 mm in diameter and fitted with a ground-glass stopper or a polytetrafluoroethylene cap and evaporate the solvent with gentle heating under a stream of *nitrogen R*. Add 2 ml of a 15 per cent *V/V* solution of *glacial acetic acid R* and 50 mg of *sodium bismuthate R*. Stopper the tube and shake the suspension in a mechanical shaker protected from light for 1 h. Add 2 ml of a 15 per cent *V/V* solution of *glacial acetic acid R* and filter into a 50 ml separating funnel, washing the filter with two quantities, each of 5 ml, of *water R*. Shake the clear filtrate with 10 ml of *methylene chloride R*. Wash the organic layer with 5 ml of *1 M sodium hydroxide* and two quantities, each of 5 ml, of *water R*. Dry over *anhydrous sodium sulphate R*.

Reference solution (a). Dissolve 25 mg of *methylprednisolone CRS* in *methanol R* and dilute to 5 ml with the same solvent. This solution is also used to prepare reference solution (b). Dilute 2 ml of the solution to 10 ml with *methylene chloride R*.

Reference solution (b). Transfer 0.4 ml of the solution obtained during preparation of reference solution (a) to a glass tube 100 mm long and 20 mm in diameter and fitted with a ground-glass stopper or a polytetrafluoroethylene cap and evaporate the solvent with gentle heating under a stream of *nitrogen R*. Add 2 ml of a 15 per cent *V/V* solution of *glacial acetic acid R* and 50 mg of *sodium bismuthate R*. Stopper the tube and shake the suspension in a mechanical shaker protected from light for 1 h. Add 2 ml of a 15 per cent *V/V* solution of *glacial acetic acid R* and filter into a 50 ml separating funnel, washing the filter with two quantities, each of 5 ml, of *water R*. Shake the clear filtrate with 10 ml of *methylene chloride R*. Wash the organic layer with 5 ml of *1 M sodium hydroxide* and two quantities, each of 5 ml, of *water R*. Dry over *anhydrous sodium sulphate R*.

Apply to the plate 5 µl of test solution (a), 5 µl of reference solution (a), 10 µl of test solution (b) and 10 µl of reference solution (b), applying the latter two in small quantities in order to obtain small spots. Develop over a path of 15 cm using a mixture of 5 volumes of *butanol R* saturated with *water R*, 10 volumes of *toluene R* and 85 volumes of *ether R*. Allow the plate to dry in air and examine in ultraviolet light at 254 nm. The principal spot in each of the chromatograms obtained with the test solutions is similar in position and size to the principal spot in the chromatogram obtained with the corresponding reference solution. Spray with *alcoholic solution of sulphuric acid R* and heat at 120 °C for 15 min. Allow to cool. Examine the plate in daylight and in ultraviolet light at 365 nm. The principal spot in each of the chromatograms obtained with the test solutions is similar in position, colour in daylight, fluorescence in ultraviolet light at 365 nm and size to the principal spot in the chromatogram obtained with the corresponding reference solution. The principal spots in the chromatograms obtained with test solution (b) and reference solution (b) have an R_f value distinctly higher than that of the principal spots in the chromatograms obtained with test solution (a) and reference solution (a).

D. Add about 2 mg to 2 ml of *sulphuric acid R* and shake to dissolve. Within 5 min, an intense red colour develops. When examined in ultraviolet light at 365 nm, brownish-red fluorescence is seen. Add the solution to 10 ml of *water R* and mix. The colour fades and there is a yellowish-green fluorescence in ultraviolet light at 365 nm.

TESTS

Specific optical rotation (*2.2.7*). Dissolve 0.250 g in *dioxan R* and dilute to 25.0 ml with the same solvent. The specific optical rotation is + 79.0 to + 86.0, calculated with reference to the dried substance.

Related substances. Examine by liquid chromatography (*2.2.29*).

Test solution. Dissolve 25.0 mg of the substance to be examined in a mixture of equal volumes of *acetonitrile R* and *methanol R* and dilute to 10.0 ml with the same mixture of solvents.

Reference solution (a). Dissolve 2 mg of *methylprednisolone CRS* and 2 mg of *betamethasone CRS* in mobile phase A and dilute to 100.0 ml with the same mobile phase.

Reference solution (b). Dilute 1.0 ml of the test solution to 100.0 ml with mobile phase A.

The chromatographic procedure may be carried out using:

– a stainless steel column 0.25 m long and 4.6 mm in internal diameter packed with *octadecylsilyl silica gel for chromatography R* (5 µm),

– as mobile phase at a flow rate of 2.5 ml/min a linear-gradient programme using the following conditions:

Mobile phase A. In a 1000 ml volumetric flask mix 250 ml of *acetonitrile R* with 700 ml of *water R* and allow to equilibrate; adjust the volume to 1000 ml with *water R* and mix again,

Mobile phase B. Acetonitrile R,

Time (min)	Mobile phase A (per cent *V/V*)	Mobile phase B (per cent *V/V*)	Comment
0	100	0	isocratic
15	100	0	begin linear gradient
40	0	100	end chromatogram, return to 100 A
41	100	0	begin equilibration with A
46 = 0	100	0	end equilibration, begin next chromatogram

– as detector a spectrophotometer set at 254 nm,

maintaining the temperature of the column at 45 °C.

Equilibrate the column with mobile phase B at a flow rate of 2.5 ml/min for at least 30 min and then with mobile phase A for 5 min. For subsequent chromatograms, use the conditions described from 40 min to 46 min. Adjust the sensitivity of the system so that the height of the principal peak in the chromatogram obtained with 20 µl of reference solution (b) is at least 50 per cent of the full scale of the recorder.

Inject 20 µl of reference solution (a). When the chromatograms are recorded in the conditions described above, the retention times are: methylprednisolone about 11.5 min and betamethasone about 12.5 min. The test is not valid unless the resolution between the peaks corresponding to methylprednisolone and betamethasone is at least 1.5; if necessary, adjust the concentration of acetonitrile in mobile phase A.

Inject separately 20 µl of a mixture of equal volumes of *acetonitrile R* and *methanol R* as a blank, 20 µl of the test solution and 20 µl of reference solution (b). In the chromatogram obtained with the test solution: the area of any peak, apart from the principal peak, is not greater than half the area of the principal peak in the chromatogram obtained with reference solution (b) (0.5 per cent); the sum of the areas of all the peaks, apart from the principal peak, is

Monographs M

not greater than twice the area of the principal peak in the chromatogram obtained with reference solution (b) (2 per cent). Disregard any peak due to the blank and any peak with an area less than 0.05 times the area of the principal peak in the chromatogram obtained with reference solution (b).

Loss on drying (*2.2.32*). Not more than 1.0 per cent, determined on 0.500 g by drying in an oven at 100 °C to 105 °C.

ASSAY

Dissolve 0.100 g in *alcohol R* and dilute to 100.0 ml with the same solvent. Dilute 2.0 ml of the solution to 100.0 ml with *alcohol R*. Measure the absorbance (*2.2.25*) at the maximum at 243 nm.

Calculate the content of $C_{22}H_{30}O_5$ taking the specific absorbance to be 395.

STORAGE

Store protected from light.

IMPURITIES

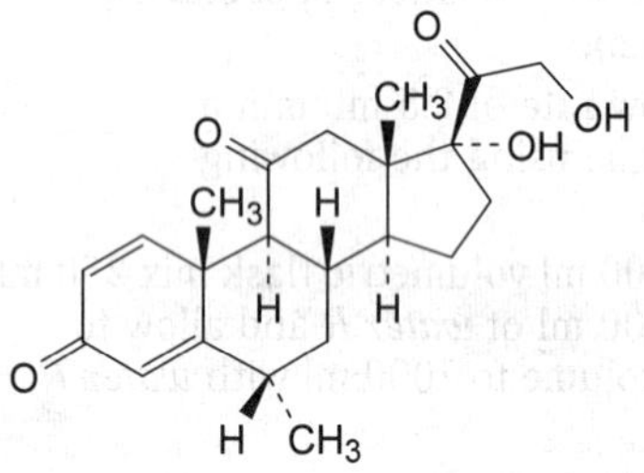

A. 17,21-dihydroxy-6α-methylpregna-1,4-diene-3,11,20-trione,

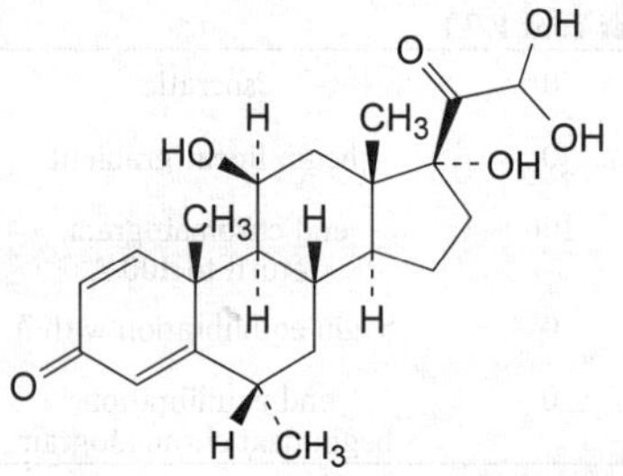

B. 11β,17,21,21-tetrahydroxy-6α-methylpregna-1,4-diene-3,20-dione,

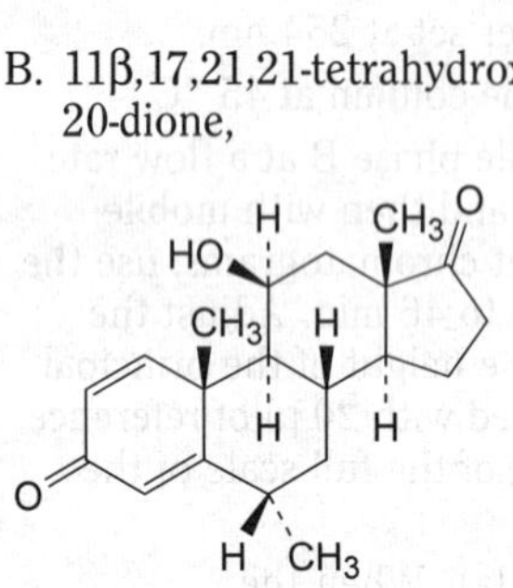

C. 11β-hydroxy-6α-methylandrosta-1,4-diene-3,17-dione,

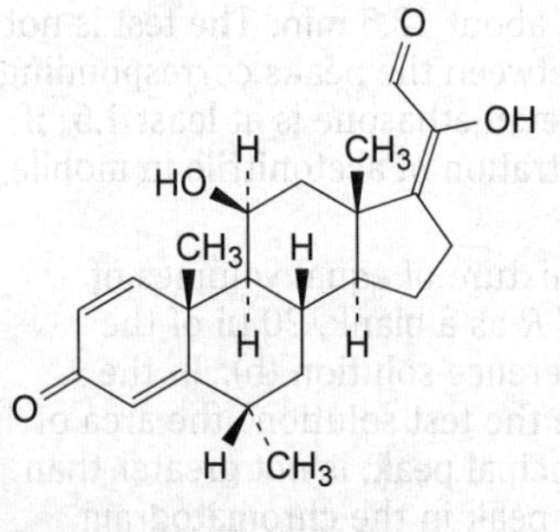

and (*Z*)-isomer

D. (*E*)- and (*Z*)-11β,20-dihydroxy-6α-methylpregna-1,4,17(20)-triene-3,21-dione.

01/2005:0933

METHYLPREDNISOLONE ACETATE

Methylprednisoloni acetas

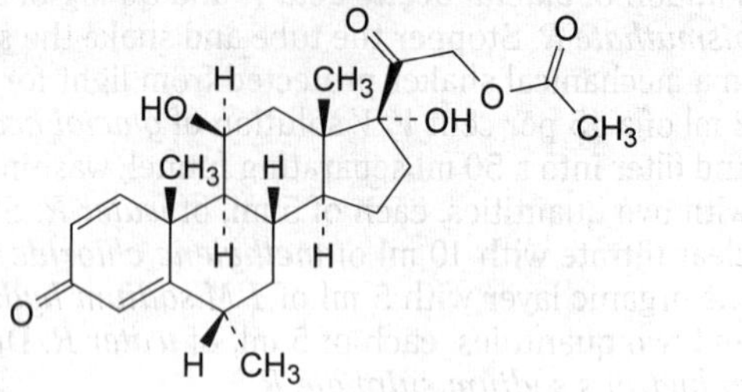

$C_{24}H_{32}O_6$ M_r 416.5

DEFINITION

Methylprednisolone acetate contains not less than 97.0 per cent and not more than the equivalent of 103.0 per cent of 11β,17-dihydroxy-6α-methyl-3,20-dioxopregna-1,4-dien-21-yl acetate, calculated with reference to the dried substance.

CHARACTERS

A white or almost white, crystalline powder, practically insoluble in water, sparingly soluble in acetone and in alcohol.

IDENTIFICATION

First identification: A, B.

Second identification: C, D, E.

A. Examine by infrared absorption spectrophotometry (*2.2.24*), comparing with the spectrum obtained with *methylprednisolone acetate CRS*. If the spectra obtained in the solid state show differences, dissolve the substance to be examined and the reference substance separately in the minimum volume of *acetone R*, evaporate to dryness and record new spectra using the residues.

B. Examine by thin-layer chromatography (*2.2.27*), using *silica gel* GF_{254} *R* as the coating substance.

Test solution. Dissolve 10 mg of the substance to be examined in a mixture of 1 volume of *methanol R* and 9 volumes of *methylene chloride R* and dilute to 10 ml with the same mixture of solvents.

Reference solution (a). Dissolve 10 mg of *methylprednisolone acetate CRS* in a mixture of 1 volume of *methanol R* and 9 volumes of *methylene chloride R* and dilute to 10 ml with the same mixture of solvents.

Reference solution (b). Dissolve 10 mg of *prednisolone acetate CRS* and 10 mg of *methylprednisolone acetate CRS* in a mixture of 1 volume of *methanol R* and 9 volumes of *methylene chloride R* and dilute to 10 ml with the same mixture of solvents.

Apply separately to the plate 5 µl of each solution. Develop over a path of 15 cm using a mixture of 5 volumes of *butanol R*, 10 volumes of *toluene R* and 85 volumes of *ether R*. Allow the plate to dry in air and examine in ultraviolet light at 254 nm. The principal spot in the chromatogram obtained with the test solution is similar in position and size to the principal spot in the chromatogram obtained with reference solution (a). Spray the plate with *alcoholic solution of sulphuric acid R*. Heat at 120 °C for 10 min or until the spots appear. Allow to cool. Examine in daylight and in ultraviolet light at 365 nm. The principal spot in the chromatogram obtained with the test solution is similar in position, colour in daylight, fluorescence in ultraviolet light at 365 nm and size to the principal spot in the chromatogram obtained with reference solution (a). The test is not valid unless the chromatogram obtained with reference solution (b) shows two spots which, when examined in ultraviolet light at 365 nm, may not be completely separated.

C. Examine by thin-layer chromatography (*2.2.27*), using *silica gel GF_{254} R* as the coating substance.

Test solution (a). Dissolve 25 mg of the substance to be examined in *methanol R* and dilute to 5 ml with the same solvent. This solution is also used to prepare test solution (b). Dilute 2 ml of the solution to 10 ml with *methylene chloride R*.

Test solution (b). Transfer 2 ml of the solution obtained during preparation of test solution (a) to a 15 ml glass tube with a ground-glass stopper or a polytetrafluoroethylene cap. Add 10 ml of *saturated methanolic potassium hydrogen carbonate solution R* and immediately pass a current of *nitrogen R* through the solution for 5 min. Stopper the tube. Heat in a water-bath at 45 °C protected from light for 1 h. Allow to cool.

Reference solution (a). Dissolve 25 mg of *methylprednisolone acetate CRS* in *methanol R* and dilute to 5 ml with the same solvent. This solution is also used to prepare reference solution (b). Dilute 2 ml of the solution to 10 ml with *methylene chloride R*.

Reference solution (b). Transfer 2 ml of the solution obtained during preparation of reference solution (a) to a 15 ml glass tube with a ground-glass stopper or a polytetrafluoroethylene cap. Add 10 ml of *saturated methanolic potassium hydrogen carbonate solution R* and immediately pass a current of *nitrogen R* through the solution for 5 min. Stopper the tube. Heat in a water-bath at 45 °C protected from light for 1 h. Allow to cool.

Apply separately to the plate 5 µl of each solution. Prepare the mobile phase by adding a mixture of 1.2 volumes of *water R* and 8 volumes of *methanol R* to a mixture of 15 volumes of *ether R* and 77 volumes of *methylene chloride R*. Develop over a path of 15 cm. Allow the plate to dry in air and examine in ultraviolet light at 254 nm. The principal spot in each of the chromatograms obtained with the test solutions is similar in position and size to the principal spot in the chromatogram obtained with the corresponding reference solution. Spray with *alcoholic solution of sulphuric acid R*. Heat at 120 °C for 10 min or until the spots appear. Allow to cool. Examine in daylight and in ultraviolet light at 365 nm. The principal spot in each of the chromatograms obtained with the test solutions is similar in position, colour in daylight, fluorescence in ultraviolet light at 365 nm and size to the principal spot in the chromatogram obtained with the corresponding reference solution. The principal spots in the chromatograms obtained with test solution (b) and reference solution (b) have an R_f value distinctly lower than that of the principal spots in the chromatograms obtained respectively with test solution (a) and reference solution (a).

D. Add about 2 mg to 2 ml of *sulphuric acid R* and shake to dissolve. Within 5 min, an intense red colour develops. When examined in ultraviolet light at 365 nm, a reddish-brown fluorescence is seen. Add the solution to 10 ml of *water R* and mix. The colour fades and there is a greenish-yellow fluorescence in ultraviolet light at 365 nm.

E. About 10 mg gives the reaction of acetyl (*2.3.1*).

TESTS

Specific optical rotation (*2.2.7*). Dissolve 0.250 g in *dioxan R* and dilute to 25.0 ml with the same solvent. The specific optical rotation is + 97 to + 105, calculated with reference to the dried substance.

Related substances. Examine by liquid chromatography (*2.2.29*).

Test solution. Dissolve 20.0 mg of the substance to be examined in 5 ml of *tetrahydrofuran R* and dilute to 10.0 ml with *water R*.

Reference solution (a). Dissolve 4 mg of *methylprednisolone acetate CRS* and 4 mg of *dexamethasone acetate CRS* in the mobile phase and dilute to 20.0 ml with the mobile phase. Dilute 2.0 ml of this solution to 10.0 ml with the mobile phase.

Reference solution (b). Dilute 1.0 ml of the test solution to 50.0 ml with the mobile phase.

The chromatographic procedure may be carried out using:

- a stainless steel column 0.25 m long and 4.6 mm in internal diameter packed with *octadecylsilyl silica gel for chromatography R* (5 µm),
- as mobile phase at a flow rate of 1 ml/min a mixture prepared as follows: in a 1000 ml volumetric flask mix 260 ml *tetrahydrofuran R* and 700 ml of *water R* and leave to equilibrate; adjust the volume to 1000 ml with *water R* and mix again,
- as detector a spectrophotometer set at 254 nm.

Equilibrate the column with the mobile phase at a flow rate of 1 ml/min for about 45 min.

Adjust the sensitivity of the system so that the height of the principal peak in the chromatogram obtained with 20 µl of reference solution (b) is at least 50 per cent of the full scale of the recorder.

Inject 20 µl of reference solution (a). When the chromatograms are recorded in the prescribed conditions, the retention times are: methylprednisolone acetate, about 43 min; dexamethasone acetate, about 57 min. The test is not valid unless the resolution between the peaks corresponding to methylprednisolone acetate and dexamethasone acetate is not less than 6.5. If necessary, adjust the concentration of *water R* in the mobile phase.

Inject separately 20 µl of the test solution and 20 µl of reference solution (b). Continue the chromatography for 1.5 times the retention time of the principal peak. In the chromatogram obtained with the test solution, the sum of the areas of all the peaks, apart from the principal peak, is not greater than half the area of the principal peak in the chromatogram obtained with reference solution (b) (1.0 per cent). Disregard any peak due to the solvent and any peak with an area less than 0.025 times the area of the principal peak in the chromatogram obtained with reference solution (b).

Loss on drying (*2.2.32*). Not more than 0.5 per cent, determined on 1.000 g by drying in an oven at 100 °C to 105 °C.

ASSAY

Dissolve 0.100 g in *alcohol R* and dilute to 100.0 ml with the same solvent. Dilute 1.0 ml of the solution to 100.0 ml with *alcohol R*. Measure the absorbance (*2.2.25*) at the maximum at 243 nm.

Calculate the content of $C_{24}H_{32}O_6$, taking the specific absorbance to be 355.

STORAGE

Store protected from light.

Monographs M

IMPURITIES

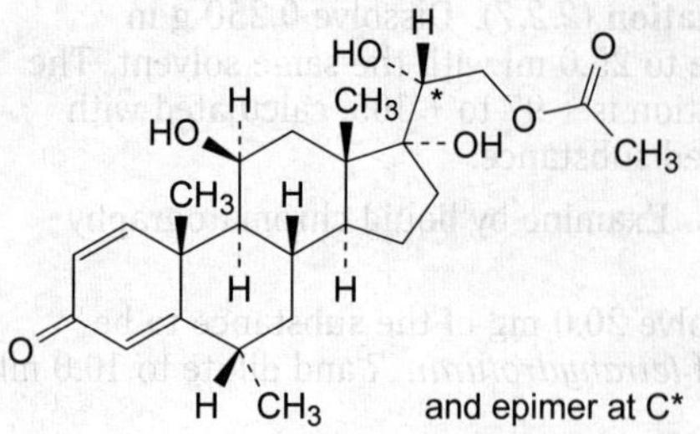

A. (20*RS*)-11β,17,20-trihydroxy-6α-methyl-3-oxopregna-1,4-dien-21-yl acetate,

B. methylprednisolone,

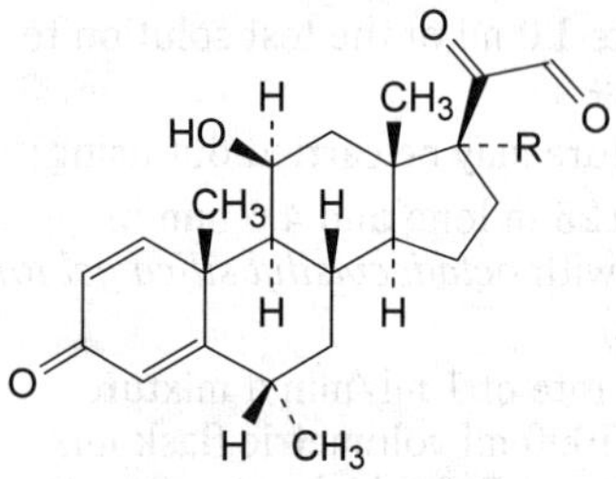

C. R = OH: 11β,17-dihydroxy-6α-methylpregna-1,4-diene-3,20,21-trione,

D. R = H: 11β-hydroxy-6α-methylpregna-1,4-diene-3,20,21-trione,

E. prednisolone acetate,

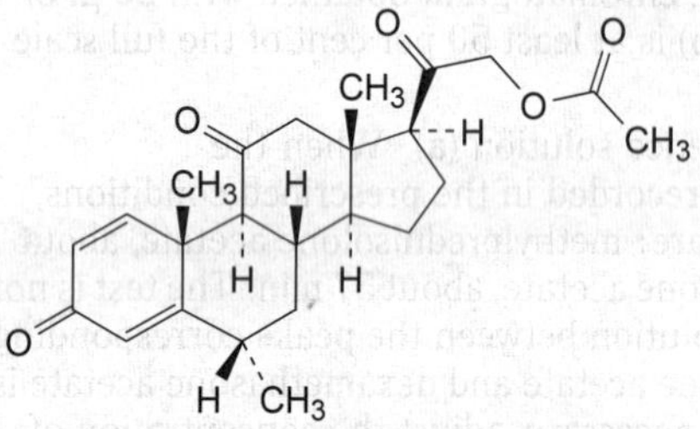

F. 6α-methyl-3,11,20-trioxopregna-1,4-dien-21-yl acetate,

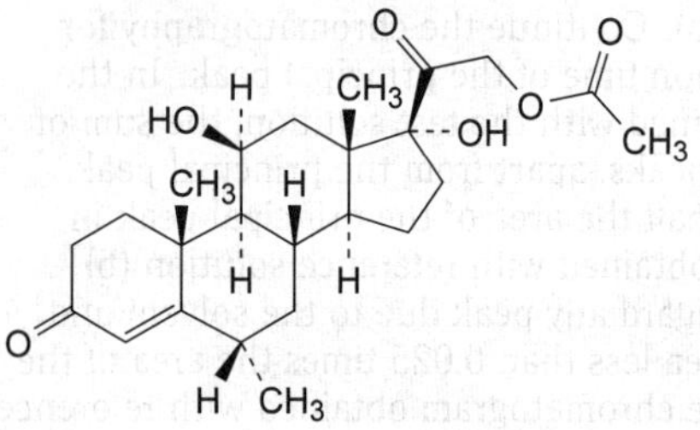

G. 11β,17-dihydroxy-6α-methyl-3,20-dioxopregn-4-en-21-yl acetate,

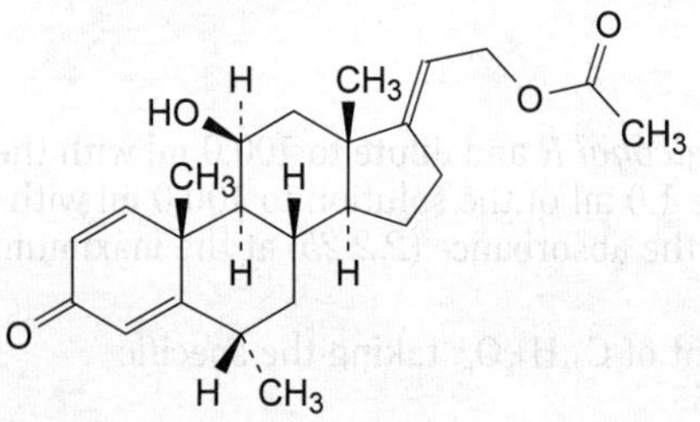

H. 11β-hydroxy-6α-methyl-3-oxopregna-1,4,17(20)-trien-21-yl acetate.

01/2005:1131
corrected

METHYLPREDNISOLONE HYDROGEN SUCCINATE

Methylprednisoloni hydrogenosuccinas

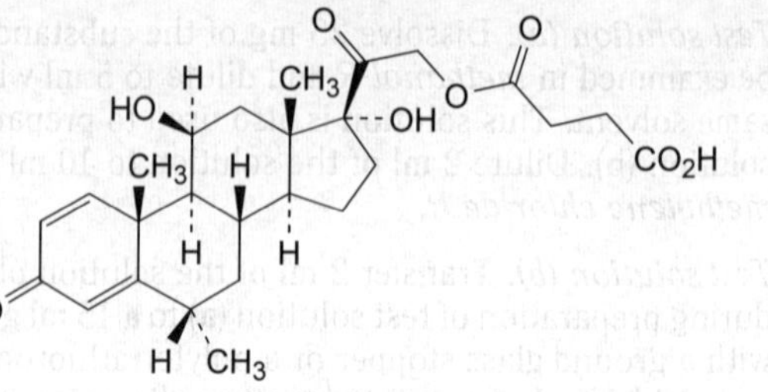

$C_{26}H_{34}O_8$ M_r 474.6

DEFINITION

Methylprednisolone hydrogen succinate contains not less than 97.0 per cent and not more than the equivalent of 103.0 per cent of 4-[(11β,17-dihydroxy-6α-methyl-3,20-dioxopregna-1,4-dien-21-yl)oxy]-4-oxobutanoic acid, calculated with reference to the dried substance.

CHARACTERS

A white or almost white, hygroscopic powder, practically insoluble in water, slightly soluble in acetone and in ethanol. It dissolves in dilute solutions of alkali hydroxides.

IDENTIFICATION

First identification: A, B.

Second identification: C, D.

A. Examine by infrared absorption spectrophotometry (*2.2.24*), comparing with the spectrum obtained with *methylprednisolone hydrogen succinate CRS*.

B. Examine by thin layer chromatography (*2.2.27*), using a *TLC silica gel F_{254} plate R*.

Test solution. Dissolve 10 mg of the substance to be examined in a mixture of 1 volume of *methanol R* and 9 volumes of *methylene chloride R* and dilute to 10 ml with the same mixture of solvents.

Reference solution (a). Dissolve 20 mg of *methylprednisolone hydrogen succinate CRS* in a mixture of 1 volume of *methanol R* and 9 volumes of *methylene chloride R* and dilute to 20 ml with the same mixture of solvents.

Reference solution (b). Dissolve 10 mg of *hydrocortisone hydrogen succinate CRS* in reference solution (a) and dilute to 10 ml with the same reference solution.

Apply to the plate 10 µl of each solution. Develop over a path of 15 cm using a mixture of 0.1 volumes of *anhydrous formic acid R*, 1 volume of *ethanol R* and 15 volumes of *methylene chloride R*. Allow the plate to dry in air and examine in ultraviolet light at 254 nm. The principal spot in the chromatogram obtained with the test solution is similar in position and size to the principal spot in the chromatogram obtained with reference solution (a). Spray the plate with *alcoholic solution of sulphuric acid R*. Heat at 120 °C for 10 min or until the spots appear. Allow to cool. Examine in daylight and in ultraviolet light at 365 nm. The principal spot in the chromatogram obtained with the test solution is similar in position, colour in daylight, fluorescence in ultraviolet light at 365 nm and size to the principal spot in the chromatogram obtained with reference solution (a).

The test is not valid unless the chromatogram obtained with reference solution (b) shows two spots which may, however, not be completely separated.

C. Examine by thin layer chromatography (*2.2.27*), using a *TLC silica gel F_{254} plate R*.

Test solution (a). Dissolve 25 mg of the substance to be examined in *methanol R* with gentle heating and dilute to 5 ml with the same solvent. This solution is also used to prepare test solution (b). Dilute 2 ml of the solution to 10 ml with *methylene chloride R*.

Test solution (b). Transfer 2 ml of the solution obtained during the preparation of test solution (a) to a 15 ml glass tube with a ground-glass stopper or a polytetrafluoroethylene cap. Add 10 ml of a 0.8 g/l solution of *sodium hydroxide R* in *methanol R* and immediately pass a stream of *nitrogen R* through the solution for 5 min. Stopper the tube. Heat in a water-bath at 45 °C, protected from light, for 30 min. Allow to cool.

Reference solution (a). Dissolve 25 mg of *methylprednisolone hydrogen succinate CRS* in *methanol R* with gentle heating and dilute to 5 ml with the same solvent. This solution is also used to prepare reference solution (b). Dilute 2 ml of the solution to 10 ml with *methylene chloride R*.

Reference solution (b). Transfer 2 ml of the solution obtained during preparation of reference solution (a) to a 15 ml glass tube with a ground-glass stopper or a polytetrafluoroethylene cap. Add 10 ml of a 0.8 g/l solution of *sodium hydroxide R* in *methanol R* and immediately pass a stream of *nitrogen R* through the solution for 5 min. Stopper the tube. Heat in a water-bath at 45 °C, protected from light, for 30 min. Allow to cool.

Apply to the plate 5 µl of each solution. Prepare the mobile phase by adding a mixture of 1.2 volumes of *water R* and 8 volumes of *methanol R* to a mixture of 15 volumes of *ether R* and 77 volumes of *methylene chloride R*. Develop over a path of 15 cm. Allow the plate to dry in air and examine in ultraviolet light at 254 nm. The principal spot in each of the chromatograms obtained with the test solutions is similar in position and size to the principal spot in the chromatogram obtained with the corresponding reference solution.

Spray the plate with *alcoholic solution of sulphuric acid R*. Heat at 120 °C for 10 min or until the spots appear. Allow to cool. Examine in daylight and in ultraviolet light at 365 nm. The principal spot in each of the chromatograms obtained with the test solutions is similar in position, colour in daylight, fluorescence in ultraviolet light at 365 nm and size to the principal spot in the chromatogram obtained with the corresponding reference solution. The principal spot in each of the chromatograms obtained with test solution (b) and reference solution (b) has an R_f value distinctly higher than that of the principal spot in each of the chromatograms obtained with test solution (a) and reference solution (a).

D. Add about 2 mg to 2 ml of *sulphuric acid R* and shake to dissolve. Within 5 min a reddish-brown colour develops. Add the solution to 10 ml of *water R* and mix. The colour fades and a precipitate is formed.

TESTS

Appearance of solution. Dissolve 0.100 g in 5 ml of *sodium hydrogen carbonate solution R*. The solution is clear (*2.2.1*).

Specific optical rotation (*2.2.7*). Dissolve 0.250 g in *dioxan R* and dilute to 25.0 ml with the same solvent. The specific optical rotation is + 87 to + 95, calculated with reference to the dried substance.

Related substances. Examine by liquid chromatography (*2.2.29*).

Test solution. Dissolve 25.0 mg of the substance to be examined in the mobile phase and dilute to 10.0 ml with the mobile phase.

Reference solution (a). Dissolve 25 mg of *methylprednisolone hydrogen succinate for performance test CRS* in the mobile phase and dilute to 10.0 ml with the mobile phase.

Reference solution (b). Dilute 1.0 ml of the test solution to 100.0 ml with the mobile phase.

The chromatographic procedure may be carried out using:

- a stainless steel column 0.25 m long and 4.0 mm in internal diameter packed with *octadecylsilyl silica gel for chromatography R* (5 µm),
- as mobile phase at a flow rate of 1 ml/min a mixture of 33 volumes of *acetonitrile R* and 67 volumes of a 3 per cent *V/V* solution of *glacial acetic acid R*,
- as detector a spectrophotometer set at 254 nm.

Equilibrate the column with the mobile phase at a flow rate of 1 ml/min for about 30 min.

Adjust the sensitivity of the system so that the height of the principal peak in the chromatogram obtained with 20 µl of reference solution (b) is at least 50 per cent of the full scale of the recorder.

Inject 20 µl of reference solution (a). When the chromatograms are recorded in the prescribed conditions, the retention times are: methylprednisolone hydrogen succinate about 22 min and methylhydrocortisone 21-(hydrogen succinate) (the impurity eluting immediately after the main peak and appearing as a shoulder) about 24 min. Measure the height (*A*) above the base-line of the peak due to methylhydrocortisone 21-(hydrogen succinate) and the height (*B*) above the base-line of the lowest point of the curve separating this peak from the peak due to methylprednisolone hydrogen succinate. The test is not valid unless *A* is greater than four times *B*. If necessary, adjust the concentration of acetonitrile in the mobile phase.

Inject separately 20 µl of the test solution and 20 µl of reference solution (b). Continue the chromatography for twice the retention time of the principal peak. In the chromatogram obtained with the test solution: the area of any peak, apart from the principal peak, is not greater than 0.5 times the area of the principal peak in the chromatogram obtained with reference solution (b) (0.5 per cent); the sum of the areas of all the peaks, apart from the principal peak, is not greater than the area of the principal peak in the chromatogram obtained with reference solution (b) (1 per cent). Disregard any peak due to the solvent and any peak with an area less than 0.05 times the area of the principal peak in the chromatogram obtained with reference solution (b).

Loss on drying (*2.2.32*). Not more than 1.0 per cent, determined on 1.000 g by drying in an oven at 100-105 °C.

Sulphated ash (*2.4.14*). Not more than 0.1 per cent, determined on 1.0 g.

ASSAY

Dissolve 50.0 mg in *alcohol R* and dilute to 100.0 ml with the same solvent. Dilute 2.0 ml of the solution to 50.0 ml with *alcohol R*. Measure the absorbance (*2.2.25*) at the maximum at 243 nm.

Calculate the content of $C_{26}H_{34}O_8$ taking the specific absorbance to be 316.

Monographs M

STORAGE

Store in an airtight container, protected from light.

IMPURITIES

A. methylprednisolone,

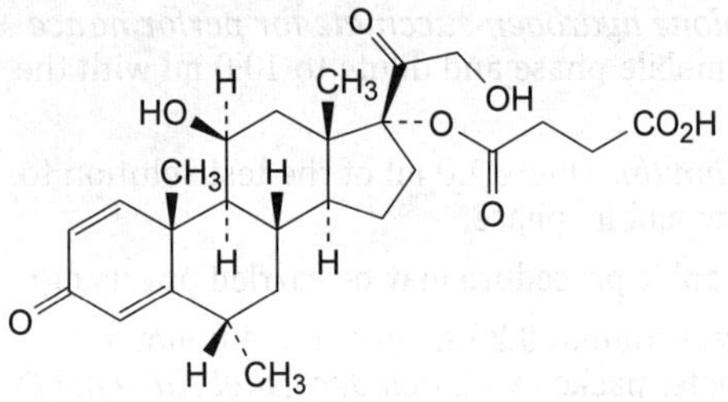

B. 4-[(11β,21-dihydroxy-6α-methyl-3,20-dioxopregna-1,4-dien-17-yl)oxy]-4-oxobutanoic acid (methylprednisolone 17-(hydrogen succinate)),

C. methylprednisolone acetate,

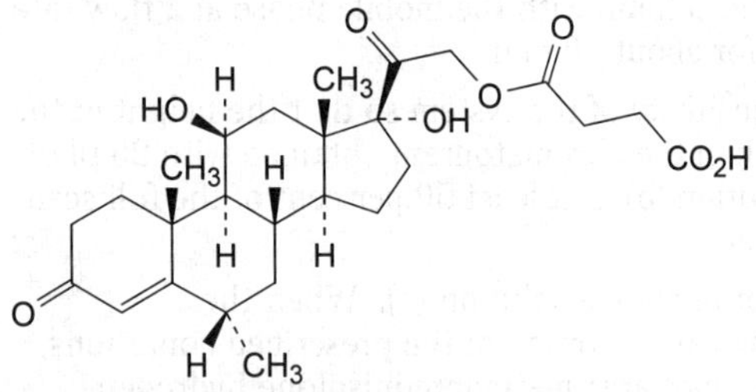

D. 4-[(11β,17-dihydroxy-6α-methyl-3,20-dioxopregn-4-en-21-yl)oxy]-4-oxobutanoic acid (methylhydrocortisone 21-(hydrogen succinate)).

Monographs M

01/2005:1675

N-METHYLPYRROLIDONE

N-Methylpyrrolidonum

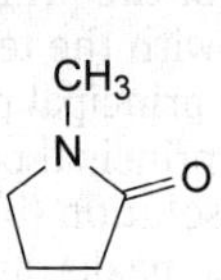

C_5H_9NO M_r 99.1

DEFINITION

1-Methylpyrrolidin-2-one.

CHARACTERS

Appearance: clear, colourless liquid.

Solubility: miscible with water and with alcohol.

bp: about 204 °C.

Relative density: about 1.034.

Refractive index: about 1.469.

IDENTIFICATION

Infrared absorption spectrophotometry (*2.2.24*).

Preparation: films.

Comparison: *Ph. Eur. reference spectrum of N-methylpyrrolidone.*

TESTS

Appearance. The substance to be examined is clear (*2.2.1*) and colourless (*2.2.2, Method II*).

Alkalinity. Dissolve 50 ml of the substance to be examined in 50 ml of *water R* previously adjusted with *0.02 M potassium hydroxide* or *0.02 M hydrochloric acid* until a yellow colour is obtained using 0.5 ml of *bromothymol blue solution R1* as indicator. Titrate with *0.02 M hydrochloric acid* to the initial coloration. Not more than 8.0 ml of *0.02 M hydrochloric acid* is required.

Related substances. Gas chromatography (*2.2.28*): use the normalisation procedure.

Test solution. The substance to be examined.

Reference solution. To 1 ml of the substance to be examined, add 1 ml of *2-pyrrolidone R* and dilute to 20 ml with *methylene chloride R*.

Column:

– *material*: fused silica,
– *size*: *l* = 30 m, Ø = 0.32 mm,
– *stationary phase*: *poly(dimethyl)siloxane R* (5 μm).

Carrier gas: *nitrogen for chromatography R*.

Linear velocity: 20 cm/s.

Split ratio: 1:100.

Temperature:

	Time (min)	Temperature (°C)
Column	0	100
	0 - 23.3	100 → 170
	23.3 - 53	170
Injection port		280
Detector		280

Detection: flame ionisation.

Injection: 1 μl.

System suitability: reference solution:

– *resolution*: minimum 2.0 between the peaks due to *N*-methylpyrrolidone and impurity G.

Limits:

– *any impurity*: maximum 0.1 per cent,
– *total*: maximum 0.3 per cent,
– *disregard limit*: 0.02 per cent.

Heavy metals (*2.4.8*): maximum 10 ppm.

Dissolve 4.0 g in *water R* and dilute to 20.0 ml with the same solvent. 12 ml of the solution complies with limit test A. Prepare the standard using *lead standard solution (2 ppm Pb) R*.

Water (*2.5.32*): maximum 0.1 per cent, determined on 1.000 g.

STORAGE

Protected from light.

IMPURITIES

A. $H_3C\text{-}NH_2$: methanamine (methylamine),

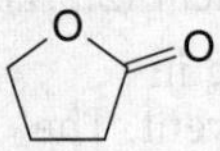

B. dihydrofuran-2(3*H*)-one (γ-butyrolactone),

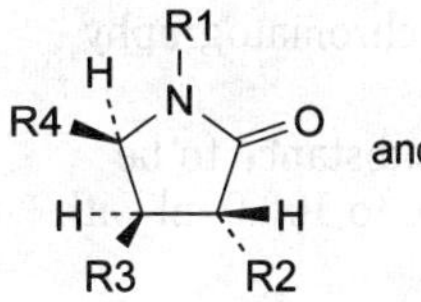

C. R1 = R2 = CH_3, R3 = R4 = H: (3*RS*)-1,3-dimethylpyrrolidin-2-one,

D. R1 = R3 = CH_3, R2 = R4 = H: (4*RS*)-1,4-dimethylpyrrolidin-2-one,

E. R1 = R4 = CH_3, R2 = R3 = H: (5*RS*)-1,5-dimethylpyrrolidin-2-one,

G. R1 = R2 = R3 = R4 = H: pyrrolidin-2-one (2-pyrrolidone),

F. HO-$[CH_2]_4$-OH: butane-1,4-diol,

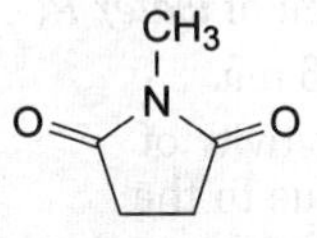

H. 1-methylpyrrolidine-2,5-dione (*N*-methylsuccinimide),

I. propylene glycol.

01/2005:0410

METHYLTESTOSTERONE

Methyltestosteronum

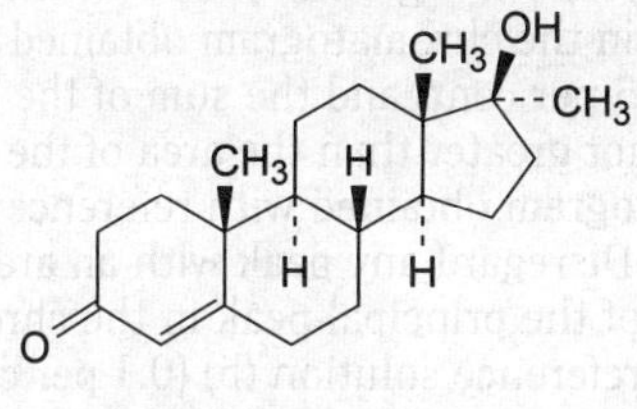

$C_{20}H_{30}O_2$ M_r 302.5

DEFINITION

Methyltestosterone contains not less than 97.0 per cent and not more than the equivalent of 103.0 per cent of 17β-hydroxy-17α-methylandrost-4-en-3-one, calculated with reference to the dried substance.

CHARACTERS

A white or slightly yellowish-white, crystalline powder, practically insoluble in water, freely soluble in alcohol.

IDENTIFICATION

First identification: B.

Second identification: A, C.

A. Melting point (*2.2.14*): 162 °C to 168 °C.

B. Examine by infrared absorption spectrophotometry (*2.2.24*), comparing with the spectrum obtained with *methyltestosterone CRS.*

C. After examination of the chromatograms obtained in the test for related substances, spray the plate with a saturated solution of *potassium dichromate R* in a mixture of 30 volumes of *water R* and 70 volumes of *sulphuric acid R* and examine immediately in daylight. The principal spot in the chromatogram obtained with the test solution is similar in position, colour and size to the principal spot in the chromatogram obtained with reference solution (a).

TESTS

Specific optical rotation (*2.2.7*). Dissolve 0.250 g in *alcohol R* and dilute to 25.0 ml with the same solvent. The specific optical rotation is + 79 to + 85, calculated with reference to the dried substance.

Related substances. Examine by thin-layer chromatography (*2.2.27*), using as the coating substance a suitable silica gel containing a fluorescent indicator having an optimal intensity at 254 nm.

Test solution. Dissolve 0.2 g of the substance to be examined in a mixture of 1 volume of *methanol R* and 9 volumes of *chloroform R* and dilute to 10 ml with the same mixture of solvents.

Reference solution (a). Dissolve 20 mg of *methyltestosterone CRS* in 1 ml of a mixture of 1 volume of *methanol R* and 9 volumes of *chloroform R.*

Reference solution (b). Dilute 1 ml of the test solution to 100 ml with a mixture of 1 volume of *methanol R* and 9 volumes of *chloroform R.*

Reference solution (c). Dilute 5 ml of reference solution (b) to 10 ml with a mixture of 1 volume of *methanol R* and 9 volumes of *chloroform R.*

Reference solution (d). Dissolve 10 mg of *testosterone CRS* in 0.5 ml of reference solution (a) and dilute to 10 ml with a mixture of 1 volume of *methanol R* and 9 volumes of *chloroform R.*

Apply separately to the plate 5 µl of each solution. Develop over a path of 15 cm using a mixture of 1 volume of *anhydrous acetic acid R*, 30 volumes of *light petroleum R* and 70 volumes of *butyl acetate R.* Allow the plate to dry in air and examine in ultraviolet light at 254 nm. Any spot in the chromatogram obtained with the test solution, apart from the principal spot, is not more intense than the spot in the chromatogram obtained with reference solution (b) (1.0 per cent) and at most one such spot is more intense than the spot in the chromatogram obtained with reference solution (c) (0.5 per cent). The test is not valid unless the chromatogram obtained with reference solution (d) shows two clearly separated spots.

Loss on drying (*2.2.32*). Not more than 2.0 per cent, determined on 0.50 g by drying in an oven at 100 °C to 105 °C for 2 h.

ASSAY

Dissolve 50.0 mg in *alcohol R* and dilute to 50.0 ml with the same solvent. Dilute 10.0 ml of the solution to 100.0 ml with *alcohol R.* Dilute 10.0 ml of this solution to 100.0 ml with *alcohol R.* Measure the absorbance (*2.2.25*) at the maximum at 241 nm.

Calculate the content of $C_{20}H_{30}O_2$ taking the specific absorbance to be 540.

STORAGE

Store protected from light.

01/2005:1132
corrected

METHYLTHIONINIUM CHLORIDE

Methylthioninii chloridum

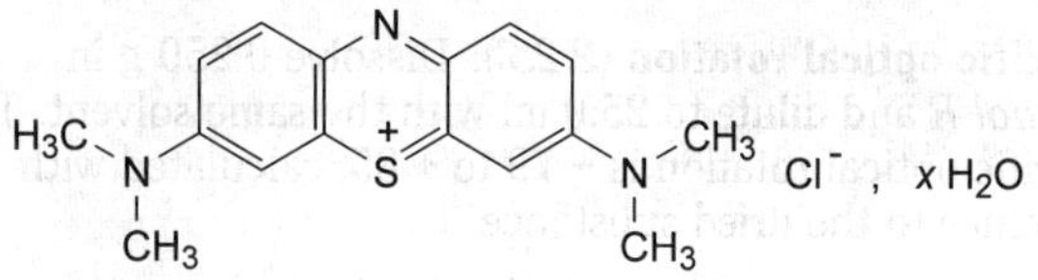

$C_{16}H_{18}ClN_3S,xH_2O$ M_r 319.9 (anhydrous substance)

DEFINITION

Methylthioninium chloride (methylene blue) contains not less than 95.0 per cent and not more than the equivalent of 101.0 per cent of 3,7-bis(dimethylamino)phenothiazin-5-ylium chloride, calculated with reference to the dried substance.

CHARACTERS

A dark blue, crystalline powder with a copper-coloured sheen, or green crystals with a bronze-coloured sheen, soluble in water, slightly soluble in alcohol.

IDENTIFICATION

A. Dissolve 10 mg in *dilute hydrochloric acid R* and dilute to 100 ml with the same acid. Dilute 5 ml of the solution to 100 ml with *dilute hydrochloric acid R*. Examined between 240 nm and 800 nm (*2.2.25*), the solution shows four absorption maxima, at 255 nm to 260 nm, 285 nm to 290 nm, 675 nm to 685 nm and 740 nm to 750 nm.

B. Examine by thin-layer chromatography (*2.2.27*), using a *TLC silica gel plate R*.

Test solution. Dissolve 10 mg of the substance to be examined in *methanol R* and dilute to 10 ml with the same solvent. Dilute 1 ml to 10 ml with *methanol R*.

Reference solution. Dissolve 10 mg of *methylthioninium chloride CRS* in *methanol R* and dilute to 10 ml with the same solvent. Dilute 1 ml to 10 ml with *methanol R*.

Apply to the plate 2 µl of each solution. Develop over a path of 8 cm using a mixture of 20 volumes of *anhydrous formic acid R* and 80 volumes of *propanol R*. Allow the plate to dry in air protected from light. Examine in daylight. The principal spot in the chromatogram obtained with the test solution is similar in position and size to the principal spot in the chromatogram obtained with the reference solution. A secondary spot may appear above the principal spot in both chromatograms.

C. Dissolve about 1 mg in 10 ml of *water R*. Add 1 ml of *glacial acetic acid R* and 0.1 g of *zinc powder R*. Heat to boiling. The solution becomes colourless. Filter and shake the filtrate. It becomes blue in contact with air.

D. Ignite 50 mg with 0.5 g of *anhydrous sodium carbonate R*. Cool and dissolve the residue in 10 ml of *dilute nitric acid R*. Filter. The filtrate, without further addition of *dilute nitric acid R*, gives reaction (a) of chlorides(*2.3.1*).

TESTS

Methanol-insoluble substances. To 1.0 g add 20 ml of *methanol R* and boil under a reflux condenser for 5 min. Filter through a tared sintered-glass filter (40) and wash the filter with *methanol R* until a colourless filtrate is obtained. Dry the filter at 100 °C and weigh. The residue weighs not more than 10.0 mg (1.0 per cent).

Related substances. Examine by liquid chromatography (*2.2.29*).

Test solution. Dissolve 15.0 mg of the substance to be examined in the mobile phase and dilute to 100.0 ml with the mobile phase.

Reference solution (a). Dissolve 15.0 mg of *methylthioninium impurity A CRS* in the mobile phase and dilute to 100.0 ml with the mobile phase. To 1.0 ml of this solution, add 1.0 ml of the test solution and dilute to 10.0 ml with the mobile phase.

Reference solution (b). Dilute 1.0 ml of the test solution to 100.0 ml with the mobile phase.

The chromatographic procedure may be carried out using:

– a stainless steel column 0.25 m long and 4 mm in internal diameter packed with *octadecylsilyl silica gel for chromatography R* (7 µm),

– as mobile phase at a flow rate of 1 ml/min a mixture of 27 volumes of *acetonitrile R* and 73 volumes of a mixture of 3.4 ml of *phosphoric acid R* and 1000 ml of *water R*,

– as detector a spectrophotometer set at 246 nm.

Inject 20 µl of each solution. Adjust the sensitivity of the detector so that the height of the peak due to the substance to be examined (retention time about 11 min) in the chromatogram obtained with reference solution (a) is at least 80 per cent of the full scale of the recorder. The test is not valid unless in the chromatogram obtained with reference solution (a), the resolution between the peaks due to impurity A and methylthioninium is at least 1.5. If necessary, adjust the concentration of acetonitrile in the mobile phase. Continue the chromatography of the test solution for twice the retention time of the principal peak. In the chromatogram obtained with the test solution the area of any peak corresponding to impurity A is not greater than five times the area of the principal peak in the chromatogram obtained with reference solution (b) (5.0 per cent); the area of any peak, apart from the principal peak and the peak due to impurity A, is not greater than half the area of the principal peak in the chromatogram obtained with reference solution (b) (0.5 per cent) and the sum of the areas of any such peaks is not greater than the area of the principal peak in the chromatogram obtained with reference solution (b) (1.0 per cent). Disregard any peak with an area less than 0.1 times that of the principal peak in the chromatogram obtained with reference solution (b) (0.1 per cent).

Metals. Examine by atomic emission spectrometry (*2.2.22*) in argon plasma, using as detector a conventional optical system or a mass spectrometer; in the case of a mass spectrometer, use indium as internal standard.

Test solution. In a 10 ml volumetric flask, dissolve with stirring 100 mg in 9 ml of *water R*, add 100.0 µl of a 10 µg/ml solution of indium prepared from indium *elementary standard solution for atomic spectrometry (1.000 g/l) R* in *nitric acid R* which has been diluted fifty-fold with *water R*. Dilute to 10.0 ml with *water R*.

Reference solutions. Into a 100 ml volumetric flask, introduce 10.0 ml of a standard solution containing 1.00 µg/ml of each of the metals to be determined and prepared by dilution, with *water R*, of each *elementary standard solution for atomic spectrometry (1.000 g/l) R* for the corresponding elements. Add 1.00 ml of a 10 µg/ml solution of indium prepared from indium *elementary standard solution for atomic spectrometry (1.000 g/l) R* in *nitric acid R* which has been diluted fifty-fold with *water R*. Dilute to 100.0 ml with *water R*.

Blank solution. Dilute one hundred-fold with *water R* the 10 µg/ml solution of indium used for the test and reference solutions.

Monographs M

Element	Optical detection			Mass detection
	Signal (nm)	Background 1 (nm)	Background 2 (nm)	Isotope
Aluminium	396.15	396.05	396.25	27
Cadmium	214.44	214.37	214.51	114
Chromium	283.56	283.49	283.64	*
Copper	327.40	327.31	327.48	65
Tin	190.00**	189.90	190.10	118
Iron	238.20	238.27	238.14	*
Manganese	260.57	260.50	260.64	55
Mercury	253.70***	253.60	253.80	200
Molybdenum	202.03	202.02	202.04	95
Nickel	231.60	231.54	231.66	60
Lead	217.00**	216.90	217.10	208
Zinc	213.86	213.80	213.91	66
Indium				115

*Element difficult, if not impossible, to be determined with a mass spectrometer as detector.

**Borderline sensitivity with conventional optical spectrometry.

***Mercury is often impossible to determine using conventional optical spectrometry;it may be quantified using a device for the determination of hydrides.

Element	Maximum content in ppm
Aluminium	100
Cadmium	1
Chromium	10
Copper	100
Tin	10
Iron	100
Manganese	10
Mercury	1
Molybdenum	10
Nickel	10
Lead	10
Zinc	100

Loss on drying (*2.2.32*): 8.0 per cent to 22.0 per cent, determined on 1.000 g by drying in an oven at 100-105 °C.

Sulphated ash (*2.4.14*). Not more than 0.25 per cent, determined on 1.0 g.

ASSAY

Dissolve 0.300 g in 30 ml of *water R* with heating. Cool, add 50.0 ml of *potassium dichromate solution R1* and dilute to 100.0 ml with *water R*. Allow to stand for 10 min. Filter and discard the first 20 ml of filtrate. Introduce 50.0 ml of the filtrate into a flask with a ground-glass neck, add 50 ml of *dilute sulphuric acid R* and 8.0 ml of *potassium iodide solution R*. Allow to stand protected from light for 5 min, then add 80 ml of *water R*. Titrate with *0.1 M sodium thiosulphate* using 2 ml of *starch solution R*, added towards the end of the titration, as indicator. Carry out a blank titration.

1 ml of *0.1 M sodium thiosulphate* is equivalent to 10.66 mg of $C_{16}H_{18}ClN_3S$.

STORAGE

Store in an airtight container, protected from light.

IMPURITIES

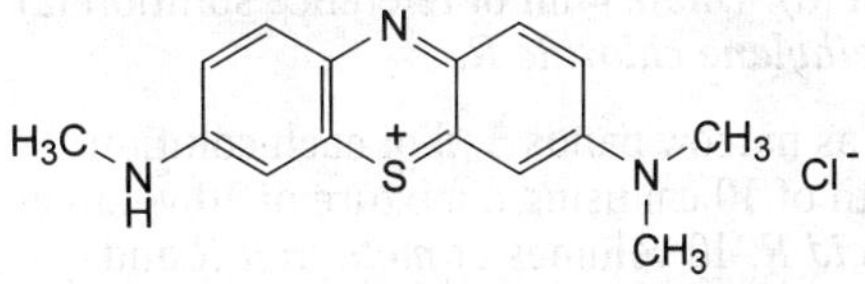

A. 3-(dimethylamino)-7-(methylamino)phenothiazin-5-ylium chloride.

01/2005:1347

METIXENE HYDROCHLORIDE

Metixeni hydrochloridum

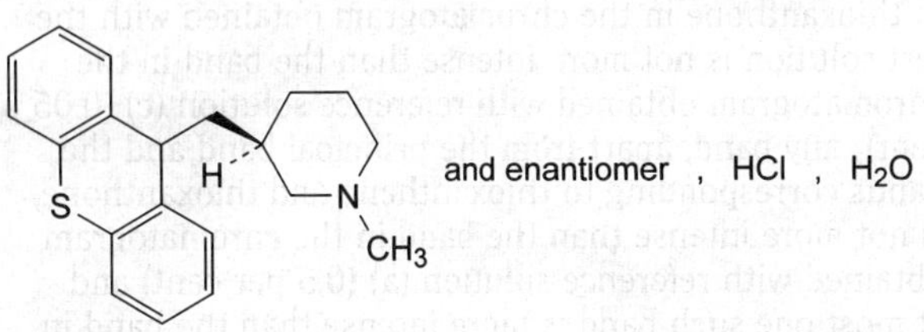

$C_{20}H_{24}ClNS,H_2O$ M_r 363.9

DEFINITION

Metixene hydrochloride contains not less than 98.0 per cent and not more than the equivalent of 102.0 per cent of (*RS*)-1-methyl-3-[(9*H*-thioxanthen-9-yl)methyl]piperidine hydrochloride, calculated with reference to the dried substance.

CHARACTERS

A white or almost white, crystalline or fine crystalline powder, soluble in water, soluble in alcohol and in methylene chloride.

IDENTIFICATION

A. Examine by infrared absorption spectrophotometry (*2.2.24*), comparing with the spectrum obtained with *metixene hydrochloride CRS*.

B. It gives reaction (a) of chlorides (*2.3.1*).

TESTS

Appearance of solution. Dissolve 0.40 g in *methanol R* and dilute to 20.0 ml with the same solvent. The solution is clear (*2.2.1*) and not more intensely coloured than reference solution Y_6 (*2.2.2, Method I*).

pH (*2.2.3*). Dissolve 0.18 g in *carbon dioxide-free water R* heating if necessary at about 50 °C, cool and dilute to 10.0 ml with the same solvent. The pH of the solution, measured immediately, is 4.4 to 5.8.

Related substances. Examine by thin-layer chromatography (*2.2.27*), using a *TLC silica gel plate R*. *Carry out the test rapidly and protected from light.*

Test solution. Dissolve 50 mg of the substance to be examined in *methylene chloride R* and dilute to 5.0 ml with the same solvent.

Reference solution (a). Dissolve 5 mg of *metixene hydrochloride CRS* in *methylene chloride R* and dilute to 100.0 ml with the same solvent.

Reference solution (b). Dissolve 20 mg of *thioxanthene CRS* in 50 ml of *methylene chloride R*. Dilute 1.0 ml of the solution to 20.0 ml with *methylene chloride R*.

Reference solution (c). Dissolve 5 mg of *thioxanthone CRS* in 50 ml of *methylene chloride R*. Dilute 1.0 ml of the solution to 20.0 ml with *methylene chloride R*.

Reference solution (d). Dilute 4 ml of reference solution (a) to 10.0 ml with *methylene chloride R*.

Apply to the plate as narrow bands 5 µl of each solution. Develop over a path of 10 cm using a mixture of 10 volumes of *glacial acetic acid R*, 10 volumes of *methanol R* and 80 volumes of *methylene chloride R*. Dry the plate in a stream of cold air. Spray with a mixture of 1 volume of *sulphuric acid R* and 9 volumes of *alcohol R* and heat at 100 °C for 10 min. Allow the plate to cool and examine in ultraviolet light at 365 nm. Thioxanthene shows orange fluorescence and thioxanthone shows greenish-blue fluorescence. Any band corresponding to thioxanthene in the chromatogram obtained with the test solution is not more intense than the band in the chromatogram obtained with reference solution (b) (0.2 per cent); any band corresponding to thioxanthone in the chromatogram obtained with the test solution is not more intense than the band in the chromatogram obtained with reference solution (c) (0.05 per cent); any band, apart from the principal band and the bands corresponding to thioxanthene and thioxanthone, is not more intense than the band in the chromatogram obtained with reference solution (a) (0.5 per cent) and at most one such band is more intense than the band in the chromatogram obtained with reference solution (d) (0.2 per cent). The test is not valid unless the bands in the chromatograms obtained with reference solutions (b) and (c) are clearly visible and differentiated.

Loss on drying (*2.2.32*). Not less than 4.0 per cent and not more than 6.0 per cent, determined on 0.500 g by drying in an oven at 138-142 °C.

Sulphated ash (*2.4.14*). Not more than 0.1 per cent, determined on 1.0 g.

ASSAY

Dissolve 0.250 g in a mixture of 5.0 ml of *0.01 M hydrochloric acid* and 50 ml of *alcohol R*. Carry out a potentiometric titration (*2.2.20*), using *0.1 M sodium hydroxide*. Read the volume added between the 2 points of inflexion.

1 ml of *0.1 M sodium hydroxide* is equivalent to 34.59 mg of $C_{20}H_{24}ClNS$.

STORAGE

Store protected from light.

IMPURITIES

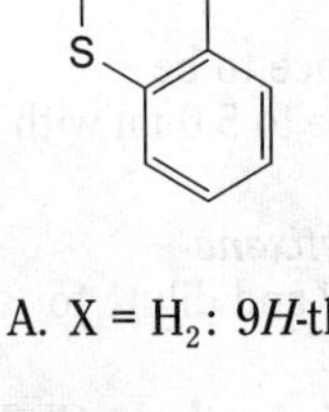

A. X = H_2: 9*H*-thioxanthene,

B. X = O: 9*H*-thioxanthen-9-one (thioxanthone).

01/2005:1348

METOCLOPRAMIDE

Metoclopramidum

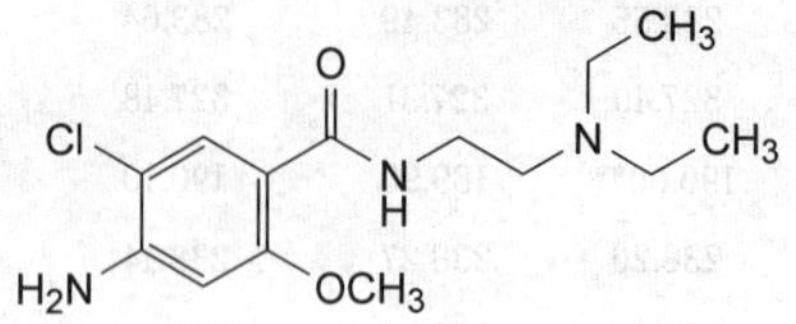

$C_{14}H_{22}ClN_3O_2$ M_r 299.8

DEFINITION

Metoclopramide contains not less than 99.0 per cent and not more than the equivalent of 101.0 per cent of 4-amino-5-chloro-*N*-[2-(diethylamino)ethyl]-2-methoxybenzamide, calculated with reference to the dried substance.

CHARACTERS

A white or almost white, fine powder, practically insoluble in water, sparingly soluble in methylene chloride, sparingly soluble to slightly soluble in alcohol.

It shows polymorphism.

IDENTIFICATION

First identification: A, B.

Second identification: A, C.

A. Melting point (*2.2.14*): 145 °C to 149 °C.

B. Examine by infrared absorption spectrophotometry (*2.2.24*), comparing with the spectrum obtained with *metoclopramide CRS*. Examine the substances prepared as discs.

C. Examine the chromatograms obtained in test A for related substances (see Tests) in ultraviolet light at 254 nm before spraying with *dimethylaminobenzaldehyde solution R1*. The principal spot in the chromatogram obtained with test solution (a) is similar in position and size to the principal spot in the chromatogram obtained with reference solution (a).

TESTS

Appearance of solution. Dissolve 2.5 g in 25 ml of *1 M hydrochloric acid*. The freshly prepared solution is clear (*2.2.1*) and not more intensely coloured than reference solution Y_6 (*2.2.2, Method II*).

Related substances

A. Examine by thin-layer chromatography (*2.2.27*), using a *TLC silica gel F_{254} plate R*.

Test solution (a). Dissolve 40 mg of the substance to be examined in *methanol R* and dilute to 10 ml with the same solvent.

Test solution (b). Dissolve 0.160 g of the substance to be examined in *methanol R* and dilute to 10 ml with the same solvent.

Reference solution (a). Dissolve 20 mg of *metoclopramide CRS* and 10 mg of *sulpiride CRS* in *methanol R* and dilute to 5 ml with the same solvent.

Reference solution (b). Dissolve 20 mg of *N,N-diethylethane-1,2-diamine R* in *methanol R* and dilute to 50 ml with the same solvent. Dilute 2 ml of the solution to 25 ml with *methanol R*.

Apply to the plate 10 µl of each solution. Develop over a path of 12 cm using a mixture of 2 volumes of *concentrated ammonia R*, 10 volumes of *dioxan R*,

14 volumes of *methanol R* and 90 volumes of *methylene chloride R*. Allow the plate to dry in air. Examine in ultraviolet light at 254 nm (identification C). Spray with *dimethylaminobenzaldehyde solution R1*. Allow the plate to dry in air. Any spot corresponding to impurity E (not visualised in ultraviolet light at 254 nm)in the chromatogram obtained with test solution (b) is not more intense than the spot in the chromatogram obtained with reference solution (b) (0.2 per cent). The test is not valid unless the chromatogram obtained with reference solution (a) shows two clearly separated spots.

B. Examine by liquid chromatography (*2.2.29*).

Test solution. Dissolve 10.0 mg of the substance to be examined in the mobile phase and dilute to 10.0 ml with the mobile phase.

Reference solution (a). Dilute 0.2 ml of the test solution to 100.0 ml with the mobile phase.

Reference solution (b). Dissolve 10.0 mg of *metoclopramide impurity A CRS* in the mobile phase and dilute to 100.0 ml with the mobile phase. Mix 1.0 ml of this solution with 0.1 ml of the test solution and dilute to 10.0 ml with the mobile phase.

The chromatographic procedure may be carried out using:

– a stainless steel column 0.25 m long and 4.6 mm in internal diameter packed with *octylsilyl silica gel for chromatography R* (5 µm),

– as mobile phase at a flow rate of 1.5 ml/min a mixture prepared as follows: dissolve 6.8 g of *potassium dihydrogen phosphate R* in 700 ml of *water R*; add 0.2 ml of *N,N-dimethyloctylamine R* and adjust to pH 4.0 with *dilute phosphoric acid R*; dilute to 1000 ml with *water R*, add 250 ml of *acetonitrile R* and mix,

– as detector a spectrophotometer set at 240 nm.

Inject 10 µl of each solution. Adjust the sensitivity of the system so that the heights of the principal peaks in the chromatogram obtained with reference solution (b) are at least 50 per cent of the full scale of the recorder. The test is not valid unless, in the chromatogram obtained with reference solution (b), the resolution between the two principal peaks is at least 2.0. Continue the chromatography of the test solution for eight times the retention time of metoclopramide. In the chromatogram obtained with the test solution: the area of any peak, apart from the principal peak, is not greater than the area of the principal peak in the chromatogram obtained with reference solution (a) (0.2 per cent) and the sum of the areas of any such peaks is not greater than three times the area of the principal peak in the chromatogram obtained with reference solution (a) (0.6 per cent). Disregard any peak with an area less than 0.1 times that of the principal peak in the chromatogram obtained with reference solution (a).

Heavy metals (*2.4.8*). 1.0 g complies with limit test C for heavy metals (20 ppm). Prepare the standard using 2 ml of *lead standard solution (10 ppm Pb) R*.

Loss on drying (*2.2.32*). Not more than 1.0 per cent, determined on 1.000 g by drying in an oven at 100-105 °C.

Sulphated ash (*2.4.14*). Not more than 0.1 per cent, determined on 1.0 g.

ASSAY

Dissolve 0.250 g in 50 ml of *anhydrous acetic acid R* and add 5 ml of *acetic anhydride R*. Titrate with *0.1 M perchloric acid*, determining the end-point potentiometrically (*2.2.20*).

1 ml of *0.1 M perchloric acid* is equivalent to 29.98 mg of $C_{14}H_{22}ClN_3O_2$.

IMPURITIES

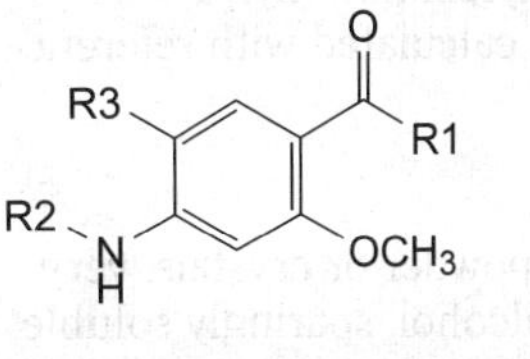

A. R1 = $NH\text{-}CH_2\text{-}CH_2\text{-}N(C_2H_5)_2$, R2 = $CO\text{-}CH_3$, R3 = Cl: 4-(acetylamino)-5-chloro-*N*-[2-(diethylamino)ethyl]-2-methoxybenzamide,

B. R1 = OCH_3, R2 = $CO\text{-}CH_3$, R3 = Cl: methyl 4-(acetylamino)-5-chloro-2-methoxybenzoate,

C. R1 = OH, R2 = H, R3 = Cl: 4-amino-5-chloro-2-methoxybenzoic acid,

D. R1 = OCH_3, R2 = $CO\text{-}CH_3$, R3 = H: methyl 4-(acetylamino)-2-methoxybenzoate,

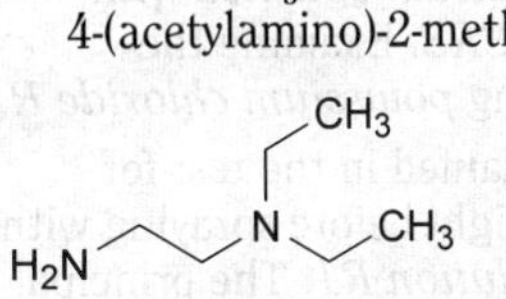

E. *N,N*-diethylethane-1,2-diamine,

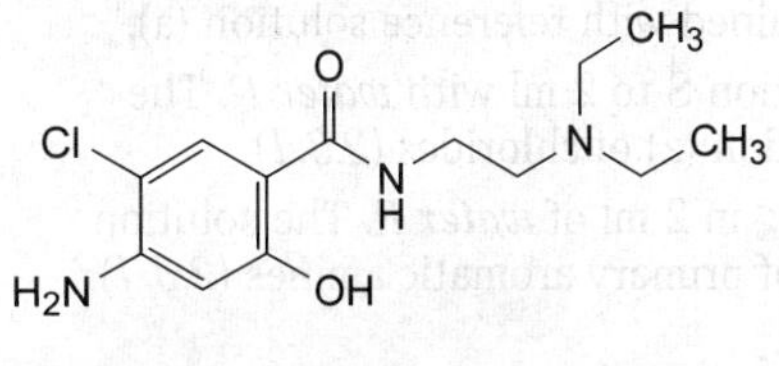

F. 4-amino-5-chloro-*N*-[2-(diethylamino)ethyl]-2-hydroxybenzamide,

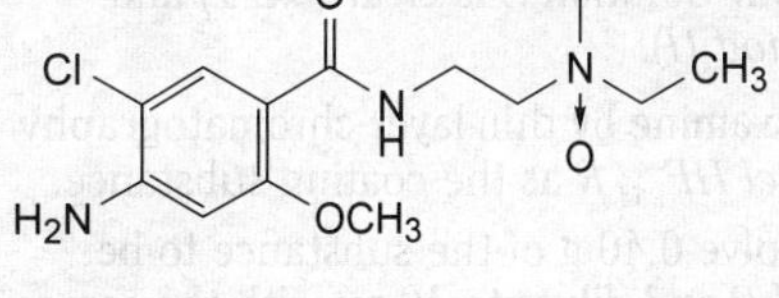

G. *N'*-(4-amino-5-chloro-2-methoxybenzoyl)-*N,N*-diethylethane-1,2-diamine *N*-oxide,

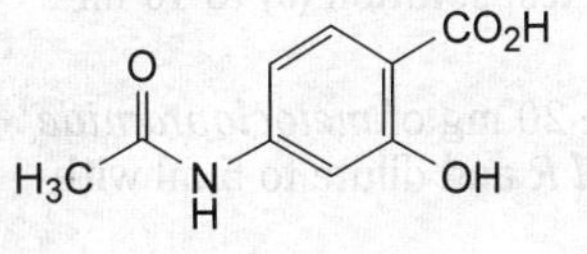

H. 4-(acetylamino)-2-hydroxybenzoic acid.

01/2005:0674

METOCLOPRAMIDE HYDROCHLORIDE

Metoclopramidi hydrochloridum

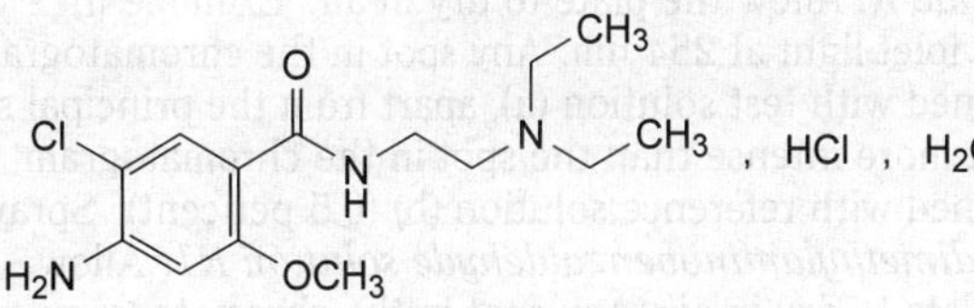

$C_{14}H_{23}Cl_2N_3O_2,H_2O$ M_r 354.3

DEFINITION

Metoclopramide hydrochloride contains not less than 99.0 per cent and not more than the equivalent of 101.0 per cent of 4-amino-5-chloro-*N*-[2-(diethylamino)ethyl]-2-methoxybenzamide hydrochloride, calculated with reference to the anhydrous substance.

CHARACTERS

White or almost white, crystalline powder or crystals, very soluble in water, freely soluble in alcohol, sparingly soluble in methylene chloride.

It melts at about 183 °C with decomposition.

IDENTIFICATION

First identification: A, B, D.

Second identification: A, C, D, E.

A. The pH (*2.2.3*) of solution S (see Tests) is 4.5 to 6.0.

B. Examine by infrared absorption spectrophotometry (*2.2.24*), comparing with the spectrum obtained with *metoclopramide hydrochloride CRS*. Examine the substances as discs prepared using *potassium chloride R*.

C. Examine the chromatograms obtained in the test for related substances in ultraviolet light before spraying with *dimethylaminobenzaldehyde solution R1*. The principal spot in the chromatogram obtained with test solution (b) is similar in position and size to the principal spot in the chromatogram obtained with reference solution (a).

D. Dilute 1 ml of solution S to 2 ml with *water R*. The solution gives reaction (a) of chlorides (*2.3.1*).

E. Dissolve about 2 mg in 2 ml of *water R*. The solution gives the reaction of primary aromatic amines (*2.3.1*).

TESTS

Solution S. Dissolve 2.5 g in *carbon dioxide-free water R* and dilute to 25 ml with the same solvent.

Appearance of solution. Solution S is clear (*2.2.1*) and colourless (*2.2.2, Method II*).

Related substances. Examine by thin-layer chromatography (*2.2.27*), using *silica gel HF_{254} R* as the coating substance.

Test solution (a). Dissolve 0.40 g of the substance to be examined in *methanol R* and dilute to 10 ml with the same solvent.

Test solution (b). Dilute 1 ml of test solution (a) to 10 ml with *methanol R*.

Reference solution (a). Dissolve 20 mg of *metoclopramide hydrochloride CRS* in *methanol R* and dilute to 5 ml with the same solvent.

Reference solution (b). Dilute 5 ml of test solution (a) to 100 ml with *methanol R*. Dilute 1 ml of this solution to 10 ml with *methanol R*.

Reference solution (c). Dissolve 10 mg of *N,N-diethylethylenediamine R* in *methanol R* and dilute to 50 ml with the same solvent.

Apply separately to the plate 5 µl of each solution. Develop over a path of 12 cm using a mixture of 2 volumes of *concentrated ammonia R*, 10 volumes of *dioxan R*, 14 volumes of *methanol R* and 90 volumes of *methylene chloride R*. Allow the plate to dry in air. Examine in ultraviolet light at 254 nm. Any spot in the chromatogram obtained with test solution (a), apart from the principal spot, is not more intense than the spot in the chromatogram obtained with reference solution (b) (0.5 per cent). Spray with *dimethylaminobenzaldehyde solution R1*. Allow the plate to dry in air. Any spot in the chromatogram obtained with test solution (a) that has not been visualised in ultraviolet light at 254 nm is not more intense than the spot in the chromatogram obtained with reference solution (c) (0.5 per cent).

Heavy metals (*2.4.8*). 12 ml of solution S complies with limit test A for heavy metals (20 ppm). Prepare the standard using *lead standard solution (2 ppm Pb) R*.

Water (*2.5.12*): 4.5 per cent to 5.5 per cent, determined on 0.500 g by the semi-micro determination of water.

Sulphated ash (*2.4.14*). Not more than 0.1 per cent, determined on 1.0 g.

ASSAY

Dissolve 0.2500 g in a mixture of 5.0 ml of *0.01 M hydrochloric acid* and 50 ml of *alcohol R*. Carry out a potentiometric titration (*2.2.20*), using *0.1 M sodium hydroxide*. Read the volume of *0.1 M sodium hydroxide* added between the two points of inflexion.

1 ml of *0.1 M sodium hydroxide* is equivalent to 33.63 mg of $C_{14}H_{23}Cl_2N_3O_2$.

STORAGE

Store protected from light.

01/2005:1448

METOPROLOL SUCCINATE

Metoprololi succinas

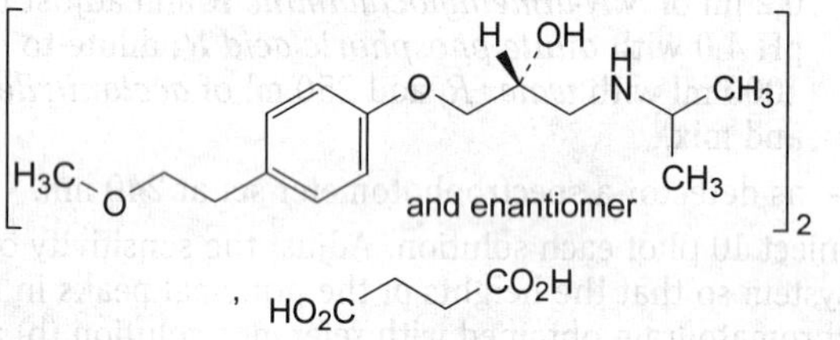

$C_{34}H_{56}N_2O_{10}$ M_r 653

DEFINITION

Bis[(2*RS*)-1-[4-(2-methoxyethyl)phenoxy]-3-[(1-methylethyl)amino]propan-2-ol] butanedioate.

Content: 99.0 per cent to 101.0 per cent (dried substance).

CHARACTERS

Appearance: white, crystalline powder.

Solubility: freely soluble in water, soluble in methanol, slightly soluble in alcohol, very slightly soluble in ethyl acetate.

IDENTIFICATION

Infrared absorption spectrophotometry (*2.2.24*).

Comparison: *Ph. Eur. reference spectrum of metoprolol succinate.*

TESTS

Solution S. Dissolve 0.500 g in *carbon dioxide-free water R* and dilute to 25.0 ml with the same solvent.

Appearance of solution. Solution S is not more opalescent than reference suspension II (*2.2.1*) and it is colourless (*2.2.2, Method II*).

pH (*2.2.3*): 7.0 to 7.6 for solution S.

Related substances

A. Thin-layer chromatography (*2.2.27*).

Test solution. Dissolve 0.50 g of the substance to be examined in *methanol R* and dilute to 10 ml with the same solvent.

Reference solution. Dilute 1 ml of the test solution to 50 ml with *methanol R*. Dilute 5 ml of this solution to 50 ml with *methanol R*.

Plate: *TLC silica gel plate R*.

Mobile phase: place 2 beakers each containing 30 volumes of *concentrated ammonia R* at the bottom of a chromatographic tank containing a mixture of 20 volumes of *methanol R* and 80 volumes of *ethyl acetate R*.

Application: 10 μl.

Development: over a path of 12 cm in a tank saturated for at least 1 h.

Drying: in air for at least 3 h.

Detection: expose the plate to iodine vapour for at least 15 h.

Limits:

- *any impurity*: any spot, apart from the principal spot, is not more intense than the spot in the chromatogram obtained with the reference solution (0.2 per cent),
- *disregard* any spot on the starting line.

B. Liquid chromatography (*2.2.29*).

Test solution. Dissolve 20.0 mg of the substance to be examined in the mobile phase and dilute to 10.0 ml with the mobile phase.

Reference solution (a). Dissolve 5.0 mg of the substance to be examined and 3.0 mg of *metoprolol impurity A CRS* in the mobile phase and dilute to 100.0 ml with the mobile phase.

Reference solution (b). Dilute 1.0 ml of the test solution to 100.0 ml with the mobile phase. Dilute 1.0 ml of the solution to 10.0 ml with the mobile phase.

Reference solution (c). *If this solution is required (see below), it is to be prepared in a fume cupboard. This solution is used only to identify the peak due to impurity C*. Dissolve 10 mg of the substance to be examined in 10 ml of *0.1 M hydrochloric acid*. Transfer this solution to an evaporating dish 10 cm in diameter. Place the dish so that the surface of the solution is 5 cm from a lamp emitting ultraviolet light (*2.1.3*) at 254 nm for 6 h. Dilute 0.5 ml of this solution to 25 ml with the mobile phase.

Column:

- *size*: *l* = 0.15 m, Ø = 3.9 mm,
- *stationary phase*: *octadecylsilyl silica gel for chromatography R1* (5 μm) with a pore size of 10 nm and a carbon loading of 19 per cent.

Mobile phase: dissolve 3.9 g of *ammonium acetate R* in 810 ml of *water R*, add 2.0 ml of *triethylamine R*, 10.0 ml of *glacial acetic acid R*, 3.0 ml of *phosphoric acid R* and 146 ml of *acetonitrile R* and mix.

Flow rate: 1 ml/min.

Detection: spectrophotometer at 280 nm.

Injection: 20 μl; inject the test solution and reference solutions (a) and (b).

Run time: 3 times the retention time of metoprolol.

Relative retention with reference to metoprolol (retention time = about 7 min): impurity C = about 0.3; impurity A = about 0.7.

System suitability: reference solution (a):

- *resolution*: minimum of 6.0 between the peaks due to impurity A and to metoprolol.

Limits:

- *any impurity*: not more than the area of the principal peak in the chromatogram obtained with reference solution (b) (0.1 per cent),
- *total*: not more than 5 times the area of the principal peak in the chromatogram obtained with reference solution (b) (0.5 per cent),
- *disregard limit*: 0.5 times the area of the principal peak in the chromatogram obtained with reference solution (b) (0.05 per cent); disregard any peak due to succinic acid.

If a peak occurs with a retention time of about 2.3 min (impurity C) which has an area greater than the area of the principal peak in the chromatogram obtained with reference solution (b), prepare and inject reference solution (c). For the chromatogram obtained with the test solution, multiply the peak area of impurity C by a correction factor of 0.1.

Heavy metals (*2.4.8*): maximum 10 ppm.

Dissolve 2.0 g in 20 ml of *water R*. 12 ml of the solution complies with limit test A. Prepare the standard using *lead standard solution (1 ppm Pb) R*.

Loss on drying (*2.2.32*): maximum 0.5 per cent, determined on 1.000 g by drying in an oven at 100-105 °C.

Sulphated ash (*2.4.14*): maximum 0.1 per cent, determined on 1.0 g.

ASSAY

Dissolve 0.250 g in 40 ml of *anhydrous acetic acid R*. Titrate with *0.1 M perchloric acid*, determining the end-point potentiometrically (*2.2.20*).

1 ml of *0.1 M perchloric acid* is equivalent to 32.64 mg of $C_{34}H_{56}N_2O_{10}$.

STORAGE

Protected from light.

IMPURITIES

By liquid chromatography: *A, B, C, D, E, F, G, H, J*.

By thin-layer chromatography: *M, N, O*.

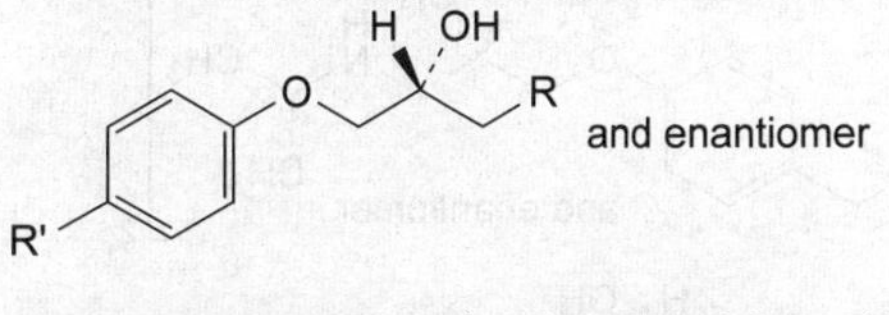

A. R = $NH-CH_2-CH_3$, R′ = $CH_2-CH_2-OCH_3$: (2*RS*)-1-(ethylamino)-3-[4-(2-methoxyethyl)phenoxy]propan-2-ol,

C. R = $NH-CH(CH_3)_2$, R′ = CHO: 4-[(2*RS*)-2-hydroxy-3-[(1-methylethyl)amino]propoxy]benzaldehyde,

D. R = OH, R′ = $CH_2-CH_2-OCH_3$: (2*RS*)-3-[4-(2-methoxyethyl)phenoxy]propane-1,2-diol,

H. R = $NH-CH(CH_3)_2$, R′ = CH_2-CH_2-OH: (2*RS*)-1-[4-(2-hydroxyethyl)phenoxy]-3-[(1-methylethyl)amino]propan-2-ol,

J. R = $O-CH_2-CHOH-CH_2-NH-CH(CH_3)_2$, R′ = $CH_2-CH_2-OCH_3$: 1-[2-hydroxy-3-[(1-methylethyl)amino]propoxy]-3-[4-(2-methoxyethyl)phenyl]propan-2-ol,

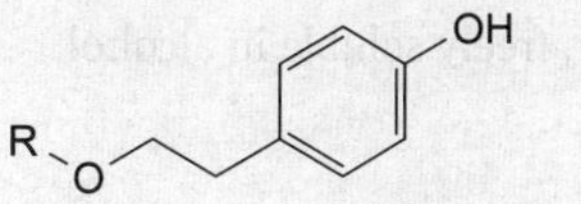

B. R = CH_3: 4-(2-methoxyethyl)phenol,

G. R = H: 2-(4-hydroxyphenyl)ethanol,

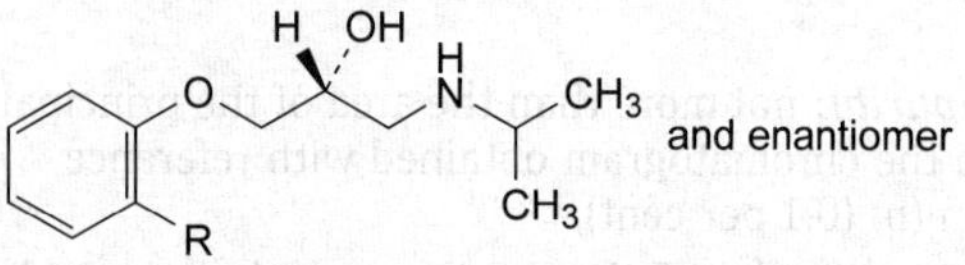

E. R = CH_2-CH_2-OCH_3: (2*RS*)-1-[2-(2-methoxyethyl)phenoxy]-3-[(1-methylethyl)amino]propan-2-ol,

F. R = H: (2*RS*)-1-[(1-methylethyl)amino]-3-phenoxypropan-2-ol,

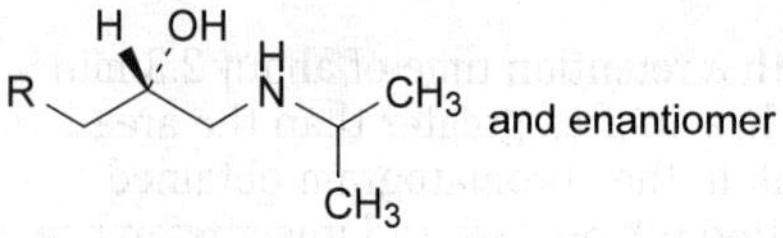

M. R = NH-CH(CH_3)$_2$: 1,3-bis[(1-methylethyl)amino]propan-2-ol,

N. R = OH: (2*RS*)-3-[(1-methylethyl)amino]propane-1,2-diol,

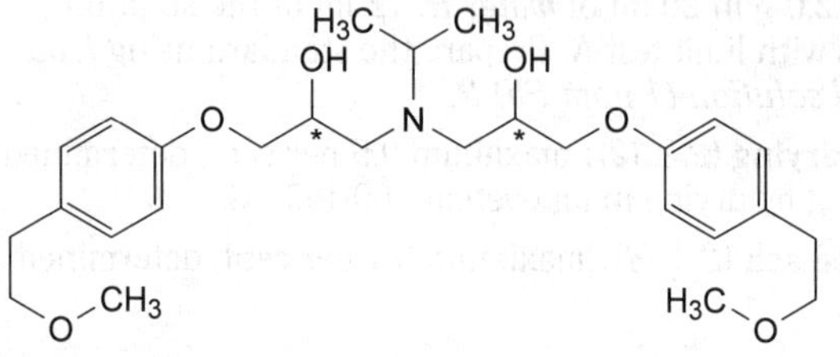

O. 1,1′-[(1-methylethyl)imino]bis[3-[4-(2-methoxyethyl)phenoxy]propan-2-ol].

01/2005:1028

METOPROLOL TARTRATE

Metoprololi tartras

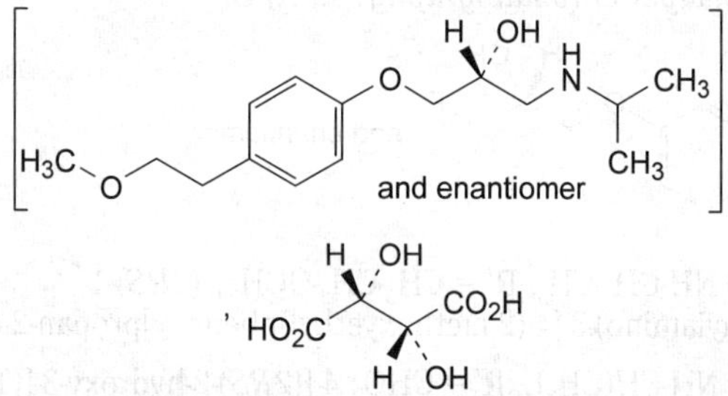

$C_{34}H_{56}N_2O_{12}$ M_r 685

DEFINITION

Bis[(2*RS*)-1-[4-(2-methoxyethyl)phenoxy]-3-[(1-methylethyl)amino]propan-2-ol] (2*R*,3*R*)-2,3-dihydroxybutanedioate.

Content: 99.0 per cent to 101.0 per cent (dried substance).

CHARACTERS

Appearance: white, crystalline powder or colourless crystals.

Solubility: very soluble in water, freely soluble in alcohol.

It shows polymorphism.

IDENTIFICATION

A. Specific optical rotation (see Tests).

B. Infrared absorption spectrophotometry (*2.2.24*).

Comparison: *metoprolol tartrate CRS.*

If the spectra obtained in the solid state show differences, record further spectra using discs prepared by placing 25 µl of a 100 g/l solution in *methylene chloride R* on a disc of *potassium bromide R* and evaporating the solvent. Examine immediately.

TESTS

Solution S. Dissolve 0.500 g in *carbon dioxide-free water R* and dilute to 25.0 ml with the same solvent.

Appearance of solution. Solution S is clear (*2.2.1*) and not more intensely coloured than reference solution B_8 (*2.2.2, Method II*).

pH (*2.2.3*): 6.0 to 7.0 for solution S.

Specific optical rotation (*2.2.7*): + 7.0 to + 10.0 (dried substance), determined on solution S.

Related substances

A. Thin-layer chromatography (*2.2.27*).

Test solution. Dissolve 0.50 g of the substance to be examined in *methanol R* and dilute to 10 ml with the same solvent.

Reference solution (a). Dilute 1 ml of the test solution to 20 ml with *methanol R*. Dilute 5 ml of this solution to 50 ml with *methanol R*.

Reference solution (b). Dilute 4 ml of reference solution (a) to 10 ml with *methanol R*.

Plate: *TLC silica gel plate R.*

Mobile phase: place 2 beakers each containing 30 volumes of *concentrated ammonia R* at the bottom of a chromatographic tank containing a mixture of 20 volumes of *methanol R* and 80 volumes of *ethyl acetate R*.

Application: 5 µl.

Development: over a path of 12 cm in a tank saturated for at least 1 h.

Drying: in air for at least 3 h.

Detection: expose the plate to iodine vapour for at least 15 h.

Limits:

– *any impurity*: any spot, apart from the principal spot, is not more intense than the spot in the chromatogram obtained with reference solution (a) (0.5 per cent) and at most 1 such spot is more intense than the spot in the chromatogram obtained with reference solution (b) (0.2 per cent),

– *disregard* any spot on the starting-line.

B. Liquid chromatography (*2.2.29*).

Test solution. Dissolve 20.0 mg of the substance to be examined in the mobile phase and dilute to 10.0 ml with the mobile phase.

Reference solution (a). Dissolve 5.0 mg of *metoprolol tartrate CRS* and 3.0 mg of *metoprolol impurity A CRS* in the mobile phase and dilute to 100.0 ml with the mobile phase.

Reference solution (b). Dilute 1.0 ml of the test solution to 20.0 ml with the mobile phase. Dilute 3.0 ml of the solution to 50.0 ml with the mobile phase.

Reference solution (c). If this solution is required (see below), it is to be prepared in a fume cupboard. This solution is used only to identify the peak due to impurity C. Dissolve 10 mg of *metoprolol tartrate CRS* in 10 ml of *0.1 M hydrochloric acid.* Transfer this solution to an evaporating dish 10 cm in diameter. Place the dish so that the surface of the solution is 5 cm from a lamp emitting ultraviolet light (*2.1.3*) at 254 nm for 6 h. Dilute 0.5 ml of this solution to 25 ml with the mobile phase.

Column:
- *size*: *l* = 0.15 m, Ø = 3.9 mm,
- *stationary phase*: *octadecylsilyl silica gel for chromatography R1* (5 µm) with a pore size of 10 nm and a carbon loading of 19 per cent.

Mobile phase: dissolve 3.9 g of *ammonium acetate R* in 810 ml of *water R*, add 2.0 ml of *triethylamine R*, 10.0 ml of *glacial acetic acid R*, 3.0 ml of *phosphoric acid R* and 146 ml of *acetonitrile R* and mix.

Flow rate: 1 ml/min.

Detection: spectrophotometer at 280 nm.

Injection: 20 µl; inject the test solution and reference solutions (a) and (b).

Run time: 3 times the retention time of metoprolol.

Relative retention with reference to metoprolol (retention time = about 7 min): impurity C = about 0.3; impurity A = about 0.7.

System suitability: reference solution (a):
- *resolution*: minimum of 6.0 between the peaks due to impurity A and to metoprolol.

Limits:
- *any impurity (A to J)*: not more than the area of the principal peak in the chromatogram obtained with reference solution (b) (0.3 per cent),
- *total*: not more than 1.7 times the area of the principal peak in the chromatogram obtained with reference solution (b) (0.5 per cent),
- *disregard limit*: 0.17 times the area of the principal peak in the chromatogram obtained with reference solution (b) (0.05 per cent); disregard any peak due to tartaric acid.

If a peak occurs with a retention time of about 2.3 min (impurity C) which has an area greater than the area of the principal peak in the chromatogram obtained with reference solution (b), prepare and inject reference solution (c). For the chromatogram obtained with the test solution, multiply the peak area of impurity C by a correction factor of 0.1.

Heavy metals (*2.4.8*): maximum 10 ppm.

Dissolve 2.0 g in 20 ml of *water R*. 12 ml of the solution complies with limit test A. Prepare the standard using *lead standard solution (1 ppm Pb) R*.

Loss on drying (*2.2.32*): maximum 0.5 per cent, determined on 1.000 g by drying *in vacuo* over *anhydrous calcium chloride R* for 4 h.

Sulphated ash (*2.4.14*): maximum 0.1 per cent, determined on 1.0 g.

ASSAY

Dissolve 0.250 g in 30 ml of *anhydrous acetic acid R*. Titrate with *0.1 M perchloric acid*, determining the end-point potentiometrically (*2.2.20*).

1 ml of *0.1 M perchloric acid* is equivalent to 34.24 mg of $C_{34}H_{56}N_2O_{12}$.

STORAGE

Protected from light.

IMPURITIES

By liquid chromatography: A, B, C, D, E, F, G, H, J.

By thin-layer chromatography: M, N, O.

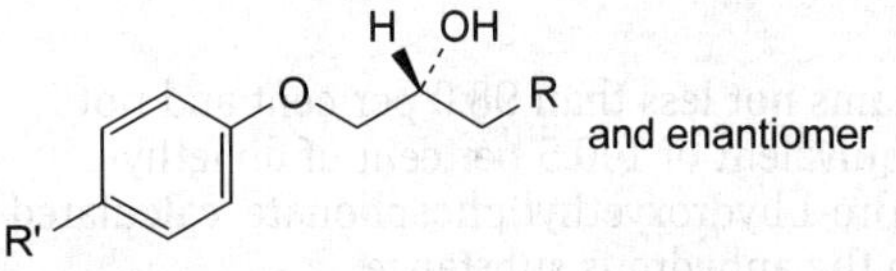

A. R = NH-CH_2-CH_3, R′ = CH_2-CH_2-OCH_3: (2*RS*)-1-(ethylamino)-3-[4-(2-methoxyethyl)phenoxy]propan-2-ol,

C. R = NH-CH(CH_3)$_2$, R′ = CHO: 4-[(2*RS*)-2-hydroxy-3-[(1-methylethyl)amino]propoxy]benzaldehyde,

D. R = OH, R′ = CH_2-CH_2-OCH_3: (2*RS*)-3-[4-(2-methoxyethyl)phenoxy]propane-1,2-diol,

H. R = NH-CH(CH_3)$_2$, R′ = CH_2-CH_2-OH: (2*RS*)-1-[4-(2-hydroxyethyl)phenoxy]-3-[(1-methylethyl)amino]propan-2-ol,

J. R = O-CH_2-CHOH-CH_2-NH-CH(CH_3)$_2$, R′ = CH_2-CH_2-OCH_3: 1-[2-hydroxy-3-[(1-methylethyl)amino]propoxy]-3-[4-(2-methoxyethyl)phenoxy]propan-2-ol,

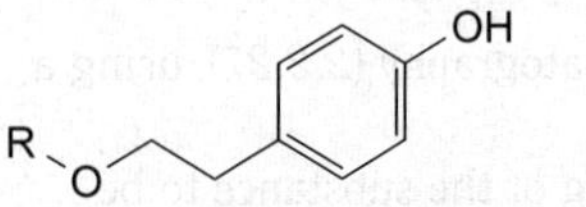

B. R = CH_3: 4-(2-methoxyethyl)phenol,

G. R = H: 2-(4-hydroxyphenyl)ethanol,

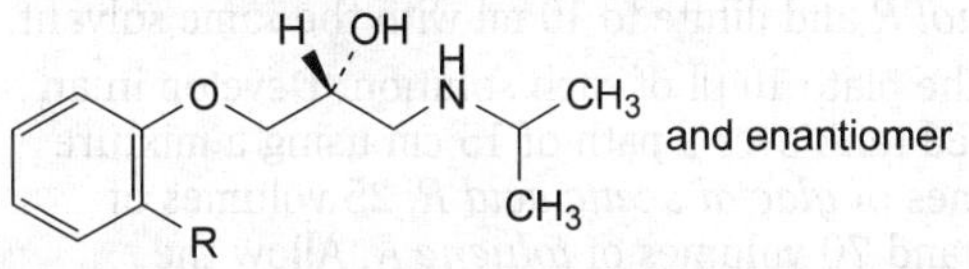

E. R = CH_2-CH_2-OCH_3: (2*RS*)-1-[2-(2-methoxyethyl)phenoxy]-3-[(1-methylethyl)amino]propan-2-ol,

F. R = H: (2*RS*)-1-[(1-methylethyl)amino]-3-phenoxypropan-2-ol,

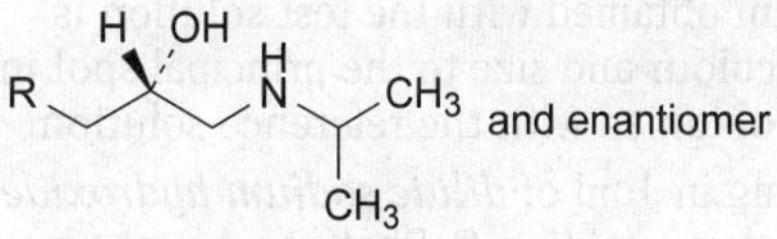

M. R = NH-CH(CH_3)$_2$: 1,3-bis[(1-methylethyl)amino]propan-2-ol,

N. R = OH: (2*RS*)-3-[(1-methylethyl)amino]propane-1,2-diol,

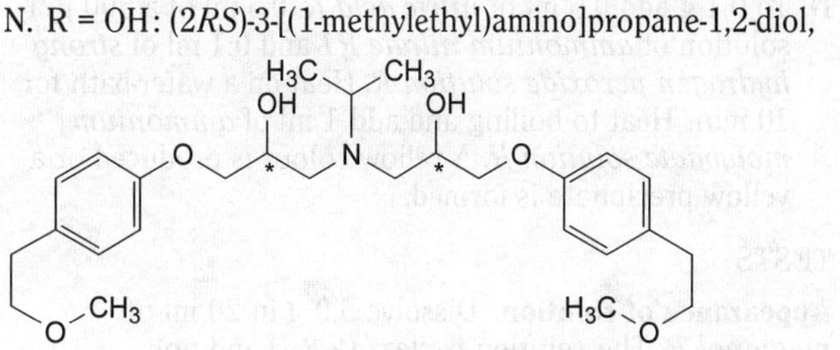

O. 1,1′-[(1-methylethyl)imino]bis[3-[4-(2-methoxyethyl)phenoxy]propan-2-ol].

01/2005:1133

METRIFONATE

Metrifonatum

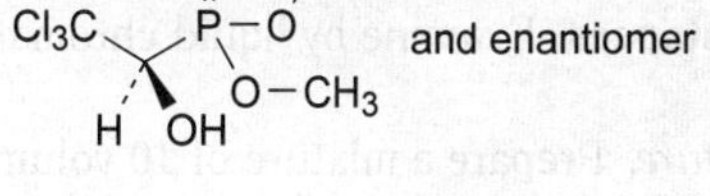

$C_4H_8Cl_3O_4P$ M_r 257.4

DEFINITION

Metrifonate contains not less than 98.0 per cent and not more than the equivalent of 100.5 per cent of dimethyl (*RS*)-(2,2,2-trichloro-1-hydroxyethyl)phosphonate, calculated with reference to the anhydrous substance.

CHARACTERS

A white, crystalline powder, freely soluble in water, very soluble in methylene chloride, freely soluble in acetone and in alcohol.

It melts between 76 °C and 81 °C.

IDENTIFICATION

First identification: A, B.

Second identification: B, C, D.

A. Examine by infrared absorption spectrophotometry (*2.2.24*), comparing with the spectrum obtained with *metrifonate CRS*. Examine the substances prepared as discs.

B. Examine by thin-layer chromatography (*2.2.27*), using a *TLC silica gel plate R*.

Test solution. Dissolve 10 mg of the substance to be examined in *methanol R* and dilute to 10 ml with the same solvent.

Reference solution. Dissolve 10 mg of *metrifonate CRS* in *methanol R* and dilute to 10 ml with the same solvent.

Apply to the plate 10 µl of each solution. Develop in an unsaturated tank over a path of 15 cm using a mixture of 5 volumes of *glacial acetic acid R*, 25 volumes of *dioxan R* and 70 volumes of *toluene R*. Allow the plate to dry in air. Spray with a 50 g/l solution of *4-(4-nitrobenzyl)pyridine R* in *acetone R* and heat at 120 °C for 15 min. Before the plate cools, spray with a 100 g/l solution of *tetraethylene pentamine R* in *acetone R*. Examine immediately. The principal spot in the chromatogram obtained with the test solution is similar in position, colour and size to the principal spot in the chromatogram obtained with the reference solution.

C. Dissolve about 20 mg in 1 ml of *dilute sodium hydroxide solution R*. Add 1 ml of *pyridine R*. Shake and heat on a water-bath for 2 min. A red colour develops in the upper layer.

D. To 0.1 g add 0.5 ml of *nitric acid R*, 0.5 ml of a 500 g/l solution of *ammonium nitrate R1* and 0.1 ml of *strong hydrogen peroxide solution R*. Heat on a water-bath for 10 min. Heat to boiling and add 1 ml of *ammonium molybdate solution R*. A yellow colour is produced or a yellow precipitate is formed.

TESTS

Appearance of solution. Dissolve 5.0 g in 20 ml of *methanol R*. The solution is clear (*2.2.1*) and not more intensely coloured than reference solution Y_7 (*2.2.2, Method II*).

Acidity. Dissolve 2.5 g in *carbon dioxide-free water R* and dilute to 50 ml with the same solvent. Add 0.1 ml of *methyl red solution R*. Not more than 1.0 ml of *0.1 M sodium hydroxide* is required to change the colour of the indicator to yellow.

Optical rotation (*2.2.7*). Dissolve 0.1 g in *alcohol R* and dilute to 10.0 ml with the same solvent. The angle of optical rotation is − 0.10° to + 0.10°.

Related substances. Examine by liquid chromatography (*2.2.29*).

Solvent mixture. Prepare a mixture of 10 volumes of mobile phase B and 90 volumes of mobile phase A.

Test solution. Dissolve 0.20 g of the substance to be examined in the solvent mixture and dilute to 10.0 ml with the solvent mixture.

Reference solution (a). Use a freshly prepared solution. Dissolve 10.0 mg of *desmethylmetrifonate CRS* in the solvent mixture and dilute to 20.0 ml with the solvent mixture. Dilute 1.0 ml of this solution to 5.0 ml with the solvent mixture.

Reference solution (b). Dissolve 0.10 g of *dichlorvos R* in the solvent mixture and dilute to 50.0 ml with the solvent mixture. Dilute 1.0 ml of this solution to 50.0 ml with the solvent mixture.

Reference solution (c). Dilute 1.0 ml of the test solution to 10.0 ml with the solvent mixture. Dilute 5.0 ml of this solution to 100.0 ml with the solvent mixture.

Reference solution (d). Use a freshly prepared solution. Mix 1.0 ml of reference solution (a), 1.0 ml of reference solution (b) and 0.025 ml of the test solution.

Reference solution (e). Dilute 4.0 ml of the test solution to 100.0 ml with the solvent mixture. Dilute 1.0 ml of this solution to 10.0 ml with the solvent mixture.

The chromatographic procedure may be carried out using:

– a stainless steel column 0.25 m long and 4.6 mm in internal diameter packed with a suitable octadecylsilyl silica gel for chromatography (10 µm),

– as mobile phase at a flow rate of 1 ml/min:

Mobile phase A. A 1.36 g/l solution of *potassium dihydrogen phosphate R*, previously adjusted to pH 2.9 with *phosphoric acid R*,

Mobile phase B. Acetonitrile R,

Time (min)	Mobile phase A (per cent *V/V*)	Mobile phase B (per cent *V/V*)
0 - 5	90	10
5 - 25	90 → 85	10 → 15
25 - end	85 → 45	15 → 55

– as detector a spectrophotometer set at 210 nm,

equilibrating the column for 5 min with the same mixture of mobile phases used for the first 5 min and maintaining the temperature of the column at 40 °C.

When the chromatograms are recorded in the prescribed conditions the peaks elute in the following order: desmethylmetrifonate, metrifonate and dichlorvos. Inject 10 µl of reference solution (e). Adjust the sensitivity of the system so that the height of the principal peak in the chromatogram obtained is 50 per cent to 70 per cent of the full scale of the recorder. Inject 50 µl of reference solution (d). The test is not valid unless the resolution between the peaks corresponding to desmethylmetrifonate and metrifonate is at least 3.0 and the resolution between the peaks corresponding to metrifonate and dichlorvos is at least 4.5.

Inject 50 µl of the test solution and 50 µl each of reference solutions (a), (b) and (c). Continue the chromatography of the test solution for three times the retention time of metrifonate. In the chromatogram obtained with the test solution: the area of any peak corresponding to desmethylmetrifonate is not greater than the area of the principal peak in the chromatogram obtained with reference solution (a) (0.5 per cent); the area of any peak corresponding to dichlorvos is not greater than the area of the principal peak in the chromatogram obtained with reference solution (b) (0.2 per cent); the area of any other peak, apart from the principal peak and the peaks corresponding to desmethylmetrifonate and dichlorvos respectively, is not greater than the area of the principal peak in the chromatogram obtained with reference solution (c) (0.5 per cent) and the sum of the areas of all these peaks is not greater than twice the area of the principal peak in the chromatogram obtained with reference solution (c) (1 per cent). Disregard any peak with an area less than 0.1 times the area of the principal peak in the chromatogram obtained with reference solution (e).

Chlorides. Not more than 500 ppm. Dissolve 5.00 g in 30 ml of *alcohol R* and add a mixture of 15 ml of *nitric acid R* and 100 ml of *water R*. Using a silver electrode, titrate with *0.01 M silver nitrate*, determining the end-point potentiometrically (*2.2.20*).

1 ml of *0.01 M silver nitrate* is equivalent to 0.3546 mg of Cl.

Heavy metals (*2.4.8*). Dissolve 2.0 g in 20 ml of *water R*. 12 ml of the solution complies with limit test A for heavy metals (10 ppm). Prepare the standard using *lead standard solution (1 ppm Pb) R*.

Water (*2.5.12*). Not more than 0.3 per cent, determined on 3.000 g by the semi-micro determination of water.

ASSAY

Dissolve 0.300 g in 30 ml of *alcohol R*. Add 10 ml of *ethanolamine R* and allow to stand for 1 h at 20-22 °C. Add a chilled mixture of 15 ml of *nitric acid R* and 100 ml of *water R* maintaining the temperature of the mixture at 20-22 °C. Maintain at that temperature and titrate with *0.1 M silver nitrate*, using a silver electrode and determining the end-point potentiometrically (*2.2.20*).

Calculate the percentage content of $C_4H_8Cl_3O_4P$, taking into account the content of chloride and using the following expression:

$$\left[\frac{V_P}{M_P} - \frac{V_{Cl} \times 0.1}{M_{Cl}}\right] \times 25.74 \times 0.1$$

V_P = volume of silver nitrate used in the assay, in millilitres,

M_P = mass of substance used in the assay, in grams,

V_{Cl} = volume of silver nitrate used in the test for chlorides in millilitres,

M_{Cl} = mass of substance used in the test for chlorides, in grams.

STORAGE

Store protected from light.

IMPURITIES

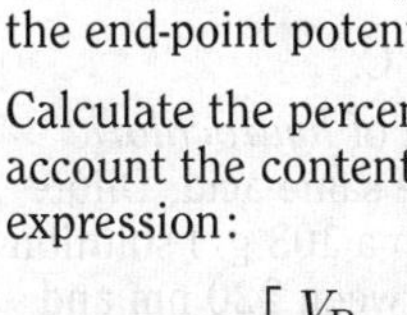

and enantiomer

A. methyl (*RS*)-(2,2,2-trichloro-1-hydroxyethyl)phosphonate acid (desmethylmetrifonate),

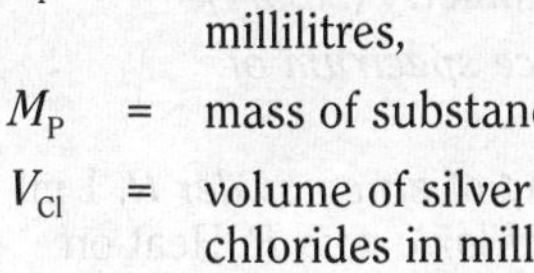

B. 2,2-dichloroethenyl dimethyl phosphate (dichlorvos).

01/2005:0675

METRONIDAZOLE

Metronidazolum

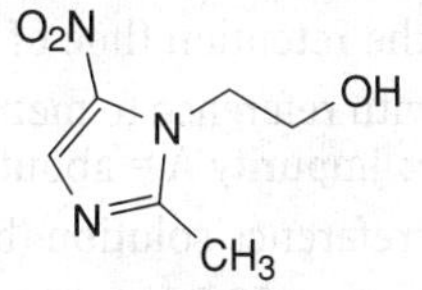

$C_6H_9N_3O_3$ M_r 171.2

DEFINITION

2-(2-Methyl-5-nitro-1*H*-imidazol-1-yl)ethanol.

Content: 99.0 per cent to 101.0 per cent (dried substance).

CHARACTERS

Appearance: white or yellowish, crystalline powder.

Solubility: slightly soluble in water, in acetone, in alcohol and in methylene chloride.

IDENTIFICATION

First identification: C.

Second identification: A, B, D.

A. Melting point (*2.2.14*): 159 °C to 163 °C.

B. Dissolve 40.0 mg in *0.1 M hydrochloric acid* and dilute to 100.0 ml with the same acid. Dilute 5.0 ml of the solution to 100.0 ml with *0.1 M hydrochloric acid*. Examined between 230 nm and 350 nm (*2.2.25*), the solution shows an absorption maximum at 277 nm and a minimum at 240 nm. The specific absorbance at the maximum is 365 to 395.

C. Infrared absorption spectrophotometry (*2.2.24*).

   Preparation: discs.

   Comparison: *metronidazole CRS*.

D. To about 10 mg add about 10 mg of *zinc powder R*, 1 ml of *water R* and 0.25 ml of *dilute hydrochloric acid R*. Heat on a water-bath for 5 min. Cool. The solution gives the reaction of primary aromatic amines (*2.3.1*).

TESTS

Appearance of solution. The solution is not more opalescent than reference suspension II (*2.2.1*) and not more intensely coloured than reference solution GY_6 (*2.2.2, Method II*).

Dissolve 1.0 g in *1 M hydrochloric acid* and dilute to 20 ml with the same acid.

Related substances. Liquid chromatography (*2.2.29*). *Prepare the solutions protected from light.*

Test solution. Dissolve 0.05 g of the substance to be examined in the mobile phase and dilute to 100.0 ml with the mobile phase.

Reference solution (a). Dilute 1.0 ml of the test solution to 100.0 ml with the mobile phase and dilute 1.0 ml of this solution to 10.0 ml with the mobile phase.

Reference solution (b). Dissolve 5.0 mg of *metronidazole impurity A CRS* in the mobile phase, add 10.0 ml of the test solution and dilute to 100.0 ml with the mobile phase. Dilute 1.0 ml to 100.0 ml with the mobile phase.

Column:

– *size*: *l* = 0.25 m, Ø = 4.6 mm,

– *stationary phase*: *octadecylsilyl silica gel for chromatography R* (5 µm).

Mobile phase: mix 30 volumes of *methanol R* and 70 volumes of a 1.36 g/l solution of *potassium dihydrogen phosphate R*,

Flow rate: 1 ml/min.

Detection: spectrophotometer at 315 nm.

Injection: 10 µl.

Run time: 3 times the retention time of metronidazole.

Relative retention with reference to metronidazole (retention time = about 7 min): impurity A = about 0.7.

System suitability: reference solution (b):

- *resolution*: minimum of 2.0 between the peaks due to metronidazole and to impurity A.

Limits:

- *any impurity*: not more than the area of the principal peak in the chromatogram obtained with reference solution (a) (0.1 per cent),
- *total*: not more than twice the area of the principal peak in the chromatogram obtained with reference solution (a) (0.2 per cent),
- *disregard limit*: 0.1 times the area of the principal peak in the chromatogram obtained with reference solution (a) (0.01 per cent).

Heavy metals (*2.4.8*): maximum 20 ppm.

1.0 g complies with limit test C. Prepare the standard using 2 ml of *lead standard solution (10 ppm Pb) R*.

Loss on drying (*2.2.32*): maximum 0.5 per cent, determined on 1.000 g by drying in an oven at 100-105 °C for 3 h.

Sulphated ash (*2.4.14*): maximum 0.1 per cent, determined on 1.0 g.

ASSAY

Dissolve 0.150 g in 50 ml of *anhydrous acetic acid R*. Titrate with *0.1 M perchloric acid*, determining the end-point potentiometrically (*2.2.20*).

1 ml of *0.1 M perchloric acid* is equivalent to 17.12 mg of $C_6H_9N_3O_3$.

STORAGE

Protected from light.

IMPURITIES

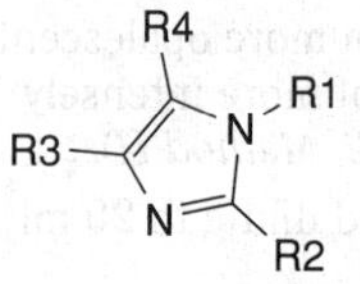

A. R1 = R4 = H, R2 = CH_3, R3 = NO_2: 2-methyl-4-nitroimidazole,

B. R1 = R2 = R4 = H, R3 = NO_2: 4-nitroimidazole,

C. R1 = CH_2-CH_2-OH, R2 = R4 = H, R3 = NO_2: 2-(4-nitro-1*H*-imidazol-1-yl)ethanol,

D. R1 = CH_2-CH_2-OH, R2 = R3 = H, R4 = NO_2: 2-(5-nitro-1*H*-imidazol-1-yl)ethanol,

E. R1 = CH_2-CH_2-OH, R2 = CH_3, R3 = NO_2, R4 = H: 2-(2-methyl-4-nitro-1*H*-imidazol-1-yl)ethanol,

F. R1 = CH_2-CH_2-O-CH_2-CH_2-OH, R2 = CH_3, R3 = H, R4 = NO_2: 2-[2-(2-methyl-5-nitro-1*H*-imidazol-1-yl)ethoxy]ethanol,

G. R1 = CH_2-CO_2H, R2 = CH_3, R3 = H, R4 = NO_2: 2-(2-methyl-5-nitro-1*H*-imidazol-1-yl)acetic acid.

01/2005:0934

METRONIDAZOLE BENZOATE

Metronidazoli benzoas

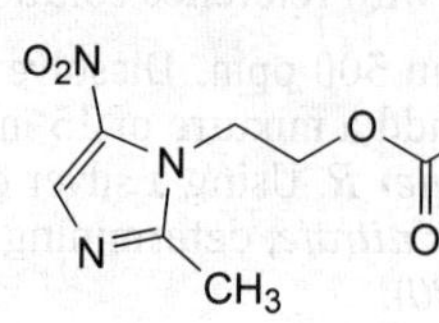

$C_{13}H_{13}N_3O_4$ M_r 275.3

DEFINITION

2-(2-Methyl-5-nitro-1*H*-imidazol-1-yl)ethyl benzoate.

Content: 98.5 per cent to 101.0 per cent (dried substance).

CHARACTERS

Appearance: white or slightly yellowish, crystalline powder or flakes.

Solubility: practically insoluble in water, freely soluble in methylene chloride, soluble in acetone, slightly soluble in alcohol.

IDENTIFICATION

First identification: C.

Second identification: A, B, D.

A. Melting point (*2.2.14*): 99 °C to 102 °C.

B. Dissolve 0.100 g in a 103 g/l solution of *hydrochloric acid R* and dilute to 100.0 ml with the same acid. Dilute 1.0 ml of the solution to 100.0 ml with a 103 g/l solution of *hydrochloric acid R*. Examined between 220 nm and 350 nm (*2.2.25*), the solution shows 2 absorption maxima, at 232 nm and 275 nm. The specific absorbance at the absorption maximum at 232 nm is 525 to 575.

C. Infrared absorption spectrophotometry (*2.2.24*).

Comparison: *Ph. Eur. reference spectrum of metronidazole benzoate*.

D. To about 10 mg add about 10 mg of *zinc powder R*, 1 ml of *water R* and 0.3 ml of *hydrochloric acid R*. Heat on a water-bath for 5 min and cool. The solution gives the reaction of primary aromatic amines (*2.3.1*).

TESTS

Appearance of solution. The solution is not more opalescent than reference suspension II (*2.2.1*) and not more intensely coloured than reference solution GY_3 (*2.2.2, Method II*).

Dissolve 1.0 g in *dimethylformamide R* and dilute to 10 ml with the same solvent.

Acidity. Dissolve 2.0 g in a mixture of 20 ml of *dimethylformamide R* and 20 ml of *water R*, previously neutralised with *0.02 M hydrochloric acid* or *0.02 M sodium hydroxide* using 0.2 ml of *methyl red solution R*. Not more than 0.25 ml of *0.02 M sodium hydroxide* is required to change the colour of the indicator.

Related substances. Liquid chromatography (*2.2.29*).

Solvent mixture. Mix 45 volumes of mobile phase B and 55 volumes of mobile phase A.

Test solution. Dissolve 0.100 g of the substance to be examined in the solvent mixture and dilute to 10.0 ml with the solvent mixture.

Reference solution (a). Dilute 1.0 ml of the test solution to 100.0 ml with the solvent mixture. Dilute 1.0 ml of the solution to 10.0 ml with the solvent mixture.

Reference solution (b). Dissolve 5.0 mg of *metronidazole CRS*, 5.0 mg of *2-methyl-5-nitroimidazole R* and 5.0 mg of *benzoic acid R* in the solvent mixture and dilute to 50.0 ml with the solvent mixture. Dilute 1.0 ml of the solution to 10.0 ml with the solvent mixture.

Column:

- *size*: *l* = 0.25 m, Ø = 4.6 mm,
- *stationary phase*: spherical *di-isobutyloctadecylsilyl silica gel for chromatography R* (5 µm) with a specific surface area of 180 m²/g, a pore size of 8 nm and a carbon loading of 10 per cent.

Mobile phase:

- *mobile phase A*: 1.5 g/l solution of *potassium dihydrogen phosphate R* adjusted to pH 3.2 with *phosphoric acid R*,
- *mobile phase B*: *acetonitrile R*,

Time (min)	Mobile phase A (per cent *V/V*)	Mobile phase B (per cent *V/V*)
0 - 5	80	20
5 - 15	80 → 55	20 → 45
15 - 40	55	45
40 - 41	55 → 80	45 → 20
41 - 45	80	20

Flow rate: 1 ml/min.

Detection: spectrophotometer at 235 nm.

Injection: 10 µl.

Relative retention with reference to metronidazole benzoate (retention time = about 20 min): impurity B = about 0.17; impurity A = about 0.20; impurity C = about 0.7.

System suitability: reference solution (b):

- *resolution*: minimum 2.0 between the peaks due to impurity A and impurity B.

Limits:

- *impurities A, B, C*: for each impurity, not more than the area of the corresponding peak in the chromatogram obtained with reference solution (b) (0.1 per cent),
- *any other impurity*: for each impurity, not more than the area of the principal peak in the chromatogram obtained with reference solution (a) (0.1 per cent),
- *total*: not more than twice the area of the principal peak in the chromatogram obtained with reference solution (a) (0.2 per cent),
- *disregard limit*: 0.1 times the area of the principal peak in the chromatogram obtained with reference solution (a) (0.01 per cent).

Heavy metals (*2.4.8*): maximum 20 ppm.

1.0 g complies with limit test C. Prepare the standard using 2 ml of *lead standard solution (10 ppm Pb) R*.

Loss on drying (*2.2.32*): maximum 0.5 per cent, determined on 1.000 g by drying in an oven at 80 °C for 3 h.

Sulphated ash (*2.4.14*): maximum 0.1 per cent, determined on 1.0 g.

ASSAY

Dissolve 0.250 g in 50 ml of *anhydrous acetic acid R*. Titrate with *0.1 M perchloric acid*, determining the end-point potentiometrically (*2.2.20*).

1 ml of *0.1 M perchloric acid* is equivalent to 27.53 mg of $C_{13}H_{13}N_3O_4$.

STORAGE

Protected from light.

IMPURITIES

Specified impurities: *A, B, C*.

A. metronidazole,

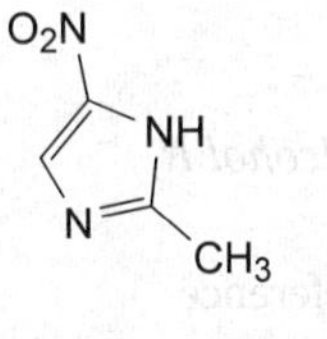

B. 2-methyl-5-nitroimidazole,

C. benzoic acid.

01/2005:1029

MEXILETINE HYDROCHLORIDE

Mexiletini hydrochloridum

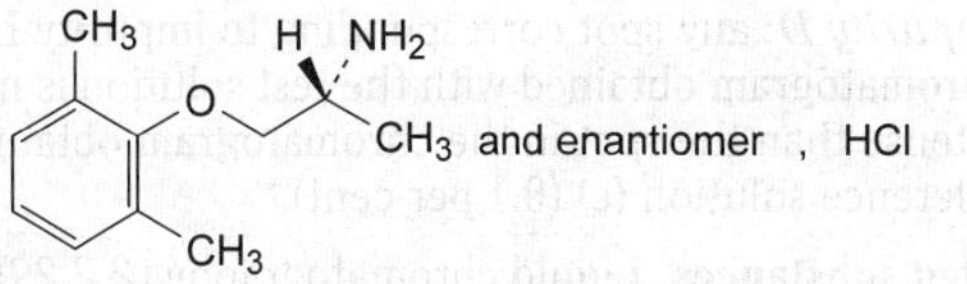

$C_{11}H_{18}ClNO$ M_r 215.7

DEFINITION

(2*RS*)-1-(2,6-Dimethylphenoxy)propan-2-amine hydrochloride.

Content: 99.0 per cent to 101.0 per cent (anhydrous substance).

CHARACTERS

Appearance: white or almost white, crystalline powder.

Solubility: freely soluble in water and in methanol, sparingly soluble in methylene chloride.

It shows polymorphism.

IDENTIFICATION

A. Infrared absorption spectrophotometry (*2.2.24*).

Comparison: *mexiletine hydrochloride CRS.*

If the spectra obtained in the solid state show differences, dissolve the substance to be examined and the reference substance separately in *methanol R*, evaporate to dryness and record new spectra using the residues.

B. Dilute 1.5 ml of solution S (see Tests) to 15 ml with *water R*. The solution gives reaction (a) of chlorides (*2.3.1*).

TESTS

Solution S. Dissolve 2.0 g in *carbon dioxide-free water R* and dilute to 20 ml with the same solvent.

Appearance of solution. The solution is clear (*2.2.1*) and colourless (*2.2.2, Method II*).

Dilute 5 ml of solution S to 10 ml with *water R*.

pH (*2.2.3*): 4.0 to 5.5 for solution S.

Impurity D. Thin-layer chromatography (*2.2.27*).

Test solution. Dissolve 0.500 g of the substance to be examined in *methanol R* and dilute to 5.0 ml with the same solvent.

Reference solution (a). Dissolve the content of a vial of *mexiletine impurity D CRS* in 4.0 ml of *methanol R*.

Reference solution (b). Dilute 1.0 ml of the test solution to 20.0 ml with *methanol R*.

Reference solution (c). Dilute 1.0 ml of reference solution (a) to 5.0 ml with *methanol R*.

Reference solution (d). Dilute 1.0 ml of reference solution (a) to 5.0 ml with reference solution (b).

Plate: *TLC silica gel plate R*.

Mobile phase: *concentrated ammonia R, alcohol R, acetone R, toluene R (3:7:45:45 V/V/V/V)*.

Application: 5 µl of the test solution and reference solutions (c) and (d).

Development: over a path of 10 cm.

Drying: in air.

Detection: spray with *ninhydrin solution R3* and heat at 100-105 °C for 15 min or until the spots appear.

System suitability: the chromatogram obtained with reference solution (b) shows 2 clearly separated spots.

Limit:

- *impurity D*: any spot corresponding to impurity D in the chromatogram obtained with the test solution is not more intense than the spot in the chromatogram obtained with reference solution (c) (0.1 per cent).

Related substances. Liquid chromatography (*2.2.29*).

Test solution. Dissolve 0.200 g of the substance to be examined in the mobile phase and dilute to 10.0 ml with the mobile phase.

Reference solution (a). Dilute 1.0 ml of the test solution to 10.0 ml with the mobile phase.

Reference solution (b). Dissolve the content of a vial of *mexiletine impurity C CRS* in the mobile phase and transfer the solution quantitatively to a volumetric flask containing 16.0 mg of *2,6-dimethylphenol R*. Dilute to 20.0 ml with the mobile phase. Mix 1.0 ml of this solution with 2.0 ml of reference solution (a) and dilute the mixture to 100.0 ml with the mobile phase.

Column:

- *size*: *l* = 0.25 m, Ø = 4.6 mm,
- *stationary phase*: *end-capped octadecylsilyl silica gel for chromatography R* (5 µm).

Mobile phase: mix 65 volumes of *methanol R2* and 35 volumes of a solution prepared as follows: dissolve 11.5 g of *anhydrous sodium acetate R* in 500 ml of *water R*, add 3.2 ml of *glacial acetic acid R*, mix and allow to cool; adjust to pH 4.8 with *glacial acetic acid R* and dilute to 1000 ml with *water R*.

Flow rate: 1.0 ml/min.

Detection: spectrophotometer at 262 nm.

Injection: 20 µl.

Run time: 5.5 times the retention time of mexiletine.

Relative retention with reference to mexiletine (retention time = about 4 min): impurity C = about 0.7; impurity A = about 1.8.

System suitability: reference solution (b):

- *resolution*: minimum 5.0 between the peaks due to mexiletine and impurity C.

Limits:

- *impurity A*: not more than 2.5 times the area of the corresponding peak in the chromatogram obtained with reference solution (b) (0.1 per cent),
- *impurity C*: not more than 20 times the area of the corresponding peak in the chromatogram obtained with reference solution (b) (0.1 per cent),
- *any other impurity*: for each impurity, not more than 0.5 times the area of the peak due to mexiletine in the chromatogram obtained with reference solution (b) (0.1 per cent),
- *total*: not more than 2.5 times the area of the peak due to mexiletine in the chromatogram obtained with reference solution (b) (0.5 per cent),
- *disregard limit*: 0.25 times the area of the peak due to mexiletine in the chromatogram obtained with reference solution (b) (0.05 per cent).

Heavy metals (*2.4.8*): maximum 10 ppm.

2.0 g complies with limit test C. Prepare the standard using 2 ml of *lead standard solution (10 ppm Pb) R*.

Water (*2.5.12*): maximum 0.5 per cent, determined on 1.00 g.

Sulphated ash (*2.4.14*): maximum 0.1 per cent, determined on 1.0 g.

ASSAY

Dissolve 0.150 g in 50 ml of a mixture of equal volumes of *anhydrous acetic acid R* and *acetic anhydride R*. Titrate immediately with *0.1 M perchloric acid*, determining the end-point potentiometrically (*2.2.20*) and completing the titration within 2 min.

1 ml of *0.1 M perchloric acid* is equivalent to 21.57 mg of $C_{11}H_{18}ClNO$.

IMPURITIES

Specified impurities: A, C, D.

Other detectable impurities: B.

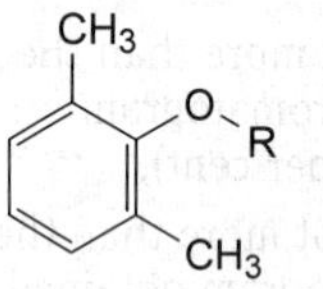

A. R = H: 2,6-dimethylphenol,

B. R = CH_2-CO-CH_3: 1-(2,6-dimethylphenoxy)propan-2-one,

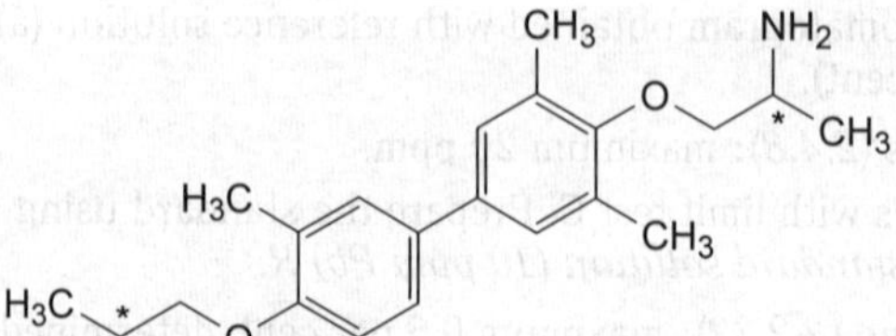

C. 1,1′-[(3,3′,5,5′-tetramethylbiphenyl-4,4′-diyl)bisoxy]dipropan-2-amine,

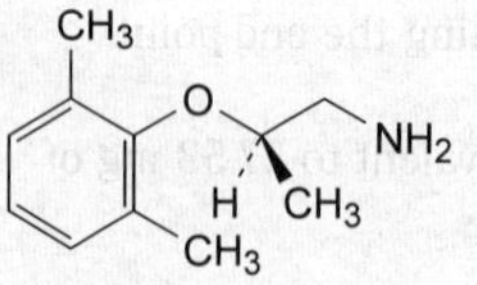

and enantiomer

D. (2*RS*)-2-(2,6-dimethylphenoxy)propan-1-amine.

01/2005:0846

MIANSERIN HYDROCHLORIDE

Mianserini hydrochloridum

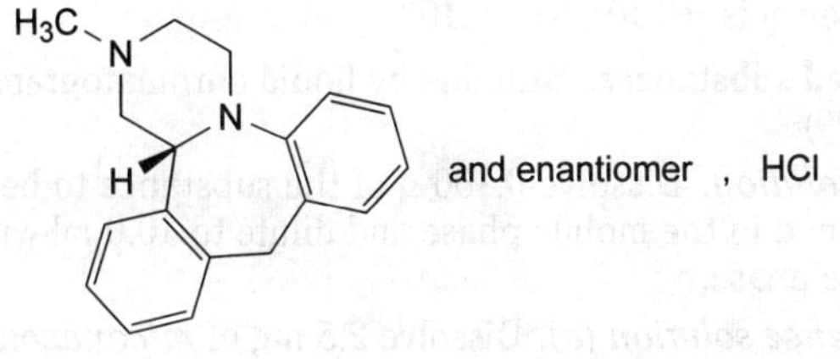

$C_{18}H_{21}ClN_2$ M_r 300.8

DEFINITION

Mianserin hydrochloride contains not less than 98.5 per cent and not more than the equivalent of 101.0 per cent of (*RS*)-2-methyl-1,2,3,4,10,14b-hexahydrodibenzo[*c,f*]pyrazino[1,2-*a*]azepine hydrochloride, calculated with reference to the dried substance.

CHARACTERS

White or almost white, crystalline powder or crystals, sparingly soluble in water, soluble in methylene chloride, slightly soluble in alcohol.

IDENTIFICATION

First identification: B, D.

Second identification: A, C, D.

A. Dissolve 50.0 mg in *water R* and dilute to 50.0 ml with the same solvent. Dilute 5.0 ml of the solution to 50.0 ml with *water R*. Examined between 230 nm and 350 nm (*2.2.25*), the solution shows an absorption maximum at 279 nm. The specific absorption at the maximum is 64 to 72.

B. Examine by infrared absorption spectrophotometry (*2.2.24*), comparing with the spectrum obtained with *mianserin hydrochloride CRS*. Examine the substances as discs prepared using *potassium chloride R*. If the spectra obtained show differences, dissolve the substance to be examined and the reference substance separately in *methanol R*, evaporate to dryness and record new spectra using the residues.

C. Examine by thin-layer chromatography (*2.2.27*), using *silica gel GF_{254} R* as the coating substance.

Test solution. Dissolve 10 mg of the substance to be examined in *methylene chloride R* and dilute to 5 ml with the same solvent.

Reference solution (a). Dissolve 10 mg of *mianserin hydrochloride CRS* in *methylene chloride R* and dilute to 5 ml with the same solvent.

Reference solution (b). Dissolve 10 mg of *mianserin hydrochloride CRS* and 10 mg of *cyproheptadine hydrochloride CRS* in *methylene chloride R* and dilute to 5 ml with the same solvent.

Apply to the plate 2 µl of each solution. Develop over a path of 15 cm using a mixture of 5 volumes of *diethylamine R*, 20 volumes of *ether R* and 75 volumes of *cyclohexane R*. Examine in ultraviolet light at 254 nm. The principal spot in the chromatogram obtained with the test solution is similar in position and size to the principal spot in the chromatogram obtained with reference solution (a). The test is not valid unless the chromatogram obtained with reference solution (b) shows two clearly separated principal spots.

D. It gives reaction (a) of chlorides (*2.3.1*).

TESTS

pH (*2.2.3*). Dissolve 0.10 g in *carbon dioxide-free water R* and dilute to 10 ml with the same solvent. The pH of the solution is 4.0 to 5.5.

Related substances. Examine by thin-layer chromatography (*2.2.27*), using *silica gel G R* as the coating substance.

Test solution. Dissolve 0.20 g of the substance to be examined in a mixture of 1 volume of *ammonia R* and 4 volumes of *methanol R* and dilute to 10 ml with the same mixture of solvents.

Reference solution (a). Dilute 1 ml of the test solution to 200 ml with a mixture of 1 volume of *ammonia R* and 4 volumes of *methanol R*.

Reference solution (b). Dilute 5 ml of reference solution (a) to 25 ml with a mixture of 1 volume of *ammonia R* and 4 volumes of *methanol R*.

Apply to the plate 5 µl of each solution. Develop over a path of 15 cm using a mixture of 10 volumes of *methanol R* and 90 volumes of *methylene chloride R*. Dry the plate in a current of cold air. Expose the plate to iodine vapour for 20 min. Any spot in the chromatogram obtained with the test solution, apart from the principal spot, is not more intense than the spot in the chromatogram obtained with reference solution (a) (0.5 per cent) and at most one such spot is more intense than the spot in the chromatogram obtained with reference solution (b) (0.1 per cent).

Loss on drying (*2.2.32*). Not more than 0.5 per cent, determined on 1.000 g by drying over *diphosphorus pentoxide R* at 65 °C at a pressure not exceeding 700 Pa for 3 h.

Sulphated ash (*2.4.14*). Not more than 0.1 per cent, determined on 1.0 g.

ASSAY

Dissolve 0.200 g in a mixture of 5.0 ml of *0.01 M hydrochloric acid* and 50 ml of *alcohol R*. Carry out a potentiometric titration (*2.2.20*), using *0.1 M sodium hydroxide*. Read the volume added between the two points of inflexion.

1 ml of *0.1 M sodium hydroxide* is equivalent to 30.08 mg of $C_{18}H_{21}ClN_2$.

STORAGE

Store protected from light.

IMPURITIES

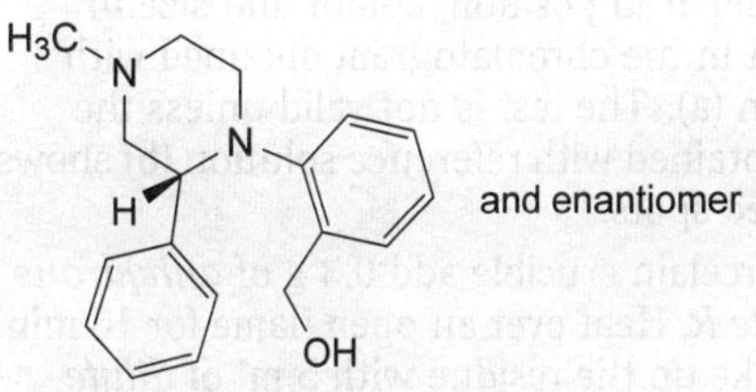

A. [2-[(2*RS*)-4-methyl-2-phenylpiperazin-1-yl]phenyl]methanol.

01/2005:0935

MICONAZOLE

Miconazolum

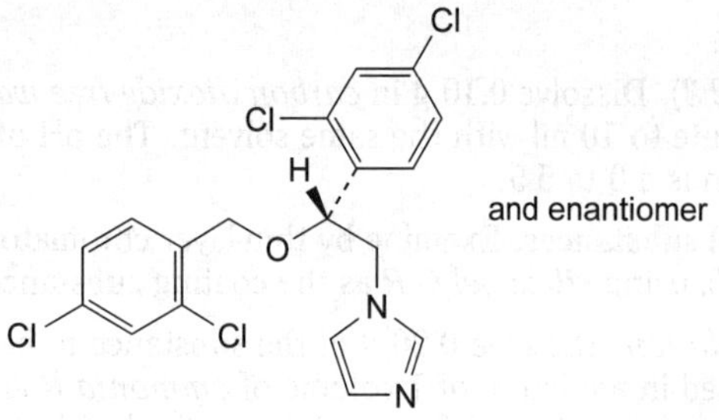

$C_{18}H_{14}Cl_4N_2O$ M_r 416.1

DEFINITION

Miconazole contains not less than 99.0 per cent and not more than the equivalent of 101.0 per cent of 1-[(2*RS*)-2-[(2,4-dichlorobenzyl)oxy]-2-(2,4-dichlorophenyl)ethyl]-1*H*-imidazole, calculated with reference to the dried substance.

CHARACTERS

A white or almost white powder, very slightly soluble in water, freely soluble in methanol, soluble in alcohol.

It shows polymorphism.

IDENTIFICATION

First identification: A, B.

Second identification: A, C, D.

A. Melting point (*2.2.14*): 83 °C to 87 °C.

B. Examine by infrared absorption spectrophotometry (*2.2.24*), comparing with the spectrum obtained with *miconazole CRS*. Examine the substances as discs prepared using *potassium bromide R*.

C. Examine by thin-layer chromatography (*2.2.27*), using a suitable octadecylsilyl silica gel as the coating substance.

Test solution. Dissolve 30 mg of the substance to be examined in the mobile phase and dilute to 5 ml with the mobile phase.

Reference solution (a). Dissolve 30 mg of *miconazole CRS* in the mobile phase and dilute to 5 ml with the mobile phase.

Reference solution (b). Dissolve 30 mg of *miconazole CRS* and 30 mg of *econazole nitrate CRS* in the mobile phase and dilute to 5 ml with the mobile phase.

Apply separately to the plate 5 µl of each solution. Develop over a path of 15 cm using a mixture of 20 volumes of *ammonium acetate solution R*, 40 volumes of *dioxan R* and 40 volumes of *methanol R*. Dry the plate in a current of warm air for 15 min and expose it to iodine vapour until the spots appear. Examine in daylight. The principal spot in the chromatogram obtained with the test solution is similar in position, colour and size to the principal spot in the chromatogram obtained with reference solution (a). The test is not valid unless the chromatogram obtained with reference solution (b) shows 2 clearly separated spots.

D. To 30 mg in a porcelain crucible add 0.3 g of *anhydrous sodium carbonate R*. Heat over an open flame for 10 min. Allow to cool. Take up the residue with 5 ml of *dilute nitric acid R* and filter. To 1 ml of the filtrate add 1 ml of *water R*. The solution gives reaction (a) of chlorides (*2.3.1*).

TESTS

Solution S. Dissolve 0.1 g in *methanol R* and dilute to 10 ml with the same solvent.

Appearance of solution. Solution S is clear (*2.2.1*) and is not more intensely coloured than reference solution Y_6 (*2.2.2, Method II*).

Optical rotation (*2.2.7*). The angle of optical rotation of solution S is − 0.10° to + 0.10°.

Related substances. Examine by liquid chromatography (*2.2.29*).

Test solution. Dissolve 0.100 g of the substance to be examined in the mobile phase and dilute to 10.0 ml with the mobile phase.

Reference solution (a). Dissolve 2.5 mg of *miconazole CRS* and 2.5 mg of *econazole nitrate CRS* in the mobile phase and dilute to 100.0 ml with the mobile phase.

Reference solution (b). Dilute 1.0 ml of the test solution to 100.0 ml with the mobile phase. Dilute 5.0 ml of this solution to 20.0 ml with the mobile phase.

The chromatographic procedure may be carried out using:

- a stainless steel column 0.10 m long and 4.6 mm in internal diameter packed with *octadecylsilyl silica gel for chromatography R* (3 µm),
- as mobile phase at a flow rate of 2 ml/min a solution of 6.0 g of *ammonium acetate R* in a mixture of 300 ml of *acetonitrile R*, 320 ml of *methanol R* and 380 ml of *water R*,
- as detector a spectrophotometer set at 235 nm.

Equilibrate the column with the mobile phase at a flow rate of 2 ml/min for about 30 min.

Adjust the sensitivity of the system so that the height of the principal peak in the chromatogram obtained with 10 µl of reference solution (b) is not less than 50 per cent of the full scale of the recorder.

Inject 10 µl of reference solution (a). When the chromatograms are recorded in the prescribed conditions, the retention times are: econazole nitrate, about 10 min; miconazole, about 20 min. The test is not valid unless the resolution between the peaks corresponding to econazole nitrate and miconazole is not less than 10; if necessary, adjust the composition of the mobile phase.

Inject separately 10 µl of the test solution and 10 µl of reference solution (b). Continue the chromatography for 1.2 times the retention time of the principal peak. In the chromatogram obtained with the test solution: the area of any peak, apart from the principal peak, is not greater than the area of the principal peak in the chromatogram obtained with reference solution (b) (0.25 per cent); the sum of the areas of all the peaks, apart from the principal peak, is not greater than twice that of the principal peak in the chromatogram obtained with reference solution (b) (0.5 per cent). Disregard any peak due to the solvent and any peak with an area less than 0.2 times the area of the principal peak in the chromatogram obtained with reference solution (b).

Loss on drying (*2.2.32*). Not more than 0.5 per cent, determined on 1.000 g by drying *in vacuo* at 60 °C for 4 h.

Sulphated ash (*2.4.14*). Not more than 0.1 per cent, determined on 1.0 g.

ASSAY

Dissolve 0.300 g in 50 ml of a mixture of 1 volume of *anhydrous acetic acid R* and 7 volumes of *methyl ethyl ketone R*. Using 0.2 ml of *naphtholbenzein solution R* as indicator, titrate with *0.1 M perchloric acid* until the colour changes from orange-yellow to green.

1 ml of *0.1 M perchloric acid* is equivalent to 41.61 mg of $C_{18}H_{14}Cl_4N_2O$.

STORAGE

Store protected from light.

IMPURITIES

Specified impurities: A, B, C, D, E, F, G.

Other detectable impurities: H, I.

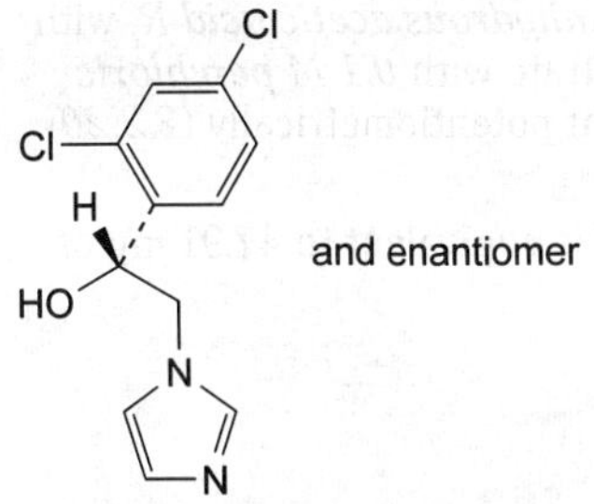

A. (1*RS*)-1-(2,4-dichlorophenyl)-2-(1*H*-imidazol-1-yl)ethanol,

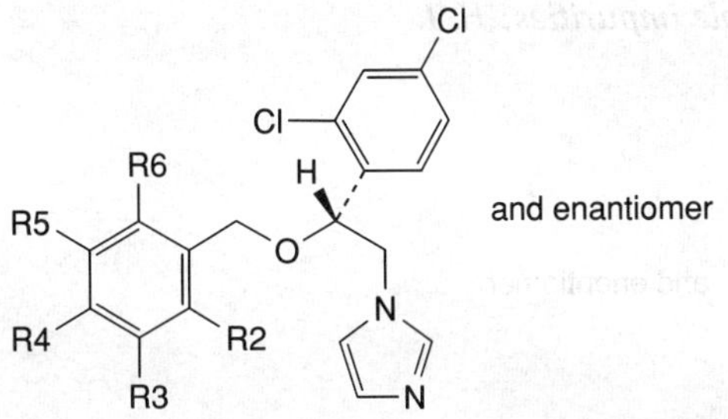

B. R2 = R3 = R5 = R6 = H, R4 = Cl: 1-[(2*RS*)-2-[(4-chlorobenzyl)oxy]-2-(2,4-dichlorophenyl)ethyl]-1*H*-imidazole,

D. R2 = R6 = Cl, R3 = R4 = R5 = H: 1-[(2*RS*)-2-[(2,6-dichlorobenzyl)oxy]-2-(2,4-dichlorophenyl)ethyl]-1*H*-imidazole,

F. R2 = R5 = R6 = H, R3 = R4 = Cl: 1-[(2*RS*)-2-[(3,4-dichlorobenzyl)oxy]-2-(2,4-dichlorophenyl)ethyl]-1*H*-imidazole,

G. R2 = R5 = Cl, R3 = R4 = R6 = H: 1-[(2*RS*)-2-[(2,5-dichlorobenzyl)oxy]-2-(2,4-dichlorophenyl)ethyl]-1*H*-imidazole,

H. R2 = R3 = R4 = R5 = R6 = H: 1-[(2*RS*)-2-benzyloxy-2-(2,4-dichlorophenyl)ethyl]-1*H*-imidazole,

I. R2 = Cl, R3 = R4 = R5 = R6 = H: 1-[(2*RS*)-2-[(2-chlorobenzyl)oxy]-2-(2,4-dichlorophenyl)ethyl]-1*H*-imidazole,

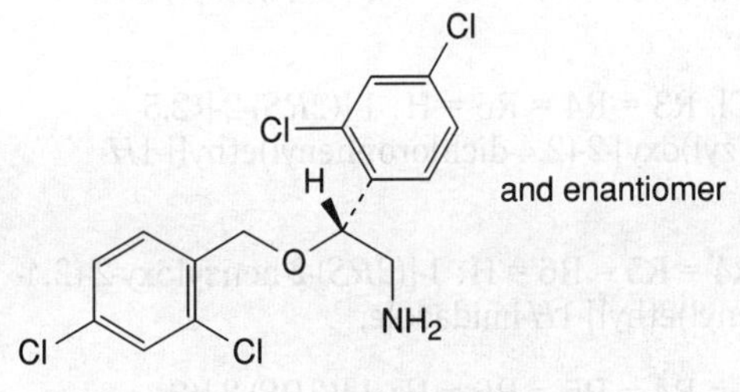

C. (2*RS*)-2-[(2,4-dichlorobenzyl)oxy]-2-(2,4-dichlorophenyl)ethanamine,

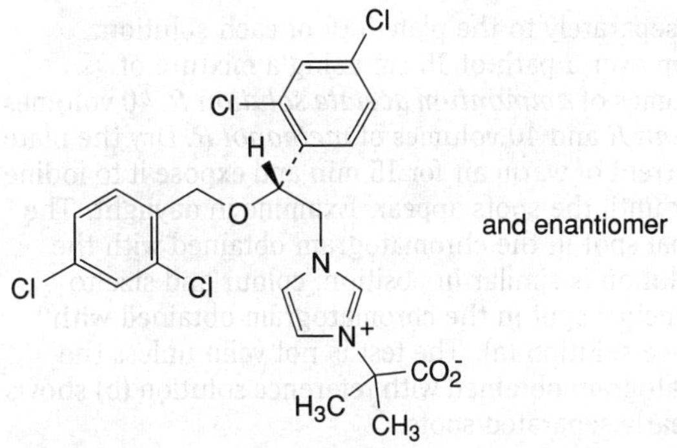

E. 2-[1-[(2*RS*)-2-[(2,4-dichlorobenzyl)oxy]-2-(2,4-dichlorophenyl)ethyl]-1*H*-imidazol-3-io]-2-methylpropanoate.

01/2005:0513

MICONAZOLE NITRATE

Miconazoli nitras

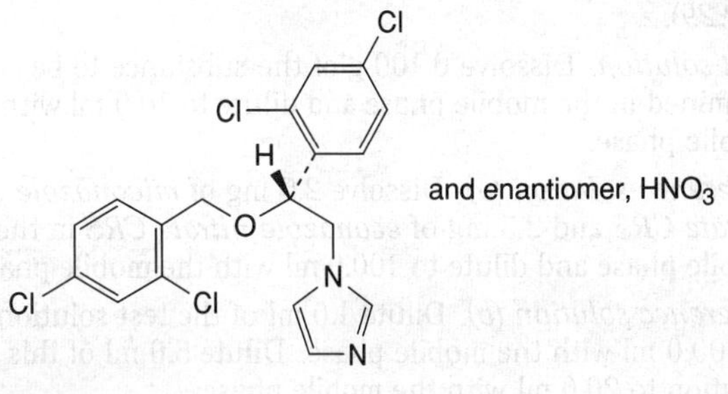

$C_{18}H_{15}Cl_4N_3O_4$ M_r 479.1

DEFINITION

Miconazole nitrate contains not less than 99.0 per cent and not more than the equivalent of 101.0 per cent of 1-[(2*RS*)-2-[(2,4-dichlorobenzyl)oxy]-2-(2,4-dichlorophenyl)ethyl]-1*H*-imidazole nitrate, calculated with reference to the dried substance.

CHARACTERS

A white or almost white powder, very slightly soluble in water, sparingly soluble in methanol, slightly soluble in alcohol.

IDENTIFICATION

First identification: A, B.

Second identification: A, C, D.

A. Melting point (*2.2.14*): 178 °C to 184 °C.

B. Examine by infrared absorption spectrophotometry (*2.2.24*), comparing with the spectrum obtained with *miconazole nitrate CRS*. Examine the substances prepared as discs using *potassium bromide R*.

C. Examine by thin-layer chromatography (*2.2.27*), using a suitable octadecylsilyl silica gel as the coating substance.
Test solution. Dissolve 30 mg of the substance to be examined in the mobile phase and dilute to 5 ml with the mobile phase.
Reference solution (a). Dissolve 30 mg of *miconazole nitrate CRS* in the mobile phase and dilute to 5 ml with the mobile phase.
Reference solution (b). Dissolve 30 mg of *miconazole nitrate CRS* and 30 mg of *econazole nitrate CRS* in the mobile phase and dilute to 5 ml with the mobile phase.

Apply separately to the plate 5 µl of each solution. Develop over a path of 15 cm using a mixture of 20 volumes of *ammonium acetate solution R*, 40 volumes of *dioxan R* and 40 volumes of *methanol R*. Dry the plate in a current of warm air for 15 min and expose it to iodine vapour until the spots appear. Examine in daylight. The principal spot in the chromatogram obtained with the test solution is similar in position, colour and size to the principal spot in the chromatogram obtained with reference solution (a). The test is not valid unless the chromatogram obtained with reference solution (b) shows two clearly separated spots.

D. It gives the reaction of nitrates (*2.3.1*).

TESTS

Solution S. Dissolve 0.1 g in *methanol R* and dilute to 10 ml with the same solvent.

Appearance of solution. Solution S is clear (*2.2.1*) and is not more intensely coloured than reference solution Y_7 (*2.2.2, Method II*).

Optical rotation (*2.2.7*). The angle of optical rotation of solution S is − 0.10° to + 0.10°.

Related substances. Examine by liquid chromatography (*2.2.29*).

Test solution. Dissolve 0.100 g of the substance to be examined in the mobile phase and dilute to 10.0 ml with the mobile phase.

Reference solution (a). Dissolve 2.5 mg of *miconazole nitrate CRS* and 2.5 mg of *econazole nitrate CRS* in the mobile phase and dilute to 100.0 ml with the mobile phase.

Reference solution (b). Dilute 1.0 ml of the test solution to 100.0 ml with the mobile phase. Dilute 5.0 ml of this solution to 20.0 ml with the mobile phase.

The chromatographic procedure may be carried out using:

– a stainless steel column 0.10 m long and 4.6 mm in internal diameter packed with *octadecylsilyl silica gel for chromatography R* (3 µm),

– as mobile phase at a flow rate of 2 ml/min a solution of 6.0 g of *ammonium acetate R* in a mixture of 300 ml of *acetonitrile R*, 320 ml of *methanol R* and 380 ml of *water R*,

– as detector a spectrophotometer set at 235 nm.

Equilibrate the column with the mobile phase at a flow rate of 2 ml/min for about 30 min.

Adjust the sensitivity of the system so that the height of the principal peak in the chromatogram obtained with 10 µl of reference solution (b) is not less than 50 per cent of the full scale of the recorder.

Inject 10 µl of reference solution (a). When the chromatogram is recorded in the prescribed conditions, the retention times are: econazole nitrate, about 10 min; miconazole nitrate, about 20 min. The test is not valid unless the resolution between the peaks corresponding to econazole nitrate and miconazole nitrate is at least 10; if necessary, adjust the composition of the mobile phase.

Inject separately 10 µl of the test solution and 10 µl of reference solution (b). Continue the chromatography for 1.2 times the retention time of the principal peak. In the chromatogram obtained with the test solution: the area of any peak apart from the principal peak is not greater than the area of the principal peak in the chromatogram obtained with reference solution (b) (0.25 per cent); the sum of the areas of the peaks apart from the principal peak is not greater than twice the area of the principal peak in the chromatogram obtained with reference solution (b) (0.5 per cent). Disregard any peak due to the nitrate ion and any peak with an area less than 0.2 times the area of the principal peak in the chromatogram obtained with reference solution (b).

Loss on drying (*2.2.32*). Not more than 0.5 per cent, determined on 1.000 g by drying in an oven at 100 °C to 105 °C for 2 h.

Sulphated ash (*2.4.14*). Not more than 0.1 per cent, determined on 1.0 g.

ASSAY

Dissolve 0.350 g in 75 ml of *anhydrous acetic acid R*, with slight heating if necessary. Titrate with *0.1 M perchloric acid* determining the end-point potentiometrically (*2.2.20*). Carry out a blank titration.

1 ml of *0.1 M perchloric acid* is equivalent to 47.91 mg of $C_{18}H_{15}Cl_4N_3O_4$.

STORAGE

Store protected from light.

IMPURITIES

Specified impurities: A, B, C, D, E, F, G.

Other detectable impurities: H, I.

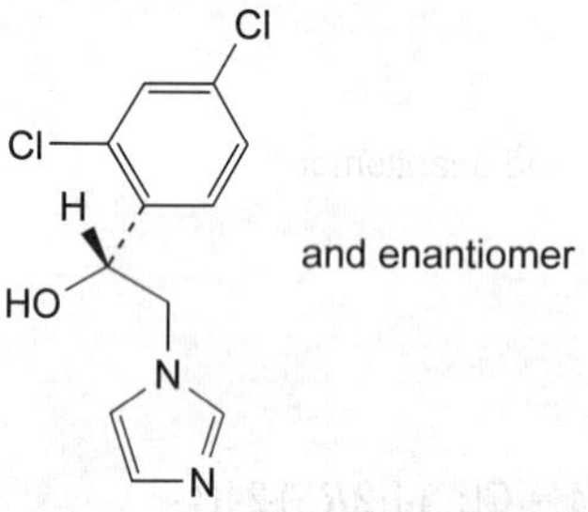

A. (1*RS*)-1-(2,4-dichlorophenyl)-2-(1*H*-imidazol-1-yl)ethanol,

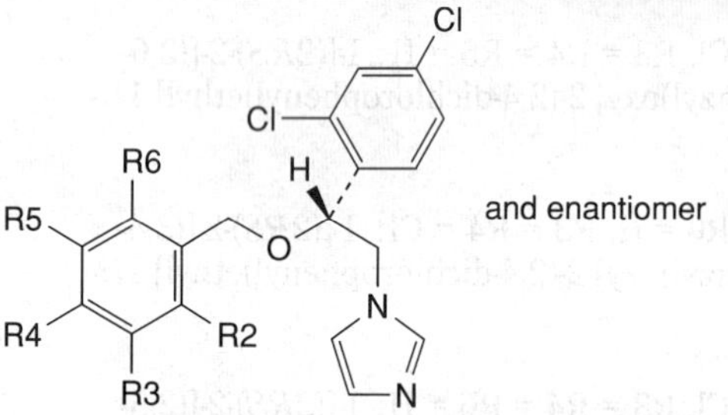

B. R2 = R3 = R5 = R6 = H, R4 = Cl: 1-[(2*RS*)-2-[(4-chlorobenzyl)oxy]-2-(2,4-dichlorophenyl)ethyl]-1*H*-imidazole,

D. R2 = R6 = Cl, R3 = R4 = R5 = H: 1-[(2*RS*)-2-[(2,6-dichlorobenzyl)oxy]-2-(2,4-dichlorophenyl)ethyl]-1*H*-imidazole,

F. R2 = R5 = R6 = H, R3 = R4 = Cl: 1-[(2*RS*)-2-[(3,4-dichlorobenzyl)oxy]-2-(2,4-dichlorophenyl)ethyl]-1*H*-imidazole,

G. R2 = R5 = Cl, R3 = R4 = R6 = H: 1-[(2*RS*)-2-[(2,5-dichlorobenzyl)oxy]-2-(2,4-dichlorophenyl)ethyl]-1*H*-imidazole,

H. R2 = R3 = R4 = R5 = R6 = H: 1-[(2*RS*)-2-benzyloxy-2-(2,4-dichlorophenyl)ethyl]-1*H*-imidazole,

I. R2 = Cl, R3 = R4 = R5 = R6 = H: 1-[(2*RS*)-2-[(2-chlorobenzyl)oxy]-2-(2,4-dichlorophenyl)ethyl]-1*H*-imidazole,

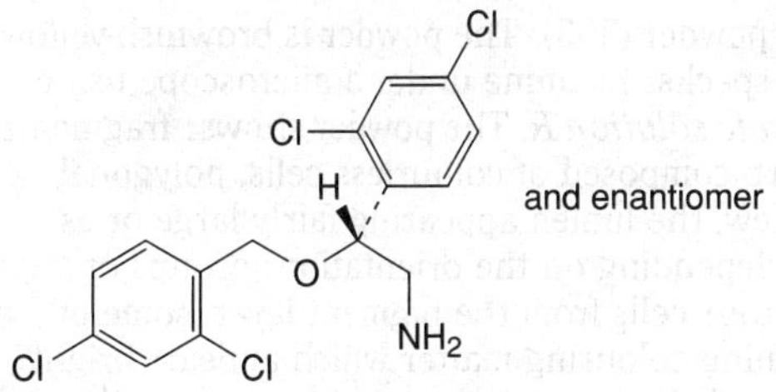

C. (2*RS*)-2-[(2,4-dichlorobenzyl)oxy]-2-(2,4-dichlorophenyl)ethanamine,

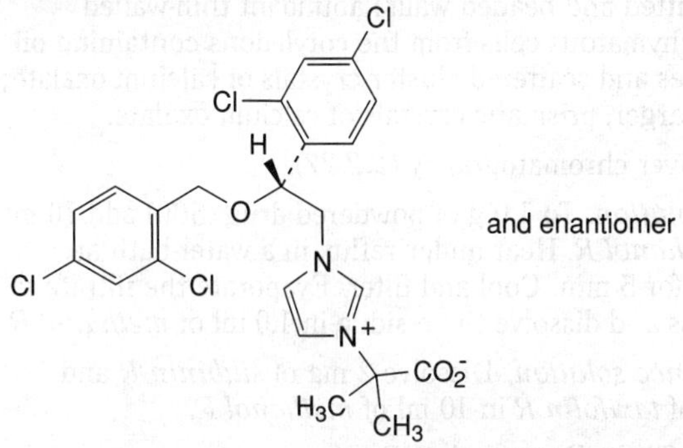

E. 2-[1-[(2*RS*)-2-[(2,4-dichlorobenzyl)oxy]-2-(2,4-dichlorophenyl)ethyl]-1*H*-imidazol-3-io]-2-methylpropanoate.

01/2005:0936

MIDAZOLAM

Midazolamum

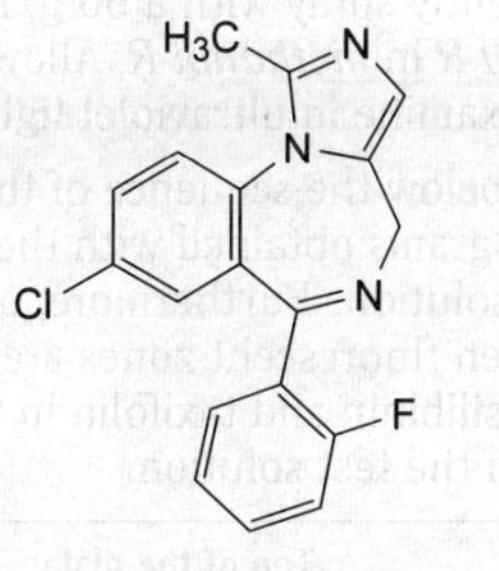

$C_{18}H_{13}ClFN_3$ M_r 325.8

DEFINITION

Midazolam contains not less than 98.5 per cent and not more than the equivalent of 101.5 per cent of 8-chloro-6-(2-fluorophenyl)-1-methyl-4*H*-imidazo[1,5-*a*][1,4]benzodiazepine, calculated with reference to the dried substance.

CHARACTERS

A white or yellowish, crystalline powder, practically insoluble in water, freely soluble in acetone and in alcohol, soluble in methanol.

IDENTIFICATION

First identification: B.

Second identification: A, C, D, E.

A. Melting point (*2.2.14*): 161 °C to 164 °C.

B. Examine by infrared absorption spectrophotometry (*2.2.24*), comparing with the spectrum obtained with *midazolam CRS*.

C. Examine the chromatograms obtained in the test for related substances in ultraviolet light at 254 nm. The principal spot in the chromatogram obtained with test solution (b) is similar in position and size to the principal spot in the chromatogram obtained with reference solution (b).

D. Mix 90 mg with 0.30 g of *anhydrous sodium carbonate R* and ignite in a crucible until an almost white residue is obtained (normally in less than 5 min). Allow to cool and dissolve the residue in 5 ml of *dilute nitric acid R*. Filter (the filtrate is also used in identification test E). Add 1.0 ml of the filtrate to a freshly prepared mixture of 0.1 ml of *alizarin S solution R* and 0.1 ml of *zirconyl nitrate solution R*. Mix, allow to stand for 5 min and compare the colour of the solution with that of a blank prepared in the same manner. The colour of the test solution is yellow and that of the blank is red.

E. To 1 ml of the filtrate obtained in identification test D add 1 ml of *water R*. The solution gives reaction (a) of chlorides (*2.3.1*).

TESTS

Appearance of solution. Dissolve 0.1 g in *0.1 M hydrochloric acid* and dilute to 10 ml with the same acid. The solution is clear (*2.2.1*) and not more intensely coloured than reference solution Y_6 (*2.2.2, Method II*).

Related substances. Examine by thin-layer chromatography (*2.2.27*), using *silica gel GF_{254} R* as the coating substance.

Test solution (a). Dissolve 0.2 g of the substance to be examined in *alcohol R* and dilute to 5 ml with the same solvent.

Test solution (b). Dilute 1 ml of test solution (a) to 50 ml with *alcohol R*.

Reference solution (a). Dilute 1 ml of test solution (a) to 10 ml with *alcohol R*. Dilute 2 ml of the solution to 100 ml with *alcohol R*.

Reference solution (b). Dissolve 8 mg of *midazolam CRS* in *alcohol R* and dilute to 10 ml with the same solvent.

Reference solution (c). Dissolve 8 mg of *midazolam CRS* and 8 mg of *chlordiazepoxide CRS* in *alcohol R* and dilute to 10 ml with the same solvent.

Apply separately to the plate 5 µl of each solution. Develop over a path of 12 cm using a mixture of 2 volumes of *glacial acetic acid R*, 15 volumes of *water R*, 20 volumes of *methanol R* and 80 volumes of *ethyl acetate R*. Allow the plate to dry in air and examine in ultraviolet light at 254 nm. Any spot in the chromatogram obtained with test solution (a), apart from the principal spot, is not more intense than the spot in the chromatogram obtained with reference solution (a) (0.2 per cent). The test is not valid unless the chromatogram obtained with reference solution (c) shows two clearly separated spots.

Loss on drying (*2.2.32*). Not more than 0.5 per cent, determined on 1.000 g by drying in an oven at 100 °C to 105 °C for 2 h.

Sulphated ash (*2.4.14*). Not more than 0.1 per cent, determined on 1.0 g in a platinum crucible.

ASSAY

Dissolve 0.120 g in 30 ml of *anhydrous acetic acid R* and add 20 ml of *acetic anhydride R*. Titrate with *0.1 M perchloric acid* determining the end-point potentiometrically (*2.2.20*). Titrate to the second point of inflexion.

1 ml of *0.1 M perchloric acid* is equivalent to 16.29 mg of $C_{18}H_{13}ClFN_3$.

STORAGE

Store protected from light.

IMPURITIES

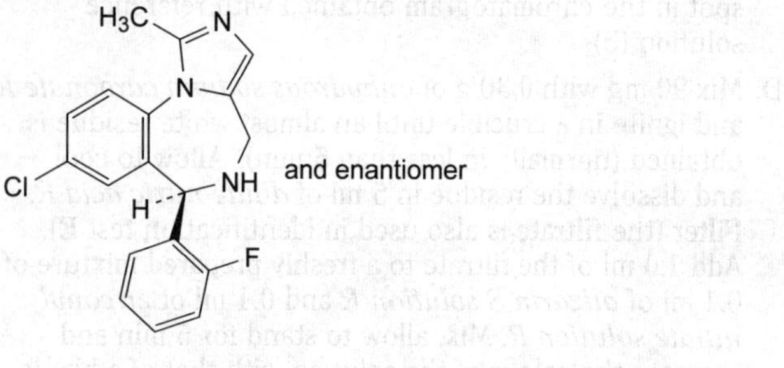

A. (6*RS*)-8-chloro-6-(2-fluorophenyl)-1-methyl-5,6-dihydro-4*H*-imidazo[1,5-*a*][1,4]benzodiazepine,

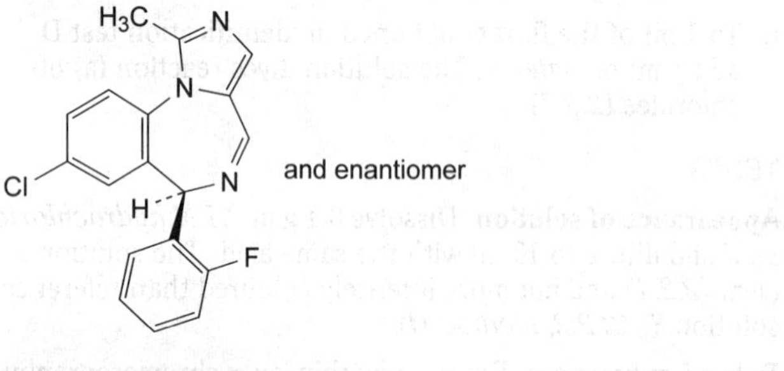

B. (6*RS*)-8-chloro-6-(2-fluorophenyl)-1-methyl-6*H*-imidazo[1,5-*a*][1,4]benzodiazepine,

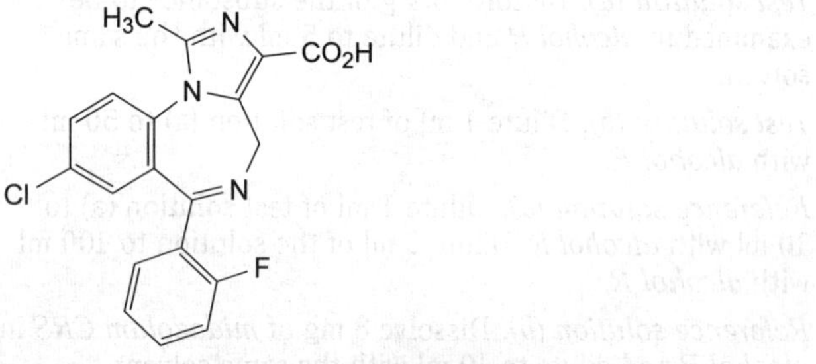

C. 8-chloro-6-(2-fluorophenyl)-1-methyl-4*H*-imdazo[1,5-*a*][1,4]benzodiazepine-3-carboxylic acid.

01/2005:1860

MILK-THISTLE FRUIT

Silybi mariani fructus

DEFINITION

Mature fruit, devoid of the pappus, of *Silybum marianum* L. Gaertner.

Content: minimum 1.5 per cent of silymarin expressed as silibinin ($C_{25}H_{22}O_{10}$; M_r 482.4) (dried drug).

CHARACTERS

No rancid odour.

Macroscopic and microscopic characters described under identification tests A and B.

IDENTIFICATION

A. Strongly compressed, elongate-obovate achenes, about 6 mm to 8 mm long, 3 mm broad and 1.5 mm thick; outer surface smooth and shiny with a grey to pale brown ground colour variably streaked dark brown longitudinally to give an overall pale greyish to brown colour; tapering at the base and crowned at the apex with a glistening, pale yellow extension forming a collar about 1 mm high surrounding the remains of the style. Cut transversely, the fruit shows a narrow, brown outer area and 2 large, dense, white oily cotyledons.

B. Reduce to a powder (355). The powder is brownish-yellow with darker specks. Examine under a microscope using *chloral hydrate solution R*. The powder shows: fragments of the epicarp composed of colourless cells, polygonal in surface view, the lumen appearing fairly large or as a small slit, depending on the orientation; groups of parenchymatous cells from the pigment layer, some of them containing colouring matter which appears bright red; very abundant groups of large sclereids from the testa with bright yellow pitted walls and a narrow lumen; occasionally fragments of small-celled parenchyma with pitted and beaded walls; abundant thin-walled parenchymatous cells from the cotyledons containing oil globules and scattered cluster crystals of calcium oxalate; a few larger, prismatic crystals of calcium oxalate.

C. Thin-layer chromatography (*2.2.27*).

Test solution. To 1.0 g of powdered drug (500) add 10 ml of *methanol R*. Heat under reflux in a water-bath at 70 °C for 5 min. Cool and filter. Evaporate the filtrate to dryness and dissolve the residue in 1.0 ml of *methanol R*.

Reference solution. Dissolve 2 mg of *silibinin R* and 5 mg of *taxifolin R* in 10 ml of *methanol R*.

Plate: *TLC silica gel plate R*.

Mobile phase: *anhydrous formic acid R, acetone R, methylene chloride R* (8.5:16.5:75 *V/V/V*).

Application: 30 µl of the test solution and 10 µl of the reference solution, as bands.

Development: over a path of 10 cm.

Drying: at 100-105 °C.

Detection: spray the warm plate with a 10 g/l solution of *diphenylboric acid aminoethyl ester R* in *methanol R* and subsequently spray with a 50 g/l solution of *macrogol 400 R* in *methanol R*. Allow the plate to dry for 30 min and examine in ultraviolet light at 365 nm.

Results: see below the sequence of the zones present in the chromatograms obtained with the reference solution and the test solution. Furthermore, other orange and yellowish-green fluorescent zones are present between the zones of silibinin and taxifolin in the chromatogram obtained with the test solution.

Top of the plate	
Silibinin: a yellowish-green fluorescent zone	A yellowish-green fluorescent zone (silibinin)
———	
Taxifolin: an orange fluorescent zone	An orange fluorescent zone (taxifolin)
	A yellowish-green fluorescent zone (silicristin)
———	———
	A light blue fluorescent zone (starting line)
Reference solution	**Test solution**

TESTS

Foreign matter (*2.8.2*): maximum 2 per cent.

Loss on drying (*2.2.32*): maximum 8.0 per cent, determined on 1.000 g of the powdered drug (500) by drying in an oven at 100-105 °C for 2 h.

Total ash (*2.4.16*): maximum 8.0 per cent.

ASSAY

Liquid chromatography (*2.2.29*).

Test solution. Place 5.00 g of the powdered drug (500) in a continuous-extraction apparatus. Add 100 ml of *light petroleum R* and heat in a water-bath for 8 h. Allow the defatted drug to dry at room temperature. In a continuous-extraction apparatus, extract the latter with 100 ml of *methanol R* in a water-bath for 5 h. Evaporate the methanolic extract *in vacuo* to a volume of about 30 ml. Filter into a 50 ml volumetric flask, rinsing the extraction flask and the filter, and diluting to 50.0 ml with *methanol R*. Dilute 5.0 ml of this solution to 50.0 ml with *methanol R*.

Reference solution (a). Dissolve 5.0 mg of *silibinin R*, dried *in vacuo*, in *methanol R* and dilute to 50.0 ml with the same solvent.

Reference solution (b). Dissolve 1.0 mg of *silicristin R* in *methanol R* and dilute to 10.0 ml with the same solvent.

Reference solution (c). Dissolve 1.0 mg of *silidianin R* in *methanol R* and dilute to 10.0 ml with the same solvent.

Reference solution (d). Dissolve 1.0 mg of *isosilibinin R* in *methanol R* and dilute to 10.0 ml with the same solvent.

Column:

- *size*: l = 0.125 m, Ø = 4 mm,
- *stationary phase*: *octadecylsilyl silica gel for chromatography R* (5 µm).

Mobile phase:

- *mobile phase A*: *phosphoric acid R, methanol R, water R* (0.5:35:65 *V/V/V*),
- *mobile phase B*: *phosphoric acid R, methanol R, water R* (0.5:50:50 *V/V/V*),

Time (min)	Mobile phase A (per cent *V/V*)	Mobile phase B (per cent *V/V*)
0 - 28	100 → 0	0 → 100
28 - 35	0	100
35 - 36	0 → 100	100 → 0
36 - 51	100	0

Flow rate: 0.8 ml/min.

Detection: spectrophotometer at 288 nm.

Injection: 10 µl.

Retention time: silibinin B = about 30 min. If necessary, adjust the time periods of the gradient.

System suitability: reference solution:

- *resolution*: minimum 1.8 between the peaks due to silibinin A and silibinin B.

Using the retention times determined from the chromatogram obtained with the reference solutions, locate the peaks of silicristin, silidianin, silibinin A, silibinin B, isosilibinin A and isosilibinin B in the chromatogram obtained with the test solution. The peak due to silidianin may vary in size, be absent or be present as the major peak. Determine the area of the peaks due to silicristin, silidianin, silibinin A, silibinin B, isosilibinin A and isosilibinin B.

Calculate the percentage content of silymarin, calculated as silibinin, from the expression:

$$\frac{(A1 + A2 + A3 + A4 + A5 + A6) \times m_1 \times p \times 1000}{(A7 + A8) \times m_2 \times (100 - d)}$$

$A1$ = area of the peak due to silicristin in the chromatogram obtained with the test solution,

$A2$ = area of the peak due to silidianin in the chromatogram obtained with the test solution,

$A3$ = area of the peak due to silibinin A in the chromatogram obtained with the test solution,

$A4$ = area of the peak due to silibinin B in the chromatogram obtained with the test solution,

$A5$ = area of the peak due to isosilibinin A in the chromatogram obtained with the test solution,

$A6$ = area of the peak due to isosilibinin B in the chromatogram obtained with the test solution,

$A7$ = area of the peak due to silibinin A in the chromatogram obtained with reference solution (a),

$A8$ = area of the peak due to silibinin B in the chromatogram obtained with reference solution (a),

m_1 = mass of *silibinin R* in the reference solution, in grams,

m_2 = mass of the drug to be examined, in grams,

p = combined percentage content of silibinin A and silibinin B in *silibinin R*,

d = percentage loss on drying of the drug.

01/2005:1030

MINOCYCLINE HYDROCHLORIDE

Minocyclini hydrochloridum

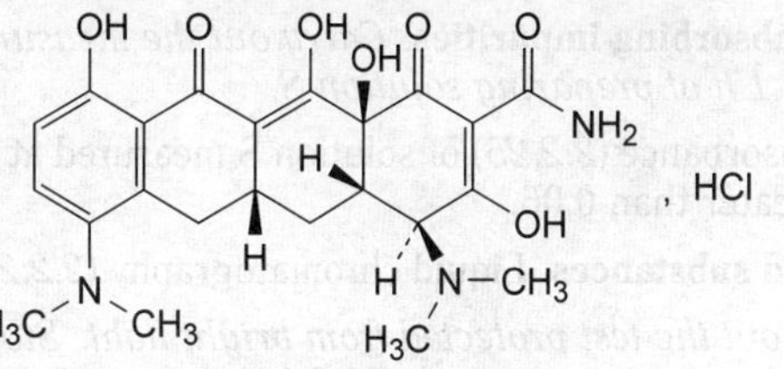

$C_{23}H_{28}ClN_3O_7$ M_r 493.9

DEFINITION

(4*S*,4a*S*,5a*R*,12a*S*)-4,7-Bis(dimethylamino)-3,10,12,12a-tetrahydroxy-1,11-dioxo-1,4,4a,5,5a,6,11,12a-octahydrotetracene-2-carboxamide hydrochloride.

Content: 96.0 per cent to 102.5 per cent (anhydrous substance).

CHARACTERS

Appearance: yellow, crystalline powder, hygroscopic.

Solubility: sparingly soluble in water, slightly soluble in alcohol. It dissolves in solutions of alkali hydroxides and carbonates.

IDENTIFICATION

A. Thin-layer chromatography (*2.2.27*).

Test solution. Dissolve 5 mg of the substance to be examined in *methanol R* and dilute to 10 ml with the same solvent.

Reference solution (a). Dissolve 5 mg of *minocycline hydrochloride CRS* in *methanol R* and dilute to 10 ml with the same solvent.

Reference solution (b). Dissolve 5 mg of *minocycline hydrochloride CRS* and 5 mg of *oxytetracycline hydrochloride CRS* in *methanol R* and dilute to 10 ml with the same solvent.

Plate: *TLC octadecylsilyl silica gel F_{254} plate R.*

Mobile phase: mix 20 volumes of *acetonitrile R*, 20 volumes of *methanol R* and 60 volumes of a 63 g/l solution of *oxalic acid R* previously adjusted to pH 2 with *concentrated ammonia R.*

Application: 1 µl

Development: over 3/4 of the plate.

Drying: in air.

Detection: examine in ultraviolet light at 254 nm.

System suitability: reference solution (b):

– the chromatogram shows 2 clearly separated spots.

Results: the principal spot in the chromatogram obtained with the test solution is similar in position and size to the principal spot in the chromatogram obtained with reference solution (a).

B. To about 2 mg add 5 ml of *sulphuric acid R*. A bright yellow colour develops. Add 2.5 ml of *water R* to the solution. The solution becomes pale yellow.

C. It gives reaction (a) of chlorides (*2.3.1*).

TESTS

Solution S. Dissolve 0.200 g in *carbon dioxide-free water R* and dilute to 20.0 ml with the same solvent.

Appearance of solution. The solution is clear (*2.2.1*) and its absorbance (*2.2.25*) at 450 nm using a 1 cm cell is not greater than 0.23.

Dilute 1.0 ml of solution S to 10.0 ml with *water R.*

pH (*2.2.3*): 3.5 to 4.5 for solution S.

Light-absorbing impurities. *Carry out the measurement within 1 h of preparing solution S.*

The absorbance (*2.2.25*) of solution S measured at 560 nm is not greater than 0.06.

Related substances. Liquid chromatography (*2.2.29*).

Carry out the test protected from bright light. Store the solutions at a temperature of 2-8 °C and use them within 3 h of preparation.

Test solution (a). Dissolve 25.0 mg of the substance to be examined in the mobile phase and dilute to 100.0 ml with the mobile phase.

Test solution (b). Dilute 10.0 ml of test solution (a) to 20.0 ml with the mobile phase.

Reference solution (a). Dissolve 12.5 mg of *minocycline hydrochloride CRS* in the mobile phase and dilute to 100.0 ml with the mobile phase.

Reference solution (b). Dilute 2.0 ml of test solution (a) to 100.0 ml with the mobile phase.

Reference solution (c). Dilute 1.2 ml of test solution (a) to 100.0 ml with the mobile phase.

Reference solution (d). Dissolve 10 mg of *minocycline hydrochloride CRS* in 1 ml of *water R*. Boil the solution on a water-bath for 20 min. Dilute to 25 ml with the mobile phase.

Column:

– *size*: *l* = 0.20 m, Ø = 4.6 mm,

– *stationary phase*: *octylsilyl silica gel for chromatography R* (5 µm).

Mobile phase: mix 25 volumes of a 4 g/l solution of *sodium edetate R*, 27 volumes of *dimethylformamide R* and 50 volumes of a 28 g/l solution of *ammonium oxalate R*, adjust to pH 7.0 using *tetrabutylammonium hydroxide solution (104 g/l) R.*

Flow rate: 1 ml/min.

Detection: spectrophotometer at 280 nm.

Injection: 20 µl; inject test solution (a) and reference solutions (a), (b), (c) and (d).

Run time: 1.5 times the retention time of minocycline.

System suitability:

– *resolution*: minimum 2.0 between the peaks due to impurity A and minocycline in the chromatogram obtained with reference solution (d),

– *number of theoretical plates*: minimum 15 000, calculated for the peak due to minocycline in the chromatogram obtained with reference solution (a).

Limits:

– *impurity A*: not more than the area of the principal peak in the chromatogram obtained with reference solution (c) (1.2 per cent),

– *any other impurity*: not more than the area of the principal peak in the chromatogram obtained with reference solution (c) (1.2 per cent),

– *total of other impurities*: not more than the area of the principal peak in the chromatogram obtained with reference solution (b) (2.0 per cent).

Heavy metals (*2.4.8*): maximum 50 ppm.

0.5 g complies with limit test C. Prepare the standard using 2.5 ml of *lead standard solution (10 ppm Pb) R.*

Water (*2.5.12*): 5.0 per cent to 8.0 per cent, determined on 0.500 g.

Sulphated ash (*2.4.14*): maximum 0.5 per cent, determined on 1.0 g.

Bacterial endotoxins (*2.6.14*): less than 1.25 IU/mg, if intended for use in the manufacture of parenteral dosage forms without a further appropriate procedure for the removal of bacterial endotoxins.

ASSAY

Liquid chromatography (*2.2.29*) as described in the test for related substances with the following modifications.

Injection: test solution (b) and reference solution (a).

System suitability:

– *repeatability*: maximum relative standard deviation of the peak area for minocycline of 1.5 per cent after 6 injections of reference solution (a).

Calculate the percentage content of $C_{23}H_{28}ClN_3O_7$.

STORAGE

In an airtight container, protected from light. If the substance is sterile, store in a sterile, airtight, tamper-proof container.

LABELLING

The label states, where applicable, that the substance is free from bacterial endotoxins.

IMPURITIES

Specified impurities: *A, B, C, D.*

Monographs M

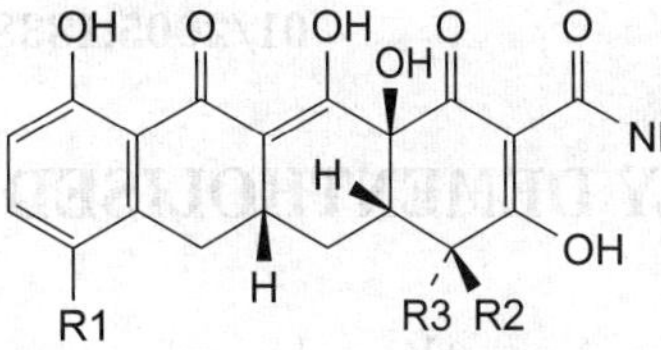

A. R1 = R3 = $N(CH_3)_2$, R2 = H: (4*R*,4a*S*,5a*R*,12a*S*)-4,7-bis(dimethylamino)-3,10,12,12a-tetrahydroxy-1,11-dioxo-1,4,4a,5,5a,6,11,12a-octahydrotetracene-2-carboxamide (4-epiminocycline),

B. R1 = R3 = H, R2 = $N(CH_3)_2$: (4*S*,4a*S*,5a*R*,12a*S*)-4-(dimethylamino)-3,10,12,12a-tetrahydroxy-1,11-dioxo-1,4,4a,5,5a,6,11,12a-octahydrotetracene-2-carboxamide (sancycline),

C. R1 = $NH\text{-}CH_3$, R2 = $N(CH_3)_2$, R3 = H: (4*S*,4a*S*,5a*R*,12a*S*)-4-(dimethylamino)-3,10,12,12a-tetrahydroxy-7-(methylamino)-1,11-dioxo-1,4,4a,5,5a,6,11,12a-octahydrotetracene-2-carboxamide (7-monodemethylminocycline),

D. R1 = NH2, R2 = $N(CH_3)_2$, R3 = H: (4*S*,4a*S*,5a*R*,12a*S*)-7-amino-4-(dimethylamino)-3,10,12,12a-tetrahydroxy-1,11-dioxo-1,4,4a,5,5a,6,11,12a-octahydrotetracene-2-carboxamide (7-aminosancycline).

01/2005:0937
corrected

MINOXIDIL

Minoxidilum

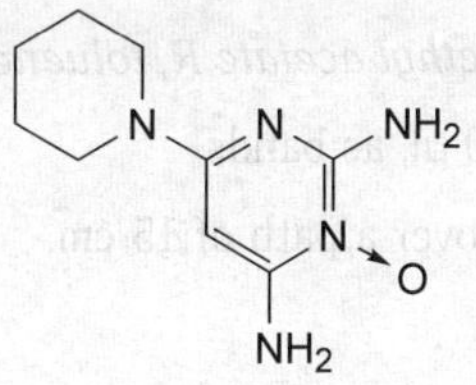

$C_9H_{15}N_5O$ M_r 209.3

DEFINITION

Minoxidil contains not less than 98.5 per cent and not more than the equivalent of 101.0 per cent of 6-(piperidin-1-yl)pyrimidine-2,4-diamine 3-oxide, calculated with reference to the dried substance.

CHARACTERS

A white or almost white, crystalline powder, slightly soluble in water, soluble in methanol and in propylene glycol.

IDENTIFICATION

First identification: A, B.

Second identification: A, C, D.

A. Dissolve 20.0 mg in *0.1 M hydrochloric acid* and dilute to 100.0 ml with the same solvent (solution a). Dilute 2.0 ml of solution (a) to 100.0 ml with *0.1 M hydrochloric acid* (solution b) and dilute 2.0 ml of solution (a) to 100.0 ml with *0.1 M sodium hydroxide* (solution c). Examine solutions (b) and (c) between 200 nm and 350 nm (*2.2.25*). Solution (b) shows two absorption maxima, at 230 nm and 281 nm. The specific absorbance at the maximum at 230 nm is 1015 to 1120 and that at the maximum at 281 nm is 1060 to 1170. Solution (c) shows three absorption maxima, at 230 nm, 262 nm and 288 nm. The specific absorbance at the maximum at 230 nm is 1525 to 1685, that at the maximum at 262 nm is 485 to 535 and that at the maximum at 288 nm is 555 to 605.

B. Examine by infrared absorption spectrophotometry (*2.2.24*), comparing with the spectrum obtained with *minoxidil CRS*.

C. Examine by thin-layer chromatography (*2.2.27*), using *silica gel GF_{254} R* as the coating substance.

Test solution. Dissolve 10 mg of the substance to be examined in *methanol R* and dilute to 10 ml with the same solvent.

Reference solution. Dissolve 10 mg of *minoxidil CRS* in *methanol R* and dilute to 10 ml with the same solvent.

Apply to the plate 2 µl of each solution. Develop over a path of 10 cm using a mixture of 1.5 volumes of *concentrated ammonia R* and 100 volumes of *methanol R*. Allow the plate to dry in air and examine in ultraviolet light at 254 nm. The principal spot in the chromatogram obtained with the test solution is similar in position and size to the principal spot in the chromatogram obtained with the reference solution.

D. Dissolve about 10 mg in 1 ml of *methanol R*. Add 0.1 ml of *copper sulphate solution R*. A green colour develops. The solution becomes greenish-yellow on the addition of 0.1 ml of *dilute hydrochloric acid R*.

TESTS

Appearance of solution. Dissolve 0.5 g in 12.5 ml of *methanol R* and dilute to 25 ml with *water R*. The solution is clear (*2.2.1*) and not more intensely coloured than reference solution Y_6 (*2.2.2, Method II*).

Related substances. Examine by liquid chromatography (*2.2.29*).

Test solution. Dissolve 25.0 mg of the substance to be examined in the mobile phase and dilute to 100.0 ml with the mobile phase.

Reference solution (a). Dilute 1.0 ml of the test solution to 100.0 ml with the mobile phase.

Reference solution (b). Dissolve 5 mg of *deoxyminoxidil CRS* (minoxidil impurity E) in the mobile phase and dilute to 20 ml with the mobile phase. To 2 ml of this solution, add 2 ml of the test solution and dilute to 10 ml with the mobile phase.

The chromatographic procedure may be carried out using:

- a stainless steel column 0.10 m long and 3 mm in internal diameter packed with *octadecylsilyl silica gel for chromatography R* (5 µm),
- as mobile phase at a flow rate of 1 ml/min a mixture prepared as follows: dissolve 3.0 g of *docusate sodium R* in a mixture of 10 ml of *glacial acetic acid R* and 300 ml of *water R*, adjust to pH 3.0 with *perchloric acid R* and add 700 ml of *methanol R*,
- as detector a spectrophotometer set at 240 nm,
- a 10 µl loop injector.

Inject 10 µl of each solution and continue the chromatography for twice the retention time of the principal peak. In the chromatogram obtained with the test solution, the sum of the areas of any peaks, apart from the principal peak, is not greater than 1.5 times the area of the principal peak in the chromatogram obtained with reference solution (a) (1.5 per cent). The test is not valid unless, in the chromatogram obtained with reference solution (b), the resolution between the peaks corresponding to minoxidil and deoxyminoxidil is at least 2.0. Disregard any peak with an area less than 0.1 times of that of the peak in the chromatogram obtained with reference solution (a).

Heavy metals (*2.4.8*). 1.0 g complies with the limit test C for heavy metals (20 ppm). Prepare the standard using 2 ml of *lead standard solution (10 ppm Pb) R*.

Loss on drying (*2.2.32*). Not more than 0.5 per cent, determined on 1.000 g by drying in an oven at 100-105 °C.

Sulphated ash (*2.4.14*). Not more than 0.1 per cent, determined on 1.0 g.

ASSAY

Dissolve 0.150 g in 50 ml of *anhydrous acetic acid R*. Titrate with *0.1 M perchloric acid*, determining the end-point potentiometrically (*2.2.20*). Carry out a blank titration.

1 ml of *0.1 M perchloric acid* is equivalent to 20.93 mg of $C_9H_{15}N_5O$.

STORAGE

Store protected from light.

IMPURITIES

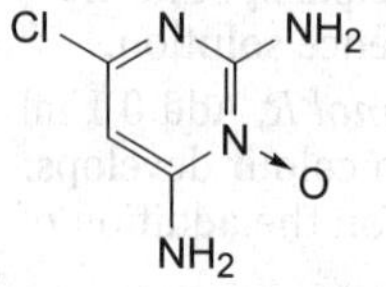

A. 6-chloropyrimidine-2,4-diamine 3-oxide,

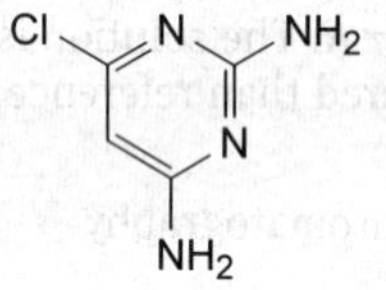

B. 6-chloropyrimidine-2,4-diamine,

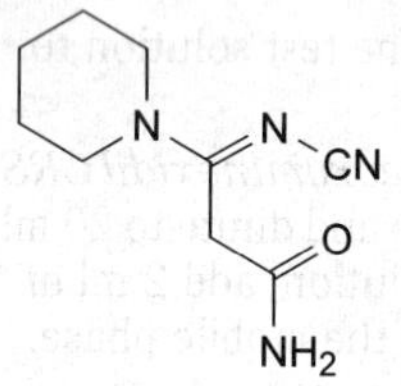

C. 3-(cyanoimino)-3-(piperidin-1-yl)propanamide,

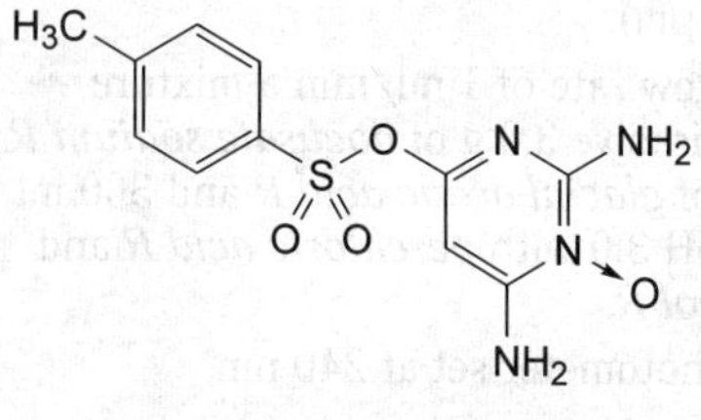

D. 6-[[(4-methylphenyl)sulphonyl]oxy]pyrimidine-2,4-diamine 3-oxide,

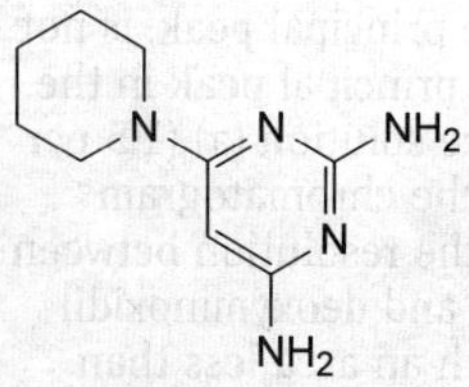

E. 6-(piperidin-1-yl)pyrimidine-2,4-diamine (desoxyminoxidil).

01/2005:1838

MINT OIL, PARTLY DEMENTHOLISED

Menthae arvensis aetheroleum partim mentholi privum

DEFINITION

Essential oil obtained by steam distillation from the fresh, flowering aerial parts, recently gathered from *Mentha canadensis* L. (syn. *M. arvensis* L. var. *glabrata* (Benth) Fern., *M. arvensis* var. *piperascens* Malinv. ex Holmes), followed by partial separation of menthol by crystallisation.

CHARACTERS

Appearance: colourless or pale yellow to greenish-yellow liquid with a characteristic odour.

IDENTIFICATION

First identification: B.

Second identification: A.

A. Thin-layer chromatography (*2.2.27*).

Test solution. Dissolve 0.1 ml of the substance to be examined in 1.0 ml of *toluene R*.

Reference solution. Dissolve 4 µl of *carvone R*, 4 µl of *pulegone R*, 10 µl of *menthyl acetate R*, 20 µl of *cineole R* and 50 mg of *menthol R* in 5 ml of *toluene R*.

Plate: *TLC silica gel F_{254} plate R.*

Mobile phase: *ethyl acetate R, toluene R (5:95 V/V).*

Application: 10 µl, as bands.

Development: over a path of 15 cm.

Drying: in air.

Detection A: examine in ultraviolet light at 254 nm.

Results A: see below the sequence of the zones present in the chromatograms obtained with the reference solution and the test solution. Furthermore, a quenching zone may be present in the upper third of the chromatogram obtained with the test solution.

Top of the plate	
Carvone and pulegone: a quenching zone	A quenching zone
	A quenching zone
Reference solution	**Test solution**

Detection B: spray with *anisaldehyde solution R* and heat at 100-105 °C for 5-10 min. Examine immediately in daylight.

Results B: see below the sequence of the zones present in the chromatograms obtained with the reference solution and the test solution. Furthermore, the zone due to cineole in the reference solution is absent in the chromatogram obtained with the test solution. No yellowish-brown zone below the intense reddish-violet zone is present in the chromatogram obtained with the test solution.

Top of the plate	
	An intense reddish-violet zone (near the solvent front)
Menthyl acetate: a bluish-violet zone	A bluish-violet zone (menthyl acetate)
	A strongly greenish zone
	A greenish zone
Carvone and pulegone: a reddish zone	A reddish zone
Cineole: a violet zone	
	A distinctly violet zone
Menthol: an intense blue zone	A very intense blue zone (menthol)
Reference solution	**Test solution**

B. Examine the chromatograms obtained in the test for chromatographic profile.
Results: the characteristic peaks in the chromatogram obtained with the test solution are approximately similar in retention time to those in the chromatogram obtained with the reference solution. Carvone may be absent from the chromatogram obtained with the test solution.

TESTS

Relative density (*2.2.5*): 0.888 to 0.910.

Refractive index (*2.2.6*): 1.456 to 1.470.

Optical rotation (*2.2.7*): − 16.0° to − 34.0°.

Acid value (*2.5.1*): maximum 1.0, determined on 5.00 g of the substance to be examined dissolved in 50 ml of the prescribed mixture of solvents.

Chromatographic profile. Gas chromatography (*2.2.28*): use the normalisation procedure.

Test solution. Dissolve 0.20 g of the substance to be examined in *hexane R* and dilute to 10.0 ml with the same solvent.

Reference solution. Dissolve 10 mg of *limonene R*, 20 mg of *cineole R*, 40 mg of *menthone R*, 10 mg of *isomenthone R*, 40 mg of *menthyl acetate R*, 20 mg of *isopulegol R*, 60 mg of *menthol R*, 20 mg of *pulegone R* and 10 mg of *carvone R* in *hexane R* and dilute to 10.0 ml with the same solvent.

Column:
– *material*: fused silica,
– *size*: l = 30 m (a film thickness of 1 μm may be used) to 60 m (a film thickness of 0.2 μm may be used), Ø = 0.25-0.53 mm,
– *stationary phase*: *macrogol 20 000 R*.

Carrier gas: *helium for chromatography R*.

Flow rate: 1.5 ml/min.

Split ratio: 1:100.

Temperature:

	Time (min)	Temperature (°C)
Column	0 - 10	60
	10 - 70	60 → 180
	70 - 75	180
Injection port		200
Detector		220

Detection: flame ionisation.

Injection: 1.0 μl.

Elution order: order indicated in the composition of the reference solution. Record the retention times of these substances.

System suitability: reference solution:
– *resolution*: minimum 1.5 between the peaks due to limonene and cineole.

Using the retention times determined from the chromatogram obtained with the reference solution, locate the components of the reference solution in the chromatogram obtained with the test solution.

Determine the percentage content of these components. The percentages are within the following ranges:
– *limonene*: 1.5 per cent to 7.0 per cent,
– *cineole*: maximum 1.5 per cent,
– *menthone*: 17.0 per cent to 35.0 per cent,
– *isomenthone*: 5.0 per cent to 13.0 per cent,
– *menthyl acetate*: 1.5 per cent to 7.0 per cent,
– *isopulegol*: 1.0 per cent to 3.0 per cent,
– *menthol*: 30.0 per cent to 50.0 per cent,
– *pulegone*: maximum 2.0 per cent,
– *carvone*: maximum 2.0 per cent.

The ratio of cineole content to limonene content is less than 1.

STORAGE

In a well-filled, airtight container, protected from light, at a temperature not exceeding 25 °C.

01/2005:1655

MITOMYCIN

Mitomycinum

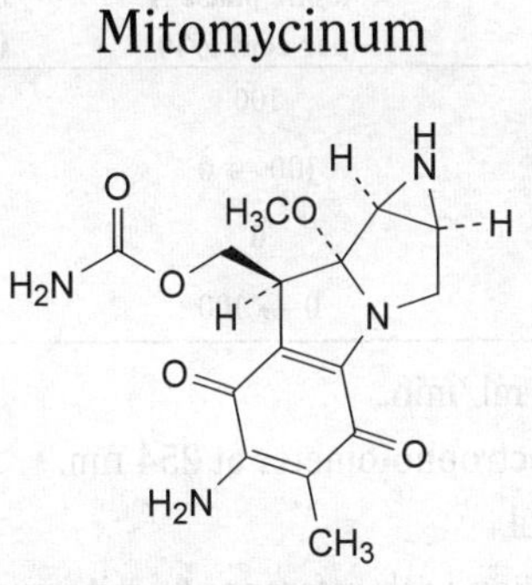

$C_{15}H_{18}N_4O_5$ *M*$_r$ 334.3

DEFINITION

[(1a*S*,8*S*,8a*R*,8b*S*)-6-Amino-8a-methoxy-5-methyl-4,7-dioxo-1,1a,2,4,7,8,8a,8b-octahydroazirino[2′,3′:3,4]pyrrolo[1,2-*a*]indol-8-yl]methyl carbamate (mitomycin C).

Substance produced by a strain of *Streptomyces caespitotus*.

Content: 97.0 per cent to 102.0 per cent (anhydrous substance).

CHARACTERS

Appearance: blue-violet crystals or crystalline powder.

Solubility: slightly soluble in water, freely soluble in dimethylacetamide, sparingly soluble in methanol, slightly soluble in acetone.

IDENTIFICATION

A. Infrared absorption spectrophotometry (*2.2.24*).
Comparison: *mitomycin CRS*.

B. Examine the chromatograms obtained in the assay.

Results: the principal peak in the chromatogram obtained with the test solution is similar in retention time and size to the principal peak in the chromatogram obtained with reference solution (a).

TESTS

pH (*2.2.3*): 5.5 to 7.5.

Dissolve 10 mg in 10 ml of *carbon dioxide-free water R*.

Related substances. Liquid chromatography (*2.2.29*). *Prepare the solutions immediately before use.*

Test solution. Dissolve 50.0 mg of the substance to be examined in *methanol R* and dilute to 10.0 ml with the same solvent.

Reference solution (a). Dilute 1.0 ml of the test solution to 100.0 ml with *methanol R*. Dilute 5.0 ml of this solution to 10.0 ml with *methanol R*.

Reference solution (b). Dissolve 10 mg of *cinnamamide R* in *methanol R* and dilute to 10 ml with the same solvent. Mix 2 ml of this solution and 1 ml of the test solution and dilute to 10 ml with *methanol R*.

Column:

- *size*: l = 0.25 m, Ø = 4.6 mm,
- *stationary phase*: spherical *base-deactivated end-capped octadecylsilyl silica gel for chromatography R* (5 µm),
- *temperature*: 30 °C.

Mobile phase:

- *mobile phase A*: *methanol R*, 0.77 g/l solution of *ammonium acetate R* (20:80 *V/V*);
- *mobile phase B*: *methanol R*, 0.77 g/l solution of *ammonium acetate R* (50:50 *V/V*);

Time (min)	Mobile phase A (per cent *V/V*)	Mobile phase B (per cent *V/V*)
0 - 10	100	0
10 - 30	100 → 0	0 → 100
30 - 45	0	100
45 - 50	0 → 100	100 → 0

Flow rate: 1.0 ml/min.

Detection: spectrophotometer at 254 nm.

Injection: 10 µl.

Relative retention with reference to mitomycin (retention time = about 21 min): impurity D = about 0.6; impurity C = about 1.2; impurity A = about 1.3; impurity B = about 1.6.

System suitability: reference solution (b):

- *resolution*: minimum 15.0 between the peaks due to mitomycin and impurity A.

Limits:

- *correction factor*: for the calculation of content, multiply the peak area of impurity A by 0.35,
- *impurities A, B, C, D*: for each impurity, not more than the area of the principal peak in the chromatogram obtained with reference solution (a) (0.5 per cent),
- *any other impurity*: for each impurity, not more than the area of the principal peak in the chromatogram obtained with reference solution (a) (0.5 per cent),
- *total*: not more than 4 times the area of the principal peak in the chromatogram obtained with reference solution (a) (2.0 per cent),
- *disregard limit*: 0.1 times the area of the principal peak in the chromatogram obtained with reference solution (a) (0.05 per cent).

Water (*2.5.12*): maximum 2.5 per cent, determined on 0.30 g.

Bacterial endotoxins (*2.6.14, Method B*): less than 10 IU/ mg, if intended for use in the manufacture of parenteral dosage forms without a further appropriate procedure for the removal of bacterial endotoxins.

ASSAY

Liquid chromatography (*2.2.29*).

Test solution. Dissolve 50.0 mg of the substance to be examined in *dimethylacetamide R* and dilute to 100.0 ml with the same solvent.

Reference solution (a). Dissolve 50.0 mg of *mitomycin CRS* in *dimethylacetamide R* and dilute to 100.0 ml with the same solvent.

Reference solution (b). Dissolve 10 mg of *cinnamamide R* in *methanol R* and dilute to 20 ml with the same solvent. Mix 2 ml of this solution with 2 ml of reference solution (a).

Column:

- *size*: l = 0.30 m, Ø = 3.9 mm,
- *stationary phase*: *end-capped phenylsilyl silica gel for chromatography R* (10 µm) with a specific surface area of 330 m^2/g, a carbon loading of 8 per cent and a pore size of 12.5 nm.

Mobile phase: mix 23 volumes of *methanol R*, 77 volumes of a solution containing 2.05 g/l of *ammonium acetate R* and 2.8 ml/l of *dilute acetic acid R*.

Flow rate: 2.0 ml/min.

Detection: variable wavelength spectrophotometer capable of operating at 365 nm and 254 nm.

Injection: 20 µl.

Run time: twice the retention time of mitomycin.

Relative retention with reference to mitomycin (retention time = about 8 min): impurity A = about 1.2.

System suitability:

- *resolution*: minimum 1.8 between the peaks due to mitomycin and impurity A in the chromatogram obtained with reference solution (b) at 254 nm,
- *symmetry factor*: maximum 1.3 for the principal peak in the chromatogram obtained with reference solution (a) at 365 nm.

Calculate the percentage content of $C_{15}H_{18}N_4O_5$, from the chromatograms obtained at 365 nm and the declared content of *mitomycin CRS*.

STORAGE

Protected from light.

LABELLING

The label states where applicable that the substance is free from bacterial endotoxins.

IMPURITIES

Specified impurities: A, B, C, D.

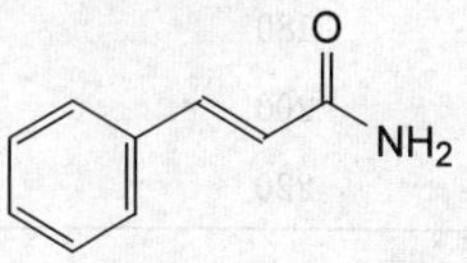

A. (*E*)-3-phenylprop-2-enamide (cinnamamide),

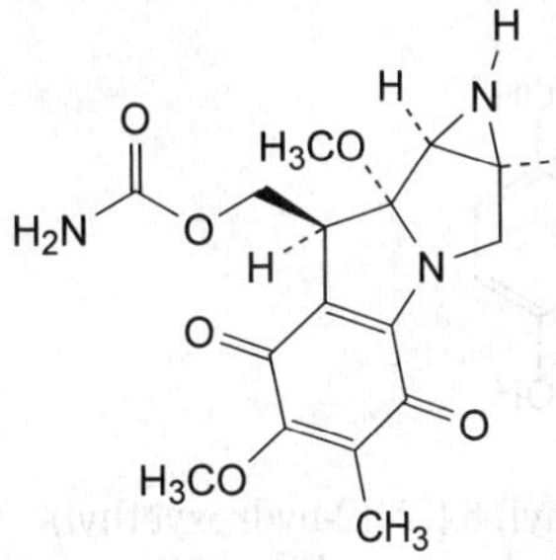

B. [(1a*S*,8*S*,8a*R*,8b*S*)-6,8a-dimethoxy-5-methyl-4,7-dioxo-1,1a,2,4,7,8,8a,8b-octahydroazirino[2′,3′:3,4]pyrrolo[1,2-*a*]indol-8-yl]methyl carbamate (mitomycin A),

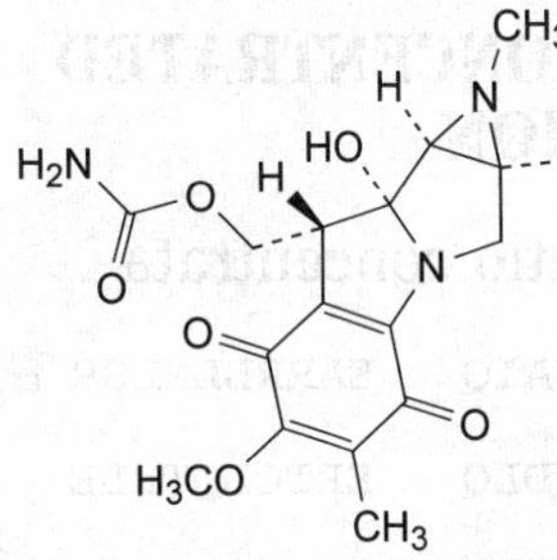

C. [(1a*S*,8*R*,8a*R*,8b*S*)-8a-hydroxy-6-methoxy-1,5-dimethyl-4,7-dioxo-1,1a,2,4,7,8,8a,8b-octahydroazirino[2′,3′:3,4]pyrrolo[1,2-*a*]indol-8-yl]methyl carbamate (mitomycin B),

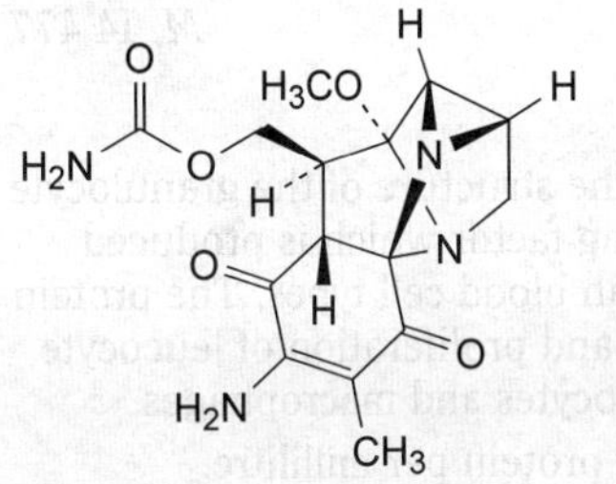

D. [(1*S*,2*S*,4*S*,5*R*,6*S*,6a*R*,10a*S*,11*S*)-8-amino-5-methoxy-9-methyl-7,10-dioxo-2,3,6,6a,7,10-hexahydro-1,2,5-metheno-1*H*,5*H*-imidazo[2,1-*i*]indol-6-yl]methyl carbamate (albomitomycin C).

01/2005:1243

MITOXANTRONE HYDROCHLORIDE

Mitoxantroni hydrochloridum

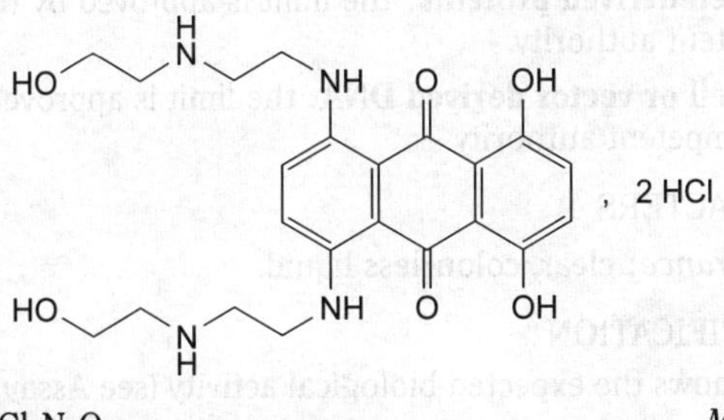

$C_{22}H_{30}Cl_2N_4O_6$ M_r 517.4

DEFINITION

Mitoxantrone hydrochloride contains not less than 97.0 per cent and not more than the equivalent of 102.0 per cent of 1,4-dihydroxy-5,8-bis[[2-[(2-hydroxyethyl)amino]ethyl]amino]anthracene-9,10-dione dihydrochloride, calculated with reference to the anhydrous, ethanol-free substance.

CHARACTERS

A dark blue, electrostatic powder, hygroscopic, sparingly soluble in water, slightly soluble in methanol, practically insoluble in acetone.

CAUTION: Mitoxantrone hydrochloride and impurity A are electrostatic. The use of an antistatic gun or other suitable method to discharge the solids before weighing or transfer is recommended.

IDENTIFICATION

A. Dissolve 2 mg to 3 mg in 1 ml of *methanol R* by warming in a water-bath at 40-50 °C. Evaporate the solution to dryness under a stream of dry nitrogen, warming gently if necessary. Examine the residue by infrared absorption spectrophotometry (*2.2.24*), comparing with the *Ph. Eur. reference spectrum of mitoxantrone hydrochloride.*

B. It gives reaction (b) of chlorides (2.3.1).

TESTS

Ethanol. Not more than 1.6 per cent *m/m* of ethanol, determined by gas chromatography (*2.2.28*), using *propanol R* as the internal standard.

Internal standard solution. Dilute 2.0 ml of *propanol R* to 100 ml with *water R*. Dilute 5.0 ml of this solution to 100 ml with *water R*.

Test solution. Mix 0.100 g of the substance to be examined with 2.0 ml of the internal standard solution and dilute to 5.0 ml with *water R*. Place the flask in a sonic bath for 2 min then shake the flask for 2 min. If necessary repeat the sonication and shaking until dissolution is complete.

Reference solution. Dilute 2.0 ml of *ethanol R* to 100.0 ml with *water R*. Dilute 5.0 ml of this solution to 100.0 ml with *water R*. Dilute 10.0 ml of this solution and 10.0 ml of the internal standard solution to 25.0 ml with *water R*.

The chromatographic procedure may be carried out using:

– a column 2 m long and 3 mm in internal diameter packed with *ethylvinylbenzene-divinylbenzene copolymer R*,
– *helium for chromatography R* as the carrier gas at a flow rate of 19 ml/min,
– a flame-ionisation detector,

maintaining the column at a temperature of 120 °C, the temperature of the injector at 175 °C and the temperature of the detector at 210 °C.

Inject 1 µl of the test solution and 1 µl of the reference solution. The retention times are about 1 min for ethanol and about 2 min for propanol. The test is not valid unless the resolution between the peaks due to ethanol and propanol in the chromatogram obtained with the reference solution is at least six. Calculate the content of ethanol taking its density (*2.2.5*) to be 0.790 g/ml at 20 °C.

Related substances. Examine by liquid chromatography (*2.2.29*) as prescribed under Assay. In the chromatogram obtained with the test solution, the area of any peak apart from the principal peak is not greater than the area of the peak in the chromatogram obtained with reference solution (b) (1 per cent) and the sum of the areas of all the peaks apart from the principal peak is not greater than twice the area of the peak in the chromatogram obtained with reference solution (b) (2 per cent). Disregard any peak with an area less than that of the principal peak in the chromatogram obtained with reference solution (d).

Water (*2.5.12*). Not more than 6.0 per cent, determined on 0.300 g by the semi-micro determination of water.

ASSAY

Examine by liquid chromatography (*2.2.29*).

Test solution. Dissolve 20.0 mg of the substance to be examined in about 40 ml of the mobile phase, if necessary with the aid of ultrasonication, and dilute to 50.0 ml with the mobile phase.

Reference solution (a). Dissolve 20.0 mg of *mitoxantrone hydrochloride CRS* in about 40 ml of the mobile phase, if necessary with the aid of ultrasonication, and dilute to 50.0 ml with the mobile phase.

Reference solution (b). Dilute 1 ml of the test solution to 100 ml with the mobile phase.

Reference solution (c). Dissolve 2.0 mg of *mitoxantrone impurity A CRS* in 1.0 ml of reference solution (a).

Reference solution (d). Dilute 1 ml of reference solution (b) to 10 ml with the mobile phase.

The chromatographic procedure may be carried out using:

- a column 0.30 m long and 3.0 mm in internal diameter packed with *phenylsilyl silica gel for chromatography R* (10 μm),
- as mobile phase at a flow rate of 3 ml/min a mixture of 750 volumes of *water R*, 250 volumes of *acetonitrile R* and 25 volumes of a solution prepared as follows: dissolve 22.0 g of *sodium heptanesulphonate R* in about 150 ml of *water R* and filter through a 0.45 μm filter; wash the filter with *water R* and combine the filtrate and washings; add 32.0 ml of *glacial acetic acid R* and dilute to 250 ml with *water R*,
- as detector a spectrophotometer set at 254 nm,
- a loop injector.

Inject separately 50 μl of each solution. The test is not valid unless the resolution between the two principal peaks in the chromatogram obtained with reference solution (c) is at least 3.0. Record the chromatogram obtained with the test solution for three times the retention time of the principal peak. Calculate the content of $C_{22}H_{30}Cl_2N_4O_6$ from the peak areas in the chromatograms obtained with the test solution and reference solution (a) and the declared content of $C_{22}H_{30}Cl_2N_4O_6$ in *mitoxantrone hydrochloride CRS*.

STORAGE

Store in an airtight container.

IMPURITIES

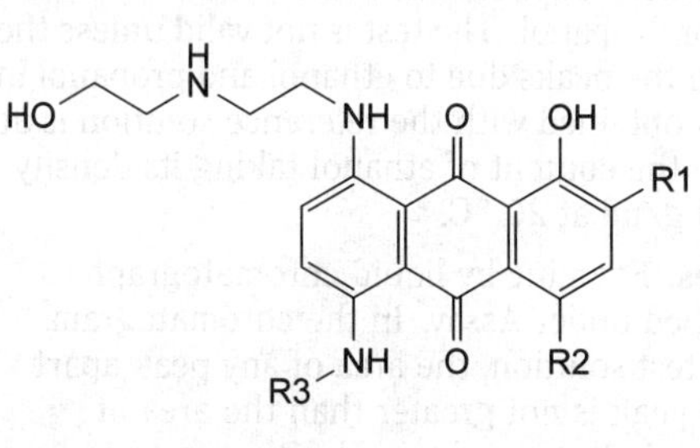

A. R1 = R3 = H, R2 = OH: 1-amino-5,8-dihydroxy-4-[[2-[(2-hydroxyethyl)amino]ethyl]amino]anthracene-9,10-dione,

B. R1 = R2 = H, R3 = CH_2-CH_2-NH-CH_2-CH_2OH: 5-hydroxy-1,4-bis[[2-[(2-hydroxyethyl)amino]ethyl]amino]anthracene-9,10-dione,

C. R1 = Cl, R2 = OH, R3 = CH_2-CH_2NH-CH_2-CH_2OH: 2-chloro-1,4-dihydroxy-5,8-bis[[2-[(2-hydroxyethyl)amino]ethyl]amino]anthracene-9,10-dione,

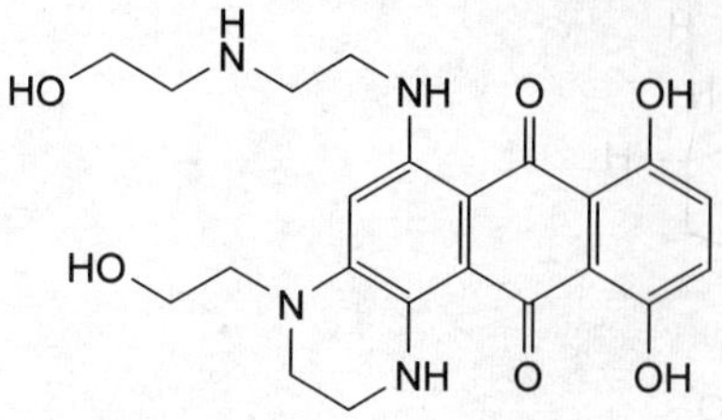

D. 8,11-dihydroxy-4-(2-hydroxyethyl)-6-[[2-[(2-hydroxyethyl)amino]ethyl]amino]-1,2,3,4-tetrahydronaphtho[2,3-*f*]quinoxaline-7,12-dione.

01/2005:1641

MOLGRAMOSTIM CONCENTRATED SOLUTION

Molgramostimi solutio concentrata

APARSPSPST	QPWEHVNAIQ	EARRLLNLSR
DTAAEMNETV	EVISEMFDLQ	EPTCLQTRLE
LYKQGLRGSL	TKLKGPLTMM	ASHYKQHCPP
TPETSCATQI	ITFESFKENL	KDFLLVIPFD
CWEPVQE		

$C_{639}H_{1007}N_{171}O_{196}S_8$ M_r 14 477

DEFINITION

Solution of a protein having the structure of the granulocyte macrophage colony stimulating factor which is produced and secreted by various human blood cell types. The protein stimulates the differentiation and proliferation of leucocyte stem cells into mature granulocytes and macrophages.

Content: minimum 2.0 mg of protein per millilitre.

Potency: minimum 0.7 × 10^7 IU per milligram of protein.

PRODUCTION

Molgramostim concentrated solution is produced by a method based on recombinant DNA (rDNA) technology, using bacteria as host cells. It is produced under conditions designed to minimise microbial contamination of the product.

Prior to release, the following tests are carried out on each batch of the final bulk product, unless exemption has been granted by the competent authority.

Host-cell derived proteins: the limit is approved by the competent authority.

Host-cell or vector derived DNA: the limit is approved by the competent authority.

CHARACTERS

Appearance: clear, colourless liquid.

IDENTIFICATION

A. It shows the expected biological activity (see Assay).

B. Isoelectric focusing (*2.2.54*).

Test solution. Dilute the preparation to be examined with *water R* to obtain a concentration of 0.25 mg/ml.

Reference solution (a). Dilute *molgramostim CRS* with *water R* to obtain a concentration of 0.25 mg/ml.

Reference solution (b). Use an isoelectric point (pI) calibration solution, in the pI range of 2.5-6.5, prepared according to the manufacturer's instructions.

Focusing:

- *pH gradient*: 4.0-6.5,
- *catholyte*: 8.91 g/l (0.1 M) solution of *β-alanine R*,
- *anolyte*: 14.7 g/l (0.1 M) solution of *glutamic acid R* in a 50 per cent *V/V* solution of *dilute phosphoric acid R* (0.5 M),
- *application*: 20 μl.

Detection: immerse the gel in a suitable volume of a solution containing 115 g/l of *trichloroacetic acid R* and 34.5 g/l of *sulphosalicylic acid R* and shake the container gently for 30 min. Transfer the gel to a mixture of 32 volumes of *glacial acetic acid R*, 100 volumes of *ethanol R* and 268 volumes of *water R* (mixture A) and rinse for 5 min. Immerse the gel for 10 min in a staining solution prewarmed to 60 °C and prepared by adding *brilliant blue R* at a concentration of 1.2 g/l to mixture A. Wash the gel in several containers with mixture A and keep the gel in this mixture until the background is clear (12-24 h). After adequate destaining, soak the gel for 1 h in a 10 per cent *V/V* solution of *glycerol R* in mixture A.

System suitability:

- in the electropherogram obtained with reference solution (b), the relevant isoelectric point markers are distributed along the entire length of the gel,
- in the electropherogram obtained with reference solution (a), the pI of the principal band is 4.9 to 5.4.

Results: the principal band in the electropherogram obtained with the test solution corresponds in position to the principal band in the electropherogram obtained with reference solution (a). Plot the migration distances of the relevant pI markers versus their pI and determine the isoelectric points of the principal component of each of the test solution and reference solution (a). They do not differ by more than 0.2 pI units.

C. Examine the electropherograms obtained under reducing conditions in the test for impurities with molecular masses differing from that of molgramostim. The principal band in the electropherogram obtained with test solution (a) is similar in position to the principal band in the electropherogram obtained with reference solution (a).

D. Peptide mapping (*2.2.55*).

Test solution. Introduce 50 μl of *tris-hydrochloride buffer solution pH 8.0 R* and 50 μl of the preparation to be examined at a concentration of 2 mg/ml into a polypropylene tube of 0.5 ml capacity. Add 4 μl of a 1 mg/ml solution of *trypsin for peptide mapping R* in a 0.01 per cent *V/V* solution of *trifluoroacetic acid R*, cap tightly and mix well. Incubate at about 37 °C for 18 h. Add 125 μl of a 764 g/l (8 M) solution of *guanidine hydrochloride R* and mix well. Add 10 μl of a 154.2 g/l (1 M) solution of *dithiothreitol R* and mix well. Place the capped tube in boiling water for 1 min. Cool to room temperature.

Reference solution. Prepare at the same time and in the same manner as for the test solution but use *molgramostim CRS* instead of the preparation to be examined.

Examine the 2 tryptic digests by liquid chromatography (*2.2.29*).

Column:

- *size*: l = 0.10 m, Ø = 4.6 mm,
- *stationary phase*: *octadecylsilyl silica gel for chromatography R* (5 μm) with a pore size of 30 nm.

Mobile phase:

- *mobile phase A*: dilute 1 ml of *trifluoroacetic acid R* in 1000 ml of *water R*;
- *mobile phase B*: dilute 1 ml of *trifluoroacetic acid R* in 100 ml of *water R*; add 900 ml of *acetonitrile for chromatography R* and mix;

Time (min)	Mobile Phase A (per cent *V/V*)	Mobile Phase B (per cent *V/V*)
0 - 35.0	100 → 65	0 → 35
35.0 - 105.0	65 → 35	35 → 65
105.0 - 107.5	35 → 100	65 → 0
107.5 - 120.0	100	0

Flow rate: 1.0 ml/min.

Detection: spectrophotometer at 214 nm.

Equilibration: at initial conditions for at least 12 min.

Injection: 200 μl.

System suitability: the chromatograms obtained with the reference solution and the test solution are qualitatively similar to the *Ph. Eur. reference chromatogram of molgramostim digest*.

Results: the profile of the chromatogram obtained with the test solution corresponds to that of the chromatogram obtained with the reference solution.

E. *N*-Terminal sequence analysis.

Perform the Edman degradation using an automated solid-phase sequencer, operated in accordance with the manufacturer's instructions.

Load about 1 nmol of the test preparation to a sequencing cartridge using the protocol provided by the manufacturer. Run 16 sequencing cycles, noting, if appropriate, the presence of proline at positions 2, 6, 8 and 12.

Identify the phenylthiohydantoin (PTH)-amino acids released at each sequencing cycle by reverse-phase liquid chromatography. The procedure may be carried out using the column and reagents recommended by the manufacturer of the sequencing equipment for the separation of PTH-amino acids.

The separation procedure is calibrated using:

- the mixture of PTH-amino acids provided by the manufacturer of the sequencer, with the gradient conditions adjusted as indicated to achieve optimum resolution of all amino acids,
- a sample obtained from a blank sequencing cycle obtained as recommended by the equipment manufacturer.

Results: the first 16 amino acids are: Ala-Pro-Ala-Arg-Ser-Pro-Ser-Pro-Ser-Thr-Gln-Pro-Trp-Glu-His-Val.

TESTS

Impurities with molecular masses differing from that of molgramostim. Polyacrylamide gel electrophoresis (*2.2.31*) under both reducing and non-reducing conditions.

Gel dimensions: 0.75 mm thick.

Resolving gel: 14 per cent acrylamide.

Sample buffer A. Mix equal volumes of *water R* and *concentrated SDS-PAGE sample buffer R*.

Sample buffer B (reducing conditions). Mix equal volumes of *water R* and *concentrated SDS-PAGE sample buffer for reducing conditions R*.

Monographs M

Test solution (a). Dilute the preparation to be examined in *water R* to obtain a concentration of 1.0 mg/ml. To 1 volume of this solution add 1 volume of *concentrated SDS-PAGE sample buffer R.*

Test solution (b) (2 per cent control). Dilute 0.020 ml of test solution (a) to 1.0 ml with sample buffer A.

Test solution (c) (1 per cent control). To 0.20 ml of test solution (b) add 0.20 ml of sample buffer A.

Test solution (d) (0.5 per cent control). To 0.20 ml of test solution (c) add 0.20 ml of sample buffer A.

Test solution (e) (0.25 per cent control). To 0.20 ml of test solution (d) add 0.20 ml of sample buffer A.

Test solution (f) (0.1 per cent control). To 0.20 ml of test solution (e) add 0.30 ml of sample buffer A.

Test solution (g) (0.05 per cent control). To 0.20 ml of test solution (f) add 0.20 ml of sample buffer A.

Test solution (h) (0.025 per cent control). To 0.20 ml of test solution (g) add 0.20 ml of sample buffer A.

Test solution (i). Prepare as for test solution (a), but using *concentrated SDS-PAGE sample buffer for reducing conditions R.*

Test solutions (j)-(p). Prepare as for test solutions (b)-(h), but using sample buffer B.

Reference solution (a). Dilute *molgramostim CRS* in *water R* to obtain a concentration of 0.02 mg/ml. Mix 1 volume of this solution with 1 volume of *concentrated SDS-PAGE sample buffer R.*

Reference solution (b). Prepare as for reference solution (a), but using *concentrated SDS-PAGE sample buffer for reducing conditions R.*

Reference solution (c). Use a solution of molecular mass markers suitable for calibrating SDS-PAGE gels in the range of 14 400-94 000. Dissolve in sample buffer or sample buffer (reducing conditions), as appropriate.

Sample treatment: boil for 3 min.

Application: 50 µl; apply reduced and non-reduced solutions to separate gels.

Detection: silver staining as described below.

Immerse the gel overnight in a mixture of 10 volumes of *acetic acid R,* 40 volumes of *water R* and 50 volumes of *methanol R.* Transfer the gel to a 100 g/l solution of *glutaraldehyde R* and shake for about 30 min. Replace the glutaraldehyde solution with *water R,* and keep the gel in *water R* for 20 min. Repeat this washing-step twice. Transfer the gel to a mixture containing 0.75 g/l of *sodium hydroxide R,* 14 g/l of *concentrated ammonia R* and 8 g/l of *silver nitrate R.* This solution is prepared immediately before use. Place the gel on a shaker in the dark for 5 min. Wash the gel for 30 s in each of 3 containers with *water R* and shake the gel in a mixture consisting of 0.05 g/l of *citric acid R,* 0.05 per cent *V/V* of *formaldehyde R* and 0.005 per cent *V/V* of *methanol R* in *water R.* Protein bands become visible during this step. Keep the gel in the solution until sufficiently stained and then rinse the gel repeatedly with *water R* in a shaking water bath. Soak gels in a solution consisting of 10 per cent *V/V* of *acetic acid R* and 1 per cent *V/V* of *glycerol R.*

System suitability:

- the validation criteria are met (*2.2.31*),
- a band is seen in the electropherogram obtained with test solution (h),
- a gradation of intensity of staining is seen in the electropherograms obtained with test solutions (a)-(h) and (i)-(p),
- the molecular mass of the principal band in the electrophoregram obtained with reference solution (a) or (b) is within the range of 15 100 to 17 100.

Limits: compare the staining intensity of each non-molgramostim band observed in the electropherogram obtained with test solution (a) to the staining intensity of the principal band in the electropherograms obtained with test solutions (b)-(h). Proceed similarly with the electropherograms obtained with test solutions (i)-(p). The impurity level is estimated as the dilution, in percentage, of the solution giving the electropherogram with the closest intensity of staining.

Reducing conditions:

- *impurity with an apparent molecular mass of 20 000*: maximum 1 per cent,
- *impurity with an apparent molecular mass of 25 000*: maximum 0.1 per cent,
- *impurity with an apparent molecular mass of 30 000*: maximum 0.3 per cent,
- *total*: maximum 2 per cent.

Non-reducing conditions:

- *total of all impurities of molecular masses higher than 30 000*: maximum 1 per cent.

Related proteins. Liquid chromatography (*2.2.29*): use the normalisation procedure.

Test solution (a). Dilute the preparation to be examined with *0.05 M phosphate buffer solution pH 7.0 R* to obtain a concentration of 0.5 mg/ml.

Test solution (b). Mix 1 volume of test solution (a) with 4 volumes of a 0.125 mg/ml solution of *human albumin R* or *bovine albumin R* in *0.05 M phosphate buffer solution pH 7.0 R.*

Reference solution (a). Dilute *molgramostim CRS* with *0.05 M phosphate buffer solution pH 7.0 R* to obtain a concentration of 0.5 mg/ml.

Reference solution (b). Mix 1 volume of reference solution (a) with 4 volumes of a 0.125 mg/ml solution of *human albumin R* or *bovine albumin R* in *0.05 M phosphate buffer solution pH 7.0 R.*

Column:

- *size*: *l* = 0.15 m, Ø = 4.6 mm,
- *stationary phase*: *butylsilyl silica gel for chromatography R* (5 µm) with a pore size of 30 nm.

Mobile phase:

- *mobile phase A*: to about 800 ml of *water R* add 1.0 ml of *trifluoroacetic acid R* and dilute to 1000 ml with *water R*;
- *mobile phase B*: to 100 ml of *water R* add 1.0 ml of *trifluoroacetic acid R* and 900 ml of *acetonitrile for chromatography R*;

Time (min)	Mobile Phase A (per cent *V/V*)	Mobile Phase B (per cent *V/V*)
0 - 30	64 → 44	36 → 56
30 - 35	44 → 0	56 → 100
35 - 45	0	100
45 - 50	0 → 64	100 → 36
50 - 60	64	36

Flow rate: 1.2 ml/min.

Detection: spectrophotometer at 214 nm.

Injection: 100 µl of test solution (a), reference solutions (a) and (b).

Monographs M

System suitability: reference solution (b):

- *retention time*: molgramostin = about 22 min,
- *repeatability*: maximum relative standard deviation of 5.0 per cent after 4 injections,
- *resolution*: minimum 2 between the peaks due to albumin and molgramostim.

Limits:

- *any impurity*: for each impurity, maximum 1.5 per cent,
- *total of impurities eluting between 5 min and 30 min*: maximum 4 per cent.

Bacterial endotoxins (*2.6.14*): less than 5 IU in the volume that contains 1.0 mg of protein.

ASSAY

Protein. Liquid chromatography (*2.2.29*) as described in the test for related proteins.

Injection: 150 µl of test solution (b) and reference solution (b).

Calculate the content of molgramostim using the declared content of molgramostim in *molgramostim CRS*.

Potency. Determination of the biological activity of molgramostim concentrated solution based on the stimulation of proliferation of TF-1 cells by molgramostim. The following method uses the conversion of tetrazolium bromide (MTT) as a staining method. Validated alternative stains such as Almar blue have also been found suitable.

TF-1 cells are incubated with varying dilutions of test and reference preparations of molgramostim. They are then incubated with a solution of MTT. This cytochemical stain is converted by cellular dehydrogenases to a purple formazan product. The formazan is then measured spectrophotometrically. The potency of the preparation to be examined is determined by comparison of the dilutions of the test preparation with the dilutions of the appropriate International Standard of molgramostim or with a reference preparation calibrated in International Units, which yield the same response (50 per cent maximal stimulation).

The International Unit is the activity contained in a stated amount of the appropriate International Standard. The equivalence in International Units of the International Standard is stated by the World Health Organisation.

Add 50 µl of dilution medium to all wells of a 96-well microtitre plate. Add an additional 50 µl of this solution to the wells designed for the blanks. Add 50 µl of each solution to be tested in triplicate (test preparation and reference preparation at a concentration of about 65 IU/ml, plus a series of 10 twofold dilutions to obtain a standard curve). Then add to each well 50 µl of a TF-1 cell suspension containing 3×10^5 cells per millilitre, maintaining the cells in a uniform suspension during addition.

Incubate the plate at 36.0-38.0 °C for a minimum of 24 h in a humidified incubator using 6 ± 1 per cent CO_2. Add 25 µl of a 5.0 g/l sterile solution of *tetrazolium bromide R* to each well. Reincubate for 5 h. Remove the plates from the incubator and add to each well 100 µl of a 240 g/l solution of *sodium dodecyl sulphate R* previously adjusted to pH 2.7 with hydrochloric acid. Reincubate overnight.

Determine the relative quantity of purple formazan product formed in each well by measuring the absorbance (*2.2.25*) using a 96-well microtitre plate reader. Read each plate at 570 nm and at 690 nm. Subtract the reading at 690 nm from the reading at 570 nm. Analyse the data by fitting a sigmoidal dose-response curve to the data obtained and by using a suitable statistical method, for example the 4-parameter model (see *5.3*).

The estimated potency is not less than 80 per cent and not more than 125 per cent of the stated potency. The confidence limits (P = 0.95) of the estimated potency are not less than 74 per cent and not more than 136 per cent of the stated potency.

STORAGE

In an airtight container, protected from light, at a temperature below − 65 °C.

LABELLING

The label states:

- the content, in milligrams of protein per millilitre,
- the potency, in International Units per milligram of protein.

01/2005:1449
corrected

MOMETASONE FUROATE

Mometasoni furoas

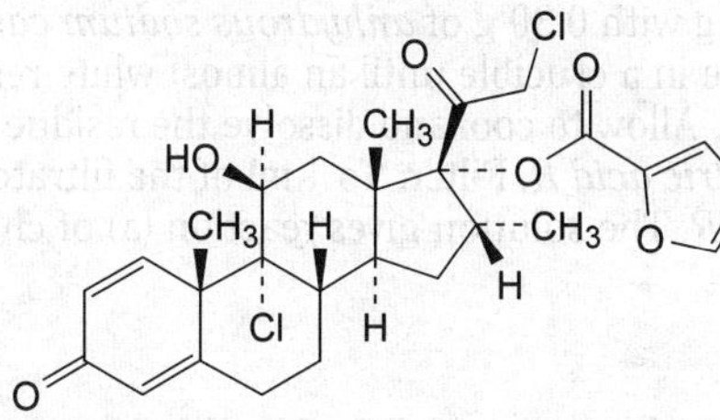

$C_{27}H_{30}Cl_2O_6$ M_r 521.4

DEFINITION

Mometasone furoate contains not less than 97.0 per cent and not more than the equivalent of 103.0 per cent of 9,21-dichloro-11β-hydroxy-16α-methyl-3,20-dioxopregna-1,4-dien-17-yl furan-2-carboxylate, calculated with reference to the dried substance.

CHARACTERS

A white or almost white powder, practically insoluble in water, soluble in acetone and in methylene chloride, slightly soluble in alcohol.

It melts at about 220 °C, with decomposition.

IDENTIFICATION

First identification: A, B.

Second identification; B, C, D.

A. Examine by infrared absorption spectrophotometry (*2.2.24*), comparing with the spectrum obtained with *mometasone furoate CRS*. Examine the substances prepared as discs.

B. Examine by thin-layer chromatography (*2.2.27*), using a *TLC silica gel F_{254} plate R*.

Test solution. Dissolve 10 mg of the substance to be examined in *methylene chloride R* and dilute to 10 ml with the same solvent.

Reference solution (a). Dissolve 20 mg of *mometasone furoate CRS* in *methylene chloride R* and dilute to 20 ml with the same solvent.

Reference solution (b). Dissolve 10 mg of *beclometasone dipropionate CRS* in reference solution (a) and dilute to 10 ml with the same solution.

Apply separately to the plate 5 µl of each solution. Prepare the mobile phase by adding a mixture of 1.2 volumes of *water R* and 8 volumes of *methanol R* to a mixture

Monographs M

of 15 volumes of *ether R* and 77 volumes of *methylene chloride R*. Develop over a path of 15 cm. Allow the plate to dry in air and examine in ultraviolet light at 254 nm. The principal spot in the chromatogram obtained with the test solution is similar in position and size to the principal spot in the chromatogram obtained with reference solution (a). Spray with *alcoholic solution of sulphuric acid R*. Heat at 120 °C for 10 min or until the spots appear. Allow to cool. Examine the chromatograms in daylight and in ultraviolet light at 365 nm. The principal spot in the chromatogram obtained with the test solution is similar in position, colour in daylight, fluorescence in ultraviolet light at 365 nm and size to the principal spot in the chromatogram obtained with reference solution (a). The test is not valid unless the chromatogram obtained with reference solution (b) shows two spots which, when examined in ultraviolet light at 365 nm, may not be completely separated.

C. Add about 2 mg to 2 ml of *sulphuric acid R* and shake to dissolve. Within 15 min a light yellow colour develops. When examined in ultraviolet light at 365 nm, no fluorescence is seen. Add the solution to 10 ml of *water R* and mix. The colour fades and there is no fluorescence.

D. Mix 80 mg with 0.30 g of *anhydrous sodium carbonate R* and ignite in a crucible until an almost white residue is obtained. Allow to cool and dissolve the residue in 5 ml of *dilute nitric acid R*. Filter. To 1 ml of the filtrate add 1 ml of *water R*. The solution gives reaction (a) of chlorides (*2.3.1*).

TESTS

Specific optical rotation (*2.2.7*). Dissolve 50.0 mg in *alcohol R* and dilute to 10.0 ml with the same solvent. The specific optical rotation is + 50 to + 55, calculated with reference to the dried substance.

Related substances. Examine by liquid chromatography (*2.2.29*). *Prepare the solutions immediately before use.*

Solvent solution. Prepare a mixture of equal volumes of *acetonitrile R* and *water R* to which is added 0.1 volumes of *acetic acid R*.

Test solution. Dissolve 20.0 mg of the substance to be examined in 4.0 ml of *acetonitrile R* and dilute to 20.0 ml with the solvent solution.

Reference solution (a). Dissolve 2 mg of *mometasone furoate CRS* and 6 mg of *beclometasone dipropionate CRS* in the solvent solution and dilute to 10.0 ml with the same solvent. Dilute 0.25 ml of the solution to 10.0 ml with the solvent solution.

Reference solution (b). Dilute 1.0 ml of the test solution to 20.0 ml with the solvent solution. Dilute 1.0 ml of the solution to 10.0 ml with the solvent solution.

The chromatographic procedure may be carried out using:

- a stainless steel column 0.25 m long and 4.6 mm in internal diameter packed with *octadecylsilyl silica gel for chromatography R* (5 µm),
- as mobile phase at a flow rate of 1 ml/min a mixture of equal volumes of *acetonitrile R* and *water R*,
- as detector a spectrophotometer set at 254 nm.

Adjust the sensitivity of the system so that the height of the principal peak in the chromatogram obtained with 20 µl of reference solution (b) is at least 50 per cent of the full scale of the recorder.

Inject 20 µl of reference solution (a). When the chromatograms are recorded in the prescribed conditions, the retention times are: mometasone furoate about 17 min and beclometasone dipropionate about 22 min. The test is not valid unless the resolution between the peaks corresponding to mometasone furoate and beclometasone dipropionate is at least 6. If necessary adjust the concentration of acetonitrile in the mobile phase.

Inject separately 20 µl of the test solution and 20 µl of reference solution (b). Continue the chromatography for twice the retention time of the principal peak in the chromatogram obtained with the test solution. In the chromatogram obtained with the test solution: the area of any peak apart from the principal peak, is not greater than 0.6 times the area of the principal peak in the chromatogram obtained with reference solution (b) (0.3 per cent); the sum of the areas of all peaks apart from the principal peak, is not greater than 1.2 times the area of the principal peak in the chromatogram obtained with reference solution (b) (0.6 per cent). Disregard any peak due to the solvent and any peak with an area less than 0.1 times the area of the principal peak in the chromatogram obtained with reference solution (b).

Loss on drying (*2.2.32*). Not more than 0.5 per cent, determined on 1.000 g by drying in an oven at 100 °C to 105 °C.

ASSAY

Dissolve 50.0 mg in *alcohol R* and dilute to 100.0 ml with the same solvent. Dilute 2.0 ml of this solution to 100.0 ml with *alcohol R*. Measure the absorbance (*2.2.25*) at the maximum at 249 nm.

Calculate the content of $C_{27}H_{30}Cl_2O_6$ taking the specific absorbance to be 481.

IMPURITIES

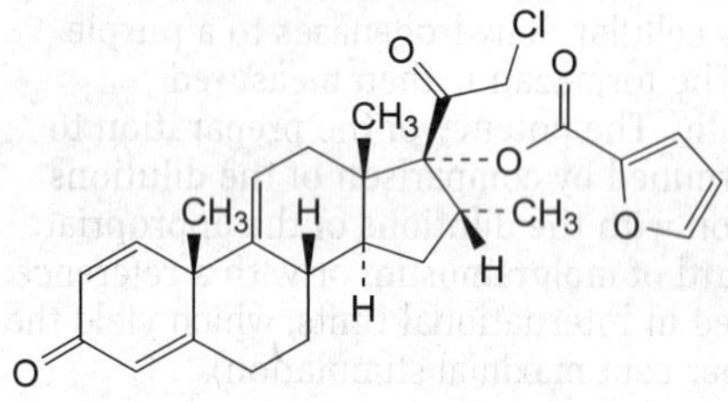

A. 21-chloro-16α-methyl-3,20-dioxopregna-1,4,9(11)-trien-17-yl furan-2-carboxylate,

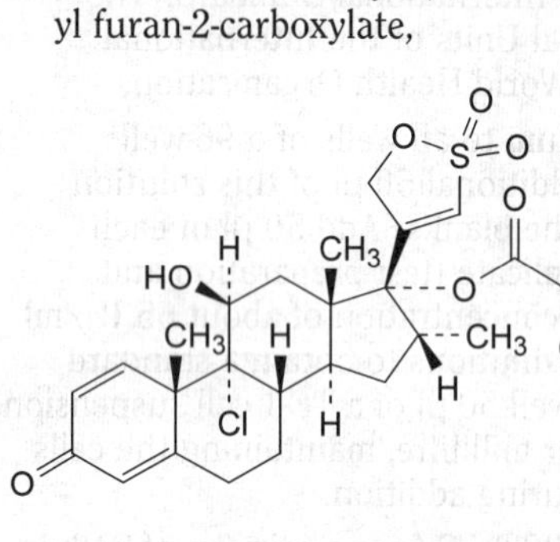

B. 4-[9-chloro-17-[(furan-2-ylcarbonyl)oxy]-11β-hydroxy-16α-methyl-3-oxoandrosta-1,4-dien-17β-yl]-5*H*-1,2-oxathiole 2,2-dioxide,

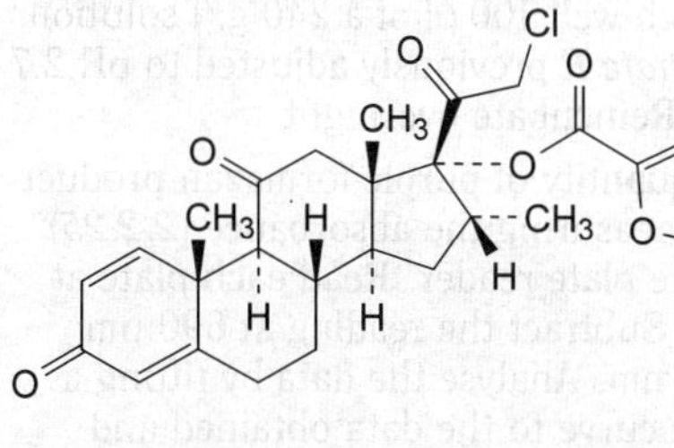

C. 21-chloro-16α-methyl-3,11,20-trioxopregna-1,4-dien-17-yl furan-2-carboxylate,

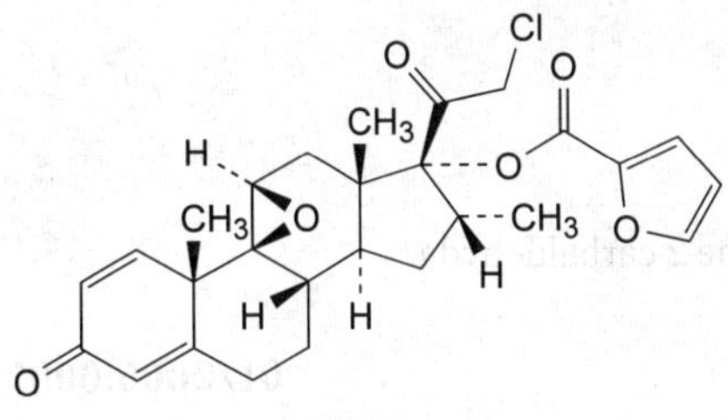

D. 21-chloro-9,11β-epoxy-16α-methyl-3,20-dioxo-9β-pregna-1,4-dien-17-yl furan-2-carboxylate,

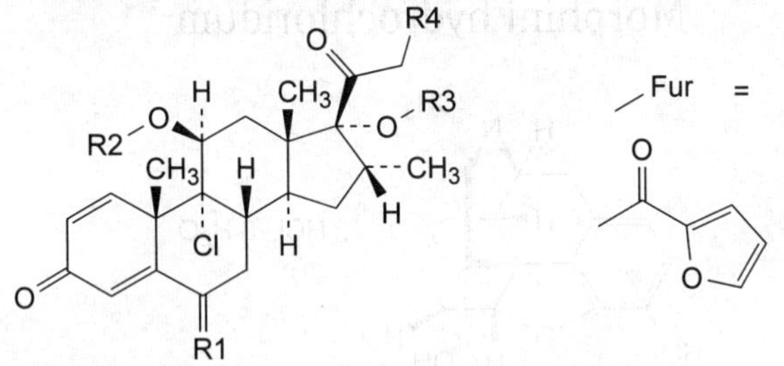

E. R1 = H_2, R2 = R3 = Fur, R4 = Cl: 9,21-dichloro-16α-methyl-3,20-dioxopregna-1,4-diene-11β,17-diyl bis(furan-2-carboxylate),

F. R1 = O, R2 = H, R3 = Fur, R4 = Cl: 9,21-dichloro-11β-hydroxy-16α-methyl-3,6,20-trioxopregna-1,4-dien-17-yl furan-2-carboxylate,

G. R1 = H_2, R2 = R3 = H, R4 = Cl: 9,21-dichloro-11β,17-dihydroxy-16α-methylpregna-1,4-diene-3,20-dione (mometasone),

H. R1 = H_2, R2 = H, R3 = Fur, R4 = OH: 9-chloro-11β,21-dihydroxy-16α-methyl-3,20-dioxopregna-1,4-dien-17-yl furan-2-carboxylate,

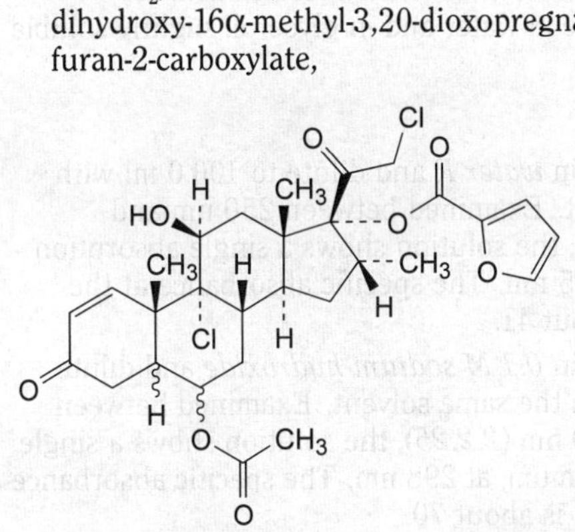

I. 9,21-dichloro-11β-hydroxy-16α-methyl-3,20-dioxo-5ξ-pregn-1-ene-6ξ,17-diyl 6-acetate 17-(furan-2-carboxylate).

01/2005:1546

MORANTEL HYDROGEN TARTRATE FOR VETERINARY USE

Moranteli hydrogenotartras ad usum veterinarium

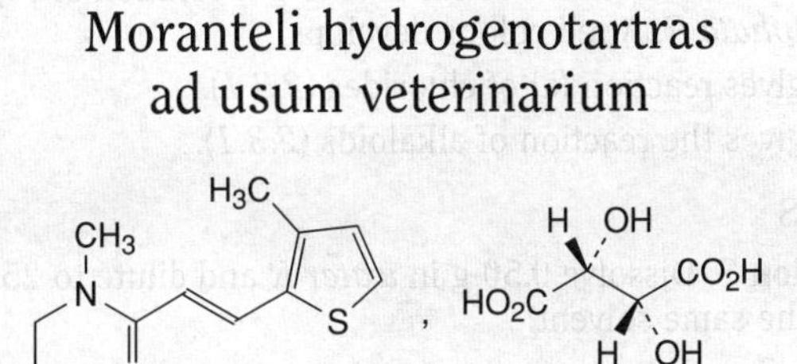

$C_{16}H_{22}N_2O_6S$ M_r 370.4

DEFINITION

1-Methyl-2-[(*E*)-2-(3-methylthiophen-2-yl)ethenyl]-1,4,5,6-tetrahydropyrimidine hydrogen tartrate.

Content: 98.5 per cent to 101.5 per cent (dried substance).

CHARACTERS

Appearance: white or pale yellow, crystalline powder.

Solubility: very soluble in water and in alcohol, practically insoluble in ethyl acetate.

IDENTIFICATION

First identification: B.

Second identification: A, C, D.

A. Melting point (*2.2.14*): 167 °C to 172 °C.

B. Infrared absorption spectrophotometry (*2.2.24*).
Comparison: *morantel hydrogen tartrate CRS.*

C. Dissolve about 10 mg in 1 ml of a 5 g/l solution of *ammonium vanadate R*. Evaporate to dryness. Add 0.1 ml of *sulphuric acid R*. A purple colour is produced.

D. Dissolve about 10 mg in 1 ml of *0.1 M sodium hydroxide*. Transfer to a separating funnel and shake with 5 ml of *methylene chloride R*. Discard the organic layer. Neutralise the aqueous layer with a few drops of *dilute hydrochloric acid R*. The solution gives reaction (b) of tartrates (*2.3.1*).

TESTS

Solution S. Dissolve 0.25 g in *carbon dioxide-free water R* and dilute to 25.0 ml with the same solvent.

Appearance of solution. Solution S is clear (*2.2.1*) and not more intensely coloured than reference solution GY_6 or Y_6 (*2.2.2, Method II*).

pH (*2.2.3*): 2.8 to 3.2 for solution S.

Related substances. Liquid chromatography (*2.2.29*).

Carry out the test protected from light.

Test solution. Dissolve 50.0 mg of the substance to be examined in the mobile phase and dilute to 100.0 ml with the mobile phase.

Reference solution (a). Dilute 1.0 ml of the test solution to 100.0 ml with the mobile phase.

Reference solution (b). Dilute 2.0 ml of reference solution (a) to 100.0 ml with the mobile phase.

Reference solution (c). Expose 10 ml of reference solution (a) to daylight for 15 min before injection.

Reference solution (d). Dissolve 15.0 mg of *tartaric acid R* in the mobile phase and dilute to 100.0 ml with the mobile phase.

Column:

– *size*: *l* = 0.25 m, Ø = 4.6 mm,

– *stationary phase*: *base-deactivated end-capped octadecylsilyl silica gel for chromatography R* (5 µm).

Mobile phase: to a mixture of 0.35 volumes of *triethylamine R* and 85 volumes of *water R* adjusted to pH 2.5 with *phosphoric acid R*, add 5 volumes of *tetrahydrofuran R* and 10 volumes of *methanol R*.

Flow rate: 0.75 ml/min.

Detection: spectrophotometer at 226 nm.

Injection: 20 µl.

Run time: twice the retention time of morantel.

System suitability: reference solution (c):

– *resolution*: minimum of 2 between the principal peak and the preceding peak ((*Z*)-isomer).

Limits:

- *any impurity apart from the peak due to tartaric acid*: not more than 0.5 times the area of the principal peak in the chromatogram obtained with reference solution (a) (0.5 per cent),
- *total*: not more than the area of the principal peak in the chromatogram obtained with reference solution (a) (1 per cent),
- *disregard limit*: the area of the principal peak in the chromatogram obtained with reference solution (b) (0.02 per cent).

Heavy metals (*2.4.8*): maximum 20 ppm.

1.0 g complies with limit test C. Prepare the standard using 2 ml of *lead standard solution (10 ppm Pb) R.*

Loss on drying (*2.2.32*): maximum 1.5 per cent, determined on 1.000 g by drying in an oven at 100-105 °C.

Sulphated ash (*2.4.14*): maximum 0.1 per cent, determined on 1.0 g.

ASSAY

Dissolve 0.280 g in 40 ml of *anhydrous acetic acid R.* Titrate with *0.1 M perchloric acid,* determining the end-point potentiometrically (*2.2.20*).

1 ml of *0.1 M perchloric acid* is equivalent to 37.04 mg of $C_{16}H_{22}N_2O_6S$.

STORAGE

Protected from light.

IMPURITIES

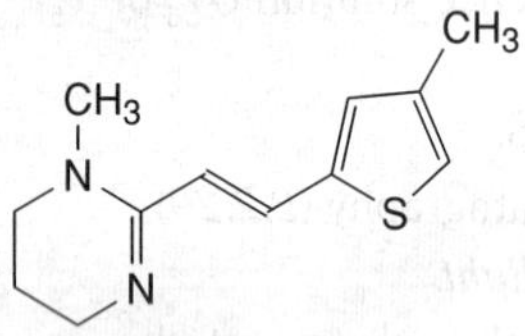

A. 1-methyl-2-[(*E*)-2-(4-methylthiophen-2-yl)ethenyl]-1,4,5,6-tetrahydropyrimidine,

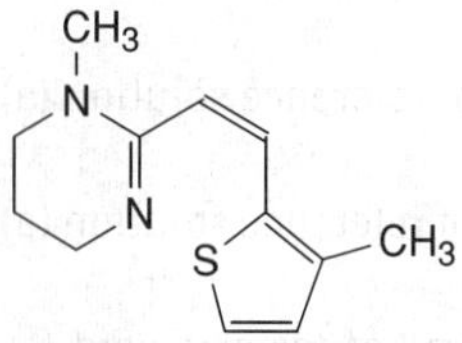

B. 1-methyl-2-[(*Z*)-2-(3-methylthiophen-2-yl)ethenyl]-1,4,5,6-tetrahydropyrimidine,

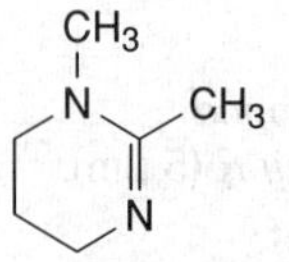

C. 1,2-dimethyl-1,4,5,6-tetrahydropyrimidine,

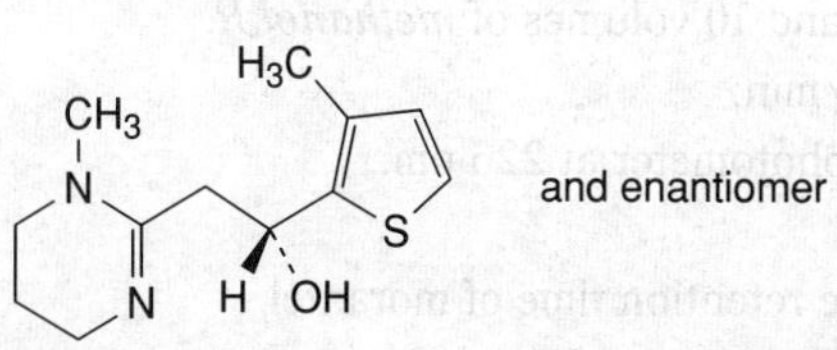

D. (1*RS*)-2-(1-methyl-1,4,5,6-tetrahydropyrimidin-2-yl)-1-(3-methylthiophen-2-yl)ethanol,

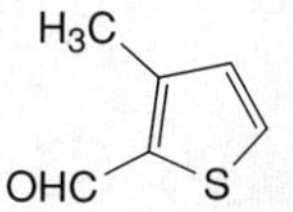

E. 3-methylthiophene-2-carbaldehyde.

01/2005:0097

MORPHINE HYDROCHLORIDE

Morphini hydrochloridum

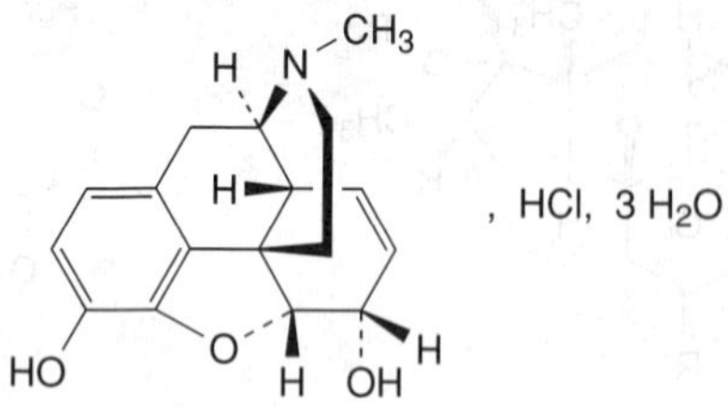

$C_{17}H_{20}ClNO_3,3H_2O$ M_r 375.8

DEFINITION

Morphine hydrochloride contains not less than 98.0 per cent and not more than the equivalent of 101.0 per cent of 7,8-didehydro-4,5α-epoxy-17-methylmorphinane-3,6α-diol hydrochloride, calculated with reference to the dried substance.

CHARACTERS

A white or almost white, crystalline powder or colourless, silky needles or cubical masses, efflorescent in a dry atmosphere, soluble in water and in glycerol, slightly soluble in alcohol.

IDENTIFICATION

A. Dissolve 10 mg in *water R* and dilute to 100.0 ml with the same solvent. Examined between 250 nm and 350 nm (*2.2.25*), the solution shows a single absorption maximum, at 285 nm. The specific absorbance at the maximum is about 41.

B. Dissolve 10 mg in *0.1 M sodium hydroxide* and dilute to 100.0 ml with the same solvent. Examined between 265 nm and 350 nm (*2.2.25*), the solution shows a single absorption maximum, at 298 nm. The specific absorbance at the maximum is about 70.

C. To about 1 mg of powdered substance in a porcelain dish add 0.5 ml of *sulphuric acid-formaldehyde reagent R.* A purple colour develops and becomes violet.

D. Dissolve about 5 mg in 5 ml of *water R* and add 0.15 ml of a freshly prepared 10 g/l solution of *potassium ferricyanide R* and 0.05 ml of *ferric chloride solution R1.* A blue colour is produced immediately.

E. Dissolve about 5 mg in 5 ml of *water R* and add 1 ml of *dilute hydrogen peroxide solution R*, 1 ml of *dilute ammonia R1* and 0.05 ml of a 40 g/l solution of *copper sulphate R.* A red colour develops.

F. It gives reaction (a) of chlorides (*2.3.1*).

G. It gives the reaction of alkaloids (*2.3.1*).

TESTS

Solution S. Dissolve 0.50 g in *water R* and dilute to 25.0 ml with the same solvent.

Appearance of solution. Solution S is clear (*2.2.1*) and not more intensely coloured than reference solution Y_6 or BY_6 (*2.2.2, Method II*).

Acidity or alkalinity. To 10 ml of solution S add 0.05 ml of *methyl red solution R*. Not more than 0.2 ml of *0.02 M sodium hydroxide* or *0.02 M hydrochloric acid* is required to change the colour of the indicator.

Specific optical rotation (*2.2.7*). − 110 to − 115, determined on solution S and calculated with reference to the dried substance.

Related substances. Examine by thin-layer chromatography (*2.2.27*), using a *TLC silica gel G plate R*.

Test solution. Dissolve 0.10 g of the substance to be examined in a mixture of equal volumes of *alcohol R* and *water R* and dilute to 10 ml with the same mixture of solvents.

Reference solution. Dissolve 50 mg of *codeine phosphate R* in 5 ml of the test solution. Dilute 0.1 ml of the solution to 10 ml with a mixture of equal volumes of *alcohol R* and *water R*.

Apply separately to the plate 10 µl of each solution. Develop over a path of 15 cm using a freshly prepared mixture of 2.5 volumes of *concentrated ammonia R*, 32.5 volumes of *acetone R*, 24.5 volumes of *ethanol R*, 10.5 volumes of *water R* and 35 volumes of *toluene R*, prepared in the order given. Dry the plate in a current of air. Spray with *potassium iodobismuthate solution R* and dry for 15 min in a current of air. Spray with *dilute hydrogen peroxide solution R*. Any spot corresponding to codeine in the chromatogram obtained with the test solution is not more intense than the corresponding spot in the chromatogram obtained with the reference solution (1 per cent); any spot apart from the principal spot and the spot corresponding to codeine, is not more intense than the spot corresponding to morphine in the chromatogram obtained with the reference solution (1 per cent). The test is not valid unless the chromatogram obtained with the reference solution shows two clearly separated spots.

Meconate. To 10 ml of solution S add 1 ml of *hydrochloric acid R* and 0.1 ml of *ferric chloride solution R1*. The absorbance (*2.2.25*) measured at 480 nm is not greater than 0.05 (0.2 per cent). Use as the compensation liquid a blank solution prepared at the same time and in the same manner using 10 ml of *water R*.

Loss on drying (*2.2.32*). 12.0 per cent to 15.0 per cent, determined on 0.500 g by drying in an oven at 130 °C.

Sulphated ash (*2.4.14*). Not more than 0.1 per cent, determined on the residue from the test for loss on drying.

ASSAY

Dissolve 0.350 g, heating if necessary, in 30 ml of *anhydrous acetic acid R*. Cool and add 6 ml of *mercuric acetate solution R*. Titrate with *0.1 M perchloric acid*, using 0.1 ml of *crystal violet solution R* as indicator.

1 ml of *0.1 M perchloric acid* is equivalent to 32.18 mg of $C_{17}H_{20}ClNO_3$.

STORAGE

Store protected from light.

IMPURITIES

A. codeine,

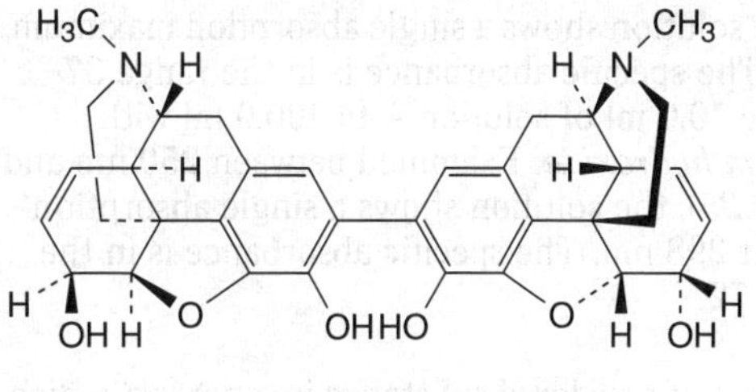

B. 2,2′-bimorphine (pseudomorphine),

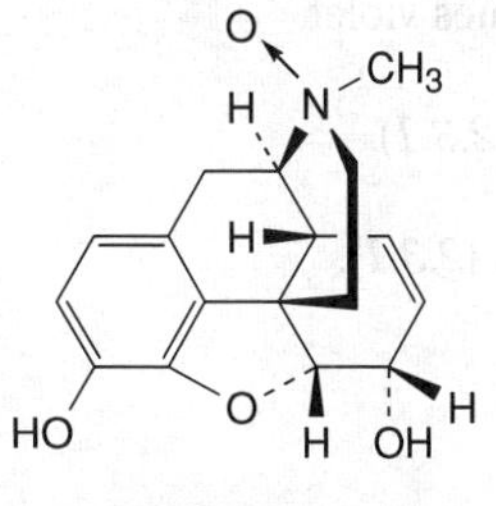

C. morphine *N*-oxide,

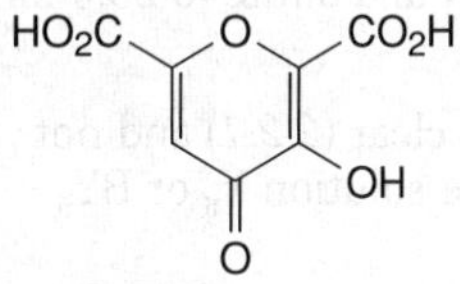

D. 3-hydroxy-4-oxo-4*H*-pyran-2,6-dicarboxylic acid (meconic acid).

01/2005:1244

MORPHINE SULPHATE

Morphini sulfas

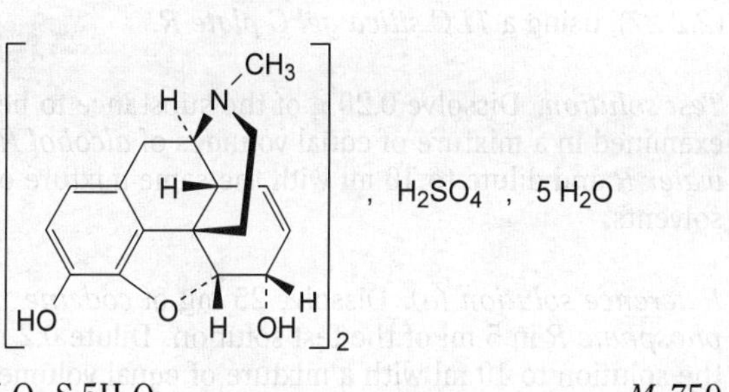

$C_{34}H_{40}N_2O_{10}S,5H_2O$ M_r 759

DEFINITION

Morphine sulphate contains not less than 98.0 per cent and not more than the equivalent of 102.0 per cent of di(7,8-didehydro-4,5α-epoxy-17-methylmorphinane-3,6α-diol) sulphate, calculated with reference to the anhydrous, ethanol-free substance.

CHARACTERS

A white or almost white, crystalline powder, soluble in water, very slightly soluble in alcohol, practically insoluble in toluene.

IDENTIFICATION

First identification: A, E.

Second identification: B, C, D, E.

A. Examine by infrared absorption spectrophotometry (*2.2.24*), after drying the substance to be examined at 145 °C for 1 h, comparing with the *Ph. Eur. reference spectrum of morphine sulphate.*

B. Dissolve 0.100 g in *water R* and dilute to 100.0 ml with the same solvent (solution A). Dilute 10.0 ml to 100.0 ml with *water R*. Examined between 250 nm and 300 nm

(*2.2.25*), the solution shows a single absorption maximum, at 285 nm. The specific absorbance is in the range 37 to 43. Dilute 10.0 ml of solution A to 100.0 ml with *0.1 M sodium hydroxide*. Examined between 250 nm and 350 nm (*2.2.25*), the solution shows a single absorption maximum, at 298 nm. The specific absorbance is in the range 64 to 72.

C. To about 1 mg of powdered substance in a porcelain dish add 0.5 ml of *sulphuric acid-formaldehyde reagent R*. A purple colour develops and becomes violet.

D. It gives the reaction of alkaloids (*2.3.1*).

E. It gives the reactions of sulphates (*2.3.1*).

TESTS

Solution S. Dissolve 0.500 g in *water R* and dilute to 25.0 ml with the same solvent.

Appearance of solution. Solution S is clear (*2.2.1*) and not more intensely coloured than reference solution Y_6 or BY_5 (*2.2.2, Method II*).

Acidity or alkalinity. To 10 ml of solution S add 0.05 ml of *methyl red solution R*. Not more than 0.2 ml of *0.02 M sodium hydroxide* or *0.02 M hydrochloric acid* is required to change the colour of the indicator.

Specific optical rotation (*2.2.7*): − 107 to − 110, determined on solution S and calculated with reference to the anhydrous, ethanol-free substance.

Related substances. Examine by thin-layer chromatography (*2.2.27*), using a *TLC silica gel G plate R*.

Test solution. Dissolve 0.20 g of the substance to be examined in a mixture of equal volumes of *alcohol R* and *water R* and dilute to 10 ml with the same mixture of solvents.

Reference solution (a). Dissolve 25 mg of *codeine phosphate R* in 5 ml of the test solution. Dilute 0.2 ml of the solution to 10 ml with a mixture of equal volumes of *alcohol R* and *water R*.

Reference solution (b). Dilute 0.1 ml of the test solution to 20 ml with a mixture of equal volumes of *alcohol R* and *water R*.

Reference solution (c). Dilute 2.0 ml of reference solution (b) to 5.0 ml with a mixture of equal volumes of *alcohol R* and *water R*.

Reference solution (d). Dilute 2.0 ml of reference solution (b) to 10.0 ml with a mixture of equal volumes of *alcohol R* and *water R*.

Apply to the plate 10 µl of each solution. Develop over a path of 10 cm using a freshly prepared mixture of 2.5 volumes of *concentrated ammonia R*, 32.5 volumes of *acetone R*, 24.5 volumes of *ethanol R*, 10.5 volumes of *water R* and 35 volumes of *toluene R*, prepared in the order given. Dry the plate in a current of air. Spray with *potassium iodobismuthate solution R* and dry for 15 min in a current of air. Spray with *dilute hydrogen peroxide solution R*. Any spot corresponding to impurity A in the chromatogram obtained with the test solution is not more intense than the corresponding spot in the chromatogram obtained with reference solution (a) (0.5 per cent). Any spot in the chromatogram obtained with the test solution, apart from the principal spot and any spot corresponding to impurity A is not more intense than the spot in the chromatogram obtained with reference solution (b) (0.5 per cent) and not more than two such spots are more intense than the spot in the chromatogram obtained with reference solution (c) (0.2 per cent). The test in not valid unless the chromatogram obtained with reference solution (a) shows two such clearly separated spots and the spot in the chromatogram obtained with reference solution (d) is clearly visible.

Ethanol (*2.4.24*). Not more than 0.5 per cent.

Iron (*2.4.9*). Dissolve the residue from the test for sulphated ash in *water R* and dilute to 10.0 ml with the same solvent. The solution complies with the limit test for iron (5 ppm).

Water (*2.5.12*): 10.4 per cent to 13.4 per cent, determined on 0.200 g by the semi-micro determination of water.

Sulphated ash (*2.4.14*). Not more than 0.1 per cent, determined on 2.0 g.

ASSAY

Dissolve 0.500 g in 120 ml of *anhydrous acetic acid R*. Titrate with *0.1 M perchloric acid*, determining the end-point potentiometrically (*2.2.20*).

1 ml of *0.1 M perchloric acid* is equivalent to 66.88 mg of $C_{34}H_{40}N_2O_{10}S$.

STORAGE

Store protected from light.

IMPURITIES

A. codeine,

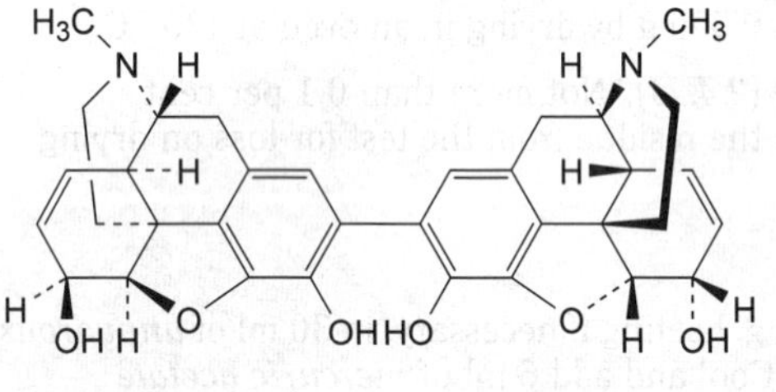

B. 2,2′-bimorphine (pseudomorphine),

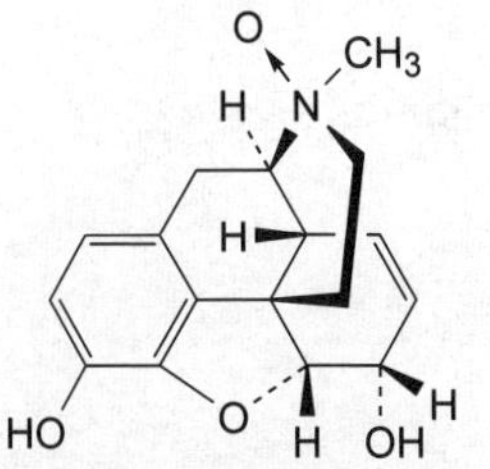

C. morphine *N*-oxide.

01/2005:1833

MOTHERWORT

Leonuri cardiacae herba

DEFINITION

Whole or cut, dried flowering aerial parts of *Leonurus cardiaca* L.

Content: minimum 0.2 per cent of flavonoids, expressed as hyperoside ($C_{21}H_{20}O_{12}$; M_r 464.4) (dried drug).

CHARACTERS

Macroscopic and microscopic characters described under identification tests A and B.

IDENTIFICATION

A. The stem pieces are hairy, longitudinally striated, quadrangular, hollow, and up to about 10 mm wide; they bear opposite and decussate, petiolate leaves and, in the axils of the upper leaves, about 6 to 12 small flowers, arranged in sessile whorls forming a long leafy spike. The lower leaves are ovate-orbicular, palmately 3 to 5-lobed, rarely 7-lobed, the lobes irregularly dentate. The upper leaves are entire or slightly trifid, lanceolate with a serrate margin and cuneate at the base. The upper surface of the leaves is green with scattered hairs, the lower surface is paler green, densely pubescent and shows a prominent palmate and reticulate venation. The flowers have a funnel-shaped calyx, 3 mm to 5 mm long with 5 stiff, recurved teeth; the corolla is 2-lipped, the upper lip pink and pubescent on the outer surface, the lower lip white with purplish spots; stamens 4, densely pubescent.

B. Reduce to a powder (355). The powder is green. Examine under a microscope using *chloral hydrate solution R*. The powder shows the following diagnostic characters: fragments of the leaf lamina with a one-layered palisade mesophyll reaching almost to the centre and a loosely arranged spongy parenchyma; fragments of leaf epidermis; upper epidermal cells with straight anticlinal walls and a striated cuticle; lower epidermal cells with sinuous anticlinal walls; stomata of the diacytic type (*2.8.3*) more numerous on the lower surface; glandular trichomes with a short unicellular stalk and a globular head composed of 8, sometimes up to 16 cells or with a unicellular head; covering trichomes conical, uniseriate, up to about 300 µm long, occasionally up to 1500 µm, composed of from 2 to 8 cells with slight swellings at the junctions and a warty or striated cuticle; fragments of the calyx containing small, cluster crystals of calcium oxalate; spherical pollen grains, about 25 µm to 30 µm in diameter, with 3 pores and 3 furrows and a smooth exine; thick-walled, lignified fibres and spirally and annularly thickened vessels from the stem; occasional brown fragments of pericarp with single crystals of calcium oxalate.

C. Thin-layer chromatography (*2.2.27*).

Test solution. To 0.5 g of the powdered drug (355) add 5 ml of *methanol R*. Heat in a water-bath at 65 °C for 5 min with shaking. Cool and filter.

Reference solution. Dissolve 5 mg of *naphthol yellow S R* and 2.0 mg of *catalpol R* in 5.0 ml of *methanol R*.

Plate: *TLC silica gel plate R.*

Mobile phase: *glacial acetic acid R, water R, ethyl acetate R* (20:20:60 *V/V/V*).

Application: 20 µl as bands.

Development: over a path of 10 cm.

Drying: in air.

Detection: spray with *dimethylaminobenzaldehyde solution R2,* using about 5 ml for a plate 200 mm square; heat at 100-105 °C for 10 min until the spots appear; examine in daylight.

Results: see below the sequence of the zones present in the chromatograms obtained with the reference solution and the test solution. Furthermore, further weak greyish-blue zones may be present in the chromatogram obtained with the test solution.

Top of the plate	
	A wide white zone
	A greyish-blue zone (iridoid)
_______	_______
Naphthol yellow S: an intense yellow zone	1 or 2 greyish-blue zones (iridoid)
Catalpol: a greyish-blue zone	
_______	
Reference solution	**Test solution**

TESTS

Foreign matter (*2.8.2*): maximum 2 per cent of brown or yellow leaves and maximum 2 per cent of other foreign matter.

Loss on drying (*2.2.32*): maximum 12.0 per cent, determined on 1.000 g of the powdered drug (355) by drying in an oven at 100-105 °C for 2 h.

Total ash (*2.4.16*): maximum 12.0 per cent.

ASSAY

Stock solution. In a 100 ml round-bottomed flask, place 1.00 g of the powdered drug (355), add 1 ml of a 5 g/l solution of *hexamethylenetetramine R*, 20 ml of *acetone R* and 2 ml of *hydrochloric acid R1.* Boil the mixture under a reflux condenser for 30 min. Filter the liquid through a plug of absorbent cotton into a flask. Add the absorbent cotton to the residue in the round-bottomed flask and extract with 2 quantities, each of 20 ml, of *acetone R*, each time boiling under a reflux condenser for 10 min. Allow to cool, filter each extract through the plug of absorbent cotton into the flask. After cooling, filter the combined acetone extracts through a paper filter into a volumetric flask, dilute to 100.0 ml with *acetone R* by rinsing the flask and the paper filter. Introduce 20.0 ml of the solution into a separating funnel, add 20 ml of *water R* and shake the mixture with 1 quantity of 15 ml and then with 3 quantities, each of 10 ml, of *ethyl acetate R.* Combine the ethyl acetate extracts in a separating funnel, wash with 2 quantities, each of 50 ml, of *water R,* and filter the extracts over 10 g of *anhydrous sodium sulphate R* into a volumetric flask and dilute to 50.0 ml with *ethyl acetate R.*

Test solution. To 10.0 ml of the stock solution add 1 ml of *aluminium chloride reagent R* and dilute to 25.0 ml with a 5 per cent *V/V* solution of *glacial acetic acid R* in *methanol R.*

Compensation liquid. Dilute 10.0 ml of the stock solution to 25.0 ml with a 5 per cent *V/V* solution of *glacial acetic acid R* in *methanol R.*

Monographs M

Measure the absorbance (*2.2.25*) of the test solution after 30 min, by comparison with the compensation liquid at 425 nm. Calculate the percentage content of flavonoids, calculated as hyperoside, from the expression:

$$\frac{A \times 1.25}{m}$$

i.e. taking the specific absorbance of hyperoside to be 500.

A = absorbance at 425 nm,

m = mass of the substance to be examined, in grams.

01/2005:1758

MOXONIDINE

Moxonidinum

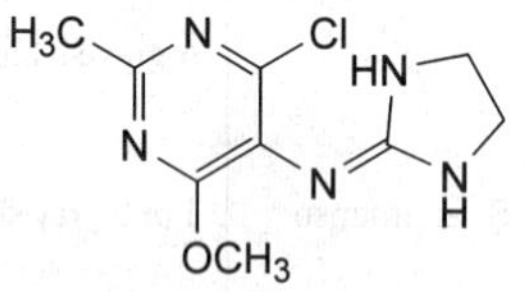

$C_9H_{12}ClN_5O$ M_r 241.7

DEFINITION

4-Chloro-*N*-(imidazolidin-2-ylidene)-6-methoxy-2-methylpyrimidin-5-amine.

Content: 97.5 per cent to 102.0 per cent (dried substance).

CHARACTERS

Appearance: white or almost white powder.

Solubility: very slightly soluble in water, sparingly soluble in methanol, slightly soluble in methylene chloride, very slightly soluble in acetonitrile.

IDENTIFICATION

Infrared absorption spectrophotometry (*2.2.24*).

Preparation: discs.

Comparison: *moxonidine CRS*.

TESTS

Related substances. Liquid chromatography (*2.2.29*).

Test solution. Dissolve 0.100 g of the substance to be examined in a mixture of equal volumes of *methanol R* and *water R* and dilute to 100.0 ml with the same mixture of solvents.

Reference solution (a). Dissolve 10.0 mg of *moxonidine CRS* in a mixture of equal volumes of *methanol R* and *water R* and dilute to 10.0 ml with the same mixture of solvents.

Reference solution (b). Dilute 1.0 ml of reference solution (a) to 100.0 ml with a mixture of equal volumes of *methanol R* and *water R*. Dilute 2.0 ml of this solution to 20.0 ml with a mixture of equal volumes of *methanol R* and *water R*.

Reference solution (c). Dissolve 5.0 mg of *moxonidine impurity A CRS* in a mixture of equal volumes of *methanol R* and *water R* and dilute to 100.0 ml with the same mixture of solvents.

Reference solution (d). Dilute 6.0 ml of reference solution (c) to 100.0 ml with a mixture of equal volumes of *methanol R* and *water R*.

Reference solution (e). Dilute 2.5 ml of reference solution (a) to 50.0 ml with reference solution (c).

Column:

- *size*: l = 0.25 m, Ø = 4 mm,
- *stationary phase*: *base-deactivated octylsilyl silica gel for chromatography R* (5 µm),
- *temperature*: 40 °C.

Mobile phase: mix 136 volumes of *acetonitrile R* with 1000 volumes of a 3.48 g/l solution of *sodium pentanesulphonate R* previously adjusted to pH 3.5 with *dilute sulphuric acid R*.

Flow rate: 1.2 ml/min.

Detection: spectrophotometer at 230 nm.

Injection: 20 µl; inject a blank, the test solution and reference solutions (b), (d) and (e).

Run time: twice the retention time of moxonidine.

Relative retentions with reference to moxonidine (retention time = about 11.6 min): impurity A = about 0.9; impurity B = about 1.7.

System suitability: reference solution (e):

- *resolution*: minimum of 2 between the peaks due to impurity A and moxonidine.

Limits:

- *impurity A*: not more than the area of the corresponding peak in the chromatogram obtained with reference solution (d) (0.3 per cent),
- *impurity B*: not more than 3 times the area of the principal peak in the chromatogram obtained with reference solution (b) (0.3 per cent),
- *any other impurity*: not more than the area of the principal peak in the chromatogram obtained with reference solution (b) (0.1 per cent),
- *total*: not more than 5 times the area of the principal peak in the chromatogram obtained with reference solution (b) (0.5 per cent),
- *disregard limit*: 0.5 times the area of the principal peak in the chromatogram obtained with reference solution (b) (0.05 per cent). Disregard any peak observed with the blank run.

Loss on drying (*2.2.32*): maximum 0.5 per cent, determined on 1.000 g by drying in an oven at 100-105 °C for 3 h.

Sulphated ash (*2.4.14*): maximum 0.1 per cent, determined on 1.0 g.

ASSAY

Liquid chromatography (*2.2.29*) as described in the test for related substances with the following modification.

Injection: test solution and reference solution (a).

Calculate the percentage content of $C_9H_{12}ClN_5O$ from the areas of the peaks and the declared content of *moxonidine CRS*.

IMPURITIES

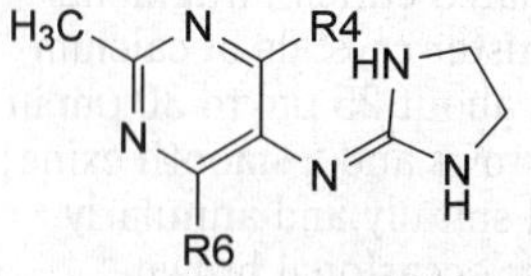

A. R4 = R6 = Cl: 4,6-dichloro-*N*-(imidazolidin-2-ylidene)-2-methylpyrimidin-5-amine (6-chloromoxonidine),

B. R4 = R6 = OCH_3: *N*-(imidazolidin-2-ylidene)-4,6-dimethoxy-2-methylpyrimidin-5-amine (4-methoxymoxonidine),

C. R4 = OH, R6 = OCH_3: 5-[(imidazolidin-2-ylidene)amino]-6-methoxy-2-methylpyrimidin-4-ol (4-hydroxymoxonidine),

D. R4 = OH, R6 = Cl: 6-chloro-5-[(imidazolidin-2-ylidene)amino]-2-methylpyrimidin-4-ol (6-desmethylmoxonidine).

01/2005:1853

MULLEIN FLOWER

Verbasci flos

DEFINITION

Dried flower, reduced to the corolla and the androecium, of *Verbascum thapsus* L., *V. densiflorum* Bertol. (*V. thapsiforme* Schrad), and *V. phlomoides* L.

CHARACTERS

Macroscopic and microscopic characters described under identification tests A and B.

IDENTIFICATION

A. The corolla of *V. thapsus* is about 20 mm in diameter, pale yellow, yellow to brown, funnel-shaped with 5 slightly unequal and spreading lobes. The corolla lobes are densely hairy on the outer surface, glabrous on the inner surface, with a fine network of light brown veins. There are 5 stamens, alternating with the petal lobes, 2 of these are long, with glabrous filaments, the other 3 shorter, with densely tormentose filaments. The anthers are attached transversely. In *V. phlomoides* the corolla is up to about 30 mm in diameter, bright yellow to orange, and the anthers are obliquely attached to the filaments. The corolla of *V. densiflorum*, about 30 mm in diameter, is almost flat and deeply divided into 5 slightly unequal lobes, with rounded apices.

B. Reduce to a powder (355). The powder is yellow or yellowish-brown. Examine under a microscope using *chloral hydrate solution R*. The powder shows many covering trichomes from the corolla, whole and fragmented; there are pluricellular, of the candelabra type with a central uniseriate axis from which whorls of branch cells arise at the position of the cross walls and at the apex. The covering trichomes from the stamen filaments are unicellular, long, thin-walled and tubular, sometimes with a club-shaped tip; they have a distinctly granular or striated surface. Numerous pollen grains, ovoid with a finely granular exine with 3 pores. Fragments of the fibrous layer of the anther with thickened walls giving a characteristic star-shaped appearance. Yellow fragments of the petals in the surface view, the epidermal cells polygonal and isodiametric; fragments of the mesophyll consisting of irregular parenchymatous cells and scattered spiral vessels.

C. Thin-layer chromatography (*2.2.27*).

Test solution. Heat 1.0 g of the powdered drug (355) in 10 ml of *methanol R* in a water-bath at 60 °C for 5 min, with stirring. Cool and filter.

Reference solution. Dissolve 1 mg of *caffeic acid R*, 2.5 mg of *hyperoside R* and 2.5 mg of *rutin R* in *methanol R* and dilute to 10 ml with the same solvent.

Plate: *TLC silica gel plate R*.

Mobile phase: *water R, anhydrous formic acid R, methyl ethyl ketone R, ethyl acetate R* (10:10:30:50 *V/V/V/V*).

Application: 10 µl of the reference solution and 30 µl of the test solution, as bands.

Development: over a path of 15 cm.

Drying: at 100-105 °C.

Detection: spray the warm plate with a 10 g/l solution of *diphenylboric acid aminoethyl ester R* in *methanol R*. Subsequently spray with a 50 g/l solution of *macrogol 400 R* in *methanol R*. Allow the plate to dry in air for 30 min and examine in ultraviolet light at 365 nm.

Results: see below the sequence of the zones present in the chromatograms obtained with the reference solution and the test solution. Furthermore, other faint zones may be present in the chromatogram obtained with the test solution.

Top of the plate	
	A yellow to yellowish-green fluorescent zone.
Caffeic acid: a greenish-blue fluorescent zone.	
	A bluish fluorescent zone.
	A greenish fluorescent zone.
	A yellowish-green fluorescent zone.
	A bluish fluorescent zone.
Hyperoside: a yellowish-brown fluorescent zone.	
	A greenish fluorescent zone.
Rutin: a yellowish-brown fluorescent zone.	
Reference solution	**Test solution**

D. Boil 1.0 g of the powdered drug (355) with 15 ml of *water R* for 1 min. Filter. Add 1 ml of *hydrochloric acid R* and boil for 1 min. A greenish-blue colour develops and, after a few minutes, cloudiness appears and then a blackish precipitate (iridoids).

TESTS

Foreign matter (*2.8.2*): maximum 5 per cent of brown petals and maximum 2 per cent of fragments of the calyx and other foreign matter, determined on 20 g.

Swelling index (*2.8.4*): minimum 9, determined on the powdered drug (710), humidified with 2 ml of *alcohol R*.

Loss on drying (*2.2.32*): maximum 12.0 per cent, determined on 1.000 g of the powdered drug (710) by drying in an oven at 100-105 °C for 2 h.

Total ash (*2.4.16*): maximum 6.0 per cent.

Ash insoluble in hydrochloric acid (*2.8.1*): maximum 2.0 per cent.

STORAGE

In an airtight container.

01/2005:1450

MUPIROCIN

Mupirocinum

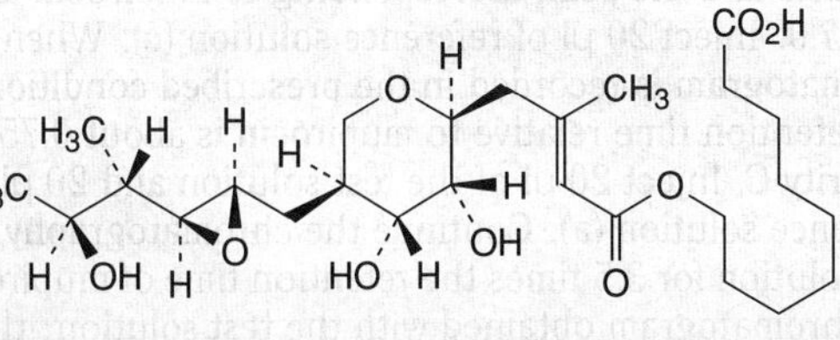

$C_{26}H_{44}O_9$ M_r 500.6

DEFINITION

Mupirocin contains not less than 93.0 per cent and not more than the equivalent of 100.5 per cent of 9-[[(2*E*)-4-[(2*S*,3*R*,4*R*,5*S*)-5-[(2*S*,3*S*,4*S*,5*S*)-2,3-epoxy-5-

hydroxy-4-methylhexyl]-3,4-dihydroxy-3,4,5,6-tetrahydro-2*H*-pyran-2-yl]-3-methylbut-2-enoyl]oxy]nonanoic acid, calculated with reference to the anhydrous substance.

CHARACTERS

A white or almost white powder, slightly soluble in water, freely soluble in acetone, in ethanol and in methylene chloride.

It shows polymorphism.

IDENTIFICATION

Examine by infrared absorption spectrophotometry (*2.2.24*), comparing with the *Ph. Eur. reference spectrum of mupirocin*.

TESTS

pH (*2.2.3*). The pH of a freshly prepared saturated solution (about 10 g/l) in *carbon dioxide-free water R* is 3.5 to 4.0.

Specific optical rotation (*2.2.7*). Dissolve 0.50 g in *methanol R* and dilute to 10.0 ml with the same solvent. The specific optical rotation is − 17 to − 21, calculated with reference to the anhydrous substance.

Related substances. Examine by liquid chromatography (*2.2.29*).

Test solution. Dissolve 50.0 mg of the substance to be examined in a mixture of equal volumes of *methanol R* and of a 13.6 g/l solution of *sodium acetate R*, adjusted to pH 4.0 with *acetic acid R* and dilute to 10.0 ml with the same mixture of solvents.

Reference solution (a). Dilute 1.0 ml of the test solution to 50.0 ml with a mixture of equal volumes of *methanol R* and of a 13.6 g/l solution of *sodium acetate R*, adjusted to pH 4.0 with *acetic acid R*.

Reference solution (b). Adjust 10 ml of reference solution (a) to pH 2.0 using *hydrochloric acid R* and allow to stand for 20 h.

Reference solution (c). Dissolve 25 mg of *mupirocin lithium CRS* in a mixture of equal volumes of *methanol R* and of a 13.6 g/l solution of *sodium acetate R*, adjusted to pH 4.0 with *acetic acid R* and dilute to 200.0 ml with the same mixture of solvents.

The chromatographic procedure may be carried out using:

– a column 0.25 m long and 4.6 mm in internal diameter packed with *octylsilyl silica gel for chromatography R* (5 µm),

– as mobile phase at a flow rate of 1 ml/min a mixture of 20 volumes of *water R*, 30 volumes of *tetrahydrofuran R* and 50 volumes of a 10.5 g/l solution of *ammonium acetate R* previously adjusted to pH 5.7 with *acetic acid R*,

– as detector a spectrophotometer set at 240 nm.

Inject 20 µl of reference solution (b). The test is not valid unless in the chromatogram obtained, the resolution between the second of the 2 peaks corresponding to hydrolysis products and the peak corresponding to mupirocin is at least 7.0. Inject 20 µl of reference solution (c). When the chromatogram is recorded in the prescribed conditions, the retention time relative to mupirocin is about 0.75 for impurity C. Inject 20 µl of the test solution and 20 µl of reference solution (a). Continue the chromatography of the test solution for 3.5 times the retention time of mupirocin. In the chromatogram obtained with the test solution: the area of any peak corresponding to impurity C is not greater than twice the area of the principal peak in the chromatogram obtained with reference solution (a) (4 per cent); the area of any peak, apart from the principal peak and any peak corresponding to impurity C, is not greater than half the area of the principal peak in the chromatogram obtained with reference solution (a) (1 per cent); the sum of the areas of all the peaks, apart from the principal peak, is not greater than 3 times the area of the principal peak in the chromatogram obtained with reference solution (a) (6 per cent). Disregard any peak with an area less than 0.05 times the area of the principal peak in the chromatogram obtained with reference solution (a).

Water (*2.5.12*). Not more than 1.0 per cent, determined on 0.500 g by the semi-micro determination of water.

ASSAY

Examine by liquid chromatography (*2.2.29*).

Test solution. Dissolve 25.0 mg of the substance to be examined in 5 ml of *methanol R* and dilute to 200.0 ml with a 7.5 g/l solution of *ammonium acetate R* adjusted to pH 5.7 with *acetic acid R*.

Reference solution (a). Dissolve 25.0 mg of *mupirocin lithium CRS* in 5 ml of *methanol R* and dilute to 200.0 ml with a 7.5 g/l solution of *ammonium acetate R* adjusted to pH 5.7 with *acetic acid R*.

Reference solution (b). Adjust 10 ml of the test solution to pH 2.0 using *hydrochloric acid R* and allow to stand for 20 h.

The chromatographic procedure may be carried out using:

– a column 0.25 m long and 4.6 mm in internal diameter packed with *octylsilyl silica gel for chromatography R* (5 µm),

– as mobile phase at a flow rate of 1 ml/min a mixture of 19 volumes of *water R*, 32 volumes of *tetrahydrofuran R* and 49 volumes of a 10.5 g/l solution of *ammonium acetate R* adjusted to pH 5.7 with *acetic acid R*,

– as detector a spectrophotometer set at 230 nm.

Inject 20 µl of reference solution (b). The test is not valid unless in the chromatogram obtained, the resolution between the second of the 2 peaks corresponding to hydrolysis products and the peak corresponding to mupirocin is at least 7.0. Inject reference solution (a) 6 times. The test is not valid unless the relative standard deviation of the peak area of mupirocin is at most 1.0 per cent. Inject the test solution and reference solution (a).

STORAGE

Protected from light.

IMPURITIES

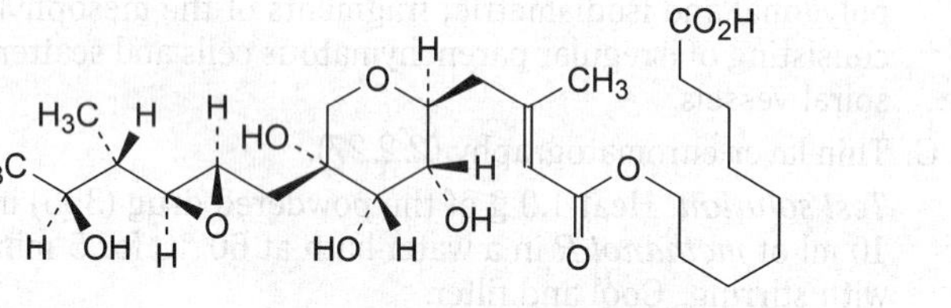

A. 9-[[(2*E*)-4-[(2*S*,3*R*,4*R*,5*S*)-5-[(2*S*,3*S*,4*S*,5*S*)-2,3-epoxy-5-hydroxy-4-methylhexyl]-3,4,5-trihydroxy-3,4,5,6-tetrahydro-2*H*-pyran-2-yl]-3-methylbut-2-enoyl]oxy]nonanoic acid (pseudomonic acid B),

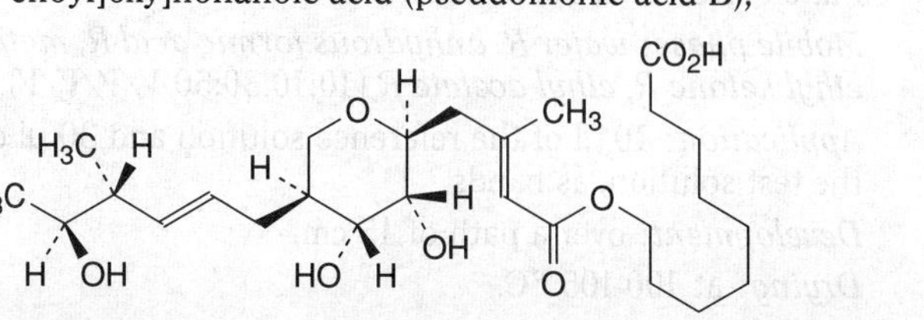

B. 9-[[(2*E*)-4-[(2*S*,3*R*,4*R*,5*S*)-3,4-dihydroxy-5-[(2*E*,4*R*,5*S*)-5-hydroxy-4-methylhex-2-enyl]-3,4,5,6-tetrahydro-2*H*-pyran-2-yl]-3-methylbut-2-enoyl]oxy]nonanoic acid (pseudomonic acid C),

Monographs M

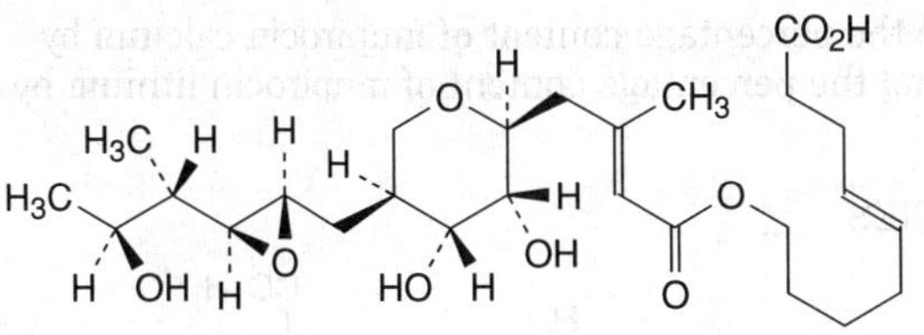

C. (4*E*)-9-[[(2*E*)-4-[(2*S*,3*R*,4*R*,5*S*)-5-[(2*S*,3*S*,4*S*,5*S*)-2,3-epoxy-5-hydroxy-4-methylhexyl]-3,4-dihydroxy-3,4,5,6-tetrahydro-2*H*-pyran-2-yl]-3-methylbut-2-enoyl]oxy]non-4-enoic acid (pseudomonic acid D),

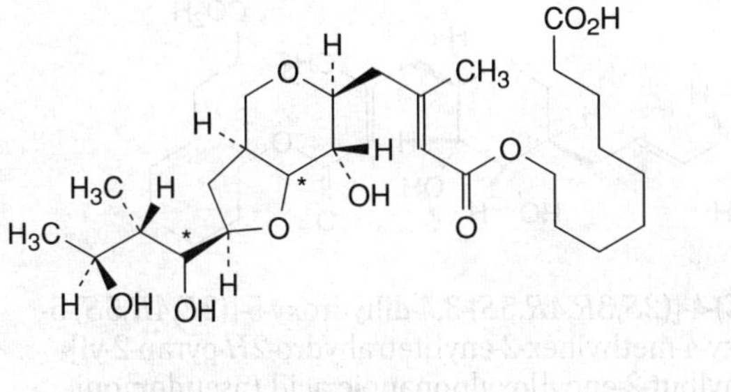

D. 9-[[(2*E*)-4-[(2*R*,3a*S*,6*S*,7*S*)-2-[(2*S*,3*S*)-1,3-dihydroxy-2-methylbutyl]-7-hydroxy-2,3,3a,6,7,7a-hexahydro-4*H*-furo[3,2-*c*]pyran-6-yl]-3-methylbut-2-enoyl]oxy]nonanoic acid,

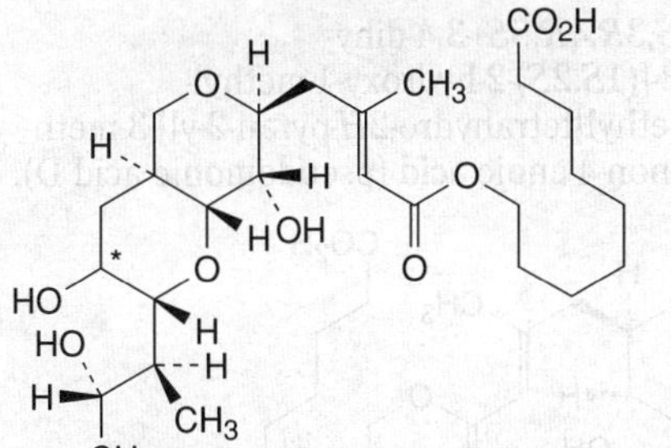

E. 9-[[(2*E*)-4-[(2*R*,3*RS*,4a*S*,7*S*,8*S*,8a*R*)-3,8-dihydroxy-2-[(1*S*,2*S*)-2-hydroxy-1-methylpropyl]-3,4,4a,7,8,8a-hexahydro-2*H*,5*H*-pyrano[4,3-*b*]pyran-7-yl]-3-methylbut-2-enoyl]oxy]nonanoic acid,

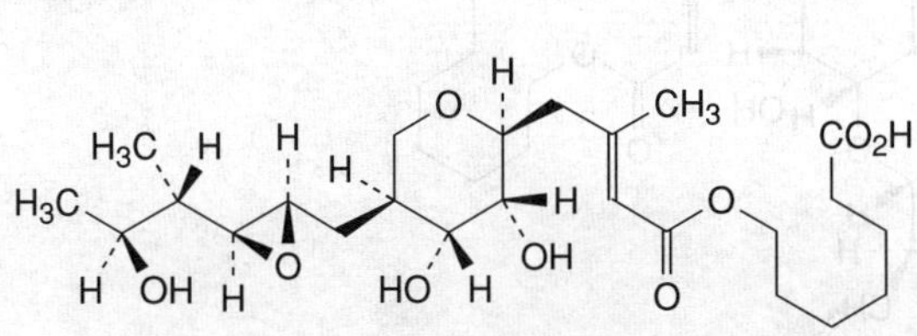

F. 7-[[(2*E*)-4-[(2*S*,3*R*,4*R*,5*S*)-5-[(2*S*,3*S*,4*S*,5*S*)-2,3-epoxy-5-hydroxy-4-methylhexyl]-3,4-dihydroxy-3,4,5,6-tetrahydro-2*H*-pyran-2-yl]-3-methylbut-2-enoyl]oxy]heptanoic acid.

01/2005:1451

MUPIROCIN CALCIUM

Mupirocinum calcicum

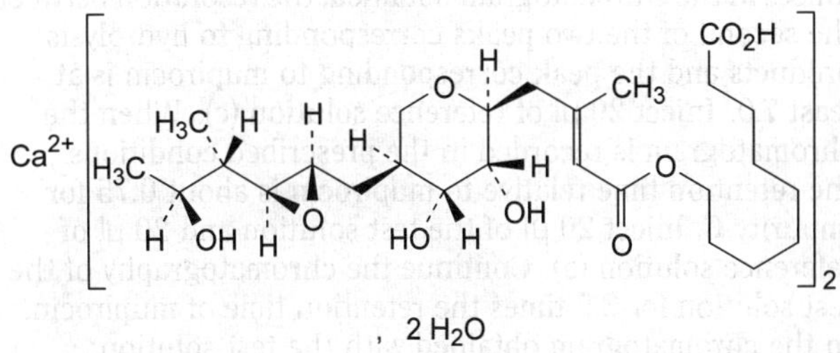

$C_{52}H_{86}O_{18}Ca,2H_2O$ M_r 1075

DEFINITION

Mupirocin calcium contains not less than 93.0 per cent and not more than the equivalent of 100.5 per cent of calcium bis[9-[[(2*E*)-4-[(2*S*,3*R*,4*R*,5*S*)-3,4-dihydroxy-5-[[(2*S*,3*S*)-3-[(1*S*,2*S*)-2-hydroxy-1-methylpropyl]oxiranyl]methyl]tetrahydro-2*H*-pyran-2-yl]-3-methylbut-2-enoyl]oxy]nonanoate], calculated with reference to the anhydrous substance.

CHARACTERS

A white or almost white powder, very slightly soluble in water, sparingly soluble in ethanol and in methylene chloride.

IDENTIFICATION

A. Examine by infrared absorption spectrophotometry (*2.2.24*), comparing with the *Ph. Eur. reference spectrum of mupirocin calcium*.

B. It gives reaction (a) of calcium (*2.3.1*).

TESTS

Specific optical rotation (*2.2.7*). Dissolve 0.50 g in *methanol R* and dilute to 10.0 ml with the same solvent. The specific optical rotation is − 16 to − 20, calculated with reference to the anhydrous substance.

Related substances. Examine by liquid chromatography (*2.2.29*).

Test solution. Dissolve 50.0 mg of the substance to be examined in a mixture of equal volumes of a 13.6 g/l solution of *sodium acetate R*, adjusted to pH 4.0 with *acetic acid R*, and *methanol R*. Dilute to 10.0 ml with the same mixture of solvents.

Reference solution (a). Dilute 1.0 ml of the test solution to 50.0 ml with a mixture of equal volumes of a 13.6 g/l solution of *sodium acetate R*, adjusted to pH 4.0 with *acetic acid R* and *methanol R*.

Reference solution (b). Adjust 10 ml of reference solution (a) to pH 2.0 using *hydrochloric acid R* and allow to stand for 20 h.

Reference solution (c). Dissolve 25 mg of *mupirocin lithium CRS* in a mixture of equal volumes of a 13.6 g/l solution of *sodium acetate R*, adjusted to pH 4.0 with *acetic acid R*, and *methanol R*. Dilute to 200.0 ml with the same mixture of solvents.

The chromatographic procedure may be carried out using:

– a column 0.25 m long and 4.6 mm in internal diameter packed with *octylsilyl silica gel for chromatography R* (5 µm),

– as mobile phase at a flow rate of 1 ml/min a mixture of 20 volumes of *water R*, 30 volumes of *tetrahydrofuran R* and 50 volumes of a 10.5 g/l solution of *ammonium acetate R* previously adjusted to pH 5.7 with *acetic acid R*,

– as detector a spectrophotometer set at 240 nm.

Inject 20 µl of reference solution (b). The test is not valid unless in the chromatogram obtained, the resolution between the second of the two peaks corresponding to hydrolysis products and the peak corresponding to mupirocin is at least 7.0. Inject 20 µl of reference solution (c). When the chromatogram is recorded in the prescribed conditions, the retention time relative to mupirocin is about 0.75 for impurity C. Inject 20 µl of the test solution and 20 µl of reference solution (a). Continue the chromatography of the test solution for 3.5 times the retention time of mupirocin. In the chromatogram obtained with the test solution: the area of any peak corresponding to impurity C is not greater than 1.25 times the area of the principal peak in the chromatogram obtained with reference solution (a) (2.5 per cent); the area of any peak, apart from the principal peak and any peak corresponding to impurity C, is not greater than half the area of the principal peak in the chromatogram obtained with reference solution (a) (1 per cent); the sum of the areas of all the peaks, apart from the principal peak, is not greater than 2.25 times the area of the principal peak in the chromatogram obtained with reference solution (a) (4.5 per cent). Disregard any peak with an area less than 0.05 times the area of the principal peak in the chromatogram obtained with reference solution (a).

Chlorides (*2.4.4*). Dissolve 10.0 mg in a mixture of 1 ml of *dilute nitric acid R* and 15 ml of *methanol R*. The solution complies with the limit test for chlorides (0.5 per cent).

Water (*2.5.12*). 3.0 per cent to 4.5 per cent, determined on 0.500 g by the semi-micro determination of water.

ASSAY

Examine by liquid chromatography (*2.2.29*).

Test solution. Dissolve 25.0 mg of the substance to be examined in 5 ml of *methanol R* and dilute to 200.0 ml with a 7.5 g/l solution of *ammonium acetate R*, adjusted to pH 5.7 with *acetic acid R*.

Reference solution (a). Dissolve 25.0 mg of *mupirocin lithium CRS* in 5 ml of *methanol R* and dilute to 200.0 ml with a 7.5 g/l solution of *ammonium acetate R*, adjusted to pH 5.7 with *acetic acid R*.

Reference solution (b). Adjust 10 ml of the test solution to pH 2.0 using *hydrochloric acid R* and allow to stand for 20 h.

The chromatographic procedure may be carried out using:

– a column 0.25 m long and 4.6 mm in internal diameter packed with *octylsilyl silica gel for chromatography R* (5 µm),

– as mobile phase at a flow rate of 1 ml/min a mixture of 19 volumes of *water R*, 32 volumes of *tetrahydrofuran R* and 49 volumes of a 10.5 g/l solution of *ammonium acetate R* adjusted to pH 5.7 with *acetic acid R*,

– as detector a spectrophotometer set at 230 nm.

Inject 20 µl of the reference solution (b). The test is not valid unless, in the chromatogram obtained, the resolution between the second of the two peaks corresponding to hydrolysis products and the peak corresponding to mupirocin is at least 7.0. Inject reference solution (a) six times. The test is not valid unless the relative standard deviation of the peak area of mupirocin is at most 1.0 per cent. Inject the test solution and the reference solution (a).

Calculate the percentage content of mupirocin calcium by multiplying the percentage content of mupirocin lithium by 1.038.

IMPURITIES

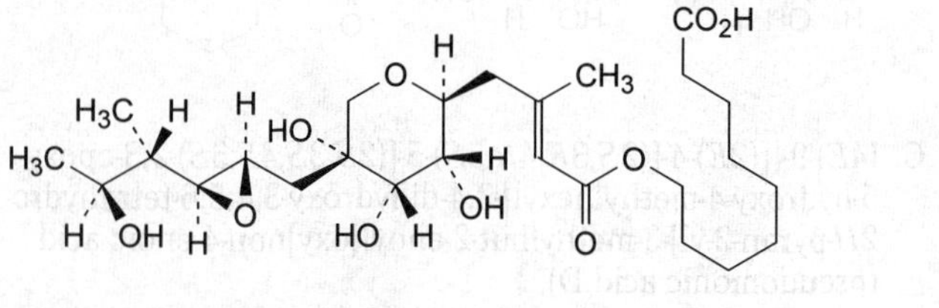

A. 9-[[(2*E*)-4-[(2*S*,3*R*,4*R*,5*R*)-3,4,5-trihydroxy-5-[[(2*S*,3*S*)-3-[(1*S*,2*S*)-2-hydroxy-1-methylpropyl]oxiranyl]methyl]tetrahydro-2*H*-pyran-2-yl]-3-methylbut-2-enoyl]oxy]nonanoic acid (pseudomonic acid B),

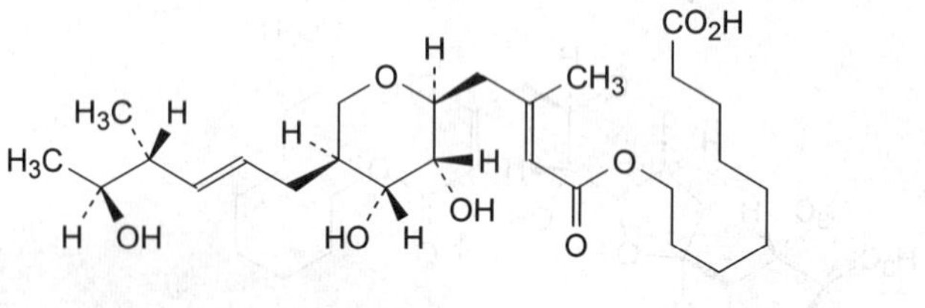

B. 9-[[(2*E*)-4-[(2*S*,3*R*,4*R*,5*S*)-3,4-dihydroxy-5-[(2*E*,4*R*,5*S*)-5-hydroxy-4-methylhex-2-enyl]tetrahydro-2*H*-pyran-2-yl]-3-methylbut-2-enoyl]oxy]nonanoic acid (pseudomonic acid C),

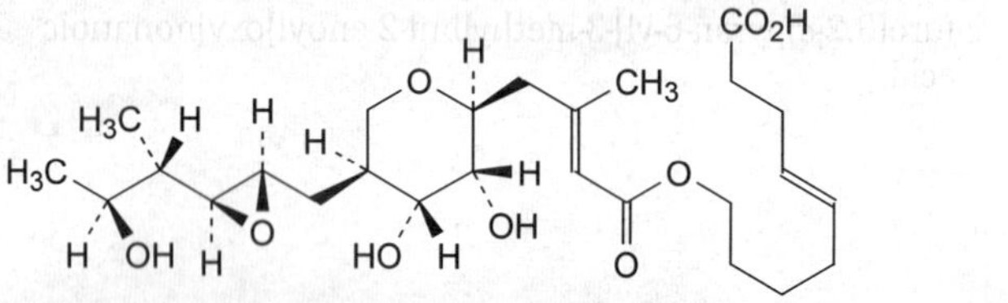

C. (4*E*)-9-[[(2*E*)-4-[(2*S*,3*R*,4*R*,5*S*)-3,4-dihydroxy-5-[[(2*S*,3*S*)-3-[(1*S*,2*S*)-2-hydroxy-1-methylpropyl]oxiranyl]methyl]tetrahydro-2*H*-pyran-2-yl]-3-methylbut-2-enoyl]oxy]non-4-enoic acid (pseudomonic acid D),

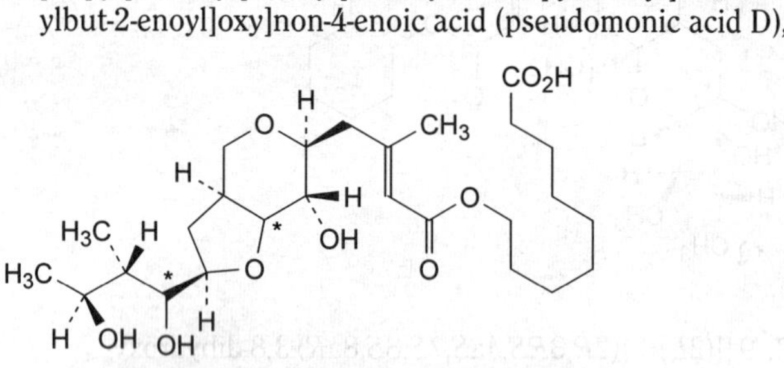

D. 9-[[(2*E*)-4-[(2*R*,3a*S*,6*S*,7*S*)-2-[(2*S*,3*S*)-1,3-dihydroxy-2-methylbutyl]-7-hydroxyhexahydro-4*H*-furo[3,2-*c*]pyran-6-yl]-3-methylbut-2-enoyl]oxy]nonanoic acid,

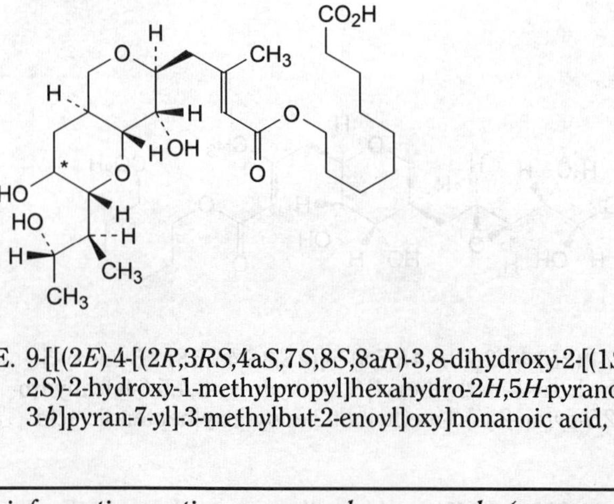

E. 9-[[(2*E*)-4-[(2*R*,3*RS*,4a*S*,7*S*,8*S*,8a*R*)-3,8-dihydroxy-2-[(1*S*,2*S*)-2-hydroxy-1-methylpropyl]hexahydro-2*H*,5*H*-pyrano[4,3-*b*]pyran-7-yl]-3-methylbut-2-enoyl]oxy]nonanoic acid,

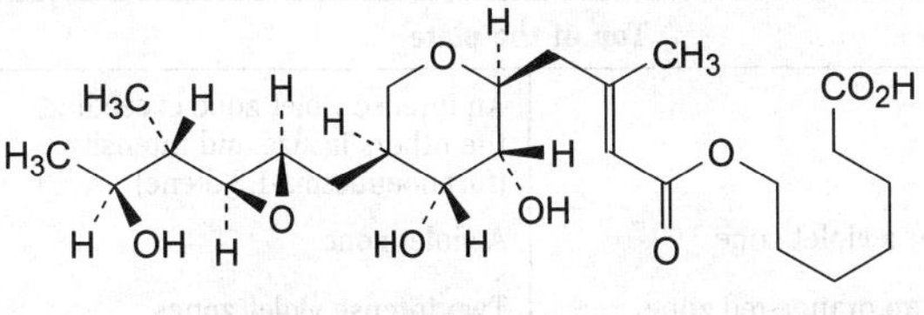

F. 7-[[(2*E*)-4-[(2*S*,3*R*,4*R*,5*S*)-3,4-dihydroxy-5-[[(2*S*,3*S*)-3-[(1*S*,2*S*)-2-hydroxy-1-methylpropyl]oxiranyl]methyl]tetrahydro-2*H*-pyran-2-yl]-3-methylbut-2-enoyl]oxy]heptanoic acid,

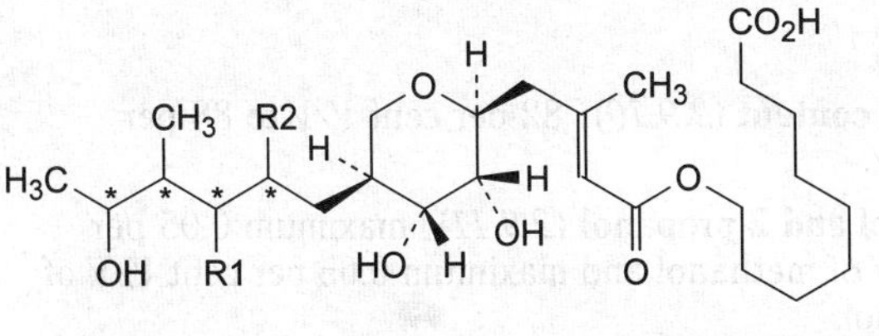

G. R1 = OH, R2 = Cl: 9-[[(2*E*)-4-[(2*S*,3*R*,4*R*,5*S*)-5-(2-chloro-3,5-dihydroxy-4-methylhexyl)-3,4-dihydroxytetrahydro-2*H*-pyran-2-yl]-3-methylbut-2-enoyl]oxy]nonanoic acid,

H. R1 = Cl, R2 = OH: 9-[[(2*E*)-4-[(2*S*,3*R*,4*R*,5*S*)-5-(3-chloro-2,5-dihydroxy-4-methylhexyl)-3,4-dihydroxytetrahydro-2*H*-pyran-2-yl]-3-methylbut-2-enoyl]oxy]nonanoic acid,

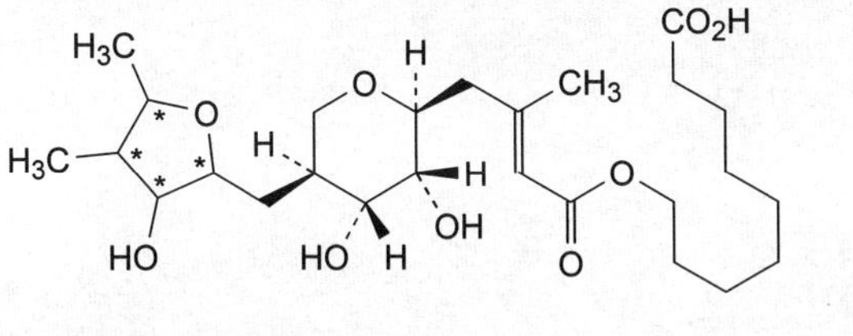

I. 9-[[(2*E*)-4-[(2*S*,3*R*,4*R*,5*S*)-3,4-dihydroxy-5-[(3-hydroxy-4,5-dimethyltetrahydrofuran-2-yl)methyl]tetrahydro-2*H*-pyran-2-yl]-3-methylbut-2-enoyl]oxy]nonanoic acid.

01/2005:1349

MYRRH

Myrrha

DEFINITION

Myrrh consists of a gum-resin, hardened in air, obtained by incision or produced by spontaneous exudation from the stem and branches of *Commiphora molmol* Engler and/or other species of *Commiphora*.

CHARACTERS

Myrrh has a bitter taste.

It has the macroscopic and microscopic characters described under identification tests A and B.

IDENTIFICATION

A. The light or dark orange-brown, irregular or roundish grains or pieces of different size show components of various colours. Their surface is mostly covered with grey to yellowish-brown dust.

B. Reduce to a powder (355). The powder is brownish-yellow to reddish-brown. Examine under a microscope, using *chloral hydrate solution R*. The powder shows only a few tissue fragments from the original plants including the following: reddish-brown cork fragments; single or grouped polyhedral to elongated stone cells with partly strongly thickened, pitted and lignified walls with a brownish content; fragments of thin-walled parenchyma and sclerenchymatous fibres; irregular prismatic to polyhedral crystals of calcium oxalate, about 10 µm to 25 µm in size.

C. Examine the chromatograms obtained in the test for *Commiphora mukul*. Spray the plate with *anisaldehyde solution R*, and examine in daylight while heating at 100 °C to 105 °C for 10 min. The chromatogram obtained with the reference solution shows in the lower third an orange-red zone (thymol) and in the middle third a violet zone (anethole).

The chromatogram obtained with the test solution shows an intense violet zone (furanoeudesma-1,3-diene), exceeding the other zones in size and intensity, above the zone of anethole in the chromatogram obtained with the reference solution; a violet zone similar in position to the zone of anethole in the chromatogram obtained with the reference solution; two intense violet zones similar in position to the zone of thymol in the chromatogram obtained with the reference solution, the upper one corresponding to curzerenone and the lower one to 2-methoxyfuranodiene. Further mostly violet zones are present in the chromatogram obtained with the test solution.

TESTS

Foreign matter (*2.8.2*). It complies with the test for foreign matter.

Commiphora mukul. Examine by thin-layer chromatography (*2.2.27*) using a *TLC silica gel plate R*.

Test solution. To 0.5 g of the powdered drug (355) add 5.0 ml of *alcohol R* and warm the mixture on a water-bath for 2 min to 3 min. Cool and filter.

Reference solution. Dissolve10 mg of *thymol R* and 40 µl of *anethole R* in 10 ml of *alcohol R*.

Apply to the plate as bands 10 µl of each solution. Develop over a path of 15 cm using a mixture of 2 volumes of *ethyl acetate R* and 98 volumes of *toluene R*. Allow the plate to dry in air. Examine in ultraviolet light at 365 nm, the chromatogram obtained with the test solution shows no blue to violet fluorescent zones in the lower third of the chromatogram.

Matter insoluble in alcohol. Not more than 70 per cent. Place 1.00 g of the powdered drug (250) in a flask. Add 30 ml of *alcohol R* and shake vigorously for 10 min. Filter the supernatant through a tared sintered-glass filter (16) avoiding the transfer of sediment from the flask. Repeat the extraction with two quantities, each of 20 ml, of *alcohol R*. Quantitatively transfer the sediment to the filter by rinsing the flask with *alcohol R*. Dry the filter and the residue in an oven at 100 °C to 105 °C and weigh.

Loss on drying (*2.2.32*). Not more than 15.0 per cent, determined on 1.000 g of powdered drug (355) by drying in an oven at 100 °C to 105 °C for 2 h.

Total ash (*2.4.16*). Not more than 7.0 per cent.

STORAGE

Store protected from light.

01/2005:1877

MYRRH TINCTURE

Myrrhae tinctura

DEFINITION

Tincture produced from *Myrrh (1349)*.

PRODUCTION

The tincture is produced from 1 part of the drug and 5 parts of ethanol (90 per cent *V/V*) by a suitable procedure.

CHARACTERS

Clear yellowish-brown or orange-brown liquid.

IDENTIFICATION

Thin-layer chromatography (*2.2.27*).

Test solution. Dilute 5 ml of the tincture to be examined to 10 ml with *alcohol R*.

Reference solution. Dissolve 10 mg of *thymol R* and 40 µl of *anethole R* in 10 ml of *ether R*.

Plate: *TLC silica gel plate R.*

Mobile phase: *ethyl acetate R, toluene R* (2:98 *V/V*).

Application: 10 µl, as bands.

Development: over a path of 15 cm.

Drying: in air.

Detection: spray with *anisaldehyde solution R* and examine in daylight whilst heating at 100-105 °C for 10 min.

Results: see below the sequence of the zones present in the chromatograms obtained with the reference solution and the test solution. Furthermore, other zones mostly violet, are present in the chromatogram obtained with the test solution.

Top of the plate	
	An intense violet zone exceeding the others in size and intensity (furanoeudesma-1,3-diene)
Anethole: a violet zone	A violet zone
Thymol: an orange-red zone	Two intense violet zones (curzerenone and below 2-methoxyfuranodiene)
Reference solution	**Test solution**

TESTS

Ethanol content (*2.9.10*): 82 per cent *V/V* to 88 per cent *V/V*.

Methanol and 2-propanol (*2.9.11*): maximum 0.05 per cent *V/V* of methanol and maximum 0.05 per cent *V/V* of 2-propanol.

Dry residue (*2.8.16*): minimum 4.0 per cent *m/m*.

STORAGE

Plastic containers are not recommended.

N

01/2005:1350

NABUMETONE

Nabumetonum

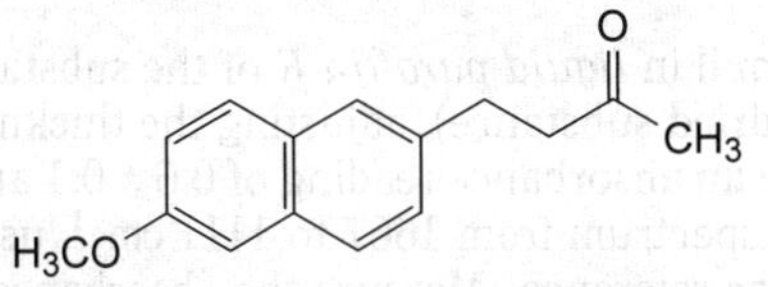

$C_{15}H_{16}O_2$ M_r 228.3

DEFINITION

Nabumetone contains not less than 97.0 per cent and not more than the equivalent of 102.0 per cent of 4-(6-methoxynaphthalen-2-yl)butan-2-one, calculated with reference to the anhydrous substance.

CHARACTERS

A white or almost white, crystalline powder, practically insoluble in water, freely soluble in acetone, slightly soluble in methanol.

IDENTIFICATION

Examine by infrared absorption spectrophotometry (*2.2.24*), comparing with the spectrum obtained with *nabumetone CRS.*

TESTS

Related substances. Examine by liquid chromatography (*2.2.29*) as described under Assay.

Inject 20 µl of test solution (a), 20 µl of reference solution (b) and 20 µl of reference solution (c). In the chromatogram obtained with test solution (a): the area of any peak due to impurity F, is not greater than the area of the principal peak in the chromatogram obtained with reference solution (c) (0.3 per cent); the sum of the areas of any other peak, apart from the principal peak and a peak due to impurity F, is not greater than the area of the principal peak in the chromatogram obtained with reference solution (b) (0.5 per cent). Disregard any peak with an area less than 0.1 times the area of the principal peak in the chromatogram obtained with reference solution (b).

Heavy metals (*2.4.8*). 2.0 g complies with limit test C for heavy metals (10 ppm). Prepare the standard using 2 ml of *lead standard solution (10 ppm Pb) R.*

Water (*2.5.12*). Not more than 0.2 per cent, determined on 1.000 g by the semi-micro determination of water.

Sulphated ash (*2.4.14*). Not more than 0.1 per cent, determined on 1.0 g.

ASSAY

Examine by liquid chromatography (*2.2.29*).

Test solution (a). Dissolve 50.0 mg of the substance to be examined in *acetonitrile R* and dilute to 10.0 ml with the same solvent.

Test solution (b). Dilute 1.0 ml of test solution (a) to 25.0 ml with *acetonitrile R.* Dilute 1.0 ml of the solution to 5.0 ml with *acetonitrile R.*

Reference solution (a). Dissolve 20.0 mg of *nabumetone CRS* in *acetonitrile R* and dilute to 10.0 ml with the same solvent. Dilute 1.0 ml of the solution to 50.0 ml with *acetonitrile R.*

Reference solution (b). Dilute 0.5 ml of test solution (a) to 100.0 ml with *acetonitrile R.*

Reference solution (c). Dissolve 1.5 mg of *nabumetone impurity F CRS* in *acetonitrile R* and dilute to 100.0 ml with the same solvent.

Reference solution (d). Dissolve 4 mg of *nabumetone impurity D CRS* in *acetonitrile R* and dilute to 100 ml with the same solvent. To 5 ml of the solution, add 5 ml of test solution (b).

The chromatographic procedure may be carried out using:

- a stainless steel column 0.15 m long and 4.6 mm in internal diameter packed with *base-deactivated octadecylsilyl silica gel for chromatography R* (4 µm),
- as mobile phase at a flow rate of 1 ml/min:

  Mobile phase A. A mixture of 12 volumes of *tetrahydrofuran R,* 28 volumes of *acetonitrile for chromatography R* and 60 volumes of a 0.1 per cent *V/V* solution of *glacial acetic acid R* in *carbon dioxide-free water R* prepared from *distilled water R,*

  Mobile phase B. A mixture of 24 volumes of *tetrahydrofuran R,* 56 volumes of *acetonitrile for chromatography R* and 20 volumes of a 0.1 per cent *V/V* solution of *glacial acetic acid R* in *carbon dioxide-free water R* prepared from *distilled water R,*

Time (min)	Mobile phase A (per cent *V/V*)	Mobile phase B (per cent *V/V*)	Comment
0 - 12	100	0	isocratic
12 - 28	100 → 0	0 → 100	linear gradient
28 - 33	0	100	isocratic
33 - 34	0 → 100	100 → 0	linear gradient
34 - 35	100	0	isocratic

- as detector a spectrophotometer set at 254 nm,

maintaining the temperature of the column at 40 °C.

Inject 20 µl of reference solution (b) and 20 µl of reference solution (d). Adjust the sensitivity of the system so that the height of the principal peak in the chromatogram obtained with reference solution (b) is at least 70 per cent of the full scale of the recorder. When the chromatograms are recorded under the prescribed conditions the retention time for nabumetone is about 11 min. The test is not valid unless, in the chromatogram obtained with reference solution (d), the resolution between the peaks corresponding to nabumetone and impurity D is at least 1.5. Inject reference solution (a) six times. The test is not valid unless the relative standard deviation of the peak area for nabumetone is at most 1.0 per cent. Inject alternately test solution (b) and reference solution (a).

Calculate the percentage content of nabumetone using the chromatogram obtained with reference solution (a).

STORAGE

Store protected from light.

IMPURITIES

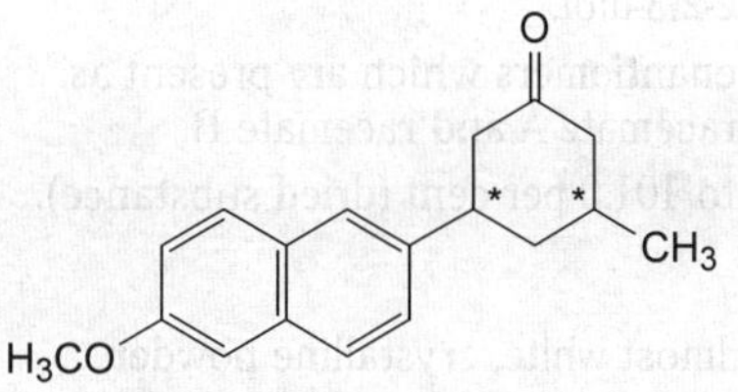

A. 3-(6-methoxynaphthalen-2-yl)-5-methylcyclohexanone,

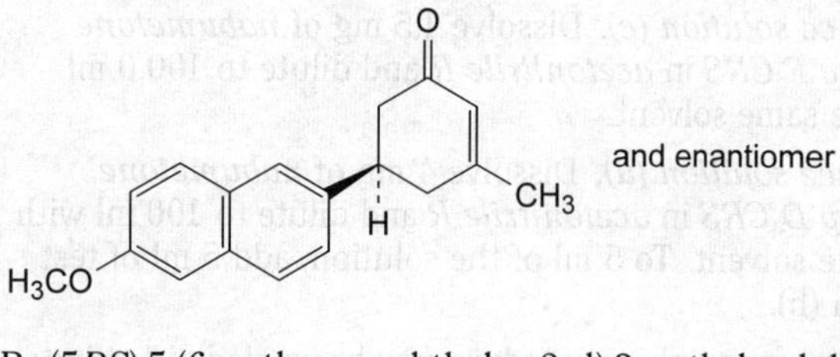

B. (5*RS*)-5-(6-methoxynaphthalen-2-yl)-3-methylcyclohex-2-enone,

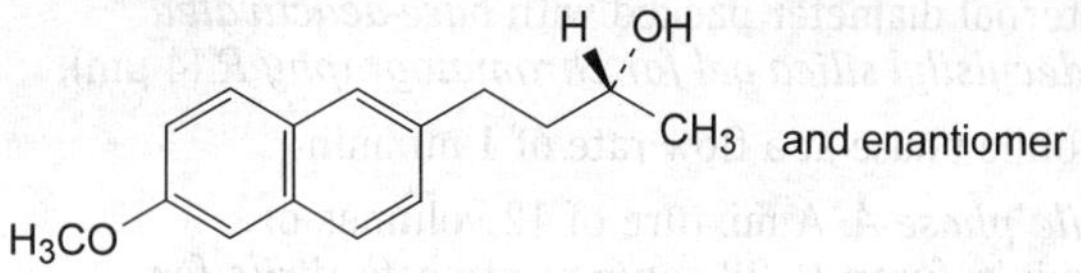

C. (2*RS*)-4-(6-methoxynaphthalen-2-yl)butan-2-ol,

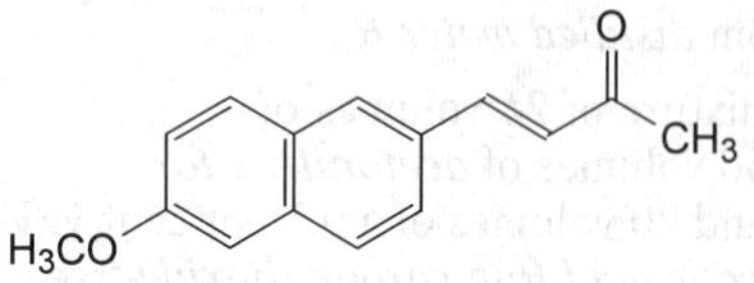

D. (*E*)-4-(6-methoxynaphthalen-2-yl)but-3-en-2-one,

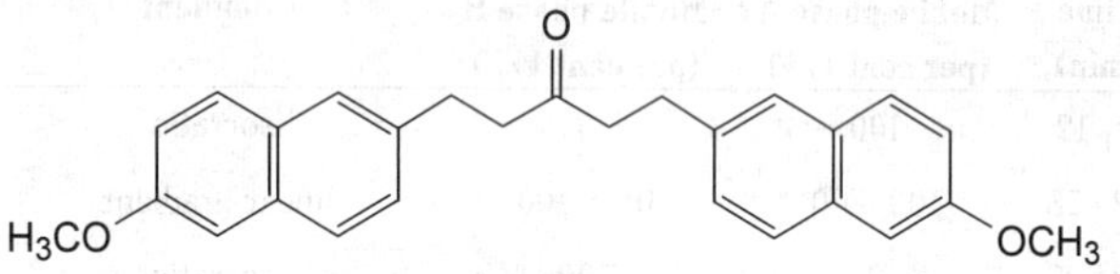

E. 1,5-bis(6-methoxynaphthalen-2-yl)pentan-3-one,

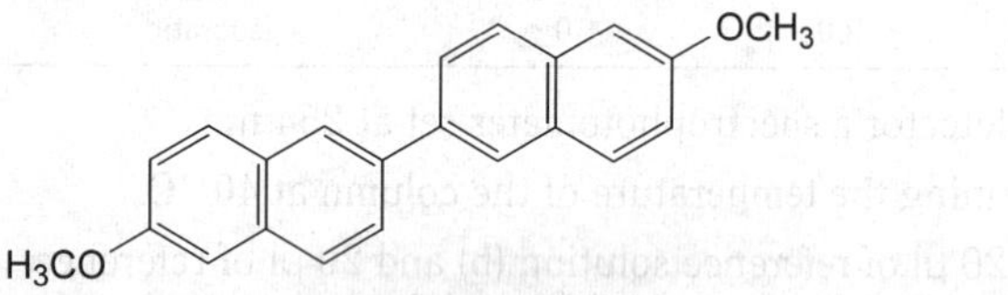

F. 6,6′-dimethoxy-2,2′-binaphthalenyl.

01/2005:1789

NADOLOL

Nadololum

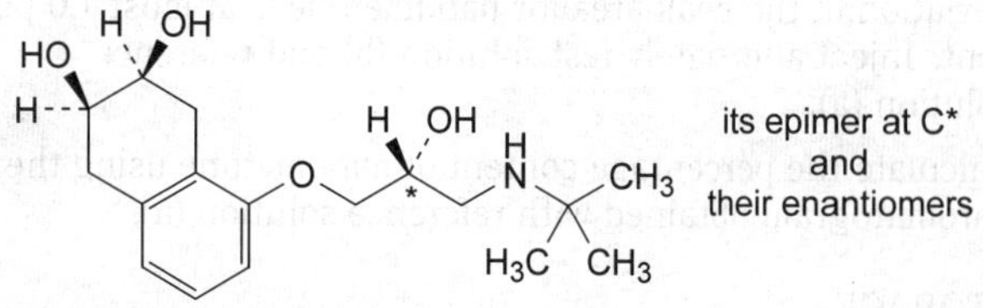

$C_{17}H_{27}NO_4$ M_r 309.4

DEFINITION

cis-5-[3-[(1,1-Dimethylethyl)amino]-2-hydroxypropoxy]-1,2,3,4-tetrahydronaphthalene-2,3-diol.

It consists of 2 pairs of enantiomers which are present as 2 racemic compounds: racemate A and racemate B.

Content: 98.5 per cent to 101.0 per cent (dried substance).

CHARACTERS

Appearance: white or almost white, crystalline powder.

Solubility: slightly soluble in water, freely soluble in alcohol, practically insoluble in acetone.

IDENTIFICATION

Infrared absorption spectrophotometry (*2.2.24*).

Comparison: *nadolol CRS*.

TESTS

Racemate content. Infrared absorption spectrophotometry (*2.2.24*).

Prepare a mull in *liquid paraffin R* of the substance to be examined (dried substance), adjusting the thickness of the mull to give an absorbance reading of 0.6 ± 0.1 at 1587 cm^{-1}. Record the spectrum from 1667 to 1111 cm^{-1}, using *liquid paraffin R* as reference. Measure the absorbance A_a, corresponding to racemate A, at the maximum at 1266 cm^{-1} and the absorbance A_b, corresponding to racemate B, at the maximum at 1250 cm^{-1}. The ratio A_a/A_b is 0.72 to 1.08 (corresponding to racemate A content of between 40 per cent and 60 per cent).

Related substances. Liquid chromatography (*2.2.29*).

Test solution. Dissolve 0.100 g of the substance to be examined in 4.0 ml of *methanol R* and dilute to 100.0 ml with a mixture of 20 volumes of *acetonitrile R* and 80 volumes of *water R*.

Reference solution (a). Dilute 1.0 ml of the test solution to 50.0 ml with a mixture of 20 volumes of *acetonitrile R* and 80 volumes of *water R*. Dilute 5.0 ml of the solution to 50.0 ml with a mixture of 20 volumes of *acetonitrile R* and 80 volumes of *water R*.

Reference solution (b). Dissolve 20 mg of *pindolol CRS* and 20 mg of the substance to be examined in 20 ml of *methanol R* and dilute to 100.0 ml with a mixture of 20 volumes of *acetonitrile R* and 80 volumes of *water R*. Dilute 1.0 ml of the solution to 100.0 ml with a mixture of 20 volumes of *acetonitrile R* and 80 volumes of *water R*.

Reference solution (c). Dilute 5.0 ml of reference solution (a) to 20.0 ml with mixture of 20 volumes of *acetonitrile R* and 80 volumes of *water R*.

Column:
- *size*: *l* = 0.30 m, Ø = 3.9 mm,
- *stationary phase*: spherical *end-capped octadecylsilyl silica gel for chromatography R* (5 µm), with a specific surface area of 700 m^2/g, a pore size of 0.9 nm and a carbon loading of 12 per cent.
- *temperature*: 40 °C.

Mobile phase:
- *mobile phase A*: 5.6 g/l solution of *sodium octanesulphonate R* adjusted to pH 3.5 with a 300 g/l solution of *phosphoric acid R*,
- *mobile phase B*: *acetonitrile R*,

Time (min)	Mobile phase A (per cent *V/V*)	Mobile phase B (per cent *V/V*)
0 - 7	77	23
7 - 30	77 → 65	23 → 35
30 - 45	65	35
45 - 50	65 → 77	35 → 23
50 - 60	77	23

Flow rate: 1 ml/min.

Detection: spectrophotometer at 206 nm.

Injection: 20 µl.

Relative retention with reference to nadolol (retention time = about 18 min): impurity A = 0.25; impurity B = 0.4; impurity C (doublet) = 0.6 and 0.7; impurity D = 1.4; impurity E = 1.6; impurity F = 2.2; impurity G = 2.6.

System suitability: reference solution (b):

- *resolution*: minimum of 8.0 between the peaks due to nadolol and to pindolol.

Limits:

- *correction factors*: for the calculation of contents, multiply the peak areas of the following impurities by the corresponding correction factor: impurity A = 1.7; impurity B = 1.7; impurity C = 1.7 (multiply the sum of the areas of the 2 peaks);
- *impurity A, B, C, D, E, F, G*: for each impurity, not more than the area of the principal peak in the chromatogram obtained with reference solution (a) (0.2 per cent);
- *any other impurity*: not more than half the area of the principal peak in the chromatogram obtained with reference solution (a) (0.1 per cent);
- *total*: not more than 2.5 times the area of the principal peak in the chromatogram obtained with reference solution (a) (0.5 per cent);
- *disregard limit*: area of the principal peak in the chromatogram obtained with reference solution (c) (0.05 per cent).

Heavy metals (*2.4.8*): maximum 30 ppm.

1.0 g complies with limit test D. Prepare the standard using 3 ml of *lead standard solution (10 ppm Pb) R*.

Loss on drying (*2.2.32*): maximum 2.0 per cent, determined on 1.000 g by drying *in vacuo* at 60 °C for 3 h.

Sulphated ash (*2.4.14*): maximum 0.1 per cent, determined on 1.0 g.

ASSAY

Dissolve 0.250 g in 100 ml of *anhydrous acetic acid R*. Titrate with *0.1 M perchloric acid*, determining the end-point potentiometrically (*2.2.20*).

1 ml of *0.1 M perchloric acid* is equivalent to 30.94 mg of $C_{17}H_{27}NO_4$.

IMPURITIES

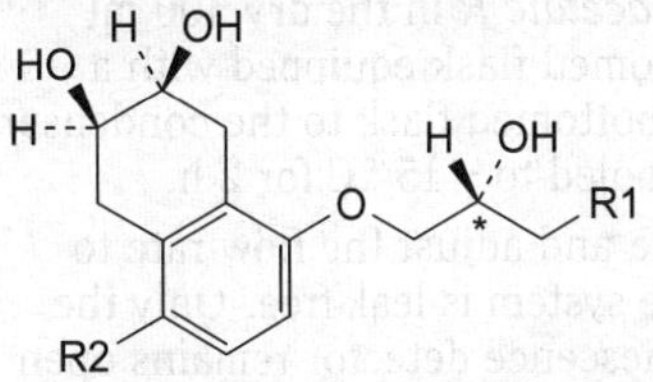

its epimer at C* and their enantiomers

A. R1 = OH, R2 = H: *cis*-5-[(2*RS*)-2,3-dihydroxypropoxy]-1,2,3,4-tetrahydronaphtalene-2,3-diol (tetraol),

B. R1 = OCH_3, R2 = H: *cis*-5-[(2*RS*)-2-hydroxy-3-methoxypropoxy]-1,2,3,4-tetrahydronaphtalene-2,3-diol,

E. R1 = NH-$C(CH_3)_3$, R2 = I: *cis*-5-[(2*RS*)-3-[(1,1-dimethylethyl)amino]-2-hydroxypropoxy]-8-iodo-1,2,3,4-tetrahydronaphtalene-2,3-diol,

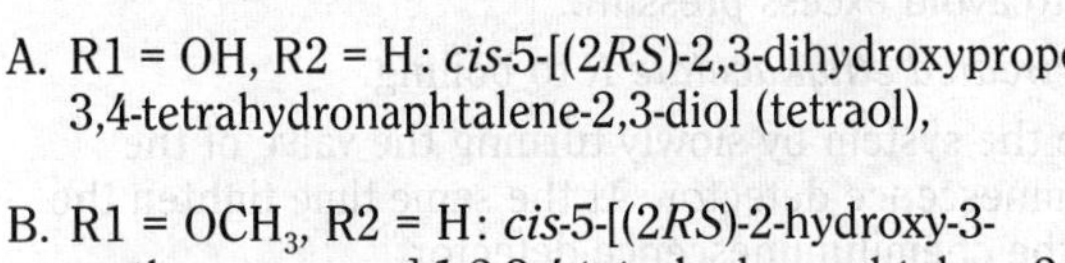

C. 5,5′-[(2-hydroxypropane-1,3-diyl)bis(oxy)]bis(*cis*-1,2,3,4-tetrahydronaphthalene-2,3-diol),

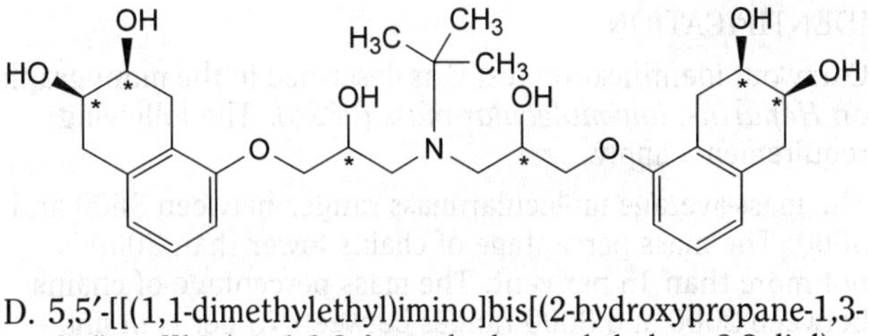

D. 5,5′-[[(1,1-dimethylethyl)imino]bis[(2-hydroxypropane-1,3-diyl)oxy]]bis(*cis*-1,2,3,4-tetrahydronaphthalene-2,3-diol),

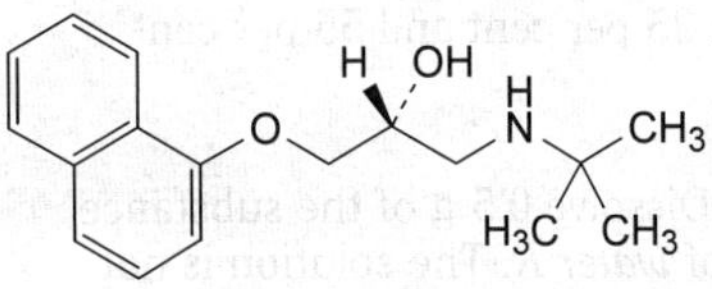

and enantiomer

F. (2*RS*)-1-[(1,1-dimethylethyl)amino]-3-(naphthalen-1-yloxy)propan-2-ol,

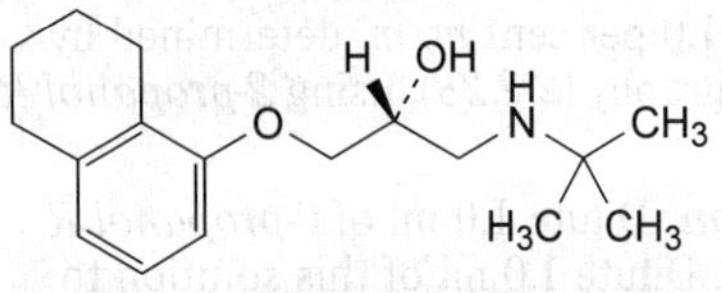

and enantiomer

G. (2*RS*)-1-[(1,1-dimethylethyl)amino]-3-[(5,6,7,8-tetrahydronaphtalen-1-yl)oxy]propan-2-ol.

01/2005:1134

NADROPARIN CALCIUM

Nadroparinum calcicum

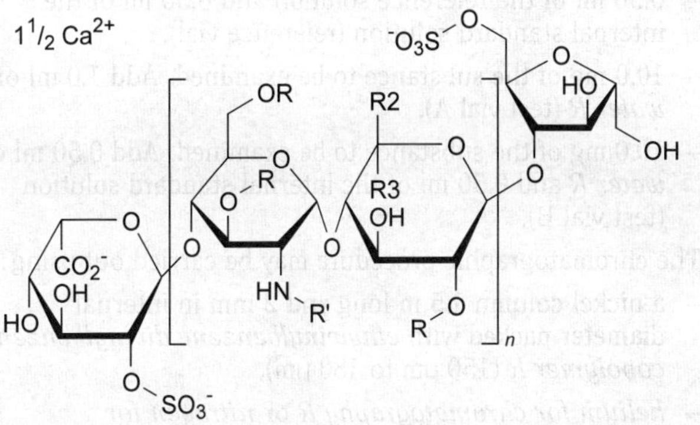

R = H or SO_3($^1/_2$ Ca) , R′ = H or SO_3($^1/_2$ Ca) or CO-CH_3

R2 = H and R3 = CO_2($^1/_2$ Ca) or R2 = CO_2($^1/_2$ Ca) and R3 = H

DEFINITION

Nadroparin calcium is the calcium salt of low-molecular-mass heparin obtained by nitrous acid depolymerisation of heparin from pork intestinal mucosa, followed by fractionation to eliminate selectively most of the chains with a molecular mass lower than 2000. The majority of the components have a 2-*O*-sulpho-α-L-idopyranosuronic acid structure at the non-reducing end and a 6-*O*-sulpho-2,5-anhydro-D-mannitol structure at the reducing end of their chain.

Nadroparin calcium complies with the monograph on *Heparins, low-molecular-mass (0828)* with the modifications and additional requirements below.

The mass-average molecular mass ranges between 3600 and 5000 with a characteristic value of about 4300.

The degree of sulphatation is about 2 per disaccharide unit.

The potency is not less than 95 IU and not more than 130 IU of anti-factor Xa activity per milligram, calculated with reference to the dried substance. The ratio of anti-factor Xa activity to anti-factor IIa activity is between 2.5 and 4.0.

IDENTIFICATION

Carry out identification test C as described in the monograph on *Heparins, low-molecular-mass (0828)*. The following requirements apply.

The mass-average molecular mass ranges between 3600 and 5000. The mass percentage of chains lower than 2000 is not more than 15 per cent. The mass percentage of chains between 2000 and 8000 ranges between 75 per cent and 95 per cent. The mass percentage of chains between 2000 and 4000 ranges between 35 per cent and 55 per cent.

TESTS

Appearance of solution. Dissolve 0.5 g of the substance to be examined in 10 ml of *water R*. The solution is not more intensely opalescent than the reference suspension II (*2.2.1*) and not more intensely coloured than the reference solution Y_5 (*2.2.2, Method II*).

Ethanol. Not more than 1.0 per cent *m/m*, determined by head-space gas chromatography (*2.2.28*), using *2-propanol R* as the internal standard.

Internal standard solution. Dilute 1.0 ml of *2-propanol R* to 100.0 ml with *water R*. Dilute 1.0 ml of this solution to 50.0 ml with *water R*.

Reference solution. Dilute 1.0 ml of *ethanol R* to 100.0 ml with *water R*. Dilute 0.5 ml of this solution to 20.0 ml with *water R*.

Vial filling. Place the following into four separate vials which can be crimp-sealed and which are compatible with the injection system:

- 1.0 ml of *water R* (blank vial),
- 0.50 ml of the reference solution and 0.50 ml of the internal standard solution (reference vial),
- 10.0 mg of the substance to be examined. Add 1.0 ml of *water R* (test vial A),
- 10.0 mg of the substance to be examined. Add 0.50 ml of *water R* and 0.50 ml of the internal standard solution (test vial B).

The chromatographic procedure may be carried out using:

- a nickel column 1.5 m long and 2 mm in internal diameter packed with *ethylvinylbenzene divinylbenzene copolymer R* (150 µm to 180 µm),
- *helium for chromatography R* or *nitrogen for chromatography R* as the carrier gas at a flow rate of 30 ml/min,
- a flame-ionisation detector.

Maintain the temperature of the column at 150 °C and that of the injection port and that of the detector at 250 °C.

Equilibrate each vial in the head-space system at 90 °C for 15 min. The pre-injection pressurisation time is 1 min.

The chromatogram obtained with the reference vial shows two peaks which correspond in order of increasing retention time to ethanol and 2-propanol (with retention times of approximately 2.5 min and 4 min). Calculate the content of ethanol (*m/m*) taking its density at 20 °C to be 0.792 g/ml.

N-NO groups. Not more than 0.25 ppm, determined by cleavage of the N-NO bond with hydrobromic acid in ethyl acetate under a reflux condenser and detection of the released NO by chemiluminescence.

Description of the apparatus (Figure 1134-1). Use a 500 ml borosilicate glass round-bottomed flask, above which is attached a condenser which is equipped with:

- on one side, a torion joint through which a stream of *argon R* can be introduced via a cannula,
- on the other side, a screw joint with a piston equipped with a septum through which the reference solution and test solution will be injected.

The round-bottomed flask is connected in series to three bubble traps which are themselves connected to two cold traps, which are in turn connected to a chemiluminescence detector. Suitable tubing ensures the junctions are leak-free.

Preparation of the chemiluminescence detector. Switch on the chemiluminescence detector 48 h before use and start the vacuum pump. The vacuum must be less than 0.5 mm Hg. 1 h before use, open the oxygen valve at a pressure of 0.2 MPa and a flow rate of 9.4 ml/min.

Preparation of the bubble trap. In each bubble trap, place 30 ml of a 300 g/l solution of *sodium hydroxide R* in *water R*.

Preparation of the cold traps.

- Trap at − 120 °C: Slowly add liquid nitrogen to an isothermic flask containing 250 ml of *ethanol R* whilst stirring with a wooden spatula until a paste is obtained. Place the cold trap in the isothermic flask prepared as described.
- Trap at − 160 °C: Slowly add liquid nitrogen to an isothermic flask containing 250 ml of *2-methylbutane R* whilst stirring with a wooden spatula until a paste is obtained. Place the cold trap in the isothermic flask prepared as described.

Drying of the 500 ml borosilicate-glass round-bottomed flask and condenser. Boil 50 ml of *ethyl acetate R* under reflux for 1 h under *argon R* without connecting the system to the chemiluminescence detector.

Test solution. Dry the substance to be examined for 12 h over *diphosphorus pentoxide R* at 60 °C under vacuum. Dissolve 0.10 g of the treated substance to be examined in 1.0 ml of *treated formamide R*. Shake the solution obtained for 30 min.

Reference solution. Dilute 0.1 ml of *nitrosodipropylamine solution R* in 6.0 ml of *ethanol R*. Dilute 0.1 ml of the solution obtained in 1.0 ml of *treated formamide R*. (This solution is equivalent to 0.05 ppm of N-NO groups).

Place 50 ml of *treated ethyl acetate R* in the dry 500 ml borosilicate glass round-bottomed flask equipped with a septum. Connect the round-bottomed flask to the condenser which has been previously cooled to − 15 °C for 2 h.

Connect the *argon R* cannula and adjust the flow rate to 0.1 litre/min. Check that the system is leak-free. Only the connector to the chemiluminescence detector remains open in order to avoid excess pressure.

Heat the *treated ethyl acetate R* to boiling.

Evacuate the system by slowly turning the valve of the chemiluminescence detector. At the same time tighten the inlet on the chemiluminescence detector.

When the system is equilibrated, the vacuum reaches 4 mm Hg.

The signal of the zero adjuster on the chemiluminescence detector is set to 10 per cent of the full scale of the recorder.

Through the septum of the 500 ml borosilicate glass round-bottomed flask, sequentially inject 0.5 ml of *water R*, 2.0 ml of *dilute hydrobromic acid R* and then another 2.0 ml of *dilute hydrobromic acid R*, making sure that the recorder pen has returned to the baseline between each injection.

Inject 50.0 µl of the reference solution, then 50.0 µl of the test solution after the recorder pen has returned to the baseline.

Calculate the content of N-NO groups of the substance to be examined.

Monographs N-O

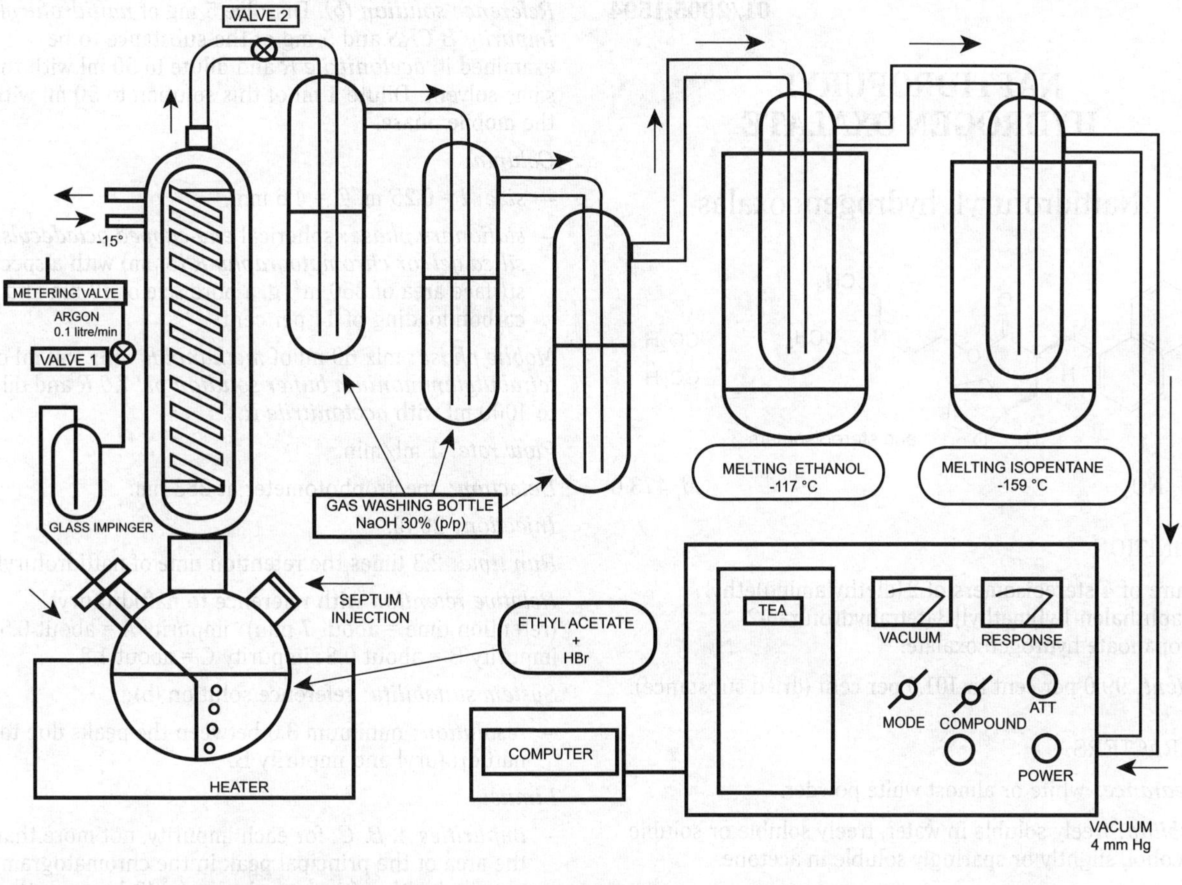

Bubble traps. Height: 24 cm, internal diameter: 2.5 cm, internal tubing 23 cm in length by 0.5 cm internal diameter. Centrally positioned Rotulex mounting. Equipped with torion joints on the inlet and outlet.

Chemiluminescence detector.

Cold trap. Height: 16.5 cm, internal diameter: 4 cm, internal tubing 14 cm in length and internal diameter 1.3 cm. Equipped with torion joints on the inlet and outlet.

Condenser. Height: 21 cm, internal diameter: 3 cm. Lower rodavis joint and upper torion joint.

Flask. Round-bottomed borosilicate glass flask equipped with a central rodavis joint, a torion joint on the left neck and a 15 cm screw joint on the right neck.

Isothermic flask. Internal depth: 22 cm, internal diameter: 8 cm.

Septum. Silicone material, diameter: 14 mm: thickness: 3.5 mm.

Torion joint.

Tubing. Polytetrafluoroethylene FEP material, internal diameter: 3.2 mm, thickness: 0.8 mm.

Figure 1134.-1. – *Apparatus used for the assay of N-NO groups*

Free sulphates. Not more than 0.5 per cent, determined by liquid chromatography (*2.2.29*) using an instrument equipped with a conductivity detector.

Test solution. Dissolve 30.0 mg of the substance to be examined in *water R* and dilute to 10.0 ml with the same solvent.

Reference solution. Dissolve 1.4787 g of *anhydrous sodium sulphate R* in *water R* and dilute to 1000.0 ml with the same solvent. Dilute 1.0 ml of this solution to 200.0 ml with *distilled water R* (5 ppm of sulphate ions).

The chromatographic procedure may be carried out using:

– an anion separation column 50 mm long and 4.6 mm in internal diameter,

– a chemical neutralisation system: neutralisation micromembrane in line with the mobile phase for anion detection,

– elute with a 1.91 g solution of *disodium tetraborate R* in 1000 ml of *water R* as mobile phase for 15 min. Change to 100 per cent of *0.1 M sodium hydroxide* for a period of 0.5 min. Elute with this solution for 10 min. Return to the initial conditions for a period of 0.5 min. The flow rate is 1.0 ml/min,

– a detector with a sensitivity of 30 μS.

Continuously pump the chemical neutralisation system in counter-flow with a 2.45 g/l solution of *sulphuric acid R*, at a flow rate of 4 ml/min.

Inject 50 μl of each solution. The chromatogram obtained with the reference solution shows a principal peak which corresponds to the sulphate ion (retention time of about 7.5 min). Change the composition of the mobile phase, if necessary, to obtain the prescribed retention time. Calculate the sulphate content of the substance to be examined.

Monographs N-O

01/2005:1594

NAFTIDROFURYL HYDROGEN OXALATE

Naftidrofuryli hydrogenooxalas

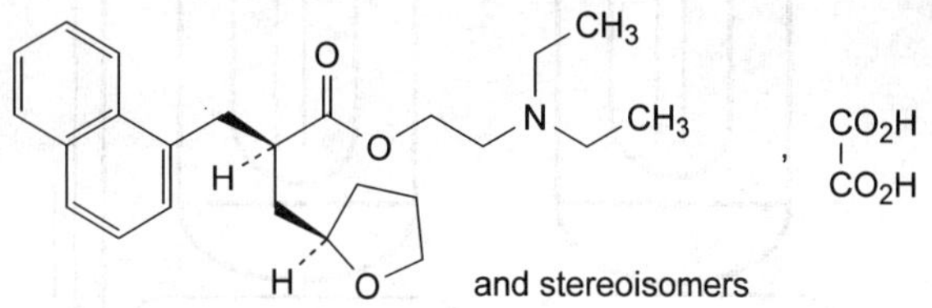

$C_{26}H_{35}NO_7$ M_r 473.6

DEFINITION

Mixture of 4 stereoisomers of 2-(diethylamino)ethyl 2-[(naphthalen-1-yl)methyl]-3-(tetrahydrofuran-2-yl)propanoate hydrogen oxalate.

Content: 99.0 per cent to 101.0 per cent (dried substance).

CHARACTERS

Appearance: white or almost white powder.

Solubility: freely soluble in water, freely soluble or soluble in alcohol, slightly or sparingly soluble in acetone.

IDENTIFICATION

A. Infrared absorption spectrophotometry (*2.2.24*).

Preparation: dissolve 1.0 g in *water R* and dilute to 50 ml with the same solvent. Add 2 ml of *concentrated ammonia R* and shake with 3 quantities, each of 10 ml, of *methylene chloride R*. To the combined lower layers, add *anhydrous sodium sulphate R*, shake, filter and evaporate the filtrate at a temperature not exceeding 30 °C, using a rotary evaporator. Use the residue obtained.

Comparison: *Ph. Eur. reference spectrum of naftidrofuryl.*

B. Dissolve 0.5 g in *water R* and dilute to 10 ml with the same solvent. Add 2.0 ml of *calcium chloride solution R*. A white precipitate is formed. The precipitate dissolves after the addition of 3.0 ml of *hydrochloric acid R*.

TESTS

Absorbance (*2.2.25*): maximum 0.1 at 430 nm.

Dissolve 1.5 g in *water R* and dilute to 10 ml with the same solvent. If necessary use an ultrasonic bath.

Related substances

A. Liquid chromatography (*2.2.29*).

Test solution. Dissolve 80.0 mg of the substance to be examined in the mobile phase and dilute to 20.0 ml with the mobile phase. Treat in an ultrasonic bath for 10 s. A precipitate is formed. Filter through a 0.45 µm membrane filter, discarding the first 5 millilitres. *Use a freshly prepared solution.*

Reference solution (a). Dissolve 5.0 mg of *naftidrofuryl impurity A CRS* in *acetonitrile R* and dilute to 25.0 ml with the same solvent. Dilute 1.0 ml of this solution to 50.0 ml with the mobile phase.

Reference solution (b). Dissolve 5 mg of *naftidrofuryl impurity B CRS* and 5 mg of the substance to be examined in *acetonitrile R* and dilute to 50 ml with the same solvent. Dilute 1 ml of this solution to 50 ml with the mobile phase.

Column:

- *size*: l = 0.25 m, Ø = 4.6 mm,
- *stationary phase*: spherical *end-capped octadecylsilyl silica gel for chromatography R* (5 µm) with a specific surface area of 350 m^2/g, a pore size of 10 nm and a carbon loading of 14 per cent.

Mobile phase: mix 60 ml of *methanol R* with 150 ml of *tetrabutylammonium buffer solution pH 7.0 R* and dilute to 1000 ml with *acetonitrile R*.

Flow rate: 1 ml/min.

Detection: spectrophotometer at 283 nm.

Injection: 20 µl.

Run time: 2.3 times the retention time of naftidrofuryl.

Relative retention with reference to naftidrofuryl (retention time = about 7 min): impurity A = about 0.5; impurity B = about 0.8; impurity C = about 1.8.

System suitability: reference solution (b):

- *resolution*: minimum 3.0 between the peaks due to naftidrofuryl and impurity B.

Limits:

- *impurities A, B, C*: for each impurity, not more than the area of the principal peak in the chromatogram obtained with reference solution (a) (0.1 per cent),
- *any other impurity*: for each impurity, not more than the area of the principal peak in the chromatogram obtained with reference solution (a) (0.1 per cent),
- *total*: not more than 3 times the area of the principal peak in the chromatogram obtained with reference solution (a) (0.3 per cent),
- *disregard limit*: 0.2 times the area of the principal peak in the chromatogram obtained with reference solution (a) (0.02 per cent).

B. Gas chromatography (*2.2.28*).

Test solution (a). Dissolve 1.0 g of the substance to be examined in *water R* and dilute to 50 ml with the same solvent. Add 2 ml of *concentrated ammonia R* and shake with 3 quantities, each of 10 ml, of *methylene chloride R*. To the combined lower layers, add *anhydrous sodium sulphate R*, shake, filter and evaporate the filtrate at a temperature not exceeding 30 °C, using a rotary evaporator. Take up the residue with *methylene chloride R* and dilute to 20.0 ml with the same solvent.

Test solution (b). Dilute 1.0 ml of test solution (a) to 10.0 ml with *methylene chloride R*.

Reference solution. Dissolve 5 mg of *naftidrofuryl impurity F CRS* in *methylene chloride R* and dilute to 50 ml with the same solvent.

Column:

- *material*: fused silica,
- *size*: l = 25 m, Ø = 0.32 mm,
- *stationary phase*: *poly(dimethyl)(diphenyl)siloxane R* (film thickness 0.45 µm).

Carrier gas: *helium for chromatography R*.

Splitter flow rate: 25 ml/min.

Flow rate: 2.9 ml/min.

Monographs N-O

Temperature:

	Time (min)	Temperature (°C)
Column	0 - 4	210
	4 - 8	210 → 230
	8 - 18	230 → 260
	18 - 30	260
Injection port		290
Detector		290

Detection: flame ionisation.

Injection: 1 µl.

Relative retention with reference to the second eluting peak of naftidrofuryl: impurity D = about 0.14; impurity B = about 0.55 (for the second eluting peak); impurity E = about 0.86; impurity F = about 1.04 (for the second eluting peak).

System suitability: test solution (b):

– *resolution*: minimum 1.0 between the 2 peaks due to the diastereoisomers of naftidrofuryl.

Limits: test solution (a):

– *impurity F*: for the sum of the areas of the 2 peaks, maximum 0.20 per cent of the sum of the areas of the 2 peaks due to naftidrofuryl (0.20 per cent),
– *impurity E*: maximum 0.20 per cent of the sum of the areas of the 2 peaks due to naftidrofuryl (0.20 per cent),
– *impurity D*: maximum 0.10 per cent of the sum of the areas of the 2 peaks due to naftidrofuryl (0.10 per cent),
– *any other impurity*: for each impurity, maximum 0.10 per cent of the sum of the areas of the 2 peaks due to naftidrofuryl (0.10 per cent),
– *total*: maximum 0.50 per cent of the sum of the areas of the 2 peaks due to naftidroduryl (0.50 per cent),
– *disregard limit*: 0.02 per cent of the sum of the areas of the 2 peaks due to naftidrofuryl (0.02 per cent); disregard any peaks due to impurity B.

Diastereoisomer ratio. Gas chromatography (*2.2.28*) as described in test B for related substances.

Limits: test solution (b):

– *first eluting naftidrofuryl diastereoisomer*: minimum 30 per cent of the sum of the areas of the 2 peaks due to naftidrofuryl.

Heavy metals (*2.4.8*): maximum 10 ppm.

In a silica crucible, mix thoroughly 1.0 g of the substance to be examined with 0.5 g of *magnesium oxide R1*. Ignite to dull redness until a homogeneous white or greyish-white mass is obtained. If after 30 min of ignition the mixture remains coloured, allow to cool, mix using a fine glass rod and repeat the ignition. If necessary repeat the operation. Heat at 800 °C for about 1 h. Take up the residue with 2 quantities, each of 5 ml, of a mixture of equal volumes of *hydrochloric acid R1* and *water R*. Add 0.1 ml of *phenolphthalein solution R* and then *concentrated ammonia R* until a pink colour is obtained. Cool, add *glacial acetic acid R* until the solution is decolorised and add 0.5 ml in excess. Filter if necessary and wash the filter. Dilute to 20 ml with *water R*. The solution complies with limit test E. Prepare the standard using 10 ml of *lead standard solution (1 ppm Pb) R*.

Loss on drying (*2.2.32*): maximum 0.5 per cent, determined on 1.000 g by drying in an oven at 100-105 °C.

Sulphated ash (*2.4.14*): maximum 0.1 per cent, determined on 1.0 g.

ASSAY

Dissolve 0.350 g in 50 ml of *anhydrous acetic acid R*. Titrate with *0.1 M perchloric acid*, determining the end-point potentiometrically (*2.2.20*).

1 ml of *0.1 M perchloric acid* is equivalent to 47.36 mg of $C_{26}H_{35}NO_7$.

IMPURITIES

Specified impurities: A, B, C, D, E, F.

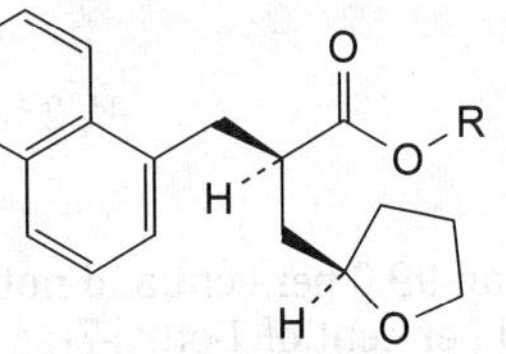

and stereoisomers

A. R = H: 2-[(naphthalen-1-yl)methyl]-3-(tetrahydrofuran-2-yl)propanoic acid,

B. R = C_2H_5: ethyl 2-[(naphthalen-1-yl)methyl]-3-(tetrahydrofuran-2-yl)propanoate,

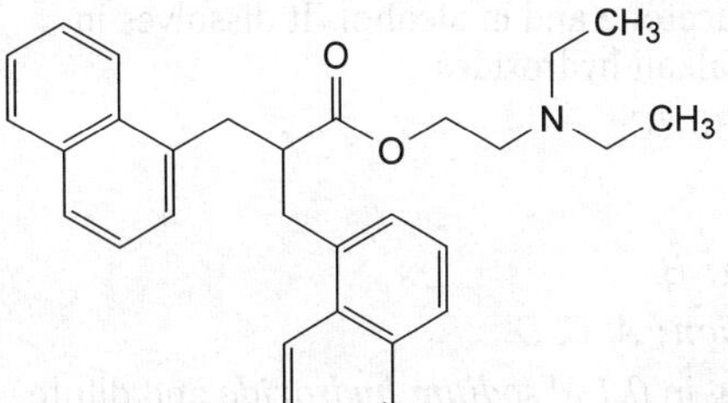

C. 2-(diethylamino)ethyl 3-(naphthalen-1-yl)-2-[(naphthalen-1-yl)methyl]propanoate,

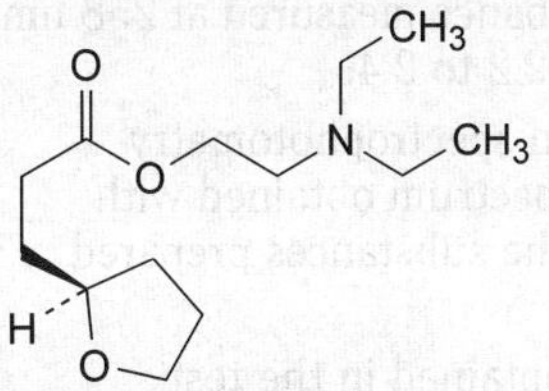

and enantiomer

D. 2-(diethylamino)ethyl 3-[(2*RS*)-tetrahydrofuran-2-yl]propanoate,

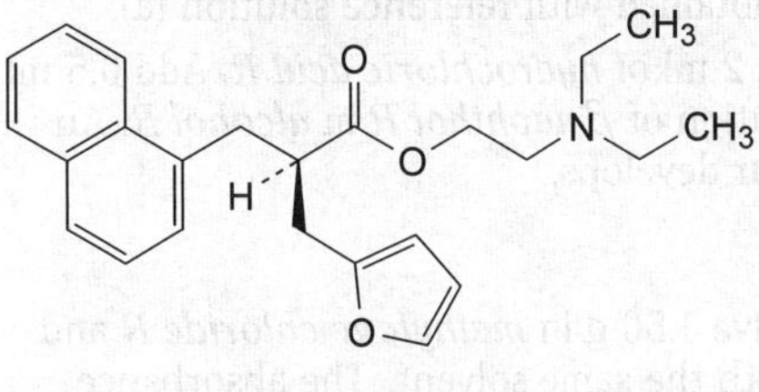

and enantiomer

E. 2-(diethylamino)ethyl (2*RS*)-2-[(furan-2-yl)methyl]-3-(naphthalen-1-yl)propanoate,

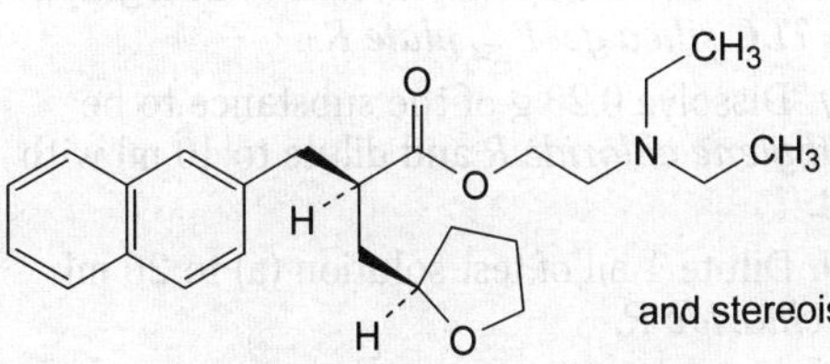

and stereoisomers

F. 2-(diethylamino)ethyl 2-[(naphthalen-2-yl)methyl]-3-(tetrahydrofuran-2-yl)propanoate.

Monographs N-O

01/2005:0701

NALIDIXIC ACID

Acidum nalidixicum

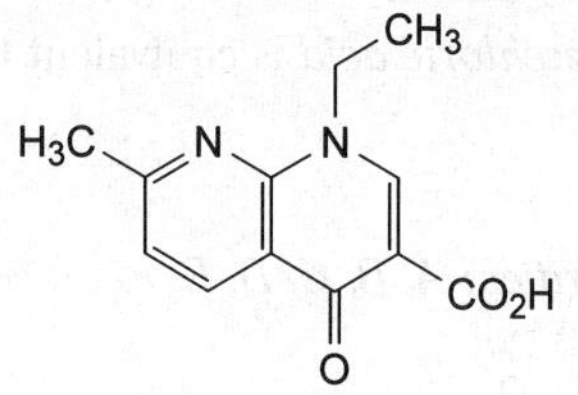

$C_{12}H_{12}N_2O_3$ M_r 232.2

DEFINITION

Nalidixic acid contains not less than 99.0 per cent and not more than the equivalent of 101.0 per cent of 1-ethyl-7-methyl-4-oxo-1,4-dihydro-1,8-naphthyridine-3-carboxylic acid, calculated with reference to the dried substance.

CHARACTERS

An almost white or pale yellow, crystalline powder, practically insoluble in water, soluble in methylene chloride, slightly soluble in acetone and in alcohol. It dissolves in dilute solutions of alkali hydroxides.

It melts at about 230 °C.

IDENTIFICATION

First identification: B.

Second identification: A, C, D.

A. Dissolve 12.5 mg in *0.1 M sodium hydroxide* and dilute to 50.0 ml with the same solvent. Dilute 2.0 ml of this solution to 100.0 ml with *0.1 M sodium hydroxide.* Examined between 230 nm and 350 nm (*2.2.25*), the solution shows two absorption maxima, at 258 nm and 334 nm. The ratio of the absorbance measured at 258 nm to that measured at 334 nm is 2.2 to 2.4.

B. Examine by infrared absorption spectrophotometry (*2.2.24*), comparing with the spectrum obtained with *nalidixic acid CRS*. Examine the substances prepared as discs.

C. Examine the chromatograms obtained in the test for related substances. The principal spot in the chromatogram obtained with the test solution (b) is similar in position and size to the principal spot in the chromatogram obtained with reference solution (a).

D. Dissolve 0.1 g in 2 ml of *hydrochloric acid R*. Add 0.5 ml of a 100 g/l solution of *β-naphthol R* in *alcohol R*. An orange-red colour develops.

TESTS

Absorbance. Dissolve 1.50 g in *methylene chloride R* and dilute to 50.0 ml with the same solvent. The absorbance (*2.2.25*) measured at 420 nm is not greater than 0.10.

Related substances. Examine by thin-layer chromatography (*2.2.27*), using a *TLC silica gel F_{254} plate R*.

Test solution (a). Dissolve 0.20 g of the substance to be examined in *methylene chloride R* and dilute to 10 ml with the same solvent.

Test solution (b). Dilute 1 ml of test solution (a) to 20 ml with *methylene chloride R*.

Reference solution (a). Dissolve 20 mg of *nalidixic acid CRS* in *methylene chloride R* and dilute to 20 ml with the same solvent.

Reference solution (b). Dilute 2 ml of test solution (b) to 10 ml with *methylene chloride R*.

Reference solution (c). Dilute 1 ml of reference solution (b) to 10 ml with *methylene chloride R*.

Reference solution (d). Dilute 1 ml of reference solution (b) to 25 ml with *methylene chloride R*.

Apply to the plate 10 µl of each solution. Develop over a path of 15 cm using a mixture of 10 volumes of *dilute ammonia R1*, 20 volumes of *methylene chloride R* and 70 volumes of *alcohol R*. Allow the plate to dry in air and examine in ultraviolet light at 254 nm. Any spot in the chromatogram obtained with the test solution (a), apart from the principal spot, is not more intense than the spot in the chromatogram obtained with reference solution (c) (0.1 per cent) and not more than one such spot is more intense than the spot in the chromatogram obtained with reference solution (d).

Heavy metals (*2.4.8*). 1.0 g complies with limit test D for heavy metals (20 ppm). Prepare the standard using 2 ml of *lead standard solution (10 ppm Pb) R*.

Loss on drying (*2.2.32*). Not more than 0.5 per cent, determined on 1.000 g by drying in an oven at 100 °C to 105 °C.

Sulphated ash (*2.4.14*). Not more than 0.1 per cent, determined on 1.0 g.

ASSAY

Dissolve 0.150 g in 10 ml of *methylene chloride R* and add 30 ml of *2-propanol R* and 10 ml of *carbon dioxide-free water R*. Keep the titration vessel covered and pass *nitrogen R* through the solution throughout the titration. Keep the temperature of the solution between 15 °C and 20 °C. Titrate with *0.1 M ethanolic sodium hydroxide*, determining the end-point potentiometrically (*2.2.20*) using a silver-silver chloride comparison electrode with a sleeve diaphragm or a capillary tip, filled with a saturated solution of *lithium chloride R* in *ethanol R*, and a glass electrode as indicator electrode.

1 ml of *0.1 M ethanolic sodium hydroxide* is equivalent to 23.22 mg of $C_{12}H_{12}N_2O_3$.

STORAGE

Store in an airtight container, protected from light.

01/2005:0729

NALOXONE HYDROCHLORIDE DIHYDRATE

Naloxoni hydrochloridum dihydricum

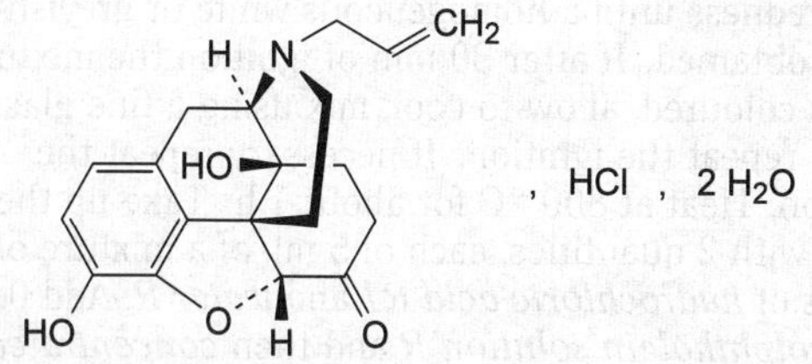

$C_{19}H_{22}ClNO_4,2H_2O$ M_r 399.9

DEFINITION

Naloxone hydrochloride dihydrate contains not less than 98.0 per cent and not more than the equivalent of 102.0 per cent of 4,5α-epoxy-3,14-dihydroxy-17-(prop-2-enyl)morphinan-6-one hydrochloride, calculated with reference to the anhydrous substance.

CHARACTERS

A white or almost white, crystalline powder, hygroscopic, freely soluble in water, soluble in alcohol, practically insoluble in toluene.

IDENTIFICATION

First identification: A, C.

Second identification: B, C.

A. Examine by infrared absorption spectrophotometry (*2.2.24*) comparing with the spectrum obtained with *naloxone hydrochloride dihydrate CRS.*

B. Examine by thin-layer chromatography (*2.2.27*), using a *TLC silica gel G plate R.*

Test solution. Dissolve 8 mg of the substance to be examined in 0.5 ml of *water R* and dilute to 1 ml with *methanol R.*

Reference solution. Dissolve 8 mg of *naloxone hydrochloride dihydrate CRS* in 0.5 ml of *water R* and dilute to 1 ml with *methanol R.*

Apply to the plate 5 µl of each solution. Develop protected from light over a path of 10 cm using a mixture of 5 volumes of *methanol R* and 95 volumes of the upper layer from a mixture of 60 ml of *dilute ammonia R2* and 100 ml of *butanol R.* Dry the plate in a current of air. Spray with a freshly prepared 5 g/l solution of *potassium ferricyanide R* in *ferric chloride solution R1.* Examine in daylight. The principal spot in the chromatogram obtained with the test solution is similar in position, colour and size to the principal spot in the chromatogram obtained with the reference solution.

C. It gives reaction (a) of chlorides (*2.3.1*).

TESTS

Solution S. Dissolve 0.50 g in *carbon dioxide-free water R* and dilute to 25.0 ml with the same solvent.

Appearance of solution. Solution S is clear (*2.2.1*) and colourless (*2.2.2, Method II*).

Acidity or alkalinity. To 10.0 ml of solution S add 0.05 ml of *methyl red solution R.* Not more than 0.2 ml of *0.02 M sodium hydroxide* or *0.02 M hydrochloric acid* is required to change the colour of the indicator.

Specific optical rotation (*2.2.7*): − 170 to − 181, determined on solution S and calculated with reference to the anhydrous substance.

Related substances. Examine by liquid chromatography (*2.2.29*).

Test solution. Dissolve 0.125 g of the substance to be examined in *0.1 M hydrochloric acid* and dilute to 25.0 ml with the same acid.

Reference solution (a). Dissolve 10.0 mg of *naloxone hydrochloride dihydrate CRS* and 10.0 mg of *naloxone impurity A CRS* in *0.1 M hydrochloric acid* and dilute to 10.0 ml with the same acid. Dilute 1.0 ml to 100.0 ml with *0.1 M hydrochloric acid.*

Reference solution (b). Dilute 1.0 ml of the test solution to 20.0 ml with *0.1 M hydrochloric acid.* Dilute 1.0 ml to 10.0 ml with *0.1 M hydrochloric acid.*

The chromatographic procedure may be carried out using:

– a stainless steel column 0.125 m long and 4.0 mm in internal diameter packed with *end-capped octylsilyl silica gel for chromatography R* (5 µm),

– as mobile phase at a flow rate of 1.5 ml/min a linear gradient programme using the following conditions:

Mobile phase A. Mix 20 ml of *acetonitrile R,* 40 ml of *tetrahydrofuran R* and 940 ml of a solution prepared as follows: dissolve 1.17 g of *sodium octanesulphonate R* in 1000 ml of *water R,* adjust the pH to 2.0 with a 50 per cent *V/V* solution of *phosphoric acid R* and filter (octanesulphonic acid solution).

Mobile phase B. Mix 170 ml of *acetonitrile R,* 40 ml of *tetrahydrofuran R* and 790 ml of the octanesulphonic acid solution.

Time (min)	Mobile phase A (per cent *V/V*)	Mobile phase B (per cent *V/V*)	Comment
0 - 40	100 → 0	0 → 100	linear gradient
40 - 50	0	100	isocratic

– as detector a spectrophotometer set at 230 nm,

maintaining the temperature of the column at 40 °C.

Inject separately 20 µl of each solution.

The test is not valid unless: the peak corresponding to naloxone in the chromatogram obtained with reference solution (a) has a signal-to-noise ratio of at least ten; in the chromatogram obtained with reference solution (a), the resolution between the peaks corresponding to impurity A and naloxone is not less than four. If necessary, adjust the chromatographic conditions.

When the chromatograms are recorded in the prescribed conditions, the retention time of naloxone is about 11 min and the relative retention time of impurity A is about 0.8 with respect to naloxone.

In the chromatogram obtained with the test solution: the area of any peak, apart from the principal peak, is not greater than the area of the principal peak in the chromatogram obtained with reference solution (b) (0.5 per cent); the sum of the areas of all the peaks, apart from the principal peak, is not greater than twice the area of the principal peak in the chromatogram obtained with reference solution (b) (1 per cent). Disregard any peak with an area less than 0.1 times that of the principal peak in the chromatogram obtained with reference solution (b).

Water (*2.5.12*): 7.5 per cent to 11.0 per cent, determined on 0.200 g by the semi-micro determination of water.

Sulphated ash (*2.4.14*). Not more than 0.2 per cent, determined on 0.50 g.

ASSAY

Dissolve 0.300 g in 50 ml of *alcohol R* and add 5.0 ml of *0.01 M hydrochloric acid.* Carry out a potentiometric titration (*2.2.20*), using *0.1 M ethanolic sodium hydroxide.* Read the volume added between the two points of inflexion.

1 ml of *0.1 M ethanolic sodium hydroxide* is equivalent to 36.38 mg of $C_{19}H_{22}ClNO_4$.

STORAGE

Store in an airtight container, protected from light.

IMPURITIES

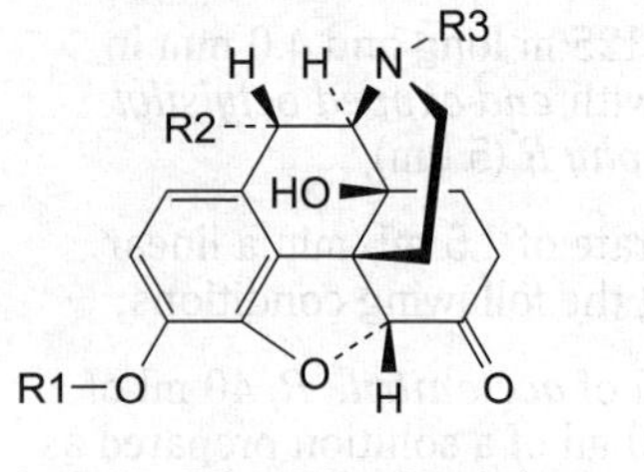

A. R1 = R2 = R3 = H: 4,5α-epoxy-3,14-dihydroxymorphinan-6-one (noroxymorphone),

B. R1 = R3 = CH_2-CH=CH_2, R2 = H: 4,5α-epoxy-14-hydroxy-17-(prop-2-enyl)-3-(prop-2-enyloxy)morphinan-6-one (3-*O*-allylnaloxone),

C. R1 = H, R2 = OH, R3 = CH_2-CH=CH_2: 4,5α-epoxy-3, 10α,14-trihydroxy-17-(prop-2-enyl)morphinan-6-one (10α-hydroxynaloxone),

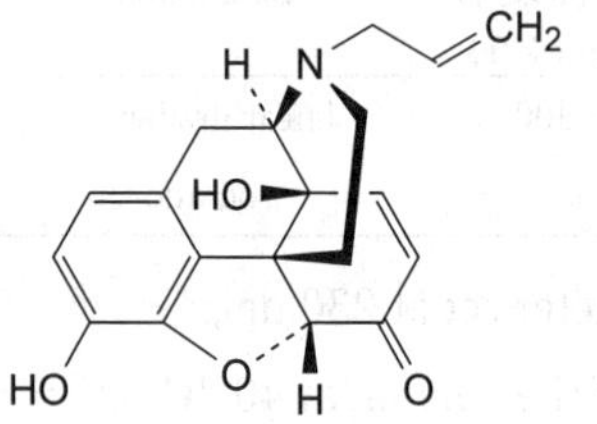

D. 7,8-didehydro-4,5α-epoxy-3,14-dihydroxy-17-(prop-2-enyl)morphinan-6-one (7,8-didehydronaloxone),

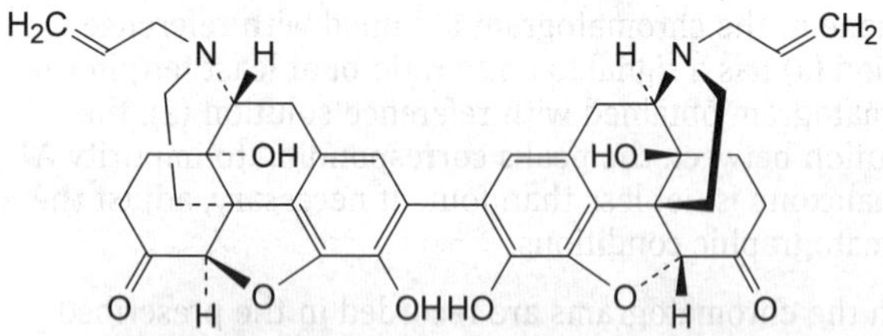

E. 4,5α:4′,5′α-diepoxy-3,3′,14,14′-tetrahydroxy-17, 17′-bis(prop-2-enyl)-2,2′-bimorphinanyl-6,6′-dione (2,2′-bisnaloxone).

01/2005:0730

NAPHAZOLINE HYDROCHLORIDE

Naphazolini hydrochloridum

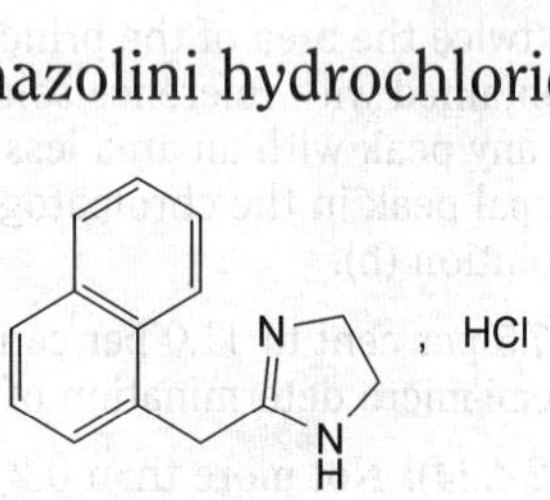

$C_{14}H_{15}ClN_2$ M_r 246.7

DEFINITION

2-(Naphthalen-1-ylmethyl)-4,5-dihydro-1*H*-imidazole hydrochloride.

Content: 99.0 per cent to 101.0 per cent (dried substance).

CHARACTERS

Appearance: white or almost white, crystalline powder.

Solubility: freely soluble in water, soluble in alcohol.

mp: about 259 °C, with decomposition.

IDENTIFICATION

First identification: B.

Second identification: A, C.

A. Dissolve 50.0 mg in *0.01 M hydrochloric acid* and dilute to 250.0 ml with the same acid. Dilute 25.0 ml of the solution to 100.0 ml with *0.01 M hydrochloric acid.* Examined between 230 nm and 350 nm (*2.2.25*), the solution shows 4 absorption maxima, at 270 nm, 280 nm, 287 nm and 291 nm. The ratios of the absorbances measured at the maxima at 270 nm, 287 nm and 291 nm to that measured at the maximum at 280 nm are 0.82 to 0.86, 0.67 to 0.70 and 0.65 to 0.69, respectively.

B. Infrared absorption spectrophotometry (*2.2.24*).

Comparison: *Ph. Eur. reference spectrum of naphazoline hydrochloride.*

C. It gives reaction (a) of chlorides (*2.3.1*).

TESTS

Solution S. Dissolve 0.5 g in *carbon dioxide-free water R* and dilute to 50 ml with the same solvent.

Appearance of solution. Solution S is clear (*2.2.1*) and colourless (*2.2.2, Method II*).

Acidity or alkalinity. To 20 ml of solution S add 0.2 ml of *0.01 M sodium hydroxide* and 0.1 ml of *methyl red solution R*. The solution is yellow. Not more than 0.6 ml of *0.01 M hydrochloric acid* is required to change the colour of the solution to red.

Related substances. Liquid chromatography (*2.2.29*).

Test solution. Dissolve 50.0 mg of the substance to be examined in the mobile phase and dilute to 100.0 ml with the mobile phase.

Reference solution (a). Dissolve 5 mg of *1-naphthylacetic acid R* in the mobile phase, add 5 ml of the test solution and dilute to 100 ml with the mobile phase.

Reference solution (b). Dissolve 5.0 mg of *naphazoline impurity A CRS* in the mobile phase and dilute to 100.0 ml with the mobile phase. Dilute 1.0 ml to 100.0 ml with the mobile phase.

Reference solution (c). Dilute 1.0 ml of the test solution to 10.0 ml with the mobile phase. Dilute 1.0 ml of this solution to 100.0 ml with the mobile phase.

Column:

- *size*: l = 0.25 m, Ø = 4.0 mm,
- *stationary phase*: *base-deactivated end-capped octylsilyl silica gel for chromatography R* (4 μm) with a pore size of 6 nm.

Mobile phase: dissolve 1.1 g of *sodium octanesulphonate R* in a mixture of 5 ml of *glacial acetic acid R*, 300 ml of *acetonitrile R* and 700 ml of *water R*.

Flow rate: 1 ml/min.

Detection: spectrophotometer at 280 nm.

Injection: 20 μl.

Run time: 3 times the retention time of naphazoline.

Retention time: naphazoline = about 14 min.

System suitability: reference solution (a):

- *resolution*: minimum 5.0 between the peaks due to naphazoline and to impurity B.

Limits:

- *impurity A*: not more than the area of the principal peak in the chromatogram obtained with reference solution (b) (0.1 per cent),
- *any other impurity*: not more than the area of the principal peak in the chromatogram obtained with reference solution (c) (0.1 per cent),

– *total*: not more than 5 times the area of the principal peak in the chromatogram obtained with reference solution (c) (0.5 per cent),
– *disregard limit*: 0.5 times the area of the principal peak in the chromatogram obtained with reference solution (c) (0.05 per cent).

Loss on drying (*2.2.32*): maximum 0.5 per cent, determined on 1.000 g by drying in an oven at 100-105 °C.

Sulphated ash (*2.4.14*): maximum 0.1 per cent, determined on 1.0 g.

ASSAY

Dissolve 0.200 g in a mixture of 5.0 ml of *0.01 M hydrochloric acid* and 50 ml of *alcohol R*. Carry out a potentiometric titration (*2.2.20*), using *0.1 M sodium hydroxide*. Read the volume added between the 2 points of inflexion.

1 ml of *0.1 M sodium hydroxide* is equivalent to 24.67 mg of $C_{14}H_{15}ClN_2$.

STORAGE

Protected from light.

IMPURITIES

Specified impurities: A.

Other detectable impurities: B, C, D.

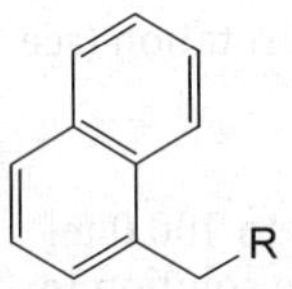

A. R = $CO\text{-}NH\text{-}[CH_2]_2\text{-}NH_2$: *N*-(2-aminoethyl)-2-(naphthalen-1-yl)acetamide (naphthylacetylethylenediamine),

B. R = CO_2H: (naphthalen-1-yl)acetic acid (1-naphthylacetic acid),

C. R = CN: (naphthalen-1-yl)acetonitrile (1-naphthylacetonitrile),

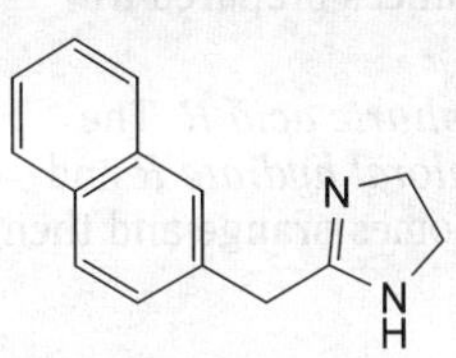

D. 2-(naphthalen-2-ylmethyl)-4,5-dihydro-1*H*-imidazole (β-naphazoline).

01/2005:0147

NAPHAZOLINE NITRATE

Naphazolini nitras

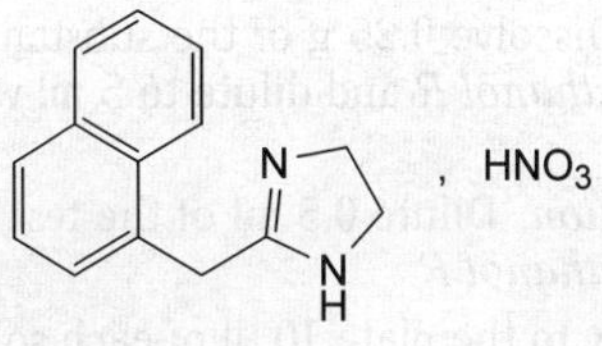

$C_{14}H_{15}N_3O_3$ M_r 273.3

DEFINITION

2-(Naphthalen-1-ylmethyl)-4,5-dihydro-1*H*-imidazole nitrate.

Content: 99.0 per cent to 101.0 per cent (dried substance).

CHARACTERS

Appearance: white or almost white, crystalline powder.

Solubility: sparingly soluble in water, soluble in alcohol.

IDENTIFICATION

First identification: C.

Second identification: A, B, D.

A. Melting point (*2.2.14*): 167 °C to 170 °C.

B. Dissolve 50.0 mg in *0.01 M hydrochloric acid* and dilute to 250.0 ml with the same acid. Dilute 25.0 ml of the solution to 100.0 ml with *0.01 M hydrochloric acid.* Examined between 230 nm and 350 nm (*2.2.25*), the solution shows 4 absorption maxima, at 270 nm, 280 nm, 287 nm and 291 nm. The ratios of the absorbances measured at the maxima at 270 nm, 287 nm and 291 nm to that measured at the maximum at 280 nm are 0.82 to 0.86, 0.67 to 0.70 and 0.65 to 0.69, respectively.

C. Infrared absorption spectrophotometry (*2.2.24*).
Comparison: *Ph. Eur. reference spectrum of naphazoline nitrate.*

D. Dissolve 45 mg of the substance to be examined in 2 ml of *water R*. Add 1 ml of *sulphuric acid R*. Shake carefully and allow to cool. Add 1 ml of *ferrous sulphate solution R2* dropwise along the walls of the container. At the junction of the 2 liquids, a brown colour develops.

TESTS

Solution S. Dissolve 0.5 g in *carbon dioxide-free water R*, warming gently, and dilute to 50 ml with the same solvent.

Appearance of solution. Solution S is clear (*2.2.1*) and colourless (*2.2.2, Method II*).

pH (*2.2.3*): 5.0 to 6.5 for solution S.

Related substances. Liquid chromatography (*2.2.29*).

Test solution. Dissolve 50.0 mg of the substance to be examined in the mobile phase and dilute to 100.0 ml with the mobile phase.

Reference solution (a). Dissolve 5 mg of *1-naphthylacetic acid R* in the mobile phase, add 5 ml of the test solution and dilute to 100 ml with the mobile phase.

Reference solution (b). Dissolve 5.0 mg of *naphazoline impurity A CRS* in the mobile phase and dilute to 100.0 ml with the same solvent. Dilute 5.0 ml to 100.0 ml with the mobile phase.

Reference solution (c). Dilute 2.0 ml of the test solution to 10.0 ml with the mobile phase. Dilute 1.0 ml of this solution to 100.0 ml with the mobile phase.

Column:
– *size*: *l* = 0.25 m, Ø = 4.0 mm,
– *stationary phase*: *end-capped base-deactivated octylsilyl silica gel for chromatography R* (4 μm) with a pore size of 6 nm.

Mobile phase: dissolve 1.1 g of *sodium octanesulphonate R* in a mixture of 5 ml of *glacial acetic acid R*, 300 ml of *acetonitrile R* and 700 ml of *water R*.

Flow rate: 1 ml/min.

Detection: spectrophotometer at 280 nm.

Injection: 20 μl.

Run time: 3 times the retention time of naphazoline.

Retention time: naphazoline = about 14 min.

System suitability: reference solution (a):
– *resolution*: minimum 5.0 between the peaks due to naphazoline and impurity B.

Limits:

- *impurity A*: not more than the area of the principal peak in the chromatogram obtained with reference solution (b) (0.5 per cent),
- *any other impurity*: not more than 0.5 times the area of the principal peak in the chromatogram obtained with reference solution (c) (0.1 per cent),
- *total*: not more than 5 times the area of the principal peak in the chromatogram obtained with reference solution (c) (1.0 per cent),
- *disregard limit*: 0.25 times the area of the principal peak in the chromatogram obtained with reference solution (c) (0.05 per cent); disregard any peak due to the nitrate ion.

Chlorides (*2.4.4*): maximum 330 ppm.

15 ml of solution S complies with the limit test for chlorides.

Loss on drying (*2.2.32*): maximum 0.5 per cent, determined on 1.000 g by drying in an oven at 100-105 °C.

Sulphated ash (*2.4.14*): maximum 0.1 per cent, determined on 1.0 g.

ASSAY

Dissolve 0.200 g in 30 ml of *anhydrous acetic acid R*. Titrate with *0.1 M perchloric acid*, determining the end-point potentiometrically (*2.2.20*).

1 ml of *0.1 M perchloric acid* is equivalent to 27.33 mg of $C_{14}H_{15}N_3O_3$.

STORAGE

Protected from light.

IMPURITIES

Specified impurities: A.

Other detectable impurities: B, C, D.

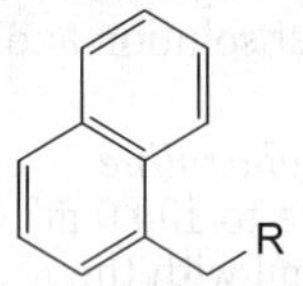

A. R = CO-NH-$[CH_2]_2$-NH_2: *N*-(2-aminoethyl)-2-(naphthalen-1-yl)acetamide (naphthylacetylethylenediamine),

B. R = CO_2H: (naphthalen-1-yl)acetic acid (1-naphthylacetic acid),

C. R = CN: (naphthalen-1-yl)acetonitrile (1-naphthylacetonitrile),

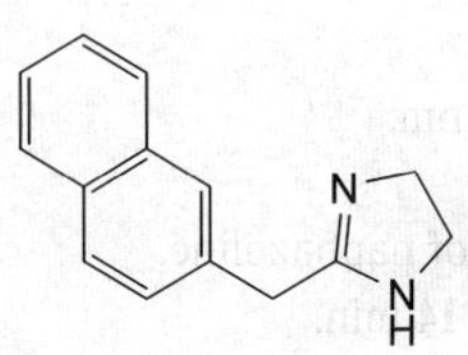

D. 2-(naphthalen-2-ylmethyl)-4,5-dihydro-1*H*-imidazole (β-naphazoline).

01/2005:0731

NAPROXEN

Naproxenum

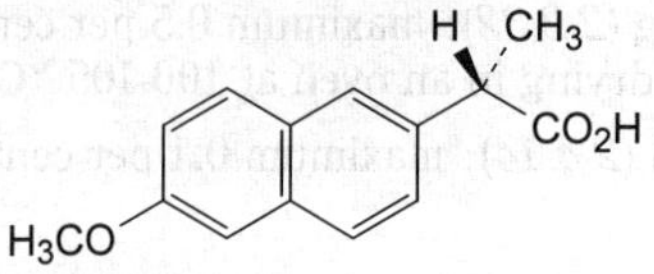

$C_{14}H_{14}O_3$ M_r 230.3

DEFINITION

Naproxen contains not less than 98.5 per cent and not more than the equivalent of 100.5 per cent of (2*S*)-2-(6-methoxynaphthalen-2-yl)propanoic acid, calculated with reference to the dried substance.

CHARACTERS

A white or almost white, crystalline powder, practically insoluble in water, soluble in alcohol and in methanol.

IDENTIFICATION

First identification: A, B, D.

Second identification: A, B, C, E.

A. It complies with the test for specific optical rotation (see Tests).

B. Melting point (*2.2.14*): 154 °C to 158 °C.

C. Dissolve 40.0 mg in *methanol R* and dilute to 100.0 ml with the same solvent. Dilute 10.0 ml of the solution to 100.0 ml with *methanol R*. Examined between 230 nm and 350 nm (*2.2.25*), the solution shows four absorption maxima, at 262 nm, 271 nm, 316 nm and 331 nm. The specific absorbances at the maxima are 216 to 238, 219 to 241, 61 to 69 and 79 to 87, respectively.

D. Examine by infrared absorption spectrophotometry (*2.2.24*) comparing with the spectrum obtained with *naproxen CRS*. Examine the substances prepared as discs, using *potassium bromide R*.

E. Dissolve about 2 mg in 2 ml of *sulphuric acid R*. The solution is yellow. Add 50 mg of *chloral hydrate R* and shake to dissolve. The solution becomes orange and then orange-red.

TESTS

Appearance of solution. Dissolve 1.25 g in *methanol R* and dilute to 25 ml with the same solvent. The solution is clear (*2.2.1*) and not more intensely coloured than reference solution BY_7 (*2.2.2, Method II*).

Specific optical rotation (*2.2.7*). Dissolve 0.500 g in *chloroform R* and dilute to 25.0 ml with the same solvent. The specific optical rotation is + 63 to + 68.5, calculated with reference to the dried substance.

Related substances. Examine by thin-layer chromatography (*2.2.27*), using *silica gel GF_{254} R* as the coating substance.

Test solution. Dissolve 0.25 g of the substance to be examined in *methanol R* and dilute to 5 ml with the same solvent.

Reference solution. Dilute 0.5 ml of the test solution to 100 ml with *methanol R*.

Apply separately to the plate 10 µl of each solution. Develop over a path of 15 cm using a mixture of 3 volumes of *glacial acetic acid R*, 9 volumes of *tetrahydrofuran R* and 90 volumes of *toluene R*. Allow the plate to dry in air and examine in ultraviolet light at 254 nm. Any spot in the chromatogram obtained with the test solution, apart from the principal spot, is not more intense than the spot in the chromatogram obtained with the reference solution (0.5 per cent).

Heavy metals (*2.4.8*). 1.0 g complies with limit test C for heavy metals (20 ppm). Prepare the standard using 2 ml of *lead standard solution (10 ppm Pb) R*.

Loss on drying (*2.2.32*). Not more than 0.5 per cent, determined on 1.000 g by drying in an oven at 100-105 °C for 3 h.

Sulphated ash (*2.4.14*). Not more than 0.1 per cent, determined on 1.0 g.

ASSAY

Dissolve 0.200 g in a mixture of 25 ml of *water R* and 75 ml of *methanol R*. Titrate with *0.1 M sodium hydroxide*, using 1 ml of *phenolphthalein solution R* as indicator.

1 ml of *0.1 M sodium hydroxide* is equivalent to 23.03 mg of $C_{14}H_{14}O_3$.

STORAGE

Store protected from light.

01/2005:1547

NEOHESPERIDIN-DIHYDROCHALCONE

Neohesperidin-dihydrochalconum

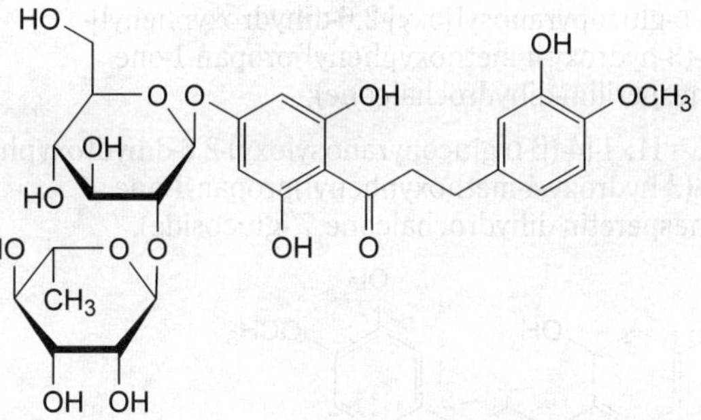

$C_{28}H_{36}O_{15}$ M_r 613

DEFINITION

1-[4-[[2-*O*-(6-Deoxy-α-L-mannopyranosyl)-β-D-glucopyranosyl]oxy]-2,6-dihydroxyphenyl]-3-(3-hydroxy-4-methoxyphenyl)propan-1-one.

Content: 96.0 per cent to 101.0 per cent (anhydrous substance).

CHARACTERS

Appearance: white or yellowish-white powder.

Solubility: practically insoluble in water, freely soluble in dimethyl sulphoxide, soluble in methanol, practically insoluble in methylene chloride.

IDENTIFICATION

A. Infrared absorption spectrophotometry (*2.2.24*).

Comparison: *neohesperidin-dihydrochalcone CRS*.

B. Examine the chromatograms obtained in the assay.

Results: the principal peak in the chromatogram obtained with test solution (b) is similar in retention time and size to the principal peak in the chromatogram obtained with reference solution (a).

TESTS

Appearance of solution. The solution is clear (*2.2.1*) and not more intensely coloured than reference solution Y_4 (*2.2.2, Method II*).

Dissolve 0.25 g in *methanol R* and dilute to 25 ml with the same solvent.

Related substances. Liquid chromatography (*2.2.29*).

Test solution (a). Dissolve 0.10 g of the substance to be examined in *dimethyl sulphoxide R* and dilute to 50.0 ml with the same solvent.

Test solution (b). Dilute 10.0 ml of test solution (a) to 20.0 ml with *dimethyl sulphoxide R*.

Reference solution (a). Dissolve 50.0 mg of *neohesperidin-dihydrochalcone CRS* in *dimethyl sulphoxide R* and dilute to 50.0 ml with the same solvent.

Reference solution (b). Dissolve 4.0 mg of *neohesperidin-dihydrochalcone impurity B CRS* in *dimethyl sulphoxide R* and dilute to 100.0 ml with the same solvent.

Reference solution (c). Dilute 1.0 ml of test solution (a) to 100.0 ml with *dimethyl sulphoxide R*.

Reference solution (d). In order to prepare *in situ* impurity F and impurity G, suspend 0.10 g of the substance to be examined in 10.0 ml of a 100 g/l solution of *sulphuric acid R*. Heat the sample for 5 min on a water-bath. Dilute immediately 1.0 ml of the resulting solution to 50.0 ml with *dimethyl sulphoxide R*.

Column:

- *size*: l = 0.15 m, Ø = 3.9 mm,
- *stationary phase*: spherical *octadecylsilyl silica gel for chromatography R* (4 µm) with a carbon loading of 7 per cent,
- *temperature*: 30 °C.

Mobile phase: mix 20 volumes of *acetonitrile R* and 80 volumes of a solution prepared by adding 5.0 ml of *glacial acetic acid R* to 1000.0 ml of *water R*.

Flow rate: 1.0 ml/min.

Detection: spectrophotometer at 282 nm.

Injection: 10 µl; inject test solution (a) and reference solutions (a), (b), (c) and (d).

Run time: 5 times the retention time of neohesperidin-dihydrochalcone which is about 10 min.

Relative retention with reference to neohesperidin-dihydrochalcone: impurity B = about 0.4; impurity D = about 0.7; impurity F = about 1.2; impurity G = about 3.7.

System suitability:

- *resolution*: minimum of 2.5 between the first peak (neohesperidin-dihydrochalcone) and the second peak (impurity F) in the chromatogram obtained with reference solution (d),
- chromatogram obtained with reference solution (a) is similar to the chromatogram provided with *neohesperidin-dihydrochalcone CRS*.

Limits:

- *impurity B*: not more than the area of the principal peak in the chromatogram obtained with reference solution (b) (2 per cent),
- *impurity D*: not more than twice the area of the principal peak in the chromatogram obtained with reference solution (c) (2 per cent),
- *any other impurity*: not more than 0.5 times the area of the principal peak in the chromatogram obtained with reference solution (c) (0.5 per cent),

- *total of all impurities apart from impurity B*: not more than 2.5 times the area of the principal peak in the chromatogram obtained with reference solution (c) (2.5 per cent),
- *disregard limit*: 0.05 times the area of the principal peak in the chromatogram obtained with reference solution (c) (0.05 per cent).

Heavy metals (*2.4.8*): maximum 10 ppm.

2.0 g complies with limit test D. Prepare the standard using 2 ml of *lead standard solution (10 ppm Pb) R*.

Water (*2.5.12*): maximum 12.0 per cent, determined on 0.200 g.

Sulphated ash (*2.4.14*): maximum 0.2 per cent, determined on 1.0 g.

ASSAY

Liquid chromatography (*2.2.29*) as described in the test for related substances.

Injection: 10 µl; inject test solution (b) and reference solutions (a) and (d).

System suitability:

- *resolution*: minimum of 2.5 between the first peak (neohesperidin-dihydrochalcone) and the second peak (impurity F) in the chromatogram obtained with reference solution (d),
- *repeatability*: reference solution (a).

Calculate the percentage content of $C_{28}H_{36}O_{15}$ using the chromatogram obtained with reference solution (a) and the stated content of $C_{28}H_{36}O_{15}$ in *neohesperidin-dihydrochalcone CRS*, correcting for the water content of the substance to be examined.

STORAGE

Protected from light.

IMPURITIES

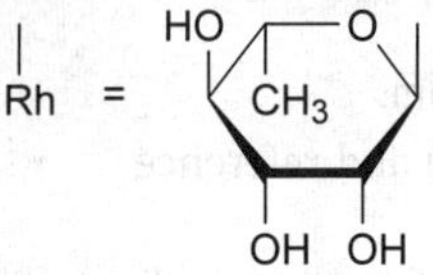

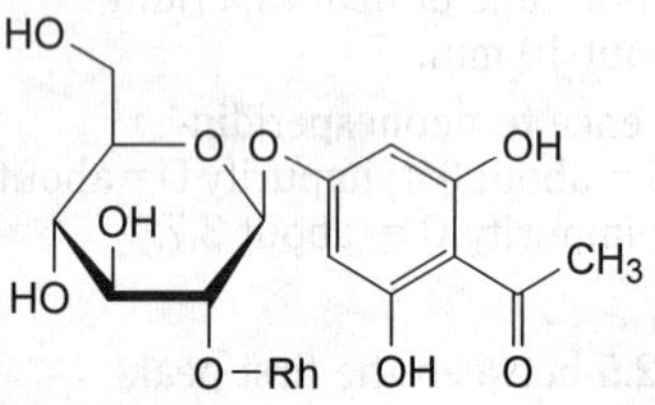

A. 1-[4-[[2-*O*-(6-deoxy-α-L-mannopyranosyl)-β-D-glucopyranosyl]oxy]-2,6-dihydroxyphenyl]ethanone (phloroacetophenone neohesperidoside),

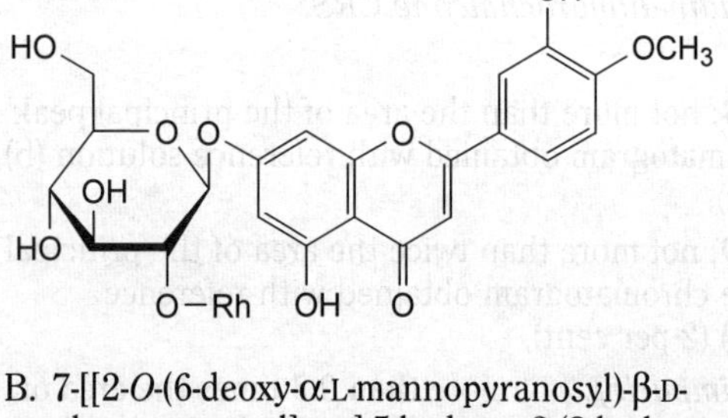

B. 7-[[2-*O*-(6-deoxy-α-L-mannopyranosyl)-β-D-glucopyranosyl]oxy]-5-hydroxy-2-(3-hydroxy-4-methoxyphenyl)-4*H*-1-benzopyran-4-one (neodiosmin),

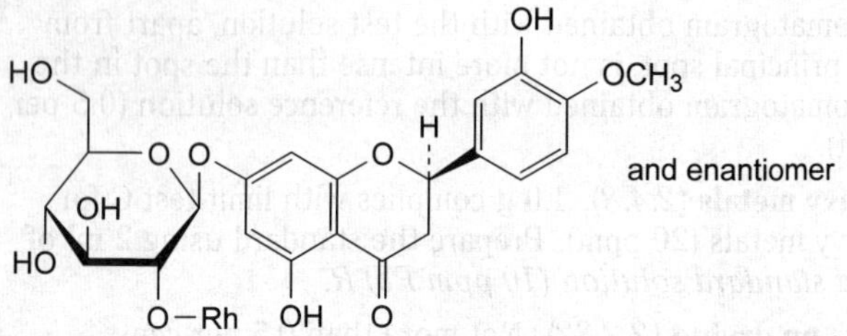

C. (2*RS*)-7-[[2-*O*-(6-deoxy-α-L-mannopyranosyl)-β-D-glucopyranosyl]oxy]-5-hydroxy-2-(3-hydroxy-4-methoxyphenyl)-2,3-dihydro-4*H*-1-benzopyran-4-one (neohesperidin),

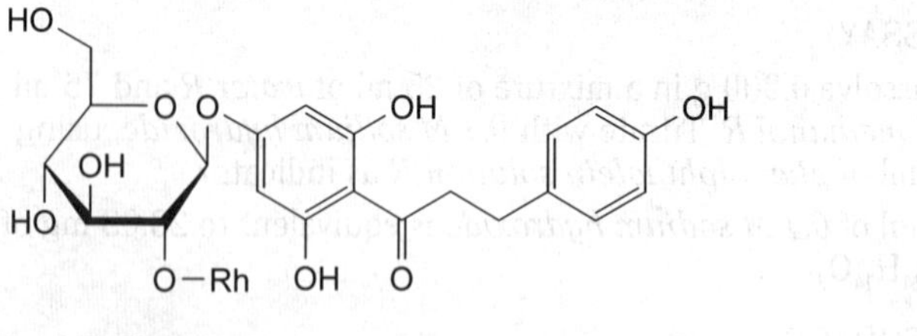

D. 1-[4-[[2-*O*-(6-deoxy-α-L-mannopyranosyl)-β-D-glucopyranosyl]oxy]-2,6-dihydroxyphenyl]-3-(4-hydroxyphenyl)propan-1-one (naringin-dihydrochalcone),

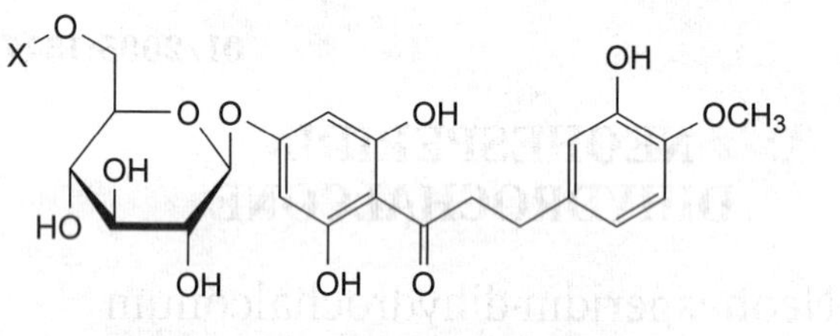

E. X = Rh: 1-[4-[[6-*O*-(6-deoxy-α-L-mannopyranosyl)-β-D-glucopyranosyl]oxy]-2,6-dihydroxyphenyl]-3-(3-hydroxy-4-methoxyphenyl)propan-1-one (hesperidin-dihydrochalcone),

F. X = H: 1-[4-(β-D-glucopyranosyloxy)-2,6-dihydroxyphenyl]-3-(3-hydroxy-4-methoxyphenyl)propan-1-one (hesperetin-dihydrochalcone 7′-glucoside),

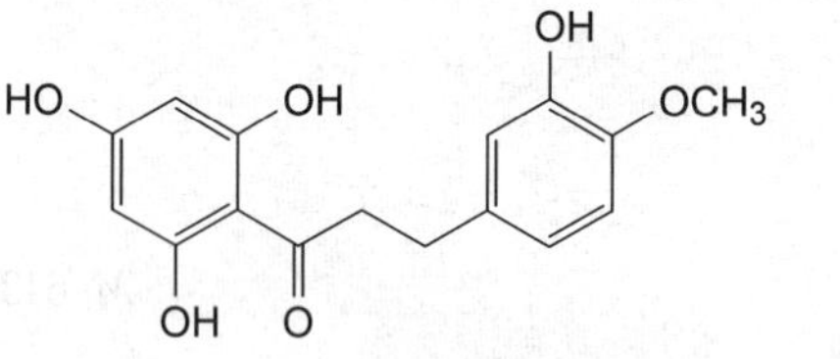

G. 3-(3-hydroxy-4-methoxyphenyl)-1-(2,4,6-trihydroxyphenyl)propan-1-one (hesperetin-dihydrochalcone).

01/2005:0197

NEOMYCIN SULPHATE

Neomycini sulfas

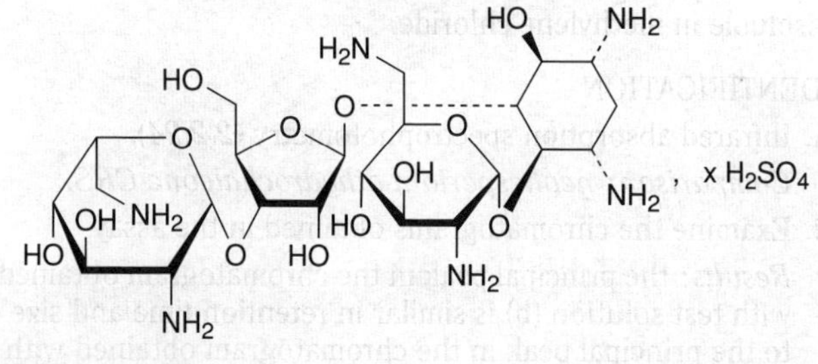

$C_{23}H_{46}N_6O_{13},xH_2SO_4$ M_r 615 (base)

DEFINITION

Mixture of sulphates of substances produced by the growth of certain selected strains of *Streptomyces fradiae*, the main component being the sulphate of 2-deoxy-4-*O*-(2,6-diamino-2,6-dideoxy-α-D-glucopyranosyl)-5-*O*-[3-*O*-(2,6-diamino-2,6-dideoxy-β-L-idopyranosyl)-β-D-ribofuranosyl]-D-streptamine (neomycin B).

Content: minimum of 680 IU/mg (dried substance).

CHARACTERS

Appearance: white or yellowish-white powder, hygroscopic.

Solubility: very soluble in water, very slightly soluble in alcohol, practically insoluble in acetone.

IDENTIFICATION

A. Examine the chromatograms obtained in the test for related substances.

Results:

- the retention time of the principal peak in the chromatogram obtained with the test solution is approximately the same as that of the principal peak in the chromatogram obtained with reference solution (e),
- it complies with the limits given for impurity C.

B. It gives reaction (a) of sulphates (*2.3.1*).

TESTS

pH (*2.2.3*): 5.0 to 7.5.

Dissolve 0.1 g in *carbon dioxide-free water R* and dilute to 10 ml with the same solvent.

Specific optical rotation (*2.2.7*): + 53.5 to + 59.0 (dried substance).

Dissolve 1.00 g in *water R* and dilute to 10.0 ml with the same solvent.

Related substances. Liquid chromatography (*2.2.29*).

Test solution. Dissolve 25.0 mg of the substance to be examined in the mobile phase and dilute to 50.0 ml with the mobile phase.

Reference solution (a). Dissolve 25.0 mg of *framycetin sulphate CRS* in the mobile phase and dilute to 50.0 ml with the mobile phase.

Reference solution (b). Dilute 5.0 ml of reference solution (a) to 100.0 ml with the mobile phase.

Reference solution (c). Dilute 1.0 ml of reference solution (a) to 100.0 ml with the mobile phase.

Reference solution (d). Dissolve the contents of a vial of *neamine CRS* (corresponding to 0.5 mg) in the mobile phase and dilute to 50.0 ml with the mobile phase.

Reference solution (e). Dissolve 10 mg of *neomycin sulphate CRS* in the mobile phase and dilute to 100.0 ml with the mobile phase.

Column:

- *size*: l = 0.25 m, Ø = 4.6 mm,
- *stationary phase*: *base-deactivated octadecylsilyl silica gel for chromatography R* (5 μm),
- *temperature*: 25 °C.

Mobile phase: mix 20.0 ml of *trifluoroacetic acid R*, 6.0 ml of *carbonate-free sodium hydroxide solution R* and 500 ml of *water R*, allow to equilibrate, dilute to 1000 ml with *water R* and degas.

Flow rate: 0.7 ml/min.

Post-column solution: *carbonate-free sodium hydroxide solution R* diluted 1 in 25 previously degassed, which is added pulse-less to the column effluent using a 375 μl polymeric mixing coil.

Flow rate: 0.5 ml/min.

Detection: pulsed amperometric detector with a gold indicator electrode, a silver-silver chloride reference electrode and a stainless steel auxiliary electrode which is the cell body, held at respectively 0.00 V detection, + 0.80 V oxidation and − 0.60 V reduction potentials, with pulse durations according to the instrument used.

Injection: 10 μl; inject the test solution and the reference solutions (b), (c), (d) and (e).

Run time: 1.5 times the retention time of neomycin B.

Relative retention with reference to neomycin B (retention time = about 10 min): impurity A = about 0.65; impurity C = about 0.9; impurity G = about 1.1.

System suitability:

- *resolution*: minimum of 2.0 between the peaks due to impurity C and to neomycin B in the chromatogram obtained with reference solution (e); if necessary, adjust the volume of the carbonate-free sodium hydroxide solution in the mobile phase,
- *signal-to-noise ratio*: minimum 10 for the principal peak in the chromatogram obtained with reference solution (c).

Limits:

- *impurity A*: not more than the area of the principal peak in the chromatogram obtained with reference solution (d) (2.0 per cent),
- *impurity C*: not more than 3 times the area of the principal peak in the chromatogram obtained with reference solution (b) (15.0 per cent) and not less than 0.6 times the area of the principal peak in the chromatogram obtained with reference solution (b) (3.0 per cent),
- *any other impurity*: not more than the area of the principal peak in the chromatogram obtained with reference solution (b) (5.0 per cent),
- *total of other impurities*: not more than 3 times the area of the principal peak in the chromatogram obtained with reference solution (b) (15.0 per cent),
- *disregard limit*: area of the principal peak in the chromatogram obtained with reference solution (c) (1.0 per cent).

Sulphate: 27.0 per cent to 31.0 per cent (dried substance). Dissolve 0.250 g in 100 ml of *water R* and adjust the solution to pH 11 using *concentrated ammonia R*. Add 10.0 ml of *0.1 M barium chloride* and about 0.5 mg of *phthalein purple R*. Titrate with *0.1 M sodium edetate* adding 50 ml of *alcohol R* when the colour of the solution begins to change, continuing the titration until the violet-blue colour disappears.

1 ml of *0.1 M barium chloride* is equivalent to 9.606 mg of SO_4.

Loss on drying (*2.2.32*): maximum 8.0 per cent, determined on 1.000 g by drying at 60 °C over *diphosphorus pentoxide R* at a pressure not exceeding 0.7 kPa for 3 h.

Sulphated ash (*2.4.14*): maximum 1.0 per cent, determined on 1.0 g.

ASSAY

Carry out the microbiological assay of antibiotics (*2.7.2*). Use *neomycin sulphate for microbiological assay CRS* as the reference substance.

Monographs N-O

STORAGE

In an airtight container, protected from light.

IMPURITIES

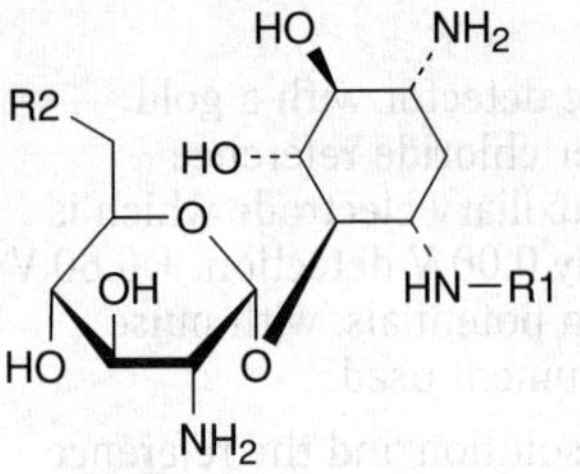

A. R1 = H, R2 = NH_2: 2-deoxy-4-*O*-(2,6-diamino-2,6-dideoxy-α-D-glucopyranosyl)-D-streptamine (neamine or neomycin A-LP),

B. R1 = CO-CH_3, R2 = NH_2: 3-*N*-acetyl-2-deoxy-4-*O*-(2,6-diamino-2,6-dideoxy-α-D-glucopyranosyl)-D-streptamine (3-acetylneamine),

D. R1 = H, R2 = OH: 4-*O*-(2-amino-2-deoxy-α-D-glucopyranosyl)-2-deoxy-D-streptamine (paromamine or neomycin D),

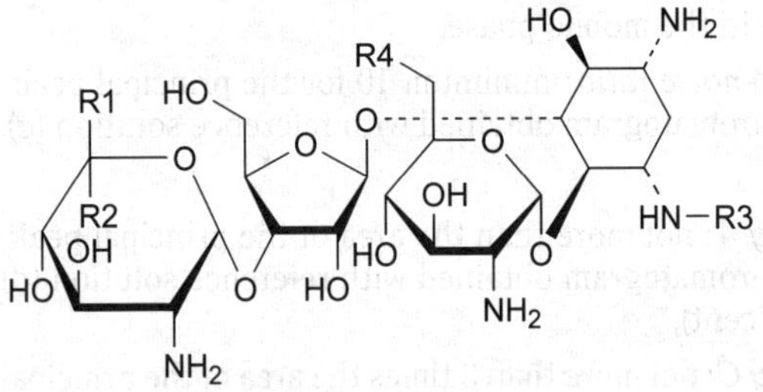

C. R1 = CH_2-NH_2, R2 = R3 = H, R4 = NH_2: 2-deoxy-4-*O*-(2,6-diamino-2,6-dideoxy-α-D-glucopyranosyl)-5-*O*-[3-*O*-(2,6-diamino-2,6-dideoxy-α-D-glucopyranosyl)-β-D-ribofuranosyl]-D-streptamine (neomycin C),

E. R1 = R3 = H, R2 = CH_2-NH_2, R4 = OH: 4-*O*-(2-amino-2-deoxy-α-D-glucopyranosyl)-2-deoxy-5-*O*-[3-*O*-(2,6-diamino-2,6-dideoxy-β-L-idopyranosyl)-β-D-ribofuranosyl]-D-streptamine (paromomycin I or neomycin E),

F. R1 = CH_2-NH_2, R2 = R3 = H, R4 = OH: 4-*O*-(2-amino-2-deoxy-α-D-glucopyranosyl)-2-deoxy-5-*O*-[3-*O*-(2,6-diamino-2,6-dideoxy-α-D-glucopyranosyl)-β-D-ribofuranosyl]-D-streptamine (paromomycin II or neomycin F),

G. R1 = H, R2 = CH_2-NH_2, R3 = CO-CH_3, R4 = NH_2: 3-*N*-acetyl-2-deoxy-4-*O*-(2,6-diamino-2,6-dideoxy-α-D-glucopyranosyl)-5-*O*-[3-*O*-(2,6-diamino-2,6-dideoxy-β-L-idopyranosyl)-β-D-ribofuranosyl]-D-streptamine (neomycin B-LP).

01/2005:0046

NEOSTIGMINE BROMIDE

Neostigmini bromidum

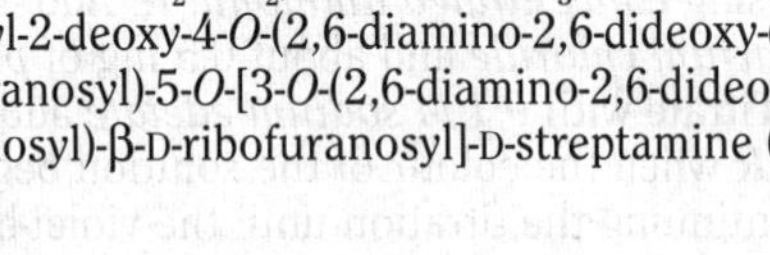

$C_{12}H_{19}BrN_2O_2$ M_r 303.2

DEFINITION

Neostigmine bromide contains not less than 98.5 per cent and not more than the equivalent of 101.0 per cent of 3-[(dimethylcarbamoyl)oxy]-*N,N,N*-trimethylanilinium bromide, calculated with reference to the dried substance.

CHARACTERS

A white, crystalline powder or colourless crystals, hygroscopic, very soluble in water, freely soluble in alcohol.

IDENTIFICATION

First identification: B, D.

Second identification: A, C, D.

A. Dissolve 20 mg in *0.5 M sulphuric acid* and dilute to 100 ml with the same acid. Examined between 230 nm and 350 nm, the solution shows 2 absorption maxima (*2.2.25*), at 260 nm and 266 nm. The specific absorbances at the maxima are about 16 and about 14, respectively.

B. Examine by infrared absorption spectrophotometry (*2.2.24*), comparing with the spectrum obtained with *neostigmine bromide CRS*.

C. Heat about 50 mg with a mixture of 0.4 g of *potassium hydroxide R* and 2 ml of *alcohol R* on a water-bath for 3 min, replacing the evaporated alcohol. Cool and add 2 ml of *water R* and 2 ml of *diazobenzenesulphonic acid solution R1*. An orange-red colour develops.

D. It gives the reactions of bromides (*2.3.1*).

TESTS

Solution S. Dissolve 2.5 g in *distilled water R* and dilute to 50 ml with the same solvent.

Appearance of solution. Solution S is clear (*2.2.1*) and colourless (*2.2.2, Method II*).

(3-Hydroxyphenyl)trimethylammonium bromide. Dissolve 50 mg in a mixture of 1 ml of *sodium carbonate solution R* and 9 ml of *water R*. The absorbance (*2.2.25*) measured immediately at 294 nm is not greater than 0.25.

Sulphates (*2.4.13*). 15 ml of solution S complies with the limit test for sulphates (200 ppm).

Loss on drying (*2.2.32*). Not more than 1.0 per cent, determined on 1.00 g by drying in an oven at 100 °C to 105 °C.

Sulphated ash (*2.4.14*). Not more than 0.1 per cent, determined on 1.0 g.

ASSAY

Dissolve 0.225 g in 2 ml of *anhydrous formic acid R*. Add 50 ml of *acetic anhydride R*. Titrate with *0.1 M perchloric acid*, determining the end-point potentiometrically (*2.2.20*).

1 ml of *0.1 M perchloric acid* is equivalent to 30.32 mg of $C_{12}H_{19}BrN_2O_2$.

STORAGE

Store protected from light.

IMPURITIES

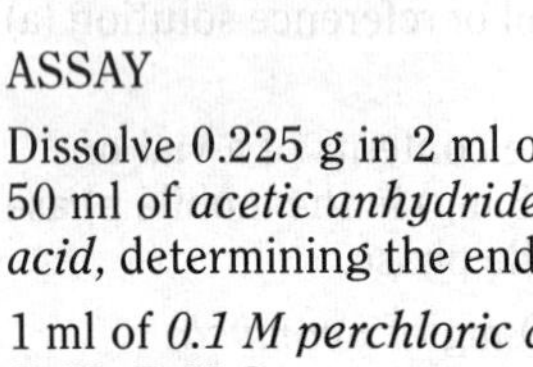

A. 3-hydroxy-*N,N,N*-trimethylanilinium bromide.

01/2005:0626

NEOSTIGMINE METILSULFATE

Neostigmini metilsulfas

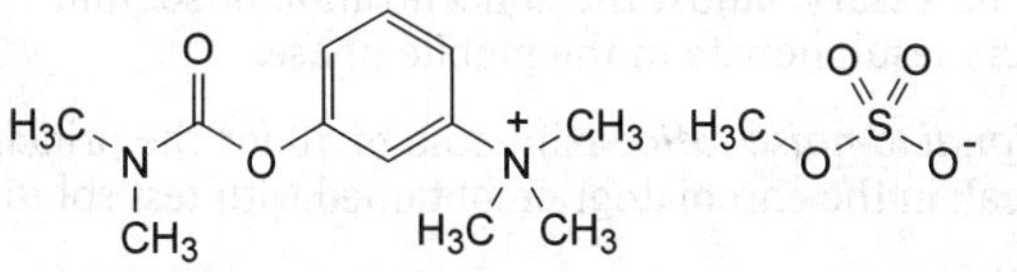

$C_{13}H_{22}N_2O_6S$ M_r 334.4

DEFINITION

Neostigmine metilsulfate contains not less than 98.5 per cent and not more than the equivalent of 101.0 per cent of 3-[(dimethylcarbamoyl)oxy]-*N,N,N*-trimethylanilinium methyl sulphate, calculated with reference to the dried substance.

CHARACTERS

A white, crystalline powder or colourless crystals, hygroscopic, very soluble in water, freely soluble in alcohol.

IDENTIFICATION

First identification: A, C.

Second identification: A, B, D, E.

A. Melting point (*2.2.14*): 144 °C to 149 °C.

B. Dissolve 50 mg in *0.5 M sulphuric acid* and dilute to 100.0 ml with the same acid. Examined between 230 nm and 350 nm (*2.2.25*), the solution shows two absorption maxima, at 261 nm and 267 nm. The ratio of the absorbance at the maximum at 267 nm to that at the maximum at 261 nm is 0.84 to 0.87. The identification is not valid unless in the test for resolution (*2.2.25*) the ratio of the absorbances is not less than 1.9.

C. Examine by infrared absorption spectrophotometry (*2.2.24*) comparing with the spectrum obtained with *neostigmine metilsulfate CRS*. Examine the substances prepared as discs.

D. To 50 mg add 0.4 g of *potassium hydroxide R* and 2 ml of *alcohol R* and heat on a water-bath for 3 min, replacing the evaporated alcohol. Cool and add 2 ml of *water R* and 2 ml of *diazobenzenesulphonic acid solution R1*. An orange-red colour develops.

E. Dissolve 0.1 g in 5 ml of *distilled water R* and add 1 ml of *barium chloride solution R1*. No precipitate is formed. Add 2 ml of *hydrochloric acid R* and heat in a water-bath for 10 min. A fine, white precipitate is formed.

TESTS

Solution S. Dissolve 2.5 g in *distilled water R* and dilute to 50 ml with the same solvent.

Appearance of solution. Solution S is clear (*2.2.1*) and colourless (*2.2.2, Method II*).

Acidity or alkalinity. To 4.0 ml of solution S add 6.0 ml of *water R* and 0.1 ml of *phenolphthalein solution R1*. The solution is colourless. Add 0.3 ml of *0.01 M sodium hydroxide*; the solution becomes red. Add 0.4 ml of *0.01 M hydrochloric acid*; the solution becomes colourless. Add 0.1 ml of *methyl red solution R*; the solution becomes red or yellowish-red.

(3-Hydroxyphenyl)trimethylammonium methyl sulphate. Dissolve 50 mg in a mixture of 1 ml of *sodium carbonate solution R* and 9 ml of *water R*. The absorbance (*2.2.25*) measured immediately at 294 nm is not greater than 0.20.

Sulphates (*2.4.13*). 15 ml of solution S complies with the limit test for sulphates (200 ppm).

Loss on drying (*2.2.32*). Not more than 0.5 per cent, determined on 1.000 g by drying in an oven at 100 °C to 105 °C.

Sulphated ash (*2.4.14*). Not more than 0.1 per cent, determined on 1.0 g.

ASSAY

Dissolve 0.300 g in 150 ml of *water R* and add 100 ml of *dilute sodium hydroxide solution R*. Distil collecting the distillate in 40 ml of a 40 g/l solution of *boric acid R* until the total volume in the collecting vessel is about 250 ml. Titrate the solution in the collecting vessel with *0.1 M hydrochloric acid*, using 0.25 ml of *methyl red mixed solution R* as indicator. Carry out a blank test.

1 ml of *0.1 M hydrochloric acid* is equivalent to 33.44 mg of $C_{13}H_{22}N_2O_6S$.

STORAGE

Store in a airtight container, protected from light.

01/2005:1351
corrected

NETILMICIN SULPHATE

Netilmicini sulfas

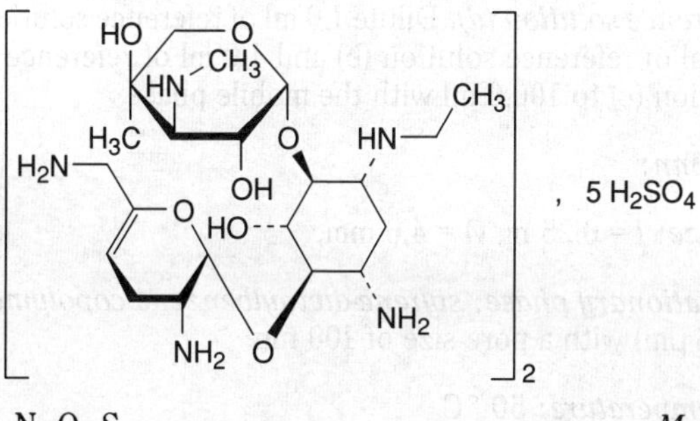

$C_{42}H_{92}N_{10}O_{34}S_5$ M_r 1442

DEFINITION

2-Deoxy-6-*O*-[3-deoxy-4-*C*-methyl-3-(methylamino)-β-L-arabinopyranosyl]-4-*O*-(2,6-diamino-2,3,4,6-tetradeoxy-α-D-*glycero*-hex-4-enopyranosyl)-1-*N*-ethyl-D-streptamine sulphate.

Substance obtained by synthesis from sisomicin.

Content: minimum 650 IU/mg (dried substance).

CHARACTERS

Appearance: white or yellowish-white powder, very hygroscopic.

Solubility: very soluble in water, practically insoluble in acetone and in alcohol.

IDENTIFICATION

A. Examine the chromatograms obtained in the test for related substances.

Results: the retention time and size of the principal peak in the chromatogram obtained with test solution (a) are approximately the same as those of the principal peak in the chromatogram obtained with reference solution (a).

B. It gives reaction (a) of sulphates (*2.3.1*).

TESTS

Solution S. Dissolve 0.80 g in *carbon dioxide-free water R* and dilute to 20.0 ml with the same solvent.

Appearance of solution. Solution S is clear (*2.2.1*) and its absorbance at 400 nm (*2.2.25*) has a maximum of 0.08.

pH (*2.2.3*): 3.5 to 5.5 for solution S.

Specific optical rotation (*2.2.7*): + 88.0 to + 96.0 (dried substance).

Dissolve 0.50 g in *water R* and dilute to 10.0 ml with the same solvent.

Related substances. Liquid chromatography (*2.2.29*).

Test solution (a). Dissolve 25.0 mg of the substance to be examined in the mobile phase and dilute to 25.0 ml with the mobile phase.

Test solution (b). Dilute 1.0 ml of test solution (a) to 100.0 ml with the mobile phase. Dilute 1.0 ml of this solution to 10.0 ml with the mobile phase.

Reference solution (a). Dissolve 25.0 mg of *netilmicin sulphate CRS* in the mobile phase and dilute to 25.0 ml with the mobile phase.

Reference solution (b). Dissolve 25.0 mg of *sisomicin sulphate CRS* in the mobile phase and dilute to 25.0 ml with the mobile phase.

Reference solution (c). Dissolve 20.5 mg of *1-N-ethylgaramine sulphate CRS* in the mobile phase and dilute to 25.0 ml with the mobile phase.

Reference solution (d). Dilute 1.0 ml of reference solution (a), 1.0 ml of reference solution (b) and 1.0 ml of reference solution (c) to 100.0 ml with the mobile phase.

Column:

- *size*: l = 0.25 m, Ø = 4.6 mm,
- *stationary phase*: *styrene-divinylbenzene copolymer R* (8 μm) with a pore size of 100 nm,
- *temperature*: 50 °C.

Mobile phase: prepare a solution in *carbon dioxide-free water R* containing 35 g/l of *anhydrous sodium sulphate R*, 0.5 g/l of *sodium octanesulphonate R*, 10 ml/l of *tetrahydrofuran R*, 50 ml/l of *0.2 M potassium dihydrogenphosphate R* previously adjusted to pH 3.0 with a 22.5 g/l solution of *phosphoric acid R* and degassed.

Flow rate: 1.0 ml/min.

Post-column solution: 20 g/l carbonate-free solution of *sodium hydroxide R* previously degassed, which is added pulse-less to the column effluent using a 375 μl polymeric mixing coil.

Flow rate: 0.3 ml/min.

Detection: pulsed amperometric detector with a gold indicator electrode, a silver-silver chloride reference electrode and a stainless steel auxiliary electrode which is the cell body, held at respectively + 0.05 V detection, + 0.75 V oxidation and − 0.15 V reduction potentials, with pulse durations according to the instrument used.

Injection: 20 μl; inject test solutions (a) and (b) and reference solution (d).

Run time: 3 times the retention time of netilmicin.

Retention time: netilmicin = about 12 min.

System suitability:

- *resolution*: minimum of 2.0 between the peaks due to impurity B (first peak) and to impurity A (second peak); minimum of 3.0 between the peaks due to impurity A (second peak) and to netilmicin (third peak) in the chromatogram obtained with reference solution (d). If necessary, adjust the concentration of sodium octanesulphonate in the mobile phase.
- *signal-to-noise ratio*: minimum of 10 for the principal peak in the chromatogram obtained with test solution (b).

Limits:

- *impurity A*: not more than the area of the second peak in the chromatogram obtained with reference solution (d) and taking into account the declared content of *sisomicin sulphate CRS* (1 per cent),
- *impurity B*: not more than the area of the first peak in the chromatogram obtained with reference solution (d) and taking into account the declared content of *1-N-ethylgaramine sulphate CRS* (1 per cent),
- *any other impurity*: not more than the area of the third peak in the chromatogram obtained with reference solution (d) (1 per cent),
- *total of other impurities*: not more than twice the area of the third peak in the chromatogram obtained with reference solution (d) (2 per cent),
- *disregard limit*: any peak with an area less than that of the principal peak in the chromatogram obtained with test solution (b) (0.1 per cent).

Sulphate: 31.5 per cent to 35.0 per cent (dried substance).

Dissolve 0.12 g in 100 ml of *water R* and adjust the solution to pH 11 using *concentrated ammonia R*. Add 30.0 ml of *0.1 M barium chloride* and about 0.5 mg of *phthalein purple R*. Titrate with *0.1 M sodium edetate* adding 50 ml of *alcohol R* when the colour of the solution begins to change and continue the titration until the violet-blue colour disappears.

1 ml of *0.1 M barium chloride* is equivalent to 9.606 mg of SO_4.

Loss on drying (*2.2.32*): maximum 15.0 per cent, determined on 0.500 g by drying at 110 °C under high vacuum for 3 h.

Sulphated ash (*2.4.14*): maximum 1.0 per cent, determined on 0.5 g.

Bacterial endotoxins (*2.6.14*): less than 1.25 IU/mg, if intended for use in the manufacture of parenteral dosage forms without a further appropriate procedure for the removal of bacterial endotoxins.

ASSAY

Carry out the microbiological assay of antibiotics (*2.7.2*), using the diffusion method.

STORAGE

In an airtight container, protected from light. If the substance is sterile, store in a sterile, airtight, tamper-proof container.

LABELLING

The label states, where applicable, that the substance is free from bacterial endotoxins.

Monographs N-O

IMPURITIES

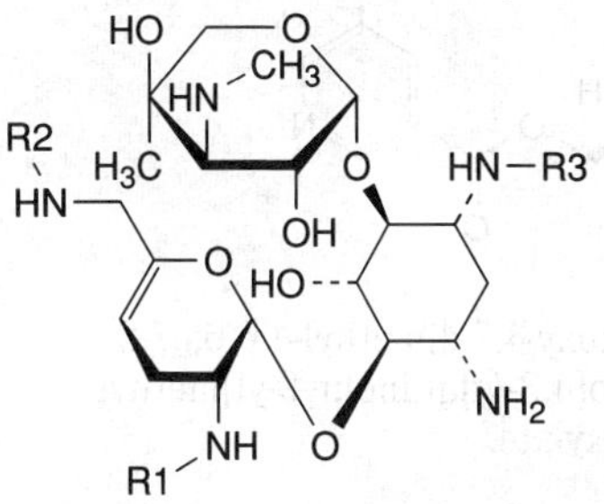

A. R1 = R2 = R3 = H: 2-deoxy-4-*O*-[3-deoxy-4-*C*-methyl-3-(methylamino)-β-L-arabinopyranosyl]-6-*O*-(2,6-diamino-2,3,4,6-tetradeoxy-α-D-*glycero*-hex-4-enopyranosyl)-L-streptamine (sisomicin),

C. R1 = R3 = C_2H_5, R2 = H: 4-*O*-[6-amino-2,3,4,6-tetradeoxy-2-(ethylamino)-α-D-*glycero*-hex-4-enopyranosyl]-2-deoxy-6-*O*-[3-deoxy-4-*C*-methyl-3-(methylamino)-β-L-arabinopyranosyl]-1-*N*-ethyl-D-streptamine (2′-*N*-ethylnetilmicin),

D. R1 = H, R2 = R3 = C_2H_5: 4-*O*-[2-amino-2,3,4,6-tetradeoxy-6-(ethylamino)-α-D-*glycero*-hex-4-enopyranosyl]-2-deoxy-6-*O*-[3-deoxy-4-*C*-methyl-3-(methylamino)-β-L-arabinopyranosyl]-1-*N*-ethyl-D-streptamine (6′-*N*-ethylnetilmicin),

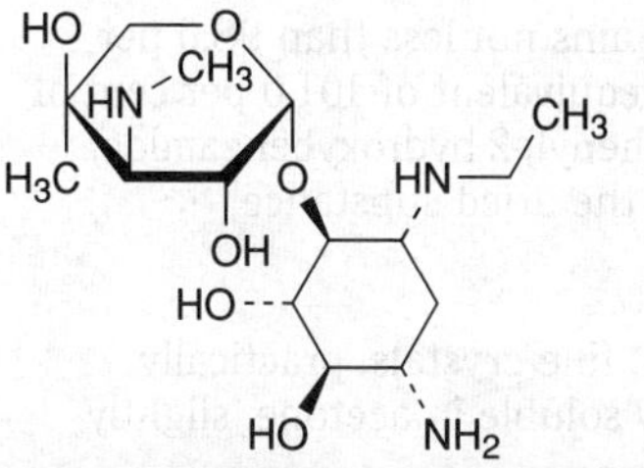

B. 2-deoxy-6-*O*-[3-deoxy-4-*C*-methyl-3-(methylamino)-β-L-arabinopyranosyl]-1-*N*-ethyl-D-streptamine (1-*N*-ethylgaramine).

01/2005:1998

NICERGOLINE

Nicergolinum

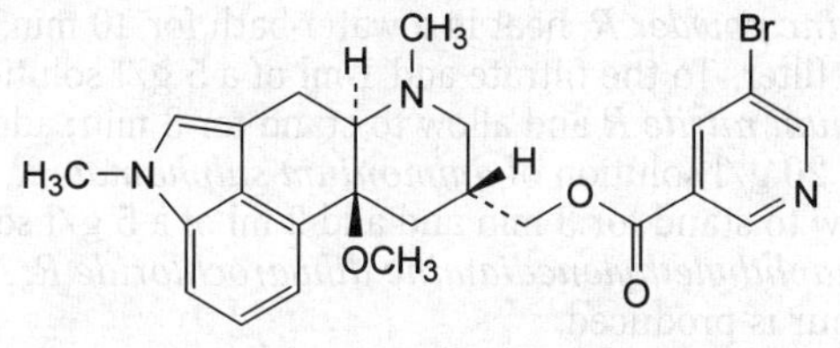

$C_{24}H_{26}BrN_3O_3$ M_r 484.4

DEFINITION

[(6a*R*,9*R*,10a*S*)-10a-Methoxy-4,7-dimethyl-4,6,6a,7,8,9,10,10a-octahydroindolo[4,3-*fg*]quinolin-9-yl]methyl 5-bromopyridine-3-carboxylate.

Content: 99.0 per cent to 101.0 per cent (anhydrous and solvent-free substance).

CHARACTERS

Appearance: fine to granular, white or yellowish powder.

Solubility: practically insoluble in water, freely soluble in methylene chloride, soluble in alcohol.

It shows polymorphism.

IDENTIFICATION

First identification: A, C.

Second identification: A, B, D.

A. Specific optical rotation (*2.2.7*): + 4.8 to + 5.8 (anhydrous substance).

Dissolve 0.50 g in *alcohol R* and dilute to 10.0 ml with the same solvent.

B. Dissolve 50.0 mg in *alcohol R* and dilute to 100.0 ml with the same solvent. Dilute 5.0 ml to 50.0 ml with *alcohol R*. Examined between 220 nm and 350 nm (*2.2.25*), the solution shows an absorption maximum at 288 nm and an absorption minimum at 251 nm. The specific absorbance at the maximum at 288 nm is 175 to 185 (anhydrous substance).

C. Infrared absorption spectrophotometry (*2.2.24*).

Preparation: discs.

Comparison: *Ph. Eur. reference spectrum of nicergoline.*

If the spectra obtained show differences, dissolve the substance to be examined in *alcohol R*, evaporate to dryness and record a further spectrum using the residue.

D. Dissolve 2 mg in 2 ml of *sulphuric acid R*. A blue colour develops.

TESTS

Appearance of solution. The solution is not more opalescent than reference suspension II (*2.2.1*) and not more intensely coloured than intensity 5 of the range of reference solutions of the most appropriate colour (*2.2.2, Method II*).

Dissolve 0.5 g in *alcohol R* and dilute to 10 ml with the same solvent.

Related substances. Liquid chromatography (*2.2.29*).

Test solution. Dissolve 25.0 mg in *acetonitrile R* and dilute to 25.0 ml with the same solvent.

Reference solution (a). Dilute 1.0 ml of the test solution to 100.0 ml with *acetonitrile R*. Dilute 10.0 ml of this solution to 50.0 ml with *acetonitrile R*.

Reference solution (b). Dissolve 25.0 mg of the substance to be examined and 10.0 mg of *nicergoline impurity A CRS* in *acetonitrile R* and dilute to 25.0 ml with the same solvent. Dilute 1.0 ml to 100.0 ml with *acetonitrile R*.

Column:

– *size*: l = 0.25 m, Ø = 4.6 mm,
– *stationary phase*: *octadecylsilyl silica gel for chromatography R* (5 µm).

Mobile phase: mix 30 volumes of *acetonitrile R*, 35 volumes of *methanol R* and 35 volumes of a freshly prepared solution of 6.8 g/l *potassium dihydrogen phosphate R* previously adjusted to pH 7.0 with *triethylamine R*.

Flow rate: 1.0 ml/min.

Detection: spectrophotometer at 288 nm.

Injection: 20 µl.

Run time: twice the retention time of nicergoline.

Relative retention with reference to nicergoline (retention time = about 25 min): impurity B = 0.5.

System suitability: reference solution (b):

– *resolution*: minimum 1.5 between the peaks due to nicergoline and impurity A.

Limits:

– *impurity B*: not more than 4 times the area of the principal peak in the chromatogram obtained with reference solution (a) (0.8 per cent),

- *any other impurity*: not more than 2.5 times the area of the principal peak in the chromatogram obtained with reference solution (a) (0.5 per cent) and not more than 2 such peaks have an area greater than the area of the principal peak in the chromatogram obtained with reference solution (a) (0.2 per cent),
- *total*: not more than 7.5 times the area of the principal peak in the chromatogram obtained with reference solution (a) (1.5 per cent),
- *disregard limit*: 0.25 times the area of the principal peak in the chromatogram obtained with reference solution (a) (0.05 per cent).

Water (*2.5.32*): maximum 0.5 per cent, determined on 0.100 g.

Sulphated ash (*2.4.14*): maximum 0.1 per cent, determined on 1.0 g.

ASSAY

Dissolve 0.400 g in 50 ml of *acetone R*. Titrate with *0.1 M perchloric acid*, determining the end-point potentiometrically (*2.2.20*). Titrate to the 1st point of inflexion.

1 ml of *0.1 M perchloric acid* is equivalent to 48.44 mg of $C_{24}H_{26}BrN_3O_3$.

IMPURITIES

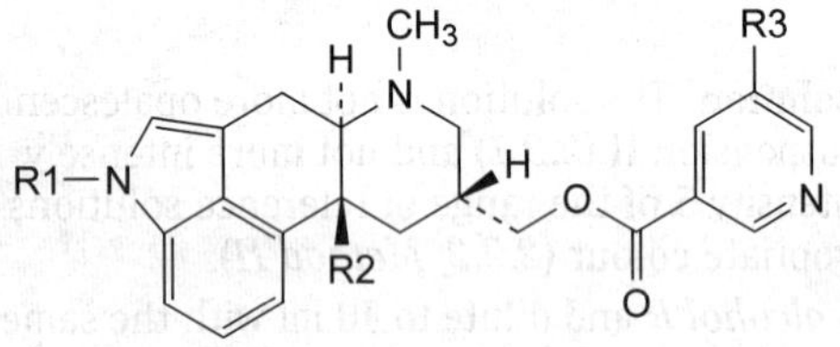

A. R1 = CH_3, R2 = OCH_3, R3 = Cl: [(6a*R*,9*R*,10a*S*)-10a-methoxy-4,7-dimethyl-4,6,6a,7,8,9,10,10a-octahydroindolo[4,3-*fg*]quinolin-9-yl]methyl 5-chloropyridine-3-carboxylate,

B. R1 = H, R2 = OCH_3, R3 = Br: [(6a*R*,9*R*,10a*S*)-10a-methoxy-7-methyl-4,6,6a,7,8,9,10,10a-octahydroindolo[4,3-*fg*]quinolin-9-yl]methyl 5-bromopyridine-3-carboxylate,

E. R1 = CH_3, R2 = OH, R3 = Br: [(6a*R*,9*R*,10a*S*)-10a-hydroxy-4,7-dimethyl-4,6,6a,7,8,9,10,10a-octahydroindolo[4,3-*fg*]quinolin-9-yl]methyl 5-bromopyridine-3-carboxylate,

G. R1 = CH_3, R2 = H, R3 = Br: [(6a*R*,9*R*,10a*R*)-4,7-dimethyl-4,6,6a,7,8,9,10,10a-octahydroindolo[4,3-*fg*]quinolin-9-yl]methyl 5-bromopyridine-3-carboxylate

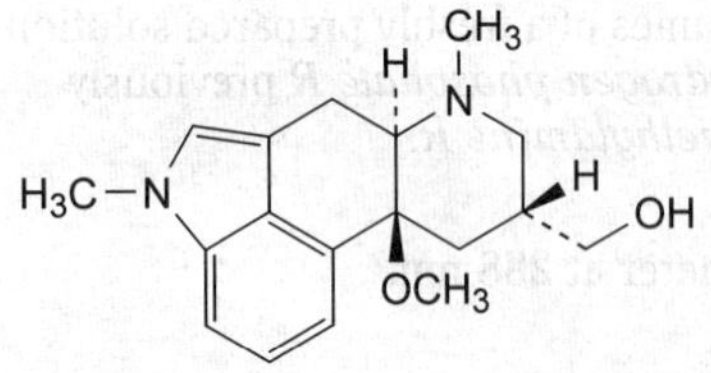

C. [(6a*R*,9*R*,10a*S*)-10a-methoxy-4,7-dimethyl-4,6,6a,7,8,9,10,10a-octahydroindolo[4,3-*fg*]quinolin-9-yl]methanol,

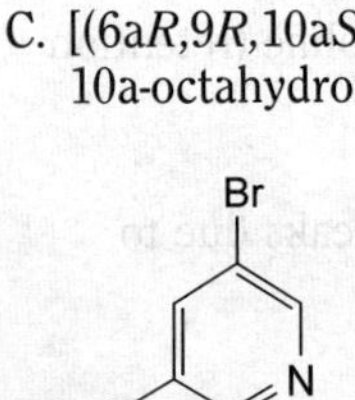

D. 5-bromopyridine-3-carboxylic acid,

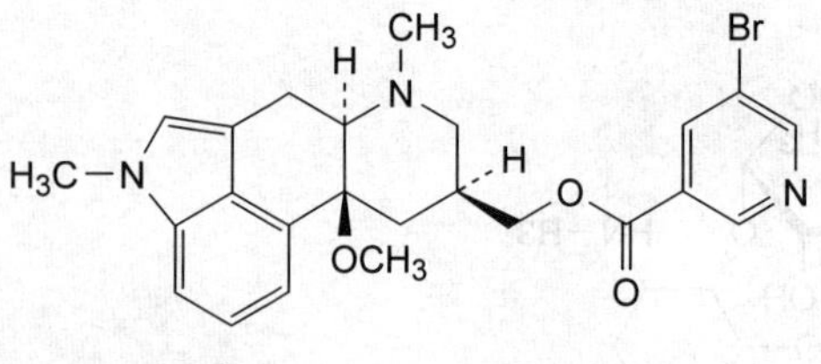

F. [(6a*R*,9*S*,10a*S*)-10a-methoxy-4,7-dimethyl-4,6,6a,7,8,9,10,10a-octahydroindolo[4,3-*fg*]quinolin-9-yl]methyl 5-bromopyridine-3-carboxylate.

01/2005:0679

NICLOSAMIDE, ANHYDROUS

Niclosamidum anhydricum

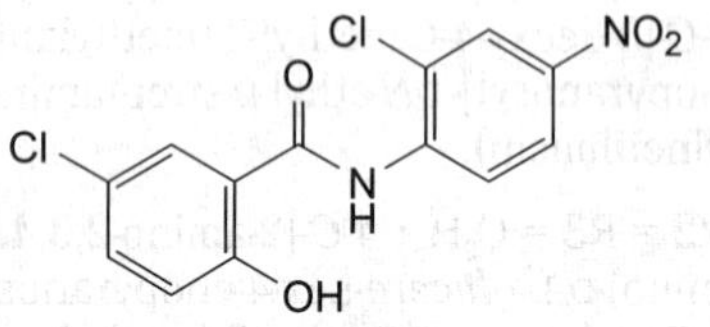

$C_{13}H_8Cl_2N_2O_4$ M_r 327.1

DEFINITION

Anhydrous niclosamide contains not less than 98.0 per cent and not more than the equivalent of 101.0 per cent of 5-chloro-*N*-(2-chloro-4-nitrophenyl)-2-hydroxybenzamide, calculated with reference to the dried substance.

CHARACTERS

Yellowish-white or yellowish, fine crystals, practically insoluble in water, sparingly soluble in acetone, slightly soluble in ethanol.

IDENTIFICATION

First identification: B, E.

Second identification: A, C, D, E.

A. Melting point (*2.2.14*): 227 °C to 232 °C.

B. Examine by infrared absorption spectrophotometry (*2.2.24*), comparing with the spectrum obtained with *anhydrous niclosamide CRS*. Examine as discs prepared using about 0.5 mg of substance and 0.3 g of *potassium bromide R*.

C. To 50 mg add 5 ml of *1 M hydrochloric acid* and 0.1 g of *zinc powder R*, heat in a water-bath for 10 min, cool and filter. To the filtrate add 1 ml of a 5 g/l solution of *sodium nitrite R* and allow to stand for 3 min; add 2 ml of a 20 g/l solution of *ammonium sulphamate R*, shake, allow to stand for 3 min and add 2 ml of a 5 g/l solution of *naphthylethylenediamine dihydrochloride R*. A violet colour is produced.

D. Heat the substance on a copper wire in a non-luminous flame. The flame becomes green.

E. It complies with the test for loss on drying (see Tests).

TESTS

Related substances. Examine by liquid chromatography (*2.2.29*).

Test solution. Dissolve 50 mg of the substance to be examined in *methanol R*, heating gently, cool and dilute to 50.0 ml with the same solvent.

Reference solution. Dilute 1.0 ml of the test solution to 100.0 ml with *acetonitrile R*. Dilute 1.0 ml of this solution to 20.0 ml with *acetonitrile R*.

The chromatographic procedure may be carried out using:

- a stainless steel column 0.125 m long and 4 mm in internal diameter packed with *octadecylsilyl silica gel for chromatography R* (5 µm),
- as mobile phase at a flow-rate of 1.0 ml/min, a mixture of equal volumes of *acetonitrile R* and a solution containing 2 g/l of *potassium dihydrogen phosphate R,* 1 g/l of *disodium hydrogen phosphate R* and 2 g/l of *tetrabutylammonium hydrogen sulphate R,*
- as detector a spectrophotometer set at 230 nm.

Adjust the sensitivity so that the height of the peak corresponding to niclosamide in the chromatogram obtained with the reference solution is not less than 20 per cent of the full scale of the recorder. Inject 20 µl of each solution and record the chromatogram for twice the retention time of niclosamide. In the chromatogram obtained with the test solution, the sum of the areas of the peaks, apart from the peak corresponding to niclosamide and the peak due to the solvent, is not greater than four times the area of the principal peak in the chromatogram obtained with the reference solution (0.2 per cent). Disregard any peak with an area less than 10 per cent of the area of the peak corresponding to niclosamide in the chromatogram obtained with the reference solution.

5-Chlorosalicylic acid

Test solution. To 1.0 g of the substance to be examined add 15 ml of *water R,* boil for 2 min, cool, filter through a membrane filter (nominal pore size: 0.45 µm), wash the filter and dilute the combined filtrate and washings to 20.0 ml with *water R.*

Reference solution. Dissolve 30 mg of *5-chlorosalicylic acid R* in 20 ml of *methanol R* and dilute to 100.0 ml with *water R.* Dilute 1.0 ml of the solution to 100.0 ml with *water R.*

To 10.0 ml of the test solution and to 10.0 ml of the reference solution add separately 0.1 ml of *ferric chloride solution R2.* Any violet colour in the test solution is not more intense than that in the reference solution (60 ppm).

2-Chloro-4-nitroaniline

Test solution. To 0.250 g of the substance to be examined add 5 ml of *methanol R,* heat to boiling, cool, add 45 ml of *1 M hydrochloric acid,* heat again to boiling, cool, filter and dilute the filtrate to 50.0 ml with *1 M hydrochloric acid.*

Reference solution. Dissolve 50 mg of *2-chloro-4-nitroaniline R* in *methanol R* and dilute to 100.0 ml with the same solvent. Dilute 1.0 ml of the solution to 100.0 ml with *methanol R.* Dilute 2.0 ml of this solution to 20.0 ml with *1 M hydrochloric acid.*

To 10.0 ml of the test solution and to 10.0 ml of the reference solution add separately 0.5 ml of a 5 g/l solution of *sodium nitrite R* and allow to stand for 3 min. Add 1 ml of a 20 g/l solution of *ammonium sulphamate R,* shake, allow to stand for 3 min and add 1 ml of a 5 g/l solution of *naphthylethylenediamine dihydrochloride R.* Any pinkish-violet colour in the test solution is not more intense than that in the reference solution (100 ppm).

Chlorides (*2.4.4*). To 2 g add a mixture of 1.2 ml of *acetic acid R* and 40 ml of *water R,* boil for 2 min, cool and filter. 2 ml of the filtrate diluted to 15 ml with *water R* complies with the limit test for chlorides (500 ppm).

Loss on drying (*2.2.32*). Not more than 0.5 per cent, determined on 1.000 g by drying in an oven at 100 °C to 105 °C for 4 h.

Sulphated ash (*2.4.14*). Not more than 0.1 per cent, determined on 1.0 g.

ASSAY

Dissolve 0.3000 g in 80 ml of a mixture of equal volumes of *acetone R* and *methanol R.* Titrate with *0.1 M tetrabutylammonium hydroxide,* determining the end-point potentiometrically (*2.2.20*).

1 ml of *0.1 M tetrabutylammonium hydroxide* is equivalent to 32.71 mg of $C_{13}H_8Cl_2N_2O_4$.

STORAGE

Store in an airtight container, protected from light.

01/2005:0680

NICLOSAMIDE MONOHYDRATE

Niclosamidum monohydricum

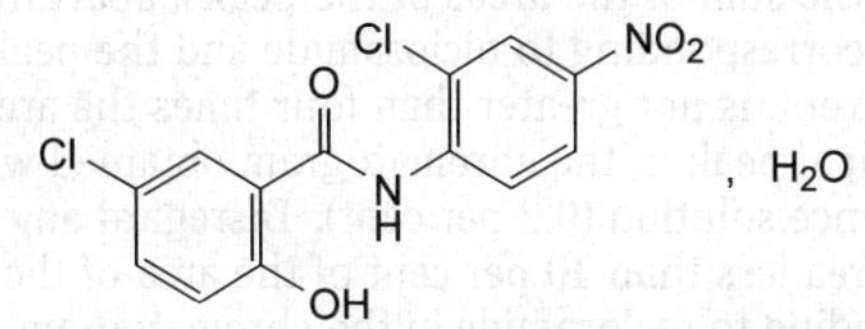

$C_{13}H_8Cl_2N_2O_4,H_2O$ M_r 345.1

DEFINITION

Niclosamide monohydrate contains not less than 98.0 per cent and not more than the equivalent of 101.0 per cent of 5-chloro-*N*-(2-chloro-4-nitrophenyl)-2-hydroxybenzamide, calculated with reference to the dried substance.

CHARACTERS

Yellowish, fine crystals, practically insoluble in water, sparingly soluble in acetone, slightly soluble in ethanol.

IDENTIFICATION

First identification: B, E.

Second identification: A, C, D, E.

A. Melting point (*2.2.14*): 227 °C to 232 °C, determined after drying at 100 °C to 105 °C for 4 h.

B. Dry the substance to be examined at 100 °C to 105 °C for 4 h. Examine by infrared absorption spectrophotometry (*2.2.24*), comparing with the spectrum obtained with *anhydrous niclosamide CRS.* Examine as discs prepared using about 0.5 mg of substance and 0.3 g of *potassium bromide R.*

C. To 50 mg add 5 ml of *1 M hydrochloric acid* and 0.1 g of *zinc powder R,* heat in a water-bath for 10 min, cool and filter. To the filtrate add 1 ml of a 5 g/l solution of *sodium nitrite R* and allow to stand for 3 min; add 2 ml of a 20 g/l solution of *ammonium sulphamate R,* shake, allow to stand for 3 min and add 2 ml of a 5 g/l solution of *naphthylethylenediamine dihydrochloride R.* A violet colour is produced.

D. Heat the substance on a copper wire in a non-luminous flame. The flame becomes green.

E. It complies with the test for loss on drying (see Tests).

TESTS

Related substances. Examine by liquid chromatography (*2.2.29*).

Test solution. Dissolve 50 mg of the substance to be examined in *methanol R,* heating gently, cool and dilute to 50.0 ml with the same solvent.

Reference solution. Dilute 1.0 ml of the test solution to 100.0 ml with *acetonitrile R.* Dilute 1.0 ml of this solution to 20.0 ml with *acetonitrile R.*

The chromatographic procedure may be carried out using:

– a stainless steel column 0.125 m long and 4 mm in internal diameter, packed with *octadecylsilyl silica gel for chromatography R* (5 µm),
– as mobile phase at a flow-rate of 1.0 ml/min, a mixture of equal volumes of *acetonitrile R* and a solution containing 2 g/l of *potassium dihydrogen phosphate R*, 1 g/l of *disodium hydrogen phosphate R* and 2 g/l of *tetrabutylammonium hydrogen sulphate R*,
– as detector a spectrophotometer set at 230 nm.

Adjust the sensitivity so that the height of the peak corresponding to niclosamide in the chromatogram obtained with the reference solution is not less than 20 per cent of full-scale of the recorder. Inject 20 µl of each solution and record the chromatogram for twice the retention time of niclosamide. In the chromatogram obtained with the test solution, the sum of the areas of the peaks, apart from the peak corresponding to niclosamide and the peak due to the solvent, is not greater than four times the area of the principal peak in the chromatogram obtained with the reference solution (0.2 per cent). Disregard any peak with an area less than 10 per cent of the area of the peak corresponding to niclosamide in the chromatogram obtained with the reference solution.

5-Chlorosalicylic acid

Test solution. To 1.0 g of the substance to be examined add 15 ml of *water R*, boil for 2 min, cool, filter through a membrane filter (nominal pore size: 0.45 µm), wash the filter and dilute the combined filtrate and washings to 20.0 ml with *water R*.

Reference solution. Dissolve 30 mg of *5-chlorosalicylic acid R* in 20 ml of *methanol R* and dilute to 100.0 ml with *water R*. Dilute 1.0 ml of the solution to 100.0 ml with *water R*.

To 10.0 ml of the test solution and to 10.0 ml of the reference solution add separately 0.1 ml of *ferric chloride solution R2*. Any violet colour produced in the test solution is not more intense than that in the reference solution (60 ppm).

2-Chloro-4-nitroaniline

Test solution. To 0.250 g of the substance to be examined add 5 ml of *methanol R*, heat to boiling, cool, add 45 ml of *1 M hydrochloric acid*, heat again to boiling, cool, filter and dilute the filtrate to 50.0 ml with *1 M hydrochloric acid*.

Reference solution. Dissolve 50 mg of *2-chloro-4-nitroaniline R* in *methanol R* and dilute to 100.0 ml with the same solvent. Dilute 1.0 ml of the solution to 100.0 ml with *methanol R*. Dilute 2.0 ml of this solution to 20.0 ml with *1 M hydrochloric acid*.

To 10.0 ml of the test solution and to 10.0 ml of the reference solution add separately 0.5 ml of a 5 g/l solution of *sodium nitrite R* and allow to stand for 3 min. Add 1 ml of a 20 g/l solution of *ammonium sulphamate R*, shake, allow to stand for 3 min and add 1 ml of a 5 g/l solution of *naphthylethylenediamine dihydrochloride R*. Any pinkish-violet colour produced in the test solution is not more intense than that in the reference solution (100 ppm).

Chlorides (*2.4.4*). To 2 g add a mixture of 1.2 ml of *acetic acid R* and 40 ml of *water R*, boil for 2 min, cool and filter. 2 ml of the filtrate diluted to 15 ml with *water R* complies with the limit test for chlorides (500 ppm).

Loss on drying (*2.2.32*): 4.5 per cent to 6.0 per cent, determined on 1.000 g by drying in an oven at 100 °C to 105 °C for 4 h.

Sulphated ash (*2.4.14*). Not more than 0.1 per cent, determined on 1.0 g.

ASSAY

Dissolve 0.3000 g in 80 ml of a mixture of equal volumes of *acetone R* and *methanol R*. Titrate with *0.1 M tetrabutylammonium hydroxide*, determining the end-point potentiometrically (*2.2.20*).

1 ml of *0.1 M tetrabutylammonium hydroxide* is equivalent to 32.71 mg of $C_{13}H_8Cl_2N_2O_4$.

STORAGE

Store protected from light.

01/2005:0047

NICOTINAMIDE

Nicotinamidum

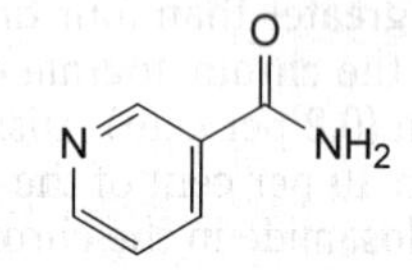

$C_6H_6N_2O$ M_r 122.1

DEFINITION

Nicotinamide contains not less than 99.0 per cent and not more than the equivalent of 101.0 per cent of pyridine-3-carboxamide, calculated with reference to the dried substance.

CHARACTERS

A white, crystalline powder or colourless crystals, freely soluble in water and in ethanol.

IDENTIFICATION

First identification: A, B.

Second identification: A, C, D.

A. Melting point (*2.2.14*): 128 °C to 131 °C.

B. Examine by infrared absorption spectrophotometry (*2.2.24*), comparing with the spectrum obtained with *nicotinamide CRS*.

C. Boil 0.1 g with 1 ml of *dilute sodium hydroxide solution R*. Ammonia is evolved which is recognisable by its odour.

D. Dilute 2 ml of solution S (see Tests) to 100 ml with *water R*. To 2 ml of the solution, add 2 ml of *cyanogen bromide solution R* and 3 ml of a 25 g/l solution of *aniline R* and shake. A yellow colour develops.

TESTS

Solution S. Dissolve 2.5 g in *carbon dioxide-free water R* and dilute to 50 ml with the same solvent.

Appearance of solution. Solution S is clear (*2.2.1*) and not more intensely coloured than reference solution BY_7 (*2.2.2, Method II*).

pH (*2.2.3*). The pH of solution S is 6.0 to 7.5.

Related substances. Examine by thin-layer chromatography (*2.2.27*), using a *TLC silica gel GF_{254} plate R*.

Test solution. Dissolve 0.4 g of the substance to be examined in a mixture of equal volumes of *alcohol R* and *water R* and dilute to 5.0 ml with the same mixture of solvents.

Reference solution. Dilute 0.5 ml of the test solution to 200 ml with a mixture of equal volumes of *alcohol R* and *water R*.

Apply to the plate 5 µl of each solution. Develop over a path of 10 cm using a mixture of 4 volumes of *water R*, 45 volumes of *ethanol R* and 48 volumes of *chloroform R*. Allow the plate to dry and examine in ultraviolet light at 254 nm. Any spot in the chromatogram obtained with the test solution, apart from the principal spot, is not more intense than the spot in the chromatogram obtained with the reference solution (0.25 per cent).

Heavy metals (*2.4.8*). Dilute 12 ml of solution S to 18 ml with *water R*. 12 ml of the solution complies with limit test A for heavy metals (30 ppm). Prepare the standard using *lead standard solution (1 ppm Pb) R*.

Loss on drying (*2.2.32*). Not more than 0.5 per cent, determined on 1.00 g by drying *in vacuo* for 18 h.

Sulphated ash (*2.4.14*). Not more than 0.1 per cent, determined on 1.0 g.

ASSAY

Dissolve 0.250 g in 20 ml of *anhydrous acetic acid R*, heating slightly if necessary, and add 5 ml of *acetic anhydride R*. Titrate with *0.1 M perchloric acid*, using *crystal violet solution R* as indicator until the colour changes to greenish-blue.

1 ml of *0.1 M perchloric acid* is equivalent to 12.21 mg of $C_6H_6N_2O$.

01/2005:1452

NICOTINE

Nicotinum

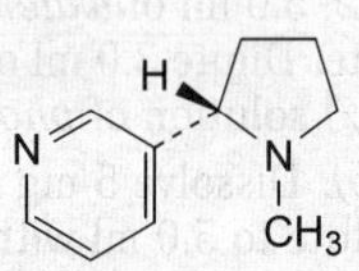

$C_{10}H_{14}N_2$ M_r 162.2

DEFINITION

Nicotine contains not less than 99.0 per cent and not more than the equivalent of 101.0 per cent of 3-[(2*S*)-1-methylpyrrolidin-2-yl]pyridine, calculated with reference to the anhydrous substance.

CHARACTERS

A colourless or brownish viscous liquid, volatile, hygroscopic, soluble in water, miscible with ethanol.

IDENTIFICATION

A. It complies with the test for specific optical rotation (see Tests).

B. Examine by infrared absorption spectrophotometry (*2.2.24*), comparing with the *Ph. Eur. reference spectrum of nicotine*.

TESTS

Appearance of solution. Dissolve 1.0 g in *water R* and dilute to 10 ml with the same solvent. The solution is clear (*2.2.1*) and not more intensely coloured than reference solution Y_5, BY_5 or R_5 (*2.2.2, Method II*).

Specific optical rotation (*2.2.7*). Dissolve 1.00 g in *ethanol R* and dilute to 50.0 ml with the same solvent. The specific optical rotation is − 140 to − 152.

Related substances. Examine by liquid chromatography (*2.2.29*).

Test solution. Dissolve 20.0 mg of the substance to be examined in the mobile phase and dilute to 25.0 ml with the mobile phase.

Reference solution (a). Dissolve 4 mg of *nicotine ditartrate CRS* and 2 mg of *myosmine R* in the mobile phase and dilute to 50.0 ml with the mobile phase.

Reference solution (b). Dilute 0.4 ml of the test solution to 100.0 ml with the mobile phase.

The chromatography may be carried out using:

– a stainless steel column 0.10 m long and 8 mm in internal diameter, packed with *octadecylsilyl silica gel for chromatography R* (4 µm),

– as mobile phase at a flow rate of 1.5 ml/min a solution prepared as follows: dissolve 2.31 g of *sodium dodecyl sulphate R* in a mixture of 250 ml of *acetonitrile R* and 750 ml of a 13.6 g/l solution of *potassium dihydrogen phosphate R*, adjusted to pH 4.5 with *sodium hydroxide R* or *phosphoric acid R*,

– as detector a spectrophotometer set at 254 nm.

Inject 25 µl of reference solution (a). When the chromatograms are recorded in the prescribed conditions the retention times are: nicotine about 13 min and impurity D about 11 min. The test is not valid unless the resolution between the impurity D peak eluting closest to the nicotine peak and the peak due to nicotine is at least 1.5; if necessary, adjust the concentration of acetonitrile in the mobile phase. Adjust the sensitivity of the system so that the height of the principal peak in the chromatogram obtained with 25 µl of reference solution (b) is at least 50 per cent of the full scale of the recorder.

Inject 25 µl of the test solution and 25 µl of reference solution (b). Continue the chromatography for twice the retention time of the principal peak. In the chromatogram obtained with the test solution: the area of any peak, apart from the principal peak, is not greater than the area of the principal peak in the chromatogram obtained with reference solution (b) (0.4 per cent); the sum of the areas of all the peaks, apart from the principal peak, is not greater than twice the area of the principal peak in the chromatogram obtained with reference solution (b) (0.8 per cent). Disregard any peak with an area less than 0.1 times the area of the principal peak in the chromatogram obtained with reference solution (b).

Water (*2.5.12*). Not more than 0.5 per cent, determined on 1.00 g by the semi-micro determination of water.

ASSAY

Dissolve 60.0 mg in 30 ml of *anhydrous acetic acid R*. Titrate with *0.1 M perchloric acid* determining the end-point potentiometrically (*2.2.20*).

1 ml of *0.1 M perchloric acid* is equivalent to 8.11 mg of $C_{10}H_{14}N_2$.

STORAGE

Store, under nitrogen, in an airtight container, protected from light.

IMPURITIES

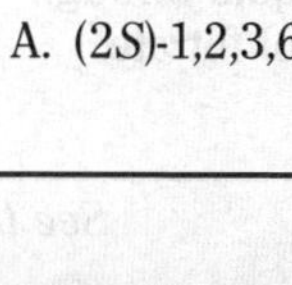

A. (2*S*)-1,2,3,6-tetrahydro-2,3′-bipyridyl (anatabine),

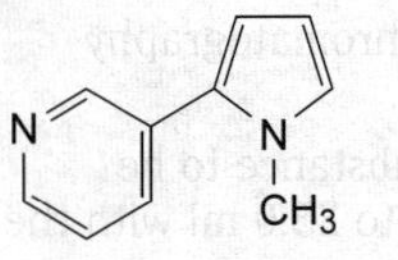

B. 3-(1-methyl-1*H*-pyrrol-2-yl)pyridine (β-nicotyrine),

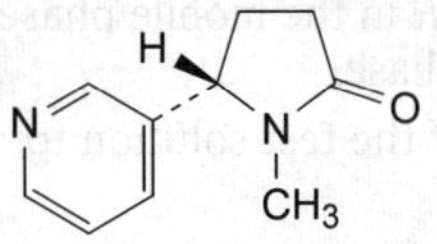

C. (5*S*)-1-methyl-5-(pyridin-3-yl)pyrrolidin-2-one (cotinine),

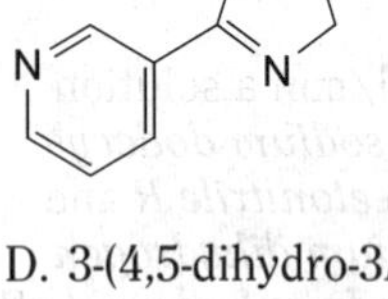

D. 3-(4,5-dihydro-3*H*-pyrrol-2-yl)pyridine (myosmine),

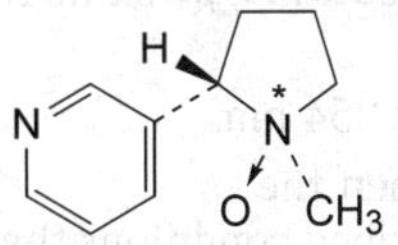

and epimer at N*

E. (1*RS*,2*S*)-1-methyl-2-(pyridin-3-yl)pyrrolidine 1-oxide (nicotine *N*-oxide).

01/2005:1792

NICOTINE RESINATE

Nicotini resinas

DEFINITION

Complex of nicotine (3-[(2*S*)-1-methylpyrrolidin-2-yl]pyridine) with a weak cationic exchange resin.

Content: 95.0 per cent to 115.0 per cent of the declared content of nicotine stated on the label (anhydrous susbtance).

It may contain glycerol.

CHARACTERS

Appearance: white or slightly yellowish powder.

Solubility: practically insoluble in water.

IDENTIFICATION

A. Infrared absorption spectrophotometry (*2.2.24*).

Preparation: shake a quantity of the substance to be examined equivalent to 100 mg of nicotine with a mixture of 10 ml of *dilute ammonia R2*, 10 ml of *water R*, 5 ml of *strong sodium hydroxide solution R* and 20 ml of *hexane R* for 5 min. Transfer the upper layer to a beaker and evaporate to produce an oily residue. Record the spectrum of the oily residue as a thin film between *sodium chloride R* plates.

Comparison: *Ph. Eur. reference spectrum of nicotine.*

B. It complies with the test for nicotine release (see Tests).

TESTS

Nicotine release: minimum 70 per cent of the content determined under Assay in 10 min.

Transfer an accurately weighed quantity of the substance to be examined equivalent to about 4 mg of nicotine, to a glass-stoppered test-tube, add 10.0 ml of a 9 g/l solution of *sodium chloride R* previously heated to 37 °C and shake vigorously for 10 min. Immediately filter the liquid through a dry filter paper discarding the first millilitre of filtrate. Transfer 1.0 ml of the filtrate to a 20 ml volumetric flask, dilute to volume with *0.1 M hydrochloric acid* and mix. Determine the absorbance (*2.2.25*) at the minima at about 236 nm and 282 nm and at the maximum at 259 nm using 1.0 ml of a 9 g/l solution of *sodium chloride R* diluted to 20 ml with *0.1 M hydrochloric acid* as compensation liquid. Calculate the percentage of nicotine release from the expression:

$$\frac{20 \times 10^6 \times (A_{259} - 0.5A_{236} - 0.5A_{282})}{323 \times C \times m}$$

323	=	specific absorbance of nicotine at 259 nm,
C	=	percentage of nicotine in the substance to be examined on the basis of the amount determined in the assay,
m	=	mass of the substance to be examined, in milligrams,
$A_{259}, A_{236}, A_{282}$	=	absorbances of the solution at the wavelength indicated by the subscript.

Related substances. Liquid chromatography (*2.2.29*).

Test solution. Accurately weigh a quantity of the substance to be examined equivalent to 20 mg of nicotine into a glass-stoppered test-tube, add 5.0 ml of *dilute ammonia R2*, 5.0 ml of *water R* and shake vigorously for 10 min. Centrifuge at about 2000 r/min for 10 min and dilute 3.0 ml of the clear solution to 10.0 ml with a 39.5 g/l solution of *phosphoric acid R*.

Reference solution (a). Weigh 60.0 mg of *nicotine ditartrate CRS* into a glass-stoppered test-tube, add 5.0 ml of *dilute ammonia R2*, 5.0 ml of *water R* and shake until dissolution is complete. Dilute 3.0 ml of the clear solution to 10.0 ml with a 39.5 g/l solution of *phosphoric acid R*.

Reference solution (b). Dissolve 5 mg of *myosmine R* in *acetonitrile R* and dilute to 5.0 ml with the same solvent. To 2.0 ml add 1.0 ml of the clear solution obtained during preparation of reference solution (a) and dilute to 10.0 ml with a 39.5 g/l solution of *phosphoric acid R*.

Reference solution (c). Dilute 1.0 ml of the test solution to 10.0 ml with a 39.5 g/l solution of *phosphoric acid R*. Dilute 1.0 ml to 20.0 ml with the mobile phase.

Column:

- *size*: *l* = 0.10 m, Ø = 8 mm,
- *stationary phase*: *octadecylsilyl silica gel for chromatography R* (4 µm).

Mobile phase: dissolve 2.31 g of *sodium dodecyl sulphate R* in a mixture of 250 ml of *acetonitrile R* and 750 ml of a 13.6 g/l solution of *potassium dihydrogen phosphate R* adjusted to pH 4.5 with *dilute sodium hydroxide R* or *dilute phosphoric acid R*.

Flow rate: 1.5 ml/min.

Detection: spectrophotometer at 254 nm.

Injection: 50 µl.

Run time: twice the retention time of nicotine.

System suitability: reference solution (b):

- *resolution*: minimum 1.5 between the peaks due to impurity D and nicotine.

Limits:

- *any impurity*: not more than the area of the principal peak in the chromatogram obtained with reference solution (c) (0.5 per cent),

– *total*: not more than twice the area of the principal peak in the chromatogram obtained with reference solution (c) (1.0 per cent),
– *disregard limit*: 0.1 times the area of the principal peak in the chromatogram obtained with reference solution (c) (0.05 per cent).

Water (*2.5.12*): maximum 5.0 per cent.

Suspend 1.0 g in 20.0 ml of *methanol R*, shake for 30 min and allow to stand for 30 min. Use 10 ml of the methanol layer for the titration. Carry out a blank titration.

ASSAY

Liquid chromatography (*2.2.29*) as described in the test for related substances.

Calculate the percentage content of nicotine using the chromatograms obtained with the test solution and reference solution (a) taking into account the declared content of *nicotine ditartrate CRS*.

STORAGE

In an airtight container, protected from light.

LABELLING

The label states the content of nicotine.

IMPURITIES

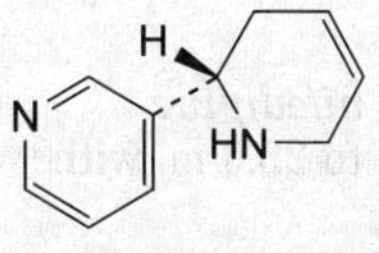

A. (2*S*)-1,2,3,6-tetrahydro-2,3′-bipyridyl (anatabine),

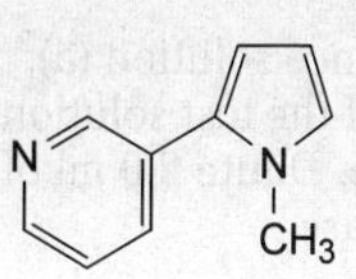

B. 3-(1-methyl-1*H*-pyrrol-2-yl)pyridine (β-nicotyrine),

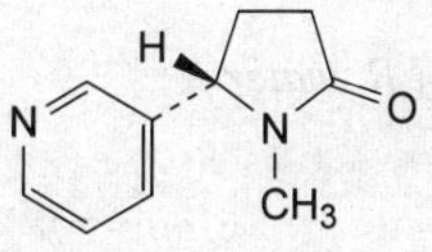

C. (5*S*)-1-methyl-5-(pyridin-3-yl)pyrrolidin-2-one (cotinine),

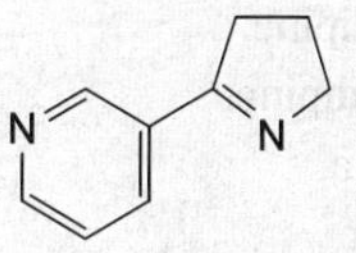

D. 3-(4,5-dihydro-3*H*-pyrrol-2-yl)pyridine (myosmine),

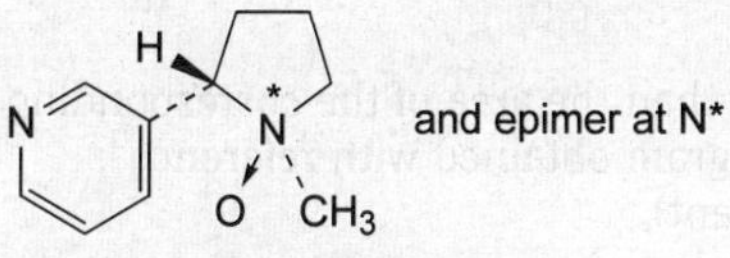

E. (1*RS*,2*S*)-1-methyl-2-(pyridin-3-yl)pyrrolidine 1-oxide (nicotine *N*-oxide).

01/2005:0459

NICOTINIC ACID

Acidum nicotinicum

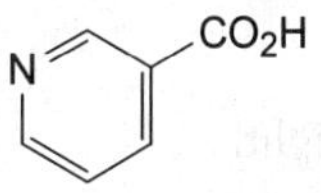

$C_6H_5NO_2$ M_r 123.1

DEFINITION

Nicotinic acid contains not less than 99.5 per cent and not more than the equivalent of 100.5 per cent of pyridine-3-carboxylic acid, calculated with reference to the dried substance.

CHARACTERS

A white, crystalline powder, soluble in boiling water and in boiling alcohol, sparingly soluble in water. It dissolves in dilute solutions of the alkali hydroxides and carbonates.

IDENTIFICATION

First identification: A, B.

Second identification: A, C.

A. Melting point (*2.2.14*): 234 °C to 240 °C.

B. Examine by infrared absorption spectrophotometry (*2.2.24*), comparing with the spectrum obtained with *nicotinic acid CRS*.

C. Dissolve about 10 mg in 10 ml of *water R*. To 2 ml of the solution add 2 ml of *cyanogen bromide solution R* and 3 ml of a 25 g/l solution of *aniline R* and shake. A yellow colour develops.

TESTS

Related substances. Examine by thin-layer chromatography (*2.2.27*), using *silica gel GF_{254} R* as the coating substance.

Test solution. Dissolve 0.5 g of the substance to be examined in *water R*, warming slightly if necessary, and dilute to 25 ml with the same solvent.

Reference solution. Dilute 0.5 ml of the test solution to 100 ml with *water R*.

Apply separately to the plate 5 µl of each solution. Develop over a path of 15 cm using a mixture of 5 volumes of *water R*, 10 volumes of *anhydrous formic acid R* and 85 volumes of *propanol R*. Dry the plate at 100 °C to 105 °C for 10 min and examine in ultraviolet light at 254 nm. Any spot in the chromatogram obtained with the test solution, apart from the principal spot, is not more intense than the spot in the chromatogram obtained with the reference solution (0.5 per cent).

Chlorides (*2.4.4*). Dissolve 0.25 g in *water R*, heating on a water-bath, and dilute to 15 ml with the same solvent. The solution complies with the limit test for chlorides (200 ppm).

Heavy metals (*2.4.8*). 1.0 g complies with limit test C for heavy metals (20 ppm). Prepare the standard using 2 ml of *lead standard solution (10 ppm Pb) R*.

Loss on drying (*2.2.32*). Not more than 1.0 per cent, determined on 1.000 g by drying in an oven at 100 °C to 105 °C for 1 h.

Sulphated ash (*2.4.14*). Not more than 0.1 per cent, determined on 1.0 g.

ASSAY

Dissolve 0.250 g in 50 ml of *water R*. Titrate with *0.1 M sodium hydroxide,* using 0.25 ml of *phenolphthalein solution R* as indicator, until a pink colour is obtained. Carry out a blank titration.

1 ml of *0.1 M sodium hydroxide* is equivalent to 12.31 mg of $C_6H_5NO_2$.

STORAGE

Store protected from light.

01/2005:0627
corrected

NIFEDIPINE

Nifedipinum

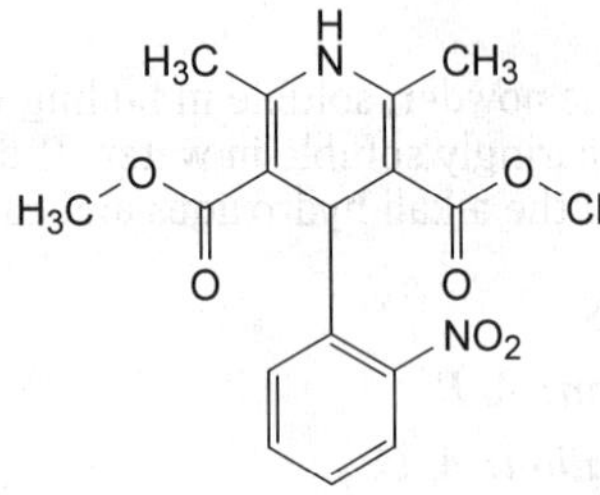

$C_{17}H_{18}N_2O_6$ M_r 346.3

DEFINITION

Dimethyl 2,6-dimethyl-4-(2-nitrophenyl)-1,4-dihydropyridine-3,5-dicarboxylate.

Content: 98.0 per cent to 102.0 per cent (dried substance).

CHARACTERS

Appearance: yellow, crystalline powder.

Solubility: practically insoluble in water, freely soluble in acetone, sparingly soluble in ethanol.

When exposed to daylight and to artificial light of certain wavelengths, it readily converts to a nitrosophenylpyridine derivative. Exposure to ultraviolet light leads to the formation of a nitrophenylpyridine derivative.

Prepare solutions immediately before use in the dark or under long-wavelength light (> 420 nm) and protect them from light.

IDENTIFICATION

First identification: B.

Second identification: A, C, D.

A. Melting point (*2.2.14*): 171 °C to 175 °C.

B. Infrared absorption spectrophotometry (*2.2.24*).
Comparison: *nifedipine CRS.*

C. Thin-layer chromatography (*2.2.27*).
Test solution. Dissolve 10 mg of the substance to be examined in *methanol R* and dilute to 10 ml with the same solvent.
Reference solution. Dissolve 10 mg of *nifedipine CRS* in *methanol R* and dilute to 10 ml with the same solvent.
Plate: *TLC silica gel* F_{254} *plate R.*
Mobile phase: *ethyl acetate R, cyclohexane R* (40:60 *V/V*).
Application: 5 µl.
Development: over 3/4 of the plate.
Drying: in air.
Detection: examine in ultraviolet light at 254 nm.
Results: the principal spot in the chromatogram obtained with the test solution is similar in position, appearance at 254 nm and size to the principal spot in the chromatogram obtained with the reference solution.

D. To 25 mg in a test tube, add 10 ml of a mixture of 1.5 volumes of *hydrochloric acid R*, 3.5 volumes of *water R* and 5 volumes of *alcohol R* and dissolve with gentle heating. Add 0.5 g of *zinc R* in granules and allow to stand for 5 min with occasional swirling. Filter into a second test tube, add 5 ml of a 10 g/l solution of *sodium nitrite R* to the filtrate and allow to stand for 2 min. Add 2 ml of a 50 g/l solution of *ammonium sulphamate R,* shake vigorously with care and add 2 ml of a 5 g/l solution of *naphthylethylenediamine dihydrochloride R.* An intense red colour develops which persists for not less than 5 min.

TESTS

Impurity D and other basic impurities. Transfer 4 g to a 250 ml conical flask and dissolve in 160 ml of *glacial acetic acid R* using an ultrasonic bath. Titrate with *0.1 M perchloric acid* using 0.25 ml of *naphtholbenzein solution R* as indicator until the colour changes from brownish-yellow to green. Not more than 0.48 ml of *0.1 M perchloric acid* is required (0.14 per cent).

Related substances. Liquid chromatography (*2.2.29*).

Test solution. Dissolve 0.200 g of the substance to be examined in 20 ml of *methanol R* and dilute to 50.0 ml with the mobile phase.

Reference solution (a). Dissolve 10 mg of *nifedipine impurity A CRS* in *methanol R* and dilute to 25.0 ml with the same solvent.

Reference solution (b). Dissolve 10 mg of *nifedipine impurity B CRS* in *methanol R* and dilute to 25.0 ml with the same solvent.

Reference solution (c). Mix 1.0 ml of reference solution (a), 1.0 ml of reference solution (b) and 0.1 ml of the test solution and dilute to 20.0 ml with the mobile phase. Dilute 2.0 ml of this solution to 10.0 ml with the mobile phase.

Column:
- *size*: l = 0.15 m, Ø = 4.6 mm,
- *stationary phase*: *octadecylsilyl silica gel for chromatography R* (5 µm).

Mobile phase: *acetonitrile R, methanol R, water R* (9:36:55 *V/V/V*).

Flow rate: 1.0 ml/min.

Detection: spectrophotometer at 235 nm.

Injection: 20 µl; inject the test solution and reference solution (c).

Run time: twice the retention time of nifedipine.

Elution order: impurity A, impurity B, nifedipine.

Retention time: nifedipine = about 15.5 min.

System suitability: reference solution (c):
- *resolution*: minimum 1.5 between the peaks due to impurity A and impurity B and minimum 1.5 between the peaks due to impurity B and nifedipine.

Limits:
- *impurity A*: not more than the area of the corresponding peak in the chromatogram obtained with reference solution (c) (0.1 per cent),
- *impurity B*: not more than the area of the corresponding peak in the chromatogram obtained with reference solution (c) (0.1 per cent),

- *any other impurity*: not more than the area of the peak due to nifedipine in the chromatogram obtained with reference solution (c) (0.1 per cent),
- *total*: not more than 0.3 per cent,
- *disregard limit*: 0.1 times the area of the peak due to nifedipine in the chromatogram obtained with reference solution (c) (0.01 per cent).

Loss on drying (*2.2.32*): maximum 0.5 per cent, determined on 1.000 g by drying in an oven at 100-105 °C for 2 h.

Sulphated ash (*2.4.14*): maximum 0.1 per cent, determined on 1.0 g.

ASSAY

Dissolve 0.1300 g in a mixture of 25 ml of *2-methyl-2-propanol R* and 25 ml of *perchloric acid solution R*. Titrate with *0.1 M cerium sulphate* using 0.1 ml of *ferroin R* as indicator, until the pink colour disappears. Titrate slowly towards the end of the titration. Carry out a blank titration.

1 ml of *0.1 M cerium sulphate* is equivalent to 17.32 mg of $C_{17}H_{18}N_2O_6$.

STORAGE

Protected from light.

IMPURITIES

Specified impurities: A, B, C, D.

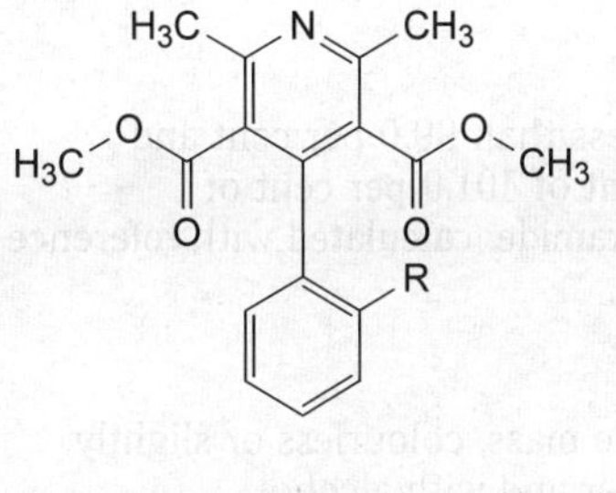

A. R = NO_2: dimethyl 2,6-dimethyl-4-(2-nitrophenyl)pyridine-3,5-dicarboxylate (nitrophenylpyridine analogue),

B. R = NO: dimethyl 2,6-dimethyl-4-(2-nitrosophenyl)pyridine-3,5-dicarboxylate (nitrosophenylpyridine analogue),

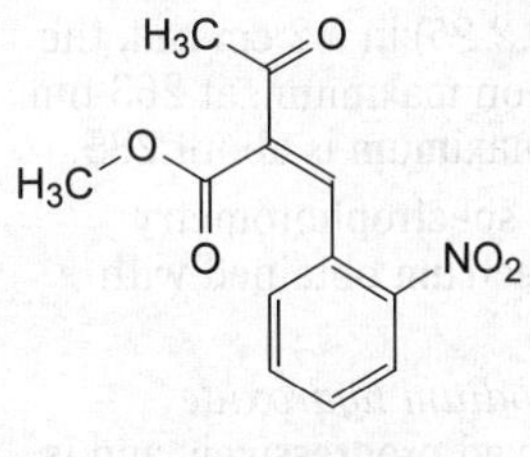

C. methyl 2-(2-nitrobenzylidene)-3-oxobutanoate,

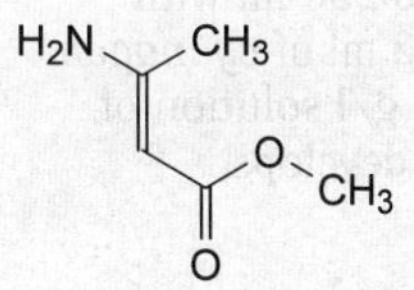

D. methyl 3-aminobut-2-enoate.

01/2005:1999
corrected

NIFUROXAZIDE

Nifuroxazidum

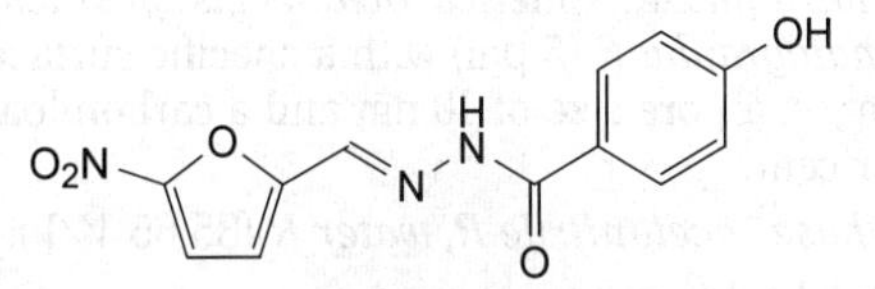

$C_{12}H_9N_3O_5$ M_r 275.2

DEFINITION

1-(4-Hydroxybenzoyl)-2-[(5-nitrofuran-2-yl)methylene]diazane.

Content: 98.5 per cent to 101.5 per cent (dried substance).

CHARACTERS

Appearance: bright yellow, crystalline powder.

Solubility: practically insoluble in water, slightly soluble in alcohol, practically insoluble in methylene chloride.

IDENTIFICATION

Infrared absorption spectrophotometry (*2.2.24*).

Comparison: *Ph. Eur. reference spectrum of nifuroxazide.*

TESTS

Specific absorbance (*2.2.25*): 940 to 1000 at the absorption maximum at 367 nm.

Protected from light, dissolve 10.0 mg in 10 ml of *ethylene glycol monomethyl ether R* and dilute to 100.0 ml with *methanol R*. Dilute 5.0 ml of this solution to 100.0 ml with *methanol R*.

Impurity A: maximum 0.05 per cent.

Test solution (a). Dissolve 1.0 g of the substance to be examined in *dimethyl sulphoxide R* and dilute to 10.0 ml with the same solvent.

Test solution (b). To 5.5 ml of test solution (a) add 50.0 ml of *water R* while stirring. Allow to stand for 15 min and filter.

Reference solution. To 0.5 ml of test solution (a) add 5.0 ml of a 50 mg/l solution of *4-hydroxybenzohydrazide R* in *dimethyl sulphoxide R*. Add 50.0 ml of *water R* while stirring. Allow to stand for 15 min and filter.

Add 0.5 ml of *phosphomolybdotungstic reagent R* and 10.0 ml of *sodium carbonate solution R* separately to 10.0 ml of test solution (b) and to 10.0 ml of the reference solution. Allow to stand for 1 h. Examine the 2 solutions at 750 nm. The absorbance (*2.2.25*) of the solution obtained with test solution (b) is not greater than that obtained with the reference solution.

Related substances. Liquid chromatography (*2.2.29*). *Use freshly prepared solutions, protected from light.*

Test solution. Dissolve 0.100 g of the substance to be examined in 15.0 ml of *dimethylformamide R* and dilute to 100.0 ml with the mobile phase. If precipitation occurs, use the supernatant liquid.

Reference solution (a). Dissolve 10.0 mg of *methyl parahydroxybenzoate R* (impurity B) in 2.0 ml of *dimethylformamide R* and dilute to 20.0 ml with the mobile phase. Dilute 1.0 ml of this solution to 100.0 ml with the mobile phase.

Reference solution (b). Dissolve 5 mg of the substance to be examined and 10 mg of *methyl parahydroxybenzoate R* in 2 ml of *dimethylformamide R* and dilute to 20 ml with the mobile phase. Dilute 1 ml of this solution to 100 ml with the mobile phase.

Column:

- *size*: *l* = 0.25 m, Ø = 4.6 mm,
- *stationary phase*: spherical *octadecylsilyl silica gel for chromatography R* (5 µm) with a specific surface area of 340 m²/g, a pore size of 10 nm and a carbon loading of 19 per cent.

Mobile phase: *acetonitrile R, water R* (35:65 *V/V*).

Flow rate: 1 ml/min.

Detection: spectrophotometer at 280 nm.

Injection: 20 µl.

Run time: 6 times the retention time of nifuroxazide.

Relative retention with reference to nifuroxazide (retention time = about 6.5 min): impurity A = about 0.4; impurity B = about 1.2; impurity C = about 2.8; impurity D = about 5.2.

System suitability: reference solution (b):

- *resolution*: minimum 3.0 between the peaks due to nifuroxazide and impurity B.

Limits:

- *any impurity*: not more than 0.6 times the area of the principal peak in the chromatogram obtained with reference solution (a) (0.3 per cent), and not more than 1 such peak has an area greater than 0.2 times the area of the principal peak in the chromatogram obtained with reference solution (a) (0.1 per cent),
- *total*: not more than the area of the principal peak in the chromatogram obtained with reference solution (a) (0.5 per cent),
- *disregard limit*: 0.1 times the area of the principal peak in the chromatogram obtained with reference solution (a) (0.05 per cent).

Heavy metals (*2.4.8*): maximum 20 ppm.

1.0 g complies with limit test D. Prepare the standard using 2 ml of *lead standard solution (10 ppm Pb) R*.

Loss on drying (*2.2.32*): maximum 0.5 per cent, determined on 1.000 g by drying in an oven at 100-105 °C for 3 h.

Sulphated ash (*2.4.14*): maximum 0.1 per cent, determined on 1.0 g.

ASSAY

Dissolve 0.200 g, if necessary with heating, in 30 ml of *dimethylformamide R* and add 20 ml of *water R*. Titrate with *0.1 M sodium hydroxide*, determining the end-point potentiometrically (*2.2.20*).

1 ml of *0.1 M sodium hydroxide* is equivalent to 27.52 mg of $C_{12}H_9N_3O_5$.

STORAGE

Protected from light.

IMPURITIES

Specified impurities: A, B, C, D.

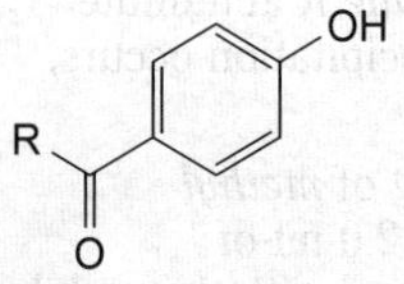

A. R = NH-NH$_2$: (4-hydroxybenzoyl)diazane (*p*-hydroxybenzohydrazide),

B. R = OCH$_3$: methyl 4-hydroxybenzoate,

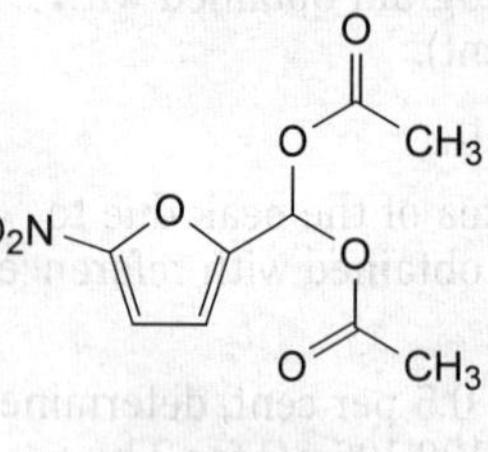

C. (5-nitrofuran-2-yl)methylene diacetate,

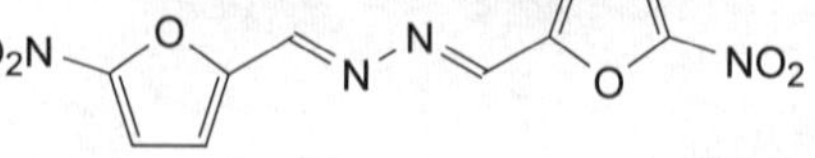

D. 1,2-bis[(5-nitrofuran-2-yl)methylene]diazane (5-nitrofurfural azine).

01/2005:0233

NIKETHAMIDE

Nicethamidum

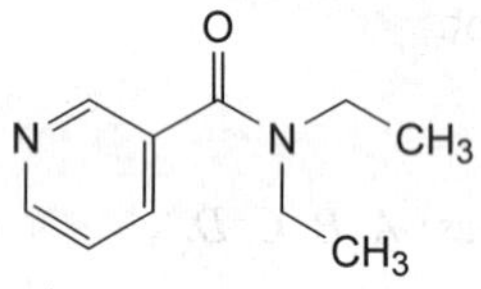

$C_{10}H_{14}N_2O$ M_r 178.2

DEFINITION

Nikethamide contains not less than 99.0 per cent and not more than the equivalent of 101.0 per cent of *N,N*-diethylpyridine-3-carboxamide, calculated with reference to the anhydrous substance.

CHARACTERS

An oily liquid or a crystalline mass, colourless or slightly yellowish, miscible with water and with alcohol.

IDENTIFICATION

First identification: A, B.

Second identification: A, C, D.

A. Dissolve 0.15 g in *0.01 M hydrochloric acid* and dilute to 100.0 ml with the same acid. Dilute 1.0 ml of this solution to 100.0 ml with *0.01 M hydrochloric acid*. Examined between 230 nm and 350 nm (*2.2.25*) in a 2 cm cell, the solution shows a single absorption maximum, at 263 nm. The specific absorbance at the maximum is about 285.

B. Examine by infrared absorption spectrophotometry (*2.2.24*), comparing with the spectrum obtained with *nikethamide CRS*.

C. Heat 0.1 g with 1 ml of *dilute sodium hydroxide solution R*. Diethylamine is evolved progressively and is recognisable by its characteristic odour and by its turning *red litmus paper R* blue.

D. Dilute 1 ml of solution S (see Tests) to 250 ml with *water R*. To 2 ml of this solution add 2 ml of *cyanogen bromide solution R*. Add 3 ml of a 25 g/l solution of *aniline R* and shake. A yellow colour develops.

TESTS

Solution S. Dissolve 2.5 g in *carbon dioxide-free water R* and dilute to 10 ml with the same solvent.

Appearance. The substance to be examined, in liquid form or liquefied by slight heating, is clear (*2.2.1*) and not more intensely coloured than reference solution Y_5 (*2.2.2, Method II*).

pH (*2.2.3*). The pH of solution S is 6.0 to 7.8.

Refractive index (*2.2.6*). 1.524 to 1.526.

Related substances. Examine by thin-layer chromatography (*2.2.27*), using *silica gel GF_{254} R* as the coating substance.

Test solution. Dissolve 0.4 g of the substance to be examined in *methanol R* and dilute to 10 ml with the same solvent.

Reference solution (a). Dissolve 40 mg of *ethylnicotinamide CRS* in *methanol R* and dilute to 100 ml with the same solvent.

Reference solution (b). Dilute 1 ml of reference solution (a) to 10 ml with *methanol R*.

Apply separately to the plate 10 µl of each solution. Develop over a path of 15 cm using a mixture of 25 volumes of *propanol R* and 75 volumes of *chloroform R*. Allow the plate to dry in air and examine in ultraviolet light at 254 nm. In the chromatogram obtained with the test solution, any spot corresponding to ethylnicotinamide is not more intense than the spot in the chromatogram obtained with reference solution (a) (1.0 per cent) and any spot, apart from the principal spot and the spot corresponding to ethylnicotinamide, is not more intense than the spot in the chromatogram obtained with reference solution (b) (0.1 per cent).

Heavy metals (*2.4.8*). Dilute 10 ml of solution S to 25 ml with *water R*. 12 ml of this solution complies with limit test A for heavy metals (10 ppm). Prepare the standard using *lead standard solution (1 ppm Pb) R*.

Water (*2.5.12*). Not more than 0.3 per cent, determined on 2.00 g by the semi-micro determination of water.

Sulphated ash (*2.4.14*). Not more than 0.1 per cent, determined on 1.0 g.

ASSAY

Dissolve 0.150 g in a mixture of 5 ml of *acetic anhydride R* and 20 ml of *anhydrous acetic acid R*. Titrate with *0.1 M perchloric acid*, determining the end-point potentiometrically (*2.2.20*).

1 ml of *0.1 M perchloric acid* is equivalent to 17.82 mg of $C_{10}H_{14}N_2O$.

01/2005:1548

NIMESULIDE

Nimesulidum

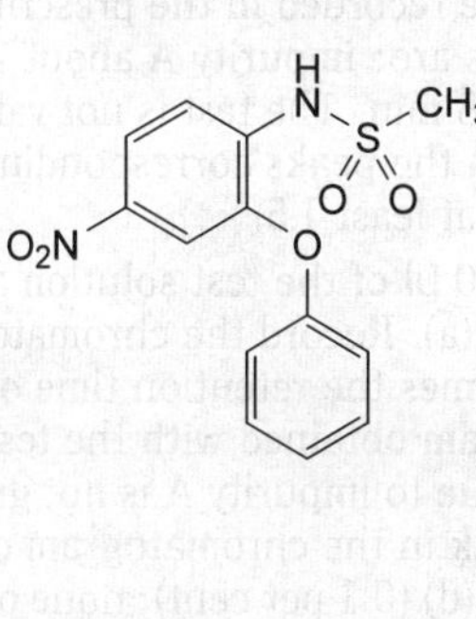

$C_{13}H_{12}N_2O_5S$ M_r 308.3

DEFINITION

N-(4-Nitro-2-phenoxyphenyl)methanesulphonamide.

Content: 98.5 per cent to 101.5 per cent (dried substance).

CHARACTERS

Appearance: yellowish crystalline powder.

Solubility: practically insoluble in water, freely soluble in acetone, slightly soluble in ethanol.

mp: about 149 °C.

It shows polymorphism.

IDENTIFICATION

Infrared absorption spectrophotometry (*2.2.24*).

Preparation: discs.

Comparison: *nimesulide CRS*.

If the spectra obtained show differences, dissolve the substance to be examined and the reference substance separately in *acetone R*, evaporate to dryness and record new spectra using the residues.

TESTS

Absorbance (*2.2.25*): maximum 0.50 at 450 nm.

Dissolve 1.0 g in *acetone R* and dilute to 10.0 ml with the same solvent.

Related substances. Liquid chromatography (*2.2.29*).

Test solution. Dissolve 20 mg of the substance to be examined in 8 ml of *acetonitrile R* and dilute to 20.0 ml with *water R*.

Reference solution (a). Dissolve 10 mg of *nimesulide impurity C CRS* and 10 mg of *nimesulide impurity D CRS* in 20 ml of *acetonitrile R* and dilute to 50.0 ml with *water R*. Dilute 1.0 ml of the solution to 50.0 ml with the mobile phase.

Reference solution (b). Dilute 1.0 ml of the test solution to 10.0 ml with the mobile phase. Dilute 1.0 ml of the solution to 100.0 ml with the mobile phase.

Column:

- *dimensions*: l = 0.125 m, Ø = 4.0 mm,
- *stationary phase*: *octadecylsilyl silica gel for chromatography R*.

Mobile phase: a mixture of 35 volumes of *acetonitrile R* and 65 volumes of a 1.15 g/l solution of *ammonium dihydrogen phosphate R* adjusted to pH 7.0 with *ammonia R*.

Flow rate: 1.3 ml/min.

Detection: spectrophotometer at 230 nm.

Injection: 20 µl.

Run time: 7 times the retention time of nimesulide.

System suitability:

- *resolution*: minimum of 2.0 between the 2 principal peaks in the chromatogram obtained with reference solution (a).

Limits:

- *any impurity*: not more than the area of the principal peak in the chromatogram obtained with reference solution (b) (0.1 per cent),
- *total*: not more than 5 times the area of the principal peak in the chromatogram obtained with reference solution (b) (0.5 per cent),
- *disregard limit*: 0.1 times the area of the principal peak in the chromatogram obtained with reference solution (b) (0.01 per cent).

Heavy metals (*2.4.8*): maximum 20 ppm.

1.0 g complies with limit test D. Prepare the standard using 2 ml of *lead standard solution (10 ppm Pb) R*.

Loss on drying (*2.2.32*): maximum 0.5 per cent, determined on 1.000 g by drying in an oven at 100-105 °C for 4 h.

Sulphated ash (*2.4.14*): maximum 0.1 per cent, determined on 1.0 g.

ASSAY

Dissolve 0.240 g in 30 ml of previously neutralised *acetone R* and add 20 ml of *water R*. Titrate with *0.1 M sodium hydroxide*, determining the end-point potentiometrically (*2.2.20*).

1 ml of *0.1 M sodium hydroxide* is equivalent to 30.83 mg of $C_{13}H_{12}N_2O_5S$.

IMPURITIES

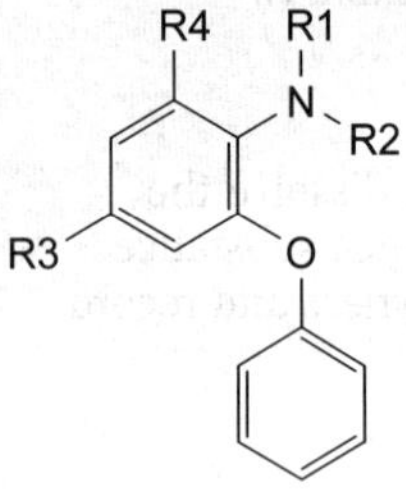

A. R1 = SO_2-CH_3, R2 = H, R3 = R4 = NO_2: *N*-(2,4-dinitro-6-phenoxyphenyl)methanesulphonamide,

B. R1 = SO_2-CH_3, R2 = R3 = R4 = H: *N*-(2-phenoxyphenyl)methanesulphonamide,

C. R1 = R2 = R3 = R4 = H: 2-phenoxyaniline,

D. R1 = R2 = R4 = H, R3 = NO_2: 4-nitro-2-phenoxyaniline,

E. R1 = R2 = SO_2-CH_3, R3 = R4 = H: *N,N*-bis(methylsulphonyl)-2-phenoxyaniline,

F. R1 = R2 = SO_2-CH_3, R3 = NO_2, R4 = H: *N,N*-bis(methylsulphonyl)-4-nitro-2-phenoxyaniline,

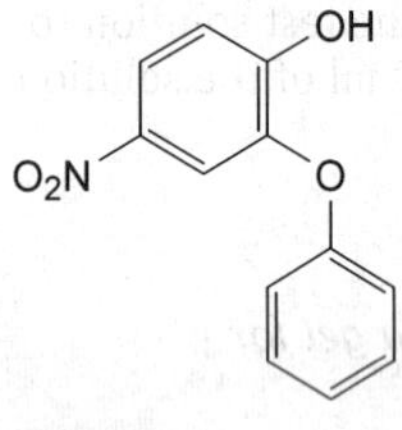

G. 4-nitro-2-phenoxyphenol.

01/2005:1245

NIMODIPINE

Nimodipinum

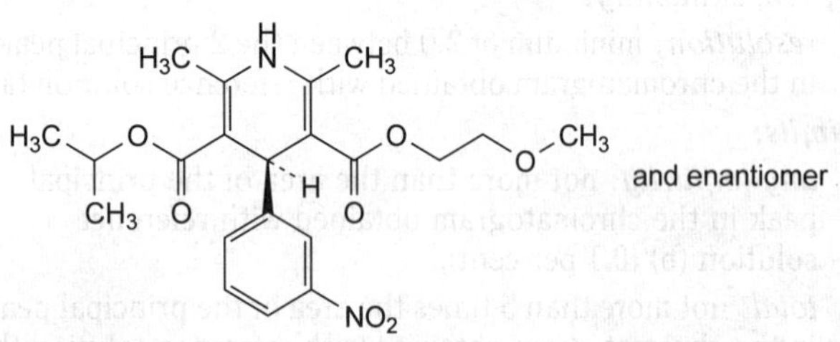

$C_{21}H_{26}N_2O_7$ M_r 418.4

DEFINITION

Nimodipine contains not less than 98.5 per cent and not more than the equivalent of 101.5 per cent of 2-methoxyethyl 1-methylethyl (4*RS*)-2,6-dimethyl-4-(3-nitrophenyl)-1,4-dihydropyridine-3,5-dicarboxylate, calculated with reference to the dried substance.

CHARACTERS

A light yellow or yellow, crystalline powder, practically insoluble in water, freely soluble in ethyl acetate, sparingly soluble in ethanol.

It shows polymorphism.

Exposure to ultraviolet light leads to the formation of a nitrophenylpyridine derivative.

Prepare solutions immediately before use either protected from light or under long-wavelength light (> 420 nm).

IDENTIFICATION

Examine by infrared absorption spectrophotometry (*2.2.24*), comparing with the spectrum obtained with *nimodipine CRS*. If the spectra obtained in the solid state show differences, record further spectra using 20 g/l solutions in *methylene chloride R* and a 0.2 mm cell.

TESTS

Solution S. Dissolve 1.0 g in *acetone R* and dilute to 20.0 ml with *acetone R*.

Appearance of solution. Solution S is clear (*2.2.1*).

Optical rotation (*2.2.7*). The angle of optical rotation, determined on solution S, is − 0.10° to + 0.10°.

Related substances. Examine by liquid chromatography (*2.2.29*).

Test solution. Dissolve 40.0 mg of the substance to be examined in 2.5 ml of *tetrahydrofuran R* and dilute to 25.0 ml with the mobile phase.

Reference solution (a). Dilute 1.0 ml of the test solution to 100.0 ml with the mobile phase. Dilute 2.0 ml of the solution to 10.0 ml with the mobile phase.

Reference solution (b). Dissolve 20.0 mg of *nimodipine impurity A CRS* in 2.5 ml of *tetrahydrofuran R* and dilute to 25.0 ml with the mobile phase. Dilute 1.0 ml of the solution to 20.0 ml with the mobile phase.

Reference solution (c). Dilute 0.5 ml of the test solution to 20.0 ml with the mobile phase.

Reference solution (d). Mix 1.0 ml of reference solution (b) and 1.0 ml of reference solution (c) and dilute to 25.0 ml with the mobile phase.

The chromatographic procedure may be carried out using:

– a stainless steel column 0.125 m long and 4.6 mm in internal diameter packed with *octadecylsilyl silica gel for chromatography R* (5 µm),

– as mobile phase at a flow rate of 2.0 ml/min a mixture of 20 volumes of *methanol R*, 20 volumes of *tetrahydrofuran R* and 60 volumes of *water R*,

– as detector a spectrophotometer set at 235 nm,

maintaining the temperature of the column at 40 °C.

Adjust the sensitivity of the system so that the height of the peak corresponding to nimodipine in the chromatogram obtained with 20 µl of reference solution (d) is at least 50 per cent of the full scale of the recorder.

Inject 20 µl of reference solution (d). When the chromatograms are recorded in the prescribed conditions, the retention times are: impurity A about 7 min and nimodipine about 8 min. The test is not valid unless the resolution between the peaks corresponding to impurity A and nimodipine is at least 1.5.

Inject separately 20 µl of the test solution and 20 µl of reference solution (a). Record the chromatogram of the test solution for four times the retention time of nimodipine. In the chromatogram obtained with the test solution: the area of the peak due to impurity A is not greater than the corresponding peak in the chromatogram obtained with reference solution (d) (0.1 per cent); none of the peaks, apart from the principal peak and the peak due to impurity A, has an area greater than the area of the principal peak in the chromatogram obtained with reference solution (a) (0.2 per cent); the sum of the areas of all the peaks, apart from the principal peak, is not greater than 2.5 times the area of the principal peak in the chromatogram obtained with reference solution (a) (0.5 per cent). Disregard any peak due to the solvent and any peak with an area less than 0.5 times the area of the principal peak in the chromatogram obtained with reference solution (d).

Loss on drying (*2.2.32*). Not more than 0.5 per cent, determined on 1.000 g by drying in an oven at 100-105 °C.

Sulphated ash (*2.4.14*). Not more than 0.1 per cent, determined on 1.0 g.

ASSAY

Dissolve 0.180 g with gentle heating in a mixture of 25 ml of *2-methyl-2-propanol R* and 25 ml of *perchloric acid solution R*. Add 0.1 ml of *ferroin R*. Titrate with *0.1 M cerium sulphate*. Titrate slowly towards the end of the titration. Carry out a blank titration.

1 ml of *0.1 M cerium sulphate* is equivalent to 20.92 mg of $C_{21}H_{26}N_2O_7$.

STORAGE

Store protected from light.

IMPURITIES

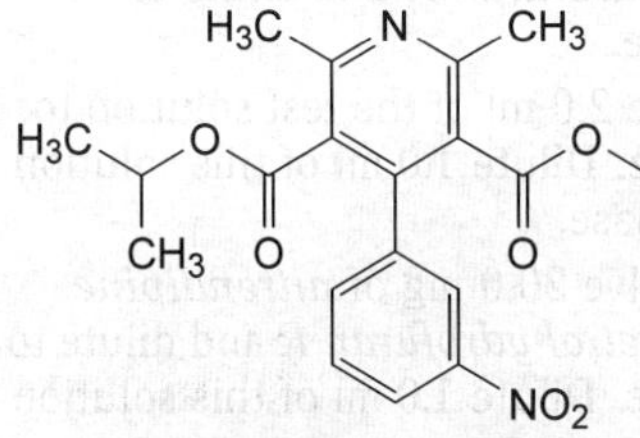

A. 2-methoxyethyl 1-methylethyl 2,6-dimethyl-4-(3-nitrophenyl)pyridine-3,5-dicarboxylate,

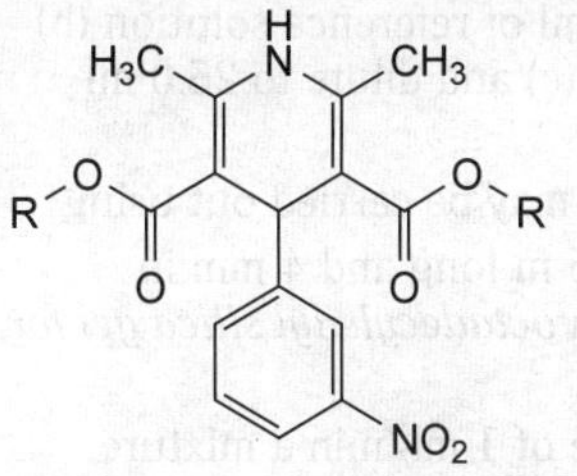

B. R = $CH(CH_3)_2$: bis(1-methylethyl) 2,6-dimethyl-4-(3-nitrophenyl)-1,4-dihydropyridine-3,5-dicarboxylate,

C. R = CH_2-CH_2-OCH_3: bis(2-methoxyethyl) 2,6-dimethyl-4-(3-nitrophenyl)-1,4-dihydropyridine-3,5-dicarboxylate.

01/2005:0415

NITRAZEPAM

Nitrazepamum

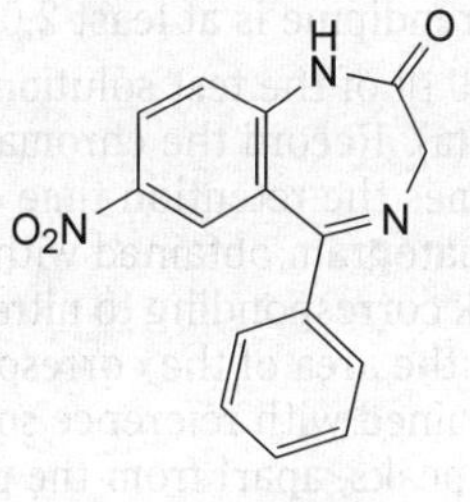

$C_{15}H_{11}N_3O_3$ M_r 281.3

DEFINITION

Nitrazepam contains not less than 99.0 per cent and not more than the equivalent of 101.0 per cent of 7-nitro-5-phenyl-1,3-dihydro-2*H*-1,4-benzodiazepin-2-one, calculated with reference to the dried substance.

CHARACTERS

A yellow, crystalline powder, practically insoluble in water, slightly soluble in alcohol.

IDENTIFICATION

First identification: A, C.

Second identification: A, B, D, E.

A. Melting point (*2.2.14*): 226 °C to 230 °C.

B. *Protect the solutions from light and measure the absorbances immediately.* Dissolve 25.0 mg in a 5 g/l solution of *sulphuric acid R* in *methanol R* and dilute to 250.0 ml with the same solvent. Dilute 5.0 ml of the solution to 100.0 ml with a 5 g/l solution of *sulphuric acid R* in *methanol R*. Examined between 230 nm and 350 nm (*2.2.25*), the solution shows an absorption maximum at 280 nm. The specific absorbance at the maximum is 890 to 950.

C. Examine by infrared absorption spectrophotometry (*2.2.24*), comparing with the spectrum obtained with *nitrazepam CRS*.

D. Dissolve about 20 mg in a mixture of 5 ml of *hydrochloric acid R* and 10 ml of *water R*. Boil for 5 min, cool and add 2 ml of a 1 g/l solution of *sodium nitrite R*. Allow to stand for 1 min and add 1 ml of a 5 g/l solution of *sulphamic acid R* and mix. Allow to stand for 1 min and add 1 ml of a 1 g/l solution of *naphthylethylenediamine dihydrochloride R*. A red colour is produced.

E. Dissolve about 10 mg in 1 ml of *methanol R*, warming if necessary, and add 0.05 ml of *dilute sodium hydroxide solution R*. An intense yellow colour is produced.

TESTS

Related substances. *Carry out the test protected from light.* Examine by thin-layer chromatography (*2.2.27*), using *silica gel GF_{254} R* as the coating substance.

Test solution. Dissolve 0.2 g of the substance to be examined in *acetone R* and dilute to 10 ml with the same solvent. Prepare the solution immediately before use.

Reference solution (a). Dissolve 10 mg of *aminonitrobenzophenone R* in *acetone R* and dilute to 100 ml with the same solvent. Dilute 10 ml of the solution to 50 ml with *acetone R*.

Reference solution (b). Dissolve 10 mg of *nitrazepam impurity A CRS* in *acetone R* and dilute to 100 ml with the same solvent. Dilute 10 ml of the solution to 50 ml with *acetone R*.

Reference solution (c). Dilute 1 ml of the test solution to 20 ml with *acetone R*. Dilute 1 ml of this solution to 50 ml with *acetone R*.

Apply separately to the plate 10 µl of each solution. Develop over a path of 12 cm using a mixture of 15 volumes of *ethyl acetate R* and 85 volumes of *nitromethane R*. Allow the plate to dry in air and examine in ultraviolet light at 254 nm. In the chromatogram obtained with the test solution: any spot corresponding to aminonitrobenzophenone is not more intense than the spot in the chromatogram obtained with reference solution (a) (0.1 per cent); any spot corresponding to nitrazepam impurity A is not more intense than the spot in the chromatogram obtained with reference solution (b) (0.1 per cent); any spot apart from the principal spot and the spots corresponding to aminonitrobenzophenone and nitrazepam impurity A is not more intense than the spot in the chromatogram obtained with reference solution (c) (0.1 per cent).

Heavy metals (*2.4.8*). 1.0 g complies with limit test D for heavy metals (20 ppm). Prepare the standard using 2 ml of *lead standard solution (10 ppm Pb) R*.

Loss on drying (*2.2.32*). Not more than 0.5 per cent, determined on 1.00 g by drying in an oven at 100 °C to 105 °C for 4 h.

Sulphated ash (*2.4.14*). Not more than 0.1 per cent, determined on 1.0 g.

ASSAY

Dissolve 0.250 g in 25 ml of *acetic anhydride R*. Titrate with *0.1 M perchloric acid*, determining the end-point potentiometrically (*2.2.20*).

1 ml of *0.1 M perchloric acid* is equivalent to 28.13 mg of $C_{15}H_{11}N_3O_3$.

STORAGE

Store protected from light.

IMPURITIES

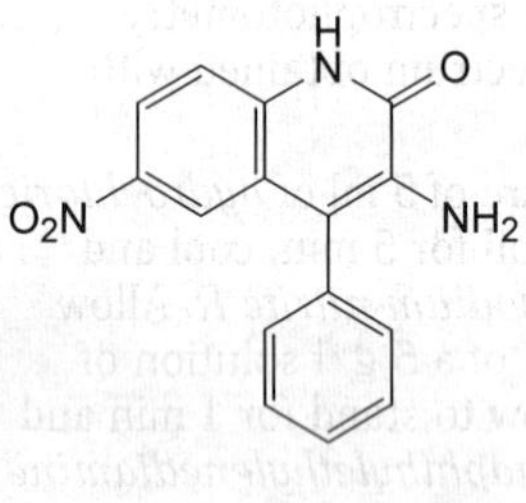

A. 3-amino-6-nitro-4-phenylquinolin-2(1*H*)-one,

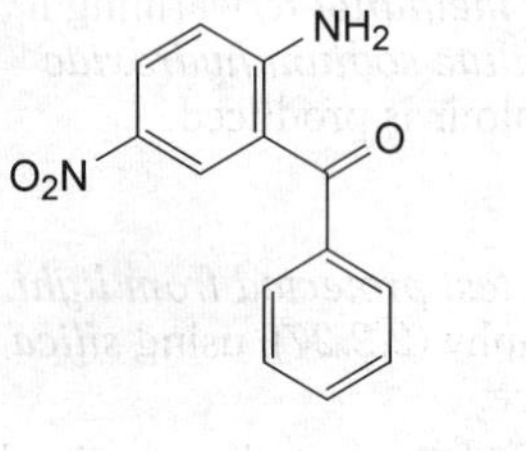

B. (2-amino-5-nitrophenyl)phenylmethanone.

01/2005:1246

NITRENDIPINE

Nitrendipinum

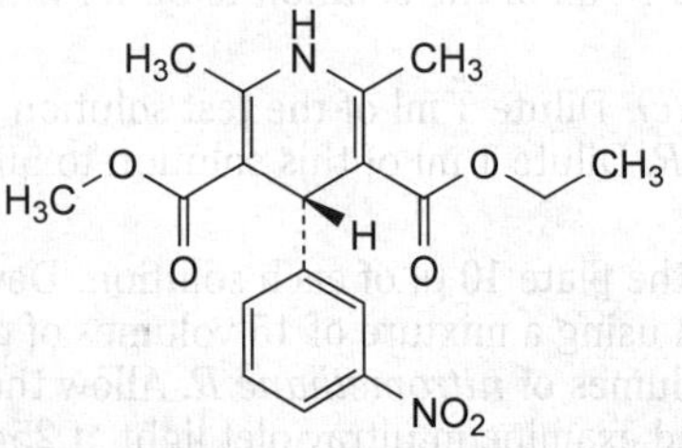

and enantiomer

$C_{18}H_{20}N_2O_6$ M_r 360.4

DEFINITION

Nitrendipine contains not less than 98.5 per cent and not more than the equivalent of 101.5 per cent of ethyl methyl (4*RS*)-2,6-dimethyl-4-(3-nitrophenyl)-1,4-dihydropyridine-3,5-dicarboxylate, calculated with reference to the dried substance.

CHARACTERS

A yellow, crystalline powder, practically insoluble in water, freely soluble in ethyl acetate, sparingly soluble in ethanol and in methanol.

It shows polymorphism.

Exposure to ultraviolet light leads to the formation of a nitrophenylpyridine derivative

Prepare solutions immediately before use either protected from light or under long-wavelength light (> 420 nm).

IDENTIFICATION

Examine by infrared absorption spectrophotometry (*2.2.24*), comparing with the spectrum obtained with *nitrendipine CRS*. If the spectra obtained in the solid state show differences, record further spectra using 20 g/l solutions in *methylene chloride R* and a 0.2 mm cell.

TESTS

Optical rotation (*2.2.7*). Dissolve 0.2 g in *acetone R* and dilute to 10.0 ml with the same solvent. The angle of optical rotation is − 0.10° to + 0.10°.

Related substances. Examine by liquid chromatography (*2.2.29*).

Test solution. Dissolve 40.0 mg of the substance to be examined in 2.5 ml of *tetrahydrofuran R* and dilute to 25.0 ml with the mobile phase.

Reference solution (a). Dilute 2.0 ml of the test solution to 10.0 ml with the mobile phase. Dilute 1.0 ml of this solution to 25.0 ml with the mobile phase.

Reference solution (b). Dissolve 20.0 mg of *nitrendipine impurity A CRS* in 2.5 ml of *tetrahydrofuran R* and dilute to 25.0 ml with the mobile phase. Dilute 1.0 ml of this solution to 20.0 ml with the mobile phase.

Reference solution (c). Dilute 0.5 ml of the test solution to 20.0 ml with the mobile phase.

Reference solution (d). Mix 1.0 ml of reference solution (b) and 1.0 ml of reference solution (c) and dilute to 25.0 ml with the mobile phase.

The chromatographic procedure may be carried out using:

- a stainless steel column 0.125 m long and 4 mm in internal diameter packed with *octadecylsilyl silica gel for chromatography R* (5 µm),
- as mobile phase at a flow rate of 1 ml/min a mixture of 14 volumes of *acetonitrile R*, 22 volumes of *tetrahydrofuran R* and 64 volumes of *water R*,
- as detector a spectrophotometer set at 235 nm,

maintaining the temperature of the column at 40 °C.

Adjust the sensitivity of the system so that the height of the nitrendipine peak in the chromatogram obtained with 20 µl of reference solution (d) is at least 50 per cent of the full scale of the recorder.

Inject 20 µl of reference solution (d). When the chromatogram is recorded in the prescribed conditions, the retention times are: nitrendipine impurity A about 6 min and nitrendipine about 8 min. The test is not valid unless the resolution between the peaks corresponding to nitrendipine impurity A and nitrendipine is at least 2.0.

Inject separately 20 µl of the test solution and 20 µl of reference solution (a). Record the chromatogram of the test solution for five times the retention time of the principal peak. In the chromatogram obtained with the test solution: the area of the peak corresponding to nitrendipine impurity A is not greater than the area of the corresponding peak in the chromatogram obtained with reference solution (d) (0.1 per cent); none of the peaks, apart from the principal peak and the peaks corresponding to nitrendipine impurity A has an area greater than that of the peak corresponding to nitrendipine in the chromatogram obtained with reference solution (a) (0.8 per cent); the sum of the areas of all the peaks, apart from the principal peak, is not greater than 1.5 times the area of the principal peak in the chromatogram obtained with reference solution (a) (1.2 per cent). Disregard any peak with an area less than 0.5 times the area of the nitrendipine peak in the chromatogram obtained with reference solution (d).

Loss on drying (*2.2.32*). Not more than 0.5 per cent, determined on 1.000 g by drying in an oven at 100-105 °C.

Sulphated ash (*2.4.14*). Not more than 0.1 per cent, determined on 1.0 g.

ASSAY

Dissolve 0.160 g with gentle heating if necessary in a mixture of 25 ml of *2-methyl-2-propanol R* and 25 ml of *perchloric acid solution R*. Titrate with *0.1 M cerium sulphate,* using 0.1 ml of *ferroin R* as indicator. Titrate slowly towards the end of the titration. Carry out a blank titration.

1 ml of *0.1 M cerium sulphate* is equivalent to 18.02 mg of $C_{18}H_{20}N_2O_6$.

STORAGE

Store protected from light.

IMPURITIES

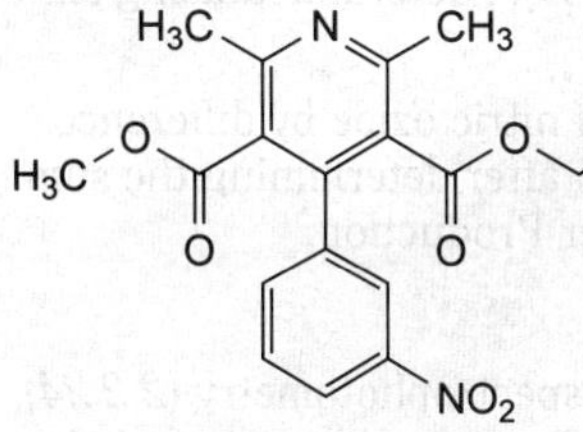

A. ethyl methyl 2,6-dimethyl-4-(3-nitrophenyl)pyridine-3,5-dicarboxylate,

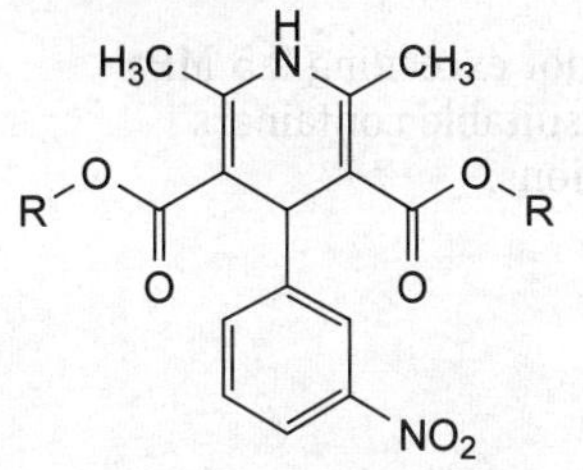

B. R = CH_3: dimethyl 2,6-dimethyl-4-(3-nitrophenyl)-1,4-dihydropyridine-3,5-dicarboxylate,

C. R = CH_2-CH_3: diethyl 2,6-dimethyl-4-(3-nitrophenyl)-1,4-dihydropyridine-3,5-dicarboxylate.

01/2005:1549

NITRIC ACID

Acidum nitricum

HNO_3 M_r 63.0

DEFINITION

Nitric acid contains not less than 68.0 per cent *m/m* and not more than 70.0 per cent *m/m* of HNO_3.

CHARACTERS

A clear, colourless to almost colourless liquid, miscible with water.

It has a relative density of about 1.41.

IDENTIFICATION

A. Dilute 1 ml to 100 ml with *water R*. The solution is strongly acid (*2.2.4*).

B. 0.2 ml of the solution obtained in identification test A gives the reaction of nitrates (*2.3.1*).

TESTS

Appearance of solution. Dilute 2 ml to 10 ml with *water R*. The solution is clear (*2.2.1*) and not more intensely coloured than reference solution Y_6 (*2.2.2, Method II*).

Chlorides (*2.4.4*). To 5 g add 10 ml of *water R* and 0.3 ml of *silver nitrate solution R2* and allow to stand for 2 min protected from light. Any opalescence is not more intense than that of a standard prepared in the same manner using 13 ml of *water R*, 0.5 ml of *nitric acid R*, 0.5 ml of *chloride standard solution (5 ppm Cl) R* and 0.3 ml of *silver nitrate solution R2* (0.5 ppm).

Sulphates (*2.4.13*). To 15 g add 0.2 g of *sodium carbonate R*. After carbon dioxide has evolved, evaporate to dryness. Dissolve the residue in 15 ml of *distilled water R*. The solution complies with the limit test for sulphates (10 ppm).

Iron (*2.4.9*). Dissolve the residue obtained in the test for sulphated ash in 1 ml of *dilute hydrochloric acid R* and dilute to 20 ml with *water R*. Dilute 1 ml to 10 ml with *water R*. The solution complies with the limit test for iron (10 ppm).

Heavy metals (*2.4.8*). Carefully evaporate 10.0 g to dryness on a water-bath. Moisten the residue with a few drops of *dilute hydrochloric acid R* and dilute to 20 ml with *water R*. 12 ml of the solution complies with limit test A for heavy metals (2 ppm). Prepare the standard using *lead standard solution (2 ppm Pb) R*.

Sulphated ash. Carefully evaporate 20.00 g to dryness. Moisten the residue with a few drops of *sulphuric acid R* and ignite to dull red. The residue does not exceed 0.01 per cent.

ASSAY

To 0.750 g add 50 ml of *water R* and titrate with *1 M sodium hydroxide,* determining the end-point potentiometrically (*2.2.20*).

1 ml of *1 M sodium hydroxide* is equivalent to 63.0 mg of HNO_3.

STORAGE

Store protected from light.

Monographs N-O

01/2005:1550

NITRIC OXIDE

Nitrogenii oxidum

NO M_r 30.01

DEFINITION

Nitric oxide contains not less than 99.0 per cent *V/V* of NO.

This monograph applies to nitric oxide for medicinal use.

CHARACTERS

A colourless gas which turns brown when exposed to air. At 20 °C and at a pressure of 101 kPa, 1 volume dissolves in about 21 volumes of water.

PRODUCTION

Carbon dioxide. Not more than 3000 ppm *V/V*, determined by gas chromatography (*2.2.28*).

Gas to be examined. The substance to be examined.

Reference gas. Use a mixture containing 3000 ppm *V/V* of *carbon dioxide R1* in *nitrogen R*.

The chromatography may be carried out using:

- a stainless steel column 3.5 m long and 2 mm in internal diameter packed with *ethylvinylbenzene-divinylbenzene copolymer R*,
- *helium for chromatography R* as the carrier gas at a flow rate of 15 ml/min,
- a thermal conductivity detector,
- a loop injector,

maintaining the temperature of the column at 50 °C.

Inject the gas to be examined and the reference gas. The test is not valid unless the chromatograms obtained show a clear separation of carbon dioxide from nitric oxide.

Calculate the carbon dioxide content in the gas to be examined from the area of the carbon dioxide peak in the chromatogram obtained with the reference gas.

Nitrogen. Not more than 3000 ppm *V/V*, determined by gas chromatography (*2.2.28*).

Gas to be examined. The substance to be examined.

Reference gas. Use a mixture containing 3000 ppm *V/V* of *nitrogen R* in *helium for chromatography R*.

The chromatography may be carried out using:

- a stainless steel column 3.5 m long and 2 mm in internal diameter packed with *molecular sieve for chromatography R* (0.5 nm),
- *helium for chromatography R* as the carrier gas at a flow rate of 15 ml/min,
- a thermal conductivity detector,
- a loop injector,

maintaining the temperature of the column at 50 °C.

Inject the gas to be examined and the reference gas. The test is not valid unless the chromatograms obtained show a clear separation of nitrogen from nitric oxide.

Calculate the nitrogen content in the gas to be examined from the area of the peak due to nitrogen in the chromatogram obtained with the reference gas.

Nitrogen dioxide. Not more than 400 ppm *V/V*, determined using an ultraviolet absorption spectrophotometry analyser.

Gas to be examined. The substance to be examined.

Reference gas (a). Use *nitrogen R1*.

Reference gas (b). Use a mixture containing 400 ppm *V/V* of *nitrogen dioxide R* in *nitrogen R*.

The apparatus consists of the following:

- an ultraviolet-visible light source (analytical wavelength about 400 nm),
- a sample gas cell through which the feed gas flows,
- a closed reference gas cell containing *nitrogen R1* in parallel with the sample gas cell,
- a rotating chopper which feeds light alternately through the reference gas cell and the sample gas cell,
- a semiconductor detector which generates a frequency modulated output whose amplitude is a measure of the difference of absorption of the sample gas and the reference gas.

Carry out the analysis in the following way:

- set the zero of the instrument using reference gas (a) through the sample gas cell at a flow rate of 1 litre/min,
- adjust the span while feeding reference gas (b) through the sample gas cell at a flow rate of 1 litre/min,
- feed the gas to be examined through the sample gas cell at a flow rate of 1 litre/min, read the value from the instrument output and calculate if necessary the concentration of nitrogen dioxide.

Nitrous oxide. Not more than 3000 ppm *V/V*, determined by gas chromatography (*2.2.28*).

Gas to be examined. The substance to be examined.

Reference gas. Use a mixture containing 3000 ppm *V/V* of *nitrous oxide R* in *nitrogen R*.

The chromatography may be carried out using:

- a stainless steel column 3.5 m long and 2 mm in internal diameter packed with *ethylvinylbenzene-divinylbenzene copolymer R*,
- *helium for chromatography R* as the carrier gas at a flow rate of 15 ml/min,
- a thermal conductivity detector,
- a loop injector,

maintaining the temperature of the column at 50 °C.

Inject the gas to be examined and the reference gas. The test is not valid unless the chromatograms obtained show a clear separation of nitrous oxide from nitric oxide.

Calculate the nitrous oxide content in the gas to be examined from the area of the peak due to nitrous oxide in the chromatogram obtained with the reference gas.

Water. Not more than 100 ppm *V/V*, determined using an electrolytic hygrometer (*2.5.28*).

Assay. Determine the content of nitric oxide by difference using the mass balance equation after determining the sum of the impurities described under Production.

IDENTIFICATION

Examine by infrared absorption spectrophotometry (*2.2.24*), comparing with the *Ph. Eur. reference spectrum of nitric oxide*.

STORAGE

Store compressed at a pressure not exceeding 2.5 MPa (25 bars) measured at 15 °C, in suitable containers complying with the legal regulations.

IMPURITIES

A. carbon dioxide,

B. nitrogen,

C. nitrogen dioxide,

D. nitrous oxide,

E. water.

01/2005:1135

NITROFURAL

Nitrofuralum

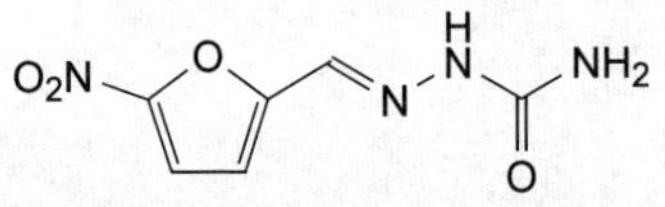

$C_6H_6N_4O_4$ M_r 198.1

DEFINITION

Nitrofural contains not less than 97.0 per cent and not more than the equivalent of 103.0 per cent of 2-[(5-nitrofuran-2-yl)methylene]diazanecarboxamide, calculated with reference to the dried substance.

CHARACTERS

A yellow or brownish-yellow, crystalline powder, very slightly soluble in water, slightly soluble in alcohol.

IDENTIFICATION

First identification: B.

Second identification: A, C, D.

A. *Carry out the test protected from bright light.* Use the solution prepared for the assay. Examined between 220 nm and 400 nm (*2.2.25*), the solution shows two absorption maxima, at 260 nm and 375 nm. The ratio of the absorbance measured at the maximum at 375 nm to that measured at the maximum at 260 nm is 1.15 to 1.30.

B. Examine by infrared absorption spectrophotometry (*2.2.24*), comparing with the spectrum obtained with *nitrofural CRS*. Examine the substances prepared as discs.

C. Examine by thin-layer chromatography (*2.2.27*), using *silica gel G R* as the coating substance.

Test solution. Dissolve 10 mg of the substance to be examined in *methanol R* and dilute to 10 ml with the same solvent.

Reference solution. Dissolve 10 mg of *nitrofural CRS* in *methanol R* and dilute to 10 ml with the same solvent.

Apply to the plate 5 µl of each solution. Develop over a path of 15 cm using a mixture of 10 volumes of *methanol R* and 90 volumes of *nitromethane R*. Allow the plate to dry in air and spray with *phenylhydrazine hydrochloride solution R*. The principal spot in the chromatogram obtained with the test solution is similar in position, colour and size to the principal spot in the chromatogram obtained with the reference solution.

D. Dissolve about 1 mg in 1 ml of *dimethylformamide R* and add 0.1 ml of *alcoholic potassium hydroxide solution R*. A violet-red colour is produced.

TESTS

pH (*2.2.3*). To 1.0 g add 100 ml of *carbon dioxide-free water R*. Shake and filter. The pH of the filtrate is 5.0 to 7.0.

Related substances. Examine by liquid chromatography (*2.2.29*).

Test solution. Dissolve 0.10 g of the substance to be examined in the mobile phase and dilute to 100.0 ml with the mobile phase.

Reference solution (a). Dissolve 10.0 mg of *(5-nitro-2-furyl)methylene diacetate R* in the mobile phase and dilute to 20.0 ml with the mobile phase. Dilute 1.0 ml of this solution to 100.0 ml with the mobile phase.

Reference solution (b). Dissolve 10 mg of *nitrofural CRS* and 10 mg of *nitrofurantoin R* in the mobile phase and dilute to 100 ml with the mobile phase. Dilute 5 ml of this solution to 100 ml with the mobile phase.

The chromatographic procedure may be carried out using:

- a stainless steel column 0.25 m long and 4.6 mm in internal diameter packed with *octadecylsilyl silica gel for chromatography R* (5 µm),
- as mobile phase at a flow rate of 1 ml per minute a mixture of 40 volumes of *acetonitrile R* and 60 volumes of *water R*,
- as detector a spectrophotometer set at 310 nm.

Inject 20 µl of reference solution (a). Adjust the sensitivity of the system so that the height of the principal peak in the chromatogram obtained is not less than 50 per cent of the full scale of the recorder. Inject 20 µl of reference solution (b). The test is not valid unless, in the chromatogram obtained, the resolution between the peaks due to nitrofurantoin and nitrofural is at least 2.0. Inject 20 µl of the test solution and 20 µl of reference solution (a). Continue the chromatography for ten times the retention time of nitrofural, which is about 3 min. In the chromatogram obtained with the test solution: the area of any peak, apart from the principal peak, is not greater than the area of the principal peak in the chromatogram obtained with reference solution (a) (0.5 per cent); the sum of the areas of all the peaks, apart from the principal peak, is not greater than twice the area of the principal peak in the chromatogram obtained with reference solution (a) (1.0 per cent). Disregard any peak with an area less than 0.05 times that of the principal peak in the chromatogram obtained with reference solution (a).

Loss on drying (*2.2.32*). Not more than 0.5 per cent, determined on 1.000 g by drying in an oven at 100-105 °C.

Sulphated ash (*2.4.14*). Not more than 0.1 per cent, determined on 1.0 g.

ASSAY

Carry out the assay protected from bright light. Dissolve 60.0 mg in 20 ml of *dimethylformamide R* and dilute to 500.0 ml with *water R*. Dilute 5.0 ml to 100.0 ml with *water R*. Prepare a reference solution in the same manner using 60.0 mg of *nitrofural CRS*. Measure the absorbances (*2.2.25*) of the two solutions at the maximum at 375 nm. Calculate the content of $C_6H_6N_4O_4$ from the absorbances measured and the concentrations of the solutions.

STORAGE

Store protected from light.

IMPURITIES

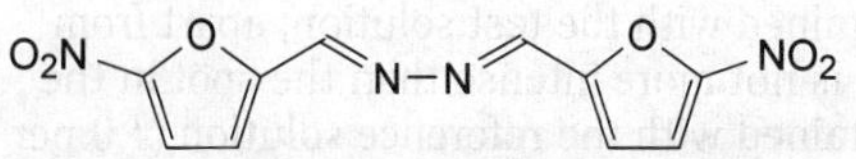

A. bis[(5-nitrofuran-2-yl)methylene]diazane,

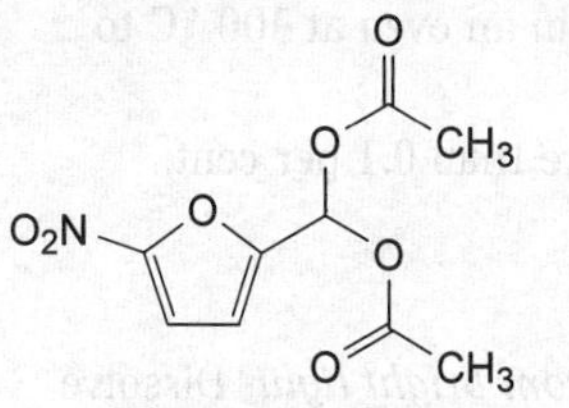

B. (5-nitrofuran-2-yl)methylene diacetate.

01/2005:0101

NITROFURANTOIN

Nitrofurantoinum

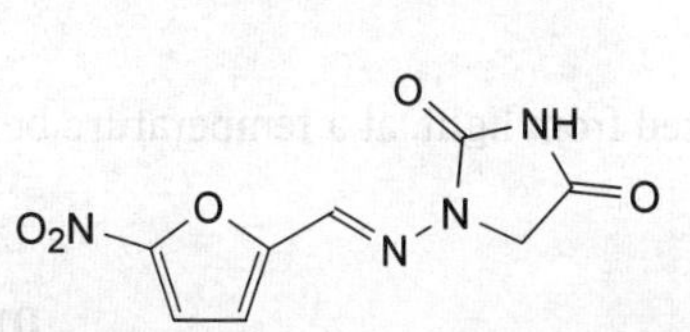

$C_8H_6N_4O_5$ M_r 238.2

DEFINITION

Nitrofurantoin contains not less than 98.0 per cent and not more than the equivalent of 102.0 per cent of 1-[[(5-nitrofuran-2-yl)methylene]amino]imidazolidine-2,4-dione, calculated with reference to the dried substance.

CHARACTERS

A yellow, crystalline powder or yellow crystals, odourless or almost odourless, very slightly soluble in water and in alcohol, soluble in dimethylformamide.

IDENTIFICATION

A. *Carry out the test protected from bright light.* Use the solution prepared for the assay. Examined between 220 nm and 400 nm (*2.2.25*), the solution shows two absorption maxima, at 266 nm and 367 nm. The ratio of the absorbance at the maximum at 367 nm to that at the maximum at 266 nm is 1.36 to 1.42.

B. Dissolve about 10 mg in 10 ml of *dimethylformamide R*. To 1 ml of the solution add 0.1 ml of *0.5 M alcoholic potassium hydroxide*. A brown colour develops.

TESTS

Related substances. Examine by thin-layer chromatography (*2.2.27*), using *silica gel HF_{254} R* as the coating substance.

Test solution. Dissolve 0.25 g of the substance to be examined in a minimum of *dimethylformamide R* and dilute to 10 ml with *acetone R*.

Reference solution. Dilute 1 ml of the test solution to 100 ml with *acetone R*.

Apply separately to the plate 10 µl of each solution. Develop over a path of 15 cm using a mixture of 10 volumes of *methanol R* and 90 volumes of *nitromethane R*. Allow the plate to dry in air and heat at 100 °C to 105 °C for 5 min. Examine in ultraviolet light at 254 nm. Spray with *phenylhydrazine hydrochloride solution R*. Heat the plate at 100 °C to 105 °C for a further 10 min. When examined in ultraviolet light and after spraying, any spot in the chromatogram obtained with the test solution, apart from the principal spot, is not more intense than the spot in the chromatogram obtained with the reference solution (1.0 per cent).

Loss on drying (*2.2.32*). Not more than 1.0 per cent, determined on 1.00 g by drying in an oven at 100 °C to 105 °C.

Sulphated ash (*2.4.14*). Not more than 0.1 per cent, determined on 1.0 g.

ASSAY

Carry out the assay protected from bright light. Dissolve 0.120 g in 50 ml of *dimethylformamide R* and dilute to 1000.0 ml with *water R*. Dilute 5.0 ml of the solution to 100.0 ml with a solution containing 18 g/l of *sodium acetate R* and 0.14 per cent *V/V* of *glacial acetic acid R*. Measure the absorbance (*2.2.25*) at the absorption maximum at 367 nm, using the sodium acetate solution described above as compensation liquid.

Calculate the content of $C_8H_6N_4O_5$, taking the specific absorbance to be 765.

STORAGE

Store protected from light, at a temperature below 25 °C.

01/2005:1247

NITROGEN

Nitrogenium

N_2 M_r 28.01

DEFINITION

Nitrogen contains not less than 99.5 per cent *V/V* of N_2.

This monograph applies to nitrogen for medicinal use.

CHARACTERS

A colourless, odourless gas. At 20 °C and at a pressure of 101 kPa, 1 volume dissolves in about 62 volumes of water and about 10 volumes of alcohol.

PRODUCTION

Carbon dioxide. Not more than 300 ppm *V/V*, determined using an infrared analyser (*2.5.24*).

Gas to be examined. The substance to be examined. It must be filtered to avoid stray light phenomena.

Reference gas (a). Use *nitrogen R1*.

Reference gas (b). Use a mixture containing 300 ppm *V/V* of *carbon dioxide R1* in *nitrogen R1*.

Calibrate the apparatus and set the sensitivity using reference gases (a) and (b). Measure the content of carbon dioxide in the gas to be examined.

Carbon monoxide. Not more than 5 ppm *V/V*, determined using an infrared analyser (*2.5.25*).

Gas to be examined. The substance to be examined. It must be filtered to avoid stray light phenomena.

Reference gas (a). Use *nitrogen R1*.

Reference gas (b). Use a mixture containing 5 ppm *V/V* of *carbon monoxide R* in *nitrogen R1*.

Calibrate the apparatus and set the sensitivity using reference gases (a) and (b). Measure the content of carbon monoxide in the gas to be examined.

Oxygen. Not more than 50 ppm *V/V*, determined using an oxygen analyser with a detector scale ranging from 0 ppm *V/V* to 100 ppm *V/V* and equipped with an electrochemical cell.

The gas to be examined passes through a detection cell containing an aqueous solution of an electrolyte, generally potassium hydroxide. The presence of oxygen in the gas to be examined produces variation in the electric signal recorded at the outlet of the cell that is proportional to the oxygen content.

Calibrate the analyser according to the instructions of the manufacturer. Pass the gas to be examined through the analyser using a suitable pressure regulator and airtight metal tubes and operating at the prescribed flow-rates until constant readings are obtained.

Water. Not more than 67 ppm *V/V*, determined using an electrolytic hygrometer (*2.5.28*).

Assay. Examine by gas chromatography (*2.2.28*).

Gas to be examined. The substance to be examined.

Reference gas (a). Use ambient air.

Reference gas (b). Use *nitrogen R1*.

The chromatographic procedure may be carried out using:

- a stainless steel column 2 m long and 2 mm in internal diameter packed with an appropriate molecular sieve for chromatography (0.5 nm),
- *helium for chromatography R* as the carrier gas at a flow rate of 40 ml/min,
- a thermal conductivity detector,
- a loop injector,

maintaining the temperature of the column at 50 °C and that of the detector at 130 °C.

Inject reference gas (a). Adjust the injected volumes and operating conditions so that the height of the peak due to nitrogen in the chromatogram obtained with the reference gas is at least 35 per cent of the full scale of the recorder. The assay is not valid unless the chromatograms obtained show a clear separation of oxygen and nitrogen.

Inject the gas to be examined and reference gas (b). Calculate the content of N_2 in the gas to be examined.

IDENTIFICATION

First identification: A.

Second identification: B, C.

A. Examine the chromatograms obtained in the Assay. The retention time of the principal peak in the chromatogram obtained with the substance to be examined is approximately the same as that of the principal peak in the chromatogram obtained with reference gas (b).

B. In a 250 ml conical flask replace the air by the substance to be examined. Place a burning or glowing splinter of wood in the flask. The splinter is extinguished.

C. In a suitable test tube, place 0.1 g of *magnesium R* in turnings. Close the tube with a two-hole stopper fitted with a glass tube reaching about 1 cm above the turnings. Pass the substance to be examined through the glass tube for 1 min without heating, then for 15 min while heating the test tube to a red glow. After cooling, add 5 ml of *dilute sodium hydroxide solution R*. The evolving vapours change the colour of moistened *red litmus paper R* blue.

TESTS

Carbon dioxide. Not more than 300 ppm *V/V*, determined using a carbon dioxide detector tube (*2.1.6*).

Carbon monoxide. Not more than 5 ppm *V/V*, determined using a carbon monoxide detector tube (*2.1.6*).

Water vapour. Not more than 67 ppm *V/V*, determined using a water vapour detector tube (*2.1.6*).

STORAGE

Store as a compressed gas or a liquid in appropriate containers complying with the legal regulations.

IMPURITIES

A. carbon dioxide,

B. carbon monoxide,

C. oxygen,

D. water.

01/2005:1685

NITROGEN, LOW-OXYGEN

Nitrogenium oxygenio depletum

N_2 M_r 28.01

DEFINITION

This monograph applies to nitrogen which is used for inerting finished medicinal products which are particularly sensitive to degradation by oxygen. It does not necessarily apply to nitrogen used in earlier production steps.

Content: minimum 99.5 per cent *V/V* of N_2, calculated by deduction of the sum of impurities found when performing the test for impurities.

CHARACTERS

Colourless and odourless gas.

Solubility: at 20 °C and at a pressure of 101 kPa, 1 volume dissolves in about 62 volumes of water and about 10 volumes of alcohol.

PRODUCTION

Oxygen: maximum 5 ppm *V/V*, determined using an oxygen analyser with a detector scale ranging from 0 ppm *V/V* to 100 ppm *V/V* and equipped with an electrochemical cell.

The gas to be examined passes through a detection cell containing an aqueous solution of an electrolyte, generally potassium hydroxide. The presence of oxygen in the gas to be examined produces variation in the electric signal recorded at the outlet of the cell that is proportional to the oxygen content.

Calibrate the analyser according to the manufacturer's instructions. Pass the gas to be examined through the analyser using a suitable pressure regulator and airtight metal tubes and operating at the prescribed flow rates until constant readings are obtained.

Impurities. Gas chromatography (*2.2.28*).

Gas to be examined. The substance to be examined.

Reference gas (a). Use ambient air.

Reference gas (b). Use *nitrogen R1*.

Column:

- *material*: stainless steel,
- *size*: l = 2 m, Ø = 2 mm,
- *stationary phase*: appropriate molecular sieve for chromatography (0.5 nm).

Carrier gas: *helium for chromatography R*.

Flow rate: 40 ml/min.

Temperature:

- *column*: 50 °C,
- *detector*: 130 °C.

Detection: thermal conductivity.

System suitability: reference gas (a): adjust the injected volumes and operating conditions so that the height of the peak due to nitrogen in the chromatogram obtained is at least 35 per cent of the full scale of the recorder:

- the chromatogram obtained shows a clear separation of oxygen and nitrogen.

Limit:

- *total*: not more than 0.5 per cent of the sum of the areas of all the peaks (0.5 per cent *V/V*).

IDENTIFICATION

First identification: A.

Second identification: B, C.

A. Examine the chromatograms obtained in the test for impurities (see Production).

Results: the principal peak in the chromatogram obtained with the gas to be examined is similar in retention time to the principal peak in the chromatogram obtained with reference gas (b).

B. In a 250 ml conical flask replace the air by the gas to be examined. Place a burning or glowing splinter of wood in the flask. The splinter is extinguished.

C. In a suitable test tube, place 0.1 g of *magnesium R* in turnings. Close the tube with a two-hole stopper fitted with a glass tube reaching about 1 cm above the turnings. Pass the gas to be examined through the glass tube for 1 min without heating, then for 15 min while heating the test tube to a red glow. After cooling, add 5 ml of *dilute sodium hydroxide solution R*. The evolving vapours turn the colour of moistened *red litmus paper R* blue.

Monographs N-O

STORAGE

Where the gas has to be stored, store as a compressed gas or a liquid in appropriate containers complying with the legal regulations.

IMPURITIES

A. oxygen,

B. argon.

01/2005:0416

NITROUS OXIDE

Dinitrogenii oxidum

N_2O M_r 44.01

DEFINITION

Content: minimum 98.0 per cent *V/V* of N_2O in the gaseous phase, when sampled at 15 °C.

This monograph applies to nitrous oxide for medicinal use.

CHARACTERS

Appearance: colourless gas.

Solubility: at 20 °C and at a pressure of 101 kPa, 1 volume dissolves in about 1.5 volumes of water.

PRODUCTION

Nitrous oxide is produced from ammonium nitrate by thermic decomposition.

Examine the gaseous phase.

If the test is performed on a cylinder, keep the cylinder at room temperature for at least 6 h before carrying out the tests. Keep the cylinder in the vertical position with the outlet valve uppermost.

Carbon dioxide. Gas chromatography (*2.2.28*).

Gas to be examined. The substance to be examined.

Reference gas. A mixture containing 300 ppm *V/V* of *carbon dioxide R1* in *nitrous oxide R*.

Column:
- *material*: stainless steel,
- *size*: l = 3.5 m, Ø = 2 mm,
- *stationary phase*: *ethylvinylbenzene-divinylbenzene copolymer R*.

Carrier gas: *helium for chromatography R*.

Flow rate: 15 ml/min.

Temperature:
- *column*: 40 °C,
- *detector*: 90 °C.

Detection: thermal conductivity.

Injection: loop injector.

Adjust the injected volumes and operating conditions so that the height of the peak due to carbon dioxide in the chromatogram obtained with the reference gas is at least 35 per cent of the full scale of the recorder. The test is not valid unless the chromatograms obtained show a clear separation of carbon dioxide from nitrous oxide.

Limit:
- *carbon dioxide*: not more than the area of the corresponding peak in the chromatogram obtained with the reference gas (300 ppm *V/V*).

Carbon monoxide. Gas chromatography (*2.2.28*). *When the test is carried out on a cylinder, use the first portion of gas to be withdrawn.*

Gas to be examined. The substance to be examined.

Reference gas. A mixture containing 5 ppm *V/V* of *carbon monoxide R* in *nitrous oxide R*.

Column:
- *material*: stainless steel,
- *size*: l = 2 m, Ø = 4 mm,
- *stationary phase*: suitable molecular sieve for chromatography (0.5 nm).

Carrier gas: *helium for chromatography R*.

Flow rate: 60 ml/min.

Temperature:
- *column*: 50 °C,
- *injection port and detector*: 130 °C.

Detection: flame ionisation with methaniser.

Injection: loop injector.

Adjust the injected volumes and the operating conditions so that the height of the peak due to carbon monoxide in the chromatogram obtained with the reference gas is at least 35 per cent of the full scale of the recorder.

Limit:
- *carbon monoxide*: not more than the area of the corresponding peak in the chromatogram obtained with the reference gas (5 ppm *V/V*).

Nitrogen monoxide and nitrogen dioxide: maximum 2 ppm *V/V* in total in the gaseous and liquid phases, determined using a chemiluminescence analyser (*2.5.26*).

Gas to be examined. The substance to be examined.

Reference gas (a). Nitrous oxide R.

Reference gas (b). A mixture containing 2 ppm *V/V* of *nitrogen monoxide R* in *nitrogen R1*.

Calibrate the apparatus and set the sensitivity using reference gases (a) and (b). Measure the content of nitrogen monoxide and nitrogen dioxide, separately examining the samples collected from the gaseous phase and the liquid phase of the gas to be examined.

Multiply the result obtained by the quenching correction factor in order to correct the quenching effect on the analyser response caused by the nitrous oxide matrix effect.

The quenching correction factor is determined by applying a known reference mixture of nitrogen monoxide in nitrous oxide and comparing the actual content with the content indicated by the analyser which has been calibrated with a NO/N_2 reference mixture.

$$\text{Quenching correction factor} = \frac{\text{actual nitrogen monoxide content}}{\text{indicated nitrogen monoxide content}}$$

Water: maximum 67 ppm *V/V*, determined using an electrolytic hygrometer (*2.5.28*).

Assay. Gas chromatography (*2.2.28*).

Gas to be examined. The substance to be examined.

Reference gas. Nitrous oxide R.

Column:
- *material*: stainless steel,
- *size*: l = 2 m, Ø = 2 mm,
- *stationary phase*: *silica gel for chromatography R* (250-355 µm).

Carrier gas: *helium for chromatography R*.

Flow rate: 50 ml/min.

Temperature:
- *column and injection port*: 60 °C,

Monographs N-O

– *detector*: 130 °C.

Detection: thermal conductivity.

Injection: loop injector.

Adjust the injected volumes and the operating conditions so that the height of the peak due to nitrous oxide in the chromatogram obtained with the reference gas is at least 35 per cent of the full scale of the recorder.

The area of the peak due to nitrous oxide in the chromatogram obtained with the gas to be examined is at least 98.0 per cent of the area of the peak due to nitrous oxide in the chromatogram obtained with the reference gas.

IDENTIFICATION

First identification: A.

Second identification: B, C.

A. Infrared absorption spectrophotometry (*2.2.24*).

Comparison: Ph. Eur. reference spectrum of nitrous oxide.

B. Place a glowing splinter of wood in the substance to be examined. The splinter bursts into flame.

C. Introduce the substance to be examined into *alkaline pyrogallol solution R*. A brown colour does not develop.

TESTS

Examine the gaseous phase.

If the test is performed on a cylinder, keep the cylinder of the substance to be examined at room temperature for at least 6 h before carrying out the tests. Keep the cylinder in the vertical position with the outlet valve uppermost.

Carbon dioxide: maximum 300 ppm *V/V*, determined using a carbon dioxide detector tube (*2.1.6*).

Carbon monoxide: maximum 5 ppm *V/V*, determined using a carbon monoxide detector tube (*2.1.6*). *When the test is carried out on a cylinder, use the first portion of the gas to be withdrawn.*

Nitrogen monoxide and nitrogen dioxide: maximum 2 ppm *V/V*, determined using a nitrogen monoxide and nitrogen dioxide detector tube (*2.1.6*).

Water vapour: maximum 67 ppm *V/V*, determined using a water vapour detector tube (*2.1.6*).

STORAGE

Store liquefied under pressure in suitable containers complying with the legal regulations. The taps and valves are not greased or oiled.

IMPURITIES

A. carbon dioxide,

B. carbon monoxide,

C. nitrogen monoxide,

D. nitrogen dioxide,

E. water.

01/2005:1453

NIZATIDINE

Nizatidinum

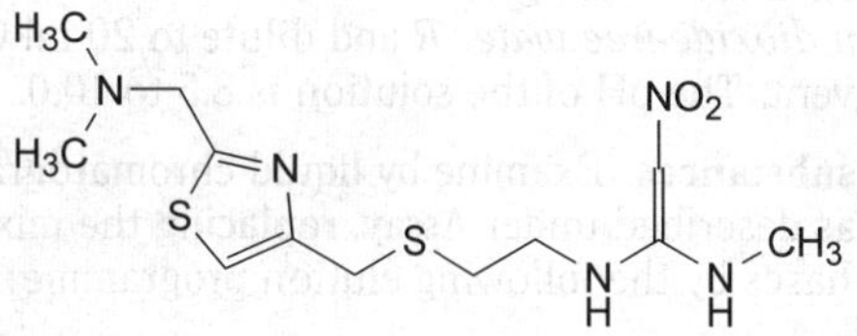

$C_{12}H_{21}N_5O_2S_2$ M_r 331.5

DEFINITION

Nizatidine contains not less than 97.0 per cent and not more than the equivalent of 101.0 per cent of (*EZ*)-*N*-[2-[[[2-[(dimethylamino)methyl]thiazol-4-yl]methyl]sulphanyl]ethyl]-*N*′-methyl-2-nitroethene-1,1-diamine, calculated with reference to the dried substance.

CHARACTERS

An almost white or slightly brownish, crystalline powder, sparingly soluble in water, soluble in methanol.

IDENTIFICATION

First identification: C.

Second identification: A, B, D.

A. Melting point (*2.2.14*): 131 °C to 134 °C.

B. Dissolve 0.10 g of the substance to be examined in *methanol R* and dilute to 100.0 ml with the same solvent. Dilute 2.0 ml of the solution to 100.0 ml with *methanol R*. Examined between 220 nm and 350 nm (*2.2.25*), the solution shows two absorption maxima, at 242 nm and 325 nm. The ratio of the absorbance measured at the maximum at 325 nm to that measured at the maximum at 242 nm is 2.2 to 2.5.

C. Examine by infrared absorption spectrophotometry (*2.2.24*), comparing with the spectrum obtained with *nizatidine CRS*. Examine the substance prepared as discs.

D. Examine by thin-layer chromatography (*2.2.27*), using a *TLC silica gel plate R*.

Test solution. Dissolve 50 mg of the substance to be examined in *methanol R* and dilute to 10 ml with the same solvent.

Reference solution (a). Dissolve 50 mg of *nizatidine CRS* in *methanol R* and dilute to 10 ml with the same solvent.

Reference solution (b). Dissolve 50 mg of *nizatidine CRS* and 50 mg of *ranitidine hydrochloride CRS* in *methanol R* and dilute to 10 ml with the same solvent.

Apply to the plate 5 µl of each solution. Develop over a path corresponding to two thirds of the height of the plate using a mixture of 2 volumes of *water R*, 4 volumes of *concentrated ammonia R1*, 15 volumes of *2-propanol R* and 25 volumes of *ethyl acetate R*. Allow the plate to dry in air and expose to iodine vapour until the spots are clearly visible. Examine in daylight. The principal spot in the chromatogram obtained with the test solution is similar in position and size to the principal spot in the chromatogram obtained with reference solution (a). The test is not valid unless the chromatogram obtained with reference solution (b) shows two clearly separated spots.

Monographs N-O

TESTS

Appearance of solution. Dissolve 0.2 g of the substance to be examined in a 10 g/l solution of *hydrochloric acid R* and dilute to 20 ml with the same acid solution. The solution is clear (*2.2.1*) and not more intensely coloured than reference solution Y_5 (*2.2.2, Method II*).

pH (*2.2.3*). Dissolve 0.2 g of the substance to be examined in *carbon dioxide-free water R* and dilute to 20 ml with the same solvent. The pH of the solution is 8.5 to 10.0.

Related substances. Examine by liquid chromatography (*2.2.29*) as described under Assay, replacing the mixture of mobile phases by the following elution programme:

Time (min)	Mobile phase A (per cent *V/V*)	Mobile phase B (per cent *V/V*)	Comment
0 - 3	76	24	isocratic
3 - 20	76 → 50	24 → 50	linear gradient
20 - 45	50	50	isocratic
45 - 50	50 → 76	50 → 24	linear gradient
50 - 60	76	24	re-equilibration

Inject 20 µl of reference solution (a). Adjust the sensitivity of the system so that the height of the principal peak in the chromatogram obtained with the reference solution is at least 50 per cent of the full scale of the recorder. The test is not valid unless the retention time of nizatidine is between 10 min and 20 min and the symmetry factor of the peak due to nizatidine is not greater than 2.0. Inject 20 µl of reference solution (c). The test is not valid unless the resolution between the peak due to nizatidine (first peak) and impurity F (second peak) is at least 2.0.

Inject 20 µl of test solution (a). In the chromatogram obtained, the area of any peak apart from the principal peak, is not greater than 0.3 times the area of the principal peak in the chromatogram obtained with reference solution (a) (0.3 per cent) and the sum of the areas of all these peaks is not greater than 1.5 times the area of the principal peak in the chromatogram obtained with reference solution (a) (1.5 per cent). Disregard any peak with an area less than 0.03 times the area of the principal peak in the chromatogram obtained with reference solution (a).

Heavy metals (*2.4.8*). 1.0 g complies with limit test C for heavy metals (20 ppm). Prepare the standard using 2 ml of *lead standard solution (10 ppm Pb) R*.

Loss on drying (*2.2.32*). Not more than 0.5 per cent, determined on 1.000 g by drying in an oven at 100 °C to 105 °C.

Sulphated ash (*2.4.14*). Not more than 0.1 per cent, determined on 1.0 g.

ASSAY

Examine by liquid chromatography (*2.2.29*).

Test solution (a). Dissolve 50.0 mg of the substance to be examined in a mixture of 24 volumes of mobile phase B and 76 volumes of mobile phase A and dilute to 10.0 ml with the same mixture of mobile phases.

Test solution (b). Dissolve 15.0 mg of the substance to be examined in a mixture of 24 volumes of mobile phase B and 76 volumes of mobile phase A and dilute to 50.0 ml with the same mixture of mobile phases.

Reference solution (a). Dilute 1.0 ml of test solution (a) to 100.0 ml with a mixture of 24 volumes of mobile phase B and 76 volumes of mobile phase A.

Reference solution (b). Dissolve 15.0 mg of *nizatidine CRS* in a mixture of 24 volumes of mobile phase B and 76 volumes of mobile phase A and dilute to 50.0 ml with the same mixture of mobile phases.

Reference solution (c). Dissolve 5 mg of *nizatidine CRS* and 0.5 mg of *nizatidine impurity F CRS* in a mixture of 24 volumes of mobile phase B and 76 volumes of mobile phase A and dilute to 100.0 ml with the same mixture of mobile phases.

The chromatographic procedure may be carried out using:

– a stainless steel column 0.25 m long and 4.6 mm in internal diameter packed with *octadecylsilyl silica gel for chromatography R* (5 µm),

– as mobile phase at a flow rate of 1.0 ml/min a mixture of 35 volumes of mobile phase B and 65 volumes of mobile phase A:

Mobile phase A. Dissolve 5.9 g of *ammonium acetate R* in 760 ml of *water R*, add 1 ml of *diethylamine R*, and adjust the pH to 7.5 with *acetic acid R*,

Mobile phase B. Methanol R,

– as detector a spectrophotometer set at 254 nm.

Inject 20 µl of reference solution (b). The test is not valid unless the retention time of nizatidine is between 8 min and 10 min and the symmetry of the peak due to nizatidine is not greater than 2.0.

Inject reference solution (b) six times. The test is not valid unless the relative standard deviation of the peak area for nizatidine is at most 2.0 per cent.

Inject 20 µl of test solution (b) and 20 µl of reference solution (b). Calculate the percentage content of nizatidine from the areas of the peaks and the declared content of *nizatidine CRS*.

IMPURITIES

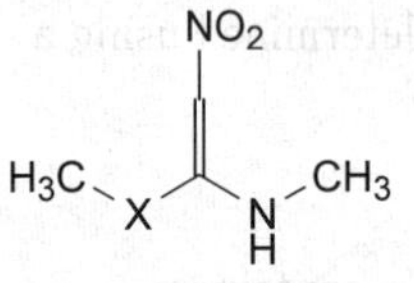

A. X = NH: *N,N'*-dimethyl-2-nitroethene-1,1-diamine,

B. X = S:(*EZ*)-*N*-methyl-1-(methylsulphanyl)-2-nitroethen-1-amine,

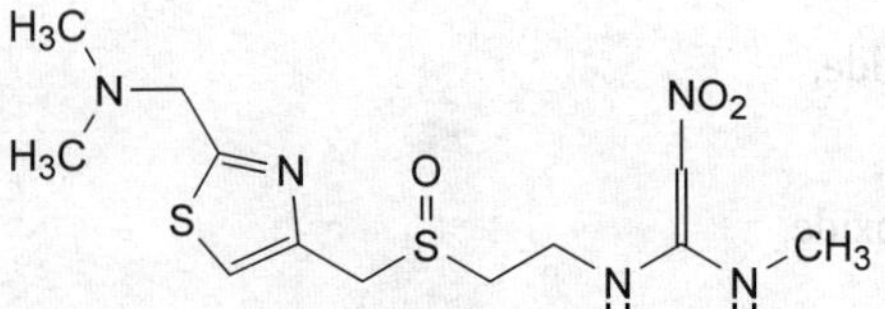

C. (*EZ*)-*N*-[2-[[[2-[(dimethylamino)methyl]thiazol-4-yl]methyl]sulphinyl]ethyl]-*N'*-methyl-2-nitroethene-1,1-diamine,

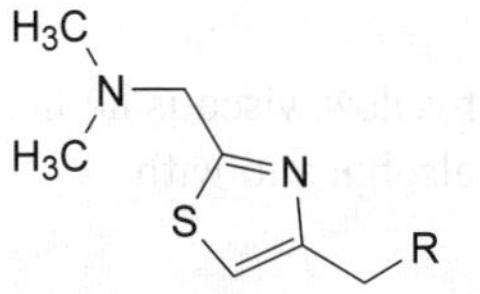

D. R = $S\text{-}CH_2\text{-}CH_2\text{-}NH_2$: 2-[[[2-[(dimethylamino)methyl]thiazol-4-yl]methyl]sulphanyl]ethanamine,

E. R = $S\text{-}CH_2\text{-}CH_2\text{-}NH\text{-}CO\text{-}CH_2\text{-}NO_2$: *N*-[2-[[[2-[(dimethylamino)methyl]thiazol-4-yl]methyl]sulphanyl]ethyl]-2-nitroacetamide,

I. R = $S\text{-}CH_2\text{-}CH_2\text{-}NH\text{-}CO\text{-}NH\text{-}CH_3$: *N*-[2-[[[2-[(dimethylamino)methyl]thiazol-4-yl]methyl]sulphanyl]ethyl]-*N′*-methylurea,

J. R = OH: [2-[(dimethylamino)methyl]thiazol-4-yl]methanol,

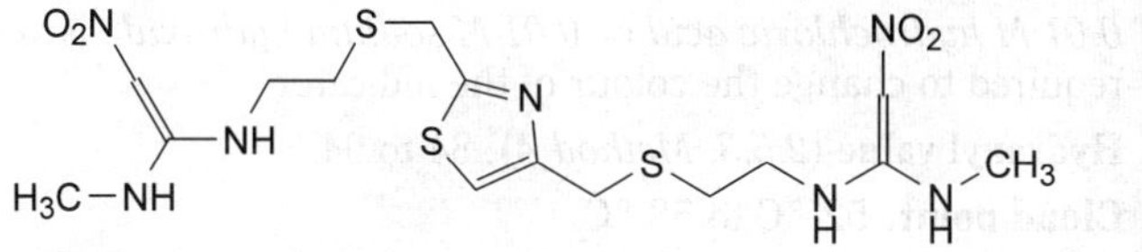

F. (*EZ*)-*N*[1],*N*[1′]-[thiazole-2,4-diylbis(methylenesulphanediylethylene)]bis(*N′*-methyl-2-nitroethene-1,1-diamine),

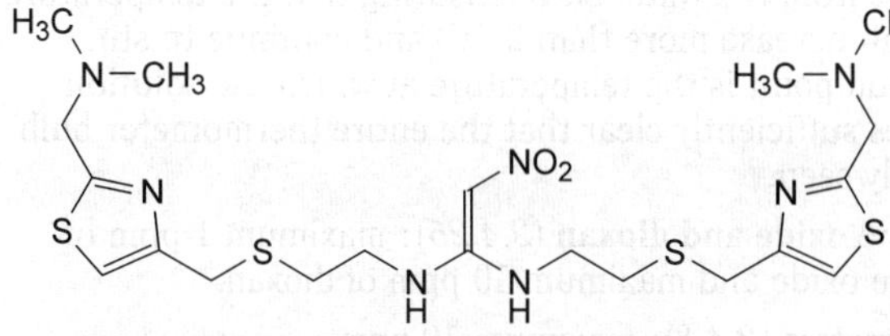

G. *N,N′*-bis[2-[[[2-[(dimethylamino)methyl]thiazol-4-yl]methyl]sulphanyl]ethyl]-2-nitroethene-1,1-diamine,

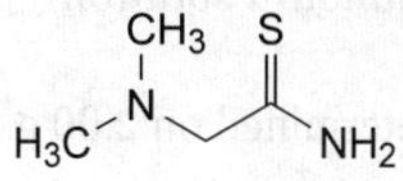

H. 2-(dimethylamino)thioacetamide,

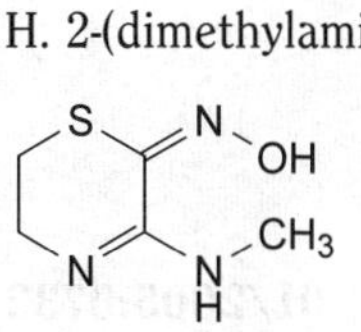

K. 3-(methylamino)-5,6-dihydro-2*H*-1,4-thiazin-2-one oxime.

01/2005:1551

NOMEGESTROL ACETATE

Nomegestroli acetas

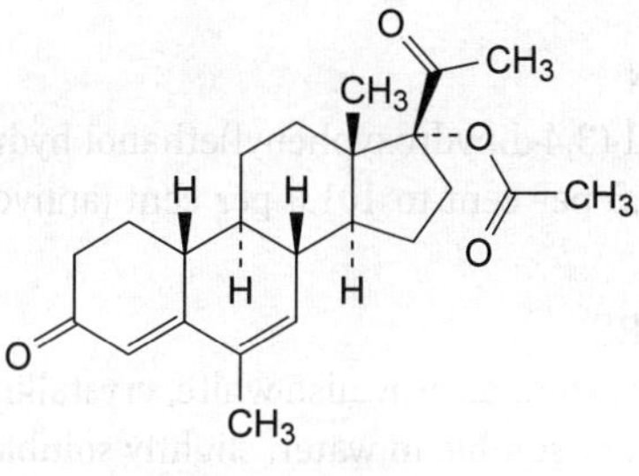

$C_{23}H_{30}O_4$ M_r 370.5

DEFINITION

Nomegestrol acetate contains not less than 97.0 per cent and not more than the equivalent of 103.0 per cent of 6-methyl-3,20-dioxo-19-norpregna-4,6-dien-17-yl acetate, calculated with reference to the dried substance.

CHARACTERS

A white or almost white, crystalline powder, practically insoluble in water, freely soluble in acetone, soluble in alcohol.

IDENTIFICATION

Examine by infrared absorption spectrophotometry (*2.2.24*), comparing with the spectrum obtained with *nomegestrol acetate CRS*.

TESTS

Appearance of solution. Dissolve 1.0 g in *methylene chloride R* and dilute to 10 ml with the same solvent. The solution is clear (*2.2.1*) and not more intensely coloured than reference solution Y_5 (*2.2.2, Method II*).

Specific optical rotation (*2.2.7*). Dissolve 0.500 g in *ethanol R* and dilute to 25.0 ml with the same solvent. The specific optical rotation is − 60.0 to − 64.0, calculated with reference to the dried substance.

Related substances. Examine by liquid chromatography (*2.2.29*).

Test solution. Dissolve 25.0 mg of the substance to be examined in *methanol R* and dilute to 50.0 ml with the same solvent.

Reference solution (a). Dilute 1.0 ml of the test solution to 200.0 ml with the mobile phase.

Reference solution (b). Dissolve 25.0 mg of *nomegestrol acetate impurity A CRS* in *methanol R* and dilute to 50.0 ml with the same solvent.

Reference solution (c). Dissolve 25.0 mg of *nomegestrol acetate CRS* in 20 ml of *methanol R*, add 0.25 ml of reference solution (b) and dilute to 50.0 ml with the mobile phase.

The chromatographic procedure may be carried out using:

- a stainless steel column 0.25 m long and 4.6 mm in internal diameter packed with *octadecylsilyl silica gel for chromatography R* (5 µm),
- as mobile phase at a flow rate of 1.3 ml/min a mixture of 24 volumes of *acetonitrile R*, 38 volumes of *methanol R* and 38 volumes of *water R*,
- as detector, a variable wavelength spectrophotometer capable of operating at 245 nm and at 290 nm.

Inject 10 µl of reference solution (c) and record the chromatogram with the detector set at 245 nm.

When the chromatogram is recorded in the prescribed conditions, the retention times are: nomegestrol acetate about 17 min and impurity A about 18.5 min. Adjust the sensitivity of the system at 245 nm so that the height of the peak due to impurity A in the chromatogram obtained with reference solution (c) is at least 50 per cent of the full scale of the recorder.

Measure the height H_p above the baseline of the peak due to impurity A and the height H_v above the baseline of the lowest point of the curve separating this peak from the peak due to nomegestrol acetate. The test is not valid unless H_p is greater than 5 times H_v.

Inject 10 µl of reference solution (a) and record the chromatogram with the detector set at 290 nm. Adjust the sensitivity of the system at 290 nm so that the height of the

Monographs N-O

principal peak in the chromatogram obtained with reference solution (a) is at least 50 per cent of the full scale of the recorder.

Inject 10 µl of the test solution and record the chromatograms at 245 nm and 290 nm for 1.5 times the retention time of the principal peak.

In the chromatogram obtained with the test solution at 290 nm: the area of any peak, apart from the principal peak, is not greater than 0.2 times the area of the principal peak in the chromatogram obtained with reference solution (a) (0.1 per cent). Disregard any peak with an area less than 0.04 times that of the principal peak in the chromatogram obtained with reference solution (a) (0.02 per cent). In the chromatogram obtained with the test solution at 245 nm: the area of any peak corresponding to impurity A is not greater than 0.4 times the area of the peak due to impurity A in the chromatogram obtained with reference solution (c) (0.2 per cent); the area of any peak, apart from the principal peak and any peak corresponding to impurity A, is not greater than 0.2 times the area of the peak due to impurity A in the chromatogram obtained with reference solution (c) (0.1 per cent). Disregard any peak with an area less than 0.1 times that of the peak due to impurity A in the chromatogram obtained with reference solution (c) (0.05 per cent).

In the chromatograms obtained at 290 nm and 245 nm, the sum of the related substances apart from impurity A is not greater than 0.3 per cent.

Loss on drying (*2.2.32*). Not more than 0.5 per cent, determined on 1.000 g by drying in an oven at 100-105 °C.

ASSAY

Dissolve 50.0 mg in *ethanol R* and dilute to 100.0 ml with the same solvent. Dilute 2.0 ml of the solution to 100.0 ml with *ethanol R*. Measure the absorbance (*2.2.25*) at the maximum at 287 nm.

Calculate the content of $C_{23}H_{30}O_4$ taking the specific absorbance to be 685.

STORAGE

Store protected from light.

IMPURITIES

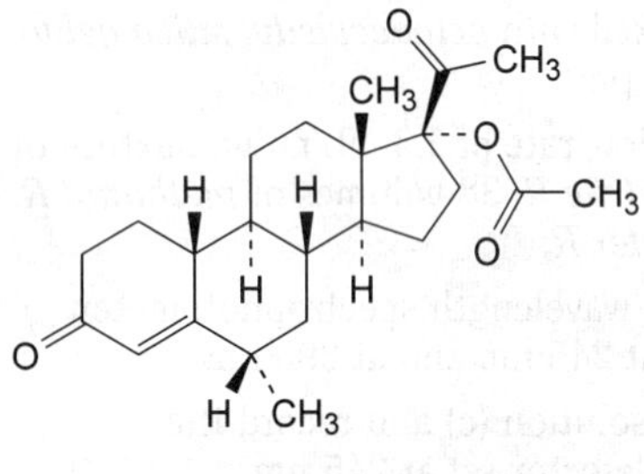

A. 6α-methyl-3,20-dioxo-19-norpregn-4-en-17-yl acetate.

01/2005:1454

NONOXINOL 9

Nonoxinolum 9

DEFINITION

α-(4-Nonylphenyl)-ω-hydroxynona(oxyethylene).

Mixture consisting mainly of monononylphenyl ethers of macrogols corresponding to the formula: $C_9H_{19}C_6H_4\text{-}[OCH_2\text{-}CH_2]_n\text{-}OH$ where the average value of *n* is 9. It may contain free macrogols.

CHARACTERS

Appearance: clear, colourless or light yellow, viscous liquid.

Solubility: miscible with water, with alcohol and with vegetable oils.

IDENTIFICATION

A. Infrared absorption spectrophotometry (*2.2.24*).
   Comparison: *Ph. Eur. reference spectrum of nonoxinol 9.*
   Preparation: film between *sodium chloride R* plates.

B. It complies with the test for cloud point (see Tests).

TESTS

Acidity or alkalinity. Boil 1.0 g with 20 ml of *carbon dioxide-free water R* for 1 min, with constant stirring. Cool and filter. To 10 ml of the filtrate, add 0.05 ml of *bromothymol blue solution R1*. Not more than 0.5 ml of *0.01 M hydrochloric acid* or *0.01 M sodium hydroxide* is required to change the colour of the indicator.

Hydroxyl value (*2.5.3, Method A*): 84 to 94.

Cloud point: 52 °C to 58 °C.

Dissolve 1.0 g in 99 g of *water R*. Transfer about 30 ml of this solution into a test-tube, heat on a water-bath and stir continuously until the solution becomes cloudy. Remove the test-tube from the water-bath (ensuring that the temperature does not increase more than 2 °C) and continue to stir. The cloud point is the temperature at which the solution becomes sufficiently clear that the entire thermometer bulb is plainly seen.

Ethylene oxide and dioxan (*2.4.25*): maximum 1 ppm of ethylene oxide and maximum 10 ppm of dioxan.

Heavy metals (*2.4.8*): maximum 10 ppm.

Dissolve 2.0 g in *distilled water R* and dilute to 20.0 ml with the same solvent. 12 ml of this solution complies with limit test A. Prepare the standard using *lead standard solution (1 ppm Pb) R*.

Water (*2.5.12*): maximum 0.5 per cent, determined on 2.00 g.

Total ash (*2.4.16*): maximum 0.4 per cent, determined on 1.0 g.

STORAGE

In an airtight container.

01/2005:0732

NORADRENALINE HYDROCHLORIDE

Noradrenalini hydrochloridum

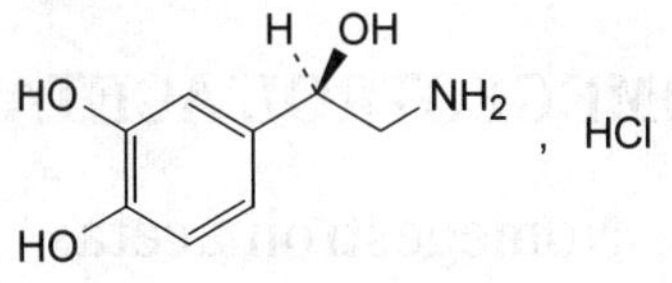

$C_8H_{12}ClNO_3$ M_r 205.6

DEFINITION

(*R*)-2-Amino-1-(3,4-dihydroxyphenyl)ethanol hydrochloride.

Content: 98.5 per cent to 101.0 per cent (anhydrous substance).

CHARACTERS

Appearance: white or brownish-white, crystalline powder.

Solubility: very soluble in water, slightly soluble in alcohol.

It becomes coloured on exposure to air and light.

IDENTIFICATION

A. Specific optical rotation (see Tests).

B. Infrared absorption spectrophotometry (*2.2.24*).

Dissolve 2 g in 20 ml of a 5 g/l solution of *sodium metabisulphite R* and make alkaline by addition of *ammonia R*. Keep in iced water for 1 h and filter. Wash the precipitate with 3 quantities, each of 2 ml, of *water R*, with 5 ml of *alcohol R* and finally with 5 ml of *ether R* and dry *in vacuo* for 3 h. Examine the noradrenaline base thus prepared, comparing with the spectrum obtained with noradrenaline base prepared by the same method from a suitable amount of *noradrenaline tartrate CRS*. Examine the substances prepared as discs.

C. 0.2 ml of solution S (see Tests) gives reaction (a) of chlorides (*2.3.1*).

TESTS

Solution S. Dissolve 0.500 g in *carbon dioxide-free water R* and dilute to 25.0 ml with the same solvent.

Appearance of solution. The solution is clear (*2.2.1*) and not more intensely coloured than a mixture of 0.2 ml of blue primary solution, 0.4 ml of yellow primary solution, 0.4 ml of red primary solution and 9 ml of a 13.7 per cent *V/V* solution of *dilute hydrochloric acid R* (*2.2.2, Method II*).

Dissolve 0.2 g in *carbon dioxide-free water R* and dilute to 10 ml with the same solvent. Examine the solution immediately.

pH (*2.2.3*): 3.5 to 4.5 for solution S.

Specific optical rotation (*2.2.7*): − 37 to − 41, determined on solution S (anhydrous substance).

Noradrenalone: maximum 0.12 per cent.

Dissolve 30.0 mg in *0.01 M hydrochloric acid* and dilute to 25.0 ml with the same acid. The absorbance (*2.2.25*) of the solution measured at 310 nm is not greater than 0.20.

Adrenaline. Thin-layer chromatography (*2.2.27*).

Test solution. Dissolve 0.15 g of the substance to be examined in *water R* and dilute to 10 ml with the same solvent. Prepare immediately before use.

Reference solution (a). Dissolve 12.5 mg of *adrenaline tartrate CRS* in *water R* and dilute to 10 ml with the same solvent. Prepare immediately before use.

Reference solution (b). Dilute 2 ml of reference solution (a) to 10 ml with *water R*.

Reference solution (c). Mix 2 ml of the test solution and 2 ml of reference solution (b).

Plate: *TLC silica gel G plate R.*

Mobile phase: *anhydrous formic acid R, acetone R, methylene chloride R* (0.5:50:50 *V/V/V*).

Application: apply as bands 20 mm by 2 mm, 6 µl of the test solution, 6 µl of reference solution (a), 6 µl of reference solution (b) and 12 µl of reference solution (c). Allow to dry in air and spray the bands with a saturated solution of *sodium hydrogen carbonate R*. Allow the plate to dry in air and spray the bands twice with *acetic anhydride R*, drying between the 2 sprayings. Heat the plate at 50 °C for 90 min.

Development: over a path of 15 cm.

Drying: in air.

Detection: spray with a solution freshly prepared by mixing 2 volumes of *ethylenediamine R* and 8 volumes of *methanol R* and adding 2 volumes of a 5 g/l solution of *potassium ferricyanide R*. Dry the plate at 60 °C for 10 min and examine in ultraviolet light at 254 nm and 365 nm.

System suitability: the chromatogram obtained with reference solution (c) shows above the most intense zone a clearly separated zone corresponding to the most intense zone in the chromatogram obtained with reference solution (a).

Limits: any zone situated immediately above the most intense zone is not more intense than the corresponding zone in the chromatogram obtained with reference solution (b) (1.0 per cent).

Water (*2.5.12*): maximum 0.5 per cent, determined on 1.000 g.

Sulphated ash (*2.4.14*): maximum 0.1 per cent, determined on 0.50 g.

ASSAY

Dissolve 0.180 g in 50 ml of *acetic anhydride R* and add 10 ml of *anhydrous formic acid R*. Titrate with *0.1 M perchloric acid*, determining the end-point potentiometrically (*2.2.20*).

1 ml of *0.1 M perchloric acid* is equivalent to 20.56 mg of $C_8H_{12}ClNO_3$.

STORAGE

Store in an airtight container, or preferably in a sealed tube under vacuum or under an inert gas, protected from light.

01/2005:0285

NORADRENALINE TARTRATE

Noradrenalini tartras

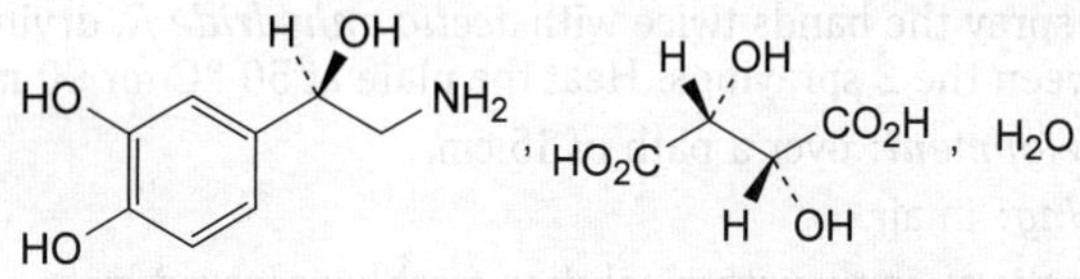

$C_{12}H_{17}NO_9,H_2O$ M_r 337.3

DEFINITION

(1*R*)-2-Amino-1-(3,4-dihydroxyphenyl)ethanol hydrogen (2*R*,3*R*)-2,3-dihydroxybutanedioate monohydrate.

Content: 98.5 per cent to 101.0 per cent (anhydrous substance).

CHARACTERS

Appearance: white or almost white, crystalline powder.

Solubility: freely soluble in water, slightly soluble in alcohol.

IDENTIFICATION

A. Dissolve 2 g in 20 ml of a 5 g/l solution of *sodium metabisulphite R* and make alkaline by addition of *ammonia R*. Keep in iced water for 1 h and filter. Reserve the filtrate for identification test C. Wash the precipitate with 3 quantities, each of 2 ml, of *water R*, with 5 ml of *alcohol R* and finally with 5 ml of *ether R* and dry *in vacuo* for 3 h. The specific optical rotation (*2.2.7*) of the precipitate (noradrenaline base) is − 44 to − 48, determined using a 20.0 g/l solution in *0.5 M hydrochloric acid*.

B. Infrared absorption spectrophotometry (*2.2.24*).

Use noradrenaline base prepared as described under identification test A and compare with the spectrum obtained with noradrenaline base prepared by the same method from a suitable amount of *noradrenaline tartrate CRS*. Examine the substances prepared as discs.

C. 0.2 ml of the filtrate obtained in identification test A gives reaction (b) of tartrates (*2.3.1*).

Monographs N-O

TESTS

Appearance of solution. The solution is clear (*2.2.1*) and not more intensely coloured than reference solution BY_5 (*2.2.2, Method II*).

Dissolve 0.2 g in *water R* and dilute to 10 ml with the same solvent. Examine the solution immediately.

Noradrenalone: the absorbance (*2.2.25*) of the solution measured at 310 nm is not greater than 0.20.

Dissolve 50.0 mg in *0.01 M hydrochloric acid* and dilute to 25.0 ml with the same acid.

Adrenaline. Thin-layer chromatography (*2.2.27*).

Test solution. Dissolve 0.25 g of the substance to be examined in *water R* and dilute to 10 ml with the same solvent. Prepare immediately before use.

Reference solution (a). Dissolve 12.5 mg of *adrenaline tartrate CRS* in *water R* and dilute to 10 ml with the same solvent. Prepare immediately before use.

Reference solution (b). Dilute 2 ml of reference solution (a) to 10 ml with *water R*.

Reference solution (c). Mix 2 ml of the test solution with 2 ml of reference solution (b).

Plate: *TLC silica gel G plate R*.

Mobile phase: *anhydrous formic acid R, acetone R, methylene chloride R* (0.5:50:50 *V/V/V*).

Application: apply as bands 20 mm by 2 mm, 6 µl of the test solution, 6 µl of reference solution (a), 6 µl of reference solution (b) and 12 µl of reference solution (c). Allow to dry in air and spray the bands with a saturated solution of *sodium hydrogen carbonate R*. Allow the plate to dry in air and spray the bands twice with *acetic anhydride R*, drying between the 2 sprayings. Heat the plate at 50 °C for 90 min.

Development: over a path of 15 cm.

Drying: in air.

Detection: spray with a solution freshly prepared by mixing 2 volumes of *ethylenediamine R* and 8 volumes of *methanol R* and adding 2 volumes of a 5 g/l solution of *potassium ferricyanide R*. Dry the plate at 60 °C for 10 min and examine in ultraviolet light at 254 nm and 365 nm.

System suitability: the chromatogram obtained with reference solution (c) shows above the most intense zone a clearly separated zone corresponding to the most intense zone in the chromatogram obtained with reference solution (a).

Limit:

– *adrenaline*: any zone situated immediately above the most intense zone is not more intense than the corresponding zone in the chromatogram obtained with reference solution (b) (1.0 per cent).

Water (*2.5.12*): 4.5 per cent to 5.8 per cent, determined on 0.500 g.

Sulphated ash (*2.4.14*): maximum 0.1 per cent, determined on 0.5 g.

ASSAY

Dissolve 0.300 g in 50 ml of *anhydrous acetic acid R*, heating gently if necessary. Titrate with *0.1 M perchloric acid* using 0.1 ml of *crystal violet solution R* as indicator, until a bluish-green colour is obtained.

1 ml of *0.1 M perchloric acid* is equivalent to 31.93 mg of $C_{12}H_{17}NO_9$.

STORAGE

In an airtight container, or preferably in a sealed tube under vacuum or under an inert gas, protected from light.

01/2005:0234

NORETHISTERONE

Norethisteronum

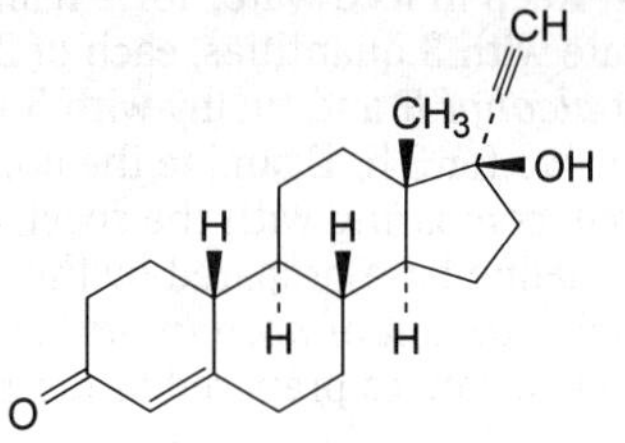

$C_{20}H_{26}O_2$ M_r 298.4

DEFINITION

Norethisterone contains not less than 98.0 per cent and not more than the equivalent of 102.0 per cent of 17-hydroxy-19-nor-17α-pregn-4-en-20-yn-3-one, calculated with reference to the dried substance.

CHARACTERS

A white or yellowish-white, crystalline powder, practically insoluble in water, slightly soluble in alcohol.

It melts at about 206 °C, with decomposition.

IDENTIFICATION

First identification: A, B, E.

Second identification: B, C, D, E.

A. Examine by infrared absorption spectrophotometry (*2.2.24*), comparing with the spectrum obtained with *norethisterone CRS*. Examine the substances prepared in the form of discs. If the spectra obtained with the substance to be examined and the reference substance show differences, dissolve the substances in *chloroform R*, evaporate to dryness on a water-bath and then record the spectra.

B. Examine by thin-layer chromatography (*2.2.27*), using *kieselguhr G R* as the coating substance. Impregnate the plate by placing it in a tank containing the necessary quantity of a mixture of 10 volumes of *formamide R* and 90 volumes of *acetone R* so that the plate dips about 5 mm into the liquid. When the front of the impregnation mixture has risen at least 1 cm above the level prescribed for the mobile phase, remove the plate and allow it to stand at room temperature until the solvent has completely evaporated (about 2 min to 5 min). Use the impregnated plate within 2 h and carry out the chromatography in the same direction as the impregnation.

Test solution. Dissolve 10 mg of the substance to be examined in *chloroform R* and dilute to 10 ml with the same solvent.

Reference solution. Dissolve 10 mg of *norethisterone CRS* in *chloroform R* and dilute to 10 ml with the same solvent.

Apply separately to the plate 2 µl of each solution. Develop over a path of 15 cm using a mixture of 20 volumes of *dioxan R* and 80 volumes of *hexane R*. Heat the plate at 120 °C for 15 min and spray with *alcoholic solution of sulphuric acid R*. Heat at 120 °C for 10 min to 15 min or until the spots appear. Allow to cool and examine in daylight and in ultraviolet light at 365 nm. The principal spot in the chromatogram obtained with the test solution is similar in position, colour, fluorescence and size to the principal spot in the chromatogram obtained with the reference solution.

C. Dissolve about 2 mg in 2 ml of *alcohol R*, add 1 ml of *ammoniacal silver nitrate solution R* and heat on a water-bath. The solution becomes turbid and a white precipitate is formed which becomes grey when heated. A silver mirror is deposited on the walls of the tube.

D. Dissolve about 2 mg in a cooled mixture of 2 ml of *ethanol R* and 2 ml of *sulphuric acid R* and heat to 70 °C. The resulting solution is dichroic, appearing blue-violet in transmitted light and red in reflected light. The solution shows a bright-red fluorescence in ultraviolet light at 365 nm.

E. Dissolve about 2 mg in 2 ml of *alcohol R*, add 1 ml of a 10 g/l solution of *butylhydroxytoluene R* in *alcohol R* and 2 ml of *1 M sodium hydroxide*. Heat in a water-bath at 80 °C for 30 min and cool to room temperature. A yellowish-pink colour is produced.

TESTS

Solution S. Dissolve 0.200 g in *dioxan R* and dilute to 10.0 ml with the same solvent.

Appearance of solution. Solution S is clear (*2.2.1*) and not more intensely coloured than reference solution Y_6 (*2.2.2, Method I*).

Specific optical rotation (*2.2.7*). Dilute 5.0 ml of solution S to 10.0 ml with *dioxan R*. The specific optical rotation is −33 to −37, calculated with reference to the dried substance.

Absorbance (*2.2.25*). Dissolve 10.0 mg in *alcohol R* and dilute to 100.0 ml with the same solvent. Dilute 10.0 ml of this solution to 100.0 ml with *alcohol R*. The solution shows an absorption maximum at 240 nm. The specific absorbance at the maximum is 550 to 590, calculated with reference to the dried substance.

Related substances. Examine by thin-layer chromatography (*2.2.27*), using a suitable silica gel as the coating substance.

Test solution. Dissolve 50 mg of the substance to be examined in a mixture of 1 volume of *methanol R* and 9 volumes of *chloroform R* and dilute to 10 ml with the same mixture of solvents.

Reference solution (a). Dilute 1.0 ml of the test solution to 200 ml with a mixture of 1 volume of *methanol R* and 9 volumes of *chloroform R*.

Reference solution (b). Dissolve 25 mg of *ethisterone CRS* in a mixture of 1 volume of *methanol R* and 9 volumes of *chloroform R*, add 5 ml of the test solution and dilute to 100 ml with the same mixture of solvents.

Apply separately to the plate, as two applications of 5 µl, 10 µl of each solution. Develop over a path of 15 cm using a mixture of 10 volumes of *acetone R* and 90 volumes of *chloroform R*. Allow the plate to dry in air, spray with *alcoholic solution of sulphuric acid R* and heat at 100 °C to 105 °C for 5 min. Examine in ultraviolet light at 365 nm.

Any spot in the chromatogram obtained with the test solution, apart from the principal spot, is not more intense than the spot in the chromatogram obtained with reference solution (a) (0.5 per cent). The test is not valid unless the chromatogram obtained with reference solution (b) shows two clearly separated spots of approximately equal intensity.

Loss on drying (*2.2.32*). Not more than 0.5 per cent, determined on 1.00 g by drying in an oven at 100 °C to 105 °C for 3 h.

ASSAY

Dissolve 0.200 g in 40 ml of *tetrahydrofuran R*. Add 10 ml of a 100 g/l solution of *silver nitrate R*. Using 2 ml of *bromocresol green solution R* as indicator, titrate with *0.1 M sodium hydroxide* until a violet colour is obtained. Carry out a blank titration.

1 ml of *0.1 M sodium hydroxide* is equivalent to 29.84 mg of $C_{20}H_{26}O_2$.

STORAGE

Store protected from light.

01/2005:0850

NORETHISTERONE ACETATE

Norethisteroni acetas

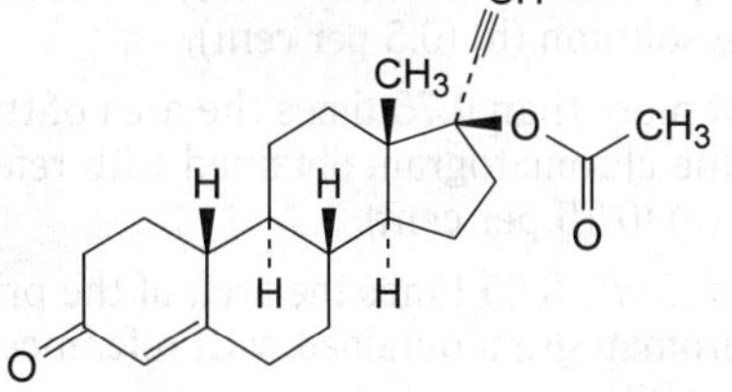

$C_{22}H_{28}O_3$ M_r 340.5

DEFINITION

3-Oxo-19-nor-17α-pregn-4-en-20-yn-17-yl acetate.

Content: 98.0 per cent to 101.0 per cent (dried substance).

CHARACTERS

Appearance: white or yellowish-white, crystalline powder.

Solubility: practically insoluble in water, freely soluble in methylene chloride, soluble in alcohol.

It shows polymorphism.

IDENTIFICATION

Infrared absorption spectrophotometry (*2.2.24*).

Preparation: discs.

Comparison: *norethisterone acetate CRS.*

If the spectra show differences, dissolve the substance to be examined and the reference substance separately in *methylene chloride R*, evaporate to dryness on a water-bath and record new spectra using the residues.

TESTS

Specific optical rotation (*2.2.7*) −30 to −35 (dried substance).

Dissolve 0.500 g in *ethanol R* and dilute to 25.0 ml with the same solvent.

Related substances. Liquid chromatography (*2.2.29*).

Test solution. Dissolve 25.0 mg of the substance to be examined in the mobile phase and dilute to 10.0 ml with the mobile phase.

Reference solution (a). Dissolve 2 mg of *desoxycortone acetate CRS* and 2 mg of *norethisterone acetate CRS* in the mobile phase and dilute to 50.0 ml with the mobile phase.

Reference solution (b). Dilute 1.0 ml of the test solution to 100.0 ml with the mobile phase.

Column:

- *size*: l = 0.25 m, Ø = 4.6 mm,
- *stationary phase*: *octadecylsilyl silica gel for chromatography R* (5 µm).

Monographs N-O

Mobile phase: *acetonitrile R*, *water R* (60:40 *V/V*).

Flow rate: 1.0 ml/min.

Detection: variable wavelength spectrophotometer capable of operating at 254 nm and at 210 nm.

Injection: 20 µl.

Run time: 3 times the retention time of norethisterone acetate.

Relative retention with reference to norethisterone acetate (retention time = about 10 min): impurity A = about 0.48; impurity D = about 0.65; impurity E = about 0.83; impurity C = about 1.35; impurity B = about 1.40.

System suitability: reference solution (a) at 254 nm:

- *resolution*: minimum of 3.5 between the peaks due to norethisterone acetate and to desoxycortone acetate.

Limits: spectrophotometer at 254 nm:

- *any impurity*: not more than 0.5 times the area of the principal peak in the chromatogram obtained with reference solution (b) (0.5 per cent),
- *total*: not more than 0.75 times the area of the principal peak in the chromatogram obtained with reference solution (b) (0.75 per cent),
- *disregard limit*: 0.05 times the area of the principal peak in the chromatogram obtained with reference solution (b) (0.05 per cent).

Limits: spectrophotometer at 210 nm:

- *any impurity* with a relative retention between 1.0 and 1.6, with reference to norethisterone acetate (retention time = about 10 min): not more than 0.3 times the area of the principal peak in the chromatogram obtained with reference solution (b) (0.3 per cent),
- *total of these impurities*: not more than 0.5 times the area of the principal peak in the chromatogram obtained with reference solution (b) (0.5 per cent),
- *disregard limit*: 0.05 times the area of the principal peak in the chromatogram obtained with reference solution (b) (0.05 per cent).

Loss on drying (*2.2.32*): maximum 0.5 per cent, determined on 1.000 g by drying in an oven at 100-105 °C.

ASSAY

Dissolve 0.200 g in 40 ml of *tetrahydrofuran R*. Add 10 ml of a 100 g/l solution of *silver nitrate R* and titrate with *0.1 M sodium hydroxide*, determining the end-point potentiometrically (*2.2.20*). Carry out a blank titration.

1 ml of *0.1 M sodium hydroxide* is equivalent to 34.05 mg of $C_{22}H_{28}O_3$.

IMPURITIES

Specified impurities: A, B, C, D, E.

Other detectable impurities: F, G.

A. norethisterone,

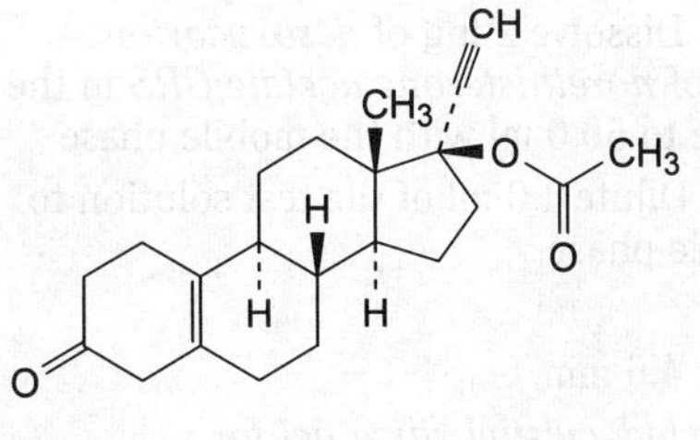

B. 3-oxo-19-nor-17α-pregn-5(10)-en-20-yn-17-yl acetate,

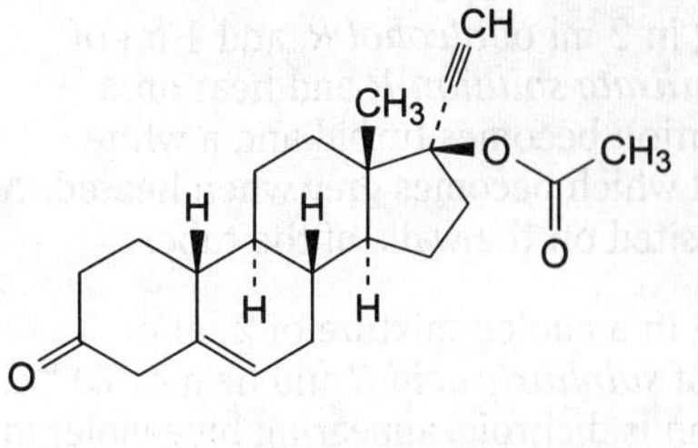

C. 3-oxo-19-nor-17α-pregn-5-en-20-yn-17-yl acetate,

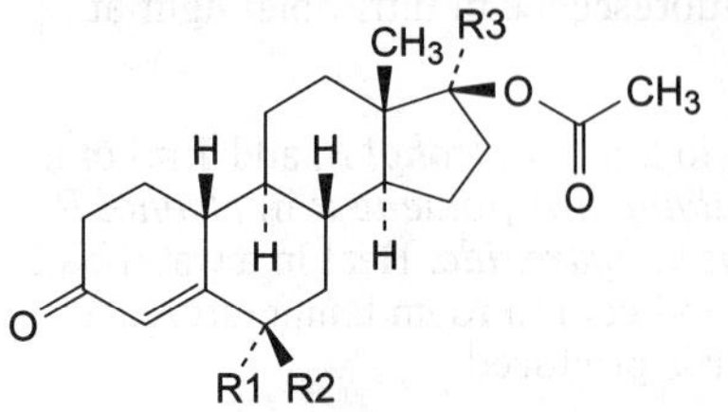

D. R1 = H, R2 = CO-CH_3, R3 = C≡CH: 6β-acetyl-3-oxo-19-nor-17α-pregn-4-en-20-yn-17-yl acetate,

E. R1 = R2 = H, R3 = CO-CH_3: 3,20-dioxo-19-nor-17α-pregn-4-en-17-yl acetate,

F. R1 = H, R2 = OH, R3 = C≡CH: 6β-hydroxy-3-oxo-19-nor-17α-pregn-4-en-20-yn-17-yl acetate,

G. R1 + R2 = O, R3 = C≡CH: 3,6-dioxo-19-nor-17α-pregn-4-en-20-yn-17-yl acetate.

01/2005:1248

NORFLOXACIN

Norfloxacinum

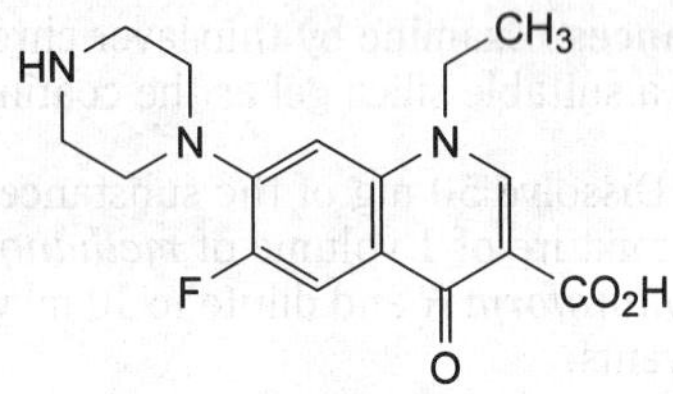

$C_{16}H_{18}FN_3O_3$ M_r 319.3

DEFINITION

Norfloxacin contains not less than 99.0 per cent and not more than the equivalent of 101.0 per cent of 1-ethyl-6-fluoro-4-oxo-7-(piperazin-1-yl)-1,4-dihydroquinoline-3-carboxylic acid, calculated with reference to the dried substance.

CHARACTERS

A white or pale-yellow, hygroscopic, photosensitive, crystalline powder, very slightly soluble in water, slightly soluble in acetone and in alcohol.

IDENTIFICATION

Examine by infrared absorption spectrophotometry (*2.2.24*), comparing with the spectrum obtained with *norfloxacin CRS*. Examine the substances prepared as discs.

TESTS

Appearance of solution. Dissolve 0.5 g in a previously filtered 4 g/l solution of *sodium hydroxide R* in *methanol R* and dilute to 50 ml with the same solution. The solution is not more opalescent than reference suspension II (*2.2.1*) and not more intensely coloured than reference solution B_7 (*2.2.2, Method II*).

Related substances. Examine by thin-layer chromatography (*2.2.27*), using a *TLC silica gel GF$_{254}$ plate R*, previously washed with *methanol R* and dried in air.

Test solution (a). Dissolve 40 mg of the substance to be examined in a mixture of equal volumes of *methanol R* and *methylene chloride R* and dilute to 5 ml with the same mixture of solvents.

Test solution (b). Dilute 1 ml of test solution (a) to 10 ml with a mixture of equal volumes of *methanol R* and *methylene chloride R*.

Reference solution (a). Dilute 1 ml of test solution (b) to 50 ml with a mixture of equal volumes of *methanol R* and *methylene chloride R*.

Reference solution (b). Dissolve 4.0 mg of *norfloxacin impurity A CRS* in a mixture of equal volumes of *methanol R* and *methylene chloride R* and dilute to 5 ml with the same mixture of solvents. Dilute 1 ml of this solution to 2 ml with test solution (b).

Apply to the plate 5 µl of test solution (a) and 5 µl of each reference solution. Develop over a path of 18 cm using a mixture of 8 volumes of *water R*, 14 volumes of *diethylamine R*, 20 volumes of *toluene R*, 40 volumes of *chloroform R* and 40 volumes of *methanol R*. Dry the plate in a current of air and examine in ultraviolet light at 254 nm and then 365 nm. Any spot in the chromatogram obtained with test solution (a), apart from the principal spot, is not more intense than the principal spot in the chromatogram obtained with reference solution (a) (0.2 per cent) and there are no more than three such spots. The test is not valid unless, in the chromatogram obtained with reference solution (b), the ratio of the R_f value of impurity A to the R_f value of norfloxacin is at least 1.2.

Heavy metals (*2.4.8*). 2.0 g complies with limit test D for heavy metals (15 ppm). Prepare the standard using 3 ml of *lead standard solution (10 ppm Pb) R*.

Loss on drying (*2.2.32*). Not more than 1.0 per cent, determined on 1.000 g by drying in an oven at 100-105 °C under high vacuum for 2 h.

Sulphated ash (*2.4.14*). Not more than 0.1 per cent, determined on 1.0 g in a platinum crucible.

ASSAY

Dissolve 0.240 g in 80 ml of *anhydrous acetic acid R*. Titrate with *0.1 M perchloric acid,* determining the end-point potentiometrically (*2.2.20*).

1 ml of *0.1 M perchloric acid* is equivalent to 31.93 mg of $C_{16}H_{18}FN_3O_3$.

STORAGE

Store in an airtight container, protected from light.

IMPURITIES

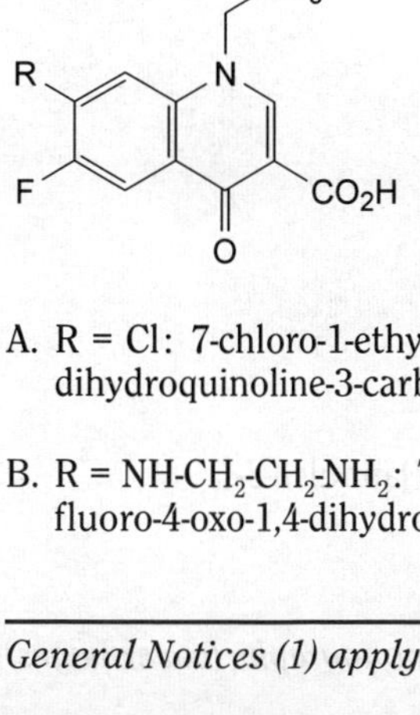

A. R = Cl: 7-chloro-1-ethyl-6-fluoro-4-oxo-1,4-dihydroquinoline-3-carboxylic acid,

B. R = NH-CH_2-CH_2-NH_2: 7-[(2-aminoethyl)amino]-1-ethyl-6-fluoro-4-oxo-1,4-dihydroquinoline-3-carboxylic acid.

01/2005:0940

NORGESTREL

Norgestrelum

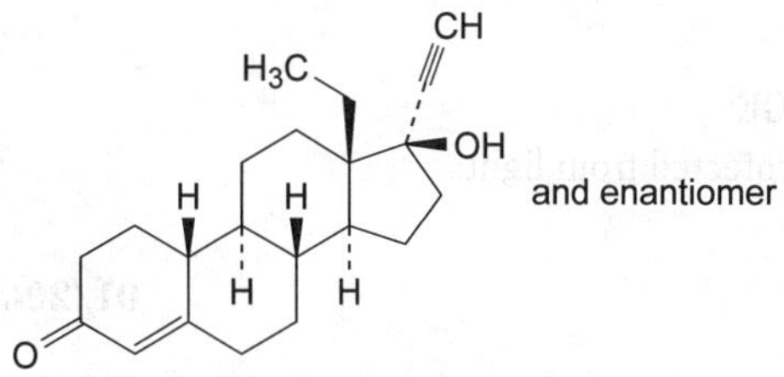

$C_{21}H_{28}O_2$ M_r 312.5

DEFINITION

Norgestrel contains not less than 98.0 per cent and not more than the equivalent of 102.0 per cent of *rac*-13-ethyl-17-hydroxy-18,19-dinor-17α-pregn-4-en-20-yn-3-one, calculated with reference to the dried substance.

CHARACTERS

A white or almost white, crystalline powder, practically insoluble in water, sparingly soluble in methylene chloride, slightly soluble in alcohol.

IDENTIFICATION

A. Dissolve 0.5 g in *methylene chloride R* and dilute to 10.0 ml with the same solvent. The angle of optical rotation (*2.2.7*) is + 0.05° to − 0.05°.

B. Examine by infrared absorption spectrophotometry (*2.2.24*), comparing with the spectrum obtained with *norgestrel CRS*.

TESTS

Related substances. Examine by thin-layer chromatography (*2.2.27*), using *silica gel G R* as the coating substance.

Test solution. Dissolve 0.2 g of the substance to be examined in *methylene chloride R* and dilute to 10 ml with the same solvent.

Reference solution (a). Dilute 1 ml of the test solution to 10 ml with *methylene chloride R*. Dilute 1 ml of this solution to 20 ml with *methylene chloride R*.

Reference solution (b). Dilute 4 ml of reference solution (a) to 10 ml with *methylene chloride R*.

Reference solution (c). Dissolve 5 mg of *norgestrel CRS* and 5 mg of *ethinylestradiol CRS* in *methylene chloride R* and dilute to 50 ml with the same solvent.

Apply to the plate 10 µl of each solution. Develop over a path of 15 cm using a mixture of 20 volumes of *ethyl acetate R* and 80 volumes of *methylene chloride R*. Allow the plate to dry in air, spray with a 100 g/l solution of *phosphomolybdic acid R* in *alcohol R*, heat at 100-105 °C for 15 min and examine immediately. Any spot in the chromatogram obtained with the test solution, apart from the principal spot, is not more intense than the principal spot in the chromatogram obtained with reference solution (a) (0.5 per cent) and at most two such spots are more intense than the spot in the chromatogram obtained with reference solution (b) (0.2 per cent). The test is not valid unless the chromatogram obtained with reference solution (c) shows two clearly separated spots.

Loss on drying (*2.2.32*). Not more than 0.5 per cent, determined on 1.000 g by drying in an oven at 100-105 °C.

Sulphated ash (*2.4.14*). Not more than 0.1 per cent, determined on 1.0 g.

Monographs N-O

ASSAY

Dissolve 0.200 g in 45 ml of *tetrahydrofuran R*. Add 10 ml of a 100 g/l solution of *silver nitrate R*. After 1 min, titrate with *0.1 M sodium hydroxide* determining the end-point potentiometrically (*2.2.20*). Carry out a blank titration.

1 ml of *0.1 M sodium hydroxide* is equivalent to 31.25 mg of $C_{21}H_{28}O_2$.

STORAGE

Store protected from light.

01/2005:0941

NORTRIPTYLINE HYDROCHLORIDE

Nortriptylini hydrochloridum

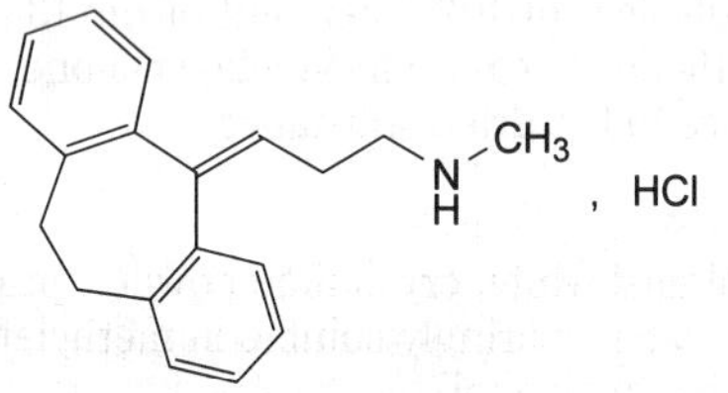

$C_{19}H_{22}ClN$ M_r 299.8

DEFINITION

Nortriptyline hydrochloride contains not less than 98.0 per cent and not more than the equivalent of 101.0 per cent of 3-(10,11-dihydro-5*H*-dibenzo[*a,d*][7]annulen-5-ylidene)-*N*-methylpropan-1-amine hydrochloride, calculated with reference to the dried substance.

CHARACTERS

A white or almost white powder, sparingly soluble in water, soluble in alcohol and in methylene chloride.

IDENTIFICATION

First identification: C, E.

Second identification: A, B, D, E.

A. Melting point (*2.2.14*): 216 °C to 220 °C.

B. Dissolve 20.0 mg in *methanol R* and dilute to 100.0 ml with the same solvent. Dilute 5.0 ml of this solution to 100.0 ml with *methanol R*. Examined between 230 nm and 350 nm (*2.2.25*), the solution shows an absorption maximum at 239 nm. The specific absorbance at the maximum is 465 to 495.

C. Examine by infrared absorption spectrophotometry (*2.2.24*), comparing with the *Ph. Eur. reference spectrum of nortriptyline hydrochloride*.

D. Dissolve 50 mg in 3 ml of warm *water R*, cool and add 0.05 ml of a 25 g/l solution of *quinhydrone R* in *methanol R*. A red colour develops slowly.

E. 50 mg gives reaction (b) of chlorides (*2.3.1*).

TESTS

Appearance of solution. Dissolve 0.5 g in *water R* with gentle heating and dilute to 25 ml with the same solvent. The solution is clear (*2.2.1*) and not more intensely coloured than reference solution B_7 (*2.2.2, Method II*).

Acidity or alkalinity. Dissolve 0.2 g with gentle heating in *carbon dioxide-free water R* and dilute to 10 ml with the same solvent. Add 0.1 ml of *methyl red solution R* and 0.2 ml of *0.01 M sodium hydroxide*. The solution is yellow. Add 0.4 ml of *0.01 M hydrochloric acid*. The solution is red.

Related substances. *Prepare the solutions in subdued light and develop the chromatograms protected from light.* Examine by thin-layer chromatography (*2.2.27*), using a *TLC silica gel plate R*.

Test solution (a). Dissolve 0.20 g of the substance to be examined in *alcohol R* and dilute to 10 ml with the same solvent.

Test solution (b). Dilute 1 ml of test solution (a) to 2 ml with *alcohol R*.

Reference solution (a). Dissolve 10 mg of *dibenzosuberone CRS* in *alcohol R* and dilute to 10 ml with the same solvent. Dilute 1 ml of the solution to 100 ml with *alcohol R*.

Reference solution (b). Dissolve 10 mg of *norcyclobenzaprine CRS* in *alcohol R* and dilute to 10 ml with the same solvent. Dilute 1 ml of the solution to 100 ml with *alcohol R*.

Reference solution (c). To 0.1 ml of test solution (b) add 10 ml of reference solution (b).

Apply to the plate 5 µl of each solution. Develop over a path of 15 cm in an unsaturated tank using a mixture of 3 volumes of *diethylamine R*, 15 volumes of *ethyl acetate R* and 85 volumes of *cyclohexane R*. Allow the plate to dry in air and spray with a freshly prepared mixture of 4 volumes of *formaldehyde solution R* and 96 volumes of *sulphuric acid R*. Examine immediately in ultraviolet light at 365 nm and then at 254 nm. In the chromatogram obtained with test solution (a): any spot corresponding to dibenzosuberone, is not more intense than the spot in the chromatogram obtained with reference solution (a) (0.05 per cent); and any spot in the chromatogram obtained with test solution (b), apart from the principal spot and any spot corresponding to dibenzosuberone, is not more intense than the spot in the chromatogram obtained with reference solution (b) (0.1 per cent). The test is not valid unless the chromatogram obtained with reference solution (c) shows two clearly separated spots.

Heavy metals (*2.4.8*). 1.0 g complies with limit test C for heavy metals (20 ppm). Prepare the standard using 2 ml of *lead standard solution (10 ppm Pb) R*.

Loss on drying (*2.2.32*). Not more than 0.5 per cent, determined on 1.000 g by drying in an oven at 100-105 °C for 2 h.

Sulphated ash (*2.4.14*). Not more than 0.1 per cent, determined on 1.0 g.

ASSAY

Dissolve 0.250 g in 30 ml of *alcohol R*. Add 1.0 ml of *0.1 M hydrochloric acid*. Carry out a potentiometric titration (*2.2.20*), using *0.1 M sodium hydroxide*. Read the volume added between the two points of inflexion.

1 ml of *0.1 M sodium hydroxide* is equivalent to 29.98 mg of $C_{19}H_{22}ClN$.

STORAGE

Store protected from light.

IMPURITIES

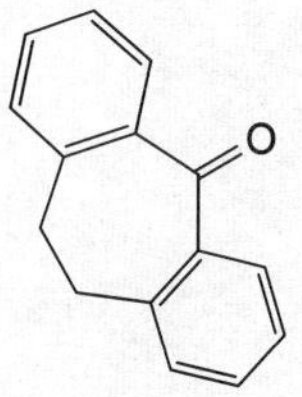

A. 10,11-dihydro-5*H*-dibenzo[*a,d*][7]annulen-5-one(dibenzosuberone),

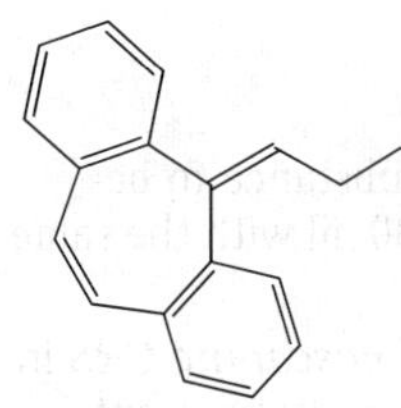

B. 3-(5*H*-dibenzo[*a*,*d*][7]annulen-5-ylidene)-*N*-methylpropan-1-amine (norcyclobenzaprine),

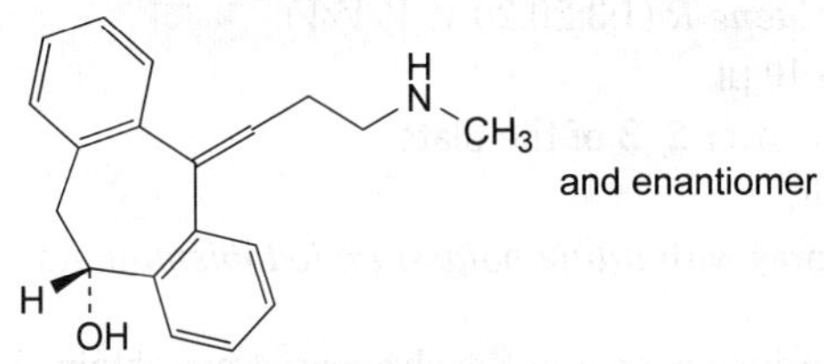

C. 10,11-dihydro-5-[3-(methylamino)propylidene]-5*H*-dibenzo[*a*,*d*][7]annulen-10-ol.

01/2005:0516

NOSCAPINE

Noscapinum

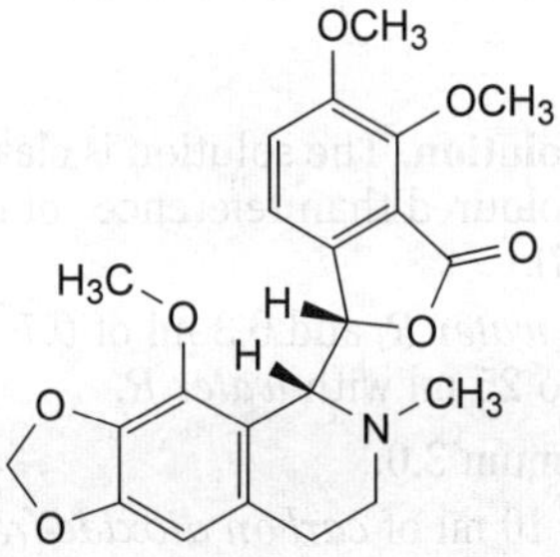

$C_{22}H_{23}NO_7$ M_r 413.4

DEFINITION

(3*S*)-6,7-Dimethoxy-3-[(5*R*)-4-methoxy-6-methyl-5,6,7,8-tetrahydro-1,3-dioxolo[4,5-*g*]isoquinolin-5-yl]isobenzofuran-1(3*H*)-one.

Content: 99.0 per cent to 101.0 per cent (dried substance).

CHARACTERS

Appearance: white, crystalline powder or colourless crystals.

Solubility: practically insoluble in water, soluble in acetone, slightly soluble in alcohol. It dissolves in strong acids; on dilution of the solution with water, the base may be precipitated.

IDENTIFICATION

First identification: *C, E.*

Second identification: *A, B, D, E.*

A. It complies with the test for specific optical rotation (see Tests).

B. Melting point (*2.2.14*): 174 °C to 177 °C.

C. Infrared absorption spectrophotometry (*2.2.24*).

Comparison: *noscapine CRS.*

D. Thin-layer chromatography (*2.2.27*).

Test solution. Dissolve 25 mg of the substance to be examined in *acetone R* and dilute to 100 ml with the same solvent.

Reference solution. Dissolve 25 mg of *noscapine CRS* in *acetone R* and dilute to 100 ml with the same solvent.

Plate: *TLC silica gel plate R.*

Mobile phase: *concentrated ammonia R, alcohol R, acetone R, toluene R* (1:3:20:20 *V/V/V/V*).

Application: 10 µl.

Development: over 2/3 of the plate.

Drying: in air.

Detection: spray with *dilute potassium iodobismuthate solution R.*

Results: the principal spot in the chromatogram obtained with the test solution is similar in position, colour and size to the principal spot in the chromatogram obtained with the reference solution.

E. To 20 mg add 10 ml of *water R* and shake. It does not dissolve.

TESTS

Appearance of solution. The solution is clear (*2.2.1*) and not more intensely coloured than reference solution Y_6 (*2.2.2, Method II*).

Dissolve 0.2 g in *acetone R* and dilute to 10 ml with the same solvent. Examine immediately after preparation.

Specific optical rotation (*2.2.7*): + 42 to + 48 (dried substance).

Dissolve 0.500 g in *0.1 M hydrochloric acid* and dilute to 25.0 ml with the same acid.

Related substances. Liquid chromatography (*2.2.29*).

Test solution. Dissolve 20.0 mg of the substance to be examined with gentle heating in 14 ml of *methanol R,* cool the solution and dilute to 20.0 ml with *phosphate buffer solution pH 6.0 R1.*

Reference solution (a). Dilute 1.0 ml of the test solution to 20.0 ml with the mobile phase. Dilute 1.0 ml of the solution to 10.0 ml with the mobile phase.

Reference solution (b). Dissolve 5 mg of *papaverine hydrochloride R* in the mobile phase and dilute to 50.0 ml with the mobile phase. Dilute 1.0 ml of the solution to 20.0 ml with the mobile phase.

Reference solution (c). Dissolve 1.5 mg of *papaverine hydrochloride R* in 10 ml of the test solution and dilute to 50 ml with the mobile phase.

Column:

- *size*: l = 0.125 m, Ø = 4.6 mm,
- *stationary phase*: *nitrile silica gel for chromatography R* (5 µm).

Mobile phase: *methanol R, phosphate buffer solution pH 6.0 R1* (350:650 *V/V*).

Flow rate: 1 ml/min.

Detection: spectrophotometer at 240 nm.

Injection: 20 µl.

Run time: 2.5 times the retention time of noscapine.

Relative retention with reference to noscapine (retention time = about 10 min): impurity A = about 1.3.

System suitability: reference solution (c):

- *resolution*: minimum 2 between the peaks due to noscapine and to impurity A.

Limits:

- *impurity A*: not more than the area of the principal peak in the chromatogram obtained with reference solution (b) (0.5 per cent),
- *any other impurity*: not more than 0.4 times the area of the principal peak in the chromatogram obtained with reference solution (a) (0.2 per cent),

– *total of other impurities*: not more than the area of the principal peak in the chromatogram obtained with reference solution (a) (0.5 per cent),
– *disregard limit*: 0.1 times the area of the principal peak in the chromatogram obtained with reference solution (a) (0.05 per cent).

Loss on drying (*2.2.32*): maximum 1.0 per cent, determined on 0.500 g by drying in an oven at 100-105 °C.

Sulphated ash (*2.4.14*): maximum 0.1 per cent, determined on 1.0 g.

ASSAY

Dissolve 0.350 g in 40 ml of *anhydrous acetic acid R*, warming gently. Titrate with *0.1 M perchloric acid*, determining the end-point potentiometrically (*2.2.20*).

1 ml of *0.1 M perchloric acid* is equivalent to 41.34 mg of $C_{22}H_{23}NO_7$.

STORAGE

Protected from light.

IMPURITIES

A. papaverine.

01/2005:0515

NOSCAPINE HYDROCHLORIDE

Noscapini hydrochloridum

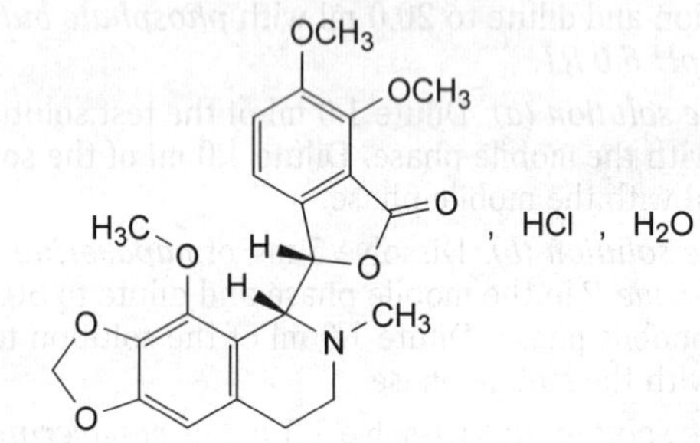

$C_{22}H_{24}ClNO_7,H_2O$ M_r 467.9

DEFINITION

(3*S*)-6,7-Dimethoxy-3-[(5*R*)-4-methoxy-6-methyl-5,6,7,8-tetrahydro-1,3-dioxolo[4,5-*g*]isoquinolin-5-yl]isobenzofuran-1(3*H*)-one hydrochloride monohydrate.

Content: 99.0 per cent to 101.0 per cent (dried substance).

CHARACTERS

Appearance: white, crystalline powder or colourless crystals, hygroscopic.

Solubility: freely soluble in water and in alcohol. Aqueous solutions are faintly acid; the base may be precipitated when the solutions are allowed to stand.

mp: about 200 °C, with decomposition.

IDENTIFICATION

First identification: C, E.

Second identification: A, B, D, E.

A. It complies with the test for specific optical rotation (see Tests).

B. Melting point (*2.2.14*) of the precipitate obtained in identification test E: 174 °C to 177 °C.

C. Infrared absorption spectrophotometry (*2.2.24*).

Preparation: examine the precipitate obtained in identification test E.

Comparison: *noscapine CRS.*

D. Thin-layer chromatography (*2.2.27*).

Test solution. Dissolve 25 mg of the substance to be examined in *alcohol R* and dilute to 100 ml with the same solvent.

Reference solution. Dissolve 22 mg of *noscapine CRS* in *acetone R* and dilute to 100 ml with the same solvent.

Plate: *TLC silica gel plate R.*

Mobile phase: *concentrated ammonia R, alcohol R, acetone R, toluene R* (1:3:20:20 *V/V/V/V*).

Application: 10 µl.

Development: over 2/3 of the plate.

Drying: in air.

Detection: spray with *dilute potassium iodobismuthate solution R.*

Results: the principal spot in the chromatogram obtained with the test solution is similar in position, colour and size to the principal spot in the chromatogram obtained with the reference solution.

E. Dissolve about 40 mg in a mixture of 2 ml of *water R* and 3 ml of *alcohol R* and add 1 ml of *dilute ammonia R2.* Heat until dissolution is complete. Allow to cool, scratching the wall of the tube with a glass rod. Filter. The filtrate gives reaction (a) of chlorides (*2.3.1*). Wash the precipitate with *water R*, dry at 100-105 °C and reserve for identification tests B and C.

TESTS

Appearance of solution. The solution is clear (*2.2.1*) and not more intensely coloured than reference solution Y_6 or BY_6 (*2.2.2, Method II*).

Dissolve 0.5 g in *water R*, add 0.3 ml of *0.1 M hydrochloric acid* and dilute to 25 ml with *water R.*

pH (*2.2.3*): minimum 3.0.

Dissolve 0.2 g in 10 ml of *carbon dioxide-free water R.*

Specific optical rotation (*2.2.7*): + 38.5 to + 44.0 (dried substance).

Dissolve 0.500 g in *0.01 M hydrochloric acid* and dilute to 25.0 ml with the same acid.

Related substances. Liquid chromatography (*2.2.29*).

Test solution. Dissolve 20.0 mg of the substance to be examined with gentle heating in 14 ml of *methanol R*, cool the solution and dilute to 20.0 ml with *phosphate buffer solution pH 6.0 R1.*

Reference solution (a). Dilute 1.0 ml of the test solution to 20.0 ml with the mobile phase. Dilute 1.0 ml of the solution to 10.0 ml with the mobile phase.

Reference solution (b). Dissolve 5 mg of *papaverine hydrochloride R* in the mobile phase and dilute to 50.0 ml with the mobile phase. Dilute 1.0 ml of the solution to 20.0 ml with the mobile phase.

Reference solution (c). Dissolve 1.5 mg of *papaverine hydrochloride R* in 10 ml of the test solution and dilute to 50 ml with the mobile phase.

Column:
– *size*: *l* = 0.125 m, Ø = 4.6 mm,
– *stationary phase*: *nitrile silica gel for chromatography R* (5 µm).

Mobile phase: *methanol R, phosphate buffer solution pH 6.0 R1* (350:650 *V/V*).

Flow rate: 1 ml/min.

Detection: spectrophotometer at 240 nm.

Injection: 20 µl.

Monographs N-O

Run time: 2.5 times the retention time of noscapine.

Relative retention with reference to noscapine (retention time = about 10 min): impurity A = about 1.3.

System suitability: reference solution (c):
- *resolution*: minimum 2 between the peaks due to noscapine and to impurity A.

Limits:
- *impurity A*: not more than the area of the principal peak in the chromatogram obtained with reference solution (b) (0.5 per cent),
- *any other impurity*: not more than 0.4 times the area of the principal peak in the chromatogram obtained with reference solution (a) (0.2 per cent),
- *total of other impurities*: not more than the area of the principal peak in the chromatogram obtained with reference solution (a) (0.5 per cent),
- *disregard limit*: 0.1 times the area of the principal peak in the chromatogram obtained with reference solution (a) (0.05 per cent).

Loss on drying (*2.2.32*): 2.5 per cent to 6.5 per cent, determined on 0.200 g by drying in an oven at 100-105 °C.

Sulphated ash (*2.4.14*): maximum 0.1 per cent, determined on 1.0 g.

ASSAY

Dissolve 0.400 g in a mixture of 5.0 ml of *0.01 M hydrochloric acid* and 50 ml of *alcohol R*. Carry out a potentiometric titration (*2.2.20*), using *0.1 M sodium hydroxide*. Read the volume added between the 2 points of inflexion.

1 ml of *0.1 M sodium hydroxide* is equivalent to 44.99 mg of $C_{22}H_{24}ClNO_7$.

STORAGE

In an airtight container, protected from light.

IMPURITIES

A. papaverine.

01/2005:1552

NUTMEG OIL

Myristicae fragrantis aetheroleum

DEFINITION

Nutmeg oil is obtained by steam distillation of the dried and crushed kernels of *Myristica fragrans* Houtt.

CHARACTERS

A colourless or pale yellow liquid, with a spicy odour.

IDENTIFICATION

First identification: B.

Second identification: A.

A. Examine by thin-layer chromatography (*2.2.27*), using a *TLC silica gel plate R*.

Test solution. Dissolve 1 ml of the substance to be examined in *toluene R* and dilute to 10 ml with the same solvent.

Reference solution. Dissolve 20 µl of *myristicine R* in 10 ml of *toluene R*.

Apply to the plate as bands 10 µl of each solution. Develop over a path of 15 cm using a mixture of 5 volumes of *ethyl acetate R* and 95 volumes of *toluene R*. Allow the plate to dry in air and spray with *vanillin reagent R*. Heat the plate at 100 °C to 105 °C for 10 min. Examine in daylight. The chromatogram obtained with the reference solution shows in the upper third a pink to reddish-brown zone (myristicine). The chromatogram obtained with the test solution shows a series of zones of which one is similar in position and colour to the zone in the chromatogram obtained with the reference solution. Above this zone a brownish zone (safrole) and a violet zone (hydrocarbons) are present. Below the myristicine zone, 5 blue zones of variable intensity are present.

B. Examine the chromatograms obtained in the test for chromatographic profile. The retention times of the principal peaks in the chromatogram obtained with the test solution are similar to those in the chromatogram obtained with the reference solution.

TESTS

Relative density (*2.2.5*): 0.885 to 0.905.

Refractive index (*2.2.6*): 1.475 to 1.485.

Optical rotation (*2.2.7*): + 8° to + 18°.

Chromatographic profile. Examine by gas chromatography (*2.2.28*).

Test solution. The substance to be examined.

Reference solution. Dissolve 15 µl of *α-pinene R*, 15 µl of *β-pinene R*, 15 µl of *sabinene R*, 5 µl of *car-3-ene R*, 5 µl of *limonene R*, 5 µl of *γ-terpinene R*, 5 µl of *terpinen-4-ol R*, 5 µl of *safrole R* and 10 µl of *myristicine R* in 1 ml of *hexane R*.

The chromatographic procedure may be carried out using:
- a fused-silica column 25 m to 60 m long and about 0.3 mm in internal diameter, coated with *macrogol 20 000 R* as the bonded phase,
- *helium for chromatography R* as the carrier gas at a flow rate of 1.5 ml/min,
- a flame-ionisation detector,
- a split ratio of 1:100.
- with the following temperature programme:

	Time (min)	Temperature (°C)	Rate (°C/min)	Comment
Column	0 - 10	50	–	isothermal
	10 - 75	50 → 180	2	linear gradient
	75 - 130	180		isothermal
Injection port		200 - 220		
Detector		240 - 250		

Inject 0.2 µl of the reference solution. When the chromatogram is recorded in the prescribed conditions, the components elute in the order indicated in the composition of the reference solution. Record the retention times of these substances.

The test is not valid unless the resolution between the peaks corresponding to β-pinene and sabinene is at least 1.5.

Inject 0.2 µl of the test solution. Using the retention times determined from the chromatogram obtained with the reference solution, locate the components of the reference solution in the chromatogram obtained with the test solution. Determine the percentage content of each of these components by the normalisation procedure.

The percentages are within the following ranges:
- *α-pinene*: 15 per cent to 28 per cent,
- *β-pinene*: 13 per cent to 18 per cent,
- *sabinene*: 14 per cent to 29 per cent,
- *car-3-ene*: 0.5 per cent to 2.0 per cent,
- *limonene*: 2.0 per cent to 7.0 per cent,
- *γ-terpinene*: 2.0 per cent to 6.0 per cent,

– *terpinen-4-ol*: 2.0 per cent to 6.0 per cent,
– *safrole*: less than 2.5 per cent,
– *myristicine*: 5.0 per cent to 12.0 per cent.

STORAGE

Store in a well-filled, airtight container, protected from light and heat.

01/2005:0517

NYSTATIN

Nystatinum

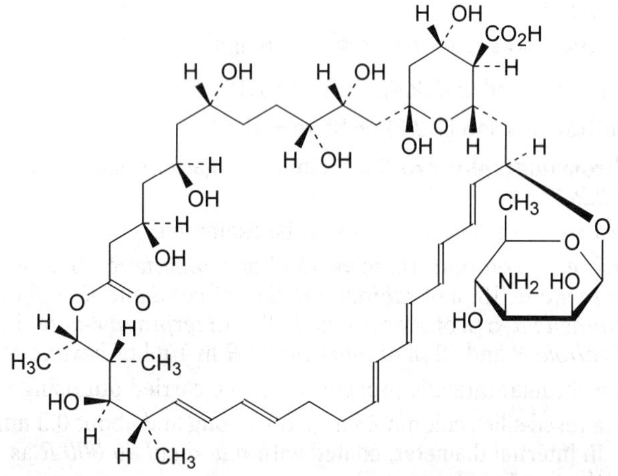

$C_{47}H_{75}NO_{17}$ M_r 926

DEFINITION

Antifungal substance obtained by fermentation using certain strains of *Streptomyces noursei* as the production micro-organism. It contains mainly tetraenes, the principal component being (1*S*,3*R*,4*R*,7*R*,9*R*,11*R*,15*S*,16*R*,17*R*,18*S*,19*E*,21*E*,25*E*,27*E*,29*E*,31*E*,33*R*,35*S*,36*R*,37*S*)-33-[(3-amino-3,6-dideoxy-β-D-mannopyranosyl)oxy]-1,3,4,7,9,11,17,37-octahydroxy-15,16,18-trimethyl-13-oxo-14,39-dioxabicyclo[33.3.1]nonatriaconta-19,21,25,27,29,31-hexaene-36-carboxylic acid (nystatin A1).

Content: minimum 4400 IU/mg (dried substance) and minimum 5000 IU/mg (dried substance) if intended for oral administration.

PRODUCTION

If nystatin is not intended for cutaneous administration, the method of manufacture is validated to demonstrate that the product, if tested, would comply with the following test.

Abnormal toxicity (*2.6.9*). Inject intraperitoneally into each mouse a quantity equivalent to not less than 600 IU suspended in 0.5 ml of a 5 g/l solution of *acacia R*.

CHARACTERS

Appearance: yellow or slightly brownish powder, hygroscopic.

Solubility: practically insoluble in water, freely soluble in dimethylformamide and in dimethyl sulphoxide, slightly soluble in methanol, practically insoluble in alcohol.

IDENTIFICATION

First identification: B, E.

Second identification: A, C, D.

A. Examine the solution prepared in the test for absorbance between 220 nm and 350 nm (*2.2.25*). The solution shows 4 absorption maxima at 230 nm, 291 nm, 305 nm and 319 nm, and a shoulder at 280 nm. The ratios of the absorbances at the absorption maxima at 291 nm and 319 nm to the absorbance at the absorption maximum at 305 nm are 0.61 to 0.73 and 0.83 to 0.96, respectively. The ratio of the absorbance measured at the absorption maximum at 230 nm to that measured at the shoulder at 280 nm is 0.83 to 1.25.

B. Infrared absorption spectrophotometry (*2.2.24*).
Comparison: *nystatin CRS*.

C. To about 2 mg add 0.1 ml of *hydrochloric acid R*. A brown colour develops.

D. To about 2 mg add 0.1 ml of *sulphuric acid R*. A brown colour develops that becomes violet on standing.

E. Examine the chromatograms obtained in the test for composition.
Results: the principal peak in the chromatogram obtained with the test solution is similar in retention time to the principal peak in the chromatogram obtained with reference solution (a).

TESTS

Absorbance (*2.2.25*). Dissolve 0.10 g in a mixture of 5.0 ml of *glacial acetic acid R* and 50 ml of *methanol R* and dilute to 100.0 ml with *methanol R*. Dilute 1.0 ml of the solution to 100.0 ml with *methanol R*. Determined at the maximum at 305 nm within 30 min of preparation of the solution, the absorbance is not less than 0.60.

Composition. Liquid chromatography (*2.2.29*): use the normalisation procedure. *Carry out the test protected from light.*

Test solution. Dissolve 20 mg of the substance to be examined in *dimethyl sulphoxide R* and dilute to 50 ml with the same solvent.

Reference solution (a). Dissolve 20 mg of *nystatin CRS* in *dimethyl sulphoxide R* and dilute to 50 ml with the same solvent.

Reference solution (b). Dissolve 20 mg of the substance to be examined in 25 ml of *methanol R* and dilute to 50 ml with *water R*. To 10.0 ml of the solution add 2.0 ml of *dilute hydrochloric acid R*. Allow to stand at room temperature for 1 h.

Reference solution (c). Dilute 1.0 ml of reference solution (a) to 100.0 ml with *dimethyl sulphoxide R*. Dilute 1.0 ml of this solution to 10.0 ml with *dimethyl sulphoxide R*.

Column:
– *size*: *l* = 0.15 m, Ø = 4.6 mm,
– *stationary phase: base-deactivated end-capped octadecylsilyl silica gel for chromatography R* (5 μm),
– *temperature*: 30 °C.

Mobile phase:
– *mobile phase A*: *acetonitrile R*, 3.85 g/l solution of *ammonium acetate R* (29:71 *V/V*),
– *mobile phase B*: 3.85 g/l solution of *ammonium acetate R*, *acetonitrile R* (40:60 *V/V*),

Time (min)	Mobile phase A (per cent *V/V*)	Mobile phase B (per cent *V/V*)
0 - 25	100	0
25 - 35	100 → 0	0 → 100
35 - 45	0	100
45 - 50	0 → 100	100 → 0
50 - 55	100	0

Flow rate: 1.0 ml/min.

Detection: spectrophotometer at 305 nm.

Injection: 20 μl

Retention time: nystatin A1 = about 14 min.

System suitability: reference solution (b):

- *resolution*: minimum 3.5 between the 2 principal peaks (retention time = about 13 min and 19 min).

Composition:

- *nystatin A1*: minimum 85.0 per cent,
- *any other compound*: maximum 4.0 per cent,
- *disregard limit*: the area of the principal peak in the chromatogram obtained with reference solution (c); disregard any peak with a retention time of less than 2 min.

Heavy metals (*2.4.8*): maximum 20 ppm.

1.0 g complies with limit test C. Prepare the standard using 2 ml of *lead standard solution (10 ppm Pb) R*.

Loss on drying (*2.2.32*): maximum 5.0 per cent, determined on 1.000 g by drying at 60 °C over *diphosphorus pentoxide R* at a pressure not exceeding 0.1 kPa for 3 h.

Sulphated ash (*2.4.14*): maximum 3.5 per cent, determined on 1.0 g.

ASSAY

Carry out the microbiological assay of antibiotics (*2.7.2*). *Protect the solutions from light throughout the assay.*

Dissolve the substance to be examined and *nystatin CRS* separately in *dimethylformamide R* and dilute with a mixture of 5 volumes of *dimethylformamide R* and 95 volumes of buffer solution pH 6.0.

STORAGE

In an airtight container, protected from light.

LABELLING

The label states where applicable, that the substance is only for cutaneous use.

O

01/2005:1887

OAK BARK

Quercus cortex

DEFINITION

Cut and dried bark from the fresh young branches of *Quercus robur* L., *Q. petraea* (Matt.) Liebl. and *Q. pubescens* Willd.

Content: minimum 3.0 per cent of tannins, expressed as pyrogallol ($C_6H_6O_3$; M_r 126.1) (dried drug).

CHARACTERS

Macroscopic and microscopic characters described under identification tests A and B.

IDENTIFICATION

A. The bark occurs in channelled or quilled pieces, not more than 3 mm thick. The outer surface is light grey or greenish-grey, rather smooth, with occasional lenticels. The inner surface is dull brown or reddish-brown and has slightly raised longitudinal striations about 0.5 mm to 1 mm wide. The fracture is splintery and fibrous.

B. Reduce to a powder (355). The powder is light brown to reddish-brown and fibrous. Examine under a microscope using *chloral hydrate solution R*. The powder shows groups of thick-walled fibres surrounded by a moderately thickened parenchymatous sheath containing prism crystals of calcium oxalate; fragments of cork composed of thin-walled tabular cells filled with brownish or reddish contents; abundant sclereids, isolated and in groups, some large with thick, stratified walls and branching pits, others smaller and thinner-walled with simple pits, often with dense brown contents; fragments of parenchyma containing cluster crystals of calcium oxalate; occasional fragments of sieve tissue, thin-walled, some showing sieve areas on the oblique end-walls.

C. To 1 g of the powdered drug (710) add 10 ml of *alcohol (30 per cent V/V) R* and heat the mixture under a reflux condenser on a water-bath for 30 min. Cool and filter. To 1 ml of the solution add 2 ml of a 10 g/l solution of *vanillin R* in *hydrochloric acid R*. A red colour develops.

TESTS

Foreign matter (*2.8.2*): maximum 2 per cent.

Loss on drying (*2.2.32*): maximum 10.0 per cent, determined on 1.000 g of the powdered drug (710) by drying in an oven at 100-105 °C for 2 h.

Total ash (*2.4.16*): maximum 8.0 per cent.

ASSAY

Carry out the determination of tannins in herbal drugs (*2.8.14*). Use 0.700 g of the powdered drug (710).

01/2005:1553

OCTOXINOL 10

Octoxinolum 10

DEFINITION

α-[4-(1,1,3,3-Tetramethylbutyl)phenyl]-ω-hydroxydeca(oxyethylene).

Mixture consisting mainly of mono-octylphenyl ethers of macrogols corresponding to the formula $C_8H_{17}C_6H_4\text{-}[OCH_2\text{-}CH_2]_n\text{-}OH$ where the average value of *n* is 10. It may contain free macrogols.

CHARACTERS

Appearance: clear, colourless or light yellow, viscous liquid.

Solubility: miscible with water, with ethanol and with vegetable oils.

IDENTIFICATION

A. Infrared absorption spectrophotometry (*2.2.24*).

Comparison: *Ph. Eur. reference spectrum of octoxinol 10.*

Preparation: film between *sodium chloride R* plates.

B. It complies with the test for cloud point (see Tests).

TESTS

Acidity or alkalinity. Boil 1.0 g with 20 ml of *carbon dioxide-free water R* for 1 min, with constant stirring. Cool and filter. To 10 ml of the filtrate, add 0.05 ml of *bromothymol blue solution R1*. Not more than 0.5 ml of *0.01 M hydrochloric acid* or *0.01 M sodium hydroxide* is required to change the colour of the indicator.

Hydroxyl value (*2.5.3, Method A*): 85 to 101.

Cloud point: 63 °C to 70 °C.

Dissolve 1.0 g in 99 g of *water R*. Transfer about 30 ml of this solution to a test-tube, heat on a water-bath and stir continuously until the solution becomes cloudy. Remove the test-tube from the water-bath (ensuring that the temperature does not increase more than 2 °C), and continue to stir. The cloud point is the temperature at which the solution becomes sufficiently clear that the entire thermometer bulb is plainly seen.

Ethylene oxide and dioxan (*2.4.25*): maximum 1 ppm of ethylene oxide and maximum 10 ppm of dioxan.

Heavy metals (*2.4.8*): maximum 10 ppm.

Dissolve 2.0 g in *distilled water R* and dilute to 20.0 ml with the same solvent. 12 ml of this solution complies with limit test A. Prepare the standard using *lead standard solution (1 ppm Pb) R*.

Water (*2.5.12*): maximum 0.5 per cent, determined on 2.00 g.

Total ash (*2.4.16*): maximum 0.4 per cent, determined on 1.0 g.

STORAGE

In an airtight container.

01/2005:2057

OCTYL GALLATE

Octylis gallas

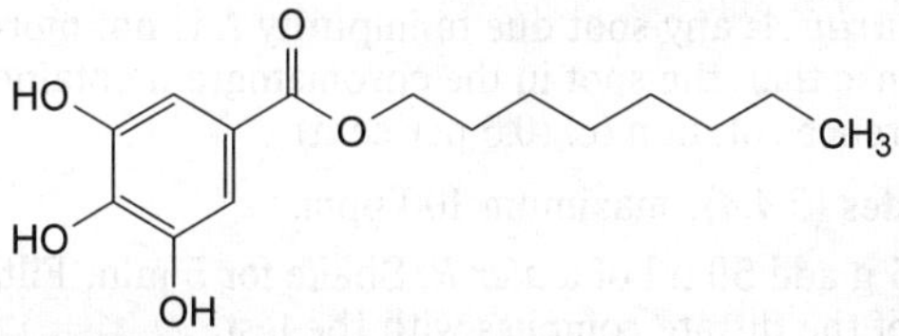

$C_{15}H_{22}O_5$ M_r 282.3

DEFINITION

Octyl 3,4,5-trihydroxybenzoate.

Content: 97.0 per cent to 103.0 per cent (dried substance).

CHARACTERS

Appearance: white or almost white, crystalline powder.

Solubility: practically insoluble in water, freely soluble in ethanol (96 per cent), practically insoluble in methylene chloride.

IDENTIFICATION

A. Melting point (*2.2.14*).

Determine the melting point of the substance to be examined. Mix equal parts of the substance to be examined and *octyl gallate CRS* and determine the melting point of the mixture. The difference between the melting points (which are about 101 °C) is not greater than 2 °C.

B. Examine the chromatograms obtained in the test for impurity A.

Results: the principal spot in the chromatogram obtained with test solution (b) is similar in position, colour and size to the principal spot in the chromatogram obtained with reference solution (a).

TESTS

Impurity A. Thin-layer chromatography (*2.2.27*).

Test solution (a). Dissolve 0.20 g of the substance to be examined in *acetone R* and dilute to 10 ml with the same solvent.

Test solution (b). Dilute 1.0 ml of test solution (a) to 20 ml with *acetone R*.

Reference solution (a). Dissolve 10 mg of *octyl gallate CRS* in *acetone R* and dilute to 10 ml with the same solvent.

Reference solution (b). Dissolve 20 mg of *gallic acid R* in *acetone R* and dilute to 20 ml with the same solvent.

Reference solution (c). Dilute 1.0 ml of reference solution (b) to 10 ml with *acetone R*.

Reference solution (d). Dilute 1.0 ml of reference solution (b) to 5 ml with test solution (a).

Plate: *TLC silica gel plate R*.

Mobile phase: *anhydrous formic acid R, ethyl formate R, toluene R* (10:40:50 *V/V/V*).

Application: 5 µl of test solutions (a) and (b) and reference solutions (a), (c) and (d).

Development: over 2/3 of the plate.

Drying: in air for 10 min.

Detection: spray with a mixture of 1 volume of *ferric chloride solution R1* and 9 volumes of *ethanol (96 per cent) R*.

System suitability: reference solution (d):

– the chromatogram shows 2 clearly separated principal spots.

Limit: test solution (a):

– *impurity A*: any spot due to impurity A is not more intense than the spot in the chromatogram obtained with reference solution (c) (0.5 per cent).

Chlorides (*2.4.4*): maximum 100 ppm.

To 1.65 g add 50 ml of *water R*. Shake for 5 min. Filter. 15 ml of the filtrate complies with the test.

Heavy metals (*2.4.8*): maximum 10 ppm.

2.0 g complies with limit test C. Prepare the reference solution using 2 ml of *lead standard solution (10 ppm Pb) R*.

Loss on drying (*2.2.32*): maximum 0.5 per cent, determined on 1.000 g by drying in an oven at 70 °C.

Sulphated ash (*2.4.14*): maximum 0.1 per cent, determined on 1.0 g.

ASSAY

Dissolve 0.100 g in *methanol R* and dilute to 250.0 ml with the same solvent. Dilute 5.0 ml of the solution to 200.0 ml with *methanol R*. Measure the absorbance (*2.2.25*) at the absorption maximum at 275 nm.

Calculate the content of $C_{15}H_{22}O_5$ taking the specific absorbance to be 387.

STORAGE

In a non-metallic container, protected from light.

IMPURITIES

Specified impurities: A.

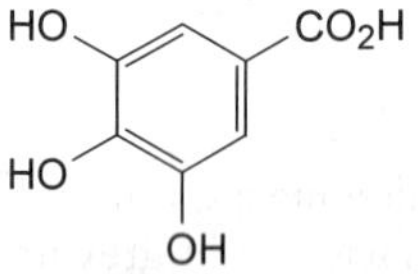

A. 3,4,5-trihydroxybenzoic acid (gallic acid).

01/2005:1136

OCTYLDODECANOL

Octyldodecanolum

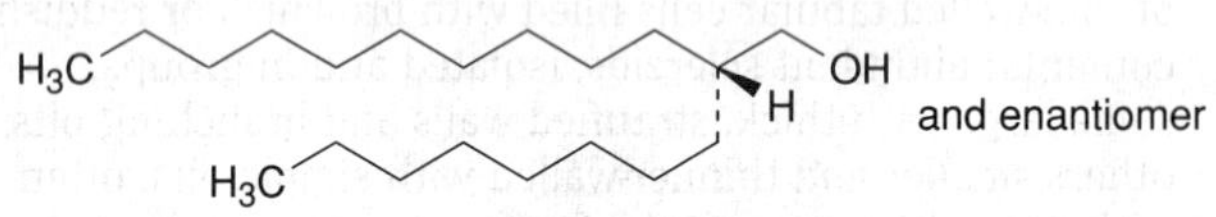

DEFINITION

Condensation product of saturated liquid fatty alcohols.

Content: not less than 90 per cent of (2*RS*)-2-octyldodecan-1-ol ($C_{20}H_{42}O$; M_r 298.6), the remainder consisting mainly of related alcohols.

CHARACTERS

Appearance: clear, colourless or yellowish, oily liquid.

Solubility: practically insoluble in water, miscible with alcohol.

Relative density: about 0.840.

Refractive index: about 1.455.

IDENTIFICATION

A. It complies with the test for hydroxyl value (see Tests).

B. Thin-layer chromatography (*2.2.27*).

Test solution. Dissolve 0.20 g of the substance to be examined in *toluene R* and dilute to 20 ml with the same solvent.

Reference solution. Dissolve 0.20 g of *octyldodecanol CRS* in *toluene R* and dilute to 20 ml with the same solvent.

Plate: suitable silica gel plate.

Mobile phase: *ethyl acetate R, toluene R* (5:95 *V/V*).

Application: 2 µl.

Development: over a path of 12 cm.

Drying: in air.

Detection: spray with about 7 ml of a mixture of 1 volume of a 25 g/l solution of *vanillin R* in *alcohol R* and 4 volumes of *sulphuric acid R* and heat at 130 °C for 5-10 min.

Results: the principal spot in the chromatogram obtained with the test solution is similar in position, colour and size to the principal spot in the chromatogram obtained with the reference solution.

TESTS

Acidity or alkalinity. Mix 5.0 g thoroughly for 1 min with a mixture of 0.1 ml of *bromothymol blue solution R1*, 2 ml of *heptane R* and 10 ml of *water R*. If the aqueous layer is blue, not more than 0.15 ml of *0.01 M hydrochloric acid* is required to change the colour of the indicator to yellow. If the aqueous layer is yellow, add 0.45 ml of *0.1 M sodium hydroxide* and shake vigorously. After standing to ensure complete separation, the aqueous layer is blue.

Optical rotation (*2.2.7*): − 0.10° to + 0.10°.

Dissolve 2.50 g in *alcohol R* and dilute to 25 ml with the same solvent.

Hydroxyl value (*2.5.3, Method A*): 175 to 190.

Iodine value (*2.5.4*): maximum 8.0.

Peroxide value (*2.5.5*): maximum 5.0.

Saponification value (*2.5.6*): maximum 5.0.

Heavy metals (*2.4.8*): maximum 10 ppm.

2.0 g complies with limit test C. Prepare the standard using 2 ml of *lead standard solution (10 ppm Pb) R*.

Water (*2.5.12*): maximum 0.5 per cent, determined on 2.00 g.

Sulphated ash (*2.4.14*): maximum 0.1 per cent, determined on 1.0 g.

ASSAY

Gas chromatography (*2.2.28*).

Internal standard solution. Dissolve 0.4 g of *tetradecane R* in *hexane R* and dilute to 100.0 ml with the same solvent.

Test solution. Dissolve 0.100 g of the substance to be examined in the internal standard solution and dilute to 10.0 ml with the same solution.

Reference solution. Dissolve 0.100 g of *octyldodecanol CRS* in the internal standard solution and dilute to 10.0 ml with the same solution.

Column:

- *material*: stainless steel,
- *size*: *l* = 60 m, Ø = 0.25 mm,
- *stationary phase*: *poly(dimethyl)(diphenyl)(divinyl)siloxane R* (film thickness 0.25 µm).

Carrier gas: *helium for chromatography R*.

Flow rate: 0.68 ml/min.

Temperature:

	Time (min)	Temperature (°C)
Column	0 - 2	180
	2 - 22	180 → 280
	22 - 52	280
Injection port		290
Detector		300

Detection: flame ionisation.

Injection: 1 µl.

Calculate the content of $C_{20}H_{42}O$ in the substance to be examined.

STORAGE

Protected from light.

01/2005:1455

OFLOXACIN

Ofloxacinum

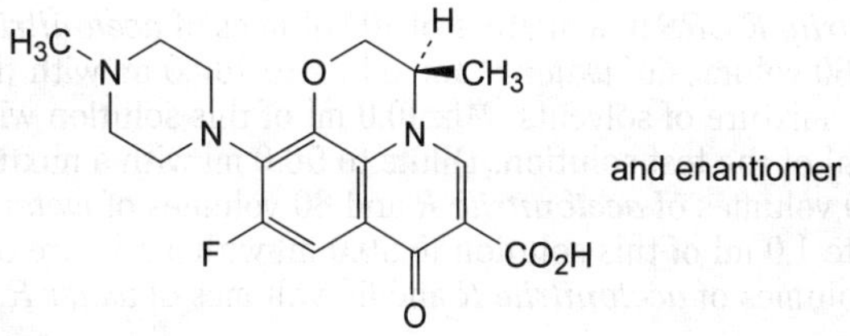

$C_{18}H_{20}FN_3O_4$ M_r 361.4

DEFINITION

Ofloxacin contains not less than 99.0 per cent and not more than the equivalent of 101.0 per cent of (*RS*)-9-fluoro-3-methyl-10-(4-methylpiperazin-1-yl)-7-oxo-2,3-dihydro-7*H*-pyrido[1,2,3-*de*]-1,4-benzoxazine-6-carboxylic acid, calculated with reference to the dried substance.

CHARACTERS

A pale yellow or bright yellow, crystalline powder, slightly soluble in water, soluble in glacial acetic acid, slightly soluble to soluble in methylene chloride, slightly soluble in methanol.

IDENTIFICATION

Examine by infrared absorption spectrophotometry (*2.2.24*), comparing with the spectrum obtained with *ofloxacin CRS*. Examine the substances prepared as discs.

TESTS

Absorbance (*2.2.25*). Dissolve 0.5 g in *0.1 M hydrochloric acid* and dilute to 100 ml with the same solvent. The absorbance of the solution measured at 440 nm is not greater than 0.25.

Optical rotation (*2.2.7*). Dissolve 0.300 g in a mixture of 10 volumes of *methanol R* and 40 volumes of *methylene chloride R* and dilute to 10 ml with the same mixture of solvents. The angle of optical rotation is − 0.10° to + 0.10°.

Impurity A. Examine by thin-layer chromatography (*2.2.27*), using a *TLC silica gel GF_{254} plate R* (2 µm to 10 µm).

Test solution. Dissolve 0.250 g of the substance to be examined in a mixture of 10 volumes of *methanol R* and 40 volumes of *methylene chloride R* and dilute to 5.0 ml with the same mixture of solvents.

Reference solution.Dissolve 10 mg of *ofloxacin impurity A CRS* in a mixture of 10 volumes of *methanol R* and 40 volumes of *methylene chloride R* and dilute to 100.0 ml with the same mixture of solvents.

Apply to the plate 10 µl of each solution. Develop over a path of 10 cm using a mixture of 1 volume of *glacial acetic acid R*, 1 volume of *water R* and 2 volumes of *ethyl acetate R*. Allow the plate to dry in air and examine in ultraviolet light at 254 nm. Any spot due to impurity A in the chromatogram obtained with the test solution is not more intense than the spot in the chromatogram obtained with the reference solution (0.2 per cent).

Related substances. Examine by liquid chromatography (*2.2.29*). *Prepare the solutions immediately before use.*

Test solution. Dissolve 10.0 mg of the substance to be examined in a mixture of 10 volumes of *acetonitrile R* and 60 volumes of *water R* and dilute to 50.0 ml with the same mixture of solvents.

Reference solution (a). Dilute 1.0 ml of the test solution to 50.0 ml with a mixture of 10 volumes of *acetonitrile R* and 60 volumes of *water R.* Dilute 1.0 ml of this solution to 10.0 ml with a mixture of 10 volumes of *acetonitrile R* and 60 volumes of *water R.*

Reference solution (b). Dissolve 10.0 mg of *ofloxacin impurity E CRS* in a mixture of 10 volumes of *acetonitrile R* and 60 volumes of *water R* and dilute to 100.0 ml with the same mixture of solvents. Mix 10.0 ml of this solution with 5.0 ml of the test solution. Dilute to 50.0 ml with a mixture of 10 volumes of *acetonitrile R* and 60 volumes of *water R.* Dilute 1.0 ml of this solution to 50.0 ml with a mixture of 10 volumes of *acetonitrile R* and 60 volumes of *water R.*

The chromatographic procedure may be carried out using:

- a stainless steel column 0.15 m long and 4.6 mm in internal diameter packed with *octadecylsilyl silica gel for chromatography R* (5 µm),
- as mobile phase a mixture prepared as follows: dissolve 4.0 g of *ammonium acetate R* and 7.0 g of *sodium perchlorate R* in 1300 ml of *water R.* Adjust to pH 2.2 with *phosphoric acid R.* Add 240 ml of *acetonitrile R.* Adjust the flow rate of the mobile phase so that a retention time of about 20 min is obtained for ofloxacin,
- as detector a spectrophotometer set at 294 nm,

maintaining the temperature of the column at 45 °C.

Inject 10 µl of reference solution (b). Adjust the sensitivity of the system so that the heights of the two principal peaks in the chromatogram obtained are at least 50 per cent of the full scale of the recorder. The test is not valid unless: in the chromatogram obtained, the resolution between the peaks corresponding to impurity E and ofloxacin is at least 2.0. Inject 10 µl of the test solution and 10 µl of reference solution (a). Continue the chromatography for 2.5 times the retention time of the principal peak. In the chromatogram obtained with the test solution, the area of any peak, apart from the principal peak, is not greater than the area of the principal peak in the chromatogram obtained with reference solution (a) (0.2 per cent); the sum of the areas of all the peaks is not greater than 2.5 times the area of the principal peak in the chromatogram obtained with reference solution (a) (0.5 per cent). Disregard any peak with an area less than 0.1 times the area of the principal peak in the chromatogram obtained with reference solution (a).

Heavy metals (*2.4.8*). 2.0 g complies with limit test C for heavy metals (10 ppm). Prepare the standard using 2 ml of *lead standard solution (10 ppm Pb) R.*

Loss on drying (*2.2.32*). Not more than 0.2 per cent, determined on 1.000 g by drying at 100 °C to 105 °C for 4 h.

Sulphated ash (*2.4.14*). Not more than 0.1 per cent, determined on 1.0 g.

ASSAY

Dissolve 0.300 g in 100 ml of *anhydrous acetic acid R.* Titrate with *0.1 M perchloric acid* determining the end-point potentiometrically (*2.2.20*).

1 ml of *0.1 M perchloric acid* is equivalent to 36.14 mg of $C_{18}H_{20}FN_3O_4$.

STORAGE

Store in an airtight container, protected from light.

IMPURITIES

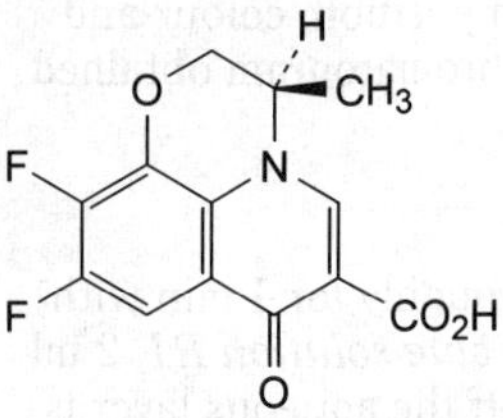

and enantiomer

A. (*RS*)-9,10-difluoro-3-methyl-7-oxo-2,3-dihydro-7*H*-pyrido[1,2,3-*de*]-1,4-benzoxazine-6-carboxylic acid (FPA),

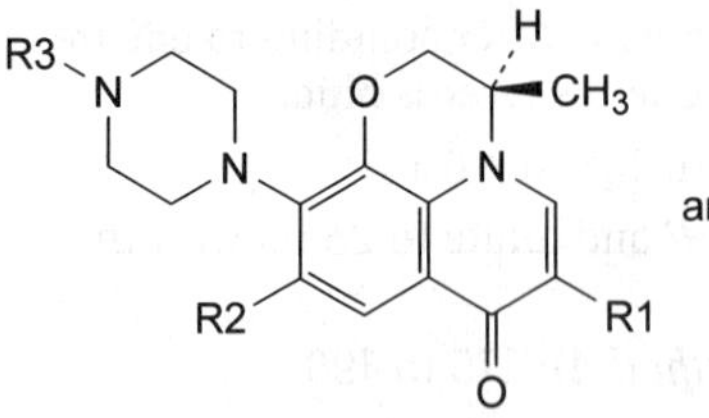

and enantiomer

B. R1 = H, R2 = F, R3 = CH_3:(*RS*)-9-fluoro-3-methyl-10-(4-methylpiperazin-1-yl)-2,3-dihydro-7*H*-pyrido[1,2,3-*de*]-1,4-benzoxazin-7-one,

C. R1 = CO_2H, R2 = H, R3 = CH_3:(*RS*)-3-methyl-10-(4-methylpiperazin-1-yl)-7-oxo-2,3-dihydro-7*H*-pyrido[1,2,3-*de*]-1,4-benzoxazine-6-carboxylic acid,

E. R1 = CO_2H, R2 = F, R3 = H: (*RS*)-9-fluoro-3-methyl-7-oxo-10-(piperazin-1-yl)-2,3-dihydro-7*H*-pyrido[1,2,3-*de*]-1,4-benzoxazine-6-carboxylic acid,

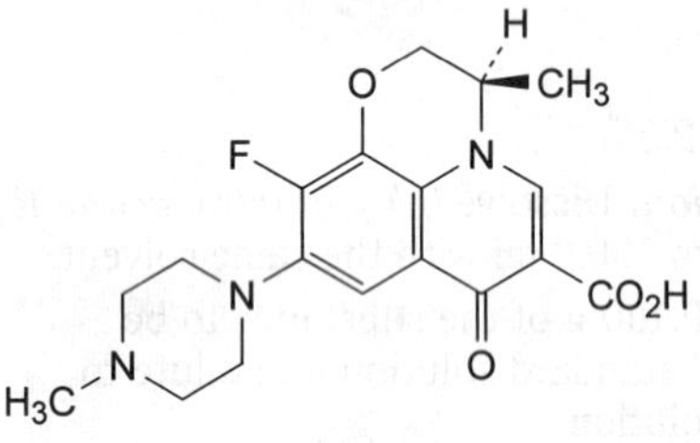

and enantiomer

D. (*RS*)-10-fluoro-3-methyl-9-(4-methylpiperazin-1-yl)-7-oxo-2,3-dihydro-7*H*-pyrido[1,2,3-*de*]-1,4-benzoxazine-6-carboxylic acid,

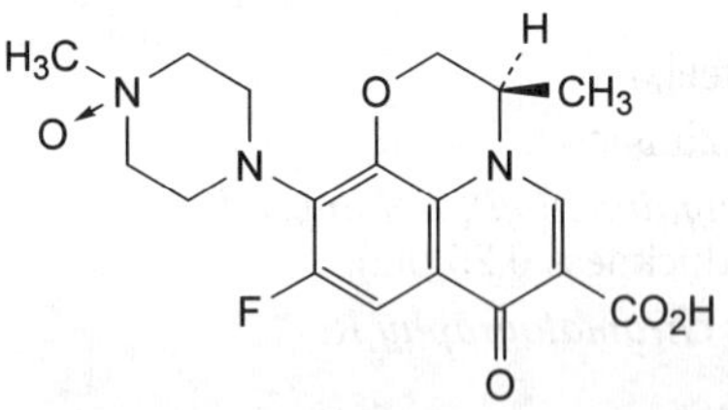

and enantiomer

F. 4-[(*RS*)-6-carboxy-9-fluoro-3-methyl-7-oxo-2,3-dihydro-7*H*-pyrido[1,2,3-*de*]-1,4-benzoxazine-10-yl]-1-methylpiperazine 1-oxide.

01/2005:0799

OLEIC ACID

Acidum oleicum

DEFINITION

(*Z*)-Octadec-9-enoic acid ($C_{18}H_{34}O_2$; M_r 282.5), together with varying amounts of saturated and other unsaturated fatty acids. A suitable antioxidant may be added.

Content: 65.0 per cent to 88.0 per cent of $C_{18}H_{34}O_2$.

CHARACTERS

Appearance: clear, yellowish or brownish, oily liquid.

Solubility: practically insoluble in water, miscible with alcohol and with methylene chloride.

Relative density: about 0.892.

IDENTIFICATION

A. It complies with the test for acid value (see Tests).

B. It complies with the test for iodine value (see Tests).

C. It complies with the test for composition of fatty acids (see Tests).

Margaric acid: maximum 0.2 per cent for oleic acid of vegetable origin and maximum 4.0 per cent for oleic acid of animal origin.

TESTS

Appearance. The substance to be examined is not more intensely coloured than reference solution Y_1 or BY_1 (*2.2.2, Method I*).

Acid value (*2.5.1*): 195 to 204, determined on 0.5 g.

Iodine value (*2.5.4*): 89 to 105.

Peroxide value (*2.5.5*): maximum 10.0.

Composition of fatty acids. Gas chromatography (*2.4.22, Method C*).

Test solution. Prepare as described in the method but omitting the initial hydrolysis.

Composition of the fatty acid fraction of the substance:

- *myristic acid*: maximum 5.0 per cent,
- *palmitic acid*: maximum 16.0 per cent,
- *palmitoleic acid*: maximum 8.0 per cent,
- *stearic acid*: maximum 6.0 per cent,
- *oleic acid*: 65.0 per cent to 88.0 per cent,
- *linoleic acid*: maximum 18.0 per cent,
- *linolenic acid*: maximum 4.0 per cent,
- *fatty acids of chain length greater than* C_{18}: maximum 4.0 per cent.

Total ash (*2.4.16*): maximum 0.1 per cent, determined on 2.00 g.

STORAGE

In an airtight, well-filled container, protected from light.

LABELLING

The label states:

- the name and concentration of any added antioxidant,
- the origin of oleic acid (animal or vegetable).

01/2005:1249

OLEOYL MACROGOLGLYCERIDES

Macrogolglyceridorum oleates

DEFINITION

Oleoyl macrogolglycerides are mixtures of monoesters, diesters and triesters of glycerol and monoesters and diesters of macrogols. They are obtained by partial alcoholysis of an unsaturated oil mainly containing triglycerides of oleic acid using macrogol with a mean relative molecular mass between 300 and 400 or by esterification of glycerol and macrogol with unsaturated fatty acids or by mixing glycerol esters and condensates of ethylene oxide with the fatty acids of this unsaturated oil.

CHARACTERS

Amber oily liquids, which may give rise to a deposit after prolonged periods at 20 °C, practically insoluble but dispersible in water, freely soluble in methylene chloride.

The viscosity at 40 °C is about 35 mPa·s, the relative density at 20 °C is about 0.95 and the refractive index at 20 °C is about 1.47.

IDENTIFICATION

A. Examine by thin-layer chromatography (*2.2.27*), using a suitable silica gel as the coating substance.

Test solution. Dissolve 1.0 g of the substance to be examined in *methylene chloride R* and dilute to 20 ml with the same solvent.

Apply to the plate 10 µl of the test solution. Develop over a path of 15 cm using a mixture of 30 volumes of *hexane R* and 70 volumes of *ether R*. Allow the plate to dry in air. Spray with a 0.1 g/l solution of *rhodamine B R* in *alcohol R* and examine in ultraviolet light at 365 nm. The chromatogram shows a spot corresponding to triglycerides with an R_f value of about 0.9 (R_{st} 1) and spots corresponding to 1,3-diglycerides (R_{st} 0.7), to 1,2-diglycerides (R_{st} 0.6), to monoglycerides (R_{st} 0.1) and to esters of macrogol (R_{st} 0).

B. They comply with the test for hydroxyl value (see Tests).

C. They comply with the test for fatty acid composition (see Tests).

D. They comply with the test for saponification value (see Tests).

TESTS

Acid value (*2.5.1*). Not more than 2.0, determined on 2.0 g.

Hydroxyl value (*2.5.3, Method A*): 45 to 65, determined on 1.0 g.

Iodine value (*2.5.4*): 75 to 95.

Peroxide value (*2.5.5*). Not more than 12.0, determined on 2.0 g.

Saponification value (*2.5.6*): 150 to 170, determined on 2.0 g.

Alkaline impurities. Introduce 5.0 g into a test-tube and carefully add a mixture, neutralised if necessary with *0.01 M hydrochloric acid* or with *0.01 M sodium hydroxide*, of 0.05 ml of a 0.4 g/l solution of *bromophenol blue R* in *alcohol R*, 0.3 ml of *water R* and 10 ml of *alcohol R*. Shake and allow to stand. Not more than 1.0 ml of *0.01 M hydrochloric acid* is required to change the colour of the upper layer to yellow.

Free glycerol. Not more than 3.0 per cent. Dissolve 1.20 g in 25.0 ml of *methylene chloride R*. Heat if necessary. After cooling, add 100 ml of *water R*. Shake and add 25.0 ml of a 6 g/l solution of *periodic acid R*. Shake and allow to stand for 30 min. Add 40 ml of a 75 g/l solution of *potassium iodide R*. Allow to stand for 1 min. Add 1 ml of *starch solution R*. Titrate the iodine with *0.1 M sodium thiosulphate*. Carry out a blank titration.

1 ml of *0.1 M sodium thiosulphate* is equivalent to 2.3 mg of glycerol.

Composition of fatty acids (*2.4.22, Method A*). The fatty-acid fraction has the following composition:

- *palmitic acid*: 4.0 per cent to 9.0 per cent,
- *stearic acid*: not more than 6.0 per cent,
- *oleic acid*: 58.0 per cent to 80.0 per cent,
- *linoleic acid*: 15.0 per cent to 35.0 per cent,
- *linolenic acid*: not more than 2.0 per cent,

Monographs N-O

– *arachidic acid*: not more than 2.0 per cent,
– *eicosenoic acid*: not more than 2.0 per cent.

Ethylene oxide and dioxan (*2.4.25*). Not more than 1 ppm of ethylene oxide and 10 ppm of dioxan.

Heavy metals (*2.4.8*). 2.0 g complies with limit test C for heavy metals (10 ppm). Prepare the standard using 2 ml of *lead standard solution (10 ppm Pb) R*.

Water (*2.5.12*). Not more than 1.0 per cent, determined on 1.0 g by the semi-micro determination of water. Use a mixture of 30 volumes of *anhydrous methanol R* and 70 volumes of *methylene chloride R* as solvent.

Total ash (*2.4.16*). Not more than 0.1 per cent, determined on 1.0 g.

STORAGE

Store protected from light and at room temperature.

LABELLING

The label states the type of macrogol used (mean relative molecular mass) or the number of units of ethylene oxide per molecule (nominal value).

01/2005:2073

OLEYL ALCOHOL

Alcohol oleicus

DEFINITION

Mixture of unsaturated and saturated long-chain fatty alcohols consisting mainly of octadec-9-enol (oleyl alcohol and elaidyl alcohol; $C_{18}H_{36}O$; M_r 268.5). It may be of vegetable or animal origin.

CHARACTERS

Appearance: colourless or light yellow liquid.

IDENTIFICATION

A. It complies with the test for hydroxyl value (see Tests).

B. It complies with the test for composition of fatty alcohols (see Tests).

TESTS

Appearance. The substance to be examined is clear (*2.2.1*) and not more intensely coloured than reference solution B_6 (*2.2.2, Method II*).

Refractive index (*2.2.6*): 1.458 to 1.460, determined at 25 °C.

Cloud point: maximum 10 °C.

Introduce about 60 g into a cylindrical flat-bottomed container, 30-33.5 mm internal diameter and 115-125 mm high. Heat to 30 °C, cool, and immerse the container in iced water with the surfaces of the water and the sample at the same level. Insert a thermometer and, using it as a stirring rod begin stirring rapidly and steadily when the temperature falls below 20 °C. Keep the thermometer immersed throughout the test, remove and examine the container at regular intervals. The cloud point is the temperature at which the immersed portion of the thermometer, positioned vertically in the centre of the container, is no longer visible when viewed horizontally through the container and sample.

Acid value (*2.5.1*): maximum 1.0, determined on 5.0 g.

Hydroxyl value (*2.5.3, Method A*): 205 to 215.

Saponification value (*2.5.6*): maximum 2.0.

Composition of fatty alcohols. Gas chromatography (*2.2.28*): use the normalisation procedure.

Test solution. Mix 25 mg of the substance to be examined with 1.0 ml of *methylene chloride R*.

Reference solution (a). Dissolve 25 mg of each of *arachidyl alcohol R, linolenyl alcohol R, linoleyl alcohol R, oleyl alcohol R, palmityl alcohol R* and *stearyl alcohol R* in *methylene chloride R* and dilute to 5 ml with the same solvent. Dilute 1 ml of this solution to 5 ml with *methylene chloride R*.

Reference solution (b). Dissolve 10 mg of *linoleyl alcohol R* and 1 g of *oleyl alcohol R* in *methylene chloride R* and dilute to 40 ml with the same solvent.

Column:
– *size*: *l* = 30 m, Ø = 0.32 mm,
– *stationary phase*: *poly(dimethyl)siloxane R* (film thickness 1 µm).

Carrier gas: *helium for chromatography R*.

Flow rate: 1 ml/min.

Split ratio: 1:11.

Temperature:

	Time (min)	Temperature (°C)
Column	0 - 1	170
	1 - 9	170 → 210
	9 - 65	210
Injection port		270
Detector		280

Detection: flame ionisation.

Injection: 1 µl.

Identify the peaks using the chromatogram obtained with reference solution (a).

Relative retention with reference to oleyl alcohol (retention time = about 30 min): palmityl alcohol = about 0.6; linolenyl alcohol = about 0.8; linoleyl alcohol = about 0.9; stearyl alcohol = about 1.1; arachidyl alcohol = about 1.9 (elaidyl alcohol co-elutes with oleyl alcohol).

System suitability: reference solution (b):
– *peak-to-valley ratio*: minimum 1.2 between the peaks due to linoleyl alcohol and oleyl alcohol.

Limits:
– *palmityl alcohol*: maximum 8.0 per cent,
– *stearyl alcohol*: maximum 5.0 per cent,
– *oleyl alcohol* (sum of oleyl and elaidyl alcohols): minimum 80.0 per cent,
– *linoleyl alcohol*: maximum 3.0 per cent,
– *linolenyl alcohol*: maximum 0.5 per cent,
– *arachidyl alcohol*: maximum 0.3 per cent.

01/2005:1878

OLIVE LEAF

Oleae folium

DEFINITION

Dried leaf of *Olea europaea* L.

Content: minimum 5.0 per cent of oleuropein ($C_{25}H_{32}O_{13}$; M_r 540.5) (dried drug).

Monographs N-O

CHARACTERS

Macroscopic and microscopic characters described under identification tests A and B.

IDENTIFICATION

A. The leaf is simple, thick and coriaceous, lanceolate to obovate, 30 mm to 50 mm long and 10 mm to 15 mm wide, with a mucronate apex and tapering at the base to a short petiole; the margins are entire and reflexed abaxially. The upper surface is greyish-green, smooth and shiny, the lower surface paler and pubescent, particularly along the midrib and main lateral veins.

B. Reduce to a powder (355). The powder is yellowish-green. Examine under a microscope using *chloral hydrate solution R*. The powder shows the following diagnostic characters: fragments of the epidermis in surface view with small, thick-walled polygonal cells and, in the lower epidermis only, small anomocytic stomata (*2.8.3*); fragments of the lamina in sectional view showing a thick cuticle, a palisade composed of 3 layers of cells and a small-celled spongy parenchyma; numerous sclereids, very thick-walled and mostly fibre-like with blunt or, occasionally, forked ends, isolated or associated with the parenchyma of the mesophyll; abundant, very large peltate trichomes, with a central unicellular stalk from which radiate some 10 to 30 thin-walled cells which become free from the adjoining cells at the margin of the shield, given an uneven, jagged appearance.

C. Thin-layer chromatography (*2.2.27*).

Test solution. To 1.0 g of the powdered drug (355) add 10 ml of *methanol R*. Boil under a reflux condenser for 15 min. Cool and filter.

Reference solution. Dissolve 10 mg of *oleuropein R* and 1 mg of *rutin R* in 1 ml of *methanol R*.

Plate: *TLC silica gel plate R*.

Mobile phase: *water R, methanol R, methylene chloride R* (1.5:15:85 *V/V/V*).

Application: 10 µl as bands.

Development: over a path of 10 cm.

Drying: in air.

Detection: spray with *vanillin reagent R* and heat at 100-105 °C for 5 min; examine in daylight.

Results: see below the sequence of the zones present in the chromatograms obtained with the reference solution and the test solution. Furthermore, other faint zones may be present in the chromatogram obtained with the test solution.

Top of the plate	
	A dark violet-blue zone (solvent front) A dark violet-blue zone
	_______
Oleuropein: a brownish-green zone	A brownish-green zone (oleuropein)
_______	_______
Rutin: a brownish-yellow zone	
Reference solution	**Test solution**

TESTS

Foreign matter (*2.8.2*): maximum 2 per cent.

Loss on drying (*2.2.32*): maximum 10.0 per cent, determined on 1.000 g of the powdered drug (355) by drying in an oven at 100-105 °C for 2 h.

Total ash (*2.4.16*): maximum 9.0 per cent.

ASSAY

Liquid chromatography (*2.2.29*).

Test solution. In a flask, place 1.000 g of the powdered drug (355) and add 50 ml of *methanol R*. Heat in a water-bath at 60 °C for 30 min with shaking. Allow to cool and filter into a 100 ml volumetric flask. Rinse the flask and the filter with *methanol R* and dilute to 100.0 ml with the same solvent. Dilute 2.0 ml of the solution to 20.0 ml with *water R*.

Reference solution. Dissolve 5.0 mg of *oleuropein R* in 5.0 ml of *methanol R*. Dilute 1.0 ml of the solution to 25.0 ml with *water R*.

Column:

- *size*: l = 0.15 m, Ø = 3.9 mm,
- *stationary phase*: *octadecylsilyl silica gel for chromatography R* (5 µm),
- *temperature*: 25 °C.

Mobile phase:

- *mobile phase A*: dilute 1.0 ml of *glacial acetic acid R* to 100 ml with *water R*,
- *mobile phase B*: *methanol R*,

Time (min)	Mobile phase A (per cent *V/V*)	Mobile phase B (per cent *V/V*)
0 - 5	85 → 40	15 → 60
5 - 12	40 → 20	60 → 80
12 - 15	20 → 85	80 → 15

Flow rate: 1 ml/min.

Detection: spectrophotometer at 254 nm.

Injection: 20 µl.

Retention time: oleuropein = about 9 min.

Calculate the percentage content of oleuropein from the expression.

$$\frac{A_1 \times m_2 \times p \times 8}{A_2 \times m_1}$$

A_1 = area of the peak due to oleuropein in the chromatogram obtained with the test solution,

A_2 = area of the peak due to oleuropein in the chromatogram obtained with the reference solution,

m_1 = mass of the drug to be examined, in grams,

m_2 = mass of *oleuropein R* in the reference solution, in grams,

p = percentage content of oleuropein in *oleuropein R*.

01/2005:1456

OLIVE OIL, REFINED

Olivae oleum raffinatum

DEFINITION

Refined olive oil is the fatty oil obtained by refining of crude olive oil, obtained by cold expression or other suitable mechanical means from the ripe drupes of *Olea europaea* L. A suitable antioxidant may be added.

CHARACTERS

A clear, colourless or greenish-yellow, transparent liquid, practically insoluble in alcohol, miscible with light petroleum (50 °C to 70 °C).

Monographs N-O

When cooled, it begins to become cloudy at 10 °C and becomes a butter-like mass at about 0 °C. It has a relative density of about 0.913.

IDENTIFICATION

A. It complies with the test for absorbance (see Tests).

B. Carry out the test for identification of fatty oils by thin-layer chromatography (*2.3.2*). The chromatogram obtained shows spots corresponding to those in the typical chromatogram for olive oil. For certain types of refined olive oil, the difference in the size of spots E and F is less pronounced than in the typical chromatogram.

TESTS

Acid value (*2.5.1*). Not more than 0.5, determined on 10.0 g.

Peroxide value (*2.5.5, Method A*). Not more than 10.0. If intended for use in the manufacture of parenteral dosage forms, not more than 5.0.

Unsaponifiable matter. Not more than 1.5 per cent. Place 5.0 g (*m* g) in a 150 ml flask fitted with a reflux condenser. Add 50 ml of *2 M alcoholic potassium hydroxide R* and heat on a water-bath for 1 h, shaking frequently. Add 50 ml of *water R* through the top of the condenser, shake, allow to cool and transfer the contents of the flask to a separating funnel. Rinse the flask with several portions to a total of 50 ml of *light petroleum R1* and add the rinsings to the separating funnel. Shake vigorously for 1 min. Allow to separate and transfer the aqueous layer to a second separating funnel. If an emulsion forms, add small quantities of *alcohol R* or a concentrated solution of *potassium hydroxide R*. Shake the aqueous layer with 2 quantities, each of 50 ml, of *light petroleum R1*. Combine the light petroleum layers in a third separating funnel and wash with 3 quantities, each of 50 ml, of *alcohol (50 per cent V/V) R*. Transfer the light petroleum layer to a tared 250 ml flask. Rinse the separating funnel with small quantities of *light petroleum R1* and add to the flask. Evaporate the light petroleum on a water-bath and dry the residue at 100 °C to 105 °C for 15 min, keeping the flask horizontal. Allow to cool in a desiccator and weigh (*a* g). Repeat the drying for successive periods of 15 min until the loss of mass between 2 successive weighings does not exceed 0.1 per cent. Dissolve the residue in 20 ml of *alcohol R*, previously neutralised to 0.1 ml of *bromophenol blue solution R*. If necessary, titrate with *0.1 M hydrochloric acid* (*b* ml).

Calculate the percentage content of unsaponifiable matter from the expression:

$$\frac{100\,(a - 0.032b)}{m}$$

If $0.032b$ is greater than 5 per cent of *a*, the test is invalid and must be repeated.

Alkaline impurities (*2.4.19*). It complies with the test for alkaline impurities in fatty oils.

Absorbance (*2.2.25*). Dissolve 1.00 g in *cyclohexane R* and dilute to 100.0 ml with the same solvent. The absorbance measured at 270 nm is 0.20 to 1.20.

Composition of fatty acids (*2.4.22, Method A*). The fatty acid fraction of the oil has the following composition:

- *saturated fatty acids of chain length less than C_{16}*: not more than 0.1 per cent,
- *palmitic acid*: 7.5 per cent to 20.0 per cent,
- *palmitoleic acid* (equivalent chain length on polyethyleneglycol adipate 16.3): not more than 3.5 per cent,
- *stearic acid*: 0.5 per cent to 5.0 per cent,
- *oleic acid* (equivalent chain length on polyethyleneglycol adipate 18.3): 56.0 per cent to 85.0 per cent,
- *linoleic acid* (equivalent chain length on polyethyleneglycol adipate 18.9): 3.5 per cent to 20.0 per cent,
- *linolenic acid* (equivalent chain length on polyethyleneglycol adipate 19.7): not more than 1.2 per cent,
- *arachidic acid*: not more than 0.7 per cent,
- *eicosenoic acid* (equivalent chain length on polyethyleneglycol adipate 20.3): not more than 0.4 per cent,
- *behenic acid*: not more than 0.2 per cent,
- *lignoceric acid*: not more than 0.2 per cent.

Sterols (*2.4.23*). The sterol fraction of the oil has the following composition:

- *sum of contents of β-sitosterol, Δ5,23-stigmastadienol, clerosterol, sitostanol, Δ5-avenasterol and Δ5,24-stigmastadienol*: not less than 93.0 per cent,
- *cholesterol*: not more than 0.5 per cent,
- *Δ7-stigmasterol*: not more than 0.5 per cent,
- *campesterol*: not more than 4.0 per cent,

and the content of stigmasterol is not more than that of campesterol.

Sesame oil. In a ground-glass-stoppered cylinder shake 10 ml for about 1 min with a mixture of 0.5 ml of a 0.35 per cent *V/V* solution of *furfural R* in *acetic anhydride R* and 4.5 ml of *acetic anhydride R*. Filter through a filter paper impregnated with *acetic anhydride R*. To the filtrate add 0.2 ml of *sulphuric acid R*. No bluish-green colour develops.

Water (*2.5.32*). If intended for use in the manufacture of parenteral dosage forms, not more than 0.1 per cent, determined on 5.0 g by the coulometric method. Use a mixture of equal volumes of *decanol R* and *anhydrous methanol R* as solvent.

STORAGE

Store in a well-filled container, protected from light, at a temperature not exceeding 25 °C. If intended for use in the manufacture of parenteral dosage forms, store under an inert gas.

LABELLING

The label states:

- where applicable, that the substance is suitable for use in the manufacture of parenteral dosage forms,
- the name and concentration of any added antioxidant,
- the name of the inert gas.

01/2005:0518

OLIVE OIL, VIRGIN

Olivae oleum virginale

DEFINITION

Virgin olive oil is the fatty oil obtained by cold expression or other suitable mechanical means from the ripe drupes of *Olea europaea* L.

CHARACTERS

A clear, yellow or greenish-yellow, transparent liquid with a characteristic odour, practically insoluble in alcohol, miscible with light petroleum (50 °C to 70 °C).

Monographs N-O

When cooled, it begins to become cloudy at 10 °C and becomes a butter-like mass at about 0 °C. It has a relative density of about 0.913.

IDENTIFICATION

Carry out the test for identification of fatty oils by thin-layer chromatography (*2.3.2*). The chromatogram obtained shows spots corresponding to those in the typical chromatogram for olive oil. For certain types of olive oil, the difference in the size of spots E and F is less pronounced than in the typical chromatogram.

TESTS

Acid value (*2.5.1*). Not more than 2.0, determined on 5.0 g.

Peroxide value (*2.5.5, Method A*). Not more than 20.0.

Unsaponifiable matter. Not more than 1.5 per cent. Place 5.0 g (*m* g) in a 150 ml flask fitted with a reflux condenser. Add 50 ml of *2 M alcoholic potassium hydroxide R* and heat on a water-bath for 1 h, shaking frequently. Add 50 ml of *water R* through the top of the condenser, shake, allow to cool and transfer the contents of the flask to a separating funnel. Rinse the flask with several portions to a total of 50 ml of *light petroleum R1* and add the rinsings to the separating funnel. Shake vigorously for 1 min. Allow to separate and transfer the aqueous layer to a second separating funnel. If an emulsion forms, add small quantities of *alcohol R* or a concentrated solution of *potassium hydroxide R*. Shake the aqueous layer with 2 quantities, each of 50 ml, of *light petroleum R1*. Combine the light petroleum layers in a third separating funnel and wash with 3 quantities, each of 50 ml, of *alcohol (50 per cent V/V) R*. Transfer the light petroleum layer to a tared 250 ml flask. Rinse the separating funnel with small quantities of *light petroleum R1* and add to the flask. Evaporate the light petroleum on a water-bath and dry the residue at 100 °C to 105 °C for 15 min, keeping the flask horizontal. Allow to cool in a desiccator and weigh (*a* g). Repeat the drying for successive periods of 15 min until the loss of mass between 2 successive weighings does not exceed 0.1 per cent. Dissolve the residue in 20 ml of *alcohol R*, previously neutralised to 0.1 ml of *bromophenol blue solution R*. If necessary, titrate with *0.1 M hydrochloric acid* (*b* ml).

Calculate the percentage content of unsaponifiable matter from the expression:

$$\frac{100\,(a - 0.032b)}{m}$$

If 0.032*b* is greater than 5 per cent of *a*, the test is invalid and must be repeated.

Absorbance (*2.2.25*). Dissolve 1.00 g in *cyclohexane R* and dilute to 100.0 ml with the same solvent. The absorbance measured at 270 nm is not greater than 0.20. The ratio of the absorbance at 232 nm to that at 270 nm is greater than 8.

Composition of fatty acids (*2.4.22, Method A*). The fatty acid fraction of the oil has the following composition:

- *saturated fatty acids of chain length less than* C_{16}: not more than 0.1 per cent,
- *palmitic acid*: 7.5 per cent to 20.0 per cent,
- *palmitoleic acid* (equivalent chain length on polyethyleneglycol adipate 16.3): not more than 3.5 per cent,
- *stearic acid*: 0.5 per cent to 5.0 per cent,
- *oleic acid* (equivalent chain length on polyethyleneglycol adipate 18.3): 56.0 per cent to 85.0 per cent,
- *linoleic acid* (equivalent chain length on polyethyleneglycol adipate 18.9): 3.5 per cent to 20.0 per cent,
- *linolenic acid* (equivalent chain length on polyethyleneglycol adipate 19.7): not more than 1.2 per cent,
- *arachidic acid*: not more than 0.7 per cent,
- *eicosenoic acid* (equivalent chain length on polyethyleneglycol adipate 20.3): not more than 0.4 per cent,
- *behenic acid*: not more than 0.2 per cent,
- *lignoceric acid*: not more than 0.2 per cent.

Sterols (*2.4.23*). The sterol fraction of the oil has the following composition:

- *sum of contents of β-sitosterol, Δ5,23-stigmastadienol, clerosterol, sitostanol, Δ5-avenasterol and Δ5,24-stigmastadienol*: not less than 93.0 per cent,
- *cholesterol*: not more than 0.5 per cent,
- *Δ7-stigmasterol*: not more than 0.5 per cent,
- *campesterol*: not more than 4.0 per cent,

and the content of stigmasterol is not more than that of campesterol.

Sesame oil. In a ground-glass-stoppered cylinder shake 10 ml for about 1 min with a mixture of 0.5 ml of a 0.35 per cent *V/V* solution of *furfural R* in *acetic anhydride R* and 4.5 ml of *acetic anhydride R*. Filter through a filter paper impregnated with *acetic anhydride R*. To the filtrate add 0.2 ml of *sulphuric acid R*. No bluish-green colour develops.

STORAGE

Store in a well-filled container, protected from light, at a temperature not exceeding 25 °C.

01/2005:1457

OLSALAZINE SODIUM

Olsalazinum natricum

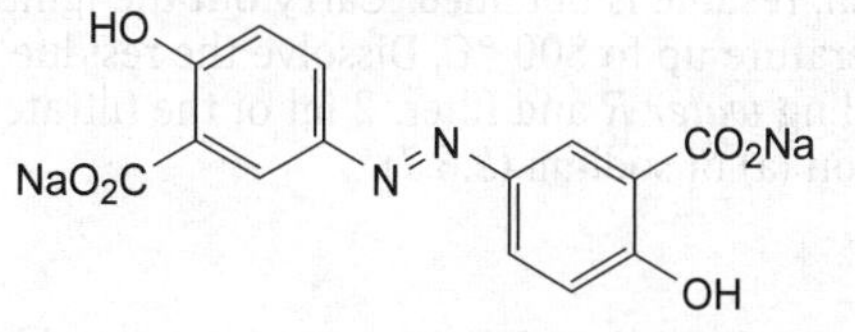

$C_{14}H_8N_2Na_2O_6$ M_r 346.2

DEFINITION

Olsalazine sodium contains not less than 98.0 per cent and not more than the equivalent of 102.0 per cent of disodium 3,3′-diazenediylbis(6-hydroxybenzoate), calculated with reference to the dried and acetate-free substance.

CHARACTERS

A yellow, fine, crystalline powder, sparingly soluble in water, soluble in dimethyl sulphoxide, very slightly soluble in methanol.

It shows polymorphism.

IDENTIFICATION

First identification: B, D.

Second identification: A, C, D.

A. Dissolve 40.0 mg in 5 ml of *0.1 M sodium hydroxide* and dilute to 100.0 ml with a 7.8 g/l solution of *sodium dihydrogen phosphate R* adjusted to pH 7.2 with *strong sodium hydroxide solution R* (buffer solution). Dilute

2.0 ml of the solution to 100.0 ml with the buffer solution. Examined between 240 nm and 400 nm (*2.2.25*), the solution shows absorption maxima at 255 nm and 362 nm. The ratio of the absorbance measured at the maximum at 255 nm to that measured at the maximum at 362 nm is 0.53 to 0.56.

B. Examine by infrared absorption spectrophotometry (*2.2.24*), comparing with the spectrum obtained with *olsalazine sodium CRS*. If the spectra obtained in the solid state show differences, dissolve the substance to be examined and the reference substance separately in *methanol R*, evaporate to dryness and record new spectra using the residues.

C. Examine by thin-layer chromatography (*2.2.27*), using a *TLC silica gel* F_{254} *plate R*.

Test solution. Dissolve 10 mg of the substance to be examined in a mixture of 1 volume of *dilute ammonia R2* and 4 volumes of *alcohol R* and dilute to 10 ml with the same mixture of solvents.

Reference solution (a). Dissolve 10 mg of *olsalazine sodium CRS* in a mixture of 1 volume of *dilute ammonia R2* and 4 volumes of *alcohol R* and dilute to 10 ml with the same mixture of solvents.

Reference solution (b). Dissolve 5 mg of *sulfasalazine CRS* in reference solution (a) and dilute to 5 ml with reference solution (a).

Apply to the plate 10 µl of each solution. Develop over a path of 15 cm using a mixture of 5 volumes of *anhydrous formic acid R*, 50 volumes of *acetone R* and 60 volumes of *methylene chloride R*. Allow the plate to dry in air and examine in ultraviolet light at 254 nm. The principal spot in the chromatogram obtained with the test solution is similar in position and size to the principal spot in the chromatogram obtained with reference solution (a). The test is not valid unless the chromatogram obtained with reference solution (b) shows two separated spots.

D. To 0.5 g of the substance to be examined add 2 ml of *sulphuric acid R*. Progressively heat to ignition and continue heating until an almost white, or at most greyish, residue is obtained. Carry out the ignition at a temperature up to 800 °C. Dissolve the residue in 10 ml of boiling *water R* and filter. 2 ml of the filtrate gives reaction (a) of sodium (*2.3.1*).

TESTS

Acetate. Not more than 1.0 per cent, determined by liquid chromatography (*2.2.29*).

Test solution. Dissolve 0.125 g of the substance to be examined in 25.0 ml of *water R* and add 1.0 ml of *dilute hydrochloric acid R*. Centrifuge and then filter the solution through a 0.45 µm filter and also through an appropriate filter for removal of chlorides.

Reference solution (a). Dissolve 0.140 g of *sodium acetate R*, 0.150 g of *sodium formate R* and 0.180 g of *potassium sulphate R* in 100.0 ml of *water R*. Dilute 1.0 ml of this solution to 100.0 ml with *water R*.

Reference solution (b). Use suitable amounts of *sodium acetate R* to prepare not fewer than five reference solutions containing 10 µg/ml to 50 µg/ml of acetate.

The ion-exclusion chromatographic procedure may be carried out using:

- a separation column 0.25 m long and 6 mm in internal diameter packed with *ion-exclusion resin for chromatography R* with a capacity of about 27 meq/column.
- a suppressor column,
- as mobile phase at a flow rate of 0.9 ml/min *0.0001 M hydrochloric acid,*
- a conductivity detector set at 10 µS·cm^{-1}.

Inject 0.1 ml of reference solution (a). The chromatogram shows three separated peaks. Inject 0.1 ml of the test solution and 0.1 ml of reference solution (b). Prepare a calibration curve from the average of the readings obtained with the reference solutions and determine the concentration of acetate in the test solution from the curve obtained. Measure the peak area for acetate. Calculate the percentage content of acetate content from the following expression:

$$\frac{2.6\,c}{m}$$

c = concentration of acetate in the test solution (µg/ml), determined by linear interpolation of the standard curve for reference solution (b),

m = mass of sample (mg).

Methanesulphonic acid. Liquid chromatography (*2.2.29*).

Test solution. Dissolve 0.25 g of the substance to be examined in 20 ml of *water R*, add 1.0 ml of *dilute hydrochloric acid R* and dilute to 25.0 ml with *water R*. Centrifuge and then filter the solution through a 0.45 µm filter and also through an appropriate filter for removal of chloride.

Reference solution (a). Dissolve 0.25 g of *methanesulphonic acid R* in 50 ml of *water R*. Add 0.58 g of *sodium acetate R* and 0.08 g of *sodium chloride R* and dilute to 100.0 ml with *water R*. Dilute 1.0 ml of the solution to 100.0 ml with *water R*.

Reference solution (b). Dissolve 0.10 g of *methanesulphonic acid R* in *water R* and dilute to 100.0 ml with *water R*. Dilute 3.0 ml of the solution to 100.0 ml with *water R*.

The reversed-phase ion chromatographic procedure may be carried out using:

- a pre-column 0.035 m long and 4 mm in internal diameter packed with *reversed-phase ion resin for chromatography R* (10 µm),
- a separation column 0.25 m long and 4 mm in internal diameter packed with *reversed-phase ion resin for chromatography R* (10 µm),
- as mobile phase at a flow rate of 1.0 ml/min, a mixture of 10 volumes of *acetonitrile for chromatography R* and 990 volumes of a solution containing 1.6 g/l of *tetrabutylammonium hydroxide R* and 0.053 g/l of *anhydrous sodium carbonate R,*
- a conductivity detector set at 50 µS·cm^{-1}.

Inject 100 µl of reference solution (a). The test is not valid unless the chromatogram shows 3 separated peaks. Inject 100 µl each of the test solution and reference solution (b). In the chromatogram obtained with the test solution, the area of the peak corresponding to methanesulphonic acid is not greater than the area of the corresponding peak in the chromatogram obtained with reference solution (b) (0.3 per cent).

Related substances. Examine by liquid chromatography (*2.2.29*).

Test solution. Dissolve 20.0 mg of the substance to be examined in mobile phase A and dilute to 25.0 ml with mobile phase A.

Reference solution (a). Dilute 0.5 ml of the test solution to 100.0 ml with the mobile phase A.

Reference solution (b). Dissolve 20.0 mg of *olsalazine sodium for performance test CRS* in mobile phase A and dilute to 25.0 ml with mobile phase A.

The chromatographic procedure may be carried out using:

- a stainless steel column 0.125 m long and 4.0 mm in internal diameter packed with *octadecylsilyl silica gel for chromatography R* (5 µm),
- as mobile phase at a flow rate of 1 ml/min, the following linear gradient programme:

  Mobile phase A. Dissolve 2.38 g of *tetrabutylammonium hydrogen sulphate R* and 3.6 g of *disodium hydrogen phosphate dihydrate R* in 900 ml of *water R*. Adjust to pH 7.6 with *dilute sodium hydroxide solution R*. Dilute to 1000.0 ml with *water R*. Mix 700 ml of this buffer solution with 300 ml of *methanol R*,

  Mobile phase B. Dissolve 4.75 g of *tetrabutylammonium hydrogen sulphate R* and 3.6 g of *disodium hydrogen phosphate dihydrate R* in 900 ml of *water R*. Adjust to pH 7.6 with *dilute sodium hydroxide solution R*. Dilute to 1000.0 ml with *water R*. Mix 350 ml of this buffer solution with 650 ml of *methanol R*,

Time (min)	Mobile phase A (per cent *V/V*)	Mobile phase B (per cent *V/V*)	Comment
0 - 15	55	45	isocratic
15 - 45	55 → 0	45 → 100	linear gradient
45 - 50	0 → 55	100 → 45	return to initial composition
50 - 65	55	45	equilibration

- as detector a spectrophotometer set at 360 nm,

maintaining the temperature of the column at 30 °C.

Inject 20 µl of reference solution (a). Adjust the sensitivity of the system so that the height of the principal peak in the chromatogram obtained is at least 50 per cent of the full scale of the recorder.

Inject 20 µl of reference solution (b). The test is not valid unless the chromatogram obtained is similar to the chromatogram obtained with *olsalazine sodium for performance test CRS*. If necessary, adjust the proportion of mobile phase A in the mobile phase (increasing the proportion of mobile phase A increases the retention time).

Inject 20 µl of the test solution. In the chromatogram obtained with the test solution: the area of any peak, apart from the principal peak, is not greater than twice the area of the principal peak in the chromatogram obtained with reference solution (a) (1 per cent), and not more than one such peak has an area greater than the area of the principal peak in the chromatogram obtained with reference solution (a) (0.5 per cent); the sum of the areas of all the peaks, apart from the principal peak, is not greater than four times the area of the principal peak in the chromatogram obtained with reference solution (a) (2 per cent). Disregard any peak with an area less than 0.05 times that of the principal peak in the chromatogram obtained with reference solution (a) (0.025 per cent).

Heavy metals (*2.4.8*). 1.0 g complies with limit test D for heavy metals (20 ppm). Prepare the standard using 2 ml of *lead standard solution (10 ppm Pb) R*.

Loss on drying (*2.2.32*). Not more than 2.0 per cent, determined on 1.000 g by drying in an oven at 150 °C.

ASSAY

Dissolve 0.100 g in 15 ml of *ethylene glycol R*. Add 40 ml of *dioxan R* and 0.2 ml of a 224 g/l solution of *potassium chloride R*. Titrate with *0.1 M hydrochloric acid*, determining the end-point potentiometrically (*2.2.20*). Carry out a blank titration.

Correct the volume consumed for the content of acetate, taking the molecular mass of acetate to be 59.0.

1 ml of *0.1 M hydrochloric acid* is equivalent to 17.31 mg of $C_{14}H_8N_2Na_2O_6$.

IMPURITIES

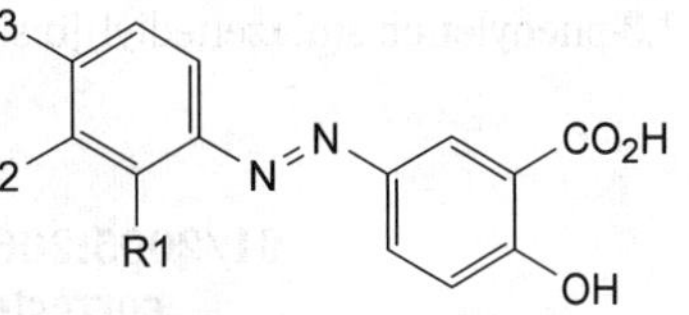

A. R1 = H, R2 = CO_2H, R3 = OCH_3: 6-hydroxy-6′-methoxy-3,3′-diazenediyldibenzoic acid,

B. R1 = OH, R2 = CO_2H, R3 = H: 2,6′-dihydroxy-3,3′-diazenediyldibenzoic acid,

C. R1 = R2 = H, R3 = OH: 2-hydroxy-5-[(4-hydroxyphenyl)diazenyl]benzoic acid,

D. R1 = H, R2 = CO_2H, R3 = Cl: 6-chloro-6′-hydroxy-3,3′-diazenediyldibenzoic acid,

E. R1 = H, R2 = $CO\text{-}CH_2\text{-}SO_3H$, R3 = OH: 2-hydroxy-5-[[4-hydroxy-3-(sulphoacetyl)phenyl]diazenyl]benzoic acid,

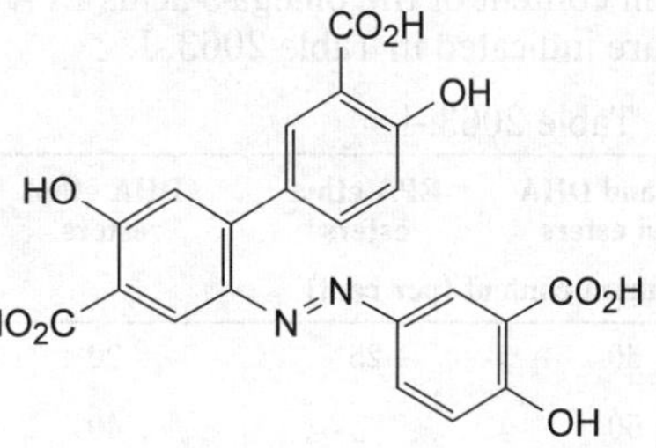

F. 2′-[(3-carboxy-4-hydroxyphenyl)diazenyl]-4,5′-dihydroxybiphenyl-3,4′-dicarboxylic acid,

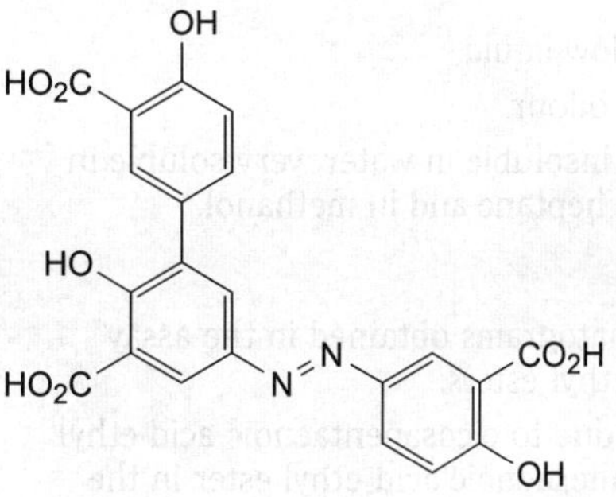

G. 5-[(3-carboxy-4-hydroxyphenyl)diazenyl]-2,4′-dihydroxybiphenyl-3,3′-dicarboxylic acid,

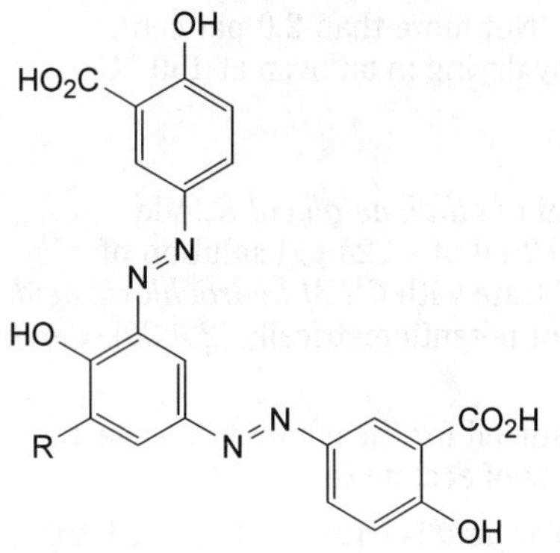

H. R = CO_2H: 3,3′-[5-carboxy-4-hydroxy-1,3-phenylenebis(diazenediyl)]bis(6-hydroxybenzoic) acid,

I. R = H: 3,3′-[4-hydroxy-1,3-phenylenebis(diazenediyl)]bis(6-hydroxybenzoic) acid.

01/2005:2063
corrected

OMEGA-3-ACID ETHYL ESTERS 60

Omega-3 acidorum esteri ethylici 60

DEFINITION

Ethyl esters of *alpha*-linolenic acid (C18:3 n-3), moroctic acid (C18:4 n-3), eicosatetraenoic acid (C20:4 n-3), timnodonic (eicosapentaenoic) acid (C20:5 n-3; EPA), heneicosapentaenoic acid (C21:5 n-3), clupanodonic acid (C22:5 n-3) and cervonic (docosahexaenoic) acid (C22:6 n-3; DHA). Omega-3-acid ethyl esters 60 are obtained by transesterification of the body oil of fat fish species coming from families like *Engraulidae, Carangidae, Clupeidae, Osmeridae, Salmonidae* and *Scombridae* and subsequent physico-chemical purification processes, including molecular distillation. The minimum content of total omega-3-acid ethyl esters and the minimum content of the omega-3-acids EPA and DHA ethyl esters are indicated in Table 2063.-1.

Table 2063.-1

Total omega-3-acid ethyl esters	EPA and DHA ethyl esters	EPA ethyl esters	DHA ethyl esters
Minimum content (per cent)			
65	50	25	20
60	50	–	40
55	50	40	–

Tocopherol may be added as an antioxidant.

CHARACTERS

Appearance: light yellow liquid.

It has a slight fish-like odour.

Solubility: practically insoluble in water, very soluble in acetone, in ethanol, in heptane and in methanol.

IDENTIFICATION

A. Examine the chromatograms obtained in the assay for EPA and DHA ethyl esters.

Results: the peaks due to eicosapentaenoic acid ethyl ester and to docosahexaenoic acid ethyl ester in the chromatogram obtained with the test solution are similar in retention time to the corresponding peaks in the chromatogram obtained with the reference solution.

B. The substance to be examined complies with the assay for Total omega-3-acid ethyl esters.

TESTS

Absorbance (*2.2.25*): maximum 0.60 at 233 nm.

Dilute 0.300 g of the substance to be examined to 50.0 ml with *trimethylpentane R*. Dilute 2.0 ml of this solution to 50.0 ml wtih *trimethylpentane R*.

Acid value (*2.5.1*): maximum 2.0, determined on 10 g in 50 ml of the prescribed mixture of solvents.

Peroxide value (*2.5.5, Method A*): maximum 10.0.

Anisidine value: maximum 20.0.

The anisidine value is defined as 100 times the absorbance measured in a 1 cm cell of a solution containing 1 g of the substance to be examined in 100 ml of a mixture of solvents and reagents according to the method described below.

Carry out the operations as rapidly as possible, avoiding exposure to actinic light.

Test solution (a). Dilute 0.500 g of the substance to be examined to 25.0 ml with *trimethylpentane R*.

Test solution (b). To 5.0 ml of test solution (a) add 1.0 ml of a 2.5 g/l solution of *p-anisidine R* in *glacial acetic acid R*, shake and protect from light.

Reference solution. To 5.0 ml of *trimethylpentane R* add 1.0 ml of a 2.5 g/l solution of *p-anisidine R* in *glacial acetic acid R*, shake and protect from light.

Measure the absorbance (*2.2.25*) of test solution (a) at 350 nm using *trimethylpentane R1* as the compensation liquid. Measure the absorbance of test solution (b) at 350 nm exactly 10 min after its preparation, using the reference solution as the compensation liquid.

Calculate the anisidine value from the expression:

$$\frac{25 \times (1.2\, A_s - A_b)}{m}$$

A_s = absorbance of test solution (b) at 350 nm,

A_b = absorbance of test solution (a) at 350 nm,

m = mass of the substance to be examined in test solution (a), in grams.

Oligomers and partial glycerides. Size exclusion chromatography (*2.2.30*).

Test solution. Dilute 10.0 mg of the substance to be examined to 10.0 ml with *tetrahydrofuran R*.

Reference solution. In a 100 ml volumetric flask dissolve 50 mg of *monodocosahexaenoin R*, 30 mg of *didocosahexaenoin R* and 20 mg of *tridocosahexaenoin R* in *tetrahydrofuran R* and dilute to 100.0 ml with the same solvent.

Column 1:

– *dimensions*: l = 0.3 m, Ø = 7.8 mm,

– *stationary phase*: *styrene-divinylbenzene copolymer R* (7 µm), with a pore size of 10 nm.

Columns 2 and 3 placed closest to the injector:

– *dimensions*: l = 0.3 m, Ø = 7.8 mm,

– *stationary phase*: *styrene-divinylbenzene copolymer R* (7 µm), with a pore size of 50 nm.

Mobile phase: *tetrahydrofuran R*.

Flow rate: 0.8 ml/min.

Detection: differential refractometer.

Injection: 40 µl.

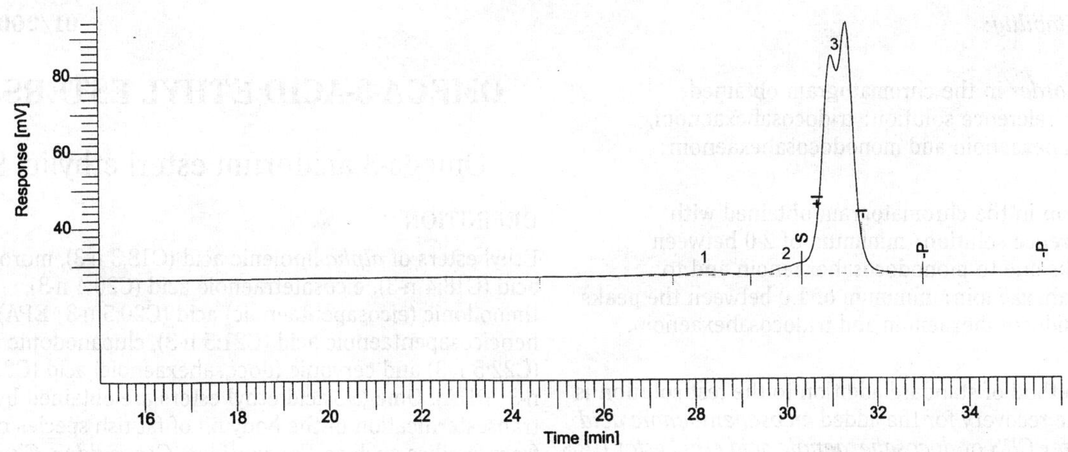

Figure 2063.-1. – *Chromatogram for the test for oligomers and partial glycerides in omega-3-acid ethyl esters 60*

Figure 2063.-2. – *Chromatogram for the assay of omega-3-acid ethyl ester in omega-3-acid ethyl esters*

Monographs N-O

System suitability:

- *elution order* in the chromatogram obtained with the reference solution: tridocosahexaenoin, didocosahexaenoin and monodocosahexaenoin;
- *resolution* in the chromatogram obtained with the reference solution: minimum of 2.0 between the peaks due to monodocosahexaenoin and to didocosahexaenoin; minimum of 1.0 between the peaks due to didocosahexaenoin and tridocosahexaenoin,
- if the method of standard addition to the test solution is used, the recovery for the added *eicosapentaenoic acid ethyl ester CRS* or *docosahexaenoic acid ethyl ester CRS* is minimum 95 per cent.

Calculate the percentage content of oligomers plus partial glycerides using the following expression:

$$\frac{B}{A} \times 100$$

A = sum of areas of all the peaks in the chromatogram,

B = sum of the areas of the peaks with a retention time smaller than those of the ethyl ester peaks.

The ethyl ester peaks, which may be present in the form of an unresolved double peak, are identified as the major peaks in the chromatogram (Figure 2063.-1).

Limit:

- *oligomers + partial glycerides*: maximum 7.0 per cent.

Monographs N-O

ASSAY

EPA and DHA ethyl esters (*2.4.29*). See Figure 2063.-2.

Total omega-3-acids ethyl esters (*2.4.29*). See Figure 2063.-2.

STORAGE

Under an inert gas, in an airtight container, protected from light.

LABELLING

The label states:

- the content of total omega-3-acid ethyl esters,
- the content of EPA ethyl ester and DHA ethyl ester,
- the concentration of any added tocopherol.

01/2005:1250

OMEGA-3-ACID ETHYL ESTERS 90

Omega-3 acidorum esteri ethylici 90

DEFINITION

Ethyl esters of *alpha*-linolenic acid (C18:3 n-3), moroctic acid (C18:4 n-3), eicosatetraenoic acid (C20:4 n-3), timnodonic (eicosapentaenoic) acid (C20:5 n-3; EPA), heneicosapentaenoic acid (C21:5 n-3), clupanodonic acid (C22:5 n-3) and cervonic (docosahexaenoic) acid (C22:6 n-3; DHA). Omega-3-acid ethyl esters are obtained by transesterification of the body oil of fat fish species coming from families such as *Engraulidae, Carangidae, Clupeidae, Osmeridae, Salmonidae* and *Scombridae* and subsequent physico-chemical purification processes, including urea fractionation followed by molecular distillation.

Content:

- EPA and DHA ethyl esters: minimum 80 per cent, with minimum 40 per cent of EPA ethyl esters and minimum 34 per cent of DHA ethyl esters,
- total omega-3-acid ethyl esters: minimum 90 per cent.

Tocopherol may be added as an antioxidant.

CHARACTERS

Appearance: light yellow liquid.

It has a slight fish-like odour.

Solubility: practically insoluble in water, very soluble in acetone, in ethanol, in heptane and in methanol.

IDENTIFICATION

Examine the chromatograms obtained in the assay for EPA and DHA ethyl esters.

Results: the peaks due to eicosapentaenoic acid ethyl ester and to docosahexaenoic acid ethyl ester in the chromatogram obtained with the test solution are similar in retention time and size to the corresponding peaks in the chromatogram obtained with the reference solution.

TESTS

Absorbance (*2.2.25*): maximum 0.55 at 233 nm.

Dilute 0.300 g of the substance to be examined to 50.0 ml with *trimethylpentane R.* Dilute 2.0 ml of this solution to 50.0 ml with *trimethylpentane R.*

Acid value (*2.5.1*): maximum 2.0, determined on 10 g in 50 ml of the prescribed mixture of solvents.

Anisidine value: maximum 20.0.

The anisidine value is defined as 100 times the absorbance measured in a 1 cm cell of a solution containing 1 g of the substance to be examined in 100 ml of a mixture of solvents and reagents according to the method described below.

Carry out the operations as rapidly as possible, avoiding exposure to actinic light.

Test solution (a). Dilute 0.500 g of the substance to be examined to 25.0 ml with *trimethylpentane R.*

Test solution (b). To 5.0 ml of test solution (a) add 1.0 ml of a 2.5 g/l solution of *p-anisidine R* in *glacial acetic acid R,* shake and protect from light.

Reference solution. To 5.0 ml of *trimethylpentane R* add 1.0 ml of a 2.5 g/l solution of *p-anisidine R* in *glacial acetic acid R,* shake and protect from light.

Measure the absorbance (*2.2.25*) of test solution (a) at 350 nm using *trimethylpentane R1* as the compensation liquid. Measure the absorbance of test solution (b) at 350 nm exactly 10 min after its preparation, using the reference solution as the compensation liquid.

Calculate the anisidine value from the expression:

$$\frac{25 \times (1.2A_s - A_b)}{m}$$

A_s = absorbance of test solution (b) at 350 nm,

A_b = absorbance of test solution (a) at 350 nm,

m = mass of the substance to be examined in test solution (a), in grams.

Peroxide value (*2.5.5, Method A*): maximum 10.0.

Oligomers. Size-exclusion chromatography (*2.2.30*).

Test solution. Dilute 10.0 mg of the substance to be examined to 10.0 ml with *tetrahydrofuran R*.

Reference solution. Into a 100 ml volumetric flask dissolve 50 mg of *monodocosahexaenoin R*, 30 mg of *didocosahexaenoin R* and 20 mg of *tridocosahexaenoin R* in *tetrahydrofuran R* and dilute to 100.0 ml with the same solvent.

Column 1:

– *size*: *l* = 0.3 m, Ø = 7.8 mm,

– *stationary phase*: *styrene-divinylbenzene copolymer R* (7 µm) with a pore size of 10 nm.

Columns 2 and 3 placed closest to the injector:

– *size*: *l* = 0.3 m, Ø = 7.8 mm,

– *stationary phase*: *styrene-divinylbenzene copolymer R* (7 µm) with a pore size of 50 nm.

Mobile phase: *tetrahydrofuran R.*

Flow rate: 0.8 ml/min.

Detection: differential refractometer.

Injection: 40 µl.

System suitability:

– *elution order* in the chromatogram obtained with the reference solution: tridocosahexaenoin, didocosahexaenoin, monodocosahexaenoin,

– *resolution* in the chromatogram obtained with the reference solution: minimum of 2.0 between the peaks due to monodocosahexaenoin and to didocosahexaenoin and minimum of 1.0 between the peaks due to didocosahexaenoin and to tridocosahexaenoin,

– if the method of standard addition to the test solution is used, the recovery for the added *eicosapentaenoic acid ethyl ester CRS* or *docosahexaenoic acid ethyl ester CRS* is minimum 95 per cent.

Calculate the percentage content of oligomers using the following expression:

$$\frac{B}{A} \times 100$$

A = sum of areas of all the peaks in the chromatogram,

B = sum of the areas of the peaks with a retention time smaller than those of the ethyl ester peaks.

The ethyl ester peaks, which may be present in the form of an unresolved double peak, are identified as the major peaks in the chromatogram (Figure 1250.-1).

Limit:

– *oligomers*: maximum 1.0 per cent.

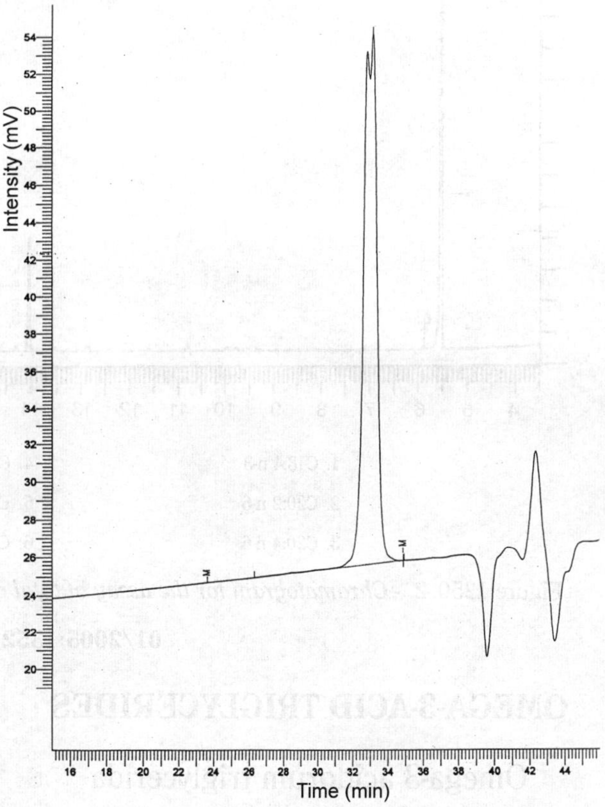

Figure 1250.-1. – *Chromatogram of the test for oligomers in omega-3-acid ethyl esters 90*

ASSAY

EPA and DHA ethyl esters (*2.4.29*). See Figure 1250.-2.

Total omega-3-acid ethyl esters (*2.4.29*). See Figure 1250.-2.

STORAGE

Under an inert gas, in an airtight container, protected from light.

LABELLING

The label states the concentration of any added tocopherol.

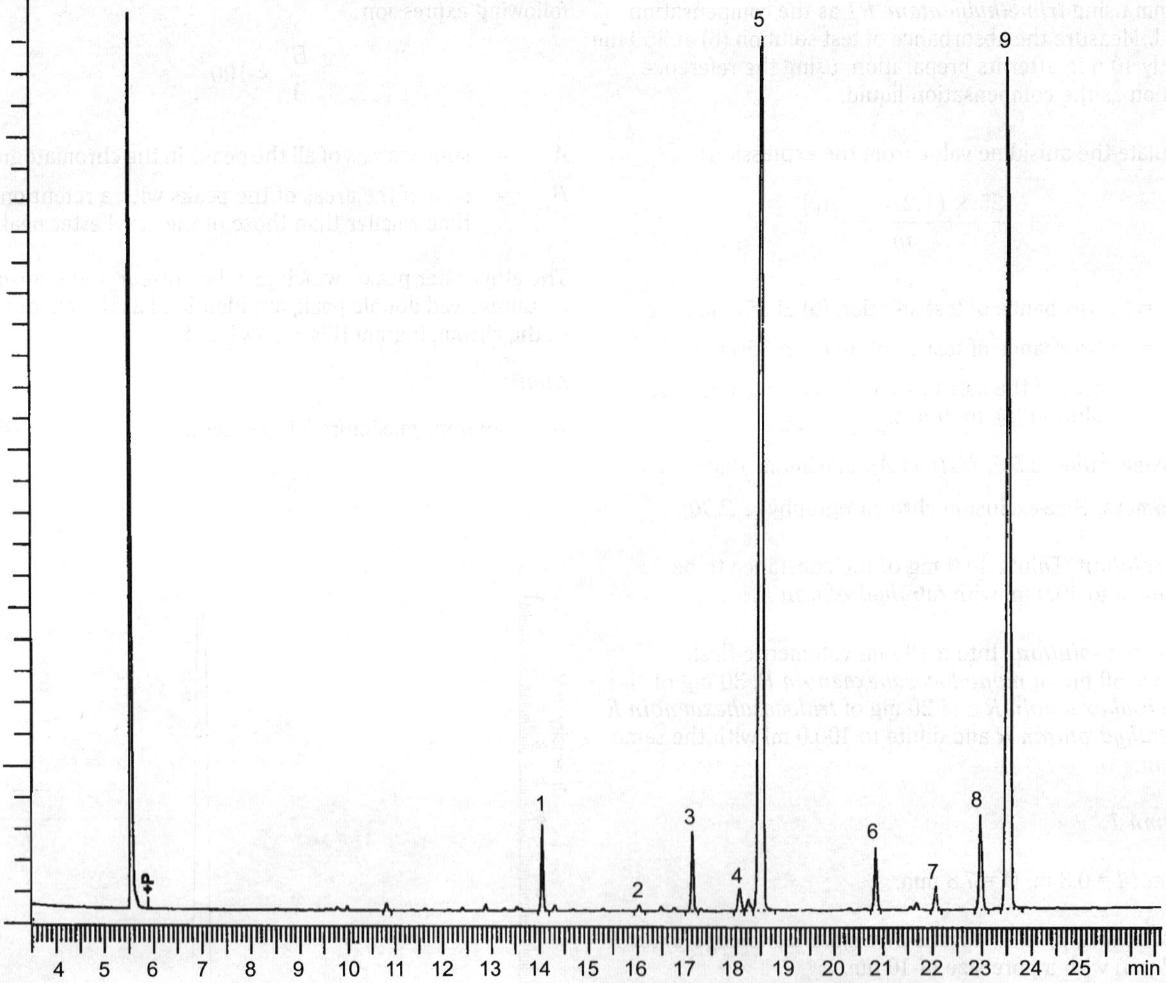

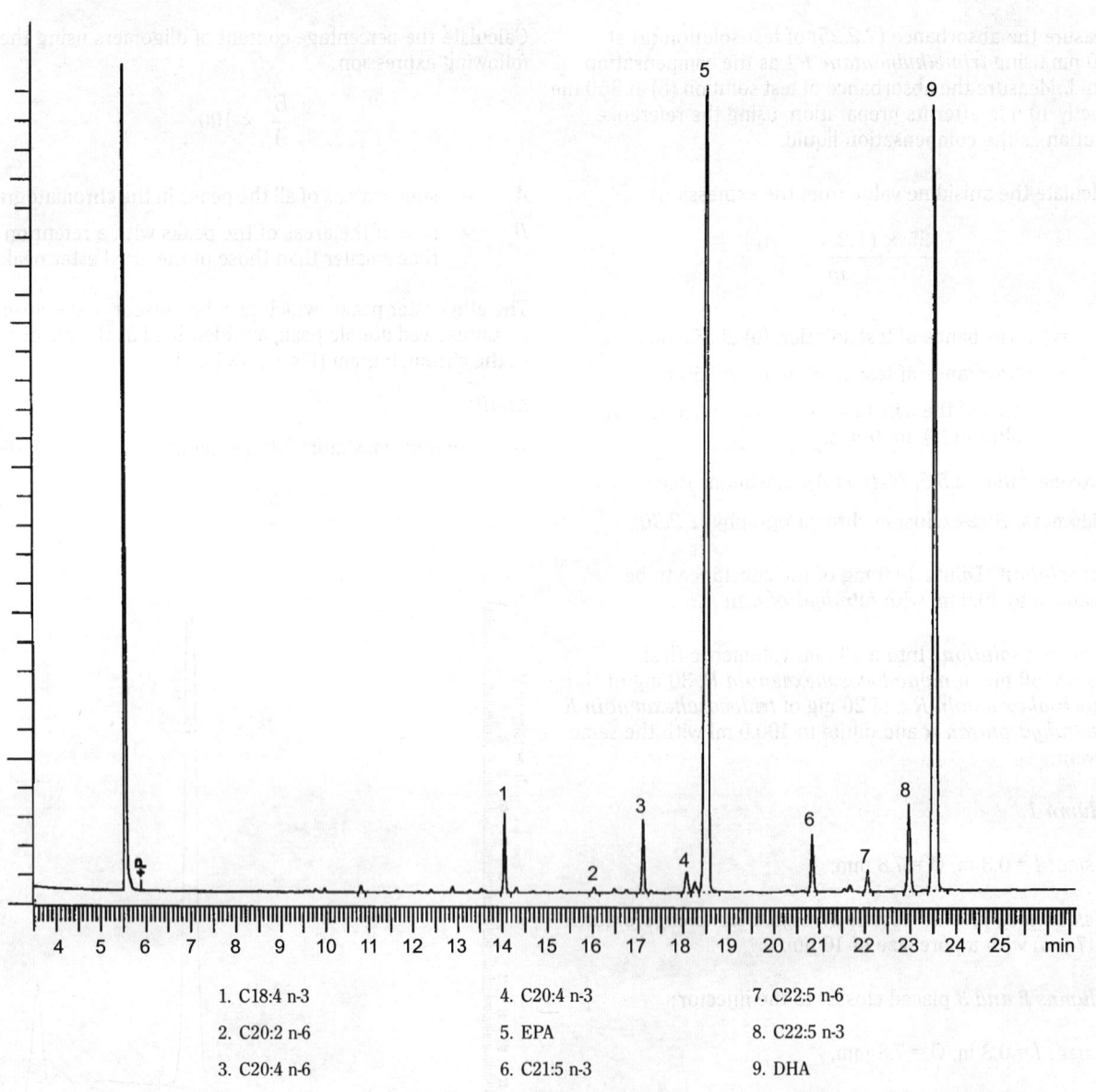

1. C18:4 n-3
2. C20:2 n-6
3. C20:4 n-6
4. C20:4 n-3
5. EPA
6. C21:5 n-3
7. C22:5 n-6
8. C22:5 n-3
9. DHA

Figure 1250.-2. - *Chromatogram for the assay of total omega-3-acid ethyl esters in omega-3-acid ethyl esters 90*

Monographs N-O

01/2005:1352

OMEGA-3-ACID TRIGLYCERIDES

Omega-3 acidorum triglycerida

DEFINITION

Mixture of mono-, di- and triesters of omega-3 acids with glycerol containing mainly triesters and obtained either by esterification of concentrated and purified omega-3 acids with glycerol or by transesterification of the omega-3 acid ethyl esters with glycerol. The origin of the omega-3 acids is the body oil from fatty fish species coming from families like *Engraulidae, Carangidae, Clupeidae, Osmeridae, Salmonidae* and *Scombridae.* The omega-3 acids are identified as the following acids: alpha-linolenic acid (C18:3 n-3), moroctic acid (C18:4 n-3), eicosatetraenoic acid (C20:4 n-3), timnodonic (eicosapentaenoic) acid (C20:5 n-3; EPA), heneicosapentaenoic acid (C21:5 n-3), clupanodonic acid (C22:5 n-3) and cervonic (docosahexaenoic) acid (C22:6 n-3; DHA).

Content:

– sum of the contents of the omega-3 acids EPA and DHA, expressed as triglycerides: minimum 45.0 per cent,
– total omega-3 acids, expressed as triglycerides: minimum 60.0 per cent.

Tocopherol may be added as an antioxidant.

CHARACTERS

Appearance: pale yellow liquid.

Solubility: practically insoluble in water, very soluble in acetone and in heptane, slightly soluble in ethanol.

IDENTIFICATION

Examine the chromatograms obtained in the assay for EPA and DHA.

Results: the peaks due to eicosapentaenoic acid methyl ester and to docosahexaenoic acid methyl ester in the chromatogram obtained with test solution (b) are similar in retention time and size to the corresponding peaks in the chromatogram obtained with reference solution (a).

TESTS

Absorbance (*2.2.25*): maximum 0.73 at 233 nm.

Dilute 0.300 g of the substance to be examined to 50.0 ml with *trimethylpentane R.* Dilute 2.0 ml of this solution to 50.0 ml with *trimethylpentane R.*

Acid value (*2.5.1*): maximum 3.0, determined on 10.0 g in 50 ml of the prescribed mixture of solvents.

Anisidine value: maximum 30.0.

The anisidine value is defined as 100 times the absorbance measured in a 1 cm cell filled with a solution containing 1 g of the substance to be examined in 100 ml of a mixture of solvents and reagents according to the method described below.

Carry out the operations as rapidly as possible, avoiding exposure to actinic light.

Test solution (a). Dilute 0.500 g of the substance to be examined to 25.0 ml with *trimethylpentane R*.

Test solution (b). To 5.0 ml of test solution (a) add 1.0 ml of a 2.5 g/l solution of *p-anisidine R* in *glacial acetic acid R*, shake and store protected from light.

Reference solution. To 5.0 ml of *trimethylpentane R* add 1.0 ml of a 2.5 g/l solution of *p-anisidine R* in *glacial acetic acid R*, shake and store protected from light.

Measure the absorbance (*2.2.25*) of test solution (a) at 350 nm using *trimethylpentane R* as the compensation liquid. Measure the absorbance of test solution (b) at 350 nm exactly 10 min after its preparation, using the reference solution as the compensation liquid.

Calculate the anisidine value from the expression:

$$\frac{25 \times (1.2A_s - A_b)}{m}$$

A_s = absorbance of test solution (b),

A_b = absorbance of test solution (a),

m = mass of the substance to be examined in test solution (a), in grams.

Peroxide value (*2.5.5, Method A*): maximum 10.0.

Oligomers and partial glycerides. Size-exclusion chromatography (*2.2.30*).

Test solution. Dilute 10.0 mg of the substance to be examined to 10.0 ml with *tetrahydrofuran R*.

Reference solution. In a 100 ml volumetric flask dissolve 50 mg of *monodocosahexaenoin R*, 30 mg of *didocosahexaenoin R* and 20 mg of *tridocosahexaenoin R* in *tetrahydrofuran R* and dilute to 100.0 ml with the same solvent.

Column 1:

- *dimensions*: l = 0.3 m, Ø = 7.8 mm,
- *stationary phase*: *styrene-divinylbenzene copolymer R* (7 µm) with a pore size of 10 nm.

Columns 2 and 3 placed closest to the injector:

- *dimensions*: l = 0.3 m, Ø = 7.8 mm,
- *stationary phase*: *styrene-divinylbenzene copolymer R* (7 µm) with a pore size of 50 nm.

Mobile phase: *tetrahydrofuran R*.

Flow rate: 0.8 ml/min.

Detection: differential refractometer.

Injection: 40 µl.

System suitability: reference solution:

- *elution order*: tridocosahexaenoin, didocosahexaenoin, monodocosahexaenoin,
- *resolution*: minimum of 2.0 between the peaks due to monodocosahexaenoin and to didocosahexaenoin and minimum of 1.0 between the peaks due to didocosahexaenoin and to tridocosahexaenoin.

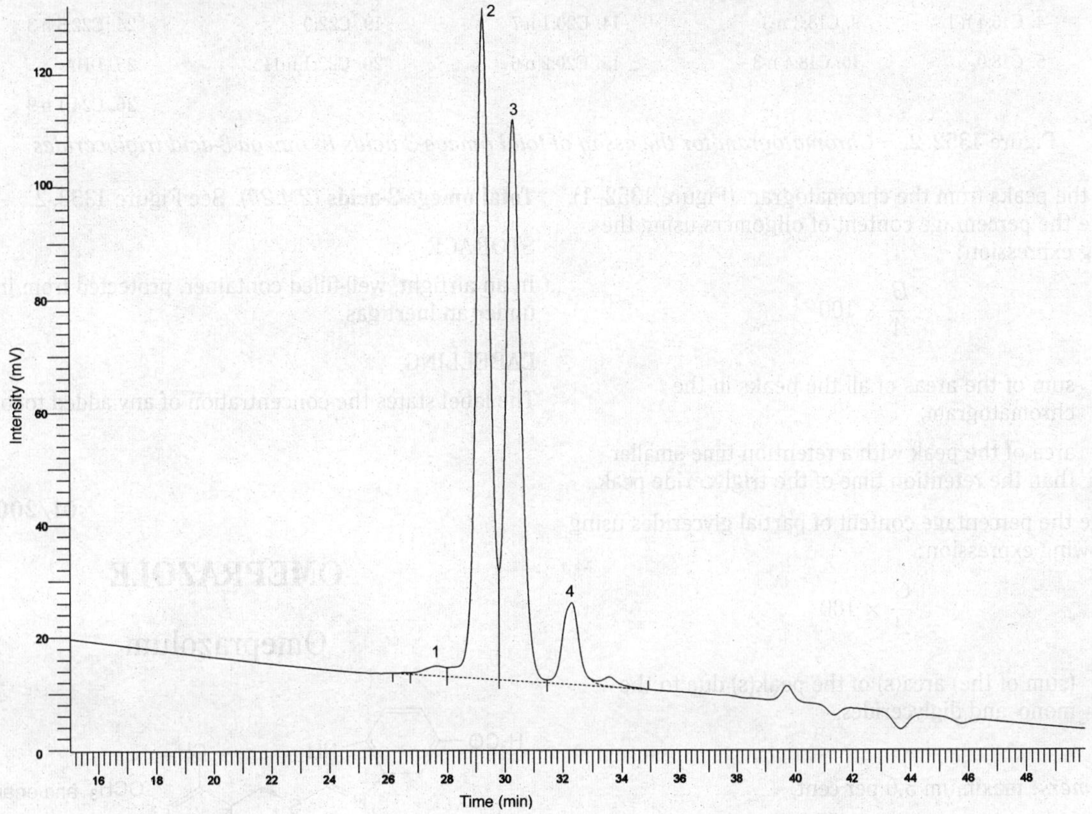

1. Oligomers 2. Triglycerides 3. Diglycerides 4. Monoglycerides

Figure 1352.-1. – *Chromatogram of the test for oligomers and partial glycerides in omega-3-acid triglycerides*

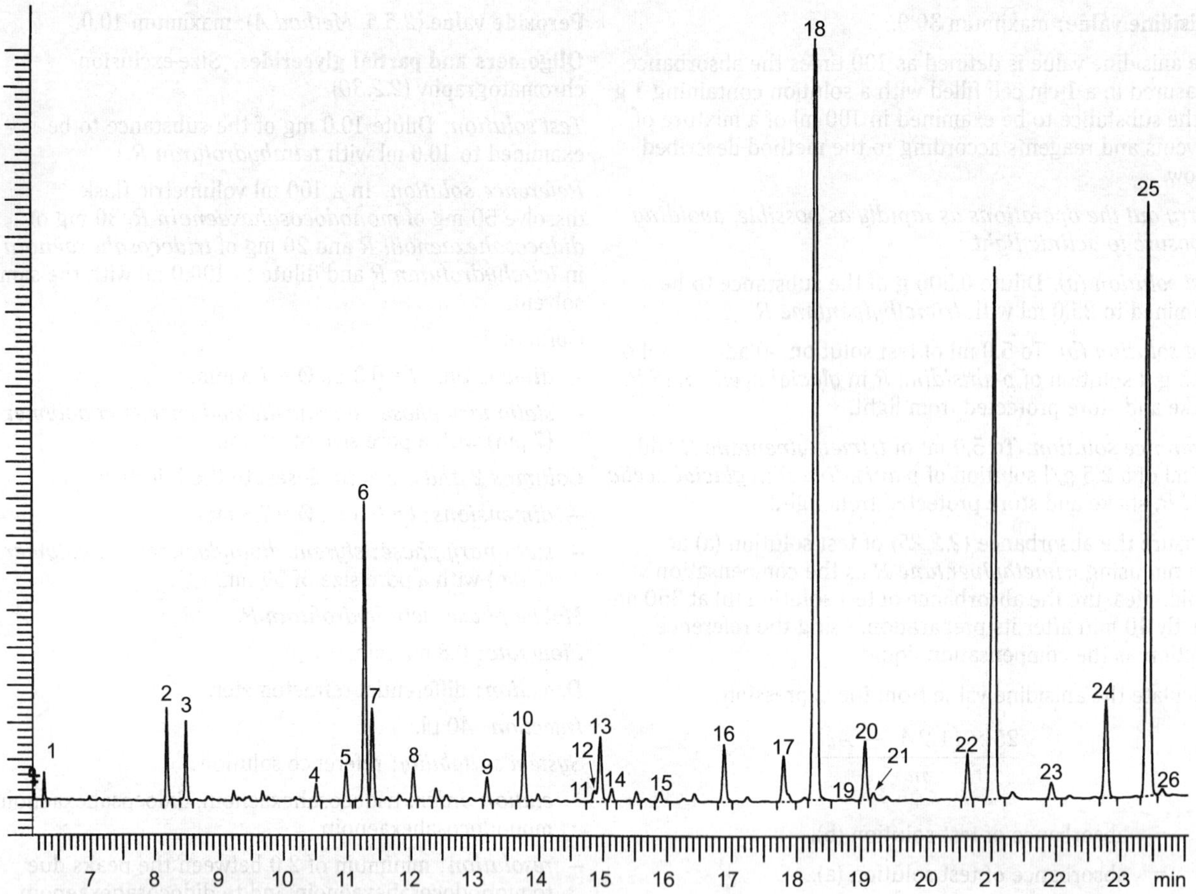

1. C14:0
2. C16:0
3. C16:1 n-7
4. C16:4 n-1
5. C18:0
6. C18:1 n-9
7. C18:1 n-7
8. C18:2 n-6
9. C18:3 n-3
10. C18:4 n-3
11. C20:0
12. C20:1 n-11
13. C20:1 n-9
14. C20:1 n-7
15. C20:2 n-6
16. C20:4 n-6
17. C20:4 n-3
18. EPA
19. C22:0
20. C22:1 n-11
21. C22:1 n-9
22. C21:5 n-3
23. C22:5 n-6
24. C22:5 n-3
25. DHA
26. C24:1 n-9

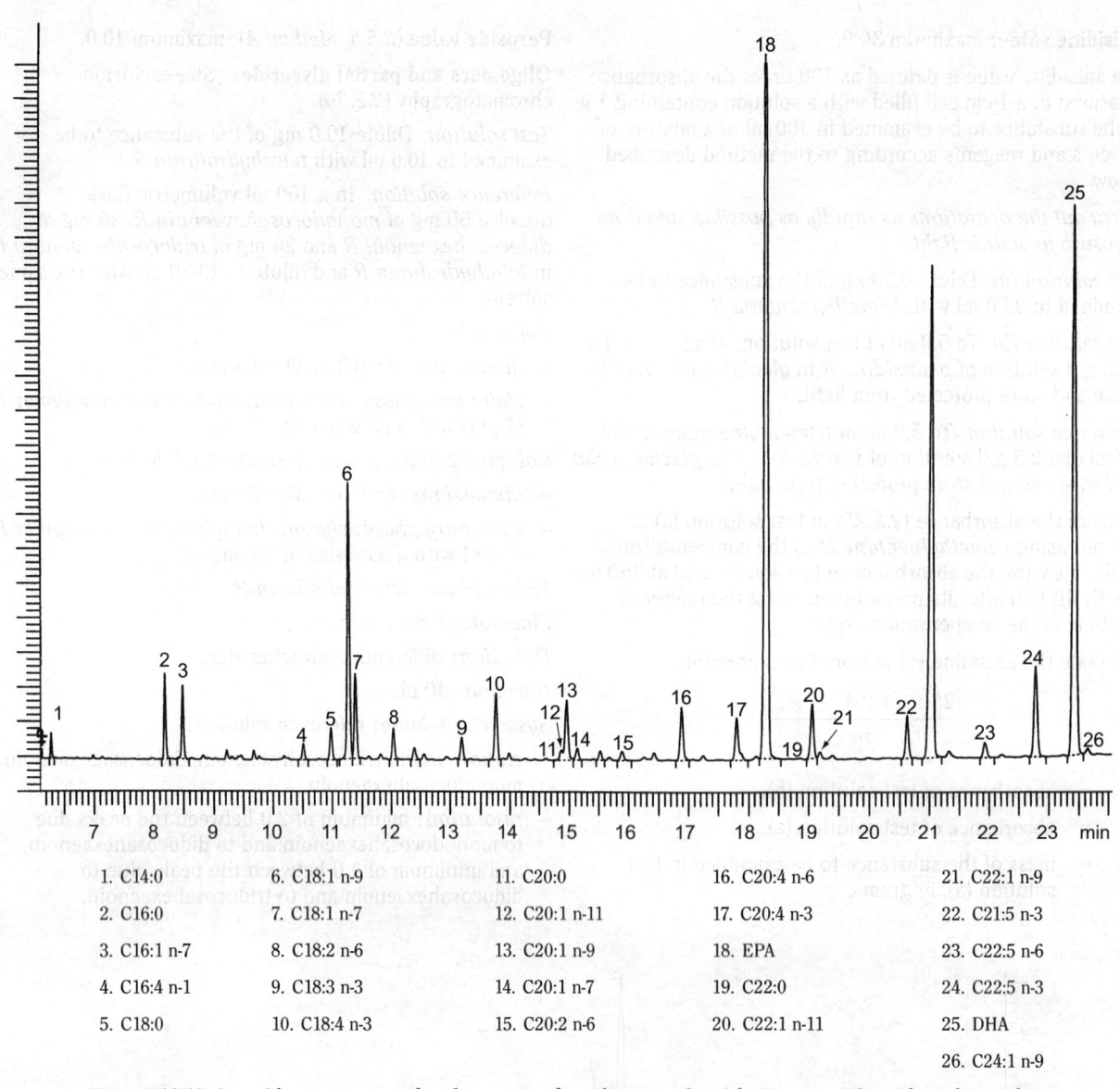

Figure 1352.-2. – *Chromatogram for the assay of total omega-3 acids in omega-3-acid triglycerides*

Identify the peaks from the chromatogram (Figure 1352.-1). Calculate the percentage content of oligomers using the following expression:

$$\frac{B}{A} \times 100$$

A = sum of the areas of all the peaks in the chromatogram,

B = area of the peak with a retention time smaller than the retention time of the triglyceride peak.

Calculate the percentage content of partial glycerides using the following expression:

$$\frac{C}{A} \times 100$$

C = (sum of the) area(s) of the peak(s) due to the mono- and diglycerides.

Limits:
- *oligomers*: maximum 3.0 per cent,
- *partial glycerides*: maximum 50.0 per cent.

ASSAY

EPA and DHA (*2.4.29*). See Figure 1352.-2.

Total omega-3-acids (*2.4.29*). See Figure 1352.-2.

STORAGE

In an airtight, well-filled container, protected from light, under an inert gas.

LABELLING

The label states the concentration of any added tocopherol.

01/2005:0942

OMEPRAZOLE

Omeprazolum

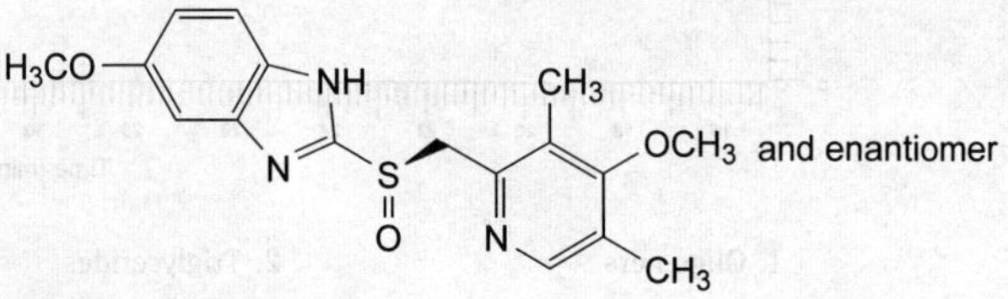

$C_{17}H_{19}N_3O_3S$ M_r 345.4

DEFINITION

Omeprazole contains not less than 99.0 per cent and not more than the equivalent of 101.0 per cent of 5-methoxy-2-[(*RS*)-[(4-methoxy-3,5-dimethylpyridin-2-yl)methyl]sulphinyl]-1*H*-benzimidazole, calculated with reference to the dried substance.

CHARACTERS

A white or almost white powder, very slightly soluble in water, soluble in methylene chloride, sparingly soluble in alcohol and in methanol. It dissolves in dilute solutions of alkali hydroxides.

It shows polymorphism.

IDENTIFICATION

First identification: B.

Second identification: A, C.

A. Dissolve 2.0 mg in *0.1 M sodium hydroxide* and dilute to 100.0 ml with the same solvent. Examined between 230 nm and 350 nm (*2.2.25*), the solution shows 2 absorption maxima at 276 nm and 305 nm. The ratio of the absorbance measured at the absorption maximum at 305 nm to that measured at the absorption maximum at 276 nm is 1.6 to 1.8.

B. Examine by infrared absorption spectrophotometry (*2.2.24*), comparing with the spectrum obtained with *omeprazole CRS*. If the spectra obtained in the solid state show differences, dissolve the substance to be examined and the reference substance separately in *methanol R*, evaporate to dryness and record new spectra using the residues.

C. Examine the chromatograms obtained in the test for impurity C. The principal spot in the chromatogram obtained with test solution (b) is similar in position and size to the principal spot in the chromatogram obtained with reference solution (a). Place the plate in a tank saturated with vapour from *acetic acid R*. The spots rapidly turn brown.

TESTS

Solution S. Dissolve 0.50 g in *methylene chloride R* and dilute to 25 ml with the same solvent.

Appearance of solution. Solution S is clear (*2.2.1*).

Absorbance (*2.2.25*). The absorbance of solution S measured at 440 nm is not more than 0.10 (this limit corresponds to 0.035 per cent of impurity F or impurity G).

Impurity C. Examine by thin-layer chromatography (*2.2.27*), using a *TLC silica gel F_{254} plate R*.

Test solution (a). Dissolve 0.10 g of the substance to be examined in 2.0 ml of a mixture of equal volumes of *methanol R* and *methylene chloride R*.

Test solution (b). Dilute 1.0 ml of test solution (a) to 10 ml with *methanol R*.

Reference solution (a). Dissolve 10 mg of *omeprazole CRS* in 2.0 ml of *methanol R*.

Reference solution (b). Dilute 1 ml of test solution (a) to 10 ml with a mixture of equal volumes of *methanol R* and *methylene chloride R*. Dilute 1 ml of this solution to 100 ml with a mixture of equal volumes of *methanol R* and *methylene chloride R*.

Apply to the plate 10 µl of each solution. Develop over a path of 15 cm using a mixture of 20 volumes of *2-propanol R*, 40 volumes of *methylene chloride R* previously shaken with *concentrated ammonia R* (shake 100 ml of *methylene chloride R* with 30 ml of *concentrated ammonia R* in a separating funnel; allow the layers to separate and use the lower layer) and 40 volumes of *methylene chloride R*. Allow the plate to dry in air. Examine in ultraviolet light at 254 nm. Any spot in the chromatogram obtained with test solution (a) with a higher R_f value than that of the spot due to omeprazole is not more intense than the spot in the chromatogram obtained with reference solution (b) (0.1 per cent).

Related substances. Examine by liquid chromatography (*2.2.29*).

Test solution. Dissolve 3.0 mg of the substance to be examined in the mobile phase and dilute to 25.0 ml with the mobile phase.

Reference solution (a). Dissolve 1.0 mg of *omeprazole CRS* and 1.0 mg of *omeprazole impurity D CRS* in the mobile phase and dilute to 10.0 ml with the mobile phase.

Reference solution (b). Dilute 1.0 ml of the test solution to 100.0 ml with the mobile phase. Dilute 1.0 ml of this solution to 10.0 ml with the mobile phase.

The chromatographic procedure may be carried out using:

- a stainless steel column 0.15 m long and 4 mm in internal diameter packed with *octylsilyl silica gel for chromatography R* (5 µm),
- as mobile phase at a flow rate of 1 ml/min a mixture of 27 volumes of *acetonitrile R* and 73 volumes of a 1.4 g/l solution of *disodium hydrogen phosphate R* previously adjusted to pH 7.6 with *phosphoric acid R*,
- as detector a spectrophotometer set at 280 nm.

When the chromatograms are recorded under the prescribed conditions, the retention time of omeprazole is about 9 min and the relative retention time of impurity D is about 0.8. Inject separately 40 µl of each solution and continue the chromatography for 3 times the retention time of omeprazole. Adjust the sensitivity of the system so that the height of the principal peak in the chromatogram obtained with reference solution (b) is at least 15 per cent of the full scale of the recorder. The test is not valid unless in the chromatogram obtained with reference solution (a), the resolution between the peaks due to impurity D and omeprazole is greater than 3. If necessary, adjust the pH of the mobile phase or the concentration of *acetonitrile R*; an increase in the pH will improve the resolution. The area of any peak, apart from the principal peak, in the chromatogram obtained with the test solution is not greater than the area of the peak in the chromatogram obtained with reference solution (b) (0.1 per cent).

Residual solvents. Examine by head-space gas chromatography (*2.2.28*), using the standard additions method. The content of chloroform is not more than 50 ppm, and the content of methylene chloride is not more than 100 ppm.

The chromatographic procedure may be carried out using:

- a fused-silica column 30 m long and 0.32 mm in internal diameter coated with a 1.8 µm film of cross-linked *poly[(cyanopropyl)(phenyl)][dimethyl]siloxane R*,
- *nitrogen for chromatography R* as the carrier gas,
- a flame-ionisation detector,
- a suitable head-space sampler.

Place 0.50 g of the substance to be examined in a 10 ml vial. Add 4.0 ml of *dimethylacetamide R* and stopper the vial. Equilibrate the vial at 80 °C for 1 h.

Loss on drying (*2.2.32*): maximum 0.2 per cent, determined on 1.000 g by drying under high vacuum at 60 °C for 4 h.

Sulphated ash (*2.4.14*): maximum 0.1 per cent, determined on 1.0 g.

Monographs N-O

ASSAY

Dissolve 1.100 g in a mixture of 10 ml of *water R* and 40 ml of *alcohol R*. Titrate with *0.5 M sodium hydroxide*, determining the end-point potentiometrically (*2.2.20*).

1 ml of *0.5 M sodium hydroxide* is equivalent to 0.1727 g of $C_{17}H_{19}N_3O_3S$.

STORAGE

In an airtight container, protected from light, at a temperature between 2 °C and 8 °C.

IMPURITIES

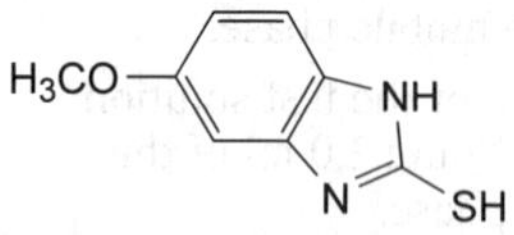

A. 5-methoxy-1*H*-benzimidazole-2-thiol,

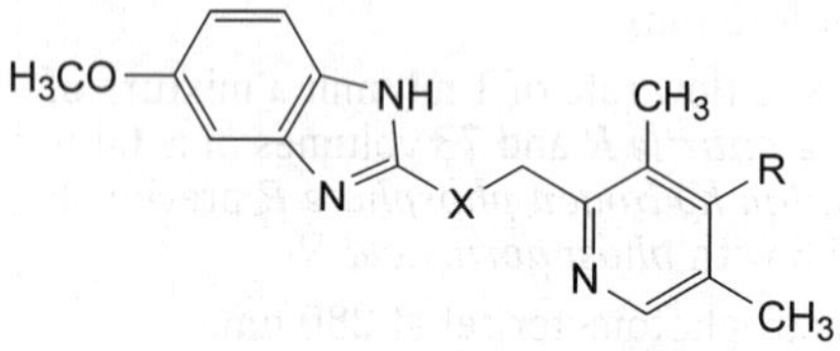

B. R = H, X = SO: 2-[(*RS*)-[(3,5-dimethylpyridin-2-yl)methyl]sulphinyl]-5-methoxy-1*H*-benzimidazole,

C. R = OCH_3, X = S: 5-methoxy-2-[[(4-methoxy-3,5-dimethylpyridin-2-yl)methyl]sulphanyl]-1*H*-benzimidazole (ufiprazole),

D. R = OCH_3, X = SO_2: 5-methoxy-2-[[(4-methoxy-3,5-dimethylpyridin-2-yl)methyl]sulphonyl]-1*H*-benzimidazole (omeprazole sulphone),

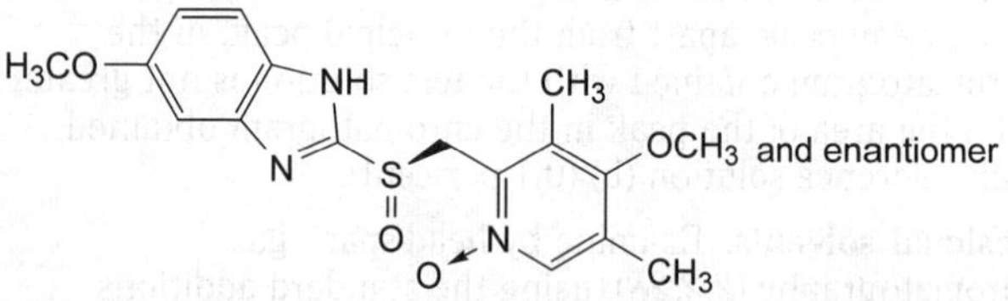

E. 4-methoxy-2-[[(*RS*)-(5-methoxy-1*H*-benzimidazol-2-yl)sulphinyl]methyl]-3,5-dimethylpyridine 1-oxide,

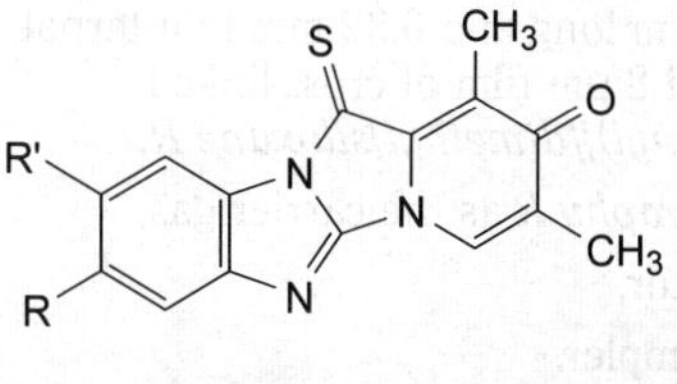

F. R = OCH_3, R′ = H: 1,3-dimethyl-8-methoxy-12-thioxopyrido[1′,2′:3,4]imidazo[1,2-*a*]benzimidazol-2(12*H*)-one,

G. R = H, R′ = OCH_3: 1,3-dimethyl-9-methoxy-12-thioxopyrido[1′,2′:3,4]imidazo[1,2-*a*]benzimidazol-2(12*H*)-one.

01/2005:1032

OMEPRAZOLE SODIUM

Omeprazolum natricum

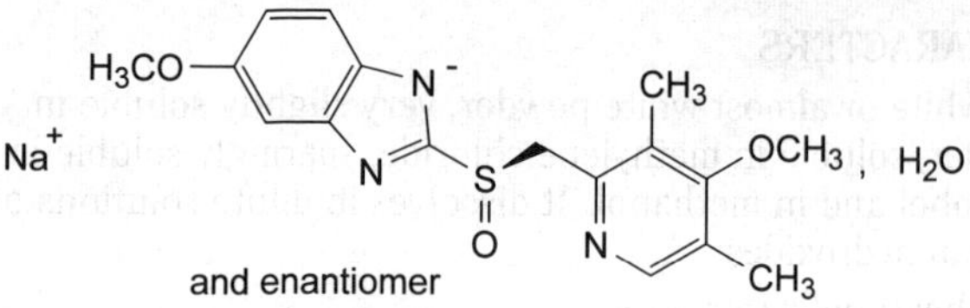

$C_{17}H_{18}N_3NaO_3S,H_2O$ M_r 385.4

DEFINITION

Omeprazole sodium contains not less than 98.0 per cent and not more than the equivalent of 101.0 per cent of sodium 5-methoxy-2-[(*RS*)-[(4-methoxy-3,5-dimethylpyridin-2-yl)methyl]sulphinyl]-1*H*-benzimidazole, calculated with reference to the anhydrous substance.

CHARACTERS

A white or almost white powder, hygroscopic, freely soluble in water and in alcohol, soluble in propylene glycol, very slightly soluble in methylene chloride.

IDENTIFICATION

A. Dissolve 2.0 mg in *0.1 M sodium hydroxide* and dilute to 100.0 ml with the same solvent. Examined between 230 nm and 350 nm (*2.2.25*), the solution shows two absorption maxima, at 276 nm and 305 nm. The ratio of the absorbance measured at the maximum at 305 nm to that measured at the maximum at 276 nm is 1.6 to 1.8.

B. Examine the chromatograms obtained in the test for omeprazole impurity C. The principal spot in the chromatogram obtained with test solution (b) is similar in position and size to the principal spot in the chromatogram obtained with reference solution (a). Place the plate in a tank saturated with vapour of *acetic acid R*. The spots rapidly turn brown.

C. Ignite 1 g and cool. Add 1 ml of *water R* to the residue and neutralise with *hydrochloric acid R*. Filter and dilute the filtrate to 4 ml with *water R*. 0.1 ml of the solution gives reaction (b) of sodium (*2.3.1*).

TESTS

Solution S. Dissolve 0.50 g in *carbon dioxide-free water R* and dilute to 25 ml with the same solvent.

Appearance of solution. Solution S is clear (*2.2.1*) and not more intensely coloured than reference solution B_6 (*2.2.2, Method II*).

pH (*2.2.3*). The pH of solution S is 10.3 to 11.3.

Omeprazole impurity C. Examine by thin-layer chromatography (*2.2.27*), using *silica gel HF_{254} R* as the coating substance.

Test solution (a). Dissolve 0.10 g of the substance to be examined in 2.0 ml of *methanol R*.

Test solution (b). Dilute 1.0 ml of test solution (a) to 10 ml with *methanol R*.

Reference solution (a). Dissolve 9 mg of *omeprazole CRS* in 2.0 ml of *methanol R*.

Reference solution (b). Dilute 1.0 ml of test solution (b) to 100 ml with *methanol R*.

Apply separately to the plate 10 µl of each solution. Develop over a path of 15 cm using a mixture of 20 volumes of *2-propanol R*, 40 volumes of *methylene chloride R* previously shaken with *concentrated ammonia R* (shake 100 ml of *methylene chloride R* with 30 ml of *concentrated ammonia R* in a separating funnel, allow the layers to separate and use the lower layer) and 40 volumes of *methylene chloride R*. Allow the plate to dry in air. Examine in ultraviolet light at 254 nm. Any spot in the chromatogram obtained with test solution (a) with a higher R_f value than that of the spot corresponding to omeprazole is not more intense than the spot in the chromatogram obtained with reference solution (b) (0.1 per cent).

Related substances. Examine by liquid chromatography (*2.2.29*).

Test solution. Dissolve 3.0 mg of the substance to be examined in the mobile phase and dilute to 25.0 ml with the mobile phase.

Reference solution (a). Dissolve 1.0 mg of *omeprazole CRS* and 1.0 mg of *omeprazole impurity D CRS* in the mobile phase and dilute to 10.0 ml with the mobile phase.

Reference solution (b). Dilute 1.0 ml of the test solution to 100.0 ml with the mobile phase. Dilute 1.0 ml of this solution to 10.0 ml with the mobile phase.

The chromatography may be carried out using:

- a stainless steel column 0.15 m long and 4 mm in internal diameter packed with *octylsilyl silica gel for chromatography R* (5 µm),
- as mobile phase at a flow rate of 1 ml/min a mixture of 27 volumes of *acetonitrile R* and 73 volumes of a 1.4 g/l solution of *disodium hydrogen phosphate R*, previously adjusted to pH 7.6 with *phosphoric acid R*,
- as detector a spectrophotometer set at 280 nm.

When the chromatograms are recorded in the prescribed conditions, the retention time of omeprazole is about 9 min and the relative retention time of omeprazole impurity D is about 0.8. Inject separately 40 µl of each solution and continue the chromatography for three times the retention time of omeprazole. Adjust the sensitivity of the detector so that the height of the principal peak in the chromatogram obtained with reference solution (b) is not less than 15 per cent of the full scale of the recorder. The test is not valid unless in the chromatogram obtained with reference solution (a), the resolution between the peaks corresponding to omeprazole impurity D and omeprazole is greater than 3. If necessary adjust the pH of the mobile phase or the concentration of *acetonitrile R*, an increase in the pH will improve the resolution. The area of any peak apart from the principal peak in the chromatogram obtained with the test solution is not greater than the area of the peak in the chromatogram obtained with reference solution (b) (0.1 per cent).

Heavy metals (*2.4.8*). 1.0 g complies with limit test C for heavy metals (20 ppm). Prepare the standard using 2 ml of *lead standard solution (10 ppm Pb) R*.

Water (*2.5.12*): 4.5 per cent to 10.0 per cent, determined on 0.300 g by the semi-micro determination of water.

ASSAY

Dissolve 0.300 g in 50 ml of *water R*. Titrate with *0.1 M hydrochloric acid*, determining the end-point potentiometrically (*2.2.20*).

1 ml of *0.1 M hydrochloric acid* corresponds to 36.74 mg of $C_{17}H_{18}N_3NaO_3S$.

STORAGE

Store in an airtight container, protected from light.

IMPURITIES

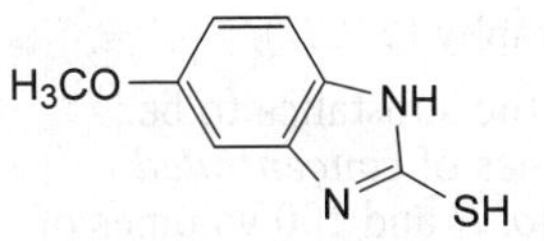

A. 5-methoxy-1*H*-benzimidazole-2-thiol,

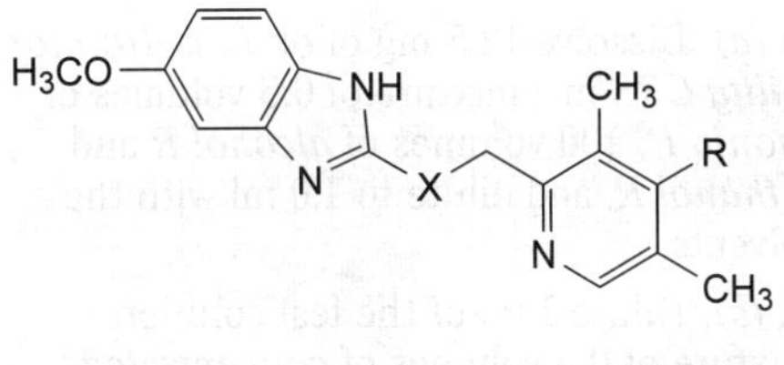

B. R = H, X = SO: 2-[(*RS*)-[(3,5-dimethylpyridin-2-yl)methyl]sulphinyl]-5-methoxy-1*H*-benzimidazole,

C. R = OCH_3, X = S: 5-methoxy-2-[[(4-methoxy-3,5-dimethylpyridin-2-yl)methyl]thio]-1*H*-benzimidazole (ufiprazole),

D. R = OCH_3, X = SO_2: 5-methoxy-2-[[(4-methoxy-3,5-dimethylpyridin-2-yl)methyl]sulfonyl]-1*H*-benzimidazole (omeprazole-sulphone),

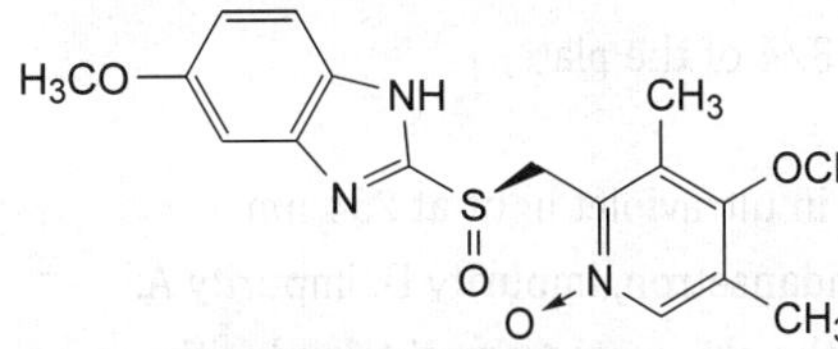

E. 4-methoxy-2-[[(*RS*)-(5-methoxy-1*H*-benzimidazol-2-yl)sulphinyl]methyl]-3,5-dimethylpyridine 1-oxide,

01/2005:2016

ONDANSETRON HYDROCHLORIDE DIHYDRATE

Ondansetroni hydrochloridum dihydricum

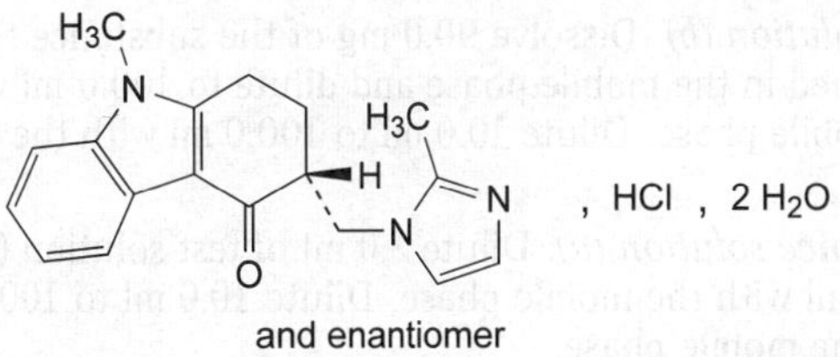

$C_{18}H_{20}ClN_3O,2H_2O$ M_r 365.9

DEFINITION

(3*RS*)-9-Methyl-3-[(2-methyl-1*H*-imidazol-1-yl)methyl]-1,2,3,9-tetrahydro-4*H*-carbazol-4-one hydrochloride dihydrate.

Content: 97.5 per cent to 102.0 per cent (anhydrous substance).

CHARACTERS

Appearance: white or almost white powder.

Solubility: sparingly soluble in water and in alcohol, soluble in methanol, slightly soluble in methylene chloride.

IDENTIFICATION

A. Infrared absorption spectrophotometry (*2.2.24*).

Comparison: *ondansetron hydrochloride dihydrate CRS.*

B. It gives reaction (a) of chlorides (*2.3.1*).

TESTS

Impurity B. Thin-layer chromatography (*2.2.27*).

Test solution. Dissolve 0.125 g of the substance to be examined in a mixture of 0.5 volumes of *concentrated ammonia R*, 100 volumes of *alcohol R* and 100 volumes of *methanol R*, and dilute to 10.0 ml with the same mixture of solvents.

Reference solution (a). Dissolve 12.5 mg of *ondansetron for TLC system suitability CRS* in a mixture of 0.5 volumes of *concentrated ammonia R*, 100 volumes of *alcohol R* and 100 volumes of *methanol R*, and dilute to 1.0 ml with the same mixture of solvents.

Reference solution (b). Dilute 1 ml of the test solution to 100 ml with a mixture of 0.5 volumes of *concentrated ammonia R*, 100 volumes of *alcohol R* and 100 volumes of *methanol R*. Dilute 4.0 ml to 10.0 ml with a mixture of 0.5 volumes of *concentrated ammonia R*, 100 volumes of *alcohol R* and 100 volumes of *methanol R*.

Plate: *TLC silica gel F_{254} plate R*.

Mobile phase: *concentrated ammonia R, methanol R, ethyl acetate R, methylene chloride R* (2:40:50:90 *V/V/V/V*).

Application: 20 µl.

Development: over 3/4 of the plate.

Drying: in air.

Detection: examine in ultraviolet light at 254 nm.

Order of elution: ondansetron, impurity B, impurity A.

System suitability: the chromatogram obtained with reference solution (a) shows 3 clearly separated spots.

Limit:

- *impurity B*: any spot corresponding to impurity B in the chromatogram obtained with the test solution is not more intense than the principal spot in the chromatogram obtained with reference solution (b) (0.4 per cent).

Related substances. Liquid chromatography (*2.2.29*).

Test solution (a). Dissolve 50.0 mg of the substance to be examined in the mobile phase and dilute to 100.0 ml with the mobile phase.

Test solution (b). Dissolve 90.0 mg of the substance to be examined in the mobile phase and dilute to 100.0 ml with the mobile phase. Dilute 10.0 ml to 100.0 ml with the mobile phase.

Reference solution (a). Dilute 2.0 ml of test solution (a) to 100.0 ml with the mobile phase. Dilute 10.0 ml to 100.0 ml with the mobile phase.

Reference solution (b). Dissolve 10.0 mg of *imidazole R* and 10.0 mg of *2-methylimidazole R* in the mobile phase and dilute to 100.0 ml with the mobile phase. Dilute 1.0 ml to 100.0 ml with the mobile phase.

Reference solution (c). Dissolve 5.0 mg of *ondansetron for LC system suitability CRS* in the mobile phase and dilute to 10.0 ml with the mobile phase.

Reference solution (d). Dissolve 5.0 mg of *ondansetron impurity D CRS* in the mobile phase and dilute to 100.0 ml with the mobile phase. Dilute 1.0 ml to 100.0 ml with the mobile phase.

Reference solution (e). Dissolve 90.0 mg of *ondansetron hydrochloride dihydrate CRS* in the mobile phase and dilute to 100.0 ml with the mobile phase. Dilute 10.0 ml to 100.0 ml with the mobile phase.

Column:

- *size*: *l* = 0.25 m, Ø = 4.6 mm,
- *stationary phase*: spherical *nitrile silica gel for chromatography R* (5 µm) with a specific surface area of 220 m^2/g and a pore size of 8 nm.

Mobile phase: mix 20 volumes of *acetonitrile R* and 80 volumes of a 2.8 g/l solution of *sodium dihydrogen phosphate monohydrate R* previously adjusted to pH 5.4 with a 40 g/l solution of *sodium hydroxide R*.

Flow rate: 1.5 ml/min.

Detection: spectrophotometer at 216 nm.

Injection: 20 µl; inject test solution (a) and reference solutions (a), (b), (c) and (d).

Run time: 1.5 times the retention time of ondansetron.

Relative retentions with reference to ondansetron (retention time = about 18 min): impurity E = about 0.1; impurity F = about 0.2; impurity C = about 0.4; impurity D = about 0.5; impurity H = about 0.7; impurity A = about 0.8; impurity G = about 0.9.

System suitability:

- *resolution*: minimum of 1.3 between the peak due to impurity E (first peak) and the peak due to impurity F (second peak) in the chromatogram obtained with reference solution (b) and minimum of 2.5 between the peak due to impurity C (first peak) and the peak due to impurity D (second peak) in the chromatogram obtained with reference solution (c).

Limits:

- *correction factor*: for the calculation of contents, multiply the peak area of impurity C by 0.6,
- *impurity C*: not more than the area of the principal peak in the chromatogram obtained with reference solution (a) (0.2 per cent),
- *impurity D*: not more than the area of the principal peak in the chromatogram obtained with reference solution (d) (0.1 per cent),
- *impurity E*: not more than the area of the corresponding peak in the chromatogram obtained with reference solution (b) (0.2 per cent),
- *impurity F*: not more than the area of the corresponding peak in the chromatogram obtained with reference solution (b) (0.2 per cent),
- *any other impurity*: not more than the area of the principal peak in the chromatogram obtained with reference solution (a) (0.2 per cent),
- *total*: not more than twice the area of the principal peak in the chromatogram obtained with reference solution (a) (0.4 per cent),
- *disregard limit*: 0.2 times the area of the principal peak in the chromatogram obtained with reference solution (a) (0.04 per cent).

Water (*2.5.12*): 9.0 per cent to 10.5 per cent, determined on 0.200 g.

Sulphated ash (*2.4.14*): maximum 0.1 per cent, determined on 1.0 g.

ASSAY

Liquid chromatography (*2.2.29*) as described in the test for related substances with the following modification.

Injection: test solution (b) and reference solution (e).

Calculate the percentage content of $C_{18}H_{20}ClN_3O$.

STORAGE

Protected from light.

Monographs N-O

IMPURITIES

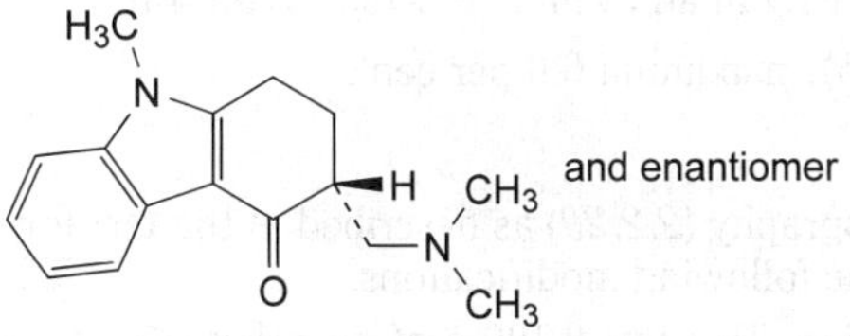

A. (3*RS*)-3-[(dimethylamino)methyl]-9-methyl-1,2,3,9-tetrahydro-4*H*-carbazol-4-one,

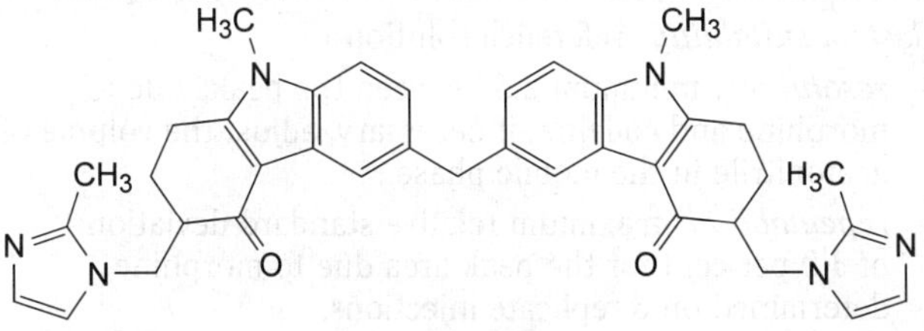

B. 6,6′-methylenebis[(3*RS*)-9-methyl-3-[(2-methyl-1*H*-imidazol-1-yl)methyl]-1,2,3,9-tetrahydro-4*H*-carbazol-4-one],

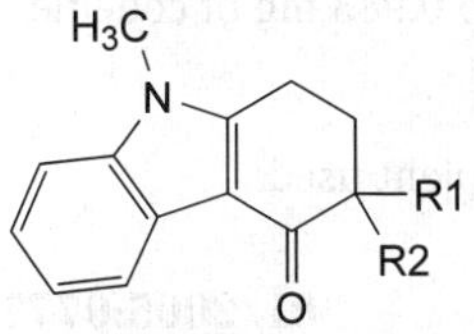

C. R1 = R2 = H: 9-methyl-1,2,3,9-tetrahydro-4*H*-carbazol-4-one,

D. R1 + R2 = CH_2: 9-methyl-3-methylene-1,2,3,9-tetrahydro-4*H*-carbazol-4-one,

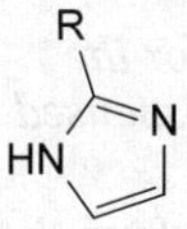

E. R = H: 1*H*-imidazole,

F. R = CH_3: 2-methyl-1*H*-imidazole,

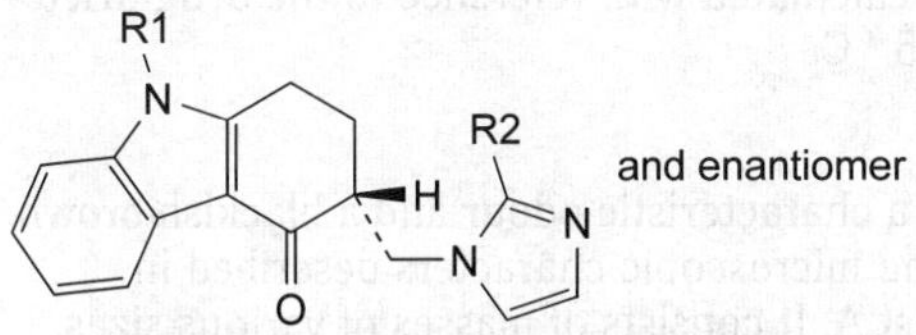

G. R1 = CH_3, R2 = H: (3*RS*)-3-[(1*H*-imidazol-1-yl)methyl]-9-methyl-1,2,3,9-tetrahydro-4*H*-carbazol-4-one (*C*-demethylondansetron),

H. R1 = H, R2 = CH_3: (3*RS*)-3-[(2-methyl-1*H*-imidazol-1-yl)methyl]-1,2,3,9-tetrahydro-4*H*-carbazol-4-one (*N*-demethylondansetron).

01/2005:1840

OPIUM, PREPARED

Opii pulvis normatus

DEFINITION

Raw opium powdered (180), and dried at a temperature not exceeding 70 °C.

Content:

– morphine ($C_{17}H_{19}NO_3$; M_r 285.3): 9.8 per cent to 10.2 per cent (drug dried at 100-105 °C for 4 h),

– codeine ($C_{18}H_{21}NO_3$; M_r 299.4): minimum 1.0 per cent (drug dried at 100-105 °C for 4 h).

Content adjusted if necessary by adding a suitable excipient or raw opium powder.

CHARACTERS

Appearance: yellowish-brown or dark brown powder.

IDENTIFICATION

A. Examine under a microscope using a 20 g/l solution of *potassium hydroxide R*. It is seen to consist of granules of latex agglomerated in irregular masses, and of light brown elongated filaments. Some fragments of vessels and rather elongated, refringent crystals are also visible, as well as a smaller number of round pollen grains and fragments of elongated fibres. Hairs of various lengths with sharp points and fragments of epicarp consisting of polygonal cells with thick walls defining a stellate lumen may be present. Examine under a microscope using *glycerol (85 per cent) R*. Particles of excipient and a few grains of starch introduced during the handling of the latex may be seen.

B. Thin-layer chromatography (*2.2.27*).

Test solution. Triturate 0.10 g of the drug to be examined with 5 ml of *alcohol (70 per cent V/V) R*, rinse with 3 ml of *alcohol (70 per cent V/V) R*, transfer to a 25 ml conical flask. Heat in a water-bath at 50-60 °C with stirring for 30 min. Cool, filter, wash the filter with *alcohol (70 per cent V/V) R* and dilute the filtrate to 10 ml with the same solvent.

Reference solution. Dissolve 2.0 mg of *papaverine hydrochloride R*, 12.0 mg of *codeine phosphate R*, 12.0 mg of *noscapine hydrochloride R* and 25.0 mg of *morphine hydrochloride R* in *alcohol (70 per cent V/V) R* and dilute to 25.0 ml with the same solvent.

Plate: *TLC silica gel G plate R*.

Mobile phase: *concentrated ammonia R, alcohol R, acetone R, toluene R (2:6:40:40 V/V/V/V)*.

Application: 20 µl, as bands of 20 mm by 3 mm.

Development: over a path of 15 cm.

Drying: at 100-105 °C for 15 min.

Detection: allow to cool and spray with *potassium iodobismuthate solution R2* and then with a 4 g/l solution of *sulphuric acid R*, examine in daylight.

Results: see below the sequence of the zones present in the chromatograms obtained with the reference solution and the test solution. Furthermore, a dark red zone (thebaine) situated between the codeine zone and the papaverine zone may be present in the chromatogram obtained with the test solution.

Top of the plate	
Noscapine: an orange-red or red zone	An orange-red or red zone (noscapine)
Papaverine: an orange-red or red zone	An orange-red or red zone (papaverine)
Codeine: an orange-red or red zone	An orange-red or red zone (codeine)
Morphine: an orange-red or red zone	An orange-red or red zone (morphine)
Reference solution	**Test solution**

C. To 1.0 g of the drug to be examined add 5 ml of *water R*, shake for 5 min and filter. To the filtrate add 0.25 ml of *ferric chloride solution R2*. A red colour develops which does not disappear on the addition of 0.5 ml of *dilute hydrochloric acid R*.

TESTS

Thebaine. Liquid chromatography (*2.2.29*).

Test solution. Suspend 1.00 g of the drug to be examined in 50 ml of *alcohol (50 per cent V/V) R*, mix using sonication for 1 h, allow to cool and dilute to 100.0 ml with the same solvent. Allow to stand. To 10.0 ml of the supernatant liquid, add 5 ml of *ammonium chloride buffer solution pH 9.5 R*, dilute to 25.0 ml with *water R* and mix. Transfer 20.0 ml of the solution to a chromatography column about 0.15 m long and about 30 mm in internal diameter containing 15 g of *kieselguhr for chromatography R*. Allow to stand for 15 min. Elute with 2 quantities, each of 40 ml, of a mixture of 15 volumes of *2-propanol R* and 85 volumes of *methylene chloride R*. Evaporate the eluate to dryness *in vacuo* at 40 °C. Transfer the residue to a volumetric flask with the aid of the mobile phase and dilute to 25.0 ml with the mobile phase.

Reference solution. Dissolve 25.0 mg of *thebaine R* in the mobile phase and dilute to 25.0 ml with the mobile phase. Dilute 10.0 ml of the solution to 100.0 ml with the mobile phase.

Precolumn:
- *size*: *l* = 40 mm, Ø = 4.6 mm,
- *stationary phase*: *octylsilyl silica gel for chromatography R* (5 µm).

Column:
- *size*: *l* = 0.25 m, Ø = 4.6 mm,
- *stationary phase*: *octylsilyl silica gel for chromatography R* (5 µm).

Mobile phase: dissolve 1.0 g of *sodium heptanesulphonate monohydrate R* in 420 ml of *water R*, adjust to pH 3.2 with phosphoric acid (4.9 g/l H_3PO_4) (about 5 ml) and add 180 ml of *acetonitrile R*.

Flow rate: 1.5 ml/min.

Detection: spectrophotometer at 280 nm.

Injection: a suitable volume with a loop injector.

System suitability: reference solution:
- *mass distribution ratio*: minimum 3.0 for the peak due to thebaine.

Calculate the percentage content of alkaloid from the expression:

$$\frac{m_1 \times A_2 \times 125}{m_2 \times A_1} \times \frac{100}{100 - h}$$

m_1 = mass of the alkaloid in the reference solution, in grams,

m_2 = mass of the substance to be examined in the test solution, in grams,

A_1 = area of the peak due to the alkaloid in the chromatogram obtained with the reference solution,

A_2 = area of the peak due to the alkaloid in the chromatogram obtained with the test solution,

h = percentage loss on drying.

Limit:
- *thebaine*: maximum 3.0 per cent (dried drug).

Loss on drying (*2.2.32*): maximum 8.0 per cent, determined on 1.000 g by drying in an oven at 100-105 °C for 4 h.

Total ash (*2.4.16*): maximum 6.0 per cent.

ASSAY

Liquid chromatography (*2.2.29*) as described in the test for thebaine with the following modifications.

Reference solution. Dissolve 0.100 g of *morphine hydrochloride R* and 25.0 mg of *codeine R* in the mobile phase and dilute to 25.0 ml with the mobile phase. Dilute 10.0 ml of the solution to 100.0 ml with the mobile phase.

System suitability: reference solution:
- *resolution*: minimum 2.5 between the peaks due to morphine and codeine; if necessary, adjust the volume of acetonitrile in the mobile phase,
- *repeatability*: maximum relative standard deviation of 1.0 per cent for the peak area due to morphine, determined on 6 replicate injections.

Calculate the percentage content of morphine and codeine from the expression given in the test for thebaine. For the calculation, 1 mg of *morphine hydrochloride R* is taken to be equivalent to 0.759 mg of morphine and 1 mg of *codeine R* is taken to be equivalent to 0.943 mg of codeine.

LABELLING

The label states the name of any excipient used.

01/2005:0777

OPIUM, RAW

Opium crudum

DEFINITION

Raw opium is intended only as starting material for the manufacture of galenical preparations. It is not dispensed as such.

Raw opium is the air-dried latex obtained by incision from the unripe capsules of *Papaver somniferum* L. It contains not less than 10.0 per cent of morphine ($C_{17}H_{19}NO_3$; M_r 285.3) and not less than 2.0 per cent of codeine ($C_{18}H_{21}NO_3$; M_r 299.4), both calculated with reference to the drug dried at 100 °C to 105 °C.

CHARACTERS

Raw opium has a characteristic odour and a blackish-brown colour. It has the microscopic characters described in identification test A. It consists of masses of various sizes, which tend to be soft and shiny and, after drying, become hard and brittle.

IDENTIFICATION

Strip off any covering, cut the substance to be examined into thin slices, if necessary, dry at about 60 °C for 48 h and reduce to a powder (500).

A. Examined under a microscope, a suspension of raw opium in a 20 g/l solution of *potassium hydroxide R* is seen to consist of granules of latex agglomerated in irregular masses, and of light-brown elongated filaments. Some fragments of vessels and rather elongated, refringent crystals are also visible, as well as a smaller number of round pollen grains and fragments of elongated fibres. Hairs of various lengths with sharp points and a few grains of starch introduced during the handling of the latex may be present. Fragments of epicarp consisting of polygonal cells with thick walls defining a stellate lumen may also be present.

B. Examine by thin-layer chromatography (*2.2.27*), using *silica gel G R* as the coating substance.

Test solution. Triturate 0.10 g of the powdered drug with 5 ml of *alcohol (70 per cent V/V) R*, add 3 ml of *alcohol (70 per cent V/V) R*, transfer to a 25 ml conical flask and heat in a water-bath at 50 °C to 60 °C with stirring for 30 min. Cool, filter, wash the filter with *alcohol (70 per cent V/V) R* and dilute the filtrate to 10 ml with the same solvent.

Reference solution. Dissolve 2.0 mg of *papaverine hydrochloride R*, 12.0 mg of *codeine phosphate R*, 12.0 mg of *noscapine hydrochloride R* and 25.0 mg of *morphine hydrochloride R* in *alcohol (70 per cent V/V) R* and dilute to 25.0 ml with the same solvent.

Apply separately to the plate as bands 20 mm by 3 mm 20 µl of each solution. Develop over a path of 15 cm using a freshly prepared mixture of 2 volumes of *concentrated ammonia R*, 6 volumes of *alcohol R*, 40 volumes of *acetone R* and 40 volumes of *toluene R*. Dry the plate at 100 °C to 105 °C for 15 min, allow to cool and spray with *potassium iodobismuthate solution R2* and then with a 4 g/l solution of *sulphuric acid R*. The chromatogram obtained with the reference solution shows in the lower part an orange-red or red zone (morphine), above it a similarly coloured zone (codeine) and in the upper part an orange-red or red zone (papaverine) and above it a similarly coloured zone (noscapine). The chromatogram obtained with the test solution shows orange-red or red zones corresponding to those in the chromatogram obtained with the reference solution. The chromatogram obtained with the test solution may also show a dark red zone (thebaine) situated between those due to codeine and to papaverine.

C. To 1.0 g of the powdered drug add 5 ml of *water R*, shake for 5 min and filter. To the filtrate add 0.25 ml of *ferric chloride solution R2*. A red colour develops which does not disappear on the addition of 0.5 ml of *dilute hydrochloric acid R*.

TESTS

Thebaine. Not more than 3.0 per cent, determined by liquid chromatography (*2.2.29*) and calculated with reference to the dried drug.

Test solution. Prepare the test solution as described in the assay.

Reference solution. Dissolve 25.0 mg of *thebaine R* in the mobile phase and dilute to 25.0 ml with the mobile phase. Dilute 10.0 ml of the solution to 100.0 ml with the mobile phase.

The chromatographic procedure is carried out as described in the assay. The test is not valid unless the mass distribution ratio for thebaine is at least 3.0 and the number of theoretical plates is at least 3000. Calculate the percentage content of thebaine from the expression given in the assay.

Loss on drying (*2.2.32*). Not more than 15.0 per cent, determined on 1.000 g of raw opium cut into thin slices, by drying in an oven at 100 °C to 105 °C for 4 h.

Total ash (*2.4.16*). Not more than 6.0 per cent.

ASSAY

Examine by liquid chromatography (*2.2.29*).

Test solution. Suspend 1.00 g of raw opium, cut into thin slices, in 50 ml of *alcohol (50 per cent V/V) R*, mix with the aid of ultrasound for 1 h, allow to cool and dilute to 100.0 ml with the same solvent. Allow to stand. To 10.0 ml of the supernatant liquid add 5 ml of *ammonium chloride buffer solution pH 9.5 R*, dilute to 25.0 ml with *water R* and mix. Transfer 20.0 ml of the solution to a chromatography column about 0.15 m long and about 30 mm in internal diameter containing 15 g of *kieselguhr for chromatography R*. Allow to stand for 15 min. Elute with two quantities, each of 40 ml, of a mixture of 15 volumes of *2-propanol R* and 85 volumes of *methylene chloride R*. Evaporate the eluate to dryness *in vacuo* at 40 °C. Transfer the residue to a volumetric flask with the aid of the mobile phase and dilute to 25.0 ml with the mobile phase.

Reference solution. Dissolve 0.100 g of *morphine hydrochloride R* and 25.0 mg of *codeine R* in the mobile phase and dilute to 25.0 ml with the mobile phase. Dilute 10.0 ml of the solution to 100.0 ml with the mobile phase.

The chromatographic procedure may be carried out using:

- a column 0.25 m long and 4.6 mm in internal diameter packed with *octylsilyl silica gel for chromatography R* (5 µm), equipped with a guard column 40 mm long and 4.6 mm in internal diameter packed with *octylsilyl silica gel for chromatography R* (5 µm),
- as mobile phase at a flow rate of 1.5 ml/min a solution prepared as follows: dissolve 1.0 g of *sodium heptanesulphonate monohydrate R* in 420 ml of *water R*, adjust to pH 3.2 by addition of phosphoric acid (4.9 g/l H_3PO_4) (about 5 ml) and add 180 ml of *acetonitrile R*,
- as detector a spectrophotometer set at 280 nm,
- an loop injector.

Inject suitable volumes of each solution.

The assay is not valid unless the resolution between the peaks corresponding to morphine and codeine is at least 2.5. If necessary, adjust the volume of acetonitrile in the mobile phase. Inject the reference solution six times. The assay is not valid unless the relative standard deviation of the peak area for morphine is at most 1.0 per cent. Inject alternately the test solution and the reference solution.

Calculate the percentage content of each alkaloid from the expression:

$$\frac{m_1 \times A_2 \times 625}{m_2 \times A_1 \times 5} \times \frac{100}{100 - h}$$

m_1 = mass in grams of the alkaloid used to prepare the reference solution,

m_2 = mass in grams of the substance to be examined used to prepare the test solution,

A_1 = area of the peak corresponding to the alkaloid in the chromatogram obtained with the reference solution,

A_2 = area of the peak corresponding to the alkaloid in the chromatogram obtained with the test solution,

h = percentage loss on drying.

For the calculation, 1 mg of *morphine hydrochloride R* is taken to be equivalent to 0.759 mg of morphine and 1 mg of *codeine R* is taken to be equivalent to 0.943 mg of codeine.

STORAGE

Store protected from light.

Monographs N-O

01/2005:1033

ORCIPRENALINE SULPHATE

Orciprenalini sulfas

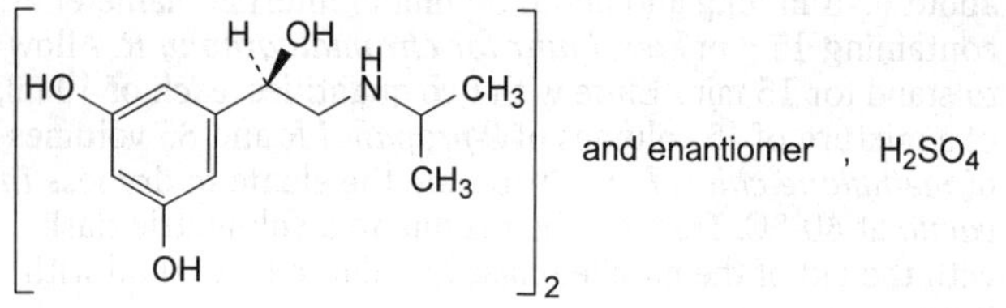

$C_{22}H_{36}N_2O_{10}S$ M_r 520.6

DEFINITION

Orciprenaline sulphate contains not less than 98.0 per cent and not more than the equivalent of 102.0 per cent of di[(*RS*)-1-(3,5-dihydroxyphenyl)-2-[(1-methylethyl)amino]ethanol] sulphate, calculated with reference to the anhydrous, solvent-free substance.

CHARACTERS

A white, crystalline powder, slightly hygroscopic, freely soluble in water and in alcohol, practically insoluble in methylene chloride.

IDENTIFICATION

First identification: B, E.

Second identification: A, C, D, E.

A. Dissolve 50.0 mg in a 0.04 per cent *V/V* solution of *hydrochloric acid R* and dilute to 50.0 ml with the same acid solution. Dilute 5.0 ml of the solution to 50.0 ml with a 0.04 per cent *V/V* solution of *hydrochloric acid R*. Examined between 240 nm and 350 nm (*2.2.25*), the solution shows an absorption maximum at 278 nm. The specific absorbance at the maximum is 68.5 to 76.0, calculated with reference to the anhydrous and solvent-free substance.

B. Examine by infrared absorption spectrophotometry (*2.2.24*), comparing with the spectrum obtained with *orciprenaline sulphate CRS*. Examine the substances prepared as discs. If the spectra obtained show differences, dissolve 50 mg of the substance to be examined and the reference substance separately in the minimum volume of *water R* with heating. Add 10 ml of *acetone R* and centrifuge. Dry the precipitate at 40 °C under reduced pressure for 3 h and record new spectra using the residues.

C. Examine by thin-layer chromatography (*2.2.27*), using *silica gel G R* as the coating substance.

Test solution. Dissolve 10 mg of the substance to be examined in *alcohol R* and dilute to 10 ml with the same solvent.

Reference solution (a). Dissolve 10 mg of *orciprenaline sulphate CRS* in *alcohol R* and dilute to 10 ml with the same solvent.

Reference solution (b). Dissolve 10 mg of *orciprenaline sulphate CRS* and 10 mg of *salbutamol CRS* in *alcohol R* and dilute to 10 ml with the same solvent.

Apply separately to the plate 2 µl of each solution. Develop over a path of 15 cm using a mixture of 1.5 volumes of *ammonia R*, 10 volumes of *water R* and 90 volumes of *aldehyde-free methanol R*. Allow the plate to dry in air and spray with a 10 g/l solution of *potassium permanganate R*. The principal spot in the chromatogram obtained with the test solution is similar in position, colour and size to the principal spot in the chromatogram obtained with reference solution (a). The test is not valid unless the chromatogram obtained with reference solution (b) shows two clearly separated principal spots.

D. Dissolve about 20 mg in 2 ml of *alcohol R*. Add 2 ml of a 1 g/l solution of *dichloroquinonechlorimide R* in *alcohol R* and 1 ml of *sodium carbonate solution R*. A violet colour is produced, turning to brown.

E. It gives reaction (a) of sulphates (*2.3.1*).

TESTS

Solution S. Dissolve 2.0 g in *carbon dioxide-free water R* and dilute to 20 ml with the same solvent.

Appearance of solution. Solution S is clear (*2.2.1*) and colourless (*2.2.2, Method II*).

pH (*2.2.3*). The pH of solution S is 4.0 to 5.5.

Related substances. Examine by thin-layer chromatography (*2.2.27*), using *silica gel G R* as the coating substance.

Test solution. Dissolve 0.20 g of the substance to be examined in a mixture of 1 volume of *water R* and 5 volumes of *methanol R* and dilute to 10 ml with the same mixture of solvents.

Reference solution (a). Dilute 1 ml of the test solution to 100 ml with a mixture of 1 volume of *water R* and 5 volumes of *methanol R*.

Reference solution (b). Dilute 5 ml of reference solution (a) to 10 ml with a mixture of 1 volume of *water R* and 5 volumes of *methanol R*.

Reference solution (c). Dilute 5 ml of reference solution (a) to 20 ml with a mixture of 1 volume of *water R* and 5 volumes of *methanol R*.

Apply separately to the plate 10 µl of each solution. Develop over a path of 15 cm using a mixture of 4 volumes of *concentrated ammonia R*, 16 volumes of *water R*, 30 volumes of *2-propanol R* and 50 volumes of *ethyl acetate R*. Allow the plate to dry in air. Expose the plate to iodine vapour. Any spot in the chromatogram obtained with the test solution, apart from the principal spot, is not more intense than the principal spot in the chromatogram obtained with reference solution (a) (1.0 per cent) and at most one such spot is more intense than the principal spot in the chromatogram obtained with reference solution (b) (0.5 per cent). The test is not valid unless the spot in the chromatogram obtained with reference solution (c) is clearly visible.

Methanol and 2-propanol. Not more than 0.1 per cent *m/m* of methanol and 0.3 per cent *m/m* of 2-propanol, determined by gas chromatography (*2.2.28*), using *ethanol R1* as internal standard.

Internal standard solution. Dilute 2 ml of *ethanol R1* to 100 ml with *water R*. Dilute 1 ml of the solution to 10 ml with *water R*.

Test solution (a). Dissolve 1.0 g of the substance to be examined in *water R* and dilute to 10.0 ml with the same solvent.

Test solution (b). Dissolve 1.0 g of the substance to be examined in *water R*, add 1.0 ml of the internal standard solution and dilute to 10.0 ml with *water R*.

Reference solution. Dilute a mixture of 1.0 ml of *methanol R* and 3.0 ml of *2-propanol R* to 100.0 ml with *water R*. Dilute 1.0 ml of the solution to 10.0 ml with *water R*. To 1.0 ml of this solution, add 1.0 ml of the internal standard solution and dilute to 10.0 ml with *water R*.

The chromatographic procedure may be carried out using:

- a glass column 2 m long and 2 mm in internal diameter packed with *ethylvinylbenzene-divinylbenzene copolymer R* (150 μm to 180 μm),
- *nitrogen for chromatography R* as the carrier gas at a flow rate of 30 ml/min,
- a flame-ionisation detector,

maintaining the temperature of the column at 140 °C and that of the injection port and of the detector at 180 °C.

Inject 1 μl of each solution. In the chromatogram obtained with test solution (a), verify that there is no peak with the same retention time as the internal standard. Calculate the content of methanol and 2-propanol taking their density at 20 °C to be 0.792 g/ml and 0.785 g/ml, respectively.

Phenone. Dissolve 0.50 g in a 0.04 per cent *V/V* solution of *hydrochloric acid R* and dilute to 25.0 ml with the same acid solution. The absorbance (*2.2.25*) of the solution measured at 328 nm is not greater than 0.16 (0.1 per cent).

Iron (*2.4.9*). The residue obtained in the test for sulphated ash complies with the limit test for iron (20 ppm). Prepare the standard using *iron standard solution (2 ppm Fe) R*.

Heavy metals. 1.0 g complies with limit test C for heavy metals (20 ppm). Prepare the standard using 2 ml of *lead standard solution (10 ppm Pb) R*.

Water (*2.5.12*). Not more than 2.0 per cent, determined on 1.00 g by the semi-micro determination of water.

Sulphated ash (*2.4.14*). Not more than 0.1 per cent, determined on 1.0 g.

ASSAY

Dissolve 0.400 g in 30 ml of *anhydrous acetic acid R*. Titrate with *0.1 M perchloric acid* using 0.1 ml of *crystal violet solution R* as indicator.

1 ml of *0.1 M perchloric acid* is equivalent to 52.06 mg of $C_{22}H_{36}N_2O_{10}S$.

STORAGE

Store protected from light.

IMPURITIES

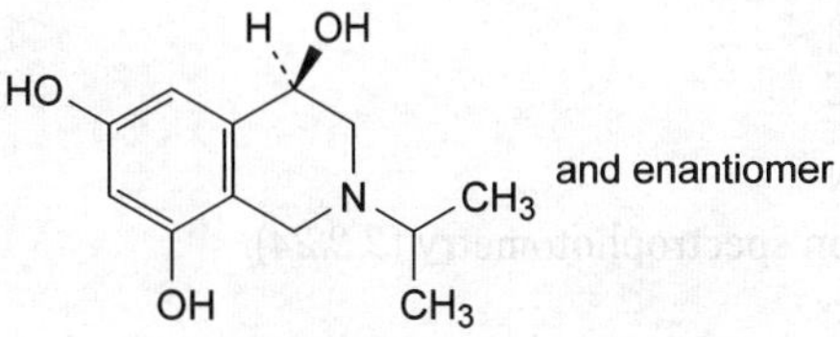

A. 2-(1-methylethyl)-1,2,3,4-tetrahydroisoquinoline-4,6,8-triol,

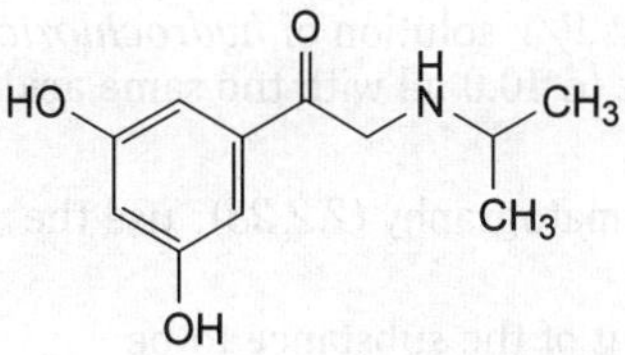

B. 1-(3,5-dihydroxyphenyl)-2-[(1-methylethyl)amino]ethanone.

01/2005:1880

OREGANO

Origani herba

DEFINITION

Dried leaves and flowers separated from the stems of *Origanum onites* L. or *Origanum vulgare* L. subsp. *hirtum* (Link) Ietsw., or a mixture of both species.

Content: minimum 25 ml/kg of essential oil and minimum 1.5 per cent of carvacrol and thymol (both $C_{10}H_{14}O$; M_r 150.2) (anhydrous drug).

CHARACTERS

Macroscopic and microscopic characters described under identification tests A and B.

IDENTIFICATION

A. *O. onites*. The leaf is yellowish-green, usually 4 mm to 22 mm long and 3 mm to 14 mm wide. It has long or short petiole or is sessile. The lamina is ovate, elliptic or ovate-lanceolate. Margins are entire or serrate, apex is acute or obtuse. The veins are yellowish and conspicuous on the adaxial surface. Flowers are solitary or seen as broken parts of the corymb. The calyx is bract-like and inconspicuous. The corolla is white, on top of inflorescenses or single flowers, or inconspicuous. The bract is imbricate and green like the leaves. The drug consists yellowish or yellowish-brown stem parts.

   O. vulgare (subsp. *hirtum*). The leaf is green and usually 3 mm to 28 mm long and 2.5 mm to 19 mm wide. It is petiolate or sessile. The lamina is ovate or ovate-eliptic. The margins are entire or serrate, the apex is acute or obtuse. Flowers are rare, found as broken parts of the corymbs. Bracts are greenish-yellow and imbricate. Calyx is corolla-like and inconspicuous. Corolla is white on top of inflorescenses, slightly conspicuous or inconspicuous.

B. Reduce to a powder (355). The powder is green (*O. vulgare*) to yellowish-green (*O. onites*). Examine under a microscope using *chloral hydrate solution R*. The covering trichomes are of lamiaceous type or short, unicellular and rarely conical; conical trichomes shaped as pointed teeth are more abundant in *O. vulgare*. Covering trichomes are thick-walled in *O. vulgare*. Covering trichomes contain prismatic crystals in *O. onites*, minute needles in *O. vulgare*. Cuticle on covering trichomes is smooth; warty in *O. vulgare*. The epidermises of the leaves have cells with walls which are sinuous and the stomata are of diacytic type (*2.8.3*); in *O. vulgare* cells of the upper epidermis are beaded; secretory trichomes with 8-16 cells (12 in *O. vulgare*); glandular trichomes are numerous in *O. onites*; rare in *O. vulgare*. They have unicellular head and unicellular, bicellular or tricellular (bicellular or tricellular in *O. vulgare*) stalk; pollen grains are smooth, spherical and more abundant in *O. onites*.

C. Thin-layer chromatography (*2.2.27*).

   Test solution. To 1.0 g of the powdered drug (355) add 5 ml of *methylene chloride R* and shake for 3 min, filter through about 2 g of *anhydrous sodium sulphate R*.

   Reference solution. Dissolve 1 mg of *thymol R* and 10 μl of *carvacrol R* in 10 ml of *methylene chloride R*.

   Plate: *TLC silica gel plate R*.

   Mobile phase: *methylene chloride R*.

   Application: 20 μl, as bands.

   Development: over a path of 15 cm.

   Drying: in air.

Detection: spray with *anisaldehyde solution R* using 10 ml for a plate 200 mm square and heat at 100-105 °C for 10 min.

Results: see below the sequence of the zones present in the chromatograms obtained with the reference solution and the test solution. Furthermore, other zones are present in the lower third and upper part of the chromatogram obtained with the test solution.

Top of the plate	
	A bluish-purple zone
———	———
	A pale green zone
Thymol: a pink zone	A pink zone (thymol)
Carvacrol: a pale violet zone	A pale violet zone (carvacrol)
———	
	A pale purple zone
	A grey zone
	A pale green zone
	A bluish-purple zone
	An intense brown zone
Reference solution	**Test solution**

TESTS

Foreign matter (*2.8.2*): maximum 2 per cent.

Water (*2.2.13*): maximum 120 ml/kg, determined on 20.0 g of the powdered drug (355).

Total ash (*2.4.16*): maximum 15.0 per cent.

Ash insoluble in hydrochloric acid (*2.8.1*): maximum 4.0 per cent.

ASSAY

Essential oil (*2.8.12*). Use 30.0 g of the drug, a 1000 ml round-bottomed flask and 400 ml of *water R* as the distillation liquid. Distil at a rate of 2-3 ml/min for 2 h without *xylene R* in the graduated tube.

Carvacrol and thymol. Gas chromatography (*2.2.28*): use the normalisation procedure.

Test solution. Filter the essential oil obtained in the assay of essential oil over a small amount of *anhydrous sodium sulphate R* and dilute to 5.0 ml with *hexane R* by rinsing the apparatus and the anhydrous sodium sulphate.

Reference solution. Dissolve 0.20 g of *thymol R* and 50 mg of *carvacrol R* in *hexane R*, dilute to 5.0 ml with the same solvent.

Column:

– *material*: fused silica,
– *size*: *l* = 60 m, Ø = 0.25 mm,
– *stationary phase*: *macrogol 20 000 R* (film thickness 0.25 µm).

Carrier gas: *nitrogen for chromatography R* or *helium for chromatography R*.

Flow rate: 1.5 ml/min.

Split ratio: 1:100.

Temperature:

	Time (min)	**Temperature (°C)**
Column	0 - 45	40 → 250
Injection port		190
Detector		210

Detection: flame ionisation.
Injection: 0.2 µl.
Elution order: order indicated in the composition of the reference solution. Record the retention times of these substances.
System suitability: reference solution:
– *resolution*: minimum of 1.5 between the peaks due to thymol and carvacrol.

Using the retention times determined from the chromatogram obtained with the reference solution, locate the components of the reference solution in the chromatogram obtained with the test solution.

Determine the percentage content of carvacrol and thymol. Disregard the peak of hexane.

01/2005:1759

ORPHENADRINE CITRATE

Orphenadrini citras

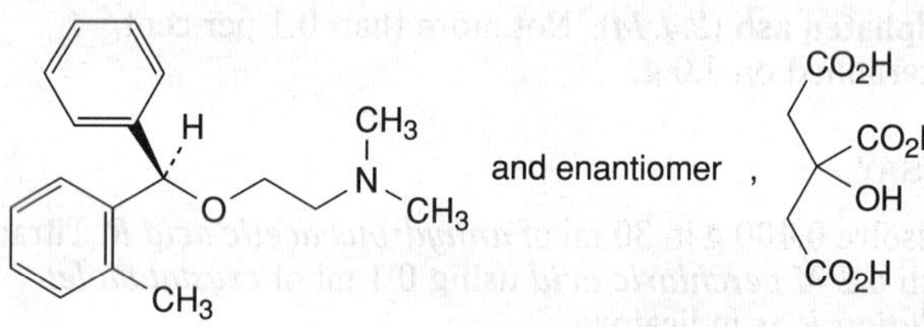

$C_{24}H_{31}NO_8$ M_r 461.5

DEFINITION

(*RS*)-*N*,*N*-Dimethyl-2-[(2-methylphenyl)phenylmethoxy]ethanamine dihydrogen 2-hydroxypropane-1,2,3-tricarboxylate.

Content: 98.5 per cent to 101.0 per cent (dried substance).

CHARACTERS

Appearance: white or almost white, crystalline powder.

Solubility: sparingly soluble in water, slightly soluble in alcohol.

mp: about 137 °C.

IDENTIFICATION

Infrared absorption spectrophotometry (*2.2.24*).

Preparation: discs.

Comparison: *orphenadrine citrate CRS.*

TESTS

Appearance of solution. The solution is clear (*2.2.1*) and its absorbance (*2.2.25*) at 436 nm has a maximum of 0.050. Dissolve 1.0 g in a 3.6 per cent *V/V* solution of *hydrochloric acid R* in *alcohol R* and dilute to 10.0 ml with the same acid solution.

Related substances. Gas chromatography (*2.2.28*): use the normalisation procedure.

Test solution. Dissolve 0.500 g of the substance to be examined in *water R* and dilute to 50 ml with the same solvent. Add 2 ml of *concentrated ammonia R* and shake with 3 quantities, each of 10 ml, of *toluene R*. To the combined upper layers add *anhydrous sodium sulphate R*, shake, filter and evaporate the filtrate, at a temperature not exceeding 50 °C, using a rotary evaporator. Take up the residue with *toluene R* and dilute to 20.0 ml with the same solvent.

Reference solution. Dissolve 30 mg of *orphenadrine citrate CRS* and 30 mg of *orphenadrine impurity E CRS* in 20 ml of *water R*. Add 1 ml of *concentrated ammonia R* and shake with 3 quantities, each of 5 ml, of *toluene R*. To the combined upper layers add *anhydrous sodium sulphate R*, shake, filter and evaporate the filtrate, at a temperature not exceeding 50 °C, using a rotary evaporator. Take up the residue with *toluene R* and dilute to 20.0 ml with the same solvent.

Column:
- *size*: *l* = 60 m, Ø = 0.32 mm,
- *stationary phase*: *poly(dimethyl)(diphenyl)siloxane R* (film thickness 1.0 µm).

Carrier gas: *helium for chromatography R*.

Flow rate: 1 ml/min.

Split ratio: 1:25.

Temperature:
- *column*: 240 °C,
- *injection port and detector*: 290 °C.

Detection: flame ionisation.

Injection: 2 µl.

Run time: 1.3 times the retention time of orphenadrine.

System suitability: reference solution:
- *resolution*: minimum of 1.5 between the peaks due to orphenadrine and to impurity E.

Limits:
- *any impurity*: maximum 0.3 per cent,
- *total*: maximum 1.0 per cent,
- *disregard limit*: 0.02 per cent.

Heavy metals (*2.4.8*): maximum 10 ppm.

2.0 g complies with limit test C. Prepare the standard using 2 ml of *lead standard solution (10 ppm Pb) R*.

Loss on drying (*2.2.32*): maximum 0.5 per cent, determined on 1.000 g by drying in an oven at 100-105 °C for 3 h.

Sulphated ash (*2.4.14*): maximum 0.1 per cent, determined on 1.0 g.

ASSAY

Dissolve 0.350 g in 50 ml of *anhydrous acetic acid R*. Titrate with *0.1 M perchloric acid*, determining the end-point potentiometrically (*2.2.20*).

1 ml of *0.1 M perchloric acid* is equivalent to 46.15 mg of $C_{24}H_{31}NO_8$.

STORAGE

Protected from light. If the substance is sterile, store in a sterile, airtight, tamper-proof container, protected from light.

IMPURITIES

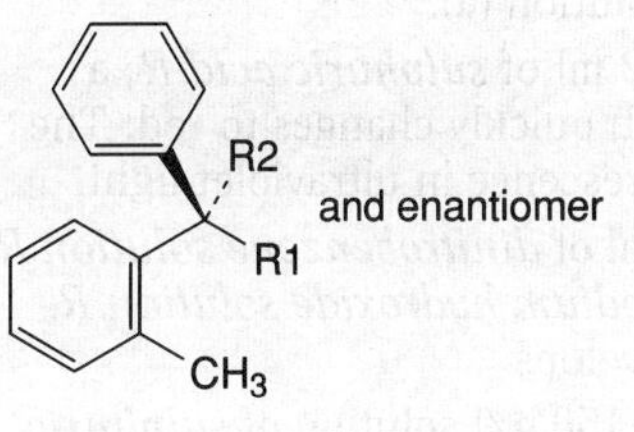

A. R1 = OH, R2 = H: (*RS*)-(2-methylphenyl)phenylmethanol (2-methylbenzhydrol),

B. R1 + R2 = O: (2-methylphenyl)phenylmethanone (2-methylbenzophenone),

C. R1 = O-CH_2-CH_2-NH_2, R2 = H: (*RS*)-2-[(2-methylphenyl)phenylmethoxy]ethanamine,

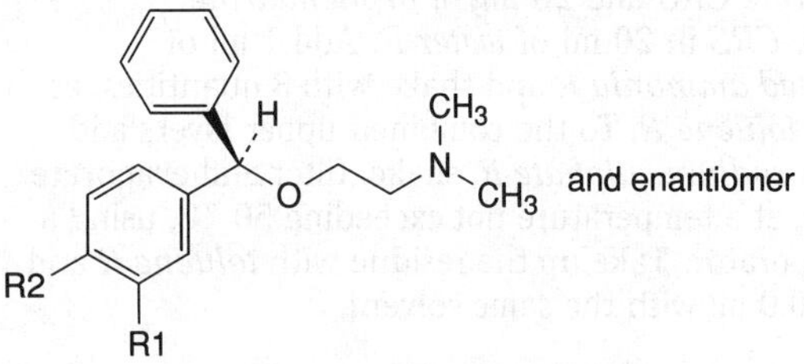

D. R1 = R2 = H: diphenhydramine,

E. R1 = CH_3, R2 = H: (*RS*)-*N*,*N*-dimethyl-2-[(3-methylphenyl)phenylmethoxy]ethanamine (*meta*-methylbenzyl isomer),

F. R1 = H, R2 = CH_3: (*RS*)-*N*,*N*-dimethyl-2-[(4-methylphenyl)phenylmethoxy]ethanamine (*para*-methylbenzyl isomer).

01/2005:1760

ORPHENADRINE HYDROCHLORIDE

Orphenadrini hydrochloridum

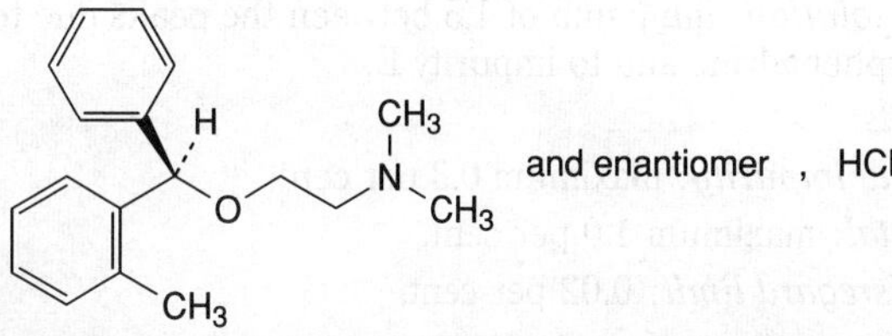

$C_{18}H_{24}ClNO$ M_r 305.9

DEFINITION

(*RS*)-*N*,*N*-Dimethyl-2-[(2-methylphenyl)phenylmethoxy]ethanamine hydrochloride.

Content: 98.5 per cent to 101.0 per cent (dried substance).

CHARACTERS

Appearance: white or almost white, crystalline powder.

Solubility: freely soluble in water and in alcohol.

mp: about 160 °C.

IDENTIFICATION

A. Infrared absorption spectrophotometry (*2.2.24*).

Preparation: discs.

Comparison: *orphenadrine hydrochloride CRS*.

B. It gives reaction (a) of chlorides (*2.3.1*).

TESTS

Appearance of solution. The solution is clear (*2.2.1*) and its absorbance (*2.2.25*) at 436 nm has a maximum of 0.050.

Dissolve 0.70 g in *alcohol R* and dilute to 10.0 ml with the same solvent.

Related substances. Gas chromatography (*2.2.28*): use the normalisation procedure.

Test solution. Dissolve 0.300 g of the substance to be examined in *water R* and dilute to 50 ml with the same solvent. Add 2 ml of *concentrated ammonia R* and shake with 3 quantities, each of 10 ml, of *toluene R*. To the combined upper layers add *anhydrous sodium sulphate R*, shake, filter and evaporate the filtrate, at a temperature not

Monographs N-O

exceeding 50 °C, using a rotary evaporator. Take up the residue with *toluene R* and dilute to 20.0 ml with the same solvent.

Reference solution. Dissolve 20 mg of *orphenadrine hydrochloride CRS* and 20 mg of *orphenadrine impurity E CRS* in 20 ml of *water R*. Add 1 ml of *concentrated ammonia R* and shake with 3 quantities, each of 5 ml, of *toluene R*. To the combined upper layers add *anhydrous sodium sulphate R*, shake, filter and evaporate the filtrate, at a temperature not exceeding 50 °C, using a rotary evaporator. Take up the residue with *toluene R* and dilute to 20.0 ml with the same solvent.

Column:

- *size*: l = 60 m, Ø = 0.32 mm,
- *stationary phase*: *poly(dimethyl)(diphenyl)siloxane R* (film thickness 1.0 μm).

Carrier gas: *helium for chromatography R*.

Flow rate: 1 ml/min.

Split ratio: 1:25.

Temperature:

- *column*: 240 °C,
- *injection port and detector*: 290 °C.

Detection: flame ionisation.

Injection: 2 μl.

Run time: 1.3 times the retention time of orphenadrine.

System suitability: reference solution:

- *resolution*: minimum of 1.5 between the peaks due to orphenadrine and to impurity E.

Limits:

- *any impurity*: maximum 0.3 per cent,
- *total*: maximum 1.0 per cent,
- *disregard limit*: 0.02 per cent.

Heavy metals (*2.4.8*): maximum 10 ppm.

2.0 g complies with limit test C. Prepare the standard using 2 ml of *lead standard solution (10 ppm Pb) R*.

Loss on drying (*2.2.32*): maximum 0.5 per cent, determined on 1.000 g by drying in an oven at 100-105 °C for 3 h.

Sulphated ash (*2.4.14*): maximum 0.1 per cent, determined on 1.0 g.

ASSAY

Dissolve 0.250 g in 50 ml of *acetic anhydride R*. Titrate with *0.1 M perchloric acid*, determining the end-point potentiometrically (*2.2.20*).

1 ml of *0.1 M perchloric acid* is equivalent to 30.59 mg of $C_{18}H_{24}ClNO$.

STORAGE

Protected from light. If the substance is sterile, store in a sterile, airtight, tamper-proof container, protected from light.

IMPURITIES

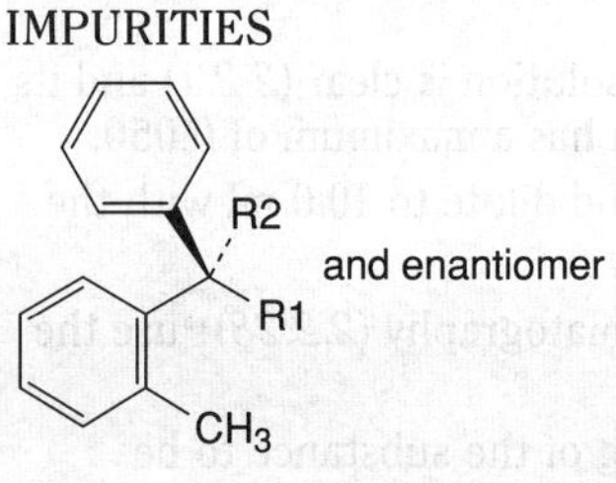

A. R1 = OH, R2 = H: (*RS*)-(2-methylphenyl)phenylmethanol (2-methylbenzhydrol),

B. R1+ R2 = O: (2-methylphenyl)phenylmethanone (2-methylbenzophenone),

C. R1 = O-CH_2-CH_2-NH_2, R2 = H: (*RS*)-2-[(2-methylphenyl)phenylmethoxy]ethanamine,

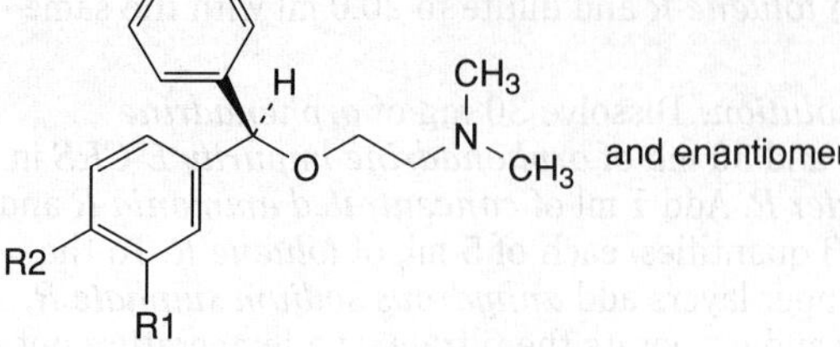

D. R1 = R2 = H: diphenhydramine,

E. R1 = CH_3, R2 = H: (*RS*)-*N,N*-dimethyl-2-[(3-methylphenyl)phenylmethoxy]ethanamine (*meta*-methylbenzyl isomer),

F. R1 = H, R2 = CH_3: (*RS*)-*N,N*-dimethyl-2-[(4-methylphenyl)phenylmethoxy]ethanamine (*para*-methylbenzyl isomer).

01/2005:0048

OUABAIN

Ouabainum

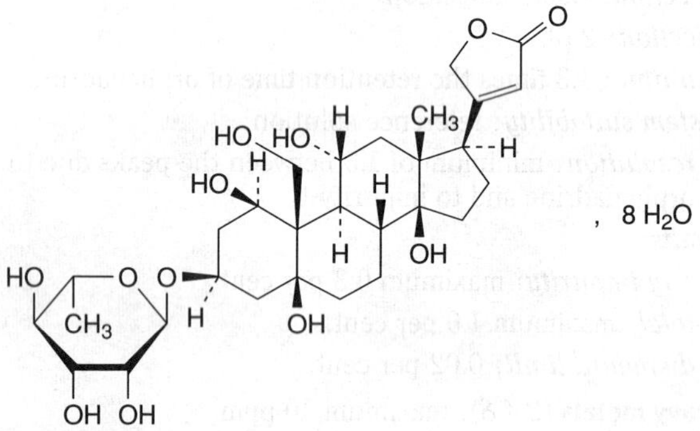

$C_{29}H_{44}O_{12},8H_2O$ M_r 729

DEFINITION

Ouabain contains not less than 96.0 per cent and not more than the equivalent of 104.0 per cent of 3β-[(6-deoxy-α-L-mannopyranosyl)oxy]-1β,5,11α,14,19-pentahydroxy-5β,14β-card-20(22)-enolide, calculated with reference to the anhydrous substance.

CHARACTERS

A white, crystalline powder or colourless crystals, sparingly soluble in water and in ethanol, practically insoluble in ethyl acetate.

IDENTIFICATION

A. Examine the chromatograms obtained in the test for related substances. The principal spot in the chromatogram obtained with the test solution is similar in position, colour and size to the spot in the chromatogram obtained with reference solution (a).

B. Dissolve 2 mg to 3 mg in 2 ml of *sulphuric acid R*; a pink colour develops which quickly changes to red. The solution shows green fluorescence in ultraviolet light.

C. Dissolve about 1 mg in 1 ml of *dinitrobenzene solution R* and add 0.2 ml of *dilute sodium hydroxide solution R*. An intense blue colour develops.

D. Dissolve 0.1 g in 5 ml of a 150 g/l solution of *sulphuric acid R* and boil for a few minutes. The solution becomes yellow and turbid. Filter and add to the filtrate 5 ml of a 120 g/l solution of *sodium hydroxide R* and 3 ml of *cupri-tartaric solution R*. Heat. A red precipitate is formed.

TESTS

Solution S. Dissolve 0.20 g in 15 ml of *water R*, heating on a water-bath. Allow to cool and dilute to 20.0 ml with the same solvent.

Appearance of solution. Solution S is clear (*2.2.1*) and colourless (*2.2.2, Method II*).

Specific optical rotation (*2.2.7*). − 30 to − 33, determined on solution S and calculated with reference to the anhydrous substance.

Related substances. Examine by thin-layer chromatography (*2.2.27*),using *silica gel G R* as the coating substance.

Test solution. Dissolve a quantity of the substance to be examined corresponding to 20 mg of the anhydrous substance in 1.0 ml of a mixture of 32 volumes of *water R*, 100 volumes of *chloroform R* and 100 volumes of *methanol R*.

Reference solution (a). Dissolve a quantity of *ouabain CRS* corresponding to 20 mg of the anhydrous substance in 1.0 ml of a mixture of 32 volumes of *water R*, 100 volumes of *chloroform R* and 100 volumes of *methanol R*.

Reference solution (b). Dissolve a quantity of *ouabain CRS* corresponding to 10 mg of the anhydrous substance in a mixture of 32 volumes of *water R*, 100 volumes of *chloroform R*, 100 volumes of *methanol R* and dilute to 25 ml with the same mixture of solvents.

Reference solution (c). Dilute 2.5 ml of reference solution (b) to 10 ml with a mixture of 32 volumes of *water R*, 100 volumes of *chloroform R* and 100 volumes of *methanol R*.

Apply separately to the plate 5 µl of each solution. Develop over a path of 13 cm using a homogeneous mixture of 4 volumes of *water R*, 15 volumes of *methanol R*, 15 volumes of *dimethyl sulphoxide R* and 70 volumes of *chloroform R*. Dry the plate immediately at 140 °C for 30 min in a ventilated drying oven. Allow to cool, spray with *alcoholic sulphuric acid solution R* and heat at 140 °C for 15 min. Any spot in the chromatogram obtained with the test solution, apart from the principal spot, is not more intense than the spot in the chromatogram obtained with reference solution (b) (2.0 per cent). The test is not valid unless the principal spot in the chromatogram obtained with reference solution (a) and the principal spot in the chromatogram obtained with the test solution migrate over a distance sufficient to give unequivocal separation of the secondary spots and the spot in the chromatogram obtained with reference solution (c) is clearly visible.

Alkaloids and strophanthin-K. To 5.0 ml of solution S add 0.5 ml of a 100 g/l solution of *tannic acid R*. No precipitate is formed.

Water (*2.5.12*). 18.0 per cent to 22.0 per cent, determined on 0.100 g by the semi-micro determination of water.

Sulphated ash (*2.4.14*). Not more than 0.1 per cent, determined on 1.0 g.

ASSAY

Dissolve 40.0 mg in *alcohol R* and dilute to 50.0 ml with the same solvent. Dilute 5.0 ml of the solution to 100.0 ml with *alcohol R*. Prepare a reference solution in the same manner using 40.0 mg of *ouabain CRS*. To 5.0 ml of each solution add 3.0 ml of *alkaline sodium picrate solution R*, allow to stand protected from bright light for 30 min and measure the absorbance (*2.2.25*) of each solution at the maximum at 495 nm using as the compensation liquid a mixture of 5.0 ml of *alcohol R* and 3.0 ml of *alkaline sodium picrate solution R* prepared at the same time.

Calculate the content of $C_{29}H_{44}O_{12}$ from the absorbances measured and the concentrations of the solutions.

STORAGE

Store protected from light.

01/2005:2017

OXALIPLATIN

Oxaliplatinum

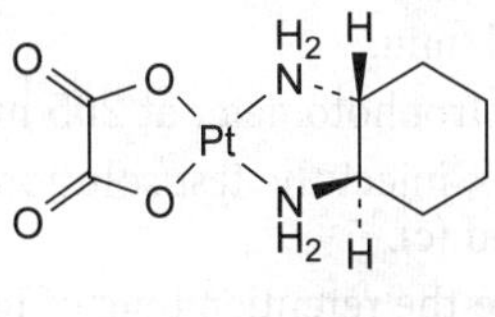

$C_8H_{14}N_2O_4Pt$ M_r 397.3

DEFINITION

(*SP*-4-2)-[(1*R*,2*R*)-Cyclohexane-1,2-diamine-κ*N*,κ*N'*][ethanedioato(2-)-κ*O*[1],κ*O*[2]]platinum.

Content: 98.0 per cent to 102.0 per cent (dried substance).

CHARACTERS

Appearance: white or almost white, crystalline powder.

Solubility: slightly soluble in water, very slightly soluble in methanol, practically insoluble in ethanol.

IDENTIFICATION

A. Infrared absorption spectrophotometry (*2.2.24*).

Comparison: *oxaliplatin CRS*.

B. It complies with the test for specific optical rotation (see Tests).

TESTS

Appearance of solution. The solution is clear (*2.2.1*) and colourless (*2.2.2, Method II*).

Dissolve 0.10 g in *water R* and dilute to 50 ml with the same solvent.

Acidity. Dissolve 0.10 g in *carbon dioxide-free water R*, dilute to 50 ml with the same solvent and add 0.5 ml of *phenolphthalein solution R1*. The solution is colourless. Not more than 0.60 ml of *0.01 M sodium hydroxide* is required to change the colour of the indicator to pink.

Specific optical rotation (*2.2.7*): + 74.5 to + 78.0 (dried substance).

Dissolve 0.250 g in *water R* and dilute to 50.0 ml with the same solvent.

Related substances

A. Impurity A. Liquid chromatography (*2.2.29*). *Use vigorous shaking and very brief sonication to dissolve the substance to be examined. Inject the test solution within 20 min of preparation.*

Test solution. Dissolve 0.100 g of the substance to be examined in *water R* and dilute to 50.0 ml with the same solvent.

Reference solution (a). Dissolve 14.0 mg of *oxalic acid R* (impurity A) in *water R* and dilute to 250.0 ml with the same solvent.

Reference solution (b). Dilute 5.0 ml of reference solution (a) to 200.0 ml with *water R*.

Reference solution (c). Dissolve 12.5 mg of *sodium nitrate R* in *water R* and dilute to 250.0 ml with the same solvent. Dilute a mixture of 2.0 ml of this solution and 25.0 ml of reference solution (a) to 100.0 ml with *water R*.

Column:

- *size*: *l* = 25 cm, Ø = 4.6 mm,
- *stationary phase*: *base-deactivated octadecylsilyl silica gel for chromatography R* (5 µm).

Temperature: 40 °C.

Mobile phase: mix 20 volumes of *acetonitrile R* with 80 volumes of a solution prepared as follows: to 10 ml of a 320 g/l solution of *tetrabutylammonium hydroxide R* add 1.36 g of *potassium dihydrogen phosphate R* and dilute to 1000 ml with *water R*; adjust this solution to pH 6.0 with *phosphoric acid R*.

Flow rate: 2 ml/min.

Detection: spectrophotometer at 205 nm.

Injection: 20 µl; inject the test solution and reference solutions (b) and (c).

Run time: twice the retention time of impurity A.

Retention times: nitrate = about 2.7 min; impurity A = about 4.7 min.

System suitability:

- *resolution*: minimum 9 between the peaks due to nitrate and impurity A in the chromatogram obtained with reference solution (c),
- *signal-to-noise ratio*: minimum of 10 for the peak due to impurity A in the chromatogram obtained with reference solution (b).

Limits:

- *impurity A*: not more than twice the area of the principal peak in the chromatogram obtained with reference solution (b) (0.1 per cent).

B. Impurity B. Liquid chromatography (*2.2.29*). *Use vigorous shaking and very brief sonication to dissolve the substance to be examined. Inject the test solution within 20 min of preparation. Use suitable polypropylene containers for the preparation and injection of all solutions. Glass pipettes may be used for diluting solutions.*

Test solution. Dissolve 0.100 g of the substance to be examined in *water R* and dilute to 50.0 ml with the same solvent.

Reference solution (a). Dissolve 12.5 mg of *oxaliplatin impurity B CRS* in 63 ml of *methanol R* and dilute to 250.0 ml with *water R*. Dilute 3.0 ml to 200.0 ml with *water R*.

Reference solution (b). In order to prepare *in situ* the degradation compound (impurity E) dissolve 12.5 mg of *oxaliplatin impurity B CRS* in 63 ml of *methanol R* and dilute to 250 ml with *water R*. Adjust to pH 6.0 with a 0.2 g/l solution of *sodium hydroxide R*. Heat for 4 h at 70 °C and allow to cool.

Column:

- *size*: *l* = 25 cm, Ø = 4.6 mm,
- *stationary phase*: *base-deactivated octadecylsilyl silica gel for chromatography R* (5 µm).

Temperature: 40 °C.

Mobile phase: mix 20 volumes of *acetonitrile R* with 80 volumes of a solution prepared as follows: dissolve 1.36 g of *potassium dihydrogen phosphate R* and 1 g of *sodium heptanesulphonate R* in 1000 ml of *water R*; adjust this solution to pH 3.0 ± 0.05 with *phosphoric acid R*.

Flow rate: 2.0 ml/min.

Detection: spectrophotometer at 215 nm.

Injection: 20 µl.

Run time: 2.5 times the retention time of impurity B.

Retention times: impurity B = about 4.3 min; impurity E = about 6.4 min.

System suitability:

- *resolution*: minimum 7 between the peaks due to impurity B and impurity E in the chromatogram obtained with reference solution (b),
- *signal-to-noise ratio*: minimum of 10 for the peak due to impurity B in the chromatogram obtained with reference solution (a).

Limits:

- *impurity B*: not more than 3.3 times the area of the principal peak in the chromatogram obtained with reference solution (a) (0.1 per cent).

C. Impurity C and other related substances. Liquid chromatography (*2.2.29*). *Use vigorous shaking and very brief sonication to dissolve the substance to be examined. Inject the test solution within 20 min of preparation.*

Test solution (a). Dissolve 0.100 g of the substance to be examined in *water R* and dilute to 50.0 ml with the same solvent.

Test solution (b). Dissolve 50.0 mg of the substance to be examined in *water R* and dilute to 500.0 ml with the same solvent.

Reference solution (a). Dissolve 10 mg of *oxaliplatin impurity C CRS* and 10 mg of *oxaliplatin CRS* in *water R* and dilute to 100.0 ml with the same solvent.

Reference solution (b). Dilute 1.0 ml of reference solution (a) to 100.0 ml with *water R*.

Reference solution (c). Dissolve 5 mg of *dichlorodiaminocyclohexaneplatinum CRS* in *methanol R* and dilute to 50.0 ml with the same solvent. To 10.0 ml of this solution add 10.0 ml of reference solution (a) and dilute to 100.0 ml with *water R*.

Reference solution (d). Dissolve 50.0 mg of *oxaliplatin CRS* in *water R* and dilute to 500.0 ml with the same solvent.

Reference solution (e). Dissolve 5.0 mg of *dichlorodiaminocyclohexaneplatinum CRS* in reference solution (d) and dilute to 50.0 ml with the same solvent.

Reference solution (f). To 0.100 g of the substance to be examined add 1.0 ml of reference solution (a) and dilute to 50.0 ml with *water R*.

Column:

- *size*: *l* = 25 cm, Ø = 4.6 mm,
- *stationary phase*: *octadecylsilyl silica gel for chromatography R* (5 µm).

Temperature: 40 °C.

Mobile phase: mixture of solutions A and B (99:1 *V/V*).

- *solution A*: dilute 0.6 ml of *dilute phosphoric acid R* in 1000 ml of *water R* and adjust to pH 3.0 with either *sodium hydroxide solution R* or *phosphoric acid R*,
- *solution B*: *acetonitrile R*.

Flow rate: 1.2 ml/min.

Detection: spectrophotometer at 210 nm.

Injection: 10 µl; inject test solution (a) and reference solutions (b), (c) and (f).

Run time: 3 times the retention time of oxaliplatin.

Monographs N-O

Retention times: impurity C = about 4.4 min; dichlorodiaminocyclohexaneplatinum = about 6.9 min; oxaliplatin = about 8.0 min.

System suitability:

- *resolution*: minimum 2.0 between the peaks due to dichlorodiaminocyclohexaneplatinum and oxaliplatin in the chromatogram obtained with reference solution (c),
- *signal-to-noise ratio*: minimum 50 for the peak due to impurity C and minimum 10 for the peak due to oxaliplatin in the chromatogram obtained with reference solution (b).

Limits:

- *impurity C*: not more than half the area of the peak due to impurity C in the chromatogram obtained with reference solution (f) (0.1 per cent),
- *any other impurity*: not more than twice the area of the peak due to oxaliplatin in the chromatogram obtained with reference solution (b) (0.1 per cent),
- *total of other impurities*: not more than twice the area of the peak due to oxaliplatin in the chromatogram obtained with reference solution (b) (0.1 per cent),
- *disregard limit*: the area of the peak due to oxaliplatin in the chromatogram obtained with reference solution (b) (0.05 per cent); disregard any peak with a retention time less than 2 min.

D. *Total of impurities*: the sum of impurities A, B, C and other related impurities is not greater than 0.30 per cent.

Impurity D. Liquid chromatography (*2.2.29*).

Test solution. Dissolve 30 mg of the substance to be examined in *methanol R* and dilute to 50.0 ml with the same solvent.

Reference solution (a). Dissolve 5 mg of *oxaliplatin impurity D CRS* in *methanol R* and dilute to 100.0 ml with the same solvent.

Reference solution (b). Dilute 15.0 ml of reference solution (a) to 50.0 ml with *methanol R*.

Reference solution (c). Dissolve 150.0 mg of *oxaliplatin CRS* in *methanol R* and dilute to 200.0 ml with the same solvent.

Reference solution (d). Dilute 5.0 ml of reference solution (c) to 100.0 ml with *methanol R*.

Reference solution (e). To 40 ml of reference solution (c) add 1.0 ml of reference solution (b) and dilute to 50.0 ml with *methanol R*.

Reference solution (f). Mix 4.0 ml of reference solution (a) and 5.0 ml of reference solution (d) and dilute to 50.0 ml with *methanol R*.

Column:

- *size*: *l* = 25 cm, Ø = 4.6 mm,
- *stationary phase*: *silica gel OC for chiral separations R*.

Temperature: 40 °C.

Mobile phase: *ethanol R, methanol R* (3:7 *V/V*).

Flow rate: 0.3 ml/min.

Detection: spectrophotometer at 254 nm.

Injection: 20 µl; inject the test solution and reference solutions (e) and (f).

Run time: twice the retention time of oxaliplatin.

Retention times: oxaliplatin = about 14 min; impurity D = about 16 min.

System suitability:

- *resolution*: minimum 1.5 between the peaks due to oxaliplatin and impurity D in the chromatogram obtained with reference solution (f),
- *signal-to-noise ratio*: minimum 10 for the peak due to impurity D in the chromatogram obtained with reference solution (e).

Limits:

- *impurity D*: not more than twice the peak height of the corresponding peak in the chromatogram obtained with reference solution (e) (0.1 per cent).

Silver: maximum 5 ppm.

Atomic absorption spectrometry (*2.2.23, Method II*).

Test solution. Dissolve 0.1000 g of the substance to be examined in *water R* and dilute to 50.0 ml with the same solvent. Dilute 20 µl of this solution to 40 µl with *0.5 M nitric acid*.

Reference solution (a). Dilute a solution of *silver nitrate R* containing 1000 ppm of silver in *0.5 M nitric acid* with *0.5 M nitric acid* to obtain a solution which contains 10 ppb of silver.

Reference solution (b). Mix 20 µl of the test solution and 8 µl of reference solution (a) and dilute to 40 µl with *0.5 M nitric acid*.

Reference solution (c). Mix 20 µl of the test solution and 16 µl of reference solution (a) and dilute to 40 µl with *0.5 M nitric acid*.

Source: silver hollow-cathode lamp.

Wavelength: 328.1 nm.

Atomisation device: furnace.

Measure the absorbance of the test solution and reference solutions (b) and (c).

Loss on drying (*2.2.32*): maximum 0.5 per cent, determined on 1.000 g by drying in an oven at 100-105 °C for 2 h.

Bacterial endotoxins (*2.6.14*): less than 1.0 IU/mg, if intended for use in the manufacture of parenteral dosage forms without a further appropriate procedure for the removal of bacterial endotoxins.

ASSAY

Liquid chromatography (*2.2.29*) as described in the test for impurity C and other related substances with the following modifications.

Injection: 20 µl; inject test solution (b) and reference solutions (d) and (e).

System suitability:

- *resolution*: minimum 2.0 between the peaks due to dichlorodiaminocyclohexaneplatinum and oxaliplatin in the chromatogram obtained with reference solution (e),
- *repeatability*: reference solution (d).

Calculate the percentage content of oxaliplatin using the chromatogram obtained with reference solution (d).

LABELLING

The label states where applicable, that the substance is free from bacterial endotoxins.

IMPURITIES

Specified impurities: A, B, C, D.

Other detectable impurities: E.

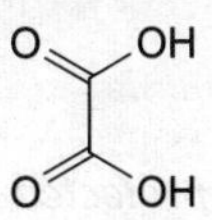

A. ethanedioic acid (oxalic acid),

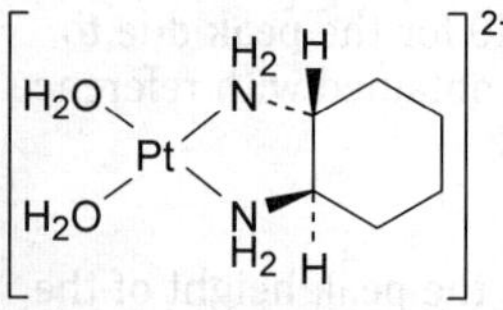

B. (*SP*-4-2)-diaqua[(1*R*,2*R*)-cyclohexane-1,2-diamine-κ*N*, κ*N*′]platinum (diaquodiaminocyclohexaneplatinum),

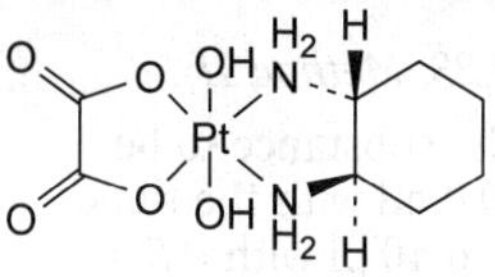

C. (*OC*-6-33)-[(1*R*,2*R*)-cyclohexane-1,2-diamine-κ*N*, κ*N*′][ethanedioato(2-)-κ*O*[1],κ*O*[2]]dihydroxyplatinum,

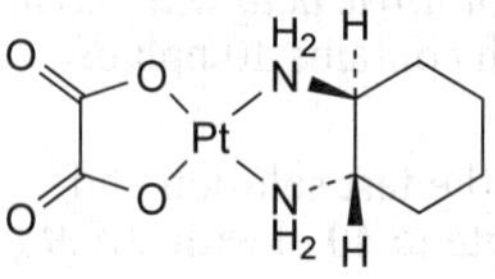

D. (*SP*-4-2)-[(1*S*,2*S*)-cyclohexane-1,2-diamine-κ*N*, κ*N*′][ethanedioato(2-)-κ*O*[1],κ*O*[2]]platinum (*S*,*S*-enantiomer of oxaliplatin),

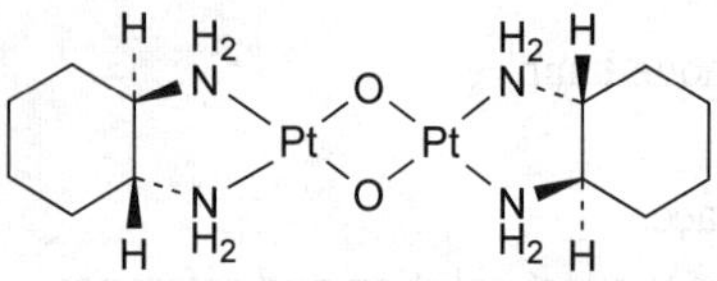

E. (*SP*-4-2)-di-μ-oxobis[(1*R*,2*R*)-cyclohexane-1,2-diamine-κ*N*, κ*N*′]diplatinum (diaquodiaminocyclohexaneplatinum dimer).

01/2005:0778

OXAZEPAM

Oxazepamum

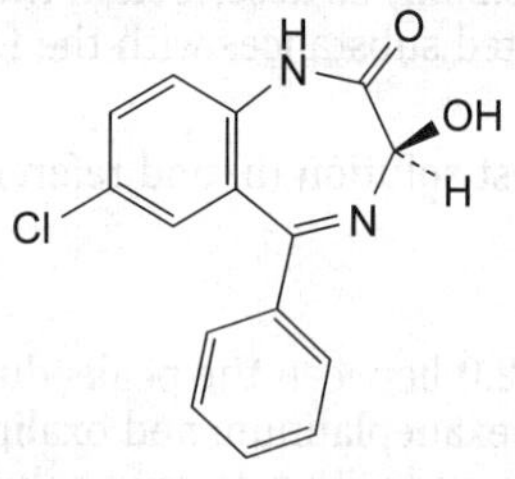

and enantiomer

$C_{15}H_{11}ClN_2O_2$ M_r 286.7

DEFINITION

Oxazepam contains not less than 98.5 per cent and not more than the equivalent of 101.0 per cent of (3*RS*)-7-chloro-3-hydroxy-5-phenyl-1,3-dihydro-2*H*-1,4-benzodiazepin-2-one, calculated with reference to the dried substance.

CHARACTERS

A white or almost white, crystalline powder, practically insoluble in water, slightly soluble in alcohol and in methylene chloride.

IDENTIFICATION

First identification: B, C.

Second identification: A, C, D.

A. *Prepare the solutions immediately before use, protected from light.* Dissolve 20.0 mg in *alcohol R* and dilute to 100.0 ml with the same solvent. Dilute 10.0 ml of the solution to 50.0 ml with *alcohol R* (solution A). Dilute 10.0 ml of solution A to 100.0 ml with *alcohol R* (solution B). Examined between 300 nm and 350 nm (*2.2.25*), solution A shows an absorption maximum at 316 nm. Examined between 220 nm and 250 nm, solution B shows an absorption maximum at 229 nm. The specific absorbance at the maximum at 229 nm is 1220 to 1300.

B. Examine by infrared absorption spectrophotometry (*2.2.24*) comparing with the spectrum obtained with *oxazepam CRS*. Examine the substances prepared as discs.

C. Examine the chromatograms obtained in the test for related substances in ultraviolet light at 254 nm. The principal spot in the chromatogram obtained with test solution (b) is similar in position and size to the principal spot in the chromatogram obtained with reference solution (a).

D. Dissolve about 20 mg in a mixture of 5 ml of *hydrochloric acid R* and 10 ml of *water R*. Heat to boiling for 5 min and cool. Add 2 ml of a 1 g/l solution of *sodium nitrite R* and allow to stand for 1 min. Add 1 ml of a 5 g/l solution of *sulphamic acid R*, mix and allow to stand for 1 min. Add 1 ml of a 1 g/l solution of *naphthylethylenediamine dihydrochloride R*. A red colour develops.

TESTS

Related substances. *Carry out the test protected from light.* Examine by thin-layer chromatography (*2.2.27*), using as the coating substance a suitable silica gel with a fluorescent indicator having an optimal intensity at 254 nm. Before use, wash the plate with *methanol R* until the solvent front has migrated at least 17 cm. Allow the plate to dry in air and heat at 100 °C to 105 °C for 30 min.

Test solution (a). Dissolve 50 mg of the substance to be examined in *acetone R* and dilute to 10 ml with the same solvent.

Test solution (b). Dilute 2 ml of test solution (a) to 10 ml with *acetone R*.

Reference solution (a). Dissolve 10 mg of *oxazepam CRS* in *acetone R* and dilute to 10 ml with the same solvent.

Reference solution (b). Dissolve 10 mg of *oxazepam CRS* and 10 mg of *bromazepam CRS* in *acetone R* and dilute to 10 ml with the same solvent.

Reference solution (c). Dilute 1 ml of test solution (b) to 100 ml with *acetone R*.

Reference solution (d). Dilute 5 ml of reference solution (c) to 10 ml with *acetone R*.

Apply separately to the plate 20 µl of each solution. Develop over a path of 15 cm, in the same direction as the washing with *methanol R*, using a mixture of 10 volumes of *methanol R* and 100 volumes of *methylene chloride R*. Allow the plate to dry in air and examine in ultraviolet light at 254 nm. Any spot in the chromatogram obtained with test solution (a), apart from the principal spot, is not more intense than the spot in the chromatogram obtained with reference solution (c) (0.2 per cent) and at most one such spot is more intense than the spot in the chromatogram obtained with reference solution (d) (0.1 per cent). The test is not valid unless the chromatogram obtained with reference solution (b) shows two clearly separated spots.

Loss on drying (*2.2.32*). Not more than 0.5 per cent, determined on 1.000 g by drying in an oven at 100 °C to 105 °C at a pressure not exceeding 0.7 kPa.

Sulphated ash (*2.4.14*). Not more than 0.1 per cent, determined on 1.0 g.

ASSAY

Dissolve 0.250 g in a mixture of 10 ml of *anhydrous acetic acid R* and 90 ml of *acetic anhydride R*. Titrate with *0.1 M perchloric acid* determining the end-point potentiometrically (*2.2.20*).

1 ml of *0.1 M perchloric acid* is equivalent to 28.67 mg of $C_{15}H_{11}ClN_2O_2$.

STORAGE

Store protected from light.

01/2005:1761

OXELADIN HYDROGEN CITRATE

Oxeladini hydrogenocitras

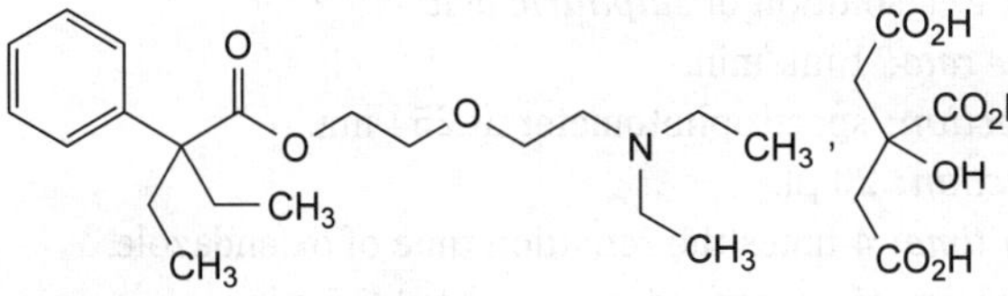

$C_{26}H_{41}NO_{10}$ M_r 527.6

DEFINITION

2-[2-(Diethylamino)ethoxy]ethyl 2-ethyl-2-phenylbutanoate dihydrogen 2-hydroxypropane-1,2,3-tricarboxylate.

Content: 99.0 per cent to 101.0 per cent (dried substance).

CHARACTERS

Appearance: white or almost white, crystalline powder.

Solubility: freely soluble in water, slightly to very slightly soluble in ethyl acetate.

It shows polymorphism.

IDENTIFICATION

Infrared absorption spectrophotometry (*2.2.24*).

Comparison: *oxeladin hydrogen citrate CRS*.

If the spectra obtained in the solid state show differences, dissolve the substance to be examined and the reference substance separately in *anhydrous ethanol R*, evaporate to dryness and record new spectra using the residues.

TESTS

Appearance of solution. The solution is clear (*2.2.1*) and not more intensely coloured than reference solution Y_6 (*2.2.2, Method II*).

Dissolve 2.0 g in *water R* and dilute to 10.0 ml with the same solvent.

Related substances. Gas chromatography (*2.2.28*): use the normalisation procedure. *Prepare the solutions immediately before use.*

Test solution. Dissolve 0.500 g of the substance to be examined in *water R* and dilute to 50 ml with the same solvent. Add 1 ml of a 10.3 g/l solution of *hydrochloric acid R* and shake with 3 quantities, each of 10 ml, of *methylene chloride R*. Combine the lower layers. Add 5 ml of *concentrated ammonia R* to the aqueous layer and shake with 3 quantities, each of 10 ml, of *methylene chloride R*. Combine the lower layers obtained to the lower layers obtained previously, add *anhydrous sodium sulphate R*, shake, filter and evaporate the filtrate, at a temperature not exceeding 30 °C, using a rotary evaporator. Take up the residue with *methylene chloride R* and dilute to 20.0 ml with the same solvent.

Reference solution (a). Dissolve 5 mg of *oxeladin impurity D CRS* in 10 ml of *water R*, add 0.5 ml of *concentrated ammonia R* and shake with 3 quantities, each of 2 ml, of *methylene chloride R*. To the combined lower layers, add 0.2 ml of the test solution and dilute to 10.0 ml with *methylene chloride R*.

Reference solution (b). Dilute 1.0 ml of the test solution to 100.0 ml with *methylene chloride R*. Dilute 1.0 ml of this solution to 20.0 ml with *methylene chloride R*.

Reference solution (c). Dissolve 5 mg of *oxeladin impurity C CRS* in 10 ml of *water R*, add 0.5 ml of *concentrated ammonia R* and shake with 3 quantities, each of 2 ml, of *methylene chloride R*. Combine the lower layers and dilute to 10 ml with *methylene chloride R*.

Column:

- *material*: fused silica,
- *size*: *l* = 25 m, Ø = 0.32 mm,
- *stationary phase*: *poly(dimethyl)(diphenyl)siloxane R* (film thickness 0.4 µm).

Carrier gas: *helium for chromatography R*.

Flow rate: 1.0 ml/min. Adjust the flow rate if necessary to obtain a retention time of about 13 min for oxeladin.

Split ratio: 1:15.

Temperature:

	Time (min)	Temperature (°C)
Column	0 - 4	160
	4 - 12	160 → 240
	12 - 21	240
	21 - 30	240 → 160
Injection port		280
Detector		280

Detection: flame ionisation.

Injection: 1 µl.

Relative retention with reference to oxeladin (retention time = about 13 min): impurity A = about 0.2; impurity B = about 0.4; impurity C = about 0.8; impurity D = about 0.9.

System suitability: reference solution (a):

- *resolution*: minimum 10 between the peaks due to impurity D and oxeladin.

Limits:

- *impurity C*: maximum 0.2 per cent,
- *impurity D*: maximum 0.3 per cent,
- *any other impurity*: for each impurity, maximum 0.1 per cent,
- *total*: maximum 1.0 per cent,
- *disregard limit*: the area of the principal peak in the chromatogram obtained with reference solution (b) (0.05 per cent).

Loss on drying (*2.2.32*): maximum 0.5 per cent, determined on 1.000 g by drying *in vacuo* at 60 °C for 3 h.

Sulphated ash (*2.4.14*): maximum 0.1 per cent, determined on 1.0 g.

ASSAY

Dissolve 0.400 g in 50 ml of *anhydrous acetic acid R*. Titrate with *0.1 M perchloric acid*, determining the end-point potentiometrically (*2.2.20*).

1 ml of *0.1 M perchloric acid* is equivalent to 52.76 mg of $C_{26}H_{41}NO_{10}$.

IMPURITIES

Specified impurities: C, D.

Other detectable impurities: A, B.

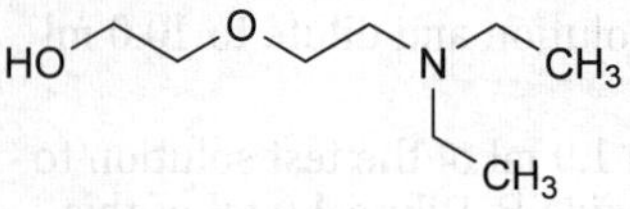

A. 2-[2-(diethylamino)ethoxy]ethanol,

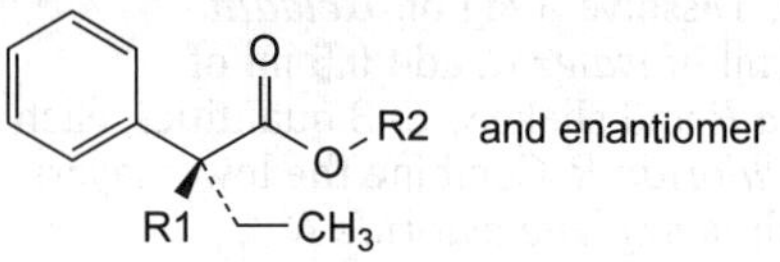

B. R1 = C_2H_5, R2 = H: 2-ethyl-2-phenylbutanoic acid,

C. R1 = C_2H_5, R2 = $[CH_2]_2$-$N(C_2H_5)_2$: 2-(diethylamino)ethyl 2-ethyl-2-phenylbutanoate,

D. R1 = H, R2 = $[CH_2]_2$-O-$[CH_2]_2$-$N(C_2H_5)_2$: 2-[2-(diethylamino)ethoxy]ethyl (2*RS*)-2-phenylbutanoate.

01/2005:1458

OXFENDAZOLE FOR VETERINARY USE

Oxfendazolum ad usum veterinarium

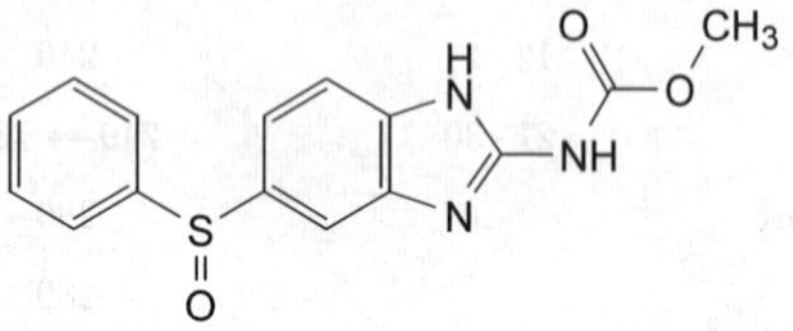

$C_{15}H_{13}N_3O_3S$ M_r 315.4

DEFINITION

Methyl [5-(phenylsulphinyl)-1*H*-benzimidazol-2-yl]carbamate.

Content: 97.5 per cent to 100.5 per cent (dried substance).

CHARACTERS

Appearance: white or almost white powder.

Solubility: practically insoluble in water, slightly soluble in alcohol and in methylene chloride.

It shows polymorphism.

IDENTIFICATION

Infrared absorption spectrophotometry (*2.2.24*).

Comparison: *oxfendazole CRS.*

If the spectra obtained in the solid state show differences, dissolve the substance to be examined and the reference substance separately in *alcohol R*, evaporate to dryness and record new spectra using the residues.

TESTS

Related substances. Liquid chromatography (*2.2.29*).

Test solution. Dissolve 25.0 mg of the substance to be examined in the mobile phase and dilute to 100.0 ml with the mobile phase.

Reference solution (a). Dilute 1.0 ml of the test solution to 100.0 ml with the mobile phase.

Reference solution (b). To 10 ml of the test solution, add 0.25 ml of *strong hydrogen peroxide solution R* and dilute to 25 ml with the mobile phase.

Reference solution (c). Dissolve 5.0 mg of *fenbendazole CRS* and 10.0 mg of *oxfendazole impurity B CRS* in the mobile phase and dilute to 100.0 ml with the mobile phase. Dilute 1.0 ml to 20.0 ml with the mobile phase.

Reference solution (d). Dissolve 5 mg of *oxfendazole with impurity D CRS* in the mobile phase and dilute to 20 ml with the mobile phase (solution used for identification of impurity D).

Column:

– *size*: *l* = 0.25 m, Ø = 4.6 mm,
– *stationary phase*: spherical *end-capped octadecylsilyl silica gel for chromatography R* (5 µm) with a specific surface area of 350 m^2/g, a pore size of 10 nm and a carbon loading of 14 per cent.

Mobile phase: mix 36 volumes of *acetonitrile R* and 64 volumes of a 2 g/l solution of *sodium pentanesulphonate R* adjusted to pH 2.7 with a 2.8 per cent *V/V* solution of *sulphuric acid R*.

Flow rate: 1 ml/min.

Detection: spectrophotometer at 254 nm.

Injection: 20 µl.

Run time: 4 times the retention time of oxfendazole.

Retention time: oxfendazole = about 6.5 min.

System suitability: reference solution (b):

– *resolution*: minimum 4.0 between the 2 principal peaks corresponding to impurity C (1st peak) and oxfendazole (2nd peak).

Limits:

– *impurity A*: not more than the area of the corresponding peak in the chromatogram obtained with reference solution (c) (1.0 per cent),
– *impurity B*: not more than the area of the corresponding peak in the chromatogram obtained with reference solution (c) (2.0 per cent),
– *impurity C or D*: for each impurity, not more than the area of the principal peak in the chromatogram obtained with reference solution (a) (1.0 per cent),
– *any other impurity*: not more than 0.1 times the area of the principal peak in the chromatogram obtained with reference solution (a) (0.1 per cent),
– *total*: not more than 3 times the area of the principal peak in the chromatogram obtained with reference solution (a) (3.0 per cent),
– *disregard limit*: 0.05 times the area of the principal peak in the chromatogram obtained with reference solution (a) (0.05 per cent).

Loss on drying (*2.2.32*): maximum 0.5 per cent, determined on 1.000 g by drying in an oven at 100-105 °C at a pressure not exceeding 0.7 kPa for 2 h.

Sulphated ash (*2.4.14*): maximum 0.2 per cent, determined on 1.0 g.

ASSAY

Dissolve 0.250 g in 3 ml of *anhydrous formic acid R.* Add 40 ml of *anhydrous acetic acid R.* Titrate with *0.1 M perchloric acid,* determining the end-point potentiometrically (*2.2.20*).

1 ml of *0.1 M perchloric acid* is equivalent to 31.54 mg of $C_{15}H_{13}N_3O_3S$.

STORAGE

Protected from light.

IMPURITIES

A. fenbendazole,

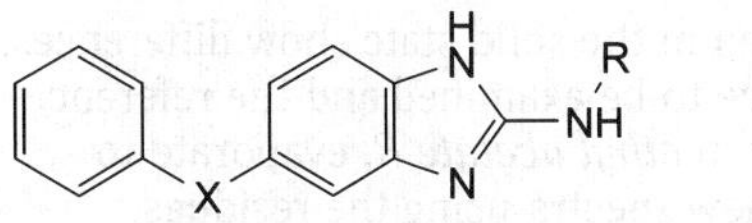

B. X = SO_2, R = CO_2-CH_3: methyl [5-(phenylsulphonyl)-1*H*-benzimidazol-2-yl]carbamate,

C. X = SO, R = H: 5-(phenylsulphinyl)-1*H*-benzimidazol-2-amine,

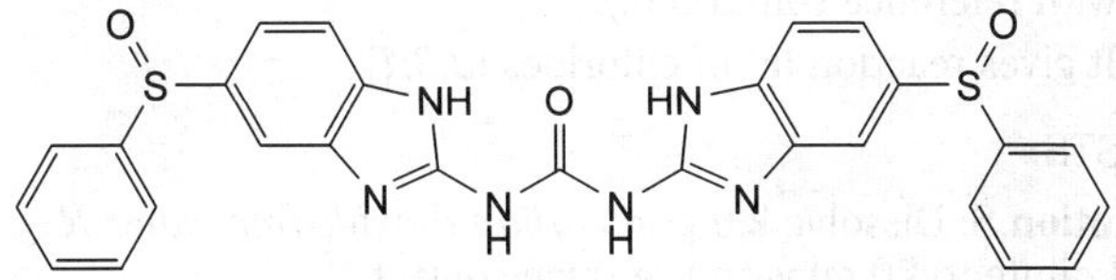

D. *N*,*N'*-bis[5-(phenylsulphinyl)-1*H*-benzimidazol-2-yl]urea.

01/2005:1353

OXOLINIC ACID

Acidum oxolinicum

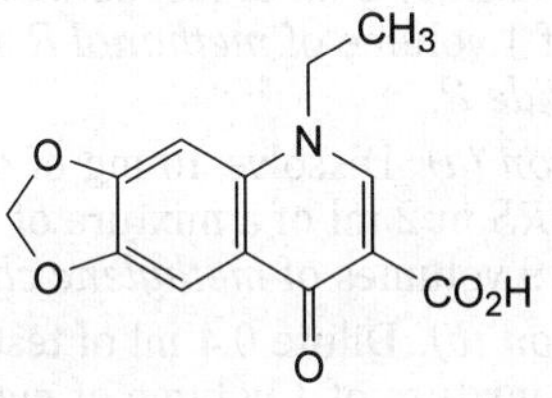

$C_{13}H_{11}NO_5$ M_r 261.2

DEFINITION

Oxolinic acid contains not less than 98.0 per cent and not more than the equivalent of 102.0 per cent of 5-ethyl-8-oxo-5,8-dihydro-1,3-dioxolo[4,5-*g*]quinoline-7-carboxylic acid, calculated with reference to the dried substance.

CHARACTERS

An almost white or pale yellow, crystalline powder, practically insoluble in water, very slightly soluble in methylene chloride, practically insoluble in alcohol. It dissolves in dilute solutions of alkali hydroxides.

IDENTIFICATION

First identification: B.

Second identification: A, C.

A. Dissolve 25.0 mg in 5 ml of *0.1 M sodium hydroxide,* heating on a water-bath. Allow to cool and dilute to 100.0 ml with *methanol R.* Dilute 2.0 ml of the solution to 100.0 ml with *0.1 M hydrochloric acid.* Examined between 220 nm and 350 nm (*2.2.25*), the solution shows three absorption maxima, at 260 nm, 322 nm and 336 nm respectively. The ratio of the absorbance measured at the maximum at 260 nm to that measured at the maximum at 336 nm is 4.9 to 5.2.

B. Examine by infrared absorption spectrophotometry (*2.2.24*), comparing with the spectrum obtained with *oxolinic acid CRS.* Examine the substances prepared as discs.

C. Examine by thin-layer chromatography (*2.2.27*), using a suitable silica gel as the coating substance.

Test solution. Dissolve 10 mg of the substance to be examined in 3 ml of *dilute sodium hydroxide solution R* and dilute to 20 ml with *alcohol R.*

Reference solution (a). Dissolve 10 mg of *oxolinic acid CRS* in 3 ml of *dilute sodium hydroxide solution R* and dilute to 20 ml with *alcohol R.*

Reference solution (b). Dissolve 5 mg of *ciprofloxacin hydrochloride CRS* in *methanol R* and dilute to 10 ml with the same solvent. Dilute 1 ml of the solution to 2 ml with reference solution (a).

Apply separately to the plate 10 µl of each solution. At the bottom of a chromatographic tank, place an evaporating disk containing 50 ml of *concentrated ammonia R.* Close the tank and expose the plate to the ammonia vapour for 15 min. Withdraw the plate and transfer to a chromatographic tank and develop over a path of 15 cm using a mixture of 10 volumes of *acetonitrile R,* 20 volumes of *concentrated ammonia R,* 40 volumes of *methanol R* and 40 volumes of *methylene chloride R.* Allow the plate to dry in air. Examine in ultraviolet light at 254 nm. The principal spot in the chromatogram obtained with the test solution is similar in position, fluorescence and size to the principal spot in the chromatogram obtained with reference solution (a). The identification is not valid unless the chromatogram obtained with reference solution (b) shows two clearly separated spots.

TESTS

Solution S. Dissolve 0.6 g in 20 ml of a 40 g/l solution of *sodium hydroxide R.*

Appearance of solution. Solution S is clear (*2.2.1*) and not more intensely coloured than reference solution B_7 (*2.2.2, Method II*).

Related substances. Examine by thin-layer chromatography (*2.2.27*), using as the coating substance a suitable cellulose with a particle size of narrow distribution.

Test solution. Dissolve 50 mg in 3 ml of *dilute sodium hydroxide solution R* and dilute to 10 ml with *alcohol R.*

Reference solution (a). Dilute 1 ml of the test solution to 50.0 ml with *alcohol R.* Dilute 1.0 ml of the solution to 5.0 ml with *alcohol R.*

Reference solution (b). Dissolve 2 mg of *oxolinic acid impurity B CRS* in *alcohol R* and dilute to 10 ml with the same solvent. Dilute 0.5 ml of the solution to 10 ml with *alcohol R.*

Reference solution (c). Dissolve 5 mg of the substance to be examined and 5 mg of *oxolinic acid impurity A CRS* in 2 ml of *dilute sodium hydroxide solution R* and dilute to 40 ml with *alcohol R.*

Apply separately to the plate 5 µl of each solution, in sufficiently small portions to obtain small spots. Develop over a path of 6 cm (corresponding to two thirds of the plate height) with a mixture of 15 volumes of *ammonia R,* 30 volumes of *water R* and 55 volumes of *propanol R.* Allow the plate to dry in air and examine in ultraviolet light at 254 nm. In the chromatogram obtained with the test solution: any spot corresponding to oxolinic acid impurity B is not more intense than the spot in the chromatogram obtained with reference solution (b) (0.2 per cent); any spot apart from the principal spot and any spot corresponding to oxolinic acid impurity B is not more intense than the spot in the chromatogram obtained with reference solution (a) (0.4 per cent). The test is not valid unless the chromatogram obtained with reference solution (c) shows two clearly separated principal spots.

Heavy metals (*2.4.8*). 2.0 g complies with limit test D for heavy metals (10 ppm). Prepare the standard using 2 ml of *lead standard solution (10 ppm Pb) R.*

Loss on drying (*2.2.32*). Not more than 0.5 per cent determined on 1.000 g by heating in an oven at 100 °C to 105 °C.

Sulphated ash (*2.4.14*). Not more than 0.1 per cent determined on 1.0 g.

ASSAY

Dissolve 0.200 g in 150 ml of *dimethylformamide R*. Titrate with *0.1 M tetrabutylammonium hydroxide*, determining the end-point potentiometrically (*2.2.20*). Use a glass indicator electrode and a calomel reference electrode containing, as the electrolyte, a saturated solution of *potassium chloride R* in *methanol R*. Carry out a blank titration.

1 ml of *0.1 M tetrabutylammonium hydroxide* is equivalent to 26.12 mg of $C_{13}H_{11}NO_5$.

STORAGE

Store protected from light.

IMPURITIES

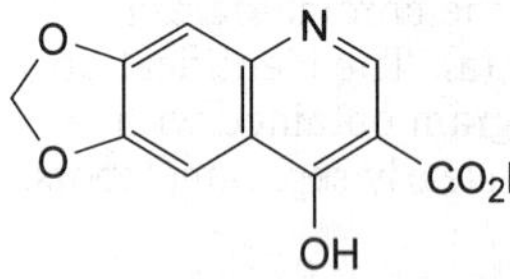

A. 8-hydroxy-1,3-dioxolo[4,5-*g*]quinoline-7-carboxylic acid,

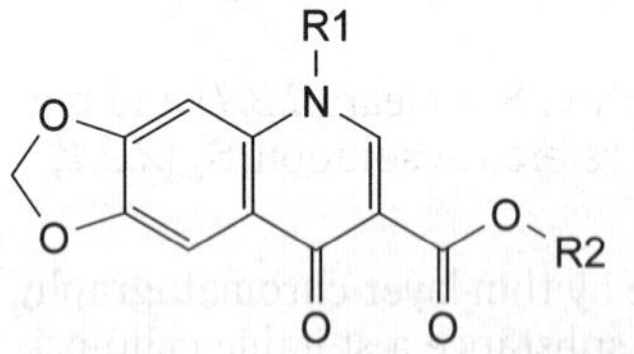

B. R1 = R2 = C_2H_5: ethyl 5-ethyl-8-oxo-5,8-dihydro-1,3-dioxolo[4,5-*g*]quinoline-7-carboxylate,

C. R1 = CH_3, R2 = H: 5-methyl-8-oxo-5,8-dihydro-1,3-dioxolo[4,5-*g*]quinoline-7-carboxylic acid.

01/2005:0628

OXPRENOLOL HYDROCHLORIDE

Oxprenololi hydrochloridum

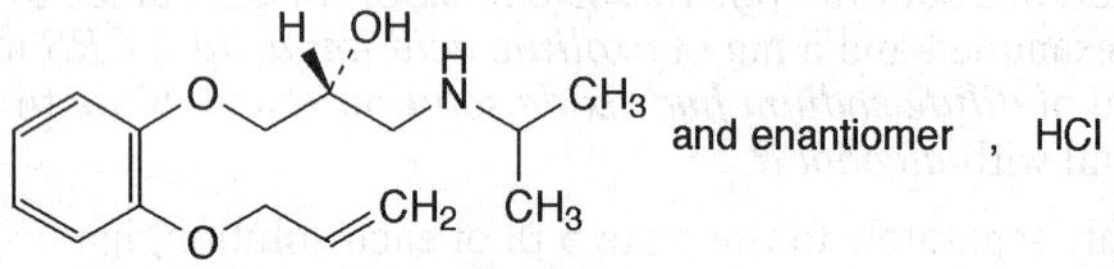

$C_{15}H_{24}ClNO_3$ M_r 301.8

DEFINITION

(2*RS*)-1-[(1-methylethyl)amino]-3-[2-(prop-2-enyloxy)phenoxy]propan-2-ol hydrochloride.

Content: 98.5 per cent to 101.5 per cent (dried substance).

CHARACTERS

Appearance: white or almost white, crystalline powder.

Solubility: very soluble in water, freely soluble in alcohol.

IDENTIFICATION

First identification: B, D.

Second identification: A, C, D.

A. Melting point (*2.2.14*): 107 °C to 110 °C.

B. Infrared absorption spectrophotometry (*2.2.24*).

Comparison: *oxprenolol hydrochloride CRS.*

If the spectra obtained in the solid state show differences, dissolve the substance to be examined and the reference substance separately in *ethyl acetate R*, evaporate to dryness and record new spectra using the residues.

C. Examine the chromatograms obtained in the test for related substances.

Results: the principal spot in the chromatogram obtained with test solution (b) is similar in position, colour and size to the principal spot in the chromatogram obtained with reference solution (a).

D. It gives reaction (a) of chlorides (*2.3.1*).

TESTS

Solution S. Dissolve 2.0 g in *carbon dioxide-free water R* and dilute to 20 ml with the same solvent.

Appearance of solution. Solution S is clear (*2.2.1*) and not more intensely coloured than reference solution GY_6 (*2.2.2, Method II*).

pH (*2.2.3*): 4.5 to 6.0 for freshly prepared solution S.

Related substances. Thin-layer chromatography (*2.2.27*).

Test solution (a). Dissolve 0.10 g of the substance to be examined in 2 ml of a mixture of 1 volume of *methanol R* and 9 volumes of *methylene chloride R*.

Test solution (b). Dilute 1 ml of test solution (a) to 10 ml with a mixture of 1 volume of *methanol R* and 9 volumes of *methylene chloride R*.

Reference solution (a). Dissolve 10 mg of *oxprenolol hydrochloride CRS* in 2 ml of a mixture of 1 volume of *methanol R* and 9 volumes of *methylene chloride R*.

Reference solution (b). Dilute 0.4 ml of test solution (a) to 100 ml with a mixture of 1 volume of *methanol R* and 9 volumes of *methylene chloride R*.

Reference solution (c). Dilute 5 ml of reference solution (b) to 10 ml with a mixture of 1 volume of *methanol R* and 9 volumes of *methylene chloride R*.

Reference solution (d). Dissolve 5 mg of *alprenolol hydrochloride CRS* in 1 ml of reference solution (a).

Plate: *TLC silica gel G plate R*.

Mobile phase: *concentrated ammonia R, methanol R, methylene chloride R* (2:12:88 *V/V/V*).

Application: 2 µl; allow the spots to dry in air for 15 min.

Development: over a path of 13 cm.

Drying: in a current of warm air for 10 min.

Detection: allow to cool and spray with *anisaldehyde solution R*. Heat at 100-105 °C for 5-10 min. Examine in daylight.

System suitability: the test is not valid unless the chromatogram obtained with reference solution (d) shows 2 clearly separated spots.

Limits: in the chromatogram obtained with test solution (a):

– *any impurity*: any spot, apart from the principal spot, is not more intense than the spot in the chromatogram obtained with reference solution (b) (0.4 per cent); not more than 1 such spot is more intense than the spot in the chromatogram obtained with reference solution (c) (0.2 per cent).

Lead: maximum 5 ppm.

Atomic absorption spectrometry (*2.2.23, Method II*).

Test solution. Dissolve 1.00 g of the substance to be examined in *water R* and dilute to 25.0 ml with the same solvent.

Reference solutions. Prepare the reference solutions using 0.5 ml and 1.0 ml respectively of *lead standard solution (10 ppm Pb) R* diluted to 25.0 ml with *water R*.

Source: lead hollow-cathode lamp.

Wavelength: 217.0 nm.

Loss on drying (*2.2.32*): maximum 0.5 per cent, determined on 1.000 g by drying *in vacuo* at 60 °C for 6 h.

Sulphated ash (*2.4.14*): maximum 0.1 per cent, determined on 1.0 g.

ASSAY

Dissolve 0.250 g in a mixture of 5.0 ml of *0.01 M hydrochloric acid* and 50 ml of *alcohol R*. Carry out a potentiometric titration (*2.2.20*), using *0.1 M sodium hydroxide*. Read the volume added between the 2 points of inflexion.

1 ml of *0.1 M sodium hydroxide* is equivalent to 30.18 mg of $C_{15}H_{24}ClNO_3$.

STORAGE

Protected from light.

01/2005:1251

OXYBUPROCAINE HYDROCHLORIDE

Oxybuprocaini hydrochloridum

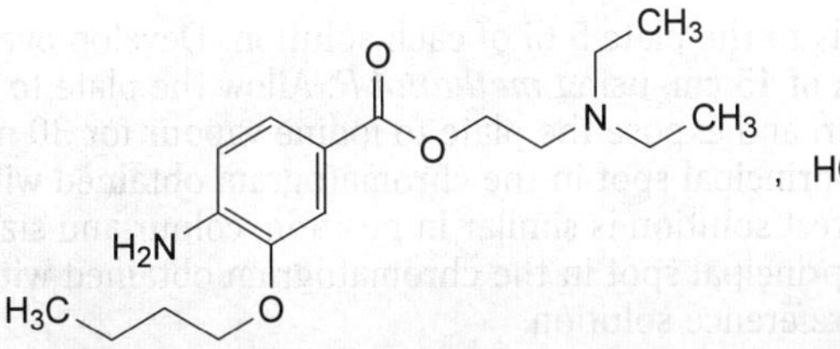

$C_{17}H_{29}ClN_2O_3$ M_r 344.9

DEFINITION

Oxybuprocaine hydrochloride contains not less than 98.5 per cent and not more than the equivalent of 101.5 per cent of 2-(diethylamino)ethyl 4-amino-3-butoxybenzoate hydrochloride, calculated with reference to the dried substance.

CHARACTERS

A white, crystalline powder or colourless crystals, very soluble in water, freely soluble in alcohol.

It shows polymorphism.

IDENTIFICATION

First identification: B, D.

Second identification: A, C, D.

A. Melting point (*2.2.14*): 158 °C to 162 °C.

B. Examine by infrared absorption spectrophotometry (*2.2.24*),comparing with the spectrum obtained with *oxybuprocaine hydrochloride CRS*. Examine the substances prepared as discs. If the spectra obtained show differences, dissolve the substance to be examined and the reference substance separately in *methanol R*, evaporate to dryness and record the spectra again using the residues.

C. Examine by thin-layer chromatography (*2.2.27*), using as the coating substance a suitable silica gel with a fluorescent indicator having an optimal intensity at 254 nm.

Test solution. Dissolve 40 mg of the substance to be examined in *methanol R* and dilute to 10 ml with the same solvent.

Reference solution (a). Dissolve 40 mg of *oxybuprocaine hydrochloride CRS* in *methanol R* and dilute to 10 ml with the same solvent.

Reference solution (b). Dissolve 20 mg of *procaine hydrochloride R* in reference solution (a) and dilute to 5 ml with the same solution.

Apply separately to the plate 5 µl of each solution. Develop over a path of 10 cm using a mixture of 10 volumes of *anhydrous formic acid R*, 15 volumes of *methanol R*, 15 volumes of *water R* and 60 volumes of *ethyl acetate R*. Dry the plate in a current of hot air for 10 min and examine in ultraviolet light at 254 nm. Spray with *dimethylaminobenzaldehyde solution R7*. The principal spot in the chromatogram obtained with the test solution is similar in position, colour and size to the principal spot in the chromatogram obtained with reference solution (a). The test is not valid unless the chromatogram obtained with reference solution (b) shows two clearly separated spots.

D. Dilute 0.2 ml of solution S (see Tests) to 2 ml with *water R*. The solution gives reaction (a) of chlorides (*2.3.1*).

TESTS

Solution S. Dissolve 5.0 g in *carbon dioxide-free water R* and dilute to 50 ml with the same solvent.

Appearance of solution. Solution S is clear (*2.2.1*) and not more intensely coloured than reference solution Y_5 (*2.2.2, Method II*).

pH (*2.2.3*). The pH of solution S is 4.5 to 6.0.

Related substances. Examine by liquid chromatography (*2.2.29*).

Buffer solution pH 2.5. Add 6 ml of *perchloric acid solution R* and 12 ml of *dilute phosphoric acid R* to 950 ml of *water R*. Adjust the pH to 2.5 with a 40 g/l solution of *sodium hydroxide R* and dilute to 1000.0 ml with *water R*.

Test solution. Dissolve 10.0 mg of the substance to be examined in the mobile phase and dilute to 25.0 ml with the mobile phase.

Reference solution (a). Dilute 1.0 ml of the test solution to 20.0 ml with the mobile phase and dilute 5.0 ml of this solution to 100.0 ml with the mobile phase.

Reference solution (b). Mix 1.0 ml of the test solution with 1 ml of a 40 g/l solution of *sodium hydroxide R* and allow to stand for 20 min. Add 1 ml of *dilute phosphoric acid R* and dilute to 100.0 ml with the mobile phase. Dilute 25 ml to 100.0 ml with the mobile phase.

The chromatographic procedure may be carried out using:

- a stainless steel column 0.15 m long and 3.9 mm in internal diameter packed with *octadecylsilyl silica gel for chromatography R1* (5 µm) with a pore size of 10 nm and a carbon loading of 19 per cent,
- as mobile phase at a flow rate of 1 ml/min a mixture of 25 volumes of *acetonitrile R* and 75 volumes of buffer solution pH 2.5,
- as detector a spectrophotometer set at 309 nm,

maintaining the temperature of the column at 35 °C.

When the chromatograms are recorded in the prescribed conditions the retention time is about 9 min for oxybuprocaine hydrochloride. Adjust the sensitivity of the system so that the height of the principal peak in the chromatogram obtained with reference solution (a) is at least 50 per cent of the full scale of the recorder.

Inject 20 µl of reference solution (b). The test is not valid unless: in the chromatogram obtained with reference solution (b), the resolution between the main peaks corresponding to oxybuprocaine and oxybuprocaine impurity B (hydrolysis product) is at least twelve.

Inject 20 µl of the test solution and 20 µl of reference solution (a). Continue the chromatography for four times the retention time of the principal peak. In the chromatogram obtained with the test solution: the area of any peak, apart from the principal peak, is not greater than 0.4 times the area of the principal peak in the chromatogram obtained with reference solution (a) (0.1 per cent); the sum of the areas of all the peaks apart from the principal peak is not greater than the area of the principal peak in the chromatogram obtained with reference solution (a) (0.25 per cent). Disregard any peak with an area less than 0.05 times that of the peak due to oxybuprocaine hydrochloride in the chromatogram obtained with reference solution (a).

Heavy metals (*2.4.8*). 12 ml of solution S complies with limit test A for heavy metals (10 ppm). Prepare the standard using *lead standard solution (1 ppm Pb) R*.

Loss on drying (*2.2.32*). Not more than 0.5 per cent determined on 1.000 g by drying in an oven at 100-105 °C.

Sulphated ash (*2.4.14*). Not more than 0.1 per cent, determined on 1.0 g.

ASSAY

Dissolve 0.300 g in a mixture of 20 ml of *anhydrous acetic acid R* and 20 ml of *acetic anhydride R*. Titrate with *0.1 M perchloric acid*, determining the end-point potentiometrically (*2.2.20*).

1 ml of *0.1 M perchloric acid* is equivalent to 34.49 mg of $C_{17}H_{29}ClN_2O_3$.

STORAGE

Store protected from light.

IMPURITIES

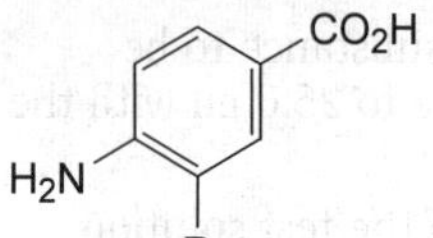

A. R = H: 4-aminobenzoic acid,

B. R = O-CH_2-CH_2-CH_2-CH_3 : 4-amino-3-butoxybenzoic acid,

C. R = OH: 4-amino-3-hydroxybenzoic acid.

01/2005:1354

OXYBUTYNIN HYDROCHLORIDE

Oxybutynini hydrochloridum

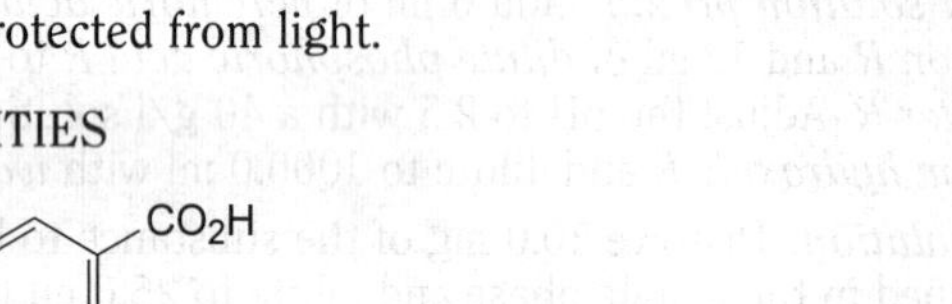

and enantiomer

$C_{22}H_{32}ClNO_3$ M_r 394.0

DEFINITION

Oxybutynin hydrochloride contains not less than 99.0 per cent and not more than the equivalent of 102.0 per cent of 4-(diethylamino)but-2-ynyl (*RS*)-2-cyclohexyl-2-hydroxy-2-phenylacetate hydrochloride, calculated with reference to the dried substance.

CHARACTERS

A white or almost white, crystalline powder, freely soluble in water and in alcohol, soluble in acetone, slightly soluble in cyclohexane.

IDENTIFICATION

First identification: B, D.

Second identification: A, C, D.

A. Melting point (*2.2.14*): 124 °C to 129 °C.

B. Examine by infrared absorption spectrophotometry (*2.2.24*), comparing with the spectrum obtained with *oxybutynin hydrochloride CRS*. Examine the substances prepared as discs.

C. Examine by thin-layer chromatography (*2.2.27*), using a *TLC silica gel plate R*.

Test solution. Dissolve 50 mg of the substance to be examined in *alcohol R* and dilute to 10 ml with the same solvent.

Reference solution. Dissolve 10 mg of *oxybutynin hydrochloride CRS* in *alcohol R* and dilute to 2 ml with the same solvent.

Apply to the plate 5 µl of each solution. Develop over a path of 15 cm, using *methanol R*. Allow the plate to dry in air, and expose the plate to iodine vapour for 30 min. The principal spot in the chromatogram obtained with the test solution is similar in position, colour and size to the principal spot in the chromatogram obtained with the reference solution.

D. It gives reaction (a) of chlorides (*2.3.1*).

TESTS

Solution S. Dissolve 2.00 g in *water R* and dilute to 20.0 ml with the same solvent.

Appearance of solution. Solution S is clear (*2.2.1*) and not more intensely coloured than reference solution BY_5 (*2.2.2, Method II*).

Optical rotation (*2.2.7*). The angle of optical rotation, determined on solution S, is − 0.10° to + 0.10°.

Related substances. Examine by liquid chromatography (*2.2.29*).

Test solution. Dissolve 50.0 mg of the substance to be examined in the mobile phase and dilute to 10.0 ml with the mobile phase.

Reference solution (a). Dissolve 50.0 mg of *oxybutynin hydrochloride CRS* and 50.0 mg of *oxybutynin impurity A CRS* in the mobile phase and dilute to 100.0 ml with the mobile phase. Dilute 10.0 ml of the solution to 100.0 ml with the mobile phase.

Reference solution (b). Dilute 1.0 ml of the test solution to 200.0 ml with the mobile phase.

The chromatographic procedure may be carried out using:

- a stainless steel column 0.15 m long and 3.9 mm in internal diameter packed with *octylsilyl silica gel for chromatography R2* (5 µm),
- as mobile phase at a flow rate of 1 ml/min a mixture of 49 volumes of a solution containing 3.4 g/l of *potassium dihydrogen phosphate R* and 4.36 g/l of *dipotassium hydrogen phosphate R* and 51 volumes of *acetonitrile R*,

– as detector a spectrophotometer set at 210 nm.

Inject 10 µl of reference solution (a). When the chromatograms are recorded in the prescribed conditions the retention times are: oxybutynin hydrochloride about 15 min and impurity A about 24 min. Adjust the sensitivity of the system so that the heights of the peaks in the chromatogram obtained are about 20 per cent of the full scale of the recorder. The test is not valid unless the resolution between the peaks due to oxybutynin hydrochloride and to impurity A is at least 11.0.

Inject 10 µl of the test solution, 10 µl of reference solution (a) and 10 µl of reference solution (b). Continue the chromatography for about twice the retention time of the principal peak. In the chromatogram obtained with the test solution: the area of any peak due to impurity A is not greater than 1.5 times the area of the peak due to impurity A in the chromatogram obtained with reference solution (a) (1.5 per cent); the sum of the areas of all the peaks, apart from the principal peak and the peak due to impurity A, is not greater than the area of the principal peak in the chromatogram obtained with reference solution (b) (0.5 per cent). Disregard any peak with an area less than 0.05 times the area of the principal peak in the chromatogram obtained with reference solution (b).

Heavy metals (*2.4.8*). 12 ml of solution S complies with limit test A for heavy metals (20 ppm). Prepare the standard using 2 ml of *lead standard solution (10 ppm Pb) R*.

Loss on drying (*2.2.32*). Not more than 3.0 per cent determined on 1.000 g by drying in an oven at 100-105 °C.

Sulphated ash (*2.4.14*). Not more than 0.1 per cent, determined on 1.0 g.

ASSAY

Dissolve 0.300 g in a mixture of 5.0 ml of *0.01 M hydrochloric acid* and 50 ml of *alcohol R*. Carry out a potentiometric titration (*2.2.20*), using *0.1 M sodium hydroxide*. Read the volume added between the two points of inflexion.

1 ml of *0.1 M sodium hydroxide* is equivalent to 39.4 mg of $C_{22}H_{32}ClNO_3$.

STORAGE

Store protected from light.

IMPURITIES

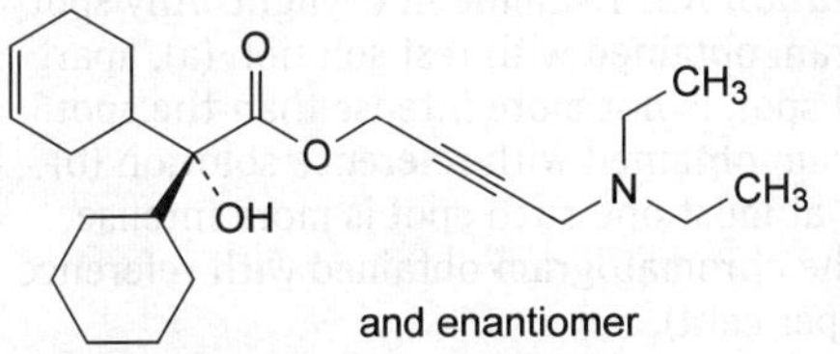

and enantiomer

A. 4-(diethylamino)but-2-ynyl (*RS*)-2-(cyclohex-3-enyl)-2-cyclohexyl-2-hydroxyacetate,

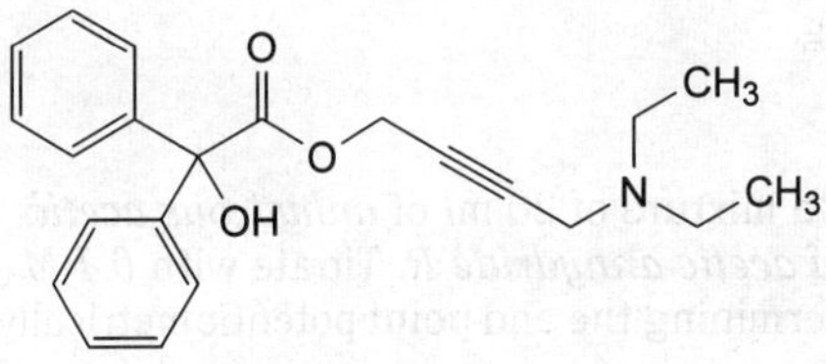

B. 4-(diethylamino)but-2-ynyl 2-hydroxy-2,2-diphenylacetate (diphenyl analogue of oxybutynin),

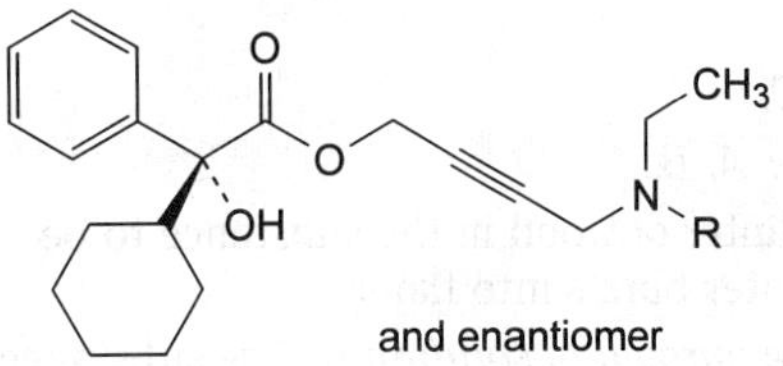

and enantiomer

C. R = CH_3: 4-(ethylmethylamino)but-2-ynyl (*RS*)-2-cyclohexyl-2-hydroxy-2-phenylacetate (methylethyl analogue of oxybutynin),

E. R = CH_2-CH_2-CH_3: 4-(ethylpropylamino)but-2-ynyl (*RS*)-2-cyclohexyl-2-hydroxy-2-phenylacetate (ethylpropyl analogue of oxybutynin),

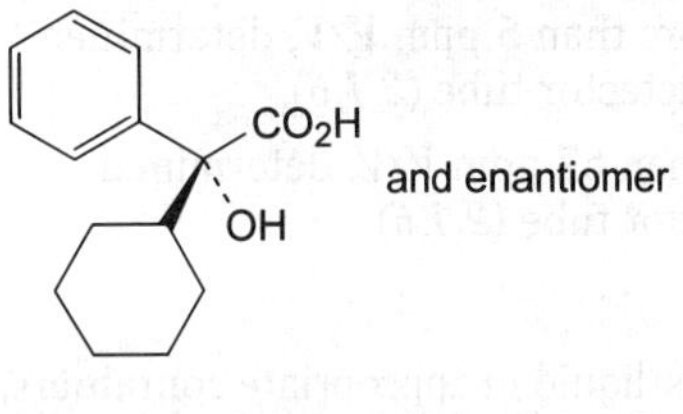

and enantiomer

D. (*RS*)-2-cyclohexyl-2-hydroxy-2-phenylacetic acid (phenylcyclohexylglycolic acid).

01/2005:0417

OXYGEN

Oxygenium

O_2 M_r 32.00

DEFINITION

Oxygen contains not less than 99.5 per cent *V/V* of O_2.

This monograph applies to oxygen for medicinal use.

CHARACTERS

A colourless, odourless gas. At 20 °C and at a pressure of 101 kPa, 1 volume dissolves in about 32 volumes of water.

PRODUCTION

Carbon dioxide. Not more than 300 ppm *V/V*, determined using an infrared analyser (*2.5.24*).

Gas to be examined. The substance to be examined. It must be filtered to avoid stray light phenomena.

Reference gas (a). Use *oxygen R*.

Reference gas (b). Use a mixture containing 300 ppm *V/V* of *carbon dioxide R1* in *nitrogen R1*.

Calibrate the apparatus and set the sensitivity using reference gases (a) and (b). Measure the content of carbon dioxide in the gas to be examined.

Carbon monoxide. Not more than 5 ppm *V/V*, determined using an infrared analyser (*2.5.25*).

Gas to be examined. The substance to be examined. It must be filtered to avoid stray light phenomena.

Reference gas (a). Use *oxygen R*.

Reference gas (b). Use a mixture containing 5 ppm *V/V* of *carbon monoxide R* in *nitrogen R1*.

Calibrate the apparatus and set the sensitivity using reference gases (a) and (b). Measure the content of carbon monoxide in the gas to be examined.

Water. Not more than 67 ppm *V/V*, determined using an electrolytic hygrometer (*2.5.28*).

Assay. Determine the concentration of oxygen using a paramagnetic analyser (*2.5.27*).

IDENTIFICATION

First identification: C.

Second identification: A, B.

A. Place a glowing splinter of wood in the substance to be examined. The splinter bursts into flame.

B. Shake with *alkaline pyrogallol solution R*. The substance to be examined is absorbed and the solution becomes dark brown.

C. It complies with the limits of the assay.

TESTS

Carbon dioxide. Not more than 300 ppm *V/V*, determined using a carbon dioxide detector tube (*2.1.6*).

Carbon monoxide. Not more than 5 ppm *V/V*, determined using a carbon monoxide detector tube (*2.1.6*).

Water vapour. Not more than 67 ppm *V/V*, determined using a water vapour detector tube (*2.1.6*).

STORAGE

Store as a compressed gas or liquid in appropriate containers, complying with the legal regulations. Taps and valves are not to be greased or oiled.

IMPURITIES

A. carbon dioxide,

B. carbon monoxide,

C. water.

01/2005:0943

OXYMETAZOLINE HYDROCHLORIDE

Oxymetazolini hydrochloridum

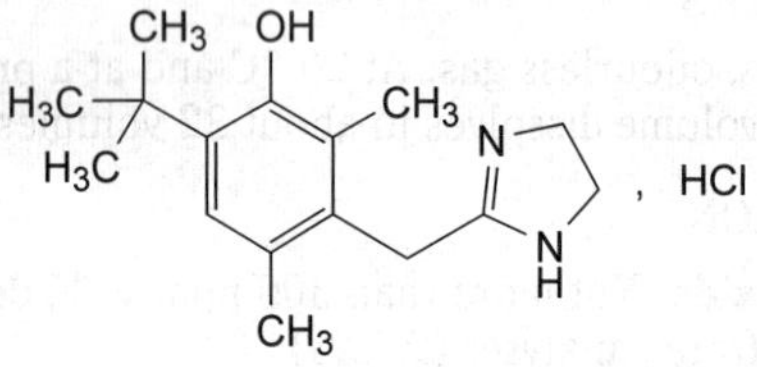

$C_{16}H_{25}ClN_2O$ M_r 296.8

DEFINITION

Oxymetazoline hydrochloride contains not less than 99.0 per cent and not more than the equivalent of 101.0 per cent of 3-[(4,5-dihydro-1*H*-imidazol-2-yl)methyl]-6-(1,1-dimethylethyl)-2,4-dimethylphenol hydrochloride, calculated with reference to the dried substance.

CHARACTERS

A white or almost white, crystalline powder, freely soluble in water and in alcohol.

IDENTIFICATION

First identification: A, D.

Second identification: B, C, D.

A. Examine by infrared absorption spectrophotometry (*2.2.24*) comparing with the spectrum obtained with *oxymetazoline hydrochloride CRS*.

B. Examine the chromatograms obtained in the test for related substances. The principal spot in the chromatogram obtained with test solution (b) is similar in position, colour and size to the principal spot in the chromatogram obtained with reference solution (a).

C. To a solution of about 2 mg in 1 ml of *water R* add 0.2 ml of a 50 g/l solution of *sodium nitroprusside R* and 0.2 ml of *dilute sodium hydroxide solution R*. Allow to stand for 10 min. Add 2 ml of *sodium hydrogen carbonate solution R*. A violet colour develops.

D. It gives reaction (a) of chlorides (*2.3.1*).

TESTS

Solution S. Dissolve 2.5 g in *water R* and dilute to 50 ml with the same solvent.

Appearance of solution. Solution S is clear (*2.2.1*) and not more intensely coloured than reference solution BY_7 (*2.2.2, Method II*).

Acidity or alkalinity. Dissolve 0.25 g in *water R* and dilute to 25 ml with the same solvent. Add 0.1 ml of *methyl red solution R* and 0.2 ml of *0.01 M hydrochloric acid*. The solution is red. Not more than 0.4 ml of *0.01 M sodium hydroxide* is required to change the colour of the indicator to yellow.

Related substances. Examine by thin-layer chromatography (*2.2.27*), using *silica gel G R* as the coating substance.

Test solution (a). Dissolve 0.40 g of the substance to be examined in a mixture of equal volumes of *ethyl acetate R* and *methanol R* and dilute to 10 ml with the same mixture of solvents.

Test solution (b). Dilute 1 ml of test solution (a) to 10 ml with a mixture of equal volumes of *ethyl acetate R* and *methanol R*.

Reference solution (a). Dissolve 40 mg of *oxymetazoline hydrochloride CRS* in a mixture of equal volumes of *ethyl acetate R* and *methanol R* and dilute to 10 ml with the same mixture of solvents.

Reference solution (b). Dilute 1 ml of test solution (b) to 20 ml with a mixture of equal volumes of *ethyl acetate R* and *methanol R*.

Reference solution (c). Dilute 1 ml of test solution (b) to 40 ml with a mixture of equal volumes of *ethyl acetate R* and *methanol R*.

Apply separately to the plate 5 µl of each solution. Develop over a path of 15 cm using a mixture of 6 volumes of *diethylamine R*, 15 volumes of *cyclohexane R* and 79 volumes of *ethanol R*. Dry the plate in a current of warm air for 5 min. Allow to cool and spray with a freshly prepared 5.0 g/l solution of *potassium ferricyanide R* in *ferric chloride solution R2*. Examine in daylight. Any spot in the chromatogram obtained with test solution (a), apart from the principal spot, is not more intense than the spot in the chromatogram obtained with reference solution (b) (0.5 per cent) and at most one such spot is more intense than the spot in the chromatogram obtained with reference solution (c) (0.25 per cent).

Loss on drying (*2.2.32*). Not more than 1.0 per cent, determined on 1.000 g by drying in an oven at 100 °C to 105 °C.

Sulphated ash (*2.4.14*). Not more than 0.1 per cent, determined on 1.0 g.

ASSAY

Dissolve 0.200 g in a mixture of 20 ml of *anhydrous acetic acid R* and 20 ml of *acetic anhydride R*. Titrate with *0.1 M perchloric acid* determining the end-point potentiometrically (*2.2.20*).

1 ml of *0.1 M perchloric acid* is equivalent to 29.68 mg of $C_{16}H_{25}ClN_2O$.

IMPURITIES

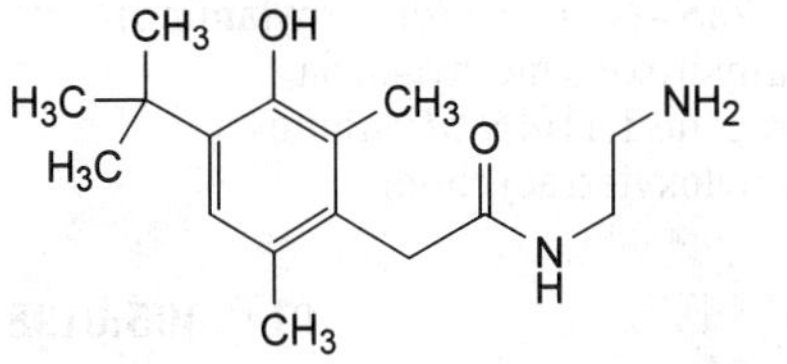

A. *N*-(2-aminoethyl)-2-[4-(1,1-dimethylethyl)-3-hydroxy-2,6-dimethylphenyl]acetamide.

01/2005:0199

OXYTETRACYCLINE DIHYDRATE

Oxytetracyclinum dihydricum

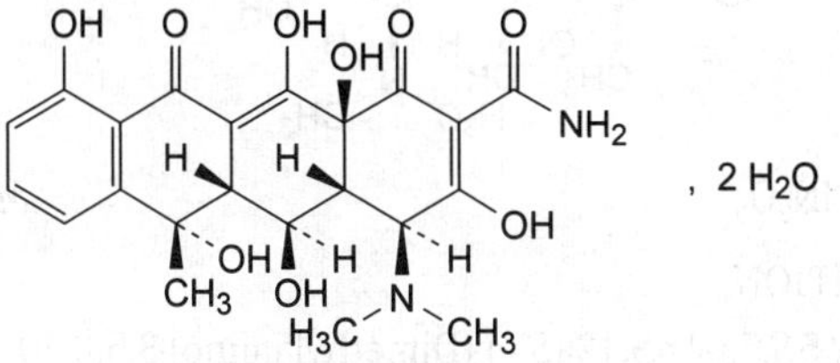

$C_{22}H_{24}N_2O_9,2\ H_2O$ M_r 496.4

DEFINITION

(4*S*,4a*R*,5*S*,5a*R*,6*S*,12a*S*)-4-(Dimethylamino)-3,5,6,10,12,12a-hexahydroxy-6-methyl-1,11-dioxo-1,4,4a,5,5a,6,11,12a-octahydrotetracene-2-carboxamide dihydrate.

Substance produced by the growth of certain strains of *Streptomyces rimosus* or obtained by any other means.

Content: 95.0 per cent to 102.0 per cent (anhydrous substance).

CHARACTERS

Appearance: yellow, crystalline powder.

Solubility: very slightly soluble in water. It dissolves in dilute acid and alkaline solutions.

IDENTIFICATION

A. Thin-layer chromatography (*2.2.27*).

Test solution. Dissolve 5 mg of the substance to be examined in *methanol R* and dilute to 10 ml with the same solvent.

Reference solution (a). Dissolve 5 mg of *oxytetracycline CRS* in *methanol R* and dilute to 10 ml with the same solvent.

Reference solution (b). Dissolve 5 mg of *oxytetracycline CRS*, 5 mg of *tetracycline hydrochloride R* and 5 mg of *minocycline hydrochloride R* in *methanol R* and dilute to 10 ml with the same solvent.

Plate: *TLC octadecylsilyl silica gel F_{254} plate R*.

Mobile phase: mix 20 volumes of *acetonitrile R*, 20 volumes of *methanol R* and 60 volumes of a 63 g/l solution of *oxalic acid R* previously adjusted to pH 2 with *concentrated ammonia R*.

Application: 1 µl.

Development: over 3/4 of the plate.

Drying: in air.

Detection: examine in ultraviolet light at 254 nm.

System suitability: the chromatogram obtained with reference solution (b) shows 3 clearly separated spots.

Results: the principal spot in the chromatogram obtained with the test solution is similar in position and size to the principal spot in the chromatogram obtained with reference solution (a).

B. To about 2 mg add 5 ml of *sulphuric acid R*. A deep red colour develops. Add the solution to 2.5 ml of *water R*. The colour becomes yellow.

C. Dissolve about 10 mg in a mixture of 1 ml of *dilute nitric acid R* and 5 ml of *water R*. Shake and add 1 ml of *silver nitrate solution R2*. Any opalescence in the solution is not more intense than that in a mixture of 1 ml of *dilute nitric acid R*, 5 ml of a 0.021 g/l solution of *potassium chloride R* and 1 ml of *silver nitrate solution R2*.

TESTS

pH (*2.2.3*): 4.5 to 7.5.

Suspend 0.1 g in 10 ml of *carbon dioxide-free water R*.

Specific optical rotation (*2.2.7*): − 203 to − 216 (anhydrous substance).

Dissolve 0.250 g in *0.1 M hydrochloric acid* and dilute to 25.0 ml with the same acid.

Specific absorbance (*2.2.25*): 290 to 310 determined at 353 nm (anhydrous substance).

Dissolve 20.0 mg in *buffer solution pH 2.0 R* and dilute to 100.0 ml with the same buffer solution. Dilute 10.0 ml of the solution to 100.0 ml with *buffer solution pH 2.0 R*.

Light-absorbing impurities. *Carry out the measurements within 1 h of preparing the solutions.*

Dissolve 20.0 mg in a mixture of 1 volume of *1 M hydrochloric acid* and 99 volumes of *methanol R* and dilute to 10.0 ml with the same mixture of solvents. The absorbance (*2.2.25*), determined at 430 nm has a maximum of 0.25 (anhydrous substance).

Dissolve 0.100 g in a mixture of 1 volume of *1 M hydrochloric acid* and 99 volumes of *methanol R* and dilute to 10.0 ml with the same mixture of solvents. The absorbance (*2.2.25*) determined at 490 nm has a maximum of 0.20 (anhydrous substance).

Related substances. Liquid chromatography (*2.2.29*).

Test solution. Dissolve 20.0 mg of the substance to be examined in *0.01 M hydrochloric acid* and dilute to 25.0 ml with the same acid.

Reference solution (a). Dissolve 20.0 mg of *oxytetracycline CRS* in *0.01 M hydrochloric acid* and dilute to 25.0 ml with the same acid.

Reference solution (b). Dissolve 20.0 mg of *4-epioxytetracycline CRS* in *0.01 M hydrochloric acid* and dilute to 25.0 ml with the same acid.

Reference solution (c). Dissolve 20.0 mg of *tetracycline hydrochloride CRS* in *0.01 M hydrochloric acid* and dilute to 25.0 ml with the same acid.

Reference solution (d). Mix 1.5 ml of reference solution (a), 1.0 ml of reference solution (b) and 3.0 ml of reference solution (c) and dilute to 25.0 ml with *0.01 M hydrochloric acid*.

Reference solution (e). Mix 1.0 ml of reference solution (b) and 4.0 ml of reference solution (c) and dilute to 200.0 ml with *0.01 M hydrochloric acid*.

Column:

– *size*: *l* = 0.25 m, Ø = 4.6 mm,
– *stationary phase*: *styrene-divinylbenzene copolymer R* (8 µm),
– *temperature*: 60 °C.

Mobile phase: weigh 60.0 g of *2-methyl-2-propanol R* and transfer to a 1000 ml volumetric flask with the aid of 200 ml of *water R*; add 60 ml of *0.33 M phosphate buffer solution pH 7.5 R*, 50 ml of a 10 g/l solution of *tetrabutylammonium hydrogen sulphate R* adjusted to pH 7.5 with *dilute sodium hydroxide solution R* and 10 ml of a 0.4 g/l solution of *sodium edetate R* adjusted to pH 7.5 with *dilute sodium hydroxide solution R*; dilute to 1000 ml with *water R*.

Flow rate: 1.0 ml/min.

Detection: spectrophotometer at 254 nm.

Injection: 20 µl; inject the test solution and reference solutions (d) and (e).

System suitability: reference solution (d):

- *resolution*: minimum 4.0 between the peaks due to impurity A (1st peak) and oxytetracycline (2nd peak) and minimum 5.0 between the peaks and due to oxytetracycline and impurity B (3rd peak); adjust the 2-methyl-2-propanol content in the mobile phase if necessary,
- *symmetry factor*: maximum 1.25 for the peak due to oxytetracycline.

Limits:

- *impurity A*: not more than the area of the corresponding peak in the chromatogram obtained with reference solution (e) (0.5 per cent),
- *impurity B*: not more than the area of the corresponding peak in the chromatogram obtained with reference solution (e) (2.0 per cent),
- *impurity C (eluting on the tail of the principal peak)*: not more than 4 times the area of the peak due to impurity A in the chromatogram obtained with reference solution (e) (2.0 per cent),
- *disregard limit*: 0.02 times the area of the peak due to oxytetracycline in the chromatogram obtained with reference solution (d) (0.1 per cent).

Heavy metals (*2.4.8*): maximum 50 ppm.

0.5 g complies with limit test F. Prepare the standard using 2.5 ml of *lead standard solution (10 ppm Pb) R*.

Water (*2.5.12*): 6.0 per cent to 9.0 per cent, determined on 0.250 g.

Sulphated ash (*2.4.14*): maximum 0.5 per cent, determined on 1.0 g.

ASSAY

Liquid chromatography (*2.2.29*) as described in the test for related substances with the following modification.

Injection: test solution and reference solution (a).

Calculate the percentage content of $C_{22}H_{24}N_2O_9$.

STORAGE

In an airtight container, protected from light.

IMPURITIES

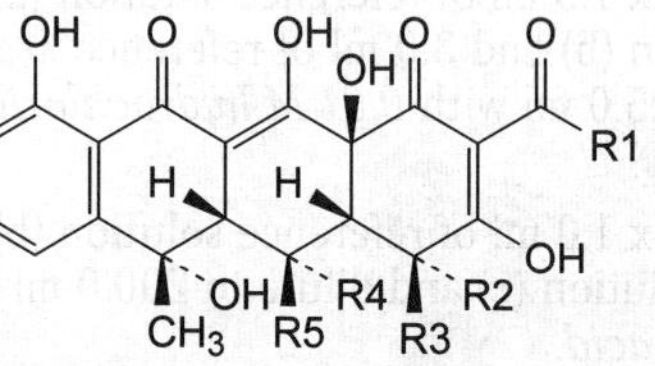

A. R1 = NH_2, R2 = $N(CH_3)_2$, R3 = R4 = H, R5 = OH: (4*R*,4a*R*,5*S*,5a*R*,6*S*,12a*S*)-4-(dimethylamino)-3,5,6,10,12,12a-hexahydroxy-6-methyl-1,11-dioxo-1,4,4a,5,5a,6,11,12a-octahydrotetracene-2-carboxamide (4-epioxytetracycline),

B. R1 = NH_2, R2 = R4 = R5 = H, R3 = $N(CH_3)_2$: tetracycline,

C. R1 = CH_3, R2 = R4 = H, R3 = $N(CH_3)_2$, R5 = OH: (4*S*,4a*R*,5*S*,5a*R*,6*S*,12a*S*)-2-acetyl-4-(dimethylamino)-3,5,6,10,12,12a-hexahydroxy-6-methyl-4a,5a,6,12a-tetrahydrotetracene-1,11(4*H*,5*H*)-dione (2-acetyl-2-decarbamoyloxytetracycline).

01/2005:0198

OXYTETRACYCLINE HYDROCHLORIDE

Oxytetracyclini hydrochloridum

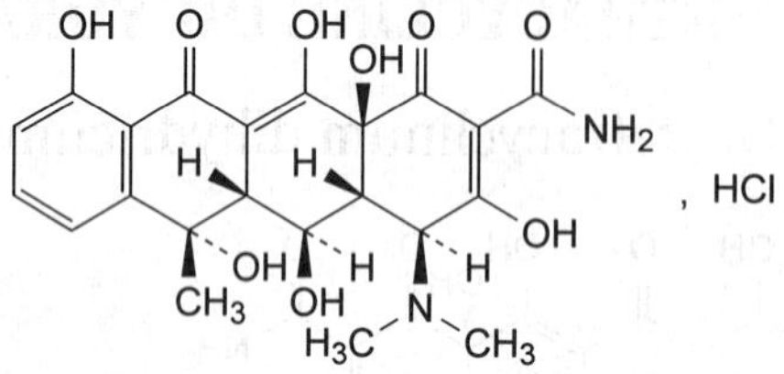

$C_{22}H_{25}ClN_2O_9$ M_r 496.9

DEFINITION

(4*S*,4a*R*,5*S*,5a*R*,6*S*,12a*S*)-4-(Dimethylamino)-3,5,6,10,12,12a-hexahydroxy-6-methyl-1,11-dioxo-1,4,4a,5,5a,6,11,12a-octahydrotetracene-2-carboxamide hydrochloride.

Substance produced by the growth of certain strains of *Streptomyces rimosus* or obtained by any other means.

Content: 95.0 per cent to 102.0 per cent (anhydrous substance).

CHARACTERS

Appearance: yellow, crystalline powder, hygroscopic.

Solubility: freely soluble in water, sparingly soluble in alcohol. Solutions in water become turbid on standing, owing to the precipitation of oxytetracycline.

IDENTIFICATION

A. Thin-layer chromatography (*2.2.27*).

Test solution. Dissolve 5 mg of the substance to be examined in *methanol R* and dilute to 10 ml with the same solvent.

Reference solution (a). Dissolve 5 mg of *oxytetracycline hydrochloride CRS* in *methanol R* and dilute to 10 ml with the same solvent.

Reference solution (b). Dissolve 5 mg of *oxytetracycline hydrochloride CRS*, 5 mg of *tetracycline hydrochloride R* and 5 mg of *minocycline hydrochloride R* in *methanol R* and dilute to 10 ml with the same solvent.

Plate: *TLC octadecylsilyl silica gel F_{254} plate R*.

Mobile phase: mix 20 volumes of *acetonitrile R*, 20 volumes of *methanol R* and 60 volumes of a 63 g/l solution of *oxalic acid R* previously adjusted to pH 2 with *concentrated ammonia R*.

Application: 1 µl.

Development: over 3/4 of the plate.

Drying: in air.

Detection: examine in ultraviolet light at 254 nm.

System suitability: the chromatogram obtained with reference solution (b) shows 3 clearly separated spots.

Results: the principal spot in the chromatogram obtained with the test solution is similar in position and size to the principal spot in the chromatogram obtained with reference solution (a).

B. To about 2 mg add 5 ml of *sulphuric acid R*. A deep red colour develops. Add the solution to 2.5 ml of *water R*. The colour becomes yellow.

C. It gives reaction (a) of chlorides (*2.3.1*).

TESTS

pH (*2.2.3*): 2.3 to 2.9.

Dissolve 0.1 g in 10 ml of *carbon dioxide-free water R*.

Specific optical rotation (*2.2.7*): − 188 to − 200 (anhydrous substance).

Dissolve 0.250 g in *0.1 M hydrochloric acid* and dilute to 25.0 ml with the same acid.

Specific absorbance (*2.2.25*): 270 to 290 determined at 353 nm (anhydrous substance).

Dissolve 20.0 mg in *buffer solution pH 2.0 R* and dilute to 100.0 ml with the same buffer solution. Dilute 10.0 ml of the solution to 100.0 ml with *buffer solution pH 2.0 R*.

Light-absorbing impurities. *Carry out the measurements within 1 h of preparing the solutions.*

Dissolve 20.0 mg in a mixture of 1 volume of *1 M hydrochloric acid* and 99 volumes of *methanol R* and dilute to 10.0 ml with the same mixture of solvents. The absorbance (*2.2.25*) determined at 430 nm has a maximum of 0.50 (anhydrous substance).

Dissolve 0.100 g in a mixture of 1 volume of *1 M hydrochloric acid* and 99 volumes of *methanol R* and dilute to 10.0 ml with the same mixture of solvents. The absorbance (*2.2.25*) determined at 490 nm has a maximum of 0.20 (anhydrous substance).

Related substances. Liquid chromatography (*2.2.29*).

Test solution. Dissolve 20.0 mg of the substance to be examined in *0.01 M hydrochloric acid* and dilute to 25.0 ml with the same acid.

Reference solution (a). Dissolve 20.0 mg of *oxytetracycline CRS* in *0.01 M hydrochloric acid* and dilute to 25.0 ml with the same acid.

Reference solution (b). Dissolve 20.0 mg of *4-epioxytetracycline CRS* in *0.01 M hydrochloric acid* and dilute to 25.0 ml with the same acid.

Reference solution (c). Dissolve 20.0 mg of *tetracycline hydrochloride CRS* in *0.01 M hydrochloric acid* and dilute to 25.0 ml with the same acid.

Reference solution (d). Dissolve 8.0 mg of *α-apo-oxytetracycline CRS* in 5 ml of *0.01 M sodium hydroxide* and dilute to 100.0 ml with *0.01 M hydrochloric acid.*

Reference solution (e). Dissolve 8.0 mg of *β-apo-oxytetracycline CRS* in 5 ml of *0.01 M sodium hydroxide* and dilute to 100.0 ml with *0.01 M hydrochloric acid.*

Reference solution (f). Mix 1.5 ml of reference solution (a), 1.0 ml of reference solution (b), 3.0 ml of reference solution (c), 3.0 ml of reference solution (d) and 3.0 ml of reference solution (e) and dilute to 25.0 ml with *0.01 M hydrochloric acid.*

Reference solution (g). Mix 1.0 ml of reference solution (b), 4.0 ml of reference solution (c) and 40.0 ml of reference solution (e) and dilute to 200.0 ml with *0.01 M hydrochloric acid.*

Column:

– *size*: *l* = 0.25 m, Ø = 4.6 mm,
– *stationary phase*: *styrene-divinylbenzene copolymer R* (8 µm),
– *temperature*: 60 °C.

Mobile phase: weigh 30.0 g (for mobile phase A) and 100.0 g (for mobile phase B) of *2-methyl-2-propanol R* and transfer separately to 1000 ml volumetric flasks with the aid of 200 ml of *water R*; to each flask add 60 ml of *0.33 M phosphate buffer solution pH 7.5 R*, 50 ml of a 10 g/l solution of *tetrabutylammonium hydrogen sulphate R* adjusted to pH 7.5 with *dilute sodium hydroxide solution R* and 10 ml of a 0.4 g/l solution of *sodium edetate R* adjusted to pH 7.5 with *dilute sodium hydroxide solution R*; dilute each solution to 1000 ml with *water R*,

Time (min)	Mobile phase A (per cent *V/V*)	Mobile phase B (per cent *V/V*)
0 - 15	70	30
15 - 30	30	70
30 - 45	70	30

Flow rate: 1 ml/min.

Detection: spectrophotometer at 254 nm.

Injection: 20 µl; inject the test solution and reference solutions (f) and (g).

System suitability: reference solution (f):

– *resolution*: minimum 4.0 between the peaks due to impurity A (1st peak) and oxytetracycline (2nd peak), minimum 5.0 between the peaks due to oxytetracycline and impurity B (3rd peak) and minimum 3.5 between the peaks due to impurity D (4th peak) and impurity E (5th peak); if necessary, adapt the ratio mobile phase A: mobile phase B and/or adjust the time programme used to produce the one-step gradient elution,
– *symmetry factor*: maximum 1.25 for the peak due to oxytetracycline.

Limits:

– *impurity A*: not more than the area of the corresponding peak in the chromatogram obtained with reference solution (g) (0.5 per cent),
– *impurity B*: not more than the area of the corresponding peak in the chromatogram obtained with reference solution (g) (2.0 per cent),
– *impurity C (eluting on the tail of the main peak)*: not more than 4 times the area of the peak due to impurity A in the chromatogram obtained with reference solution (g) (2.0 per cent),
– *total of impurities D, E and F (eluting between the latter two)*: not more than the area of the peak due to impurity E in the chromatogram obtained with reference solution (g) (2.0 per cent),
– *disregard limit*: 0.02 times the area of the peak due to oxytetracycline in the chromatogram obtained with reference solution (f) (0.1 per cent).

Heavy metals (*2.4.8*): maximum 50 ppm.

0.5 g complies with limit test F. Prepare the standard using 2.5 ml of *lead standard solution (10 ppm Pb) R*.

Water (*2.5.12*): maximum 2.0 per cent, determined on 0.500 g.

Sulphated ash (*2.4.14*): maximum 0.5 per cent, determined on 1.0 g.

Bacterial endotoxins (*2.6.14*): less than 0.4 IU/mg, if intended for use in the manufacture of parenteral dosage forms without a further appropriate procedure for the removal of bacterial endotoxins.

ASSAY

Liquid chromatography (*2.2.29*) as described in the test for related substances with the following modification.

Monographs N-O

Injection: test solution and reference solution (a).

Calculate the percentage content of $C_{22}H_{25}ClN_2O_9$ taking 1 mg of oxytetracycline as equivalent to 1.079 mg of oxytetracycline hydrochloride.

STORAGE

In an airtight container, protected from light. If the substance is sterile, store in a sterile, airtight, tamper-proof container.

LABELLING

The label states, where applicable, that the substance is free from bacterial endotoxins.

IMPURITIES

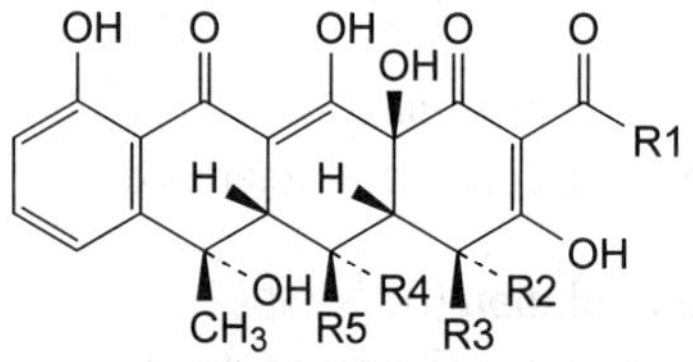

A. R1 = NH_2, R2 = $N(CH_3)_2$, R3 = R4 = H, R5 = OH: (4*R*,4a*R*,5*S*,5a*R*,6*S*,12a*S*)-4-(dimethylamino)-3,5,6,10,12,12a-hexahydroxy-6-methyl-1,11-dioxo-1,4,4a,5,5a,6,11,12a-octahydrotetracene-2-carboxamide (4-epioxytetracycline),

B. R1 = NH_2, R2 = R4 = R5 = H, R3 = $N(CH_3)_2$: tetracycline,

C. R1 = CH_3, R2 = R4 = H, R3 = $N(CH_3)_2$, R5 = OH: (4*S*,4a*R*,5*S*,5a*R*,6*S*,12a*S*)-2-acetyl-4-(dimethylamino)-3,5,6,10,12,12a-hexahydroxy-6-methyl-4a,5a,6,12a-tetrahydrotetracene-1,11(4*H*,5*H*)-dione (2-acetyl-2-decarbamoyloxytetracycline),

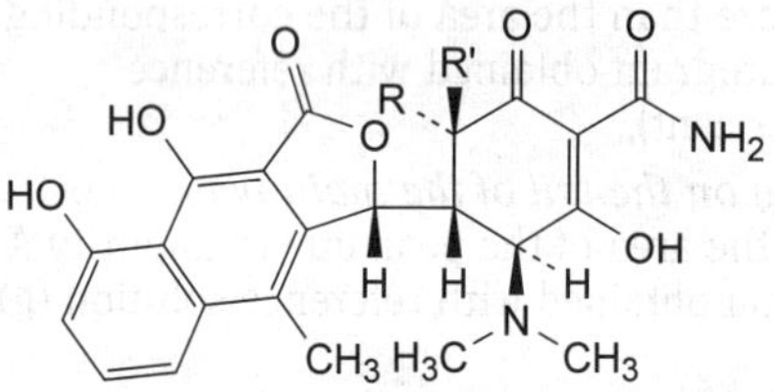

D. R = OH, R′ = H: (3*S*,4*S*,5*S*)-4-[(1*R*)-4,5-dihydroxy-9-methyl-3-oxo-1,3-dihydronaphtho[2,3-*c*]furan-1-yl]-3-(dimethylamino)-2,5-dihydroxy-6-oxocyclohex-1-enecarboxamide (α-apo-oxytetracycline),

E. R = H, R′ = OH: (3*S*,4*S*,5*R*)-4-[(1*R*)-4,5-dihydroxy-9-methyl-3-oxo-1,3-dihydronaphtho[2,3-*c*]furan-1-yl]-3-(dimethylamino)-2,5-dihydroxy-6-oxocyclohex-1-enecarboxamide (β-apo-oxytetracycline),

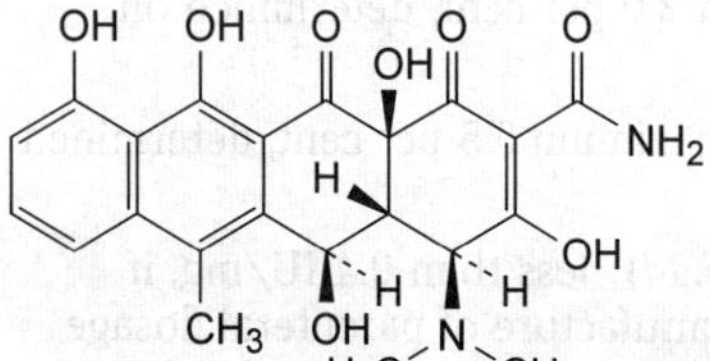

F. (4*S*,4a*R*,5*R*,12a*S*)-4-(dimethylamino)-3,5,10,11,12a-pentahydroxy-6-methyl-1,12-dioxo-1,4,4a,5,12,12a-hexahydrotetracene-2-carboxamide (anhydro-oxytetracycline).

01/2005:0780

OXYTOCIN

Oxytocinum

H-Cys–Tyr–Ile–Gln–Asn–Cys–Pro–Leu–Gly-NH_2

$C_{43}H_{66}N_{12}O_{12}S_2$ M_r 1007

DEFINITION

Oxytocin is a cyclic nonapeptide having the structure of the hormone produced by the posterior lobe of the pituitary gland that stimulates contraction of the uterus and milk ejection in receptive mammals. It is obtained by chemical synthesis and is available in the freeze-dried form as an acetate. It contains not less than 93.0 per cent and not more than the equivalent of 102.0 per cent of the peptide $C_{43}H_{66}N_{12}O_{12}S_2$, calculated with reference to the anhydrous, acetic acid-free substance.

By convention, for the purpose of labelling oxytocin preparations, 1 mg of oxytocin peptide ($C_{43}H_{66}N_{12}O_{12}S_2$) is equivalent to 600 IU of biological activity.

CHARACTERS

A white or almost white powder, hygroscopic, very soluble in water and in dilute solutions of acetic acid and of ethanol.

IDENTIFICATION

Examine the chromatograms obtained in the assay. The retention time of the principal peak in the chromatogram obtained with the test solution is approximately the same as that of the principal peak in the chromatogram obtained with the reference solution.

TESTS

pH (*2.2.3*). Dissolve 0.200 g in *carbon dioxide-free water R* and dilute to 10.0 ml with the same solvent. The pH of the solution is 3.0 to 6.0.

Amino acids. Examine by means of an amino-acid analyser. Standardise the apparatus with a mixture containing equimolar amounts of ammonia, glycine and the L-form of the following amino acids:

lysine	threonine	alanine	leucine
histidine	serine	valine	tyrosine
arginine	glutamic acid	methionine	phenylalanine
aspartic acid	proline	isoleucine	

together with half the equimolar amount of L-cystine. For the validation of the method, an appropriate internal standard, such as *DL-norleucine R*, is used.

Test solution. Place 1.0 mg of the substance to be examined in a rigorously cleaned hard-glass tube 100 mm long and 6 mm in internal diameter. Add a suitable amount of a 50 per cent *V/V* solution of *hydrochloric acid R*. Immerse the tube in a freezing mixture at − 5 °C, reduce the pressure to below 133 Pa and seal. Heat at 110 °C to 115 °C for 16 h. Cool, open the tube, transfer the contents to a 10 ml flask with the aid of five quantities, each of 0.2 ml, of *water R* and evaporate to dryness over *potassium hydroxide R* under reduced pressure. Take up the residue in *water R* and evaporate to dryness over *potassium hydroxide R* under reduced pressure; repeat these operations once. Take up the residue in a buffer solution suitable for the amino-acid analyser used and dilute to a suitable volume with the same buffer solution. Apply a suitable volume to the amino-acid analyser.

Express the content of each amino acid in moles. Calculate the relative proportions of the amino acids, taking one-sixth of the sum of the number of moles of aspartic acid, glutamic acid, proline, glycine, isoleucine and leucine as equal to one. The values fall within the following limits: aspartic acid 0.95 to 1.05; glutamic acid 0.95 to 1.05; proline 0.95 to 1.05; glycine 0.95 to 1.05; leucine 0.90 to 1.10; isoleucine 0.90 to 1.10; tyrosine 0.7 to 1.05; half-cystine 1.4 to 2.1; not more than traces of other amino acids are present.

Related peptides. Examine by liquid chromatography (*2.2.29*) as described under Assay.

Inject 50 µl of the test solution. In the chromatogram obtained the area of any peak, apart from the principal peak, is not greater than 1.5 per cent of the total area of the peaks; the sum of the areas of all the peaks, apart from the principal peak, is not greater than 5 per cent of the total area of the peaks. Disregard any peak due to the solvent and any peak with an area less than 0.1 per cent of that of the principal peak.

Acetic acid (*2.5.34*): 6.0 per cent to 10.0 per cent.

Test solution. Dissolve 15.0 mg of the substance to be examined in a mixture of 5 volumes of mobile phase B and 95 volumes of mobile phase A and dilute to 10.0 ml with the same mixture of solvents.

Water (*2.5.12*). Not more than 5.0 per cent, determined on at least 50 mg by the semi-micro determination of water.

Bacterial endotoxins (*2.6.14*): less than 300 IU/mg, if intended for use in the manufacture of parenteral dosage forms without a further appropriate procedure for removal of bacterial endotoxins.

ASSAY

Examine by liquid chromatography (*2.2.29*).

Test solution. Prepare a 0.25 mg/ml solution of the substance to be examined in a 15.6 g/l solution of *sodium dihydrogen phosphate R*.

Reference solution. Dissolve the contents of a vial of *oxytocin CRS* in a 15.6 g/l solution of *sodium dihydrogen phosphate R* to obtain a concentration of 0.25 mg/ml.

Resolution solution. Dissolve the contents of a vial of *oxytocin/desmopressin validation mixture CRS* in 500 µl of a 15.6 g/l solution of *sodium dihydrogen phosphate R*.

The chromatographic procedure may be carried out using:

- a stainless steel column 0.125 m long and 4.6 mm in internal diameter packed with *octadecylsilyl silica gel for chromatography R* (5 µm),
- as mobile phase at a flow rate of 1 ml/min:

  Mobile phase A. A 15.6 g/l solution of *sodium dihydrogen phosphate R*,

  Mobile phase B. Mix 1 volume of *acetonitrile for chromatography R* with 1 volume of *water R*,

Time (min)	Mobile phase A (per cent *V/V*)	Mobile phase B (per cent *V/V*)	Comment
0 - 30	70 → 40	30 → 60	linear gradient
30 - 30.1	40 → 70	60 → 30	switch to initial eluent composition
30.1 - 45	70	30	re-equilibration

- as detector a spectrophotometer set at 220 nm.

Equilibrate the column with a mixture of 30 volumes of mobile phase B and 70 volumes of mobile phase A.

Inject 25 µl of the resolution solution. When the chromatograms are recorded in the prescribed conditions, the retention times are: oxytocin about 7.5 min and desmopressin about 10 min. The test is not valid unless the resolution between the peaks corresponding to desmopressin and oxytocin is at least 5.0.

Inject 25 µl of the test solution and 25 µl of the reference solution.

Calculate the content of oxytocin ($C_{43}H_{66}N_{12}O_{12}S_2$) from the peak areas in the chromatograms obtained with the test solution and the reference solution and the declared content of $C_{43}H_{66}N_{12}O_{12}S_2$ in *oxytocin CRS*.

STORAGE

Store in an airtight container, protected from light, at a temperature of 2 °C to 8 °C. If the substance is sterile, store in a sterile, airtight, tamper-proof container.

LABELLING

The label states:

- the oxytocin peptide content ($C_{43}H_{66}N_{12}O_{12}S_2$),
- where applicable, that the substance is free from bacterial endotoxins.

01/2005:0779

OXYTOCIN BULK SOLUTION

Oxytocini solutio

DEFINITION

Oxytocin bulk solution is a solution of oxytocin, a cyclic nonapeptide having the structure of the hormone produced by the posterior lobe of the pituitary gland that stimulates contraction of the uterus and milk ejection in receptive mammals. It is obtained by chemical synthesis. It is available as a bulk solution with a stated concentration of not less than 0.25 mg of oxytocin per millilitre, in a solvent that may contain an appropriate antimicrobial preservative. It contains not less than 95.0 per cent and not more than 105.0 per cent of the amount of the peptide $C_{43}H_{66}N_{12}O_{12}S_2$ stated per millilitre.

By convention, for the purpose of labelling oxytocin preparations, 1 mg of oxytocin peptide ($C_{43}H_{66}N_{12}O_{12}S_2$) is equivalent to 600 IU of biological activity.

CHARACTERS

A clear, colourless liquid.

IDENTIFICATION

Examine the chromatograms obtained under Assay. The retention time of the principal peak in the chromatogram obtained with the test solution is similar to that of the principal peak in the chromatogram obtained with the reference solution.

TESTS

pH (*2.2.3*). The pH of the preparation to be examined is 3.0 to 5.0.

Amino acids. Examine by means of an amino-acid analyser. Standardise the apparatus with a mixture containing equimolar amounts of ammonia, glycine and the L-form of the following amino acids:

lysine	threonine	alanine	leucine
histidine	serine	valine	tyrosine
arginine	glutamic acid	methionine	phenylalanine
aspartic acid	proline	isoleucine	

Monographs N-O

together with half the equimolar amount of L-cystine. For the validation of the method, an appropriate internal standard, such as *DL-norleucine R*, is used.

Test solution. Place a volume of the preparation to be examined containing 0.25 mg of peptide in a rigorously cleaned hard-glass tube 100 mm long and 6 mm in internal diameter. Evaporate to dryness. Add a suitable amount of a 50 per cent *V/V* solution of *hydrochloric acid R*. Immerse the tube in a freezing mixture at −5 °C, reduce the pressure to below 133 Pa and seal. Heat at 110 °C to 115 °C for 16 h. Cool, open the tube, transfer the contents to a 10 ml flask with the aid of five quantities, each of 0.2 ml, of *water R* and evaporate to dryness over *potassium hydroxide R* under reduced pressure. Take up the residue in *water R* and evaporate to dryness over *potassium hydroxide R* under reduced pressure; repeat these operations once. Take up the residue in a buffer solution suitable for the amino-acid analyser used and dilute to a suitable volume with the same buffer solution.

Apply to the amino-acid analyser a suitable, accurately measured volume of the test solution such that the peak given by the amino acid present in the largest amount occupies most of the available chart height of the recorder.

Express the content of each amino acid in moles. Calculate the relative proportions of the amino acids taking one sixth of the sum of the number of moles of aspartic acid, glutamic acid, proline, glycine, isoleucine and leucine as equal to 1. The values fall within the following limits: aspartic acid 0.95 to 1.05; glutamic acid 0.95 to 1.05; proline 0.95 to 1.05; glycine 0.95 to 1.05; leucine 0.90 to 1.10; isoleucine 0.90 to 1.10; tyrosine 0.7 to 1.05; half cystine 1.4 to 2.1; not more than traces of other amino acids are present.

Related peptides. Examine by liquid chromatography (*2.2.29*) as described under Assay.

Inject 50 µl of the test solution. In the chromatogram obtained, the area of any peak apart from the principal peak is not greater than 1.5 per cent of the total area of the peaks; the sum of the areas of all peaks, apart from the principal peak, is not greater than 5 per cent of the total area of the peaks. Disregard any peak due to the solvent or to the antimicrobial preservative and any peak with an area less than 0.1 per cent of that of the principal peak.

Bacterial endotoxins (*2.6.14*): less than 300 IU in the volume that contains 1 mg of oxytocin, if intended for use in the manufacture of parenteral dosage forms without a further appropriate procedure for the removal of bacterial endotoxins.

Monographs N-O

ASSAY

Examine by liquid chromatography (*2.2.29*).

Test solution. Use the preparation to be examined.

Reference solution. Dissolve the contents of a vial of *oxytocin CRS* in a 15.6 g/l solution of *sodium dihydrogen phosphate R* to obtain a concentration of 0.25 mg/ml.

Resolution solution. Dissolve the contents of a vial of *oxytocin/desmopressin validation mixture CRS* with 500 µl of a 15.6 g/l solution of *sodium dihydrogen phosphate R*.

The chromatographic procedure may be carried out using:

- a stainless steel column 0.125 m long and 4.6 mm in internal diameter packed with *octadecylsilyl silica gel for chromatography R* (5 µm),
- as mobile phases at a flow rate of 1 ml/min:

  Mobile phase A. A 15.6 g/l solution of *sodium dihydrogen phosphate R,*

  Mobile phase B. Mix 1 volume of *acetonitrile for chromatography R* with 1 volume of *water R,*

Time (min)	Mobile phase A (per cent *V/V*)	Mobile phase B (per cent *V/V*)	Comment
0 - 30	70 → 40	30 → 60	linear gradient
30 - 30.1	40 → 70	60 → 30	return to initial conditions
30.1 - 45	70	30	re-equilibration

- as detector a spectrophotometer set at 220 nm.

Equilibrate the column with a mixture of 30 volumes of mobile phase B and 70 volumes of mobile phase A.

Inject 25 µl of the resolution solution. When the chromatograms are recorded in the prescribed conditions, the retention times are: oxytocin about 7.5 min and desmopressin about 10 min. The test is not valid unless the resolution between the desmopressin peak and the oxytocin peak is at least 5.0.

Inject 25 µl of the reference solution and 25 µl of the test solution. Calculate the content of oxytocin ($C_{43}H_{66}N_{12}O_{12}S_2$) from the peak areas in the chromatograms obtained with the test solution and the reference solution and the declared content of $C_{43}H_{66}N_{12}O_{12}S_2$ in *oxytocin CRS*.

STORAGE

Store at a temperature between 2 °C and 8 °C, protected from light. If the substance is sterile, store in a sterile, airtight, tamper-proof container.

LABELLING

The label states:

- the oxytocin peptide content in milligrams of $C_{43}H_{66}N_{12}O_{12}S_2$ per millilitre,
- where applicable, that the preparation is free from bacterial endotoxins,
- the name of any added antimicrobial preservative.

P

01/2005:1904

PALMITIC ACID

Acidum palmiticum

DEFINITION

Hexadecanoic acid ($C_{16}H_{32}O_2$; M_r 256.4), obtained from fats or oils of vegetable or animal origin.

Content: minimum 92.0 per cent.

CHARACTERS

Appearance: white, waxy solid.

Solubility: practically insoluble in water, soluble in alcohol.

IDENTIFICATION

A. It complies with the test for freezing point (see Tests).

B. Acid value (*2.5.1*): 216 to 220, determined on 0.1 g.

C. Examine the chromatograms obtained in the assay.

Results: the principal peak in the chromatogram obtained with the test solution is similar in retention time to the principal peak in the chromatogram obtained with the reference solution.

TESTS

Appearance. Heat the substance to be examined to about 75 °C. The resulting liquid is not more intensely coloured than reference solution Y_7 or BY_7 (*2.2.2, Method I*).

Acidity. Melt 5.0 g, stir for 2 min in 10 ml of hot *carbon dioxide-free water R*, cool slowly and filter. To the filtrate add 0.05 ml of *methyl orange solution R*. No red colour develops.

Freezing point (*2.2.18*): 60 °C to 66 °C.

Iodine value (*2.5.4*): maximum 1.

Stearic acid: maximum 6.0 per cent, determined as prescribed in the assay.

Nickel (*2.4.27*): maximum 1 ppm.

ASSAY

Gas chromatography (*2.4.22, Method C*). Prepare the solutions as described in the method but omitting the initial hydrolysis.

Reference solution. Prepare the reference solution in the same manner as the test solution using a mixture of 50 mg of *palmitic acid R* and 50 mg of *stearic acid R* instead of the substance to be examined.

Relative retention with reference to methyl stearate: methyl palmitate = about 0.9.

System suitability:

– *resolution*: minimum 5.0 between the peaks due to methyl stearate and methyl palmitate.

01/2005:0350

PANCREAS POWDER

Pancreatis pulvis

DEFINITION

Pancreas powder is prepared from the fresh or frozen pancreases of mammals. It contains various enzymes having proteolytic, lipolytic and amylolytic activities.

1 milligram of pancreas powder contains not less than 1.0 European Pharmacopoeia Unit (Ph. Eur. U.) of total proteolytic activity, 15 European Pharmacopoeia Units of lipolytic activity and 12 European Pharmacopoeia Units of amylolytic activity.

Pancreas powder is prepared in conditions designed to minimise the degree of microbial contamination.

CHARACTERS

A slightly brown, amorphous powder, partly soluble in water, practically insoluble in alcohol.

IDENTIFICATION

A. Triturate 0.5 g with 10 ml of *water R* and adjust to pH 8 by the addition of *0.1 M sodium hydroxide,* using 0.1 ml of *cresol red solution R* as indicator. Divide the suspension into two equal parts (suspension (a) and suspension (b)). Boil suspension (a). To each suspension add 10 mg of *fibrin congo red R,* heat to 38 °C to 40 °C and maintain at this temperature for 1 h. Suspension (a) is colourless or slightly pink and suspension (b) is distinctly more red.

B. Triturate 0.25 g with 10 ml of *water R* and adjust to pH 8 by the addition of *0.1 M sodium hydroxide,* using 0.1 ml of *cresol red solution R* as indicator. Divide the suspension into two equal parts (suspension (a) and suspension (b)). Boil suspension (a). Dissolve 0.1 g of *soluble starch R* in 100 ml of boiling *water R,* boil for 2 min, cool and dilute to 150 ml with *water R.* To 75 ml of the starch solution add suspension (a) and to the remaining 75 ml add suspension (b). Heat each mixture to 38 °C to 40 °C and maintain at this temperature for 5 min.

To 1 ml of each mixture add 10 ml of *iodine solution R2.* The mixture obtained with suspension (a) has an intense blue-violet colour; the mixture obtained with suspension (b) has the colour of the iodine solution.

TESTS

Fat content. In an extraction apparatus, treat 1.0 g with *light petroleum R1* for 3 h. Evaporate the solvent and dry the residue at 100 °C to 105 °C for 2 h. The residue weighs not more than 50 mg (5.0 per cent).

Loss on drying (*2.2.32*). Not more than 5.0 per cent, determined on 0.50 g by drying at 60 °C at a pressure not exceeding 670 Pa for 4 h.

Microbial contamination. Total viable aerobic count (*2.6.12*) not more than 10^4 micro-organisms per gram, determined by plate count. It complies with the tests for *Escherichia coli* and *Salmonella* (*2.6.13*).

ASSAY

Total proteolytic activity. The total proteolytic activity of pancreas powder is determined by comparing the quantity of peptides non-precipitable by a 50 g/l solution of *trichloroacetic acid R* released per minute from a substrate of casein solution with the quantity of such peptides released by *pancreas powder (protease) BRP* from the same substrate in the same conditions.

Casein solution. Suspend a quantity of *casein BRP* equivalent to 1.25 g of dried substance in 5 ml of *water R,* add 10 ml of *0.1 M sodium hydroxide* and stir for 1 min. (Determine the water content of *casein BRP* prior to the test by heating at 60 °C *in vacuo* for 4 h.) Add 60 ml of *water R* and stir with a magnetic stirrer until the solution is practically clear. Adjust to pH 8.0 with *0.1 M sodium hydroxide* or *0.1 M hydrochloric acid.* Dilute to 100.0 ml with *water R.* Use the solution on the day of preparation.

Monographs P

Enterokinase solution. Dissolve 50 mg of *enterokinase BRP* in *0.02 M calcium chloride solution R* and dilute to 50.0 ml with the same solvent. Use the solution on the day of preparation.

For the test suspension and the reference suspension, prepare the suspension and carry out the dilution at 0 °C to 4 °C.

Test suspension. Triturate 0.100 g of the substance to be examined for 5 min adding gradually 25 ml of *0.02 M calcium chloride solution R*. Transfer completely to a volumetric flask and dilute to 100.0 ml with *0.02 M calcium chloride solution R*. To 10.0 ml of this suspension add 10.0 ml of enterokinase solution and heat on a water-bath at 35 ± 0.5 °C for 15 min. Cool and dilute with *borate buffer solution pH 7.5 R* at 5 ± 3 °C to a final concentration of about 0.065 Ph. Eur. U. of total proteolytic activity per millilitre calculated on the basis of the stated activity.

Reference suspension. Prepare a suspension of *pancreas powder (protease) BRP* as described for the test suspension but without the addition of enterokinase so as to obtain a known final concentration of about 0.065 Ph. Eur. U. per millilitre calculated on the basis of the stated activity.

Designate tubes in duplicate T, T_b, S_1, S_{1b}, S_2, S_{2b}, S_3, S_{3b}; designate a tube B.

Add *borate buffer solution pH 7.5 R* to the tubes as follows:

B: 3.0 ml,

S_1 and S_{1b}: 2.0 ml,

S_2, S_{2b}, T and T_b: 1.0 ml.

Add the reference suspension to the tubes as follows:

S_1 and S_{1b}: 1.0 ml,

S_2 and S_{2b}: 2.0 ml,

S_3 and S_{3b}: 3.0 ml.

Add 2.0 ml of the test suspension to tubes T and T_b.

Add 5.0 ml of a 50 g/l solution of *trichloroacetic acid R* to tubes B, S_{1b}, S_{2b}, S_{3b} and T_b. Mix by shaking.

Place the tubes and the casein solution in a water-bath at 35 ± 0.5 °C. Place a glass rod in each tube. When temperature equilibrium is reached, add 2.0 ml of the casein solution to tubes B, S_{1b}, S_{2b}, S_{3b} and T_b. Mix. At time zero, add 2.0 ml of casein solution successively and at intervals of 30 s to tubes S_1, S_2, S_3 and T. Mix immediately after each addition. Exactly 30 min after addition of the casein solution, taking into account the regular interval adopted, add 5.0 ml of a 50 g/l solution of *trichloroacetic acid R* to tubes S_1, S_2, S_3 and T. Mix. Withdraw the tubes from the water-bath and allow to stand at room temperature for 20 min.

Filter the contents of each tube twice through the same suitable filter paper previously washed with a 50 g/l solution of *trichloroacetic acid R*, then with *water R* and dried.

A suitable filter paper complies with the following test: filter 5 ml of a 50 g/l of *trichloroacetic acid R* on a 7 cm disc of white filter paper; the absorbance (*2.2.25*) of the filtrate, measured at 275 nm using unfiltered trichloroacetic acid solution as the compensation liquid, is less than 0.04.

A schematic presentation of the above operations is shown in Table 0350.-1.

Table 0350.-1

	Tubes								
	S_1	S_{1b}	S_2	S_{2b}	S_3	S_{3b}	T	T_b	B
Buffer solution	2	2	1	1			1	1	3
Reference solution	1	1	2	2	3	3			
Suspension test							2	2	
Trichloroacetic acid solution		5		5		5		5	5
Mix		+		+		+		+	+
Water-bath 35 °C	+	+	+	+	+	+	+	+	+
Casein solution		2		2		2		2	2
Mix		+		+		+		+	+
Casein solution	2		2		2		2		
Mix	+		+		+		+		
Water-bath 35 °C 30 min	+	+	+	+	+	+	+	+	+
Trichloroacetic solution	5		5		5		5		
Mix	+		+		+		+		
Room temperature 20 min	+	+	+	+	+	+	+	+	+
Filter	+	+	+	+	+	+	+	+	+

Measure the absorbance (*2.2.25*) of the filtrates at 275 nm using the filtrate obtained from tube B as the compensation liquid.

Correct the average absorbance values for the filtrates obtained from tubes S_1, S_2 and S_3 by subtracting the average values obtained for the filtrates from tubes S_{1b}, S_{2b} and S_{3b} respectively. Draw a calibration curve of the corrected values against volume of reference suspension used.

Determine the activity of the substance to be examined using the corrected absorbance for the test suspension ($T - T_b$) and the calibration curve and taking into account the dilution factors.

The test is not valid unless the corrected absorbance values are between 0.15 and 0.60.

Lipolytic activity. The lipolytic activity is determined by comparing the rate at which a suspension of pancreas powder hydrolyses a substrate of olive oil emulsion with the rate at which a suspension of *pancreas powder (amylase and lipase) BRP* hydrolyses the same substrate under the same conditions. *The test is carried out under nitrogen.*

Olive oil stock emulsion. In an 800 ml beaker 9 cm in diameter, place 40 ml of *olive oil R*, 330 ml of *acacia solution R* and 30 ml of *water R*. Place an electric mixer at the bottom of the beaker. Place the beaker in a vessel containing *alcohol R* and a sufficient quantity of ice as a cooling mixture. Emulsify using the mixer at an average speed of 1000 r/min to 2000 r/min. Cool to 5 °C to 10 °C. Increase the mixing speed to 8000 r/min. Mix for 30 min keeping the temperature below 25 °C by the continuous addition of crushed ice into the cooling mixture. (A mixture of calcium chloride and crushed ice is also suitable). Store the stock emulsion in a refrigerator and use within 14 days. The emulsion must not separate into two distinct layers. Check the diameter of the globules of the emulsion under a microscope. At least 90 per cent have a diameter below 3 μm and none has a diameter greater than 10 μm. Shake the emulsion thoroughly before preparing the emulsion substrate.

Olive oil emulsion. For ten determinations, mix the following solutions in the order indicated: 100 ml of stock emulsion, 80 ml of *tris(hydroxymethyl)aminomethane solution R1*, 20 ml of a freshly prepared 80 g/l of *sodium taurocholate BRP* and 95 ml of *water R*. Use on the day of preparation.

Apparatus. Use a reaction vessel of about 50 ml capacity provided with:

- a device that will maintain a temperature of 37 ± 0.5 °C,
- a magnetic stirrer,
- a lid with holes for the insertion of electrodes, the tip of a burette, a tube for the admission of nitrogen and the introduction of reagents.

An automatic or manual titration apparatus may be used. In the latter case, the burette is graduated in 0.005 ml and the pH-meter is provided with a wide reading scale and glass-calomel electrodes. After each test the reaction vessel is evacuated by suction and washed several times with *water R*, the washings being removed each time by suction.

Test suspension. In a small mortar cooled to 0 °C to 4 °C, triturate carefully a quantity of the substance to be examined equivalent to about 2500 Ph. Eur. U. of lipolytic activity with 1 ml of cooled *maleate buffer solution pH 7.0 R* (lipase solvent) until a very fine suspension is obtained. Dilute the suspension with cold *maleate buffer solution pH 7.0 R*, transfer quantitatively to a volumetric flask and dilute to 100.0 ml with the cold buffer solution. Keep the flask containing the test suspension in iced water during the titration.

Reference suspension. To avoid absorption of water formed by condensation, allow the reference preparation to reach room temperature before opening the container. Prepare a suspension of *pancreas powder (amylase and lipase) BRP* as described for the test suspension using a quantity equivalent to about 2500 Ph. Eur. U.

Carry out the titrations immediately after preparation of the test suspension and the reference suspension. Place 29.5 ml of olive oil emulsion in the reaction vessel equilibrated at 37 ± 0.5 °C. Fit the vessel with the electrodes, a stirrer and the burette (the tip being immersed in the olive oil emulsion).

Put the lid in place and switch on the apparatus. Carefully add *0.1 M sodium hydroxide* with stirring. Adjust to pH 9.2. Using a rapid-flow graduated pipette transfer about 0.5 ml of the previously homogenised reference suspension, start the chronometer and add continuously *0.1 M sodium hydroxide* to maintain the pH at 9.0. After exactly 1 min, note the volume of *0.1 M sodium hydroxide* used. Carry out the measurement a further four times. Discard the first reading and determine the average of the four others (S_1). Make two further determinations (S_2 and S_3). Calculate the average of the values S_1, S_2 and S_3. The average volume of *0.1 M sodium hydroxide* used should be about 0.12 ml/min with limits of 0.08 ml to 0.16 ml.

Carry out three determinations in the same manner for the test suspension (T_1, T_2 and T_3). If the quantity of *0.1 M sodium hydroxide* used is outside the limits 0.08 ml to 0.16 ml per minute, the assay is repeated with a quantity of test suspension which is more suitable but situated between 0.4 ml and 0.6 ml. Otherwise the quantity of the substance to be examined is adjusted to comply with the conditions of the test. Calculate the average of the values T_1, T_2 and T_3.

Calculate the activity in Ph. Eur. Units per milligram from the expression:

$$\frac{n \times m_1}{n_1 \times m} \times A$$

n = average volume of *0.1 M sodium hydroxide* used per minute during the titration of the test suspension,

n_1 = average volume of *0.1 M sodium hydroxide* used per minute during the titration of the reference suspension,

m = mass in milligrams of the substance to be examined,

m_1 = mass in milligrams of the reference preparation,

A = activity of *pancreas powder (amylase and lipase) BRP* in Ph. Eur. Units per milligram.

Amylolytic activity. The amylolytic activity is determined by comparing the rate at which a suspension of pancreas powder hydrolyses a substrate of starch solution with the rate at which a suspension of *pancreas powder (amylase and lipase) BRP* hydrolyses the same substrate under the same conditions.

Starch solution. To a quantity of *starch BRP* equivalent to 2.0 g of the dried substance add 10 ml of *water R* and mix. (Determine the water content of *starch BRP* prior to the test by heating at 120 °C for 4 h). Add this suspension, whilst stirring continuously, to 160 ml of boiling *water R*. Wash the container several times with successive quantities, each of 10 ml, of *water R* and add the washings to the hot starch solution. Heat to boiling, stirring continuously. Cool to room temperature and dilute to 200 ml with *water R*. Use the solution on the day of preparation.

For the test suspension and the reference suspension, prepare the suspension and carry out the dilution at 0 °C to 4 °C.

Test suspension. Triturate a quantity of the substance to be examined equivalent to about 1500 Ph. Eur. U. of amylolytic activity with 60 ml of *phosphate buffer solution pH 6.8 R1* for 15 min. Transfer quantitatively to a volumetric flask and dilute to 100.0 ml with *phosphate buffer solution pH 6.8 R1*.

Reference suspension. Prepare a suspension of *pancreas powder (amylase and lipase) BRP* as described for the test suspension, using a quantity equivalent to about 1500 Ph. Eur. U.

In a test tube 200 mm long and 22 mm in diameter, fitted with a ground-glass stopper, place 25.0 ml of starch solution, 10.0 ml of *phosphate buffer solution pH 6.8 R1* and 1.0 ml of a 11.7 g/l solution of *sodium chloride R*. Close the tube, shake and place in a water-bath at 25.0 ± 0.1 °C. When the temperature equilibrium has been reached, add 1.0 ml of the test suspension and start the chronometer. Mix and place the tube in the water-bath. After exactly 10 min, add 2 ml of *1 M hydrochloric acid.* Transfer the mixture quantitatively to a 300 ml conical flask fitted with a ground-glass stopper. Whilst shaking continuously, add 10.0 ml of *0.05 M iodine* and immediately, 45 ml of *0.1 M sodium hydroxide.* Allow to stand in the dark at a temperature between 15 °C and 25 °C for 15 min. Add 4 ml of a mixture of 1 volume of *sulphuric acid R* and 4 volumes of *water R*. Titrate the excess of iodine with *0.1 M sodium thiosulphate* using a microburette. Carry out a blank titration adding the 2 ml of *1 M hydrochloric acid*before introducing the test suspension. Carry out the titration of the reference suspension in the same manner.

Monographs P

Calculate the amylolytic activity in Ph. Eur. Units per milligram from the expression:

$$\frac{(n' - n)\, m_1}{(n'_1 - n_1)\, m} \times A$$

n = number of millilitres of *0.1 M sodium thiosulphate* used in the titration of the test suspension,

n_1 = number of millilitres of *0.1 M sodium thiosulphate* used in the titration of the reference suspension,

n' = number of millilitres of *0.1 M sodium thiosulphate* used in the blank titration of the test suspension,

n'_1 = number of millilitres of *0.1 M sodium thiosulphate* used in the blank titration of the reference suspension,

m = mass in milligrams of the substance to be examined,

m_1 = mass in milligrams of the reference preparation,

A = activity of *pancreas powder (amylase and lipase) BRP* in Ph. Eur. Units per milligram.

STORAGE

Store in an airtight container, at a temperature of 2 °C to 8 °C.

01/2005:0681

PANCURONIUM BROMIDE

Pancuronii bromidum

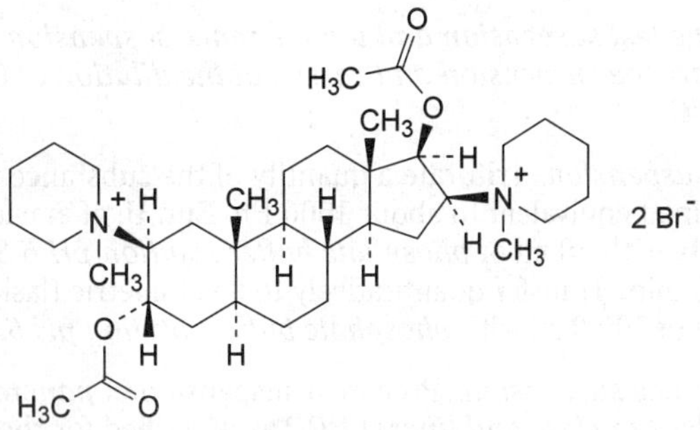

$C_{35}H_{60}Br_2N_2O_4$ M_r 733

DEFINITION

1,1′-[3α,17β-Bis(acetyloxy)-5α-androstane-2β,16β-diyl]bis(1-methylpiperidinium) dibromide.

Content: 98.0 per cent to 102.0 per cent (anhydrous substance).

CHARACTERS

Appearance: white or almost white, crystalline powder, hygroscopic.

Solubility: very soluble to freely soluble in water, very soluble in methylene chloride, freely soluble in alcohol.

IDENTIFICATION

A. Infrared absorption spectrophotometry (*2.2.24*).

Preparation: discs.

Comparison: *pancuronium bromide CRS*.

B. Examine the chromatograms obtained in the test for related substances.

Results: the principal spot in the chromatogram obtained with the test solution is similar in position, colour and size to the principal spot in the chromatogram obtained with reference solution (a).

C. It gives reaction (a) of bromides (*2.3.1*).

TESTS

Appearance of solution. The solution is clear (*2.2.1*) and colourless (*2.2.2, Method II*).

Dissolve 50 mg in *water R* and dilute to 25 ml with the same solvent.

Specific optical rotation (*2.2.7*): + 38 to + 42 (anhydrous substance).

Dissolve 0.75 g in *water R* and dilute to 25.0 ml with the same solvent.

Related substances. Thin-layer chromatography (*2.2.27*). *Prepare the solutions immediately before use.*

Test solution. Dissolve 50 mg of the substance to be examined in *methylene chloride R* and dilute to 5 ml with the same solvent.

Reference solution (a). Dissolve 50 mg of *pancuronium bromide CRS* in *methylene chloride R* and dilute to 5 ml with the same solvent.

Reference solution (b). Dilute 0.1 ml of the test solution to 20 ml with *methylene chloride R*.

Reference solution (c). Dissolve 5 mg of *pancuronium impurity A CRS* in *methylene chloride R* and dilute to 50 ml with the same solvent.

Reference solution (d). Dissolve 5 mg of *pancuronium bromide CRS* in 1 ml of reference solution (c).

Plate: *TLC silica gel plate R*.

Mobile phase: 400 g/l solution of *sodium iodide R, acetonitrile R, 2-propanol R* (5:10:85 *V/V/V*).

Application: 2 µl.

Development: in an unlined and unsaturated tank over a path of 12 cm.

Drying: in a current of cold air.

Detection: expose the plate to iodine vapour for about 10 min and cover the plate with a glass plate.

System suitability:

- the chromatogram obtained with reference solution (d) shows 2 distinct spots and the ratio of the R_f values of impurity A and of pancuronium bromide is at least 1.2,
- a spot is clearly visible in the chromatogram obtained with reference solution (b).

Limits:

- *impurity A*: any spot corresponding to impurity A is not more intense than the principal spot in the chromatogram obtained with reference solution (c) (1.0 per cent),
- *any other impurity*: any spot, apart from the principal spot and any spot corresponding to impurity A, is not more intense than the spot in the chromatogram obtained with reference solution (b) (0.5 per cent).

Water (*2.5.12*): maximum 8.0 per cent, determined on 0.300 g.

Sulphated ash (*2.4.14*): maximum 0.1 per cent, determined on 1.0 g.

ASSAY

Dissolve 0.2000 g in 50 ml of *acetic anhydride R*, heating if necessary. Titrate with *0.1 M perchloric acid*, determining the end-point potentiometrically (*2.2.20*).

1 ml of *0.1 M perchloric acid* is equivalent to 36.63 mg of $C_{35}H_{60}Br_2N_2O_4$.

STORAGE

In an airtight container, protected from light.

IMPURITIES

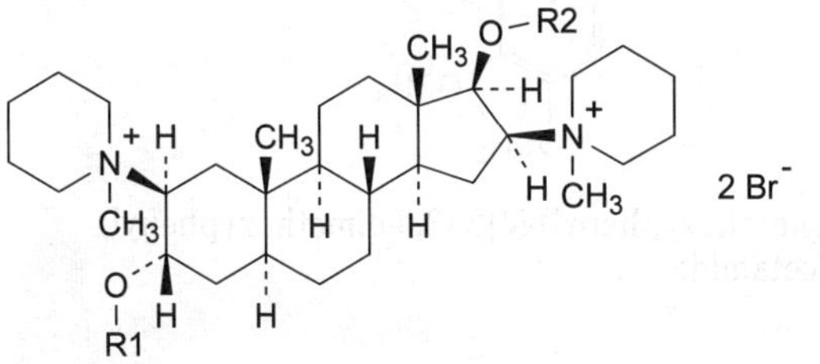

A. R1 = CO-CH_3, R2 = H: 1,1′-[3α-(acetyloxy)-17β-hydroxy-5α-androstane-2β,16β-diyl]bis(1-methylpiperidinium) dibromide (dacuronium bromide),

B. R1 = H, R2 = CO-CH_3: 1,1′-[17β-(acetyloxy)-3α-hydroxy-5α-androstane-2β,16β-diyl]bis(1-methylpiperidinium) dibromide,

C. R1 = R2 = H: 1,1′-(3α,17β-dihydroxy-5α-androstane-2β,16β-diyl)bis(1-methylpiperidinium) dibromide.

01/2005:0102
corrected

PAPAVERINE HYDROCHLORIDE

Papaverini hydrochloridum

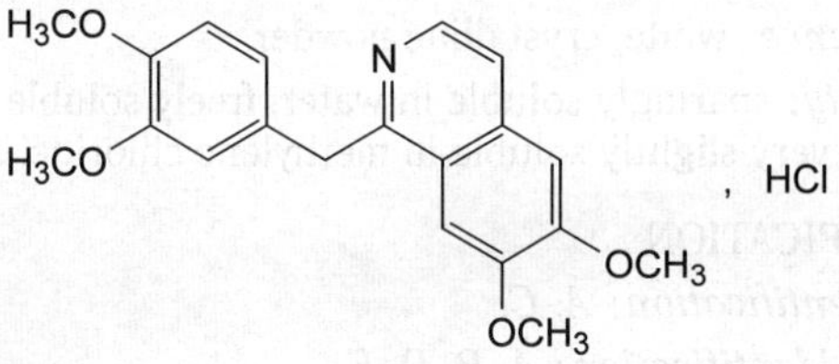

$C_{20}H_{22}ClNO_4$ M_r 375.9

DEFINITION

1-(3,4-Dimethoxybenzyl)-6,7-dimethoxyisoquinoline hydrochloride.

Content: 99.0 per cent to 101.0 per cent (dried substance).

CHARACTERS

Appearance: white or almost white, crystalline powder or white or almost white crystals.

Solubility: sparingly soluble in water, slightly soluble in alcohol.

IDENTIFICATION

First identification: A, D.

Second identification: B, C, D.

A. Infrared absorption spectrophotometry (*2.2.24*).

Comparison: *papaverine hydrochloride CRS.*

B. Thin-layer chromatography (*2.2.27*).

Test solution. Dissolve 5 mg of the substance to be examined in *methanol R* and dilute to 10 ml with the same solvent.

Reference solution. Dissolve 5 mg of *papaverine hydrochloride CRS* in *methanol R* and dilute to 10 ml with the same solvent.

Plate: *TLC silica gel GF_{254} plate R.*

Mobile phase: *diethylamine R, ethyl acetate R, toluene R* (10:20:70 *V/V/V*).

Application: 10 µl.

Development: over 2/3 of the plate.

Drying: at 100-105 °C for 2 h.

Detection: examine in ultraviolet light at 254 nm.

Results: the principal spot in the chromatogram obtained with the test solution is similar in position and size to the principal spot in the chromatogram obtained with the reference solution.

C. To 10 ml of solution S (see Tests) add 5 ml of *ammonia R* dropwise and allow to stand for 10 min. The precipitate, washed and dried, melts (*2.2.14*) at 146 °C to 149 °C.

D. It gives reaction (a) of chlorides (*2.3.1*).

TESTS

Solution S. Dissolve 0.4 g in *carbon dioxide-free water R*, heating gently if necessary, and dilute to 20 ml with the same solvent.

Appearance of solution. Solution S is clear (*2.2.1*) and not more intensely coloured than reference solution BY_6 (*2.2.2, Method II*).

pH (*2.2.3*): 3.0 to 4.0 for solution S.

Related substances. Liquid chromatography (*2.2.29*).

Solvent mixture: *acetonitrile R*, mobile phase A (20:80 *V/V*).

Test solution. Dissolve 20.0 mg of the substance to be examined in the solvent mixture and dilute to 10.0 ml with the solvent mixture.

Reference solution (a). Dilute 1.0 ml of the test solution to 100.0 ml with the solvent mixture. Dilute 1.0 ml of this solution to 10.0 ml with the solvent mixture.

Reference solution (b). Dissolve 12 mg of *noscapine CRS* in 1.0 ml of the test solution and dilute to 100.0 ml with the solvent mixture.

Column:

- *size*: *l* = 0.25 m, Ø = 4.0 mm,
- *stationary phase*: *base-deactivated octylsilyl silica gel for chromatography R* (5 µm).

Mobile phase:

- *mobile phase A*: 3.4 g/l solution of *potassium dihydrogen phosphate R* adjusted to pH 3.0 with *dilute phosphoric acid R*,
- *mobile phase B*: *acetonitrile R*,
- *mobile phase C*: *methanol R*,

Time (min)	Mobile phase A (per cent *V/V/V*)	Mobile phase B (per cent *V/V/V*)	Mobile phase C (per cent *V/V/V*)
0 - 5	85	5	10
5 - 12	85 → 60	5	10 → 35
12 - 20	60	5	35
20 - 24	60 → 40	5 → 20	35 → 40
24 - 27	40	20	40
27 - 32	40 → 85	20 → 5	40 → 10
32 - 40	85	5	10

Flow rate: 1 ml/min.

Detection: spectrophotometer at 238 nm.

Injection: 10 µl.

Relative retention with reference to papaverine (retention time = about 23.4 min): impurity E = about 0.7; impurity C = about 0.75; impurity B = about 0.8; impurity A = about 0.9; impurity F = about 1.1; impurity D = about 1.2.

Monographs P

System suitability: reference solution (b):
- *resolution*: minimum 1.5 between the peaks due to impurity A and papaverine.

Limits:
- *correction factors*: for the calculation of contents, multiply the peak areas of the following impurities by the corresponding correction factor: impurity C = 2.7; impurity D = 0.5; impurity A = 6.2;
- *any impurity*: not more than the area of the principal peak in the chromatogram obtained with reference solution (a) (0.1 per cent);
- *total*: not more than 5 times the area of the principal peak in the chromatogram obtained with reference solution (a) (0.5 per cent);
- *disregard limit*: 0.5 times the area of the principal peak in the chromatogram obtained with reference solution (a) (0.05 per cent).

Loss on drying (*2.2.32*): maximum 0.5 per cent, determined on 1.000 g by drying in an oven at 100-105 °C.

Sulphated ash (*2.4.14*): maximum 0.1 per cent, determined on the residue from the test for loss on drying.

ASSAY

Dissolve 0.300 g in a mixture of 5.0 ml of *0.01 M hydrochloric acid* and 50 ml of *alcohol R*. Carry out a potentiometric titration (*2.2.20*), using *0.1 M sodium hydroxide*. Read the volume added between the 2 points of inflexion.

1 ml of *0.1 M sodium hydroxide* is equivalent to 37.59 mg of $C_{20}H_{22}ClNO_4$.

IMPURITIES

A. noscapine,

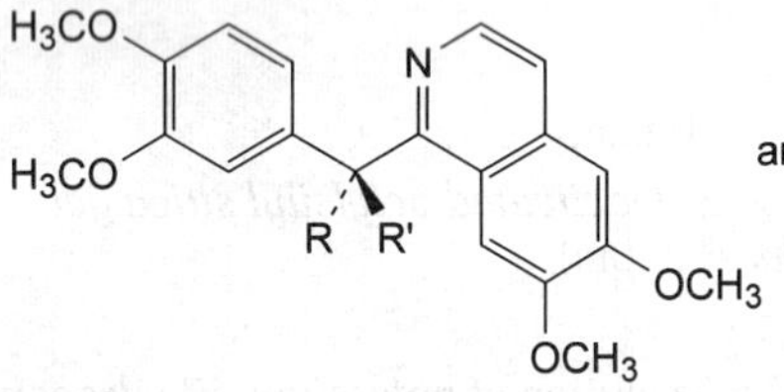

and enantiomer

B. R = OH, R′ = H: (*RS*)-(3,4-dimethoxyphenyl)(6,7-dimethoxyisoquinolin-1-yl)methanol (papaverinol),

D. R + R′ = O: (3,4-dimethoxyphenyl)(6,7-dimethoxyisoquinolin-1-yl)methanone (papaveraldine),

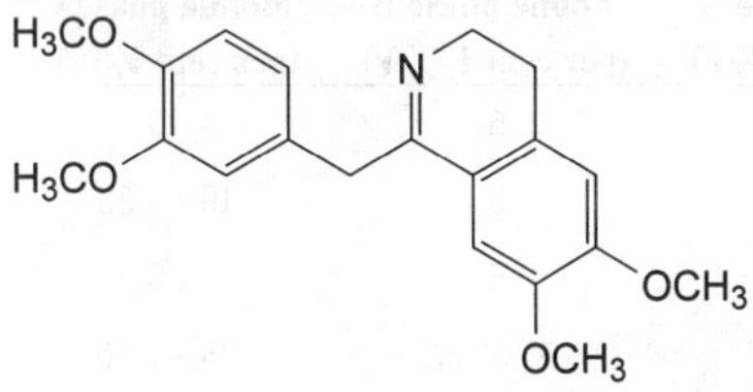

C. 1-(3,4-dimethoxybenzyl)-6,7-dimethoxy-3,4-dihydroisoquinoline (dihydropapaverine),

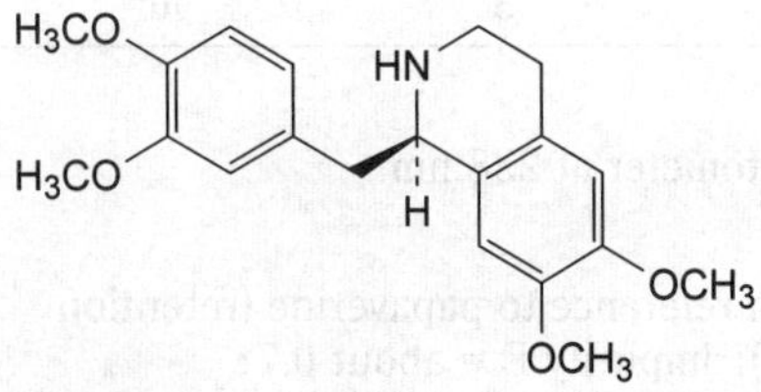

and enantiomer

E. (1*RS*)-1-(3,4-dimethoxybenzyl)-6,7-dimethoxy-1,2,3,4-tetrahydroisoquinoline (tetrahydropapaverine),

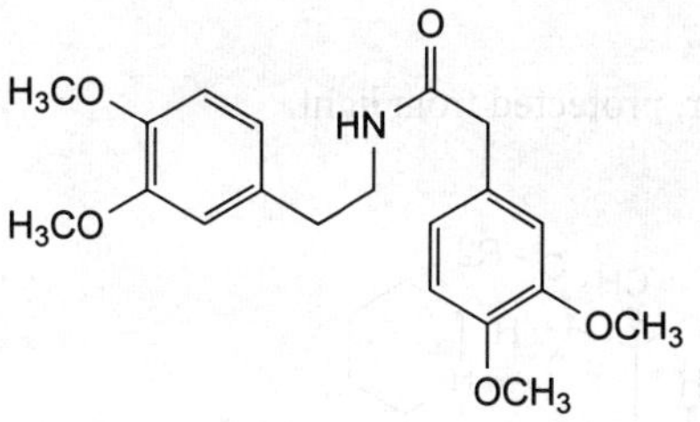

F. 2-(3,4-dimethoxyphenyl)-*N*-[2-(3,4-dimethoxyphenyl)-ethyl]acetamide.

01/2005:0049

PARACETAMOL

Paracetamolum

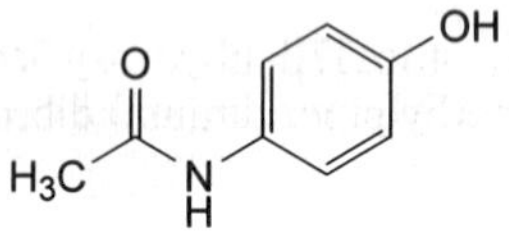

$C_8H_9NO_2$ M_r 151.2

DEFINITION

N-(4-Hydroxyphenyl)acetamide.

Content: 99.0 per cent to 101.0 per cent (dried substance).

CHARACTERS

Appearance: white, crystalline powder.

Solubility: sparingly soluble in water, freely soluble in alcohol, very slightly soluble in methylene chloride.

IDENTIFICATION

First identification: A, C.

Second identification: A, B, D, E.

A. Melting point (*2.2.14*): 168 °C to 172 °C.

B. Dissolve 0.1 g in *methanol R* and dilute to 100.0 ml with the same solvent. To 1.0 ml of the solution add 0.5 ml of a 10.3 g/l solution of *hydrochloric acid R* and dilute to 100.0 ml with *methanol R*. Protect the solution from bright light and immediately measure the absorbance (*2.2.25*) at the absorption maximum at 249 nm. The specific absorbance at the maximum is 860 to 980.

C. Infrared absorption spectrophotometry (*2.2.24*).
Preparation: discs.
Comparison: *paracetamol CRS.*

D. To 0.1 g add 1 ml of *hydrochloric acid R*, heat to boiling for 3 min, add 1 ml of *water R* and cool in an ice bath. No precipitate is formed. Add 0.05 ml of a 4.9 g/l solution of *potassium dichromate R*. A violet colour develops which does not change to red.

E. It gives the reaction of acetyl (*2.3.1*). Heat over a naked flame.

TESTS

Related substances. Liquid chromatography (*2.2.29*). *Prepare the solutions immediately before use.*

Test solution. Dissolve 0.200 g of the substance to be examined in 2.5 ml of *methanol R* containing 4.6 g/l of a 400 g/l solution of *tetrabutylammonium hydroxide R* and dilute to 10.0 ml with a mixture of equal volumes of a 17.9 g/l solution of *disodium hydrogen phosphate R* and of a 7.8 g/l solution of *sodium dihydrogen phosphate R.*

Reference solution (a). Dilute 1.0 ml of the test solution to 50.0 ml with the mobile phase. Dilute 5.0 ml of this solution to 100.0 ml with the mobile phase.

Reference solution (b). Dilute 1.0 ml of reference solution (a) to 10.0 ml with the mobile phase.

Reference solution (c). Dissolve 5.0 mg of *4-aminophenol R*, 5 mg of *paracetamol CRS* and 5.0 mg of *chloroacetanilide R* in *methanol R* and dilute to 20.0 ml with the same solvent. Dilute 1.0 ml to 250.0 ml with the mobile phase.

Reference solution (d). Dissolve 20.0 mg of *4-nitrophenol R* in *methanol R* and dilute to 50.0 ml with the same solvent. Dilute 1.0 ml to 20.0 ml with the mobile phase.

Column:

- *size*: l = 0.25 m, Ø = 4.6 mm,
- *stationary phase*: *octylsilyl silica gel for chromatography R* (5 µm),
- *temperature*: 35 °C.

Mobile phase: mix 375 volumes of a 17.9 g/l solution of *disodium hydrogen phosphate R*, 375 volumes of a 7.8 g/l solution of *sodium dihydrogen phosphate R* and 250 volumes of *methanol R* containing 4.6 g/l of a 400 g/l solution of *tetrabutylammonium hydroxide R*.

Flow rate: 1.5 ml/min.

Detection: spectrophotometer at 245 nm.

Injection: 20 µl.

Run time: 12 times the retention time of paracetamol.

Relative retentions with reference to paracetamol (retention time = about 4 min): impurity K = about 0.8; impurity F = about 3; impurity J = about 7.

System suitability: reference solution (c):

- *resolution*: minimum 4.0 between the peaks due to impurity K and to paracetamol,
- *signal-to-noise ratio*: minimum 50 for the peak due to impurity J.

Limits:

- *impurity J*: not more than 0.2 times the area of the corresponding peak in the chromatogram obtained with reference solution (c) (10 ppm),
- *impurity K*: not more than the area of the corresponding peak in the chromatogram obtained with reference solution (c) (50 ppm),
- *impurity F*: not more than half the area of the corresponding peak in the chromatogram obtained with reference solution (d) (0.05 per cent),
- *any other impurity*: not more than half the area of the principal peak in the chromatogram obtained with reference solution (a) (0.05 per cent),
- *total of other impurities*: not more than the area of the principal peak in the chromatogram obtained with reference solution (a) (0.1 per cent),
- *disregard limit* for the calculation of the total of other impurities: the area of the principal peak in the chromatogram obtained with reference solution (b) (0.01 per cent).

Heavy metals (*2.4.8*): maximum 20 ppm.

Dissolve 1.0 g in a mixture of 15 volumes of *water R* and 85 volumes of *acetone R* and dilute to 20 ml with the same mixture of solvents. 12 ml of the solution complies with limit test B. Prepare the standard using lead standard solution (1 ppm Pb) obtained by diluting *lead standard solution (100 ppm Pb) R* with a mixture of 15 volumes of *water R* and 85 volumes of *acetone R*.

Loss on drying (*2.2.32*): maximum 0.5 per cent, determined on 1.000 g by drying in an oven at 100-105 °C.

Sulphated ash (*2.4.14*): maximum 0.1 per cent, determined on 1.0 g.

ASSAY

Dissolve 0.300 g in a mixture of 10 ml of *water R* and 30 ml of *dilute sulphuric acid R*. Boil under a reflux condenser for 1 h, cool and dilute to 100.0 ml with *water R*. To 20.0 ml of the solution add 40 ml of *water R*, 40 g of ice, 15 ml of *dilute hydrochloric acid R* and 0.1 ml of *ferroin R*. Titrate with *0.1 M cerium sulphate* until a greenish-yellow colour is obtained. Carry out a blank titration.

1 ml of *0.1 M cerium sulphate* is equivalent to 7.56 mg of $C_8H_9NO_2$.

STORAGE

Protected from light.

IMPURITIES

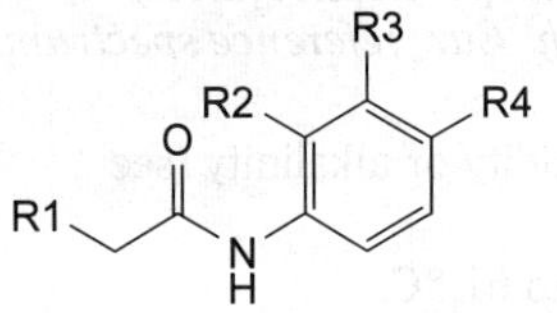

A. R1 = R3 = R4 = H, R2 = OH: *N*-(2-hydroxyphenyl)acetamide,

B. R1 = CH_3, R2 = R3 = H, R4 = OH: *N*-(4-hydroxyphenyl)propanamide,

C. R1 = R2 = H, R3 = Cl, R4 = OH: *N*-(3-chloro-4-hydroxyphenyl)acetamide,

D. R1 = R2 = R3 = R4 = H: *N*-phenylacetamide,

H. R1 = R2 = R3 = H, R4 = O-CO-CH_3: 4-(acetylamino)phenyl acetate,

J. R1 = R2 = R3 = H, R4 = Cl: *N*-(4-chlorophenyl)acetamide (chloroacetanilide),

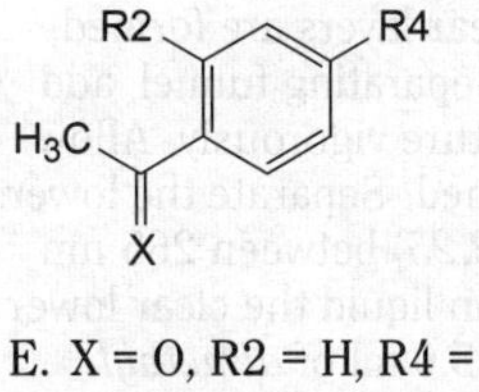

E. X = O, R2 = H, R4 = OH: 1-(4-hydroxyphenyl)ethanone,

G. X = N-OH, R2 = H, R4 = OH: 1-(4-hydroxyphenyl)ethanone oxime,

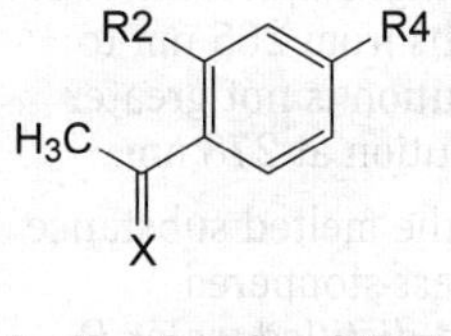

I. X = O, R2 = OH, R4 = H: 1-(2-hydroxyphenyl)ethanone,

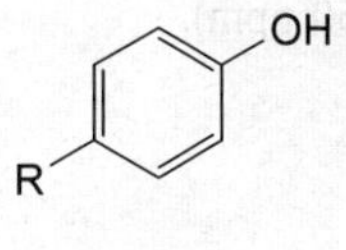

F. R = NO_2: 4-nitrophenol,

K. R = NH_2: 4-aminophenol.

01/2005:1034

PARAFFIN, HARD

Paraffinum solidum

DEFINITION

Hard paraffin is a purified mixture of solid saturated hydrocarbons generally obtained from petroleum. It may contain a suitable antioxidant.

CHARACTERS

A colourless or white mass, practically insoluble in water, freely soluble in methylene chloride, practically insoluble in alcohol. The melted substance is free from fluorescence in daylight.

IDENTIFICATION

First identification: A, C.

Second identification: B, C.

A. Examine by infrared absorption spectrophotometry (*2.2.24*), comparing with the *Ph. Eur. reference spectrum of hard paraffin*.

B. It complies with the test for acidity or alkalinity (see Tests).

C. Melting point (*2.2.16*): 50 °C to 61 °C.

TESTS

Acidity or alkalinity. To 15 g add 30 ml of boiling *water R* and shake vigorously for 1 min. Allow to cool and to separate. To 10 ml of the aqueous layer add 0.1 ml of *phenolphthalein solution R*. The solution is colourless. Not more than 1.0 ml of *0.01 M sodium hydroxide* is required to change the colour of the indicator to red. To a further 10 ml of the aqueous layer add 0.1 ml of *methyl red solution R*. The solution is yellow. Not more than 0.5 ml of *0.01 M hydrochloric acid* is required to change the colour of the indicator to red.

Polycyclic aromatic hydrocarbons. *Use reagents for ultraviolet absorption spectrophotometry.* Dissolve 0.50 g in 25 ml of *heptane R* and place in a 125 ml separating funnel with unlubricated ground-glass parts (stopper, stopcock). Add 5.0 ml of *dimethyl sulphoxide R*. Shake vigorously for 1 min and allow to stand until two clear layers are formed. Transfer the lower layer to a second separating funnel, add 2 ml of *heptane R* and shake the mixture vigorously. Allow to stand until two clear layers are formed. Separate the lower layer and measure its absorbance (*2.2.25*) between 265 nm and 420 nm using as the compensation liquid the clear lower layer obtained by vigorously shaking 5.0 ml of *dimethyl sulphoxide R* with 25 ml of *heptane R* for 1 min. Prepare a 7.0 mg/l reference solution of *naphthalene R* in *dimethyl sulphoxide R* and measure the absorbance of this solution at the maximum at 278 nm using *dimethyl sulphoxide R* as the compensation liquid. At wavelengths from 265 nm to 420 nm, the absorbance of the test solution is not greater than one-third that of the reference solution at 278 nm.

Sulphates (*2.4.13*). Introduce 2.0 g of the melted substance to be examined into a 50 ml ground-glass-stoppered separating funnel. Add 30 ml of boiling *distilled water R* and shake vigorously for 1 min. Filter. 15 ml of the filtrate complies with the limit test for sulphates (150 ppm).

STORAGE

Store protected from light.

LABELLING

The label states, where applicable, the name and concentration of any added antioxidant.

01/2005:0240

PARAFFIN, LIGHT LIQUID

Paraffinum perliquidum

DEFINITION

Light liquid paraffin is a purified mixture of liquid saturated hydrocarbons obtained from petroleum.

CHARACTERS

A colourless, transparent, oily liquid, free from fluorescence in daylight. Practically insoluble in water, slightly soluble in ethanol (96 per cent), miscible with hydrocarbons.

IDENTIFICATION

First identification: A, C.

Second identification: B, C.

A. Examine by infrared absorption spectrophotometry (*2.2.24*), comparing with the *Ph. Eur. reference spectrum of liquid paraffin*.

B. In a test tube cautiously boil 1 ml with 1 ml of *0.1 M sodium hydroxide*, with continuous shaking, for about 30 s. On cooling to room temperature, 2 phases separate. To the aqueous phase add 0.1 ml of *phenolphthalein solution R*. The colour turns to red.

C. It complies with the test for viscosity (see Tests).

TESTS

Acidity or alkalinity. To 10 ml add 20 ml of boiling *water R* and shake vigorously for 1 min. Separate the aqueous layer and filter. To 10 ml of the filtrate, add 0.1 ml of *phenolphthalein solution R*. The solution is colourless. Not more than 0.1 ml of *0.1 M sodium hydroxide* is required to change the colour of the indicator to pink.

Relative density (*2.2.5*): 0.810 to 0.875.

Viscosity (*2.2.9*): 25 mPa·s to 80 mPa·s.

Polycyclic aromatic hydrocarbons. *Use reagents for ultraviolet spectrophotometry.*

Introduce 25.0 ml into a 125 ml separating funnel with unlubricated ground-glass parts (stopper, stopcock). Add 25 ml of *hexane R* which has been previously shaken twice with one-fifth its volume of *dimethyl sulphoxide R*. Mix and add 5.0 ml of *dimethyl sulphoxide R*. Shake vigorously for 1 min and allow to stand until 2 clear layers are formed. Transfer the lower layer to a second separating funnel, add 2 ml of *hexane R* and shake the mixture vigorously. Allow to stand until 2 clear layers are formed. Separate the lower layer and measure its absorbance (*2.2.25*) between 260 nm and 420 nm, using as the compensation liquid the clear lower layer obtained by vigorously shaking 5.0 ml of *dimethyl sulphoxide R* with 25 ml of *hexane R* for 1 min. Prepare a 7.0 mg/l reference solution of *naphthalene R* in *trimethylpentane R* and measure the absorbance of the solution at the maximum at 275 nm, using *trimethylpentane R* as the compensation liquid. At no wavelength between 260 nm and 420 nm does the absorbance of the test solution exceed one-third that of the reference solution at 275 nm.

Readily carbonisable substances. Use a ground-glass-stoppered tube about 125 mm long and 18 mm in internal diameter, graduated at 5 ml and 10 ml; wash with hot *water R* (temperature at least 60 °C), *acetone R*, *heptane R* and finally with *acetone R*, dry at 100-110 °C. Cool in a desiccator. Introduce 5 ml of the substance to be examined and add 5 ml of *nitrogen-free sulphuric acid R1*. Insert the stopper and shake as vigorously as possible, in the

Monographs P

longitudinal direction of the tube, for 5 s. Loosen the stopper, immediately place the tube in a water-bath, avoiding contact of the tube with the bottom or side of the bath, and heat for 10 min. After 2 min, 4 min, 6 min and 8 min, remove the tube from the bath and shake as vigorously as possible, in the longitudinal direction of the tube for 5 s. At the end of 10 min of heating, remove the tube from the water-bath and allow to stand for 10 min. Centrifuge at 2000 *g* for 5 min. The lower layer is not more intensely coloured (*2.2.2, Method I*) than a mixture of 0.5 ml of blue primary solution, 1.5 ml of red primary solution, 3.0 ml of yellow primary solution and 2 ml of a 10 g/l solution of *hydrochloric acid R*.

Solid paraffins. Dry a suitable quantity of the substance to be examined by heating at 100 °C for 2 h and cool in a desiccator over *sulphuric acid R*. Place in a glass tube with an internal diameter of about 25 mm, close the tube and immerse in a bath of iced water. After 4 h, the liquid is sufficiently clear for a black line, 0.5 mm wide, to be easily seen against a white background held vertically behind the tube.

STORAGE

Protected from light.

01/2005:0239

PARAFFIN, LIQUID

Paraffinum liquidum

DEFINITION

Liquid paraffin is a purified mixture of liquid saturated hydrocarbons obtained from petroleum.

CHARACTERS

A colourless, transparent, oily liquid, free from fluorescence in daylight. Practically insoluble in water, slightly soluble in ethanol (96 per cent), miscible with hydrocarbons.

IDENTIFICATION

First identification: A, C.

Second identification: B, C.

A. Examine by infrared absorption spectrophotometry (*2.2.24*), comparing with the *Ph. Eur. reference spectrum of liquid paraffin.*

B. In a test tube cautiously boil 1 ml with 1 ml of *0.1 M sodium hydroxide*, with continuous shaking, for about 30 s. On cooling to room temperature, 2 phases separate. To the aqueous phase add 0.1 ml of *phenolphthalein solution R*. The colour turns to red.

C. It complies with the test for viscosity (see Tests).

TESTS

Acidity or alkalinity. To 10 ml add 20 ml of boiling *water R* and shake vigorously for 1 min. Separate the aqueous layer and filter. To 10 ml of the filtrate, add 0.1 ml of *phenolphthalein solution R*. The solution is colourless. Not more than 0.1 ml of *0.1 M sodium hydroxide* is required to change the colour of the indicator to pink.

Relative density (*2.2.5*): 0.827 to 0.890.

Viscosity (*2.2.9*): 110 mPa·s to 230 mPa·s.

Polycyclic aromatic hydrocarbons. *Use reagents for ultraviolet spectrophotometry.*

Introduce 25.0 ml into a 125 ml separating funnel with unlubricated ground-glass parts (stopper, stopcock). Add 25 ml of *hexane R* which has been previously shaken twice with one-fifth its volume of *dimethyl sulphoxide R*. Mix and add 5.0 ml of *dimethyl sulphoxide R*. Shake vigorously for 1 min and allow to stand until 2 clear layers are formed. Transfer the lower layer to a second separating funnel, add 2 ml of *hexane R* and shake the mixture vigorously. Allow to stand until 2 clear layers are formed. Separate the lower layer and measure its absorbance (*2.2.25*) between 260 nm and 420 nm, using as the compensation liquid the clear lower layer obtained by vigorously shaking 5.0 ml of *dimethyl sulphoxide R* with 25 ml of *hexane R* for 1 min. Prepare a 7.0 mg/l reference solution of *naphthalene R* in *trimethylpentane R* and measure the absorbance of the solution at the maximum at 275 nm, using *trimethylpentane R* as the compensation liquid. At no wavelength between 260 nm and 420 nm does the absorbance of the test solution exceed one-third that of the reference solution at 275 nm.

Readily carbonisable substances. Use a ground-glass-stoppered tube about 125 mm long and 18 mm in internal diameter, graduated at 5 ml and 10 ml; wash with hot *water R* (temperature at least 60 °C), *acetone R, heptane R* and finally with *acetone R*, dry at 100-110 °C. Cool in a desiccator. Introduce 5 ml of the substance to be examined and add 5 ml of *nitrogen-free sulphuric acid R1*. Insert the stopper and shake as vigorously as possible, in the longitudinal direction of the tube, for 5 s. Loosen the stopper, immediately place the tube in a water-bath, avoiding contact of the tube with the bottom or side of the bath, and heat for 10 min. After 2 min, 4 min, 6 min and 8 min, remove the tube from the bath and shake as vigorously as possible, in the longitudinal direction of the tube for 5 s. At the end of 10 min of heating, remove the tube from the water-bath and allow to stand for 10 min. Centrifuge at 2000 *g* for 5 min. The lower layer is not more intensely coloured (*2.2.2, Method I*) than a mixture of 0.5 ml of blue primary solution, 1.5 ml of red primary solution, 3.0 ml of yellow primary solution and 2 ml of a 10 g/l solution of *hydrochloric acid R*.

Solid paraffins. Dry a suitable quantity of the substance to be examined by heating at 100 °C for 2 h and cool in a desiccator over *sulphuric acid R*. Place in a glass tube with an internal diameter of about 25 mm, close the tube and immerse in a bath of iced water. After 4 h, the liquid is sufficiently clear for a black line, 0.5 mm wide, to be easily seen against a white background held vertically behind the tube.

STORAGE

Protected from light.

01/2005:1799

PARAFFIN, WHITE SOFT

Vaselinum album

DEFINITION

Purified and wholly or nearly decolorised mixture of semi-solid hydrocarbons, obtained from petroleum. It may contain a suitable antioxidant. White soft paraffin described in this monograph is not suitable for oral use.

CHARACTERS

Appearance: white or almost white, translucent, soft unctuous mass, slightly fluorescent in daylight when melted.

Solubility: practically insoluble in water, soluble in methylene chloride, practically insoluble in alcohol and in glycerol.

Monographs P

IDENTIFICATION

First identification: A, B, D.

Second identification: A, C, D.

A. The drop point is between 35 °C and 70 °C and does not differ by more than 5 °C from the value stated on the label, according to method (*2.2.17*) with the following modification to fill the cup: heat the substance to be examined at a temperature not exceeding 80 °C, with stirring to ensure uniformity. Warm the metal cup at a temperature not exceeding 80 °C in an oven, remove it from the oven, place on a clean plate or ceramic tile and pour a sufficient quantity of the melted sample into the cup to fill it completely. Allow the filled cup to cool for 30 min on the plate or the ceramic tile and place it in a water bath at 24-26 °C for 30-40 min. Level the surface of the sample with a single stroke of a knife or razor blade, avoiding compression of the sample.

B. Infrared absorption spectrophotometry (*2.2.24*).

Comparison: *Ph. Eur. reference spectrum of white soft paraffin.*

C. Melt 2 g and when a homogeneous phase is obtained, add 2 ml of *water R* and 0.2 ml of *0.05 M iodine*. Shake. Allow to cool. The solid upper layer is violet-pink.

D. It complies with the test for appearance (see Tests).

TESTS

Appearance. The substance is white. Melt 12 g on a water-bath. The melted mass is not more intensely coloured than a mixture of 1 volume of yellow primary solution and 9 volumes of a 1 per cent *m/V* solution of *hydrochloric acid R* (*2.2.2, Method II*).

Acidity or alkalinity. To 10 g add 20 ml of boiling *water R* and shake vigorously for 1 min. Allow to cool and decant. To 10 ml of the aqueous layer add 0.1 ml of *phenolphthalein solution R*. The solution is colourless. Not more than 0.5 ml of *0.01 M sodium hydroxide* is required to change the colour of the indicator to red.

Consistency (*2.9.9*): 60 to 300.

Polycyclic aromatic hydrocarbons: maximum 300 ppm.

Use reagents for ultraviolet spectrophotometry. Dissolve 1.0 g in 50 ml of *hexane R* which has been previously shaken twice with 10 ml of *dimethyl sulphoxide R*. Transfer the solution to a 125 ml separating funnel with unlubricated ground-glass parts (stopper, stopcock). Add 20 ml of *dimethyl sulphoxide R*. Shake vigorously for 1 min and allow to stand until 2 clear layers are formed. Transfer the lower layer to a second separating funnel. Repeat the extraction with a further 20 ml of *dimethyl sulphoxide R*. Shake vigorously the combined lower layers with 20 ml of *hexane R* for 1 min. Allow to stand until 2 clear layers are formed. Separate the lower layer and dilute to 50.0 ml with *dimethyl sulphoxide R*. Measure the absorbance (*2.2.25*) over the range 260 nm to 420 nm using a path length of 4 cm and as compensation liquid the clear lower layer obtained by vigorously shaking 10 ml of *dimethyl sulphoxide R* with 25 ml of *hexane R* for 1 min. Prepare a reference solution in *dimethyl sulphoxide R* containing 6.0 mg of *naphthalene R* per litre and measure the absorbance of the solution at the maximum at 278 nm using a path length of 4 cm and *dimethyl sulphoxide R* as compensation liquid. At no wavelength in the range 260 nm to 420 nm does the absorbance of the test solution exceed that of the reference solution at 278 nm.

Sulphated ash (*2.4.14*): maximum 0.05 per cent, determined on 2.0 g.

STORAGE

Protected from light.

LABELLING

The label states:

– the nominal drop point,

– where applicable, the name and concentration of any added antioxidant.

01/2005:1554

PARAFFIN, YELLOW SOFT

Vaselinum flavum

DEFINITION

Yellow soft paraffin is a purified mixture of semi-solid hydrocarbons, obtained from petroleum. It may contain a suitable antioxidant.

CHARACTERS

A yellow, translucent, unctuous mass, slightly fluorescent in daylight when melted, practically insoluble in water, soluble in methylene chloride, practically insoluble in alcohol and in glycerol.

IDENTIFICATION

First identification: A, B, D.

Second identification: A, C, D.

A. The drop point (*2.2.17*) is 40 °C to 60 °C and does not differ by more than 5 °C from the value stated on the label, with the following modification to fill the cup: heat the substance to be examined at 118 °C to 122 °C, with stirring to ensure uniformity, then cool to 100 °C to 107 °C. Warm the metal cup at 103 °C to 107 °C in an oven, remove it from the oven, place on a clean plate or ceramic tile and pour a sufficient quantity of the melted sample into the cup to fill it completely. Allow the filled cup to cool for 30 min on the ceramic tile and place it in a water-bath at 24 °C to 26 °C for a further 30 min to 40 min. Level the surface of the sample with a single stroke of a knife or razor blade, avoiding compression of the sample.

B. Examine by infrared absorption spectrophotometry (*2.2.24*) comparing with the *Ph. Eur. reference spectrum of yellow soft paraffin*. The spectrum obtained shows major peaks similar in position and intensity to the Ph. Eur. reference spectrum.

C. Melt 2 g and when a homogenous phase is obtained, add 2 ml of *water R* and 0.2 ml of *0.05 M iodine*. Shake. Allow to cool. The solid upper layer is violet-pink.

D. It complies with the test for appearance (see Tests).

TESTS

Appearance. The substance is yellow. Melt 12 g on a water-bath. The melted mass is not more intensely coloured than a mixture of 7.6 volumes of yellow primary solution and 2.4 volumes of red primary solution (*2.2.2, Method II*).

Acidity or alkalinity. To 10 g add 20 ml of boiling *water R* and shake vigorously for 1 min. Allow to cool and decant. To 10 ml of the aqueous layer add 0.1 ml of *phenolphthalein solution R*. The solution is colourless. Not more than 0.5 ml of *0.01 M sodium hydroxide* is required to change the colour of the indicator to red.

Consistency (*2.9.9*). The consistency is 100 to 300.

Polycyclic aromatic hydrocarbons. *Use reagents for ultraviolet absorption spectrophotometry.* Dissolve 1.0 g in 50 ml of *hexane R* which has been previously shaken twice with one-fifth its volume of *dimethyl sulphoxide R*. Transfer the solution to a 125 ml separating funnel with unlubricated ground-glass parts (stopper, stopcock). Add 20 ml of *dimethyl sulphoxide R*. Shake vigorously for 1 min and allow to stand until two clear layers are formed. Transfer the lower layer to a second separating funnel. Repeat the extraction with a further 20 ml of *dimethyl sulphoxide R*. Shake vigorously the combined lower layers with 20 ml of *hexane R* for 1 min. Allow to stand until two clear layers are formed. Separate the lower layer and dilute to 50.0 ml with *dimethyl sulphoxide R*. Measure the absorbance (*2.2.25*) between 260 nm and 420 nm using a path length of 4 cm and using as the compensation liquid the clear lower layer obtained by vigorously shaking 10 ml of *dimethyl sulphoxide R* with 25 ml of *hexane R* for 1 min. Prepare a 9.0 mg/l reference solution of *naphthalene R* in *dimethyl sulphoxide R* and measure the absorbance of this solution at the maximum at 278 nm using a path length of 4 cm and using *dimethyl sulphoxide R* as the compensation liquid. At no wavelength in the range of 260 nm to 420 nm does the absorbance of the test solution exceed that of the reference solution at 278 nm.

Sulphated ash (*2.4.14*). Not more than 0.05 per cent, determined on 2.0 g.

STORAGE

Store protected from light.

LABELLING

The label states:

- the nominal drop point,
- where applicable, the name and concentration of any added antioxidant.

01/2005:0351

PARALDEHYDE

Paraldehydum

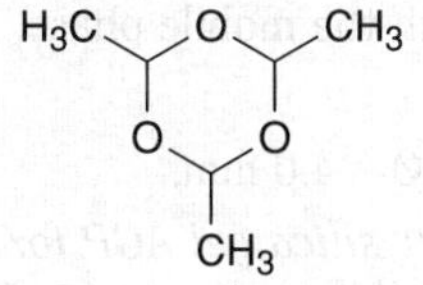

$C_6H_{12}O_3$ M_r 132.2

DEFINITION

Paraldehyde is 2,4,6-trimethyl-1,3,5-trioxane, the cyclic trimer of acetaldehyde. It may contain a suitable quantity of an antioxidant.

CHARACTERS

A colourless or slightly yellow, transparent liquid. It solidifies on cooling to form a crystalline mass. Soluble in water, but less soluble in boiling water, miscible with alcohol and with essential oils.

IDENTIFICATION

A. Solution S (see Tests) is clear (*2.2.1*) but becomes turbid on warming.

B. To 5 ml add 0.1 ml of *dilute sulphuric acid R* and heat. Acetaldehyde, recognisable by its odour, is evolved.

C. To 5 ml of solution S in a test-tube add 5 ml of *ammoniacal silver nitrate solution R* and heat in a water-bath. Silver is deposited as a mirror on the wall of the tube.

TESTS

Solution S. Dissolve 20.0 ml in *carbon dioxide-free water R* and dilute to 200.0 ml with the same solvent.

Acidity. To 50.0 ml of solution S add 0.05 ml of *phenolphthalein solution R*. Not more than 1.5 ml of *0.1 M sodium hydroxide* is required to change the colour of the indicator.

Refractive index (*2.2.6*): 1.403 to 1.406.

Relative density (*2.2.5*): 0.991 to 0.996.

Distillation range (*2.2.11*). Not more than 10 per cent distils below 123 °C and not less than 95 per cent distils below 126 °C.

Freezing point (*2.2.18*): 10 °C to 13 °C.

Acetaldehyde. To 5.0 ml add a mixture of 0.2 ml of *methyl orange solution R*, 5 ml of *alcohol (60 per cent V/V) R* and 5 ml of *alcoholic hydroxylamine solution R* and shake. Not more than 0.8 ml of *0.5 M sodium hydroxide* is required to change the colour of the indicator to pure yellow.

Peroxides. Place 50.0 ml of solution S in a ground-glass-stoppered flask, add 5 ml of *dilute sulphuric acid R* and 10 ml of *potassium iodide solution R*, close the flask and allow to stand protected from light for 15 min. Titrate with *0.1 M sodium thiosulphate* using 1 ml of *starch solution R* as indicator. Allow to stand for 5 min and, if necessary complete the titration. Not more than 2.0 ml of *0.1 M sodium thiosulphate* is required.

Non-volatile residue. Heat 5.0 ml in a tared evaporating dish on a water-bath and dry at 105 °C for 1 h. The residue weighs not more than 3 mg (0.6 g/l).

STORAGE

Store in a small, well-filled, airtight container, protected from light. If the substance has solidified the whole contents of the container must be liquefied before use.

LABELLING

The label states the name and quantity of any added antioxidant.

01/2005:1252

PARNAPARIN SODIUM

Parnaparinum natricum

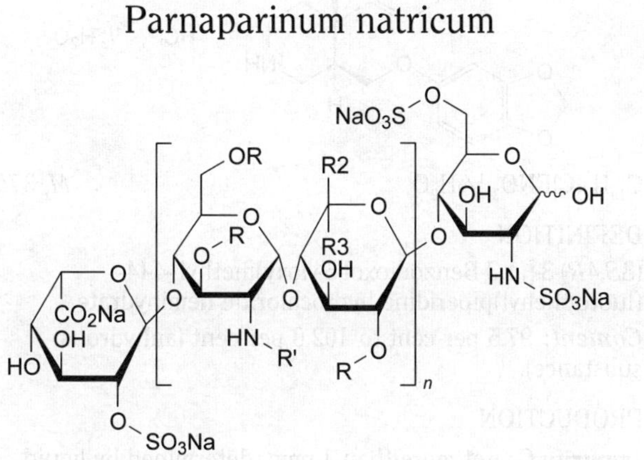

n = 1 to 21 , R = H or SO_3Na , R' = SO_3Na or $CO\text{-}CH_3$
R2 = H and R3 = CO_2Na or R2 = CO_2Na and R3 = H

DEFINITION

Sodium salt of a low-molecular-mass heparin that is obtained by radical-catalysed depolymerisation, with hydrogen peroxide and with a cupric salt, of heparin from bovine or porcine intestinal mucosa. The majority of the components have a 2-*O*-sulpho-α-L-idopyranosuronic acid structure at the non-reducing end and a 2-*N*,6-*O*-disulpho-D-glucosamine structure at the reducing end of their chain.

Parnaparin sodium complies with the monograph on *Low-molecular-mass heparins (0828)*, with the modifications and additional requirements below.

The mass-average molecular mass ranges between 4000 and 6000 with a characteristic value of about 5000.

The degree of sulphatation is 2.0 to 2.6 per disaccharide unit.

The potency is not less than 75 IU and not more than 110 IU of anti-factor Xa activity per milligram calculated with reference to the dried substance. The ratio of anti-factor Xa activity to anti-factor IIa activity is between 1.5 and 3.0.

IDENTIFICATION

Carry out identification test C as described in the monograph on *Low-molecular-mass heparins (0828)*. In order to verify the suitability of the system in the lower molecular mass ranges (for example M_r 2000), a suitable reference preparation is used. The following requirements apply.

The mass-average molecular mass ranges between 4000 and 6000. The mass percentage of chains lower than 3000 is not more than 30 per cent. The mass percentage of chains between 3000 and 8000 ranges between 50 per cent and 60 per cent.

TESTS

Appearance of solution. The solution is clear (*2.2.1*) and not more intensely coloured than reference solution Y_5 (*2.2.2, Method II*).

Dissolve 1.5 g in 10 ml of *water R*.

Copper: maximum 10 ppm, determined by atomic absorption spectrometry (*2.2.23, Method I*) and calculated with reference to the dried substance.

01/2005:2018

PAROXETINE HYDROCHLORIDE HEMIHYDRATE

Paroxetini hydrochloridum hemihydricum

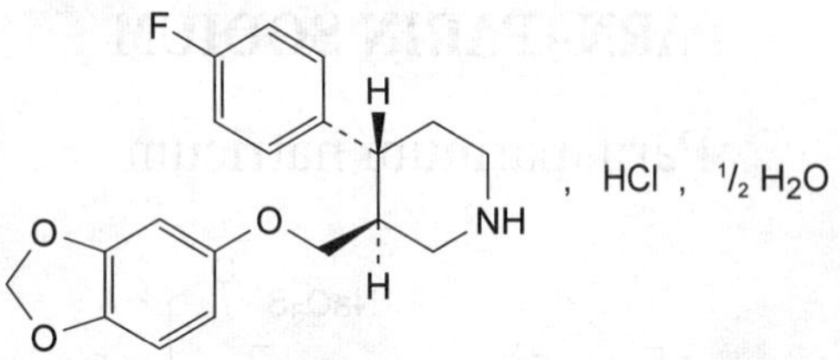

$C_{19}H_{21}ClFNO_3,{}^1/_2H_2O$ M_r 374.8

DEFINITION

(3*S*,4*R*)-3-[(1,3-Benzodioxol-5-yloxy)methyl]-4-(4-fluorophenyl)piperidine hydrochloride hemihydrate.

Content: 97.5 per cent to 102.0 per cent (anhydrous substance).

PRODUCTION

Impurity G: not more than 1 ppm, determined by liquid chromatography, coupled with tandem mass spectrometry using a suitable, validated method.

CHARACTERS

Appearance: white or almost white, crystalline powder.

Solubility: slightly soluble in water, freely soluble in methanol, sparingly soluble in alcohol and in methylene chloride.

It shows pseudopolymorphism.

IDENTIFICATION

A. Infrared absorption spectrophotometry (*2.2.24*).

Comparison: *paroxetine hydrochloride hemihydrate CRS*.

If the spectra obtained show differences, dissolve 1 part of the substance to be examined and 1 part of the reference substance separately in 10 parts of a mixture of 1 volume of *water R* and 9 volumes of *2-propanol R*, heat to 70 °C to dissolve. Recrystallise and record new spectra using the residues.

B. Examine the chromatograms obtained in the test for impurity D.

Injection: test solution and reference solution (c).

Results: the principal peak in the chromatogram obtained with the test solution is similar in retention time and size to the principal peak in the chromatogram obtained with reference solution (c).

C. It complies with the test for water (see Tests).

D. It gives reaction (b) of chlorides (*2.3.1*).

TESTS

Impurity D. Liquid chromatography (*2.2.29*).

Test solution. Dissolve 0.1000 g of the substance to be examined in 20 ml of *methanol R* and dilute to 100.0 ml with the mobile phase.

Reference solution (a). Dilute 1.0 ml of the test solution to 100.0 ml with the mobile phase. Dilute 1.0 ml to 10.0 ml with the mobile phase.

Reference solution (b). Dissolve 5 mg of *paroxetine impurity D CRS* and 5 mg of *paroxetine hydrochloride hemihydrate CRS* in 2 ml of *methanol R* and dilute to 100.0 ml with the mobile phase.

Reference solution (c). Dissolve 10 mg of *paroxetine hydrochloride hemihydrate CRS* in 2 ml of *methanol R* and dilute to 10.0 ml with the mobile phase.

Column:

– *size*: *l* = 0.10 m, Ø = 4.0 mm,

– *stationary phase*: *silica gel AGP for chiral chromatography R* (5 µm).

Mobile phase: mix 2 volumes of *methanol R* and 8 volumes of a 5.8 g/l solution of *sodium chloride R*.

Flow rate: 0.5 ml/min.

Detection: spectrophotometer at 295 nm.

Injection: 10 µl; inject the test solution and reference solutions (a) and (b).

Run time: 2.5 times the retention time of paroxetine.

Retention time: paroxetine = about 30 min.

System suitability: reference solution (b):

– *resolution*: minimum 2.2 between the peaks due to impurity D and paroxetine.

Limit:

– *impurity D*: not more than twice the area of the principal peak in the chromatogram obtained with reference solution (a) (0.2 per cent).

Related subtances. Liquid chromatography (*2.2.29*).

Solvent mixture. Mix 1 volume of *tetrahydrofuran R* and 9 volumes of *water R*.

Test solution. Dissolve 50.0 mg of the substance to be examined in the solvent mixture and dilute to 50.0 ml with the same solvent mixture.

Reference solution (a). Dilute 5.0 ml of the test solution to 50.0 ml with the solvent mixture.

Reference solution (b). Dissolve 2 mg of *paroxetine impurity C CRS* in the solvent mixture and dilute to 20.0 ml with the same solvent mixture.

Reference solution (c). To 2.0 ml of reference solution (a) add 2.0 ml of reference solution (b) and dilute to 20.0 ml with the solvent mixture.

Reference solution (d). Dilute 2.0 ml of reference solution (a) to 200.0 ml with the solvent mixture.

Reference solution (e). Dissolve 2 mg of *paroxetine impurity A CRS* in the solvent mixture and dilute to 20 ml with the same solvent mixture.

Column:
- *size*: *l* = 0.25 m, Ø = 4.6 mm,
- *stationary phase*: *end-capped octylsilyl silica gel for chromatography R* (5 µm),
- *temperature*: 40 °C.

Mobile phase:
- *mobile phase A*: *trifluoroacetic acid R, tetrahydrofuran R, water R* (5:100:900 *V/V/V*),
- *mobile phase B*: *trifluoroacetic acid R, tetrahydrofuran R, acetonitrile R* (5:100:900 *V/V/V*),

Time (min)	Mobile phase A (per cent *V/V*)	Mobile phase B (per cent *V/V*)
0 - 30	80	20
30 - 50	80 → 20	20 → 80
50 - 60	20	80
60 - 65	20 → 80	80 → 20
65 - 70	80	20

Flow rate: 1 ml/min.

Detection: spectrophotometer at 295 nm.

Injection: 20 µl; inject the test solution and reference solutions (c), (d) and (e).

Relative retention with reference to paroxetine: impurity A = about 0.8.

System suitability: reference solution (c):
- *resolution*: minimum 3.5 between the peaks due to impurity C and paroxetine.

Limits:
- *impurity A*: not more than 3 times the area of the principal peak in the chromatogram obtained with reference solution (d) (0.3 per cent),
- *any other impurity*: not more than the area of the principal peak in the chromatogram obtained with reference solution (d) (0.1 per cent),
- *total*: not more than 5 times the area of the principal peak in the chromatogram obtained with reference solution (d) (0.5 per cent),
- *disregard limit*: 0.5 times the area of the principal peak in the chromatogram obtained with reference solution (d) (0.05 per cent).

Heavy metals (*2.4.8*): maximum 20 ppm.

1.0 g complies with limit test C. Use a platinum crucible. Prepare the standard using 2 ml of *lead standard solution (10 ppm Pb) R*.

Water (*2.5.12*): 2.2 per cent to 2.7 per cent, determined on 0.300 g.

Sulphated ash (*2.4.14*): maximum 0.1 per cent, determined on 1.0 g in a platinum crucible.

ASSAY

Liquid chromatography (*2.2.29*).

Test solution. Dissolve 50.0 mg of the substance to be examined in *water R* and dilute to 100.0 ml with the same solvent.

Reference solution (a). Dissolve 50.0 mg of *paroxetine hydrochloride hemihydrate CRS* in *water R* and dilute to 100.0 ml with the same solvent.

Reference solution (b). Dissolve 5.0 mg of *paroxetine hydrochloride hemihydrate CRS* and 5 mg of *paroxetine impurity A CRS* in *water R* and dilute to 10.0 ml with the same solvent.

Column:
- *size*: *l* = 0.25 m, Ø = 4.6 mm,
- *stationary phase*: *trimethylsilyl silica gel for chromatography R* (5 µm).

Mobile phase: dissolve 3.85 g of *ammonium acetate R* in *water R*, adjust to pH 5.5 with *anhydrous acetic acid R* and dilute to 600 ml with the same solvent; add 400 ml of *acetonitrile R*; slowly add with stirring, 10 ml of *triethylamine R* and readjust to pH 5.5 with *anhydrous acetic acid R*.

Flow rate: 1 ml/min.

Detection: spectrophotometer at 295 nm.

Injection: 10 µl.

Run time: twice the retention time of paroxetine.

System suitability: reference solution (b):
- *resolution*: minimum 2 between the peaks due to paroxetine and impurity A.

Calculate the percentage content of paroxetine hydrochloride using the chromatogram obtained with reference solution (a).

STORAGE

Protected from light.

IMPURITIES

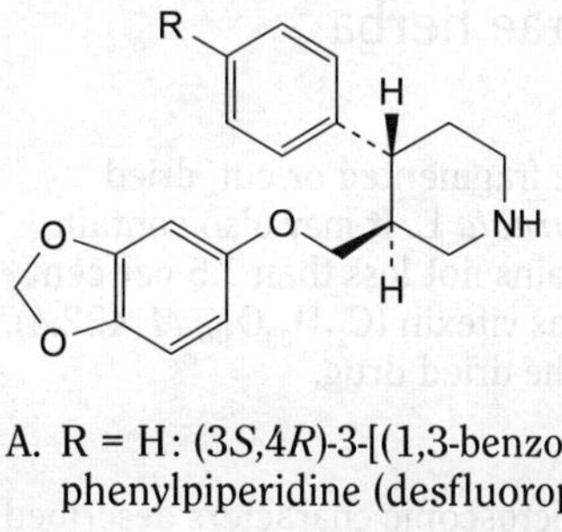

A. R = H: (3*S*,4*R*)-3-[(1,3-benzodioxol-5-yloxy)methyl]-4-phenylpiperidine (desfluoroparoxetine),

B. R = OCH_3: (3*S*,4*R*)-3-[(1,3-benzodioxol-5-yloxy)methyl]-4-(4-methoxyphenyl)piperidine,

C. R = OC_2H_5: (3*S*,4*R*)-3-[(1,3-benzodioxol-5-yloxy)methyl]-4-(4-ethoxyphenyl)piperidine,

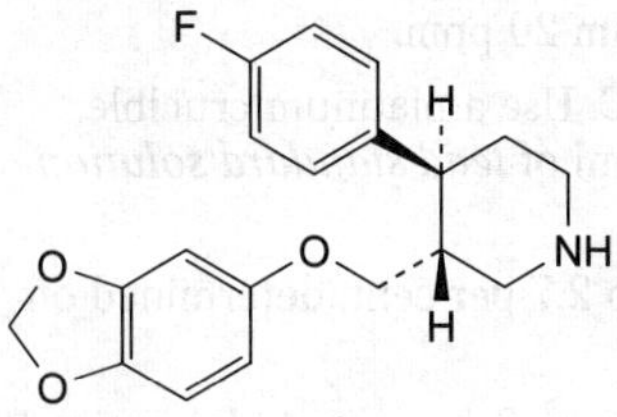

D. (3*R*,4*S*)-3-[(1,3-benzodioxol-5-yloxy)methyl]-4-(4-fluorophenyl)piperidine ((+)-*trans*-paroxetine),

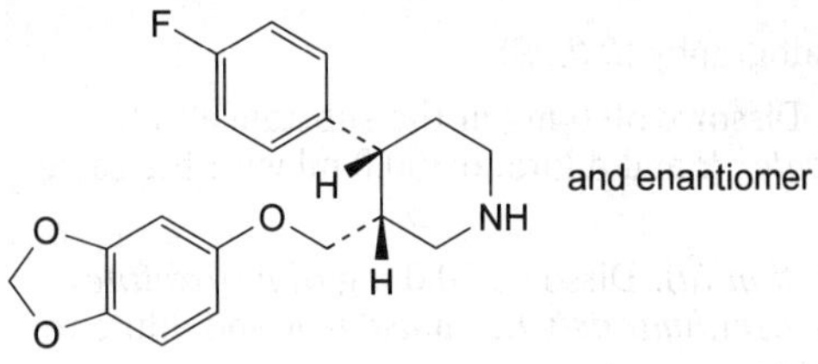

E. (3*RS*,4*RS*)-3-[(1,3-benzodioxol-5-yloxy)methyl]-4-(4-fluorophenyl)piperidine (*cis*-paroxetine),

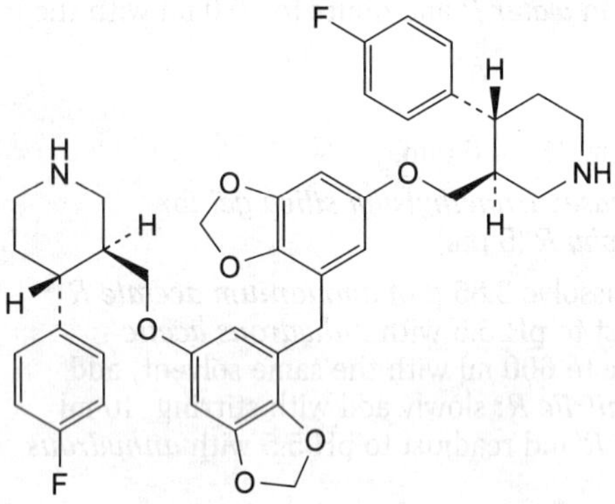

F. 3,3′-[methylenebis(1,3-benzodioxole-6,4-diyloxymethylene)]bis[4-(4-fluorophenyl)piperidine],

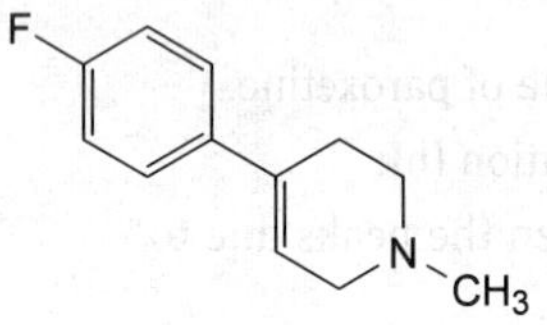

G. 4-(4-fluorophenyl)-1-methyl-1,2,3,6-tetrahydropyridine.

01/2005:1459

PASSION FLOWER

Passiflorae herba

DEFINITION

Passion flower consists of the fragmented or cut, dried aerial parts of *Passiflora incarnata* L. It may also contain flowers and/or fruits. It contains not less than 1.5 per cent of total flavonoids expressed as vitexin ($C_{21}H_{20}O_{10}$; M_r 432.4), calculated with reference to the dried drug.

CHARACTERS

It has the macroscopic and microscopic characters described under Identification tests A and B.

IDENTIFICATION

A. The green to greenish-grey or brownish stem is ligneous, hollow, longitudinally striated, glabrous or very slightly pubescent, with a diameter that is generally less than 8 mm. The green or greenish-brown leaves are alternate, finely dentate and pubescent, deeply divided into three acute lobes of which the central lobe is the largest. The midrib is much more prominent on the lower surface. The petiole is pubescent and bears two dark-coloured nectaries near the lamina. The tendrils are very numerous and grow from the axils of the leaves; they are fine, smooth, round and terminated in cylindrical spirals. The radiate flowers, if present, have three small bracts and a corolla consisting of five white, elongated petals with several rows of filiform, petaloid appendices. If present, the greenish to brownish fruit is flattened and oval; it contains several flattened, brownish-yellow, pitted seeds.

B. Reduce to a powder (355). The powder is light green. Examine under a microscope using *chloral hydrate solution R*. The powder shows fragments of the leaf epidermis with sinuous walls and anomocytic stomata (*2.8.3*); numerous cluster crystals of calcium oxalate isolated or aligned along the veins; many isolated or grouped fibres from the stems associated with pitted vessels and tracheids; uniseriate trichomes with one to three thin-walled cells, straight or slightly curved, ending in a point or sometimes a hook. In addition the powder shows, if flowers are present, papillose epidermises of the petals and appendages and pollen grains with a reticulate exine; and if mature fruits are present, scattered brown tannin cells and brownish-yellow, pitted fragments of the testa.

C. Examine the chromatograms obtained in the test for other species of *Passiflora*.

The chromatogram obtained with the test solution shows below the zone due to rutin in the chromatogram obtained with the reference solution a zone of intense yellow fluorescence, above it a zone of green fluorescence (diglycosylflavone), below the zone due to hyperoside in the chromatogram obtained with the reference solution a zone of yellow fluorescence (iso-orientin) and above a zone of green fluorescence (isovitexin), above the zone due to hyperoside in the chromatogram obtained with the reference solution a zone of brownish-yellow fluorescence (orientin) and above it a zone of green fluorescence (vitexin). These latter two zones may be absent. Further zones may be present.

TESTS

Foreign matter (*2.8.2*). It complies with the test for foreign matter.

Other species of *Passiflora*. Examine by thin-layer chromatography (*2.2.27*), using a *TLC silica gel plate R*.

Test solution. To 1.0 g of the powdered drug (355) add 5 ml of *methanol R*. Heat to boiling under a reflux condenser for 10 min. Cool and filter.

Reference solution. Dissolve with heating 2.0 mg of *rutin R* and 2.0 mg of *hyperoside R* in 10 ml of *methanol R*.

Apply separately to the plate as bands 10 µl of each solution. Develop over a path of 15 cm using a mixture of 10 volumes of *anhydrous formic acid R*, 10 volumes of *water R*, 30 volumes of *methyl ethyl ketone R* and 50 volumes of *ethyl acetate R*. Allow the plate to dry in air. Spray with a 10 g/l solution of *diphenylboric acid aminoethyl ester R* in *methanol R* and then with a 50 g/l solution of *macrogol 400 R* in *methanol R*. Allow the plate to dry in air for 30 min. Examine the plate in ultraviolet light at 365 nm. The chromatogram obtained with the reference solution shows in the lower third a zone of yellowish-brown fluorescence due to rutin and in the middle third a zone of yellowish-brown fluorescence due to hyperoside.

The chromatogram obtained with the test solution shows no intense zones of greenish-yellow or orange-yellow fluorescence between the zone due to diglycosylflavones and that due to iso-orientin (*P. coerulea* and *P. edulis*).

Total ash (*2.4.16*). Not more than 13.0 per cent.

Loss on drying (*2.2.32*). Not more than 10.0 per cent, determined on 1.000 g of the powdered drug (355) by drying in an oven at 100 °C to 105 °C for 2 h.

ASSAY

Stock solution. In a 100 ml round-bottomed flask, introduce 0.200 g of the powdered drug (250) and add 40 ml of *alcohol (60 per cent V/V) R*. Heat in a water-bath at 60 °C under a reflux condenser for 30 min while shaking frequently. Allow to cool and filter the mixture through a plug of absorbent cotton in a 100 ml flask. Transfer the absorbent cotton with the drug residue into the round-bottomed flask. Add 40 ml of *alcohol (60 per cent V/V) R* and heat again in a water-bath at 60 °C under reflux for 10 min. Allow to cool and filter the mixture and the first filtrate from the 100 ml flask through a paper filter in the 100 ml volumetric flask. Dilute to 100 ml with the same solvent, while rinsing the flask, round-bottomed flask and filter.

Test solution. Introduce 5.0 ml of stock solution into a flask. Evaporate to dryness under reduced pressure and take up the residue with 10 ml of a mixture of 10 volumes of *methanol R* and 100 volumes of *glacial acetic acid R*. Add 10 ml of a solution consisting of 25 g/l of *boric acid R* and 20 g/l of oxalic acid in *anhydrous formic acid R* and dilute to 25.0 ml with *anhydrous acetic acid R*.

Compensation solution. Into a second flask introduce 5.0 ml of the stock solution. Evaporate to dryness under reduced pressure and take up the residue with 10 ml of a mixture of 10 volumes of *methanol R* and 100 volumes of *glacial acetic acid R*. Add 10 ml of *anhydrous formic acid R* and dilute to 25.0 ml with *anhydrous acetic acid R*.

Measure the absorbance (*2.2.25*) of the test solution after 30 min by comparison with the compensation solution at 401 nm.

Calculate the percentage content of total flavonoids, expressed as vitexin, from the expression:

$$\frac{A \times 0.8}{m}$$

taking the value of the specific absorbance to be 628.

A = absorbance of the test solution at 401 nm,

m = mass of the substance to be examined, in grams.

STORAGE

Store protected from light.

01/2005:1460
corrected

PEFLOXACIN MESILATE DIHYDRATE

Pefloxacini mesilas dihydricus

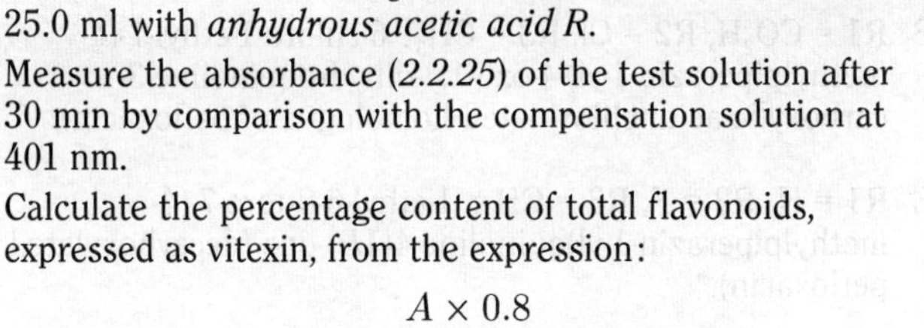

$C_{18}H_{24}FN_3O_6S,2H_2O$ M_r 465.5

DEFINITION

Pefloxacin mesilate dihydrate contains not less than 98.5 per cent and not more than the equivalent of 101.5 per cent of 1-ethyl-6-fluoro-7-(4-methylpiperazin-1-yl)-4-oxo-1,4-dihydroquinoline-3-carboxylic acid methanesulphonate, calculated with reference to the anhydrous substance.

PRODUCTION

The production method must be evaluated to determine the potential for formation of alkyl mesilates, which is particularly likely to occur if the reaction medium contains lower alcohols. Where necessary, the production method is validated to demonstrate that alkyl mesilates are not detectable in the final product.

CHARACTERS

A fine, white or almost white powder, freely soluble in water, slightly soluble in alcohol, very slightly soluble in methylene chloride.

IDENTIFICATION

A. Dissolve separately 0.1 g of the substance to be examined and 0.1 g of *pefloxacin mesilate dihydrate CRS* in 10 ml of *water R*. Add 5 ml of *1 M sodium hydroxide*. Adjust the pH of the solution to 7.4 ± 0.1 with *phosphoric acid R* and shake with 2 quantities, each of 30 ml, of *methylene chloride R*. Combine the organic layers and dry over *anhydrous sodium sulphate R*. Evaporate to dryness. Examine the residues by infrared absorption spectrophotometry (*2.2.24*), comparing the spectra obtained. Examine the residues as discs prepared using *potassium bromide R*.

B. Examine by thin-layer chromatography (*2.2.27*), using a *TLC silica gel plate R*.

Test solution. Dissolve 40 mg in *water R* and dilute to 1 ml with the same solvent.

Reference solution. Dissolve 60 mg of *methanesulphonic acid R* in *water R* and dilute to 10 ml with the same solvent.

Apply to the plate 10 µl of each solution. Develop over a path of 15 cm using a mixture of 5 volumes of *water R*, 10 volumes of *ammonia R*, 20 volumes of *butanol R* and 65 volumes of *acetone R*. Allow the plate to dry in air. Spray with a 0.4 g/l solution of *bromocresol purple R* in *alcohol (50 per cent V/V) R*, adjusted to pH 10 using *1 M sodium hydroxide*. The spot in the chromatogram obtained with the test solution is similar in position, colour and size to the spot in the chromatogram obtained with the reference solution.

TESTS

Solution S. Dissolve 1.0 g in *carbon dioxide-free water R* and dilute to 10.0 ml with the same solvent.

Appearance of solution. Examined within 1 h after its preparation, solution S is not more opalescent than reference suspension II (*2.2.1*) and not more intensely coloured than intensity 3 of the range of reference solutions of the most appropriate colour (*2.2.2, Method II*).

pH (*2.2.3*). Dilute 1 ml of solution S to 10 ml with *carbon dioxide-free water R*. The pH of the solution is 3.5 to 4.5.

Related substances. Examine by liquid chromatography (*2.2.29*).

Test solution. Dissolve 20.0 mg of the substance to be examined in the mobile phase and dilute to 100.0 ml with the mobile phase.

Monographs P

Reference solution (a). Dissolve 5.0 mg of *pefloxacin impurity B CRS* in the mobile phase and dilute to 50.0 ml with the mobile phase. Dilute 1.0 ml of this solution to 100.0 ml with the mobile phase. In 2.0 ml of the solution obtained, dissolve the contents of a vial of *pefloxacin impurity C CRS*.

Reference solution (b). Dissolve 10.0 mg of *norfloxacin impurity A CRS* (pefloxacin impurity F) in the mobile phase and dilute to 100.0 ml with the mobile phase. Dilute 1.0 ml of this solution to 100.0 ml with the mobile phase.

The chromatographic procedure may be carried out using:

- a stainless steel column 0.15 m long and 6 mm in internal diameter packed with *octadecylsilyl vinyl polymer for chromatography R* (5 µm),
- as mobile phase at a flow rate of 1 ml/min a mixture prepared as follows: 30 volumes of *acetonitrile R*, 70 volumes of a solution containing 2.70 g/l of *cetyltrimethylammonium bromide R* and 6.18 g/l of *boric acid R* (exactly adjusted to pH 8.30 with *1 M sodium hydroxide*), and 0.2 volumes of *thiodiethylene glycol R*,
- as detector a spectrophotometer set at 258 nm and 273 nm.

Inject 20 µl of reference solution (a). Record the chromatogram at 273 nm. The test is not valid unless the resolution between the peaks corresponding to impurity B and impurity C is at least 1.5. Inject 20 µl of the test solution and 20 µl of reference solution (b). Record the chromatograms of the test solution at 258 nm and 273 nm for 4 times the retention time of pefloxacin (about 60 min). Record the chromatogram of reference solution (b) at 258 nm. When the chromatograms are recorded in the prescribed conditions, the relative retentions are indicated in the following table.

	Approximate relative retention	Correction factor
Impurity E	0.2	–
Impurity D	0.3	–
Impurity A	0.5	–
Impurity G	0.8	1.4
Pefloxacin	1	–
Impurity C	1.7	2.4
Impurity B	1.8	–
Impurity H	2.4	1.8
Impurity F	3.5	–

From the chromatogram obtained at 258 nm with the test solution, calculate the percentage content of impurity C, F, G and H using the area of the principal peak in the chromatogram obtained at 258 nm with reference solution (b) (external standardisation) taking into account the correction factors indicated in the table.

From the chromatogram obtained at 273 nm with the test solution, calculate the percentage content of impurity A, B, D and E and of any unknown impurity from the areas of the peaks in the chromatogram obtained with the test solution by the normalisation procedure, disregarding the peaks with an area less than 0.0005 times that of the principal peak in the chromatogram obtained at 273 nm with the test solution.

None of the impurities has a content of more than 0.5 per cent and not more than 3 impurities have a content between 0.2 per cent and 0.5 per cent. The sum of the contents of the impurities is not more than 1.0 per cent.

Heavy metals (*2.4.8*). 1.0 g complies with limit test E for heavy metals (10 ppm). Prepare the standard using 10.0 ml of *lead standard solution (1 ppm Pb) R*.

Water (*2.5.12*): 7.0 per cent to 8.5 per cent, determined on 50.0 mg by the semi-micro determination of water using a mixture of 10 volumes of *methanol R* and 50 volumes of *methylene chloride R*.

Sulphated ash (*2.4.14*). Not more than 0.1 per cent, determined on 1.0 g.

ASSAY

Dissolve 0.200 g in 15.0 ml of *anhydrous acetic acid R* and add 75.0 ml of *acetic anhydride R*. Titrate with *0.1 M perchloric acid*, determining the end-point potentiometrically (*2.2.20*).

1 ml of *0.1 M perchloric acid* is equivalent to 21.48 mg of $C_{18}H_{24}FN_3O_6S$.

STORAGE

Store in an airtight container, protected from light.

IMPURITIES

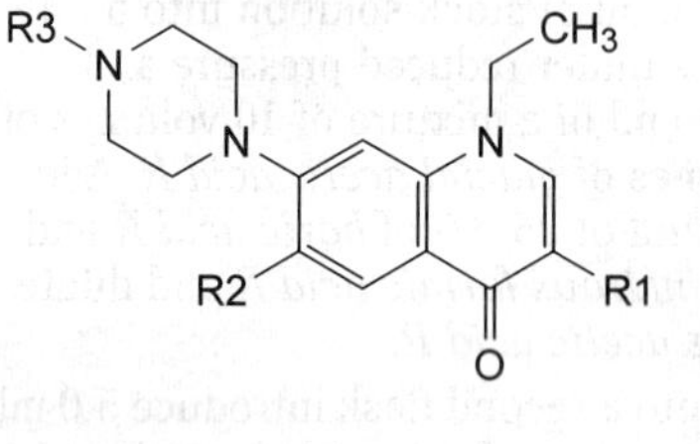

A. R1 = CO_2H, R2 = F, R3 = H: 1-ethyl-6-fluoro-4-oxo-7-(piperazin-1-yl)-1,4-dihydroquinoline-3-carboxylic acid (demethylated pefloxacin or norfloxacin),

B. R1 = CO_2H, R2 = Cl, R3 = CH_3: 6-chloro-1-ethyl-7-(4-methylpiperazin-1-yl)-4-oxo-1,4-dihydroquinoline-3-carboxylic acid (chlorinated homologue of pefloxacin),

E. R1 = H, R2 = F, R3 = CH_3: 1-ethyl-6-fluoro-7-(4-methylpiperazin-1-yl)quinoline-4(1*H*)-one (decarboxylated pefloxacin),

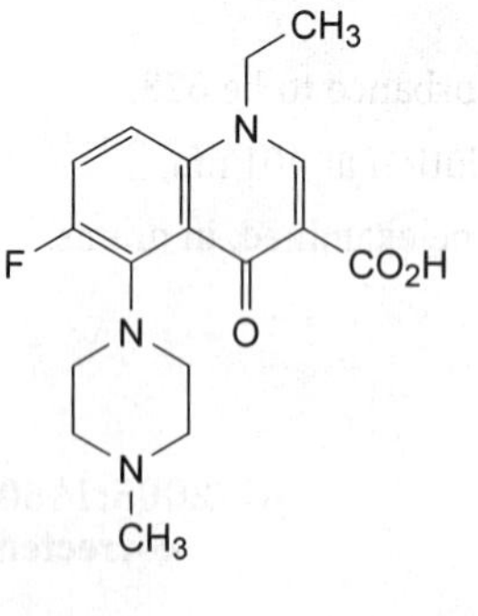

C. 1-ethyl-6-fluoro-5-(4-methylpiperazin-1-yl)-4-oxo-1,4-dihydroquinoline-3-carboxylic acid (isopefloxacin),

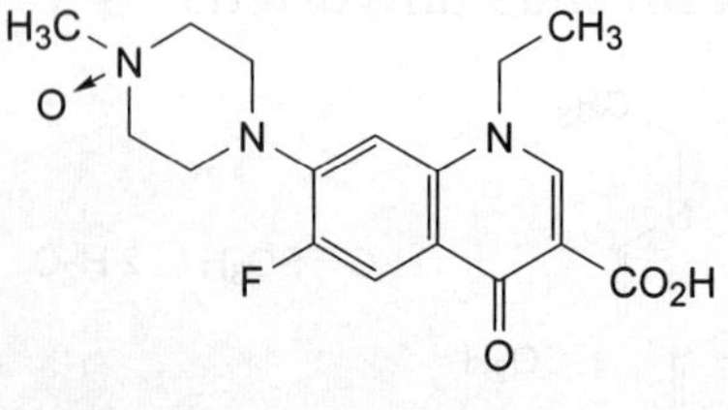

D. 4-(3-carboxy-1-ethyl-6-fluoro-4-oxo-1,4-dihydroquinolin-7-yl)-1-methylpiperazine 1-oxide (*N*-oxide of pefloxacin),

Monographs P

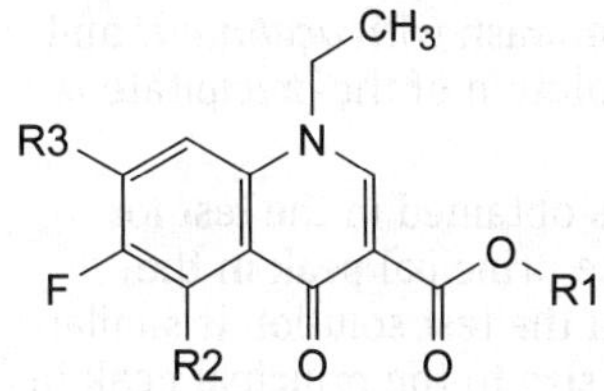

F. R1 = R2 = H, R3 = Cl: 7-chloro-1-ethyl-6-fluoro-4-oxo-1,4-dihydroquinoline-3-carboxylic acid (*N*-ethyl acid) (norfloxacin impurity A),

G. R1 = C_2H_5, R2 = H, R3 = Cl: ethyl 7-chloro-1-ethyl-6-fluoro-4-oxo-1,4-dihydroquinoline-3-carboxylate (*N*-ethyl ester),

H. R1 = R3 = H, R2 = Cl: 5-chloro-1-ethyl-6-fluoro-4-oxo-1,4-dihydroquinoline-3-carboxylic acid (iso-*N*-ethyl acid).

01/2005:1461

PENBUTOLOL SULPHATE

Penbutololi sulfas

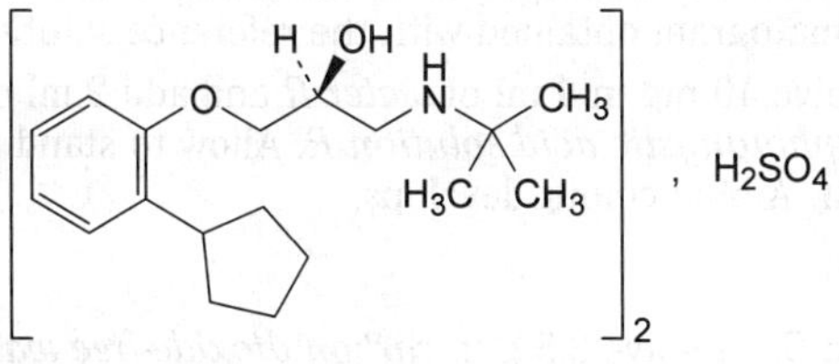

$C_{36}H_{60}N_2O_8S$ M_r 681

DEFINITION

Penbutolol sulphate contains not less than 99.0 per cent and not more than the equivalent of 101.0 per cent of di[(2*S*)-1-(2-cyclopentylphenoxy)-3-[(1,1-dimethylethyl)amino]propan-2-ol] sulphate, calculated with reference to the dried substance.

CHARACTERS

A white or almost white, crystalline powder, slightly soluble in water, soluble in methanol, practically insoluble in cyclohexane.

IDENTIFICATION

First identification: A, C, D.

Second identification: B, C, D.

A. Examine by infrared absorption spectrophotometry (*2.2.24*), comparing with the spectrum obtained with *penbutolol sulphate CRS*.

B. Examine by thin-layer chromatography (*2.2.27*), using a *TLC silica gel F_{254} plate R*.

Test solution. Dissolve 40 mg of the substance to be examined in 1 ml of *methanol R*.

Reference solution. Dissolve 40 mg of *penbutolol sulphate CRS* in 1 ml of *methanol R*.

Apply to the plate 5 µl of each solution. Develop over a path of 15 cm using a mixture of 10 volumes of *glacial acetic acid R*, 20 volumes of *water R*, 35 volumes of *butanol R* and 35 volumes of *ethyl acetate R*. Allow the plate to dry in air and examine in ultraviolet light at 254 nm. The principal spot in the chromatogram obtained with the test solution is similar in position and size to the principal spot in the chromatogram obtained with the reference solution.

C. Dissolve 50 mg in a mixture of 5 ml of *water R* and 1 ml of *0.1 M hydrochloric acid*. The solution gives reaction (a) of sulphates (*2.3.1*).

D. It complies with the test for specific optical rotation (see Tests).

TESTS

Solution S. Dissolve 1.00 g in *methanol R* and dilute to 20.0 ml with the same solvent.

Acidity or alkalinity. To 4 ml of solution S add 4 ml of *carbon dioxide-free water R*. Add 0.1 ml of *methyl red solution R* and 0.2 ml of *0.01 M sodium hydroxide*. The solution is yellow. Add 0.4 ml of *0.01 M hydrochloric acid*. The solution is red.

Specific optical rotation (*2.2.7*): − 23 to − 25 determined on solution S, calculated with reference to the dried substance.

Related substances. Examine by liquid chromatography (*2.2.29*).

Test solution. Dissolve 40.0 mg of the substance to be examined in a mixture of 40 volumes of mobile phase B and 60 volumes of mobile phase A and dilute to 10.0 ml with the same mixture of solvents.

Reference solution (a). Dissolve 4.0 mg of the substance to be examined and 1.0 mg of *penbutolol impurity A CRS* in 5.0 ml of a mixture of 40 volumes of mobile phase B and 60 volumes of mobile phase A.

Reference solution (b). Dilute 1.0 ml of the test solution to 200.0 ml with a mixture of 40 volumes of mobile phase B and 60 volumes of mobile phase A.

Reference solution (c). Dilute 1.0 ml of reference solution (b) to 10.0 ml with a mixture of 40 volumes of mobile phase B and 60 volumes of mobile phase A.

Reference solution (d). Dissolve 5.0 mg of *penbutolol impurity A CRS* in a mixture of 40 volumes of mobile phase B and 60 volumes of mobile phase A and dilute to 50.0 ml with the same mixture of solvents. Dilute 2.0 ml to 10.0 ml with the same mixture of solvents.

The chromatographic procedure may be carried out using:

– a stainless steel column 0.25 m long and 4.6 mm in internal diameter, packed with *octadecylsilyl silica gel for chromatography R* (5 µm),

– as mobile phase at a flow rate of 1.0 ml/min:

Mobile phase A. Mix 39 volumes of *acetonitrile for chromatography R* and 61 volumes of *methanol R*,

Mobile phase B. Dissolve 11 g of *sodium heptanesulphonate R* in 1000 ml of *water R*, add 5.0 ml of *triethylamine R* and adjust to pH 2.7 with *phosphoric acid R*,

Time (min)	Mobile phase A (per cent *V/V*)	Mobile phase B (per cent *V/V*)	Comment
0 - 15	60	40	isocratic
15 - 35	60 → 80	40 → 20	linear gradient
35 - 36	80 → 60	20 → 40	linear gradient

– as detector a spectrophotometer set at 270 nm.

Inject 10 µl of reference solution (b) and adjust the sensitivity of the system so that the height of the second peak (penbutolol) is at least 20 per cent of the full scale of the recorder. The resolution between the 2 principal peaks must be at least 3.0.

Inject 10 µl of each of the other solutions. In the chromatogram obtained with the test solution, the area of any peak corresponding to impurity A is not greater than the area of the principal peak in the chromatogram obtained with reference solution (d) (0.5 per cent), the area of any peak, apart from the principal peak and that of impurity A, is not greater than the area of the principal peak in the chromatogram obtained with reference solution (b) (0.5 per cent) and the sum of the areas of all the peaks, apart from the principal peak and the peak corresponding to impurity A, is not greater than twice the area of the principal peak in the chromatogram obtained with reference solution (b) (1 per cent). Disregard any peak with an area less than that of the principal peak in the chromatogram obtained with reference solution (c).

Heavy metals (*2.4.8*). 1.0 g complies with limit test F for heavy metals (10 ppm). Prepare the reference solution using 1 ml of *lead standard solution (10 ppm Pb) R*.

Loss on drying (*2.2.32*). Not more than 0.5 per cent, determined on 1.000 g by drying in an oven at 100-105 °C.

Sulphated ash (*2.4.14*). Not more than 0.1 per cent, determined on 1.0 g.

ASSAY

Dissolve 0.500 g in 40 ml of *anhydrous acetic acid R*. Titrate with *0.1 M perchloric acid* determining the end-point potentiometrically (*2.2.20*).

1 ml of *0.1 M perchloric acid* is equivalent to 68.10 mg of $C_{36}H_{60}N_2O_8S$.

STORAGE

Store protected from light.

IMPURITIES

Specified impurities: A.

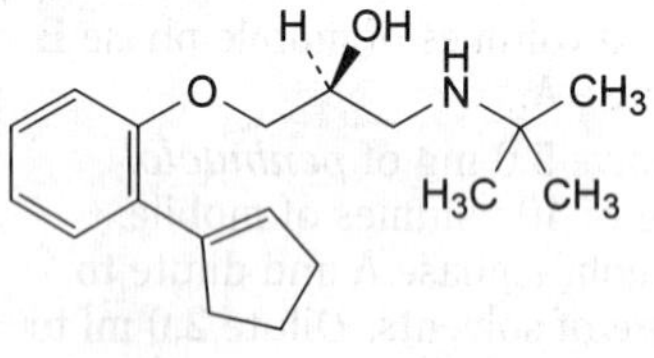

A. (2*S*)-1-[2-(cyclopent-1-enyl)phenoxy]-3-[(1,1-dimethylethyl)amino]propan-2-ol.

01/2005:0566

PENICILLAMINE

Penicillaminum

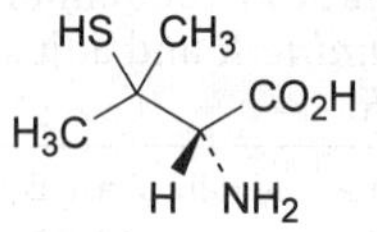

$C_5H_{11}NO_2S$ M_r 149.2

DEFINITION

Penicillamine contains not less than 98.0 per cent and not more than the equivalent of 101.0 per cent of (2*S*)-2-amino-3-methyl-3-sulphanylbutanoic acid, calculated with reference to the dried substance.

CHARACTERS

A white or almost white, crystalline powder, freely soluble in water, slightly soluble in alcohol.

IDENTIFICATION

First identification: A, B, D.

Second identification: A, C, D.

A. Dissolve 0.5 g in a mixture of 0.5 ml of *hydrochloric acid R* and 4 ml of warm *acetone R*, cool in iced water and initiate crystallisation by scratching the wall of the tube with a glass rod. A white precipitate is formed. Filter with the aid of vacuum, wash with *acetone R* and dry with suction. A 10 g/l solution of the precipitate is dextrorotatory.

B. Examine the chromatograms obtained in the test for penicillamine disulphide. The principal peak in the chromatogram obtained with the test solution is similar in position and approximate size to the principal peak in the chromatogram obtained with reference solution (a).

C. Examine by thin-layer chromatography (*2.2.27*), using *silica gel G R* as the coating substance.

   Test solution. Dissolve 10 mg of the substance to be examined in 4 ml of *water R*.

   Reference solution. Dissolve 10 mg of *penicillamine CRS* in 4 ml of *water R*.

   Apply separately to the plate 2 µl of each solution. Develop over a path of 10 cm using a mixture of 18 volumes of *glacial acetic acid R*, 18 volumes of *water R* and 72 volumes of *butanol R*. Dry the plate at 100 °C to 105 °C for 5 min to 10 min and expose to iodine vapour for 5 min to 10 min. The principal spot in the chromatogram obtained with the test solution is similar in position, colour and size to the principal spot in the chromatogram obtained with the reference solution.

D. Dissolve 40 mg in 4 ml of *water R* and add 2 ml of *phosphotungstic acid solution R*. Allow to stand for 5 min. A blue colour develops.

TESTS

Solution S. Dissolve 2.5 g in *carbon dioxide-free water R* and dilute to 25 ml with the same solvent.

Appearance of solution. Solution S is clear (*2.2.1*) and not more intensely coloured than intensity 6 of the range of reference solutions of the most appropriate colour (*2.2.2, Method II*).

pH (*2.2.3*). Dilute 1 ml of solution S to 10 ml with *carbon dioxide-free water R*. The pH of this solution is 4.5 to 5.5.

Specific optical rotation (*2.2.7*). Dissolve 0.500 g in *1 M sodium hydroxide* and dilute to 10.0 ml with the same solvent. The specific optical rotation is − 61.0 to − 65.0, calculated with reference to the dried substance.

Penicillamine disulphide. Examine by liquid chromatography (*2.2.29*).

Test solution. Dissolve 40 mg of the substance to be examined in the mobile phase and dilute to 10.0 ml with the mobile phase.

Reference solution (a). Dissolve 40 mg of *penicillamine CRS* in the mobile phase and dilute to 10.0 ml with the mobile phase.

Reference solution (b). Dissolve 20 mg of *penicillamine disulphide CRS* in the mobile phase and dilute to 50.0 ml with the mobile phase. Dilute 1.0 ml of this solution to 10.0 ml with the mobile phase.

The chromatographic procedure may be carried out using:

- a stainless steel column 0.25 m long and 5 mm in internal diameter packed with *octylsilyl silica gel for chromatography R* (10 µm),
- as mobile phase at a flow rate of 2.0 ml/min a solution containing 0.1 g/l of *sodium edetate R* and 2 g/l of *methanesulphonic acid R*,
- as detector a spectrophotometer set at 220 nm.

In the chromatogram obtained with the test solution the area of any peak due to penicillamine disulphide is not greater than the area of the corresponding peak in the chromatogram obtained with reference solution (b) (1 per cent).

Ultraviolet-absorbing substances. Dissolve 0.100 g in *water R* and dilute to 50.0 ml with the same solvent. The absorbance (*2.2.25*) of the solution at 268 nm is not greater than 0.07 (about 0.5 per cent of penilloic acid).

Heavy metals (*2.4.8*). 12 ml of solution S complies with limit test A for heavy metals (20 ppm). Prepare the standard using *lead standard solution (2 ppm Pb) R*.

Mercury. Not more than 10 ppm of Hg, determined by atomic absorption spectrometry (*2.2.23, Method I*).

Test solution. To 1.00 g of the substance to be examined add 10 ml of *water R* and 0.15 ml of *perchloric acid R* and swirl until dissolution is complete. Add 1.0 ml of a 10 g/l solution of *ammonium pyrrolidinedithiocarbamate R* which has been washed immediately before use three times, each time with an equal volume of *methyl isobutyl ketone R*. Mix and add 2.0 ml of *methyl isobutyl ketone R* and shake for 1 min. Dilute to 25.0 ml with *water R* and allow the layers to separate; use the methyl isobutyl ketone layer.

Reference solutions. Dissolve a quantity of *mercuric oxide R* equivalent to 0.108 g of HgO in the smallest necessary volume of *dilute hydrochloric acid R* and dilute to 1000.0 ml with *water R* (100 ppm Hg). Prepare the reference solutions in the same manner as the test solution but using instead of the substance to be examined suitable volumes of the solution containing 100 ppm of Hg.

Measure the absorbance at 254 nm using a mercury hollow-cathode lamp as source of radiation and an air-acetylene flame. Set the zero of the instrument using a methyl isobutyl ketone layer obtained as described for the test solution but omitting the substance to be examined.

Penicillin. *Carry out all the operations in a penicillin-free atmosphere and with equipment reserved for this test. Sterilise the equipment at 180 °C for 3 h and the buffer solutions at 121 °C for 20 min before use.*

Test solution (a). Dissolve 1.000 g of the substance to be examined in 8 ml of *buffer solution pH 2.5 R* and add 8 ml of *ether R*. Shake vigorously for 1 min. Repeat the extraction and combine the ether layers. Add 8 ml of *buffer solution pH 2.5 R*. Shake for 1 min, allow to settle and quantitatively separate the upper layer, taking care to eliminate the aqueous phase completely (*penicillin is unstable at pH 2.5; carry out operations at this pH within 6 min to 7 min*). Add 8 ml of *phosphate buffer solution pH 6.0 R2*; shake for 5 min, allow to settle, separate the aqueous layer and check that the pH is 6.0.

Test solution (b). To 2 ml of test solution (a) add 20 µl of *penicillinase solution R* and incubate at 37 °C for 1 h.

Reference solution (a). Dissolve 5 mg of *benzylpenicillin sodium R* in 500 ml of *phosphate buffer solution pH 6.0 R2*. Dilute 0.25 ml of this solution to 200.0 ml with *buffer solution pH 2.5 R*. Carry out the extraction using 8 ml of this solution as described for test solution (a).

Reference solution (b). To 2 ml of reference solution (a), add 20 µl of *penicillinase solution R* and incubate at 37 °C for 1 h.

Reference solution (c). Prepare the solution as described for test solution (a) but omitting the substance to be examined (blank).

Liquefy a suitable nutrient medium such as that described below and inoculate it at a suitable temperature with a culture of *Micrococcus flavus* (ATCC 9341) to give 5 × 10^4 micro-organisms per millilitre or a different quantity if necessary to obtain the required sensitivity and formation of clearly defined inhibition zones of suitable diameter. Immediately pour the inoculated medium into five Petri dishes 10 cm in diameter to give uniform layers 2 mm to 5 mm deep. The medium may alternatively consist of two layers, only the upper layer being inoculated. Store the dishes so that no appreciable growth or death of the micro-organisms occurs before use and so that the surface of the medium is dry at the time of use. In each dish, place five stainless steel hollow cylinders 6 mm in diameter on the surface of the agar evenly spaced on a circle with a radius of about 25 mm and concentric with the dish. For each dish, place in separate cylinders 0.15 ml of test solutions (a) and (b) and reference solutions (a), (b) and (c). Maintain at 30 °C for at least 24 h. Measure the diameters of the inhibition zones to at least 0.1 mm. The test is valid if reference solution (a) gives a clear inhibition zone and if reference solutions (b) and (c) give no inhibition zone. If test solution (a) gives an inhibition zone, this is caused by penicillin if test solution (b) gives no inhibition zone. If this is so, the average diameter of the inhibition zones given by test solution (a) for the five Petri dishes is less than the average diameter of the inhibition zones given by reference solution (a) (0.1 ppm).

Nutrient medium (pH 6.0)

Peptone	5 g
Yeast extract	1.5 g
Meat extract	1.5 g
Sodium chloride	3.5 g
Agar	15 g
Distilled water R	1000 ml

Loss on drying (*2.2.32*). Not more than 0.5 per cent, determined on 1.000 g by drying over *diphosphorus pentoxide R* at 60 °C at a pressure not exceeding 670 Pa.

Sulphated ash (*2.4.14*). Not more than 0.1 per cent, determined on 1.0 g.

ASSAY

Dissolve 0.1000 g in 30 ml of *anhydrous acetic acid R*. Titrate with *0.1 M perchloric acid*, determining the end-point potentiometrically (*2.2.20*).

1 ml of *0.1 M perchloric acid* is equivalent to 14.92 mg of $C_5H_{11}NO_2S$.

IMPURITIES

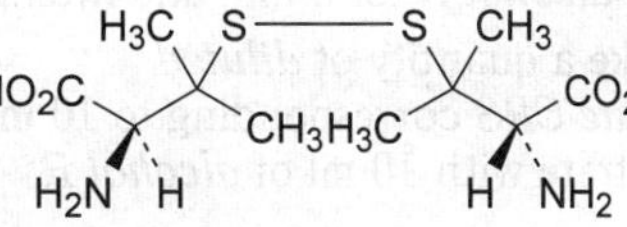

A. 3,3′-(disulphanediyl)bis[(2*S*)-2-amino-3-methylbutanoic] acid (penicillamine disulphide),

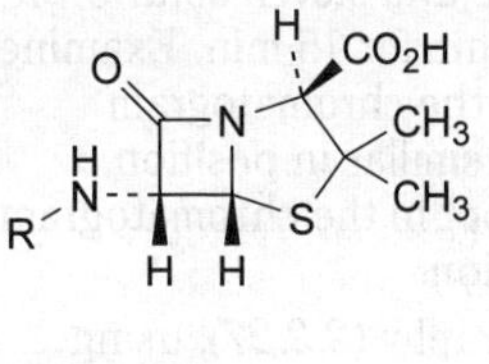

B. penicillin.

01/2005:1355

PENTAERYTHRITYL TETRANITRATE, DILUTED

Pentaerythrityli tetranitras dilutus

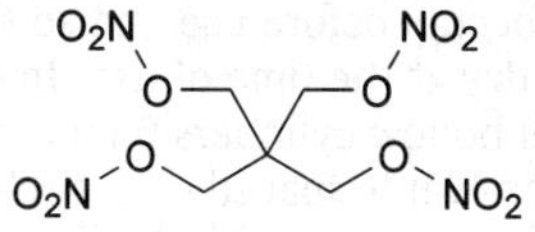

$C_5H_8N_4O_{12}$ M_r 316.1

DEFINITION

Diluted pentaerythrityl tetranitrate is a dry mixture of pentaerythrityl tetranitrate and *Lactose monohydrate (0187)* or *Mannitol (0559)*. It contains not less than 95.0 per cent *m/m* and not more than 105.0 per cent *m/m* of the declared content of 2,2-bis(hydroxymethyl)propane-1,3-diol tetranitrate.

CHARACTERS

Undiluted pentaerythrityl tetranitrate is a white or slightly yellowish powder, practically insoluble in water, soluble in acetone, slightly soluble in alcohol.

The solubility of the diluted product depends on the diluent and its concentration.

IDENTIFICATION

First identification: A, B, D.

Second identification: A, C, D.

A. The melting point (*2.2.14*) of the residue obtained with the substance to be examined in identification test B is 138 °C to 142 °C.

B. Shake a quantity of the substance to be examined and a quantity of *diluted pentaerythrityl tetranitrate CRS*, each corresponding to 25 mg of pentaerythrityl tetranitrate with 10 ml of *acetone R* for 5 min. Filter, evaporate to dryness at a temperature below 40 °C and dry the residue over *diphosphorus pentoxide R* at a pressure of 0.7 kPa for 16 h. Examine the residue obtained with the substance to be examined by infrared absorption spectrophotometry (*2.2.24*), comparing with the spectrum of the residue obtained with *diluted pentaerythrityl tetranitrate CRS*. Examine the residues prepared as discs.

C. Examine by thin-layer chromatography (*2.2.27*), using a *TLC silica gel G plate R*.

Test solution. Shake a quantity of the substance to be examined corresponding to 10 mg of pentaerythrityl tetranitrate with 10 ml of *alcohol R* for 5 min and filter.

Reference solution. Shake a quantity of *diluted pentaerythrityl tetranitrate CRS* corresponding to 10 mg of pentaerythrityl tetranitrate with 10 ml of *alcohol R* for 5 min and filter.

Apply separately to the plate 10 µl of each solution. Develop over a path of 15 cm using a mixture of 20 volumes of *ethyl acetate R* and 80 volumes of *toluene R*. Dry the plate in a current of air. Spray with freshly prepared *potassium iodide and starch solution R*. Expose to ultraviolet light at 254 nm for 15 min. Examine in daylight. The principal spot in the chromatogram obtained with the test solution is similar in position, colour and size to the principal spot in the chromatogram obtained with the reference solution.

D. Examine by thin-layer chromatography (*2.2.27*), using a *TLC silica gel G plate R*.

Test solution. Shake a quantity of the substance to be examined corresponding to 0.10 g of lactose or mannitol with 10 ml of *water R*. Filter if necessary.

Reference solution (a) Dissolve 0.10 g of *lactose R* in *water R* and dilute to 10 ml with the same solvent.

Reference solution (b). Dissolve 0.10 g of *mannitol R* in *water R* and dilute to 10 ml with the same solvent.

Reference solution (c). Mix equal volumes of reference solutions (a) and (b).

Apply separately to the plate 1 µl of each solution and thoroughly dry the starting points. Develop over a path of 15 cm using a mixture of 10 volumes of *water R*, 15 volumes of *methanol R*, 25 volumes of *anhydrous acetic acid R* and 50 volumes of *ethylene chloride R*, measured accurately since a slight excess of water produces cloudiness. Dry the plate in a current of warm air. Repeat immediately the development after renewing the mobile phase. Dry the plate in a current of warm air. Spray with *4-aminobenzoic acid solution R*. Dry the plate in a current of cold air until the acetone is removed. Heat the plate at 100 °C for 15 min. Allow to cool and spray with a 2 g/l solution of *sodium periodate R*. Dry the plate in a current of cold air. Heat the plate at 100 °C for 15 min. The principal spot in the chromatogram obtained with the test solution is similar in position, colour and size to the principal spot in the chromatogram obtained with reference solution (a) for lactose or to the principal spot in the chromatogram obtained with reference solution (b) for mannitol. The test is not valid unless the chromatogram obtained with reference solution (c) shows two clearly separated spots.

TESTS

Inorganic nitrates. Examine by thin-layer chromatography (*2.2.27*), using a *TLC silica gel plate R*.

Test solution. Shake a quantity of the substance to be examined corresponding to 0.10 g of pentaerythrityl tetranitrate with 5 ml of *alcohol R* and filter.

Reference solution. Dissolve 10 mg of *potassium nitrate R* in 1 ml of *water R* and dilute to 100 ml with *alcohol R*.

Apply separately to the plate 10 µl of each solution. Develop over a path of 15 cm using a mixture of 15 volumes of *glacial acetic acid R*, 30 volumes of *acetone R* and 60 volumes of *toluene R*. Dry the plate thoroughly in a current of air until the acetic acid is completely removed. Spray copiously with freshly prepared *potassium iodide and starch solution R*. Expose the plate to ultraviolet light at 254 nm for 15 min. Examine in daylight. Any spot corresponding to nitrate ion in the chromatogram obtained with the test solution is not more intense than the spot in the chromatogram obtained with the reference solution (0.5 per cent, calculated as potassium nitrate).

Related substances. Examine by liquid chromatography (*2.2.29*) as described under Assay.

Adjust the sensitivity of the system so that the height of the principal peak in the chromatogram obtained with reference solution (c) is at least 20 per cent of the full scale of the recorder.

The test is not valid unless in the chromatogram obtained with reference solution (e), the resolution between the peaks corresponding to glyceryl trinitrate and to pentaerythrityl tetranitrate is at least 2.0.

Inject 20 µl of test solution (a) and 20 µl of reference solution (c) and record the chromatogram of test solution (a) for at least five times the retention time of pentaerythrityl tetranitrate. In the chromatogram obtained with test solution (a); the area of any peak, apart from the principal peak is not greater than the area of the principal peak in the chromatogram obtained with reference solution (c) (0.3 per cent); the sum of the areas of all the peaks, apart from the principal peak, is not greater than twice the area of the principal peak in the chromatogram obtained with reference solution (c) (0.6 per cent). Disregard any peak with an area less than 0.2 times that of the principal peak in the chromatogram obtained with reference solution (c).

ASSAY

Examine by liquid chromatography (*2.2.29*).

Test solution (a). Sonicate for 15 min a quantity of the substance to be examined corresponding to 25.0 mg of pentaerythrityl tetranitrate in 20 ml of *methanol R* and dilute to 25.0 ml with the mobile phase. Filter through a suitable membrane filter.

Test solution (b). Dilute 1.0 ml of test solution (a) to 10.0 ml with the mobile phase.

Reference solution (a). Sonicate for 15 min a quantity of *diluted pentaerythrityl tetranitrate CRS* corresponding to 25.0 mg of pentaerythrityl tetranitrate in 20 ml of *methanol R* and dilute to 25.0 ml with the mobile phase. Filter through a suitable membrane filter.

Reference solution (b). Dilute 1.0 ml of reference solution (a) to 10.0 ml with the mobile phase.

Reference solution (c). Dilute 0.3 ml of reference solution (b) to 10.0 ml with the mobile phase.

Reference solution (d). Sonicate for 15 min a quantity of *glyceryl trinitrate solution CRS* corresponding to 20.0 mg of glyceryl trinitrate in 20 ml of *methanol R* and dilute to 25.0 ml with the mobile phase. Filter through a suitable membrane filter. Dilute 1.0 ml of the filtrate to 10.0 ml with the mobile phase.

Reference solution (e). To 1 ml of reference solution (b), add 1 ml of reference solution (d) and dilute to 10 ml with the mobile phase.

The chromatographic procedure may be carried out using:

- a stainless steel column 0.25 m long and 4.6 mm in internal diameter packed with *octadecylsilyl silica gel for chromatography R* (10 μm),
- as mobile phase at a flow rate of 2 ml/min a mixture of 40 volumes of *water R* and 60 volumes of *methanol R*,
- as detector a spectrophotometer set at 230 nm.

When the chromatograms are recorded in the prescribed conditions the retention time of pentaerythrityl tetranitrate is about 8 min. Inject 20 μl of reference solution (b). Adjust the sensitivity of the system so that the height of the principal peak in the chromatogram obtained is at least 50 per cent of the full scale of the recorder. Inject reference solution (b) six times. The assay is not valid unless the relative standard deviation for the area of the principal peak is at most 2.0 per cent. Inject test solution (b) and reference solution (b) alternately.

STORAGE

Store protected from light and heat.

LABELLING

The label states:

- the content of pentaerythrityl tetranitrate as a percentage,
- the diluent used.

IMPURITIES

A. inorganic nitrates,

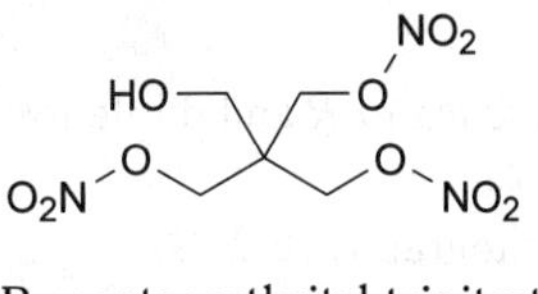

B. pentaerythrityl trinitrate,

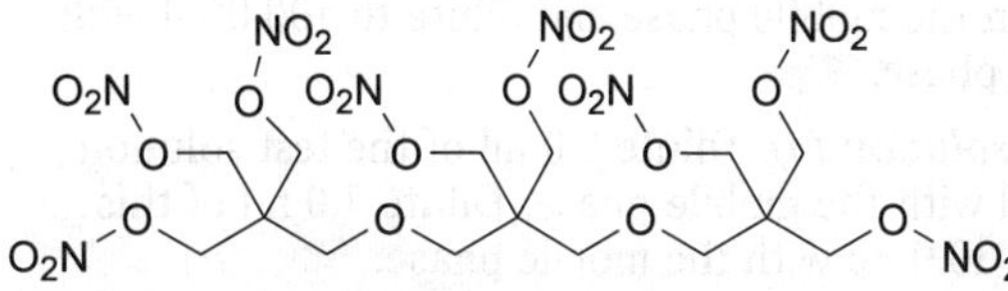

C. tripentaerythrityl octanitrate,

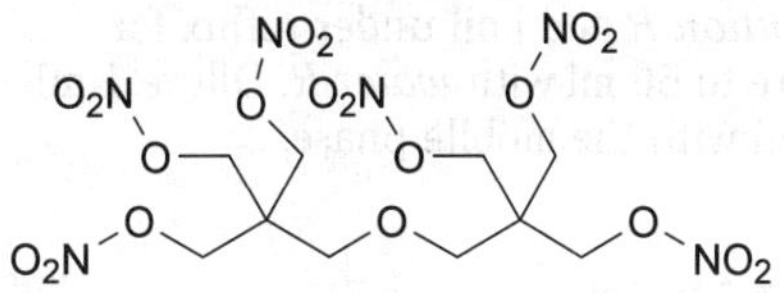

D. dipentaerythrityl hexanitrate.

01/2005:1137

PENTAMIDINE DIISETIONATE

Pentamidini diisetionas

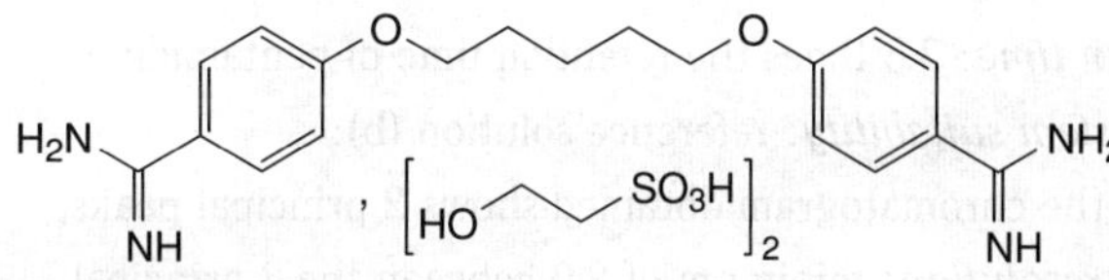

$C_{23}H_{36}N_4O_{10}S_2$ M_r 592.7

DEFINITION

4,4′-[Pentane-1,5-diylbis(oxy)]dibenzamidine di(2-hydroxyethanesulphonate).

Content: 98.5 per cent to 101.5 per cent (dried substance).

CHARACTERS

Appearance: white or almost white powder or colourless crystals, hygroscopic.

Solubility: freely soluble in water, sparingly soluble in alcohol, practically insoluble in methylene chloride.

IDENTIFICATION

A. Infrared absorption spectrophotometry (*2.2.24*).
   Preparation: discs.
   Comparison: *pentamidine diisetionate CRS*.

B. Dissolve about 40 mg in 5 ml of *water R* and add dropwise with shaking 1 ml of a 10 g/l solution of *sodium chloride R*. Allow to stand for 5 min. The mixture remains clear.

C. Treat 0.15 g by the oxygen-flask method (*2.5.10*). Use 10 ml of *dilute hydrogen peroxide solution R* to absorb the combustion products. The solution gives reaction (a) of sulphates (*2.3.1*).

TESTS

Appearance of solution. The solution is not more opalescent than reference suspension II (*2.2.1*) and not more intensely coloured than intensity 6 of the range of reference solutions of the most appropriate colour (*2.2.2, Method II*).

Dissolve 2.0 g in *water R* and dilute to 20 ml with the same solvent.

pH (*2.2.3*): 4.5 to 6.5.

Dissolve 0.5 g in *carbon dioxide-free water R* and dilute to 10 ml with the same solvent.

Related substances. Liquid chromatography (*2.2.29*).

Test solution. Dissolve 0.100 g of the substance to be examined in the mobile phase and dilute to 100.0 ml with the mobile phase.

Reference solution (a). Dilute 2.0 ml of the test solution to 100.0 ml with the mobile phase. Dilute 1.0 ml of this solution to 10.0 ml with the mobile phase.

Reference solution (b). To 0.1 g in a conical flask, add 40 ml of *water R* and glass beads. Adjust to pH 10.5 with *dilute sodium hydroxide solution R* and boil under reflux for 20 min. Cool and dilute to 50 ml with *water R*. Dilute 1 ml of the solution to 50 ml with the mobile phase.

Column:

- *size*: l = 0.25 m, Ø = 4.6 mm,
- *stationary phase*: *octadecylsilyl silica gel for chromatography R* (5 µm).

Mobile phase: mix 65 volumes of *methanol R* and 35 volumes of a 30 g/l solution of *ammonium acetate R* previously adjusted to pH 7.5 using *triethylamine R*.

Flow rate: 1 ml/min.

Detection: spectrophotometer at 265 nm.

Injection: 10 µl.

Run time: 3.5 times the retention time of pentamidine.

System suitability: reference solution (b):

- the chromatogram obtained shows 2 principal peaks,
- *resolution*: minimum of 2.0 between the 2 principal peaks.

Limits:

- *any impurity*: not more than the area of the principal peak in the chromatogram obtained with reference solution (a) (0.2 per cent),
- *total*: not more than twice the area of the principal peak in the chromatogram obtained with reference solution (a) (0.4 per cent),
- *disregard limit*: 0.1 times the area of the principal peak in the chromatogram obtained with reference solution (a) (0.02 per cent).

Heavy metals (*2.4.8*): maximum 20 ppm.

1.0 g complies with limit test C. Prepare the standard using 2 ml of *lead standard solution (10 ppm Pb) R*.

Loss on drying (*2.2.32*): maximum 4.0 per cent, determined on 1.000 g by drying in an oven at 100-105 °C.

Sulphated ash (*2.4.14*): maximum 0.1 per cent, determined on 1.0 g.

ASSAY

Dissolve 0.250 g in 50 ml of *dimethylformamide R*. Add 0.25 ml of *thymol blue solution R*. Titrate with *0.1 M tetrabutylammonium hydroxide*, under a current of *nitrogen R*, until the colour of the indicator changes to blue. Carry out a blank titration.

1 ml of *0.1 M tetrabutylammonium hydroxide* is equivalent to 29.63 mg of $C_{23}H_{36}N_4O_{10}S_2$.

STORAGE

In an airtight container.

IMPURITIES

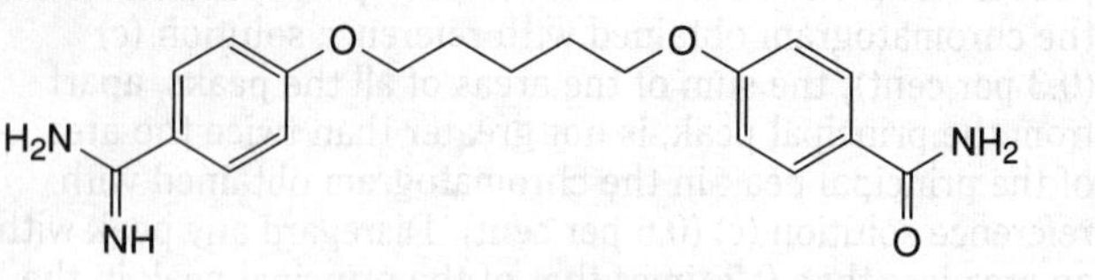

A. 4-[[5-(4-amidinophenoxy)pentyl]oxy]benzenecarboxamide.

01/2005:1462

PENTAZOCINE

Pentazocinum

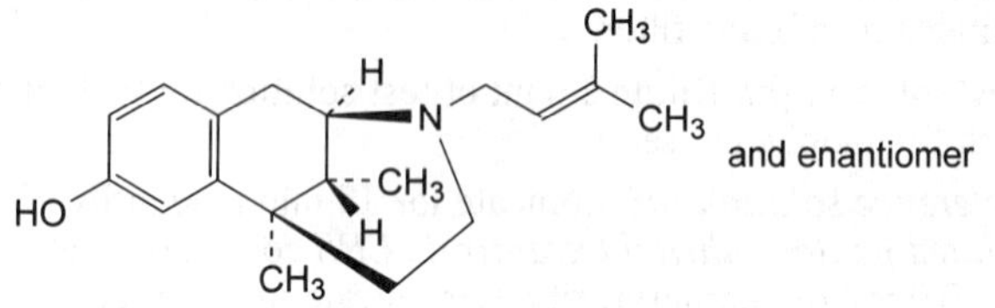

$C_{19}H_{27}NO$ M_r 285.4

DEFINITION

Pentazocine contains not less than 99.0 per cent and not more than the equivalent of 101.0 per cent of (2*RS*,6*RS*,11*RS*)-6,11-dimethyl-3-(3-methylbut-2-enyl)-1,2,3,4,5,6-hexahydro-2,6-methano-3-benzazocin-8-ol, calculated with reference to the dried substance.

CHARACTERS

A white or almost white powder, practically insoluble in water, freely soluble in methylene chloride and soluble in alcohol.

It shows polymorphism.

IDENTIFICATION

Examine by infrared absorption spectrophotometry (*2.2.24*), comparing with the *Ph. Eur. reference spectrum for pentazocine (form A)*.

TESTS

Absorbance (*2.2.25*). Dissolve 0.100 g in a mixture of 20 ml of *water R* and 1 ml of *1 M hydrochloric acid*, and dilute to 100.0 ml with *water R*. To 10.0 ml add 1 ml of *1 M hydrochloric acid* and dilute to 100.0 ml with *water R*. The specific absorbance at the maximum at 278 nm is 0.67 to 0.71, calculated with reference to the dried substance.

Related substances. Examine by thin-layer chromatography (*2.2.27*), using a *TLC silica gel F_{254} plate R*.

Test solution. Dissolve 0.20 g of the substance to be examined in *methylene chloride R* and dilute to 10 ml with the same solvent.

Reference solution (a). Dilute 1 ml of the test solution to 100 ml with *methylene chloride R*.

Reference solution (b). Dilute 5 ml of reference solution (a) to 10 ml with *methylene chloride R*.

Reference solution (c). Dilute 5 ml of reference solution (a) to 20 ml with *methylene chloride R*.

Apply to the plate 10 µl of each solution. Develop over a path corresponding to two thirds of the plate height using a mixture of 3 volumes of *isopropylamine R*, 3 volumes of *methanol R* and 94 volumes of *methylene chloride R*. Allow the plate to dry in air and examine in ultraviolet light at 254 nm. Heat the plate at 100 °C to 105 °C for 15 min, allow to cool, expose to iodine vapour and re-examine under ultraviolet light at 254 nm. By each method of visualisation: any spot in the chromatogram obtained with the test solution, apart from the principal spot, is not more intense than the spot obtained with reference solution (a) (1 per cent); not more than one such spot is more intense than the spot in the chromatogram obtained with reference solution (b) (0.5 per cent) and not more than four such spots are more intense than the spot in the chromatogram obtained with reference solution (c) (0.25 per cent).

Loss on drying (*2.2.32*). Not more than 0.5 per cent, determined on 1.000 g by drying at 60 °C at a pressure not exceeding 0.7 kPa for 4 h.

Sulphated ash (*2.4.14*). Not more than 0.1 per cent, determined on 1.0 g.

ASSAY

Dissolve 0.200 g in 50 ml of *anhydrous acetic acid R*. Titrate with *0.1 M perchloric acid*, determining the end-point potentiometrically (*2.2.20*).

1 ml of *0.1 M perchloric acid* is equivalent to 28.54 mg of $C_{19}H_{27}NO$.

STORAGE

Store protected from light.

01/2005:1463

PENTAZOCINE HYDROCHLORIDE

Pentazocini hydrochloridum

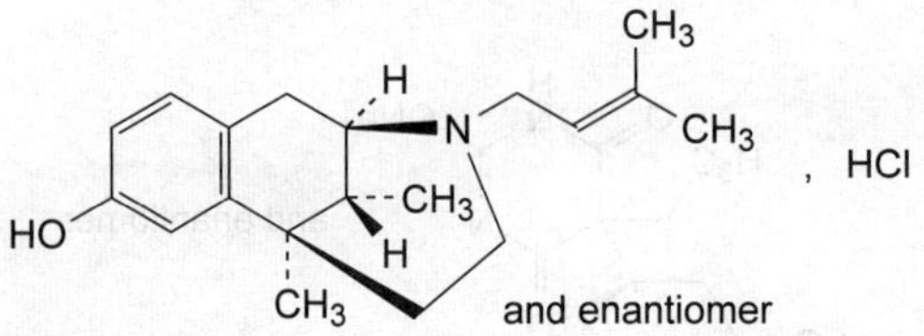

$C_{19}H_{28}ClNO$ M_r 321.9

DEFINITION

Pentazocine hydrochloride contains not less than 99.0 per cent and not more than the equivalent of 101.0 per cent of (2*RS*,6*RS*,11*RS*)-6,11-dimethyl-3-(3-methylbut-2-enyl)-1,2,3,4,5,6-hexahydro-2,6-methano-3-benzazocin-8-ol hydrochloride, calculated with reference to the dried substance.

CHARACTERS

A white or almost white powder, sparingly soluble in water, soluble in alcohol and sparingly soluble in methylene chloride.

It shows polymorphism.

IDENTIFICATION

A. Examine by infrared absorption spectrophotometry (*2.2.24*), comparing with the *Ph. Eur. reference spectrum of pentazocine hydrochloride*.

B. It gives reaction (a) of chlorides (*2.3.1*).

TESTS

pH (*2.2.3*). Dissolve 0.1 g in 10 ml of *carbon dioxide-free water R*. The pH of the solution is 4.0 to 6.0.

Absorbance (*2.2.25*). Dissolve 0.100 g in a mixture of 20 ml of *water R* and 1 ml of *1 M hydrochloric acid*, and dilute to 100.0 ml with *water R*. To 10.0 ml add 1 ml of *1 M hydrochloric acid* and dilute to 100.0 ml with *water R*. The specific absorbance at the maximum at 278 nm is 0.59 to 0.63, calculated with reference to the dried substance.

Related substances. Examine by thin-layer chromatography (*2.2.27*), using a *TLC silica gel F_{254} plate R*.

Test solution. Dissolve 0.20 g in 3 ml of *methanol R* and dilute to 10 ml with *methylene chloride R*.

Reference solution (a). Dilute 1 ml of the test solution to 100 ml with *methylene chloride R*.

Reference solution (b). Dilute 5 ml of reference solution (a) to 10 ml with *methylene chloride R*.

Reference solution (c). Dilute 5 ml of reference solution (a) to 20 ml with *methylene chloride R*.

Apply to the plate 10 µl of each solution. Develop over a path corresponding to two-thirds of the plate height using a mixture of 3 volumes of *isopropylamine R*, 3 volumes of *methanol R* and 94 volumes of *methylene chloride R*. Allow the plate to dry in air and examine in ultraviolet light at 254 nm. Heat the plate at 100 °C to 105 °C for 15 min, allow to cool, expose to iodine vapour and re-examine under ultraviolet light at 254 nm. By each method of visualisation: any spot in the chromatogram obtained with the test solution, apart from the principal spot, is not more intense than the spot obtained with reference solution (a) (1 per cent); not more than one such spot is more intense than the spot in the chromatogram obtained with reference solution (b) (0.5 per cent); and not more than four such spots are more intense than the spot in the chromatogram obtained with reference solution (c) (0.25 per cent).

Loss on drying (*2.2.32*). Not more than 0.5 per cent, determined on 1.000 g by drying at 60 °C at a pressure not exceeding 0.7 kPa for 4 h.

Sulphated ash (*2.4.14*). Not more than 0.1 per cent, determined on 1.0 g.

ASSAY

Dissolve 0.250 g in 50 ml of *alcohol R*. Add 5 ml of *0.01 M hydrochloric acid*. Carry out a potentiometric titration (*2.2.20*), using *0.1 M sodium hydroxide*. Read the volume added between the two points of inflection.

1 ml of *0.1 M sodium hydroxide* is equivalent to 32.19 mg of $C_{19}H_{28}ClNO$.

STORAGE

Store protected from light.

01/2005:0200

PENTOBARBITAL

Pentobarbitalum

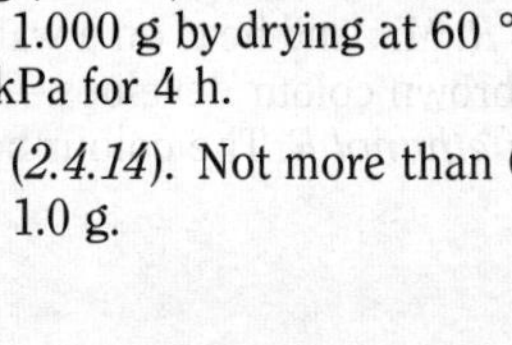

$C_{11}H_{18}N_2O_3$ M_r 226.3

DEFINITION

Pentobarbital contains not less than 99.0 per cent and not more than the equivalent of 101.0 per cent of 5-ethyl-5-[(1*RS*)-1-methylbutyl]pyrimidine-2,4,6(1*H*,3*H*,5*H*)-trione, calculated with reference to the dried substance.

CHARACTERS

A white, crystalline powder or colourless crystals, very slightly soluble in water, freely soluble in ethanol. It forms water-soluble compounds with alkali hydroxides and carbonates and with ammonia.

IDENTIFICATION

A. Determine the melting point (*2.2.14*) of the substance to be examined. Mix equal parts of the substance to be examined and *pentobarbital CRS* and determine the melting point of the mixture. The difference between the melting points (which are about 133 °C) is not greater than 2 °C.

B. Examine by thin-layer chromatography (*2.2.27*), using *silica gel GF_{254} R* as the coating substance.

Test solution. Dissolve 0.1 g of the substance to be examined in *alcohol R* and dilute to 100 ml with the same solvent.

Reference solution. Dissolve 0.1 g of *pentobarbital CRS* in *alcohol R* and dilute to 100 ml with the same solvent.

Apply to the plate 10 µl of each solution. Develop over a path of 18 cm using the lower layer of a mixture of 5 volumes of *concentrated ammonia R*, 15 volumes of *alcohol R* and 80 volumes of *chloroform R*. Examine immediately in ultraviolet light at 254 nm. The principal spot in the chromatogram obtained with the test solution is similar in position and size to the principal spot in the chromatogram obtained with the reference solution.

C. To about 10 mg add about 10 mg of *vanillin R* and 2 ml of *sulphuric acid R*. Mix and heat on a water-bath for 2 min. A reddish-brown colour develops. Cool and add cautiously 5 ml of *ethanol R*. The colour becomes violet and then blue.

TESTS

Appearance of solution. Dissolve 1.0 g in a mixture of 4 ml of *dilute sodium hydroxide solution R* and 6 ml of *water R*. The solution is clear (*2.2.1*) and not more intensely coloured than reference solution Y_6 (*2.2.2, Method II*).

Acidity. Boil 1.0 g with 50 ml of *water R* for 2 min, allow to cool and filter. To 10 ml of the filtrate add 0.15 ml of *methyl red solution R*. The solution is orange-yellow. Not more than 0.1 ml of *0.1 M sodium hydroxide* is required to produce a pure yellow colour.

Related substances. Examine by thin-layer chromatography (*2.2.27*), using *silica gel GF_{254} R* as the coating substance.

Test solution. Dissolve 1.0 g of the substance to be examined in *alcohol R* and dilute to 100 ml with the same solvent.

Reference solution. Dilute 0.5 ml of the test solution to 100 ml with *alcohol R*.

Apply to the plate 20 µl of each solution. Develop over a path of 15 cm using the lower layer of a mixture of 5 volumes of *concentrated ammonia R*, 15 volumes of *alcohol R* and 80 volumes of *chloroform R*. Examine immediately in ultraviolet light at 254 nm. Spray with *diphenylcarbazone mercuric reagent R*. Allow the plate to dry in air and spray with freshly prepared *alcoholic potassium hydroxide solution R* diluted 1 in 5 with *aldehyde-free alcohol R*. Heat at 100 °C to 105 °C for 5 min and examine immediately. When examined in ultraviolet light and after spraying, any spot in the chromatogram obtained with the test solution, apart from the principal spot, is not more intense than the spot in the chromatogram obtained with the reference solution (0.5 per cent).

Isomer. Dissolve 0.3 g in 5 ml of a 50 g/l solution of *anhydrous sodium carbonate R*, heating slightly if necessary. Add a solution of 0.3 g of *nitrobenzyl chloride R* in 10 ml of *alcohol R* and heat under a reflux condenser for 30 min. Cool to 25 °C, filter and wash the precipitate with five quantities, each of 5 ml, of *water R*. In a small flask, heat the precipitate with 25 ml of *alcohol R* under a reflux condenser until dissolved (about 10 min). Cool to 25 °C, if necessary scratching the wall of the flask with a glass rod to induce crystallisation, and filter. The precipitate, washed with two quantities, each of 5 ml, of *water R* and dried at 100 °C to 105 °C for 30 min, melts (*2.2.14*) at 136 °C to 148 °C.

Loss on drying (*2.2.32*). Not more than 0.5 per cent, determined on 1.000 g by drying in an oven at 100 °C to 105 °C.

Sulphated ash (*2.4.14*). Not more than 0.1 per cent, determined on 1.0 g.

ASSAY

Dissolve 0.100 g in 5 ml of *pyridine R*. Add 0.5 ml of *thymolphthalein solution R* and 10 ml of *silver nitrate solution in pyridine R*. Titrate with *0.1 M ethanolic sodium hydroxide* until a pure blue colour is obtained. Carry out a blank titration.

1 ml of *0.1 M ethanolic sodium hydroxide* is equivalent to 11.31 mg of $C_{11}H_{18}N_2O_3$.

01/2005:0419

PENTOBARBITAL SODIUM

Pentobarbitalum natricum

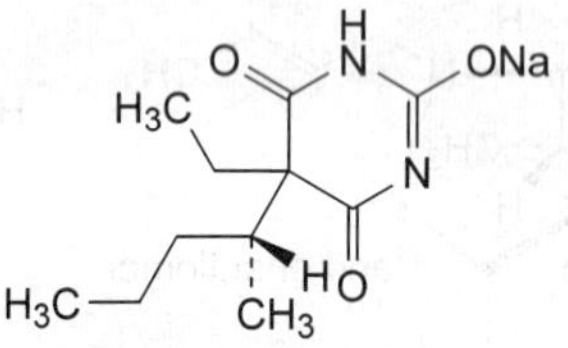

and enantiomer

$C_{11}H_{17}N_2NaO_3$ M_r 248.3

DEFINITION

Pentobarbital sodium contains not less than 99.0 per cent and not more than the equivalent of 101.5 per cent of the sodium derivative of 5-ethyl-5-[(1*RS*)-1-methylbutyl]pyrimidine-2,4,6(1*H*,3*H*,5*H*)-trione, calculated with reference to the dried substance.

CHARACTERS

A white, crystalline powder, hygroscopic, very soluble in water.

IDENTIFICATION

A. Dissolve 1 g in 10 ml of *water R* and add 5 ml of *dilute acetic acid R*. A white, crystalline precipitate is formed. Filter, wash the precipitate with *water R* and dry at 100 °C to 105 °C. Determine the melting point (*2.2.14*) of the precipitate. Mix equal parts of the precipitate and *pentobarbital CRS* and determine the melting point of the mixture. The difference between the melting points (which are about 131 °C) is not greater than 2 °C.

B. Examine by thin-layer chromatography (*2.2.27*), using a *TLC silica gel F_{254} plate R*.

Test solution. Dissolve 25 mg of the precipitate obtained in identification test A in *alcohol R* and dilute to 25 ml with the same solvent.

Reference solution. Dissolve 25 mg of *pentobarbital CRS* in *alcohol R* and dilute to 25 ml with the same solvent.

Apply to the plate 10 µl of each solution. Develop over a path of 18 cm using the lower layer from a mixture of 5 volumes of *concentrated ammonia R*, 15 volumes of *alcohol R* and 80 volumes of *chloroform R*. Examine immediately in ultraviolet light at 254 nm. The principal spot in the chromatogram obtained with the test solution is similar in position and size to the principal spot in the chromatogram obtained with the reference solution.

C. To about 10 mg add about 10 mg of *vanillin R* and 2 ml of *sulphuric acid R*. Mix and heat on a water-bath for 2 min. A reddish-brown colour develops. Cool and add cautiously 5 ml of *ethanol R*. The colour becomes violet and then blue.

D. Ignite 1 g. The residue gives reaction (a) of sodium (*2.3.1*).

TESTS

pH (*2.2.3*). Dissolve 1.0 g in *carbon dioxide-free water R* and dilute to 10 ml with the same solvent. The pH measured immediately after preparation of the solution is 9.6 to 11.0.

Related substances. Examine by thin-layer chromatography (*2.2.27*), using a *TLC silica gel GF_{254} plate R*.

Test solution. Dissolve 0.2 g of the substance to be examined in *alcohol R* and dilute to 10 ml with the same solvent.

Reference solution. Dilute 0.5 ml of the test solution to 100 ml with *alcohol R*.

Apply to the plate 10 µl of each solution. Develop over a path of 15 cm using the lower layer from a mixture of 5 volumes of *concentrated ammonia R*, 15 volumes of *alcohol R* and 80 volumes of *chloroform R*. Examine immediately in ultraviolet light at 254 nm. Any spot in the chromatogram obtained with the test solution, apart from the principal spot, is not more intense than the spot in the chromatogram obtained with the reference solution (0.5 per cent). Spray with *diphenylcarbazone mercuric reagent R*. Allow the plate to dry in air and spray with freshly prepared *alcoholic potassium hydroxide solution R* diluted 1 in 5 with *aldehyde-free alcohol R*. Heat at 100 °C to 105 °C for 5 min and examine immediately in daylight. Any spot in the chromatogram obtained with the test solution, apart from the principal spot, is not more intense than the spot in the chromatogram obtained with the reference solution (0.5 per cent).

Free pentobarbital. Not more than 3.5 per cent. Dissolve 2.00 g in 75 ml of *dimethylformamide R*, heating gently if necessary. Titrate with *0.1 M sodium methoxide* until the colour changes from olive-green to blue, using 0.25 ml of a 10 g/l solution of *thymol blue R* in *dimethylformamide R* as indicator. Carry out a blank titration.

1 ml of *0.1 M sodium methoxide* is equivalent to 22.63 mg of pentobarbital.

Isomer. Dissolve 0.3 g in 5 ml of a 50 g/l solution of *anhydrous sodium carbonate R*. Add a solution of 0.3 g of *nitrobenzyl chloride R* in 10 ml of *alcohol R* and heat under a reflux condenser for 30 min. Cool to 25 °C, if necessary scratching the wall of the container with a glass rod to induce crystallisation. Filter and wash the precipitate with five quantities, each of 5 ml, of *water R*. In a small flask, heat the precipitate with 25 ml of *alcohol R* under a reflux condenser until dissolved (about 10 min). Cool to 25 °C, if necessary scratching the wall of the flask with a glass rod to induce crystallisation, and filter. The precipitate, washed with two quantities, each of 5 ml, of *water R* and dried at 100 °C to 105 °C for 30 min, melts (*2.2.14*) at 136 °C to 148 °C.

Heavy metals (*2.4.8*). Dissolve 1.0 g in *water R* and dilute to 10.0 ml with the same solvent. To 9 ml of the solution, add 3 ml of *dilute acetic acid R* and 3 ml of *buffer solution pH 3.5 R* and filter. Dilute the filtrate to 18 ml with *water R*. 12 ml of the solution complies with limit test A for heavy metals (20 ppm). In preparing the test solution, replace the buffer solution with *water R*. Prepare the standard using *lead standard solution (1 ppm Pb) R*.

Loss on drying (*2.2.32*). Not more than 3.0 per cent, determined on 1.00 g by drying in an oven at 100 °C to 105 °C.

ASSAY

Dissolve 0.200 g in 15 ml of a 127.5 g/l solution of *silver nitrate R* in *pyridine R*. Titrate with *0.1 M ethanolic sodium hydroxide* until a pure blue colour is obtained, using 0.5 ml of *thymolphthalein solution R* as indicator. Carry out a blank titration.

1 ml of *0.1 M ethanolic sodium hydroxide* is equivalent to 24.83 mg of $C_{11}H_{17}N_2NaO_3$.

STORAGE

Store in an airtight container.

01/2005:0851

PENTOXIFYLLINE

Pentoxifyllinum

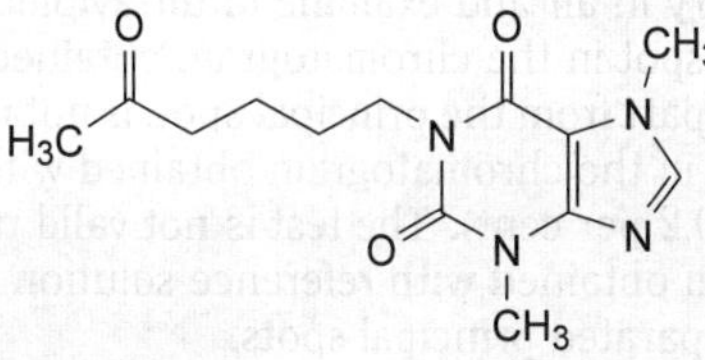

$C_{13}H_{18}N_4O_3$ M_r 278.3

DEFINITION

Pentoxifylline contains not less than 99.0 per cent and not more than the equivalent of 101.0 per cent of 3,7-dimethyl-1-(5-oxohexyl)-3,7-dihydro-1*H*-purine-2,6-dione, calculated with reference to the dried substance.

CHARACTERS

A white or almost white, crystalline powder, soluble in water, freely soluble in methylene chloride, sparingly soluble in alcohol.

IDENTIFICATION

First identification: A, B.

Second identification: A, C, D.

A. Melting point (*2.2.14*): 103 °C to 107 °C.

B. Examine by infrared absorption spectrophotometry (*2.2.24*), comparing with the spectrum obtained with *pentoxifylline CRS*. Examine the substances prepared as discs.

C. Examine the chromatograms obtained in the test for related substances in ultraviolet light at 254 nm. The principal spot in the chromatogram obtained with test solution (b) is similar in position and size to the principal spot in the chromatogram obtained with reference solution (a).

D. It gives the reaction of xanthines (*2.3.1*).

Monographs P

TESTS

Solution S. Dissolve 2.5 g in *carbon dioxide-free water R* prepared from *distilled water R* and dilute to 50 ml with the same solvent.

Appearance of solution. Dilute 4 ml of solution S to 10 ml with *water R*. The solution is clear (*2.2.1*) and not more intensely coloured than reference solution Y_7 (*2.2.2, Method II*).

Acidity. To 8 ml of solution S add 12 ml of *water R* and 0.05 ml of *bromothymol blue solution R1*. The solution is green or yellow. Not more than 0.2 ml of *0.01 M sodium hydroxide* is required to change the colour of the indicator to blue.

Related substances. Examine by thin-layer chromatography (*2.2.27*), using *silica gel GF_{254} R* as the coating substance.

Test solution (a). Dissolve 0.10 g of the substance to be examined in *methanol R* and dilute to 5 ml with the same solvent.

Test solution (b). Dilute 1 ml of test solution (a) to 10 ml with *methanol R*.

Reference solution (a). Dissolve 20 mg of *pentoxifylline CRS* in *methanol R* and dilute to 10 ml with the same solvent.

Reference solution (b). Dilute 1 ml of test solution (b) to 50 ml with *methanol R*.

Reference solution (c). Dissolve 20 mg of *pentoxifylline CRS* and 20 mg of *theophylline CRS* in *methanol R* and dilute to 10 ml with the same solvent.

Apply separately to the plate 20 µl of each solution. Develop over a path of 10 cm using a mixture of 15 volumes of *methanol R* and 85 volumes of *ethyl acetate R*. Allow the plate to dry in air and examine in ultraviolet light at 254 nm. Any spot in the chromatogram obtained with test solution (a), apart from the principal spot, is not more intense than the spot in the chromatogram obtained with reference solution (b) (0.2 per cent). The test is not valid unless the chromatogram obtained with reference solution (c) shows two clearly separated principal spots.

Chlorides (*2.4.4*). Place 20 ml of solution S in a separating funnel and shake with two quantities, each of 20 ml, of *2-methylpropan-1-ol R*. Dilute 10 ml of the aqueous layer to 15 ml with *water R*. The solution complies with the limit test for chlorides (100 ppm).

Sulphates (*2.4.13*). 15 ml of solution S complies with the limit test for sulphates (200 ppm).

Heavy metals (*2.4.8*). 2.0 g complies with the limit test C for heavy metals (10 ppm). Prepare the standard using 2 ml of *lead standard solution (10 ppm Pb) R*.

Loss on drying (*2.2.32*). Not more than 0.5 per cent, determined on 1.000 g by drying over *diphosphorus pentoxide R* at 60 °C at a pressure not exceeding 700 Pa.

Sulphated ash (*2.4.14*). Not more than 0.1 per cent, determined on 1.0 g.

ASSAY

Dissolve 0.200 g in 5 ml of *anhydrous acetic acid R*. Add 20 ml of *acetic anhydride R*. Titrate with *0.1 M perchloric acid* determining the end-point potentiometrically (*2.2.20*).

1 ml of *0.1 M perchloric acid* is equivalent to 27.83 mg of $C_{13}H_{18}N_4O_3$.

STORAGE

Store protected from light.

IMPURITIES

A. theobromine.

01/2005:1621

PENTOXYVERINE HYDROGEN CITRATE

Pentoxyverini hydrogenocitras

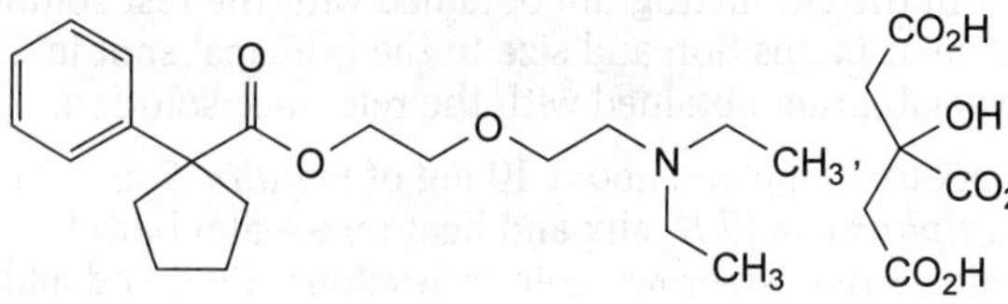

$C_{26}H_{39}NO_{10}$ M_r 525.6

DEFINITION

2-[2-(Diethylamino)ethoxy]ethyl 1-phenylcyclopentanecarboxylate dihydrogen 2-hydroxypropane-1,2,3-tricarboxylate.

Content: 98.5 per cent to 101.0 per cent (dried substance).

CHARACTERS

Appearance: white or almost white, crystalline powder.

Solubility: freely soluble in water, very soluble in glacial acetic acid, freely soluble in methanol, soluble in alcohol and in methylene chloride.

mp: about 93 °C.

IDENTIFICATION

A. Infrared absorption spectrophotometry (*2.2.24*).
   Comparison: *Ph. Eur. reference spectrum of pentoxyverine hydrogen citrate.*

B. Dissolve 0.25 g in 5 ml of *water R*. The solution gives the reaction of citrates (*2.3.1*).

TESTS

Solution S. Dissolve 5.0 g in *carbon dioxide-free water R* and dilute to 50 ml with the same solvent.

Appearance of solution. Solution S is clear (*2.2.1*) and not more intensely coloured than reference solution Y_6 (*2.2.2, Method II*).

pH (*2.2.3*): 3.3 to 3.7 for solution S.

Related substances. Liquid chromatography (*2.2.29*).

Test solution. Dissolve 25.0 mg of the substance to be examined in the mobile phase and dilute to 25.0 ml with the mobile phase.

Reference solution. Introduce 5.0 mg of *pentoxyverine impurity A CRS* and 5.0 mg of *pentoxyverine impurity B CRS* in a conical flask, add 5.0 ml of the test solution and dilute to 100.0 ml with the mobile phase. Dilute 3.0 ml of the solution to 50.0 ml with the mobile phase.

Column:
- *size*: l = 0.15 m, Ø = 3.9 mm,
- *stationary phase*: *end-capped octylsilyl silica gel for chromatography R* (5 µm) with a pore size of 10 nm and a carbon loading of 12 per cent,
- *temperature*: 50 °C.

Mobile phase: mix 35 volumes of *acetonitrile R* and 65 volumes of a 0.15 per cent (*m/V*) solution of *sodium heptanesulphonate R* adjusted to pH 3.0 with *dilute sulphuric acid R*.

Flow rate: 1.0 ml/min.

Detection: spectrophotometer at 205 nm.

Injection: 20 µl.

Run time: 3 times the retention time of pentoxyverine.

Monographs P

Relative retention with reference to pentoxyverine (retention time = about 6 min): impurity B = about 0.8; impurity A = about 1.5.

System suitability: reference solution:

– *resolution*: minimum of 5.0 between the peaks due to pentoxyverine and to impurity A,
– *signal-to-noise ratio*: minimum of 100 for the peak due to pentoxyverine,
– *symmetry factor*: maximum of 2.0 for the peak due to pentoxyverine.

Limits:

– *impurity A*: not more than the area of the corresponding peak in the chromatogram obtained with the reference solution (0.3 per cent),
– *impurity B*: not more than the area of the corresponding peak in the chromatogram obtained with the reference solution (0.3 per cent),
– *any other impurity*: not more than one-third of the area of the peak due to pentoxyverine in the chromatogram obtained with the reference solution (0.1 per cent),
– *total of any other impurity*: not more than the area of the peak due to pentoxyverine in the chromatogram obtained with the reference solution (0.3 per cent),
– *disregard limit*: 0.1 times the area of the peak due to pentoxyverine in the chromatogram obtained with the reference solution (0.03 per cent); disregard any peak with a retention time less than or equal to 2.5 min.

Loss on drying (*2.2.32*): maximum 0.5 per cent, determined on 1.000 g by drying *in vacuo* at 60 °C for 4 h.

Sulphated ash (*2.4.14*): maximum 0.1 per cent, determined on 1.0 g.

ASSAY

Dissolve 0.400 g in 70 ml of *anhydrous acetic acid R*. Titrate with *0.1 M perchloric acid*, determining the end-point potentiometrically (*2.2.20*).

1 ml of *0.1 M perchloric acid* is equivalent to 52.56 mg of $C_{26}H_{39}NO_{10}$.

STORAGE

Protected from light.

IMPURITIES

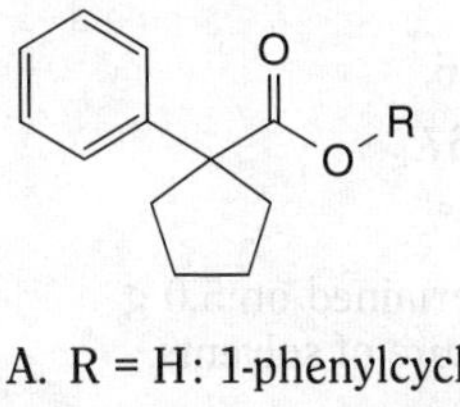

A. R = H: 1-phenylcyclopentanecarboxylic acid,

B. R = CH_2-CH_2-N(CH_2-CH_3)$_2$: 2-(diethylamino)ethyl 1-phenylcyclopentanecarboxylate (caramiphen).

01/2005:0406

PEPPERMINT LEAF

Menthae piperitae folium

DEFINITION

Peppermint leaf consists of the whole or cut dried leaves of *Mentha × piperita* L. The whole drug contains not less than 12 ml/kg of essential oil. The cut drug contains not less than 9 ml/kg of essential oil.

CHARACTERS

Peppermint leaf has a characteristic and penetrating odour and a characteristic aromatic taste; it is green to brownish-green, with brownish-violet veins in some varieties. The petioles are green to brownish-violet.

It has the macroscopic and microscopic characters described under Identification tests A and B.

IDENTIFICATION

A. The leaf is entire, broken or cut, thin, fragile; the entire leaf is 3 cm to 9 cm long and 1 cm to 3 cm wide and often crumpled. The lamina is oval or lanceolate, the apex acuminate, the margin sharply dentate and the base asymmetrical. Venation is pinnate, prominent on the lower surface, with lateral veins leaving the midrib at about 45°. The lower surface is slightly pubescent and secretory trichomes are visible under a lens (6×) as bright yellowish points. The petiole is grooved, usually up to 1 mm in diameter and 0.5 cm to 1 cm long.

B. Reduce to a powder (355). The powder is brownish-green. Examine under a microscope using *chloral hydrate solution R*. The powder shows the following diagnostic characteristics: leaf-tissue fragments with cells of the epidermis having sinuous-wavy walls and the cuticle striated over the veins and diacytic stomata predominantly present on the lower epidermis; epidermis fragments from near the leaf margin with isodiametric cells straighter-walled showing distinct beading and pitting in anticlinal walls; covering trichomes short, conical, unicellular or bicellular, or elongated, uniseriate with three to eight cells with striated cuticle; glandular trichomes of two types: (a) unicellular base with small, rounded unicellular head 15 µm to 25 µm in diameter; (b) unicellular base with enlarged oval head 55 µm to 70 µm in diameter composed of eight radiating cells; dorsiventral mesophyll fragment with a single palisade layer and four to six layers of spongy parenchyma; yellowish crystals of menthol under the cuticle of secretory cells. Calcium oxalate crystals are absent.

C. Examine by thin-layer chromatography (*2.2.27*), using *silica gel* GF_{254} *R* as the coating substance.

Test solution. To 0.2 g of the recently powdered drug add 2 ml of *methylene chloride R*, shake for a few minutes and filter. Evaporate the filtrate to dryness at about 40 °C and dissolve the residue in 0.1 ml of *toluene R*.

Reference solution. Dissolve 50 mg of *menthol R*, 20 µl of *cineole R*, 10 mg of *thymol R* and 10 µl of *menthyl acetate R* in *toluene R* and dilute to 10 ml with the same solvent.

Apply separately to the plate as bands 10 µl of the reference solution and 20 µl of the test solution. Develop over a path of 15 cm using a mixture of 5 volumes of *ethyl acetate R* and 95 volumes of *toluene R*. Allow the plate to dry in air until the solvent has evaporated and examine in ultraviolet light at 254 nm. The chromatogram obtained with the test solution may show a light quenching zone situated just below the level of the zone (thymol) in the chromatogram obtained with the reference solution (carvone, pulegone). Spray with *anisaldehyde solution R* and examine in daylight while heating for 5 min to 10 min at 100 °C to 105 °C. The chromatogram obtained with the reference solution shows, in order of increasing R_f value: in the lower third a deep-blue to violet zone (menthol); a violet-blue to brown zone (cineole); a pink zone (thymol); and a bluish-violet zone (menthyl acetate). The chromatogram obtained with the test solution shows: a zone due to menthol (the most intense); a faint zone due to cineole; at R_f values between those of the cineole and thymol zones in the chromatogram obtained with the reference solution, it may show light pink, or bluish-grey or greyish-green zones (carvone, pulegone, isomenthone); in the middle of the chromatogram, a bluish-violet zone (menthyl acetate) and just below it a greenish-blue zone (menthone); an intense reddish-violet zone (hydrocarbons) appears near the solvent front; other less intensely coloured zones also appear.

TESTS

Foreign matter (*2.8.2*). Carry out the determinations using 10 g of the drug.

Foreign organs. Not more than 5 per cent of stems; the diameter of the stems is not greater than 1.5 mm.

Foreign elements. Not more than 2 per cent. Not more than 8 per cent of the leaves show brown stains due to *Puccinia menthae*.

Water (*2.2.13*). Not more than 110 ml/kg, determined on 20.0 g by distillation.

Total ash (*2.4.16*). Not more than 15.0 per cent.

Ash insoluble in hydrochloric acid (*2.8.1*). Not more than 1.5 per cent.

ASSAY

Carry out the determination of essential oils in vegetable drugs (*2.8.12*). Use 20.0 g of crushed drug, a 500 ml flask, 200 ml of *water R* as the distillation liquid and 0.50 ml of *xylene R* in the graduated tube. Distil at a rate of 3-4 ml/min for 2 h.

STORAGE

Store protected from light.

01/2005:0405

PEPPERMINT OIL

Menthae piperitae aetheroleum

DEFINITION

Essential oil obtained by steam distillation from the fresh aerial parts of the flowering plant of *Mentha × piperita* L.

CHARACTERS

Appearance: a colourless, pale yellow or pale greenish-yellow liquid.

It has a characteristic odour and taste followed by a sensation of cold.

Solubility: miscible with alcohol and with methylene chloride.

IDENTIFICATION

First identification: B.

Second identification: A.

A. Examine the chromatograms obtained in the test for mint oil.

Results A: see below the sequence of the zones present in the chromatograms obtained with the reference solution and the test solution.

Top of the plate	
—	—
Thymol: a quenching zone	
	Quenching zones may be present (carvone, pulegone)
—	—
Reference solution	**Test solution**

Results B: see below the sequence of the zones present in the chromatograms obtained with the reference solution and the test solution. Furthermore, other less intensely coloured zones may be present in the chromatogram obtained with the test solution.

Top of the plate	
	An intense violet-red zone (near the solvent front) (hydrocarbons) A brownish-yellow zone (menthofuran)
—	—
Menthyl acetate: a violet-blue zone	A violet-blue zone (menthyl acetate) A greenish-blue zone (menthone)
Thymol: a pink zone	
	Light pink or greyish-blue or greyish-green zones may be present (carvone, pulegone, isomenthone)
Cineole: a violet-blue to brown zone	A faint violet-blue to brown zone (cineole)
—	—
Menthol: an intense blue to violet zone	An intense blue to violet zone (menthol)
Reference solution	**Test solution**

B. Examine the chromatograms obtained in the test for chromatographic profile.

Results: the characteristic peaks in the chromatogram obtained with the test solution are similar in retention time to those in the chromatogram obtained with the reference solution. Carvone and pulegone may be present in the chromatogram obtained with the test solution.

TESTS

Relative density (*2.2.5*): 0.900 to 0.916.

Refractive index (*2.2.6*): 1.457 to 1.467.

Optical rotation (*2.2.7*): − 10° to − 30°.

Acid value (*2.5.1*): maximum 1.4, determined on 5.0 g diluted in 50 ml of the prescribed mixture of solvents.

Fatty oils and resinified essential oils (*2.8.7*). It complies with the test for fatty oils and resinified essential oils.

Mint oil

A. Thin-layer chromatography (*2.2.27*).

Test solution. Mix 0.1 g of the substance to be examined with *toluene R* and dilute to 10 ml with the same solvent.

Reference solution. Dissolve 50 mg of *menthol R*, 20 µl of *cineole R*, 10 mg of *thymol R* and 10 µl of *menthyl acetate R* in *toluene R* and dilute to 10 ml with the same solvent.

Plate: TLC silica gel F_{254} plate R.

Mobile phase: ethyl acetate R, toluene R (5:95 V/V).

Application: 10 µl of the reference solution and 20 µl of the test solution, as bands.

Development: over a path of 15 cm.

Drying: in air.

Detection A: examine in ultraviolet light at 254 mm.

Detection B: spray with *anisaldehyde solution R* and heat at 100-105 °C for 5-10 min. Examine immediately in daylight.

Result B: the chromatogram obtained with the test solution shows no blue zone between the zones due to cineole and menthol.

B. Examine the chromatograms obtained in the test for chromatographic profile.

Results: the chromatogram obtained with the test solution does not show a peak with the retention time of isopulegol that has an area of more than 0.2 per cent of the total area.

Chromatographic profile. Gas chromatography (*2.2.28*): use the normalisation procedure.

Test solution. Mix 0.20 g of the substance to be examined with *hexane R* and dilute to 10.0 ml with the same solvent.

Reference solution (a). Dissolve 10 µl of *limonene R*, 20 µl of *cineole R*, 40 µl of *menthone R*, 10 µl of *menthofuran R*, 10 µl of *isomenthone R*, 40 µl of *menthyl acetate R*, 20 µl of *isopulegol R*, 60 mg of *menthol R*, 20 µl of *pulegone R*, 10 µl of *piperitone R* and 10 µl of *carvone R* in *hexane R* and dilute to 10.0 ml with the same solvent.

Reference solution (b). Dissolve 5 µl of *isopulegol R* in *hexane R* and dilute to 10 ml with the same solvent. Dilute 0.1 ml to 5 ml with *hexane R*.

Column:

- *material*: fused silica,
- *size*: l = 60 m, Ø = 0.25 mm,
- *stationary phase*: *macrogol 20 000 R* (film thickness 0.25 µm).

Carrier gas: *helium for chromatography R*.

Flow rate: 1.5 ml/min.

Split ratio: 1:50.

Temperature:

	Time (min)	Temperature (°C)
Column	0 - 10	60
	10 - 70	60 - 180
	70 - 75	180
Injection port		200
Detector		220

Detection: flame ionisation.

Injection: 1 µl.

Elution order: order indicated in the composition of reference solution (a); record the retention times of these substances.

System suitability: reference solution (a):

- *resolution*: minimum 1.5 between the peaks due to limonene and cineole and minimum 1.5 between the peaks due to piperitone and carvone.

Using the retention times determined from the chromatogram obtained with reference solution (a), locate the components of the reference solution in the chromatogram obtained with the test solution (disregard the peak due to hexane).

Determine the percentage content of the components. The limits are within the following ranges:

- *limonene*: 1.0 per cent to 5.0 per cent,
- *cineole*: 3.5 per cent to 14.0 per cent,
- *menthone*: 14.0 per cent to 32.0 per cent,
- *menthofuran*: 1.0 per cent to 9.0 per cent,
- *isomenthone*: 1.5 per cent to 10.0 per cent,
- *menthyl acetate*: 2.8 per cent to 10.0 per cent,
- *isopulegol*: maximum 0.2 per cent,
- *menthol*: 30.0 per cent to 55.0 per cent,
- *pulegone*: maximum 4.0 per cent,
- *carvone*: maximum 1.0 per cent,
- *disregard limit*: peak area obtained with reference solution (b) (0.05 per cent).

The ratio of cineole content to limonene content is minimum 2.

STORAGE

In a well-filled, airtight container, protected from light, at a temperature not exceeding 25 °C.

01/2005:0682
corrected

PEPSIN POWDER

Pepsini pulvis

DEFINITION

Pepsin powder is prepared from the gastric mucosa of pigs, cattle or sheep. It contains gastric proteinases, active in acid medium (pH 1 to 5). It has an activity not less than 0.5 Ph. Eur. U./mg, calculated with reference to the dried substance.

PRODUCTION

The animals from which pepsin powder is derived must fulfil the requirements for the health of animals suitable for human consumption to the satisfaction of the competent authority.

It must have been shown to what extent the method of production allows inactivation or removal of any contamination by viruses or other infectious agents.

CHARACTERS

A white or slightly yellow, crystalline or amorphous powder, hygroscopic, soluble in water, practically insoluble in alcohol. The solution in water may be slightly opalescent with a weak acidic reaction.

IDENTIFICATION

In a mortar, pound 30 mg of *fibrin blue R*. Suspend in 20 ml of *dilute hydrochloric acid R2*. Filter the suspension on a filter paper and wash with *dilute hydrochloric acid R2* until a colourless filtrate is obtained. Perforate the filter paper and wash the *fibrin blue R* through it into a conical flask using 20 ml of *dilute hydrochloric acid R2*. Shake before use. Dissolve a quantity of the substance to be examined, equivalent to not less than 20 Ph. Eur. U., in 2 ml of *dilute hydrochloric acid R2* and adjust to pH 1.6 ± 0.1. Add 1 ml of this solution to a test-tube containing 4 ml of the fibrin blue suspension, mix and place in a water-bath at 25 °C with gentle shaking. Prepare a blank solution at the same time and in the same manner using 1 ml of *water R*. After 15 min of incubation the blank solution is colourless and the test solution is blue.

TESTS

Loss on drying (*2.2.32*). Not more than 5.0 per cent, determined on 0.500 g by drying at 60 °C over *diphosphorus pentoxide R* at a pressure not exceeding 670 Pa for 4 h.

Monographs P

Microbial contamination. Total viable aerobic count (*2.6.12*) not more than 10^4 micro-organisms per gram, determined by plate-count. It complies with the tests for *Escherichia coli* and *Salmonella* (*2.6.13*).

ASSAY

The activity of pepsin powder is determined by comparing the quantity of peptides, non-precipitable by *trichloroacetic acid solution R* and assayed using the *phosphomolybdotungstic reagent R*, which are released per minute from a substrate of *haemoglobin solution R*, with the quantity of such peptides released by *pepsin powder BRP* from the same substrate in the same conditions.

For the test solution and the reference solution, prepare the solution and carry out the dilution at 0 °C to 4 °C.

Avoid shaking and foaming during preparation of the test and reference solutions.

Test solution. Immediately before use, prepare a solution of the substance to be examined expected to contain 0.5 Ph. Eur. U./ml in *dilute hydrochloric acid R2*; before dilution to volume, adjust to pH 1.6 ± 0.1, if necessary, using *1 M hydrochloric acid.*

Reference solution. Less than 15 min before use, prepare a solution of *pepsin powder BRP* containing 0.5 Ph. Eur. U./ml in *dilute hydrochloric acid R2*; before dilution to volume, adjust to pH 1.6 ± 0.1, if necessary, using *1 M hydrochloric acid.*

Designate tubes in duplicate T, T_b, S_1, S_{1b}, S_2, S_{2b}, S_3, S_{3b}; designate a tube B.

Add *dilute hydrochloric acid R2* to the tubes as follows:

B: 1.0 ml

S_1 and S_{1b}: 0.5 ml

S_2, S_{2b} and T and T_b: 0.25 ml

Add the reference solution to the tubes as follows:

S_1 and S_{1b}: 0.5 ml

S_2 and S_{2b}: 0.75 ml

S_3 and S_{3b}: 1.0 ml

Add 0.75 ml of the test solution to tubes T and T_b.

Add 10.0 ml of *trichloroacetic acid solution R* to tubes S_{1b}, S_{2b}, S_{3b}, T_b and B. Mix by shaking.

Place the tubes and *haemoglobin solution R* in a water bath at 25 ± 0.1 °C. When temperature equilibrium is reached, add 5.0 ml of *haemoglobin solution R* to tubes B, S_{1b}, S_{2b}, S_{3b} and T_b. Mix.

At time zero add 5.0 ml of *haemoglobin solution R* successively and at intervals of 30 s to tubes S_1, S_2, S_3 and T. Mix immediately after each addition.

Exactly 10 min after adding the *haemoglobin solution R*, stop the reaction by adding, at intervals of 30 s, 10.0 ml of *trichloroacetic acid solution R* to tubes S_1, S_2, S_3 and T (the use of a fast-flowing or blow-out pipette is recommended) and mix.

Filter the contents of each tube (samples and blanks) twice through the same suitable filter paper previously washed with a 50 g/l solution of *trichloroacetic acid R*, then with *water R* and dried. Discard the first 5 ml of filtrate. Place 3.0 ml of each filtrate separately in a tube containing 20 ml of *water R*. Mix.

A suitable filter paper complies with the following test: filter 5 ml of a 50 g/l solution of *trichloroacetic acid R* through a 7 cm disc of white filter paper: the absorbance (*2.2.25*) of the filtrate, measured at 275 nm using unfiltered *trichloroacetic acid R* solution as the compensation liquid, is less than 0.04.

Add to each tube 1.0 ml of *sodium hydroxide solution R* and 1.0 ml of *phosphomolybdotungstic reagent R*, beginning with the blanks and then the samples of each set, in a known order.

A schematic presentation of the above operations is shown in Table 0682.-1.

After 15 min measure the absorbance (*2.2.25*) of solutions S_1, S_2, S_3, S_{1b}, S_{2b}, S_{3b} and T at 540 nm using the filtrate obtained from tube B as the compensation liquid. Correct the average absorbance values for the filtrates obtained from tubes S_1, S_2 and S_3 by subtracting the average values obtained for the filtrates from tubes S_{1b}, S_{2b}, S_{3b} respectively.

Draw a calibration curve of the corrected values against volume of reference solution used. Determine the activity of the substance to be examined using the corrected absorbance for the test solution ($T - T_b$) together with the calibration curve and taking into account the dilution factors.

Table 0682.-1

	Tubes								
	S_1	S_{1b}	S_2	S_{2b}	S_3	S_{3b}	T	T_b	B
Dilute hydrochloric acid R2 (ml)	0.5	0.5	0.25	0.25			0.25	0.25	1.0
Reference solution (ml)	0.5	0.5	0.75	0.75	1.0	1.0			
Test solution (ml)							0.75	0.75	
Trichloroacetic acid solution R (ml)		10.0		10.0		10.0		10.0	10.0
Mix		+		+		+		+	+
Water bath at 25 °C	+	+	+	+	+	+	+	+	+
Haemoglobin solution R (ml)		5.0		5.0		5.0		5.0	5.0
Mix		+		+		+		+	+
Haemoglobin solution R (ml)	5.0		5.0		5.0		5.0		
Mix	+		+		+		+		
Water bath at 25 °C, 10 min	+	+	+	+	+	+	+	+	+
Trichloroacetic acid solution R (ml)	10.0		10.0		10.0		10.0		
Mix	+		+		+		+		
Filter	+	+	+	+	+	+	+	+	+

STORAGE

Store in an airtight container, protected from light, at a temperature of 2 °C to 8 °C.

LABELLING

The label states the activity in European Pharmacopoeia Units per milligram.

01/2005:1555

PERGOLIDE MESILATE

Pergolidi mesilas

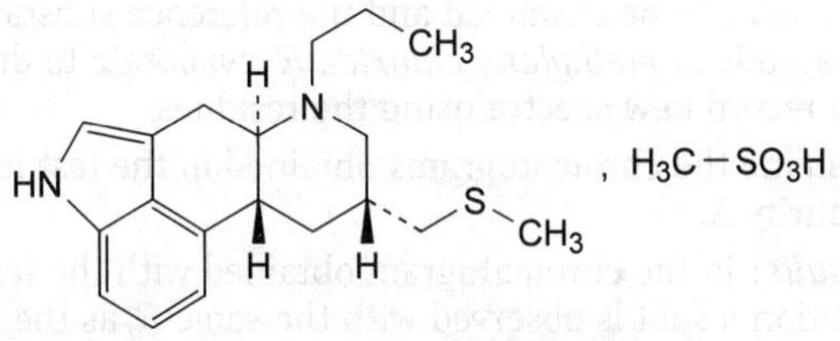

$C_{20}H_{30}N_2O_3S_2$ M_r 410.6

DEFINITION

Pergolide mesilate contains not less than 97.5 per cent and not more than 102.0 per cent of (6a*R*,9*R*,10a*R*)-9-[(methylsulphanyl)methyl]-7-propyl-4,6,6a,7,8,9,10,10a-octahydroindolo[4,3-*fg*]quinoline monomethanesulphonate, calculated with reference to the dried substance.

PRODUCTION

The production method must be evaluated to determine the potential for formation of alkyl mesilates, which is particularly likely to occur if the reaction medium contains lower alcohols. Where necessary, the production method is validated to demonstrate that alkyl mesilates are not detectable in the final product.

CHARACTERS

A white or almost white, crystalline powder, slightly soluble in water, sparingly soluble in methanol, slightly soluble in alcohol and in methylene chloride, very slightly soluble in acetone.

IDENTIFICATION

A. The specific optical rotation (*2.2.7*) is − 17 to − 23, calculated with reference to the dried substance and determined on a solution prepared as follows: dissolve 0.25 g in *dimethylformamide R* and dilute to 25.0 ml with the same solvent.

B. Examine by infrared absorption spectrophotometry (*2.2.24*), comparing with the spectrum obtained with *pergolide mesilate CRS*. Examine the substances prepared as discs.

TESTS

Related substances. Examine by liquid chromatography (*2.2.29*).

Test solution. Dissolve 30.0 mg of the substance to be examined in *methanol R* and dilute to 10.0 ml with the same solvent.

Reference solution (a). Dilute 1.0 ml of the test solution to 100.0 ml with *methanol R*. Dilute 1.0 ml of this solution to 10.0 ml with *methanol R*.

Reference solution (b). Dissolve 10 mg of *4,4′-dimethoxybenzophenone R* in *methanol R* and dilute to 10 ml with the same solvent. To 1 ml of this solution add 2 ml of the test solution and dilute to 100 ml with *methanol R*. Dilute 1 ml of this solution to 10 ml with *methanol R*.

The chromatographic procedure may be carried out using:
- a stainless steel column 0.25 m long and 4.6 mm in internal diameter packed with *base-deactivated octadecylsilyl silica gel for chromatography R* (5 µm),
- as mobile phase at a flow rate of 1 ml/min:

  Mobile phase A. Mix 5.0 ml of *morpholine for chromatography R* with 995 ml of *water R* and adjust to pH 7.0 with *phosphoric acid R*. Use within 24 h,

  Mobile phase B. Mix equal volumes of *acetonitrile R*, *methanol R* and *tetrahydrofuran R*,

Time (min)	Mobile phase A (per cent *V/V*)	Mobile phase B (per cent *V/V*)	Comment
0 - 35	70 → 0	30 → 100	linear gradient
35 - 40	0 → 70	100 → 30	return to initial conditions
40 - 50	70	30	re-equilibration

- as detector a spectrophotometer set at 280 nm,

maintaining the temperature of the column at 40 °C.

Adjust the sensitivity of the system so that the height of the principal peak in the chromatogram obtained with 20 µl of reference solution (a) is at least 90 per cent of the full scale of the recorder.

Inject 20 µl of reference solution (b). The test is not valid unless, in the chromatogram obtained, the resolution between the peaks corresponding to 4,4′-dimethoxybenzophenone (first peak) and pergolide (second peak) is at least 2.0.

Inject 20 µl of the test solution and 20 µl of reference solution (a).

In the chromatogram obtained with the test solution: the area of any peak, apart from the principal peak, is not greater than the area of the principal peak in the chromatogram obtained with reference solution (a) (0.1 per cent); the sum of the areas of all the peaks, apart from the principal peak, is not greater than 5 times the area of the principal peak in the chromatogram obtained with reference solution (a) (0.5 per cent). Disregard any peak with an area less than 0.2 times that of the principal peak in the chromatogram obtained with reference solution (a) (0.02 per cent).

Loss on drying (*2.2.32*). Not more than 0.5 per cent, determined on 1.000 g by drying *in vacuo* at 100-105 °C for 1 h.

Sulphated ash (*2.4.14*). Not more than 0.1 per cent, determined on 1.0 g.

ASSAY

Examine by liquid chromatography (*2.2.29*).

Solution A. Dissolve 5.0 mg of *DL-methionine R* in 500 ml of *0.01 M hydrochloric acid*. Add 500 ml of *methanol R* and mix.

Test solution. Dissolve 65.0 mg of the substance to be examined in solution A and dilute to 100.0 ml with the same solution. Dilute 10.0 ml to 100.0 ml with solution A.

Reference solution. Dissolve 65.0 mg of *pergolide mesilate CRS* in solution A and dilute to 100.0 ml with the same solution. Dilute 10.0 ml to 100.0 ml with solution A.

The chromatographic procedure may be carried out using:
- a stainless steel column 0.25 m long and 4.6 mm in internal diameter packed with *base-deactivated octylsilyl silica gel for chromatography R* (5 µm),

Monographs P

- as mobile phase at a flow rate of 1 ml/min a mixture of 1 volume of *acetonitrile R*, 1 volume of *methanol R* and 2 volumes of a mixture prepared as follows: dissolve 2.0 g of *sodium octanesulphonate R* in *water R*, add 1.0 ml of *anhydrous acetic acid R* and dilute to 1000 ml with *water R*,
- as detector a spectrophotometer set at 280 nm,

maintaining the temperature of the column at 40 °C.

Inject 20 µl of the reference solution. When the chromatogram is recorded in the prescribed conditions, the retention time of pergolide is about 9 min. Adjust the sensitivity of the system so that the height of the principal peak in the chromatogram obtained with the reference solution is at least 50 per cent of the full scale of the recorder.

The assay is not valid unless the symmetry factor of the peak due to pergolide is at most 1.5.

Inject 20 µl of the test solution.

Calculate the percentage content of $C_{20}H_{30}N_2O_3S_2$ from the areas of the peaks and the declared content of *pergolide mesilate CRS*.

STORAGE

Store protected from light.

IMPURITIES

Specified impurities: A.

Other detectable impurities: B.

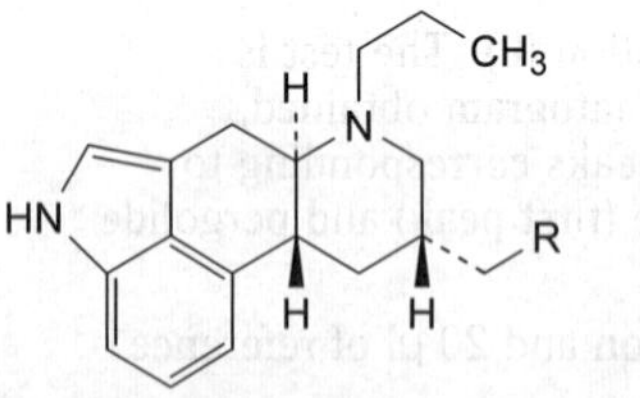

A. R = SO-CH_3: (6a*R*,9*R*,10a*R*)-9-[(methylsulphinyl)methyl]-7-propyl-4,6,6a,7,8,9,10,10a-octahydroindolo[4,3-*fg*]quinoline (pergolide sulphoxide),

B. R = SO_2-CH_3: (6a*R*,9*R*,10a*R*)-9-[(methylsulphonyl)methyl]-7-propyl-4,6,6a,7,8,9,10,10a-octahydroindolo[4,3-*fg*]quinoline (pergolide sulphone).

01/2005:2019

PERINDOPRIL *tert*-BUTYLAMINE

tert-Butylamini perindoprilum

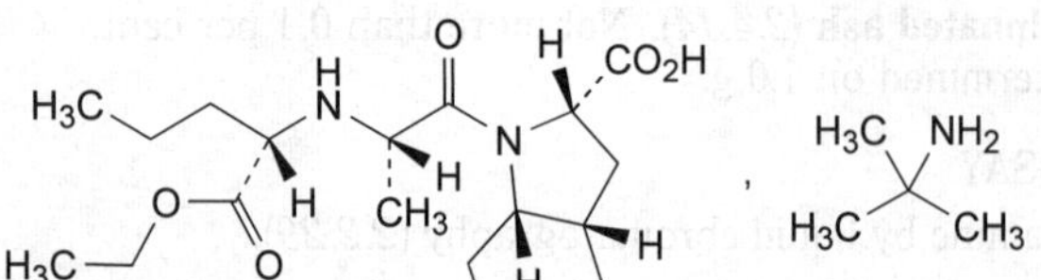

$C_{23}H_{43}N_3O_5$ M_r 441.6

DEFINITION

2-Methylpropan-2-amine (2*S*,3a*S*,7a*S*)-1-[(2*S*)-2-[[(1*S*)-1-(ethoxycarbonyl)butyl]amino]propanoyl]octahydro-1*H*-indole-2-carboxylate.

Content: 99.0 per cent to 101.0 per cent (anhydrous substance).

CHARACTERS

Appearance: white or almost white, crystalline powder, slightly hygroscopic.

Solubility: freely soluble in water and in alcohol, sparingly soluble in methylene chloride.

It shows polymorphism.

IDENTIFICATION

A. Specific optical rotation (*2.2.7*): − 66 to − 69 (anhydrous substance).

Dissolve 0.250 g in *alcohol R* and dilute to 25.0 ml with the same solvent.

B. Infrared absorption spectrophotometry (*2.2.24*).

Preparation: discs.

Comparison: *perindopril tert-butylamine CRS.*

If the spectra obtained show differences, dissolve the substance to be examined and the reference substance separately in *methylene chloride R*, evaporate to dryness and record new spectra using the residues.

C. Examine the chromatograms obtained in the test for impurity A.

Results: in the chromatogram obtained with the test solution a spot is observed with the same R_f as the spot with the higher R_f in the chromatogram with reference solution (c) (*tert*-butylamine).

TESTS

Impurity A. Thin-layer chromatography (*2.2.27*).

Test solution. Dissolve 0.20 g of the substance to be examined in *methanol R* and dilute to 10 ml with the same solvent.

Reference solution (a). Dissolve 5 mg of *perindopril impurity A CRS* in *methanol R* and dilute to 25.0 ml with the same solvent.

Reference solution (b). Dilute 5 ml of reference solution (a) to 20 ml with *methanol R.*

Reference solution (c). To 5 ml of reference solution (a) add 5 ml of a 20 g/l solution of *1,1-dimethylethylamine R* in *methanol R.*

Plate: *TLC silica gel plate R.*

Mobile phase: *glacial acetic acid R, toluene R, methanol R* (1:40:60 *V/V/V*).

Application: 10 µl; apply the test solution and reference solutions (b) and (c).

Development: in a saturated tank, over 2/3 of the plate.

Drying: in a current of warm air.

Detection: expose to iodine vapour for at least 20 h.

System suitability: the chromatogram obtained with reference solution (c) shows 2 clearly separated spots.

Limit:

- *impurity A*: any spot due to impurity A is not more intense than the spot in the chromatogram obtained with reference solution (b) (0.25 per cent).

Stereochemical purity. Liquid chromatography (*2.2.29*).

Test solution. Dissolve 20 mg of the substance to be examined in *alcohol R* and dilute to 10.0 ml with the same solvent.

Reference solution (a). Dilute 1.0 ml of the test solution to 200.0 ml with *alcohol R.*

Reference solution (b). Dissolve 10 mg of *perindopril for stereochemical purity CRS* in *alcohol R* and dilute to 5.0 ml with the same solvent.

Reference solution (c). Dilute 10.0 ml of reference solution (a) to 50.0 ml with *alcohol R.*

Column:

- *size*: *l* = 0.25 m, Ø = 4.6 mm,

– *stationary phase*: spherical *octadecylsilyl silica gel for chromatography R* (5 µm) with a specific surface area of 450 m^2/g and a pore size of 10 nm,

– *temperature*: 50 °C for the column and at least 30 cm of the tubing preceding the column.

Mobile phase: mix, in the following order, 21.7 volumes of *acetonitrile R*, 0.3 volumes of *pentanol R* and 78 volumes of a 1.50 g/l solution of *sodium heptanesulphonate R*, previously adjusted to pH 2.0 with a mixture of equal volumes of *perchloric acid R* and *water R*.

Flow rate: 0.8 ml/min.

Detection: spectrophotometer at 215 nm.

Equilibration: minimum 4 h.

Injection: 10 µl.

Run time: 1.5 times the retention time of perindopril.

Retention time: perindopril = about 100 min.

System suitability:
– *signal-to-noise ratio*: minimum 3 for the principal peak in the chromatogram obtained with reference solution (c),

– *peak-to-valley ratio*: minimum 3, where H_p = height above the baseline of the peak due to impurity I and H_v = height above the baseline of the lowest point of the curve separating this peak from the peak due to perindopril in the chromatogram obtained with reference solution (b),

– the chromatogram obtained with reference solution (b) is similar to the chromatogram provided with *perindopril for stereochemical purity CRS*.

Limits:
– *any impurity*: not more than 0.2 times the area of the principal peak in the chromatogram obtained with reference solution (a) (0.1 per cent); disregard any peak with a retention time less than 0.6 times the retention time of perindopril and any peak with a retention time greater than 1.4 times the retention time of perindopril.

Related subtances. Liquid chromatography (*2.2.29*).

Test solution. Dissolve 60 mg of the substance to be examined in mobile phase A and dilute to 20.0 ml with mobile phase A.

Reference solution (a). Dissolve 15 mg of *perindopril for system suitability CRS* in mobile phase A and dilute to 5.0 ml with mobile phase A.

Reference solution (b). Dilute 1.0 ml of the test solution to 200.0 ml with mobile phase A.

Column:

– *size*: l = 0.25 m, Ø = 4 mm,

– *stationary phase*: spherical *octylsilyl silica gel for chromatography R* (4 µm) with a pore size of 6 nm,

– *temperature*: 70 °C.

Mobile phase:

– *mobile phase A*: dissolve 0.92 g of *sodium heptanesulphonate R* in 1000 ml of *water R*, add 1 ml of *triethylamine R* and adjust to pH 2.0 with a mixture of equal volumes of *perchloric acid R* and *water R*,

– *mobile phase B*: *acetonitrile R1*,

Time (min)	Mobile phase A (per cent *V/V*)	Mobile phase B (per cent *V/V*)
0 - 1	70	30
1 - 20	70 → 40	30 → 60
20 - 25	40	60
25 - 35	40 → 20	60 → 80
35 - 40	20 → 0	80 → 100
40 - 45	0 → 70	100 → 30

Flow rate: 1.5 ml/min.

Detection: spectrophotometer at 215 nm.

Injection: 20 µl.

Relative retention with reference to perindopril (retention time = about 8 min): impurity B = about 0.4; impurity C = about 0.8; impurity D = about 0.9; impurity E = about 1.4; impurity F = about 1.7; impurity G = about 2.2 and 2.3; impurity H = about 3.6 and 3.7.

System suitability: reference solution (a):

– *peak-to-valley ratio*: minimum 10, where H_p = height above the baseline of the peak due to impurity D and H_v = height above the baseline of the lowest point of the curve separating this peak from the peak due to perindopril.

Limits:

– *impurity B*: not more than 0.6 times the area of the principal peak in the chromatogram obtained with reference solution (b) (0.3 per cent),

– *impurity E*: not more than 0.8 times the area of the principal peak in the chromatogram obtained with reference solution (b) (0.4 per cent),

– *impurities F, H*: for each impurity, not more than 0.4 times the area of the principal peak in the chromatogram obtained with reference solution (b) (0.2 per cent),

– *any other impurity*: not more than 0.2 times the area of the principal peak in the chromatogram obtained with reference solution (b) (0.1 per cent),

– *total*: not more than twice the area of the principal peak in the chromatogram obtained with reference solution (b) (1 per cent),

– *disregard limit*: 0.1 times the area of the principal peak in the chromatogram obtained with reference solution (b) (0.05 per cent).

Water (*2.5.12*): maximum 1.0 per cent, determined on 0.50 g.

Sulphated ash (*2.4.14*): maximum 0.1 per cent, determined on 1.0 g.

ASSAY

Dissolve 0.160 g in 50 ml of *anhydrous acetic acid R*. Titrate with *0.1 M perchloric acid*, determining the end-point potentiometrically (*2.2.20*).

1 ml of *0.1 M perchloric acid* is equivalent to 22.08 mg of $C_{23}H_{43}N_3O_5$.

STORAGE

In an airtight container.

IMPURITIES

Specified impurities: A, B, E, F, H, I.

Other detectable impurities: C, D, G.

Monographs P

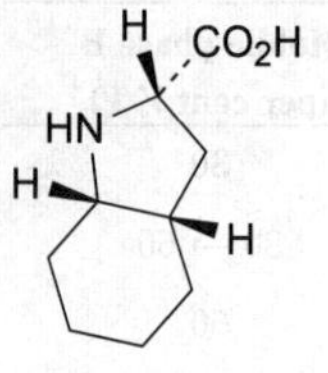

A. (2*S*,3a*S*,7a*S*)-octahydro-1*H*-indole-2-carboxylic acid,

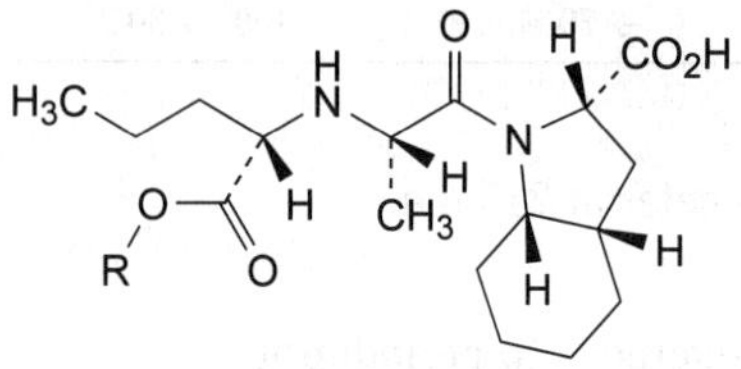

B. R = H: (2*S*,3a*S*,7a*S*)-1-[(2*S*)-2-[[(1*S*)-1-carboxybutyl]amino]propanoyl]octahydro-1*H*-indole-2-carboxylic acid,

E. R = $CH(CH_3)_2$: (2*S*,3a*S*,7a*S*)-1-[(2*S*)-2-[[(1*S*)-1-[(1-methylethoxy)carbonyl]butyl]amino]propanoyl]octahydro-1*H*-indole-2-carboxylic acid,

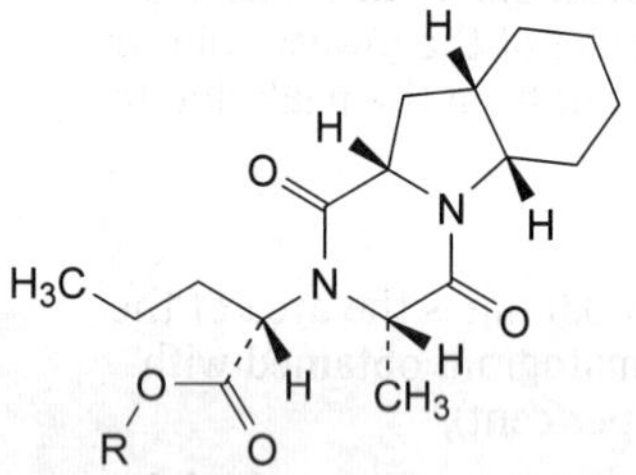

C. R = H: (2*S*)-2-[(3*S*,5a*S*,9a*S*,10a*S*)-3-methyl-1,4-dioxodecahydropyrazino[1,2-*a*]indol-2(1*H*)-yl]pentanoic acid,

F. R = C_2H_5: ethyl (2*S*)-2-[(3*S*,5a*S*,9a*S*,10a*S*)-3-methyl-1,4-dioxodecahydropyrazino[1,2-*a*]indol-2(1*H*)-yl]pentanoate,

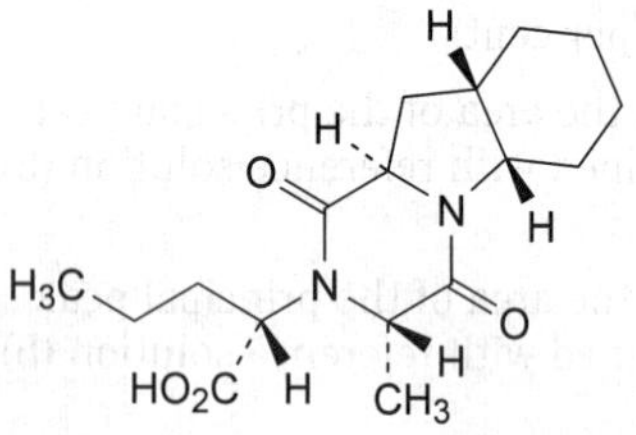

D. (2*S*)-2-[(3*S*,5a*S*,9a*S*,10a*R*)-3-methyl-1,4-dioxodecahydropyrazino[1,2-*a*]indol-2(1*H*)-yl]pentanoic acid,

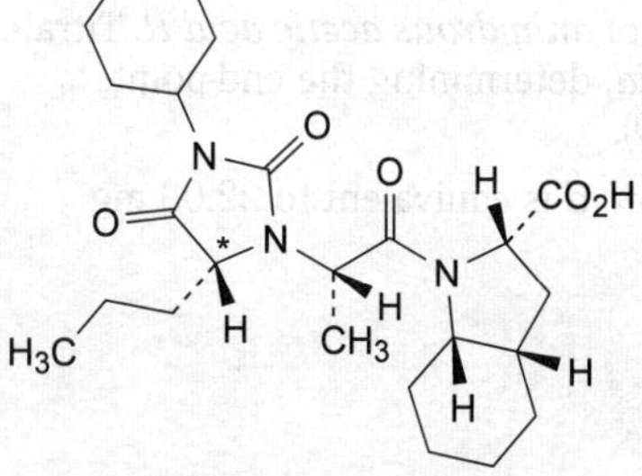

and epimer at C*

G. (2*S*,3a*S*,7a*S*)-1-[(2*S*)-2-[(5*RS*)-3-cyclohexyl-2,4-dioxo-5-propylimidazolidin-1-yl]propanoyl]octahydro-1*H*-indole-2-carboxylic acid,

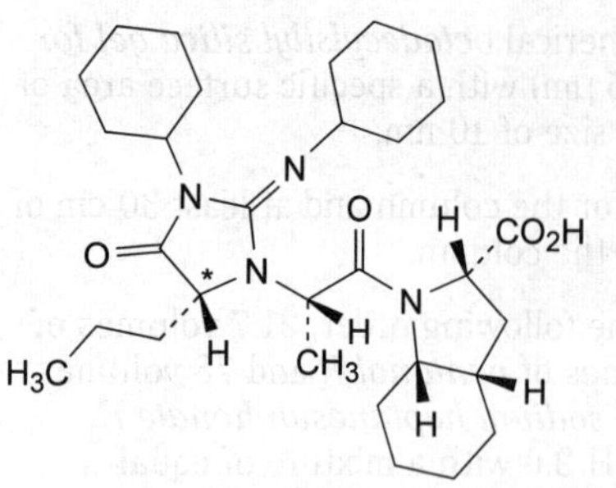

and epimer at C*

H. (2*S*,3a*S*,7a*S*)-1-[(2*S*)-2-[(5*RS*)-3-cyclohexyl-2-(cyclohexylimino)-4-oxo-5-propylimidazolidin-1-yl]propanoyl]octahydro-1*H*-indole-2-carboxylic acid,

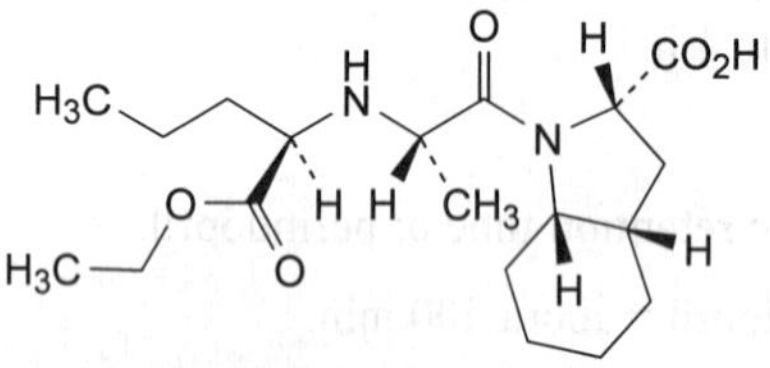

I. (2*S*,3a*S*,7a*S*)-1-[(2*S*)-2-[[(1*R*)-1-(ethoxycarbonyl)butyl]amino]propanoyl]octahydro-1*H*-indole-2-carboxylic acid.

01/2005:0862

PERITONEAL DIALYSIS, SOLUTIONS FOR

Solutiones ad peritonealem dialysim

DEFINITION

Solutions for peritoneal dialysis are preparations for intraperitoneal use containing electrolytes with a concentration close to the electrolytic composition of plasma. They contain glucose in varying concentrations or other suitable osmotic agents.

Solutions for peritoneal dialysis are supplied in:

– rigid or semi-rigid plastic containers,
– flexible plastic containers fitted with a special connecting device; these are generally filled to a volume below their nominal capacity and presented in closed protective envelopes,
– glass containers.

The containers and closures comply with the requirements for containers for preparations for parenteral use (*3.2.1* and *3.2.2*).

Several formulations are used. The concentrations of the components per litre of solution are usually in the following range:

Table 0862.-1

	Expression in mmol	Expression in mEq
Sodium	125 - 150	125 - 150
Potassium	0 - 4.5	0 - 4.5
Calcium	0 - 2.5	0 - 5.0
Magnesium	0.25 - 1.5	0.50 - 3.0
Acetate and/or lactate and/or hydrogen carbonate	30 - 60	30 - 60
Chloride	90 - 120	90 - 120
Glucose	25 - 250	

Monographs P

When hydrogen carbonate is present, the solution of sodium hydrogen carbonate is supplied in a container or a separate compartment and is added to the electrolyte solution immediately before use.

Unless otherwise justified and authorised, antioxidants such as metabisulphite salts are not added to the solutions.

IDENTIFICATION

According to the stated composition, the solution to be examined gives the following identification reactions (*2.3.1*):

- potassium: reaction (b);
- calcium: reaction (a);
- sodium: reaction (b);
- chlorides: reaction (a);
- acetates: to 5 ml of the solution to be examined add 1 ml of *hydrochloric acid R* in a test-tube fitted with a stopper and a bent tube, heat and collect a few millilitres of distillate; carry out reaction (b) of acetates on the distillate;
- lactates, hydrogen carbonates; the identification is carried out together with the assay;
- magnesium: to 0.1 ml of *titan yellow solution R* add 10 ml of *water R*, 2 ml of the solution to be examined and 1 ml of *1 M sodium hydroxide*; a pink colour is produced;
- glucose: to 5 ml of the solution to be examined, add 2 ml of *dilute sodium hydroxide solution R* and 0.05 ml of *copper sulphate solution R*; the solution is blue and clear; heat to boiling; an abundant red precipitate is formed.

TESTS

Appearance of solution. The solution is clear (*2.2.1*) and not more intensely coloured than reference solution Y_4 (*2.2.2, Method I*).

pH (*2.2.3*). The pH of the solution is 5.0 to 6.5. If the solution contains hydrogen carbonate, the pH is 6.5 to 8.0.

Hydroxymethylfurfural. To a volume of the solution containing the equivalent of 25 mg of glucose, add 5.0 ml of a 100 g/l solution of *p-toluidine R* in *2-propanol R* containing 10 per cent *V/V* of *glacial acetic acid R* and 1.0 ml of a 5 g/l solution of *barbituric acid R*. The absorbance (*2.2.25*) determined at 550 nm after allowing the mixture to stand for 2 min to 3 min is not greater than that of a standard prepared at the same time in the same manner using a solution containing 10 µg of *hydroxymethylfurfural R* in the same volume as the solution to be examined. If the solution contains hydrogen carbonate, use as the standard a solution containing 20 µg of *hydroxymethylfurfural R*.

Aluminium (*2.4.17*). Take 400 ml, adjust to pH 6.0 and add 10 ml of *acetate buffer solution pH 6.0 R*. The solution complies with the limit test for aluminium (15 µg/l). Use as the reference solution a mixture of 3 ml of *aluminium standard solution (2 ppm Al) R*, 10 ml of *acetate buffer solution pH 6.0 R* and 9 ml of *water R*. To prepare the blank use a mixture of 10 ml of *acetate buffer solution pH 6.0 R* and 10 ml of *water R*.

Particulate contamination. Carry out the test for sub-visible particles (*2.9.19*) using 50 ml of solution.

Table 0862.-2

Particles larger than	10 µm	25 µm
Maximum number of particles per millilitre	25	3

Extractable volume (*2.9.17*). The solution complies with the test prescribed for parenteral infusions.

Sterility (*2.6.1*). The solution complies with the test for sterility.

Bacterial endotoxins (*2.6.14*): less than 0.25 IU/ml.

Pyrogens (*2.6.8*). Solutions for which a validated test for bacterial endotoxins cannot be carried out comply with the test for pyrogens. Inject per kilogram of the rabbit's mass 10 ml of the solution.

ASSAY

Sodium: 97.5 per cent to 102.5 per cent of the content of sodium (Na) stated on the label, determined by atomic absorption spectrometry (*2.2.23, Method II*).

Test solution. If necessary, dilute the solution to be examined with *water R* to a concentration suitable for the instrument to be used.

Reference solutions. Prepare the reference solutions using *sodium standard solution (200 ppm Na) R*.

Measure the absorbance at 589.0 nm using a sodium hollow-cathode lamp as source of radiation and an air-propane or an air-acetylene flame.

Potassium. 95.0 per cent to 105.0 per cent of the content of potassium (K) stated on the label, determined by atomic absorption spectrometry (*2.2.23, Method I*).

Test solution. If necessary, dilute the solution to be examined with *water R* to a concentration suitable for the instrument to be used. To 100 ml of the solution add 10 ml of a 22 g/l solution of *sodium chloride R*.

Reference solutions. Prepare the reference solutions using *potassium standard solution (100 ppm K) R*. To 100 ml of each reference solution add 10 ml of a 22 g/l solution of *sodium chloride R*.

Measure the absorbance at 766.5 nm, using a potassium hollow-cathode lamp as source of radiation and an air-propane or an air-acetylene flame.

Calcium. 95.0 per cent to 105.0 per cent of the content of calcium (Ca) stated on the label, determined by atomic absorption spectrometry (*2.2.23, Method I*).

Test solution. If necessary, dilute the solution to be examined with *water R* to a concentration suitable for the instrument to be used.

Reference solutions. Prepare the reference solutions using *calcium standard solution (400 ppm Ca) R*.

Measure the absorbance at 422.7 nm using a calcium hollow-cathode lamp as source of radiation and an air-propane or an air-acetylene flame.

Magnesium: 95.0 per cent to 105.0 per cent of the content of magnesium (Mg) stated on the label, determined by atomic absorption spectrometry (*2.2.23, Method I*).

Test solution. If necessary, dilute the solution to be examined with *water R* to a concentration suitable for the instrument to be used.

Reference solutions. Prepare the reference solutions using *magnesium standard solution (100 ppm Mg) R*.

Measure the absorbance at 285.2 nm using a magnesium hollow-cathode lamp as source of radiation and an air-propane or an air-acetylene flame.

Total chloride. 95.0 per cent to 105.0 per cent of the content of chloride (Cl) stated on the label. Dilute to 50 ml with *water R* an accurately measured volume of the solution to be examined containing the equivalent of about 60 mg of chloride. Add 5 ml of *dilute nitric acid R*, 25.0 ml of *0.1 M silver nitrate* and 2 ml of *dibutyl phthalate R*. Shake.

Monographs P

Using 2 ml of *ferric ammonium sulphate solution R2* as indicator, titrate with *0.1 M ammonium thiocyanate* until a reddish-yellow colour is obtained.

1 ml of *0.1 M silver nitrate* is equivalent to 3.545 mg of Cl.

Acetate: 95.0 per cent to 105.0 per cent of the content of acetate stated on the label. To a volume of the solution to be examined, corresponding to about 0.7 mmol of acetate, add 10.0 ml of *0.1 M hydrochloric acid.* Carry out a potentiometric titration (*2.2.20*), using *0.1 M sodium hydroxide.* Read the volume added between the two points of inflexion.

1 ml of *0.1 M sodium hydroxide* is equivalent to 0.1 mmol of acetate.

Lactate: 95.0 per cent to 105.0 per cent of the content of lactate stated on the label. To a volume of the solution to be examined, corresponding to about 0.7 mmol of lactate, add 10.0 ml of *0.1 M hydrochloric acid.* Then add 50 ml of *acetonitrile R.* Carry out a potentiometric titration (*2.2.20*), using *0.1 M sodium hydroxide.* Read the volume added between the two points of inflexion.

1 ml of *0.1 M sodium hydroxide* is equivalent to 0.1 mmol of lactate.

Sodium hydrogen carbonate: 95.0 per cent to 105.0 per cent of the content of sodium hydrogen carbonate stated on the label. Titrate with *0.1 M hydrochloric acid,* a volume of the solution to be examined corresponding to about 0.1 g of sodium hydrogen carbonate, determining the end-point potentiometrically (*2.2.20*).

1 ml of *0.1 M hydrochloric acid* is equivalent to 8.40 mg of $NaHCO_3$.

Lactate and hydrogen carbonate: 95.0 per cent to 105.0 per cent of the content of lactates and/or hydrogen carbonates stated on the label. Examine by liquid chromatography (*2.2.29*).

Test solution. Solution to be examined.

Reference solution. Dissolve in 100 ml of *water for chromatography R* quantities of lactates and hydrogen carbonates, accurately weighed, in order to obtain solutions having concentrations representing about 90 per cent, 100 per cent and 110 per cent of the concentrations indicated on the label.

The chromatographic procedure may be carried out using:

- a column 0.30 m long and 7.8 mm in internal diameter packed with *cation exchange resin R* (9 μm),
- as mobile phase at a flow rate of 0.6 ml/min *0.005 M sulphuric acid* previously degassed with *helium R,*
- a differential refractometer detector,

maintaining the temperature of the column at 85 °C.

Inject in duplicate 20 μl of test solution and 20 μl of each reference solution. When the chromatograms are recorded in the prescribed conditions, the peaks elute in the following order: lactates then hydrogen carbonates.

Determine the concentration of lactates and hydrogen carbonates in the test solution by interpolating the peak area for lactate and the peak height for hydrogen carbonate from the linear regression curve obtained with the reference solutions.

Reducing sugars (expressed as anhydrous glucose). 95.0 per cent to 105.0 per cent of the content of glucose stated on the label. Transfer a volume of solution to be examined containing the equivalent of 25 mg of glucose to a 250 ml conical flask with a ground-glass neck and add 25.0 ml of *cupri-citric solution R.* Add a few grains of pumice, fit a reflux condenser, heat so that boiling occurs within 2 min and boil for exactly 10 min. Cool and add 3 g of *potassium iodide R* dissolved in 3 ml of *water R.* Carefully add, in small amounts, 25 ml of a 25 per cent *m/m* solution of *sulphuric acid R.* Titrate with *0.1 M sodium thiosulphate* using *starch solution R,* added towards the end of the titration, as indicator. Carry out a blank titration using 25.0 ml of *water R.*

Calculate the content of reducing sugars expressed as anhydrous glucose ($C_6H_{12}O_6$), by means of Table 0862.-3:

Table 0862.-3

Volume of 0.1 M sodium thiosulphate (ml)	Anhydrous glucose (mg)
8	19.8
9	22.4
10	25.0
11	27.6
12	30.3
13	33.0
14	35.7
15	38.5
16	41.3

STORAGE

Store at a temperature not below 4 °C.

LABELLING

The label states:

- the formula of the solution for peritoneal dialysis, expressed in grams per litre and in millimoles per litre,
- the calculated osmolarity, expressed in milliosmoles per litre,
- the nominal volume of the solution for peritoneal dialysis in the container,
- that the solution is free from bacterial endotoxins, or where applicable, that it is apyrogenic,
- the storage conditions,
- that the solution is not to be used for intravenous infusion,
- that any unused portion of solution is to be discarded.

01/2005:0629

PERPHENAZINE

Perphenazinum

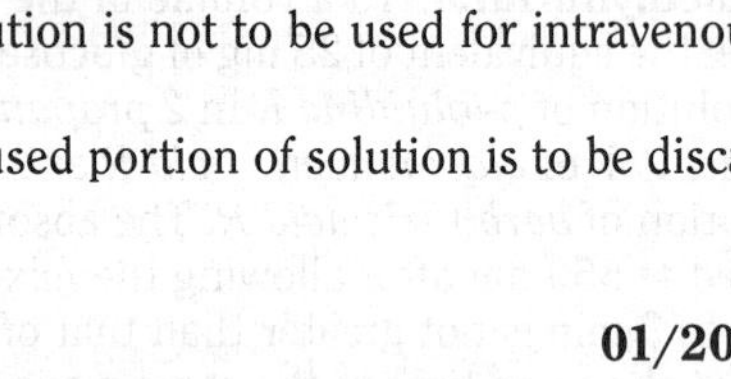

$C_{21}H_{26}ClN_3OS$ M_r 404.0

DEFINITION

Perphenazine contains not less than 99.0 per cent and not more than the equivalent of 101.0 per cent of 2-[4-[3-(2-chlorophenothiazin-10-yl)propyl]piperazin-1-yl]ethanol, calculated with reference to the dried substance.

CHARACTERS

A white or yellowish-white, crystalline powder, practically insoluble in water, freely soluble in methylene chloride, soluble in alcohol. It dissolves in dilute solutions of hydrochloric acid.

IDENTIFICATION

First identification: A, C

Second identification: A, B, D.

A. Melting point (*2.2.14*): 96 °C to 100 °C.

B. Dissolve 10 mg in *methanol R* and dilute to 100 ml with the same solvent. Dilute 10 ml of the solution to 100 ml with *methanol R*. Examined between 230 nm and 350 nm (*2.2.25*), the solution shows two absorption maxima, at 257 nm and 313 nm. The ratio of the absorbance measured at the maximum at 313 nm to that measured at the maximum at 257 nm is 0.120 to 0.128.

C. Examine by infrared absorption spectrophotometry (*2.2.24*), comparing with the spectrum obtained with *perphenazine CRS*. Examine the substances prepared as discs.

D. Examine by thin-layer chromatography (*2.2.27*), using *kieselguhr G R* as the coating substance. Impregnate the plate by placing it in a closed tank containing the necessary quantity of the impregnation mixture containing 2.5 per cent *V/V* of *phenoxyethanol R* and 7.5 per cent *V/V* of *formamide R* in *acetone R* so that the plate dips about 5 mm beneath the surface of the liquid. When the impregnation mixture has risen at least 17 cm from the lower edge of the plate, remove the plate and use immediately for chromatography. Carry out the chromatography in the same direction as the impregnation.

Test solution. Dissolve 20 mg of the substance to be examined in *chloroform R* and dilute to 10 ml with the same solvent.

Reference solution. Dissolve 20 mg of *perphenazine CRS* in *chloroform R* and dilute to 10 ml with the same solvent.

Apply separately to the plate 2 µl of each solution. Develop in the dark over a path of 15 cm using a mixture of 2 volumes of *diethylamine R* and 100 volumes of *light petroleum R*, saturated with phenoxyethanol (add *phenoxyethanol R* - 6 volumes to 8 volumes - to the above mixture of solvents until there is a persistent cloudiness after shaking, decant, and use the supernatant liquid, even if it is cloudy). Expose the plate to ultraviolet light at 365 nm and examine after a few minutes. The principal spot in the chromatogram obtained with the test solution is similar in position, fluorescence and size to the principal spot in the chromatogram obtained with the reference solution. Dry the plate at 120 °C for 20 min, allow to cool and spray with a 10 per cent *V/V* solution of *sulphuric acid R* in *alcohol R*. The principal spot in the chromatogram obtained with the test solution is of the same colour as the principal spot in the chromatogram obtained with the reference solution.

TESTS

Appearance of solution. Dissolve 0.20 g in 10 ml of *methanol R*. The solution is clear (*2.2.1*).

Related substances. Examine by thin-layer chromatography (*2.2.27*), using *silica gel GF_{254} R* as the coating substance. Prepare the solutions immediately before use.

Test solution. Dissolve 0.1 g of the substance to be examined in *methanol R* and dilute to 10 ml with the same solvent.

Reference solution. Dilute 0.5 ml of the test solution to 100 ml with *methanol R*.

Apply separately to the plate 10 µl of each solution. Develop over a path of 15 cm using a mixture of 1 volume of *concentrated ammonia R*, 14 volumes of *water R* and 85 volumes of *butanol R*. Allow the plate to dry in air. Examine in ultraviolet light at 254 nm. Any spot in the chromatogram obtained with the test solution, apart from the principal spot, is not more intense than the spot in the chromatogram obtained with the reference solution (0.5 per cent).

Loss on drying (*2.2.32*). Not more than 0.5 per cent, determined on 1.000 g by drying *in vacuo* at 65 °C for 4 h.

Sulphated ash (*2.4.14*). Not more than 0.1 per cent, determined on 1.0 g.

ASSAY

Dissolve 0.1500 g in 25 ml of *anhydrous acetic acid R*. Titrate with *0.1 M perchloric acid* determining the end-point potentiometrically (*2.2.20*).

1 ml of *0.1 M perchloric acid* is equivalent to 20.20 mg of $C_{21}H_{26}ClN_3OS$.

STORAGE

Store protected from light.

01/2005:0754

PERU BALSAM

Balsamum peruvianum

DEFINITION

Peru balsam is the balsam obtained from the scorched and wounded trunk of *Myroxylon balsamum* (L.) Harms var. *pereirae* (Royle) Harms. It contains not less than 45.0 per cent *m/m* and not more than 70.0 per cent *m/m* of esters, mainly benzyl benzoate and benzyl cinnamate.

CHARACTERS

A dark brown, viscous liquid which is transparent and yellowish-brown when viewed in a thin layer; the liquid is not sticky, it is non-drying and does not form threads; practically insoluble in water, freely soluble in ethanol, not miscible with fatty oils, except for castor oil.

IDENTIFICATION

A. Dissolve 0.20 g in 10 ml of *alcohol R*. Add 0.2 ml of *ferric chloride solution R1*. A green to olive-green colour develops.

B. Examine by thin-layer chromatography (*2.2.27*), using *silica gel GF_{254} R* as the coating substance.

Test solution. Dissolve 0.5 g of the substance to be examined in 10 ml of *ethyl acetate R*.

Reference solution. Dissolve 4 mg of *thymol R*, 30 mg of *benzyl cinnamate R* and 80 µl of *benzyl benzoate R* in 5 ml of *ethyl acetate R*.

Apply separately to the plate as bands 20 mm by 3 mm 10 µl of each solution. Develop twice over a path of 10 cm using a mixture of 0.5 volumes of *glacial acetic acid R*, 10 volumes of *ethyl acetate R* and 90 volumes of *hexane R*. Allow the plate to dry in air, examine in ultraviolet light at 254 nm and mark the quenching zones. The chromatogram obtained with the reference solution shows in the upper third two quenching zones, the higher one corresponding to benzyl benzoate and the lower one to benzyl cinnamate. The chromatogram obtained with the test solution shows two quenching zones at the same levels and of approximately the same size. Spray the plate with a freshly prepared 200 g/l

Monographs P

solution of *phosphomolybdic acid R* in *alcohol R*, using 10 ml for a plate 200 mm square and examine the plate in daylight while heating at 100 °C to 105 °C for 5 min to 10 min. The zones due to benzyl benzoate and benzyl cinnamate are coloured blue against a yellow background. The chromatogram obtained with the reference solution shows at about the middle a violet-grey zone (thymol). In the chromatogram obtained with the test solution, a blue zone (nerolidol) is seen just below the level of the zone due to thymol in the chromatogram obtained with the reference solution. Just below the zone due to nerolidol, no blue zone is seen corresponding to a quenching zone seen when examined in ultraviolet light at 254 nm (colophony). In the upper and lower part of the chromatogram obtained with the test solution, other faint blue zones may be seen.

TESTS

Relative density (*2.2.5*): 1.14 to 1.17.

Saponification value (*2.5.6*): 230 to 255, determined on the residue obtained in the assay.

Artificial balsams. Shake 0.20 g with 6 ml of *light petroleum R1*. The light petroleum solution is clear and colourless and the whole of the insoluble parts of the balsam stick to the wall of the test-tube.

Fatty oils. Shake 1 g with 3 ml of a 1000 g/l solution of *chloral hydrate R*. The resulting solution is as clear as the 1000 g/l solution of *chloral hydrate R*.

Turpentine. Evaporate to dryness 4 ml of the solution obtained in the test for artificial balsams. The residue has no odour of turpentine.

ASSAY

To 2.50 g in a separating funnel add 7.5 ml of *dilute sodium hydroxide solution R* and 40 ml of *peroxide-free ether R* and shake vigorously for 10 min. Separate the lower layer and shake it with three quantities, each of 15 ml, of *peroxide-free ether R*. Combine the ether layers, dry over 10 g of *anhydrous sodium sulphate R* and filter. Wash the sodium sulphate with two quantities, each of 10 ml, of *peroxide-free ether R*. Combine the ether layers and evaporate to dryness. Dry the residue (esters) at 100 °C to 105 °C for 30 min and weigh.

STORAGE

Store protected from light.

01/2005:0420

PETHIDINE HYDROCHLORIDE

Pethidini hydrochloridum

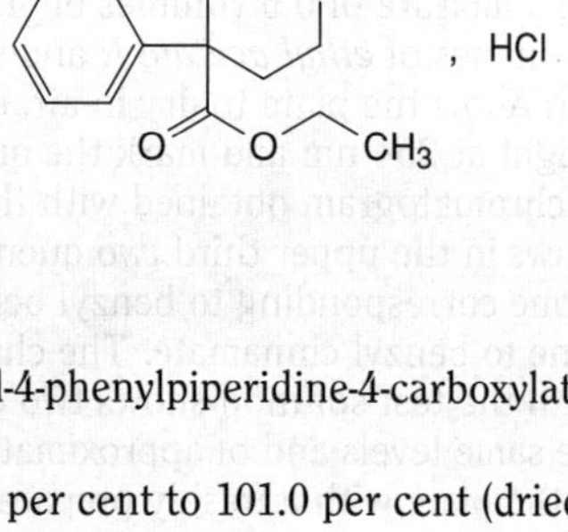

$C_{15}H_{22}ClNO_2$ M_r 283.8

DEFINITION

Ethyl 1-methyl-4-phenylpiperidine-4-carboxylate hydrochloride.

Content: 99.0 per cent to 101.0 per cent (dried substance).

PRODUCTION

If intended for use in the manufacture of parenteral dosage forms, the manufacturing process is validated to show that the content of impurity B is not more than 0.1 ppm.

CHARACTERS

Appearance: white, crystalline powder.

Solubility: very soluble in water, freely soluble in alcohol.

IDENTIFICATION

First identification: B, D.

Second identification: A, C, D.

A. Melting point (*2.2.14*): 187 °C to 190 °C.

B. Infrared absorption spectrophotometry (*2.2.24*).
Comparison: *Ph. Eur. reference spectrum of pethidine hydrochloride.*

C. Dissolve 0.1 g in 10 ml of *ethanol R* and add 10 ml of *picric acid solution R*. A crystalline precipitate is formed which, when washed with *water R* and dried at 100-105 °C, melts (*2.2.14*) at 186 °C to 193 °C. Mix equal quantities of the precipitate and the substance to be examined and determine the melting point of the mixture. The melting point is at least 20 °C lower than that of the precipitate.

D. To 5 ml of solution S (see Tests) add 5 ml of *water R*. The solution gives reaction (a) of chlorides (*2.3.1*).

TESTS

Solution S. Dissolve 0.5 g in *carbon dioxide-free water R* and dilute to 25 ml with the same solvent.

Appearance of solution. Solution S is clear (*2.2.1*) and colourless (*2.2.2, Method II*).

Acidity or alkalinity. To 10 ml of solution S add 0.2 ml of *methyl red solution R* and 0.2 ml of *0.01 M sodium hydroxide*. The solution is yellow. Add 0.3 ml of *0.01 M hydrochloric acid*. The solution is red.

Impurity B. Liquid chromatography (*2.2.29*).

Test solution (a). Dissolve 0.100 g of the substance to be examined in a mixture of 20 volumes of *acetonitrile R* and 80 volumes of *water R* and dilute to 25.0 ml with the same mixture of solvents.

Test solution (b). Dissolve 0.125 g of the substance to be examined in a mixture of 20 volumes of *acetonitrile R* and 80 volumes of *water R* and dilute to 10.0 ml with the same mixture of solvents.

Reference solution (a). Dilute 0.5 ml of test solution (a) to 100.0 ml with a mixture of 20 volumes of *acetonitrile R* and 80 volumes of *water R*.

Reference solution (b). Dissolve 10.0 mg of *pethidine impurity A CRS* in a mixture of 20 volumes of *acetonitrile R* and 80 volumes of *water R* and dilute to 100.0 ml with the same mixture of solvents.

Reference solution (c). Dissolve 12.5 mg of *1-methyl-4-phenyl-1,2,3,6-tetrahydropyridine R* in a mixture of 20 volumes of *acetonitrile R* and 80 volumes of *water R* and dilute to 10.0 ml with the same mixture of solvents. Dilute 1.0 ml of the solution to 100.0 ml with a mixture of 20 volumes of *acetonitrile R* and 80 volumes of *water R*.

Reference solution (d). Dilute 5.0 ml of reference solution (b) and 1.0 ml of reference solution (c) to 100.0 ml with a mixture of 20 volumes of *acetonitrile R* and 80 volumes of *water R*.

Column:

– *size*: l = 0.25 m, Ø = 4.0 mm,

– *stationary phase*: spherical *end-capped octadecylsilyl silica gel for chromatography R* (5 µm) with a specific surface area of 340 m^2/g, a pore size of 10 nm and a carbon loading of 19 per cent.

Mobile phase:
– *mobile phase A*: mix equal volumes of a 42.0 g/l solution of *sodium perchlorate R* and of a 11.6 g/l solution of *phosphoric acid R*, adjust to pH 2.0 with *triethylamine R*,
– *mobile phase B*: *acetonitrile R*,

Time (min)	Mobile phase A (per cent *V/V*)	Mobile phase B (per cent *V/V*)
0 - 15	80 → 75	20 → 25
15 - 31	75 → 55	25 → 45
31 - 40	55	45
40 - 41	55 → 80	45 → 20
41 - 50	80	20

Flow rate: 1.0 ml/min.
Detection: spectrophotometer at 210 nm.
Injection: 50 µl; inject test solution (b) and reference solution (d).
Relative retention with reference to pethidine (retention time = about 24 min): impurity B = about 0.66; impurity A = about 0.68.
System suitability: reference solution (d):
– *signal-to-noise ratio*: minimum 10 for the first peak,
– *peak-to-valley ratio*: minimum 4, where H_p = height above the baseline of the peak due to impurity B, and H_v = height above the baseline of the lowest point of the curve separating this peak from the peak due to impurity A.

Limit:
– *impurity B*: not more than the area of the corresponding peak in the chromatogram obtained with reference solution (d) (10 ppm) if intended for non-parenteral use.

Related substances. Liquid chromatography (*2.2.29*) as described in the test for impurity B with the following modifications.
Injection: 20 µl; inject test solution (a) and reference solution (a).
Limits:
– *any impurity*: not more than the area of the principal peak in the chromatogram obtained with reference solution (a) (0.5 per cent),
– *total*: not more than twice the area of the principal peak in the chromatogram obtained with reference solution (a) (1.0 per cent),
– *disregard limit*: 0.1 times the area of the principal peak in the chromatogram obtained with reference solution (a) (0.05 per cent).

Loss on drying (*2.2.32*): maximum 0.5 per cent, determined on 1.000 g by drying in an oven at 100-105 °C.

Sulphated ash (*2.4.14*): maximum 0.1 per cent, determined on 1.0 g.

ASSAY

Dissolve 0.220 g in 50 ml of *alcohol R*. Add 5.0 ml of *0.01 M hydrochloric acid*. Titrate with *0.1 M sodium hydroxide* determining the end-point potentiometrically (*2.2.20*). Read the volume added between the 2 points of inflexion.
1 ml of *0.1 M sodium hydroxide* is equivalent to 28.38 mg of $C_{15}H_{22}ClNO_2$.

STORAGE

In an airtight container, protected from light.

LABELLING

The label states, where applicable, that the substance is suitable for use in the manufacture of parenteral dosage forms.

IMPURITIES

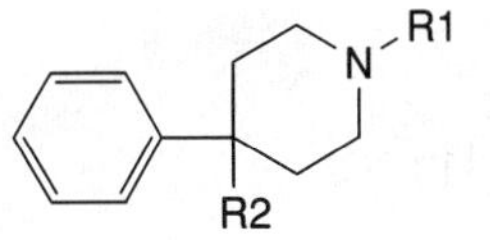

A. R1 = CH_3, R2 = H: 1-methyl-4-phenylpiperidine (MPP),
C. R1 = CH_3, R2 = CO_2H: 1-methyl-4-phenylpiperidine-4-carboxylic acid,
D. R1 = CH_3, R2 = CO_2-CH_3: methyl 1-methyl-4-phenylpiperidine-4-carboxylate,
E. R1 = H, R2 = CO_2-CH_2-CH_3: ethyl 4-phenylpiperidine-4-carboxylate,
F. R1 = CH_2-C_6H_5, R2 = CO_2H: 1-benzyl-4-phenylpiperidine-4-carboxylic acid,
G. R1 = CH_3, R2 = CO_2-$CH(CH_3)_2$: 1-methylethyl 1-methyl-4-phenylpiperidine-4-carboxylate,
H. R1 = CH_2-C_6H_5, R2 = CO_2-CH_2-CH_3: ethyl 1-benzyl-4-phenylpiperidine-4-carboxylate,
J. R1 = CH_2-CH_3, R2 = CO_2-CH_2-CH_3: ethyl 1-ethyl-4-phenylpiperidine-4-carboxylate,

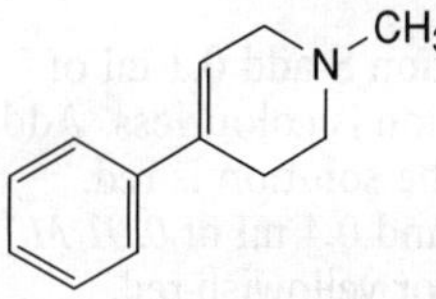

B. 1-methyl-4-phenyl-1,2,3,6-tetrahydropyridine (MPTP),

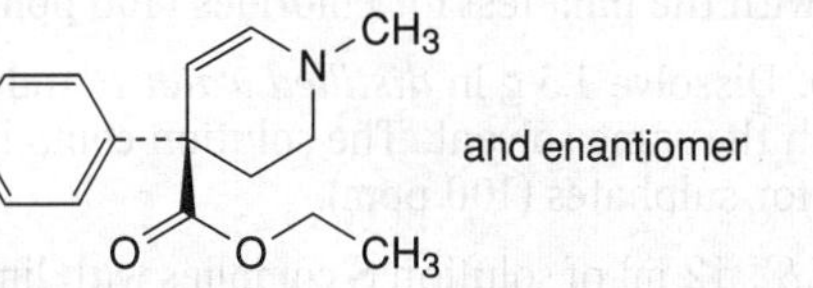

I. ethyl (4*RS*)-1-methyl-4-phenyl-1,2,3,4-tetrahydropyridine-4-carboxylate.

01/2005:0421

PHENAZONE

Phenazonum

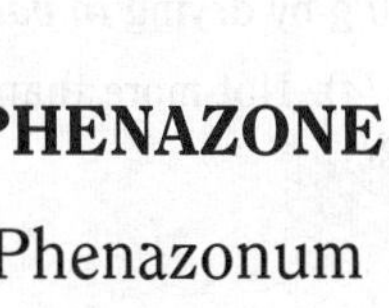

$C_{11}H_{12}N_2O$ M_r 188.2

DEFINITION

Phenazone contains not less than 99.0 per cent and not more than the equivalent of 100.5 per cent of 1,5-dimethyl-2-phenyl-1,2-dihydro-3*H*-pyrazol-3-one, calculated with reference to the dried substance.

CHARACTERS

A white or almost white, crystalline powder or colourless crystals, very soluble in water, in alcohol and in methylene chloride.

IDENTIFICATION

First identification: A, B.

Second identification: A, C, D.

A. Melting point (*2.2.14*): 109 °C to 113 °C.

B. Examine by infrared absorption spectrophotometry (*2.2.24*), comparing with the spectrum obtained with *phenazone CRS*. Examine the substances prepared as discs using *potassium bromide R*.

C. To 1 ml of solution S (see Tests) add 4 ml of *water R* and 0.25 ml of *dilute sulphuric acid R*. Add 1 ml of *sodium nitrite solution R*. A green colour develops.

D. To 1 ml of solution S add 4 ml of *water R* and 0.5 ml of *ferric chloride solution R2*. A red colour develops which is discharged on the addition of *dilute sulphuric acid R*.

TESTS

Solution S. Dissolve 2.5 g in *carbon dioxide-free water R* and dilute to 50 ml with the same solvent.

Appearance of solution. Solution S is clear (*2.2.1*) and colourless (*2.2.2, Method II*).

Acidity or alkalinity. To 10 ml of solution S add 0.1 ml of *phenolphthalein solution R*. The solution is colourless. Add 0.2 ml of *0.01 M sodium hydroxide*. The solution is red. Add 0.25 ml of *methyl red solution R* and 0.4 ml of *0.01 M hydrochloric acid*. The solution is red or yellowish-red.

Chlorides (*2.4.4*). 10 ml of solution S diluted to 15 ml with *water R* complies with the limit test for chlorides (100 ppm).

Sulphates (*2.4.13*). Dissolve 1.5 g in *distilled water R* and dilute to 15 ml with the same solvent. The solution complies with the limit test for sulphates (100 ppm).

Heavy metals (*2.4.8*). 12 ml of solution S complies with limit test A for heavy metals (20 ppm). Prepare the standard using *lead standard solution (1 ppm Pb) R*.

Loss on drying (*2.2.32*). Not more than 1.0 per cent, determined on 1.000 g by drying *in vacuo* at 60 °C for 6 h.

Sulphated ash (*2.4.14*). Not more than 0.1 per cent, determined on 1.0 g.

ASSAY

Dissolve 0.150 g in 20 ml of *water R*. Add 2 g of *sodium acetate R* and 25.0 ml of *0.05 M iodine*. Allow to stand protected from light for 30 min. Add 25 ml of *methylene chloride R* and shake until the precipitate dissolves. Titrate with *0.1 M sodium thiosulphate*, using 1 ml of *starch solution R*, added towards the end of the titration, as indicator. Carry out a blank titration.

1 ml of *0.05 M iodine* is equivalent to 9.41 mg of $C_{11}H_{12}N_2O$.

STORAGE

Store protected from light.

01/2005:1357

PHENIRAMINE MALEATE

Pheniramini maleas

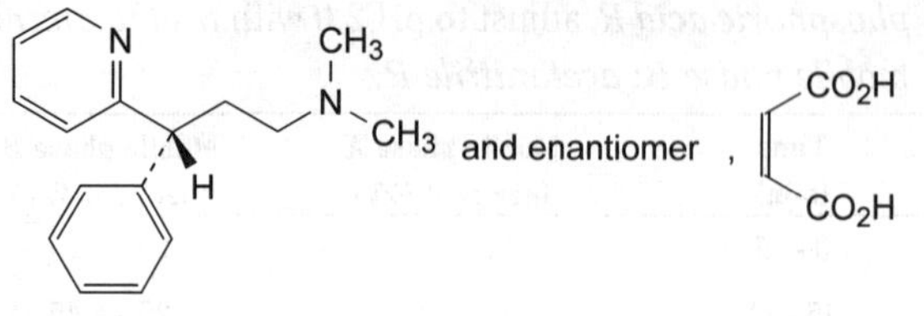

$C_{20}H_{24}N_2O_4$ M_r 356.4

DEFINITION

Pheniramine maleate contains not less than 98.0 per cent and not more than the equivalent of 102.0 per cent of (3*RS*)-*N*,*N*-dimethyl-3-phenyl-3-(pyridin-2-yl)propan-1-amine (*Z*)-butenedioate, calculated with reference to the dried substance.

CHARACTERS

A white, crystalline powder, very soluble in water, freely soluble in alcohol, in methanol and in methylene chloride.

IDENTIFICATION

First identification: C, D.

Second identification: A, B, D.

A. Melting point (*2.2.14*): 106 °C to 109 °C.

B. Dissolve 40.0 mg in *0.1 M hydrochloric acid* and dilute to 100.0 ml with the same acid. Dilute 5.0 ml of this solution to 50.0 ml with *0.1 M hydrochloric acid*. Examined between 220 nm and 320 nm (*2.2.25*), the solution shows a shoulder at 261 nm and an absorption maximum at 265 nm. The specific absorbance at the maximum is 200 to 220.

C. Examine by infrared absorption spectrophotometry (*2.2.24*), comparing with the spectrum obtained with *pheniramine maleate CRS*. Examine the substances prepared as discs.

D. Examine by thin-layer chromatography (*2.2.27*), using as the coating substance a suitable silica gel with a fluorescent indicator having an optimal intensity at 254 nm.

Test solution. Dissolve 0.10 g of the substance to be examined in *methanol R* and dilute to 5.0 ml with the same solvent.

Reference solution (a). Dissolve 65 mg of *maleic acid R* in *methanol R* and dilute to 10 ml with the same solvent.

Reference solution (b). Dissolve 0.10 g of *pheniramine maleate CRS* in *methanol R* and dilute to 5.0 ml with the same solvent.

Apply to the plate 5 µl of each solution. Develop over a path of 12 cm using a mixture of 3 volumes of *water R*, 7 volumes of *anhydrous formic acid R*, 20 volumes of *methanol R* and 70 volumes of *di-isopropyl ether R*. Examine in ultraviolet light at 254 nm. The chromatogram obtained with the test solution shows two clearly separated spots. The upper spot is similar in position and size to the spot in the chromatogram obtained with reference solution (a). The lower spot is similar in position and size to the spot in the chromatogram obtained with reference solution (b).

TESTS

Solution S. Dissolve 2.0 g in *water R* and dilute to 20 ml with the same solvent.

Appearance of solution. Solution S is clear (*2.2.1*)and not more intensely coloured than reference solution BY_6 (*2.2.2, Method II*).

pH (*2.2.3*). Dissolve 0.20 g in 20.0 ml of *carbon dioxide-free water R*. The pH of the solution is 4.5 to 5.5.

Optical rotation (*2.2.7*). The angle of optical rotation, determined on solution S, is − 0.10° to + 0.10°.

Related substances. Examine by liquid chromatography (*2.2.29*).

Test solution. Dissolve 20.0 mg of the substance to be examined in a mixture of 1 volume of *acetonitrile R* and 9 volumes of mobile phase A and dilute to 20.0 ml with the same mixture of solvents.

Reference solution (a). Dissolve 10.0 mg of *2-benzylpyridine R* in 10.0 ml of the test solution. Dilute to 100.0 ml with a mixture of 1 volume of *acetonitrile R* and 9 volumes of mobile phase A.

Reference solution (b). Dilute 2.0 ml of the test solution to 100.0 ml with a mixture of 1 volume of *acetonitrile R* and 9 volumes of mobile phase A. Dilute 1.0 ml of this solution to 10.0 ml with a mixture of 1 volume of *acetonitrile R* and 9 volumes of mobile phase A.

The chromatographic procedure may be carried out using:

– a stainless steel column 0.30 m long and 3.9 mm in internal diameter packed with *dimethyloctadecylsilyl silica gel for chromatography R* (10 µm),

– as mobile phase at a flow rate of 1 ml/min:

Mobile phase A. A 5.056 g/l solution of *sodium heptanesulphonate R* adjusted to pH 2.5 with *phosphoric acid R*,

Mobile phase B. Acetonitrile R,

Time (min)	Mobile phase A (per cent *V/V*)	Mobile phase B (per cent *V/V*)	Comment
0	90	10	equilibration
0 - 35	90 → 62	10 → 38	linear gradient
35 - 37	62 → 90	38 → 10	linear gradient

– as detector a spectrophotometer set at 264 nm.

Inject 20 µl of each solution. Adjust the sensitivity of the system so that the height of the principal peak in the chromatogram obtained with reference solution (b) is at least 50 per cent of the full scale of the recorder.

The test is not valid unless: the chromatogram obtained with reference solution (a) shows three principal peaks (maleic acid, 2-benzylpyridine and pheniramine in order of elution); the resolution between the peaks corresponding to 2-benzylpyridine and pheniramine is at least 8. In the chromatogram obtained with the test solution: the area of any peak, apart from the principal peak and the peak due to maleic acid, is not greater than the principal peak in the chromatogram obtained with reference solution (b) (0.2 per cent); the sum of the areas of all the peaks, apart from the principal peak and the peak due to maleic acid, is not greater than five times the area of the principal peak in the chromatogram obtained with reference solution (b) (1 per cent). Disregard any peak with an area less than 0.5 times the area of the principal peak in the chromatogram obtained with reference solution (b).

Heavy metals (*2.4.8*). 1.0 g complies with limit test C for heavy metals (20 ppm). Prepare the standard using 2 ml of *lead standard solution (10 ppm Pb) R*.

Loss on drying (*2.2.32*). Not more than 0.5 per cent, determined on 1.000 g by drying in an oven at 60 °C *in vacuo* for 3 h.

Sulphated ash (*2.4.14*). Not more than 0.1 per cent, determined on 1.0 g.

ASSAY

Dissolve 0.260 g in 50 ml of *anhydrous acetic acid R*. Titrate with *0.1 M perchloric acid*, determining the end-point potentiometrically (*2.2.20*).

1 ml of *0.1 M perchloric acid* is equivalent to 17.82 mg of $C_{20}H_{24}N_2O_4$.

STORAGE

Store protected from light.

IMPURITIES

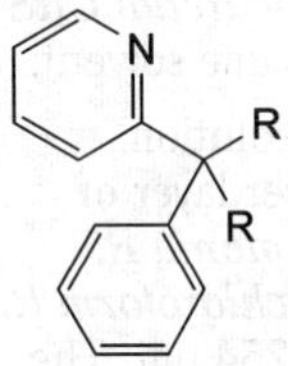

A. R = H: 2-benzylpyridine,

D. R = CH_2-CH_2-N(CH_3)$_2$: *N,N,N′,N′*-tetramethyl-3-phenyl-3-(pyridin-2-yl)pentane-1,5-diamine.

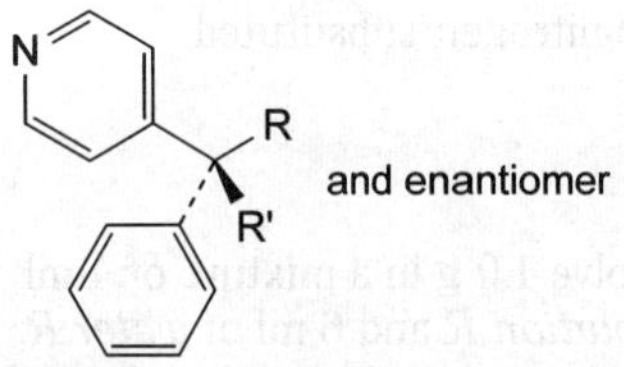

B. R = R′ = H: 4-benzylpyridine,

C. R = CH_2-CH_2-N(CH_3)$_2$, R′ = H: (3*RS*)-*N,N*-dimethyl-3-phenyl-3-(pyridin-4-yl)propan-1-amine.

01/2005:0201

PHENOBARBITAL

Phenobarbitalum

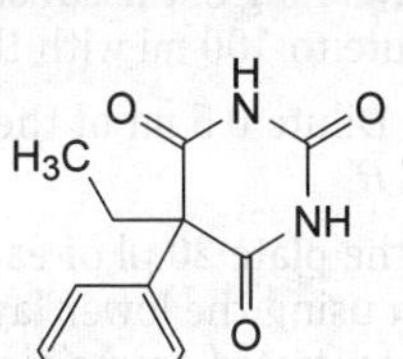

$C_{12}H_{12}N_2O_3$ M_r 232.2

DEFINITION

Phenobarbital contains not less than 99.0 per cent and not more than the equivalent of 101.0 per cent of 5-ethyl-5-phenylpyrimidine-2,4,6(1*H*,3*H*,5*H*)-trione, calculated with reference to the dried substance.

CHARACTERS

A white, crystalline powder or colourless crystals, very slightly soluble in water, freely soluble in alcohol. It forms water-soluble compounds with alkali hydroxides and carbonates and with ammonia.

IDENTIFICATION

First identification: A, B.

Second identification: A, C, D.

A. Determine the melting point (*2.2.14*) of the substance to be examined. Mix equal parts of the substance to be examined and *phenobarbital CRS* and determine the melting point of the mixture. The difference between the melting points (which are about 176 °C) is not greater than 2 °C.

B. Examine by infrared absorption spectrophotometry (*2.2.24*), comparing with the spectrum obtained with *phenobarbital CRS.*

C. Examine by thin-layer chromatography (*2.2.27*), using *silica gel* GF_{254} *R* as the coating substance.

Test solution. Dissolve 0.1 g of the substance to be examined in *alcohol R* and dilute to 100 ml with the same solvent.

Reference solution. Dissolve 0.1 g of *phenobarbital CRS* in *alcohol R* and dilute to 100 ml with the same solvent.

Apply separately to the plate 10 µl of each solution. Develop over a path of 18 cm using the lower layer of a mixture of 5 volumes of *concentrated ammonia R,* 15 volumes of *alcohol R* and 80 volumes of *chloroform R.* Examine immediately in ultraviolet light at 254 nm. The principal spot in the chromatogram obtained with the test solution is similar in position and size to the principal spot in the chromatogram obtained with the reference solution.

D. It gives the reaction of non-nitrogen substituted barbiturates (*2.3.1*).

TESTS

Appearance of solution. Dissolve 1.0 g in a mixture of 4 ml of *dilute sodium hydroxide solution R* and 6 ml of *water R.* The solution is clear (*2.2.1*) and not more intensely coloured than reference solution Y_6 (*2.2.2, Method II*).

Acidity. Boil 1.0 g with 50 ml of *water R* for 2 min, allow to cool and filter. To 10 ml of the filtrate add 0.15 ml of *methyl red solution R.* The solution is orange-yellow. Not more than 0.1 ml of *0.1 M sodium hydroxide* is required to produce a pure yellow colour.

Related substances. Examine by thin-layer chromatography (*2.2.27*), using *silica gel* GF_{254} *R* as the coating substance.

Test solution. Dissolve 1.0 g of the substance to be examined in *alcohol R* and dilute to 100 ml with the same solvent.

Reference solution. Dilute 0.5 ml of the test solution to 100 ml with *alcohol R.*

Apply separately to the plate 20 µl of each solution. Develop over a path of 15 cm using the lower layer of a mixture of 5 volumes of *concentrated ammonia R,* 15 volumes of *alcohol R* and 80 volumes of *chloroform R.* Examine immediately in ultraviolet light at 254 nm. Spray with *diphenylcarbazone mercuric reagent R.* Allow the plate to dry in air and spray with freshly prepared *alcoholic potassium hydroxide solution R* diluted 1 in 5 with *aldehyde-free alcohol R.* Heat at 100 °C to 105 °C for 5 min and examine immediately. When examined in ultraviolet light and after spraying, any spot in the chromatogram obtained with the test solution, apart from the principal spot, is not more intense than the spot in the chromatogram obtained with the reference solution (0.5 per cent).

Loss on drying (*2.2.32*). Not more than 0.5 per cent, determined on 1.00 g by drying in an oven at 100 °C to 105 °C.

Sulphated ash (*2.4.14*). Not more than 0.1 per cent, determined on 1.0 g.

ASSAY

Dissolve 0.100 g in 5 ml of *pyridine R.* Add 0.5 ml of *thymolphthalein solution R* and 10 ml of *silver nitrate solution in pyridine R.* Titrate with *0.1 M ethanolic sodium hydroxide* until a pure blue colour is obtained. Carry out a blank titration.

1 ml of *0.1 M ethanolic sodium hydroxide* is equivalent to 11.61 mg of $C_{12}H_{12}N_2O_3$.

01/2005:0630

PHENOBARBITAL SODIUM

Phenobarbitalum natricum

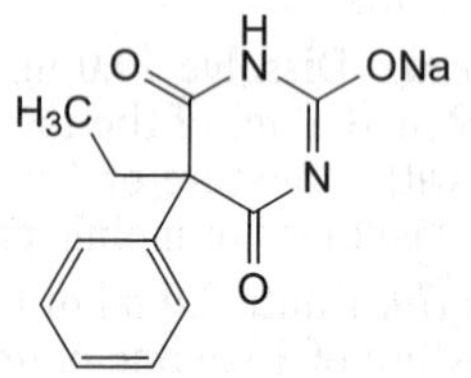

$C_{12}H_{11}N_2NaO_3$ M_r 254.2

DEFINITION

Phenobarbital sodium contains not less than 99.0 per cent and not more than the equivalent of 101.0 per cent of the sodium derivative of 5-ethyl-5-phenylpyrimidine-2,4,6(1*H*,3*H*,5*H*)-trione, calculated with reference to the dried substance.

CHARACTERS

A white, crystalline powder, hygroscopic, freely soluble in carbon dioxide-free water (a small fraction may be insoluble), soluble in alcohol, practically insoluble in methylene chloride.

IDENTIFICATION

First identification: A, B, E.

Second identification: A, C, D, E.

A. Acidify 10 ml of solution S (see Tests) with *dilute hydrochloric acid R* and shake with 20 ml of *ether R.* Separate the ether layer, wash with 10 ml of *water R,* dry over *anhydrous sodium sulphate R* and filter. Evaporate the filtrate to dryness and dry the residue at 100 °C to 105 °C. Determine the melting point (*2.2.14*) of the test residue. Mix equal parts of the residue and of *phenobarbital CRS* and determine the melting point of the mixture. The difference between the two melting points (which are about 176 °C) is not greater than 2 °C.

B. Examine by infrared absorption spectrophotometry (*2.2.24*), comparing the residue obtained during identification test A with the spectrum obtained with *phenobarbital CRS.* If the spectra obtained in the solid state show differences, dissolve the test residue and the reference substance separately in *ethanol R,* evaporate to dryness and record the spectra again.

C. Examine by thin-layer chromatography (*2.2.27*), using *silica gel* GF_{254} *R* as the coating substance.

Test solution. Dissolve 0.10 g of the substance to be examined in *alcohol (50 per cent V/V) R* and dilute to 100 ml with the same solvent.

Reference solution. Dissolve 90 mg of *phenobarbital CRS* in *alcohol (50 per cent V/V) R* and dilute to 100 ml with the same solvent.

Apply separately to the plate 10 µl of each solution. Develop over a path of 18 cm using the lower layer from a mixture of 5 volumes of *concentrated ammonia R*, 15 volumes of *alcohol R* and 80 volumes of *chloroform R*. Examine immediately in ultraviolet light at 254 nm. The principal spot in the chromatogram obtained with the test solution is similar in position and size to the principal spot in the chromatogram obtained with the reference solution.

D. It gives the reaction of non-nitrogen substituted barbiturates (*2.3.1*).

E. It gives reaction (a) of sodium (*2.3.1*).

TESTS

Solution S. Dissolve 5.0 g in *alcohol (50 per cent V/V) R* and dilute to 50 ml with the same solvent.

Appearance of solution. Solution S is clear (*2.2.1*) and not more intensely coloured than reference solution Y_7 (*2.2.2, Method II*).

pH (*2.2.3*). Dissolve 5.0 g as completely as possible in *carbon dioxide-free water R* and dilute to 50 ml with the same solvent. The pH of the solution is not greater than 10.2.

Related substances. Examine by thin-layer chromatography (*2.2.27*), using *silica gel GF_{254} R* as the coating substance.

Test solution. Dissolve 1.0 g of the substance to be examined in *alcohol (50 per cent V/V) R* and dilute to 100 ml with the same solvent.

Reference solution. Dilute 0.5 ml of the test solution to 100 ml with *alcohol (50 per cent V/V) R*.

Apply separately to the plate 20 µl of each solution. Develop over a path of 15 cm using the lower layer from a mixture of 5 volumes of *concentrated ammonia R*, 15 volumes of *alcohol R* and 80 volumes of *chloroform R*. Examine immediately in ultraviolet light at 254 nm. Spray with *diphenylcarbazone mercuric reagent R*. Allow the plate to dry in air and spray with freshly prepared *alcoholic potassium hydroxide solution R* diluted 1 in 5 with *aldehyde-free alcohol R*. Heat at 100 °C to 105 °C for 5 min and examine immediately. When examined in ultraviolet light and after spraying, any spot in the chromatogram obtained with the test solution, apart from the principal spot, is not more intense than the spot in the chromatogram obtained with the reference solution (0.5 per cent). Disregard any spot at the starting-point.

Loss on drying (*2.2.32*). Not more than 7.0 per cent, determined on 0.500 g by drying in an oven at 150 °C for 4 h.

ASSAY

Dissolve 0.150 g in 2 ml of *water R* and add 8 ml of *0.05 M sulphuric acid.* Heat to boiling and cool. Add 30 ml of *methanol R* and shake until dissolution is complete. Carry out a potentiometric titration (*2.2.20*), using *0.1 M sodium hydroxide.* After the first point of inflexion, interrupt the addition of sodium hydroxide, add 10 ml of *pyridine R*, mix and continue the titration. Read the volume added between the two points of inflexion.

1 ml of *0.1 M sodium hydroxide* is equivalent to 25.42 mg of $C_{12}H_{11}N_2NaO_3$.

STORAGE

Store in an airtight container.

01/2005:0631

PHENOL

Phenolum

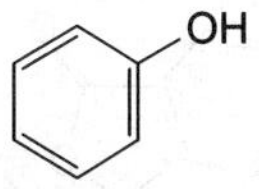

C_6H_6O M_r 94.1

DEFINITION

Phenol contains not less than 99.0 per cent and not more than the equivalent of 100.5 per cent of C_6H_6O.

CHARACTERS

Colourless or faintly pink or faintly yellowish crystals or crystalline masses, deliquescent, soluble in water, very soluble in alcohol, in glycerol and in methylene chloride.

IDENTIFICATION

A. Dissolve 0.5 g in 2 ml of *concentrated ammonia R*. The substance dissolves completely. Dilute to about 100 ml with *water R*. To 2 ml of the dilute solution add 0.05 ml of *strong sodium hypochlorite solution R*. A blue colour develops and becomes progressively more intense.

B. To 1 ml of solution S (see Tests) add 10 ml of *water R* and 0.1 ml of *ferric chloride solution R1*. A violet colour is produced which disappears on addition of 5 ml of *2-propanol R*.

C. To 1 ml of solution S add 10 ml of *water R* and 1 ml of *bromine water R*. A pale-yellow precipitate is formed.

TESTS

Solution S. Dissolve 1.0 g in *water R* and dilute to 15 ml with the same solvent.

Appearance of solution. Solution S is clear (*2.2.1*) and not more intensely coloured than reference solution B_6 (*2.2.2, Method II*).

Acidity. To 2 ml of solution S add 0.05 ml of *methyl orange solution R*. The solution is yellow.

Freezing point (*2.2.18*). Not less than 39.5 °C.

Residue on evaporation. Not more than 0.05 per cent, determined by evaporating 5.000 g to dryness on a water-bath and drying the residue at 100 °C to 105 °C for 1 h.

ASSAY

Dissolve 2.000 g in *water R* and dilute to 1000.0 ml with the same solvent. Transfer 25.0 ml of the solution to a ground-glass-stoppered flask and add 50.0 ml of *0.0167 M bromide-bromate* and 5 ml of *hydrochloric acid R*, close the flask, allow to stand with occasional swirling for 30 min and then allow to stand for a further 15 min. Add 5 ml of a 200 g/l solution of *potassium iodide R*, shake and titrate with *0.1 M sodium thiosulphate* until a faint yellow colour remains. Add 0.5 ml of *starch solution R* and 10 ml of *chloroform R* and continue the titration with vigorous shaking. Carry out a blank titration.

1 ml of *0.0167 M bromide-bromate* is equivalent to 1.569 mg of C_6H_6O.

STORAGE

Store in an airtight container, protected from light.

01/2005:1584

PHENOLPHTHALEIN

Phenolphthaleinum

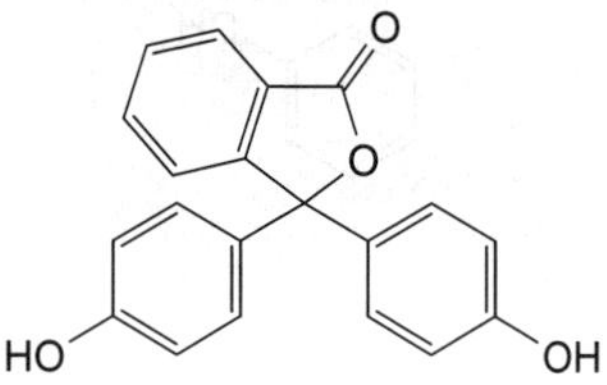

$C_{20}H_{14}O_4$ M_r 318.3

DEFINITION

Phenolphthalein contains not less than 98.0 per cent and not more than the equivalent of 101.0 per cent of 3,3-bis(4-hydroxyphenyl)isobenzofuran-1(3*H*)-one, calculated with reference to the dried substance.

CHARACTERS

A white or almost white powder, practically insoluble in water, soluble in alcohol.

It melts at about 260 °C.

IDENTIFICATION

A. Dissolve 25.0 mg in *alcohol R* and dilute to 100.0 ml with the same solvent (solution A). To 2.0 ml of solution A add 5.0 ml of *1 M hydrochloric acid*and dilute to 50.0 ml with *alcohol R* (solution A_1). To 10.0 ml of solution A add 5.0 ml of *1 M hydrochloric acid* and dilute to 50.0 ml with *alcohol R* (solution A_2). To 2.0 ml of solution A add 5.0 ml of *1 M sodium hydroxide* and dilute to 50.0 ml with *alcohol R* (solution B). Examined between 220 nm and 250 nm (*2.2.25*), solution A_1 shows an absorption maximum at 229 nm. The specific absorbance at the maximum at 229 nm is 922 to 1018. Examined between 250 nm and 300 nm, solution A_2 shows an absorption maximum at 276 nm. The specific absorbance at the maximum at 276 nm is 142 to 158. Examined between 230 nm and 270 nm, solution B shows an absorption maximum at 249 nm. The specific absorbance at the maximum at 249 nm is 744 to 822.

B. Dissolve about 10 mg in *alcohol R*. Add 1 ml of *dilute sodium hydroxide solution R*. The solution is red. Add 5 ml of *dilute sulphuric acid R*. The colour disappears.

TESTS

Solution S. To 2.0 g add 40 ml of *distilled water R* and heat to boiling. Cool and filter.

Appearance of solution. Dissolve 0.20 g in 5 ml of *alcohol R*. The solution is clear (*2.2.1*) and not more intensely coloured than reference solution Y_7 (*2.2.2, Method II*).

Acidity or alkalinity. To 10 ml of solution S add 0.15 ml of *bromothymol blue solution R1*. Add 0.05 ml of *0.01 M hydrochloric acid,* the solution is yellow. Add 0.10 ml of *0.01 M sodium hydroxide,* the solution is blue.

Related substances. Examine by thin-layer chromatography (*2.2.27*), using a *TLC silica gel F_{254} plate R.*

Test solution. Dissolve 0.5 g of the substance to be examined in *alcohol R* and dilute to 10 ml with the same solvent.

Reference solution (a). Dilute 1 ml of the test solution to 10 ml with *alcohol R*. Dilute 5 ml of this solution to 100 ml with *alcohol R*.

Reference solution (b). Dissolve 25 mg of *fluorene R* in *alcohol R,* add 0.5 ml of the test solution and dilute to 10 ml with *alcohol R*.

Apply to the plate 5 µl of the test solution and 5 µl of each of the reference solutions. Develop over a path corresponding to two-thirds of the plate height using a mixture of 50 volumes of *acetone R* and 50 volumes of *methylene chloride R*. Allow the plate to dry in air. Examine in ultraviolet light at 254 nm and re-examine after exposure to ammonia vapour. Any spot in the chromatogram obtained with the test solution, apart from the principal spot, is not more intense than the spot in the chromatogram obtained with reference solution (a) (0.5 per cent). The test is not valid unless the chromatogram obtained with reference solution (b) shows 2 clearly separated spots.

Chlorides (*2.4.4*). Dilute 10 ml of solution S to 15 ml with *water R*. The solution complies with the limit test for chlorides (100 ppm).

Sulphates (*2.4.13*). 15 ml of solution S complies with the limit test for sulphates (200 ppm).

Heavy metals (*2.4.8*). Heat 3 g with 50 ml of *dilute hydrochloric acid R* on a water-bath for 5 min and filter. Evaporate the filtrate almost to dryness and dissolve the residue in 30 ml of *water R*. 12 ml of this solution complies with limit test A for heavy metals (10 ppm). Prepare the standard using 10 ml of *lead standard solution (1 ppm Pb) R*.

Loss on drying (*2.2.32*). Not more than 0.5 per cent, determined on 1.000 g by drying in an oven at 100 °C to 105 °C.

Sulphated ash (*2.4.14*). Not more than 0.1 per cent, determined on 1.0 g.

ASSAY

Dissolve 0.100 g in 5 ml of *dimethylformamide R*. Add 5 ml of *sodium carbonate solution R,* 10 ml of *sodium hydrogen carbonate solution R,* 35 ml of *water R* and 50.0 ml of *0.05 M iodine*. Add 10 ml of *methylene chloride R* and 20 ml of *dilute sulphuric acid R*. Titrate the excess of iodine with *0.1 M sodium thiosulphate,* using 0.3 ml of *starch solution R* added towards the end of the titration, as indicator. Carry out a blank titration.

1 ml of *0.05 M iodine* is equivalent to 3.979 mg of $C_{20}H_{14}O_4$.

STORAGE

Store protected from light.

01/2005:0242

PHENOLSULFONPHTHALEIN

Phenolsulfonphthaleinum

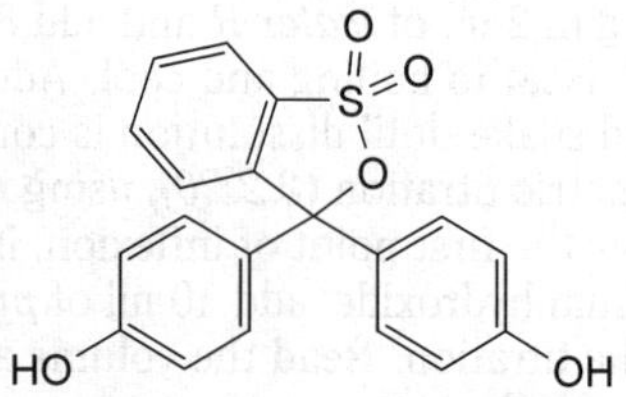

$C_{19}H_{14}O_5S$ M_r 354.4

DEFINITION

Phenolsulfonphthalein (phenol red) contains not less than 98.0 per cent and not more than the equivalent of 102.0 per cent of 3,3-bis(4-hydroxyphenyl)-3*H*-2,1-benzoxathiole 1,1-dioxide, calculated with reference to the dried substance.

CHARACTERS

A bright-red to dark-red, crystalline powder, very slightly soluble in water, slightly soluble in alcohol.

IDENTIFICATION

A. Dissolve 10 mg in a 10 g/l solution of *sodium carbonate R* and dilute to 200.0 ml with the sodium carbonate solution. Dilute 5.0 ml of the solution to 100.0 ml with a 10 g/l solution of *sodium carbonate R*. Examined between 400 nm and 630 nm (*2.2.25*), the solution shows an absorption maximum at 558 nm. The specific absorbance at the maximum is 1900 to 2100.

B. Dissolve about 10 mg in 1 ml of *dilute sodium hydroxide solution R* and add 9 ml of *water R*. The solution is deep red. To 5 ml of the solution add a slight excess of *dilute sulphuric acid R*. The colour becomes orange.

C. To 5 ml of the solution prepared for identification test B add 1 ml of *0.0167 M bromide-bromate* and 1 ml of *dilute hydrochloric acid R*, shake and allow to stand for 15 min. Make alkaline with *dilute sodium hydroxide solution R*. An intense violet-blue colour is produced.

TESTS

Related substances. Examine by thin-layer chromatography (*2.2.27*), using *silica gel GF_{254} R* as the coating substance.

Test solution. Dissolve 0.1 g of the substance to be examined in *0.1 M sodium hydroxide* and dilute to 5 ml with the same solvent.

Reference solution. Dilute 0.5 ml of the test solution to 100 ml with *0.1 M sodium hydroxide*.

Apply separately to the plate 10 µl of each solution. Develop over a path of 15 cm using a mixture of 25 volumes of *glacial acetic acid R*, 25 volumes of *water R* and 100 volumes of *tert-pentyl alcohol R*. Allow the plate to dry in air until the solvent has evaporated and expose the plate to the vapour from *concentrated ammonia R*. Examine in ultraviolet light at 254 nm. Not more than one spot, apart from the principal spot, appears in the chromatogram obtained with the test solution and this spot is not more intense than the spot in the chromatogram obtained with the reference solution (0.5 per cent).

Insoluble matter. To 1.0 g of the finely powdered substance to be examined add 12 ml of *sodium hydrogen carbonate solution R*. Allow to stand for 1 h, shaking frequently. Dilute to 100 ml with *water R* and allow to stand for 15 h. Centrifuge at 2000 *g* to 3000 *g*, for 30 min, decant the supernatant liquid and wash the residue with 25 ml of a 10 g/l solution of *sodium hydrogen carbonate R* and then 25 ml of *water R*. Dry at 100 °C to 105 °C. The residue weighs not more than 5 mg (0.5 per cent).

Loss on drying (*2.2.32*). Not more than 1.0 per cent, determined on 1.00 g of the powdered substance to be examined by drying in an oven at 100 °C to 105 °C.

Sulphated ash (*2.4.14*). Not more than 0.2 per cent, determined on 0.5 g.

ASSAY

Dissolve 0.900 g in 15 ml of *1 M sodium hydroxide* and dilute to 250.0 ml with *water R*. To 10.0 ml of the solution in a glass-stoppered flask add 25 ml of *glacial acetic acid R*, 20.0 ml of *0.0167 M potassium bromate*, 5 ml of a 100 g/l solution of *potassium bromide R* and 5 ml of *hydrochloric acid R*. Allow to stand protected from light for 15 min, add 10 ml of a 100 g/l solution of *potassium iodide R* and titrate immediately with *0.1 M sodium thiosulphate*, using 0.1 ml of *starch solution R* as indicator.

1 ml of *0.0167 M potassium bromate* is equivalent to 4.43 mg of $C_{19}H_{14}O_5S$.

01/2005:0781

PHENOXYETHANOL

Phenoxyethanolum

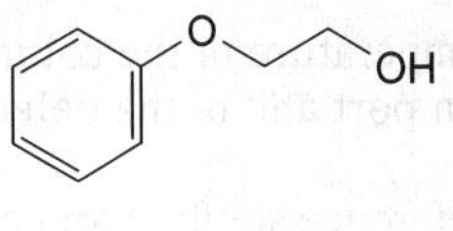

$C_8H_{10}O_2$ M_r 138.2

DEFINITION

Phenoxyethanol contains not less than 99.0 per cent and not more than the equivalent of 100.5 per cent *m/m* of 2-phenoxyethanol.

CHARACTERS

A colourless, slightly viscous liquid, slightly soluble in water, miscible with acetone, with alcohol and with glycerol, slightly soluble in arachis oil and in olive oil.

IDENTIFICATION

First identification: C.

Second identification: A, B, D.

A. Refractive index (*2.2.6*): 1.537 to 1.539.

B. Dissolve 80.0 mg in *water R* and dilute to 100.0 ml with the same solvent. Dilute 10.0 ml of the solution to 100.0 ml with *water R*. Examined between 240 nm and 350 nm (*2.2.25*), the solution shows two absorption maxima, at 269 nm and at 275 nm. The specific absorbances at the maxima are 95 to 105 and 75 to 85 respectively.

C. Examine by infrared absorption spectrophotometry (*2.2.24*), comparing with the spectrum obtained with *phenoxyethanol CRS*.

D. Shake 2 ml with a mixture of 4 g of *potassium permanganate R*, 5.4 g of *sodium carbonate R* and 75 ml of *water R* for 30 min. Add 25 g of *sodium chloride R* and stir continuously for 60 min, filter and acidify with *hydrochloric acid R* to about pH 1.7. The melting point of the precipitate, after recrystallisation from *water R*, is 96 °C to 99 °C (*2.2.14*).

TESTS

Relative density (*2.2.5*): 1.105 to 1.110.

Related substances. Examine by gas chromatography (*2.2.28*), using *methyl laurate R* as internal standard.

Internal standard solution. Dissolve 1.25 g of *methyl laurate R* in *methylene chloride R* and dilute to 25 ml with the same solvent.

Test solution (a). Dissolve 5.0 g of the substance to be examined in *methylene chloride R* and dilute to 10.0 ml with the same solvent.

Test solution (b). Dissolve 5.0 g of the substance to be examined in *methylene chloride R*, add 1.0 ml of the internal standard solution and dilute to 10.0 ml with *methylene chloride R*.

Reference solution. To 1.0 ml of test solution (a), add 10.0 ml of the internal standard solution and dilute to 100.0 ml with *methylene chloride R*.

The chromatographic procedure may be carried out using:

- a glass column 1.5 m long and 4 mm in internal diameter packed with *silanised diatomaceous earth for gas chromatography R* (150 µm to 180 µm) impregnated with 3 per cent *m/m* of *polymethylphenylsiloxane R,*
- *nitrogen for chromatography R* as the carrier gas at a flow rate of 30 ml/min,
- a flame-ionisation detector,

maintaining the temperature of the column at 130 °C and that of the injection port and of the detector at 200 °C.

Inject 1 µl of the reference solution and adjust the sensitivity of the detector so that the heights of the two peaks, apart from the solvent peak, are not less than 70 per cent of the full scale of the recorder. The substances elute in the following order: phenoxyethanol and methyl laurate. The test is not valid unless, in the chromatogram obtained with the reference solution, the resolution between the peaks corresponding to phenoxyethanol and methyl laurate is not less than twelve.

Inject 1 µl of test solution (a). In the chromatogram obtained, verify that there is no peak with the same retention time as the internal standard.

Inject separately 1 µl of test solution (b) and the reference solution. Continue the chromatography for five times the retention time of phenoxyethanol (which is about 5 min). From the chromatogram obtained with the reference solution, calculate the ratio (*R*) of the area of the peak due to phenoxyethanol to the area of the peak due to the internal standard. From the chromatogram obtained with test solution (b), calculate the ratio of the sum of the areas of any peaks, apart from the principal peak, the peak due to the internal standard and the peak due to the solvent, to the area of the peak due to the internal standard: this ratio is not greater than *R* (1.0 per cent).

Phenol. Dissolve 1.00 g in 50 ml of *methylene chloride R,* add 1 ml of *dilute sodium hydroxide solution R* and 10 ml of *water R.* Shake. Wash the upper layer with two quantities, each of 20 ml, of *methylene chloride R* and dilute to 100.0 ml with *water R.* The absorbance (*2.2.25*) of the resulting solution at the maximum at 287 nm is not more than 0.27 (0.1 per cent).

ASSAY

To 2.000 g in an acetylation flask fitted with an air condenser, add 10.0 ml of freshly prepared *acetic anhydride solution R1* and heat with frequent shaking in a water-bath for 45 min. Cool and carefully add 10 ml of *water R.* Heat for a further 2 min. Cool, add 10 ml of *butanol R,* shake vigorously and titrate the excess of acetic acid with *1 M sodium hydroxide* using 0.2 ml of *phenolphthalein solution R* as indicator. Repeat the procedure without the substance to be examined. The difference between the volumes used in the titrations represents the amount of acetic anhydride required for the acetylation of the substance to be examined.

1 ml of *1 M sodium hydroxide* is equivalent to 0.1382 g of $C_8H_{10}O_2$.

01/2005:0148
corrected

PHENOXYMETHYLPENICILLIN

Phenoxymethylpenicillinum

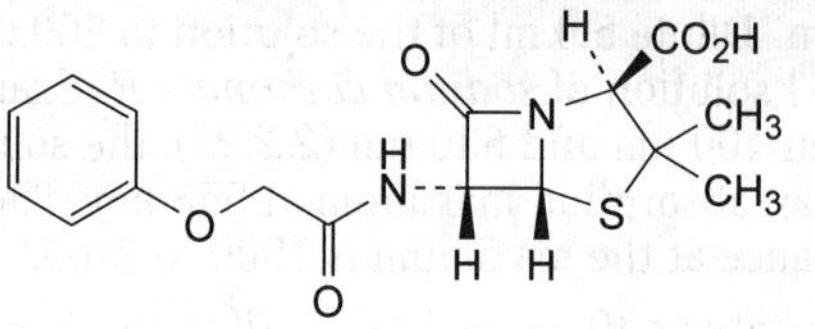

$C_{16}H_{18}N_2O_5S$ M_r 350.4

DEFINITION

Phenoxymethylpenicillin is (2*S*,5*R*,6*R*)-3,3-dimethyl-7-oxo-6-[(phenoxyacetyl)amino]-4-thia-1-azabicyclo[3.2.0]heptane-2-carboxylic acid, a substance produced by the growth of certain strains of *Penicillium notatum* or related organisms on a culture medium containing an appropriate precursor, or obtained by any other means. The sum of the percentage contents of phenoxymethylpenicillin and 4-hydroxyphenoxymethylpenicillin is not less than 95.0 per cent and not more than the equivalent of 100.5 per cent, calculated with reference to the anhydrous substance.

CHARACTERS

A white or almost white, crystalline powder, slightly hygroscopic, very slightly soluble in water, soluble in alcohol.

IDENTIFICATION

First identification: B.

Second identification: A, C, D.

A. It complies with the test for pH (see Tests).
B. Examine by infrared absorption spectrophotometry (*2.2.24*), comparing with the spectrum obtained with *phenoxymethylpenicillin CRS.*
C. Examine by thin-layer chromatography (*2.2.27*), using *silanised silica gel H R* as the coating substance.
   Test solution. Dissolve 25 mg of the substance to be examined in 5 ml of *acetone R.*
   Reference solution (a). Dissolve 25 mg of *phenoxymethylpenicillin CRS* in 5 ml of *acetone R.*
   Reference solution (b). Dissolve 25 mg of *benzylpenicillin potassium CRS* and 25 mg of *phenoxymethylpenicillin potassium CRS* in 5 ml of *water R.*
   Apply to the plate 1 µl of each solution. Develop over a path of 15 cm using a mixture of 30 volumes of *acetone R* and 70 volumes of a 154 g/l solution of *ammonium acetate R,* adjusted to pH 5.0 with *glacial acetic acid R.* Allow the plate to dry in air and expose it to iodine vapour until the spots appear. Examine in daylight. The principal spot in the chromatogram obtained with the test solution is similar in position, colour and size to the principal spot in the chromatogram obtained with reference solution (a). The test is not valid unless the chromatogram obtained with reference solution (b) shows 2 clearly separated spots.
D. Place about 2 mg in a test-tube about 150 mm long and 15 mm in diameter. Moisten with 0.05 ml of *water R* and add 2 ml of *sulphuric acid-formaldehyde reagent R.* Mix the contents of the tube by swirling; the solution is reddish-brown. Place the test-tube on a water-bath for 1 min; a dark reddish-brown colour develops.

TESTS

pH (*2.2.3*). Suspend 50 mg in 10 ml of *carbon dioxide-free water R*. The pH of the suspension is 2.4 to 4.0.

Specific optical rotation (*2.2.7*). Dissolve 0.250 g in *butanol R* and dilute to 25.0 ml with the same solvent. The specific optical rotation is + 186 to + 200, calculated with reference to the anhydrous substance.

Related substances. Examine by liquid chromatography (*2.2.29*) as described under Assay. Inject 20 µl of reference solution (d) and elute isocratically with the chosen mobile phase until elution of the phenoxymethylpenicillin peak. Adjust the sensitivity of the system to obtain a peak with a signal-to-noise ratio of at least 3. Inject 20 µl of reference solution (e). Inject 20 µl of test solution (b) and start the elution isocratically. Immediately after elution of the phenoxymethylpenicillin peak start the following linear gradient.

Time (min)	Mobile phase A (per cent *V/V*)	Mobile phase B (per cent *V/V*)	Comment
0 - 20	60 $\rightarrow$ 0	40 $\rightarrow$ 100	linear gradient
20 - 35	0	100	isocratic
35 - 50	0 $\rightarrow$ 60	100 $\rightarrow$ 40	re-equilibration

Inject the dissolution mixture and use the same elution pattern to obtain a blank. In the chromatogram obtained with test solution (b), the area of any peak, apart from the principal peak and any peak corresponding to 4-hydroxyphenoxymethylpenicillin, is not greater than the area of the principal peak in the chromatogram obtained with reference solution (e) (1 per cent).

4-Hydroxyphenoxymethylpenicillin. Not more than 4.0 per cent, calculated with reference to the anhydrous substance and determined by liquid chromatography (*2.2.29*), as described under Assay.

Water (*2.5.12*). Not more than 0.5 per cent, determined on 1.000 g by the semi-micro determination of water.

ASSAY

Examine by liquid chromatography (*2.2.29*).

Dissolution mixture. To 250 ml of *0.2 M potassium dihydrogen phosphate R* add 500 ml of *water R* and adjust to pH 6.5 with an 8.4 g/l solution of *sodium hydroxide R*. Dilute to 1000 ml with *water R*.

Test solution (a). Dissolve 50.0 mg of the substance to be examined in the dissolution mixture and dilute to 50.0 ml with the same mixture.

Test solution (b). Prepare immediately before use. Dissolve 80.0 mg of the substance to be examined in the dissolution mixture and dilute to 20.0 ml with the same mixture.

Reference solution (a). Dissolve 55.0 mg of *phenoxymethylpenicillin potassium CRS* in the dissolution mixture and dilute to 50.0 ml with the same mixture.

Reference solution (b). Dissolve 10.0 mg of *4-hydroxyphenoxymethylpenicillin CRS* in the dissolution mixture and dilute to 25.0 ml with the same mixture. Dilute 5.0 ml of the solution to 100.0 ml with the dissolution mixture.

Reference solution (c). Dissolve 10 mg of *phenoxymethylpenicillin potassium CRS* and 10 mg of *benzylpenicillin sodium CRS* in the dissolution mixture and dilute to 50 ml with the same mixture.

Reference solution (d). Dilute 1.0 ml of reference solution (a) to 20 ml with the dissolution mixture. Dilute 1.0 ml of the solution to 50 ml with the dissolution mixture.

Reference solution (e). Dilute 1.0 ml of reference solution (a) to 25.0 ml with the dissolution mixture.

The chromatographic procedure may be carried out using:

– a column 0.25 m long and 4.6 mm in internal diameter packed with *octadecylsilyl silica gel for chromatography R* (5 µm),
– as mobile phase at a flow rate of 1.0 ml/min:
  Mobile phase A. Mix 10 volumes of *phosphate buffer solution pH 3.5 R*, 30 volumes of *methanol R* and 60 volumes of *water R*,
  Mobile phase B. Mix 10 volumes of *phosphate buffer solution pH 3.5 R*, 35 volumes of *water R* and 55 volumes of *methanol R*,
– as detector a spectrophotometer set at 254 nm.

Equilibrate the column with a mobile phase ratio A:B of 60:40. Inject 20 µl of reference solution (c). The test is not valid unless, in the chromatogram obtained, the resolution between the 2 principal peaks is at least 6.0 (if necessary, adjust the ratio A:B of the mobile phase) and the mass distribution ratio for the second peak (phenoxymethylpenicillin) is 5.0 to 7.0. Inject reference solution (a) 6 times. The test is not valid unless the relative standard deviation for the area of the principal peak is at most 1.0 per cent. Inject alternately test solution (a) and reference solutions (a) and (b).

Calculate the percentage content of phenoxymethylpenicillin by multiplying the percentage content of phenoxymethylpenicillin potassium by 0.902. Calculate the percentage content of 4-hydroxyphenoxymethylpenicillin by multiplying if necessary by the correction factor supplied with the CRS.

STORAGE

Store in an airtight container.

IMPURITIES

A. benzylpenicillin,

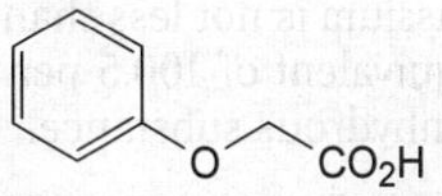

B. phenoxyacetic acid,

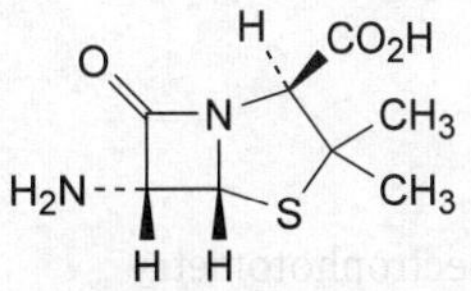

C. (2*S*,5*R*,6*R*)-6-amino-3,3-dimethyl-7-oxo-4-thia-1-azabicyclo[3.2.0]heptane-2-carboxylic acid (6-aminopenicillanic acid),

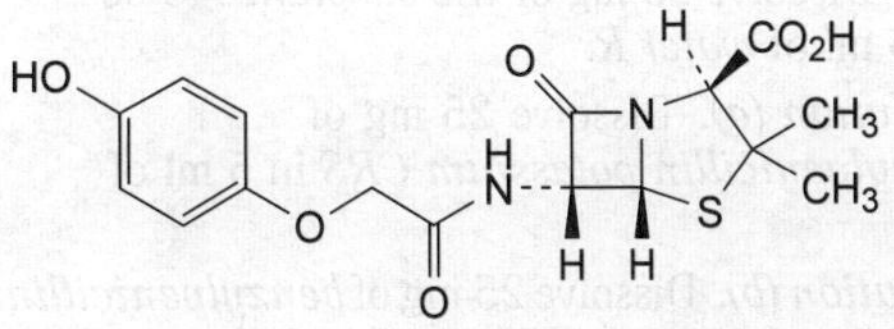

D. (2*S*,5*R*,6*R*)-3,3-dimethyl-7-oxo-6-[[2-(4-hydroxyphenoxy)acetyl]amino]-4-thia-1-azabicyclo[3.2.0]heptane-2-carboxylic acid (4-hydroxyphenoxymethylpenicillin),

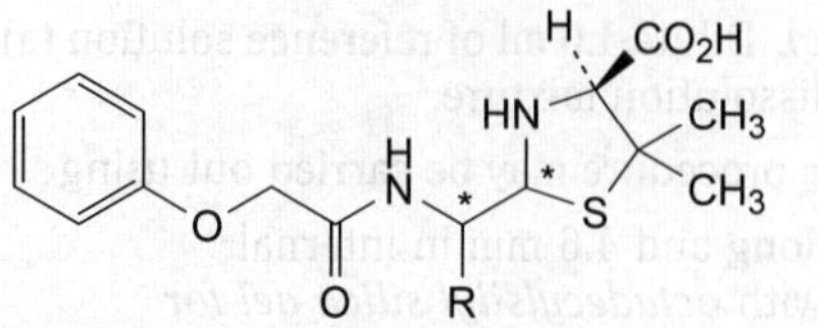

E. R = CO_2H: (4*S*)-2-[carboxy[(phenoxyacetyl)amino]methyl]-5,5-dimethylthiazolidine-4-carboxylic acid (penicilloic acids of phenoxymethylpenicillin),

F. R = H: (2*RS*,4*S*)-5,5-dimethyl-2-[[(phenoxyacetyl)amino]methyl]thiazolidine-4-carboxylic acid (penilloic acids of phenoxymethylpenicillin).

01/2005:0149
corrected

PHENOXYMETHYLPENICILLIN POTASSIUM

Phenoxymethylpenicillinum kalicum

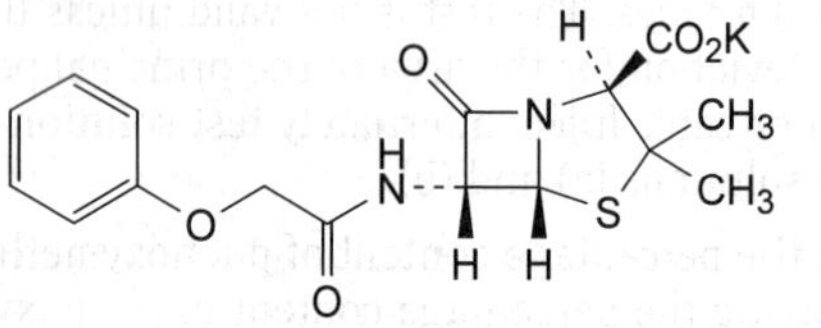

$C_{16}H_{17}KN_2O_5S$ M_r 388.5

DEFINITION

Phenoxymethylpenicillin potassium is the potassium salt of (2*S*,5*R*,6*R*)-3,3-dimethyl-7-oxo-6-[(phenoxyacetyl)amino]-4-thia-1-azabicyclo[3.2.0]heptane-2-carboxylic acid, a substance produced by the growth of certain strains of *Penicillium notatum* or related organisms on a culture medium containing an appropriate precursor, or obtained by any other means. The sum of the percentage contents of phenoxymethylpenicillin potassium and 4-hydroxyphenoxymethylpenicillin potassium is not less than 95.0 per cent and not more than the equivalent of 100.5 per cent, calculated with reference to the anhydrous substance.

CHARACTERS

A white or almost white, crystalline powder, freely soluble in water, practically insoluble in alcohol.

IDENTIFICATION

First identification: A, D.

Second identification: B, C, D.

A. Examine by infrared absorption spectrophotometry (*2.2.24*), comparing with the spectrum obtained with *phenoxymethylpenicillin potassium CRS.*

B. Examine by thin-layer chromatography (*2.2.27*), using *silanised silica gel H R* as the coating substance.

Test solution. Dissolve 25 mg of the substance to be examined in 5 ml of *water R.*

Reference solution (a). Dissolve 25 mg of *phenoxymethylpenicillin potassium CRS* in 5 ml of *water R.*

Reference solution (b). Dissolve 25 mg of *benzylpenicillin potassium CRS* and 25 mg of *phenoxymethylpenicillin potassium CRS* in 5 ml of *water R.*

Apply to the plate 1 µl of each solution. Develop over a path of 15 cm using a mixture of 30 volumes of *acetone R* and 70 volumes of a 154 g/l solution of *ammonium acetate R*, adjusted to pH 5.0 with *glacial acetic acid R.* Allow the plate to dry in air and expose it to iodine vapour until the spots appear. Examine in daylight. The principal spot in the chromatogram obtained with the test solution is similar in position, colour and size to the principal spot in the chromatogram obtained with reference solution (a). The test is not valid unless the chromatogram obtained with reference solution (b) shows 2 clearly separated spots.

C. Place about 2 mg in a test-tube about 150 mm long and 15 mm in diameter. Moisten with 0.05 ml of *water R* and add 2 ml of *sulphuric acid-formaldehyde reagent R.* Mix the contents of the tube by swirling; the solution is reddish-brown. Place the test-tube in a water-bath for 1 min; a dark reddish-brown colour develops.

D. It gives reaction (a) of potassium (*2.3.1*).

TESTS

pH (*2.2.3*). Dissolve 50 mg in *carbon dioxide-free water R* and dilute to 10 ml with the same solvent. The pH of the solution is 5.5 to 7.5.

Specific optical rotation (*2.2.7*). Dissolve 0.250 g in *carbon dioxide-free water R* and dilute to 25.0 ml with the same solvent. The specific optical rotation is + 215 to + 230, calculated with reference to the anhydrous substance.

Related substances. Examine by liquid chromatography (*2.2.29*) as described under Assay. Inject 20 µl of reference solution (d) and elute isocratically with the chosen mobile phase until elution of the phenoxymethylpenicillin peak. Adjust the sensitivity of the system to obtain a peak with a signal-to-noise ratio of at least 3. Inject 20 µl of reference solution (e). Inject 20 µl of test solution (b) and start the elution isocratically. Immediately after elution of the phenoxymethylpenicillin peak start the following linear gradient.

Time (min)	Mobile phase A (per cent *V/V*)	Mobile phase B (per cent *V/V*)	Comment
0 - 20	60 → 0	40 → 100	linear gradient
20 - 35	0	100	isocratic
35 - 50	0 → 60	100 → 40	re-equilibration

Inject the dissolution mixture and use the same elution pattern to obtain a blank. In the chromatogram obtained with test solution (b), the area of any peak, apart from the principal peak and any peak corresponding to 4-hydroxyphenoxymethylpenicillin, is not greater than the area of the principal peak in the chromatogram obtained with reference solution (e) (1 per cent).

4-Hydroxyphenoxymethylpenicillin potassium. Not more than 4.0 per cent, calculated with reference to the anhydrous substance and determined by liquid chromatography (*2.2.29*), as described under Assay.

Water (*2.5.12*). Not more than 1.0 per cent, determined on 1.000 g by the semi-micro determination of water.

ASSAY

Examine by liquid chromatography (*2.2.29*).

Dissolution mixture. To 250 ml of *0.2 M potassium dihydrogen phosphate R* add 500 ml of *water R* and adjust to pH 6.5 with an 8.4 g/l solution of *sodium hydroxide R.* Dilute to 1000 ml with *water R.*

Test solution (a). Dissolve 50.0 mg of the substance to be examined in the dissolution mixture and dilute to 50.0 ml with the same mixture.

Test solution (b). Prepare immediately before use. Dissolve 80.0 mg of the substance to be examined in the dissolution mixture and dilute to 20.0 ml with the same mixture.

Reference solution (a). Dissolve 50.0 mg of *phenoxymethylpenicillin potassium CRS* in the dissolution mixture and dilute to 50.0 ml with the same mixture.

Reference solution (b). Dissolve 10.0 mg of *4-hydroxyphenoxymethylpenicillin CRS* in the dissolution mixture and dilute to 25.0 ml with the same mixture. Dilute 5.0 ml of the solution to 100.0 ml with the dissolution mixture.

Reference solution (c). Dissolve 10 mg of *phenoxymethylpenicillin potassium CRS* and 10 mg of *benzylpenicillin sodium CRS* in the dissolution mixture and dilute to 50 ml with the same mixture.

Reference solution (d). Dilute 1.0 ml of reference solution (a) to 20 ml with the dissolution mixture. Dilute 1.0 ml of the solution to 50 ml with the dissolution mixture.

Reference solution (e). Dilute 1.0 ml of reference solution (a) to 25.0 ml with the dissolution mixture.

The chromatographic procedure may be carried out using:

- a column 0.25 m long and 4.6 mm in internal diameter packed with *octadecylsilyl silica gel for chromatography R* (5 µm),
- as mobile phase at a flow rate of 1.0 ml/min:

  Mobile phase A. Mix 10 volumes of *phosphate buffer solution pH 3.5 R*, 30 volumes of *methanol R* and 60 volumes of *water R*,

  Mobile phase B. Mix 10 volumes of *phosphate buffer solution pH 3.5 R*, 35 volumes of *water R* and 55 volumes of *methanol R*,
- as detector a spectrophotometer set at 254 nm.

Equilibrate the column with a mobile phase ratio A:B of 60:40. Inject 20 µl of reference solution (c). The test is not valid unless, in the chromatogram obtained, the resolution between the 2 principal peaks is at least 6.0 (if necessary, adjust the ratio A:B of the mobile phase) and the mass distribution ratio for the second peak (phenoxymethylpenicillin) is 5.0 to 7.0. Inject reference solution (a) 6 times. The test is not valid unless the relative standard deviation for the area of the principal peak is at most 1.0 per cent. Inject alternately test solution (a) and reference solutions (a) and (b).

Calculate the percentage content of phenoxymethylpenicillin potassium. Calculate the percentage content of 4-hydroxyphenoxymethylpenicillin potassium by multiplying the percentage content of 4-hydroxyphenoxymethylpenicillin if necessary by the correction factor supplied with the CRS.

IMPURITIES

A. benzylpenicillin,

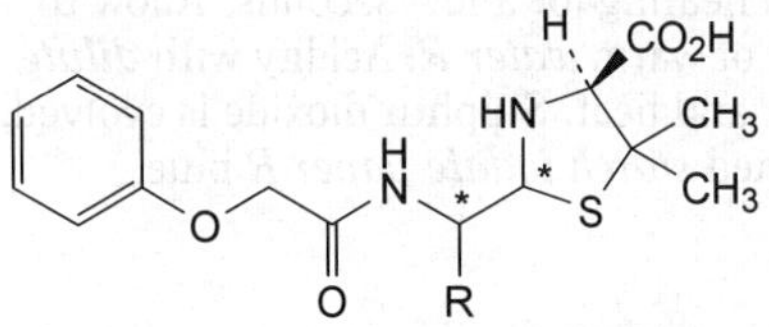

B. phenoxyacetic acid,

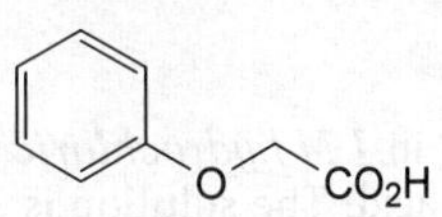

C. (2*S*,5*R*,6*R*)-6-amino-3,3-dimethyl-7-oxo-4-thia-1-azabicyclo[3.2.0]heptane-2-carboxylic acid (6-aminopenicillanic acid),

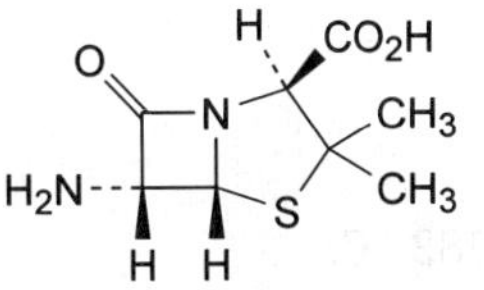

D. (2*S*,5*R*,6*R*)-3,3-dimethyl-7-oxo-6-[[2-(4-hydroxyphenoxy)acetyl]amino]-4-thia- 1-azabicyclo[3.2.0]heptane-2-carboxylic acid (4-hydroxyphenoxymethylpenicillin),

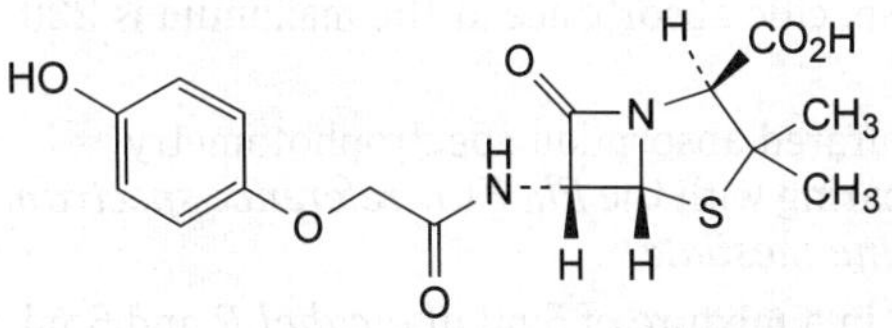

E. R = CO_2H: (4*S*)-2-[carboxy[(phenoxyacetyl)amino]methyl]-5,5dimethylthiazolidine-4-carboxylic acid (penicilloic acids of phenoxymethylpenicillin),

F. R = H: (2*RS*,4*S*)-5,5-dimethyl-2-[[(phenoxyacetyl)amino]methyl]thiazolidine-4-carboxylic acid (penilloic acids of phenoxymethylpenicillin).

01/2005:1138

PHENTOLAMINE MESILATE

Phentolamini mesilas

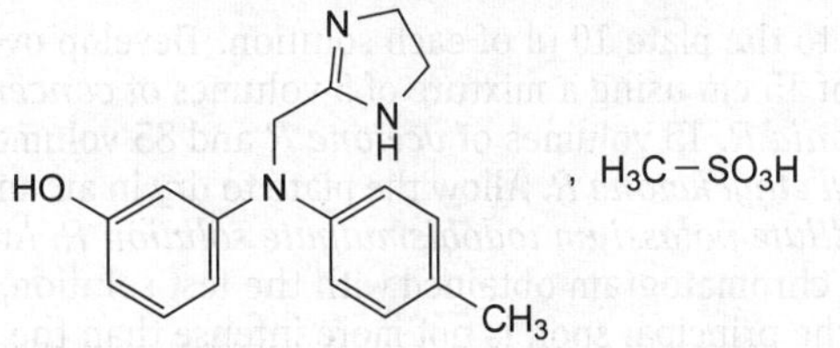

$C_{18}H_{23}N_3O_4S$ M_r 377.5

DEFINITION

Phentolamine mesilate contains not less than 98.0 per cent and not more than the equivalent of 100.5 per cent of 3-[[(4,5-dihydro-1*H*-imidazol-2-yl)methyl](4-methylphenyl)amino]phenol methanesulphonate, calculated with reference to the dried substance.

PRODUCTION

The production method must be evaluated to determine the potential for formation of alkyl mesilates, which is particularly likely to occur if the reaction medium contains lower alcohols. Where necessary, the production method is validated to demonstrate that alkyl mesilates are not detectable in the final product.

CHARACTERS

A white, crystalline powder, slightly hygroscopic, freely soluble in water and in alcohol, practically insoluble in methylene chloride.

IDENTIFICATION

First identification: C, E

Second identification: A, B, D, E.

A. Melting point (*2.2.14*): 178 °C to 182 °C.

B. Dissolve 60.0 mg in *water R* and dilute to 100.0 ml with the same solvent. Dilute 5.0 ml of the solution to 100.0 ml with *water R*. Examined between 230 nm and 350 nm (*2.2.25*), the solution shows an absorption maximum at 278 nm. The specific absorbance at the maximum is 220 to 245.

C. Examine by infrared absorption spectrophotometry (*2.2.24*), comparing with the *Ph. Eur. reference spectrum of phentolamine mesilate.*

D. Dissolve 0.5 g in a mixture of 5 ml of *alcohol R* and 5 ml of a 10 g/l solution of *hydrochloric acid R* and add 0.5 ml of a 5 g/l solution of *ammonium vanadate R*. A light green precipitate is produced.

E. Mix 50 mg with 0.2 g of *sodium hydroxide R*, heat to fusion and continue heating for a few seconds. Allow to cool and add 0.5 ml of warm *water R*. Acidify with *dilute hydrochloric acid R* and heat. Sulphur dioxide is evolved, which turns moistened *starch iodate paper R* blue.

TESTS

Acidity. Dissolve 0.1 g in *carbon dioxide-free water R* and dilute to 10 ml with the same solvent. Add 0.1 ml of *methyl red solution R*. If the solution is red, not more than 0.05 ml of *0.1 M sodium hydroxide* is required to change the colour of the indicator to yellow.

Related substances. Examine by thin-layer chromatography (*2.2.27*), using *silica gel G R* as the coating substance.

Test solution. Dissolve 0.10 g of the substance to be examined in *alcohol R* and dilute to 5 ml with the same solvent.

Reference solution (a). Dilute 0.5 ml of the test solution to 100 ml with *alcohol R*.

Reference solution (b). Dilute 5 ml of reference solution (a) to 10 ml with *alcohol R*.

Apply to the plate 10 µl of each solution. Develop over a path of 15 cm using a mixture of 5 volumes of *concentrated ammonia R*, 15 volumes of *acetone R* and 85 volumes of *methyl ethyl ketone R*. Allow the plate to dry in air and spray with *dilute potassium iodobismuthate solution R*. Any spot in the chromatogram obtained with the test solution, apart from the principal spot, is not more intense than the spot in the chromatogram obtained with reference solution (a) (0.5 per cent) and at most one such spot is more intense than the spot in the chromatogram obtained with reference solution (b) (0.25 per cent).

Loss on drying (*2.2.32*). Not more than 0.5 per cent, determined on 1.000 g by drying in an oven at 100-105 °C.

Sulphated ash (*2.4.14*). Not more than 0.1 per cent, determined on 1.0 g.

ASSAY

Dissolve 0.300 g in 100 ml of *2-propanol R1*. Titrate under a current of nitrogen with *0.1 M tetrabutylammonium hydroxide in 2-propanol*. Determine the end-point potentiometrically (*2.2.20*), using a glass electrode as indicator electrode and a calomel electrode containing a saturated solution of *tetramethylammonium chloride R* in *2-propanol R1* as the comparison electrode. Carry out a blank titration.

1 ml of *0.1 M tetrabutylammonium hydroxide in 2-propanol* is equivalent to 37.75 mg of $C_{18}H_{23}N_3O_4S$.

STORAGE

In an airtight container, protected from light.

IMPURITIES

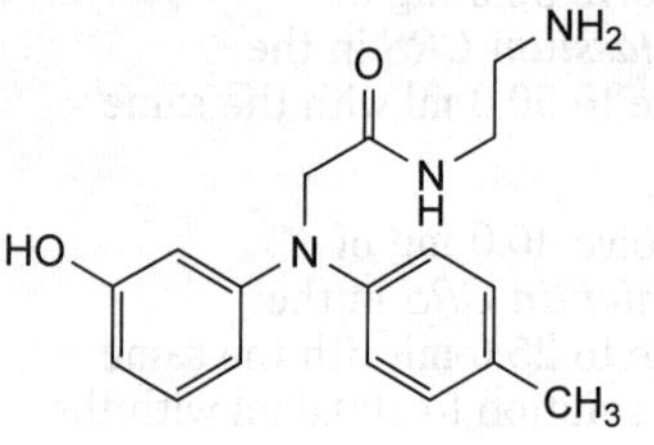

A. *N*-(2-aminoethyl)-2-[(3-hydroxyphenyl)(4-methylphenyl)amino]acetamide.

01/2005:0782

PHENYLALANINE

Phenylalaninum

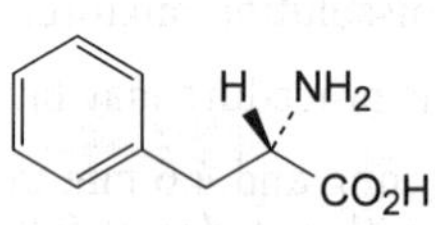

$C_9H_{11}NO_2$ M_r 165.2

DEFINITION

Phenylalanine contains not less than 98.5 per cent and not more than the equivalent of 101.0 per cent of (*S*)-2-amino-3-phenylpropanoic acid, calculated with reference to the dried substance.

CHARACTERS

A white or almost white, crystalline powder, or shiny, white flakes, sparingly soluble in water, very slightly soluble in alcohol. It dissolves in dilute mineral acids and in dilute solutions of alkali hydroxides.

IDENTIFICATION

First identification: A, B.

Second identification: A, C, D.

A. It complies with the test for specific optical rotation (see Tests).

B. Examine by infrared absorption spectrophotometry (*2.2.24*), comparing with the spectrum obtained with *phenylalanine CRS*. Examine the substances prepared as discs.

C. Examine the chromatograms obtained in the test for ninhydrin-positive substances. The principal spot in the chromatogram obtained with test solution (b) is similar in position, colour and size to the principal spot in the chromatogram obtained with reference solution (a).

D. To about 10 mg add 0.5 g of *potassium nitrate R* and 2 ml of *sulphuric acid R*. Heat on a water-bath for 20 min. Allow to cool. Add 5 ml of a 50 g/l solution of *hydroxylamine hydrochloride R* and allow to stand in iced water for 10 min. Add 9 ml of *strong sodium hydroxide solution R*. A violet-red to violet-brown colour develops.

TESTS

Appearance of solution. Dissolve 0.5 g in *1 M hydrochloric acid* and dilute to 10 ml with the same acid. The solution is clear (*2.2.1*) and not more intensely coloured than reference solution BY_6 (*2.2.2, Method II*).

Specific optical rotation (*2.2.7*). Dissolve 0.50 g in *water R* and dilute to 25.0 ml with the same solvent. The specific optical rotation is − 33.0 to − 35.5, calculated with reference to the dried substance.

Ninhydrin-positive substances. Examine by thin-layer chromatography (*2.2.27*), using a *TLC silica gel plate R*.

Test solution (a). Dissolve 0.10 g of the substance to be examined in a mixture of equal volumes of *glacial acetic acid R* and *water R* and dilute to 10 ml with the same mixture of solvents.

Test solution (b). Dilute 1 ml of test solution (a) to 50 ml with a mixture of equal volumes of *glacial acetic acid R* and *water R*.

Reference solution (a). Dissolve 10 mg of *phenylalanine CRS* in a mixture of equal volumes of *glacial acetic acid R* and *water R* and dilute to 50 ml with the same mixture of solvents.

Reference solution (b). Dilute 5 ml of test solution (b) to 20 ml with a mixture of equal volumes of *glacial acetic acid R* and *water R*.

Reference solution (c). Dissolve 10 mg of *phenylalanine CRS* and 10 mg of *tyrosine CRS* in a mixture of equal volumes of *glacial acetic acid R* and *water R* and dilute to 25 ml with the same mixture of solvents.

Apply separately to the plate 5 µl of each solution. Develop over a path of 15 cm using a mixture of 20 volumes of *glacial acetic acid R*, 20 volumes of *water R* and 60 volumes of *butanol R*. Allow the plate to dry in air, spray with *ninhydrin solution R* and heat at 100 °C to 105 °C for 15 min. Any spot in the chromatogram obtained with test solution (a), apart from the principal spot, is not more intense than the spot in the chromatogram obtained with reference solution (b) (0.5 per cent). The test is not valid unless the chromatogram obtained with reference solution (c) shows two clearly separated spots.

Chlorides (*2.4.4*). Dissolve 0.25 g in 3 ml of *dilute nitric acid R* and dilute to 15 ml with *water R*. The solution complies with the limit test for chlorides, without any further addition of nitric acid (200 ppm).

Sulphates (*2.4.13*). Dissolve 0.5 g in a mixture of 5 volumes of *dilute hydrochloric acid R* and 25 volumes of *distilled water R* and dilute to 15 ml with the same mixture of solvents. The solution complies with the limit test for sulphates (300 ppm).

Ammonium (*2.4.1*). 50 mg complies with limit test B for ammonium (200 ppm). Prepare the standard using 0.1 ml of *ammonium standard solution (100 ppm NH_4) R*.

Iron (*2.4.9*). In a separating funnel, dissolve 1.0 g in 10 ml of *dilute hydrochloric acid R*. Shake with three quantities, each of 10 ml, of *methyl isobutyl ketone R1*, shaking for 3 min each time. To the combined organic layers add 10 ml of *water R* and shake for 3 min. The aqueous layer complies with the limit test for iron (10 ppm).

Heavy metals (*2.4.8*). 2.0 g complies with limit test D for heavy metals (10 ppm). Prepare the standard using 2 ml of *lead standard solution (10 ppm Pb) R*.

Loss on drying (*2.2.32*). Not more than 0.5 per cent, determined on 1.000 g by drying in an oven at 100 °C to 105 °C.

Sulphated ash (*2.4.14*). Not more than 0.1 per cent, determined on 1.0 g.

ASSAY

Dissolve 0.100 g in 3 ml of *anhydrous formic acid R*. Add 30 ml of *anhydrous acetic acid R*. Titrate with *0.1 M perchloric acid* using 0.1 ml of *naphtholbenzein solution R* as indicator, until the colour changes from yellow to green.

1 ml of *0.1 M perchloric acid* is equivalent to 16.52 mg of $C_9H_{11}NO_2$.

STORAGE

Store protected from light.

01/2005:0422

PHENYLBUTAZONE

Phenylbutazonum

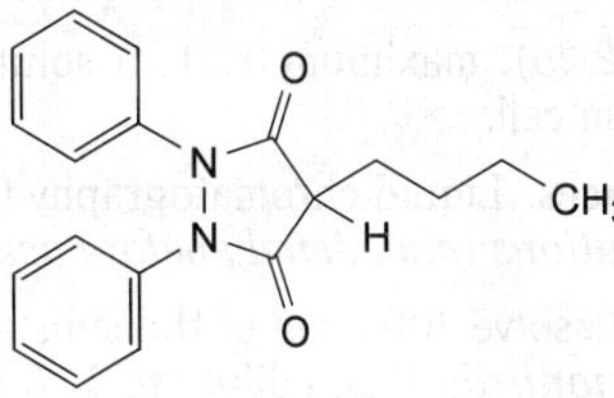

$C_{19}H_{20}N_2O_2$ M_r 308.4

DEFINITION

4-Butyl-1,2-diphenylpyrazolidine-3,5-dione.

Content: 99.0 per cent to 101.0 per cent (dried substance).

CHARACTERS

Appearance: white or almost white, crystalline powder.

Solubility: practically insoluble in water, sparingly soluble in alcohol. It dissolves in alkaline solutions.

IDENTIFICATION

First identification: A, C.

Second identification: A, B, D.

A. Melting point (*2.2.14*): 104 °C to 107 °C.

B. Thin-layer chromatography (*2.2.27*).

Test solution. Dissolve 25 mg of the substance to be examined in a mixture of equal volumes of *ethanol R* and *methylene chloride R* and dilute to 25 ml with the same mixture of solvents.

Reference solution. Dissolve 25 mg of *phenylbutazone CRS* in a mixture of equal volumes of *ethanol R* and *methylene chloride R* and dilute to 25 ml with the same mixture of solvents.

Plate: *TLC silica gel GF_{254} plate R*.

Mobile phase: *acetone R, methylene chloride R* (20:80 *V/V*).

Application: 5 µl.

Development: over a path of 10 cm.

Drying: in air.

Detection: examine in ultraviolet light at 254 nm.

Results: the principal spot in the chromatogram obtained with the test solution is similar in position and size to the principal spot in the chromatogram obtained with the reference solution.

C. Infrared absorption spectrophotometry (*2.2.24*).

Comparison: *phenylbutazone CRS.*

D. To 0.1 g add 1 ml of *glacial acetic acid R* and 2 ml of *hydrochloric acid R* and heat the mixture under a reflux condenser for 30 min. Cool, add 10 ml of *water R* and filter. To the filtrate add 3 ml of a 7 g/l solution of *sodium nitrite R*. A yellow colour is produced. To 1 ml of the solution add a solution of 10 mg of *β-naphthol R* in 5 ml of *sodium carbonate solution R*. A brownish-red to violet-red precipitate is formed.

TESTS

Solution S. Dissolve 1.0 g with shaking in 20 ml of *dilute sodium hydroxide solution R* and maintain the solution at 25 °C for 3 h.

Appearance of solution. Solution S is clear (*2.2.1*).

Acidity or alkalinity. Heat to boiling 1.0 g in 50 ml of *water R*, cool with shaking in a closed flask and filter. To 25 ml of the filtrate add 0.5 ml of *phenolphthalein solution R*. The solution is colourless. Not more than 0.5 ml of *0.01 M sodium hydroxide* is required to change the colour of the indicator. Add 0.6 ml of *0.01 M hydrochloric acid* and 0.1 ml of *methyl red solution R*; the solution is red or orange.

Absorbance (*2.2.25*): maximum 0.20 for solution S at 420 nm in a 4 cm cell.

Related substances. Liquid chromatography (*2.2.29*). *Prepare the solutions immediately before use.*

Test solution. Dissolve 100.0 mg of the substance to be examined in *acetonitrile R* and dilute to 10.0 ml with the same solvent.

Reference solution (a). Dilute 1.0 ml of the test solution to 100.0 ml with *acetonitrile R*. Dilute 1.0 ml to 10.0 ml with *acetonitrile R*.

Reference solution (b). Dissolve 5 mg of *phenylbutazone impurity B CRS* and 5 mg of *1,2-diphenylhydrazine R* in *acetonitrile R*, add 0.5 ml of the test solution and dilute to 50 ml with *acetonitrile R*. Dilute 2.5 ml to 10 ml with *acetonitrile R*.

Reference solution (c). Dissolve 1.0 mg of *benzidine R* in *acetonitrile R* and dilute to 100.0 ml with the same solvent. Dilute 1.0 ml to 100.0 ml with *acetonitrile R*. Dilute 5.0 ml to 10.0 ml with *acetonitrile R*.

Column:
- *size*: l = 0.125 m, Ø = 4.0 mm,
- *stationary phase*: *octadecylsilyl silica gel for chromatography R* (5 µm),
- *temperature*: 30 °C.

Mobile phase:
- *mobile phase A*: dissolve 1.36 g of *sodium acetate R* in *water R*, adjust to pH 5.2 with a 52.5 g/l solution of *citric acid R* and dilute to 1000 ml with *water R*,
- *mobile phase B*: *acetonitrile R*,

Time (min)	Mobile phase A (per cent *V/V*)	Mobile phase B (per cent *V/V*)
0 - 10	70	30
10 - 20	70 → 40	30 → 60
20 - 35	40	60
35 - 40	40 → 70	60 → 30

Flow rate: 1.5 ml/min.

Detection: spectrophotometer at 240 nm.

Injection: 20 µl; inject the test solution and reference solutions (a) and (b).

Relative retentions with reference to phenylbutazone (retention time = about 13 min): impurity E = about 0.2; impurity A = about 0.5; impurity B = about 1.2; impurity C = about 1.3; impurity D = about 1.7.

System suitability: reference solution (b):
- *resolution*: minimum 2.0 between the peaks due to phenylbutazone and to impurity B.

Limits:
- *correction factor*: for the calculation of content, multiply the peak area of impurity C by 0.55,
- *impurities A, B*: for each impurity, not more than 2.5 times the area of the principal peak in the chromatogram obtained with reference solution (a) (0.25 per cent),
- *impurity C*: not more than twice the area of the principal peak in the chromatogram obtained with reference solution (a) (0.20 per cent),
- *any other impurity*: not more than the area of the principal peak in the chromatogram obtained with reference solution (a) (0.1 per cent),
- *total*: not more than 5 times the area of the principal peak in the chromatogram obtained with reference solution (a) (0.5 per cent),
- *disregard limit*: 0.25 times the area of the principal peak in the chromatogram obtained with reference solution (a) (0.025 per cent); disregard any peak due to impurity E.

Impurity E. Liquid chromatography (*2.2.29*) as described in the test for related substances with the following modifications.

Detection: spectrophotometer at 280 nm.

Injection: test solution and reference solution (c).

System suitability: reference solution (c):
- *signal-to-noise ratio*: minimum 10 for the principal peak.

Limit:
- *impurity E*: not more than the area of the principal peak in the chromatogram obtained with reference solution (c) (5 ppm).

Heavy metals (*2.4.8*): maximum 20 ppm.

1.0 g complies with limit test C. Prepare the standard using 2 ml of *lead standard solution (10 ppm Pb) R*.

Loss on drying (*2.2.32*): maximum 0.2 per cent, determined on 1.000 g by drying *in vacuo* at 80 °C for 4 h.

Sulphated ash (*2.4.14*): maximum 0.1 per cent, determined on 1.0 g.

ASSAY

Dissolve 0.250 g in 25 ml of *acetone R* and add 0.5 ml of *bromothymol blue solution R1*. Titrate with *0.1 M sodium hydroxide* until a blue colour is obtained which persists for 15 s. Carry out a blank titration.

1 ml of *0.1 M sodium hydroxide* is equivalent to 30.84 mg of $C_{19}H_{20}N_2O_2$.

STORAGE

Protected from light.

IMPURITIES

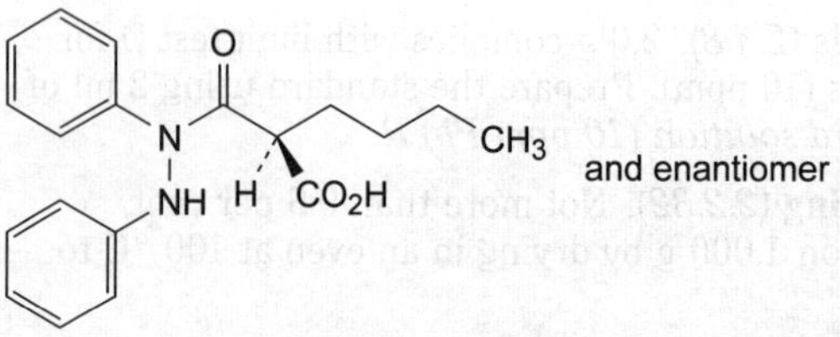

A. (2*RS*)-2-[(1,2-diphenyldiazanyl)carbonyl]hexanoic acid,

Monographs P

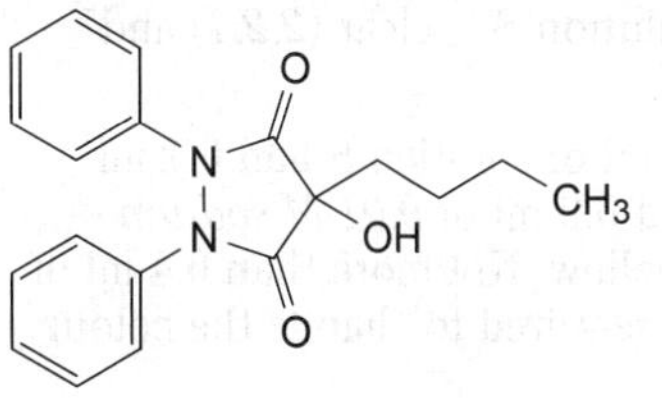

B. 4-butyl-4-hydroxy-1,2-diphenylpyrazolidine-3,5-dione,

C. C_6H_5-NH-NH-C_6H_5: 1,2-diphenyldiazane, (1,2-diphenylhydrazine),

D. C_6H_5-N=N-C_6H_5: 1,2-diphenyldiazene,

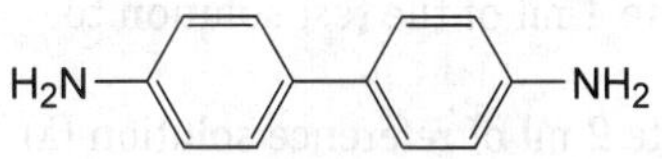

E. biphenyl-4,4′-diamine (benzidine).

01/2005:1035

PHENYLEPHRINE

Phenylephrinum

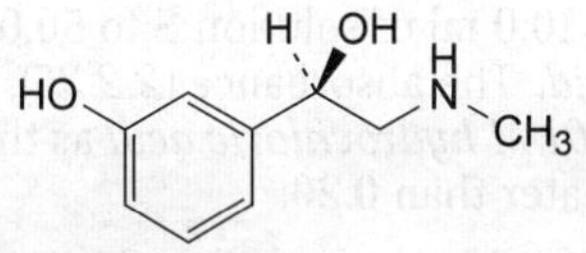

$C_9H_{13}NO_2$ M_r 167.2

DEFINITION

Phenylephrine contains not less than 99.0 per cent and not more than the equivalent of 100.5 per cent of (1*R*)-1-(3-hydroxyphenyl)-2-(methylamino)ethanol, calculated with reference to the dried substance.

CHARACTERS

A white or almost white, crystalline powder, slightly soluble in water, sparingly soluble in methanol, slightly soluble in alcohol. It dissolves in dilute mineral acids and in dilute solutions of alkali hydroxides.

It melts at about 174 °C.

IDENTIFICATION

First identification: A, B.

Second identification: A, C, D.

A. It complies with the test for specific optical rotation (see Tests).

B. Examine by infrared absorption spectrophotometry (*2.2.24*), comparing with the spectrum obtained with *phenylephrine CRS*.

C. Examine the chromatograms obtained in the test for related substances. The principal spot in the chromatogram obtained with the test solution is similar in position, colour and size to the principal spot in the chromatogram obtained with reference solution (a).

D. Dissolve about 10 mg in 1 ml of *1 M hydrochloric acid*, add 0.05 ml of *copper sulphate solution R* and 1 ml of a 200 g/l solution of *sodium hydroxide R*. A violet colour develops. Add 1 ml of *ether R* and shake. The upper layer remains colourless.

TESTS

Appearance of solution. Dissolve 1 g in *1 M hydrochloric acid* and dilute to 10 ml with the same acid. The solution is clear (*2.2.1*) and not more intensely coloured than reference solution Y_7 (*2.2.2, Method II*).

Specific optical rotation (*2.2.7*). Dissolve 1.250 g in *1 M hydrochloric acid* and dilute to 25.0 ml with the same acid. The specific optical rotation is − 53 to − 57, calculated with reference to the dried substance.

Absorbance. Dissolve 0.50 g in *0.1 M hydrochloric acid* and dilute to 200 ml with the same solvent. Measure the absorbance (*2.2.25*) at 315 nm using *0.1 M hydrochloric acid* as the compensation liquid. The absorbance is not more than 0.15 (0.4 per cent, calculated as impurity C).

Related substances. Examine by thin-layer chromatography (*2.2.27*), using *silica gel HF_{254} R* as the coating substance.

Solvent mixture. Prepare a mixture of equal volumes of *methylene chloride R* and methanolic hydrochloric acid *hydrochloric acid R* diluted to 10 volumes with *methanol R*.

Test solution. Dissolve 0.1 g of the substance to be examined in the solvent mixture and dilute to 5 ml with the same solvent mixture.

Reference solution (a). Dissolve 20 mg of *phenylephrine CRS* in the solvent mixture and dilute to 1 ml with the same solvent mixture.

Reference solution (b). Dilute 0.1 ml of the test solution to 20 ml with the solvent mixture.

Reference solution (c). Dilute 0.1 ml of the test solution to 50 ml with the solvent mixture.

Apply separately to the plate 10 µl of each solution and develop over a path of 15 cm using a mixture of 0.5 volumes of *concentrated ammonia R*, 25 volumes of *methanol R* and 70 volumes of *methylene chloride R*. Dry the plate in a current of cold air. Examine in ultraviolet light at 254 nm. Spray with a 1 g/l solution of *fast red B salt R* in a 50 g/l solution of *sodium carbonate R* and examine in daylight. Any spot in the chromatogram obtained with the test solution, apart from the principal spot, is not more intense than the spot in the chromatogram obtained with reference solution (b) (0.5 per cent) and at most two such spots are more intense than the spot in the chromatogram obtained with reference solution (c) (0.2 per cent).

Loss on drying (*2.2.32*). Not more than 0.5 per cent, determined on 1.000 g by drying in an oven at 100 °C to 105 °C.

Sulphated ash (*2.4.14*). Not more than 0.1 per cent, determined on 1.0 g.

ASSAY

Dissolve 0.150 g in 60 ml of *anhydrous acetic acid R*. Titrate with *0.1 M perchloric acid* determining the end-point potentiometrically (*2.2.20*).

1 ml of *0.1 M perchloric acid* is equivalent to 16.72 mg of $C_9H_{13}NO_2$.

STORAGE

Store in an airtight container, protected from light.

IMPURITIES

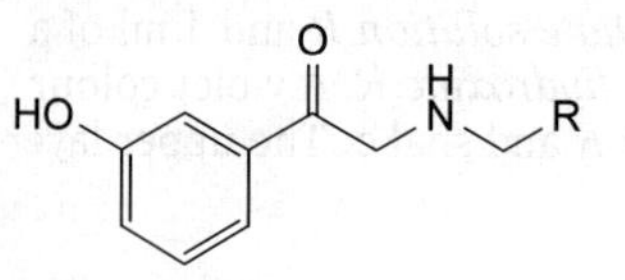

A. R = C_6H_5: 2-(benzylamino)-1-(3-hydroxyphenyl)ethanone,

C. R = H: 1-(3-hydroxyphenyl)-2-(methylamino)ethanone,

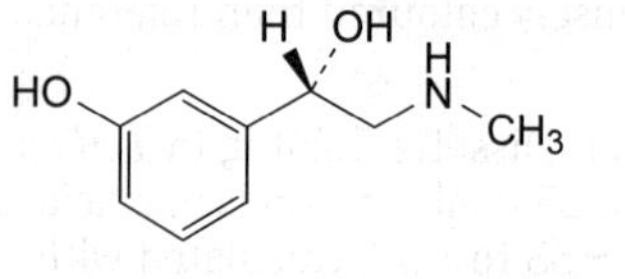

B. (1*S*)-1-(3-hydroxyphenyl)-2-(methylamino)ethanol.

01/2005:0632

PHENYLEPHRINE HYDROCHLORIDE

Phenylephrini hydrochloridum

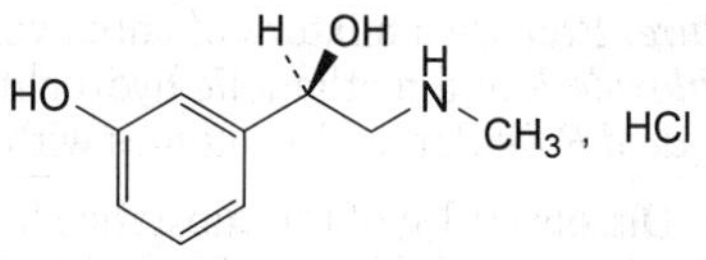

$C_9H_{14}ClNO_2$ M_r 203.7

DEFINITION

Phenylephrine hydrochloride contains not less than 98.5 per cent and not more than the equivalent of 101.0 per cent of (1*R*)-1-(3-hydroxyphenyl)-2-(methylamino)ethanol hydrochloride, calculated with reference to the dried substance.

CHARACTERS

A white or almost white, crystalline powder, freely soluble in water and in alcohol.

It melts at about 143 °C.

IDENTIFICATION

First identification: A, B, E.

Second identification: A, C, D, E.

A. It complies with the test for specific optical rotation (see Tests).

B. Examine by infrared absorption spectrophotometry (*2.2.24*), comparing with the spectrum obtained with *phenylephrine hydrochloride CRS*. Examine the substances prepared as discs.

C. Dissolve 0.3 g in 3 ml of *water R*, add 1 ml of *dilute ammonia R1* and initiate crystallisation by scratching the wall of the tube with a glass rod. The crystals, washed with iced *water R* and dried at 105 °C for 2 h, melt (*2.2.14*) at 171 °C to 176 °C.

D. Dissolve about 10 mg in 1 ml of *water R* and add 0.05 ml of a 125 g/l solution of *copper sulphate R* and 1 ml of a 200 g/l solution of *sodium hydroxide R*. A violet colour is produced. Add 1 ml of *ether R* and shake; the ether layer remains colourless.

E. It gives reaction (a) of chlorides (*2.3.1*).

TESTS

Solution S. Dissolve 2.00 g in *carbon dioxide-free water R* prepared from *distilled water R* and dilute to 100.0 ml with the same solvent.

Appearance of solution. Solution S is clear (*2.2.1*) and colourless (*2.2.2, Method II*).

Acidity or alkalinity. To 10 ml of solution S add 0.1 ml of *methyl red solution R* and 0.2 ml of *0.01 M sodium hydroxide*. The solution is yellow. Not more than 0.4 ml of *0.01 M hydrochloric acid* is required to change the colour of the indicator to red.

Specific optical rotation (*2.2.7*): − 43 to − 47, determined on solution S and calculated with reference to the dried substance.

Related substances. Examine by thin-layer chromatography (*2.2.27*), using *silica gel H R* as the coating substance.

Test solution. Dissolve 0.10 g of the substance to be examined in *methanol R* and dilute to 5 ml with the same solvent.

Reference solution (a). Dilute 1 ml of the test solution to 200 ml with *methanol R*.

Reference solution (b). Dilute 2 ml of reference solution (a) to 5 ml with *methanol R*.

Apply separately to the plate 5 µl of each solution. Develop over a path of 15 cm using a mixture of 5 volumes of *chloroform R*, 15 volumes of *ammonia R* and 80 volumes of *2-propanol R*. Dry the plate in a current of cold air, spray with *ninhydrin solution R* and heat at 100 °C to 105 °C for 5 min to 10 min. Examine in daylight. Any spot in the chromatogram obtained with the test solution, apart from the principal spot, is not more intense than the spot in the chromatogram obtained with the reference solution (a) (0.5 per cent) and at most two such spots are more intense than the spot in the chromatogram obtained with reference solution (b) (0.2 per cent).

Ketones. Dilute 10.0 ml of solution S to 50.0 ml with *0.01 M hydrochloric acid*. The absorbance (*2.2.25*), measured at 310 nm using *0.01 M hydrochloric acid* as the compensation liquid, is not greater than 0.20.

Sulphates (*2.4.13*). 15 ml of solution S complies with the limit test for sulphates (500 ppm).

Loss on drying (*2.2.32*). Not more than 1.0 per cent, determined on 1.000 g by drying in an oven at 100 °C to 105 °C.

Sulphated ash (*2.4.14*). Not more than 0.1 per cent, determined on 1.0 g.

ASSAY

Dissolve 0.1500 g in a mixture of 0.5 ml of *0.1 M hydrochloric acid* and 80 ml of *alcohol R*. Carry out a potentiometric titration (*2.2.20*) using *0.1 M ethanolic sodium hydroxide*. Read the volume added between the two points of inflexion.

1 ml of *0.1 M ethanolic sodium hydroxide* is equivalent to 20.37 mg of $C_9H_{14}ClNO_2$.

01/2005:2042

PHENYLMERCURIC ACETATE

Phenylhydrargyri acetas

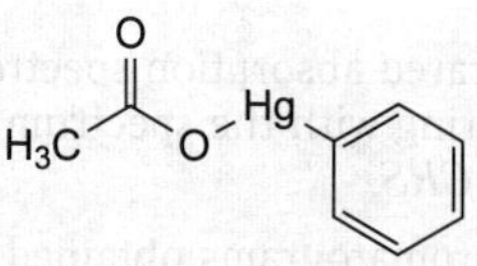

$C_8H_8HgO_2$ M_r 336.7

DEFINITION

Content: 98.0 per cent to 100.5 per cent (dried substance).

CHARACTERS

Appearance: white or yellowish, crystalline powder or small, colourless crystals.

Solubility: slightly soluble in water, soluble in acetone and in alcohol.

IDENTIFICATION

First identification: A.

Second identification: B, C.

A. Infrared absorption spectrophotometry (*2.2.24*).

Comparison: *Ph. Eur. reference spectrum of phenylmercuric acetate.*

B. To 5 ml of solution S (see Tests) add 5 ml of *water R* and 0.1 ml of *sodium sulphide solution R.* A white precipitate is formed that darkens slowly on heating.

C. To 10 ml of solution S add 2 ml of *potassium iodide solution R* and shake vigorously. Filter. The filtrate gives reaction (b) of acetates (*2.3.1*).

TESTS

Solution S. Dissolve 0.250 g in 40 ml of *water R* by heating to boiling. Allow to cool and dilute to 50 ml with *water R.* Prepare the solution immediately before use.

Appearance of solution. Solution S is not more opalescent than reference suspension II (*2.2.1*) and is colourless (*2.2.2, Method II*).

Ionised mercury: maximum 0.2 per cent.

To 2 ml of solution S add 8 ml of *water R,* 2 ml of *potassium iodide solution R* and 3 ml of *dilute hydrochloric acid R.* Filter. The filtrate is not more coloured than the potassium iodide solution used. Wash the precipitate with 3 ml of *water R.* Combine the filtrate and the washings, add 2 ml of *dilute sodium hydroxide solution R* and dilute to 20 ml with *water R.* 12 ml of this solution complies with limit test A for heavy metals (*2.4.8*). Prepare the standard using *lead standard solution (1 ppm Pb) R.*

Polymercuric benzene compounds: maximum 1.5 per cent. Shake 0.2 g with 10 ml of *acetone R.* Filter. Wash the residue twice with 5 ml of *acetone R.* Dry the residue at 105 °C for 1 h. The residue weighs a maximum of 3 mg.

Loss on drying (*2.2.32*): maximum 0.5 per cent, determined on 0.500 g by drying in an oven at 45 °C for 15 h.

ASSAY

Dissolve with heating 0.300 g in 100 ml of *water R.* Cool and add 3 ml of *nitric acid R.* Titrate with *0.1 M ammonium thiocyanate* using 2 ml of *ferric ammonium sulphate solution R2* as indicator, until a persistent reddish-yellow colour is obtained.

1 ml of *0.1 M ammonium thiocyanate* is equivalent to 33.67 mg of phenylmercuric acetate.

STORAGE

Protected from light.

01/2005:0103

PHENYLMERCURIC BORATE

Phenylhydrargyri boras

DEFINITION

Phenylmercuric borate is a compound consisting of equimolecular proportions of phenylmercuric orthoborate and phenylmercuric hydroxide ($C_{12}H_{13}BHg_2O_4$; M_r 633) or of the dehydrated form (metaborate, $C_{12}H_{11}BHg_2O_3$; M_r 615) or a mixture of the two compounds. It contains not less than 64.5 per cent and not more than 66.0 per cent of Hg (A_r 200.6) and not less than the equivalent of 9.8 per cent and not more than the equivalent of 10.3 per cent of borates, expressed as H_3BO_3, both calculated with reference to the dried substance.

CHARACTERS

A white or slightly yellowish, crystalline powder or colourless, shiny crystals, slightly soluble in water and in alcohol.

IDENTIFICATION

A. Examine by infrared absorption spectrophotometry (*2.2.24*), comparing with the *Ph. Eur. reference spectrum of phenylmercuric borate.* Examine the substance as a disc.

B. To 2 ml of solution S (see Tests) add 8 ml of *water R* and 0.1 ml of *sodium sulphide solution R.* A white precipitate is formed that darkens slowly on heating.

C. Dissolve about 20 mg in 2 ml of *methanol R.* The solution is clear and colourless. Ignite; the solution burns with a green-edged flame.

TESTS

Solution S. Dissolve 0.25 g by sprinkling it on the surface of 25 ml of boiling *water R,* cool and dilute to 25 ml with *water R.*

Appearance of solution. Solution S is clear (*2.2.1*) and colourless (*2.2.2, Method II*).

Ionised mercury. To 10 ml of solution S add 2 ml of *potassium iodide solution R* and 3 ml of *dilute hydrochloric acid R.* Filter. The filtrate is colourless. Wash the precipitate with 3 ml of *water R.* Combine the filtrate and the washings, add 2 ml of *dilute sodium hydroxide solution R* and dilute to 20 ml with *water R.* 12 ml of this solution complies with limit test A for heavy metals (*2.4.8*). Prepare the standard using a mixture of 2.5 ml of *lead standard solution (2 ppm Pb) R* and 7.5 ml of *water R.*

Loss on drying (*2.2.32*). Not more than 3.5 per cent, determined on 0.50 g by drying in an oven at 45 °C for 15 h (± 30 min).

ASSAY

Mercury. Dissolve 0.300 g in 100 ml of *water R* and add 3 ml of *nitric acid R.* Titrate with *0.1 M ammonium thiocyanate,* using 2 ml of *ferric ammonium sulphate solution R2* as indicator, until a persistent reddish-yellow colour is obtained.

1 ml of *0.1 M ammonium thiocyanate* is equivalent to 20.06 mg of Hg.

Borates. Dissolve 0.600 g with heating in 25 ml of *water R.* Dissolve 10 g of *sorbitol R* in the hot solution and cool. Titrate with *0.1 M sodium hydroxide,* using 0.5 ml of *phenolphthalein solution R* as indicator, until a persistent pink colour is obtained. Carry out a blank titration.

1 ml of *0.1 M sodium hydroxide* is equivalent to 6.18 mg of H_3BO_3.

STORAGE

Store protected from light.

Monographs P

01/2005:0783

PHENYLMERCURIC NITRATE

Phenylhydrargyri nitras

DEFINITION

Phenylmercuric nitrate is a mixture of phenylmercuric nitrate ($C_6H_5HgNO_3$; M_r 339.7) and phenylmercuric hydroxide (C_6H_5HgOH; M_r 294.7). It contains not less than 62.5 per cent and not more than 64.0 per cent of Hg (A_r 200.6), calculated with reference to the dried substance.

CHARACTERS

A white or pale yellow powder, very slightly soluble in water and in alcohol, slightly soluble in hot water. It dissolves in glycerol and in fatty oils.

IDENTIFICATION

A. To 5 ml of solution S (see Tests) add 8 ml of *water R* and 0.1 ml of *sodium sulphide solution R*. A white precipitate is formed that darkens slowly on heating.

B. To 1 ml of a saturated solution of the substance to be examined add 1 ml of *dilute hydrochloric acid R*. A white, flocculent precipitate is formed.

C. To 5 ml of solution S add 1 ml of *dilute hydrochloric acid R*, 2 ml of *methylene chloride R* and 0.2 ml of *dithizone solution R*. Shake. The lower layer is orange-yellow.

D. About 10 mg gives the reaction of nitrates (*2.3.1*).

TESTS

Solution S. To 0.1 g add 45 ml of *water R* and heat to boiling with shaking. Cool, filter and dilute to 50 ml with *water R*.

Appearance of solution. Solution S is colourless (*2.2.2, Method II*).

Inorganic mercuric compounds. To 10 ml of solution S add 2 ml of *potassium iodide solution R* and 3 ml of *dilute hydrochloric acid R*. Filter. The filtrate is colourless. Wash the precipitate with 2 ml of *water R*. Combine the filtrate and washings, add 2 ml of *dilute sodium hydroxide solution R* and dilute to 20 ml with *water R*. 12 ml of the solution complies with limit test A for heavy metals (0.1 per cent) (*2.4.8*). Prepare the standard using *lead standard solution (1 ppm Pb) R*.

Loss on drying (*2.2.32*). Not more than 1.0 per cent, determined on 1.000 g by drying *in vacuo* for 24 h.

ASSAY

Dissolve 0.150 g in a mixture of 10 ml of *dilute nitric acid R* and 90 ml of *water R*, heating to boiling. Cool to 15 °C to 20 °C. Titrate with *0.1 M ammonium thiocyanate* using 2 ml of *ferric ammonium sulphate solution R2* as indicator, until a persistent reddish-yellow colour is obtained. Carry out a blank titration.

1 ml of *0.1 M ammonium thiocyanate* is equivalent to 20.06 mg of Hg.

STORAGE

Store protected from light.

01/2005:0683

PHENYLPROPANOLAMINE HYDROCHLORIDE

Phenylpropanolamini hydrochloridum

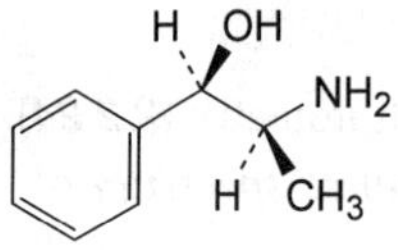

and enantiomer , HCl

$C_9H_{14}ClNO$ M_r 187.7

DEFINITION

Phenylpropanolamine hydrochloride contains not less than 99.0 per cent and not more than the equivalent of 101.5 per cent of (1*RS*,2*SR*)-2-amino-1-phenylpropan-1-ol hydrochloride, calculated with reference to the dried substance.

CHARACTERS

A white or almost white, crystalline powder, freely soluble in water and in alcohol, practically insoluble in methylene chloride.

IDENTIFICATION

First identification: B, E.

Second identification: A, C, D, E.

A. Melting point (*2.2.14*): 194 °C to 197 °C.

B. Examine by infrared absorption spectrophotometry (*2.2.24*), comparing with the spectrum obtained with *phenylpropanolamine hydrochloride CRS*. Examine the substances prepared as discs without recrystallisation.

C. Examine the chromatograms obtained in the test for related substances. The principal spot in the chromatogram obtained with test solution (b) is similar in position, colour and size to the principal spot in the chromatogram obtained with reference solution (a).

D. Dissolve 50 mg in 5 ml of *water R*, add 0.2 ml of *copper sulphate solution R* and 0.3 ml of *dilute sodium hydroxide solution R*. A violet colour develops. Add 2 ml of *ether R* and shake. A violet precipitate is formed between the two layers.

E. It gives reaction (a) of chlorides (*2.3.1*).

TESTS

Solution S. Dissolve 1.25 g in *water R* and dilute to 25 ml with the same solvent.

Appearance of solution. Solution S is clear (*2.2.1*) and colourless (*2.2.2, Method II*).

Acidity or alkalinity. To 10 ml of solution S add 0.1 ml of *methyl red solution R* and 0.2 ml of *0.01 M sodium hydroxide*. The solution is yellow. Add 0.4 ml of *0.01 M hydrochloric acid*. The solution is red.

Related substances. Examine by thin-layer chromatography (*2.2.27*), using *silica gel H R* as the coating substance.

Test solution (a). Dissolve 0.20 g of the substance to be examined in *alcohol R* and dilute to 10 ml with the same solvent.

Test solution (b). Dilute 1 ml of test solution (a) to 10 ml with *alcohol R*.

Reference solution (a). Dissolve 20 mg of *phenylpropanolamine hydrochloride CRS* in *alcohol R* and dilute to 10 ml with the same solvent.

Reference solution (b). Dilute 1 ml of reference solution (a) to 10 ml with *alcohol R.*

Reference solution (c). Dissolve 20 mg of *norpseudoephedrine hydrochloride CRS* in *alcohol R,* add 1 ml of test solution (a) and dilute to 10 ml with *alcohol R.*

Reference solution (d). Dissolve 60 mg of *ammonium chloride R* in *methanol R* and dilute to 10 ml with the same solvent.

Before applying the solutions, spray the plate with a 20 g/l solution of *disodium tetraborate R,* using 8 ml for a plate 100 mm by 200 mm and dry in a stream of cold air for 30 min. Apply separately to the plate as bands about 10 mm by 3 mm 10 µl of each solution. Develop over a path of 10 cm using a mixture of 6 volumes of *concentrated ammonia R,* 24 volumes of *alcohol R* and 70 volumes of *butanol R.* Dry the plate in a current of warm air until the solvents have evaporated, allow to cool, spray with a 2 g/l solution of *ninhydrin R* in *alcohol R* and heat at 110 °C for 15 min. Any spot in the chromatogram obtained with test solution (a) apart from the principal spot and the spot corresponding to ammonium chloride is not more intense than the spot in the chromatogram obtained with reference solution (b) (1.0 per cent). The test is not valid unless the chromatogram obtained with reference solution (c) shows two clearly separated spots.

Phenylpropanonamine. Dissolve 1.0 g in *0.01 M hydrochloric acid* and dilute to 50.0 ml with the same acid. The absorbance (*2.2.25*) of the solution measured at 283 nm is not greater than 0.10.

Heavy metals (*2.4.8*). 12 ml of solution S complies with limit test A for heavy metals (20 ppm). Prepare the standard using *lead standard solution (1 ppm Pb) R.*

Loss on drying (*2.2.32*). Not more than 0.5 per cent, determined on 1.000 g by drying in an oven at 100 °C to 105 °C.

Sulphated ash (*2.4.14*). Not more than 0.1 per cent, determined on 1.0 g.

ASSAY

Dissolve 0.1500 g in a mixture of 5 ml of *0.01 M hydrochloric acid* and 50 ml of *alcohol R.* Carry out a potentiometric titration (*2.2.20*), using *0.1 M sodium hydroxide.* Read the volume added between the two points of inflexion.

1 ml of *0.1 M sodium hydroxide* is equivalent to 18.77 mg of $C_9H_{14}ClNO$.

01/2005:1253

PHENYTOIN

Phenytoinum

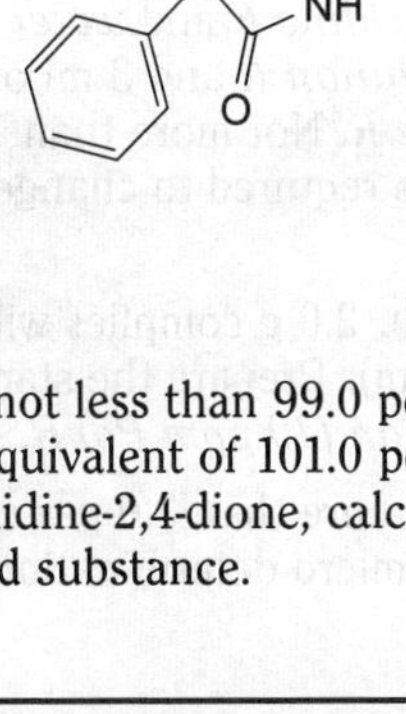

$C_{15}H_{12}N_2O_2$ M_r 252.3

DEFINITION

Phenytoin contains not less than 99.0 per cent and not more than the equivalent of 101.0 per cent of 5,5-diphenylimidazolidine-2,4-dione, calculated with reference to the dried substance.

CHARACTERS

A white or almost white, crystalline powder, practically insoluble in water, sparingly soluble in alcohol, very slightly soluble in methylene chloride. It dissolves in dilute solutions of alkali hydroxides.

IDENTIFICATION

First identification: A.

Second identification: B, C, D.

A. Examine by infrared absorption spectrophotometry (*2.2.24*), comparing with the spectrum obtained with *phenytoin CRS.*

B. Examine the chromatograms obtained in the test for related substances. The principal spot in the chromatogram obtained with test solution (b) is similar in position and size to the principal spot in the chromatogram obtained with reference solution (a).

C. To about 10 mg add 1 ml of *water R* and 0.05 ml of *ammonia R.* Heat until boiling begins. Add 0.05 ml of a 50 g/l solution of *copper sulphate R* in *dilute ammonia R2* and shake. A pink, crystalline precipitate is formed.

D. It complies with the test for sulphated ash (see Tests).

TESTS

Appearance of solution. Dissolve 1.0 g in a mixture of 5 ml of *1 M sodium hydroxide* and 20 ml of *water R.* The solution is clear (*2.2.1*) and not more intensely coloured than reference solution BY_6 (*2.2.2, Method II*).

Acidity or alkalinity. To 1.0 g add 45 ml of *water R* and boil for 2 min. Allow to cool and filter. Wash the filter with *carbon dioxide-free water R* and dilute the combined filtrate and washings to 50 ml with the same solvent. To 10 ml of the solution add 0.15 ml of *methyl red solution R.* Not more than 0.5 ml of *0.01 M hydrochloric acid* is required to change the colour of the indicator to red. To 10 ml of the solution add 0.15 ml of *bromothymol blue solution R1.* Not more than 0.5 ml of *0.01 M sodium hydroxide* is required to change the colour of the indicator to blue.

Related substances. Examine by thin-layer chromatography (*2.2.27*), using as the coating substance a suitable silica gel with a fluorescent indicator having an optimal intensity at 254 nm. Before use, wash the plate with a mixture of 30 volumes of *dioxan R* and 75 volumes of *hexane R.* Allow the plate to dry in air.

Test solution (a). Dissolve 0.40 g of the substance to be examined in a mixture of equal volumes of *acetone R* and *methanol R* and dilute to 10 ml with the same mixture of solvents.

Test solution (b). Dilute 1 ml of test solution (a) to 20 ml with a mixture of equal volumes of *acetone R* and *methanol R.*

Reference solution (a). Dissolve 20 mg of *phenytoin CRS* in a mixture of equal volumes of *acetone R* and *methanol R* and dilute to 10 ml with the same mixture of solvents.

Reference solution (b). Dissolve 8 mg of *benzophenone R* in a mixture of equal volumes of *acetone R* and *methanol R* and dilute to 100 ml with the same mixture of solvents.

Reference solution (c). Dissolve 8 mg of *benzil R* in a mixture of equal volumes of *acetone R* and *methanol R* and dilute to 100 ml with the same mixture of solvents.

Reference solution (d). Dilute 1 ml of test solution (a) to 100 ml with a mixture of equal volumes of *acetone R* and *methanol R.*

Reference solution (e). Mix 1 ml of reference solution (b) and 1 ml of reference solution (c).

Apply separately to the plate 10 µl of each solution and dry the plate in a stream of cold air for 2 min. Develop over a path of 15 cm using a mixture of 30 volumes of *dioxan R* and 75 volumes of *hexane R*. Allow the plate to dry in air and examine in ultraviolet light at 254 nm. In the chromatogram obtained with test solution (a): any spot corresponding to benzophenone is not more intense than the spot in the chromatogram obtained with reference solution (b) (0.2 per cent); any spot corresponding to benzil is not more intense than the spot in the chromatogram obtained with reference solution (c) (0.2 per cent) and any spot, apart from the principal spot and any spot corresponding to benzo-phenone and benzil, is not more intense than the spot in the chromatogram obtained with reference solution (d) (1 per cent). The test is not valid unless the chromatogram obtained with reference solution (e) shows two clearly separated principal spots.

Heavy metals (*2.4.8*). 2.0 g complies with limit test C for heavy metals (10 ppm). Prepare the standard using 2 ml of *lead standard solution (10 ppm Pb) R*.

Loss on drying(*2.2.32*). Not more than 0.5 per cent, determined on 1.000 g by drying in an oven at 100 °C to 105 °C.

Sulphated ash (*2.4.14*). Not more than 0.1 per cent, determined on 1.0 g.

ASSAY

Dissolve 0.200 g in 50 ml of *dimethylformamide R*. Titrate with *0.1 M sodium methoxide*, determining the end-point potentiometrically (*2.2.20*).

1 ml of *0.1 M sodium methoxide* is equivalent to 25.23 mg of $C_{15}H_{12}N_2O_2$.

IMPURITIES

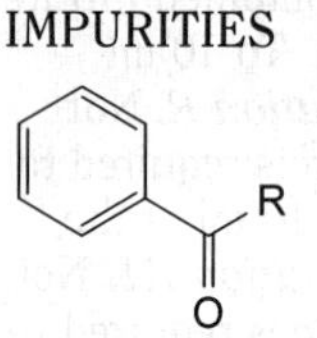

A. R = C_6H_5: diphenylmethanone (benzophenone),

B. R = CO-C_6H_5: diphenylethanedione (benzil).

01/2005:0521

PHENYTOIN SODIUM

Phenytoinum natricum

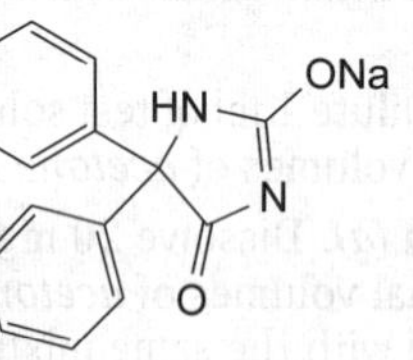

$C_{15}H_{11}N_2NaO_2$ M_r 274.3

DEFINITION

Phenytoin sodium contains not less than 98.5 per cent and not more than the equivalent of 100.5 per cent of sodium 4-oxo-5,5-diphenyl-4,5-dihydro-1*H*-imidazol-2-olate, calculated with reference to the anhydrous substance.

CHARACTERS

A white, crystalline powder, slightly hygroscopic, soluble in water and in alcohol, practically insoluble in methylene chloride.

IDENTIFICATION

First identification: A, C.

Second identification: B, C.

A. Dissolve 0.1 g in 20 ml of *water R*. Acidify with *dilute hydrochloric acid R* and shake with three quantities, each of 30 ml, of *chloroform R*. Wash the combined chloroform layers with *water R*, evaporate to dryness and dry the residue at 100 °C to 105 °C (test residue). Repeat the operations using 0.1 g of *phenytoin sodium CRS* (reference residue). Examine by infrared absorption spectrophotometry (*2.2.24*), comparing with the spectrum obtained with *phenytoin sodium CRS*. Examine as discs prepared using *potassium bromide R*.

B. To about 10 mg add 1 ml of *water R* and 0.05 ml of *ammonia R*. Heat until boiling begins. Add 0.05 ml of a 50 g/l solution of *copper sulphate R* in *dilute ammonia R2* and shake. A pink, crystalline precipitate is formed.

C. Ignite 1 g and cool. Add 2 ml of *water R* to the residue and neutralise the solution with *hydrochloric acid R*. Filter and dilute the filtrate to 4 ml with *water R*. 0.1 ml of the solution gives reaction (b) of sodium (*2.3.1*).

TESTS

Appearance of solution. Suspend 1.0 g in 5 ml of *water R* and dilute to 20 ml with *0.1 M sodium hydroxide*. The solution is clear (*2.2.1*) and not more intensely coloured than reference solution BY_6 (*2.2.2, Method II*).

Related substances. Examine by thin-layer chromatography (*2.2.27*), using as the coating substance a suitable silica gel containing a fluorescent indicator having an optimal intensity at 254 nm.

Test solution. Dissolve 0.4 g of the substance to be examined in *methanol R* and dilute to 10 ml with the same solvent.

Reference solution (a). Dilute 1 ml of the test solution to 100 ml with *methanol R*.

Reference solution (b). Dissolve 20 mg of *benzophenone R* in *methanol R* and dilute to 100 ml with the same solvent.

Apply separately to the plate 10 µl of each solution and dry the plate in a stream of cold air for 2 min. Develop over a path of 15 cm using a mixture of 10 volumes of *concentrated ammonia R*, 45 volumes of *chloroform R* and 45 volumes of *2-propanol R*. Dry the plate in an oven at 80 °C for 5 min and examine in ultraviolet light at 254 nm. In the chromatogram obtained with the test solution, any spot corresponding to benzophenone is not more intense than the spot in the chromatogram obtained with reference solution (b) (0.5 per cent) and any spot, apart from the principal spot and the spot corresponding to benzophenone, is not more intense than the spot in the chromatogram obtained with reference solution (a) (1.0 per cent).

Free phenytoin. Dissolve 0.30 g in 10 ml of a mixture of equal volumes of *pyridine R* and *water R*. Add 0.5 ml of *phenolphthalein solution R* and 3 ml of *silver nitrate solution in pyridine R*. Not more than 1.0 ml of *0.1 M sodium hydroxide* is required to change the colour of the indicator to pink.

Heavy metals (*2.4.8*). 2.0 g complies with limit test C for heavy metals (10 ppm). Prepare the standard using 2 ml of *lead standard solution (10 ppm Pb) R*.

Water (*2.5.12*). Not more than 3.0 per cent, determined on 1.000 g by the semi-micro determination of water.

ASSAY

Suspend 0.180 g in 2 ml of *water R*. Add 8.0 ml of *0.05 M sulphuric acid* and heat gently for 1 min. Add 30 ml of *methanol R* and cool. Carry out a potentiometric titration (*2.2.20*), using *0.1 M sodium hydroxide*. After reaching the first point of inflexion, interrupt the addition of *0.1 M sodium hydroxide*, add 5 ml of *silver nitrate solution in pyridine R*, mix and continue the titration. Read the volume of *0.1 M sodium hydroxide* added between the two points of inflexion.

1 ml of *0.1 M sodium hydroxide* is equivalent to 27.43 mg of $C_{15}H_{11}N_2NaO_2$.

STORAGE

Store in an airtight container.

01/2005:0522

PHOLCODINE

Pholcodinum

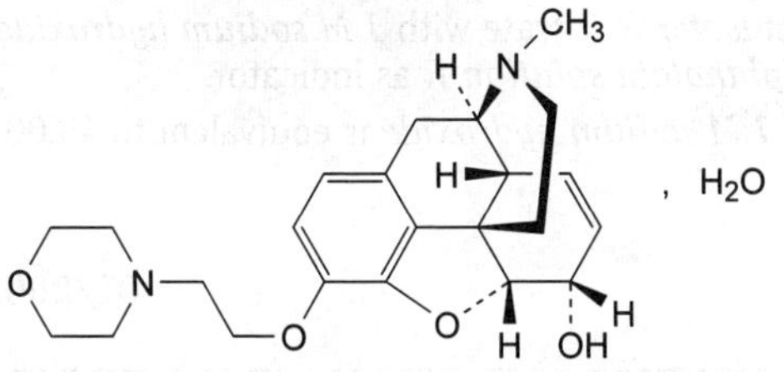

$C_{23}H_{30}N_2O_4,H_2O$ M_r 416.5

DEFINITION

Pholcodine contains not less than 98.5 per cent and not more than the equivalent of 100.5 per cent of 7,8-didehydro-4,5α-epoxy-17-methyl-3-[2-(morpholin-4-yl)ethoxy]morphinan-6α-ol, calculated with reference to the dried substance.

CHARACTERS

A white or almost white, crystalline powder or colourless crystals, sparingly soluble in water, freely soluble in acetone and in alcohol. It dissolves in dilute mineral acids.

IDENTIFICATION

First identification: A.

Second identification: B, C.

A. Examine by infrared absorption spectrophotometry (*2.2.24*), comparing with the *Ph. Eur. reference spectrum of pholcodine*.

B. Dissolve 0.100 g in *water R* and dilute to 100.0 ml with the same solvent. To 10.0 ml of this solution add 75 ml of *water R* and 10 ml of *1 M sodium hydroxide* and dilute to 100.0 ml with *water R*. Examined between 230 nm and 350 nm (*2.2.25*), the solution shows an absorption maximum at 284 nm. The specific absorbance at the maximum is 36 to 38.

C. Dissolve 50 mg in 1 ml of *sulphuric acid R* and add 0.05 ml of *ammonium molybdate solution R*. A pale-blue colour is produced which becomes deep blue on gentle warming. Add 0.05 ml of *dilute nitric acid R*. The colour becomes brownish-red.

TESTS

Specific optical rotation (*2.2.7*). Dissolve 1.000 g in *alcohol R* and dilute to 50.0 ml with the same solvent. The specific optical rotation is − 94 to − 98, calculated with reference to the dried substance.

Related substances. Examine by thin-layer chromatography (*2.2.27*), using *silica gel G R* as the coating substance.

Test solution. Dissolve 0.25 g of the substance to be examined in *chloroform R* and dilute to 10 ml with the same solvent.

Reference solution (a). Dilute 0.5 ml of the test solution to 50 ml with *chloroform R*.

Reference solution (b). Dilute 5 ml of reference solution (a) to 10 ml with *chloroform R*.

Apply separately to the plate 10 µl of each solution. Develop over a path of 15 cm using a mixture of 2.5 volumes of *concentrated ammonia R*, 32.5 volumes of *acetone R*, 35 volumes of *alcohol R* and 35 volumes of *toluene R*. Dry the plate in a current of air and spray with *dilute potassium iodobismuthate solution R*. In the chromatogram obtained with the test solution, any spot apart from the principal spot is not more intense than the spot in the chromatogram obtained with reference solution (a) (1.0 per cent) and not more than one such spot situated above the principal spot is more intense than the spot in the chromatogram obtained with reference solution (b) (0.5 per cent).

Morphine. Dissolve 0.10 g in *0.1 M hydrochloric acid* and dilute to 5 ml with the same acid. Add 2 ml of a 10 g/l solution of *sodium nitrite R*, allow to stand for 15 min and add 3 ml of *dilute ammonia R1*. The solution is not more intensely coloured than reference solution B_4 (*2.2.2, Method II*) (about 0.13 per cent of morphine).

Loss on drying (*2.2.32*): 3.9 per cent to 4.5 per cent, determined on 0.500 g by drying in an oven at 100 °C to 105 °C.

Sulphated ash (*2.4.14*). Not more than 0.1 per cent, determined on 1.0 g.

ASSAY

Dissolve 0.180 g in 50 ml of *anhydrous acetic acid R*, warming gently. Titrate with *0.1 M perchloric acid* determining the end-point potentiometrically (*2.2.20*) at the second point of inflexion.

1 ml of *0.1 M perchloric acid* is equivalent to 19.93 mg of $C_{23}H_{30}N_2O_4$.

01/2005:0004

PHOSPHORIC ACID, CONCENTRATED

Acidum phosphoricum concentratum

H_3PO_4 M_r 98.0

DEFINITION

Concentrated phosphoric acid contains not less than 84.0 per cent *m/m* and not more than 90.0 per cent *m/m* of H_3PO_4.

CHARACTERS

A clear, colourless, syrupy liquid, corrosive, miscible with water and with alcohol. When stored at a low temperature it may solidify into a mass of colourless crystals which do not melt at a temperature below 28 °C.

It has a relative density of about 1.7.

IDENTIFICATION

A. Dilute with *water R*. The solution is strongly acid (*2.2.4*).

B. Solution S (see Tests) neutralised with *dilute sodium hydroxide solution R* gives the reactions of phosphates (*2.3.1*).

TESTS

Solution S. Dilute 10.0 g to 150 ml with *water R*.

Appearance of solution. Solution S is clear (*2.2.1*) and colourless (*2.2.2, Method II*).

Substances precipitated with ammonia. To 10 ml of solution S add 8 ml of *dilute ammonia R1*. Any opalescence in the solution is not more intense than that in a mixture of 10 ml of solution S and 8 ml of *water R*.

Hypophosphorous acid and phosphorous acid. To 5 ml of solution S add 2 ml of *silver nitrate solution R2* and heat on a water-bath for 5 min. The solution shows no change in appearance.

Chlorides (*2.4.4*). 15 ml of solution S complies with the limit test for chlorides (50 ppm).

Sulphates (*2.4.13*). 1.5 g diluted to 15 ml with *distilled water R* complies with the limit test for sulphates (100 ppm).

Arsenic (*2.4.2*). 7.5 ml of solution S complies with limit test A for arsenic (2 ppm).

Iron (*2.4.9*). 3 ml of solution S diluted to 10 ml with *water R* complies with the limit test for iron (50 ppm).

Heavy metals (*2.4.8*). To 2.5 g add 4 ml of *dilute ammonia R1* and dilute to 25 ml with *water R*. 12 ml of the solution complies with limit test A for heavy metals (10 ppm). Prepare the standard using *lead standard solution (1 ppm Pb) R*.

ASSAY

To 1.000 g add a solution of 10 g of *sodium chloride R* in 30 ml of *water R*. Titrate with *1 M sodium hydroxide*, using *phenolphthalein solution R* as indicator.

1 ml of *1 M sodium hydroxide* is equivalent to 49.00 mg of H_3PO_4.

STORAGE

Store in a glass container.

01/2005:0005

PHOSPHORIC ACID, DILUTE

Acidum phosphoricum dilutum

DEFINITION

Dilute phosphoric acid contains 9.5 per cent *m/m* to 10.5 per cent *m/m* of H_3PO_4 (M_r 98.0).

PREPARATION

To 115 g of concentrated phosphoric acid add 885 g of *water R* and mix.

IDENTIFICATION

A. It is strongly acid (*2.2.4*).

B. Solution S (see Tests), neutralised with *dilute sodium hydroxide solution R*, gives the reactions of phosphates (*2.3.1*).

TESTS

Solution S. Dilute 86 g to 150 ml with *water R*.

Appearance of solution. Solution S is clear (*2.2.1*) and colourless (*2.2.2, Method II*).

Substances precipitated with ammonia. To 10 ml of solution S add 8 ml of *dilute ammonia R1*. Any opalescence in the solution is not more intense than that in a mixture of 10 ml of solution S and 8 ml of *water R*.

Hypophosphorous acid and phosphorous acid. To 5 ml of solution S add 2 ml of *silver nitrate solution R2* and heat on a water-bath for 5 min. The solution shows no change in appearance.

Chlorides (*2.4.4*). 15 ml of solution S complies with the limit test for chlorides (6 ppm).

Sulphates (*2.4.13*). 15 ml of the substance to be examined complies with the limit test for sulphates (10 ppm).

Arsenic (*2.4.2*). 7.5 ml of solution S complies with limit test A for arsenic (0.2 ppm).

Iron (*2.4.9*). 3 ml of solution S diluted to 10 ml with *water R* complies with the limit test for iron (6 ppm).

Heavy metals (*2.4.8*). To 20 g of the substance to be examined add 4 ml of *dilute ammonia R1* and dilute to 25 ml with *water R*. 12 ml of the solution complies with limit test A for heavy metals (1 ppm). Prepare the standard using a mixture of 8 ml of *lead standard solution (1 ppm Pb) R* and 2 ml of *water R*.

ASSAY

To 8.60 g add a solution of 10 g of *sodium chloride R* in 30 ml of *water R*. Titrate with *1 M sodium hydroxide*, using *phenolphthalein solution R* as indicator.

1 ml of *1 M sodium hydroxide* is equivalent to 49.00 mg of H_3PO_4.

01/2005:0352

PHTHALYLSULFATHIAZOLE

Phthalylsulfathiazolum

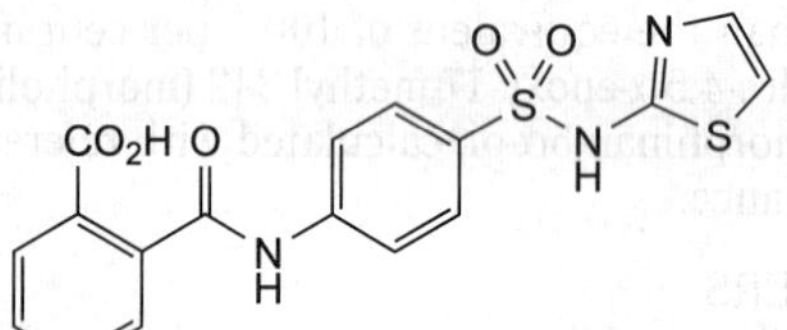

$C_{17}H_{13}N_3O_5S_2$ M_r 403.4

DEFINITION

Phthalylsulfathiazole contains not less than 98.5 per cent and not more than the equivalent of 101.5 per cent of 2-[[4-(thiazol-2-ylsulphamoyl)phenyl]carbamoyl]benzoic acid, calculated with reference to the dried substance.

CHARACTERS

A white or yellowish-white, crystalline powder, practically insoluble in water, freely soluble in dimethylformamide, slightly soluble in acetone and in alcohol.

IDENTIFICATION

First identification: A, B, E.

Second identification: B, C, D, E.

A. Examine by infrared absorption spectrophotometry (*2.2.24*), comparing with the spectrum obtained with *phthalylsulfathiazole CRS*.

B. To 1 g add 8.5 ml of *dilute sodium hydroxide solution R* and boil under a reflux condenser for 30 min. Cool and add 17.5 ml of *dilute hydrochloric acid R*. Shake vigorously and filter. Neutralise the filtrate with *dilute sodium hydroxide solution R*. Filter, wash the precipitate with *water R*, recrystallise from *water R* and dry the crystals at 100 °C to 105 °C. The crystals melt (*2.2.14*) at 200 °C to 203 °C.

C. To 0.1 g in a test-tube add 3 ml of *dilute sulphuric acid R* and 0.5 g of *zinc powder R*. Fumes are evolved which produce a black stain on *lead acetate paper R*.

D. To 0.1 g add 0.5 g of *resorcinol R* and 0.3 ml of *sulphuric acid R* and heat on a water-bath until a homogeneous mixture is obtained. Allow to cool. Add 5 ml of *dilute sodium hydroxide solution R*. Dilute 0.1 ml of this brownish-red mixture to 25 ml with *water R*. An intense green fluorescence appears which disappears on acidification.

E. Dissolve about 10 mg of the crystals obtained in identification test B in 200 ml of *0.1 M hydrochloric acid.* 2 ml of the solution gives the reaction of primary aromatic amines (*2.3.1*) with formation of an orange precipitate.

TESTS

Appearance of solution. Dissolve 1.0 g in *1 M sodium hydroxide* and dilute to 20 ml with the same solvent. The solution is clear (*2.2.1*) and not more intensely coloured than reference solution BY_5 (*2.2.2, Method II*).

Acidity. To 2.0 g add 20 ml of *water R*, shake continuously for 30 min and filter. To 10 ml of the filtrate add 0.1 ml of *phenolphthalein solution R*. Not more than 0.2 ml of *0.1 M sodium hydroxide* is required to change the colour of the indicator.

Sulfathiazole and other primary aromatic amines. Dissolve 5 mg in a mixture of 3.5 ml of *water R*, 6 ml of *dilute hydrochloric acid R* and 25 ml of *alcohol R*, previously cooled to 15 °C. Place immediately in iced water and add 1 ml of a 2.5 g/l solution of *sodium nitrite R*. Allow to stand for 3 min, add 2.5 ml of a 40 g/l solution of *sulphamic acid R* and allow to stand for 5 min. Add 1 ml of a 4 g/l solution of *naphthylethylenediamine dihydrochloride R* and dilute to 50 ml with *water R*. Measured at 550 nm, the absorbance (*2.2.25*) is not greater than that of a standard prepared at the same time and in the same manner using a mixture of 1 ml of a solution containing in 100 ml; 10 mg of *sulfathiazole R* and 0.5 ml of *hydrochloric acid R*, 2.5 ml of *water R*, 6 ml of *dilute hydrochloric acid R* and 25 ml of *alcohol R*.

Heavy metals (*2.4.8*). 1.0 g complies with limit test C for heavy metals (20 ppm). Prepare the standard using 2 ml of *lead standard solution (10 ppm Pb) R*.

Loss on drying (*2.2.32*). Not more than 2 per cent, determined on 1.00 g by drying in an oven at 100 °C to 105 °C.

Sulphated ash (*2.4.14*). Not more than 0.1 per cent, determined on 1.0 g.

ASSAY

Dissolve 0.300 g in 40 ml of *dimethylformamide R*. Titrate with *0.1 M sodium hydroxide* until the colour becomes blue. using 0.2 ml of *thymolphthalein solution R* as indicator. Carry out a blank titration.

1 ml of *0.1 M sodium hydroxide* is equivalent to 20.17 mg of $C_{17}H_{13}N_3O_5S_2$.

STORAGE

Store protected from light.

01/2005:0286

PHYSOSTIGMINE SALICYLATE

Physostigmini salicylas

Eserini salicylas

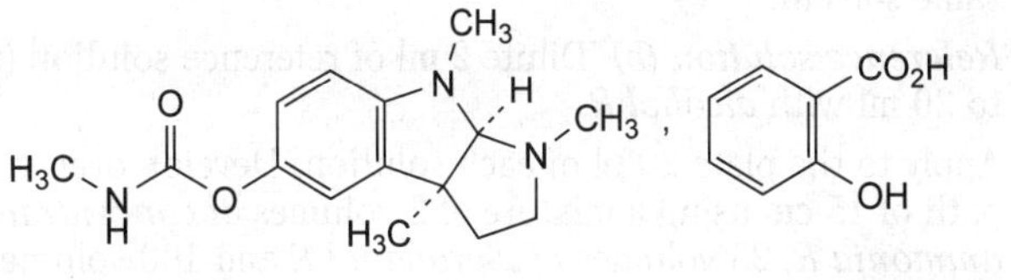

$C_{22}H_{27}N_3O_5$ M_r 413.5

DEFINITION

Physostigmine salicylate contains not less than 98.5 per cent and not more than the equivalent of 101.0 per cent of (3a*S*,8a*R*)-1,2,3,3a,8,8a-hexahydro-1,3a,8-trimethylpyrrolo[2,3-*b*]indol-5-yl methylcarbamate salicylate, calculated with reference to the dried substance.

CHARACTERS

Colourless or almost colourless crystals, sparingly soluble in water, soluble in alcohol. The crystals gradually become red when exposed to air and light; the colour develops more quickly when the crystals are also exposed to moisture. Aqueous solutions are unstable.

It melts at about 182 °C, with decomposition.

IDENTIFICATION

First identification: A, B.

Second identification: B, C, D.

A. Examine by infrared absorption spectrophotometry (*2.2.24*), comparing with the spectrum obtained with *physostigmine salicylate CRS*.

B. Examine the chromatograms obtained in the test for related substances. The principal spot in the chromatogram obtained with test solution (b) is similar in position, colour and size to the principal spot in the chromatogram obtained with reference solution (a).

C. Heat about 10 mg in a porcelain dish with a few drops of *dilute ammonia R1*. An orange colour develops. Evaporate the solution to dryness. The residue dissolves in *alcohol R* giving a blue solution. Add 0.1 ml of *glacial acetic acid R*. The colour becomes violet. Dilute with *water R*. An intense red fluorescence appears.

D. Solution S (see Tests) gives reaction (a) of salicylates (*2.3.1*).

TESTS

Solution S. Dissolve 0.900 g, without heating, in 95 ml of *carbon dioxide-free water R* prepared from *distilled water R* and dilute to 100.0 ml with the same solvent. Prepare immediately before use.

Appearance of solution. Solution S is clear (*2.2.1*) and colourless (*2.2.2, Method II*).

pH (*2.2.3*). The pH of solution S is 5.1 to 5.9.

Specific optical rotation (*2.2.7*): − 90 to − 94, determined on solution S and calculated with reference to the dried substance.

Related substances. Examine by thin-layer chromatography (*2.2.27*), using *silica gel G R* as the coating substance.

Test solution (a). Dissolve 0.2 g of the substance to be examined in *alcohol R* and dilute to 10 ml with the same solvent.

Test solution (b). Dilute 2.5 ml of test solution (a) to 50 ml with *alcohol R*.

Reference solution (a). Dissolve 10 mg of *physostigmine salicylate CRS* in *alcohol R* and dilute to 10 ml with the same solvent.

Reference solution (b). Dilute 2 ml of reference solution (a) to 20 ml with *alcohol R*.

Apply to the plate 20 µl of each solution. Develop over a path of 15 cm using a mixture of 2 volumes of *concentrated ammonia R*, 23 volumes of *2-propanol R* and 100 volumes of *cyclohexane R*. Dry the plate in a current of cold air and carry out a second development in the same direction. Allow the plate to dry in air and spray with freshly prepared *potassium iodobismuthate solution R* and then with *dilute hydrogen peroxide solution R*. Examine the plate within 2 min. Any spot in the chromatogram obtained with test solution (a), apart from the principal spot, is not more intense than the spot in the chromatogram obtained with reference solution (b) (0.5 per cent).

Eseridine. To 5 ml of solution S add a few crystals of *potassium iodate R*, 0.05 ml of *dilute hydrochloric acid R* and 2 ml of *chloroform R*. Shake. No violet colour develops in the chloroform layer within 1 min.

Sulphates (*2.4.13*). 15 ml of solution S complies with the limit test for sulphates (0.1 per cent).

Loss on drying (*2.2.32*). Not more than 1.0 per cent, determined on 1.00 g by drying in an oven at 100 °C to 105 °C.

Sulphated ash (*2.4.14*). Not more than 0.1 per cent, determined on the residue obtained in the test for loss on drying.

ASSAY

Dissolve 0.350 g in 50 ml of a mixture of equal volumes of *anhydrous acetic acid R* and *chloroform R*. Titrate with *0.1 M perchloric acid* determining the end-point potentiometrically (*2.2.20*).

1 ml of *0.1 M perchloric acid* is equivalent to 41.35 mg of $C_{22}H_{27}N_3O_5$.

STORAGE

Store in an airtight container, protected from light.

01/2005:0684

PHYSOSTIGMINE SULPHATE

Physostigmini sulfas

Eserini sulfas

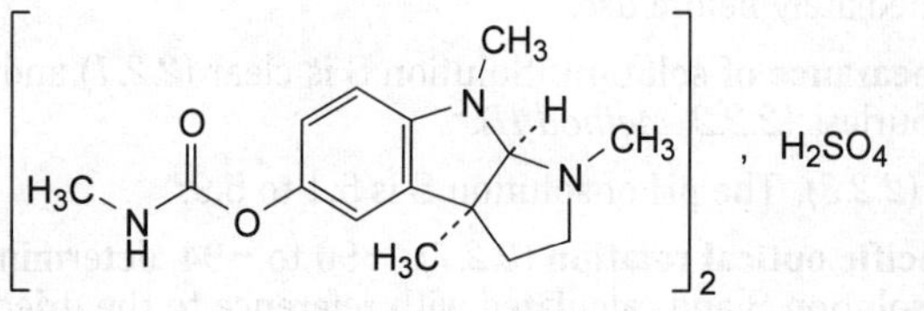

$C_{30}H_{44}N_6O_8S$ M_r 649

DEFINITION

Physostigmine sulphate contains not less than 97.0 per cent and not more than the equivalent of 101.0 per cent of di[(3a*S*,8a*R*)-1,2,3,3a,8,8a-hexahydro-1,3a,8-trimethylpyrrolo[2,3-*b*]indol-5-yl methylcarbamate] sulphate, calculated with reference to the dried substance.

CHARACTERS

A white or almost white, crystalline powder, hygroscopic, very soluble in water, freely soluble in alcohol. It gradually becomes red when exposed to air and light; the colour develops more quickly when the substance is also exposed to moisture. Aqueous solutions are unstable.

It melts at about 145 °C, with decomposition.

IDENTIFICATION

First identification: A, D.

Second identification: B, C, D.

A. Examine by infrared absorption spectrophotometry (*2.2.24*), comparing with the spectrum obtained with *physostigmine sulphate CRS*. Examine the substances prepared as discs using *potassium bromide R*.

B. Examine the chromatograms obtained in the test for related substances. The principal spot in the chromatogram obtained with test solution (b) is similar in position, colour and size to the principal spot in the chromatogram obtained with reference solution (a).

C. Heat about 10 mg in a porcelain dish with 0.5 ml of *dilute ammonia R1*. An orange colour develops. Evaporate the solution to dryness. The residue dissolves in *alcohol R* giving a blue solution. Add 0.1 ml of *glacial acetic acid R*. The colour becomes violet. Dilute with water. An intense red fluorescence appears.

D. It gives reaction (a) of sulphates (*2.3.1*).

TESTS

Solution S. Dissolve 0.500 g without heating in *carbon dioxide-free water R* and dilute to 50.0 ml with the same solvent. Prepare immediately before use.

Appearance of solution. Solution S is clear (*2.2.1*) and colourless (*2.2.2, Method II*).

pH (*2.2.3*). The pH of solution S is 3.5 to 5.5.

Specific optical rotation (*2.2.7*): − 116 to − 120, determined on solution S and calculated with reference to the dried substance.

Related substances. Examine by thin-layer chromatography (*2.2.27*), using *silica gel G R* as the coating substance.

Test solution (a). Dissolve 0.15 g of the substance to be examined in *alcohol R* and dilute to 5 ml with the same solvent.

Test solution (b). Dilute 1 ml of test solution (a) to 10 ml with *alcohol R*.

Reference solution (a). Dissolve 30 mg of *physostigmine sulphate CRS* in *alcohol R* and dilute to 10 ml with the same solvent.

Reference solution (b). Dilute 5 ml of test solution (b) to 100 ml with *alcohol R*.

Apply separately to the plate 10 µl of each solution. Develop over a path of 15 cm using a mixture of 2 volumes of *concentrated ammonia R*, 23 volumes of *2-propanol R* and 100 volumes of *cyclohexane R*. Dry the plate in a current of cold air and carry out a second development in the same direction. Allow the plate to dry in air and spray with freshly prepared *potassium iodo-bismuthate solution R* and then with *dilute hydrogen peroxide solution R*. Examine the plate within 2 min. Any spot in the chromatogram obtained with test solution (a), apart from the principal spot, is not more intense than the spot in the chromatogram obtained with reference solution (b) (0.5 per cent).

Eseridine. To 5 ml of solution S add a few crystals of *potassium iodate R*, 0.05 ml of *dilute hydrochloric acid R* and 2 ml of *chloroform R* and shake. After 1 min, the chloroform layer is not more intensely coloured than a reference solution prepared at the same time in the same manner using 5 ml of *water R* instead of solution S.

Loss on drying (*2.2.32*). Not more than 1.0 per cent, determined on 1.000 g by drying in an oven at 100 °C to 105 °C.

Sulphated ash (*2.4.14*). Not more than 0.1 per cent, determined on the residue obtained in the test for loss on drying.

ASSAY

Dissolve 0.5000 g in a mixture of 20 ml of *anhydrous acetic acid R* and 40 ml of *acetic anhydride R*. Titrate with *0.1 M perchloric acid* determining the end-point potentiometrically (*2.2.20*) at the first inflexion point.

1 ml of *0.1 M perchloric acid* is equivalent to 64.88 mg of $C_{30}H_{44}N_6O_8S$.

STORAGE

Store in a well-filled, airtight glass container, protected from light.

01/2005:1036

PHYTOMENADIONE

Phytomenadionum

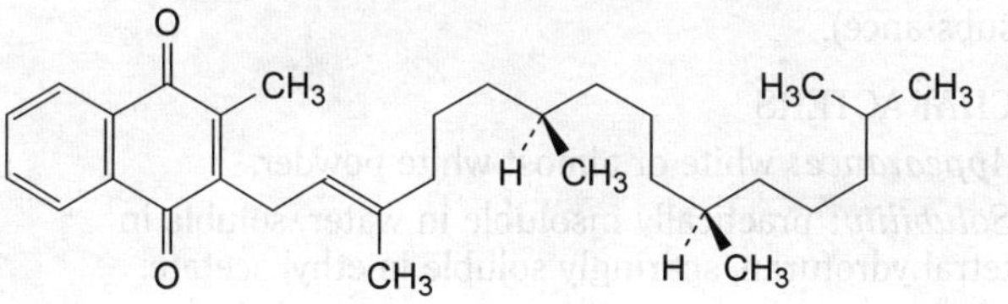

$C_{31}H_{46}O_2$ M_r 450.7

DEFINITION

Phytomenadione is a mixture of 2-methyl-3-[(2*E*)-(7*R*,11*R*)-3,7,11,15-tetramethylhexadec-2-enyl]naphthalene-1,4-dione (*trans*-phytomenadione), 2-methyl-3-[(2*Z*)-(7*R*,11*R*)-3,7,11,15-tetramethylhexadec-2-enyl]naphthalene-1,4-dione (*cis*-phytomenadione) and 2,3-epoxy-2-methyl-3-[(2*E*)-(7*R*,11*R*)-3,7,11,15-tetramethylhexadec-2-enyl]-2,3-dihydronaphthalene-1,4-dione (*trans*-epoxyphytomenadione). It contains not more than 4.0 per cent of *trans*-epoxyphytomenadione and not less than 75.0 per cent of *trans*-phytomenadione. The total of the three components is not less than 97.0 per cent and not more than the equivalent of 103.0 per cent.

CHARACTERS

A clear, intense yellow, viscous, oily liquid, practically insoluble in water, sparingly soluble in alcohol, miscible with fatty oils.

It decomposes on exposure to actinic light.

The refractive index is about 1.526.

IDENTIFICATION

Carry out all operations as rapidly as possible avoiding exposure to actinic light.

A. Dissolve 10.0 mg in *trimethylpentane R* and dilute to 100.0 ml with the same solvent. Examined between 275 nm and 340 nm (*2.2.25*), the solution shows an absorption maximum at 327 nm and an absorption minimum at 285 nm. The specific absorbance at the maximum is 67 to 73. Dilute 10.0 ml of the solution to 50.0 ml with *trimethylpentane R*. Examined between 230 nm and 280 nm, the solution shows four absorbance maxima, at 243 nm, 249 nm, 261 nm and 270 nm respectively.

B. Examine the chromatograms obtained in the test for menadione and other related substances. The principal spot in the chromatogram obtained with test solution (b) is similar in position, colour and size to the principal spot in the chromatogram obtained with reference solution (a).

C. Dissolve 50 mg in 10 ml of *methanol R* and add 1 ml of a200 g/l solution of *potassium hydroxide R* in *methanol R*. A green colour is produced which becomes violet-red on heating in a water-bath at 40 °C and then reddish-brown on standing.

TESTS

Appearance of solution. Dissolve 2.5 g in *trimethylpentane R* and dilute to 25 ml with the same solvent. The solution is clear (*2.2.1*).

Acid value (*2.5.1*). Not more than 2.0, determined on 2.00 g.

Menadione and other related substances. Examine by thin-layer chromatography (*2.2.27*), using a *TLC silica gel* F_{254} *plate R*.

Test solution (a). Dissolve 0.40 g of the substance to be examined in *cyclohexane R* and dilute to 10 ml with the same solvent.

Test solution (b). Dilute 1 ml of test solution (a) to 10 ml with *cyclohexane R*.

Reference solution (a). Dissolve 40 mg of *phytomenadione CRS* in *cyclohexane R* and dilute to 10 ml with the same solvent.

Reference solution (b). Dilute 1 ml of test solution (b) to 20 ml with *cyclohexane R*.

Reference solution (c). Dissolve 4.0 mg of *menadione R* in *cyclohexane R* and dilute to 50 ml with the same solvent.

Apply to the plate 10 µl of each solution. Develop over a path of 15 cm using a mixture of 20 volumes of *cyclohexane R* and 80 volumes of *toluene R*. Allow the plate to dry in air for 5 min. Examine in ultraviolet light at 254 nm and spray with a 100 g/l solution of *phosphomolybdic acid R* in *ethanol R*. Heat at 120 °C for 5 min. Examine in daylight. In the chromatogram obtained with test solution (a): any spot corresponding to menadione is not more intense that the spot in the chromatogram obtained with reference solution (c) (0.2 per cent); any spot, apart from the principal spot and any spot corresponding to menadione, is not more intense than the spot in the chromatogram obtained with reference solution (b) (0.5 per cent). Disregard any spot below the principal spot, which may not be completely separated from the principal spot.

Sulphated ash (*2.4.14*). Not more than 0.1 per cent, determined on 1.0 g.

ASSAY

Examine by liquid chromatography (*2.2.29*).

Test solution. Dissolve 15.0 mg of the substance to be examined in the mobile phase and dilute to 10.0 ml with the mobile phase.

Reference solution (a). Dissolve 15.0 mg of *phytomenadione CRS* in the mobile phase and dilute to 10.0 ml with the mobile phase.

Reference solution (b). Dissolve 15.0 mg of *phytomenadione CRS* and 4.0 mg of *trans-epoxyphytomenadione CRS* in the mobile phase and dilute to 10.0 ml with the mobile phase.

The chromatographic procedure may be carried out using:

- a stainless steel column 0.25 m long and 4.6 mm in internal diameter packed with spherical *silica gel for chromatography R* (5 µm) with a porosity of 8 nm,
- as mobile phase at a flow rate of 0.4 ml/min a mixture of 0.67 volumes of *octanol R*, 3.3 volumes of *di-isopropyl ether R* and 1000 volumes of *heptane R*,
- as detector a spectrophotometer set at 254 nm,
- a 20 µl loop injector.

Inject reference solution (b). When using a recorder, adjust the sensitivity of the system so that the height of the principal peak is at least 50 per cent of the full scale of the recorder. The test is not valid unless the order of elution of the peaks is: *trans*-epoxyphytomenadione, *cis*-phytomenadione and *trans*-phytomenadione. Carry out six replicate injections of reference solution (a). The assay is not valid unless the relative standard deviation of the peak area of the *trans*-isomer is less than 1.0 per cent and the resolution between the peaks corresponding to *trans*-phytomenadione and *cis*-phytomenadione is at least 2.5. Inject the test solution and reference solution (a) and calculate the percentage contents of *trans*-phytomenadione, *cis*-phytomenadione and *trans*-epoxyphytomenadione using the following expressions:

$$trans\text{-phytomenadione} = \frac{m' \times A'_{trans} \times S_{trans}}{m \times S'_{trans}}$$

$$cis\text{-phytomenadione} = \frac{m' \times A'_{cis} \times S_{cis}}{m \times S'_{cis}}$$

$$trans\text{-epoxyphytomenadione} = \frac{m' \times A'_{epoxy} \times S_{epoxy}}{m \times S'_{epoxy}}$$

m' = mass of the reference substance in reference solution (a), in milligrams,

m = mass of the substance to be examined in the test solution, in milligrams,

A'_{trans} = percentage content of *trans*-phytomenadione in *phytomenadione CRS*,

A'_{cis} = percentage content of *cis*-phytomenadione in *phytomenadione CRS*,

A'_{epoxy} = percentage content of *trans*-epoxyphytomenadione in *phytomenadione CRS*,

S_{trans} = area of the peak corresponding to the *trans*-isomer in the chromatogram obtained with the test solution,

S_{cis} = area of the peak corresponding to the *cis*-isomer in the chromatogram obtained with the test solution,

S_{epoxy} = area of the peak corresponding to *trans*-epoxyphytomenadione in the chromatogram obtained with the test solution,

S'_{trans} = area of the peak corresponding to the *trans*-isomer in the chromatogram obtained with reference solution (a),

S'_{cis} = area of the peak corresponding to the *cis*-isomer in the chromatogram obtained with reference solution (a),

S'_{epoxy} = area of the peak corresponding to *trans*-epoxyphytomenadione in the chromatogram obtained with reference solution (a).

STORAGE

Store protected from light.

IMPURITIES

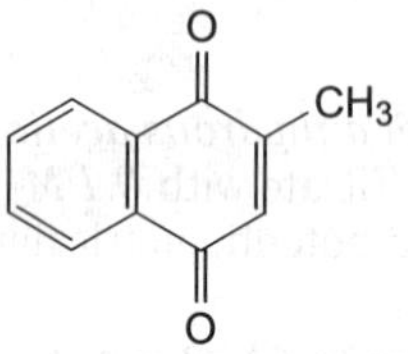

A. 2-methylnaphthalene-1,4-dione (menadione).

01/2005:1911

PHYTOSTEROL

Phytosterolum

DEFINITION

Natural mixture of sterols obtained from plants of the genuses *Hypoxis, Pinus* and *Picea.*

Content: minimum 70.0 per cent of β-sitosterol (dried substance).

CHARACTERS

Appearance: white or almost white powder.

Solubility: practically insoluble in water, soluble in tetrahydrofuran, sparingly soluble in ethyl acetate.

IDENTIFICATION

A. Mix 1 ml of *acetic anhydride R* with 0.5 ml of solution S (see Tests). After the addition of 0.1 ml of *sulphuric acid R* a red colour is produced which changes rapidly to violet then to blue and finally to green.

B. Examine the chromatograms obtained in the assay.

Results: the principal peak in the chromatogram obtained with the test solution is similar in retention time to the peak in the chromatogram obtained with reference solution (b).

TESTS

Solution S. Dissolve 1.0 g in *tetrahydrofuran R* and dilute to 20 ml with the same solvent.

Appearance of solution. Solution S is clear (*2.2.1*) and not more intensely coloured than reference solution Y_6 (*2.2.2, Method II*).

Acidity or alkalinity. Shake 0.20 g with a mixture of 4.0 ml of *ethyl acetate R* and 10.0 ml of *carbon dioxide-free water R* for 3 min. Allow the layers to separate. To the aqueous layer add 0.1 ml of *bromothymol blue solution R1.* If the solution is yellow not more than 0.5 ml of *0.01 M sodium hydroxide* is required to change the colour to blue. If the solution is blue not more than 0.5 ml of *0.01 M hydrochloric acid* is required to change the colour to yellow.

Specific optical rotation (*2.2.7*): − 15 to − 28 (dried substance).

Dissolve 0.500 g in *ethyl acetate R* and dilute to 10.0 ml with the same solvent.

Acid value (*2.5.1*): maximum 1.0, determined on 2.0 g.

Peroxide value (*2.5.5*): maximum 10.0.

Saponification value (*2.5.6*): maximum 3.

Other sterols. Examine the chromatogram obtained with the test solution in the assay (Figure 1911.-1).

Composition of the other sterols:

– *cholesterol*: maximum 0.5 per cent,
– *brassicasterol*: maximum 0.5 per cent,
– *campesterol*: maximum 15.0 per cent,
– *campestanol*: maximum 5.0 per cent,
– *stigmasterol*: maximum 5.0 per cent,
– *sitostanol*: maximum 15.0 per cent,
– *Δ7-stigmastenol*: maximum 5.0 per cent.

Loss on drying (*2.2.32*): maximum 4.0 per cent, determined on 0.250 g by drying in an oven at 100-105 °C for 2 h.

Total ash (*2.4.16*): maximum 0.5 per cent, determined on 1.0 g.

ASSAY

Gas chromatography (*2.2.28*): use the normalisation procedure.

Test solution. Dissolve 0.100 g in *tetrahydrofuran R* and dilute to 10.0 ml with the same solvent. Introduce 100 µl of this solution into a 3 ml flask and evaporate to dryness under *nitrogen R*. Add 100 µl of a freshly prepared mixture of 50 µl of *1-methylimidazole R* and 1.0 ml of *heptafluoro-N-methyl-N-trimethylsilyl)butanamide R*, close the flask tightly and heat to 100 °C for 15 min. Allow to cool.

Reference solution (a). Dissolve 25 mg of *β-sitosterol R* and 25 mg of *sitostanol R* in *tetrahydrofuran R* and dilute to 10.0 ml with the same solvent. Introduce 100 µl of this solution into a 3 ml flask and evaporate to dryness under *nitrogen R*. Add 100 µl of a freshly prepared mixture of 50 µl of *1-methylimidazole* and 1.0 ml of *heptafluoro-N-methyl-N-(trimethylsilyl)butanamide R*. Close the flask tightly and heat to 100 °C for 15 min. Allow to cool.

Reference solution (b). Dissolve 0.100 g of *β-sitosterol R* in *tetrahydrofuran R* and dilute to 10.0 ml with the same solvent. Introduce 100 µl of this solution into a 3 ml flask and evaporate to dryness under *nitrogen R*. Add 100 µl of a freshly prepared mixture of 50 µl of *1-methylimidazole R* and 1.0 ml of *heptafluoro-N-methyl-N-(trimethylsilyl)butanamide R*. Close the flask tightly and heat to 100 °C for 15 min. Allow to cool.

Column:

– *material*: quartz,
– *size*: l = 25 m, Ø = 0.3 mm,
– *stationary phase*: *poly(dimethyl)(diphenyl)(divinyl)siloxane R* (1 µm).

Carrier gas: *hydrogen for chromatography R*.

Flow rate: 2 ml/min.

Split ratio: 1:20.

Temperature:

– *column*: 280 °C,
– *injection port and detector*: 300 °C.

Detection: flame ionisation.

Injection: 1 µl.

Relative retentions with reference to β-sitosterol (retention time = about 16 min): cholesterol = about 0.7; brassicasterol = about 0.77; campesterol = about 0.84; campestanol = about 0.86; stigmasterol = about 0.9; sitostanol = about 1.02; Δ7-stigmastenol = about 1.1.

System suitability: reference solution (a):

– *resolution*: minimum of 1.0 between the peaks due to β-sitosterol and sitostanol.

STORAGE

In an airtight container, protected from light.

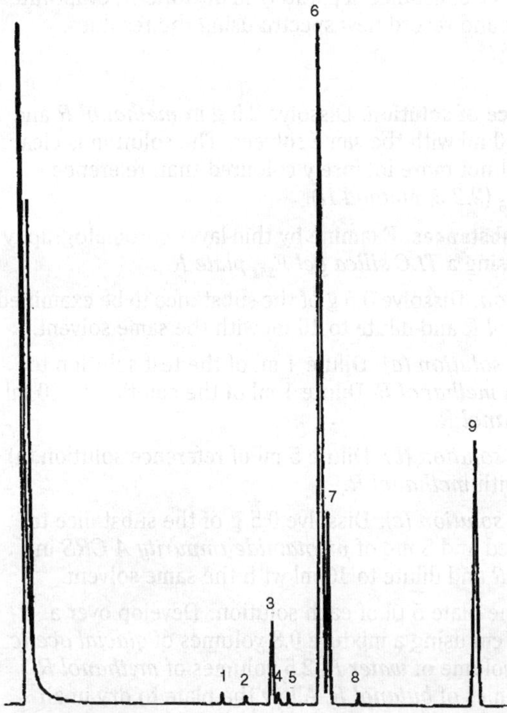

1. cholesterol	5. stigmasterol
2. brassicasterol	6. β-sitosterol
3. campesterol	7. sitostanol
4. campestanol	8. Δ7-stigmastenol

Figure 1911.-1. – *Assay of phytosterol (trimethylsilane derivatives)*

01/2005:1358

PICOTAMIDE MONOHYDRATE

Picotamidum monohydricum

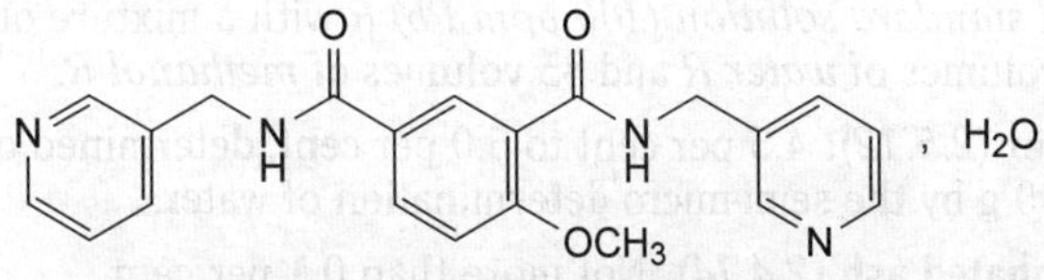

$C_{21}H_{20}N_4O_3,H_2O$ M_r 394.4

DEFINITION

Picotamide monohydrate contains not less than 98.0 per cent and not more than 101.0 per cent of 4-methoxy-*N,N'*-bis(pyridin-3-ylmethyl)benzene-1,3-dicarboxamide, calculated with reference to the anhydrous substance.

CHARACTERS

A white or almost white, crystalline powder, slightly soluble in water, soluble in ethanol and in methylene chloride. It dissolves in dilute mineral acids.

It shows polymorphism.

IDENTIFICATION

Examine by infrared spectrophotometry (*2.2.24*), comparing with the spectrum obtained with *picotamide monohydrate CRS*. If the spectra obtained in the solid state shows differences, dissolve the substance to be examined and the reference substance separately in *acetone R*, evaporate to dryness and record new spectra using the residues.

TESTS

Appearance of solution. Dissolve 2.5 g in *methanol R* and dilute to 50 ml with the same solvent. The solution is clear (*2.2.1*) and not more intensely coloured than reference solution Y_6 (*2.2.2, Method II*).

Related substances. Examine by thin-layer chromatography (*2.2.27*), using a *TLC silica gel F_{254} plate R*.

Test solution. Dissolve 0.5 g of the substance to be examined in *methanol R* and dilute to 10 ml with the same solvent.

Reference solution (a). Dilute 1 ml of the test solution to 10 ml with *methanol R*. Dilute 1 ml of the solution to 20 ml with *methanol R*.

Reference solution (b). Dilute 5 ml of reference solution (a) to 10 ml with *methanol R*.

Reference solution (c). Dissolve 0.5 g of the substance to be examined and 5 mg of *picotamide impurity A CRS* in *methanol R* and dilute to 10 ml with the same solvent.

Apply to the plate 5 µl of each solution. Develop over a path of 15 cm using a mixture 0.8 volumes of *glacial acetic acid R*, 1 volume of *water R*, 2.5 volumes of *methanol R* and 8 volumes of *butanol R*. Allow the plate to dry in air and examine in ultraviolet light at 254 nm. Any spot in the chromatogram obtained with the test solution, apart from the principal spot, is not more intense than the principal spot in the chromatogram obtained with reference solution (a) (0.5 per cent) and not more than one such spot is more intense than the spot in the chromatogram obtained with reference solution (b) (0.25 per cent). The test is not valid unless the chromatogram obtained with reference solution (c) shows two clearly separated principal spots.

Chlorides (*2.4.4*). Dissolve 0.25 g in a mixture of 2.5 ml of *dilute nitric acid R* and 12.5 ml of *water R*. The solution complies with the limit test for chlorides (200 ppm).

Heavy metals (*2.4.8*). Dissolve 1.0 g by gently heating in a mixture of 15 volumes of *water R* and 85 volumes of *methanol R* and dilute to 20 ml with the same mixture of solvents. 12 ml of the solution complies with limit test B for heavy metals (20 ppm). Prepare the standard, using lead standard solution (1 ppm Pb) obtained by diluting *lead standard solution (100 ppm Pb) R* with a mixture of 15 volumes of *water R* and 85 volumes of *methanol R*.

Water (*2.5.12*): 4.5 per cent to 5.0 per cent, determined on 0.300 g by the semi-micro determination of water.

Sulphated ash (*2.4.14*). Not more than 0.1 per cent, determined on 1.0 g.

ASSAY

Dissolve 0.150 g in a mixture of 20 ml of *anhydrous acetic acid R* and 20 ml of *acetic anhydride R*. Titrate with *0.1 M perchloric acid*, determining the end-point potentiometrically (*2.2.20*).

1 ml of *0.1 M perchloric acid* is equivalent to 18.82 mg of $C_{21}H_{20}N_4O_3$.

IMPURITIES

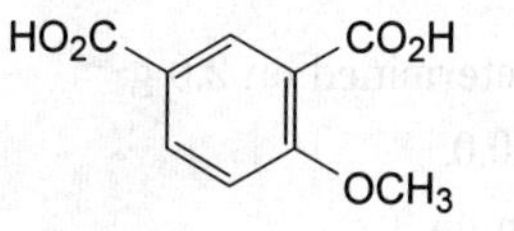

A. 4-methoxybenzene-1,3-dicarboxylic acid,

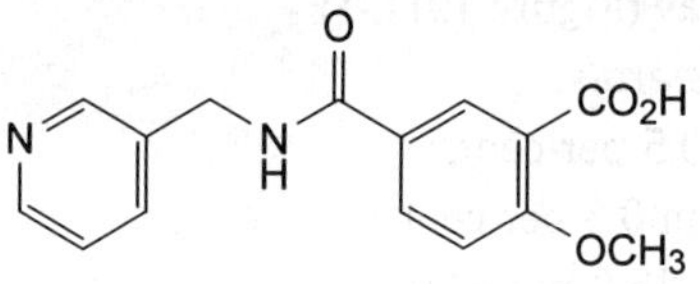

B. 2-methoxy-5-[[(pyridin-3-ylmethyl)amino]carbonyl]benzoic acid,

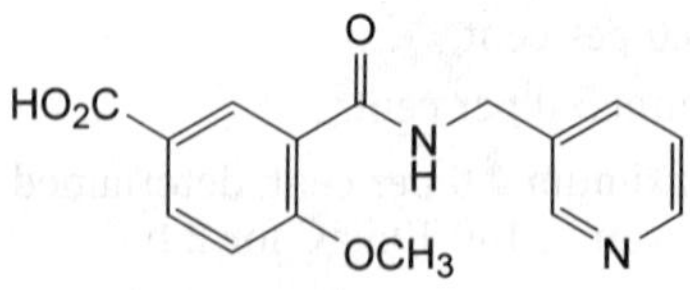

C. 4-methoxy-3-[[(pyridin-3-ylmethyl)amino]carbonyl]benzoic acid,

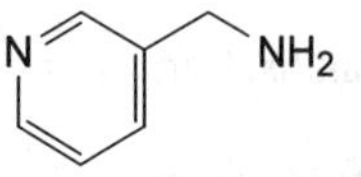

D. (pyridin-3-yl)methanamine.

01/2005:0633

PILOCARPINE HYDROCHLORIDE

Pilocarpini hydrochloridum

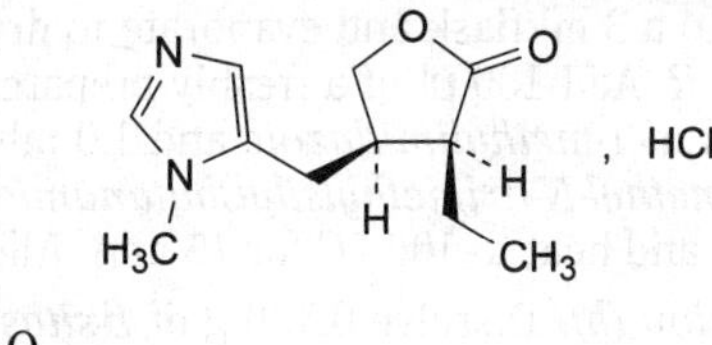

$C_{11}H_{17}ClN_2O_2$ M_r 244.7

DEFINITION

Pilocarpine hydrochloride contains not less than 99.0 per cent and not more than the equivalent of 101.0 per cent of (3*S*,4*R*)-3-ethyl-4-[(1-methyl-1*H*-imidazol-5-yl)methyl]dihydrofuran-2(3*H*)-one hydrochloride, calculated with reference to the dried substance.

CHARACTERS

A white or almost white, crystalline powder or colourless crystals, hygroscopic, very soluble in water and in alcohol. It melts at about 203 °C.

IDENTIFICATION

First identification: A, B, E.

Second identification: A, C, D, E.

A. It complies with the test for specific optical rotation (see Tests).

B. Examine by infrared absorption spectrophotometry (*2.2.24*), comparing with the spectrum obtained with *pilocarpine hydrochloride CRS*. If the substances are examined as discs, prepare using *potassium chloride R*.

C. Examine by thin-layer chromatography (*2.2.27*), using a *TLC silica gel G plate R*.

Test solution. Dissolve 10 mg in *methanol R* and dilute to 2 ml with the same solvent.

Reference solution. Dissolve 10 mg of *pilocarpine hydrochloride CRS* in *methanol R* and dilute to 2 ml with the same solvent.

Apply to the plate 2 µl of each solution. Develop over a path of 15 cm using a mixture of 1 volume of *concentrated ammonia R*, 14 volumes of *methanol R* and 85 volumes of *methylene chloride R*. Dry the plate at 100-105 °C for 10 min, allow to cool and spray with *dilute potassium iodobismuthate solution R*. The principal spot in the chromatogram obtained with the test solution is similar in position, colour and size to the principal spot in the chromatogram obtained with the reference solution.

D. Dilute 0.2 ml of solution S (see Tests) to 2 ml with *water R*. Add 0.05 ml of a 50 g/l solution of *potassium dichromate R*, 1 ml of *dilute hydrogen peroxide solution R* and 2 ml of *methylene chloride R* and shake. A violet colour develops in the organic layer.

E. It gives reaction (a) of chlorides (*2.3.1*).

TESTS

Solution S. Dissolve 2.50 g in *carbon dioxide-free water R* and dilute to 50.0 ml with the same solvent.

Appearance of solution. Solution S is clear (*2.2.1*) and not more intensely coloured than reference solution Y_7 (*2.2.2, Method II*).

pH (*2.2.3*). The pH of solution S is 3.5 to 4.5.

Specific optical rotation (*2.2.7*): + 89 to + 93, determined on solution S and calculated with reference to the dried substance.

Related substances. Examine by liquid chromatography (*2.2.29*).

Test solution. Dissolve 0.100 g of the substance to be examined in *water R* and dilute to 100.0 ml with the same solvent.

Reference solution (a). Dilute 5.0 ml of the test solution to 100.0 ml with *water R*. Dilute 2.0 ml of the solution to 20.0 ml with *water R*.

Reference solution (b). Dissolve 5.0 mg of *pilocarpine nitrate for system suitability CRS* in *water R* and dilute to 50.0 ml with the same solvent.

Reference solution (c). To 5 ml of the test solution, add 0.1 ml of *ammonia R* and heat the solution on a water-bath for 30 min, cool and dilute to 25 ml with *water R*. Take 3 ml of this solution and dilute to 25 ml with *water R*. Mainly pilocarpic acid is formed.

The chromatographic procedure may be carried out using:

- a stainless steel column 0.15 m long and 4.6 mm in internal diameter packed with *octadecylsilyl silica gel for chromatography R1* (5 µm) with a pore size of 10 nm and a carbon loading of 19 per cent,
- as mobile phase at a flow rate of 1.2 ml/min a solution prepared as follows: mix 55 volumes of *methanol R*, 60 volumes of *acetonitrile R* and 885 volumes of a 0.679 g/l solution of *tetrabutylammonium dihydrogen phosphate R*, previously adjusted to pH 7.7 with *dilute ammonia R2*,
- as detector a spectrophotometer set at 220 nm.

Inject 20 µl of each solution. Continue the chromatography for twice the retention time of the principal component (about 40 min). When the chromatograms are recorded in the prescribed conditions, the substances are eluted in the following sequence: pilocarpic acid, isopilocarpic acid, isopilocarpine and pilocarpine. The test is not valid unless the resolution between the peaks corresponding to isopilocarpine and pilocarpine in the chromatogram obtained with reference solution (b) is at least 1.6. In the chromatogram obtained with the test solution: the area of the peak corresponding to isopilocarpine is not greater than twice the area of the principal peak in the chromatogram obtained with reference solution (a) (1 per cent); the sum of the areas of the peaks corresponding to isopilocarpine and pilocarpic acid is not greater than 3 times the area of the principal peak in the chromatogram obtained with reference solution (a) (1.5 per cent); and the sum of the areas of any peaks apart from the principal peak and the peaks corresponding to isopilocarpine and pilocarpic acid is not greater than the principal peak in the chromatogram obtained with reference solution (a) (0.5 per cent). Disregard any peak with an area less than 0.4 times the area of the principal peak in the chromatogram obtained with reference solution (a).

Iron (*2.4.9*). 10 ml of solution S complies with the limit test for iron (10 ppm). Prepare the standard using 5 ml of *iron standard solution (1 ppm Fe) R* and 5 ml of *water R*.

Loss on drying (*2.2.32*). Not more than 0.5 per cent, determined on 1.000 g by drying in an oven at 100-105 °C.

Sulphated ash (*2.4.14*). Not more than 0.1 per cent, determined on 1.0 g.

ASSAY

Dissolve 0.200 g in 50 ml of *alcohol R* and add 5 ml of *0.01 M hydrochloric acid*.Titrate with *0.1 M sodium hydroxide*, determining the end-point potentiometrically (*2.2.20*). Read the volume added between the two points of inflexion.

1 ml of *0.1 M sodium hydroxide* is equivalent to 24.47 mg of $C_{11}H_{17}ClN_2O_2$.

STORAGE

Store in an airtight container, protected from light.

IMPURITIES

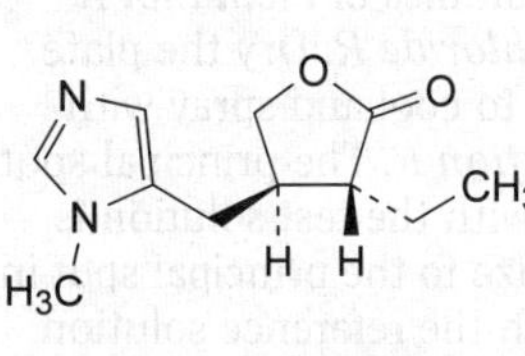

A. (3*R*,4*R*)-3-ethyl-4-[(1-methyl-1*H*-imidazol-5-yl)methyl]dihydrofuran-2(3*H*)-one (isopilocarpine),

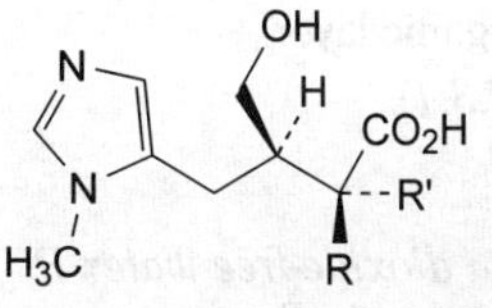

B. R = C_2H_5, R′ = H: (2*S*,3*R*)-2-ethyl-3-(hydroxymethyl)-4-(1-methyl-1*H*-imidazol-5-yl)butanoic acid (pilocarpic acid),

C. R = H, R′ = C_2H_5: (2*R*,3*R*)-2-ethyl-3-(hydroxymethyl)-4-(1-methyl-1*H*-imidazol-5-yl)butanoic acid (isopilocarpic acid).

01/2005:0104

PILOCARPINE NITRATE

Pilocarpini nitras

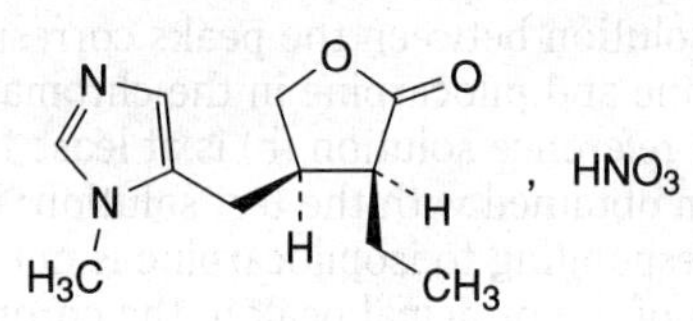

$C_{11}H_{17}N_3O_5$ M_r 271.3

DEFINITION

Pilocarpine nitrate contains not less than 98.5 per cent and not more than the equivalent of 101.0 per cent of (3*S*,4*R*)-3-ethyl-4-[(1-methyl-1*H*-imidazol-5-yl)methyl]dihydrofuran-2(3*H*)-one nitrate, calculated with reference to the dried substance.

CHARACTERS

A white or almost white, crystalline powder or colourless crystals, sensitive to light, freely soluble in water, sparingly soluble in alcohol.

It melts at about 174 °C with decomposition.

IDENTIFICATION

First identification: A, B, E.

Second identification: A, C, D, E.

A. It complies with the test for specific optical rotation (see Tests).

B. Examine by infrared absorption spectrophotometry (*2.2.24*), comparing with the spectrum obtained with *pilocarpine nitrate CRS*.

C. Examine thin-layer chromatography (*2.2.27*), using a *TLC silica gel G plate R*.

Test solution. Dissolve 10 mg of the substance to be examined in *water R* and dilute to 10 ml with the same solvent.

Reference solution. Dissolve 10 mg of *pilocarpine nitrate CRS* in *water R* and dilute to 10 ml with the same solvent.

Apply to the plate 10 µl of each solution. Develop over a path of 15 cm using a mixture of 1 volume of *concentrated ammonia R*, 14 volumes of *methanol R* and 85 volumes of *methylene chloride R*. Dry the plate at 100-105 °C for 10 min, allow to cool and spray with *potassium iodobismuthate solution R*. The principal spot in the chromatogram obtained with the test solution is similar in position, colour and size to the principal spot in the chromatogram obtained with the reference solution.

D. Dilute 0.2 ml of solution S (see Tests) to 2 ml with *water R*. Add 0.05 ml of a 50 g/l solution of *potassium dichromate R*, 1 ml of *dilute hydrogen peroxide solution R* and 2 ml of *methylene chloride R* and shake. A violet colour develops in the organic layer.

E. It gives the reaction of nitrates (*2.3.1*).

TESTS

Solution S. Dissolve 2.50 g in *carbon dioxide-free water R* and dilute to 50.0 ml with the same solvent. *Prepare immediately before use.*

Appearance of solution. Solution S is clear (*2.2.1*) and not more intensely coloured than reference solution Y_6 (*2.2.2, Method II*).

pH (*2.2.3*). The pH of solution S is 3.5 to 4.5.

Specific optical rotation (*2.2.7*). + 80 to + 83, determined on solution S and calculated with reference to the dried substance.

Related substances. Examine by liquid chromatography (*2.2.29*).

Test solution. Dissolve 0.100 g of the substance to be examined in *water R* and dilute to 100.0 ml with the same solvent.

Reference solution (a). Dissolve 5.0 ml of the test solution to 100.0 ml with *water R*. Dilute 2.0 ml of this solution to 20.0 ml with *water R*.

Reference solution (b). Dissolve 5.0 mg of *pilocarpine nitrate for system suitability CRS* in *water R* and dilute to 50.0 ml with the same solvent.

Reference solution (c). To 5 ml of the test solution, add 0.1 ml of *ammonia R* and heat the solution on a water-bath for 30 min, cool and dilute to 25 ml with *water R*. Take 3 ml of this solution and dilute to 25 ml with *water R*. Mainly pilocarpic acid is formed.

The chromatographic procedure may be carried out using:

- a stainless steel column 0.15 m long and 4.6 mm in internal diameter packed with *octadecylsilyl silica gel for chromatography R1* (5 µm) with a pore size of 10 nm and a carbon loading of 19 per cent,
- as mobile phase at a flow rate of 1.2 ml/min a solution prepared as follows: mix 55 volumes of *methanol R*, 60 volumes of *acetonitrile R* and 885 volumes of a 0.679 g/l solution of *tetrabutylammonium dihydrogen phosphate R*, previously adjusted to pH 7.7 with *diluted ammonia R2*,
- as detector a spectrophotometer set at 220 nm.

Inject 20 µl of each solution. Continue the chromatography for twice the retention time of the principal peak (about 40 min). When the chromatograms are recorded in the prescribed conditions, the substances are eluted in the following sequence: pilocarpic acid, isopilocarpic acid, isopilocarpine and pilocarpine. The test is not valid unless the resolution between the peaks corresponding to isopilocarpine and pilocarpine in the chromatogram obtained with reference solution (b) is at least 1.6. In the chromatogram obtained with the test solution: the area of the peak corresponding to isopilocarpine is not greater than twice the area of the principal peak in the chromatogram obtained with reference solution (a) (1 per cent); the sum of the area of the peaks corresponding to isopilocarpine and pilocarpic acid is less than 3 times the area of the principal peak in the chromatogram obtained with reference solution (a) (1.5 per cent); and the sum of the areas of any peaks apart from the principal peak and the peaks corresponding to isopilocarpine and pilocarpic acid is not greater than the principal peak in the chromatogram obtained with reference solution (a) (0.5 per cent). Disregard any peak with an area less than 0.4 times the area of the principal peak in the chromatogram obtained with reference solution (a) and any peak due to the nitrate ion with a relative retention time relative to pilocarpine of about 0.3.

Chlorides (*2.4.4*). 15 ml of solution S complies with the limit test for chlorides (70 ppm).

Iron (*2.4.9*). 10 ml of solution S complies with the limit test for iron (10 ppm). Prepare the standard using 5 ml of *iron standard solution (1 ppm Fe) R* and 5 ml of *water R*.

Loss on drying (*2.2.32*). Not more than 0.5 per cent, determined on 1.000 g by drying in an oven at 100-105 °C.

Sulphated ash (*2.4.14*). Not more than 0.1 per cent, determined on 1.0 g.

ASSAY

Dissolve 0.250 g in 30 ml of *anhydrous acetic acid R*. Titrate with *0.1 M perchloric acid* determining the end-point potentiometrically (*2.2.20*).

1 ml of *0.1 M perchloric acid* is equivalent to 27.13 mg of $C_{11}H_{17}N_3O_5$.

STORAGE

Store protected from light.

IMPURITIES

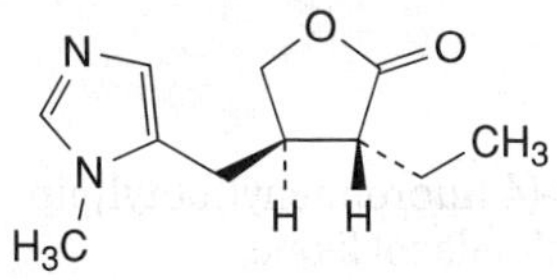

A. (3*R*,4*R*)-3-ethyl-4-[(1-methyl-1*H*-imidazol-5-yl)methyl]dihydrofuran-2(3*H*)-one (isopilocarpine),

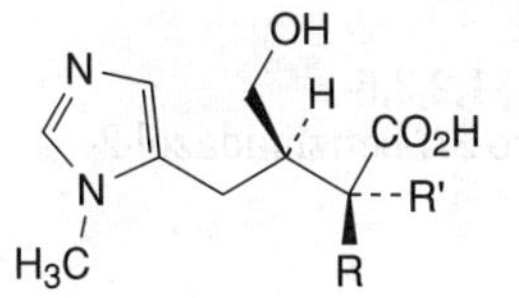

B. R = C_2H_5, R′ = H: (2*S*,3*R*)-2-ethyl-3-(hydroxymethyl)-4-(1-methyl-1*H*-imidazol-5-yl)butanoic acid (pilocarpic acid),

C. R = H, R′ = C_2H_5: (2*R*,3*R*)-2-ethyl-3-(hydroxymethyl)-4-(1-methyl-1*H*-imidazol-5-yl)butanoic acid (isopilocarpic acid).

01/2005:1254

PIMOZIDE

Pimozidum

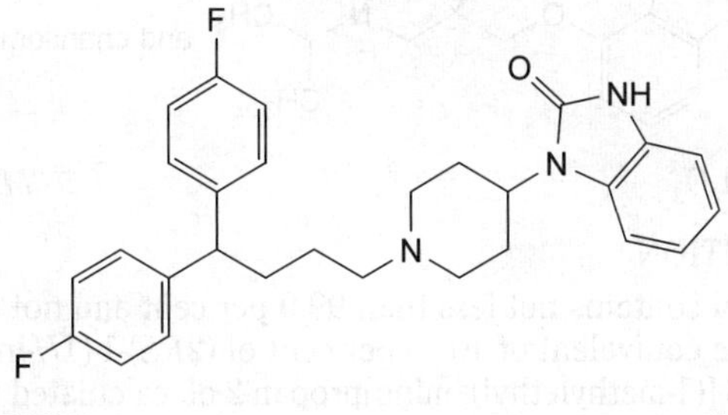

$C_{28}H_{29}F_2N_3O$ M_r 461.6

DEFINITION

Pimozide contains not less than 99.0 per cent and not more than the equivalent of 101.0 per cent of 1-[1-[4,4-bis(4-fluorophenyl)butyl]piperidin-4-yl]-1,3-dihydro-2*H*-benzimidazol-2-one, calculated with reference to the dried substance.

CHARACTERS

A white or almost white powder, practically insoluble in water, soluble in methylene chloride, sparingly soluble in methanol, slightly soluble in alcohol.

IDENTIFICATION

First identification: B.

Second identification: A, C, D.

A. Melting point (*2.2.14*): 216 °C to 220 °C.

B. Examine by infrared absorption spectrophotometry (*2.2.24*), comparing with the spectrum obtained with *pimozide CRS*. Examine the substances prepared as discs.

C. Examine by thin-layer chromatography (*2.2.27*), using a suitable silica gel as the coating substance.

Test solution. Dissolve 30 mg of the substance to be examined in a mixture of 1 volume of *acetone R* and 9 volumes of *methanol R* and dilute to 10 ml with the same mixture of solvents.

Reference solution (a). Dissolve 30 mg of *pimozide CRS* in a mixture of 1 volume of *acetone R* and 9 volumes of *methanol R* and dilute to 10 ml with the same mixture of solvents.

Reference solution (b). Dissolve 30 mg of *pimozide CRS* and 30 mg of *benperidol CRS* in a mixture of 1 volume of *acetone R* and 9 volumes of *methanol R* and dilute to 10 ml with the same mixture of solvents.

Apply separately to the plate 10 µl of each solution. Develop over a path of 15 cm using a mixture of 1 volume of *acetone R* and 9 volumes of *methanol R*. Allow the plate to dry in a current of warm air for 15 min and expose it to iodine vapour until the spots appear. The principal spot in the chromatogram obtained with the test solution is similar in position and size to the principal spot in the chromatogram obtained with reference solution (a). The test is not valid unless the chromatogram obtained with reference solution (b) shows two clearly separated spots.

D. Mix about 5 mg with 45 mg of *heavy magnesium oxide R* and ignite in a crucible until an almost white residue is obtained (usually less than 5 min). Allow to cool, add 1 ml of *water R*, 0.05 ml of *phenolphthalein solution R1* and about 1 ml of *dilute hydrochloric acid R* to render the solution colourless. Filter. To a freshly prepared mixture of 0.1 ml of *alizarin S solution R* and 0.1 ml of *zirconyl nitrate solution R*, add 1.0 ml of the filtrate. Mix, allow to stand for 5 min and compare the colour of the solution with that of a blank prepared in the same manner. The test solution is yellow and the blank is red.

TESTS

Appearance of solution. Dissolve 0.2 g in *methanol R* and dilute to 20 ml with the same solvent. The solution is clear (*2.2.1*) and not more intensely coloured than reference solution Y_7 (*2.2.2, Method II*).

Related substances. Examine by liquid chromatography (*2.2.29*).

Test solution. Dissolve 0.10 g of the substance to be examined in *methanol R* and dilute to 10.0 ml with the same solvent.

Reference solution (a). Dissolve 5.0 mg of *pimozide CRS* and 2.0 mg of *mebendazole CRS* in *methanol R* and dilute to 100.0 ml with the same solvent.

Reference solution (b). Dilute 5.0 ml of the test solution to 100.0 ml with *methanol R*. Dilute 1.0 ml of this solution to 10.0 ml with *methanol R*.

The chromatographic procedure may be carried out using:

– a stainless steel column 0.1 m long and 4.6 mm in internal diameter packed with *octadecylsilyl silica gel for chromatography R* (3 µm),

– as mobile phase at a flow rate of 2.0 ml/min:

Mobile phase A. A solution containing 2.5 g/l of *ammonium acetate R* and 8.5 g/l of *tetrabutylammonium hydrogen sulphate R*,

Mobile phase B. Acetonitrile R,

Time (min)	Mobile phase A (per cent *V/V*)	Mobile phase B (per cent *V/V*)	Comment
0 - 10	80 → 70	20 → 30	linear gradient
10 - 15	70	30	isocratic elution
15 - 20	80	20	switch to initial eluent composition
20 = 0	80	20	restart gradient

– as detector a spectrophotometer set at 280 nm.

Equilibrate the column for at least 10 min at the initial elution composition.

Adjust the sensitivity of the system so that the height of the principal peak in the chromatogram obtained with 10 µl of reference solution (b) is at least 50 per cent of the full scale of the recorder.

Inject 10 µl of reference solution (a). When the chromatogram is recorded in the prescribed conditions, the retention times are: mebendazole, about 7 min and pimozide, about 8 min. The test is not valid unless the resolution between the peaks due to mebendazole and pimozide is at least 5.0. If necessary, adjust the concentration of acetonitrile in the mobile phase or adjust the time programme for the linear-gradient elution.

Inject separately 10 µl of *methanol R* as a blank, 10 µl of the test solution and 10 µl of reference solution (b). In the chromatogram obtained with the test solution: the area of any peak, apart from the principal peak, is not greater than the area of the principal peak in the chromatogram obtained with reference solution (b) (0.5 per cent); the sum of the areas of all peaks, apart from the principal peak, is not greater than 1.5 times the area of the principal peak in the chromatogram obtained with reference solution (b) (0.75 per cent). Disregard any peak in the chromatogram obtained with the blank run and any peak with an area less than 0.1 times the area of the principal peak in the chromatogram obtained with reference solution (b).

Loss on drying (*2.2.32*). Not more than 0.5 per cent, determined on 1.000 g by drying in an oven at 100-105 °C.

Sulphated ash (*2.4.14*). Not more than 0.1 per cent, determined on 1.0 g in a platinum crucible.

ASSAY

Dissolve 0.300 g in 50 ml of a mixture of 1 volume of *anhydrous acetic acid R* and 7 volumes of *methyl ethyl ketone R* and titrate with *0.1 M perchloric acid*, using 0.2 ml of *naphtholbenzein solution R* as indicator.

1 ml *0.1 M perchloric acid* is equivalent to 46.16 mg of $C_{28}H_{29}F_2N_3O$.

STORAGE

Store protected from light.

IMPURITIES

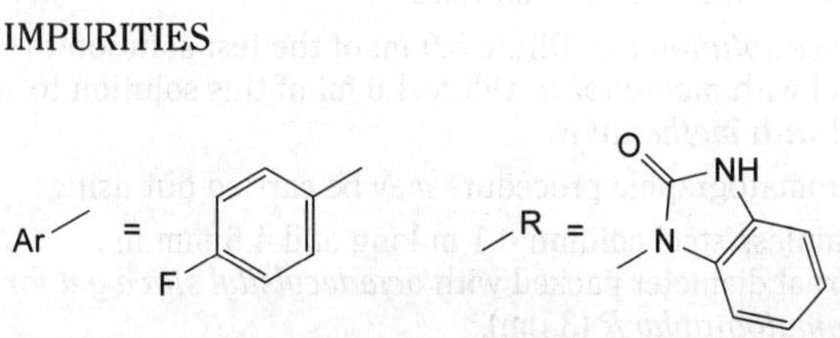

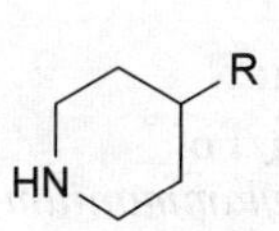

A. 1-(piperidin-4-yl)-1,3-dihydro-2*H*-benzimidazol-2-one,

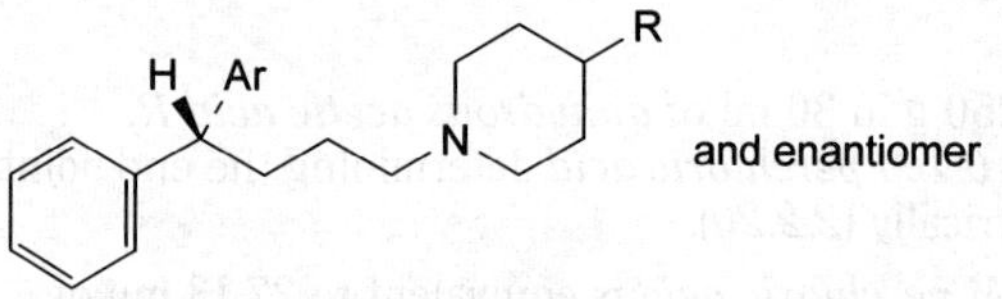

B. 1-[1-[(4*RS*)-4-(4-fluorophenyl)-4-phenylbutyl]piperidin-4-yl]-1,3-dihydro-2*H*-benzimidazol-2-one,

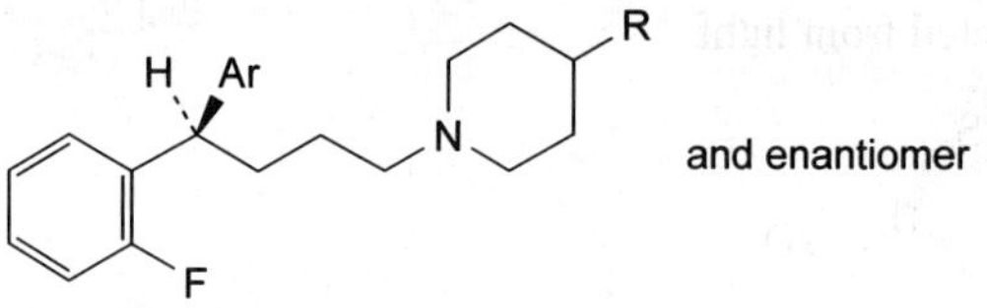

C. 1-[1-[(4*RS*)-4-(2-fluorophenyl)-4-(4-fluorophenyl)butyl]piperidin-4-yl]-1,3-dihydro-2*H*-benzimidazol-2-one,

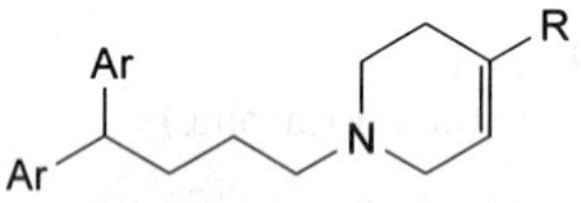

D. 1-[1-[4,4-bis(4-fluorophenyl)butyl]-1,2,3,6-tetrahydropyridin-4-yl]-1,3-dihydro-2*H*-benzimidazol-2-one,

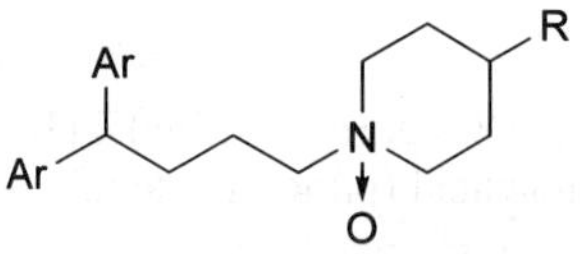

E. 1-[1-[4,4-bis(4-fluorophenyl)butyl]piperidin-4-yl 1-oxide]-1,3-dihydro-2*H*-benzimidazol-2-one.

01/2005:0634

PINDOLOL

Pindololum

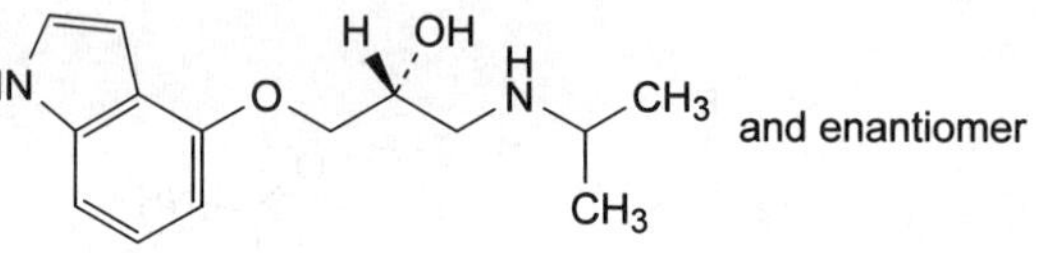

$C_{14}H_{20}N_2O_2$ M_r 248.3

DEFINITION

Pindolol contains not less than 99.0 per cent and not more than the equivalent of 101.0 per cent of (2*RS*)-1-(1*H*-indol-4-yloxy)-3-[(1-methylethyl)amino]propan-2-ol, calculated with reference to the dried substance.

CHARACTERS

A white or almost white, crystalline powder, practically insoluble in water, slightly soluble in methanol. It dissolves in dilute mineral acids.

IDENTIFICATION

First identification: A, C.

Second identification: A, B, D.

A. Melting point (*2.2.14*): 169 °C to 174 °C.

B. Dissolve 20.0 mg in a 0.085 per cent *V/V* solution of *hydrochloric acid R* in *methanol R* and dilute to 100.0 ml with the same solution. Dilute 10.0 ml of the solution to 100.0 ml with a 0.085 per cent *V/V* solution of *hydrochloric acid R* in *methanol R*. Examined between 230 nm and 320 nm (*2.2.25*), the solution shows two absorption maxima, at 264 nm and at 287 nm, and a shoulder at 275 nm. The specific absorbance at the maxima are 330 to 350 and 170 to 190, respectively.

C. Examine by infrared absorption spectrophotometry (*2.2.24*), comparing with the spectrum obtained with *pindolol CRS*.

D. Examine in daylight the chromatograms on plate A obtained in the test for related substances. The principal spot in the chromatogram obtained with test solution (b) is similar in position, colour and size to the principal spot in the chromatogram obtained with reference solution (a).

TESTS

Appearance of solution. Dissolve 0.5 g in *dilute acetic acid R* and dilute to 10 ml with the same acid. The solution is clear (*2.2.1*) and not more intensely coloured than reference solution BY_5 or B_5 (*2.2.2, Method II*).

Related substances. Examine by thin-layer chromatography (*2.2.27*), using *silica gel GF_{254} R* as the coating substance. *Carry out all operations as rapidly as possible, protected from light.*

Test solution (a). Dissolve 0.10 g of the substance to be examined in a mixture of 1 volume of *anhydrous acetic acid R* and 99 volumes of *methanol R* and dilute to 5 ml with the same mixture of solvents. Prepare immediately before use and apply this solution to the plate last.

Test solution (b). Dilute 1 ml of test solution (a) to 10 ml with a mixture of 1 volume of *anhydrous acetic acid R* and 99 volumes of *methanol R*.

Reference solution (a). Dissolve 20 mg of *pindolol CRS* in a mixture of 1 volume of *anhydrous acetic acid R* and 99 volumes of *methanol R* and dilute to 10 ml with the same mixture of solvents.

Reference solution (b). Dilute 1.5 ml of reference solution (a) to 50 ml with a mixture of 1 volume of *anhydrous acetic acid R* and 99 volumes of *methanol R*.

A. Apply separately 5 µl of each solution. Develop the plate without delay over a path of 10 cm using a freshly prepared mixture of 4 volumes of *concentrated ammonia R*, 50 volumes of *ethyl acetate R* and 50 volumes of *methanol R*. Dry the plate briefly in a current of cold air. Spray the plate without delay with *dimethylaminobenzaldehyde solution R7* and heat to 50 °C for 20 min. Any spot in the chromatogram obtained with test solution (a), apart from the principal spot, is not more intense than the spot in the chromatogram obtained with reference solution (b) (0.3 per cent).

B. Apply separately 10 µl of each solution. Develop the plate without delay over a path of 10 cm using a freshly prepared mixture of 4 volumes of *concentrated ammonia R*, 50 volumes of *ethyl acetate R* and 50 volumes of *methanol R*. Dry the plate briefly in a current of cold air. Examine the plate without delay in ultraviolet light at 254 nm. Any spot in the chromatogram obtained with test solution (a), apart from the principal spot and the spots detected on plate A, is not more intense than the spot in the chromatogram obtained with reference solution (b) (0.3 per cent).

Heavy metals (*2.4.8*). 1.0 g complies with limit test C for heavy metals (20 ppm). Prepare the standard using 2 ml of *lead standard solution (10 ppm Pb) R*.

Loss on drying (*2.2.32*). Not more than 0.5 per cent, determined on 1.000 g by drying in an oven at 100 °C to 105 °C.

Sulphated ash (*2.4.14*). Not more than 0.1 per cent, determined on 1.0 g.

ASSAY

Dissolve 0.200 g in 80 ml of *methanol R*. Titrate with *0.1 M hydrochloric acid*, determining the end-point potentiometrically (*2.2.20*).

1 ml of *0.1 M hydrochloric acid* is equivalent to 24.83 mg of $C_{14}H_{20}N_2O_2$.

STORAGE

Store protected from light.

IMPURITIES

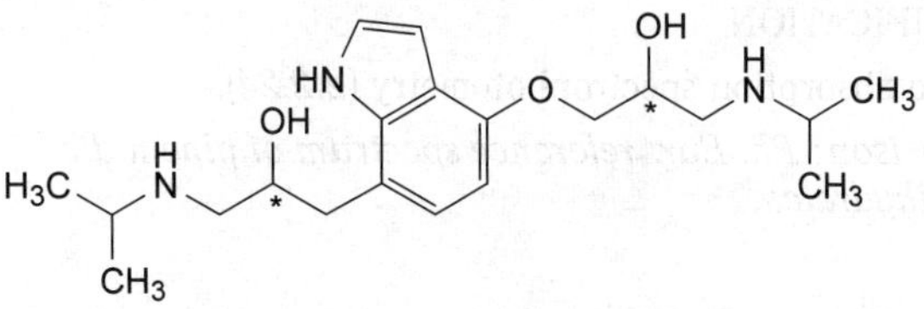

A. 1-[[7-[2-hydroxy-3-[(1-methylethyl)amino]propyl]-1*H*-indol-4-yl]oxy]-3-[(1-methylethyl)amino]propan-2-ol,

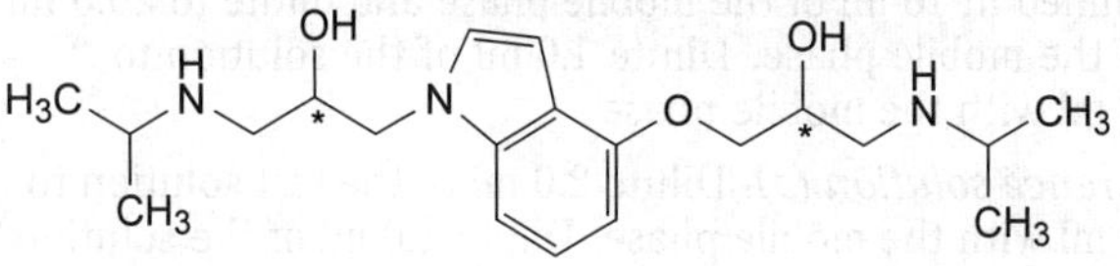

B. 1-[4-[2-hydroxy-3-[(1-methylethyl)amino]propoxy]-1*H*-indol-1-yl]-3-[(1-methylethyl)amino]propan-2-ol,

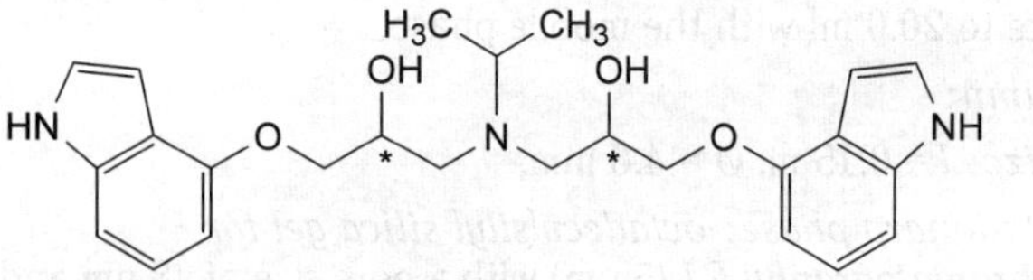

C. 1,1′-[(1-methylethyl)imino]bis[3-(1*H*-indol-4-yloxy)propan-2-ol],

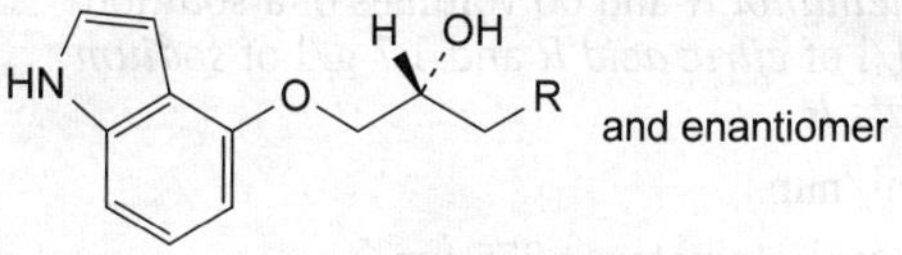

D. R = OH: (2*RS*)-3-(1*H*-indol-4-yloxy)propane-1,2-diol,

F. R = Cl: (2*RS*)-1-chloro-3-(1*H*-indol-4-yloxy)propan-2-ol,

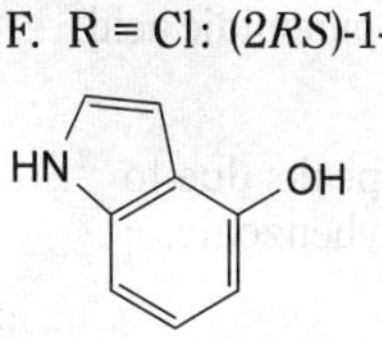

E. 1*H*-indol-4-ol.

01/2005:1743

PIPEMIDIC ACID TRIHYDRATE

Acidum pipemidicum trihydricum

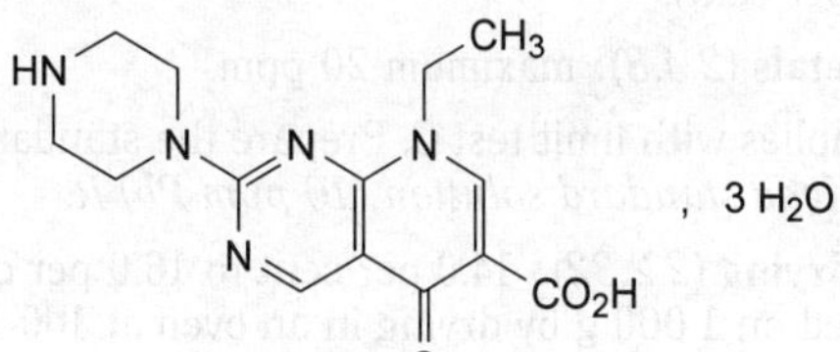

$C_{14}H_{17}N_5O_3,3H_2O$ M_r 357.4

DEFINITION

8-Ethyl-5-oxo-2-(piperazin-1-yl)-5,8-dihydropyrido[2,3-*d*]pyrimidine-6-carboxylic acid trihydrate.

Content: 98.5 per cent to 101.0 per cent (dried substance).

CHARACTERS

Appearance: pale yellow or yellow, crystalline powder.

Solubility: very slightly soluble in water. It dissolves in dilute solutions of acids and of alkali hydroxides.

IDENTIFICATION

Infrared absorption spectrophotometry (*2.2.24*).

Comparison: *Ph. Eur. reference spectrum of pipemidic acid trihydrate.*

TESTS

Related substances. Liquid chromatography (*2.2.29*).

Test solution. Dissolve 20 mg of the substance to be examined in 10 ml of the mobile phase and dilute to 20.0 ml with the mobile phase. Dilute 1.0 ml of the solution to 10.0 ml with the mobile phase.

Reference solution (a). Dilute 2.0 ml of the test solution to 10.0 ml with the mobile phase. Dilute 1.0 ml of the solution to 100.0 ml with the mobile phase.

Reference solution (b). Dissolve 10.0 mg of *ethyl parahydroxybenzoate R* in 2.0 ml of the test solution and dilute to 20.0 ml with the mobile phase.

Column:

- *size*: *l* = 0.15 m, Ø = 4.6 mm,
- *stationary phase*: *octadecylsilyl silica gel for chromatography R1* (5 µm) with a pore size of 18 nm and a carbon loading of 13 per cent.

Mobile phase: mix 20 volumes of *acetonitrile R*, 20 volumes of *methanol R* and 60 volumes of a solution containing 5.7 g/l of *citric acid R* and 1.7 g/l of *sodium decanesulphonate R*.

Flow rate: 0.8 ml/min.

Detection: spectrophotometer at 275 nm.

Injection: 20 µl.

Run time: 2.5 times the retention time of pipemidic acid.

System suitability: reference solution (b):

- *resolution*: minimum 4.0 between the peaks due to pipemidic acid and to ethyl parahydroxybenzoate.

Limits:

- *any impurity*: not more than the area of the principal peak in the chromatogram obtained with reference solution (a) (0.2 per cent),
- *total*: not more than 5 times the area of the principal peak in the chromatogram obtained with reference solution (a) (1.0 per cent),
- *disregard limit*: 0.25 times the area of the principal peak in the chromatogram obtained with reference solution (a) (0.05 per cent).

Heavy metals (*2.4.8*): maximum 20 ppm.

1.0 g complies with limit test C. Prepare the standard using 2.0 ml of *lead standard solution (10 ppm Pb) R*.

Loss on drying (*2.2.32*): 14.0 per cent to 16.0 per cent, determined on 1.000 g by drying in an oven at 100-105 °C.

Sulphated ash (*2.4.14*): maximum 0.1 per cent, determined on 1.0 g.

ASSAY

Dissolve 0.240 g in 50 ml of *anhydrous acetic acid R*. Titrate with *0.1 M perchloric acid*, determining the end-point potentiometrically (*2.2.20*).

1 ml of *0.1 M perchloric acid* is equivalent to 30.33 mg of $C_{14}H_{17}N_5O_3$.

STORAGE

Protected from light.

IMPURITIES

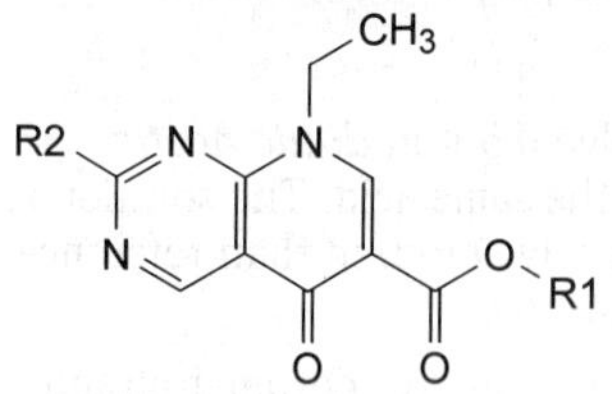

A. R1 = H, R2 = OH: 8-ethyl-2-hydroxy-5-oxo-5,8-dihydropyrido[2,3-*d*]pyrimidine-6-carboxylic acid,

B. R1 = H, R2 = OCH_3: 8-ethyl-2-methoxy-5-oxo-5,8-dihydropyrido[2,3-*d*]pyrimidine-6-carboxylic acid,

C. R1 = H, R2 = OC_2H_5: 2-ethoxy-8-ethyl-5-oxo-5,8-dihydropyrido[2,3-*d*]pyrimidine-6-carboxylic acid,

D. R1 = C_2H_5, R2 = Cl: ethyl 2-chloro-8-ethyl-5-oxo-5,8-dihydropyrido[2,3-*d*]pyrimidine-6-carboxylate,

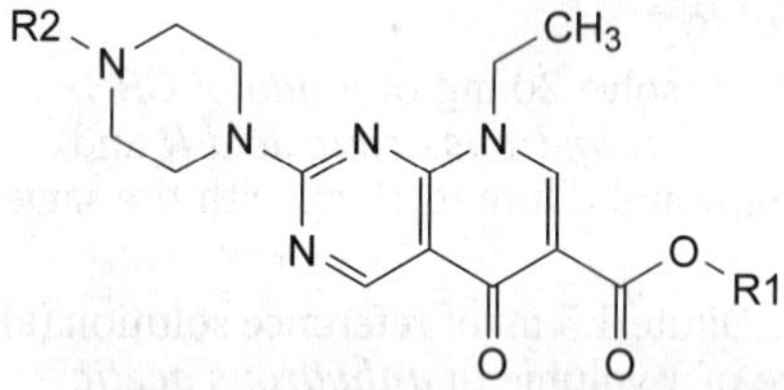

E. R1 = C_2H_5, R_2 = H: ethyl 8-ethyl-5-oxo-2-(piperazin-1-yl)-5,8-dihydropyrido[2,3-*d*]pyrimidine-6-carboxylate,

F. R1 = H, R2 = $CO\text{-}CH_3$: 2-(4-acetylpiperazin-1-yl)-8-ethyl-5-oxo-5,8-dihydropyrido[2,3-*d*]pyrimidine-6-carboxylic acid (acetylpipemidic acid).

01/2005:1169

PIPERACILLIN

Piperacillinum

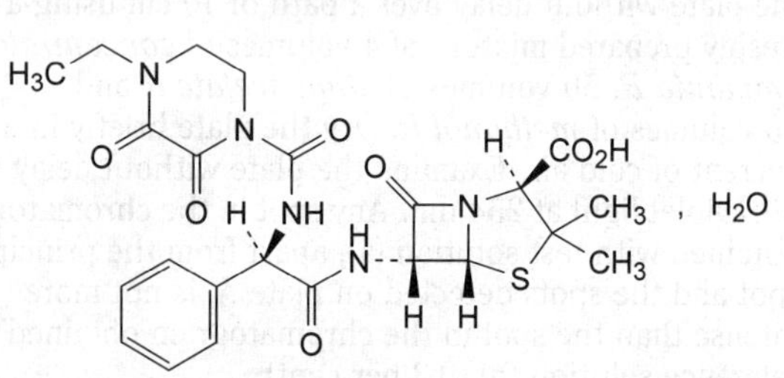

$C_{23}H_{27}N_5O_7S,H_2O$ M_r 535.6

DEFINITION

Piperacillin contains not less than 96.0 per cent and not more than the equivalent of 101.0 per cent of (2*S*,5*R*,6*R*)-6-[[(2*R*)-2-[[(4-ethyl-2,3-dioxopiperazin-1-yl)carbonyl]amino]-2-phenylacetyl]amino]-3,3-dimethyl-7-oxo-4-thia-1-azabicyclo[3.2.0]heptane-2-carboxylic acid, calculated with reference to the anhydrous substance.

CHARACTERS

A white or almost white powder, slightly soluble in water, freely soluble in methanol, slightly soluble in ethyl acetate.

IDENTIFICATION

Examine by infrared absorption spectrophotometry (*2.2.24*), comparing with the spectrum obtained with *piperacillin CRS.*

TESTS

Solution S. Dissolve 2.50 g in *sodium carbonate solution R* and dilute to 25 ml with the same solvent.

Appearance of solution. Solution S is not more opalescent than reference suspension II (*2.2.1*). The absorbance of solution S measured at 430 nm (*2.2.25*) is not greater than 0.10.

Specific optical rotation (*2.2.7*). Dissolve 0.250 g in *methanol R* and dilute to 25.0 ml with the same solvent. The specific optical rotation is + 165 to + 175, calculated with reference to the anhydrous substance.

Related substances. Examine by liquid chromatography (*2.2.29*) as prescribed under Assay. Inject 20 µl of reference solution (b) and elute isocratically with the chosen mobile phase. Inject 20 µl of test solution (b). Start the elution isocratically. Immediately after elution of the piperacillin peak start the following linear gradient.

Time (min)	Mobile phase A (per cent *V/V*)	Mobile phase B (per cent *V/V*)	Comment
0 - 30	88 → 0	12 → 100	linear gradient
30 - 45	0 → 88	100 → 12	re-equilibration

In the chromatogram obtained with test solution (b), the area of any peak, apart from the principal peak, is not greater than twice the area of the principal peak in the chromatogram obtained with reference solution (b) (2 per cent). Disregard any peak due to the solvent.

***N,N*-Dimethylaniline** (*2.4.26, Method A*). Not more than 20 ppm.

Heavy metals (*2.4.8*). 1.0 g complies with limit test C for heavy metals (20 ppm). Prepare the standard using 2 ml of *lead standard solution (10 ppm Pb) R.*

Water (*2.5.12*): 2.0 per cent to 4.0 per cent, determined on 0.500 g by the semi-micro determination of water.

ASSAY

Examine by liquid chromatography (*2.2.29*).

Solvent mixture. Mix 25 volumes of *acetonitrile R* and 75 volumes of a 31.2 g/l solution of *sodium dihydrogen phosphate R.*

Test solution (a). Dissolve 25.0 mg of the substance to be examined in the solvent mixture and dilute to 50.0 ml with the solvent mixture.

Test solution (b). Prepare the solution immediately before use. Dissolve 40.0 mg of the substance to be examined in the solvent mixture and dilute to 20.0 ml with the solvent mixture.

Reference solution (a). Dissolve 25.0 mg of *piperacillin CRS* in the solvent mixture and dilute to 50.0 ml with the solvent mixture.

Reference solution (b). Dilute 1.0 ml of reference solution (a) to 25.0 ml with the solvent mixture.

Reference solution (c). Dissolve 10.0 mg of *piperacillin CRS* and 10.0 mg of *anhydrous ampicillin CRS* in the solvent mixture and dilute to 50.0 ml with the solvent mixture.

Reference solution (d). Dilute 1.0 ml of reference solution (a) to 100.0 ml with the solvent mixture. Dilute 1.0 ml of the solution to 50.0 ml with the solvent mixture.

The chromatographic procedure may be carried out using:

– a column 0.25 m long and 4.6 mm in internal diameter packed with *octadecylsilyl silica gel for chromatography R* (5 µm),

– as mobile phase at a flow rate of 1.0 ml/min a mixture of 88 volumes of mobile phase A and 12 volumes of mobile phase B:

Mobile phase A. Mix 576 ml of *water R*, 200 ml of a 31.2 g/l solution of *sodium dihydrogen phosphate R* and 24 ml of an 80 g/l solution of *tetrabutylammonium hydroxide R.* If necessary, adjust to pH 5.5 with *dilute phosphoric acid R* or *dilute sodium hydroxide solution R*; then add 200 ml of *acetonitrile R,*

Mobile phase B. Mix 126 ml of *water R*, 200 ml of a 31.2 g/l solution of *sodium dihydrogen phosphate R* and 24 ml of an 80 g/l solution of *tetrabutylammonium hydroxide R.* If necessary, adjust to pH 5.5 with *dilute phosphoric acid R* or *dilute sodium hydroxide solution R*; then add 650 ml of *acetonitrile R,*

– as detector a spectrophotometer set at 220 nm.

Inject 20 µl of reference solution (c). The test is not valid unless in the chromatogram obtained, the resolution between the peaks corresponding to ampicillin and to piperacillin is at least 10 (if necessary, adjust the ratio A:B of the mobile phase) and the mass distribution ratio for the second peak (piperacillin) is 2.0 to 3.0. Inject 20 µl of reference solution (d). Adjust the sensitivity of the system to obtain a peak with a signal-to-noise ratio of at least 3. Inject reference solution (a) 6 times. The test is not valid unless the relative standard deviation of the peak area of piperacillin is at most 1.0 per cent. Inject alternately test solution (a) and reference solution (a).

IMPURITIES

A. ampicillin,

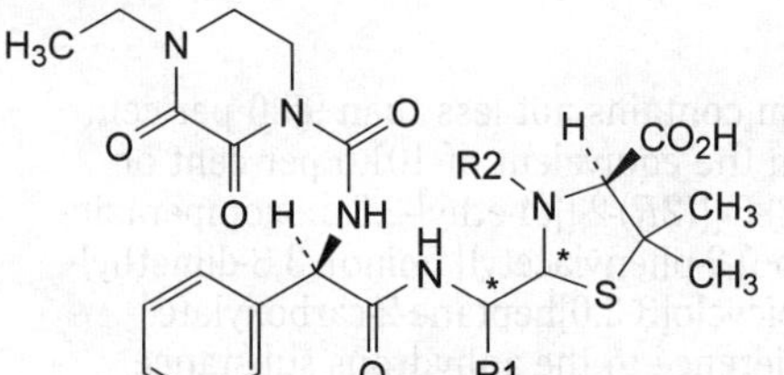

B. R1 = CO_2H, R2 = H: (4*S*)-2-[carboxy[[(2*R*)-2-[[(4-ethyl-2,3-dioxopiperazin-1-yl)carbonyl]amino]-2-phenylacetyl]amino]methyl]-5,5-dimethylthiazolidine-4-carboxylic acid (penicilloic acids of piperacillin),

C. R1 = R2 = H: (2*RS*,4*S*)-2-[[[(2*R*)-2-[[(4-ethyl-2,3-dioxopiperazin-1-yl)carbonyl]amino]-2-phenylacetyl]amino]methyl]-5,5-dimethylthiazolidine-4-carboxylic acid (penilloic acids of piperacillin),

F. R1 = CO_2H, R2 = $CO\text{-}CH_3$: (4*S*)-3-acetyl-2-[carboxy[[(2*R*)-2-[[(4-ethyl-2,3-dioxopiperazin-1-yl)carbonyl]amino]-2-phenylacetyl]amino]methyl]-5,5-dimethylthiazolidine-4-carboxylic acid (acetylated penicilloic acids of piperacillin),

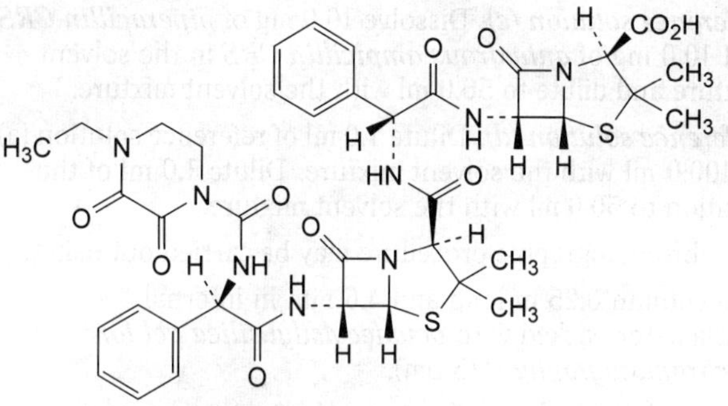

D. (2*S*,5*R*,6*R*)-6-[[(2*R*)-2-[[[(2*S*,5*R*,6*R*)-6-[[(2*R*)-2-[[(4-ethyl-2,3-dioxopiperazin-1-yl)carbonyl]amino]-2-phenylacetyl]amino]-3,3-dimethyl-7-oxo-4-thia-1-azabicyclo[3.2.0]hept-2-yl]carbonyl]amino]-2-phenylacetyl]amino]-3,3-dimethyl-7-oxo-4-thia-1-azabicyclo[3.2.0]heptane-2-carboxylic acid (piperacillinylampicillin),

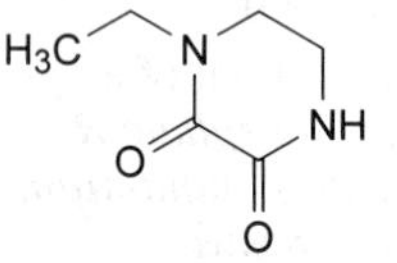

E. 1-ethylpiperazine-2,3-dione.

01/2005:1168

PIPERACILLIN SODIUM

Piperacillinum natricum

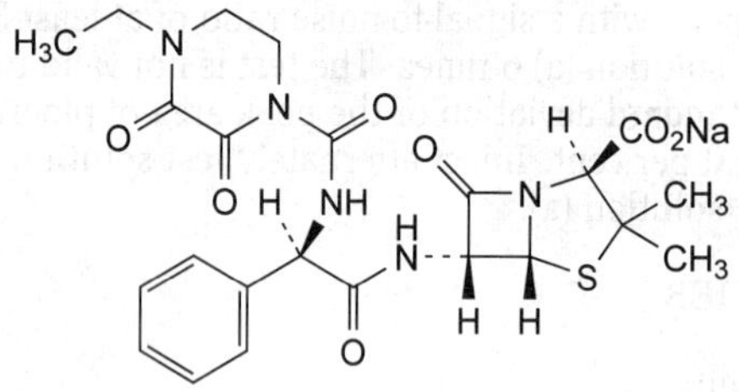

$C_{23}H_{26}N_5NaO_7S$ M_r 539.5

DEFINITION

Piperacillin sodium contains not less than 95.0 per cent and not more than the equivalent of 101.0 per cent of sodium (2*S*,5*R*,6*R*)-6-[[(2*R*)-2-[[(4-ethyl-2,3-dioxopiperazin-1-yl)carbonyl]amino]-2-phenylacetyl]amino]- 3,3-dimethyl-7-oxo-4-thia-1-azabicyclo[3.2.0]heptane-2-carboxylate, calculated with reference to the anhydrous substance.

CHARACTERS

A white or almost white powder, hygroscopic, freely soluble in water and in methanol, practically insoluble in ethyl acetate.

IDENTIFICATION

A. Dissolve 0.250 g in *water R*, add 0.5 ml of *dilute hydrochloric acid R* and 5 ml of *ethyl acetate R*; stir and allow to stand for 10 min in iced water. Filter the crystals through a small sintered-glass filter (40), applying suction. Wash with 5 ml of *water R* and 5 ml of *ethyl acetate R* and dry in an oven at 60 °C for 60 min. Examine the crystals by infrared absorption spectrophotometry (*2.2.24*), comparing with the spectrum obtained with *piperacillin CRS*.

B. It gives reaction (a) of sodium (*2.3.1*).

TESTS

Solution S. Dissolve 2.50 g in *carbon dioxide-free water R* and dilute to 25 ml with the same solvent.

Appearance of solution. Solution S is clear (*2.2.1*). The absorbance of solution S measured at 430 nm (*2.2.25*) is not greater than 0.10.

pH (*2.2.3*). The pH of solution S is 5.0 to 7.0.

Specific optical rotation (*2.2.7*). Dissolve 0.250 g in *water R* and dilute to 25.0 ml with the same solvent. The specific optical rotation is + 175 to + 190, calculated with reference to the anhydrous substance.

Related substances. Examine by liquid chromatography (*2.2.29*) as prescribed under Assay. Inject 20 µl of reference solution (b) and elute isocratically with the chosen mobile phase. Inject 20 µl of test solution (b). Start the elution isocratically. Immediately after elution of the piperacillin peak start the following linear gradient.

Time (min)	Mobile phase A (per cent *V/V*)	Mobile phase B (per cent *V/V*)	Comment
0 - 30	88 → 0	12 → 100	linear gradient
30 - 45	0 → 88	100 → 12	re-equilibration

In the chromatogram obtained with test solution (b), the area of any peak, apart from the principal peak, is not greater than twice the area of the principal peak in the chromatogram obtained with reference solution (b) (2 per cent). Disregard any peak due to the solvent.

***N,N*-Dimethylaniline** (*2.4.26, Method A*). Not more than 20 ppm.

Heavy metals (*2.4.8*). 1.0 g complies with the limit test C for heavy metals (20 ppm). Prepare the standard using 2 ml of *lead standard solution (10 ppm Pb) R*.

Water (*2.5.12*). Not more than 2.0 per cent, determined on 0.500 g by the semi-micro determination of water.

Bacterial endotoxins (*2.6.14*): less than 0.07 IU/mg, if intended for use in the manufacture of parenteral dosage forms without a further appropriate procedure for the removal of bacterial endotoxins.

ASSAY

Examine by liquid chromatography (*2.2.29*).

Solvent mixture. Mix 25 volumes of *acetonitrile R* and 75 volumes of a 31.2 g/l solution of *sodium dihydrogen phosphate R*.

Test solution (a). Dissolve 25.0 mg of the substance to be examined in the solvent mixture and dilute to 50.0 ml with the solvent mixture.

Test solution (b). Prepare the solution immediately before use. Dissolve 40.0 mg of the substance to be examined in the solvent mixture and dilute to 20.0 ml with the solvent mixture.

Reference solution (a). Dissolve 25.0 mg of *piperacillin CRS* in the solvent mixture and dilute to 50.0 ml with the solvent mixture.

Reference solution (b). Dilute 1.0 ml of reference solution (a) to 25.0 ml with the solvent mixture.

Reference solution (c). Dissolve 10.0 mg of *piperacillin CRS* and 10.0 mg of *anhydrous ampicillin CRS* in the solvent mixture and dilute to 50.0 ml with the solvent mixture.

Reference solution (d). Dilute 1.0 ml of reference solution (a) to 100.0 ml with the solvent mixture. Dilute 1.0 ml of the solution to 50.0 ml with the solvent mixture.

The chromatographic procedure may be carried out using:

– a column 0.25 m long and 4.6 mm in internal diameter packed with *octadecylsilyl silica gel for chromatography R* (5 µm),
– as mobile phase at a flow rate of 1.0 ml/min a mixture of 88 volumes of mobile phase A and 12 volumes of mobile phase B:

Mobile phase A. Mix 576 ml of *water R*, 200 ml of a 31.2 g/l solution of *sodium dihydrogen phosphate R* and 24 ml of a 80 g/l solution of *tetrabutylammonium hydroxide R*. If necessary, adjust to pH 5.5 with *dilute phosphoric acid R* or *dilute sodium hydroxide solution R*; then add 200 ml of *acetonitrile R*,

Mobile phase B. Mix 126 ml of *water R*, 200 ml of a 31.2 g/l solution of *sodium dihydrogen phosphate R* and 24 ml of a 80 g/l solution of *tetrabutylammonium hydroxide R*. If necessary, adjust to pH 5.5 with *dilute phosphoric acid R* or *dilute sodium hydroxide solution R*; then add 650 ml of *acetonitrile R*,

– as detector a spectrophotometer set at 220 nm.

Inject 20 µl of reference solution (c). The test is not valid unless in the chromatogram obtained, the resolution between the peaks corresponding to ampicillin and to piperacillin is at least ten (if necessary, adjust the A:B ratio of the mobile phase) and the mass distribution ratio for the second peak (piperacillin) is 2.0 to 3.0. Inject 20 µl of reference solution (d). Adjust the sensitivity of the system to obtain a peak with a signal-to-noise ratio of at least 3. Inject reference solution (a) six times. The test is not valid unless the relative standard deviation of the peak area of piperacillin is at most 1.0 per cent. Inject alternately test solution (a) and reference solution (a).

Calculate the percentage content of piperacillin sodium multiplying the result by 1.042.

STORAGE

Store in an airtight container. If the substance is sterile, store in a sterile, airtight, tamper-proof container.

LABELLING

The label states, where applicable, that the substance is free from bacterial endotoxins.

IMPURITIES

Specified impurities: A, B, C, D, E, F, G.

Other detectable impurities: H.

A. ampicillin,

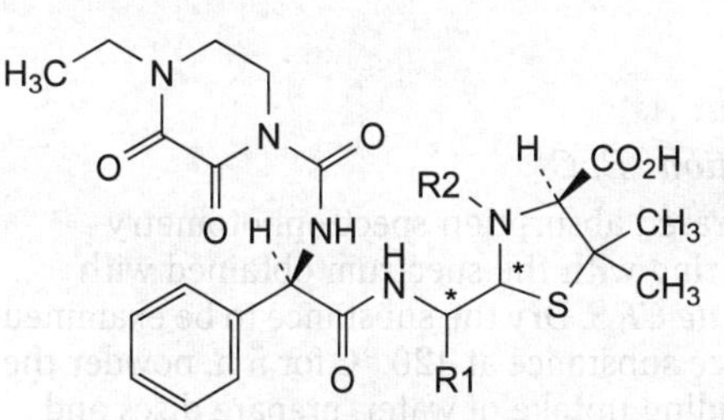

B. R1 = CO_2H, R2 = H: (4*S*)-2-[carboxy[[(2*R*)-2-[[(4-ethyl-2,3-dioxopiperazin-1-yl)carbonyl]amino]-2-phenylacetyl]amino]methyl]-5,5-dimethylthiazolidine-4-carboxylic acid (penicilloic acids of piperacillin),

C. R1 = R2 = H: (2*RS*,4*S*)-2-[[[(2*R*)-2-[[(4-ethyl-2,3-dioxopiperazin-1-yl)carbonyl]amino]-2-phenylacetyl]amino]methyl]-5,5-dimethylthiazolidine-4-carboxylic acid (penilloic acids of piperacillin),

F. R1 = CO_2H, R2 = $CO\text{-}CH_3$: (4*S*)-3-acetyl-2-[carboxy[[(2*R*)-2-[[(4-ethyl-2,3-dioxopiperazin-1-yl)carbonyl]amino]-2-phenylacetyl]amino]methyl]-5,5-dimethylthiazolidine-4-carboxylic acid (acetylated penicilloic acids of piperacillin).

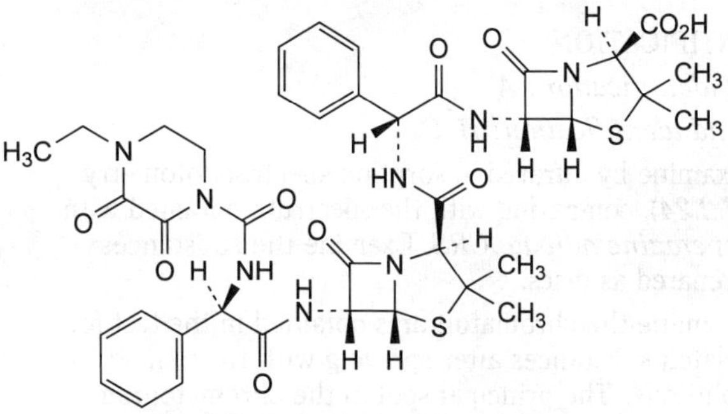

D. (2*S*,5*R*,6*R*)-6-[[(2*R*)-2-[[[(2*S*,5*R*,6*R*)-6-[[(2*R*)-2-[[(4-ethyl-2,3-dioxopiperazin-1-yl)carbonyl]amino]-2-phenylacetyl]amino]-3,3-dimethyl-7-oxo-4-thia-1-azabicyclo[3.2.0]hept-2-yl]carbonyl]amino]-2-phenylacetyl]amino]-3,3-dimethyl-7-oxo-4-thia-1-azabicyclo[3.2.0]heptane-2-carboxylic acid (piperacillinylampicillin),

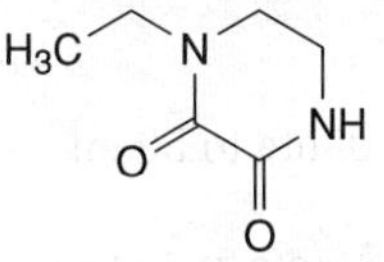

E. 1-ethylpiperazine-2,3-dione,

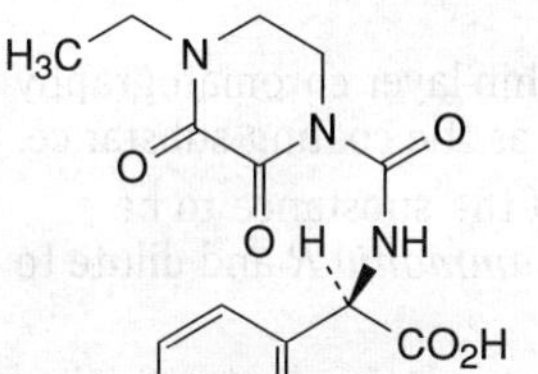

G. (2*R*)-2-[[(4-ethyl-2,3-dioxopiperazin-1-yl)carbonyl]amino]-2-phenylacetic acid,

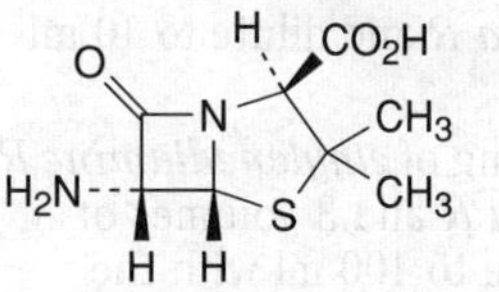

H. (2*S*,5*R*,6*R*)-6-amino-3,3-dimethyl-7-oxo-4-thia-1-azabicyclo[3.2.0]heptane-2-carboxylic acid (6-aminopenicillanic acid).

01/2005:0423

PIPERAZINE ADIPATE

Piperazini adipas

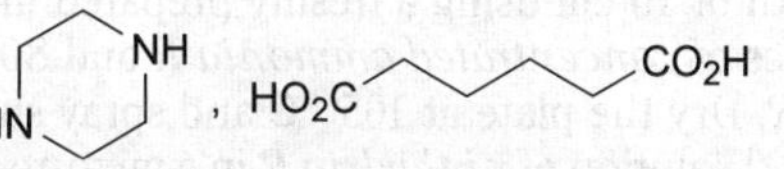

$C_{10}H_{20}N_2O_4$ M_r 232.3

DEFINITION

Piperazine adipate contains not less than 98.0 per cent and not more than the equivalent of 101.0 per cent of piperazine hexanedioate, calculated with reference to the anhydrous substance.

CHARACTERS

A white crystalline powder, soluble in water, practically insoluble in alcohol. It melts at about 250 °C, with decomposition.

IDENTIFICATION

First identification: A.

Second identification: B, C.

A. Examine by infrared absorption spectrophotometry (*2.2.24*), comparing with the spectrum obtained with *piperazine adipate CRS*. Examine the substances prepared as discs.

B. Examine the chromatograms obtained in the test for related substances after spraying with the ninhydrin solutions. The principal spot in the chromatogram obtained with test solution (b) is similar in position, colour and size to the principal spot in the chromatogram obtained with reference solution (a).

C. To 10 ml of solution S (see Tests) add 5 ml of *hydrochloric acid R* and shake with three quantities, each of 10 ml, of *ether R*. Evaporate the combined ether layers to dryness. The residue, washed with 5 ml of *water R* and dried at 100 °C to 105 °C, melts (*2.2.14*) at 150 °C to 154 °C.

TESTS

Solution S. Dissolve 2.5 g in *water R* and dilute to 50 ml with the same solvent.

Appearance of solution. Solution S is clear (*2.2.1*) and not more intensely coloured than reference solution B_8 (*2.2.2, Method II*).

Related substances. Examine by thin-layer chromatography (*2.2.27*), using a suitable silica gel as the coating substance.

Test solution (a). Dissolve 1.0 g of the substance to be examined in 6 ml of *concentrated ammonia R* and dilute to 10 ml with *ethanol R*.

Test solution (b). Dilute 1 ml of test solution (a) to 10 ml with a mixture of 2 volumes of *ethanol R* and 3 volumes of *concentrated ammonia R*.

Reference solution (a). Dissolve 0.1 g of *piperazine adipate CRS* in a mixture of 2 volumes of *ethanol R* and 3 volumes of *concentrated ammonia R* and dilute to 10 ml with the same mixture of solvents.

Reference solution (b). Dissolve 25 mg of *ethylenediamine R* in a mixture of 2 volumes of *ethanol R* and 3 volumes of *concentrated ammonia R* and dilute to 100 ml with the same mixture of solvents.

Reference solution (c). Dissolve 25 mg of *triethylenediamine R* in a mixture of 2 volumes of *ethanol R* and 3 volumes of *concentrated ammonia R* and dilute to 100 ml with the same mixture of solvents.

Reference solution (d). Dissolve 12.5 mg of *triethylenediamine R* in 5.0 ml of test solution (a) and dilute to 50 ml with a mixture of 2 volumes of *ethanol R* and 3 volumes of *concentrated ammonia R*.

Apply separately to the plate 5 µl of each solution. Develop over a path of 15 cm using a freshly prepared mixture of 20 volumes of *concentrated ammonia R* and 80 volumes of *acetone R*. Dry the plate at 105 °C and spray successively with a 3 g/l solution of *ninhydrin R* in a mixture of 3 volumes of *anhydrous acetic acid R* and 100 volumes of *butanol R* and a 1.5 g/l solution of *ninhydrin R* in *ethanol R*. Dry the plate at 105 °C for 10 min. Any spot in the chromatogram obtained with test solution (a), apart from the principal spot, is not more intense than the spot in the chromatogram obtained with reference solution (b) (0.25 per cent). Spray the plate with *0.05 M iodine* and allow to stand for about 10 min. Any spot corresponding to triethylenediamine in the chromatogram obtained with test solution (a) is not more intense than the spot in the chromatogram obtained with reference solution (c) (0.25 per cent). The test is not valid unless the chromatogram obtained with reference solution (d) shows two clearly separated spots. Disregard any spots remaining on the starting line.

Heavy metals (*2.4.8*). 12 ml of solution S complies with limit test A for heavy metals (20 ppm). Prepare the standard using *lead standard solution (1 ppm Pb) R*.

Water (*2.5.12*). Not more than 0.5 per cent, determined on 1.00 g by the semi-micro determination of water.

Sulphated ash (*2.4.14*). Not more than 0.1 per cent, determined on 1.0 g.

ASSAY

Dissolve 0.100 g in 10 ml of *anhydrous acetic acid R* with gentle heating and dilute to 70 ml with the same acid. Titrate with *0.1 M perchloric acid* using 0.25 ml of *naphtholbenzein solution R* as indicator until the colour changes from brownish-yellow to green.

1 ml of *0.1 M perchloric acid* is equivalent to 11.61 mg of $C_{10}H_{20}N_2O_4$.

01/2005:0424

PIPERAZINE CITRATE

Piperazini citras

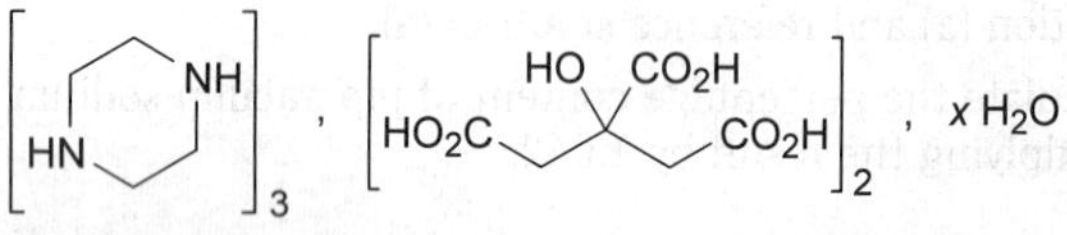

$C_{24}H_{46}N_6O_{14},xH_2O$ M_r 643 (anhydrous substance)

DEFINITION

Piperazine citrate contains not less than 98.0 per cent and not more than the equivalent of 101.0 per cent of tripiperazine bis(2-hydroxy-propane-1,2,3-tricarboxylate), calculated with reference to the anhydrous substance. It contains a variable quantity of water.

CHARACTERS

A white granular powder, freely soluble in water, practically insoluble in alcohol.

After drying at 100 °C to 105 °C, it melts at about 190 °C.

IDENTIFICATION

First identification: A.

Second identification: B, C.

A. Examine by infrared absorption spectrophotometry (*2.2.24*), comparing with the spectrum obtained with *piperazine citrate CRS*. Dry the substance to be examined and the reference substance at 120 °C for 5 h, powder the substances avoiding uptake of water, prepare discs and record the spectra without delay.

B. Examine the chromatograms obtained in the test for related substances after spraying with the ninhydrin solutions. The principal spot in the chromatogram obtained with test solution (b) is similar in position, colour and size to the principal spot in the chromatogram obtained with reference solution (a).

C. Dissolve 0.5 g in *water R* and dilute to 5 ml with the same solvent. The solution gives the reaction of citrates (*2.3.1*).

Monographs P

TESTS

Solution S. Dissolve 1.25 g in *water R* and dilute to 25 ml with the same solvent.

Appearance of solution. Solution S is clear (*2.2.1*) and not more intensely coloured than reference solution B_8 (*2.2.2, Method II*).

Related substances. Examine by thin-layer chromatography (*2.2.27*), using a suitable silica gel as the coating substance.

Test solution (a). Dissolve 1.0 g of the substance to be examined in 6 ml of *concentrated ammonia R* and dilute to 10 ml with *ethanol R*.

Test solution (b). Dilute 1 ml of test solution (a) to 10 ml with a mixture of 2 volumes of *ethanol R* and 3 volumes of *concentrated ammonia R*.

Reference solution (a). Dissolve 0.1 g of *piperazine citrate CRS* in a mixture of 2 volumes of *ethanol R* and 3 volumes of *concentrated ammonia R* and dilute to 10 ml with the same mixture of solvents.

Reference solution (b). Dissolve 25 mg of *ethylenediamine R* in a mixture of 2 volumes of *ethanol R* and 3 volumes of *concentrated ammonia R* and dilute to 100 ml with the same mixture of solvents.

Reference solution (c). Dissolve 25 mg of *triethylenediamine R* in a mixture of 2 volumes of *ethanol R* and 3 volumes of *concentrated ammonia R* and dilute to 100 ml with the same mixture of solvents.

Reference solution (d). Dissolve 12.5 mg of *triethylenediamine R* in 5.0 ml of test solution (a) and dilute to 50 ml with a mixture of 2 volumes of *ethanol R* and 3 volumes of *concentrated ammonia R*.

Apply separately to the plate 5 µl of each solution. Develop over a path of 15 cm using a freshly prepared mixture of 20 volumes of *concentrated ammonia R* and 80 volumes of *acetone R*. Dry the plate at 105 °C and spray successively with a 3 g/l solution of *ninhydrin R* in a mixture of 3 volumes of *anhydrous acetic acid R* and 100 volumes of *butanol R* and a 1.5 g/l solution of *ninhydrin R* in *ethanol R*. Dry the plate at 105 °C for 10 min. Any spot in the chromatogram obtained with test solution (a), apart from the principal spot, is not more intense than the spot in the chromatogram obtained with reference solution (b) (0.25 per cent). Spray the plate with *0.05 M iodine* and allow to stand for about 10 min. Any spot corresponding to triethylenediamine in the chromatogram obtained with test solution (a) is not more intense than the spot in the chromatogram obtained with reference solution (c) (0.25 per cent). The test is not valid unless the chromatogram obtained with reference solution (d) shows two clearly separated spots. Disregard any spots remaining on the starting line.

Heavy metals (*2.4.8*). 12 ml of solution S complies with limit test A for heavy metals (20 ppm). Prepare the standard using *lead standard solution (1 ppm Pb) R*.

Water (*2.5.12*). 10.0 per cent to 14.0 per cent, determined on 0.300 g by the semi-micro determination of water.

Sulphated ash (*2.4.14*). Not more than 0.1 per cent, determined on 1.0 g.

ASSAY

Dissolve 0.100 g in 10 ml of *anhydrous acetic acid R* with gentle heating and dilute to 70 ml with the same acid. Titrate with *0.1 M perchloric acid* using 0.25 ml of *naphtholbenzein solution R* as indicator until the colour changes from brownish-yellow to green.

1 ml of *0.1 M perchloric acid* is equivalent to 10.71 mg of $C_{24}H_{46}N_6O_{14}$.

01/2005:0425

PIPERAZINE HYDRATE

Piperazinum hydricum

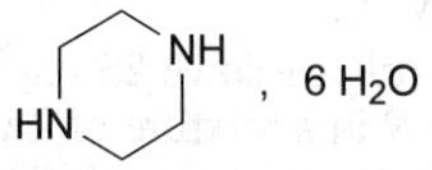

$C_4H_{10}N_2,6H_2O$ M_r 194.2

DEFINITION

Piperazine hydrate contains not less than 98.0 per cent and not more than the equivalent of 101.0 per cent of piperazine hexahydrate.

CHARACTERS

Colourless, deliquescent crystals, freely soluble in water and in alcohol.

It melts at about 43 °C.

IDENTIFICATION

First identification: A.

Second identification: B, C.

A. Examine by infrared absorption spectrophotometry (*2.2.24*), comparing with the spectrum obtained with *piperazine hydrate CRS*. Dry the substance to be examined and the reference substance over *diphosphorus pentoxide R in vacuo* for 48 h, powder the substances avoiding uptake of water, prepare discs and record the spectra without delay.

B. Examine the chromatograms obtained in the test for related substances after spraying with the ninhydrin solutions. The principal spot in the chromatogram obtained with test solution (b) is similar in position, colour and size to the principal spot in the chromatogram obtained with reference solution (a).

C. Dissolve 0.5 g in 5 ml of *dilute sodium hydroxide solution R*. Add 0.2 ml of *benzoyl chloride R* and mix. Continue to add *benzoyl chloride R* in portions of 0.2 ml until no further precipitate is formed. Filter and wash the precipitate with a total of 10 ml of *water R* added in small portions. Dissolve the precipitate in 2 ml of hot *alcohol R* and pour the solution into 5 ml of *water R*. Allow to stand for 4 h, filter, wash the crystals with *water R* and dry at 100 °C to 105 °C. The crystals melt (*2.2.14*) at 191 °C to 196 °C.

TESTS

Solution S. Dissolve 1.0 g in *carbon dioxide-free water R* and dilute to 20 ml with the same solvent.

Appearance of solution. Solution S is clear (*2.2.1*) and not more intensely coloured than reference solution B_8 (*2.2.2, Method II*).

pH (*2.2.3*). The pH of solution S is 10.5 to 12.0.

Related substances. Examine by thin-layer chromatography (*2.2.27*), using a suitable silica gel as the coating substance.

Test solution (a). Dissolve 1.0 g of the substance to be examined in 6 ml of *concentrated ammonia R* and dilute to 10 ml with *ethanol R*.

Test solution (b). Dilute 1 ml of test solution (a) to 10 ml with a mixture of 2 volumes of *ethanol R* and 3 volumes of *concentrated ammonia R*.

Reference solution (a). Dissolve 0.1 g of *piperazine hydrate CRS* in a mixture of 2 volumes of *ethanol R* and 3 volumes of *concentrated ammonia R* and dilute to 10 ml with the same mixture of solvents.

Reference solution (b). Dissolve 25 mg of *ethylenediamine R* in a mixture of 2 volumes of *ethanol R* and 3 volumes of *concentrated ammonia R* and dilute to 100 ml with the same mixture of solvents.

Reference solution (c). Dissolve 25 mg of *triethylenediamine R* in a mixture of 2 volumes of *ethanol R* and 3 volumes of *concentrated ammonia R* and dilute to 100 ml with the same mixture of solvents.

Reference solution (d). Dissolve 12.5 mg of *triethylenediamine R* in 5.0 ml of test solution (a) and dilute to 50 ml with a mixture of 2 volumes of *ethanol R* and 3 volumes of *concentrated ammonia R.*

Apply separately to the plate 5 µl of each solution. Develop over a path of 15 cm using a freshly prepared mixture of 20 volumes of *concentrated ammonia R* and 80 volumes of *acetone R*. Dry the plate at 105 °C and spray successively with a 3 g/l solution of *ninhydrin R* in a mixture of 3 volumes of *anhydrous acetic acid R* and 100 volumes of *butanol R* and a 1.5 g/l solution of *ninhydrin R* in *ethanol R*. Dry the plate at 105 °C for 10 min. Any spot in the chromatogram obtained with test solution (a), apart from the principal spot, is not more intense than the spot in the chromatogram obtained with reference solution (b) (0.25 per cent). Spray the plate with *0.05 M iodine* and allow to stand for about 10 min. Any spot corresponding to triethylenediamine in the chromatogram obtained with test solution (a) is not more intense than the spot in the chromatogram obtained with reference solution (c) (0.25 per cent). The test is not valid unless the chromatogram obtained with reference solution (d) shows two clearly separated spots.

Heavy metals (*2.4.8*). 12 ml of solution S complies with limit test A for heavy metals (20 ppm). Prepare the standard using *lead standard solution (1 ppm Pb) R*.

Sulphated ash (*2.4.14*). Not more than 0.1 per cent, determined on 1.0 g.

ASSAY

Dissolve 80.0 mg in 10 ml of *anhydrous acetic acid R* with gentle heating and dilute to 70 ml with the same acid. Titrate with *0.1 M perchloric acid* using 0.25 ml of *naphtholbenzein solution R* as indicator until the colour changes from brownish-yellow to green.

1 ml of *0.1 M perchloric acid* is equivalent to 9.705 mg of $C_4H_{10}N_2,6H_2O$.

STORAGE

Store in an airtight container, protected from light.

01/2005:1733

PIRACETAM

Piracetamum

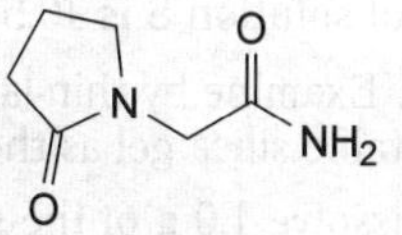

$C_6H_{10}N_2O_2$ M_r 142.2

DEFINITION

2-(2-Oxopyrrolidin-1-yl)acetamide.

Content: 98.0 per cent to 102.0 per cent (dried substance).

CHARACTERS

Appearance: white or almost white powder.

Solubility: freely soluble in water, soluble in alcohol.

It shows polymorphism.

IDENTIFICATION

Infrared absorption spectrophotometry (*2.2.24*).

Comparison: *piracetam CRS*.

If the spectra obtained in the solid state show differences, dissolve the substance to be examined and the reference substance separately in *alcohol R*, evaporate to dryness on a water-bath and record new spectra using the residues.

TESTS

Appearance of solution. The solution is clear (*2.2.1*) and colourless (*2.2.2, Method II*).

Dissolve 2.0 g in *water R* and dilute to 10 ml with the same solvent.

Related substances. Liquid chromatography (*2.2.29*).

Test solution. Dissolve 50.0 mg of the substance to be examined in a mixture of 10 volumes of *acetonitrile R* and 90 volumes of *water R* and dilute to 100.0 ml with the same mixture of solvents.

Reference solution (a). Dissolve 5 mg of the substance to be examined and 10 mg of *2-pyrrolidone R* in a mixture of 10 volumes of *acetonitrile R* and 90 volumes of *water R* and dilute to 100.0 ml with the same mixture of solvents.

Reference solution (b). Dilute 1.0 ml of the test solution to 100.0 ml with a mixture of 10 volumes of *acetonitrile R* and 90 volumes of *water R*. Dilute 5.0 ml to 50.0 ml with a mixture of 10 volumes of *acetonitrile R* and 90 volumes of *water R*.

Column:

– *size*: l = 0.25 m, Ø = 4.6 mm,
– *stationary phase*: *end-capped octadecylsilyl silica gel for chromatography R* (5 µm).

Mobile phase: mix 10 volumes of *acetonitrile R* and 90 volumes of a 1.0 g/l solution of *dipotassium hydrogen phosphate R*, adjust to pH 6.0 with *dilute phosphoric acid R.*

Flow rate: 1.0 ml/min.

Detection: spectrophotometer at 205 nm.

Injection: 20 µl.

Run time: 8 times the retention time of piracetam.

Retention time: piracetam = about 4 min.

System suitability: reference solution (a):

– *resolution*: minimum 3.0 between the peaks due to piracetam and impurity A.
– *symmetry factor*: maximum 2.0 for the peak due to piracetam.

Limits:

– *any impurity*: not more than the area of the principal peak in the chromatogram obtained with reference solution (b) (0.1 per cent),
– *total*: not more than 3 times the area of the principal peak in the chromatogram obtained with reference solution (b) (0.3 per cent),
– *disregard limit*: half the area of the principal peak in the chromatogram obtained with reference solution (b) (0.05 per cent).

Heavy metals (*2.4.8*): maximum 10 ppm.

Dissolve 2 g in 20 ml of *water R*. 12 ml of the solution complies with limit test A. Prepare the standard using *lead standard solution (1 ppm Pb) R*.

Loss on drying (*2.2.32*): maximum 1.0 per cent, determined on 1.000 g by drying in an oven at 100-105 °C.

Sulphated ash (*2.4.14*): maximum 0.1 per cent, determined on 1.0 g.

ASSAY

Dissolve 0.750 g in 50 ml of *carbon dioxide-free water R*. Add 20.0 ml of *1 M sodium hydroxide* and heat to boiling for 15 min. Allow to cool and add 25.0 ml of *1 M hydrochloric acid*. Heat to boiling for 2 min and allow to cool. Add 0.1 ml of *phenolphthalein solution R1*. Titrate with *1 M sodium hydroxide* until a pink colour is obtained.

1 ml of *1 M sodium hydroxide* is equivalent to 142.2 mg of $C_6H_{10}N_2O_2$.

STORAGE

Protected from light.

IMPURITIES

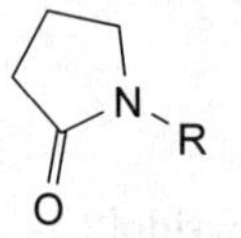

A. R = H: pyrrolidin-2-one (2-pyrrolidone),

B. R = CH_2-CO-O-CH_3: methyl (2-oxopyrrolidin-1-yl)acetate,

C. R = CH_2-CO-O-C_2H_5: ethyl (2-oxopyrrolidin-1-yl)acetate,

D. R = CH_2-CO_2H: (2-oxopyrrolidin-1-yl)acetic acid.

01/2005:2001

PIRENZEPINE DIHYDROCHLORIDE MONOHYDRATE

Pirenzepini dihydrochloridum monohydricum

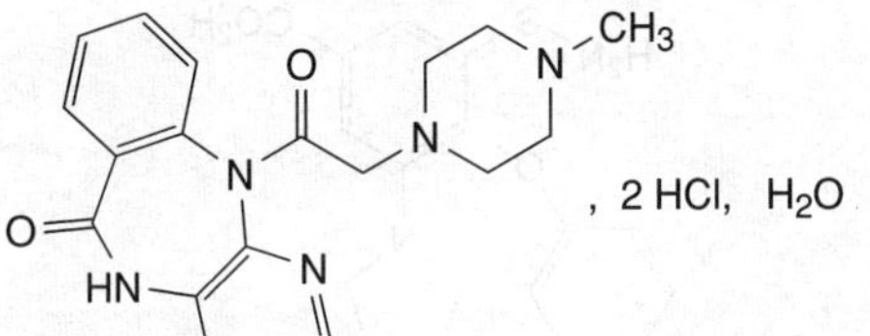

$C_{19}H_{23}Cl_2N_5O_2,H_2O$ M_r 442.3

DEFINITION

11-[(4-Methylpiperazin-1-yl)acetyl]-5,11-dihydro-6*H*-pyrido[2,3-*b*][1,4]benzodiazepin-6-one dihydrochloride monohydrate.

Content: 98.0 per cent to 102.0 per cent (anhydrous substance).

CHARACTERS

Appearance: white or yellowish, crystalline powder.

Solubility: freely soluble in water, slightly soluble in methanol, very slightly soluble in ethanol, practically insoluble in methylene chloride.

IDENTIFICATION

First identification: B, D.

Second identification: A, C, D.

A. Dissolve 30.0 mg in *methanol R* and dilute to 100.0 ml with the same solvent. Dilute 10.0 ml of the solution to 100.0 ml with *methanol R*. Examined between 240 nm and 360 nm (*2.2.25*), the solution shows an absorption maximum at 283 nm. The specific absorbance at the maximum is 190 to 205 (anhydrous substance).

B. Infrared absorption spectrophotometry (*2.2.24*).

Comparison: pirenzepine dihydrochloride monohydrate CRS.

C. Examine the chromatograms obtained in the test for impurity D.

Results: the principal band obtained in the chromatogram obtained with test solution (b) is similar in position, colour and size to the principal band in the chromatogram obtained with reference solution (d).

D. To 0.2 ml of solution S (see Tests) add 1.8 ml of *water R*. The solution gives reaction (a) of chlorides (*2.3.1*).

TESTS

Solution S. Dissolve 2.5 g in *carbon dioxide-free water R* and dilute to 25 ml with the same solvent.

Appearance of solution. Solution S is clear (*2.2.1*) and not more intensely coloured than reference solution GY_5 (*2.2.2, Method II*).

pH (*2.2.3*): 1.0 to 2.0 for solution S.

Impurity D. Thin-layer chromatography (*2.2.27*).

Test solution (a). To 0.10 g add 0.1 ml of *concentrated ammonia R* and dilute to 10 ml with *methanol R*.

Test solution (b). Dilute 1 ml of test solution (a) to 10 ml with *methanol R*.

Reference solution (a). To 0.1 g of *pirenzepine dihydrochloride monohydrate CRS* add 0.1 ml of *concentrated ammonia R* and dilute to 10 ml with *methanol R*.

Reference solution (b). Dissolve 25 mg of *methylpiperazine R* in *methanol R* and dilute to 25 ml with the same solvent. Dilute 2.0 ml of the solution to 100 ml with *methanol R*.

Reference solution (c). Dilute 5 ml of test solution (a) to 100 ml with *methanol R*. Dilute 4 ml of this solution to 100 ml with *methanol R*. Mix 1 ml with 1 ml of reference solution (b).

Reference solution (d). Dilute 1 ml of reference solution (a) to 10 ml with *methanol R*.

Plate: *TLC silica gel plate R.*

Mobile phase: *concentrated ammonia R, methanol R, ethyl acetate R, toluene R* (7:25:28:40 *V/V/V/V*).

Application: 20 µl as bands of 20 mm by 2 mm.

Development: over 2/3 of the plate.

Drying: in air.

Detection: expose the plate to iodine vapour until the band in the chromatogram obtained with reference solution (b) is clearly visible (at most 60 min).

System suitability: the test is not valid unless the chromatogram obtained with reference solution (c) shows 2 clearly separated bands.

Limit:

– *impurity D*: any band corresponding to impurity D in the chromatogram obtained with test solution (a) is not more intense than the band in the chromatogram obtained with reference solution (b) (0.2 per cent).

Related substances. Liquid chromatography (*2.2.29*).

Test solution. Dissolve 0.30 g of the substance to be examined in *water R* and dilute to 10.0 ml with the same solvent. To 1.0 ml of the solution add 5 ml of *methanol R* and dilute to 10.0 ml with mobile phase A.

Reference solution (a). Dilute 2.0 ml of the test solution to 100.0 ml with mobile phase A. Dilute 1.0 ml of this solution to 10.0 ml with mobile phase A.

Reference solution (b). Dissolve 0.1 g of *1-phenylpiperazine R* in *methanol R* and dilute to 10 ml with the same solvent. Mix 1 ml of the solution with 1 ml of the test solution, add 5 ml of *methanol R* and dilute to 10 ml with mobile phase A.

Column:

- *size*: *l* = 0.125 m, Ø = 4.6 mm,
- *stationary phase*: *octadecylsilyl silica gel for chromatography R* (5 µm).

Mobile phase:

- *mobile phase A*: dissolve 2.0 g of *sodium dodecyl sulphate R* in *water R*, adjust to pH 3.2 with *acetic acid R* and dilute to 1000 ml with *water R*,
- *mobile phase B*: *methanol R*,
- *mobile phase C*: *acetonitrile R*,

Time (min)	Mobile phase A (per cent *V/V*)	Mobile phase B (per cent *V/V*)	Mobile phase C (per cent *V/V*)
0 - 15	55 → 25	30	15 → 45
15 - 18	25 → 20	30→ 0	45 → 80
18 - 20	20 → 55	0 → 30	80 → 15
20 - 25	55	30	15

Flow rate: 1 ml/min.

Detection: spectrophotometer at 283 nm.

Injection: 10 µl.

System suitability: reference solution (b):

- *resolution*: minimum of 5.0 between the peaks corresponding to pirenzepine and to 1-phenylpiperazine.

Limits:

- *any impurity*: not more than the peak area of the principal peak in the chromatogram obtained with reference solution (a) (0.2 per cent),
- *total*: not more than 2.5 times the area of the principal peak in the chromatogram obtained with reference solution (a) (0.5 per cent),
- *disregard limit*: 0.2 times the area of the principal peak in the chromatogram obtained with reference solution (a) (0.04 per cent).

Water (*2.5.12*): 3.5 per cent to 5.0 per cent, determined on 0.250 g.

Sulphated ash (*2.4.14*): maximum 0.1 per cent, determined on 1.0 g.

ASSAY

Dissolve 0.300 g in 50 ml of *water R*. Carry out a potentiometric titration (*2.2.20*), using *0.1 M sodium hydroxide*. Read the volume at the first point of inflection.

1 ml of *0.1 M sodium hydroxide* is equivalent to 42.43 mg of $C_{19}H_{23}Cl_2N_5O_2$.

STORAGE

Protected from light.

Monographs P

IMPURITIES

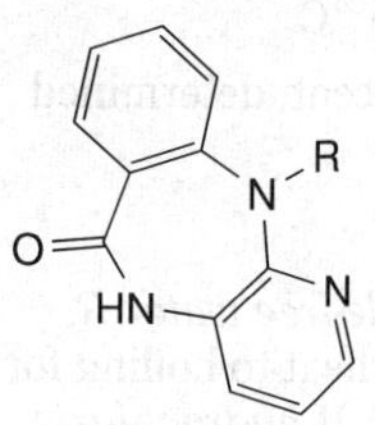

A. R = CO-CH_2-Cl: 11-(chloroacetyl)-5,11-dihydro-6*H*-pyrido[2,3-*b*][1,4]benzodiazepin-6-one,

B. R = H: 5,11-dihydro-6*H*-pyrido[2,3-*b*][1,4]benzodiazepin-6-one,

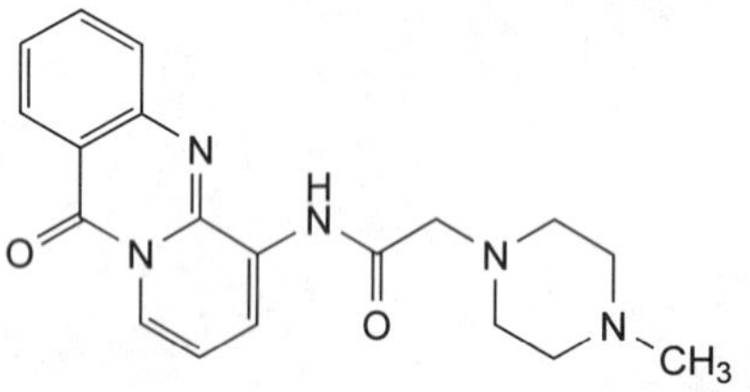

C. 6-[[(4-methylpiperazin-1-yl)acetyl]amino]-11*H*-pyrido[2,1-*b*]quinazolin-11-one,

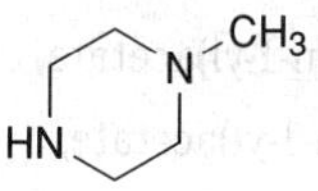

D. 1-methylpiperazine.

01/2005:1556

PIRETANIDE

Piretanidum

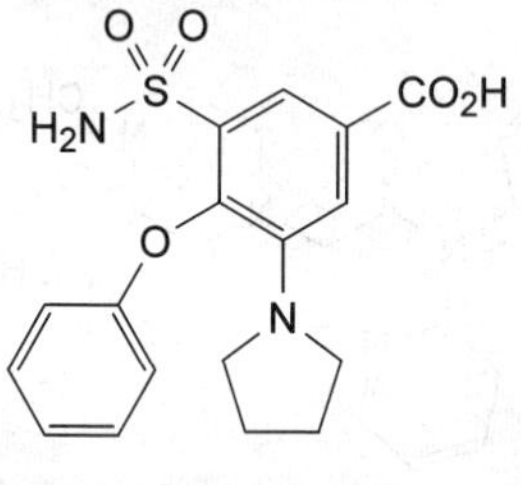

$C_{17}H_{18}N_2O_5S$ M_r 362.4

DEFINITION

Piretanide contains not less than 99.0 per cent and not more than the equivalent of 101.0 per cent of 4-phenoxy-3-(pyrrolidin-1-yl)-5-sulphamoylbenzoic acid, calculated with reference to the dried substance.

CHARACTERS

A yellowish-white to yellowish powder, very slightly soluble in water, sparingly soluble in ethanol.

It shows polymorphism.

IDENTIFICATION

Examine by infrared absorption spectrophotometry (*2.2.24*), comparing with the spectrum obtained with *piretanide CRS*. Examine the substances prepared as discs. If the spectra obtained show differences, dissolve the substance to be examined and the reference substance separately in *acetone R*, evaporate to dryness and record new spectra using the residues.

TESTS

Appearance of solution. Dissolve 0.1 g in *methanol R* and dilute to 10 ml with the same solvent. The solution is clear (*2.2.1*) and not more intensely coloured than reference solution GY_4 (*2.2.2, Method II*).

Related substances. Examine by liquid chromatography (*2.2.29*).

Test solution. Dissolve 20 mg of the substance to be examined in a mixture of 10 volumes of *ethanol R*, 45 volumes of *acetonitrile R* and 45 volumes of *water R* and dilute to 20.0 ml with the same mixture of solvents.

Reference solution (a). Dissolve 10 mg of *piretanide CRS* and 3 mg of *piretanide impurity A CRS* in a mixture of 10 volumes of *ethanol R*, 45 volumes of *acetonitrile R* and 45 volumes of *water R* and dilute to 10.0 ml with the same mixture of solvents.

Reference solution (b). Dilute 0.3 ml of the test solution to 100.0 ml with a mixture of 10 volumes of *ethanol R*, 45 volumes of *acetonitrile R* and 45 volumes of *water R*.

The chromatographic procedure may be carried out using:

– a stainless steel column 0.125 m long and 4 mm in internal diameter packed with *octylsilyl silica gel for chromatography R* (5 µm),
– as mobile phase at a flow rate of 1 ml/min a mixture of 35 volumes of *acetonitrile R* and 65 volumes of a solution prepared as follows: add 1 ml of *trifluoroacetic acid R* to 500 ml of *water R*, add 1 ml of *triethylamine R* and dilute to 1000 ml with *water R*,
– as detector a spectrophotometer set at 232 nm.

Inject 10 µl of reference solution (a). When the chromatograms are recorded in the conditions described the relative retention of impurity A is about 0.9. The test is not valid unless the resolution between the peaks corresponding to impurity A and piretanide is not less than 2.

Inject 10 µl of the test solution and 10 µl of reference solution (b). Continue the chromatography of the test solution for 5 times the retention time of the principal peak. In the chromatogram obtained with the test solution: the area of any peak, apart from the principal peak, is not greater than the area of the principal peak in the chromatogram obtained with reference solution (b) (0.3 per cent); the sum of the areas of all the peaks, apart from the principal peak, is not greater than 3.33 times the area of the principal peak in the chromatogram obtained with reference solution (b) (1.0 per cent). Disregard any peak with an area less than 0.1 times the area of the principal peak in the chromatogram obtained with reference solution (b).

Heavy metals (*2.4.8*). 2.0 g complies with limit test C for heavy metals (10 ppm). Prepare the standard using 2 ml of *lead standard solution (10 ppm Pb) R*.

Loss on drying (*2.2.32*). Not more than 0.5 per cent, determined on 1.000 g by drying in an oven at 100 °C to 105 °C for 4 h.

Sulphated ash (*2.4.14*). Not more than 0.1 per cent, determined on 1.0 g.

ASSAY

Dissolve 0.300 g in 25 ml of *anhydrous acetic acid R*. Titrate with *0.1 M perchloric acid* determining the end-point potentiometrically (*2.2.20*).

1 ml of *0.1 M perchloric acid* is equivalent to 36.24 mg of $C_{17}H_{18}N_2O_5S$.

STORAGE

Store protected from light.

IMPURITIES

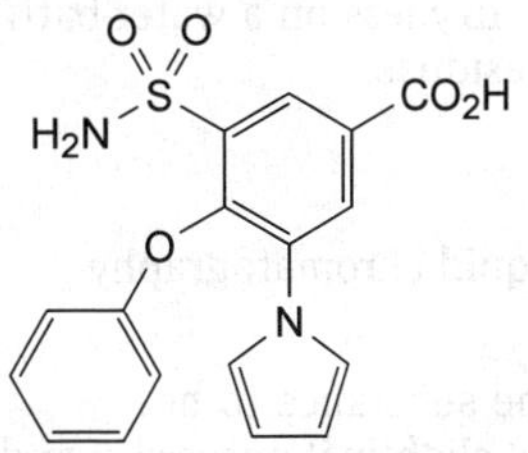

A. 4-phenoxy-3-(1*H*-pyrrol-1-yl)-5-sulphamoylbenzoic acid,

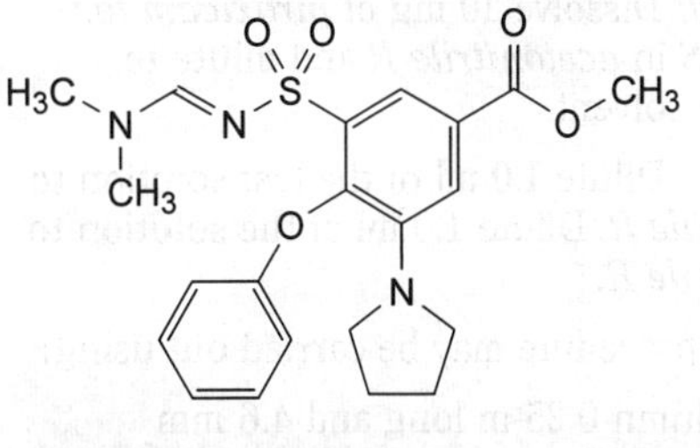

B. methyl-3-[[(dimethylamino)methylene]sulphamoyl]-4-phenoxy-5-(pyrrolidin-1-yl)benzoate,

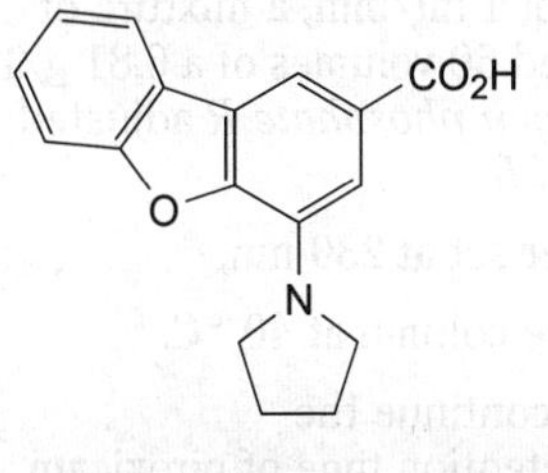

C. 4-(pyrrolidin-1-yl)dibenzo[*b,d*]furan-2-carboxylic acid.

01/2005:0944
corrected

PIROXICAM

Piroxicamum

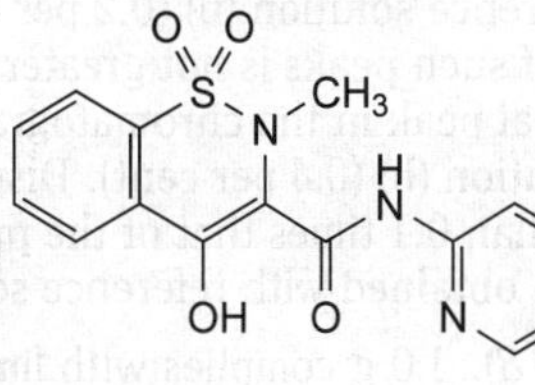

$C_{15}H_{13}N_3O_4S$ M_r 331.4

DEFINITION

Piroxicam contains not less than 98.5 per cent and not more than the equivalent of 101.0 per cent of 4-hydroxy-2-methyl-*N*-(pyridin-2-yl)-2*H*-1,2-benzothiazine-3-carboxamide 1,1-dioxide, calculated with reference to the dried substance.

CHARACTERS

A white or slightly yellow, crystalline powder, practically insoluble in water, soluble in methylene chloride, slightly soluble in ethanol.

It shows polymorphism.

IDENTIFICATION

Examine by infrared absorption spectrophotometry (*2.2.24*), comparing with the spectrum obtained with *piroxicam CRS*. Examine the substances as discs prepared using *potassium bromide R*. If the spectra obtained in the solid state show differences, dissolve the substance to be examined and the reference substance separately in the minimum volume of *methylene chloride R*, evaporate to dryness on a water-bath and record new spectra using the residues.

TESTS

Related substances. Examine by liquid chromatography (*2.2.29*).

Test solution. Dissolve 75 mg of the substance to be examined in *acetonitrile R* warming slightly if necessary and dilute to 50.0 ml with the same solvent.

Reference solution (a). Dissolve 10 mg of *piroxicam for system suitability CRS* in *acetonitrile R* and dilute to 50.0 ml with the same solvent.

Reference solution (b). Dilute 1.0 ml of the test solution to 10.0 ml with *acetonitrile R*. Dilute 1.0 ml of the solution to 50.0 ml with *acetonitrile R*.

The chromatographic procedure may be carried out using:

– a stainless steel column 0.25 m long and 4.6 mm in internal diameter packed with *base-deactivated octadecylsilyl silica gel for chromatography R* (5 µm),

– as mobile phase at a flow rate of 1 ml/min, a mixture of 40 volumes of *acetonitrile R* and 60 volumes of a 6.81 g/l solution of *potassium dihydrogen phosphate R* adjusted to pH 3.0 with *phosphoric acid R*,

– as detector a spectrophotometer set at 230 nm,

maintaining the temperature of the column at 40 °C.

Inject 20 µl of each solution and continue the chromatography for 5 times the retention time of piroxicam. The test is not valid unless the chromatogram obtained with reference solution (a) has a similar profile to the chromatogram supplied with *piroxicam for system suitability CRS* and shows a peak due to impurity B with a relative retention of about 0.85 and a symmetry factor of at most 1.5.

In the chromatogram obtained with the test solution: the area of any peak, apart from the principal peak, is not greater than the area of the principal peak in the chromatogram obtained with reference solution (b) (0.2 per cent) and the sum of the areas of such peaks is not greater than twice the area of the principal peak in the chromatogram obtained with reference solution (b) (0.4 per cent). Disregard any peak with an area less than 0.1 times that of the principal peak in the chromatogram obtained with reference solution (b).

Heavy metals (*2.4.8*). 1.0 g complies with limit test C (20 ppm). Prepare the standard using 2 ml of *lead standard solution (10 ppm Pb) R*.

Loss on drying (*2.2.32*). Not more than 0.5 per cent, determined on 1.000 g by drying *in vacuo* at 100-105 °C for 4 h.

Sulphated ash (*2.4.14*). Not more than 0.1 per cent, determined on 1.0 g.

ASSAY

Dissolve 0.250 g in 60 ml of a mixture of equal volumes of *acetic anhydride R* and *anhydrous acetic acid R*. Titrate with *0.1 M perchloric acid*, determining the end-point potentiometrically (*2.2.20*).

1 ml of *0.1 M perchloric acid* is equivalent to 33.14 mg of $C_{15}H_{13}N_3O_4S$.

STORAGE

In an airtight container, protected from light.

IMPURITIES

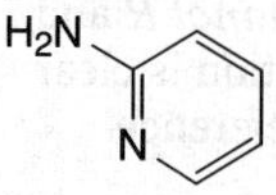

A. pyridin-2-amine,

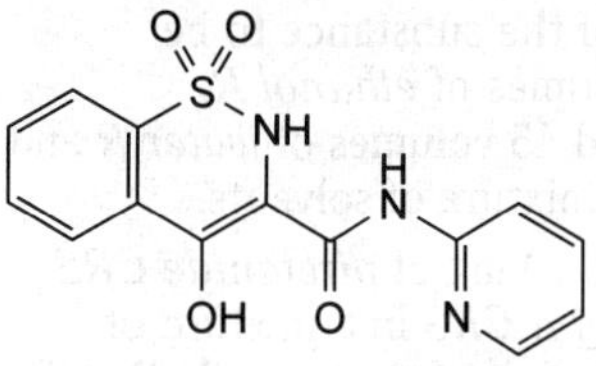

B. 4-hydroxy-*N*-(pyridin-2-yl)-2*H*-1,2-benzothiazine-3-carboxamide 1,1-dioxide,

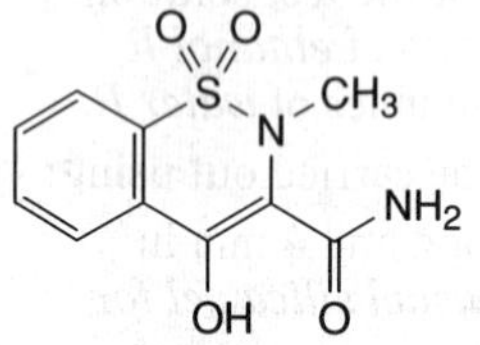

C. 4-hydroxy-2-methyl-2*H*-1,2-benzothiazine-3-carboxamide 1,1-dioxide,

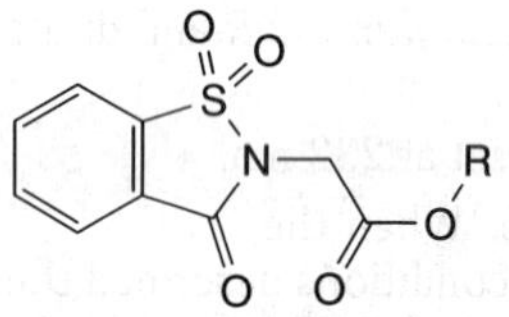

D. R = CH_3: methyl (1,1-dioxido-3-oxo-1,2-benzisothiazol-2(3*H*)-yl)acetate,

E. R = C_2H_5: ethyl (1,1-dioxido-3-oxo-1,2-benzisothiazol-2(3*H*)-yl)acetate,

F. R = $CH(CH_3)_2$: 1-methylethyl (1,1-dioxido-3-oxo-1,2-benzisothiazol-2(3*H*)-yl)acetate,

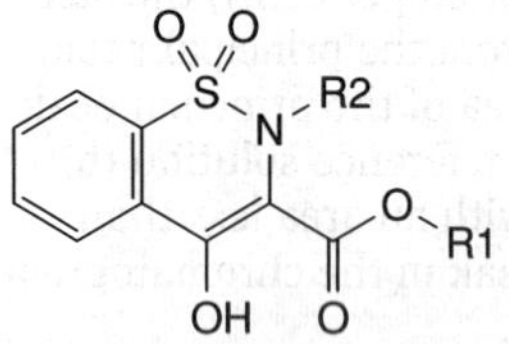

G. R1 = CH_3, R2 = H: methyl 4-hydroxy-2*H*-1,2-benzothiazine-3-carboxylate 1,1-dioxide,

H. R1 = C_2H_5, R2 = H: ethyl 4-hydroxy-2*H*-1,2-benzothiazine-3-carboxylate 1,1-dioxide,

I. R1 = $CH(CH_3)_2$, R2 = H: 1-methylethyl 4-hydroxy-2*H*-1,2-benzothiazine-3-carboxylate 1,1-dioxide,

J. R1 = R2 = CH_3: methyl 4-hydroxy-2-methyl-2*H*-1,2-benzothiazine-3-carboxylate 1,1-dioxide,

K. R1 = C_2H_5, R2 = CH_3: ethyl 4-hydroxy-2-methyl-2*H*-1,2-benzothiazine-3-carboxylate 1,1-dioxide,

L. R1 = $CH(CH_3)_2$, R2 = CH_3: 1-methylethyl 4-hydroxy-2-methyl-2*H*-1,2-benzothiazine-3-carboxylate 1,1-dioxide.

01/2005:0852

PIVAMPICILLIN

Pivampicillinum

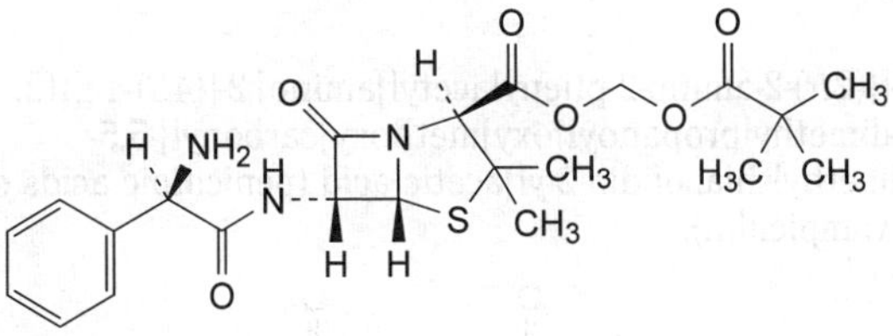

$C_{22}H_{29}N_3O_6S$ M_r 463.6

DEFINITION

Pivampicillin contains not less than 95.0 per cent and not more than the equivalent of 101.0 per cent of methylene (2*S*,5*R*,6*R*)-6-[[(2*R*)-2-amino-2-phenylacetyl]amino]-3,3-dimethyl-7-oxo-4-thia-1-azabicyclo[3.2.0]heptane-2-carboxylate 2,2-dimethylpropanoate, calculated with reference to the anhydrous substance.

CHARACTERS

A white or almost white, crystalline powder, practically insoluble in water, freely soluble in methanol, soluble in ethanol. It dissolves in dilute acids.

IDENTIFICATION

First identification: A.

Second identification: B, C.

A. Examine by infrared absorption spectrophotometry (*2.2.24*), comparing with the spectrum obtained with *pivampicillin CRS*.

B. Examine by thin-layer chromatography (*2.2.27*), using *silanised silica gel H R* as the coating substance.

Test solution. Dissolve 10 mg of the substance to be examined in 2 ml of *methanol R*.

Reference solution (a). Dissolve 10 mg of *pivampicillin CRS* in 2 ml of *methanol R*.

Reference solution (b). Dissolve 10 mg of *bacampicillin hydrochloride CRS*, 10 mg of *pivampicillin CRS* and 10 mg of *talampicillin hydrochloride CRS* in 2 ml of *methanol R*.

Apply to the plate 1 µl of each solution. Develop over a path of 15 cm using a mixture of 10 volumes of a 272 g/l solution of *sodium acetate R*, adjusted to pH 5.0 with *glacial acetic acid R*, 40 volumes of *water R* and 50 volumes of *alcohol R*. Dry the plate in a current of warm air, spray with *ninhydrin solution R1* and heat the plate at 60 °C for 10 min. The principal spot in the chromatogram obtained with the test solution is similar in position, colour and size to the principal spot in the chromatogram obtained with reference solution (a). The test is not valid unless the chromatogram obtained with reference solution (b) shows 3 clearly separated spots.

C. Place about 2 mg in a test-tube about 150 mm long and 15 mm in diameter. Moisten with 0.05 ml of *water R* and add 2 ml of *sulphuric acid-formaldehyde reagent R*. Mix the contents of the tube by swirling; the solution is almost colourless. Place the test-tube in a water-bath for 1 min; a dark yellow colour develops.

TESTS

Appearance of solution. Dissolve 50 mg in 12 ml of *0.1 M hydrochloric acid*. The solution is not more opalescent than reference suspension II (*2.2.1*) and not more intensely coloured than reference solution B_7 (*2.2.2, Method I*).

Specific optical rotation (*2.2.7*). Dissolve 0.100 g in 5.0 ml of *alcohol R* and dilute to 10.0 ml with *0.1 M hydrochloric acid*. The specific optical rotation is + 208 to + 222, calculated with reference to the anhydrous substance.

Related substances. Examine by liquid chromatography (*2.2.29*). *Prepare the solutions immediately before use.*

Test solution. Dissolve 50.0 mg of the substance to be examined in 10.0 ml of *acetonitrile R* and dilute to 20 ml with a 1 g/l solution of *phosphoric acid R*.

Reference solution. Mix 2.0 ml of the test solution with 9.0 ml of *acetonitrile R* and 9.0 ml of a 1 g/l solution of *phosphoric acid R*.

The chromatographic procedure may be carried out using:

– a column 0.125 m long and 4 mm in internal diameter packed with *end-capped octylsilyl silica gel for chromatography R*,

– as mobile phase at a flow rate of 1.5 ml/min:

Mobile phase A. A mixture of 50 volumes of a 1.32 g/l solution of *ammonium phosphate R*, adjusted to pH 2.5 with a 100 g/l solution of *phosphoric acid R*, and 50 volumes of *acetonitrile R*,

Mobile phase B. A mixture of 15 volumes of a 1.32 g/l solution of *ammonium phosphate R*, adjusted to pH 2.5 with a 100 g/l solution of *phosphoric acid R*, and 85 volumes of *acetonitrile R*,

Time (min)	Mobile phase A (per cent *V/V*)	Mobile phase B (per cent *V/V*)	Comment
0 - 10	100	0	isocratic
10 - 12	0	100	isocratic
12 - 17	100	0	re-equilibration

– as detector a spectrophotometer set at 220 nm.

Inject 50 µl of the test solution and 50 µl of the reference solution. The test is not valid unless the ratio of the mass distribution ratio of pivampicillin dimer (which has a retention time of about 5 min) to that of pivampicillin (principal peak) is at least 12. In the chromatogram obtained with the test solution, the sum of the areas of all the peaks, apart from the principal peak, is not greater than 0.3 times the area of the principal peak in the chromatogram obtained with the reference solution (3 per cent). Disregard any peak due to the solvent and any peak with an area less than 0.01 times the area of the principal peak in the chromatogram obtained with the reference solution.

***N,N*-Dimethylaniline** (*2.4.26, Method B*). Not more than 20 ppm.

Test solution. To 1.00 g of the substance to be examined in a ground-glass-stoppered tube add 10 ml of *0.5 M sulphuric acid*. Heat the tube for 10 min in a water-bath, cool and add 15 ml of *1 M sodium hydroxide* and 1.0 ml of the internal standard solution. Stopper the tube and shake vigorously for 1 min. Centrifuge if necessary and use the upper layer.

Triethanolamine. Examine by thin-layer chromatography (*2.2.27*), using *silica gel H R* as the coating substance.

Test solution. Dissolve 0.100 g of the substance to be examined in 1.0 ml of a mixture of 1 volume of *water R* and 9 volumes of *acetonitrile R*.

Reference solution. Dissolve 5.0 mg of *triethanolamine R* in a mixture of 1 volume of *water R* and 9 volumes of *acetonitrile R* and dilute to 100 ml with the same mixture of solvents.

Apply to the plate 10 µl of each solution. Develop over a path of 12 cm using a mixture of 5 volumes of *methanol R*, 15 volumes of *butanol R*, 24 volumes of *phosphate buffer solution pH 5.8 R*, 40 volumes of *glacial acetic acid R* and 80 volumes of *butyl acetate R*. Dry the plate at 110 °C for 10 min and allow to cool. Place in a chromatographic tank an evaporating dish containing a mixture of 1 volume of *hydrochloric acid R1*, 1 volume of *water R* and 2 volumes of a 15 g/l solution of *potassium permanganate R*. Close the tank and allow to stand for 15 min. Place the dried plate in the tank and close the tank. Leave the plate in contact with the chlorine vapour in the tank for 15-20 min. Remove the plate, allow it to stand in air for 2-3 min and spray with *tetramethyldiaminodiphenylmethane reagent R*. Any spot corresponding to triethanolamine in the chromatogram obtained with the test solution is not more intense than the spot in the chromatogram obtained with the reference solution (0.05 per cent).

Water (*2.5.12*). Not more than 1.0 per cent, determined on 0.30 g by the semi-micro determination of water.

Sulphated ash (*2.4.14*). Not more than 0.5 per cent, determined on 1.0 g.

ASSAY

Examine by liquid chromatography (*2.2.29*). *Use the solutions within 2 h of preparation.*

Test solution. Dissolve 50.0 mg of the substance to be examined in the mobile phase and dilute to 50.0 ml with the mobile phase. Dilute 10.0 ml of the solution to 50.0 ml with the mobile phase.

Reference solution (a). Dissolve 50.0 mg of *pivampicillin CRS* in the mobile phase and dilute to 50.0 ml with the mobile phase. Dilute 10.0 ml of the solution to 50.0 ml with the mobile phase.

Reference solution (b). Dissolve 25.0 mg of *propyl parahydroxybenzoate CRS* in the mobile phase and dilute to 50.0 ml with the mobile phase. Dilute 10.0 ml of the solution to 50.0 ml with the mobile phase. Mix 5.0 ml of this solution with 5.0 ml of reference solution (a).

The chromatographic procedure may be carried out using:

- a stainless steel column 0.125 m long and 4 mm in internal diameter packed with *octadecylsilyl silica gel for chromatography R* (5 µm),
- as mobile phase at a flow rate of 1.5 ml/min a mixture of 40 volumes of *acetonitrile R* and 60 volumes of a 2.22 g/l solution of *phosphoric acid R* adjusted to pH 2.5 with *triethylamine R*,
- as detector a spectrophotometer set at 220 nm.

Inject 20 µl of reference solution (b). Adjust the sensitivity of the system so that the height of each of the 2 principal peaks in the chromatogram obtained is at least 50 per cent of the full scale of the recorder. The test is not valid unless the resolution between the first peak (pivampicillin) and the second peak (propyl parahydroxybenzoate) is at least 5.0 and the symmetry factor for the pivampicillin peak is at most 2.0. Inject 20 µl of reference solution (a) 6 times. The test is not valid unless the relative standard deviation for the area of the principal peak is at most 1.0 per cent. Inject alternately the test solution and reference solution (a).

STORAGE

Store in an airtight container.

IMPURITIES

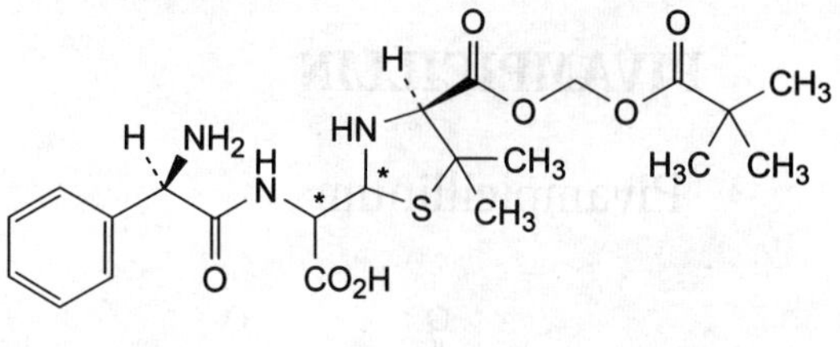

A. 2-[[(2*R*)-2-amino-2-phenylacetyl]amino]-2-[(4*S*)-4-[[[(2,2-dimethylpropanoyl)oxy]methoxy]carbonyl]-5,5-dimethylthiazolidin-2-yl]acetic acid (penicilloic acids of pivampicillin),

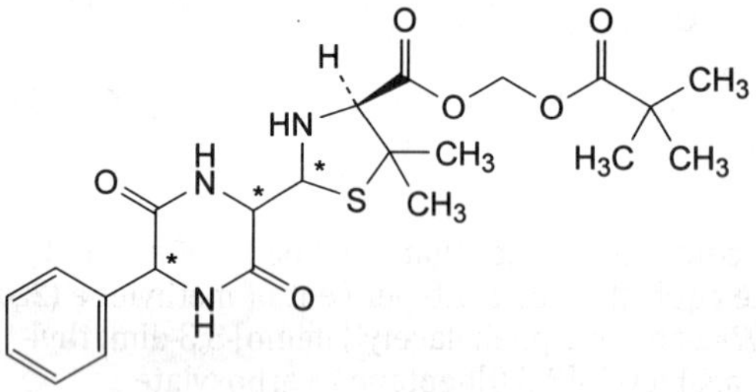

B. methylene (4*S*)-5,5-dimethyl-2-(3,6-dioxo-5-phenylpiperazin-2-yl)thiazolidine-4-carboxylate 2,2-dimethylpropanoate (diketopiperazines of pivampicillin),

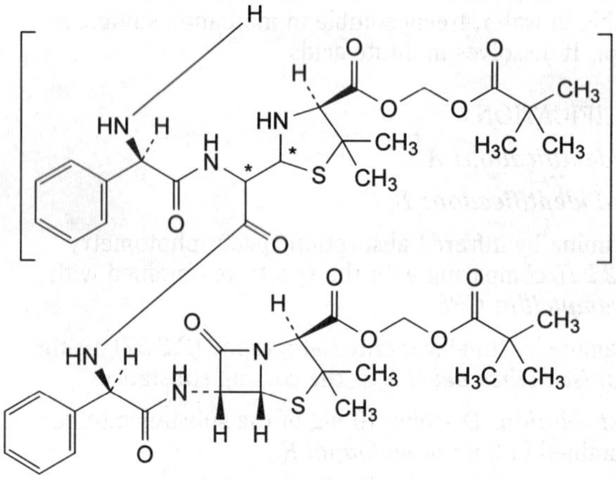

C. co-oligomers of pivampicillin and of penicilloic acids of pivampicillin.

01/2005:1359

PIVMECILLINAM HYDROCHLORIDE

Pivmecillinami hydrochloridum

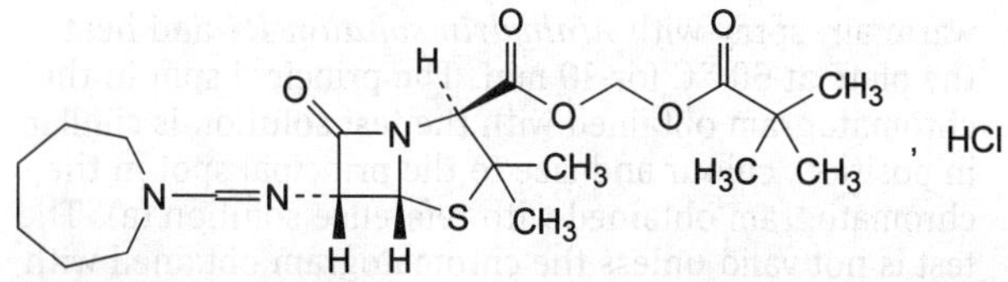

$C_{21}H_{34}ClN_3O_5S$ M_r 476.0

DEFINITION

Pivmecillinam hydrochloride contains not less than 97.0 per cent and not more than the equivalent of 101.5 per cent of methylene 2,2-dimethylpropanoate (2*S*,5*R*,6*R*)-6-[[(hexahydro-1*H*-azepin-1-yl)methylene]amino]-3,3-dimethyl-

7-oxo-4-thia-1-azabicyclo[3.2.0]heptane-2-carboxylate hydrochloride, calculated with reference to the anhydrous substance.

CHARACTERS

A white or almost white, crystalline powder, freely soluble in water, in ethanol and in methanol, slightly soluble in acetone.

IDENTIFICATION

A. Examine by infrared absorption spectrophotometry (*2.2.24*), comparing with the spectrum obtained with *pivmecillinam hydrochloride CRS*. Examine the substances prepared as discs.

B. It gives reaction (a) of chlorides (*2.3.1*).

TESTS

Appearance of solution. Dissolve 0.5 g in *water R* and dilute to 10 ml with the same solvent. The solution is not more opalescent than reference suspension II (*2.2.1*) and not more intensely coloured than reference solution B_8 (*2.2.2, Method I*).

pH (*2.2.3*). Dissolve 1.0 g in *carbon dioxide-free water R* and dilute to 10 ml with the same solvent. The pH of the solution is 2.8 to 3.8.

Related substances. Examine by liquid chromatography (*2.2.29*) as prescribed under Assay. Inject 20 µl of reference solution (b). Adjust the sensitivity of the system so that the height of the principal peak in the chromatogram obtained is at least 50 per cent of the full-scale of the recorder. Inject 20 µl of test solution (b) and continue the chromatography for 3 times the retention time of the principal peak. In the chromatogram obtained with test solution (b): the area of any peak, apart from the principal peak, is not greater than 1.5 times the area of the principal peak in the chromatogram obtained with reference solution (b) (1.5 per cent); the sum of the areas of all the peaks, apart from the principal peak, is not greater than 3 times the area of the principal peak in the chromatogram obtained with reference solution (b) (3 per cent). Disregard any peak with an area less than 0.1 times that of the principal peak in the chromatogram obtained with reference solution (b).

***N,N*-Dimethylaniline** (*2.4.26, Method A*): maximum 20 ppm.

Test solution. Prepare as described in the general method but heat at about 27 °C after the addition of *strong sodium hydroxide solution R*, to dissolve the precipitate formed, then add the *trimethylpentane R*.

Heavy metals (*2.4.8*). Dissolve 1.0 g in *water R* and dilute to 20 ml with the same solvent. 12 ml of the solution complies with limit test A for heavy metals (20 ppm). Prepare the standard using *lead standard solution (1 ppm Pb) R*.

Water (*2.5.12*). Not more than 0.5 per cent, determined on 1.00 g by the semi-micro determination of water.

Sulphated ash (*2.4.14*). Not more than 0.1 per cent, determined on 1.0 g.

ASSAY

Examine by liquid chromatography (*2.2.29*). *Prepare the test and reference solutions immediately before use.*

Solvent mixture. To 45 volumes of *acetonitrile R* add 55 volumes of a 13.5 g/l solution of *potassium dihydrogen phosphate R* previously adjusted to pH 3.0 with *dilute phosphoric acid R*.

Test solution (a). Dissolve 20.0 mg of the substance to be examined in the solvent mixture and dilute to 200.0 ml with the solvent mixture.

Test solution (b). Dissolve 25.0 mg of the substance to be examined in the solvent mixture and dilute to 25.0 ml with the solvent mixture.

Reference solution (a). Dissolve 20.0 mg of *pivmecillinam hydrochloride CRS* in the solvent mixture and dilute to 200.0 ml with the solvent mixture.

Reference solution (b). Dilute 5.0 ml of reference solution (a) to 50.0 ml with the solvent mixture.

Reference solution (c). Dissolve 5 mg of *pivmecillinam hydrochloride CRS* and 5 mg of *pivmecillinam impurity C CRS* in the solvent mixture and dilute to 50 ml with the solvent mixture.

The chromatographic procedure may be carried out using:

- a stainless steel column 0.25 m long and 4.0 mm in internal diameter packed with *octadecylsilyl silica gel for chromatography R* (5 µm),
- as mobile phase at a flow rate of 1.0 ml/min a mixture prepared as follows: dissolve 0.55 g of *tetraethylammonium hydrogen sulphate R* and 1.0 g of *tetramethylammonium hydrogen sulphate R* in the solvent mixture and dilute to 1000 ml with the solvent mixture,
- as detector a spectrophotometer set at 220 nm.

Inject 20 µl of reference solution (c). Adjust the sensitivity of the system so that the heights of the 2 principal peaks in the chromatogram obtained are at least 50 per cent of the full scale of the recorder. The test is not valid unless, in the chromatogram obtained, the resolution between the first peak (pivmecillinam) and the second peak (impurity C) is at least 3.5. Inject reference solution (a) 6 times. The test is not valid unless the relative standard deviation of the peak area for pivmecillinam is at most 1.0 per cent. Inject alternately test solution (a) and reference solution (a).

STORAGE

Store protected from light, at a temperature of 2 °C to 8 °C.

IMPURITIES

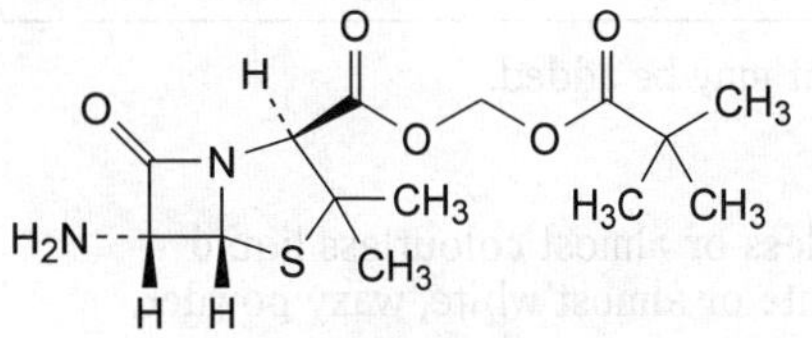

A. methylene (2*S*,5*R*,6*R*)-6-amino-3,3-dimethyl-7-oxo-4-thia-1-azabicyclo[3.2.0]heptane-2-carboxylate 2,2-dimethylpropanoate (pivaloyloxymethyl 6-aminopenicillanate),

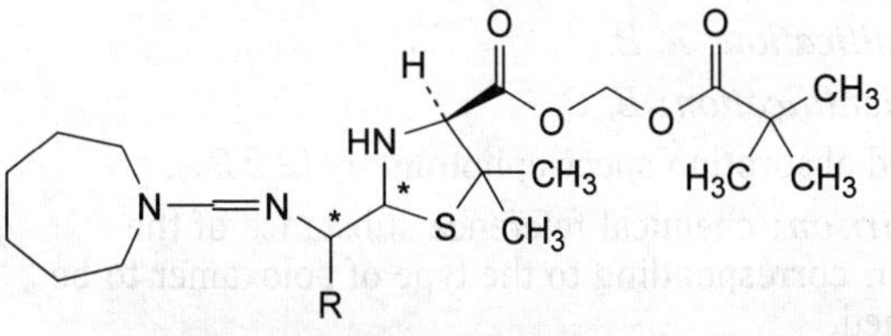

B. R = CO_2H: 2-[[(hexahydro-1*H*-azepin-1-yl)methylene]amino]-2-[(4*S*)-4-[[(2,2-dimethylpropanoyl)oxy]methoxy]carbonyl]-5,5-dimethylthiazolidin-2-yl]acetic acid (penicilloic acids of pivmecillinam),

C. R = H: methylene 2,2-dimethylpropanoate (2*RS*,4*S*)-2-[[[(hexahydro-1*H*-azepin-1-yl)methylene]amino]methyl]-5,5-dimethylthiazolidin-4-carboxylate,

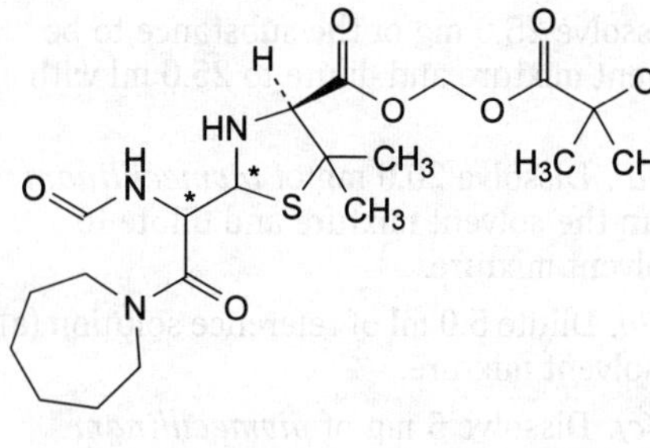

D. methylene 2,2-dimethylpropanoate (4*S*)-2-[1-(formylamino)-2-(hexahydro-1*H*-azepin-1-yl)-2-oxoethyl]-5,5-dimethylthiazolidin-4-carboxylate.

01/2005:1464

POLOXAMERS

Poloxamera

DEFINITION

Synthetic block copolymer of ethylene oxide and propylene oxide, represented by the following general formula:

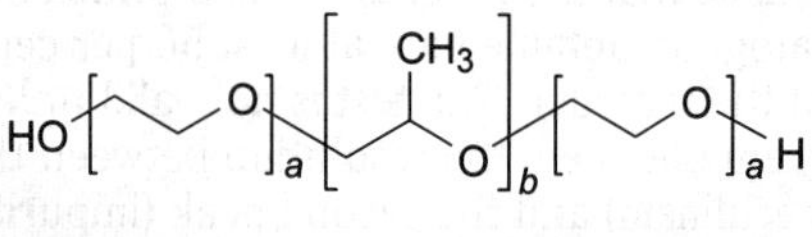

Poloxamer type	Ethylene oxide units (a)	Propylene oxide units (b)	Content of oxyethylene (per cent)	Average molecular mass
124	10 - 15	18 - 23	44.8 - 48.6	2090 - 2360
188	75 - 85	25 - 30	79.9 - 83.7	7680 - 9510
237	60 - 68	35 - 40	70.5 - 74.3	6840 - 8830
338	137 - 146	42 - 47	81.4 - 84.9	12 700 - 17 400
407	95 - 105	54 - 60	71.5 - 74.9	9840 - 14 600

A suitable antioxidant may be added.

CHARACTERS

Appearance: colourless or almost colourless liquid (poloxamer 124); white or almost white, waxy powder, microbeads or flakes.

Solubility: very soluble in water and in alcohol, practically insoluble in light petroleum (50-70 °C).

mp: about 50 °C for poloxamers 188, 237, 338 and 407.

IDENTIFICATION

First identification: A, B.

Second identification: B, C.

A. Infrared absorption spectrophotometry (*2.2.24*).

Comparison: chemical reference substance of the Ph. Eur. corresponding to the type of poloxamer to be examined.

B. It complies with the test for average molecular mass (see Tests).

C. It complies with the test for oxypropylene:oxyethylene ratio (see Tests).

TESTS

Solution S. Dissolve 10.0 g in *carbon dioxide-free water R* and dilute to 100 ml with the same solvent.

Appearance of solution. Solution S is not more intensely coloured than reference solution BY_7 (*2.2.2, Method II*).

pH (*2.2.3*): 5.0 to 7.5 for solution S.

Ethylene oxide, propylene oxide and dioxan. Head-space gas chromatography (*2.2.28*).

Ethylene oxide stock solution. Introduce 0.5 g of *ethylene oxide solution R5* in a vial and dilute to 50.0 ml with *dimethyl sulphoxide R1*. Mix carefully.

Ethylene oxide solution. Dilute 1.0 ml of ethylene oxide stock solution to 250 ml with *dimethyl sulphoxide R1*.

Propylene oxide stock solution. Introduce about 7 ml of *methylene chloride R* in a volumetric flask and add 0.500 g (*m*) of *propylene oxide R*. Dilute to 10.0 ml with *methylene chloride R*. Dilute 0.5 ml of this solution to 50.0 ml with *dimethyl sulphoxide R1*. Mix carefully. Calculate the exact concentration of propylene oxide in mg/ml using the following expression:

$$\frac{m \times 1000 \times 0.5}{10 \times 50}$$

Propylene oxide solution. Dilute 1.0 ml of propylene oxide stock solution to 50.0 ml with *dimethyl sulphoxide R1*.

Calculate the exact concentration of propylene oxide in µg/ml using the following expression:

$$\frac{C \times 1000 \times 1}{50}$$

C = concentration of the propylene oxide stock solution in mg/ml.

Dioxan solution. Introduce 0.100 g (*m*) of *dioxan R* in a flask and dilute to 50.0 ml with *dimethyl sulphoxide R1*. Dilute 2.50 ml of this solution to 100.0 ml with *dimethyl sulphoxide R1*.

Calculate the exact concentration of dioxan in µg/ml using the following expression:

$$\frac{m \times 2.50 \times 1000 \times 1000}{50 \times 100}$$

Mixture solution. Dilute a mixture of 6.0 ml of ethylene oxide solution, 6.0 ml of propylene oxide solution and 2.5 ml of dioxan solution to 25.0 ml with *dimethyl sulphoxide R1*.

Test solution. To 1.000 g of the substance to be examined in a head-space vial, add 4.0 ml of *dimethyl sulphoxide R1* and close the vial immediately.

Reference solution. To 1.000 g of the substance to be examined in a head-space vial, add 2.0 ml of *dimethyl sulphoxide R1* and 2.0 ml of the mixture solution. Close the vial immediately.

Column:

– *material*: fused silica,
– *size*: *l* = 50 m, Ø = 0.32 mm,
– *stationary phase*: *poly(dimethyl)(diphenyl)siloxane R* (film thickness 5 µm).

Carrier gas: *helium for chromatography R.*

Flow rate: 1.4 ml/min.

Static head-space conditions:

– *equilibrium temperature*: 110 °C,
– *equilibration time*: 30 min,
– *transfer-line temperature*: 140 °C,
– *pressurisation time*: 1 min,
– *injection time*: 0.05 min.

Temperature:

	Time (min)	Temperature (°C)
	0 - 10	70
Column	10 - 27	70 → 240
Injection port		250
Detector		250

Detection: flame ionisation.

Injection: inject a suitable volume of the gaseous phase, for example 1 ml.

Relative retention with reference to ethylene oxide (retention time = about 6 min): propylene oxide = about 1.3; methylene chloride = about 1.6; dioxan = about 3.0; dimethyl sulphoxide = about 3.7.

Limits:

– *ethylene oxide*: not more than half the area of the corresponding peak in the chromatogram obtained with the reference solution (1 ppm),
– *propylene oxide*: not more than half the area of the corresponding peak in the chromatogram obtained with the reference solution (5 ppm),
– *dioxan*: not more than half the area of the corresponding peak in the chromatogram obtained with the reference solution (10 ppm).

Average molecular mass. Weigh 15 g (*m*) of the substance to be examined into a 250 ml ground-glass-stoppered flask, add 25.0 ml of *phthalic anhydride solution R* and a few glass beads and swirl to dissolve. Boil gently under a reflux condenser for 1 h, allow to cool and add 2 quantities, each of 10 ml, of *pyridine R*, through the condenser. Add 10 ml of *water R*, mix and allow to stand for 10 min. Add 40.0 ml of *0.5 M sodium hydroxide* and 0.5 ml of a 10 g/l solution of *phenolphthalein R* in *pyridine R*. Titrate with *0.5 M sodium hydroxide* to a light pink endpoint that persists for 15 s and record the volume of sodium hydroxide used (*S*). Prepare a blank in the same manner but omitting the substance to be examined. Record the volume of sodium hydroxide used (*B*).

Calculate the average molecular mass using the expression:

$$\frac{4000m}{B - S}$$

Oxypropylene:oxyethylene ratio. Nuclear magnetic resonance spectrometry (*2.2.33*).

Use a 100 g/l solution of the substance to be examined in *deuterated chloroform R*. Record the average area of the doublet appearing at about 1.08 ppm due to the methyl groups of the oxypropylene units (A_1) and the average area of the composite band from 3.2 ppm to 3.8 ppm due to CH_2O groups of both the oxyethylene and oxypropylene units and the CHO groups of the oxypropylene units (A_2) with reference to the internal standard.

Calculate the percentage of oxyethylene, by weight, in the sample being examined using the following expression:

$$\frac{3300\alpha}{33\alpha + 58}$$

$$\text{where } \alpha = \frac{A_2}{A_1} - 1$$

Water (*2.5.12*): maximum 1.0 per cent, determined on 1.000 g.

Total ash (*2.4.16*): maximum 0.4 per cent, determined on 1.0 g.

STORAGE

In an airtight container.

LABELLING

The label states:

– the type of poloxamer,
– the name and concentration of any added antioxidant.

01/2005:0733

POLYACRYLATE DISPERSION 30 PER CENT

Polyacrylatis dispersio 30 per centum

DEFINITION

Polyacrylate dispersion 30 per cent is a dispersion in water of a copolymer of ethyl acrylate and methyl methacrylate having a mean relative molecular mass of about 800 000. It may contain a suitable emulsifier. The residue on evaporation is not less than 28.5 per cent *m/m* and not more than 31.5 per cent *m/m*.

CHARACTERS

An opaque, white, slightly viscous liquid, miscible with water, soluble in acetone, in ethanol and in 2-propanol.

IDENTIFICATION

First identification: A.

Second identification: B, C, D, E.

A. Examine by infrared absorption spectrophotometry (*2.2.24*), comparing with the *Ph. Eur. reference spectrum of polyacrylate*.

B. To 1 g add 5 ml of *water R* and mix; the mixture remains opaque. Take three 1 g portions and mix separately with 5 g each of *ethanol R*, *acetone R* and *2-propanol R*. Transparent solutions are obtained.

C. To 1 g add 10 ml of *0.1 M sodium hydroxide*. The mixture remains opaque.

D. It complies with the test for appearance of a film (see Tests).

E. Dry 4 g in a Petri dish at 60 °C in an oven for 4 h and transfer the resulting clear film to a small test-tube (100 mm × 12 mm). Heat over a flame and collect the fumes that evolve in a second test-tube held over the mouth of the first tube. The condensate gives the reaction of esters (*2.3.1*).

TESTS

Relative density (*2.2.5*): 1.037 to 1.047.

Apparent viscosity. Determine the viscosity (*2.2.10*) using a rotating viscometer at 20 °C. At a shear rate of 10 s^{-1}, the apparent viscosity is not more than 50 mPa·s.

Appearance of a film. Pour 1 ml on a glass plate and allow to dry. A clear elastic film is formed.

Particulate matter. Filter 100.0 g through a tared stainless steel sieve (90). Rinse with *water R* until a clear filtrate is obtained and dry at 80 °C to constant mass. The mass of the residue is not more than 0.500 g.

Residual monomers. Not more than 100 ppm, determined by liquid chromatography (*2.2.29*).

Test solution. Dissolve 1.00 g of the substance to be examined in *tetrahydrofuran R* and dilute to 50.0 ml with the same solvent. To 5.0 ml of a 35 g/l solution of *sodium perchlorate R* add 10.0 ml of the solution dropwise whilst stirring continuously. Centrifuge and filter the clear supernatant liquid. Dilute 5.0 ml to 10.0 ml with *water R*.

Reference solution. Dissolve 10 mg each of *ethyl acrylate R* and *methyl methacrylate R* in *tetrahydrofuran R* and dilute to 50.0 ml with the same solvent. Dilute 1.0 ml of this solution to 100.0 ml with *tetrahydrofuran R*. To 10.0 ml of the final solution add 5.0 ml of a 35 g/l solution of *sodium perchlorate R* and mix. Dilute 5.0 ml of the mixture to 10.0 ml with *water R*.

The chromatographic procedure may be carried out using:

- a column 0.12 m long and 4.6 mm in internal diameter packed with *octadecylsilyl silica gel for chromatography R* (5 µm to 10 µm),
- as mobile phase at a flow rate of 2 ml/min a mixture of 15 volumes of *acetonitrile R* and 85 volumes of *water R*,
- as detector a spectrophotometer set at 205 nm.

Inject separately equal volumes (about 50 µl) of each solution.

Calculate the percentage content of monomers from the area of the peaks in the chromatograms obtained with the test solution and the reference solution and from the content of monomers in the reference solution.

Heavy metals (*2.4.8*). 1.0 g complies with limit test C for heavy metals (20 ppm). Prepare the standard using 2 ml of *lead standard solution (10 ppm Pb) R*.

Sulphated ash (*2.4.14*). Not more than 0.4 per cent, determined on 1.0 g.

Microbial contamination. Total viable aerobic count (*2.6.12*) not more than 10^3 micro-organisms per gram, determined by plate count.

ASSAY

Dry 1.000 g at 110 °C for 3 h and weigh the mass of the residue.

STORAGE

Store at a temperature of 5 °C to 25 °C. Protect from freezing. Handle the substance so as to minimise microbial contamination.

LABELLING

The label states, where applicable, the name and concentration of any added emulsifier.

Monographs P

01/2005:0203
corrected

POLYMYXIN B SULPHATE

Polymyxini B sulfas

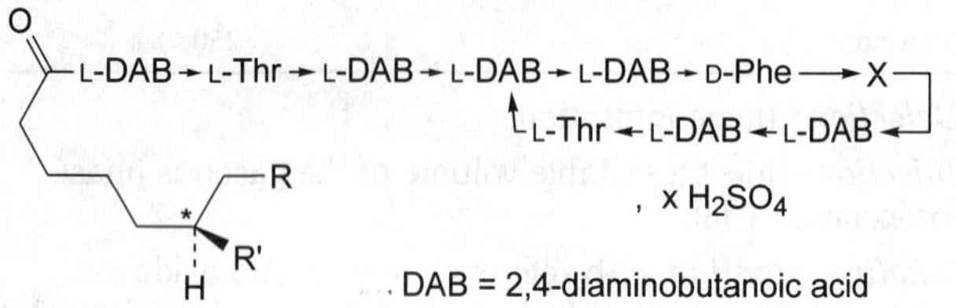

polymyxin	R	R′	X	Molecular formula	M_r
B1	CH_3	CH_3	L-Leu	$C_{56}H_{98}N_{16}O_{13}$	1204
B2	H	CH_3	L-Leu	$C_{55}H_{96}N_{16}O_{13}$	1190
B3	CH_3	H	L-Leu	$C_{55}H_{96}N_{16}O_{13}$	1190
B1-I	CH_3	CH_3	L-Ile	$C_{56}H_{98}N_{16}O_{13}$	1204

DEFINITION

Mixture of the sulphates of polypeptides produced by the growth of certain strains of *Paenibacillus polymyxa*, or obtained by any other means, the main component being polymyxin B1.

Content:

- sum of polymyxins B1, B2, B3 and B1-I: minimum 80.0 per cent (dried substance),
- polymyxin B3: maximum 6.0 per cent (dried substance),
- polymyxin B1-I: maximum 15.0 per cent (dried substance).

CHARACTERS

Appearance: white or almost white powder, hygroscopic.

Solubility: soluble in water, slightly soluble in alcohol.

IDENTIFICATION

First identification: B, D.

Second identification: A, C, D.

A. Thin-layer chromatography (*2.2.27*).

Test solution. Dissolve 5 mg of the substance to be examined in 1 ml of a mixture of equal volumes of *hydrochloric acid R* and *water R*. Heat at 135 °C in a sealed tube for 5 h. Evaporate to dryness on a water-bath and continue the heating until the hydrochloric acid has evaporated. Dissolve the residue in 0.5 ml of *water R*.

Reference solution (a). Dissolve 20 mg of *leucine R* in *water R* and dilute to 10 ml with the same solvent.

Reference solution (b). Dissolve 20 mg of *threonine R* in *water R* and dilute to 10 ml with the same solvent.

Reference solution (c). Dissolve 20 mg of *phenylalanine R* in *water R* and dilute to 10 ml with the same solvent.

Reference solution (d). Dissolve 20 mg of *serine R* in *water R* and dilute to 10 ml with the same solvent.

Plate: *TLC silica gel G plate R*.

Mobile phase: *water R, phenol R* (25:75 *V/V*).

Carry out the following procedures protected from light.

Application: 5 µl, as bands of 10 mm.

Place the plate in the chromatographic tank, so that it is not in contact with the mobile phase, and allow to become impregnated with the vapour of the solvent for at least 12 h.

Development: over a path of 12 cm using the same mobile phase.

Drying: at 100-105 °C.

Detection: spray with *ninhydrin solution R1* and heat at 110 °C for 5 min.

Results: the chromatogram obtained with the test solution shows bands corresponding to those in the chromatograms obtained with reference solutions (a), (b) and (c), but shows no band corresponding to that in the chromatogram obtained with reference solution (d). The chromatogram obtained with the test solution also shows a band with a very low R_f value (2,4-diaminobutyric acid).

B. Examine the chromatograms obtained in the assay.

Results: the peaks due to polymyxins B1, B2, B3 and B1-I in the chromatogram obtained with the test solution are similar in retention time to the corresponding peaks in the chromatogram obtained with reference solution (a).

C. Dissolve about 2 mg in 5 ml of *water R* and add 5 ml of a 100 g/l solution of *sodium hydroxide R*. Shake and add dropwise 0.25 ml of a 10 g/l solution of *copper sulphate R*, shaking after each addition. A reddish-violet colour develops.

D. It gives reaction (a) of sulphates (*2.3.1*).

TESTS

pH (*2.2.3*): 5.0 to 7.0.

Dissolve 0.2 g in *carbon dioxide-free water R* and dilute to 10 ml with the same solvent.

Specific optical rotation (*2.2.7*): − 78 to − 90 (dried substance).

Dissolve 0.50 g in *water R* and dilute to 25.0 ml with the same solvent.

Related substances. Liquid chromatography (*2.2.29*): use the normalisation procedure.

Test solution. Dissolve 50.0 mg of the substance to be examined in a mixture of 20 volumes of *acetonitrile R* and 80 volumes of *water R* and dilute to 100.0 ml with the same mixture of solvents.

Reference solution (a). Dissolve 50.0 mg of *polymyxin B sulphate CRS* in a mixture of 20 volumes of *acetonitrile R* and 80 volumes of *water R* and dilute to 100.0 ml with the same mixture of solvents.

Reference solution (b). Dilute 1.0 ml of reference solution (a) to 100.0 ml with a mixture of 20 volumes of *acetonitrile R* and 80 volumes of *water R*.

Column:

- *size*: l = 0.25 m, Ø = 4.6 mm,
- *stationary phase*: *base-deactivated end-capped octadecylsilyl silica gel for chromatography R* (5 µm),
- *temperature*: 30 °C.

Mobile phase: mix 20 volumes of *acetonitrile R* and 80 volumes of a solution prepared as follows: dissolve 4.46 g of *anhydrous sodium sulphate R* in 900 ml of *water R*, adjust to pH 2.3 using *dilute phosphoric acid R* and dilute to 1000 ml with *water R*.

Flow rate: 1.0 ml/min.

Detection: spectrophotometer at 215 nm.

Injection: 20 µl.

Run time: 1.4 times the retention time of polymyxin B1.

Relative retention with reference to polymyxin B1 (retention time = about 35 min): polymyxin B2 = about 0.5; polymyxin B3 = about 0.6; polymyxin B1-I = about 0.8.

System suitability: reference solution (a):

- *resolution*: minimum of 3.0 between the peaks due to polymyxin B2 and polymyxin B3.

Limits:

- *any impurity*: maximum 3.0 per cent,
- *total*: maximum 17.0 per cent,
- *disregard limit*: 0.7 times the area of the principal peak in the chromatogram obtained with reference solution (b).

Sulphate: 15.5 per cent to 17.5 per cent (dried substance).

Dissolve 0.250 g in 100 ml of *water R* and adjust the solution to pH 11 using *concentrated ammonia R*. Add 10.0 ml of *0.1 M barium chloride* and about 0.5 mg of *phthalein purple R*. Titrate with *0.1 M sodium edetate*, adding 50 ml of *alcohol R* when the colour of the solution begins to change and continuing the titration until the violet-blue colour disappears.

1 ml of *0.1 M barium chloride* is equivalent to 9.606 mg of SO_4.

Loss on drying (*2.2.32*): maximum 6.0 per cent, determined on 1.000 g by drying at 60 °C over *diphosphorus pentoxide R* at a pressure not exceeding 670 Pa for 3 h.

Sulphated ash (*2.4.14*): maximum 0.75 per cent, determined on 1.0 g.

Pyrogens (*2.6.8*). If intended for use in the manufacture of parenteral dosage forms without a further appropriate procedure for the removal of pyrogens, it complies with the test for pyrogens. Inject, per kilogram of the rabbit's mass, 1 ml of a solution in *water for injections R* containing 1.5 mg of the substance to be examined per millilitre.

ASSAY

Liquid chromatography (*2.2.29*) as described in the test for related substances with the following modification.

Injection: test solution and reference solution (a).

Calculate the percentage content of polymyxin B3 and B1-I, and the sum of polymyxins B1, B2, B3 and B1-I using the corresponding declared contents of *polymyxin sulphate CRS*.

STORAGE

In an airtight container, protected from light. If the substance is sterile, store in a sterile, airtight, tamper-proof container.

LABELLING

The label states, where applicable, that the substance is apyrogenic.

Monographs P

01/2005:0426
corrected

POLYSORBATE 20

Polysorbatum 20

DEFINITION

Mixture of partial esters of fatty acids, mainly lauric acid, with sorbitol and its anhydrides ethoxylated with approximately 20 moles of ethylene oxide for each mole of sorbitol and sorbitol anhydrides.

CHARACTERS

Appearance: oily, yellow to brownish-yellow, clear or slightly opalescent liquid.

Solubility: soluble in water, in ethanol, in ethyl acetate and in methanol, practically insoluble in fatty oils and in liquid paraffin.

Relative density: about 1.10.

Viscosity: about 400 mPa·s at 25 °C.

IDENTIFICATION

First identication: A, D.

Second identification: B, C, D, E.

A. Infrared absorption spectrophotometry (*2.2.24*).
Comparison: *Ph. Eur. reference spectrum of polysorbate 20.*

B. It complies with the test for hydroxyl value (see Tests).

C. It complies with the test for saponification value (see Tests).

D. It complies with the test for composition of fatty acids (see Tests).

E. Dissolve 0.1 g in 5 ml of *methylene chloride R*. Add 0.1 g of *potassium thiocyanate R* and 0.1 g of *cobalt nitrate R*. Stir with a glass rod. The solution becomes blue.

TESTS

Acid value (*2.5.1*): maximum 2.0.

Dissolve 5.0 g in 50 ml of the prescribed mixture of solvent.

Hydroxyl value (*2.5.3, Method A*): 96 to 108.

Peroxide value: maximum 10.0.

Introduce 10.0 g into a 100 ml beaker, dissolve with *glacial acetic acid R* and dilute to 20 ml with the same solvent. Add 1 ml of *saturated potassium iodide solution R* and allow to stand for 1 min. Add 50 ml of *carbon dioxide-free water R* and a magnetic stirring bar. Titrate with *0.01 M sodium thiosulphate*, determining the end-point potentiometrically (*2.2.20*). Carry out a blank titration.

Determine the peroxide value using the following expression:

$$\frac{(n_1 - n_2) \times M \times 1000}{m}$$

n_1 = volume of *0.01 M sodium thiosulphate* required for the substance to be examined, in millilitres,

n_2 = volume of *0.01 M sodium thiosulphate* required for the blank, in millilitres,

M = molarity of the sodium thiosulphate solution, in moles per litre,

m = mass of substance to be examined, in grams.

Saponification value (*2.5.6*): 40 to 50, determined on 4.0 g.

Use 15.0 ml of *0.5 M alcoholic potassium hydroxide* and dilute with 50 ml of *alcohol R* before carrying out the titration. Heat under reflux for 60 min.

Composition of fatty acids (*2.4.22, Method C*). Prepare reference solution (a) as indicated in Table 2.4.22.-2.

Column:
- *material*: fused silica,
- *dimensions*: l = 30 m, Ø = 0.32 mm,
- *stationary phase*: *macrogol 20 000 R* (film thickness 0.5 µm).

Carrier gas: *helium for chromatography R*.

Linear velocity: 50 cm/s.

Temperature:

	Time (min)	Temperature (°C)
Column	0 - 14	80 → 220
	14 - 54	220
Injection port		250
Detector		250

Detection: flame ionisation.

Injection: 1 µl.

Composition of the fatty acid fraction of the substance:
- *caproic acid*: maximum 1.0 per cent,
- *caprylic acid*: maximum 10.0 per cent,
- *capric acid*: maximum 10.0 per cent,
- *lauric acid*: 40.0 per cent to 60.0 per cent,
- *myristic acid*: 14.0 per cent to 25.0 per cent,
- *palmitic acid*: 7.0 per cent to 15.0 per cent,
- *stearic acid*: maximum 7.0 per cent,
- *oleic acid*: maximum 11.0 per cent,
- *linoleic acid*: maximum 3.0 per cent.

Ethylene oxide and dioxan (*2.4.25, Method A*): maximum 1 ppm of ethylene oxide and 10 ppm of dioxan.

Heavy metals (*2.4.8*): maximum 10 ppm.

2.0 g complies with limit test C. Prepare the standard using 2 ml of *lead standard solution (10 ppm Pb) R*.

Water (*2.5.12*): maximum 3.0 per cent, determined on 1.00 g.

Total ash (*2.4.16*): maximum 0.25 per cent, determined on 2.0 g.

STORAGE

In an airtight container, protected from light.

01/2005:1914

POLYSORBATE 40

Polysorbatum 40

DEFINITION

Mixture of partial esters of fatty acids, mainly *Palmitic acid (1904)*, with sorbitol and its anhydrides ethoxylated with approximately 20 moles of ethylene oxide for each mole of sorbitol and sorbitol anhydrides.

CHARACTERS

Appearance: oily, viscous, yellowish or brownish-yellow liquid.

Solubility: miscible with water, with ethanol, with ethyl acetate and with methanol, practically insoluble in fatty oils and in liquid paraffin.

Relative density: about 1.10.

Viscosity: about 400 mPa·s at 30 °C.

IDENTIFICATION

First identication: A, D.

Second identification: B, C, D, E.

A. Infrared absorption spectrophotometry (*2.2.24*).
Comparison: *Ph. Eur. reference spectrum of polysorbate 40.*

B. It complies with the test for hydroxyl value (see Tests).

C. It complies with the test for saponification value (see Tests).

Monographs P

D. It complies with the test for composition of fatty acids (see Tests).

E. Dissolve 0.1 g in 5 ml of *methylene chloride R*. Add 0.1 g of *potassium thiocyanate R* and 0.1 g of *cobalt nitrate R*. Stir with a glass rod. The solution becomes blue.

TESTS

Acid value (*2.5.1*): maximum 2.0.

Dissolve 5.0 g in 50 ml of the prescribed mixture of solvents.

Hydroxyl value (*2.5.3, Method A*): 89 to 105.

Peroxide value: maximum 10.0.

Introduce 10.0 g into a 100 ml beaker, dissolve with *glacial acetic acid R* and dilute to 20 ml with the same solvent. Add 1 ml of *saturated potassium iodide solution R* and allow to stand for 1 min. Add 50 ml of *carbon dioxide-free water R* and a magnetic stirring bar. Titrate with *0.01 M sodium thiosulphate*, determining the end-point potentiometrically (*2.2.20*). Carry out a blank titration.

Determine the peroxide value using the following expression:

$$\frac{(n_1 - n_2) \times M \times 1000}{m}$$

n_1 = volume of *0.01 M sodium thiosulphate* required for the substance to be examined, in millilitres,

n_2 = volume of *0.01 M sodium thiosulphate* required for the blank, in millilitres,

M = molarity of the sodium thiosulphate solution, in moles per litre,

m = mass of substance to be examined, in grams.

Saponification value (*2.5.6*): 41 to 52, determined on 4.0 g.

Use 15.0 ml of *0.5 M alcoholic potassium hydroxide* and dilute with 50 ml of *alcohol R* before carrying out the titration. Heat under reflux for 60 min.

Composition of fatty acids (*2.4.22, Method C*). Prepare reference solution (a) as indicated in Table 2.4.22.-1.

Column:

- *material*: fused silica,
- *size*: l = 30 m, Ø = 0.32 mm,
- *stationary phase*: *macrogol 20 000 R* (film thickness 0.5 µm).

Carrier gas: *helium for chromatography R*.

Linear velocity: 50 cm/s.

Temperature:

	Time (min)	Temperature (°C)
Column	0 - 14	80 → 220
	14 - 54	220
Injection port		250
Detector		250

Detection: flame ionisation.

Injection: 1 µl.

Composition of the fatty acid fraction of the substance:

- *palmitic acid*: minimum 92.0 per cent.

Ethylene oxide and dioxan (*2.4.25, Method A*): maximum 1 ppm of ethylene oxide and maximum 10 ppm of dioxan.

Heavy metals (*2.4.8*): maximum 10 ppm.

2.0 g complies with limit test C. Prepare the standard using 2 ml of *lead standard solution (10 ppm Pb) R*.

Water (*2.5.12*): maximum 3.0 per cent, determined on 1.00 g.

Total ash (*2.4.16*): maximum 0.25 per cent, determined on 2.0 g.

STORAGE

In an airtight container, protected from light.

01/2005:0427

POLYSORBATE 60

Polysorbatum 60

DEFINITION

Mixture of partial esters of fatty acids, mainly *Stearic acid 50 (1474)*, with sorbitol and its anhydrides ethoxylated with approximately 20 moles of ethylene oxide for each mole of sorbitol and sorbitol anhydrides.

CHARACTERS

Appearance: yellowish-brown gelatinous mass which becomes a clear liquid at temperatures above 25 °C.

Solubility: soluble in water, in ethanol, in ethyl acetate and in methanol, practically insoluble in fatty oils and in liquid paraffin.

Relative density: about 1.10.

Viscosity: about 400 mPa·s at 30 °C.

IDENTIFICATION

First identication: A, D.

Second identification: B, C, D, E.

A. Infrared absorption spectrophotometry (*2.2.24*).

Comparison: *Ph. Eur. reference spectrum of polysorbate 60.*

B. It complies with the test for hydroxyl value (see Tests).

C. It complies with the test for saponification value (see Tests).

D. It complies with the test for composition of fatty acids (see Tests).

E. Dissolve 0.1 g in 5 ml of *methylene chloride R*. Add 0.1 g of *potassium thiocyanate R* and 0.1 g of *cobalt nitrate R*. Stir with a glass rod. The solution becomes blue.

TESTS

Acid value (*2.5.1*): maximum 2.0.

Dissolve 5.0 g in 50 ml of the prescribed mixture of solvents.

Hydroxyl value (*2.5.3, Method A*): 81 to 96.

Peroxide value: maximum 10.0.

Introduce 10.0 g into a 100 ml beaker, dissolve with *glacial acetic acid R* and dilute to 20 ml with the same solvent. Add 1 ml of *saturated potassium iodide solution R* and allow to stand for 1 min. Add 50 ml of *carbon dioxide-free water R* and a magnetic stirring bar. Titrate with *0.01 M sodium thiosulphate*, determining the end-point potentiometrically (*2.2.20*). Carry out a blank titration.

Determine the peroxide value using the following expression:

$$\frac{(n_1 - n_2) \times M \times 1000}{m}$$

n_1 = volume of *0.01 M sodium thiosulphate* required for the substance to be examined, in millilitres,

n_2 = volume of *0.01 M sodium thiosulphate* required for the blank, in millilitres,

Monographs P

M = molarity of the sodium thiosulphate solution, in moles per litre,

m = mass of substance to be examined, in grams.

Saponification value (*2.5.6*): 45 to 55, determined on 4.0 g. Use 15.0 ml of *0.5 M alcoholic potassium hydroxide* and dilute with 50 ml of *alcohol R* before carrying out the titration. Heat under reflux for 60 min.

Composition of fatty acids (*2.4.22, Method C*). Prepare reference solution (a) as indicated in Table 2.4.22.-1.

Column:
- *material*: fused silica,
- *size*: l = 30 m, Ø = 0.32 mm,
- *stationary phase*: *macrogol 20 000 R* (film thickness 0.5 µm).

Carrier gas: *helium for chromatography R*.

Linear velocity: 50 cm/s.

Temperature:

	Time (min)	Temperature (°C)
Column	0 - 14	80 → 220
	14 - 54	220
Injection port		250
Detector		250

Detection: flame ionisation.

Injection: 1 µl.

Composition of the fatty acid fraction of the substance:
- *stearic acid*: 40.0 per cent to 60.0 per cent,
- *sum of the contents of palmitic and stearic acids*: minimum 90.0 per cent.

Ethylene oxide and dioxan (*2.4.25, Method A*): maximum 1 ppm of ethylene oxide and maximum 10 ppm of dioxan.

Heavy metals (*2.4.8*): maximum 10 ppm.

2.0 g complies with limit test C. Prepare the standard using 2 ml of *lead standard solution (10 ppm Pb) R*.

Water (*2.5.12*): maximum 3.0 per cent, determined on 1.00 g.

Total ash (*2.4.16*): maximum 0.25 per cent, determined on 2.0 g.

STORAGE

In an airtight container, protected from light.

01/2005:0428

POLYSORBATE 80

Polysorbatum 80

DEFINITION

Mixture of partial esters of fatty acids, mainly *Oleic acid (0799)*, with sorbitol and its anhydrides ethoxylated with approximately 20 moles of ethylene oxide for each mole of sorbitol and sorbitol anhydrides.

CHARACTERS

Appearance: oily, yellowish or brownish-yellow, clear liquid.

Solubility: miscible with water, with ethanol, with ethyl acetate and with methanol, practically insoluble in fatty oils and in liquid paraffin.

Relative density: about 1.10.

Viscosity: about 400 mPa·s at 25 °C.

IDENTIFICATION

First identication: *A, D.*

Second identification: *B, C, D, E.*

A. Infrared absorption spectrophotometry (*2.2.24*).
   Comparison: *Ph. Eur. reference spectrum of polysorbate 80.*

B. It complies with the test for hydroxyl value (see Tests).

C. It complies with the test for saponification value (see Tests).

D. It complies with the test for composition of fatty acids (see Tests).

E. Dissolve 0.1 g in 5 ml of *methylene chloride R*. Add 0.1 g of *potassium thiocyanate R* and 0.1 g of *cobalt nitrate R*. Stir with a glass rod. The solution becomes blue.

TESTS

Acid value (*2.5.1*): maximum 2.0.

Dissolve 5.0 g in 50 ml of the prescribed mixture of solvents.

Hydroxyl value (*2.5.3, Method A*): 65 to 80.

Peroxide value: maximum 10.0.

Introduce 10.0 g into a 100 ml beaker, dissolve with *glacial acetic acid R* and dilute to 20 ml with the same solvent. Add 1 ml of *saturated potassium iodide solution R* and allow to stand for 1 min. Add 50 ml of *carbon dioxide-free water R* and a magnetic stirring bar. Titrate with *0.01 M sodium thiosulphate*, determining the end-point potentiometrically (*2.2.20*). Carry out a blank titration.

Determine the peroxide value using the following expression:

$$\frac{(n_1 - n_2) \times M \times 1000}{m}$$

n_1 = volume of *0.01 M sodium thiosulphate* required for the substance to be examined, in millilitres,

n_2 = volume of *0.01 M sodium thiosulphate* required for the blank, in millilitres,

M = molarity of the sodium thiosulphate solution, in moles per litre,

m = mass of substance to be examined, in grams.

Saponification value (*2.5.6*): 45 to 55, determined on 4.0 g. Use 15.0 ml of *0.5 M alcoholic potassium hydroxide* and dilute with 50 ml of *alcohol R* before carrying out the titration. Heat under reflux for 60 min.

Composition of fatty acids (*2.4.22, Method C*). Prepare reference solution (a) as indicated in Table 2.4.22.-3.

Column:
- *material*: fused silica,
- *size*: l = 30 m, Ø = 0.32 mm,
- *stationary phase*: *macrogol 20 000 R* (film thickness 0.5 µm).

Carrier gas: *helium for chromatography R*.

Linear velocity: 50 cm/s.

Temperature:

	Time (min)	Temperature (°C)
Column	0 - 14	80 → 220
	14 - 54	220
Injection port		250
Detector		250

Detection: flame ionisation.

Injection: 1 µl.

Composition of the fatty acid fraction of the substance:
- *myristic acid*: maximum 5.0 per cent,
- *palmitic acid*: maximum 16.0 per cent,
- *palmitoleic acid*: maximum 8.0 per cent,
- *stearic acid*: maximum 6.0 per cent,
- *oleic acid*: 58.0 per cent to 85.0 per cent,
- *linoleic acid*: maximum 18.0 per cent,
- *linolenic acid*: maximum 4.0 per cent,

Ethylene oxide and dioxan (*2.4.25, Method A*): maximum 1 ppm of ethylene oxide and maximum 10 ppm of dioxan.

Heavy metals (*2.4.8*): maximum 10 ppm.

2.0 g complies with limit test C. Prepare the standard using 2 ml of *lead standard solution (10 ppm Pb) R*.

Water (*2.5.12*): maximum 3.0 per cent, determined on 1.00 g.

Total ash (*2.4.16*): maximum 0.25 per cent, determined on 2.0 g.

STORAGE

In an airtight container, protected from light.

01/2005:1962

POLY(VINYL ACETATE)

Poly(vinylis acetas)

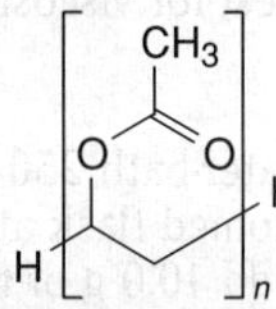

DEFINITION

Poly(vinyl acetate) is a thermoplastic polymer obtained by polymerisation of vinyl acetate using a suitable starter, without solvent or with water or 2-propanol. The vast majority of the acetate moieties are attached to non-neighbouring carbon atoms of the chain.

The index *n* is about 100 - 17 000. The relative molecular mass lies between 10 000 and 1500 000. The viscosity is 4 to 250 mPa·s. The ester value, which characterises the degree of hydrolysis, is 615 to 675.

CHARACTERS

Appearance: white powder or colourless granules or beads.

Solubility: practically insoluble in water, freely soluble in ethyl acetate, soluble in alcohol. It is hygroscopic and swells in water.

It softens at temperatures above 40-50 °C.

IDENTIFICATION

A. Infrared absorption spectrophotometry (*2.2.24*).

   Preparation: discs prepared as follows: dissolve about 200 mg in 5 ml of *acetone R*, place 2 drops on a *potassium bromide R* disc and dry to evaporate the solvent.

   The spectrum obtained shows absorption maxima corresponding to poly(vinyl acetate) at 1750 cm^{-1}, 1400 cm^{-1} and 1020 cm^{-1}.

B. It complies with the test for viscosity (see Tests).

C. Saponify 0.500 g in a mixture of 25.0 ml of *0.5 M alcoholic potassium hydroxide R* and 25.0 ml of *water R* (*2.5.6*). The solution obtained gives the reaction of acetates (*2.3.1*).

TESTS

Solution S. Suspend 50.0 g in 100 ml of *ethyl acetate R* in a borosilicate glass flask with a ground-glass neck. Heat under a reflux condenser with constant stirring for 30 min. Allow to cool. Filter through a tared sintered glass filter (No. 16) and wash the residue with 50.0 ml of *ethyl acetate R*, pour the filtrate into a 250 ml graduated flask. Dilute to 250 ml with *ethyl acetate R*.

Appearance of solution. Solution S is clear (*2.2.1*) and colourless (*2.2.2, Method I*).

Viscosity (*2.2.49*): 85 per cent to 115 per cent of the value stated on the label.

Determine the viscosity immediately after preparation of solution S at 20 ± 0.1 °C by using a rolling ball viscosimeter.

Acid value (*2.5.1*): maximum 2.0, determined on 5.0 g dissolved in 50 ml of *alcohol R* by shaking for 3 h.

Ester value (*2.5.2*): 615 to 675.

Saponify 0.500 g in a mixture of 25.0 ml of *0.5 M alcoholic potassium hydroxide* and 25.0 ml of *water R* (*2.5.6*).

Residual peroxides: maximum 100 ppm, calculated as hydrogen peroxide.

Place 0.85 g in a borosilicate glass flask with a ground-glass neck. Add 10 ml of *ethyl acetate R* and heat under a reflux condenser with constant agitation. Allow to cool. Replace the air in the container with *oxygen-free nitrogen R* and add a solution of 1 ml of *glacial acetic acid R* and 0.5 g of *sodium iodide R* in 40 ml of *water R*. Shake thoroughly and allow to stand protected from light for 20 min. Titrate with *0.005 M sodium thiosulphate R* until the yellow colour is discharged. Carry out a blank titration. The difference between the titration volumes is not greater than 1.0 ml.

Vinyl acetate. Head-space gas chromatography (*2.2.28*).

Reference solution. Place 15 ml of *dimethylformamide R* in a 20 ml vial, add 45 µl of *vinyl acetate R* and 50.0 µl of *butanal R* and dilute to volume with *dimethylformamide R*. Dilute 1 ml of the solution to 10 ml with *dimethylformamide R*.

Test solution (a). Place 0.2000 g of the substance to be examined in a 20 ml vial and add 1.00 ml of *dimethylformamide R*. Close the vial and secure the stopper. Shake, avoiding contact between the stopper and the liquid.

Test solution (b). Place 0.2000 g of the substance to be examined in a 20 ml vial and add 1.00 ml of the reference solution. Close the vial and secure the stopper. Shake, avoiding contact between the stopper and the liquid.

Column:
- *material*: fused silica,
- *size*: *l* = 25 m, Ø = 0.32 mm,
- *stationary phase*: *poly(dimethyl)(diphenyl)(divinyl)siloxane R* (film thickness: 0.32 µm),

Carrier gas: *nitrogen for chromatography R*.

Flow rate: 20 ml/min.

Static head-space conditions which may be used:
- *equilibration temperature*: 60 °C,
- *equilibration time*: 20 min,
- *transfer-line temperature*: 120 °C,
- *carrier gas*: *nitrogen for chromatography R*.

Temperature:
- *column*: 155 °C,
- *injection port*: 120 °C,
- *detector*: 180 °C.

Detection: flame ionisation.

Injection: 1.6 ml of the gaseous phase of test solutions (a) and (b).

System suitability: test solution (b):

– *resolution*: minimum of 2.0 between the peaks due to vinyl acetate and butanal,
– *signal-to-noise ratio*: minimum of 5 for the vinyl acetate peak.

Calculate the percentage of vinyl acetate from the expression:

$$\frac{V \times S_1 \times 0.931}{(m_1 S_2 - m_2 S_1) \times 2000}$$

S_1 = peak area or height for vinyl acetate in the chromatogram obtained with test solution (a),

S_2 = peak area or height for vinyl acetate in the chromatogram obtained with test solution (b),

m_1 = mass of the substance to be examined used to prepare test solution (a), in grams,

m_2 = mass of the substance to be examined used to prepare test solution (b), in grams,

0.931 = density of vinyl acetate, in grams per millilitre,

V = volume of vinyl acetate used to prepare the reference solution, in microlitres.

Limit:

– *vinyl acetate*: maximum 0.3 per cent.

Heavy metals (*2.4.8*): maximum 10 ppm.

1.0 g complies with limit test D. Prepare the standard using 1 ml of *lead standard solution (10 ppm Pb) R*.

Loss on drying (*2.2.32*): maximum 1.0 per cent, determined on 1.000 g by drying in an oven at 100-105 °C.

Sulphated ash (*2.4.14*): maximum 0.1 per cent, determined on 1.0 g.

The following test concerning the pharmacotechnological properties may be carried out depending on the intended formulation. It is not a mandatory requirement.

Infrared absorption spectrum (*2.2.24*). The determination of the spectrum and comparison with a suitable sample is useful for ensuring suitable functionality-related properties.

LABELLING

The label states:

– the nominal relative molecular mass,
– the viscosity.

Monographs P

01/2005:1961

POLY(VINYL ALCOHOL)

Poly(alcohol vinylicus)

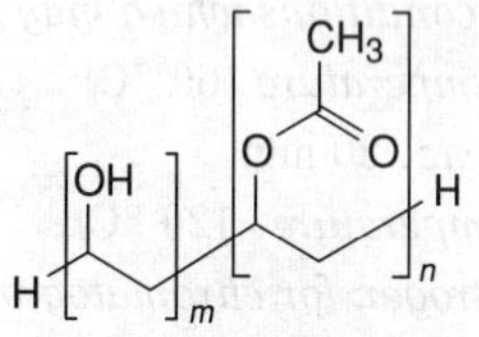

DEFINITION

Poly(vinyl alcohol) is obtained by polymerisation of vinyl acetate, followed by partial or almost complete hydrolysis of poly(vinyl acetate) in the presence of catalytic amounts of alkali or mineral acids.

Poly(vinyl alcohol) polymers comply with the following indices:

$$0 \leq \frac{n}{m} \leq 0.35$$

The mean relative molecular mass lies between 20 000 and 150 000. The viscosity is 3 to 70 mPa·s. The ester value which characterises the degree of hydrolysis is not greater than 280.

CHARACTERS

Appearance: yellowish-white powder or translucent granules.

Solubility: soluble in water, slightly soluble in ethanol, practically insoluble in acetone.

Various grades of poly(vinyl alcohol) are available. They differ in their degree of polymerisation and their degree of hydrolysis which determine the physical properties of the different grades. They are characterised by the viscosity and the ester value of the substance.

IDENTIFICATION

A. Infrared absorption spectrophotometry (*2.2.24*).

Preparation: discs; in some cases, the sample has to be milled, after cooling if necessary, before preparing the discs.

The spectrum obtained shows absorption maxima corresponding to poly(vinyl alcohol) at 2940 cm^{-1} and 2920 cm^{-1}.

B. It complies with the test for viscosity (see Tests).

TESTS

Solution S. Heat on a water-bath 250 ml of *water R* in a borosilicate round-bottomed flask attached to a reflux condenser with stirrer, add 10.0 g of the substance to be examined and continue heating for 30 min with continuous stirring. Remove the flask from the water-bath and continue stirring until room temperature is reached.

Appearance of solution. Solution S is clear (*2.2.1*) and not more intensely coloured than reference solution Y_7 (*2.2.2, Method II*).

pH (*2.2.3*): 4.5 to 6.5 for solution S.

Viscosity (*2.2.49*): 85 per cent to 115 per cent of the value stated on the label.

Determine the viscosity using a falling ball viscometer immediately after preparation of solution S at 20 ± 0.1 °C.

Acid value: maximum 3.0.

Add 1 ml of *phenolphthalein solution R* to 50 ml of solution S and titrate with *0.05 M potassium hydroxide* until the pink colour persists for 15 s. Calculate the acid value from the expression:

$$\frac{2.805V}{2}$$

V = number of millilitres of *0.05 M potassium hydroxide* used.

Ester value (*2.5.2*): 90 per cent to 110 per cent of the value stated on the label.

Saponify 1.00 g in a mixture of 25.0 ml of *0.5 M alcoholic potassium hydroxide* and 25.0 ml of *water R* (*2.5.6*).

Heavy metals (*2.4.8*): maximum 10 ppm.

1.0 g complies with limit test D. Prepare the standard using 1 ml of *lead standard solution (10 ppm Pb) R*.

Loss on drying (*2.2.32*): maximum 5.0 per cent, determined on 1.000 g by drying in an oven at 100-105 °C for 3 h.

Sulphated ash (*2.4.14*): maximum 1.0 per cent, determined on 1.0 g.

The following test concerning the pharmacotechnological properties may be carried out depending on the intended formulation. It is not a mandatory requirement.

Infrared absorption spectrum (*2.2.24*). The determination of the spectrum and comparison with a suitable sample is useful for ensuring suitable functionality-related properties. The intensities of the absorption maxima at 1720 cm^{-1} and 1260 cm^{-1} are inversely proportional to the degree of hydrolysis.

LABELLING

The label states:

– the viscosity for a 40 g/l solution,

– the ester value.

01/2005:1139
corrected

POTASSIUM ACETATE

Kalii acetas

$C_2H_3KO_2$ M_r 98.1

DEFINITION

Potassium acetate contains not less than 99.0 per cent and not more than the equivalent of 101.0 per cent of $C_2H_3KO_2$, calculated with reference to the dried substance.

CHARACTERS

A white, crystalline powder or colourless crystals, deliquescent, very soluble in water, freely soluble in alcohol.

IDENTIFICATION

A. It gives reaction (a) of acetates (*2.3.1*).

B. It gives reaction (a) of potassium (*2.3.1*).

TESTS

Solution S. Dissolve 10.0 g in *distilled water R* and dilute to 100 ml with the same solvent.

Appearance of solution. Solution S is clear (*2.2.1*) and colourless (*2.2.2, Method II*).

pH (*2.2.3*). Dissolve 1.0 g in *carbon dioxide-free water R* and dilute to 20 ml with the same solvent. The pH of the solution is 7.5 to 9.0.

Reducing substances. Dilute 10 ml of solution S to 100 ml with *water R*. Add 5 ml of *dilute sulphuric acid R* and 0.5 ml of a 0.32 g/l solution of *potassium permanganate R*. Mix and boil gently for 5 min. The solution remains pink.

Chlorides (*2.4.4*). Dilute 2.5 ml of solution S to 15 ml with *water R*. The solution complies with the limit test for chlorides (200 ppm).

Sulphates (*2.4.13*). Dilute 7.5 ml of solution S to 15 ml with *distilled water R*. The solution complies with the limit test for sulphates (200 ppm).

Aluminium (*2.4.17*). If intended for use in the manufacture of peritoneal dialysis solutions, haemofiltration solutions or haemodialysis solutions, it complies with the test for aluminium. Dissolve 2.0 g in 50 ml of *water R* and add 5 ml of *acetate buffer solution pH 6.0 R*. The solution complies with the limit test for aluminium (1 ppm). Use as a reference solution a mixture of 1 ml of *aluminium standard solution (2 ppm Al) R*, 5 ml of *acetate buffer solution pH 6.0 R* and 49 ml of *water R*. To prepare the blank use a mixture of 5 ml of *acetate buffer solution pH 6.0 R* and 50 ml of *water R*.

Iron (*2.4.9*). Dilute 5 ml of solution S to 10 ml with *water R*. The solution complies with the limit test for iron (20 ppm).

Heavy metals (*2.4.8*). Dissolve 5.0 g in *water R* and dilute to 20 ml with the same solvent. 12 ml of the solution complies with limit test A for heavy metals (4 ppm). Prepare the standard using *lead standard solution (1 ppm Pb) R*.

Sodium. Not more than 0.5 per cent of Na, determined by atomic emission spectrometry (*2.2.22, Method II*).

Test solution. Dissolve 1.00 g in *water R* and dilute to 100.0 ml with the same solvent.

Reference solutions. Prepare the reference solutions using *sodium standard solution (200 ppm Na) R*, diluted as necessary with *water R*.

Measure the emission intensity at 589 nm.

Loss on drying (*2.2.32*). Not more than 3.0 per cent, determined on 1.000 g by drying in an oven at 100 °C to 105 °C.

ASSAY

Dissolve 80.0 mg in 20 ml of *anhydrous acetic acid R*. Add 0.2 ml of *naphtholbenzein solution R*. Titrate with *0.1 M perchloric acid*. Carry out a blank titration.

1 ml of *0.1 M perchloric acid* is equivalent to 9.81 mg of $C_2H_3KO_2$.

STORAGE

Store in an airtight container.

01/2005:0184

POTASSIUM BROMIDE

Kalii bromidum

KBr M_r 119.0

DEFINITION

Content: 98.0 per cent to 100.5 per cent (dried substance).

CHARACTERS

Appearance: white, crystalline powder or colourless crystals.

Solubility: freely soluble in water and in glycerol, slightly soluble in alcohol.

IDENTIFICATION

A. It gives reaction (a) of bromides (*2.3.1*).

B. Solution S (see Tests) gives the reactions of potassium (*2.3.1*).

TESTS

Solution S. Dissolve 10.0 g in *carbon dioxide-free water R* prepared from *distilled water R* and dilute to 100 ml with the same solvent.

Appearance of solution. Solution S is clear (*2.2.1*) and colourless (*2.2.2, Method II*).

Acidity or alkalinity. To 10 ml of solution S add 0.1 ml of *bromothymol blue solution R1*. Not more than 0.5 ml of *0.01 M hydrochloric acid* or *0.01 M sodium hydroxide* is required to change the colour of the indicator.

Bromates. To 10 ml of solution S add 1 ml of *starch solution R*, 0.1 ml of a 100 g/l solution of *potassium iodide R* and 0.25 ml of *0.5 M sulphuric acid* and allow to stand protected from light for 5 min. No blue or violet colour develops.

Chlorides: maximum 0.6 per cent.

In a conical flask, dissolve 1.000 g in 20 ml of *dilute nitric acid R*. Add 5 ml of *strong hydrogen peroxide solution R* and heat on a water-bath until the solution is completely decolorised. Wash down the sides of the flask with a little *water R* and heat on a water-bath for 15 min. Allow to cool, dilute to 50 ml with *water R* and add 5.0 ml of *0.1 M silver nitrate* and 1 ml of *dibutyl phthalate R*. Shake and titrate with *0.1 M ammonium thiocyanate,* using 5 ml of *ferric ammonium sulphate solution R2* as indicator. Not more than 1.7 ml of *0.1 M silver nitrate* is used. Note the volume of *0.1 M silver nitrate* used (see Assay). Carry out a blank test.

Iodides. To 5 ml of solution S add 0.15 ml of *ferric chloride solution R1* and 2 ml of *methylene chloride R*. Shake and allow to separate. The lower layer is colourless (*2.2.2, Method I*).

Sulphates (*2.4.13*): maximum 100 ppm.

15 ml of solution S complies with the limit test for sulphates.

Iron (*2.4.9*): maximum 20 ppm.

5 ml of solution S diluted to 10 ml with *water R* complies with the limit test for iron.

Magnesium and alkaline-earth metals (*2.4.7*): maximum 200 ppm, calculated as Ca.

10.0 g complies with the limit test for magnesium and alkaline-earth metals. The volume of *0.01 M sodium edetate* used does not exceed 5.0 ml.

Heavy metals (*2.4.8*): maximum 10 ppm.

12 ml of solution S complies with limit test A. Prepare the standard using *lead standard solution (1 ppm Pb) R*.

Loss on drying (*2.2.32*): maximum 1.0 per cent, determined on 1.000 g by drying in an oven at 100-105 °C for 3 h.

ASSAY

Dissolve 2.000 g in *water R* and dilute to 100.0 ml with the same solvent. To 10.0 ml of the solution add 50 ml of *water R*, 5 ml of *dilute nitric acid R*, 25.0 ml of *0.1 M silver nitrate* and 2 ml of *dibutyl phthalate R*. Shake. Titrate with *0.1 M ammonium thiocyanate,* using 2 ml of *ferric ammonium sulphate solution R2* as indicator and shaking vigorously towards the end-point.

1 ml of *0.1 M silver nitrate* is equivalent to 11.90 mg of KBr.

Calculate the percentage content of KBr from the expression:

$$a - 3.357\,b$$

a = percentage content of KBr and KCl obtained in the assay and calculated as KBr,

b = percentage content of Cl in the test for chlorides.

01/2005:1557

POTASSIUM CARBONATE

Kalii carbonas

K_2CO_3 M_r 138.2

DEFINITION

Potassium carbonate contains not less than 99.0 per cent and not more than the equivalent of 101.0 per cent of K_2CO_3, calculated with reference to the dried substance.

CHARACTERS

A white granular powder, hygroscopic, freely soluble in water, practically insoluble in alcohol.

IDENTIFICATION

A. Dissolve 1 g in 10 ml of *water R*. The solution is strongly alkaline (*2.2.4*).

B. 2 ml of the solution prepared for identification test A gives the reaction of carbonates and bicarbonates (*2.3.1*).

C. 1 ml of the solution prepared for identification test A gives reaction (b) of potassium (*2.3.1*).

TESTS

Solution S. Dissolve 10.0 g in 25 ml of *distilled water R*. Slowly add 14 ml of *hydrochloric acid R*. When the effervescence has ceased, boil for a few minutes. Allow to cool and dilute to 50 ml with *distilled water R*.

Appearance of solution. Solution S is not more opalescent than reference suspension II (*2.2.1*) and not more intensely coloured than reference solution Y_6 (*2.2.2, Method II*).

Chlorides (*2.4.4*). Dissolve 0.50 g in 10 ml of *water R*. Carefully add dropwise 1 ml of *nitric acid R*. Boil. Cool, add 5 ml of *dilute nitric acid R* and dilute to 15 ml with *water R*. The solution complies with the limit test for chlorides (100 ppm).

Sulphates (*2.4.13*). Dilute 7.50 ml of solution S to 15 ml with *distilled water R*. The solution complies with the limit test for sulphates (100 ppm).

Calcium (*2.4.3*). To 5 ml of solution S, add 1 ml of *concentrated ammonia R*. Boil. Cool. Dilute to 15 ml with *distilled water R*. The solution complies with the limit test for calcium (100 ppm).

Iron (*2.4.9*). 5 ml of solution S diluted to 10 ml with *water R* complies with the limit test for iron (10 ppm).

Heavy metals (*2.4.8*). Dilute 10 ml of solution S to 20 ml with *water R*. 12 ml of the solution complies with limit test A for heavy metals (20 ppm). Prepare the standard using *lead standard solution (2 ppm Pb) R*.

Loss on drying (*2.2.32*). Not more than 5.0 per cent, determined on 0.300 g by drying in an oven at 120 °C to 125 °C for 5 h.

ASSAY

Dissolve 0.500 g in 50 ml of *carbon dioxide-free water R*. Carry out a potentiometric titration (*2.2.20*), using *1 M hydrochloric acid*. Read the volume added at the second point of inflexion.

1 ml of *1 M hydrochloric acid* is equivalent to 69.1 mg of K_2CO_3.

STORAGE

Store in an airtight container.

Monographs P

01/2005:0185

POTASSIUM CHLORIDE

Kalii chloridum

KCl M_r 74.6

DEFINITION

Potassium chloride contains not less than 99.0 per cent and not more than the equivalent of 100.5 per cent of KCl, calculated with reference to the dried substance.

CHARACTERS

A white, crystalline powder or colourless crystals, freely soluble in water, practically insoluble in ethanol.

IDENTIFICATION

A. It gives the reactions of chlorides (*2.3.1*).

B. Solution S (see Tests) gives the reactions of potassium (*2.3.1*).

TESTS

Solution S. Dissolve 10.0 g in *carbon dioxide-free water R* prepared from *distilled water R* and dilute to 100 ml with the same solvent.

Appearance of solution. Solution S is clear (*2.2.1*) and colourless (*2.2.2, Method II*).

Acidity or alkalinity. To 50 ml of solution S add 0.1 ml of *bromothymol blue solution R1*. Not more than 0.5 ml of *0.01 M hydrochloric acid* or *0.01 M sodium hydroxide* is required to change the colour of the indicator.

Bromides. Dilute 1.0 ml of solution S to 50 ml with *water R*. To 5.0 ml of the solution add 2.0 ml of *phenol red solution R2* and 1.0 ml of *chloramine solution R1* and mix immediately. After exactly 2 min add 0.15 ml of *0.1 M sodium thiosulphate*, mix and dilute to 10.0 ml with *water R*. The absorbance (*2.2.25*) of the solution measured at 590 nm, using *water R* as the compensation liquid, is not greater than that of a standard prepared at the same time and in the same manner using 5 ml of a 3.0 mg/l solution of *potassium bromide R* (0.1 per cent).

Iodides. Moisten 5 g by the dropwise addition of a freshly prepared mixture of 0.15 ml of *sodium nitrite solution R*, 2 ml of *0.5 M sulphuric acid*, 25 ml of *iodide-free starch solution R* and 25 ml of *water R*. After 5 min, examine in daylight. The substance shows no blue colour.

Sulphates (*2.4.13*). 5 ml of solution S diluted to 15 ml with *distilled water R* complies with the limit test for sulphates (300 ppm).

Barium. To 5 ml of solution S add 5 ml of *distilled water R* and 1 ml of *dilute sulphuric acid R*. After 15 min, any opalescence in the solution is not more intense than that in a mixture of 5 ml of solution S and 6 ml of *distilled water R*.

Heavy metals (*2.4.8*). 12 ml of solution S complies with limit test A for heavy metals (10 ppm). Prepare the standard using *lead standard solution (1 ppm Pb) R*.

Iron (*2.4.9*). 5 ml of solution S diluted to 10 ml with *water R* complies with the limit test for iron (20 ppm).

Magnesium and alkaline-earth metals (*2.4.7*). 10.0 g complies with the limit test for magnesium and alkaline-earth metals. The volume of *0.01 M sodium edetate* used does not exceed 5.0 ml (200 ppm, calculated as Ca).

Sodium. If intended for use in the manufacture of parenteral dosage forms or haemodialysis solutions, it complies with the test for sodium. Not more than 0.1 per cent of Na, determined by atomic emission spectrometry (*2.2.22*).

Test solution. Dissolve 1.00 g of the substance to be examined in *water R* and dilute to 100.0 ml with the same solvent.

Reference solutions. Dissolve in *water R* 0.5084 g of *sodium chloride R*, previously dried at 100 °C to 105 °C for 3 h, and dilute to 1000.0 ml with the same solvent (200 µg of Na per millilitre). Dilute as required.

Measure the emission intensity at 589 nm.

Aluminium (*2.4.17*). If intended for use in the manufacture of haemodialysis solutions, it complies with the test for aluminium. Dissolve 4 g in 100 ml of *water R* and add 10 ml of *acetate buffer solution pH 6.0 R*. The solution complies with the limit test for aluminium (1 ppm). Use as the reference solution a mixture of 2 ml of *aluminium standard solution (2 ppm Al) R*, 10 ml of *acetate buffer solution pH 6.0 R* and 98 ml of *water R*. To prepare the blank use a mixture of 10 ml of *acetate buffer solution pH 6.0 R* and 100 ml of *water R*.

Loss on drying (*2.2.32*). Not more than 1.0 per cent, determined on 1.000 g by drying in an oven at 100-105 °C for 3 h.

ASSAY

Dissolve 1.300 g in *water R* and dilute to 100.0 ml with the same solvent. To 10.0 ml of the solution add 50 ml of *water R*, 5 ml of *dilute nitric acid R*, 25.0 ml of *0.1 M silver nitrate* and 2 ml of *dibutyl phthalate R*. Shake. Titrate with *0.1 M ammonium thiocyanate*, using 2 ml of *ferric ammonium sulphate solution R2* as indicator and shaking vigorously towards the end-point.

1 ml of *0.1 M silver nitrate* is equivalent to 7.46 mg of KCl.

LABELLING

The label states:

– where applicable, that the substance is suitable for use in the manufacture of parenteral dosage forms,

– where applicable, that the substance is suitable for use in the manufacture of haemodialysis solutions.

01/2005:0400

POTASSIUM CITRATE

Kalii citras

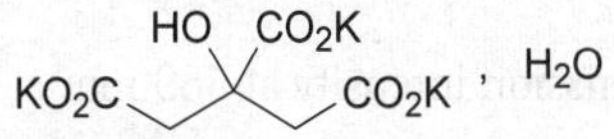

$C_6H_5K_3O_7,H_2O$ M_r 324.4

DEFINITION

Potassium citrate contains not less than 99.0 per cent and not more than the equivalent of 101.0 per cent of tripotassium 2-hydroxypropane-1,2,3-tricarboxylate, calculated with reference to the anhydrous substance.

CHARACTERS

A white, granular powder or transparent crystals, hygroscopic, very soluble in water, practically insoluble in alcohol.

IDENTIFICATION

A. To 1 ml of solution S (see Tests) add 4 ml of *water R*. The solution gives the reaction of citrates (*2.3.1*).

B. 0.5 ml of solution S gives reaction (b) of potassium (*2.3.1*).

TESTS

Solution S. Dissolve 10.0 g in *carbon dioxide-free water R* prepared from *distilled water R* and dilute to 100 ml with the same solvent.

Appearance of solution. Solution S is clear (*2.2.1*) and colourless (*2.2.2, Method II*).

Acidity or alkalinity. To 10 ml of solution S add 0.1 ml of *phenolphthalein solution R*. Not more than 0.2 ml of *0.1 M hydrochloric acid* or *0.1 M sodium hydroxide* is required to change the colour of the indicator.

Readily carbonisable substances. To 0.20 g of the powdered substance to be examined add 10 ml of *sulphuric acid R* and heat in a water-bath at 90 ± 1 °C for 60 min. Cool rapidly. The solution is not more intensely coloured than reference solution Y_2 or GY_2 (*2.2.2, Method II*).

Chlorides (*2.4.4*). Dilute 10 ml of solution S to 15 ml with *water R*. The solution complies with the limit test for chlorides (50 ppm).

Oxalates. Dissolve 0.50 g in 4 ml of *water R*, add 3 ml of *hydrochloric acid R* and 1 g of granulated *zinc R* and heat on a water-bath for 1 min. Allow to stand for 2 min, decant the liquid into a test-tube containing 0.25 ml of a 10 g/l solution of *phenylhydrazine hydrochloride R* and heat to boiling. Cool rapidly, transfer to a graduated cylinder and add an equal volume of *hydrochloric acid R* and 0.25 ml of *potassium ferricyanide solution R*. Shake and allow to stand for 30 min. Any pink colour in the solution is not more intense than that in a standard prepared at the same time and in the same manner using 4 ml of a 0.05 g/l solution of *oxalic acid R* (300 ppm).

Sulphates (*2.4.13*). To 10 ml of solution S add 2 ml of *hydrochloric acid R1* and dilute to 15 ml with *distilled water R*. The solution complies with the limit test for sulphates (150 ppm).

Heavy metals (*2.4.8*). 12 ml of solution S complies with limit test A for heavy metals (10 ppm). Prepare the standard using *lead standard solution (1 ppm Pb) R*.

Sodium. Not more than 0.3 per cent of Na, determined by atomic emission spectrometry (*2.2.22, Method II*).

Test solution. To 10 ml of solution S add 1 ml of *dilute hydrochloric acid R* and dilute to 100 ml with *distilled water R*.

Reference solutions. Dilute as necessary with *distilled water R* a solution of *sodium chloride R* containing 1 mg of Na per millilitre.

Measure the emission intensity at 589 nm.

Water (*2.5.12*): 4.0 per cent to 7.0 per cent, determined on 0.500 g by the semi-micro determination of water. After adding the substance to be examined, stir for 15 min before titrating.

ASSAY

Dissolve 0.150 g in 20 ml of *anhydrous acetic acid R*, heating to about 50 °C. Allow to cool. Titrate with *0.1 M perchloric acid* using 0.25 ml of *naphtholbenzein solution R* as indicator until a green colour is obtained.

1 ml of *0.1 M perchloric acid* is equivalent to 10.21 mg of $C_6H_5K_3O_7$.

STORAGE

Store in an airtight container.

01/2005:1140

POTASSIUM CLAVULANATE

Kalii clavulanas

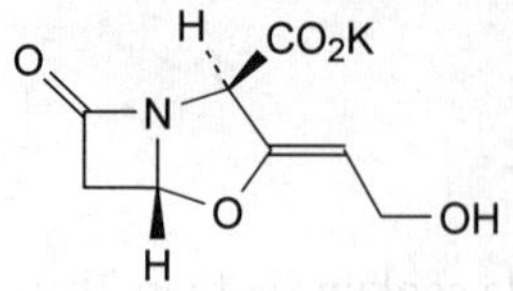

$C_8H_8KNO_5$ M_r 237.3

DEFINITION

Potassium (2*R*,3*Z*,5*R*)-3-(2-hydroxyethylidene)-7-oxo-4-oxa-1-azabicyclo[3.2.0]heptane-2-carboxylate, the potassium salt of a substance produced by the growth of certain strains of *Streptomyces clavuligerus* or obtained by any other means.

Content: 96.5 per cent to 102.0 per cent (anhydrous substance).

CHARACTERS

Appearance: white or almost white, crystalline powder, hygroscopic.

Solubility: freely soluble in water, slightly soluble in alcohol, very slightly soluble in acetone.

PRODUCTION

The method of production, extraction and purification are such that clavam-2-carboxylate is eliminated or present at a level not exceeding 0.01 per cent.

IDENTIFICATION

A. Infrared absorption spectrophotometry (*2.2.24*).

Comparison: *Ph. Eur. reference spectrum of potassium clavulanate*.

B. It gives reaction (b) of potassium (*2.3.1*).

TESTS

Solution S. Dissolve 0.400 g in *carbon dioxide-free water R* and dilute to 20.0 ml with the same solvent.

pH (*2.2.3*): 5.5 to 8.0.

Dilute 5 ml of solution S to 10 ml with *carbon dioxide-free water R*.

Specific optical rotation (*2.2.7*): + 53 to + 63 (anhydrous substance), determined on solution S.

Absorbance (*2.2.25*): maximum 0.40 at 278 nm.

Dissolve 50.0 mg in *0.1 M phosphate buffer solution pH 7.0 R* and dilute to 50.0 ml with the same solution. Measure immediately the absorbance of this solution.

Related substances. Liquid chromatography (*2.2.29*). *Prepare the solutions immediately before use.*

Test solution. Dissolve 0.250 g of the substance to be examined in mobile phase A and dilute to 25.0 ml with mobile phase A.

Reference solution (a). Dilute 1.0 ml of the test solution to 100.0 ml with mobile phase A.

Reference solution (b). Dissolve 10 mg of *lithium clavulanate CRS* and 10 mg of *amoxicillin trihydrate CRS* in mobile phase A and dilute to 100 ml with mobile phase A.

Column:

– *size*: *l* = 0.10 m, Ø = 4.6 mm,
– *stationary phase*: *octadecylsilyl silica gel for chromatography R* (5 μm),
– *temperature*: 40 °C.

Monographs P

Mobile phase:

- *mobile phase A*: a 7.8 g/l solution of *sodium dihydrogen phosphate R* adjusted to pH 4.0 with *phosphoric acid R* and filtered through a 0.5 µm filter,
- *mobile phase B*: a mixture of equal volumes of mobile phase A and *methanol R,*

Time (min)	Mobile phase A (per cent *V/V*)	Mobile phase B (per cent *V/V*)
0 - 4	100	0
4 - 15	100 → 50	0 → 50
15 - 18	50	50
18 - 24	50 → 100	50 → 0
24 - 39	100	0

Flow rate: 1 ml/min.

Detection: spectrophotometer at 230 nm.

Injection: 20 µl.

System suitability: reference solution (b):

- *resolution*: minimum 13 between the first peak (clavulanate) and the second peak (amoxicillin).

Limits:

- *any impurity*: not more than the area of the principal peak in the chromatogram obtained with reference solution (a) (1.0 per cent),
- *total*: not more than twice the area of the principal peak in the chromatogram obtained with reference solution (a) (2.0 per cent),
- *disregard limit*: 0.05 times the area of the principal peak in the chromatogram obtained with reference solution (a) (0.05 per cent).

Aliphatic amines. Gas chromatography (*2.2.28*).

The method shown below can be used to determine the following aliphatic amines: 1,1-dimethylethylamine; diethylamine; *N,N,N′,N′*-tetramethylethylenediamine; 1,1,3,3-tetramethylbutylamine; *N,N′*-diisopropylethylenediamine; 2,2′-oxydi(*N,N*)dimethylethylamine.

Internal standard solution: dissolve 50 µl of *3-methylpentan-2-one R* in *water R* and dilute to 100.0 ml with the same solvent.

Test solution. Weigh 1.00 g of the substance to be examined into a centrifuge tube. Add 5.0 ml of the internal standard solution, 5.0 ml of *dilute sodium hydroxide solution R,* 10.0 ml of *water R*, 5.0 ml of *2-methylpropanol R* and 5 g of *sodium chloride R*. Shake vigorously for 1 min. Centrifuge to separate the layers.

Reference solution. Dissolve 80.0 mg of each of the following amines *1,1-dimethylethylamine R*; *diethylamine R*; *tetramethylethylenediamine R*; *1,1,3,3-tetramethylbutylamine R*; *N,N′-diisopropylethylenediamine R* and *2,2′-oxybis(N,N-dimethylethylamine) R* in *dilute hydrochloric acid R* and dilute to 200.0 ml with the same acid. Introduce 5.0 ml of this solution into a centrifuge tube. Add 5.0 ml of the internal standard solution, 10.0 ml of *dilute sodium hydroxide solution R*, 5.0 ml of *2-methylpropanol R* and 5 g of *sodium chloride R*. Shake vigorously for 1 min. Centrifuge to separate the layers.

Column:

- *material*: fused silica,
- *size*: *l* = 50 m, Ø = 0.53 mm,
- *stationary phase*: *poly(dimethyl)(diphenyl)siloxane R* (film thickness 5 µm).

Carrier gas: *helium for chromatography R.*

Flow rate: 8 ml/min.

Split ratio: 1:10.

Temperature:

	Time (min)	Temperature (°C)
Column	0 - 7	35
	7 - 10.8	35 → 150
	10.8 - 25.8	150
Injection port		200
Detector		250

Detection: flame ionisation.

Injection: 1 µl of the upper layers obtained from test solution and reference solution.

Relative retention with reference to 3-methylpentan-2-one (retention time = about 11.4 min): impurity H = about 0.55; impurity I = about 0.76; impurity J = about 1.07; impurity K = about 1.13; impurity L = about 1.33; impurity M = about 1.57.

Limit:

- *aliphatic amines*: maximum 0.2 per cent.

2-Ethylhexanoic acid (*2.4.28*): maximum 0.8 per cent.

Water (*2.5.12*): maximum 0.5 per cent, determined on 1.00 g.

Bacterial endotoxins (*2.6.14*): less than 0.03 IU/mg if intended for use in the manufacture of parenteral dosage forms without a further appropriate procedure for the removal of bacterial endotoxins.

ASSAY

Liquid chromatography (*2.2.29*). *Prepare the solutions immediately before use.*

Test solution. Dissolve 50.0 mg of the substance to be examined in a 4.1 g/l solution of *sodium acetate R* previously adjusted to pH 6.0 with *glacial acetic acid R,* and dilute to 50.0 ml with the same solution.

Reference solution (a). Dissolve 50.0 mg of *lithium clavulanate CRS* in a 4.1 g/l solution of *sodium acetate R* previously adjusted to pH 6.0 with *glacial acetic acid R* and dilute to 50.0 ml with the same solution.

Reference solution (b). Dissolve 50.0 mg of *lithium clavulanate CRS* and 50.0 mg of *amoxicillin trihydrate CRS* in a 4.1 g/l solution of *sodium acetate R* previously adjusted to pH 6.0 with *glacial acetic acid R* and dilute to 50.0 ml with the same solution.

Column:

- *size*: *l* = 0.3 m, Ø = 4.6 mm,
- *stationary phase*: *octadecylsilyl silica gel for chromatography R* (5 µm).

Mobile phase: mix 5 volumes of *methanol R1* and 95 volumes of a 15 g/l solution of *sodium dihydrogen phosphate R* previously adjusted to pH 4.0 with *dilute phosphoric acid R.*

Flow rate: 1 ml/min.

Detection: spectrophotometer at 230 nm.

Injection: 10 µl.

System suitability: reference solution (b):

- *resolution*: minimum 3.5 between the first peak (clavulanate) and the second peak (amoxicillin).

1 mg of clavulanate ($C_8H_9NO_5$) is equivalent to 1.191 mg of $C_8H_8KNO_5$.

Monographs P

STORAGE

In an airtight container, at a temperature of 2 °C to 8 °C. If the substance is sterile, store in a sterile, airtight, tamper-proof container.

LABELLING

The label states, where applicable, that the substance is free from bacterial endotoxins.

IMPURITIES

Specified impurities: A, B, C, D, G, H, I, J, K, L, M.

Other detectable impurities: E, F.

By liquid chromatography: A, B, C, D, E, F, G.

By gas chromatography: H, I, J, K, L, M.

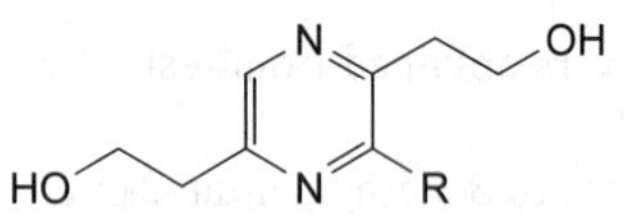

A. R = H: 2,2′-(pyrazine-2,5-diyl)diethanol,

B. R = CH_2-CH_2-CO_2H: 3-[3,6-bis(2-hydroxyethyl)pyrazin-2-yl]propanoic acid,

C. R = CH_2-CH_3: 2,2′-(3-ethylpyrazine-2,5-diyl)diethanol,

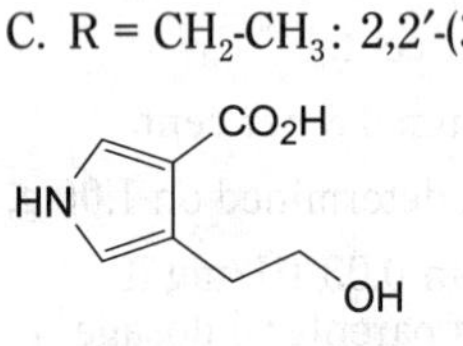

D. 4-(2-hydroxyethyl)pyrrole-3-carboxylic acid,

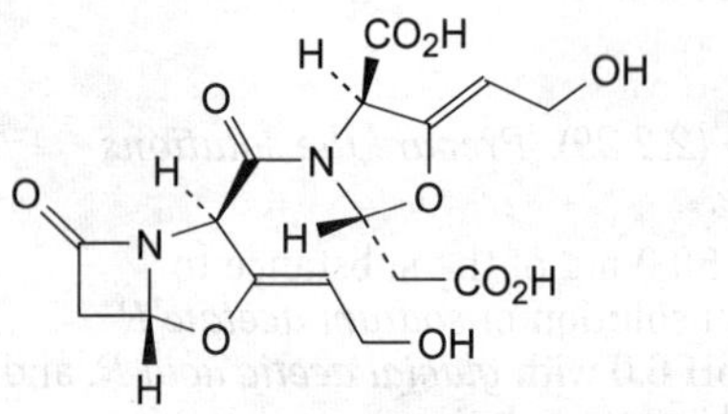

E. (2*R*,4*R*,5*Z*)-2-(carboxymethyl)-5-(2-hydroxyethylidene)-3-[[(2*R*,3*Z*,5*R*)-3-(2-hydroxyethylidene)-7-oxo-4-oxa-1-azabibyclo[3.2.0]hept-2-yl]carbonyl]oxazolidine-4-carboxylic acid,

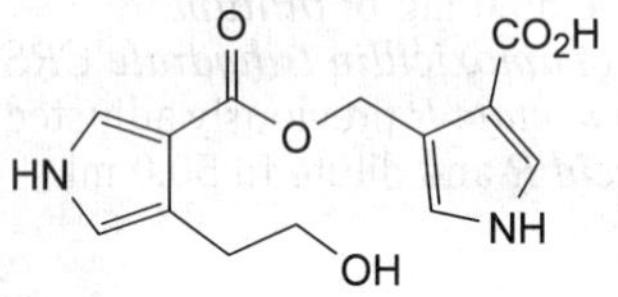

F. 4-[[[[4-(2-hydroxyethyl)-1*H*-pyrrol-3-yl]carbonyl]oxy]methyl]-1*H*-pyrrole-3-carboxylic acid,

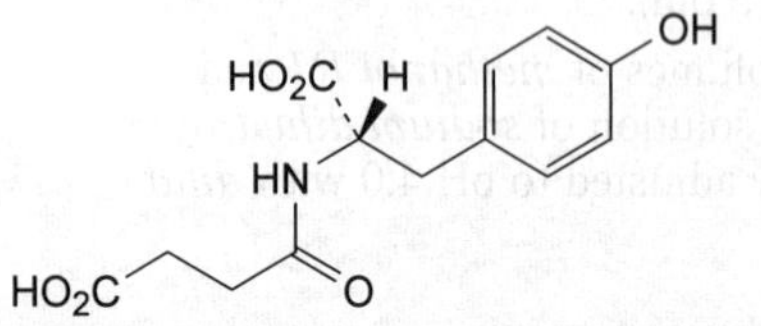

G. 4-[[(1*S*)-1-carboxy-2-(4-hydroxyphenyl)ethyl]amino]-4-oxobutanoic acid (*N*-succinyltyrosine),

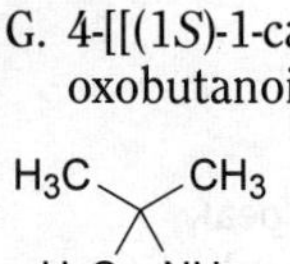

H. 2-amino-2-methylpropane (1,1-dimethylethylamine),

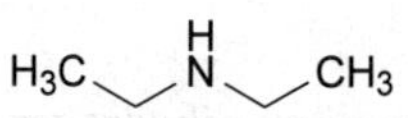

I. diethylamine,

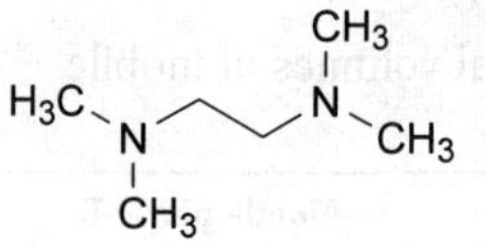

J. 1,2-bis(dimethylamino)ethane (*N,N,N′,N′*-tetramethylethylenediamine),

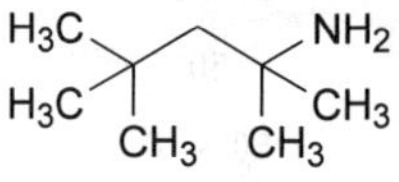

K. 2-amino-2,4,4-trimethylpentane (1,1,3,3-tetramethylbutylamine),

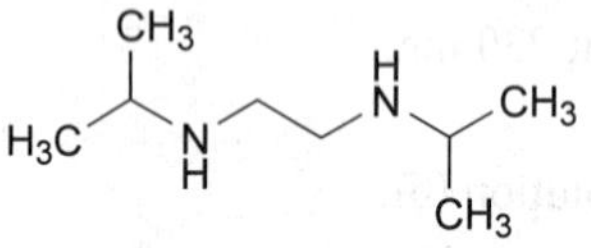

L. *N,N′*-bis(1-methylethyl)-1,2-ethanediamine (*N,N′*-diisopropylethylenediamine),

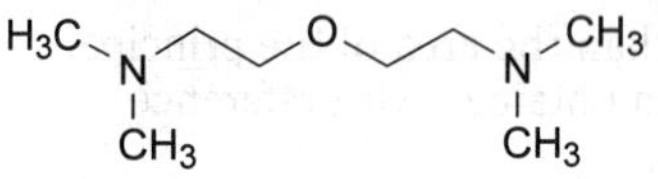

M. bis(2-dimethylamino)ethyl ether [2,2′-oxybis(*N,N*-dimethylethylamine)].

01/2005:1653
corrected

POTASSIUM CLAVULANATE, DILUTED

Kalii clavulanas dilutus

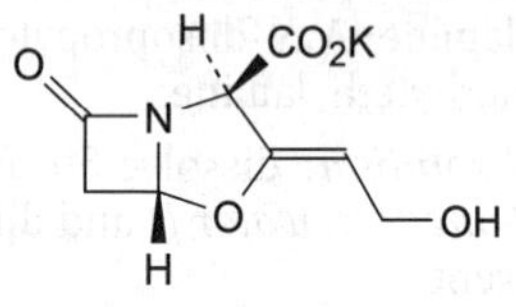

$C_8H_8KNO_5$ M_r 237.3

DEFINITION

Dry mixture of *Potassium clavulanate (1140)* and *Cellulose, microcrystalline (0316)* or *Silica, colloidal anhydrous (0434)* or *Silica, colloidal hydrated (0738).*

Content: 91.2 per cent to 107.1 per cent of the content of potassium clavulanate stated on the label.

CHARACTERS

Appearance of diluted potassium clavulanate: white or almost white powder, hygroscopic.

Solubility of potassium clavulanate: freely soluble in water, slightly soluble in alcohol, very slightly soluble in acetone.

The solubility of the diluted product depends on the diluent and its concentration.

IDENTIFICATION

A. Examine the chromatograms obtained in the assay.

Results: the principal peak in the chromatogram obtained with the test solution is similar in retention time to the principal peak in the chromatogram obtained with reference solution (a).

B. It gives reaction (b) of potassium (*2.3.1*).

C. Depending on the diluent used, carry out the corresponding identification test (a) or (b).

(a) A quantity of the substance to be examined, corresponding to 20 mg of cellulose, when placed on a watch-glass and dispersed in 4 ml of *iodinated zinc chloride solution R*, becomes violet-blue.

(b) It gives the reaction of silicates (*2.3.1*).

TESTS

pH (*2.2.3*): 4.8 to 8.0.

Suspend a quantity of the substance to be examined corresponding to 0.200 g of potassium clavulanate in 20 ml of *carbon dioxide-free water R*.

Absorbance (*2.2.25*): maximum 0.40 measured immediately at 278 nm.

Disperse a quantity of the substance to be examined corresponding to 50.0 mg of potassium clavulanate in 10 ml of *0.1 M phosphate buffer solution pH 7.0 R*, dilute to 50.0 ml with the same buffer solution and filter.

Related substances. Liquid chromatography (*2.2.29*). *Prepare the solutions immediately before use.*

Test solution. Disperse a quantity of the substance to be examined corresponding to 0.250 g of potassium clavulanate in 5 ml of mobile phase A, dilute to 25.0 ml with mobile phase A and filter.

Reference solution (a). Dilute 1.0 ml of the test solution to 100.0 ml with mobile phase A.

Reference solution (b). Dissolve 10 mg of *amoxicillin trihydrate CRS* in 1 ml of the test solution and dilute to 100 ml with mobile phase A.

Column:

- *size*: *l* = 0.10 m, Ø = 4.6 mm,
- *stationary phase*: *octadecylsilyl silica gel for chromatography R* (5 µm),
- *temperature*: 40 °C.

Mobile phase:

- *mobile phase A*: 7.8 g/l solution of *sodium dihydrogen phosphate R* adjusted to pH 4.0 with *dilute phosphoric acid R*,
- *mobile phase B*: mixture of equal volumes of mobile phase A and *methanol R*,

Time (min)	Mobile phase A (per cent *V/V*)	Mobile phase B (per cent *V/V*)
0 - 4	100	0
4 - 15	100 → 50	0 → 50
15 - 18	50	50
18 - 24	50 → 100	50 → 0
24 - 39	100	0

Flow rate: 1 ml/min.

Detection: spectrophotometer at 230 nm.

Injection: 20 µl.

System suitability: reference solution (b):

- *resolution*: minimum of 13 between the peak due to clavulanate (1st peak) and the peak due to amoxicillin (2nd peak).

Limits:

- *any impurity*: not more than the area of the principal peak in the chromatogram obtained with reference solution (a) (1.0 per cent),
- *total*: not more than twice the area of the principal peak in the chromatogram obtained with reference solution (a) (2.0 per cent),
- *disregard limit*: 0.05 times the area of the principal peak in the chromatogram obtained with reference solution (a) (0.05 per cent).

Water (*2.5.12*): maximum 2.5 per cent, determined on 1.000 g.

ASSAY

Liquid chromatography (*2.2.29*). *Prepare the solutions immediately before use.*

Test solution. Disperse a quantity of the substance to be examined corresponding to 50.0 mg of potassium clavulanate in a 4.1 g/l solution of *sodium acetate R* previously adjusted to pH 6.0 with *glacial acetic acid R*, dilute to 50.0 ml with the same solution and filter.

Reference solution (a). Dissolve 50.0 mg of *lithium clavulanate CRS* in a 4.1 g/l solution of *sodium acetate R* previously adjusted to pH 6.0 with *glacial acetic acid R* and dilute to 50.0 ml with the same solution.

Reference solution (b). Dissolve 10 mg of *amoxicillin trihydrate CRS* in 10 ml of reference solution (a).

Column:

- *size*: *l* = 0.3 m, Ø = 4.6 mm,
- *stationary phase*: *octadecylsilyl silica gel for chromatography R* (10 µm).

Mobile phase: mix 5 volumes of *methanol R1* and 95 volumes of a 15 g/l solution of *sodium dihydrogen phosphate R* previously adjusted to pH 4.0 with *dilute phosphoric acid R*.

Flow rate: 1 ml/min.

Detection: spectrophotometer at 230 nm.

Injection: 10 µl.

System suitability: reference solution (b):

- *resolution*: minimum 3.5 between the peak due to clavulanate (1st peak) and the peak due to amoxicillin (2nd peak).

1 mg of $C_8H_9NO_5$ is equivalent to 1.191 mg of $C_8H_8KNO_5$.

STORAGE

In an airtight container.

LABELLING

The label states the *m/m* percentage content of potassium clavulanate and the diluent used to prepare the mixture.

IMPURITIES

Specified impurities: A, B, C, D, G.

Other detectable impurities: E, F.

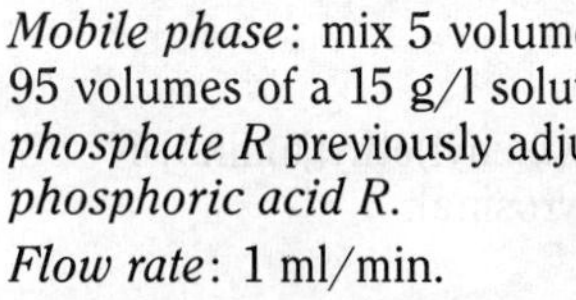

A. R = H: 2,2′-(pyrazine-2,5-diyl)diethanol,

B. R = CH_2-CH_2-CO_2H: 3-[3,6-bis(2-hydroxyethyl)pyrazin-2-yl]propanoic acid,

C. R = CH_2-CH_3: 2,2′-(3-ethylpyrazine-2,5-diyl)diethanol,

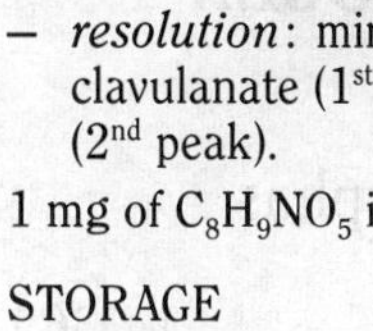

D. 4-(2-hydroxyethyl)-1*H*-pyrrole-3-carboxylic acid,

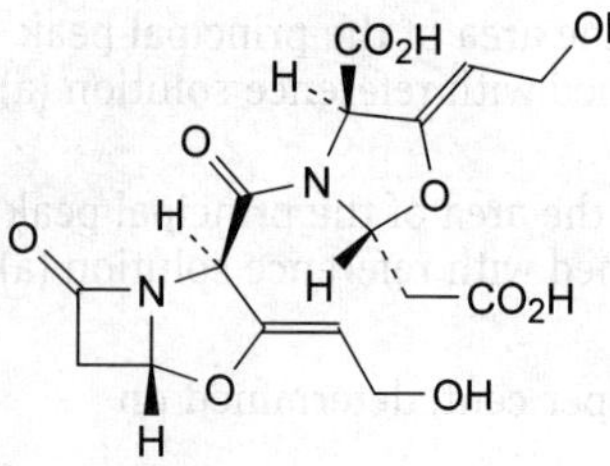

E. (2*R*,4*R*,5*Z*)-2-(carboxymethyl)-5-(2-hydroxyethylidene)-3-[[(2*R*,3*Z*,5*R*)-3-(2-hydroxyethylidene)-7-oxo-4-oxa-1-azabicyclo[3.2.0]hept-2-yl]carbonyl]oxazolidine-4-carboxylic acid,

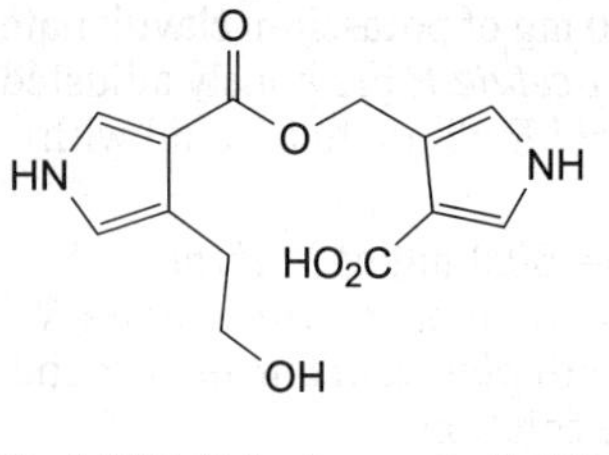

F. 4-[[[[4-(2-hydroxyethyl)-1*H*-pyrrol-3-yl]carbonyl]oxy]methyl]-1*H*-pyrrole-3-carboxylic acid,

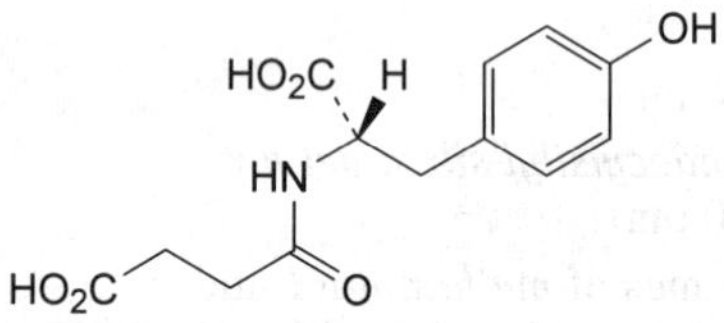

G. 4-[[(1*S*)-1-carboxy-2-(4-hydroxyphenyl)ethyl]amino]-4-oxobutanoic acid (*N*-succinyltyrosine).

01/2005:0920

POTASSIUM DIHYDROGEN PHOSPHATE

Kalii dihydrogenophosphas

KH_2PO_4 — M_r 136.1

DEFINITION

Potassium dihydrogen phosphate contains not less than 98.0 per cent and not more than the equivalent of 100.5 per cent of KH_2PO_4, calculated with reference to the dried substance.

CHARACTERS

A white, crystalline powder or colourless crystals, freely soluble in water, practically insoluble in alcohol.

IDENTIFICATION

A. Solution S (see Tests) is faintly acid (*2.2.4*).

B. Solution S gives reaction (b) of phosphates (*2.3.1*).

C. 0.5 ml of solution S gives reaction (b) of potassium (*2.3.1*).

TESTS

Solution S. Dissolve 10.0 g in *carbon dioxide-free water R* prepared from *distilled water R* and dilute to 100 ml with the same solvent.

Appearance of solution. Solution S is clear (*2.2.1*) and colourless (*2.2.2, Method II*).

pH (*2.2.3*). To 5 ml of solution S add 5 ml of *carbon dioxide-free water R*. The pH of the solution is 4.2 to 4.5.

Reducing substances. To 5 ml of solution S add 5 ml of *dilute sulphuric acid R* and 0.25 ml of *0.02 M potassium permanganate*. Heat on a water-bath for 5 min. The colour of the permanganate is not completely discharged.

Chlorides (*2.4.4*). Dilute 2.5 ml of solution S to 15 ml with *water R*. The solution complies with the limit test for chlorides (200 ppm).

Sulphates (*2.4.13*). To 5 ml of solution S add 0.5 ml of *hydrochloric acid R* and dilute to 15 ml with *distilled water R*. The solution complies with the limit test for sulphates (300 ppm).

Arsenic (*2.4.2*). 0.5 g complies with limit test A for arsenic (2 ppm).

Iron (*2.4.9*). 10 ml of solution S complies with the limit test for iron (10 ppm).

Sodium. If intended for use in the manufacture of parenteral dosage forms, it complies with the test for sodium. Not more than 0.1 per cent of Na, determined by atomic emission spectrometry (*2.2.22, Method I*).

Test solution. Dissolve 1.00 g of the substance to be examined in *water R* and dilute to 100.0 ml with the same solvent.

Reference solution. Dissolve in *water R* 0.5084 g of *sodium chloride R*, previously dried at 100 °C to 105 °C for 3 h, and dilute to 1000.0 ml with the same solvent (200 µg of Na per millilitre). Dilute as necessary.

Measure the emission intensity at 589 nm.

Heavy metals (*2.4.8*). 12 ml of solution S complies with limit test A for heavy metals (10 ppm). Prepare the standard using *lead standard solution (1 ppm Pb) R*.

Loss on drying (*2.2.32*). Not more than 2.0 per cent, determined on 1.000 g by drying in an oven at 125 °C to 130 °C.

ASSAY

Dissolve 1.000 g in 50 ml of *carbon dioxide-free water R*. Titrate with carbonate-free *1 M sodium hydroxide*, determining the end-point potentiometrically (*2.2.20*).

1 ml of *1 M sodium hydroxide* is equivalent to 0.1361 g of KH_2PO_4.

LABELLING

The label states, where applicable, that the substance is suitable for use in the manufacture of parenteral dosage forms.

01/2005:2076

POTASSIUM HYDROGEN ASPARTATE HEMIHYDRATE

Kalii hydrogenoaspartas hemihydricus

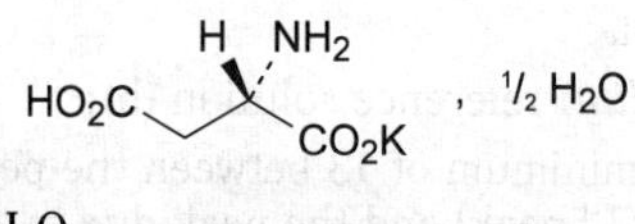

$C_4H_6KNO_4, {}^1/_2H_2O$ — M_r 180.2

DEFINITION

Potassium hydrogen (2*S*)-2-aminobutanedioate hemihydrate.

Content: 99.0 per cent to 101.0 per cent (anhydrous substance).

CHARACTERS

Appearance: white powder, or white crystalline powder or colourless crystals.

Solubility: very soluble in water, practically insoluble in alcohol and in methylene chloride.

IDENTIFICATION

A. It complies with the test for specific optical rotation (see Tests).

B. Examine the chromatograms obtained in the test for ninhydrin-positive substances.

Results: the principal spot in the chromatogram obtained with test solution (b) is similar in position, colour and size to the principal spot in the chromatogram obtained with reference solution (a).

C. It gives reaction (b) of potassium (*2.3.1*).

TESTS

Solution S. Dissolve 2.5 g in *carbon dioxide-free water R* prepared from *distilled water R* and dilute to 100 ml with the same solvent.

Appearance of solution. Solution S is clear (*2.2.1*) and colourless (*2.2.2, Method II*).

pH (*2.2.3*): 6.0 to 7.5 for solution S.

Specific optical rotation (*2.2.7*): + 18.0 to + 20.5 (anhydrous substance).

Dissolve 0.50 g in a mixture of equal volumes of *hydrochloric acid R* and *water R* and dilute to 25.0 ml with the same mixture of solvents.

Ninhydrin-positive substances. Thin-layer chromatography (*2.2.27*).

Test solution (a). Solution S.

Test solution (b). Dilute 1.0 ml of solution S to 10.0 ml with *water R*.

Reference solution (a). Dissolve 25 mg of *potassium hydrogen aspartate hemihydrate CRS* in *water R* and dilute to 10 ml with the same solvent.

Reference solution (b). Dilute 1.0 ml of test solution (b) to 20.0 ml with *water R*.

Reference solution (c). Dissolve 10 mg of *glutamic acid CRS* and 10 mg of the substance to be examined in *water R* and dilute to 25 ml with the same solvent.

Plate: *TLC silica gel plate R*.

Mobile phase: *glacial acetic acid R, water R, butanol R* (20:20:60 *V/V/V*).

Application: 5 µl.

Development: over 2/3 of the plate.

Drying: in air.

Detection: spray with *ninhydrin solution R* and heat at 100-105 °C for 15 min.

System suitability: reference solution (c):

– the chromatogram shows 2 clearly separated principal spots.

Limits: test solution (a):

– *any impurity*: any spot, apart from the principal spot, is not more intense than the spot in the chromatogram obtained with reference solution (b) (0.5 per cent).

Chlorides (*2.4.4*): maximum 200 ppm.

To 10 ml of solution S add 5 ml of *water R*.

Sulphates (*2.4.13*): maximum 500 ppm.

To 12 ml of solution S add 3 ml of *distilled water R*.

Ammonium (*2.4.1, Method B*): maximum 200 ppm, determined on 50 mg.

Prepare the standard using 0.1 ml of *ammonium standard solution (100 ppm NH_4) R*.

Iron (*2.4.9*): maximum 30 ppm.

In a separating funnel, dissolve 0.33 g in 10 ml of *dilute hydrochloric acid R*. Shake with 3 quantities, each of 10 ml, of *methyl isobutyl ketone R1*, shaking for 3 min each time. To the combined organic layers add 10 ml of *water R* and shake for 3 min. The aqueous layer complies with the limit test for iron.

Heavy metals (*2.4.8*): maximum 10 ppm.

Dissolve 2.0 g in *water R* and dilute to 20 ml with the same solvent. 12 ml of the solution complies with limit test A. Prepare the standard using *lead standard solution (1 ppm Pb) R*.

Water (*2.5.12*): 4.0 per cent to 6.0 per cent, determined on 0.200 g.

Dissolve the substance to be examined in 10 ml of *formamide R1* and add 10 ml of *anhydrous methanol R*.

ASSAY

Dissolve 70.0 mg in 5 ml of *anhydrous formic acid R*, add 50 ml of *anhydrous acetic acid R*. Titrate with *0.1 M perchloric acid*, determining the end-point potentiometrically (*2.2.20*).

1 ml of *0.1 M perchloric acid* is equivalent to 8.56 mg of $C_4H_6KNO_4$.

01/2005:1141

POTASSIUM HYDROGEN CARBONATE

Kalii hydrogenocarbonas

$KHCO_3$ M_r 100.1

DEFINITION

Potassium hydrogen carbonate contains not less than 99.0 per cent and not more than the equivalent of 101.0 per cent of $KHCO_3$.

CHARACTERS

A white, crystalline powder or colourless crystals, freely soluble in water, practically insoluble in alcohol. When heated in the dry state or in solution, it is gradually converted to potassium carbonate.

IDENTIFICATION

A. To 5 ml of solution S (see Tests) add 0.1 ml of *phenolphthalein solution R*. A pale pink colour is produced. Heat; gas is evolved and the colour becomes red.

B. It gives the reaction of carbonates and bicarbonates (*2.3.1*).

C. 1 ml of solution S gives reaction (b) of potassium (*2.3.1*).

TESTS

Solution S. Dissolve 5.0 g in 90 ml of *carbon dioxide-free water R* prepared from *distilled water R* and dilute to 100 ml with the same solvent.

Appearance of solution. Solution S is clear (*2.2.1*) and colourless (*2.2.2, Method II*).

Carbonates. The pH (*2.2.3*) of freshly prepared solution S is not more than 8.6.

Monographs P

Chlorides (*2.4.4*). Dilute 7 ml of solution S to 15 ml with *dilute nitric acid R*. The solution complies with the limit test for chlorides (150 ppm).

Sulphates (*2.4.13*). Dilute 10 ml of solution S to 15 ml with *acetic acid R*. The solution complies with the limit test for sulphates (150 ppm). Prepare the standard using a mixture of 7.5 ml of *sulphate standard solution (10 ppm SO_4) R* and 7.5 ml of *distilled water R*.

Ammonium (*2.4.1*). 10 ml of solution S diluted to 15 ml with *water R* complies with the limit test for ammonium (20 ppm). Prepare the standard using a mixture of 5 ml of *water R* and 10 ml of *ammonium standard solution (1 ppm NH_4) R*.

Calcium (*2.4.3*). Dilute 10 ml of solution S to 15 ml with *acetic acid R*. The solution complies with the limit test for calcium (100 ppm). Prepare the standard using 5 ml of *calcium standard solution (10 ppm Ca) R* and 10 ml of *distilled water R*.

Heavy metals (*2.4.8*). Dissolve 2.0 g in a mixture of 2 ml of *hydrochloric acid R* and 18 ml of *water R*. 12 ml of the solution complies with limit test A for heavy metals (10 ppm). Prepare the standard using *lead standard solution (1 ppm Pb) R*.

Iron (*2.4.9*). 10 ml of solution S complies with the limit test for iron (20 ppm).

Sodium. Not more than 0.5 per cent of Na, determined by atomic emission spectrometry (*2.2.22, Method II*).

Test solution. Dissolve 1.00 g in *water R* and dilute to 100.0 ml with the same solvent.

Reference solutions. Prepare the reference solutions using *sodium standard solution (200 ppm Na) R*, diluted as necessary with *water R*.

Measure the emission intensity at 589 nm.

ASSAY

Dissolve 0.800 g in 50 ml of *carbon dioxide-free water R*. Add 0.1 ml of *methyl orange solution R*. Titrate with *1 M hydrochloric acid* until the yellow colour begins to change to yellowish-pink. Heat cautiously and boil for at least 2 min. The solution becomes yellow. Cool and titrate until a yellowish-red colour is obtained.

1 ml of *1 M hydrochloric acid* is equivalent to 0.1001 g of $KHCO_3$.

01/2005:1984

POTASSIUM HYDROGEN TARTRATE

Kalii hydrogenotartras

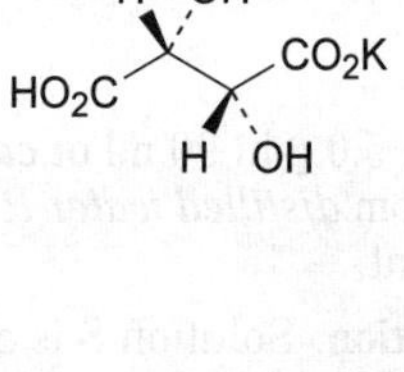

$C_4H_5KO_6$ M_r 188.2

DEFINITION

Potassium hydrogen (2*R*,3*R*)-2,3-dihydroxybutane-1,4-dioate.

Content: 99.5 per cent to 100.5 per cent (dried substance).

CHARACTERS

Appearance: white, crystalline powder or colourless crystals.

Solubility: slightly soluble in water, practically insoluble in alcohol. It dissolves in dilute solutions of mineral acids and alkali hydroxides.

IDENTIFICATION

A. It complies with the test for specific optical rotation (see Tests).

B. Suspend 0.5 g in 50 ml of *water R* and boil until dissolution is complete. Allow to cool (solution A). To 5 ml of solution A, add 0.1 ml of *methyl red solution R*. The solution is red.

C. Solution A gives reaction (a) of tartrates (*2.3.1*).

D. Solution A gives reaction (b) of potassium (*2.3.1*).

TESTS

Specific optical rotation (*2.2.7*): + 8.0 to + 9.2 (dried substance).

Dissolve 2.50 g in 20 ml of *1 M hydrochloric acid* with heating. Allow to cool. Dilute to 25.0 ml with *water R*.

Oxalic acid: maximum 500 ppm.

Dissolve 0.43 g in 4 ml of *water R*. Add 3 ml of *hydrochloric acid R* and 1 g of *zinc R* in granules and boil for 1 min. Allow to stand for 2 min. Collect the liquid in a test-tube containing 0.25 ml of a 10 g/l solution of *phenylhydrazine hydrochloride R* and heat to boiling. Cool rapidly, transfer to a graduated cylinder and add an equal volume of *hydrochloric acid R* and 0.25 ml of a 50 g/l solution of *potassium ferricyanide R*. Shake and allow to stand for 30 min. Any pink colour in the solution is not more intense than that in a standard prepared at the same time in the same manner using a mixture of 1 ml of *water R* and 3 ml of a 0.1 g/l solution of *oxalic acid R*.

Chlorides (*2.4.4*): maximum 500 ppm.

Dissolve 1.0 g with heating in a mixture of 3 ml of *dilute nitric acid R* and 50 ml of *water R*. Dilute to 100 ml with *water R*. Dilute 10 ml of the solution to 15 ml with *water R*. The solution complies with the limit test for chlorides.

Sulphates (*2.4.13*): maximum 500 ppm.

Suspend 0.30 g in 3.0 ml of *dilute hydrochloric acid R* and dilute to 15 ml with *distilled water R*. Heat until dissolution is complete. The solution complies with the limit test for sulphates.

Barium. Suspend 0.50 g in a mixture of 1.5 ml of *dilute hydrochloric acid R* and 8.5 ml of *water R*. Heat until dissolution is complete. Allow to cool. Add 1 ml of *dilute sulphuric acid R*. The solution remains clear (*2.2.1*) on standing for 15 min.

Heavy metals (*2.4.8*): maximum 10 ppm.

2.0 g complies with limit test C. Prepare the standard using 2 ml of *lead standard solution (10 ppm Pb) R*.

Loss on drying (*2.2.32*): maximum 0.5 per cent, determined on 1.000 g by drying in an oven at 100-105 °C.

ASSAY

Dissolve 0.170 g in 100 ml of *water R* at 100 °C. Titrate the hot solution with *0.1 M sodium hydroxide*, using 0.3 ml of *phenolphthalein solution R* as indicator.

1 ml of *0.1 M sodium hydroxide* is equivalent to 18.82 mg of $C_4H_5KO_6$.

01/2005:0840

POTASSIUM HYDROXIDE

Kalii hydroxidum

KOH M_r 56.11

DEFINITION

Potassium hydroxide contains not less than 85.0 per cent and not more than the equivalent of 100.5 per cent of total alkali, calculated as KOH.

CHARACTERS

White, crystalline, hard masses, supplied as sticks, pellets or irregularly shaped pieces, deliquescent in air, hygroscopic, absorbing carbon dioxide, very soluble in water, freely soluble in alcohol.

IDENTIFICATION

A. Dissolve 0.1 g in 10 ml of *water R* (this solution is used for identification test B). Dilute 1 ml of the solution to 100 ml with *water R*. The pH (*2.2.3*) of this solution is not less than 10.5.

B. 1 ml of the initial solution prepared in identification test A gives reaction (b) of potassium (*2.3.1*).

TESTS

Solution S1. Dissolve 2.5 g in 10 ml of *water R*. Carefully add 2 ml of *nitric acid R*, with cooling, and dilute to 25 ml with *dilute nitric acid R*.

Solution S2. Dissolve 10 g in 15 ml of *distilled water R*. Carefully add 12 ml of *hydrochloric acid R*, with cooling, and dilute to 50 ml with *dilute hydrochloric acid R*.

Appearance of solution. Dissolve 5 g in *carbon dioxide-free water R* and dilute to 50 ml with the same solvent. The solution is clear (*2.2.1*) and colourless (*2.2.2, Method II*).

Carbonates. Not more than 2.0 per cent, calculated as K_2CO_3, as determined in the assay.

Chlorides (*2.4.4*). Dilute 10 ml of solution S1 to 15 ml with *water R*. The solution complies with the limit test for chlorides (50 ppm).

Phosphates (*2.4.11*). Dilute 5 ml of solution S1 to 100 ml with *water R*. The solution complies with the limit test for phosphates (20 ppm).

Sulphates (*2.4.13*). 15 ml of solution S2 complies with the limit test for sulphates (50 ppm).

Aluminium (*2.4.17*). If intended for use in the manufacture of haemodialysis solutions, it complies with the test for aluminium. Dissolve 20 g in 100 ml of *water R* and add 10 ml of *acetate buffer solution pH 6.0 R*. The solution complies with the limit test for aluminium (0.2 ppm). Use as the reference solution a mixture of 2 ml of *aluminium standard solution (2 ppm Al) R*, 10 ml of *acetate buffer solution pH 6.0 R* and 98 ml of *water R*. To prepare the blank use a mixture of 10 ml of *acetate buffer solution pH 6.0 R* and 100 ml of *water R*.

Iron (*2.4.9*). Dilute 5 ml of solution S2 to 10 ml with *water R*. The solution complies with the limit test for iron (10 ppm).

Sodium. Not more than 1.0 per cent of Na, determined by atomic absorption spectrometry (*2.2.23, Method II*).

Test solution. Dissolve 1.00 g in 50 ml of *water R*, add 5 ml of *sulphuric acid R* and dilute to 100.0 ml with *water R*. Dilute 1.0 ml of the solution to 10.0 ml with *water R*.

Reference solutions. Prepare the reference solutions using *sodium standard solution (200 ppm Na) R*, diluted as necessary with *water R*.

Measure the absorbance at 589 nm using a sodium hollow-cathode lamp as a source of radiation and an air-acetylene flame.

Heavy metals (*2.4.8*). Dilute 10 ml of solution S2 to 20 ml with *water R*. 12 ml of the solution complies with limit test A for heavy metals (10 ppm). Prepare the standard using *lead standard solution (1 ppm Pb) R*.

ASSAY

Dissolve 2.000 g in 25 ml of *carbon-dioxide free water R*. Add 25 ml of freshly prepared *barium chloride solution R1* and 0.3 ml of *phenolphthalein solution R*. Add slowly with shaking 25.0 ml of *1 M hydrochloric acid* and continue the titration with *1 M hydrochloric acid* until the colour changes from pink to colourless. Add 0.3 ml of *bromophenol blue solution R* and continue the titration with *1 M hydrochloric acid* until the colour changes from violet-blue to yellow.

1 ml of *1 M hydrochloric acid* used in the second part of the titration is equivalent to 69.11 mg of K_2CO_3.

1 ml of *1 M hydrochloric acid* used in the combined titrations is equivalent to 56.11 mg of total alkali, calculated as KOH.

STORAGE

Store in an airtight, non-metallic container.

LABELLING

The label states, where applicable, that the substance is suitable for use in the manufacture of haemodialysis solutions.

01/2005:0186

POTASSIUM IODIDE

Kalii iodidum

KI 166.0

DEFINITION

Potassium iodide contains not less than 99.0 per cent and not more than the equivalent of 100.5 per cent of KI, calculated with reference to the dried substance.

CHARACTERS

A white powder or colourless crystals, very soluble in water, freely soluble in glycerol, soluble in alcohol.

IDENTIFICATION

A. Solution S (see Tests) gives the reactions of iodides (*2.3.1*).

B. Solution S gives the reactions of potassium (*2.3.1*).

TESTS

Solution S. Dissolve 10.0 g in *carbon dioxide-free water R* prepared from *distilled water R* and dilute to 100 ml with the same solvent.

Appearance of solution. Solution S is clear (*2.2.1*) and colourless (*2.2.2, Method II*).

Alkalinity. To 12.5 ml of solution S add 0.1 ml of *bromothymol blue solution R1*. Not more than 0.5 ml of *0.01 M hydrochloric acid* is required to change the colour of the indicator.

Monographs P

Iodates. To 10 ml of solution S add 0.25 ml of *iodide-free starch solution R* and 0.2 ml of *dilute sulphuric acid R* and allow to stand protected from light for 2 min. No blue colour develops.

Sulphates (*2.4.13*). 10 ml of solution S diluted to 15 ml with *distilled water R* complies with the limit test for sulphates (150 ppm).

Thiosulphates. To 10 ml of solution S add 0.1 ml of *starch solution R* and 0.1 ml of *0.005 M iodine*. A blue colour is produced.

Heavy metals (*2.4.8*). 12 ml of solution S complies with limit test A for heavy metals (10 ppm). Prepare the standard using *lead standard solution (1 ppm Pb) R*.

Iron (*2.4.9*). 5 ml of solution S diluted to 10 ml with *water R* complies with the limit test for iron (20 ppm).

Loss on drying (*2.2.32*). Not more than 1.0 per cent, determined on 1.00 g of previously powdered substance by drying in an oven at 100-105 °C for 3 h.

ASSAY

Dissolve 1.500 g in *water R* and dilute to 100.0 ml with the same solvent. To 20.0 ml of the solution add 40 ml of *hydrochloric acid R* and titrate with *0.05 M potassium iodate* until the colour changes from red to yellow. Add 5 ml of *chloroform R* and continue the titration, shaking vigorously, until the chloroform layer is decolourised.

1 ml of *0.05 M potassium iodate* is equivalent to 16.60 mg of KI.

STORAGE

Store protected from light.

01/2005:2075

POTASSIUM METABISULPHITE

Kalii metabisulfis

$K_2S_2O_5$ M_r 222.3

DEFINITION

Potassium metabisulphite (potassium disulphite).

Content: 95.0 per cent to 101.0 per cent.

CHARACTERS

Appearance: white powder or colourless crystals.

Solubility: freely soluble in water, slightly soluble in alcohol.

IDENTIFICATION

A. It complies with the test for pH (see Tests).

B. To 5 ml of solution S (see Tests), add 0.5 ml of *0.05 M iodine*. The mixture is colourless and gives reaction (a) of sulphates (*2.3.1*).

C. Solution S gives reaction (a) of potassium (*2.3.1*).

TESTS

Solution S. Dissolve 5.0 g in *carbon dioxide-free water R* and dilute to 100 ml with the same solvent.

Appearance of solution. Solution S is clear (*2.2.1*) and colourless (*2.2.2, Method I*).

pH (*2.2.3*): 3.0 to 4.5 for solution S.

Thiosulphates. To 2.00 g add 25 ml of a 42.5 g/l solution of *sodium hydroxide R* and 75 ml of *water R*. Shake until dissolved and add 10 ml of *formaldehyde R* and 10 ml of *acetic acid R*. After 5 min, titrate with *0.03 M iodine* using 1 ml of *starch solution R*. Carry out a blank titration. The difference between the volumes consumed in the 2 titrations is maximum 0.15 ml.

Iron: maximum 10 ppm.

Atomic absorption spectrometry (*2.2.23, Method I*).

Test solution. Dilute 20 ml of solution S to 50 ml with *water R*.

Reference solutions. Prepare the reference solutions using *iron standard solution (20 ppm Fe) R*, diluted as necessary with *water R*.

Source: iron hollow-cathode lamp.

Wavelength: 248.3 nm.

Atomisation device: air-acetylene flame.

Selenium: maximum 10 ppm.

To 3.0 g add 10 ml of *formaldehyde R*. Carefully add 2 ml of *hydrochloric acid R* in small portions. Heat on a water-bath for 20 min. Any pink colour in the solution is not more intense than that of a reference solution prepared at the same time in the same manner using 1.0 g of the substance to be examined to which 0.2 ml of *selenium standard solution (100 ppm Se) R* has been added.

Zinc: maximum 25 ppm.

Atomic absorption spectrometry (*2.2.23, Method I*).

Test solution. Dilute 20 ml of solution S to 50 ml with *water R*.

Reference solutions. Prepare the reference solutions using *zinc standard solution (100 ppm Zn) R*, diluted as necessary with *water R*.

Source: zinc hollow-cathode lamp.

Wavelength: 213.9 nm.

Atomisation device: air-acetylene flame.

Heavy metals (*2.4.8*): maximum 10 ppm.

Introduce 40 ml of solution S into a silica crucible, add 10 ml of *hydrochloric acid R* and evaporate to dryness. Dissolve the residue in 19 ml of *water R* and add 1 ml of a 40 g/l solution of *sodium fluoride R*. The solution complies with limit test E. Prepare the standard using 20 ml of *lead standard solution (1 ppm Pb) R*.

ASSAY

In a 500 ml conical flask containing 50.0 ml of *0.05 M iodine* introduce 0.150 g and add 5 ml of *hydrochloric acid R*. Titrate the excess of iodine with *0.1 M sodium thiosulphate* using 0.1 ml of *starch solution R*.

1 ml of *0.05 M iodine* is equivalent to 5.558 mg of $K_2S_2O_5$.

STORAGE

In an airtight container, protected from light.

01/2005:1465

POTASSIUM NITRATE

Kalii nitras

KNO_3 M_r 101.1

DEFINITION

Potassium nitrate contains not less than 99.0 per cent and not more than the equivalent of 101.0 per cent of KNO_3, calculated with reference to the dried substance.

Monographs P

CHARACTERS

A white, crystalline powder or colourless crystals, freely soluble in water, very soluble in boiling water, practically insoluble in alcohol.

IDENTIFICATION

A. It gives the reaction of nitrates (*2.3.1*).

B. Solution S (see Tests) gives the reactions of potassium (*2.3.1*).

TESTS

Solution S. Dissolve 10.0 g in *carbon dioxide-free water R* prepared from *distilled water R* and dilute to 100 ml with the same solvent.

Appearance of solution. Solution S is clear (*2.2.1*) and colourless (*2.2.2, Method II*).

Acidity or alkalinity. To 10 ml of solution S add 0.05 ml of *bromothymol blue solution R1*. Not more than 0.5 ml of *0.01 M hydrochloric acid* or *0.01 M sodium hydroxide* is required to change the colour of the indicator.

Reducible substances. To 10 ml of solution S, add 0.5 ml of *dilute sulphuric acid R* and 2 ml of *zinc iodide and starch solution R*. The solution does not become blue within 2 min.

Chlorides (*2.4.4*). If intended for ophthalmic use, it complies with the test for chlorides. Dissolve 2.5 g in *water R* and dilute to 15 ml with the same solvent. The solution complies with the limit test for chlorides (20 ppm).

Sulphates (*2.4.13*). Dilute 10 ml of solution S to 15 ml with *distilled water R*. The solution complies with the limit test for sulphates (150 ppm).

Ammonium (*2.4.1*). 1 ml of solution S complies with the limit test (A) for ammonium (100 ppm). If intended for ophthalmic use, not more than 50 ppm of ammonium.

Calcium (*2.4.3*). Dilute 10 ml of solution S to 15 ml with *distilled water R*. The solution complies with the limit test for calcium (100 ppm). If intended for ophthalmic use, not more than 50 ppm of calcium.

Iron (*2.4.9*). Dilute 5 ml of solution S to 10 ml with *water R*. The solution complies with the limit test for iron (20 ppm). If intended for ophthalmic use, not more than 10 ppm of iron.

Sodium. Not more than 0.1 per cent of Na, determined by atomic emission spectrometry (*2.2.22, Method II*).

Test solution. Dissolve 1.00 g in *water R* and dilute to 100.0 ml with the same solvent.

Reference solutions. Prepare the reference solutions using *sodium standard solution (200 ppm Na) R*, diluted as necessary with *water R*.

Measure the emission intensity at 589 nm.

Heavy metals (*2.4.8*). 12 ml of solution S complies with limit test A for heavy metals (10 ppm). Prepare the standard using *lead standard solution (1 ppm Pb) R*.

Loss on drying (*2.2.32*). Not more than 0.5 per cent determined on 1.000 g by drying in an oven at 100 °C to 105 °C.

ASSAY

Prepare a chromatography column 0.3 m long and 10 mm in internal diameter and filled with 10 g of *strongly acidic cation-exchange resin R* covered with *carbon dioxide-free water R*. Maintain a 1 cm layer of liquid above the resin at all times. Allow 100 ml of *dilute hydrochloric acid R* to run through the column at a flow rate of about 5 ml/min. Wash the column (with the tap completely open) with *carbon dioxide-free water R* until neutral to *blue litmus paper R*. Dissolve 0.200 g of the substance to be examined in 2 ml of *carbon dioxide-free water R* in a beaker and transfer it to the column reservoir, allow the solution to run through the column at a flow rate of about 3 ml/min and collect the eluate. Wash the beaker with 10 ml of *carbon dioxide-free water R* and transfer this solution at the same flow rate to the column before it runs dry. Finally wash the column with 200 ml of *carbon dioxide-free water R* (with the tap completely open) until neutral to *blue litmus paper R*. Titrate the combined eluate and washings with *0.1 M sodium hydroxide*, using 1 ml of *phenolphthalein solution R* as indicator.

1 ml of *0.1 M sodium hydroxide* is equivalent to 10.11 mg of KNO_3.

LABELLING

The label states, where applicable, that the substance is suitable for ophthalmic use.

01/2005:1987

POTASSIUM PERCHLORATE

Kalii perchloras

$KClO_4$ M_r 138.6

DEFINITION

Content: 99.0 per cent to 102.0 per cent.

CHARACTERS

Appearance: white, crystalline powder or colourless crystals.

Solubility: sparingly soluble in water, practically insoluble in alcohol.

IDENTIFICATION

A. Dissolve 0.1 g in 5 ml of *water R*. Add 5 ml of *indigo carmine solution R* and heat to boiling. The colour of the solution does not disappear.

B. It complies with the test for chlorates and chlorides (see Tests).

C. Heat 10 mg over a flame for 2 min. Dissolve the residue in 2 ml of *water R*. The solution gives reaction (a) of chlorides (*2.3.1*).

D. Dissolve 50 mg with heating in 5 ml of *water R*. Allow to cool to room temperature. The solution gives reaction (a) of potassium (*2.3.1*).

TESTS

Solution S. Suspend 5.0 g in 90 ml of *distilled water R* and heat to boiling. Allow to cool. Filter. Dilute the filtrate to 100 ml with *carbon dioxide-free water R*.

Appearance of solution. The solution is clear (*2.2.1*) and colourless (*2.2.2, Method II*).

Dissolve 0.20 g in *water R* and dilute to 20 ml with the same solvent.

Acidity or alkalinity. To 5 ml of solution S add 5 ml of *water R* and 0.1 ml of *phenolphthalein solution R*. Not more than 0.25 ml of *0.01 M sodium hydroxide* is required to change the colour of the indicator. To 5 ml of solution S, add 5 ml of *water R* and 0.1 ml of *bromocresol green solution R*. Not more than 0.25 ml of *0.01 M hydrochloric acid* is required to change the colour of the indicator.

Chlorates and chlorides (*2.4.4*): maximum 100 ppm (calculated as chlorides).

To 5 ml of solution S, add 5 ml of *water R* and heat to boiling. Add 1 ml of *nitric acid R* and 0.1 g of *sodium nitrite R*. Allow to cool to room temperature. Dilute to 15 ml

Monographs P

with *water R*. The solution complies with the limit test for chlorides. Prepare the standard using 5 ml of *chloride standard solution (5 ppm Cl) R* and 10 ml of *water R*, and adding only 1 ml of *dilute nitric acid R*.

Sulphates (*2.4.13*): maximum 100 ppm.

15 ml of solution S complies with the limit test for sulphates. Prepare the standard using a mixture of 7.5 ml of *sulphate standard solution (10 ppm SO_4) R* and 7.5 ml of *water R*.

Calcium (*2.4.3*): maximum 100 ppm.

15 ml of solution S complies with the limit test for calcium. Prepare the standard using a mixture of 7.5 ml of *calcium standard solution (10 ppm Ca) R*, 1 ml of *dilute acetic acid R* and 7.5 ml of *distilled water R*.

Heavy metals (*2.4.8*): maximum 20 ppm.

12 ml of solution S complies with limit test A. Prepare the standard using *lead standard solution (1 ppm Pb) R*.

ASSAY

Prepare a chromatography column 0.3 m long and 10 mm in internal diameter and filled with 10 g of *strongly acidic ion-exchange resin R* covered with *carbon dioxide-free water R*. Maintain a 1 cm layer of liquid above the resin throughout the determination. Allow 100 ml of *dilute hydrochloric acid R* to run through the column at a flow rate of about 5 ml/min. Wash the column (with the tap completely open) with *carbon dioxide-free water R* until the eluate is neutral to *blue litmus paper R*. Dissolve 0.100 g of the substance to be examined in 10 ml of *carbon dioxide-free water R* in a beaker and transfer it to the column reservoir, allow the solution to run through the column at a flow rate of about 3 ml/min and collect the eluate. Wash the beaker 3 times with 10 ml of *carbon dioxide-free water R* and transfer this solution at the same flow rate to the column before it runs dry. Finally, wash the column with 200 ml of *carbon dioxide-free water R* (with the tap completely open) until the eluate is neutral to *blue litmus paper R*. Titrate the combined eluate and washings with *0.1 M sodium hydroxide*, using 1 ml of *phenolphthalein solution R* as indicator.

1 ml of *0.1 M sodium hydroxide* is equivalent to 13.86 mg of $KClO_4$.

01/2005:0121

POTASSIUM PERMANGANATE

Kalii permanganas

$KMnO_4$ M_r 158.0

DEFINITION

Potassium permanganate contains not less than 99.0 per cent and not more than the equivalent of 100.5 per cent of $KMnO_4$.

CHARACTERS

A dark purple or brownish-black, granular powder or dark purple or almost black crystals, usually having a metallic lustre, soluble in cold water, freely soluble in boiling water. It decomposes on contact with certain organic substances.

IDENTIFICATION

A. Dissolve about 50 mg in 5 ml of *water R* and add 1 ml of *alcohol R* and 0.3 ml of *dilute sodium hydroxide solution R*. A green colour develops. Heat to boiling. A dark brown precipitate is formed.

B. Filter the mixture obtained in identification test A. The filtrate gives reaction (b) of potassium (*2.3.1*).

TESTS

Solution S. Dissolve 0.75 g in 25 ml of *distilled water R*, add 3 ml of *alcohol R* and boil for 2 min to 3 min. Cool, dilute to 30 ml with *distilled water R* and filter.

Appearance of solution. Solution S is colourless (*2.2.2, Method II*).

Substances insoluble in water. Dissolve 0.5 g in 50 ml of *water R* and heat to boiling. Filter through a tared sintered-glass filter (16). Wash with *water R* until the filtrate is colourless and collect the residue on the filter. The residue, dried in an oven at 100 °C to 105 °C, weighs not more than 5 mg (1.0 per cent).

Chlorides (*2.4.4*). 10 ml of solution S diluted to 15 ml with *water R* complies with the limit test for chlorides (200 ppm).

Sulphates (*2.4.13*). 12 ml of solution S diluted to 15 ml with *distilled water R* complies with the limit test for sulphates (500 ppm).

ASSAY

Dissolve 0.300 g in *water R* and dilute to 100.0 ml with the same solvent. To 20.0 ml of the solution add 20 ml of *water R*, 1 g of *potassium iodide R* and 10 ml of *dilute hydrochloric acid R*. Titrate the liberated iodine with *0.1 M sodium thiosulphate*, using 1 ml of *starch solution R* as indicator.

1 ml of *0.1 M sodium thiosulphate* is equivalent to 3.160 mg of $KMnO_4$.

01/2005:1986

POTASSIUM SODIUM TARTRATE TETRAHYDRATE

Kalii natrii tartras tetrahydricus

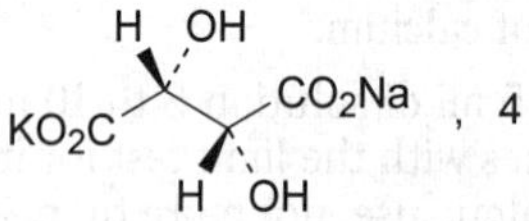

$C_4H_4KNaO_6,4H_2O$ M_r 282.2

DEFINITION

Potassium sodium (+)-(2*R*,3*R*)-2,3-dihydroxybutanedioate tetrahydrate.

Content: 98.0 per cent to 101.0 per cent (anhydrous substance).

CHARACTERS

Appearance: white, crystalline powder or colourless, transparent crystals.

Solubility: very soluble in water, practically insoluble in alcohol.

IDENTIFICATION

A. It complies with the test for specific optical rotation (see Tests).

B. It gives reaction (b) of tartrates (*2.3.1*).

C. It gives reaction (b) of potassium (*2.3.1*).

D. It gives reaction (a) of sodium (*2.3.1*).

TESTS

Solution S. Dissolve 5.000 g in *carbon dioxide-free water R*, prepared from *distilled water R*, and dilute to 100.0 ml with the same solvent.

Appearance of solution. Solution S is clear (*2.2.1*) and colourless (*2.2.2, Method II*).

Acidity or alkalinity. To 5 ml of solution S, add 0.1 ml of *phenolphthalein solution R*. Not more than 0.5 ml of *0.01 M hydrochloric acid* or *0.01 M sodium hydroxide* is required to change the colour of the indicator.

Specific optical rotation (*2.2.7*): + 28.0 to + 30.0 (anhydrous substance), determined on solution S.

Chlorides (*2.4.4*): maximum 100 ppm.

Dilute 10 ml of solution S to 15 ml with *water R*. The solution complies with the limit test for chlorides.

Sulphates (*2.4.13*): maximum 50 ppm.

Dissolve 1.0 g in *distilled water R* and dilute to 15 ml with the same solvent. The solution complies with the limit test for sulphates. Prepare the reference solution with a mixture of 5 ml of *sulphate standard solution (10 ppm SO_4) R* and 10 ml of *distilled water R*.

Ammonium (*2.4.1*): maximum 40 ppm.

5 ml of solution S complies with the limit test for ammonium.

Barium and oxalates. To 5 ml of solution S, add 3 ml of *calcium sulphate solution R*. Allow to stand for 5 min. Any opalescence in the solution is not more intense than that in a mixture of 3 ml of *calcium sulphate solution R* and 5 ml of *distilled water R*.

Calcium (*2.4.3*): maximum 200 ppm.

Dilute 10 ml of solution S to 15 ml with *distilled water R*. The solution complies with the limit test for calcium.

Heavy metals (*2.4.8*): maximum 10 ppm.

Dissolve 2.0 g in *water R* and dilute to 20 ml with the same solvent. 12 ml of the solution complies with limit test A. Prepare the standard using *lead standard solution (1 ppm Pb) R*

Water (*2.5.12*): 24.0 per cent to 26.5 per cent, determined on 50.0 mg. Use 50 ml of *anhydrous methanol R*. Titrate slowly.

ASSAY

To 0.100 g of finely powdered substance add 40 ml of *anhydrous acetic acid R* and 20 ml of *acetic anhydride R*. Titrate slowly with *0.1 M perchloric acid*, determining the end-point potentiometrically (*2.2.20*).

1 ml of *0.1 M perchloric acid* is equivalent to 10.51 mg of $C_4H_4KNaO_6$.

01/2005:0618

POTASSIUM SORBATE

Kalii sorbas

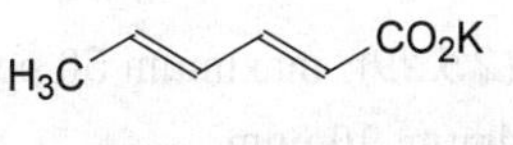

$C_6H_7KO_2$ M_r 150.2

DEFINITION

Potassium sorbate contains not less than 99.0 per cent and not more than the equivalent of 101.0 per cent of potassium (*E,E*)-hexa-2,4-dienoate, calculated with reference to the dried substance.

CHARACTERS

White or almost white powder or granules, very soluble in water, slightly soluble in alcohol.

IDENTIFICATION

First identification: B, D.

Second identification: A, C, D.

A. Dissolve 50.0 mg in *water R* and dilute to 250.0 ml with the same solvent. Dilute 2.0 ml of this solution to 200.0 ml with *0.1 M hydrochloric acid*. Examined between 230 nm and 350 nm (*2.2.25*), the solution shows a maximum at 264 nm. The specific absorbance at the maximum is 1650 to 1900.

B. Examine by infrared absorption spectrophotometry (*2.2.24*), comparing with the spectrum obtained with *potassium sorbate CRS*.

C. Dissolve 1.0 g in 50 ml of *water R*, add 10 ml of *dilute hydrochloric acid R* and shake. Filter the crystalline precipitate, wash with *water R* and dry in a vacuum over *sulphuric acid R* for 4 h. The residue obtained melts (*2.2.14*) at 132 °C to 136 °C.

D. Dissolve 0.2 g in 2 ml of *water R* and add 2 ml of *dilute acetic acid R*. Filter. The solution gives reaction (b) of potassium (*2.3.1*).

TESTS

Solution S. Dissolve 2.5 g in *carbon dioxide-free water R* and dilute to 50 ml with the same solvent.

Appearance of solution. Solution S is clear (*2.2.1*) and not more intensely coloured than reference solution Y_5 (*2.2.2, Method II*).

Acidity or alkalinity. To 20 ml of solution S add 0.1 ml of *phenolphthalein solution R*. Not more than 0.25 ml of *0.1 M sodium hydroxide* or *0.1 M hydrochloric acid* is required to change the colour of the indicator.

Aldehydes. Dissolve 1.0 g in a mixture of 30 ml of *water R* and 50 ml of *2-propanol R*, adjust the solution to pH 4 with *1 M hydrochloric acid* and dilute to 100 ml with *water R*. To 10 ml of the solution add 1 ml of *decolorised fuchsin solution R* and allow to stand for 30 min. Any colour in the solution is not more intense than that in a standard prepared at the same time by adding 1 ml of *decolorised fuchsin solution R* to a mixture of 1.5 ml of *acetaldehyde standard solution (100 ppm C_2H_4O) R*, 4 ml of *2-propanol R* and 4.5 ml of *water R* (0.15 per cent, calculated as C_2H_4O).

Heavy metals (*2.4.8*). 2.0 g complies with limit test D for heavy metals (10 ppm). Prepare the standard using 2 ml of *lead standard solution (10 ppm Pb) R*.

Loss on drying (*2.2.32*). Not more than 1.0 per cent, determined on 1.000 g by drying in an oven at 100 °C to 105 °C for 3 h.

ASSAY

Dissolve 0.120 g in 20 ml of *anhydrous acetic acid R*. Titrate with *0.1 M perchloric acid* using 0.1 ml of *crystal violet solution R* as indicator until the colour changes from violet to bluish-green.

1 ml of *0.1 M perchloric acid* is equivalent to 15.02 mg of $C_6H_7KO_2$.

STORAGE

Store protected from light.

Monographs P

01/2005:1622

POTASSIUM SULPHATE

Kalii sulfas

K_2SO_4 M_r 174.3

DEFINITION

Content: 98.5 per cent to 101.0 per cent of K_2SO_4 (dried substance).

CHARACTERS

Appearance: white, crystalline powder or colourless crystals.

Solubility: soluble in water, practically insoluble in ethanol.

IDENTIFICATION

A. It gives the reactions of sulphates (*2.3.1*).

B. It gives the reactions of potassium (*2.3.1*).

TESTS

Solution S. Dissolve 10.0 g in 90 ml of *carbon dioxide-free water R* prepared from *distilled water R*, heating gently. Allow to cool and dilute to 100 ml with *carbon dioxide-free water R* prepared from *distilled water R*.

Appearance of solution. Solution S is clear (*2.2.1*) and colourless (*2.2.2, Method II*).

Acidity or alkalinity. To 10 ml of solution S add 0.1 ml of *bromothymol blue solution R1*. Not more than 0.5 ml of *0.01 M hydrochloric acid* or *0.01 M sodium hydroxide* is required to change the colour of the indicator.

Chlorides (*2.4.4*): maximum 40 ppm.

Dilute 12.5 ml of solution S to 15 ml with *water R*.

Calcium (*2.4.3*): maximum 200 ppm.

Dilute 5 ml of solution S to 15 ml with *distilled water R*.

Iron (*2.4.9*): maximum 10 ppm, determined on 10 ml of solution S.

Magnesium: maximum 20 ppm.

To 5 ml of solution S add 5 ml of *water R*, 1 ml of *glycerol (85 per cent) R*, 0.15 ml of *titan yellow solution R*, 0.25 ml of *ammonium oxalate solution R* and 5 ml of *dilute sodium hydroxide solution R* and shake. Any pink colour in the test solution is not more intense than that in a standard prepared at the same time and in the same manner using a mixture of 1 ml of *magnesium standard solution (10 ppm Mg) R* and 9 ml of *water R*.

Sodium: maximum 0.10 per cent.

Atomic emission spectrometry (*2.2.22, Method I*).

Test solution. Dissolve 1.00 g of the substance to be examined in *water R* and dilute to 100.0 ml with the same solvent.

Reference solutions. Dissolve in *water R* 0.50 g of *sodium chloride R*, previously dried at 100-105 °C for 3 h, and dilute to 1000.0 ml with the same solvent (200 μg of Na per millilitre). Dilute as required.

Wavelength: 589 nm.

Heavy metals (*2.4.8*): maximum 20 ppm.

12 ml of solution S complies with limit test A. Prepare the standard using *lead standard solution (2 ppm Pb) R*.

Loss on drying (*2.2.32*): maximum 1.0 per cent, determined on 1.000 g by drying in an oven at 130 °C for 4 h.

ASSAY

Dissolve 0.150 g in 40 ml of *water R*. Add 0.2 ml of *0.1 M hydrochloric acid* and 80 ml of *methanol R*. Carry out a potentiometric titration (*2.2.20*), using *0.1 M lead nitrate* and as indicator electrode a lead-selective electrode and as reference electrode a silver-silver chloride electrode.

1 ml of *0.1 M lead nitrate* is equivalent to 17.43 mg of K_2SO_4.

01/2005:0355

POTATO STARCH

Solani amylum

DEFINITION

Potato starch is obtained from the tuber of *Solanum tuberosum* L.

CHARACTERS

Appearance: very fine, white powder which creaks when pressed between the fingers.

Solubility: practically insoluble in cold water and in alcohol.

Potato starch does not contain starch grains of any other origin. It may contain a minute quantity, if any, of tissue fragments of the original plant.

IDENTIFICATION

A. Examined under a microscope using a mixture of equal volumes of *glycerol R* and *water R*, it presents granules, either irregularly shaped, ovoid or pear-shaped, usually 30 μm to 100 μm in size but occasionally exceeding 100 μm, or rounded, 10 μm to 35 μm in size. There are occasional compound granules having 2 to 4 components. The ovoid and pear-shaped granules have an eccentric hilum and the rounded granules acentric or slightly eccentric hilum. All granules show clearly visible concentric striations. Between crossed nicol prisms, the granules show a distinct black cross intersecting at the hilum.

B. Suspend 1 g in 50 ml of *water R*, boil for 1 min and cool. A thick, opalescent mucilage is formed.

C. To 1 ml of the mucilage obtained in identification test B, add 0.05 ml of *iodine solution R1*. An orange-red to dark blue colour is produced which disappears on heating.

TESTS

pH (*2.2.3*): 5.0 to 8.0.

Shake 5.0 g with 25.0 ml of *carbon dioxide-free water R* for 60 s. Allow to stand for 15 min.

Foreign matter. Examined under a microscope using a mixture of equal volumes of *glycerol R* and *water R*, not more than traces of matter other than starch granules are present. No starch grains of any other origin are present.

Oxidising substances (*2.5.30*): maximum 20 ppm, calculated as H_2O_2.

Sulphur dioxide (*2.5.29*): maximum 50 ppm.

Iron (*2.4.9*): maximum 10 ppm.

Shake 1.5 g with 15 ml of *dilute hydrochloric acid R*. Filter. The filtrate complies with the limit test for iron.

Loss on drying (*2.2.32*): maximum 20.0 per cent, determined on 1.000 g by drying in an oven at 130 °C for 90 min.

Sulphated ash (*2.4.14*): maximum 0.6 per cent, determined on 1.0 g.

Microbial contamination. Total viable aerobic count (*2.6.12*) not more than 10^3 bacteria and not more than 10^2 fungi per gram, determined by plate count. It complies with the test for *Escherichia coli* (*2.6.13*).

01/2005:0685
corrected

POVIDONE

Povidonum

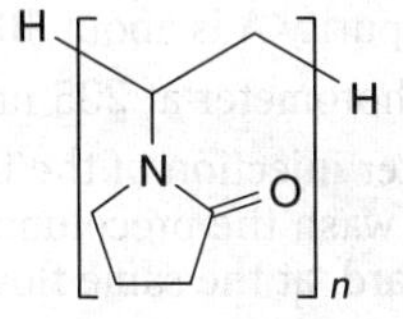

$C_{6n}H_{9n+2}N_nO_n$

DEFINITION

α-Hydro-ω-hydropoly[1-(2-oxopyrrolidin-1-yl)ethylene]. It consists of linear polymers of 1-ethenylpyrrolidin-2-one.

Content: 11.5 per cent to 12.8 per cent of nitrogen (N; A_r 14.01) (anhydrous substance).

The different types of povidone are characterised by their viscosity in solution, expressed as a *K*-value.

The *K*-value of povidone having a stated *K*-value of 15 or less is 85.0 per cent to 115.0 per cent of the stated value.

The *K*-value of povidone having a stated *K*-value or a stated *K*-value range with an average of more than 15 is 90.0 per cent to 108.0 per cent of the stated value or of the average of the stated range.

CHARACTERS

Appearance: white or yellowish-white powder or flakes, hygroscopic.

Solubility: freely soluble in water, in alcohol and in methanol, slightly soluble in acetone.

IDENTIFICATION

First identification: A, E.

Second identification: B, C, D, E.

A. Infrared absorption spectrophotometry (*2.2.24*).

Preparation: dry the substances previously at 105 °C for 6 h. Record the spectra using 4 mg of substance.
Comparison: *povidone CRS*.

B. To 0.4 ml of solution S1 (see Tests) add 10 ml of *water R*, 5 ml of *dilute hydrochloric acid R* and 2 ml of *potassium dichromate solution R*. An orange-yellow precipitate is formed.

C. To 1 ml of solution S1 add 0.2 ml of *dimethylaminobenzaldehyde solution R1* and 0.1 ml of *sulphuric acid R*. A pink colour is produced.

D. To 0.1 ml of solution S1 add 5 ml of *water R* and 0.2 ml of *0.05 M iodine*. A red colour is produced.

E. It is freely soluble in *water R*.

TESTS

Solution S. Dissolve 1.0 g in *carbon dioxide-free water R* and dilute to 20 ml with the same solvent. Add the substance to be examined to the water in small portions with magnetic stirring.

Solution S1. Dissolve 2.5 g in *carbon dioxide-free water R* and dilute to 25 ml with the same solvent. Add the substance to be examined to the water in small portions with magnetic stirring.

Appearance of solution. Solution S is clear (*2.2.1*) and not more intensely coloured than reference solution B_6, BY_6 or R_6 (*2.2.2, Method II*).

pH (*2.2.3*): 3.0 to 5.0 for solution S, for povidone having a stated *K*-value of at most 30; 4.0 to 7.0 for solution S, for povidone having a stated *K*-value of more than 30.

Viscosity, expressed as *K*-value. For povidone having a stated value of 18 or less, use a 50 g/l solution. For povidone having a declared value of more than 18, use a 10 g/l solution. For povidone having a declared value of more than 95, use a 1.0 g/l solution. Allow to stand for 1 h and determine the viscosity (*2.2.9*) of the solution at 25 °C, using viscometer No.1 with a minimum flow time of 100 s. Calculate the *K*-value from the expression:

$$\frac{1.5\log\eta - 1}{0.15 + 0.003c} + \frac{\sqrt{300c\log\eta + (c + 1.5c\log\eta)^2}}{0.15c + 0.003c^2}$$

c = concentration of the substance to be examined, calculated with reference to the anhydrous substance, in grams per 100 ml,

η = viscosity of the solution relative to that of *water R*.

Aldehydes: maximum 500 ppm, expressed as acetaldehyde.

Test solution. Dissolve 1.0 g of the substance to be examined in *phosphate buffer solution pH 9.0 R* and dilute to 100.0 ml with the same solvent. Stopper the flask and heat at 60 °C for 1 h. Allow to cool.

Reference solution. Dissolve 0.140 g of *acetaldehyde ammonia trimer trihydrate R* in *water R* and dilute to 200.0 ml with the same solvent. Dilute 1.0 ml of this solution to 100.0 ml with *phosphate buffer solution pH 9.0 R*.

Into 3 identical spectrophotometric cells with a path length of 1 cm, introduce separately 0.5 ml of the test solution, 0.5 ml of the reference solution and 0.5 ml of *water R* (blank). To each cell, add 2.5 ml of *phosphate buffer solution pH 9.0 R* and 0.2 ml of *nicotinamide-adenine dinucleotide solution R*. Mix and stopper tightly. Allow to stand at 22 ± 2 °C for 2-3 min and measure the absorbance (*2.2.25*) of each solution at 340 nm, using *water R* as the compensation liquid. To each cell, add 0.05 ml of *aldehyde dehydrogenase solution R*, mix and stopper tightly. Allow to stand at 22 ± 2 °C for 5 min. Measure the absorbance of each solution at 340 nm using *water R* as the compensation liquid.

Monographs P

Determine the content of aldehydes using the expression:

$$\frac{(A_{t2} - A_{t1}) - (A_{b2} - A_{b1})}{(A_{s2} - A_{s1}) - (A_{b2} - A_{b1})} \times \frac{100\,000 \times C}{m}$$

A_{t1} = absorbance of the test solution before the addition of aldehyde dehydrogenase,

A_{t2} = absorbance of the test solution after the addition of aldehyde dehydrogenase,

A_{s1} = absorbance of the reference solution before the addition of aldehyde dehydrogenase,

A_{s2} = absorbance of the reference solution after the addition of aldehyde dehydrogenase,

A_{b1} = absorbance of the blank before the addition of aldehyde dehydrogenase,

A_{b2} = absorbance of the blank after the addition of aldehyde dehydrogenase,

m = mass of povidone calculated with reference to the anhydrous substance, in grams,

C = concentration of acetaldehyde in the reference solution, calculated from the weight of the acetaldehyde ammonia trimer trihydrate with the factor 0.72, in milligrams per millilitre.

Peroxides: maximum 400 ppm, expressed as H_2O_2.

Dissolve 2.0 g in 50 ml of *water R*. To 25 ml of this solution, add 2 ml of *titanium trichloride-sulphuric acid reagent R*. Allow to stand for 30 min. The absorbance (*2.2.25*) of the solution, measured at 405 nm using a mixture of 25 ml of a 40 g/l solution of the substance to be examined and 2 ml of a 13 per cent *V/V* solution of *sulphuric acid R* as the compensation liquid, is not greater than 0.35.

Hydrazine. Thin-layer chromatography (*2.2.27*). *Use freshly prepared solutions.*

Test solution. Dissolve 2.5 g of the substance to be examined in 25 ml of *water R*. Add 0.5 ml of a 50 g/l solution of *salicylaldehyde R* in *methanol R*, mix and heat in a water-bath at 60 °C for 15 min. Allow to cool, add 2.0 ml of *toluene R*, shake for 2 min and centrifuge. Use the clear supernatant layer.

Reference solution. Dissolve 9 mg of *salicylaldehyde azine R* in *toluene R* and dilute to 100 ml with the same solvent. Dilute 1 ml of the solution to 10 ml with *toluene R*.

Plate: *TLC silanised silica gel plate R*.

Mobile phase: *water R, methanol R* (1:2 *V/V*).

Application: 10 μl.

Development: over a path of 15 cm.

Drying: in air.

Detection: examine in ultraviolet light at 365 nm.

Limit:

– *hydrazine*: any spot corresponding to salicylaldehyde azine in the chromatogram obtained with the test solution is not more intense than the spot in the chromatogram obtained with the reference solution (1 ppm).

Impurity A. Liquid chromatography (*2.2.29*).

Test solution. Dissolve 0.25 g of the substance to be examined in the mobile phase and dilute to 10.0 ml with the mobile phase.

Reference solution (a). Dissolve 50 mg of *1-vinylpyrrolidin-2-one R* in *methanol R* and dilute to 100.0 ml with the same solvent. Dilute 1.0 ml of the solution to 100.0 ml with *methanol R*. Dilute 5.0 ml of this solution to 100.0 ml with the mobile phase.

Reference solution (b). Dissolve 10 mg of *1-vinylpyrrolidin-2-one R* and 0.5 g of *vinyl acetate R* in *methanol R* and dilute to 100.0 ml with the same solvent. Dilute 1.0 ml of the solution to 100.0 ml with the mobile phase.

Precolumn:

– *size*: *l* = 0.025 m, Ø = 4 mm,

– *stationary phase*: *octadecylsilyl silica gel for chromatography R* (5 μm).

Column:

– *size*: *l* = 0.25 m, Ø = 4 mm,

– *stationary phase*: *octadecylsilyl silica gel for chromatography R* (5 μm),

– *temperature*: 40 °C.

Mobile phase: *acetonitrile R, water R* (10:90 *V/V*).

Flow rate: adjusted so that the retention time of the peak corresponding to impurity A is about 10 min.

Detection: spectrophotometer at 235 nm.

Injection: 50 μl. After injection of the test solution, wait for about 2 min and wash the precolumn by passing the mobile phase backward, at the same flow rate applied in the test, for 30 min.

System suitability:

– *resolution*: minimum 2.0 between the peaks due to impurity A and to vinyl acetate in the chromatogram obtained with reference solution (b),

– *repeatability*: maximum relative standard deviation of 2.0 per cent after 5 injections of reference solution (a).

Limit:

– *impurity A*: not more than the area of the principal peak in the chromatogram obtained with reference solution (a) (10 ppm).

Impurity B. Liquid chromatography (*2.2.29*).

Test solution. Dissolve 100 mg of the substance to be examined in *water R* and dilute to 50.0 ml with the same solvent.

Reference solution. Dissolve 100 mg of *2-pyrrolidone R* in *water R* and dilute to 100 ml with the same solvent. Dilute 3.0 ml to 50.0 ml with *water R*.

Precolumn:

– *size*: *l* = 0.025 m, Ø = 4 mm,

– *stationary phase*: *end-capped octadecylsilyl silica gel for chromatography R* (5 μm).

Column:

– *size*: *l* = 0.25 m, Ø = 4 mm,

– *stationary phase*: spherical *aminohexadecylsilyl silica gel for chromatography R* (5 μm),

– *temperature*: 30 °C.

Mobile phase: *water R*, adjusted to pH 2.4 with *phosphoric acid R*.

Flow rate: 1 ml/min.

Detection: spectrophotometer at 205 nm. A detector is placed between the precolumn and the analytical column. A second detector is placed after the analytical column.

Injection: 10 μl. When impurity B has left the precolumn (after about 1.2 min) switch the flow directly from the pump to the analytical column. Before the next chromatogram is run, wash the precolumn by reversed flow.

System suitability:

– *symmetry factor*: maximum 2.0 for the peak due to impurity B.

Limit:

– *impurity B*: not more than the area of the principal peak in the chromatogram obtained with the reference solution (3.0 per cent).

Heavy metals (*2.4.8*): maximum 10 ppm.

2.0 g complies with limit test D. Prepare the standard using 2.0 ml of *lead standard solution (10 ppm Pb) R*.

Water (*2.5.12*): maximum 5.0 per cent, determined on 0.500 g.

Sulphated ash (*2.4.14*): maximum 0.1 per cent, determined on 1.0 g.

ASSAY

Place 100.0 mg of the substance to be examined (*m* mg) in a combustion flask, add 5 g of a mixture of 1 g of *copper sulphate R*, 1 g of *titanium dioxide R* and 33 g of *dipotassium sulphate R*, and 3 glass beads. Wash any adhering particles from the neck into the flask with a small quantity of *water R*. Add 7 ml of *sulphuric acid R*, allowing it to run down the sides of the flask, and mix the contents by rotation. Close the mouth of the flask loosely, for example by means of a glass bulb with a short stem, to avoid excessive loss of sulphuric acid. Heat gradually at first, then increase the temperature until there is vigorous boiling with condensation of sulphuric acid in the neck of the flask; precautions are to be taken to prevent the upper part of the flask from becoming overheated. Continue the heating for 45 min. Cool, dissolve the solid material by cautiously adding to the mixture 20 ml of *water R*, cool again and place in a steam-distillation apparatus. Add 30 ml of *strong sodium hydroxide solution R* through the funnel, rinse cautiously the funnel with 10 ml of *water R* and distil immediately by passing steam through the mixture. Collect about 80-100 ml of distillate in a mixture of 30 ml of a 40 g/l solution of *boric acid R* and 3 drops of *bromocresol green-methyl red solution R* and enough *water R* to cover the tip of the condenser. Towards the end of the distillation lower the receiver so that the tip of the condenser is above the surface of the acid solution and rinse the end part of the condenser with a small quantity of *water R*. Titrate the distillate with *0.025 M sulphuric acid* until the colour of the solution changes from green through pale greyish-blue to pale greyish-red-purple (n_1 ml of *0.025 M sulphuric acid*).

Repeat the test using about 100.0 mg of *glucose R* in place of the substance to be examined (n_2 ml of *0.025 M sulphuric acid*).

$$\text{percentage content of nitrogen} = \frac{0.7004\ (n_1 - n_2)}{m} \times 100$$

STORAGE

In an airtight container.

LABELLING

The label indicates the nominal *K*-value.

IMPURITIES

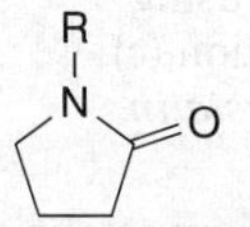

A. R = $CH{=}CH_2$: 1-ethenylpyrrolidin-2-one (1-vinylpyrrolidin-2-one),

B. R = H: pyrrolidin-2-one (2-pyrrolidone).

01/2005:1142

POVIDONE, IODINATED

Povidonum iodinatum

DEFINITION

Complex of iodine and povidone.

Content: 9.0 per cent to 12.0 per cent of available iodine (dried substance).

PRODUCTION

It is produced using povidone that complies with the monograph on *Povidone (0685)*, except that the povidone used may contain not more than 2.0 per cent of formic acid and not more than 8.0 per cent of water.

CHARACTERS

Appearance: yellowish-brown or reddish-brown, amorphous powder.

Solubility: soluble in water and in ethanol (96 per cent), practically insoluble in acetone.

IDENTIFICATION

A. Infrared absorption spectrophotometry (*2.2.24*).

Comparison: *iodinated povidone CRS*.

B. Dissolve 10 mg in 10 ml of *water R* and add 1 ml of *starch solution R*. An intense blue colour is produced.

C. Dissolve 0.1 g in 5 ml of *water R* and add a 10 g/l solution of *sodium sulphite R* dropwise, until the solution becomes colourless. Add 2 ml of *potassium dichromate solution R* and 1 ml of *hydrochloric acid R*. A light brown precipitate is formed.

TESTS

pH (*2.2.3*): 1.5 to 5.0.

Dissolve 1.0 g in 10 ml of *carbon dioxide-free water R*.

Iodide: maximum 6.0 per cent (dried substance).

Dissolve 0.500 g in 100 ml of *water R*. Add *sodium metabisulphite R* until the colour of the iodine has disappeared. Add 25.0 ml of *0.1 M silver nitrate*, 10 ml of *nitric acid R* and 5 ml of *ferric ammonium sulphate solution R2*. Titrate with *0.1 M ammonium thiocyanate*. Carry out a blank titration.

1 ml of *0.1 M silver nitrate* is equivalent to 12.69 mg of total iodine. From the percentage of total iodine, calculated with reference to the dried substance, subtract the percentage of available iodine as determined in the assay to obtain the percentage of iodide.

Loss on drying (*2.2.32*): maximum 8.0 per cent, determined on 0.500 g by drying in an oven at 100-105 °C for 3 h.

Sulphated ash (*2.4.14*): maximum 0.1 per cent, determined on 1.0 g.

ASSAY

Transfer 1.000 g into a ground-glass-stoppered flask containing 150 ml of *water R* and stir for 1 h. Add 0.1 ml of *dilute acetic acid R* and titrate with *0.1 M sodium thiosulphate* using *starch solution R* as indicator.

1 ml of *0.1 M sodium thiosulphate* is equivalent to 12.69 mg of available iodine.

STORAGE

Protected from light.

01/2005:2059
corrected

PRAVASTATIN SODIUM

Pravastatinum natricum

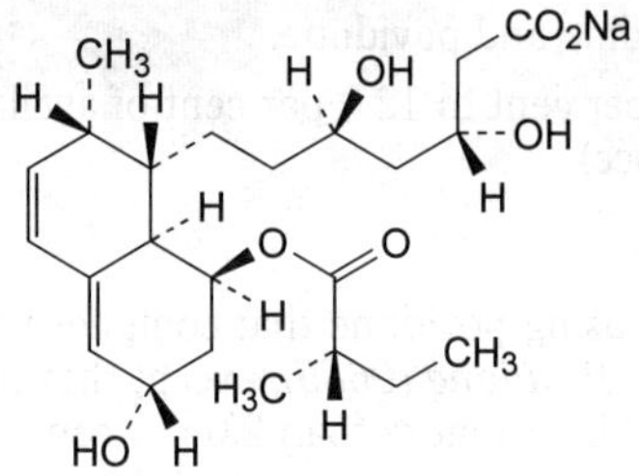

$C_{23}H_{35}NaO_7$ M_r 446.5

DEFINITION

Sodium (3*R*,5*R*)-3,5-dihydroxy-7-[(1*S*,2*S*,6*S*,8*S*,8a*R*)-6-hydroxy-2-methyl-8-[[(2*S*)-2-methylbutanoyl]oxy]-1,2,6,7,8,8a-hexahydronaphthalen-1-yl]heptanoate.

Content: 97.0 per cent to 102.0 per cent (anhydrous and ethanol-free substance).

CHARACTERS

Appearance: white to yellowish white powder or crystalline powder, hygroscopic.

Solubility: freely soluble in water and in methanol, soluble in ethanol.

IDENTIFICATION

A. Specific optical rotation (see Tests).

B. Infrared absorption spectrophotometry (*2.2.24*).

Comparison: *Ph. Eur. reference spectrum of pravastatin sodium.*

C. 1 ml of solution S (see Tests) gives reaction (a) of sodium (*2.3.1*).

TESTS

Solution S. Dissolve 1.00 g in *carbon dioxide free water R* and dilute to 20.0 ml with the same solvent.

Appearance of solution. The solution is clear (*2.2.1*) and not more intensely coloured than reference solution BY_6 (*2.2.2, Method II*).

Dilute 2.0 ml of solution S to 10.0 ml with *water R.*

pH (*2.2.3*): 7.2 to 9.0 for solution S.

Specific optical rotation (*2.2.7*): + 153 to + 159 (anhydrous and ethanol-free substance).

Dilute 2.0 ml of solution S to 20.0 ml with *water R.*

Related substances. Liquid chromatography (*2.2.29*).

Solvent mixture. Mix 9 volumes of *methanol R* with 11 volumes of *water R.*

Test solution (a). Dissolve 0.1000 g of the substance to be examined in the solvent mixture and dilute to 100.0 ml with the solvent mixture.

Test solution (b). Dilute 10.0 ml of test solution (a) to 100.0 ml with the solvent mixture.

Reference solution (a). Dissolve 5.0 mg of the substance to be examined and 5.0 mg of *pravastatin impurity A CRS* in the solvent mixture and dilute to 50.0 ml with the solvent mixture.

Reference solution (b). Dilute 2.0 ml of test solution (a) to 100.0 ml with the solvent mixture. Dilute 1.0 ml to 10.0 ml with the solvent mixture.

Reference solution (c). Dissolve 12.4 mg of *pravastatin 1,1,3,3-tetramethylbutylamine CRS* in the solvent mixture and dilute to 100.0 ml with the solvent mixture.

Column:

– *size*: l = 0.15 m, Ø = 4.6 mm,
– *stationary phase*: *octadecylsilyl silica gel for chromatography R* (5 µm),
– *temperature*: 25 °C.

Mobile phase: *glacial acetic acid R, triethylamine R, methanol R, water R* (1:1:450:550 *V/V/V/V*).

Flow rate: 1.3 ml/min.

Detection: spectrophotometer at 238 nm.

Injection: 10 µl; inject test solution (a) and reference solutions (a) and (b).

Run time: 2.5 times the retention time of pravastatin.

Relative retention with reference to pravastatin (retention time = about 21 min): impurity B = about 0.2; impurity A = about 0.6; impurity C = about 2.1.

System suitability: reference solution (a):

– *resolution*: minimum 7.0 between the peaks due to impurity A and to pravastatin.

Limits:

– *impurity A*: not more than 1.5 times the area of the principal peak in the chromatogram obtained with reference solution (b) (0.3 per cent),
– *any impurity*: not more than the area of the principal peak in the chromatogram obtained with reference solution (b) (0.2 per cent),
– *total*: not more than 3 times the area of the principal peak in the chromatogram obtained with reference solution (b) (0.6 per cent),
– *disregard limit*: 0.25 times the area of the principal peak in the chromatogram obtained with reference solution (b) (0.05 per cent).

Ethanol (*2.4.24, System A*): maximum 3.0 per cent *m/m*.

Heavy metals (*2.4.8*): maximum 20 ppm.

Dissolve 2.0 g of substance to be examined in a mixture of 15 volumes of *water R* and 85 volumes of *methanol R* and dilute to 20 ml with the same mixture of solvents. 12 ml of this solution complies with limit test B. Prepare the standard using lead standard solution (2 ppm Pb) prepared by diluting *lead standard solution (100 ppm Pb) R* with a mixture of 15 volumes of *water R* and 85 volumes of *methanol R*.

Water (*2.5.12*): maximum 4.0 per cent, determined on 0.500 g.

ASSAY

Liquid chromatography (*2.2.29*) as described in the test for related substances.

Injection: test solution (b) and reference solution (c).

Calculate the percentage content of $C_{23}H_{35}NaO_7$ using the chromatogram obtained with reference solution (c) and the declared content of pravastatin in *pravastatin 1,1,3,3-tetramethylbutylamine CRS.*

1 mg of pravastatin is equivalent to 1.052 mg of pravastatin sodium.

STORAGE

In an airtight container.

Monographs P

IMPURITIES

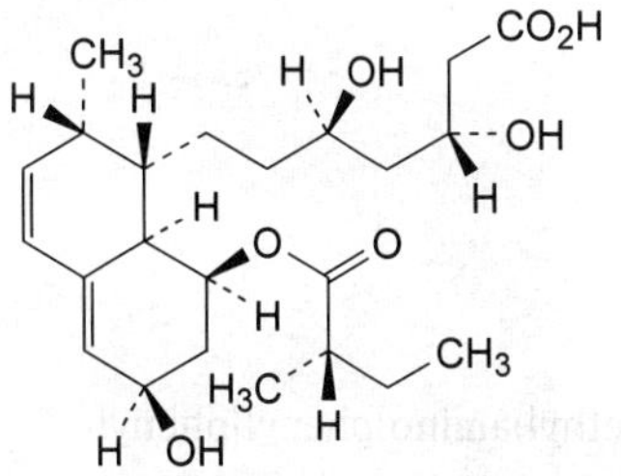

A. (3*R*,5*R*)-3,5-dihydroxy-7-[(1*S*,2*S*,6*R*,8*S*,8a*R*)-6-hydroxy-2-methyl-8-[[(2*S*)-2-methylbutanoyl]oxy]-1,2,6,7,8,8a-hexahydronaphthalen-1-yl]heptanoic acid (6′-epipravastatin),

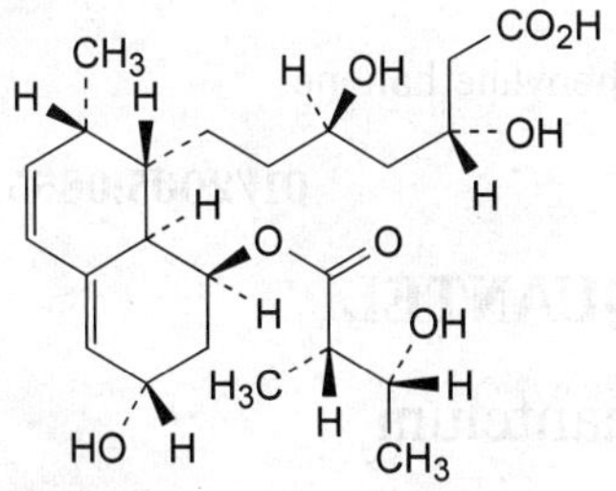

B. (3*R*,5*R*)-3,5-dihydroxy-7-[(1*S*,2*S*,6*S*,8*S*,8a*R*)-6-hydroxy-8-[[(2*S*,3*R*)-3-hydroxy-2-methylbutanoyl]oxy]-2-methyl-1,2,6,7,8,8a-hexahydronaphthalen-1-yl]heptanoic acid (3″-hydroxypravastatin),

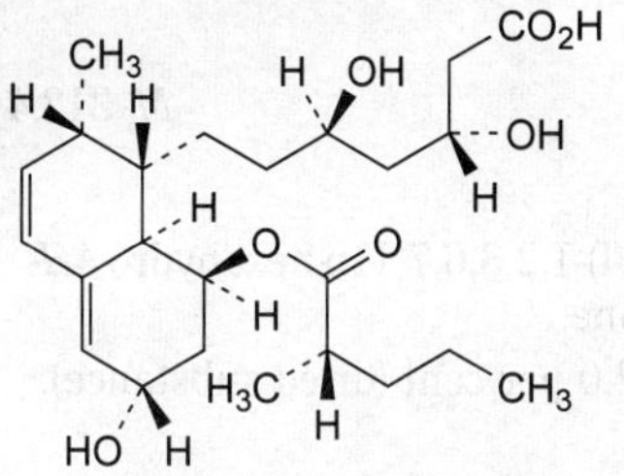

C. (3*R*,5*R*)-3,5-dihydroxy-7-[(1*S*,2*S*,6*S*,8*S*,8a*R*)-6-hydroxy-2-methyl-8-[[(2*S*)-2-methylpentanoyl]oxy]-1,2,6,7,8,8a-hexahydronaphthalen-1-yl]heptanoic acid,

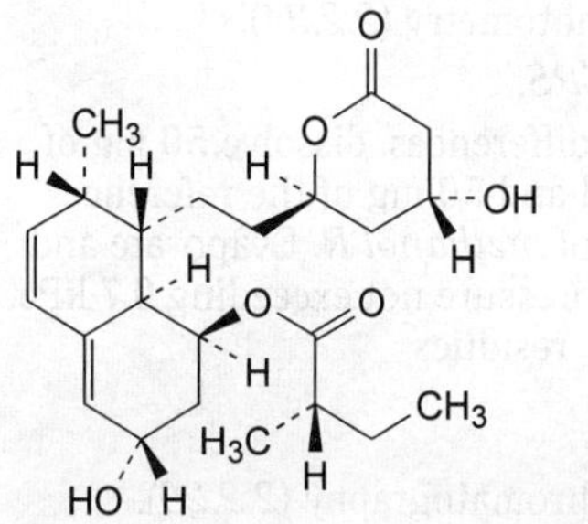

D. (1*S*,3*S*,7*S*,8*S*,8a*R*)-3-hydroxy-8-[2-[(2*R*,4*R*)-4-hydroxy-6-oxotetrahydro-2*H*-pyran-2-yl]ethyl]-7-methyl-1,2,3,7,8,8a-hexahydronaphthalen-1-yl (2*S*)-2-methylbutanoate (pravastatin lactone).

01/2005:1466

PRAZEPAM

Prazepamum

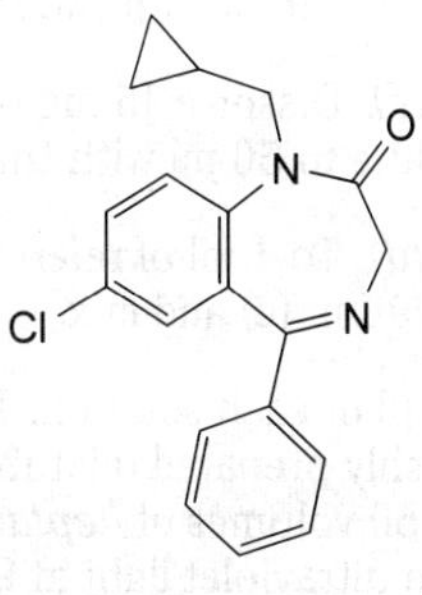

$C_{19}H_{17}ClN_2O$ M_r 324.8

DEFINITION

Prazepam contains not less than 98.5 per cent and not more than the equivalent of 101.0 per cent of 7-chloro-1-(cyclopropylmethyl)-5-phenyl-1,3-dihydro-2*H*-1,4-benzodiazepin-2-one, calculated with reference to the dried substance.

CHARACTERS

A white or almost white, crystalline powder, practically insoluble in water, freely soluble in methylene chloride, sparingly soluble in ethanol.

It melts at about 145 °C.

IDENTIFICATION

First identification: B.

Second identification: A, C.

A. Dissolve 30.0 mg in *alcohol R* and dilute to 100.0 ml with the same solvent. Dilute 20.0 ml of the solution to 100.0 ml (solution A) and 2.0 ml of the solution to 100.0 ml (solution B) with the same solvent. Examined between 300 nm and 350 nm (*2.2.25*), solution A shows an absorption maximum at 312 nm. Examined between 210 nm and 300 nm, solution B shows an absorption maximum at 228 nm and a point of inflexion at about 252 nm. The specific absorbance at the maximum at 228 nm is 900 to 940. The specific absorbance at the maximum at 312 nm is 59 to 63.

B. Examine by infrared absorption spectrophotometry (*2.2.24*), comparing with the spectrum obtained with *prazepam CRS*.

C. Examine the chromatograms obtained in the test for related substances. The principal spot in the chromatogram obtained with test solution (b) is similar in position, fluorescence at 365 nm and size to the principal spot in the chromatogram obtained with reference solution (b).

TESTS

Appearance of solution. Dissolve 0.25 g in *alcohol R* and dilute to 10 ml with the same solvent. The solution is clear (*2.2.1*) and colourless (*2.2.2, Method II*).

Related substances. Examine by thin-layer chromatography (*2.2.27*), using as the coating substance a suitable silica gel with a fluorescent indicator having an optimal intensity at 254 nm.

Test solution (a). Dissolve 0.50 g of the substance to be examined in *acetone R* and dilute to 5 ml with the same solvent.

Test solution (b). Dilute 1 ml of test solution (a) to 100 ml with *acetone R*.

Reference solution (a). Dilute 1 ml of test solution (b) to 10 ml with *acetone R*.

Reference solution (b). Dissolve 10 mg of *prazepam CRS* in *acetone R* and dilute to 10 ml with the same solvent.

Reference solution (c). Dissolve 15 mg of *nordazepam CRS* in *acetone R* and dilute to 50 ml with the same solvent.

Reference solution (d). To 1 ml of reference solution (a) add 1 ml of reference solution (c) and mix.

Apply to the plate 5 µl of each solution. Develop over a path of 10 cm using a freshly prepared mixture of 50 volumes of *ethyl acetate R* and 50 volumes of *heptane R*. Dry the plate in air and examine in ultraviolet light at 254 nm and 365 nm. In the chromatogram obtained with test solution (a): any spot corresponding to nordazepam is not more intense than the spot in the chromatogram obtained with reference solution (c) (0.3 per cent); not more than four additional spots are present, none of which are more intense than the spot in the chromatogram obtained with reference solution (a) (0.1 per cent). The test is not valid unless the chromatogram obtained with reference solution (d) shows two clearly separated spots.

Heavy metals (*2.4.8*). 1.0 g complies with limit test C for heavy metals (20 ppm). Prepare the standard using 2 ml of *lead standard solution (10 ppm Pb) R*.

Loss on drying (*2.2.32*). Not more than 0.5 per cent, determined on 1.000 g by drying in an oven at 100 °C to 105 °C.

Sulphated ash (*2.4.14*). Not more than 0.1 per cent, determined on 1.0 g.

ASSAY

Dissolve 0.250 g in 25 ml of *anhydrous acetic acid R*. Titrate with *0.1 M perchloric acid*, determining the end-point potentiometrically (*2.2.20*).

1 ml of *0.1 M perchloric acid* is equivalent to 32.48 mg of $C_{19}H_{17}ClN_2O$.

STORAGE

Store protected from light.

IMPURITIES

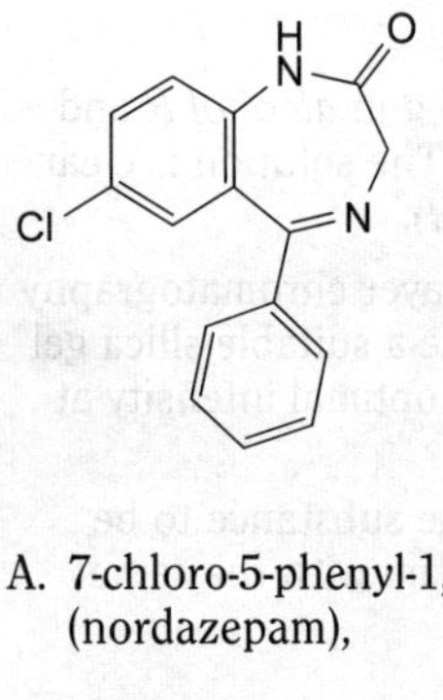

A. 7-chloro-5-phenyl-1,3-dihydro-2*H*-1,4-benzodiazepin-2-one (nordazepam),

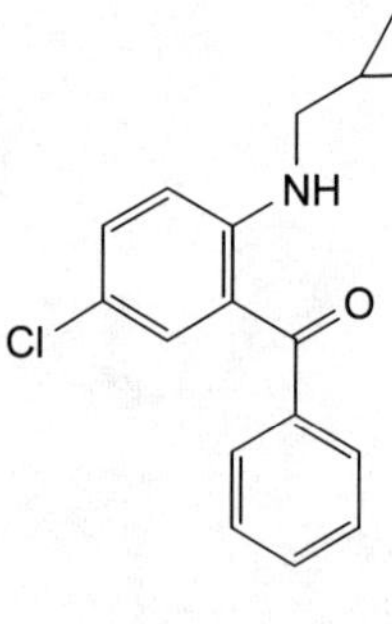

B. [5-chloro-2-[(cyclopropylmethyl)amino]phenyl]phenylmethanone,

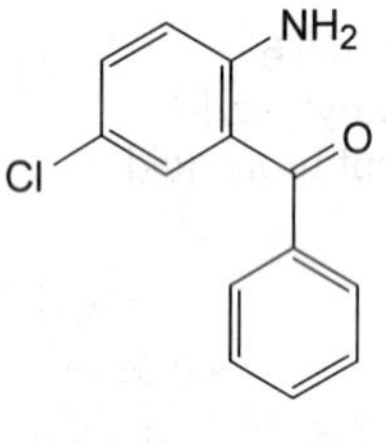

C. (2-amino-5-chlorophenyl)phenylmethanone.

01/2005:0855

PRAZIQUANTEL

Praziquantelum

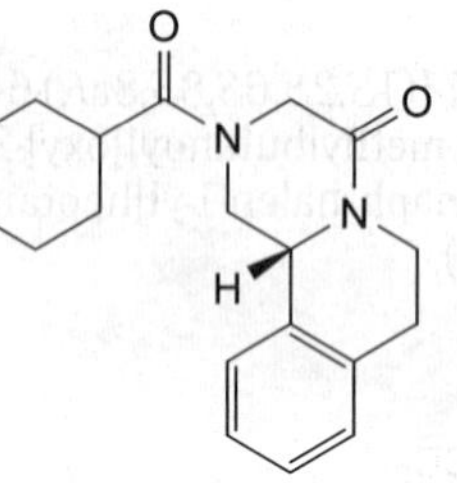

and enantiomer

$C_{19}H_{24}N_2O_2$ M_r 312.4

DEFINITION

(11b*RS*)-2-(Cyclohexylcarbonyl)-1,2,3,6,7,11b-hexahydro-4*H*-pyrazino[2,1-*a*]isoquinolin-4-one.

Content: 97.5 per cent to 102.0 per cent (dried substance).

CHARACTERS

Appearance: white or almost white, crystalline powder.

Solubility: very slightly soluble in water, freely soluble in alcohol and in methylene chloride.

It shows polymorphism.

IDENTIFICATION

Infrared absorption spectrophotometry (*2.2.24*).

Comparison: *praziquantel CRS.*

If the spectra obtained show differences, dissolve 50 mg of the substance to be examined and 50 mg of the reference substance separately in 2 ml of *methanol R*. Evaporate and dry the residue at 60 °C at a pressure not exceeding 0.7 kPa. Record new spectra using the residues.

TESTS

Related substances. Liquid chromatography (*2.2.29*).

Test solution (a). Dissolve 40.0 mg of the substance to be examined in the mobile phase and dilute to 10.0 ml with the mobile phase.

Test solution (b). Dilute 1.0 ml of test solution (a) to 20.0 ml with the mobile phase.

Reference solution (a). Dissolve 40.0 mg of *praziquantel CRS* in the mobile phase and dilute to 10.0 ml with the mobile phase. Dilute 1.0 ml to 20.0 ml with the mobile phase.

Reference solution (b). Dissolve 5 mg of *praziquantel impurity A CRS* in reference solution (a) and dilute to 25.0 ml with reference solution (a). Dilute 2.0 ml of this solution to 20.0 ml with the mobile phase.

Reference solution (c). Dilute 1.0 ml of test solution (a) to 20.0 ml with the mobile phase. Dilute 5.0 ml of this solution to 50.0 ml with the mobile phase.

Column:

- *size*: *l* = 0.25 m, Ø = 4.0 mm,
- *stationary phase*: *octadecylsilyl silica gel for chromatography R* (5 µm).

Mobile phase: *acetonitrile R, water R* (45:55 *V/V*).

Flow rate: 1 ml/min.

Detection: spectrophotometer at 210 nm.

Injection: 20 µl; inject test solution (a) and reference solutions (b) and (c).

Run time: 5 times the retention time of praziquantel (retention time = about 9 min).

System suitability: reference solution (b):

- *resolution*: minimum 3.0 between the peaks corresponding to impurity A and praziquantel.

Limits:

- *any impurity*: not more than the area of the principal peak in the chromatogram obtained with reference solution (c) (0.5 per cent), not more than 1 such peak having an area greater than 0.4 times the area of the principal peak in the chromatogram obtained with reference solution (c) (0.2 per cent),
- *total*: not more than the area of the principal peak in the chromatogram obtained with reference solution (c) (0.5 per cent),
- *disregard limit*: 0.1 times the area of the principal peak in the chromatogram obtained with reference solution (c) (0.05 per cent).

Heavy metals (*2.4.8*): maximum 20 ppm.

1.0 g complies with limit test C. Prepare the standard using 2 ml of *lead standard solution (10 ppm Pb) R*.

Loss on drying (*2.2.32*): maximum 0.5 per cent, determined on 1.000 g by drying in an oven at 50 °C over *diphosphorus pentoxide R* at a pressure not exceeding 0.7 kPa for 2 h.

Sulphated ash (*2.4.14*): maximum 0.1 per cent, determined on 1.0 g.

ASSAY

Liquid chromatography (*2.2.29*) as described in the test for related substances with the following modification.

Injection: test solution (b) and reference solution (a).

Calculate the percentage content of $C_{19}H_{24}N_2O_2$.

STORAGE

Protected from light.

IMPURITIES

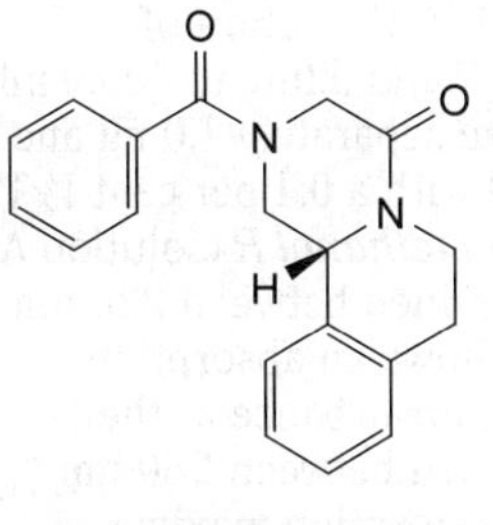

and enantiomer

A. (11b*RS*)-2-benzoyl-1,2,3,6,7,11b-hexahydro-4*H*-pyrazino[2,1-*a*]isoquinolin-4-one,

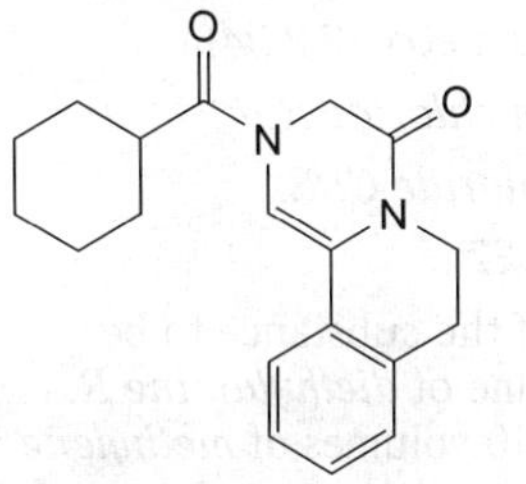

B. 2-(cyclohexylcarbonyl)-2,3,6,7-tetrahydro-4*H*-pyrazino[2,1-*a*]isoquinolin-4-one,

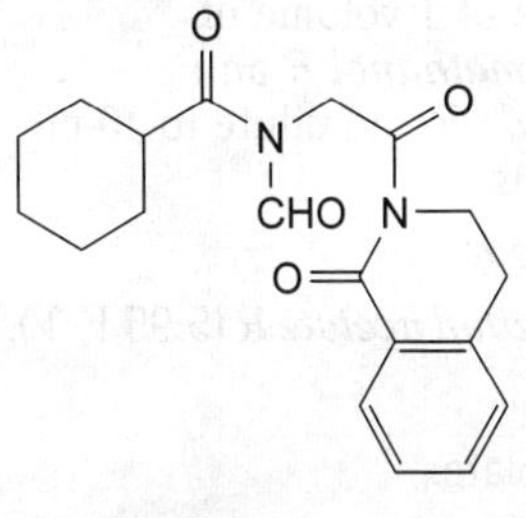

C. *N*-formyl-*N*-[2-oxo-2-(1-oxo-3,4-dihydroisoquinolin-2(1*H*)-yl)ethyl]cyclohexanecarboxamide.

01/2005:0856

PRAZOSIN HYDROCHLORIDE

Prazosini hydrochloridum

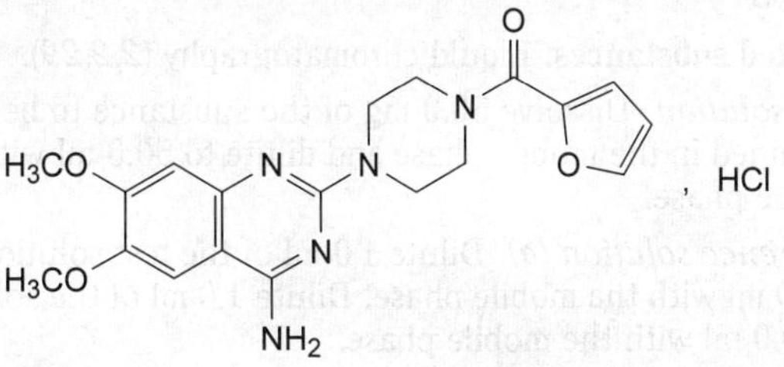

$C_{19}H_{22}ClN_5O_4$ M_r 419.9

DEFINITION

1-(4-Amino-6,7-dimethoxyquinazolin-2-yl)-4-(furan-2-ylcarbonyl)piperazine hydrochloride.

Content: 98.5 per cent to 101.0 per cent (anhydrous substance).

CHARACTERS

Appearance: white or almost white powder.

Solubility: very slightly soluble in water, slightly soluble in alcohol and in methanol, practically insoluble in acetone.

IDENTIFICATION

First identification: B, D.

Second identification: *A, C, D.*

A. Dissolve 50.0 mg in a 0.1 per cent *V/V* solution of *hydrochloric acid R* in *methanol R* and dilute to 100.0 ml with the same acid solution. Dilute separately 1.0 ml and 5.0 ml of this solution to 100.0 ml with a 0.1 per cent *V/V* solution of *hydrochloric acid R* in *methanol R* (solution A and solution B, respectively). Examined between 220 nm and 280 nm (*2.2.25*), solution A shows an absorption maximum at 247 nm. The specific absorbance at the maximum is 1320 to 1400. Examined between 280 nm and 400 nm, solution B shows 2 absorption maxima, at 330 nm and 343 nm. The specific absorbances at the maxima are 260 to 280 and 240 to 265, respectively.

B. Infrared absorption spectrophotometry (*2.2.24*).

Preparation: discs of *potassium chloride R*.

Comparison: *prazosin hydrochloride CRS*.

C. Thin-layer chromatography (*2.2.27*).

Test solution. Dissolve 10 mg of the substance to be examined in a mixture of 1 volume of *diethylamine R*, 10 volumes of *methanol R* and 10 volumes of *methylene chloride R* and dilute to 10 ml with the same mixture of solvents.

Reference solution. Dissolve 10 mg of *prazosin hydrochloride CRS* in a mixture of 1 volume of *diethylamine R*, 10 volumes of *methanol R* and 10 volumes of *methylene chloride R* and dilute to 10 ml with the same mixture of solvents.

Plate: *TLC silica gel* GF_{254} *plate R*.

Mobile phase: *diethylamine R*, *ethyl acetate R* (5:95 *V/V*).

Application: 10 µl.

Development: over 2/3 of the plate.

Drying: in a current of warm air.

Detection: examine in ultraviolet light at 254 nm.

Results: the principal spot in the chromatogram obtained with the test solution is similar in position and size to the principal spot in the chromatogram obtained with the reference solution.

D. Dissolve about 2 mg in 2 ml of *water R*. The solution gives reaction (a) of chlorides (*2.3.1*).

TESTS

Related substances. Liquid chromatography (*2.2.29*).

Test solution. Dissolve 50.0 mg of the substance to be examined in the mobile phase and dilute to 50.0 ml with the mobile phase.

Reference solution (a). Dilute 1.0 ml of the test solution to 100.0 ml with the mobile phase. Dilute 1.0 ml of the solution to 10.0 ml with the mobile phase.

Reference solution (b). Dissolve 8 mg of *metoclopramide hydrochloride CRS* in 1 ml of the test solution and dilute to 25.0 ml with the mobile phase. Dilute 1.0 ml of the solution to 10.0 ml with the mobile phase.

Column:

- *size*: l = 0.25 m, Ø = 4.6 mm,
- *stationary phase*: *octadecylsilyl silica gel for chromatography R* (5 µm),

Mobile phase: mix 50 volumes of *methanol R* and 50 volumes of a solution containing 3.484 g/l of *sodium pentanesulphonate R* and 3.64 g/l of *tetramethylammonium hydroxide R* adjusted to pH 5.0 with *glacial acetic acid R*.

Flow rate: 1 ml/min.

Detection: spectrophotometer at 254 nm.

Injection: 20 µl.

Run time: 6 times the retention time of prazosin.

Retention times: prazosin = about 9 min; metoclopramide = about 5 min.

System suitability: reference solution (b):

- *resolution*: minimum 8 between the peaks due to metoclopramide and to prazosin.

Limits:

- *any impurity*: not more than twice the area of the principal peak in the chromatogram obtained with reference solution (a) (0.2 per cent),
- *total*: not more than 5 times the area of the principal peak in the chromatogram obtained with reference solution (a) (0.5 per cent),
- *disregard limit*: 0.5 times the area of the principal peak in the chromatogram obtained with reference solution (a) (0.05 per cent).

Iron: maximum 100 ppm.

Atomic absorption spectrometry (*2.2.23, Method I*).

Test solution. To 1.0 g add dropwise about 1.5 ml of *nitric acid R*. After fuming has subsided, evaporate on a water-bath and ignite by gradually raising the temperature from 150 °C to 1000 °C, maintaining the final temperature for 1 h. Cool, dissolve the residue in 20 ml of *dilute hydrochloric acid R*, evaporate to about 5 ml and dilute to 25.0 ml with *dilute hydrochloric acid R*.

Reference solutions. Prepare the reference solutions using *iron standard solution (8 ppm Fe) R*, diluted as necessary with *water R*.

Source: iron hollow-cathode lamp.

Wavelength: 248 nm.

Flame: air-acetylene.

Nickel: maximum 50 ppm.

Atomic absorption spectrometry (*2.2.23, Method I*).

Test solution. Use the test solution prepared in the test for iron.

Reference solutions. Prepare the reference solutions using *nickel standard solution (10 ppm Ni) R*, diluted as necessary with *water R*.

Source: nickel hollow-cathode lamp.

Wavelength: 232 nm.

Flame: air-acetylene.

Water (*2.5.12*): maximum 0.5 per cent, determined on 1.000 g. Use a mixture of equal volumes of *methanol R* and *methylene chloride R* as the solvent.

Sulphated ash (*2.4.14*): maximum 0.1 per cent, determined on 1.0 g.

ASSAY

In order to avoid overheating in the reaction medium, mix thoroughly throughout and stop the titration immediately after the end-point has been reached.

Dissolve 0.350 g in a mixture of 20 ml of *anhydrous formic acid R* and 30 ml of *acetic anhydride R*. Titrate quickly with *0.1 M perchloric acid*, determining the end-point potentiometrically (*2.2.20*).

1 ml of *0.1 M perchloric acid* is equivalent to 41.99 mg of $C_{19}H_{22}ClN_5O_4$.

STORAGE

Protected from light.

IMPURITIES

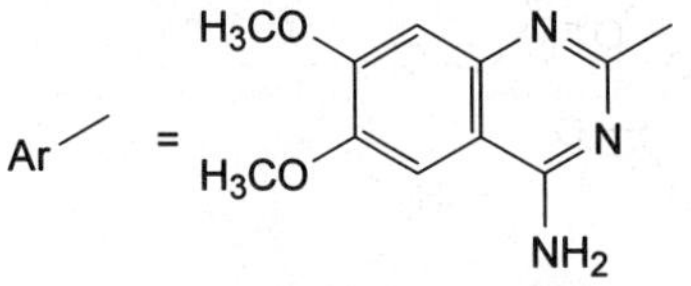

A. Ar-Cl: 2-chloro-6,7-dimethoxyquinazolin-4-amine,

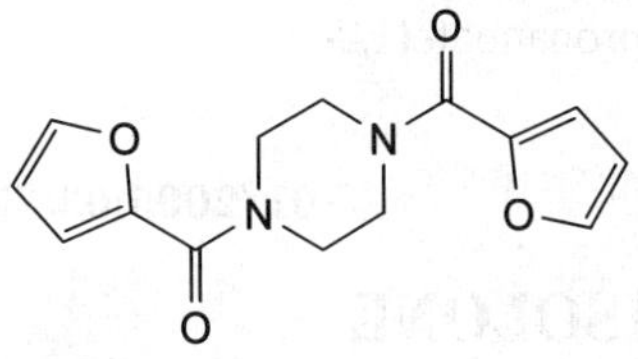

B. 1,4-bis(furan-2-ylcarbonyl)piperazine,

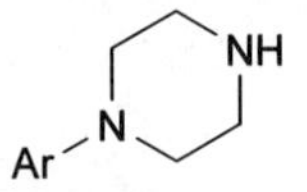

C. 6,7-dimethoxy-2-(piperazin-1-yl)quinazolin-4-amine,

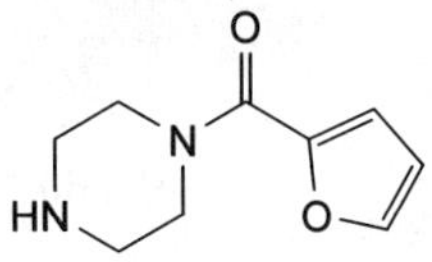

D. 1-(furan-2-ylcarbonyl)piperazine,

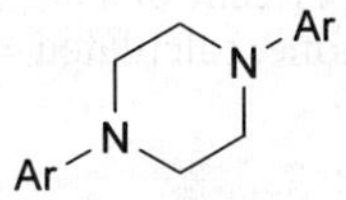

E. 2,2′-(piperazin-1,4-diyl)bis(6,7-dimethoxyquinazolin-4-amine).

01/2005:1467

PREDNICARBATE

Prednicarbatum

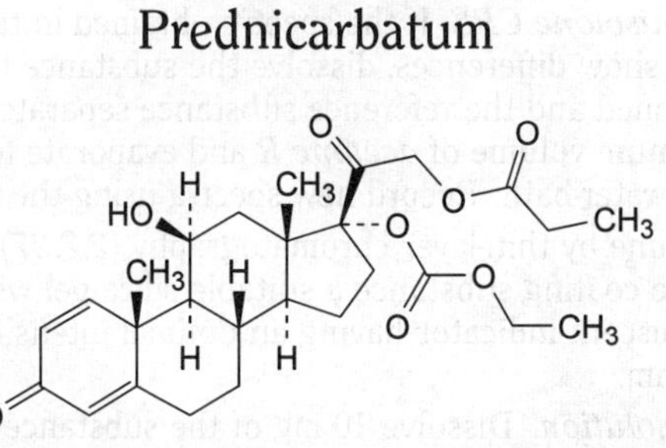

$C_{27}H_{36}O_8$ M_r 488.6

DEFINITION

Prednicarbate contains not less than 97.0 per cent and not more than the equivalent of 102.0 per cent of 11β-hydroxy-3,20-dioxopregna-1,4-diene-17,21-diyl 17-ethylcarbonate 21-propanoate, calculated with reference to the dried substance.

CHARACTERS

A white or almost white, crystalline powder, practically insoluble in water, freely soluble in alcohol and in acetone, sparingly soluble in propylene glycol.

It shows polymorphism.

IDENTIFICATION

A. Examine by infrared absorption spectrophotometry (*2.2.24*), comparing with the spectrum obtained with *prednicarbate CRS*. If the spectra obtained in the solid state show differences, dissolve the substance to be examined and the reference substance separately in the minimum volume of *alcohol R*, evaporate to dryness on a water-bath and record the spectra again using the residues.

B. Examine by thin-layer chromatography (*2.2.27*), using a *TLC silica gel F_{254} plate R*.

Test solution. Dissolve 10 mg of the substance to be examined in a mixture of 1 volume of *methanol R* and 9 volumes of *methylene chloride R* and dilute to 10 ml with the same mixture of solvents.

Reference solution (a). Dissolve 10 mg of *prednicarbate CRS* in a mixture of 1 volume of *methanol R* and 9 volumes of *methylene chloride R* and dilute to 10 ml with the same mixture of solvents.

Reference solution (b). Dissolve 5 mg of *prednisolone acetate CRS* in 5 ml of reference solution (a).

Apply to the plate 5 µl of each solution. Prepare the mobile phase by adding a mixture of 1.2 volumes of *water R* and 8 volumes of *methanol R* to a mixture of 15 volumes of *ether R* and 77 volumes of *methylene chloride R*. Develop over a path of 15 cm. Allow the plate to dry in air and examine in ultraviolet light at 254 nm. The principal spot in the chromatogram obtained with the test solution is similar in position and size to the principal spot in the chromatogram obtained with reference solution (a). Spray the plate with *alcoholic solution of sulphuric acid R*. Heat at 120 °C for 10 min or until the spots appear. Allow to cool. Examine in daylight and in ultraviolet light at 365 nm. The principal spot in the chromatogram obtained with the test solution is similar in position, colour in daylight, fluorescence in ultraviolet light at 365 nm and size to the principal spot in the chromatogram obtained with reference solution (a). The test is not valid unless the chromatogram obtained with reference solution (b) shows two clearly separated spots.

TESTS

Specific optical rotation (*2.2.7*). Dissolve 0.250 g in *alcohol R* and dilute to 25.0 ml with the same solvent. The specific optical rotation is + 60 to + 66, calculated with reference to the dried substance.

Related substances. Examine by liquid chromatography (*2.2.29*) as described under Assay.

Inject 20 µl of reference solution (a). Adjust the sensitivity of the system so that the heights of the two principal peaks in the chromatogram obtained are about 50 per cent of the full scale of the recorder. When the chromatograms are recorded in the conditions described above, the retention times are: prednicarbate about 17 min and impurity F about 19 min. The test is not valid unless the resolution between the peaks corresponding to prednicarbate and impurity F is at least 3.0; if this resolution is not achieved, adjust the composition of the mobile phase.

Inject 20 µl of the test solution and 20 µl of reference solution (b). Continue the chromatography for twice the retention time of the principal peak. In the chromatogram obtained with the test solution: the area of any peak corresponding to impurity F is not greater than twice the area of the principal peak in the chromatogram obtained with reference solution (b) (1 per cent); the area of any peak, apart from the principal peak and a peak corresponding to impurity F, is not greater than the area of the principal peak in the chromatogram obtained with reference solution (b) (0.5 per cent); the sum of the areas of all the peaks, apart from the principal peak, is not greater than four times the area of the principal peak in the chromatogram obtained with reference solution (b) (2 per cent). Disregard any peak with an area less than 0.025 times the area of the principal peak in the chromatogram obtained with reference solution (b).

Loss on drying (*2.2.32*). Not more than 0.5 per cent, determined on 1.000 g by drying in an oven at 100 °C to 105 °C.

ASSAY

Examine by liquid chromatography (*2.2.29*). *Prepare the solutions immediately before use.*

Test solution. Dissolve 30.0 mg of the substance to be examined in the mobile phase and dilute to 50.0 ml with the mobile phase.

Reference solution (a). Dissolve 3 mg of *prednicarbate impurity F CRS* in the mobile phase, add 5.0 ml of the test solution and dilute to 100.0 ml with the mobile phase. Dilute 1.0 ml to 10.0 ml with the mobile phase.

Reference solution (b). Dilute 1.0 ml of the test solution to 200.0 ml with the mobile phase.

Reference solution (c). Dissolve 30.0 mg of *prednicarbate CRS* in the mobile phase and dilute to 50.0 ml with the mobile phase.

The chromatographic procedure may be carried out using:

– a stainless steel column 0.125 m long and 4 mm in internal diameter packed with *octadecylsilyl silica gel for chromatography R* (5 µm),
– as mobile phase at a flow rate of 0.7 ml/min a mixture of 5 volumes of *acetonitrile R* and 6 volumes of *water R*,
– as detector a spectrophotometer set at 243 nm.

Inject 20 µl of reference solution (a). When the chromatograms are recorded in the prescribed conditions the retention times are: prednicarbate about 17 min and impurity F about 19 min. The test is not valid unless the resolution between the peaks corresponding to prednicarbate and impurity F is not less than 3.0; if this resolution is not achieved, adjust the composition of the mobile phase.

Inject 20 µl of reference solution (c). Adjust the sensitivity of the system so that the height of the principal peak in the chromatogram obtained is at least 50 per cent of the full scale of the recorder.

Inject 20 µl of the test solution.

Calculate the percentage content of prednicarbate.

STORAGE

Store protected from light.

IMPURITIES

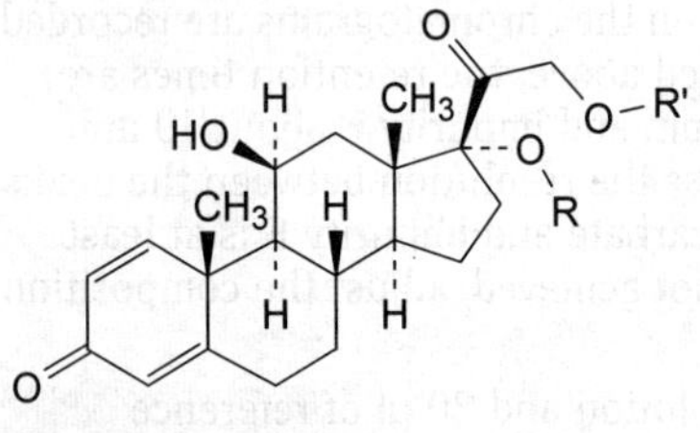

A. R = R′ = H: prednisolone,

B. R = CO-O-C_2H_5, R′ = H: prednisolone 17-ethylcarbonate,

C. R = H, R′ = CO-C_2H_5: prednisolone 21-propanoate,

D. R = H, R′ = CO-O-C_2H_5: prednisolone 21-ethylcarbonate,

E. R = CO-O-C_2H_5, R′ = CO-CH_3: prednisolone 21-acetate 17-ethylcarbonate,

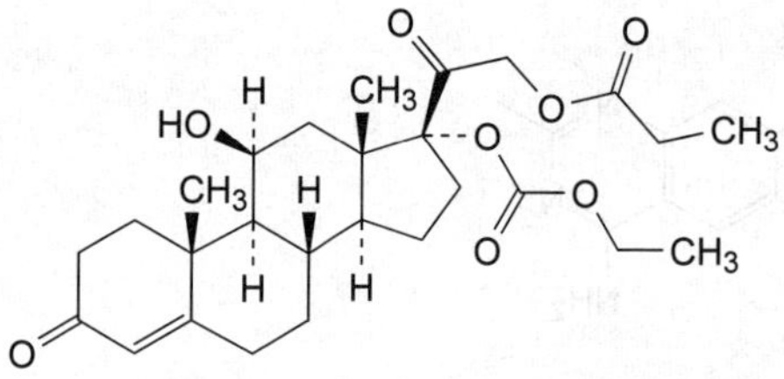

F. 11β-hydroxy-3,20-dioxopregn-4-ene-17,21-diyl 17-ethylcarbonate 21-propanoate(1,2-dihydroprednicarbate).

01/2005:0353

PREDNISOLONE

Prednisolonum

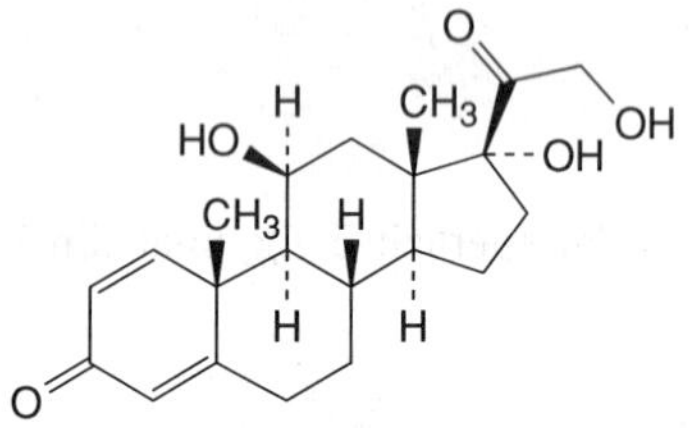

$C_{21}H_{28}O_5$ M_r 360.4

DEFINITION

Prednisolone contains not less than 97.0 per cent and not more than the equivalent of 103.0 per cent of 11β,17,21-trihydroxypregna-1,4-diene-3,20-dione, calculated with reference to the dried substance.

CHARACTERS

A white or almost white, crystalline powder, hygroscopic, very slightly soluble in water, soluble in alcohol and in methanol, sparingly soluble in acetone, slightly soluble in methylene chloride.

It shows polymorphism.

IDENTIFICATION

A. Examine by infrared absorption spectrophotometry (*2.2.24*), comparing with the spectrum obtained with *prednisolone CRS*. If the spectra obtained in the solid state show differences, dissolve the substance to be examined and the reference substance separately in the minimum volume of *acetone R* and evaporate to dryness on a water-bath. Record new spectra using the residues.

B. Examine by thin-layer chromatography (*2.2.27*), using as the coating substance a suitable silica gel with a fluorescent indicator having an optimal intensity at 254 nm.

Test solution. Dissolve 10 mg of the substance to be examined in a mixture of 1 volume of *methanol R* and 9 volumes of *methylene chloride R* and dilute to 10 ml with the same mixture of solvents.

Reference solution (a). Dissolve 20 mg of *prednisolone CRS* in a mixture of 1 volume of *methanol R* and 9 volumes of *methylene chloride R* and dilute to 20 ml with the same mixture of solvents.

Reference solution (b). Dissolve 10 mg of *hydrocortisone CRS* in reference solution (a) and dilute to 10 ml with reference solution (a).

Apply to the plate 5 µl of each solution. Develop over a path of 15 cm using a mixture of 10 volumes of *methanol R* and 90 volumes of *methylene chloride R*. Allow the plate to dry in air and examine in ultraviolet

Monographs P

light at 254 nm. The principal spot in the chromatogram obtained with the test solution is similar in position and size to the principal spot in the chromatogram obtained with reference solution (a). Spray with *alcoholic solution of sulphuric acid R*. Heat at 120 °C for 10 min or until the spots appear. Allow to cool. Examine the chromatograms in daylight and in ultraviolet light at 365 nm. The principal spot in the chromatogram obtained with the test solution is similar in position, colour in daylight, fluorescence in ultraviolet light at 365 nm and size to the principal spot in the chromatogram obtained with reference solution (a). The test is not valid unless the chromatogram obtained with reference solution (b) shows 2 clearly separated spots.

TESTS

Specific optical rotation (*2.2.7*). Dissolve 0.250 g in *dioxan R* and dilute to 25.0 ml with the same solvent. The specific optical rotation is + 96 to + 102, calculated with reference to the dried substance.

Related substances. Examine by liquid chromatography (*2.2.29*).

Test solution. Dissolve 25.0 mg of the substance to be examined in 2 ml of *tetrahydrofuran R* and dilute to 10.0 ml with *water R*.

Reference solution (a). Dissolve 2 mg of *prednisolone CRS* and 2 mg of *hydrocortisone CRS* in the mobile phase and dilute to 100.0 ml with the mobile phase.

Reference solution (b). Dilute 1.0 ml of the test solution to 100.0 ml with the mobile phase.

The chromatographic procedure may be carried out using:

- a stainless steel column 0.25 m long and 4.6 mm in internal diameter packed with *base-deactivated end-capped octadecylsilyl silica gel for chromatography R* (5 μm),
- as mobile phase at a flow rate of 1 ml/min a mixture prepared as follows: in a 1000 ml volumetric flask mix 220 ml of *tetrahydrofuran R* with 700 ml of *water R* and allow to equilibrate; dilute to 1000 ml with *water R* and mix again,
- as detector a spectrophotometer set at 254 nm,

maintaining the temperature of the column at 45 °C.

Equilibrate the column with the mobile phase at a flow rate of 1 ml/min for about 30 min.

Adjust the sensitivity of the system so that the height of the principal peak in the chromatogram obtained with 20 μl of reference solution (b) is at least 50 per cent of the full scale of the recorder.

Inject 20 μl of reference solution (a). When the chromatograms are recorded in the prescribed conditions, the retention times are: prednisolone about 14 min and hydrocortisone about 15.5 min. The test is not valid unless in the chromatogram obtained with reference solution (a) the resolution between the peaks due to prednisolone and hydrocortisone is at least 2.2. If necessary, adjust the concentration of *tetrahydrofuran R* in the mobile phase.

Inject separately 20 μl of the solvent mixture of the test solution as a blank, 20 μl of the test solution and 20 μl of reference solution (b). Continue the chromatography of the test solution for 4.5 times the retention time of the principal peak. In the chromatogram obtained with the test solution: the area of any peak, apart from the principal peak, is not greater than the area of the principal peak in the chromatogram obtained with reference solution (b) (1 per cent) and not more than one such peak has an area greater than half the area of the principal peak in the chromatogram obtained with reference solution (b) (0.5 per cent); the sum of the areas of all the peaks, apart from the principal peak, is not greater than 2.0 times the area of the principal peak in the chromatogram obtained with reference solution (b) (2 per cent). Disregard any peak obtained with the blank run and any peak with an area less than 0.05 times the area of the principal peak in the chromatogram obtained with reference solution (b).

Loss on drying (*2.2.32*). Not more than 1.0 per cent, determined on 0.500 g by drying in an oven at 100-105 °C.

ASSAY

Dissolve 0.100 g in *alcohol R* and dilute to 100.0 ml with the same solvent. Dilute 2.0 ml of the solution to 100.0 ml with *alcohol R*. Measure the absorbance (*2.2.25*) at the maximum at 243.5 nm.

Calculate the content of $C_{21}H_{28}O_5$ taking the specific absorbance to be 415.

STORAGE

Store in an airtight container, protected from light.

IMPURITIES

A. hydrocortisone.

01/2005:0734

PREDNISOLONE ACETATE

Prednisoloni acetas

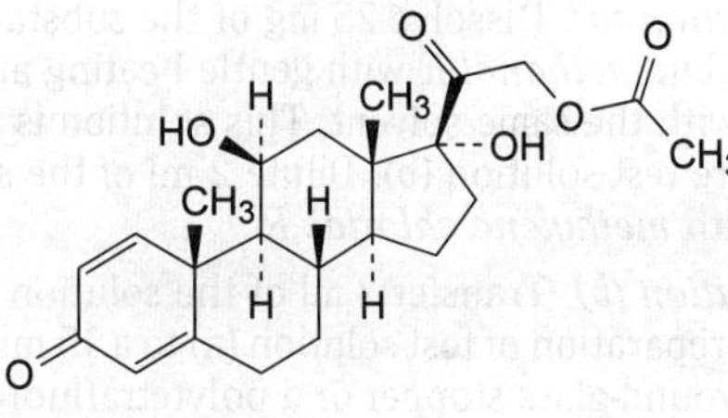

$C_{23}H_{30}O_6$ M_r 402.5

DEFINITION

Prednisolone acetate contains not less than 97.0 per cent and not more than the equivalent of 103.0 per cent of 11β,17-dihydroxy-3,20-dioxopregna,-1,4-dien-21-yl acetate, calculated with reference to the dried substance.

CHARACTERS

A white or almost white, crystalline powder, practically insoluble in water, slightly soluble in alcohol and in methylene chloride.

It melts at about 230 °C, with decomposition.

IDENTIFICATION

First identification: A, B.

Second identification: C, D, E.

A. Examine by infrared absorption spectrophotometry (*2.2.24*), comparing with the spectrum obtained with *prednisolone acetate CRS*. Examine the substances prepared as discs.

B. Examine by thin-layer chromatography (*2.2.27*), using as the coating substance a suitable silica gel with a fluorescent indicator having an optimal intensity at 254 nm.

Test solution. Dissolve 10 mg of the substance to be examined in a mixture of 1 volume of *methanol R* and 9 volumes of *methylene chloride R* and dilute to 10 ml with the same mixture of solvents.

Monographs P

Reference solution (a). Dissolve 20 mg of *prednisolone acetate CRS* in a mixture of 1 volume of *methanol R* and 9 volumes of *methylene chloride R* and dilute to 20 ml with the same mixture of solvents.

Reference solution (b). Dissolve 10 mg of *prednisolone pivalate CRS* in reference solution (a) and dilute to 10 ml with the same solution.

Apply separately to the plate 5 µl of each solution. Prepare the mobile phase by adding a mixture of 1.2 volumes of *water R* and 8 volumes of *methanol R* to a mixture of 15 volumes of *ether R* and 77 volumes of *methylene chloride R*. Develop over a path of 15 cm. Allow the plate to dry in air and examine in ultraviolet light at 254 nm. The principal spot in the chromatogram obtained with the test solution is similar in position and size to the principal spot in the chromatogram obtained with reference solution (a). Spray the plate with *alcoholic solution of sulphuric acid R*. Heat at 120 °C for 10 min or until the spots appear. Allow to cool. Examine in daylight and in ultraviolet light at 365 nm. The principal spot in the chromatogram obtained with the test solution is similar in position, colour in daylight, fluorescence in ultraviolet light at 365 nm and size to the principal spot in the chromatogram obtained with reference solution (a). The test is not valid unless the chromatogram obtained with reference solution (b) shows two clearly separated spots.

C. Examine by thin-layer chromatography (*2.2.27*), using as the coating substance a suitable silica gel with a fluorescent indicator having an optimal intensity at 254 nm.

Test solution (a). Dissolve 25 mg of the substance to be examined in *methanol R* with gentle heating and dilute to 5 ml with the same solvent. This solution is also used to prepare test solution (b). Dilute 2 ml of the solution to 10 ml with *methylene chloride R*.

Test solution (b). Transfer 2 ml of the solution obtained during preparation of test solution (a) to a 15 ml glass tube with a ground-glass stopper or a polytetrafluoroethylene cap. Add 10 ml of *saturated methanolic potassium hydrogen carbonate solution R* and immediately pass a stream of *nitrogen R* briskly through the solution for 5 min. Stopper the tube. Heat in a water-bath at 45 °C, protected from light, for 2 h 30 min. Allow to cool.

Reference solution (a). Dissolve 25 mg of *prednisolone acetate CRS* in *methanol R* with gentle heating and dilute to 5 ml with the same solvent. This solution is also used to prepare reference solution (b). Dilute 2 ml of the solution to 10 ml with *methylene chloride R*.

Reference solution (b). Transfer 2 ml of the solution obtained during preparation of reference solution (a) to a 15 ml glass tube with a ground-glass stopper or a polytetrafluoroethylene cap. Add 10 ml of *saturated methanolic potassium hydrogen carbonate solution R* and immediately pass a stream of *nitrogen R* briskly through the solution for 5 min. Stopper the tube. Heat in a water-bath at 45 °C, protected from light, for 2 h 30 min. Allow to cool.

Apply separately to the plate 5 µl of each solution. Prepare the mobile phase by adding a mixture of 1.2 volumes of *water R* and 8 volumes of *methanol R* to a mixture of 15 volumes of *ether R* and 77 volumes of *methylene chloride R*. Develop over a path of 15 cm. Allow the plate to dry in air and examine in ultraviolet light at 254 nm. The principal spot in each of the chromatograms obtained with the test solutions is similar in position and size to the principal spot in the chromatogram obtained with the corresponding reference solution. Spray the plate with *alcoholic solution of sulphuric acid R*. Heat at 120 °C for 10 min or until the spots appear. Allow to cool. Examine in daylight and in ultraviolet light at 365 nm. The principal spot in each of the chromatograms obtained with the test solutions is similar in position, colour in daylight, fluorescence in ultraviolet light at 365 nm and size to the principal spot in the chromatogram obtained with the corresponding reference solution. The principal spot in each of the chromatograms obtained with test solution (b) and reference solution (b) has an R_f value distinctly lower than that of the principal spots in each of the chromatograms obtained with test solution (a) and reference solution (a).

D. Add about 2 mg to 2 ml of *sulphuric acid R* and shake to dissolve. Within 5 min, an intense red colour develops. When examined in ultraviolet light at 365 nm, a reddish-brown fluorescence is seen. Add the solution to 10 ml of *water R* and mix. The colour fades and there is greenish-yellow fluorescence in ultraviolet light at 365 nm.

E. About 10 mg gives the reaction of acetyl (*2.3.1*).

TESTS

Specific optical rotation (*2.2.7*). Dissolve 0.250 g in *dioxan R* and dilute to 25.0 ml with the same solvent. The specific optical rotation is + 112 to + 119, calculated with reference to the dried substance.

Related substances. Examine by liquid chromatography (*2.2.29*).

Test solution. Dissolve 25.0 mg of the substance to be examined in *methanol R* and dilute to 10.0 ml with the same solvent.

Reference solution (a). Dissolve 2 mg of *prednisolone acetate CRS* and 2 mg of *hydrocortisone acetate CRS* in the mobile phase and dilute to 100.0 ml with the mobile phase.

Reference solution (b). Dilute 1.0 ml of the test solution to 100.0 ml with the mobile phase.

The chromatographic procedure may be carried out using:

– a stainless steel column 0.25 m long and 4.6 mm in internal diameter, packed with *base-deactivated end-capped octadecylsilyl silica gel for chromatography R* (5 µm),
– as mobile phase at a flow rate of 1 ml/min a mixture prepared as follows: in a 1000 ml volumetric flask mix 350 ml of *acetonitrile R* with 600 ml of *water R* and allow to equilibrate; adjust the volume to 1000 ml with *water R* and mix again,
– as detector a spectrophotometer set at 254 nm.

Equilibrate the column with the mobile phase at a flow rate of 1 ml/min for about 30 min.

Adjust the sensitivity of the system so that the height of the principal peak in the chromatogram obtained with 20 µl of reference solution (b) is at least 50 per cent of the full scale of the recorder.

Inject 20 µl of reference solution (a). When the chromatograms are recorded in the prescribed conditions, the retention times are: prednisolone acetate, about 24 min and hydrocortisone acetate, about 26 min. The test is not valid unless the resolution between the peaks corresponding to prednisolone acetate and hydrocortisone acetate is at least 2.5; if necessary, adjust the concentration of acetonitrile in the mobile phase.

Inject separately 20 µl of the test solution and 20 µl of reference solution (b). Continue the chromatography for 2.5 times the retention time of the principal peak in the chromatogram obtained with the test solution. In the chromatogram obtained with the test solution: the area of

Monographs P

any peak, apart from the principal peak, is not greater than the area of the principal peak in the chromatogram obtained with reference solution (b) (1 per cent) and not more than one such peak has an area greater than half the area of the principal peak in the chromatogram obtained with reference solution (b) (0.5 per cent); the sum of the areas of all the peaks, apart from the principal peak, is not greater than twice the area of the principal peak in the chromatogram obtained with reference solution (b) (2 per cent). Disregard any peak due to the solvent and any peak with an area less than 0.05 times the area of the principal peak in the chromatogram obtained with reference solution (b).

Loss on drying (*2.2.32*). Not more than 0.5 per cent, determined on 1.000 g by drying in an oven at 100 °C to 105 °C.

ASSAY

Dissolve 0.100 g in *alcohol R* and dilute to 100.0 ml with the same solvent. Dilute 2.0 ml of the solution to 100.0 ml with *alcohol R*. Measure the absorbance (*2.2.25*) at the maximum at 243 nm.

Calculate the content of $C_{23}H_{30}O_6$ taking the specific absorbance to be 370.

STORAGE

Store protected from light.

IMPURITIES

A. hydrocortisone acetate,

B. prednisolone.

01/2005:0736

PREDNISOLONE PIVALATE

Prednisoloni pivalas

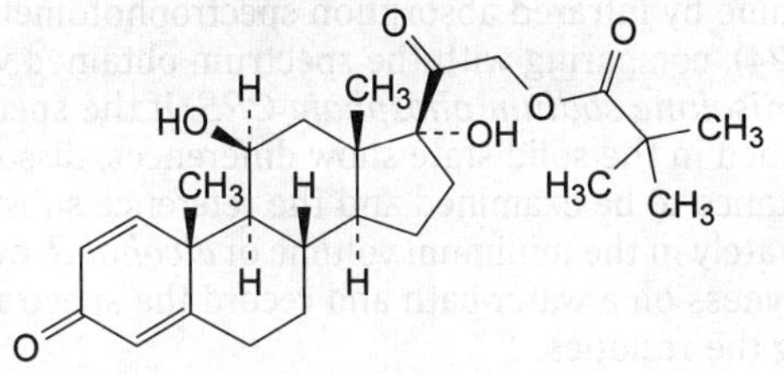

$C_{26}H_{36}O_6$ M_r 444.6

DEFINITION

Prednisolone pivalate contains not less than 97.0 per cent and not more than the equivalent of 103.0 per cent of 11β,17-dihydroxy-3,20-dioxopregna-1,4-dien-21-yl 2,2-dimethylpropanoate, calculated with reference to the dried substance.

CHARACTERS

A white or almost white, crystalline powder, practically insoluble in water, slightly soluble in alcohol, soluble in methylene chloride.

It melts at about 229 °C, with decomposition.

IDENTIFICATION

First identification: B, C.

Second identification: A, C, D.

A. Dissolve 10.0 mg in *ethanol R* and dilute to 100.0 ml with the same solvent. Place 2.0 ml of this solution in a ground-glass-stoppered tube, add 10.0 ml of *phenylhydrazine-sulphuric acid solution R*, mix and heat in a water-bath at 60 °C for 20 min. Cool immediately. The absorbance (*2.2.25*) of the solution at the maximum at 415 nm is 0.20 to 0.30.

B. Examine by infrared absorption spectrophotometry (*2.2.24*), comparing with the spectrum obtained with *prednisolone pivalate CRS*. If the spectra obtained in the solid state show differences, dissolve the substance to be examined and the reference substance separately in the minimum volume of *alcohol R*, evaporate to dryness on a water-bath and record the spectra again using the residues.

C. Examine by thin-layer chromatography (*2.2.27*), using as the coating substance a suitable silica gel with a fluorescent indicator having an optimal intensity at 254 nm.

Test solution. Dissolve 10 mg of the substance to be examined in a mixture of 1 volume of *methanol R* and 9 volumes of *methylene chloride R* and dilute to 10 ml with the same mixture of solvents.

Reference solution (a). Dissolve 10 mg of *prednisolone pivalate CRS* in a mixture of 1 volume of *methanol R* and 9 volumes of *methylene chloride R* and dilute to 10 ml with the same mixture of solvents.

Reference solution (b). Dissolve 10 mg of *prednisolone acetate CRS* in a mixture of 1 volume of *methanol R* and 9 volumes of *methylene chloride R* and dilute to 10 ml with the same mixture of solvents. Dilute 5 ml of this solution to 10 ml with reference solution (a).

Apply separately to the plate 5 µl of each solution. Prepare the mobile phase by adding a mixture of 1.2 volumes of *water R* and 8 volumes of *methanol R* to a mixture of 15 volumes of *ether R* and 77 volumes of *methylene chloride R*. Develop over a path of 15 cm. Allow the plate to dry in air and examine in ultraviolet light at 254 nm. The principal spot in the chromatogram obtained with the test solution is similar in position and size to the principal spot in the chromatogram obtained with reference solution (a). Spray the plate with *alcoholic solution of sulphuric acid R*. Heat at 120 °C for 10 min or until the spots appear. Allow to cool. Examine in daylight and in ultraviolet light at 365 nm. The principal spot in the chromatogram obtained with the test solution is similar in position, colour in daylight, fluorescence in ultraviolet light at 365 nm and size to the principal spot in the chromatogram obtained with reference solution (a). The test is not valid unless the chromatogram obtained with reference solution (b) shows two clearly separated spots.

D. Add about 2 mg to 2 ml of *sulphuric acid R* and shake to dissolve. Within 5 min, an intense red colour develops. When examined in ultraviolet light at 365 nm, a reddish-brown fluorescence is seen. Add the solution to 10 ml of *water R* and mix. The colour fades and there is greenish-yellow fluorescence in ultraviolet light at 365 nm.

TESTS

Specific optical rotation (*2.2.7*). Dissolve 0.250 g in *dioxan R* and dilute to 25.0 ml with the same solvent. The specific optical rotation is + 104 to + 112, calculated with reference to the dried substance.

Related substances. Examine by liquid chromatography (*2.2.29*).

Test solution. Dissolve 62.5 mg of the substance to be examined in 2 ml of a mixture of 1 volume of *water R* and 4 volumes of *tetrahydrofuran R* and dilute to 25.0 ml with the mobile phase.

Monographs P

Reference solution (a). Dissolve 25 mg of *prednisolone acetate CRS*, 25 mg of *cortisone acetate CRS* and 25 mg of *prednisolone pivalate CRS* in 2 ml of a mixture of 1 volume of *water R* and 4 volumes of *tetrahydrofuran R* and dilute to 25.0 ml with the mobile phase. Dilute 1.0 ml of this solution to 25.0 ml with the mobile phase.

Reference solution (b). Dilute 1.0 ml of the test solution to 50.0 ml with the mobile phase.

The chromatographic procedure may be carried out using:

– a stainless steel column 0.15 m long and 4.6 mm in internal diameter packed with *octadecylsilyl silica gel for chromatography R* (5 µm),

– as mobile phase at a flow rate of 1 ml/min a mixture prepared as follows: mix 19 ml of *butyl acetate R1* carefully with 37 ml of *tetrahydrofuran R* and 213 ml of *ethylene glycol monomethyl ether R* and then with 231 ml of *water R*, leave to equilibrate for 1 h and filter through a 0.45 µm filter,

– as detector a spectrophotometer set at 254 nm.

Adjust the sensitivity so that the height of the principal peak in the chromatogram obtained with reference solution (b) is 70 per cent to 90 per cent of the full scale.

Equilibrate the column with the mobile phase at a flow rate of 1 ml/min for about 30 min.

Inject 20 µl of reference solution (a). When the chromatograms are recorded in the conditions described above the retention times are: prednisolone acetate about 3.5 min, cortisone acetate about 4.5 min and prednisolone pivalate about 13 min. The test is not valid unless the resolution between the peaks corresponding to prednisolone acetate and cortisone acetate is at least 2.5; if this resolution is not achieved, adjust the concentration of water in the mobile phase.

Inject separately 20 µl of the test solution and 20 µl of reference solution (b). Continue the chromatography for 1.5 times the retention time of the principal peak. In the chromatogram obtained with the test solution: the area of any peak apart from the principal peak is not greater than the area of the principal peak in the chromatogram obtained with reference solution (b) (2.0 per cent) and not more than one such peak has an area greater than half the area of the principal peak in the chromatogram obtained with reference solution (b) (1.0 per cent); the sum of the areas of all the peaks apart from the principal peak is not greater than 1.25 times the area of the principal peak in the chromatogram obtained with reference solution (b) (2.5 per cent). Disregard any peak due to the solvent and any peak with an area less than 0.025 times the area of the principal peak in the chromatogram obtained with reference solution (b).

Loss on drying (*2.2.32*). Not more than 0.5 per cent, determined on 1.000 g by drying in an oven at 100 °C to 105 °C.

ASSAY

Dissolve 0.100 g in *alcohol R* and dilute to 100.0 ml with the same solvent. Dilute 5.0 ml of the solution to 250.0 ml with *alcohol R*. Measure the absorbance (*2.2.25*) at the maximum at 243 nm.

Calculate the content of $C_{26}H_{36}O_6$ taking the specific absorbance to be 337.

STORAGE

Store protected from light.

01/2005:0735

PREDNISOLONE SODIUM PHOSPHATE

Prednisoloni natrii phosphas

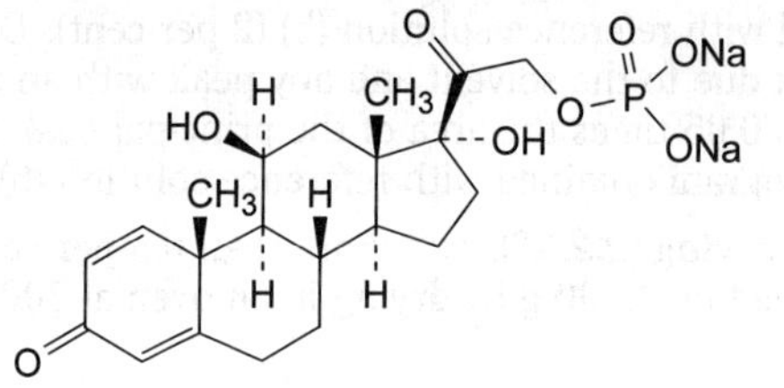

$C_{21}H_{27}Na_2O_8P$ M_r 484.4

DEFINITION

Prednisolone sodium phosphate contains not less than 96.0 per cent and not more than the equivalent of 103.0 per cent of 11β,17-dihydroxy-3,20-dioxopregna-1,4-dien-21-yl disodium phosphate, calculated with reference to the anhydrous substance.

CHARACTERS

A white or almost white, crystalline powder, hygroscopic, freely soluble in water, very slightly soluble in alcohol.

IDENTIFICATION

First identification: B, C.

Second identification: A, C, D, E.

A. Dissolve 10.0 mg in 5 ml of *water R* and dilute to 100.0 ml with *ethanol R*. Place 2.0 ml of this solution in a ground-glass-stoppered tube, add 10.0 ml of *phenylhydrazine-sulphuric acid solution R*, mix and heat in a water-bath at 60 °C for 20 min. Cool immediately. The absorbance (*2.2.25*) of the solution at the maximum at 415 nm is 0.10 to 0.20.

B. Examine by infrared absorption spectrophotometry (*2.2.24*), comparing with the spectrum obtained with *prednisolone sodium phosphate CRS*. If the spectra obtained in the solid state show differences, dissolve the substance to be examined and the reference substance separately in the minimum volume of *alcohol R*, evaporate to dryness on a water-bath and record the spectra again using the residues.

C. Examine by thin-layer chromatography (*2.2.27*), using as the coating substance a suitable silica gel with a fluorescent indicator having an optimal intensity at 254 nm.

Test solution. Dissolve 10 mg of the substance to be examined in *methanol R* and dilute to 10 ml with the same solvent.

Reference solution (a). Dissolve 10 mg of *prednisolone sodium phosphate CRS* in *methanol R* and dilute to 10 ml with the same solvent.

Reference solution (b). Dissolve 10 mg of *dexamethasone sodium phosphate CRS* in *methanol R* and dilute to 10 ml with the same solvent. Dilute 5 ml of this solution to 10 ml with reference solution (a).

Apply separately to the plate 5 µl of each solution. Develop over a path of 15 cm using a mixture of 20 volumes of *glacial acetic acid R*, 20 volumes of *water R* and 60 volumes of *butanol R*. Allow the plate to dry in air and examine in ultraviolet light at 254 nm. The principal spot in the chromatogram obtained with the test solution is similar in position and size to the

Monographs P

principal spot in the chromatogram obtained with reference solution (a). Spray the plate with *alcoholic solution of sulphuric acid R*. Heat at 120 °C for 10 min or until the spots appear. Allow to cool. Examine in daylight and in ultraviolet light at 365 nm. The principal spot in the chromatogram obtained with the test solution is similar in position, colour in daylight, fluorescence in ultraviolet light at 365 nm and size to the principal spot in the chromatogram obtained with reference solution (a). The test is not valid unless the chromatogram obtained with reference solution (b) shows two spots which may however not be completely separated.

D. Add about 2 mg to 2 ml of *sulphuric acid R* and shake to dissolve. Within 5 min, an intense red colour develops. When examined in ultraviolet light at 365 nm, a reddish-brown fluorescence is seen. Add the solution to 10 ml of *water R* and mix. The colour fades and there is greenish-yellow fluorescence in ultraviolet light at 365 nm.

E. To about 40 mg add 2 ml of *sulphuric acid R* and heat gently until white fumes are evolved. Add *nitric acid R* dropwise, continue the heating until the solution is almost colourless and cool. Add 2 ml of *water R*, heat until white fumes are again evolved, cool, add 10 ml of *water R* and neutralise to *red litmus paper R* with *dilute ammonia R1*. The solution gives reaction (a) of sodium (*2.3.1*) and reaction (b) of phosphates (*2.3.1*).

TESTS

Solution S. Dissolve 1.0 g in *carbon dioxide-free water R* and dilute to 20 ml with the same solvent.

Appearance of solution. Solution S is clear (*2.2.1*) and not more intensely coloured than reference solution B_7 (*2.2.2, Method II*).

pH (*2.2.3*). The pH of solution S is 7.5 to 9.0.

Specific optical rotation (*2.2.7*). Dissolve 0.250 g in *water R* and dilute to 25.0 ml with the same solvent. The specific optical rotation is + 94 to + 100, calculated with reference to the anhydrous substance.

Related substances. Examine by liquid chromatography (*2.2.29*).

Test solution. Dissolve 62.5 mg of the substance to be examined in the mobile phase and dilute to 25.0 ml with the mobile phase.

Reference solution (a). Dissolve 25 mg of *prednisolone sodium phosphate CRS* and 25 mg of *prednisolone CRS* in the mobile phase and dilute to 25.0 ml with the same solvent. Dilute 1.0 ml of this solution to 25.0 ml with the mobile phase.

Reference solution (b). Dilute 1.0 ml of the test solution to 50.0 ml with the mobile phase.

The chromatographic procedure may be carried out using:

– a stainless steel column 0.15 m long and 4.6 mm in internal diameter packed with *octadecylsilyl silica gel for chromatography R* (5 µm),
– as mobile phase at a flow rate of 1 ml/min a mixture prepared as follows: in a 250 ml conical flask weigh 1.360 g of *potassium dihydrogen phosphate R* and 0.600 g of *hexylamine R*, mix and allow to stand for 10 min and then dissolve in 185 ml of *water R*; add 65 ml of *acetonitrile R*, mix and filter through a 0.45 µm filter,
– as detector a spectrophotometer set at 254 nm.

Inject 20 µl of reference solution (b). Adjust the sensitivity of the system so that the height of the principal peak in the chromatogram obtained with reference solution (b) is 70 per cent to 90 per cent of the full scale of the recorder.

Equilibrate the column with the mobile phase at a flow rate of 1 ml/min for about 30 min.

Inject 20 µl of reference solution (a). When the chromatograms are recorded in the conditions described above the retention times are: prednisolone sodium phosphate, about 6.5 min and prednisolone, about 8.5 min. The test is not valid unless the resolution between the peaks corresponding to prednisolone sodium phosphate and prednisolone is at least 4.5; if this resolution is not achieved, increase the concentration of *acetonitrile R* or increase the concentration of *water R* in the mobile phase.

Inject separately 20 µl of the test solution and 20 µl of reference solution (b). Continue the chromatography for three times the retention time of the principal peak. In the chromatogram obtained with the test solution: the area of any peak apart from the principal peak is not greater than the area of the principal peak in the chromatogram obtained with reference solution (b) (2 per cent) and not more than one such peak has an area greater than half the area of the principal peak in the chromatogram obtained with reference solution (b) (1 per cent); the sum of the areas of all the peaks apart from the principal peak is not greater than 1.5 times the area of the principal peak in the chromatogram obtained with reference solution (b) (3 per cent). Disregard any peak due to the solvent and any peak with an area less than 0.025 times the area of the principal peak in the chromatogram obtained with reference solution (b).

Inorganic phosphate. Dissolve 50 mg in *water R* and dilute to 100 ml with the same solvent. To 10 ml of this solution add 5 ml of *molybdovanadic reagent R*, mix and allow to stand for 5 min. Any yellow colour in the solution is not more intense than that in a standard prepared at the same time in the same manner using 10 ml of *phosphate standard solution (5 ppm PO_4) R* (1 per cent).

Water (*2.5.12*). Not more than 8.0 per cent, determined on 0.200 g by the semi-micro determination of water.

ASSAY

Dissolve 0.100 g in *water R* and dilute to 100.0 ml with the same solvent. Dilute 5.0 ml of the solution to 250.0 ml with *water R*. Measure the absorbance (*2.2.25*) at the maximum at 247 nm.

Calculate the content of $C_{21}H_{27}Na_2O_8P$ taking the specific absorbance to be 312.

STORAGE

Store protected from light.

01/2005:0354

PREDNISONE

Prednisonum

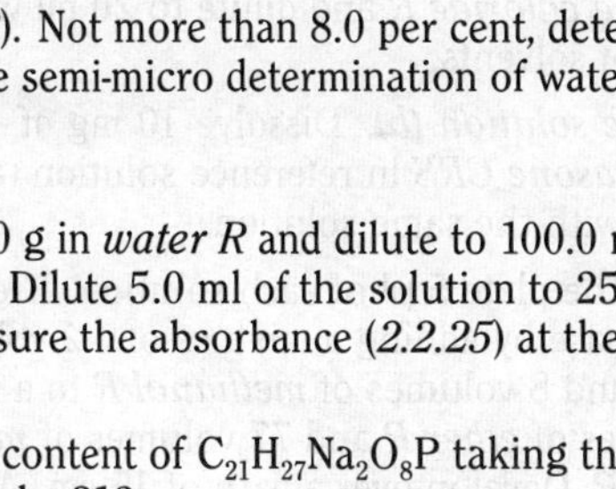

$C_{21}H_{26}O_5$ M_r 358.4

DEFINITION

Prednisone contains not less than 97.0 per cent and not more than the equivalent of 103.0 per cent of 17,21-dihydroxypregna-1,4-diene-3,11,20-trione, calculated with reference to the dried substance.

CHARACTERS

A white or almost white, crystalline powder, practically insoluble in water, slightly soluble in alcohol and in methylene chloride.

It shows polymorphism.

IDENTIFICATION

First identification: A, B.

Second identification: C, D.

A. Examine by infrared absorption spectrophotometry (*2.2.24*), comparing with the spectrum obtained with *prednisone CRS*. If the spectra obtained in the solid state show differences, dissolve the substance to be examined and the reference substance separately in the minimum volume of *acetone R*, evaporate to dryness on a water-bath and record new spectra using the residues.

B. Examine by thin-layer chromatography (*2.2.27*), using as the coating substance a suitable silica gel with a fluorescent indicator having an optimal intensity at 254 nm.

Test solution. Dissolve 10 mg of the substance to be examined in a mixture of 1 volume of *methanol R* and 9 volumes of *methylene chloride R* and dilute to 10 ml with the same mixture of solvents.

Reference solution (a). Dissolve 20 mg of *prednisone CRS* in a mixture of 1 volume of *methanol R* and 9 volumes of *methylene chloride R* and dilute to 20 ml with the same mixture of solvents.

Reference solution (b). Dissolve 10 mg of *betamethasone CRS* in reference solution (a) and dilute to 10 ml with the same solution.

Apply to the plate 5 µl of each solution. Prepare the mobile phase by adding a mixture of 1.2 volumes of *water R* and 8 volumes of *methanol R* to a mixture of 15 volumes of *ether R* and 77 volumes of *methylene chloride R*. Develop over a path of 15 cm. Allow the plate to dry in air and examine in ultraviolet light at 254 nm. The principal spot in the chromatogram obtained with the test solution is similar in position and size to the principal spot in the chromatogram obtained with reference solution (a). Spray with *alcoholic solution of sulphuric acid R*. Heat at 120 °C for 10 min or until the spots appear. Allow to cool. Examine the plate in daylight and in ultraviolet light at 365 nm. The principal spot in the chromatogram obtained with the test solution is similar in position, colour in daylight, fluorescence in ultraviolet light at 365 nm and size to the principal spot in the chromatogram obtained with reference solution (a). The test is not valid unless the chromatogram obtained with reference solution (b) shows two clearly separated spots.

C. Examine by thin-layer chromatography (*2.2.27*), using as the coating substance a suitable silica gel with a fluorescent indicator having an optimal intensity at 254 nm.

Test solution (a). Dissolve 25 mg of the substance to be examined in *methanol R* and dilute to 5 ml with the same solvent. This solution is also used to prepare test solution (b). Dilute 2 ml of the solution to 10 ml with *methylene chloride R*.

Test solution (b). Transfer 0.4 ml of the solution obtained during preparation of test solution (a) to a glass tube 100 mm long and 20 mm in diameter and fitted with a ground-glass stopper or a polytetrafluoroethylene cap and evaporate the solvent with gentle heating under a stream of *nitrogen R*. Add 2 ml of a 15 per cent *V/V* solution of *glacial acetic acid R* and 50 mg of *sodium bismuthate R*. Stopper the tube and shake the suspension in a mechanical shaker, protected from light, for 1 h. Add 2 ml of a 15 per cent *V/V* solution of *glacial acetic acid R* and filter into a 50 ml separating funnel, washing the filter with two quantities, each of 5 ml, of *water R*. Shake the clear filtrate with 10 ml of *methylene chloride R*. Wash the organic layer with 5 ml of *1 M sodium hydroxide* and two quantities, each of 5 ml, of *water R*. Dry over *anhydrous sodium sulphate R*.

Reference solution (a). Dissolve 25 mg of *prednisone CRS* in *methanol R* and dilute to 5 ml with the same solvent. This solution is also used to prepare reference solution (b). Dilute 2 ml of the solution to 10 ml with *methylene chloride R*.

Reference solution (b). Transfer 0.4 ml of the solution obtained during preparation of reference solution (a) to a glass tube 100 mm long and 20 mm in diameter and fitted with a ground-glass stopper or a polytetrafluoroethylene cap and evaporate the solvent with gentle heating under a stream of *nitrogen R*. Add 2 ml of a 15 per cent *V/V* solution of *glacial acetic acid R* and 50 mg of *sodium bismuthate R*. Stopper the tube and shake the suspension in a mechanical shaker, protected from light, for 1 h. Add 2 ml of a 15 per cent *V/V* solution of *glacial acetic acid R* and filter into a 50 ml separating funnel, washing the filter with two quantities, each of 5 ml, of *water R*. Shake the clear filtrate with 10 ml of *methylene chloride R*. Wash the organic layer with 5 ml of *1 M sodium hydroxide* and two quantities, each of 5 ml, of *water R*. Dry over *anhydrous sodium sulphate R*.

Apply to the plate 5 µl of test solution (a) and reference solution (a) and 50 µl of test solution (b) and reference solution (b), applying the latter two in small quantities in order to obtain small spots. Prepare the mobile phase by adding a mixture of 1.2 volumes of *water R* and 8 volumes of *methanol R* to a mixture of 15 volumes of *ether R* and 77 volumes of *methylene chloride R*. Develop over a path of 15 cm. Allow the plate to dry in air and examine in ultraviolet light at 254 nm. The principal spot in each of the chromatograms obtained with the test solutions is similar in position and size to the principal spot in the chromatogram obtained with the corresponding reference solution. Spray with *alcoholic solution of sulphuric acid R*. Heat at 120 °C for 10 min or until the spots appear. Allow to cool. Examine the chromatograms in daylight and in ultraviolet light at 365 nm. The principal spot in each of the chromatograms obtained with the test solutions is similar in position, colour in daylight, fluorescence in ultraviolet light at 365 nm and size to the principal spot in the chromatogram obtained with the corresponding reference solution. The principal spots in the chromatograms obtained with test solution (b) and reference solution (b) have an R_f value distinctly higher than that of the principal spots in the chromatograms obtained with test solution (a) and reference solution (a).

D. Add about 2 mg to 2 ml of *sulphuric acid R* and shake to dissolve. Within 5 min, a yellow colour develops with a blue fluorescence in ultraviolet light at 365 nm. Add the solution to 10 ml of *water R* and mix. The colour fades but the blue fluorescence in ultraviolet light does not disappear.

TESTS

Specific optical rotation (*2.2.7*). Dissolve 0.125 g in *dioxan R* and dilute to 25.0 ml with the same solvent. The specific optical rotation is + 167 to + 175, calculated with reference to the dried substance.

Related substances. Examine by liquid chromatography (*2.2.29*).

Test solution. Dissolve 25.0 mg of the substance to be examined in *methanol R* and dilute to 10.0 ml with the same solvent.

Reference solution (a). Dissolve 2 mg of *prednisone CRS* and 2 mg of *prednisolone CRS* in *methanol R* and dilute to 100.0 ml with the same solvent.

Reference solution (b). Dilute 1.0 ml of the test solution to 100.0 ml with *methanol R*.

The chromatographic procedure may be carried out using:

– a stainless steel column 0.25 m long and 4.6 mm in internal diameter, packed with *octadecylsilyl silica gel for chromatography R* (5 μm),

– as mobile phase at a flow rate of 2.5 ml/min a linear gradient programme using the following conditions:

Mobile phase A. In a 1000 ml volumetric flask mix 100 ml of *acetonitrile R* with 200 ml of *methanol R* and 650 ml of *water R* and allow to equilibrate; adjust the volume to 1000 ml with *water R* and mix again,

Mobile phase B. Acetonitrile R,

Time (min)	Mobile phase A (per cent *V/V*)	Mobile phase B (per cent *V/V*)	Comment
0	100	0	isocratic
25	100	0	begin linear gradient
40	40	60	end chromatogram, change to 100B
41	0	100	begin treatment with B
46	0	100	end treatment, return to 100A
47	100	0	begin equilibration with A
52 = 0	100	0	end equilibration, begin next chromatogram

– as detector a spectrophotometer set at 254 nm,

maintaining the temperature of the column at 45 °C.

Equilibrate the column for at least 30 min with mobile phase B at a flow rate of 2.5 ml/min and then with the mobile phase A for 5 minutes. For subsequent chromatograms, use the conditions described from 40.0 to 52.0 min. Adjust the sensitivity of the system so that the height of the principal peak in the chromatogram obtained with 20 μl of reference solution (b) is not less than 50 per cent of the full scale of the recorder.

Inject 20 μl of reference solution (a). When the chromatograms are recorded in the prescribed conditions, the retention times are: prednisone, about 19 minutes and prednisolone, about 23 minutes. The test is not valid unless the resolution between the peaks corresponding to prednisone and prednisolone is at least 2.7; if necessary, adjust the concentration of acetonitrile in mobile phase A.

Inject separately 20 μl of *methanol R* as a blank, 20 μl of the test solution and 20 μl of reference solution (b). In the chromatogram obtained with the test solution: the area of any peak apart from the principal peak is not greater than 0.25 times the area of the principal peak in the chromatogram obtained with reference solution (b) (0.25 per cent); the sum of the areas of all the peaks, apart from the principal peak, is not greater than 0.75 times the area of the principal peak in the chromatogram obtained with reference solution (b) (0.75 per cent). Disregard any peak due to the blank run and any peak with an area less than 0.05 times the area of the principal peak in the chromatogram obtained with reference solution (b).

Loss on drying (*2.2.32*). Not more than 1.0 per cent, determined on 0.500 g by drying in an oven at 100 °C to 105 °C.

ASSAY

Dissolve 0.100 g in *alcohol R* and dilute to 100.0 ml with the same solvent. Dilute 2.0 ml of the solution to 100.0 ml with *alcohol R*. Measure the absorbance (*2.2.25*) at the maximum at 238 nm.

Calculate the content of $C_{21}H_{26}O_5$ taking the specific absorbance to be 425.

STORAGE

Store protected from light.

01/2005:1362

PRILOCAINE

Prilocainum

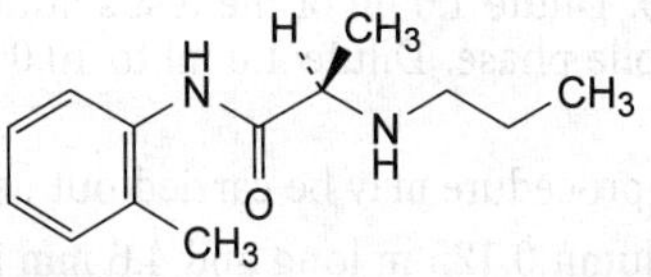

and enantiomer

$C_{13}H_{20}N_2O$ M_r 220.3

DEFINITION

Prilocaine contains not less than 99.0 per cent and not more than the equivalent of 101.0 per cent of (*RS*)-*N*-(2-methylphenyl)-2-(propylamino)propanamide, calculated with reference to the anhydrous substance.

CHARACTERS

A white or almost white, crystalline powder, slightly soluble in water, very soluble in acetone and in alcohol.

IDENTIFICATION

First identification: B.

Second identification: A, C.

A. Melting point (*2.2.14*): 36 °C to 39 °C, determined without previous drying.

B. Examine by infrared absorption spectrophotometry (*2.2.24*), comparing with the spectrum obtained with *prilocaine CRS*. Examine the substances by applying 50 μl of a 30 g/l solution in *ether R* to *potassium bromide R* discs and evaporating the solvent.

C. Examine by thin-layer chromatography (*2.2.27*), using a *TLC silica gel GF_{254} plate R.*

Test solution. Dissolve 20.0 mg of the substance to be examined in *alcohol R* and dilute to 5 ml with the same solvent.

Reference solution (a). Dissolve 20.0 mg of *prilocaine CRS* in *alcohol R* and dilute to 5 ml with the same solvent.

Reference solution (b). Dissolve 20.0 mg of *prilocaine CRS* and 20.0 mg of *lidocaine CRS* in *alcohol R* and dilute to 5 ml with the same solvent.

Apply to the plate 10 μl of each solution. Develop over a path of 12 cm, using a mixture of 1 volume of *concentrated ammonia R*, 5 volumes of *methanol R* and

100 volumes of *ether R*. Allow the plate to dry in air and examine in ultraviolet light at 254 nm. The principal spot in the chromatogram obtained with the test solution is similar in position and size to the principal spot in the chromatogram obtained with reference solution (a). The test is not valid unless the chromatogram obtained with reference solution (b) shows two clearly separated spots.

TESTS

Solution S. Dissolve 2.50 g in 15 ml of *dilute hydrochloric acid R* and dilute to 50.0 ml with *water R*.

Appearance of solution. Solution S is clear (*2.2.1*) and colourless (*2.2.2, Method II*).

Optical rotation (*2.2.7*). The angle of optical rotation, determined on solution S, is − 0.10° to + 0.10°.

Related substances. Examine by liquid chromatography (*2.2.29*).

Test solution. Dissolve 25.0 mg of the substance to be examined in the mobile phase and dilute to 10.0 ml with the mobile phase.

Reference solution (a). Dissolve 2.5 mg of the substance to be examined and 3.0 mg of *prilocaine impurity E CRS* in the mobile phase and dilute to 100.0 ml with the mobile phase. Dilute 1.0 ml to 10.0 ml with the mobile phase.

Reference solution (b). Dilute 1.0 ml of the test solution to 100.0 ml with the mobile phase. Dilute 1.0 ml to 10.0 ml with the mobile phase.

The chromatographic procedure may be carried out using:

– a stainless steel column 0.125 m long and 4.6 mm in internal diameter packed with *octadecylsilyl silica gel for chromatography R* (5 µm),

– as mobile phase at a flow rate of 1 ml/min a mixture of 40 volumes of *acetonitrile R* and 60 volumes of a solution prepared as follows: dissolve 0.180 g of *sodium dihydrogen phosphate monohydrate R* and 2.89 g of *disodium hydrogen phosphate dihydrate R* in 1000 ml of *water R* (pH 8.0),

– as detector a spectrophotometer set at 240 nm.

Inject 20 µl of reference solution (a). Adjust the sensitivity of the system so that the heights of the two principal peaks in the chromatogram obtained are at least 20 per cent of the full scale of the recorder. The test is not valid unless the resolution between the peaks corresponding to impurity E and prilocaine is at least 3.0. Inject 20 µl of the test solution and 20 µl of reference solution (b). Continue the chromatography of the test solution for twice the retention time of prilocaine, which is about 7 min. In the chromatogram obtained with the test solution: the area of any peak, apart from the principal peak, is not greater than twice the area of the principal peak in the chromatogram obtained with reference solution (b) (0.2 per cent) and not more than one such peak has an area greater than the area of the principal peak in the chromatogram obtained with reference solution (b) (0.1 per cent); the sum of the areas of all the peaks, apart from the principal peak, is not greater than five times the area of the principal peak in the chromatogram obtained with reference solution (b) (0.5 per cent). Disregard any peak with an area less than 0.2 times the area of the principal peak in the chromatogram obtained with reference solution (b).

***o*-Toluidine**. *Use freshly prepared solutions.* Examine by liquid chromatography (*2.2.29*).

Test solution. Dissolve 0.100 g of the substance to be examined in the mobile phase and dilute to 10.0 ml with the mobile phase.

Reference solution. Dissolve 10.0 mg of *o-toluidine hydrochloride R* in the mobile phase and dilute to 100.0 ml with the mobile phase. Dilute 1.0 ml of this solution to 100.0 ml with the mobile phase.

Carry out the chromatography using the same system as described under Related substances. Inject 20 µl of the reference solution. Adjust the sensitivity of the system so that the height of the peak in the chromatogram obtained is at least 50 per cent of the full scale of the recorder. Inject 20 µl of the test solution. Continue the chromatography of the test solution for twice the retention time of prilocaine. In the chromatogram obtained with the test solution, the area of any peak corresponding to *o*-toluidine is not greater than the area of the principal peak in the chromatogram obtained with the reference solution (100 ppm).

Heavy metals (*2.4.8*). 1.0 g complies with limit test C for heavy metals (20 ppm). Prepare the standard using 2 ml of *lead standard solution (10 ppm Pb) R*.

Water (*2.5.12*). Not more than 0.5 per cent, determined on 1.00 g by the semi-micro determination of water.

Sulphated ash (*2.4.14*). Not more than 0.1 per cent, determined on 1.0 g.

ASSAY

Dissolve 0.400 g in 20 ml of *anhydrous acetic acid R*. Titrate with *0.1 M perchloric acid*, determining the end-point potentiometrically (*2.2.20*).

1 ml of *0.1 M perchloric acid* is equivalent to 22.03 mg of $C_{13}H_{20}N_2O$.

IMPURITIES

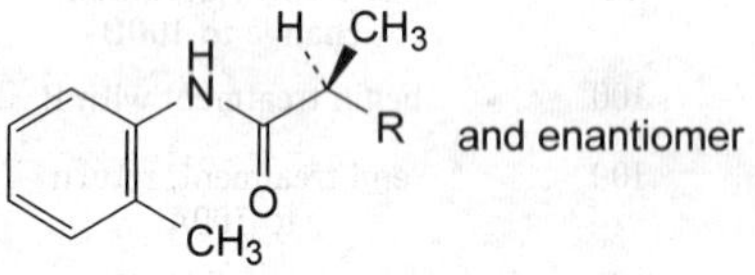

A. R = Cl: (*RS*)-2-chloro-*N*-(2-methylphenyl)propanamide,

C. R = NH-C_2H_5: (*RS*)-2-(ethylamino)-*N*-(2-methylphenyl)propanamide,

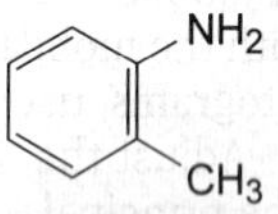

B. 2-methylbenzenamine (*o*-toluidine),

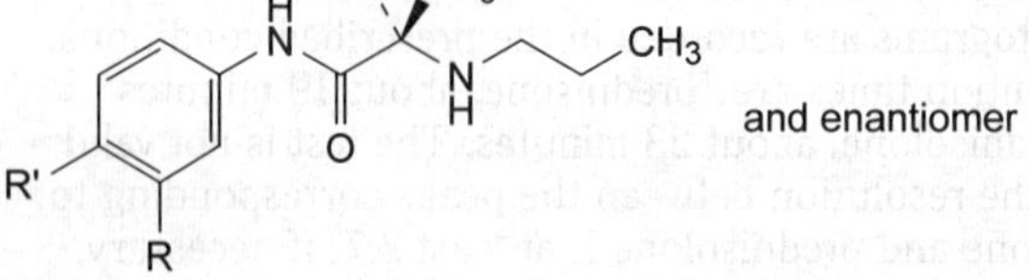

D. R = CH_3, R′ = H: (*RS*)-*N*-(3-methylphenyl)-2-(propylamino)propanamide,

E. R = H, R′ = CH_3: (*RS*)-*N*-(4-methylphenyl)-2-(propylamino)propanamide,

F. R = R′ = H: (*RS*)-*N*-phenyl-2-(propylamino)propanamide.

01/2005:1363

PRILOCAINE HYDROCHLORIDE

Prilocaini hydrochloridum

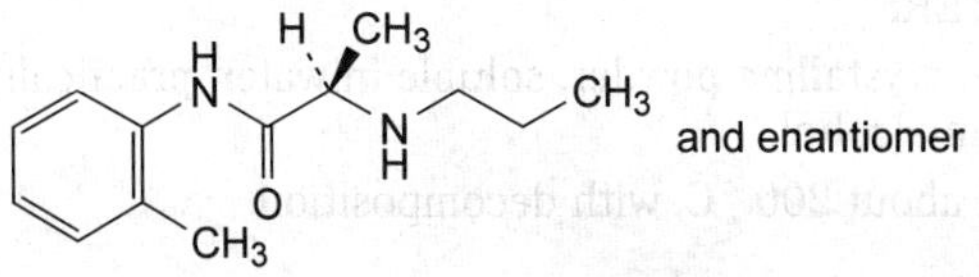

$C_{13}H_{21}ClN_2O$ M_r 256.8

DEFINITION

Prilocaine hydrochloride contains not less than 99.0 per cent and not more than the equivalent of 101.0 per cent of (*RS*)-*N*-(2-methylphenyl)-2-(propylamino)propanamide hydrochloride, calculated with reference to the dried substance.

CHARACTERS

A white, crystalline powder or colourless crystals, freely soluble in water and in alcohol, very slightly soluble in acetone.

IDENTIFICATION

First identification: B, D.

Second identification: A, C, D.

A. Melting point (*2.2.14*): 168 °C to 171 °C.

B. Examine by infrared absorption spectrophotometry (*2.2.24*), comparing with the spectrum obtained with *prilocaine hydrochloride CRS*. Examine the substances prepared as discs.

C. Examine by thin-layer chromatography (*2.2.27*), using a *TLC silica gel GF_{254} plate R*.

Test solution. Dissolve 20.0 mg of the substance to be examined in *alcohol R* and dilute to 5 ml with the same solvent.

Reference solution (a). Dissolve 20.0 mg of *prilocaine hydrochloride CRS* in *alcohol R* and dilute to 5 ml with the same solvent.

Reference solution (b). Dissolve 20.0 mg of *prilocaine hydrochloride CRS* and 20.0 mg of *lidocaine hydrochloride CRS* in *alcohol R* and dilute to 5 ml with the same solvent.

Apply to the plate 10 µl of each solution. Develop over a path of 12 cm, using a mixture of 1 volume of *concentrated ammonia R*, 5 volumes of *methanol R* and 100 volumes of *ether R*. Allow the plate to dry in air and examine in ultraviolet light at 254 nm. The principal spot in the chromatogram obtained with the test solution is similar in position and size to the principal spot in the chromatogram obtained with reference solution (a). The test is not valid unless the chromatogram obtained with reference solution (b) shows two clearly separated spots.

D. It gives reaction (a) of chlorides (*2.3.1*).

TESTS

Solution S. Dissolve 2.50 g in *carbon dioxide-free water R* and dilute to 50.0 ml with the same solvent.

Appearance of solution. Solution S is clear (*2.2.1*) and colourless (*2.2.2, Method II*).

Optical rotation (*2.2.7*). The angle of optical rotation, determined on solution S, is − 0.10° to + 0.10°.

Acidity or alkalinity. Dilute 4 ml of solution S to 10 ml with *carbon dioxide-free water R*. Add 0.1 ml of *bromocresol green solution R* and 0.40 ml of *0.01 M sodium hydroxide*. The solution is blue. Add 0.80 ml of *0.01 M hydrochloric acid*. The solution is yellow.

Related substances. Examine by liquid chromatography (*2.2.29*).

Test solution. Dissolve 30.0 mg of the substance to be examined in the mobile phase and dilute to 10.0 ml with the mobile phase.

Reference solution (a). Dissolve 3.0 mg of the substance to be examined and 3.0 mg of *prilocaine impurity E CRS* in the mobile phase and dilute to 100.0 ml with the mobile phase. Dilute 1.0 ml of this solution to 10.0 ml with the mobile phase.

Reference solution (b). Dilute 1.0 ml of the test solution to 100.0 ml with the mobile phase. Dilute 1.0 ml of this solution to 10.0 ml with the mobile phase.

The chromatographic procedure may be carried out using:

- a stainless steel column 0.125 m long and 4.6 mm in internal diameter packed with *octadecylsilyl silica gel for chromatography R* (5 µm),
- as mobile phase at a flow rate of 1 ml/min a mixture of 40 volumes of *acetonitrile R* and 60 volumes of a solution prepared as follows: dissolve 0.180 g of *sodium dihydrogen phosphate monohydrate R* and 2.89 g of *disodium hydrogen phosphate dihydrate R* in 1000 ml of *water R* (pH 8.0),
- as detector a spectrophotometer set at 240 nm.

Inject 20 µl of reference solution (a). Adjust the sensitivity of the system so that the heights of the two principal peaks in the chromatogram obtained are at least 20 per cent of the full scale of the recorder. The test is not valid unless the resolution between the peaks corresponding to impurity E and prilocaine is at least 3.0. Inject 20 µl of the test solution and 20 µl of reference solution (b). Continue the chromatography of the test solution for twice the retention time of prilocaine, which is about 7 min. In the chromatogram obtained with the test solution: the area of any peak, apart from the principal peak, is not greater than twice the area of the principal peak in the chromatogram obtained with reference solution (b) (0.2 per cent) and not more than one such peak has an area greater than the area of the principal peak in the chromatogram obtained with reference solution (b) (0.1 per cent); the sum of the areas of all the peaks, apart from the principal peak, is not greater than five times the area of the principal peak in the chromatogram obtained with reference solution (b) (0.5 per cent). Disregard any peak with an area less than 0.2 times the area of the principal peak in the chromatogram obtained with reference solution (b).

***o*-Toluidine**. *Use freshly prepared solutions*. Examine by liquid chromatography (*2.2.29*).

Test solution. Dissolve 0.100 g of the substance to be examined in the mobile phase and dilute to 10.0 ml with the mobile phase.

Reference solution. Dissolve 10.0 mg of *o-toluidine hydrochloride R* in the mobile phase and dilute to 100.0 ml with the mobile phase. Dilute 1.0 ml of this solution to 100.0 ml with the mobile phase.

Carry out the chromatography using the same system as described under Related substances. Inject 20 µl of the reference solution. Adjust the sensitivity of the system so that the height of the peak in the chromatogram obtained is at least 50 per cent of the full scale of the recorder. Inject 20 µl of the test solution. Continue the chromatography of

Monographs P

the test solution for twice the retention time of prilocaine. In the chromatogram obtained with the test solution, the area of any peak corresponding to *o*-toluidine is not greater than the area of the principal peak in the chromatogram obtained with the reference solution (100 ppm).

Heavy metals (*2.4.8*). 1.0 g complies with limit test C for heavy metals (20 ppm). Prepare the standard using 2 ml of *lead standard solution (10 ppm Pb) R.*

Loss on drying (*2.2.32*). Not more than 0.5 per cent, determined on 1.000 g by drying in an oven at 100 °C to 105 °C.

Sulphated ash (*2.4.14*). Not more than 0.1 per cent, determined on 1.0 g.

ASSAY

Dissolve 0.400 g in a mixture of 5.0 ml of *0.01 M hydrochloric acid* and 50 ml of *alcohol R*. Carry out a potentiometric titration (*2.2.20*), using *0.1 M sodium hydroxide*. Read the volume added between the two points of inflexion.

1 ml of *0.1 M sodium hydroxide* is equivalent to 25.68 mg of $C_{13}H_{21}ClN_2O$.

IMPURITIES

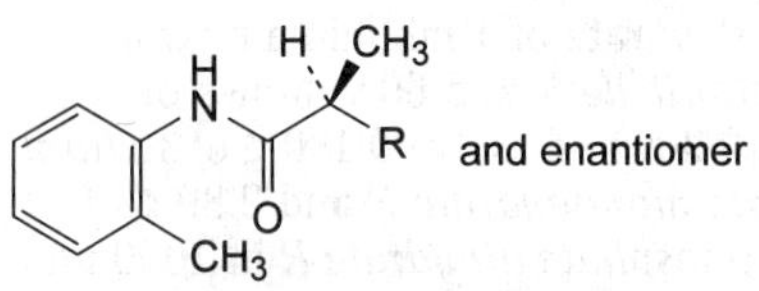

A. R = Cl: (*RS*)-2-chloro-*N*-(2-methylphenyl)propanamide,

C. R = NH-C_2H_5: (*RS*)-2-ethylamino-*N*-(2-methylphenyl)propanamide,

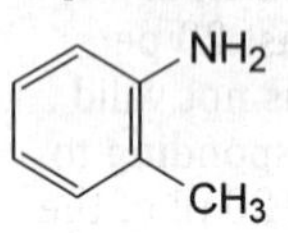

B. 2-methylbenzenamine (*o*-toluidine),

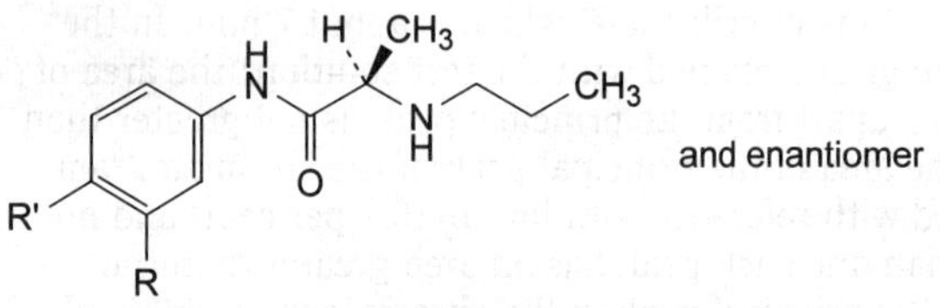

D. R = CH_3, R′ = H: (*RS*)-*N*-(3-methylphenyl)-2-(propylamino)propanamide,

E. R = H, R′ = CH_3: (*RS*)-*N*-(4-methylphenyl)-2-(propylamino)propanamide,

F. R = R′ = H: (*RS*)-*N*-phenyl-2-(propylamino)propanamide.

01/2005:0635
corrected

PRIMAQUINE DIPHOSPHATE

Primaquini diphosphas

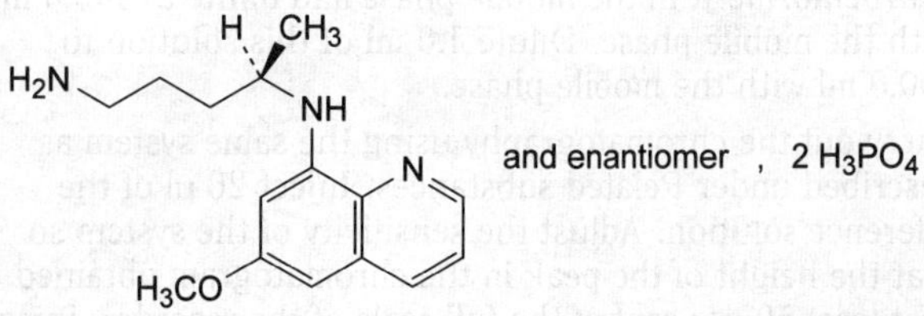

$C_{15}H_{27}N_3O_9P_2$ M_r 455.3

DEFINITION

Primaquine diphosphate contains not less than 98.5 per cent and not more than the equivalent of 101.5 per cent of (4*RS*)-*N*[4]-(6-methoxyquinolin-8-yl)pentane-1,4-diamine bisphosphate, calculated with reference to the dried substance.

CHARACTERS

An orange, crystalline powder, soluble in water, practically insoluble in alcohol.

It melts at about 200 °C, with decomposition.

IDENTIFICATION

First identification: B, D.

Second identification: A, C, D.

A. Dissolve 15 mg in *0.01 M hydrochloric acid* and dilute to 100.0 ml with the same acid. Examined between 310 nm and 450 nm (*2.2.25*), the solution shows two absorption maxima, at 332 nm and 415 nm. The specific absorbances at the maxima are 45 to 52 and 27 to 35, respectively. Dilute 5.0 ml of the solution to 50.0 ml with *0.01 M hydrochloric acid.* Examined between 215 nm and 310 nm, the solution shows three absorption maxima, at 225 nm, 265 nm and 282 nm. The specific absorbances at the maxima are 495 to 515, 335 to 350 and 330 to 345, respectively.

B. Examine by infrared absorption spectrophotometry (*2.2.24*), comparing with the spectrum obtained with *primaquine diphosphate CRS*. Examine the substances as discs prepared as follows: dissolve separately 0.1 g of the substance to be examined and 0.1 g of the reference substance in 5 ml of *water R*, add 2 ml of *dilute ammonia R2* and 5 ml of *methylene chloride R* and shake; dry the methylene chloride layer over 0.5 g of *anhydrous sodium sulphate R*; prepare a blank disc using about 0.3 g of *potassium bromide R*; apply dropwise to the disc 0.1 ml of the methylene chloride layer, allowing the methylene chloride to evaporate between applications; dry the disc at 50 °C for 2 min.

C. Examine by thin-layer chromatography (*2.2.27*), using a *TLC silica gel GF_{254} plate R*.

Carry out all operations as rapidly as possible, protected from light. Prepare the test and reference solutions immediately before use.

Test solution. Dissolve 0.20 g of the substance to be examined in 5 ml of *water R* and dilute to 10 ml with *methanol R*. Dilute 1 ml of the solution to 10 ml with a mixture of equal volumes of *methanol R* and *water R*.

Reference solution. Dissolve 20 mg of *primaquine diphosphate CRS* in 5 ml of *water R* and dilute to 10 ml with *methanol R*.

Carry out pre-washing of the plate with a mixture of 1 volume of *concentrated ammonia R*, 40 volumes of *methanol R* and 60 volumes of *methylene chloride R*. Allow the plate to dry in air. Apply to the plate 5 µl of each solution. Develop over a path of 15 cm using the mixture of solvents prescribed for pre-washing. Allow the plate to dry in air and examine in ultraviolet light at 254 nm. The principal spot in the chromatogram obtained with the test solution is similar in position and size to the principal spot in the chromatogram obtained with the reference solution.

D. Dissolve 50 mg in 5 ml of *water R*. Add 2 ml of *dilute sodium hydroxide solution R* and shake with two quantities, each of 5 ml, of *methylene chloride R*. The aqueous layer, acidified by addition of *nitric acid R*, gives reaction (b) of phosphates (*2.3.1*).

TESTS

Related substances. Examine by liquid chromatography (*2.2.29*).

Test solution. Dissolve 50 mg of the substance to be examined in *water R* and dilute to 5.0 ml with the same solvent. To 1.0 ml of the solution add 0.2 ml of *concentrated ammonia R* and shake with 10.0 ml of the mobile phase. Use the clear lower layer.

Reference solution (a). Dissolve 50 mg of *primaquine diphosphate CRS* in *water R* and dilute to 5.0 ml with the same solvent. To 1.0 ml of the solution add 0.2 ml of *concentrated ammonia R* and shake with 10.0 ml of the mobile phase. Use the clear lower layer.

Reference solution (b). Dilute 3.0 ml of the test solution to 100.0 ml with the mobile phase.

Reference solution (c). Dilute 1.0 ml of the test solution to 10.0 ml with the mobile phase. Dilute 1.0 ml of this solution to 50.0 ml with the mobile phase.

The chromatographic procedure may be carried out using:

- a column 0.2 m long and 4.6 mm in internal diameter packed with *silica gel for chromatography R* (10 µm),
- as mobile phase at a flow rate of 3.0 ml/min a mixture of 0.1 volumes of *concentrated ammonia R*, 10 volumes of *methanol R*, 45 volumes of *methylene chloride R* and 45 volumes of *hexane R*,
- as detector a spectrophotometer set at 261 nm,
- a loop injector.

Inject 20 µl of each solution and continue the chromatography for at least twice the retention time of primaquine. The test is not valid unless in the chromatogram obtained with reference solution (a), just before the principal peak there is a peak whose area is about 6 per cent of that of the principal peak and the resolution between these peaks is not less than 2.0; in the chromatogram obtained with reference solution (c) the signal-to-noise ratio of the principal peak is not less than five. In the chromatogram obtained with the test solution, the sum of the areas of any peaks, apart from the principal peak, is not greater than the area of the principal peak in the chromatogram obtained with reference solution (b) (3.0 per cent). Disregard the peak due to the solvent and any peak whose area is less than that of the principal peak in the chromatogram obtained with reference solution (c).

Loss on drying (*2.2.32*). Not more than 0.5 per cent, determined on 1.000 g by drying in an oven at 100 °C to 105 °C.

ASSAY

Dissolve 0.2000 g in 40 ml of *anhydrous acetic acid R*, heating gently. Allow to cool and titrate with *0.1 M perchloric acid*, determining the end-point potentiometrically (*2.2.20*).

1 ml of *0.1 M perchloric acid* is equivalent to 22.77 mg of $C_{15}H_{27}N_3O_9P_2$.

STORAGE

Store protected from light.

01/2005:0584

PRIMIDONE

Primidonum

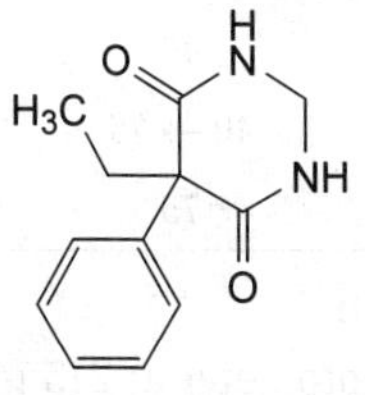

$C_{12}H_{14}N_2O_2$ M_r 218.3

DEFINITION

5-Ethyl-5-phenyldihydropyrimidine-4,6(1*H*,5*H*)-dione.

Content: 98.0 per cent to 102.0 per cent (dried substance).

CHARACTERS

Appearance: white or almost white, crystalline powder.

Solubility: very slightly soluble in water, slightly soluble in ethanol (96 per cent). It dissolves in alkaline solutions.

IDENTIFICATION

First identification: B.

Second identification: A, C, D.

A. Use the solution prescribed for the assay. Examined between 240 nm and 300 nm (*2.2.25*), the solution shows 3 absorption maxima, at 252 nm, 257 nm and 264 nm, and 2 absorption minima, at 254 nm and 261 nm. The ratio of the absorbance measured at the absorption maximum at 257 nm to that measured at the absorption minimum at 261 nm is 2.00 to 2.20. The identification is valid if, in the test for resolution (*2.2.25*), the ratio of the absorbances is not less than 2.0.

B. Infrared absorption spectrophotometry (*2.2.24*).
Preparation: discs of *potassium bromide R*.
Comparison: *primidone CRS*.

C. Dissolve 0.1 g in 5 ml of a 5 g/l solution of *chromotropic acid, sodium salt R* in a mixture of 4 volumes of *water R* and 9 volumes of *sulphuric acid R*. A pinkish-blue colour develops on heating.

D. Mix 0.2 g and 0.2 g of *anhydrous sodium carbonate R*. Heat until the mixture melts. Ammonia is evolved which is detectable by its alkaline reaction (*2.2.4*).

TESTS

Related substances. Liquid chromatography (*2.2.29*).

Test solution. Dissolve 50.0 mg of the substance to be examined in *methanol R1* and dilute to 50.0 ml with the same solvent.

Reference solution (a). Dilute 1.0 ml of the test solution to 100.0 ml with *methanol R1*. Dilute 1.0 ml of this solution to 10.0 ml with *methanol R1*.

Reference solution (b). Dissolve 5 mg of *primidone for peak identification CRS* (containing impurities A, B, C, D, E and F) in *methanol R1* and dilute to 5 ml with the same solvent.

Column:
- *size*: *l* = 0.10 m, Ø = 4.6 mm,
- *stationary phase*: *monolithic octadecylsilyl silica gel for chromatography R.*

Mobile phase:
- *mobile phase A*: 1.36 g/l solution of *potassium dihydrogen phosphate R*,

– *mobile phase B*: *methanol R1*,

Time (min)	Mobile phase A (per cent *V/V*)	Mobile phase B (per cent *V/V*)
0 - 1	75	25
1 - 6	75 → 40	25 → 60
6 - 8	40	60
8 - 8.5	40 → 75	60 → 25
8.5 - 10	75	25

Flow rate: 3.2 ml/min.

Detection: spectrophotometer at 215 nm.

Injection: 10 µl.

Identification of impurities: use the chromatogram supplied with *primidone for peak identification CRS* and the chromatogram obtained with reference solution (b) to identify the peaks.

Relative retention with reference to primidone (retention time = about 2.2 min): impurity A = about 0.5; impurity B = about 1.4; impurity C = about 1.6; impurity D = about 1.75; impurity E = about 2.0; impurity F = about 2.8.

System suitability: reference solution (b):

– *resolution*: minimum 2.5 between the peaks due to impurity B and impurity C.

Limits:

– *correction factors*: for the calculation of contents, multiply the peak areas of the following impurities by the corresponding correction factor: impurity A = 1.5; impurity C = 1.5; impurity D = 1.4; impurity E = 1.3;
– *impurity F*: not more than 3 times the area of the principal peak in the chromatogram obtained with reference solution (a) (0.3 per cent);
– *impurities A, B, C, D, E*: for each impurity, not more than the area of the principal peak in the chromatogram obtained with reference solution (a) (0.1 per cent);
– *any other impurity*: for each impurity, not more than the area of the principal peak in the chromatogram obtained with reference solution (a) (0.1 per cent);
– *total*: not more than 5 times the area of the principal peak in the chromatogram obtained with reference solution (a) (0.5 per cent);
– *disregard limit*: 0.5 times the area of the principal peak in the chromatogram obtained with reference solution (a) (0.05 per cent).

Heavy metals (*2.4.8*): maximum 10 ppm.

2.0 g complies with limit test D. Prepare the reference solution using 2 ml of *lead standard solution (10 ppm Pb) R*.

Loss on drying (*2.2.32*): maximum 0.5 per cent, determined on 1.000 g by drying in an oven at 100-105 °C for 2 h.

Sulphated ash (*2.4.14*): maximum 0.1 per cent, determined on 1.0 g.

ASSAY

Dissolve 60.0 mg with heating in 70 ml of *ethanol (96 per cent) R*, cool and dilute to 100.0 ml with the same solvent. Prepare a reference solution in the same manner using 60.0 mg of *primidone CRS*. Measure the absorbance (*2.2.25*) of the 2 solutions at the absorption maximum at 257 nm.

Calculate the content of $C_{12}H_{14}N_2O_2$ from the absorbances measured and the concentrations of the solutions.

IMPURITIES

Specified impurities: *A, B, C, D, E, F*.

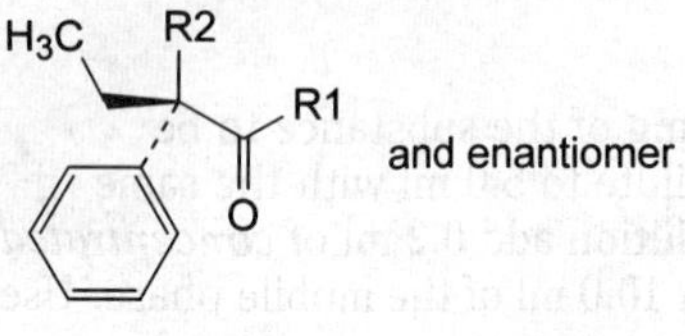

A. R1 = NH_2, R2 = CO-NH_2: 2-ethyl-2-phenylpropanediamide (ethylphenylmalonamide),

C. R1 = NH_2, R2 = H: (2*RS*)-2-phenylbutanamide,

D. R1 = NH_2, R2 = CN: (2*RS*)-2-cyano-2-phenylbutanamide,

E. R1 = OH, R2 = H: (2*RS*)-2-phenylbutanoic acid,

B. phenobarbital,

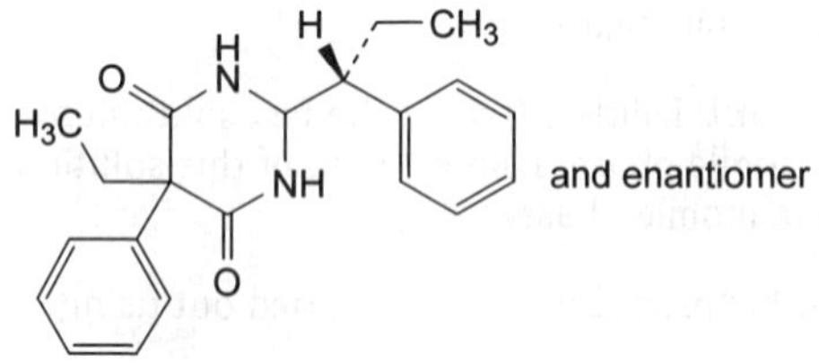

F. 5-ethyl-5-phenyl-2-[(1*RS*)-1-phenylpropyl]dihydropyrimidine-4,6(1*H*,5*H*)-dione.

01/2005:1364

PRIMULA ROOT

Primulae radix

DEFINITION

Primula root consists of the whole or cut, dried rhizome and root of *Primula veris* L. or *P. elatior* (L.) Hill.

CHARACTERS

Primula root has a bitter taste.

It has the macroscopic and microscopic characters described under identification tests A and B.

IDENTIFICATION

A. The coarsely torose, greyish-brown rhizome is straight or slightly curved, about 1 cm to 5 cm long and about 2 mm to 4 mm thick. The rhizome crown often bears the remains of stems and leaves. Attached to the rhizome are numerous brittle roots, about 1 mm thick and usually 6 cm to 8 cm long. The root of *P. elatior* is light brown to reddish-brown, that of *P. veris* light yellow to yellowish-white. The fracture is smooth.

B. Reduce to a powder (355). The powder is greyish-brown. Examine under a microscope, using *chloral hydrate solution R*. The powder shows fragments of parenchyma from the root bark, medulla and bark of the rhizome consisting of rounded cells with thickened and pitted walls; brownish fragments from the surface tissue showing root hairs; vessels with reticulate thickening. Yellowish-green groups of strongly pitted stone cells are characteristic of the presence of *P. elatior*. Examine under a microscope using a 50 per cent *V/V* solution of *glycerol R*. The powder shows single or compound starch grains of various size and shape.

C. Use the chromatograms obtained in the test for *Vincetoxicum hirundinaria medicus* root. Spray the plate with *anisaldehyde solution R*. Heat at 100 °C to 105 °C for 5 min to 10 min. Examine in daylight. The main zone (aescin) in the chromatogram obtained with the reference solution is bluish-violet and is situated near the boundary between the lower and middle thirds. The chromatogram obtained with the test solution shows one or two strong dark violet zones a little below the aescin zone in the chromatogram obtained with the reference solution; further pale violet, yellowish or brownish-green zones may be visible.

TESTS

Foreign matter (*2.8.2*). It complies with the test for foreign matter.

Vincetoxicum hirundinaria medicus root. Examine by thin-layer chromatography (*2.2.27*), using a *TLC silica gel F_{254} plate R*.

Test solution. To 1.0 g of the powdered drug (500) add 10 ml of *alcohol (70 per cent V/V) R* and heat under a reflux condenser for 15 min. Cool and filter.

Reference solution. Dissolve 10 mg of *aescin R* in 1.0 ml of *alcohol (70 per cent V/V) R.*

Apply to the plate as bands 20 µl of each solution. Develop over a path of 12 cm using the upper phase of a mixture of 10 volumes of *glacial acetic acid R*, 40 volumes of *water R* and 50 volumes of *butanol R*. Allow the plate to dry in an oven at 100 °C to 105 °C. Examine in ultraviolet light at 254 nm. The chromatograms obtained with the reference solution and the test solution show a quenching zone (aescin) near the boundary between the lower and the middle thirds. Mark this zone. Examine in ultraviolet light at 365 nm. In the chromatogram obtained with the test solution no zones of light-blue or greenish fluorescence occur below the main zone of aescin in the chromatogram obtained with the reference solution.

Loss on drying (*2.2.32*). Not more than 10.0 per cent, determined on 1.000 g of powdered drug (355) by drying in an oven at 100 °C to 105 °C for 2 h.

Total ash (*2.4.16*). Not more than 9.0 per cent.

Ash insoluble in hydrochloric acid (*2.8.1*). Not more than 3.0 per cent.

STORAGE

Store protected from light.

01/2005:0243

PROBENECID

Probenecidum

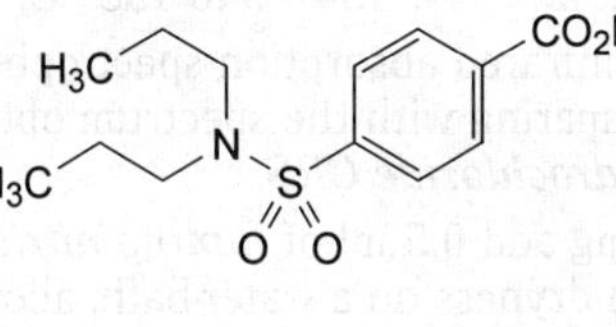

$C_{13}H_{19}NO_4S$ M_r 285.4

DEFINITION

Probenecid contains not less than 99.0 per cent and not more than the equivalent of 101.0 per cent of 4-(dipropylsulphamoyl)benzoic acid, calculated with reference to the dried substance.

CHARACTERS

A white or almost white, crystalline powder or small crystals, practically insoluble in water, soluble in acetone, sparingly soluble in ethanol.

IDENTIFICATION

First identification: A, C.

Second identification: A, B, D.

A. Melting point (*2.2.14*): 197 °C to 202 °C.

B. Dissolve 20 mg in a mixture of 1 volume of *0.1 M hydrochloric acid* and 9 volumes of *alcohol R* and dilute to 100.0 ml with the same mixture of solvents. Dilute 5.0 ml of the solution to 100.0 ml with a mixture of 1 volume of *0.1 M hydrochloric acid* and 9 volumes of *alcohol R*. Examined between 220 nm and 350 nm (*2.2.25*), the solution shows two absorption maxima, at 223 nm and 248 nm. The specific absorbance at the maximum at 248 nm is 310 to 350.

C. Examine by infrared absorption spectrophotometry (*2.2.24*), comparing with the spectrum obtained with *probenecid CRS*.

D. Dissolve 0.2 g in the smallest necessary quantity of *dilute ammonia R2* (about 0.6 ml). Add 3 ml of *silver nitrate solution R2*. A white precipitate is formed which dissolves in an excess of ammonia.

TESTS

Appearance of solution. Dissolve 1.0 g in *1 M sodium hydroxide* and dilute to 10 ml with the same solvent. The solution is clear (*2.2.1*) and not more intensely coloured than reference solution Y_6 (*2.2.2, Method II*).

Acidity. To 2.0 g add 100 ml of *water R* and heat on a water-bath for 30 min. Make up to the original volume with *water R*, allow to cool to room temperature and filter. To 50 ml of the filtrate add 0.1 ml of *phenolphthalein solution R*. Not more than 0.5 ml of *0.1 M sodium hydroxide* is required to change the colour of the indicator.

Related substances. Examine by thin-layer chromatography (*2.2.27*), using *silica gel GF_{254} R* as the coating substance.

Test solution. Dissolve 0.1 g of the substance to be examined in *acetone R* and dilute to 10 ml with the same solvent.

Reference solution. Dilute 0.5 ml of the test solution to 100 ml with *acetone R*.

Apply separately to the plate 20 µl of each solution. Develop over a path of 15 cm using a mixture of 10 volumes of *glacial acetic acid R*, 15 volumes of *chloroform R*, 20 volumes of *di-isopropyl ether R* and 55 volumes of *toluene R*. Allow the plate to dry in air and examine in ultraviolet light at 254 nm. Any spot in the chromatogram obtained with the test solution, apart from the principal spot, is not more intense than the spot in the chromatogram obtained with the reference solution (0.5 per cent).

Heavy metals (*2.4.8*). 1.0 g complies with limit test C for heavy metals (20 ppm). Prepare the standard using 2 ml of *lead standard solution (10 ppm Pb) R*.

Loss on drying (*2.2.32*). Not more than 0.5 per cent, determined on 1.00 g by drying in an oven at 100 °C to 105 °C.

Sulphated ash (*2.4.14*). Not more than 0.1 per cent, determined on 1.0 g.

ASSAY

Dissolve 0.250 g in 50 ml of *alcohol R*, shaking and heating slightly if necessary. Titrate with *0.1 M sodium hydroxide*, determining the end-point potentiometrically (*2.2.20*).

1 ml of *0.1 M sodium hydroxide* is equivalent to 28.54 mg of $C_{13}H_{19}NO_4S$.

01/2005:0567

PROCAINAMIDE HYDROCHLORIDE

Procainamidi hydrochloridum

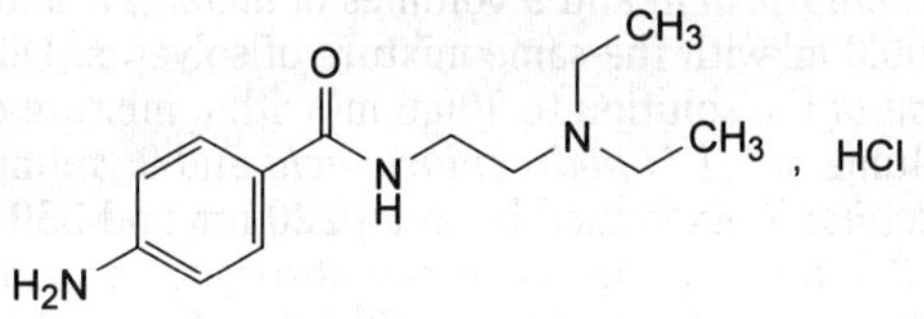

$C_{13}H_{22}ClN_3O$ — M_r 271.8

DEFINITION

Procainamide hydrochloride contains not less than 98.0 per cent and not more than the equivalent of 101.0 per cent of 4-amino-*N*-[2-(diethylamino)ethyl]benzamide hydrochloride, calculated with reference to the dried substance.

CHARACTERS

A white or very slightly yellow, crystalline powder, hygroscopic, very soluble in water, freely soluble in alcohol, slightly soluble in acetone.

IDENTIFICATION

First identification: C, D.

Second identification: A, B, D, E.

A. Melting point (*2.2.14*): 166 °C to 170 °C.

B. Dissolve 10.0 mg in *0.1 M sodium hydroxide* and dilute to 100.0 ml with the same solvent. Dilute 10.0 ml of the solution to 100.0 ml with *0.1 M sodium hydroxide*. Examined between 220 nm and 350 nm (*2.2.25*), the solution shows an absorption maximum at 273 nm. The specific absorbance at the maximum is 580 to 610.

C. Examine by infrared absorption spectrophotometry (*2.2.24*), comparing with the spectrum obtained with *procainamide hydrochloride CRS*.

D. Dilute 1 ml of solution S to 5 ml with *water R*. The solution gives reaction (a) of chlorides (*2.3.1*).

E. Dilute 1 ml of solution S (see Tests) to 2 ml with *water R*. 1 ml of this solution gives the reaction of primary aromatic amines (*2.3.1*).

TESTS

Solution S. Dissolve 2.5 g in *carbon dioxide-free water R* and dilute to 25 ml with the same solvent.

Appearance of solution. Solution S is clear (*2.2.1*) and not more intensely coloured than reference solution B_6 (*2.2.2, Method II*).

pH (*2.2.3*). The pH of solution S is 5.6 to 6.3.

Related substances. Examine by thin-layer chromatography (*2.2.27*), using *silica gel GF_{254} R* as the coating substance.

Test solution. Dissolve 0.10 g of the substance to be examined in *alcohol R* and dilute to 10 ml with the same solvent.

Reference solution. Dilute 1 ml of the test solution to 200 ml with *alcohol R*.

Apply to the plate 5 µl of each solution. Develop over a path of 12 cm using a mixture of 15 volumes of *glacial acetic acid R*, 30 volumes of *water R* and 60 volumes of *butanol R*. Place the plate in a stream of cold air until the plate appears dry. Examine in ultraviolet light at 254 nm. Any spot in the chromatogram obtained with the test solution, apart from the principal spot, is not more intense than the spot in the chromatogram obtained with the reference solution (0.5 per cent).

Heavy metals (*2.4.8*). 1.0 g complies with limit test C for heavy metals (20 ppm). Prepare the standard using 2 ml of *lead standard solution (10 ppm Pb) R*.

Loss on drying (*2.2.32*). Not more than 0.5 per cent, determined on 1.000 g by drying in an oven at 100 °C to 105 °C.

Sulphated ash (*2.4.14*). Not more than 0.1 per cent, determined on 1.0 g.

ASSAY

Dissolve 0.2500 g in 50 ml of *dilute hydrochloric acid R*. Carry out the determination of primary aromatic amino-nitrogen (*2.5.8*).

1 ml of *0.1 M sodium nitrite* is equivalent to 27.18 mg of $C_{13}H_{22}ClN_3O$.

STORAGE

Store in an airtight container, protected from light.

01/2005:0050

PROCAINE HYDROCHLORIDE

Procaini hydrochloridum

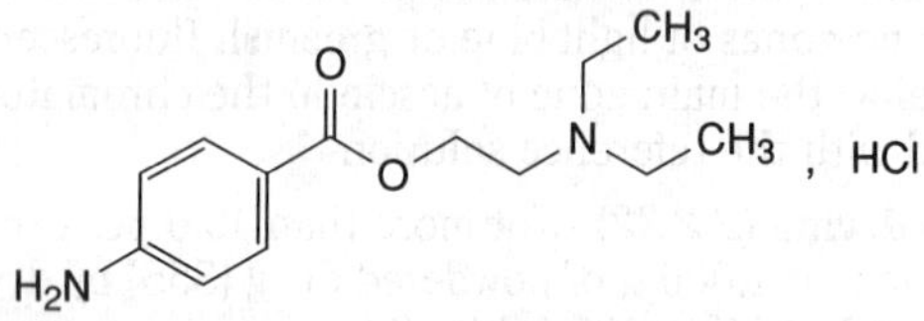

$C_{13}H_{21}ClN_2O_2$ — M_r 272.8

DEFINITION

Procaine hydrochloride contains not less than 99.0 per cent and not more than the equivalent of 101.0 per cent of 2-(diethylamino)ethyl 4-aminobenzoate hydrochloride, calculated with reference to the dried substance.

CHARACTERS

A white, crystalline powder or colourless crystals, very soluble in water, soluble in alcohol.

IDENTIFICATION

First identification: A, B, E.

Second identification: A, C, D, E, F.

A. Melting point (*2.2.14*): 154 °C to 158 °C.

B. Examine by infrared absorption spectrophotometry (*2.2.24*), comparing with the spectrum obtained with *procaine hydrochloride CRS*.

C. To about 5 mg add 0.5 ml of *fuming nitric acid R*. Evaporate to dryness on a water-bath, allow to cool and dissolve the residue in 5 ml of *acetone R*. Add 1 ml of *0.1 M alcoholic potassium hydroxide*. Only a brownish-red colour develops.

D. To 0.2 ml of solution S (see Tests) add 2 ml of *water R* and 0.5 ml of *dilute sulphuric acid R* and shake. Add 1 ml of a 1 g/l solution of *potassium permanganate R*. The colour is immediately discharged.

E. It gives reaction (a) of chlorides (*2.3.1*).

F. Dilute 1 ml of solution S to 100 ml with *water R*. 2 ml of this solution gives the reaction of primary aromatic amines (*2.3.1*).

TESTS

Solution S. Dissolve 2.5 g in *carbon dioxide-free water R* and dilute to 50 ml with the same solvent.

Appearance of solution. Solution S is clear (*2.2.1*) and colourless (*2.2.2, Method II*).

pH (*2.2.3*). Dilute 4 ml of solution S to 10 ml with *carbon dioxide-free water R*. The pH of the solution is 5.0 to 6.5.

Related substances. Examine by thin-layer chromatography (*2.2.27*), using *silica gel* GF_{254} *R* as the coating substance.

Test solution. Dissolve 1.0 g of the substance to be examined in *water R* and dilute to 10 ml with the same solvent.

Reference solution. Dissolve 50 mg of *4-aminobenzoic acid R* in *water R* and dilute to 100 ml with the same solvent. Dilute 1 ml of the solution to 10 ml with *water R*.

Apply separately to the plate 5 µl of each solution. Develop over a path of 10 cm using a mixture of 4 volumes of *glacial acetic acid R*, 16 volumes of *hexane R* and 80 volumes of *dibutyl ether R*. Dry the plate at 100 °C to 105 °C for 10 min and examine in ultraviolet light at 254 nm. Any spot in the chromatogram obtained with the test solution, apart from the principal spot, is not more intense than the spot in the chromatogram obtained with the reference solution (0.05 per cent). The principal spot in the chromatogram obtained with the test solution remains on the starting point.

Heavy metals (*2.4.8*). Dissolve 1.0 g in *water R* and dilute to 25.0 ml with the same solvent. Carry out the prefiltration. 10 ml of the prefiltrate complies with limit test E for heavy metals (5 ppm). Prepare the standard using 2 ml of *lead standard solution (1 ppm Pb) R*.

Loss on drying (*2.2.32*). Not more than 0.5 per cent, determined on 1.00 g by drying in an oven at 100 °C to 105 °C.

Sulphated ash (*2.4.14*). Not more than 0.1 per cent, determined on 1.0 g.

ASSAY

Dissolve 0.400 g in 50 ml of *dilute hydrochloric acid R*. Carry out the determination of primary aromatic amino nitrogen (*2.5.8*).

1 ml of *0.1 M sodium nitrite* is equivalent to 27.28 mg of $C_{13}H_{21}ClN_2O_2$.

STORAGE

Store protected from light.

01/2005:0244

PROCHLORPERAZINE MALEATE

Prochlorperazini maleas

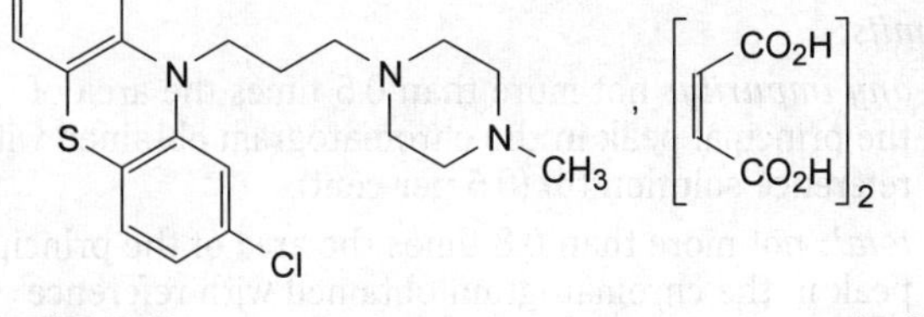

$C_{28}H_{32}ClN_3O_8S$ M_r 606

DEFINITION

Prochlorperazine maleate contains not less than 98.0 per cent and not more than the equivalent of 101.0 per cent of 2-chloro-10-[3-(4-methylpiperazin-1-yl)propyl]-10*H*-phenothiazine bis[hydrogen (*Z*)-butenedioate], calculated with reference to the dried substance.

CHARACTERS

A white or pale-yellow, crystalline powder, very slightly soluble in water and in alcohol.

IDENTIFICATION

First identification: B, C, D.

Second identification: A, C, D.

A. *Carry out the test protected from light.* Dissolve 50 mg in *0.1 M hydrochloric acid* and dilute to 500.0 ml with the same acid. Examined immediately between 280 nm and 350 nm (*2.2.25*), the solution shows an absorption maximum at 305 nm. Dilute 10.0 ml of the solution to 100.0 ml with *0.1 M hydrochloric acid*. Examined immediately between 230 nm and 280 nm, the solution shows an absorption maximum at 255 nm. The specific absorbance at the maximum is 525 to 575.

B. Examine by infrared absorption spectrophotometry (*2.2.24*), comparing with the spectrum obtained with *prochlorperazine maleate CRS*.

C. It complies with the identification of phenothiazines by thin-layer chromatography (*2.3.3*), with the following modifications:

Test solution. Dissolve 20 mg of the substance to be examined in a mixture of equal volumes of *chloroform R* and *methanol R* and dilute to 20 ml with the same mixture of solvents.

Reference solution. Dissolve 20 mg of *prochlorperazine maleate CRS* in a mixture of equal volumes of *chloroform R* and *methanol R* and dilute to 20 ml with the same mixture of solvents.

Apply separately to the plate 4 µl of each solution.

D. Triturate 0.2 g with a mixture of 1 ml of *strong sodium hydroxide solution R* and 3 ml of *water R*. Shake with three quantities, each of 5 ml, of *ether R*. To 0.1 ml of the aqueous layer add a solution of 10 mg of *resorcinol R* in 3 ml of *sulphuric acid R*. Heat in a water-bath for 15 min. No colour develops. To the remainder of the aqueous layer add 2 ml of *bromine solution R*. Heat in a water-bath for 15 min and then heat to boiling. Cool. To 0.1 ml of the solution add a solution of 10 mg of *resorcinol R* in 3 ml of *sulphuric acid R*. Heat in a water-bath for 15 min. A blue colour develops.

TESTS

pH (*2.2.3*). The pH of a freshly prepared saturated solution in *carbon dioxide-free water R* is 3.0 to 4.0.

Related substances. *Carry out the test protected from light.* Examine by thin-layer chromatography (*2.2.27*), using *silica gel* GF_{254} *R* as the coating substance.

Test solution. Dissolve 0.2 g of the substance to be examined in a mixture of 5 volumes of *diethylamine R* and 95 volumes of *methanol R* and dilute to 10 ml with the same mixture of solvents. Prepare immediately before use.

Reference solution. Dilute 1 ml of the test solution to 200 ml with a mixture of 5 volumes of *diethylamine R* and 95 volumes of *methanol R*.

Apply separately to the plate 10 µl of each solution. Develop over a path of 12 cm using a mixture of 10 volumes of *acetone R*, 10 volumes of *diethylamine R* and 80 volumes of *cyclohexane R*. Allow the plate to dry in air and examine in ultraviolet light at 254 nm. Any spot in the chromatogram obtained with the test solution, apart from the principal spot, is not more intense than the spot in the chromatogram obtained with the reference solution (0.5 per cent). Disregard any spots remaining at the starting-points.

Loss on drying (*2.2.32*). Not more than 1.0 per cent, determined on 1.00 g by drying in an oven at 100 °C to 105 °C.

Sulphated ash (*2.4.14*). Not more than 0.1 per cent, determined on 1.0 g.

ASSAY

Dissolve 0.200 g of the powdered substance to be examined in 50 ml of *anhydrous acetic acid R*, warming on a water-bath. Allow to cool to room temperature. Titrate with *0.1 M perchloric acid* determining the end-point potentiometrically (*2.2.20*).

1 ml of *0.1 M perchloric acid* is equivalent to 30.31 mg of $C_{28}H_{32}ClN_3O_8S$.

STORAGE

Store protected from light.

01/2005:0429

PROGESTERONE

Progesteronum

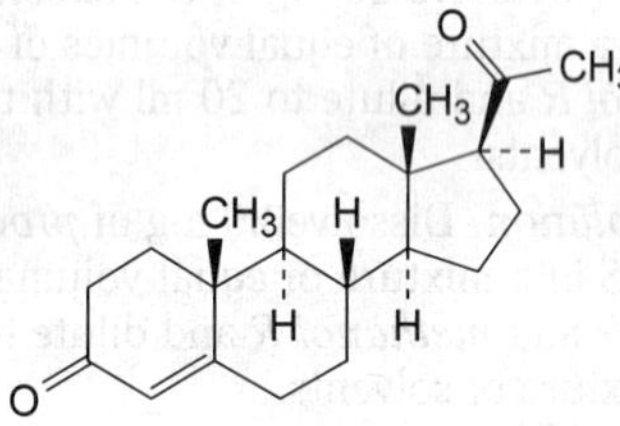

$C_{21}H_{30}O_2$ M_r 314.5

DEFINITION

Pregn-4-ene-3,20-dione.

Content: 97.0 per cent to 103.0 per cent (dried substance).

CHARACTERS

Appearance: white or almost white, crystalline powder or colourless crystals.

Solubility: practically insoluble in water, freely soluble in ethanol, sparingly soluble in acetone and in fatty oils.

It shows polymorphism.

IDENTIFICATION

A. Infrared absorption spectrophotometry (*2.2.24*).

Comparison: *progesterone CRS.*

If the spectra obtained in the solid state show differences, dissolve the substance to be examined and the reference substance separately in *ethanol R*, evaporate to dryness and record new spectra using the residues.

B. Thin-layer chromatography (*2.2.27*)

Test solution. Dissolve 10 mg of the substance to be examined in a mixture of 1 volume of *methanol R* and 9 volumes of *methylene chloride R* and dilute to 10 ml with the same mixture of solvents.

Reference solution. Dissolve 10 mg of *progesterone CRS* in a mixture of 1 volume of *methanol R* and 9 volumes of *methylene chloride R* and dilute to 10 ml with the same mixture of solvents.

Plate: *TLC silica gel F_{254} plate R.*

Mobile phase: *ethyl acetate R, methylene chloride R* (33:66 *V/V*).

Application: 5 µl.

Development: over 3/4 of the plate.

Drying: in air.

Detection A: examine in ultraviolet light at 254 nm.

Detection B: spray with *alcoholic solution of sulphuric acid R*, heat at 120 °C for 15 min and allow to cool. Examine in daylight and in ultraviolet light at 365 nm.

Results A: the principal spot in the chromatogram obtained with the test solution is similar in position, colour and size to the principal spot in the chromatogram obtained with the reference solution.

Results B: the principal spot in the chromatogram obtained with the test solution is similar in position, fluorescence in ultraviolet light at 365 nm and size to the principal spot in the chromatogram obtained with the reference solution.

TESTS

Specific optical rotation (*2.2.7*): + 186 to + 194 (dried substance).

Dissolve 0.250 g in *ethanol R* and dilute to 25.0 ml with the same solvent.

Related substances. Liquid chromatography (*2.2.29*).

Test solution. Dissolve 20.0 mg of the substance to be examined in *methanol R* and dilute to 50.0 ml with the same solvent.

Reference solution (a). Dissolve 2.0 mg of *progesterone CRS* and 2.0 mg of *progesterone impurity C CRS* in *methanol R* and dilute to 50.0 ml with the same solvent.

Reference solution (b). Dilute 1.0 ml of the test solution to 100.0 ml with *methanol R.*

Column:

- *size*: *l* = 0.15 m, Ø = 4.6 mm,
- *stationary phase*: spherical *end-capped octadecylsilyl silica gel for chromatography R* (5 µm).

Mobile phase:

- *mobile phase A*: *water R,*
- *mobile phase B*: *acetonitrile R.*

Time (min)	Mobile phase A (per cent *V/V*)	Mobile phase B (per cent *V/V*)
0 - 20	50	50
20 - 27	50 → 20	50 → 80
27 - 45	20	80
45 - 50	50	50

Flow rate: 0.8 ml/min.

Detection: spectrophotometer at 241 nm.

Injection: 10 µl.

System suitability: reference solution (a):

- *resolution*: minimum 1.5 between the peaks due to impurity C and to progesterone.

Limits:

- *any impurity*: not more than 0.5 times the area of the principal peak in the chromatogram obtained with reference solution (b) (0.5 per cent),
- *total*: not more than 0.8 times the area of the principal peak in the chromatogram obtained with reference solution (b) (0.8 per cent),

– *disregard limit*: 0.05 times the area of the principal peak in the chromatogram obtained with reference solution (b) (0.05 per cent).

Loss on drying (*2.2.32*): maximum 0.5 per cent, determined on 0.500 g by drying in an oven at 100-105 °C for 2 h.

ASSAY

Dissolve 25.0 mg in *alcohol R* and dilute to 250.0 ml with the same solvent. Dilute 5.0 ml of the solution to 50.0 ml with *alcohol R*. Measure the absorbance (*2.2.25*) at the maximum at 241 nm.

Calculate the content of $C_{21}H_{30}O_2$ taking the specific absorbance to be 535.

STORAGE

Protected from light.

IMPURITIES

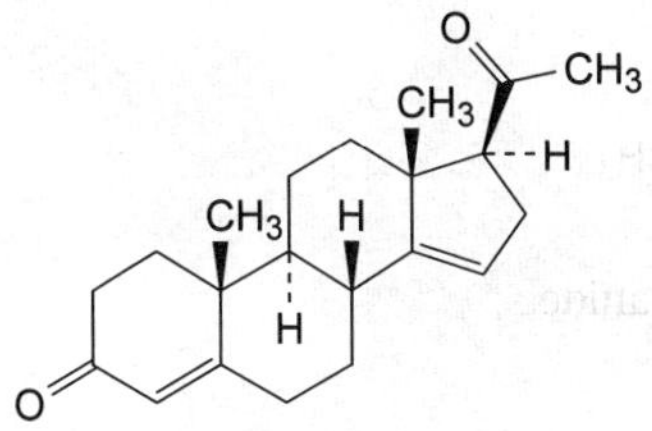

A. pregna-4,14-diene-3,20-dione,

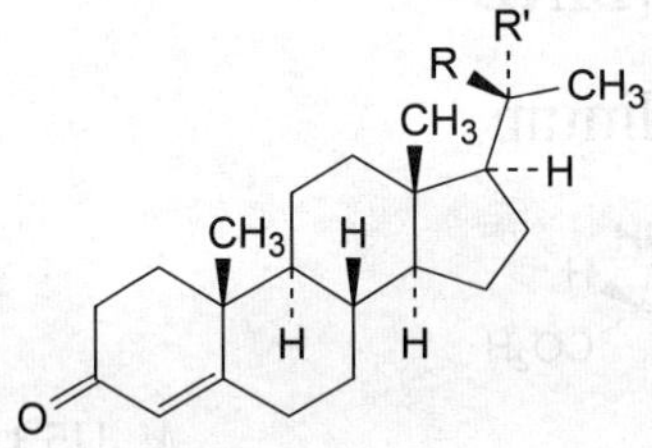

B. R = OH, R′ = H: (20*S*)-20-hydroxypregn-4-en-3-one,

C. R = H, R′ = OH: (20*R*)-20-hydroxypregn-4-en-3-one,

D. R = O-CO-CH_3, R′ = H: (20*S*)-3-oxopregn-4-en-20-yl acetate,

E. R = H, R′ = O-CO-CH_3: (20*R*)-3-oxopregn-4-en-20-yl acetate,

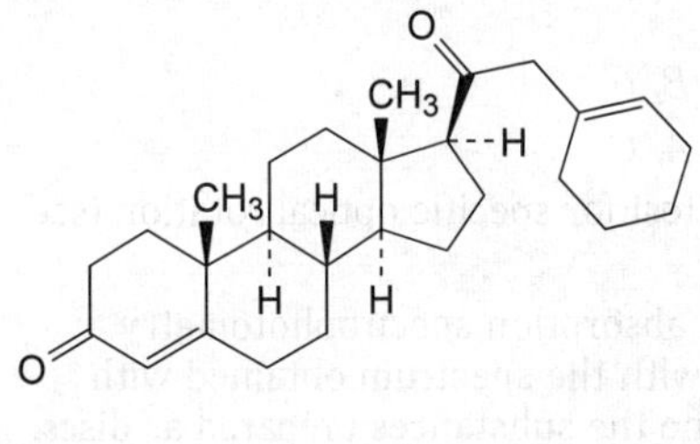

F. 21-(cyclohex-1-enyl)pregn-4-ene-3,20-dione,

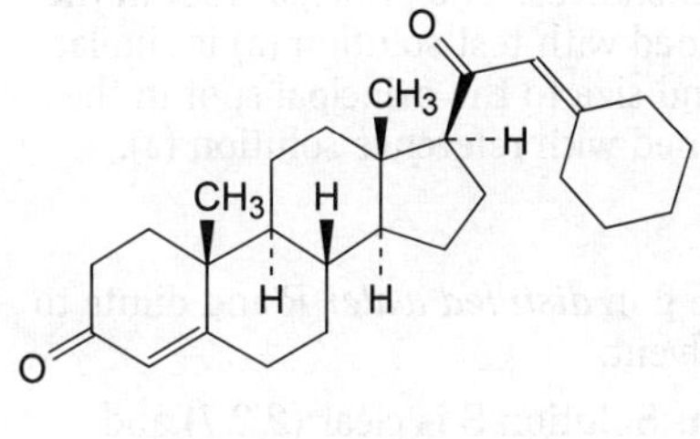

G. 21-(cyclohexylidene)pregn-4-ene-3,20-dione.

01/2005:2002

PROGUANIL HYDROCHLORIDE

Proguanili hydrochloridum

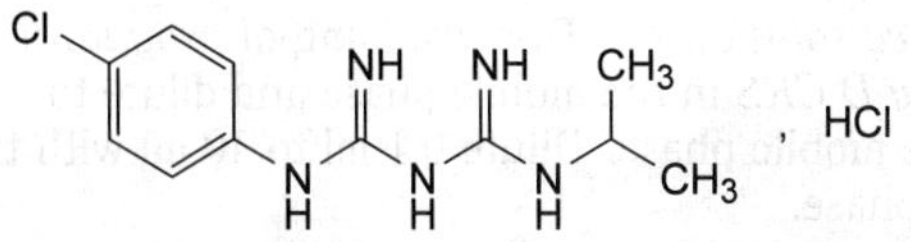

$C_{11}H_{17}Cl_2N_5$ M_r 290.2

DEFINITION

1-(4-Chlorophenyl)-5-(1-methylethyl)biguanide hydrochloride.

Content: 98.5 per cent to 101.0 per cent (dried substance).

CHARACTERS

Appearance: white, crystalline powder.

Solubility: slightly soluble in water, sparingly soluble in ethanol, practically insoluble in methylene chloride.

IDENTIFICATION

First identification: A, D.

Second identification: B, C, D.

A. Infrared absorption spectrophotometry (*2.2.24*).

Comparison: *Ph. Eur. reference spectrum of proguanil hydrochloride.*

B. Dissolve 0.4 g in 50 ml of *water R* (solution A). To 15 ml of solution A add 2 ml of *dilute sodium hydroxide solution R*. Extract with 20 ml of *ethyl acetate R*. Wash the organic layer with *water R*, evaporate to dryness and dry at 105 °C. The melting point (*2.2.14*) of the residue is 130 °C to 133 °C.

C. To 10 ml of solution A, add 1 drop of *copper sulphate solution R* and 2 ml of *dilute ammonia R1*. Add 5 ml of *toluene R* and stir. Allow to stand until separation of the layers is obtained. The upper layer is violet-red.

D. It gives reaction (a) of chlorides (*2.3.1*).

TESTS

Acidity or alkalinity. To 35 ml of *water R* maintained at 60-65 °C, add 0.2 ml of *methyl red mixed solution R*. Neutralise to a grey colour with either *0.01 M sodium hydroxide* or *0.01 M hydrochloric acid*. Add 0.4 g of the substance to be examined and stir until completely dissolved. The solution is grey or green. Not more than 0.2 ml of *0.01 M hydrochloric acid* is required to change the colour of the solution to reddish-violet.

Chloroaniline: maximum 250 ppm.

Dissolve 0.10 g in 1 ml of *2 M hydrochloric acid* and dilute to 20 ml with *water R*. Cool to 5 °C. Add 1 ml of a 3.45 g/l solution of *sodium nitrite R* and allow to stand at 5 °C for 5 min. Add 2 ml of a 50 g/l solution of *ammonium sulphamate R* and allow to stand for 10 min. Add 2 ml of *naphthylethylenediamine dihydrochloride solution R*, dilute to 50 ml with *water R* and allow to stand for 30 min. Any red colour produced is not more intense than that of a standard prepared at the same time and in the same manner, using 20 ml of a 1.25 mg/l solution of *chloroaniline R*.

Related substances. Liquid chromatography (*2.2.29*).

Test solution. Dissolve 10.0 mg of the substance to be examined in the mobile phase and dilute to 100.0 ml with the mobile phase.

Reference solution (a). Dilute 1.0 ml of the test solution to 50.0 ml with the mobile phase. Dilute 1.0 ml of this solution to 10.0 ml with the mobile phase.

Reference solution (b). Dissolve 5 mg of *proguanil impurity C CRS* in the mobile phase and dilute to 100 ml with the mobile phase. Dilute 0.1 ml to 10 ml with the mobile phase.

Reference solution (c). Dissolve 5 mg of *proguanil impurity D CRS* in the mobile phase and dilute to 100 ml with the mobile phase. Dilute 0.1 ml to 10 ml with the mobile phase.

Reference solution (d). Dilute 1 ml of the test solution to 200 ml with the mobile phase. To 1 ml add 1 ml of reference solution (c) and mix.

Column:
- *size*: l = 0.125 m, Ø = 4.6 mm,
- *stationary phase*: *octadecylsilyl silica gel for chromatography R* (5 µm).

Mobile phase: dissolve 3.78 g of *sodium hexanesulphonate R* in a mixture of 10 volumes of *glacial acetic acid R*, 800 volumes of *water R* and 1200 volumes of *methanol R*.

Flow rate: 1 ml/min.

Detection: spectrophotometer at 230 nm and 254 nm.

Injection: 20 µl.

Run time: 5 times the retention time of proguanil.

Retention time: proguanil = about 6 min.

System suitability: reference solution (d) at 230 nm:
- *resolution*: minimum 5 between the peaks due to impurity D and proguanil.

Limits:
- *impurity C*: not more than 3.5 times the area of the principal peak in the chromatogram obtained with reference solution (a) at 230 nm (0.7 per cent),
- *impurity D*: not more than the area of the principal peak in the chromatogram obtained with reference solution (a) at 230 nm (0.2 per cent),
- *any other impurity*: not more than 0.5 times the area of the principal peak in the chromatogram obtained with reference solution (a) at 230 nm and at 254 nm (0.1 per cent),
- *total*: the sum of the calculated percentage contents of known and unknown impurities is not greater than 1 per cent, considering each peak at the wavelength at which the peak shows the higher value,
- *disregard limit*: 0.25 times the area of the principal peak in the chromatogram obtained with reference solution (a) (0.05 per cent).

Loss on drying (*2.2.32*): maximum 0.5 per cent, determined on 1.000 g by drying in an oven at 100-105 °C.

Sulphated ash (*2.4.14*): maximum 0.1 per cent, determined on 1.0 g.

ASSAY

Suspend 0.100 g in 20 ml of *anhydrous acetic acid R*, shake and heat at 50 °C for 5 min. Cool to room temperature and add 40 ml of *acetic anhydride R*. Titrate with *0.1 M perchloric acid*, determining the end-point potentiometrically (*2.2.20*).

1 ml of *0.1 M perchloric acid* is equivalent to 14.51 mg of $C_{11}H_{17}Cl_2N_5$.

STORAGE

Protected from light.

IMPURITIES

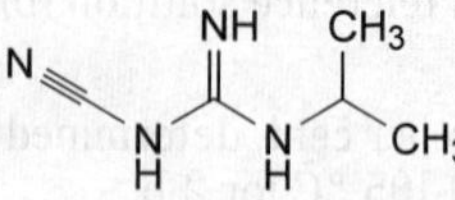

A. 1-cyano-3-(1-methylethyl)guanidine,

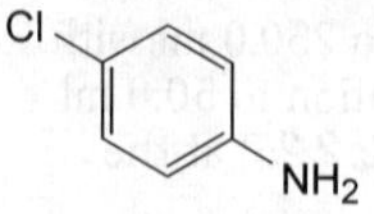

B. 4-chloroaniline,

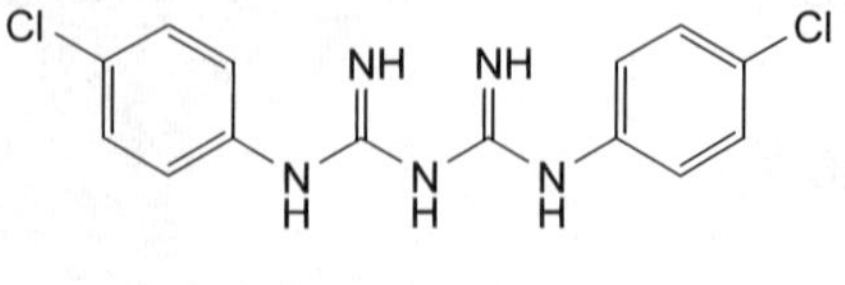

C. 1,5-bis(4-chlorophenyl)biguanide,

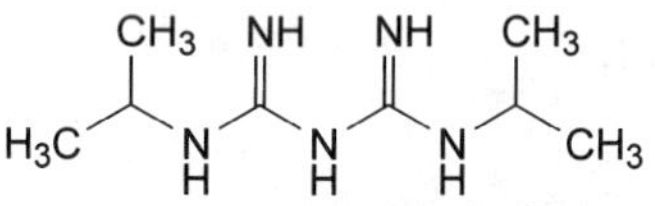

D. 1,5-bis(1-methylethyl)biguanide.

01/2005:0785

PROLINE

Prolinum

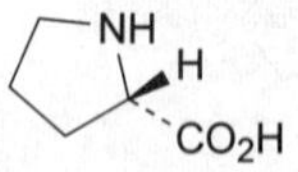

$C_5H_9NO_2$ M_r 115.1

DEFINITION

Proline contains not less than 98.5 per cent and not more than the equivalent of 101.0 per cent of (*S*)-pyrrolidine-2-carboxylic acid, calculated with reference to the dried substance.

CHARACTERS

White or almost white, crystalline powder or colourless crystals, very soluble in water, freely soluble in alcohol.

IDENTIFICATION

First identification: *A, B.*

Second identification: *A, C.*

A. It complies with the test for specific optical rotation (see Tests).

B. Examine by infrared absorption spectrophotometry (*2.2.24*), comparing with the spectrum obtained with *proline CRS*. Examine the substances prepared as discs.

C. Examine the chromatograms obtained in the test for ninhydrin-positive substances. The principal spot in the chromatogram obtained with test solution (b) is similar in position, colour and size to the principal spot in the chromatogram obtained with reference solution (a).

TESTS

Solution S. Dissolve 2.5 g in *distilled water R* and dilute to 50 ml with the same solvent.

Appearance of solution. Solution S is clear (*2.2.1*) and colourless (*2.2.2, Method II*).

Specific optical rotation (*2.2.7*). Dissolve 1.00 g in *water R* and dilute to 25.0 ml with the same solvent. The specific optical rotation is − 84.0 to − 86.0, calculated with reference to the dried substance.

Ninhydrin-positive substances. Examine by thin-layer chromatography (*2.2.27*), using a *TLC silica gel plate R*.

Test solution (a). Dissolve 0.10 g of the substance to be examined in *0.1 M hydrochloric acid* and dilute to 10 ml with the same acid.

Test solution (b). Dilute 1 ml of test solution (a) to 50 ml with *water R*.

Reference solution (a). Dissolve 10 mg of *proline CRS* in *0.1 M hydrochloric acid* and dilute to 50 ml with the same acid.

Reference solution (b). Dilute 5 ml of test solution (b) to 20 ml with *water R*.

Reference solution (c). Dissolve 10 mg of *proline CRS* and 10 mg of *threonine CRS* in *0.1 M hydrochloric acid* and dilute to 25 ml with the same acid.

Apply to the plate 5 µl of each solution. Allow the plate to dry in air. Develop over a path of 15 cm using a mixture of 20 volumes of *glacial acetic acid R*, 20 volumes of *water R* and 60 volumes of *butanol R*. Allow the plate to dry in air, spray with *ninhydrin solution R* and heat at 100 °C to 105 °C for 15 min. Any spot in the chromatogram obtained with test solution (a), apart from the principal spot, is not more intense than the spot in the chromatogram obtained with reference solution (b) (0.5 per cent). The test is not valid unless the chromatogram obtained with reference solution (c) shows two clearly separated spots.

Chlorides (*2.4.4*). Dilute 5 ml of solution S to 15 ml with *water R*. The solution complies with the limit test for chlorides (200 ppm).

Sulphates (*2.4.13*). Dilute 10 ml of solution S to 15 ml with *distilled water R*. The solution complies with the limit test for sulphates (300 ppm).

Ammonium (*2.4.1*). 50 mg complies with limit test B for ammonium (200 ppm). Prepare the standard using 0.1 ml of *ammonium standard solution (100 ppm NH_4) R*.

Iron (*2.4.9*). In a separating funnel, dissolve 1.0 g in 10 ml of *dilute hydrochloric acid R*. Shake with three quantities, each of 10 ml, of *methyl isobutyl ketone R1*, shaking for 3 min each time. To the combined organic layers add 10 ml of *water R* and shake for 3 min. The aqueous layer complies with the limit test for iron (10 ppm).

Heavy metals (*2.4.8*). Dissolve 2.0 g in *water R* and dilute to 20 ml with the same solvent. 12 ml of the solution complies with limit test A for heavy metals (10 ppm). Prepare the standard using the *lead solution (1 ppm Pb) R*.

Loss on drying (*2.2.32*). Not more than 0.5 per cent, determined on 1.000 g by drying in an oven at 100 °C to 105 °C.

Sulphated ash (*2.4.14*). Not more than 0.1 per cent, determined on 1.0 g.

ASSAY

Dissolve 0.100 g in 3 ml of *anhydrous formic acid R*. Add 30 ml of *anhydrous acetic acid R*. Titrate with *0.1 M perchloric acid* using 0.1 ml of *naphtholbenzein solution R* as indicator, until the colour changes from brownish-yellow to green.

1 ml of *0.1 M perchloric acid* is equivalent to 11.51 mg of $C_5H_9NO_2$.

STORAGE

Store protected from light.

01/2005:1365

PROMAZINE HYDROCHLORIDE

Promazini hydrochloridum

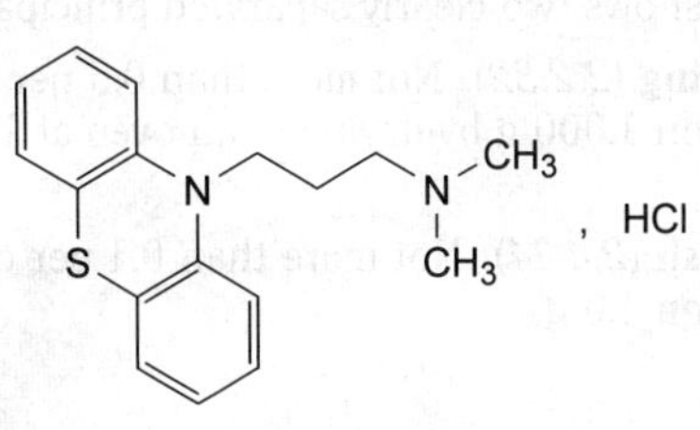

$C_{17}H_{21}ClN_2S$ M_r 320.9

DEFINITION

Promazine hydrochloride contains not less than 99.0 per cent and not more than the equivalent of 101.0 per cent of 3-(10*H*-phenothiazin-10-yl)-*N*,*N*-dimethylpropan-1-amine hydrochloride, calculated with reference to the dried substance.

CHARACTERS

A white or almost white, crystalline powder, slightly hygroscopic, very soluble in water, in alcohol and in methylene chloride.

It melts at about 179 °C.

IDENTIFICATION

First identification: A, B, D.

Second identification: B, C, D.

A. Examine by infrared absorption spectrophotometry (*2.2.24*), comparing with the spectrum obtained with *promazine hydrochloride CRS*.

B. It complies with the identification test for phenothiazines by thin-layer chromatography (*2.3.3*). Use *promazine hydrochloride CRS* to prepare the reference solution.

C. Dissolve about 5 mg in 2 ml of *sulphuric acid R* and allow to stand for 5 min. An orange colour is produced.

D. It gives reaction (b) of chlorides (*2.3.1*).

TESTS

pH (*2.2.3*). Dissolve 0.5 g in *carbon dioxide-free water R* and dilute to 10 ml with the same solvent. The pH of the freshly prepared solution is 4.2 to 5.2.

Related substances. *Carry out the test protected from bright light. Prepare the solutions immediately before use.*

Examine by thin layer chromatography (*2.2.27*), using a *TLC silica gel F_{254} plate R*.

Test solution. Dissolve 0.10 g of the substance to be examined in a mixture of 5 volumes of *diethylamine R* and 95 volumes of *methanol R* and dilute to 10 ml with the same mixture of solvents.

Reference solution (a). Dilute 1 ml of the test solution to 200 ml with a mixture of 5 volumes of *diethylamine R* and 95 volumes of *methanol R*.

Reference solution (b). Dissolve 10 mg of *chlorprothixene hydrochloride CRS* in a mixture of 5 volumes of *diethylamine R* and 95 volumes of *methanol R*, add 1 ml of the test solution and dilute to 10 ml with the same mixture of solvents.

Monographs P

Apply to the plate 10 µl of each solution. Develop over a path of 15 cm using a mixture of 10 volumes of *acetone R*, 10 volumes of *diethylamine R* and 80 volumes of *cyclohexane R*. Allow the plate to dry in air and examine in ultraviolet light at 254 nm. Any spot in the chromatogram obtained with the test solution, apart from the principal spot, is not more intense than the spot in the chromatogram obtained with the reference solution (a) (0.5 per cent). Disregard any spot at the starting point. The test is not valid unless the chromatogram obtained with reference solution (b) shows two clearly separated principal spots.

Loss on drying (*2.2.32*). Not more than 0.5 per cent, determined on 1.000 g by drying in an oven at 100 °C to 105 °C.

Sulphated ash (*2.4.14*). Not more than 0.1 per cent, determined on 1.0 g.

ASSAY

Dissolve 0.250 g in a mixture of 5.0 ml of *0.01 M hydrochloric acid* and 50 ml of *alcohol R*. Carry out a potentiometric titration (*2.2.20*), using *0.1 M sodium hydroxide*. Read the volume added between the two points of inflexion.

1 ml of *0.1 M sodium hydroxide* is equivalent to 32.09 mg of $C_{17}H_{21}ClN_2S$.

STORAGE

Store protected from light.

IMPURITIES

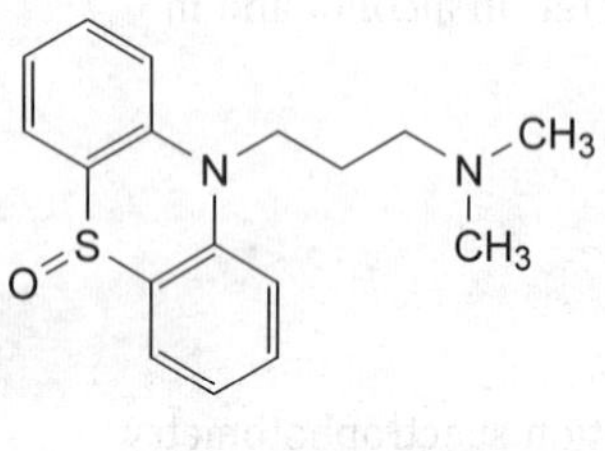

A. 3-(10*H*-phenothiazin-10-yl)-*N*,*N*-dimethylpropan-1-amine *S*-oxide (promazine sulphoxide).

01/2005:0524

PROMETHAZINE HYDROCHLORIDE

Promethazini hydrochloridum

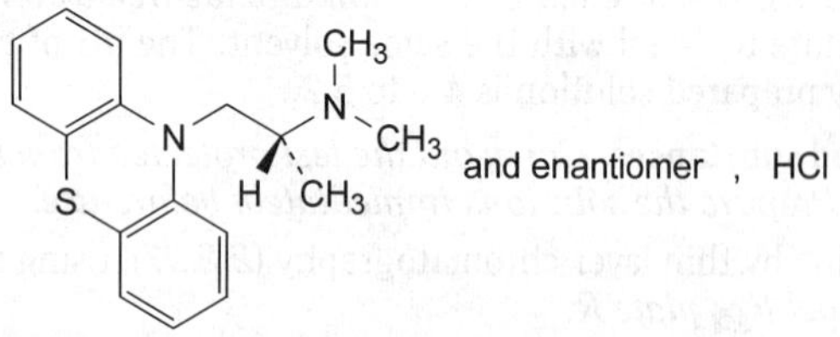

$C_{17}H_{21}ClN_2S$ M_r 320.9

DEFINITION

Promethazine hydrochloride contains not less than 99.0 per cent and not more than the equivalent of 101.0 per cent of (2*RS*)-*N*,*N*-dimethyl-1-(10*H*-phenothiazin-10-yl)propan-2-amine hydrochloride, calculated with reference to the dried substance.

CHARACTERS

A white or faintly yellowish, crystalline powder, very soluble in water, freely soluble in alcohol and in methylene chloride.

It melts at about 222 °C, with decomposition.

IDENTIFICATION

First identification: A, B, D.

Second identification: B, C, D.

A. Examine by infrared absorption spectrophotometry (*2.2.24*), comparing with the spectrum obtained with *promethazine hydrochloride CRS*.

B. It complies with the identification test for phenothiazines by thin-layer chromatography (*2.3.3*).

C. Dissolve 0.1 g in 3 ml of *water R*. Add dropwise 1 ml of *nitric acid R*. A precipitate is formed which rapidly dissolves to give a red solution, becoming orange and then yellow. Heat to boiling. The solution becomes orange and an orange-red precipitate is formed.

D. It gives reaction (b) of chlorides (*2.3.1*).

TESTS

pH (*2.2.3*). Dissolve 1.0 g in *carbon dioxide-free water R* and dilute to 10 ml with the same solvent. The pH of the solution measured immediately after preparation is 4.0 to 5.0.

Related substances. *Carry out the test protected from bright light. Prepare the solutions immediately before use.* Examine by thin-layer chromatography (*2.2.27*), using a suitable silica gel as the coating substance.

Test solution. Dissolve 0.20 g of the substance to be examined in a mixture of 5 volumes of *diethylamine R* and 95 volumes of *methanol R* and dilute to 10 ml with the same mixture of solvents.

Reference solution (a). Dissolve 20 mg of *isopromethazine hydrochloride CRS* in a mixture of 5 volumes of *diethylamine R* and 95 volumes of *methanol R* and dilute to 100 ml with the same mixture of solvents.

Reference solution (b). Dilute 0.5 ml of the test solution to 100 ml with a mixture of 5 volumes of *diethylamine R* and 95 volumes of *methanol R*.

Reference solution (c). Dilute 0.2 ml of the test solution to 100 ml with a mixture of 5 volumes of *diethylamine R* and 95 volumes of *methanol R*.

Apply separately to the plate 10 µl of the test solution and 10 µl of each reference solution. Develop in an unsaturated tank over a path of 12 cm using a mixture of 5 volumes of *diethylamine R*, 10 volumes of *acetone R* and 85 volumes of *cyclohexane R*. Allow the plate to dry in air and examine in ultraviolet light at 254 nm. Disregard any spot at the starting point.

In the chromatogram obtained with the test solution: any spot corresponding to isopromethazine hydrochloride is not more intense that the spot in the chromatogram obtained with reference solution (a) (1 per cent); any spot, apart from the principal spot and the spot corresponding to isopromethazine hydrochloride, is not more intense than the spot in the chromatogram obtained with reference solution (b) (0.5 per cent) and at most three such spots are more intense than the spot in the chromatogram obtained with reference solution (c) (0.2 per cent).

Heavy metals (*2.4.8*). Dissolve 1.0 g in 5 ml of *water R*, add 5 ml of *acetone R* and 5 ml of *buffer solution pH 3.5 R*. Carry out the prefiltration. The prefiltrate complies with limit test E for heavy metals (10 ppm). Prepare the standard using 5 ml of *lead standard solution (2 ppm Pb) R*.

Loss on drying (*2.2.32*). Not more than 0.5 per cent, determined on 1.000 g by drying in an oven at 100 °C to 105 °C.

Sulphated ash (*2.4.14*). Not more than 0.1 per cent, determined on 1.0 g.

ASSAY

Dissolve 0.250 g in a mixture of 5.0 ml of *0.01 M hydrochloric acid* and 50 ml of *alcohol R*. Carry out a potentiometric titration (*2.2.20*), using *0.1 M sodium hydroxide*. Read the volume added between the two points of inflexion.

1 ml of *0.1 M sodium hydroxide* is equivalent to 32.09 mg of $C_{17}H_{21}ClN_2S$.

STORAGE

Store protected from light.

IMPURITIES

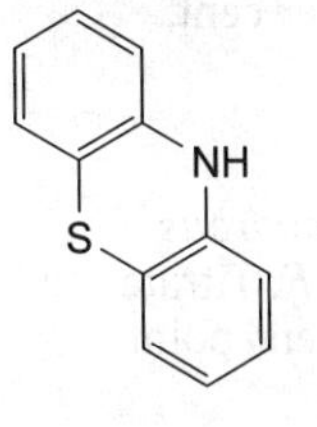

A. phenothiazine,

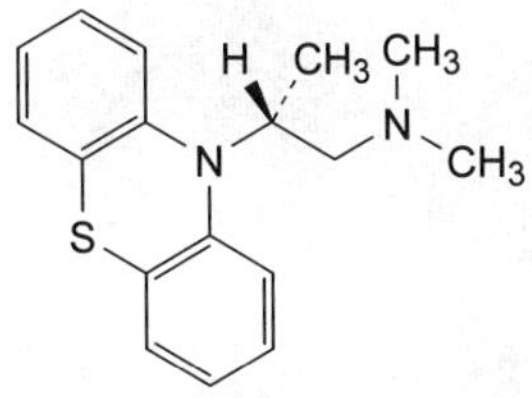

and enantiomer

B. (2*RS*)-*N*,*N*-dimethyl-2-(10*H*-phenothiazin-10-yl)propan-1-amine (isopromethazine),

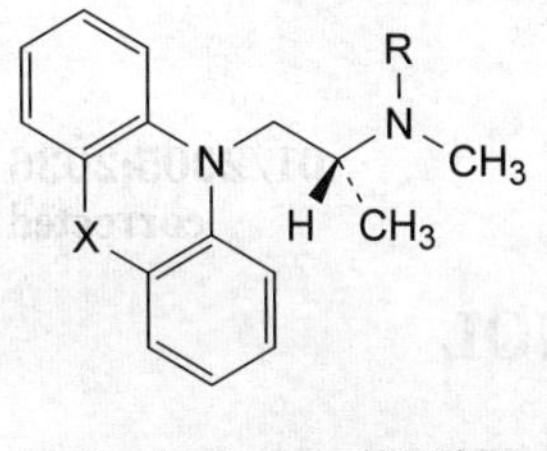

and enantiomer

C. R = H, X = S: (2*RS*)-*N*-methyl-1-(10*H*-phenothiazin-10-yl)propan-2-amine,

D. R = CH_3, X = SO: (2*RS*)-*N*,*N*-dimethyl-1-(10*H*-phenothiazin-10-yl)propan-2-amine *S*-oxide.

01/2005:1366

PROPACETAMOL HYDROCHLORIDE

Propacetamoli hydrochloridum

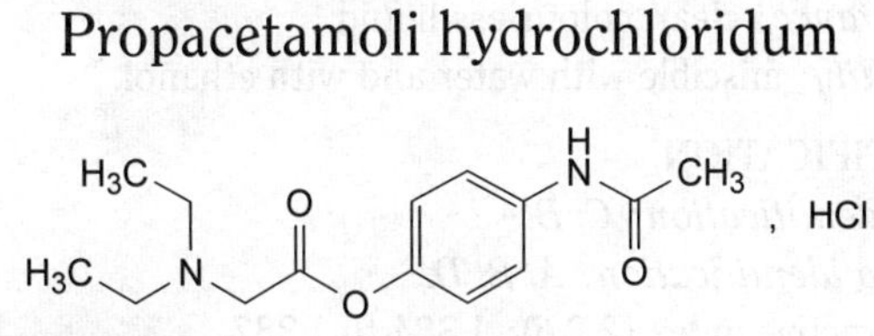

$C_{14}H_{21}ClN_2O_3$ M_r 300.8

DEFINITION

Propacetamol hydrochloride contains not less than 98.0 per cent and not more than the equivalent of 102.0 per cent of 4-(acetylamino)phenyl (diethylamino)acetate hydrochloride, calculated with reference to the dried substance.

CHARACTERS

A white or almost white, crystalline powder, freely soluble in water, slightly soluble in ethanol, practically insoluble in acetone.

IDENTIFICATION

A. Examine by infrared absorption spectrophotometry (*2.2.24*), comparing with the *Ph. Eur. reference spectrum of propacetamol hydrochloride*.

B. It gives reaction (a) of chlorides (*2.3.1*).

TESTS

Solution S. *Prepare the solution immediately before use.* Dissolve 1.75 g in *water R* and dilute to 10.0 ml with the same solvent.

Appearance of solution. Solution S is clear (*2.2.1*) and not more intensely coloured than reference solution Y_6 or BY_6 (*2.2.2, Method II*).

Absorbance. The absorbance (*2.2.25*) of solution S measured at 390 nm is not greater than 0.05.

Related substances. Examine by liquid chromatography (*2.2.29*).

Solution A. Dissolve 2.16 g of *sodium octanesulphonate R* in 900 ml of *water R* and dilute to 1000 ml with the same solvent. Adjust to pH 3.0 with *acetic acid R*.

Test solution. Suspend 1.00 g of the substance to be examined in 10.0 ml of *acetonitrile R*. Shake for 10 min. Allow to stand. Take 3.0 ml of the supernatant solution and dilute to 10.0 ml with solution A. *Inject this solution immediately after preparation.*

Reference solution (a). Dissolve 50 mg of *paracetamol R* in *acetonitrile R* and dilute to 50.0 ml with the same solvent. Dilute 1.0 ml of the solution to 50.0 ml with *acetonitrile R*. Dilute 3.0 ml of the latter solution to 10.0 ml with solution A.

Reference solution (b). Dissolve 10 mg of *paracetamol R* and 0.100 g of *4-aminophenol R* in *acetonitrile R* and dilute to 50.0 ml with the same solvent. Dilute 1.0 ml of the solution to 50.0 ml with *acetonitrile R*. Dilute 3.0 ml of the latter solution to 10.0 ml with solution A.

The chromatographic procedure may be carried out using:

– a stainless steel column 0.25 m long and 4.6 mm in internal diameter packed with *octadecylsilyl silica gel for chromatography R* (5 µm),

– as mobile phase at a flow rate of 1 ml/min a mixture of 30 volumes of *acetonitrile R* and 70 volumes of solution A,

– as detector a spectrophotometer set at 246 nm.

Inject 20 µl of reference solution (b). The chromatogram obtained shows a peak corresponding to paracetamol (first peak) and a peak corresponding to 4-aminophenol (second peak) with a retention time relative to paracetamol of about 1.6. Adjust the sensitivity of the system so that the height of the two principal peaks is at least 20 per cent of the full scale of the recorder.

Inject 20 µl of the test solution and 20 µl of reference solution (a). Continue the chromatography of the test solution for twice the retention time of the principal peak. In the chromatogram obtained with the test solution: the area of any peak corresponding to paracetamol is not greater than that of the peak due to paracetamol in the chromatogram obtained with reference solution (a) (200 ppm); the area of any peak, apart from the principal peak and the peak due to paracetamol, is not greater than 3.2 times the area of the principal peak in the chromatogram obtained with reference solution (a) (0.1 per cent taking into account the response factor of paracetamol of 1.6); the sum of the areas of any peak, apart from the principal peak, is not greater than 6.4 times the area of the paracetamol peak in the chromatogram obtained with reference solution (a) (0.2 per cent taking into account the relative response factor of paracetamol of 1.6). Disregard any peak with an area less than 0.01 times the area of the principal peak in the chromatogram obtained with reference solution (a).

4-Aminophenol. Examine by thin-layer chromatography (*2.2.27*), using a *TLC silica gel F_{254} plate R*.

Test solution. Suspend 4.00 g of the substance to be examined in 8 ml of *acetonitrile R*. Shake for 30 min and filter. Dilute to 10 ml with *acetonitrile R*.

Reference solution (a). Dissolve 25 mg of *4-aminophenol R* in *acetonitrile R* and dilute to 50 ml with the same solvent. Dilute 10 ml of the solution to 50 ml with *acetonitrile R*.

Reference solution (b). Dilute 5 ml of reference solution (a) to 50 ml with *acetonitrile R*.

Reference solution (c). Dilute 0.2 ml of reference solution (a) to 5 ml with the test solution.

Apply to the plate 50 µl of the test solution and 50 µl each of reference solutions (b) and (c). Develop over a path of 15 cm using a mixture of 3 volumes of *anhydrous formic acid R*, 4 volumes of *water R*, 30 volumes of *methanol R* and 64 volumes of *methylene chloride R*. Allow the plate to dry in air and examine in ultraviolet light at 254 nm. Spray with a 10 g/l solution of *dimethylaminobenzaldehyde R* in *alcohol R*. Reference solution (c) shows two spots: one visible in ultraviolet light and corresponding to propacetamol hydrochloride and the other one yellow, visible after spraying and corresponding to 4-aminophenol. An additional spot may appear in ultraviolet light and corresponds to paracetamol. In the chromatogram obtained with the test solution, any yellow spot corresponding to 4-aminophenol and not visible in ultraviolet light is not more intense than the spot in the chromatogram obtained with reference solution (b) (25 ppm). The test is not valid unless the chromatogram obtained with reference solution (c) shows two clearly separated spots.

Methanol. Examine by gas chromatography (*2.2.28*), using *propanol R* as the internal standard.

Internal standard solution. Dilute 2.0 ml of *propanol R* to 20.0 ml with *water R*. Dilute 1.0 ml of the solution to 25.0 ml with *water R*. Dilute 1.0 ml of this solution to 25.0 ml with *water R*.

Test solution. Dissolve 2.00 g of the substance to be examined in *water R*, add 2.0 ml of the internal standard solution and dilute to 10.0 ml with *water R*.

Reference solution. Dilute 0.8 ml of *methanol R* to 50.0 ml with *water R*. Dilute 1.0 ml of the solution to 25.0 ml with *water R*. To 2.0 ml of the solution, add 2.0 of the internal standard solution and dilute to 10.0 ml with *water R*.

The chromatographic procedure may be carried out using:

– a glass column 2 m long and 2 mm in internal diameter packed with carbon molecular sieve impregnated with 0.2 per cent of macrogol 1500,
– *nitrogen for chromatography R* as the carrier gas,
– a flame-ionisation detector,

with the following temperature programme:

	Time (min)	Temperature (°C)	Rate (°C/min)	Comment
Column	0 - 1.5	60	-	isothermal
	1.5 - 5.5	60 → 80	5	linear gradient
	5.5 - 15.5	80	-	isothermal
Injection port		170		
Detector		220		

Inject 2 µl of the test solution and 2 µl of the reference solution.

Calculate the ratio of the area of the peak due to methanol to the area of the peak due to propanol for both chromatograms. The ratio for the test solution is not greater than that for the reference solution (500 ppm).

Heavy metals (*2.4.8*). Dissolve 2.0 g in *water R* and dilute to 20 ml with the same solvent. 12 ml of the solution complies with limit test A for heavy metals (10 ppm). Prepare the standard using *lead standard solution 1 ppm (Pb) R*.

Loss on drying (*2.2.32*). Not more than 0.5 per cent, determined on 1.000 g by drying in an oven at 100-105 °C for 3 h.

Sulphated ash (*2.4.14*). Not more than 0.1 per cent, determined on 1.0 g.

ASSAY

Dissolve 0.250 g in a mixture of 25 ml of *anhydrous acetic acid R* and 25 ml of *acetic anhydride R*. Titrate with *0.1 M perchloric acid*, determining the end-point potentiometrically (*2.2.20*).

1 ml of *0.1 M perchloric acid* is equivalent to 30.08 mg of $C_{14}H_{21}ClN_2O_3$.

STORAGE

Store protected from humidity.

IMPURITIES

A. paracetamol,

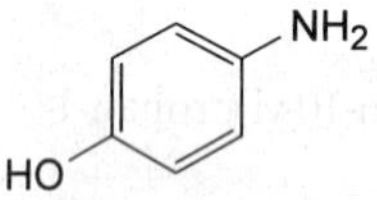

B. 4-aminophenol.

01/2005:2036
corrected

PROPANOL

Propanolum

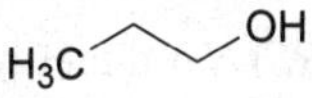

C_3H_8O M_r 60.1

DEFINITION

Propan-1-ol.

CHARACTERS

Appearance: clear, colourless liquid.

Solubility: miscible with water and with ethanol.

IDENTIFICATION

First identification: C, B.

Second identification: A, B, D.

A. Refractive index (*2.2.6*): 1.384 to 1.387.

B. Boiling point (*2.2.12*): 96 °C to 98 °C.

C. Infrared absorption spectrophotometry (*2.2.24*).
Comparison: *Ph. Eur. reference spectrum of propanol.*

D. To 1.0 ml add 0.10 g of *dinitrobenzoyl chloride R* and 0.05 ml of *sulphuric acid R*. Boil under reflux for 30 min. Evaporate until the excess of propanol is removed, add 5 ml of *heptane R* to the residue and heat to boiling. Filter the hot solution. Wash the crystals formed on cooling with *heptane R* and dry in vacuum (2 kPa, at room temperature for 24 h). The small, colourless, shiny plates melt (*2.2.14*) between 71 °C and 74 °C.

TESTS

Solution S. Dissolve the residue obtained in the test for non-volatile matter in 1 ml of *1 M hydrochloric acid* and dilute to 50.0 ml with *water R*.

Appearance. The substance to be examined is clear (*2.2.1*) and colourless (*2.2.2, Method II*). Dilute 2 ml to 10 ml with *water R*. After 5 min, the solution is clear (*2.2.1*).

Acidity or alkalinity. To 10.0 ml of *carbon dioxide-free water R* add 0.1 ml of *phenolphthalein solution R* and *0.01 M sodium hydroxide* until the solution becomes pale pink. After addition of 5.0 ml of the substance to be examined the colour of the solution does not become more intense. If the colour fades, add 0.2 ml of *0.01 M sodium hydroxide*. The solution is pink.

Absorbance (*2.2.25*). Measure the absorbance between 230 nm and 310 nm using *water R* as the compensation liquid. The absorbance *A* is not greater than the following values.

Wavelength (nm)	Absorbance *A*
230	0.300
250	0.100
270	0.030
290	0.020
310	0.010

The absorption curve does not show any peaks.

Reducing substances. Place 10.0 ml in a test tube of about 20 mm in diameter in a water bath at 20 °C. Keep protected from actinic light and add 1.0 ml of a freshly prepared 0.16 g/l solution of *potassium permanganate R*. The mixture, maintained at 20 °C, slowly changes its colour from violet to red. After 30 min, the test solution is not less intensely coloured (*2.2.2, Method II*) than 10.0 ml of a reference solution prepared as follows: to 5.5 ml of primary solution yellow, add 13.0 ml of primary solution red and dilute to 100.0 ml with *water R*.

Related substances. Gas chromatography (*2.2.28*).

Test solution. The substance to be examined.

Reference solution (a). Dilute 1.0 ml of the test solution to 100.0 ml with *heptane R*. Dilute 1.0 ml of the solution to 10.0 ml with *heptane R*.

Reference solution (b). Mix 0.1 ml of *acetone R* with 0.1 ml of *2-propanol R* and dilute to 100 ml with the test solution.

Column:

– *material*: fused silica,
– *size*: *l* = 30 m, Ø = 0.25 mm,
– *stationary phase*: *poly[(cyanopropyl)(phenyl)][dimethyl]siloxane R* (film thickness 1.4 µm).

Carrier gas: *helium for chromatography R.*

Linear velocity: 25 cm/s.

Split ratio: 1:200.

Temperature:

	Time (min)	Temperature (°C)
Column	0 - 12	40
	12 - 28	40 → 200
	28 - 38	200
Injection port		240
Detector		240

Detection: flame ionisation.

Injection: 1 µl.

System suitability: reference solution (b):

– *resolution*: minimum 2.0 between the peaks due to impurity D and impurity E.

Limits:

– *any impurity*: not more than the area of the peak due to propanol in the chromatogram obtained with reference solution (a) (0.1 per cent),
– *total*: not more than 3 times the area of the peak due to propanol in the chromatogram obtained with reference solution (a) (0.3 per cent),
– *disregard limit*: 0.1 times the area of the peak due to propanol in the chromatogram obtained with reference solution (a) (0.01 per cent).

Non-volatile matter: maximum 0.004 per cent.

Evaporate 50 ml of the substance to be examined to dryness at 100 °C and dry the residue in an oven at 100-105 °C to constant mass. The residue weighs a maximum of 2 mg. The residue is used for the preparation of solution S.

Water (*2.5.12*): maximum 0.2 per cent, determined on 10 g.

STORAGE

Protected from light.

IMPURITIES

A. CH_3-OH: methanol,

B. ethanol,

C. CH_3-CH_2-CHO: propanal,

D. acetone,

E. isopropyl alcohol (2-propanol),

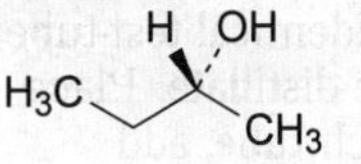

and enantiomer

F. butan-2-ol (*sec*-butanol),

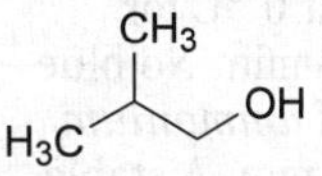

G. 2-methylpropan-1-ol (isobutanol),

H. CH_3-$[CH_2]_3$-OH: butan-1-ol (*n*-butanol),

I. CH_3-$[CH_2]_4$-OH: pentan-1-ol (*n*-pentanol),

J. CH_3-$[CH_2]_5$-OH: hexan-1-ol (*n*-hexanol).

01/2005:0857

PROPANTHELINE BROMIDE

Propanthelini bromidum

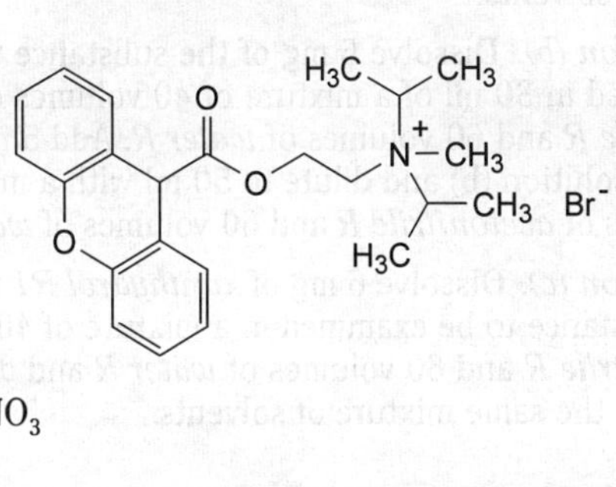

$C_{23}H_{30}BrNO_3$ M_r 448.4

DEFINITION

Propantheline bromide contains not less than 98.5 per cent and not more than the equivalent of 101.0 per cent of *N*-methyl-*N*,*N*-bis(1-methylethyl)-2-[(9*H*-xanthen-9-ylcarbonyl)oxy]ethanaminium bromide, calculated with reference to the dried substance.

CHARACTERS

A white or yellowish-white powder, slightly hygroscopic, very soluble in water, in alcohol and in methylene chloride.

IDENTIFICATION

A. Dissolve 60 mg in *methanol R* and dilute to 100.0 ml with the same solvent. Dilute 10.0 ml of the solution to 100.0 ml with *methanol R*. Examined between 230 nm and 350 nm (*2.2.25*), the solution shows two absorption maxima, at 246 nm and 282 nm. The specific absorbances at the maxima are 115 to 125 and 57 to 63, respectively.

B. Dissolve 0.2 g in 15 ml of *water R* and add 1 ml of *strong sodium hydroxide solution R*. Boil for 2 min and cool slightly. Add 7.5 ml of *dilute hydrochloric acid R* and filter. Wash the residue with *water R* and recrystallise from *alcohol (50 per cent V/V) R*. Dry at 100 °C to 105 °C for 1 h. Dissolve about 10 mg of the residue in 5 ml of *sulphuric acid R*. The solution has an intense yellow colour and shows an intense yellowish-green fluorescence when examined in ultraviolet light at 365 nm.

C. Dissolve 50 mg in 0.1 ml of *water R* in a 25 ml flask and add 1 ml of a saturated solution of *potassium permanganate R*. Attach a fractionating column and a condenser, with the end of the delivery tube immersed in 1 ml of *water R* in a test-tube placed in a bath of iced water. Distil fairly vigorously and continue heating for 1 min after a dry residue has been obtained in the flask. Prepare a blank by introducing into an identical test-tube a volume of *water R* equal to that of the distillate. Place the tubes in a bath of iced water. To each tube, add 0.5 ml of a 20 per cent *V/V* solution of *morpholine R* and 0.5 ml of a freshly prepared 50 g/l solution of *sodium nitroprusside R*. Mix and allow to stand at 0 °C for 5 min and then at room temperature for 3 min. No blue colour develops in either tube. Add 1 g of *ammonium sulphate R*, mix and allow to stand for 15 min. A stable, intense pink colour develops in the test solution. A brownish-yellow colour develops in the blank.

D. It gives reaction (a) of bromides (*2.3.1*).

TESTS

Appearance of solution. Dissolve 0.6 g in *water R* and dilute to 20 ml with the same solvent. The solution is clear (*2.2.1*).

Related substance. Examine by liquid chromatography (*2.2.29*).

Test solution (a). Dissolve 6 mg of the substance to be examined in a mixture of 40 volumes of *acetonitrile R* and 60 volumes of *water R* and dilute to 50 ml with the same mixture of solvents.

Test solution (b). Dissolve 6 mg of the substance to be examined in 30 ml of a mixture of 40 volumes of *acetonitrile R* and 60 volumes of *water R*. Add 5 ml of reference solution (b) and dilute to 50 ml with a mixture of 40 volumes of *acetonitrile R* and 60 volumes of *water R*.

Test solution (c). Dissolve 6 mg of *xanthydrol R1* and 6 mg of the substance to be examined in a mixture of 40 volumes of *acetonitrile R* and 60 volumes of *water R* and dilute to 50 ml with the same mixture of solvents.

Reference solution (a). Dissolve 6 mg of *xanthydrol R1* in a mixture of 40 volumes of *acetonitrile R* and 60 volumes of *water R* and dilute to 50 ml with the same mixture of solvents.

Reference solution (b). Dilute 5 ml of reference solution (a) to 50 ml with a mixture of 40 volumes of *acetonitrile R* and 60 volumes of *water R*.

The chromatographic procedure may be carried out using:

- a stainless steel column 0.25 m long and 4.6 mm in internal diameter, packed with *octadecylsilyl silica gel for chromatography R* (5 µm),
- as mobile phase at a flow rate of 1 ml/min a mixture of equal volumes of *acetonitrile R* and a solution containing 28 g/l of *sodium perchlorate R* and 11 g/l of *phosphoric acid R*, adjusted to pH 3.8 with *strong sodium hydroxide solution R* and then with *0.1 M sodium hydroxide*,
- as detector a spectrophotometer set at 206 nm,
- a loop injector.

Inject 20 µl of test solution (c). The test is not valid unless the resolution between the peaks corresponding to propantheline and xanthydrol is at least 8.0. Inject 20 µl of test solution (a), 20 µl of reference solution (a) and 20 µl of test solution (b). Continue the chromatography for twice the retention time of the propantheline peak. In the chromatogram obtained with test solution (a), there is no peak corresponding to the principal peak in the chromatogram obtained with reference solution (a). In the chromatogram obtained with test solution (b), the area of any peak, apart from the principal peak and the xanthydrol peak, is not greater than the area of the xanthydrol peak (1.0 per cent) and not more than one such peak has an area greater than or equal to half the area of the xanthydrol peak (0.5 per cent). Disregard any peak with a retention time relative to that of the propantheline peak, less than 0.2 (bromide).

Loss on drying (*2.2.32*). Not more than 1.0 per cent, determined on 1.000 g by drying in an oven at 100 °C to 105 °C.

Sulphated ash (*2.4.14*). Not more than 0.1 per cent, determined on 1.0 g.

ASSAY

Dissolve 0.400 g in 50 ml of *acetic anhydride R*. Titrate with *0.1 M perchloric acid*, determining the end-point potentiometrically (*2.2.20*).

1 ml of *0.1 M perchloric acid* corresponds to 44.84 mg of $C_{23}H_{30}BrNO_3$.

STORAGE

Store in an airtight container.

01/2005:1558

PROPOFOL

Propofolum

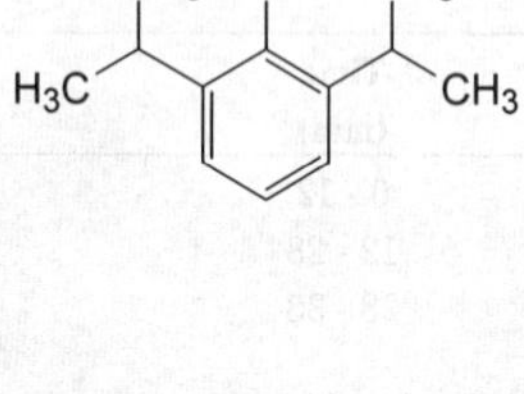

$C_{12}H_{18}O$ M_r 178.3

DEFINITION

Propofol contains not less than 98.0 per cent and not more than the equivalent of 102.0 per cent of 2,6-bis(1-methylethyl)phenol.

CHARACTERS

A colourless or very light yellow, clear liquid, very slightly soluble in water, miscible with hexane and with methanol.

IDENTIFICATION

Examine by infrared absorption spectrophotometry (*2.2.24*) as a thin film between potassium bromide plates, comparing with the spectrum obtained with the *propofol CRS*.

TESTS

Refractive index (*2.2.6*). The refractive index is not less than 1.5125 and not more than 1.5145.

Impurity J. Examine by liquid chromatography (*2.2.29*).

Prepare the solutions immediately before use and protect from light.

Test solution. Dissolve 0.5 g of the substance to be examined in *hexane R* and dilute to 10.0 ml with the same solvent.

Reference solution. Dissolve 5 µl of *propofol impurity J CRS* (corresponding to 5 mg) in *hexane R* and dilute to 50.0 ml with the same solvent. Dilute 5.0 ml of this solution to 100.0 ml with *hexane R*.

The chromatographic procedure used in the test for related substances may be used, by monitoring the eluate of the column at 254 nm in place of 275 nm.

Inject 20 µl of the test solution and 20 µl of the reference solution and continue the chromatography for 6 times the retention time of the propofol peak. In the chromatogram obtained with the test solution the area of any peak due to impurity J is not greater than 5 times the area of the peak due to impurity J in the chromatogram obtained with the reference solution (0.05 per cent).

Related substances. Examine by liquid chromatography (*2.2.29*) as described under Assay.

Inject 10 µl of reference solution (a) and continue the chromatography for 15 min. The resolution of the 2 principal peaks observed (impurity J, approximate retention time 2.5 min and propofol, approximate retention time 3 min) is at least 4.0.

Inject 10 µl of reference solution (b) and locate the peaks due to impurity G (relative retention about 0.5) and impurity E (relative retention about 5), both with respect to propofol.

Inject 10 µl of reference solution (c) and adjust the sensitivity of the system so that the height of the peak due to propofol is at least 50 per cent of the full scale of the recorder.

Inject separately 10 µl of test solution (a) and reference solution (c) and record the chromatogram of test solution (a) for 6 times the retention time of the peak due to propofol. In the chromatogram obtained with test solution (a): the area of any peak due to impurity G is not greater than 0.4 times the area of the peak due to propofol in the chromatogram obtained with reference solution (c) (0.2 per cent taking into account a response factor of 0.2); and the area of any peak due to impurity E is not greater than 0.4 times the area of the peak due to propofol in the chromatogram obtained with reference solution (c) (0.01 per cent taking into account a response factor of 4.0). The area of any other peak apart from that due to propofol and the 2 impurities is not greater than 0.5 times the area of the peak due to propofol in the chromatogram obtained with reference solution (c) (0.05 per cent). The sum of all impurities including impurity G and impurity E is not greater than 0.3 per cent. Disregard any peak with an area less than 0.25 times the area of the peak due to propofol in the chromatogram obtained with reference solution (c) (0.025 per cent).

ASSAY

Examine by liquid chromatography (*2.2.29*).

Test solution (a). Dissolve 1.00 g of the substance to be examined in *hexane R* and dilute to 10.0 ml with the same solvent.

Test solution (b). Dissolve 0.240 g of the substance to be examined in *hexane R* and dilute to 100.0 ml with the same solvent.

Reference solution (a). Dissolve 5 µl of the substance to be examined and 15 µl of *propofol impurity J CRS* in *hexane R* and dilute to 50.0 ml with the same solvent.

Reference solution (b). Dilute 0.1 ml of *propofol for system suitability CRS* to 1.0 ml with *hexane R*.

Reference solution (c). Dilute 1.0 ml of test solution (a) to 100.0 ml with *hexane R*. Dilute 1.0 ml of this solution to 10.0 ml with *hexane R*.

Reference solution (d). Dissolve 0.240 g of *propofol CRS* in *hexane R* and dilute to 100.0 ml with the same solvent.

The chromatographic procedure may be carried out using:

– a stainless steel column 0.20 m long and 5 mm in internal diameter packed with *silica gel for chromatography R* (5 µm),

– as mobile phase at a flow rate of 2.0 ml/min a mixture of 1.0 volumes of *ethanol R*, 7.5 volumes of *acetonitrile R* and 990 volumes of *hexane R*,

– as detector a spectrophotometer set at 275 nm.

Inject 10 µl of test solution (b) and 10 µl of reference solution (d). Continue the chromatography for 5 times the retention time of the peak due to propofol.

STORAGE

Store protected from light under an inert atmosphere of gas.

IMPURITIES

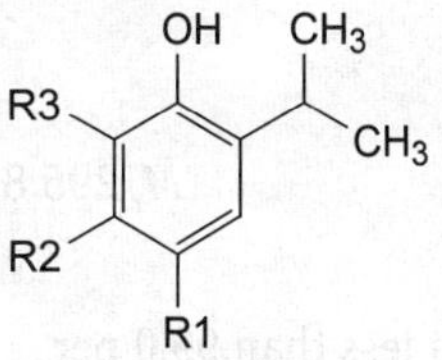

A. R1 = $CH(CH_3)_2$, R2 = R3 = H: 2,4-bis(1-methylethyl)phenol,

B. R1 = R2 = H, R3 = $CCH_3{=}CH_2$: 2-(1-methylethenyl)-6-(1-methylethyl)phenol,

C. R1 = R2 = R3 = H: 2-(1-methylethyl)phenol,

D. R1 = R3 = H, R2 = $CH(CH_3)_2$: 2,5-bis(1-methylethyl)phenol,

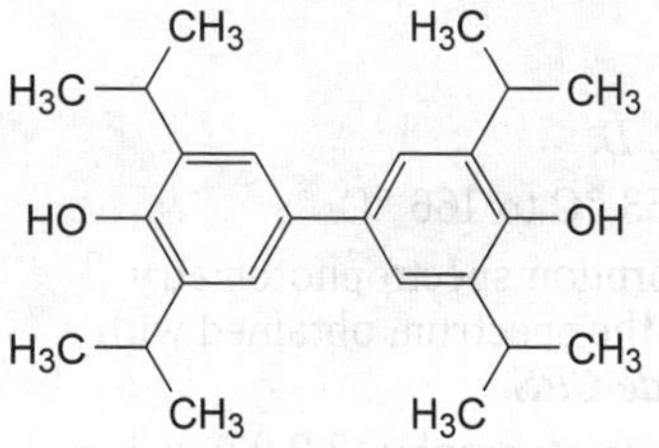

E. 3,3′,5,5′-tetrakis(1-methylethyl)biphenyl-4,4′-diol,

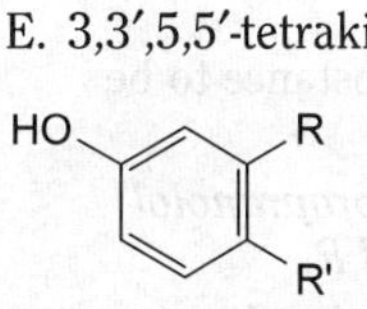

F. R = $CH(CH_3)_2$, R′ = H: 3-(1-methylethyl)phenol,

H. R = H, R′ = $CH(CH_3)_2$: 4-(1-methylethyl)phenol,

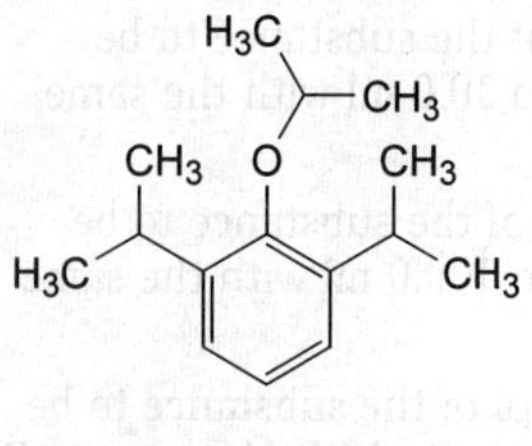

G. 2-(1-methylethoxy)-1,3-bis(1-methylethyl)benzene,

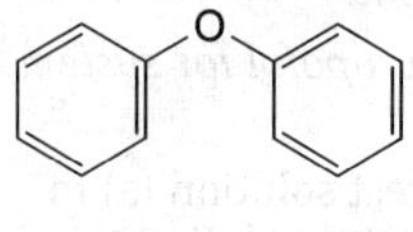

I. oxydibenzene,

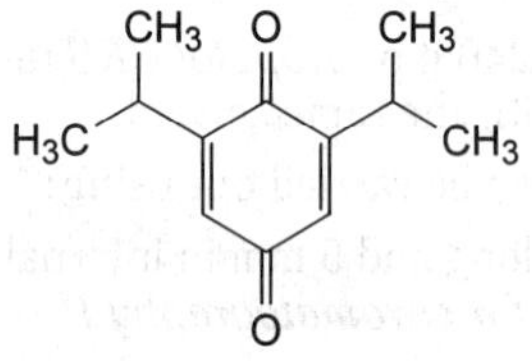

J. 2,6-bis(1-methylethyl)-1,4-benzoquinone.

01/2005:0568
corrected

PROPRANOLOL HYDROCHLORIDE

Propranololi hydrochloridum

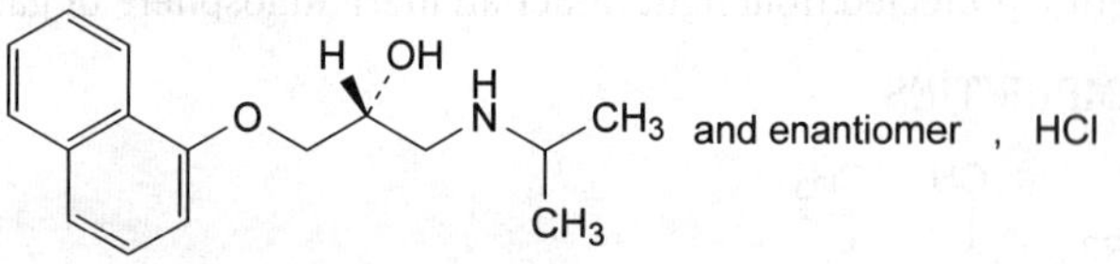

$C_{16}H_{22}ClNO_2$ M_r 295.8

DEFINITION

Propranolol hydrochloride contains not less than 99.0 per cent and not more than the equivalent of 101.0 per cent of (2*RS*)-1-[(1-methylethyl)amino]-3-(naphthalen-1-yloxy)propan-2-ol hydrochloride, calculated with reference to the dried substance.

CHARACTERS

A white or almost white powder, soluble in water and in alcohol.

IDENTIFICATION

First identification: B, D.

Second identification: A, C, D.

A. Melting point (*2.2.14*): 163 °C to 166 °C.

B. Examine by infrared absorption spectrophotometry (*2.2.24*), comparing with the spectrum obtained with *propranolol hydrochloride CRS*.

C. Examine by thin-layer chromatography (*2.2.27*), using *silica gel G R* as the coating substance.

Test solution. Dissolve 10 mg of the substance to be examined in 1 ml of *methanol R*.

Reference solution. Dissolve 10 mg of *propranolol hydrochloride CRS* in 1 ml of *methanol R*.

Apply separately to the plate 10 µl of each solution. Develop over a path of 15 cm using a mixture of 1 volume of *concentrated ammonia R1* and 99 volumes of *methanol R*. Dry the plate at 100 °C to 105 °C and spray with *anisaldehyde solution R*. Heat the plate at 100 °C to 105 °C until the colour of the spots reaches maximum intensity (10 min to 15 min). The principal spot in the chromatogram obtained with the test solution is similar in position, colour and size to the principal spot in the chromatogram obtained with the reference solution.

D. It gives reaction (a) of chlorides (*2.3.1*).

TESTS

Appearance of solution. Dissolve 2.0 g in *methanol R* and dilute to 20 ml with the same solvent. The solution is clear (*2.2.1*) and not more intensely coloured than intensity 6 of the range of reference solutions of the most appropriate colour (*2.2.2, Method II*).

Acidity or alkalinity. Dissolve 0.20 g in *carbon dioxide-free water R* and dilute to 20 ml with the same solvent. Add 0.2 ml of *methyl red solution R* and 0.2 ml of *0.01 M hydrochloric acid*. The solution is red. Add 0.4 ml of *0.01 M sodium hydroxide*. The solution is yellow.

Related substances. Examine by liquid chromatography (*2.2.29*).

Test solution. Dissolve 20.0 mg of the substance to be examined in the mobile phase and dilute to 10.0 ml with the mobile phase.

Reference solution (a). Dissolve 10.0 mg of *propranolol hydrochloride for performance test CRS* in the mobile phase and dilute to 10.0 ml with the mobile phase.

Reference solution (b). Dilute 2.0 ml of the test solution to 100.0 ml with the mobile phase. Dilute 1.0 ml of the solution to 10.0 ml with the mobile phase.

The chromatographic procedure may be carried out using:

- a stainless steel column 0.25 m long and 4.6 mm in internal diameter packed with *octadecylsilyl silica gel for chromatography R* (5 µm),
- as mobile phase at a flow rate of 1.8 ml/min a mixture prepared as follows: mix 1.6 g of *sodium laurilsulfate R* and 0.31 g of *tetrabutylammonium dihydrogen phosphate R* in a mixture of 1 ml of *sulphuric acid R*, 450 ml of *water R* and 550 ml of *acetonitrile R*; adjust to pH 3.3 using *dilute sodium hydroxide solution R*,
- as detector a spectrophotometer set at 292 nm.

Equilibrate the column for at least 30 min.

Inject 20 µl of reference solution (a). As a system suitability requirement, baseline separation is obtained between the peaks due to impurity A and propranolol; use the chromatogram supplied with *propranolol hydrochloride for performance test CRS* to identify the peak due to impurity A. Inject 20 µl of reference solution (b). Adjust the sensitivity of the system so that the height of the principal peak in the chromatogram obtained is at least 50 per cent of the full scale of the recorder.

Inject 20 µl of the test solution. Continue the chromatography for five times the retention time of the principal peak. In the chromatogram obtained with the test solution, the area of any peak apart from the principal peak, is not greater than half the area of the principal peak in the chromatogram obtained with reference solution (b) (0.1 per cent) and the sum of the area of all peaks, apart from the principal peak, is not greater than twice the area of the principal peak in the chromatogram obtained with reference solution (b) (0.4 per cent).

Heavy metals (*2.4.8*). Dissolve 1.0 g in a mixture of 15 volumes of *water R* and 85 volumes of *methanol R* and dilute to 20 ml with the same mixture of solvents. 12 ml of the solution complies with limit test B for heavy metals (20 ppm). Prepare the standard using lead standard solution

(1 ppm Pb) prepared by diluting *lead standard solution (100 ppm Pb) R* with a mixture of 15 volumes of *water R* and 85 volumes of *methanol R.*

Loss on drying (*2.2.32*). Not more than 0.5 per cent, determined on 1.000 g by drying in an oven at 100 °C to 105 °C.

Sulphated ash (*2.4.14*). Not more than 0.1 per cent, determined on 1.0 g.

ASSAY

Dissolve 0.250 g in 25 ml of *alcohol R.* Titrate with *0.1 M sodium hydroxide,* determining the end-point potentiometrically (*2.2.20*).

1 ml of *0.1 M sodium hydroxide* is equivalent to 29.58 mg of $C_{16}H_{22}ClNO_2$.

IMPURITIES

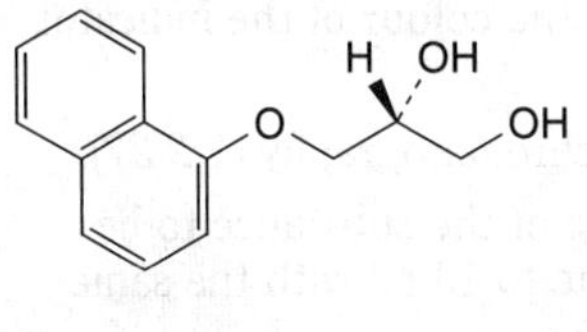

A. 3-(naphthalen-1-yloxy)propane-1,2-diol (diol derivative),

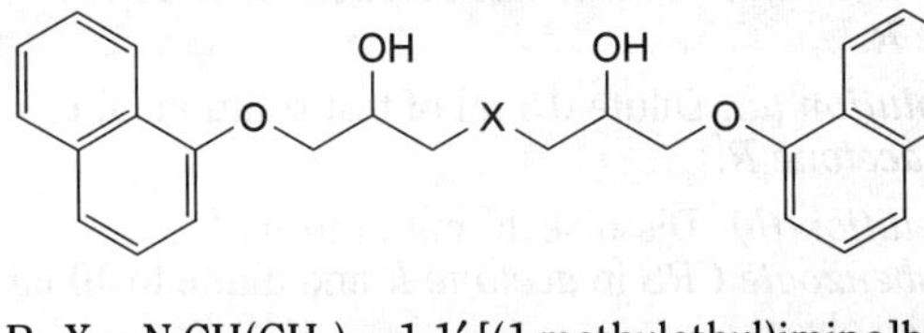

B. X = N-CH(CH_3)$_2$: 1,1′-[(1-methylethyl)imino]bis[3-(naphthalen-1-yloxy)propan-2-ol] (tertiary amine derivative),

C. X = O: 1,1′-oxybis[3-(naphthalen-1-yloxy)propan-2-ol] (bis-ether derivative).

01/2005:1039

PROPYL GALLATE

Propylis gallas

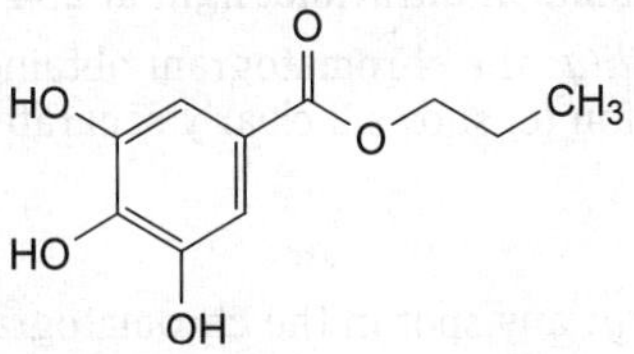

$C_{10}H_{12}O_5$ M_r 212.2

DEFINITION

Propyl gallate contains not less than 97.0 per cent and not more than the equivalent of 103.0 per cent of propyl 3,4,5-trihydroxybenzoate, calculated with reference to the dried substance.

CHARACTERS

A white or almost white, crystalline powder, very slightly soluble in water, freely soluble in ethanol (96 per cent). It dissolves in dilute solutions of alkali hydroxides.

IDENTIFICATION

First identification: B.

Second identification: A, C, D.

A. Melting point (*2.2.14*): 148 °C to 151 °C.

B. Examine by infrared absorption spectrophotometry (*2.2.24*), comparing with the spectrum obtained with *propyl gallate CRS.*

C. Examine the chromatograms obtained in the test for gallic acid. The principal spot in the chromatogram obtained with test solution (b) is similar in position, colour and size to the principal spot in the chromatogram obtained with reference solution (a).

D. Dissolve about 10 mg in 10 ml of *water R* by heating to about 70 °C. Cool and add 1 ml of *bismuth subnitrate solution R.* A bright yellow precipitate is formed.

TESTS

Appearance of solution. Dissolve 1.0 g in *ethanol (96 per cent) R* and dilute to 20 ml with the same solvent. The solution is clear (*2.2.1*) and not more intensely coloured than reference solution BY_5 (*2.2.2, Method II*).

Gallic acid. Examine by thin-layer chromatography (*2.2.27*), using *silica gel G R* as the coating substance.

Test solution (a). Dissolve 0.20 g of the substance to be examined in *acetone R* and dilute to 10 ml with the same solvent.

Test solution (b). Dilute 1 ml of test solution (a) to 20 ml with *acetone R.*

Reference solution (a). Dissolve 10 mg of *propyl gallate CRS* in *acetone R* and dilute to 10 ml with the same solvent.

Reference solution (b). Dissolve 20 mg of *gallic acid R* in *acetone R* and dilute to 20 ml with the same solvent. Dilute 1 ml of the solution to 10 ml with *acetone R.*

Reference solution (c). Dilute 0.5 ml of test solution (b) to 5 ml with reference solution (b).

Apply separately to the plate 5 µl of each solution. Develop over a path of 8 cm using a mixture of 10 volumes of *anhydrous formic acid R,* 40 volumes of *ethyl formate R* and 50 volumes of *toluene R.* Allow the plate to dry in air for 10 min and spray with a mixture of 1 volume of *ferric chloride solution R1* and 9 volumes of *ethanol (96 per cent) R.* Any spot due to gallic acid in the chromatogram obtained with test solution (a) is not more intense than the spot in the chromatogram obtained with reference solution (b) (0.5 per cent). The test is not valid unless the chromatogram obtained with reference solution (c) shows 2 clearly separated principal spots.

Total chlorine. Mix 0.5 g with 2 g of *calcium carbonate R1.* Dry and ignite at 700 °C. Take up the residue with 20 ml of *dilute nitric acid R* and dilute to 30 ml with *water R.* 15 ml of the solution, without further addition of *dilute nitric acid R,* complies with the limit test for chlorides (*2.4.4*) (200 ppm).

Chlorides (*2.4.4*). To 1.65 g add 50 ml of *water R.* Shake for 5 min. Filter. 15 ml of the filtrate complies with the limit test for chlorides (100 ppm).

Zinc. Not more than 25 ppm of Zn, determined by atomic absorption spectrometry (*2.2.23, Method II*).

Test solution. To 2.5 ml of the solution obtained in the test for heavy metals, add 2.5 ml of *water R.*

Reference solutions. Prepare the reference solutions using *zinc standard solution (10 ppm Zn) R,* diluted as necessary with *water R.*

Measure the absorbance at 213.9 nm using a zinc hollow-cathode lamp as the source of radiation and an air-acetylene flame.

Heavy metals (*2.4.8*). 2.0 g complies with limit test C for heavy metals (10 ppm). Prepare the reference solution using 2 ml of *lead standard solution (10 ppm Pb) R.*

Loss on drying (*2.2.32*). Not more than 0.5 per cent, determined on 1.000 g by drying in an oven at 100-105 °C.

Sulphated ash (*2.4.14*). Not more than 0.1 per cent, determined on 1.0 g.

ASSAY

Dissolve 0.100 g in *methanol R* and dilute to 250.0 ml with the same solvent. Dilute 5.0 ml of the solution to 200.0 ml with *methanol R*. Measure the absorbance (*2.2.25*) at the absorption maximum at 275 nm.

Calculate the content of $C_{10}H_{12}O_5$ taking the specific absorbance to be 503.

STORAGE

Protected from light.

IMPURITIES

Specified impurities: A.

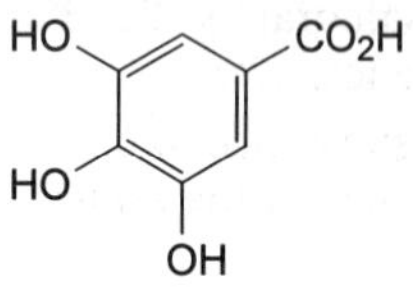

A. 3,4,5-trihydroxybenzoic acid (gallic acid).

01/2005:0431

PROPYL PARAHYDROXYBENZOATE

Propylis parahydroxybenzoas

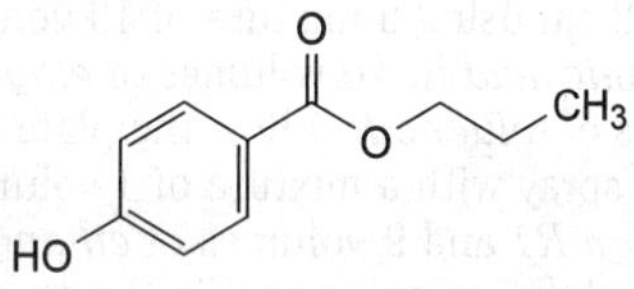

$C_{10}H_{12}O_3$ M_r 180.2

DEFINITION

Propyl 4-hydroxybenzoate.

Content: 98.0 per cent to 102.0 per cent.

CHARACTERS

Appearance: white, crystalline powder.

Solubility: very slightly soluble in water, freely soluble in alcohol and in methanol.

IDENTIFICATION

First identification: A, B.

Second identification: A, C, D.

A. Melting point (*2.2.14*): 96 °C to 99 °C.

B. Infrared absorption spectrophotometry (*2.2.24*).

Comparison: *propyl parahydroxybenzoate CRS.*

C. Examine the chromatograms obtained in the test for related substances.

Results: the principal spot in the chromatogram obtained with test solution (b) is similar in position and size to the principal spot in the chromatogram obtained with reference solution (b).

D. To about 10 mg in a test-tube add 1 ml of *sodium carbonate solution R*, boil for 30 s and cool (solution A). To a further 10 mg in a similar test-tube add 1 ml of *sodium carbonate solution R*; the substance partly dissolves (solution B). Add at the same time to solution A and solution B 5 ml of *aminopyrazolone solution R* and 1 ml of *potassium ferricyanide solution R* and mix. Solution B is yellow to orange-brown. Solution A is orange to red, the colour being clearly more intense than any similar colour which may be obtained with solution B.

TESTS

Solution S. Dissolve 1.0 g in *alcohol R* and dilute to 10 ml with the same solvent.

Appearance of solution. Solution S is clear (*2.2.1*) and not more intensely coloured than reference solution BY_6 (*2.2.2, Method II*).

Acidity. To 2 ml of solution S add 3 ml of *alcohol R*, 5 ml of *carbon dioxide-free water R* and 0.1 ml of *bromocresol green solution R*. Not more than 0.1 ml of *0.1 M sodium hydroxide* is required to change the colour of the indicator to blue.

Related substances. Thin-layer chromatography (*2.2.27*).

Test solution (a). Dissolve 0.10 g of the substance to be examined in *acetone R* and dilute to 10 ml with the same solvent.

Test solution (b). Dilute 1 ml of test solution (a) to 10 ml with *acetone R*.

Reference solution (a). Dilute 0.5 ml of test solution (a) to 100 ml with *acetone R*.

Reference solution (b). Dissolve 10 mg of *propyl parahydroxybenzoate CRS* in *acetone R* and dilute to 10 ml with the same solvent.

Reference solution (c). Dissolve 10 mg of *ethyl parahydroxybenzoate CRS* in 1 ml of test solution (a) and dilute to 10 ml with *acetone R*.

Plate: suitable octadecylsilyl silica gel with a fluorescent indicator having an optimal intensity at 254 nm as the coating substance.

Mobile phase: *glacial acetic acid R, water R, methanol R* (1:30:70 *V/V/V*).

Application: 2 µl.

Development: over a path of 15 cm.

Drying: in air.

Detection: examine in ultraviolet light at 254 nm.

System suitability: the chromatogram obtained with reference solution (c) shows 2 clearly separated principal spots.

Limits:

– *any impurity*: any spot in the chromatogram obtained with test solution (a), apart from the principal spot, is not more intense than the spot in the chromatogram obtained with reference solution (a) (0.5 per cent).

Sulphated ash (*2.4.14*): maximum 0.1 per cent, determined on 1.0 g.

ASSAY

To 1.000 g add 20.0 ml of *1 M sodium hydroxide*. Heat at about 70 °C for 1 h. Cool rapidly in an ice bath. Prepare a blank in the same manner. Carry out the titration on the solutions at room temperature. Titrate the excess sodium hydroxide with *0.5 M sulphuric acid*, continuing the titration until the second point of inflexion and determining the end-point potentiometrically (*2.2.20*).

1 ml of *1 M sodium hydroxide* is equivalent to 180.2 mg of $C_{10}H_{12}O_3$.

Monographs P

IMPURITIES

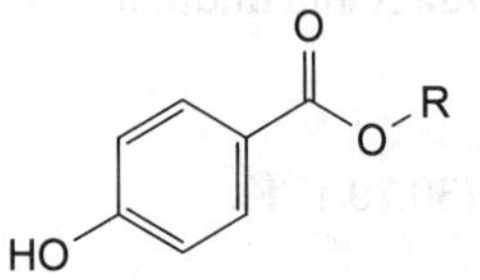

A. R = H: 4-hydroxybenzoic acid,

B. R = CH_3: methyl 4-hydroxybenzoate,

C. R = CH_2-CH_3: ethyl 4-hydroxybenzoate,

D. R = CH_2-CH_2-CH_2-CH_3: butyl 4-hydroxybenzoate.

01/2005:0430

PROPYLENE GLYCOL

Propylenglycolum

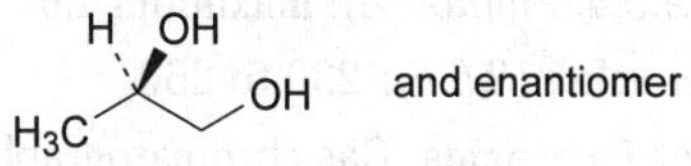

$C_3H_8O_2$ M_r 76.1

DEFINITION

Propylene glycol is (*RS*)-propane-1,2-diol.

CHARACTERS

A viscous, clear, colourless, hygroscopic liquid, miscible with water and with ethanol (96 per cent).

IDENTIFICATION

A. It complies with the test for relative density (see Tests).

B. It complies with the test for refractive index (see Tests).

C. Boiling point (*2.2.12*): 184 °C to 189 °C.

D. To 0.5 ml add 5 ml of *pyridine R* and 2 g of finely ground *nitrobenzoyl chloride R*. Boil for 1 min and pour into 15 ml of cold *water R* with shaking. Filter, wash the precipitate with 20 ml of a saturated solution of *sodium hydrogen carbonate R* and then with *water R* and dry. Dissolve in boiling *ethanol (80 per cent V/V) R* and filter the hot solution. On cooling, crystals are formed which, after drying at 100-105 °C, melt (*2.2.14*) at 121 °C to 128 °C.

TESTS

Appearance. It is clear (*2.2.1*) and colourless (*2.2.2, Method II*).

Relative density (*2.2.5*): 1.035 to 1.040.

Refractive index (*2.2.6*): 1.431 to 1.433.

Acidity. To 10 ml add 40 ml of *water R* and 0.1 ml of *bromothymol blue solution R1*. The solution is greenish-yellow. Not more than 0.05 ml of *0.1 M sodium hydroxide* is required to change the colour of the indicator to blue.

Oxidising substances. To 10 ml add 5 ml of *water R*, 2 ml of *potassium iodide solution R* and 2 ml of *dilute sulphuric acid R* and allow to stand in a ground-glass-stoppered flask protected from light for 15 min. Titrate with *0.05 M sodium thiosulphate*, using 1 ml of *starch solution R* as indicator. Not more than 0.2 ml of *0.05 M sodium thiosulphate* is required.

Reducing substances. To 1 ml add 1 ml of *dilute ammonia R1* and heat in a water-bath at 60 °C for 5 min. The solution is not yellow. Immediately add 0.15 ml of *0.1 M silver nitrate* and allow to stand for 5 min. The solution does not change its appearance.

Heavy metals (*2.4.8*). Mix 4 ml with 16 ml of *water R*. 12 ml of the solution complies with limit test A for heavy metals (5 ppm *m/V*). Prepare the reference solution using *lead standard solution (1 ppm Pb) R*.

Water (*2.5.12*). Not more than 0.2 per cent, determined on 5.00 g by the semi-micro determination of water.

Sulphated ash (*2.4.14*). Heat 50 g until it burns and ignite. Allow to cool. Moisten the residue with *sulphuric acid R* and ignite; repeat the operations. The residue weighs not more than 5 mg (0.01 per cent).

STORAGE

Store in an airtight container.

01/2005:2122

PROPYLENE GLYCOL DICAPRYLOCAPRATE

Propylenglycoli dicaprylocapras

DEFINITION

Propylene glycol diesters of saturated fatty acids, mainly caprylic acid (octanoic acid; $C_8H_{16}O_2$) and capric acid (decanoic acid; $C_{10}H_{20}O_2$), of vegetable origin.

CHARACTERS

Appearance: almost colourless to light yellow, oily liquid.

Solubility: practically insoluble in water, soluble in fatty oils and in light petroleum, slightly soluble in anhydrous ethanol.

IDENTIFICATION

A. Refractive index (*2.2.6*): 1.439 to 1.442.

B. Relative density (*2.2.5*): 0.910 to 0.930.

C. Viscosity (*2.2.9*): 9 mPa·s to 12 mPa·s.

D. It complies with the test for composition of fatty acids (see Tests).

TESTS

Appearance. The substance to be examined is clear (*2.2.1*) and not more intensely coloured than reference solution BY_6 (*2.2.2, Method II*).

Acid value (*2.5.1*): maximum 0.2.

Hydroxyl value (*2.5.3, Method A*): maximum 10.

Iodine value (*2.5.4*): maximum 1.0.

Peroxide value (*2.5.5, Method A*): maximum 1.0.

Saponification value (*2.5.6*): 320 to 340.

Unsaponifiable matter (*2.5.7*): maximum 0.3 per cent, determined on 5.0 g.

Alkaline impurities. Dissolve 2.00 g of the substance to be examined in a mixture of 1.5 ml of *ethanol (96 per cent) R* and 3.0 ml of *ether R*. Add 0.05 ml of *bromophenol blue solution R*. Not more than 0.15 ml of *0.01 M hydrochloric acid* is required to change the colour of the indicator to yellow.

Composition of fatty acids. Gas chromatography (*2.4.22, Method C*). Prepare reference solution (a) as indicated in Table 2.4.22.-2.

Column:

- *material*: fused silica,
- *size*: *l* = 30 m, Ø = 0.32 mm,
- *stationary phase*: *macrogol 20 000 R* (film thickness 0.5 µm),

Carrier gas: *helium for chromatography R*.

Flow rate: 1.3 ml/min.

Split ratio: 1:100.

Temperature:

	Time (min)	Temperature (°C)
Column	0 - 1	70
	1 - 35	70 → 240
	35 - 50	240
Injection port		250
Detector		250

Detection: flame ionisation.

Composition of the fatty acid fraction of the substance to be examined:

- *caproic acid*: maximum 2.0 per cent,
- *caprylic acid*: 50.0 per cent to 80.0 per cent,
- *capric acid*: 20.0 per cent to 50.0 per cent,
- *lauric acid*: maximum 3.0 per cent,
- *myristic acid*: maximum 1.0 per cent.

Water (*2.5.12*): maximum 0.1 per cent, determined on 5.00 g.

Total ash (*2.4.16*): maximum 0.1 per cent, determined on 2.0 g.

STORAGE

Protected from light.

01/2005:2087
corrected

PROPYLENE GLYCOL DILAURATE

Propylenglycoli dilauras

DEFINITION

Mixture of propylene glycol mono- and diesters of lauric acid.

Content: minimum 70.0 per cent of diesters and maximum 30.0 per cent of monoesters.

CHARACTERS

Appearance: clear, oily liquid at 20 °C, colourless or slightly yellow.

Solubility: practically insoluble in water, very soluble in alcohol, in methanol and in methylene chloride.

IDENTIFICATION

A. Thin-layer chromatography (*2.2.27*).

Test solution. Dissolve 0.1 g of the substance to be examined in *methylene chloride R* and dilute to 2 ml with the same solvent.

Reference solution. Dissolve 0.1 g of *propylene glycol dilaurate CRS* in *methylene chloride R* and dilute to 2 ml with the same solvent.

Plate: *TLC silica gel plate R*.

Mobile phase: *hexane R, ether R* (30:70 *V/V*).

Application: 10 µl.

Development: over a path of 15 cm.

Drying: in air.

Detection: spray with a 0.1 g/l solution of *rhodamine 6 G R* in *alcohol R*. Examine in ultraviolet light at 365 nm.

Results: the spots in the chromatogram obtained with the test solution are similar in position to those in the chromatogram obtained with the reference solution.

B. It complies with the test for composition of fatty acids (see Tests).

C. It complies with the assay (content of diesters).

TESTS

Acid value (*2.5.1*): maximum 4.0, determined on 5.00 g.

Iodine value (*2.5.4, Method A*): maximum 1.0.

Saponification value (*2.5.6*): 230 to 250.

Composition of fatty acids. Gas chromatography (*2.4.22, Method C*). Use the mixture of calibrating substances in Table 2.4.22.-2.

Composition of the fatty acid fraction of the substance:

- *caprylic acid*: maximum 0.5 per cent,
- *capric acid*: maximum 2.0 per cent,
- *lauric acid*: minimum 95.0 per cent,
- *myristic acid*: maximum 3.0 per cent,
- *palmitic acid*: maximum 1.0 per cent.

Free propylene glycol: maximum 2.0 per cent, determined as prescribed under Assay.

Water (*2.5.12*): maximum 1.0 per cent, determined on 1.00 g.

Total ash (*2.4.16*): maximum 0.1 per cent, determined on 1.0 g.

ASSAY

Size-exclusion chromatography (*2.2.30*).

Stock solution. Introduce 0.100 g of *propylene glycol R* into a flask and dilute to 25.0 ml with *tetrahydrofuran R*.

Test solution. In a 15 ml flask, weigh 0.200 g (*m*). Add 5.0 ml of *tetrahydrofuran R* and shake to dissolve. Reweigh the flask and calculate the total mass of solvent and substance (*M*).

Reference solutions. Into four 15 ml flasks, introduce respectively 0.25 ml, 0.5 ml, 1.0 ml and 2.5 ml of stock solution and add 5.0 ml of *tetrahydrofuran R*. Weigh each flask and calculate the concentration of propylene glycol in milligrams per gram for each reference solution.

Column:

- *size*: *l* = 0.6 m, Ø = 7 mm,
- *stationary phase*: *styrene-divinylbenzene copolymer R* (5 µm) with a pore size of 10 nm.

Mobile phase: *tetrahydrofuran R*.

Flow rate: 1 ml/min.

Detection: differential refractometer.

Injection: 40 µl.

Relative retention with reference to propylene glycol: diesters = about 0.85; monoesters = about 0.90.

Calculations:

- *free propylene glycol*: from the calibration curve obtained with the reference solutions, determine the concentration (*C*) in milligrams per gram in the test solution and calculate the percentage content in the substance to be examined using the following expression:

$$\frac{C \times M}{m \times 10}$$

- *monoesters*: calculate the percentage content of monoesters using the following expression:

$$\frac{A}{A+B} \times (100 - D)$$

A = area of the peak due to the monoesters,

B = area of the peak due to the diesters,

D = percentage content of free propylene glycol + percentage content of free fatty acids.

Calculate the percentage content of free fatty acids using the expression:

$$\frac{I_A \times 200}{561.1}$$

I_A = acid value.

- *diesters*: calculate the percentage content of diesters using the following expression:

$$\frac{B}{A+B} \times (100 - D)$$

STORAGE

Protected from moisture.

01/2005:1915
corrected

PROPYLENE GLYCOL MONOLAURATE

Propylenglycoli monolauras

DEFINITION

Mixture of propylene glycol mono- and diesters of lauric acid.

Content:

- propylene glycol monolaurate (type I): 45.0 per cent to 70.0 per cent of monoesters and 30.0 per cent to 55.0 per cent of diesters,
- propylene glycol monolaurate (type II): minimum 90.0 per cent of monoesters and maximum 10.0 per cent of diesters.

CHARACTERS

Appearance: clear, oily liquid at 20 °C, colourless or slightly yellow.

Solubility: practically insoluble in water, very soluble in alcohol, in methanol and in methylene chloride.

IDENTIFICATION

A. Thin-layer chromatography (*2.2.27*).

Test solution. Dissolve 0.1 g of the substance to be examined in *methylene chloride R* and dilute to 2 ml with the same solvent.

Reference solution. Dissolve 0.1 g of *propylene glycol monolaurate CRS* in *methylene chloride R* and dilute to 2 ml with the same solvent.

Plate: *TLC silica gel plate R.*

Mobile phase: *hexane R, ether R* (30:70 *V/V*).

Application: 10 µl.

Development: over a path of 15 cm.

Drying: in air.

Detection: spray with a 0.1 g/l solution of *rhodamine 6 G R* in *alcohol R*. Examine in ultraviolet light at 365 nm.

Results: the spots in the chromatogram obtained with the test solution are similar in position to those in the chromatogram obtained with the reference solution.

B. It complies with the test for composition of fatty acids (see Tests).

C. It complies with the assay (content of monoesters).

TESTS

Acid value (*2.5.1*): maximum 4.0, determined on 5.00 g.

Iodine value (*2.5.4, Method A*): maximum 1.0.

Saponification value (*2.5.6*): 210 to 245 for propylene glycol monolaurate (type I) and 200 to 230 for propylene glycol monolaurate (type II).

Composition of fatty acids. Gas chromatography (*2.4.22, Method C*). Use the mixture of calibrating substances in Table 2.4.22.-2.

Composition of the fatty acid fraction of the substance:

- *caprylic acid*: maximum 0.5 per cent,
- *capric acid*: maximum 2.0 per cent,
- *lauric acid*: minimum 95.0 per cent,
- *myristic acid*: maximum 3.0 per cent,
- *palmitic acid*: maximum 1.0 per cent.

Free propylene glycol: maximum 5.0 per cent for propylene glycol monolaurate (type I) and maximum 1.0 per cent for propylene glycol monolaurate (type II), determined as prescribed under Assay.

Water (*2.5.12*): maximum 1.0 per cent, determined on 1.00 g.

Total ash (*2.4.16*): maximum 0.1 per cent, determined on 1.0 g.

ASSAY

Size-exclusion chromatography (*2.2.30*).

Stock solution. Introduce 0.100 g of *propylene glycol R* into a vial and dilute to 25.0 ml with *tetrahydrofuran R.*

Test solution. In a 15 ml flask, weigh 0.200 g (*m*). Add 5.0 ml of *tetrahydrofuran R* and shake to dissolve. Reweigh the flask and calculate the total mass of solvent and substance (*M*).

Reference solutions. Into four 15 ml flasks, introduce respectively 0.25 ml, 0.5 ml, 1.0 ml and 2.5 ml of stock solution and add 5.0 ml of *tetrahydrofuran R.* In a fifth 15 ml flask, introduce 5.0 ml of stock solution. Weigh each flask and calculate the concentration of propylene glycol in milligrams per gram for each reference solution.

Column:

- *size*: *l* = 0.6 m, Ø = 7 mm,
- *stationary phase*: *styrene-divinylbenzene copolymer R* (5 µm) with a pore size of 10 nm.

Mobile phase: *tetrahydrofuran R.*

Flow rate: 1 ml/min.

Detection: differential refractometer.

Injection: 40 µl.

Relative retention with reference to propylene glycol: diesters = about 0.85; monoesters = about 0.90.

Monographs P

Calculations:

– *free propylene glycol*: from the calibration curve obtained with the reference solutions, determine the concentration (C) in milligrams per gram in the test solution and calculate the percentage content in the substance to be examined using the following expression:

$$\frac{C \times M}{m \times 10}$$

– *monoesters*: calculate the percentage content of monoesters using the following expression:

$$\frac{A}{A+B} \times (100 - D)$$

A = area of the peak due to the monoesters,

B = area of the peak due to the diesters,

D = percentage content of free propylene glycol + percentage content of free fatty acids.

Calculate the percentage content of free fatty acids using the expression:

$$\frac{I_A \times 200}{561.1}$$

I_A = acid value.

– *diesters*: calculate the percentage content of diesters using the following expression:

$$\frac{B}{A+B} \times (100 - D)$$

STORAGE

Protected from moisture.

LABELLING

The label states the type of propylene glycol monolaurate (type I or type II).

01/2005:1469

PROPYLENE GLYCOL MONOPALMITOSTEARATE

Propylenglycoli monopalmitostearas

DEFINITION

Mixture of propylene glycol mono- and diesters and of stearic and palmitic acids, produced by the condensation of propylene glycol and stearic acid 50 of vegetable or animal origin (see *Stearic acid (1474)*).

Content: minimum of 50.0 per cent of monoesters.

CHARACTERS

Appearance: white or almost white, waxy solid.

Solubility: practically insoluble in water, soluble in acetone and in hot alcohol.

IDENTIFICATION

A. It complies with the test for melting point (see Tests).

B. It complies for the test for composition of fatty acids (see Tests).

C. It complies with the assay (monoesters content).

TESTS

Melting point (*2.2.15*): 33 °C to 40 °C.

Acid value (*2.5.1*): maximum 4.0, determined on 10.0 g.

Iodine value (*2.5.4*): maximum 3.0.

Saponification value (*2.5.6*): 170 to 185, determined on 2.0 g.

Composition of fatty acids (*2.4.22, Method A*). The fatty acid fraction has the following composition:

– *stearic acid*: 40.0 per cent to 60.0 per cent,

– *sum of contents of palmitic acid and stearic acid*: minimum 90.0 per cent.

Free propylene glycol: maximum 5.0 per cent, determined as prescribed under Assay.

Total ash (*2.4.16*): maximum 0.1 per cent, determined on 1.0 g.

ASSAY

Size-exclusion chromatography (*2.2.30*).

Test solution. In a 15 ml flask, weigh about 0.2 g (m), to the nearest 0.1 mg. Add 5.0 ml of *tetrahydrofuran R* and shake to dissolve. Heat gently, if necessary. Reweigh the flask and calculate the total mass of solvent and substance (M).

Reference solutions. In four 15 ml flasks, weigh, to the nearest 0.1 mg, about 2.5 mg, 5.0 mg, 10.0 mg and 20.0 mg of *propylene glycol R*. Add 5.0 ml of *tetrahydrofuran R* and shake to dissolve. Weigh the flasks again and calculate the concentration of propylene glycol in milligrams per gram for each reference solution.

Column:

– *size*: l = 0.6 m, Ø = 7 mm,

– *stationary phase*: *styrene-divinylbenzene copolymer R* (particle diameter 5 µm, pore size 10 nm).

Mobile phase: *tetrahydrofuran R*.

Flow rate: 1 ml/min.

Detection: differential refractometer.

Injection: 40 µl.

Relative retention with reference to propylene glycol: diesters = about 0.78, monoesters = about 0.84.

Limits:

– *free propylene glycol*: from the calibration curve obtained with the reference solutions, determine the concentration (C) in milligrams per gram in the test solution and calculate the percentage content in the substance to be examined using the following expression:

$$\frac{C \times M}{m \times 10}$$

– *monoesters*: calculate the percentage content of monoesters using the following expression:

$$\frac{A}{A+B} \times (100 - D)$$

Monographs P

A = area of the peak due to the monoesters,

B = area of the peak due to the diesters,

D = percentage content of free propylene glycol + percentage content of free fatty acids which is determined using the following expression:

$$\frac{I_A \times 270}{561.1}$$

I_A = acid value.

STORAGE

Protected from light.

01/2005:0525

PROPYLTHIOURACIL

Propylthiouracilum

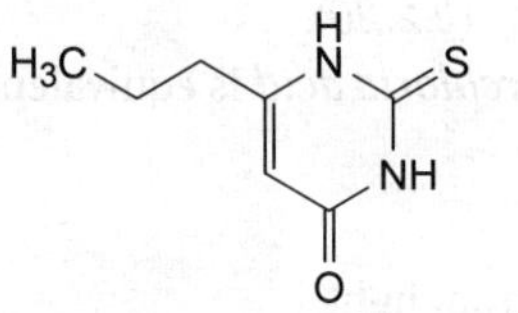

$C_7H_{10}N_2OS$ M_r 170.2

DEFINITION

Propylthiouracil contains not less than 98.0 per cent and not more than the equivalent of 100.5 per cent of 2,3-dihydro-6-propyl-2-thioxopyrimidin-4(1*H*)-one, calculated with reference to the dried substance.

CHARACTERS

White or almost white, crystalline powder or crystals, very slightly soluble in water, sparingly soluble in alcohol. It dissolves in solutions of alkali hydroxides.

IDENTIFICATION

First identification: A, B.

Second identification: A, C, D.

A. Melting point (*2.2.14*): 217 °C to 221 °C.

B. Examine by infrared absorption spectrophotometry (*2.2.24*), comparing with the spectrum obtained with *propylthiouracil CRS*. Examine as discs prepared using 1 mg of substance and 0.3 g of *potassium bromide R*.

C. Examine the chromatograms obtained in the test for impurity A and related substances in ultraviolet light at 254 nm before exposure of the plate to iodine vapour. The principal spot in the chromatogram obtained with test solution (b) is similar in position and size to the principal spot in the chromatogram obtained with reference solution (a).

D. To about 20 mg add 8 ml of *bromine water R* and shake for a few minutes. Boil until the mixture is decolourised, allow to cool and filter. To the filtrate add 2 ml of *barium chloride solution R1*. A white precipitate is formed whose colour does not become violet on the addition of 5 ml of *dilute sodium hydroxide solution R*.

TESTS

Impurity A and related substances. Examine by thin-layer chromatography (*2.2.27*), using a *TLC silica gel* GF_{254} *plate R*.

Test solution (a). Dissolve 0.1 g of the substance to be examined in *methanol R* and dilute to 10 ml with the same solvent.

Test solution (b). Dilute 1 ml of test solution (a) to 10 ml with *methanol R*.

Reference solution (a). Dissolve 10 mg of *propylthiouracil CRS* in *methanol R* and dilute to 10 ml with the same solvent.

Reference solution (b). Dissolve 50 mg of *thiourea R* in *methanol R* and dilute to 100 ml with the same solvent. Dilute 1 ml of this solution to 100 ml with *methanol R*.

Reference solution (c). Dilute 1 ml of test solution (a) to 100 ml with *methanol R*.

Apply separately to the plate 10 µl of each solution. Develop over a path of 15 cm using a mixture of 0.1 volumes of *glacial acetic acid R*, 6 volumes of *2-propanol R* and 50 volumes of *chloroform R*. Allow the plate to dry in air. Examine in ultraviolet light at 254 nm. Expose the plate to iodine vapour for 10 min. In the chromatogram obtained with test solution (a), any spot corresponding to impurity A is not more intense than the spot in the chromatogram obtained with reference solution (b) (0.05 per cent) and any spot apart from the principal spot and any spot corresponding to impurity A is not more intense than the spot in the chromatogram obtained with reference solution (c) (1.0 per cent).

Heavy metals (*2.4.8*). 1.0 g complies with limit test F for heavy metals (20 ppm). Prepare the standard using 2 ml of *lead standard solution (10 ppm Pb) R*.

Loss on drying (*2.2.32*). Not more than 0.5 per cent, determined on 1.000 g by drying in an oven at 100 °C to 105 °C.

Sulphated ash (*2.4.14*). Not more than 0.1 per cent, determined on 1.0 g.

ASSAY

To 0.300 g add 30 ml of *water R* and 30.0 ml of *0.1 M sodium hydroxide*. Boil and shake until dissolution is complete. Add 50 ml of *0.1 M silver nitrate* while stirring, boil gently for 5 min and cool. Titrate with *0.1 M sodium hydroxide*, determining the end-point potentiometrically (*2.2.20*). The volume of *0.1 M sodium hydroxide* used is equal to the sum of the volume added initially and the volume used in the final titration.

1 ml of *0.1 M sodium hydroxide* is equivalent to 8.511 mg of $C_7H_{10}N_2OS$.

STORAGE

Store protected from light.

IMPURITIES

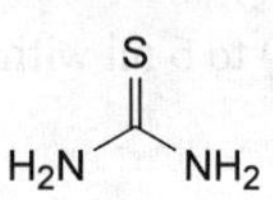

A. thiourea.

01/2005:0636

PROPYPHENAZONE

Propyphenazonum

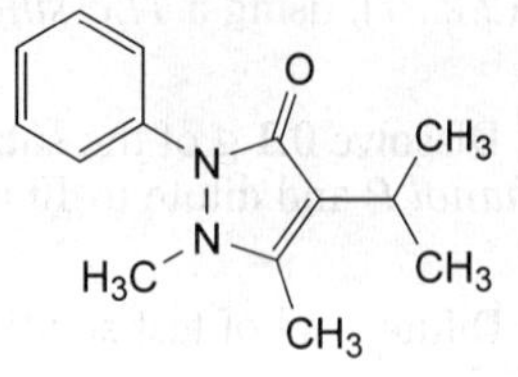

$C_{14}H_{18}N_2O$ M_r 230.3

DEFINITION

Propyphenazone contains not less than 99.0 per cent and not more than the equivalent of 101.0 per cent of 1,5-dimethyl-4-(1-methylethyl)-2-phenyl-1,2-dihydro-3*H*-pyrazol-3-one, calculated with reference to the dried substance.

CHARACTERS

A white or slightly yellowish, crystalline powder, slightly soluble in water, freely soluble in alcohol and in methylene chloride.

IDENTIFICATION

First identification: A, B.

Second identification: A, C, D.

A. Melting point (*2.2.14*): 102 °C to 106 °C.

B. Examine by infrared absorption spectrophotometry (*2.2.24*), comparing with the spectrum obtained with *propyphenazone CRS*. Examine the substances prepared as discs.

C. Examine the chromatograms obtained in the test for related substances. The principal spot in the chromatogram obtained with test solution (b) is similar in position, colour and size to the principal spot in the chromatogram obtained with reference solution (a).

D. To 1 ml of solution S (see Tests) add 0.1 ml of *ferric chloride solution R1*. A brownish-red colour appears which becomes yellow on addition of 1 ml of *dilute hydrochloric acid R*.

TESTS

Solution S. Dissolve 2 g in a mixture of equal volumes of *alcohol R* and *carbon dioxide-free water R* and dilute to 50 ml with the same mixture of solvents.

Appearance of solution. Solution S is clear (*2.2.1*) and colourless (*2.2.2, Method II*).

Acidity or alkalinity. To 10 ml of solution S add 0.1 ml of *phenolphthalein solution R*. The solution is colourless. Add 0.2 ml of *0.01 M sodium hydroxide*; the solution becomes pink. Add 0.4 ml of *0.01 M hydrochloric acid*; the solution becomes colourless. Add 0.2 ml of *methyl red solution R*. The solution becomes orange or red.

Related substances. Examine by thin-layer chromatography (*2.2.27*), using *silica gel HF_{254} R* as the coating substance.

Test solution (a). Dissolve 0.40 g of the substance to be examined in *methanol R* and dilute to 5 ml with the same solvent.

Test solution (b). Dilute 1 ml of test solution (a) to 5 ml with *methanol R*.

Reference solution (a). Dissolve 80 mg of *propyphenazone CRS* in *methanol R* and dilute to 5 ml with the same solvent.

Reference solution (b). Dilute 1 ml of test solution (b) to 100 ml with *methanol R*.

Apply to the plate 5 µl of each solution. Develop over a path of 15 cm using a mixture of 10 volumes of *butanol R*, 45 volumes of *cyclohexane R* and 45 volumes of *ethyl acetate R*. Dry the plate in a current of hot air for 15 min and examine in ultraviolet light at 254 nm. Any spot in the chromatogram obtained with test solution (a), apart from the principal spot, is not more intense than the spot in the chromatogram obtained with reference solution (b) (0.2 per cent). Spray with a mixture of equal volumes of *potassium ferricyanide solution R* and *ferric chloride solution R1*. Any spot in the chromatogram obtained with test solution (a), apart from the principal spot, is not more intense than the spot in the chromatogram obtained with reference solution (b) (0.2 per cent).

Heavy metals (*2.4.8*). 1.0 g complies with limit test C (10 ppm). Prepare the standard using 1 ml of *lead standard solution (10 ppm Pb) R*.

Loss on drying (*2.2.32*). Not more than 0.5 per cent, determined on 1.000 g by drying *in vacuo* at 60 °C for 4 h.

Sulphated ash (*2.4.14*). Not more than 0.1 per cent, determined on 0.5 g.

ASSAY

Dissolve 0.2000 g in 10 ml of *anhydrous acetic acid R* and add 75 ml of *ethylene chloride R*. Titrate with *0.1 M perchloric acid*, determining the end-point potentiometrically (*2.2.20*).

1 ml of *0.1 M perchloric acid* is equivalent to 23.03 mg of $C_{14}H_{18}N_2O$.

STORAGE

Store protected from light.

IMPURITIES

A. phenazone,

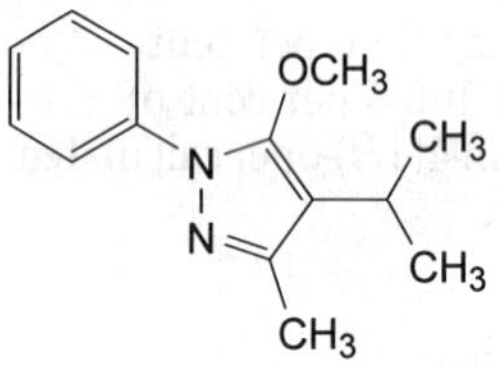

B. 5-methoxy-3-methyl-4-(1-methylethyl)-1-phenyl-1*H*-pyrazole,

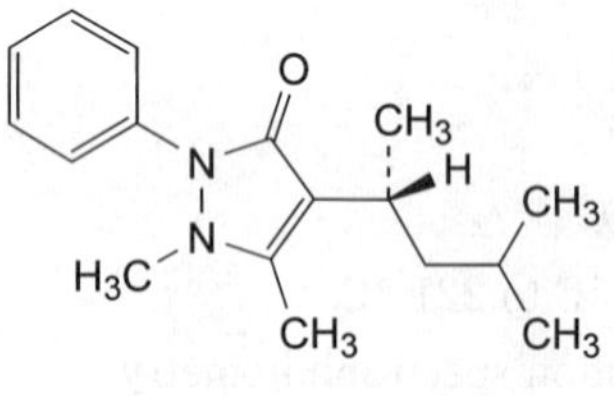

and enantiomer

C. 4-[(1*RS*)-1,3-dimethylbutyl]-1,5-dimethyl-2-phenyl-1,2-dihydro-3*H*-pyrazol-3-one.

01/2005:0686

PROTAMINE HYDROCHLORIDE

Protamini hydrochloridum

DEFINITION

Protamine hydrochloride consists of the hydrochlorides of basic peptides extracted from the sperm or roe of fish, usually species of *Salmonidae* and *Clupeidae*. It binds with heparin in solution, inhibiting its anticoagulant activity; in the conditions of the assay this binding gives rise to a precipitate. Calculated with reference to the dried substance, 1 mg of protamine hydrochloride precipitates not less than 100 IU of heparin.

PRODUCTION

Protamine hydrochloride is prepared in conditions designed to minimise the risk of microbial contamination.

The method of manufacture is validated to demonstrate that the product, if tested, would comply with the following test:

Abnormal toxicity (*2.6.9*). Inject into each mouse 0.5 mg dissolved in 0.5 ml of *water for injections R*.

CHARACTERS

Appearance: white or almost white powder, hygroscopic.

Solubility: soluble in water, practically insoluble in alcohol.

IDENTIFICATION

A. Specific optical rotation (*2.2.7*): − 40 to − 60 (dried substance).

   Dissolve 1.000 g in *0.1 M hydrochloric acid* and dilute to 100.0 ml with the same solvent.

B. In the conditions of the assay, protamine hydrochloride forms a precipitate.

C. To 0.5 ml of solution S (see Tests) add 4.5 ml of *water R*, 1.0 ml of a 100 g/l solution of *sodium hydroxide R* and 1.0 ml of a 0.2 g/l solution of *α-naphthol R* and mix. Cool the mixture to 5 °C. Add 0.5 ml of *sodium hypobromite solution R*. An intense red colour is produced.

D. Heat 2 ml of solution S in a water-bath at 60 °C and add 0.1 ml of *mercuric sulphate solution R*. Mix. No precipitate is formed. Cool the mixture in iced water. A precipitate is formed.

E. It gives reaction (a) of chlorides (*2.3.1*).

TESTS

Solution S. Dissolve 0.50 g in *water R* and dilute to 25.0 ml with the same solvent.

Appearance of solution. The solution is not more opalescent than reference suspension II (*2.2.1*) and not more intensely coloured than reference solution BY_6 or Y_6 (*2.2.2, Method II*).

To 2.5 ml of solution S add 7.5 ml of *water R*.

Absorbance (*2.2.25*): maximum 0.1 between wavelengths of 260 nm to 280 nm.

Dilute 2.5 ml of solution S to 5.0 ml with *water R*.

Chloride: 12.3 per cent to 19.0 per cent (dried substance).

Dissolve 0.400 g in 50 ml of *water R*. Add 5 ml of *dilute nitric acid R*, 25.0 ml of *0.1 M silver nitrate* and 2 ml of *dibutyl phthalate R* and shake. Titrate with *0.1 M ammonium thiocyanate* using 2 ml of *ferric ammonium sulphate solution R2* as indicator; shake vigorously when approaching the end-point.

1 ml of *0.1 M silver nitrate* is equivalent to 3.545 mg of chloride (Cl).

Sulphates: maximum 4.0 per cent (dried substance).

Dissolve 0.500 g in 200 ml of *distilled water R*, add 5.0 ml of *dilute hydrochloric acid R* and heat to boiling. Add dropwise 10 ml of a hot 100 g/l solution of *barium chloride R* while stirring with a glass rod, cover the beaker with a watch glass and allow to stand on a water-bath for 2 h to obtain a coarse granular precipitate. Add 0.1 ml of a 100 g/l solution of *barium chloride R* to the clear supernatant liquid. If a turbidity develops, repeat the precipitation procedure. Transfer the precipitate quantitatively to a previously ignited and tared porcelain crucible and wash with hot *distilled water R* until the addition of *silver nitrate solution R1* to the washings produces no opalescence. Ignite the precipitate at 600 °C for 1 h. Allow to cool in a desiccator and weigh.

1 mg of residue is equivalent to 0.412 mg of sulphate (SO_4).

Barium: maximum 10 ppm.

Atomic absorption spectrometry (*2.2.23, Method I*).

Test solution. Dissolve 1.0 g of the substance to be examined in *distilled water R*, add 1 ml of a 250 g/l solution of *caesium chloride R* and 0.2 ml of *hydrochloric acid R* and dilute to 20.0 ml with *distilled water R*.

Reference solution. To 1.0 ml of *barium standard solution (50 ppm Ba) R* add 5 ml of a 250 g/l solution of *caesium chloride R* and 1 ml of *hydrochloric acid R* and dilute to 100.0 ml with *distilled water R*.

Source: hollow-cathode lamp.

Wavelength: 553.3 nm.

Flame: air-acetylene-nitrous oxide flame of suitable composition.

Iron (*2.4.9*): maximum 10 ppm.

Dissolve 1.0 g with heating in *water R* and dilute to 10 ml with the same solvent.

Mercury: maximum 10 ppm.

Introduce 2.0 g of the substance to be examined into a ground-glass-stoppered 250 ml conical flask and add 20 ml of a mixture of equal volumes of *nitric acid R* and *sulphuric acid R*. Boil under a reflux condenser for 1 h, cool and cautiously dilute with *water R*. Boil until nitrous fumes are no longer seen. Cool the solution, cautiously dilute to 200.0 ml with *water R*, mix and filter. Transfer 50.0 ml of the filtrate to a separating funnel. Shake with successive small portions of *chloroform R* until the chloroform layer remains colourless. Discard the chloroform layers. To the aqueous layer add 25 ml of *dilute sulphuric acid R*, 115 ml of *water R* and 10 ml of a 200 g/l solution of *hydroxylamine hydrochloride R*. Titrate with *dithizone solution R2*; after each addition, shake the mixture 20 times and towards the end of the titration allow to separate and discard the chloroform layer. Titrate until a bluish-green colour is obtained. Calculate the content of mercury using the equivalent in micrograms of mercury per millilitre of titrant determined in the standardisation of the *dithizone solution R2*.

Nitrogen: 23.0 per cent to 27.0 per cent (dried substance).

Carry out the determination of nitrogen by sulphuric acid digestion (*2.5.9*), using 10.0 mg and heating for 3-4 h.

Heavy metals (*2.4.8*): maximum 20 ppm.

1.0 g complies with limit test D. Prepare the standard using 2 ml of *lead standard solution (10 ppm Pb) R*.

Loss on drying (*2.2.32*): maximum 5.0 per cent, determined on 1.000 g by drying in an oven at 100-105 °C for 3 h.

Bacterial endotoxins (*2.6.14*): less than 7.0 IU/mg, if intended for use in the manufacture of parenteral dosage forms without a further appropriate procedure for the removal of bacterial endotoxins.

ASSAY

Test solution (a). Dissolve 15.0 mg of the substance to be examined in *water R* and dilute to 100.0 ml with the same solvent.

Test solution (b). Dilute 2.0 ml of test solution (a) to 3.0 ml with *water R*.

Test solution (c). Dilute 1.0 ml of test solution (a) to 3.0 ml with *water R*.

Monographs P

Use as titrant a 1 in 6 dilution of *heparin sodium BRP* in *water R* (for example, 1.7 ml diluted to 10.0 ml with *water R*). Titrate each test solution in duplicate as follows: introduce an accurately measured volume of the solution to be titrated, for example, 1.5 ml, into the cell of a suitable colorimeter, set the apparatus for measurement at a suitable wavelength (none is critical) in the visible range, add the titrant in small volumes until there is a sharp increase in the absorbance and note the volume of titrant added.

Carry out 3 independent assays. For each individual titration, calculate the number of International Units of heparin in the volume of titrant added at the end-point per milligram of the substance to be examined. Calculate the potency of the substance as the average of the 18 values. Test the linearity of the response by the usual statistical methods. Calculate the 3 standard deviations for the results obtained with each of the 3 test solutions. Calculate the three standard deviations for the results obtained with each of the 3 independent assays. The assay is not valid unless each of the 6 standard deviations is less than 5 per cent of the average result.

STORAGE

In an airtight, tamper-proof container. If the substance is sterile, store in a sterile, airtight, tamper-proof container.

LABELLING

The label states, where applicable, that the substance is free from bacterial endotoxins.

01/2005:0569

PROTAMINE SULPHATE

Protamini sulfas

DEFINITION

Protamine sulphate consists of the sulphates of basic peptides extracted from the sperm or roe of fish, usually species of *Salmonidae* and *Clupeidae*. It binds with heparin in solution, inhibiting its anticoagulant activity; in the conditions of the assay this binding gives rise to a precipitate. Calculated with reference to the dried substance, 1 mg of protamine sulphate precipitates not less than 100 IU of heparin.

PRODUCTION

Protamine sulphate is prepared in conditions designed to minimise the risk of microbial contamination.

The method of manufacture is validated to demonstrate that the product, if tested, would comply with the following test:

Abnormal toxicity (*2.6.9*). Inject into each mouse 0.5 mg dissolved in 0.5 ml of *water for injections R*.

CHARACTERS

Appearance: white or almost white powder, hygroscopic.

Solubility: sparingly soluble in water, practically insoluble in alcohol.

IDENTIFICATION

A. Specific optical rotation (*2.2.7*): − 65 to − 85 (dried substance).

Dissolve 1.000 g in *0.1 M hydrochloric acid* and dilute to 100.0 ml with the same solvent.

B. In the conditions of the assay, protamine sulphate forms a precipitate.

C. To 0.5 ml of solution S (see Tests) add 4.5 ml of *water R*, 1.0 ml of a 100 g/l solution of *sodium hydroxide R* and 1.0 ml of a 0.2 g/l solution of *α-naphthol R* and mix. Cool the mixture to 5 °C. Add 0.5 ml of *sodium hypobromite solution R*. An intense red colour is produced.

D. Heat 2 ml of solution S in a water-bath at 60 °C and add 0.1 ml of *mercuric sulphate solution R*. Mix. No precipitate is formed. Cool the mixture in iced water. A precipitate is formed.

E. It gives reaction (a) of sulphates (*2.3.1*).

TESTS

Solution S. Dissolve 0.20 g in *water R* and dilute to 10.0 ml with the same solvent.

Appearance of solution. The solution is not more opalescent than reference suspension II (*2.2.1*) and not more intensely coloured than reference solution BY_6 or Y_6 (*2.2.2, Method II*). To 2.5 ml of solution S add 7.5 ml of *water R*.

Absorbance (*2.2.25*): maximum 0.1 between wavelengths of 260 nm to 280 nm.

Dilute 2.5 ml of solution S to 5.0 ml with *water R*.

Sulphate: 16 per cent to 24 per cent (dried substance).

Dissolve 0.150 g in 15 ml of *distilled water R* in a beaker. Add 5 ml of *dilute hydrochloric acid R*. Heat to boiling and slowly add to the boiling solution 10 ml of a 100 g/l solution of *barium chloride R*. Cover the beaker and heat on a water-bath for 1 h. Filter. Wash the precipitate several times with small quantities of hot *water R*. Dry and ignite the residue at 600 °C to constant mass.

1.0 g of residue is equivalent to 0.4117 g of sulphate (SO_4).

Iron (*2.4.9*): maximum 10 ppm.

Dissolve 1.0 g with heating in *water R* and dilute to 10 ml with the same solvent.

Mercury: maximum 10 ppm.

Introduce 2.0 g of the substance to be examined into a 250 ml ground-glass-stoppered conical flask and add 20 ml of a mixture of equal volumes of *nitric acid R* and *sulphuric acid R*. Boil under a reflux condenser for 1 h, cool and cautiously dilute with *water R*. Boil until nitrous fumes are no longer seen. Cool the solution, cautiously dilute to 200.0 ml with *water R*, mix and filter. Transfer 50.0 ml of the filtrate to a separating funnel. Shake with successive small portions of *chloroform R* until the chloroform layer remains colourless. Discard the chloroform layers. To the aqueous layer add 25 ml of *dilute sulphuric acid R*, 115 ml of *water R* and 10 ml of a 200 g/l solution of *hydroxylamine hydrochloride R*. Titrate with *dithizone solution R2*; after each addition, shake the mixture 20 times and towards the end of the titration allow to separate and discard the chloroform layer. Titrate until a bluish-green colour is obtained. Calculate the content of mercury using the equivalent in micrograms of mercury per millilitre of titrant, determined in the standardisation of the *dithizone solution R2*.

Nitrogen: 21.0 per cent to 26.0 per cent (dried substance).

Carry out the determination of nitrogen by sulphuric acid digestion (*2.5.9*), using 10.0 mg and heating for 3-4 h.

Heavy metals (*2.4.8*): maximum 20 ppm.

1.0 g complies with limit test D. Prepare the standard using 2 ml of *lead standard solution (10 ppm Pb) R*.

Loss on drying (*2.2.32*): maximum 5.0 per cent, determined on 1.000 g by drying in an oven at 100-105 °C for 3 h.

Monographs P

Bacterial endotoxins (*2.6.14*): less than 7.0 IU/mg, if intended for use in the manufacture of parenteral dosage forms without a further appropriate procedure for the removal of bacterial endotoxins.

ASSAY

Test solution (a). Dissolve 15.0 mg of the substance to be examined in *water R* and dilute to 100.0 ml with the same solvent.

Test solution (b). Dilute 2.0 ml of test solution (a) to 3.0 ml with *water R*.

Test solution (c). Dilute 1.0 ml of test solution (a) to 3.0 ml with *water R*.

Use as titrant a 1 to 6 dilution of *heparin sodium BRP* in *water R* (for example, 1.7 ml diluted to 10.0 ml with *water R*). Titrate each test solution in duplicate as follows: introduce an accurately measured volume of the solution to be titrated, for example 1.5 ml, into the cell of a suitable colorimeter and set the apparatus for measurement at a suitable wavelength (none is critical) in the visible range. Add the titrant in small volumes until there is a sharp increase in the absorbance and note the volume of titrant added.

Carry out 3 independent assays. For each individual titration, calculate the number of International Units of heparin in the volume of titrant added at the end-point per milligram of the substance to be examined. Calculate the potency of the substance as the average of the 18 values. Test the linearity of the response by the usual statistical methods. Calculate the 3 standard deviations for the results obtained with each of the 3 test solutions. Calculate the 3 standard deviations for the results obtained with each of the 3 independent assays. The assay is not valid unless each of the 6 standard deviations is less than 5 per cent of the average result.

STORAGE

In an airtight, tamper-proof container. If the substance is sterile, store in a sterile, airtight, tamper-proof container.

LABELLING

The label states, where applicable, that the substance is free from bacterial endotoxins.

01/2005:1144

PROTIRELIN

Protirelinum

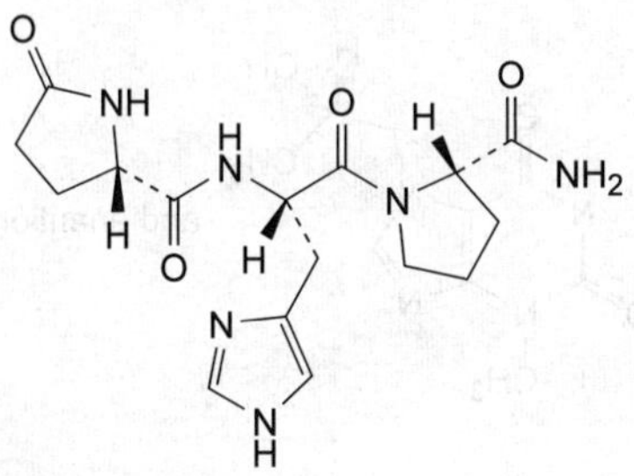

$C_{16}H_{22}N_6O_4$ M_r 362.4

DEFINITION

5-Oxo-L-prolyl-L-histidyl-L-prolinamide.

Synthetic tripeptide with the same sequence of amino acids as the natural hypothalamic neurohormone, which stimulates the release and synthesis of thyrotropin.

Content: 97.0 per cent to 102.0 per cent (anhydrous and acetic acid-free substance).

CHARACTERS

Appearance: white or yellowish-white powder, hygroscopic.

Solubility: very soluble in water, freely soluble in methanol.

IDENTIFICATION

A. Infrared absorption spectrophotometry (*2.2.24*).
Comparison: *protirelin CRS*.

B. Examine the chromatograms obtained in the assay.
Results: the principal peak in the chromatogram obtained with the test solution is similar in retention time and size to the principal peak in the chromatogram obtained with the reference solution.

TESTS

Appearance of solution. A 10 g/l solution is clear (*2.2.1*) and not more intensely coloured than reference solution Y_5 (*2.2.2, Method II*).

Specific optical rotation (*2.2.7*): − 62 to − 70 (anhydrous and acetic acid-free substance).

Dissolve 10 mg in 1.0 ml of *water R*.

Related substances. Liquid chromatography (*2.2.29*).

Test solution. Dissolve 5.0 mg of the substance to be examined in mobile phase A and dilute to 5.0 ml with mobile phase A.

Reference solution (a). Dissolve the contents of a vial of *D-His-protirelin CRS* in an appropriate volume of mobile phase A to obtain a concentration of 1 mg/ml. Mix equal volumes of this solution and the test solution.

Reference solution (b). Dilute 0.2 ml of the test solution to 10.0 ml with mobile phase A.

Column:
- *size*: l = 0.25 m, Ø = 4.0 mm,
- *stationary phase*: spherical *octadecylsilyl silica gel for chromatography R* (5 µm) with a pore size of 12 nm.

Mobile phase:
- *mobile phase A*: a mixture of 100 ml of *acetonitrile for chromatography R*, 1900 ml of *water R* and 2.0 g of *sodium octanesulphonate R*, containing 2.5 ml/l of *tetraethylammonium hydroxide solution R*; adjust to pH 3.5 with *phosphoric acid R*,
- *mobile phase B*: a mixture of 300 ml of *acetonitrile for chromatography R*, 1700 ml of *water R* and 2.0 g of *sodium octanesulphonate R*, containing 2.5 ml/l of *tetraethylammonium hydroxide solution R*; adjust to pH 3.5 with *phosphoric acid R*,

Time (min)	Mobile phase A (per cent *V/V*)	Mobile phase B (per cent *V/V*)
0 - 30	74 → 41	26 → 59
30 - 35	41 → 74	59 → 26
35 - 50	74	26

Flow rate: 1 ml/min.

Detection: spectrophotometer at 210 nm.

Injection: 10 µl.

Relative retention with reference to protirelin (retention time = about 18 min): impurity C = about 0.2; impurity D = about 0.68; impurity A = about 0.91; impurity B = about 0.95; impurity E = about 1.08.

System suitability: reference solution (a):
- *resolution*: minimum 2.5 between the peaks due to impurity A and protirelin,
- *symmetry factor*: 0.9 to 1.2 for the peak due to protirelin.

Limits:

- *any impurity*: for each impurity, not more than the area of the principal peak in the chromatogram obtained with reference solution (b) (2 per cent),
- *total*: not more than 1.5 times the area of the principal peak in the chromatogram obtained with reference solution (b) (3 per cent),
- *disregard limit*: 0.05 times the area of the principal peak in the chromatogram obtained with reference solution (b) (0.1 per cent).

Acetic acid (*2.5.34*): maximum 2.0 per cent.

Test solution. Dissolve 40.0 mg of the substance to be examined in a mixture of 5 volumes of mobile phase B and 95 volumes of mobile phase A and dilute to 10.0 ml with the same mixture of solvents.

Water (*2.5.12*): maximum 7.0 per cent, determined on 0.200 g.

Bacterial endotoxins (*2.6.14*): less than 0.7 IU/mg, if intended for use in the manufacture of parenteral dosage forms without a further appropriate procedure for the removal of bacterial endotoxins.

ASSAY

Liquid chromatography (*2.2.29*) as described in the test for related substances with the following modification.

Reference solution. Dissolve the contents of a vial of *protirelin CRS* in an appropriate volume of mobile phase A to obtain a concentration of 1.0 mg/ml.

Calculate the content of protirelin ($C_{16}H_{22}N_6O_4$) using the peak areas of the chromatograms obtained with the test solution and the reference solution and the declared content of $C_{16}H_{22}N_6O_4$ in *protirelin CRS*.

STORAGE

In an airtight container, protected from light at a temperature of 2 °C to 8 °C. If the substance is sterile, store in a sterile, airtight, tamper-proof container.

LABELLING

The label states:

- the mass of peptide in the container,
- where applicable, that the substance is free from bacterial endotoxins.

IMPURITIES

Specified impurities: A, B, C, D, E.

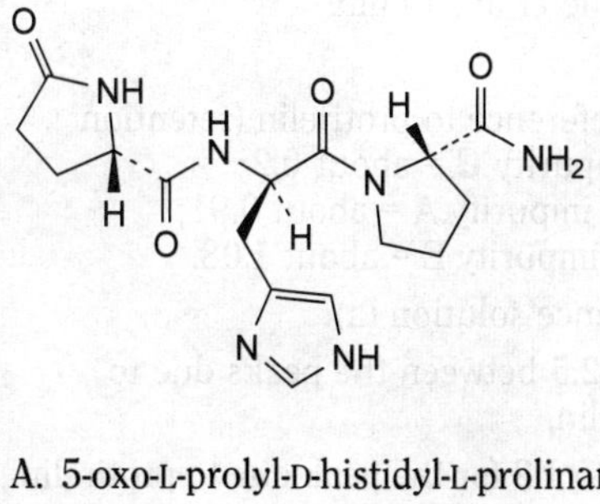

A. 5-oxo-L-prolyl-D-histidyl-L-prolinamide,

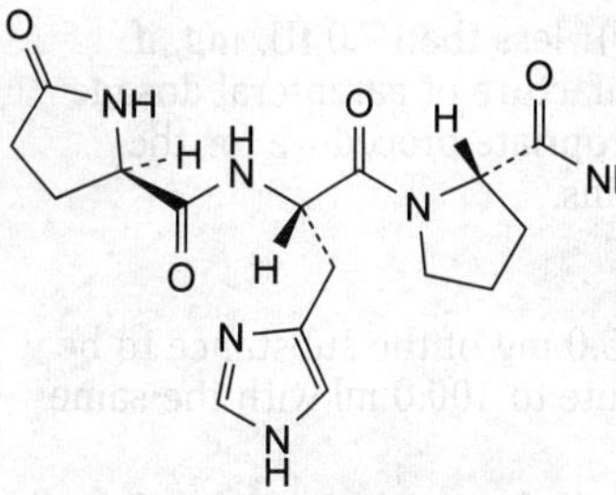

B. 5-oxo-D-prolyl-L-histidyl-L-prolinamide,

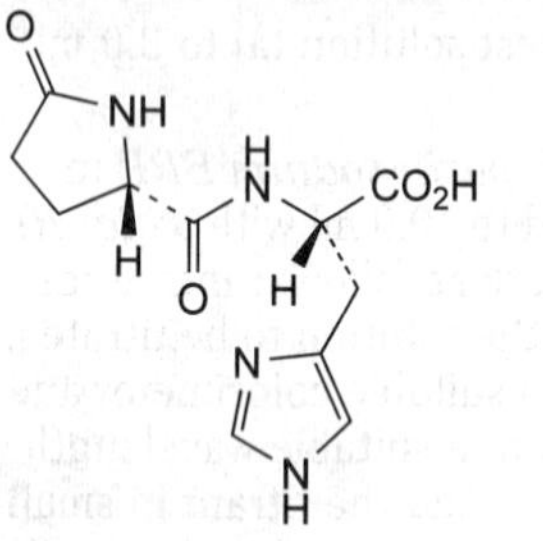

C. 5-oxo-L-prolyl-L-histidine,

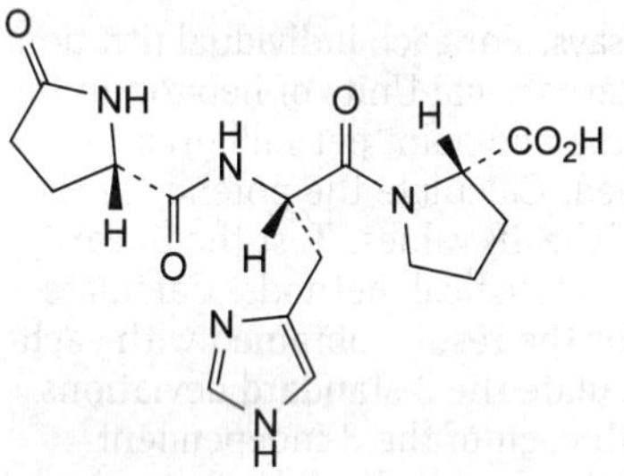

D. 5-oxo-L-prolyl-L-histidyl-L-proline,

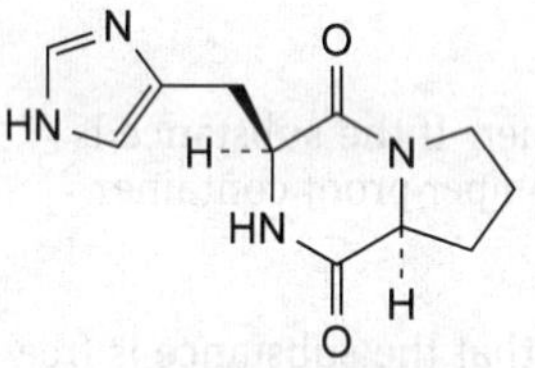

E. (3*S*,8a*S*)-3-(1*H*-imidazol-4-ylmethyl)hexahydropyrrolo[1,2-*a*]pyrazine-1,4-dione (cyclo(-L-histidyl-L-prolyl-)).

01/2005:0526

PROXYPHYLLINE

Proxyphyllinum

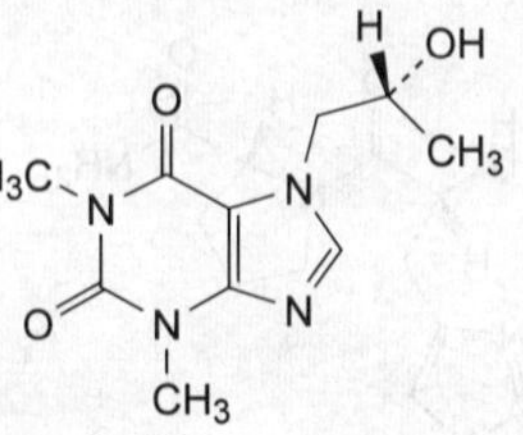

and enantiomer

$C_{10}H_{14}N_4O_3$ M_r 238.2

DEFINITION

Proxyphylline contains not less than 98.5 per cent and not more than the equivalent of 101.0 per cent of 7-[(2*RS*)-2-hydroxypropyl]-1,3-dimethyl-3,7-dihydro-1*H*-purine-2,6-dione, calculated with reference to the dried substance.

CHARACTERS

A white, crystalline powder, very soluble in water, soluble in alcohol.

IDENTIFICATION

First identification: B, C.

Second identification: A, C, D.

A. Melting point (*2.2.14*): 134 °C to 136 °C.

B. Examine by infrared absorption spectrophotometry (*2.2.24*), comparing with the spectrum obtained with *proxyphylline CRS*. Examine the substances as discs prepared using 0.5 mg to 1 mg of the substance to be examined in 0.3 g of *potassium bromide R*.

C. Dissolve 1 g in 5 ml of *acetic anhydride R* and boil under a reflux condenser for 15 min. Allow to cool and add 100 ml of a mixture of 20 volumes of *ether R* and 80 volumes of *light petroleum R*. Cool in iced water for at least 20 min, shaking from time to time. Filter, wash the precipitate with a mixture of 20 volumes of *ether R* and 80 volumes of *light petroleum R*, recrystallise from *alcohol R* and dry *in vacuo*. The crystals melt (*2.2.14*) at 87 °C to 92 °C.

D. It gives the reaction of xanthines (*2.3.1*).

TESTS

Solution S. Dissolve 2.5 g in *carbon dioxide-free water R* and dilute to 50 ml with the same solvent.

Appearance of solution. Solution S is clear (*2.2.1*) and colourless (*2.2.2, Method II*).

Acidity or alkalinity. To 10 ml of solution S add 0.25 ml of *bromothymol blue solution R1*. The solution is yellow or green. Not more than 0.4 ml of *0.01 M sodium hydroxide* is required to change the colour of the indicator to blue.

Related substances. Examine by thin-layer chromatography (*2.2.27*), using *silica gel HF_{254} R* as the coating substance.

Test solution. Dissolve 0.3 g of the substance to be examined in a mixture of 20 volumes of *water R* and 30 volumes of *methanol R* and dilute to 10 ml with the same mixture of solvents. Prepare immediately before use.

Reference solution (a). Dilute 1 ml of the test solution to 100 ml with *methanol R*.

Reference solution (b). Dilute 0.2 ml of the test solution to 100 ml with *methanol R*.

Reference solution (c). Dissolve 10 mg of *theophylline R* in *methanol R*, add 0.3 ml of the test solution and dilute to 10 ml with *methanol R*.

Apply separately to the plate 10 µl of each solution. Develop over a path of 15 cm using a mixture of 1 volume of *concentrated ammonia R*, 10 volumes of *ethanol R* and 90 volumes of *chloroform R*. Allow the plate to dry in air and examine in ultraviolet light at 254 nm. Any spot in the chromatogram obtained with the test solution, apart from the principal spot, is not more intense than the spot in the chromatogram obtained with reference solution (a) (1 per cent) and at most one such spot is more intense than the spot in the chromatogram obtained with reference solution (b) (0.2 per cent). The test is not valid unless the chromatogram obtained with reference solution (c) shows two clearly separated spots.

Chlorides (*2.4.4*). Dilute 2.5 ml of solution S to 15 ml with *water R*. The solution complies with the limit test for chlorides (400 ppm).

Heavy metals (*2.4.8*). 12 ml of solution S complies with limit test A for heavy metals (20 ppm). Prepare the standard using *lead standard solution (1 ppm Pb) R*.

Loss on drying (*2.2.32*). Not more than 0.5 per cent, determined on 1.000 g by drying in an oven at 100 °C to 105 °C.

Sulphated ash (*2.4.14*). Not more than 0.1 per cent, determined on 1.0 g.

ASSAY

In order to avoid overheating in the reaction medium, mix thoroughly throughout and stop the titration immediately after the end-point has been reached.

Dissolve 0.200 g in 3.0 ml of *anhydrous formic acid R* and add 50.0 ml of *acetic anhydride R*. Titrate with *0.1 M perchloric acid* determining the end-point potentiometrically (*2.2.20*).

1 ml of *0.1 M perchloric acid* is equivalent to 23.82 mg of $C_{10}H_{14}N_4O_3$.

STORAGE

Store protected from light.

01/2005:1367
corrected

PSEUDOEPHEDRINE HYDROCHLORIDE

Pseudoephedrini hydrochloridum

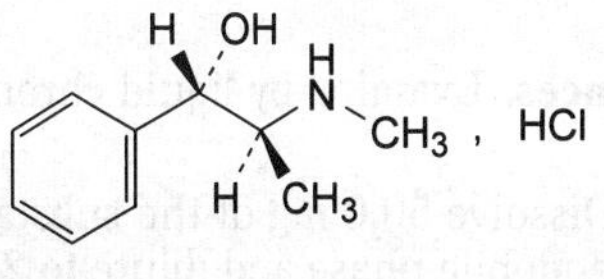

$C_{10}H_{16}ClNO$ M_r 201.7

DEFINITION

Pseudoephedrine hydrochloride contains not less than 99.0 per cent and not more than the equivalent of 101.0 per cent of (1*S*,2*S*)-2-(methylamino)-1-phenylpropan-1-ol hydrochloride, calculated with reference to the dried substance.

CHARACTERS

A white or almost white, crystalline powder or colourless crystals, freely soluble in water and in alcohol, sparingly soluble in methylene chloride.

It melts at about 184 °C.

IDENTIFICATION

First identification: A, B, D.

Second identification: A, C, D.

A. It complies with the test for specific optical rotation (see Tests).

B. Examine by infrared absorption spectrophotometry (*2.2.24*), comparing with the spectrum obtained with *pseudoephedrine hydrochloride CRS*. Examine the substances prepared as discs.

C. Examine by thin-layer chromatography (*2.2.27*), using a suitable silica gel as the coating substance.

Test solution. Dissolve 20 mg of the substance to be examined in *methanol R* and dilute to 10 ml with the same solvent.

Reference solution (a). Dissolve 20 mg of *pseudoephedrine hydrochloride CRS* in *methanol R* and dilute to 10 ml with the same solvent.

Reference solution (b). Dissolve 10 mg of *ephedrine hydrochloride CRS* in reference solution (a) and dilute to 5 ml with the same solution.

Apply to the plate 10 µl of each solution. Develop over a path of 15 cm using a mixture of 5 volumes of *methylene chloride R*, 15 volumes of *concentrated ammonia R* and 80 volumes of *2-propanol R*. Allow the plate to dry in air and spray with *ninhydrin solution R*. Heat at 110 °C for 5 min. The principal spot in the chromatogram obtained with the test solution is similar in position, colour and size to the principal spot in the chromatogram obtained with reference solution (a). The test is not valid unless the chromatogram obtained with reference solution (b) shows two clearly separated spots.

D. Solution S (see Tests) gives reaction (a) of chlorides (*2.3.1*).

TESTS

Solution S. Dissolve 1.25 g in *carbon dioxide-free water R* and dilute to 25.0 ml with the same solvent.

Appearance of solution. Solution S is clear (*2.2.1*) and colourless (*2.2.2, Method II*).

Acidity or alkalinity. Dilute 2 ml of solution S to 10 ml with *carbon dioxide-free water R*. Add 0.1 ml of *methyl red solution R* and 0.1 ml of *0.01 M sodium hydroxide*; the solution is yellow. Add 0.2 ml of *0.01 M hydrochloric acid*; the solution is red.

Specific optical rotation (*2.2.7*): + 61.0 to + 62.5, determined on solution S and calculated with reference to the dried substance.

Related substances. Examine by liquid chromatography (*2.2.29*).

Test solution. Dissolve 50.0 mg of the substance to be examined in the mobile phase and dilute to 25.0 ml with the mobile phase.

Reference solution (a). Dissolve 20.0 mg of *ephedrine hydrochloride CRS* in the mobile phase and dilute to 20.0 ml with the mobile phase. Dilute 1.0 ml of the solution to 50.0 ml with the mobile phase.

Reference solution (b). Dilute 1.0 ml of the test solution to 200.0 ml with the mobile phase.

Reference solution (c). Dissolve 10 mg of *ephedrine hydrochloride CRS* in 5 ml of the test solution and dilute to 100 ml with the mobile phase.

The chromatographic procedure may be carried out using:

- a stainless steel column 0.25 m long and 4.6 mm in internal diameter packed with *phenylsilyl silica gel for chromatography R* (5 µm),
- as mobile phase at a flow rate of 1 ml/min a mixture of 6 volumes of *methanol R* and 94 volumes of a 11.6 g/l solution of *ammonium acetate R* adjusted to pH 4.0 with *glacial acetic acid R*,
- as detector a spectrophotometer set at 257 nm.

Inject 20 µl of reference solution (c). Adjust the sensitivity of the system so that the heights of the two peaks in the chromatogram obtained are at least 50 per cent of the full scale of the recorder. The test is not valid unless the resolution between the peaks corresponding to ephedrine and pseudoephedrine is at least 2.0. If necessary reduce the content of methanol in the mobile phase. Inject 20 µl of the test solution, 20 µl of reference solution (a) and 20 µl of reference solution (b). Continue the chromatography of the test solution for 1.5 times the retention time of pseudoephedrine. In the chromatogram obtained with the test solution: the area of any peak due to ephedrine is not greater than the area of the principal peak in the chromatogram obtained with reference solution (a) (1 per cent); the area of any peak, apart from the principal peak and any peak due to ephedrine, is not greater than the area of the principal peak in the chromatogram obtained with reference solution (b) (0.5 per cent) and the sum of the areas of such peaks is not greater than twice the area of the principal peak in the chromatogram obtained with reference solution (b) (1 per cent). Disregard any peak with an area less than 0.1 times that of the principal peak in the chromatogram obtained with reference solution (b).

Loss on drying (*2.2.32*). Not more than 0.5 per cent, determined on 1.000 g by drying in an oven at 100-105 °C.

Sulphated ash (*2.4.14*). Not more than 0.1 per cent, determined on 1.0 g.

ASSAY

Dissolve 0.170 g in 30 ml of *alcohol R*. Add 5.0 ml of *0.01 M hydrochloric acid.* Carry out a potentiometric titration (*2.2.20*), using *0.1 M sodium hydroxide*. Read the volume added between the two points of inflexion.

1 ml of *0.1 M sodium hydroxide* is equivalent to 20.17 mg of $C_{10}H_{16}ClNO$.

STORAGE

Store protected from light.

IMPURITIES

A. ephedrine.

01/2005:0858

PSYLLIUM SEED

Psyllii semen

DEFINITION

Psyllium seed consists of the ripe, whole, dry seeds of *Plantagoafra* L. (*Plantago psyllium* L.) or *Plantago indica* L. (*Plantago arenaria* Waldstein and Kitaibel).

CHARACTERS

Psyllium seed has a sweet taste.

It has the macroscopic characters described under Identification.

IDENTIFICATION

P. afra seeds are light brown to very dark brown but never black, smooth and shiny having an elliptical oblong shape. They are 2 mm to 3 mm long and 0.8 mm to 1.0 mm wide, one end being wider than the other. Towards the middle of the dorsal surface there is a fairly marked transverse constriction of light colour. On the ventral surface, there is a linear lighter-coloured groove in the middle of which is a clear spot corresponding to the hilum and bounded by swollen edges.

P. indica seeds are almost identical to the seeds of *P. afra*, but a little less shiny; they are 2 mm to 3 mm long and have a maximum diameter of 1.5 mm.

TESTS

Swelling index (*2.8.4*). Not less than 10.

Foreign matter (*2.8.2*). Not more than 1.0 per cent, determined on 10.0 g of the drug, including greenish unripe seeds. Psyllium seed does not contain seeds having a dark central spot on the groove (*Plantago lanceolata* L. and *P. major* L.) or seeds with brownish-grey or pinkish outer coats (*P. ovata* Forssk. and *P. sempervirens* Crantz).

Loss on drying (*2.2.32*). Not more than 14.0 per cent, determined on 1.000 g of drug by drying in an oven at 100 °C to 105 °C for 2 h.

Total ash (*2.4.16*). Not more than 4.0 per cent.

STORAGE

Store protected from light and moisture.

01/2005:1886

PYGEUM AFRICANUM BARK

Pruni africanae cortex

DEFINITION

Whole or cut, dried bark of the stems and branches of *Prunus africana* (Hook f.) Kalkm. (syn. *Pygeum africanum* Hook f.).

CHARACTERS

Macroscopic and microscopic characters described under identification tests A and B.

IDENTIFICATION

A. The dark brown to reddish-brown bark occurs in curved, hard, irregular pieces. The outer surface has a wrinkled dark reddish-brown cork with areas of adhering lichen. The reddish-brown to dark brown inner surface bears longitudinal striations. It may also occur in rolled fragments with a fibrous fracture.

B. Reduce to a powder (355). The powder is reddish-brown. Examine under a microscope using *chloral hydrate solution R*. The powdered drug shows thick-walled sclereids, solitary or in groups; calcium oxalate cluster crystals of different size; numerous lignified fibres, thick-walled and with narrow lumen, some of them solitary and most in groups with forked ends; fragments of pigmented polygonal cells of reddish-brown colour; fragments of cork. Examine under a microscope using a 50 per cent *V/V* solution of *glycerol R*, the powder shows some isolated small starch grains that stain bluish-black against *iodine solution R1*.

C. Thin-layer chromatography (*2.2.27*).

Test solution. Extract 15.0 g of powdered drug (250) with *methylene chloride R* for 30 min in a continuous extraction apparatus (Soxhlet type). Filter. Evaporate the solvent to dryness under reduced pressure. Dissolve the residue in 1 ml of *methylene chloride R*.

Reference solution. Dissolve 20 mg of *β-sitosterol R* and 20 mg of *ursolic acid R* in 10 ml of a mixture of equal volumes of *methanol R* and *methylene chloride R*.

Plate: *TLC silica gel plate R*.

Mobile phase: *methanol R, methylene chloride R* (10:90 *V/V*).

Application: 10 μl, as 1 cm bands.

Development: over a path of 15 cm.

Drying: in air.

Detection: spray with *vanillin reagent R*. Heat the plate at 100-105 °C for 10 min and allow to cool; examine in daylight.

Results: see below the sequence of the zones present in the chromatograms obtained with the reference solution and the test solution. Furthermore, other zones may be present in the chromatogram obtained with the test solution.

Top of the plate	
	A violet zone
	Several weak violet, blue or grey zones
———	———
β-Sitosterol: a violet zone	A violet zone (β-sitosterol)
Ursolic acid: a blue zone	A blue zone (ursolic acid)
	Several weak violet, blue or grey zones
———	———
	A violet zone (β-sitosterol glucoside)
Reference solution	**Test solution**

TESTS

Foreign matter (*2.8.2*): maximum 3.0 per cent.

Loss on drying (*2.2.32*): maximum 12.0 per cent, determined on 1.000 g of powdered drug (355) by drying in an oven at 100-105 °C for 2 h.

Total ash (*2.4.16*): maximum 10.0 per cent.

Extractable matter: minimum 0.5 per cent.

Extract 20.0 g of the powdered drug (250) with *methylene chloride R* for 4 h in a continuous extraction apparatus (Soxhlet type). Evaporate the solution to dryness on a water-bath *in vacuo* and then dry the residue at 80 °C for 2 h. The residue weighs a minimum of 0.10 g.

01/2005:1680

PYRANTEL EMBONATE

Pyranteli embonas

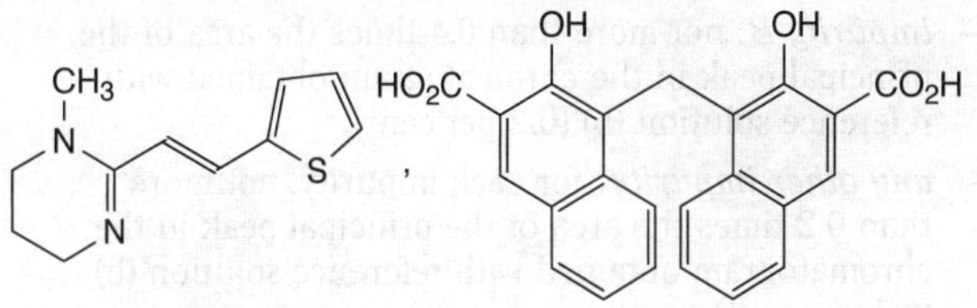

$C_{34}H_{30}N_2O_6S$ M_r 594.7

DEFINITION

1-Methyl-2-[(*E*)-2-(thiophen-2-yl)ethenyl]-1,4,5,6-tetrahydropyrimidine hydrogen 4,4′-methylenebis(3-hydroxynaphthalene-2-carboxylate).

Content: 98.0 per cent to 102.0 per cent (dried substance).

CHARACTERS

Appearance: pale yellow or yellow powder.

Solubility: pratically insoluble in water, soluble in dimethyl sulphoxide, pratically insoluble in methanol.

IDENTIFICATION

Infrared absorption spectrophotometry (*2.2.24*).

Comparison: *pyrantel embonate CRS*.

TESTS

Related substances. Liquid chromatography (*2.2.29*). *Prepare the solutions immediately before use and strictly protect from light at all stages.*

Solvent mixture. Mix 5 volumes of *glacial acetic R* with 5 volumes of *water R* and add 2 volumes of *diethylamine R* with cooling.

Monographs P

Test solution. Dissolve 80 mg in 7 ml of the solvent mixture and dilute to 100.0 ml with *acetonitrile R*.

Reference solution (a). Dissolve 10.0 mg of *pyrantel impurity A CRS* in the solvent mixture, add 2.5 ml of the test solution and dilute to 50.0 ml with the solvent mixture. Dilute 2.0 ml of this solution to 100.0 ml with the solvent mixture.

Reference solution (b). Dilute 1.0 ml of the test solution to 200.0 ml with the mobile phase.

Column:

– *size*: l = 0.25 m, Ø = 4.6 mm,

– *stationary phase*: *silica gel for chromatography R* (5 µm).

Mobile phase: solvent mixture, *acetonitrile for chromatography R* (72:928 *V/V*).

Flow rate: 1 ml/min.

Detection: spectrophotometer at 288 nm.

Injection: 20 µl.

Run time: 4 times the retention time of pyrantel.

Relative retention with reference to pyrantel (retention time = about 11 min): embonic acid = about 0.5; impurity A = about 1.3; impurity B = about 1.8 (impurity A also gives rise to an embonate peak).

System suitability: reference solution (a):

– *resolution*: minimum 4.0 between the peaks due to pyrantel and impurity A.

Limits:

– *correction factor*: for the calculation of content, multiply the peak area of impurity B by 0.4,

– *impurity A*: not more than the area of the corresponding peak in the chromatogram obtained with reference solution (a) (0.5 per cent),

– *impurity B*: not more than 0.4 times the area of the principal peak in the chromatogram obtained with reference solution (b) (0.2 per cent),

– *any other impurity*: for each impurity, not more than 0.2 times the area of the principal peak in the chromatogram obtained with reference solution (b) (0.1 per cent),

– *sum of impurities other than A and B*: not more than 0.6 times the area of the principal peak in the chromatogram obtained with reference solution (b) (0.3 per cent),

– *disregard limit*: 0.1 times the area of the principal peak in the chromatogram obtained with reference solution (b) (0.05 per cent).

Chlorides (*2.4.4*): maximum 360 ppm.

To 0.46 g add 10 ml of *dilute nitric acid R* and 30 ml of *water R*. Heat on a water-bath for 5 min. Cool, dilute to 50 ml with *water R*, mix well and filter. 15 ml complies with the limit test for chlorides.

Sulphates (*2.4.13*): maximum 0.1 per cent.

To 0.50 g add 2.5 ml of *dilute nitric acid R* and dilute to 50 ml with *distilled water R*. Heat on a water-bath for 5 min, shake for 2 min, cool and filter. 15 ml complies with the limit test for sulphates.

Iron (*2.4.9*): maximum 75 ppm.

Ignite 0.66 g at 800 °C for 2 h. Dissolve the residue in 2.5 ml of *dilute hydrochloric acid R* with gentle heating for 10 min. Cool and dilute to 50 ml with *water R*. 10 ml complies with the limit test for iron.

Heavy metals (*2.4.8*): maximum 20 ppm.

1.0 g complies with limit test D. Prepare the reference solution using 2.0 ml of *lead standard solution (10 ppm Pb) R*.

Loss on drying (*2.2.32*): maximum 1.0 per cent, determined on 1.000 g by drying *in vacuo* at 60 °C for 3 h.

Sulphated ash (*2.4.14*): maximum 0.1 per cent, determined on 1.0 g.

ASSAY

To 0.450 g add 10 ml of *acetic anhydride R* and 50 ml *glacial acetic acid R*, heat at 50 °C and stir for 10 min. Allow to cool (a clear solution is not obtained). Titrate with *0.1 M perchloric acid*, determining the end-point potentiometrically (*2.2.20*). Carry out a blank titration.

1 ml of *0.1 M perchloric acid* is equivalent to 59.47 mg of $C_{34}H_{30}N_2O_6S$.

STORAGE

Protected from light.

IMPURITIES

Specified impurities: A, B.

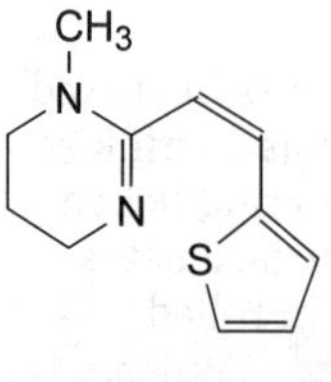

A. 1-methyl-2-[(*Z*)-2-(thiophen-2-yl)ethenyl]-1,4,5,6-tetrahydropyrimidine,

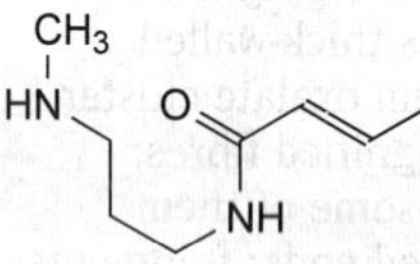

B. (*E*)-*N*-[3-(methylamino)propyl]-3-(thiophen-2-yl)prop-2-enamide.

01/2005:0859

PYRAZINAMIDE

Pyrazinamidum

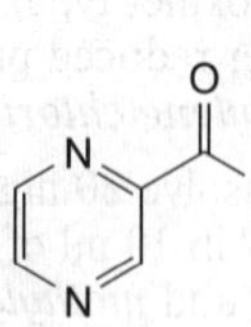

$C_5H_5N_3O$ M_r 123.1

DEFINITION

Pyrazinamide contains not less than 99.0 per cent and not more than the equivalent of 100.5 per cent of pyrazine-2-carboxamide, calculated with reference to the anhydrous substance.

CHARACTERS

A white, crystalline powder, sparingly soluble in water, slightly soluble in alcohol and in methylene chloride.

IDENTIFICATION

First identification: C.

Second identification: A, B, D.

A. Melting point (*2.2.14*): 188 °C to 191 °C.

B. Dissolve 50.0 mg in *water R* and dilute to 100.0 ml with the same solvent (solution (a)). Dilute 1.0 ml of solution (a) to 10.0 ml with *water R*. Examined between 290 nm and 350 nm (*2.2.25*), the solution shows an absorption maximum at 310 nm. Dilute 2.0 ml of solution (a) to 100.0 ml with *water R*. Examined between 230 nm and 290 nm, the solution shows an absorption maximum at 268 nm. The specific absorbance at the maximum is 640 to 680.

C. Examine by infrared absorption spectrophotometry (*2.2.24*), comparing with the spectrum obtained with *pyrazinamide CRS*. Examine the substances prepared as discs. If the spectra obtained show differences, dissolve the substance to be examined and the reference substance separately in *alcohol R*, evaporate to dryness and record new spectra using the residues.

D. Dissolve 0.1 g in 5 ml of *water R*. Add 1 ml of *ferrous sulphate solution R2*. The solution becomes orange. Add 1 ml of *dilute sodium hydroxide solution R*. The solution becomes dark blue.

TESTS

Solution S. Dissolve 0.5 g in *carbon dioxide-free water R* and dilute to 50 ml with the same solvent.

Appearance of solution. Solution S is clear (*2.2.1*) and colourless (*2.2.2, Method II*).

Acidity or alkalinity. To 25 ml of solution S add 0.05 ml of *phenolphthalein solution R1* and 0.2 ml of *0.01 M sodium hydroxide*. The solution is red. Add 1.0 ml of *0.01 M hydrochloric acid*. The solution is colourless. Add 0.15 ml of *methyl red solution R*. The solution is red.

Related substances. Examine by thin-layer chromatography (*2.2.27*), using *silica gel GF_{254} R* as the coating substance.

Test solution. Dissolve 0.1 g of the substance to be examined in a mixture of 1 volume of *methanol R* and 9 volumes of *methylene chloride R* and dilute to 10 ml with the same mixture of solvents.

Reference solution (a). Dilute 1 ml of the test solution to 50 ml with a mixture of 1 volume of *methanol R* and 9 volumes of *methylene chloride R*. Dilute 1 ml of the solution to 10 ml with a mixture of 1 volume of *methanol R* and 9 volumes of *methylene chloride R*.

Reference solution (b). Dissolve 10 mg of *nicotinic acid CRS* in a mixture of 1 volume of *methanol R* and 9 volumes of *methylene chloride R*, add 1 ml of the test solution and dilute to 10 ml with the same mixture of solvents.

Apply separately to the plate 20 µl of each solution. Develop over a path of 10 cm using a mixture of 20 volumes of *glacial acetic acid R*, 20 volumes of *water R* and 60 volumes of *butanol R*. Allow the plate to dry in air and examine immediately in ultraviolet light at 254 nm. Any spot in the chromatogram obtained with the test solution, apart from the principal spot, is not more intense than the spot in the chromatogram obtained with reference solution (a) (0.2 per cent). The test is not valid unless the chromatogram obtained with reference solution (b) shows two clearly separated principal spots.

Heavy metals (*2.4.8*). 1.0 g complies with limit test C for heavy metals (10 ppm). Prepare the standard using 1 ml of *lead standard solution (10 ppm Pb) R*.

Water (*2.5.12*). Not more than 0.5 per cent, determined on 2.00 g by the semi-micro determination of water.

Sulphated ash (*2.4.14*). Not more than 0.1 per cent, determined on 1.0 g.

ASSAY

Dissolve 0.100 g in 50 ml of *acetic anhydride R*. Titrate with *0.1 M perchloric acid*, determining the end-point potentiometrically (*2.2.20*).

1 ml of *0.1 M perchloric acid* is equivalent to 12.31 mg of $C_5H_5N_3O$.

IMPURITIES

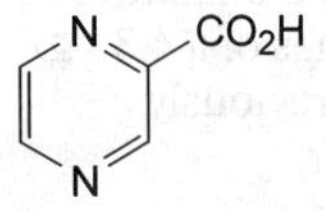

A. pyrazine-2-carboxylic acid.

01/2005:1255

PYRIDOSTIGMINE BROMIDE

Pyridostigmini bromidum

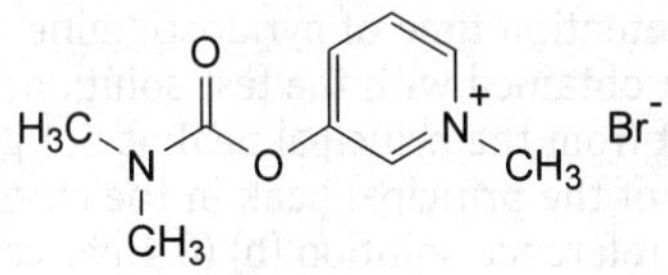

$C_9H_{13}BrN_2O_2$ M_r 261.1

DEFINITION

Pyridostigmine bromide contains not less than 98.5 per cent and not more than the equivalent of 101.0 per cent of 3-(dimethylcarbamoyloxy)-1-methylpyridinium bromide, calculated with reference to the dried substance.

CHARACTERS

A white or almost white, crystalline, deliquescent powder, very soluble in water and in alcohol.

IDENTIFICATION

A. Examine by infrared absorption spectrophotometry (*2.2.24*), comparing with the spectrum obtained with *pyridostigmine bromide CRS*.

B. It gives reaction (a) of bromides (*2.3.1*).

TESTS

Solution S. Dissolve 1.0 g in *carbon dioxide-free water R* and dilute to 100 ml with the same solvent.

Appearance of solution. Solution S is clear (*2.2.1*) and colourless (*2.2.2, Method II*).

Acidity or alkalinity. To 40 ml of solution S add a few drops of *methyl red solution R*. To 20 ml of this solution add 0.2 ml of *0.02 M sodium hydroxide*. The solution is yellow. To the other 20 ml add 0.2 ml of *0.02 M hydrochloric acid*. The solution is red.

Related substances. Examine by liquid chromatography (*2.2.29*).

Test solution. Dissolve 50 mg of the substance to be examined in the mobile phase at about 40 °C. Allow to cool and dilute to 50.0 ml with the same solvent.

Reference solution (a). Dissolve 4 mg of *pyridostigmine impurity A CRS* and 4 mg of *pyridostigmine bromide CRS* in the mobile phase and dilute to 100.0 ml with the same solvent. Dilute 5.0 ml to 100.0 ml with the mobile phase.

Reference solution (b). Dilute 1.0 ml of the test solution to 100.0 ml with the mobile phase. Dilute 10.0 ml to 50.0 ml with the mobile phase.

Monographs P

Reference solution (c). Dilute 5.0 ml of reference solution (b) to 20.0 ml with the mobile phase.

The chromatographic procedure may be carried out using:

– a stainless steel column 0.25 m long and 4.0 mm in internal diameter packed with *base-deactivated octadecylsilyl silica gel for chromatography R* (5 μm to 10 μm),
– as mobile phase at a flow rate of 1.1 ml/min a mixture of 30 volumes of *acetonitrile R* and 70 volumes of a 4.33 g/l solution of *sodium dodecyl sulphate R*, previously adjusted to pH 2.0 with *phosphoric acid R*,
– as detector a spectrophotometer set at 220 nm.

Inject 20 μl of reference solution (b). Adjust the sensitivity of the system so that the height of the principal peak in the chromatogram obtained is at least 50 per cent of the full scale of the recorder. Inject 20 μl of reference solution (a). The test is not valid unless in the chromatogram obtained, the resolution between the peaks due to pyridostigmine and pyridostigmine impurity A is at least 1.5. Inject separately 20 μl of the test solution, 20 μl of reference solution (b) and 20 μl of reference solution (c). Continue the chromatography for twice the retention time of pyridostigmine. In the chromatogram obtained with the test solution: the area of any peak apart from the principal peak is not greater than twice the area of the principal peak in the chromatogram obtained with reference solution (b) (0.4 per cent), at most one such peak has an area greater than the area of the principal peak in the chromatogram obtained with reference solution (b) (0.2 per cent) and at most one further peak has an area greater than half of the area of the principal peak in the chromatogram obtained with reference solution (b) (0.1 per cent); the sum of the area of all of the peaks apart from the principal peak is not greater than 2.5 times the area of the principal peak in the chromatogram obtained with reference solution (b) (0.5 per cent). Disregard any peak due to the solvent and any peak with an area less than the area of the principal peak in the chromatogram obtained with reference solution (c).

Heavy metals (*2.4.8*). 1.0 g complies with limit test C for heavy metals (20 ppm). Prepare the standard using 2 ml of *lead standard solution (10 ppm Pb) R*.

Loss on drying (*2.2.32*). Not more than 0.5 per cent, determined on 1.000 g by drying in an oven at 100 °C to 105 °C.

Sulphated ash (*2.4.14*). Not more than 0.1 per cent, determined on 1.0 g.

ASSAY

Dissolve 0.230 g in 10 ml of *anhydrous acetic acid R*. Add 40 ml of *acetic anhydride R*. Titrate with *0.1 M perchloric acid*, determining the end-point potentiometrically (*2.2.20*).

1 ml of *0.1 M perchloric acid* is equivalent to 26.11 mg of $C_9H_{13}BrN_2O_2$.

STORAGE

Store in an airtight container, protected from light. If the substance is sterile, store in a sterile, airtight, tamper-proof container, protected from light.

IMPURITIES

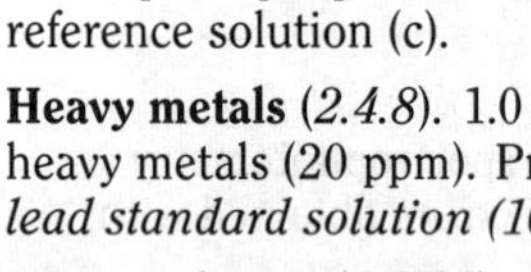

A. pyridin-3-yl dimethylcarbamate,

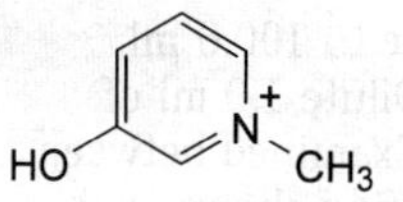

B. 3-hydroxy-1-methylpyridinium.

01/2005:0245

PYRIDOXINE HYDROCHLORIDE

Pyridoxini hydrochloridum

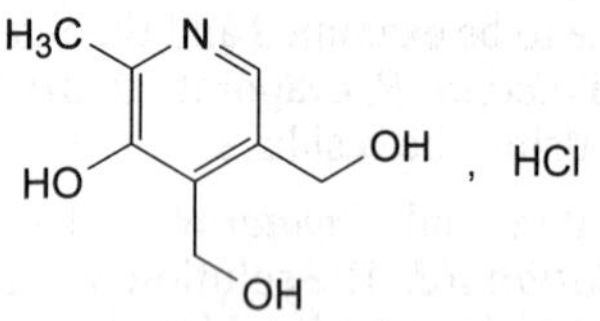

$C_8H_{12}ClNO_3$ M_r 205.6

DEFINITION

Pyridoxine hydrochloride contains not less than 99.0 per cent and not more than the equivalent of 101.0 per cent of (5-hydroxy-6-methylpyridine-3,4-diyl)dimethanol hydrochloride, calculated with reference to the dried substance.

CHARACTERS

A white or almost white, crystalline powder, freely soluble in water, slightly soluble in alcohol.

It melts at about 205 °C, with decomposition.

IDENTIFICATION

First identification: B, D.

Second identification: A, C, D.

A. Dilute 1.0 ml of solution S (see Tests) to 50.0 ml with *0.1 M hydrochloric acid* (solution A). Dilute 1.0 ml of solution A to 100.0 ml with *0.1 M hydrochloric acid.* Examined between 250 nm and 350 nm (*2.2.25*), the solution shows an absorption maximum at 288 nm to 296 nm. The specific absorbance at the maximum is 425 to 445. Dilute 1.0 ml of solution A to 100.0 ml with a mixture of equal volumes of *0.025 M potassium dihydrogen phosphate solution* and *0.025 M disodium hydrogen phosphate solution* (*2.2.3*). Examined between 220 nm and 350 nm, the solution shows 2 absorption maxima, at 248 nm to 256 nm and at 320 nm to 327 nm. The specific absorbances at the maxima are 175 to 195 and 345 to 365, respectively.

B. Examine by infrared absorption spectrophotometry (*2.2.24*), comparing with the spectrum obtained with *pyridoxine hydrochloride CRS.*

C. Examine the chromatograms obtained in the test for related substances. The principal spot in the chromatogram obtained with test solution (b) is similar in position, colour and size to the principal spot in the chromatogram obtained with reference solution (a).

D. Solution S gives reaction (a) of chlorides (*2.3.1*).

TESTS

Solution S. Dissolve 2.50 g in *carbon dioxide-free water R* and dilute to 50.0 ml with the same solvent.

Appearance of solution. Solution S is clear (*2.2.1*) and not more intensely coloured than reference solution Y_7 (*2.2.2, Method II*).

pH (*2.2.3*). The pH of solution S is 2.4 to 3.0.

Related substances. Examine by thin-layer chromatography (*2.2.27*), using a *TLC silica gel G plate R*.

Test solution (a). Dissolve 1.0 g of the substance to be examined in *water R* and dilute to 10 ml with the same solvent.

Test solution (b). Dilute 1 ml of test solution (a) to 10 ml with *water R*.

Reference solution (a). Dissolve 0.10 g of *pyridoxine hydrochloride CRS* in *water R* and dilute to 10 ml with the same solvent.

Reference solution (b). Dilute 2.5 ml of test solution (a) to 100 ml with *water R*. Dilute 1 ml of this solution to 10 ml with *water R*.

Apply to the plate 2 µl of each solution. Develop in an unsaturated tank over a path of 15 cm using a mixture of 9 volumes of *concentrated ammonia R*, 13 volumes of *methylene chloride R*, 13 volumes of *tetrahydrofuran R* and 65 volumes of *acetone R*. Allow the plate to dry in air and spray with a 50 g/l solution of *sodium carbonate R* in a mixture of 30 volumes of *alcohol R* and 70 volumes of *water R*. Dry the plate in a current of air, spray with a 1 g/l solution of *dichloroquinonechlorimide R* in *alcohol R* and examine the chromatograms immediately. Any spot in the chromatogram obtained with test solution (a), apart from the principal spot, is not more intense than the spot in the chromatogram obtained with reference solution (b) (0.25 per cent). Disregard any spots remaining on the starting line.

Heavy metals (*2.4.8*). 12 ml of solution S complies with limit test A (20 ppm). Prepare the standard using *lead standard solution (1 ppm Pb) R*.

Loss on drying (*2.2.32*). Not more than 0.5 per cent, determined on 1.000 g by drying in an oven at 100-105 °C.

Sulphated ash (*2.4.14*). Not more than 0.1 per cent, determined on 1.0 g.

ASSAY

In order to avoid overheating in the reaction medium, mix thoroughly throughout and stop the titration immediately after the end-point has been reached.

Dissolve 0.150 g in 5 ml of *anhydrous formic acid R*. Add 50 ml of *acetic anhydride R*. Titrate with *0.1 M perchloric acid*, determining the end-point potentiometrically (*2.2.20*). Carry out a blank titration.

1 ml of *0.1 M perchloric acid* is equivalent to 20.56 mg of $C_8H_{12}ClNO_3$.

STORAGE

Store protected from light.

IMPURITIES

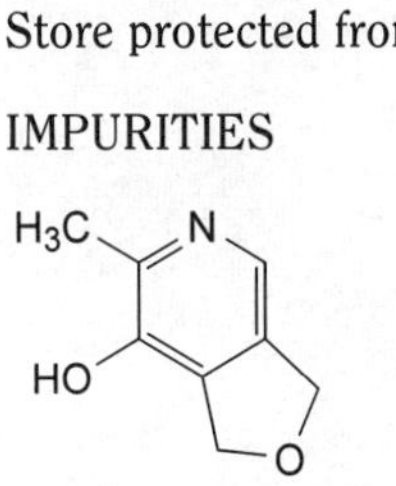

A. 6-methyl-1,3-dihydrofuro[3,4-*c*]pyridin-7-ol,

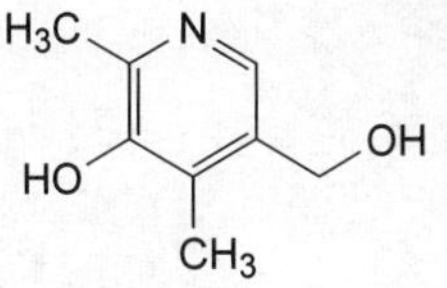

B. 5-(hydroxymethyl)-2,4-dimethylpyridin-3-ol.

01/2005:0288

PYRIMETHAMINE

Pyrimethaminum

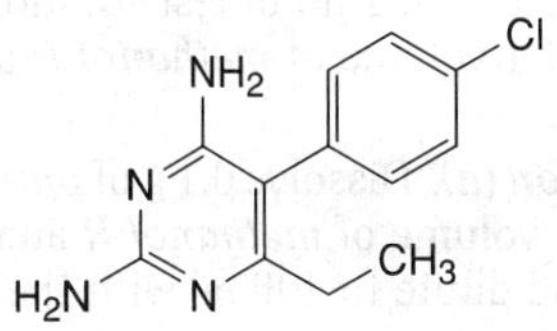

$C_{12}H_{13}ClN_4$ M_r 248.7

DEFINITION

Pyrimethamine contains not less than 99.0 per cent and not more than the equivalent of 101.0 per cent of 5-(4-chlorophenyl)-6-ethylpyrimidine-2,4-diamine, calculated with reference to the dried substance.

CHARACTERS

An almost white, crystalline powder or colourless crystals, practically insoluble in water, slightly soluble in alcohol.

IDENTIFICATION

First identification: C.

Second identification: A, B, D.

A. Melting point (*2.2.14*): 239 °C to 243 °C.

B. Dissolve 0.14 g in *ethanol R* and dilute to 100.0 ml with the same solvent. Dilute 10.0 ml of this solution to 100.0 ml with *0.1 M hydrochloric acid*. Dilute 10.0 ml of this solution to 100.0 ml with *0.1 M hydrochloric acid*. Examined between 250 nm and 300 nm (*2.2.25*), the solution shows an absorption maximum at 272 nm and an absorption minimum at 261 nm. The specific absorbance at the maximum is 310 to 330.

C. Examine by infrared absorption spectrophotometry (*2.2.24*), comparing with the spectrum obtained with *pyrimethamine CRS*.

D. Examine the chromatograms obtained in the test for related substances in ultraviolet light at 254 nm. The principal spot in the chromatogram obtained with test solution (b) is similar in position and size to the principal spot in the chromatogram obtained with reference solution (a).

TESTS

Solution S. Shake 1.0 g with 50 ml of *distilled water R* for 2 min and filter.

Appearance of solution. *Prepare the solution immediately before use.*

Dissolve 0.25 g in a mixture of 1 volume of *methanol R* and 3 volumes of *methylene chloride R* and dilute to 10 ml with the same mixture of solvents. The solution is clear (*2.2.1*) and not more intensely coloured than reference solution BY_6 (*2.2.2, Method II*).

Acidity or alkalinity. To 10 ml of solution S add 0.05 ml of *phenolphthalein solution R1*. The solution is colourless. Not more than 0.2 ml of *0.01 M sodium hydroxide* is required to change the colour of the indicator to pink. Add 0.4 ml of *0.01 M hydrochloric acid* and 0.05 ml of *methyl red solution R*. The solution is red or orange.

Related substances. Examine by thin-layer chromatography (*2.2.27*), using *silica gel GF$_{254}$ R* as the coating substance. *Prepare the solutions immediately before use.*

Test solution (a). Dissolve 0.25 g of the substance to be examined in a mixture of 1 volume of *methanol R* and 9 volumes of *chloroform R* and dilute to 25 ml with the same mixture of solvents.

Test solution (b). Dilute 1 ml of test solution (a) to 10 ml with a mixture of 1 volume of *methanol R* and 9 volumes of *chloroform R*.

Reference solution (a). Dissolve 0.1 g of *pyrimethamine CRS* in a mixture of 1 volume of *methanol R* and 9 volumes of *chloroform R* and dilute to 100 ml with the same mixture of solvents.

Reference solution (b). Dilute 2.5 ml of test solution (a) to 100 ml with a mixture of 1 volume of *methanol R* and 9 volumes of *chloroform R*. Dilute 1 ml of the solution to 10 ml with a mixture of 1 volume of *methanol R* and 9 volumes of *chloroform R*.

Apply to the plate 20 µl of each solution. Develop over a path of 10 cm using a mixture of 4 volumes of *chloroform R*, 8 volumes of *propanol R*, 12 volumes of *glacial acetic acid R* and 76 volumes of *toluene R*. Allow the plate to dry in air. Examine in ultraviolet light at 254 nm. Any spot in the chromatogram obtained with test solution (a), apart from the principal spot, is not more intense than the spot in the chromatogram obtained with reference solution (b) (0.25 per cent).

Sulphates (*2.4.13*). 15 ml of solution S complies with the limit test for sulphates (80 ppm). Prepare the standard using a mixture of 2.5 ml of *sulphate standard solution (10 ppm SO_4) R* and 12.5 ml of *distilled water R*.

Loss on drying (*2.2.32*). Not more than 0.5 per cent, determined on 0.50 g by drying in an oven at 100 °C to 105 °C for 4 h.

Sulphated ash (*2.4.14*). Not more than 0.1 per cent, determined on 1.0 g.

ASSAY

Dissolve 0.200 g in 25 ml of *anhydrous acetic acid R*, heating gently. Cool. Titrate with *0.1 M perchloric acid* determining the end-point potentiometrically (*2.2.20*).

1 ml of *0.1 M perchloric acid* is equivalent to 24.87 mg of $C_{12}H_{13}ClN_4$.

STORAGE

Store protected from light.

Q

01/2005:0017

QUINIDINE SULPHATE

Chinidini sulfas

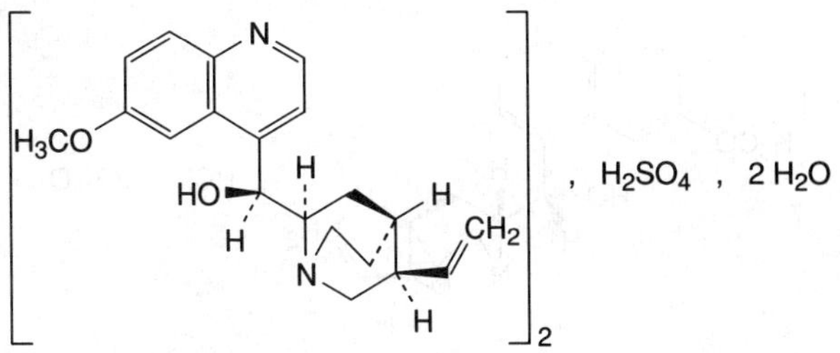

$C_{40}H_{50}N_4O_8S,2H_2O$ M_r 783

DEFINITION

Quinidine sulphate contains not less than 99.0 per cent and not more than the equivalent of 101.0 per cent of alkaloid monosulphates, calculated as bis[(*S*)-[(2*R*,4*S*,5*R*)-5-ethenyl-1-azabicyclo[2.2.2]oct-2-yl](6-methoxyquinolin-4-yl)methanol] sulphate, with reference to the dried substance.

CHARACTERS

A white or almost white, crystalline powder or silky, colourless needles, slightly soluble in water, soluble in boiling water and in alcohol, practically insoluble in acetone.

IDENTIFICATION

A. Examine by thin-layer chromatography (*2.2.27*), using a *TLC silica gel G plate R.*

Test solution. Dissolve 0.10 g of the substance to be examined in *methanol R* and dilute to 10 ml with the same solvent.

Reference solution. Dissolve 0.10 g of *quinidine sulphate CRS* in *methanol R* and dilute to 10 ml with the same solvent.

Apply to the plate 5 µl of each solution. Develop over a path of 15 cm using a mixture of 10 volumes of *diethylamine R*, 24 volumes of *ether R* and 40 volumes of *toluene R*. Dry the plate in a current of air for 15 min and repeat the development. Dry the plate at 105 °C for 30 min, allow to cool and spray with *iodoplatinate reagent R*. The principal spot in the chromatogram obtained with the test solution is similar in position, colour and size to the principal spot in the chromatogram obtained with the reference solution.

B. Dissolve about 5 mg in 5 ml of *water R*. Add 0.2 ml of *bromine water R* and 1 ml of *dilute ammonia R2*. A green colour develops.

C. Dissolve 0.1 g in 3 ml of *dilute sulphuric acid R* and dilute to 100 ml with *water R*. When examined in ultraviolet light at 366 nm, an intense blue fluorescence appears which disappears almost completely on addition of 1 ml of *hydrochloric acid R*.

D. Dissolve about 50 mg in 5 ml of hot *water R*, cool, add 1 ml of *silver nitrate solution R1* and stir with a glass rod. After a few minutes, a white precipitate is formed that dissolves on the addition of *dilute nitric acid R*.

E. It gives reaction (a) of sulphates (*2.3.1*).

F. It complies with the test for pH (see Tests).

TESTS

Solution S. Dissolve 0.500 g in *0.1 M hydrochloric acid* and dilute to 25.0 ml with the same acid.

Appearance of solution. Solution S is clear (*2.2.1*) and not more intensely coloured than reference solution GY_6 (*2.2.2, Method II*).

pH (*2.2.3*). Dissolve 0.10 g in *carbon dioxide-free water R* and dilute to 10 ml with the same solvent. The pH of the solution is 6.0 to 6.8.

Specific optical rotation (*2.2.7*): + 275 to + 290, determined on solution S and calculated with reference to the dried substance.

Other cinchona alkaloids. Examine by liquid chromatography (*2.2.29*).

Test solution. Dissolve 20 mg of the substance to be examined, with gentle heating if necessary, in 5 ml of the mobile phase and dilute to 10 ml with the mobile phase.

Reference solution (a). Dissolve 20 mg of *quinine sulphate CRS*, with gentle heating if necessary, in 5 ml of the mobile phase and dilute to 10 ml with the mobile phase.

Reference solution (b). Dissolve 20 mg of *quinidine sulphate CRS*, with gentle heating if necessary, in 5 ml of the mobile phase and dilute to 10 ml with the mobile phase.

Reference solution (c). To 1 ml of reference solution (a) add 1 ml of reference solution (b).

Reference solution (d). Dilute 1.0 ml of reference solution (a) to 10.0 ml with the mobile phase. Dilute 1.0 ml of this solution to 50.0 ml with the mobile phase.

Reference solution (e). Dissolve 10 mg of *thiourea R* in the mobile phase and dilute to 10 ml with the mobile phase.

The chromatographic procedure may be carried out using:

– a stainless steel column 0.15 m to 0.25 m long and 4.6 mm in internal diameter packed with *octadecylsilyl silica gel for chromatography R* (5 µm or 10 µm),

– as mobile phase at a flow rate of 1.5 ml/min a mixture prepared as follows: dissolve 6.8 g of *potassium dihydrogen phosphate R* and 3.0 g of *hexylamine R* in 700 ml of *water R*, adjust to pH 2.8 with *dilute phosphoric acid R*, add 60 ml of *acetonitrile R* and dilute to 1000 ml with *water R*,

– as detector a spectrophotometer set at 250 nm for recording the chromatogram obtained with reference solution (e) and at 316 nm for the other solutions.

Inject 10 µl of reference solution (b) and 10 µl of reference solution (e). If necessary, adjust the concentration of acetonitrile in the mobile phase so that, in the chromatogram obtained with reference solution (b), the mass distribution factor of the peak corresponding to quinidine is 3.5 to 4.5, $t_{R'}$ being calculated from the peak corresponding to thiourea in the chromatogram obtained with reference solution (e).

Inject 10 µl each of reference solutions (a), (b), (c) and (d). The chromatogram obtained with reference solution (a) shows a principal peak corresponding to quinine and a peak corresponding to dihydroquinine, with a retention time relative to quinine of about 1.4. The chromatogram obtained with reference solution (b) shows a principal peak corresponding to quinidine and a peak corresponding to dihydroquinidine, with a retention time relative to quinidine of about 1.5. The chromatogram obtained with reference solution (c) shows 4 peaks corresponding to quinidine, quinine, dihydroquinidine and dihydroquinine which are identified by comparison of their retention times with those of the corresponding peaks in the chromatograms obtained with reference solutions (a) and (b).

The test is not valid unless: in the chromatogram obtained with reference solution (c), the resolution between the peaks corresponding to quinine and quinidine is at least 3.0 and the resolution between the peaks corresponding to dihydroquinidine and quinine is at least 2.0; and the chromatogram obtained with reference solution (d) shows a principal peak with a signal-to-noise ratio of at least 4.

Inject 10 µl of the test solution and record the chromatogram for 2.5 times the retention time of the principal peak. Calculate the percentage content of related substances from the areas of the peaks in the chromatogram obtained with the test solution by the normalisation procedure, disregarding any peaks with an area less than that of the peak in the chromatogram obtained with reference solution (d). The content of dihydroquinidine is not greater than 15 per cent, the content of any related substance eluted before quinidine is not greater than 5 per cent and the content of any other related substance is not greater than 2.5 per cent.

Boron. *Avoid where possible the use of glassware.*

Test solution. Dissolve 1.00 g in a mixture of 0.5 ml of *hydrochloric acid R* and 4.0 ml of *water R.*

Reference solution. Dissolve 0.572 g of *boric acid R* in *water R* and dilute to 1000.0 ml with the same solvent. Dilute 5.0 ml to 100.0 ml with *water R.* To 1.0 ml of this solution add 3.0 ml of *water R* and 0.5 ml of *hydrochloric acid R.*

Blank solution. Add 0.5 ml of *hydrochloric acid R* to 4.0 ml of *water R.*

Add 3.0 ml of a 100 g/l solution of *2-ethylhexane-1,3-diol R* in *methylene chloride R* to the test solution, to the reference solution and to the blank solution and shake for 1 min. Allow to stand for 6 min. To 1.0 ml of the lower layer, add 2.0 ml of a 3.75 g/l solution of *curcumin R* in *anhydrous acetic acid R* and 0.3 ml of *sulphuric acid R.* Mix and after 20 min add 25.0 ml of *alcohol R.* Mix. The colour of the blank solution is yellow. Any red colour in the test solution is not more intense than that in the reference solution (5 ppm of B).

Loss on drying (*2.2.32*). 3.0 per cent to 5.0 per cent, determined on 1.000 g by drying in an oven at 130 °C.

Sulphated ash (*2.4.14*). Not more than 0.1 per cent, determined on 1.0 g.

ASSAY

Dissolve 0.200 g in 20 ml of *acetic anhydride R.* Titrate with *0.1 M perchloric acid,* using 0.15 ml of *naphtholbenzein solution R* as indicator.

1 ml of *0.1 M perchloric acid* is equivalent to 24.90 mg of $C_{40}H_{50}N_4O_8S$.

STORAGE

Store protected from light.

IMPURITIES

A. quinine,

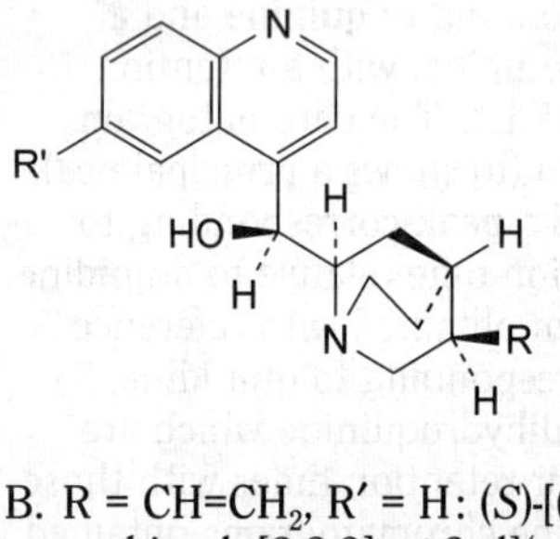

B. R = CH=CH$_2$, R′ = H: (*S*)-[(2*R*,4*S*,5*R*)-5-ethenyl-1-azabicyclo[2.2.2]oct-2-yl](quinolin-4-yl)methanol (cinchonine),

C. R = C$_2$H$_5$, R′ = OCH$_3$: (*S*)-[(2*R*,4*S*,5*R*)-5-ethyl-1-azabicyclo[2.2.2]oct-2-yl](6-methoxyquinolin-4-yl)methanol (dihydroquinidine).

01/2005:0018

QUININE HYDROCHLORIDE

Chinini hydrochloridum

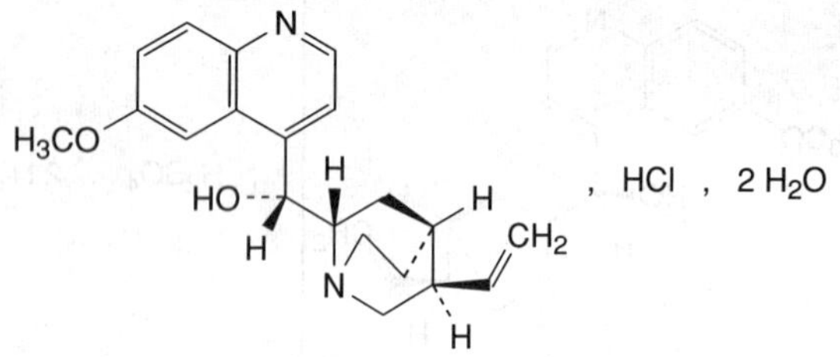

$C_{20}H_{25}ClN_2O_2,2H_2O$ M_r 396.9

DEFINITION

Quinine hydrochloride contains not less than 99.0 per cent and not more than the equivalent of 101.0 per cent of alkaloid monohydrochlorides, calculated as (*R*)-[(2*S*,4*S*,5*R*)-5-ethenyl-1-azabicyclo[2.2.2]oct-2-yl](6-methoxyquinolin-4-yl)methanol hydrochloride, with reference to the dried substance.

CHARACTERS

Fine, silky needles, often in clusters, colourless, soluble in water, freely soluble in alcohol.

IDENTIFICATION

A. Examine by thin-layer chromatography (*2.2.27*), using a *TLC silica gel G plate R.*

Test solution. Dissolve 0.10 g of the substance to be examined in *methanol R* and dilute to 10 ml with the same solvent.

Reference solution. Dissolve 0.10 g of *quinine sulphate CRS* in *methanol R* and dilute to 10 ml with the same solvent.

Apply separately to the plate 5 µl of each solution. Develop over a path of 15 cm using a mixture of 10 volumes of *diethylamine R,* 24 volumes of *ether R* and 40 volumes of *toluene R.* Dry the plate in a current of air for 15 min and repeat the development. Dry the plate at 105 °C for 30 min, allow to cool and spray with *iodoplatinate reagent R.* The principal spot in the chromatogram obtained with the test solution is similar in position, colour and size to the principal spot in the chromatogram obtained with the reference solution.

B. Dissolve about 10 mg in *water R* and dilute to 10 ml with the same solvent. To 5 ml of the solution add 0.2 ml of *bromine water R* and 1 ml of *dilute ammonia R2.* A green colour develops.

C. Dissolve 0.1 g in 3 ml of *dilute sulphuric acid R* and dilute to 100 ml with *water R.* When examined in ultraviolet light at 366 nm, an intense blue fluorescence appears which disappears almost completely on the addition of 1 ml of *hydrochloric acid R.*

D. It gives the reactions of chlorides (*2.3.1*).

E. It complies with the test for pH (see Tests).

TESTS

Solution S. Dissolve 1.0 g in *carbon dioxide-free water R* prepared from *distilled water R* and dilute to 50 ml with the same solvent.

Appearance of solution. Solution S is clear (*2.2.1*) and not more intensely coloured than reference solution Y_6 (*2.2.2, Method II*).

pH (*2.2.3*). Dilute 10 ml of solution S to 20 ml with *carbon dioxide-free water R*. The pH of the solution is 6.0 to 6.8.

Specific optical rotation (*2.2.7*). Dissolve 0.500 g in *0.1 M hydrochloric acid* and dilute to 25.0 ml with the same acid. The specific optical rotation is − 245 to − 258, calculated with reference to the dried substance.

Other cinchona alkaloids. Examine by liquid chromatography (*2.2.29*).

Test solution. Dissolve 20 mg of the substance to be examined, with gentle heating if necessary, in 5 ml of the mobile phase and dilute to 10 ml with the mobile phase.

Reference solution (a). Dissolve 20 mg of *quinine sulphate CRS*, with gentle heating if necessary, in 5 ml of the mobile phase and dilute to 10 ml with the mobile phase.

Reference solution (b). Dissolve 20 mg of *quinidine sulphate CRS*, with gentle heating if necessary, in 5 ml of the mobile phase and dilute to 10 ml with the mobile phase.

Reference solution (c). To 1 ml of reference solution (a) add 1 ml of reference solution (b).

Reference solution (d). Dilute 1.0 ml of reference solution (a) to 10.0 ml with the mobile phase. Dilute 1.0 ml of this solution to 50.0 ml with the mobile phase.

Reference solution (e). Dissolve 10 mg of *thiourea R* in the mobile phase and dilute to 10 ml with the mobile phase.

The chromatographic procedure may be carried out using:

– a stainless steel column 0.15 m to 0.25 m long and 4.6 mm in internal diameter packed with *octadecylsilyl silica gel for chromatography R* (5 µm or 10 µm),

– as mobile phase at a flow rate of 1.5 ml/min a mixture prepared as follows: dissolve 6.8 g of *potassium dihydrogen phosphate R* and 3.0 g of *hexylamine R* in 700 ml of *water R*, adjust to pH 2.8 with *dilute phosphoric acid R*, add 60 ml of *acetonitrile R* and dilute to 1000 ml with *water R*,

– as detector a spectrophotometer set at 250 nm for recording the chromatogram obtained with reference solution (e) and at 316 nm for the other solutions.

Inject 10 µl of reference solution (b) and 10 µl of reference solution (e). If necessary, adjust the concentration of acetonitrile in the mobile phase so that, in the chromatogram obtained with reference solution (b), the mass distribution factor of the peak corresponding to quinidine is 3.5 to 4.5, $t_{R'}$ being calculated from the peak corresponding to thiourea in the chromatogram obtained with reference solution (e).

Inject 10 µl each of reference solutions (a), (b), (c) and (d). The chromatogram obtained with reference solution (a) shows a principal peak corresponding to quinine and a peak corresponding to dihydroquinine, with a retention time relative to quinine of about 1.4. The chromatogram obtained with reference solution (b) shows a principal peak corresponding to quinidine and a peak corresponding to dihydroquinidine with a retention time relative to quinidine of about 1.5. The chromatogram obtained with reference solution (c) shows 4 peaks corresponding to quinidine, quinine, dihydroquinidine and dihydroquinine, which are identified by comparison of their retention times with those of the corresponding peaks in the chromatograms obtained with reference solutions (a) and (b).

The chromatographic system is not satisfactory unless in the chromatogram obtained with reference solution (c), the resolution between the peaks corresponding to quinine and quinidine is at least 3.0 and the resolution between the peaks corresponding to dihydroquinidine and quinine is at least 2.0 and the chromatogram obtained with reference solution (d) shows a principal peak with a signal-to-noise ratio of at least 4.

Inject 10 µl of the test solution. Record the chromatograms for 2.5 times the retention time of the principal peak. Calculate the percentage content of related substances from the areas of the peaks in the chromatogram obtained with the test solution by the normalisation procedure, ignoring any peaks with an area less than that of the peak in the chromatogram obtained with reference solution (d). The content of dihydroquinine is not greater than 10 per cent, the content of any related substance eluted before quinine is not greater than 5 per cent and the content of any other related substance is not greater than 2.5 per cent.

Sulphates (*2.4.13*). 15 ml of solution S complies with the limit test for sulphate (500 ppm).

Barium. To 15 ml of solution S add 1 ml of *dilute sulphuric acid R*. After at least 15 min, any opalescence in the solution is not more intense than that in a mixture of 15 ml of solution S and 1 ml of *distilled water R*.

Loss on drying (*2.2.32*). 6.0 per cent to 10.0 per cent, determined on 1.000 g by drying in an oven at 100 °C to 105 °C.

Sulphated ash (*2.4.14*). Not more than 0.1 per cent, determined on 1.0 g.

ASSAY

Dissolve 0.250 g in 50 ml of *alcohol R* and add 5.0 ml of *0.01 M hydrochloric acid*. Titrate with *0.1 M sodium hydroxide*, determining the end-point potentiometrically (*2.2.20*). Read the volume added between the 2 inflexion points.

1 ml of *0.1 M sodium hydroxide* is equivalent to 36.09 mg of $C_{20}H_{25}ClN_2O_2$

STORAGE

Store protected from light.

IMPURITIES

A. quinidine,

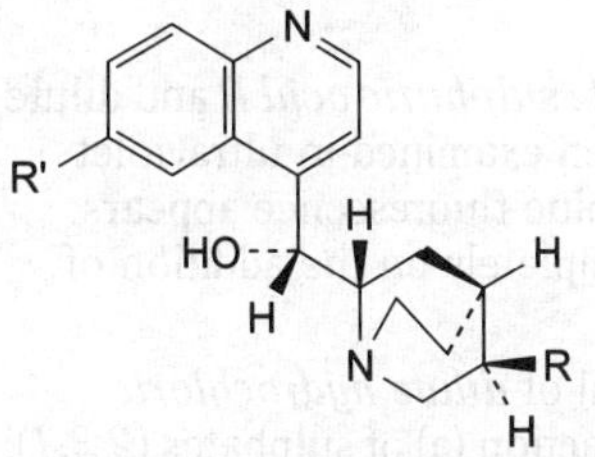

B. R = CH=CH$_2$, R′ = H: (*R*)-[(2*S*,4*S*,5*R*)-5-ethenyl-1-azabicyclo[2.2.2]oct-2-yl](quinolin-4-yl)methanol (cinchonidine),

C. R = C$_2$H$_5$, R′ = OCH$_3$: (*R*)-[(2*S*,4*S*,5*R*)-5-ethyl-1-azabicyclo[2.2.2]oct-2-yl](6-methoxyquinolin-4-yl)methanol (dihydroquinine).

01/2005:0019

QUININE SULPHATE

Chinini sulfas

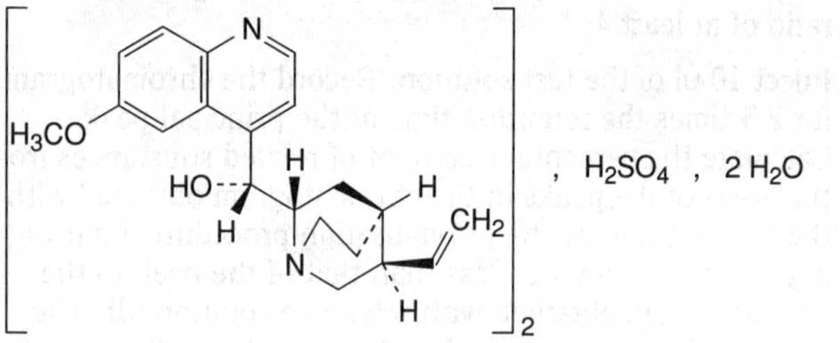

$C_{40}H_{50}N_4O_8S,2H_2O$ M_r 783

DEFINITION

Quinine sulphate contains not less than 99.0 per cent and not more than the equivalent of 101.0 per cent of alkaloid monosulphates, calculated as bis[(*R*)-[(2*S*,4*S*,5*R*)-5-ethenyl-1-azabicyclo[2.2.2]oct-2-yl](6-methoxyquinolin-4-yl)methanol] sulphate, with reference to the dried substance.

CHARACTERS

A white or almost white, crystalline powder or fine, colourless needles, slightly soluble in water, sparingly soluble in boiling water and in alcohol.

IDENTIFICATION

A. Examine by thin-layer chromatography (*2.2.27*), using a *TLC silica gel G plate R*.

Test solution. Dissolve 0.10 g of the substance to be examined in *methanol R* and dilute to 10 ml with the same solvent.

Reference solution. Dissolve 0.10 g of *quinine sulphate CRS* in *methanol R* and dilute to 10 ml with the same solvent.

Apply to the plate 5 µl of each solution. Develop over a path of 15 cm using a mixture of 10 volumes of *diethylamine R*, 24 volumes of *ether R* and 40 volumes of *toluene R*. Dry the plate in a current of air for 15 min and repeat the development. Dry the plate at 105 °C for 30 min, allow to cool and spray with *iodoplatinate reagent R*. The principal spot in the chromatogram obtained with the test solution is similar in position, colour and size to the principal spot in the chromatogram obtained with the reference solution.

B. Dissolve about 5 mg in 5 ml of *water R*. Add 0.2 ml of *bromine water R* and 1 ml of *dilute ammonia R2*. A green colour develops.

C. Dissolve 0.1 g in 3 ml of *dilute sulphuric acid R* and dilute to 100 ml with *water R*. When examined in ultraviolet light at 366 nm, an intense blue fluorescence appears which disappears almost completely on the addition of 1 ml of *hydrochloric acid R*.

D. Dissolve about 45 mg in 5 ml of *dilute hydrochloric acid R*. The solution gives reaction (a) of sulphates (*2.3.1*).

E. It complies with the test for pH (see Tests).

TESTS

Solution S. Dissolve 0.500 g in *0.1 M hydrochloric acid* and dilute to 25.0 ml with the same acid.

Appearance of solution. Solution S is clear (*2.2.1*) and not more intensely coloured than reference solution GY_6 (*2.2.2, Method II*).

pH (*2.2.3*). The pH of a 10 g/l suspension in *water R* is 5.7 to 6.6.

Specific optical rotation (*2.2.7*). − 237 to − 245, determined on solution S and calculated with reference to the dried substance.

Other cinchona alkaloids. Examine by liquid chromatography (*2.2.29*).

Test solution. Dissolve 20 mg of the substance to be examined, with gentle heating if necessary, in 5 ml of the mobile phase and dilute to 10 ml with the mobile phase.

Reference solution (a). Dissolve 20 mg of *quinine sulphate CRS*, with gentle heating if necessary, in 5 ml of the mobile phase and dilute to 10 ml with the mobile phase.

Reference solution (b). Dissolve 20 mg of *quinidine sulphate CRS*, with gentle heating if necessary, in 5 ml of the mobile phase and dilute to 10 ml with the mobile phase.

Reference solution (c). To 1 ml of reference solution (a) add 1 ml of reference solution (b).

Reference solution (d). Dilute 1.0 ml of reference solution (a) to 10.0 ml with the mobile phase. Dilute 1.0 ml of this solution to 50.0 ml with the mobile phase.

Reference solution (e). Dissolve 10 mg of *thiourea R* in the mobile phase and dilute to 10 ml with the mobile phase.

The chromatographic procedure may be carried out using:

– a stainless steel column 0.15 m to 0.25 m long and 4.6 mm in internal diameter packed with *octadecylsilyl silica gel for chromatography R* (5 µm or 10 µm),
– as mobile phase at a flow rate of 1.5 ml/min a mixture prepared as follows: dissolve 6.8 g of *potassium dihydrogen phosphate R* and 3.0 g of *hexylamine R* in 700 ml of *water R*, adjust to pH 2.8 with *dilute phosphoric acid R*, add 60 ml of *acetonitrile R* and dilute to 1000 ml with *water R*,
– as detector a spectrophotometer set at 250 nm for recording the chromatogram obtained with reference solution (e) and at 316 nm for the other solutions.

Inject 10 µl of reference solution (b) and 10 µl of reference solution (e). If necessary, adjust the concentration of acetonitrile in the mobile phase so that, in the chromatogram obtained with reference solution (b), the mass distribution factor of the peak corresponding to quinidine is 3.5 to 4.5, $t_{R'}$ being calculated from the peak corresponding to thiourea in the chromatogram obtained with reference solution (e).

Inject 10 µl each of reference solutions (a), (b), (c) and (d). The chromatogram obtained with reference solution (a) shows a principal peak corresponding to quinine and a peak, corresponding to dihydroquinine, with a retention time relative to quinine of about 1.4. The chromatogram obtained with reference solution (b) shows a principal peak corresponding to quinidine and a peak, corresponding to dihydroquinidine, with a retention time relative to quinidine of about 1.5. The chromatogram obtained with reference solution (c) shows 4 peaks corresponding to quinidine, quinine, dihydroquinidine and dihydroquinine which are identified by comparison of their retention times with those of the corresponding peaks in the chromatograms obtained with reference solutions (a) and (b).

The test is not valid unless: in the chromatogram obtained with reference solution (c), the resolution between the peaks corresponding to quinine and quinidine is at least 3.0 and the resolution between the peaks corresponding to dihydroquinidine and quinine is at least 2.0; and the chromatogram obtained with reference solution (d) shows a principal peak with a signal-to-noise ratio of at least 4.

Monographs Q-S

Inject 10 µl of the test solution. Record the chromatograms for 2.5 times the retention time of the principal peak. Calculate the percentage content of related substances from the areas of the peaks in the chromatogram obtained with the test solution by the normalisation procedure, disregarding any peaks with an area less than that of the peak in the chromatogram obtained with reference solution (d). The content of dihydroquinine is not greater than 10 per cent, the content of any related substance eluted before quinine is not greater than 5 per cent and the content of any other related substance is not greater than 2.5 per cent.

Loss on drying (*2.2.32*): 3.0 per cent to 5.0 per cent, determined on 1.000 g by drying in an oven at 100 °C to 105 °C.

Sulphated ash (*2.4.14*). Not more than 0.1 per cent, determined on 1.0 g.

ASSAY

Dissolve 0.300 g in a mixture of 10 ml of *chloroform R* and 20 ml of *acetic anhydride R*. Titrate with *0.1 M perchloric acid*, determining the end-point potentiometrically (*2.2.20*).

1 ml of *0.1 M perchloric acid* is equivalent to 24.90 mg of $C_{40}H_{50}N_4O_8S$.

STORAGE

Store protected from light.

IMPURITIES

A. quinidine,

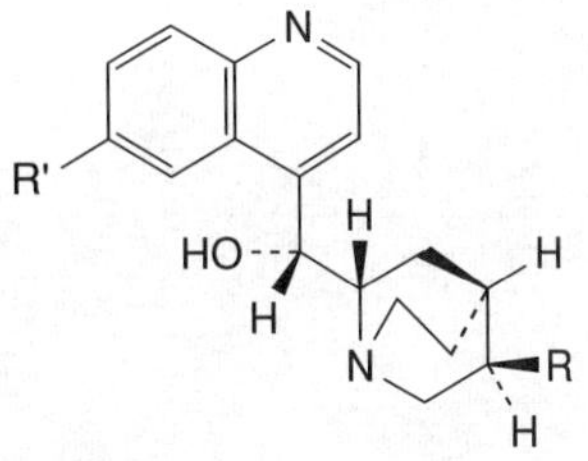

B. R = CH=CH_2, R′ = H: (*R*)-[(2*S*,4*S*,5*R*)-5-ethenyl-1-azabicyclo[2.2.2]oct-2-yl](quinolin-4-yl)methanol (cinchonidine),

C. R = C_2H_5, R′ = OCH_3: (*R*)-[(2*S*,4*S*,5*R*)-5-ethyl-1-azabicyclo[2.2.2]oct-2-yl](6-methoxyquinolin-4-yl)methanol (dihydroquinine).

R

01/2005:1368

RAMIPRIL

Ramiprilum

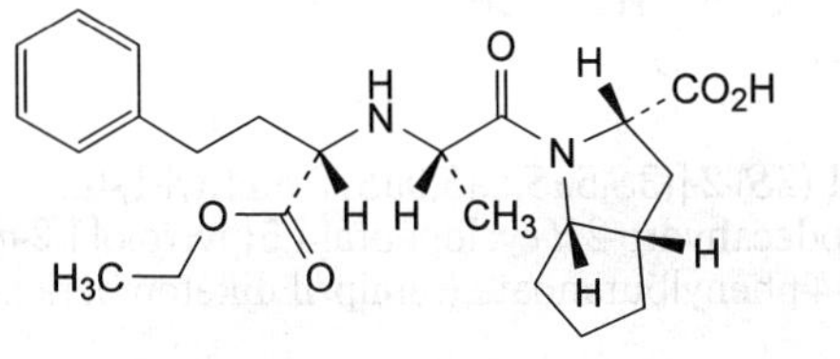

$C_{23}H_{32}N_2O_5$ M_r 416.5

DEFINITION

Ramipril contains not less than 98.0 per cent and not more than the equivalent of 101.0 per cent of (2*S*,3a*S*,6a*S*)-1-[(*S*)-2-[[(*S*)-1-(ethoxycarbonyl)-3-phenylpropyl]amino]propanoyl]octahydrocyclopenta[*b*]pyrrole-2-carboxylic acid, calculated with reference to the dried substance.

CHARACTERS

A white or almost white, crystalline powder, sparingly soluble in water, freely soluble in methanol.

IDENTIFICATION

A. It complies with the test for specific optical rotation (see Tests).

B. Examine by infrared absorption spectrophotometry (*2.2.24*), comparing with the spectrum obtained with *ramipril CRS*.

TESTS

Appearance of solution. Dissolve 0.1 g in *methanol R* and dilute to 10 ml with the same solvent. The solution is clear (*2.2.1*) and colourless (*2.2.2, Method II*).

Specific optical rotation (*2.2.7*). Dissolve 0.250 g in a mixture of 14 volumes of *hydrochloric acid R1* and 86 volumes of *methanol R* and dilute to 25.0 ml with the same mixture of solvents. The specific optical rotation is + 32.0 to + 38.0, calculated with reference to the dried substance.

Related substances. Examine by liquid chromatography (*2.2.29*).

Test solution. Dissolve 20.0 mg of the substance to be examined in mobile phase A and dilute to 20.0 ml with the same mobile phase.

Reference solution (a). Dissolve 5 mg each of *ramipril impurity A CRS, ramipril impurity B CRS, ramipril impurity C CRS* and *ramipril impurity D CRS* in 5 ml of the test solution and dilute to 10 ml with mobile phase B.

Reference solution (b). Dilute 5.0 ml of the test solution to 100.0 ml with mobile phase B. Dilute 5.0 ml of the solution to 50.0 ml with mobile phase B.

Reference solution (c). Dilute 1.0 ml of reference solution (b) to 10.0 ml with mobile phase B.

The chromatographic procedure may be carried out using:

– a stainless steel column 0.25 m long and 4.0 mm in internal diameter packed with *octadecylsilyl silica gel for chromatography R* (3 µm),

– as mobile phase at a flow rate of 1.0 ml/min:

Mobile phase A. Dissolve 2.0 g of *sodium perchlorate R* in a mixture of 0.5 ml of *triethylamine R* and 800 ml of *water R*; adjust to pH 3.6 with *phosphoric acid R* and add 200 ml of *acetonitrile R*,

Mobile phase B. Dissolve 2.0 g of *sodium perchlorate R* in a mixture of 0.5 ml of *triethylamine R* and 300 ml of *water R*; adjust to pH 2.6 with *phosphoric acid R* and add 700 ml of *acetonitrile R*,

Time (min)	Mobile phase A (per cent *V/V*)	Mobile phase B (per cent *V/V*)	Comment
0 - 6	90	10	isocratic
6 - 7	90 → 75	10 → 25	linear gradient
7 - 20	75 → 65	25 → 35	linear gradient
20 - 30	65 → 25	35 → 75	linear gradient
30 - 40	25	75	isocratique
40 - 45	25 → 90	75 → 10	linear gradient
45 - 55	90	10	re-equilibration

– as detector a spectrophotometer set at 210 nm,

maintaining the temperature of the column at 65 °C.

Equilibrate the column with a mixture of 90 per cent mobile phase A and 10 per cent mobile phase B for at least 35 min. If a suitable baseline cannot be obtained, use another grade of triethylamine.

Inject 10 µl of reference solution (c). Adjust the sensitivity of the system so that the chromatogram obtained shows a visible peak. Inject 10 µl of reference solution (a), 10 µl of reference solution (b) and 10 µl of the test solution. The test is not valid unless: in the chromatogram obtained with reference solution (a) the resolution between the peaks corresponding to ramipril impurity A and ramipril is at least 3.0; in the chromatogram obtained with reference solution (c) the principal peak has a signal-to-noise ratio of at least three; and in the chromatogram obtained with the test solution, the symmetry factor of the principal peak is 0.8 to 2.0.

When the chromatograms are recorded in the prescribed conditions, the retention times are: ramipril impurity A about 14 min, ramipril about 18 min, ramipril impurity B about 22 min, toluene about 24 min, ramipril impurity C about 26 min and ramipril impurity D about 28 min.

In the chromatogram obtained with the test solution, multiply the area of any peak corresponding to ramipril impurity C by a correction factor of 2.4.

In the chromatogram obtained with the test solution: the area of each peak corresponding to ramipril impurity A, ramipril impurity B, ramipril impurity C and ramipril impurity D is not greater than the area of the principal peak in the chromatogram obtained with reference solution (b) (0.5 per cent); the area of any peak, apart from the principal peak and any peak corresponding to the impurities A, B, C and D, is not greater than 0.2 times the area of the principal peak in the chromatogram obtained with reference solution (b) (0.1 per cent); the sum of the areas of all peaks, apart from the principal peak, is not greater than twice the area of the principal peak in the chromatogram obtained with reference solution (b) (1 per cent). Disregard any peak with an area less than that of the principal peak in the chromatogram obtained with reference solution (c).

Palladium. Not more than 20 ppm of Pd, determined by atomic absorption spectrometry (*2.2.23, Method I*).

Test solution. Dissolve 0.200 g of the substance to be examined in a mixture of 0.3 volumes of *nitric acid R* and 99.7 volumes of *water R* and dilute to 100.0 ml with the same mixture of solvents.

Monographs Q-S

Reference solutions. Use solutions containing 0.02 µg, 0.03 µg and 0.05 µg of palladium per millilitre, freshly prepared by dilution of *palladium standard solution (0.5 ppm Pd) R* with a mixture of 0.3 volumes of *nitric acid R* and 99.7 volumes of *water R*.

Modifier solution. Dissolve 0.150 g of *magnesium nitrate R* in a mixture of 0.3 volumes of *nitric acid R* and 99.7 volumes of *water R* and dilute to 100.0 ml with the same mixture of solvents.

Inject separately 20 µl of the test solution and 20 µl of the reference solution, and 10 µl of the modifier solution. Measure the absorbance at 247.6 nm using a palladium hollow-cathode lamp as a source of radiation, a transmission band of preferably 1 nm and a graphite tube.

Loss on drying (*2.2.32*). Not more than 0.2 per cent, determined on 1.000 g by drying in an oven under high vacuum at 60 °C for 4 h.

Sulphated ash (*2.4.14*). Not more than 0.1 per cent, determined on 1.0 g.

ASSAY

Dissolve 0.300 g in 25 ml of *methanol R* and add 25 ml of *water R*. Titrate with *0.1 M sodium hydroxide*, determining the end-point potentiometrically (*2.2.20*). Carry out a blank titration.

1 ml of *0.1 M sodium hydroxide* is equivalent to 41.65 mg of $C_{23}H_{32}N_2O_5$.

STORAGE

Store protected from light.

IMPURITIES

Specified impurities: A, B, C, D.

Other detectable impurities: E, F, G, H, I, J, K, L, M, N.

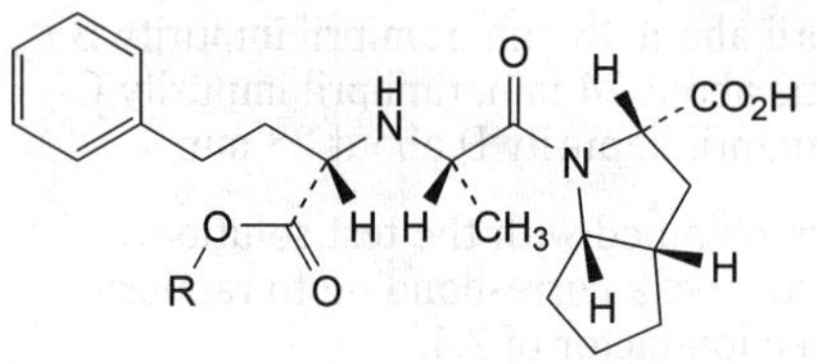

A. R = CH_3: (2*S*,3a*S*,6a*S*)-1-[(*S*)-2-[[(*S*)-1-(methoxycarbonyl)-3-phenylpropyl]amino]propanoyl]octahydrocyclopenta[*b*]pyrrole-2-carboxylic acid (ramipril methyl ester),

B. R = $CH(CH_3)_2$: (2*S*,3a*S*,6a*S*)-1-[(*S*)-2-[[(*S*)-1-[(1-methylethoxy)carbonyl]-3-phenylpropyl]amino]propanoyl]octahydrocyclopenta[*b*]pyrrole-2-carboxylic acid (ramipril isopropyl ester),

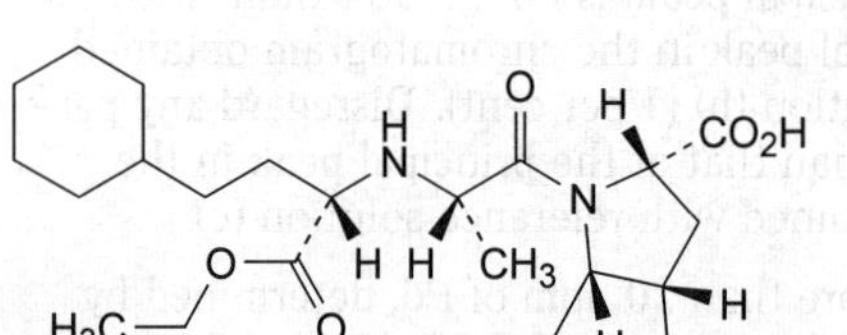

C. (2*S*,3a*S*,6a*S*)1-[(*S*)-2-[[(*S*)-3-cyclohexyl-1-(ethoxycarbonyl)propyl]amino]propanoyl]octahydrocyclopenta[*b*]pyrrole-2-carboxylic acid (hexahydroramipril),

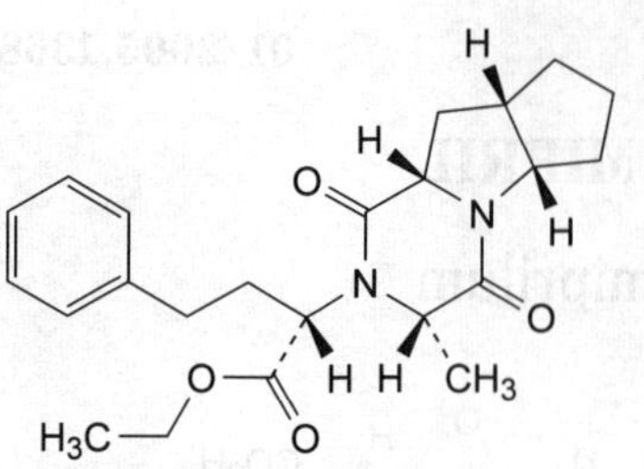

D. ethyl (2*S*)-2-[(3*S*,5a*S*,8a*S*,9a*S*)-3-methyl-1,4-dioxodecahydro-2*H*-cyclopenta[4,5]pyrrolo[1,2-*a*]pyrazin-2-yl]-4-phenylbutanoate (ramipril diketopiperazine),

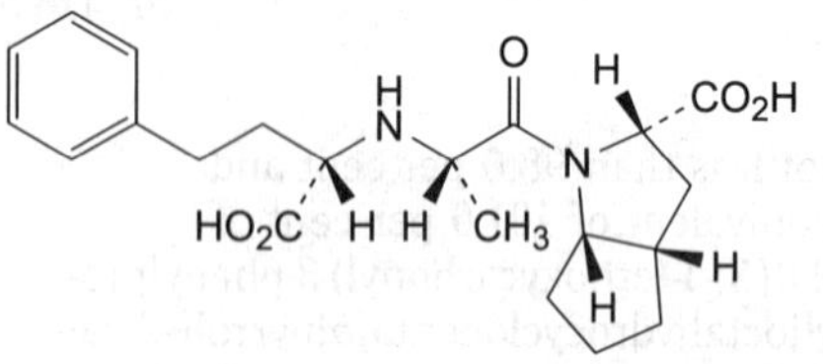

E. (2*S*,3a*S*,6a*S*)-1-[(*S*)-2-[[(*S*)-1-carboxy-3-phenylpropyl]amino]propanoyl]octahydrocyclopenta[*b*]pyrrole-2-carboxylic acid (ramipril diacid),

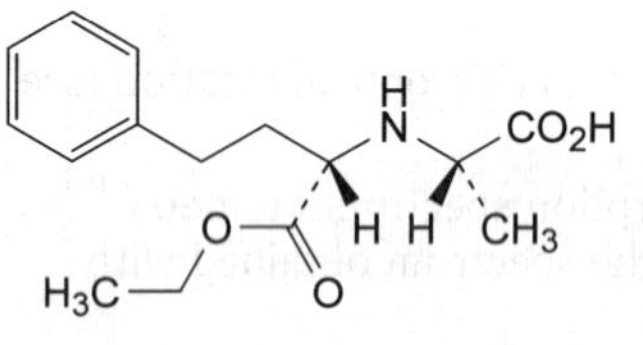

F. (*S*)-2-[[(*S*)-1-(ethoxycarbonyl)-3-phenylpropyl]amino]propanoic acid,

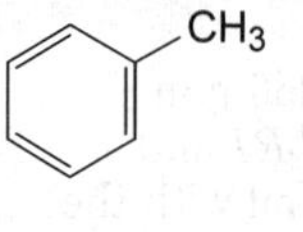

G. toluene,

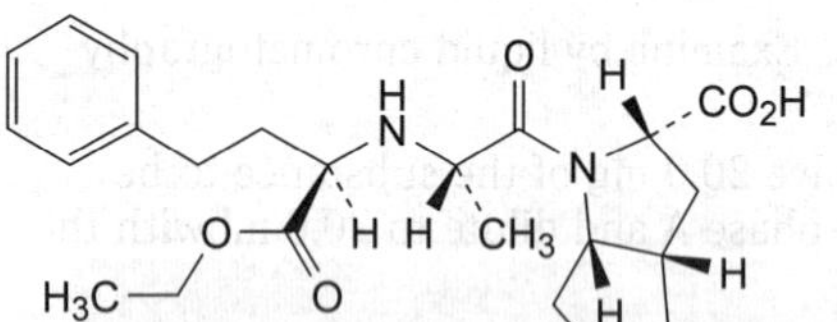

H. (2*S*,3a*S*,6a*S*)-1-[(*R*)-2-[[(*S*)-1-(ethoxycarbonyl)-3-phenylpropyl]amino]propanoyl]octahydrocyclopenta[*b*]pyrrole-2-carboxylic acid ((*R*,*S*-*S*,*S*,*S*) isomer of ramipril),

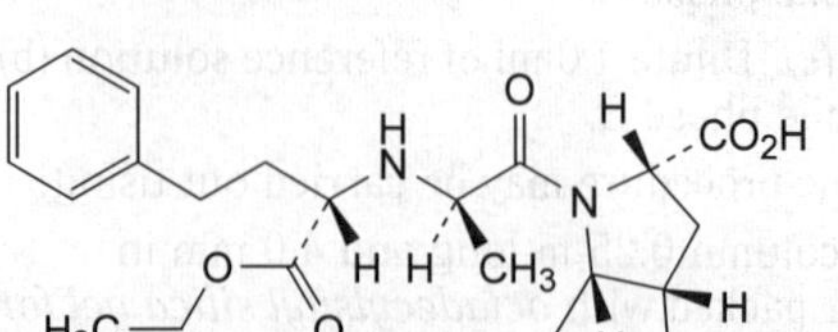

I. (2*S*,3a*S*,6a*S*)-1-[(*S*)-2-[[(*R*)-1-(ethoxycarbonyl)-3-phenylpropyl]amino]propanoyl]octahydrocyclopenta[*b*]pyrrole-2-carboxylic acid ((*S*,*R*-*S*,*S*,*S*) isomer of ramipril),

Monographs Q-S

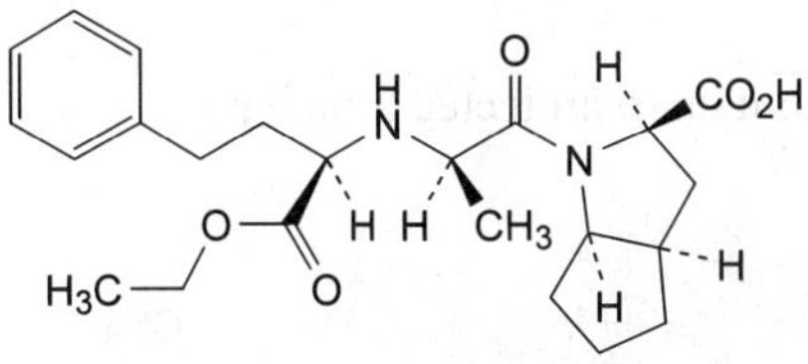

J. (2*R*,3a*R*,6a*R*)-1-[(*R*)-2-[[(*R*)-1-(ethoxycarbonyl)-3-phenylpropyl]amino]propanoyl]octahydrocyclopenta[*b*]pyrrole-2-carboxylic acid ((*R*,*R*-*R*,*R*,*R*) isomer of ramipril),

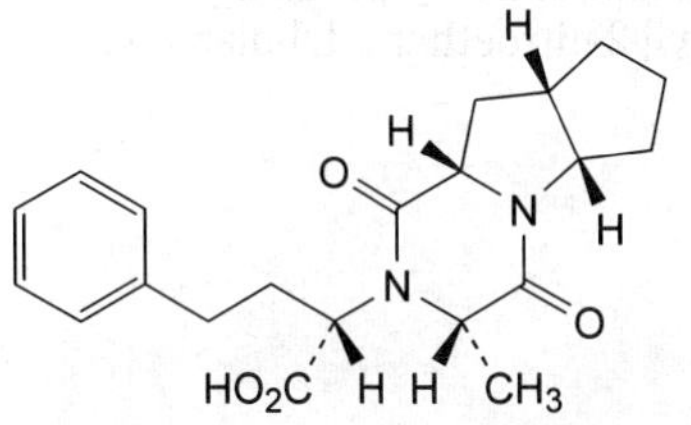

K. (2*S*)-2-[(3*S*,5a*S*,8a*S*,9a*S*)-3-methyl-1,4-dioxodecahydro-2*H*-cyclopenta[4,5]pyrrolo[1,2-*a*]pyrazin-2-yl]-4-phenylbutanoic acid (ramipril diketopiperazine acid),

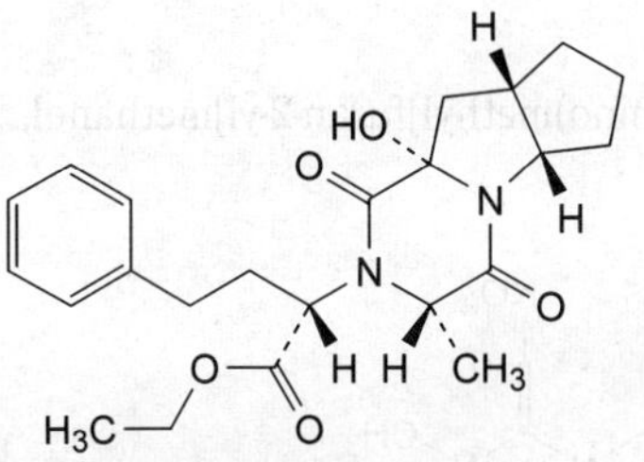

L. ethyl (2*S*)-2-[(3*S*,5a*S*,8a*S*,9a*S*)-9a-hydroxy-3-methyl-1,4-dioxodecahydro-2*H*-cyclopenta[4,5]pyrrolo[1,2-*a*]pyrazin-2-yl]-4-phenylbutanoate (ramipril hydroxydiketopiperazine),

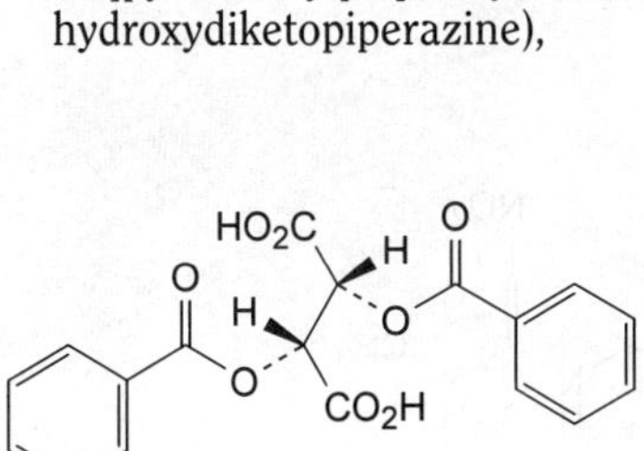

M. (2*R*,3*R*)-2,3-di(benzoyloxy)butanedioic acid (dibenzoyltartric acid),

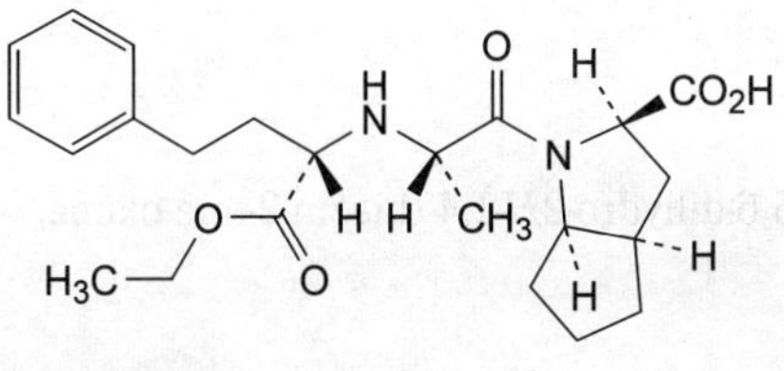

N. (2*R*,3a*R*,6a*R*)-1-[(*S*)-2-[[(*S*)-1-(ethoxycarbonyl)-3-phenylpropyl]amino]propanoyl]octahydrocyclopenta[*b*]pyrrole-2-carboxylic acid ((*S*,*S*-*R*,*R*,*R*) isomer of ramipril).

01/2005:0946

RANITIDINE HYDROCHLORIDE

Ranitidini hydrochloridum

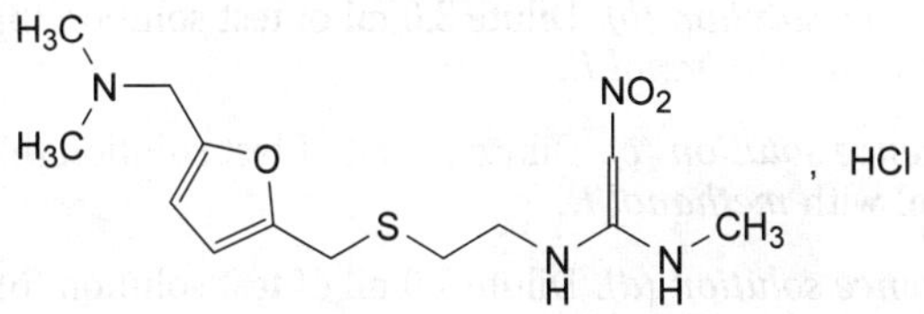

$C_{13}H_{23}ClN_4O_3S$ M_r 350.9

DEFINITION

Ranitidine hydrochloride contains not less than 98.5 per cent and not more than the equivalent of 101.0 per cent of *N*-[2-[[[5-[(dimethylamino)methyl]furan-2-yl]methyl]sulphanyl]ethyl]-*N'*-methyl-2-nitroethene-1,1-diamine hydrochloride, calculated with reference to the dried substance.

CHARACTERS

A white or pale yellow, crystalline powder, freely soluble in water and in methanol, sparingly soluble in ethanol, very slightly soluble in methylene chloride.

It shows polymorphism.

IDENTIFICATION

First identification: B, D.

Second identification: A, C, D.

A. Dissolve 10 mg in *water R* and dilute to 100.0 ml with the same solvent. Dilute 5.0 ml of the solution to 50.0 ml with *water R*. Examined between 220 nm and 360 nm (*2.2.25*), the solution shows two absorption maxima, at 229 nm and 315 nm. The ratio of the absorbance measured at the maximum at 229 nm to that measured at the maximum at 315 nm is 1.01 to 1.07.

B. Examine by infrared absorption spectrophotometry (*2.2.24*), comparing with the spectrum obtained with *ranitidine hydrochloride CRS*. Examine the substances as mulls in *liquid paraffin R*. If the spectra show differences, dissolve 20 mg of the substance to be examined and 20 mg of the reference substance separately in 5 ml of *methanol R*. Evaporate to dryness in a water-bath at 40 °C under reduced pressure and with constant stirring. Dry the residues under high vacuum at 60 °C for 1 h and record new spectra using the residues.

C. Examine the chromatograms obtained in the test for related substances (see Tests). The principal spot in the chromatogram obtained with test solution (b) is similar in position, colour and size to the principal spot in the chromatogram obtained with reference solution (a).

D. It gives reaction (a) of chlorides (*2.3.1*).

TESTS

Solution S. Dissolve 1.0 g in *carbon dioxide-free water R* and dilute to 100.0 ml with the same solvent.

Appearance of solution. Solution S is clear (*2.2.1*) and not more intensely coloured than reference solution BY_5 (*2.2.2, Method II*).

pH (*2.2.3*). The pH of solution S is 4.5 to 6.0.

Related substances. Examine by thin-layer chromatography (*2.2.27*), using *silica gel G R* as the coating substance.

Test solution (a). Dissolve 0.50 g of the substance to be examined in *methanol R* and dilute to 25 ml with the same solvent.

Test solution (b). Dilute 1 ml of test solution (a) to 10 ml with *methanol R.*

Reference solution (a). Dissolve 20 mg of *ranitidine hydrochloride CRS* in *methanol R* and dilute to 10 ml with the same solvent.

Reference solution (b). Dilute 3.0 ml of test solution (b) to 100 ml with *methanol R.*

Reference solution (c). Dilute 2.0 ml of test solution (b) to 100 ml with *methanol R.*

Reference solution (d). Dilute 1.0 ml of test solution (b) to 100 ml with *methanol R.*

Reference solution (e). Dilute 0.5 ml of test solution (b) to 100 ml with *methanol R.*

Reference solution (f). Dissolve 10 mg of *ranitidine impurity A CRS* in *methanol R* and dilute to 100 ml with the same solvent.

Reference solution (g). Dissolve 10 mg of *ranitidine impurity B CRS* in *methanol R* and dilute to 10 ml with the same solvent.

Reference solution (h). Dissolve 10 mg of *ranitidine impurity B CRS* in test solution (a) and dilute to 10 ml with the same solution.

Apply to the plate 10 µl of each solution. Develop over a path of 15 cm using a mixture of 2 volumes of *water R,* 4 volumes of *concentrated ammonia R1,* 15 volumes of *2-propanol R* and 25 volumes of *ethyl acetate R.* Allow the plate to dry in air and expose to iodine vapour until the spots are clearly visible. Examine in daylight. In the chromatogram obtained with test solution (a): any spot corresponding to ranitidine impurity A is not more intense than the spot in the chromatogram obtained with reference solution (f) (0.5 per cent); any spot apart from the principal spot and any spot corresponding to ranitidine impurity A is not more intense than the spot in the chromatogram obtained with reference solution (b) (0.3 per cent); at most three such spots are more intense than the spot in the chromatogram obtained with reference solution (d) (0.1 per cent) and at most one of these is more intense than the spot in the chromatogram obtained with reference solution (c) (0.2 per cent). The test is not valid unless the chromatogram obtained with reference solution (h) shows two clearly separated spots, corresponding to ranitidine impurity B (whose R_f value is obtained from the chromatogram obtained with reference solution (g)) and ranitidine, and the chromatogram obtained with reference solution (e) shows a clearly visible spot.

Heavy metals (*2.4.8*). 1.0 g complies with limit test C for heavy metals (20 ppm). Prepare the standard using 2 ml of *lead standard solution (10 ppm Pb) R.*

Loss on drying (*2.2.32*). Not more than 0.75 per cent, determined on 1.000 g by drying under high vacuum at 60 °C.

Sulphated ash (*2.4.14*). Not more than 0.1 per cent, determined on 1.0 g.

ASSAY

Dissolve 0.280 g in 35 ml of *water R.* Titrate with *0.1 M sodium hydroxide,* determining the end-point potentiometrically (*2.2.20*).

1 ml of *0.1 M sodium hydroxide* is equivalent to 35.09 mg of $C_{13}H_{23}ClN_4O_3S$.

STORAGE

Store in an airtight container, protected from light.

IMPURITIES

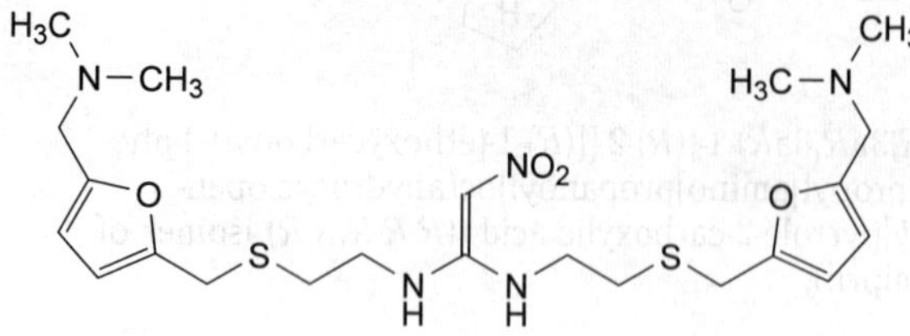

A. *N,N'*-bis[2-[[[5-[(dimethylamino)methyl]furan-2-yl]methyl]sulphanyl]ethyl]-2-nitroethene-1,1-diamine,

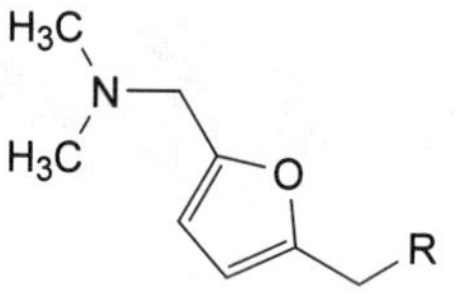

B. R = $S-CH_2-CH_2-NH_2$: 2-[[[5-[(dimethylamino)methyl]furan-2-yl]methyl]sulphanyl]ethanamine,

D. R = $S-CH_2-CH_2-NH-CO-CH_2-NO_2$: *N*-[2-[[[5-[(dimethylamino)methyl]furan-2-yl]methyl]sulphanyl]ethyl]-2-nitroacetamide,

F. R = OH: [5-[(dimethylamino)methyl]furan-2-yl]methanol,

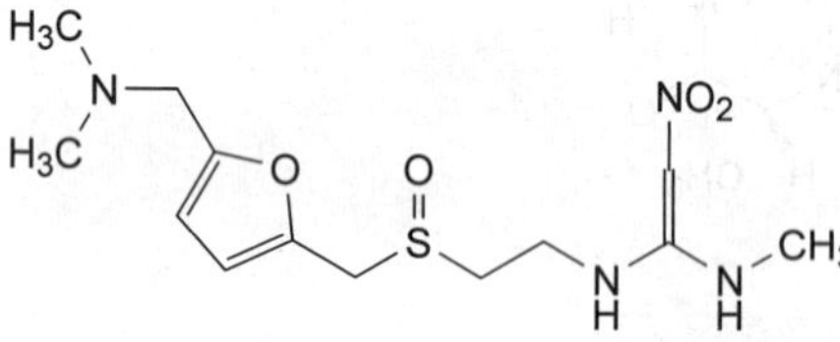

C. *N*-[2-[[[5-[(dimethylamino)methyl]furan-2-yl]methyl]sulphinyl]ethyl]-*N'*-methyl-2-nitroethene-1,1-diamine,

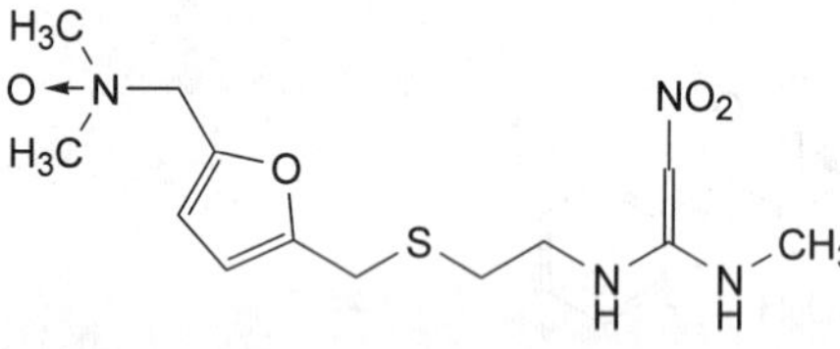

E. *N,N*-dimethyl[5-[[[2-[[1-(methylamino)-2-nitroethenyl]amino]ethyl]sulphanyl]methyl]furan-2-yl]methanamine *N*-oxide,

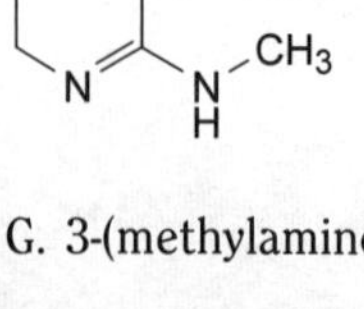

G. 3-(methylamino)-5,6-dihydro-2*H*-1,4-thiazin-2-one oxime,

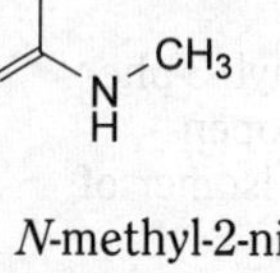

H. *N*-methyl-2-nitroacetamide.

01/2005:1369

RAPESEED OIL, REFINED

Rapae oleum raffinatum

DEFINITION

Refined rapeseed oil is the fatty oil obtained from the seeds of *Brassica napus* L. and *Brassica campestris* L. by mechanical expression or by extraction. It is then refined. A suitable antioxidant may be added.

CHARACTERS

A clear, light yellow liquid, practically insoluble in water and in alcohol, miscible with light petroleum (bp: 40 °C to 60 °C).

It has a relative density of about 0.917 and a refractive index of about 1.473.

IDENTIFICATION

Carry out the identification of fatty oils by thin-layer chromatography (*2.3.2*). The chromatogram obtained is similar to the typical chromatogram for rapeseed oil.

TESTS

Acid value (*2.5.1*). Not more than 0.5, determined on 10.0 g.

Peroxide value (*2.5.5*). Not more than 10.0.

Unsaponifiable matter (*2.5.7*). Not more than 1.5 per cent, determined on 5.0 g.

Alkaline impurities (*2.4.19*). It complies with the test for alkaline impurities in fatty oils.

Composition of fatty acids (*2.4.22, Method A*). The fatty acid fraction of the oil has the following composition:

- *palmitic acid*: 2.5 per cent to 6.0 per cent,
- *stearic acid*: not more than 3.0 per cent,
- *oleic acid*: 50.0 per cent to 67.0 per cent,
- *linoleic acid*: 16.0 per cent to 30.0 per cent,
- *linolenic acid*: 6.0 per cent to 14.0 per cent,
- *eicosenoic acid*: not more than 5.0 per cent,
- *erucic acid*: not more than 2.0 per cent.

STORAGE

Store in an airtight, well-filled container, protected from light.

LABELLING

The label states:

- the name and concentration of any added antioxidant,
- whether the oil is obtained by mechanical expression or by extraction.

01/2005:1881

RED POPPY PETALS

Papaveris rhoeados flos

DEFINITION

Dried, whole or fragmented petals of *Papaver rhoeas* L.

CHARACTERS

Macroscopic and microscopic characters described under identification tests A and B.

IDENTIFICATION

A. The petal is dark red to dark violet-brown, very thin, floppy, wrinkled, often crumpled into a ball and velvety to the touch. It is broadly ovate with an entire margin, about 6 cm long and 4 cm to 6 cm wide, narrowing at the base where there is a black spot. The vascular bundles radiate from the base and they anastomose in a continuous arc, all at the same short distance from the margin.

B. Reduce to a powder (355). Examine under a microscope using *chloral hydrate solution R*. The powder is an intense reddish-pink and shows fragments of epidermis composed of elongated, sinuous-walled cells with small, rounded, anomocytic stomata (*2.8.3*), numerous vascular bundles with spiral vessels embedded in the parenchyma; occasional fragments of the fibrous layer of the anthers; rounded pollen grains, about 30 µm in diameter, with 3 pores and a finely verrucose exine.

C. Thin-layer chromatography (*2.2.27*).

Test solution. To 1.0 g of the powdered drug (355) add 10 ml of *alcohol (60 per cent V/V) R*. Stir for 15 min. Filter through a filter paper.

Reference solution. Dissolve 1 mg of *quinaldine red R* and 1 mg of *sulphan blue R* in 2 ml of *methanol R*.

Plate: *TLC silica gel plate R.*

Mobile phase: *anhydrous formic acid R, water R, butanol R* (10:12:40 *V/V/V*).

Application: 10 µl, as bands.

Development: over a path of 10 cm.

Drying: in air.

Detection: examine in daylight.

Results: see below the sequence of zones present in the chromatograms obtained with the reference solution and the test solution. Furthermore, other bands may be present in the chromatogram obtained with the test solution.

Top of the plate	
	2 yellow zones
Quinaldine red: an orange-red zone	
_______	_______
	A violet principal zone A violet zone A yellow zone
Sulphan blue: a blue zone	
_______	_______
	A compact group of violet zones
Reference solution	**Test solution**

TESTS

Foreign matter (*2.8.2*): maximum 2.0 per cent of capsules and maximum 1.0 per cent of other foreign matter.

Loss on drying (*2.2.32*): maximum 12.0 per cent, determined on 1.000 g of the powdered drug (355) by drying in an oven at 100-105 °C for 2 h.

Total ash (*2.4.16*): maximum 11.0 per cent.

Colouring capacity. Place 1.0 g of the powdered drug (355) in a 250 ml flask and add 100 ml of *ethanol (30 per cent V/V) R*. Allow to macerate for 4 h with frequent stirring. Filter and discard the first 10 ml. Transfer 10.0 ml of the filtrate to a 100 ml volumetric flask and add 2 ml of *hydrochloric acid R*. Dilute to 100.0 ml with *ethanol (30 per*

Monographs Q-S

cent V/V) R. Allow to stand for 10 min. The absorbance (*2.2.25*) measured at 523 nm using *ethanol (30 per cent V/V) R* as compensation liquid is not less than 0.6.

01/2005:0528

RESERPINE

Reserpinum

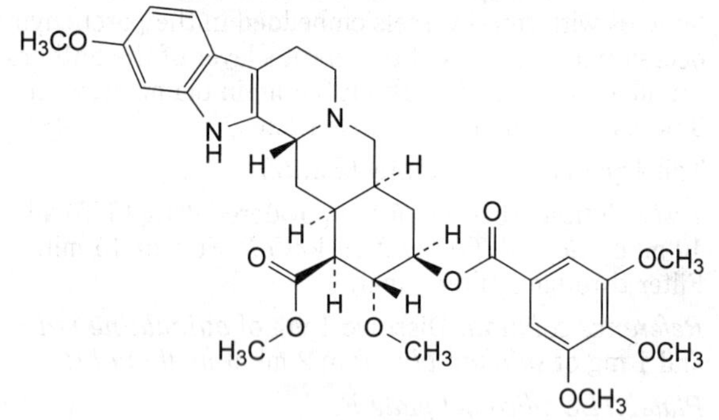

$C_{33}H_{40}N_2O_9$ M_r 609

DEFINITION

Reserpine contains not less than 99.0 per cent and not more than the equivalent of 101.0 per cent of total alkaloids and not less than 98.0 per cent and not more than the equivalent of 102.0 per cent of methyl 11,17α-dimethoxy-18β-[(3,4,5-trimethoxybenzoyl)oxy]-3β,20α-yohimban-16β-carboxylate, both calculated with reference to the dried substance.

CHARACTERS

A crystalline powder or small, white to slightly yellow crystals, darkening slowly on exposure to light, practically insoluble in water, very slightly soluble in alcohol.

IDENTIFICATION

First identification: B.

Second identification: A, C, D, E.

A. Dissolve 20.0 mg in *chloroform R* and dilute to 10.0 ml with the same solvent. Dilute 1.0 ml of this solution to 100.0 ml with *alcohol R*. Examined immediately between 230 nm and 350 nm (*2.2.25*), the solution shows a maximum at 268 nm. The specific absorbance at the maximum is 265 to 285. Over the range 288 nm to 295 nm, the curve shows a slight absorption minimum followed by a shoulder or a slight absorption maximum; over this range, the specific absorbance is about 170.

B. Examine by infrared absorption spectrophotometry (*2.2.24*), comparing with the spectrum obtained with *reserpine CRS*. Examine the substances prepared as discs.

C. To about 1 mg add 0.1 ml of a 1 g/l solution of *sodium molybdate R* in *sulphuric acid R*. A yellow colour is produced which becomes blue within 2 min.

D. To about 1 mg add 0.2 ml of a freshly prepared 10 g/l solution of *vanillin R* in *hydrochloric acid R*. A pink colour develops within 2 min.

E. Mix about 0.5 mg with 5 mg of *dimethylaminobenzaldehyde R* and 0.2 ml of *glacial acetic acid R* and add 0.2 ml of *sulphuric acid R*. A green colour is produced. Add 1 ml of *glacial acetic acid R*. The colour becomes red.

TESTS

Specific optical rotation (*2.2.7*). *Carry out the determination immediately after preparing the solution.* Dissolve 0.250 g in *chloroform R* and dilute to 25.0 ml with the same solvent. The specific optical rotation is − 116 to − 128, calculated with reference to the dried substance.

Oxidation products. Dissolve 20 mg in *glacial acetic acid R* and dilute to 100.0 ml with the same acid. The absorbance (*2.2.25*) measured immediately at 388 nm is not greater than 0.10.

Loss on drying (*2.2.32*). Not more than 0.5 per cent, determined on 0.500 g by drying at 60 °C over *diphosphorus pentoxide R* at a pressure not exceeding 667 Pa for 3 h.

Sulphated ash (*2.4.14*). Not more than 0.1 per cent, determined on 0.5 g.

ASSAY

Total alkaloids. Dissolve 0.500 g in a mixture of 6 ml of *acetic anhydride R* and 40 ml of *anhydrous acetic acid R*. Titrate with *0.1 M perchloric acid*, determining the end-point potentiometrically (*2.2.20*).

1 ml of *0.1 M perchloric acid* is equivalent to 60.9 mg of total alkaloids.

Reserpine. *Protect the solutions from light.* Moisten 25.0 mg with 2 ml of *alcohol R*, add 2 ml of *0.25 M sulphuric acid* and 10 ml of *alcohol R*, and warm gently to effect solution. Cool and dilute to 100.0 ml with *alcohol R*. Dilute 5.0 ml of this solution to 50.0 ml with *alcohol R*. Prepare a reference solution in the same manner using 25.0 mg of *reserpine CRS*. Place 10.0 ml of each solution separately in two boiling-tubes, add 2.0 ml of *0.25 M sulphuric acid* and 2.0 ml of a freshly prepared 3 g/l solution of *sodium nitrite R*. Mix and heat in a water-bath at 55 °C for 35 min. Cool, add 1.0 ml of a freshly prepared 50 g/l solution of *sulphamic acid R* and dilute to 25.0 ml with *alcohol R*. Measure the absorbance (*2.2.25*) of each solution at the maximum at 388 nm, using as the compensation liquid 10.0 ml of the same solution treated at the same time in the same manner, but omitting the sodium nitrite.
Calculate the content of $C_{33}H_{40}N_2O_9$ from the absorbances measured and the concentrations of the solutions.

STORAGE

Store protected from light.

01/2005:0290

RESORCINOL

Resorcinolum

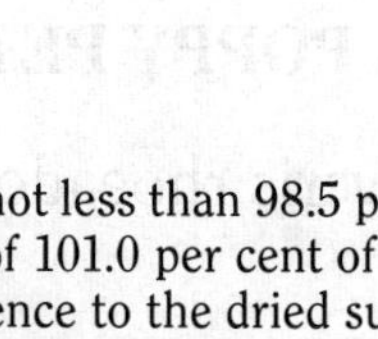

$C_6H_6O_2$ M_r 110.1

DEFINITION

Resorcinol contains not less than 98.5 per cent and not more than the equivalent of 101.0 per cent of benzene-1,3-diol, calculated with reference to the dried substance.

CHARACTERS

A colourless or slightly pinkish-grey, crystalline powder or crystals, turning red on exposure to light and air, very soluble in water and in alcohol.

IDENTIFICATION

A. Melting point (*2.2.14*): 109 °C to 112 °C.

B. Dissolve 0.1 g in 1 ml of *water R*, add 1 ml of *strong sodium hydroxide solution R* and 0.1 ml of *chloroform R*, heat and allow to cool. An intense, deep-red colour develops which becomes pale yellow on the addition of a slight excess of *hydrochloric acid R*.

C. Thoroughly mix about 10 mg with about 10 mg of *potassium hydrogen phthalate R*, both finely powdered. Heat over a naked flame until an orange-yellow colour is obtained. Cool and add 1 ml of *dilute sodium hydroxide solution R* and 10 ml of *water R* and shake to dissolve. The solution shows an intense green fluorescence.

TESTS

Solution S. Dissolve 2.5 g in *carbon dioxide-free water R* and dilute to 25 ml with the same solvent.

Appearance of solution. Solution S is clear (*2.2.1*) and not more intensely coloured than reference solution B_5 or R_5 (*2.2.2, Method II*) and remains so when heated in a water-bath for 5 min.

Acidity or alkalinity. To 10 ml of solution S add 0.05 ml of *bromophenol blue solution R2*. Not more than 0.05 ml of *0.1 M hydrochloric acid* or *0.1 M sodium hydroxide* is required to change the colour of the indicator.

Related substances. Examine by thin-layer chromatography (*2.2.27*), using *silica gel G R* as the coating substance.

Test solution. Dissolve 0.5 g of the substance to be examined in *methanol R* and dilute to 10 ml with the same solvent.

Reference solution. Dilute 0.1 ml of the test solution to 20 ml with *methanol R*.

Apply separately to the plate 2 µl of each solution. Develop over a path of 15 cm using a mixture of 40 volumes of *ethyl acetate R* and 60 volumes of *hexane R*. Allow the plate to dry in air for 15 min and expose it to iodine vapour. Any spot in the chromatogram obtained with the test solution, apart from the principal spot, is not more intense than the spot in the chromatogram obtained with the reference solution (0.5 per cent).

Pyrocatechol. To 2 ml of solution S add 1 ml of *ammonium molybdate solution R2* and mix. Any yellow colour in the solution is not more intense than that in a standard prepared at the same time in the same manner using 2 ml of a 0.1 g/l solution of *pyrocatechol R*.

Loss on drying (*2.2.32*). Not more than 1.0 per cent, determined on 1.00 g of powdered substance by drying in a desiccator for 4 h.

Sulphated ash (*2.4.14*). Not more than 0.1 per cent, determined on 1.0 g.

ASSAY

Dissolve 0.500 g in *water R* and dilute to 250.0 ml with the same solvent. To 25.0 ml of the solution in a ground-glass-stoppered flask add 1.0 g of *potassium bromide R*, 50.0 ml of *0.0167 M potassium bromate*, 15 ml of *chloroform R* and 15.0 ml of *hydrochloric acid R1*. Stopper the flask, shake and allow to stand in the dark for 15 min, shaking occasionally. Add 10 ml of a 100 g/l solution of *potassium iodide R*, shake thoroughly, allow to stand for 5 min and titrate with *0.1 M sodium thiosulphate*, using 1 ml of *starch solution R* as indicator.

1 ml of *0.0167 M potassium bromate* is equivalent to 1.835 mg of $C_6H_6O_2$.

STORAGE

Store protected from light.

01/2005:1879

RESTHARROW ROOT

Ononidis radix

DEFINITION

Whole or cut, dried root of *Ononis spinosa* L.

CHARACTERS

Macroscopic and microscopic characters described under identification tests A and B.

IDENTIFICATION

A. The root is more or less flattened, twisted and branched, deeply wrinkled, brown in colour and grooved longitudinally. The transversely cut surface shows a thin bark and a xylem cylinder with a conspicuously radiate structure. The fracture of the root is short and fibrous.

B. Reduce to a powder (355). The powder is light brown or brown. Examine under a microscope using *chloral hydrate solution R*. The powder shows brown fragments of cork composed of thin-walled polygonal cells; groups of thick-walled narrow fibres, often accompanied by a parenchymatous crystal sheath containing prisms of calcium oxalate; fragments of vessels with numerous small bordered pits; parenchymatous cells with single prisms of calcium oxalate. Examine under a microscope using a mixture of equal volumes of *glycerol R* and *water R*. The powder shows numerous simple, round starch granules, 5 µm to 10 µm in diameter.

C. Thin-layer chromatography (*2.2.27*).

Test solution. To 1.0 g of the powdered drug (180) add 15.0 ml of *methanol R* and boil under a reflux condenser for 30 min. Cool and filter.

Reference solution. Dissolve 10 mg of *resorcinol R* and 50 mg of *vanillin R* in 10 ml of *methanol R*.

Plate: *TLC silica gel F_{254} plate R.*

Mobile phase: *alcohol R, methylene chloride R, toluene R (10:45:45 V/V/V).*

Application: 20 µl, as bands.

Development: over a path of 15 cm.

Drying: in air.

Detection A: examine in ultraviolet light at 254 nm and 365 nm.

Results A: see below the sequence of the zones present in the chromatograms obtained with the reference solution and the test solution. Furthermore, other fluorescent zones are present in the middle third of the chromatogram obtained with the test solution.

Top of the plate	
Vanillin: a zone visible at 254 nm	
_______	_______
Resorcinol: a zone visible at 254 nm	An intense blue fluorescent zone visible at 365 nm
_______	_______
Reference solution	**Test solution**

Detection B: spray with *anisaldehyde solution R*. Heat at 100-105 °C for 5-10 min. Examine in daylight.

Monographs Q-S

Results B: see below the sequence of the zones present in the chromatograms obtained with the reference solution and the test solution.

Top of the plate	
Vanillin: a greyish-violet zone	
	A violet zone (onocol)
Resorcinol: a red zone	
Reference solution	**Test solution**

TESTS

Extractable matter: minimum 15.0 per cent.

To 2.00 g of the powdered drug (250) add a mixture of 8 g of *water R* and 12 g of *alcohol R* and allow to macerate for 2 h, shaking frequently. Filter, evaporate 5 g of the filtrate to dryness on a water-bath and dry at 100-105 °C for 2 h. The residue weighs a minimum of 75 mg.

Foreign matter (*2.8.2*). It complies with the test for foreign matter.

Loss on drying (*2.2.32*): maximum 10.0 per cent, determined on 1.000 g of the powdered drug (355) by drying in an oven at 100-105 °C for 2 h.

Total ash (*2.4.16*): maximum 8.0 per cent.

01/2005:0289

RHATANY ROOT

Ratanhiae radix

DEFINITION

Rhatany root, known as Peruvian rhatany, consists of the dried, usually fragmented, underground organs of *Krameria triandra* Ruiz and Pavon. It contains not less than 5.0 per cent of tannins, expressed as pyrogallol ($C_6H_6O_3$; M_r 126.1), calculated with reference to the dried drug.

CHARACTERS

It has the macroscopic and microscopic characters described under identification tests A and B.

IDENTIFICATION

A. The taproot is dark red-brown and has a thick, knotty crown. The secondary roots are the same colour and nearly straight or somewhat tortuous. The bark is rugged to scaly in the older pieces and smooth with sharp, transverse fissures in the younger pieces; it separates readily from the wood. The fracture is fibrous in the bark and splintery in the wood. The smooth, transversely cut surface shows a dark brown-red bark about one third of the radius in thickness; a dense, pale red-brown and finely porous wood is present with numerous fine medullary rays; the central heartwood is often darker.

B. Reduce to a powder (355). The powder is brown-red. Examine under a microscope using *chloral hydrate solution R*. The powder shows cork cells containing dark brown phlobaphenes; fragments of unlignified phloem fibres, usually 12 µm to 30 µm in diameter with moderately thick walls; phloem parenchyma cells in files containing prisms and microcrystals of calcium oxalate; fragments of vessels usually 20 µm to 60 µm in diameter with bordered pits; fragments of tracheids up to 20 µm wide with slit-shaped pits. Examine under a microscope using a 50 per cent *V/V* solution of *glycerol R*. The powder shows rounded starch granules, simple or two- to four-compound, an individual granule measuring up to 30 µm in diameter and some granules being found in the cells of the medullary rays and in the parenchyma.

C. Examine by thin-layer chromatography (*2.2.27*), using a *TLC silica gel plate R*.

Test solution. To 1.0 g of the powdered drug (355) add 10 ml of a mixture of 3 volumes of *water R* and 7 volumes of *alcohol R*, shake for 10 min and filter. To the filtrate add 10 ml of *light petroleum R* and shake. Separate the light petroleum layer, add 2 g of *anhydrous sodium sulphate R*, shake and filter. Evaporate the filtrate to dryness. Dissolve the residue in 0.5 ml of *methanol R*.

Reference solution. Dissolve 5.0 mg of *Sudan red G R* in 10 ml of *methanol R*.

Apply to the plate as bands 10 µl of each solution. Develop over a path of 15 cm using a mixture of 2 volumes of *ethyl acetate R* and 98 volumes of *toluene R*. Allow the plate to dry in air and spray the plate with a 5 g/l solution of *fast blue B salt R*. Allow the plate to dry in air and spray the plate with *0.1 M ethanolic sodium hydroxide*. Examine in daylight. The chromatogram obtained with the reference solution shows in the lower third a red zone due to Sudan red G. The chromatogram obtained with the test solution shows a violet zone due to rhatany phenol I similar in position to the zone of Sudan red G in the chromatogram obtained with the reference solution, below it the brownish zone due to rhatany phenol II and below it the bluish-grey zone due to rhatany phenol III. Further zones may be present.

TESTS

Foreign matter (*2.8.2*). Not more than 2 per cent of foreign matter and not more than 5 per cent of fragments of crown or root exceeding 25 mm in diameter. Root without bark may be present in very small quantities.

Loss on drying (*2.2.32*). Not more than 12.0 per cent, determined on 1.000 g of the powdered drug (355) by drying in an oven at 100 °C to 105 °C.

Total ash (*2.4.16*). Not more than 5.5 per cent.

ASSAY

Carry out the determination of tannins in herbal drugs (*2.8.14*). Use 0.750 g of powdered drug (180).

STORAGE

Store protected from light.

01/2005:1888

RHATANY TINCTURE

Ratanhiae tinctura

DEFINITION

Tincture produced from *Rhatany root (0289)*.

Content: minimum 1.0 per cent *m/m* of tannins, expressed as pyrogallol ($C_6H_6O_3$; M_r 126.1).

PRODUCTION

The tincture is produced from 1 part of the drug and 5 parts of ethanol (70 per cent *V/V*) by a suitable procedure.

CHARACTERS

Appearance: reddish-brown liquid.

IDENTIFICATION

Thin-layer chromatography (*2.2.27*).

Test solution. To 5 ml of the tincture to be examined, add 10 ml of *light petroleum R* and shake. Separate the light petroleum layer, add 2 g of *anhydrous sodium sulphate R*, shake and filter. Evaporate the filtrate to dryness. Dissolve the residue in 0.5 ml of *methylene chloride R.*

Reference solution. Dissolve 5 mg of *thymol R* and 10 mg of *dichlorophenolindophenol, sodium salt R* in 10 ml of *alcohol (60 per cent V/V) R.*

Plate: *TLC silica gel plate R.*

Mobile phase: *methylene chloride R.*

Application: 10 µl, as bands.

Development: over a path of 10 cm.

Drying: in air.

Detection: spray with a 5 g/l solution of *fast blue B salt R*; allow the plate to dry in air and spray with *0.1 M ethanolic sodium hydroxide*; examine in daylight.

Results: see below the sequence of the zones present in the chromatograms obtained with the reference solution and the test solution. Furthermore, other zones may be present in the chromatogram obtained with the test solution.

Top of the plate	
_______	_______
Thymol: an orange brownish-yellow zone	A violet zone
_______	_______
	A greenish-grey zone
	A bluish-grey zone
	A yellowish-brown zone
Dichlorophenolindophenol: a greyish-blue zone	A violet zone
Reference solution	**Test solution**

TESTS

Ethanol (*2.9.10*): 63 per cent *V/V* to 67 per cent *V/V*.

Methanol and 2-propanol (*2.9.11*): maximum 0.05 per cent *V/V* of methanol and maximum 0.05 per cent *V/V* of 2-propanol.

ASSAY

Carry out the determination of tannins in herbal drugs (*2.8.14*) using 2.500 g of the tincture to be examined.

01/2005:0291

RHUBARB

Rhei radix

DEFINITION

Rhubarb consists of the whole or cut, dried underground parts of *Rheum palmatum* L. or of *Rheum officinale* Baillon or of hybrids of these two species or of a mixture. The underground parts are often divided; the stem and most of the bark with the rootlets are removed. It contains not less than 2.2 per cent of hydroxyanthracene derivatives, expressed as rhein ($C_{15}H_8O_6$, M_r 284.2), calculated with reference to the dried drug.

CHARACTERS

Rhubarb has a characteristic, aromatic odour.

It has the macroscopic and microscopic characters described under identification tests A and B.

IDENTIFICATION

A. The appearance is variable: disc-shaped pieces up to 10 cm in diameter and 1 cm to 5 cm in thickness; cylindrical pieces; oval or planoconvex pieces. The surface has a pinkish tinge and is usually covered with a layer of brownish-yellow powder. It shows, especially after moistening, a reticulum of darker lines. This structure causes the marbled appearance of the drug. The fracture is granular. The transverse section of the rhizome shows a narrow outer zone of radiating brownish-red lines. These medullary rays are crossed perpendicularly by a dark cambial ring. Inside this zone is a ring of small star-spot formations of anomalous vascular bundles. The root shows a more radiate structure.

B. Reduce to a powder (355). The powder is orange to brownish-yellow. Examine under a microscope using *chloral hydrate solution R*. The powder shows the following diagnostic characters: large calcium oxalate cluster crystals, which may measure more than 100 µm, and their fragments; reticulately thickened non-lignified vessels measuring up to 175 µm. Numerous groups of rounded or polygonal, thin-walled parenchyma cells. Sclereids and fibres are absent. Examine under a microscope using a 50 per cent *V/V* solution of *glycerol R*. The powder shows simple, rounded or compound (2 to 4) starch granules with a star-shaped hilum.

C. Examine by thin-layer chromatography (*2.2.27*), using a suitable silica gel as the coating substance.

Test solution. Heat 50 mg of the powdered drug (180) in a water-bath for 15 min with a mixture of 1 ml of *hydrochloric acid R* and 30 ml of *water R.* Allow to cool and shake the liquid with 25 ml of *ether R.* Dry the ether layer over *anhydrous sodium sulphate R* and filter. Evaporate the ether layer to dryness and dissolve the residue in 0.5 ml of *ether R.*

Reference solution. Dissolve 5 mg of *emodin R* in 5 ml of *ether R.*

Apply separately to the plate as bands 20 µl of each solution. Develop over a path of 10 cm using a mixture of 1 volume of *anhydrous formic acid R*, 25 volumes of *ethyl acetate R* and 75 volumes of *light petroleum R.* Allow the plate to dry in air and examine in ultraviolet light at 365 nm. The chromatogram obtained with the reference solution shows in its central part a zone of orange fluorescence (emodin). The chromatogram obtained with the test solution shows: a zone due to emodin; above the emodin zone, two zones of similar fluorescence (physcione and chrysophanol, in order of increasing R_f value); below the emodin zone, also two zones of similar fluorescence (rhein and aloe-emodin, in order of decreasing R_f value). Spray with a 100 g/l solution of *potassium hydroxide R* in *methanol R.* All the zones become red to violet.

D. To about 50 mg of the powdered drug (180) add 25 ml of *dilute hydrochloric acid R* and heat the mixture on a water-bath for 15 min. Allow to cool, shake with 20 ml of *ether R* and discard the aqueous layer. Shake the ether layer with 10 ml of *dilute ammonia R1.* The aqueous layer becomes red to violet.

TESTS

Rheum rhaponticum. Examine by thin-layer chromatography (*2.2.27*), using *silica gel G R* as the coating substance.

Test solution. To 0.2 g of the powdered drug (180) add 2 ml of *methanol R* and boil for 5 min under a reflux condenser. Allow to cool and filter. Use the filtrate as the test solution.

Reference solution. Dissolve 10 mg of *rhaponticin R* in 10 ml of *methanol R*.

Apply separately to the plate, as bands not more than 20 mm by 3 mm, 20 µl of each solution. Develop over a path of 12 cm using a mixture of 20 volumes of *methanol R* and 80 volumes of *methylene chloride R*. Allow the plate to dry in air and spray with *phosphomolybdic acid solution R*. The chromatogram obtained with the test solution does not show a blue zone near the starting-line (rhaponticin) corresponding to the zone in the chromatogram obtained with the reference solution.

Foreign matter (*2.8.2*). It complies with the test for foreign matter.

Loss on drying (*2.2.32*). Not more than 12.0 per cent, determined on 1.000 g of the powdered drug (180) by drying in an oven at 100 °C to 105 °C.

Total ash (*2.4.16*). Not more than 12.0 per cent.

Ash insoluble in hydrochloric acid (*2.8.1*). Not more than 2.0 per cent.

ASSAY

Carry out the assay protected from bright light.

Introduce 0.100 g of the powdered drug (180) into a 100 ml flask. Add 30.0 ml of *water R*, mix and weigh. Heat in a water-bath under a reflux condenser for 15 min. Allow to cool, add 50 mg of *sodium hydrogen carbonate R*, weigh and adjust to the original mass with *water R*. Centrifuge and transfer 10.0 ml of the liquid to a 100 ml round-bottomed flask with a ground-glass neck. Add 20 ml of *ferric chloride solution R1* and mix. Heat under a reflux condenser on a water-bath for 20 min, add 1 ml of *hydrochloric acid R* and heat for a further 20 min, shaking frequently. Cool, transfer to a separating funnel and shake with three quantities, each of 25 ml, of *ether R* previously used to rinse the flask. Combine the ether extracts and wash with two quantities, each of 15 ml, of *water R*. Filter the ether extracts through a plug of absorbent cotton into a volumetric flask and dilute to 100.0 ml with *ether R*. Evaporate 10.0 ml carefully to dryness on a water-bath and dissolve the residue in 10.0 ml of a 5 g/l solution of *magnesium acetate R* in *methanol R*. Measure the absorbance (*2.2.25*) at 515 nm, using *methanol R* as the compensation liquid.

Calculate the percentage content of rhein from the expression:

$$\frac{A \times 0.64}{m}$$

i.e. taking the specific absorbance of rhein to be 468, calculated on the basis of the specific absorbance of barbaloin.

A = absorbance at 515 nm,

m = mass of the drug used, in grams.

STORAGE

Store protected from light.

01/2005:2109

RIBAVIRIN

Ribavirinum

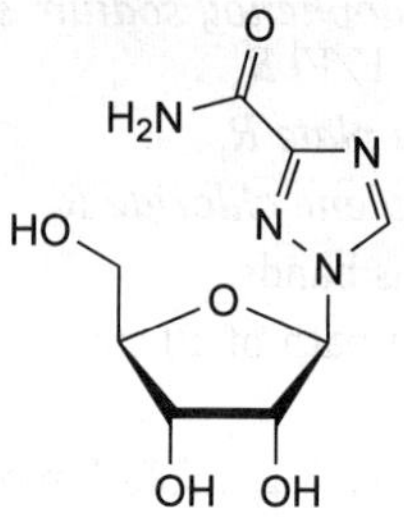

$C_8H_{12}N_4O_5$ M_r 244.2

DEFINITION

1-β-D-Ribofuranosyl-1*H*-1,2,4-triazole-3-carboxamide.

Content: 98.0 per cent to 102.0 per cent (dried substance).

CHARACTERS

Appearance: white or almost white, crystalline powder.

Solubility: freely soluble in water, slightly soluble in ethanol (96 per cent), slightly soluble or very slightly soluble in methylene chloride.

It shows polymorphism.

IDENTIFICATION

Infrared absorption spectrophotometry (*2.2.24*).

Comparison: *ribavirin CRS*.

If the spectra obtained in the solid state show differences, dissolve the substance to be examined and the reference substance separately in *methylene chloride R*, evaporate to dryness and record new spectra using the residues.

TESTS

pH (*2.2.3*): 4.0 to 6.5.

Dissolve 0.200 g in *carbon dioxide-free water R* and dilute to 10.0 ml with the same solvent.

Specific optical rotation (*2.2.7*): − 33 to − 37 (dried substance).

Dissolve 0.250 g in *water R* and dilute to 25.0 ml with the same solvent. Determine the specific optical rotation within 10 min of preparing the solution.

Related substances. Liquid chromatography (*2.2.29*).

Test solution. Dissolve 25.0 mg of the substance to be examined in the mobile phase and dilute to 100.0 ml with the mobile phase. Dilute 10.0 ml of the solution to 100.0 ml with the mobile phase.

Reference solution (a). Dilute 1.0 ml of the test solution to 100.0 ml with the mobile phase. Dilute 1.0 ml of this solution to 10.0 ml with the mobile phase.

Reference solution (b). Dissolve the contents of a vial of *ribavirin for system suitability CRS* in 2.0 ml of the mobile phase.

Reference solution (c). Dissolve 25.0 mg of *ribavirin CRS* in the mobile phase and dilute to 100.0 ml with the mobile phase. Dilute 10.0 ml of the solution to 100.0 ml with the mobile phase.

Column:

– *size*: l = 0.10 m, Ø = 7.8 mm,
– *stationary phase*: *strong cation-exchange resin R* (9 µm),
– *temperature*: 40 °C.

Monographs Q-S

Mobile phase: *water R* adjusted to pH 2.5 with *sulphuric acid R*.

Flow rate: 1 ml/min.

Detection: spectrophotometer at 207 nm.

Injection: 10 µl of the test solution and reference solutions (a) and (b).

Run time: 11 times the retention time of ribavirin.

Relative retention with reference to ribavirin (retention time = about 4 min): impurity F = about 1.2.

System suitability: reference solution (b):

- *peak-to-valley ratio*: minimum 1.2, where H_p = height above the baseline of the peak due to impurity F and H_v = height above the baseline of the lowest point of the curve separating this peak from the peak due to ribavirin.

Limits:

- *impurity F*: not more than the area of the principal peak in the chromatogram obtained with reference solution (a) (0.1 per cent),
- *any other impurity*: for each impurity, not more than the area of the principal peak in the chromatogram obtained with reference solution (a) (0.1 per cent),
- *total*: not more than twice the area of the principal peak in the chromatogram obtained with reference solution (a) (0.2 per cent),
- *disregard limit*: 0.5 times the area of the principal peak in the chromatogram obtained with reference solution (a) (0.05 per cent).

Heavy metals (*2.4.8*): maximum 10 ppm.

Dissolve 4.0 g in 20 ml of *water R*. 12 ml of the solution complies with limit test A. Prepare the reference solution using 10 ml of *lead standard solution (2 ppm Pb) R*.

Loss on drying (*2.2.32*): maximum 0.5 per cent, determined on 1.000 g by drying in an oven at 100-105 °C for 5 h.

Sulphated ash (*2.4.14*): maximum 0.1 per cent, determined on 1.0 g.

ASSAY

Liquid chromatography (*2.2.29*) as described in the test for related substances with the following modification.

Injection: test solution and reference solution (c).

Calculate the percentage content of $C_8H_{12}N_4O_5$ using the declared content of $C_8H_{12}N_4O_5$ in *ribavirin CRS*.

STORAGE

Protected from light.

IMPURITIES

Specified impurities: F.

Other detectable impurities: A, B, C, D, E, G.

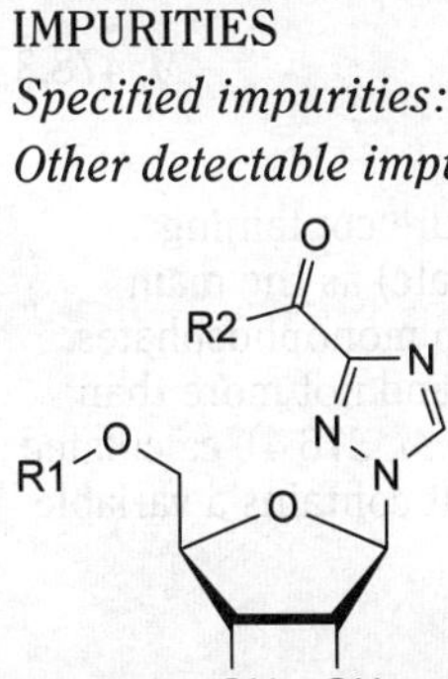

A. R1 = H, R2 = OH: 1-β-D-ribofuranosyl-1*H*-1,2,4-triazole-3-carboxylic acid,

E. R1 = CO-C_6H_5, R2 = NH_2: 1-(5-*O*-benzoyl-β-D-ribofuranosyl)-1*H*-1,2,4-triazole-3-carboxamide (5′-*O*-benzoylribavirin),

F. R1 = CO-CH_3, R2 = NH_2: 1-(5-*O*-acetyl-β-D-ribofuranosyl)-1*H*-1,2,4-triazole-3-carboxamide (5′-*O*-acetylribavirin),

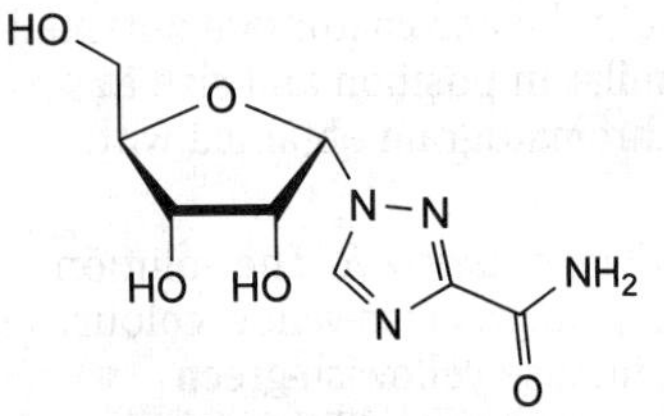

B. 1-α-D-ribofuranosyl-1*H*-1,2,4-triazole-3-carboxamide (anomer),

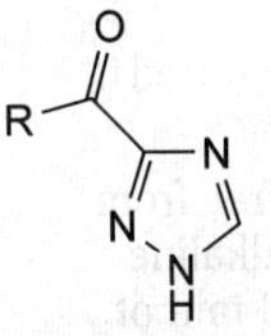

C. R = OH: 1*H*-1,2,4-triazole-3-carboxylic acid,

D. R = NH_2: 1*H*-1,2,4-triazole-3-carboxamide,

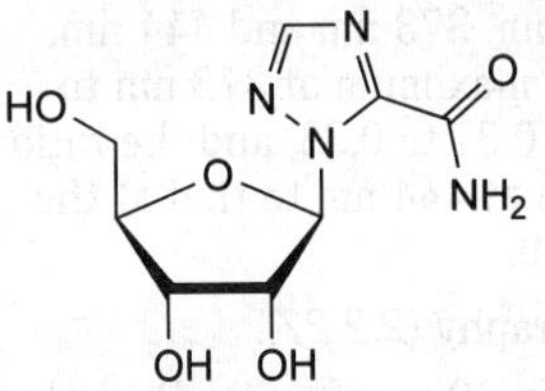

G. 1-β-D-ribofuranosyl-1*H*-1,2,4-triazole-5-carboxamide (*N*-isomer).

01/2005:0292

RIBOFLAVIN

Riboflavinum

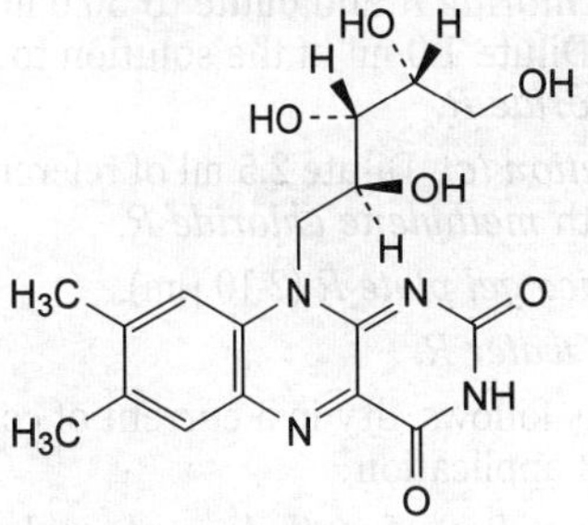

$C_{17}H_{20}N_4O_6$ M_r 376.4

DEFINITION

7,8-Dimethyl-10-[(2*S*,3*S*,4*R*)-2,3,4,5-tetrahydroxypentyl]benzo[*g*]pteridine-2,4(3*H*,10*H*)-dione.

Contents: 97.0 per cent to 103.0 per cent (dried substance).

CHARACTERS

Appearance: yellow or orange-yellow, crystalline powder.

Solubility: very slightly soluble in water, practically insoluble in alcohol.

Solutions deteriorate on exposure to light, especially in the presence of alkali.

It shows polymorphism.

IDENTIFICATION

A. It complies with the test for specific optical rotation (see Tests).

Monographs Q-S

B. Examine the chromatogram obtained in the test for lumiflavin.

Results: the principal spot in the chromatogram obtained with test solution (a) is similar in position and size to the principal spot in the chromatogram obtained with reference solution (a).

C. Dissolve about 1 mg in 100 ml of *water R*. The solution has, by transmitted light, a pale greenish-yellow colour, and, by reflected light, an intense yellowish-green fluorescence which disappears on the addition of mineral acids or alkalis.

TESTS

Specific optical rotation (*2.2.7*): − 115 to − 135 (dried substance).

Dissolve 50.0 mg in *0.05 M sodium hydroxide* free from carbonate and dilute to 10.0 ml with the same alkaline solution. Measure the optical rotation within 30 min of dissolution.

Absorbance (*2.2.25*). Dilute the final solution prepared for the assay with an equal volume of *water R*. The solution shows 4 maxima, at 223 nm, 267 nm, 373 nm and 444 nm. The ratio of the absorbance at the maximum at 373 nm to that at the maximum at 267 nm is 0.31 to 0.33, and the ratio of the absorbance at the maximum at 444 nm to that at the maximum at 267 nm is 0.36 to 0.39.

Lumiflavin. Thin-layer chromatography (*2.2.27*).

Test solution (a). Suspend 25 mg in 10 ml of *water R*; shake for 5 min and filter the suspension to remove the undissolved material.

Test solution (b). Shake 25 mg of the substance to be examined with 10.0 ml of *methylene chloride R* and filter the suspension to remove the undissolved material.

Reference solution (a). Suspend 25 mg of *riboflavin CRS* in 10 ml of *water R*; shake for 5 min and filter the suspension to remove the undissolved material.

Reference solution (b). Dissolve 25 mg of *lumiflavin R* in *methylene chloride R* and dilute to 50.0 ml with the same solvent. Dilute 1.0 ml of the solution to 20.0 ml with *methylene chloride R.*

Reference solution (c). Dilute 2.5 ml of reference solution (b) to 100.0 ml with *methylene chloride R.*

Plate: *TLC silica gel plate R* (2-10 μm).

Mobile phase: *water R.*

Application: as follows, dry in a current of cold air after each individual application:

- 1st application: 2 μl of *methylene chloride R* followed by 2 μl of test solution (a),
- 2nd application: 2 μl of *methylene chloride R* followed by 2 μl of reference solution (a),
- 3rd application: 2 μl of reference solution (b) followed by 2 μl of reference solution (a),
- 4th application: 10 μl of test solution (b),
- 5th application: 10 μl of reference solution (c).

Development: over a path of 6 cm.

Drying: in a current of cold air.

Detection: examine in ultraviolet light at 365 nm.

System suitability: the chromatogram obtained with the 3rd application shows 2 clearly separated spots.

Limit: in the chromatogram obtained with test solution (b):

- *lumiflavin*: any spot corresponding to lumiflavin is not more intense than the principal spot in the chromatogram obtained with reference solution (c) (0.025 per cent).

Loss on drying (*2.2.32*): maximum 1.5 per cent, determined on 1.000 g by drying in an oven at 100-105 °C.

Sulphated ash (*2.4.14*): maximum 0.1 per cent, determined on the residue obtained in the test for loss on drying.

ASSAY

Carry out the assay protected from light.

In a brown-glass 500 ml volumetric flask, suspend 65.0 mg in 5 ml of *water R* ensuring that it is completely wetted and dissolve in 5 ml of *dilute sodium hydroxide solution R*. As soon as dissolution is complete, add 100 ml of *water R* and 2.5 ml of *glacial acetic acid R* and dilute to 500.0 ml with *water R*. Place 20.0 ml of this solution in a 200 ml brown-glass volumetric flask, add 3.5 ml of a 14 g/l solution of *sodium acetate R* and dilute to 200.0 ml with *water R*. Measure the absorbance (*2.2.25*) at the maximum at 444 nm.

Calculate the content of $C_{17}H_{20}N_4O_6$ taking the specific absorbance to be 328.

STORAGE

In an airtight container, protected from light.

IMPURITIES

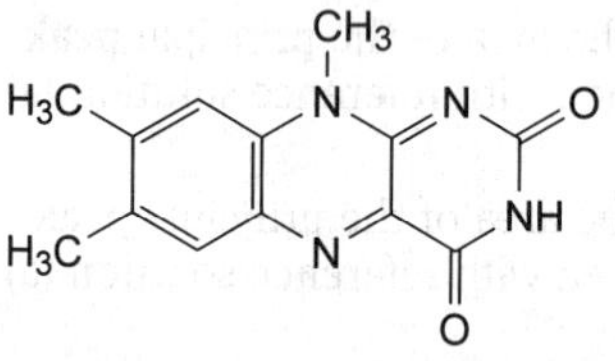

A. 7,8,10-trimethylbenzo[*g*]pteridine-2,4(3*H*,10*H*)-dione (lumiflavin).

01/2005:0786

RIBOFLAVIN SODIUM PHOSPHATE

Riboflavini natrii phosphas

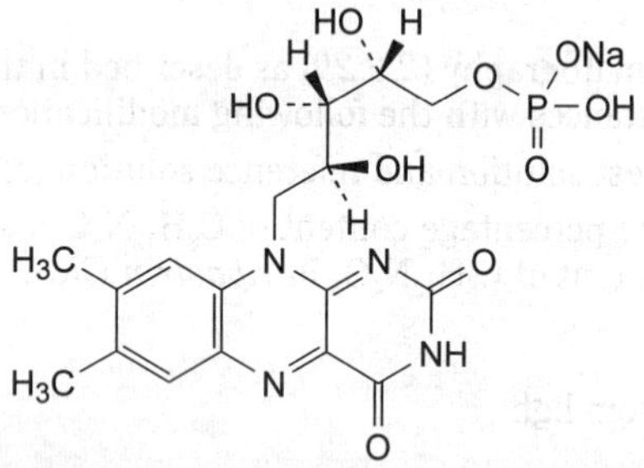

$C_{17}H_{20}N_4NaO_9P$ M_r 478.3

DEFINITION

Riboflavin sodium phosphate is a mixture containing riboflavin 5′-(sodium hydrogen phosphate) as the main component and other riboflavin sodium monophosphates. It contains not less than 73.0 per cent and not more than 79.0 per cent of riboflavin ($C_{17}H_{20}N_4O_6$; M_r 376.4), calculated with reference to the dried substance. It contains a variable amount of water.

CHARACTERS

A yellow or orange-yellow, crystalline powder, hygroscopic, soluble in water, very slightly soluble in alcohol.

IDENTIFICATION

A. Dissolve 50.0 mg in *phosphate buffer solution pH 7.0 R* and dilute to 100.0 ml with the same buffer solution. Dilute 2.0 ml of the solution to 100.0 ml with *phosphate buffer solution pH 7.0 R*. Examined between 230 nm and 350 nm (*2.2.25*), the solution shows an absorption maximum at 266 nm. The specific absorbance at the maximum is 580 to 640.

B. Examine the chromatograms obtained in the test for related substances. The principal peak in the chromatogram obtained with the test solution is similar in position and approximate size to the principal peak in the chromatogram obtained with reference solution (b).

C. Dissolve about 10 mg in *dilute sodium hydroxide solution R* and dilute to 100 ml with the same solution. Expose 1 ml to ultraviolet light at 254 nm for 5 min, add sufficient *acetic acid R* to make the solution acidic to *blue litmus paper R* and shake with 2 ml of *methylene chloride R*. The lower layer shows yellow fluorescence.

D. To 0.5 g add 10 ml of *nitric acid R*, evaporate the mixture to dryness on a water-bath. Ignite the residue until it becomes white, dissolve the residue in 5 ml of *water R* and filter. The filtrate gives reaction (a) of sodium and reaction (b) of phosphates (*2.3.1*).

TESTS

pH (*2.2.3*). Dissolve 0.5 g in *carbon dioxide-free water R* and dilute to 50 ml with the same solvent. The pH of the solution is 5.0 to 6.5.

Specific optical rotation (*2.2.7*). Dissolve 0.300 g in 18.2 ml of *hydrochloric acid R1* and dilute to 25.0 ml with *water R*. The specific optical rotation is + 38.0 to + 43.0, calculated with reference to the dried substance.

Lumiflavin. To about 35 mg add 10 ml of *methylene chloride R*, shake for 5 min and filter. The filtrate is not more intensely coloured than reference solution BY_6 (*2.2.2, Method II*).

Related substances. Examine by liquid chromatography (*2.2.29*). *Carry out the test protected from actinic light.*

Test solution. Dissolve 0.100 g of the substance to be examined in 50 ml of *water R* and dilute to 100.0 ml with the mobile phase. Dilute 8.0 ml of this solution to 50.0 ml with the mobile phase.

Reference solution (a). Dissolve 60 mg of *riboflavin CRS* in 1 ml of *hydrochloric acid R* and dilute to 250.0 ml with *water R*. Dilute 4.0 ml to 100.0 ml with the mobile phase.

Reference solution (b). Dissolve 0.100 g of *riboflavin sodium phosphate CRS* in 50 ml of *water R* and dilute to 100.0 ml with the mobile phase. Dilute 8.0 ml of this solution to 50.0 ml with the mobile phase.

The chromatographic procedure may be carried out using:

- a stainless steel column 0.25 m long and 4.6 mm in internal diameter packed with *octadecylsilyl silica gel for chromatography R* (5 µm),
- as mobile phase at a flow rate of 2 ml/min a mixture of 150 volumes of *methanol R* and 850 volumes of a 7.35 g/l solution of *potassium dihydrogen phosphate R*,
- as detector a spectrophotometer set at 266 nm.

When the chromatograms are recorded in the prescribed conditions, the retention time of riboflavin 5′-monophosphate is about 20 min and the relative retention times are: riboflavin 3′,4′-diphosphate about 0.2, riboflavin 3′,5′-diphosphate about 0.3, riboflavin 4′,5′-diphosphate about 0.5, riboflavin 3′-monophosphate about 0.7, riboflavin 4′-mono-phosphate about 0.9, riboflavin 5′-monophosphate 1, riboflavin about 2.

Inject 100 µl of reference solution (a). Adjust the sensitivity of the system so that the height of the principal peak in the chromatogram obtained is at least 50 per cent of the full scale of the recorder. Inject 100 µl of reference solution (b). Continue the chromatography until the peak corresponding to riboflavin can be clearly evaluated. The test is not valid unless in the chromatogram obtained with reference solution (b), the resolution between the peaks corresponding to riboflavin 4′-monophosphate and riboflavin 5′-monophosphate is at least 1.5.

Inject 100 µl of the test solution, 100 µl of reference solution (a) and 100 µl of reference solution (b). Calculate the percentage content of free riboflavin and of riboflavin in the form of the diphosphates of riboflavin from the areas of the peaks in the chromatogram obtained with the test solution and the amount of free riboflavin in reference solution (a). The content of free riboflavin is not greater than 6.0 per cent and the content of riboflavin in the form of the diphosphates of riboflavin is not greater than 6.0 per cent, both calculated with reference to dried material.

Inorganic phosphate. Dissolve 0.10 g in *water R* and dilute to 100 ml with the same solvent. To 5 ml of the solution, add 10 ml of *water R*, 5 ml of *buffered copper sulphate solution pH 4.0 R*, 2 ml of a 30 g/l solution of *ammonium molybdate R*, 1 ml of a freshly prepared solution containing 20 g/l of *4-methylaminophenol sulphate R* and 50 g/l of *sodium metabisulphite R* and 1 ml of a 3 per cent *V/V* solution of *perchloric acid R*. Dilute to 25.0 ml with *water R* and measure, within 15 min of its preparation, the absorbance of the solution at 800 nm (*2.2.25*) using as the compensation liquid a solution prepared in the same manner but without the substance to be examined. The absorbance is not greater than that of a solution prepared as follows: to 15 ml of *phosphate standard solution (5 ppm PO_4) R*, add 5 ml of *buffered copper sulphate solution pH 4.0 R*, 2 ml of a 30 g/l solution of *ammonium molybdate R*, 1 ml of a freshly prepared solution containing 20 g/l of *4-methylaminophenol sulphate R* and 50 g/l of *sodium metabisulphite R* and 1 ml of a 3 per cent *V/V* solution of *perchloric acid R*; dilute to 25.0 ml with *water R* (1.5 per cent).

Heavy metals (*2.4.8*). To 2.0 g in a silica crucible add 2 ml of *nitric acid R*, dropwise, followed by 0.25 ml of *sulphuric acid R*. Heat cautiously until white fumes are evolved and ignite. Extract the cooled residue with two quantities, each of 2 ml, of *hydrochloric acid R* and evaporate the extracts to dryness. Dissolve the residue in 2 ml of *dilute acetic acid R* and dilute to 20 ml with *water R*. 12 ml of the solution complies with limit test A for heavy metals (10 ppm). Prepare the standard using 10 ml of *lead standard solution (1 ppm Pb) R*.

Loss on drying (*2.2.32*). Not more than 8.0 per cent, determined on 1.000 g by drying in an oven at 100 °C to 105 °C at a pressure not exceeding 0.7 kPa for 5 h.

ASSAY

Carry out the assay protected from light.

Dissolve 0.100 g in 150 ml of *water R*, add 2 ml of *glacial acetic acid R* and dilute to 1000.0 ml with *water R*. To 10.0 ml add 3.5 ml of a 14 g/l solution of *sodium acetate R* and dilute to 50.0 ml with *water R*. Measure the absorbance (*2.2.25*) at the maximum at 444 nm.

Calculate the content of $C_{17}H_{20}N_4O_6$ taking the specific absorbance to be 328.

STORAGE

Store in an airtight container, protected from light.

IMPURITIES

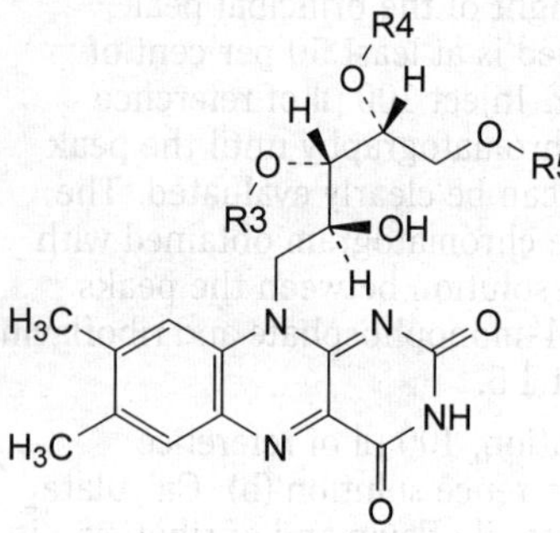

A. R3 = R4 = PO_3H_2, R5 = H: riboflavin 3′,4′-diphosphate,

B. R3 = R5 = PO_3H_2, R4 = H: riboflavin 3′,5′-diphosphate,

C. R3 = H, R4 = R5 = PO_3H_2: riboflavin 4′,5′-diphosphate,

D. R3 = R4 = R5 = H: riboflavin,

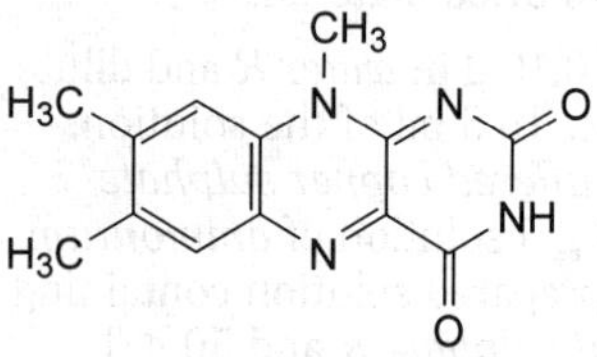

E. 7,8,10-trimethylbenzo[*g*]pteridine-2,4(3*H*,10*H*)-dione (lumiflavin).

01/2005:1884

RIBWORT PLANTAIN

Plantaginis lanceolatae folium

DEFINITION

Whole or fragmented, dried leaf and scape of *Plantago lanceolata* L. s. l.

Content: minimum 1.5 per cent of total *ortho*-dihydroxycinnamic acid derivatives expressed as acteoside ($C_{29}H_{36}O_{15}$; M_r 624.6) (dried drug).

CHARACTERS

Macroscopic and microscopic characters described under identification tests A and B.

IDENTIFICATION

A. The leaf is up to 30 cm long and 4 cm wide, yellowish-green to brownish-green, with a prominent, whitish-green, almost parallel venation on the abaxial surface. It consists of a lanceolate lamina narrowing at the base into a channelled petiole. The margin is indistinctly dentate and often undulate. It has 3, 5 or 7 primary veins, nearly equal in length and running almost parallel. Hairs may be almost absent, sparsely scattered or sometimes abundant, especially on the lower surface and over the veins. The scape is brownish-green, longer than the leaves, 3 mm to 4 mm in diameter and is deeply grooved longitudinally, with 5 to 7 conspicuous ribs. The surface is usually covered with fine hairs.

B. Reduce to a powder (355). The powder is yellowish-green. Examine under a microscope using *chloral hydrate solution R*. The powder shows the following diagnostic characters: fragments of epidermis, composed of cells with irregularly sinuous anticlinal walls, the fragments from the scape with thickened outer walls and a coarsely ridged cuticle; stomata mostly of the diacytic type (*2.8.3*) and sometimes anomocytic; the multicellular, uniseriate, conical covering trichomes are highly characteristic, with a basal cell larger than the other epidermal cells followed by a short cell supporting 2 or more elongated cells with the lumen narrow and variable, occluded at intervals corresponding to slight swellings in the trichome and giving a jointed appearance; the terminal cell has an acute apex and a filiform lumen; the glandular trichomes have a unicellular cylindrical stalk and a multicellular, elongated, conical head consisting of several rows of small cells and a single terminal cell; dense groups of lignified fibro-vascular tissue with narrow, spirally and annularly thickened vessels and slender, moderately thickened fibres.

C. Examine the chromatograms obtained for *Digitalis lanata* leaves.

Results A: see below the sequence of the zones present in the chromatograms obtained with the reference solution and the test solution. Furthermore, other zones may be present in the chromatograms obtained with the test solution.

Top of the plate	
Acteoside: a yellow zone	A yellow zone (acteoside)
Aucubin: a blue zone	A blue zone (aucubin)
Reference solution	**Test solution**

TESTS

***Digitalis lanata* leaves.** Thin layer chromatography (*2.2.27*).

Test solution. Use a freshly prepared solution. To 1 g of the powdered drug (355) in a 25 ml flask, add 10 ml of a mixture of 30 volumes of *water R* and 70 volumes of *methanol R* and shake for 30 min. Filter, rinse the flask and filter with 2 quantities, each of 5 ml, with the mixture of 30 volumes of *water R* and 70 volumes of *methanol R*. Dilute to 25 ml with a mixture of 30 volumes of *water R* and 70 volumes of *methanol R*.

Reference solution. Dissolve 1 mg of *acteoside R* and 1 mg of *aucubin R* in 1 ml of a mixture of 30 volumes of *water R* and 70 volumes of *methanol R*.

Plate: *TLC silica gel F_{254} plate R*.

Mobile phase: *acetic acid R, anhydrous formic acid R, water R, ethyl acetate R* (11:11:27:100 *V/V/V/V*).

Application: 10 μl as bands.

Development: over a path of 8 cm; heat immediately after development at about 120 °C for 5-10 min.

Detection A: examine in daylight.

Detection B: examine in ultraviolet light at 365 nm.

Results B: the chromatogram obtained with the test solution shows no bright blue fluorescent zone just below the reddish-brown fluorescent zone corresponding to aucubin in the chromatogram obtained with the reference solution.

Foreign matter (*2.8.2*): maximum 5 per cent of leaves of different colour and maximum 2 per cent of other foreign matter.

Loss on drying (*2.2.32*): maximum 10.0 per cent, determined on 1.000 g of the powdered drug (355) by drying in an oven at 100-105 °C for 2 h.

Total ash (*2.4.16*): maximum 14.0 per cent.

ASSAY

Stock solution. In a flask, place 1.000 g of the powdered drug (355) and add 90 ml of *alcohol (50 per cent V/V) R.* Boil in a water-bath under a reflux condenser for 30 min. Allow to cool and filter into a 100 ml volumetric flask. Rinse the flask and the filter with 10 ml of *alcohol (50 per cent V/V) R.* Combine the filtrate and the rinsings and dilute to 100.0 ml with *alcohol (50 per cent V/V) R.*

Test solution. To a 10 ml volumetric flask add, mixing after each addition, 1.0 ml of stock solution, 2 ml of *0.5 M hydrochloric acid,* 2 ml of a solution prepared by dissolving 10 g of *sodium nitrite R* and 10 g of *sodium molybdate R* in 100 ml of *water R* and then add 2 ml of *dilute sodium hydroxide solution R.* Dilute to 10.0 ml with *water R.*

Immediately measure the absorbance (*2.2.25*) of the test solution at 525 nm using as compensation liquid a solution prepared as follows: to a 10 ml volumetric flask, add 1.0 ml of stock solution, 2 ml of *0.5 M hydrochloric acid,* 2 ml of *dilute sodium hydroxide solution R* and dilute to 10.0 ml with *water R.*

Calculate the percentage content of total *ortho*-dihydroxycinnamic acid derivatives, expressed as acteoside, from the expression:

$$\frac{A \times 1000}{185 \times m}$$

i.e. taking the specific absorbance to be 185 for acteoside at 525 nm.

A = absorbance of the test solution at 525 nm,

m = mass of the substance to be examined, in grams.

01/2005:0349

RICE STARCH

Oryzae amylum

DEFINITION

Rice starch is obtained from the caryopsis of *Oryza sativa* L.

CHARACTERS

A very fine, white powder which creaks when pressed between the fingers, tasteless, practically insoluble in cold water and in alcohol. The presence of granules with cracks or irregularities on the edge is exceptional.

DESCRIPTION

Examined under a microscope it presents polyhedral granules 2 µm to 5 µm in size, either isolated or aggregated in ovoid masses of 10 µm to 20 µm in size. The granules have a poorly visible central hilum and there are no concentric striations. Between crossed nicol prisms, the starch granules show a distinct black cross intersecting at the hilum.

IDENTIFICATION

A. Suspend 1 g in 50 ml of *water R,* boil for 1 min and cool. A thin, cloudy mucilage is formed.

B. To 1 ml of the mucilage obtained in identification test A add 0.05 ml of *iodine solution R1.* A dark-blue colour is produced which disappears on heating.

TESTS

Acidity. Add 10 g to 100 ml of *alcohol (70 per cent V/V) R* previously neutralised to 0.5 ml of *phenolphthalein solution R* and shake for 1 h. Filter and take 50 ml of the filtrate. Not more than 2.0 ml of *0.1 M sodium hydroxide* is required to change the colour of the indicator.

Foreign matter. Not more than traces of cell membranes and protoplasm are present.

Loss on drying (*2.2.32*). Not more than 15.0 per cent, determined on 1.00 g by drying in an oven at 100-105 °C.

Sulphated ash (*2.4.14*). Not more than 1.0 per cent, determined on 1.0 g.

Microbial contamination. Total viable aerobic count (*2.6.12*) not more than 10^3 bacteria and 10^2 fungi per gram, determined by plate count. It complies with the test for *Escherichia coli* (*2.6.13*).

STORAGE

In an airtight container.

01/2005:1657
corrected

RIFABUTIN

Rifabutinum

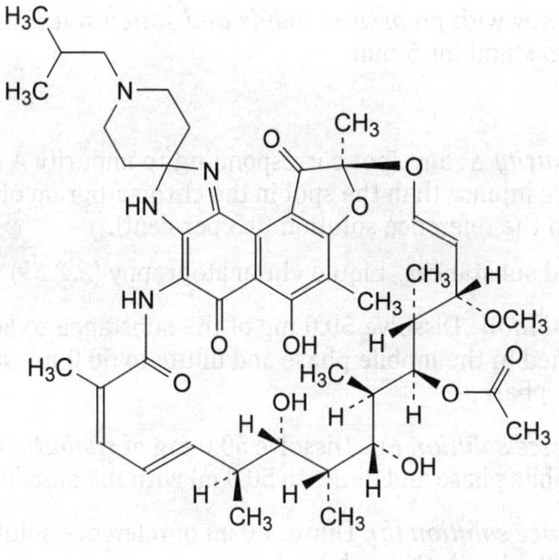

$C_{46}H_{62}N_4O_{11}$ M_r 847

DEFINITION

(9*S*,12*E*,14*S*,15*R*,16*S*,17*R*,18*R*,19*R*,20*S*,21*S*,22*E*,24*Z*)-6,18,20-trihydroxy-14-methoxy-7,9,15,17,19,21,25-heptamethyl-1′-(2-methylpropyl)-5,10,26-trioxo-3,5,9,10-tetrahydrospiro[9,4-(epoxypentadeca[1,11,13]trienimino)-2*H*-furo[2′,3′:7,8]naphtho[1,2-*d*]imidazole-2,4′-piperidine]-16-yl acetate.

Content: 96.0 per cent to 102.0 per cent (anhydrous substance).

CHARACTERS

Appearance: reddish-violet amorphous powder.

Solubility: slightly soluble in water, soluble in methanol, slightly soluble in alcohol.

IDENTIFICATION

A. Infrared absorption spectrophotometry (*2.2.24*).

Preparation: discs.

Comparison: *rifabutin CRS.*

B. Examine the chromatograms obtained in the test for related substances.

Monographs Q-S

Results: the principal peak in the chromatogram obtained with the test solution is similar in retention time and size to the principal peak in the chromatogram obtained with reference solution (a).

TESTS

Impurity A. Thin-layer chromatography (*2.2.27*).

Test solution. Dissolve 0.100 g of the substance to be examined in a mixture of equal volumes of *methanol R* and *methylene chloride R* and dilute to 10 ml with the same mixture of solvents.

Reference solution. Dissolve 10 mg of *rifabutin impurity A CRS* in a mixture of equal volumes of *methanol R* and *methylene chloride R* and dilute to 10 ml with the same mixture of solvents. Dilute 3 ml of the solution to 100 ml with a mixture of equal volumes of *methanol R* and *methylene chloride R*.

Plate: *TLC silica gel F_{254} plate R*.

Mobile phase: *acetone R, light petroleum R* (23:77 *V/V*).

Application: 10 µl.

Development: over 2/3 of the plate.

Drying: in air.

Detection: expose the plate to iodine vapour for about 5 min, then spray with *potassium iodide and starch solution R* and allow to stand for 5 min.

Limit:

- *impurity A*: any spot corresponding to impurity A is not more intense than the spot in the chromatogram obtained with the reference solution (0.3 per cent).

Related substances. Liquid chromatography (*2.2.29*).

Test solution. Dissolve 50.0 mg of the substance to be examined in the mobile phase and dilute to 50.0 ml with the mobile phase.

Reference solution (a). Dissolve 50.0 mg of *rifabutin CRS* in the mobile phase and dilute to 50.0 ml with the mobile phase.

Reference solution (b). Dilute 1.0 ml of reference solution (a) to 100.0 ml with the mobile phase.

Reference solution (c). Dissolve about 10 mg of *rifabutin CRS* in 2 ml of *methanol R*, add 1 ml of *dilute sodium hydroxide solution R* and allow to stand for about 4 min. Add 1 ml of *dilute hydrochloric acid R* and dilute to 50 ml with the mobile phase.

Column:

- *size*: l = 0.110 m, Ø = 4.6 mm,
- *stationary phase*: *octylsilyl silica gel for chromatography R* (5 µm).

Mobile phase: mix equal volumes of *acetonitrile R* and a 13.6 g/l solution of *potassium dihydrogen phosphate R* adjusted to pH 6.5 with *dilute sodium hydroxide solution R*.

Flow rate: 1 ml/min.

Detection: spectrophotometer at 254 nm.

Injection: 20 µl.

Run time: 2.5 times the retention time of rifabutin.

Relative retention with reference to rifabutin (retention time = about 9 min): impurity E = about 0.5; impurity B = about 0.6; impurity D = about 0.9; impurity C = about 1.3.

System suitability: reference solution (c):

- *resolution*: minimum 2.0 between the second peak of the 3 peaks due to degradation products and the peak due to rifabutin.

Limits:

- *any impurity*: not more than the area of the principal peak in the chromatogram obtained with reference solution (b) (1.0 per cent); not more than 1 such peak has an area greater than half the area of the principal peak in the chromatogram obtained with reference solution (b) (0.5 per cent),
- *total*: not more than 3 times the area of the principal peak in the chromatogram obtained with reference solution (b) (3.0 per cent),
- *disregard limit*: 0.05 times the area of the principal peak in the chromatogram obtained with reference solution (b) (0.05 per cent).

Water (*2.5.12*): maximum 2.5 per cent, determined on 0.200 g.

Sulphated ash (*2.4.14*): maximum 0.3 per cent, determined on 1.0 g.

ASSAY

Liquid chromatography (*2.2.29*) as described in the test for related substances with the following modification.

Injection: test solution and reference solution (a).

Calculate the percentage content of ribabutin.

IMPURITIES

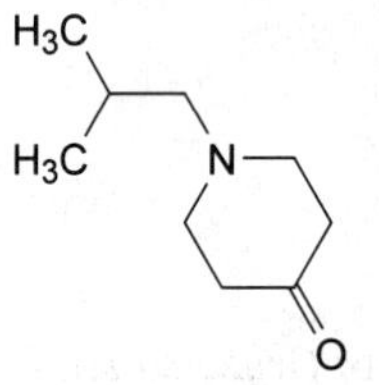

A. 1-(2-methylpropyl)piperidin-4-one,

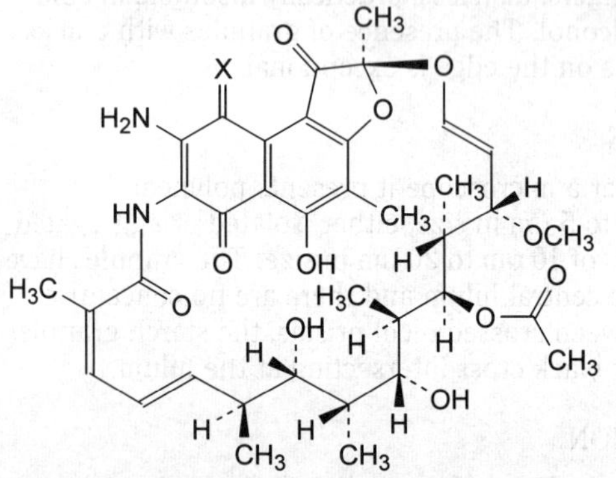

B. X = O: 3-aminorifamycin S,

D. X = NH: 3-amino-4-imidorifamycin S,

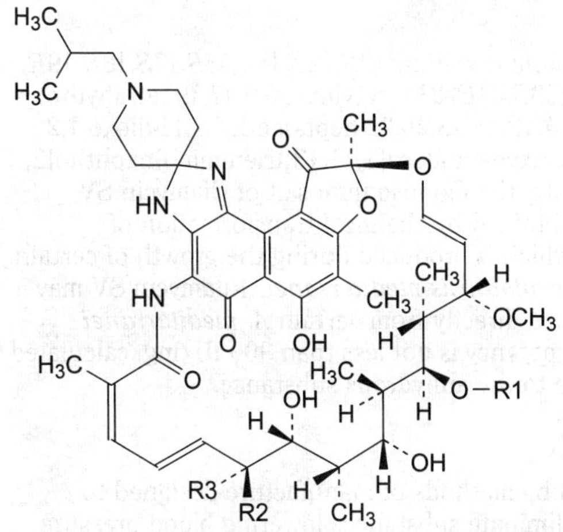

C. R1 = CO-CH_3, R2 + R3 = CH_2: 21,31-didehydrorifabutin,

E. R1 = R3 = H, R2 = CH_3: 16-deacetylrifabutin.

01/2005:0052

RIFAMPICIN

Rifampicinum

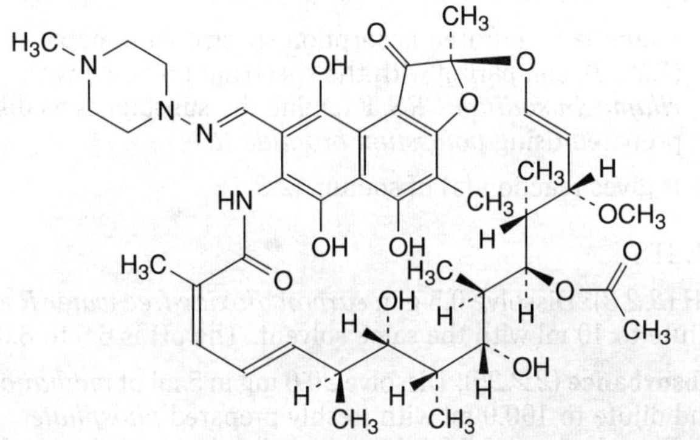

$C_{43}H_{58}N_4O_{12}$ M_r 823

DEFINITION

Rifampicin is (2*S*,12*Z*,14*E*,16*S*,17*S*,18*R*,19*R*,20*R*,21*S*,22*R*,23*S*,24*E*)-5,6,9,17,19-pentahydroxy-23-methoxy-2,4,12,16,18,20,22-heptamethyl-8-[[(4-methylpiperazin-1-yl)imino]methyl]-1,11-dioxo-1,2-dihydro-2,7-(epoxypentadeca[1,11,13]trienimino)naphto[2,1-*b*]furan-21-yl acetate, a semisynthetic antibiotic obtained from rifamycin SV. It contains not less than 97.0 per cent and not more than the equivalent of 102.0 per cent of $C_{43}H_{58}N_4O_{12}$, calculated with reference to the dried substance.

CHARACTERS

A reddish-brown or brownish-red, crystalline powder, slightly soluble in water, soluble in methanol, slightly soluble in acetone and in alcohol.

IDENTIFICATION

A. Dissolve 50 mg in 50 ml of *methanol R*. Dilute 1 ml of the solution to 50 ml with *phosphate buffer solution pH 7.4 R*. Examined between 220 nm and 500 nm, the solution shows 4 absorption maxima (*2.2.25*), at 237 nm, 254 nm, 334 nm and 475 nm. The ratio of the absorbance at the maximum at 334 nm to that at 475 nm is about 1.75.

B. Examine by infrared absorption spectrophotometry (*2.2.24*), comparing with the spectrum obtained with *rifampicin CRS*. Examine the substances prepared as mulls in *liquid paraffin R*.

C. Suspend about 25 mg in 25 ml of *water R*, shake for 5 min and filter. To 5 ml of the filtrate add 1 ml of a 100 g/l solution of *ammonium persulphate R* in *phosphate buffer solution pH 7.4 R* and shake for a few minutes. The colour changes from orange-yellow to violet-red and no precipitate is formed.

TESTS

pH (*2.2.3*). The pH of a 10 g/l suspension in *carbon dioxide-free water R* is 4.5 to 6.5.

Related substances. Examine by liquid chromatography (*2.2.29*). *Prepare the test solution and the reference solution immediately before use.*

Solvent mixture. To 10 volumes of a 210.1 g/l solution of *citric acid R* add 23 volumes of a 136.1 g/l solution of *potassium dihydrogen phosphate R*, 77 volumes of a 174.2 g/l solution of *dipotassium hydrogen phosphate R*, 250 volumes of *acetonitrile R* and 640 volumes of *water R*.

Test solution. Dissolve 20.0 mg of the substance to be examined in *acetonitrile R* and dilute to 10.0 ml with the same solvent. Dilute 5.0 ml to 50.0 ml with the solvent mixure.

Reference solution. Dissolve 20.0 mg of *rifampicin quinone CRS* in *acetonitrile R* and dilute to 100.0 ml with the same solvent. To 1.0 ml of the solution add 1.0 ml of the test solution and dilute to 100.0 ml with the solvent mixture.

The chromatographic procedure may be carried out using:

- a stainless steel column 0.12 m long and 4.6 mm in internal diameter packed with *octylsilyl silica gel for chromatography R* (5 µm),
- as mobile phase at a flow rate of 1.5 ml/min a mixture of 35 volumes of *acetonitrile R* and 65 volumes of a solution containing 0.1 per cent *V/V* of *phosphoric acid R*, 1.9 g/l of *sodium perchlorate R*, 5.9 g/l of *citric acid R* and 20.9 g/l of *potassium dihydrogen phosphate R*,
- as detector a spectrophotometer set at 254 nm,
- a 20 µl loop injector.

Inject the reference solution. Adjust the sensitivity of the detector so that the height of the 2 principal peaks is not less than half the full scale of the recorder. The test is not valid unless the resolution between the 2 principal peaks is at least 4.0. Adjust the concentration of acetonitrile in the mobile phase, if necessary. Inject the test solution and continue the chromatography for at least twice the retention time of rifampicin: the area of any peak corresponding to rifampicin quinone is not greater than 1.5 times the area of the corresponding peak in the chromatogram obtained with the reference solution (1.5 per cent); the area of any peak, apart from the principal peak and the peak corresponding to rifampicin quinone, is not greater than the area of the rifampicin peak in the chromatogram obtained with the reference solution (1.0 per cent) and the sum of the areas of any such peaks is not greater than 3.5 times the area of the rifampicin peak in the chromatogram obtained with the reference solution (3.5 per cent). Disregard any peak due to the solvent and any peak with an area less than 0.05 times that of the peak corresponding to rifampicin in the chromatogram obtained with the reference solution.

Heavy metals (*2.4.8*). 1.0 g complies with limit test C for heavy metals (20 ppm). Prepare the standard using 2 ml of *lead standard solution (10 ppm Pb) R*.

Loss on drying (*2.2.32*). Not more than 1.0 per cent, determined on 1.000 g by drying at 80 °C at a pressure not exceeding 670 Pa for 4 h.

Sulphated ash (*2.4.14*). Not more than 0.1 per cent, determined on 2.0 g.

ASSAY

Dissolve 0.100 g in *methanol R* and dilute to 100.0 ml with the same solvent. Dilute 2.0 ml of the solution to 100.0 ml with *phosphate buffer solution pH 7.4 R*. Measure the absorbance (*2.2.25*) at the maximum at 475 nm, using *phosphate buffer solution pH 7.4 R* as the compensation liquid.

Calculate the content of $C_{43}H_{58}N_4O_{12}$, taking the specific absorbance to be 187.

STORAGE

Store under nitrogen in an airtight container, protected from light at a temperature not exceeding 25 °C.

IMPURITIES

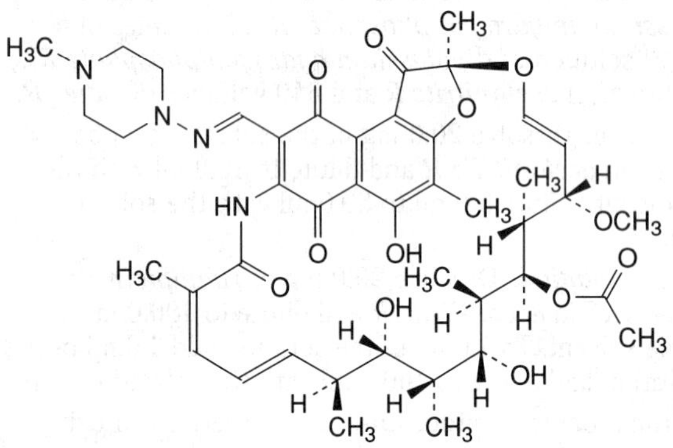

A. rifampicin quinone,

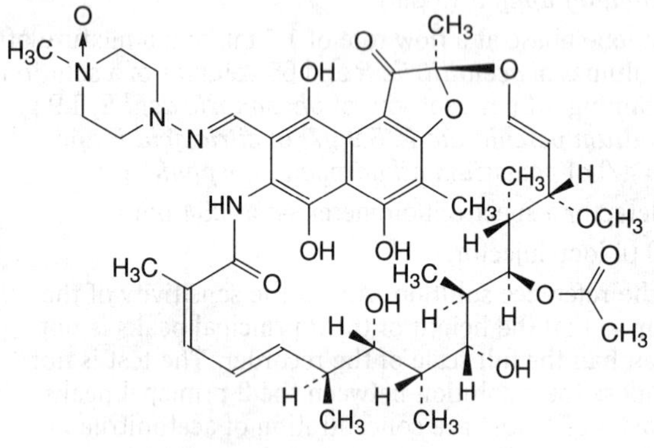

B. rifampicin *N*-oxide.

01/2005:0432

RIFAMYCIN SODIUM

Rifamycinum natricum

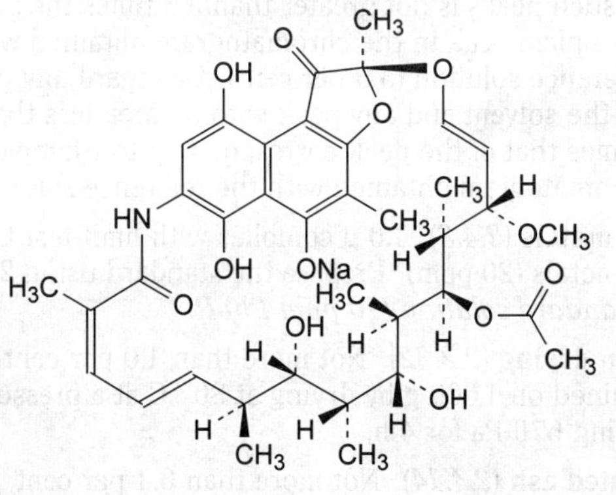

$C_{37}H_{46}NNaO_{12}$ M_r 720

DEFINITION

Rifamycin sodium is sodium (2*S*,12*Z*,14*E*,16*S*,17*S*,18*R*,19*R*,20*R*,21*S*,22*R*,23*S*,24*E*)-21-(acetyloxy)-6,9,17,19-tetrahydroxy-23-methoxy-2,4,12,16,18,20,22-heptamethyl-1,11-dioxo-1,2-dihydro-2,7-(epoxypentadeca[1,11,13]trienimino)naphtho[2,1-*b*]furan-5-olate, the monosodium salt of rifamycin SV, a substance obtained by chemical transformation of rifamycin B, which is produced during the growth of certain strains of *Amycolatopsis mediterranei*. Rifamycin SV may also be obtained directly from certain *A. mediterranei* mutants. The potency is not less than 900 IU/mg, calculated with reference to the anhydrous substance.

PRODUCTION

It is produced by methods of manufacture designed to minimise or eliminate substances lowering blood pressure. The method of manufacture is validated to demonstrate that the product if tested would comply with the following test.

Abnormal toxicity (*2.6.9*). Inject into each mouse 4 mg dissolved in 0.5 ml of *water for injections R*.

CHARACTERS

A fine or slightly granular, red powder, soluble in water, freely soluble in ethanol.

IDENTIFICATION

A. Examine by infrared absorption spectrophotometry (*2.2.24*), comparing with the spectrum obtained with *rifamycin sodium CRS*. Examine the substances as discs prepared using *potassium bromide R*.

B. It gives reaction (a) of sodium (*2.3.1*).

TESTS

pH (*2.2.3*). Dissolve 0.5 g in *carbon dioxide-free water R* and dilute to 10 ml with the same solvent. The pH is 6.5 to 8.0.

Absorbance (*2.2.25*). Dissolve 20.0 mg in 5 ml of *methanol R* and dilute to 100.0 ml with freshly prepared *phosphate buffer solution pH 7.0 R1* to which 1 g/l of *ascorbic acid R* has been added immediately before use. Dilute 5.0 ml of the solution to 50.0 ml with the same phosphate buffer solution containing ascorbic acid. Allow to stand for 30 min. The solution shows an absorption maximum at 445 nm. The specific absorbance at the maximum is 190 to 210, calculated with reference to the anhydrous substance.

Rifamycin B, rifamycin S and other related substances. Examine by liquid chromatography (*2.2.29*). *Prepare the solutions immediately before use.*

Test solution. Dissolve 50.0 mg of the substance to be examined in a mixture of equal volumes of a 3.9 g/l solution of *sodium dihydrogen phosphate R*, adjusted to pH 3.0 with *phosphoric acid R*, and *acetonitrile R* and dilute to 50.0 ml with the same mixture of solvents.

Reference solution (a). Dissolve 10.0 mg of *rifamycin B CRS* and 40.0 mg of *rifamycin S CRS* in a mixture of equal volumes of a 3.9 g/l solution of *sodium dihydrogen phosphate R*, adjusted to pH 3.0 with *phosphoric acid R*, and *acetonitrile R* and dilute to 200.0 ml with the same mixture of solvents. Dilute 5.0 ml of the solution to 50.0 ml with the same mixture of solvents.

Reference solution (b). Dissolve 25 mg of the substance to be examined and 8 mg of *rifamycin S CRS* in a mixture of equal volumes of a 3.9 g/l solution of *sodium dihydrogen phosphate R*, adjusted to pH 3.0 with *phosphoric acid R*, and *acetonitrile R* and dilute to 250.0 ml with the same mixture of solvents.

The chromatographic procedure may be carried out using:
- a stainless steel column 0.25 m long and 4.6 mm in internal diameter packed with *octadecylsilyl silica gel for chromatography R* (5 µm),
- as mobile phase at a flow rate of 1 ml/min the following solutions, prepared and maintained at a temperature not lower than 20 °C:

  Mobile phase A. Mix 10 volumes of *acetonitrile R* and 90 volumes of a 3.9 g/l solution of *sodium dihydrogen phosphate R*, adjusted to pH 7.5 with *dilute sodium hydroxide solution R*,

  Mobile phase B. Mix 70 volumes of *acetonitrile R* and 30 volumes of a 3.9 g/l solution of *sodium dihydrogen phosphate R*, adjusted to pH 7.5 with *dilute sodium hydroxide solution R*,

Time (min)	Mobile phase A (per cent *V/V*)	Mobile phase B (per cent *V/V*)	Comment
0 - 40	80 → 20	20 → 80	linear gradient
40 - 45	20	80	isocratic
45 - 47	20 → 80	80 → 20	linear gradient
47 - 55	80	20	re-equilibration

- as detector a spectrophotometer set at 254 nm,
- a 20 µl loop injector.

Inject reference solution (a). When the chromatogram is recorded in the prescribed conditions, the substances elute in the following order: rifamycin B, rifamycin SV, rifamycin S. Inject reference solution (b). Adjust the sensitivity of the system so that the height of the peak corresponding to rifamycin S in the chromatogram obtained is at least 50 per cent of the full scale of the recorder. The test is not valid unless the resolution between the peaks corresponding to rifamycin SV and rifamycin S is at least 5.0. Inject the test solution and reference solution (a). In the chromatogram obtained with the test solution: the area of any peak corresponding to rifamycin B is not greater than that of the peak due to rifamycin B in the chromatogram obtained with reference solution (a) (0.5 per cent); the area of any peak corresponding to rifamycin S is not greater than that of the peak due to rifamycin S in the chromatogram obtained with reference solution (a) (2 per cent); the sum of the areas of all the peaks, apart from the principal peak and any peaks corresponding to rifamycin B and rifamycin S, is not greater than the area of the peak corresponding to rifamycin S in the chromatogram obtained with reference solution (a) (2 per cent). Disregard any peak with an area less than 0.05 times that of the area of the peak corresponding to rifamycin S in the chromatogram obtained with reference solution (a).

Heavy metals (*2.4.8*). 2.0 g complies with limit test C for heavy metals (10 ppm). Prepare the standard using 2 ml of *lead standard solution (10 ppm Pb) R*.

Water (*2.5.12*): 12.0 per cent to 17.0 per cent, determined on 0.200 g by the semi-micro determination of water.

Bacterial endotoxins (*2.6.14*): less than 0.50 IU/mg, if intended for use in the manufacture of parenteral dosage forms without a further appropriate procedure for removal of bacterial endotoxins.

ASSAY

Carry out the microbiological assay of antibiotics (*2.7.2*).

STORAGE

Store in an airtight container, protected from light at a temperature of 2 °C to 8 °C. If the substance is sterile, store in a sterile, airtight, tamper-proof container.

LABELLING

The label states, where applicable, that the substance is free from bacterial endotoxins.

IMPURITIES

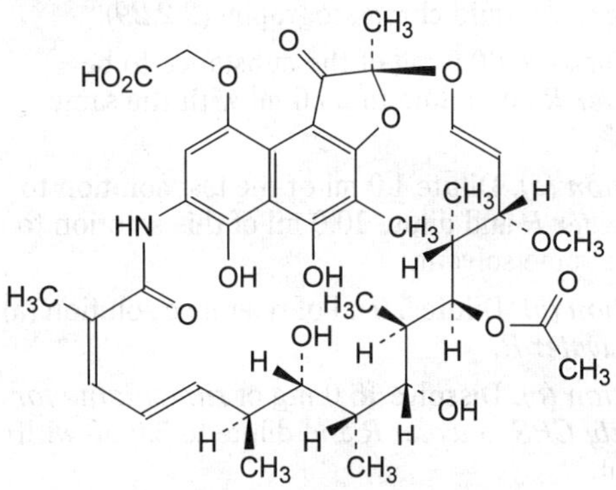

A. rifamycin B,

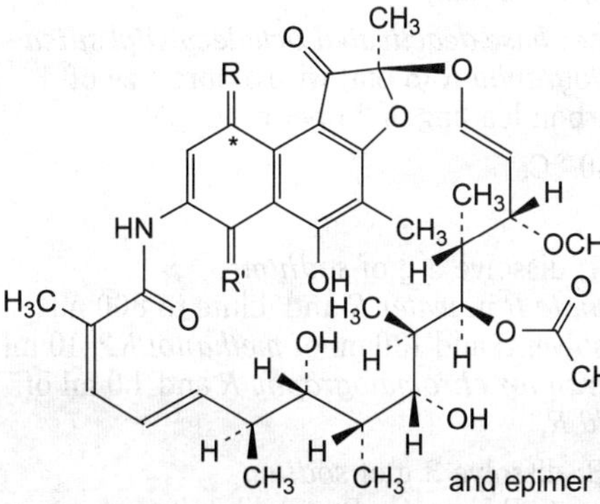

and epimer at C*

B. R = R′ = =O: rifamycin S,

C. -R- = -O-CO-CH_2-O-, R′ = =O: rifamycin O.

01/2005:2020

RILMENIDINE DIHYDROGEN PHOSPHATE

Rilmenidini dihydrogenophosphas

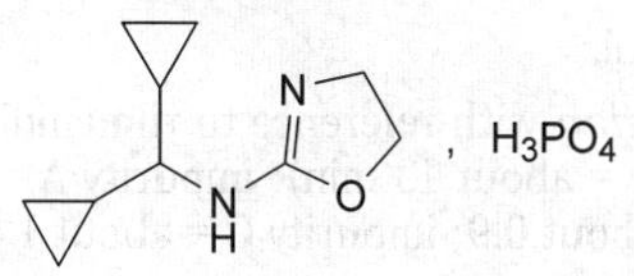

$C_{10}H_{19}N_2O_5P$ M_r 278.2

DEFINITION

N-(Dicyclopropylmethyl)-4,5-dihydro-oxazol-2-amine dihydrogen phosphate.

Content: 99.0 per cent to 101.0 per cent (dried substance).

CHARACTERS

Appearance: white or almost white powder.

Solubility: freely soluble in water, slightly soluble in alcohol, practically insoluble in methylene chloride.

IDENTIFICATION

A. Infrared absorption spectrophotometry (*2.2.24*).

Comparison: *Ph. Eur. reference spectrum of rilmenidine dihydrogen phosphate.*

B. Dissolve 10 mg in *water R* and dilute to 1 ml with the same solvent. The solution gives reaction (b) of phosphates (*2.3.1*).

TESTS

Related substances. Liquid chromatography (*2.2.29*).

Test solution. Dissolve 60.0 mg of the substance to be examined in *water R* and dilute to 20.0 ml with the same solvent.

Reference solution (a). Dilute 1.0 ml of the test solution to 100.0 ml with *water R* and dilute 10.0 ml of this solution to 50.0 ml with the same solvent.

Reference solution (b). Dilute 5.0 ml of reference solution (a) to 20.0 ml with *water R.*

Reference solution (c). Dissolve 15.0 mg of *rilmenidine for system suitability CRS* in *water R* and dilute to 5.0 ml with the same solvent.

Column:

- *size*: l = 0.15 m, Ø = 3 mm,
- *stationary phase*: *base-deactivated octadecylsilyl silica gel for chromatography R* (5 μm) with a pore size of 10 nm and a carbon loading of 25 per cent,
- *temperature*: 40 °C.

Mobile phase:

- *mobile phase A*: dissolve 3 g of *sodium heptanesulphonate R* in *water R* and dilute to 860 ml with the same solvent; add 130 ml of *methanol R2,* 10 ml of *tetrahydrofuran for chromatography R* and 1.0 ml of *phosphoric acid R,*
- *mobile phase B*: dissolve 3 g of *sodium heptanesulphonate R* in *water R* and dilute to 600 ml with the same solvent; add 350 ml of *acetonitrile for chromatography R,* 50 ml of *tetrahydrofuran for chromatography R* and 1.0 ml of *phosphoric acid R,*

Time (min)	Mobile phase A (per cent *V/V*)	Mobile phase B (per cent *V/V*)
0 - 14	100 → 0	0 → 100
14 - 15	0 → 100	100 → 0
15 - 30	100	0

Flow rate: 1 ml/min.

Detection: spectrophotometer at 205 nm.

Injection: 20 μl.

Relative retention with reference to rilmenidine (retention time = about 13 min): impurity A = about 0.6; impurity B = about 0.9; impurity C = about 1.4.

With these conditions the inflexion of the baseline, corresponding to the beginning of the gradient, appears on the recorder after a minimum time t of 5 min. If this is not the case (t < 5 min) modify the chromatographic sequence by adding an isocratic elution with 100 per cent of mobile phase A for a time corresponding to (5-t) min before the linear gradient.

System suitability: reference solution (c):

- *peak-to-valley ratio*: minimum 3, where H_p = height above the baseline of the peak due to impurity B and H_v = height above the baseline of the lowest point of the curve separating this peak from the peak due to rilmenidine.

Limits:

- *any impurity*: not more than 0.5 times the area of the principal peak in the chromatogram obtained with reference solution (a) (0.1 per cent),
- *total*: not more than the area of the principal peak in the chromatogram obtained with reference solution (a) (0.2 per cent),
- *disregard limit*: area of the principal peak in the chromatogram obtained with reference solution (b) (0.05 per cent).

Loss on drying (*2.2.32*): maximum 0.5 per cent, determined on 1.000 g by drying in an oven *in vacuo* at 50 °C over *diphosphorus pentoxide R* for 2 h.

ASSAY

Dissolve 0.200 g in 50 ml of *anhydrous acetic acid R.* Titrate with *0.1 M perchloric acid,* determining the end-point potentiometrically (*2.2.20*).

1 ml of *0.1 M perchloric acid* is equivalent to 27.82 mg of $C_{10}H_{19}N_2O_5P$.

IMPURITIES

Specified impurities: A, B, C.

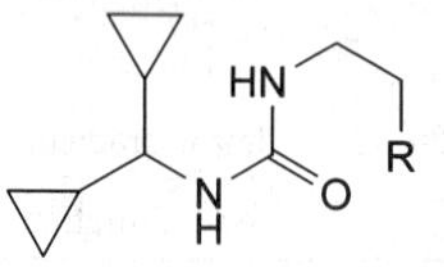

A. R = OH: 1-(dicyclopropylmethyl)-3-(2-hydroxyethyl)urea,

B. R = Cl: 1-(2-chloroethyl)-3-(dicyclopropylmethyl)urea,

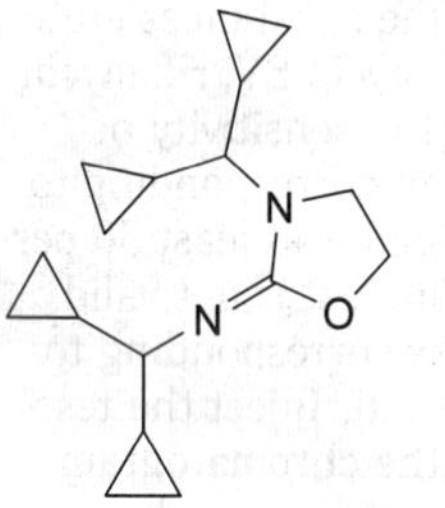

C. *N*,3-bis(dicyclopropylmethyl)oxazolidin-2-imine.

01/2005:1559

RISPERIDONE

Risperidonum

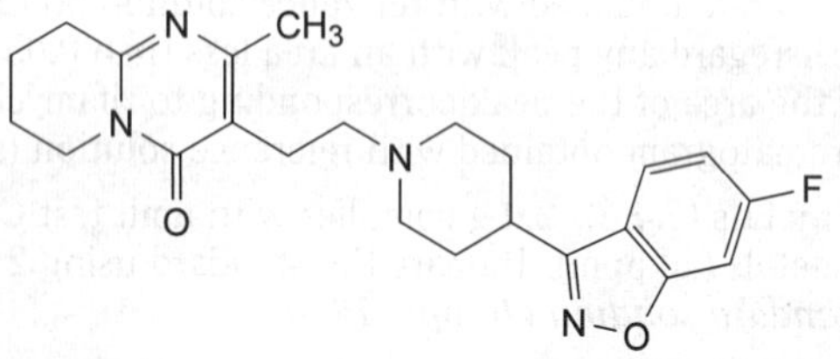

$C_{23}H_{27}FN_4O_2$ M_r 410.5

DEFINITION

3-[2-[4-(6-Fluoro-1,2-benzisoxazol-3-yl)piperidin-1-yl]ethyl]-2-methyl-6,7,8,9-tetrahydro-4*H*-pyrido[1,2-*a*]pyrimidin-4-one.

Content: 99.0 per cent to 101.0 per cent (dried substance).

CHARACTERS

Appearance: white or almost white powder.

Solubility: practically insoluble in water, freely soluble in methylene chloride, sparingly soluble in ethanol (96 per cent). It dissolves in dilute acid solutions.

It shows polymorphism.

IDENTIFICATION

Infrared absorption spectrophotometry (*2.2.24*).

Preparation: discs.

Comparison: *risperidone CRS.*

If the spectra obtained show differences, dissolve the substance to be examined and the reference substance separately in *acetone R*, evaporate to dryness and record new spectra using the residues.

TESTS

Appearance of solution. The solution is clear (*2.2.1*) and colourless (*2.2.2, Method II*).

Dissolve 0.1 g in a 7.5 g/l solution of *tartaric acid R* and dilute to 100 ml with the same acid solution.

Related substances. Liquid chromatography (*2.2.29*).

Test solution. Dissolve 0.100 g of the substance to be examined in *methanol R* and dilute to 10.0 ml with the same solvent.

Reference solution (a). Dissolve 10 mg of *risperidone for system suitability CRS* (containing impurities A, B, C, D and E) in *methanol R* and dilute to 1.0 ml with the same solvent.

Reference solution (b). Dilute 1.0 ml of the test solution to 100.0 ml with *methanol R*. Dilute 5.0 ml of this solution to 25.0 ml with *methanol R*.

Column:

- *size*: l = 0.10 m, Ø = 4.6 mm,
- *stationary phase*: *base-deactivated octadecylsilyl silica gel for chromatography R* (3 µm).

Mobile phase:

- *mobile phase A*: 5 g/l solution of *ammonium acetate R*,
- *mobile phase B*: *methanol R*,

Time (min)	Mobile phase A (per cent *V/V*)	Mobile phase B (per cent *V/V*)
0 - 2	70	30
2 - 17	70 → 30	30 → 70
17 - 22	30	70
22 - 23	30 → 70	70 → 30
23 - 27	70	30

Flow rate: 1.5 ml/min.

Detection: spectrophotometer at 260 nm.

Injection: 10 µl.

Relative retention with reference to risperidone (retention time = about 12 min): impurity A = about 0.69; impurity B = about 0.75; impurity C = about 0.81; impurity D = about 0.94; impurity H = about 0.96; impurity G = about 1.04; impurity E = about 1.12; impurity F = about 1.32; impurity I = about 1.60.

System suitability: reference solution (a):

- *peak-to-valley ratio*: minimum 1.5, where H_p = height above the baseline of the peak due to impurity D and H_v = height above the baseline of the lowest point of the curve separating this peak from the peak due to risperidone,
- the chromatogram obtained is similar to the chromatogram supplied with *risperidone for system suitability CRS.*

Limits:

- *impurities A, B, C, D, E*: for each impurity, not more than the area of the principal peak in the chromatogram obtained with reference solution (b) (0.2 per cent),
- *any other impurity*: for each impurity, not more than 0.5 times the area of the principal peak in the chromatogram obtained with reference solution (b) (0.1 per cent),
- *total*: not more than 1.5 times the area of the principal peak in the chromatogram obtained with reference solution (b) (0.3 per cent),
- *disregard limit*: 0.25 times the area of the principal peak in the chromatogram obtained with reference solution (b) (0.05 per cent).

Loss on drying (*2.2.32*): maximum 0.5 per cent, determined on 1.000 g by drying in an oven at 100-105 °C for 4 h.

Sulphated ash (*2.4.14*): maximum 0.1 per cent, determined on 1.0 g in a platinum crucible.

ASSAY

Dissolve 0.160 g in 70 ml of a mixture of 1 volume of *anhydrous acetic acid R* and 7 volumes of *methyl ethyl ketone R* and titrate with *0.1 M perchloric acid.* Determine the end-point potentiometrically (*2.2.20*).

1 ml of *0.1 M perchloric acid* is equivalent to 20.53 mg of $C_{23}H_{27}FN_4O_2$.

STORAGE

Protected from light.

IMPURITIES

Specified impurities: A, B, C, D, E.

Other detectable impurities: F, G, H, I.

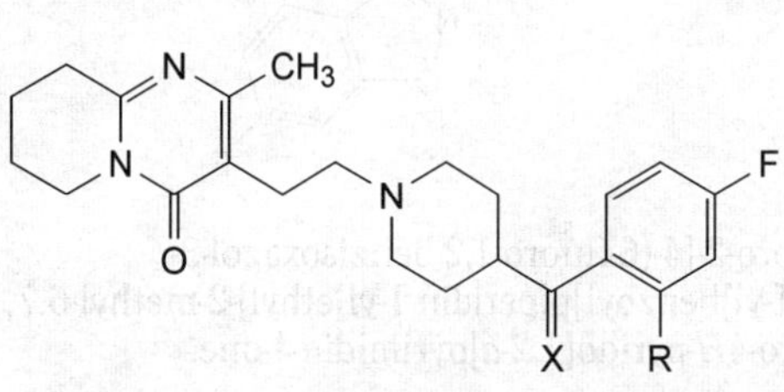

A. R = F, X = N-OH: 3-[2-[4-[(*E*)-(2,4-difluorophenyl)(hydroxyimino)methyl]piperidin-1-yl]ethyl]-2-methyl-6,7,8,9-tetrahydro-4*H*-pyrido[1,2-*a*]pyrimidin-4-one,

B. R = F, X = N-OH: 3-[2-[4-[(*Z*)-(2,4-difluorophenyl)(hydroxyimino)methyl]piperidin-1-yl]ethyl]-2-methyl-6,7,8,9-tetrahydro-4*H*-pyrido[1,2-*a*]pyrimidin-4-one,

G. R = OH, X = O: 3-[2-[4-(4-fluoro-2-hydroxybenzoyl)piperidin-1-yl]ethyl]-2-methyl-6,7,8,9-tetrahydro-4*H*-pyrido[1,2-*a*]pyrimidin-4-one,

H. R = F, X = O: 3-[2-[4-(2,4-difluorobenzoyl)piperidin-1-yl]ethyl]-2-methyl-6,7,8,9-tetrahydro-4*H*-pyrido[1,2-*a*]pyrimidin-4-one,

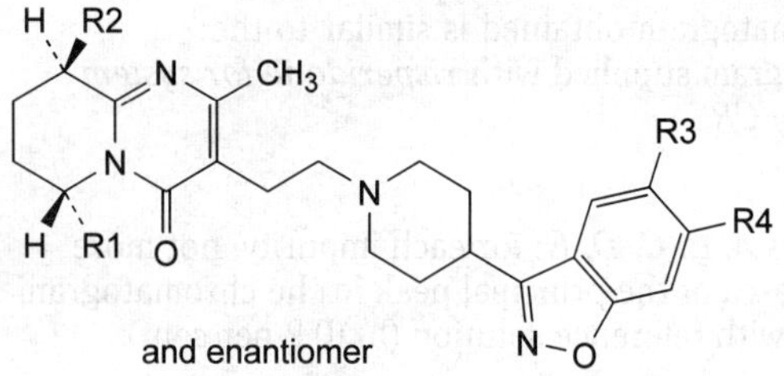

C. R1 = R3 = H, R2 = OH, R4 = F: (9*RS*)-3-[2-[4-(6-fluoro-1,2-benzisoxazol-3-yl)piperidin-1-yl]ethyl]-9-hydroxy-2-methyl-6,7,8,9-tetrahydro-4*H*-pyrido[1,2-*a*]pyrimidin-4-one,

D. R1 = R2 = R4 = H, R3 = F: 3-[2-[4-(5-fluoro-1,2-benzisoxazol-3-yl)piperidin-1-yl]ethyl]-2-methyl-6,7,8,9-tetrahydro-4*H*-pyrido[1,2-*a*]pyrimidin-4-one,

E. R1 = CH_3, R2 = R3 = H, R4 = F: (6*RS*)-3-[2-[4-(6-fluoro-1,2-benzisoxazol-3-yl)piperidin-1-yl]ethyl]-2,6-dimethyl-6,7,8,9-tetrahydro-4*H*-pyrido[1,2-*a*]pyrimidin-4-one,

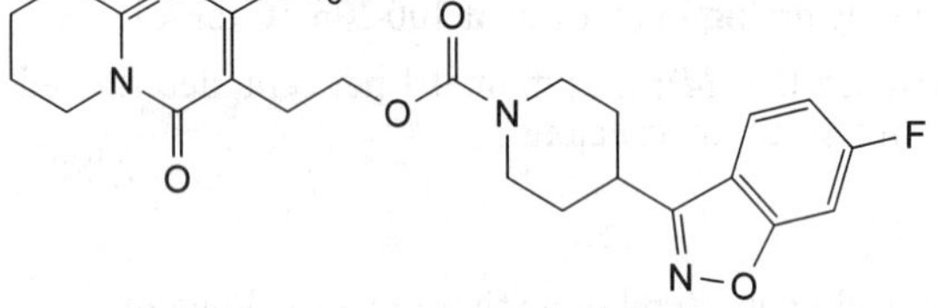

F. 2-[2-methyl-4-oxo-6,7,8,9-tetrahydro-4*H*-pyrido[1,2-*a*]pyrimidin-3-yl]ethyl 4-(6-fluoro-1,2-benzisoxazol-3-yl)piperidin-1-carboxylate,

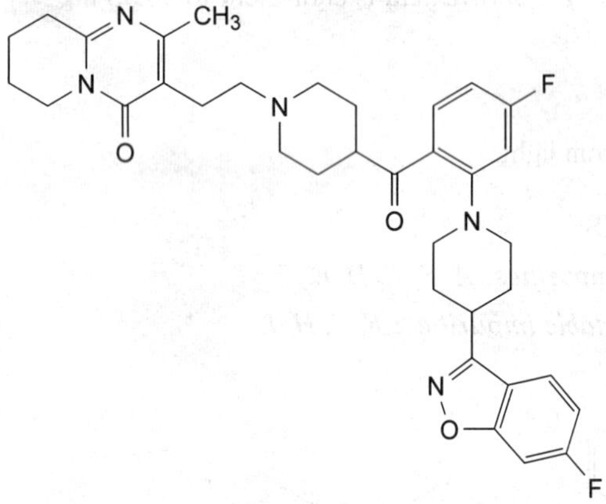

I. 3-[2-[4-[4-fluoro-2-[4-(6-fluoro-1,2-benzisoxazol-3-yl)piperidin-1-yl]benzoyl]piperidin-1-yl]ethyl]-2-methyl-6,7,8,9-tetrahydro-4*H*-pyrido[1,2-*a*]pyrimidin-4-one.

01/2005:1623

ROSELLE

Hibisci sabdariffae flos

DEFINITION

Whole or cut dried calyces and epicalyces of *Hibiscus sabdariffa* L. collected during fruiting.

Content: minimum 13.5 per cent of acids, expressed as citric acid ($C_6H_8O_7$; M_r 192.1) (dried drug).

CHARACTERS

Acidic taste.

Macroscopic and microscopic characters described under identification tests A and B.

IDENTIFICATION

A. The calyx is joined in the lower half to form an urceolate structure, the upper half dividing to form 5 long acuminate recurved tips. The tips have a prominent, slightly protruding midrib and a large, thick nectary gland about 1 mm in diameter. The epicalyx consist of 8 to 12 small, obovate leaflets which are adnate to the base of the calyx. The calyx and epicalyx are fleshy, dry, easily fragmented and coloured bright-red to deep-purple, somewhat lighter at the base of the inner side.

B. Reduce to a powder (355). The powder is red to purplish-red. Examine under a microscope using *chloral hydrate solution R*. The powder shows predominantly red coloured fragments of the parenchyme containing numerous crystal clusters of calcium oxalate and, sporadically, mucilage filled cavities, sometimes associated with polygonal epidermal cells and anisocytic stomata (*2.8.3*); numerous fragments of vascular bundles with spiral and reticulate vessels; sclerenchymatous fibres with a wide lumen; rarely, rectangular, pitted parenchymatous cells; fragments of unicellular, smooth, bent covering trichomes and occasional glandular trichomes; rounded pollen grains with spiny exine.

C. Thin-layer chromatography (*2.2.27*).

Test solution. To 1.0 g of the powdered drug (355) add 10 ml of *alcohol (60 per cent) V/V R*. Shake for 15 min and filter.

Reference solution. Dissolve 2.5 mg of *quinaldine red R* in 10 ml of *alcohol R*.

Plate: *TLC silica gel plate R*.

Mobile phase: *acetic acid R, water R, butanol R* (15:30:60 *V/V/V*).

Application: 20 µl, as bands.

Development: over a path of 10 cm.

Drying: in air.

Detection: examine in daylight.

Results: see below the sequence of the zones present in the chromatograms obtained with the reference and test solutions.

Top of the plate	
Quinaldine red: an orange red zone	
	A pale violet zone
	A violet-blue zone
	A violet-blue zone
	A violet-blue zone
Reference solution	**Test solution**

TESTS

Foreign matter (*2.8.2*): maximum 2 per cent of fragments of fruits: red funicles and parts of the 5 caverned capsule with yellowish-grey pericarp, whose thin walls consist of several layers of differently directed fibres; flattened, reniform seeds with a dotted surface.

Loss on drying (*2.2.32*): maximum 11.0 per cent, determined on 1.000 g of the powdered drug (355) by drying in an oven at 100-105 °C for 2 h.

Total ash (*2.4.16*): maximum 10.0 per cent.

Colouring power: reduce the drug to a coarse powder (1400) and mix 100 g of drug. Reduce about 10 g of this mixture to a powder (355). To 1.0 g of the powdered drug (355) add 25 ml of boiling *water R* in a 100 ml flask and heat for 15 min on a water-bath with frequent shaking. Filter the hot mixture into a 50 ml graduated flask; rinse successively the 100 ml flask and the filter 3 times with 5 ml of warm *water R*. After cooling dilute to 50 ml with *water R*.

Dilute 5 ml of this solution to 50 ml with *water R*. Measure the absorbance (*2.2.25*) at 520 nm using *water R* as the compensation liquid. The absorbance is not less than 0.350 for the whole drug and not less than 0.250 for the cut drug.

ASSAY

Shake 1.000 g of the powdered drug (355) with 100 ml of *carbon dioxide free water R* for 15 min. Filter. To 50.0 ml of the filtrate add 100 ml of *carbon dioxide free water R*. Titrate with *0.1 M sodium hydroxide* until pH 7.0, determining the end-point potentiometrically (*2.2.20*).

1 ml of *0.1 M sodium hydroxide* is equivalent to 6.4 mg of citric acid.

01/2005:1560

ROSEMARY LEAF

Rosmarini folium

DEFINITION

Whole, dried leaf of *Rosmarinus officinalis* L.

Content:

– minimum 12 ml/kg of essential oil (anhydrous drug),
– minimum 3 per cent of total hydroxycinnamic derivatives, expressed as rosmarinic acid ($C_{18}H_{16}O_8$; M_r 360) (anhydrous drug).

CHARACTERS

Strongly aromatic odour.

Macroscopic and microscopic characters described under identification tests A and B.

IDENTIFICATION

A. The leaves are sessile, tough, linear to linear-lanceolate, 1 cm to 4 cm long and 2 mm to 4 mm wide, with recurved edges. The upper surface is dark green, glabrous and grainy, the lower surface is greyish-green and densely tomentose with a prominent midrib.

B. Reduce to a powder (355). The powder is greyish-green to yellowish-green. Examine under a microscope using *chloral hydrate solution R*. The powder shows fragments of lower epidermis with straight to sinuous-walled cells and numerous diacytic stomata (*2.8.3*); fragments of the upper epidermis with straight-walled cells, slightly thickened and pitted, and an underlying hypodermis composed of large, irregular cells with thickened and beaded anticlinal walls; fragments in sectional view showing the hypodermal cells extending across the lamina at intervals, separating the one or two-layered palisade into large, crescent-shaped areas; numerous multicellular, extensively branched, covering trichomes of the lower epidermis and rare conical covering trichomes of the upper epidermis; glandular trichomes of 2 types, the majority with a short, unicellular stalk and a radiate head composed of 8 cells, others, less abundant, with a unicellular stalk and a spherical, unicellular or bicellular head.

C. Thin-layer chromatography (*2.2.27*).

*Test solution.*Dissolve 20 µl of the oil obtained in the assay in 1 ml of *hexane R*.

Reference solution. Dissolve 5 mg of *borneol R*, 5 mg of *bornyl acetate R* and 10 µl of *cineole R* in 1 ml of *hexane R*.

Plate: *TLC silica gel G plate R.*

Mobile phase: *ethyl acetate R, toluene R* (5:95 *V/V*).

Application: 10 µl, as bands.

Development: over a path of 15 cm.

Drying: in air.

Detection: spray with *anisaldehyde solution R.* Heat at 100-105 °C for 10 min. Examine in daylight.

Results: see below the sequence of the zones present in the chromatograms obtained with the reference solution and the test solution.

Top of the plate	
	A red zone
Bornyl acetate: a yellowish-brown zone	A yellowish-brown zone of low intensity
	A coloured zone of low intensity
Cineole: a violet zone	A violet zone
	Coloured zones of low intensity
Borneol: a violet-brown zone	A violet-brown zone
	A coloured zone of low intensity
Reference solution	**Test solution**

D. Thin-layer chromatography (*2.2.27*).

Test solution. Grind 1.0 g of the drug in 10 ml of *methanol R* and filter.

Reference solution. Dissolve 5.0 mg of *rosmarinic acid R* and 1.0 mg of *caffeic acid R* in 10 ml of *methanol R.*

Plate: *TLC silica gel plate R.*

Mobile phase: *anhydrous formic acid R, acetone R, methylene chloride R* (8.5:25:85 *V/V/V*).

Application: 10 µl of the test solution and 20 µl of the reference solution, as bands.

Development: over a path of 8 cm.

Drying: in air.

Detection: examine in ultraviolet light at 365 nm.

Results: see below the sequence of the zones present in the chromatograms obtained with the reference solution and the test solution.

Top of the plate	
	A pink fluorescent zone
Caffeic acid: a light blue fluorescent zone	A blue fluorescent zone of low intensity
Rosmarinic acid: a light blue fluorescent zone	An intense light blue fluorescent zone
Reference solution	**Test solution**

TESTS

Foreign matter (*2.8.2*): maximum 5 per cent of stems and maximum 2 per cent of other foreign matter.

Water (*2.2.13*): maximum 100 ml/kg, determined on 20.0 g of the powdered drug (355).

Total ash (*2.4.16*): maximum 9.0 per cent.

ASSAY

Total hydroxycinnamic derivatives

Stock solution. To 0.200 g of the powdered drug (355) add 80 ml of *alcohol (50 per cent V/V) R*. Boil in a water-bath under a reflux condenser for 30 min. Allow to cool and filter. Rinse the filter with 10 ml of *alcohol (50 per cent V/V) R.* Combine the filtrate and the rinsings in a volumetric flask and dilute to 100.0 ml with *alcohol (50 per cent V/V) R.*

Monographs Q-S

Test solution. To 1.0 ml of the stock solution add 2 ml of *0.5 M hydrochloric acid,* 2 ml of a solution prepared by dissolving 10 g of *sodium nitrite R* and 10 g of *sodium molybdate R* in 100 ml of *water R* and then add 2 ml of *dilute sodium hydroxide solution R* and dilute to 10.0 ml with *water R*; mix.

Compensation solution. Dilute 1.0 ml of the stock solution to 10.0 ml with *water R.*

Measure immediately the absorbance (*2.2.25*) of the test solution at 505 nm.

Calculate the percentage content of total hydroxycinnamic derivatives, expressed as rosmarinic acid, from the expression:

$$\frac{A \times 2.5}{m}$$

i.e. taking the specific absorbance of rosmarinic acid to be 400.

A = absorbance of the test solution at 505 nm,

m = mass of the substance to be examined, in grams.

Essential oil (*2.8.12*). Use 25.0 g of the crushed drug, a 1000 ml flask and 300 ml of *water R* as the distillation liquid. Distil at a rate of 2-3 ml/min for 3 h.

01/2005:1846

ROSEMARY OIL

Rosmarini aetheroleum

DEFINITION

Essential oil obtained by steam distillation from the flowering aerial parts of *Rosmarinus officinalis* L.

CHARACTERS

Appearance: clear, mobile, colourless to pale yellow liquid with a characteristic odour.

IDENTIFICATION

First identification: B.

Second identification: A.

A. Thin-layer chromatography (*2.2.27*).

Test solution. Dissolve 0.5 ml of the substance to be examined in *toluene R* and dilute to 10 ml with the same solvent.

Reference solution. Dissolve 50 mg of *borneol R,* 50 mg of *bornyl acetate R* and 100 µl of *cineole R* in *toluene R* and dilute to 10 ml with the same solvent.

Plate: *TLC silica gel plate R.*

Mobile phase: *ethyl acetate R, toluene R* (5:95 *V/V*).

Application: 10 µl, as bands.

Development: over a path of 15 cm.

Drying: in air.

Detection: spray the plate with *vanillin reagent R* and heat the plate at 100-105 °C for 10 min. Examine immediately in daylight.

Results: see below the sequence of the zones present in the chromatograms obtained with the reference solution and the test solution. Furthermore, several violet-blue to violet-grey zones of medium intensity (terpene alcohols) are present in the lower third of the chromatogram obtained with the test solution.

Top of the plate	
	An intense violet zone
	A violet-grey zone
———	———
Bornyl acetate: a bluish-grey zone of low intensity	A bluish-grey zone of low intensity (bornyl acetate)
	A violet-pink zone
———	———
Cineole: an intense blue zone	An intense blue zone (cineole)
Borneol: a violet-blue zone of medium intensity	A violet -blue zone of medium intensity (borneol)
Reference solution	**Test solution**

B. Examine the chromatograms obtained in the test for chromatographic profile.

Results: the characteristic peaks in the chromatogram obtained with the test solution are similar in retention time to those in the chromatogram obtained with the reference solution.

TESTS

Relative density (*2.2.5*): 0.895 to 0.920.

Refractive index (*2.2.6*): 1.464 to 1.473.

Optical rotation (*2.2.7*): −5° to + 8°.

Acid value (*2.5.1*): maximum 1.0.

Chromatographic profile. Gas chromatography (*2.2.28*): use the normalisation procedure.

Test solution. Dissolve 0.20 ml of the substance to be examined in *hexane R* and dilute to 10.0 ml with the same solvent.

Reference solution. Dissolve 20 µl of *α-pinene R,* 10 mg of *camphene R,* 20 µl of *β-pinene R,* 10 µl of *β-myrcene R,* 20 µl of *limonene R,* 50 µl of *cineole R,* 10 µl of *p-cymene R,* 50 mg of *camphor R,* 30 mg of *bornyl acetate R,* 10 mg of *α-terpineol R,* 10 mg of *borneol R* and 10 µl of *verbenone R* in *hexane R* and dilute to 10.0 ml with the same solvent.

Column:

– *material*: fused silica,
– *size*: *l* = 30 m (a film thickness of 1 µm may be used) to 60 m (a film thickness of 0.2 µm may be used), Ø = 0.25-0.53 mm,
– *stationary phase*: *macrogol 20 000 R.*

Carrier gas: *helium for chromatography R.*

Flow rate: 1 ml/min.

Split ratio: 1:50.

Temperature:

	Time (min)	Temperature (°C)
Column	0 - 10	50
	10 - 85	50 → 200
	85 - 110	200
Injection port		200
Detector		250

Detection: flame ionisation.

Injection: 1 µl.

Elution order: order indicated in the composition of the reference solution. Record the retention times of these substances.

Monographs Q-S

System suitability: reference solution:

- *resolution*: minimum 1.5 between the peaks due to limonene and cineole and minimum 1.5 between the peaks due to α-terpineol and borneol.

Using the retention times determined from the chromatogram obtained with the reference solution, locate the components of the reference solution in the chromatogram obtained with the test solution.

Determine the percentage content of these components.

For rosemary oil, Spanish type, the percentages are within the following ranges:

- *α-pinene*: 18 per cent to 26 per cent,
- *camphene*: 8.0 per cent to 12.0 per cent,
- *β-pinene*: 2.0 per cent to 6.0 per cent,
- *β-myrcene*: 1.5 per cent to 5.0 per cent,
- *limonene*: 2.5 per cent to 5.0 per cent,
- *cineole*: 16.0 per cent to 25.0 per cent,
- *p-cymene*: 1.0 per cent to 2.2 per cent,
- *camphor*: 13.0 per cent to 21.0 per cent,
- *bornyl acetate*: 0.5 per cent to 2.5 per cent,
- *α-terpineol*: 1.0 per cent to 3.5 per cent,
- *borneol*: 2.0 per cent to 4.5 per cent,
- *verbenone*: 0.7 per cent to 2.5 per cent.

For rosemary oil, Moroccan and Tunisian type, the percentages are within the following ranges:

- *α-pinene*: 9.0 per cent to 14.0 per cent,
- *camphene*: 2.5 per cent to 6.0 per cent,
- *β-pinene*: 4.0 per cent to 9.0 per cent,
- *β-myrcene*: 1.0 per cent to 2.0 per cent,
- *limonene*: 1.5 per cent to 4.0 per cent,
- *cineole*: 38.0 per cent to 55.0 per cent,
- *p-cymene*: 0.8 per cent to 2.5 per cent,
- *camphor*: 5.0 per cent to 15.0 per cent,
- *bornyl acetate*: 0.1 per cent to 1.5 per cent,
- *α-terpineol*: 1.0 per cent to 2.6 per cent,
- *borneol*: 1.5 per cent to 5.0 per cent,
- *verbenone*: maximum 0.4 per cent.

STORAGE

In a well-filled, airtight container, protected from light, at a temperature not exceeding 25 °C.

LABELLING

The label states that the content is Spanish type or Moroccan and Tunisian type.

01/2005:1146

ROXITHROMYCIN

Roxithromycinum

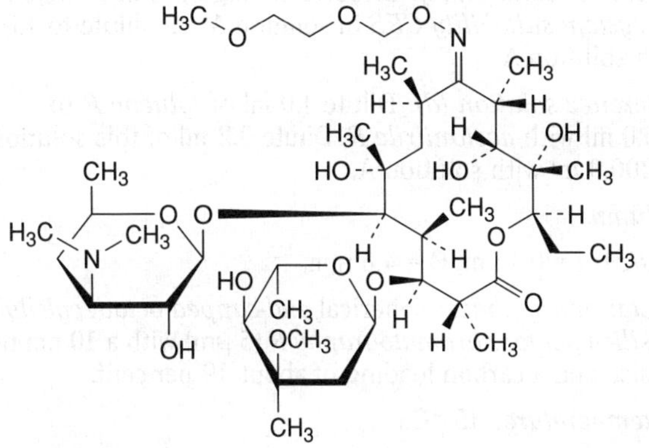

$C_{41}H_{76}N_2O_{15}$ M_r 837

DEFINITION

(3*R*,4*S*,5*S*,6*R*,7*R*,9*R*,11*S*,12*R*,13*S*,14*R*)-4-[(2,6-Dideoxy-3-*C*-methyl-3-*O*-methyl-α-L-*ribo*-hexopyranosyl)oxy]-14-ethyl-7,12,13-trihydroxy-10-[(*E*)-[(2-methoxyethoxy)methoxy]imino]-3,5,7,9,11,13-hexamethyl-6-[[3,4,6-trideoxy-3-(dimethylamino)-β-D-*xylo*-hexopyranosyl]oxy]oxacyclotetradecan-2-one (erythromycin 9-(*E*)-[*O*-[(2-methoxyethoxy)methyl]oxime]).

Content: 96.0 per cent to 102.0 per cent (anhydrous substance).

CHARACTERS

Appearance: white, crystalline powder.

Solubility: very slightly soluble in water, freely soluble in acetone, in alcohol and in methylene chloride. It is slightly soluble in dilute hydrochloric acid.

It shows polymorphism.

IDENTIFICATION

A. Infrared absorption spectrophotometry (*2.2.24*).

Comparison: *roxithromycin CRS.*

If the spectra obtained shows differences, prepare further spectra using 90 g/l solutions in *methylene chloride R*.

B. Examine the chromatograms obtained in the assay.

Results: the principal peak in the chromatogram obtained with the test solution is similar in retention time and size to the principal peak in the chromatogram obtained with reference solution (a).

TESTS

Appearance of solution. The solution is clear (*2.2.1*) and colourless (*2.2.2, Method II*).

Dissolve 0.2 g in *methanol R* and dilute to 20 ml with the same solvent.

Specific optical rotation (*2.2.7*): − 93 to − 96 (anhydrous substance).

Dissolve 0.500 g in *acetone R* and dilute to 50.0 ml with the same solvent.

Related substances. Liquid chromatography (*2.2.29*).

Solution A. Mix 30 volumes of *acetonitrile R* and 70 volumes of a 48.6 g/l solution of *ammonium dihydrogen phosphate R*, adjusted to pH 5.3 with *dilute sodium hydroxide solution R.*

Test solution. Dissolve 50.0 mg of the substance to be examined in solution A and dilute to 25.0 ml with solution A.

Reference solution (a). Dissolve 50.0 mg of *roxithromycin CRS* in solution A and dilute to 25.0 ml with solution A.

Reference solution (b). Dilute 1.0 ml of reference solution (a) to 100.0 ml with solution A.

Reference solution (c). Dissolve 2.0 mg of *roxithromycin for system suitability CRS* in solution A and dilute to 1.0 ml with solution A.

Reference solution (d). Dilute 1.0 ml of *toluene R* to 100.0 ml with *acetonitrile R*. Dilute 0.2 ml of this solution to 200.0 ml with solution A.

Column:

- *size*: l = 0.15 m, Ø = 4.6 mm,
- *stationary phase*: spherical *end-capped octadecylsilyl silica gel for chromatography R* (5 µm) with a 10 nm pore size and a carbon loading of about 19 per cent,
- *temperature*: 15 °C.

Mobile phase:

- *mobile phase A*: mix 26 volumes of *acetonitrile R* and 74 volumes of a 59.7 g/l solution of *ammonium dihydrogen phosphate R*, adjusted to pH 4.3 with *dilute sodium hydroxide solution R*,
- *mobile phase B*: *water R*, *acetonitrile R* (30:70 *V/V*),

Time (min)	Mobile phase A (per cent *V/V*)	Mobile phase B (per cent *V/V*)
0 - 50	100	0
50 - 51	100 → 90	0 → 10
51 - 80	90	10
80 - 81	90 → 100	10 → 0
81 - 100	100	0

Flow rate: 1.1 ml/min.

Detection: spectrophotometer at 205 nm.

Injection: 20 µl, using an injector maintained at 8 °C, of the test solution and reference solutions (b), (c) and (d).

Relative retention with reference to roxithromycin (retention time = about 22 min): impurity A = about 0.28; impurity B = about 0.31; impurity C = about 0.33; impurity D = about 0.62; impurity E = about 0.67; impurity F = about 0.83; impurity G = about 1.15; impurity K = about 1.7; impurity H = about 1.85; impurity J = about 2.65; impurity I = about 3.1.

System suitability: reference solution (c):

- *peak-to-valley ratio*: minimum 2.0, where H_p = height above the baseline of the peak due to impurity G and H_v = height above the baseline of the lowest point of the curve separating this peak from the peak due to roxithromycin.

Limits:

- *impurity G*: not more than the area of the principal peak in the chromatogram obtained with reference solution (b) (1.0 per cent),
- *impurities A, B, C, D, E, F, H, I, J*: for each impurity, not more than 0.5 times the area of the principal peak in the chromatogram obtained with reference solution (b) (0.5 per cent),
- *total*: not more than 3 times the area of the principal peak in the chromatogram obtained with reference solution (b) (3.0 per cent),
- *disregard limit*: 0.05 times the area of the principal peak in the chromatogram obtained with reference solution (b) (0.05 per cent). Disregard any peak due to toluene (use reference solution (d) to identify it).

Heavy metals (*2.4.8*): maximum 10 ppm.

Dissolve 2.0 g in a mixture of 15 volumes of *water R* and 85 volumes of *acetone R* and dilute to 20 ml with the same mixture of solvents. 12 ml of the solution complies with the limit test B. Prepare the standard using lead standard solution (1 ppm Pb) obtained by diluting *lead standard solution (100 ppm Pb) R* with a mixture of 15 volumes of *water R* and 85 volumes of *acetone R*.

Water (*2.5.12*): maximum 3.0 per cent, determined on 0.200 g.

Sulphated ash (*2.4.14*): maximum 0.1 per cent, determined on 1.0 g.

ASSAY

Liquid chromatography (*2.2.29*) as described in the test for related substances, with the following modifications.

Column:

- *size*: l = 0.25 m.

Mobile phase: mix 307 volumes of *acetonitrile R* and 693 volumes of a 49.1 g/l solution of *ammonium dihydrogen phosphate R* adjusted to pH 5.3 with *dilute sodium hydroxide solution R*.

Flow rate: 1.5 ml/min.

Injection: test solution and reference solutions (a) and (c).

Retention time: roxithromycin = about 12 min.

System suitability: reference solution (c):

- *peak-to-valley ratio*: minimum 1.5, where H_p = height above the baseline of the peak due to impurity G and H_v = height above the baseline of the lowest point of the curve separating this peak from the peak due to roxithromycin.

STORAGE

In an airtight container.

IMPURITIES

Specified impurities: A, B, C, D, E, F, G, H, I, J.

Other detectable impurities: K.

A. (3*R*,4*S*,5*S*,6*R*,7*R*,9*R*,11*R*,12*R*,13*S*,14*R*)-4-[(2,6-dideoxy-3-*C*-methyl-3-*O*-methyl-α-L-*ribo*-hexopyranosyl)oxy]-14-ethyl-7,12,13-trihydroxy-3,5,7,9,11,13-hexamethyl-6-[[3,4,6-trideoxy-3-(dimethylamino)-β-D-*xylo*-hexopyranosyl]oxy]oxacyclotetradecane-2,10-dione (erythromycin A),

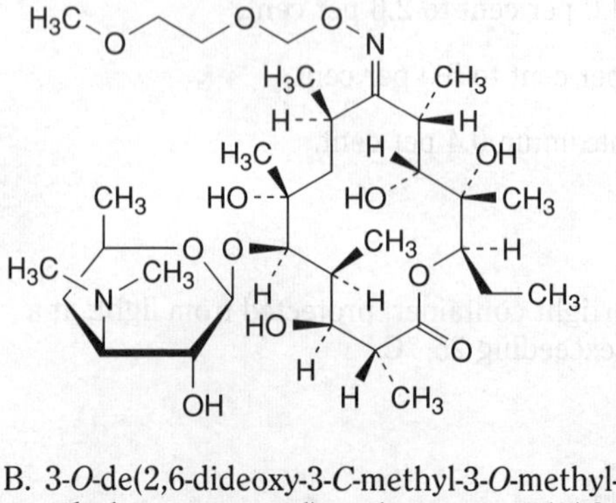

B. 3-*O*-de(2,6-dideoxy-3-*C*-methyl-3-*O*-methyl-α-L-*ribo*-hexopyranosyl)erythromycin 9-(*E*)-[*O*-[(2-methoxyethoxy)methyl]oxime],

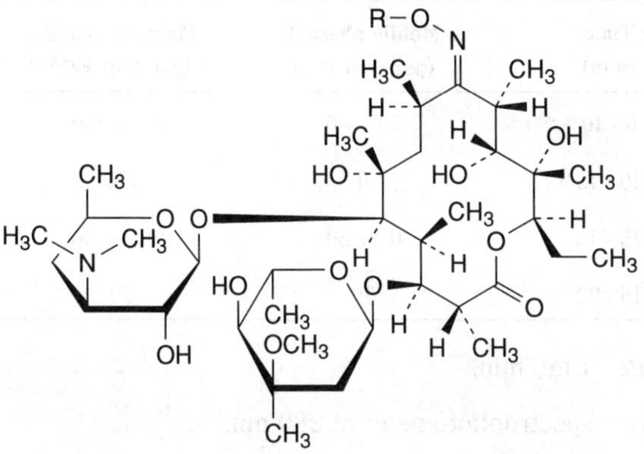

C. R = H: erythromycin 9-(*E*)-oxime,

G. R = CH_2-O-CH_2-O-CH_2-CH_2-OCH_3: erythromycin 9-(*E*)-[*O*-[[(2-methoxyethoxy)methoxy]methyl]oxime],

J. R = CH_2-O-CH_2-CH_2Cl: erythromycin 9-(*E*)-[*O*-[(2-chloroethoxy)methyl]oxime],

K. R = CH_2-O-CH_2-CH_2-O-CH_2OH: erythromycin 9-(*E*)-[*O*-[[2-(hydroxymethoxy)ethoxy]methyl]oxime],

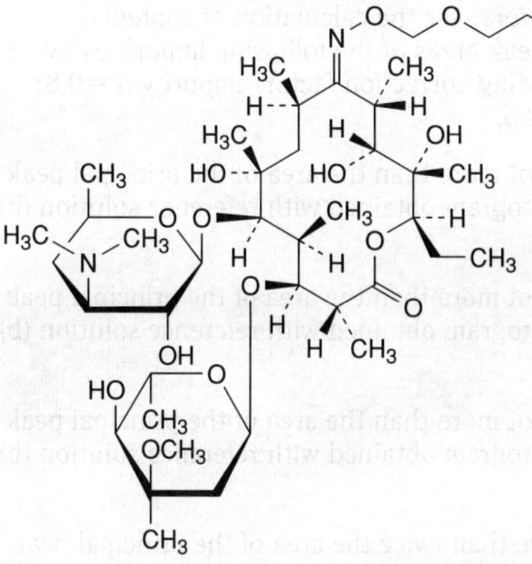

D. erythromycin 9-(*Z*)-[*O*-[(2-methoxyethoxy)methyl]oxime],

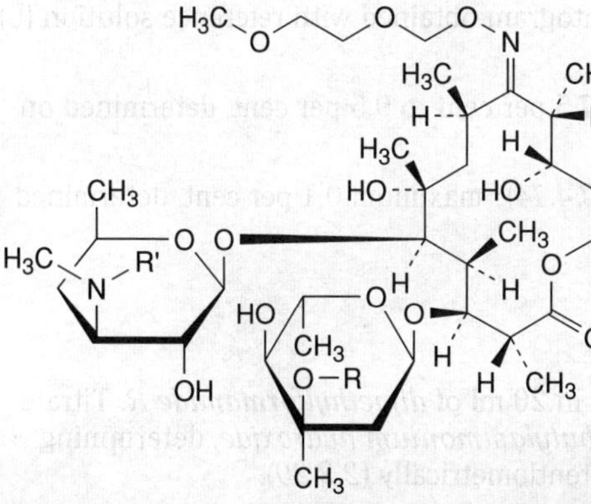

E. R = H, R′ = CH_3: 3″-*O*-demethylerythromycin 9-(*E*)-[*O*-[(2-methoxyethoxy)methyl]oxime],

F. R = CH_3, R′ = H: 3′-*N*-demethylerythromycin 9-(*E*)-[*O*-[(2-methoxyethoxy)methyl]oxime],

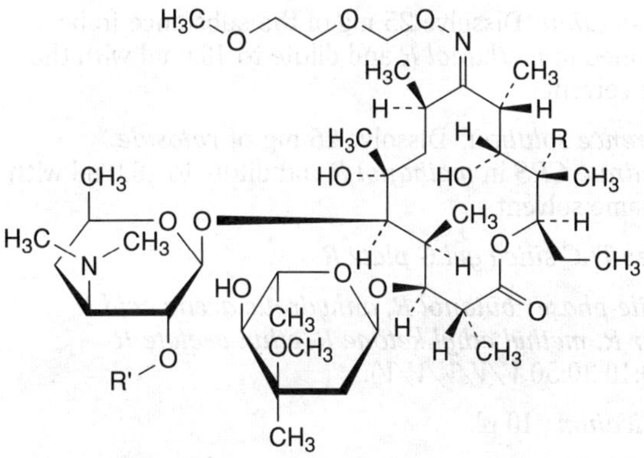

H. R = R′ = H: 12-deoxyerythromycin 9-(*E*)-[*O*-[(2-methoxyethoxy)methyl]oxime],

I. R = OH, R′ = CH_2-O-CH_2-CH_2-OCH_3: 2′-*O*-[(2-methoxyethoxy)methyl]erythromycin 9-(*E*)-[*O*-[(2-methoxyethoxy)methyl]oxime].

01/2005:1795

RUTOSIDE TRIHYDRATE

Rutosidum trihydricum

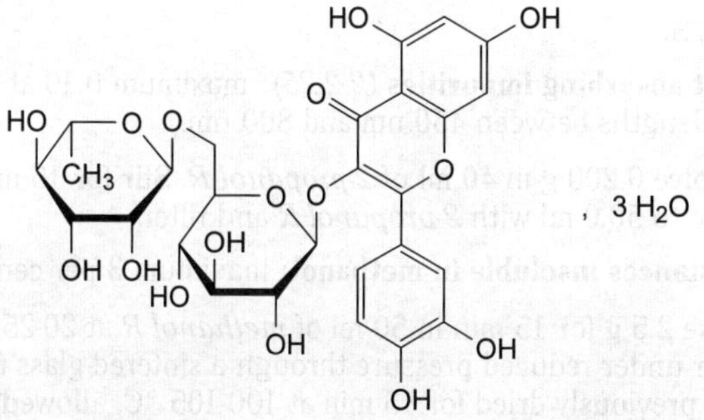

$C_{27}H_{30}O_{16},3H_2O$ M_r 665

DEFINITION

3-[[6-*O*-(6-Deoxy-α-L-mannopyranosyl)-β-D-glucopyranosyl]oxy]-2-(3,4-dihydroxyphenyl)-5,7-dihydroxy-4*H*-1-benzopyran-4-one.

Content: 95.0 per cent to 101.0 per cent (anhydrous substance).

CHARACTERS

Appearance: yellow or greenish-yellow, crystalline powder.

Solubility: practically insoluble in water, soluble in methanol, sparingly soluble in ethanol, practically insoluble in methylene chloride. It dissolves in solutions of alkali hydroxides.

IDENTIFICATION

First identification: B.

Second identification: A, C, D.

A. Dissolve 50.0 mg in *methanol R*, dilute to 250.0 ml with the same solvent and filter if necessary. Dilute 5.0 ml of the solution to 50.0 ml with *methanol R*. Examined between 210 nm and 450 nm (*2.2.25*), the solution shows 2 absorption maxima, at 257 nm and 358 nm. The specific absorbance at the maximum at 358 nm is 305 to 330, calculated with reference to the anhydrous substance.

B. Infrared absorption spectrophotometry (*2.2.24*).
Comparison: *rutoside trihydrate CRS*.

C. Thin-layer chromatography (*2.2.27*).

Test solution. Dissolve 25 mg of the substance to be examined in *methanol R* and dilute to 10.0 ml with the same solvent.

Reference solution. Dissolve 25 mg of *rutoside trihydrate CRS* in *methanol R* and dilute to 10.0 ml with the same solvent.

Plate: *TLC silica gel G plate R.*

Mobile phase: *butanol R, anhydrous acetic acid R, water R, methyl ethyl ketone R, ethyl acetate R* (5:10:10:30:50 *V/V/V/V/V*).

Application: 10 µl.

Development: over a path of 10 cm.

Drying: in air.

Detection: spray with a mixture of 7.5 ml of a 10 g/l solution of *potassium ferricyanide R* and 2.5 ml of *ferric chloride solution R1* and examine for 10 min.

Results: the principal spot in the chromatogram obtained with the test solution is similar in position, colour and size to the principal spot in the chromatogram obtained with the reference solution.

D. Dissolve 10 mg in 5 ml of *alcohol R*, add 1 g of *zinc R* and 2 ml of *hydrochloric acid R1*. A red colour develops.

TESTS

Light absorbing impurities (*2.2.25*): maximum 0.10 at wavelengths between 450 nm and 800 nm.

Dissolve 0.200 g in 40 ml of *2-propanol R*. Stir for 15 min, dilute to 50.0 ml with *2-propanol R* and filter.

Substances insoluble in methanol: maximum 3 per cent.

Shake 2.5 g for 15 min in 50 ml of *methanol R* at 20-25 °C. Filter under reduced pressure through a sintered-glass filter (1.6) previously dried for 15 min at 100-105 °C, allowed to cool in a desiccator and tared. Wash the filter 3 times with 20 ml of *methanol R*. Dry the filter for 30 min at 100-105 °C. Allow to cool and weigh. The residue weighs a maximum of 75 mg.

Related substances. Liquid chromatography (*2.2.29*).

Test solution. Dissolve 0.10 g of the substance to be examined in 20 ml of *methanol R* and dilute to 100.0 ml with mobile phase B.

Reference solution (a). Dissolve 10.0 mg of *rutoside trihydrate CRS* in 10.0 ml of *methanol R*.

Reference solution (b). Dilute 1.0 ml of reference solution (a) to 50.0 ml with mobile phase B.

Column:

- *size*: *l* = 0.25 m, Ø = 4.0 mm,
- *stationary phase*: *octylsilyl silica gel for chromatography R* (5 µm),
- *temperature*: 30 °C.

Mobile phase:

- *mobile phase A*: mix 5 volumes of *tetrahydrofuran R* with 95 volumes of a 15.6 g/l solution of *sodium dihydrogen phosphate R* adjusted to pH 3.0 with *phosphoric acid R*,
- *mobile phase B*: mix 40 volumes of *tetrahydrofuran R* with 60 volumes of a 15.6 g/l solution of *sodium dihydrogen phosphate R* adjusted to pH 3.0 with *phosphoric acid R*,

Time (min)	Mobile phase A (per cent *V/V*)	Mobile phase B (per cent *V/V*)
0 - 10	50 → 0	50 → 100
10 - 15	0	100
15 - 16	0 → 50	100 → 50
16 - 20	50	50

Flow rate: 1 ml/min.

Detection: spectrophotometer at 280 nm.

Injection: 20 µl.

Relative retention with reference to rutoside (retention time = about 7 min): impurity B = about 1.1; impurity A = about 1.2; impurity C = about 2.5.

System suitability: reference solution (a):

- *peak-to-valley ratio*: minimum 10, where H_p = height above the baseline of the peak due to impurity B and H_v = height above the baseline of the lowest point of the curve separating this peak from the peak due to rutoside.

Limits: locate the impurities by comparison with the chromatogram provided with *rutoside trihydrate CRS.*

- *correction factors*: for the calculation of contents, multiply the peak areas of the following impurities by the corresponding correction factor: impurity A = 0.8; impurity C = 0.5,
- *impurity A*: not more than the area of the principal peak in the chromatogram obtained with reference solution (b) (2.0 per cent),
- *impurity B*: not more than the area of the principal peak in the chromatogram obtained with reference solution (b) (2.0 per cent),
- *impurity C*: not more than the area of the principal peak in the chromatogram obtained with reference solution (b) (2.0 per cent),
- *total*: not more than twice the area of the principal peak in the chromatogram obtained with reference solution (b) (4.0 per cent),
- *disregard limit*: 0.05 times the area of the principal peak in the chromatogram obtained with reference solution (b) (0.1 per cent).

Water (*2.5.12*): 7.5 per cent to 9.5 per cent, determined on 0.100 g.

Sulphated ash (*2.4.14*): maximum 0.1 per cent, determined on 1.0 g.

ASSAY

Dissolve 0.200 g in 20 ml of *dimethylformamide R*. Titrate with *0.1 M tetrabutylammonium hydroxide*, determining the end-point potentiometrically (*2.2.20*).

1 ml of *0.1 M tetrabutylammonium hydroxide* is equivalent to 30.53 mg of $C_{27}H_{30}O_{16}$.

STORAGE

Protected from light.

IMPURITIES

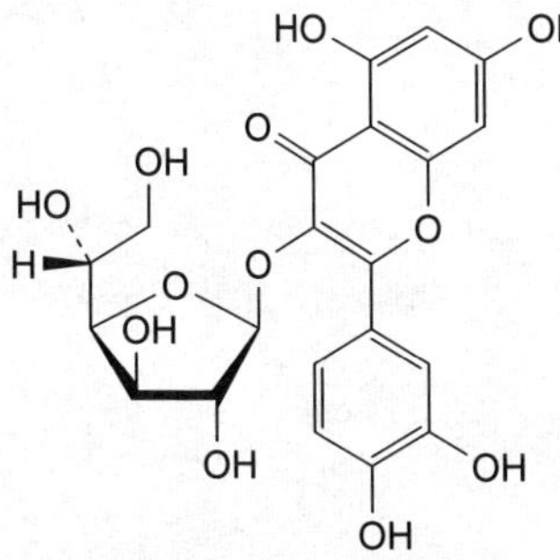

A. 2-(3,4-dihydroxyphenyl)-3-(β-D-glucofuranosyloxy)-5,7-dihydroxy-4*H*-1-benzopyran-4-one (isoquercitroside),

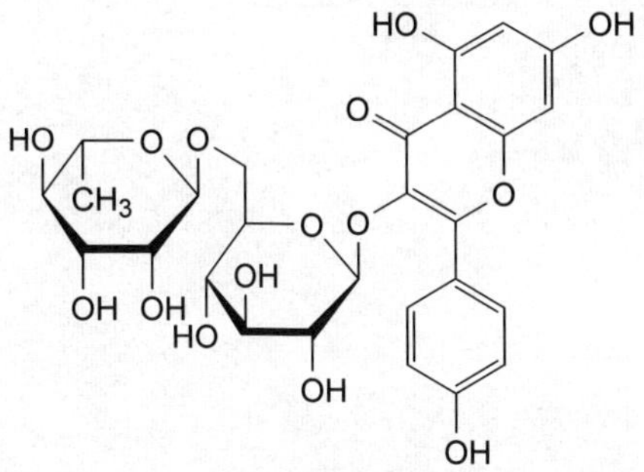

B. 3-[[6-*O*-(6-deoxy-α-L-mannopyranosyl)-β-D-glucopyranosyl]oxy]-5,7-dihydroxy-2-(4-hydroxyphenyl)-4*H*-1-benzopyran-4-one (kaempferol 3-rutinoside),

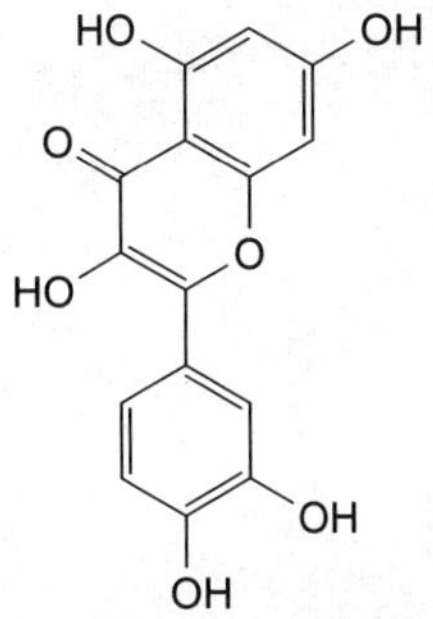

C. 2-(3,4-dihydroxyphenyl)-3,5,7-trihydroxy-4*H*-1-benzopyran-4-one (quercetin).

Monographs Q-S

S

01/2005:0947

SACCHARIN

Saccharinum

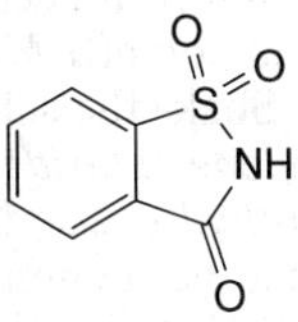

$C_7H_5NO_3S$ M_r 183.2

DEFINITION

1,2-Benzisothiazol-3(2*H*)-one 1,1-dioxide.

Content: 98.0 per cent to 101.0 per cent (dried substance).

CHARACTERS

Appearance: white, crystalline powder or colourless crystals.

Solubility: sparingly soluble in boiling water and in alcohol, slightly soluble in cold water. It dissolves in dilute solutions of alkali hydroxides and carbonates.

IDENTIFICATION

First identification: C.

Second identification: A, B, D, E.

A. A saturated solution, prepared without heating, turns *blue litmus paper R* red.

B. Melting point (*2.2.14*): 226 °C to 230 °C.

C. Infrared absorption spectrophotometry (*2.2.24*).

Preparation: discs.

Comparison: *saccharin CRS.*

D. Mix about 10 mg with about 10 mg of *resorcinol R*, add 0.25 ml of *sulphuric acid R* and carefully heat the mixture over a naked flame until a dark green colour is produced. Allow to cool, add 10 ml of *water R* and *dilute sodium hydroxide solution R* until an alkaline reaction is produced. An intense green fluorescence develops.

E. To 0.2 g add 1.5 ml of *dilute sodium hydroxide solution R*, evaporate to dryness and heat the residue carefully until it melts, avoiding carbonisation. Allow to cool, dissolve the mass in about 5 ml of *water R*, add *dilute hydrochloric acid R* until a weak acid reaction is produced and filter, if necessary. To the filtrate add 0.2 ml of *ferric chloride solution R2.* A violet colour develops.

TESTS

Solution S. Dissolve 5.0 g in 20 ml of a 200 g/l solution of *sodium acetate R* and dilute to 25 ml with the same solution.

Appearance of solution. Solution S is clear (*2.2.1*) and colourless (*2.2.2, Method II*).

o- and p-Toluenesulphonamide. Gas chromatography (*2.2.28*).

Internal standard solution. Dissolve 25 mg of *caffeine R* in *methylene chloride R* and dilute to 100 ml with the same solvent.

Test solution. Suspend 10.0 g of the substance to be examined in 20 ml of *water R* and dissolve using 5 ml to 6 ml of *strong sodium hydroxide solution R*. If necessary adjust the solution to pH 7-8 with *1 M sodium hydroxide* or *1 M hydrochloric acid* and dilute to 50 ml with *water R*. Shake the solution with 4 quantities, each of 50 ml, of *methylene chloride R*. Combine the lower layers, dry over *anhydrous sodium sulphate R* and filter. Wash the filter and the sodium sulphate with 10 ml of *methylene chloride R*. Combine the solution and the washings and evaporate almost to dryness in a water-bath at a temperature not exceeding 40 °C. Using a small quantity of *methylene chloride R*, quantitatively transfer the residue into a suitable 10 ml tube, evaporate to dryness in a current of nitrogen and dissolve the residue in 1.0 ml of the internal standard solution.

Blank solution. Evaporate 200 ml of *methylene chloride R* to dryness in a water-bath at a temperature not exceeding 40 °C. Dissolve the residue in 1 ml of *methylene chloride R.*

Reference solution. Dissolve 20.0 mg of *o-toluenesulphonamide R* and 20.0 mg of *p-toluenesulphonamide R* in *methylene chloride R* and dilute to 100.0 ml with the same solvent. Dilute 5.0 ml of the solution to 50.0 ml with *methylene chloride R*. Evaporate 5.0 ml of the final solution to dryness in a current of nitrogen. Dissolve the residue in 1.0 ml of the internal standard solution.

Column:

- *material*: fused silica,
- *size*: *l* = 10 m, Ø = 0.53 mm,
- *stationary phase*: *polymethylphenylsiloxane R* (film thickness 2 µm).

Carrier gas: *nitrogen for chromatography R.*

Flow rate: 10 ml/min.

Split ratio: 1:2.

Temperature:

- *column*: 180 °C,
- *injection port and detector*: 250 °C.

Detection: flame ionisation.

Injection: 1 µl.

Order of elution: *o*-toluenesulphonamide, *p*-toluenesulphonamide, caffeine.

System suitability: reference solution:

- *resolution*: minimum of 1.5 between the peaks due to *o*-toluenesulphonamide and *p*-toluenesulphonamide.

Limits:

- *o-toluenesulphonamide*: the ratio of its area to that of the internal standard is not greater than the corresponding ratio in the chromatogram obtained with the reference solution (10 ppm),
- *p-toluenesulphonamide*: the ratio of its area to that of the internal standard is not greater than the corresponding ratio in the chromatogram obtained with the reference solution (10 ppm).

Heavy metals (*2.4.8*): maximum 20 ppm.

Dilute 10 ml of solution S to 20 ml with *water R*. 12 ml of the solution complies with limit test A. Prepare the standard using *lead standard solution (2 ppm Pb) R.*

Loss on drying (*2.2.32*): maximum 1.0 per cent, determined on 1.000 g by drying in an oven at 100-105 °C for 4 h.

Sulphated ash (*2.4.14*): maximum 0.1 per cent, determined on 1.0 g.

ASSAY

Dissolve 0.150 g in 25 ml of *alcohol R*, with slight heating if necessary. Add 25 ml of *water R* and 0.25 ml of *phenolphthalein solution R1*. Titrate with *0.1 M sodium hydroxide*. Carry out a blank titration.

1 ml of *0.1 M sodium hydroxide* is equivalent to 18.32 mg of $C_7H_5NO_3S$.

Monographs Q-S

01/2005:0787

SACCHARIN SODIUM

Saccharinum natricum

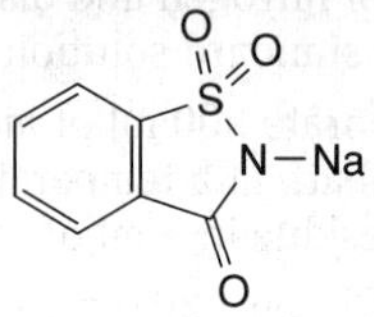

$C_7H_4NNaO_3S$ M_r 205.2

DEFINITION

2-Sodio-1,2-benzisothiazol-3(2*H*)-one 1,1-dioxide.

Content: 99.0 per cent to 101.0 per cent (anhydrous substance). It may contain a variable quantity of water.

CHARACTERS

Appearance: white, crystalline powder or colourless crystals, efflorescent in dry air.

Solubility: freely soluble in water, sparingly soluble in alcohol.

IDENTIFICATION

First identification: *B, E.*

Second identification: *A, C, D, E.*

A. To 5 ml of solution S (see Tests) add 3 ml of *dilute hydrochloric acid R*. A white precipitate is formed. Filter and wash with *water R*. Dry the precipitate at 100-105 °C. The melting point (*2.2.14*) is 226 °C to 230 °C.

B. Infrared absorption spectrophotometry (*2.2.24*).

Preparation: discs; dry the substances at 100-105 °C before use.

Comparison: *saccharin sodium CRS*.

C. Mix about 10 mg with about 10 mg of *resorcinol R*, add 0.25 ml of *sulphuric acid R* and carefully heat the mixture over a naked flame until a dark green colour is produced. Allow to cool, add 10 ml of *water R* and *dilute sodium hydroxide solution R* until an alkaline reaction is produced. An intense green fluorescence develops.

D. To 0.2 g add 1.5 ml of *dilute sodium hydroxide solution R*, evaporate to dryness and heat the residue carefully until it melts, avoiding carbonisation. Allow to cool, dissolve the mass in about 5 ml of *water R*, add *dilute hydrochloric acid R* until a weak acid reaction is produced and filter, if necessary. To the filtrate add 0.2 ml of *ferric chloride solution R2*. A violet colour develops.

E. 0.5 ml of solution S gives reaction (a) of sodium (*2.3.1*).

TESTS

Solution S. Dissolve 5.0 g in *carbon dioxide-free water R* and dilute to 50.0 ml with the same solvent.

Appearance of solution. The solution is clear (*2.2.1*) and colourless (*2.2.2, Method II*).

Dissolve 5.0 g in 25 ml of *carbon dioxide-free water R*.

Acidity or alkalinity. To 10.0 ml of solution S add 5.0 ml of *0.005 M sulphuric acid*. Heat to boiling and cool. Add 0.1 ml of *phenolphthalein solution R*. Not less than 4.5 ml and not more than 5.5 ml of *0.01 M sodium hydroxide* is required to change the colour of the indicator to pink.

***o*- and *p*-Toluenesulphonamide.** Gas chromatography (*2.2.28*).

Internal standard solution. Dissolve 25 mg of *caffeine R* in *methylene chloride R* and dilute to 100 ml with the same solvent.

Test solution. Dissolve 10.0 g of the substance to be examined in 50 ml of *water R*. If necessary adjust the solution to pH 7-8 by addition of *1 M sodium hydroxide* or *1 M hydrochloric acid*. Shake the solution with 4 quantities, each of 50 ml, of *methylene chloride R*. Combine the lower layers, dry over *anhydrous sodium sulphate R* and filter. Wash the filter and the sodium sulphate with 10 ml of *methylene chloride R*. Combine the solution and the washings and evaporate almost to dryness in a water-bath at a temperature not exceeding 40 °C. Using a small quantity of *methylene chloride R*, quantitatively transfer the residue into a suitable 10 ml tube, evaporate to dryness in a current of *nitrogen R* and add 1.0 ml of the internal standard solution.

Blank solution. Evaporate 200 ml of *methylene chloride R* to dryness in a water-bath at a temperature not exceeding 40 °C. Dissolve the residue in 1 ml of *methylene chloride R*.

Reference solution. Dissolve 20.0 mg of *o-toluenesulphonamide R* and 20.0 mg of *p-toluenesulphonamide R* in *methylene chloride R* and dilute to 100.0 ml with the same solvent. Dilute 5.0 ml of the solution to 50.0 ml with *methylene chloride R*. Evaporate 5.0 ml of the final solution to dryness in a current of *nitrogen R*. Take up the residue using 1.0 ml of the internal standard solution.

Column:

- *material*: fused silica,
- *size*: l = 10 m, Ø = 0.53 mm,
- *stationary phase*: *polymethylphenylsiloxane R* (film thickness 2 μm).

Carrier gas: *nitrogen for chromatography R*.

Flow rate: 10 ml/min.

Split ratio: 1:2.

Temperature:

- *column*: 180 °C,
- *injection port and detector*: 250 °C.

Detection: flame ionisation.

Injection: 1 μl.

Elution order: *o*-toluenesulphonamide, *p*-toluenesulphonamide, caffeine.

System suitability: reference solution:

- *resolution*: minimum of 1.5 between the peaks due to *o*-toluenesulphonamide and *p*-toluenesulphonamide.

Limits:

- *o-toluenesulphonamide*: the ratio of its area to that of the internal standard is not greater than the corresponding ratio in the chromatogram obtained with the reference solution (10 ppm),
- *p-toluenesulphonamide*: the ratio of its area to that of the internal standard is not greater than the corresponding ratio in the chromatogram obtained with the reference solution (10 ppm).

Heavy metals (*2.4.8*): maximum 20 ppm.

12 ml of solution S complies with limit test A. Prepare the standard using *lead standard solution (2 ppm Pb) R*.

Water (*2.5.12*): maximum 15.0 per cent, determined on 0.200 g.

Monographs Q-S

ASSAY

Dissolve 0.150 g in 50 ml of *anhydrous acetic acid R*, with slight heating if necessary. Titrate with *0.1 M perchloric acid*, determining the end-point potentiometrically (*2.2.20*).

1 ml of *0.1 M perchloric acid* is equivalent to 20.52 mg of $C_7H_4NNaO_3S$.

STORAGE

In an airtight container.

01/2005:2088

SAFFLOWER OIL, REFINED

Carthami oleum raffinatum

DEFINITION

Fatty oil obtained from seeds of *Carthamus tinctorius* L. (type I) or from seeds of hybrids of *Carthamus tinctorius* L. (type II), by expression and/or extraction followed by refining. Type II refined safflower oil is rich in oleic acid. It may contain a suitable antioxidant.

CHARACTERS

Appearance: clear, viscous, yellow to pale yellow liquid.

Solubility: miscible with light petroleum (bp: 40-60 °C), practically insoluble in alcohol.

	Refined safflower oil (type I)	Refined safflower oil (type II)
Relative density	about 0.922	about 0.914
Refractive index	about 1.476	about 1.472

IDENTIFICATION

First identification: B.

Second identification: A.

A. Carry out the identification of fatty oils by thin-layer chromatography (*2.3.2*). The chromatogram obtained is comparable with the type chromatogram for type I or type II refined safflower oil.

B. It complies with the test for composition of fatty acids (see Tests).

TESTS

Acid value (*2.5.1*): maximum 0.5.

Peroxide value (*2.5.5*): maximum 10.0. Maximum 5.0, if intended for the manufacture of parenteral dosage forms.

Unsaponifiable matter (*2.5.7*): maximum 1.5 per cent, determined on 5.0 g.

Alkaline impurities (*2.4.19*). It complies with the test for alkaline impurities in fatty oils.

Composition of fatty acids (*2.4.22, Method A*). Use the mixture of calibrating substances in Table 2.4.22.-3.

Composition of the fatty acid fraction of type I refined safflower oil:

- *saturated fatty acids of chain length less than C14*: maximum 0.2 per cent,
- *myristic acid*: maximum 0.2 per cent,
- *palmitic acid*: 4.0 per cent to 10.0 per cent,
- *stearic acid*: 1.0 per cent to 5.0 per cent,
- *oleic acid* (equivalent chain length on polyethyleneglycol adipate 18.3): 8.0 per cent to 21.0 per cent,
- *linoleic acid* (equivalent chain length on polyethyleneglycol adipate 18.9): 68.0 per cent to 83.0 per cent,
- *linolenic acid* (equivalent chain length on polyethyleneglycol adipate 19.7): maximum 0.5 per cent,
- *arachidic acid*: maximum 0.5 per cent,
- *eicosenoic acid* (equivalent chain length on polyethyleneglycol adipate 20.3): maximum 0.5 per cent,
- *behenic acid*: maximum 1.0 per cent.

Composition of the fatty acid fraction of type II refined safflower oil:

- *saturated fatty acids of chain length less than C14*: maximum 0.2 per cent,
- *myristic acid*: maximum 0.2 per cent,
- *palmitic acid*: 3.6 per cent to 6.0 per cent,
- *stearic acid*: 1.0 per cent to 5.0 per cent,
- *oleic acid* (equivalent chain length on polyethyleneglycol adipate 18.3): 70.0 per cent to 84.0 per cent,
- *linoleic acid* (equivalent chain length on polyethyleneglycol adipate 18.9): 7.0 per cent to 23.0 per cent,
- *linolenic acid* (equivalent chain length on polyethyleneglycol adipate 19.7): maximum 0.5 per cent,
- *arachidic acid*: maximum 1.0 per cent,
- *eicosenoic acid* (equivalent chain length on polyethyleneglycol adipate 20.3): maximum 1.0 per cent,
- *behenic acid*: maximum 1.2 per cent.

Brassicasterol (*2.4.23*): maximum 0.3 per cent of brassicasterol in the sterol fraction of the oil.

Water (*2.5.32*): maximum 0.1 per cent, determined on 5.00 g, if intended for use in the manufacture of parenteral dosage forms.

STORAGE

In a well-filled, airtight container, protected from light.

LABELLING

The label states:

- where applicable, that the substance is suitable for use in the manufacture of parenteral dosage forms,
- the name and concentration of any added antioxidant,
- the type of oil (type I or type II).

01/2005:1370

SAGE LEAF (SALVIA OFFICINALIS)

Salviae officinalis folium

DEFINITION

Whole or cut dried leaves of *Salvia officinalis* L.

Content: minimum 15 ml/kg of essential oil for the whole drug and minimum 10 ml/kg of essential oil for the cut drug (anhydrous drug).

CHARACTERS

Sage leaf (*Salvia officinalis*) oil is rich in thujone.

Macroscopic and microscopic characters described under identification tests A and B.

IDENTIFICATION

A. The lamina of whole sage leaf (Salvia officinalis) is about 2 cm to 10 cm long and 1 cm to 2 cm wide, oblong-ovate, elliptical. The margin is finely crenate to smooth. The apex is rounded or subacute and the base is shrunken at the petiole and rounded or cordate. The upper surface

Monographs Q-S

is greenish-grey and finely granular; the lower surface is white and pubescent and shows a dense network of raised veinlets.

B. Reduce to a powder (355). The powder is light grey to brownish-green. Examine under a microscope using *chloral hydrate solution R*. The powder shows the following diagnostic characters: very numerous articulated and bent trichomes with narrow elongated cells and a very thick cell at the base as well as fragments of these trichomes; fragments of the upper epidermis with pitted, somewhat polygonal cells; fragments of the lower epidermis with sinuous cells and numerous diacytic stomata (*2.8.3*); rare single glandular trichomes with a uni- or bicellular head and a stalk consisting of 1 to 4 cells; abundant glandular trichomes with a unicellular stalk and a head composed of 8 radiating cells with a raised common cuticle.

C. Thin-layer chromatography (*2.2.27*).

Test solution. Shake 0.5 g of the freshly powdered drug (355) with 5 ml of *ethanol R* for 5 min.

Reference solution. Dissolve 20 µl of *thujone R* and 25 µl of *cineole R* in 20 ml of *ethanol R*.

Plate: *TLC silica gel plate R*.

Mobile phase: *ethyl acetate R, toluene R* (5:95 *V/V*).

Application: 20 µl, as bands.

Development: over a path of 15 cm.

Drying: in air.

Detection: spray the plate with a 200 g/l solution of *phosphomolybdic acid R* in *ethanol R* and heat at 100-105 °C for 10 min. Examine in daylight.

Results: see below the sequence of the zones present in the chromatograms obtained with the reference solution and the test solution. Furthermore, other zones are present in the chromatogram obtained with the test solution.

Top of the plate	
	A blue zone (near the solvent front)
———	———
α-Thujone and β-thujone: 2 pinkish-violet zones	2 pinkish-violet zones (α-thujone and β-thujone)
Cineole: a blue zone	A blue zone (cineole)
———	———
	Blue zones
Reference solution	**Test solution**

TESTS

Foreign matter (*2.8.2*): maximum 3 per cent of stems and maximum 2 per cent of other foreign matter.

Water (*2.2.13*): maximum 100 ml/kg, determined on 20.0 g.

Total ash (*2.4.16*): maximum 10.0 per cent.

ASSAY

Carry out the determination of essential oils in vegetable drugs (*2.8.12*). Use 20.0 g of the substance to be examined, cut, if necessary, immediately before the assay, a 500 ml flask, 250 ml of *water R* as the distillation liquid and 0.5 ml of *xylene R* in the graduated tube. Distil at a rate of 2-3 ml/min for 2 h.

01/2005:1561

SAGE LEAF, THREE-LOBED

Salviae trilobae folium

DEFINITION

Three-lobed sage leaf consists of the whole or cut, dried leaves of *Salvia fructicosa* Mill. (*S. triloba* L. fil). The whole drug contains not less than 18 ml/kg of essential oil, and the cut drug not less than 12 ml/kg of essential oil, both calculated with reference to the anhydrous drug.

CHARACTERS

Three-lobed sage leaf has a spicy odour when ground, similar to eucalyptus oil.

It has the macroscopic and microscopic characters described under identification tests A and B.

IDENTIFICATION

A. The lamina of the whole three-lobed sage leaf is about 8 mm to 50 mm long and about 4 mm to 20 mm wide, and oblong-ovate to lanceolate. The margin is finely crenate and undulate but indistinct owing to the dense hairy covering on both surfaces. The base is obtuse and sometimes bears one or two more or less developed lobes. The upper surface is grey-tomentose pubescent, the lower surface is densely white-tomentose pubescent; the venation is indistinct. The densely white-tomentose pubescent petiole is about 1 mm in diameter.

B. Reduce to a powder (355). The powder is greyish-green and tomentose. Examine under a microscope using *chloral hydrate solution R*. The powder shows very numerous, whole and fragmented, covering and glandular trichomes, scattered and attached to fragments of the epidermises; covering trichomes articulated, uniseriate, thick-walled and bluntly tapering, those on the upper epidermis straight, those on the lower epidermis longer, tortuous and more densely packed; glandular trichomes, some with a unicellular or bicellular head and a stalk consisting of from one to four cells, the majority having a short, unicellular stalk and a head composed of eight radiating cells with a raised common cuticle; the upper epidermis with pitted and beaded cells, somewhat polygonal, with a few diacytic stomata (*2.8.3*); the lower epidermis with sinuous- to wavy-walled cells and numerous diacytic stomata.

C. Examine the chromatogram obtained in the test for thujone. The chromatogram obtained with the test solution shows a blue zone corresponding to cineole, equal or greater in size and intensity to the zone in the chromatogram obtained with the reference solution. Further zones are present.

TESTS

Thujone. Examine by thin-layer chromatography (*2.2.27*), using a *TLC silica gel plate R*.

Test solution. Shake 0.3 g of the freshly powdered drug (355) with 5.0 ml of *ethanol R* for 5 min.

Reference solution. Dissolve 20 µl of *thujone R* and 25 µl of *cineole R* in 20 ml of *ethanol R*.

Apply to the plate as bands 20 µl of each solution. Develop over a path of 15 cm using a mixture of 5 volumes of *ethyl acetate R* and 95 volumes of *toluene R*. Allow the plate to dry in air. Spray with a 200 g/l solution of *phosphomolybdic acid R* in *ethanol R* and heat at 100 °C to 105 °C for 10 min. Examine in daylight. The chromatogram obtained with the reference solution shows in the middle part a blue zone (cineole) and in the upper part a pink-blue zone (thujone). The chromatogram obtained with the test solution shows no zone or a very faint pink-blue zone corresponding to thujone.

Foreign matter (*2.8.2*). Not more than 8 per cent of stems and not more than 2 per cent of other foreign matter.

Water (*2.2.13*). Not more than 100 ml/kg, determined on 20.0 g by distillation.

Total ash (*2.4.16*). Not more than 10.0 per cent.

ASSAY

Carry out the determination of essential oils in vegetable drugs (*2.8.12*). Use 20.0 g of drug, if necessary cut immediately before the assay, a 500 ml flask, 250 ml of *water R* as the distillation liquid and 0.50 ml of *xylene R* in the graduated tube. Distil at a rate of 2 ml/min to 3 ml/min for 2 h.

STORAGE

Store protected from light.

01/2005:1889

SAGE TINCTURE

Salviae tinctura

DEFINITION

Tincture produced from *Sage leaf (Salvia officinalis) (1370)*.

Content: minimum 0.1 per cent *m/m* of essential oil.

PRODUCTION

The tincture is produced from 1 part of comminuted drug and 10 parts of ethanol (70 per cent *V/V*) by a suitable procedure.

CHARACTERS

Appearance: brownish liquid with a characteristic odour.

IDENTIFICATION

Thin-layer chromatography (*2.2.27*).

Test solution. The tincture to be examined.

Reference solution. Dissolve 20 µl of *thujone R* and 25 µl of *cineole R* in 20 ml of *ethanol R*.

Plate: *TLC silica gel plate R*.

Mobile phase: *ethyl acetate R, toluene R (5:95 V/V)*.

Application: 20 µl, as bands.

Development: over a path of 15 cm.

Drying: in air.

Detection: spray with a 200 g/l solution of *phosphomolybdic acid R* in *ethanol R* and heat at 100-105 °C for 10 min. Examine in daylight.

Results: see below the sequence of the zones present in the chromatograms obtained with the reference solution and the test solution. Furthermore, other zones are present in the chromatogram obtained with the test solution.

Top of the plate	
	A blue zone (near the solvent front)
———	
α-Thujone and β-thujone: 2 pinkish-violet zones	2 pinkish-violet zones (α-thujone and β-thujone)
Cineole: a blue zone	A blue zone (cineole)
———	———
	Blue zones
Reference solution	**Test solution**

TESTS

Ethanol content (*2.9.10*): 64 per cent *V/V* to 69 per cent *V/V*.

Methanol and 2-propanol (*2.9.11*): maximum 0.05 per cent *V/V* of methanol and maximum 0.05 per cent of 2-propanol.

Dry residue (*2.8.16*): minimum 2.0 per cent *m/m*, determined on 3.00 g.

ASSAY

In a 500 ml round-bottomed flask, place 30.0 g of the tincture and add 100 ml of *water R*. Distil, using a descending condenser, into a separating funnel which has been marked beforehand at 50 ml. Stop the distillation process as soon as the distillate reaches the 50 ml mark. Rinse the condenser with 10 ml of *pentane R*. Dissolve in the distillate sufficient *sodium chloride R* to produce a saturated solution. Shake with 3 quantities, each of 20 ml, of *pentane R*. Dry the combined pentane layers, including the pentane from rinsing the condenser, over *anhydrous sodium sulphate R* and filter through a plug of absorbent cotton into a weighed 100 ml round-bottomed flask. Wash the sodium sulphate several times with small quantities of *pentane R*. Remove the pentane carefully at a temperature not exceeding 40 °C. Dry the residue in a desiccator over *diphosphorus pentoxide R* and hard paraffin at atmospheric pressure and at room temperature for 2 h. Weigh the residue (essential oil).

01/2005:0529

SALBUTAMOL

Salbutamolum

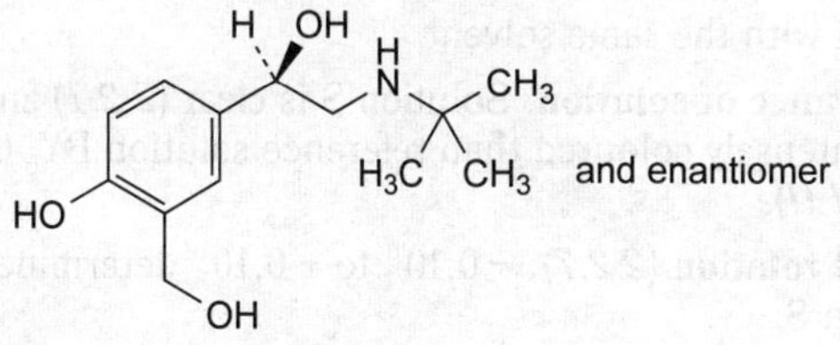

$C_{13}H_{21}NO_3$ M_r 239.3

DEFINITION

(1*RS*)-2-[(1,1-Dimethylethyl)amino]-1-[4-hydroxy-3-(hydroxymethyl)phenyl]ethanol.

Content: 98.0 per cent to 101.0 per cent (dried substance).

CHARACTERS

Appearance: white or almost white, crystalline powder.

Solubility: sparingly soluble in water, soluble in alcohol.

mp: about 155 °C, with decomposition.

IDENTIFICATION

First identification: B.

Second identification: A, C, D.

A. Dissolve 80.0 mg in a 10 g/l solution of *hydrochloric acid R* and dilute to 100.0 ml with the same acid. Dilute 10.0 ml of the solution to 100.0 ml with a 10 g/l solution of *hydrochloric acid R*. Examined between 230 nm and 350 nm (*2.2.25*), the solution shows an absorption maximum at 276 nm. The specific absorbance at the maximum is 66 to 75.

B. Infrared absorption spectrophotometry (*2.2.24*).
Comparison: *salbutamol CRS*.

C. Thin-layer chromatography (*2.2.27*).

Test solution. Dissolve 10 mg of the substance to be examined in *methanol R* and dilute to 50 ml with the same solvent.

Reference solution. Dissolve 10 mg of *salbutamol CRS* in *methanol R* and dilute to 50 ml with the same solvent.

Plate: *TLC silica gel plate R*.

Mobile phase: *concentrated ammonia R, water R, ethyl acetate R, 2-propanol R, methyl isobutyl ketone R* (3:18:35:45:50 *V/V/V/V/V*).

Application: 5 µl.

Development: over a path of 18 cm.

Drying: in air.

Detection: spray with a 1 g/l solution of *methylbenzothiazolone hydrazone hydrochloride R* in a 90 per cent *V/V* solution of *methanol R*, followed by a 20 g/l solution of *potassium ferricyanide R* in a mixture of 1 volume of *concentrated ammonia R1* and 3 volumes of *water R*, followed by a further spraying with a 1 g/l solution of *methylbenzothiazolone hydrazone hydrochloride R* in a 90 per cent *V/V* solution of *methanol R*.

Results: the principal spot in the chromatogram obtained with the test solution is similar in position, colour and size to the principal spot in the chromatogram obtained with the reference solution.

D. Dissolve about 10 mg in 50 ml of a 20 g/l solution of *disodium tetraborate R*. Add 1 ml of a 30 g/l solution of *aminopyrazolone R*, 10 ml of *methylene chloride R* and 10 ml of a 20 g/l solution of *potassium ferricyanide R*. Shake and allow to separate. An orange-red colour develops in the methylene chloride layer.

TESTS

Solution S. Dissolve 0.50 g in *methanol R* and dilute to 25.0 ml with the same solvent.

Appearance of solution. Solution S is clear (*2.2.1*) and not more intensely coloured than reference solution BY_5 (*2.2.2, Method II*).

Optical rotation (*2.2.7*): − 0.10° to + 0.10° determined on solution S.

Related substances. Liquid chromatography (*2.2.29*).

Test solution. Dissolve 0.100 g of the substance to be examined in the mobile phase and dilute to 50.0 ml with the mobile phase.

Reference solution. Dissolve 2.0 mg of *salbutamol CRS*, 2.0 mg of *salbutamol impurity B CRS*, 3.0 mg of *salbutamol impurity D CRS*, 3.0 mg of *salbutamol impurity F CRS*, 3.0 mg of *salbutamol impurity G CRS* and 3.0 mg of *salbutamol impurity I CRS* in the mobile phase and dilute to 10.0 ml with the mobile phase. Dilute 2.0 ml of the solution to 100.0 ml with the mobile phase.

Column:

- *size*: l = 0.15 m, Ø = 3.9 mm,
- *stationary phase*: spherical *end-capped octylsilyl silica gel for chromatography R* (5 µm) with a specific surface of 335 m^2/g, a pore size of 10 nm and a carbon loading of 11.7 per cent.

Mobile phase: mix 22 volumes of *acetonitrile R* and 78 volumes of a solution containing 2.87 g/l of *sodium heptanesulphonate R* and 2.5 g/l of *potassium dihydrogen phosphate R* ajusted to pH 3.65 with *dilute phosphoric acid R*.

Flow rate: 1 ml/min.

Detection: spectrophotometer at 220 nm.

Injection: 20 µl.

Run time: 25 times the retention time of salbutamol.

Relative retention with reference to salbutamol (retention time = about 1.9 min): impurity B = about 1.3, impurity A = about 1.7, impurity C = about 2.0, impurity D = about 2.7, impurity H = about 3.0, impurity E = about 3.1, impurity G = about 4.1, impurity F = about 6.2, impurity I = about 23.2.

System suitability: reference solution:

- *resolution*: minimum of 3.0 between the peaks due to salbutamol and to impurity B.

Limits:

- *impurity D*: not more than the area of the corresponding peak in the chromatogram obtained with reference solution (0.3 per cent),
- *impurity F*: not more than the area of the corresponding peak in the chromatogram obtained with reference solution (0.3 per cent),
- *impurity G*: not more than the area of the corresponding peak in the chromatogram obtained with reference solution (0.3 per cent),
- *impurity I*: not more than the area of the corresponding peak in the chromatogram obtained with reference solution (0.3 per cent),
- *any other impurity*: not more than 1.5 times the area of the peak due to salbutamol in the chromatogram obtained with reference solution (0.3 per cent),
- *total*: maximum 1.0 per cent,
- *disregard limit*: 0.05 per cent.

Impurity J: maximum 0.2 per cent.

Dissolve 50.0 mg in a 1 g/l solution of *hydrochloric acid R* and dilute to 25.0 ml with the same solvent. The absorbance (*2.2.25*) of the solution measured at 310 nm is not greater than 0.10.

Boron: maximum 50 ppm.

Test solution. To 50 mg of the substance to be examined add 5 ml of a solution containing 13 g/l of *anhydrous sodium carbonate R* and 17 g/l of *potassium carbonate R*. Evaporate to dryness on a water-bath and dry at 120 °C. Ignite the residue rapidly until the organic matter has been destroyed, allow to cool and add 0.5 ml of *water R* and 3.0 ml of a freshly prepared 1.25 g/l solution of *curcumin R* in *glacial acetic acid R*. Warm gently to effect solution, allow to cool and add 3.0 ml of a mixture prepared by adding 5 ml of *sulphuric acid R*, slowly and with stirring, to 5 ml of *glacial acetic acid R*. Mix and allow to stand for 30 min. Dilute to 100.0 ml with *alcohol R*, filter and use the filtrate.

Reference solution. Dissolve 0.572 g of *boric acid R* in 1000.0 ml of *water R*. Dilute 1.0 ml to 100.0 ml with *water R*. To 2.5 ml of the solution add 5 ml of a solution containing 13 g/l of *anhydrous sodium carbonate R* and 17 g/l of *potassium carbonate R*, and treat this mixture in the same manner as the test solution.

Measure the absorbance (*2.2.25*) of the test solution and of the reference solution at the maximum at about 555 nm. The absorbance of the test solution is not greater than that of the reference solution.

Loss on drying (*2.2.32*): maximum 0.5 per cent, determined on 1.000 g by drying in an oven at 100-105 °C.

Sulphated ash (*2.4.14*): maximum 0.1 per cent, determined on 1.0 g.

ASSAY

Dissolve 0.200 g in 30 ml of *anhydrous acetic acid R*. Titrate with *0.1 M perchloric acid*, determining the end-point potentiometrically (*2.2.20*).

Monographs Q-S

1 ml of *0.1 M perchloric acid* is equivalent to 23.93 mg of $C_{13}H_{21}NO_3$.

STORAGE

Protected from light.

IMPURITIES

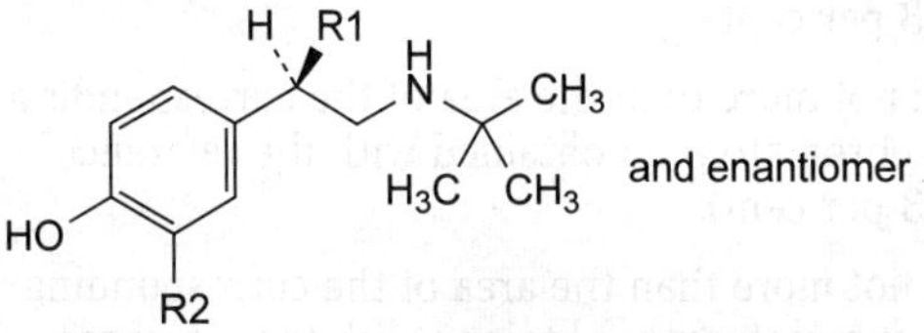

A. R1 = OCH_3, R2 = CH_2OH: [5-[(1*RS*)-2-[(1,1-dimethylethyl)amino]-1-methoxyethyl]-2-hydroxyphenyl]methanol,

B. R1 = OH, R2 = H: (1*RS*)-2-[(1,1-dimethylethyl)amino]-1-(4-hydroxyphenyl)ethanol,

C. R1 = OH, R2 = CH_3: (1*RS*)-2-[(1,1-dimethylethyl)amino]-1-(4-hydroxy-3-methylphenyl)ethanol,

D. R1 = OH, R2 = CHO : 5-[(1*RS*)-2-[(1,1-dimethylethyl)amino]-1-hydroxyethyl]-2-hydroxybenzaldehyde,

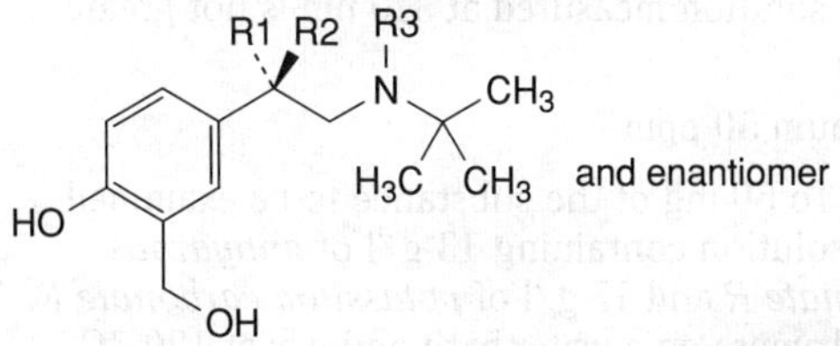

E. R1 = H, R2 = OH, R3 = CH_2-C_6H_5: (1*RS*)-2-[benzyl(1,1-dimethylethyl)amino]-1-[4-hydroxy-3-(hydroxymethyl)phenyl]ethanol,

G. R1+R2 = O, R3 = CH_2-C_6H_5: 2-[benzyl(1,1-dimethylethyl)amino]-1-[4-hydroxy-3-(hydroxymethyl)phenyl]ethanone,

J. R1+R2 = O, R3 = H: 2-[(1,1-dimethylethyl)amino]-1-[4-hydroxy-3-(hydroxymethyl)phenyl]ethanone (salbutamone),

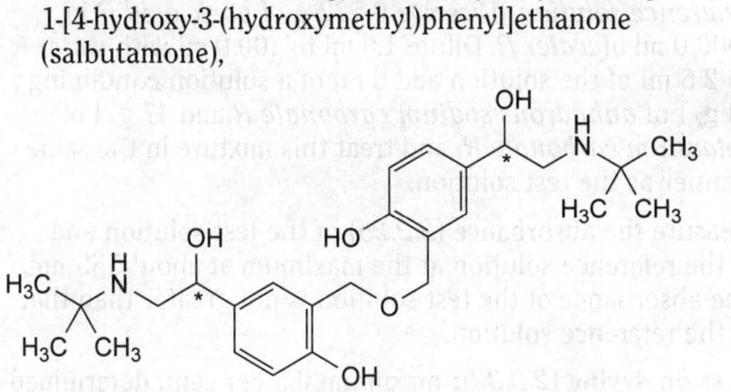

F. 1,1′-[oxybis[methylene(4-hydroxy-1,3-phenylene)]]bis[2-[(1,1-dimethylethyl)amino]ethanol],

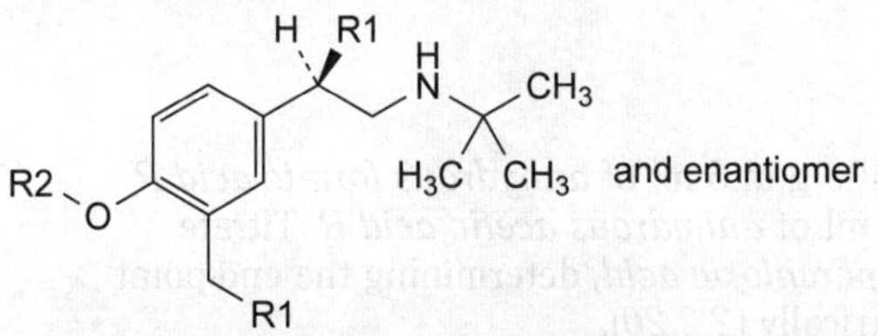

H. R1 = R2 = H: 4-[2-[(1,1-dimethylethyl)amino]ethyl]-2-methylphenol,

I. R1 = OH, R2 = CH_2-C_6H_5: (1*RS*)-2-[(1,1-dimethylethyl)amino]-1-[3-(hydroxymethyl)-4-benzyloxyphenyl]ethanol.

01/2005:0687

SALBUTAMOL SULPHATE

Salbutamoli sulfas

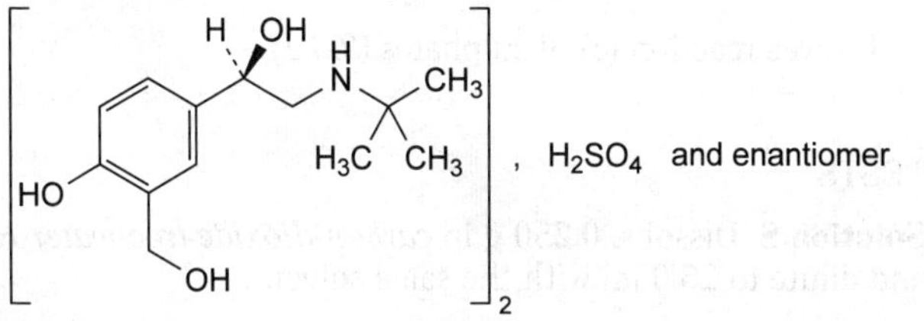

$C_{26}H_{44}N_2O_{10}S$ M_r 576.7

DEFINITION

Bis[(1*RS*)-2-[(1,1-dimethylethyl)amino]-1-[4-hydroxy-3-(hydroxymethyl)phenyl]ethanol] sulphate.

Content: 98.0 per cent to 101.0 per cent (dried substance).

CHARACTERS

Appearance: white or almost white, crystalline powder.

Solubility: freely soluble in water, practically insoluble or very slightly soluble in alcohol and in methylene chloride.

IDENTIFICATION

First identification: B, E.

Second identification: A, C, D, E.

A. Dissolve 80.0 mg in a 10 g/l solution of *hydrochloric acid R* and dilute to 100.0 ml with the same acid. Dilute 10.0 ml of the solution to 100.0 ml with a 10 g/l solution of *hydrochloric acid R*. Examined between 230 nm and 350 nm (*2.2.25*), the solution shows an absorption maximum at 276 nm. The specific absorbance at the maximum is 55 to 64.

B. Infrared absorption spectrophotometry (*2.2.24*).

Preparation: discs of *potassium bromide R*.

Comparison: *salbutamol sulphate CRS*.

C. Thin-layer chromatography (*2.2.27*).

Test solution. Dissolve 12 mg of the substance to be examined in *water R* and dilute to 10 ml with the same solvent.

Reference solution. Dissolve 12 mg of *salbutamol sulphate CRS* in *water R* and dilute to 10 ml with the same solvent.

Plate: *TLC silica gel plate R*.

Mobile phase: *concentrated ammonia R, water R, ethyl acetate R, 2-propanol R, methyl isobutyl ketone R* (3:18:35:45:50 *V/V/V/V/V*).

Application: 1 µl.

Development: over a path of 18 cm.

Drying: in air.

Detection: spray with a 1 g/l solution of *methylbenzothiazolone hydrazone hydrochloride R* in a 90 per cent *V/V* solution of *methanol R*, followed by a 20 g/l solution of *potassium ferricyanide R* in a mixture of 1 volume of *concentrated ammonia R1* and 3 volumes of *water R*, followed by a further spraying with a 1 g/l solution of *methylbenzothiazolone hydrazone hydrochloride R* in a 90 per cent *V/V* solution of *methanol R*.

Results: the principal spot in the chromatogram obtained with the test solution is similar in position, colour and size to the principal spot in the chromatogram obtained with the reference solution.

D. Dissolve about 10 mg in 50 ml of a 20 g/l solution of *disodium tetraborate R*. Add 1 ml of a 30 g/l solution of *aminopyrazolone R*, 10 ml of *methylene chloride R* and 10 ml of a 20 g/l solution of *potassium ferricyanide R*. Shake and allow to separate. An orange-red colour develops in the methylene chloride layer.

E. It gives reaction (a) of sulphates (*2.3.1*).

TESTS

Solution S. Dissolve 0.250 g in *carbon dioxide-free water R* and dilute to 25.0 ml with the same solvent.

Appearance of solution. Solution S is clear (*2.2.1*) and not more intensely coloured than reference solution BY_6 (*2.2.2, Method II*).

Optical rotation (*2.2.7*): − 0.10° to + 0.10°, determined on solution S.

Acidity or alkalinity. To 10 ml of solution S add 0.15 ml of *methyl red solution R* and 0.2 ml of *0.01 M sodium hydroxide*. The solution is yellow. Not more than 0.4 ml of *0.01 M hydrochloric acid* is required to change the colour of the indicator to red.

Related substances. Liquid chromatography (*2.2.29*).

Test solution. Dissolve 0.100 g of the substance to be examined in the mobile phase and dilute to 50.0 ml with the mobile phase.

Reference solution. Dissolve 2.4 mg of *salbutamol sulphate CRS*, 2.0 mg of *salbutamol impurity B CRS*, 3.0 mg of *salbutamol impurity D CRS*, 3.0 mg of *salbutamol impurity F CRS*, 3.0 mg of *salbutamol impurity G CRS* and 3.0 mg of *salbutamol impurity I CRS* in the mobile phase and dilute to 10.0 ml with the mobile phase. Dilute 2.0 ml of the solution to 100.0 ml with the mobile phase.

Column:

- *size*: l = 0.15 m, Ø = 3.9 mm,
- *stationary phase*: spherical *end-capped octylsilyl silica gel for chromatography R* (5 µm) with a specific surface area of 335 m^2/g, a pore size of 10 nm and a carbon loading of 11.7 per cent.

Mobile phase: mix 22 volumes of *acetonitrile R* and 78 volumes of a solution containing 2.87 g/l of *sodium heptanesulphonate R* and 2.5 g/l of *potassium dihydrogen phosphate R* adjusted to pH 3.65 with *dilute phosphoric acid R*.

Flow rate: 1 ml/min.

Detection: spectrophotometer at 220 nm.

Injection: 20 µl.

Run time: 25 times the retention time of salbutamol.

Relative retention with reference to salbutamol (retention time = about 1.9 min): impurity B = about 1.3, impurity A = about 1.7, impurity C = about 2.0, impurity D = about 2.7, impurity H = about 3.0, impurity E = about 3.1, impurity G = about 4.1, impurity F = about 6.2, impurity I = about 23.2.

System suitability: reference solution:

- *resolution*: minimum of 3.0 between the peaks due to salbutamol and to impurity B.

Limits:

- *impurity D*: not more than the area of the corresponding peak in the chromatogram obtained with the reference solution (0.3 per cent),
- *impurity F*: not more than the area of the corresponding peak in the chromatogram obtained with the reference solution (0.3 per cent),
- *impurity G*: not more than the area of the corresponding peak in the chromatogram obtained with the reference solution (0.3 per cent),
- *impurity I*: not more than the area of the corresponding peak in the chromatogram obtained with the reference solution (0.3 per cent),
- *any other impurity*: not more than 1.5 times the area of the peak due to salbutamol in the chromatogram obtained with the reference solution (0.3 per cent),
- *total*: maximum 1.0 per cent,
- *disregard limit*: 0.05 per cent.

Impurity J: maximum 0.2 per cent.

Dissolve 60.0 mg in a 1 g/l solution of *hydrochloric acid R* and dilute to 25.0 ml with the same solvent. The absorbance (*2.2.25*) of the solution measured at 310 nm is not greater than 0.10.

Boron: maximum 50 ppm.

Test solution. To 50 mg of the substance to be examined add 5 ml of a solution containing 13 g/l of *anhydrous sodium carbonate R* and 17 g/l of *potassium carbonate R*. Evaporate to dryness on a water-bath and dry at 120 °C. Ignite the residue rapidly until the organic matter has been destroyed, allow to cool and add 0.5 ml of *water R* and 3.0 ml of a freshly prepared 1.25 g/l solution of *curcumin R* in *glacial acetic acid R*. Warm gently to effect solution, allow to cool and add 3.0 ml of a mixture prepared by adding 5 ml of *sulphuric acid R*, slowly and with stirring, to 5 ml of *glacial acetic acid R*. Mix and allow to stand for 30 min. Dilute to 100.0 ml with *alcohol R*, filter and use the filtrate.

Reference solution. Dissolve 0.572 g of *boric acid R* in 1000.0 ml of *water R*. Dilute 1.0 ml to 100.0 ml with *water R*. To 2.5 ml of the solution add 5 ml of a solution containing 13 g/l of *anhydrous sodium carbonate R* and 17 g/l of *potassium carbonate R*, and treat this mixture in the same manner as the test solution.

Measure the absorbance (*2.2.25*) of the test solution and of the reference solution at the maximum at about 555 nm. The absorbance of the test solution is not greater than that of the reference solution.

Loss on drying (*2.2.32*): maximum 0.5 per cent, determined on 1.000 g by drying in an oven at 100-105 °C.

Sulphated ash (*2.4.14*): maximum 0.1 per cent, determined on 1.0 g.

ASSAY

Dissolve 0.400 g in 5 ml of *anhydrous formic acid R* and add 35 ml of *anhydrous acetic acid R*. Titrate with *0.1 M perchloric acid*, determining the end-point potentiometrically (*2.2.20*).

1 ml of *0.1 M perchloric acid* is equivalent to 57.67 mg of $C_{26}H_{44}N_2O_{10}S$.

STORAGE

Protected from light.

Monographs Q-S

IMPURITIES

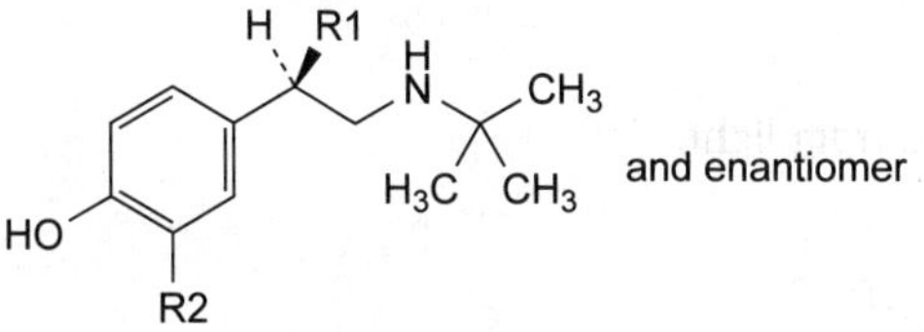

A. R1 = OCH_3, R2 = CH_2OH: [5-[(1*RS*)-2-[(1,1-dimethylethyl)amino]-1-methoxyethyl]-2-hydroxyphenyl]methanol,

B. R1 = OH, R2 = H: (1*RS*)-2-[(1,1-dimethylethyl)amino]-1-(4-hydroxyphenyl)ethanol,

C. R1 = OH, R2 = CH_3: (1*RS*)-2-[(1,1-dimethylethyl)amino]-1-(4-hydroxy-3-methylphenyl)ethanol,

D. R1 = OH, R2 = CHO: 5-[(1*RS*)-2-[(1,1-dimethylethyl)amino]-1-hydroxyethyl]-2-hydroxybenzaldehyde,

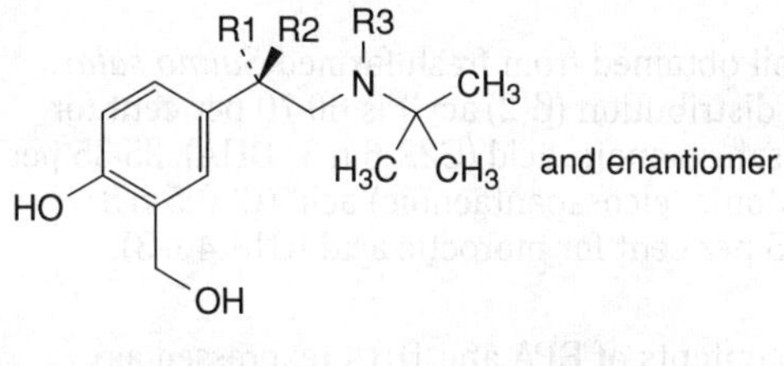

E. R1 = H, R2 = OH, R3 = CH_2-C_6H_5: (1*RS*)-2-[benzyl(1,1-dimethylethyl)amino]-1-[4-hydroxy-3-(hydroxymethyl)phenyl]ethanol,

G. R1+R2 = O, R3 = CH_2-C_6H_5: 2-[benzyl(1,1-dimethylethyl)amino]-1-[4-hydroxy-3-(hydroxymethyl)phenyl]ethanone,

J. R1+R2 = O, R3 = H: 2-[(1,1-dimethylethyl)amino]-1-[4-hydroxy-3-(hydroxymethyl)phenyl]ethanone (salbutamone),

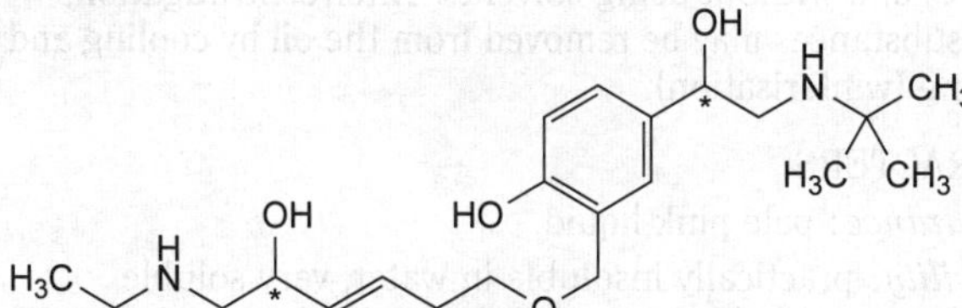

F. 1,1′-[oxybis[methylene(4-hydroxy-1,3-phenylene)]]bis[2-[(1,1-dimethylethyl)amino]ethanol],

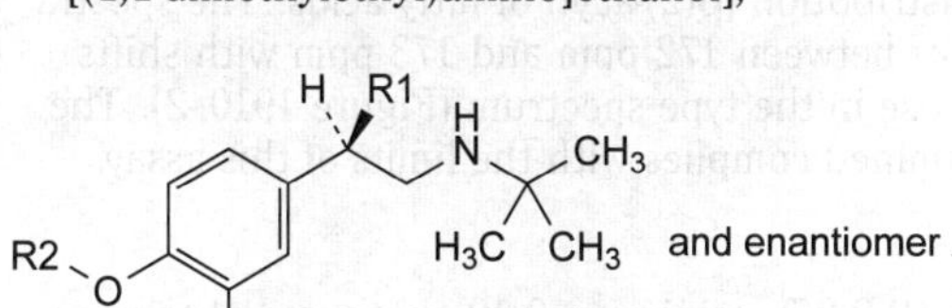

H. R1 = R2 = H: 4-[2-[(1,1-dimethylethyl)amino]ethyl]-2-methylphenol,

I. R1 = OH, R2 = CH_2-C_6H_5: (1*RS*)-2-[(1,1-dimethylethyl)amino]-1-[3-(hydroxymethyl)-4-benzyloxyphenyl]ethanol.

01/2005:0366

SALICYLIC ACID

Acidum salicylicum

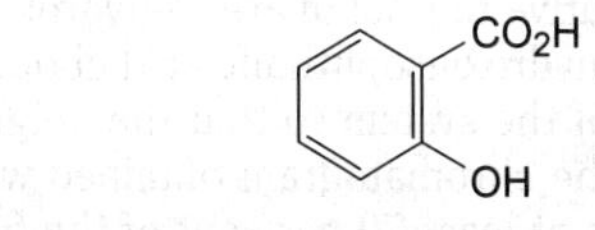

$C_7H_6O_3$ M_r 138.1

DEFINITION

Salicylic acid contains not less than 99.0 per cent and not more than the equivalent of 100.5 per cent of 2-hydroxybenzenecarboxylic acid, calculated with reference to the dried substance.

CHARACTERS

A white, crystalline powder or white or colourless, acicular crystals, slightly soluble in water, freely soluble in alcohol, sparingly soluble in methylene chloride.

IDENTIFICATION

First identification: A, B.

Second identification: A, C.

A. Melting point (*2.2.14*): 158 °C to 161 °C.

B. Examine by infrared absorption spectrophotometry (*2.2.24*), comparing with the spectrum obtained with *salicylic acid CRS*.

C. Dissolve about 30 mg in 5 ml of *0.05 M sodium hydroxide*, neutralise if necessary and dilute to 20 ml with *water R*. 1 ml of the solution gives reaction (a) of salicylates (*2.3.1*).

TESTS

Solution S. Dissolve 2.5 g in 50 ml of boiling *distilled water R*, cool and filter.

Appearance of solution. Dissolve 1 g in 10 ml of *alcohol R*. The solution is clear (*2.2.1*) and colourless (*2.2.2, Method II*).

Related substances. Examine by liquid chromatography (*2.2.29*).

Test solution. Dissolve 0.50 g of the substance to be examined in the mobile phase and dilute to 100.0 ml with the mobile phase.

Reference solution (a). Dissolve 10 mg of *phenol R* in the mobile phase and dilute to 100.0 ml with the mobile phase.

Reference solution (b). Dissolve 25 mg of *4-hydroxyisophthalic acid R* in the mobile phase and dilute to 100.0 ml with the mobile phase.

Reference solution (c). Dissolve 50 mg of *4-hydroxybenzoic acid R* in the mobile phase and dilute to 100.0 ml with the mobile phase.

Reference solution (d). Dilute 1.0 ml of reference solution (a) to 10.0 ml with the mobile phase.

Reference solution (e). Dilute a mixture of 1.0 ml of each of reference solutions (a), (b) and (c) to 10.0 ml with the mobile phase.

Reference solution (f). Dilute a mixture of 0.1 ml of each of reference solutions (a), (b) and (c) to 10.0 ml with the mobile phase.

The chromatographic procedure may be carried out using:

– a stainless steel column 0.15 m long and 4.6 mm in internal diameter packed with non-deactivated *octadecylsilyl silica gel for chromatography R* (5 µm),

Monographs Q-S

– as mobile phase at a flow rate of 0.5 ml/min a mixture of 1 volume of *glacial acetic acid R*, 40 volumes of *methanol R* and 60 volumes of *water R*,
– as detector a spectrophotometer set at 270 nm.

Inject 10 μl of reference solutions (d) and (e). When the chromatograms are recorded in the prescribed conditions, the retention times relative to phenol are: 4-hydroxybenzoic acid about 0.70 and 4-hydroxyisophthalic acid about 0.90. Adjust the sensitivity of the system so that the height of the principal peak in the chromatogram obtained with reference solution (f) is at least 70 per cent of the full scale of the recorder. The test is not valid unless: in the chromatogram obtained with reference solution (e), the third peak corresponds to the phenol peak in the chromatogram obtained with reference solution (d) and the resolution between the peaks corresponding to 4-hydroxyisophthalic acid and to phenol is at least 1.0. If this resolution is not obtained adjust the quantity of acetic acid in the mobile phase.

Inject 10 μl of the test solution and 10 μl of reference solution (f). In the chromatogram obtained with the test solution: the areas of the peaks due to 4-hydroxybenzoic acid, 4-hydroxyisophthalic acid and phenol are not greater than the areas of the corresponding peaks in the chromatogram obtained with reference solution (f) (0.1 per cent for 4-hydroxybenzoic acid; 0.05 per cent for 4-hydroxyisophthalic acid and 0.02 per cent for phenol).

In the chromatogram obtained with the test solution: the area of any peak, apart from the principal peak and the peaks due to 4-hydroxybenzoic acid, 4-hydroxyisophthalic acid and phenol, is not greater than that of the peak due to 4-hydroxyisophthalic acid in the chromatogram obtained with reference solution (f) (0.05 per cent); the sum of the areas of all the peaks, apart from the principal peak, is not greater than twice the area of the peak due to 4-hydroxybenzoic acid in the chromatogram obtained with reference solution (f) (0.2 per cent). Disregard any peak with an area less than 0.01 times that of the principal peak in the chromatogram obtained with reference solution (f).

Chlorides (*2.4.4*). 10 ml of solution S diluted to 15 ml with *water R* complies with the limit test for chlorides (100 ppm).

Sulphates. Not more than 200 ppm. Dissolve 1.0 g in 5 ml of *dimethylformamide R* and add 4 ml of *water R*. Mix thoroughly. Add 0.2 ml of *dilute hydrochloric acid R* and 0.5 ml of a 25 per cent *m/m* solution of *barium chloride R*. After 15 min any opalescence in the solution is not more intense than that in a standard prepared as follows: to 2 ml of *sulphate standard solution (100 ppm SO_4) R* add 0.2 ml of *dilute hydrochloric acid R*, 0.5 ml of a 25 per cent *m/m* solution of *barium chloride R*, 3 ml of *water R* and 5 ml of *dimethylformamide R*.

Heavy metals (*2.4.8*). Dissolve 2.0 g in 15 ml of *alcohol R* and add 5 ml of *water R*. 12 ml of the solution complies with limit test B for heavy metals (20 ppm). Prepare the standard using lead standard solution (2 ppm Pb) prepared by diluting *lead standard solution (100 ppm Pb) R* with a mixture of 5 volumes of *water R* and 15 volumes of *alcohol R*.

Loss on drying (*2.2.32*). Not more than 0.5 per cent, determined on 1.000 g by drying in a desiccator.

Sulphated ash (*2.4.14*). Not more than 0.1 per cent, determined on 2.0 g.

ASSAY

Dissolve 0.120 g in 30 ml of *alcohol R* and add 20 ml of *water R*. Titrate with *0.1 M sodium hydroxide*, using 0.1 ml of *phenol red solution R* as indicator.

1 ml of *0.1 M sodium hydroxide* is equivalent to 13.81 mg of $C_7H_6O_3$.

STORAGE

Store protected from light.

IMPURITIES

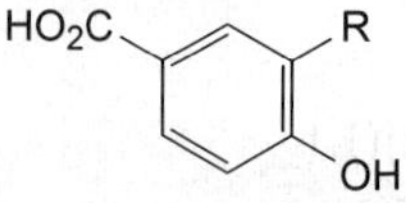

A. R = H: 4-hydroxybenzoic acid,

B. R = CO_2H: 4-hydroxyisophthalic acid,

C. phenol.

01/2005:1910

SALMON OIL, FARMED

Salmonis domestici oleum

DEFINITION

Purified fatty oil obtained from fresh farmed *Salmo salar*. The positional distribution (β(2)-acyl) is 60-70 per cent for cervonic (docosahexaenoic) acid (C22:6 n-3; DHA), 25-35 per cent for timnodonic (eicosapentaenoic) acid (C20:5 n-3; EPA) and 40-55 per cent for moroctic acid (C18:4 n-3).

Content:

– sum of the contents of EPA and DHA (expressed as triglycerides): 10.0 per cent to 28.0 per cent.

Authorised antioxidants in concentrations not exceeding the levels specified by the competent authority may be added.

PRODUCTION

The fish shall only be given feed with a composition that is in accordance with the relevant EU or other applicable regulations.

The oil is produced by mechanical expression of fresh raw materials, either from the whole fish, or fish where the fillets have been removed, at a temperature not exceeding 100 °C, and without using solvents. After centrifugation, solid substances may be removed from the oil by cooling and filtering (winterisation).

CHARACTERS

Appearance: pale pink liquid.

Solubility: practically insoluble in water, very soluble in acetone and in heptane, slightly soluble in anhydrous ethanol.

IDENTIFICATION

Examine the ^{13}C NMR spectra obtained in the assay for positional distribution (β(2)-acyl) of fatty acids. The spectra contain peaks between 172 ppm and 173 ppm with shifts similar to those in the type spectrum (Figure 1910.-2). The oil to be examined complies with the limits of this assay.

TESTS

Absorbance (*2.2.25*): minimum 0.10, measured at the maximum between 470 nm and 480 nm.

Dissolve 5.0 ml in 5.0 ml of *trimethylpentane R*.

Acid value (*2.5.1*): maximum 2.0.

Anisidine value (*2.5.36*): maximum 10.0.

Peroxide value (*2.5.5, Method A*): maximum 5.0.

Unsaponifiable matter (*2.5.7*): maximum 1.5 per cent, determined on 5.0 g.

Linoleic acid (*2.4.29*): maximum 11.0 per cent.

Identify the peak due to linoleic acid using the chromatogram in Figure 1910.-1. Determine the percentage content by normalisation.

ASSAY

Positional distribution (β(2)-acyl) of fatty acids (*2.2.33*) Use a high resolution FT-NMR spectrometer operating at minimum 300 MHz.

Test solution. Dissolve 190-210 mg of fresh salmon oil in 500 µl of *deuterated chloroform R*. Prepare at least 3 samples and examine within 3 days.

Acquisition of ^{13}*C NMR spectra.* The following parameters may be used.

- *sweep width*: 200 ppm (−5 to 195 ppm),
- *irradiation frequency offset*: 95 ppm,
- *time domain*: 64 K,
- *pulse delay*: 2 s,
- *pulse program*: zgig 30 (inverse gated, 30° excitation pulse),
- *dummy scans*: 4,
- *number of scans*: 4096.

Processing and plotting. The following parameters may be used:

- *size*: 64 K (zero-filling),
- *window multiplication*: exponential,
- *Lorentzian broadening factor*: 0.2 Hz.

Use the $CDCl_3$ signal for shift referencing. The shift of the central peak of the 1:1:1 triplet is set to 77.16 ppm.

Plot the spectral region δ 171.5-173.5 ppm. Compare the spectrum with the reference spectrum in Figure 1910.-2. The shift values lie within the ranges given in Table 1910.-1.

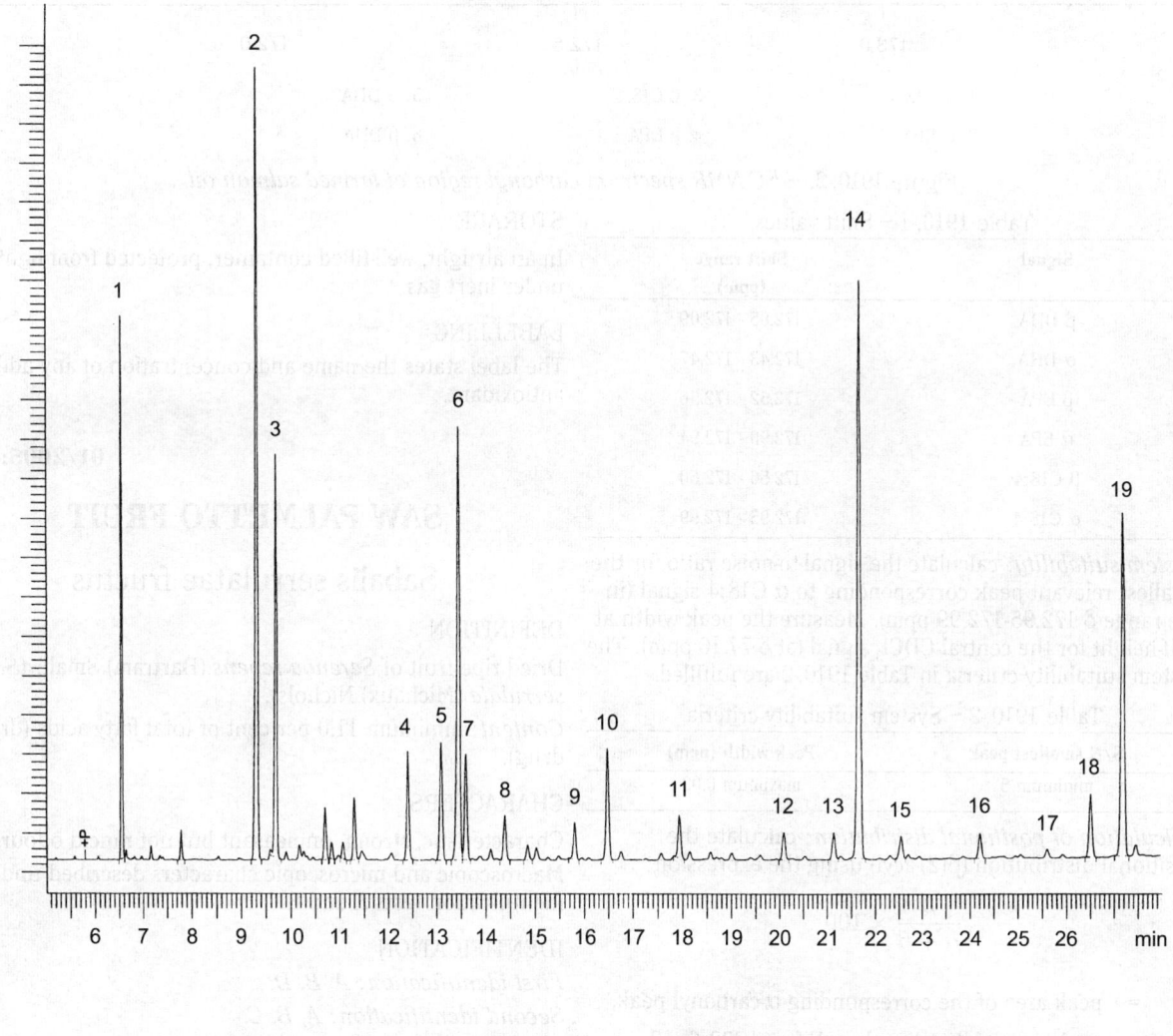

1. C14:0	6. C18:1 n-9	11. C20:1 n-9	16. C21:5 n-3
2. C16:0	7. C18:1 n-7	12. C20:4 n-6	17. C22:5 n-6
3. C16:1 n-7	8. C18:2 n-6	13. C20:4 n-3	18. C22:5 n-3
4. C16:4 n-1	9. C18:3 n-3	14. EPA	19. DHA
5. C18:0	10. C18:4 n-3	15. C22:1 n-11	

Figure 1910.-1. – *Chromatogram for the composition of fatty acids in farmed salmon oil*

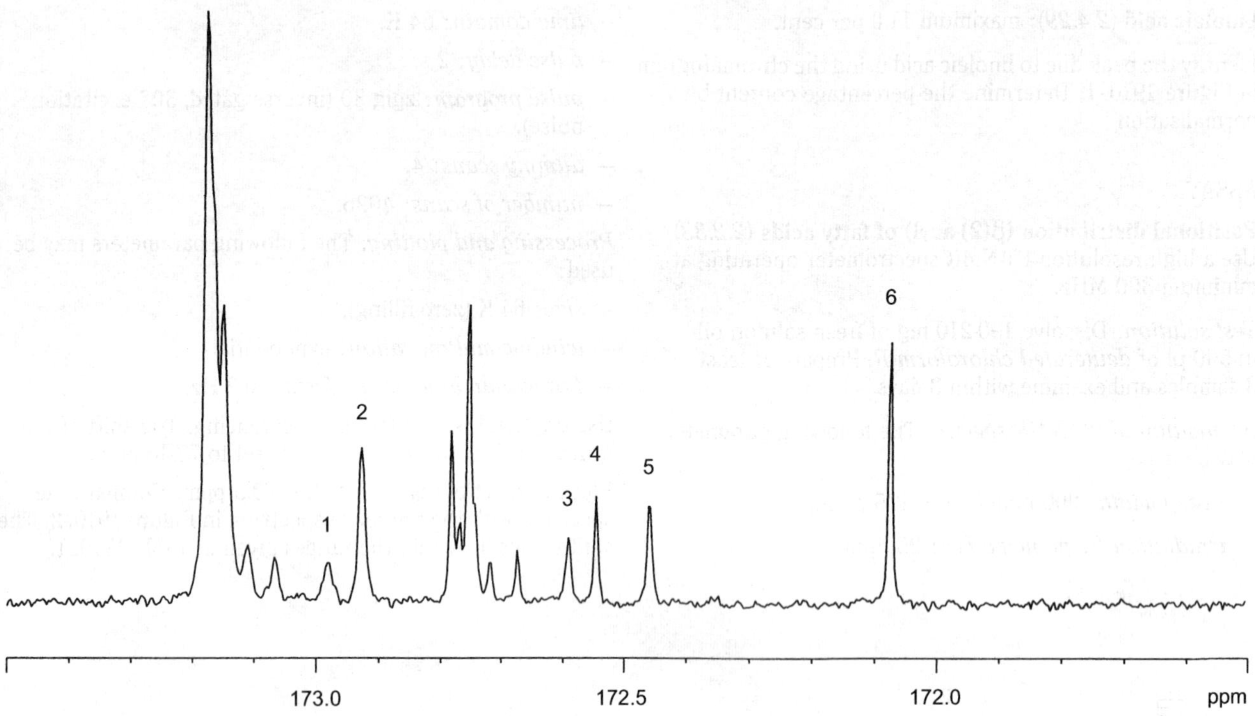

1. α C18:4	3. β C18:4	5. α DHA
2. α EPA	4. β EPA	6. β DHA

Figure 1910.-2. – *^{13}C NMR spectrum carbonyl region of farmed salmon oil*

Table 1910.-1 – Shift values

Signal	Shift range (ppm)
β DHA	172.05 - 172.09
α DHA	172.43 - 172.47
β EPA	172.52 - 172.56
α EPA	172.90 - 172.94
β C18:4	172.56 - 172.60
α C18:4	172.95 - 172.99

System suitability: calculate the signal-to-noise ratio for the smallest relevant peak corresponding to α C18:4 signal (in the range δ 172.95-172.99 ppm). Measure the peak width at half-height for the central $CDCl_3$ signal (at δ 77.16 ppm). The system suitability criteria in Table 1910.-2 are fulfilled.

Table 1910.-2 – System suitability criteria

S/N smallest peak	Peak width (ppm)
minimum 5	maximum 0.02

Calculation of positional distribution: calculate the positional distribution (β(2)-acyl) using the expression:

$$\frac{\beta}{\alpha + \beta} \times 100$$

α = peak area of the corresponding α-carbonyl peak,

β = peak area of β-carbonyl peak from C22:6 n-3, C20:5 n-3 or C18:4 n-3, respectively.

Limits:

	Positional distribution (mole (%))		
	β DHA	β EPA	β C18:4
Limits	60 - 70	25 - 35	40 - 55

EPA and DHA (*2.4.29*). See Figure 1910.-1.

STORAGE

In an airtight, well-filled container, protected from light, under inert gas.

LABELLING

The label states the name and concentration of any added antioxidant.

01/2005:1848

SAW PALMETTO FRUIT

Sabalis serrulatae fructus

DEFINITION

Dried ripe fruit of *Serenoa repens* (Bartram) Small. (*Sabal serrulata* (Michaux) Nichols).

Content: minimum 11.0 per cent of total fatty acids (dried drug).

CHARACTERS

Characteristic, strong, unpleasant but not rancid odour.

Macroscopic and microscopic characters described under identification tests A and B.

IDENTIFICATION

First identification: A, B, D.

Second identification: A, B, C.

A. The fruit is an ovoid to subspherical drupe, with a dark brown to blackish, roughly wrinkled surface and more or less coppery sheen, up to 2.5 cm long and 1.5 cm in diameter. The apex sometimes bears the remains of the style and tubular calyx, with 3 teeth, and the base bears a small depression with the scar of the stalk. The epicarp and underlying mesocarp form a thin fragile layer, which partially peels off, revealing the thin, hard, pale brown endocarp, which is fibrous and easily separable. The seed is irregularly spherical to ovoid, up to 12 mm long and 8 mm in diameter, with a hard, smooth or finely pitted surface which is reddish-brown with a paler, raised and membranous area over the raphe and micropyle; cut transversely, the seed has a thin testa, narrow perisperm and a large area of dense, horny, greyish-white endosperm, with the embryo positioned to one side.

B. Reduce to a powder (710). The powder is reddish or blackish-brown and oily. Examine under a microscope using *chloral hydrate solution R*. The powder shows fragments of epicarp composed of several layers of thin-walled, reddish-brown, pigmented, polyhedral cells (10 µm to 40 µm) which are strongly cuticularised; those of the outer layers are much smaller than those of the inner layers. Parenchyma cells of the mesocarp may be large and filled with oil droplets, or smaller and containing nodules of silica. Groups of xylem tissue of the mesocarp show small lignified, annular or spirally thickened vessels. Stone cells of the mesocarp (20 µm to 200 µm) may be found scattered, usually singly but sometimes in small groups, the walls are moderately thickened, distinctly striated and finely pitted. Fragments of endocarp contain groups of elongated sclereids about 300 µm long, with strongly thickened walls and numerous pits. The seed testa consists of small, thin-walled cells with brownish contents and underlying sclereids; albumen cells are thick-walled with large conspicuous pits and contain aleurone grains and fixed oil.

C. Thin-layer chromatography (*2.2.27*).

Test solution. To 1.5 g of the powdered drug (710), add 20 ml of *alcohol R* and stir for 15 min. Filter.

Reference solution. Dissolve 4 mg of *β-amyrin R* and 10 mg of *β-sitosterol R* in 10 ml of *alcohol R*.

Plate: *TLC silica gel plate R* (2-10 µm).

Mobile phase: *acetic acid R, ethyl acetate R, toluene R* (1:30:70 *V/V/V*).

Application: 8 µl of the test solution and 2 µl of the reference solution, as bands.

Development: over a path of 10 cm.

Drying: in air.

Detection: spray with *anisaldehyde solution R*; dry the plate at 100-105 °C for 5-10 min; examine in daylight.

Results: see below the sequence of the zones present in the chromatograms obtained with the reference solution and the test solution. Furthermore, other faint zones are present, especially in the lower third, in the chromatogram obtained with the test solution.

Top of the plate	
	A strong blue zone
	A faint blue zone
β-Amyrin: a blue zone	A faint blue zone
	A strong bluish-violet zone
β-Sitosterol: a blue zone	
	A faint blue zone
	A faint blue zone
Reference solution	**Test solution**

D. Examine the chromatograms obtained in the assay of total fatty acids.

Results: the characteristic peaks in the chromatogram obtained with the test solution are similar in retention time to the characteristic peaks in the chromatogram obtained with the reference solution. The principal peak is due to lauric acid.

TESTS

Foreign matter (*2.8.2*): maximum 2.0 per cent.

Loss on drying (*2.2.32*): maximum 12.0 per cent, determined on 1.000 g of the powdered drug (710) by drying in an oven at 100-105 °C for 2 h.

Total ash (*2.4.16*): maximum 5.0 per cent.

ASSAY

Total fatty acids. Gas chromatography (*2.2.28*).

Internal standard solution. Dissolve 0.47 g of *methyl pelargonate R* and 0.47 g of *methyl margarate R* in 20.0 ml of *dimethylformamide R* and dilute to 100.0 ml with the same solvent.

Test solution. Reduce 50 g of the drug to a powder (200). Place 4.0 g of the powdered drug in a 100 ml volumetric flask. Add 60.0 ml of *dimethylformamide R*. Mix using sonication for 15 min and then shake for 30 min. Dilute to 100.0 ml with *dimethylformamide R*. Allow to stand for a few minutes and filter. To 20.0 ml of this solution add 4.0 ml of the internal standard solution and dilute to 25.0 ml with *dimethylformamide R*. To 0.4 ml of this solution add 0.6 ml of an 18.84 g/l solution of *trimethylsulphonium hydroxide R* in *methanol R* and mix.

Reference solution. Dissolve 32.0 mg of *caproic acid R*, 62.0 mg of *caprylic acid R*, 68.0 mg of *capric acid R*, 0.699 g of *lauric acid R*, 0.267 g of *myristic acid R*, 10.0 mg of *palmitoleic acid R*, 0.217 g of *palmitic acid R*, 0.115 g of *linoleic acid R*, 18.0 mg of *linolenic acid R*, 0.870 g of *oleic acid R* and 49.0 mg of *stearic acid R* in *dimethylformamide R* and dilute to 10.0 ml with the same solvent. To 1.0 ml of the solution add 4.0 ml of the internal standard solution and dilute to 25.0 ml with *dimethylformamide R*. To 0.4 ml of this solution add 0.6 ml of an 18.84 g/l solution of *trimethylsulphonium hydroxide R* in *methanol R* and mix.

Column:

- *material*: fused silica,
- *size*: l = 25 m (a film thickness of 1 µm may be used) to 60 m (a film thickness of 0.2 µm may be used), Ø = 0.20-0.53 mm,
- *stationary phase*: *poly(dimethyl)siloxane R*.

Carrier gas: *helium for chromatography R*.

Flow rate: 0.5 ml/min.

Split ratio: 1:40.

Temperature:

	Time (min)	Temperature (°C)
Column	0 - 2	150
	2 - 7	150 → 190
	7 - 22	190 → 220
Injection port		300
Detector		300

Detection: flame ionisation.

Injection: 1.0 µl.

Using the retention times determined from the chromatogram obtained with the reference solution, locate the components of the reference solution on the chromatogram obtained with the test solution.

Monographs Q-S

Use the expression below to determine the percentage content of the different fatty acids. Determine the content of caproic acid, caprylic acid, capric acid and lauric acid using methyl pelargonate as the internal standard. Determine the content of myristic acid, palmitoleic acid, palmitic acid, linoleic acid, linolenic acid, oleic acid and stearic acid using methyl margarate as the internal standard. The peak area of lauric acid is not less than 20 per cent of the total area of the peaks.

$$\frac{A_1}{A_3} \times \frac{A_2}{A_4} \times \frac{m_2}{m_1} \times p \times 0.5$$

- A_1 = area of the peak due to the considered derivatised fatty acid in the chromatogram obtained with the test solution,
- A_2 = area of the peak due to methyl pelargonate or methyl margarate in the chromatogram obtained with the reference solution,
- A_3 = area of the peak due to methyl pelargonate or methyl margarate in the chromatogram obtained with the test solution,
- A_4 = area of the peak due to the considered derivatised fatty acid in the chromatogram obtained with the reference solution,
- m_1 = mass of the test sample, in grams,
- m_2 = mass of the considered fatty acid in the reference solution, in grams,
- p = percentage purity of the considered fatty acid in the reference solution.

01/2005:1260

SELEGILINE HYDROCHLORIDE

Selegilini hydrochloridum

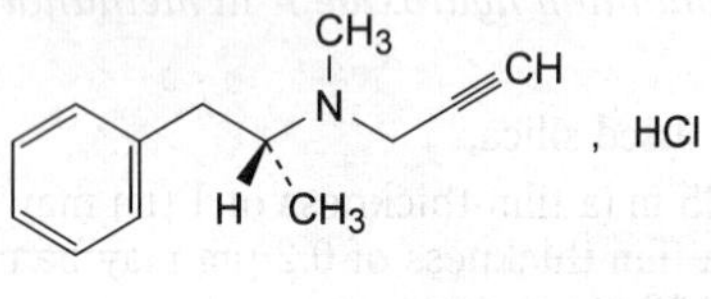

$C_{13}H_{18}ClN$ M_r 223.7

DEFINITION

Selegiline hydrochloride contains not less than 99.0 per cent and not more than the equivalent of 101.0 per cent of *N*-methyl-*N*-[(1*R*)-1-methyl-2-phenylethyl]prop-2-yn-1-amine hydrochloride, calculated with reference to the dried substance.

CHARACTERS

A white or almost white, crystalline powder, freely soluble in water and in methanol, slightly soluble in acetone.

It melts at about 143 °C.

IDENTIFICATION

A. Dissolve 2.000g in *carbon dioxide-free water R* and dilute to 20.0 ml with the same solvent. The specific optical rotation (*2.2.7*) is − 10.0 to − 12.0, calculated with reference to the dried substance.

B. Examine by infrared absorption spectrophotometry (*2.2.24*), comparing with the spectrum obtained with *selegiline hydrochloride CRS*. Examine the substances as discs prepared using *potassium chloride R*.

C. It gives reaction (a) of chlorides (*2.3.1*).

TESTS

pH (*2.2.3*). Dissolve 0.20 g in *carbon dioxide-free water R* and dilute to 10 ml with the same solvent. The pH of the solution is 3.5 to 4.5.

Related substances. Examine by liquid chromatography (*2.2.29*).

Test solution. Dissolve 20 mg of the substance to be examined in the mobile phase and dilute to 10.0 ml with the mobile phase.

Reference solution (a). Dissolve 50.0 mg of *selegiline hydrochloride CRS* and 10.0 mg of *butyl parahydroxybenzoate R* in the mobile phase and dilute to 50.0 ml with the mobile phase. Dilute 1.0 ml to 20.0 ml with the mobile phase.

Reference solution (b). Dilute 1.0 ml of the test solution to 10.0 ml with the mobile phase. Dilute 1.0 ml to 50.0 ml with the mobile phase.

The chromatographic procedure may be carried out using:

– a stainless steel column 0.25 m long and 4.6 mm in internal diameter packed with *octylsilyl silica gel for chromatography R* (5 µm),
– as mobile phase at a flow rate of 1 ml/min a mixture prepared as follows: dilute 500 ml of *acetonitrile R* to 1000.0 ml with a butylammonium acetate buffer solution pH 6.5 prepared by dissolving 4 ml of *butylamine R* in 900 ml of *water R* and adjusting to pH 6.5 with *acetic acid R* before diluting to 1000.0 ml with *water R*,
– as detector a spectrophotometer set at 215 nm.

Inject 20 µl of reference solution (a). The test is not valid unless, in the chromatogram obtained with reference solution (a), the resolution between the peaks corresponding to selegiline and butyl parahydroxybenzoate is greater than three. Inject 20 µl of the test solution and 20 µl of reference solution (b). Continue the chromatography for 1.7 times the retention time of selegiline. In the chromatogram obtained with the test solution: the area of any peak apart from the principal peak is not greater than that of the peak in the chromatogram obtained with reference solution (b) (0.2 per cent); and the sum of the areas of such peaks is not greater than 2.5 times the area of the principal peak in the chromatogram obtained with reference solution (b) (0.5 per cent). Disregard any peak due to chlorides and any peak with an area less than 0.1 times that of the principal peak in the chromatogram obtained with reference solution (b) (0.02 per cent).

(*S*)-Selegiline. Examine by liquid chromatography (*2.2.29*).

Test solution. Dissolve 20.0 mg of the substance to be examined in a mixture of 1 ml of *2-propanol R* and 10 µl of *butylamine R* and dilute to 10.0 ml with the mobile phase.

Reference solution (a). Dissolve 8.0 mg of *(RS)-selegiline hydrochloride CRS* in a mixture of 10 µl of *butylamine R* and 1 ml of *2-propanol R* and dilute to 10.0 ml with the mobile phase.

Reference solution (b). Dilute 0.5 ml of reference solution (a) to 20.0 ml with the mobile phase.

The chromatographic procedure may be carried out using:

– a stainless steel column 0.25 m long and 4.6 mm in internal diameter packed with *silica gel OD for chiral separation R*,
– as the mobile phase at a flow rate of 1 ml/min a mixture of 0.2 volumes of *2-propanol R* and 99.8 volumes of *cyclohexane R*,
– as detector a spectrophotometer set at 220 nm.

Inject 20 µl of each solution. When the chromatograms are recorded in the prescribed conditions, the retention time of (*S*)-selegiline is about 10 min. Adjust the sensitivity of the system so that the height of the peaks in the chromatogram obtained with reference solution (b) is about 10 per cent of the full scale of the recorder. The test is not valid unless in the chromatogram obtained with reference solution (a) the resolution between the peaks corresponding to (*S*)-selegiline and (*R*)-selegiline is at least 1.5. If necessary, adjust the concentration of 2-propanol in the mobile phase. In the chromatogram obtained with the test solution, any peak due to (*S*)-selegiline is not greater than the area of the corresponding peak in the chromatogram obtained with reference solution (b) (0.5 per cent).

Loss on drying (*2.2.32*). Not more than 0.5 per cent, determined on 1.000 g by drying at 60 °C at a pressure not exceeding 0.5 kPa.

Sulphated ash (*2.4.14*). Not more than 0.1 per cent, determined on 1.0 g.

ASSAY

Dissolve 0.180 g in 50 ml of *acetic anhydride R*. Titrate with *0.1 M perchloric acid*, determining the end-point potentiometrically (*2.2.20*).

1 ml of *0.1 M perchloric acid* is equivalent to 22.37 mg of $C_{13}H_{18}ClN$.

STORAGE

Store protected from light.

IMPURITIES

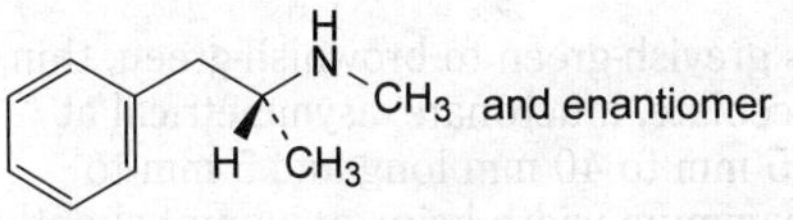

A. (2*RS*)-*N*-methyl-1-phenylpropan-2-amine [(*RS*)-metamphetamine],

B. (2*R*)-1-phenylpropan-2-amine (amphetamine),

C. (1*RS*,2*SR*)-2-amino-1-phenylpropan-1-ol (phenylpropanolamine),

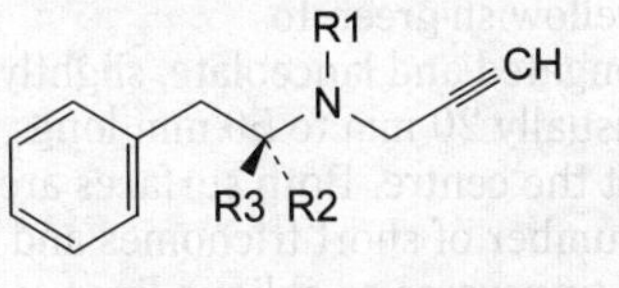

D. R1 = R3 = H, R2 = CH_3: *N*-[(1*R*)-1-methyl-2-phenylethyl]prop-2-yn-1-amine (demethylselegiline),

E. R1 = R3 = CH_3, R2 = H: *N*-methyl-*N*-[(1*S*)-1-methyl-2-phenylethyl]prop-2-yn-1-amine [(*S*)-selegiline].

01/2005:1147

SELENIUM DISULPHIDE

Selenii disulfidum

SeS_2 M_r 143.1

DEFINITION

Selenium disulphide contains not less than 52.0 per cent and not more than 55.5 per cent of Se.

CHARACTERS

A bright-orange or reddish-brown powder, practically insoluble in water.

IDENTIFICATION

A. Gently boil about 50 mg with 5 ml of *nitric acid R* for 30 min. Dilute to 50 ml with *water R* and filter. To 5 ml of the filtrate add 10 ml of *water R* and 5 g of *urea R*. Heat to boiling, cool and add 1.5 ml of *potassium iodide solution R*. A yellow to orange colour is produced which darkens rapidly on standing. This solution is used in identification test B.

B. Allow the coloured solution obtained under identification A to stand for 10 min and filter through *kieselguhr for chromatography R*. 5 ml of the filtrate give reaction (a) of sulphates (*2.3.1*).

TESTS

Soluble selenium compounds. To 10 g add 100 ml of *water R*, mix well, allow to stand for 1 h with frequent shaking and filter. To 10 ml of the filtrate add 2 ml of a 115 g/l solution of *anhydrous formic acid R*, dilute to 50 ml with *water R* and adjust to pH 2.0 to 3.0 with an 115 g/l solution of *anhydrous formic acid R*. Add 2 ml of a 5 g/l solution of *3,3′-diaminobenzidine tetrahydrochloride R*. Allow to stand for 45 min and then adjust to pH 6.0 to 7.0 with *dilute ammonia R1*. Shake the solution for 1 min with 10 ml of *toluene R* and allow the phases to separate. The absorbance (*2.2.25*) of the upper layer measured at 420 nm is not greater than that of a standard prepared at the same time and in the same manner beginning at the words "add 2 ml of an 115 g/l solution of *anhydrous formic acid R*" and using 5 ml of *selenium standard solution (1 ppm Se) R* (5 ppm, calculated as Se).

ASSAY

To 0.100 g add 25 ml of *fuming nitric acid R* and heat on a water-bath for 1 h; a small insoluble residue may remain. Cool and dilute to 100.0 ml with *water R*. To 25.0 ml add 50 ml of *water R* and 5 g of *urea R* and heat to boiling. Cool, add 7 ml of *potassium iodide solution R*, 3 ml of *starch solution R* and titrate immediately with *0.1 M sodium thiosulphate*. Carry out a blank titration.

1 ml of *0.1 M sodium thiosulphate* is equivalent to 1.974 mg of Se.

01/2005:0202

SENEGA ROOT

Polygalae radix

DEFINITION

Senega root consists of the dried and usually fragmented root and root crown of *Polygala senega* L. or of certain other closely related species or of a mixture of these *Polygala* species.

CHARACTERS

Senega root has a faint, sweet odour, slightly rancid or reminiscent of methyl salicylate.

Reduced to a powder, it is irritant and sternutatory. Shaken with water, the powder produces a copious froth.

It has the macroscopic and microscopic characters described under identification tests A, B and C.

IDENTIFICATION

A. The root crown is greyish-brown and wider than the root; it forms an irregular head consisting of numerous remains of stems and tightly packed purplish-brown buds. The taproot is brown to yellow, occasionally branched, sometimes flexuous, usually tortous without secondary roots, except in the Japanese varieties and species, which contain numerous fibrous rootlets. The diameter is usually 1 mm to 8 mm at the crown, gradually tapering to the tip; the surface is transversely and longitudinally striated and often shows a more or less distinct decurrent, elongated spiral keel. The fracture is short and shows a yellowish cortex of varying thickness surrounding a paler central woody area somewhat circular or irregular in shape depending on the species.

B. Examine under a microscope using *chloral hydrate solution R*. The transverse section of the root shows cork formed from several layers of thin-walled cells, phelloderm of slightly collenchymatous cells containing droplets of oil; the phloem and xylem arrangement is usually normal, especially near the crown but where a keel is present this is formed by increased development of phloem; other anomalous secondary development sometimes occurs, resulting in the formation of one or two large wedge-shaped rays in the phloem and xylem, the parenchymatous cells of which contain droplets of oil. The xylem is usually central and consists of vessels up to 60 µm in diameter associated with numerous thin-walled tracheids and a few small lignified parenchymatous cells.

C. Reduce to a powder (355). The powder is light brown. Examine under a microscope using *chloral hydrate solution R*. The powder shows the following diagnostic characters: longitudinal fragments of lignified tissue made up of pitted tracheids and somewhat larger vessels with numerous bordered pits or with reticulate thickening; yellowish parenchyma and collenchymatous cells containing droplets of oil; occasional fragments of cork, and of epidermal tissue with stomata and unicellular trichomes from the bud scales. Crystals and stone cells are absent.

D. Examine by thin-layer chromatography (*2.2.27*), using *silica gel G R* as the coating substance.

Test solution. To 1.0 g of the powdered drug (355) add 10 ml of *alcohol (70 per cent V/V) R*, boil under a reflux condenser for 15 min, filter and allow to cool.

Reference solution. Dissolve 10 mg of *aescin R* in *alcohol (70 per cent V/V) R* and dilute to 10 ml with the same solvent.

Apply to the plate as bands 20 mm by 3 mm 10 µl of the test solution and 10 µl and 40 µl of the reference solution. Develop over a path of 12 cm using the upper layer of a mixture of 10 volumes of *glacial acetic acid R*, 40 volumes of *water R* and 50 volumes of *butanol R*. Dry the plate at 100-105 °C, spray with about 10 ml of *anisaldehyde solution R* for a plate 200 mm square and heat again at 100-105 °C, observing the chromatogram obtained with the test solution until red zones (corresponding to saponosides) appear. In the chromatogram obtained with the test solution, three to five red zones appear in the lower and middle parts, similar in position to the grey-violet zones corresponding to aescin in the chromatogram obtained with the reference solution. Spray the plate with about 10 ml of a 200 g/l solution of *phosphomolybdic acid R* in *ethanol R* and heat at 100-105 °C, observing the chromatograms, until the zones corresponding to saponosides become blue. The intensity and size of the zones in the chromatogram obtained with the test solution are between those of the two bands corresponding to aescin in the chromatograms obtained respectively with 10 µl and 40 µl of the reference solution.

TESTS

Foreign matter (*2.8.2*). It complies with the test for foreign matter.

Total ash (*2.4.16*). Not more than 6.0 per cent.

Ash insoluble in hydrochloric acid (*2.8.1*). Not more than 3.0 per cent.

STORAGE

Store protected from light and humidity.

01/2005:0206

SENNA LEAF

Sennae folium

DEFINITION

Senna leaf consists of the dried leaflets of *Cassia senna* L. (*C. acutifolia* Delile), known as Alexandrian or Khartoum senna, or *Cassia angustifolia* Vahl, known as Tinnevelly senna, or a mixture of the two species. It contains not less than 2.5 per cent of hydroxyanthracene glycosides, calculated as sennoside B ($C_{42}H_{38}O_{20}$; M_r 863) with reference to the dried drug.

CHARACTERS

Senna leaf has a slight characteristic odour.

It has the macroscopic and microscopic characters described under identification tests A and B.

IDENTIFICATION

A. *C. senna* occurs as greyish-green to brownish-green, thin, fragile leaflets, lanceolate, mucronate, asymmetrical at the base, usually 15 mm to 40 mm long and 5 mm to 15 mm wide, the maximum width being at a point slightly below the centre; the lamina is slightly undulant with both surfaces covered with fine, short trichomes. Pinnate venation is visible mainly on the lower surface, with lateral veins leaving the midrib at an angle of about 60° and anastomosing to form a ridge near the margin.

Stomatal index (*2.8.3*): 10-12.5-15.

C. angustifolia occurs as yellowish-green to brownish-green leaflets, elongated and lanceolate, slightly asymmetrical at the base, usually 20 mm to 50 mm long and 7 mm to 20 mm wide at the centre. Both surfaces are smooth with a very small number of short trichomes and are frequently marked with transverse or oblique lines.

Stomatal index (*2.8.3*): 14-17.5-20

B. Reduce to a powder (355). The powder is light green to greenish-yellow. Examine under a microscope using *chloral hydrate solution R*. The powder shows the following diagnostic characters: polygonal epidermal cells showing paracytic stomata (*2.8.3*); unicellular trichomes, conical in shape, with warted walls, isolated or attached to fragments of epidermis; fragments of vascular bundles with a crystal sheath of prismatic crystals of calcium oxalate; cluster crystals isolated or in fragments of parenchyma.

C. Examine by thin-layer chromatography (*2.2.27*), using *silica gel G R* as the coating substance.

Test solution. To 0.5 g of the powdered drug (180) add 5 ml of a mixture of equal volumes of *alcohol R* and *water R* and heat to boiling. Centrifuge and use the supernatant liquid.

Reference solution. Dissolve 10 mg of *senna extract CRS* in 1 ml of a mixture of equal volumes of *alcohol R* and *water R* (a slight residue remains).

ASSAY

Carry out the assay protected from bright light.

Place 0.150 g of the powdered drug (180) in a 100 ml flask. Add 30.0 ml of *water R*, mix, weigh and place in a water-bath. Heat under a reflux condenser for 15 min. Allow to cool, weigh and adjust to the original mass with *water R*. Centrifuge and transfer 20.0 ml of the supernatant liquid to a 150 ml separating funnel. Add 0.1 ml of *dilute hydrochloric acid R* and shake with three quantities, each of 15 ml, of *chloroform R*. Allow to separate and discard the chloroform layer. Add 0.10 g of *sodium hydrogen carbonate R* and shake for 3 min. Centrifuge and transfer 10.0 ml of the supernatant liquid to a 100 ml round-bottomed flask with a ground-glass neck. Add 20 ml of *ferric chloride solution R1* and mix. Heat for 20 min under a reflux condenser in a water-bath with the water level above that of the liquid in the flask; add 1 ml of *hydrochloric acid R* and heat for a further 20 min, with frequent shaking, to dissolve the precipitate. Cool, transfer the mixture to a separating funnel and shake with three quantities, each of 25 ml, of *ether R* previously used to rinse the flask. Combine the ether layers and wash with two quantities, each of 15 ml, of *water R*. Transfer the ether layers to a volumetric flask and dilute to 100.0 ml with *ether R*. Evaporate 10.0 ml carefully to dryness and dissolve the residue in 10.0 ml of a 5 g/l solution of *magnesium acetate R* in *methanol R*. Measure the absorbance (*2.2.25*) at 515 nm using *methanol R* as the compensation liquid.

Calculate the percentage content of sennoside B from the expression:

$$\frac{A \times 1.25}{m}$$

i.e. taking the specific absorbance to be 240.

A = absorbance at 515 nm,

m = mass of the substance to be examined, in grams.

STORAGE

Store protected from light and moisture.

01/2005:0208

SENNA PODS, TINNEVELLY

Sennae fructus angustifoliae

DEFINITION

Tinnevelly senna pods consist of the dried fruit of *Cassia angustifolia* Vahl. They contain not less than 2.2 per cent of hydroxyanthracene glycosides, calculated as sennoside B ($C_{42}H_{38}O_{20}$; M_r 863) with reference to the dried drug.

CHARACTERS

Tinnevelly senna pods have a slight odour.

They have the macroscopic and microscopic characters described under identification tests A and B.

IDENTIFICATION

A. They occur as flattened, slightly reniform pods, yellowish-brown to brown with dark brown patches at the positions corresponding to the seeds, usually 35 mm to 60 mm long and 14 mm to 18 mm wide. At one end is a stylar point and at the other a short stalk. The pods contain five to eight flattened and obovate seeds, green to pale brown, with incomplete, wavy, transverse ridges on the testa.

B. Reduce to a powder (355). The powder is brown. Examine under a microscope using *chloral hydrate solution R*. The powder shows the following diagnostic characters: epicarp with polygonal cells and a small number of conical warty trichomes and occasional anomocytic or paracytic stomata (*2.8.3*); fibres in two crossed layers accompanied by a crystal sheath of calcium oxalate prisms; characteristic palisade cells in the seed and stratified cells in the endosperm; clusters and prisms of calcium oxalate.

C. Examine by thin-layer chromatography (*2.2.27*), using *silica gel g R* as the coating substance.

Test solution. To 0.5 g of the powdered drug (180) add 5 ml of a mixture of equal volumes of *alcohol R* and *water R* and heat to boiling. Centrifuge and use the supernatant liquid.

Reference solution. Dissolve 10 mg of *senna extract CRS* in 1 ml of a mixture of equal volumes of *alcohol R* and *water R* (a slight residue remains).

Apply to the plate as bands 20 mm by 2 mm 10 µl of each solution. Develop over a path of 10 cm using a mixture of 1 volume of *glacial acetic acid R*, 30 volumes of *water R*, 40 volumes of *ethyl acetate R* and 40 volumes of *propanol R*. Allow the plate to dry in air, spray with a 20 per cent *V/V* solution of *nitric acid R* and heat at 120 °C for 10 min. Allow to cool and spray with a 50 g/l solution of *potassium hydroxide R* in *alcohol (50 per cent V/V) R* until the zones appear. The principal zones in the chromatogram obtained with the test solution are similar in position (sennosides B, A, D and C in the order of increasing R_f value), colour and size to the principal zones in the chromatogram obtained with the reference solution. Between the zones corresponding to sennosides D and C a red zone corresponding to rhein-8-glucoside may be visible. The zones corresponding to sennosides D and C are faint in the chromatogram obtained with the test solution.

D. Place about 25 mg of the powdered drug (180) in a conical flask and add 50 ml of *water R* and 2 ml of *hydrochloric acid R*. Heat in a water-bath for 15 min, cool and shake with 40 ml of *ether R*. Separate the ether, dry over *anhydrous sodium sulphate R*, evaporate 5 ml to dryness and to the cooled residue add 5 ml of *dilute ammonia R1*. A yellow or orange colour develops. Heat on a water-bath for 2 min. A reddish-violet colour develops.

TESTS

Foreign matter (*2.8.2*). Not more than 1 per cent.

Loss on drying (*2.2.32*). Not more than 12.0 per cent, determined on 1.000 g of the powdered drug (355) by drying in an oven at 100-105 °C for 2 h.

Total ash (*2.4.16*). Not more than 9.0 per cent.

Ash insoluble in hydrochloric acid (*2.8.1*). Not more than 2.0 per cent.

ASSAY

Carry out the assay protected from bright light.

Place 0.150 g of the powdered drug (180) in a 100 ml flask. Add 30.0 ml of *water R*, mix, weigh and place in a water-bath. Heat under a reflux condenser for 15 min. Allow to cool, weigh and adjust to the original mass with *water R*. Centrifuge and transfer 20.0 ml of the supernatant liquid to a 150 ml separating funnel. Add 0.1 ml of *dilute hydrochloric acid R* and shake with three quantities, each of 15 ml, of *chloroform R*. Allow to separate and discard the chloroform layer. Add 0.10 g of *sodium hydrogen carbonate R* and shake for 3 min. Centrifuge and transfer 10.0 ml of the supernatant liquid to a 100 ml round-bottomed flask with a ground-glass neck. Add 20 ml of *ferric chloride solution R1* and mix. Heat for 20 min under a reflux condenser in a water-bath with the water level above that of the liquid in the flask; add 1 ml of *hydrochloric acid R* and heat for a further 20 min, with frequent shaking, to dissolve the precipitate. Cool, transfer the mixture to a separating funnel and shake with three quantities, each of 25 ml, of *ether R* previously used to rinse the flask. Combine the ether layers and wash with two quantities, each of 15 ml, of *water R*. Transfer the ether layers to a volumetric flask and dilute to 100.0 ml with *ether R*. Evaporate 10.0 ml carefully to dryness and dissolve the residue in 10.0 ml of a 5 g/l solution of *magnesium acetate R* in *methanol R*. Measure the absorbance (*2.2.25*) at 515 nm using *methanol R* as the compensation liquid.

Calculate the percentage content of sennoside B from the expression:

$$\frac{A \times 1.25}{m}$$

i.e. taking the specific absorbance to be 240.

A = absorbance at 515 nm,

m = mass of the substance to be examined, in grams.

STORAGE

Store protected from light and moisture.

01/2005:0788

SERINE

Serinum

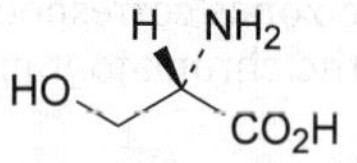

$C_3H_7NO_3$ M_r 105.1

DEFINITION

Serine contains not less than 98.5 per cent and not more than the equivalent of 101.0 per cent of (*S*)-2-amino-3-hydroxypropanoic acid, calculated with reference to the dried substance.

CHARACTERS

A white or almost white, crystalline powder or colourless crystals, freely soluble in water, practically insoluble in alcohol.

IDENTIFICATION

First identification: A, B.

Second identification: A, C, D.

A. It complies with the test for specific optical rotation (see Tests).

B. Examine by infrared absorption spectrophotometry (*2.2.24*), comparing with the spectrum obtained with *serine CRS*. Examine the substances prepared as discs.

C. Examine the chromatograms obtained in the test for ninhydrin-positive substances. The principal spot in the chromatogram obtained with test solution (b) is similar in position, colour and size to the principal spot in the chromatogram obtained with reference solution (a).

D. To 1 ml of a 10 g/l solution of the substance to be examined in a test-tube, add 5 ml of a 20 g/l solution of *sodium periodate R*. Heat on a water-bath and collect the vapour on glass wool moistened with *water R* and inserted in the opening of the test tube. After heating for 5 min, transfer the glass wool to a test-tube containing 1 ml of a 15 g/l solution of *chromotropic acid, sodium salt R* and 3 ml of *sulphuric acid R*. Heat on a water-bath for 10 min. A violet-red colour is produced.

TESTS

Solution S. Dissolve 2.5 g in *distilled water R* and dilute to 50 ml with the same solvent.

Appearance of solution. Solution S is clear (*2.2.1*) and not more intensely coloured than reference solution BY_6 (*2.2.2, Method II*).

Specific optical rotation (*2.2.7*). Dissolve 2.50 g in *dilute hydrochloric acid R* and dilute to 25.0 ml with the same acid. The specific optical rotation is + 14.0 to + 16.0, calculated with reference to the dried substance.

Ninhydrin-positive substances. Examine by thin-layer chromatography (*2.2.27*), using a *TLC silica gel plate R*.

Test solution (a). Dissolve 0.10 g of the substance to be examined in *0.1 M hydrochloric acid* and dilute to 10 ml with the same acid.

Test solution (b). Dilute 1 ml of test solution (a) to 50 ml with *water R*.

Reference solution (a). Dissolve 10 mg of *serine CRS* in *0.1 M hydrochloric acid* and dilute to 50 ml with the same acid.

Reference solution (b). Dilute 5 ml of test solution (b) to 20 ml with *water R*.

Reference solution (c). Dissolve 10 mg of *methionine CRS* and 10 mg of *serine CRS* in *0.1 M hydrochloric acid* and dilute to 25 ml with the same acid.

Apply to the plate 5 µl of each solution. Develop over a path of 15 cm using a mixture of 20 volumes of *glacial acetic acid R*, 20 volumes of *water R* and 60 volumes of *butanol R*. Allow the plate to dry in air, spray with *ninhydrin solution R* and heat at 100 °C to 105 °C for 15 min. Any spot in the chromatogram obtained with test solution (a), apart from the principal spot, is not more intense than the spot in the chromatogram obtained with reference solution (b) (0.5 per cent). The test is not valid unless the chromatogram obtained with reference solution (c) shows two clearly separated spots.

Chlorides (*2.4.4*). Dilute 5 ml of solution S to 15 ml with *water R*. The solution complies with the limit test for chlorides (200 ppm).

Sulphates (*2.4.13*). Dilute 10 ml of solution S to 15 ml with *distilled water R*. The solution complies with the limit test for sulphates (300 ppm).

Ammonium (*2.4.1*). 50 mg complies with limit test B for ammonium (200 ppm). Prepare the standard using 0.1 ml of *ammonium standard solution (100 ppm NH_4) R*.

Iron (*2.4.9*). In a separating funnel, dissolve 1.0 g in 10 ml of *dilute hydrochloric acid R*. Shake with three quantities, each of 10 ml, of *methyl isobutyl ketone R1*, shaking for 3 min each time. To the combined organic layers add 10 ml of *water R* and shake for 3 min. The aqueous layer complies with the limit test for iron (10 ppm).

Heavy metals (*2.4.8*). Dissolve 2.0 g in *water R* and dilute to 20 ml with the same solvent. 12 ml of the solution complies with limit test A for heavy metals (10 ppm). Prepare the standard using *lead standard solution (1 ppm Pb) R*.

Loss on drying (*2.2.32*). Not more than 0.5 per cent, determined on 1.000 g by drying in an oven at 100 °C to 105 °C.

Sulphated ash (*2.4.14*). Not more than 0.1 per cent, determined on 1.0 g.

ASSAY

Dissolve 0.100 g in 3 ml of *anhydrous formic acid R*. Add 30 ml of *anhydrous acetic acid R*. Using 0.1 ml of *naphtholbenzein solution R* as indicator, titrate with *0.1 M perchloric acid* until the colour changes from brownish-yellow to green.

1 ml of *0.1 M perchloric acid* is equivalent to 10.51 mg of $C_3H_7NO_3$.

STORAGE

Store protected from light.

01/2005:1148

SERTACONAZOLE NITRATE

Sertaconazoli nitras

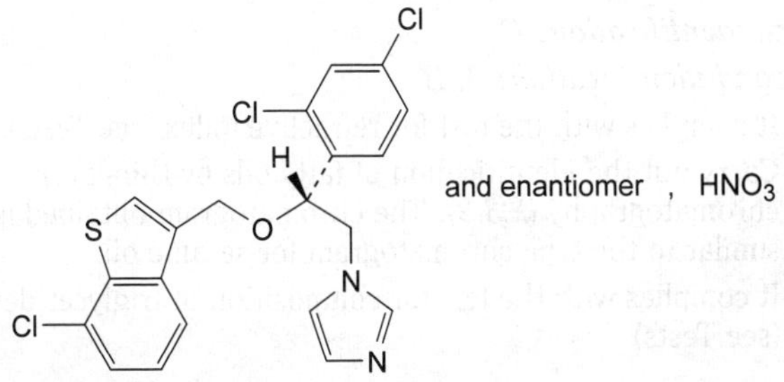

$C_{20}H_{16}Cl_3N_3O_4S$ M_r 500.8

DEFINITION

Sertaconazole nitrate contains not less than 98.5 per cent and not more than the equivalent of 101.0 per cent of (*RS*)-1-[2-[(7-chloro-1-benzothiophen-3-yl)methoxy]-2-(2,4-dichlorophenyl)ethyl]-1*H*-imidazole nitrate, calculated with reference to the anhydrous substance.

CHARACTERS

A white or almost white powder, practically insoluble in water, soluble in methanol, sparingly soluble in alcohol and in methylene chloride.

IDENTIFICATION

First identification: A, C.

Second identification: A, B, D, E.

A. Melting point (*2.2.14*): 156 °C to 161 °C.

B. Dissolve 0.1 g in *methanol R* and dilute to 100 ml with the same solvent. Dilute 10 ml of the solution to 100 ml with *methanol R*. Examined between 240 nm and 320 nm (*2.2.25*), the solutions shows three absorption maxima, at 260 nm, 293 nm and 302 nm. The ratio of the absorbance measured at the maximum at 302 nm to that measured at the maximum at 293 nm is 1.16 to 1.28.

C. Examine by infrared absorption spectrophotometry (*2.2.24*), comparing with the spectrum obtained with *sertaconazole nitrate CRS*. Dry the substances at 100-105 °C for 2 h and examine as discs prepared using *potassium bromide R*.

D. Examine by thin-layer chromatography (*2.2.27*), using *silica gel G R* as the coating substance.

Test solution. Dissolve 40 mg of the substance to be examined in a mixture of 1 volume of *concentrated ammonia R* and 9 volumes of *methanol R* and dilute to 10 ml with the same mixture of solvents.

Reference solution (a). Dissolve 40 mg of *sertaconazole nitrate CRS* in a mixture of 1 volume of *concentrated ammonia R* and 9 volumes of *methanol R* and dilute to 10 ml with the same mixture of solvents.

Reference solution (b). Dissolve 20 mg of *miconazole nitrate CRS* in reference solution (a) and dilute to 5 ml with the same solution.

Apply to the plate 5 µl of each solution. Develop over a path of 15 cm using a mixture of 1 volume of *concentrated ammonia R*, 40 volumes of *toluene R* and 60 volumes of *dioxan R*. Dry the plate in a current of air for 15 min and expose the plate to iodine vapour for 30 min. The principal spot in the chromatogram obtained with the test solution is similar in position, colour and size to the spot in the chromatogram obtained with reference solution (a). The test is not valid unless the chromatogram obtained with reference solution (b) shows two clearly separated spots.

E. About 1 mg gives the reaction of nitrates (*2.3.1*).

TESTS

Appearance of solution. Dissolve 0.1 g in *alcohol R* and dilute to 10 ml with the same solvent. The solution is clear (*2.2.1*) and not more intensely coloured than reference solution Y_5 (*2.2.2, Method II*).

Related substances. Examine by liquid chromatography (*2.2.29*).

Test solution. Dissolve 10.0 mg of the substance to be examined in the mobile phase and dilute to 10.0 ml with the mobile phase.

Reference solution (a). Dilute 5.0 ml of the test solution to 100.0 ml with the mobile phase. Dilute 1.0 ml of the solution to 20.0 ml with the mobile phase.

Reference solution (b). Dissolve 5.0 mg of *sertaconazole nitrate CRS* and 5.0 mg of *miconazole nitrate CRS* in the mobile phase and dilute to 20.0 ml with the mobile phase. Dilute 1.0 ml of the solution to 50.0 ml with the mobile phase.

The chromatographic procedure may be carried out using:

- a stainless steel column 0.25 m long and 4.0 mm in internal diameter packed with *nitrile silica gel for chromatography R1* (10 µm),
- as mobile phase at a flow rate of 1.6 ml/min a mixture of 37 volumes of *acetonitrile R* and 63 volumes of a 1.5 g/l solution of *sodium dihydrogen phosphate R*,
- as detector a spectrophotometer set at 220 nm.

Inject 20 µl of reference solution (a) and 20 µl of reference solution (b). When the chromatograms are recorded in the prescribed conditions, the retention times are: nitrate ion, about 1 min; miconazole, about 17 min; sertaconazole, about 19 min. When using a recorder, adjust the sensitivity of the system so that the height of the principal peak in the chromatogram obtained with reference solution (a) is not less than 25 per cent of the full scale of the recorder. The test is not valid unless in the chromatogram obtained with reference solution (b), the resolution between the peaks due to miconazole and sertaconazole is at least 2.0.

Inject separately 20 µl of the test solution and 20 µl of reference solution (a). Continue the chromatography for 1.3 times the retention time of the principal peak. In the chromatogram obtained with the test solution: the area of any peak, apart from the principal peak and the peak due to nitrate ion, is not greater than the area of the principal peak in the chromatogram obtained with reference solution (a) (0.25 per cent) and the sum of the areas of such peaks, is not greater than twice the area of the principal peak in the chromatogram obtained with the reference solution (a) (0.5 per cent). Disregard any peak with an area less than 0.2 times the area of the principal peak in the chromatogram obtained with reference solution (a).

Water (*2.5.12*). Not more than 1.0 per cent, determined on 0.50 g by the semi-micro determination of water.

Sulphated ash (*2.4.14*). Not more than 0.1 per cent, determined on 1.0 g.

ASSAY

Dissolve 0.400 g in 50 ml of a mixture of equal volumes of *anhydrous acetic acid R* and *methyl ethyl ketone R*. Titrate with *0.1 M perchloric acid,* determining the end-point potentiometrically (*2.2.20*). Carry out a blank titration.

1 ml of *0.1 M perchloric acid* is equivalent to 50.08 mg of $C_{20}H_{16}Cl_3N_3O_4S$.

STORAGE

Store protected from light.

IMPURITIES

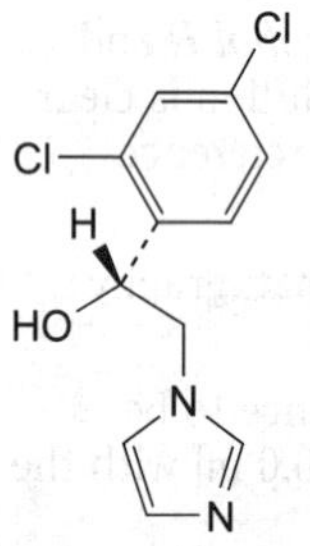

and enantiomer

A. (1*RS*)-1-(2,4-dichlorophenyl)-2-(1*H*-imidazol-1-yl)ethanol,

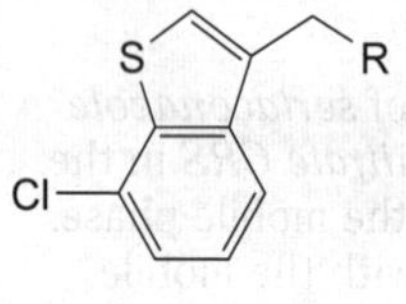

B. R = Br: 3-(bromomethyl)-7-chloro-1-benzothiophen,

C. R = OH: (7-chloro-1-benzothiophen-3-yl)methanol.

01/2005:0433

SESAME OIL, REFINED

Sesami oleum raffinatum

DEFINITION

Refined sesame oil is the fatty oil obtained from the ripe seeds of *Sesamum indicum* L. by expression or extraction, then refined. Improved colour and odour may be obtained by further refining. It may contain a suitable antioxidant.

CHARACTERS

A clear, light yellow liquid, almost colourless, practically insoluble in alcohol, miscible with light petroleum.

It has a relative density of about 0.919.

It solidifies to a soft mass at about −4 °C.

IDENTIFICATION

First identification: C.

Second identification: A, B.

A. It complies with the test for refractive index (see Tests).

B. Carry out the identification of fatty oils by thin-layer chromatography (*2.3.2*). The chromatogram obtained is similar to the type chromatogram for sesame oil.

C. It complies with the test for composition of triglycerides (see Tests).

TESTS

Refractive index (*2.2.6*): 1.470 to 1.476.

Acid value (*2.5.1*). Not more than 0.6, determined on 10.0 g. If intended for use in the manufacture of parenteral dosage forms, not more than 0.3.

Peroxide value (*2.5.5*). Not more than 10.0. If intended for use in the manufacture of parenteral dosage forms, not more than 5.0.

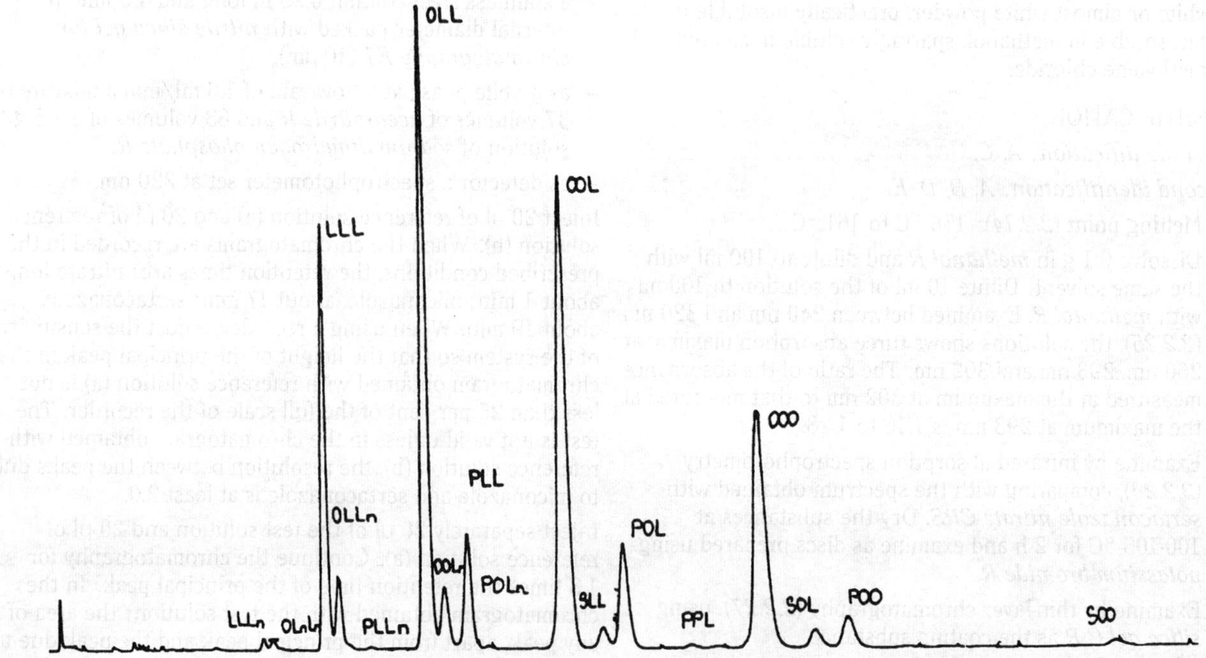

Figure 0433.-1. – *Chromatogram for the composition of triglycerides in sesame oil*

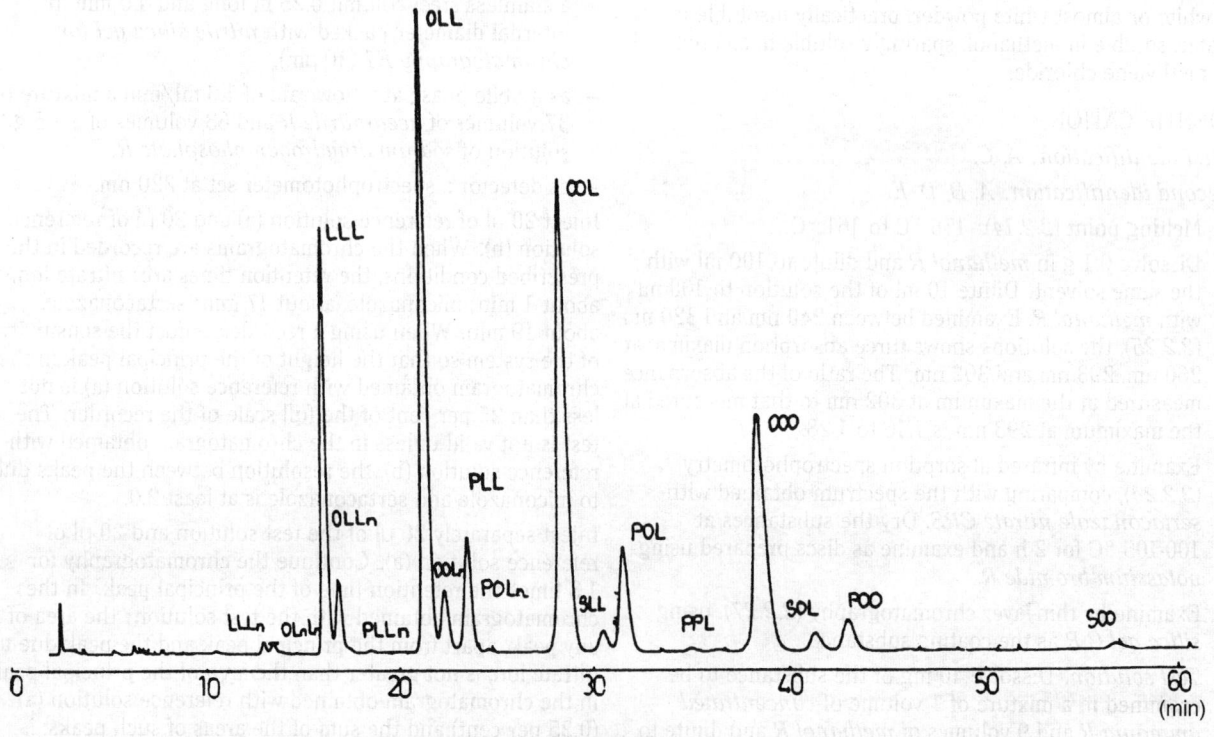

Unsaponifiable matter (*2.5.7*). Not more than 2.0 per cent, determined on 5.0 g.

Alkaline impurities (*2.4.19*). It complies with the test for alkaline impurities in fatty oils.

Cottonseed oil. Mix 5 ml in a test-tube with 5 ml of a mixture of equal volumes of *pentanol R* and a 10 g/l solution of *sulphur R* in *carbon disulphide R*. Warm the mixture carefully until the carbon disulphide is expelled, and immerse the tube to one-third of its depth in boiling *saturated sodium chloride solution R*. No reddish colour develops within 15 min.

Composition of triglycerides. Examine by liquid chromatography (*2.2.29*).

Test solution. Into a 10 ml volumetric flask, weigh 0.200 g and dilute to 10.0 ml with the mobile phase.

The chromatographic procedure may be carried out using:

- two stainless steel columns 0.25 m long and 4.6 mm in internal diameter packed with *octadecylsilyl silica gel for chromatography R* (5 µm) in series,
- as mobile phase at a flow rate of 1.0 ml/min a mixture of 1 volume of *methylene chloride R* and 2 volumes of *acetonitrile R*,
- as detector a refractometer.

Inject 20 µl of the test solution. Identify the peaks from the type chromatogram (Figure 0433.-1). The fatty acid radicals are designated as linolenic (Ln), linoleic (L), oleic (O), palmitic (P) and stearic (S).

Calculate the percentage content of triglycerides from the areas of the peaks in the chromatogram obtained with the test solution by the normalisation procedure.

The composition of triglycerides is the following:

- LLL: 7.0 per cent to 19.0 per cent,
- OLL: 13.0 per cent to 30.0 per cent,
- PLL: 5.0 per cent to 9.0 per cent,
- OOL: 14.0 per cent to 25.0 per cent,
- POL: 8.0 per cent to 16.0 per cent,
- OOO: 5.0 per cent to 14.0 per cent,
- SOL: 2.0 per cent to 8.0 per cent,
- POO: 2.0 per cent to 10.0 per cent.

Water (*2.5.12*). If intended for use in the manufacture of parenteral dosage forms, not more than 0.05 per cent, determined on 5.0 g by the semi-micro determination of water.

STORAGE

Store in an airtight, well-filled container, protected from light.

Refined sesame oil intended for use in the manufacture of parenteral dosage forms is stored under an inert gas in an airtight container.

When the container has been opened, its contents are to be used as soon as possible. Any part of the contents not used at once is protected by an atmosphere of an inert gas.

LABELLING

The label states:

- whether the oil is obtained by expression or extraction,
- where applicable, the name and amount of any added antioxidant,
- where applicable, that the substance is suitable for use in the manufacture of parenteral dosage forms,
- where applicable, the name of the inert gas used.

01/2005:1149

SHELLAC

Lacca

DEFINITION

Shellac is a purified material obtained from the resinous secretion of the female insect *Kerria lacca* (Kerr) Lindinger (*Laccifer lacca* Kerr). There are four types of shellac depending on the nature of the treatment of crude secretion (seedlac): wax-containing shellac, bleached shellac, dewaxed shellac and bleached, dewaxed shellac.

Wax-containing shellac is obtained from seedlac; it is purified by filtration of the molten substance and/or by hot extraction using a suitable solvent.

Bleached shellac is obtained from seedlac by treatment with sodium hypochlorite after dissolution in a suitable alkaline solution, precipitation by dilute acid and drying.

Dewaxed shellac is obtained from wax-containing shellac or seedlac by treatment with a suitable solvent and removal of the insoluble wax by filtering.

Bleached, dewaxed shellac is obtained from wax-containing shellac or seedlac by treatment with sodium hypochlorite after dissolution in a suitable alkaline solution; the insoluble wax is removed by filtration. It is precipitated by dilute acid and dried.

CHARACTERS

Shellac occurs as brownish-orange or yellow, shining, translucent, hard or brittle, more or less thin flakes (wax-containing shellac and dewaxed shellac), or a creamy white or brownish-yellow powder (bleached shellac and bleached, dewaxed shellac).

Shellac is practically insoluble in water. With ethanol, it gives a more or less opalescent solution (wax containing shellac and bleached shellac) or a clear solution (dewaxed shellac and bleached, dewaxed shellac). When warmed, it is sparingly soluble or soluble in alkaline solutions.

IDENTIFICATION

A. Examine by thin-layer chromatography (*2.2.27*), using as the coating substance a suitable silica gel with a fluorescent indicator having an optimal intensity at 254 nm.

   Test solution. Heat 0.25 g of the powdered substance (500) on a water-bath with 2 ml of *dilute sodium hydroxide solution R* for 5 min. Cool, add 5 ml of *ethyl acetate R* and slowly, with stirring, 2 ml of *dilute acetic acid R*. Shake and filter the upper layer through *anhydrous sodium sulphate R*.

   Reference solution. Dissolve 6.0 mg of *aleuritic acid R* in 1.0 ml of *methanol R*, heating slightly if necessary.

   Apply to the plate as bands 10 µl of each solution. Develop twice over a path of 15 cm using a mixture of 1 volume of *acetic acid R*, 8 volumes of *methanol R*, 32 volumes of *methylene chloride R* and 60 volumes of *ethyl acetate R*. Allow the plate to dry in air. Spray the plate with *anisaldehyde solution R*. Heat the plate at 100° C to 105 °C for 5 min to 10 min and examine in daylight. The chromatogram obtained with the test solution shows several coloured zones, one of which is similar in position and colour to the zone in the chromatogram obtained with the reference solution. Above this zone the chromatogram obtained with the test solution shows a pink zone and below it several violet zones. Below the zone corresponding to aleuritic acid, there is a light blue zone (shellolic acid) accompanied by zones of the same colour but of lower intensity. Other faint grey and violet zones may be visible.

B. Examine the chromatograms obtained in the test for colophony. For wax-containing shellac, in the chromatogram obtained with the test solution, a more or less strong bluish-grey zone is visible, just above the zone due to thymolphthalein in the chromatogram obtained with the reference solution. For dewaxed shellac, no such zone is visible just above the zone due to thymolphthalein in the chromatogram obtained with the reference solution.

TESTS

Colophony. Examine by thin-layer chromatography (*2.2.27*), as described under identification test A with the following modifications.

Test solution. Dissolve 50 mg of the powdered substance (500), while heating, in a mixture of 0.5 ml of *methylene chloride R* and 0.5 ml of *methanol R*.

Reference solution. Dissolve 2.0 mg of *thymolphthalein R* in 1.0 ml of *methanol R*.

Examine the plate in ultraviolet light at 254 nm. Mark the quenching zones in the chromatogram obtained with the test solution that have similar R_f values to that of the quenching zone of thymolphthalein in the chromatogram obtained with the reference solution. Spray with *anisaldehyde solution R*, heat the plate at 100 °C to 105 °C for 5 min to 10 min and examine in daylight. The chromatogram obtained with the reference solution shows a principal zone with a reddish- violet colour (thymolphthalein). None of the quenching zones in the chromatogram obtained with the test solution that have an R_f value similar to the zone due to thymolphthalein in the reference solution show a more or less strong violet or brownish colour (colophony). Disregard any faint violet zone at this level that does not show quenching before spraying and heating.

Acid value (*2.5.1*): 65 to 95, calculated with reference to the dried substance. Examine 1.00 g of the coarsely ground substance. Determine the end-point by potentiometry (*2.2.20*).

Arsenic (*2.4.2*). Introduce 0.33 g of the substance to be examined and 5 ml of *sulphuric acid R* into a combustion flask. Carefully add a few millilitres of *strong hydrogen peroxide solution R* and heat to boiling until a clear, colourless solution is obtained. Continue heating to eliminate the water and as much sulphuric acid as possible and dilute to 25 ml with *water R*. The solution complies with limit test A for arsenic (3 ppm).

Heavy metals (*2.4.8*). 2.0 g complies with limit test D for heavy metals (10 ppm). Prepare the standard using 2 ml of *lead standard solution (10 ppm Pb) R*.

Loss on drying (*2.2.32*). Not more than 2.0 per cent for unbleached shellac and not more than 6.0 per cent for bleached shellac, determined on 1.000 g of the powdered substance (500) by drying in an oven at 40 °C to 45 °C for 24 h.

STORAGE

Store protected from light. Store bleached shellac and bleached, dewaxed shellac at a temperature not exceeding 15 °C.

LABELLING

The label indicates the type of shellac.

Monographs Q-S

01/2005:0434

SILICA, COLLOIDAL ANHYDROUS

Silica colloidalis anhydrica

SiO_2 M_r 60.1

DEFINITION

Colloidal anhydrous silica contains not less than 99.0 per cent and not more than the equivalent of 100.5 per cent of SiO_2, determined on the ignited substance.

CHARACTERS

A light, fine, white, amorphous powder, with a particle size of about 15 nm, practically insoluble in water and in mineral acids except hydrofluoric acid. It dissolves in hot solutions of alkali hydroxides.

IDENTIFICATION

About 20 mg gives the reaction of silicates (*2.3.1*).

TESTS

pH (*2.2.3*). Shake 1.0 g with 30 ml of *carbon dioxide-free water R*. The pH of the suspension is 3.5 to 5.5.

Chlorides (*2.4.4*). To 1.0 g add a mixture of 20 ml of *dilute nitric acid R* and 30 ml of *water R* and heat on a water-bath for 15 min, shaking frequently. Dilute to 50 ml with *water R* if necessary, filter and cool. 10 ml of the filtrate diluted to 15 ml with *water R* complies with the limit test for chlorides (250 ppm).

Heavy metals (*2.4.8*). Suspend 2.5 g in sufficient *water R* to produce a semi-fluid slurry. Dry at 140 °C. When the dried substance is white, break up the mass with a glass rod. Add 25 ml of *1 M hydrochloric acid* and boil gently for 5 min, stirring frequently with the glass rod. Centrifuge for 20 min and filter the supernatant liquid through a membrane filter. To the residue in the centrifuge tube add 3 ml of *dilute hydrochloric acid R* and 9 ml of *water R* and boil. Centrifuge for 20 min and filter the supernatant liquid through the same membrane filter. Wash the residue with small quantities of *water R*, combine the filtrates and washings and dilute to 50 ml with *water R*. To 20 ml of the solution add 50 mg of *ascorbic acid R* and 1 ml of *concentrated ammonia R*. Neutralise with *dilute ammonia R2*. Dilute to 25 ml with *water R*. 12 ml of the solution complies with limit test A for heavy metals (25 ppm). Prepare the standard using *lead standard solution (1 ppm Pb) R*.

Loss on ignition. Not more than 5.0 per cent, determined on 0.200 g by ignition in a platinum crucible at 900 °C for 2 h. Allow to cool in a desiccator before weighing.

ASSAY

To the residue obtained in the test for loss on ignition add 0.2 ml of *sulphuric acid R* and sufficient *alcohol R* to moisten the residue completely. Add 6 ml of *hydrofluoric acid R* and evaporate to dryness on a hot-plate at 95 °C to 105 °C, taking care to avoid loss from sputtering. Wash down the sides of the dish with 6 ml of *hydrofluoric acid R* and evaporate to dryness. Ignite at 900 °C, allow to cool in a desiccator and weigh.

The difference between the mass of the final residue and the mass of the residue obtained in the test for loss on ignition gives the amount of SiO_2 in the quantity of the substance to be examined used.

01/2005:0738

SILICA, COLLOIDAL HYDRATED

Silica colloidalis hydrica

DEFINITION

Colloidal hydrated silica contains not less than 98.0 per cent and not more than the equivalent of 100.5 per cent of SiO_2 (M_r 60.1), determined on the ignited substance.

CHARACTERS

A white or almost white, light, fine, amorphous powder, practically insoluble in water and in mineral acids, with the exception of hydrofluoric acid. It dissolves in hot solutions of alkali hydroxides.

IDENTIFICATION

A. About 20 mg gives the reaction of silicates (*2.3.1*).

B. When heated in an oven at 100 °C to 105 °C for 2 h, it shows a loss of mass greater than 3 per cent.

TESTS

Solution S. To 2.5 g add 50 ml of *hydrochloric acid R* and mix. Heat on a water-bath for 30 min, stirring from time to time. Maintain the original volume by adding *dilute hydrochloric acid R*. Evaporate to dryness. Add to the residue a mixture of 8 ml of *dilute hydrochloric acid R* and 24 ml of *water R*. Heat to boiling and filter under reduced pressure through a sintered-glass filter (16). Wash the residue on the filter with a hot mixture of 3 ml of *dilute hydrochloric acid R* and 9 ml of *water R*. Wash with small quantities of *water R*, combine the filtrate and washings and dilute to 50 ml with *water R*.

pH (*2.2.3*). Suspend 1.0 g in 30 ml of a 75 g/l solution of *potassium chloride R*. The pH of the suspension is 4.0 to 7.0.

Water-absorption capacity. In a mortar, triturate 5 g with 5 ml of *water R*, added drop by drop. The mixture remains powdery.

Substances soluble in hydrochloric acid. In a platinum dish, evaporate to dryness 10.0 ml of solution S and dry to constant mass at 100 °C to 105 °C. The mass of the residue is not more than 10 mg (2.0 per cent).

Chlorides (*2.4.4*). Heat 0.5 g with 50 ml of *water R* on a water-bath for 15 min. Dilute to 100 ml with *water R* and centrifuge at 1500 *g* for 5 min. 10 ml of the supernatant solution diluted to 15 ml with *water R* complies with the limit test for chlorides (0.1 per cent).

Sulphates (*2.4.13*). Dilute 2 ml of solution S to 100 ml with *distilled water R*. 15 ml of the solution complies with the limit test for sulphates (1 per cent).

Iron (*2.4.9*). To 2 ml of solution S add 28 ml of *water R*. 10 ml of the solution complies with the limit test for iron (300 ppm).

Heavy metals (*2.4.8*). To 20 ml of solution S add 50 mg of *hydroxylamine hydrochloride R* and 1 ml of *concentrated ammonia R*. Adjust to pH 3.5 by adding *dilute ammonia R2*, monitoring the pH potentiometrically. Dilute to 25 ml with *water R*. 12 ml of the solution complies with limit test A for heavy metals (25 ppm). Prepare the standard using *lead standard solution (1 ppm Pb) R*.

Loss on ignition. Not more than 20.0 per cent, determined on 0.200 g in a platinum crucible by heating at 100 °C to 105 °C for 1 h and then at 900 °C for 2 h.

ASSAY

To the residue obtained in the test for loss on ignition add 0.2 ml of *sulphuric acid R* and a quantity of *alcohol R* sufficient to moisten the residue completely. Add 6 ml of *hydrofluoric acid R* and evaporate to dryness at 95 °C to 105 °C, taking care to avoid loss from sputtering. Wash the inside of the dish with 6 ml of *hydrofluoric acid R* and evaporate to dryness again. Ignite at 900 °C, allow to cool in a desiccator and weigh. The difference between the mass of the final residue and that of the mass obtained in the test for loss on ignition corresponds to the mass of SiO_2 in the test sample.

01/2005:1562

SILICA, DENTAL TYPE

Silica ad usum dentalem

DEFINITION

Dental type silica is an amorphous silica (precipitated, gel or obtained by flame hydrolysis). It contains not less than 94.0 per cent and not more than 100.5 per cent of SiO_2 determined on the ignited substance.

CHARACTERS

A white or almost white, light, fine amorphous powder, practically insoluble in water and in mineral acids. It dissolves in hydrofluoric acid and hot solutions of alkali hydroxides.

IDENTIFICATION

About 20 mg gives the reaction of silicates (*2.3.1*).

TESTS

Solution S. To 2.5 g add 50 ml of *hydrochloric acid R* and mix. Heat on a water-bath for 30 min, stirring from time to time. Evaporate to dryness. Add to the residue a mixture of 8 ml of *dilute hydrochloric acid R* and 24 ml of *water R*. Heat to boiling and filter under reduced pressure through a sintered-glass filter (16). Wash the residue on the filter with a hot mixture of 3 ml of *dilute hydrochloric acid R* and 9 ml of *water R*. Wash with small quantities of *water R*, combine the washings and the filtrate and dilute to 50 ml with *water R*.

pH (*2.2.3*). Suspend 5 g in a mixture of 5 ml of a 7.46 g/l solution of *potassium chloride R* and 90 ml of *carbon dioxide-free water R*. The pH of the suspension is 3.2 to 8.9.

Chlorides. Examine by liquid chromatography (*2.2.29*) as prescribed under sulphates.

Inject 25 µl of the test solution and 25 µl of the reference solution. In the chromatogram obtained with the test solution the area of any peak corresponding to chloride is not greater than that of the corresponding peak in the chromatogram obtained with the reference solution (0.3 per cent).

Sulphates. Examine by liquid chromatography (*2.2.29*).

Test solution. To 0.625 g add 30 ml of *water R* and boil for 2 h. Allow to cool and quantitatively transfer to a 50 ml graduated flask. Dilute to 50.0 ml with *water R*. Dilute 5.0 ml of the supernatant to 50.0 ml with *water R* and filter through a membrane filter (nominal pore size: 0.45 µm).

Reference solution. Dissolve 0.50 g of *anhydrous sodium sulphate R* and 0.062 g of *sodium chloride R* in *water R* and dilute to 1000.0 ml with *water R*. Dilute 5.0 ml of this solution to 50.0 ml with *water R*.

The chromatographic procedure may be carried out using:
- a non-metallic column 0.25 m long and 4.6 mm in internal diameter packed with a suitable anion-exchange resin (30 µm to 50 µm),
- as mobile phase at a flow rate of 1.2 ml/min a solution prepared as follows: dissolve 0.508 g of *sodium carbonate R* and 0.05 g of *sodium hydrogen carbonate R* in *water R* and dilute to 1000 ml with the same solvent,
- a conductivity detector,
- a loop injector.

Inject 25 µl of the test solution and 25 µl of the reference solution. When the chromatograms are recorded in the prescribed conditions, the retention times are: sulphate about 8 min and chloride about 4 min.

In the chromatogram obtained with the test solution the area of any peak corresponding to sulphate is not greater than that of the corresponding peak in the chromatogram obtained with the reference solution (4.0 per cent calculated as sodium sulphate).

Iron (*2.4.9*). Dilute 2 ml of solution S to 40 ml with *water R*. 10 ml of the solution complies with the limit test for iron (400 ppm).

Heavy metals (*2.4.8*). To 20 ml of solution S, add 50 mg of *hydroxylamine hydrochloride R* and 1 ml of *concentrated ammonia R*. Adjust to pH 3.5 by adding *dilute ammonia R2*, monitoring the pH potentiometrically. Dilute to 25 ml with *water R*. 12 ml of the solution complies with limit test A for heavy metals (25 ppm). Prepare the standard using *lead standard solution (1 ppm Pb) R*.

Loss on ignition. Not more than 25.0 per cent, determined on 0.200 g in a platinum crucible by heating at 100 °C to 105 °C for 1 h and then at 1000 °C for 2 h.

ASSAY

To the residue obtained in the test for loss on ignition add 0.2 ml of *sulphuric acid R* and a quantity of *alcohol R* sufficient to moisten the residue completely. Add 6 ml of *hydrofluoric acid R* and evaporate to dryness at 95 °C to 105 °C, taking care to avoid loss from sputtering. Wash the inside of the crucible with 6 ml of *hydrofluoric acid R* and evaporate to dryness again. Ignite at 900 °C, allow to cool in a desiccator and weigh. The difference between the mass of the final residue and that of the mass obtained in the test for loss on ignition corresponds to the mass of SiO_2 in the test sample.

01/2005:0009

SILVER NITRATE

Argenti nitras

$AgNO_3$ M_r 169.9

DEFINITION

Silver nitrate contains not less than 99.0 per cent and not more than the equivalent of 100.5 per cent of $AgNO_3$.

CHARACTERS

A white, crystalline powder or transparent, colourless crystals, very soluble in water, soluble in alcohol.

IDENTIFICATION

A. 10 mg gives the reaction of nitrates (*2.3.1*).

B. 10 mg gives the reaction of silver (*2.3.1*).

TESTS

Solution S. Dissolve 2.0 g in *water R* and dilute to 50 ml with the same solvent.

Appearance of solution. Solution S is clear (*2.2.1*) and colourless (*2.2.2, Method II*).

Acidity or alkalinity. To 2 ml of solution S add 0.1 ml of *bromocresol green solution R*. The solution is blue. To 2 ml of solution S add 0.1 ml of *phenol red solution R*. The solution is yellow.

Foreign salts. To 30 ml of solution S, add 7.5 ml of *dilute hydrochloric acid R*, shake vigorously, heat for 5 min on a water-bath and filter. Evaporate 20 ml of the filtrate to dryness on a water-bath and dry at 100-105 °C. The residue weighs not more than 2 mg (0.3 per cent).

Aluminium, lead, copper and bismuth. Dissolve 1.0 g in a mixture of 4 ml of *concentrated ammonia R* and 6 ml of *water R*. The solution is clear (*2.2.1*) and colourless (*2.2.2, Method II*).

ASSAY

Dissolve 0.300 g in 50 ml of *water R* and add 2 ml of *dilute nitric acid R* and 2 ml of *ferric ammonium sulphate solution R2*. Titrate with *0.1 M ammonium thiocyanate* until a reddish-yellow colour is obtained.

1 ml of *0.1 M ammonium thiocyanate* is equivalent to 16.99 mg of $AgNO_3$.

STORAGE

Store in a non-metallic container, protected from light.

01/2005:1470

SIMETICONE

Simeticonum

DEFINITION

Simeticone is prepared by incorporation of 4 per cent to 7 per cent silica into poly(dimethylsiloxane) with a degree of polymerisation between 20 and 400. Simeticone contains 90.5 per cent to 99.0 per cent of poly(dimethylsiloxane).

PRODUCTION

Poly(dimethylsiloxane) is obtained by hydrolysis and polycondensation of dichlorodimethylsilane and chlorotrimethylsilane and the silica is modified at the surface by incorporation of methylsilyl groups.

CHARACTERS

A viscous, greyish-white, opalescent liquid, practically insoluble in water, very slightly soluble to practically insoluble in ethanol, practically insoluble in methanol, partly miscible with ethyl acetate, with methylene chloride, with methyl ethyl ketone and with toluene.

IDENTIFICATION

A. Examine by infrared absorption spectrophotometry (*2.2.24*). Absorption maxima are observed at 2964 cm^{-1}, 2905 cm^{-1}, 1412 cm^{-1}, 1260 cm^{-1} and 1020 cm^{-1}. Examine the substances as thin films between *sodium chloride R* plates.

B. Heat 0.5 g in a test-tube over a small flame until white fumes begin to appear. Invert the tube over a second tube containing 1 ml of a 1 g/l solution of *chromotropic acid, sodium salt R* in *sulphuric acid R* so that the fumes reach the solution. Shake the second tube for about 10 s and heat on a water-bath for 5 min. The solution is violet.

C. The residue obtained in the test for silica under Assay, gives the reaction of silicates (*2.3.1*).

TESTS

Acidity. To 2.0 g add 25 ml of a mixture of equal volumes of *ethanol R* and *ether R* previously neutralised to 0.2 ml of *bromothymol blue solution R1*, and shake. Not more than 3.0 ml of *0.01 M sodium hydroxide* is required to change the colour of the solution to blue.

Defoaming activity

Foaming solution. Dissolve 5.0 g of *docusate sodium R* in 1 litre of *water R* (warm to 50 °C if necessary).

Defoaming solution. To 50 ml of *methyl ethyl ketone R* add 0.250 g of simeticone, warm to not more than 50 °C with shaking.

Into a 250 ml cylindrical tube about 5 cm in diameter introduce 100 ml of foaming solution and 1 ml of defoaming solution. Close tightly and fix the tube on a suitable oscillating shaker that complies with the following conditions:

- 250 to 300 oscillations per minute,
- angle of oscillation of about 10°,
- oscillation radius of about 10 cm.

Shake for 10 s and record the time between the end of the shaking and the instant the first portion of foam-free liquid surface appears.

This duration does not exceed 15 s.

Mineral oils. Place 2.0 g in a test-tube and examine in ultraviolet light at 365 nm. The fluorescence is not more intense than that of a solution containing 0.1 ppm of *quinine sulphate R* in *0.005 M sulphuric acid* examined in the same conditions.

Phenylated compounds. Dissolve 5.0 g with shaking in 10.0 ml of *cyclohexane R*. Determine the absorbance of the solution between 200 nm and 350 nm (*2.2.25*) using *cyclohexane R* as the compensation liquid. The corrected absorbance (absorbance measured at the maximum between 250 nm and 270 nm minus the absorbance measured at 300 nm) is not greater than 0.2.

Heavy metals. Mix 1.0 g with *methylene chloride R* and dilute to 20 ml with the same solvent. Add 1.0 ml of a freshly prepared 0.02 g/l solution of *dithizone R* in *methylene chloride R*, 0.5 ml of *water R* and 0.5 ml of a mixture of 1 volume of *dilute ammonia R2* and 9 volumes of a 2 g/l solution of *hydroxylamine hydrochloride R*. At the same time, prepare a standard as follows: to 20 ml of *methylene chloride R* add 1.0 ml of a freshly prepared 0.02 g/l solution of *dithizone R* in *methylene chloride R*, 0.5 ml of *lead standard solution (10 ppm Pb) R* and 0.5 ml of a mixture of 1 volume of *dilute ammonia R2* and 9 volumes of a 2 g/l solution of *hydroxylamine hydrochloride R*. Immediately shake each solution vigorously for 1 min. Any red colour in the test solution is not more intense than that in the standard (5 ppm).

Volatile matter. Not more than 1.0 per cent, determined on 1.00 g by heating in an oven at 150 °C for 2 h. Carry out the test using a dish 60 mm in diameter and 10 mm deep.

ASSAY

Silica. Not more than 7 per cent, determined on not less than 20.0 mg. Heat the substance to be examined to 800 °C increasing the temperature by 20 °C/min under a current of *nitrogen R* at a flow rate of 200 ml/min and weigh the residue (silica).

Dimeticone

Test solution. Place about 50 mg (*E*) in a screw-capped 125 ml cylindrical tube, add 25.0 ml of *toluene R*, swirl manually to disperse and add 50 ml of *dilute hydrochloric acid R*, close the tube and place on a vortex mixer; shake for 5 min. Transfer the contents of the tube to a separating funnel, allow to settle and transfer 5 ml of the upper layer to a screw-capped test tube containing 0.5 g of *anhydrous sodium sulphate R*. Cap and shake vigorously manually. Centrifuge to obtain a clear test solution.

Reference solution. Introduce about 0.20 g of *dimeticone CRS* in 100.0 ml of *toluene R*. Prepare the reference solution in the same way as for the test solution, using 25.0 ml of the dimeticone solution obtained above. Prepare a blank by shaking 10 ml of *toluene R* with 1 g of *anhydrous sodium sulphate R*. Centrifuge the resulting suspension.

Record the infrared absorption spectra for the test solution and the reference solution in 0.5 mm cells, from 1330 cm^{-1} to 1180 cm^{-1}, and determine the absorbance of the band at 1260 cm^{-1} (*2.2.24*).

Calculate the percentage content of dimeticone using the expression:

$$\frac{25C \times A_M \times 100}{A_E \times E}$$

A_M = absorbance of the test solution,

A_E = absorbance of the reference solution,

C = concentration of the reference solution, in milligrams per millilitre,

E = mass of the substance to be examined, in milligrams.

01/2005:1563

SIMVASTATIN

Simvastatinum

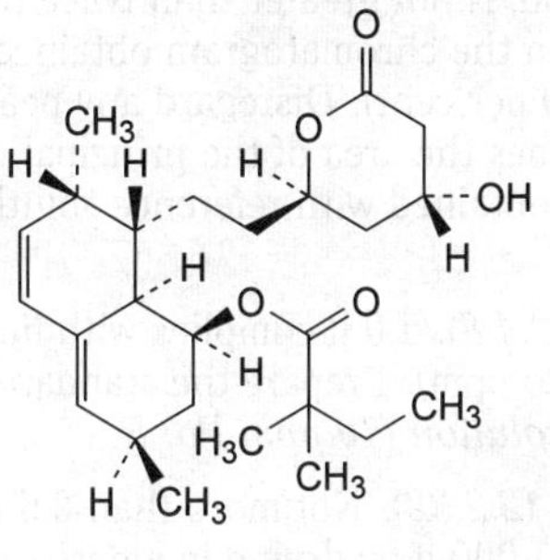

$C_{25}H_{38}O_5$ M_r 418.6

DEFINITION

Simvastatin contains not less than 97.0 per cent and not more than the equivalent of 102.0 per cent of (1*S*,3*R*,7*S*,8*S*,8a*R*)-8-[2-[(2*R*,4*R*)-4-hydroxy-6-oxotetrahydro-2*H*-pyran-2-yl]ethyl]-3,7-dimethyl-1,2,3,7,8,8a-hexahydronaphthalen-1-yl 2,2-dimethylbutanoate, calculated with reference to the dried substance. A suitable antioxidant may be added.

CHARACTERS

A white or almost white, crystalline powder, practically insoluble in water, very soluble in methylene chloride, freely soluble in alcohol.

Monographs Q-S

IDENTIFICATION

A. It complies with the test for specific optical rotation (see Tests).

B. Examine by infrared absorption spectrophotometry (*2.2.24*), comparing with the spectrum obtained with *simvastatin CRS*. Examine the substances prepared as discs.

TESTS

Appearance of solution. Dissolve 0.200 g in *methanol R* and dilute to 20 ml with the same solvent. The solution is clear (*2.2.1*) and not more intensely coloured than reference solution BY_7 (*2.2.2, Method II*).

Specific optical rotation (*2.2.7*). Dissolve 0.125 g in *acetonitrile R* and dilute to 25.0 ml with the same solvent. The specific optical rotation is + 285 to + 300, calculated with reference to the dried substance.

Related substances. Examine by liquid chromatography (*2.2.29*) as prescribed under Assay.

Inject 5 µl of reference solution (b). Adjust the sensitivity of the system so that the height of the principal peak in the chromatogram obtained is at least 20 per cent of the full scale of the recorder. Inject 5 µl of test solution (a) and continue the chromatography for five times the retention time of simvastatin. When the chromatograms are recorded under the prescribed conditions the relative retentions are: impurity A about 0.45, lovastatin (impurity E) and epilovastatin (impurity F) about 0.60, impurity G about 0.80, impurity B about 2.38, impurity C about 2.42 and impurity D about 3.80 (retention time of simvastatin: about 2.6 min). In the chromatogram obtained with test solution (a): the area of the peak due to lovastatin and epilovastatin is not greater than twice the area of the principal peak in the chromatogram obtained with reference solution (b) (1.0 per cent); the area of any peak apart from the principal peak and the peak due to lovastatin and epilovastatin is not greater than 0.8 times the area of the principal peak in the chromatogram obtained with reference solution (b) (0.4 per cent); the sum of the areas of all peaks, apart from the principal peak and the peak due to lovastatin and epilovastatin, is not greater than twice the area of the principal peak in the chromatogram obtained with reference solution (b) (1.0 per cent). Disregard any peak with an area less than 0.1 times the area of the principal peak in the chromatogram obtained with reference solution (b) (0.05 per cent).

Heavy metals (*2.4.8*). 1.0 g complies with limit test C for heavy metals (20 ppm). Prepare the standard using 2 ml of *lead standard solution (10 ppm Pb) R*.

Loss on drying (*2.2.32*). Not more than 0.5 per cent, determined on 1.000 g by drying in a desiccator under high vacuum at 60 °C for 3 h.

Sulphated ash (*2.4.14*). Not more than 0.1 per cent, determined on 1.0 g.

ASSAY

Examine by liquid chromatography (*2.2.29*). *Prepare the solutions immediately before use.*

Solvent mixture. Prepare a mixture of 40 volumes of a solution of a 1.4 g/l solution of *potassium dihydrogen phosphate R*, adjusted to pH 4.0 with *phosphoric acid R*, and 60 volumes of *acetonitrile R*. Filter.

Test solution (a). Dissolve 75.0 mg of the substance to be examined in the solvent mixture and dilute to 50.0 ml with the solvent mixture.

Test solution (b). Dissolve 40.0 mg of the substance to be examined in the solvent mixture and dilute to 50.0 ml with the solvent mixture.

Reference solution (a). Dissolve 1.0 mg of *simvastatin CRS* and 1.0 mg of *lovastatin CRS* in the solvent mixture and dilute to 50.0 ml with the solvent mixture.

Reference solution (b). Dilute 0.5 ml of test solution (a) to 100.0 ml with the solvent mixture.

Reference solution (c). Dissolve 40.0 mg of *simvastatin CRS* in the solvent mixture and dilute to 50.0 ml with the solvent mixture.

The chromatographic procedure may be carried out using:

– a stainless steel column 0.033 m long and 4.6 mm in internal diameter packed with *end-capped octadecylsilyl silica gel for chromatography R* (3 µm),

– as mobile phase at a flow rate of 3.0 ml/min:

Mobile phase A. Mix 50 volumes of *acetonitrile R* and 50 volumes of a 0.1 per cent *V/V* solution of *phosphoric acid R*,

Mobile phase B. A 0.1 per cent *V/V* solution of *phosphoric acid R* in *acetonitrile R*,

Time (min)	Mobile phase A (per cent *V/V*)	Mobile phase B (per cent *V/V*)	Comment
0 - 4.5	100	0	isocratic
4.5 - 4.6	100 → 95	0 → 5	linear gradient
4.6 - 8.0	95 → 25	5 → 75	linear gradient
8.0 - 11.5	25	75	isocratic
11.5 - 11.6	25 → 100	75 → 0	linear gradient
11.6 - 13	100	0	re-equilibration

– as detector a spectrophotometer set at 238 nm.

Inject 5 µl of reference solution (a). The test and the assay are not valid unless, in the chromatogram obtained, the resolution between the peak corresponding to lovastatin and epilovastatin and the peak corresponding to simvastatin is at least 5.0. When the chromatograms are recorded under the prescribed conditions the retention times are: lovastatin and epilovastatin about 1.6 min and simvastatin about 2.6 min. Inject 5 µl of reference solution (c). Adjust the sensitivity of the system so that the height of the principal peak is at least 50 per cent of the full scale of the recorder. Inject 5 µl of test solution (b).

Calculate the content of simvastatin from the peak areas in the chromatograms obtained with test solution (b) and reference solution (c) and the declared content of *simvastatin CRS*.

STORAGE

Store under nitrogen, in an airtight container, protected from light.

LABELLING

The label states the name and concentration of any added antioxidant.

IMPURITIES

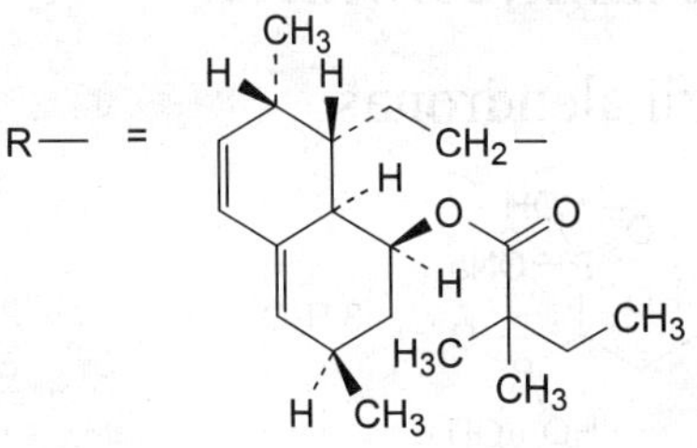

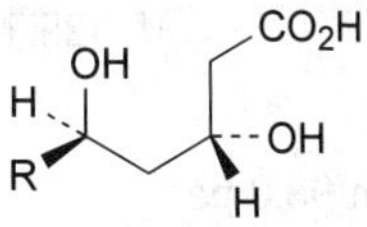

A. (3*R*,5*R*)-7-[(1*S*,2*S*,6*R*,8*S*,8a*R*)-8-[(2,2-dimethylbutanoyl)oxy]-2,6-dimethyl-1,2,6,7,8,8a-hexahydronaphthalen-1-yl]-3,5-dihydroxyheptanoic acid (hydroxy acid),

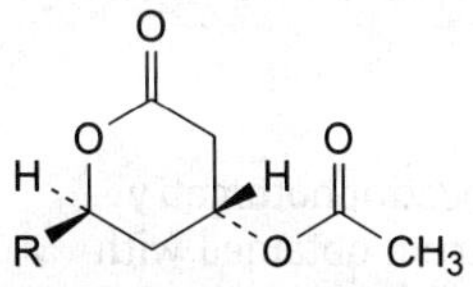

B. (1*S*,3*R*,7*S*,8*S*,8a*R*)-8-[2-[(2*R*,4*R*)-4-(acetyloxy)-6-oxotetrahydro-2*H*-pyran-2-yl]ethyl]-3,7-dimethyl-1,2,3,7,8,8a-hexahydronaphthalen-1-yl 2,2-dimethylbutanoate (acetate ester),

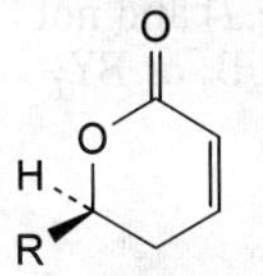

C. (1*S*,3*R*,7*S*,8*S*,8a*R*)-3,7-dimethyl-8-[2-[(2*R*)-6-oxo-3,6-dihydro-2*H*-pyran-2-yl]ethyl]-1,2,3,7,8,8a-hexahydronaphthalen-1-yl 2,2-dimethylbutanoate (anhydrosimvastatin),

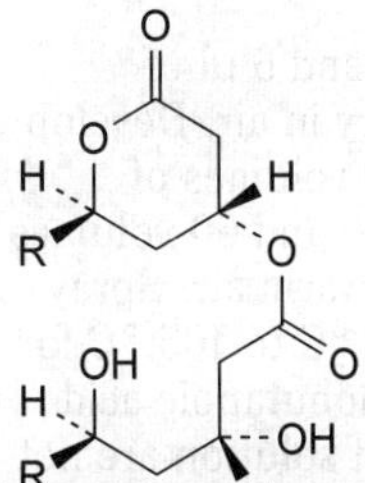

D. (2*R*,4*R*)-2-[[(1*S*,2*S*,6*R*,8*S*,8a*R*)-8-[(2,2-dimethylbutanoyl)oxy]-2,6-dimethyl-1,2,6,7,8,8a-hexahydronaphthalen-1-yl]ethyl]-6-oxotetrahydro-2*H*-pyran-4-yl (3*R*,5*R*)-7-[(1*S*,2*S*,6*R*,8*S*,8a*R*)-8-[(2,2-dimethylbutanoyl)oxy]-2,6-dimethyl-1,2,6,7,8,8a-hexahydronaphthalen-1-yl]-3,5-dihydroxyheptanoate (dimer),

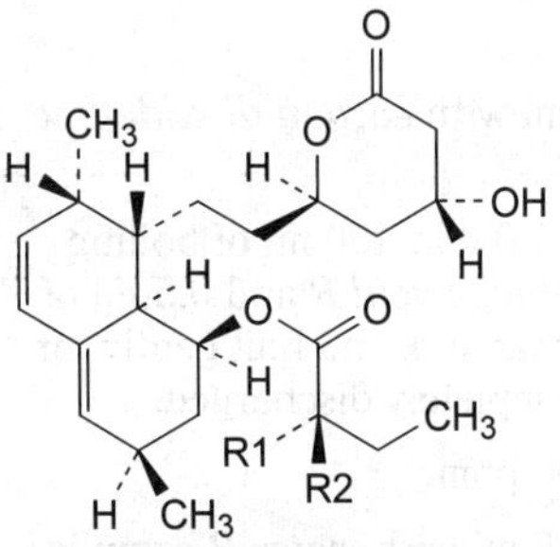

E. R1 = CH_3, R2 = H: (1*S*,3*R*,7*S*,8*S*,8a*R*)-8-[2-[(2*R*,4*R*)-4-hydroxy-6-oxotetrahydro-2*H*-pyran-2-yl]ethyl]-3,7-dimethyl-1,2,3,7,8,8a-hexahydronaphthalen-1-yl (2*S*)-2-methylbutanoate (lovastatin),

F. R1 = H, R2 = CH_3: (1*S*,3*R*,7*S*,8*S*,8a*R*)-8-[2-[(2*R*,4*R*)-4-hydroxy-6-oxotetrahydro-2*H*-pyran-2-yl]ethyl]-3,7-dimethyl-1,2,3,7,8,8a-hexahydronaphthalen-1-yl (2*R*)-2-methylbutanoate (epilovastatin),

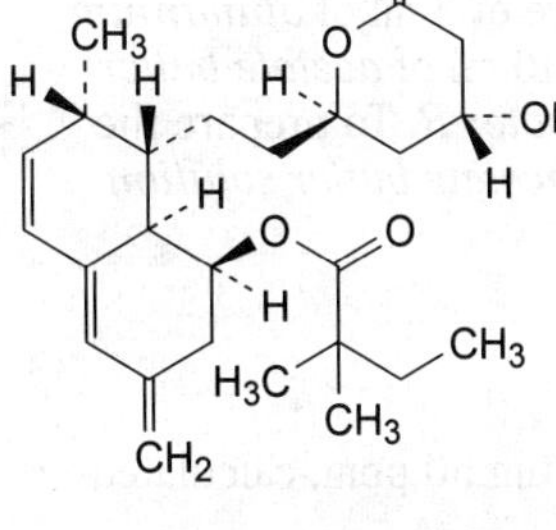

G. (1*S*,7*S*,8*S*,8a*R*)-8-[2-[(2*R*,4*R*)-4-hydroxy-6-oxotetrahydro-2*H*-pyran-2-yl]ethyl]-7-methyl-3-methylene-1,2,3,7,8,8a-hexahydronaphthalen-1-yl 2,2-dimethylbutanoate.

01/2005:0411

SODIUM ACETATE TRIHYDRATE

Natrii acetas trihydricus

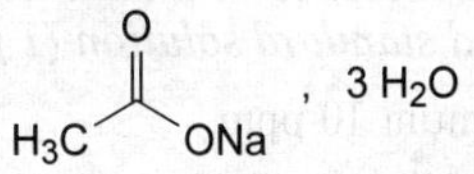

$C_2H_3NaO_2,3H_2O$ M_r 136.1

DEFINITION

Sodium ethanoate trihydrate.

Content: 99.0 per cent to 101.0 per cent (dried substance).

CHARACTERS

Appearance: colourless crystals.

Solubility: very soluble in water, soluble in alcohol.

IDENTIFICATION

A. 1 ml of solution S (see Tests) gives reaction (b) of acetates (*2.3.1*).

B. 1 ml of solution S gives reaction (a) of sodium (*2.3.1*).

C. It complies with the test for loss on drying (see Tests).

TESTS

Solution S. Dissolve 10.0 g in *carbon dioxide-free water R* prepared from *distilled water R* and dilute to 100 ml with the same solvent.

Appearance of solution. Solution S is clear (*2.2.1*) and colourless (*2.2.2, Method II*).

pH (*2.2.3*): 7.5 to 9.0.

Dilute 5 ml of solution S to 10 ml with *carbon dioxide-free water R*.

Reducing substances. Dissolve 1.0 g in 100 ml of boiling *water R*, add 5 ml of *dilute sulphuric acid R* and 0.5 ml of *0.002 M potassium permanganate*, mix and boil gently for 5 min. The pink colour is not completely discharged.

Chlorides (*2.4.4*): maximum 200 ppm.

2.5 ml of solution S diluted to 15 ml with *water R* complies with the limit test for chlorides.

Sulphates (*2.4.13*): maximum 200 ppm.

7.5 ml of solution S diluted to 15 ml with *distilled water R* complies with the limit test for sulphates.

Aluminium (*2.4.17*): maximum 0.2 ppm, if intended for use in the manufacture of dialysis solutions.

Dissolve 20 g in 100 ml of *water R* and adjust to pH 6.0 by the addition of *1 M hydrochloric acid* (about 10 ml). The solution complies with the limit test for aluminium. Use as the reference solution a mixture of 2 ml of *aluminium standard solution (2 ppm Al) R*, 10 ml of *acetate buffer solution pH 6.0 R* and 98 ml of *water R*. To prepare the blank, use a mixture of 10 ml of *acetate buffer solution pH 6.0 R* and 100 ml of *water R*.

Arsenic (*2.4.2*): maximum 2 ppm.

0.5 g complies with limit test A.

Calcium and magnesium: maximum 50 ppm, calculated as Ca.

To 200 ml of *water R* add 10 ml of *ammonium chloride buffer solution pH 10.0 R*, 0.1 g of *mordant black 11 triturate R*, 2.0 ml of *0.05 M zinc chloride* and, dropwise, *0.02 M sodium edetate* until the colour changes from violet to blue. Add to the solution 10.0 g of the substance to be examined and shake to dissolve. Titrate with *0.02 M sodium edetate* until the blue colour is restored. Not more than 0.65 ml of *0.02 M sodium edetate* is required.

Heavy metals (*2.4.8*): maximum 10 ppm.

12 ml of solution S complies with limit test A. Prepare the standard using *lead standard solution (1 ppm Pb) R*.

Iron (*2.4.9*): maximum 10 ppm.

10 ml of solution S complies with the limit test for iron.

Loss on drying (*2.2.32*): 39.0 per cent to 40.5 per cent, determined on 1.000 g by drying in an oven at 130 °C. Introduce the substance to be examined into the oven while the latter is cold.

ASSAY

Dissolve 0.250 g in 50 ml of *anhydrous acetic acid R*, add 5 ml of *acetic anhydride R*, mix and allow to stand for 30 min. Using 0.3 ml of *naphtholbenzein solution R* as indicator, titrate with *0.1 M perchloric acid* until a green colour is obtained.

1 ml of *0.1 M perchloric acid* is equivalent to 8.20 mg of $C_2H_3NaO_2$.

STORAGE

In an airtight container.

LABELLING

The label states, where applicable, that the substance is suitable for use in the manufacture of dialysis solutions.

Monographs Q-S

01/2005:1564
corrected

SODIUM ALENDRONATE

Natrii alendronas

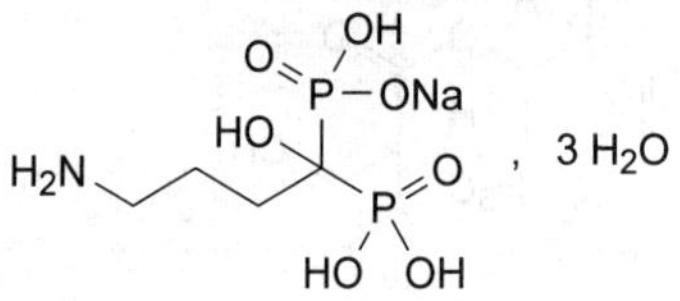

$C_4H_{12}NNaO_7P_2,3H_2O$ M_r 325.1

DEFINITION

Sodium alendronate contains not less than 98.0 per cent and not more than the equivalent of 102.0 per cent of (4-amino-1-hydroxybutylidene)bisphosphonic acid monosodium salt, calculated with reference to the dried substance.

CHARACTERS

A white or almost white, crystalline powder, soluble in water, very slightly soluble in methanol, practically insoluble in methylene chloride.

IDENTIFICATION

A. Examine by infrared absorption spectrophotometry (*2.2.24*), comparing with the spectrum obtained with *sodium alendronate CRS*. Examine the substances prepared as discs.

B. It gives reaction (a) of sodium (*2.3.1*).

TESTS

Solution S. Dissolve 0.5 g in *carbon dioxide-free water R* prepared from *distilled water R* and dilute to 50 ml with the same solvent.

Appearance of solution. Solution S is clear (*2.2.1*) and not more intensely coloured than reference solution B_7 or BY_7 (*2.2.2, Method II*).

pH (*2.2.3*). The pH of solution S is 4.0 to 5.0.

4-aminobutanoic acid. Examine by thin-layer chromatography (*2.2.27*), using a *TLC silica gel plate R*.

Test solution. Dissolve 0.10 g of the substance to be examined in *water R* and dilute to 10 ml with the same solvent.

Reference solution (a). Dissolve 0.10 g of *4-aminobutanoic acid R* in *water R* and dilute to 200 ml with the same solvent.

Reference solution (b). Dilute 1 ml of reference solution (a) to 10 ml with *water R*.

Apply to the plate 5 µl of the test solution and 5 µl of reference solution (b). Allow the plate to dry in air. Develop over a path of 15 cm using a mixture of 20 volumes of *water R*, 20 volumes of *glacial acetic acid R* and 60 volumes of *butanol R*. Dry the plate in a current of warm air. Spray with *ninhydrin solution R* and heat at 100 °C to 105 °C for 15 min. Any spots corresponding to 4-aminobutanoic acid in the chromatogram obtained with the test solution are not more intense than the spot in the chromatogram obtained with reference solution (b) (0.5 per cent).

Phosphate and phosphite. Examine the chromatograms obtained in the assay. In the chromatogram obtained with the test solution: the area of any peak corresponding to phosphate is not greater than that of the peak due to phosphate in the chromatogram obtained with reference solution (d) (0.5 per cent); the area of any peak corresponding to phosphite is not greater than that of the peak due to phosphite in the chromatogram obtained with reference solution (d) (0.5 per cent).

Heavy metals (*2.4.8*). 1.0 g complies with limit test F for heavy metals (20 ppm). Prepare the standard using 2 ml of *lead standard solution (10 ppm Pb) R*.

Loss on drying (*2.2.32*): 16.1 per cent to 17.1 per cent, determined on 1.000 g by drying in an oven at 140 °C to 145 °C.

ASSAY

Examine by liquid chromatography (*2.2.29*).

Test solution. Dissolve 50.0 mg of the substance to be examined in *water R* and dilute to 25.0 ml with the same solvent.

Reference solution (a). Dissolve 50.0 mg of *sodium alendronate CRS* in *water R* and dilute to 25.0 ml with the same solvent.

Reference solution (b). Dissolve 3.0 g of *phosphoric acid R* in *water R* and dilute to 100.0 ml with the same solvent. Dilute 1.0 ml of the solution to 100.0 ml with *water R*.

Reference solution (c). Dissolve 2.5 g of *phosphorous acid R* in *water R* and dilute to 100.0 ml with the same solvent. Dilute 1.0 ml of the solution to 100.0 ml with *water R*.

Reference solution (d). Mix 2.0 ml of reference solution (b) and 2.0 ml of reference solution (c) and dilute to 50.0 ml with *water R*.

The chromatographic procedure may be carried out using:

- a column 0.15 m long and 4.6 mm in internal diameter packed with *anion exchange resin R1* (7 µm),
- as mobile phase at a flow rate of 1.2 ml/min a solution of 0.2 ml of *anhydrous formic acid R* in 1000 ml of *water R*, adjusted to pH 3.5 with *2 M sodium hydroxide solution*,
- as detector a refractometer,
- a 100 µl loop injector,

maintaining the temperature of the column at 35 °C.

Inject reference solution (a) six times. The assay is not valid unless the relative standard deviation of the peak area of sodium alendronate is at most 1.0 per cent. Inject the test solution, reference solution (a) and reference solution (d). The retention time of sodium alendronate is about 16 min and the relative retention times are: phosphate about 1.3 and phosphite about 1.6. Record the chromatograms for twice the retention time of the principal peak in the chromatogram obtained with the test solution.

Calculate the percentage content of $C_4H_{12}NNaO_7P_2$ from the peak areas and the declared content of *sodium alendronate CRS*.

IMPURITIES

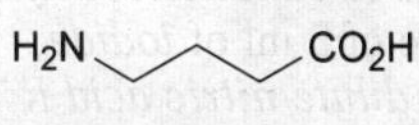

A. 4-aminobutanoic acid,

B. phosphate,

C. phosphite.

01/2005:0625

SODIUM ALGINATE

Natrii alginas

DEFINITION

Sodium alginate consists mainly of the sodium salt of alginic acid, which is a mixture of polyuronic acids $[C_6H_8O_6]_n$ composed of residues of D-mannuronic acid and L-guluronic acid, and is obtained mainly from algae belonging to the Phaeophyceae.

CHARACTERS

A white or pale yellowish-brown powder, slowly soluble in water forming a viscous, colloidal solution, practically insoluble in alcohol.

IDENTIFICATION

A. Dissolve 0.2 g with shaking in 20 ml of *water R*. To 5 ml of this solution add 1 ml of *calcium chloride solution R*. A voluminous gelatinous mass is formed.

B. To 10 ml of the solution prepared in identification test A add 1 ml of *dilute sulphuric acid R*. A gelatinous mass is formed.

C. To 5 mg add 5 ml of *water R*, 1 ml of a freshly prepared 10 g/l solution of *1,3-dihydroxynaphthalene R* in *alcohol R* and 5 ml of *hydrochloric acid R*. Boil for 3 min, cool, add 5 ml of *water R*, and shake with 15 ml of *di-isopropyl ether R*. Carry out a blank test. The upper layer obtained with the substance to be examined exhibits a deeper bluish-red colour than that obtained with the blank.

D. It complies with the test for sulphated ash. The residue obtained, dissolved in 2 ml of *water R*, gives reaction (a) of sodium (*2.3.1*).

TESTS

Solution S. Dissolve 0.10 g in *water R*, with constant stirring, dilute to 30 ml with the same solvent and allow to stand for 1 h.

Appearance of solution. Dilute 1 ml of solution S to 10 ml with *water R*. The solution is not more opalescent than reference suspension II (*2.2.1*) and not more intensely coloured than intensity 6 of the range of reference solutions of the most appropriate colour (*2.2.2, Method II*).

Chlorides. Not more than 1.0 per cent. To 2.50 g add 50 ml of *dilute nitric acid R*, shake for 1 h and dilute to 100.0 ml with *dilute nitric acid R*. Filter. To 50.0 ml of the filtrate add 10.0 ml of *0.1 M silver nitrate* and 5 ml of *toluene R*. Titrate with *0.1 M ammonium thiocyanate*, using 2 ml of *ferric ammonium sulphate solution R2* as indicator and shaking vigorously towards the end point.

1 ml of *0.1 M silver nitrate* is equivalent to 3.545 mg of Cl.

Calcium. Not more than 1.5 per cent of Ca, determined by atomic absorption spectrometry (*2.2.23, Method II*).

Test solution. Dissolve 0.10 g of the substance to be examined in 50 ml of *dilute ammonia R2*, heating on a water-bath. Allow to cool and dilute to 100.0 ml with *distilled water R* (solution (a)). Dilute 3.0 ml of solution (a) to 100.0 ml with *distilled water R*.

Reference solutions. Prepare three reference solutions in the same manner as the test solution but add 0.75 ml, 1.0 ml and 1.5 ml respectively of *calcium standard solution (100 ppm Ca) R* to the 3.0 ml of solution (a).

Set the zero of the instrument using a mixture of 1.5 volumes of *dilute ammonia R2* and 98.5 volumes of *distilled water R*. Measure the absorbance at 422.7 nm using a calcium hollow-cathode lamp as source of radiation and an air-acetylene flame.

Heavy metals (*2.4.8*). 1.0 g complies with the limit test F for heavy metals (20 ppm). Prepare the standard using 2 ml of *lead standard solution (10 ppm Pb) R*.

Loss on drying (*2.2.32*). Not more than 15.0 per cent, determined on 0.1000 g by drying in an oven at 100 °C to 105 °C for 4 h.

Sulphated ash (*2.4.14*): 30.0 per cent to 36.0 per cent, determined on 0.1000 g and calculated with reference to the dried substance.

Microbial contamination. Total viable aerobic count (*2.6.12*) not more than 10^3 micro-organisms per gram, determined by plate-count. It complies with the tests for *Escherichia coli* and *Salmonella* (*2.6.13*).

01/2005:1150

SODIUM AMIDOTRIZOATE

Natrii amidotrizoas

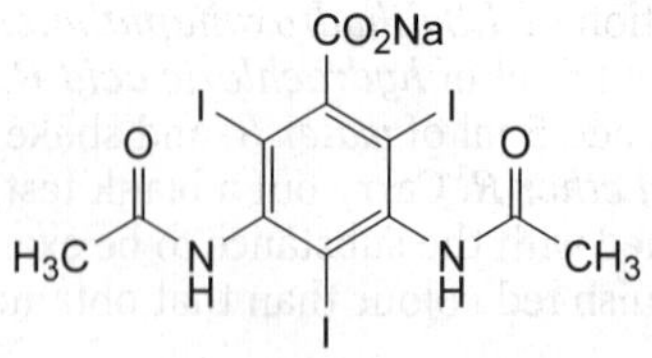

$C_{11}H_8I_3N_2NaO_4$ M_r 636

DEFINITION

Sodium amidotrizoate contains not less than 98.0 per cent and not more than the equivalent of 101.0 per cent of sodium 3,5-bis(acetylamino)-2,4,6-tri-iodobenzoate, calculated with reference to the anhydrous substance.

CHARACTERS

A white or almost white powder, freely soluble in water, slightly soluble in alcohol, practically insoluble in acetone. It melts at about 261 °C with decomposition.

IDENTIFICATION

First identification: A, D.

Second identification: B, C, D.

A. Examine by infrared absorption spectrophotometry (*2.2.24*), comparing with the spectrum obtained with *sodium amidotrizoate CRS*. Dry both the substance to be examined and the reference substance at 100 °C to 105 °C for 3 h.

B. Examine the chromatograms obtained in the test for related substances. The principal spot in the chromatogram obtained with test solution (b) is similar in position and size to the principal spot in the chromatogram obtained with reference solution (b).

C. Heat 50 mg gently in a small porcelain dish over a naked flame. Violet vapour is evolved.

D. It gives reaction (a) of sodium (*2.3.1*).

TESTS

Solution S. Dissolve 10 g in *carbon dioxide-free water R* and dilute to 20 ml with the same solvent.

Appearance of solution. Dilute 1 ml of solution S to 10 ml with *water R*. The solution is clear (*2.2.1*) and colourless (*2.2.2, Method II*).

pH (*2.2.3*). The pH of solution S is 7.5 to 9.5.

Related substances. Examine by thin-layer chromatography (*2.2.27*), using a *TLC silica gel GF_{254} plate R. Prepare the solutions in subdued light and develop the chromatograms protected from light.*

Test solution (a). Dissolve 0.50 g of the substance to be examined in a 3 per cent *V/V* solution of *ammonia R* in *methanol R* and dilute to 10 ml with the same solution.

Test solution (b). Dilute 1 ml of test solution (a) to 10 ml with a 3 per cent *V/V* solution of *ammonia R* in *methanol R*.

Reference solution (a). Dilute 1 ml of test solution (b) to 50 ml with a 3 per cent *V/V* solution of *ammonia R* in *methanol R*.

Reference solution (b). Dissolve 50 mg of *sodium amidotrizoate CRS* in a 3 per cent *V/V* solution of *ammonia R* in *methanol R* and dilute to 10 ml with the same solution.

Apply separately to the plate 2 µl of each solution. Develop over a path of 15 cm using a mixture of 20 volumes of *anhydrous formic acid R*, 25 volumes of *methyl ethyl ketone R* and 60 volumes of *toluene R*. Allow the plate to dry until the solvents have evaporated and examine in ultraviolet light at 254 nm. Any spot in the chromatogram obtained with test solution (a), apart from the principal spot, is not more intense than the spot in the chromatogram obtained with reference solution (a) (0.2 per cent).

Free aromatic amines. *Maintain the solutions and reagents in iced water, protected from light.* To 0.50 g in a 50 ml volumetric flask add 15 ml of *water R*. Shake and add 1 ml of *dilute sodium hydroxide solution R*. Cool in iced water, add 5 ml of a freshly prepared 5 g/l solution of *sodium nitrite R* and 12 ml of *dilute hydrochloric acid R*. Shake gently and allow to stand for exactly 2 min after adding the hydrochloric acid. Add 10 ml of a 20 g/l solution of *ammonium sulphamate R*. Allow to stand for 5 min, shaking frequently, and add 0.15 ml of a 100 g/l solution of *α-naphthol R* in *alcohol R*. Shake and allow to stand for 5 min. Add 3.5 ml of *buffer solution pH 10.9 R*, mix and dilute to 50.0 ml with *water R*. The absorbance (*2.2.25*), measured within 20 min at 485 nm using as the compensation liquid a solution prepared at the same time and in the same manner but omitting the substance to be examined, is not greater than 0.30.

Free iodine and iodides. Not more than 50 ppm. Dissolve 1.0 g in *distilled water R* and dilute to 10 ml with the same solvent. Add dropwise *dilute nitric acid R* until the precipitation is complete, then add 3 ml of *dilute nitric acid R*. Filter and wash the precipitate with 5 ml of *water R*. Collect the filtrate and washings. Add 1 ml of *strong hydrogen peroxide solution R* and 1 ml of *methylene chloride R*. Shake. The lower layer is not more intensely coloured than a reference solution prepared simultaneously and in the same manner, using a mixture of 5 ml of *iodide standard solution (10 ppm I) R*, 3 ml of *dilute nitric acid R* and 15 ml of *water R*.

Heavy metals (*2.4.8*). Dilute 4 ml of solution S to 20 ml with *water R*. 12 ml of this solution complies with limit test A for heavy metals (20 ppm). Prepare the standard using *lead standard solution (2 ppm Pb) R*.

Water (*2.5.12*). Not more than 11.0 per cent, determined on 0.400 g by the semi-micro determination of water.

ASSAY

To 0.150 g in a 250 ml round-bottomed flask add 5 ml of *strong sodium hydroxide solution R*, 20 ml of *water R*, 1 g of *zinc powder R* and a few glass beads. Boil under a reflux condenser for 30 min. Allow to cool and rinse the condenser with 20 ml of *water R*, adding the rinsings to the flask. Filter through a sintered-glass filter and wash the filter with several quantities of *water R*. Collect the filtrate and washings. Add 40 ml of *dilute sulphuric acid R* and titrate immediately with *0.1 M silver nitrate*. Determine the end-point potentiometrically (*2.2.20*), using a suitable electrode system such as silver-mercurous sulphate.

1 ml of *0.1 M silver nitrate* is equivalent to 21.20 mg of $C_{11}H_8I_3N_2NaO_4$.

STORAGE

Store protected from light.

IMPURITIES

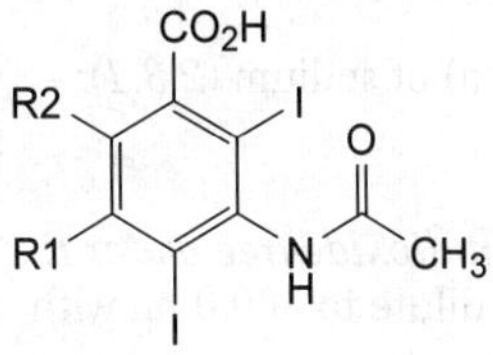

A. R1 = NH_2, R2 = I: 3-acetylamino-5-amino-2,4,6-triiodobenzoic acid,

B. R1 = $NHCOCH_3$, R2 = H: 3,5-bis(acetylamino)-2,4-diiodobenzoic acid.

01/2005:1993

SODIUM AMINOSALICYLATE DIHYDRATE

Natrii aminosalicylas dihydricus

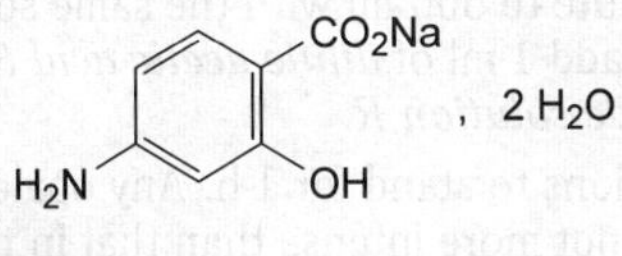

$C_7H_6NNaO_3,2H_2O$ M_r 211.2

DEFINITION

Sodium 4-amino-2-hydroxybenzoate dihydrate.

Content: 99.0 per cent to 101.0 per cent (dried substance).

CHARACTERS

Appearance: white, crystalline powder or white or almost white crystals, slightly hygroscopic.

Solubility: freely soluble in water, sparingly soluble in alcohol, practically insoluble in methylene chloride.

IDENTIFICATION

First identification: A, E.

Second identification: B, C, D, E.

A. Infrared absorption spectrophotometry (*2.2.24*).

Comparison: *Ph. Eur. reference spectrum of sodium aminosalicylate dihydrate.*

B. Introduce 0.3 g into a porcelain crucible. Cautiously heat on a small flame until vapour is evolved. Cover the crucible with a watch glass and collect the white sublimate. The melting point (*2.2.14*) of the sublimate is 120 °C to 124 °C.

C. To 0.1 ml of solution S (see Tests) add 5 ml of *water R* and 0.1 ml of *ferric chloride solution R1*. A reddish-brown colour develops.

D. 2 ml of solution S gives the reaction of primary aromatic amines (*2.3.1*).

E. 0.5 ml of solution S gives reaction (a) of sodium (*2.3.1*).

TESTS

Solution S. Dissolve 0.50 g in *carbon dioxide-free water R* and dilute to 25 ml with the same solvent.

Appearance of solution. The freshly prepared solution is clear (*2.2.1*) and not more intensely coloured than reference solution B_5 (*2.2.2, Method II*).

Dissolve 2.5 g in *water R* and dilute to 25 ml with the same solvent.

pH (*2.2.3*): 6.5 to 8.5 for solution S.

Related substances. Liquid chromatography (*2.2.29*). *Use freshly prepared solutions and mobile phases.*

Test solution. Dissolve 50.0 mg of the substance to be examined in *water R* and dilute to 50.0 ml with the same solvent.

Reference solution (a). Dissolve 5.0 mg of *3-aminophenol R* in *water R* and dilute to 100.0 ml with the same solvent.

Reference solution (b). Dissolve 5.0 mg of *mesalazine CRS* in *water R* and dilute to 100.0 ml with the same solvent. To 10.0 ml of this solution add 1.0 ml of reference solution (a) and dilute to 50.0 ml with *water R*.

Column:

- *size*: l = 0.25 m, Ø = 4.6 mm,
- *stationary phase*: spherical *base-deactivated octylsilyl silica gel for chromatography R* (5 µm).

Mobile phase:

- *mobile phase A*: dissolve 2.2 g of *perchloric acid R* and 1.0 g of *phosphoric acid R* in *water R* and dilute to 1000.0 ml with the same solvent,
- *mobile phase B*: dissolve 1.7 g of *perchloric acid R* and 1.0 g of *phosphoric acid R* in *acetonitrile R* and dilute to 1000.0 ml with the same solvent,

Time (min)	Mobile phase A (per cent *V/V*)	Mobile phase B (per cent *V/V*)
0 - 15	100	0
15 - 30	100 → 40	0 → 60
30 - 35	40 → 100	60 → 0
35 - 45	100	0

Flow rate: 1.25 ml/min.

Detection: spectrophotometer at 220 nm.

Injection: 10 µl.

Relative retention with reference to 4-aminosalicylate (retention time = about 12 min): impurity A = about 0.30; impurity B = about 0.37.

System suitability: reference solution (b):

- *resolution*: minimum 4.0 between the peaks due to impurity A and impurity B.

Limits:

- *impurity A*: not more than the area of the corresponding peak in the chromatogram obtained with reference solution (b) (0.1 per cent),
- *impurity B*: not more than the area of the corresponding peak in the chromatogram obtained with reference solution (b) (1.0 per cent),

- *any other impurity*: for each impurity, not more than 0.1 times the area of the peak due to impurity B in the chromatogram obtained with reference solution (b) (0.1 per cent),
- *total*: not more than the area of the peak due to impurity B in the chromatogram obtained with reference solution (b) (1.0 per cent),
- *disregard limit*: 0.05 times the area of the peak due to impurity B in the chromatogram obtained with reference solution (b) (0.05 per cent).

Heavy metals (*2.4.8*): maximum 10 ppm.

2.0 g complies with limit test C. Prepare the standard using 2 ml of *lead standard solution (10 ppm Pb) R*.

Loss on drying (*2.2.32*): 16.0 per cent to 17.5 per cent, determined on 1.000 g by drying in an oven at 100-105 °C.

Pyrogens (*2.6.8*). If intended for use in the manufacture of parenteral dosage forms without a further appropriate procedure for the removal of pyrogens, it complies with the test for pyrogens. Inject per kilogram of the rabbit's mass, 10 ml of a 20 mg/ml solution of the substance to be examined in *water for injections R*.

ASSAY

Dissolve 0.150 g in 20 ml of *water R*. Add 10 ml of a 500 g/l solution of *sodium bromide R* and 25 ml of *glacial acetic acid R*. Add 5 ml of *0.1 M sodium nitrite* rapidly and continue the titration with the same titrant, determining the end-point potentiometrically (*2.2.20*).

1 ml of *0.1 M sodium nitrite* is equivalent to 17.52 mg of $C_7H_6NNaO_3$.

STORAGE

In an airtight container, protected from light. If the substance is sterile, store in a sterile, airtight, tamper-proof container.

LABELLING

The label states, where applicable, that the substance is apyrogenic.

IMPURITIES

Specified impurities: A, B.

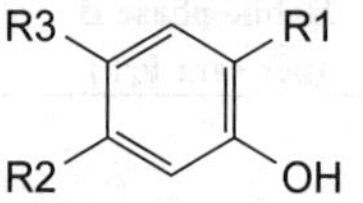

A. R1 = R3 = H, R2 = NH_2: 3-aminophenol,

B. R1 = CO_2H, R2 = H, R3 = NH_2: 5-amino-2-hydroxybenzoic acid (mesalazine).

Monographs Q-S

01/2005:1791

SODIUM ASCORBATE

Natrii ascorbas

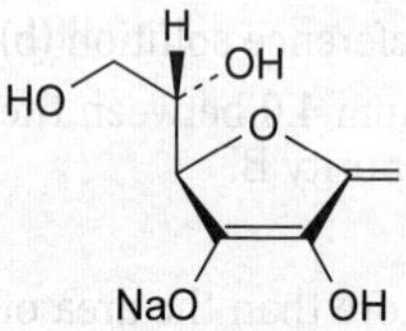

$C_6H_7NaO_6$ M_r 198.1

DEFINITION

Sodium (2*R*)-2-[(1*S*)-1,2-dihydroxyethyl]-4-hydroxy-5-oxo-2,5-dihydrofuran-3-olate.

Content: 99.0 per cent to 101.0 per cent (dried substance).

CHARACTERS

Appearance: white or yellowish, crystalline powder or crystals.

Solubility: freely soluble in water, sparingly soluble in alcohol, practically insoluble in methylene chloride.

IDENTIFICATION

First identification: B, D.

Second identification: A, C, D.

A. Specific optical rotation (*2.2.7*) (see Tests).

B. Infrared absorption spectrophotometry (*2.2.24*).

Preparation: discs.

Comparison: *sodium ascorbate CRS*.

C. To 1 ml of solution S (see Tests) add 0.2 ml of *dilute nitric acid R* and 0.2 ml of *silver nitrate solution R2*. A grey precipitate is formed.

D. 1 ml of solution S gives reaction (a) of sodium (*2.3.1*).

TESTS

Solution S. Dissolve 10.0 g in *carbon dioxide-free water R* prepared from *distilled water R* and dilute to 100.0 ml with the same solvent.

Appearance of solution. Solution S is clear (*2.2.1*) and not more intensely coloured than reference solution Y_6 or BY_6 (*2.2.2, Method II*). Examine the colour immediately after preparation of the solution.

pH (*2.2.3*): 7.0 to 8.0 for solution S.

Specific optical rotation (*2.2.7*): + 103 to + 108 (dried substance), determined on freshly prepared solution S.

Oxalic acid: maximum 0.3 per cent.

Test solution. Dissolve 0.25 g in 5 ml of *water R*. Add 1 ml of *dilute acetic acid R* and 0.5 ml of *calcium chloride solution R*.

Reference solution. Dissolve 70 mg of *oxalic acid R* in *water R* and dilute to 500 ml with the same solvent; to 5 ml of the solution add 1 ml of *dilute acetic acid R* and 0.5 ml of *calcium chloride solution R*.

Allow the solutions to stand for 1 h. Any opalescence in the test solution is not more intense than that in the reference solution.

Benzene (*2.4.24, System A*): maximum 2 ppm.

Sulphates (*2.4.13*): maximum 150 ppm.

To 10 ml of solution S add 2 ml of *hydrochloric acid R1* and dilute to 15 ml with *distilled water R*. The solution complies with the limit test for sulphates.

Copper: maximum 5 ppm.

Atomic absorption spectrometry (*2.2.23, Method I*).

Test solution. Dissolve 2.0 g in *0.1 M nitric acid* and dilute to 25.0 ml with the same solvent.

Reference solutions. Prepare reference solutions (0.2 ppm, 0.4 ppm and 0.6 ppm) by diluting *copper standard solution (10 ppm Cu) R* with *0.1 M nitric acid*.

Source: copper hollow-cathode lamp.

Wavelength: 324.8 nm.

Flame: air-acetylene.

Iron: maximum 2 ppm.

Atomic absorption spectrometry (*2.2.23, Method I*).

Test solution. Dissolve 5.0 g in *0.1 M nitric acid* and dilute to 25.0 ml with the same solvent.

Reference solutions. Prepare reference solutions (0.2 ppm, 0.4 ppm and 0.6 ppm) by diluting *iron standard solution (20 ppm Fe) R* with *0.1 M nitric acid*.

Source: iron hollow-cathode lamp.

Wavelength: 248.3 nm.

Flame: air-acetylene.

Nickel: maximum 1 ppm.

Atomic absorption spectrometry (*2.2.23, Method I*).

Test solution. Dissolve 10.0 g in *0.1 M nitric acid* and dilute to 25.0 ml with the same solvent.

Reference solutions. Prepare reference solutions (0.2 ppm, 0.4 ppm and 0.6 ppm) by diluting *nickel standard solution (10 ppm Ni) R* with *0.1 M nitric acid*.

Source: nickel hollow-cathode lamp.

Wavelength: 232.0 nm.

Flame: air-acetylene.

Heavy metals (*2.4.8*): maximum 10 ppm.

Dissolve 2.0 g in *water R* and dilute to 20 ml with the same solvent. 12 ml of the solution complies with limit test A. Prepare the standard using *lead standard solution (1 ppm Pb) R*.

Loss on drying (*2.2.32*): maximum 0.25 per cent, determined on 1.000 g by drying in an oven at 100-105 °C.

ASSAY

Dissolve 80 mg in a mixture of 10 ml of *dilute sulphuric acid R* and 80 ml of *carbon dioxide-free water R*. Add 1 ml of *starch solution R*. Titrate with *0.05 M iodine* until a persistent violet-blue colour is obtained.

1 ml of *0.05 M iodine* is equivalent to 9.91 mg of $C_6H_7NaO_6$.

STORAGE

Non-metallic container, protected from light.

01/2005:0123

SODIUM BENZOATE

Natrii benzoas

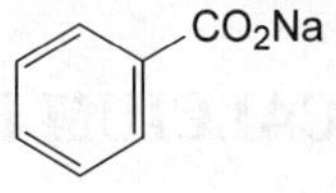

$C_7H_5NaO_2$ M_r 144.1

DEFINITION

Sodium benzoate contains not less than 99.0 per cent and not more than the equivalent of 100.5 per cent of sodium benzenecarboxylate, calculated with reference to the dried substance.

CHARACTERS

A white, crystalline or granular powder or flakes, slightly hygroscopic, freely soluble in water, sparingly soluble in alcohol (90 per cent *V/V*).

IDENTIFICATION

A. It gives reactions (b) and (c) of benzoates (*2.3.1*).

B. It gives reaction (a) of sodium (*2.3.1*).

TESTS

Solution S. Dissolve 10.0 g in *carbon dioxide-free water R* and dilute to 100 ml with the same solvent.

Appearance of solution. Solution S is clear (*2.2.1*) and not more intensely coloured than reference solution Y_6 (*2.2.2, Method II*).

Acidity or alkalinity. To 10 ml of solution S add 10 ml of *carbon dioxide-free water R* and 0.2 ml of *phenolphthalein solution R*. Not more than 0.2 ml of *0.1 M sodium hydroxide* or *0.1 M hydrochloric acid* is required to change the colour of the indicator.

Halogenated compounds. *All glassware used must be chloride-free and may be prepared by soaking overnight in a 500 g/l solution of nitric acid R, rinsed with water R and stored full of water R. It is recommended that glassware be reserved exclusively for this test.*

To 20.0 ml of solution S add 5 ml of *water R* and dilute to 50.0 ml with *alcohol R* (test solution).

Determination of ionised chlorine. In three 25 ml volumetric flasks, prepare the following solutions.

Solution (a). To 4.0 ml of the test solution add 3 ml of *dilute sodium hydroxide solution R* and 3 ml of *alcohol R*. This solution is used to prepare solution A.

Solution (b). To 3 ml of *dilute sodium hydroxide solution R* add 2 ml of *water R* and 5 ml of *alcohol R*. This solution is used to prepare solution B.

Solution (c). To 4.0 ml of *chloride standard solution (8 ppm Cl) R* add 6.0 ml of *water R*. This solution is used to prepare solution C.

In a fourth 25 ml volumetric flask, place 10 ml of *water R*. To each flask add 5 ml of *ferric ammonium sulphate solution R5*, mix and add dropwise and with swirling 2 ml of *nitric acid R* and 5 ml of *mercuric thiocyanate solution R*. Shake. Dilute the contents of each flask to 25.0 ml with *water R* and allow the solutions to stand in a water-bath at 20 °C for 15 min. Measure at 460 nm in a 2 cm cell the absorbance (*2.2.25*) of solution A using solution B as the compensation liquid, and the absorbance of solution C using the solution obtained with 10 ml of *water R* as the compensation liquid. The absorbance of solution A is not greater than that of solution C (200 ppm).

Determination of total chlorine

Solution (a). To 10.0 ml of the test solution add 7.5 ml of *dilute sodium hydroxide solution R* and 0.125 g of *nickel-aluminium alloy R* and heat on a water-bath for 10 min. Allow to cool to room temperature, filter into a 25 ml volumetric flask and wash the filter with 3 quantities, each of 2 ml, of *alcohol R* (a slight precipitate may form that disappears on acidification). Dilute the filtrate and washings to 25.0 ml with *water R*. This solution is used to prepare solution A.

Solution (b). In the same manner, prepare a similar solution replacing the test solution by a mixture of 5 ml of *alcohol R* and 5 ml of *water R*. This solution is used to prepare solution B.

Solution (c). To 6.0 ml of *chloride standard solution (8 ppm Cl) R* add 4.0 ml of *water R*. This solution is used to prepare solution C.

In four 25 ml volumetric flasks, place separately 10 ml of solution (a), 10 ml of solution (b), 10 ml of solution (c) and 10 ml of *water R*. To each flask add 5 ml of *ferric ammonium sulphate solution R5*, mix and add dropwise and with swirling 2 ml of *nitric acid R* and 5 ml of *mercuric thiocyanate solution R*. Shake. Dilute the contents of each flask to 25.0 ml with *water R* and allow the solutions to stand in a water-bath at 20 °C for 15 min. Measure at 460 nm in a 2 cm cell the absorbance (*2.2.25*) of solution A using solution B as the compensation liquid, and the absorbance of

Monographs Q-S

solution C using the solution obtained with 10 ml of *water R* as the compensation liquid. The absorbance of solution A is not greater than that of solution C (300 ppm).

Heavy metals (*2.4.8*). 2.0 g complies with limit test C for heavy metals (10 ppm). Prepare the standard using 2 ml of *lead standard solution (10 ppm Pb) R*.

Loss on drying (*2.2.32*). Not more than 2.0 per cent, determined on 1.00 g by drying in an oven at 100 °C to 105 °C.

ASSAY

Dissolve 0.250 g in 20 ml of *anhydrous acetic acid R*, heating to 50 °C if necessary. Cool. Using 0.05 ml of *naphtholbenzein solution R* as indicator, titrate with *0.1 M perchloric acid* until a green colour is obtained.

1 ml of *0.1 M perchloric acid* is equivalent to 14.41 mg of $C_7H_5NaO_2$.

01/2005:0190

SODIUM BROMIDE

Natrii bromidum

NaBr M_r 102.9

DEFINITION

Content: 98.0 per cent to 100.5 per cent (dried substance).

CHARACTERS

Appearance: white, granular powder or small, colourless, transparent or opaque crystals, slightly hygroscopic.

Solubility: freely soluble in water, soluble in alcohol.

IDENTIFICATION

A. It gives reaction (a) of bromides (*2.3.1*).

B. Solution S (see Tests) gives the reactions of sodium (*2.3.1*).

TESTS

Solution S. Dissolve 10.0 g in *carbon dioxide-free water R* prepared from *distilled water R* and dilute to 100 ml with the same solvent.

Appearance of solution. Solution S is clear (*2.2.1*) and colourless (*2.2.2, Method II*).

Acidity or alkalinity. To 10 ml of solution S add 0.1 ml of *bromothymol blue solution R1*. Not more than 0.5 ml of *0.01 M hydrochloric acid* or *0.01 M sodium hydroxide* is required to change the colour of the indicator.

Bromates. To 10 ml of solution S add 1 ml of *starch solution R*, 0.1 ml of a 100 g/l solution of *potassium iodide R* and 0.25 ml of *0.5 M sulphuric acid* and allow to stand protected from light for 5 min. No blue or violet colour develops.

Chlorides: maximum 0.6 per cent.

In a conical flask, dissolve 1.000 g in 20 ml of *dilute nitric acid R*. Add 5 ml of *strong hydrogen peroxide solution R* and heat on a water-bath until the solution is completely decolourised. Wash down the sides of the flask with a little *water R* and heat on a water-bath for 15 min. Allow to cool, dilute to 50 ml with *water R* and add 5.0 ml of *0.1 M silver nitrate* and 1 ml of *dibutyl phthalate R*. Shake and titrate with *0.1 M ammonium thiocyanate*, using 5 ml of *ferric ammonium sulphate solution R2* as indicator. Not more than 1.7 ml of *0.1 M silver nitrate* is used. Note the volume of *0.1 M silver nitrate* used (see Assay). Carry out a blank test.

Iodides. To 5 ml of solution S add 0.15 ml of *ferric chloride solution R1* and 2 ml of *methylene chloride R*. Shake and allow to separate. The lower layer is colourless (*2.2.2, Method I*).

Sulphates (*2.4.13*): maximum 100 ppm.

15 ml of solution S complies with the limit test for sulphates.

Iron (*2.4.9*): maximum 20 ppm.

5 ml of solution S diluted to 10 ml with *water R* complies with the limit test for iron.

Magnesium and alkaline-earth metals (*2.4.7*): maximum 200 ppm, calculated as Ca.

10.0 g complies with the limit test for magnesium and alkaline-earth metals. The volume of *0.01 M sodium edetate* used does not exceed 5.0 ml.

Heavy metals (*2.4.8*): maximum 10 ppm.

12 ml of solution S complies with limit test A. Prepare the standard using *lead standard solution (1 ppm Pb) R*.

Loss on drying (*2.2.32*): maximum 3.0 per cent, determined on 1.000 g by drying in an oven at 100-105 °C for 3 h.

ASSAY

Dissolve 2.000 g in *water R* and dilute to 100.0 ml with the same solvent. To 10.0 ml of the solution add 50 ml of *water R*, 5 ml of *dilute nitric acid R*, 25.0 ml of *0.1 M silver nitrate* and 2 ml of *dibutyl phthalate R*. Shake. Titrate with *0.1 M ammonium thiocyanate*, using 2 ml of *ferric ammonium sulphate solution R2* as indicator and shaking vigorously towards the end-point.

1 ml of *0.1 M silver nitrate* is equivalent to 10.29 mg of NaBr.

Calculate the percentage content of NaBr from the expression:

$$a - 2.902\,b$$

a = percentage content of NaBr and NaCl obtained in the assay and calculated as NaBr,

b = percentage content of Cl in the test for chlorides.

STORAGE

In an airtight container.

01/2005:0231

SODIUM CALCIUM EDETATE

Natrii calcii edetas

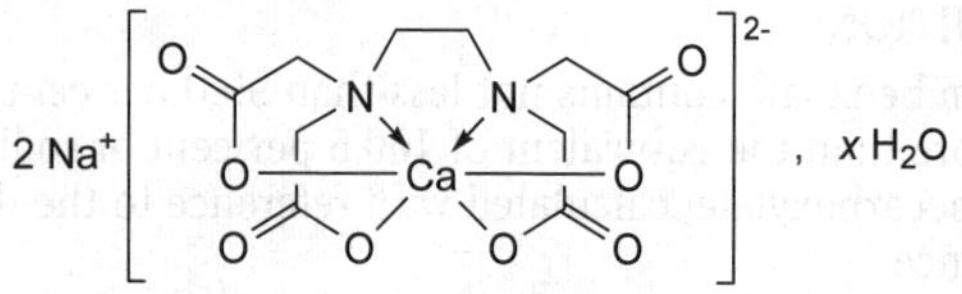

$C_{10}H_{12}CaN_2Na_2O_8,xH_2O$ M_r 374.3 (anhydrous substance)

DEFINITION

Disodium [(ethylenedinitrilo)tetraacetato]calciate(2−).

Content: 98.0 per cent to 102.0 per cent (anhydrous substance).

It contains a variable amount of water of crystallisation.

CHARACTERS

Appearance: white or almost white powder, hygroscopic.

Solubility: freely soluble in water, practically insoluble in alcohol.

IDENTIFICATION

First identification: A, C, D.

Second identification: B, C, D.

A. Infrared absorption spectrophotometry (*2.2.24*).
   Preparation: discs.
   Comparison: *sodium calcium edetate CRS.*

B. Dissolve 2 g in 10 ml of *water R*, add 6 ml of *lead nitrate solution R*, shake and add 3 ml of *potassium iodide solution R*. No yellow precipitate is formed. Make alkaline to *red litmus paper R* by the addition of *dilute ammonia R2* and add 3 ml of *ammonium oxalate solution R*. A white precipitate is formed.

C. Ignite. The residue gives the reactions of calcium (*2.3.1*).

D. The residue obtained in identification test C gives the reactions of sodium (*2.3.1*).

TESTS

Solution S. Dissolve 5.0 g in *water R* and dilute to 100 ml with the same solvent.

Appearance of solution. Solution S is clear (*2.2.1*) and colourless (*2.2.2, Method II*).

pH (*2.2.3*): 6.5 to 8.0.

Dissolve 5.0 g in *carbon dioxide-free water R* and dilute to 25 ml with the same solvent.

Impurity A. Liquid chromatography (*2.2.29*). *Carry out the test protected from light.*

Solvent mixture. Dissolve 10.0 g of *ferric sulphate pentahydrate R* in 20 ml of *0.5 M sulphuric acid* and add 780 ml of *water R*. Adjust to pH 2.0 with *1 M sodium hydroxide* and dilute to 1000 ml with *water R*.

Test solution. Dissolve 0.100 g of the substance to be examined in the solvent mixture and dilute to 25.0 ml with the solvent mixture.

Reference solution. Dissolve 40.0 mg of *nitrilotriacetic acid R* in the solvent mixture and dilute to 100.0 ml with the solvent mixture. To 1.0 ml of the solution add 0.1 ml of the test solution and dilute to 100.0 ml with the solvent mixture.

Column:

– *size*: l = 0.10 m, Ø = 4.6 mm,

– *stationary phase*: spherical *graphitised carbon for chromatography R1* (5 µm) with a specific surface area of 120 m^2/g and a pore size of 25 nm.

Mobile phase: dissolve 50.0 mg of *ferric sulphate pentahydrate R* in 50 ml of *0.5 M sulphuric acid* and add 750 ml of *water R*. Adjust to pH 1.5 with *0.5 M sulphuric acid* or *1 M sodium hydroxide*, add 20 ml of *ethylene glycol R* and dilute to 1000 ml with *water R*.

Flow rate: 1 ml/min.

Detection: spectrophotometer at 273 nm.

Injection: 20 µl; filter the solutions and inject immediately.

Run time: 4 times the retention time of the iron complex of impurity A.

Retention time: iron complex of impurity A = about 5 min; iron complex of edetic acid = about 10 min.

System suitability: reference solution:

– *resolution*: minimum 7 between the peaks due to the iron complex of impurity A and the iron complex of edetic acid,

– *signal-to-noise ratio*: minimum 50 for the peak due to impurity A.

Limit:

– *impurity A*: not more than the area of the corresponding peak in the chromatogram obtained with the reference solution (0.1 per cent).

Disodium edetate: maximum 1.0 per cent.

Dissolve 5.0 g in 250 ml of *water R*. Add 10 ml of *ammonium chloride buffer solution pH 10.0 R* and about 50 mg of *mordant black 11 triturate R*. Not more than 1.5 ml of *0.1 M magnesium chloride* is required to change the colour of the indicator to violet.

Chlorides (*2.4.4*): maximum 0.1 per cent.

To 20 ml of solution S add 30 ml of *dilute nitric acid R*, allow to stand for 30 min and filter. Dilute 2.5 ml of the filtrate to 15 ml with *water R*.

Iron (*2.4.9*): maximum 80 ppm.

Dilute 2.5 ml of solution S to 10 ml with *water R*. Add 0.25 g of *calcium chloride R* to the test solution and the standard before the addition of the *thioglycollic acid R*.

Heavy metals (*2.4.8*): maximum 20 ppm.

1.0 g complies with limit test D. Prepare the standard using 2 ml of *lead standard solution (10 ppm Pb) R*.

Water (*2.5.12, Method B*): 5.0 per cent to 13.0 per cent, determined on 0.100 g.

ASSAY

Dissolve 0.300 g in *water R* and dilute to 300 ml with the same solvent. Add 2 g of *hexamethylenetetramine R* and 2 ml of *dilute hydrochloric acid R*. Titrate with *0.1 M lead nitrate*, using about 50 mg of *xylenol orange triturate R* as indicator.

1 ml of *0.1 M lead nitrate* is equivalent to 37.43 mg of $C_{10}H_{12}CaN_2Na_2O_8$.

STORAGE

In an airtight container, protected from light.

IMPURITIES

Specified impurities: A.

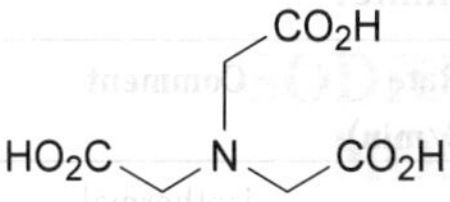

A. nitrilotriacetic acid.

01/2005:1471

SODIUM CAPRYLATE

Natrii caprylas

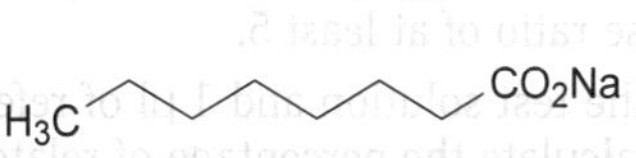

$C_8H_{15}NaO_2$ M_r 166.2

DEFINITION

Sodium caprylate contains not less than 99.0 per cent and not more than the equivalent of 101.0 per cent of sodium octanoate, calculated with reference to the anhydrous substance.

CHARACTERS

A white, crystalline powder, very soluble or freely soluble in water, freely soluble in acetic acid, sparingly soluble in alcohol, practically insoluble in acetone.

IDENTIFICATION

A. Examine the chromatograms obtained in the test for related substances. The retention time and size of the principal peak in the chromatogram obtained with the

Calculate the percentage content of sodium stearyl sulphate in the substance to be examined, using the expression:

$$\frac{(B \times 1.377) \times m'_H \times 100}{S_{Hc(corr)} \times m'}$$

B = area of the peak corresponding to stearyl alcohol in the chromatogram obtained with test solution (c).

The percentage content of sodium cetostearyl sulphate corresponds to the sum of the percentage content of sodium cetyl sulphate and the percentage content of sodium stearyl sulphate.

LABELLING

The label states, where appropriate, the name and concentration of any added buffer.

01/2005:0193

SODIUM CHLORIDE

Natrii chloridum

NaCl M_r 58.44

DEFINITION

Sodium chloride contains not less than 99.0 per cent and not more than the equivalent of 100.5 per cent of NaCl, calculated with reference to the dried substance.

CHARACTERS

A white, crystalline powder or colourless crystals or white pearls, freely soluble in water, practically insoluble in ethanol.

IDENTIFICATION

A. It gives the reactions of chlorides (*2.3.1*).

B. It gives the reactions of sodium (*2.3.1*).

TESTS

If the substance is in the form of pearls crush before use.

Solution S. Dissolve 20.0 g in *carbon dioxide-free water R* prepared from *distilled water R* and dilute to 100.0 ml with the same solvent.

Appearance of solution. Solution S is clear (*2.2.1*) and colourless (*2.2.2, Method II*).

Acidity or alkalinity. To 20 ml of solution S add 0.1 ml of *bromothymol blue solution R1*. Not more than 0.5 ml of *0.01 M hydrochloric acid* or *0.01 M sodium hydroxide* is required to change the colour of the indicator.

Bromides. To 0.5 ml of solution S add 4.0 ml of *water R*, 2.0 ml of *phenol red solution R2* and 1.0 ml of a 0.1 g/l solution of *chloramine R* and mix immediately. After exactly 2 min, add 0.15 ml of *0.1 M sodium thiosulphate*, mix and dilute to 10.0 ml with *water R*. The absorbance (*2.2.25*) of the solution measured at 590 nm, using *water R* as the compensation liquid, is not greater than that of a standard prepared at the same time and in the same manner, using 5.0 ml of a 3.0 mg/l solution of *potassium bromide R* (100 ppm).

Ferrocyanides. Dissolve 2.0 g in 6 ml of *water R*. Add 0.5 ml of a mixture of 5 ml of a 10 g/l solution of *ferric ammonium sulphate R* in a 2.5 g/l solution of *sulphuric acid R* and 95 ml of a 10 g/l solution of *ferrous sulphate R*. No blue colour develops within 10 min.

Iodides. Moisten 5 g by the dropwise addition of a freshly prepared mixture of 0.15 ml of *sodium nitrite solution R*, 2 ml of *0.5 M sulphuric acid*, 25 ml of *iodide-free starch solution R* and 25 ml of *water R*. After 5 min, examine in daylight. The substance shows no blue colour.

Nitrites. To 10 ml of solution S add 10 ml of *water R*. Measure the absorbance (*2.2.25*) of the solution at 354 nm. The absorbance is not greater than 0.01.

Phosphates (*2.4.11*). Dilute 2 ml of solution S to 100 ml with *water R*. The solution complies with the limit test for phosphates (25 ppm).

Sulphates (*2.4.13*). Dilute 7.5 ml of solution S to 30 ml with *distilled water R*. 15 ml of the solution complies with the limit test for sulphates (200 ppm).

Aluminium (*2.4.17*). If intended for use in the manufacture of peritoneal dialysis solutions, haemodialysis solutions or haemofiltration solutions, it complies with the test for aluminium. Dissolve 20.0 g in 100 ml of *water R* and add 10 ml of *acetate buffer solution pH 6.0 R*. The solution complies with the limit test for aluminium (0.2 ppm). Use as the reference solution a mixture of 2 ml of *aluminium standard solution (2 ppm Al) R*, 10 ml of *acetate buffer solution pH 6.0 R* and 98 ml of *water R*. To prepare the blank, use a mixture of 10 ml of *acetate buffer solution pH 6.0 R* and 100 ml of *water R*.

Arsenic (*2.4.2*). 5 ml of solution S complies with limit test A for arsenic (1 ppm).

Barium. To 5 ml of solution S add 5 ml of *distilled water R* and 2 ml of *dilute sulphuric acid R*. After 2 h, any opalescence in the solution is not more intense than that in a mixture of 5 ml of solution S and 7 ml of *distilled water R*.

Iron (*2.4.9*). 10 ml of solution S complies with the limit test for iron (2 ppm). Prepare the standard using a mixture of 4 ml of *iron standard solution (1 ppm Fe) R* and 6 ml of *water R*.

Magnesium and alkaline-earth metals (*2.4.7*). 10.0 g complies with the limit test for magnesium and alkaline-earth metals (use 150 mg of *mordant black 11 triturate R*. The volume of *0.01 M sodium edetate* used does not exceed 2.5 ml (100 ppm, calculated as Ca).

Potassium. If intended for use in the manufacture of parenteral dosage forms or haemodialysis, haemofiltration or peritoneal dialysis solutions, it contains not more than 500 ppm of K, determined by atomic emission spectrometry (*2.2.22, Method I*).

Test solution. Dissolve 1.00 g of the substance to be examined in *water R* and dilute to 100.0 ml with the same solvent.

Reference solutions. Dissolve 1.144 g of *potassium chloride R*, previously dried at 100-105 °C for 3 h, in *water R* and dilute to 1000.0 ml with the same solvent (600 µg of K per millilitre). Dilute as required.

Measure the emission intensity at 766.5 nm.

Heavy metals (*2.4.8*). 12 ml of solution S complies with limit test A for heavy metals (5 ppm). Prepare the standard using *lead standard solution (1 ppm Pb) R*.

Loss on drying (*2.2.32*). Not more than 0.5 per cent, determined on 1.000 g by drying in an oven at 100-105 °C for 2 h.

Bacterial endotoxins (*2.6.14*): less than 5 IU/g, if intended for use in the manufacture of parenteral dosage forms without a further appropriate procedure for removal of bacterial endotoxins.

ASSAY

Dissolve 50.0 mg in *water R* and dilute to 50 ml with the same solvent. Titrate with *0.1 M silver nitrate* determining the end-point potentiometrically (*2.2.20*).

1 ml of *0.1 M silver nitrate* is equivalent to 5.844 mg of NaCl.

LABELLING

The label states:

- where applicable, that the substance is suitable for use in the manufacture of parenteral dosage forms,
- where applicable, that the substance is free from bacterial endotoxins,
- where applicable, that the substance is suitable for use in the manufacture of peritoneal dialysis solutions, haemodialysis solutions or haemofiltration solutions.

01/2005:0412

SODIUM CITRATE

Natrii citras

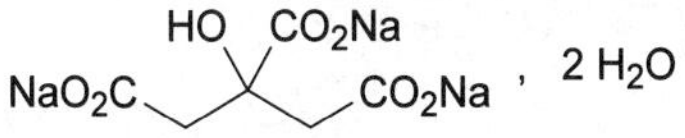

$C_6H_5Na_3O_7,2H_2O$ M_r 294.1

DEFINITION

Sodium citrate contains not less than 99.0 per cent and not more than the equivalent of 101.0 per cent of trisodium 2-hydroxypropane-1,2,3-tricarboxylate, calculated with reference to the anhydrous substance.

CHARACTERS

A white, crystalline powder or white, granular crystals, slightly deliquescent in moist air, freely soluble in water, practically insoluble in alcohol.

IDENTIFICATION

A. To 1 ml of solution S (see Tests) add 4 ml of *water R*. The solution gives the reaction of citrates (*2.3.1*).

B. 1 ml of solution S gives reaction (a) of sodium (*2.3.1*).

TESTS

Solution S. Dissolve 10.0 g in *carbon dioxide-free water R* prepared from *distilled water R* and dilute to 100 ml with the same solvent.

Appearance of solution. Solution S is clear (*2.2.1*) and colourless (*2.2.2, Method II*).

Acidity or alkalinity. To 10 ml of solution S add 0.1 ml of *phenolphthalein solution R*. Not more than 0.2 ml of *0.1 M hydrochloric acid* or *0.1 M sodium hydroxide* is required to change the colour of the indicator.

Readily carbonisable substances. To 0.20 g of the powdered substance to be examined add 10 ml of *sulphuric acid R* and heat in a water-bath at 90 ± 1 °C for 60 min. Cool rapidly. The solution is not more intensely coloured than reference solution Y_2 or GY_2 (*2.2.2, Method II*).

Chlorides (*2.4.4*). Dilute 10 ml of solution S to 15 ml with *water R*. The solution complies with the limit test for chlorides (50 ppm).

Oxalates. Dissolve 0.50 g in 4 ml of *water R*, add 3 ml of *hydrochloric acid R* and 1 g of granulated *zinc R* and heat on a water-bath for 1 min. Allow to stand for 2 min, decant the liquid into a test-tube containing 0.25 ml of a 10 g/l solution of *phenylhydrazine hydrochloride R* and heat to boiling. Cool rapidly, transfer to a graduated cylinder and add an equal volume of *hydrochloric acid R* and 0.25 ml of *potassium ferricyanide solution R*. Shake and allow to stand for 30 min. Any pink colour in the solution is not more intense than that in a standard prepared at the same time in the same manner using 4 ml of a 50 mg/l solution of *oxalic acid R* (300 ppm).

Sulphates (*2.4.13*). To 10 ml of solution S add 2 ml of *hydrochloric acid R1* and dilute to 15 ml with *distilled water R*. The solution complies with the limit test for sulphates (150 ppm).

Heavy metals (*2.4.8*). 12 ml of solution S complies with limit test A for heavy metals (10 ppm). Prepare the standard using *lead standard solution (1 ppm Pb) R*.

Water (*2.5.12*): 11.0 per cent to 13.0 per cent, determined on 0.300 g by the semi-micro determination of water. After adding the substance to be examined, stir for 15 min before titrating.

Pyrogens (*2.6.8*). If intended for use in large-volume preparations for parenteral use, the competent authority may require that it comply with the test for pyrogens. Inject per kilogram of the rabbit's mass 10 ml of a freshly prepared solution in *water for injections R* containing per millilitre 10.0 mg of the substance to be examined and 7.5 mg of pyrogen-free *calcium chloride R*.

ASSAY

Dissolve 0.150 g in 20 ml of *anhydrous acetic acid R*, heating to about 50 °C. Allow to cool. Using 0.25 ml of *naphtholbenzein solution R* as indicator, titrate with *0.1 M perchloric acid* until a green colour is obtained.

1 ml of *0.1 M perchloric acid* is equivalent to 8.602 mg of $C_6H_5Na_3O_7$.

STORAGE

Store in an airtight container.

01/2005:0562

SODIUM CROMOGLICATE

Natrii cromoglicas

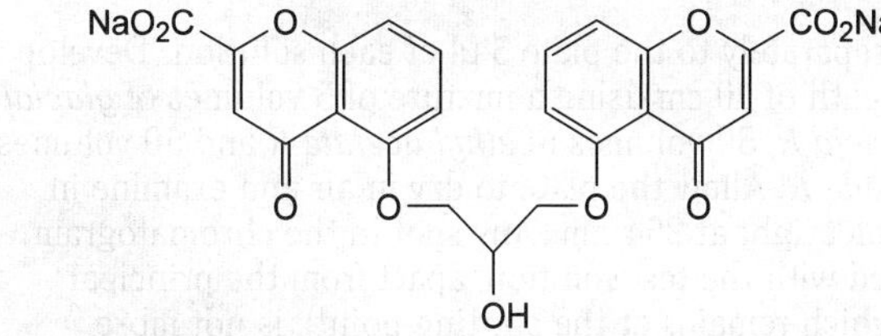

$C_{23}H_{14}Na_2O_{11}$ M_r 512.3

DEFINITION

Sodium cromoglicate contains not less than 98.0 per cent and not more than the equivalent of 101.0 per cent of disodium 5,5′-[(2-hydroxypropane-1,3-diyl)bis(oxy)]bis(4-oxo-4*H*-1-benzopyran-2-carboxylate, calculated with reference to the dried substance.

CHARACTERS

A white or almost white, crystalline powder, hygroscopic, soluble in water, practically insoluble in alcohol.

IDENTIFICATION

First identification: B, D.

Second identification: A, C, D.

Monographs Q-S

A. Dissolve 10.0 mg in *phosphate buffer solution pH 7.4 R* and dilute to 100.0 ml with the same solvent. Dilute 10.0 ml of this solution to 100.0 ml with the same solvent. Examined between 230 nm and 350 nm (*2.2.25*), the solution shows two absorption maxima, at 239 nm and 327 nm. The ratio of the absorbance at the maximum at 327 nm to that at the maximum at 239 nm is 0.25 to 0.30.

B. Examine by infrared absorption spectrophotometry (*2.2.24*), comparing with the spectrum obtained with *sodium cromoglicate CRS*. Examine the substances prepared as discs.

C. Dissolve about 5 mg in 0.5 ml of *methanol R*. Add 3 ml of a solution in *methanol R* containing 5 g/l of *aminopyrazolone R* and 1 per cent *V/V* of *hydrochloric acid R*. Allow to stand for 5 min. The solution shows an intense yellow colour.

D. It gives reaction (a) of sodium (*2.3.1*).

TESTS

Solution S. Dissolve 0.5 g in *carbon dioxide-free water R* and dilute to 25 ml with the same solvent.

Appearance of solution. Solution S is not more opalescent than reference suspension II (*2.2.1*) and not more intensely coloured than reference solution BY_5 (*2.2.2, Method II*).

Acidity or alkalinity. To 10 ml of solution S add 0.1 ml of *phenolphthalein solution R*. The solution is colourless. Add 0.2 ml of *0.01 M sodium hydroxide*. The solution is pink. Add 0.4 ml of *0.01 M hydrochloric acid*. The solution is colourless. Add 0.25 ml of *methyl red solution R*. The solution is red.

Related substances. Examine by thin-layer chromatography (*2.2.27*), using *silica gel GF_{254} R* as the coating substance.

Test solution. Dissolve 0.2 g of the substance to be examined in a mixture of 1 volume of *acetone R*, 4 volumes of *tetrahydrofuran R* and 6 volumes of *water R* and dilute to 10 ml with the same mixture of solvents.

Reference solution. Dissolve 10 mg of *1,3-bis(2-acetyl-3-hydroxyphenoxy)-2-propanol CRS* in *chloroform R* and dilute to 100 ml with the same solvent.

Apply separately to the plate 5 µl of each solution. Develop over a path of 10 cm using a mixture of 5 volumes of *glacial acetic acid R*, 50 volumes of *ethyl acetate R* and 50 volumes of *toluene R*. Allow the plate to dry in air and examine in ultraviolet light at 254 nm. Any spot in the chromatogram obtained with the test solution, apart from the principal spot (which remains at the starting point), is not more intense than the spot in the chromatogram obtained with the reference solution (0.5 per cent).

Oxalate. Dissolve 0.10 g in 20 ml of *water R*, add 5.0 ml of *iron salicylate solution R* and dilute to 50.0 ml with *water R*. Determine the absorbance (*2.2.25*) at 480 nm. The absorbance is not less than that of a standard prepared in the same manner using 0.35 mg of *oxalic acid R* instead of the substance to be examined.

Heavy metals (*2.4.8*). 1.0 g complies with limit test C for heavy metals (20 ppm). Prepare the standard using 2 ml of *lead standard solution (10 ppm Pb) R*.

Loss on drying (*2.2.32*). Not more than 10.0 per cent, determined on 1.000 g by drying over *diphosphorus pentoxide R* at 100 °C to 105 °C and at a pressure of 300 Pa to 600 Pa.

ASSAY

Dissolve 0.200 g with heating in a mixture of 5 ml of *2-propanol R* and 25 ml of *ethylene glycol R*. Cool and add 30 ml of *dioxan R*. Titrate with *0.1 M perchloric acid*, determining the end-point potentiometrically (*2.2.20*).

1 ml of *0.1 M perchloric acid* is equivalent to 25.62 mg of $C_{23}H_{14}Na_2O_{11}$.

STORAGE

Store in an airtight container, protected from light.

01/2005:0774

SODIUM CYCLAMATE

Natrii cyclamas

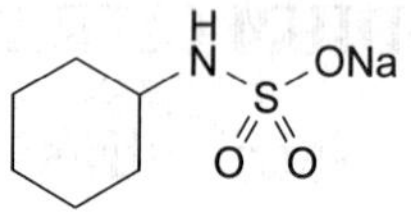

$C_6H_{12}NNaO_3S$ M_r 201.2

DEFINITION

Sodium cyclamate contains not less than 98.5 per cent and not more than the equivalent of 101.0 per cent of sodium *N*-cyclohexylsulphamate, calculated with reference to the dried substance.

CHARACTERS

A white, crystalline powder or colourless crystals, freely soluble in water, slightly soluble in alcohol.

IDENTIFICATION

First identification: A, E.

Second identification: B, C, D, E.

A. Examine by infrared absorption spectrophotometry (*2.2.24*), comparing with the spectrum obtained with *sodium cyclamate CRS*.

B. Examine the chromatograms obtained in the test for sulphamic acid. The principal spot in the chromatogram obtained with test solution (b) is similar in position, colour and size to the principal spot in the chromatogram obtained with reference solution (a).

C. To 1 ml of solution S (see Tests), add 1 ml of *water R* and 2 ml of *silver nitrate solution R1* and shake. A white, crystalline precipitate is formed.

D. To 1 ml of solution S add 5 ml of *water R*, 2 ml of *dilute hydrochloric acid R* and 4 ml of *barium chloride solution R1* and mix. The solution is clear. Add 2 ml of *sodium nitrite solution R*. A voluminous white precipitate is formed and gas is given off.

E. A mixture of 1 ml of solution S and 1 ml of *water R* gives reaction (a) of sodium (*2.3.1*).

TESTS

Solution S. Dissolve 5 g in *carbon dioxide-free water R* prepared from *distilled water R* and dilute to 50 ml with the same solvent.

Appearance of solution. Solution S is clear (*2.2.1*) and colourless (*2.2.2, Method II*).

pH (*2.2.3*). The pH of solution S is 5.5 to 7.5.

Absorbance (*2.2.25*). The absorbance of solution S, measured at 270 nm, is not greater than 0.10.

Monographs Q-S

Sulphamic acid. Examine by thin-layer chromatography (*2.2.27*), using a *TLC silica gel G plate R*.

Test solution (a). Use solution S.

Test solution (b). Dilute 1 ml of test solution (a) to 10 ml with *water R*.

Reference solution (a). Dissolve 0.10 g of *sodium cyclamate CRS* in *water R* and dilute to 10 ml with the same solvent.

Reference solution (b). Dissolve 10 mg of *sulphamic acid R* in *water R* and dilute to 100 ml with the same solvent.

Apply to the plate 2 µl of each solution. Develop over a path of 12 cm using a mixture of 10 volumes of *concentrated ammonia R*, 10 volumes of *water R*, 20 volumes of *ethyl acetate R* and 70 volumes of *propanol R*. Dry the plate in a current of warm air, heat at 105 °C for 5 min and spray the hot plate with *strong sodium hypochlorite solution R* diluted to a concentration of 5 g/l of active chlorine. Place the plate in a current of cold air until an area of coating below the points of application gives at most a faint blue colour with a drop of *potassium iodide and starch solution R*; avoid prolonged exposure to cold air. Spray with *potassium iodide and starch solution R* and examine the chromatograms within 5 min. Any spot corresponding to sulphamic acid in the chromatogram obtained with test solution (a) is not more intense than the spot in the chromatogram obtained with reference solution (b) (0.1 per cent).

Aniline, cyclohexylamine and dicyclohexylamine. Not more than 1 ppm of aniline, not more than 10 ppm of cyclohexylamine and not more than 1 ppm of dicyclohexylamine determined by gas chromatography (*2.2.28*) using *tetradecane R* as the internal standard.

Internal standard solution. Dissolve 2 µl of *tetradecane R* in *methylene chloride R* and dilute to 100 ml with the same solvent.

Test solution. Dissolve 2.00 g of the substance to be examined in 20 ml of *water R* and add 0.5 ml of *strong sodium hydroxide solution R* and shake with 30 ml of *toluene R*. Shake 20 ml of the upper layer with 4 ml of a mixture of equal volumes of *dilute acetic acid R* and *water R*. Separate the lower layer and add 0.5 ml of *strong sodium hydroxide solution R* and 0.5 ml of the internal standard solution. Shake and use the lower layer for chromatography immediately after separation.

Reference solution. Dissolve 10.0 mg (about 12 µl) of *cyclohexylamine R*, 1.0 mg (about 1.1 µl) of *dicyclohexylamine R* and 1.0 mg (about 1 µl) of *aniline R* in *water R* and dilute to 1000 ml with the same solvent. Dilute 10.0 ml of this solution to 100.0 ml with *water R* (solution A). To 20.0 ml of solution A, add 0.5 ml of *strong sodium hydroxide solution R* and extract with 30 ml of *toluene R*. Shake 20 ml of the upper layer with 4 ml of a mixture of equal volumes of *dilute acetic acid R* and *water R*. Separate the lower layer and add 0.5 ml of *strong sodium hydroxide solution R* and 0.5 ml of the internal standard solution. Shake and use the lower layer for chromatography immediately after separation.

The chromatographic procedure may be carried out using:

– a fused silica column 25 m long and 0.32 mm in internal diameter coated with *poly(dimethyl)(diphenyl)siloxane R* (0.51 µm),

– *helium for chromatography R* as the carrier gas at a flow rate of 1.8 ml/min,

– a flame-ionisation detector,

– a split vent at a flow rate of 20 ml/min,

with the following temperature programme:

	Time (min)	Temperature (°C)	Rate (°C/min)	Comment
Column	0 - 1	85		isothermal
	1 - 9	85 → 150	8	linear gradient
	9 - 13	150		isothermal
Injection port		250		
Detector		270		

Inject 1.5 µl of each solution. When the chromatograms are recorded in the conditions prescribed, the retention times relative to cyclohexylamine (about 2.3 min) are the following: aniline about 1.4, tetradecane about 4.3 and dicyclohexylamine about 4.5.

Sulphates (*2.4.13*). Dilute 1.5 ml of solution S to 15 ml with *distilled water R*. The solution complies with the limit test for sulphates (0.1 per cent).

Heavy metals (*2.4.8*). 12 ml of solution S complies with limit test A for heavy metals (10 ppm). Prepare the standard using *lead standard solution (1 ppm Pb) R*.

Loss on drying (*2.2.32*). Not more than 1.0 per cent, determined on 1.000 g in an oven at 100 °C to 105 °C for 4 h.

ASSAY

Dissolve without heating 0.150 g in 60 ml of *anhydrous acetic acid R*. Titrate with *0.1 M perchloric acid*, determining the end-point potentiometrically (*2.2.20*).

1 ml of *0.1 M perchloric acid* is equivalent to 20.12 mg of $C_6H_{12}NNaO_3S$.

IMPURITIES

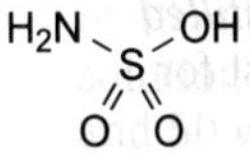

A. sulphamic acid,

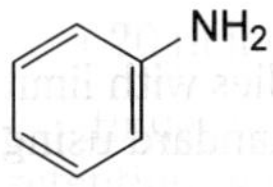

B. aniline (phenylamine),

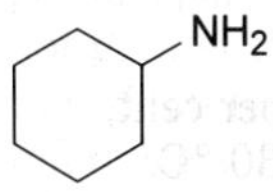

C. cyclohexanamine,

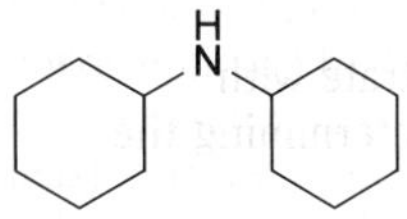

D. *N*-cyclohexylcyclohexanamine.

01/2005:0194

SODIUM DIHYDROGEN PHOSPHATE DIHYDRATE

Natrii dihydrogenophosphas dihydricus

$NaH_2PO_4,2H_2O$ M_r 156.0

DEFINITION

Sodium dihydrogen phosphate dihydrate contains not less than 98.0 per cent and not more than the equivalent of 100.5 per cent of NaH_2PO_4, calculated with reference to the dried substance.

01/2005:1995

SODIUM GLYCEROPHOSPHATE, HYDRATED

Natrii glycerophosphas hydricus

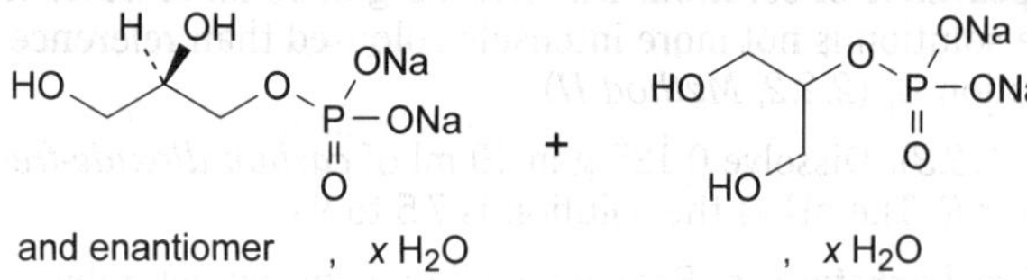

$C_3H_7Na_2O_6P, xH_2O$ M_r 216.0 (anhydrous substance)

DEFINITION

Mixture of variable proportions of sodium (2*RS*)-2,3-dihydroxypropyl phosphate and sodium 2-hydroxy-1-(hydroxymethyl)ethyl phosphate. The degree of hydration is 4 to 6.

Content: 98.0 per cent to 102.0 per cent (anhydrous substance).

CHARACTERS

Appearance: white, crystalline powder or crystals.

Solubility: freely soluble in water, practically insoluble in acetone and in alcohol.

IDENTIFICATION

A. Solution S (see Tests) gives reaction (a) of sodium (*2.3.1*).

B. To 0.1 g add 5 ml of *dilute nitric acid R*. Heat to boiling and boil for 1 min. Cool. The solution gives reaction (b) of phosphates (*2.3.1*).

C. In a test-tube fitted with a glass tube, mix 0.1 g with 5 g of *potassium hydrogen sulphate R*. Heat strongly and direct the white vapour into 5 ml of *decolorised fuchsin solution R*. A violet-red colour develops which becomes violet upon heating for 30 min on a water-bath.

TESTS

Solution S. Dissolve 10.0 g in *carbon dioxide-free water R* prepared from *distilled water R* and dilute to 100 ml with the same solvent.

Appearance of solution. Solution S is not more opalescent than reference suspension II (*2.2.1*) and not more intensely coloured than reference solution Y_6 (*2.2.2, Method II*).

Alkalinity. To 10 ml of solution S add 0.2 ml of *phenolphthalein solution R*. Not more than 1.0 ml of *0.1 M hydrochloric acid* is required to change the colour of the indicator, (n_2).

Glycerol and alcohol-soluble substances: maximum 1.0 per cent.

Shake 1.000 g with 25 ml of *alcohol R* for 10 min. Filter. Evaporate the filtrate on a water-bath and dry the residue at 70 °C for 1 h. The residue weighs not more than 10 mg.

Chlorides (*2.4.4*): maximum 200 ppm.

Dilute 2.5 ml of solution S to 15 ml with *water R*.

Phosphates (*2.4.11*): maximum 0.1 per cent.

Dilute 1 ml of solution S to 10 ml with *water R*. Dilute 1 ml of this solution to 100 ml with *water R*.

Sulphates (*2.4.13*): maximum 500 ppm.

Dilute 3 ml of solution S to 15 ml with *water R*.

Iron (*2.4.9*): maximum 20 ppm.

Dilute 5 ml of solution S to 10 ml with *water R*.

Heavy metals (*2.4.8*): maximum 20 ppm.

Dilute 10 ml of solution S to 20 ml with *water R*. 12 ml of the solution complies with limit test A. Prepare the standard using 10 ml of *lead standard solution (1 ppm Pb) R*.

Water (*2.5.12*): 25.0 per cent to 35.0 per cent, determined on 0.100 g.

ASSAY

Dissolve 0.250 g in 30 ml of *water R*. Titrate with *0.05 M sulphuric acid*, determining the end-point potentiometrically (*2.2.20*), (n_1).

Calculate the percentage content of sodium glycerophosphate (anhydrous substance) from the expression:

$$\frac{216.0\left(n_1 - \frac{n_2}{4}\right)}{m\,(100 - a)}$$

a = percentage content of water,

n_1 = volume of *0.05 M sulphuric acid* used in the assay, in millilitres,

n_2 = volume of *0.1 M hydrochloric acid* used in the test for alkalinity, in millilitres,

m = mass of the substance to be examined, in grams.

01/2005:1472
corrected

SODIUM HYALURONATE

Natrii hyaluronas

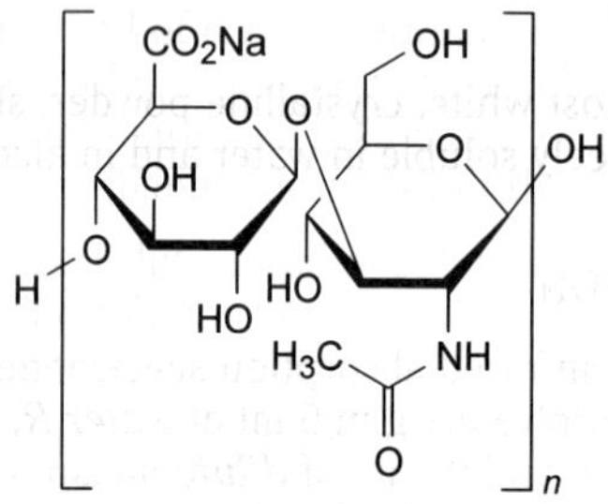

$(C_{14}H_{20}NNaO_{11})_n$

DEFINITION

Sodium hyaluronate is the sodium salt of hyaluronic acid, a glycosaminoglycan consisting of D-glucuronic acid and *N*-acetyl-D-glucosamine disaccharide units. It contains not less than 95.0 per cent and not more than the equivalent of 105.0 per cent of sodium hyaluronate, calculated with reference to the dried substance. It has an intrinsic viscosity of not less than 90 per cent and not more than 120 per cent of the value stated on the label.

PRODUCTION

Sodium hyaluronate is extracted from cocks' combs or obtained by fermentation from *Streptococci*, Lancefield Groups A and C. It is produced by methods of manufacture designed to minimise or eliminate infectious agents. When produced by fermentation of gram-positive bacteria, the process must be shown to reduce or eliminate pyrogenic or inflammatory components of the cell wall.

CHARACTERS

A white or almost white, very hygroscopic powder or a fibrous aggregate, sparingly soluble to soluble in water, practically insoluble in acetone and in ethanol.

IDENTIFICATION

A. Examine by infrared absorption spectrophotometry (*2.2.24*), comparing with the *Ph. Eur. reference spectrum of sodium hyaluronate.*

B. It gives reaction (a) of sodium (*2.3.1*).

TESTS

Solution S. Weigh a quantity of the substance to be examined equivalent to 0.10 g of the dried substance and add 30.0 ml of a 9 g/l solution of *sodium chloride R*. Mix gently on a shaker until dissolved (about 12 h).

Appearance of solution. Solution S is clear (*2.2.1*). The absorbance of solution S measured at 600 nm (*2.2.25*) is not greater than 0.01.

pH (*2.2.3*). Dissolve the substance to be examined in *carbon dioxide-free water R* to obtain a solution containing a quantity equivalent to 5 mg of the dried substance per millilitre. The pH of the solution is 5.0 to 8.5.

Intrinsic viscosity. *Sodium hyaluronate is very hygroscopic and must be protected from moisture during weighing.*

Buffer solution (0.15 M sodium chloride in 0.01 M phosphate buffer solution pH 7.0). Dissolve 0.78 g of *sodium dihydrogen phosphate R* and 4.50 g of *sodium chloride R* in *water R* and dilute to 500.0 ml with the same solvent (solution A). Dissolve 1.79 g of *disodium hydrogen phosphate R* and 4.50 g of *sodium chloride R* in *water R* and dilute to 500.0 ml with the same solvent (solution B). Mix solutions A and B until a pH of 7.0 is reached. Filter through a sintered-glass filter (4).

Test solution (a) (concentration c_1 of sodium hyaluronate). Weigh 0.200 g (m_{0p}) *(NOTE: this value is only indicative and should be adjusted after an initial measurement of the viscosity of test solution (a))* of the substance to be examined and dilute with 50.0 g (m_{0s}) of buffer solution at 4 °C. Mix the solution by shaking at 4 °C during 24 h. Weigh 5.00 g (m_{1p}) of this solution and dilute with 100.0 g (m_{1s}) of buffer solution at 25 °C. Mix this solution by shaking for 20 min. Filter the solution through a sintered-glass filter (100), and discard the first 10 ml.

Test solution (b) (concentration c_2 of sodium hyaluronate). Weigh 30.0 g (m_{2p}) of test solution (a) and dilute with 10.0 g (m_{2s}) of buffer solution at 25 °C. Mix this solution by shaking for 20 min. Filter the solution through a sintered-glass filter (100) and discard the first 10 ml.

Test solution (c) (concentration c_3 of sodium hyaluronate). Weigh 20.0 g (m_{3p} of test solution (a) and dilute with 20.0 g (m_{3s}) of buffer solution at 25 °C. Mix this solution by shaking for 20 min. Filter the solution through a sintered-glass filter (100) and discard the first 10 ml.

Test solution (d) (concentration c_4 of sodium hyaluronate). Weigh 10.0 g (m_{4p} of test solution (a) and dilute with 30.0 g (m_{4s}) of buffer solution at 25 °C. Mix this solution by shaking for 20 min. Filter the solution through a sintered-glass filter (100) and discard the first 10 ml.

Determine the flow-time for the buffer solution (t_0) and the flow times for the four test solutions (t_1, t_2, t_3 and t_4), at 25.00 ± 0.03 °C (*2.2.9*). Use an appropriate suspended level viscometer (specifications: viscometer constant about 0.005 mm²/s², kinematic viscosity range 1 to 5 mm²/s², internal diameter of tube *R* 0.53 mm, volume of bulb *C* 5.6 ml, internal diameter of tube *N* 2.8 mm to 3.2 mm) with a funnel-shaped lower capillary end. Use the same viscometer for all measurements; measure all outflow times in triplicate. The test is not valid unless the results do not differ by more than 0.35 per cent from the mean and if the flow time t_1 is not less than 1.6 and not more than 1.8 times t_0. If this is not the case, adjust the value of m_{0p} and repeat the procedure.

Calculation of the relative viscosities

Since the densities of the sodium hyaluronate solutions and of the solvent are almost equal, the relative viscosities η_{ri} (being η_{r1}, η_{r2}, η_{r3} and η_{r4}) can be calculated from the ratio of the flow times for the respective solutions t_i (being t_1, t_2, $t_3$and t_4) to the flow time of the solvent t_0, but taking into account the kinetic energy correction factor for the capillary (B = 30 800 s³), as shown below:

$$\eta_{ri} = \frac{t_i - \dfrac{B}{t_i^2}}{t_0 - \dfrac{B}{t_0^2}}$$

Calculation of the concentrations

Calculation of the concentration c_1 (expressed in kg/m³) of sodium hyaluronate in test solution (a)

$$c_1 = m_{0p} \times \frac{x}{100} \times \frac{100 - h}{100} \times \frac{1}{m_{0p} + m_{0s}} \times \frac{m_{1p}}{m_{1p} + m_{1s}} \times \rho_{25}$$

x = percentage content of sodium hyaluronate as determined under Assay,

h = loss on drying as a percentage,

ρ_{25} = 1005 kg/m³ (density of the test solution at 25 °C).

Calculation of the other concentrations

$$c_2 = c_1 \times \frac{m_{2p}}{m_{2s} + m_{2p}}$$

$$c_3 = c_1 \times \frac{m_{3p}}{m_{3s} + m_{3p}}$$

$$c_4 = c_1 \times \frac{m_{4p}}{m_{4s} + m_{4p}}$$

Calculation of the intrinsic viscosity

The intrinsic viscosity $[\eta]$ is calculated by linear least-squares regression analysis using the Martin equation:

$$\log\left(\frac{\eta_r - 1}{c}\right) = \log\,[\eta] + k\,[\eta]\,c$$

The decimal antilogarithm of the intercept is the intrinsic viscosity expressed in m³/kg.

Sulphated glycosaminoglycans. *If the product is extracted from cocks' combs, it complies with the following requirement. Appropriate safety precautions are to be taken when handling perchloric acid at elevated temperature.*

Test solution. Introduce a quantity of the substance to be examined equivalent to 50.0 mg of the dried substance into a test-tube 150 mm long and 16 mm in internal diameter and dissolve in 1.0 ml of *perchloric acid R*.

Reference solution. Dissolve 0.149 g of *anhydrous sodium sulphate R* in *water R* and dilute to 100.0 ml with the same solvent. Dilute 10.0 ml to 100.0 ml with *water R*. Evaporate 1.0 ml in a test-tube 150 mm long and 16 mm in internal diameter in a heating block at 90 °C to 95 °C, and dissolve the residue in 1.0 ml of *perchloric acid R*.

Plug each test-tube with a piece of glass wool. Place the test-tubes in a heating block or a silicone oil bath maintained at 180 °C and heat until clear, colourless solutions are obtained (about 12 h). Remove the test-tubes and cool to room temperature. Add to each test-tube 3.0 ml of a 33.3 g/l solution of *barium chloride R*, cap and shake vigorously.

Allow the test-tubes to stand for 30 min. Shake each test-tube once again, and determine the absorbance (*2.2.25*) at 660 nm, using *water R* as a blank.

The absorbance obtained with the test solution is not greater than the absorbance obtained with the reference solution (1 per cent).

Nucleic acids. The absorbance (*2.2.25*) of solution S at 260 nm is not greater than 0.5.

Protein. Not more than 0.3 per cent. If intended for use in the manufacture of parenteral dosage forms, not more than 0.1 per cent.

Test solution (a). Dissolve the substance to be examined in *water R* to obtain a solution containing a quantity equivalent to about 10 mg of the dried substance per millilitre.

Test solution (b). Mix equal volumes of test solution (a) and *water R.*

Reference solutions .Prepare a 0.5 mg/ml stock solution of *bovine albumin R* in *water R*. Prepare five dilutions of the stock solution containing between 5 μg/ml and 50 μg/ml of *bovine albumin R.*

Add 2.5 ml of freshly prepared *cupri-tartaric solution R3* to test-tubes containing 2.5 ml of *water R* (blank), 2.5 ml of the test solutions (a) or (b) or 2.5 ml of the reference solutions. Mix after each addition. After about 10 min, add to each test-tube 0.50 ml of a mixture of equal volumes of *water R* and *phosphomolybdotungstic reagent R* prepared immediately before use. Mix after each addition. After 30 min, measure the absorbance (*2.2.25*) of each solution at 750 nm against the blank. From the calibration curve obtained with the five reference solutions determine the content of protein in the test solutions.

Chlorides (*2.4.4*). Dissolve 67 mg in 100 ml of *water R*. 15 ml of the solution complies with the limit test for chlorides (0.5 per cent).

Iron. Not more than 80 ppm of Fe, determined by atomic absorption spectrometry (*2.2.23, Method II*).

Test solution. Dissolve a quantity of the substance to be examined equivalent to 0.25 g of the dried substance in 1 ml of *nitric acid R* by heating on a water-bath. Cool and dilute to 10.0 ml with *water R.*

Reference solutions. Prepare two reference solutions in the same manner as the test solution, adding 1.0 ml and 2.0 ml respectively of *iron standard solution (10 ppm Fe) R* to the dissolved substance to be examined.

Measure the absorbance at 248.3 nm, using an iron hollow-cathode lamp as source of radiation, a transmission band of 0.2 nm and an air-acetylene flame.

Loss on drying (*2.2.32*). Not more than 20.0 per cent, determined on 0.500 g by drying at 100-110 °C over *diphosphorus pentoxide R* for 6 h.

Microbial contamination. Total aerobic viable count (*2.6.12*) not more than 10^2 micro-organisms per gram. Use 1 g of the substance to be examined.

Bacterial endotoxins (*2.6.14*): if intended for use in the manufacture of parenteral dosage forms without a further appropriate procedure for the removal of bacterial endotoxins, less than 0.5 IU/mg. If intended for use in the manufacture of intra-ocular preparations or intra-articular preparations without a further appropriate procedure for the removal of bacterial endotoxins, less than 0.05 IU/mg.

ASSAY

Determine the glucuronic acid content by reaction with carbazole as described below.

Reagent A. Dissolve 0.95 g of *disodium tetraborate R* in 100.0 ml of *sulphuric acid R.*

Reagent B. Dissolve 0.125 g of *carbazole R* in 100.0 ml of *ethanol R.*

Test solution. Prepare this solution in triplicate. Dissolve 0.170 g of the substance to be examined in *water R* and dilute to 100.0 g with the same solvent. Dilute 10.0 g of this solution to 200.0 g with *water R.*

Reference stock solution. Dissolve 0.100 g of *D-glucuronic acid R*, previously dried to constant mass in vacuum over *diphosphorus pentoxide R* (*2.2.32*), in *water R* and dilute to 100.0 g with the same solvent.

Reference solutions. Prepare five dilutions of the reference stock solution containing between 6.5 μg/g and 65 μg/g of *D-glucuronic acid R.*

Place 25 test-tubes, numbered 1 to 25, in iced water. Add 1.0 ml of the five reference solutions in triplicate to the test-tubes 1 to 15 (reference tubes), 1.0 ml of the three test solutions in triplicate to the test-tubes 16 to 24 (sample tubes), and 1.0 ml of *water R* to test-tube 25 (blank). Add 5.0 ml of freshly prepared reagent A to each test-tube. Tightly close the test-tubes with plastic caps, shake the contents, and place on a water bath for exactly 15 min. Cool in iced water, and add to each test tube 0.20 ml of reagent B. Recap the tubes, shake, and put them again on a water-bath for exactly 15 min. Cool to room temperature and measure the absorbance (*2.2.25*) of the solutions at 530 nm, against the blank.

From the calibration curve obtained with the mean absorbances read for each reference solution, determine the mean concentrations of D-glucuronic acid in the test solutions.

Calculate the percentage content of sodium hyaluronate from the expression:

$$\frac{c_g}{c_s} \times Z \times \frac{100}{100 - h} \times \frac{401.3}{194.1}$$

c_g = mean of concentrations of D-glucuronic acid in the test solutions, in milligrams per gram,

c_s = mean of concentrations of the substance to be examined in the test solutions, in milligrams per gram,

Z = determined percentage content of $C_6H_{10}O_7$ in *D-glucuronic acid R,*

h = loss on drying as a percentage,

401.3 = relative molecular mass of the disaccharide fragment,

194.1 = relative molecular mass of glucuronic acid.

STORAGE

Store in an airtight container, protected from light and humidity. If the substance is sterile, store in a sterile, airtight, tamper-proof container.

LABELLING

The label states:

- the intrinsic viscosity,
- the origin of the substance,
- the intended use of the substance,
- where applicable, that the substance is suitable for parenteral administration other than intra-articular administration,

– where applicable, that the substance is suitable for parenteral administration, including intra-articular administration,
– where applicable that the material is suitable for intra-ocular use.

01/2005:0195

SODIUM HYDROGEN CARBONATE

Natrii hydrogenocarbonas

$NaHCO_3$ M_r 84.0

DEFINITION

Sodium hydrogen carbonate contains not less than 99.0 per cent and not more than the equivalent of 101.0 per cent of $NaHCO_3$.

CHARACTERS

A white, crystalline powder, soluble in water, practically insoluble in alcohol. When heated in the dry state or in solution, it gradually changes into sodium carbonate.

IDENTIFICATION

A. To 5 ml of solution S (see Tests) add 0.1 ml of *phenolphthalein solution R*. A pale pink colour is produced. Heat; gas is evolved and the solution becomes red.

B. It gives the reaction of carbonates and bicarbonates (*2.3.1*).

C. Solution S gives reaction (a) of sodium (*2.3.1*).

TESTS

Solution S. Dissolve 5.0 g in 90 ml of *carbon dioxide-free water R* and dilute to 100.0 ml with the same solvent.

Appearance of solution. Solution S is clear (*2.2.1*) and colourless (*2.2.2, Method II*).

Carbonates. The pH (*2.2.3*) of freshly prepared solution S is not more than 8.6.

Chlorides (*2.4.4*). To 7 ml of solution S add 2 ml of *nitric acid R* and dilute to 15 ml with *water R*. The solution complies with the limit test for chlorides (150 ppm).

Sulphates (*2.4.13*). To a suspension of 1.0 g in 10 ml of *distilled water R* add *hydrochloric acid R* until neutral and about 1 ml in excess. Dilute to 15 ml with *distilled water R*. The solution complies with the limit test for sulphates (150 ppm).

Ammonium (*2.4.1*). 10 ml of solution S diluted to 15 ml with *water R* complies with the limit test for ammonium (20 ppm). Prepare the standard using a mixture of 5 ml of *water R* and 10 ml of *ammonium standard solution (1 ppm NH_4) R*.

Arsenic (*2.4.2*). 0.5 g complies with limit test A for arsenic (2 ppm).

Calcium (*2.4.3*). To a suspension of 1.0 g in 10 ml of *distilled water R* add *hydrochloric acid R* until neutral and dilute to 15 ml with *distilled water R*. The solution complies with the limit test for calcium (100 ppm).

Iron (*2.4.9*). Dissolve 0.5 g in 5 ml of *dilute hydrochloric acid R* and dilute to 10 ml with *water R*. The solution complies with the limit test for iron (20 ppm).

Heavy metals (*2.4.8*). Dissolve 2.0 g in a mixture of 2 ml of *hydrochloric acid R* and 18 ml of *water R*. 12 ml of the solution complies with limit test A for heavy metals (10 ppm). Prepare the standard using *lead standard solution (1 ppm Pb) R*.

ASSAY

Dissolve 1.500 g in 50 ml of *carbon dioxide-free water R*. Titrate with *1 M hydrochloric acid*, using 0.2 ml of *methyl orange solution R* as indicator.

1 ml of *1 M hydrochloric acid* is equivalent to 84.0 mg of $NaHCO_3$.

01/2005:0677

SODIUM HYDROXIDE

Natrii hydroxidum

NaOH M_r 40.00

DEFINITION

Sodium hydroxide contains not less than 97.0 per cent and not more than the equivalent of 100.5 per cent of total alkali, calculated as NaOH.

CHARACTERS

White, crystalline masses, supplied as pellets, sticks or slabs, deliquescent, readily absorbing carbon dioxide, very soluble in water, freely soluble in alcohol.

IDENTIFICATION

A. Dissolve 0.1 g in 10 ml of *water R*. Dilute 1 ml of the solution to 100 ml with *water R*. The pH (*2.2.3*) of the final solution is not less than 11.0.

B. 2 ml of solution S (see Tests) gives reaction (a) of sodium (*2.3.1*).

TESTS

Solution S. *Carry out the procedure described below with caution.* Dissolve 5.0 g in 12 ml of *distilled water R*. Add 17 ml of *hydrochloric acid R1*, adjust to pH 7 with *1 M hydrochloric acid* and dilute to 50 ml with *distilled water R*.

Appearance of solution. Dissolve 1.0 g in 10 ml of *water R*. The solution is clear (*2.2.1*) and colourless (*2.2.2, Method II*).

Carbonates. Not more than 2.0 per cent, calculated as Na_2CO_3, as determined in the assay.

Chlorides (*2.4.4*). Dissolve 1.0 g in 5 ml of *water R*, acidify the solution with about 4 ml of *nitric acid R* and dilute to 15 ml with *water R*. The solution, without addition of *dilute nitric acid R*, complies with the limit test for chlorides (50 ppm).

Sulphates (*2.4.13*). Dissolve 3.0 g in 6 ml of *distilled water R*, adjust to pH 7 with *hydrochloric acid R* (about 7.5 ml) and dilute to 15 ml with *distilled water R*. The solution complies with the limit test for sulphates (50 ppm).

Iron (*2.4.9*). 10 ml of solution S complies with the limit test for iron (10 ppm).

Heavy metals (*2.4.8*). 12 ml of solution S complies with limit test A for heavy metals (20 ppm). Prepare the standard using *lead standard solution (2 ppm Pb) R*.

ASSAY

Dissolve 2.000 g in about 80 ml of *carbon dioxide-free water R*. Add 0.3 ml of *phenolphthalein solution R* and titrate with *1 M hydrochloric acid*. Add 0.3 ml of *methyl orange solution R* and continue the titration with *1 M hydrochloric acid*.

1 ml of *1 M hydrochloric acid* used in the second part of the titration is equivalent to 0.1060 g of Na_2CO_3.

1 ml of *1 M hydrochloric acid* used in the combined titrations is equivalent to 40.00 mg of total alkali, calculated as NaOH.

STORAGE

Store in an airtight, non-metallic container.

01/2005:0196

SODIUM IODIDE

Natrii iodidum

NaI M_r 149.9

DEFINITION

Sodium iodide contains not less than 99.0 per cent and not more than the equivalent of 100.5 per cent of NaI, calculated with reference to the dried substance.

CHARACTERS

A white, crystalline powder or colourless crystals, hygroscopic, very soluble in water, freely soluble in alcohol.

IDENTIFICATION

A. Solution S (see Tests) gives the reactions of iodides (*2.3.1*).

B. Solution S gives the reactions of sodium (*2.3.1*).

TESTS

Solution S. Dissolve 10.0 g in *carbon dioxide-free water R* prepared from *distilled water R* and dilute to 100 ml with the same solvent.

Appearance of solution. Solution S is clear (*2.2.1*) and colourless (*2.2.2, Method II*).

Alkalinity. To 12.5 ml of solution S add 0.1 ml of *bromothymol blue solution R1*. Not more than 0.7 ml of *0.01 M hydrochloric acid* is required to change the colour of the indicator.

Iodates. To 10 ml of solution S add 0.25 ml of *iodide-free starch solution R* and 0.2 ml of *dilute sulphuric acid R* and allow to stand protected from light for 2 min. No blue colour develops.

Sulphates (*2.4.13*). 10 ml of solution S diluted to 15 ml with *distilled water R* complies with the limit test for sulphates (150 ppm).

Thiosulphates. To 10 ml of solution S add 0.1 ml of *starch solution R* and 0.1 ml of *0.005 M iodine*. A blue colour is produced.

Heavy metals (*2.4.8*). 12 ml of solution S complies with limit test A for heavy metals (10 ppm). Prepare the standard using *lead standard solution (1 ppm Pb) R*.

Iron (*2.4.9*). 5 ml of solution S diluted to 10 ml with *water R* complies with the limit test for iron (20 ppm).

Loss on drying (*2.2.32*). Not more than 3.0 per cent, determined on 1.00 g by drying in an oven at 100 °C to 105 °C for 3 h.

ASSAY

Dissolve 1.300 g in *water R* and dilute to 100.0 ml with the same solvent. To 20.0 ml of the solution add 40 ml of *hydrochloric acid R* and titrate with *0.05 M potassium iodate* until the colour changes from red to yellow. Add 5 ml of *chloroform R* and continue the titration, shaking vigorously, until the chloroform layer is decolorised.

1 ml of *0.05 M potassium iodate* is equivalent to 14.99 mg of NaI.

STORAGE

Store protected from light.

01/2005:1151

SODIUM LACTATE SOLUTION

Natrii lactatis solutio

DEFINITION

Solution of a mixture of the enantiomers of sodium 2-hydroxyproponate in approximately equal proportions.

Content: minimum 50.0 per cent *m/m* of sodium 2-hydroxypropanoate ($C_3H_5NaO_3$; M_r 112.1); 96.0 per cent to 104.0 per cent of the content of sodium lactate stated on the label.

CHARACTERS

Appearance: clear, colourless, slightly syrupy liquid.

Solubility: miscible with water and with alcohol.

IDENTIFICATION

A. To 0.1 ml add 10 ml of *water R*. 5 ml of the solution gives the reaction of lactates (*2.3.1*).

B. It gives reaction (a) of sodium (*2.3.1*).

TESTS

Solution S. Dilute a quantity of the substance to be examined corresponding to 40.0 g of sodium lactate to 200 ml with *distilled water R*.

Appearance of solution. The substance to be examined is clear (*2.2.1*) and not more intensely coloured than reference solution BY_7 (*2.2.2, Method II*).

pH (*2.2.3*): 6.5 to 9.0 for the substance to be examined.

Reducing sugars and sucrose. To 5 ml of the substance to be examined add 2 ml of *dilute sodium hydroxide solution R* and 0.2 ml of *copper sulphate solution R*. The solution is clear and blue and remains so on boiling. Add to the hot solution 4 ml of *hydrochloric acid R*. Boil for 1 min. Add 6 ml of *strong sodium hydroxide solution R* and heat to boiling again. The solution is clear and blue.

Methanol. Gas chromatography (*2.4.24*).

Limit:

– *methanol*: maximum 50 ppm, calculated with reference to sodium lactate, if intended for use in the manufacture of parenteral dosage forms, dialysis, haemodialysis or haemofiltration solutions.

Chlorides (*2.4.4*): maximum 50 ppm calculated with reference to sodium lactate.

Dilute 5 ml of solution S to 15 ml with *water R*. The solution complies with the limit test for chlorides.

Oxalates and phosphates. To 1 ml of the substance to be examined add 15 ml of *alcohol R* and 2 ml of *calcium chloride solution R*. Heat at 75 °C for 5 min. Any opalescence in the solution is not more intense than that of a standard prepared at the same time and in the same manner using a mixture of 1 ml of the substance to be examined, 15 ml of *alcohol R* and 2 ml of *water R*.

Sulphates (*2.4.13*): maximum 100 ppm calculated with reference to sodium lactate.

To 7.5 ml of solution S, add 1.9 ml of *hydrochloric acid R1* and dilute to 15 ml with *distilled water R*. The solution complies with the limit test for sulphates without addition of 0.5 ml of *acetic acid R*. Acidify the standard solution with 0.05 ml of *hydrochloric acid R1* instead of 0.5 ml of *acetic acid R*.

Aluminium: maximum 0.1 ppm, if intended for use in the manufacture of parenteral dosage forms, dialysis, haemodialysis or haemofiltration solutions.

Atomic absorption spectrometry (*2.2.23, Method I*). For the preparation of the solutions, use equipment that is aluminium-free or that will not release aluminium under the conditions of use (glass, polyethylene, etc).

Modifier solution. Dissolve 100.0 g of *ammonium nitrate R* in a mixture of 50 ml of *water R* and 4 ml of *nitric acid R* and dilute to 200 ml with *water R*.

Blank solution. Dilute to 2.0 ml of the modifier solution to 25.0 ml with *water R*.

Test solution. To 1.25 g add 2.0 ml of the modifier solution and dilute to 25.0 ml with *water R*.

Reference solutions. Prepare the reference solutions immediately before use (0.010 ppm to 0.050 ppm of aluminium) using *aluminium standard solution (200 ppm Al) R*.

Source: aluminium hollow-cathode lamp.

Wavelength: 309.3 nm.

Atomisation device: a graphite furnace.

Carrier gas: *argon R*.

Conditions: the device is equipped with a non-specific absorption correction system. Heat the oven to 120 °C for as many seconds as there are microlitres of solution introduced into the apparatus, then heat at 1000 °C for 30 s and finally at 2700 °C for 6 s.

Barium. To 10 ml of solution S add 10 ml of *calcium sulphate solution R*. Allow to stand for 30 min. Any opalescence (*2.2.1*) in the solution is not more intense than that of a standard prepared at the same time and in the same manner using a mixture of 10 ml of solution S and 10 ml of *distilled water R*.

Iron (*2.4.9*): maximum 10 ppm calculated with reference to sodium lactate.

Dilute 5 ml of solution S to 10 ml with *water R*. The solution complies with the limit test for iron.

Heavy metals (*2.4.8*): maximum 10 ppm calculated with reference to sodium lactate.

12 ml of solution S complies with limit test A. Prepare the standard using *lead standard solution (2 ppm Pb) R*.

Bacterial endotoxins (*2.6.14*): less than 5 IU/g, if intended for use in the manufacture of parenteral dosage forms without a further appropriate procedure for the removal of bacterial endotoxins.

ASSAY

Dissolve a quantity of the substance to be examined corresponding to 75.0 mg of sodium lactate in a mixture of 10 ml of *glacial acetic acid R* and 20 ml of *acetic anhydride R*. Allow to stand for 15 min. Add 1 ml of *naphtholbenzein solution R* and titrate with *0.1 M perchloric acid*.

1 ml of *0.1 M perchloric acid* is equivalent to 11.21 mg of $C_3H_5NaO_3$.

LABELLING

The label states:

- where applicable, that the substance is suitable for use in the manufacture of dialysis, haemodialysis and haemofiltration solutions,
- where applicable, that the substance is suitable for use in the manufacture of parenteral dosage forms,
- the declared content of sodium lactate.

01/2005:2033

SODIUM (*S*)-LACTATE SOLUTION

Natrii (*S*)-lactatis solutio

DEFINITION

Content: minimum 50.0 per cent *m/m* of sodium (*S*)-2-hydroxypropanoate ($C_3H_5NaO_3$; M_r 112.1); 96.0 per cent to 104.0 per cent of the content of sodium lactate stated on the label, not less than 95.0 per cent of which is the (*S*)-enantiomer.

CHARACTERS

Appearance: clear, colourless, slightly syrupy liquid.

Solubility: miscible with water and with alcohol.

IDENTIFICATION

A. To 0.1 ml add 10 ml of *water R*. 5 ml of the solution gives the reaction of lactates (*2.3.1*).

B. It gives reaction (a) of sodium (*2.3.1*).

C. It complies with the limits of the assay.

TESTS

Solution S. Dilute a quantity of the substance to be examined corresponding to 40.0 g of sodium lactate to 200 ml with *distilled water R*.

Appearance of solution. The substance to be examined is clear (*2.2.1*) and not more intensely coloured than reference solution BY_7 (*2.2.2, Method II*).

pH (*2.2.3*): 6.5 to 9.0 for the substance to be examined.

Reducing sugars and sucrose. To 5 ml of the substance to be examined add 2 ml of *dilute sodium hydroxide solution R* and 0.2 ml of *copper sulphate solution R*. The solution is clear and blue and remains so on boiling. Add to the hot solution 4 ml of *hydrochloric acid R*. Boil for 1 min. Add 6 ml of *strong sodium hydroxide solution R* and heat to boiling again. The solution is clear and blue.

Methanol. Gas chromatography (*2.4.24*).

Limit:

- *methanol*: maximum 50 ppm, calculated with reference to sodium lactate, if intended for use in the manufacture of parenteral dosage forms, dialysis, haemodialysis or haemofiltration solutions.

Chlorides (*2.4.4*): maximum 50 ppm calculated with reference to sodium lactate.

Dilute 5 ml of solution S to 15 ml with *water R*. The solution complies with the limit test for chlorides.

Oxalates and phosphates. To 1 ml of the substance to be examined add 15 ml of *alcohol R* and 2 ml of *calcium chloride solution R*. Heat at 75 °C for 5 min. Any opalescence in the solution is not more intense than that of a standard prepared at the same time and in the same manner using a mixture of 1 ml of the substance to be examined, 15 ml of *alcohol R* and 2 ml of *water R*.

Sulphates (*2.4.13*): maximum 100 ppm calculated with reference to sodium lactate.

To 7.5 ml of solution S, add 1.9 ml of *hydrochloric acid R1* and dilute to 15 ml with *distilled water R*. The solution complies with the limit test for sulphates without addition of 0.5 ml of *acetic acid R*. Acidify the standard solution with 0.05 ml of *hydrochloric acid R1* instead of 0.5 ml of *acetic acid R*.

Monographs Q-S

Aluminium: maximum 0.1 ppm, if intended for use in the manufacture of parenteral dosage forms, dialysis, haemodialysis or haemofiltration solutions.

Atomic absorption spectrometry (*2.2.23, Method I*). For the preparation of the solutions, use equipment that is aluminium-free or that will not release aluminium under the conditions of use (glass, polyethylene, etc).

Modifier solution. Dissolve 100.0 g of *ammonium nitrate R* in a mixture of 50 ml of *water R* and 4 ml of *nitric acid R* and dilute to 200 ml with *water R.*

Blank solution. Dilute 2.0 ml of the modifier solution to 25.0 ml with *water R.*

Test solution. To 1.25 g add 2.0 ml of the modifier solution and dilute to 25.0 ml with *water R.*

Reference solutions. Prepare the reference solutions immediately before use (0.010 ppm to 0.050 ppm of aluminium) using *aluminium standard solution (200 ppm Al) R.*

Source: aluminium hollow-cathode lamp.

Wavelength: 309.3 nm.

Atomisation device: a graphite furnace.

Carrier gas: *argon R.*

Conditions: the device is equipped with a non-specific absorption correction system. Heat the oven to 120 °C for as many seconds as there are microlitres of solution introduced into the apparatus, then heat at 1000 °C for 30 s and finally at 2700 °C for 6 s.

Barium. To 10 ml of solution S add 10 ml of *calcium sulphate solution R.* Allow to stand for 30 min. Any opalescence (*2.2.1*) in the solution is not more intense than that of a standard prepared at the same time and in the same manner using a mixture of 10 ml of solution S and 10 ml of *distilled water R.*

Iron (*2.4.9*): maximum 10 ppm calculated with reference to sodium lactate.

Dilute 5 ml of solution S to 10 ml with *water R.* The solution complies with the limit test for iron.

Heavy metals (*2.4.8*): maximum 10 ppm calculated with reference to sodium lactate.

12 ml of solution S complies with limit test A. Prepare the standard using *lead standard solution (2 ppm Pb) R.*

Bacterial endotoxins (*2.6.14*): less than 5 IU/g if intended for use in the manufacture of parenteral dosage forms without a further appropriate procedure for the removal of bacterial endotoxins.

ASSAY

Dissolve a quantity of the substance to be examined corresponding to 75.0 mg of sodium lactate in a mixture of 10 ml of *glacial acetic acid R* and 20 ml of *acetic anhydride R.* Allow to stand for 15 min. Add 1 ml of *naphtholbenzein solution R* and titrate with *0.1 M perchloric acid.*

1 ml of *0.1 M perchloric acid* is equivalent to 11.21 mg of $C_3H_5NaO_3$.

(*S*)-enantiomer. Transfer a quantity of the substance to be examined corresponding to 2.50 g of sodium lactate into a 50 ml volumetric flask, dilute with about 30 ml of *water R* and add 5.0 g of *ammonium molybdate R.* Dissolve and dilute with *water R* to 50.0 ml. Measure the angle of optical rotation (*2.2.7*). Calculate the percentage content of (*S*)-enantiomer using the expression:

$$50 + \left(24.04 \times \alpha \times \frac{5.0}{m} \times \frac{50}{c}\right)$$

α = angle of optical rotation (absolute value),

m = mass of the substance to be examined, in grams,

c = percentage content of $C_3H_5NaO_3$ in the substance to be examined.

The complex of sodium (*S*)-lactate formed under these test conditions is leavorotatory.

LABELLING

The label states:

- where applicable, that the substance is suitable for use in the manufacture of dialysis, haemodialysis and haemofiltration solutions,
- where applicable, that the substance is suitable for use in the manufacture of parenteral dosage forms,
- the declared content of sodium lactate.

01/2005:0098

SODIUM LAURILSULFATE

Natrii laurilsulfas

DEFINITION

Sodium laurilsulfate is a mixture of sodium alkyl sulphates consisting chiefly of sodium dodecyl sulphate, $C_{12}H_{25}NaO_4S$ (*M*r 288.4). It contains not less than 85.0 per cent of sodium alkyl sulphates, calculated as $C_{12}H_{25}NaO_4S$.

CHARACTERS

A white or pale yellow powder or crystals, freely soluble in water giving an opalescent solution, partly soluble in alcohol.

IDENTIFICATION

A. Dissolve 0.1 g in 10 ml of *water R* and shake. A copious foam is formed.

B. To 0.1 ml of the solution prepared for identification test A, add 0.1 ml of a 1 g/l solution of *methylene blue R* and 2 ml of *dilute sulphuric acid R.* Add 2 ml of *methylene chloride R* and shake. An intense blue colour develops in the methylene chloride layer.

C. Mix about 10 mg with 10 ml of *ethanol R.* Heat to boiling on a water-bath, shaking frequently. Filter immediately and evaporate the ethanol. Dissolve the residue in 8 ml of *water R*, add 3 ml of *dilute hydrochloric acid R*, evaporate the solution to half its volume and allow to cool. Separate the congealed fatty alcohols by filtration. To the filtrate add 1 ml of *barium chloride solution R1.* A white, crystalline precipitate is formed.

D. Ignite 0.5 g. The residue gives reaction (a) of sodium (*2.3.1*).

TESTS

Alkalinity. Dissolve 1.0 g in 100 ml of *carbon dioxide-free water R* and add 0.1 ml of *phenol red solution R.* Not more than 0.5 ml of *0.1 M hydrochloric acid* is required to change the colour of the indicator.

Non-esterified alcohols. Dissolve 10 g in 100 ml of *water R*, add 100 ml of *alcohol R* and shake the solution with 3 quantities, each of 50 ml, of *pentane R*, adding *sodium chloride R*, if necessary, to promote separation of the 2 layers. Wash the combined organic layers with 3 quantities, each of 50 ml, of *water R*, dry over *anhydrous sodium sulphate R*, filter and evaporate on a water-bath until the solvent has evaporated. Heat the residue at 105 °C for 15 min and cool. The residue weighs not more than 0.4 g (4 per cent).

Sodium chloride and sodium sulphate. Not more than a total of 8.0 per cent of NaCl and Na_2SO_4.

Sodium chloride. Dissolve 5.00 g in 50 ml of *water R*, add *dilute nitric acid R* dropwise until the solution is neutral to *blue litmus paper R*, add 2 ml of *potassium chromate solution R* and titrate with *0.1 M silver nitrate.*

1 ml of *0.1 M silver nitrate* is equivalent to 5.844 mg of NaCl.

Sodium sulphate. Dissolve 0.500 g in 20 ml of *water R*, warming gently if necessary, and add 1 ml of a 0.5 g/l solution of *dithizone R1* in *acetone R*. If the solution is red, add *1 M nitric acid,* dropwise, until the solution becomes bluish-green. Add 2.0 ml of *dichloroacetic acid solution R* and 80 ml of *acetone R*. Titrate with *0.01 M lead nitrate* until a persistent violet-red or orange-red colour is obtained. Carry out a blank titration.

1 ml of *0.01 M lead nitrate* is equivalent to 1.420 mg of Na_2SO_4.

ASSAY

Dissolve 1.15 g in *water R*, warming if necessary, and dilute to 1000.0 ml with the same solvent. To 20.0 ml of the solution add 15 ml of *chloroform R* and 10 ml of *dimidium bromide-sulphan blue mixed solution R.* Titrate with *0.004 M benzethonium chloride,* shaking vigorously and allowing the layers to separate before each addition, until the pink colour of the chloroform layer is completely discharged and a greyish-blue colour is obtained.

1 ml of *0.004 M benzethonium chloride* is equivalent to 1.154 mg of sodium alkyl sulphates, calculated as $C_{12}H_{25}NaO_4S$.

01/2005:0849

SODIUM METABISULPHITE

Natrii metabisulfis

$Na_2S_2O_5$ M_r 190.1

DEFINITION

Sodium metabisulphite (sodium disulphite) contains not less than 95.0 per cent and not more than the equivalent of 100.5 per cent of $Na_2S_2O_5$.

CHARACTERS

A white or almost white, crystalline powder or colourless crystals, freely soluble in water, slightly soluble in alcohol.

IDENTIFICATION

A. Solution S (see Tests) complies with the test for pH (see Tests).

B. To 0.4 ml of *iodinated potassium iodide solution R* add 8 ml of *distilled water R* and 1 ml of a 1 to 10 dilution of solution S in *distilled water R*. The solution is colourless and gives reaction (a) of sulphates (*2.3.1*).

C. Solution S gives reaction (a) of sodium (*2.3.1*).

TESTS

Solution S. Dissolve 5.0 g in *carbon dioxide-free water R* prepared from *distilled water R* and dilute to 100 ml with the same solvent.

Appearance of solution. Solution S is clear (*2.2.1*) and colourless (*2.2.2, Method II*).

pH (*2.2.3*). The pH of solution S is 3.5 to 5.0.

Thiosulphates. To 5 ml of solution S add 5 ml of *dilute hydrochloric acid R*. The solution remains clear (*2.2.1*) for not less than 15 min.

Arsenic (*2.4.2*). Mix 0.20 g with 2 ml of *water R* in a dish. Add, drop by drop, 1.5 ml of *nitric acid R*. Evaporate the mixture to dryness on a water-bath. Heat over a flame until no more vapour is evolved. Take up the residue in 25 ml of *water R*. The solution complies with limit test A for arsenic (5 ppm).

Iron (*2.4.9*). 10 ml of solution S complies with the limit test for iron (20 ppm).

Heavy metals (*2.4.8*). To 40 ml of solution S in a silica crucible, add 10 ml of *hydrochloric acid R* and evaporate to dryness. Dissolve the residue in 19 ml of *water R* and add 1 ml of a 40 g/l solution of *sodium fluoride R*. 12 ml of the solution complies with limit test A for heavy metals (20 ppm). Prepare the standard using *lead standard solution (2 ppm Pb) R*.

ASSAY

Dissolve 0.200 g in 50.0 ml of *0.05 M iodine*. Add 5 ml of *dilute hydrochloric acid R*. Titrate with *0.1 M sodium thiosulphate* using 1 ml of *starch solution R*, added towards the end of the titration, as indicator.

1 ml of *0.05 M iodine* is equivalent to 4.753 mg of $Na_2S_2O_5$.

STORAGE

Store protected from light.

01/2005:1262

SODIUM METHYL PARAHYDROXYBENZOATE

Methylis parahydroxybenzoas natricum

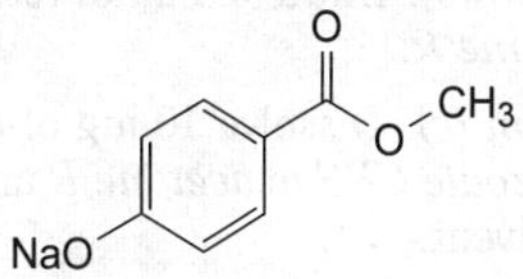

$C_8H_7NaO_3$ M_r 174.1

DEFINITION

Sodium methyl parahydroxybenzoate contains not less than 99.0 per cent and not more than the equivalent of 102.0 per cent of sodium 4-(methoxycarbonyl)phenolate, calculated with reference to the anhydrous substance.

CHARACTERS

A white, crystalline powder, freely soluble in water, sparingly soluble in alcohol, practically insoluble in methylene chloride.

IDENTIFICATION

First identification: A, B, E.

Second identification: A, C, D, E.

A. Dissolve 0.5 g in 50 ml of *water R*. Immediately add 5 ml of *hydrochloric acid R1*. Filter and wash the precipitate with *water R*. Dry under vacuum at 80 °C for 2 h. The precipitate obtained melts (*2.2.14*) at 125 °C to 128 °C.

B. Examine the precipitate obtained in identification test A by infrared absorption spectrophotometry (*2.2.24*), comparing with the spectrum obtained with *methyl parahydroxybenzoate CRS*.

C. Examine the chromatograms obtained in the test for related substances. The principal spot in the chromatogram obtained with test solution (b) is similar in position and size to the principal spot in the chromatogram obtained with reference solution (c).

D. To about 10 mg in a test-tube add 1 ml of *sodium carbonate solution R*, boil for 30 s and cool. Add 5 ml of *aminopyrazolone solution R* and 1 ml of *potassium ferricyanide solution R* and mix. An orange to red colour develops.

E. To 1 ml of solution S (see Tests) add 1 ml of *water R*. The solution gives reaction (a) of sodium (*2.3.1*).

TESTS

Solution S. Dissolve 5.0 g in *carbon dioxide-free water R* prepared from *distilled water R* and dilute to 50 ml with the same solvent.

Appearance of solution. Solution S examined immediately after preparation is clear (*2.2.1*) and not more intensely coloured than reference solution BY_6 (*2.2.2, Method I*).

pH (*2.2.3*). Dilute 1 ml of solution S to 100 ml with *carbon dioxide-free water R*. The pH of the solution is 9.5 to 10.5.

Related substances. Examine by thin-layer chromatography (*2.2.27*), using as the coating substance a suitable octadecylsilyl silica gel with a fluorescent indicator having an optimal intensity at 254 nm.

Test solution (a). Dissolve 0.100 g in 10 ml of *water R*. Immediately add 2 ml of *hydrochloric acid R* and shake with 50 ml of *ether R*. Evaporate the upper layer to dryness and dissolve the residue to 10 ml with *acetone R*.

Test solution (b). Dilute 1 ml of test solution (a) to 10 ml with *acetone R*.

Reference solution (a). Dissolve 34.3 mg of *4-hydroxybenzoic acid R* in *acetone R* and dilute to 100 ml with the same solvent.

Reference solution (b). Dilute 0.5 ml of test solution (a) to 100 ml with *acetone R*.

Reference solution (c). Dissolve 10 mg of *methyl parahydroxybenzoate CRS* in *acetone R* and dilute to 10 ml with the same solvent.

Reference solution (d). Dissolve 10 mg of *ethyl parahydroxybenzoate CRS* in 1 ml of test solution (a) and dilute to 10 ml with *acetone R*.

Apply separately to the plate 5 µl of each solution. Develop over a path of 15 cm using a mixture of 1 volume of *glacial acetic acid R*, 30 volumes of *water R* and 70 volumes of *methanol R*. Allow the plate to dry in air and examine in ultraviolet light at 254 nm. In the chromatogram obtained with test solution (a): any spot due to 4-hydroxybenzoic acid is not more intense than the spot in the chromatogram obtained with reference solution (a) (4 per cent) and any spot, apart from the principal spot and the spot due to 4-hydroxybenzoic acid, is not more intense than the spot in the chromatogram obtained with reference solution (b) (0.5 per cent). The test is not valid unless the chromatogram obtained with reference solution (d) shows two clearly separated principal spots.

Chlorides (*2.4.4*). To 10 ml of solution S, add 30 ml of *water R* and 1 ml of *nitric acid R* and dilute to 50 ml with *water R*. Shake and filter. Dilute 10 ml of the filtrate to 15 ml with *water R*. The solution complies with the limit test for chlorides (350 ppm). Prepare the standard using 14 ml of *chloride standard solution (5 ppm Cl) R* to which 1 ml of *water R* has been added.

Sulphates (*2.4.13*). To 25 ml of solution S, add 5 ml of *distilled water R* and 10 ml of *hydrochloric acid R* and dilute to 50 ml with *distilled water R*. Shake and filter. Dilute 10 ml of the filtrate to 15 ml with *distilled water R*. The solution complies with the limit test for sulphates (300 ppm).

Heavy metals (*2.4.8*). 2.0 g complies with limit test C for heavy metals (10 ppm). Prepare the standard using 2 ml of *lead standard solution (10 ppm Pb) R*.

Water (*2.5.12*). Not more than 5.0 per cent, determined on 0.500 g by the semi-micro determination of water.

ASSAY

Dissolve 0.150 g in 50 ml of *anhydrous acetic acid R*. Titrate with *0.1 M perchloric acid*, determining the end-point potentiometrically (*2.2.20*).

1 ml of *0.1 M perchloric acid* is equivalent to 17.41 mg of $C_8H_7NaO_3$.

IMPURITIES

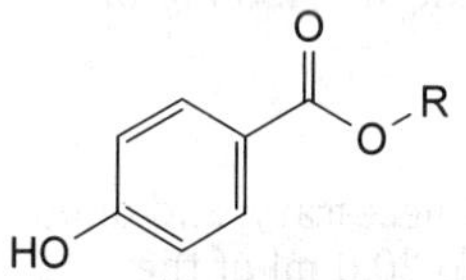

A. R = H: 4-hydroxybenzoic acid,

B. R = CH_2-CH_3: ethyl 4-hydroxybenzoate,

C. R = CH_2-CH_2-CH_3: propyl 4-hydroxybenzoate,

D. R = CH_2-CH_2-CH_2-CH_3: butyl 4-hydroxybenzoate.

01/2005:1565

SODIUM MOLYBDATE DIHYDRATE

Natrii molybdas dihydricus

$Na_2MoO_4,2H_2O$ M_r 241.9

DEFINITION

Sodium molybdate dihydrate contains not less than 98.0 per cent and not more than the equivalent of 100.5 per cent of Na_2MoO_4, calculated with reference to the dried substance.

CHARACTERS

A white powder or colourless crystals, freely soluble in water.

IDENTIFICATION

A. It complies with the test for loss on drying (see Tests).

B. Dissolve 0.2 g in 5 ml of a mixture of equal volumes of *nitric acid R* and *water R* and add 0.1 g of *ammonium chloride R*. Add 0.3 ml of *disodium hydrogen phosphate solution R* and heat slowly at 50 °C to 60 °C. A yellow precipitate is formed.

C. Dissolve 0.15 g in 2 ml of *water R*, the solution gives reaction (a) of sodium (*2.3.1*).

TESTS

Solution S. Dissolve 10.0 g in *water R* and dilute to 50 ml with the same solvent.

Appearance of solution. Solution S is clear (*2.2.1*) and colourless (*2.2.2, Method II*).

Chlorides. To 10 ml of a mixture of equal volumes of *nitric acid R* and *water R* add 10 ml of solution S with shaking. Add 1 ml of *0.1 M silver nitrate*. Any opalescence in the solution is not more intense after 5 min than that of a standard solution prepared at the same time in the same manner with 2 ml of *chloride standard solution (50 ppm Cl) R* (50 ppm).

Phosphates. Dissolve 2.0 g by heating in 13 ml of *water R*. In the still hot solution, dissolve 8.0 g of *ammonium nitrate R1*. Add this solution to 27 ml of a mixture of equal volumes of *nitric acid R* and *water R*. Any yellow colour or opalescence in the solution is not more intense within 3 h than that in a standard solution prepared at the same time as follows: dissolve 1.0 g in 12 ml of *water R* and add 1 ml of *phosphate standard solution (200 ppm PO_4) R* (200 ppm).

Ammonium (*2.4.1*). 0.10 g complies with limit test B for ammonium (10 ppm). Prepare the standard using 1 ml of *ammonium standard solution (1 ppm NH_4) R*.

Heavy metals. To 10 ml of solution S, add 2 ml of *water R*, 6 ml of a 168 g/l solution of *sodium hydroxide R* and 2 ml of *concentrated ammonia R* (solution A). To 0.5 ml of *thioacetamide reagent R* add a mixture of 15 ml of solution A and 5 ml of *water R*. Any coloration of the solution is not more intense after 2 min than that of a standard solution prepared at the same time as follows: to 0.5 ml of *thioacetamide reagent R* add a mixture of 5 ml of solution A, 1 ml of *lead standard solution (10 ppm Pb) R* and 14 ml of *water R* (10 ppm).

Loss on drying (*2.2.32*): 14.0 per cent to 16.0 per cent, determined on 1.000 g by drying in an oven at 140 °C for 3 h.

ASSAY

Dissolve 0.100 g in 30 ml of *water R*, add 0.5 g of *hexamethylenetetramine R* and 0.1 ml of a 250 g/l solution of *nitric acid R*. Heat to 60 °C. Titrate with *0.05 M lead nitrate* using *4-(2-pyridylazo)resorcinol monosodium salt R* as indicator.

1 ml of *0.05 M lead nitrate* is equivalent to 10.30 mg of Na_2MoO_4.

01/2005:1996

SODIUM NITRITE

Natrii nitris

$NaNO_2$ M_r 69.0

DEFINITION

Content: 98.5 per cent to 100.5 per cent (dried substance).

CHARACTERS

Appearance: colourless crystals or mass or yellowish rods, hygroscopic.

Solubility: freely soluble in water, soluble in alcohol.

IDENTIFICATION

A. Dilute 1 ml of solution S1 (see Tests) to 25 ml with *water R*. To 0.1 ml of the solution add 1 ml of *sulphanilic acid solution R1*. Allow to stand for 2-3 min. Add 1 ml of *β-naphthol solution R* and 1 ml of *dilute sodium hydroxide solution R*. An intense red colour develops.

B. To 1 ml of the solution prepared for identification test A add 3 ml of a 20 g/l solution of *phenazone R* and 0.4 ml of *dilute sulphuric acid R*. An intense green colour develops.

C. To 0.15 ml of solution S1, add 0.35 ml of *water R*. The solution gives reaction (b) of sodium (*2.3.1*).

TESTS

Solution S1. Dissolve 2.5 g in *carbon dioxide-free water R* and dilute to 50 ml with the same solvent.

Solution S2. Dissolve 3 g in *distilled water R*. Cautiously add 10 ml of *nitric acid R* and evaporate to dryness. Dissolve the residue in 10 ml of *distilled water R*, neutralise with *dilute sodium hydroxide solution R* and dilute to 30 ml with *distilled water R*.

Appearance of solution. Solution S1 is clear (*2.2.1*) and not more intensely coloured than reference solution B_6 (*2.2.2, Method II*).

Acidity or alkalinity. To 10 ml of solution S1, add 0.05 ml of *phenol red solution R*. Add 0.1 ml of *0.01 M sodium hydroxide*. The solution is red. Add 0.3 ml of *0.01 M hydrochloric acid*. The solution is yellow.

Chlorides (*2.4.4*): maximum 50 ppm.

Dilute 10 ml of solution S2 to 15 ml with *water R*. The solution complies with the limit test for chlorides.

Sulphates (*2.4.13*): maximum 200 ppm.

Dilute 7.5 ml of solution S2 to 15 ml with *distilled water R*. The solution complies with the limit test for sulphates.

Heavy metals (*2.4.8*): maximum 20 ppm.

Dilute 10 ml of solution S2 to 20 ml with *water R*. 12 ml of the solution complies with limit test A. Prepare the standard using *lead standard solution (1 ppm Pb) R*.

Loss on drying (*2.2.32*): maximum 1.0 per cent, determined on 1.000 g by drying *in vacuo*.

ASSAY

Dissolve 0.400 g in 100.0 ml of *water R*. Introduce 20.0 ml of the solution, while stirring continuously and keeping the tip of the pipette below the surface of the liquid, into a conical flask containing 30.0 ml of *0.1 M cerium sulphate*. Immediately stopper the flask and allow to stand for 2 min. Add 10 ml of a 200 g/l solution of *potassium iodide R* and 2 ml of *starch solution R*.

While stirring continuously, titrate with *0.1 M sodium thiosulphate* until the blue colour disappears. Carry out a blank titration.

1 ml of *0.1 M cerium sulphate* is equivalent to 3.45 mg of $NaNO_2$.

STORAGE

In an airtight container.

01/2005:0565

SODIUM NITROPRUSSIDE

Natrii nitroprussias

$Na_2[Fe(CN)_5NO],2H_2O$ M_r 298.0

DEFINITION

Sodium nitroprusside contains not less than 99.0 per cent and not more than the equivalent of 100.5 per cent of sodium pentacyanonitrosylferrate (III), calculated with reference to the anhydrous substance.

CHARACTERS

Reddish-brown powder or crystals, freely soluble in water, slightly soluble in alcohol.

IDENTIFICATION

A. Dissolve 0.700 g in *water R* and dilute to 100.0 ml with the same solvent. Examined between 350 nm and 600 nm (*2.2.25*) immediately after preparation, the solution shows an absorption maximum at 395 nm, a shoulder at about 510 nm and a minimum at 370 nm. The specific absorbance at the maximum is 0.65 to 0.80.

B. Dissolve about 20 mg in 2 ml of *water R* and add 0.1 ml of *sodium sulphide solution R*. A deep violet-red colour is produced.

C. Dissolve 50 mg in 1 ml of *water R* and acidify the solution by the addition of *hydrochloric acid R*. Place a drop of the solution in an oxidising flame. A persistent yellow colour is produced.

TESTS

Insoluble matter. Dissolve 10 g without heating in 50 ml of *water R*. Allow to stand for 30 min and filter through a sintered-glass filter (16). Wash the filter with cold *water R* until the filtrate is colourless. Dry the residue on the filter at 105 °C. The residue weighs not more than 1 mg (100 ppm).

Chlorides (*2.4.4*). In a metallic crucible (nickel) mix 1.0 g of the substance to be examined with 8 ml of a 200 g/l solution of *sodium hydroxide R*. Heat slowly and evaporate carefully to dryness over a small flame, then heat to a dull red colour for 30 min. Allow to cool and transfer the solid residue with three successive portions, each of 8 ml of *dilute sulphuric acid R*. Filter the sulphuric acid extracts on a filter paper and collect the filtrates. Render the filtrate acid to *litmus paper R* by adding, if necessary, a few drops of *dilute sulphuric acid R*. Wash the crucible and the filter paper with three successive portions of 10 ml of *water R*, add the washings to the main sulphuric acid solution and dilute to 60 ml with *water R*. Mix. 15 ml of the solution complies with the limit test for chlorides (200 ppm).

Ferricyanides. Dissolve 1.25 g in *acetate buffer solution pH 4.6 R* and dilute to 50.0 ml with the same buffer solution. Use three 50 ml volumetric flasks (*A*, *B*, *C*). To flask *B* add 1.0 ml of *ferricyanide standard solution (50 ppm* $Fe(CN)_6$*) R*. To flasks *A* and *B* add 1 ml of a 5 g/l solution of *ferrous ammonium sulphate R*. To the three flasks add 10.0 ml of the solution of the substance to be examined. Dilute the contents of each flask to 50.0 ml with *water R*. Allow to stand for 30 min. The absorbance (*2.2.25*) of the solution in flask *A* measured at 720 nm using the solution in flask *C* as the compensation liquid is not greater than the absorbance of the solution in flask *B* measured at 720 nm using the solution in flask *A* as the compensation liquid (200 ppm).

Ferrocyanides. Dissolve 4.0 g in *water R* and dilute to 100.0 ml with the same solvent. Use three 50 ml volumetric flasks (*A*, *B*, *C*). To flask *B* add 2.0 ml of *ferrocyanide standard solution (100 ppm* $Fe(CN)_6$*) R*. To flasks *A* and *B* add 1 ml of *ferric chloride solution R2*. To the three flasks add 25.0 ml of the solution of the substance to be examined. Dilute the contents of each flask to 50.0 ml with *water R*. Allow to stand for 30 min. The absorbance (*2.2.25*) of the solution in flask *A* measured at 695 nm using the solution in flask *C* as the compensation liquid is not greater than the absorbance of the solution in flask *B* measured at 695 nm using the solution in flask *A* as the compensation liquid (200 ppm).

Sulphates. For the preparation and dilution of the solutions use *distilled water R*.

Test solution. Dissolve 3.6 g in 120 ml of water, add with mixing 4 ml of *sulphate standard solution (10 ppm* SO_4*) R* and 20 ml of a 250 g/l solution of *cupric chloride R* and dilute to 150.0 ml with water. Allow to stand for 16 h and filter or centrifuge until a clear light-blue solution is obtained.

Reference solution. To 40 ml of *sulphate standard solution (10 ppm* SO_4*) R* add 80 ml of water and 12 ml to 13 ml of a 250 g/l solution of *cupric chloride R*. Dilute to 150.0 ml with water. The volume of cupric chloride solution added is such that the colour of the final solution matches that of the test solution.

Allow the solutions to stand. Filter both solutions, discarding the first 25 ml of filtrate. To 100 ml of each filtrate, add 0.5 ml of *acetic acid R*. Mix and add 2 ml of a 250 g/l solution of *barium chloride R* and mix again. The test solution is not more opalescent than the reference solution (100 ppm).

Water (*2.5.12*): 9.0 per cent to 15.0 per cent, determined on 0.250 g by the semi-micro determination of water.

ASSAY

Dissolve 0.250 g in 100 ml of *water R* and add 0.1 ml of *dilute sulphuric acid R*. Titrate with *0.1 M silver nitrate*, determining the end-point potentiometrically (*2.2.20*) with a silver-mercurous sulphate electrode system.

1 ml of *0.1 M silver nitrate* is equivalent to 13.10 mg of $Na_2[Fe(CN)_5NO]$.

STORAGE

Store protected from light.

01/2005:1997

SODIUM PERBORATE, HYDRATED

Natrii perboras hydricus

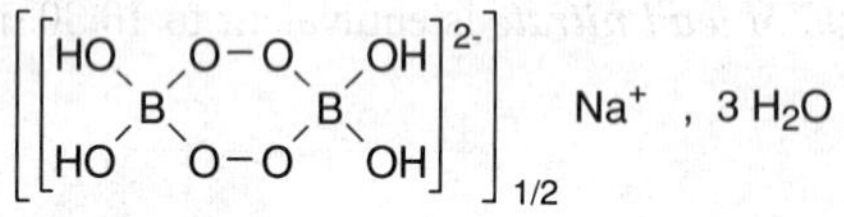

$NaBO_3,4H_2O$ or $NaBO_2,H_2O_2,3H_2O$ M_r 153.9

DEFINITION

Content: 96.0 per cent to 103.0 per cent.

CHARACTERS

Appearance: colourless, prismatic crystals or white powder, stable in the crystalline form.

Solubility: sparingly soluble in water, with slow decomposition. It dissolves in dilute mineral acids.

IDENTIFICATION

A. Mix 1 ml of a saturated solution with a mixture of 1 ml of *dilute sulphuric acid R* and 0.2 ml of a 70 g/l solution of *potassium dichromate R*, shake with 2 ml of *ether R* and allow to stand. A blue colour is produced in the ether layer.

B. The mixture obtained by treating about 100 mg with 0.1 ml of *sulphuric acid R* and 5 ml of *methanol R* burns with a greenish flame when ignited.

C. It gives reaction (a) of sodium (*2.3.1*).

TESTS

Chlorides (*2.4.4*): maximum 330 ppm.

Dissolve 0.15 g in 15 ml of *water R*. The solution complies with the limit test for chlorides.

Sulphates (*2.4.13*): maximum 1.2 per cent.

Dissolve 0.13 g in 150 ml of *distilled water R*. 15 ml of the solution complies with the limit test for sulphates.

Iron (*2.4.9*): maximum 20 ppm.

Dissolve 2.5 g in 10 ml of *dilute hydrochloric acid R* with heating, evaporate to dryness, with stirring, and dissolve the residue in 25 ml of hot *water R*. Dilute 5 ml of the obtained solution to 10 ml with *water R*. The solution complies with the limit test for iron.

Heavy metals (*2.4.8*): maximum 10 ppm.

12 ml of the solution obtained in the test for iron complies with limit test A. Prepare the standard using *lead standard solution (1 ppm Pb) R*.

ASSAY

Dissolve 0.300 g in 50.0 ml of *water R*. Dilute 10.0 ml of the solution to 50 ml with *water R* and add 10 ml of *dilute sulphuric acid R*. Titrate with *0.02 M potassium permanganate*.

1 ml of *0.02 M potassium permanganate* is equivalent to 7.693 mg of NaH_8BO_7.

STORAGE

In an airtight container.

01/2005:1031

SODIUM PICOSULFATE

Natrii picosulfas

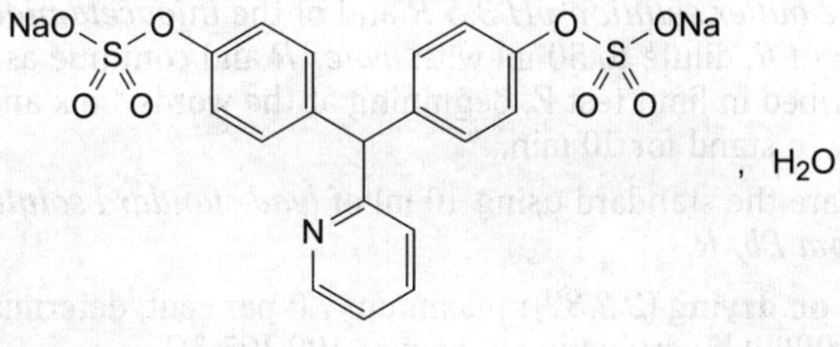

$C_{18}H_{13}NNa_2O_8S_2,H_2O$ M_r 499.4

DEFINITION

Sodium picosulfate contains not less than 98.5 per cent and not more than the equivalent of 100.5 per cent of 4,4′-(pyridin-2-ylmethylene)bisphenyl bis(sodium sulphate), calculated with reference to the anhydrous substance.

CHARACTERS

A white or almost white, crystalline powder, freely soluble in water, slightly soluble in alcohol.

IDENTIFICATION

First identification: A, E.

Second identification: B, C, D, E.

A. Examine by infrared absorption spectrophotometry (*2.2.24*), comparing with the spectrum obtained with *sodium picosulfate CRS*. Examine the substances prepared as discs.

B. Examine the chromatograms obtained in the test for related substances in ultraviolet light at 254 nm. The principal spot in the chromatogram obtained with test solution (b) is similar in position and size to the principal spot in the chromatogram obtained with reference solution (a).

C. To 5 ml of solution S (see Tests) add 1 ml of *dilute hydrochloric acid R* and heat to boiling. Add 1 ml of *barium chloride solution R1*. A white precipitate is formed.

D. To about 10 mg add 3 ml of *sulphuric acid R* and 0.1 ml of *potassium dichromate solution R1*. A violet colour develops.

E. The solution S gives reaction (a) of sodium (*2.3.1*).

TESTS

Solution S. Dissolve 2.5 g in *distilled water R* and dilute to 50 ml with the same solvent.

Appearance of solution. Solution S is clear (*2.2.1*) and not more intensely coloured than reference solution GY_7 (*2.2.2, Method II*).

Acidity or alkalinity. To 10 ml of solution S add 0.05 ml of *phenolphthalein solution R*. The solution is colourless. Not more than 0.25 ml of *0.01 M sodium hydroxide* is required to change the colour of the indicator to pink.

Related substances. Examine by thin-layer chromatography (*2.2.27*), using *silica gel GF_{254} R* as the coating substance.

Test solution (a). Dissolve 0.20 g of the substance to be examined in *methanol R* and dilute to 5 ml with the same solvent.

Test solution (b). Dilute 1 ml of test solution (a) to 10 ml with *methanol R*.

Reference solution (a). Dissolve 20 mg of *sodium picosulfate CRS* in *methanol R* and dilute to 5 ml with the same solvent.

Reference solution (b). Dilute 2 ml of test solution (b) to 100 ml with *methanol R*.

Reference solution (c). Dissolve 0.20 g of the substance to be examined in 2 ml of a 103 g/l solution of *hydrochloric acid R*. Heat rapidly to boiling and maintain boiling for 10 s. Cool in iced water and dilute to 10 ml with *methanol R*.

Apply to the plate 5 µl of each solution. Develop over a path of 10 cm using a mixture of 2.5 volumes of *anhydrous formic acid R*, 12.5 volumes of *water R*, 25 volumes of *methanol R* and 60 volumes of *ethyl acetate R*. Dry the plate in a current of hot air for 15 min and examine in ultraviolet light at 254 nm. Spray with a 200 g/l solution of *hydrochloric acid R* in *methanol R* and heat at 110 °C for 10 min. Spray the hot plate with a freshly prepared solution containing 50 g/l of *ferric chloride R* and 1 g/l of *potassium ferricyanide R*. Examine the wet plate. Any spot in the chromatogram obtained with test solution (a), apart from the principal spot, is not more intense than the spot in the chromatogram obtained with reference solution (b) (0.2 per cent). The test is not valid unless the chromatogram obtained with reference solution (c) shows three clearly separated spots. A fourth spot may be present on the starting-line.

Chlorides (*2.4.4*). Dilute 5 ml of solution S to 15 ml with *water R*. The solution complies with the limit test for chlorides (200 ppm).

Sulphates (*2.4.13*). Dilute 7.5 ml of solution S to 15 ml with *distilled water R*. The solution complies with the limit test for sulphates (400 ppm).

Heavy metals (*2.4.8*). 12 ml of solution S complies with limit test A for heavy metals (20 ppm). Prepare the standard using 10 ml of *lead standard solution (1 ppm Pb) R*.

Water (*2.5.12*): 3.0 per cent to 5.0 per cent, determined on 0.500 g by the semi-micro determination of water.

ASSAY

Dissolve 0.400 g in 80 ml of *methanol R*. Titrate with *0.1 M perchloric acid*, determining the end-point potentiometrically (*2.2.20*).

1 ml of *0.1 M perchloric acid* is equivalent to 48.14 mg of $C_{18}H_{13}NNa_2O_8S_2$.

Monographs Q-S

IMPURITIES

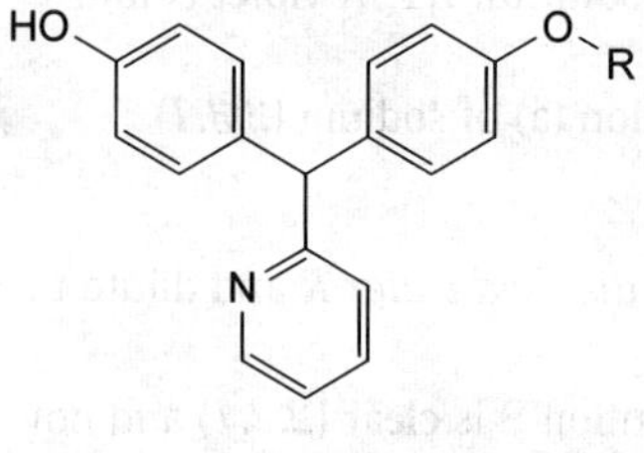

A. R = SO_3Na: 4-[(pyridin-2-yl)(4-hydroxyphenyl)methyl]phenyl sodium sulphate,

B. R = H: 4,4′-[(pyridin-2-yl)methylene]bisphenol.

01/2005:1909
corrected

SODIUM POLYSTYRENE SULPHONATE

Natrii polystyrenesulfonas

DEFINITION

Polystyrene sulphonate resin prepared in the sodium form.

Exchange capacity: 2.8 mmol to 3.4 mmol of potassium per gram (dried substance).

Content: 9.4 per cent to 11.0 per cent of Na (dried substance).

CHARACTERS

Appearance: almost white or light brown powder.

Solubility: practically insoluble in water, in alcohol and in methylene chloride.

IDENTIFICATION

A. Infrared absorption spectrophotometry (*2.2.24*).
   Preparation: discs using finely ground substance.
   Comparison: *Ph. Eur. reference spectrum of sodium polystyrene sulphonate.*

B. Suspend 0.1 g in *water R*, add 2 ml of a 150 g/l solution of *potassium carbonate R*, and heat to boiling. Allow to cool and filter. To the filtrate add 4 ml of *potassium pyroantimonate solution R* and heat to boiling. Allow to cool in iced water and if necessary rub the inside of the test-tube with a glass rod. A dense white precipitate is formed.

TESTS

Styrene. Liquid chromatography (*2.2.29*).

Test solution. Shake 10.0 g of the substance to be examined with 10 ml of *acetone R* for 30 min, centrifuge and use the supernatant liquid.

Reference solution. Dissolve 10 mg of *styrene R* in *acetone R* and dilute to 100 ml with the same solvent. Dilute 1 ml of this solution to 100 ml with *acetone R*.

Column:

- *size*: *l* = 0.25 m, Ø = 4 mm,
- *stationary phase*: *octadecylsilyl silica gel for chromatography R* (5 µm).

Mobile phase: *acetonitrile R, water R* (1:1 *V/V*).

Flow rate: 2 ml/min.

Detection: spectrophotometer at 254 nm.

Injection: 20 µl.

Limit:

- *styrene*: not more than the area of the principal peak in the chromatogram obtained with the reference solution (1 ppm).

Calcium: maximum 0.10 per cent.

Atomic emission spectrometry (*2.2.22, Method I*).

Test solution. To 1.10 g add 5 ml of *hydrochloric acid R*, heat to boiling, cool and add 10 ml of *water R*. Filter, wash the filter and residue with *water R* and dilute the filtrate and washing to 25.0 ml with *water R*.

Reference solutions. Prepare the reference solutions using *calcium standard solution (400 ppm Ca) R*, diluted as necessary with *water R*.

Wavelength: 422.7 nm.

Potassium: maximum 0.10 per cent.

Atomic emission spectrometry (*2.2.22, Method I*).

Test solution. To 1.10 g add 5 ml of *hydrochloric acid R*, heat to boiling, cool and add 10 ml of *water R*. Filter, wash the filter and residue with *water R* and dilute the filtrate and washings to 25.0 ml with *water R*.

Reference solutions. Prepare the reference solutions using *potassium standard solution (100 ppm K) R*, diluted as necessary with *water R*.

Wavelength: 766.5 nm.

Heavy metals (*2.4.8*): maximum 10 ppm.

Treat 1.0 g as described in limit test F. After the addition of the *buffer solution pH 3.5 R* and of the *thioacetamide reagent R*, dilute to 50 ml with *water R* and continue as described in limit test E, beginning at the words "mix and allow to stand for 10 min...".

Prepare the standard using 10 ml of *lead standard solution (1 ppm Pb) R*.

Loss on drying (*2.2.32*): maximum 7.0 per cent, determined on 1.000 g by drying in an oven at 100-105 °C.

Microbial contamination (*2.6.13*): not more than 10^2 enterobacteria and certain other gram-negative bacteria per gram.

ASSAY

Sodium. Atomic emission spectrometry (*2.2.22, Method I*).

Test solution. In a platinum crucible moisten 0.90 g with a few drops of *sulphuric acid R*, ignite very gently and allow to cool. Moisten with a few drops of *sulphuric acid R* again, ignite at 800 °C until a carbon-free ash is obtained and allow to cool.

Add 20 ml of *water R* to the crucible, warm gently on a water-bath until dissolution, cool, transfer quantitatively to a 100 ml graduated flask and dilute to 100.0 ml with *water R*. Dilute 5 ml of this solution to 1000.0 ml with *water R*.

Reference solutions. Prepare the reference solutions using *sodium standard solution (200 ppm Na) R*, diluted as necessary with *water R*.

Wavelength: 589 nm.

Exchange capacity. Atomic emission spectrometry (*2.2.22, Method I*).

Solution A. 9.533 g/l solution of *potassium chloride R*.

Test solution. To 1.6 g of the substance to be examined in a dry 250 ml ground-glass-stoppered flask add 100 ml of solution A, stopper and shake for 15 min. Filter, discard the first 20 ml of the filtrate and dilute 4 ml of the filtrate to 1000 ml with *water R*.

Reference solutions. Prepare the reference solutions by diluting 0, 1, 2, 3 and 4 ml of solution A respectively and 4, 3, 2, 1 and 0 ml of a 7.63 g/l solution of *sodium chloride R* to 1000 ml with *water R.*

Wavelength: 766.5 nm.

Prepare a calibration curve using the reference solutions and calculate the potassium exchange capacity of the substance to be examined in millimoles per gram taking the concentration of potassium in solution A as 128 mmoles of K per litre.

STORAGE

In an airtight container.

IMPURITIES

Specified impurities: A.

A. styrene.

01/2005:2041

SODIUM PROPIONATE

Natrii propionas

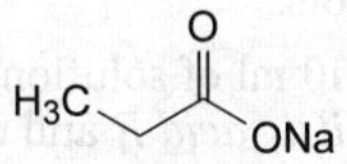

$C_3H_5NaO_2$ M_r 96.1

DEFINITION

Sodium propanoate.

Content: 99.0 per cent to 101.0 per cent (dried substance).

CHARACTERS

Appearance: colourless crystals or white powder, slightly hygroscopic.

Solubility: freely soluble in water, sparingly soluble in alcohol, practically insoluble in methylene chloride.

IDENTIFICATION

First identification: A, D.

Second identification: B, C, D.

A. Infrared absorption spectrophotometry (*2.2.24*).

Comparison: *Ph. Eur. reference spectrum of sodium propionate.*

B. Dissolve 0.1 g in a mixture of 2 ml of *copper sulphate solution R* and 2 ml of *methylene chloride R.* Shake vigorously and allow to stand. Both the upper and the lower layer show a blue colour.

C. To 5 ml of solution S (see Tests) add 2 ml of *0.1 M silver nitrate.* A white precipitate is formed.

D. Solution S gives reaction (a) of sodium (*2.3.1*).

TESTS

Solution S. Dissolve 10 g in *carbon dioxide-free water R* prepared from *distilled water R* and dilute to 100 ml with the same solvent.

Appearance of solution. Solution S is clear (*2.2.1*) and colourless (*2.2.2, Method II*).

pH (*2.2.3*): 7.8 to 9.2.

Dilute 1 ml of solution S to 5 ml with *water R.*

Related substances. Liquid chromatography (*2.2.29*).

Test solution. Dissolve 0.250 g of the substance to be examined in *water R* and dilute to 100 ml with the same solvent.

Reference solution (a). Dissolve 10 mg of the substance to be examined and 10 mg of *sodium acetate R* in *water R* and dilute to 100 ml with the same solvent.

Reference solution (b). Dilute 1.0 ml of the test solution to 100 ml with *water R.*

Column:

- *size*: *l* = 0.25 m, Ø = 4.6 mm,
- *stationary phase*: *octadecylsilyl silica gel for chromatography R* (5 µm).

Mobile phase: dilute 1 ml of *phosphoric acid R* to 1000 ml with *water R.*

Flow rate: 1 ml/min.

Detection: spectrophotometer at 210 nm.

Injection: 20 µl.

System suitability: reference solution (a):

- *resolution*: minimum 5 between the peaks due to sodium acetate and sodium propionate.

Limits:

- *any impurity*: not more than 0.1 times the area of the principal peak in the chromatogram obtained with reference solution (b) (0.1 per cent),
- *total*: not more than half the area of the principal peak in the chromatrogram obtained with reference solution (b) (0.5 per cent),
- *disregard limit*: 0.05 times the area of the principal peak in the chromatogram obtained with reference solution (b) (0.05 per cent).

Readily oxidisable substances. In a ground-glass-stoppered conical flask introduce 10 g of the substance to be examined. Add 100 ml of *water R* and stir to dissolve. Add 25 ml of *sodium hypobromite solution R* and 10 ml of a 200 g/l solution of *sodium acetate R,* stopper the flask and allow to stand for 15 min. Add 10 ml of *potassium iodide solution R* and 20 ml of *hydrochloric acid R* while cooling. Titrate with *0.2 M sodium thiosulphate,* adding 2 ml of *starch solution R* towards the end of the titration. Carry out a blank titration. The difference between the volumes used in the 2 titrations is not greater than 2.2 ml.

Iron (*2.4.9*): maximum 10 ppm.

10 ml of solution S complies with the limit test for iron.

Heavy metals (*2.4.8*): maximum 10 ppm.

12 ml of solution S complies with limit test A. Prepare the standard using *lead standard solution (1 ppm Pb) R.*

Loss on drying (*2.2.32*): maximum 0.5 per cent, determined on 1.000 g by heating in an oven at 100-105 °C for 3 h.

ASSAY

Dissolve 80.0 mg in 30 ml of *anhydrous acetic acid R.* Titrate with *0.1 M perchloric acid,* determining the end-point potentiometrically (*2.2.20*).

1 ml of *0.1 M perchloric acid* is equivalent to 9.61 mg of $C_3H_5NaO_2$.

STORAGE

In an airtight container.

Monographs Q-S

01/2005:1263

SODIUM PROPYL PARAHYDROXYBENZOATE

Propylis parahydroxybenzoas natricum

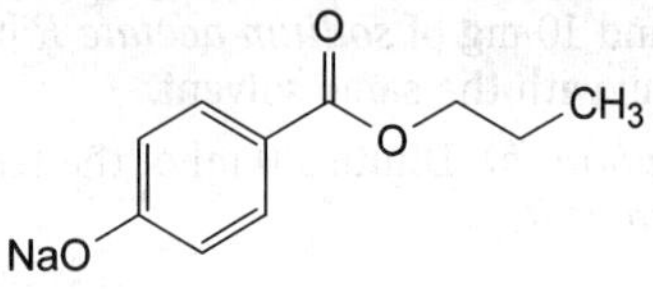

$C_{10}H_{11}NaO_3$ M_r 202.2

DEFINITION

Sodium propyl parahydroxybenzoate contains not less than 99.0 per cent and not more than the equivalent of 104.0 per cent of sodium 4-(propoxycarbonyl)phenolate, calculated with reference to the anhydrous substance.

CHARACTERS

A white, crystalline powder, freely soluble in water, sparingly soluble in alcohol, practically insoluble in methylene chloride.

IDENTIFICATION

First identification: A, B, E.

Second identification: A, C, D, E.

A. Dissolve 0.5 g in 50 ml of *water R*. Immediately add 5 ml of *hydrochloric acid R1*. Filter, and wash the precipitate with *water R*. Dry at 80 °C *in vacuo* for 2 h. The melting point (*2.2.14*) of the precipitate is 96 °C to 99 °C.

B. Examine the precipitate obtained in identification test A by infrared absorption spectrophotometry (*2.2.24*), comparing with the spectrum obtained with *propyl parahydroxybenzoate CRS*.

C. Examine the chromatograms obtained in the test for related substances. The principal spot in the chromatogram obtained with test solution (b) is similar in position and size to the principal spot in the chromatogram obtained with reference solution (c).

D. To about 10 mg in a test-tube add 1 ml of *sodium carbonate solution R*, boil for 30 s and cool. Add 5 ml of *aminopyrazolone solution R* and 1 ml of *potassium ferricyanide solution R* and mix. An orange to red colour develops.

E. To 1 ml of solution S (see Tests) add 1 ml of *water R*. The solution gives reaction (a) of sodium (*2.3.1*).

TESTS

Solution S. Dissolve 5.0 g in *carbon dioxide-free water R* prepared from *distilled water R*, and dilute to 50 ml with the same solvent.

Appearance of solution. Solution S, examined immediately after preparation, is clear (*2.2.1*) and not more intensely coloured than reference solution BY_6 (*2.2.2, Method II*).

pH (*2.2.3*). Dilute 1 ml of solution S to 100 ml with *carbon dioxide-free water R*. The pH of the solution is 9.5 to 10.5.

Related substances. Examine by thin-layer chromatography (*2.2.27*), using as the coating substance a suitable octadecylsilyl silica gel with a fluorescent indicator having an optimal intensity at 254 nm.

Test solution (a). Dissolve 0.100 g of the substance to be examined in 10 ml of *water R*. Immediately add 2 ml of *hydrochloric acid R* and shake with 50 ml of *ether R*. Evaporate the upper layer to dryness and take up the residue with 10 ml of *acetone R*.

Test solution (b). Dilute 1 ml of test solution (a) to 10 ml with *acetone R*.

Reference solution (a). Dissolve 34.3 mg of *4-hydroxybenzoic acid R* in *acetone R* and dilute to 100 ml with the same solvent.

Reference solution (b). Dilute 0.5 ml of test solution (a) to 100 ml with *acetone R*.

Reference solution (c). Dissolve 10 mg of *propyl parahydroxybenzoate CRS* in *acetone R* and dilute to 10 ml with the same solvent.

Reference solution (d). Dissolve 10 mg of *ethyl parahydroxybenzoate CRS* in 1 ml of test solution (a) and dilute to 10 ml with *acetone R*.

Apply separately to the plate 5 µl of each solution. Develop over a path of 15 cm using a mixture of 1 volume of *glacial acetic acid R*, 30 volumes of *water R* and 70 volumes of *methanol R*. Allow the plate to dry in air and examine in ultraviolet light at 254 nm. In the chromatogram obtained with test solution (a): any spot due to 4-hydroxybenzoic acid is not more intense than the spot in the chromatogram obtained with reference solution (a) (4 per cent); and any spot, apart from the principal spot and the spot due to 4-hydroxybenzoic acid, is not more intense than the spot in the chromatogram obtained with reference solution (b) (0.5 per cent). The test is not valid unless the chromatogram obtained with reference solution (d) shows two clearly separated principal spots.

Chlorides (*2.4.4*). To 10 ml of solution S add 30 ml of *water R* and 1 ml of *nitric acid R* and dilute to 50 ml with *water R*. Shake and filter. Dilute 10 ml of the filtrate to 15 ml with *water R*. The solution complies with the limit test for chlorides (350 ppm). Prepare the standard using 14 ml of *chloride standard solution (5 ppm Cl) R* to which 1 ml of *water R* has been added.

Sulphates (*2.4.13*). To 25 ml of solution S add 5 ml of *distilled water R* and 10 ml of *hydrochloric acid R* and dilute to 50 ml with *distilled water R*. Shake and filter. Dilute 10 ml of the filtrate to 15 ml with *distilled water R*. The solution complies with the limit test for sulphates (300 ppm).

Heavy metals (*2.4.8*). 2.0 g complies with limit test C for heavy metals (10 ppm). Prepare the standard using 2 ml of *lead standard solution (10 ppm Pb) R*.

Water (*2.5.12*). Not more than 5.0 per cent, determined on 0.500 g by the semi-micro determination of water.

ASSAY

Dissolve 0.150 g in 50 ml of *anhydrous acetic acid R*. Titrate with *0.1 M perchloric acid*, determining the end-point potentiometrically (*2.2.20*).

1 ml of *0.1 M perchloric acid* is equivalent to 20.22 mg of $C_{10}H_{11}NaO_3$.

IMPURITIES

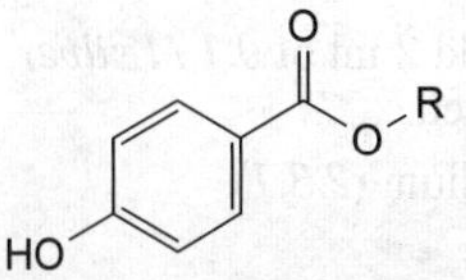

A. R = H: 4-hydroxybenzoic acid,

B. R = CH_3 : methyl 4-hydroxybenzoate,

C. R = CH_2-CH_3: ethyl 4-hydroxybenzoate,

D. R = CH_2-CH_2-CH_2-CH_3: butyl 4-hydroxybenzoate.

01/2005:0413

SODIUM SALICYLATE

Natrii salicylas

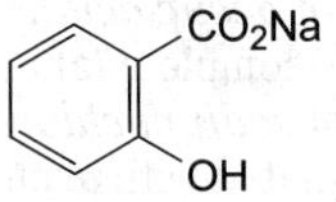

$C_7H_5NaO_3$ M_r 160.1

DEFINITION

Sodium salicylate contains not less than 99.0 per cent and not more than the equivalent of 101.0 per cent of sodium 2-hydroxybenzenecarboxylate, calculated with reference to the dried substance.

CHARACTERS

A white, crystalline powder or small, colourless crystals or shiny flakes, freely soluble in water, sparingly soluble in alcohol.

IDENTIFICATION

First identification: A, C.

Second identification: B, C.

A. Examine by infrared absorption spectrophotometry (*2.2.24*), comparing with the spectrum obtained with *sodium salicylate CRS*.

B. Solution S (see Tests) gives the reactions of salicylates (*2.3.1*).

C. It gives reaction (b) of sodium (*2.3.1*).

TESTS

Solution S. Dissolve 5.0 g in *carbon dioxide-free water R* prepared from *distilled water R* and dilute to 50 ml with the same solvent.

Appearance of solution. Solution S is clear (*2.2.1*) and not more intensely coloured than reference solution BY_6 (*2.2.2, Method II*).

Acidity. To 20 ml of solution S add 0.1 ml of *phenol red solution R*. The solution is yellow. Not more than 2.0 ml of *0.01 M sodium hydroxide* is required to change the colour of the indicator to reddish-violet.

Chlorides (*2.4.4*). To 5 ml of solution S add 5 ml of *water R* and 10 ml of *dilute nitric acid R* and filter. 10 ml of the filtrate diluted to 15 ml with *water R* complies with the limit test for chlorides (200 ppm).

Sulphates (*2.4.13*). 2.5 ml of solution S diluted to 15 ml with *distilled water R* complies with the limit test for sulphates (600 ppm).

Heavy metals (*2.4.8*). Dissolve 1.6 g in 16 ml of a mixture of 5 volumes of *water R* and 10 volumes of *alcohol R*. 12 ml of the solution complies with limit test B for heavy metals (20 ppm). Prepare the standard using lead standard solution (2 ppm Pb) prepared by diluting *lead standard solution (100 ppm Pb) R* with a mixture of 5 volumes of *water R* and 10 volumes of *alcohol R*.

Loss on drying (*2.2.32*). Not more than 0.5 per cent, determined on 1.00 g by drying in an oven at 100 °C to 105 °C.

ASSAY

Dissolve 0.130 g in 30 ml of *anhydrous acetic acid R*. Titrate with *0.1 M perchloric acid*, determining the end-point potentiometrically (*2.2.20*).

1 ml of *0.1 M perchloric acid* is equivalent to 16.01 mg of $C_7H_5NaO_3$.

STORAGE

Store in an airtight container, protected from light.

01/2005:1677

SODIUM SELENITE PENTAHYDRATE

Natrii selenis pentahydricus

$Na_2SeO_3,5H_2O$ M_r 263.0

DEFINITION

Content: 98.5 per cent to 101.5 per cent.

CHARACTERS

Appearance: white, crystalline powder, hygroscopic.

Solubility: freely soluble in water, practically insoluble in alcohol.

IDENTIFICATION

A. Dissolve 50 mg in 5 ml of a mixture of equal volumes of *dilute hydrochloric acid R* and *water R* and heat to boiling. Add 0.05 g of *ascorbic acid R*; a red precipitate is formed which may become black.

B. Dissolve 50 mg in a mixture of 1 ml of *dilute hydrochloric acid R* and 5 ml of *water R*. Add 1 ml of *barium chloride solution R1*; the solution remains clear.

C. It gives reaction (a) of sodium (*2.3.1*).

D. It complies with the limits of the assay.

TESTS

Solution S. Dissolve 5.0 g in *carbon dioxide-free water R* and dilute to 50.0 ml with the same solvent.

Appearance of solution. Solution S is clear (*2.2.1*) and colourless (*2.2.2, Method II*).

Acidity or alkalinity. To 10 ml of solution S, add 0.1 ml of *thymolphthalein solution R*; the solution is blue. Not more than 0.3 ml of *1 M hydrochloric acid* is required to change the colour of the indicator from blue to colourless.

Chlorides (*2.4.4*): maximum 50 ppm.

To 10 ml of solution S, add 2 ml of *nitric acid R* and dilute to 15 ml with *water R*.

Sulphates and selenates (*2.4.13*): maximum 300 ppm (determined as sulphates).

Dissolve 0.5 g in 10 ml of *distilled water R*. Add 0.5 ml of *hydrochloric acid R1* and dilute to 15 ml with *distilled water R*.

Iron: maximum 50 ppm.

To 2 ml of solution S, add 2 ml of a 200 g/l solution of *sulphosalicylic acid R*, 5 ml of *concentrated ammonia R* and dilute to 10 ml with *water R*. The solution is not more intensely coloured than a reference solution prepared in the same manner using 1 ml of *iron standard solution (10 ppm Fe) R*.

ASSAY

Dissolve 0.120 g in 50 ml of *water R*, add 7 ml of *glacial acetic acid R*, 25.0 ml of *0.1 M sodium thiosulphate* and 0.5 g of *potassium iodide R*. Titrate immediately with *0.05 M iodine solution* using *starch solution R* as indicator.

1 ml of *0.1 M sodium thiosulphate* is equivalent to 6.575 mg of $Na_2SeO_3,5H_2O$.

STORAGE

In an airtight container.

01/2005:0983

SODIUM STARCH GLYCOLATE (TYPE A)

Carboxymethylamylum natricum A

DEFINITION

Sodium starch glycolate (type A) is the sodium salt of a cross-linked partly *O*-carboxymethylated potato starch.
It contains not less than 2.8 per cent and not more than 4.2 per cent of Na (A_r 22.99), calculated with reference to the substance washed with alcohol (80 per cent *V/V*) and dried.

CHARACTERS

A white or almost white, fine, free-flowing powder, very hygroscopic, practically insoluble in methylene chloride. It gives a translucent suspension in water.

Examined under a microscope it is seen to consist of: granules, irregularly shaped, ovoid or pear-shaped, 30 µm to 100 µm in size, or rounded, 10 µm to 35 µm in size; compound granules consisting of two to four components occur occasionally; the granules have an eccentric hilum and clearly visible concentric striations; between crossed nicol prisms, the granules show a distinct black cross intersecting at the hilum; small crystals are visible at the surface of the granules. The granules show considerable swelling in contact with water.

IDENTIFICATION

A. It complies with the test for pH (see Tests).

B. Prepare with shaking and without heating a mixture of 4.0 g and 20 ml of *carbon dioxide-free water R*. The mixture has the appearance of a gel. Add 100 ml of *carbon dioxide-free water R* and shake. A suspension forms that settles after standing.

C. To 5 ml of the suspension obtained in identification test B add 0.05 ml of *iodine solution R1*. A dark blue colour is produced.

D. Solution S2 (see Tests) gives reaction (a) of sodium (*2.3.1*).

TESTS

Solution S1. Centrifuge the suspension obtained in identification test B at 2500 *g* for 10 min. Collect carefully the supernatant liquid.

Solution S2. Place 2.5 g in a silica or platinum crucible and add 2 ml of a 500 g/l solution of *sulphuric acid R*. Heat on a water-bath, then cautiously over a naked flame, raising the temperature progressively, and then incinerate in a muffle furnace at 600 ± 25 °C. Continue heating until all black particles have disappeared. Allow to cool, add a few drops of *dilute sulphuric acid R* and heat and incinerate as above. Allow to cool, add a few drops of *ammonium carbonate solution R*, evaporate to dryness and incinerate cautiously. Allow to cool and dissolve the residue in 50 ml of *water R*.

Appearance of solution S1. Solution S1 is clear (*2.2.1*) and colourless (*2.2.2, Method II*).

pH (*2.2.3*). The pH of solution S1 is 5.5 to 7.5.

Sodium glycolate. *Carry out the test protected from light.*

Test solution. Place 0.20 g of the substance to be examined in a beaker. Add 5 ml of *acetic acid R* and 5 ml of *water R*. Stir until dissolution is complete (about 10 min). Add 50 ml of *acetone R* and 1 g of *sodium chloride R*. Filter through a fast filter paper impregnated with *acetone R*, rinse the beaker and filter with *acetone R*. Combine the filtrate and washings and dilute to 100.0 ml with *acetone R*. Allow to stand for 24 h without shaking. Use the clear supernatant liquid.

Reference solution. Dissolve 0.310 g of *glycollic acid R*, previously dried *in vacuo* over *diphosphorus pentoxide R*, in *water R* and dilute to 500.0 ml with the same solvent. To 5.0 ml of this solution, add 5 ml of *acetic acid R* and allow to stand for about 30 min. Add 50 ml of *acetone R* and 1 g of *sodium chloride R* and dilute to 100.0 ml with *acetone R*.

Heat 2.0 ml of the test solution on a water-bath for 20 min. Cool to room temperature and add 20.0 ml of *2,7-dihydroxynaphthalene solution R*. Shake and heat in a water-bath for 20 min. Cool under running water, transfer to a volumetric flask and dilute to 25.0 ml with *sulphuric acid R*, maintaining the flask under running water. Within 10 min, measure the absorbance at 540 nm (*2.2.25*) using *water R* as the compensation liquid. The absorbance of the solution prepared with the test solution is not greater than that of a solution prepared at the same time and in the same manner with 2.0 ml of the reference solution (2.0 per cent).

Sodium chloride. Not more than 7.0 per cent. Shake 1.00 g with 20 ml of *alcohol (80 per cent V/V) R* for 10 min and filter. Repeat the operation four times. Dry the residue to constant mass at 100 °C and set aside for the assay. Combine the filtrates. Evaporate to dryness, take up the residue with *water R* and dilute to 25.0 ml with the same solvent. To 10.0 ml of the solution add 30 ml of *water R* and 5 ml of *dilute nitric acid R*. Titrate with *0.1 M silver nitrate*, determining the end-point potentiometrically (*2.2.20*), using a silver indicator electrode.

1 ml of *0.1 M silver nitrate* is equivalent to 5.844 mg of NaCl.

Iron (*2.4.9*). 10 ml of solution S2 complies with the limit test for iron (20 ppm).

Heavy metals (*2.4.8*). 1.0 g complies with limit test D for heavy metals (20 ppm). Prepare the standard using 2 ml of *lead standard solution (10 ppm Pb) R*.

Loss on drying (*2.2.32*). Not more than 10.0 per cent, determined on 1.000 g by drying in an oven at 100 °C to 105 °C for 4 h.

Microbial contamination. It complies with the test for *Escherichia coli* and Salmonella (*2.6.13*).

ASSAY

To 0.500 g of the dried and crushed residue obtained in the test for sodium chloride add 80 ml of *anhydrous acetic acid R* and heat under a reflux condenser for 2 h. Cool the solution to room temperature. Titrate with *0.1 M perchloric acid*, determining the end-point potentiometrically (*2.2.20*). Carry out a blank test.

1 ml of *0.1 M perchloric acid* is equivalent to 2.299 mg of Na.

STORAGE

Store in an airtight container, protected from light.

01/2005:0984

SODIUM STARCH GLYCOLATE (TYPE B)

Carboxymethylamylum natricum B

DEFINITION

Sodium starch glycolate (type B) is the sodium salt of a cross-linked partly *O*-carboxymethylated potato starch.

It contains not less than 2.0 per cent and not more than 3.4 per cent of Na (A_r 22.99), calculated with reference to the substance washed with alcohol (80 per cent *V/V*) and dried.

CHARACTERS

A white or almost white, fine, free-flowing powder, very hygroscopic, practically insoluble in methylene chloride. It gives a translucent suspension in water.

Examined under a microscope it is seen to consist of: granules, irregularly shaped, ovoid or pear shaped, 30 µm to 100 µm in size, or rounded, 10 µm to 35 µm in size; compound granules consisting of two to four components occur occasionally; the granules have an eccentric hilum and clearly visible concentric striations; between crossed nicol prisms, the granules show a distinct black cross intersecting at the hilum; small crystals are visible at the surface of the granules. The granules show considerable swelling in contact with water.

IDENTIFICATION

A. It complies with the test for pH (see Tests).

B. Prepare with shaking and without heating a mixture of 4.0 g and 20 ml of *carbon dioxide-free water R*. The mixture has the appearance of a gel. Add 100 ml of *carbon dioxide-free water R* and shake. A suspension forms that settles after standing.

C. To 5 ml of the suspension obtained in identification test B add 0.05 ml of *iodine solution R1*. A dark blue colour is produced.

D. Solution S2 (see Tests) gives reaction (a) of sodium (*2.3.1*).

TESTS

Solution S1. Centrifuge the suspension obtained in identification test B at 2500 *g* for 10 min. Collect carefully the supernatant liquid.

Solution S2. Place 2.5 g in a silica or platinum crucible and add 2 ml of a 500 g/l solution of *sulphuric acid R*. Heat on a water-bath, then cautiously over a naked flame, raising the temperature progressively, and then incinerate in a muffle furnace at 600 ± 25 °C. Continue heating until all black particles have disappeared. Allow to cool, add a few drops of *dilute sulphuric acid R* and heat and incinerate as above. Allow to cool, add a few drops of *ammonium carbonate solution R*, evaporate to dryness and incinerate cautiously. Allow to cool and dissolve the residue in 50 ml of *water R*.

Appearance of solution S1. Solution S1 is clear (*2.2.1*) and colourless (*2.2.2, Method II*).

pH (*2.2.3*). The pH of solution S1 is 3.0 to 5.0.

Sodium glycolate. *Carry out the test protected from light.*

Test solution. Place 0.20 g of the substance to be examined in a beaker. Add 5 ml of *acetic acid R* and 5 ml of *water R*. Stir until dissolution is complete (about 10 min). Add 50 ml of *acetone R* and 1 g of *sodium chloride R*. Filter through a fast filter paper impregnated with *acetone R*, rinse the beaker and filter with *acetone R*. Combine the filtrate and washings and dilute to 100.0 ml with *acetone R*. Allow to stand for 24 h without shaking. Use the clear supernatant liquid.

Reference solution. Dissolve 0.310 g of *glycollic acid R*, previously dried *in vacuo* over *diphosphorus pentoxide R*, in *water R* and dilute to 500.0 ml with the same solvent. To 5.0 ml of this solution, add 5 ml of *acetic acid R* and allow to stand for about 30 min. Add 50 ml of *acetone R* and 1 g of *sodium chloride R* and dilute to 100.0 ml with *acetone R*.

Heat 2.0 ml of the test solution on a water-bath for 20 min. Cool to room temperature and add 20.0 ml of *2,7-dihydroxynaphthalene solution R*. Shake and heat in a water-bath for 20 min. Cool under running water, transfer quantitatively to a volumetric flask and dilute to 25.0 ml with *sulphuric acid R*, maintaining the flasks under running water. Within 10 min, measure the absorbance at 540 nm (*2.2.25*) using *water R* as the compensation liquid. The absorbance of the solution prepared with the test solution is not greater than that of a solution prepared at the same time and in the same manner with 2.0 ml of the reference solution (2.0 per cent).

Sodium chloride. Not more than 7.0 per cent. Shake 1.00 g with 20 ml of *alcohol (80 per cent V/V) R* for 10 min and filter. Repeat the operation four times. Dry the residue to constant mass at 100 °C and set aside for the assay. Combine the filtrates. Evaporate to dryness, take up the residue with *water R* and dilute to 25.0 ml with the same solvent. To 10.0 ml of the solution add 30 ml of *water R* and 5 ml of *dilute nitric acid R*. Titrate with *0.1 M silver nitrate*, determining the end-point potentiometrically (*2.2.20*) using a silver indicator electrode.

1 ml of *0.1 M silver nitrate* is equivalent to 5.844 mg of NaCl.

Iron (*2.4.9*). 10 ml of solution S2 complies with the limit test for iron (20 ppm).

Heavy metals (*2.4.8*). 1.0 g complies with limit test D for heavy metals (20 ppm). Prepare the standard using 2 ml of *lead standard solution (10 ppm Pb) R*.

Loss on drying (*2.2.32*). Not more than 10.0 per cent, determined on 1.000 g by drying in an oven at 100 °C to 105 °C for 4 h.

Microbial contamination. It complies with the test for *Escherichia coli* and *Salmonella* (*2.6.13*).

ASSAY

To 0.500 g of the dried and crushed residue obtained in the test for sodium chloride add 80 ml of *anhydrous acetic acid R* and heat under a reflux condenser for 2 h. Cool the solution to room temperature. Titrate with *0.1 M perchloric acid*, determining the end-point potentiometrically (*2.2.20*). Carry out a blank test.

1 ml of *0.1 M perchloric acid* is equivalent to 2.299 mg of Na.

STORAGE

Store in an airtight container, protected from light.

01/2005:1566

SODIUM STARCH GLYCOLATE (TYPE C)

Carboxymethylamylum natricum C

DEFINITION

Sodium starch glycolate (type C) is the sodium salt of a cross-linked by physical dehydration, partly *O*-carboxymethylated starch. It contains not less than

2.8 per cent and not more than 5.0 per cent of Na (A_r 22.99), calculated with reference to the substance washed with alcohol (80 per cent *V/V*) and dried.

CHARACTERS

A white or almost white, fine, free-flowing powder, very hygroscopic, soluble in water, practically insoluble in methylene chloride. It gives a translucent gel-like product in water.

Examined under a microscope it is seen to consist of granules, irregularly shaped, ovoid or pear-shaped, 30 μm to 100 μm in size, or rounded, 10 μm to 35 μm in size; compound granules consisting of two to four components occur occasionally; the granules have an eccentric hilum and clearly visible concentric striations; between crossed nicol prisms, the granules show a distinct black cross intersecting at the hilum; small crystals are visible at the surface of the granules. The granules show considerable swelling in contact with water.

IDENTIFICATION

A. It complies with the test for pH (see Tests).

B. Mix with shaking and without heating 4.0 g and 20 ml of *carbon dioxide-free water R*. The mixture has the appearance of a gel. Add 100 ml of *carbon dioxide-free water R* and shake: the gel remains stable (difference from types A and B). Keep the gel for the tests for appearance of gel and pH.

C. To 5 ml of the gel obtained in identification test B add 0.05 ml of *iodine solution R1*. A dark blue colour is produced.

D. Solution S (see Tests) gives reaction (a) of sodium (*2.3.1*).

TESTS

Solution S. Place 2.5 g in a silica or platinum crucible and add 2 ml of a 500 g/l solution of *sulphuric acid R*. Heat on a water-bath, then cautiously over a naked flame, raising the temperature progressively, and then incinerate in a muffle furnace at 600 ± 25 °C. Continue heating until all black particles have disappeared. Allow to cool, add a few drops of *sulphuric acid R* and heat and incinerate as described above. Allow to cool, add a few drops of *ammonium carbonate solution R*, evaporate to dryness and incinerate cautiously. Allow to cool and dissolve the residue in 50 ml of *water R*.

Appearance of gel. The gel prepared under identification test B is colourless (*2.2.2, Method II*).

pH (*2.2.3*). The pH of the gel prepared under identification test B is 5.5 to 7.5.

Sodium glycolate. *Carry out the test protected from light.*

Test solution. Place 0.20 g of the substance to be examined in a beaker. Add 5 ml of *acetic acid R* and 5 ml of *water R*. Stir until dissolution is complete (about 10 min). Add 50 ml of *acetone R* and 1 g of *sodium chloride R*. Filter through a fast filter paper impregnated with *acetone R*, rinse the beaker and filter with *acetone R*. Combine the filtrate and washings and dilute to 100.0 ml with *acetone R*. Allow to stand for 24 h without shaking. Use the clear supernatant liquid.

Reference solution. Dissolve 0.310 g of *glycollic acid R*, previously dried *in vacuo* over *diphosphorus pentoxide R*, in *water R* and dilute to 500.0 ml with the same solvent. To 5.0 ml of this solution, add 5 ml of *acetic acid R* and allow to stand for about 30 min. Add 50 ml of *acetone R* and 1 g of *sodium chloride R* and dilute to 100.0 ml with *acetone R*.

Heat 2.0 ml of the test solution on a water-bath for 20 min. Cool to room temperature and add 20.0 ml of *2,7-dihydroxynaphthalene solution R*. Shake and heat on a water-bath for 20 min. Cool under running water, transfer to a volumetric flask and dilute to 25.0 ml with *sulphuric acid R*, maintaining the flask under running water. Within 10 min, measure the absorbance at 540 nm (*2.2.25*) using *water R* as the compensation liquid. The absorbance of the solution prepared with the test solution is not greater than that of a solution prepared at the same time and in the same manner with 2.0 ml of the reference solution (2.0 per cent).

Sodium chloride. Not more than 1 per cent. Shake 1.00 g with 20 ml of *alcohol (80 per cent V/V) R* for 10 min and filter. Repeat the operation four times. Dry the residue to constant mass at 100 °C and set aside for the assay. Combine the filtrates. Evaporate to dryness, take up the residue with *water R* and dilute to 25.0 ml with the same solvent. To 10.0 ml of the solution add 30 ml of *water R* and 5 ml of *dilute nitric acid R*. Titrate with *0.1 M silver nitrate*, determining the end-point potentiometrically (*2.2.20*), using a silver indicator electrode.

1 ml of *0.1 M silver nitrate* is equivalent to 5.844 mg of NaCl.

Iron (*2.4.9*). 10 ml of solution S complies with the limit test for iron (20 ppm).

Heavy metals (*2.4.8*). 1.0 g complies with limit test D for heavy metals (20 ppm). Prepare the standard using 2 ml of *lead standard solution (10 ppm Pb) R*.

Loss on drying (*2.2.32*). Not more than 7.0 per cent, determined on 1.000 g by drying in an oven at 100 °C to 105 °C for 4 h.

Microbial contamination. It complies with the test for *Escherichia coli* and *Salmonella* (*2.6.13*).

ASSAY

To 0.500 g of the dried and crushed residue obtained in the test for sodium chloride add 80 ml of *anhydrous acetic acid R* and heat under a reflux condenser for 2 h. Cool the solution to room temperature. Titrate with *0.1 M perchloric acid*, determining the end-point potentiometrically (*2.2.20*). Carry out a blank test.

1 ml of *0.1 M perchloric acid* is equivalent to 2.299 mg of Na.

STORAGE

Store in an airtight container, protected from light.

01/2005:2058

SODIUM STEARATE

Natrii stearas

DEFINITION

Mixture of sodium salts of different fatty acids consisting mainly of stearic acid [$C_{17}H_{35}COONa$; M_r 306.5] and palmitic acid [$C_{15}H_{31}COONa$; M_r 278.4].

Content:

- sodium: 7.4 per cent to 8.5 per cent (A_r 22.99) (dried substance),
- stearic acid in the fatty acid fraction: minimum 40 per cent,
- sum of stearic acid and palmitic acid in the fatty acid fraction: minimum 90 per cent.

CHARACTERS

Appearance: white or yellowish, fine powder, with a greasy touch.

Solubility: slightly soluble in water and in alcohol.

IDENTIFICATION

First identification: C, D.

Monographs Q-S

Second identification: A, B, D.

A. Freezing point (*2.2.18*): minimum 53 °C for the residue obtained in the preparation of solution S (see Tests).

B. Acid value (*2.5.1*): 195 to 210, determined on 0.200 g of the residue obtained in the preparation of solution S dissolved in 25 ml of the prescribed mixture of solvents.

C. Examine the chromatograms obtained in the assay of stearic acid and palmitic acid.

Results: the 2 principal peaks in the chromatogram obtained with the test solution are similar in retention time and size to the 2 principal peaks in the chromatogram obtained with the reference solution.

D. Solution S gives reaction (b) of sodium (*2.3.1*).

TESTS

Solution S. To 10.0 g add 100 ml of *peroxide-free ether R* and 80 ml of *acetic acid R.* Boil under a reflux condenser until dissolution is complete. Allow to cool. In a separating funnel, separate the aqueous layer and shake the ether layer with 2 quantities, each of 8 ml, of *acetic acid R.* Combine the aqueous layers, wash with 30 ml of *peroxide-free ether R* and dilute to 100 ml with *distilled water R* (solution S). Evaporate the ether layers to dryness on a water-bath and dry the residue at 100-105 °C.

Acidity or alkalinity. Dissolve 2.0 g in 50 ml of previously neutralised *alcohol R* and add 3 drops of *phenolphthalein solution R*; the solution is colourless. Not less than 0.60 ml and not more than 0.85 ml of *0.1 M sodium hydroxide* is required to change the colour of the indicator.

Chlorides (*2.4.4*): maximum 0.1 per cent.

Dilute 0.5 ml of solution S to 15 ml with *water R.*

Sulphates (*2.4.13*): maximum 0.3 per cent.

Dilute 0.5 ml of solution S to 15 ml with *distilled water R.*

Nickel: maximum 5 ppm.

Atomic absorption spectrometry (*2.2.23, Method II*).

Test solution. Place 50.0 mg of the substance to be examined in a polytetrafluoroethylene digestion flask and add 0.5 ml of a mixture of 1 volume of *heavy metal-free hydrochloric acid R* and 5 volumes of *heavy metal-free nitric acid R.* Allow to digest at 170 °C for 5 h. Allow to cool. Dissolve the residue in *water R* and dilute to 5.0 ml with the same solvent.

Reference solutions. Prepare the reference solutions using *nickel standard solution (10 ppm Ni) R*, diluted as necessary with *water R.*

Source: nickel hollow-cathode lamp.

Wavelength: 232.0 nm.

Atomisation device: air-acetylene flame.

Loss on drying (*2.2.32*): maximum 5.0 per cent.

In a weighing glass introduce 1.0 g of previously washed *sand R*, dry at 100-105 °C and weigh. Add 0.500 g of the substance to be examined and 10 ml of *alcohol R.* Evaporate the alcohol at 80 °C and dry the residue at 100-105 °C for 4 h.

Microbial contamination. Total viable aerobic count (*2.6.12*) not more than 10^3 micro-organisms per gram, determined by plate count. It complies with the test for *Escherichia coli* (*2.6.13*).

ASSAY

Sodium. Dissolve 0.250 g with gentle heating in a mixture of 5 ml of *acetic anhydride R* and 20 ml of *anhydrous acetic acid R.* Cool and add 20 ml of *dioxan R.* Titrate with *0.1 M perchloric acid,* determining the end-point potentiometrically (*2.2.20*).

1 ml of *0.1 M perchloric acid* is equivalent to 2.299 mg of Na.

Stearic acid and palmitic acid. Gas chromatography (*2.2.28*): use the normalisation procedure.

Test solution. In a conical flask fitted with a reflux condenser, dissolve 0.10 g of the substance to be examined in 5 ml of *boron trifluoride-methanol solution R.* Boil under a reflux condenser for 10 min. Add 4 ml of *heptane R* through the condenser and boil again under a reflux condenser for 10 min. Allow to cool. Add 20 ml of *saturated sodium chloride solution R.* Shake and allow the layers to separate. Remove about 2 ml of the organic layer and dry over 0.2 g of *anhydrous sodium sulphate R.* Dilute 1.0 ml of the solution to 100.0 ml with *heptane R.*

Reference solution. Prepare the reference solution in the same manner as the test solution using 50.0 mg of *palmitic acid CRS* and 50.0 mg of *stearic acid CRS* instead of the substance to be examined.

Column:
- *material*: fused silica,
- *size*: *l* = 30 m, Ø = 0.32 mm,
- *stationary phase*: *macrogol 20 000 R* (film thickness 0.5 µm).

Carrier gas: *helium for chromatography R.*

Flow rate: 2.4 ml/min.

Temperature:

	Time (min)	Temperature (°C)
Column	0 - 2	70
	2 - 36	70 → 240
	36 - 41	240
Injection port		220
Detector		260

Detection: flame ionisation.

Injection: 1 µl.

Relative retention with reference to methyl stearate (retention time = about 40 min): methyl palmitate = about 0.88.

System suitability: reference solution:
- *resolution*: minimum 5.0 between the peaks due to methyl stearate and methyl palmitate.

Calculate the content of stearic acid and palmitic acid.

STORAGE

In an airtight container, protected from light.

01/2005:1567

SODIUM STEARYL FUMARATE

Natrii stearylis fumaras

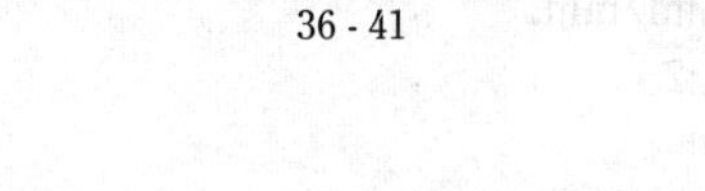

$C_{22}H_{39}NaO_4$ M_r 390.5

DEFINITION

Sodium octadecyl (*E*)-butenedioate.

Content: 99.0 per cent to 101.5 per cent (anhydrous substance).

CHARACTERS

Appearance: white or almost white, fine powder with agglomerates of flat, circular particles.

Solubility: practically insoluble in water, slightly soluble in methanol, practically insoluble in acetone and in ethanol.

IDENTIFICATION

Infrared absorption spectrophotometry (*2.2.24*).

Comparison: *sodium stearyl fumarate CRS.*

TESTS

Related substances. Gas chromatography (*2.2.28*): use the normalisation procedure.

Silylation solution. To 2 ml of *N,O-bis(trimethylsilyl)trifluoroacetamide R* add 0.02 ml of *chlorotrimethylsilane R* and mix.

Test solution. Introduce 15.0 mg of the substance to be examined in a vial with a screw cap and add 1 ml of the silylation solution. Seal the vial and heat at about 70 °C for 1 h. After the reaction a precipitate remains in the vial; filter the solution through a nylon filter (pore size 0.45 µm).

Reference solution. Introduce 1.0 mg of *sodium stearyl maleate CRS* and 1.0 mg of *sodium stearyl fumarate CRS* into a vial with a screw cap and add 1 ml of the silylation solution. Seal the vial and heat at about 70 °C for 1 h.

Column:

– *material*: fused silica,
– *size*: *l* = 15 m, Ø = 0.53 mm,
– *stationary phase*: *poly(dimethyl)siloxane R* (film thickness 0.15 µm).

Carrier gas: *helium for chromatography R.*

Flow rate: 2 ml/min.

Split ratio: 1:25.

Temperature:

	Time (min)	Temperature (°C)
Column	0 - 1	180
	1 - 21	180 → 320
	21 - 26	320
Injection port		250
Detector		320

Detection: flame ionisation.

Injection: 2 µl.

Relative retention with reference to stearyl trimethylsilyl fumarate (retention time = about 9 min): stearyl alcohol = 0.30; stearyl trimethylsilyl ether = 0.35; palmityl trimethylsilyl fumarate = 0.80; heptadecyl trimethylsilyl fumarate = 0.85; stearyl trimethylsilyl maleate = 0.90; nonadecyl trimethylsilyl fumarate = 1.05; eicos-11-enyl trimethylsilyl fumarate = 1.15; distearyl fumarate = 2.25.

System suitability:

– *resolution*: minimum 1.5 between the peaks in the chromatogram obtained with the reference solution.

Limits:

– *any impurity*: maximum 0.5 per cent,
– *total*: maximum 5.0 per cent.

Water (*2.5.12*): maximum 5.0 per cent, determined on 0.250 g.

ASSAY

Dissolve 0.250 g, accurately weighed, in 10 ml of *methylene chloride R* and add 30 ml of *anhydrous acetic acid R.* Titrate with *0.1 M perchloric acid,* determining the end-point potentiometrically (*2.2.20*).

1 ml of *0.1 M perchloric acid* is equivalent to 39.05 mg of $C_{22}H_{39}NaO_4$.

01/2005:0099

SODIUM SULPHATE, ANHYDROUS

Natrii sulfas anhydricus

Na_2SO_4 M_r 142.0

DEFINITION

Content: 98.5 per cent to 101.0 per cent (dried substance).

CHARACTERS

Appearance: white powder, hygroscopic.

Solubility: freely soluble in water.

IDENTIFICATION

A. It gives the reactions of sulphates (*2.3.1*).

B. It gives the reactions of sodium (*2.3.1*).

C. It complies with the test for loss on drying (see Tests).

TESTS

Solution S. Dissolve 2.2 g in *carbon dioxide-free water R* prepared from *distilled water R* and dilute to 100 ml with the same solvent.

Appearance of solution. Solution S is clear (*2.2.1*) and colourless (*2.2.2, Method II*).

Acidity or alkalinity. To 10 ml of solution S add 0.1 ml of *bromothymol blue solution R1.* Not more than 0.5 ml of *0.01 M hydrochloric acid* or *0.01 M sodium hydroxide* is required to change the colour of the indicator.

Chlorides (*2.4.4*): maximum 450 ppm.

5 ml of solution S diluted to 15 ml with *water R* complies with the limit test for chlorides.

Calcium (*2.4.3*): maximum 450 ppm, if intended for use in the manufacture of parenteral dosage forms.

10 ml of solution S diluted to 15 ml with *distilled water R* complies with the limit test for calcium.

Iron (*2.4.9*): maximum 90 ppm, if intended for use in the manufacture of parenteral dosage forms.

5 ml of solution S diluted to 10 ml with *water R* complies with the limit test for iron.

Magnesium: maximum 200 ppm, if intended for use in the manufacture of parenteral dosage forms.

To 10 ml of solution S add 1 ml of *glycerol (85 per cent) R*, 0.15 ml of *titan yellow solution R*, 0.25 ml of *ammonium oxalate solution R* and 5 ml of *dilute sodium hydroxide solution R* and shake. Any pink colour in the test solution is not more intense than that in a standard prepared at the same time in the same manner using a mixture of 5 ml of *magnesium standard solution (10 ppm Mg) R* and 5 ml of *water R.*

Heavy metals (*2.4.8*): maximum 45 ppm.

12 ml of solution S complies with limit test A. Prepare the standard using *lead standard solution (1 ppm Pb) R.*

Monographs Q-S

Loss on drying (*2.2.32*): maximum 0.5 per cent, determined on 1.000 g by drying in an oven at 130 °C.

ASSAY

Dissolve 0.100 g in 40 ml of *water R*. Add a mixture of 0.2 ml of *0.1 M hydrochloric acid* and 80 ml of *methanol R*. Carry out a potentiometric titration (*2.2.20*), using *0.1 M lead nitrate* and as indicator electrode a lead-selective electrode and as reference electrode a silver-silver chloride electrode.

1 ml of *0.1 M lead nitrate* is equivalent to 14.20 mg of Na_2SO_4.

STORAGE

Store in an airtight container.

LABELLING

The label states, where applicable, that the substance is suitable for use in the manufacture of parenteral dosage forms.

01/2005:0100

SODIUM SULPHATE DECAHYDRATE

Natrii sulfas decahydricus

$Na_2SO_4,10H_2O$ M_r 322.2

DEFINITION

Content: 98.5 per cent to 101.0 per cent (dried substance).

CHARACTERS

Appearance: white, crystalline powder or colourless, transparent crystals.

Solubility: freely soluble in water, practically insoluble in alcohol. It partly dissolves in its own water of crystallisation at about 33 °C.

IDENTIFICATION

A. It gives the reactions of sulphates (*2.3.1*).

B. It gives the reactions of sodium (*2.3.1*).

C. It complies with the test for loss on drying (see Tests).

TESTS

Solution S. Dissolve 5.0 g in *carbon dioxide-free water R* prepared from *distilled water R* and dilute to 100 ml with the same solvent.

Appearance of solution. Solution S is clear (*2.2.1*) and colourless (*2.2.2, Method II*).

Acidity or alkalinity. To 10 ml of solution S add 0.1 ml of *bromothymol blue solution R1*. Not more than 0.5 ml of *0.01 M hydrochloric acid* or *0.01 M sodium hydroxide* is required to change the colour of the indicator.

Chlorides (*2.4.4*): maximum 200 ppm.

5 ml of solution S diluted to 15 ml with *water R* complies with the limit test for chlorides.

Calcium (*2.4.3*): maximum 200 ppm, if intended for use in the manufacture of parenteral dosage forms.

10 ml of solution S diluted to 15 ml with *distilled water R* complies with the limit test for calcium.

Iron (*2.4.9*): maximum 40 ppm, if intended for use in the manufacture of parenteral dosage forms.

5 ml of solution S diluted to 10 ml with *water R* complies with the limit test for iron.

Magnesium: maximum 100 ppm, if intended for use in the manufacture of parenteral dosage forms.

To 10 ml of solution S add 1 ml of *glycerol (85 per cent) R*, 0.15 ml of *titan yellow solution R*, 0.25 ml of *ammonium oxalate solution R* and 5 ml of *dilute sodium hydroxide solution R* and shake. Any pink colour in the test solution is not more intense than that in a standard prepared at the same time in the same manner using a mixture of 5 ml of *magnesium standard solution (10 ppm Mg) R* and 5 ml of *water R*.

Heavy metals (*2.4.8*): maximum 20 ppm.

12 ml of solution S complies with limit test A. Prepare the standard using *lead standard solution (1 ppm Pb) R*.

Loss on drying (*2.2.32*): 52.0 per cent to 57.0 per cent, determined on 1.000 g by drying at 30 °C for 1 h, then at 130 °C.

ASSAY

Dissolve 0.250 g in 40 ml of *water R*. Add a mixture of 0.2 ml of *0.1 M hydrochloric acid* and 80 ml of *methanol R*. Carry out a potentiometric titration (*2.2.20*), using *0.1 M lead nitrate* and as indicator electrode a lead-selective electrode and as reference electrode a silver-silver chloride electrode.

1 ml of *0.1 M lead nitrate* is equivalent to 14.20 mg of Na_2SO_4.

LABELLING

The label states, where applicable, that the substance is suitable for use in the manufacture of parenteral dosage forms.

01/2005:0775

SODIUM SULPHITE, ANHYDROUS

Natrii sulfis anhydricus

Na_2SO_3 M_r 126.0

DEFINITION

Anhydrous sodium sulphite contains not less than 95.0 per cent and not more than the equivalent of 100.5 per cent of Na_2SO_3.

CHARACTERS

A white powder, freely soluble in water, very slightly soluble in alcohol.

IDENTIFICATION

A. Solution S (see Tests) is slightly alkaline (*2.2.4*).

B. To 5 ml of solution S, add 0.5 ml of *0.05 M iodine*. The solution is colourless and gives reaction (a) of sulphates (*2.3.1*).

C. Solution S gives reaction (a) of sodium (*2.3.1*).

D. It complies with the limits of the assay.

TESTS

Solution S. Dissolve 5 g in *water R* and dilute to 100 ml with the same solvent.

Solution S1. To 10.0 g add 25 ml of *water R*. Shake until mostly dissolved and carefully and progressively add 15 ml of *hydrochloric acid R*. Heat to boiling. Cool and dilute to 100.0 ml with *water R*.

Appearance of solution. Solution S is clear (*2.2.1*) and colourless (*2.2.2, Method I*).

Monographs Q-S

Thiosulphates. To 2.00 g add 100 ml of *water R*. Shake and add 10 ml of *formaldehyde solution R* and 10 ml of *acetic acid R*. Allow to stand for 5 min. Add 0.5 ml of *starch solution R* and titrate with *0.05 M iodine*. Carry out a blank titration. The difference between the volumes used in the titrations is not more than 0.15 ml (0.1 per cent).

Iron (*2.4.9*). 10 ml of solution S1 complies with the limit test for iron (10 ppm).

Selenium. To 3.0 g add 10 ml of *formaldehyde solution R* and carefully and progressively add 2 ml of *hydrochloric acid R*. Heat on a water-bath for 20 min. Any pink colour in the solution is not more intense than that of a standard prepared at the same time and in the same manner using 1.0 g of the substance to be examined to which has been added 0.2 ml of *selenium standard solution (100 ppm Se) R* (10 ppm).

Zinc. Not more than 25 ppm of Zn, determined by atomic absorption spectrometry (*2.2.23, Method I*).

Test solution. Dilute 2.0 ml of solution S1 to 10.0 ml with *water R*.

Reference solutions. Prepare the reference solutions using *zinc standard solution (100 ppm Zn) R*, diluted as necessary with *water R*.

Measure the absorbance at 213.9 nm using a zinc hollow-cathode lamp as source of radiation and an air-acetylene flame.

Heavy metals (*2.4.8*). 12 ml of solution S1 complies with limit test A for heavy metals (10 ppm). Prepare the standard using *lead standard solution (1 ppm Pb) R*.

ASSAY

Introduce 0.250 g into a 500 ml conical flask containing 50.0 ml of *0.05 M iodine*. Shake until completely dissolved. Add 1 ml of *starch solution R* and titrate the excess of iodine with *0.1 M sodium thiosulphate*. Carry out a blank titration.

1 ml of *0.05 M iodine* is equivalent to 6.30 mg of Na_2SO_3.

STORAGE

Store in an airtight container.

01/2005:0776

SODIUM SULPHITE HEPTAHYDRATE

Natrii sulfis heptahydricus

$Na_2SO_3,7H_2O$ M_r 252.2

DEFINITION

Sodium sulphite heptahydrate contains not less than 48.0 per cent and not more than the equivalent of 52.5 per cent of Na_2SO_3.

CHARACTERS

Colourless crystals, freely soluble in water, very slightly soluble in alcohol.

IDENTIFICATION

A. Solution S (see Tests) is slightly alkaline (*2.2.4*).

B. To 5 ml of solution S, add 0.5 ml of *0.05 M iodine*. The solution is colourless and gives reaction (a) of sulphates (*2.3.1*).

C. Solution S gives reaction (a) of sodium (*2.3.1*).

D. It complies with the limits of the assay.

TESTS

Solution S. Dissolve 10 g in *water R* and dilute to 100 ml with the same solvent.

Solution S1. To 20.0 g add 25 ml of *water R*. Shake until mostly dissolved and carefully and progressively add 15 ml of *hydrochloric acid R*. Heat to boiling. Cool and dilute to 100.0 ml with *water R*.

Appearance of solution. Solution S is clear (*2.2.1*) and colourless (*2.2.2, Method I*).

Thiosulphates. To 4.00 g add 100 ml of *water R*. Shake to dissolve and add 10 ml of *formaldehyde solution R* and 10 ml of *acetic acid R*. Allow to stand for 5 min. Add 0.5 ml of *starch solution R* and titrate with *0.05 M iodine*. Carry out a blank titration. The difference between the volumes used in the titrations is not more than 0.15 ml (0.05 per cent).

Iron (*2.4.9*). 10 ml of solution S1 complies with the limit test for iron (5 ppm).

Selenium. To 6.0 g add 10 ml of *formaldehyde solution R* and carefully and progressively add 2 ml of *hydrochloric acid R*. Heat on a water-bath for 20 min. Any pink colour in the solution is not more intense than that of a standard prepared at the same time and in the same manner using 2.0 g of the substance to be examined to which has been added 0.2 ml of *selenium standard solution (100 ppm Se) R* (5 ppm).

Zinc. Not more than 12 ppm of Zn, determined by atomic absorption spectrometry (*2.2.23, Method I*).

Test solution. Dilute 2.0 ml of solution S1 to 10.0 ml with *water R*.

Reference solutions. Prepare the reference solutions using *zinc standard solution (100 ppm Zn) R*, diluted as necessary with *water R*.

Measure the absorbance at 213.9 nm using a zinc hollow-cathode lamp as source of radiation and an air-acetylene flame.

Heavy metals (*2.4.8*). 12 ml of solution S1 complies with limit test A for heavy metals (5 ppm). Prepare the standard using *lead standard solution (1 ppm Pb) R*.

ASSAY

Introduce 0.500 g into a 500 ml conical flask containing 50.0 ml of *0.05 M iodine*. Shake until completely dissolved. Add 1 ml of *starch solution R* and titrate the excess of iodine with *0.1 M sodium thiosulphate*. Carry out a blank titration.

1 ml of *0.05 M iodine* is equivalent to 6.30 mg of Na_2SO_3.

01/2005:0414

SODIUM THIOSULPHATE

Natrii thiosulfas

$Na_2S_2O_3,5H_2O$ M_r 248.2

DEFINITION

Sodium thiosulphate contains not less than 99.0 per cent and not more than the equivalent of 101.0 per cent of $Na_2S_2O_3,5H_2O$.

CHARACTERS

Transparent, colourless crystals, efflorescent in dry air, very soluble in water, practically insoluble in alcohol. It dissolves in its water of crystallisation at about 49 °C.

IDENTIFICATION

A. It decolourises *iodinated potassium iodide solution R*.

B. To 0.5 ml of solution S (see Tests) add 0.5 ml of *water R* and 2 ml of *silver nitrate solution R2*. A white precipitate is formed which rapidly becomes yellowish and then black.

C. To 2.5 ml of solution S add 2.5 ml of *water R* and 1 ml of *hydrochloric acid R*. A precipitate of sulphur is formed and gas is evolved which gives a blue colour to *starch iodate paper R*.

D. 1 ml of solution S gives reaction (a) of sodium (*2.3.1*).

TESTS

Solution S. Dissolve 10.0 g in *carbon dioxide-free water R* prepared from *distilled water R* and dilute to 100 ml with the same solvent.

Appearance of solution. Solution S is clear (*2.2.1*) and colourless (*2.2.2, Method II*).

pH (*2.2.3*). The pH of solution S is 6.0 to 8.4.

Sulphates and sulphites. Dilute 2.5 ml of solution S to 10 ml with *distilled water R*. To 3 ml of this solution first add 2 ml of *iodinated potassium iodide solution R* and continue the addition dropwise until a very faint persistent yellow colour appears. Dilute to 15 ml with *distilled water R*. The solution complies with the limit test for sulphates (*2.4.13*) (0.2 per cent).

Sulphides. To 10 ml of solution S add 0.05 ml of a freshly prepared 50 g/l solution of *sodium nitroprusside R*. The solution does not become violet.

Heavy metals. To 10 ml of solution S add 0.05 ml of *sodium sulphide solution R*. After 2 min, any brown colour in the solution is not more intense than that in a standard prepared at the same time and in the same manner using 10 ml of *lead standard solution (1 ppm Pb) R* (10 ppm).

ASSAY

Dissolve 0.500 g in 20 ml of *water R* and titrate with *0.05 M iodine*, using 1 ml of *starch solution R*, added towards the end of the titration, as indicator.

1 ml of *0.05 M iodine* is equivalent to 24.82 mg of $Na_2S_2O_3,5H_2O$.

STORAGE

Store in an airtight container.

01/2005:0678

SODIUM VALPROATE

Natrii valproas

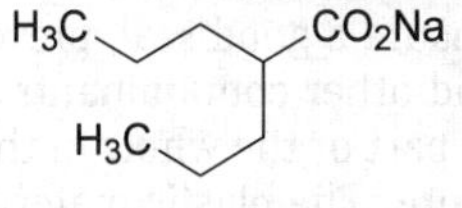

$C_8H_{15}NaO_2$ M_r 166.2

DEFINITION

Sodium valproate contains not less than 98.5 per cent and not more than the equivalent of 101.0 per cent of sodium 2-propylpentanoate, calculated with reference to the dried substance.

CHARACTERS

A white or almost white, crystalline powder, hygroscopic, very soluble in water, slightly to freely soluble in alcohol.

IDENTIFICATION

A. Examine by infrared absorption spectrophotometry (*2.2.24*), comparing with the spectrum obtained with *sodium valproate CRS*. If the spectra obtained in the solid state for the substance to be examined and the reference substance show differences, record further spectra using discs prepared by placing 50 µl of a 100 g/l solution in *methanol R* on a disc of *potassium bromide R* and evaporating the solvent *in vacuo*. Use the discs immediately.

B. Examine the chromatograms obtained in the test for related substances. The retention time of the principal peak in the chromatogram obtained with test solution (b) corresponds to that of the principal peak in the chromatogram obtained with reference solution (b).

C. 2 ml of solution S (see Tests) gives reaction (a) of sodium (*2.3.1*).

TESTS

Solution S. Dissolve 1.25 g in 20 ml of *distilled water R* in a separating funnel, add 5 ml of *dilute nitric acid R* and shake. Allow the mixture to stand for 12 h. Use the lower layer.

Appearance of solution. Dissolve 2.0 g in *water R* and dilute to 10 ml with the same solvent. The solution is not more opalescent than reference suspension II (*2.2.1*) and not more intensely coloured than reference solution Y_6 (*2.2.2, Method II*).

Acidity or alkalinity. Dissolve 1.0 g in 10 ml of *water R*. Add 0.1 ml of *phenolphthalein solution R*. Not more than 0.75 ml of *0.1 M hydrochloric acid* or *0.1 M sodium hydroxide* is required to change the colour of the indicator.

Related substances. Examine by gas chromatography (*2.2.28*), using *butyric acid R* as the internal standard.

Internal standard solution. Dissolve 10 mg of *butyric acid R* in *heptane R* and dilute to 200 ml with the same solvent.

Test solution (a). Dissolve 0.500 g of the substance to be examined in 10 ml of *water R*. Add 5 ml of *dilute sulphuric acid R* and shake with three quantities, each of 20 ml, of *heptane R*. Add 10.0 ml of the internal standard solution to the combined upper layers, shake with *anhydrous sodium sulphate R*, filter and evaporate the filtrate, at a temperature not exceeding 30 °C, using a rotary evaporator. Take up the residue with *heptane R* and dilute to 10.0 ml with the same solvent. Dilute 1.0 ml of the solution to 10.0 ml with *heptane R*.

Test solution (b). Dissolve 40 mg of the substance to be examined in 100 ml of *water R*. To 10 ml of the solution add 0.5 ml of *dilute sulphuric acid R* and shake with three quantities, each of 5 ml, of *heptane R*. Shake with *anhydrous sodium sulphate R*, filter and evaporate the filtrate, at a temperature not exceeding 30 °C, to a volume of about 10 ml, using a rotary evaporator.

Reference solution (a). Dissolve 20 mg of *2-(1-methylethyl)pentanoic acid CRS* in 5.0 ml of test solution (b)and dilute to 10 ml with *heptane R*. Dilute 1 ml of the solution to 10 ml with *heptane R*.

Reference solution (b). Prepare as prescribed for test solution (b), using *sodium valproate CRS* instead of the substance to be examined.

The chromatographic procedure may be carried out using:

– a wide-bore fused-silica column 30 m long and 0.53 mm in internal diameter coated with *macrogol 20 000 2-nitroterephthalate R* (film thickness 0.5 µm),
– *helium for chromatography R* as the carrier gas at a flow rate of 8 ml/min,
– a flame-ionisation detector,

Monographs Q-S

with the following temperature programme:

	Time (min)	Temperature (°C)	Rate (°C/min)	Comment
Column	0 - 10	130	-	isothermal
	10 - 30	130 → 190	3	linear gradient
Injection port		220		
Detector		220		

Inject 1 µl of each solution. Adjust the sensitivity of the system so that the height of the peak due to the internal standard is at least 20 per cent of the full scale of the recorder. The test is not valid unless, in the chromatogram obtained with reference solution (a), the resolution between the peaks corresponding to 2-(1-methylethyl)pentanoic acid and valproic acid is at least 3.0. In the chromatogram obtained with test solution (a): the sum of the areas of the peaks, apart from the principal peak is not greater than three times the area of the peak due to the internal standard (0.3 per cent); none of the peaks, apart from the principal peak, has an area greater than that of the peak due to the internal standard (0.1 per cent). Disregard any peak with an area less than 0.1 times the area of the peak due to the internal standard.

Chlorides (*2.4.4*). To 5 ml of solution S add 10 ml of *water R*. The solution complies with the limit test for chlorides (200 ppm).

Sulphates (*2.4.13*). Solution S complies with the limit test for sulphates (200 ppm).

Heavy metals (*2.4.8*). 1.0 g complies with limit test C for heavy metals (20 ppm). Prepare the standard using 2 ml of *lead standard solution (10 ppm Pb) R*.

Loss on drying (*2.2.32*). Not more than 2.0 per cent, determined on 1.000 g by drying in an oven at 100 °C to 105 °C.

ASSAY

Dissolve 0.1500 g in 25 ml of *anhydrous acetic acid R*. Titrate with *0.1 M perchloric acid* determining the end-point potentiometrically (*2.2.20*).

1 ml of *0.1 M perchloric acid*, is equivalent to 16.62 mg of $C_8H_{15}NaO_2$.

STORAGE

Store in an airtight container.

IMPURITIES

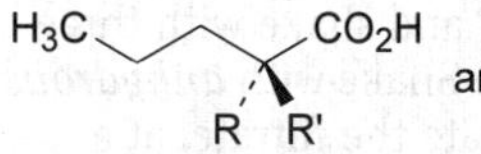

and enantiomer

A. R = R′ = H: pentanoic acid (valeric acid),

B. R = H, R′ = CH_2-CH_3: (*2RS*)-2-ethylpentanoic acid,

C. R = H, R′ = $CH(CH_3)_2$: (*2RS*)-2-(1-methylethyl)pentanoic acid,

D. R = R′ = CH_2-CH_2-CH_3: 2,2-dipropylpentanoic acid,

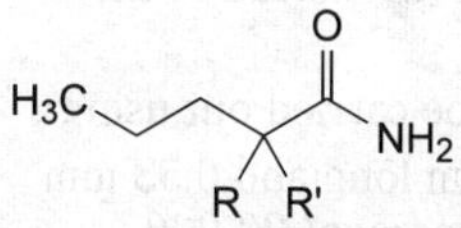

E. R = R′ = H: pentanamide (valeramide),

F. R = H, R′ = CH_2-CH_2-CH_3: 2-propylpentanamide,

G. R = R′ = CH_2-CH_2-CH_3: 2,2-dipropylpentanamide,

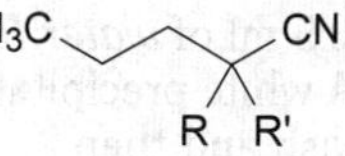

H. R = R′ = H: pentanenitrile (valeronitrile),

I. R = H, R′ = CH_2-CH_2-CH_3: 2-propylpentanenitrile,

J. R = R′ = CH_2-CH_2-CH_3: 2,2-dipropylpentanenitrile.

01/2005:1264

SOLUTIONS FOR ORGAN PRESERVATION

Solutiones ad conservationem partium corporis

DEFINITION

Solutions for organ preservation are sterile, aqueous preparations, intended for storage, protection and/or perfusion of mammalian body organs that are in particular destined for transplantation.

They contain electrolytes that are typically at a concentration close to the intracellular electrolyte composition.

They may contain carbohydrates (such as glucose or mannitol), amino acids, calcium-complexing agents (such as citrate or phosphate), hydrocolloids (such as starch or gelatin derivatives) and other excipients, for example to make the preparation isotonic with blood, to adjust or buffer the pH, to prevent deterioration of the ingredients, but not to adversely affect the intended action of the preparation or, at the concentration used, to cause toxicity or undue local irritation. Solutions for organ preservation may also contain active substances or these may be added immediately before use.

Solutions for organ preservation, examined under suitable conditions of visibility, are clear and practically free from particles.

Solutions for organ preservation may also be presented as concentrated solutions. They are diluted to the prescribed volume with a prescribed liquid immediately before use. After dilution, they comply with the requirements for solutions for organ preservation.

Before use, the solutions for organ preservation are cooled below room temperature, typically to 2 °C to 6 °C, to reduce the temperature of the body organ and its metabolism.

Where applicable, the containers for solutions for organ preservation comply with the requirements for *Materials used for the manufacture of containers* (*3.1* and subsections) and *Containers* (*3.2* and subsections). Solutions for organ preservation are supplied in glass containers (*3.2.1*) or in other containers such as plastic containers (*3.2.2* and *3.2.8*). The tightness of the container is ensured by suitable means. Closures ensure a good seal, prevent the access of micro-organisms and other contaminants and usually permit the withdrawal of a part or the whole of the contents without removal of the closure. The plastic materials or elastomers of which the closure is composed are sufficiently firm and elastic to allow the passage of a needle with the least possible shedding of particles.

PRODUCTION

Solutions for organ preservation are prepared using materials and methods designed to ensure their sterility and to avoid the introduction of contaminants and the growth of micro-organisms; recommendations on this aspect are provided in the text on *Methods of preparation of sterile products* (*5.1.1*).

Unless otherwise justified and authorised, solutions for organ preservation are prepared from *water for injections R* and do not contain antimicrobial preservatives.

TESTS

pH (*2.2.3*). *Carry out the test at room temperature*. The pH of the solution is 5.0 to 8.0.

Osmolality (*2.2.35*). The osmolality of the solution is 250 mosmol/kg to 380 mosmol/kg.

Hydroxymethylfurfural. If the solution contains glucose, it complies with the following test: to a volume of the preparation to be examined containing the equivalent of 25 mg of glucose, add 5.0 ml of a 100 g/l solution of *p-toluidine R* in *2-propanol R* containing 10 per cent *V/V* of *glacial acetic acid R* and 1.0 ml of a 5 g/l solution of *barbituric acid R*. The absorbance (*2.2.25*), determined at 550 nm after allowing the mixture to stand for 2 min to 3 min, is not greater than that of a standard prepared at the same time in the same manner using a solution containing 10 μg of *hydroxymethylfurfural R* in the same volume as the preparation to be examined.

Particulate contamination. Carry out the test for sub-visible particles (*2.9.19*) using 50 ml of preparation to be examined. The solution contains not more than 50 particles per millilitre larger than 10 μm and not more than 5 particles per millilitre larger than 25 μm.

Products for which the label states that the product is to be used with a final filter are exempted from these requirements.

Sterility (*2.6.1*). The solution complies with the test for sterility.

Bacterial endotoxins (*2.6.14*): less than 0.5 IU/ml.

Pyrogens (*2.6.8*). Solutions for which a validated test for bacterial endotoxins cannot be carried out comply with the test for pyrogens. Inject per kilogram of the rabbit's mass 10 ml of the solution, unless otherwise justified and authorised.

LABELLING

The label states:

- that the solution is not to be used for injection,
- the formula of the solution for organ preservation expressed in grams per litre and in millimoles per litre,
- the nominal volume of the solution for organ preservation in the container,
- the osmolality, expressed in milliosmoles per kilogram,
- that any unused portion of the ready-to-use solution, of the concentrated solution or of the diluted solution must be discarded,
- the storage conditions,
- if applicable, that the solution is to be used in conjunction with a final filter.

In addition, for concentrated solutions the label states that the solution must be diluted with a suitable liquid immediately before use.

01/2005:0949

SOMATOSTATIN

Somatostatinum

H-Ala-Gly-Cys-Lys-Asn-Phe-Phe-Trp-Lys-Thr-Phe-Thr-Ser-Cys-OH

$C_{76}H_{104}N_{18}O_{19}S_2$ M_r 1638

DEFINITION

Somatostatin is a cyclic tetradecapeptide having the structure of the hypothalamic hormone that inhibits the release of human growth hormone. It is obtained by chemical synthesis. It contains a variable amount of acetic acid. It is available in the freeze-dried form.

Content: 95.0 per cent to 103.0 per cent of somatostatin (anhydrous and acetic acid-free substance).

CHARACTERS

Appearance: white, amorphous powder.

Solubility: freely soluble in water and in acetic acid, practically insoluble in methylene chloride.

IDENTIFICATION

A. Thin-layer chromatography (*2.2.27*).

Test solution. Dissolve 1.0 mg of the substance to be examined in 1.0 ml of *water R*.

Reference solution. Dissolve the contents of a vial of *somatostatin CRS* in *water R* and dilute with the same solvent to obtain a final concentration of 1 mg/ml.

Plate: *TLC silica gel plate R*.

Mobile phase: *glacial acetic acid R, pyridine R, water R, butanol R* (10:15:20:45 *V/V/V/V*).

Application: 20 μl.

Development: over a path of 15 cm.

Drying: in a current of warm air.

Detection: spray with a 1 g/l solution of *ninhydrin R* and heat the plate in an oven at 110 °C for about 5 min.

Results: the principal spot in the chromatogram obtained with the test solution is similar in position, colour and size to the principal spot in the chromatogram obtained with the reference solution.

B. Examine the chromatograms obtained in the assay.

Results: the principal peak in the chromatogram obtained with the test solution is similar in retention time to the principal peak in the chromatogram obtained with the reference solution.

TESTS

Specific optical rotation (*2.2.7*): − 37 to − 47 (anhydrous and acetic acid-free substance).

Dissolve 2.0 mg in 1.0 ml of a 1.0 per cent *V/V* solution of *glacial acetic acid R*.

Absorbance (*2.2.25*): maximum 0.20 at 280 nm (calculated with reference to the peptide content as determined in the assay).

Dissolve 5.0 mg in a 9 g/l solution of *sodium chloride R* and dilute to 100.0 ml with the same solvent.

Amino acids. Examine by means of an amino-acid analyser. Standardise the apparatus with a mixture containing equimolar amounts of ammonia, glycine and the L-form of the following amino acids:

Lysine	Threonine	Alanine	Leucine
Histidine	Serine	Valine	Tyrosine
Arginine	Glutamic acid	Methionine	Phenylalanine
Aspartic acid	Proline	Isoleucine	

together with half the equimolar amount of L-cystine. For the validation of the method, an appropriate internal standard, such as *DL-norleucine R*, is used.

Test solution. Place 1.0 mg of the substance to be examined in a rigorously cleaned hard-glass tube 100 mm long and 6 mm in internal diameter. Add a suitable amount of a

50 per cent *V/V* solution of *hydrochloric acid R*. Immerse the tube in a freezing mixture at − 5 °C, reduce the pressure to below 133 Pa and seal. Heat at 110-115 °C for 16 h. Cool, open the tube, transfer the contents to a 10 ml flask with the aid of 5 quantities, each of 0.2 ml, of *water R* and evaporate to dryness over *potassium hydroxide R* under reduced pressure. Take up the residue in *water R* and evaporate to dryness over *potassium hydroxide R* under reduced pressure; repeat these operations once. Take up the residue in a buffer solution suitable for the amino-acid analyser used and dilute to a suitable volume with the same buffer solution.

Apply a suitable volume to the amino-acid analyser.

Express the content of each amino acid in moles. Calculate the relative proportions of the amino acids taking one eighth of the sum of the number of moles of aspartic acid, alanine, lysine, glycine and phenylalanine as equal to one. The values fall within the following limits: aspartic acid 0.95 to 1.05; glycine 0.95 to 1.05; alanine 0.95 to 1.05; phenylalanine 2.85 to 3.15; serine 0.7 to 1.05; threonine 1.4 to 2.1; half-cystine 1.4 to 2.1; lysine 1.9 to 2.1. Not more than traces of other amino acids are present.

Related peptides. Liquid chromatography (*2.2.29*): use the normalisation procedure.

Test solution. Dissolve 5.0 mg of the substance to be examined in *water R* and dilute to 10.0 ml with the same solvent.

Column:

- *size*: *l* = 0.05 m, Ø = 4.6 mm,
- *stationary phase*: *octadecylsilyl silica gel for chromatography R* (5 µm).

Mobile phase:

- *mobile phase A*: dilute 11 ml of *phosphoric acid R* with *water R*, adjust to pH 2.3 with *triethylamine R* and dilute to 1000 ml with *water R*,
- *mobile phase B*: *acetonitrile for chromatography R*,

Time (min)	Mobile phase A (per cent *V/V*)	Mobile phase B (per cent *V/V*)
0 - 18	79 → 60	21 → 40
18 - 20	60	40
20 - 21	60 → 79	40 → 21
21 - 26	79	21

Flow rate: 1.5 ml/min.

Detection: spectrophotometer at 215 nm.

Injection: 25 µl.

Limits:

- *any impurity*: maximum 1 per cent,
- *total*: maximum 2 per cent,
- *disregard limit*: 0.03 per cent.

Acetic acid (*2.5.34*): 3.0 per cent to 15.0 per cent.

Test solution. Dissolve 7.0 mg of the substance to be examined in a mixture of 5 volumes of mobile phase B and 95 volumes of mobile phase A and dilute to 10.0 ml with the same mixture of solvents.

Water (*2.5.12*): maximum 8.0 per cent, determined on 10.0 mg.

Bacterial endotoxins (*2.6.14*): less than 10 IU/mg, if intended for use in the manufacture of parenteral dosage forms without a further appropriate procedure for the removal of bacterial endotoxins.

ASSAY

Liquid chromatography (*2.2.29*).

Test solution. Dissolve 5.0 mg of the substance to be examined in *water R* and dilute to 10.0 ml with the same solvent.

Reference solution. Dissolve the contents of a vial of *somatostatin CRS* in *water R* and dilute with the same solvent to obtain a final concentration of 0.5 mg/ml.

Column:

- *size*: *l* = 0.05 m, Ø = 4.6 mm,
- *stationary phase*: *octadecylsilyl silica gel for chromatography R* (5 µm).

Mobile phase: mix 25 volumes of mobile phase B and 75 volumes of mobile phase A,

- *mobile phase A*: dilute 11 ml of *phosphoric acid R* with *water R*, adjust to pH 2.3 with *triethylamine R* and dilute to 1000 ml with *water R*,
- *mobile phase B*: *acetonitrile for chromatography R*.

Flow rate: 1.5 ml/min.

Detection: spectrophotometer at 215 nm.

Injection: 25 µl.

Run time: 15 min.

Calculate the content of somatostatin ($C_{76}H_{104}N_{18}O_{19}S_2$) using the chromatograms obtained with the test solution and the reference solution and the declared content of $C_{76}H_{104}N_{18}O_{19}S_2$ in *somatostatin CRS*.

STORAGE

In an airtight container protected from light, at a temperature of 2 °C to 8 °C. If the substance is sterile, store in a sterile, airtight, tamper-proof container.

LABELLING

The label states, where applicable, that the substance is free from bacterial endotoxins.

01/2005:0951
corrected

SOMATROPIN

Somatropinum

$C_{990}H_{1528}N_{262}O_{300}S_7$ M_r 22 125

DEFINITION

Somatropin is a protein having the structure (191 amino-acid residues) of the major component of growth hormone produced by the human pituitary. It contains not less than 91.0 per cent and not more than the equivalent of 105.0 per cent of somatropin(1) ($C_{990}H_{1528}N_{262}O_{300}S_7$), calculated with reference to the anhydrous substance.

PRODUCTION

Somatropin is produced by a method based on recombinant DNA (rDNA) technology. During the course of product development, it must be demonstrated that the manufacturing process produces a product having a biological activity of not less than 2.5 IU/mg, using a validated bioassay based on growth promotion and approved by the competent authority.

Somatropin complies with the following additional requirements.

(1) 1 mg of anhydrous somatropin ($C_{990}H_{1528}N_{262}O_{300}S_7$) is equivalent to 3.0 IU of biological activity.

Monographs Q-S

Host-cell-derived proteins. The limit is approved by the competent authority.

Host-cell- and vector-derived DNA. The limit is approved by the competent authority.

CHARACTERS

A white or almost white powder.

IDENTIFICATION

A. Examine the electropherograms obtained in the test for isoform distribution. In the electropherogram obtained with test solution (a), the principal band corresponds in position to that in the electropherogram obtained with reference solution (a).

B. Examine the chromatograms obtained in the test for related proteins. The retention time of the principal peak in the chromatogram obtained with the test solution is similar to that of the principal peak in the chromatogram obtained with the reference solution.

C. Examine by peptide mapping.

Test solution. Prepare a solution of the substance to be examined in *0.05 M tris-hydrochloride buffer solution pH 7.5 R* to obtain a solution containing 2.0 mg/ml of somatropin and transfer about 1.0 ml to a tube made from suitable material such as polypropylene. Prepare a 1 mg/ml solution of *trypsin for peptide mapping R* in *0.05 M tris-hydrochloride buffer solution pH 7.5 R* and add 30 µl to the solution of the substance to be examined. Cap the tube and place in a water-bath at 37 °C for 4 h. Remove from the water-bath and stop the reaction immediately, for example by freezing. If analysed immediately using an automatic injector, maintain the temperature at 2 °C to 8 °C.

Reference solution. Prepare at the same time and in the same manner as for the test solution but using *somatropin CRS* instead of the substance to be examined.

Examine by liquid chromatography (*2.2.29*).

The chromatographic procedure may be carried out using:

– a stainless steel column 0.25 m long and 4.6 mm in internal diameter packed with *octylsilyl silica gel for chromatography R* (5 µm to 10 µm),

– as mobile phase at a flow rate of 1 ml/min:

Mobile phase A. Dilute 1 ml of *trifluoroacetic acid R* to 1000 ml with *water R*,

Mobile phase B. To 100 ml of *water R* add 1 ml of *trifluoroacetic acid R* and dilute to 1000 ml with *acetonitrile for chromatography R*,

following the elution conditions as described in the table below (if necessary, the gradient or the temperature of the column may be modified to improve separation of the digest):

Time (min)	Mobile phase A (per cent *V/V*)	Mobile phase B (per cent *V/V*)
0 - 20	100 → 80	0 → 20
20 - 40	80 → 75	20 → 25
40 - 65	75 → 50	25 → 50
65 - 70	50 → 20	50 → 80
70 - 71	20 → 100	80 → 0
71 - 85	100	0

– as detector a spectrophotometer set at 214 nm,

maintaining the temperature of the column at 30 °C.

Equilibrate the column with mobile phase A for at least 15 min. Carry out a blank run using the above-mentioned gradient.

Inject 100 µl of the test solution and 100 µl of the reference solution. The test is not valid unless the chromatogram obtained with each solution is qualitatively similar to the chromatogram of somatropin digest supplied with *somatropin CRS*. The profile of the chromatogram obtained with the test solution corresponds to that of the chromatogram obtained with the reference solution.

D. Examine the chromatograms obtained in the assay. The retention time of the principal peak in the chromatogram obtained with the test solution is similar to that of the principal peak in the chromatogram obtained with the reference solution.

TESTS

Related proteins. Examine by liquid chromatography (*2.2.29*).

Test solution. Prepare a solution of the substance to be examined in *0.05 M tris-hydrochloride buffer solution pH 7.5 R*, containing 2.0 mg/ml of somatropin.

Reference solution. Prepare a solution of *somatropin CRS* in *0.05 M tris-hydrochloride buffer solution pH 7.5 R*, containing 2.0 mg/ml of somatropin.

Resolution solution (somatropin/desamido-somatropin resolution mixture). Prepare a solution of *somatropin CRS* in *0.05 M tris-hydrochloride buffer solution pH 7.5 R* to obtain a 2.0 mg/ml solution of somatropin. Either filter through a sterile filter or add *sodium azide R* to a concentration of 0.1 mg/ml and allow to stand at room temperature for 24 h.

Maintain the solutions at 2 °C to 8 °C and use within 24 h. If an automatic injector is used, maintain the temperature at 2 °C to 8 °C.

The chromatographic procedure may be carried out using:

– a stainless steel column 0.25 m long and 4.6 mm in internal diameter packed with a suitable singly end-capped butylsilyl silica gel, with a granulometry of 5 µm and a porosity of 30 nm. A silica saturation column is to be placed between the pump and the injector valve,

– as mobile phase at a flow rate of 0.5 ml/min a mixture of 29 volumes of *propanol R* and 71 volumes of *0.05 M tris-hydrochloride buffer solution pH 7.5 R*,

– as detector a spectrophotometer set at 220 nm,

maintaining the temperature of the column at 45 °C.

Prior to use, rinse the column with 200 ml to 500 ml of a 0.1 per cent *V/V* solution of *trifluoroacetic acid R* in a 50 per cent *V/V* solution of *acetonitrile R*. Repeat as necessary, to improve column performance.

Inject 20 µl of the reference solution. If necessary, adjust the concentration of *propanol R* in the mobile phase so that the retention time of the principal peak is about 33 min.

Inject 20 µl of the resolution solution. Desamido-somatropin appears as a small peak at a retention time of about 0.85 relative to the principal peak. The test is not valid unless the resolution between the peaks corresponding to somatropin and desamido-somatropin is at least 1.0 and the symmetry factor of the somatropin peak is 0.9 to 1.8.

Inject 20 µl of the test solution. In the chromatogram obtained, the sum of the areas of all the peaks, apart from the principal peak, is not greater than 6.0 per cent of the total area of the peaks. Disregard any peak due to the solvent.

Monographs Q-S

Dimer and related substances of higher molecular mass. Examine by size-exclusion chromatography (*2.2.30*) as described under Assay.

Inject 20 µl of the test solution. In the chromatogram obtained with the test solution, the sum of the areas of any peak with a retention time less than that of the principal peak is not greater than 4.0 per cent of the total area of the peaks. Disregard any peak due to the solvent.

Isoform distribution. Examine by isoelectric focusing.

Test solution (a). Prepare a solution of the substance to be examined in *0.025 M phosphate buffer solution pH 7.0 R*, containing 2.0 mg/ml of somatropin.

Test solution (b). Add 0.1 ml of test solution (a) to 1.9 ml of *0.025 M phosphate buffer solution pH 7.0 R.*

Reference solution (a). Prepare a solution of *somatropin CRS* in *0.025 M phosphate buffer solution pH 7.0 R*, containing 2.0 mg/ml of somatropin.

Reference solution (b). Use an isoelectric point calibration solution in the pH range of 2.5 to 6.5, prepared and used according to the manufacturer's instructions.

Operate the apparatus in accordance with the manufacturer's instructions. The isoelectric focusing procedure may be carried out using a pre-cast gel 245 mm × 110 mm × 1 mm, with a pH in the range 4.0 to 6.5. Apply to the gel 15 µl of each solution. Use as the anode solution a 14.7 g/l solution of *glutamic acid R* in phosphoric acid (50 g/l H_3PO_4) and as the cathode solution an 89.1 g/l solution of *β-alanine R.* Adjust the operating conditions to 2000 V and 25 mA. Allow focusing to take place for 2.5 h at a constant voltage and at a power of not more than 25 W. Immerse the gel for 30 min in a solution containing 115 g/l of *trichloroacetic acid R* and 34.5 g/l of *sulphosalicylic acid R*, and then for 5 min in a mixture of 8 volumes of *acetic acid R*, 25 volumes of *ethanol R* and 67 volumes of deionised *water R* (de-stain solution). Stain the gel by immersion in a 1.15 g/l solution of *acid blue 83 R* in de-stain solution at 60 °C for 10 min, and then place the gel in de-stain solution until excess stain is removed.

The test is not valid unless the distribution of bands in the electropherogram obtained with reference solution (b) corresponds to the manufacturer's indications. The electropherogram obtained with reference solution (a) contains a major band with an isoelectric point of approximately five, and a slightly more acidic minor band at approximately 4.8. In the electropherogram obtained with test solution (a), no band apart from the major band is more intense than the major band in the electropherogram obtained with test solution (b) (5 per cent).

Water (*2.5.32*). Not more than 10.0 per cent, determined by the micro determination of water.

Bacterial endotoxins (*2.6.14*): less than 5 IU/mg, if intended for use in the manufacture of parenteral dosage forms without a further appropriate procedure for removal of bacterial endotoxins.

ASSAY

Examine by size-exclusion chromatography (*2.2.30*).

Test solution. Prepare a solution of the substance to be examined in *0.025 M phosphate buffer solution pH 7.0 R*, containing 1.0 mg/ml of somatropin.

Reference solution. Dissolve the contents of a vial of *somatropin CRS* in *0.025 M phosphate buffer solution pH 7.0 R* and dilute with the same solvent to obtain a concentration of 1.0 mg/ml.

Resolution solution. Place one vial of *somatropin CRS* in an oven at 50 °C for a period (typically between 12 and 24 h) sufficient to generate 1 per cent to 2 per cent of dimer. Dissolve its contents in *0.025 M phosphate buffer solution pH 7.0 R* and dilute with the same solvent to obtain a concentration of 1.0 mg/ml.

The chromatographic procedure may be carried out using:

- a stainless steel column 0.30 m long and 7.8 mm in internal diameter packed with *hydrophilic silica gel for chromatography R* of a grade suitable for fractionation of globular proteins in the molecular mass range 5000 to 150 000,
- as mobile phase at a flow rate of 0.6 ml/min a mixture (filtered and degassed) consisting of 3 volumes of *2-propanol R* and 97 volumes of *0.063 M phosphate buffer solution pH 7.0 R,*
- as detector a spectrophotometer set at 214 nm.

Inject 20 µl of the resolution solution. In the chromatogram obtained, the main peak elutes at a retention time of approximately 12 min to 17 min and the peaks corresponding to the somatropin dimer and to the higher molecular weight proteins at relative retention times of 0.90 and 0.65 respectively, relative to the main peak. The resolution, defined by the ratio of the height above the baseline of the valley separating the monomer and dimer peaks to the height of the dimer peak, is not greater than 0.4.

Inject 20 µl of the test solution and 20 µl of the reference solution.

Calculate the content of somatropin ($C_{990}H_{1528}N_{262}O_{300}S_7$) from the peak areas in the chromatograms obtained with the test solution and the reference solution and the declared content of ($C_{990}H_{1528}N_{262}O_{300}S_7$) in *somatropin CRS.*

STORAGE

Store in an airtight container at a temperature of 2 °C to 8 °C. If the substance is sterile, store in a sterile, airtight, tamper-proof container.

LABELLING

The label states, where applicable, that the substance is free from bacterial endotoxins.

01/2005:0950
corrected

SOMATROPIN BULK SOLUTION

Somatropini solutio ad praeparationem

DEFINITION

Somatropin bulk solution is a solution containing a protein having the structure (191 amino-acid residues) of the major component of growth hormone produced by the human pituitary. It may contain buffer salts and other auxiliary substances. It contains not less than 91.0 per cent and not more than 105.0 per cent of the amount of somatropin[(2)] ($C_{990}H_{1528}N_{262}O_{300}S_7$) stated on the label.

PRODUCTION

Somatropin bulk solution is produced by a method based on recombinant DNA (rDNA) technology. During the course of product development, it must be demonstrated that the manufacturing process produces a product having a biological activity of at least 2.5 IU/mg, using a validated bioassay based on growth promotion and approved by the competent authority.

(2) 1 mg of anhydrous somatropin ($C_{990}H_{1528}N_{262}O_{300}S_7$) is equivalent to 3.0 IU of biological activity.

Monographs Q-S

Somatropin bulk solution complies with the following additional requirements.

Host-cell-derived proteins. The limit is approved by the competent authority.

Host-cell- and vector-derived DNA. The limit is approved by the competent authority.

CHARACTERS

A clear or slightly turbid, colourless solution.

IDENTIFICATION

A. Examine the electropherograms obtained in the test for isoform distribution. In the electropherogram obtained with test solution (a), the principal band corresponds in position to that in the electropherogram obtained with reference solution (a).

B. Examine the chromatograms obtained in the test for related proteins. The retention time of the principal peak in the chromatogram obtained with the test solution is similar to that of the principal peak in the chromatogram obtained with the reference solution.

C. Examine by peptide mapping.

Test solution. Dilute the solution to be examined with *0.05 M tris-hydrochloride buffer solution pH 7.5 R* so that it contains 2.0 mg/ml of somatropin, and transfer about 1.0 ml to a tube made from suitable material such as polypropylene. Prepare a 1 mg/ml solution of *trypsin for peptide mapping R* in *0.05 M tris-hydrochloride buffer solution pH 7.5 R* and add 30 µl to the solution of the substance to be examined. Cap the tube and place in a water-bath at 37 °C for 4 h. Remove from the water-bath and stop the reaction immediately, for example by freezing. If analysed immediately using an automatic injector, maintain the temperature at 2 °C to 8 °C.

Note: If a 2 mg/ml somatropin concentration is not obtainable, a similar digest relationship (µg of trypsin per mg of somatropin) may be used.

Reference solution. Prepare a solution of *somatropin CRS* in *0.05 M tris-hydrochloride buffer solution pH 7.5 R* containing 2.0 mg/ml of somatropin and treat at the same time and in the same manner as for the test solution.

Examine by liquid chromatography (*2.2.29*).

The chromatographic procedure may be carried out using:

- a stainless steel column 0.25 m long and 4.6 mm in internal diameter packed with *octylsilyl silica gel for chromatography R* (5 µm to 10 µm),
- as mobile phase at a flow rate of 1 ml/min:

Mobile phase A. Dilute 1 ml of *trifluoroacetic acid R* to 1000 ml with *water R*,

Mobile phase B. To 100 ml of *water R* add 1 ml of *trifluoroacetic acid R* and dilute to 1000 ml with *acetonitrile for chromatography R*,

following the elution conditions as described in the table below (if necessary, the gradient or the temperature of the column may be modified to improve separation of the digest):

Time (min)	Mobile phase A (per cent *V/V*)	Mobile phase B (per cent *V/V*)
0 - 20	100 → 80	0 → 20
20 - 40	80 → 75	20 → 25
40 - 65	75 → 50	25 → 50
65 - 70	50 → 20	50 → 80
70 - 71	20 → 100	80 → 0
71 - 85	100	0

- as detector a spectrophotometer set at 214 nm,

maintaining the temperature of the column at 30 °C.

Equilibrate the column with mobile phase A for at least 15 min. Carry out a blank run using the above-mentioned gradient.

Inject 100 µl of the test solution and 100 µl of the reference solution. The test is not valid unless the chromatogram obtained with each solution is qualitatively similar to the chromatogram of somatropin digest supplied with *somatropin CRS*. The profile of the chromatogram obtained with the test solution corresponds to that of the chromatogram obtained with the reference solution.

D. Examine the chromatograms obtained in the assay. The retention time of the principal peak in the chromatogram obtained with the test solution is similar to that of the principal peak in the chromatogram obtained with the reference solution.

TESTS

Related proteins. Examine by liquid chromatography (*2.2.29*).

Test solution. Dilute the solution to be examined with *0.05 M tris-hydrochloride buffer solution pH 7.5 R* so as to contain 2.0 mg/ml of somatropin or less, but then correct the injection volume accordingly.

Reference solution. Prepare a solution of *somatropin CRS* in *0.05 M tris-hydrochloride buffer solution pH 7.5 R*, containing 2.0 mg/ml of somatropin.

Resolution solution (somatropin/desamido-somatropin resolution mixture). Prepare a solution of *somatropin CRS* in *0.05 M tris-hydrochloride buffer solution pH 7.5 R*, containing 2.0 mg/ml of somatropin. Either filter through a sterile filter or add *sodium azide R* to a concentration of 0.1 mg/ml and allow to stand at room temperature for 24 h.

Maintain the solutions at 2 °C to 8 °C and use within 24 h. If an automatic injector is used, maintain the temperature at 2 °C to 8 °C.

The chromatographic procedure may be carried out using:

- a stainless steel column 0.25 m long and 4.6 mm in internal diameter packed with a suitable singly end-capped butylsilyl silica gel, with a granulometry of 5 µm and a porosity of 30 nm. A silica saturation column is to be placed between the pump and the injector valve,
- as mobile phase at a flow rate of 0.5 ml/min a mixture of 29 volumes of *propanol R* and 71 volumes of *0.05 M tris-hydrochloride buffer solution pH 7.5 R*,
- as detector a spectrophotometer set at 220 nm,

maintaining the temperature of the column at 45 °C.

Prior to use, rinse the column with 200 ml to 500 ml of a 0.1 per cent *V/V* solution of *trifluoroacetic acid R* in a 50 per cent *V/V* solution of *acetonitrile R*. Repeat as necessary, to improve column performance.

Inject 20 µl of the reference solution. If necessary, adjust the concentration of *propanol R* in the mobile phase so that the retention time of the principal peak is about 33 min.

Monographs Q-S

Inject 20 µl of the resolution solution. Desamido-somatropin appears as a small peak at a retention time of about 0.85 relative to the principal peak. The test is not valid unless the resolution between the peaks corresponding to somatropin and desamido-somatropin is at least 1.0 and the symmetry factor of the somatropin peak is 0.9 to 1.8.

Inject 20 µl of the test solution. In the chromatogram obtained, the sum of the areas of all the peaks, apart from the principal peak, is not greater than 6.0 per cent of the total area of the peaks. Disregard any peak due to the solvent.

Dimer and related substances of higher molecular mass. Examine by size-exclusion chromatography (*2.2.30*) as described under Assay.

Inject 20 µl of the test solution. In the chromatogram obtained with the test solution, the sum of the areas of any peak with a retention time less than that of the principal peak is not greater than 4.0 per cent of the total area of the peaks. Disregard any peak due to the solvent.

Isoform distribution. Examine by isoelectric focusing.

Test solution (a). Dilute the solution to be examined with *0.025 M phosphate buffer solution pH 7.0 R* so as to contain 2.0 mg/ml of somatropin.

Test solution (b). Add 0.1 ml of test solution (a) to 1.9 ml of *0.025 M phosphate buffer solution pH 7.0 R.*

Reference solution (a). Prepare a solution of *somatropin CRS* in *0.025 M phosphate buffer solution pH 7.0 R*, containing 2.0 mg/ml of somatropin.

Reference solution (b). Use an isoelectric point calibration solution in the pH range of 2.5 to 6.5, prepared and used according to the manufacturer's instructions.

Operate the apparatus in accordance with the manufacturer's instructions. The isoelectric focusing procedure may be carried out using a pre-cast gel 245 mm × 110 mm × 1 mm, with a pH in the range 4.0 to 6.5. Apply to the gel 15 µl of each solution. Use as the anode solution a 14.7 g/l solution of *glutamic acid R* in phosphoric acid (50 g/l H_3PO_4) and as the cathode solution an 89.1 g/l solution of *β-alanine R*. Adjust the operating conditions to 2000 V and 25 mA. Allow focusing to take place for 2.5 h at a constant voltage and at a power of not more than 25 W. Immerse the gel for 30 min in a solution containing 115 g/l of *trichloroacetic acid R* and 34.5 g/l of *sulphosalicylic acid R*, and then for 5 min in a mixture of 8 volumes of *acetic acid R*, 25 volumes of *ethanol R* and 67 volumes of deionised *water R* (de-stain solution). Stain the gel by immersion in a 1.15 g/l solution of *acid blue 83 R* in de-stain solution at 60 °C for 10 min, and then place the gel in de-stain solution until excess stain is removed.

The test is not valid unless the distribution of bands in the electropherogram obtained with reference solution (b) corresponds to the manufacturer's indications. The electropherogram obtained with reference solution (a) contains a major band with an isoelectric point of approximately five, and a slightly more acidic minor band at approximately 4.8. In the electropherogram obtained with test solution (a), no band apart from the major band is more intense than the major band in the electropherogram obtained with test solution (b) (5 per cent).

Bacterial endotoxins (*2.6.14*): less than 5 IU in the volume that contains 1 mg of somatropin, if intended for use in the manufacture of parenteral dosage forms without a further appropriate procedure for removal of bacterial endotoxins.

ASSAY

Examine by size-exclusion chromatography (*2.2.30*).

Test solution. Dilute the solution to be examined with *0.025 M phosphate buffer solution pH 7.0 R* so as to contain 1.0 mg/ml of somatropin.

Reference solution. Dissolve the contents of a vial of *somatropin CRS* in *0.025 M phosphate buffer solution pH 7.0 R* and dilute with the same solvent to obtain a concentration of 1.0 mg/ml.

Resolution solution. Place one vial of *somatropin CRS* in an oven at 50 °C for a period (typically between 12 h and 24 h) sufficient to generate 1 per cent to 2 per cent of dimer. Dissolve its contents in *0.025 M phosphate buffer solution pH 7.0 R* and dilute with the same solvent to obtain a concentration of 1.0 mg/ml.

The chromatographic procedure may be carried out using:

- a stainless steel column 0.30 m long and 7.8 mm in internal diameter packed with *hydrophilic silica gel for chromatography R* of a grade suitable for fractionation of globular proteins in the molecular mass range 5000 to 150 000,
- as mobile phase at a flow rate of 0.6 ml/min a mixture (filtered and degassed) consisting of 3 volumes of *2-propanol R* and 97 volumes of *0.063 M phosphate buffer solution pH 7.0 R*,
- as detector a spectrophotometer set at 214 nm.

Inject 20 µl of the resolution solution. In the chromatogram obtained, the main peak elutes at a retention time of approximately 12 min to 17 min and the peaks corresponding to the somatropin dimer and to the higher molecular weight proteins at relative retention times of 0.90 and 0.65 respectively, relative to the main peak. The resolution, defined by the ratio of the height above the baseline of the valley separating the monomer and dimer peaks to the height of the dimer peak, is not greater than 0.4.

Inject 20 µl of the test solution and 20 µl of the reference solution.

Calculate the content of somatropin ($C_{990}H_{1528}N_{262}O_{300}S_7$) from the peak areas in the chromatograms obtained with the test solution and the reference solution and the declared content of ($C_{990}H_{1528}N_{262}O_{300}S_7$) in *somatropin CRS.*

STORAGE

Store in an airtight container at a temperature of − 20 °C. Avoid repeated freezing and thawing. If the solution is sterile, store in a sterile, airtight, tamper-proof container.

LABELLING

The label states:

- the content of somatropin in milligrams per millilitre,
- the name and concentration of any auxiliary substance,
- where applicable, that the solution is free from bacterial endotoxins.

Monographs Q-S

01/2005:0952
corrected

SOMATROPIN FOR INJECTION

Somatropinum ad iniectabilium

DEFINITION

Somatropin for injection is a freeze-dried, sterile preparation of a protein having the structure (191 amino-acid residues) of the major component of growth hormone produced by the human pituitary. It contains not less than 89.0 per cent and not more than 105.0 per cent of the amount of somatropin(3) ($C_{990}H_{1528}N_{262}O_{300}S_7$) stated on the label. It complies with the requirements of the monographs on *Parenteral preparations (0520)*.

PRODUCTION

Somatropin for injection is prepared either from *Somatropin (0951)* or from *Somatropin bulk solution (0950)*, or by a method based on recombinant DNA (rDNA) technology in which the injectable preparation is produced without the isolation of an intermediate solid or liquid bulk. In the latter case, during the course of product development, it must be demonstrated that the manufacturing process produces a product having a biological activity of not less than 2.5 IU/mg, using a validated bioassay based on growth promotion and approved by the competent authority. The purified preparation, to which buffers and stabilisers may be added, is filtered through a bacteria-retentive filter, aseptically distributed in sterile containers of glass type I (*3.2.1*) and freeze-dried. The containers are immediately sealed so as to exclude microbial contamination and moisture.

Somatropin for injection complies with the following additional requirements.

Host-cell-derived proteins. The limit is approved by the competent authority.

Host-cell- and vector-derived DNA. The limit is approved by the competent authority.

Where somatropin for injection is prepared from Somatropin (0951) or from Somatropin bulk solution (0950), compliance with the requirements for host-cell-derived proteins, host-cell- and vector-derived DNA and with identification test C need not be reconfirmed by the manufacturer during subsequent production of somatropin for injection.

CHARACTERS

A white or almost white powder.

IDENTIFICATION

A. Examine the electropherograms obtained in the test for isoform distribution. In the electropherogram obtained with test solution (a), the principal band corresponds in position to that in the electropherogram obtained with reference solution (a).

B. Examine the chromatograms obtained in the test for related proteins. The retention time of the principal peak in the chromatogram obtained with the test solution is similar to that of the principal peak in the chromatogram obtained with the reference solution.

C. Examine by peptide mapping.

Test solution. Prepare a solution of the substance to be examined in *0.05 M tris-hydrochloride buffer solution pH 7.5 R* to obtain a solution containing 2.0 mg/ml of somatropin, and transfer about 1.0 ml to a tube made from suitable material such as polypropylene. Prepare a 1 mg/ml solution of *trypsin for peptide mapping R* in *0.05 M tris-hydrochloride buffer solution pH 7.5 R* and add 30 µl to the solution of the substance to be examined. Cap the tube and place in a water-bath at 37 °C for 4 h. Remove from the water-bath and stop the reaction immediately, for example by freezing. If analysed immediately using an automatic injector, maintain the temperature at 2 °C to 8 °C.

Reference solution. Prepare at the same time and in the same manner as for the test solution but using *somatropin CRS* instead of the substance to be examined.

Examine by liquid chromatography (*2.2.29*).

The chromatographic procedure may be carried out using:

– a stainless steel column 0.25 m long and 4.6 mm in internal diameter packed with *octylsilyl silica gel for chromatography R* (5 µm to 10 µm),

– as mobile phase at a flow rate of 1 ml/min:

Mobile phase A. Dilute 1 ml of *trifluoroacetic acid R* to 1000 ml with *water R*,

Mobile phase B. To 100 ml of *water R* add 1 ml of *trifluoroacetic acid R* and dilute to 1000 ml with *acetonitrile for chromatography R*,

following the elution conditions as described in the table below (if necessary, the gradient or the temperature of the column may be modified to improve separation of the digest):

Time (min)	Mobile phase A (per cent V/V)	Mobile phase B (per cent V/V)
0 - 20	100 → 80	0 → 20
20 - 40	80 → 75	20 → 25
40 - 65	75 → 50	25 → 50
65 - 70	50 → 20	50 → 80
70 - 71	20 → 100	80 → 0
71 - 85	100	0

– as detector a spectrophotometer set at 214 nm, maintaining the temperature of the column at 30 °C.

Equilibrate the column with mobile phase A for at least 15 min. Carry out a blank run using the above-mentioned gradient.

Inject 100 µl of the test solution and 100 µl of the reference solution. The test is not valid unless the chromatogram obtained with each solution is qualitatively similar to the chromatogram of somatropin digest supplied with *somatropin CRS*. The profile of the chromatogram obtained with the test solution corresponds to that of the chromatogram obtained with the reference solution.

D. Examine the chromatograms obtained in the assay. The retention time of the principal peak in the chromatogram obtained with the test solution is similar to that of the principal peak in the chromatogram obtained with the reference solution.

TESTS

Related proteins. Examine by liquid chromatography (*2.2.29*).

Test solution. Prepare a solution of the substance to be examined in *0.05 M tris-hydrochloride buffer solution pH 7.5 R*, containing 2.0 mg/ml of somatropin.

Reference solution. Prepare a solution of *somatropin CRS* in *0.05 M tris-hydrochloride buffer solution pH 7.5 R*, containing 2.0 mg/ml of somatropin.

Resolution solution (somatropin/desamido-somatropin resolution mixture). Prepare a solution of *somatropin CRS* in *0.05 M tris-hydrochloride buffer solution pH 7.5 R*, containing 2.0 mg/ml of somatropin. Either filter through a sterile filter or add *sodium azide R* to a concentration of 0.1 mg/ml and allow to stand at room temperature for 24 h.

Maintain the solutions at 2 °C to 8 °C and use within 24 h. If an automatic injector is used, maintain the temperature at 2 °C to 8 °C.

(3) 1 mg of anhydrous somatropin ($C_{990}H_{1528}N_{262}O_{300}S_7$) is equivalent to 3.0 IU of biological activity.

Monographs Q-S

The chromatographic procedure may be carried out using:

- a stainless steel column 0.25 m long and 4.6 mm in internal diameter packed with a suitable singly end-capped butylsilyl silica gel, with a granulometry of 5 µm and a porosity of 30 nm. A silica saturation column is to be placed between the pump and the injector valve,
- as mobile phase at a flow rate of 0.5 ml/min a mixture of 29 volumes of *propanol R* and 71 volumes of *0.05 M tris-hydrochloride buffer solution pH 7.5 R,*
- as detector a spectrophotometer set at 220 nm,

maintaining the temperature of the column at 45 °C.

Prior to use, rinse the column with 200 ml to 500 ml of a 0.1 per cent *V/V* solution of *trifluoroacetic acid R* in a 50 per cent *V/V* solution of *acetonitrile R*. Repeat as necessary, to improve column performance.

Inject 20 µl of the reference solution. If necessary, adjust the concentration of *propanol R* in the mobile phase so that the retention time of the principal peak is about 33 min.

Inject 20 µl of the resolution solution. Desamido-somatropin appears as a small peak at a retention time of about 0.85 relative to the principal peak. The test is not valid unless the resolution between the peaks corresponding to somatropin and desamido-somatropin is at least 1.0 and the symmetry factor of the somatropin peak is 0.9 to 1.8.

Inject 20 µl of the test solution. In the chromatogram obtained, the sum of areas of all the peaks, apart from the principal peak, is not greater than 13 per cent of the total area of the peaks. Disregard any peak due to the solvent.

Dimer and related substances of higher molecular mass. Examine by size-exclusion chromatography (*2.2.30*) as described under Assay.

Inject 20 µl of the test solution. In the chromatogram obtained with the test solution, the sum of the areas of any peak with a retention time less than that of the principal peak is not greater than 6.0 per cent of the total area of the peaks. Disregard any peak due to the solvent.

Isoform distribution. Examine by isoelectric focusing.

Test solution (a). Prepare a solution of the substance to be examined in *0.025 M phosphate buffer solution pH 7.0 R,* containing 2.0 mg/ml of somatropin.

Test solution (b). Add 0.1 ml of test solution (a) to 1.5 ml of *0.025 M phosphate buffer solution pH 7.0 R.*

Reference solution (a). Prepare a solution of *somatropin CRS* in *0.025 M phosphate buffer solution pH 7.0 R,* containing 2.0 mg/ml of somatropin.

Reference solution (b). Use an isoelectric point calibration solution in the pH range of 2.5 to 6.5, prepared and used according to the manufacturer's instructions.

Operate the apparatus in accordance with the manufacturer's instructions. The isoelectric focusing procedure may be carried out using a pre-cast gel 245 mm × 110 mm × 1 mm, with a pH in the range 4.0 to 6.5. Apply to the gel 15 µl of each solution. Use as the anode solution a 14.7 g/l solution of *glutamic acid R* in phosphoric acid (50 g/l H_3PO_4) and as the cathode solution an 89.1 g/l solution of *β-alanine R.* Adjust the operating conditions to 2000 V and 25 mA. Allow focusing to take place for 2.5 h at a constant voltage and at a power of not more than 25 W. Immerse the gel for 30 min in a solution containing 115 g/l of *trichloroacetic acid R* and 34.5 g/l of *sulphosalicylic acid R,* and then for 5 min in a mixture of 8 volumes of *acetic acid R,* 25 volumes of *ethanol R* and 67 volumes of deionised *water R* (de-stain solution). Stain the gel by immersion in a 1.15 g/l solution of *acid blue 83 R* in de-stain solution at 60 °C for 10 min, and then place the gel in de-stain solution until excess stain is removed.

The test is not valid unless the distribution of bands in the electropherogram obtained with reference solution (b) corresponds to the manufacturer's indications. The electropherogram obtained with reference solution (a) contains a major band with an isoelectric point of approximately five, and a slightly more acidic minor band at approximately 4.8. In the electropherogram obtained with test solution (a), no band apart from the major band is more intense than the major band in the electropherogram obtained with test solution (b) (6.25 per cent).

Water (*2.5.32*). Not more than 3.0 per cent, unless otherwise justified and authorised, determined by the micro determination of water.

Bacterial endotoxins (*2.6.14*): less than 5 IU/mg.

ASSAY

Examine by size-exclusion chromatography (*2.2.30*).

Test solution. Prepare a solution of the substance to be examined in *0.025 M phosphate buffer solution pH 7.0 R,* containing 1.0 mg/ml of somatropin.

Reference solution. Dissolve the contents of a vial of *somatropin CRS* in *0.025 M phosphate buffer solution pH 7.0 R* and dilute with the same solvent to obtain a concentration of 1.0 mg/ml.

Resolution solution. Place one vial of *somatropin CRS* in an oven at 50 °C for a period (typically between 12 h and 24 h) sufficient to generate 1 per cent to 2 per cent of dimer. Dissolve its contents in *0.025 M phosphate buffer solution pH 7.0 R* and dilute with the same solvent to obtain a concentration of 1.0 mg/ml.

The chromatographic procedure may be carried out using:

- a stainless steel column 0.30 m long and 7.8 mm in internal diameter packed with *hydrophilic silica gel for chromatography R* of a grade suitable for fractionation of globular proteins in the molecular mass range 5000 to 150 000,
- as mobile phase at a flow rate of 0.6 ml/min a mixture (filtered and degassed) consisting of 3 volumes of *2-propanol R* and 97 volumes of *0.063 M phosphate buffer solution pH 7.0 R,*
- as detector a spectrophotometer set at 214 nm.

Inject 20 µl of the resolution solution. In the chromatogram obtained, the main peak elutes at a retention time of approximately 12 min to 17 min and the peaks corresponding to the somatropin dimer and to the higher molecular weight proteins at relative retention times of 0.90 and 0.65 respectively, relative to the main peak. The resolution defined by the ratio of the height above the baseline of the valley separating the monomer and dimer peaks, to the height of the dimer peak, is not greater than 0.4.

Inject 20 µl of the test solution and 20 µl of the reference solution.

Calculate the content of somatropin ($C_{990}H_{1528}N_{262}O_{300}S_7$) from the peak areas in the chromatograms obtained with the test solution and the reference solution and the declared content of ($C_{990}H_{1528}N_{262}O_{300}S_7$)in *somatropin CRS*.

STORAGE

Store in a sterile, airtight, tamper-proof container, at a temperature of 2 °C to 8 °C.

LABELLING

The label states:

- the content of somatropin in the container, in milligrams,
- the composition and volume of the liquid to be added for reconstitution,

Monographs Q-S

– the time within which the reconstituted solution shall be used and the storage conditions during this period,
– the name and quantity of any added substance,
– the storage temperature,
– that the preparation shall not be shaken during reconstitution.

01/2005:0592

SORBIC ACID

Acidum sorbicum

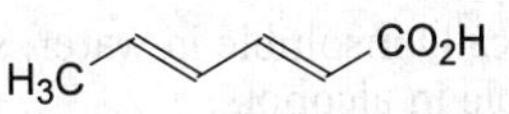

$C_6H_8O_2$ M_r 112.1

DEFINITION

Sorbic acid contains not less than 99.0 per cent and not more than the equivalent of 101.0 per cent of (*E,E*)-hexa-2,4-dienoic acid, calculated with reference to the anhydrous substance.

CHARACTERS

A white or almost white, crystalline powder, slightly soluble in water, freely soluble in alcohol.

IDENTIFICATION

First identification: A, C.

Second identification: A, B, D.

A. Melting point (*2.2.14*): 132 °C to 136 °C.

B. Dissolve 50.0 mg in *water R* and dilute to 250.0 ml with the same solvent. Dilute 2.0 ml of this solution to 200.0 ml with *0.1 M hydrochloric acid.* Examined between 230 nm and 350 nm (*2.2.25*), the solution shows a maximum at 264 nm. The specific absorbance at the maximum is 2150 to 2550.

C. Examine by infrared absorption spectrophotometry (*2.2.24*), comparing with the spectrum obtained with *sorbic acid CRS.*

D. Dissolve 0.2 g in 2 ml of *alcohol R* and add 0.2 ml of *bromine water R.* The solution is decolorised.

TESTS

Solution S. Dissolve 1.25 g in *alcohol R* and dilute to 25 ml with the same solvent.

Appearance of solution. Solution S is clear (*2.2.1*) and colourless (*2.2.2, Method II*).

Aldehydes. Dissolve 1.0 g in a mixture of 30 ml of *water R* and 50 ml of *2-propanol R*, adjust the solution to pH 4 with *0.1 M hydrochloric acid* or *0.1 M sodium hydroxide* and dilute to 100 ml with *water R.* To 10 ml of the solution add 1 ml of *decolorised fuchsin solution R* and allow to stand for 30 min. Any colour in the solution is not more intense than that in a standard prepared at the same time by adding 1 ml of *decolorised fuchsin solution R* to a mixture of 1.5 ml of *acetaldehyde standard solution (100 ppm C_2H_4O) R*, 4 ml of *2-propanol R* and 4.5 ml of *water R* (0.15 per cent, calculated as C_2H_4O).

Heavy metals (*2.4.8*). 12 ml of solution S complies with limit test B for heavy metals (10 ppm). Prepare the standard using 5 ml of *lead standard solution (1 ppm Pb) R* and 5 ml of *alcohol R.*

Water (*2.5.12*). Not more than 1.0 per cent, determined on 2.000 g by the semi-micro determination of water.

Sulphated ash (*2.4.14*). Not more than 0.2 per cent, determined on 1.0 g.

ASSAY

Dissolve 0.1000 g in 20 ml of *alcohol R.* Using 0.2 ml of *phenolphthalein solution R* as indicator, titrate with *0.1 M sodium hydroxide* until a pink colour is obtained.

1 ml of *0.1 M sodium hydroxide* is equivalent to 11.21 mg of $C_6H_8O_2$.

STORAGE

Store protected from light.

01/2005:1040

SORBITAN LAURATE

Sorbitani lauras

DEFINITION

Mixture usually obtained by partial esterification of sorbitol and its mono- and di-anhydrides with lauric acid.

CHARACTERS

Appearance: brownish-yellow, viscous liquid.

Solubility: practically insoluble, but dispersible in water, miscible with alcohol.

Relative density: about 0.98.

IDENTIFICATION

A. It complies with the test for hydroxyl value (see Tests).

B. It complies with the test for iodine value (see Tests).

C. It complies with the test for composition of fatty acids (see Tests).

TESTS

Acid value (*2.5.1*): maximum 7.0, determined on 5.0 g.

Hydroxyl value (*2.5.3, Method A*): 330 to 358.

Iodine value (*2.5.4*): maximum 10.

Peroxide value (*2.5.5*): maximum 5.0.

Saponification value (*2.5.6*): 158 to 170.

Carry out the saponification for 1 h.

Composition of fatty acids. Gas chromatography (*2.4.22, Method C*).

Prepare reference solution (a) as indicated in tables 2.4.22.-1 and 2.4.22.-2.

Composition of the fatty acid fraction of the substance:

– *caproic acid*: maximum 1.0 per cent,
– *caprylic acid*: maximum 10.0 per cent,
– *capric acid*: maximum 10.0 per cent,
– *lauric acid*: 40.0 per cent to 60.0 per cent,
– *myristic acid*: 14.0 per cent to 25.0 per cent,
– *palmitic acid*: 7.0 per cent to 15.0 per cent,
– *stearic acid*: maximum 7.0 per cent,
– *oleic acid*: maximum 11.0 per cent,
– *linoleic acid*: maximum 3.0 per cent.

Heavy metals (*2.4.8*): maximum 10 ppm.

2.0 g complies with limit test D. Prepare the standard using 2 ml of *lead standard solution (10 ppm Pb) R.*

Water (*2.5.12*): maximum 1.5 per cent, determined on 1.00 g.

Total ash (*2.4.16*): maximum 0.5 per cent.

STORAGE

Protected from light.

01/2005:1041

SORBITAN OLEATE

Sorbitani oleas

DEFINITION

Mixture usually obtained by esterification of 1 mole of sorbitol and its mono-and di-anhydrides per mole of oleic acid. A suitable antioxidant may be added.

CHARACTERS

Appearance: brownish-yellow, viscous liquid.

Solubility: practically insoluble but dispersible in water, soluble in fatty oils producing a hazy solution, miscible with alcohol.

Relative density: about 0.99.

IDENTIFICATION

A. It complies with the test for hydroxyl value (see Tests).

B. It complies with the test for iodine value (see Tests).

C. It complies with the test for composition of fatty acids (see Tests).

Margaric acid: maximum 0.2 per cent for oleic acid of vegetable origin and maximum 4.0 per cent for oleic acid of animal origin.

TESTS

Acid value (*2.5.1*): maximum 8.0, determined on 5.0 g.

Hydroxyl value (*2.5.3, Method A*): 190 to 210.

Iodine value (*2.5.4*): 62 to 76.

Peroxide value (*2.5.5*): maximum 10.0.

Saponification value (*2.5.6*): 145 to 160.

Carry out the saponification for 1 h.

Composition of fatty acids. Gas chromatography (*2.4.22, Method C*).

Composition of the fatty acid fraction of the substance:

- *myristic acid*: maximum 5.0 per cent,
- *palmitic acid*: maximum 16.0 per cent,
- *palmitoleic acid*: maximum 8.0 per cent,
- *stearic acid*: maximum 6.0 per cent,
- *oleic acid*: 65.0 per cent to 88.0 per cent,
- *linoleic acid*: maximum 18.0 per cent,
- *linolenic acid*: maximum 4.0 per cent,
- *fatty acids with chain length greater than* C_{18}: maximum 4.0 per cent.

Heavy metals (*2.4.8*): maximum 10 ppm.

2.0 g complies with limit test D. Prepare the standard using 2 ml of *lead standard solution (10 ppm Pb) R*.

Water (*2.5.12*): maximum 1.5 per cent, determined on 1.000 g.

Total ash (*2.4.16*): maximum 0.5 per cent, determined on 1.5 g.

STORAGE

Protected from light.

LABELLING

The label states:

- the name and concentration of any added antioxidant,
- the origin of the oleic acid used (animal or vegetable).

01/2005:1042

SORBITAN PALMITATE

Sorbitani palmitas

DEFINITION

Mixture usually obtained by partial esterification of sorbitol and its mono- and di-anhydrides with palmitic acid.

CHARACTERS

Appearance: yellow or yellowish powder, waxy flakes or hard masses.

Solubility: practically insoluble in water, soluble in fatty oils, slightly soluble in alcohol.

IDENTIFICATION

A. Melting point (*2.2.15*): 44 °C to 51 °C.

Introduce the melted substance into the glass capillary tubes and allow to stand at a temperature below 10 °C for 24 h.

B. It complies with the test for hydroxyl value (see Tests).

C. It complies with the test for composition of fatty acids (see Tests).

TESTS

Acid value (*2.5.1*): maximum 8.0, determined on 5.0 g.

Hydroxyl value (*2.5.3, Method A*): 270 to 305.

Peroxide value (*2.5.5*): maximum 5.0.

Saponification value (*2.5.6*): 140 to 155.

Carry out the saponification for 1 h.

Composition of fatty acids. Gas chromatography (*2.4.22, Method C*).

Composition of the fatty acid fraction of the substance:

- *palmitic acid*: minimum 92.0 per cent,
- *stearic acid*: maximum 6.0 per cent.

Heavy metals (*2.4.8*): maximum 10 ppm.

2.0 g complies with limit test D. Prepare the standard using 2 ml of *lead standard solution (10 ppm Pb) R*.

Water (*2.5.12*): maximum 1.5 per cent, determined on 1.00 g.

Total ash (*2.4.16*): maximum 0.5 per cent.

STORAGE

Protected from light.

01/2005:1916

SORBITAN SESQUIOLEATE

Sorbitani sesquioleas

DEFINITION

Mixture usually obtained by esterification of 2 moles of sorbitol and its mono- and di-anhydrides per 3 moles of oleic acid. A suitable antioxidant may be added.

CHARACTERS

Appearance: pale yellow or slightly brownish-yellow paste, which becomes a viscous, oily, brownish-yellow liquid at about 25 °C.

Solubility: dispersible in water, soluble in fatty oils, slightly soluble in ethanol.

Relative density: about 0.99.

Monographs Q-S

IDENTIFICATION

A. It complies with the test for hydroxyl value (see Tests).

B. It complies with the test for iodine value (see Tests).

C. It complies with the test for composition of fatty acids (see Tests).

Margaric acid: maximum 0.2 per cent for oleic acid of vegetable origin and maximum 4.0 per cent for oleic acid of animal origin.

TESTS

Acid value (*2.5.1*): maximum 16.0, determined on 5.0 g.

Hydroxyl value (*2.5.3, Method A*): 180 to 215.

Iodine value (*2.5.4*): 70 to 95.

Peroxide value (*2.5.5*): maximum 10.0.

Saponification value (*2.5.6*): 145 to 166.

Carry out the saponification for 1 h.

Composition of fatty acids. Gas chromatography (*2.4.22, Method C*).

Composition of the fatty acid fraction of the substance:

- *myristic acid*: maximum 5.0 per cent,
- *palmitic acid*: maximum 16.0 per cent,
- *palmitoleic acid*: maximum 8.0 per cent,
- *stearic acid*: maximum 6.0 per cent,
- *oleic acid*: 65.0 per cent to 88.0 per cent,
- *linoleic acid*: maximum 18.0 per cent,
- *linolenic acid*: maximum 4.0 per cent,
- *fatty acids with chain length greater than* C_{18}: maximum 4.0 per cent.

Heavy metals (*2.4.8*): maximum 10 ppm.

2.0 g complies with limit test D. Prepare the standard using 2 ml of *lead standard solution (10 ppm Pb) R*.

Water (*2.5.12*): maximum 1.5 per cent, determined on 1.000 g.

Total ash (*2.4.16*): maximum 0.5 per cent, determined on 1.5 g.

STORAGE

Protected from light.

LABELLING

The label states:

- the name and concentration of any added antioxidant,
- the origin of the oleic acid used (animal or vegetable).

01/2005:1043

SORBITAN STEARATE

Sorbitani stearas

DEFINITION

Mixture usually obtained by partial esterification of sorbitol and its mono- and di-anhydrides with *Stearic acid 50 (1474)* or *Stearic acid 70 (1474).*

CHARACTERS

Appearance: pale yellow, waxy solid.

Solubility: practically insoluble, but dispersible in water, slightly soluble in alcohol.

IDENTIFICATION

A. Melting point (*2.2.15*): 50 °C to 60 °C.

Introduce the melted substance into the capillary tubes and allow to stand at a temperature below 10 °C for 24 h.

B. It complies with the test for hydroxyl value (see Tests).

C. It complies with the test for composition of fatty acids (see Tests).

TESTS

Acid value (*2.5.1*): maximum 10.0, determined on 5.0 g.

Hydroxyl value (*2.5.3, Method A*): 235 to 260.

Peroxide value (*2.5.5*): maximum 5.0.

Saponification value (*2.5.6*): 147 to 157.

Carry out the saponification for 1 h.

Composition of fatty acids. Gas chromatography (*2.4.22, Method C*).

Composition of the fatty acid fraction of the subtance:

	Type of fatty acid used	Composition of fatty acids
Sorbitan stearate (type I)	Stearic acid 50	*Stearic acid*: 40.0 per cent to 60.0 per cent, *Sum of the contents of palmitic and stearic acids*: minimum 90.0 per cent.
Sorbitan stearate (type II)	Stearic acid 70	*Stearic acid*: 60.0 per cent to 80.0 per cent, *Sum of the contents of palmitic and stearic acids*: minimum 90.0 per cent.

Heavy metals (*2.4.8*): maximum 10 ppm.

2.0 g complies with limit test D. Prepare the standard using 2 ml of *lead standard solution (10 ppm Pb) R*.

Water (*2.5.12*): maximum 1.5 per cent, determined on 1.00 g.

Total ash (*2.4.16*): maximum 0.5 per cent.

STORAGE

Protected from light.

LABELLING

The label states the type of sorbitan stearate.

01/2005:1044

SORBITAN TRIOLEATE

Sorbitani trioleas

DEFINITION

Mixture usually obtained by esterification of 1 mole of sorbitol and its mono-anhydride per 3 moles of oleic acid. A suitable antioxidant may be added.

CHARACTERS

Appearance: pale yellow, light yellowish or brown solid, which becomes a viscous, oily, brownish-yellow liquid at about 25 °C.

Solubility: practically insoluble but dispersible in water, soluble in fatty oils, slightly soluble in alcohol.

Relative density: about 0.98.

IDENTIFICATION

A. It complies with the test for hydroxyl value (see Tests).

B. It complies with the test for iodine value (see Tests).

C. It complies with the test for composition of fatty acids (see Tests).

Margaric acid: maximum 0.2 per cent for oleic acid of vegetable origin and maximum 4.0 per cent for oleic acid of animal origin.

Monographs Q-S

TESTS

Acid value (*2.5.1*): maximum 16.0, determined on 5.0 g.

Hydroxyl value (*2.5.3, Method A*): 55 to 75.

Iodine value (*2.5.4*): 76 to 90.

Peroxide value (*2.5.5*): maximum 10.0.

Saponification value (*2.5.6*): 170 to 190.

Carry out the saponification for 1 h.

Composition of fatty acids. Gas chromatography (*2.4.22, Method C*).

Composition of the fatty acid fraction of the substance:

- *myristic acid*: maximum 5.0 per cent,
- *palmitic acid*: maximum 16.0 per cent,
- *palmitoleic acid*: maximum 8.0 per cent,
- *stearic acid*: maximum 6.0 per cent,
- *oleic acid*: 65.0 per cent to 88.0 per cent,
- *linoleic acid*: maximum 18.0 per cent,
- *linolenic acid*: maximum 4.0 per cent,
- *fatty acids with chain length greater than* C_{18}: maximum 4.0 per cent.

Heavy metals (*2.4.8*): maximum 10 ppm.

2.0 g complies with limit test D. Prepare the standard using 2 ml of *lead standard solution (10 ppm Pb) R*.

Water (*2.5.12*): maximum 1.5 per cent, determined on 1.000 g.

Total ash (*2.4.16*): maximum 0.5 per cent, determined on 1.5 g.

STORAGE

Protected from light.

LABELLING

The label states:

- the name and concentration of any added antioxidant,
- the origin of the oleic acid used (animal or vegetable).

01/2005:0435

SORBITOL

Sorbitolum

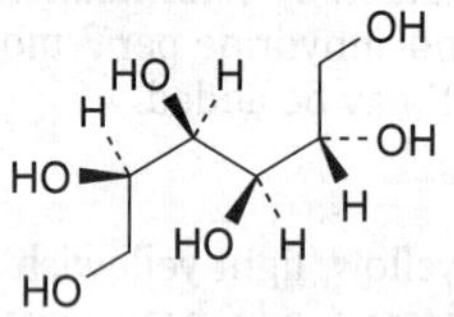

$C_6H_{14}O_6$ M_r 182.2

DEFINITION

Sorbitol contains not less than 97.0 per cent and not more than the equivalent of 102.0 per cent of D-glucitol (D-sorbitol), calculated with reference to the anhydrous substance.

CHARACTERS

A white or almost white, crystalline powder, very soluble in water, practically insoluble in alcohol.

It shows polymorphism.

IDENTIFICATION

First identification: A.

Second identification: B, C, D.

A. Examine the chromatograms obtained in the assay.

Results: the principal peak in the chromatogram obtained with the test solution is similar in retention time and size to the principal peak in the chromatogram obtained with reference solution (a).

B. Dissolve 0.5 g with heating in a mixture of 0.5 ml of *pyridine R* and 5 ml of *acetic anhydride R*. After 10 min, pour the solution into 25 ml of *water R* and allow to stand in iced water for 2 h. The precipitate, recrystallised from a small volume of *alcohol R* and dried *in vacuo*, melts (*2.2.14*) at 98 °C to 104 °C.

C. Examine by thin-layer chromatography (*2.2.27*), using a *TLC silica gel G plate R*.

Test solution. Dissolve 25 mg of the substance to be examined in *water R* and dilute to 10 ml with the same solvent.

Reference solution (a). Dissolve 25 mg of *sorbitol CRS* in *water R* and dilute to 10 ml with the same solvent.

Reference solution (b). Dissolve 25 mg of *mannitol CRS* and 25 mg of *sorbitol CRS* in *water R* and dilute to 10 ml with the same solvent.

Apply to the plate 2 µl of each solution. Develop over a path of 17 cm using a mixture of 10 volumes of *water R*, 20 volumes of *ethyl acetate R* and 70 volumes of *propanol R*. Allow the plate to dry in air and spray with *4-aminobenzoic acid solution R*. Dry the plate in a current of cold air until the acetone is removed. Heat the plate at 100 °C for 15 min. Allow to cool and spray with a 2 g/l solution of *sodium periodate R*. Dry the plate in a current of cold air. Heat the plate at 100 °C for 15 min. The principal spot in the chromatogram obtained with the test solution is similar in position, colour and size to the principal spot in the chromatogram obtained with reference solution (a). The test is not valid unless the chromatogram obtained with reference solution (b) shows 2 clearly separated spots.

D. Dissolve 5.00 g of the substance to be examined and 6.4 g of *disodium tetraborate R* in 40 ml of *water R*. Allow to stand for 1 h, shaking occasionally, and dilute to 50.0 ml with *water R*. Filter if necessary. The specific optical rotation (*2.2.7*) is + 4.0 to + 7.0, calculated with reference to the anhydrous substance.

TESTS

Appearance of solution. Dissolve 5 g in *water R* and dilute to 50 ml with the same solvent. The solution is clear (*2.2.1*) and colourless (*2.2.2, Method II*).

Conductivity (*2.2.38*). Not more than 20 µS·cm^{-1}.

Dissolve 20.0 g in *carbon dioxide-free water R* prepared from *distilled water R* and dilute to 100.0 ml with the same solvent. Measure the conductivity of the solution while gently stirring with a magnetic stirrer.

Reducing sugars. Dissolve 5.0 g in 6 ml of *water R* with the aid of gentle heat. Cool and add 20 ml of *cupri-citric solution R* and a few glass beads. Heat so that boiling begins after 4 min and maintain boiling for 3 min. Cool rapidly and add 100 ml of a 2.4 per cent *V/V* solution of *glacial acetic acid R* and 20.0 ml of *0.025 M iodine*. With continuous shaking, add 25 ml of a mixture of 6 volumes of *hydrochloric acid R* and 94 volumes of *water R* and, when the precipitate has dissolved, titrate the excess of iodine with *0.05 M sodium thiosulphate* using 1 ml of *starch solution R*, added towards the end of the titration, as indicator. Not less than 12.8 ml of *0.05 M sodium thiosulphate* is required (0.2 per cent, calculated as glucose equivalent).

Related products. Examine by liquid chromatography (*2.2.29*) as described in the assay. Inject 20 µl of reference solution (b). Adjust the sensitivity of the system so that the height of the peak due to sorbitol is at least 50 per cent of the full scale of the recorder. Inject 20 µl of the test solution and 20 µl of reference solution (c) and continue the chromatography for twice the retention time of sorbitol. In the chromatogram obtained with the test solution: the area of any peak, apart from the principal peak, is not greater than the area of the principal peak in the chromatogram obtained with reference solution (b) (2 per cent); the sum of the areas of all the peaks, apart from the principal peak, is not greater than 1.5 times the area of the principal peak in the chromatogram obtained with reference solution (b) (3 per cent). Disregard any peak with an area less than the area of the principal peak in the chromatogram obtained with reference solution (c) (0.1 per cent).

Lead (*2.4.10*). It complies with the limit test for lead in sugars (0.5 ppm).

Nickel (*2.4.15*). It complies with the limit test for nickel in polyols (1 ppm). Dissolve the substance to be examined in 150.0 ml of the prescribed mixture of solvents.

Water (*2.5.12*). Not more than 1.5 per cent, determined on 1.00 g by the semi-micro determination of water.

Microbial contamination. If intended for use in the manufacture of parenteral dosage forms the total viable aerobic count (*2.6.12*) is not more than 10^2 bacteria and 10^2 fungi per gram, determined by plate count. It complies with the tests for *Escherichia coli* and *Salmonella* (*2.6.13*).

Bacterial endotoxins (*2.6.14*): if intended for use in the manufacture of parenteral dosage forms without a further appropriate procedure for the removal of bacterial endotoxins, less than 4 IU/g for parenteral dosage forms having a concentration of less than 100 g/l of sorbitol, and less than 2.5 IU/g for parenteral dosage forms having a concentration of 100 g/l or more of sorbitol.

ASSAY

Examine by liquid chromatography (*2.2.29*).

Test solution. Dissolve 5.0 g of the substance to be examined in 20 ml of *water R* and dilute to 100.0 ml with the same solvent.

Reference solution (a). Dissolve 0.50 g of *sorbitol CRS* in 2 ml of *water R* and dilute to 10.0 ml with the same solvent.

Reference solution (b). Dilute 2.0 ml of the test solution to 100.0 ml with *water R*.

Reference solution (c). Dilute 5.0 ml of reference solution (b) to 100.0 ml with *water R*.

Reference solution (d). Dissolve 0.5 g of *sorbitol R* and 0.5 g of *mannitol R* in 5 ml of *water R* and dilute to 10.0 ml with the same solvent.

The chromatography may be carried out using:

- a stainless steel column 0.3 m long and 7.8 mm in internal diameter packed with *strong cation exchange resin (calcium form) R* (9 µm) and maintained at a temperature of 85 ± 1 °C,
- as mobile phase at a flow rate of 0.5 ml/min, degassed *water R*,
- as detector, a refractometer maintained at a constant temperature.

Inject 20 µl of reference solution (d). Continue the chromatography for 3 times the retention time of sorbitol.

When the chromatograms are recorded in the prescribed conditions, the retention time of sorbitol is about 27 min and the relative retentions with reference to sorbitol are: maltitol about 0.6, mannitol about 0.8 and iditol about 1.1. The test is not valid unless the resolution between the peaks due to sorbitol and to mannitol is at least 2 in the chromatogram obtained with reference solution (d).

Inject 20 µl of the test solution and 20 µl of reference solution (a). Continue the chromatography for twice the retention time of sorbitol.

Calculate the percentage content of D-sorbitol from the areas of the peaks and the declared content of *sorbitol CRS*.

LABELLING

The label states:

- where applicable, the maximum concentration of bacterial endotoxins,
- where applicable, that the substance is suitable for use in the manufacture of parenteral dosage forms.

IMPURITIES

A. mannitol,

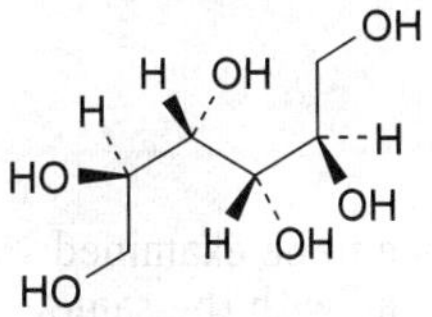

B. iditol,

C. maltitol.

01/2005:0436
corrected

SORBITOL, LIQUID (CRYSTALLISING)

Sorbitolum liquidum cristallisabile

DEFINITION

Aqueous solution of a hydrogenated, partly hydrolysed starch.

Content:

- anhydrous substance: 68.0 per cent *m/m* to 72.0 per cent *m/m*,
- D-glucitol (D-sorbitol, $C_6H_{14}O_6$): 92.0 per cent to 101.0 per cent (anhydrous substance).

CHARACTERS

Appearance: clear, colourless, syrupy liquid, miscible with water.

IDENTIFICATION

A. Examine the chromatograms obtained in the assay.

Results: the principal peak in the chromatogram obtained with the test solution is similar in retention time to the principal peak in the chromatogram obtained with reference solution (a).

B. To 7.0 g add 40 ml of *water R* and 6.4 g of *disodium tetraborate R*, allow to stand for 1 h, shaking occasionally, and dilute to 50.0 ml with *water R*. Filter if necessary. The angle of rotation (*2.2.7*) is 0° to + 1.5°.

C. It is a clear, syrupy liquid at a temperature of 25 °C.

TESTS

Appearance of solution. The solution is clear (*2.2.1*) and colourless (*2.2.2, Method II*).

Dilute 7.0 g to 50 ml with *water R*.

Conductivity (*2.2.38*): maximum 10 µS·cm^{-1} measured on the undiluted liquid sorbitol (crystallising) while gently stirring with a magnetic stirrer.

Reducing sugars: maximum 0.2 per cent calculated as glucose equivalent.

To 5.0 g add 6 ml of *water R*, 20 ml of *cupri-citric solution R* and a few glass beads. Heat so that boiling begins after 4 min and maintain boiling for 3 min. Cool rapidly and add 100 ml of a 2.4 per cent *V/V* solution of *glacial acetic acid R* and 20.0 ml of *0.025 M iodine*. With continuous shaking, add 25 ml of a mixture of 6 volumes of *hydrochloric acid R* and 94 volumes of *water R* and, when the precipitate has dissolved, titrate the excess of iodine with *0.05 M sodium thiosulphate* using 1 ml of *starch solution R*, added towards the end of the titration, as indicator. Not less than 12.8 ml of *0.05 M sodium thiosulphate* is required.

Lead (*2.4.10*): maximum 0.5 ppm.

Nickel (*2.4.15*): maximum 1 ppm.

Water (*2.5.12*): 28.0 per cent to 32.0 per cent *m/m*, determined on 0.1 g.

ASSAY

Liquid chromatography (*2.2.29*).

Test solution. Mix 1.00 g of the substance to be examined with 20 ml of *water R* and dilute to 50.0 ml with the same solvent.

Reference solution (a). Dissolve 65.0 mg of *sorbitol CRS* in 2 ml of *water R* and dilute to 5.0 ml with the same solvent.

Reference solution (b). Dissolve 65 mg of *mannitol R* and 65 mg of *sorbitol R* in 2 ml of *water R* and dilute to 5.0 ml with the same solvent.

Column:

- *size*: l = 0.3 m, Ø = 7.8 mm,
- *stationary phase*: *strong cation exchange resin (calcium form) R* (9 µm),
- *temperature*: 85 ± 1 °C.

Mobile phase: degassed *water R*.

Flow rate: 0.5 ml/min.

Detection: refractometer maintained at a constant temperature.

Injection: 20 µl.

Run time: 3 times the retention time of sorbitol.

Relative retention with reference to sorbitol (retention time = about 27 min): mannitol = about 0.8.

System suitability: reference solution (b):

- *resolution*: minimum 2 between the peaks due to mannitol and to sorbitol.

Calculate the percentage content of D-sorbitol from the areas of the peaks and the declared content of *sorbitol CRS*.

01/2005:0437 corrected

SORBITOL, LIQUID (NON-CRYSTALLISING)

Sorbitolum liquidum non cristallisabile

DEFINITION

Aqueous solution of a hydrogenated, partly hydrolysed starch.

Content:

- anhydrous substance: 68.0 per cent *m/m* to 72.0 per cent *m/m*,
- D-glucitol (D-sorbitol, $C_6H_{14}O_6$): 72.0 per cent to 92.0 per cent (anhydrous substance).

CHARACTERS

Appearance: clear, colourless, syrupy liquid, miscible with water.

IDENTIFICATION

A. Examine the chromatograms obtained in the assay.
   Results: the principal peak in the chromatogram obtained with the test solution is similar in retention time to the principal peak in the chromatogram obtained with reference solution (a).

B. To 7.0 g add 40 ml of *water R* and 6.4 g of *disodium tetraborate R*. Allow to stand for 1 h, shaking occasionally, and dilute to 50.0 ml with *water R*. Filter if necessary. The angle of rotation (*2.2.7*) is + 1.5° to + 3.5°.

C. It is a clear, syrupy liquid at 25 °C.

TESTS

Appearance of solution. The solution is clear (*2.2.1*) and colourless (*2.2.2, Method II*).

Dilute 7.0 g to 50 ml with *water R*.

Conductivity (*2.2.38*): maximum 10 µS·cm^{-1} measured on the undiluted liquid sorbitol (non crystallising) while gently stirring with a magnetic stirrer.

Reducing sugars: maximum 0.2 per cent calculated as glucose equivalent.

To 5.0 g add 6 ml of *water R*, 20 ml of *cupri-citric solution R* and a few glass beads. Heat so that boiling begins after 4 min and maintain boiling for 3 min. Cool rapidly and add 100 ml of a 2.4 per cent *V/V* solution of *glacial acetic acid R* and 20.0 ml of *0.025 M iodine*. With continuous shaking, add 25 ml of a mixture of 6 volumes of *hydrochloric acid R* and 94 volumes of *water R* and, when the precipitate has dissolved, titrate the excess of iodine with *0.05 M sodium thiosulphate* using 1 ml of *starch solution R*, added towards the end of the titration, as indicator. Not less than 12.8 ml of *0.05 M sodium thiosulphate* is required.

Reducing sugars after hydrolysis: maximum 9.3 per cent calculated as glucose equivalent.

To 6.0 g add 35 ml of *water R*, 40 ml of *1 M hydrochloric acid* and a few glass beads. Boil under a reflux condenser for 4 h. Cool and neutralise with *dilute sodium hydroxide solution R* using 0.2 ml of *bromothymol blue solution R1* as indicator. Cool and dilute to 100.0 ml with *water R*. To 3.0 ml of the solution add 5 ml of *water R*, 20 ml of *cupri-citric solution R* and a few glass beads. Heat so that boiling begins after 4 min and maintain boiling for 3 min. Cool rapidly and add 100 ml of a 2.4 per cent *V/V* solution of *glacial acetic acid R* and 20.0 ml of *0.025 M iodine*. With continuous shaking, add 25 ml of a mixture of 6 volumes of *hydrochloric acid R* and 94 volumes of *water R*. When the precipitate has dissolved, titrate the excess of iodine with *0.05 M sodium thiosulphate* using 1 ml of *starch solution R*, added towards the end of the titration, as indicator. Not less than 8.0 ml of *0.05 M sodium thiosulphate* is required.

Lead (*2.4.10*): maximum 0.5 ppm.

Nickel (*2.4.15*): maximum 1 ppm.

Water (*2.5.12*): 28.0 per cent to 32.0 per cent *m/m*, determined on 0.1 g.

ASSAY

Liquid chromatography (*2.2.29*).

Test solution. Mix 1.00 g of the substance to be examined with 20 ml of *water R* and dilute to 50.0 ml with the same solvent.

Reference solution (a). Dissolve 55.0 mg of *sorbitol CRS* in 2 ml of *water R* and dilute to 5.0 ml with the same solvent.

Reference solution (b). Dissolve 55 mg of *mannitol R* and 55 mg of *sorbitol R* in 2 ml of *water R* and dilute to 5.0 ml with the same solvent.

Column:

- *size*: l = 0.3 m, Ø = 7.8 mm,
- *stationary phase*: *strong cation exchange resin (calcium form) R* (9 μm),
- *temperature*: 85 ± 1 °C.

Mobile phase: degassed *water R*.

Flow rate: 0.5 ml/min.

Detection: refractometer maintained at a constant temperature.

Injection: 20 μl.

Run time: 3 times the retention time of sorbitol.

Relative retention with reference to sorbitol (retention time = about 27 min): mannitol = about 0.8.

System suitability: reference solution (b):

- *resolution*: minimum 2 between the peaks due to mannitol and to sorbitol.

Calculate the percentage content of D-sorbitol from the areas of the peaks and the declared content of *sorbitol CRS*.

01/2005:2048

SORBITOL, LIQUID, PARTIALLY DEHYDRATED

Sorbitolum liquidum partim deshydricum

DEFINITION

Liquid sorbitol, partially dehydrated is obtained by acid-catalysed partial internal dehydration of liquid sorbitol. It contains not less than 68.0 per cent *m/m* and not more than 85.0 per cent *m/m* of anhydrous substances, composed of a mixture of mainly D-sorbitol and 1,4-sorbitan with mannitol, hydrogenated oligo- and disaccharides, and sorbitans.

Content (nominal value):

- 1,4-sorbitan ($C_6H_{12}O_5$): minimum 15.0 per cent (anhydrous substance),
- D-sorbitol ($C_6H_{14}O_6$): minimum 25.0 per cent (anhydrous substance).

The contents of 1,4-sorbitan and D-sorbitol are within 95.0 per cent to 105.0 per cent of the nominal values.

CHARACTERS

Appearance: clear, colourless, syrupy liquid.

Solubility: miscible with water, practically insoluble in mineral oils and vegetable oils.

IDENTIFICATION

Examine the chromatograms obtained in the assay.

Results: the 2 principal peaks in the chromatogram obtained with the test solution are similar in retention time and size to the peaks in the chromatogram obtained with reference solution (a).

TESTS

Solution S. Dilute the substance to be examined with *carbon dioxide-free water R* prepared from *distilled water R* to obtain a solution containing 50.0 per cent *m/m* of anhydrous substance.

Appearance of solution. Solution S is clear (*2.2.1*) and colourless (*2.2.2, Method II*).

Conductivity (*2.2.38*): maximum 20 $\mu S \cdot cm^{-1}$.

Measure the conductivity of solution S, while gently stirring with a magnetic stirrer.

Reducing sugars: maximum 0.3 per cent, calculated as glucose (anhydrous substance).

To an amount of the substance to be examined equivalent to 3.3 g of anhydrous substance, add 3 ml of *water R*, 20.0 ml of *cupri-citric solution R* and a few glass beads. Heat so that boiling begins after 4 min. Maintain boiling for 3 min. Cool rapidly and add 100 ml of a 2.4 per cent *V/V* solution of *glacial acetic acid R* and 20.0 ml of *0.025 M iodine*. With continuous shaking, add 25 ml of a mixture of 6 ml of *hydrochloric acid R* and 94 ml of *water R*. When the precipitate has dissolved, titrate the excess of iodine with *0.05 M sodium thiosulphate* using 2 ml of *starch solution R*, added towards the end of the titration, as indicator. Not less than 12.8 ml of *0.05 M sodium thiosulphate* is required.

Nickel (*2.4.15*): maximum 1 ppm (anhydrous substance).

Water (*2.5.12*): 15.0 per cent to 32.0 per cent, determined on 0.10 g.

Microbial contamination. Total viable aerobic count (*2.6.12*) not more than 10^3 micro-organisms per gram and not more than 10^2 fungi per gram, determined by plate count. It complies with the tests for *Escherichia coli* and *Salmonella* (*2.6.13*).

ASSAY

Liquid chromatography (*2.2.29*).

Test solution. Dissolve 0.400 g of the substance to be examined in *water R* and dilute to 20.0 ml with the same solvent.

Reference solution (a). Dissolve 50.0 mg of *sorbitol CRS* and 20.0 mg of *1,4-sorbitan CRS* in *water R* and dilute to 5.0 ml with the same solvent.

Reference solution (b). Dissolve 0.100 g of *mannitol R* and 0.100 g of *sorbitol R* in *water R* and dilute to 10.0 ml with the same solvent.

Column:

- *size*: l = 0.3 m, Ø = 7.8 mm,
- *stationary phase*: *strong cation exchange resin (calcium form) R* (9 μm),
- *temperature*: 80 ± 5 °C.

Mobile phase: degassed *water R*.

Flow rate: 0.5 ml/min.

Detection: refractometer maintained at a constant temperature of about 30-35 °C.

Injection: 40 μl.

Relative retention with reference to D-sorbitol (retention time = about 25 min): 1,4-sorbitan = about 0.5; mannitol = about 0.8.

System suitability: reference solution (b):

- *resolution*: minimum 2.0 between the peaks due to mannitol and D-sorbitol.

Calculate the percentage contents of 1,4-sorbitan and D-sorbitol using the chromatogram obtained with reference solution (a) and the declared contents of *1,4-sorbitan CRS* and of *sorbitol CRS*.

LABELLING

The label states the content of D-sorbitol and the content of 1,4-sorbitan (= nominal values).

01/2005:2004

SOTALOL HYDROCHLORIDE

Sotaloli hydrochloridum

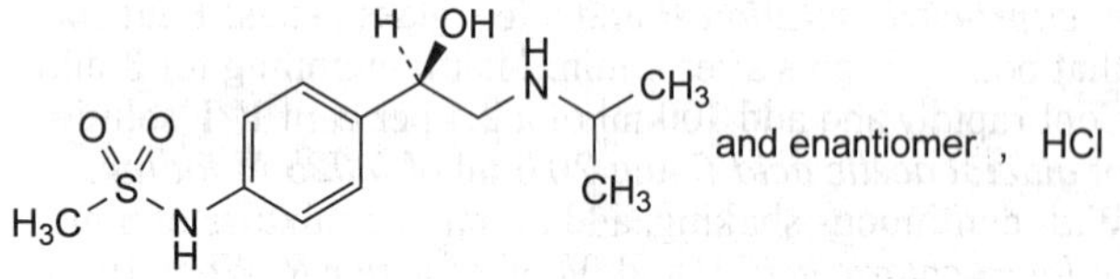

$C_{12}H_{21}ClN_2O_3S$ M_r 308.8

DEFINITION

N-[4-[(1*RS*)-1-hydroxy-2-[(1-methylethyl)amino]ethyl]phenyl]methanesulphonamide hydrochloride.

Content: 99.0 per cent to 101.0 per cent (dried substance).

CHARACTERS

Appearance: white or almost white powder.

Solubility: freely soluble in water, soluble in alcohol, practically insoluble in methylene chloride.

IDENTIFICATION

A. Infrared absorption spectrophotometry (*2.2.24*).

Comparison: *sotalol hydrochloride CRS*.

B. It gives reaction (a) of chlorides (*2.3.1*).

TESTS

Solution S. Dissolve 5.0 g in *carbon dioxide-free water R* and dilute to 50.0 ml with the same solvent.

Appearance of solution. Solution S is not more opalescent than reference suspension III (*2.2.1*) and not more intensely coloured than reference solution Y_6 (*2.2.2, Method II*).

pH (*2.2.3*): 4.0 to 5.0.

Dilute 5.0 ml of solution S to 10.0 ml with *carbon dioxide-free water R*.

Optical rotation (*2.2.7*): −0.10° to + 0.10°.

Dilute 25.0 ml of solution S to 50.0 ml with *water R*.

Related substances. Liquid chromatography (*2.2.29*).

Test solution. Dissolve 20.0 mg of the substance to be examined in the mobile phase and dilute to 10.0 ml with the mobile phase.

Reference solution (a). Dilute 1.0 ml of the test solution to 100.0 ml with the mobile phase. Dilute 3.0 ml of this solution to 10.0 ml with the mobile phase.

Reference solution (b). Dissolve 8.0 mg of *sotalol impurity B CRS* in the mobile phase and dilute to 10.0 ml with the mobile phase.

Reference solution (c). Dilute 1.0 ml of reference solution (b) to 100.0 ml with the mobile phase.

Reference solution (d). Dilute 1.5 ml of reference solution (b) to 100 ml with the mobile phase. To 1 ml of this solution add 1 ml of reference solution (a).

Column:

- *size*: *l* = 0.25 m, Ø = 4.6 mm,
- *stationary phase*: *octadecylsilyl silica gel for chromatography R* (5 µm).

Mobile phase: dissolve 2 g of *sodium octanesulphonate R* in 790 ml of *water R*. Adjust to pH 3.0 with *phosphoric acid R* and add 210 ml of *acetonitrile R*.

Flow rate: 1 ml/min.

Detection: spectrophotometer at 228 nm.

Injection: 10 µl; inject the test solution and reference solutions (a), (c) and (d).

Run time: 2.5 times the retention time of sotalol.

System suitability: reference solution (d):

- *resolution*: minimum 4.0 between the peaks due to sotalol and to impurity B.

Limits:

- *impurity B*: not more than 0.25 times the area of the principal peak in the chromatogram obtained with reference solution (c) (0.1 per cent),
- *any other impurity*: not more than the area of the principal peak in the chromatogram obtained with reference solution (a) (0.3 per cent), and not more than 1 such peak has an area greater than 0.3 times the area of the principal peak in the chromatogram obtained with reference solution (a) (0.1 per cent),
- *total of other impurities*: not more than 1.65 times the area of the principal peak in the chromatogram obtained with reference solution (a) (0.5 per cent),
- *disregard limit*: 0.17 times the area of the principal peak in the chromatogram obtained with reference solution (a) (0.05 per cent).

Palladium: maximum 0.5 ppm.

Atomic absorption spectrometry (*2.2.23, Method I*).

Test solution. Dissolve 1.00 g in a mixture of 0.25 volumes of *nitric acid R*, 0.75 volumes of *hydrochloric acid R* and 99.0 volumes of *water R* and dilute to 20.0 ml with the same mixture of solvents.

Reference solutions. Use solutions containing 0.02 µg, 0.03 µg and 0.05 µg of palladium per millilitre, freshly prepared by dilution of *palladium standard solution (0.5 ppm Pd) R* with a mixture of 0.25 volumes of *nitric acid R*, 0.75 volumes of *hydrochloric acid R* and 99.0 volumes of *water R*.

Source: palladium hollow-cathode lamp.

Wavelength: 247.6 nm.

Use a graphite tube.

Heavy metals (*2.4.8*): maximum 20 ppm.

To 10 ml of solution S add 10 ml of *water R*. 12 ml of the solution complies with limit test A. Prepare the standard using *lead standard solution (1 ppm Pb) R*.

Loss on drying (*2.2.32*): maximum 0.5 per cent, determined on 1.000 g by drying in an oven at 100-105 °C.

Sulphated ash (*2.4.14*): maximum 0.1 per cent, determined on 1.0 g.

ASSAY

In order to avoid overheating during the titration, mix thoroughly throughout and stop the titration immediately after the end-point has been reached.

Dissolve 0.250 g in 10 ml of *anhydrous formic acid R*, if necessary with the aid of ultrasound. Add 40 ml of *acetic anhydride R* and titrate immediately with *0.1 M perchloric acid*. Determine the end-point potentiometrically (*2.2.20*).

Monographs Q-S

1 ml of *0.1 M perchloric acid* is equivalent to 30.88 mg of $C_{12}H_{21}ClN_2O_3S$.

STORAGE

Protected from light.

IMPURITIES

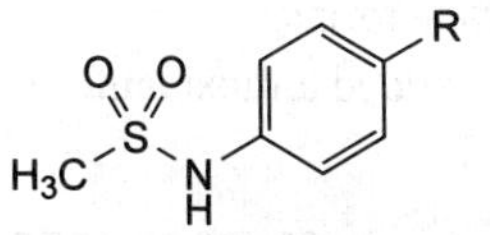

A. R = CH_2-CH_2-NH-CH$(CH_3)_2$: *N*-[4-[2-[(1-methylethyl)amino]ethyl]phenyl]methanesulphonamide,

B. R = CO-CH_2-NH-CH$(CH_3)_2$: *N*-[4-[[(1-methylethyl)amino]acetyl]phenyl]methanesulphonamide,

C. R = CHO: *N*-(4-formylphenyl)methanesulphonamide,

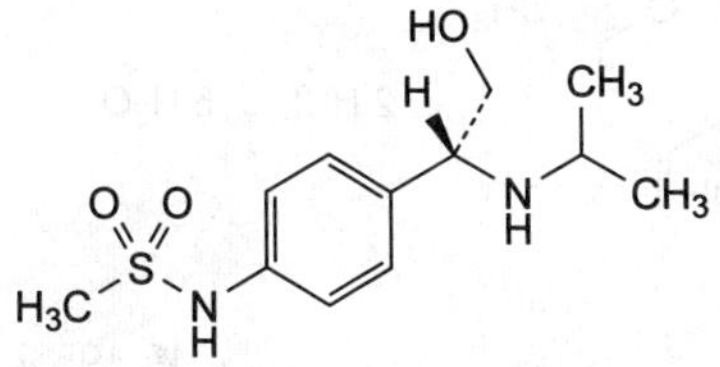

and enantiomer

D. *N*-[4-[(1*RS*)-2-hydroxy-1-[(1-methylethyl)amino]ethyl]phenyl]methanesulphonamide.

01/2005:1265

SOYA-BEAN OIL, HYDROGENATED

Soiae oleum hydrogenatum

DEFINITION

Hydrogenated soya-bean oil is the product obtained by refining, bleaching, hydrogenation and deodorisation of oil obtained from seeds of *Glycine soja* Sieb. and Zucc. and *Glycine max* (L.) Merr. (*G. hispida* (Moench) Maxim.). The product consists mainly of triglycerides of palmitic and stearic acids.

CHARACTERS

A white mass or powder which melts to a clear, pale yellow liquid when heated, practically insoluble in water, freely soluble in methylene chloride, in light petroleum (bp: 65 °C to 70 °C) after heating and in toluene, very slightly soluble in alcohol.

IDENTIFICATION

A. It complies with the test for melting point (see Tests).

B. It complies with the test for foreign fatty oils (see Tests).

TESTS

Melting point (*2.2.15*): 66 °C to 72 °C.

Acid value (*2.5.1*). Not more than 0.5, determined on 10.0 g. Dissolve the substance to be examined in 50 ml of a hot mixture of equal volumes of *alcohol R* and *toluene R*, previously neutralised with *0.1 M potassium hydroxide* using 0.5 ml of *phenolphthalein solution R1* as indicator. Titrate the solution immediately while still hot.

Peroxide value (*2.5.5*). Not more than 5.0.

Unsaponifiable matter (*2.5.7*). Not more than 1.0 per cent, determined on 5.0 g.

Alkaline impurities in fatty oils (*2.4.19*). Dissolve 2.0 g with gentle heating in a mixture of 1.5 ml of *alcohol R* and 3 ml of *toluene R*. Add 0.05 ml of a 0.4 g/l solution of *bromophenol blue R* in *alcohol R*. Not more than 0.4 ml of *0.01 M hydrochloric acid* is required to change the colour to yellow.

Composition of fatty acids (*2.4.22, Method A*).

The chromatographic procedure may be carried out using:

- a fused-silica column 25 m long and 0.25 mm in internal diameter coated with *poly(cyanopropyl)siloxane R* (film thickness 0.2 µm),
- *helium for chromatography R* as the carrier gas at a flow rate of 0.65 ml/min,
- a flame-ionisation detector,
- a split injector (1:100),

maintaining the temperature of the column at 180 °C for 20 min and that of the injection port and the detector at 250 °C.

The fatty acid fraction of the oil has the following composition:

- *saturated fatty acids of chain length less than* C_{14}: not more than 0.1 per cent,
- *myristic acid*: not more than 0.5 per cent,
- *palmitic acid*: 9.0 per cent to 16.0 per cent,
- *stearic acid*: 79.0 per cent to 89.0 per cent,
- *oleic acid and isomers* ($C_{18:1}$ *equivalent chain length on poly(cyanopropyl)siloxane 18.5 to 18.8)*: not more than 4.0 per cent,
- *linoleic acid and isomers* ($C_{18:2}$ *equivalent chain length on poly(cyanopropyl)siloxane 19.4 to 19.8)*: not more than 1.0 per cent,
- *linolenic acid and isomers* ($C_{18:3}$ *equivalent chain length on poly(cyanopropyl)siloxane 20.3 to 20.7)*: not more than 0.2 per cent,
- *arachidic acid*: not more than 1.0 per cent,
- *behenic acid*: not more than 1.0 per cent.

Nickel. Not more than 1 ppm of Ni, determined by atomic absorption spectrometry (*2.2.23, Method II*).

Test solution. Introduce 5.0 g into a platinum or silica crucible, previously tared after calcination. Cautiously heat and introduce into the substance a wick formed from twisted ashless filter paper. Light the wick. When the substance is alight stop heating. After combustion, ignite in a muffle furnace at about 600 °C. Continue the ignition until white ash is obtained. After cooling, take up the residue with two quantities, each of 2 ml, of *dilute hydrochloric acid R* and transfer into a 25 ml graduated flask. Add 0.3 ml of *nitric acid R* and dilute to 25.0 ml with *water R*.

Reference solutions. Prepare three reference solutions by adding 1.0 ml, 2.0 ml and 4.0 ml of *nickel standard solution (0.2 ppm Ni) R* to 2.0 ml of the test solution and diluting to 10.0 ml with *water R*.

Measure the absorbance at 232 nm using a nickel hollow-cathode lamp as a source of radiation, a graphite furnace as an atomic generator and *argon R* as the carrier gas.

Water (*2.5.12*). Not more than 0.3 per cent, determined on 1.000 g by the semi-micro determination of water.

STORAGE

Store protected from light.

01/2005:1473

SOYA-BEAN OIL, REFINED

Soiae oleum raffinatum

DEFINITION

Refined soya-bean oil is the fatty oil obtained from seeds of *Glycine soja* Sieb. and Zucc. and *Glycine max* (L.) Merr. (*G. hispida* (Moench) Maxim.) by extraction and subsequent refining. It may contain a suitable antioxidant.

CHARACTERS

A clear, pale yellow, liquid, miscible with light petroleum (50 °C to 70 °C), practically insoluble in alcohol.

It has a relative density of about 0.922 and a refractive index of about 1.475.

IDENTIFICATION

Carry out the identification of fatty oils by thin-layer chromatography (*2.3.2*). The chromatogram obtained is similar to the typical chromatogram for soya-bean oil.

TESTS

Acid value (*2.5.1*). Not more than 0.5, determined on 10.0 g.

Peroxide value (*2.5.5, Method A*). Not more than 10.0. If intended for use in the manufacture of parenteral dosage forms, the peroxide value is not more than 5.0.

Unsaponifiable matter (*2.5.7*). Not more than 1.5 per cent, determined on 5.0 g.

Alkaline impurities (*2.4.19*). It complies with the test for alkaline impurities in fatty oils.

Composition of fatty acids (*2.4.22, Method A*). The fatty acid fraction of the oil has the following composition:

- *saturated fatty acids of chain length less than* C_{14}: not more than 0.1 per cent,
- *myristic acid*: not more than 0.2 per cent,
- *palmitic acid*: 9.0 per cent to 13.0 per cent,
- *palmitoleic acid* (equivalent chain length on polyethyleneglycol adipate 16.3): not more than 0.3 per cent,
- *stearic acid*: 3.0 per cent to 5.0 per cent,
- *oleic acid* (equivalent chain length on polyethyleneglycol adipate 18.3): 17.0 per cent to 30.0 per cent,
- *linoleic acid* (equivalent chain length on polyethyleneglycol adipate 18.9): 48.0 per cent to 58.0 per cent,
- *linolenic acid* (equivalent chain length on polyethyleneglycol adipate 19.7): 5.0 per cent to 11.0 per cent,
- *arachidic acid*: not more than 1.0 per cent,
- *eicosenoic acid* (equivalent chain length on polyethyleneglycol adipate 20.3): not more than 1.0 per cent,
- *behenic acid*: not more than 1.0 per cent.

Brassicasterol (*2.4.23*). The sterol fraction of the oil contains not more than 0.3 per cent of brassicasterol.

Water (*2.5.32*). If intended for use in the manufacture of parenteral dosage forms, not more than 0.1 per cent, determined on 5.00 g by the coulometric determination of water. Use a mixture of equal volumes of *decanol R* and *anhydrous methanol R* as the solvent.

STORAGE

Store in a well-filled container, protected from light, at a temperature not exceeding 25 °C.

LABELLING

The label states:

- where applicable, that the substance is suitable for use in the manufacture of parenteral dosage forms,
- the name and concentration of any added antioxidant.

01/2005:1152

SPECTINOMYCIN HYDROCHLORIDE

Spectinomycini hydrochloridum

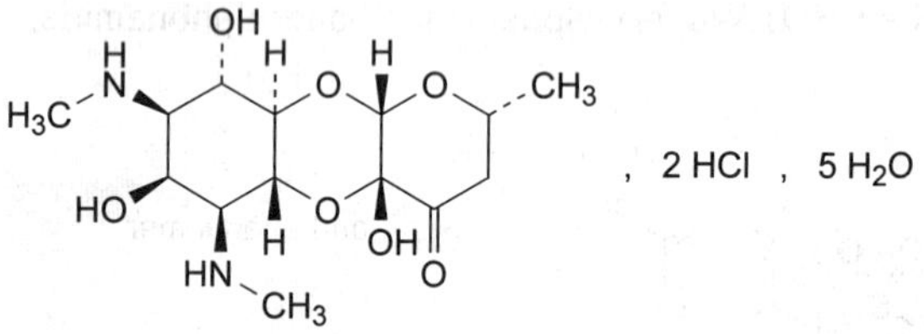

$C_{14}H_{26}Cl_2N_2O_7,5H_2O$ M_r 495.4

DEFINITION

Spectinomycin hydrochloride is the pentahydrate of the dihydrochloride of (2*R*,4a*R*,5a*R*,6*S*,7*S*,8*R*,9*S*,9a*R*,10a*S*)-4a,7,9-trihydroxy-2-methyl-6,8-bis(methylamino)decahydro-4*H*-pyrano[2,3-*b*][1,4]benzodioxin-4-one dihydrochloride, an antimicrobial substance produced by *Streptomyces spectabilis* or by any other means. It contains not less than 95.0 per cent and not more than the equivalent of 100.5 per cent of $C_{14}H_{26}Cl_2N_2O_7$ calculated with reference to the anhydrous substance.

CHARACTERS

A white or almost white powder, slightly hygroscopic, freely soluble in water, very slightly soluble in alcohol.

IDENTIFICATION

A. Examine by infrared absorption spectrophotometry (*2.2.24*), comparing with the spectrum obtained with *spectinomycin hydrochloride CRS*.

B. Dilute 1.0 ml of solution S (see Tests) to 10 ml with *water R*. The solution gives reaction (a) of chlorides (*2.3.1*).

TESTS

Solution S. Dissolve 2.0 g in *carbon dioxide-free water R* and dilute to 20.0 ml with the same solvent.

Appearance of solution. Dilute 2.0 ml of solution S to 20.0 ml with *water R*. The solution is clear (*2.2.1*) and colourless (*2.2.2, Method II*).

pH (*2.2.3*).The pH of solution S is 3.8 to 5.6.

Specific optical rotation (*2.2.7*): + 15 to + 21, determined on solution S within 20 min of preparation and calculated with reference to the anhydrous substance.

Related substances. Examine by thin-layer chromatography (*2.2.27*), using *silica gel G R* as the coating substance.

Test solution. Dilute 2.0 ml of solution S to 10 ml with *water R*.

Reference solution. Dilute 1.0 ml of the test solution to 100 ml with *water R*.

Apply separately to the plate 10 µl of each solution. Develop over a path of 12 cm using a mixture of 5 volumes of *glacial acetic acid R*, 5 volumes of *pyridine R*, 40 volumes of *water R* and 50 volumes of *propanol R*. Dry the plate in a current of warm air and spray with a 50 g/l solution of *potassium permanganate R*. Allow the plate to stand for 2 min to 3 min. Any spot in the chromatogram obtained with the test solution, apart from the principal spot, is not more intense than the spot in the chromatogram obtained with the reference solution (1.0 per cent).

Water (*2.5.12*): 16.0 per cent to 20.0 per cent, determined on 0.200 g by the semi-micro determination of water.

Sulphated ash (*2.4.14*). Not more than 1.0 per cent, determined on 1.000 g.

Bacterial endotoxins (*2.6.14*): less than 0.09 IU/mg, if intended for use in the manufacture of parenteral dosage forms without a further appropriate procedure for the removal of bacterial endotoxins. Prepare the solutions using a 0.42 per cent *m/m* solution of *sodium hydrogen carbonate R*.

ASSAY

Examine by gas chromatography (*2.2.28*), using *phenazone R* as the internal standard.

Internal standard solution. Dissolve 0.150 g of *phenazone R* in *dimethylformamide R* and dilute to 100 ml with the same solvent.

Allow the test solutions and the reference solution to stand for 1 h. Carry out the assay immediately.

Test solution (a). To 60.0 mg of the substance to be examined in a volumetric flask, add 10 ml of *dimethylformamide R* and 2.0 ml of *hexamethyldisilazane R*. Shake to dissolve and dilute to 20.0 ml with *dimethylformamide R*.

Test solution (b). To 60.0 mg of the substance to be examined in a volumetric flask add 10.0 ml of the internal standard solution and 2.0 ml of *hexamethyldisilazane R*. Shake to dissolve and dilute to 20.0 ml with *dimethylformamide R*.

Reference solution. To 60.0 mg of *spectinomycin hydrochloride CRS* in a volumetric flask add 10.0 ml of the internal standard solution and 2.0 ml of *hexamethyldisilazane R*. Shake to dissolve and dilute to 20.0 ml with *dimethylformamide R*.

The chromatographic procedure may be carried out using:

- a glass column 1.5 m long and 4 mm in internal diameter packed with *silanised diatomaceous earth for gas chromatography R* (125 µm to 150 µm) impregnated with 3 per cent *m/m* of a mixture of *polyphenylmethylsiloxane R*,
- *nitrogen for chromatography R* as the carrier gas at a flow rate of 45 ml/min,
- a flame-ionisation detector,
- an electronic integrator.

Maintain the temperature of the column at 200 °C and that of the injection port and of the detector between 200 °C and 230 °C. Inject the chosen volumes of the test solutions. The assay is not valid unless in the chromatogram obtained with test solution (b) the resolution between the main peak and the peak corresponding to the internal standard is at least 8.0. Inject alternately test solution (b) and the reference solution.

Calculate the percentage content of spectinomycin.

STORAGE

Store in an airtight container, at a temperature not exceeding 30 °C. If the substance is sterile, store in a sterile, airtight, tamper-proof container.

LABELLING

The label states, where applicable, that the substance is free from bacterial endotoxins.

IMPURITIES

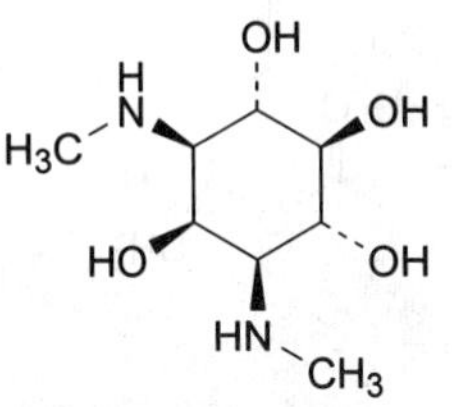

A. 1,3-dideoxy-1,3-bis(methylamino)-*myo*-inositol (actinamine),

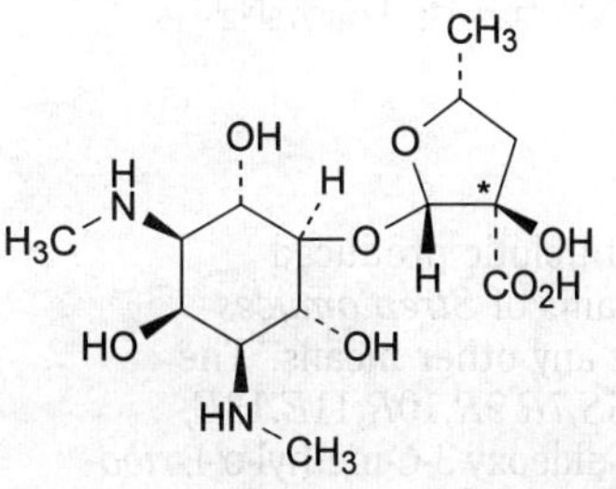

and epimer at C*

B. (2*S*,3*RS*,5*R*)-3-hydroxy-5-methyl-2-[[(1*r*,2*R*,3*S*,4*r*,5*R*,6*S*)-2,4,6-trihydroxy-3,5-bis(methylamino)cyclohexyl]oxy]tetrahyrofuran-3-carboxylic acid (actinospectinoic acid),

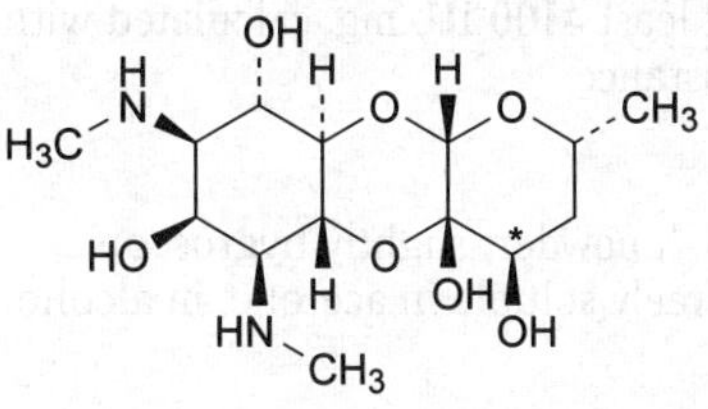

and epimer at C*

C. (2*R*,4*RS*,4a*S*,5a*R*,6*S*,7*S*,8*R*,9*S*,9a*R*,10a*S*)-2-methyl-6,8-bis(methylamino)decahydro-2*H*-pyrano[2,3-*b*][1,4]benzodioxine-4,4a,7,9-tetrol (dihydrospectinomycins),

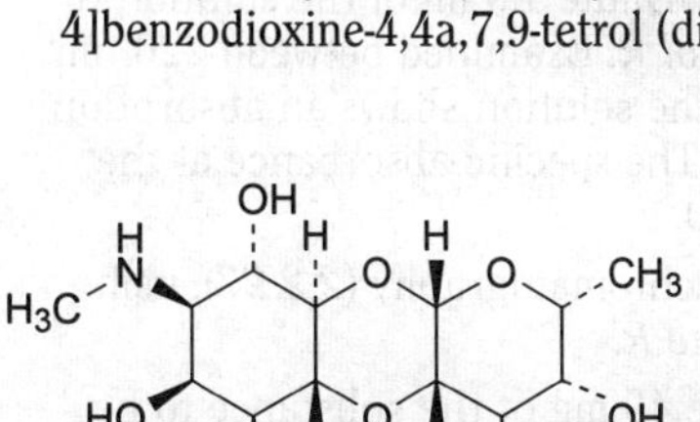

D. (2*R*,3*R*,4*S*,4a*S*,5a*R*,6*S*,7*S*,8*R*,9*S*,9a*R*,10a*S*)-2-methyl-6,8-bis(methylamino)decahydro-2*H*-pyrano[2,3-*b*][1,4]benzodioxine-3,4,4a,7,9-pentol (dihydroxyspectinomycin).

01/2005:0293
corrected

SPIRAMYCIN

Spiramycinum

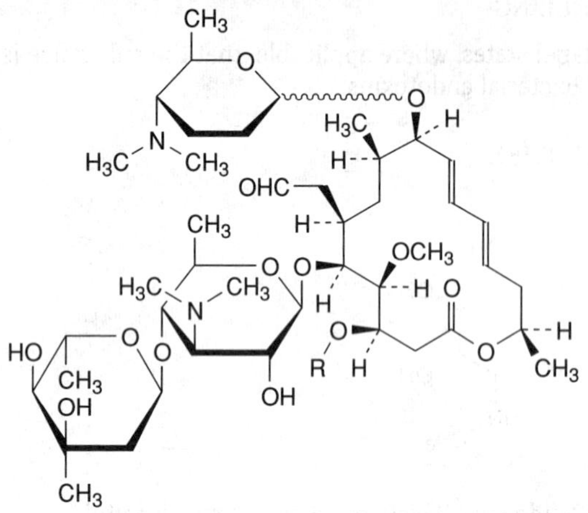

Spiramycin I	R = H	$C_{43}H_{74}N_2O_{14}$
Spiramycin II	R = CO-CH$_3$	$C_{45}H_{76}N_2O_{15}$
Spiramycin III	R = CO-CH$_2$-CH$_3$	$C_{46}H_{78}N_2O_{15}$

$C_{43}H_{74}N_2O_{14}$

DEFINITION

Spiramycin is a macrolide antibiotic produced by the growth of certain strains of *Streptomyces ambofaciens* or obtained by any other means. The main component is (4*R*,5*S*,6*S*,7*R*,9*R*,10*R*,11*E*,13*E*,16*R*)-6-[[3,6-dideoxy-4-*O*-(2,6-dideoxy-3-*C*-methyl-α-L-*ribo*-hexopyranosyl)-3-(dimethylamino)-β-D-glucopyranosyl]oxy]-4-hydroxy-5-methoxy-9,16-dimethyl-7-(2-oxoethyl)-10-[[2,3,4,6-tetradeoxy-4-(dimethylamino)-D-*erythro*-hexopyranosyl]oxy]oxacyclohexadeca-11,13-dien-2-one (spiramycin I, M_r 843). Spiramycin II (4-*O*-acetylspiramycin I) and spiramycin III (4-*O*-propanoylspiramycin I) are also present. The potency is at least 4100 IU/mg, calculated with reference to the dried substance.

CHARACTERS

A white or slightly yellowish powder, slightly hygroscopic, slightly soluble in water, freely soluble in acetone, in alcohol and in methanol.

IDENTIFICATION

A. Dissolve 0.10 g in *methanol R* and dilute to 100.0 ml with the same solvent. Dilute 1.0 ml of the solution to 100.0 ml with *methanol R*. Examined between 220 nm and 350 nm (*2.2.25*), the solution shows an absorption maximum at 232 nm. The specific absorbance at the maximum is about 340.

B. Examine by thin-layer chromatography (*2.2.27*), using a *TLC silica gel G plate R*.

Test solution. Dissolve 40 mg of the substance to be examined in *methanol R* and dilute to 10 ml with the same solvent.

Reference solution (a). Dissolve 40 mg of *spiramycin CRS* in *methanol R* and dilute to 10 ml with the same solvent.

Reference solution (b). Dissolve 40 mg of *erythromycin A CRS* in *methanol R* and dilute to 10 ml with the same solvent.

Apply to the plate 5 µl of each solution. Develop over a path of 15 cm using the upper layer of a mixture of 4 volumes of *2-propanol R*, 8 volumes of a 150 g/l solution of *ammonium acetate R* previously adjusted to pH 9.6 with *strong sodium hydroxide solution R*, and 9 volumes of *ethyl acetate R*. Allow the plate to dry in air, spray with *anisaldehyde solution R1* and heat at 110 °C for 5 min. The principal spot in the chromatogram obtained with the test solution is similar in position, colour and size to the principal spot in the chromatogram obtained with reference solution (a). If in the chromatogram obtained with the test solution one or two spots occur with R_f values slightly higher than that of the principal spot, these spots are similar in position and colour to the secondary spots in the chromatogram obtained with reference solution (a) and differ from the spots in the chromatogram obtained with reference solution (b).

C. Dissolve 0.5 g in 10 ml of *0.05 M sulphuric acid* and add 25 ml of *water R*. Adjust to about pH 8 with *0.1 M sodium hydroxide* and dilute to 50 ml with *water R*. To 5 ml of this solution add 2 ml of a mixture of 1 volume of *water R* and 2 volumes of *sulphuric acid R*. A brown colour develops.

TESTS

pH (*2.2.3*). Dissolve 0.5 g in 5 ml of *methanol R* and dilute to 100 ml with *carbon dioxide-free water R*. The pH of the solution is 8.5 to 10.5.

Specific optical rotation (*2.2.7*). Dissolve 1.00 g in a 10 per cent *V/V* solution of *dilute acetic acid R* and dilute to 50.0 ml with the same acid. The specific optical rotation is − 80 to − 85, calculated with reference to the dried substance.

Composition. Not less than 80.0 per cent of spiramycin I, not more than 5.0 per cent of spiramycin II and not more than 10.0 per cent of spiramycin III; the sum of the contents of spiramycin I, spiramycin II and spiramycin III is not less than 90.0 per cent, all contents are calculated with reference to the dried substance. Examine by liquid chromatography (*2.2.29*) as prescribed in the test for related substances. Inject reference solution (a) 6 times. The test is not valid unless the relative standard deviation of the peak area for spiramycin I is at most 1.0 per cent. Inject alternately the test solution and reference solution (a). Continue the chromatography of the test solution for 3 times the retention time of spiramycin I. Calculate the percentage content of spiramycin I, spiramycin II and spiramycin III using the declared contents of *spiramycin CRS*.

Related substances. Examine by liquid chromatography (*2.2.29*). *Prepare the solutions immediately before use.*

Test solution. Dissolve 25.0 mg of the substance to be examined in a mixture of 3 volumes of *acetonitrile R* and 7 volumes of *water R* and dilute to 100.0 ml with the same mixture of solvents.

Reference solution (a). Dissolve 25.0 mg of *spiramycin CRS* in a mixture of 3 volumes of *acetonitrile R* and 7 volumes of *water R* and dilute to 100.0 ml with the same mixture of solvents.

Reference solution (b). Dilute 2.0 ml of reference solution (a) to 100.0 ml with a mixture of 3 volumes of *acetonitrile R* and 7 volumes of *water R*.

Reference solution (c). Dilute 5.0 ml of reference solution (a) to 100.0 ml with a mixture of 3 volumes of *acetonitrile R* and 7 volumes of *water R*.

Reference solution (d). Dissolve 5 mg of *spiramycin CRS* in 25 ml of the mobile phase, then heat in a water-bath at 60 °C for 30 min.

Monographs Q-S

The chromatographic procedure may be carried out using:

– a stainless steel column 0.25 m long and 4.6 mm in internal diameter packed with spherical *octylsilyl silica gel for chromatography R* (5 µm) with a specific surface area of 350 m²/g and a pore size of 10 nm,

– as mobile phase at a flow rate of 0.8 ml/min a mixture of 30 volumes of *acetonitrile R* and 70 volumes of *buffer solution pH 2.2 R* containing 9.3 g/l of *sodium perchlorate R*,

– as detector a spectrophotometer set at 232 nm.

Inject 20 µl of reference solution (b). Adjust the sensitivity of the system so that the height of the principal peak in the chromatogram obtained is at least 50 per cent of the full scale of the recorder. Inject 20 µl of reference solution (c) and 20 µl of reference solution (d). The test is not valid unless: in the chromatogram obtained with reference solution (c), there is no significant peak with a retention time, relative to spiramycin I, of about 1.1; in the chromatogram obtained with reference solution (d), the resolution between impurity A (eluting first) and spiramycin I (eluting at 13 min to 17 min) is at least 6.3 (see Figure 0293.-1). If necessary, adjust the concentration of acetonitrile in the mobile phase (increasing the concentration to decrease the retention time or decreasing the concentration to increase the retention time).

Inject 20 µl of the test solution and 20 µl of reference solution (b). Continue the chromatography of the test solution for 3 times the retention time of spiramycin I. In the chromatogram obtained with the test solution: the area of any peak, apart from the peaks corresponding to spiramycin I, spiramycin II and spiramycin III, is not greater than the area of the principal peak in the chromatogram obtained with reference solution (b) (2 per cent). Disregard any peak with an area less than 0.05 times that of the principal peak in the chromatogram obtained with reference solution (b).

Heavy metals (*2.4.8*). 1.0 g complies with limit test C (20 ppm). Prepare the standard using 2 ml of *lead standard solution (10 ppm Pb) R*.

Loss on drying (*2.2.32*). Not more than 3.5 per cent, determined on 0.50 g by drying over *diphosphorus pentoxide R* at 80 °C at a pressure not exceeding 670 Pa for 6 h.

Sulphated ash (*2.4.14*). Not more than 0.1 per cent, determined on 1.0 g.

ASSAY

Carry out the microbiological assay of antibiotics (*2.7.2*).

STORAGE

Store in an airtight container.

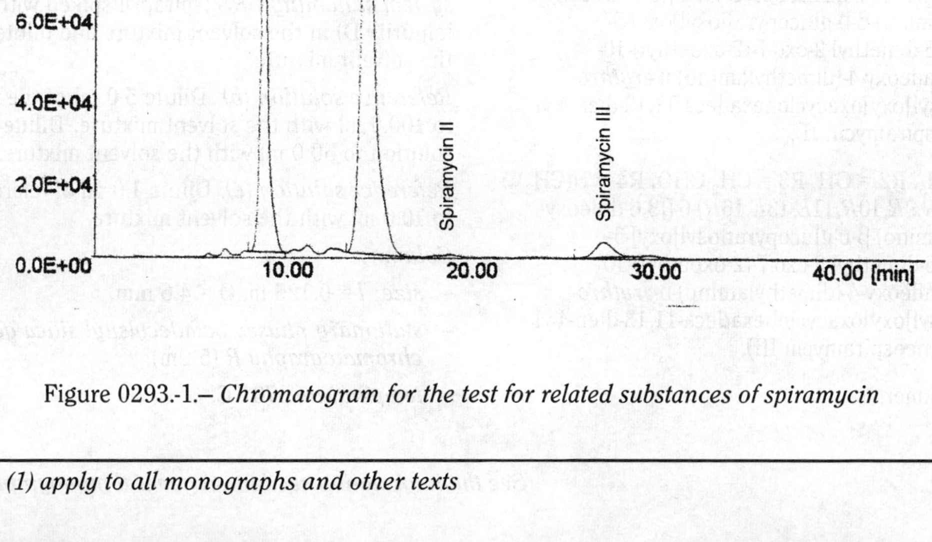

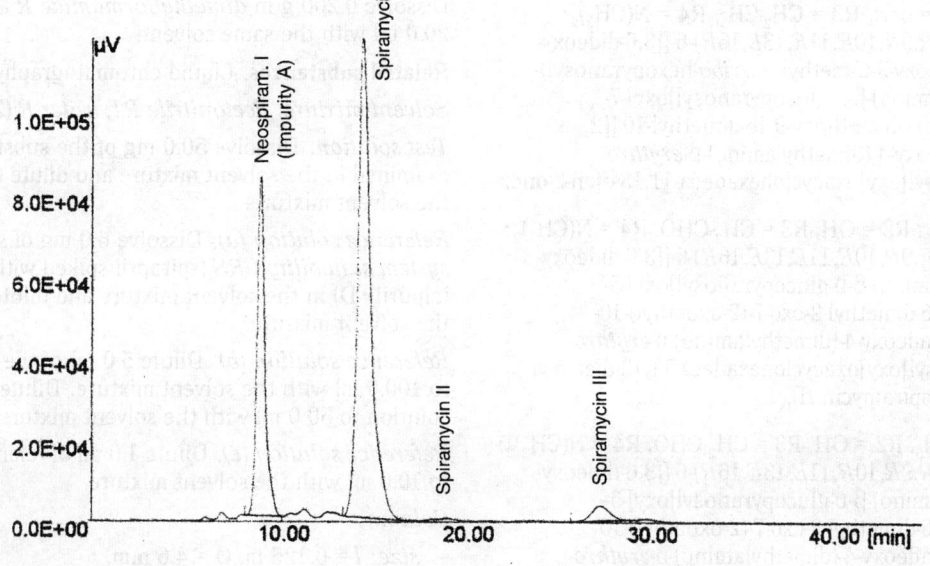

Figure 0293.-1.– *Chromatogram for the test for related substances of spiramycin*

IMPURITIES

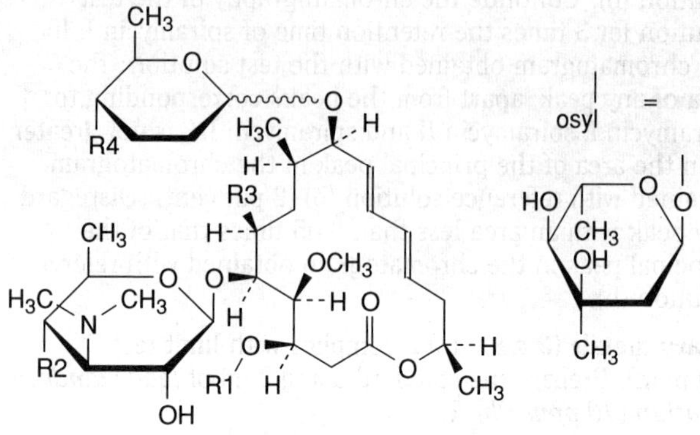

A. R1 = H, R2 = OH, R3 = CH_2-CHO, R4 = $N(CH_3)_2$: (4*R*,5*S*,6*S*,7*R*,9*R*,10*R*,11*E*,13*E*,16*R*)-6-[[3,6-dideoxy-3-(dimethylamino)-β-D-glucopyranosyl]oxy]-4-hydroxy-5-methoxy-9,16-dimethyl-7-(2-oxoethyl)-10-[[2,3,4,6-tetradeoxy-4-(dimethylamino)-D-*erythro*-hexopyranosyl]oxy]oxacyclohexadeca-11,13-dien-2-one (neospiramycin I),

B. R1 = H, R2 = osyl, R3 = CH_2-CH_2OH, R4 = $N(CH_3)_2$: (4*R*,5*S*,6*S*,7*R*,9*R*,10*R*,11*E*,13*E*,16*R*)-6-[[3,6-dideoxy-4-*O*-(2,6-dideoxy-3-*C*-methyl-α-L-*ribo*-hexopyranosyl)-3-(dimethylamino)-β-D-glucopyranosyl]oxy]-4-hydroxy-7-(2-hydroxyethyl)-5-methoxy-9,16-dimethyl-10-[[2,3,4,6-tetradeoxy-4-(dimethylamino)-D-*erythro*-hexopyranosyl]oxy]oxacyclohexadeca-11,13-dien-2-one,

C. R1 = H, R2 = osyl, R3 = CH_2-CH_2-CHO, R4 = $N(CH_3)_2$: (4*R*,5*S*,6*S*,7*S*,9*R*,10*R*,11*E*,13*E*,16*R*)-6-[[3,6-dideoxy-4-*O*-(2,6-dideoxy-3-*C*-methyl-α-L-*ribo*-hexopyranosyl)-3-(dimethylamino)-β-D-glucopyranosyl]oxy]-4-hydroxy-5-methoxy-9,16-dimethyl-7-(2-oxopropyl)-10-[[2,3,4,6-tetradeoxy-4-(dimethylamino)-D-*erythro*-hexopyranosyl]oxy]oxacyclohexadeca-11,13-dien-2-one,

D. R1 = H, R2 = osyl, R3 = CH_2-CHO, R4 = OH: (4*R*,5*S*,6*S*,7*R*,9*R*,10*R*,11*E*,13*E*,16*R*)-6-[[3,6-dideoxy-4-*O*-(2,6-dideoxy-3-*C*-methyl-α-L-*ribo*-hexopyranosyl)-3-(dimethylamino)-β-D-glucopyranosyl]oxy]-4-hydroxy-5-methoxy-9,16-dimethyl-7-(2-oxoethyl)-10-[(2,3,6-trideoxy-D-*erythro*-hexopyranosyl)oxy]oxacyclohexadeca-11,13-dien-2-one,

E. R1 = H, R2 = osyl, R3 = CH_2-CH_3, R4 = $N(CH_3)_2$: (4*R*,5*S*,6*S*,7*R*,9*R*,10*R*,11*E*,13*E*,16*R*)-6-[[3,6-dideoxy-4-*O*-(2,6-dideoxy-3-*C*-methyl-α-L-*ribo*-hexopyranosyl)-3-(dimethylamino)-β-D-glucopyranosyl]oxy]-7-ethyl-4-hydroxy-5-methoxy-9,16-dimethyl-10-[[2,3,4,6-tetradeoxy-4-(dimethylamino)-D-*erythro*-hexopyranosyl]oxy]oxacyclohexadeca-11,13-dien-2-one,

G. R1 = CO-CH_3, R2 = OH, R3 = CH_2-CHO, R4 = $N(CH_3)_2$: (4*R*,5*S*,6*S*,7*R*,9*R*,10*R*,11*E*,13*E*,16*R*)-6-[[3,6-dideoxy-3-(dimethylamino)-β-D-glucopyranosyl]oxy]-5-methoxy-9,16-dimethyl-2-oxo-7-(2-oxoethyl)-10-[[2,3,4,6-tetradeoxy-4-(dimethylamino)-D-*erythro*-hexopyranosyl]oxy]oxacyclohexadeca-11,13-dien-4-yl acetate (neospiramycin II),

H. R1 = CO-C_2H_5, R2 = OH, R3 = CH_2-CHO, R4 = $N(CH_3)_2$: (4*R*,5*S*,6*S*,7*R*,9*R*,10*R*,11*E*,13*E*,16*R*)-6-[[3,6-dideoxy-3-(dimethylamino)-β-D-glucopyranosyl]oxy]-5-methoxy-9,16-dimethyl-2-oxo-7-(2-oxoethyl)-10-[[2,3,4,6-tetradeoxy-4-(dimethylamino)-D-*erythro*-hexopyranosyl]oxy]oxacyclohexadeca-11,13-dien-4-yl propanoate (neospiramycin III),

F. spiramycin dimer.

01/2005:1766

SPIRAPRIL HYDROCHLORIDE MONOHYDRATE

Spiraprili hydrochloridum monohydricum

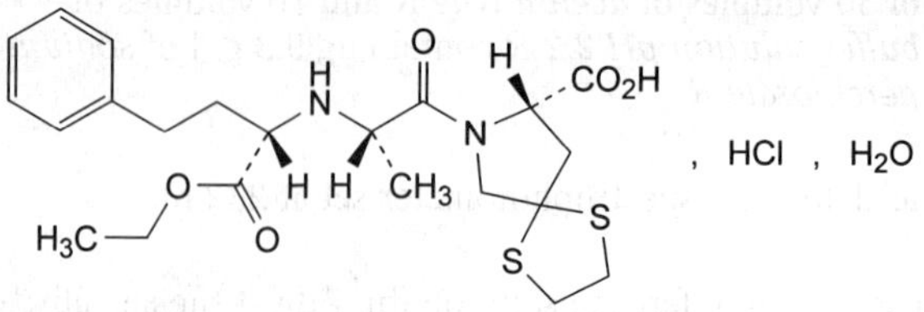

$C_{22}H_{31}ClN_2O_5S_2,H_2O$ M_r 521.1

DEFINITION

(8*S*)-7-[(2*S*)-2-[[(1*S*)-1-(Ethoxycarbonyl)-3-phenylpropyl]amino]propanoyl]-1,4-dithia-7-azaspiro[4.4]nonane-8-carboxylic acid hydrochloride monohydrate.

Content: 97.0 per cent to 102.0 per cent (anhydrous substance).

CHARACTERS

Appearance: white or almost white, fine crystalline powder.

Solubility: very slightly soluble in water, soluble in methanol, slightly soluble in acetonitrile, practically insoluble in methylene chloride.

IDENTIFICATION

A. Specific optical rotation (see Tests).

B. Infrared absorption spectrophotometry (*2.2.24*).

Preparation: discs of *potassium bromide R*.

Comparison: *spirapril hydrochloride monohydrate CRS*.

C. It gives the reactions of chlorides (*2.3.1*).

TESTS

Specific optical rotation (*2.2.7*): − 11.0 to − 13.0 (anhydrous substance).

Dissolve 0.200 g in *dimethylformamide R* and dilute to 20.0 ml with the same solvent.

Related substances. Liquid chromatography (*2.2.29*).

Solvent mixture: *acetonitrile R1*, *water R* (2:8 *V/V*).

Test solution. Dissolve 50.0 mg of the substance to be examined in the solvent mixture and dilute to 20.0 ml with the solvent mixture.

Reference solution (a). Dissolve 6.0 mg of *spirapril for system suitability CRS* (spirapril spiked with impurity B and impurity D) in the solvent mixture and dilute to 20 ml with the solvent mixture.

Reference solution (b). Dilute 5.0 ml of the test solution to 100.0 ml with the solvent mixture. Dilute 5.0 ml of this solution to 50.0 ml with the solvent mixture.

Reference solution (c). Dilute 1.0 ml of reference solution (b) to 10.0 ml with the solvent mixture.

Column:

– *size*: *l* = 0.125 m, Ø = 4.6 mm,

– *stationary phase*: *octadecylsilyl silica gel for chromatography R* (5 µm),

– *temperature*: 70 °C.

Mobile phase:

- *mobile phase A*: dissolve 4.5 g of *tetramethylammonium hydroxide R* in 900 ml of *water R*, add 100 ml of *acetonitrile R1* and adjust to pH 2.2 with *phosphoric acid R*,
- *mobile phase B*: dissolve 4.5 g of *tetramethylammonium hydroxide R* in 400 ml of *water R*, add 600 ml of *acetonitrile R1* and adjust to pH 2.2 with *phosphoric acid R*,

Time (min)	Mobile phase A (per cent *V/V*)	Mobile phase B (per cent *V/V*)
0 - 4	90	10
4 - 14	90 → 10	10 → 90
14 - 20	10	90
20 - 23	10 → 90	90 → 10
23 - 33	90	10

Flow rate: 2.0 ml/min.

Detection: spectrophotometer at 210 nm.

Injection: 20 µl.

Relative retention with reference to spirapril (retention time = about 10 min): impurity C = about 0.6; impurity B = about 0.7; impurity A = about 1.26; impurity D = about 1.38.

System suitability: reference solution (a):

- *resolution*: minimum 3.5 between the peaks due to impurity B and spirapril, and minimum 5.5 between the peaks due to spirapril and impurity D.

Limits:

- *impurities A, C*: for each impurity, not more than 0.4 times the area of the principal peak in the chromatogram obtained with reference solution (b) (0.2 per cent),
- *impurity B*: not more than 0.6 times the area of the principal peak in the chromatogram obtained with reference solution (b) (0.3 per cent),
- *impurity D*: not more than 0.8 times the area of the principal peak in the chromatogram obtained with reference solution (b) (0.4 per cent),
- *any other impurity*: for each impurity, not more than 0.2 times the area of the principal peak in the chromatogram obtained with reference solution (b) (0.1 per cent),
- *total*: not more than twice the area of the principal peak in the chromatogram obtained with reference solution (b) (1.0 per cent),
- *disregard limit*: area of the principal peak in the chromatogram obtained with reference solution (c) (0.05 per cent); disregard any peak due to the blank (solvent mixture).

Water (*2.5.12*): 3.0 per cent to 4.0 per cent, determined on 0.200 g.

Sulphated ash (*2.4.14*): maximum 0.1 per cent, determined on 1.0 g.

ASSAY

Liquid chromatography (*2.2.29*).

Solvent mixture. Mix equal volumes of *acetonitrile R1* and *water R*.

Test solution. Dissolve 20.0 mg of the substance to be examined in the solvent mixture and dilute to 100.0 ml with the solvent mixture.

Reference solution (a). Dissolve 20.0 mg of *spirapril hydrochloride monohydrate CRS* in the solvent mixture and dilute to 100.0 ml with the solvent mixture.

Reference solution (b). Dissolve 6.0 mg of *spirapril for system suitability CRS* (spirapril spiked with impurity B and impurity D) in a mixture of 2 volumes of *acetonitrile R* and 8 volumes of *water R* and dilute to 20 ml with the same mixture of solvents.

Solution A. Dissolve 4.5 g of *tetramethylammonium hydroxide R* in 900 ml of *water R*, adjust to pH 1.75 with *phosphoric acid R* and add 100 ml of *acetonitrile R1*.

Solution B. Dissolve 4.5 g of *tetramethylammonium hydroxide R* in 400 ml of *water R*, adjust to pH 1.75 with *phosphoric acid R* and add 600 ml of *acetonitrile R1*.

Column:

- *size*: l = 0.125 m, Ø = 4.6 mm,
- *stationary phase*: *octadecylsilyl silica gel for chromatography R* (5 µm),
- *temperature*: 70 °C.

Mobile phase: solution A, solution B (45:55 *V/V*).

Flow rate: 2.0 ml/min.

Detection: spectrophotometer at 210 nm.

Injection: 20 µl.

Retention time: spirapril = 1.6 min to 2.9 min; impurity D = about 13 min. Adjust the proportion of solution B in the mobile phase if necessary.

System suitability: reference solution (b):

- *resolution*: minimum 15 between the peaks due to spirapril and impurity D.

Calculate the percentage content of $C_{22}H_{31}ClN_2O_5S_2$ from the chromatograms obtained with the test solution and reference solution (a) and the declared content of *spirapril hydrochloride monohydrate CRS*.

STORAGE

In an airtight container, protected from light.

IMPURITIES

Specified impurities: A, B, C, D.

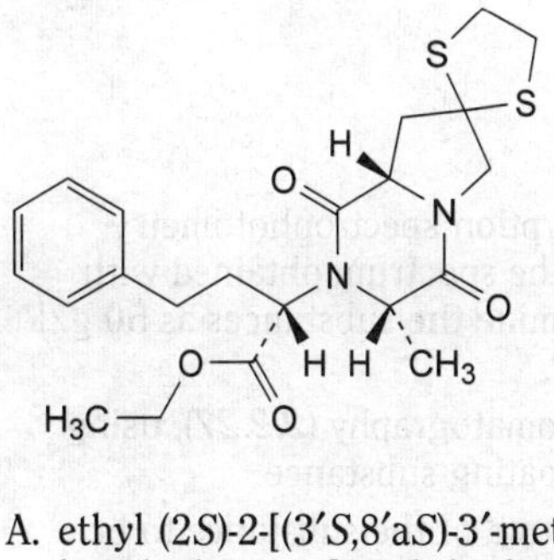

A. ethyl (2*S*)-2-[(3′*S*,8′a*S*)-3′-methyl-1′,4′-dioxo-hexahydrospiro[1,3-dithiolane-2,7′(6′*H*)-pyrrolo[1,2-*a*]pyrazin]-2′-yl]-4-phenylbutanoate,

Monographs Q-S

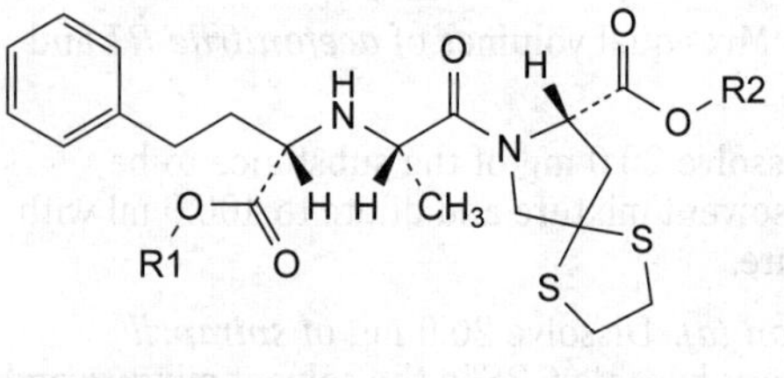

B. R1 = R2 = H: (8*S*)-7-[(2*S*)-2-[[(1*S*)-1-carboxy-3-phenylpropyl]amino]propanoyl]-1,4-dithia-7-azaspiro[4.4]nonane-8-carboxylic acid (spiraprilat),

D. R1 = C_2H_5, R2 = $CH(CH_3)_2$: 1-methylethyl (8*S*)-7-[(2*S*)-2-[[(1*S*)-1-(ethoxycarbonyl)-3-phenylpropyl]amino]propanoyl]-1,4-dithia-7-azaspiro[4.4]nonane-8-carboxylate,

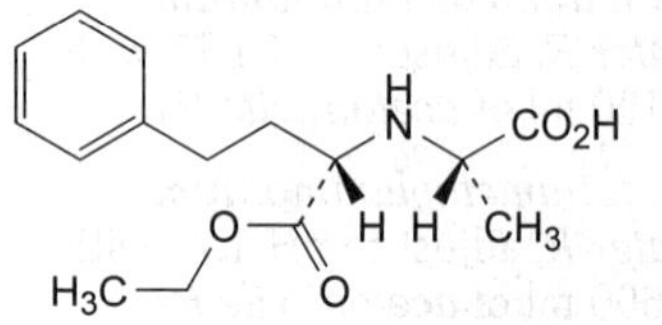

C. (2*S*)-2-[[(1*S*)-1-(ethoxycarbonyl)-3-phenylpropyl]amino]propanoic acid.

01/2005:0688

SPIRONOLACTONE

Spironolactonum

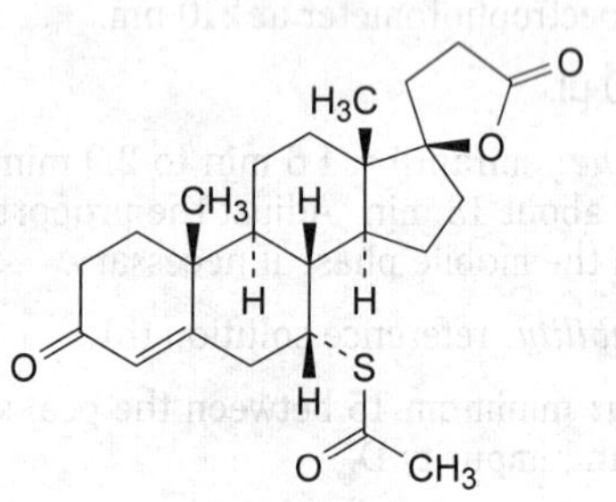

$C_{24}H_{32}O_4S$ M_r 416.6

DEFINITION

Spironolactone contains not less than 97.0 per cent and not more than the equivalent of 102.0 per cent of 7α-(acetylsulfanyl)-3′,4′-dihydrospiro[androst-4-ene-17,2′(5′*H*)-furan]-3,5′-dione, calculated with reference to the dried substance.

CHARACTERS

A white or yellowish-white powder, practically insoluble in water, soluble in alcohol.

It shows polymorphism.

IDENTIFICATION

First identification: A, C.

Second identification: B, C.

A. Examine by infrared absorption spectrophotometry (*2.2.24*), comparing with the spectrum obtained with *spironolactone CRS*. Examine the substances as 50 g/l solutions in *chloroform R*.

B. Examine by thin-layer chromatography (*2.2.27*), using *silica gel GF_{254} R* as the coating substance.

Test solution. Dissolve 20 mg of the substance to be examined in *methylene chloride R* and dilute to 10 ml with the same solvent.

Reference solution. Dissolve 20 mg of *spironolactone CRS* in *methylene chloride R* and dilute to 10 ml with the same solvent.

Apply separately to the plate 5 µl of each solution. Develop over a path of 15 cm using a mixture of 1 volume of *water R*, 24 volumes of *cyclohexane R* and 75 volumes of *ethyl acetate R*. Allow the plate to dry in air and examine in ultraviolet light at 254 nm. The principal spot in the chromatogram obtained with the test solution is similar in position and size to the principal spot in the chromatogram obtained with the reference solution.

C. To about 10 mg add 2 ml of a 50 per cent *V/V* solution of *sulphuric acid R* and shake. An orange solution with an intense yellowish-green fluorescence is produced. Heat the solution gently; the colour becomes deep red and hydrogen sulphide, which blackens *lead acetate paper R*, is evolved. Add the solution to 10 ml of *water R*; a greenish-yellow solution is produced which shows opalescence or a precipitate.

TESTS

Specific optical rotation (*2.2.7*). Dissolve 0.100 g in *chloroform R* and dilute to 10.0 ml with the same solvent. The specific optical rotation is − 33 to − 37, calculated with reference to the dried substance.

Related substances. Examine by liquid chromatography (*2.2.29*).

Test solution. Dissolve 62.5 mg of the substance to be examined in 2.5 ml of *tetrahydrofuran R* and dilute to 25.0 ml with the mobile phase.

Reference solution (a). Dilute 1.0 ml of the test solution to 100.0 ml with the mobile phase.

Reference solution (b). Dissolve 25.0 mg of *canrenone CRS* in 1 ml of *tetrahydrofuran R* and dilute to 10.0 ml with the mobile phase.

Reference solution (c). Dilute 1.0 ml of reference solution (b) to 100.0 ml with the mobile phase.

Reference solution (d). Mix 1 ml of the test solution with 1 ml of reference solution (b) and dilute to 100 ml with the mobile phase.

Reference solution (e). Dilute 0.50 ml of reference solution (a) to 10.0 ml with the mobile phase.

The chromatographic procedure may be carried out using:

- a stainless steel column 0.15 m long and 4.6 mm in internal diameter packed with *octylsilyl silica gel for chromatography R* (5 µm),
- a mixture of 8 volumes of *acetonitrile R*, 18 volumes of *tetrahydrofuran R* and 74 volumes of *water R* as the mobile phase at a flow rate of 1.8 ml/min,
- a variable wavelength spectrophotometer capable of operating at 254 nm and at 283 nm as detector.

Inject separately 20 µl of the test solution and 20 µl of reference solution (a), 20 µl of reference solution (d) and 20 µl of reference solution (e) and record the chromatograms with the detector set for recording at 254 nm. Continue the chromatography for twice the retention time of spironolactone. In the chromatogram obtained with the test solution, the sum of the areas of the peaks, except those corresponding to spironolactone and canrenone, is not greater than the area of the peak corresponding to spironolactone in the chromatogram obtained with reference solution (a) (1.0 per cent). Disregard any peak whose area is less than that of the principal peak in the chromatogram obtained with reference solution (e) (0.05 per cent). Inject 20 µl of the test solution and 20 µl of reference solution (c) and record the chromatogram with the detector set for recording at 283 nm. In the chromatogram obtained with the test solution, the area of any peak corresponding to canrenone is not greater than the area of the peak corresponding to canrenone in the chromatogram obtained with reference solution (c) (1.0 per cent). Calculate the percentage content of canrenone found when recording at 283 nm and the percentage content of the other related substances found when recording at 254 nm. Add together these percentages. The sum is not greater than 1.0 per cent. The test is not valid unless: the chromatogram obtained with reference solution (d) shows peaks, corresponding to canrenone and spironolactone, with a resolution greater than 1.4; the principal peak in the chromatogram obtained with reference solution (e) has a signal-to-noise ratio of at least 6.

Free mercapto compounds. To 2.0 g add 20 ml of *water R*, shake for 1 min and filter. To 10 ml of the filtrate add 0.05 ml of *0.01 M iodine* and 0.1 ml of *starch solution R* and mix. A blue colour develops.

Chromium. To 0.20 g in a platinum crucible add 1 g of *potassium carbonate R* and 0.3 g of *potassium nitrate R*. Heat gently until fused, and ignite at 600 °C to 650 °C until carbon is removed. Cool, dissolve the residue as completely as possible in 10 ml of *water R* with the aid of gentle heat, filter, and dilute to 20 ml with *water R*. To 10 ml of this solution add 0.5 g of *urea R*, and add a 14 per cent *V/V* solution of *sulphuric acid R* until the solution is just acid. When effervescence ceases, add a further 1 ml of the sulphuric acid, dilute to 20 ml with *water R* and add 0.5 ml of *diphenylcarbazide solution R*. The solution is not more intensely coloured than a standard prepared by adding 1 ml of a 14 per cent *V/V* solution of *sulphuric acid R* to 0.50 ml of a freshly prepared 28.3 mg/l solution of *potassium dichromate R*, diluting to 20 ml with *water R* and adding 0.5 ml of *diphenylcarbazide solution R* (50 ppm).

Loss on drying (*2.2.32*). Not more than 0.5 per cent, determined on 1.000 g by drying in an oven at 100 °C to 105 °C for 3 h.

Sulphated ash (*2.4.14*). Not more than 0.1 per cent, determined on 1.0 g.

ASSAY

Dissolve 50.0 mg in *methanol R* and dilute to 250.0 ml with the same solvent. Dilute 5.0 ml of this solution to 100.0 ml with *methanol R*. Measure the absorbance (*2.2.25*) of the solution at the maximum at 238 nm.

Calculate the content of $C_{24}H_{32}O_4S$, taking the specific absorbance to be 470.

STORAGE

Store protected from light.

01/2005:1630

SQUALANE

Squalanum

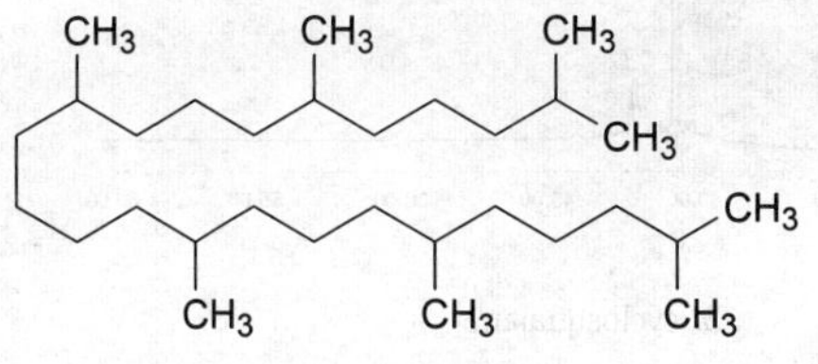

$C_{30}H_{62}$ M_r 422.8

DEFINITION

2,6,10,15,19,23-Hexamethyltetracosane (perhydrosqualene). It may be of vegetable (unsaponifiable matter of olive oil) or animal (shark liver oil) origin.

Content: 96.0 per cent to 103.0 per cent.

CHARACTERS

Appearance: clear, colourless, oily liquid.

Solubility: practically insoluble in water, miscible with most fats and oils, freely soluble in acetone and in cyclohexane, practically insoluble in alcohol.

Relative density: about 0.815.

IDENTIFICATION

A. Infrared absorption spectrophotometry (*2.2.24*).

Comparison: *squalane CRS*.

B. It complies with the test for refractive index (see Tests).

C. Examine the chromatograms obtained in the assay.

Results: the principal peak in the chromatogram obtained with the test solution is similar in retention time and size to the principal peak in the chromatogram obtained with reference solution (a).

The chromatogram obtained with squalane of vegetable origin shows a peak corresponding to cyclosqualane (Figure 1630.-1 and Figure 1630.-2).

TESTS

Appearance. The substance to be examined is clear (*2.2.1*) and colourless (*2.2.2, Method II*).

Refractive index (*2.2.6*): 1.450 to 1.454.

Acid value (*2.5.1*): maximum 0.2.

Iodine value (*2.5.4*): maximum 4.0.

Saponification value (*2.5.6*): maximum 3.0.

Nickel (*2.4.27*): maximum 1 ppm.

Total ash (*2.4.16*): maximum 0.5 per cent, determined on 1.000 g.

ASSAY

Gas chromatography (*2.2.28*).

Internal standard solution. To 1.0 ml of *dimethylacetamide R*, add 100.0 ml of *heptane R*.

Test solution. Dissolve 0.100 g in the internal standard solution and dilute to 25.0 ml with the same solution.

Reference solution (a). Dissolve 0.100 g of *squalane CRS* in the internal standard solution and dilute to 25.0 ml with the same solution.

Reference solution (b). To 0.1 ml of *methyl erucate R* add 0.100 g of the substance to be examined, dissolve in the internal standard solution and dilute to 25.0 ml with the same solution.

Column:

- *material*: fused silica,
- *size*: l = 30 m, Ø = 0.32 mm,
- *stationary phase*: *poly(dimethyl)siloxane R* (film thickness 1 μm).

Carrier gas: *helium for chromatography R*.

Flow rate: 1.7 ml/min.

Split ratio: 1:12.

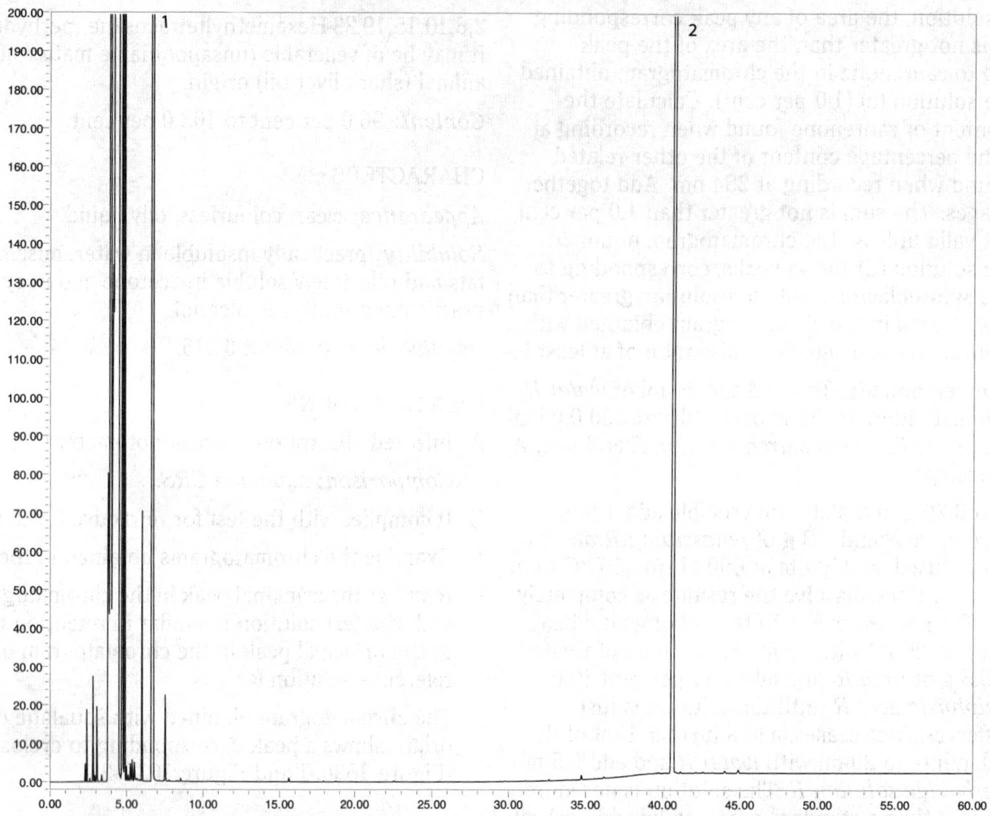

1. DMA 2. squalane

Figure 1630.-1. – *Chromatogram of squalane of animal origin*

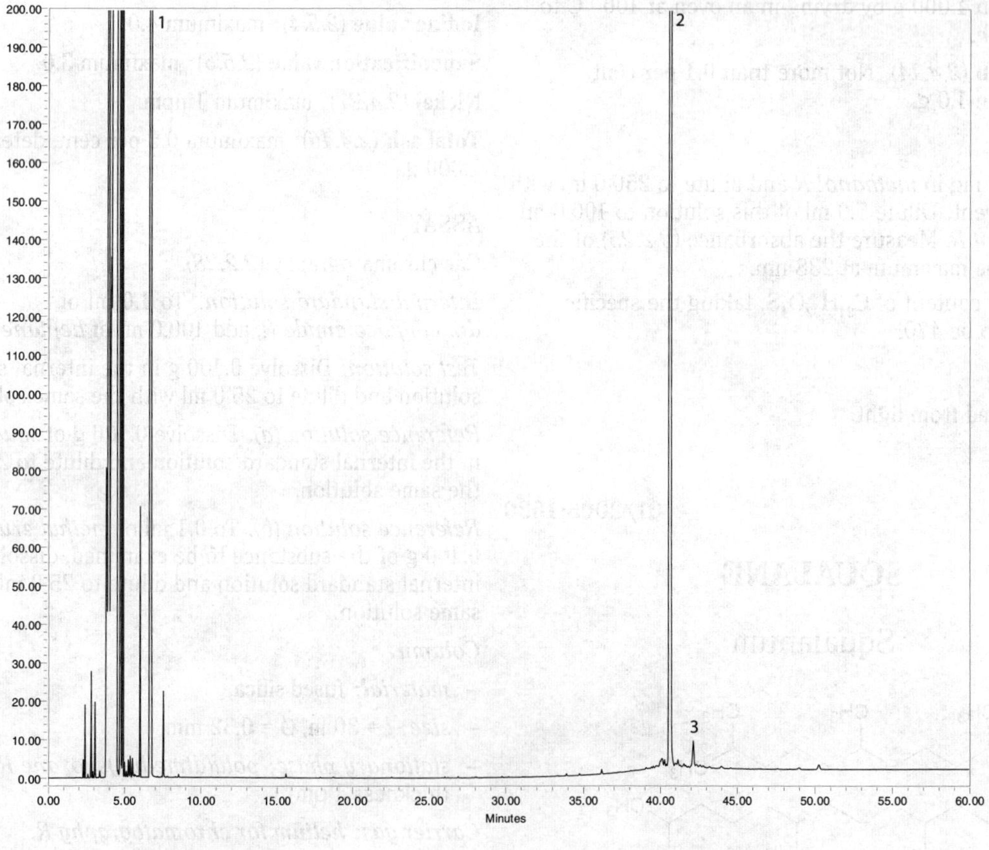

1. DMA 2. squalane 3. cyclosqualane

Figure 1630.-2. – *Chromatogram of squalane of vegetable origin*

Temperature:

	Time (min)	Temperature (°C)
Column	0 - 39	60 - 290
	39 - 50	290
Injection port		275
Detector		300

Detection: flame ionisation.

Injection: 1 µl.

Relative retentions with reference to squalane (retention time = about 41 min): internal standard = about 0.2; methyl erucate = about 0.9; cyclosqualane = 1.05.

System suitability: reference solution (b):

– *resolution*: minimum 5 between the peaks due to methyl erucate and squalane.

Calculate the percentage content of squalane from the areas of the peaks and the declared content of *squalane CRS*.

LABELLING

The label states the origin of squalane (vegetable or animal).

01/2005:1438

St. JOHN'S WORT

Hyperici herba

DEFINITION

St. John's wort consists of the whole or cut, dried flowering tops of *Hypericum perforatum* L., harvested during flowering time. It contains not less than 0.08 per cent of total hypericins expressed as hypericin ($C_{30}H_{16}O_8$; M_r 504.4), calculated with reference to the dried drug.

CHARACTERS

It has the macroscopic and microscopic characters described under identification tests A and B.

IDENTIFICATION

A. The branched and bare stem shows 2 more-or-less prominent longitudinal ridges. The leaves are opposite, sessile, exstipulate, oblong-oval and 15 mm to 30 mm long; present on the leaf margins are glands which appear as black dots and over all the surface of the leaves many small, strongly translucent excretory glands which are visible in transmitted light. The flowers are regular and form corymbose clusters at the apex of the stem. They have 5 green, acute sepals, with black secretory glands on the margins; 5 orange-yellow petals, also with black secretory glands on the margins; 3 staminal blades, each divided into many orange-yellow stamens and 3 carpels surmounted by red styles.

B. Reduce to a powder (355). The powder is greenish-yellow. Examine under a microscope using *chloral hydrate solution R*. The powder shows the following diagnostic characters: fragments of polygonal cells of the epidermis with thickened and beaded walls and paracytic or anomocytic stomata (*2.8.3*); fragments of the leaf and sepal with large oil glands and red pigment cells; thin-walled, elongated cells of the petal epidermis with straight or wavy anticlinal walls; tracheids and tracheidal vessels with pitted walls and groups of thick-walled fibres; fragments of rectangular, lignified and pitted parenchyma; fibrous layer of the anther and elongated, thin-walled cells of the filament with a striated cuticle; numerous pollen grains with 3 pores and a smooth exine, occur singly or in dense groups, and calcium oxalate cluster crystals.

C. Examine by thin-layer chromatography (*2.2.27*), using a *TLC silica gel plate R*.

Test solution. Stir 0.5 g of the powdered drug (500) in 10 ml of *methanol R* in a water-bath at 60 °C for 10 min and filter.

Reference solution. Dissolve 5 mg of *rutin R* and 5 mg of *hyperoside R* in *methanol R* and dilute to 5 ml with the same solvent.

Apply to the plate as 10 mm bands 10 µl of the test solution and 5 µl of the reference solution. Develop over a path of 10 cm using a mixture of 6 volumes of *anhydrous formic acid R*, 9 volumes of *water R* and 90 volumes of *ethyl acetate R*. Allow the plate to dry at 100-105 °C for 10 min. Spray the plate with a 10 g/l solution of *diphenylboric acid aminoethyl ester R* in *methanol R* and then with a 50 g/l solution of *macrogol 400 R* in *methanol R*. Examine the plate after about 30 min in ultraviolet light at 365 nm. The chromatogram obtained with the reference solution shows in the lower third the zone due to rutin and above it the zone due to hyperoside, both with yellow-orange fluorescence. The chromatogram obtained with the test solution shows in the lower third the reddish-orange fluorescent zones of rutin and hyperoside and in the lower part of the upper third the zone of pseudohypericin and above it the zone of hypericin, both with red fluorescence. Other yellow or blue fluorescent zones are visible.

TESTS

Foreign matter (*2.8.2*). Not more than 3 per cent of stems with a diameter greater than 5 mm, and not more than 2 per cent of other foreign matter.

Loss on drying (*2.2.32*). Not more than 10.0 per cent, determined on 1.000 g of the powdered drug (500) by drying in an oven at 100-105 °C for 2 h.

Total ash (*2.4.16*). Not more than 7.0 per cent.

ASSAY

Test solution. In a 100 ml round-bottomed flask, introduce 0.800 g of the powdered drug (500), 60 ml of a mixture of 20 volumes of *water R* and 80 volumes of *tetrahydrofuran R* and a magnetic stirrer. Boil the mixture in a water-bath at 70 °C under a reflux condenser for 30 min. Centrifuge (2 min at 700 *g*) and decant the supernatant into a 250 ml flask. Take up the residue with 60 ml of a mixture of 20 volumes of *water R* and 80 volumes of *tetrahydrofuran R*. Heat again under a reflux condenser for 30 min. Centrifuge (2 min at 700 *g*) and decant the supernatant. Combine the extracts and evaporate to dryness. Take up the residue with 15 ml of *methanol R* with the help of ultrasound and transfer to a 25 ml measuring flask. Rinse the 250 ml flask with *methanol R* and dilute to 25.0 ml with the same solvent. Centrifuge again, filter 10 ml through a syringe filter (0.2 µm). Discard the first 2 millilitres of the filtrate. Introduce 5.0 ml of the filtrate into a measuring flask and dilute to 25.0 ml with *methanol R*.

Compensation liquid. *Methanol R*.

Measure the absorbance (*2.2.25*) of the test solution at 590 nm by comparison with the compensation liquid.

Monographs Q-S

Calculate the percentage content of total hypericins, expressed as hypericin, from the expression:

$$\frac{A \times 125}{m \times 870}$$

i.e. taking the specific absorbance of hypericin to be 870.

A = absorbance at 590 nm,

m = mass of the drug to be examined, in grams.

STORAGE

Protected from light.

01/2005:1266

STANNOUS CHLORIDE DIHYDRATE

Stannosi chloridum dihydricum

$SnCl_2,2H_2O$ M_r 225.6

DEFINITION

Stannous chloride dihydrate contains not less than 98.0 per cent and not more than the equivalent of 101.0 per cent of $SnCl_2,2H_2O$.

CHARACTERS

A white, crystalline powder or colourless crystals, efflorescent in air, freely soluble in water (the solution becomes cloudy after standing or on dilution), freely soluble in alcohol. It dissolves in dilute hydrochloric acid.

IDENTIFICATION

A. To 1 ml of solution S1 (see Tests) add a mixture of 5 ml of *water R* and 0.05 ml of *mercuric chloride solution R*. A blackish-grey precipitate forms.

B. Dissolve 1.0 g in 3.0 ml of *water R*. Add 0.5 ml of *dilute sodium hydroxide solution R* to the cloudy solution; a yellowish flocculent precipitate is formed. Add 6.5 ml of *water R*. To 1.0 ml of the previously shaken suspension add 1.0 ml of *strong sodium hydroxide solution R*; the precipitate dissolves and the resulting solution is clear and colourless.

C. Dissolve 10 mg in 2 ml of *dilute nitric acid R*. The solution gives reaction (a) of chlorides (*2.3.1*).

TESTS

Solution S1. To 0.40 g add 1 ml of *dilute hydrochloric acid R* and dilute to 20 ml with *distilled water R*.

Solution S2. Dissolve 1.0 g in *dilute hydrochloric acid R* and dilute to 30 ml with the same acid. Heat to boiling. Add 30 ml of *thioacetamide solution R* and boil for 15 min (solution A). Use 5 ml, filter and heat the filtrate to boiling. Add 5 ml of *thioacetamide solution R* and boil for 15 min. If a precipitate is formed, add the remainder of solution A (solution A′) to the mixture. Add 10 ml of *thioacetamide solution R* and boil. Repeat the series of operations from "Use 5 ml,..." until a precipitate is no longer formed on addition of *thioacetamide solution R* to the filtrate obtained from the 5 ml of solution A (solution A′, solution A″,...., respectively). If no precipitate is formed or if no more precipitate is formed combine the solution obtained with the remainder of solution A (solution A′, solution A″,...., respectively), filter and wash the precipitate with 10 ml of *water R*. Heat the filtrate until the resulting vapour no longer turns a moistened piece of *lead acetate paper R* blackish-grey. Allow to cool and dilute to 50 ml with *water R*.

Appearance of solution. Dissolve 10.0 g in *dilute hydrochloric acid R* and dilute to 20 ml with the same acid. The solution is clear (*2.2.1*) and colourless (*2.2.2, Method II*).

Substances not precipitated by thioacetamide. Evaporate 25 ml of solution S2 to dryness and ignite at 600 °C. The residue weighs not more than 1 mg (0.2 per cent).

Sulphates (*2.4.13*). 15 ml of solution S1 complies with the limit test for sulphates (500 ppm).

Iron(*2.4.9*). Dilute 5 ml of solution S2 to 10 ml with *water R*. The solution complies with the limit test for iron (100 ppm).

Heavy metals. Dissolve 1.0 g in 2 ml of a mixture of 1 volume of *nitric acid R* and 3 volumes of *hydrochloric acid R*. Heat the solution on a water-bath until nitrous vapour is no longer evolved. Dissolve the residue in *water R* and dilute to 25 ml with the same solvent. To 5 ml of the solution add 3 ml of *strong sodium hydroxide solution R* and 2 ml of *water R*. Heat until a clear solution is obtained, then cool and add 0.5 ml of *thioacetamide reagent R*. After 2 min, any colour in the solution is not more intense than that of a mixture of 1.0 ml of *lead standard solution (10 ppm Pb) R*, 6 ml of *water R*, 3 ml of *strong sodium hydroxide solution R* and 0.5 ml of *thioacetamide reagent R* (50 ppm).

ASSAY

Dissolve 0.100 g in 1.5 ml of *hydrochloric acid R1* and dilute to 50 ml with *water R*. Add 5 g of *sodium potassium tartrate R*, 10 g of *sodium hydrogen carbonate R* and 1 ml of *starch solution R*. Titrate immediately with *0.05 M iodine*. Carry out a blank titration.

1 ml of *0.05 M iodine* is equivalent to 11.28 mg of $SnCl_2,2H_2O$.

STORAGE

Store in an airtight container.

01/2005:1568

STANOZOLOL

Stanozololum

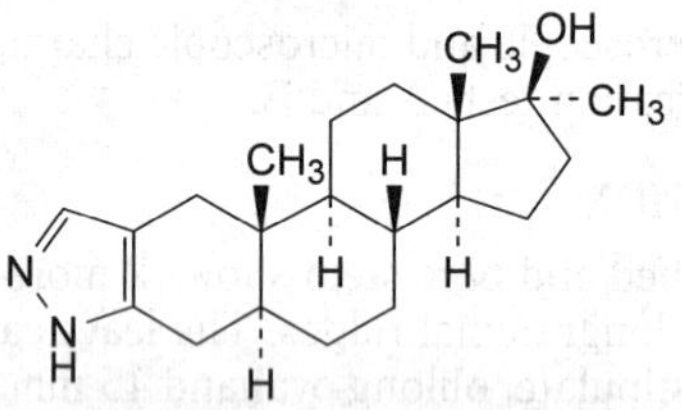

$C_{21}H_{32}N_2O$ M_r 328.5

DEFINITION

Stanozolol contains not less than 98.5 per cent and not more than the equivalent of 101.0 per cent of 17-methyl-2′*H*-5α-androst-2-eno[3,2-*c*]pyrazol-17β-ol, calculated with reference to the dried substance.

CHARACTERS

A white or almost white crystalline powder, hygroscopic, practically insoluble in water, soluble in dimethylformamide, slightly soluble in alcohol, very slightly soluble in methylene chloride.

It shows polymorphism.

IDENTIFICATION

A. Examine by infrared spectrophotometry (*2.2.24*), comparing with the spectrum obtained with *stanozolol CRS*. If the spectra obtained in the solid state show differences, dissolve the substance to be examined and the reference substance separately in the minimum volume of methylene chloride, evaporate to dryness at room temperature under an air-stream and record new spectra using the residues.

B. Examine the chromatograms obtained in the test for related substances. The principal spot in the chromatogram obtained with test solution (b) is similar in position, colour and size to the principal spot in the chromatogram obtained with reference solution (c).

TESTS

Specific optical rotation (*2.2.7*). Dissolve 0.10 g in *chloroform R* and dilute to 10.0 ml with the same solvent. The specific optical rotation is + 34 to + 40, calculated with reference to the dried substance.

Related substances. Examine by thin-layer chromatography (*2.2.27*), using a *TLC silica gel F_{254} plate R*.

Test solution (a). Dissolve 0.10 g of the substance to be examined in a mixture of 1 volume of *methanol R* and 9 volumes of *methylene chloride R* and dilute to 5 ml with the same mixture of solvents.

Test solution (b). Dilute 1 ml of test solution (a) to 10 ml with a mixture of 1 volume of *methanol R* and 9 volumes of *methylene chloride R*.

Reference solution (a). Dilute 1.0 ml of test solution (a) to 200 ml with a mixture of 1 volume of *methanol R* and 9 volumes of *methylene chloride R*.

Reference solution (b). Dissolve 5 mg of *stanozolol impurity A CRS* in reference solution (a) and dilute to 50 ml with the same solution.

Reference solution (c). Dissolve 10 mg of *stanozolol CRS* in a mixture of 1 volume of *methanol R* and 9 volumes of *methylene chloride R* and dilute to 5 ml with the same mixture of solvents.

Apply to the plate 5 µl of each solution. Develop over a path corresponding to two thirds of the plate height using a mixture of 10 volumes of *methanol R* and 90 volumes of *methylene chloride R*. Allow the plate to dry in air, spray with *alcoholic solution of sulphuric acid R*, heat at 105 °C for 15 min and examine under ultraviolet light at 365 nm. Any secondary spot in the chromatogram obtained with test solution (a) is not more intense than the spot in the chromatogram obtained with reference solution (a) (0.5 per cent). The test is not valid unless the chromatogram obtained with reference solution (b) shows two clearly separated spots.

Loss on drying (*2.2.32*). Not more than 1.0 per cent, determined on 1.000 g by drying at 100 °C at a pressure not exceeding 0.7 kPa.

ASSAY

Dissolve 0.250 g in 50 ml of *anhydrous acetic acid R*. Titrate with *0.1 M perchloric acid*, determining the end-point potentiometrically (*2.2.20*).

1 ml of *0.1 M perchloric acid* is equivalent to 32.85 mg of $C_{21}H_{32}N_2O$.

STORAGE

Store in an airtight container, protected from light.

IMPURITIES

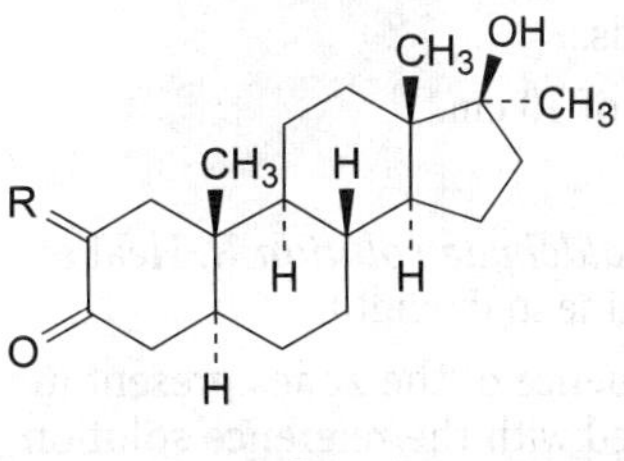

A. R = H_2: 17β-hydroxy-17-methyl-5α-androstan-3-one (mestanolone),

B. R = CH-OH: 17β-hydroxy-2-(hydroxymethylene)-17-methyl-5α-androstan-3-one (oxymetholone).

01/2005:1153

STAR ANISE

Anisi stellati fructus

DEFINITION

Dried composite fruit of *Illicium verum* Hooker fil.

Content: minimum 70 ml/kg of essential oil (anhydrous drug).

CHARACTERS

The fruit carpels are brown.

Odour of anethole.

Macroscopic and microscopic characters described under identification tests A and B.

IDENTIFICATION

A. The fruit consists of 6 to 11 (usually 8), often unequally developed, boat-shaped follicles, each 12 mm to 20 mm long and 6 mm to 11 mm thick, radially arranged around a short, central, blunt-ending columella. The follicles are bluntly peaked at the apex, flat at the base and the outer surface is greyish-brown, roughly wrinkled. The ventral suture is frequently open exposing a single, hard, ovoid, laterally compressed, shiny, reddish-brown seed about 8 mm long. The pedicel, if present, is distinctly curved and thickened at the apex. Separated follicles and seeds may be present.

B. Reduce to a powder (355). The powder is reddish-brown. Examine under a microscope using *chloral hydrate solution R*. The powder shows the following diagnostic characters: brown epicarpal cells, polygonal in surface view, with strongly striated cuticles and occasional anomocytic stomata (*2.8.3*); fragments of the endocarp with palisade-like cells up to about 600 µm long; fragments of the mesocarp with large parenchymatous cells, vessels, oil-containing cells and groups of large very elongated stone cells with thickened and pitted walls; fragments of the testa with palisade-like, yellow stone cells up to 200 µm long, with strongly pitted walls; fragments of the endosperm containing droplets of oil and aleurone grains; fragments of the columella and the fruit stalk with strongly thickened irregular stone cells up to 400 µm long and about 150 µm wide, with pointed, star-shaped projections (astrosclereids); rhomboidal or rectangular crystals of calcium oxalate.

C. Thin-layer chromatography (*2.2.27*).

Test solution. Shake 0.20 g of the freshly powdered drug (710) with 2.0 ml of *toluene R* for 15 min and filter.

Reference solution. Dissolve 3 µl of *anethole R* and 20 µl of *olive oil R* in 1 ml of *toluene R*.

Plate: *TLC silica gel plate R.*

Monographs Q-S

Mobile phase: *toluene R*.

Application: 20 µl, as bands.

Development: over a path of 10 cm.

Drying: in air.

Detection: spray with *anisaldehyde solution R*. Heat at 120 °C for 5 min and examine in daylight.

Results: see below the sequence of the zones present in the chromatograms obtained with the reference solution and the test solution. Furthermore, other weaker zones may be present in the chromatogram obtained with the test solution.

Top of the plate	
———	———
Anethole: a reddish-violet zone	A reddish-violet zone (anethole)
———	———
Triglycerides of olive oil: a bluish-violet zone	A bluish-violet zone
Reference solution	**Test solution**

TESTS

***Illicium anisatum* (= *I. religiosum*)**. The fruit must not contain follicles with an upwardly turned beak nor straight fruit stalks that are not curved at the distal end. Fragments of the endocarp with palisade-like cells less than about 360 µm long and fragments of the columella, previously separated from the fruit, with strongly thickened rounded stone cells without star-shaped projections must be absent.

Foreign matter (*2.8.2*): maximum 2 per cent.

Water (*2.2.13*): maximum 100 ml/kg, determined by distillation on 20.0 g of the powdered drug (710).

Total ash (*2.4.16*): maximum 4.0 per cent.

ASSAY

Carry out the determination of essential oils in vegetable drugs (*2.8.12*). Use a 250 ml round-bottomed flask and 100 ml of *water R* as the distillation liquid. Immediately before the determination, reduce 50.0 g of the drug to a coarse powder (1400) and mix. Further reduce about 10.0 g of this mixture to a finer powder (710). Use 2.50 g of the powder for the determination. Introduce 0.50 ml of *xylene R* into the graduated tube. Distil at a rate of 2-3 ml/min for 2 h.

01/2005:2108
corrected

STAR ANISE OIL

Anisi stellati aetheroleum

DEFINITION

Essential oil obtained by steam distillation from the dry ripe fruits of *Illicium verum* Hook. fil.

CHARACTERS

Appearance: clear, colourless or pale yellow liquid.

IDENTIFICATION

First identification: B.

Second identification: A.

A. Thin-layer chromatography (*2.2.27*).

Test solution. Dissolve 1 g of the substance to be examined in *toluene R* and dilute to 10 ml with the same solvent.

Reference solution. Dissolve 10 µl of *linalol R*, 30 µl of *anisaldehyde R* and 200 µl of *anethole R* and in *toluene R* and dilute to 15 ml with the same solvent. Dilute 1 ml of this solution to 5 ml with *toluene R*.

Plate: *TLC silica gel F_{254} plate R*.

Mobile phase: *ethyl acetate R, toluene R* (7:93 *V/V*).

Application: 5 µl as bands of 10 mm (for normal TLC plates) or 2 µl as bands of 10 mm (for fine particle TLC plates).

Development: over a path of 15 cm (for normal TLC plates) or over a path of 6 cm (for fine particle size plates).

Drying: in air.

Detection A: examine in ultraviolet light at 254 nm.

Results A: see below the sequence of zones present in the chromatograms obtained with the reference solution and the test solution. Furthermore, other zones may be present in the chromatogram obtained with the test solution.

Top of the plate	
	A quenching zone, partly separated
Anethole: a quenching zone	A very strong quenching zone (anethole)
———	
Anisaldehyde: a quenching zone	A quenching zone (anisaldehyde)
———	———
Reference solution	**Test solution**

Detection B: spray with *methyl 4-acetylbenzoate reagent R* and heat at 100-105 °C for 10 min; examine the still hot plate in daylight within 10 min.

Results B: see below the sequence of zones present in the chromatograms obtained with the reference solution and the test solution. Furthermore, other zones may be present in the chromatogram obtained with the test solution.

Top of the plate	
	A violet-brown zone, not fully separated
Anethole: a brown zone	A very strong brown zone (anethole)
———	
Anisaldehyde: a yellow zone	A yellow zone (anisaldehyde)
———	———
Linalol: a grey zone	A grey zone (linalol)
Reference solution	**Test solution**

B. Examine the chromatograms obtained in the test for chromatographic profile.

Results: the characteristic peaks in the chromatogram obtained with the test solution are similar in retention time to those in the chromatogram obtained with the reference solution.

TESTS

Relative density (*2.2.5*): 0.979 to 0.985.

Refractive index (*2.2.6*): 1.553 to 1.556.

Freezing point (*2.2.18*): 15 °C to 19 °C.

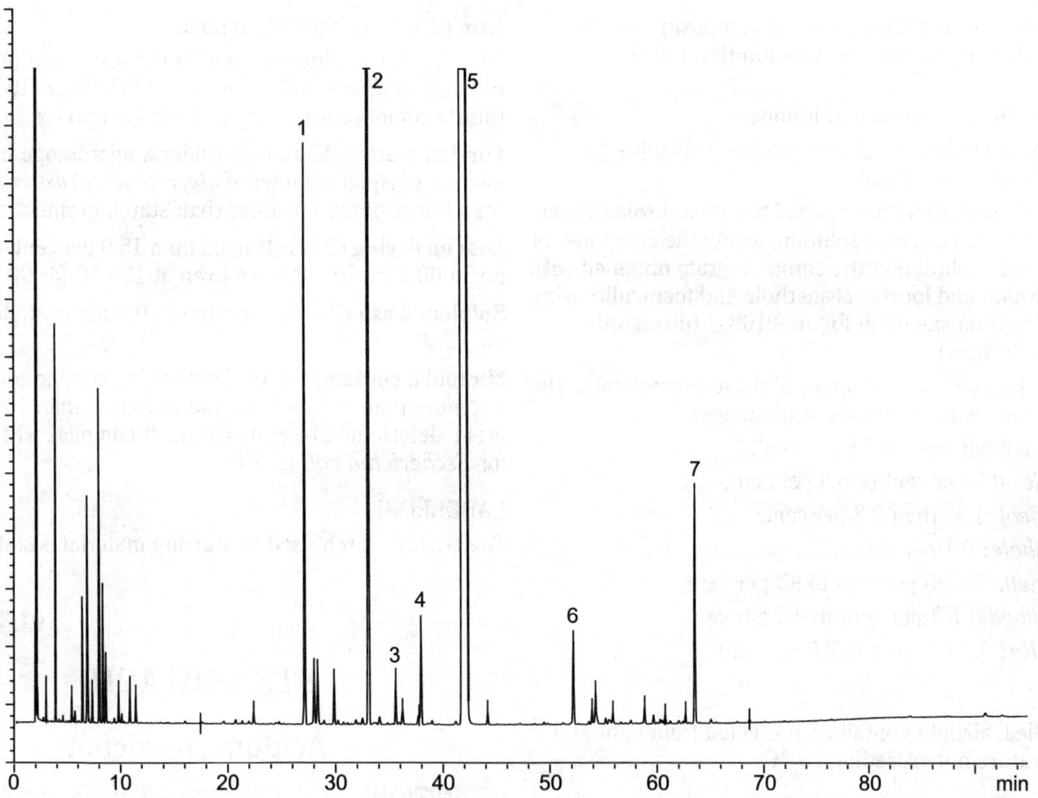

1. linalol
2. estragole
3. α-terpineol
4. *cis*-anethole
5. *trans*-anethole
6. anisaldehyde
7. foeniculin

Figure 2108.-1. – *Chromatogram for the test for chromatographic profile of star anise oil*

Fenchone. Gas chromatography (*2.2.28*) as described in the test for chromatographic profile with the following modifications.

Test solution. Dissolve 400 μl of the substance to be examined in 2.0 ml of *hexane R*.

Reference solution (a). Dilute 10 μl of *fenchone R* to 1.2 g with *hexane R*.

Reference solution (b). Dilute 100 μl of reference solution (a) to 100 ml with *hexane R*.

System suitability: reference solution (b):

– *signal-to-noise ratio*: minimum 10 for the principal peak.

Limit:

– *fenchone*: maximum 0.01 per cent.

Pseudoisoeugenyl 2-methylbutyrate. Gas chromatography (*2.2.28*) as described in the test for chromatographic profile with the following modifications.

Test solution. The substance to be examined.

Reference solution (a). Dilute 10 mg of the test solution to 1.000 g with *hexane R*. Dilute 0.5 ml of this solution to 100 ml with *hexane R*.

Reference solution (b). *Pseudoisoeugenyl 2-methylbutyrate for peak identification CRS*.

System suitability:

– the chromatogram obtained with reference solution (b) is similar to the chromatogram provided with *pseudoisoeugenyl 2-methylbutyrate for peak identification CRS*.

– *signal-to-noise ratio*: minimum 10 for the principal peak in the chromatogram obtained with reference solution (a).

Limit: locate the peak due to pseudoisoeugenyl 2-methylbutyrate by comparison with the chromatogram provided with *pseudoisoeugenyl 2-methylbutyrate for peak identification CRS*.

– *pseudoisoeugenyl 2-methylbutyrate*: maximum 0.01 per cent.

Fatty oils and resinified essential oils (*2.8.7*). It complies with the test for fatty oils and resinified essential oils.

Chromatographic profile. Gas chromatography (*2.2.28*): use the normalisation procedure.

Test solution. Dissolve 200 μl of the substance to be examined in 1.0 ml of *hexane R*.

Reference solution. To 1.0 ml of *hexane R*, add 20 μl of *linalol R*, 20 μl of *estragole R*, 20 μl of *α-terpineol R*, 60 μl of *anethole R* and 30 μl of *anisaldehyde R*.

Column:

– *material*: fused silica,

– *size*: *l* = 30 m, Ø = 0.25 mm,

– *stationary phase*: *macrogol 20 000 R* (film thickness 0.25 μm).

Carrier gas: *helium for chromatography R*.

Flow rate: 1.0 ml/min.

Split ratio: 1:100.

Temperature:

	Time (min)	Temperature (°C)
Column	0 - 5	60
	5 - 80	60 → 210
	80 - 95	210
Injection port		200
Detector		220

Detection: flame ionisation.

Injection: 0.2 μl.

Elution order: order indicated in the composition of the reference solution; record the retention times of these substances.

System suitability: reference solution:

– *resolution*: minimum 1.5 between the peaks due to estragole and α-terpineol.

Using the retention times determined from the chromatogram obtained with the reference solution, locate the components of the reference solution in the chromatogram obtained with the test solution and locate *cis*-anethole and foeniculin using the chromatogram shown in Figure 2108.-1 (disregard any peak due to hexane).

Determine the percentage content of these components. The percentages are within the following ranges:

– *linalol*: 0.2 per cent to 2.5 per cent,
– *estragole*: 0.5 per cent to 6.0 per cent,
– *α-terpineol*: less than 0.3 per cent,
– *cis-anethole*: 0.1 per cent to 0.5 per cent,
– *trans-anethole*: 86 per cent to 93 per cent,
– *anisaldehyde*: 0.1 per cent to 0.5 per cent,
– *foeniculin*: 0.1 per cent to 3.0 per cent.

STORAGE

In a well-filled, airtight container, protected from light and at a temperature not exceeding 25 °C.

01/2005:1267

STARCH, PREGELATINISED

Amylum pregelificatum

DEFINITION

Pregelatinised starch is prepared from *Maize starch (0344), Potato starch (0355)* or *Rice starch (0349)* by mechanical processing in the presence of water, with or without heat, to rupture all or part of the starch granules and subsequent drying. It contains no added substances but it may be modified to render it compressible and to improve its flow characteristics.

CHARACTERS

Appearance: white or yellowish-white powder.

It swells in cold water.

IDENTIFICATION

A. Examined under a microscope using a mixture of equal volumes of *glycerol R* and *water R* it presents irregular, translucent, white or yellowish-white flakes or pieces with an uneven surface. Under polarised light (between crossed nicol prisms), starch granules with a distinct black cross intersecting at the hilum may be seen.

B. Disperse 0.5 g in 2 ml of *water R* without heating and add 0.05 ml of *iodine solution R1*. A reddish-violet to blue colour is produced.

TESTS

pH (*2.2.3*): 4.5 to 7.0.

Progressively add 3.0 g to 100.0 ml of *carbon dioxide-free water R,* stirring continuously. Determine the pH when a homogeneous solution is obtained.

Oxidising substances (*2.5.30*). It complies with the test for oxidising substances. Use a mixture of equal volumes of *water R* and *methanol R* as solvent.

Sulphur dioxide (*2.5.29*): maximum 50 ppm.

Iron (*2.4.9*): maximum 20 ppm.

Dissolve the residue obtained in the test for sulphated ash in 20 ml of *dilute hydrochloric acid R*. Filter. 10 ml of the filtrate complies with the limit test for iron

Foreign matter. Examined under a microscope using a mixture of equal volumes of *glycerol R* and *water R*, not more than traces of matter other than starch granules are present.

Loss on drying (*2.2.32*): maximum 15.0 per cent, determined on 1.000 g by drying in an oven at 130 °C for 90 min.

Sulphated ash (*2.4.14*): maximum 0.6 per cent, determined on 1.0 g.

Microbial contamination. Total viable aerobic count (*2.6.12*) not more than 10^3 bacteria and not more than 10^2 fungi per gram, determined by plate-count. It complies with the test for *Escherichia coli* (*2.6.13*).

LABELLING

The type of starch used as starting material is stated.

01/2005:1474

STEARIC ACID

Acidum stearicum

DEFINITION

Mixture consisting mainly of stearic acid ($C_{18}H_{36}O_2$; M_r 284.5) and palmitic acid ($C_{16}H_{32}O_2$; M_r 256.4) obtained from fats or oils of vegetable or animal origin.

Content:

Stearic acid 50	*Stearic acid*: 40.0 per cent to 60.0 per cent. *Sum of the contents of stearic and palmitic acids*: minimum 90.0 per cent.
Stearic acid 70	*Stearic acid*: 60.0 per cent to 80.0 per cent. *Sum of the contents of stearic and palmitic acids*: minimum 90.0 per cent.
Stearic acid 95	*Stearic acid*: minimum 90.0 per cent. *Sum of the contents of stearic and palmitic acids*: minimum 96.0 per cent.

CHARACTERS

Appearance: white, waxy, flaky crystals, white hard masses or white or yellowish-white powder.

Solubility: practically insoluble in water, soluble in alcohol and in light petroleum (50-70 °C).

IDENTIFICATION

A. It complies with the test for freezing point (see Tests).

B. Acid value (*2.5.1*): 194 to 212, determined on 0.1 g.

C. Examine the chromatograms obtained in the assay.

Results: the retention times of the principal peaks in the chromatogram obtained with the test solution are approximately the same as those of the principal peaks in the chromatogram obtained with the reference solution.

TESTS

Appearance. Heat the substance to be examined to about 75 °C. The resulting liquid is not more intensely coloured than reference solution Y_7 or BY_7 (*2.2.2, Method I*).

Acidity. Melt 5.0 g, shake for 2 min with 10 ml of hot *carbon dioxide-free water R,* cool slowly and filter. To the filtrate add 0.05 ml of *methyl orange solution R*. No red colour develops.

Iodine value (*2.5.4*). See Table 1474.-1.

Monographs Q-S

Freezing point (*2.2.18*). See Table 1474.-1.

Table 1474.-1.

Type	Iodine value	Freezing point (°C)
Stearic acid 50	maximum 4.0	53 - 59
Stearic acid 70	maximum 4.0	57 - 64
Stearic acid 95	maximum 1.5	64 - 69

Nickel (*2.4.27*): maximum 1 ppm.

ASSAY

Gas chromatography (*2.2.28*): use the normalisation procedure.

Test solution. In a conical flask fitted with a reflux condenser, dissolve 0.100 g of the substance to be examined in 5 ml of *boron trifluoride-methanol solution R*. Boil under reflux for 10 min. Add 4.0 ml of *heptane R* through the condenser and boil again under reflux for 10 min. Allow to cool. Add 20 ml of a saturated solution of *sodium chloride R*. Shake and allow the layers to separate. Remove about 2 ml of the organic layer and dry it over 0.2 g of *anhydrous sodium sulphate R*. Dilute 1.0 ml of this solution to 10.0 ml with *heptane R*.

Reference solution. Prepare the reference solution in the same manner as the test solution using 50 mg of *palmitic acid R* and 50 mg of *stearic acid R* instead of the substance to be examined.

Column:

- *material*: fused silica,
- *size*: l = 30 m, Ø = 0.32 mm,
- *stationary phase*: *macrogol 20 000 R* (film thickness 0.5 µm).

Carrier gas: *helium for chromatography R*.

Flow rate: 2.4 ml/min.

Temperature:

	Time (min)	Temperature (°C)
Column	0 - 2	70
	2 - 36	70 → 240
	36 - 41	240
Injection port		220
Detector		260

Detection: flame ionisation.

Injection: 1 µl.

Relative retention with reference to methyl stearate: methyl palmitate = about 0.88.

System suitability: reference solution:

- *resolution*: minimum 5.0 between the peaks due to methyl stearate and methyl palmitate.

LABELLING

The label states the type of stearic acid (50, 70, 95).

01/2005:1268

STEAROYL MACROGOLGLYCERIDES

Macrogolglyceridorum stearates

DEFINITION

Stearoyl macrogolglycerides are mixtures of monoesters, diesters and triesters of glycerol and monoesters and diesters of macrogols with a mean relative molecular mass between 300 and 4000. They are obtained by partial alcoholysis of saturated oils containing mainly triglycerides of stearic acid using macrogol or by esterification of glycerol and macrogol with saturated fatty acids or by mixture of glycerol esters and condensates of ethylene oxide with the fatty acids of these hydrogenated oils. The hydroxyl value does not differ by more than 15 units from the nominal value. The saponification value does not differ by more than 10 units from the nominal value.

CHARACTERS

Pale yellow waxy solids, dispersible in warm water and in warm liquid paraffin, freely soluble in methylene chloride, soluble in warm ethanol.

IDENTIFICATION

A. Examine by thin-layer chromatography (*2.2.27*), using a suitable silica gel as the coating substance.

   Test solution. Dissolve 1.0 g of the substance to be examined in *methylene chloride R* and dilute to 20 ml with the same solvent.

   Apply to the plate 10 µl of the test solution. Develop over a path of 15 cm using a mixture of 30 volumes of *hexane R* and 70 volumes of *ether R*. Allow the plate to dry in air. Spray with a 0.1 g/l solution of *rhodamine B R* in *alcohol R* and examine in ultraviolet light at 365 nm. The chromatogram shows a spot corresponding to triglycerides with an R_f value of about 0.9 (R_{st} 1) and spots corresponding to 1,3-diglycerides (R_{st} 0.7), to 1,2-diglycerides (R_{st} 0.6), to monoglycerides (R_{st} 0.1) and to esters of macrogol (R_{st} 0).

B. They comply with the test for hydroxyl value (see Tests).

C. They comply with the test for saponification value (see Tests).

D. They comply with the test for fatty acid composition (see Tests).

TESTS

Acid value (*2.5.1*). Not more than 2.0, determined on 2.0 g.

Hydroxyl value (*2.5.3, Method A*). Determined on 1.0 g, the hydroxyl value does not differ by more than 15 units from the nominal value.

Peroxide value (*2.5.5*). Not more than 6.0, determined on 2.0 g.

Saponification value (*2.5.6*). Determined on 2.0 g, the saponification value does not differ by more than 10 units from the nominal value.

Alkaline impurities. Into a test-tube introduce 5.0 g and carefully add a mixture, neutralised if necessary with *0.01 M hydrochloric acid* or with *0.01 M sodium hydroxide*, of 0.05 ml of a 0.4 g/l solution of *bromophenol blue R* in *alcohol R*, 0.3 ml of *water R* and 10 ml of *alcohol R*. Shake and allow to stand. Not more than 1.0 ml of *0.01 M hydrochloric acid* is required to change the colour of the upper layer to yellow.

Free glycerol. Not more than 3.0 per cent. Dissolve 1.20 g in 25.0 ml of *methylene chloride R*. Heat if necessary. After cooling, add 100 ml of *water R*. Shake and add 25.0 ml of a 6 g/l solution of *periodic acid R*. Shake and allow to stand for 30 min. Add 40 ml of a 75 g/l solution of *potassium iodide R*. Allow to stand for 1 min. Add 1 ml of *starch solution R*. Titrate the iodine with *0.1 M sodium thiosulphate*. Carry out a blank titration.

1 ml of *0.1 M sodium thiosulphate* is equivalent to 2.3 mg of glycerol.

Composition of fatty acids (*2.4.22, Method A*). The constitutive fatty acid composition is the following:

- lauric acid: not more than 5.0 per cent,
- myristic acid: not more than 5.0 per cent,
- different nominal amounts of stearic acid and of palmitic acid. The sum of $C_{18}H_{36}O_2$ and $C_{16}H_{32}O_2$ is not less than 90.0 per cent.

Ethylene oxide and dioxan (*2.4.25*). Not more than 1 ppm of ethylene oxide and not more than 10 ppm of dioxan.

Heavy metals (*2.4.8*). 2.0 g complies with limit test C for heavy metals (10 ppm). Prepare the standard using 2 ml of *lead standard solution (10 ppm Pb) R*.

Water (*2.5.12*). Not more than 1.0 per cent, determined on 1.0 g by the semi-micro determination of water using a mixture of 30 volumes of *anhydrous methanol R* and 70 volumes of *methylene chloride R* as solvent.

Total ash (*2.4.16*). Not more than 0.2 per cent, determined on 1.0 g.

LABELLING

The label states the nominal hydroxyl value, the nominal saponification value and the type of the macrogol used (mean relative molecular mass) or the number of ethylene oxide units per molecule (nominal value).

01/2005:0753

STEARYL ALCOHOL

Alcohol stearylicus

DEFINITION

Stearyl alcohol is a mixture of solid alcohols; it contains not less than 95.0 per cent of octadecanol ($C_{18}H_{38}O$; M_r 270.5).

CHARACTERS

White, unctuous flakes, granules or mass, practically insoluble in water, soluble in alcohol. When melted, it is miscible with fatty oils, with liquid paraffin and with melted wool fat.

IDENTIFICATION

Examine the chromatograms obtained in the Assay. The retention time and size of the principal peak in the chromatogram obtained with the test solution are approximately the same as those of the principal peak in the chromatogram obtained with reference solution (a).

TESTS

Appearance of solution. Dissolve 0.50 g in 20 ml of *alcohol R* by heating to boiling. Allow to cool. The solution is clear (*2.2.1*) and not more intensely coloured than reference solution B_6 (*2.2.2, Method II*).

Melting point (*2.2.14*): 57 °C to 60 °C.

Acid value (*2.5.1*). Not more than 1.0.

Hydroxyl value (*2.5.3, Method A*): 197 to 217.

Iodine value (*2.5.4*). Not more than 2.0, determined on 2.00 g dissolved in 25 ml of *chloroform R*, warming if necessary.

Saponification value (*2.5.6*). Not more than 2.0.

ASSAY

Examine by gas chromatography (*2.2.28*).

Test solution. Dissolve 0.100 g of the substance to be examined in *ethanol R* and dilute to 10.0 ml with the same solvent.

Reference solution (a). Dissolve 0.100 g of *stearyl alcohol CRS* in *ethanol R* and dilute to 10.0 ml with the same solvent.

Reference solution (b). Dissolve 5 mg of *cetyl alcohol CRS* in 4.5 ml of reference solution (a) and dilute to 5.0 ml with *ethanol R*.

The chromatographic procedure may be carried out using:

- a stainless steel column 2 m long and 2 mm in internal diameter packed with *diatomaceous earth for gas chromatography R* impregnated with 10 per cent *m/m* of *poly(dimethyl)siloxane R*,
- *nitrogen for chromatography R* as the carrier gas at a flow rate of 30 ml/min,
- a flame-ionisation detector,

maintaining the temperature of the column at 220 °C, that of the injection port at 275 °C and that of the detector at 250 °C. Inject 2 µl of reference solution (b). The assay is not valid unless the resolution between the peaks corresponding to cetyl alcohol and stearyl alcohol is at least 4.0. Inject 2 µl of the test solution and 2 µl of reference solution (a). Calculate the percentage content of octadecanol using the normalisation procedure.

01/2005:0246

STRAMONIUM LEAF

Stramonii folium

DEFINITION

Stramonium leaf consists of the dried leaf or of the dried leaf, flowering tops and occasionally, fruit-bearing tops of *Datura stramonium* L. and its varieties. It contains not less than 0.25 per cent of total alkaloids, calculated as hyoscyamine ($C_{17}H_{23}NO_3$; M_r 289.4) with reference to the drug dried at 100 °C to 105 °C. The alkaloids consist mainly of hyoscyamine with varying proportions of hyoscine (scopolamine).

CHARACTERS

Stramonium leaf has an unpleasant odour.

It has the macroscopic and microscopic characters described under identification tests A and B.

IDENTIFICATION

A. The leaves are dark brownish-green to dark greyish-green, often much twisted and shrunken during drying, thin and brittle, ovate or triangular-ovate, dentately lobed with an acuminate apex and often unequal at the base. Young leaves are pubescent on the veins, older leaves are nearly glabrous. Stems are green or purplish-green, slender, curved and twisted, wrinkled longitudinally and sometimes wrinkled transversely, branched dichasially, with a single flower or an immature fruit in the fork. Flowers, on short pedicels, have a gamosepalous calyx with 5 lobes and trumpet-shaped brownish-white or purplish corolla. The fruit is a capsule, usually covered with numerous short, stiff emergences; seeds are brown to black with a minutely pitted testa.

B. Reduce to a powder (355). The powder is greyish-green. Examine under a microscope using *chloral hydrate solution R*. The powder shows the following diagnostic characters: fragments of leaf lamina showing epidermal cells with slightly wavy anticlinal walls and smooth cuticle; stomata are more frequent on the lower epidermis (anisocytic and anomocytic) (*2.8.3*); covering trichomes are conical, uniseriate with 3 to 5 cells and warty walls; glandular trichomes are short and clavate with heads formed by 2 to 7 cells; dorsiventral mesophyll, with a single layer of palisade cells and a spongy parenchyma containing cluster crystals of calcium oxalate; annularly and spirally thickened vessels. The powdered drug may also show the following: fibres and reticulately thickened vessels from the stem; subspherical pollen grains usually about 60 µm to 80 µm in diameter with 3 germinal pores and nearly smooth exine; fragments of the corolla with papillose epidermis; seed fragments containing yellowish-brown, sinuous, thick-walled sclereids of testa; occasional prisms and microsphenoidal crystals of calcium oxalate.

C. Examine the chromatograms obtained in the chromatography test. The principal zones in the chromatogram obtained with the test solution are similar in position, colour and size to the principal zones in the chromatogram obtained with the same volume of the reference solution.

D. Shake 1 g of the powdered drug (180) with 10 ml of *0.05 M sulphuric acid* for 2 min. Filter and add to the filtrate 1 ml of *concentrated ammonia R* and 5 ml of *water R*. Shake cautiously with 15 ml of *peroxide-free ether R* to avoid the formation of an emulsion. Separate the ether layer and dry over *anhydrous sodium sulphate R*. Filter and evaporate the ether in a porcelain dish. Add 0.5 ml of *nitric acid R* and evaporate to dryness on a water-bath. Add 10 ml of *acetone R* and, dropwise, a 30 g/l solution of *potassium hydroxide R* in *alcohol R*. A deep violet colour develops.

TESTS

Chromatography. Examine by thin-layer chromatography (*2.2.27*), using *silica gel G R* as the coating substance.

Test solution. To 1.0 g of the powdered drug (180) add 10 ml of *0.05 M sulphuric acid*, shake for 15 min and filter. Wash the filter with *0.05 M sulphuric acid* until 25 ml of filtrate is obtained. To the filtrate add 1 ml of *concentrated ammonia R* and shake with 2 quantities, each of 10 ml, of *peroxide-free ether R*. If necessary, separate by centrifugation. Dry the combined ether layers over *anhydrous sodium sulphate R*, filter and evaporate to dryness on a water-bath. Dissolve the residue in 0.5 ml of *methanol R*.

Reference solution. Dissolve 50 mg of *hyoscyamine sulphate R* in 9 ml of *methanol R*. Dissolve 15 mg of *hyoscine hydrobromide R* in 10 ml of *methanol R*. Mix 3.8 ml of the hyoscyamine sulphate solution and 4.2 ml of the hyoscine hydrobromide solution and dilute to 10 ml with *methanol R*.

Apply separately to the plate as bands 20 mm by 3 mm 10 µl and 20 µl of each solution, leaving 1 cm between the bands. Develop over a path of 10 cm using a mixture of 3 volumes of *concentrated ammonia R*, 7 volumes of *water R* and 90 volumes of *acetone R*. Dry the plate at 100-105 °C for 15 min, allow to cool and spray with *potassium iodobismuthate solution R2*, using about 10 ml for a plate 200 mm square, until the orange or brown zones become visible against a yellow background. The zones in the chromatograms obtained with the test solution are similar to those in the chromatograms obtained with the reference solution with respect to their position (hyoscyamine in the lower third, hyoscine in the upper third of the chromatogram) and their colour. The zones in the chromatograms obtained with the test solution are at least equal in size to the corresponding zones in the chromatogram obtained with the same volume of the reference solution. Faint secondary zones may appear, particularly in the middle of the chromatogram obtained with 20 µl of the test solution or near the starting point in the chromatogram obtained with 10 µl of the test solution. Spray the plate with *sodium nitrite solution R* until the coating is transparent. Examine after 15 min. The zones corresponding to hyoscyamine in the chromatograms obtained with the test solution and the reference solution change from brown to reddish-brown but not to greyish-blue (atropine) and any secondary zones disappear.

Foreign matter (*2.8.2*). Not more than 3 per cent of stem having a diameter exceeding 5 mm.

Total ash (*2.4.16*). Not more than 20.0 per cent.

Ash insoluble in hydrochloric acid (*2.8.1*). Not more than 4.0 per cent.

ASSAY

Take about 50 g of the drug and completely reduce it to a powder (180). Using the powder, determine the loss on drying and the total alkaloids.

a) Determine the loss on drying (*2.2.32*) on 2.000 g by drying in an oven at 100 °C to 105 °C.

b) Moisten 10.0 g of the powder with a mixture of 5 ml of *ammonia R*, 10 ml of *alcohol R* and 30 ml of *peroxide-free ether R* and mix thoroughly. Transfer the mixture to a suitable percolator, if necessary with the aid of the extracting mixture. Allow to macerate for 4 h and percolate with a mixture of 1 volume of *chloroform R* and 3 volumes of *peroxide-free ether R* until the alkaloids are completely extracted. Evaporate to dryness a few millilitres of the liquid flowing from the percolator, dissolve the residue in *0.25 M sulphuric acid* and verify the absence of alkaloids using *potassium tetraiodomercurate solution R*. Concentrate the percolate to about 50 ml by distilling on a water-bath and transfer it to a separating funnel, rinsing with *peroxide-free ether R*. Add a quantity of *peroxide-free ether R* equal to at least 2.1 times the volume of the percolate to produce a liquid of a density well below that of water. Shake the solution with no fewer than 3 quantities, each of 20 ml, of *0.25 M sulphuric acid*, separate the 2 layers by centrifugation if necessary and transfer the acid layers to a second separating funnel. Make the acid layer alkaline with *ammonia R* and shake with 3 quantities, each of 30 ml, of *chloroform R*. Combine the chloroform layers, add 4 g of *anhydrous sodium sulphate R* and allow to stand for 30 min with occasional shaking. Decant the chloroform and wash the sodium sulphate with 3 quantities, each of 10 ml, of *chloroform R*. Add the washings to the chloroform extract, evaporate to dryness on a water-bath and heat in an oven at 100-105 °C for 15 min. Dissolve the residue in a few millilitres of *chloroform R*, add 20.0 ml of *0.01 M sulphuric acid* and remove the chloroform by evaporation on a water-bath. Titrate the excess of acid with *0.02 M sodium hydroxide* using *methyl red mixed solution R* as indicator.

Calculate the percentage content of total alkaloids, expressed as hyoscyamine, from the expression:

$$\frac{57.88\,(20 - n)}{(100 - d)\,m}$$

d = loss on drying as a percentage,

n = volume of *0.02 M sodium hydroxide* used in millilitres,

m = mass of drug used, in grams.

STORAGE

Protected from moisture.

01/2005:0247

STRAMONIUM, PREPARED

Stramonii pulvis normatus

DEFINITION

Prepared stramonium is stramonium leaf powder (180) adjusted, if necessary, by the addition of powdered lactose or stramonium leaf of lower alkaloidal content to contain 0.23 per cent to 0.27 per cent of total alkaloids, calculated as hyoscyamine ($C_{17}H_{23}NO_3$; M_r 289.4) with reference to the dried drug.

CHARACTERS

Greyish-green powder with an unpleasant odour.

IDENTIFICATION

A. Examine under a microscope using *chloral hydrate solution R*. The powder shows the following diagnostic characters: fragments of leaf lamina showing epidermal cells with slightly wavy anticlinal walls and smooth cuticle; stomata are more frequent on the lower epidermis (anisocytic and anomocytic) (*2.8.3*); covering trichomes are conical, uniseriate with three to five cells and warty walls; glandular trichomes are short and clavate with heads formed by 2 to 7 cells; dorsiventral mesophyll, with a single layer of palisade cells and a spongy parenchyma containing cluster crystals of calcium oxalate; annularly and spirally thickened vessels. The powdered drug may also show the following: fibres and reticulately thickened vessels from the stem; subspherical pollen grains usually about 60 µm to 80 µm in diameter with three germinal pores and nearly smooth exine; fragments of the corolla with papillose epidermis; seed fragments containing yellowish-brown, sinuous, thick-walled sclereids of testa; occasional prisms and microsphenoidal crystals of calcium oxalate. Examined in *glycerol (85 per cent) R*, it may be seen to contain lactose crystals.

B. Examine the chromatograms obtained in the chromatography test. The principal zones in the chromatogram obtained with the test solution are similar in position, colour and size to the principal zones in the chromatogram obtained with the same volume of the reference solution.

C. Shake 1 g with 10 ml of *0.05 M sulphuric acid* for 2 min. Filter and add to the filtrate 1 ml of *concentrated ammonia R* and 5 ml of *water R*. Shake cautiously with 15 ml of *peroxide-free ether R* to avoid the formation of an emulsion. Separate the ether layer and dry over *anhydrous sodium sulphate R*. Filter and evaporate the ether in a porcelain dish. Add 0.5 ml of *nitric acid R* and evaporate to dryness on a water-bath. Add 10 ml of *acetone R* and, dropwise, a 30 g/l solution of *potassium hydroxide R* in *alcohol R*. A deep violet colour develops.

TESTS

Chromatography. Examine by thin-layer chromatography (*2.2.27*), using *silica gel G R* as the coating substance.

Test solution. To 1.0 g add 10 ml of *0.05 M sulphuric acid*, shake for 15 min and filter. Wash the filter with *0.05 M sulphuric acid* until 25 ml of filtrate is obtained. To the filtrate add 1 ml of *concentrated ammonia R* and shake with two quantities, each of 10 ml, of *peroxide-free ether R*. If necessary, separate by centrifugation. Dry the combined ether layers over *anhydrous sodium sulphate R*, filter and evaporate to dryness on a water-bath. Dissolve the residue in 0.5 ml of *methanol R*.

Reference solution. Dissolve 50 mg of *hyoscyamine sulphate R* in 9 ml of *methanol R*. Dissolve 15 mg of *hyoscine hydrobromide R* in 10 ml of *methanol R*. Mix 3.8 ml of the hyoscyamine sulphate solution and 4.2 ml of the hyoscine hydrobromide solution and dilute to 10 ml with *methanol R*.

Apply separately to the plate as bands 20 mm by 3 mm 10 µl and 20 µl of each solution, leaving 1 cm between the bands. Develop over a path of 10 cm using a mixture of 3 volumes of *concentrated ammonia R*, 7 volumes of *water R* and 90 volumes of *acetone R*. Dry the plate at 100 °C to 105 °C for 15 min, allow to cool and spray with *potassium iodobismuthate solution R2*, using about 10 ml for a plate 200 mm square, until the orange or brown zones become visible against a yellow background. The zones in the chromatograms obtained with the test solution are similar to those in the chromatograms obtained with the reference solution with respect to their position (hyoscyamine in the lower third, hyoscine in the upper third of the chromatogram) and their colour. The zones in the chromatograms obtained with the test solution are at least equal in size to the corresponding zones in the chromatogram obtained with the same volume of the reference solution. Faint secondary zones may appear, particularly in the middle of the chromatogram obtained with 20 µl of the test solution or near the starting point in the chromatogram obtained with 10 µl of the test solution. Spray the plate with *sodium nitrite solution R* until the coating is transparent. Examine after 15 min. The zones corresponding to hyoscyamine in the chromatograms obtained with the test solution and the reference solution change from brown to reddish-brown but not to greyish-blue (atropine) and any secondary zones disappear.

Loss on drying (*2.2.32*). Not more than 5.0 per cent, determined on 1.000 g by drying in an oven at 100 °C to 105 °C.

Total ash (*2.4.16*). Not more than 20.0 per cent.

Ash insoluble in hydrochloric acid (*2.8.1*). Not more than 4.0 per cent.

ASSAY

a) Determine the loss on drying (*2.2.32*) on 2.000 g by drying in an oven at 100 °C to 105 °C.

b) Moisten 10.0 g with a mixture of 5 ml of *ammonia R*, 10 ml of *alcohol R* and 30 ml of *peroxide-free ether R* and mix thoroughly. Transfer the mixture to a suitable percolator, if necessary with the aid of the extracting mixture. Allow to macerate for 4 h and percolate with a mixture of 1 volume of *chloroform R* and 3 volumes of *peroxide-free ether R* until the alkaloids are completely extracted. Evaporate to dryness a few millilitres of the liquid flowing from the percolator, dissolve the residue in *0.25 M sulphuric acid* and verify the absence of alkaloids using *potassium tetraiodomercurate solution R*. Concentrate the percolate to about 50 ml by distilling on a water-bath and transfer it to a separating funnel, rinsing with *peroxide-free ether R*. Add a quantity of *peroxide-free ether R* equal to at least 2.1 times the volume of the percolate to produce a liquid of a density well below that of water. Shake the solution with no fewer than three quantities, each of 20 ml, of *0.25 M sulphuric acid*, separate the two layers by centrifugation if necessary and transfer the acid layers to a second separating funnel. Make the acid layer alkaline with *ammonia R* and shake with three quantities, each of 30 ml, of *chloroform R*. Combine the chloroform layers, add 4 g of *anhydrous sodium sulphate R* and allow to stand for 30 min with occasional shaking. Decant the chloroform and wash the sodium sulphate with three quantities, each of 10 ml, of *chloroform R*. Add the washings to the chloroform extract, evaporate to dryness on a water-bath and heat in an oven at 100 °C to 105 °C for 15 min. Dissolve the residue in a few millilitres of *chloroform R*, add 20.0 ml of *0.01 M sulphuric acid* and remove the chloroform by evaporation on a water-bath. Titrate the excess of acid with *0.02 M sodium hydroxide* using *methyl red mixed solution R* as indicator.

Calculate the percentage content of total alkaloids, expressed as hyoscyamine, from the expression:

$$\frac{57.88\,(20 - n)}{(100 - d)\,m}$$

d = loss on drying as a percentage,

n = volume of *0.02 M sodium hydroxide* used in millilitres,

m = mass of drug used in grams.

STORAGE

Store in an airtight container, protected from light.

01/2005:0356

STREPTOKINASE BULK SOLUTION

Streptokinasi solutio ad praeparationem

DEFINITION

Streptokinase bulk solution is a preparation of a protein obtained from culture filtrates of certain strains of haemolytic *Streptococcus* group C; it has the property of combining with human plasminogen to form plasminogen activator. It may contain buffer salts and other auxiliary substances. The potency is not less than 96 000 IU per milligram of protein.

PRODUCTION

If intended for use in the manufacture of parenteral dosage forms, the method of manufacture is validated to demonstrate that the product, if tested, would comply with the following test.

Abnormal toxicity (*2.6.9*). Inject into each mouse a quantity of the preparation to be examined (if necessary, dilute with *water for injections R*) equivalent to 50 000 IU of streptokinase activity in 0.5 ml, the injection lasting 15-20 s.

CHARACTERS

Appearance: clear, colourless liquid.

IDENTIFICATION

A. Place 0.5 ml of citrated human plasma in a haemolysis tube maintained in a water-bath at 37 °C. Add 0.1 ml of a dilution of the preparation to be examined containing 10 000 IU of streptokinase activity per millilitre in *phosphate buffer solution pH 7.2 R* and 0.1 ml of a solution of *human thrombin R* containing 20 IU/ml in *phosphate buffer solution pH 7.2 R*. Mix immediately. A clot forms and lyses within 30 min. Repeat the procedure using citrated bovine plasma. The clot does not lyse within 60 min.

B. Dissolve 0.6 g of agar in 50.0 ml of *barbital buffer solution pH 8.6 R1*, heating until a clear solution is obtained. Use glass plates 50 mm square (transparency mounts) free from traces of grease. Using a pipette, apply to each plate 4 ml of the agar solution. Maintain the plates horizontal. Allow to cool. Pierce a cavity 6 mm in diameter in the centre of the agar and an appropriate number of cavities (not exceeding 6) at distances of 11 mm from the central cavity. Remove the residual agar from the cavities using a cannula connected to a vacuum pump. Using pipettes graduated in microlitres, place in the central cavity about 80 µl of goat or rabbit antistreptokinase serum containing 10 000 units of antistreptokinase activity per millilitre; place in each of the surrounding cavities about 80 µl of a dilution of the preparation to be examined containing 125 000 IU of streptokinase activity per millilitre. Allow the plates to stand in a humidified tank for 24 h. Only one precipitation arc appears and it is well defined and localised between the application point of the serum and each cavity containing the solution of the preparation to be examined.

TESTS

pH (*2.2.3*): 6.8 to 7.5.

Dilute the preparation to be examined in *carbon dioxide-free water R* to obtain a solution containing 5000 IU of streptokinase activity per millilitre.

Streptodornase: maximum 10 IU of streptodornase activity per 100 000 IU of streptokinase activity.

Test solution. Dilute the preparation to be examined in *imidazole buffer solution pH 6.5 R* to obtain a solution containing 150 000 IU of streptokinase activity per millilitre.

Reference solution. Dissolve in *imidazole buffer solution pH 6.5 R* a reference preparation of streptodornase, calibrated in International Units against the International Standard of streptodornase, to obtain a solution containing 20 IU of streptodornase activity per millilitre. The equivalence in International Units of the International Standard is stated by the World Health Organisation.

To each of 8 numbered centrifuge tubes, add 0.5 ml of a 1 g/l solution of *sodium deoxyribonucleate R* in *imidazole buffer solution pH 6.5 R*. To tube number 1 and tube number 2 add 0.25 ml of *imidazole buffer solution pH 6.5 R*, 0.25 ml of the test solution and, immediately, 3.0 ml of perchloric acid (25 g/l $HClO_4$). Mix, centrifuge at about 3000 *g* for 5 min and measure the absorbances (*2.2.25*) of the supernatant liquids at 260 nm, using as the compensation liquid a mixture of 1.0 ml of *imidazole buffer solution pH 6.5 R* and 3.0 ml of perchloric acid (25 g/l $HClO_4$) (absorbances A_1 and A_2). To the other 6 tubes (numbers 3 to 8) add 0.25 ml, 0.25 ml, 0.125 ml, 0.125 ml, 0 ml and 0 ml respectively of *imidazole buffer solution pH 6.5 R*; add to each tube 0.25 ml of the test solution and 0 ml, 0 ml, 0.125 ml, 0.125 ml, 0.25 ml and 0.25 ml respectively of the reference solution. Mix the contents of each tube and heat at 37 °C for 15 min. To each tube add 3.0 ml of perchloric acid (25 g/l $HClO_4$), mix and centrifuge. Measure the absorbances (*2.2.25*) of the

Monographs Q-S

supernatant liquids at 260 nm using the compensation liquid described above (absorbances A_3 to A_8). The absorbances comply with the following requirement:

$$(A_3 + A_4) - (A_1 + A_2) < \frac{(A_5 + A_6 + A_7 + A_8)}{2} - (A_3 + A_4)$$

Streptolysin. In a haemolysis tube, use a quantity of the preparation to be examined equivalent to 500 000 IU of streptokinase activity and dilute to 0.5 ml with a mixture of 1 volume of *phosphate buffer solution pH 7.2 R* and 9 volumes of a 9 g/l solution of *sodium chloride R*. Add 0.4 ml of a 23 g/l solution of *sodium thioglycollate R*. Heat in a water-bath at 37 °C for 10 min. Add 0.1 ml of a solution of a reference preparation of human antistreptolysin O containing 5 IU/ml. Heat at 37 °C for 5 min. Add 1 ml of *rabbit erythrocyte suspension R*. Heat at 37 °C for 30 min. Centrifuge at about 1000 *g*. In the same manner, prepare a haemolysis tube in which the solution of the preparation to be examined has been replaced by 0.5 ml of a mixture of 1 volume of *phosphate buffer solution pH 7.2 R* and 9 volumes of a 9 g/l solution of *sodium chloride R*. Measure the absorbances (*2.2.25*) of the supernatant liquids at 550 nm. The absorbance of the test solution is not more than 50 per cent greater than that of the reference solution.

Bacterial endotoxins (*2.6.14*): less than 0.02 IU per 100 IU of streptokinase activity, if intended for use in the manufacture of parenteral dosage forms without a further appropriate procedure for the removal of bacterial endotoxins.

ASSAY

Protein. (*2.5.33, Method 7, Procedure A*). 1 mg of N is equivalent to 6.25 mg of protein.

Potency

The potency of streptokinase is determined by comparing its capacity to activate plasminogen to form plasmin with the same capacity of a reference preparation of streptokinase calibrated in International Units; the formation of plasmin is determined using a suitable chromogenic substrate.

The International Unit is the activity of a stated amount of the International Standard for streptokinase. The equivalence in International Units of the International Standard is stated by the World Health Organisation.

Reference and test solutions

Prepare 2 independent series of 4 dilutions of each of the substance to be examined and of the reference preparation of streptokinase in *tris(hydroxymethyl)aminomethane sodium chloride buffer solution pH 7.4 R1*, in the range of 0.5-4.0 IU/ml. Prepare and maintain all solutions at 37 °C.

Substrate solution

Mix 1.0 ml of *tris(hydroxymethyl)aminomethane buffer solution pH 7.4 R* with 1.0 ml of *chromophore substrate R3*. Add 5 µl of a 100 g/l solution of *polysorbate 20 R*. Keep at 37 °C in a water-bath. Immediately before commencing the activation assay, add 45 µl of a 1 mg/ml solution of *human plasminogen R*.

Method

Analyse each streptokinase dilution, maintained at 37 °C, in duplicate. Initiate the activation reaction by adding 60 µl of each dilution to 40 µl of substrate solution. For blank wells, use 60 µl of *tris(hydroxymethyl)aminomethane sodium chloride buffer solution pH 7.4 R1* instead of the reference and test solutions. Allow the reaction to proceed at 37 °C for 20 min and read the absorbance (*2.2.25*) at 405 nm. If a suitable thermostatted plate reader is available, this may be used to monitor the reaction. Alternatively, it may be necessary to stop the reaction after 20 min using 50 µl of a 50 per cent *V/V* solution of *glacial acetic acid R*. Best results are obtained when the absorbance for the highest streptokinase concentration is between 0.1 and 0.2 (after blank subtraction). If necessary, adjust the time of incubation in order to reach this range of absorbances.

Calculate the regression of the absorbance on log concentrations of the solutions of the substance to be examined and of the reference preparation of streptokinase and calculate the potency of the substance to be examined using the usual statistical methods for parallel-line assays.

The estimated potency is not less than 90 per cent and not more than 111 per cent of the stated potency. The confidence limits ($P = 0.95$) of the estimated potency are not less than 80 per cent and not more than 125 per cent of the stated potency.

STORAGE

In a sealed container, protected from light and at a temperature of − 20 °C. If the substance is sterile, store in a sterile, airtight, tamper-proof container.

LABELLING

The label states:

- the number of International Units of streptokinase activity per milligram, calculated with reference to the dried preparation,
- the name and quantity of any added substance,
- where applicable, that the substance is free from bacterial endotoxins,
- where applicable, that the substance is suitable for use in the manufacture of parenteral dosage forms.

01/2005:0053

STREPTOMYCIN SULPHATE

Streptomycini sulfas

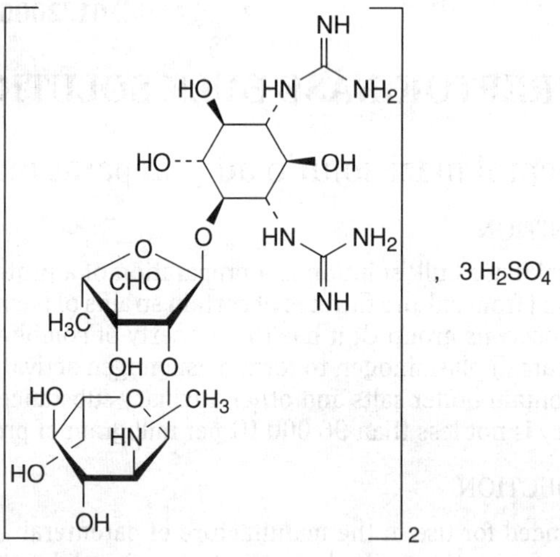

$C_{42}H_{84}N_{14}O_{36}S_3$ M_r 1457

DEFINITION

Streptomycin sulphate is bis[*N,N′*-bis(aminoiminomethyl)-4-*O*-[5-deoxy-2-*O*-[2-deoxy-2-(methylamino)-α-L-glucopyranosyl]-3-*C*-formyl-α-L-lyxofuranosyl]-D-streptamine] trisulphate, a substance produced by the growth of certain strains of *Streptomyces griseus* or obtained by any other means. Stabilisers may be added. The potency is not less than 720 IU/mg, calculated with reference to the dried substance.

PRODUCTION

It is produced by methods of manufacture designed to eliminate or minimise substances lowering blood pressure. The method of manufacture is validated to demonstrate that the product if tested would comply with the following test:

Abnormal toxicity (*2.6.9*). Inject into each mouse 1 mg of the substance to be examined dissolved in 0.5 ml of *water for injections R*.

CHARACTERS

A white or almost white powder, hygroscopic, very soluble in water, practically insoluble in ethanol.

IDENTIFICATION

A. Examine by thin-layer chromatography (*2.2.27*), using a plate coated with a 0.75 mm layer of the following mixture: mix 0.3 g of *carbomer R* with 240 ml of *water R* and allow to stand, with moderate shaking, for 1 h; adjust to pH 7 by the gradual addition, with continuous shaking, of *dilute sodium hydroxide solution R* and add 30 g of *silica gel H R*.
Heat the plate at 110 °C for 1 h, allow to cool and use immediately.
Test solution. Dissolve 10 mg of the substance to be examined in *water R* and dilute to 10 ml with the same solvent.
Reference solution (a). Dissolve 10 mg of *streptomycin sulphate CRS* in *water R* and dilute to 10 ml with the same solvent.
Reference solution (b). Dissolve 10 mg of *kanamycin monosulphate CRS*, 10 mg of *neomycin sulphate CRS* and 10 mg of *streptomycin sulphate CRS* in *water R* and dilute to 10 ml with the same solvent.
Apply separately to the plate 10 µl of each solution. Develop over a path of 12 cm using a 70 g/l solution of *potassium dihydrogen phosphate R*. Dry the plate in a current of warm air, and spray with a mixture of equal volumes of a 2 g/l solution of *1,3-dihydroxynaphthalene R* in *alcohol R* and a 460 g/l solution of *sulphuric acid R*. Heat at 150 °C for 5 min to 10 min. The principal spot in the chromatogram obtained with the test solution is similar in position, colour and size to the spot in the chromatogram obtained with reference solution (a). The test is not valid unless the chromatogram obtained with reference solution (b) shows three clearly separated spots.

B. Dissolve 5 mg to 10 mg in 4 ml of *water R* and add 1 ml of *1 M sodium hydroxide*. Heat in a water-bath for 4 min. Add a slight excess of *dilute hydrochloric acid R* and 0.1 ml of *ferric chloride solution R1*. A violet colour develops.

C. Dissolve 0.1 g in 2 ml of *water R*, add 1 ml of *α-naphthol solution R* and 2 ml of a mixture of equal volumes of *strong sodium hypochlorite solution R* and *water R*. A red colour develops.

D. Dissolve about 10 mg in 5 ml of *water R* and add 1 ml of *1 M hydrochloric acid*. Heat in a water-bath for 2 min. Add 2 ml of a 5 g/l solution of *α-naphthol R* in *1 M sodium hydroxide* and heat in a water-bath for 1 min. A faint yellow colour develops.

E. It gives the reactions of sulphates (*2.3.1*).

TESTS

Solution S. Dissolve 2.5 g in *carbon dioxide-free water R* and dilute to 10 ml with the same solvent.

Appearance of solution. Solution S is not more intensely coloured than intensity 3 of the range of reference solutions of the most appropriate colour (*2.2.2, Method II*). Allow to stand protected from light, at a temperature of about 20 °C for 24 h. Solution S is not more opalescent than reference suspension II (*2.2.1*).

pH (*2.2.3*). The pH of solution S is 4.5 to 7.0.

Methanol. Examine by gas chromatography (*2.2.28*).

Test solution. Dissolve 1.00 g of the substance to be examined in *water R* and dilute to 25.0 ml with the same solvent.

Reference solution. Dilute 12.0 mg of *methanol R* to 100 ml with *water R*.

The chromatographic procedure may be carried out using:
– a column 1.5 m to 2.0 m long and 2 mm to 4 mm in internal diameter, packed with *ethylvinylbenzene-divinylbenzene copolymer R* (150 µm to 180 µm),
– *nitrogen for chromatography R* as the carrier gas at a constant flow rate of 30 ml to 40 ml per minute,
– a flame-ionisation detector.

Maintain the column at a constant temperature between 120 °C and 140 °C and the injection port and the detector at a temperature at least 50 °C higher than that of the column. Inject the test solution and the reference solution. The area of the peak corresponding to methanol in the chromatogram obtained with the test solution is not greater than the area of the peak in the chromatogram obtained with the reference solution (0.3 per cent).

Streptomycin B. Examine by thin-layer chromatography (*2.2.27*), using *silica gel G R* as the coating substance.

Test solution. Dissolve 0.2 g of the substance to be examined in a freshly prepared mixture of 3 volumes of *sulphuric acid R* and 97 volumes of *methanol R* and dilute to 5 ml with the same mixture of solvents. Heat under a reflux condenser for 1 h, cool, rinse the condenser with *methanol R* and dilute to 20 ml with the same solvent (10 g/l solution).

Reference solution. Dissolve 36 mg of *mannose R* in a freshly prepared mixture of 3 volumes of *sulphuric acid R* and 97 volumes of *methanol R* and dilute to 5 ml with the same mixture of solvents. Heat under a reflux condenser for 1 h, cool, rinse the condenser with *methanol R* and dilute to 50 ml with the same solvent. Dilute 5 ml of the solution to 50 ml with *methanol R* (0.3 g/l solution expressed as strepto-mycin B; 1 mg of *mannose R* is equivalent to 4.13 mg of streptomycin B).

Apply separately to the plate 10 µl of each solution. Develop over a path of 13 cm to 15 cm using a mixture of 25 volumes of *glacial acetic acid R*, 25 volumes of *methanol R* and 50 volumes of *toluene R*. Allow the plate to dry in air and spray with a freshly prepared mixture of equal volumes of a 2 g/l solution of *1,3-dihydroxynaphthalene R* in *alcohol R* and a 20 per cent *V/V* solution of *sulphuric acid R* and heat at 110 °C for 5 min. Any spot corresponding to streptomycin B in the chromatogram obtained with the test solution is not more intense than the spot in the chromatogram obtained with the reference solution (3.0 per cent).

Loss on drying (*2.2.32*). Not more than 7.0 per cent, determined on 1.000 g by drying at 60 °C over *diphosphorus pentoxide R* at a pressure not exceeding 0.1 kPa for 24 h.

Sulphated ash (*2.4.14*). Not more than 1.0 per cent, determined on 1.000 g.

Sulphate. 18.0 per cent to 21.5 per cent of sulphate (SO_4), calculated with reference to the dried substance. Dissolve 0.250 g in 100 ml of *water R* and adjust the solution to pH 11 using *concentrated ammonia R*. Add 10.0 ml of *0.1 M barium chloride* and about 0.5 mg of *phthalein purple R*. Titrate with *0.1 M sodium edetate* adding 50 ml of *alcohol R* when the colour of the solution begins to change and continue the titration until the violet-blue colour disappears.

1 ml of *0.1 M barium chloride* is equivalent to 9.606 mg of sulphate (SO_4).

Colorimetric test. Dry the substance to be examined and *streptomycin sulphate CRS* at 60 °C over *diphosphorus pentoxide R* at a pressure not exceeding 0.1 kPa for 24 h. Dissolve 0.100 g of the dried substance to be examined in *water R* and dilute to 100.0 ml with the same solvent. Prepare a reference solution in the same manner using 0.100 g of the dried *streptomycin sulphate CRS*. Place 5.0 ml of each solution separately in two volumetric flasks and in a third flask place 5 ml of *water R*. To each flask add 5.0 ml of *0.2 M sodium hydroxide* and heat for exactly 10 min in a water-bath. Cool in ice for exactly 5 min, add 3 ml of a 15 g/l solution of *ferric ammonium sulphate R* in *0.5 M sulphuric acid*, dilute to 25.0 ml with *water R* and mix. Exactly 20 min after the addition of the ferric ammonium sulphate solution measure the absorbance (*2.2.25*) of the test solution and the reference solution in a 2 cm cell at the maximum at 525 nm, using as compensation liquid the solution prepared from 5 ml of *water R*. The absorbance of the test solution is not less than 90.0 per cent of that of the reference solution.

Bacterial endotoxins (*2.6.14*): less than 0.25 IU/mg, if intended for use in the manufacture of parenteral dosage forms without a further appropriate procedure for removal of bacterial endotoxins.

ASSAY

Carry out the microbiological assay of antibiotics (*2.7.2*).

STORAGE

Store in an airtight container. If the substance is sterile, store in a sterile, airtight, tamper-proof container.

LABELLING

The label states:

- where applicable, the name and quantity of any added stabiliser,
- where applicable, that the substance is free from bacterial endotoxins.

01/2005:0357

SUCCINYLSULFATHIAZOLE

Succinylsulfathiazolum

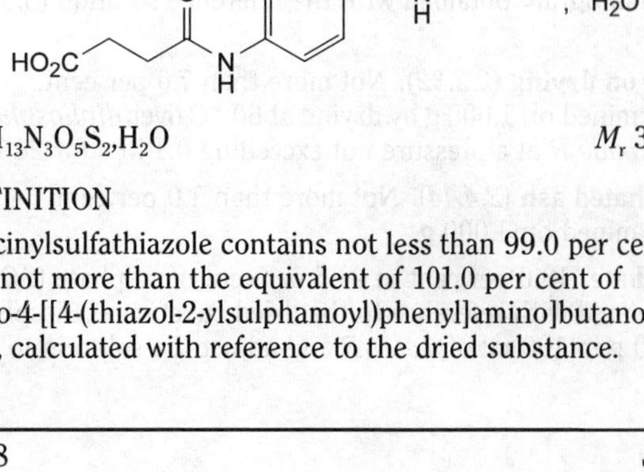

$C_{13}H_{13}N_3O_5S_2,H_2O$ M_r 373.4

DEFINITION

Succinylsulfathiazole contains not less than 99.0 per cent and not more than the equivalent of 101.0 per cent of 4-oxo-4-[[4-(thiazol-2-ylsulphamoyl)phenyl]amino]butanoic acid, calculated with reference to the dried substance.

CHARACTERS

A white or yellowish-white, crystalline powder, very slightly soluble in water, slightly soluble in acetone and in alcohol. It dissolves in solutions of alkali hydroxides and carbonates.

IDENTIFICATION

First identification: A, D.

Second identification: B, C, D, E.

A. Examine by infrared absorption spectrophotometry (*2.2.24*), comparing with the spectrum obtained with *succinylsulfathiazole CRS*. If the spectra obtained in the solid state with the substance to be examined and the reference substance show differences, dissolve in hot *water R*, allow to crystallise, dry the crystals carefully between two sheets of filter paper and prepare new discs.

B. To 2 g add 10 ml of *water R* and 10 ml of *strong sodium hydroxide solution R* and boil for 10 min. Cool and adjust to pH 3.0 with *hydrochloric acid R1*. Cool, adjust to pH 7.0 with *sodium hydrogen carbonate solution R* and filter. The precipitate, washed with *water R* and dried at 100 °C to 105 °C, melts (*2.2.14*) at 196 °C to 204 °C. Introduce the capillary containing the precipitate into the bath at a temperature of 190 °C.

C. Heat 0.1 g in a test-tube over a small flame. Fumes are evolved which blacken *lead acetate paper R*.

D. Place 0.1 g in a borosilicate-glass tube of about 30 ml capacity and add 0.5 g of *hydroquinone R* and 1 ml of *sulphuric acid R*. Heat in a glycerin bath at 135 °C for 10 min, mixing at the beginning of heating to obtain a homogeneous liquid phase. Allow to cool and place in iced water. Add carefully and with shaking 15 ml of *water R*. Add 5 ml of *toluene R*, shake for 5 s to 10 s and allow to stand for 2 min; promote separation of the two layers using a stirrer. The upper (toluene) layer shows an intense pink colour.

E. Dissolve about 10 mg of the precipitate obtained in identification test B in 200 ml of *0.1 M hydrochloric acid*. 2 ml of the solution gives the reaction of primary aromatic amines (*2.3.1*) with formation of an orange precipitate.

TESTS

Appearance of solution. Dissolve 1.0 g in a mixture of 5 ml of *dilute sodium hydroxide solution R* and 15 ml of *water R*. The solution is clear (*2.2.1*) and not more intensely coloured than reference solution Y_4 or BY_4 (*2.2.2, Method II*).

Acidity. To 2.0 g add 20 ml of *water R*, shake continuously for 30 min and filter. To 10 ml of the filtrate add 0.1 ml of *phenolphthalein solution R*. Not more than 2 ml of *0.1 M sodium hydroxide* is required to change the colour of the indicator.

Sulfathiazole and other primary aromatic amines. Dissolve 20 mg in a mixture of 3.5 ml of *water R*, 6 ml of *dilute hydrochloric acid R* and 25 ml of *alcohol R*, previously cooled to 15 °C. Place immediately in iced water and add 1 ml of a 2.5 g/l solution of *sodium nitrite R*. Allow to stand for 3 min, add 2.5 ml of a 40 g/l solution of *sulphamic acid R* and allow to stand for 5 min. Add 1 ml of a 4 g/l solution of *naphthylethylenediamine dihydrochloride R* and dilute to 50 ml with *water R*. Measured at 550 nm, the absorbance (*2.2.25*) is not greater than that of a standard prepared at the same time and in the same manner using a mixture of 1.5 ml of a solution containing 10 mg of *sulfathiazole R* and 0.5 ml of *hydrochloric acid R* per 100 ml; 2 ml of *water R*; 6 ml of *dilute hydrochloric acid R*; and 25 ml of *alcohol R*.

Heavy metals (*2.4.8*). 1.0 g complies with limit test D for heavy metals (20 ppm). Prepare the standard using 2 ml of *lead standard solution (10 ppm Pb) R*.

Loss on drying (*2.2.32*): 4.0 per cent to 5.5 per cent, determined on 1.00 g by drying in an oven at 100 °C to 105 °C.

Sulphated ash (*2.4.14*). Not more than 0.1 per cent, determined on 1.0 g.

ASSAY

Dissolve 0.300 g in 100 ml of a mixture of 1 volume of *hydrochloric acid R* and 2 volumes of *water R*. Heat under a reflux condenser for 1 h. Carry out the determination of primary aromatic amino-nitrogen (*2.5.8*), determining the end-point electrometrically.

1 ml of *0.1 M sodium nitrite* is equivalent to 35.54 mg of $C_{13}H_{13}N_3O_5S_2$.

STORAGE

Store protected from light.

01/2005:0204
corrected

SUCROSE

Saccharum

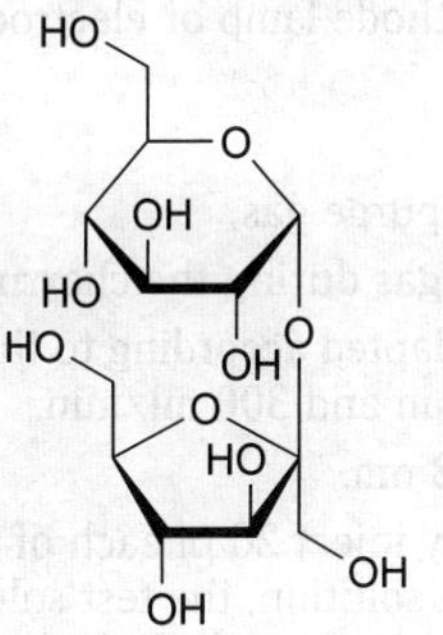

$C_{12}H_{22}O_{11}$ M_r 342.3

DEFINITION

β-D-Fructofuranosyl α-D-glucopyranoside.

It contains no additives.

CHARACTERS

Appearance: white or almost white, crystalline powder, or shiny, colourless or white or almost white crystals.

Solubility: very soluble in water, slightly soluble in alcohol, practically insoluble in ethanol.

IDENTIFICATION

First identification: A.

Second identification: B, C.

A. Infrared absorption spectrophotometry (*2.2.24*).

Comparison: *sucrose CRS*.

B. Thin-layer chromatography (*2.2.27*).

Test solution. Dissolve 10 mg of the substance to be examined in a mixture of 2 volumes of *water R* and 3 volumes of *methanol R* and dilute to 20 ml with the same mixture of solvents.

Reference solution (a). Dissolve 10 mg of *sucrose CRS* in a mixture of 2 volumes of *water R* and 3 volumes of *methanol R* and dilute to 20 ml with the same mixture of solvents.

Reference solution (b). Dissolve 10 mg each of *fructose CRS, glucose CRS, lactose CRS* and *sucrose CRS* in a mixture of 2 volumes of *water R* and 3 volumes of *methanol R* and dilute to 20 ml with the same mixture of solvents.

Plate: *TLC silica gel G plate R.*

Mobile phase: *cold saturated boric acid solution R*, 60 per cent *V/V* solution of *glacial acetic acid R*, *ethanol R*, *acetone R*, *ethyl acetate R* (10:15:20:60:60 *V/V/V/V/V*).

Application: 2 µl.

Development: in an unsaturated tank over a path of 15 cm.

Drying: in a current of warm air.

Detection: spray with a solution of 0.5 g of *thymol R* in a mixture of 5 ml of *sulphuric acid R* and 95 ml of *alcohol R*. Heat the plate at 130 °C for 10 min.

System suitability: the chromatogram obtained with reference solution (b) shows 4 clearly separated spots.

Results: the principal spot in the chromatogram obtained with the test solution is similar in position, colour and size to the principal spot in the chromatogram obtained with reference solution (a).

C. Dilute 1 ml of solution S (see Tests) to 100 ml with *water R*. To 5 ml of the solution add 0.15 ml of freshly prepared *copper sulphate solution R* and 2 ml of freshly prepared *dilute sodium hydroxide solution R*. The solution is blue and clear and remains so after boiling. To the hot solution add 4 ml of *dilute hydrochloric acid R* and boil for 1 min. Add 4 ml of *dilute sodium hydroxide solution R*. An orange precipitate is formed immediately.

TESTS

Solution S. Dissolve 50.0 g in *carbon dioxide-free water R* prepared from *distilled water R* and dilute to 100 ml with the same solvent.

Appearance of solution. Solution S is clear (*2.2.1*).

Conductivity (*2.2.38*): maximum 35 µS·cm^{-1}.

Dissolve 31.3 g in *carbon dioxide-free water R* prepared from *distilled water R* and dilute to 100 ml with the same solvent. Measure the conductivity of the solution (C_1), while gently stirring with a magnetic stirrer, and that of the water used for preparing the solution (C_2). The readings must be stable within 1 per cent over a period of 30 s. Calculate the conductivity of the solution of the substance to be examined from the following expression:

$$C_1 - 0.35\ C_2$$

Specific optical rotation (*2.2.7*): + 66.3 to + 67.0.

Dissolve 26.0 g in *water R* and dilute to 100.0 ml with the same solvent.

Colour value: maximum 45.

Dissolve 50.0 g in 50.0 ml of *water R*. Mix, filter (diameter of pores 0.45 µm) and degas. Measure the absorbance (*2.2.25*) at 420 nm, using a cell of at least 4 cm (a cell length of 10 cm or more is preferred).

Calculate the colour value using the following expression:

$$\frac{A \times 1000}{b \times c}$$

A = absorbance measured at 420 nm,

b = path length in centimetres,

c = concentration of the solution, in grams per millilitre, calculated from the refractive index (*2.2.6*) of the solution; use Table 0204.-1 and interpolate the values if necessary.

Table 0204.-1

n_D^{20}	c (g/ml)
1.4138	0.570
1.4159	0.585
1.4179	0.600
1.4200	0.615
1.4221	0.630
1.4243	0.645
1.4264	0.661

System suitability:

- *repeatability*: the absolute difference between 2 results is maximum 3.

Dextrins. If intended for use in the preparation of large-volume infusions, it complies with the test for dextrins. To 2 ml of solution S add 8 ml of *water R*, 0.05 ml of *dilute hydrochloric acid R* and 0.05 ml of *0.05 M iodine*. The solution remains yellow.

Reducing sugars. To 5 ml of solution S in a test-tube about 150 mm long and 16 mm in diameter add 5 ml of *water R*, 1.0 ml of *1 M sodium hydroxide* and 1.0 ml of a 1 g/l solution of *methylene blue R*. Mix and place in a water-bath. After exactly 2 min, take the tube out of the bath and examine the solution immediately. The blue colour does not disappear completely. Ignore any blue colour at the air/solution interface.

Sulphites: maximum 10 ppm, calculated as SO_2.

Determine the sulphites content by a suitable enzymatic method based on the following reactions. Sulphite is oxidised by sulphite oxidase to sulphate and hydrogen peroxide which in turn is reduced by nicotinamide-adenine dinucleotide-peroxidase in the presence of reduced nicotinamide-adenine dinucleotide (NADH). The amount of NADH oxidised is proportional to the amount of sulphite.

Test solution. Dissolve 4.0 g of the substance to be examined in freshly prepared *distilled water R* and dilute to 10.0 ml with the same solvent.

Reference solution. Dissolve 4.0 g of the substance to be examined in freshly prepared *distilled water R*, add 0.5 ml of *sulphite standard solution (80 ppm SO_2) R* and dilute to 10.0 ml with freshly prepared *distilled water R*.

Blank solution. Freshly prepared *distilled water R*.

Separately introduce 2.0 ml each of the test solution, the reference solution and the blank in 10 mm cuvettes and add the reagents as described in the instructions in the kit for sulphite determination. Measure the absorbance (*2.2.25*) at the absorption maximum at about 340 nm before and at the end of the reaction time and subtract the value obtained with the blank.

The absorbance difference of the test solution is not greater than half the absorbance difference of the reference solution.

Lead: maximum 0.5 ppm.

Atomic absorption spectrometry (*2.2.23, Method II*).

Test solution. Dissolve 1.5 g of the substance to be examined in 1.5 ml of *deionised distilled water R* in a digestion tube[(4)]. Add 0.75 ml of *lead-free nitric acid R1* and slowly warm to 90-95 °C, avoiding spattering. Heat for about 60 min, add again 0.75 ml of *lead-free nitric acid R1*. Heat until all brown vapours have dissipated and any reddish tint is gone (about 60 min). Cool. Add 0.5 ml of *strong hydrogen peroxide solution R* dropwise and heat at 90-95 °C for 15 min. Cool. Add again 0.5 ml of *strong hydrogen peroxide solution R* dropwise, heat at 90-95 °C for 60 min and cool. Repeat these operations until a clear, light yellow solution is obtained. Dilute to 10.0 ml with *deionised distilled water R*. Store in capped plastic vials.

Reference solutions. Prepare 3 reference solutions in the same manner as the test solution but adding 0.5 ml, 1.0 ml and 1.5 ml respectively of *lead standard solution (0.5 ppm Pb) R* in addition to the 1.5 g of the substance to be examined.

Blank solution. Prepare a blank in the same manner as for the test solution but without the substance to be examined.

Zero-setting solution. Deionised distilled water R.

Apparatus. Suitable graphite furnace atomic absorption spectrometer equipped with a background compensation system, an autosampler and pyrolytically-coated tubes or with pyrolytic graphite platforms.

Source: hollow-cathode lamp or electrodeless discharge lamp.

Gas:

- *argon R* as the purge gas,
- air as alternate gas during the charring step.

Flow rate: to be adapted according to the apparatus; usually between 200 ml/min and 300 ml/min.

Wavelength: 283.3 nm.

Method. Separately inject 20 µl each of the zero-setting solution, the blank solution, the test solution, the reference solutions, and add immediately 5 µl of *magnesium nitrate solution R1*, which is used as matrix modifier, to each of the solutions. Inject each solution in triplicate.

The ashing and atomisation temperatures and times vary according to the apparatus, the background compensation system, and the graphite tube etc. The following parameters are given for guidance and have to be adjusted.

Heat the furnace progressively to 200 °C and maintain the drying temperature at 200 °C for 30 s, the ashing temperature at 750 °C for 40 s after a 40 s temperature rise, and the atomisation temperature at 1800 °C for 10 s (0 s temperature rise). Clean out at 2600 °C for 7 s after a 1 s temperature rise. Use the zero-setting solution to set the instrument zero. Calculate the mean readings of the test solution and of the reference solutions subtracting the mean blank. If necessary, dilute with the zero-setting solution to obtain a reading within the linear range.

System suitability:

- the relative standard deviation of the 3 readings obtained for the triplicate injections of the test solution and the reference solutions to which the mean blank has been subtracted is not greater than 15 per cent.

Loss on drying (*2.2.32*): maximum 0.1 per cent, determined on 2.000 g by drying in an oven at 100-105 °C for 3 h.

(4) An acid-cleaned high density polyethylene tube, a polypropylene tube, a teflon tube or a quartz tube is suitable.

Monographs Q-S

Bacterial endotoxins (*2.6.14*): less than 0.25 IU/mg, if intended for use in the preparation of large-volume infusions.

LABELLING

The label states, where applicable, that the substance is suitable for use in the manufacture of large-volume parenteral dosage forms.

01/2005:1569

SUFENTANIL

Sufentanilum

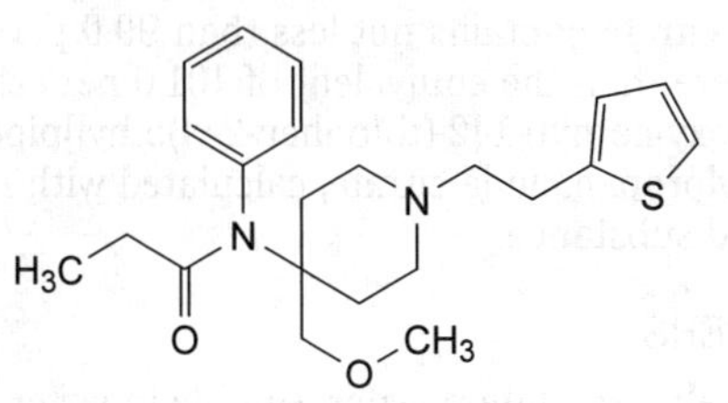

$C_{22}H_{30}N_2O_2S$ M_r 386.6

DEFINITION

Sufentanil contains not less than 99.0 per cent and not more than the equivalent of 101.0 per cent of *N*-[4-(methoxymethyl)-1-[2-(thiophen-2-yl)ethyl]piperidin-4-yl]-*N*-phenylpropanamide, calculated with reference to the dried substance.

CHARACTERS

A white or almost white powder, practically insoluble in water, freely soluble in alcohol and in methanol.

It melts at about 98 °C.

IDENTIFICATION

Examine by infrared absorption spectrophotometry (*2.2.24*),comparing with the *Ph. Eur. reference spectrum of sufentanil.*

TESTS

Appearance of solution. Dissolve 0.10 g in *methanol R* and dilute to 20 ml with the same solvent. The solution is clear (*2.2.1*) and colourless (*2.2.2, Method II*).

Related substances. Examine by liquid chromatography (*2.2.29*).

Test solution. Dissolve 0.100 g of the substance to be examined in *methanol R* and dilute to 10.0 ml with the same solvent.

Reference solution (a). In order to prepare *in situ* the degradation compound (sufentanil impurity E), dissolve 10 mg of the substance to be examined in 10.0 ml of *dilute hydrochloric acid R.* Heat on a water-bath under a reflux condenser for 4 h. Add 10.0 ml of *dilute sodium hydroxide solution R.* Evaporate to dryness on a water-bath. Cool and take up the residue in 10 ml of *methanol R.* Filter.

Reference solution (b). Dilute 1.0 ml of the test solution to 100.0 ml with *methanol R.* Dilute 5.0 ml of this solution to 20.0 ml with *methanol R.*

The chromatographic procedure may be carried out using:

- a stainless steel column 0.1 m long and 4.6 mm in internal diameter packed with *octadecylsilyl silica gel for chromatography R* (3 µm),
- as mobile phase at a flow rate of 1.5 ml/min:

  Mobile phase A. A 5 g/l solution of *ammonium carbonate R* in a mixture of 10 volumes of *tetrahydrofuran R* and 90 volumes of *water R,*

  Mobile phase B. Acetonitrile R,

Time (min)	Mobile phase A (per cent *V/V*)	Mobile phase B (per cent *V/V*)	Comment
0 - 15	90 → 40	10 → 60	linear gradient
15 - 20	40	60	isocratic
20 - 21	40 → 90	60 → 10	switch to initial eluent composition
21 - 25	90	10	re-equilibration

- as detector a spectrophotometer set at 220 nm.

Equilibrate the column for at least 30 min with *acetonitrile R* and then equilibrate with the initial eluent composition for at least 5 min.

Adjust the sensitivity of the system so that the height of the principal peak in the chromatogram obtained with 10 µl of reference solution (b) is at least 50 per cent of the full scale of the recorder.

Inject 10 µl of reference solution (a). When the chromatogram is recorded in the prescribed conditions, the retention times are: impurity E about 12 min and sufentanil about 13 min. The test is not valid unless the resolution between the peaks corresponding to sufentanil and impurity E is at least 4.0. If necessary, adjust the concentration of acetonitrile in the mobile phase or adjust the time programme for the linear gradient elution.

Inject 10 µl of *methanol R* as a blank, 10 µl of the test solution and 10 µl of reference solution (b). In the chromatogram obtained with the test solution: the area of any peak, apart from the principal peak, is not greater than the area of the principal peak in the chromatogram obtained with reference solution (b) (0.25 per cent); the sum of the areas of all the peaks, apart from the principal peak, is not greater than twice the area of the principal peak in the chromatogram obtained with reference solution (b) (0.5 per cent). Disregard any peak due to the blank and any peak with an area less than 0.2 times the area of the principal peak in the chromatogram obtained with reference solution (b) (0.05 per cent).

Loss on drying (*2.2.32*). Not more than 0.5 per cent, determined on 1.000 g by drying *in vacuo* at 60 °C for 2 h.

ASSAY

Dissolve 0.300 g in 50 ml of a mixture of 1 volume of *anhydrous acetic acid R* and 7 volumes of *methyl ethyl ketone R* and titrate with *0.1 M perchloric acid,* using 0.2 ml of *naphtholbenzein solution R* as indicator.

1 ml of *0.1 M perchloric acid* is equivalent to 38.66 mg of $C_{22}H_{30}N_2O_2S$.

STORAGE

Store protected from light.

IMPURITIES

Specified impurities: D, F, H.

Other detectable impurities: A, B, C, E, G, I.

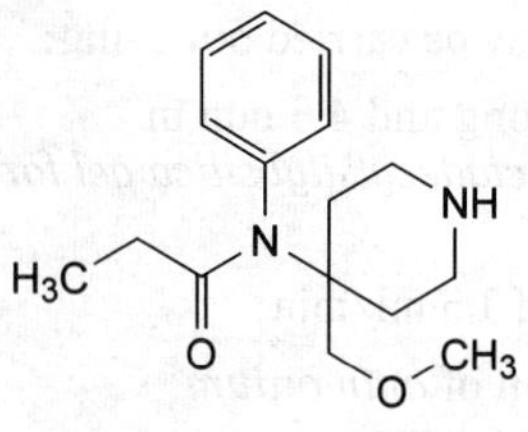

A. *N*-[4-(methoxymethyl)piperidin-4-yl]-*N*-phenylpropanamide,

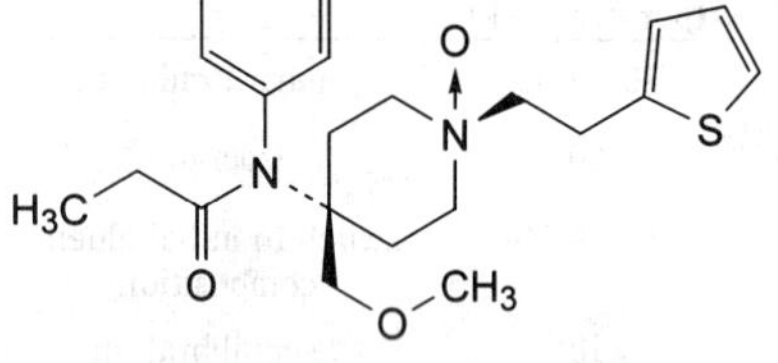

B. *cis*-4-(methoxymethyl)-4-(phenylpropanoylamino)-1-[2-(thiophen-2-yl)ethyl]piperidine 1-oxide,

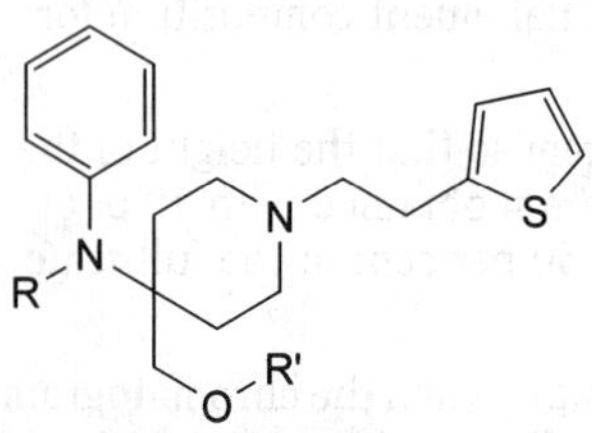

C. R = R′ = H: [4-(phenylamino)-1-[2-(thiophen-2-yl)ethyl]piperidin-4-yl]methanol,

D. R = CO-CH_3, R′ = CH_3: *N*-[4-(methoxymethyl)-1-[2-(thiophen-2-yl)ethyl]piperidin-4-yl]-*N*-phenylacetamide,

E. R = H, R′ = CH_3: 4-(methoxymethyl)-*N*-phenyl-1-[2-(thiophen-2-yl)ethyl]piperidin-4-amine,

G. R = R′ = CO-CH_2-CH_3: [4-(phenylpropanoylamino)-1-[2-(thiophen-2-yl)ethyl]piperidin-4-yl]methyl propanoate,

H. R = CO-CH_2-CH_2-CH_3, R′ = CH_3: *N*-[4-(methoxymethyl)-1-[2-(thiophen-2-yl)ethyl]piperidin-4-yl]-*N*-phenylbutanamide,

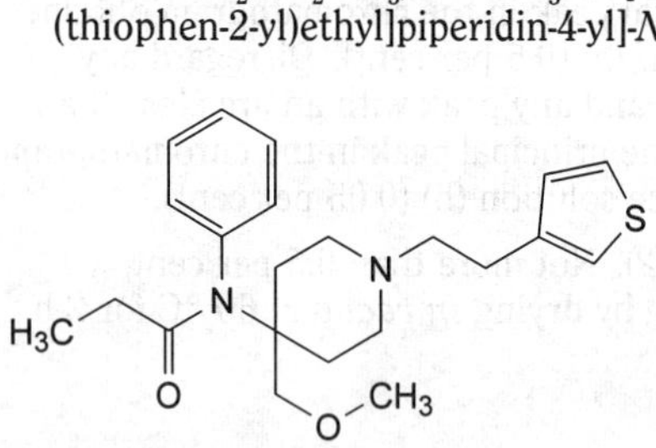

F. *N*-[4-(methoxymethyl)-1-[2-(thiophen-3-yl)ethyl]piperidin-4-yl]-*N*-phenylpropanamide,

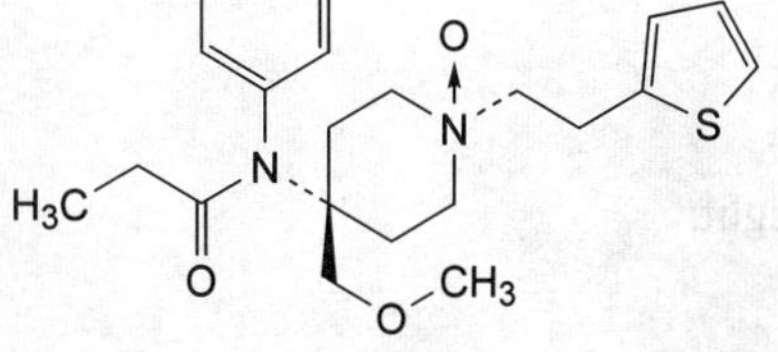

I. *trans*-4-(methoxymethyl)-4-(phenylpropanoylamino)-1-[2-(thiophen-2-yl)ethyl]piperidine 1-oxide.

01/2005:1269

SUFENTANIL CITRATE

Sufentanili citras

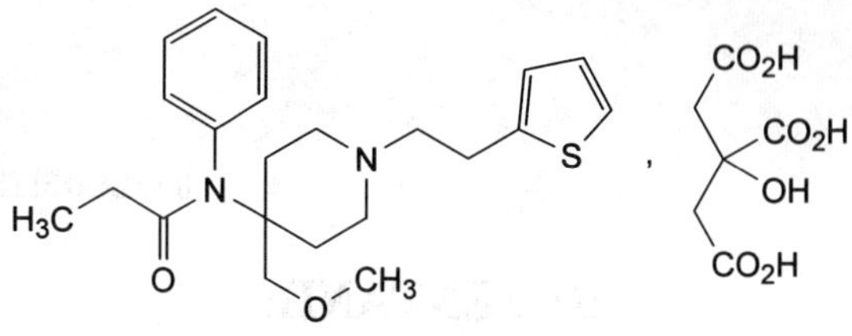

$C_{28}H_{38}N_2O_9S$ M_r 578.7

DEFINITION

Sufentanil citrate contains not less than 99.0 per cent and not more than the equivalent of 101.0 per cent of *N*-[4-(methoxymethyl)-1-[2-(thiophen-2-yl)ethyl]piperidin-4-yl]-*N*-phenylpropanamide citrate, calculated with reference to the dried substance.

CHARACTERS

A white or almost white powder, soluble in water and in alcohol, freely soluble in methanol.

It melts at about 140 °C, with decomposition.

IDENTIFICATION

Examine by infrared absorption spectrophotometry (*2.2.24*), comparing with the *Ph. Eur. reference spectrum of sufentanil citrate.*

TESTS

Appearance of solution. Dissolve 0.2 g of the substance to be examined in *water R* and dilute to 20 ml with the same solvent. The solution is clear (*2.2.1*) and colourless (*2.2.2, Method II*).

Related substances. Examine by liquid chromatography (*2.2.29*).

Test solution. Dissolve 0.100 g of the substance to be examined in *methanol R* and dilute to 10.0 ml with the same solvent.

Reference solution (a). In order to prepare *in situ* the degradation compound (sufentanil impurity E), dissolve 10 mg of the substance to be examined in 10.0 ml of *dilute hydrochloric acid R.* Heat on a water-bath under a reflux condenser for 4 h. Add 10.0 ml of *dilute sodium hydroxide solution R.* Evaporate to dryness on a water-bath. Cool and take up the residue in 10 ml of *methanol R.* Filter.

Reference solution (b). Dilute 5.0 ml of the test solution to 100.0 ml with *methanol R.* Dilute 1.0 ml of this solution to 10.0 ml with *methanol R.*

The chromatographic procedure may be carried out using:

– a stainless steel column 0.1 m long and 4.6 mm in internal diameter packed with *octadecylsilyl silica gel for chromatography R* (3 µm),

– as mobile phase at a flow rate of 1.5 ml/min the following mixtures:

Mobile phase A. A 5 g/l solution of *ammonium carbonate R* in a mixture of 10 volumes of *tetrahydrofuran R* and 90 volumes of *water R,*

Mobile phase B. Acetonitrile R,

Time (min)	Mobile phase A (per cent *V/V*)	Mobile phase B (per cent *V/V*)	Comment
0 - 15	90 → 40	10 → 60	linear gradient
15 - 20	40	60	isocratic elution
20 - 25	90	10	switch to initial eluent composition
25 = 0	90	10	restart gradient

– as detector a spectrophotometer set at 220 nm.

Equilibrate the column for at least 30 min with *acetonitrile R* and then equilibrate at the initial eluent composition for at least 5 min.

Adjust the sensitivity of the system so that the height of the principal peak in the chromatogram obtained with 10 μl of reference solution (b) is at least 50 per cent of the full scale of the recorder.

Inject 10 μl of reference solution (a). When the chromatograms are recorded in the prescribed conditions, the retention times are: sufentanil impurity E about 12 min and sufentanil about 13 min. The test is not valid unless the resolution between the peaks corresponding to sufentanil and sufentanil impurity E is at least 4.0. If necessary, adjust the concentration of acetonitrile in the mobile phase or adjust the time programme for the linear gradient elution.

Inject separately 10 μl of *methanol R* as a blank, 10 μl of the test solution and 10 μl of reference solution (b). In the chromatogram obtained with the test solution: the area of any peak, apart from the principal peak, is not greater than the area of the principal peak in the chromatogram obtained with reference solution (b) (0.5 per cent); the sum of the areas of all of the peaks, apart from the principal peak, is not greater than twice the area of the principal peak in the chromatogram obtained with reference solution (b) (1 per cent). Disregard any peak obtained with the blank run, any peak with a retention time relative to the main compound of 0.05 or less, and any peak with an area less than 0.1 times the area of the principal peak in the chromatogram obtained with reference solution (b).

Loss on drying (*2.2.32*). Not more than 0.5 per cent, determined on 1.000 g by drying *in vacuo* at 60 °C.

ASSAY

Dissolve 0.400 g in 50 ml of a mixture of 1 volume of *anhydrous acetic acid R* and 7 volumes of *methyl ethyl ketone R* and titrate with *0.1 M perchloric acid*, using 0.2 ml of *naphtholbenzein solution R* as indicator.

1 ml of *0.1 M perchloric acid* is equivalent to 57.87 mg of $C_{28}H_{38}N_2O_9S$.

STORAGE

Store protected from light.

IMPURITIES

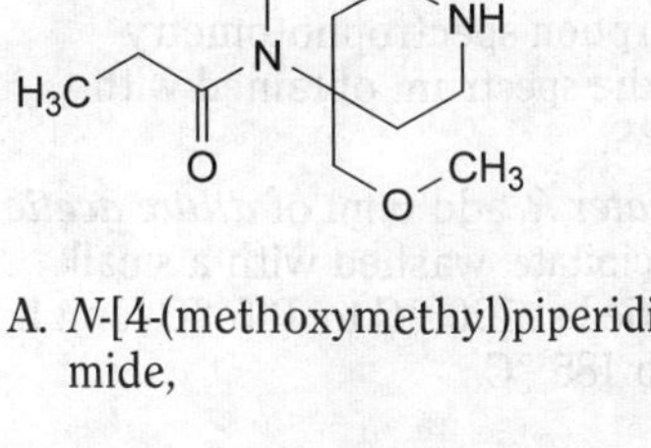

A. *N*-[4-(methoxymethyl)piperidin-4-yl]-*N*-phenylpropanamide,

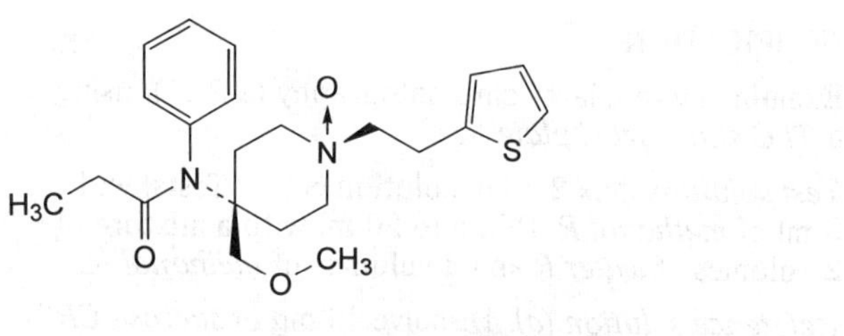

B. *cis*-4-(methoxymethyl)-4-(phenylpropanoylamino)-1-[2-(thiophen-2-yl)ethyl]piperidine 1-oxide,

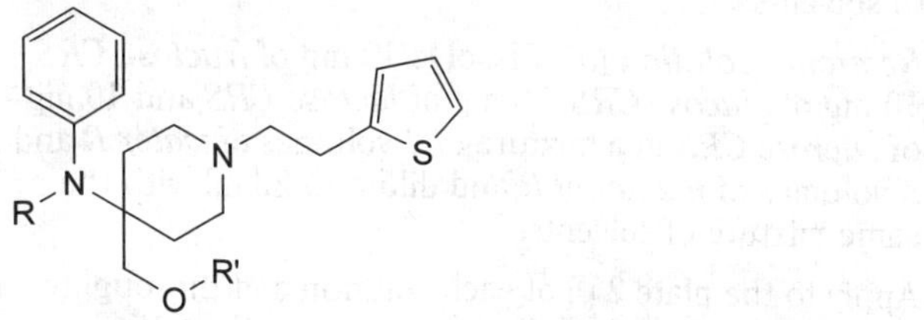

C. R = R′ = H: [4-(phenylamino)-1-[2-(thiophen-2-yl)ethyl]piperidin-4-yl]methanol,

D. R = CO-CH_3, R′ = CH_3: *N*-[4-(methoxymethyl)-1-[2-(thiophen-2-yl)ethyl]piperidin-4-yl]-*N*-phenylacetamide,

E. R = H, R′ = CH_3: 4-(methoxymethyl)-*N*-phenyl-1-[2-(thiophen-2-yl)ethyl] piperidin-4-amine,

G. R = R′ = CO-CH_2-CH_3: [4-(phenylpropanoylamino)-1-[2-(thiophen-2-yl)ethyl] piperidin-4-yl]methyl propanoate,

H. R = CO-CH_2-CH_2-CH_3, R′ = CH_3: *N*-[4-(methoxymethyl)-1-[2-(thiophen-2-yl)ethyl]piperidin-4-yl]-*N*-phenylbutanamide,

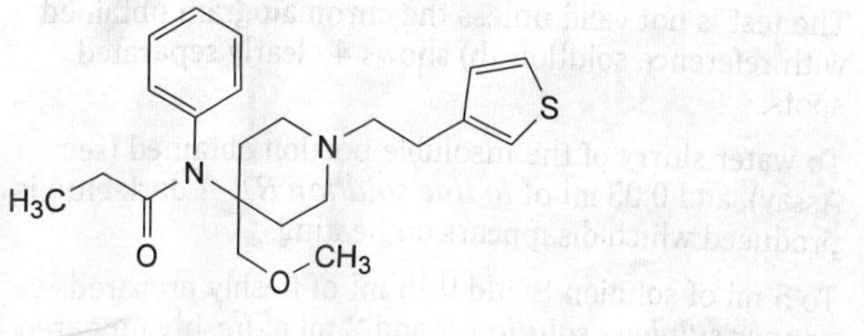

F. *N*-[4-(methoxymethyl)-1-[2-(thiophen-3-yl)ethyl]piperidin-4-yl]-*N*-phenylpropanamide,

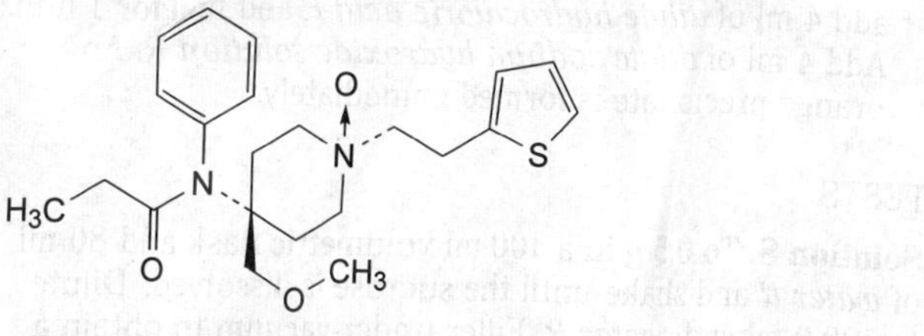

I. *trans*-4-(methoxymethyl)-4-(phenylpropanoylamino)-1-[2-(thiophen-2-yl)ethyl]piperidine 1-oxide.

01/2005:1570

SUGAR SPHERES

Sacchari spheri

DEFINITION

Sugar spheres contain not more than 92 per cent of sucrose, calculated on the dried basis. The remainder consists of maize starch and may also contain starch hydrolysates and colour additives. The diameter of sugar spheres varies usually from 200 μm to 2000 μm and the upper and lower limits of the size of the sugar spheres are stated on the label.

IDENTIFICATION

A. Examine by thin-layer chromatography (*2.2.27*), using a *TLC silica gel G plate R*.

Test solution. Mix 2 ml of solution S (see Tests) with 3 ml of *methanol R*. Dilute to 20 ml with a mixture of 2 volumes of *water R* and 3 volumes of *methanol R*.

Reference solution (a). Dissolve 10 mg of *sucrose CRS* in a mixture of 2 volumes of *water R* and 3 volumes of *methanol R* and dilute to 20 ml with the same mixture of solvents.

Reference solution (b). Dissolve 10 mg of *fructose CRS*, 10 mg of *glucose CRS*, 10 mg of *lactose CRS* and 10 mg of *sucrose CRS* in a mixture of 2 volumes of *water R* and 3 volumes of *methanol R* and dilute to 20 ml with the same mixture of solvents.

Apply to the plate 2 µl of each solution and thoroughly dry the starting points. Develop over a path of 15 cm using a mixture of 10 volumes of *water R*, 15 volumes of *methanol R*, 25 volumes of *anhydrous acetic acid R* and 50 volumes of *ethylene chloride R*, measured accurately as a slight excess of water causes cloudiness of the solution. Dry the plate in a current of warm air. Repeat the development immediately after renewing the mobile phase. Dry the plate in a current of warm air and spray evenly with a 5 g/l solution of *thymol R* in a mixture of 5 volumes of *sulphuric acid R* and 95 volumes of *alcohol R*. Heat at 130 °C for 10 min. The principal spot in the chromatogram obtained with the test solution is similar in position, colour and size to the principal spot in the chromatogram obtained with reference solution (a). The test is not valid unless the chromatogram obtained with reference solution (b) shows 4 clearly separated spots.

B. To water slurry of the insoluble portion obtained (see Assay), add 0.05 ml of *iodine solution R1*. A dark-blue is produced which disappears on heating.

C. To 5 ml of solution S add 0.15 ml of freshly prepared *copper sulphate solution R* and 2 ml of freshly prepared *dilute sodium hydroxide solution R*. The solution is blue and clear and remains so after boiling. To the hot solution add 4 ml of *dilute hydrochloric acid R* and boil for 1 min. Add 4 ml of *dilute sodium hydroxide solution R*. An orange precipitate is formed immediately.

TESTS

Solution S. To 0.5 g in a 100 ml volumetric flask add 80 ml of *water R* and shake until the sucrose is dissolved. Dilute to 100.0 ml with *water R*. Filter under vacuum to obtain a clear solution.

Fineness (*2.9.12*). Minimum of 90 per cent (*m/m*) of the sugar spheres are between the lower and the upper limits of the size of the sugar spheres stated on the label.

Heavy metals (*2.4.8*). 2.0 g complies with limit test C for heavy metals (5 ppm). Prepare the standard using 1.0 ml of *lead standard solution (10 ppm Pb) R*.

Loss on drying (*2.2.32*). Not more than 5.0 per cent, determined on 1.000 g by drying in an oven at 100 °C to 105 °C for 4 h.

Sulphated ash (*2.4.14*). Not more than 0.2 per cent, determined on 2 g.

Microbial contamination. Total viable aerobic count (*2.6.12*) not more than 10^3 bacteria and 10^2 fungi per gram, determined by plate count. It complies with the tests for *Escherichia coli* and *Salmonella* (*2.6.13*).

ASSAY

Sucrose content

Weigh 10.000 g of ground sugar spheres in a 100 ml graduated flask and complete to 100.0 ml with *water R*. Stir and decant. Filter under vacuum to obtain a clear solution (the insoluble portion is used for the identification test B). Measure the angle of optical rotation (*2.2.7*) and calculate the sucrose percentage content as follows:

$$\frac{10^6 \times \alpha}{66.5 \times l \times m \times (100 - H)}$$

α = angle of rotation,

l = length of the polarimeter tube, in decimetres,

m = exact weight of the granules sample, in grams,

H = loss on drying.

LABELLING

The label states:

– the upper and the lower limits of the size of the sugar spheres,
– any added colour additives,
– any added starch hydrolysates.

01/2005:0107

SULFACETAMIDE SODIUM

Sulfacetamidum natricum

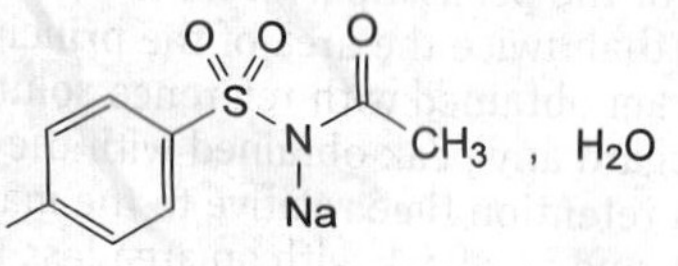

$C_8H_9N_2NaO_3S,H_2O$ M_r 254.2

DEFINITION

Sulfacetamide sodium contains not less than 99.0 per cent and not more than the equivalent of 101.0 per cent of the sodium derivative of *N*-[(4-aminophenyl)sulphonyl]acetamide, calculated with reference to the anhydrous substance.

CHARACTERS

A white or yellowish-white, crystalline powder, freely soluble in water, slightly soluble in ethanol.

IDENTIFICATION

First identification: B, F.

Second identification: A, C, D, E, F.

A. Dissolve 0.1 g in *phosphate buffer solution pH 7.0 R* and dilute to 100.0 ml with the same buffer solution. Dilute 1.0 ml of the solution to 100.0 ml with *phosphate buffer solution pH 7.0 R*. Examined between 230 nm and 350 nm (*2.2.25*), the solution shows an absorption maximum at 255 nm. The specific absorbance at the maximum is 660 to 720, calculated with reference to the anhydrous substance.

B. Examine by infrared absorption spectrophotometry (*2.2.24*), comparing with the spectrum obtained with *sulfacetamide sodium CRS*.

C. Dissolve 1 g in 10 ml of *water R*, add 6 ml of *dilute acetic acid R* and filter. The precipitate, washed with a small quantity of *water R* and dried at 100 °C to 105 °C for 4 h, melts (*2.2.14*) at 181 °C to 185 °C.

D. Dissolve 0.1 g of the precipitate obtained in identification test C in 5 ml of *alcohol R*. Add 0.2 ml of *sulphuric acid R* and heat. The odour of ethyl acetate is perceptible.

E. Dissolve about 1 mg of the precipitate obtained in identification test C, with heating, in 1 ml of *water R*. The solution gives the reaction of primary aromatic amines (*2.3.1*) with formation of an orange-red precipitate.

F. Solution S (see Tests) gives the reactions of sodium (*2.3.1*).

TESTS

Solution S. Dissolve 1.25 g in *carbon dioxide-free water R* and dilute to 25 ml with the same solvent.

Appearance of solution. Solution S is clear (*2.2.1*) and not more intensely coloured than reference solution GY_4 (*2.2.2, Method II*).

pH (*2.2.3*). The pH of solution S is 8.0 to 9.5.

Related substances. Examine by thin-layer chromatography (*2.2.27*), using *silica gel HF_{254} R* as the coating substance.

Test solution. Dissolve 1.5 g of the substance to be examined in *water R* and dilute to 15 ml with the same solvent.

Reference solution (a). Dissolve 5 mg of *sulfanilamide R* in *water R* and dilute to 10 ml with the same solvent.

Reference solution (b). Dilute 5 ml of reference solution (a) to 10 ml with *water R*.

Reference solution (c). Dissolve 5 mg of *sulfanilamide R* in 10 ml of the test solution.

Apply to the plate 5 µl of each solution. Develop over a path of 15 cm using a mixture of 10 volumes of *concentrated ammonia R*, 25 volumes of *ethanol R*, 25 volumes of *water R* and 50 volumes of *butanol R*. Allow the plate to dry in air and spray with *dimethylaminobenzaldehyde solution R2*. Any spot in the chromatogram obtained with the test solution, apart from the principal spot, is not more intense than the spot in the chromatogram obtained with reference solution (a) (0.5 per cent), and not more than one such spot is more intense than the spot in the chromatogram obtained with reference solution (b) (0.25 per cent). The test is not valid unless the chromatogram obtained with reference solution (c) shows two clearly separated spots.

Sulphates (*2.4.13*). Dissolve 2.5 g in *distilled water R* and dilute to 25 ml with the same solvent. Add 25 ml of *dilute acetic acid R*, shake for 30 min and filter. 15 ml of the filtrate complies with the limit test for sulphates (200 ppm).

Heavy metals (*2.4.8*). 12 ml of the filtrate obtained in the test for sulphates complies with limit test A for heavy metals (20 ppm). Prepare the standard using *lead standard solution (1 ppm Pb) R*.

Water (*2.5.12*). 6.0 per cent to 8.0 per cent, determined on 0.200 g by the semi-micro determination of water.

ASSAY

Dissolve 0.500 g in a mixture of 50 ml of *water R* and 20 ml of *dilute hydrochloric acid R*. Cool the solution in iced water and carry out the determination of primary aromatic amino-nitrogen (*2.5.8*), determining the end-point electrometrically.

1 ml of *0.1 M sodium nitrite* is equivalent to 23.62 mg of $C_8H_9N_2NaO_3S$.

STORAGE

Store protected from light.

01/2005:0294

SULFADIAZINE

Sulfadiazinum

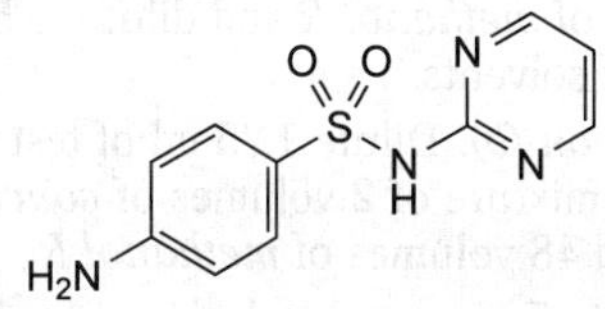

$C_{10}H_{10}N_4O_2S$ M_r 250.3

DEFINITION

Sulfadiazine contains not less than 99.0 per cent and not more than the equivalent of 101.0 per cent of 4-amino-*N*-pyrimidin-2-ylbenzenesulphonamide, calculated with reference to the dried substance.

CHARACTERS

White, yellowish-white or pinkish-white, crystalline powder or crystals, practically insoluble in water, slightly soluble in acetone, very slightly soluble in alcohol. It dissolves in solutions of alkali hydroxides and in dilute mineral acids.

It melts at about 255 °C, with decomposition.

IDENTIFICATION

First identification: A, B.

Second identification: B, C, D.

A. Examine by infrared absorption spectrophotometry (*2.2.24*), comparing with the spectrum obtained with *sulfadiazine CRS*. Examine the substances prepared as discs.

B. Examine the chromatograms obtained in the test for related substances. The principal spot in the chromatogram obtained with test solution (a) corresponds in position and size to the principal spot in the chromatogram obtained with reference solution (a).

C. Place 3 g in a dry tube. Immerse the lower part of the tube, inclined at 45°, in a silicone oil bath and heat to about 270 °C. The substance to be examined decomposes and a white or yellowish-white sublimate is formed which, after recrystallisation from *toluene R* and drying at 100 °C, melts (*2.2.14*) at 123 °C to 127 °C.

D. Dissolve about 5 mg in 10 ml of *1 M hydrochloric acid*. Dilute 1 ml of the solution to 10 ml with *water R*. The solution, without further acidification, gives the reaction of primary aromatic amines (*2.3.1*).

TESTS

Appearance of solution. Dissolve 0.8 g in a mixture of 5 ml of *dilute sodium hydroxide solution R* and 5 ml of *water R*. The solution is not more intensely coloured than reference solution Y_5, BY_5 or GY_5 (*2.2.2, Method II*).

Acidity. To 1.25 g, finely powdered, add 25 ml of *carbon dioxide-free water R*. Heat at about 70 °C for 5 min. Cool in iced water for about 15 min and filter. To 20 ml of the filtrate add 0.1 ml of *bromothymol blue solution R1*. Not more than 0.2 ml of *0.1 M sodium hydroxide* is required to change the colour of the indicator.

Related substances. Examine by thin-layer chromatography (*2.2.27*), using *silica gel GF_{254} R* as the coating substance.

Test solution (a). Dissolve 20 mg of the substance to be examined in 3 ml of a mixture of 2 volumes of *concentrated ammonia R* and 48 volumes of *methanol R* and dilute to 5.0 ml with the same mixture of solvents.

Test solution (b). Dissolve 0.10 g of the substance to be examined in 0.5 ml of *concentrated ammonia R* and dilute to 5.0 ml with *methanol R*. If the solution is not clear, heat gently until dissolution is complete.

Reference solution (a). Dissolve 20 mg of *sulfadiazine CRS* in 3 ml of a mixture of 2 volumes of *concentrated ammonia R* and 48 volumes of *methanol R* and dilute to 5.0 ml with the same mixture of solvents.

Reference solution (b). Dilute 1.25 ml of test solution (a) to 50 ml with a mixture of 2 volumes of *concentrated ammonia R* and 48 volumes of *methanol R*.

Apply to the plate 5 µl of each solution. Develop over a path of 15 cm using a mixture of 3 volumes of *dilute ammonia R1*, 5 volumes of *water R*, 40 volumes of *nitromethane R* and 50 volumes of *dioxan R*. Dry the plate at 100 °C to 105 °C and examine in ultraviolet light at 254 nm. Any spot in the chromatogram obtained with test solution (b), apart from the principal spot, is not more intense than the spot in the chromatogram obtained with reference solution (b) (0.5 per cent).

Heavy metals (*2.4.8*). 1.0 g complies with limit test D for heavy metals (20 ppm). Prepare the standard using 2 ml of *lead standard solution (10 ppm Pb) R*.

Loss on drying (*2.2.32*). Not more than 0.5 per cent, determined on 1.00 g by drying in an oven at 100 °C to 105 °C.

Sulphated ash (*2.4.14*). Not more than 0.1 per cent, determined on 1.0 g.

ASSAY

Dissolve 0.200 g in a mixture of 20 ml of *dilute hydrochloric acid R* and 50 ml of *water R*. Cool the solution in iced water. Carry out the determination of primary aromatic amino-nitrogen (*2.5.8*), determining the end-point electrometrically.

1 ml of *0.1 M sodium nitrite* is equivalent to 25.03 mg of $C_{10}H_{10}N_4O_2S$.

STORAGE

Store protected from light.

01/2005:0295

SULFADIMIDINE

Sulfadimidinum

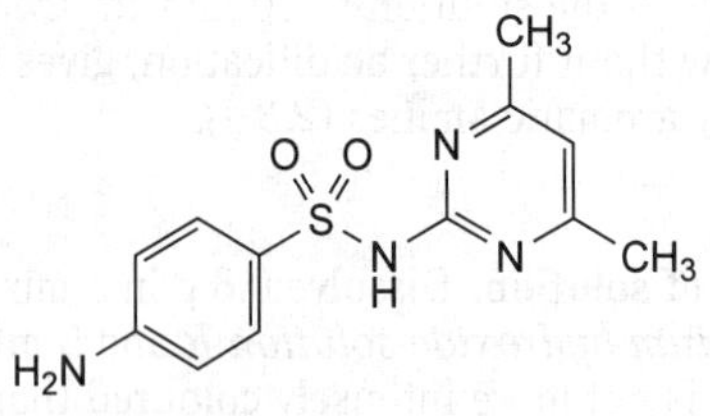

$C_{12}H_{14}N_4O_2S$ M_r 278.3

DEFINITION

Sulfadimidine contains not less than 99.0 per cent and not more than the equivalent of 101.0 per cent of 4-amino-*N*-(4,6-dimethylpyrimidin-2-yl)benzenesulphonamide, calculated with reference to the dried substance.

CHARACTERS

White or almost white powder or crystals, very slightly soluble in water, soluble in acetone, slightly soluble in alcohol. It dissolves in solutions of alkali hydroxides and in dilute mineral acids.

It melts at about 197 °C, with decomposition.

IDENTIFICATION

First identification: A, B.

Second identification: B, C, D.

A. Examine by infrared absorption spectrophotometry (*2.2.24*), comparing with the spectrum obtained with *sulfadimidine CRS*. Examine the substances prepared as discs.

B. Examine the chromatograms obtained in the test for related substances. The principal spot in the chromatogram obtained with test solution (a) corresponds in position and size to the principal spot in the chromatogram obtained with reference solution (a).

C. Place 3 g in a dry tube. Immerse the lower part of the tube, inclined at 45°, in a silicone oil bath and heat to about 270 °C. The substance to be examined decomposes and a white or yellowish-white sublimate is formed which, after recrystallisation from *toluene R* and drying at 100 °C, melts (*2.2.14*) at 150 °C to 154 °C.

D. Dissolve about 5 mg in 10 ml of *1 M hydrochloric acid*. Dilute 1 ml of the solution to 10 ml with *water R*. The solution, without further acidification, gives the reaction of primary aromatic amines (*2.3.1*).

TESTS

Appearance of solution. Dissolve 0.5 g in a mixture of 5 ml of *dilute sodium hydroxide solution R* and 5 ml of *water R*. The solution is not more intensely coloured than reference solution Y_5, BY_5 or GY_5 (*2.2.2, Method II*).

Acidity. To 1.25 g, finely powdered, add 25 ml of *carbon dioxide-free water R*. Heat at about 70 °C for 5 min. Cool in iced water for about 15 min and filter. To 20 ml of the filtrate add 0.1 ml of *bromothymol blue solution R1*. Not more than 0.2 ml of *0.1 M sodium hydroxide* is required to change the colour of the indicator.

Related substances. Examine by thin-layer chromatography (*2.2.27*), using *silica gel GF_{254} R* as the coating substance.

Test solution (a). Dissolve 20 mg of the substance to be examined in 3 ml of a mixture of 2 volumes of *concentrated ammonia R* and 48 volumes of *methanol R* and dilute to 5.0 ml with the same mixture of solvents.

Test solution (b). Dissolve 0.10 g of the substance to be examined in 0.5 ml of *concentrated ammonia R* and dilute to 5.0 ml with *methanol R*. If the solution is not clear, heat gently until dissolution is complete.

Reference solution (a). Dissolve 20 mg of *sulfadimidine CRS* in 3 ml of a mixture of 2 volumes of *concentrated ammonia R* and 48 volumes of *methanol R* and dilute to 5.0 ml with the same mixture of solvents.

Reference solution (b). Dilute 1.25 ml of test solution (a) to 50 ml with a mixture of 2 volumes of *concentrated ammonia R* and 48 volumes of *methanol R*.

Apply to the plate 5 µl of each solution. Develop over a path of 15 cm using a mixture of 3 volumes of *dilute ammonia R1*, 5 volumes of *water R*, 40 volumes of *nitromethane R* and 50 volumes of *dioxan R*. Dry the plate at 100 °C to 105 °C and examine in ultraviolet light at 254 nm. Any spot in the chromatogram obtained with test solution (b), apart from the principal spot, is not more intense than the spot in the chromatogram obtained with reference solution (b) (0.5 per cent).

Heavy metals (*2.4.8*). 1.0 g complies with limit test D for heavy metals (20 ppm). Prepare the standard using 2 ml of *lead standard solution (10 ppm Pb) R*.

Loss on drying (*2.2.32*). Not more than 0.5 per cent, determined on 1.00 g by drying in an oven at 100 °C to 105 °C.

Sulphated ash (*2.4.14*). Not more than 0.1 per cent, determined on 1.0 g.

ASSAY

Dissolve 0.250 g in a mixture of 20 ml of *dilute hydrochloric acid R* and 50 ml of *water R*. Cool the solution in iced water. Carry out the determination of primary aromatic amino-nitrogen (*2.5.8*), determining the end-point electrometrically.

1 ml of *0.1 M sodium nitrite* is equivalent to 27.83 mg of $C_{12}H_{14}N_4O_2S$.

STORAGE

Store protected from light.

01/2005:0740

SULFADOXINE

Sulfadoxinum

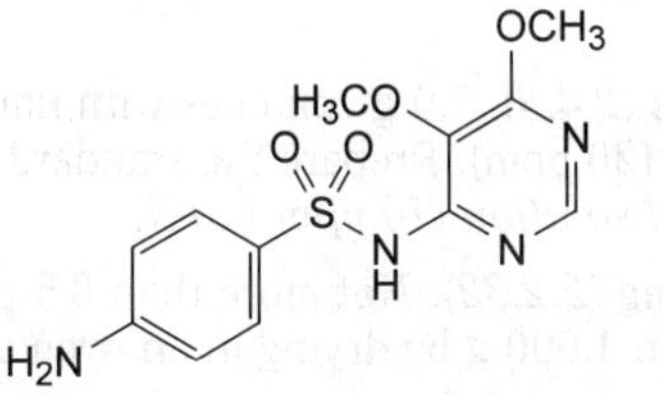

$C_{12}H_{14}N_4O_4S$ — M_r 310.3

DEFINITION

Sulfadoxine contains not less than 99.0 per cent and not more than the equivalent of 101.0 per cent of 4-amino-*N*-(5,6-dimethoxypyrimidin-4-yl)benzenesulphonamide, calculated with reference to the dried substance.

CHARACTERS

White or yellowish-white crystalline powder or crystals, very slightly soluble in water, slightly soluble in alcohol and in methanol. It dissolves in solutions of alkali hydroxides and in dilute mineral acids.

It melts at about 198 °C, with decomposition.

IDENTIFICATION

First identification: A, C.

Second identification: B, C, D.

A. Examine by infrared absorption spectrophotometry (*2.2.24*), comparing with the spectrum obtained with *sulfadoxine CRS*. Examine the substances prepared as discs.

B. Examine the chromatograms obtained in the test for related substances. The principal spot in the chromatogram obtained with test solution (b) is similar in position and size to the principal spot in the chromatogram obtained with reference solution (a).

C. Dissolve 0.5 g in 1 ml of a 40 per cent *V/V* solution of *sulphuric acid R*, heating gently. Continue heating until a crystalline precipitate appears (about 2 min). Allow to cool and add 10 ml of *dilute sodium hydroxide solution R*. Cool again. Add 25 ml of *ether R* and shake for 5 min. Separate the ether layer, dry over *anhydrous sodium sulphate R* and filter. Evaporate the solvent by heating in a water-bath. The residue melts (*2.2.14*) at 80 °C to 82 °C or at 90 °C to 92 °C.

D. Dissolve about 5 mg in 10 ml of *1 M hydrochloric acid*. Dilute 1 ml of the solution to 10 ml with *water R*. The solution, without further acidification, gives the reaction of primary aromatic amines (*2.3.1*).

TESTS

Appearance of solution. Dissolve 1.0 g in a mixture of 5 ml of *dilute sodium hydroxide solution R* and 5 ml of *water R*. The solution is not more intensely coloured than reference solution Y_5, BY_5 or GY_5 (*2.2.2, Method II*).

Acidity. To 1.25 g, finely powdered, add 25 ml of *carbon dioxide-free water R*. Heat at 70 °C for 5 min. Cool in a bath of iced water for about 15 min and filter. To 20 ml of the filtrate add 0.1 ml of *bromothymol blue solution R1*. Not more than 0.2 ml of *0.1 M sodium hydroxide* is required to change the colour of the indicator.

Related substances. Examine by thin-layer chromatography (*2.2.27*), using *silica gel GF_{254} R* as the coating substance.

Test solution (a). Dissolve 0.10 g of the substance to be examined in 3 ml of a mixture of 2 volumes of *concentrated ammonia R* and 48 volumes of *methanol R* and dilute to 5 ml with the same mixture of solvents.

Test solution (b). Dilute 1 ml of test solution (a) to 5 ml with a mixture of 2 volumes of *concentrated ammonia R* and 48 volumes of *methanol R*.

Reference solution (a). Dissolve 20 mg of *sulfadoxine CRS* in 3 ml of a mixture of 2 volumes of *concentrated ammonia R* and 48 volumes of *methanol R* and dilute to 5 ml with the same mixture of solvents.

Reference solution (b). Dilute 2.5 ml of test solution (b) to 100 ml with a mixture of 2 volumes of *concentrated ammonia R* and 48 volumes of *methanol R*.

Apply to the plate 5 µl of each solution. Develop over a path of 15 cm using a mixture of 3 volumes of *dilute ammonia R1*, 5 volumes of *water R*, 40 volumes of *nitromethane R* and 50 volumes of *dioxan R*. Dry the plate at 100 °C to 105 °C and examine in ultraviolet light at 254 nm. Any spot in the chromatogram obtained with test solution (a), apart from the principal spot, is not more intense than the spot in the chromatogram obtained with reference solution (b) (0.5 per cent).

Heavy metals (*2.4.8*). 1.0 g complies with limit test D for heavy metals (20 ppm). Prepare the standard using 2 ml of *lead standard solution (10 ppm Pb) R*.

Loss on drying (*2.2.32*). Not more than 0.5 per cent, determined on 1.000 g by drying in an oven at 100 °C to 105 °C.

Sulphated ash (*2.4.14*). Not more than 0.1 per cent, determined on 1.0 g.

ASSAY

Carry out the determination of primary aromatic amino-nitrogen (*2.5.8*), using 0.250 g and determining the end-point electrometrically.

1 ml of *0.1 M sodium nitrite* is equivalent to 31.03 mg of $C_{12}H_{14}N_4O_4S$.

STORAGE

Store protected from light.

01/2005:0741

SULFAFURAZOLE

Sulfafurazolum

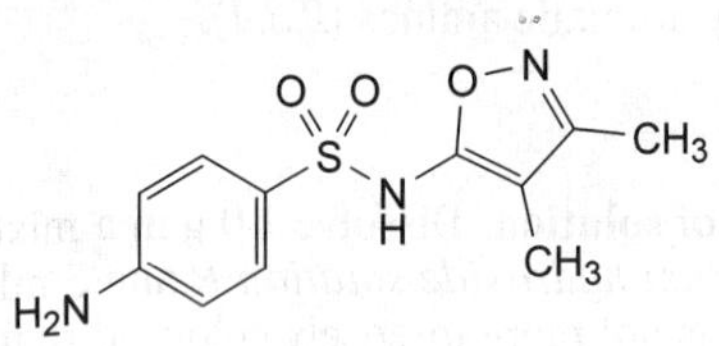

$C_{11}H_{13}N_3O_3S$ M_r 267.3

DEFINITION

Sulfafurazole contains not less than 99.0 per cent and not more than the equivalent of 101.0 per cent of 4-amino-*N*-(3,4-dimethylisoxazol-5-yl)benzenesulphonamide, calculated with reference to the dried substance.

CHARACTERS

White or yellowish-white, crystalline powder or crystals, practically insoluble in water, sparingly soluble in alcohol, slightly soluble in methylene chloride. It dissolves in solutions of alkali hydroxides and in dilute mineral acids.

It melts at about 197 °C, with decomposition.

IDENTIFICATION

First identification: A, C.

Second identification: B, C, D.

A. Examine by infrared absorption spectrophotometry (*2.2.24*), comparing with the spectrum obtained with *sulfafurazole CRS*. Examine the substances prepared as discs.

B. Examine the chromatograms obtained in the test for related substances. The principal spot in the chromatogram obtained with test solution (b) is similar in position and size to the principal spot in the chromatogram obtained with reference solution (a).

C. To 0.5 g add 1 ml of a 40 per cent *V/V* solution of *sulphuric acid R* and heat over a low flame to dissolve. Continue heating until a crystalline precipitate appears (about 2 min). Allow to cool and add 10 ml of *dilute sodium hydroxide solution R*. Cool. Shake the solution for 5 min with 25 ml of *ether R*. Separate the ether layer, dry over *anhydrous sodium sulphate R* and filter. Evaporate the solvent by heating on a water-bath. The residue melts (*2.2.14*) at 119 °C to 123 °C.

D. Dissolve about 5 mg in 10 ml of *1 M hydrochloric acid*. Dilute 1 ml of the solution to 10 ml with *water R*. The solution, without further acidification, gives the reaction of primary aromatic amines (*2.3.1*).

TESTS

Appearance of solution. Dissolve 0.4 g in a mixture of 5 ml of *dilute sodium hydroxide solution R* and 5 ml of *water R*, with gently warming if necessary. The solution is not more intensely coloured than reference solution Y_6, BY_6 or GY_6 (*2.2.2, Method II*).

Acidity. To 1.25 g, finely powdered, add 25 ml of *carbon dioxide-free water R*. Heat at 70 °C for 5 min. Cool in iced water for about 15 min and filter. To 20 ml of the filtrate add 0.1 ml of *bromothymol blue solution R1*. Not more than 0.2 ml of *0.1 M sodium hydroxide* is required to change the colour of the indicator.

Related substances. Examine by thin-layer chromatography (*2.2.27*), using *silica gel GF_{254} R* as the coating substance.

Test solution (a). Dissolve 0.10 g of the substance to be examined in 3 ml of a mixture of 2 volumes of *concentrated ammonia R* and 48 volumes of *methanol R* and dilute to 5 ml with the same mixture of solvents.

Test solution (b). Dilute 1 ml of test solution (a) to 5 ml with a mixture of 2 volumes of *concentrated ammonia R* and 48 volumes of *methanol R*.

Reference solution (a). Dissolve 20 mg of *sulfafurazole CRS* in 3 ml of a mixture of 2 volumes of *concentrated ammonia R* and 48 volumes of *methanol R* and dilute to 5 ml with the same mixture of solvents.

Reference solution (b). Dilute 1.25 ml of test solution (b) to 50 ml with a mixture of 2 volumes of *concentrated ammonia R* and 48 volumes of *methanol R*.

Apply to the plate 5 µl of each solution. Develop over a path of 15 cm using a mixture of 1 volume of *concentrated ammonia R*, 25 volumes of *methanol R* and 75 volumes of *methylene chloride R*. Dry the plate at 100 °C to 105 °C and examine in ultraviolet light at 254 nm. Any spot in the chromatogram obtained with test solution (a), apart from the principal spot, is not more intense than the spot in the chromatogram obtained with reference solution (b) (0.5 per cent).

Heavy metals (*2.4.8*). 1.0 g complies with limit test D for heavy metals (20 ppm). Prepare the standard using 2 ml of *lead standard solution (10 ppm Pb) R*.

Loss on drying (*2.2.32*). Not more than 0.5 per cent, determined on 1.000 g by drying in an oven at 100 °C to 105 °C.

Sulphated ash (*2.4.14*). Not more than 0.1 per cent, determined on 1.0 g.

ASSAY

Dissolve 0.200 g in 50 ml of *acetone R*. Titrate with *0.1 M tetrabutylammonium hydroxide* using a 4 g/l solution of *thymol blue R* in *methanol R* as indicator.

1 ml of *0.1 M tetrabutylammonium hydroxide* is equivalent to 26.73 mg of $C_{11}H_{13}N_3O_3S$.

STORAGE

Store protected from light.

01/2005:1476

SULFAGUANIDINE

Sulfaguanidinum

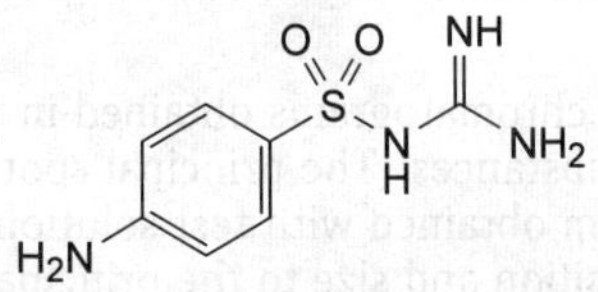

$C_7H_{10}N_4O_2S$ M_r 214.3

DEFINITION

Sulfaguanidine contains not less than 99.0 per cent and not more than the equivalent of 101.0 per cent of (4-aminophenylsulphonyl)guanidine, calculated with reference to the dried substance.

CHARACTERS

A white or almost white, fine crystalline powder, very slightly soluble in water, slightly soluble in acetone, very slightly soluble in alcohol, practically insoluble in methylene chloride. It dissolves in dilute solutions of mineral acids.

IDENTIFICATION

First identification: A, B.

Second identification: A, C, D, E.

A. Melting point (*2.2.14*): 189 °C to 193 °C, determined on the dried substance.

B. Examine by infrared absorption spectrophotometry (*2.2.24*), comparing with the spectrum obtained with *sulfaguanidine CRS*.

C. Examine the chromatograms obtained in the test for related substances. The principal spot in the chromatogram obtained with test solution (b) is similar in position and size to the principal spot in the chromatogram obtained with reference solution (a).

D. Dissolve about 5 mg in 10 ml of *1 M hydrochloric acid*. Dilute 1 ml of the solution to 10 ml with *water R*. The solution, without further acidification, gives the reaction of primary aromatic amines (*2.3.1*).

E. Suspend 0.1 g in 2 ml of *water R*, add 1 ml of *α-naphthol solution R* and 2 ml of a mixture of equal volumes of *water R* and *strong sodium hypochlorite solution R*. A red colour develops.

TESTS

Solution S. To 2.5 g, add 40 ml of *carbon dioxide-free water R*. Heat at about 70 °C for 5 min. Cool while stirring in iced water for about 15 min, filter and dilute to 50 ml with *carbon dioxide-free water R*.

Acidity. To 20 ml of solution S, add 0.1 ml of *bromothymol blue solution R1*. Not more than 0.2 ml of *0.1 M sodium hydroxide* is required to change the colour of the indicator.

Related substances. Examine by thin layer chromatography (*2.2.27*), using a *TLC silica gel GF_{254} plate R*.

Test solution (a). Dissolve 50 mg of the substance to be examined in *acetone R* and dilute to 5 ml with the same solvent.

Test solution (b). Dilute 2 ml of test solution (a) to 10 ml with *acetone R*.

Reference solution (a). Dissolve 10 mg of *sulfaguanidine CRS* in *acetone R* and dilute to 5 ml with the same solvent.

Reference solution (b). Dilute 5 ml of test solution (b) to 200 ml with *acetone R*.

Reference solution (c). Dilute 5 ml of reference solution (b) to 10 ml with *acetone R*.

Reference solution (d). Dissolve 10 mg of *sulfanilamide R* in test solution (b) and dilute to 5 ml with the same solution.

Apply to the plate 10 µl of each solution. Develop over a path of 15 cm using a mixture of 10 volumes of *anhydrous formic acid R*, 20 volumes of *methanol R* and 70 volumes of *methylene chloride R*. Allow the plate to dry in air and examine in ultraviolet light at 254 nm. Any spot in the chromatogram obtained with test solution (a), apart from the principal spot, is not more intense than the spot in the chromatogram obtained with reference solution (b) (0.5 per cent) and at most one such spot is more intense that the spot in the chromatogram obtained with reference solution (c) (0.25 per cent). The test is not valid unless the chromatogram obtained with reference solution (d) shows two clearly separated principal spots.

Heavy metals (*2.4.8*). 12 ml of solution S complies with limit test F for heavy metals (20 ppm). Prepare the standard using of *lead standard solution (1 ppm Pb) R*.

Loss on drying (*2.2.32*). Not more than 8.0 per cent, determined on 1.000 g by drying in an oven at 100 °C to 105 °C.

Sulphated ash (*2.4.14*). Not more than 0.1 per cent, determined on 1.0 g.

ASSAY

Dissolve 0.175 g in 50 ml of *dilute hydrochloric acid R*. Cool the solution in iced water. Carry out the determination of primary aromatic amino-nitrogen (*2.5.8*), determining the end-point electrometrically.

1 ml of *0.1 M sodium nitrite* is equivalent to 21.42 mg of $C_7H_{10}N_4O_2S$.

STORAGE

Store protected from light.

IMPURITIES

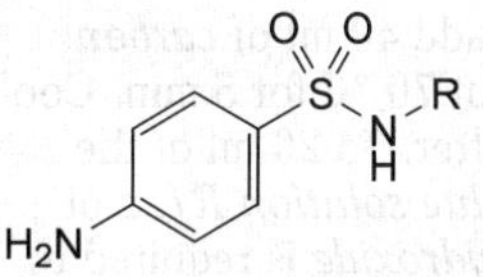

A. R = H: 4-aminobenzenesulphonamide (sulphanilamide),

B. R = CO-NH_2: *N*-[(4-aminophenyl)sulphonyl]urea (sulphacarbamide).

01/2005:0358

SULFAMERAZINE

Sulfamerazinum

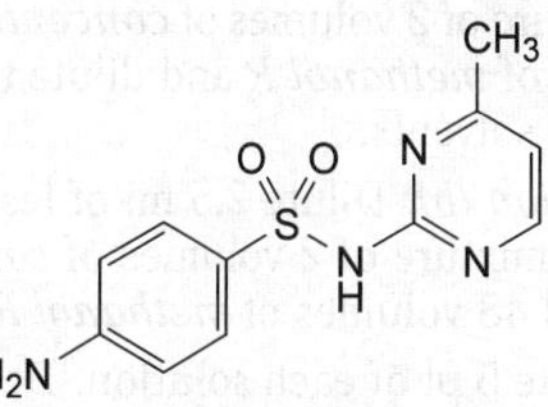

$C_{11}H_{12}N_4O_2S$ M_r 264.3

DEFINITION

Sulfamerazine contains not less than 99.0 per cent and not more than the equivalent of 101.0 per cent of 4-amino-*N*-(4-methyl-2-pyrimidinyl)benzenesulphonamide, calculated with reference to the dried substance.

CHARACTERS

White, yellowish-white or pinkish-white, crystalline powder or crystals, very slightly soluble in water, sparingly soluble in acetone, slightly soluble in alcohol, very slightly soluble in methylene chloride. It dissolves in solutions of alkali hydroxides and in dilute mineral acids.

It melts at about 235 °C, with decomposition.

IDENTIFICATION

First identification: A, B.

Second identification: B, C, D.

A. Examine by infrared absorption spectrophotometry (*2.2.24*), comparing with the spectrum obtained with *sulfamerazine CRS*. Examine the substances as discs.

B. Examine the chromatograms obtained in the test for related substances. The principal spot in the chromatogram obtained with test solution (b) is similar in position, colour and size to the principal spot in the chromatogram obtained with reference solution (a).
C. Place 3 g in a dry tube. Incline the tube by about 45°, immerse the bottom of the tube in a silicone-oil bath and heat to about 270 °C. The substance decomposes, producing a white or yellowish-white sublimate which, after recrystallisation from *toluene R* and drying at 100 °C, melts (*2.2.14*) at 157 °C to 161 °C.
D. Dissolve about 20 mg in 0.5 ml of *dilute hydrochloric acid R* and add 1 ml of *water R*. The solution gives, without further addition of acid, the identification reaction of primary aromatic amines (*2.3.1*).

TESTS

Appearance of solution. Dissolve 0.8 g in a mixture of 5 ml of *dilute sodium hydroxide solution R* and 5 ml of *water R*. The solution is not more intensely coloured than reference solution Y_4, BY_4 or GY_4 (*2.2.2, Method II*).

Acidity. To 1.25 g, finely powdered, add 40 ml of *carbon dioxide-free water R* and heat at about 70 °C for 5 min. Cool for about 15 min in iced water and filter. To 20 ml of the filtrate add 0.1 ml of *bromothymol blue solution R1*. Not more than 0.2 ml of *0.1 M sodium hydroxide* is required to change the colour of the indicator.

Related substances. Examine by thin-layer chromatography (*2.2.27*) using *silica gel* GF_{254} *R* as the coating substance.

Test solution (a). Dissolve 0.10 g of the substance to be examined in 3 ml of a mixture of 2 volumes of *concentrated ammonia R* and 48 volumes of *methanol R* and dilute to 5 ml with the same mixture of solvents.

Test solution (b). Dilute 1 ml of test solution (a) to 10 ml with a mixture of 2 volumes of *concentrated ammonia R* and 48 volumes of *methanol R*.

Reference solution (a). Dissolve 10 mg of *sulfamerazine CRS* in 3 ml of a mixture of 2 volumes of *concentrated ammonia R* and 48 volumes of *methanol R* and dilute to 5 ml with the same mixture of solvents.

Reference solution (b). Dilute 2.5 ml of test solution (b) to 50 ml with a mixture of 2 volumes of *concentrated ammonia R* and 48 volumes of *methanol R*.

Apply to the plate 5 µl of each solution. Develop over a path of 15 cm with a mixture of 3 volumes of *dilute ammonia R1*, 5 volumes of *water R*, 40 volumes of *nitromethane R* and 50 volumes of *dioxan R*. Dry the plate at 100 °C to 105 °C and examine in ultraviolet light at 254 nm. Any spot in the chromatogram obtained with test solution (a), apart from the principal spot, is not more intense that the spot in the chromatogram obtained with reference solution (b) (0.5 per cent).

Heavy metals (*2.4.8*). 1.0 g complies with limit test C for heavy metals (20 ppm). Prepare the standard using 2 ml of *lead standard solution (10 ppm Pb) R*.

Loss on drying (*2.2.32*). Not more than 0.5 per cent, determined on 1.000 g by drying in an oven at 100 °C to 105 °C.

Sulphated ash (*2.4.14*). Not more than 0.1 per cent, determined on 1.0 g.

ASSAY

Dissolve 0.2500 g in a mixture of 20 ml of *dilute hydrochloric acid R* and 50 ml of *water R*. Cool the solution in iced water. Carry out the determination of primary aromatic amino-nitrogen (*2.5.8*), determining the end-point electrometrically.

1 ml of *0.1 M sodium nitrite* is equivalent to 26.43 mg of $C_{11}H_{12}N_4O_2S$.

STORAGE

Store protected from light.

01/2005:0637

SULFAMETHIZOLE

Sulfamethizolum

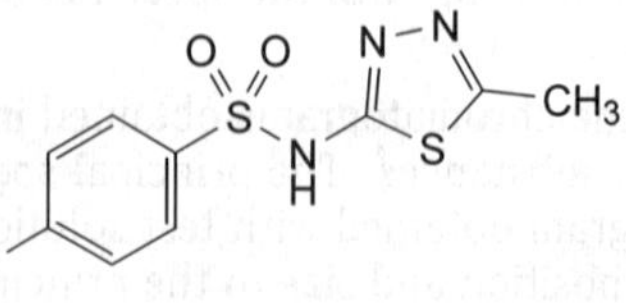

$C_9H_{10}N_4O_2S_2$ M_r 270.3

DEFINITION

Sulfamethizole contains not less than 99.0 per cent and not more than the equivalent of 101.0 per cent of 4-amino-*N*-(5-methyl-1,3,4-thiadiazol-2-yl)benzenesulphonamide, calculated with reference to the dried substance.

CHARACTERS

White or yellowish-white crystalline powder or crystals, very slightly soluble in water, soluble in acetone, sparingly soluble in alcohol. It dissolves in dilute solutions of alkali hydroxides and in dilute mineral acids.

It melts at about 210 °C.

IDENTIFICATION

First identification: A, B.

Second identification: B, C, D.

A. Examine by infrared absorption spectrophotometry (*2.2.24*), comparing with the spectrum obtained with *sulfamethizole CRS*. Examine the substances prepared as discs.
B. Examine the chromatograms obtained in the test for related substances. The principal spot in the chromatogram obtained with test solution (b) is similar in position and size to the principal spot in the chromatogram obtained with reference solution (a).
C. Dissolve 50 mg in 4 ml of *methanol R* and add 0.2 ml of a 40 g/l solution of *copper acetate R*. A flocculent, yellowish-green precipitate is formed, changing to dark green.
D. Dissolve about 5 mg in *1 M hydrochloric acid* and dilute to 10 ml with the same solvent. Dilute 1 ml of this solution to 10 ml with *water R*. The solution, without further acidification, gives the reaction of primary aromatic amines (*2.3.1*).

TESTS

Appearance of solution. Dissolve 1.0 g in a mixture of 5 ml of *dilute sodium hydroxide solution R* and 5 ml of *water R*. The solution is not more intensely coloured than reference solution Y_5, BY_5 or GY_5 (*2.2.2, Method II*).

Acidity. To 1.25 g add 25 ml of *carbon dioxide-free water R* and heat at 70 °C for 5 min. Cool for about 15 min in iced water and filter. To 20 ml of the filtrate add 0.1 ml of *bromothymol blue solution R1*. Not more than 0.5 ml of *0.1 M sodium hydroxide* is required to change the colour of the indicator.

Related substances. Examine by thin-layer chromatography (*2.2.27*), using *silica gel GF_{254} R* as the coating substance.

Test solution (a). Dissolve 0.30 g of the substance to be examined in *acetone R* and dilute to 10 ml with the same solvent.

Test solution (b). Dilute 1 ml of test solution (a) to 10 ml with *acetone R.*

Reference solution (a). Dissolve 30 mg of *sulfamethizole CRS* in *acetone R* and dilute to 10 ml with the same solvent.

Reference solution (b). Dilute 1 ml of test solution (b) to 20 ml with *acetone R.*

Apply to the plate 2 µl of each solution. Develop over a path of 15 cm using a mixture of 15 volumes of *methanol R* and 80 volumes of *chloroform R.* Dry the plate at 100 °C to 105 °C and examine in ultraviolet light at 254 nm. Any spot in the chromatogram obtained with test solution (a), apart from the principal spot, is not more intense than the spot in the chromatogram obtained with reference solution (b) (0.5 per cent).

Heavy metals (*2.4.8*). 1.0 g complies with limit test D for heavy metals (20 ppm). Prepare the standard using 2 ml of *lead standard solution (10 ppm Pb) R.*

Loss on drying (*2.2.32*). Not more than 0.5 per cent, determined on 1.000 g by drying in an oven at 100 °C to 105 °C.

Sulphated ash (*2.4.14*). Not more than 0.1 per cent, determined on 1.0 g.

ASSAY

Carry out the determination of primary aromatic amino-nitrogen (*2.5.8*), using 0.2500 g and determining the end-point electrometrically.

1 ml of *0.1 M sodium nitrite* is equivalent to 27.03 mg of $C_9H_{10}N_4O_2S_2$.

STORAGE

Store protected from light.

01/2005:0108

SULFAMETHOXAZOLE

Sulfamethoxazolum

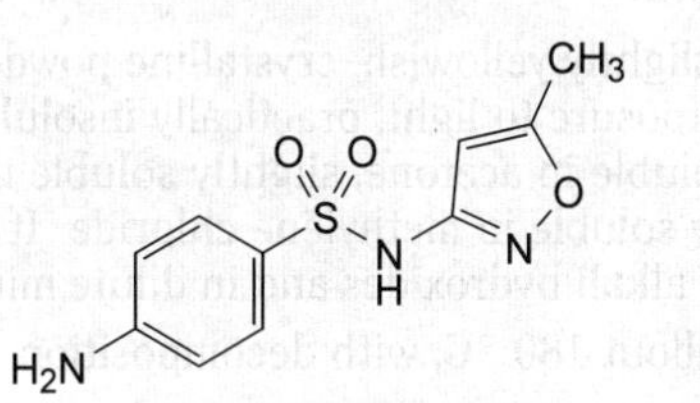

$C_{10}H_{11}N_3O_3S$ M_r 253.3

DEFINITION

4-Amino-*N*-(5-methylisoxazol-3-yl)benzenesulphonamide.

Content: 99.0 per cent to 101.0 per cent (dried substance).

CHARACTERS

Appearance: white or almost white, crystalline powder.

Solubility: practically insoluble in water, freely soluble in acetone, sparingly soluble in ethanol (96 per cent). It dissolves in dilute solutions of sodium hydroxide and in dilute acids.

IDENTIFICATION

First identification: A, B.

Second identification: A, C, D.

A. Melting point (*2.2.14*): 169 °C to 172 °C.

B. Infrared absorption spectrophotometry (*2.2.24*).
Comparison: *sulfamethoxazole CRS.*

C. Thin-layer chromatography (*2.2.27*).
Test solution. Dissolve 20 mg of the substance to be examined in 3 ml of a mixture of 2 volumes of *concentrated ammonia R* and 48 volumes of *methanol R* and dilute to 5 ml with the same mixture of solvents.
Reference solution. Dissolve 20 mg of *sulfamethoxazole CRS* in 3 ml of a mixture of 2 volumes of *concentrated ammonia R* and 48 volumes of *methanol R* and dilute to 5 ml with the same mixture of solvents.
Plate: *TLC silica gel F_{254} plate R.*
Mobile phase: *dilute ammonia R1, water R, nitromethane R, dioxan R* (3:5:41:51 *V/V/V/V*).
Application: 5 µl.
Development: over 3/4 of the plate.
Drying: at 100-105 °C.
Detection: examine in ultraviolet light at 254 nm.
Results: the principal spot in the chromatogram obtained with the test solution is similar in position and size to the principal spot in the chromatogram obtained with the reference solution.

D. Dissolve about 5 mg in 10 ml of *1 M hydrochloric acid.* Dilute 1 ml of the solution to 10 ml with *water R.* The solution, without further acidification, gives the reaction of primary aromatic amines (*2.3.1*).

TESTS

Appearance of solution. The solution is clear (*2.2.1*) and not more intensely coloured than reference solution Y_5, BY_5 or GY_5 (*2.2.2, Method II*).

Dissolve 1.0 g in a mixture of 5 ml of *dilute sodium hydroxide solution R* and 5 ml of *water R.*

Acidity. To 1.25 g, finely powdered, add 25 ml of *water R.* Heat at 70 °C for 5 min. Cool in iced water for about 15 min and filter. To 20 ml of the filtrate add 0.1 ml of *bromothymol blue solution R1.* Not more than 0.3 ml of *0.1 M sodium hydroxide* is required to change the colour of the indicator.

Related substances. Liquid chromatography (*2.2.29*).

Test solution. Dissolve 50.0 mg of the substance to be examined in 45 ml of the mobile phase, sonicate at about 45 °C for 10 min, cool and dilute to 50.0 ml with the mobile phase.

Reference solution (a). Dilute 1.0 ml of the test solution to 10.0 ml with the mobile phase. Dilute 1.0 ml of this solution to 100.0 ml with the mobile phase.

Reference solution (b). Dissolve 1 mg of the substance to be examined and 1 mg of *sulfamethoxazole impurity A CRS* in the mobile phase and dilute to 10.0 ml with the mobile phase.

Reference solution (c). Dissolve 1.0 mg of *sulfamethoxazole impurity F CRS* in the mobile phase and dilute to 10.0 ml with the mobile phase. Dilute 1.0 ml of this solution to 100.0 ml with the mobile phase.

Column:

- *size*: l = 0.25 m, Ø = 4.0 mm,
- *stationary phase*: *octylsilyl silica gel for chromatography R* (5 µm),
- *temperature*: 30 °C.

Mobile phase: mix 35 volumes of *methanol R2* and 65 volumes of a 13.6 g/l solution of *potassium dihydrogen phosphate R*, then adjust to pH 6.0 with a 100 g/l solution of *potassium hydroxide R*.

Flow rate: 0.9 ml/min.

Detection: spectrophotometer at 210 nm.

Injection: 20 μl.

Run time: 3 times the retention time of sulfamethoxazole.

Relative retentions with reference to sulfamethoxazole (retention time = about 10 min): impurity D = about 0.3; impurity E = about 0.35; impurity F = about 0.45; impurity C = about 0.5; impurity A = about 1.2; impurity B = about 2.0.

System suitability: reference solution (b):

- *resolution*: minimum 3.5 between the peaks due to sulfamethoxazole and impurity A.

Limits:

- *impurities A, B, C, D, E*: for each impurity, not more than the area of the principal peak in the chromatogram obtained with reference solution (a) (0.1 per cent),
- *impurity F*: not more than the area of the principal peak in the chromatogram obtained with reference solution (c) (0.1 per cent),
- *any other impurity*: for each impurity, not more than the area of the principal peak in the chromatogram obtained with reference solution (a) (0.1 per cent),
- *total*: not more than 3 times the area of the principal peak in the chromatogram obtained with reference solution (a) (0.3 per cent),
- *disregard limit*: 0.25 times the area of the principal peak in the chromatogram obtained with reference solution (a) (0.025 per cent).

Heavy metals (*2.4.8*): maximum 20 ppm.

1.0 g complies with limit test D. Prepare the reference solution using 2 ml of *lead standard solution (10 ppm Pb) R*.

Loss on drying (*2.2.32*): maximum 0.5 per cent, determined on 1.000 g by drying in an oven at 100-105 °C.

Sulphated ash (*2.4.14*): maximum 0.1 per cent, determined on 1.0 g.

ASSAY

Carry out the assay of primary aromatic amino-nitrogen (*2.5.8*), using 0.200 g and determining the end-point electrometrically.

1 ml of *0.1 M sodium nitrite* is equivalent to 25.33 mg of $C_{10}H_{11}N_3O_3S$.

STORAGE

Protected from light.

IMPURITIES

Specified impurities: A, B, C, D, E, F.

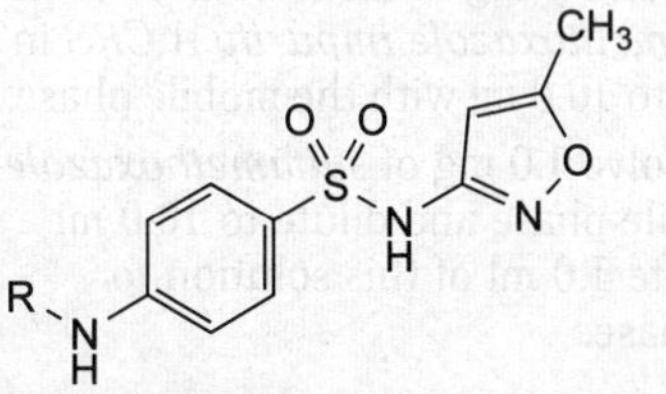

A. R = $CO\text{-}CH_3$: *N*-[4-[(5-methylisoxazol-3-yl)sulphamoyl]phenyl]acetamide,

B. R = $SO_2\text{-}C_6H_4\text{-}p\text{NH}_2$: 4-[[(4-aminophenyl)sulphonyl]amino]-*N*-(5-methylisoxazol-3-yl)benzenesulphonamide,

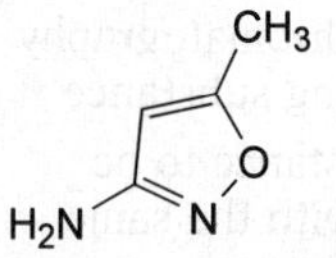

C. 5-methylisoxazol-3-amine,

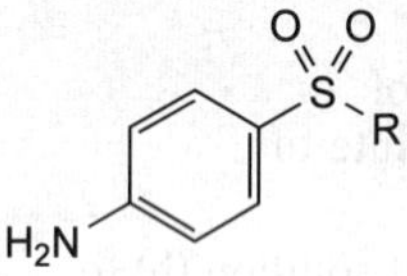

D. R = OH: 4-aminobenzenesulphonic acid (sulphanilic acid),

E. R = NH_2: 4-aminobenzenesulphonamide (sulphanilamide),

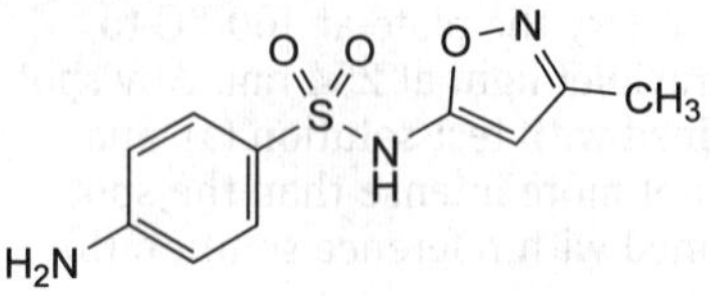

F. 4-amino-*N*-(3-methylisoxazol-5-yl)benzenesulphonamide.

01/2005:0638

SULFAMETHOXYPYRIDAZINE FOR VETERINARY USE

Sulfamethoxypyridazinum ad usum veterinarium

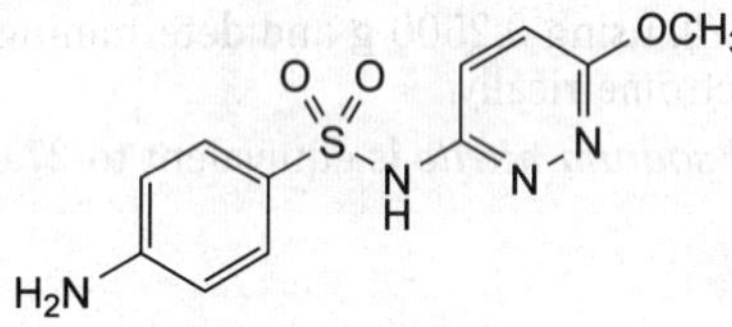

$C_{11}H_{12}N_4O_3S$ M_r 280.3

DEFINITION

Sulfamethoxypyridazine for veterinary use contains not less than 99.0 per cent and not more than the equivalent of 101.0 per cent of 4-amino-*N*-(6-methoxypyridazin-3-yl)benzenesulphonamide, calculated with reference to the dried substance.

CHARACTERS

A white or slightly yellowish, crystalline powder, colouring slowly on exposure to light, practically insoluble in water, sparingly soluble in acetone, slightly soluble in alcohol, very slightly soluble in methylene chloride. It dissolves in solutions of alkali hydroxides and in dilute mineral acids.

It melts at about 180 °C, with decomposition.

IDENTIFICATION

First identification: A, B.

Second identification: B, C, D.

A. Examine by infrared absorption spectrophotometry (*2.2.24*), comparing with the spectrum obtained with *sulfamethoxypyridazine CRS*. Examine the substances prepared as discs.

B. Examine the chromatograms obtained in the test for related substances. The principal spot in the chromatogram obtained with test solution (b) is similar in position and size to the principal spot in the chromatogram obtained with reference solution (a).

C. Dissolve 0.5 g in 1 ml of a 40 per cent *V/V* solution of *sulphuric acid R*, heating gently. Continue heating until a crystalline precipitate appears (about 2 min). Cool and add 10 ml of *dilute sodium hydroxide solution R*. Cool again, add 25 ml of *ether R* and shake the solution for 5 min. Separate the ether layer, dry over *anhydrous sodium sulphate R* and filter. Evaporate the ether by heating in a water-bath. An oily residue is obtained which becomes crystalline on cooling; if necessary, scratch the wall of the container with a glass rod. The residue melts (*2.2.14*) at 102 °Cto 106 °C.

D. Dissolve about 5 mg in 10 ml of *1 M hydrochloric acid*. Dilute 1 ml of the solution to 10 ml with *water R*. The solution, without further acidification, gives the reaction of primary aromatic amines (*2.3.1*).

TESTS

Appearance of solution. Dissolve 1.0 g in a mixture of 10 ml of *1 M sodium hydroxide* and 15 ml of *water R*. The solution is clear (*2.2.1*) and not more intensely coloured than reference solution Y_4 or BY_4 (*2.2.2, Method II*).

Acidity. To 1.25 g, finely powdered, add 25 ml of *carbon dioxide-free water R*. Heat at 70 °C for 5 min. Cool in iced water for about 15 min and filter. To 20 ml of the filtrate add 0.1 ml of *bromothymol blue solution R1*. Not more than 0.5 ml of *0.1 M sodium hydroxide* is required to change the colour of the indicator.

Related substances. Examine by thin layer chromatography (*2.2.27*), using *TLC silica gel* GF_{254} *plate R*.

Test solution (a). Dissolve 0.10 g of the substance to be examined in *acetone R* and dilute to 5 ml with the same solvent.

Test solution (b). Dilute 1 ml of test solution (a) to 10 ml with *acetone R*.

Reference solution (a). Dissolve 20 mg of *sulfamethoxypyridazine CRS* in *acetone R* and dilute to 10 ml with the same solvent.

Reference solution (b). Dilute 2.5 ml of test solution (b) to 50 ml with *acetone R*.

Apply separately to the plate 5 µl of each solution. Develop over a path of 15 cm using a mixture of 1 volume of *dilute ammonia R1*, 9 volumes of *water R*, 30 volumes of *2-propanol R* and 50 volumes of *ethyl acetate R*. Dry the plate at 100-105 °C and examine in ultraviolet light at 254 nm. Any spot in the chromatogram obtained with test solution (a), apart from the principal spot, is not more intense than the spot in the chromatogram obtained with reference solution (b) (0.5 per cent).

Heavy metals (*2.4.8*). 1.0 g complies with limit test D for heavy metals (20 ppm). Prepare the standard using 2 ml of *lead standard solution (10 ppm Pb) R*.

Loss on drying (*2.2.32*). Not more than 0.5 per cent, determined on 1.000 g by drying in an oven at 100-105 °C.

Sulphated ash (*2.4.14*). Not more than 0.1 per cent, determined on 1.0 g.

ASSAY

Carry out the assay of primary aromatic amino-nitrogen (*2.5.8*), using 0.2500 g, determining the end-point electrometrically.

1 ml of *0.1 M sodium nitrite* is equivalent to 28.03 mg of $C_{11}H_{12}N_4O_3S$.

STORAGE

Protected from light.

01/2005:1571

SULFANILAMIDE

Sulfanilamidum

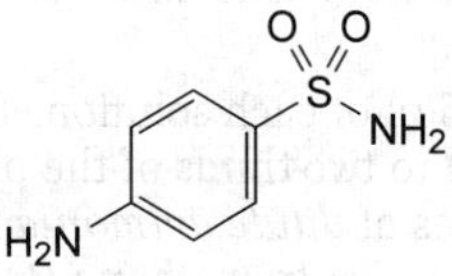

$C_6H_8N_2O_2S$ M_r 172.2

DEFINITION

Sulfanilamide contains not less than 99.0 per cent and not more than the equivalent of 101.0 per cent of 4-aminobenzenesulphonamide, calculated with reference to the dried substance.

CHARACTERS

White or yellowish-white crystals or fine powder, slightly soluble in water, freely soluble in acetone, sparingly soluble in alcohol, practically insoluble in methylene chloride. It dissolves in solutions of alkali hydroxides and in dilute mineral acids.

IDENTIFICATION

First identification: B.

Second identification: A, C, D.

A. Melting point (*2.2.14*): 164.5 °C to 166.0 °C.

B. Examine by infrared absorption spectrophotometry (*2.2.24*), comparing with the spectrum obtained with *sulfanilamide CRS*. Examine the substances prepared as discs.

C. Examine the chromatograms obtained in the test for related substances. The principal spot in the chromatogram obtained with test solution (a) is similar in position and size to the principal spot in the chromatogram obtained with reference solution (a).

D. Dissolve about 5 mg in 10 ml of *1 M hydrochloric acid*. Dilute 1 ml of the solution to 10 ml with *water R*. The solution, without further acidification, gives the reaction of primary aromatic amines (*2.3.1*).

TESTS

Solution S. To 2.5 g add 50 ml of *carbon dioxide-free water R*. Heat at about 70 °C for about 5 min. Cool in iced water for 15 min and filter.

Acidity. To 20 ml of solution S add 0.1 ml of *bromothymol blue solution R1*. Not more than 0.2 ml of *0.1 M sodium hydroxide* is required to change the colour of the indicator.

Related substances. Examine by thin-layer chromatography (*2.2.27*), using a *TLC silica gel* F_{254} *plate R*.

Test solution (a). Dissolve 20 mg of the substance to be examined in 3 ml of a mixture of 2 volumes of *concentrated ammonia R* and 48 volumes of *methanol R* and dilute to 5 ml with the same mixture of solvents.

Test solution (b). Dissolve 0.10 g of the substance to be examined in 0.5 ml of *concentrated ammonia R* and dilute to 5 ml with *methanol R*. If the solution is not clear, heat gently until dissolution is complete.

Reference solution (a). Dissolve 20 mg of *sulfanilamide CRS* in 3 ml of a mixture of 2 volumes of *concentrated ammonia R* and 48 volumes of *methanol R* and dilute to 5 ml with the same mixture of solvents.

Reference solution (b). Dilute 1.25 ml of test solution (a) to 50 ml with a mixture of 2 volumes of *concentrated ammonia R* and 48 volumes of *methanol R*.

Reference solution (c). Dissolve 20 mg of the substance to be examined and 20 mg of *sulfamerazine CRS* in 3 ml of a mixture of 2 volumes of *concentrated ammonia R* and 48 volumes of *methanol R* and dilute to 5 ml with the same mixture of solvents.

Apply to the plate 5 µl of each solution. Develop over a path corresponding to two-thirds of the plate height using a mixture of 3 volumes of *dilute ammonia R1*, 5 volumes of *water R*, 40 volumes of *nitromethane R* and 50 volumes of *dioxan R*. Dry the plate at 100 °C to 105 °C and examine in ultraviolet light at 254 nm. Any spot in the chromatogram obtained with test solution (b), apart from the principal spot, is not more intense than the spot in the chromatogram obtained with reference solution (b) (0.5 per cent). The test is not valid unless the chromatogram obtained with reference solution (c) shows two clearly separated principal spots.

Heavy metals (*2.4.8*). 12 ml of solution S complies with limit test A for heavy metals (20 ppm). Prepare the standard using *lead standard solution (1 ppm Pb) R*.

Loss on drying (*2.2.32*). Not more than 0.5 per cent, determined on 1.000 g by drying in an oven at 100 °C to 105 °C.

Sulphated ash (*2.4.14*). Not more than 0.1 per cent, determined on 1.0 g.

ASSAY

Carry out the determination of primary aromatic amino-nitrogen (*2.5.8*), using 0.140 g and determining the end-point electrometrically.

1 ml of *0.1 M sodium nitrite* is equivalent to 17.22 mg of $C_6H_8N_2O_2S$.

STORAGE

Store protected from light.

01/2005:0863

SULFASALAZINE

Sulfasalazinum

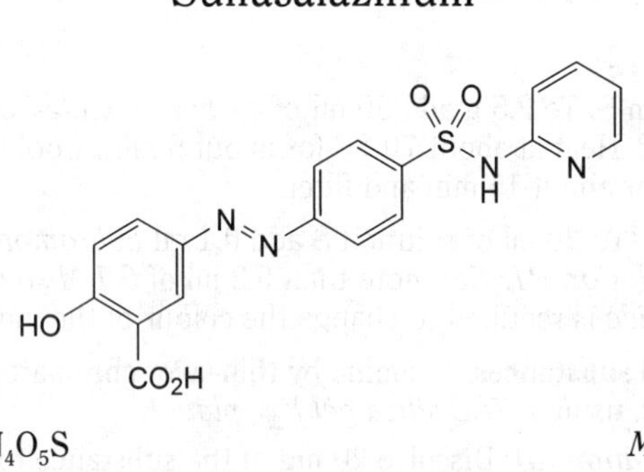

$C_{18}H_{14}N_4O_5S$ M_r 398.4

DEFINITION

Sulfasalazine contains not less than 97.0 per cent and not more than the equivalent of 101.5 per cent of 2-hydroxy-5-[2-[4-(pyridin-2-ylsulphamoyl)phenyl]diazenyl]benzoic acid, calculated with reference to the dried substance.

CHARACTERS

A bright yellow or brownish-yellow, fine powder, practically insoluble in water, very slightly soluble in alcohol, practically insoluble in methylene chloride. It dissolves in dilute solutions of alkali hydroxides.

IDENTIFICATION

Examine by infrared absorption spectrophotometry (*2.2.24*), comparing with the spectrum obtained with *sulfasalazine CRS*. Examine the substances prepared as discs.

TESTS

Related substances. Examine by liquid chromatography (*2.2.29*).

Test solution. Dissolve 25.0 mg of the substance to be examined in *dilute ammonia R3* and dilute to 25.0 ml with the same solvent.

Reference solution (a). Dilute 1.0 ml of the test solution to 100.0 ml with *dilute ammonia R3*.

Reference solution (b). Dissolve 1.0 mg of *sulfasalazine derivative for resolution CRS* in 10.0 ml of reference solution (a). Dilute 1.0 ml of this solution to 10.0 ml with reference solution (a).

The chromatographic procedure may be carried out using:

- a stainless steel column 0.25 m long and 4.6 mm in internal diameter, packed with *octadecylsilyl silica gel for chromatography R* (5 µm),
- as mobile phase at a flow rate of 1 ml/min:

  Mobile phase A. In a 1000 ml volumetric flask dissolve 1.13 g of *sodium dihydrogen phosphate R* and 2.5 g of *sodium acetate R* in 900 ml of *water R*. Adjust to pH 4.8 with *glacial acetic acid R* and adjust the volume to 1000 ml with *water R*,

  Mobile phase B. Mix 1 volume of mobile phase A with 4 volumes of *methanol R*,

Time (min)	Mobile phase A (per cent *V/V*)	Mobile phase B (per cent *V/V*)	Comment
0 - 15	60 → 45	40 → 55	linear gradient
15 - 25	45	55	isocratic
25 - 60	45 → 0	55 → 100	linear gradient
60 - 65	0	100	isocratic
65 - 67	0 → 60	100 → 40	switch to initial composition
67 - 77	60	40	re-equilibration

- as detector a spectrophotometer set at 320 nm.

Inject 20 µl of reference solution (a). Adjust the sensitivity of the detector so that the height of the principal peak in the chromatogram obtained is at least 50 per cent of the full scale of the recorder. Inject 20 µl of reference solution (b). The test is not valid unless the resolution between the peaks corresponding to sulfasalazine and sulfasalazine derivative for resolutionis at least 3.0.

Inject 20 µl of the test solution and 20 µl of reference solution (a). When the chromatograms are recorded in the prescribed conditions, the approximate retention times relative to sulfasalazine are the following: impurity A = 2.00; impurity B = 1.85; impurity C = 0.80; impurity D = 1.90; impurity E = 1.63; impurity F = 0.85; impurity G = 1.39; impurity H = 0.16; impurity I = 0.28.

In the chromatogram obtained with the test solution: the area of any peak, apart from the principal peak, is not greater than the area of the principal peak in the chromatogram obtained with reference solution (a) (1 per cent); the sum of the areas of all peaks, apart from the principal peak is not greater than four times the area of the principal peak in the chromatogram obtained with reference solution (a) (4 per cent). Disregard any peak with a retention time shorter than 6 min (corresponding to salicylic acid and sulfapyridine) and any peak with an area less than 0.05 times the area of the principal peak in the chromatogram obtained with reference solution (a).

Salicylic acid and sulfapyridine. Examine by liquid chromatography (*2.2.29*).

Test solution. Dissolve 25.0 mg of the substance to be examined in *dilute ammonia R3* and dilute to 25.0 ml with the same solvent.

Reference solution (a). Dissolve 5.0 mg of *salicylic acid R* and 5.0 mg and *sulfapyridine CRS* in *dilute ammonia R3* and dilute to 10.0 ml with the same solvent.

Reference solution (b). Dilute 2.0 ml of *reference solution (a)* to 100.0 ml with *dilute ammonia R3*.

The chromatographic procedure may be carried out using:

- a stainless steel column 0.25 m long and 4.6 mm in internal diameter, packed with *octadecylsilyl silica gel for chromatography R* (5 µm),
- as mobile phase at a flow rate of 1 ml/min a mixture of 70 volumes of mobile phase A (described in the test for related substances) and 30 volumes of mobile phase B (described in the test for related substances),
- as detector a spectrophotometer set at 300 nm.

Inject 20 µl of reference solution (b). Adjust the sensitivity of the system so that the height of the principal peaks in the chromatogram obtained is at least 50 per cent of the full scale of the recorder. When the chromatogram is recorded in the prescribed conditions, the retention times are: salicylic acid about 6 min and sulfapyridine about 7 min. The test is not valid unless the resolution between the peaks corresponding to salicylic acid and sulfapyridine is at least 2. Inject 20 µl of the test solution and 20 µl of reference solution (b). Continue the chromatography for 10 min. In the chromatogram obtained with the test solution the area of the peak corresponding to salicylic acid is not greater than 0.5 times the area of the first peak in the chromatogram obtained with reference solution (b) (0.5 per cent) and the peak corresponding to sulfapyridine is not greater than 0.5 times the area of the second peak in the chromatogram obtained with reference solution (b) (0.5 per cent). Disregard any peak with an area less than 0.05 times the area of the principal peak in the chromatogram obtained with reference solution (b).

Chlorides (*2.4.4.*). To 1.25 g add 50 ml of *distilled water R*. Heat at about 70 °C for 5 min. Cool and filter. To 20 ml of the filtrate add 1 ml of *nitric acid R*, allow to stand for 5 min and filter to obtain a clear solution. 15 ml of the filtrate complies with the limit test for chlorides (140 ppm).

Sulphates (*2.4.13*). To 20 ml of the filtrate prepared for the test for chlorides add 1 ml of *dilute hydrochloric acid R*, allow to stand for 5 min and filter. 15 ml of the filtrate complies with the limit test for sulphates (400 ppm).

Heavy metals (*2.4.8*). 2.0 g complies with limit test D for heavy metals (10 ppm). Prepare the standard using 2 ml of *lead standard solution (10 ppm Pb) R*.

Loss on drying (*2.2.32*). Not more than 1.0 per cent, determined on 1.000 g by drying in an oven at 100 °C to 105 °C for 2 h.

Sulphated ash (*2.4.14*). Not more than 0.5 per cent, determined on 1.0 g.

ASSAY

Dissolve 0.150 g in *0.1 M sodium hydroxide* and dilute to 100.0 ml with the same solvent. Transfer 5.0 ml of this solution to a 1000 ml volumetric flask containing about 750 ml of *water R*. Add 20.0 ml of *0.1 M acetic acid* and dilute to 1000.0 ml with *water R*. Prepare a standard solution at the same time and in the same manner using 0.150 g of *sulfasalazine CRS*. Measure the absorbance (*2.2.25*) of the two solutions at the maximum at 359 nm.

Calculate the content of $C_{18}H_{14}N_4O_5S$ from the absorbances measured and the concentration of the solutions.

STORAGE

Store protected from light.

IMPURITIES

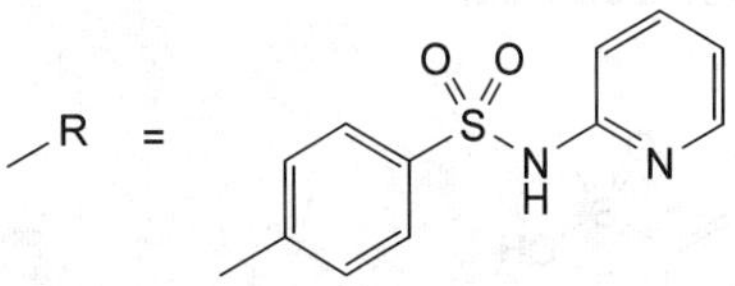

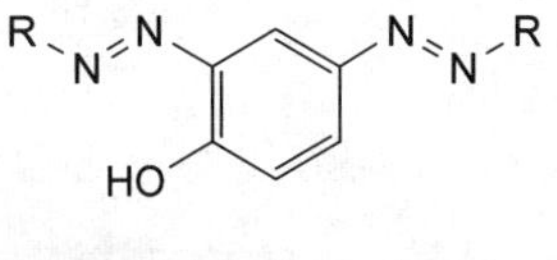

A. 4,4′-[(4-hydroxy-1,3-phenylene)bis(diazenediyl)]bis[*N*-(pyridin-2-yl)benzenesulphonamide],

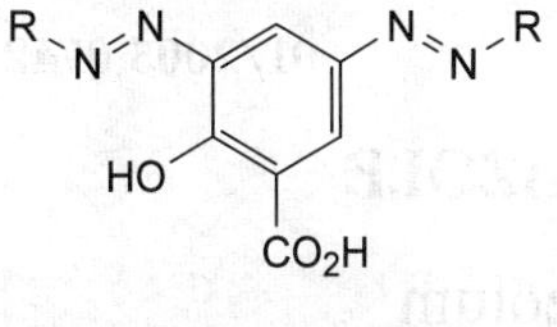

B. 2-hydroxy-3,5-bis[2-[4-(pyridin-2-ylsulphamoyl)phenyl]diazenyl]benzoic acid,

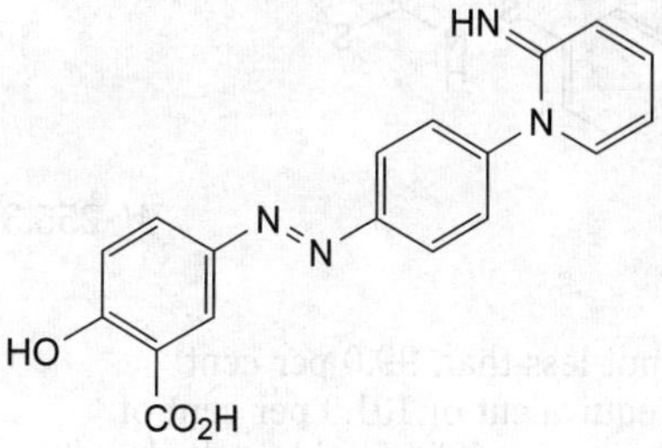

C. 2-hydroxy-5-[2-[4-(2-iminopyridin-1(2*H*)-yl)phenyl]diazenyl]benzoic acid,

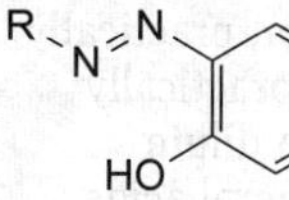

D. 4-[2-(2-hydroxyphenyl)diazenyl]-*N*-(pyridin-2-yl)benzenesulphonamide,

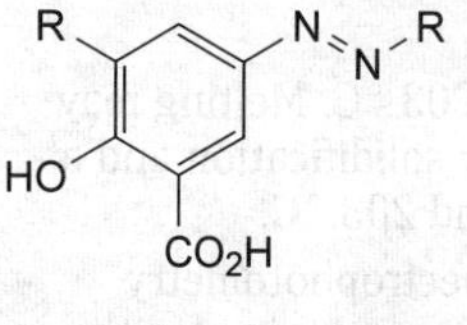

E. 2-hydroxy-4′-(pyridin-2-ylsulphamoyl)-5-[2-[4-(pyridin-2-ylsulphamoyl)phenyl]diazenyl]biphenyl-3-carboxylic acid,

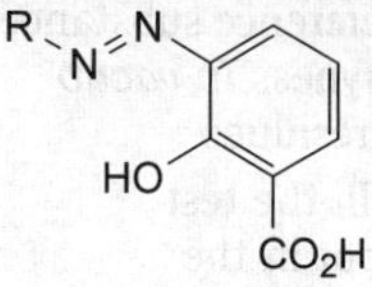

F. 2-hydroxy-3-[2-[4-(pyridin-2-ylsulphamoyl)phenyl]diazenyl]benzoic acid,

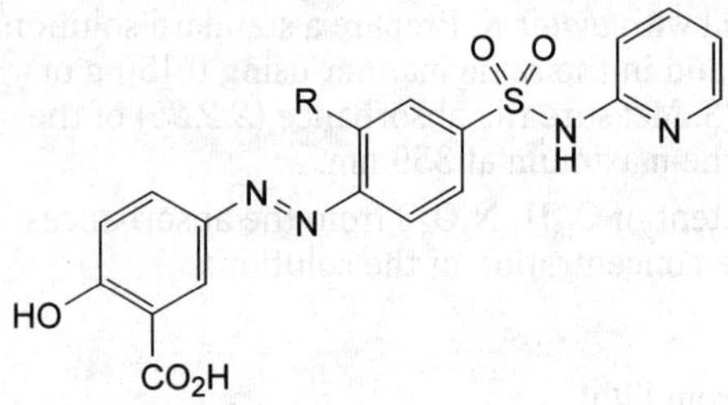

G. 5-[2-[4′,5-bis(pyridin-2-ylsulphamoyl)biphenyl-2-yl]diazenyl]-2-hydroxybenzoic acid,

H. salicylic acid,

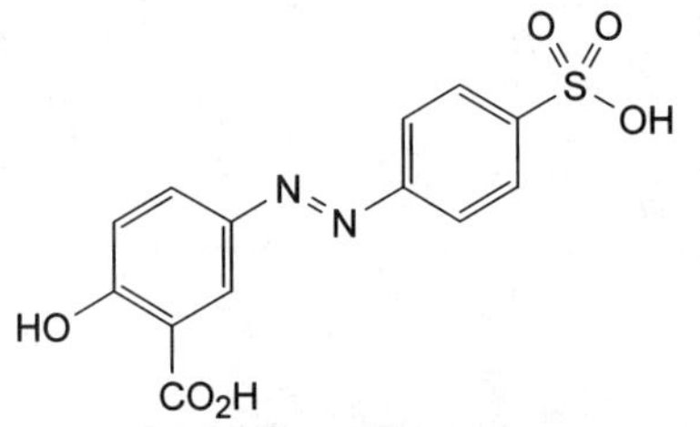

I. 2-hydroxy-5-[2-(4-sulphophenyl)diazenyl]benzoic acid.

01/2005:0742

SULFATHIAZOLE

Sulfathiazolum

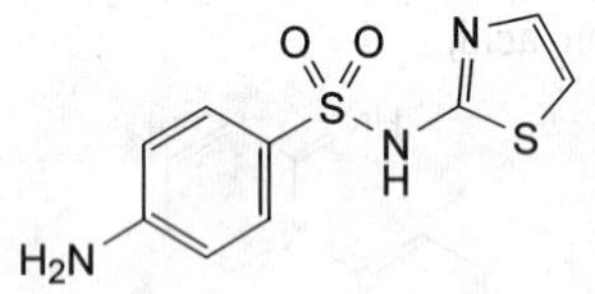

$C_9H_9N_3O_2S_2$ M_r 255.3

DEFINITION

Sulfathiazole contains not less than 99.0 per cent and not more than the equivalent of 101.0 per cent of 4-amino-*N*-(thiazol-2-yl)benzenesulphonamide, calculated with reference to the dried substance.

CHARACTERS

A white or slightly yellowish, crystalline powder, practically insoluble in water, slightly soluble in alcohol, practically insoluble in methylene chloride. It dissolves in dilute solutions of alkali hydroxides and in dilute mineral acids.

IDENTIFICATION

First identification: A, B.

Second identification: A, C, D, E.

A. Melting point (*2.2.14*): 200 °C to 203 °C. Melting may occur at about 175 °C, followed by solidification and a second melting between 200 °C and 203 °C.

B. Examine by infrared absorption spectrophotometry (*2.2.24*), comparing with the spectrum obtained with *sulfathiazole CRS*. Examine the substances prepared as discs. If the spectra obtained show differences, dissolve the substance to be examined and the reference substance separately in *alcohol R*, evaporate to dryness *in vacuo* and record the spectra again using the residues.

C. Examine the chromatograms obtained in the test for related substances. The principal spot in the chromatogram obtained with test solution (b) is similar in position, colour and size to the principal spot in the chromatogram obtained with reference solution (a).

D. Dissolve about 10 mg in a mixture of 10 ml of *water R* and 2 ml of *0.1 M sodium hydroxide* and add 0.5 ml of *copper sulphate solution R*. A greyish-blue or purple precipitate is formed.

E. Dissolve about 5 mg in 10 ml of *1 M hydrochloric acid.* Dilute 1 ml of the solution to 10 ml with *water R*. The solution, without further addition of acid, gives the reaction of primary aromatic amines (*2.3.1*).

TESTS

Appearance of solution. Dissolve 1.0 g in 10 ml of *1 M sodium hydroxide*. The solution is clear (*2.2.1*) and not more intensely coloured than reference solution GY_4 (*2.2.2, Method II*).

Acidity. To 1.0 g add 50 ml of *carbon dioxide-free water R*. Heat to 70 °C for 5 min. Cool rapidly to 20 °C and filter. To 25 ml of the filtrate add 0.1 ml of *bromothymol blue solution R1*. Not more than 0.1 ml of *0.1 M sodium hydroxide* is required to change the colour of the indicator.

Related substances. Examine by thin-layer chromatography (*2.2.27*), using *silica gel H R* as the coating substance.

Test solution (a). Dissolve 0.10 g of the substance to be examined in a mixture of 1 volume of *concentrated ammonia R* and 9 volumes of *alcohol R* and dilute to 10 ml with the same mixture of solvents.

Test solution (b). Dilute 1 ml of test solution (a) to 5 ml with a mixture of 1 volume of *concentrated ammonia R* and 9 volumes of *alcohol R*.

Reference solution (a). Dissolve 20 mg of *sulfathiazole CRS* in a mixture of 1 volume of *concentrated ammonia R* and 9 volumes of *alcohol R* and dilute to 10 ml with the same mixture of solvents.

Reference solution (b). Dissolve 50 mg of *sulfanilamide R* in a mixture of 1 volume of *concentrated ammonia R* and 9 volumes of *alcohol R* and dilute to 100 ml with the same mixture of solvents. Dilute 1 ml of this solution to 10 ml with the same mixture of solvents.

Apply to the plate 10 µl of each solution. Develop over a path of 15 cm using a mixture of 18 volumes of *ammonia R* and 90 volumes of *butanol R*. Dry the plate at 100 °C to 105 °C for 10 min and spray with a 1 g/l solution of *dimethylaminobenzaldehyde R* in *alcohol R* containing 1 per cent *V/V* of *hydrochloric acid R*. Any spot in the chromatogram obtained with test solution (a), apart from the principal spot, is not more intense than the spot in the chromatogram obtained with reference solution (b) (0.5 per cent).

Heavy metals (*2.4.8*). 1.0 g complies with limit test C for heavy metals (20 ppm). Prepare the standard using 2 ml of *lead standard solution (10 ppm Pb) R*.

Loss on drying (*2.2.32*). Not more than 0.5 per cent, determined on 1.000 g by drying in an oven at 100 °C to 105 °C.

Sulphated ash (*2.4.14*). Not more than 0.1 per cent, determined on 1.0 g.

ASSAY

Carry out the determination of primary aromatic amino-nitrogen (*2.5.8*), using 0.200 g, determining the end-point electrometrically.

1 ml of *0.1 M sodium nitrite* is equivalent to 25.53 mg of $C_9H_9N_3O_2S_2$.

STORAGE

Store protected from light.

01/2005:0790

SULFINPYRAZONE

Sulfinpyrazonum

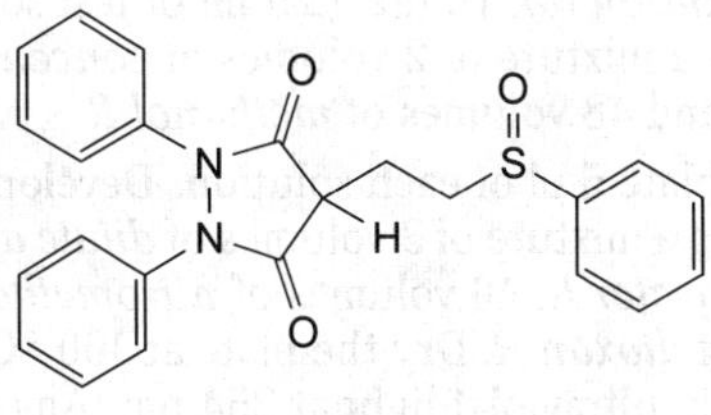

$C_{23}H_{20}N_2O_3S$ M_r 404.5

DEFINITION

Sulfinpyrazone contains not less than 99.0 per cent and not more than the equivalent of 101.0 per cent of 1,2-diphenyl-4-[2-(phenylsulphinyl)ethyl]pyrazolidine-3,5-dione, calculated with reference to the dried substance.

CHARACTERS

A white or almost white powder, very slightly soluble in water, sparingly soluble in alcohol. It dissolves in dilute solutions of alkali hydroxides.

IDENTIFICATION

First identification: A, C.

Second identification: A, B, D.

A. Melting point (*2.2.16*): 131 °C to 135 °C.

B. Dissolve 30.0 mg in *0.01 M sodium hydroxide* and dilute to 100.0 ml with the same alkaline solution. Dilute 1.0 ml of this solution to 20.0 ml with *0.01 M sodium hydroxide*. Examined between 230 nm and 350 nm (*2.2.25*), the solution shows an absorption maximum at 260 nm. The specific absorbance at the maximum is 530 to 580.

C. Examine by infrared absorption spectrophotometry (*2.2.24*), comparing with the spectrum obtained with *sulfinpyrazone CRS*. Examine the substances prepared as discs.

D. Dissolve about 10 mg in 3 ml of *acetone R* and add a mixture of 0.2 ml of *ferric chloride solution R2* and 3 ml of *water R*. A red to violet colour develops.

TESTS

Appearance of solution in acetone. Dissolve 1.25 g in *acetone R* and dilute to 25 ml with the same solvent. The solution is clear (*2.2.1*). The absorbance (*2.2.25*) of the solution, measured at 420 nm with a path-length of 4 cm, is not greater than 0.10.

Appearance of solution in 1 M sodium hydroxide. Dissolve 1.25 g, heating gently if necessary, in 25 ml of *1 M sodium hydroxide*. The solution is clear (*2.2.1*). The absorbance (*2.2.25*) of the solution, measured at 420 nm with a path-length of 4 cm, is not greater than 0.15.

Related substances. Examine by thin-layer chromatography (*2.2.27*), using a suitable silica gel with a fluorescent indicator having an optimal intensity at 254 nm. Expose the plate, in a tank, to the vapour from *glacial acetic acid R*. After 10 min, remove the plate and heat at 60 °C for 40 min. Cool and pass a current of nitrogen over the plate for 10 min.

Prepare the solutions immediately before use.

Test solution. Dissolve 0.25 g of the substance to be examined in *acetone R* and dilute to 5 ml with the same solvent.

Reference solution (a). Dilute 2 ml of the test solution to 100 ml with *acetone R*. Dilute 1 ml of this solution to 10 ml with *acetone R*.

Reference solution (b). Dissolve 10 mg of *sulfinpyrazone impurity A CRS* in *acetone R* and dilute to 10 ml with the same solvent.

Reference solution (c). Dilute 5 ml of reference solution (b) to 10 ml with *acetone R*.

Reference solution (d). Dissolve 10 mg of *sulfinpyrazone impurity B CRS* in *acetone R* and dilute to 10 ml with the same solvent.

Reference solution (e). Dilute 5 ml of reference solution (d) to 10 ml with *acetone R*.

Apply to the plate, under an atmosphere of nitrogen, 2 µl of each solution. Develop over a path of 15 cm using a mixture of 20 volumes of *glacial acetic acid R* and 80 volumes of *chloroform R*. Allow the plate to dry in air and examine in ultraviolet light at 254 nm. In the chromatogram obtained with the test solution: any spots corresponding to sulfinpyrazone impurity A and sulfinpyrazone impurity B are not more intense than the spots in the chromatograms obtained with reference solutions (b) (2.0 per cent) and (d) (2.0 per cent), respectively, and at most one of the spots is more intense than the corresponding spot in the chromatogram obtained with reference solution (c) (1.0 per cent) or (e) (1.0 per cent); any spot apart from the principal spot and the two spots previously cited is not more intense than the spot in the chromatogram obtained with reference solution (a) (0.2 per cent).

Heavy metals (*2.4.8*). 1.0 g complies with limit test C for heavy metals (10 ppm). Prepare the standard using 1 ml of *lead standard solution (10 ppm Pb) R*.

Loss on drying (*2.2.32*). Not more than 0.5 per cent, determined on 1.000 g by drying in an oven at 100 °C to 105 °C.

Sulphated ash (*2.4.14*). Not more than 0.1 per cent, determined on 1.0 g.

ASSAY

Dissolve 0.300 g in 25 ml of *acetone R*. Add 0.5 ml of *bromothymol blue solution R1*. Titrate with *0.1 M sodium hydroxide* until the colour changes from yellow to blue.

1 ml of *0.1 M sodium hydroxide* is equivalent to 40.45 mg of $C_{23}H_{20}N_2O_3S$.

STORAGE

Store protected from light.

IMPURITIES

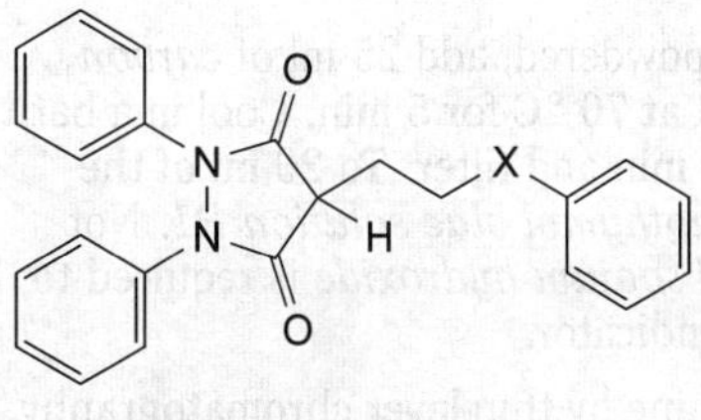

A. X = SO_2: 1,2-diphenyl-4-[2-(phenylsulphonyl)ethyl]pyrazolidine-3,5-dione,

B. X = S: 1,2-diphenyl-4-[2-(phenylsulphanyl)ethyl]pyrazolidine-3,5-dione.

01/2005:0639

SULFISOMIDINE

Sulfisomidinum

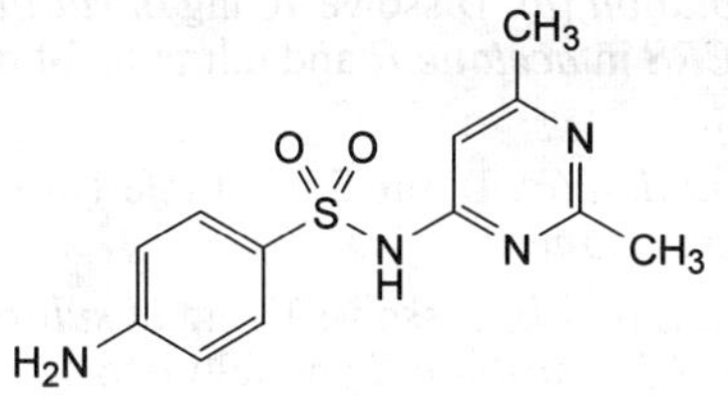

$C_{12}H_{14}N_4O_2S$ M_r 278.3

DEFINITION

Sulfisomidine contains not less than 99.0 per cent and not more than the equivalent of 101.0 per cent of 4-amino-*N*-(2, 6-dimethylpyrimidin-4-yl)benzenesulphonamide, calculated with reference to the dried substance.

CHARACTERS

White or yellowish-white powder or crystals, very slightly soluble in water, slightly soluble in acetone and in alcohol. It dissolves in dilute solutions of the alkali hydroxides and in dilute mineral acids.

It melts at about 240 °C with decomposition.

IDENTIFICATION

First identification: A, B.

Second identification: B, C, D.

A. Examine by infrared absorption spectrophotometry (*2.2.24*), comparing with the spectrum obtained with *sulfisomidine CRS*. Examine the substances prepared as discs.

B. Examine the chromatograms obtained in the test for related substances. The principal spot in the chromatogram obtained with test solution (b) is similar in position and size to the principal spot in the chromatogram obtained with reference solution (a).

C. Dissolve 50 mg with heating in 4 ml of *methanol R*. Cool and filter. Add to the filtrate 0.2 ml of a 40 g/l solution of *copper acetate R*. The solution becomes yellowish-green.

D. Dissolve about 5 mg in 10 ml of *1 M hydrochloric acid*. Dilute 1 ml of the solution to 10 ml with *water R*. The solution, without further acidification, gives the reaction of primary aromatic amines (*2.3.1*).

TESTS

Appearance of solution. Dissolve 1.0 g in a mixture of 5 ml of *dilute sodium hydroxide solution R* and 5 ml of *water R*. The solution is not more intensely coloured than reference solution Y_5, BY_5 or GY_5 (*2.2.2, Method II*).

Acidity. To 1.25 g, finely powdered, add 25 ml of *carbon dioxide-free water R*. Heat at 70 °C for 5 min. Cool in a bath of iced water for about 15 min and filter. To 20 ml of the filtrate add 0.1 ml of *bromothymol blue solution R1*. Not more than 0.2 ml of *0.1 M sodium hydroxide* is required to change the colour of the indicator.

Related substances. Examine by thin-layer chromatography (*2.2.27*), using *silica gel* GF_{254} *R* as the coating substance.

Test solution (a). Dissolve 0.10 g of the substance to be examined in 3 ml of a mixture of 2 volumes of *concentrated ammonia R* and 48 volumes of *methanol R* and dilute to 5 ml with the same mixture of solvents.

Test solution (b). Dilute 1 ml of test solution (a) to 5 ml with a mixture of 2 volumes of *concentrated ammonia R* and 48 volumes of *methanol R*.

Reference solution (a). Dissolve 20 mg of *sulfisomidine CRS* in 3 ml of a mixture of 2 volumes of *concentrated ammonia R* and 48 volumes of *methanol R* and dilute to 5 ml with the same mixture of solvents.

Reference solution (b). Dilute 1.25 ml of test solution (b) to 50 ml with a mixture of 2 volumes of *concentrated ammonia R* and 48 volumes of *methanol R*.

Apply to the plate 5 µl of each solution. Develop over a path of 15 cm using a mixture of 3 volumes of *dilute ammonia R1*, 5 volumes of *water R*, 40 volumes of *nitromethane R* and 50 volumes of *dioxan R*. Dry the plate at 100 °C to 105 °C and examine in ultraviolet light at 254 nm. Any spot in the chromatogram obtained with test solution (a), apart from the principal spot, is not more intense than the spot in the chromatogram obtained with reference solution (b) (0.5 per cent).

Heavy metals (*2.4.8*). 1.0 g complies with limit test D for heavy metals (20 ppm). Prepare the standard using 2 ml of *lead standard solution (10 ppm Pb) R*.

Loss on drying (*2.2.32*). Not more than 0.5 per cent, determined on 1.000 g by drying in an oven at 100 °C to 105 °C.

Sulphated ash (*2.4.14*). Not more than 0.1 per cent, determined on 1.0 g.

ASSAY

Carry out the determination of primary aromatic amino-nitrogen (*2.5.8*), using 0.2500 g and determining the end-point electrometrically.

1 ml of *0.1 M sodium nitrite* is equivalent to 27.83 mg of $C_{12}H_{14}N_4O_2S$.

STORAGE

Store protected from light.

01/2005:0864

SULINDAC

Sulindacum

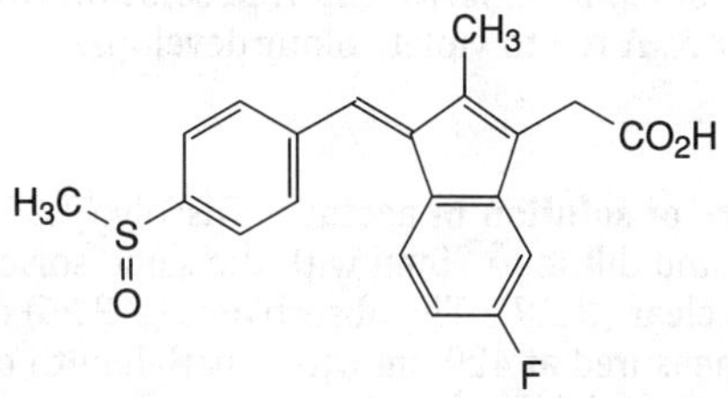

$C_{20}H_{17}FO_3S$ M_r 356.4

DEFINITION

Sulindac contains not less than 99.0 per cent and not more than the equivalent of 101.0 per cent of (*Z*)-[5-fluoro-2-methyl-1-[4-(methylsulphinyl)benzylidene]-1*H*-inden-3-yl]acetic acid, calculated with reference to the dried substance.

CHARACTERS

A yellow, crystalline powder, very slightly soluble in water, soluble in methylene chloride, sparingly soluble in alcohol. It dissolves in dilute solutions of alkali hydroxides.

It shows polymorphism.

IDENTIFICATION

First identification: C.

Second identification: A, B, D, E.

A. Melting point (*2.2.14*): 182 °C to 186 °C.

B. Dissolve 50 mg in a 0.3 per cent *V/V* solution of *hydrochloric acid R* in *methanol R* and dilute to 100 ml with the same acid solution. Dilute 2 ml of the solution to 50 ml with a 0.3 per cent *V/V* solution of *hydrochloric acid R* in *methanol R*. Examined between 230 nm and 350 nm (*2.2.25*), the solution shows 2 absorption maxima, at 284 nm and 327 nm, and a shoulder at about 258 nm. The ratio of the absorbance measured at the maximum at 284 nm to that measured at the maximum at 327 nm is 1.10 to 1.20.

C. Examine by infrared absorption spectrophotometry (*2.2.24*), comparing with the spectrum obtained with *sulindac CRS*. Examine the substances prepared as discs. If the spectra obtained show differences, dissolve the substance to be examined and the reference substance separately in the minimum volume of hot *methanol R*, evaporate to dryness and record new spectra using the residues.

D. Examine by thin-layer chromatography (*2.2.27*), using *silica gel* GF_{254} *R* as the coating substance.

Test solution. Dissolve 10 mg of the substance to be examined in *methylene chloride R* and dilute to 10 ml with the same solvent.

Reference solution (a). Dissolve 10 mg of *sulindac CRS* in *methylene chloride R* and dilute to 10 ml with the same solvent.

Reference solution (b). Dissolve 10 mg of *diflunisal CRS* in *methylene chloride R* and dilute to 10 ml with the same solvent. Dilute 1 ml of the solution to 2 ml with reference solution (a).

Apply to the plate 5 µl of each solution. Develop over a path of 15 cm using a mixture of 1 volume of *glacial acetic acid R*, 49 volumes of *methylene chloride R* and 50 volumes of *acetone R*. Dry the plate in a current of warm air and examine in ultraviolet light at 254 nm. The principal spot in the chromatogram obtained with the test solution is similar in position and size to the principal spot in the chromatogram obtained with reference solution (a). The test is not valid unless the chromatogram obtained with reference solution (b) shows 2 clearly separated principal spots.

E. Mix about 5 mg with 45 mg of *heavy magnesium oxide R* and ignite in a crucible until an almost white residue is obtained (usually less than 5 min). Allow to cool, add 1 ml of *water R*, 0.05 ml of *phenolphthalein solution R1* and about 1 ml of *dilute hydrochloric acid R* to render the solution colourless. Filter. Add 1.0 ml of the filtrate to a freshly prepared mixture of 0.1 ml of *alizarin S solution R* and 0.1 ml of *zirconyl nitrate solution R*. Mix, allow to stand for 5 min and compare the colour of the solution with that of a blank prepared in the same manner. The test solution is yellow and the blank is red.

TESTS

Related substances. Examine by liquid chromatography (*2.2.29*).

Test solution. Dissolve 0.10 g of the substance to be examined in the mobile phase and dilute to 50.0 ml with the mobile phase.

Reference solution (a). Dilute 1.0 ml of the test solution to 100.0 ml with the mobile phase. Dilute 5.0 ml to 10.0 ml with the mobile phase.

Reference solution (b). Dissolve 20.0 mg of *sulindac CRS* (which has an assigned content of *E*-isomer) in the mobile phase and dilute to 10.0 ml with the mobile phase.

The chromatographic procedure may be carried out using:

– a stainless steel column 0.25 m long and 4.6 mm in internal diameter packed with *silica gel for chromatography R* (10 µm),

– as mobile phase at a flow rate of 2 ml/min a mixture of 1 volume of *glacial acetic acid R*, 4 volumes of *alcohol R*, 100 volumes of *ethyl acetate R* and 400 volumes of *ethanol-free chloroform R*,

– as detector a spectrophotometer set at 280 nm.

Inject 20 µl of reference solution (a) and adjust the sensitivity of the system so that the height of the principal peak in the chromatogram obtained is at least 50 per cent of the full scale of the recorder. Inject 20 µl of reference solution (b) and continue the chromatography for twice the retention time of the principal peak. The chromatogram obtained shows a principal peak corresponding to sulindac and a peak corresponding to the *E*-isomer, with a retention time relative to sulindac of about 1.75.

Inject 20 µl of the test solution, 20 µl of reference solution (a) and 20 µl of reference solution (b). From the chromatograms obtained with the test solution and reference solution (b), determine the percentage content of *E*-isomer, taking into account the assigned content of this isomer in *sulindac CRS*: the value found is not more than 0.5 per cent. In the chromatogram obtained with the test solution: the area of any peak, apart from the principal peak and any peak corresponding to *E*-isomer, is not greater than the area of the principal peak in the chromatogram obtained with reference solution (a) (0.5 per cent); the sum of the areas of all the peaks, apart from the principal peak, is not greater than twice the area of the principal peak in the chromatogram obtained with reference solution (a) (1 per cent).

Heavy metals (*2.4.8*). 2.0 g complies with limit test D (10 ppm). Prepare the standard using 2 ml of *lead standard solution (10 ppm Pb) R*.

Loss on drying (*2.2.32*). Not more than 0.5 per cent, determined on 1.000 g by drying in an oven at 100-105 °C at a pressure not exceeding 700 Pa.

Sulphated ash (*2.4.14*). Not more than 0.1 per cent, determined on 1.0 g.

ASSAY

Dissolve 0.300 g in 50 ml of *methanol R*. Titrate with *0.1 M sodium hydroxide*, determining the end-point potentiometrically (*2.2.20*).

1 ml of *0.1 M sodium hydroxide* is equivalent to 35.64 mg of $C_{20}H_{17}FO_3S$.

STORAGE

Protected from light.

IMPURITIES

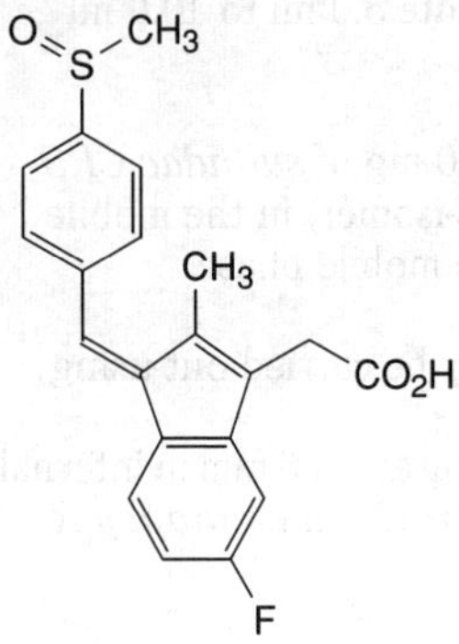

A. (*E*)-[5-fluoro-2-methyl-1-[4-(methylsulphinyl)benzylidene]-1*H*-inden-3-yl]acetic acid,

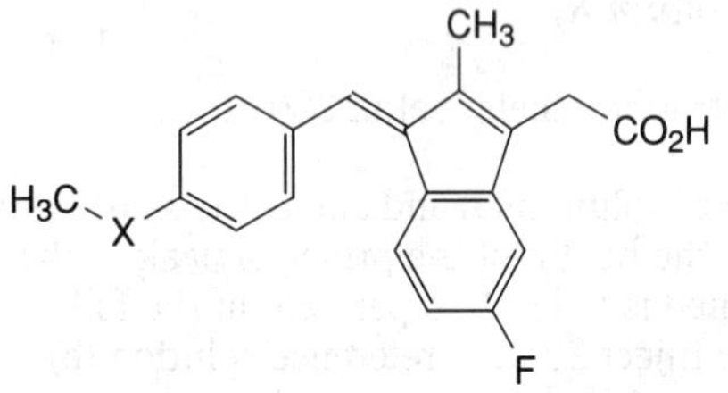

B. X = SO_2: (*Z*)-[5-fluoro-2-methyl-1-[4-(methylsulphonyl)benzylidene]-1*H*-inden-3-yl]acetic acid,

C. X = S: (*Z*)-[5-fluoro-2-methyl-1-[4-methylsulphanyl)benzylidene]-1*H*-inden-3-yl]acetic acid.

01/2005:0953

SULPHUR FOR EXTERNAL USE

Sulfur ad usum externum

S A_r 32.07

DEFINITION

Sulphur contains not less than 99.0 per cent and not more than the equivalent of 101.0 per cent of S.

CHARACTERS

A yellow powder, practically insoluble in water, soluble in carbon disulphide, slightly soluble in vegetable oils. The size of most of the particles is not greater than 20 µm and that of almost all the particles is not greater than 40 µm.

It melts at about 120 °C.

IDENTIFICATION

A. Heated in the presence of air, it burns with a blue flame, emitting sulphur dioxide which changes the colour of moistened *blue litmus paper R* to red.

B. Heat 0.1 g with 0.5 ml of *bromine water R* until decolourised. Add 5 ml of *water R* and filter. The solution gives reaction (a) of sulphates (*2.3.1*).

TESTS

Solution S. To 5 g add 50 ml of *carbon dioxide-free water R* prepared from *distilled water R*. Allow to stand for 30 min with frequent shaking and filter.

Appearance of solution. Solution S is colourless (*2.2.2, Method II*).

Odour (*2.3.4*). The substance to be examined has no perceptible odour of hydrogen sulphide.

Acidity or alkalinity. To 5 ml of solution S add 0.1 ml of *phenolphthalein solution R1*. The solution is colourless. Add 0.2 ml of *0.01 M sodium hydroxide*. The solution is red. Add 0.3 ml of *0.01 M hydrochloric acid*. The solution is colourless. Add 0.15 ml of *methyl red solution R*. The solution is orange-red.

Chlorides (*2.4.4*). Dilute 5 ml of solution S to 15 ml with *water R*. The solution complies with the limit test for chlorides (100 ppm).

Sulphates (*2.4.13*). 15 ml of solution S complies with the limit test for sulphates (100 ppm).

Sulphides. To 10 ml of solution S add 2 ml of *buffer solution pH 3.5 R* and 1 ml of a freshly prepared 1.6 g/l solution of *lead nitrate R* in *carbon dioxide-free water R*. Shake. After 1 min any colour in the solution is not more intense than that in a reference solution prepared at the same time using 1 ml of *lead standard solution (10 ppm Pb) R*, 9 ml of *carbon dioxide-free water R*, 2 ml of *buffer solution pH 3.5 R* and 1.2 ml of *thioacetamide reagent R*.

Sulphated ash (*2.4.14*). Not more than 0.2 per cent, determined on 1.0 g.

ASSAY

Carry out the oxygen-flask method (*2.5.10*), using 60.0 mg of the substance to be examined in a 1000 ml combustion flask. Absorb the combustion products in a mixture of 5 ml of *dilute hydrogen peroxide solution R* and 10 ml of *water R*. Heat to boiling, boil gently for 2 min and cool. Using 0.2 ml of *phenolphthalein solution R* as indicator, titrate with *0.1 M sodium hydroxide* until the colour changes from colourless to red. Carry out a blank titration under the same conditions.

1 ml of *0.1 M sodium hydroxide* is equivalent to 1.603 mg of S.

STORAGE

Store protected from light.

01/2005:1572

SULPHURIC ACID

Acidum sulfuricum

H_2SO_4 M_r 98.1

DEFINITION

Sulphuric acid contains not less than 95.0 per cent *m/m* and not more than 100.5 per cent *m/m* of H_2SO_4.

CHARACTERS

A colourless, oily liquid, very hygroscopic, miscible with water and with alcohol producing intense heat.

The relative density is about 1.84.

IDENTIFICATION

A. Carefully add 1 ml to 100 ml of *water R*. The solution is strongly acid (*2.2.4*).

B. The solution obtained in identification test A gives reaction (a) of sulphates (*2.3.1*).

TESTS

Appearance of solution. Carefully pour, while cooling, 5 ml into 30 ml of *water R* and dilute to 50 ml with the same solvent. The solution is clear (*2.2.1*) and colourless (*2.2.2, Method II*).

Chlorides (*2.4.4*). Mix carefully, while cooling, 3.3 g with 30 ml of *water R*. Neutralise with *ammonia R* and dilute to 50 ml with *water R*. 15 ml of the solution complies with the limit test for chlorides (50 ppm).

Nitrates. Add 5 ml to 5 ml of *water R*. Cool to room temperature and add 0.5 ml of *indigo carmine solution R*. The blue colour persists for at least 1 min.

Arsenic (*2.4.2*). Mix, while cooling, 1 g with 20 ml of *water R* and dilute to 25 ml with the same solvent. The solution complies with limit test A for arsenic (1 ppm).

Iron (*2.4.9*). Cautiously evaporate 10.0 g and ignite to dull redness. Dissolve the ignition residue in 1 ml of *dilute hydrochloric acid R* with gentle heating and dilute to 25 ml with *water R*. Dilute 1 ml of the solution to 10 ml with *water R*. The solution complies with the limit test for iron (25 ppm).

Heavy metals (*2.4.8*). 4.0 g complies with limit test F for heavy metals (5 ppm). Prepare the standard using 2 ml of *lead standard solution (10 ppm Pb) R*.

ASSAY

Weigh accurately a ground-glass-stoppered flask containing 30 ml of *water R*. Introduce 0.2 ml of the acid, cool and weigh again. Titrate with *1 M sodium hydroxide*, determining the end-point potentiometrically (*2.2.20*).

1 ml of *1 M sodium hydroxide* is equivalent to 49.04 mg of H_2SO_4.

STORAGE

Store in an airtight container.

01/2005:1045

SULPIRIDE

Sulpiridum

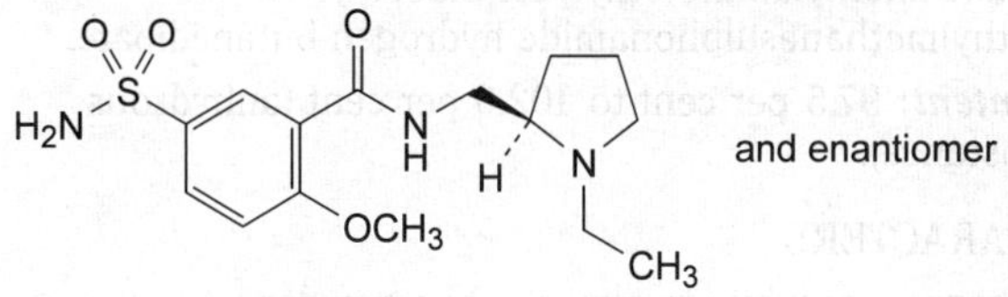

$C_{15}H_{23}N_3O_4S$ M_r 341.4

DEFINITION

Sulpiride contains not less than 98.5 per cent and not more than the equivalent of 101.0 per cent of (*RS*)-*N*-[(1-ethylpyrrolidin-2-yl)methyl]-2-methoxy-5-sulphamoylbenzamide, calculated with reference to the dried substance.

CHARACTERS

A white or almost white, crystalline powder, practically insoluble in water, sparingly soluble in methanol, slightly soluble in alcohol and in methylene chloride. It dissolves in dilute solutions of mineral acids and alkali hydroxides.

IDENTIFICATION

First identification: A, B.

Second identification: A, C, D.

A. Melting point (*2.2.14*): 177 °C to 181 °C.

B. Examine by infrared absorption spectrophotometry (*2.2.24*), comparing with the spectrum obtained with *sulpiride CRS*. Examine the substances prepared as discs.

C. Examine the chromatograms obtained in test A for related substances (see Tests) in ultraviolet light at 254 nm. The principal spot in the chromatogram obtained with test solution (b) is similar in position and size to the principal spot in the chromatogram obtained with reference solution (a).

D. To about 1 mg in a porcelain dish, add 0.5 ml of *sulphuric acid R* and 0.05 ml of *formaldehyde solution R*. Examined in ultraviolet light at 365 nm, the solution shows blue fluorescence.

TESTS

Appearance of solution. Dissolve 1.0 g in *dilute acetic acid R* and dilute to 10 ml with the same acid. The solution is clear (*2.2.1*) and not more intensely coloured than reference solution Y_6 (*2.2.2, Method I*).

Related substances

A. Examine by thin-layer chromatography (*2.2.27*), using *silica gel* HF_{254} *R* as the coating substance.

Test solution (a). Dissolve 0.20 g in *methanol R* and dilute to 10 ml with the same solvent.

Test solution (b). Dilute 1 ml of test solution (a) to 10 ml with *methanol R*.

Reference solution (a). Dissolve 20 mg of *sulpiride CRS* in *methanol R* and dilute to 10 ml with the same solvent.

Reference solution (b). Dissolve 5 mg of *sulpiride impurity A CRS* in *methanol R* and dilute to 25 ml with the same solvent.

Reference solution (c). Dilute 1.0 ml of reference solution (b) to 10 ml with *methanol R*.

Apply to the plate 10 µl of each solution. Develop over a path of 10 cm using a mixture of 2 volumes of *concentrated ammonia R*, 10 volumes of *dioxan R*, 14 volumes of *methanol R* and 90 volumes of *methylene chloride R*. Allow the plate to dry in air. Examine in ultraviolet light at 254 nm for identification test C and then spray with *ninhydrin solution R*. Heat at 100-105 °C for 15 min. Examine in daylight. Any spot in the chromatogram obtained with test solution (a) corresponding to the principal spot in the chromatogram obtained with reference solution (b) is not more intense than the spot in the chromatogram obtained with reference solution (c) (0.1 per cent).

B. Examine by liquid chromatography (*2.2.29*).

Test solution. Dissolve 0.100 g in the mobile phase and dilute to 100.0 ml with the mobile phase.

Reference solution (a). Dilute 3.0 ml of the test solution to 100.0 ml with the mobile phase. Dilute 1.0 ml of the solution to 10.0 ml with the mobile phase.

Reference solution (b). Dissolve 10 mg of *sulpiride CRS* and 10 mg of *sulpiride impurity B CRS* in the mobile phase and dilute to 100.0 ml with the same solvent.

The chromatography may be carried out using:

- a column 0.25 m long and 4.6 mm in internal diameter, packed with *octylsilyl silica gel for chromatography R* (5 µm) in spherical micro-particles,
- as mobile phase at a flow rate of 1.5 ml/min a mixture of 10 volumes of *acetonitrile R*, 10 volumes of *methanol R* and 80 volumes of a solution containing 6.8 g/l of *potassium dihydrogen phosphate R* and 1 g/l of *sodium octanesulphonate R*, adjusted to pH 3.3 using *phosphoric acid R*,
- as detector a spectrophotometer set at 240 nm,
- a loop injector.

Adjust the sensitivity of the detector so that the height of the principal peak in the chromatogram obtained with reference solution (a) is not less than 5 per cent of the full scale of the recorder. Inject 10 µl of reference solution (b). The test is not valid unless in the chromatogram obtained the resolution between the two principal peaks is at least 2.5. Inject separately 10 µl of the test solution and 10 µl of reference solution (a). Continue the chromatography for 2.5 times the retention time of sulpiride. In the chromatogram obtained with the test solution, the sum of the areas of any peaks, apart from the principal peak, is not greater than the area of the peak in the chromatogram obtained with reference solution (a) (0.3 per cent).

Chlorides (*2.4.4*). Shake 1.0 g with 20 ml of *water R*. Filter through a sintered-glass filter (40). To 10 ml of the solution add 5 ml of *water R*. The solution complies with the limit test for chlorides (100 ppm).

Iron (*2.4.9*). Ignite 1.0 g in a silica crucible. To the residue add 1 ml of *1 M hydrochloric acid*, 3 ml of *water R* and 0.1 ml of *nitric acid R*. Heat on a water-bath for a few minutes. Place the solution in a test-tube. Rinse the crucible with 4 ml of *water R*. Collect the rinsings in the test-tube and dilute to 10 ml with *water R*. The solution complies with the limit test for iron (10 ppm).

Heavy metals (*2.4.8*). 1.0 g complies with limit test C for heavy metals (10 ppm). Prepare the standard using 1 ml of *lead standard solution (10 ppm Pb) R*.

Loss on drying (*2.2.32*). Not more than 0.5 per cent, determined on 1.000 g by drying in an oven at 100-105 °C.

Sulphated ash (*2.4.14*). Not more than 0.1 per cent, determined on 1.0 g.

ASSAY

Dissolve 0.250 g in 80 ml of *anhydrous acetic acid R*. Titrate with *0.1 M perchloric acid*, determining the end-point potentiometrically (*2.2.20*).

1 ml of *0.1 M perchloric acid* is equivalent to 34.14 mg of $C_{15}H_{23}N_3O_4S$.

IMPURITIES

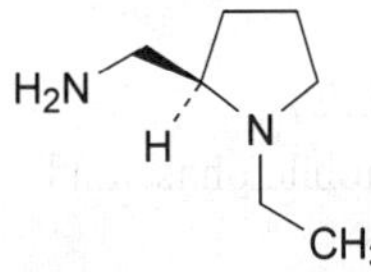

A. [(2*RS*)-1-ethylpyrrolidin-2-yl]methanamine,

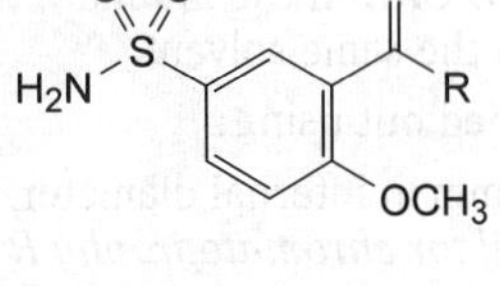

B. R = O-CH_3: methyl 2-methoxy-5-sulphamoylbenzoate,

C. R = O-C_2H_5: ethyl 2-methoxy-5-sulphamoylbenzoate,

D. R = OH: 2-methoxy-5-sulphamoylbenzoic acid,

E. R = NH_2: 2-methoxy-5-sulphamoylbenzamide,

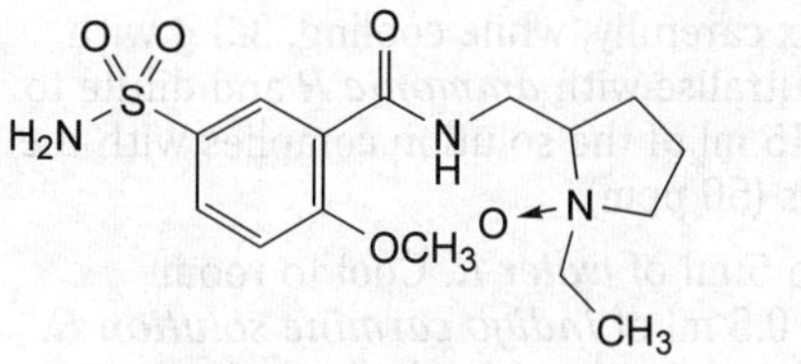

F. 1-ethyl-2-[[(2-methoxy-5-sulphamoylbenzoyl)amino]methyl]pyrrolidine 1-oxide,

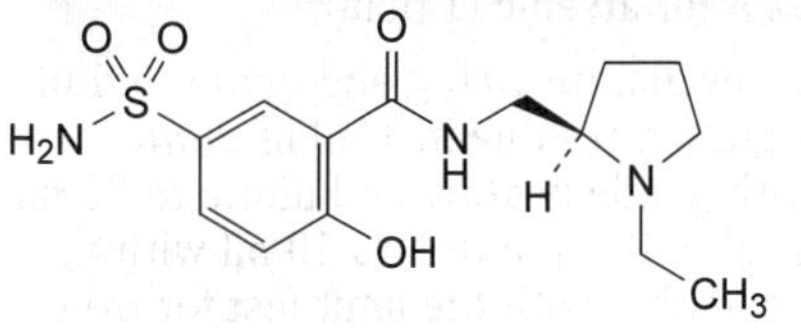

G. (*RS*)-*N*-[(1-ethylpyrrolidin-2-yl)methyl]-2-hydroxy-5-sulphamoylbenzamide.

01/2005:1573

SUMATRIPTAN SUCCINATE

Sumatriptani succinas

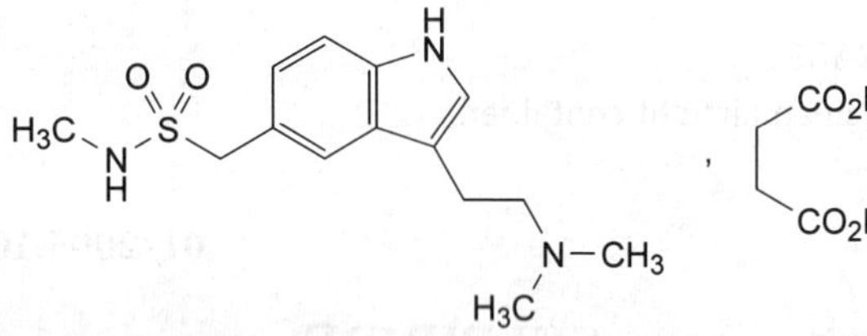

$C_{18}H_{27}N_3O_6S$ M_r 413.5

DEFINITION

[3-[2-(Dimethylamino)ethyl]-1*H*-indol-5-yl]-*N*-methylmethanesulphonamide hydrogen butanedioate.

Content: 97.5 per cent to 102.0 per cent (anhydrous substance).

CHARACTERS

Appearance: white to almost white powder.

Solubility: freely soluble in water, sparingly soluble in methanol, practically insoluble in methylene chloride.

IDENTIFICATION

Infrared absorption spectrophotometry (*2.2.24*).

Preparation: discs.

Comparison: *sumatriptan succinate CRS*.

TESTS

Solution S. Dissolve 1.0 g in *carbon dioxide-free water R* and dilute to 25.0 ml with the same solvent.

pH (*2.2.3*): 4.5 to 5.3.

Dilute 2.5 ml of solution S to 10 ml with *carbon dioxide-free water R*.

Absorbance (*2.2.25*): maximum 0.10, measured at 440 nm on solution S.

Impurity A and impurity H. Liquid chromatography (*2.2.29*).

Test solution. Dissolve 30.0 mg of the substance to be examined in the mobile phase and dilute to 10.0 ml with the mobile phase.

Reference solution (a). Dissolve 2 mg of *sumatriptan impurity A CRS* in the mobile phase, add 1 ml of the test solution and dilute to 100 ml with the mobile phase. Dilute 1 ml to 10 ml with the mobile phase.

Reference solution (b). Dilute 1.0 ml of the test solution to 100.0 ml with the mobile phase. Dilute 1.0 ml to 10.0 ml with the mobile phase.

Reference solution (c). Dissolve 3 mg of *sumatriptan for system suitability CRS* in the mobile phase and dilute to 1 ml with the mobile phase.

Column:

- *size*: l = 0.25 m, Ø = 4.6 mm,
- *stationary phase*: *silica gel for chromatography R* (5 µm).

Mobile phase: mix 10 volumes of a 771 g/l solution of *ammonium acetate R* and 90 volumes of *methanol R.*

Flow rate: 2.0 ml/min.

Detection: spectrophotometer at 282 nm.

Injection: 20 µl.

Run time: 5 times the retention time of sumatriptan.

System suitability:

- *resolution*: minimum of 1.5 between the peaks due to sumatriptan and to impurity A in the chromatogram obtained with reference solution (a),
- the chromatogram obtained with reference solution (c) is similar to the chromatogram provided with *sumatriptan for system suitability CRS.*

Limits:

- *impurity A*: not more than 6 times the area of the principal peak in the chromatogram obtained with reference solution (b) (0.6 per cent),
- *impurity H*: not more than 3 times the area of the principal peak in the chromatogram obtained with reference solution (b) (0.3 per cent).

Related substances. Liquid chromatography (*2.2.29*).

Solution A. Dissolve 2.925 g of *sodium dihydrogen phosphate R* in 600 ml of *water R,* adjust to pH 6.5 with *strong sodium hydroxide solution R,* dilute to 750 ml with *water R,* add 250 ml of *acetonitrile R* and mix.

Test solution (a). Dissolve 30.0 mg of the substance to be examined in the mobile phase and dilute to 10.0 ml with the mobile phase.

Test solution (b). Dissolve 15.0 mg of the substance to be examined in solution A and dilute to 100.0 ml with solution A.

Reference solution (a). Dissolve 2 mg of *sumatriptan impurity C CRS* in the mobile phase, add 1 ml of the test solution and dilute to 100 ml with the mobile phase. Dilute 1 ml to 10 ml with the mobile phase.

Reference solution (b). Dilute 1.0 ml of the test solution to 100.0 ml with the mobile phase. Dilute 1.0 ml to 10.0 ml with the mobile phase.

Reference solution (c). Dissolve 30 mg of *sumatriptan impurity mixture CRS* in the mobile phase and dilute to 10 ml with the mobile phase.

Reference solution (d). Dissolve 2 mg of *sumatriptan impurity D CRS* in the mobile phase and dilute to 100 ml with the mobile phase. Dilute 1 ml to 10 ml with the mobile phase.

Reference solution (e). Dissolve 15.0 mg of *sumatriptan succinate CRS* in solution A and dilute to 100.0 ml with solution A.

Reference solution (f). Dissolve 3 mg of *sumatriptan impurity C CRS* in solution A, add 40 ml of reference solution (e) and dilute to 100 ml with solution A.

Column:

- *size*: l = 0.25 m, Ø = 4 mm,
- *stationary phase*: *octadecylsilyl silica gel for chromatography R* (5 µm).

Mobile phase: mix 25 volumes of *acetonitrile R* with 75 volumes of a solution prepared as follows: dissolve 0.970 g of *dibutylamine R,* 0.735 g of *phosphoric acid R* and 2.93 g of *sodium dihydrogen phosphate R* in 750 ml of *water R,* adjust to pH 6.5 with *strong sodium hydroxide solution R* and dilute to 1000 ml with *water R.*

Flow rate: 1.5 ml/min.

Detection: spectrophotometer at 282 nm.

Injection: 10 µl; inject test solution (a) and reference solutions (a), (b), (c) and (d).

Run time: 4 times the retention time of sumatriptan.

System suitability:

- *resolution*: minimum of 1.5 between the peaks due to sumatriptan and to impurity C in the chromatogram obtained with reference solution (a),
- the chromatogram obtained with reference solution (c) shows 5 clearly separated peaks.

Limits:

The chromatogram obtained with reference solution (c) shows 5 peaks: 1 major peak due to sumatriptan, 3 peaks of about equal area due to impurities B, C and D and 1 peak due to impurity E with an area of about twice the area of the peaks due to impurities B, C or D.

Determine the retention times of impurities B, C, D and E using the chromatograms obtained with reference solutions (a), (c) and (d).

- *impurities B, C, D*: for each impurity, not more than 5 times the area of the principal peak in the chromatogram obtained with reference solution (b) (0.5 per cent),
- *impurity E or any other impurity*: for each impurity, not more than the area of the principal peak in the chromatogram obtained with reference solution (b) (0.1 per cent),
- *total*: not more than 6 times the area of the principal peak in the chromatogram obtained with reference solution (b) (0.6 per cent),
- *disregard limit*: 0.5 times the area of the principal peak in the chromatogram obtained with reference solution (b) (0.05 per cent).

Water (*2.5.12*): maximum 1.0 per cent, determined on 0.500 g.

Sulphated ash (*2.4.14*): maximum 0.1 per cent, determined on 1.0 g.

ASSAY

Liquid chromatography (*2.2.29*) as described in the test for related substances.

Injection: 10 µl; inject test solution (b) and reference solutions (e) and (f).

System suitability: reference solution (f):

- *resolution*: minimum of 1.5 between the peaks due to sumatriptan and to impurity C.

Calculate the percentage content of sumatriptan succinate using the chromatogram obtained with reference solution (e).

STORAGE

Protected from light.

IMPURITIES

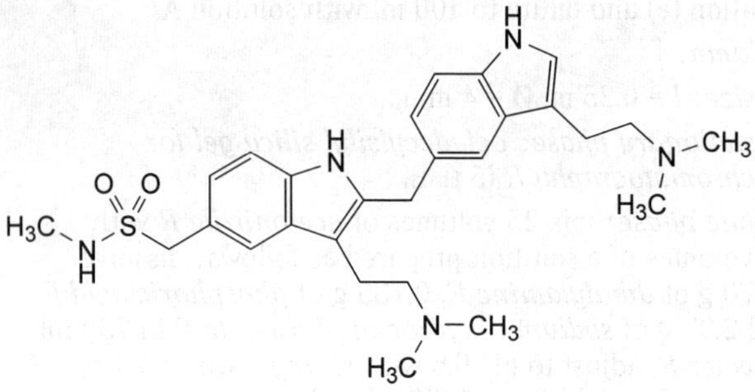

A. [3-[2-(dimethylamino)ethyl]-2-[[3-[2-(dimethylamino)ethyl]-1*H*-indol-5-yl]methyl]-1*H*-indol-5-yl]-*N*-methylmethanesulphonamide,

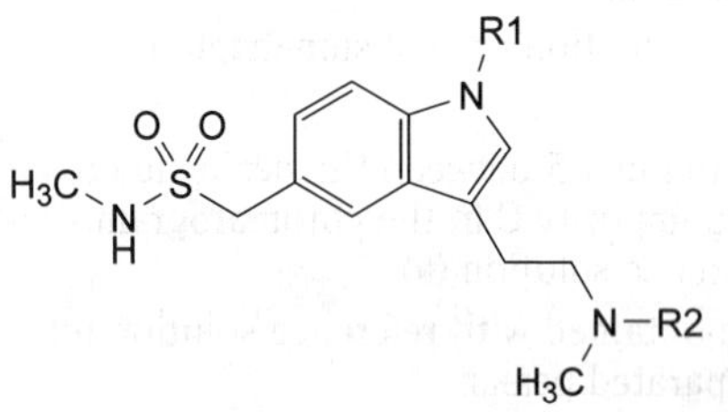

B. R1 = R2 = H: *N*-methyl[3-[2-(methylamino)ethyl]-1*H*-indol-5-yl]methanesulphonamide,

C. R1 = CH_2-OH, R2 = CH_3: [3-[2-(dimethylamino)ethyl]-1-(hydroxymethyl)-1*H*-indol-5-yl]-*N*-methylmethanesulphonamide,

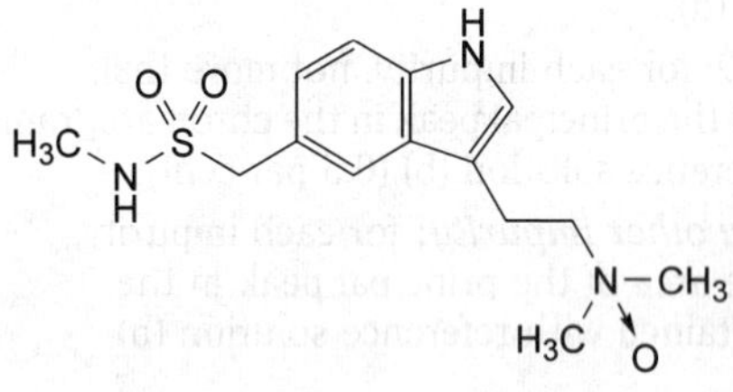

D. *N*,*N*-dimethyl-2-[5-[(methylsulphamoyl)methyl]-1*H*-indol-3-yl]ethanamine *N*-oxide,

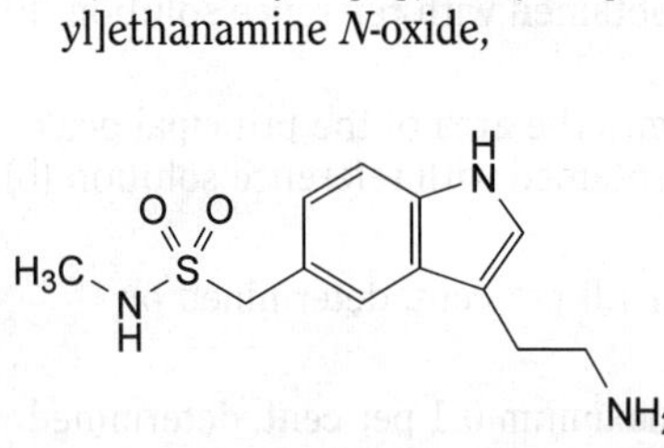

E. [3-(2-aminoethyl)-1*H*-indol-5-yl]-*N*-methylmethanesulphonamide,

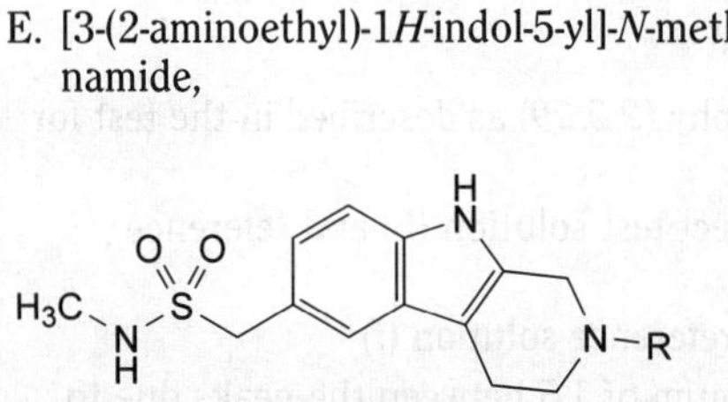

F. R = H: *N*-methyl(2,3,4,9-tetrahydro-1*H*-pyrido[3,4-*b*]indol-6-yl)methanesulphonamide,

G. R = CH_3: *N*-methyl(2-methyl-2,3,4,9-tetrahydro-1*H*-pyrido[3,4-*b*]indol-6-yl)methanesulphonamide,

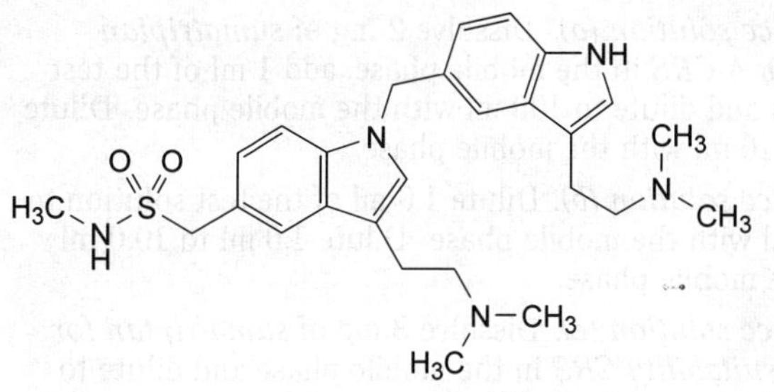

H. [3-[2-(dimethylamino)ethyl]-1-[[3-[2-(dimethylamino)ethyl]-1*H*-indol-5-yl]methyl]-1*H*-indol-5-yl]-*N*-methylmethanesulphonamide.

01/2005:1371

SUNFLOWER OIL, REFINED

Helianthi annui oleum raffinatum

DEFINITION

Sunflower oil is the fatty oil obtained from the seeds of *Helianthus annuus* L. by mechanical expression or by extraction. It is then refined. A suitable antioxidant may be added.

CHARACTERS

A clear, light yellow liquid, practically insoluble in water and in alcohol, miscible with light petroleum (bp: 40 °C to 60 °C).

It has a relative density of about 0.921 and a refractive index of about 1.474.

IDENTIFICATION

Carry out the identification of fatty oils by thin-layer chromatography (*2.3.2*). The chromatogram obtained is similar to the typical chromatogram for sunflower oil.

TESTS

Acid value (*2.5.1*). Not more than 0.5, determined on 10.0 g.

Peroxide value (*2.5.5*). Not more than 10.0.

Unsaponifiable matter (*2.5.7*). Not more than 1.5 per cent, determined on 5.0 g.

Alkaline impurities (*2.4.19*). It complies with the test for alkaline impurities in fatty oils.

Composition of fatty acids (*2.4.22, Method A*). The fatty-acid fraction of the oil has the following composition:

- *palmitic acid*: 4.0 per cent to 9.0 per cent,
- *stearic acid*: 1.0 per cent to 7.0 per cent,
- *oleic acid*: 14.0 per cent to 40.0 per cent,
- *linoleic acid*: 48.0 per cent to 74.0 per cent.

STORAGE

Store in an airtight, well-filled container, protected from light.

LABELLING

The label states:

- the name and concentration of any added antioxidant,
- whether the oil is obtained by mechanical expression or by extraction.

01/2005:0248

SUXAMETHONIUM CHLORIDE

Suxamethonii chloridum

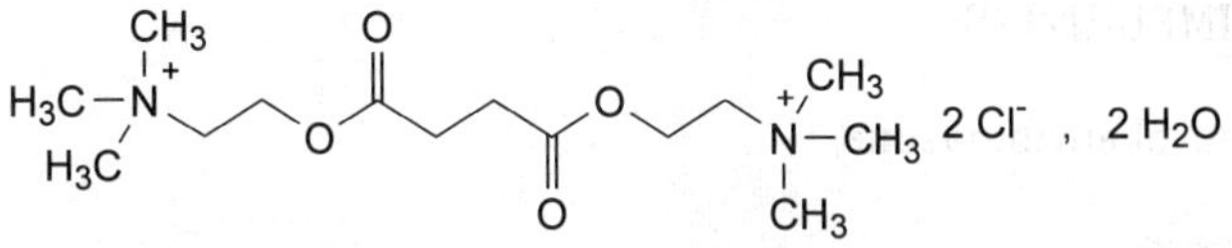

$C_{14}H_{30}Cl_2N_2O_4,2H_2O$ M_r 397.3

DEFINITION

Suxamethonium chloride contains not less than 98.0 per cent and not more than the equivalent of 102.0 per cent of 2,2′-[butanedioylbis(oxy)]bis(*N,N,N*-trimethylethanaminium) dichloride, calculated with reference to the anhydrous substance.

CHARACTERS

A white or almost white, crystalline powder, hygroscopic, freely soluble in water, slightly soluble in alcohol.

It melts at about 160 °C, determined without previous drying.

IDENTIFICATION

First identification: A, D.

Second identification: B, C, D.

A. Examine by infrared absorption spectrophotometry (*2.2.24*), comparing with the spectrum obtained with *suxamethonium chloride CRS*. Examine the substances prepared as discs.

B. To 1 ml of solution S (see Tests) add 9 ml of *water R*, 10 ml of *dilute sulphuric acid R* and 30 ml of *ammonium reineckate solution R*. A pink precipitate is formed. Allow to stand for 30 min, filter, wash with *water R*, with *alcohol R* and then with *ether R* and dry at 80 °C. The melting point (*2.2.14*) of the precipitate is 180 °C to 185 °C.

C. Dissolve about 25 mg in 1 ml of *water R* and add 0.1 ml of a 10 g/l solution of *cobalt chloride R* and 0.1 ml of *potassium ferrocyanide solution R*. A green colour is produced.

D. About 20 mg gives reaction (a) of chlorides (*2.3.1*).

TESTS

Solution S. Dissolve 1.0 g in *carbon dioxide-free water R* and dilute to 20 ml with the same solvent.

Appearance of solution. Solution S is clear (*2.2.1*). Dilute 4 ml of solution S to 10 ml with *water R*. The solution is colourless (*2.2.2, Method II*).

pH (*2.2.3*). Dilute 1 ml of solution S to 10 ml with *carbon dioxide-free water R*. The pH of the solution is 4.0 to 5.0.

Choline chloride. Examine by thin-layer chromatography (*2.2.27*), using *cellulose for chromatography R1* as the coating substance.

Test solution. Dissolve 0.4 g of the substance to be examined in *methanol R* and dilute to 10 ml with the same solvent.

Reference solution. Dissolve 0.4 g of *suxamethonium chloride CRS* and 2 mg of *choline chloride R* in *methanol R* and dilute to 10 ml with the same solvent.

Apply to the plate 5 µl of each solution. Prepare the mobile phase as follows: shake together for 10 min, 10 volumes of *anhydrous formic acid R*, 40 volumes of *water R* and 50 volumes of *butanol R*; allow to stand and use the upper layer. Develop over a path of 15 cm. Dry the plate in a current of air and spray with *potassium iodobismuthate solution R*. Any spot in the chromatogram obtained with the test solution, apart from the principal spot, is not more intense than the spot corresponding to choline chloride in the chromatogram obtained with the reference solution (0.5 per cent). The test is not valid unless the chromatogram obtained with the reference solution shows two clearly separated spots.

Water (*2.5.12*). 8.0 per cent to 10.0 per cent, determined on 0.30 g by the semi-micro determination of water.

Sulphated ash (*2.4.14*). Not more than 0.1 per cent, determined on 1.0 g.

ASSAY

Dissolve 0.150 g in 50 ml of *acetic anhydride R*. Titrate with *0.1 M perchloric acid*, determining the end-point potentiometrically (*2.2.20*).

1 ml of *0.1 M perchloric acid* is equivalent to 18.07 mg of $C_{14}H_{30}Cl_2N_2O_4$.

STORAGE

Store in an airtight container, protected from light.

01/2005:1574

SUXIBUZONE

Suxibuzonum

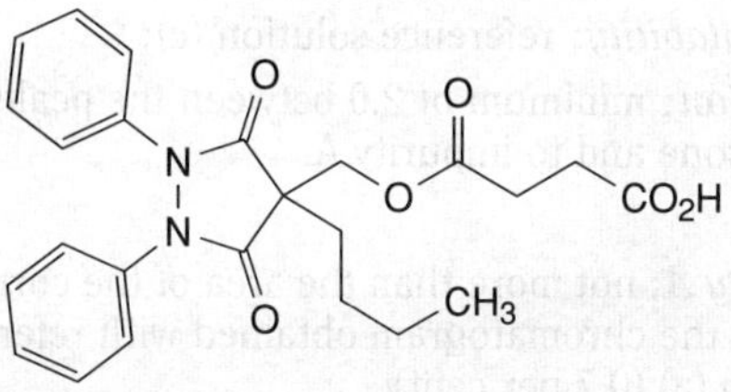

$C_{24}H_{26}N_2O_6$ M_r 438.5

DEFINITION

4-[(4-Butyl-3,5-dioxo-1,2-diphenylpyrazolidin-4-yl)methoxy]-4-oxobutanoic acid.

Content: 99.0 per cent to 101.0 per cent (dried substance).

CHARACTERS

Appearance: white, crystalline powder.

Solubility: practically insoluble in water, freely soluble in acetone, soluble in alcohol, practically insoluble in cyclohexane.

IDENTIFICATION

Infrared absorption spectrophotometry (*2.2.24*).

Comparison: *suxibuzone CRS*.

TESTS

Appearance of solution. The solution is clear (*2.2.1*) and colourless (*2.2.2, Method II*).

Dissolve 1 g in *ethanol R* and dilute to 20 ml with the same solvent.

Related substances. Liquid chromatography (*2.2.29*).

Test solution. Dissolve 0.10 g of the substance to be examined in *acetonitrile R* and dilute to 25.0 ml with the same solvent.

Reference solution (a). Dissolve 2.8 mg of *phenylbutazone CRS* (impurity A of suxibuzone), 2.8 mg of *suxibuzone impurity B CRS* and 2.8 mg of

Monographs Q-S

suxibuzone impurity C CRS in *acetonitrile R* and dilute to 10.0 ml with the same solvent. Dilute 1.0 ml of the solution to 10.0 ml with *acetonitrile R*.

Reference solution (b). Dissolve 4 mg of *phenylbutazone CRS* (impurity A of suxibuzone) in *acetonitrile R* and dilute to 100.0 ml with the same solvent. Dilute 1.0 ml of the solution to 10.0 ml with *acetonitrile R*.

Reference solution (c). Dissolve 10 mg of *phenylbutazone CRS* (impurity A of suxibuzone) in *acetonitrile R* and dilute to 25.0 ml with the same solvent. Mix 10.0 ml of this solution with 1.0 ml of the test solution and dilute the mixture to 25.0 ml with *acetonitrile R*.

Column:
- *size*: *l* = 0.125 m, Ø = 4.0 mm,
- *stationary phase*: *octadecylsilyl silica gel for chromatography R* (5 µm).

Mobile phase: mix 44 volumes of *acetonitrile R* and 56 volumes of a solution prepared as follows: dissolve 6.7 g of *citric acid R* and 2.4 g of *tris(hydroxymethyl)aminomethane R* in 950 ml of *water R*, adjust to pH 3.0 with *citric acid R* and dilute to 1000 ml with *water R*.

Flow rate: 1 ml/min.

Detection: spectrophotometer at 250 nm.

Injection: 10 µl.

Relative retention with reference to suxibuzone (retention time = about 7 min): impurity C = 0.7; impurity A = 1.4; impurity B = 3.3.

System suitability: reference solution (c):
- *resolution*: minimum of 2.0 between the peaks due to suxibuzone and to impurity A.

Limits:
- *impurity A*: not more than the area of the corresponding peak in the chromatogram obtained with reference solution (a) (0.7 per cent),
- *impurity B*: not more than the area of the corresponding peak in the chromatogram obtained with reference solution (a) (0.7 per cent),
- *impurity C*: not more than the area of the corresponding peak in the chromatogram obtained with reference solution (a) (0.7 per cent),
- *any other impurity*: not more than the area of the principal peak in the chromatogram obtained with reference solution (b) (0.1 per cent),
- *total*: not more than 10 times the area of the principal peak in the chromatogram obtained with reference solution (b) (1.0 per cent),
- *disregard limit*: 0.1 times the area of the peak due to impurity A in the chromatogram obtained with reference solution (a) (0.07 per cent).

Heavy metals (*2.4.8*): maximum 10 ppm.

2.0 g complies with limit test C. Prepare the standard using 2 ml of *lead standard solution (10 ppm Pb) R*.

Loss on drying (*2.2.32*): maximum 0.5 per cent, determined on 1.000 g by drying in an oven *in vacuo* at 60 °C.

Sulphated ash (*2.4.14*): maximum 0.1 per cent, determined on 1.0 g.

ASSAY

Dissolve 0.400 g in previously neutralised *ethanol R* and dilute to 10 ml with the same solvent. Carry out a potentiometric titration (*2.2.20*) using *0.1 M sodium hydroxide*.

1 ml of *0.1 M sodium hydroxide* is equivalent to 43.85 mg of $C_{24}H_{26}N_2O_6$.

STORAGE

Protected from light.

IMPURITIES

A. phenylbutazone,

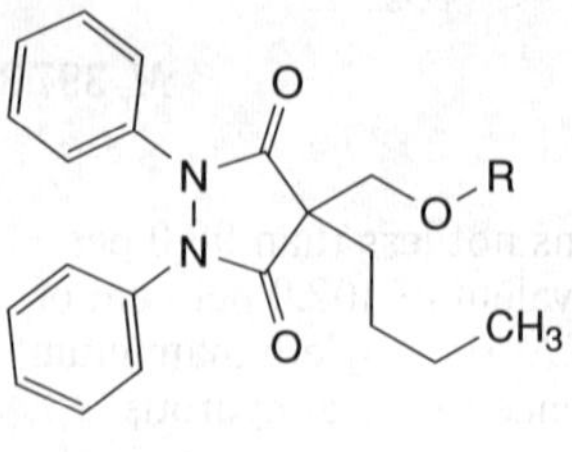

B. R = $CO\text{-}CH_2\text{-}CH_2\text{-}CO\text{-}O\text{-}CH_2\text{-}CH_3$: (4-butyl-3,5-dioxo-1,2-diphenylpyrazolidin-4-yl)methyl ethyl butanedioate,

C. R = H: 4-butyl-4-(hydroxymethyl)-1,2-diphenyl-1,2-dihydro-4*H*-pyrazole-3,5-dione.

01/2005:1811

SWEET ORANGE OIL

Aurantii dulcis aetheroleum

DEFINITION

Essential oil obtained without heating, by suitable mechanical treatment from the fresh peel of the fruit of *Citrus sinensis* (L.) Osbeck (*Citrus aurantium* L. var. *dulcis* L.). A suitable antioxidant may be added.

CHARACTERS

Appearance: clear, pale yellow to orange, mobile liquid, which may become cloudy when chilled.

It has a characteristic odour of fresh orange peel.

IDENTIFICATION

First identification: B.

Second identification: A.

A. Thin-layer chromatography (*2.2.27*).

Examine the chromatograms obtained in the test for bergapten.

Results A: see below the sequence of the zones present in the chromatograms obtained with the reference solution and the test solution.

Top of the plate	
———	———
Bergaptene: a greenish-yellow fluorescent zone	
———	———
	Many blue fluorescent zones
Reference solution	**Test solution**

Results B: see below the sequence of the zones present in the chromatograms obtained with the reference solution and the test solution.

Monographs Q-S

Top of the plate	
	A brown fluorescent zone
Linalyl acetate: a brownish-orange fluorescent zone	A faint brownish-orange fluorescent zone (linalyl acetate)
_______	_______
	Many orange fluorescent zones
Linalol: a brownish-orange fluorescent zone	A brownish-orange fluorescent zone (linalol)
Bergaptene: a faint greenish-yellow fluorescent zone	
	Many brownish-orange fluorescent zones
_______	_______
	Many blue fluorescent zones
Reference solution	**Test solution**

B. Examine the chromatograms obtained in the test for chromatographic profile.

Results: the characteristic peaks in the chromatogram obtained with the test solution are similar in retention time to those in the chromatogram obtained with the reference solution.

TESTS

Relative density (*2.2.5*): 0.842 to 0.850.

Refractive index (*2.2.6*): 1.470 to 1.476.

Optical rotation (*2.2.7*): + 94° to + 99°.

Peroxide value (*2.5.5, Method B*): maximum 20.

Fatty oils and resinified essential oils (*2.8.7*). It complies with the test for fatty oils and resinified essential oils.

Bergaptene. Thin-layer chromatography (*2.2.27*).

Test solution. Dilute 0.2 ml of the substance to be examined in 1 ml of *alcohol R*.

Reference solution. Dissolve 2 mg of *bergaptene R*, 10 µl of *linalol R* and 20 µl of *linalyl acetate R* in 10 ml of *alcohol R*.

Plate: *TLC silica gel plate R*.

Mobile phase: *ethyl acetate R, toluene R* (15:85 *V/V*).

Application: 10 µl, as bands.

Development: over a path of 15 cm.

Drying: in air.

Detection A: examine in ultraviolet light at 365 nm.

Results A: the chromatogram obtained with the test solution shows no greenish-yellow fluorescent zone present in the chromatogram obtained with the reference solution.

Detection B: spray with *anisaldehyde solution R* and heat at 100-105 °C for 10 min; examine the plate in ultraviolet light at 365 nm.

Chromatographic profile. Gas chromatography (*2.2.28*): use the normalisation procedure.

Test solution. Dilute 300 µl of the substance to be examined to 1 ml with *acetone R*.

Reference solution (a). Dilute 10 µl of *α-pinene R*, 10 µl of *β-pinene R*, 10 µl of *sabinene R*, 20 µl of *β-myrcene R*, 800 µl of *limonene R*, 10 µl of *octanal*, 10 µl of *decanal R*, 10 µl of *linalol R*, 10 µl of *citral R* (composed of neral and geranial) and 10 µl of *valencene R* in 1 ml of *acetone R*.

Reference solution (b). Dissolve 5 µl of *β-pinene R* in 10 ml of *acetone R*. Dilute 0.5 ml to 10 ml with *acetone R*.

Column:
- *material*: fused silica,
- *size*: l = 30 m, Ø = 0.53 mm,
- *stationary phase*: *macrogol 20 000 R* (film thickness 1 µm).

Carrier gas: *helium for chromatography R*.

Flow rate: 1 ml/min.

Split ratio: 1:100.

Temperature:

	Time (min)	Temperature (°C)
Column	0 - 6	50
	6 - 31	50 → 150
	31 - 41	150 → 180
	41 - 55	180
Injection port		250
Detector		250

Detection: flame ionisation.

Injection: 0.5 µl.

Elution order: order indicated in the composition of reference solution (a). Record the retention times of these substances.

System suitability: reference solution (a)
- *resolution*: minimum 3.9 between the peaks due to β-pinene and sabinene and minimum 1.5 between the peaks due to valencene and geranial.

Using the retention times determined from the chromatogram obtained with reference solution (a), locate the components of reference solution (a) in the chromatogram obtained with the test solution.

Determine the percentage content of these components. The limits are within the following ranges:
- *α-pinene*: 0.4 per cent to 0.6 per cent,
- *β-pinene*: 0.02 per cent to 0.3 per cent,
- *sabinene*: 0.2 per cent to 1.1 per cent,
- *β-myrcene*: 1.7 per cent to 2.5 per cent,
- *limonene*: 92.0 per cent to 97.0 per cent,
- *octanal*: 0.1 per cent to 0.4 per cent,
- *decanal*: 0.1 per cent to 0.4 per cent,
- *linalol*: 0.2 per cent to 0.7 per cent,
- *neral*: 0.02 per cent to 0.10 per cent,
- *valencene*: 0.02 per cent to 0.5 per cent,
- *geranial*: 0.03 per cent to 0.20 per cent.

Disregard limit: area of the peak in the chromatogram obtained with reference solution (b) (0.01 per cent).

Residue on evaporation: 1.0 per cent to 5.0 per cent.

Evaporate 5.0 g to dryness on a water-bath and dry at 100-105 °C for 4 h.

STORAGE

In a well-filled, airtight container, protected from light, at a temperature not exceeding 25 °C.

LABELLING

The label states the name and concentration of any added antioxidant.

T

01/2005:0438

TALC

Talcum

DEFINITION

Talc is a powdered, selected, natural, hydrated magnesium silicate. Pure talc has the formula $[Mg_3Si_4O_{10}(OH)_2]$; M_r 379.3]. It may contain variable amounts of associated minerals among which chlorites (hydrated aluminium and magnesium silicates), magnesite (magnesium carbonate), calcite (calcium carbonate) and dolomite (calcium and magnesium carbonate) are predominant.

PRODUCTION

Talc derived from deposits that are known to contain associated asbestos is not suitable for pharmaceutical use. The manufacturer is responsible for demonstrating by the test for amphiboles and serpentines that the product is free from asbestos. The presence of amphiboles and of serpentines is revealed by X-ray diffraction or by infrared spectrophotometry (see A and B). If detected, the specific morphological criteria of asbestos are investigated by a suitable method of optical microscopy to determine whether tremolite asbestos or chrysotile is present, as described below.

A. Examine by infrared spectrophotometry (*2.2.24*). In the range 740 cm^{-1} to 760 cm^{-1} using scale expansion, any absorption band at 758 ± 1 cm^{-1} may indicate the presence of tremolite or of chlorite. If the absorption band remains after ignition of the substance at 850 °C for at least 30 min, it indicates the presence of the tremolite. In the range 600 cm^{-1} to 650 cm^{-1} using scale expansion, any absorption band or shoulder may indicate the presence of serpentines. Examine the substance prepared as discs using *potassium bromide R*.

B. Examine by X-ray diffraction employing the following conditions:
   - Cu Kα monochromatic 40 kV radiation, 24 mA to 30 mA,
   - incident slit: 1°,
   - detection slit: 0.2°,
   - goniometer speed: 1/10° 2θ/min,
   - scanning range: 10° to 13° 2θ and 24° to 26° 2θ,
   - the sample is not oriented.

   Place the sample on the sample holder; pack and smooth its surface with a polished glass microscope slide. Record the diffractograms.

   The presence of amphiboles is detected by a diffraction peak at 10.5 ± 0.1° 2θ, the presence of serpentines is detected by diffraction peaks at 24.3 ± 0.1° 2θ and at 12.1 ± 0.1° 2θ.

   If, by one of the 2 methods, amphiboles and/or serpentine are detected, examine by a suitable method of optical microscopy to determine the asbestos character.

   Examined by optical microscopy, the presence of asbestos is shown if the following criteria are met:
   - a range of length to width ratios of 20:1 to 100:1, or higher for fibres longer than 5 μm,
   - capability of splitting into very thin fibrils,

   and if 2 or more of the following 4 criteria are met:
   - parallel fibres occurring in bundles,
   - fibre bundles displaying frayed ends,
   - fibres in the form of thin needles,
   - matted masses of individual fibres and/or fibres showing curvature.

CHARACTERS

A light, homogeneous, white or almost white powder, greasy to the touch (non abrasive), practically insoluble in water, in alcohol and in dilute solutions of acids and alkali hydroxides.

IDENTIFICATION

First identification: A.

Second identification: B, C.

A. Examine by infrared absorption spectrophotometry (*2.2.24*). The spectrum shows absorption bands at 3677 ± 2 cm^{-1}, at 1018 ± 2 cm^{-1} and at 669 ± 2 cm^{-1}. Examine the substance as discs prepared using *potassium bromide R*.

B. In a platinum crucible, melt a mixture of 0.2 g of *anhydrous sodium carbonate R* and 2.0 g of *potassium carbonate R*. To the melted mass add 0.1 g of the substance to be examined and heat until the mixture is completely melted. Allow to cool and transfer the melted mass into an evaporating dish with 50 ml of hot *water R*. Add *hydrochloric acid R* until effervescence ceases. Add 10 ml of *hydrochloric acid R* and evaporate to dryness on a water-bath. Allow to cool. Add 20 ml of *water R*, heat to boiling and filter. (The residue is used for identification test C). To 5 ml of the filtrate add 1 ml of *ammonia R* and 1 ml of *ammonium chloride solution R* and filter. To the filtrate add 1 ml of *disodium hydrogen phosphate solution R*. A white, crystalline precipitate is formed.

C. The residue obtained in identification test B gives the reaction of silicates (*2.3.1*).

TESTS

Solution S1. Weigh 10.0 g of the substance to be examined into a conical flask fitted with a reflux condenser, add 50 ml of *0.5 M hydrochloric acid* gradually while stirring and heat on a water-bath for 30 min. Allow to cool. Transfer the mixture to a beaker and allow the undissolved material to settle. Filter the supernatant through medium-speed filter paper into a 100 ml volumetric flask, retaining as much as possible of the insoluble material in the beaker. Wash the residue and the beaker with 3 quantities, each of 10 ml, of hot *water R*. Wash the filter with 15 ml of hot *water R*, allow the filtrate to cool and dilute to 100.0 ml with the same solvent.

Solution S2. Weigh 0.5 g of the substance to be examined in a 100 ml polytetrafluoroethylene dish, add 5 ml of *hydrochloric acid R*, 5 ml of *lead-free nitric acid R* and 5 ml of *perchloric acid R*. Stir gently then add 35 ml of *hydrofluoric acid R* and evaporate slowly to dryness on a hot plate. To the residue, add 5 ml of *hydrochloric acid R*, cover with a watch-glass, heat to boiling and allow to cool. Rinse the watch-glass and the dish with *water R*. Transfer into a volumetric flask, rinse the dish with *water R* and dilute to 50.0 ml with the same solvent.

pH (*2.2.3*). The pH of the filtrate obtained in the test for water-soluble substances is 7.0 to 9.0. Read the pH 1 min after inserting the electrode.

Water-soluble substances. To 10.0 g add 50 ml of *carbon dioxide-free water R*, heat to boiling and maintain boiling under a reflux condenser for 30 min. Allow to cool, filter through a medium-speed filter paper and dilute to 50.0 ml with *carbon dioxide-free water R*. Take 25.0 ml of the filtrate, evaporate to dryness and heat at 105 °C for 1 h. The residue weighs not more than 10 mg (0.2 per cent).

Aluminium. Not more than 2.0 per cent of Al, determined by atomic absorption spectrometry (*2.2.23, Method I*).

Test solution. To 5.0 ml of solution S2 add 10 ml of a 25.34 g/l solution of *caesium chloride R*, 10.0 ml of *hydrochloric acid R* and dilute to 100.0 ml with *water R.*

Reference solutions. Into 4 identical volumetric flasks, each containing 10.0 ml of *hydrochloric acid R* and 10 ml of a 25.34 g/l solution of *caesium chloride R*, introduce respectively 5.0 ml, 10.0 ml, 15.0 ml and 20.0 ml of *aluminium standard solution (100 ppm Al) R* and dilute to 100.0 ml with *water R.*

Measure the absorbance at 309.3 nm, using an aluminium hollow-cathode lamp as the radiation source and a nitrous oxide-acetylene flame.

Calcium. Not more than 0.9 per cent of Ca, determined by atomic absorption spectrometry (*2.2.23, Method I*).

Test solution. To 5.0 ml of solution S2 add 10.0 ml of *hydrochloric acid R*, 10 ml of *lanthanum chloride solution R* and dilute to 100.0 ml with *water R.*

Reference solutions. Into 4 identical volumetric flasks, each containing 10.0 ml of *hydrochloric acid R* and 10 ml of *lanthanum chloride solution R*, introduce respectively 1.0 ml, 2.0 ml, 3.0 ml and 4.0 ml of *calcium standard solution (100 ppm Ca) R1* and dilute to 100.0 ml with *water R.*

Measure the absorbance at 422.7 nm using a calcium hollow-cathode lamp as the radiation source and a nitrous oxide-acetylene flame.

Iron. Not more than 0.25 per cent of Fe, determined by atomic absorption spectrometry (*2.2.23, Method I*).

Test solution. To 2.5 ml of solution S1, add 50.0 ml of *0.5 M hydrochloric acid* and dilute to 100.0 ml with *water R.*

Reference solutions. Into 4 identical volumetric flasks, each containing 50.0 ml of *0.5 M hydrochloric acid,* introduce respectively 2.0 ml, 2.5 ml, 3.0 ml and 4.0 ml of *iron standard solution (250 ppm Fe) R* and dilute to 100.0 ml with *water R.*

Measure the absorbance at 248.3 nm using an iron hollow-cathode lamp as the radiation source and an air-acetylene flame. Make a correction using a deuterium lamp.

Lead. Not more than 10 ppm of Pb, determined by atomic absorption spectrometry (*2.2.23, Method I*).

Test solution. Use solution S1.

Reference solutions. Into 4 identical volumetric flasks, each containing 50.0 ml of *0.5 M hydrochloric acid,* introduce respectively 5.0 ml, 7.5 ml, 10.0 ml and 12.5 ml of *lead standard solution (10 ppm Pb) R1* and dilute to 100.0 ml with *water R.*

Measure the absorbance at 217.0 nm using a lead hollow-cathode lamp as the radiation source and an air-acetylene flame.

Magnesium. 17.0 per cent to 19.5 per cent of Mg, determined by atomic absorption spectrometry (*2.2.23, Method I*).

Test solution. Dilute 0.5 ml of solution S2 to 100.0 ml with *water R.* To 4.0 ml of the solution, add 10.0 ml of *hydrochloric acid R*, 10 ml of *lanthanum chloride solution R* and dilute to 100.0 ml with *water R.*

Reference solutions. Into 4 identical volumetric flasks, each containing 10.0 ml of *hydrochloric acid R* and 10 ml of *lanthanum chloride solution R*, introduce respectively 2.5 ml, 3.0 ml, 4.0 ml and 5.0 ml of *magnesium standard solution (10 ppm Mg) R1* and dilute to 100.0 ml with *water R.*

Measure the absorbance at 285.2 nm using a magnesium hollow-cathode lamp as the radiation source and an air-acetylene flame.

Loss on ignition. Not more than 7.0 per cent, determined on 1.00 g by ignition to constant weight at 1050-1100 °C.

Microbial contamination. If intended for topical administration, the total viable aerobic count (*2.6.12*) is not more than a total of 10^2 aerobic bacteria and fungi per gram. If intended for oral administration, the total viable aerobic count (*2.6.12*) is not more than a total of 10^3 aerobic bacteria and not more than 10^2 fungi per gram.

LABELLING

The label states, where applicable, that the substance is suitable for oral or topical administration.

01/2005:1046
corrected

TAMOXIFEN CITRATE

Tamoxifeni citras

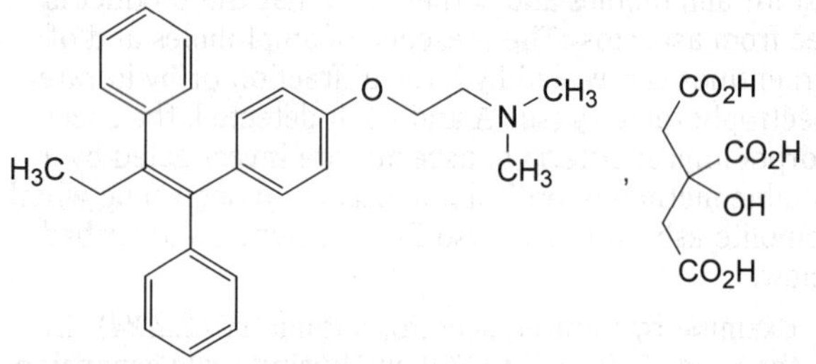

$C_{32}H_{37}NO_8$ M_r 563.6

DEFINITION

Tamoxifen citrate contains not less than 99.0 per cent and not more than the equivalent of 101.0 per cent of 2-[4-[(*Z*)-1,2-diphenylbut-1-enyl]phenoxy]-*N,N*-dimethylethanamine dihydrogen 2-hydroxypropane-1,2,3-tricarboxylate, calculated with reference to the dried substance.

CHARACTERS

A white or almost white, crystalline powder, slightly soluble in water, soluble in methanol, slightly soluble in acetone.

It shows polymorphism.

IDENTIFICATION

First identification: B.

Second identification: A, C, D.

A. Dissolve 20 mg in *methanol R* and dilute to 50.0 ml with the same solvent. Dilute 5.0 ml of the solution to 100.0 ml with *methanol R.* Examined between 220 nm and 350 nm (*2.2.25*), the solution shows two absorption maxima, at 237 nm and 275 nm. The ratio of the absorbance measured at the maximum at 237 nm to that measured at the maximum at 275 nm is 1.45 to 1.65.

B. Examine by infrared absorption spectrophotometry (*2.2.24*), comparing with the spectrum obtained with *tamoxifen citrate CRS.* Examine the substances prepared as discs. If the spectra obtained in the solid state show differences, dissolve the substance to be examined and the reference substance separately in *acetone R*, evaporate to dryness and record new spectra using the residues.

C. Examine by thin-layer chromatography (*2.2.27*), using as the coating substance a suitable silica gel with a fluorescent indicator having an optimal intensity at 254 nm.

Test solution. Dissolve 10 mg of the substance to be examined in *methanol R* and dilute to 10 ml with the same solvent.

Monographs T-Z

Reference solution (a). Dissolve 10 mg of *tamoxifen citrate CRS* in *methanol R* and dilute to 10 ml with the same solvent.

Reference solution (b). Dissolve 10 mg of *tamoxifen citrate CRS* and 10 mg of *clomifene citrate CRS* in *methanol R* and dilute to 10 ml with the same solvent.

Apply separately to the plate 5 µl of each solution. Develop over a path of 15 cm using a mixture of 10 volumes of *triethylamine R* and 90 volumes of *toluene R*. Allow the plate to dry in air and examine in ultraviolet light at 254 nm. The principal spot in the chromatogram obtained with the test solution is similar in position and size to the principal spot in the chromatogram obtained with reference solution (a). The test is not valid unless the chromatogram obtained with reference solution (b) shows two clearly separated spots.

D. Dissolve about 10 mg in 4 ml of *pyridine R* with shaking and add 2 ml of *acetic anhydride R*. A yellow colour is produced. Heat on a water-bath for 2 min. A pink to red colour is produced.

TESTS

***E*-isomer and related substances.** Examine by liquid chromatography (*2.2.29*). *Prepare the solutions immediately before use and protect from light.*

Test solution. Dissolve 15.0 mg of the substance to be examined in the mobile phase and dilute to 10.0 ml with the mobile phase.

Reference solution (a). Dissolve 15.0 mg of *tamoxifen citrate for performance test CRS* in the mobile phase and dilute to 10.0 ml with the mobile phase.

Reference solution (b). Dilute 1.0 ml of the test solution to 100.0 ml with the mobile phase.

The chromatographic procedure may be carried out using:

- a stainless steel column 0.25 m long and 4.6 mm in internal diameter packed with *octadecylsilyl silica gel for chromatography R* (5 µm),
- as mobile phase at a flow rate of 1.2 ml/min a mixture of 40 volumes of *acetonitrile R* and 60 volumes of *water R* containing 0.9 g/l of *sodium dihydrogen phosphate R* and 4.8 g/l of *N,N-dimethyloctylamine R*, adjusted to pH 3.0 with *phosphoric acid R*,
- as detector a spectrophotometer set at 240 nm.

Equilibrate the column with the mobile phase at a flow rate of 1.2 ml/min for about 30 min.

Adjust the sensitivity of the system so that the height of the peak due to the *E*-isomer in the chromatogram obtained with 10 µl of reference solution (a) is not less than 40 per cent of the full scale of the recorder. The test is not valid unless the chromatogram obtained resembles that of the specimen chromatogram provided with the *tamoxifen citrate for performance test CRS* in that the resolution between the peaks due to the *E*-isomer and to tamoxifen impurity F is at least three and there is base-line separation of the peak due to tamoxifen impurity F from the following peak of the principal component.

Inject separately 10 µl of the test solution and 10 µl of reference solution (b). Continue the chromatography for twice the retention time of the tamoxifen peak. In the chromatogram obtained with the test solution: the area of any peak, apart from the principal peak, is not greater than 0.3 times that of the principal peak in the chromatogram obtained with reference solution (b) (0.3 per cent); the sum of the areas of all the peaks, apart from the principal peak and any peak due to the *E*-isomer, is not greater than 0.5 times the area of the principal peak in the chromatogram of reference solution (b) (0.5 per cent). Disregard any peak due to the citrate (retention time = about 2.5 min) and any peak with an area less than 0.05 times the area of the principal peak in the chromatogram obtained with reference solution (b) (0.05 per cent).

Loss on drying (*2.2.32*). Not more than 0.5 per cent, determined on 1.000 g by drying *in vacuo* at 65 °C for 4 h.

Sulphated ash (*2.4.14*). Not more than 0.1 per cent, determined on 1.0 g.

ASSAY

Dissolve 0.400 g in 75 ml of *anhydrous acetic acid R*. Titrate with *0.1 M perchloric acid* using 0.1 ml of *naphtholbenzein solution R* as indicator.

1 ml of *0.1 M perchloric acid* is equivalent to 56.36 mg of $C_{32}H_{37}NO_8$.

IMPURITIES

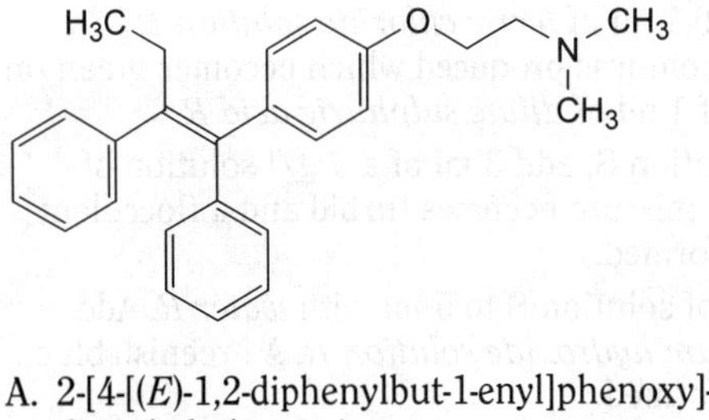

A. 2-[4-[(*E*)-1,2-diphenylbut-1-enyl]phenoxy]-*N,N*-dimethylethanamine,

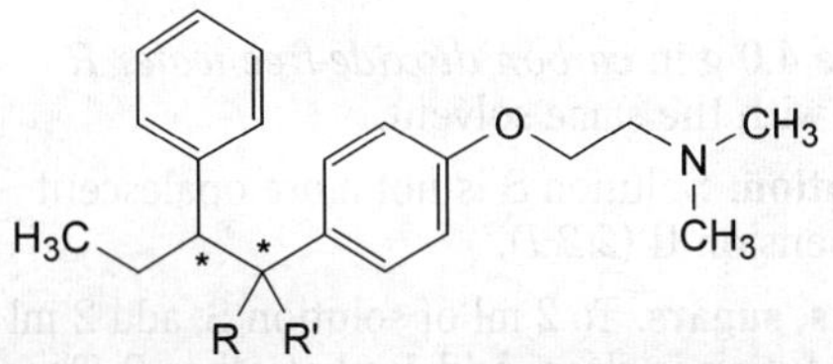

B. R = OH, R′ = C_6H_5: 1-[4-[2-(dimethylamino)ethoxy]phenyl]-1,2-diphenylbutan-1-ol,

G. R + R′ = O: (2*RS*)-1-[4-[2-(dimethylamino)ethoxy]phenyl]-2-phenylbutan-1-one,

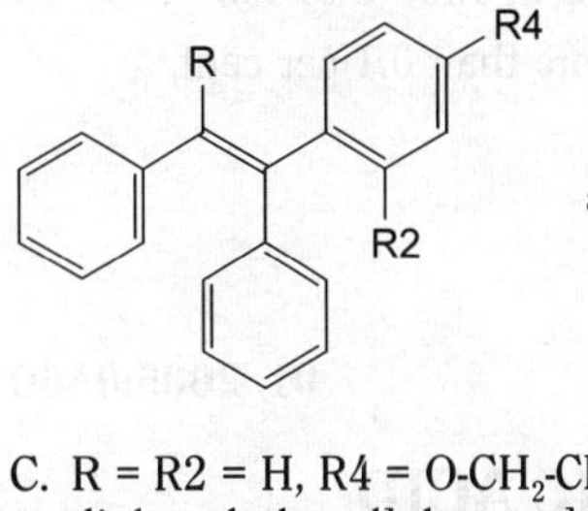

and (*Z*)-isomer

C. R = R2 = H, R4 = O-CH_2-CH_2-N$(CH_3)_2$: 2-[4-[(*EZ*)-1,2-diphenylethenyl]phenoxy]-*N,N*-dimethylethanamine,

D. R = CH_3, R2 = H, R4 = O-CH_2-CH_2-N$(CH_3)_2$: 2-[4-[(*EZ*)-1,2-diphenylprop-1-enyl]phenoxy]-*N,N*-dimethylethanamine,

E. R = C_2H_5, R2 = O-CH_2-CH_2-N$(CH_3)_2$, R4 = H: 2-[2-[(*EZ*)-1,2-diphenylbut-1-enyl]phenoxy]-*N,N*-dimethylethanamine,

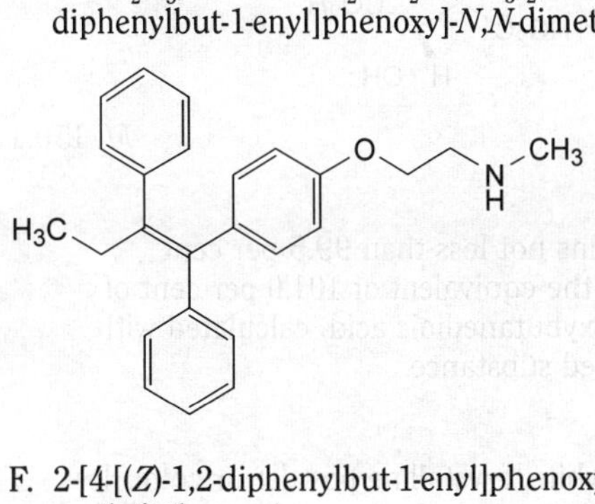

F. 2-[4-[(*Z*)-1,2-diphenylbut-1-enyl]phenoxy]-*N*-methylethanamine.

Monographs T-Z

01/2005:1477

TANNIC ACID

Tanninum

DEFINITION

Tannic acid is a mixture of esters of glucose with gallic acid and 3-galloylgallic acid.

CHARACTERS

A yellowish-white or slightly brown amorphous light powder or shiny plates, very soluble in water, freely soluble in acetone, in alcohol and in glycerol (85 per cent), practically insoluble in methylene chloride.

IDENTIFICATION

A. Dilute 0.1 ml of solution S (see Tests) to 5 ml with *water R*. Add 0.1 ml of *ferric chloride solution R1*. A blackish-blue colour is produced which becomes green on the addition of 1 ml of *dilute sulphuric acid R*.

B. To 1 ml of solution S, add 3 ml of a 1 g/l solution of *gelatin R*. The mixture becomes turbid and a flocculent precipitate is formed.

C. Dilute 0.1 ml of solution S to 5 ml with *water R*. Add 0.3 ml of *barium hydroxide solution R*. A greenish-blue precipitate is formed.

TESTS

Solution S. Dissolve 4.0 g in *carbon dioxide-free water R* and dilute to 20 ml with the same solvent.

Appearance of solution. Solution S is not more opalescent than reference suspension II (*2.2.1*).

Dextrins, gum, salts, sugars. To 2 ml of solution S, add 2 ml of *alcohol R*. The solution is clear. Add 1 ml of *ether R*. The solution remains clear for at least 10 min.

Resins. To 5 ml of solution S, add 5 ml of *water R*. The mixture remains clear for at least 15 min (*2.2.1*).

Loss on drying (*2.2.32*). Not more than 12.0 per cent, determined on 0.200 g by drying at 100 °C to 105 °C.

Sulphated ash (*2.4.14*). Not more than 0.1 per cent, determined on 1.0 g.

STORAGE

Store protected from light.

01/2005:0460

TARTARIC ACID

Acidum tartaricum

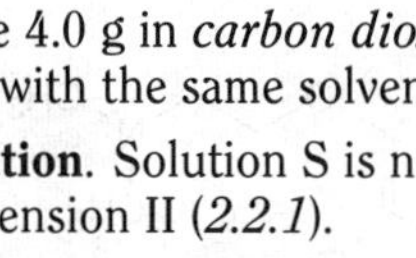

$C_4H_6O_6$ M_r 150.1

DEFINITION

Tartaric acid contains not less than 99.5 per cent and not more than the equivalent of 101.0 per cent of (2*R*,3*R*)-2,3-dihydroxybutanedioic acid, calculated with reference to the dried substance.

CHARACTERS

A white or almost white, crystalline powder or colourless crystals, very soluble in water, freely soluble in alcohol.

IDENTIFICATION

A. Solution S (see Tests) is strongly acid (*2.2.4*).

B. It gives the reactions of tartrates (*2.3.1*).

TESTS

Solution S. Dissolve 5.0 g in *distilled water R* and dilute to 50 ml with the same solvent.

Appearance of solution. Solution S is clear (*2.2.1*) and not more intensely coloured than reference solution Y_6 (*2.2.2, Method II*).

Specific optical rotation (*2.2.7*). Dissolve 5.00 g in *water R* and dilute to 25.0 ml with the same solvent. The specific optical rotation is + 12.0 to + 12.8.

Oxalic acid. Dissolve 0.80 g in 4 ml of *water R*. Add 3 ml of *hydrochloric acid R* and 1 g of *zinc R* in granules and boil for 1 min. Allow to stand for 2 min. Collect the liquid in a test-tube containing 0.25 ml of a 10 g/l solution of *phenylhydrazine hydrochloride R* and heat to boiling. Cool rapidly, transfer to a graduated cylinder and add an equal volume of *hydrochloric acid R* and 0.25 ml of a 50 g/l solution of *potassium ferricyanide R*. Shake and allow to stand for 30 min. Any pink colour in the solution is not more intense than that in a standard prepared at the same time in the same manner using 4 ml of a 0.1 g/l solution of *oxalic acid R* (350 ppm calculated as anhydrous oxalic acid).

Chlorides (*2.4.4*). 5 ml of solution S diluted to 15 ml with *water R* complies with the limit test for chlorides (100 ppm).

Sulphates (*2.4.13*). 10 ml of solution S diluted to 15 ml with *distilled water R* complies with the limit test for sulphates (150 ppm).

Calcium (*2.4.3*). To 5 ml of solution S add 10 ml of a 50 g/l solution of *sodium acetate R* in *distilled water R*. The solution complies with the limit test for calcium (200 ppm).

Heavy metals (*2.4.8*). 2.0 g complies with limit test C for heavy metals (10 ppm). Prepare the standard using 2 ml of *lead standard solution (10 ppm Pb) R*.

Loss on drying (*2.2.32*). Not more than 0.2 per cent, determined on 1.000 g by drying in an oven at 100 °C to 105 °C.

Sulphated ash (*2.4.14*). Not more than 0.1 per cent, determined on 1.0 g.

ASSAY

Dissolve 0.650 g in 25 ml of *water R*. Titrate with *1 M sodium hydroxide* using 0.5 ml of *phenolphthalein solution R* as indicator, until a pink colour is obtained.

1 ml of *1 M sodium hydroxide* is equivalent to 75.05 mg of $C_4H_6O_6$.

01/2005:1837

TEA TREE OIL

Melaleucae aetheroleum

DEFINITION

Essential oil obtained by steam distillation from the foliage and terminal branchlets of *Melaleuca alternifolia* (Maiden and Betch) Cheel, *M. linariifolia* Smith, *M. dissitiflora* F. Mueller and/or other species of *Melaleuca.*

CHARACTERS

Appearance: clear, mobile, colourless to pale yellow liquid with a characteristic odour.

IDENTIFICATION

First identification: B.

Second identification: A.

A. Thin-layer chromatography (*2.2.27*).

Test solution. Dissolve 0.1 ml of the substance to be examined in 5 ml of *heptane R*.

Reference solution. Dissolve 30 µl of *cineole R*, 60 µl of *terpinen-4-ol R* and 10 mg of *α-terpineol R* in 10 ml of *heptane R*.

Plate: *TLC silica gel plate R*.

Mobile phase: *ethyl acetate R, heptane R* (20:80 *V/V*).

Application: 10 µl, as bands.

Development: over a path of 10 cm.

Drying: in air.

Detection: spray with *anisaldehyde solution R*. Heat at 100-105 °C for 5-10 min while observing. Examine in daylight.

Results: see below the sequence of the zones present in the chromatograms obtained with the reference solution and the test solution. Furthermore, other zones are present in the chromatogram obtained with the test solution.

Top of the plate	
Cineole: a violet-brown zone	A violet-brown zone, less intense (cineole)
Terpinen-4-ol: a brownish-violet zone	A brownish-violet zone terpinen-4-ol)
α-terpineol: a violet or brownish-violet zone	A violet or brownish-violet zone (α-terpineol)
Reference solution	**Test solution**

B. Examine the chromatograms obtained in the test for chromatographic profile.

Results: the characteristic peaks in the chromatogram obtained with the test solution are similar in retention time to those in the chromatogram obtained with the reference solution.

TESTS

Relative density (*2.2.5*): 0.885 to 0.906.

Refractive index (*2.2.6*): 1.475 to 1.482.

Optical rotation (*2.2.7*): + 5° to + 15°.

Chromatographic profile. Gas chromatography (*2.2.28*): use the normalisation procedure.

Test solution. Dissolve 0.15 ml of the substance to be examined in 10 ml of *hexane R*.

Reference solution. Dissolve 5 µl of *α-pinene R*, 5 µl of *sabinene R*, 15 µl of *α-terpinene R*, 5 µl of *limonene R*, 5 µl of *cineole R*, 30 µl of *γ-terpinene R*, 5 µl of *p-cymene R*, 5 µl of *terpinolene R*, 60 µl of *terpinen-4-ol R*, 5 µl of *aromadendrene R* and 5 mg of *α-terpineol R* in 10 ml of *hexane R*.

Column:
- *material*: fused silica,
- *size*: *l* = 30 m (a film thickness of 1 µm may be used) to 60 m (a film thickness of 0.2 µm may be used), Ø = 0.25-0.53 mm,
- *stationary phase*: *macrogol 20 000 R*.

Carrier gas: *helium for chromatography R*.

Flow rate: 1.3 ml/min.

Split ratio: 1:50.

Temperature:

	Time (min)	Temperature (°C)
Column	0 - 1	50
	1 - 37	50 → 230
	37 - 45	230
Injection port		240
Detector		240

Detection: flame ionisation.

Injection: 1 µl.

Elution order: order indicated in the composition of the reference solution. Record the retention times of these substances.

System suitability: reference solution:
- *resolution*: minimum 2.7 between the peaks due to terpinen-4-ol and aromadendrene.

Using the retention times determined from the chromatogram obtained with the reference solution, locate the components of the reference solution in the chromatogram obtained with the test solution. Disregard the peak due to hexane.

Determine the percentage content of these components. The percentages are within the following ranges:
- *α-pinene*: 1.0 per cent to 6.0 per cent,
- *sabinene*: less than 3.5 per cent,
- *α-terpinene*: 5.0 per cent to 13.0 per cent,
- *limonene*: 0.5 per cent to 4.0 per cent,
- *cineole*: less than 15.0 per cent,
- *γ-terpinene*: 10.0 per cent to 28.0 per cent,
- *p-cymene*: 0.5 per cent to 12.0 per cent,
- *terpinolene*: 1.5 per cent to 5.0 per cent,
- *terpinen-4-ol*: minimum 30.0 per cent,
- *aromadendrene*: less than 7.0 per cent,
- *α-terpineol*: 1.5 per cent to 8.0 per cent.

STORAGE

In an airtight, well-filled container, protected from light, at a temperature not exceeding 25 °C.

01/2005:0954

TEMAZEPAM

Temazepamum

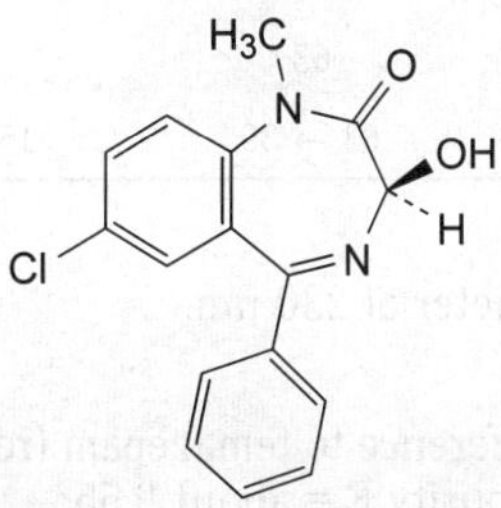

and enantiomer

$C_{16}H_{13}ClN_2O_2$ M_r 300.7

DEFINITION

(3*RS*)-7-Chloro-3-hydroxy-1-methyl-5-phenyl-1,3-dihydro-2*H*-1,4-benzodiazepin-2-one.

Content: 99.0 per cent to 101.0 per cent (dried substance).

Monographs T-Z

CHARACTERS

Appearance: white or almost white, crystalline powder.

Solubility: practically insoluble in water, freely soluble in methylene chloride, sparingly soluble in alcohol.

IDENTIFICATION

Infrared absorption spectrophotometry (*2.2.24*).

Comparison: *Ph. Eur. reference spectrum of temazepam.*

TESTS

Impurity A: maximum 0.05 per cent.

Dissolve 0.400 g in *methylene chloride R* and dilute to 20.0 ml with the same solvent. The absorbance (*2.2.25*) is maximum 0.30 at 409 nm.

Related substances. Liquid chromatography (*2.2.29*).

Test solution. Dissolve 10.0 mg of the substance to be examined in a mixture of 1 volume of *water R* and 9 volumes of *methanol R* and dilute to 50.0 ml with the same mixture of solvents.

Reference solution (a). Dilute 1.0 ml of the test solution to 100.0 ml with a mixture of 1 volume of *water R* and 9 volumes of *methanol R*. Dilute 2.0 ml of the solution to 10.0 ml with a mixture of 1 volume of *water R* and 9 volumes of *methanol R*.

Reference solution (b). Dissolve 1 mg of *oxazepam R*, 1 mg of *temazepam impurity F CRS* and 1 mg of *temazepam impurity G CRS* in a mixture of 1 volume of *water R* and 9 volumes of *methanol R* and dilute to 25 ml with the same mixture of solvents.

Reference solution (c). Dissolve 1 mg of *temazepam impurity C CRS* and 1 mg of *temazepam impurity D CRS* with a mixture of 1 volume of *water R* and 9 volumes of *methanol R* and dilute to 25 ml with the same mixture of solvents.

Column:

- *size*: l = 0.15 m, Ø = 4.6 mm,
- *stationary phase*: *end-capped octadecylsilyl silica gel for chromatography R* (3.5 µm).

Mobile phase:

- *mobile phase A*: solution containing 4.9 g/l of *sodium dihydrogen phosphate R* and 0.63 g/l of *disodium hydrogen phosphate R* (pH 5.6),
- *mobile phase B*: *methanol R*,
- *mobile phase C*: *acetonitrile R*,

Time (min)	Mobile phase A (per cent *V/V*)	Mobile phase B (per cent *V/V*)	Mobile phase C (per cent *V/V*)
0 - 18	54	39	7
18 - 25	54 → 22	39 → 63	7 → 15
25 - 31	22	63	15
31 - 37	22 → 54	63 → 39	15 → 7

Flow rate: 1.5 ml/min.

Detection: spectrophotometer at 230 nm.

Injection: 20 µl.

Relative retention with reference to temazepam (retention time = about 16 min): impurity E = about 0.55; impurity F = about 0.67; impurity G = about 0.73; impurity B = about 0.8; impurity D = about 1.2; impurity C = about 1.3; impurity A = about 1.5.

System suitability: reference solution (b):

- *resolution*: minimum 1.5 between the peaks due to impurity F and impurity G,
- *peak-to-valley ratio*: minimum 1.7, where H_p = height above the baseline of the peak due to impurity G and H_v = height above the baseline of the lowest point of the curve separating this peak from the peak due to impurity B.

Limits:

- *correction factors*: for the calculation of contents, multiply the peak areas of the following impurities by the corresponding correction factor: impurity F = 3.2; impurity G = 3.1;
- *impurities B, C, D, E, F, G*: for each impurity, not more than the area of the principal peak in the chromatogram obtained with reference solution (a) (0.2 per cent);
- *any other impurity*: for each impurity, not more than 0.5 times the area of the principal peak in the chromatogram obtained with reference solution (a) (0.1 per cent);
- *total*: not more than 2.5 times the area of the principal peak in the chromatogram obtained with reference solution (a) (0.5 per cent);
- *disregard limit*: 0.25 times the area of the principal peak in the chromatogram obtained with reference solution (a) (0.05 per cent).

Loss on drying (*2.2.32*): maximum 0.5 per cent, determined on 1.000 g by drying in an oven at 100-105 °C for 4 h.

Sulphated ash (*2.4.14*): maximum 0.1 per cent, determined on 1.0 g.

ASSAY

Dissolve 0.250 g in 50 ml of *nitroethane R*. Titrate with *0.1 M perchloric acid*, determining the end-point potentiometrically (*2.2.20*).

1 ml of *0.1 M perchloric acid* is equivalent to 30.07 mg of $C_{16}H_{13}ClN_2O_2$.

STORAGE

Protected from light.

IMPURITIES

Specified impurities: *A, B, C, D, E, F, G.*

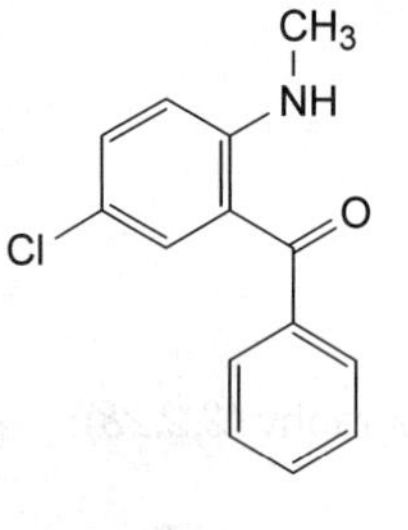

A. [5-chloro-2-(methylamino)phenyl]phenylmethanone,

B. oxazepam,

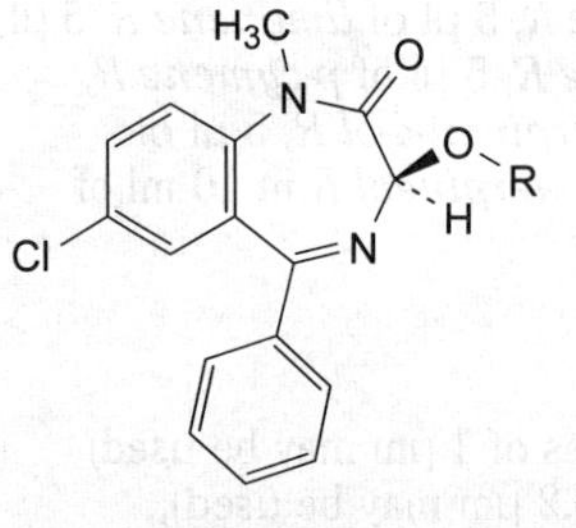

and enantiomer

C. R = $CO\text{-}CH_3$: (3*RS*)-7-chloro-1-methyl-2-oxo-5-phenyl-2,3-dihydro-1*H*-1,4-benzodiazepin-3-yl acetate,

D. R = CH_3: (3*RS*)-7-chloro-3-methoxy-1-methyl-5-phenyl-1,3-dihydro-2*H*-1,4-benzodiazepin-2-one,

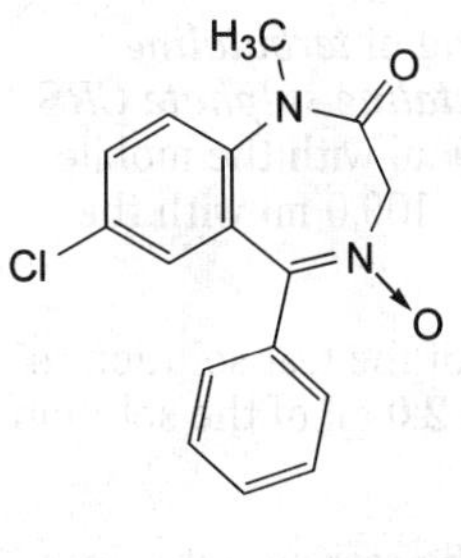

E. 7-chloro-1-methyl-5-phenyl-1,3-dihydro-2*H*-1,4-benzodiazepin-2-one 4-oxide,

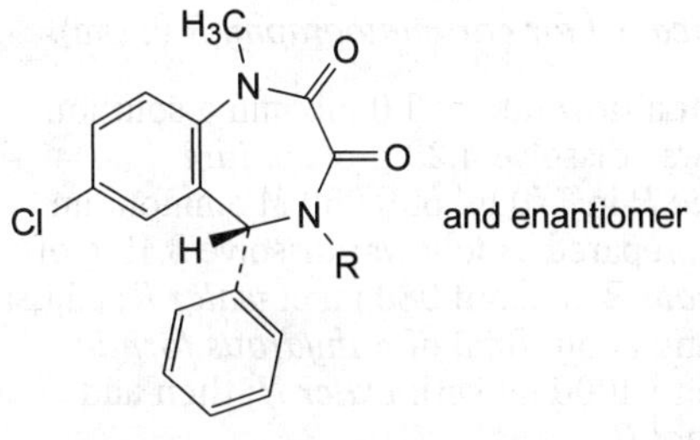

F. R = H: (5*RS*)-7-chloro-1-methyl-5-phenyl-4,5-dihydro-1*H*-1,4-benzodiazepine-2,3-dione,

G. R = CH_3: (5*RS*)-7-chloro-1,4-dimethyl-5-phenyl-4,5-dihydro-1*H*-1,4-benzodiazepine-2,3-dione.

01/2005:1156

TENOXICAM

Tenoxicamum

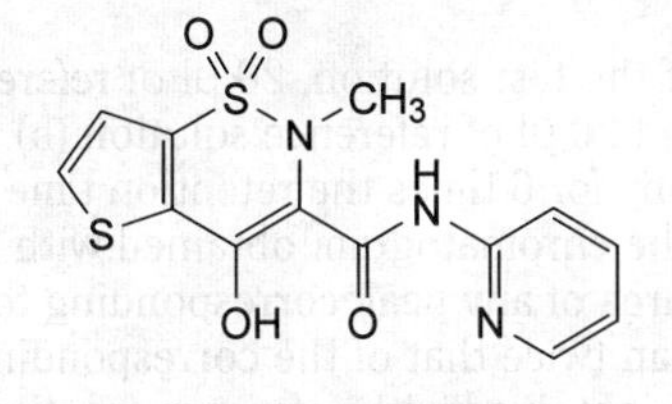

$C_{13}H_{11}N_3O_4S_2$ M_r 337.4

DEFINITION

Tenoxicam contains not less than 99.0 per cent and not more than the equivalent of 101.0 per cent of 4-hydroxy-2-methyl-*N*-(pyridin-2-yl)-2*H*-thieno[2,3-*e*]1,2-thiazine-3-carboxamide 1,1-dioxide, calculated with reference to the anhydrous substance.

CHARACTERS

A yellow, crystalline powder, practically insoluble in water, sparingly soluble in methylene chloride, very slightly soluble in ethanol. It dissolves in solutions of acids and alkalis.

It shows polymorphism.

IDENTIFICATION

Examine by infrared absorption spectrophotometry (*2.2.24*), comparing with the spectrum obtained with *tenoxicam CRS*. If the spectra obtained in the solid state show differences, dissolve the substance to be examined and the reference substance separately in the minimum quantity of *methylene chloride R*, evaporate to dryness on a water-bath and record new spectra using the residues.

TESTS

Appearance of solution. Dissolve 0.10 g in 20 ml of *methylene chloride R*. The solution is clear (*2.2.1*).

Related substances. Examine by thin-layer chromatography (*2.2.27*), using *silica gel GF_{254} R* as the coating substance.

Test solution. Dissolve 0.4 g in a mixture of 4 volumes of *concentrated ammonia R* and 96 volumes of *methanol R* and dilute to 5 ml with the same mixture of solvents.

Reference solution (a). Dilute 1 ml of the test solution to 20 ml with a mixture of 4 volumes of *concentrated ammonia R* and 96 volumes of *methanol R*. Dilute 1 ml of the solution to 20 ml with the same mixture of solvents.

Reference solution (b). Dissolve 20 mg of *tenoxicam CRS* and 20 mg of *salicylic acid CRS* in a mixture of 4 volumes of *concentrated ammonia R* and 96 volumes of *methanol R* and dilute to 5 ml with the same mixture of solvents.

Reference solution (c). Dissolve 20 mg of *pyridin-2-amine R* in a mixture of 4 volumes of *concentrated ammonia R* and 96 volumes of *methanol R* and dilute to 5 ml with the same mixture of solvents. Dilute 2 ml of the solution to 50 ml with the same mixture of solvents.

Apply separately to the plate 10 µl of each solution. Develop over a path of 15 cm with a mixture of 5 volumes of *anhydrous formic acid R*, 5 volumes of *methanol R*, 20 volumes of *acetone R* and 70 volumes of *methylene chloride R*. Allow the plate to dry in air. Examine in ultraviolet light at 254 nm. Any spot corresponding to pyridin-2-amine in the chromatogram obtained with the test solution is not more intense than the spot in the chromatogram obtained with reference solution (c) (0.2 per cent). Any spot in the chromatogram obtained with the test solution apart from the principal spot and any spot corresponding to pyridin-2-amine, is not more intense than the spot in the chromatogram obtained with reference solution (a) (0.25 per cent). The test is not valid unless the chromatogram obtained with reference solution (b) shows two clearly separated spots.

Heavy metals (*2.4.8*). 0.5 g complies with limit test C for heavy metals (20 ppm). Prepare the standard using 5 ml of *lead standard solution (2 ppm Pb) R*.

Water (*2.5.12*). Not more than 0.5 per cent, determined on 1.000 g by the semi-micro determination of water.

Sulphated ash (*2.4.14*). Not more than 0.1 per cent, determined on 1.0 g.

ASSAY

Dissolve 0.250 g in 5 ml of *anhydrous formic acid R*. Add 70 ml of *anhydrous acetic acid R*. Titrate with *0.1 M perchloric acid*, determining the end-point potentiometrically (*2.2.20*).

1 ml of *0.1 M perchloric acid* is equivalent to 33.74 mg of $C_{13}H_{11}N_3O_4S_2$.

STORAGE

Store protected from light.

IMPURITIES

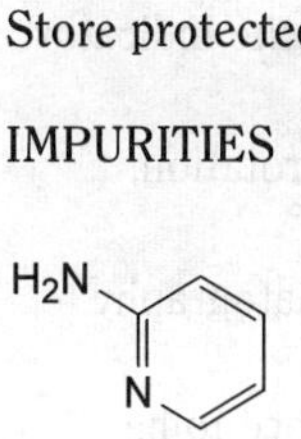

A. pyridin-2-amine,

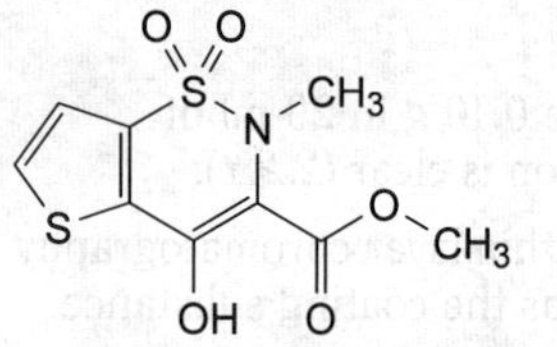

B. methyl 4-hydroxy-2-methyl-2*H*-thieno[2,3-*e*]1,2-thiazine-3-carboxylate 1,1-dioxide.

01/2005:0690

TERBUTALINE SULPHATE

Terbutalini sulfas

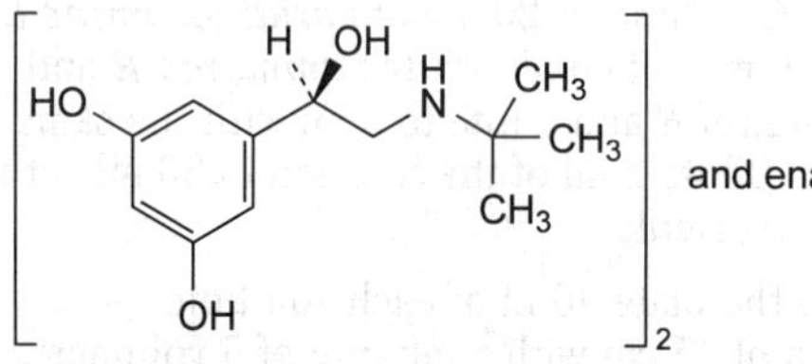

$C_{24}H_{40}N_2O_{10}S$ M_r 548.7

DEFINITION

Terbutaline sulphate contains not less than 98.0 per cent and not more than the equivalent of 101.0 per cent of bis[(1*RS*)-1-(3,5-dihydroxyphenyl)-2-[(1,1-dimethylethyl)amino]ethanol] sulphate, calculated with reference to the dried substance.

CHARACTERS

A white or almost white, crystalline powder, freely soluble in water, slightly soluble in alcohol.

It shows polymorphism.

IDENTIFICATION

A. Examine by infrared absorption spectrophotometry (*2.2.24*), comparing with the spectrum obtained with *terbutaline sulphate CRS*. If the spectra obtained in the solid state show differences, dissolve the substance to be examined and the reference substance separately in *aldehyde-free methanol R*, evaporate to dryness and record new spectra using the residues.

B. 5 ml of solution S (see Tests) gives reaction (a) of sulphates (*2.3.1*).

TESTS

Solution S. Dissolve 1.0 g in *carbon dioxide-free water R* and dilute to 50 ml with the same solvent.

Appearance of solution. Solution S is clear (*2.2.1*). The absorbance (*2.2.25*) of solution S measured at 400 nm in a 2 cm cell is not greater than 0.11.

Acidity. To 10 ml of solution S add 0.05 ml of *methyl red solution R*. Not more than 1.2 ml of *0.01 M sodium hydroxide* is required to change the colour of the indicator to yellow.

Optical rotation (*2.2.7*). The angle of optical rotation, determined on solution S, is − 0.10° to + 0.10°.

Related substances. Examine by liquid chromatography (*2.2.29*).

Test solution. Dissolve 75.0 mg of the substance to be examined in the mobile phase and dilute to 50.0 ml with the mobile phase.

Reference solution (a). Dissolve 7.5 mg of *terbutaline impurity C CRS* and 22.5 mg of *terbutaline sulphate CRS* in the mobile phase and dilute to 50.0 ml with the mobile phase. Dilute 1.0 ml of the solution to 100.0 ml with the mobile phase.

Reference solution (b). Dilute 1.0 ml of the test solution to 50.0 ml with the mobile phase. Dilute 2.0 ml of the solution to 20.0 ml with the mobile phase.

The chromatographic procedure may be carried out using:

- a stainless steel column 0.15 m long and 4.6 mm in internal diameter packed with *base-deactivated octadecylsilyl silica gel for chromatography R* (5 µm),
- as mobile phase at a flow rate of 1.0 ml/min a solution prepared as follows: dissolve 4.23 g of *sodium hexanesulphonate R* in 770 ml of 0.050 M ammonium formate solution prepared as follows: dissolve 3.15 g of *ammonium formate R* in about 980 ml of *water R*; adjust to pH 3.0 by adding about 8 ml of *anhydrous formic acid R* and dilute to 1000 ml with *water R*; then add 230 ml of *methanol R*,
- as detector a spectrophotometer set at 276 nm.

Adjust the sensitivity of the system so that the height of the principal peak in the chromatogram obtained with reference solution (b) is at least 50 per cent of the full scale of the recorder.

Inject 20 µl of reference solution (a). When the chromatograms are recorded under the prescribed conditions, the retention times are: impurity C about 9 min and terbutaline sulphate about 11 min. The test is not valid unless the resolution between the 2 peaks corresponding to terbutaline sulphate and impurity C is at least 2.0. If necessary adjust the composition of the mobile phase. Decrease the content of methanol to increase the retention time.

Inject 20 µl of the test solution, 20 µl of reference solution (a) and 20 µl of reference solution (b). Continue the chromatography for 6 times the retention time of terbutaline sulphate. In the chromatogram obtained with the test solution, the area of any peak corresponding to impurity C is not greater than twice that of the corresponding peak in the chromatogram obtained with reference solution (a) (0.2 per cent); the area of any other peak, apart from the principal peak, is not greater than that of the principal peak in the chromatogram obtained with reference solution (b) (0.2 per cent); the sum of the areas of all the peaks, apart from the principal peak and the peak corresponding to impurity C, is not greater than twice the area of the principal peak in the chromatogram obtained with reference solution (b) (0.4 per cent). Disregard any peak due to the mobile phase and any peak with an area less than 0.1 times the area of the principal peak in the chromatogram obtained with reference solution (b).

Loss on drying (*2.2.32*). Not more than 0.5 per cent, determined on 1.000 g by drying in an oven at 100-105 °C for 3 h.

ASSAY

Dissolve 0.400 g in 70 ml of *anhydrous acetic acid R* with heating. Titrate with *0.1 M perchloric acid*, determining the end-point potentiometrically (*2.2.20*).

1 ml of *0.1 M perchloric acid* is equivalent to 54.87 mg of $C_{24}H_{40}N_2O_{10}S$.

IMPURITIES

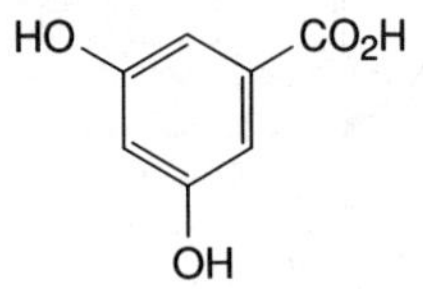

A. 3,5-dihydroxybenzoic acid (α-resorcylic acid),

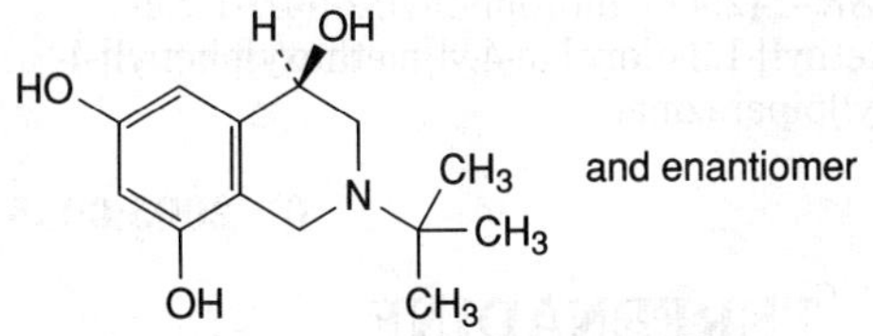

B. (4*RS*)-2-(1,1-dimethylethyl)-1,2,3,4-tetrahydroisoquinoline-4,6,8-triol,

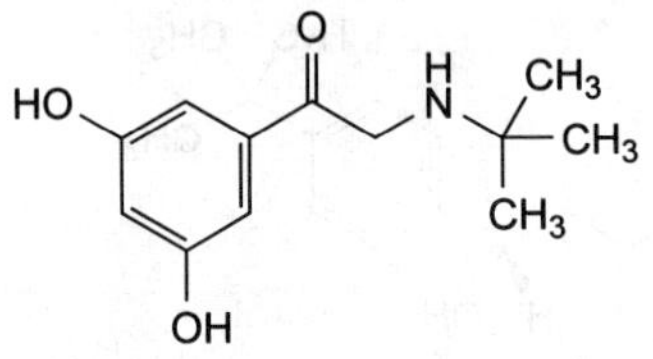

C. 1-(3,5-dihydroxyphenyl)-2-[(1,1-dimethylethyl)amino]ethanone,

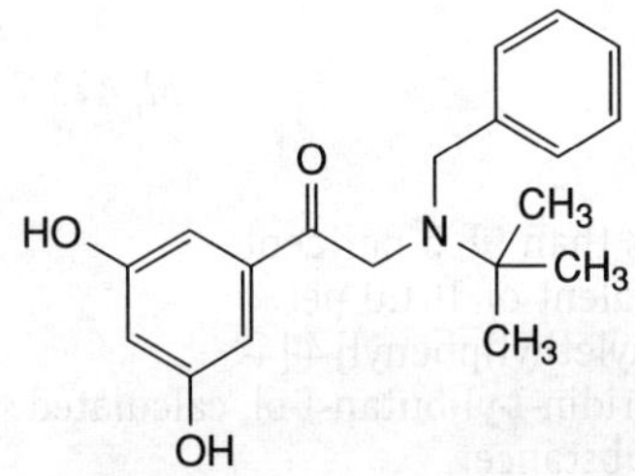

D. 2-[benzyl-(1,1-dimethylethyl)amino]-1-(3,5-dihydroxyphenyl)ethanone.

01/2005:1270

TERCONAZOLE

Terconazolum

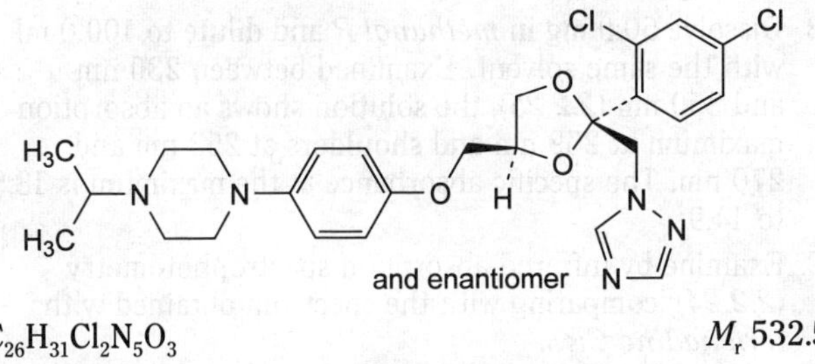

$C_{26}H_{31}Cl_2N_5O_3$ M_r 532.5

DEFINITION

Terconazole contains not less than 99.0 per cent and not more than the equivalent of 101.0 per cent of 1-[4-[[(2*RS*,4*SR*)-2-(2,4-dichlorophenyl)-2-[(1*H*-1,2,4-triazol-1-yl)methyl]-1,3-dioxolan-4-yl]methoxy]phenyl]-4-(1-methylethyl)piperazine, calculated with reference to the dried substance.

CHARACTERS

A white or almost white powder, practically insoluble in water, freely soluble in methylene chloride, soluble in acetone, sparingly soluble in alcohol.

It shows polymorphism.

IDENTIFICATION

First identification: A.

Second identification: B, C.

A. Examine by infrared absorption spectrophotometry (*2.2.24*), comparing with the spectrum obtained with *terconazole CRS*. If the spectra obtained in the solid state show differences, dissolve the substance to be examined and the reference substance separately in the minimum volume of *acetone R*, evaporate to dryness in a current of air and record new spectra using the residues.

B. Examine by thin-layer chromatography (*2.2.27*), using as the coating substance a suitable octadecylsilyl silica gel.

Test solution. Dissolve 30 mg of the substance to be examined in *methanol R* and dilute to 5 ml with the same solvent.

Reference solution (a). Dissolve 30 mg of *terconazole CRS* in *methanol R* and dilute to 5 ml with the same solvent.

Reference solution (b). Dissolve 30 mg of *terconazole CRS* and 30 mg of *ketoconazole CRS* in *methanol R* and dilute to 5 ml with the same solvent.

Apply separately to the plate 5 µl of each solution. Develop in an unsaturated tank over a path of 10 cm using a mixture of 20 volumes of *ammonium acetate solution R*, 40 volumes of *dioxan R* and 40 volumes of *methanol R*. Dry the plate in a current of warm air for 15 min and expose it to iodine vapour until the spots appear. Examine in daylight. The principal spot in the chromatogram obtained with the test solution is similar in position, colour and size to the principal spot in the chromatogram obtained with reference solution (a). The test is not valid unless the chromatogram obtained with reference solution (b) shows two clearly separated spots.

C. To 30 mg in a porcelain crucible add 0.3 g of *anhydrous sodium carbonate R*. Heat over an open flame for 10 min. Allow to cool. Take up the residue with 5 ml of *dilute nitric acid R* and filter. To 1 ml of the filtrate add 1 ml of *water R*. The solution gives reaction (a) of chlorides (*2.3.1*).

TESTS

Optical rotation (*2.2.7*). Dissolve 1.0 g in *methylene chloride R* and dilute to 10 ml with the same solvent. The angle of optical rotation is −0.10° to + 0.10°.

Related substances. Examine by liquid chromatography (*2.2.29*).

Test solution. Dissolve 0.100 g of the substance to be examined in *methanol R* and dilute to 10.0 ml with the same solvent.

Reference solution (a). Dissolve 2.5 mg of *terconazole CRS* and 2.0 mg of *ketoconazole CRS* in *methanol R* and dilute to 100.0 ml with the same solvent.

Reference solution (b). Dilute 1.0 ml of the test solution to 100.0 ml with *methanol R*. Dilute 5.0 ml of this solution to 20.0 ml with *methanol R*.

The chromatographic procedure may be carried out using:

- a stainless steel column 0.1 m long and 4.6 mm in internal diameter packed with *base-deactivated octadecylsilyl silica gel for chromatography R* (3 µm),
- as mobile phase at a flow rate of 2 ml/min:

Mobile phase A. A 3.4 g/l solution of *tetrabutylammonium hydrogen sulphate R*,

Mobile phase B. Acetonitrile R,

Time (min)	Mobile phase A (per cent V/V)	Mobile phase B (per cent V/V)	Comment
0 - 10	95 → 50	5 → 50	linear gradient
10 - 15	50	50	isocratic elution
15 - 20	95	5	switch to initial eluent composition
20 = 0	95	5	restart gradient

– as detector a spectrophotometer set at 220 nm.

Equilibrate the column for at least 30 min with *acetonitrile R* at a flow rate of 2 ml/min and then equilibrate at the initial elution composition for at least 5 min.

Adjust the sensitivity of the system so that the height of the principal peak in the chromatogram obtained with 10 µl of reference solution (b) is at least 50 per cent of the full scale of the recorder.

Inject 10 µl of reference solution (a). When the chromatograms are recorded in the prescribed conditions, the retention times are: ketoconazole about 6 min and terconazole about 7.5 min. The test is not valid unless the resolution between the peaks corresponding to ketoconazole and terconazole is at least 13. If necessary, adjust the concentration of acetonitrile in the mobile phase or adjust the time programme for the linear gradient elution.

Inject separately 10 µl of *methanol R* as a blank, 10 µl of the test solution and 10 µl of reference solution (b). In the chromatogram obtained with the test solution: the area of any peak, apart from the principal peak, is not greater than that of the principal peak in the chromatogram obtained with reference solution (b) (0.25 per cent); the sum of the areas of all the peaks, apart from the principal peak, is not greater than twice the area of the principal peak in the chromatogram obtained with reference solution (b) (0.5 per cent). Disregard any peak obtained with the blank run and any peak with an area less than 0.2 times the area of the principal peak in the chromatogram obtained with reference solution (b).

Loss on drying (*2.2.32*). Not more than 0.5 per cent, determined on 1.000 g by drying in an oven at 100-105 °C.

Sulphated ash (*2.4.14*). Not more than 0.1 per cent, determined on 1.0 g.

ASSAY

Dissolve 0.150 g in 70 ml of a mixture of 1 volume of *anhydrous acetic acid R* and 7 volumes of *methyl ethyl ketone R*. Titrate with *0.1 M perchloric acid* determining the end-point potentiometrically at the second point of inflexion (*2.2.20*).

1 ml of *0.1 M perchloric acid* is equivalent to 17.75 mg of $C_{26}H_{31}Cl_2N_5O_3$.

STORAGE

Store protected from light.

IMPURITIES

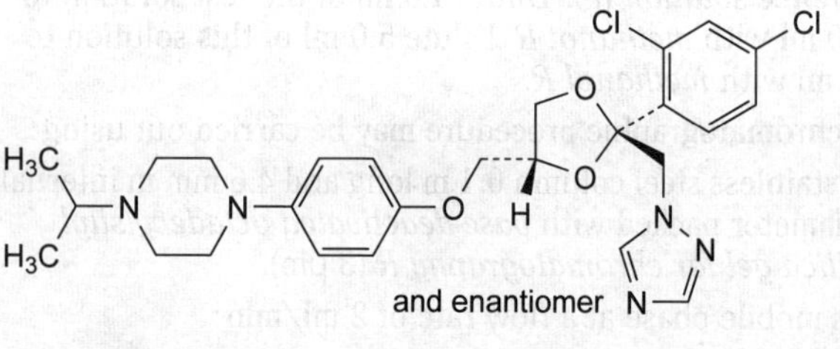

A. 1-[4-[[(2*RS*,4*RS*)2-(2,4-dichlorophenyl)-2-[(1*H*-1,2,4-triazol-1-yl)methyl]-1,3-dioxolan-4-yl]methoxy]phenyl]-4-(1-methylethyl)piperazine,

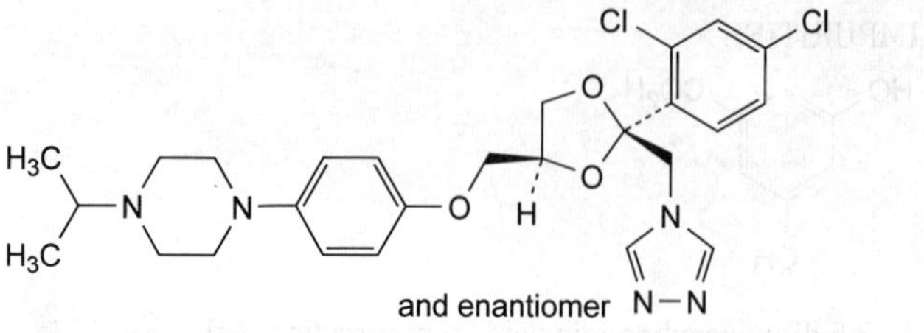

B. 1-[4-[[(2*RS*,4*SR*)-2-(2,4-dichlorophenyl)-2-[(4*H*-1,2,4-triazol-4-yl)methyl]-1,3-dioxolan-4-yl]methoxy]phenyl]-4-(1-methylethyl)piperazine.

01/2005:0955

TERFENADINE

Terfenadinum

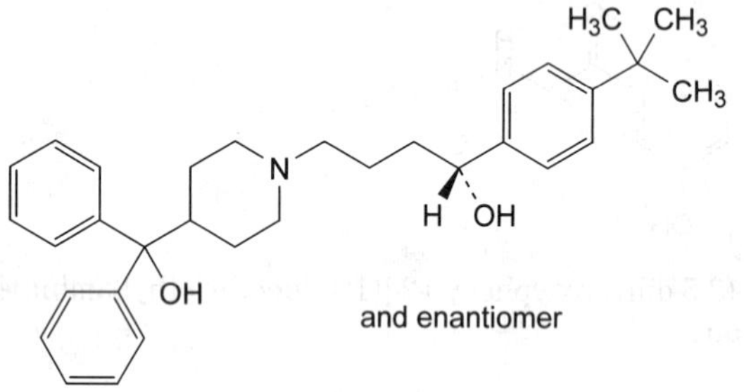

$C_{32}H_{41}NO_2$ M_r 471.7

DEFINITION

Terfenadine contains not less than 98.5 per cent and not more than the equivalent of 101.0 per cent of (1*RS*)-1-[4-(1,1-dimethylethyl)phenyl]-4-[4-(hydroxydiphenylmethyl)piperidin-1-yl]butan-1-ol, calculated with reference to the dried substance.

CHARACTERS

A white, crystalline powder, very slightly soluble in water and in dilute hydrochloric acid, freely soluble in methylene chloride, soluble in methanol.

It shows polymorphism.

IDENTIFICATION

First identification: C.

Second identification: A, B, D.

A. Melting point (*2.2.14*): 146 °C to 152 °C.

B. Dissolve 50.0 mg in *methanol R* and dilute to 100.0 ml with the same solvent. Examined between 230 nm and 350 nm (*2.2.25*), the solution shows an absorption maximum at 259 nm and shoulders at 253 nm and 270 nm. The specific absorbance at the maximum is 13.5 to 14.9.

C. Examine by infrared absorption spectrophotometry (*2.2.24*), comparing with the spectrum obtained with *terfenadine CRS*.

D. Examine by thin-layer chromatography (*2.2.27*), using *silica gel HF_{254} R* as the coating substance.

Test solution. Dissolve 50 mg of the substance to be examined in *methylene chloride R* and dilute to 10 ml with the same solvent.

Reference solution. Dissolve 50 mg of *terfenadine CRS* in *methylene chloride R* and dilute to 10 ml with the same solvent.

Apply to the plate 10 µl of each solution. Develop over a path of 15 cm using a mixture of 10 volumes of *methanol R* and 90 volumes of *methylene chloride R*.

Allow the plate to dry in air and examine in ultraviolet light at 254 nm. The principal spot in the chromatogram obtained with the test solution is similar in position and size to the principal spot in the chromatogram obtained with the reference solution.

TESTS

Related substances. Examine by liquid chromatography (*2.2.29*).

Test solution. Dissolve 15 mg of the substance to be examined in the mobile phase and dilute to 10.0 ml with the mobile phase.

Reference solution (a). Dilute 1.0 ml of the test solution to 10.0 ml with the mobile phase. Dilute 1.0 ml of this solution to 20.0 ml with the mobile phase.

Reference solution (b). Dissolve 15 mg of *terfenadine impurity A CRS* in the mobile phase and dilute to 10.0 ml with the mobile phase. To 5.0 ml of the solution, add 5.0 ml of the test solution and dilute to 50.0 ml with the mobile phase.

Reference solution (c). Dilute 10.0 ml of reference solution (a) to 25.0 ml with the mobile phase.

Reference solution (d). Dissolve 0.1 g of *potassium iodide R* in the mobile phase and dilute to 100 ml with the mobile phase. Dilute 1 ml to 100 ml with the mobile phase.

The chromatographic procedure may be carried out using:

– a stainless steel column 0.25 m long and 4.6 mm in internal diameter packed with *octylsilyl silica gel for chromatography R* (5 µm),
– as mobile phase at a flow rate of 1 ml/min a mixture prepared as follows: dilute 600 ml of *acetonitrile R* to 1 litre with *diethylammonium phosphate buffer solution pH 6.0 R*,
– as detector a spectrophotometer set at 217 nm,
– a loop injector.

Inject 20 µl of each solution and continue the chromatography for 5 times the retention time of terfenadine. The test is not valid unless, in the chromatogram obtained with reference solution (b), the resolution between the peaks corresponding to terfenadine and impurity A is greater than 5.0 and the mass distribution ratio of the peak corresponding to terfenadine is greater than 2.0. Determine the mass distribution ratio using, as unretained compound, *potassium iodide R*. In the chromatogram obtained with the test solution, the area of any peak apart from the principal peak is not greater than that of the peak in the chromatogram obtained with reference solution (c) (0.2 per cent) and the sum of the areas of all the peaks apart from the principal peak is not greater than the area of the peak in the chromatogram obtained with reference solution (a) (0.5 per cent). Disregard any peak with an area less than 2.5 per cent of that of the peak in the chromatogram obtained with reference solution (c).

Loss on drying (*2.2.32*). Not more than 0.5 per cent, determined on 1.000 g by drying at 60 °C under a pressure not exceeding 0.5 kPa.

Sulphated ash (*2.4.14*). Not more than 0.1 per cent, determined on 1.0 g.

ASSAY

Dissolve 0.400 g in 50 ml of *anhydrous acetic acid R*. Titrate with *0.1 M perchloric acid*, determining the end-point potentiometrically (*2.2.20*).

1 ml of *0.1 M perchloric acid* is equivalent to 47.17 mg of $C_{32}H_{41}NO_2$.

STORAGE

Protected from light.

IMPURITIES

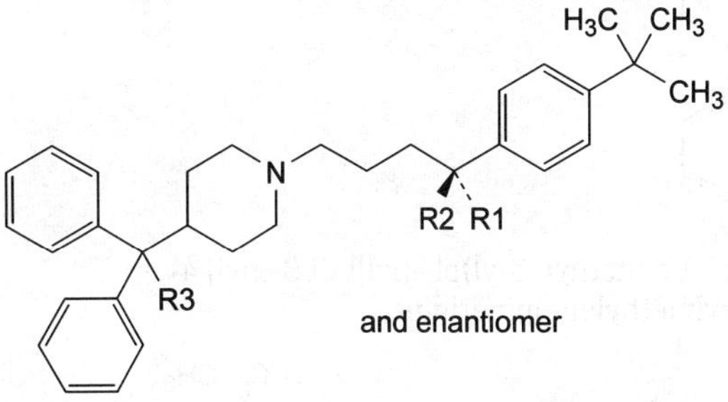

A. R1 + R2 = O, R3 = OH: 1-[4-(1,1-dimethylethyl)phenyl]-4-[4-(hydroxydiphenylmethyl)piperidin-1-yl]butan-1-one,

B. R1 = OH, R2 = R3 = H: (1*RS*)-1-[4-(1,1-dimethylethyl)phenyl]-4-[4-(diphenylmethyl)piperidin-1-yl]butan-1-ol,

H. R1 = R2 = H, R3 = OH: [1-[4-[4-(1,1-dimethylethyl)phenyl]butyl]piperidin-4-yl]diphenylmethanol,

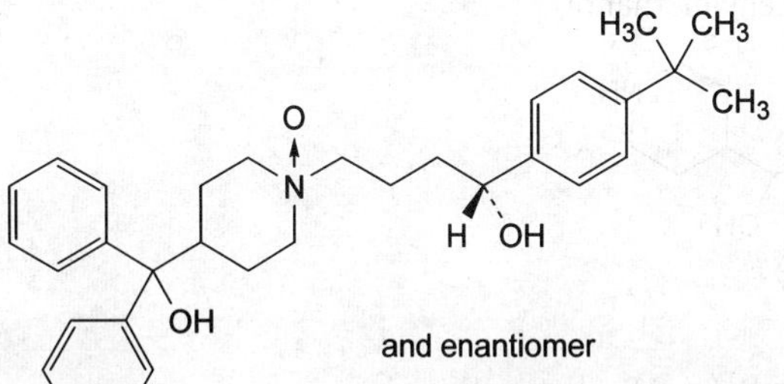

C. 1-[(4*RS*)-4-[4-(1,1-dimethylethyl)phenyl]-4-hydroxybutyl]-4-(hydroxydiphenylmethyl)piperidine 1-oxide,

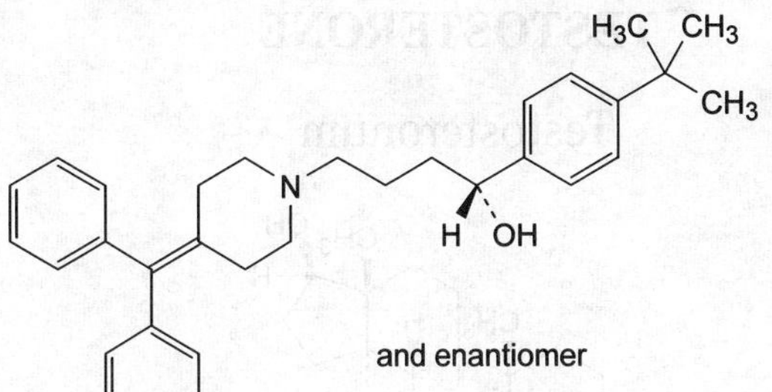

D. (1*RS*)-1-[4-(1,1-dimethylethyl)phenyl]-4-[4-(diphenylmethylene)piperidin-1-yl]butan-1-ol,

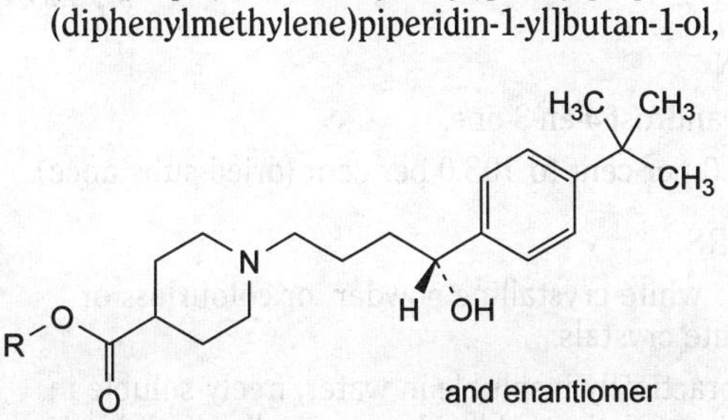

E. R = H: 1-[(4*RS*)-4-[4-(1,1-dimethylethyl)phenyl]-4-hydroxybutyl]piperidine-4-carboxylic acid,

J. R = C_2H_5: ethyl 1-[(4*RS*)-4-[4-(1,1-dimethylethyl)phenyl]-4-hydroxybutyl]piperidine-4-carboxylate,

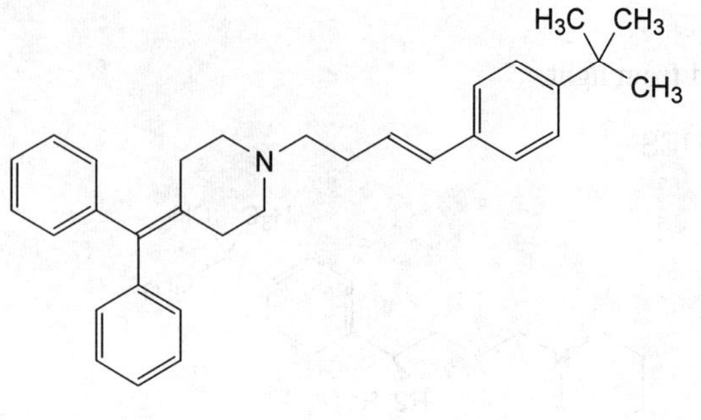

F. 1-[4-[4-(1,1-dimethylethyl)phenyl]but-3-enyl]-4-(diphenylmethylene)piperidine,

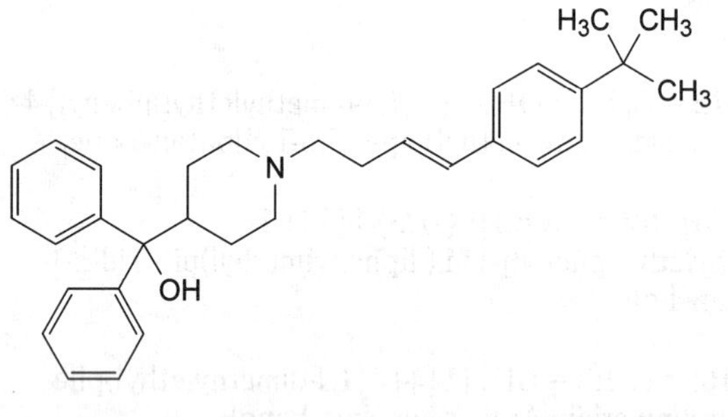

G. [1-[4-[4-(1,1-dimethylethyl)phenyl]but-3-enyl]piperidin-4-yl]diphenylmethanol,

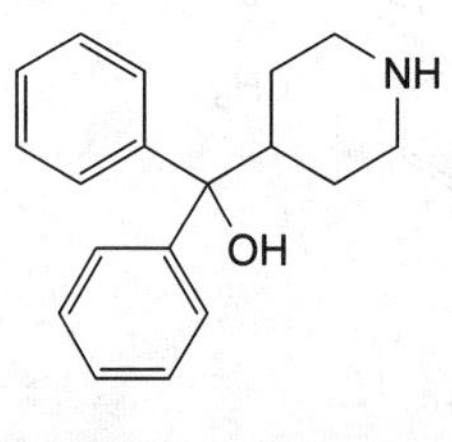

I. diphenyl(piperidin-4-yl)methanol.

01/2005:1373

TESTOSTERONE

Testosteronum

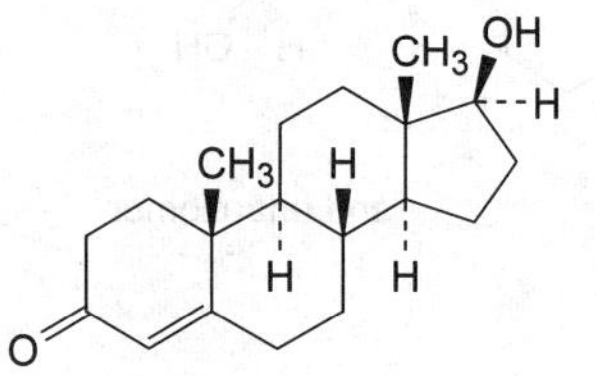

$C_{19}H_{28}O_2$ M_r 288.4

DEFINITION

17β-Hydroxyandrost-4-en-3-one.

Content: 97.0 per cent to 103.0 per cent (dried substance).

CHARACTERS

Appearance: white crystalline powder, or colourless or yellowish-white crystals.

Solubility: practically insoluble in water, freely soluble in alcohol and in methylene chloride, practically insoluble in fatty oils.

mp: about 155 °C.

IDENTIFICATION

Infrared absorption spectrophotometry (*2.2.24*).

Comparison: *testosterone CRS.*

TESTS

Specific optical rotation (*2.2.7*): + 106 to + 114 (dried substance).

Dissolve 0.250 g in *ethanol R* and dilute to 25.0 ml with the same solvent.

Impurities D and F. Thin-layer chromatography (*2.2.27*).

Test solution. Dissolve 0.100 g of the substance to be examined in *methanol R* and dilute to 10 ml with the same solvent.

Reference solution (a). Dissolve 1 mg of *stanolone R* in *methanol R* and dilute to 10 ml with the same solvent. In 1 ml of this solution, dissolve 10 mg of *testosterone for impurity D identification CRS* (testosterone spiked with about 1 per cent of impurity D).

Reference solution (b). Dilute 1.0 ml of the test solution to 100.0 ml with *methanol R.*

Reference solution (c). Dilute 2.0 ml of reference solution (b) to 10.0 ml with *methanol R.*

Reference solution (d). Dilute 1.0 ml of reference solution (b) to 10.0 ml with *methanol R.*

Plate: *TLC silica gel F_{254} plate R* (6-8 μm).

Preconditioning (in the dark): add about 5 g of powdered *silver nitrate R* to 100 ml of *methanol R*. Stir the suspension for 30 min. Filter or decant the suspension and immerse the plate in the silver nitrate solution for at least 30 min. Dry at 75 °C for 30 min.

A pre-conditioned plate can be stored in the dark for 5-7 days.

Mobile phase: *acetic acid R, ethanol R, dioxan R, methylene chloride R* (1:2:10:90 *V/V/V/V*).

Application: 2 μl.

Development: in a saturated tank over 3/4 of the plate.

Drying: allow to stand at room temperature and protected from light for 30 min.

Detection: spray with a 200 g/l solution of *toluenesulphonic acid R* in *ethanol R* and heat at 105 °C for 10 min. Examine in ultraviolet light at 365 nm.

System suitability: the chromatogram obtained with reference solution (a) shows 3 clearly separated spots; impurity D Rf = about 0.5; testosterone Rf = about 0.65; impurity F Rf = about 0.7.

Limits:

- *impurity D*: any spot due to impurity D is not more intense than the spot in the chromatogram obtained with reference solution (c) (0.2 per cent),
- *impurity F*: any spot due to impurity F is not more intense than the spot in the chromatogram obtained with reference solution (d) (0.1 per cent).

Related substances. Liquid chromatography (*2.2.29*).

Test solution. Dissolve 0.100 g of the substance to be examined in *methanol R* and dilute to 10.0 ml with the same solvent.

Reference solution (a). Dissolve 10 mg of *testosterone for system suitability CRS* (containing impurities C and I) in 1 ml of *methanol R.*

Reference solution (b). Dilute 1.0 ml of the test solution to 20.0 ml with *methanol R*. Dilute 1.0 ml of this solution to 10.0 ml with *methanol R.*

Reference solution (c). Dilute 2.0 ml of reference solution (b) to 10.0 ml with *methanol R.*

Column:

- *size*: *l* = 0.25 m, Ø = 4.6 mm,

- *stationary phase*: spherical *end-capped octadecylsilyl silica gel for chromatography R* (5 µm) with a pore size of 15 nm,
- *temperature*: 40 °C.

Mobile phase:
- *mobile phase A*: *water for chromatography R*, *methanol R* (45:55 *V/V*),
- *mobile phase B*: *methanol R*,

Time (min)	Mobile phase A (per cent *V/V*)	Mobile phase B (per cent *V/V*)
0 - 4	100	0
4 - 24	100 → 60	0 → 40
24 - 53	60 → 0	40 → 100
53 - 55	0	100
55 - 56	0 → 100	100 → 0
56 - 75	100	0

Flow rate: 1.0 ml/min.

Detection: spectrophotometer at 254 nm.

Injection: 20 µl.

Relative retention with reference to testosterone (retention time = about 18 min): impurity G = about 0.6; impurity H = about 0.8; impurity A = about 0.9; impurity I = about 0.95; impurity C = about 1.2; impurity E = about 1.7; impurity J = about 2.1; impurity B = about 2.5.

System suitability: reference solution (a):
- *resolution*: minimum baseline separation between the peaks due to impurity I and testosterone.

Limits: use the chromatogram obtained with reference solution (a) to identify the peaks due to impurities C and I:
- *correction factor*: for the calculation of content, multiply the peak area of impurity I by 2.9,
- *impurity C*: not more than the area of the principal peak in the chromatogram obtained with reference solution (b) (0.5 per cent),
- *impurity I*: not more than twice the area of the principal peak in the chromatogram obtained with reference solution (c) (0.2 per cent),
- *impurities A, B, E, G, H, J*: for each impurity, not more than the area of the principal peak in the chromatogram obtained with reference solution (c) (0.1 per cent),
- *any other impurity*: for each impurity, not more than the area of the principal peak in the chromatogram obtained with reference solution (c) (0.1 per cent),
- *total*: not more than 1.2 times the area of the principal peak in the chromatogram obtained with reference solution (b) (0.6 per cent),
- *disregard limit*: 0.5 times the area of the principal peak in the chromatogram obtained with reference solution (c) (0.05 per cent).

Loss on drying (*2.2.32*): maximum 1.0 per cent, determined on 0.500 g by drying in an oven at 100-105 °C for 2 h.

ASSAY

Dissolve 50.0 mg in *alcohol R* and dilute to 100.0 ml with the same solvent. Dilute 2.0 ml to 100.0 ml with *alcohol R*. Measure the absorbance (*2.2.25*) at the absorption maximum at 241 nm.

Calculate the content of $C_{19}H_{28}O_2$ taking the specific absorbance to be 569.

STORAGE

Protected from light.

IMPURITIES

Specified impurities: *A, B, C, D, E, F, G, H, I, J.*

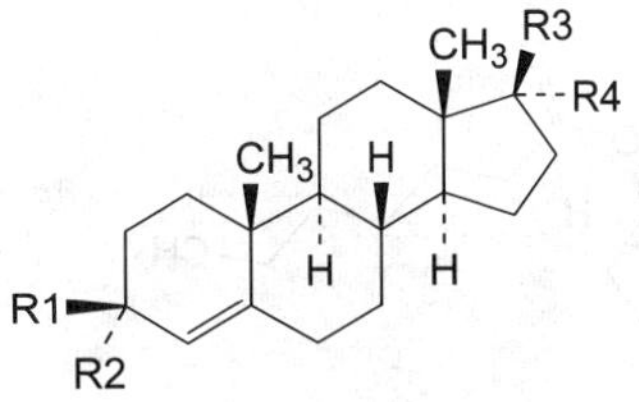

A. R1 + R2 = R3 + R4 = O: androst-4-ene-3,17-dione (androstenedione),

C. R1 + R2 = O, R3 = H, R4 = OH: 17α-hydroxyandrost-4-en-3-one (epitestosterone),

D. R1 = R3 = OH, R2 = R4 = H: androst-4-ene-3β,17β-diol (Δ4-androstenediol),

E. R1 + R2 = O, R3 = O-CO-CH_3, R4 = H: 3-oxoandrost-4-en-17β-yl acetate (testosterone acetate),

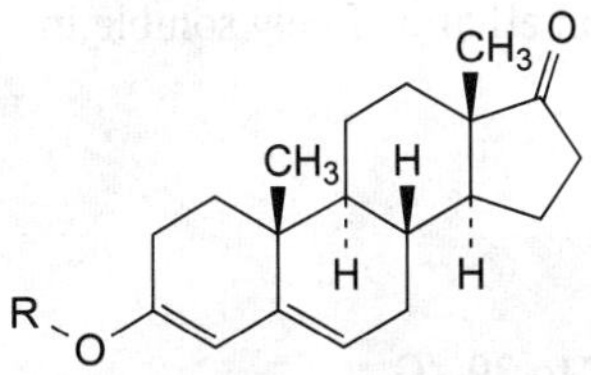

B. R = C_2H_5: 3-ethoxyandrosta-3,5-dien-17-one (androstenedione ethylenolether),

J. R = CH_3: 3-methoxyandrosta-3,5-dien-17-one (androstenedione methylenolether),

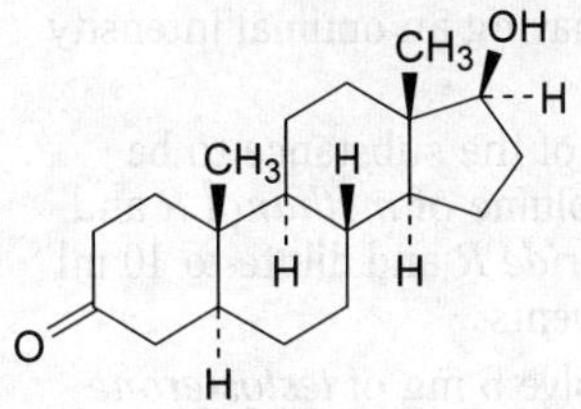

F. 17β-hydroxy-5α-androstan-3-one (androstanolone, stanolone),

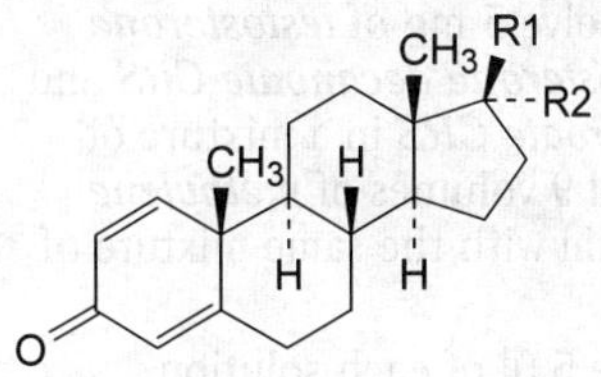

G. R1 + R2 = O: androsta-1,4-diene-3,17-dione (androstadienedione).

H. R1 = OH, R2 = H: 17β-hydroxyandrosta-1,4-dien-3-one (boldenone),

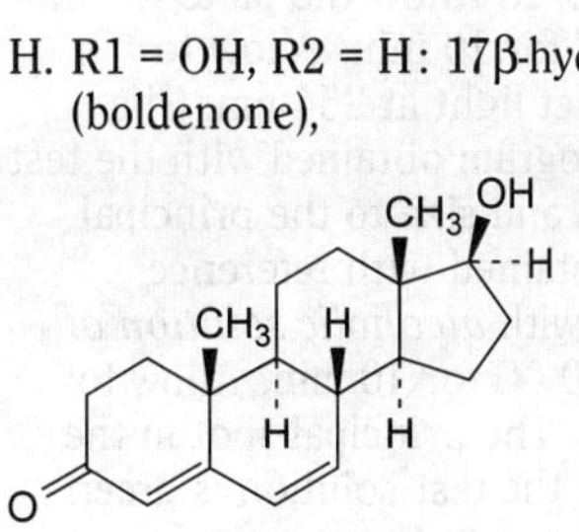

I. 17β-hydroxyandrosta-4,6-dien-3-one (Δ6-testosterone).

01/2005:1048

TESTOSTERONE ENANTATE

Testosteroni enantas

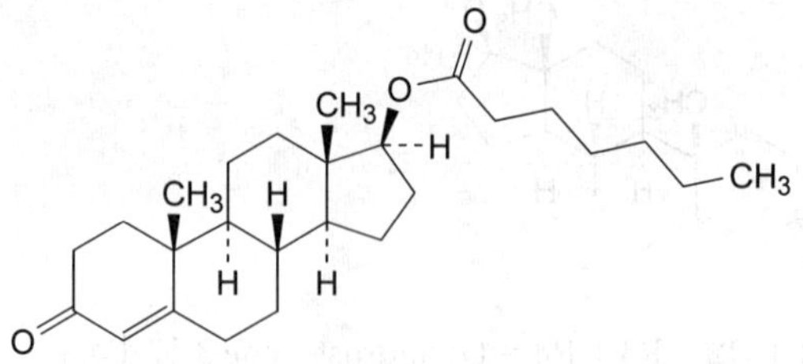

$C_{26}H_{40}O_3$ M_r 400.6

DEFINITION

Testosterone enantate contains not less than 97.0 per cent and not more than the equivalent of 103.0 per cent of 3-oxoandrost-4-en-17β-yl heptanoate, calculated with reference to the dried substance.

CHARACTERS

A white or yellowish-white, crystalline powder, practically insoluble in water, very soluble in ethanol, freely soluble in fatty oils.

IDENTIFICATION

First identification: B.

Second identification: A, C, D.

A. Melting point (*2.2.14*): 34 °C to 39 °C.

B. Examine by infrared absorption spectrophotometry (*2.2.24*), comparing with the spectrum obtained with *testosterone enantate CRS*.

C. Examine by thin-layer chromatography (*2.2.27*), using as the coating substance a suitable octadecylsilyl silica gel with a fluorescent indicator having an optimal intensity at 254 nm.

Test solution. Dissolve 5 mg of the substance to be examined in a mixture of 1 volume of *methanol R* and 9 volumes of *methylene chloride R* and dilute to 10 ml with the same mixture of solvents.

Reference solution (a). Dissolve 5 mg of *testosterone enantate CRS* in a mixture of 1 volume of *methanol R* and 9 volumes of *methylene chloride R* and dilute to 10 ml with the same mixture of solvents.

Reference solution (b). Dissolve 5 mg of *testosterone enantate CRS*, 5 mg of *testosterone decanoate CRS* and 5 mg of *testosterone isocaproate CRS* in a mixture of 1 volume of *methanol R* and 9 volumes of *methylene chloride R* and dilute to 10 ml with the same mixture of solvents.

Apply separately to the plate 5 µl of each solution. Develop over a path of 15 cm using a mixture of 20 volumes of *water R*, 40 volumes of *acetonitrile R* and 60 volumes of *2-propanol R*. Allow the plate to dry in air and heat at 100 °C for 10 min. Allow to cool and examine in ultraviolet light at 254 nm. The principal spot in the chromatogram obtained with the test solution is similar in position and size to the principal spot in the chromatogram obtained with reference solution (a). Spray the plate with *alcoholic solution of sulphuric acid R*. Heat at 120 °C for 10 min. Allow to cool and examine in daylight. The principal spot in the chromatogram obtained with the test solution is green and is similar in position and size to the principal spot in the chromatogram obtained with reference solution (a). The test is not valid unless the chromatogram obtained with reference solution (b) shows three clearly separated principal spots by each method of visualisation.

D. To about 25 mg add 2 ml of a 10 g/l solution of *potassium hydroxide R* in *methanol R* and boil under a reflux condenser for 1 h. Cool. Add 10 ml of *water R*. Acidify with *dilute hydrochloric acid R* until *blue litmus paper R* turns red. Filter and wash the precipitate with a small quantity of *water R*. The residue, after drying at 60 °C at a pressure not exceeding 0.7 kPa for 3 h, melts (*2.2.14*) at 150 °C to 153 °C.

TESTS

Specific optical rotation (*2.2.7*). Dissolve 0.250 g in *dioxan R* and dilute to 25.0 ml with the same solvent. The specific optical rotation is + 77 to + 82, calculated with reference to the dried substance.

Related substances. Examine by thin-layer chromatography (*2.2.27*), using *silica gel G R* as the coating substance.

Test solution. Dissolve 0.20 g of the substance to be examined in a mixture of 1 volume of *methanol R* and 9 volumes of *methylene chloride R* and dilute to 10 ml with the same mixture of solvents.

Reference solution (a). Dilute 1 ml of the test solution to 100 ml with a mixture of 1 volume of *methanol R* and 9 volumes of *methylene chloride R*.

Reference solution (b). Dissolve 20 mg of *testosterone propionate CRS* in a mixture of 1 volume of *methanol R* and 9 volumes of *methylene chloride R*, add 1 ml of the test solution and dilute to 100 ml with the same mixture of solvents.

Apply separately to the plate 5 µl of each solution. Develop over a path of 15 cm using a mixture of 20 volumes of *ethyl acetate R* and 80 volumes of *toluene R*. Allow the plate to dry in air. Spray with *alcoholic solution of sulphuric acid R* and heat at 120 °C for 10 min. Any spot in the chromatogram obtained with the test solution, apart from the principal spot, is not more intense than the principal spot in the chromatogram obtained with reference solution (a) (1.0 per cent). The test is not valid unless the chromatogram obtained with reference solution (b) shows two clearly separated principal spots.

Testosterone caproate. Examine by liquid chromatography (*2.2.29*).

Test solution. Dissolve 50.0 mg of the substance to be examined in the mobile phase and dilute to 50.0 ml with the mobile phase.

Reference solution (a). Dissolve 10.0 mg of *testosterone caproate CRS* in the mobile phase and dilute to 20.0 ml with the mobile phase. Dilute 1.0 ml to 50.0 ml with the mobile phase.

Reference solution (b). Dilute 1.0 ml of the test solution to 100.0 ml with the mobile phase. To 1 ml of this solution add 1 ml of reference solution (a).

The chromatographic procedure may be carried out using:

- a stainless steel column 0.12 m long and 4 mm in internal diameter packed with *octadecylsilyl silica gel for chromatography R* (5 µm),
- as mobile phase at a flow rate of 1.0 ml/min a mixture of 30 volumes of *water R* and 70 volumes of *acetonitrile R*,
- as detector a spectrophotometer set at 240 nm.

Inject 20 µl of reference solution (b). When using a recorder, adjust the sensitivity of the system so that the height of the two peaks in the chromatogram obtained with reference solution (b) is at least 50 per cent of the full scale of the recorder. The test is not valid unless in the chromatogram

Monographs T-Z

obtained the peak corresponding to testosterone caproate has a retention time of about 0.7 relative to the second peak, which corresponds to testosterone enantate.

Inject 20 µl of the test solution and 20 µl of reference solution (a). In the chromatogram obtained with the test solution, the area of any peak corresponding to testosterone caproate is not greater than the area of the peak in the chromatogram obtained with reference solution (a) (1.0 per cent).

Heptanoic acid. Dissolve 0.50 g of the substance to be examined in 10 ml of *alcohol R* previously neutralised to *bromothymol blue solution R3*. Titrate immediately with *0.01 M sodium hydroxide*. Not more than 0.6 ml of *0.01 M sodium hydroxide* is required to change the colour of the indicator to blue (0.16 per cent).

Loss on drying (*2.2.32*). Not more than 0.5 per cent, determined on 1.000 g by drying in a desiccator over *diphosphorus pentoxide R* at a pressure not exceeding 0.7 kPa.

ASSAY

Dissolve 50.0 mg in *ethanol R* and dilute to 100.0 ml with the same solvent. Dilute 2.0 ml to 100.0 ml with *ethanol R*. Measure the absorbance (*2.2.25*) at the maximum at 241 nm.

Calculate the content of $C_{26}H_{40}O_3$ taking the specific absorbance to be 422.

STORAGE

Store protected from light at a temperature of 2 °C to 8 °C.

IMPURITIES

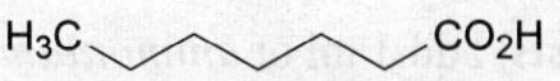

A. heptanoic acid,

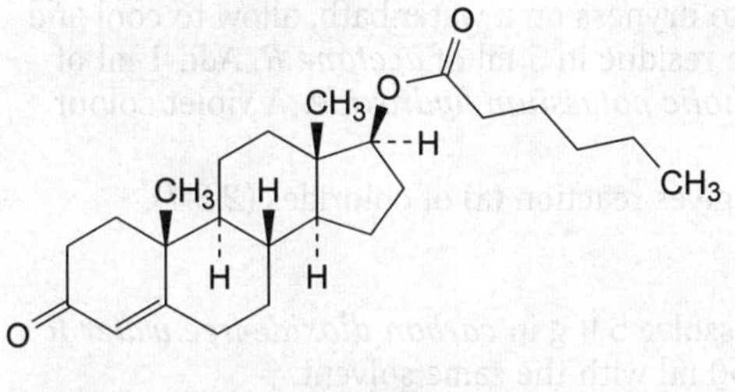

B. 3-oxoandrost-4-en-17β-yl hexanoate (testosterone caproate),

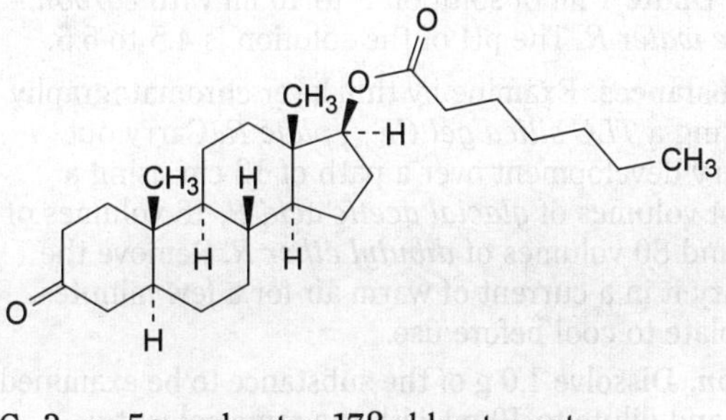

C. 3-oxo-5α-androstan-17β-yl heptanoate,

D. 17β-hydroxyandrost-4-en-3-one (testosterone).

01/2005:0297

TESTOSTERONE PROPIONATE

Testosteroni propionas

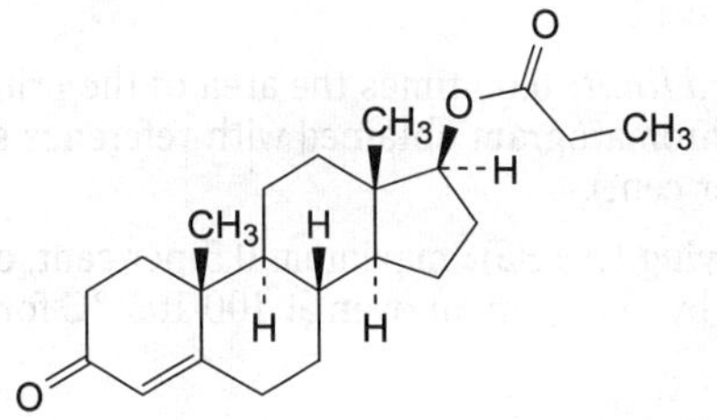

$C_{22}H_{32}O_3$ M_r 344.5

DEFINITION

3-Oxoandrost-4-en-17β-yl propanoate.

Content: 97.0 per cent to 103.0 per cent (dried substance).

CHARACTERS

Appearance: white or almost white powder or colourless crystals.

Solubility: practically insoluble in water, freely soluble in acetone and in alcohol, soluble in fatty oils.

IDENTIFICATION

Infrared absorption spectrophotometry (*2.2.24*).

Comparison: *Ph. Eur. reference spectrum of testosterone propionate.*

TESTS

Specific optical rotation (*2.2.7*): + 84 to + 90 (dried substance).

Dissolve 0.250 g in *ethanol R* and dilute to 25.0 ml with the same solvent.

Related substances. Liquid chromatography (*2.2.29*).

Test solution. Dissolve 50.0 mg of the substance to be examined in *methanol R* and dilute to 50.0 ml with the same solvent.

Reference solution (a). Dissolve 2 mg of the substance to be examined and 2 mg of *testosterone acetate CRS* in *methanol R* and dilute to 50.0 ml with the same solvent.

Reference solution (b). Dilute 1.0 ml of the test solution to 100.0 ml with *methanol R*.

Column:

- *size*: l = 0.25 m, Ø = 4.6 mm,
- *stationary phase*: *octadecylsilyl silica gel for chromatography R* (5 µm).

Mobile phase: *water R, methanol R* (20:80 *V/V*).

Flow rate: 1.5 ml/min.

Detection: spectrophotometer at 254 nm.

Injection: 20 µl.

Run time: twice the retention time of testosterone propionate.

Relative retention with reference to testosterone propionate (retention time = about 9 min): impurity C = about 0.5; impurity A = about 0.7; impurity D = about 0.8; impurity B = about 1.4.

System suitability: reference solution (a):

- *resolution*: minimum 4.0 between the peaks due to testosterone propionate and to impurity A.

Limits:

- *any impurity*: not more than 0.5 times the area of the principal peak in the chromatogram obtained with reference solution (b) (0.5 per cent),
- *total*: not more than the area of the principal peak in the chromatogram obtained with reference solution (b) (1.0 per cent),
- *disregard limit*: 0.05 times the area of the principal peak in the chromatogram obtained with reference solution (b) (0.05 per cent).

Loss on drying (*2.2.32*): maximum 0.5 per cent, determined on 0.500 g by drying in an oven at 100-105 °C for 2 h.

ASSAY

Dissolve 25.0 mg in *ethanol R* and dilute to 250.0 ml with the same solvent. Dilute 10.0 ml of the solution to 100.0 ml with *ethanol R*. Measure the absorbance (*2.2.25*) at the maximum at 240 nm.

Calculate the content of $C_{22}H_{32}O_3$ taking the specific absorbance to be 490.

IMPURITIES

Specified impurities: A, B, C, D.

Other detectable impurities: E.

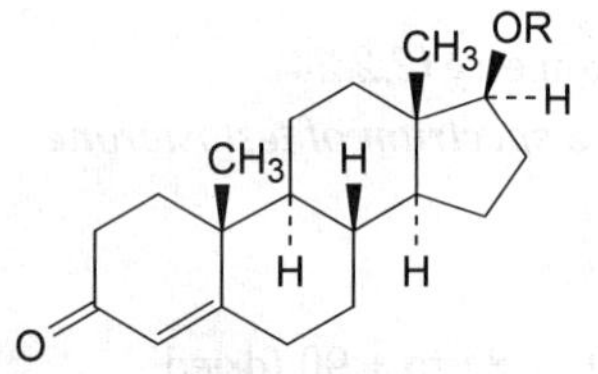

A. R = $CO\text{-}CH_3$: 3-oxoandrost-4-en-17β-yl acetate (testosterone acetate),

B. R = $CO\text{-}CH(CH_3)_2$: 3-oxoandrost-4-en-17β-yl 2-methylpropanoate (testosterone isobutyrate),

C. R = H: testosterone,

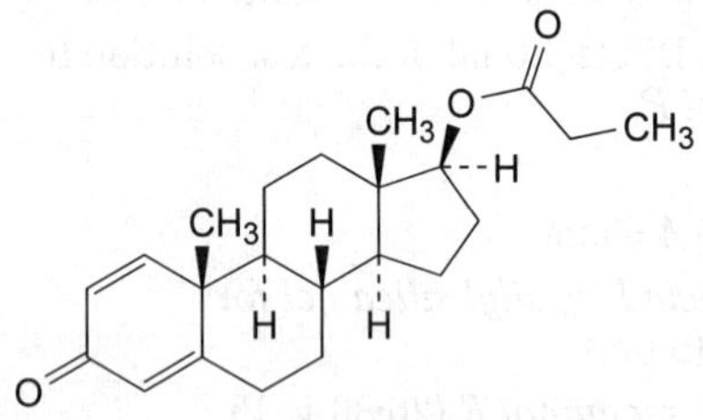

D. 3-oxoandrosta-1,4-dien-17β-yl propanoate,

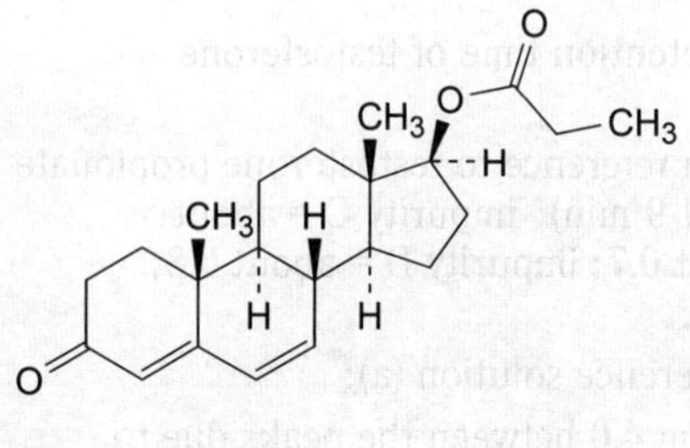

E. 3-oxoandrosta-4,6-dien-17β-yl propanoate.

01/2005:0057

TETRACAINE HYDROCHLORIDE

Tetracaini hydrochloridum

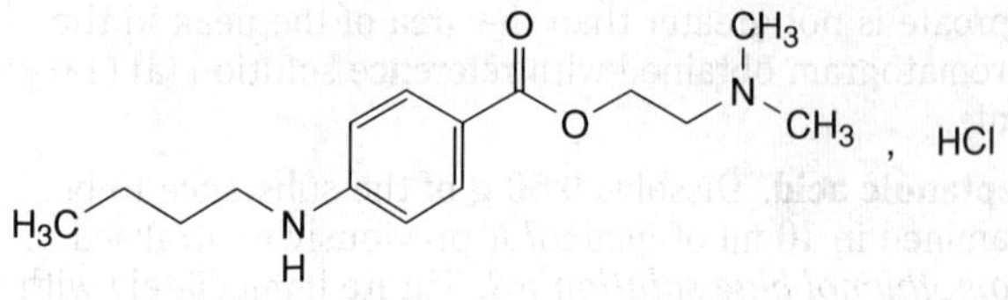

$C_{15}H_{25}ClN_2O_2$ M_r 300.8

DEFINITION

Tetracaine hydrochloride contains not less than 99.0 per cent and not more than the equivalent of 101.0 per cent of 2-(dimethylamino)ethyl 4-(butylamino)benzoate hydrochloride, calculated with reference to the dried substance.

CHARACTERS

A white, crystalline powder, slightly hygroscopic, freely soluble in water, soluble in alcohol.

It melts at about 148 °C or it may occur in either of 2 other crystalline forms which melt respectively at about 134 °C and 139 °C. Mixtures of these forms melt within the range 134 °C to 147 °C.

IDENTIFICATION

First identification: A, B, D.

Second identification: B, C, D.

A. Examine by infrared absorption spectrophotometry (*2.2.24*), comparing with the spectrum obtained with *tetracaine hydrochloride CRS.*

B. To 10 ml of solution S (see Tests) add 1 ml of *ammonium thiocyanate solution R*. A white, crystalline precipitate is formed which, after recrystallisation from *water R* and drying at 80 °C for 2 h, melts (*2.2.14*) at about 131 °C.

C. To about 5 mg add 0.5 ml of *fuming nitric acid R*. Evaporate to dryness on a water-bath, allow to cool and dissolve the residue in 5 ml of *acetone R*. Add 1 ml of *0.1 M alcoholic potassium hydroxide.* A violet colour develops.

D. Solution S gives reaction (a) of chlorides (*2.3.1*).

TESTS

Solution S. Dissolve 5.0 g in *carbon dioxide-free water R* and dilute to 50 ml with the same solvent.

Appearance of solution. Dilute 2 ml of solution S to 10 ml with *water R*. The solution is clear (*2.2.1*) and colourless (*2.2.2, Method II*).

pH (*2.2.3*). Dilute 1 ml of solution S to 10 ml with *carbon dioxide-free water R*. The pH of the solution is 4.5 to 6.5.

Related substances. Examine by thin-layer chromatography (*2.2.27*), using a *TLC silica gel* GF_{254} *plate R*. Carry out a preliminary development over a path of 12 cm using a mixture of 4 volumes of *glacial acetic acid R*, 16 volumes of *hexane R* and 80 volumes of *dibutyl ether R*. Remove the plate and dry it in a current of warm air for a few minutes. Allow the plate to cool before use.

Test solution. Dissolve 1.0 g of the substance to be examined in *water R* and dilute to 10 ml with the same solvent.

Reference solution. Dissolve 50 mg of *4-aminobenzoic acid R* in *water R* and dilute to 100 ml with the same solvent. Dilute 1 ml of the solution to 10 ml with *water R*.

Apply to the plate 5 µl of each solution. Develop over a path of 10 cm using a mixture of 4 volumes of *glacial acetic acid R*, 16 volumes of *hexane R* and 80 volumes of *dibutyl ether R*. Dry the plate at 100 °C to 105 °C for 10 min and examine in ultraviolet light at 254 nm. Any spot in the chromatogram obtained with the test solution, apart from the principal spot, is not more intense than the spot in the chromatogram obtained with the reference solution (0.05 per cent). The principal spot in the chromatogram obtained with the test solution remains at the starting point.

Heavy metals (*2.4.8*). 12 ml of solution S complies with limit test A for heavy metals (10 ppm). Prepare the standard using *lead standard solution (1 ppm Pb) R*.

Loss on drying (*2.2.32*). Not more than 1.0 per cent, determined on 1.000 g by drying in an oven at 100 °C to 105 °C.

Sulphated ash (*2.4.14*). Not more than 0.1 per cent, determined on 1.0 g.

ASSAY

Dissolve 0.250 g in 50 ml of *alcohol R* and add 5.0 ml of *0.01 M hydrochloric acid*. Carry out a potentiometric titration (*2.2.20*), using *0.1 M sodium hydroxide*. Read the volume added between the 2 points of inflexion.

1 ml of *0.1 M sodium hydroxide* is equivalent to 30.08 mg of $C_{15}H_{25}ClN_2O_2$.

STORAGE

Store protected from light.

01/2005:0644

TETRACOSACTIDE

Tetracosactidum

H-Ser–Tyr–Ser–Met–Glu–His–Phe–Arg–Trp–Gly–
Lys–Pro–Val–Gly–Lys–Lys–Arg–Arg–Pro–Val–
Lys–Val–Tyr–Pro-OH

$C_{136}H_{210}N_{40}O_{31}S$ M_r 2933

DEFINITION

Tetracosactide is a synthetic tetracosapeptide in which the sequence of amino acids is the same as that of the first twenty-four residues of human corticotropin. It is available as an acetate and contains water. It increases the rate at which corticoid hormones are secreted by the adrenal glands. The potency is not less than 800 International Units per milligram, calculated with reference to the anhydrous, acetic acid-free substance.

CHARACTERS

A white or yellow, amorphous powder, sparingly soluble in water.

IDENTIFICATION

A. It increases the amount of corticosterone produced by isolated rat adrenal cells in the conditions of the assay.

B. Examine by electrophoresis (*2.2.31*) and thin-layer chromatography (*2.2.27*) to obtain a two-dimensional separation using two plates with *cellulose for chromatography R1* as the coating substance.

Test solution. Dissolve 1 mg of the substance to be examined in 0.2 ml of a 15.4 g/l solution of *ammonium acetate R* adjusted to pH 8.2 with *dilute ammonia R2*. Add 10 µl of a 2 g/l solution of *trypsin R*, maintain the mixture at 37 °C to 38 °C for 40 min, heat on a water-bath for 3 min and add 5 µl of *glacial acetic acid R*. Evaporate to dryness at 40 °C at a pressure not exceeding 3 kPa, dry the glassy residue at 40 °C for 1 h and dissolve in 0.1 ml of *glacial acetic acid R*. Dry the solution from the frozen state, dissolve the residue in 0.1 ml of *water R* and dry again from the frozen state. Dry the final residue at 45 °C for 1 h at a pressure not exceeding 3 kPa and dissolve in 50 µl of *water R*.

Reference solution. Prepare at the same time and in the same manner as the test solution, using *tetracosactide CRS* instead of the substance to be examined.

Spray the plates with the electrolyte solution which consists of a solution containing 0.2 per cent *V/V* of *glacial acetic acid R* and 0.2 per cent *V/V* of *pyridine R*. Place the filter paper tongues to connect the plates with the appropriate compartment of each trough so that each tongue covers an area 1.5 cm wide at one end of the plate. Close the tank and allow to stand for 30 min. Apply the solutions on the anodic side. Apply to the first plate, at a point about 2.5 cm from each of two adjacent edges, 4 µl of the test solution. Apply to the second plate, at a similar position, 4 µl of the reference solution. Apply to both plates a potential of 280 V for a plate 200 mm long and allow electrophoresis to proceed for 90 min. Allow the plates to dry in air for 30 min and then dry in a current of air at 30 °C for 30 min. Carry out a second separation on each plate by thin-layer chromatography. Develop at right angles to the direction of electrophoresis over a path of 15 cm using a mixture of 8 volumes of *glacial acetic acid R*, 24 volumes of *pyridine R*, 30 volumes of *water R* and 38 volumes of *butanol R*. Dry the plates in a current of air and spray with *ninhydrin solution R1*. The principal spots in the chromatogram obtained with the test solution are similar in position to those in the chromatogram obtained with the reference solution, but their intensity may differ.

TESTS

Specific optical rotation (*2.2.7*). Dissolve 10.0 mg in 1.0 ml of a mixture of 1 volume of *glacial acetic acid R* and 99 volumes of *water R*. The specific optical rotation is − 99 to − 109, calculated with reference to the anhydrous, acetic acid-free substance.

Absorbance (*2.2.25*). Dissolve 1.0 mg in *0.1 M hydrochloric acid* and dilute to 5.0 ml with the same acid. Examined between 240 nm and 280 nm, the solution shows an absorption maximum at 276 nm. The absorbance at the maximum is 0.51 to 0.61, calculated with reference to the anhydrous, acetic acid-free substance. The ratio of the absorbance at the maximum at 276 nm to the absorbance at 248 nm is 2.4 to 2.9.

Amino acids. Examine by means of an amino-acid analyser. Standardise the apparatus with a mixture containing equimolar amounts of ammonia, glycine and the L-form of the following amino acids:

Lysine	Threonine	Alanine	Leucine
Histidine	Serine	Valine	Tyrosine
Arginine	Glutamic acid	Methionine	Phenylalanine
Aspartic acid	Proline	Isoleucine	

together with half the equimolar amount of L-cystine. For the validation of the method, an appropriate internal standard, such as *DL-norleucine R*, is used.

Test solution. Place 1.0 mg of the substance to be examined in a rigorously cleaned hard-glass tube, 100 mm long and 6 mm in internal diameter. Add a suitable amount of a

Monographs T-Z

50 per cent *V/V* solution of *hydrochloric acid R*. Immerse the tube in a freezing mixture at −5 °C, reduce the pressure to below 133 Pa and seal. Heat at 110 °C to 115 °C for 16 h. Cool, open the tube, transfer the contents to a 10 ml flask with the aid of five quantities, each of 0.2 ml, of *water R* and evaporate to dryness over *potassium hydroxide R* under reduced pressure. Take up the residue in *water R* and evaporate to dryness over *potassium hydroxide R* under reduced pressure; repeat these operations once. Take up the residue in a buffer solution suitable for the amino-acid analyser used and dilute to a suitable volume with the same buffer solution. Apply a suitable volume to the amino-acid analyser.

Express the content of each amino acid in moles. Calculate the relative proportions of the amino acids, taking that for valine to be equivalent to three. The values fall within the following limits: lysine 3.5 to 4.7; histidine 0.9 to 1.1; arginine 2.7 to 3.3; serine 1.1 to 2.2; glutamic acid 0.9 to 1.1; proline 2.5 to 3.5; glycine 1.8 to 2.2; methionine 0.9 to 1.1; tyrosine 1.7 to 2.2; phenylalanine 0.9 to 1.1. Not more than traces of other amino acids are present, with the exception of tryptophan.

Related peptides

A. Examine by liquid chromatography (*2.2.29*). Use degassed solvents.

Test solution. Dissolve 1.0 mg of the substance to be examined in 1 ml of *water R*.

Reference solution (a). Dissolve 1.0 mg of the substance to be examined in 1 ml of a 1 per cent *V/V* solution of *glacial acetic acid R* and add 50 µl of a mixture of 1 volume of *strong hydrogen peroxide solution R* and 999 volumes of *water R*. Allow to stand for 2 h.

Reference solution (b). Dissolve 1.0 mg of *tetracosactide CRS* in 1 ml of *water R*.

The chromatographic procedure may be carried out using:

– a stainless steel column 0.25 m long and 4.6 mm in internal diameter packed with *octadecylsilyl silica gel for chromatography R* (10 µm),

– as mobile phase at a flow rate of 2.0 ml/min, a mixture of 365 ml of *acetonitrile R*, 10.0 ml of *glacial acetic acid R* and 10.0 g of *ammonium sulphate R*, diluted to 2000 ml with *water R*,

– as detector a spectrophotometer set at 280 nm.

Inject 20 µl of each solution ensuring that the syringe used to inject the test solution is not contaminated with peroxide. The chromatogram obtained with reference solution (a) shows a peak due to tetracosactide corresponding to the principal peak in the chromatogram obtained with the test solution and a peak with a lower retention time, due to tetracosactide sulphoxide, of significantly greater area than any corresponding peak in the chromatogram obtained with the test solution. The test is not valid unless in the chromatogram obtained with reference solution (a), the resolution between the peaks corresponding to tetracosactide and tetracosactide sulphoxide is at least 7. In the chromatogram obtained with the test solution, the area of the peak corresponding to tetracosactide sulphoxide is not greater than 4 per cent of the sum of the areas of all the peaks, disregarding any peaks due to the solvent and the mobile phase.

B. Examine by thin-layer chromatography (*2.2.27*), using *cellulose for chromatography R* as the coating substance.

Test solution. Dissolve 3.0 mg of the substance to be examined in 1.5 ml of a mixture of equal volumes of *dilute acetic acid R* and *water R*.

Reference solution (a). Dilute 0.5 ml of the test solution to 10 ml with a mixture of equal volumes of *dilute acetic acid R* and *water R*.

Reference solution (b). Dilute 5 ml of reference solution (a) to 10 ml with a mixture of equal volumes of *dilute acetic acid R* and *water R*.

Reference solution (c). To 0.5 ml of the test solution add 50 µl of a mixture of 1 volume of *strong hydrogen peroxide solution R* and 999 volumes of *water R*. Allow to stand for 2 h.

Apply to the plate as 1 cm bands 10 µl of each solution. Develop over a path of 15 cm using a mixture of 4 volumes of *glacial acetic acid R*, 24 volumes of *pyridine R*, 30 volumes of *water R* and 42 volumes of *butanol R*. Dry the plate in a current of air and spray with *ninhydrin solution R1*. In the chromatogram obtained with reference solution (c), the band corresponding in position to the principal band in the chromatogram obtained with the test solution is reduced in intensity, and a prominent band, due to tetracosactide sulphoxide, of lower R_f is present. In the chromatogram obtained with the test solution, any band, apart from the principal band and any band due to tetracosactide sulphoxide, is not more intense than the band in the chromatogram obtained with reference solution (a) (5.0 per cent) and at most one such band is more intense than the band in the chromatogram obtained with reference solution (b) (2.5 per cent).

Peptide. Not less than 85.0 per cent of peptide, expressed as $C_{136}H_{210}N_{40}O_{31}S$, calculated with reference to the anhydrous, acetic acid-free substance.

Examine the chromatograms obtained in test A for related peptides. Calculate the content of $C_{136}H_{210}N_{40}O_{31}S$ from the peak heights or areas in the chromatograms obtained with the test solution and reference solution (b), and the declared content of $C_{136}H_{210}N_{40}O_{31}S$ in *tetracosactide CRS*.

Acetic acid (*2.5.34*): 8.0 per cent to 13.0 per cent.

Test solution. Dissolve 10.0 mg of the substance to be examined in a mixture of 5 volumes of mobile phase B and 95 volumes of mobile phase A and dilute to 10.0 ml with the same mixture of solvents.

Water (*2.5.12*): 5.0 per cent to 16.0 per cent, determined on 80.0 mg by the semi-micro determination of water.

ASSAY

The potency of tetracosactide is estimated by comparing in given conditions its activity in increasing the amount of corticosterone produced by isolated rat adrenal cells with that of the International Reference Preparation of tetracosactide or a reference preparation calibrated in International Units.

The International Unit is the activity contained in a stated amount of the International Reference Preparation which consists of a quantity of synthetic tetracosactide with mannitol. The equivalence in International Units of the International Reference Preparation is stated by the World Health Organisation.

The estimated potency is not less than 80 per cent and not more than 125 per cent of the stated potency. The confidence limits ($P = 0.95$) of the estimated potency are not less than 64 per cent and not more than 156 per cent of the stated potency.

Use siliconised glassware and rinse well with *water R* before use. Kill four male rats, each weighing between 200 g and 400 g, by exsanguination. Remove the adrenal glands, carefully free them of adhering fat and immerse in solution B maintained at 4 °C. Cut each gland into four equal pieces and transfer to a suitable plastic stirring apparatus (see

Figure 0644.-1) containing 5 ml of solution C maintained at 37 °C. Disperse the adrenal cells by stirring the mixture at 500 r/min. After 20 min, remove the supernatant liquid, cool to 4 °C, add 5 ml of solution C and repeat the dispersal procedure. Repeat the operation a further three times. Combine the five supernatant liquids, centrifuge at 4 °C in a polyethylene test-tube for 30 min after slow acceleration to 100 *g*. Suspend the resulting pellet in 8 ml of solution D and centrifuge for 30 min at 100 *g*. Again suspend the residue in 8 ml of solution D and filter the mixture through nylon gauze with 100 µm pores into a polyethylene beaker and add a suitable volume of solution D to the filtrate (a total volume of 65 ml to 105 ml has been found suitable). Maintain the resulting suspension at 4 °C.

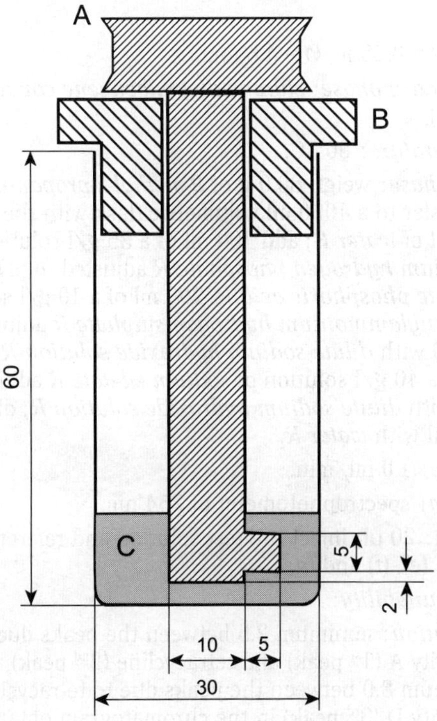

A - pulley and stirring paddle,

B - bearing,

C - incubation medium.

Figure 0644.-1. – *Stirring Apparatus*
Dimensions in millimetres

Prepare four independent dilutions, with two-fold dose intervals, from solutions of suitable concentrations of the substance to be examined and of the reference preparation using solution E as diluent. Pipette 0.1 ml of each dilution into each of four polystyrene test-tubes and add 1.0 ml of the cell suspension prepared above to each tube. Incubate at 37 °C for 2 h and then cool to 4 °C. Transfer 1 ml of the contents of each tube to a glass tube containing 1.4 ml of *methylene chloride R*, mix in a vortex mixer for 10 s and centrifuge at 3000 *g* for 5 min. Transfer 1 ml of each of the methylene chloride layers, avoiding taking up aqueous phase, to a glass tube containing 0.6 ml of a mixture of 15 volumes of *alcohol R* and 35 volumes of *sulphuric acid R*. Mix in a vortex mixer for 10 s and centrifuge at 1500 *g* for 5 min. Allow each tube to stand for 30 min. Examine by fluorimetry (*2.2.21*), irradiating the lower layer with an excitant beam of suitable wavelength such as 436 nm or 470 nm and measuring the fluorescence at the maximum between 530 nm and 545 nm. If the solutions are not transferred to spectrophotometric measurement cells, select glass tubes that give fluorescence values for a standard corticosterone which do not differ from each other by more than 5 per cent. Calculate the result of the assay by the usual statistical methods using the linear portion of the log dose-response curve.

Solution A

Sodium chloride R	6.60 g
Potassium chloride R	0.353 g
Sodium hydrogen carbonate R	0.840 g
Potassium dihydrogen phosphate R	0.161 g
Magnesium sulphate R	0.291 g
Calcium chloride R	0.373 g
2-[4-(2-Hydroxyethyl)piperazin-1-yl]ethane sulphonic acid R	4.77 g

Dissolve the above ingredients in about 950 ml of *water R*, adjust to pH 7.4 with *1 M sodium hydroxide* and add 60 mg of *benzylpenicillin sodium R* and a quantity of *streptomycin sulphate R* equivalent to 100 mg of streptomycin. Dilute to 1000 ml with *water R*.

Solution B

Add 2 g/l of *glucose R* to solution A.

Solution C

To solution B add 1 g/l of a preparation of collagenase obtained from *Clostridium histolyticum* and of a grade suitable for the preparation of dispersed cells.

Solution D

Add 5 g/l of *bovine albumin R* to solution B.

Solution E

A 9 g/l sterile solution of *sodium chloride R* containing 1 g/l of *bovine albumin R* and adjusted to pH 2.0 with *1 M hydrochloric acid.*

STORAGE

Store under nitrogen, protected from light, at a temperature between 2 °C and 8 °C.

LABELLING

The label states:

– the potency in International Units per milligram,
– the peptide content per container,
– the storage conditions.

01/2005:0211

TETRACYCLINE

Tetracyclinum

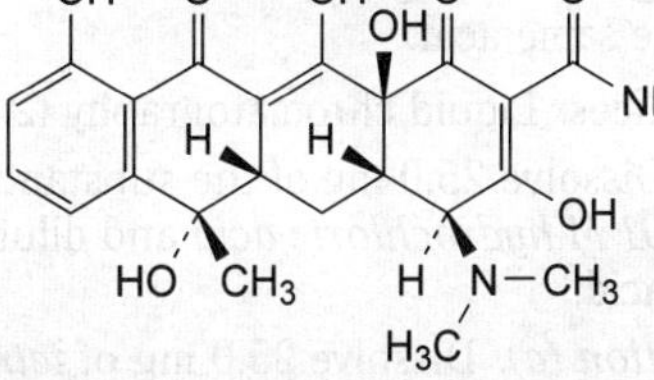

$C_{22}H_{24}N_2O_8$ M_r 444.4

DEFINITION

(4*S*,4a*S*,5a*S*,6*S*,12a*S*)-4-(Dimethylamino)-3,6,10,12,12a-pentahydroxy-6-methyl-1,11-dioxo-1,4,4a,5,5a,6,11,12a-octahydrotetracene-2-carboxamide.

Content: 88.0 per cent to 102.0 per cent (dried substance).

CHARACTERS

Appearance: yellow, crystalline powder.

Solubility: very slightly soluble in water, soluble in alcohol and in methanol, sparingly soluble in acetone. It dissolves in dilute acid and alkaline solutions.

IDENTIFICATION

A. Thin-layer chromatography (*2.2.27*).

Test solution. Dissolve 5 mg of the substance to be examined in *methanol R* and dilute to 10 ml with the same solvent.

Reference solution (a). Dissolve 5 mg of *tetracycline hydrochloride CRS* in *methanol R* and dilute to 10 ml with the same solvent.

Reference solution (b). Dissolve 5 mg of *tetracycline hydrochloride CRS*, 5 mg of *demeclocycline hydrochloride R* and 5 mg of *oxytetracycline hydrochloride R* in *methanol R* and dilute to 10 ml with the same solvent.

Plate: *TLC octadecylsilyl silica gel F_{254} plate R.*

Mobile phase: mix 20 volumes of *acetonitrile R*, 20 volumes of *methanol R* and 60 volumes of a 63 g/l solution of *oxalic acid R* previously adjusted to pH 2 with *concentrated ammonia R.*

Application: 1 µl.

Development: over 3/4 of the plate.

Drying: in air.

Detection: examine in ultraviolet light at 254 nm.

System suitability: the chromatogram obtained with reference solution (b) shows 3 clearly separated spots.

Results: the principal spot in the chromatogram obtained with the test solution is similar in position and size to the principal spot in the chromatogram obtained with reference solution (a).

B. To about 2 mg add 5 ml of *sulphuric acid R*. A violet-red colour develops. Add the solution to 2.5 ml of *water R*. The colour becomes yellow.

C. Dissolve about 10 mg in a mixture of 1 ml of *dilute nitric acid R* and 5 ml of *water R*. Shake and add 1 ml of *silver nitrate solution R2*. Any opalescence in the solution is not more intense than that in a mixture of 1 ml of *dilute nitric acid R*, 5 ml of *water R* and 1 ml of *silver nitrate solution R2*.

TESTS

pH (*2.2.3*): 3.5 to 6.0.

Suspend 0.1 g in 10 ml of *carbon dioxide-free water R*.

Specific optical rotation (*2.2.7*): − 260 to − 280 (dried substance).

Dissolve 0.250 g in *0.1 M hydrochloric acid* and dilute to 50.0 ml with the same acid.

Related substances. Liquid chromatography (*2.2.29*).

Test solution. Dissolve 25.0 mg of the substance to be examined in *0.01 M hydrochloric acid* and dilute to 25.0 ml with the same acid.

Reference solution (a). Dissolve 25.0 mg of *tetracycline hydrochloride CRS* in *0.01 M hydrochloric acid* and dilute to 25.0 ml with the same acid.

Reference solution (b). Dissolve 12.5 mg of *4-epitetracycline hydrochloride CRS* in *0.01 M hydrochloric acid* and dilute to 50.0 ml with the same acid.

Reference solution (c). Dissolve 10.0 mg of *anhydrotetracycline hydrochloride CRS* in *0.01 M hydrochloric acid* and dilute to 100.0 ml with the same acid.

Reference solution (d). Dissolve 10.0 mg of *4-epianhydrotetracycline hydrochloride CRS* in *0.01 M hydrochloric acid* and dilute to 50.0 ml with the same acid.

Reference solution (e). Mix 1.0 ml of reference solution (a), 2.0 ml of reference solution (b) and 5.0 ml of reference solution (d) and dilute to 25.0 ml with *0.01 M hydrochloric acid.*

Reference solution (f). Mix 40.0 ml of reference solution (b), 20.0 ml of reference solution (c) and 5.0 ml of reference solution (d) and dilute to 200.0 ml with *0.01 M hydrochloric acid.*

Reference solution (g). Dilute 1.0 ml of reference solution (c) to 50.0 ml with *0.01 M hydrochloric acid.*

Column:

- *size*: l = 0.25 m, Ø = 4.6 mm,
- *stationary phase*: *styrene-divinylbenzene copolymer R* (8 µm),
- *temperature*: 60 °C.

Mobile phase: weigh 80.0 g of *2-methyl-2-propanol R* and transfer to a 1000 ml volumetric flask with the aid of 200 ml of *water R*; add 100 ml of a 35 g/l solution of *dipotassium hydrogen phosphate R* adjusted to pH 9.0 with *dilute phosphoric acid R*, 200 ml of a 10 g/l solution of *tetrabutylammonium hydrogen sulphate R* adjusted to pH 9.0 with *dilute sodium hydroxide solution R* and 10 ml of a 40 g/l solution of *sodium edetate R* adjusted to pH 9.0 with *dilute sodium hydroxide solution R*; dilute to 1000.0 ml with *water R*.

Flow rate: 1.0 ml/min.

Detection: spectrophotometer at 254 nm.

Injection: 20 µl; inject the test solution and reference solutions (e), (f) and (g).

System suitability:

- *resolution*: minimum 2.5 between the peaks due to impurity A (1st peak) and tetracycline (2nd peak) and minimum 8.0 between the peaks due to tetracycline and impurity D (3rd peak) in the chromatogram obtained with reference solution (e); if necessary, adjust the concentration of 2-methyl-2-propanol in the mobile phase,
- *signal-to-noise ratio*: minimum 3 for the principal peak in the chromatogram obtained with reference solution (g),
- *symmetry factor*: maximum 1.25 for the peak due to tetracycline in the chromatogram obtained with reference solution (e).

Limits:

- *impurity A*: not more than the area of the corresponding peak in the chromatogram obtained with reference solution (f) (5.0 per cent),
- *impurity B* (eluting on the tail of the principal peak): not more than 0.4 times the area of the peak due to impurity A in the chromatogram obtained with reference solution (f) (2.0 per cent),
- *impurity C*: not more than the area of the corresponding peak in the chromatogram obtained with reference solution (f) (1.0 per cent),
- *impurity D*: not more than the area of the corresponding peak in the chromatogram obtained with reference solution (f) (0.5 per cent).

Heavy metals (*2.4.8*): maximum 50 ppm.

0.5 g complies with limit test C. Prepare the standard using 2.5 ml of *lead standard solution (10 ppm Pb) R*.

Loss on drying (*2.2.32*): maximum 13.0 per cent, determined on 1.000 g by drying in an oven at 100-105 °C.

Sulphated ash (*2.4.14*): maximum 0.5 per cent, determined on 1.0 g.

ASSAY

Liquid chromatography (*2.2.29*) as described in the test for related substances with the following modification.

Injection: test solution and reference solution (a).

Calculate the percentage content of $C_{22}H_{24}N_2O_8$.

STORAGE

Protected from light.

IMPURITIES

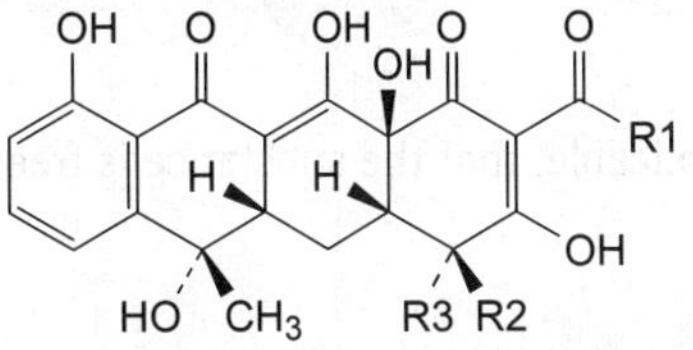

A. R1 = NH_2, R2 = H, R3 = $N(CH_3)_2$: (4*R*,4a*S*,5a*S*,6*S*,12a*S*)-4-(dimethylamino)-3,6,10,12,12a-pentahydroxy-6-methyl-1,11-dioxo-1,4,4a,5,5a,6,11,12a-octahydrotetracene-2-carboxamide (4-epitetracycline),

B. R1 = CH_3, R2 = $N(CH_3)_2$, R3 = H: (4*S*,4a*S*,5a*S*,6*S*,12a*S*)-2-acetyl-4-(dimethylamino)-3,6,10,12,12a-pentahydroxy-6-methyl-4a,5a,6,12a-tetrahydrotetracene-1,11(4*H*,5*H*)-dione (2-acetyl-2-decarbamoyltetracycline),

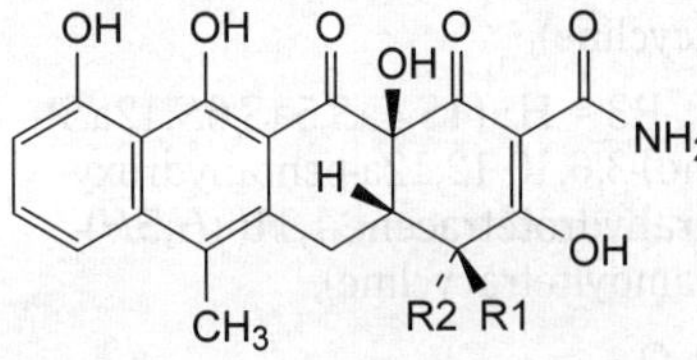

C. R1 = $N(CH_3)_2$, R2 = H: (4*S*,4a*S*,12a*S*)-4-(dimethylamino)-3,10,11,12a-tetrahydroxy-6-methyl-1,12-dioxo-1,4,4a,5,12,12a-hexahydrotetracene-2-carboxamide (anhydrotetracycline),

D. R1 = H, R2 = $N(CH_3)_2$: (4*R*,4a*S*,12a*S*)-4-(dimethylamino)-3,10,11,12a-tetrahydroxy-6-methyl-1,12-dioxo-1,4,4a,5,12,12a-hexahydrotetracene-2-carboxamide (4-epianhydrotetracycline).

01/2005:0210

TETRACYCLINE HYDROCHLORIDE

Tetracyclini hydrochloridum

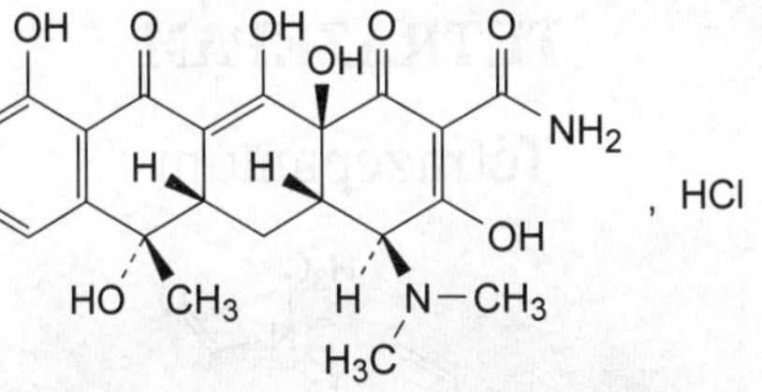

$C_{22}H_{25}ClN_2O_8$ M_r 480.9

DEFINITION

(4*S*,4a*S*,5a*S*,6*S*,12a*S*)-4-(Dimethylamino)-3,6,10,12,12a-pentahydroxy-6-methyl-1,11-dioxo-1,4,4a,5,5a,6,11,12a-octahydrotetracene-2-carboxamide hydrochloride.

Content: 95.0 per cent to 102.0 per cent (dried substance).

CHARACTERS

Appearance: yellow, crystalline powder.

Solubility: soluble in water, slightly soluble in alcohol, practically insoluble in acetone. It dissolves in solutions of alkali hydroxides and carbonates. Solutions in water become turbid on standing, owing to the precipitation of tetracycline.

IDENTIFICATION

A. Thin-layer chromatography (*2.2.27*).

Test solution. Dissolve 5 mg of the substance to be examined in *methanol R* and dilute to 10 ml with the same solvent.

Reference solution (a). Dissolve 5 mg of *tetracycline hydrochloride CRS* in *methanol R* and dilute to 10 ml with the same solvent.

Reference solution (b). Dissolve 5 mg of *tetracycline hydrochloride CRS*, 5 mg of *demeclocycline hydrochloride R* and 5 mg of *oxytetracycline hydrochloride R* in *methanol R* and dilute to 10 ml with the same solvent.

Plate: *TLC octadecylsilyl silica gel F_{254} plate R.*

Mobile phase: mix 20 volumes of *acetonitrile R*, 20 volumes of *methanol R* and 60 volumes of a 63 g/l solution of *oxalic acid R* previously adjusted to pH 2 with *concentrated ammonia R.*

Application: 1 µl.

Development: over 3/4 of the plate.

Drying: in air.

Detection: examine in ultraviolet light at 254 nm.

System suitability: the chromatogram obtained with reference solution (b) shows 3 clearly separated spots.

Results: the principal spot in the chromatogram obtained with the test solution is similar in position and size to the principal spot in the chromatogram obtained with reference solution (a).

B. To about 2 mg add 5 ml of *sulphuric acid R*. A violet-red colour develops. Add the solution to 2.5 ml of *water R*. The colour becomes yellow.

C. It gives reaction (a) of chlorides (*2.3.1*).

TESTS

pH (*2.2.3*): 1.8 to 2.8.

Dissolve 0.1 g in 10 ml of *carbon dioxide-free water R.*

Specific optical rotation (*2.2.7*): − 240 to − 255 (dried substance).

Dissolve 0.250 g in *0.1 M hydrochloric acid* and dilute to 25.0 ml with the same acid.

Related substances. Liquid chromatography (*2.2.29*).

Test solution. Dissolve 25.0 mg of the substance to be examined in *0.01 M hydrochloric acid* and dilute to 25.0 ml with the same acid.

Reference solution (a). Dissolve 25.0 mg of *tetracycline hydrochloride CRS* in *0.01 M hydrochloric acid* and dilute to 25.0 ml with the same acid.

Reference solution (b). Dissolve 15.0 mg of *4-epitetracycline hydrochloride CRS* in *0.01 M hydrochloric acid* and dilute to 50.0 ml with the same acid.

Reference solution (c). Dissolve 10.0 mg of *anhydrotetracycline hydrochloride CRS* in *0.01 M hydrochloric acid* and dilute to 100.0 ml with the same acid.

Reference solution (d). Dissolve 10.0 mg of *4-epianhydrotetracycline hydrochloride CRS* in *0.01 M hydrochloric acid* and dilute to 50.0 ml with the same acid.

Reference solution (e). Mix 1.0 ml of reference solution (a), 2.0 ml of reference solution (b) and 5.0 ml of reference solution (d) and dilute to 25.0 ml with *0.01 M hydrochloric acid.*

Reference solution (f). Mix 20.0 ml of reference solution (b), 10.0 ml of reference solution (c) and 5.0 ml of reference solution (d) and dilute to 200.0 ml using *0.01 M hydrochloric acid.*

Reference solution (g). Dilute 1.0 ml of reference solution (c) to 50.0 ml with *0.01 M hydrochloric acid.*

Column:

- *size*: l = 0.25 m, Ø = 4.6 mm,
- *stationary phase*: *styrene-divinylbenzene copolymer R* (8 µm),
- *temperature*: 60 °C.

Mobile phase: weigh 80.0 g of *2-methyl-2-propanol R* and transfer to a 1000 ml volumetric flask with the aid of 200 ml of *water R*; add 100 ml of a 35 g/l solution of *dipotassium hydrogen phosphate R* adjusted to pH 9.0 with *dilute phosphoric acid R*, 200 ml of a 10 g/l solution of *tetrabutylammonium hydrogen sulphate R* adjusted to pH 9.0 with *dilute sodium hydroxide solution R* and 10 ml of a 40 g/l solution of *sodium edetate R* adjusted to pH 9.0 with *dilute sodium hydroxide solution R*; dilute to 1000.0 ml with *water R*.

Flow rate: 1.0 ml/min.

Detection: spectrophotometer at 254 nm.

Injection: 20 µl; inject the test solution and reference solutions (e), (f) and (g).

System suitability:

- *resolution*: minimum 2.5 between the peaks due to impurity A (1st peak) and tetracycline (2nd peak) and minimum 8.0 between the peaks due to tetracycline and impurity D (3rd peak) in the chromatogram obtained with reference solution (e); if necessary, adjust the concentration of 2-methyl-2-propanol in the mobile phase,
- *signal-to-noise ratio*: minimum 3 for the principal peak in the chromatogram obtained with reference solution (g),
- *symmetry factor*: maximum 1.25 for the peak due to tetracycline in the chromatogram obtained with reference solution (e).

Limits:

- *impurity A*: not more than the area of the corresponding peak in the chromatogram obtained with reference solution (f) (3.0 per cent),
- *impurity B* (eluting on the tail of the principal peak): not more than half the area of the peak due to impurity A in the chromatogram obtained with reference solution (f) (1.5 per cent),
- *impurity C*: not more than the area of the corresponding peak in the chromatogram obtained with reference solution (f) (0.5 per cent),
- *impurity D*: not more than the area of the corresponding peak in the chromatogram obtained with reference solution (f) (0.5 per cent).

Heavy metals (*2.4.8*): maximum 50 ppm.

0.5 g complies with limit test C. Prepare the standard using 2.5 ml of *lead standard solution (10 ppm Pb) R*.

Loss on drying (*2.2.32*): maximum 2.0 per cent, determined on 1.000 g by drying at 60 °C over *diphosphorus pentoxide R* at a pressure not exceeding 670 Pa for 3 h.

Sulphated ash (*2.4.14*): maximum 0.5 per cent, determined on 1.0 g.

Bacterial endotoxins (*2.6.14*): less than 0.5 IU/mg, if intended for use in the manufacture of parenteral dosage forms without a further appropriate procedure for the removal of bacterial endotoxins.

ASSAY

Liquid chromatography (*2.2.29*) as described in the test for related substances with the following modification.

Injection: test solution and reference solution (a).

Calculate the percentage content of $C_{22}H_{25}ClN_2O_8$.

STORAGE

Protected from light. If the substance is sterile, store in a sterile, tamper-proof container.

LABELLING

The label states, where applicable, that the substance is free from bacterial endotoxins.

IMPURITIES

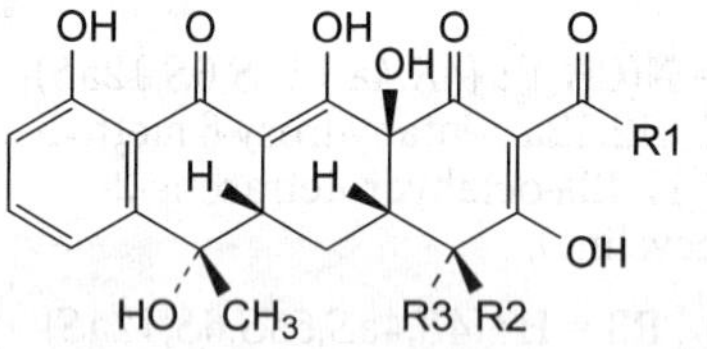

A. R1 = NH_2, R2 = H, R3 = $N(CH_3)_2$: (4*R*,4a*S*,5a*S*,6*S*,12a*S*)-4-(dimethylamino)-3,6,10,12,12a-pentahydroxy-6-methyl-1,11-dioxo-1,4,4a,5,5a,6,11,12a-octahydrotetracene-2-carboxamide (4-epitetracycline),

B. R1 = CH_3, R2 = $N(CH_3)_2$, R3 = H: (4*S*,4a*S*,5a*S*,6*S*,12a*S*)-2-acetyl-4-(dimethylamino)-3,6,10,12,12a-pentahydroxy-6-methyl-4a,5a,6,12a-tetrahydrotetracene-1,11(4*H*,5*H*)-dione (2-acetyl-2-decarbamoyltetracycline),

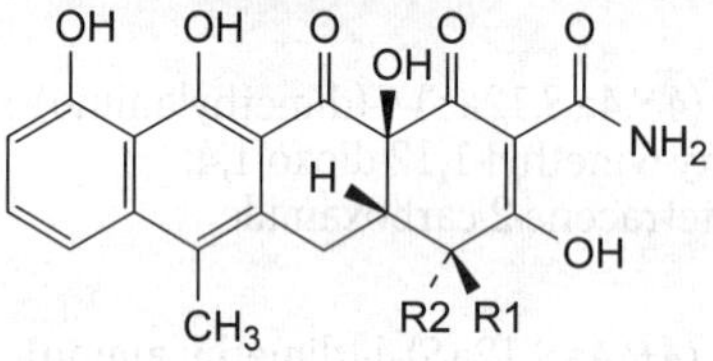

C. R1 = $N(CH_3)_2$, R2 = H: (4*S*,4a*S*,12a*S*)-4-(dimethylamino)-3,10,11,12a-tetrahydroxy-6-methyl-1,12-dioxo-1,4,4a,5,12,12a-hexahydrotetracene-2-carboxamide (anhydrotetracycline),

D. R1 = H, R2 = $N(CH_3)_2$: (4*R*,4a*S*,12a*S*)-4-(dimethylamino)-3,10,11,12a-tetrahydroxy-6-methyl-1,12-dioxo-1,4,4a,5,12,12a-hexahydrotetracene-2-carboxamide (4-epianhydrotetracycline).

01/2005:1738

TETRAZEPAM

Tetrazepamum

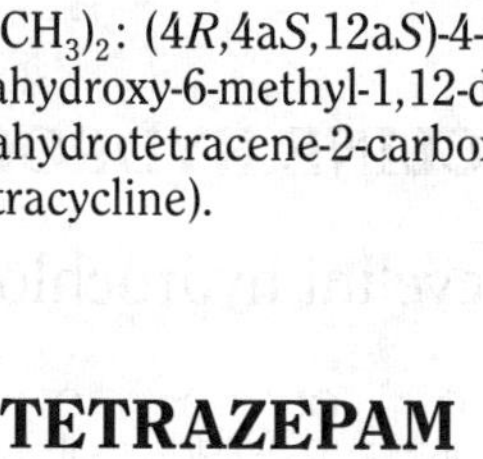

$C_{16}H_{17}ClN_2O$ M_r 288.8

DEFINITION

7-Chloro-5-(cyclohex-1-enyl)-1-methyl-1,3-dihydro-2*H*-1,4-benzodiazepin-2-one.

Content: 99.0 per cent to 101.0 per cent (dried substance).

CHARACTERS

Appearance: light yellow or yellow crystalline powder.

Solubility: practically insoluble in water, freely soluble in methylene chloride, soluble in acetonitrile.

IDENTIFICATION

Infrared absorption spectrophotometry (*2.2.24*).

Comparison: *Ph. Eur. reference spectrum of tetrazepam.*

TESTS

Related substances. Liquid chromatography (*2.2.29*).

Test solution. Dissolve 25.0 mg of the substance to be examined in *acetonitrile R* and dilute to 25.0 ml with the same solvent.

Reference solution (a). Dissolve 5.0 mg of the substance to be examined and 5.0 mg of *tetrazepam impurity C CRS* in *acetonitrile R* and dilute to 10.0 ml with the same solvent. Dilute 1.0 ml of the solution to 10.0 ml with *acetonitrile R.*

Reference solution (b). Dilute 1.0 ml of the test solution to 50.0 ml with *acetonitrile R.* Dilute 1.0 ml of this solution to 10.0 ml with *acetonitrile R.*

Column:
- *size*: l = 0.25 m, Ø = 4.6 mm,
- *stationary phase*: *octadecylsilyl silica gel for chromatography R* (5 µm).

Mobile phase:
- *mobile phase A*: mix 40 volumes of *acetonitrile R* and 60 volumes of a 3.4 g/l solution of *potassium dihydrogen phosphate R,*
- *mobile phase B*: *acetonitrile R,*

Time (min)	Mobile phase A (per cent *V/V*)	Mobile phase B (per cent *V/V*)
0 - 35	100	0
35 - 40	100 → 55	0 → 45
40 - 50	55	45
50 - 60	55 → 100	45 → 0

Flow rate: 1.5 ml/min.

Detection: a spectrophotometer at 229 nm.

Injection: 20 µl.

System suitability: reference solution (a):
- *resolution*: minimum 2.0 between the peaks due to tetrazepam and to impurity C.

Limits:
- *any impurity*: not more than the area of the principal peak in the chromatogram obtained with reference solution (b) (0.2 per cent),
- *total*: not more than 5 times the area of the principal peak in the chromatogram obtained with reference solution (b) (1.0 per cent),
- *disregard limit*: 0.25 times the area of the principal peak in the chromatogram obtained with reference solution (b) (0.05 per cent).

Chlorides (*2.4.4*): maximum 100 ppm.

Dissolve 0.750 g in 10 ml of *methylene chloride R* and add 15 ml of *water R*. Shake and separate the 2 layers. Dilute 10 ml of the aqueous layer to 15 ml with *water R*. The solution obtained complies with the limit test for chlorides.

Loss on drying (*2.2.32*): maximum 0.5 per cent, determined on 1.000 g by drying in an oven at 100-105 °C.

Sulphated ash (*2.4.14*): maximum 0.1 per cent, determined on 1.0 g.

ASSAY

Dissolve 0.230 g in 50.0 ml of *anhydrous acetic acid R*. Titrate with *0.1 M perchloric acid*, determining the end-point potentiometrically (*2.2.20*).

1 ml of *0.1 M perchloric acid* is equivalent to 28.88 mg of $C_{16}H_{17}ClN_2O$.

STORAGE

Protected from light.

IMPURITIES

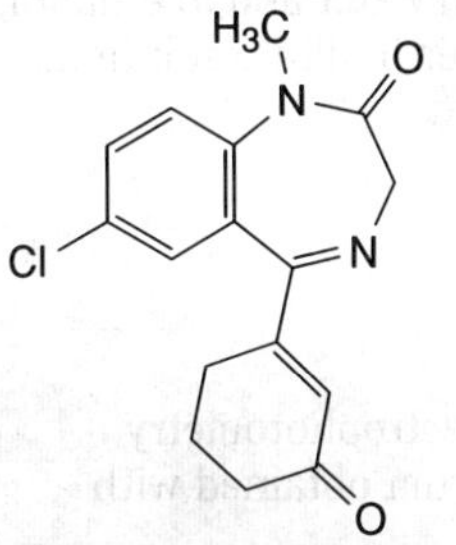

A. 7-chloro-5-(3-oxocyclohex-1-enyl)-1-methyl-1,3-dihydro-2*H*-1,4-benzodiazepin-2-one,

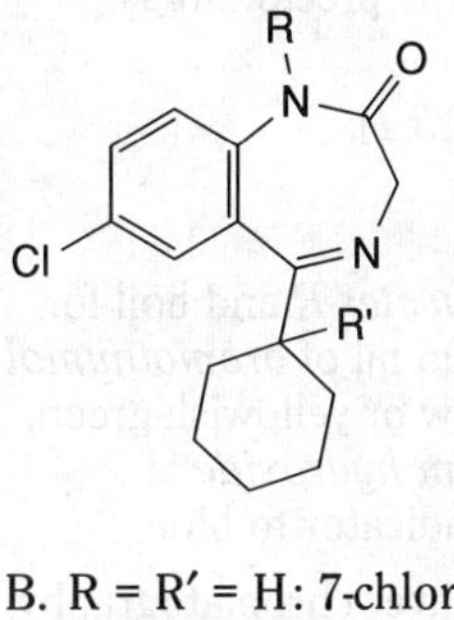

B. R = R′ = H: 7-chloro-5-cyclohexyl-1,3-dihydro-2*H*-1,4-benzodiazepin-2-one,

C. R = CH_3, R′ = H: 7-chloro-5-cyclohexyl-1-methyl-1,3-dihydro-2*H*-1,4-benzodiazepin-2-one,

D. R = CH_3, R′ = Cl: 7-chloro-5-(1-chlorocyclohexyl)-1-methyl-1,3-dihydro-2*H*-1,4-benzodiazepin-2-one,

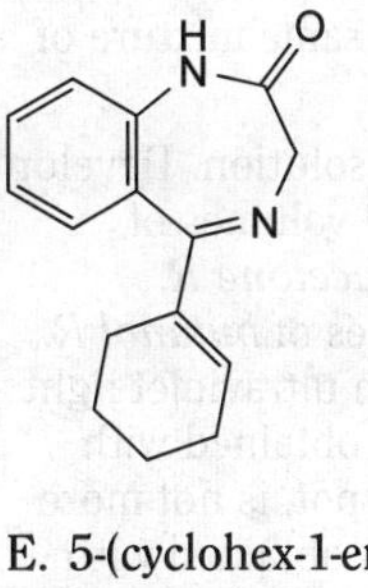

E. 5-(cyclohex-1-enyl)-1,3-dihydro-2*H*-1,4-benzodiazepin-2-one.

01/2005:0298

THEOBROMINE

Theobrominum

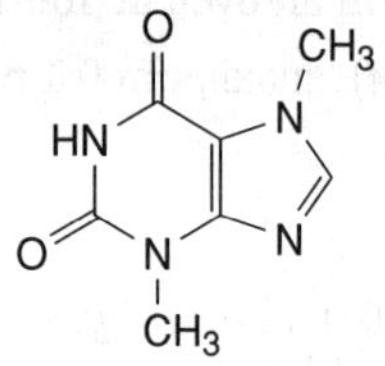

$C_7H_8N_4O_2$ M_r 180.2

DEFINITION

Theobromine contains not less than 99.0 per cent and not more than the equivalent of 101.0 per cent of 3,7-dimethyl-3,7-dihydro-1*H*-purine-2,6-dione, calculated with reference to the dried substance.

CHARACTERS

A white powder, very slightly soluble in water and in ethanol, slightly soluble in ammonia. It dissolves in dilute solutions of alkali hydroxides and in mineral acids.

IDENTIFICATION

First identification: A, C.

Second identification: B, C.

A. Examine by infrared absorption spectrophotometry (*2.2.24*), comparing with the spectrum obtained with *theobromine CRS*.

B. Dissolve about 20 mg in 2 ml of *dilute ammonia R1*, warming slightly, and cool. Add 2 ml of *silver nitrate solution R2*. The solution remains clear. Boil the solution for a few minutes. A white, crystalline precipitate is formed.

C. It gives the reaction of xanthines (*2.3.1*).

TESTS

Acidity. To 0.4 g add 20 ml of boiling *water R* and boil for 1 min. Allow to cool and filter. Add 0.05 ml of *bromothymol blue solution R1*. The solution is yellow or yellowish-green. Not more than 0.2 ml of *0.01 M sodium hydroxide* is required to change the colour of the indicator to blue.

Related substances. Examine by thin-layer chromatography (*2.2.27*), using *silica gel* GF_{254} *R* as the coating substance.

Test solution. To 0.2 g of the finely powdered substance to be examined add 10 ml of a mixture of 4 volumes of *methanol R* and 6 volumes of *chloroform R*. Heat under a reflux condenser on a water-bath for 15 min, shaking occasionally. Cool and filter.

Reference solution. Dissolve 5 mg of *theobromine CRS* in a mixture of 4 volumes of *methanol R* and 6 volumes of *chloroform R* and dilute to 50 ml with the same mixture of solvents.

Apply separately to the plate 10 µl of each solution. Develop over a path of 15 cm using a mixture of 10 volumes of *concentrated ammonia R*, 30 volumes of *acetone R*, 30 volumes of *chloroform R* and 40 volumes of *butanol R*. Allow the plate to dry in air and examine in ultraviolet light at 254 nm. Any spot in the chromatogram obtained with the test solution, apart from the principal spot, is not more intense than the spot in the chromatogram obtained with the reference solution (0.5 per cent).

Heavy metals (*2.4.8*). 1.0 g complies with limit test C for heavy metals (20 ppm). Prepare the standard using 2 ml of *lead standard solution (10 ppm Pb) R*.

Loss on drying (*2.2.32*). Not more than 0.5 per cent, determined on 1.000 g by drying in an oven at 100 °C to 105 °C.

Sulphated ash (*2.4.14*). Not more than 0.1 per cent, determined on 1.0 g.

ASSAY

Dissolve 0.150 g in 125 ml of boiling *water R*, cool to 50 °C to 60 °C and add 25 ml of *0.1 M silver nitrate*. Using 1 ml of *phenolphthalein solution R* as indicator, titrate with *0.1 M sodium hydroxide* until a pink colour is obtained.

1 ml of *0.1 M sodium hydroxide* is equivalent to 18.02 mg of $C_7H_8N_4O_2$.

01/2005:0299

THEOPHYLLINE

Theophyllinum

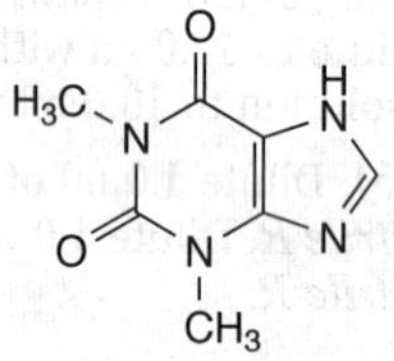

$C_7H_8N_4O_2$ M_r 180.2

DEFINITION

1,3-Dimethyl-3,7-dihydro-1*H*-purine-2,6-dione.

Content: 99.0 per cent to 101.0 per cent (dried substance).

CHARACTERS

Appearance: white, crystalline powder.

Solubility: slightly soluble in water, sparingly soluble in ethanol. It dissolves in solutions of alkali hydroxides, in ammonia and in mineral acids.

IDENTIFICATION

First identification: B, D.

Second identification: A, C, D, E.

A. Melting point (*2.2.14*): 270 °C to 274 °C, determined after drying at 100-105 °C.

B. Infrared absorption spectrophotometry (*2.2.24*).

Comparison: Ph. Eur. reference spectrum of theophylline.

C. Heat 10 mg with 1.0 ml of a 360 g/l solution of *potassium hydroxide R* in a water-bath at 90 °C for 3 min, then add 1.0 ml of *diazotised sulphanilic acid solution R*. A red colour slowly develops. Carry out a blank test.

D. It complies with the test for loss on drying (see Tests).

E. It gives the reaction of xanthines (*2.3.1*).

TESTS

Solution S. Dissolve 0.5 g with heating in *carbon dioxide-free water R*, cool and dilute to 75 ml with the same solvent.

Appearance of solution. Solution S is clear (*2.2.1*) and colourless (*2.2.2, Method II*).

Acidity. To 50 ml of solution S add 0.1 ml of *methyl red solution R*. The solution is red. Not more than 1.0 ml of *0.01 M sodium hydroxide* is required to change the colour of the indicator to yellow.

Monographs T-Z

Related substances. Liquid chromatography (*2.2.29*).

Test solution. Dissolve 40.0 mg of the substance to be examined in the mobile phase and dilute to 20.0 ml with the mobile phase.

Reference solution (a). Dilute 1.0 ml of the test solution to 100.0 ml with the mobile phase. Dilute 1.0 ml of this solution to 10.0 ml with the mobile phase.

Reference solution (b). Dissolve 10 mg of *theobromine R* in the mobile phase, add 5 ml of the test solution and dilute to 100 ml with the mobile phase. Dilute 5 ml of this solution to 50 ml with the mobile phase.

Column:

- *size*: *l* = 0.25 m, Ø = 4 mm,
- *stationary phase*: *octadecylsilyl silica gel for chromatography R* (7 µm).

Mobile phase: mix 7 volumes of *acetonitrile for chromatography R* and 93 volumes of a 1.36 g/l solution of *sodium acetate R* containing 5.0 ml/l of *glacial acetic acid R*.

Flow rate: 2.0 ml/min.

Detection: spectrophotometer at 272 nm.

Injection: 20 µl.

Run time: 3.5 times the retention time of theophylline.

Relative retention with reference to theophylline (retention time = about 6 min): impurity C = about 0.3; impurity B = about 0.4; impurity D = about 0.5; impurity A = about 2.5.

System suitability: reference solution (b):

- *resolution*: minimum 2.0 between the peaks due to theobromine and theophylline.

Limits:

- *impurities A, B, C, D*: for each impurity, not more than the area of the principal peak in the chromatogram obtained with reference solution (a) (0.1 per cent),
- *any other impurity*: for each impurity, not more than the area of the principal peak in the chromatogram obtained with reference solution (a) (0.1 per cent),
- *total*: not more than 5 times the area of the principal peak in the chromatogram obtained with reference solution (a) (0.5 per cent),
- *disregard limit*: 0.5 times the area of the principal peak in the chromatogram obtained with reference solution (a) (0.05 per cent).

Heavy metals (*2.4.8*): maximum 20 ppm.

1.0 g complies with limit test C. Prepare the standard using 2 ml of *lead standard solution (10 ppm Pb) R*.

Loss on drying (*2.2.32*): maximum 0.5 per cent, determined on 1.000 g by drying in an oven at 100-105 °C.

Sulphated ash (*2.4.14*): maximum 0.1 per cent, determined on 1.0 g.

ASSAY

Dissolve 0.150 g in 100 ml of *water R*, add 20 ml of *0.1 M silver nitrate* and shake. Add 1 ml of *bromothymol blue solution R1*. Titrate with *0.1 M sodium hydroxide*.

1 ml of *0.1 M sodium hydroxide* is equivalent to 18.02 mg of $C_7H_8N_4O_2$.

IMPURITIES

Specified impurities: A, B, C, D.

Other detectable impurities: E, F.

A. caffeine,

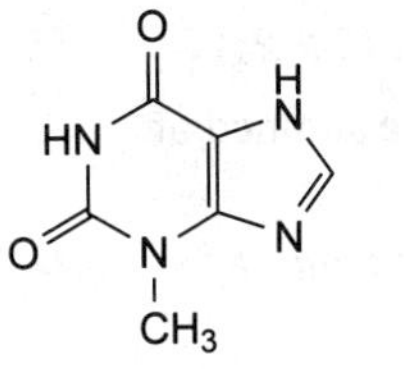

B. 3-methyl-3,7-dihydro-1*H*-purine-2,6-dione,

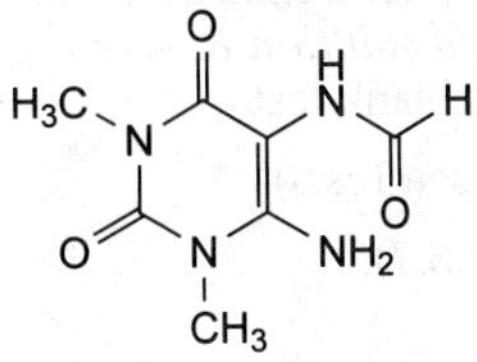

C. *N*-(6-amino-1,3-dimethyl-2,4-dioxo-1,2,3,4-tetrahydropyrimidin-5-yl)formamide,

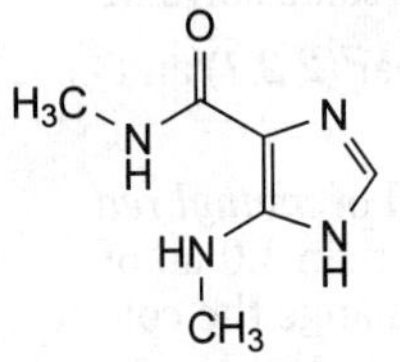

D. *N*-methyl-5-(methylamino)-1*H*-imidazole-4-carboxamide,

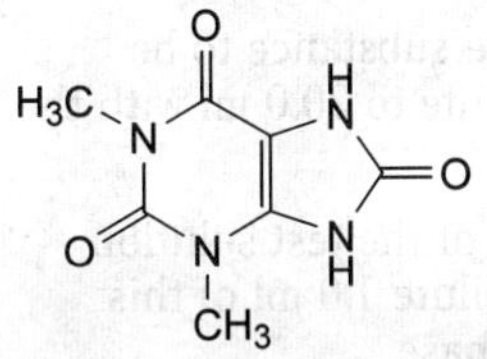

E. 1,3-dimethyl-7,9-dihydro-1*H*-purine-2,6,8(3*H*)-trione,

F. etofylline.

01/2005:0302

THEOPHYLLINE MONOHYDRATE

Theophyllinum monohydricum

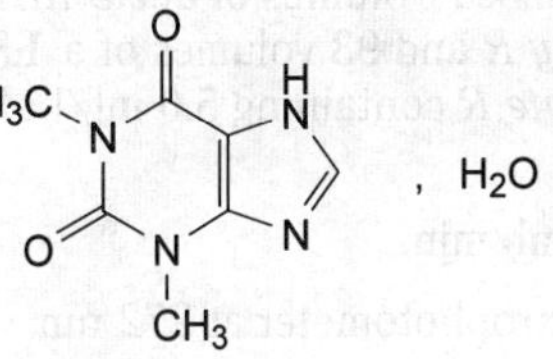

$C_7H_8N_4O_2,H_2O$ M_r 198.2

DEFINITION

1,3-Dimethyl-3,7-dihydro-1*H*-purine-2,6-dione monohydrate.

Content: 99.0 per cent to 101.0 per cent (anhydrous substance).

CHARACTERS

Appearance: white, crystalline powder.

Solubility: slightly soluble in water, sparingly soluble in ethanol. It dissolves in solutions of alkali hydroxides, in ammonia and in mineral acids.

IDENTIFICATION

First identification: B, D.

Second identification: A, C, D, E.

A. Melting point (*2.2.14*): 270 °C to 274 °C, determined after drying at 100-105 °C.

B. Infrared absorption spectrophotometry (*2.2.24*).

Preparation: dry the substance to be examined at 100-105 °C before use.

Comparison: *Ph. Eur. reference spectrum of theophylline.*

C. Heat 10 mg with 1.0 ml of a 360 g/l solution of *potassium hydroxide R* in a water-bath at 90 °C for 3 min, then add 1.0 ml of *diazotised sulphanilic acid solution R*. A red colour slowly develops. Carry out a blank test.

D. It complies with the test for water (see Tests).

E. It gives the reaction of xanthines (*2.3.1*).

TESTS

Solution S. Dissolve 0.5 g with heating in *carbon dioxide-free water R*, cool and dilute to 75 ml with the same solvent.

Appearance of solution. Solution S is clear (*2.2.1*) and colourless (*2.2.2, Method II*).

Acidity. To 50 ml of solution S add 0.1 ml of *methyl red solution R*. The solution is red. Not more than 1.0 ml of *0.01 M sodium hydroxide* is required to change the colour of the indicator to yellow.

Related substances. Liquid chromatography (*2.2.29*).

Test solution. Dissolve 40.0 mg of the substance to be examined in the mobile phase and dilute to 20.0 ml with the mobile phase.

Reference solution (a). Dilute 1.0 ml of the test solution to 100.0 ml with the mobile phase. Dilute 1.0 ml of this solution to 10.0 ml with the mobile phase.

Reference solution (b). Dissolve 10 mg of *theobromine R* in the mobile phase, add 5 ml of the test solution and dilute to 100 ml with the mobile phase. Dilute 5 ml of this solution to 50 ml with the mobile phase.

Column:

- *size*: l = 0.25 m, Ø = 4 mm,
- *stationary phase*: *octadecylsilyl silica gel for chromatography R* (7 µm).

Mobile phase: mix 7 volumes of *acetonitrile for chromatography R* and 93 volumes of a 1.36 g/l solution of *sodium acetate R* containing 5.0 ml/l of *glacial acetic acid R*.

Flow rate: 2.0 ml/min.

Detection: spectrophotometer at 272 nm.

Injection: 20 µl.

Run time: 3.5 times the retention time of theophylline.

Relative retention with reference to theophylline (retention time = about 6 min): impurity C = about 0.3; impurity B = about 0.4; impurity D = about 0.5; impurity A = about 2.5.

System suitability: reference solution (b):

- *resolution*: minimum 2.0 between the peaks due to theobromine and theophylline.

Limits:

- *impurities A, B, C, D*: for each impurity, not more than the area of the principal peak in the chromatogram obtained with reference solution (a) (0.1 per cent),
- *any other impurity*: for each impurity, not more than the area of the principal peak in the chromatogram obtained with reference solution (a) (0.1 per cent),
- *total*: not more than 5 times the area of the principal peak in the chromatogram obtained with reference solution (a) (0.5 per cent),
- *disregard limit*: 0.5 times the area of the principal peak in the chromatogram obtained with reference solution (a) (0.05 per cent).

Heavy metals (*2.4.8*): maximum 20 ppm.

1.0 g complies with limit test C. Prepare the standard using 2 ml of *lead standard solution (10 ppm Pb) R*.

Water (*2.5.12*): 8.0 per cent to 9.5 per cent, determined on 0.20 g.

Sulphated ash (*2.4.14*): maximum 0.1 per cent, determined on 1.0 g.

ASSAY

Dissolve 0.160 g in 100 ml of *water R*, add 20 ml of *0.1 M silver nitrate* and shake. Add 1 ml of *bromothymol blue solution R1*. Titrate with *0.1 M sodium hydroxide*.

1 ml of *0.1 M sodium hydroxide* is equivalent to 18.02 mg of $C_7H_8N_4O_2$.

IMPURITIES

Specified impurities: A, B, C, D.

Other detectable impurities: E, F.

A. caffeine,

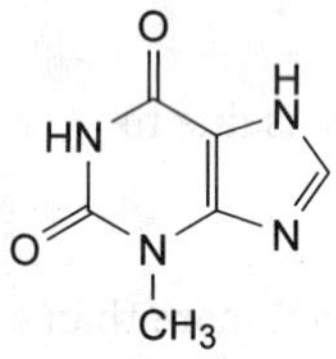

B. 3-methyl-3,7-dihydro-1*H*-purine-2,6-dione,

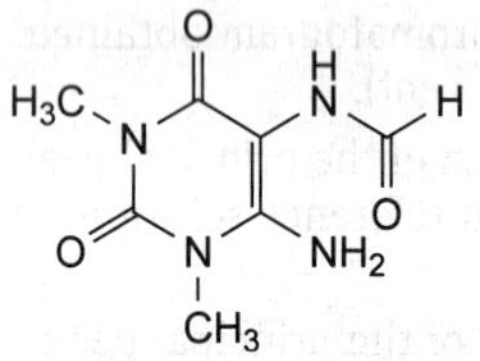

C. *N*-(6-amino-1,3-dimethyl-2,4-dioxo-1,2,3,4-tetrahydropyrimidin-5-yl)formamide,

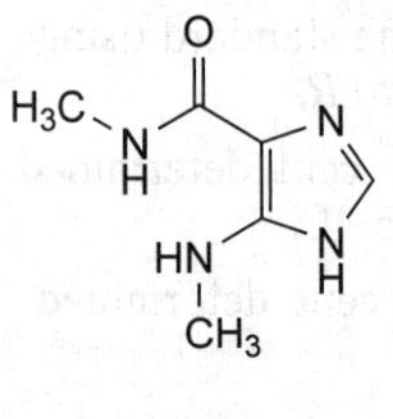

D. *N*-methyl-5-(methylamino)-1*H*-imidazole-4-carboxamide,

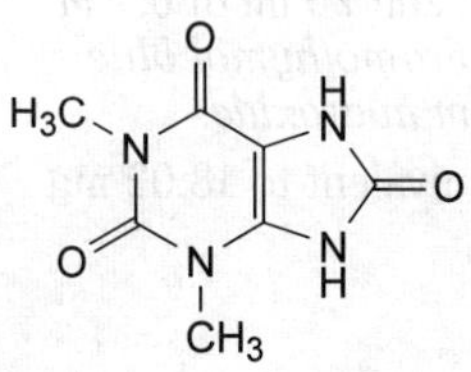

E. 1,3-dimethyl-7,9-dihydro-1*H*-purine-2,6,8(3*H*)-trione,

F. etofylline.

01/2005:0300

THEOPHYLLINE-ETHYLENEDIAMINE

Theophyllinum et ethylenediaminum

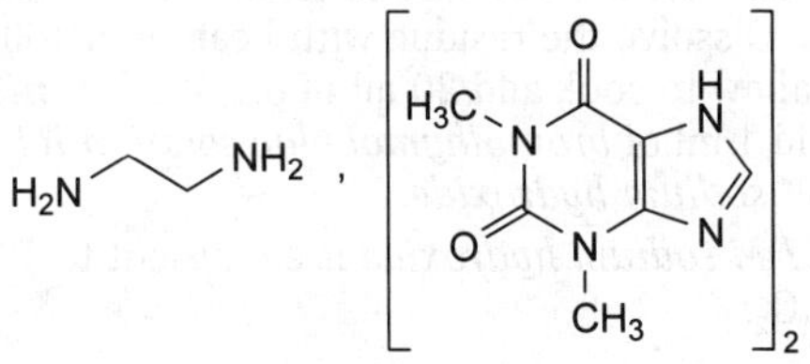

$C_{16}H_{24}N_{10}O_4$ M_r 420.4

DEFINITION

Theophylline-ethylenediamine contains not less than 84.0 per cent and not more than the equivalent of 87.4 per cent of theophylline ($C_7H_8N_4O_2$; M_r 180.2) and not less than 13.5 per cent and not more than the equivalent of 15.0 per cent of ethylenediamine ($C_2H_8N_2$; M_r 60.1), both calculated with reference to the anhydrous substance.

CHARACTERS

A white or slightly yellowish powder, sometimes granular, freely soluble in water (the solution becomes cloudy through absorption of carbon dioxide), practically insoluble in ethanol.

IDENTIFICATION

First identification: B, C, E.

Second identification: A, C, D, E, F.

Dissolve 1.0 g in 10 ml of *water R* and add 2 ml of *dilute hydrochloric acid R* dropwise with shaking. Filter. Use the precipitate for identification tests A, B, D and F and the filtrate for identification test C.

A. The precipitate, washed with *water R* and dried at 100 °C to 105 °C, melts (*2.2.14*) at 270 °C to 274 °C.

B. Examine the precipitate, washed with *water R* and dried at 100 °C to 105 °C, by infrared absorption spectrophotometry (*2.2.24*), comparing with the spectrum obtained with *theophylline CRS*.

C. To the filtrate add 0.2 ml of *benzoyl chloride R*, make alkaline with *dilute sodium hydroxide solution R* and shake vigorously. Filter the precipitate, wash with 10 ml of *water R*, dissolve in 5 ml of hot *alcohol R* and add 5 ml of *water R*. A precipitate is formed, which when washed and dried at 100 °C to 105 °C, melts (*2.2.14*) at 248 °C to 252 °C.

D. Heat about 10 mg of the precipitate with 1.0 ml of a 360 g/l solution of *potassium hydroxide R* in a water-bath at 90 °C for 3 min, then add 1.0 ml of *diazotised sulphanilic acid solution R*. A red colour slowly develops. Carry out a blank test.

E. It complies with the test for water (see Tests).

F. The precipitate gives the reaction of xanthines (*2.3.1*).

TESTS

Appearance of solution. Dissolve 0.5 g with gentle warming in 10 ml of *carbon dioxide-free water R*. The solution is not more opalescent than reference suspension II (*2.2.1*) and not more intensely coloured than reference solution GY_6 (*2.2.2, Method II*).

Related substances. Examine by thin-layer chromatography (*2.2.27*), using as the coating substance a suitable silica gel with a fluorescent indicator having an optimal intensity at 254 nm.

Test solution. Dissolve 0.2 g of the substance to be examined in 2 ml of *water R* with heating and dilute to 10 ml with *methanol R*.

Reference solution. Dilute 0.5 ml of the test solution to 100 ml with *methanol R*.

Apply to the plate 10 µl of each solution. Develop over a path of 15 cm using a mixture of 10 volumes of *concentrated ammonia R*, 30 volumes of *acetone R*, 30 volumes of *chloroform R* and 40 volumes of *butanol R*. Allow the plate to dry in air and examine in ultraviolet light at 254 nm. Any spot in the chromatogram obtained with the test solution, apart from the principal spot, is not more intense than the spot in the chromatogram obtained with the reference solution (0.5 per cent).

Heavy metals (*2.4.8*). 1.0 g complies with limit test C for heavy metals (20 ppm). Prepare the standard using 2 ml of *lead standard solution (10 ppm Pb) R*.

Water (*2.5.12*). Not more than 1.5 per cent, determined on 2.00 g dissolved in 20 ml of *anhydrous pyridine R*, by the semi-micro determination of water.

Sulphated ash (*2.4.14*). Not more than 0.1 per cent, determined on 1.0 g.

ASSAY

Ethylenediamine. Dissolve 0.250 g in 30 ml of *water R*. Add 0.1 ml of *bromocresol green solution R*. Titrate with *0.1 M hydrochloric acid* until a green colour is obtained.

1 ml of *0.1 M hydrochloric acid* is equivalent to 3.005 mg of $C_2H_8N_2$.

Theophylline. Heat 0.200 g to constant mass in an oven at 135 °C. Dissolve the residue with heating in 100 ml of *water R*, allow to cool, add 20 ml of *0.1 M silver nitrate* and shake. Add 1 ml of *bromothymol blue solution R1*. Titrate with *0.1 M sodium hydroxide*.

1 ml of *0.1 M sodium hydroxide* is equivalent to 18.02 mg of $C_7H_8N_4O_2$.

STORAGE

Store in airtight container, protected from light.

01/2005:0301

THEOPHYLLINE-ETHYLENEDIAMINE HYDRATE

Theophyllinum et ethylenediaminum hydricum

DEFINITION

Theophylline-ethylenediamine hydrate contains not less than 84.0 per cent and not more than the equivalent of 87.4 per cent of theophylline ($C_7H_8N_4O_2$; M_r 180.2) and not less than 13.5 per cent and not more than the equivalent of 15.0 per cent of ethylenediamine ($C_2H_8N_2$; M_r 60.1), both calculated with reference to the anhydrous substance.

CHARACTERS

A white or slightly yellowish powder, sometimes granular, freely soluble in water (the solution becomes cloudy through absorption of carbon dioxide), practically insoluble in ethanol.

Monographs T-Z

IDENTIFICATION

First identification: B, C, E.

Second identification: A, C, D, E, F.

Dissolve 1.0 g in 10 ml of *water R* and add 2 ml of *dilute hydrochloric acid R* dropwise with shaking. Filter. Use the precipitate for identification tests A, B, D and F and the filtrate for identification test C.

A. The precipitate, washed with *water R* and dried at 100 °C to 105 °C, melts (*2.2.14*) at 270 °C to 274 °C.

B. Examine the precipitate, washed with *water R* and dried at 100 °C to 105 °C, by infrared absorption spectrophotometry (*2.2.24*), comparing with the spectrum obtained with *theophylline CRS*.

C. To the filtrate add 0.2 ml of *benzoyl chloride R*, make alkaline with *dilute sodium hydroxide solution R* and shake vigorously. Filter the precipitate, wash with 10 ml of *water R*, dissolve in 5 ml of hot *alcohol R* and add 5 ml of *water R*. A precipitate is formed, which when washed and dried at 100 °C to 105 °C, melts (*2.2.14*) at 248 °C to 252 °C.

D. Heat about 10 mg of the precipitate with 1.0 ml of a 360 g/l solution of *potassium hydroxide R* in a water-bath at 90 °C for 3 min, then add 1.0 ml of *diazotised sulphanilic acid solution R*. A red colour slowly develops. Carry out a blank test.

E. It contains 3.0 per cent to 8.0 per cent of water (see Tests).

F. The precipitate gives the reaction of xanthines (*2.3.1*).

TESTS

Appearance of solution. Dissolve 0.5 g with gentle warming in 10 ml of *carbon dioxide-free water R*. The solution is not more opalescent than reference suspension II (*2.2.1*) and not more intensely coloured than reference solution GY_6 (*2.2.2, Method II*).

Related substances. Examine by thin-layer chromatography (*2.2.27*), using as the coating substance a suitable silica gel with a fluorescent indicator having an optimal intensity at 254 nm.

Test solution. Dissolve 0.2 g of the substance to be examined in 2 ml of *water R* with heating and dilute to 10 ml with *methanol R*.

Reference solution. Dilute 0.5 ml of the test solution to 100 ml with *methanol R*.

Apply separately to the plate 10 µl of each solution. Develop over a path of 15 cm using a mixture of 10 volumes of *concentrated ammonia R*, 30 volumes of *acetone R*, 30 volumes of *chloroform R* and 40 volumes of *butanol R*. Allow the plate to dry in air and examine in ultraviolet light at 254 nm. Any spot in the chromatogram obtained with the test solution, apart from the principal spot, is not more intense than the spot in the chromatogram obtained with the reference solution (0.5 per cent).

Heavy metals (*2.4.8*). 1.0 g complies with limit test C for heavy metals (20 ppm). Prepare the standard using 2 ml of *lead standard solution (10 ppm Pb) R*.

Water (*2.5.12*): 3.0 per cent to 8.0 per cent, determined on 0.50 g dissolved in 20 ml of *pyridine R*, by the semi-micro determination of water.

Sulphated ash (*2.4.14*). Not more than 0.1 per cent, determined on 1.0 g.

ASSAY

Ethylenediamine. Dissolve 0.250 g in 30 ml of *water R*. Add 0.1 ml of *bromocresol green solution R*. Titrate with *0.1 M hydrochloric acid* until a green colour is obtained.

1 ml of *0.1 M hydrochloric acid* is equivalent to 3.005 mg of $C_2H_8N_2$.

Theophylline. Heat 0.200 g to constant mass in an oven at 135 °C. Dissolve the residue with heating in 100 ml of *water R*, allow to cool, add 20 ml of *0.1 M silver nitrate* and shake. Add 1 ml of *bromothymol blue solution R1*. Titrate with *0.1 M sodium hydroxide*.

1 ml of *0.1 M sodium hydroxide* is equivalent to 18.02 mg of $C_7H_8N_4O_2$.

STORAGE

Store in a well-filled airtight container, protected from light.

01/2005:1706

THIAMAZOLE

Thiamazolum

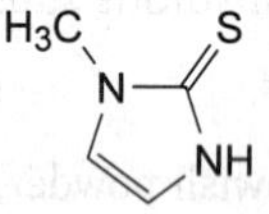

$C_4H_6N_2S$ M_r 114.2

DEFINITION

1-Methyl-1,3-dihydro-2*H*-imidazole-2-thione.

Content: 98.0 per cent to 101.0 per cent (dried substance).

CHARACTERS

Appearance: white or pale brown, crystalline powder.

Solubility: freely soluble in water, freely soluble in methylene chloride, freely soluble or soluble in ethanol (96 per cent).

IDENTIFICATION

First identification: A, C.

Second identification: A, B, D.

A. Melting point (*2.2.14*): 143 °C to 146 °C.

B. Dissolve 25 mg in 10 ml of a 0.28 per cent *V/V* solution of *sulphuric acid R* and dilute to 50.0 ml with the same solution. Dilute 1.0 ml of this solution to 100.0 ml with a 0.28 per cent *V/V* solution of *sulphuric acid R*. Examined between 200 nm and 300 nm (*2.2.25*), the solution shows 2 absorption maxima, at 211 nm and 251 nm. The ratio of the absorbance measured at the absorption maximum at 251 nm to that measured at the absorption maximum at 211 nm is 2.5 to 2.7.

C. Infrared absorption spectrophotometry (*2.2.24*).

Preparation: discs.

Comparison: *thiamazole CRS*.

D. Thin-layer chromatography (*2.2.27*).

Test solution. Dissolve 5.0 mg of the substance to be examined in *methanol R* and dilute to 5.0 ml with the same solvent.

Reference solution (a). Dissolve 5.0 mg of *thiamazole CRS* in *methanol R* and dilute to 5.0 ml with the same solvent.

Reference solution (b). Dissolve 5.0 mg of *2-methylimidazole R* in *methanol R* and dilute to 5.0 ml with the same solvent. Dilute 1.0 ml of this solution to 2.0 ml with the test solution.

Plate: *TLC silica gel F_{254} plate R.*

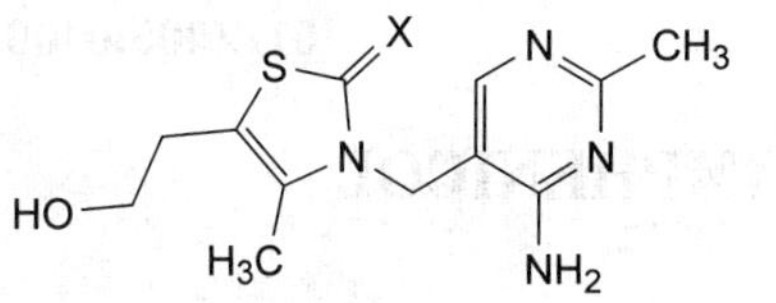

D. X = O: 3-[(4-amino-2-methylpyrimidin-5-yl)methyl]-5-(2-hydroxyethyl)-4-methylthiazol-2(3*H*)-one (oxothiamine),

E. X = S: 3-[(4-amino-2-methylpyrimidin-5-yl)methyl]-5-(2-hydroxyethyl)-4-methylthiazol-2(3*H*)-thione (thioxothiamine),

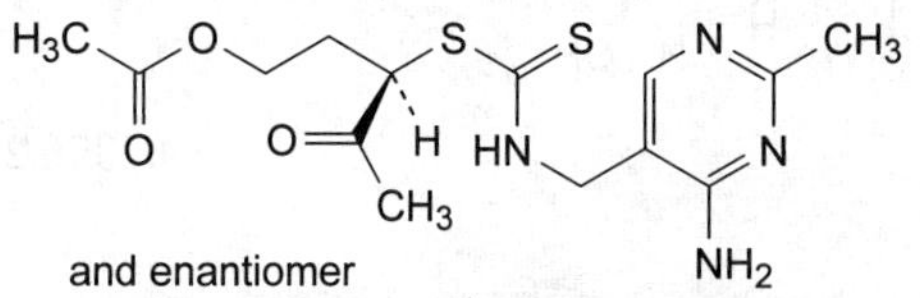

H. (3*RS*)-3-[[[(4-amino-2-methylpyrimidin-5-yl)methyl]thiocarbamoyl]sulphanyl]-4-oxopentyl acetate (ketodithiocarbamate).

01/2005:0531

THIAMINE NITRATE

Thiamini nitras

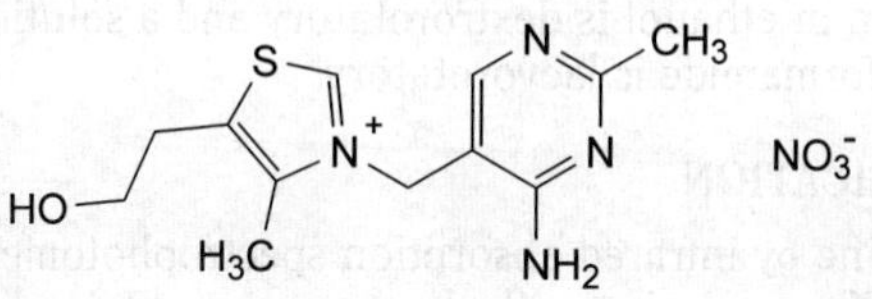

$C_{12}H_{17}N_5O_4S$ M_r 327.4

DEFINITION

3-[(4-Amino-2-methylpyrimidin-5-yl)methyl]-5-(2-hydroxyethyl)-4-methylthiazolium nitrate.

Content: 98.0 per cent to 101.0 per cent (dried substance).

CHARACTERS

Appearance: white or almost white, crystalline powder or small, colourless crystals.

Solubility: sparingly soluble in water, freely soluble in boiling water, slightly soluble in alcohol and in methanol.

IDENTIFICATION

First identification: A, C.

Second identification: B, C.

A. Infrared absorption spectrophotometry (*2.2.24*).

Comparison: *Ph. Eur. reference spectrum of thiamine nitrate.*

B. Dissolve about 20 mg in 10 ml of *water R*, add 1 ml of *dilute acetic acid R* and 1.6 ml of *1 M sodium hydroxide*, heat on a water-bath for 30 min and allow to cool. Add 5 ml of *dilute sodium hydroxide solution R*, 10 ml of *potassium ferricyanide solution R* and 10 ml of *butanol R* and shake vigorously for 2 min. The upper alcoholic layer shows an intense light-blue fluorescence, especially in ultraviolet light at 365 nm. Repeat the test using 0.9 ml of *1 M sodium hydroxide* and 0.2 g of *sodium sulphite R* instead of 1.6 ml of *1 M sodium hydroxide*. Practically no fluorescence is produced.

C. About 5 mg gives the reaction of nitrates (*2.3.1*).

TESTS

Solution S. Dissolve 1.0 g in *carbon dioxide-free water R* and dilute to 50 ml with the same solvent.

Appearance of solution. Solution S is clear (*2.2.1*) and not more intensely coloured than reference solution Y_7 (*2.2.2, Method II*).

pH (*2.2.3*): 6.8 to 7.6 for solution S.

Related substances. Liquid chromatography (*2.2.29*).

Solution A. Add 5 volumes of *glacial acetic acid R* to 95 volumes of *water R* and mix.

Test solution. Dissolve 0.35 g of the substance to be examined in 15.0 ml of solution A and dilute to 100.0 ml with *water R*.

Reference solution (a). Dissolve 5 mg of the substance to be examined and 5 mg of *thiamine impurity E CRS* in 4 ml of solution A and dilute to 25.0 ml with *water R*. Dilute 5.0 ml of the solution to 25.0 ml with *water R*.

Reference solution (b). Dilute 1.0 ml of the test solution to 100.0 ml with *water R*.

Column:

– *size*: l = 0.25 m, Ø = 4.0 mm,
– *stationary phase*: spherical *end-capped octadecylsilyl silica gel for chromatography R* (4 µm) with a specific surface area of 350 m^2/g and a pore size of 10 nm,
– *temperature*: 45 °C.

Mobile phase:

– *mobile phase A*: 3.764 g/l solution of *sodium hexanesulphonate R* adjusted to pH 3.1 with *phosphoric acid R*,
– *mobile phase B*: *methanol R2*,

Time (min)	Mobile phase A (per cent *V/V*)	Mobile phase B (per cent *V/V*)
0 - 25	90 → 70	10 → 30
25 - 33	70 → 50	30 → 50
33 - 40	50	50
40 - 45	50 → 90	50 → 10

Flow rate: 1.0 ml/min.

Detection: spectrophotometer at 248 nm.

Injection: 25 µl.

Relative retention with reference to thiamine (retention time = about 30 min): impurity A = about 0.3; impurity B = about 0.9; impurity C = about 1.2.

System suitability: reference solution (a):

– *resolution*: minimum 1.6 between the peaks due to impurity E and to thiamine.

Limits:

– *any impurity*: not more than the area of the principal peak in the chromatogram obtained with reference solution (b) (1.0 per cent),
– *total*: not more than 1.5 times the area of the principal peak in the chromatogram obtained with reference solution (b) (1.5 per cent),
– *disregard limit*: 0.05 times the area of the principal peak in the chromatogram obtained with reference solution (b) (0.05 per cent).

Heavy metals (*2.4.8*): maximum 20 ppm.

1.0 g complies with limit test D. Prepare the standard using 2 ml of *lead standard solution (10 ppm Pb) R*.

Loss on drying (*2.2.32*): maximum 1.0 per cent, determined on 1.000 g by drying in an oven at 100-105 °C.

Sulphated ash (*2.4.14*): maximum 0.1 per cent, determined on 1.0 g.

ASSAY

Dissolve 0.140 g in 5 ml of *anhydrous formic acid R* and add 50 ml of *acetic anhydride R*. Titrate immediately with *0.1 M perchloric acid*, determining the end-point potentiometrically (*2.2.20*) and carrying out the titration within 2 min. Carry out a blank titration.

1.0 ml of *0.1 M perchloric acid* is equivalent to 16.37 mg of $C_{12}H_{17}N_5O_4S$.

STORAGE

In a non-metallic container, protected from light.

IMPURITIES

Specified impurities: A, B, C.

Other detectable impurities: D, E, F, G, H.

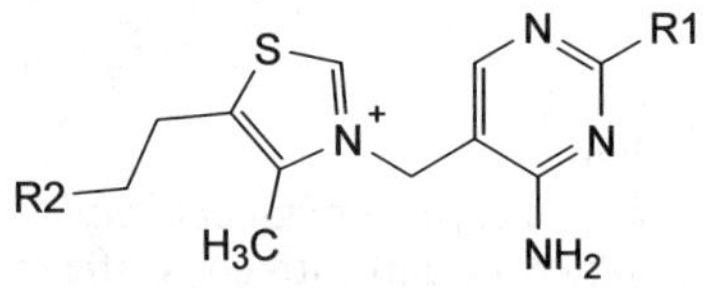

A. R1 = CH_3, R2 = $O\text{-}SO_3^-$: 3-[(4-amino-2-methylpyrimidin-5-yl)methyl]-4-methyl-5-[2-(sulphonatooxy)ethyl]thiazolium (thiamine sulphate ester),

B. R1 = H, R2 = OH: 3-[(4-aminopyrimidin-5-yl)methyl]-5-(2-hydroxyethyl)-4-methylthiazolium (desmethylthiamine),

C. R1 = CH_3, R2 = Cl: 3-[(4-amino-2-methylpyrimidin-5-yl)methyl]-5-(2-chloroethyl)-4-methylthiazolium (chlorothiamine),

F. R1 = C_2H_5, R2 = OH: 3-[(4-amino-2-ethylpyrimidin-5-yl)methyl]-5-(2-hydroxyethyl)-4-methylthiazolium (ethylthiamine),

G. R1 = CH_3, R2 = $O\text{-}CO\text{-}CH_3$: 5-[2-(acetyloxy)ethyl]-3-[(4-amino-2-methylpyrimidin-5-yl)methyl]-4-methylthiazolium (acetylthiamine),

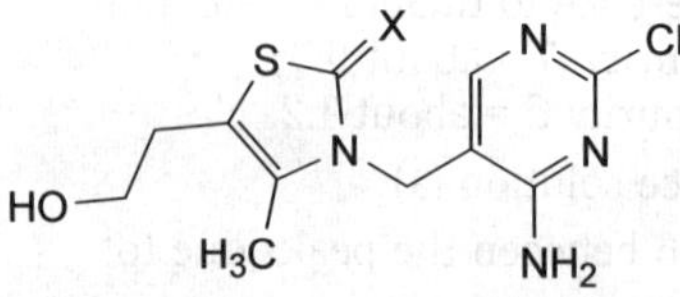

D. X = O: 3-[(4-amino-2-methylpyrimidin-5-yl)methyl]-5-(2-hydroxyethyl)-4-methylthiazol-2(3*H*)-one (oxothiamine),

E. X = S: 3-[(4-amino-2-methylpyrimidin-5-yl)methyl]-5-(2-hydroxyethyl)-4-methylthiazol-2(3*H*)-thione (thioxothiamine),

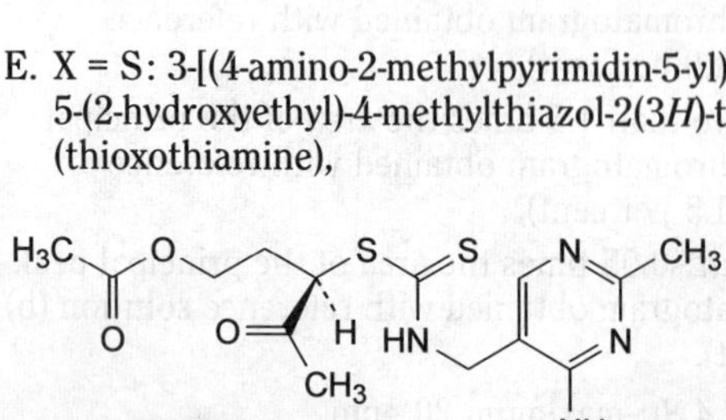

H. (3*RS*)-3-[[[(4-amino-2-methylpyrimidin-5-yl)methyl]thiocarbamoyl]sulphanyl]-4-oxopentyl acetate (ketodithiocarbamate).

01/2005:0109

THIAMPHENICOL

Thiamphenicolum

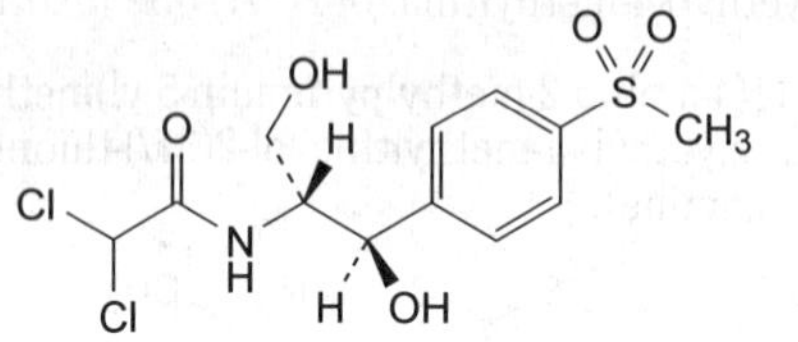

$C_{12}H_{15}Cl_2NO_5S$ M_r 356.2

DEFINITION

Thiamphenicol contains not less than 98.0 per cent and not more than the equivalent of 100.5 per cent of 2,2-dichloro-*N*-[(1*R*,2*R*)-2-hydroxy-1-(hydroxymethyl)-2-[4-(methylsulphonyl)phenyl]ethyl]acetamide, calculated with reference to the dried substance.

CHARACTERS

A fine, white or yellowish-white, crystalline powder or crystals, slightly soluble in water and in ethyl acetate, very soluble in dimethylacetamide, freely soluble in acetonitrile and in dimethylformamide, soluble in methanol, sparingly soluble in acetone and in ethanol.

A solution in ethanol is dextrorotatory and a solution in dimethylformamide is laevorotatory.

IDENTIFICATION

A. Examine by infrared absorption spectrophotometry (*2.2.24*), comparing with the spectrum obtained with *thiamphenicol CRS*. Dry the substances at 100 °C to 105 °C for 2 h and examine in the form of discs prepared using *potassium bromide R*.

B. Examine by thin-layer chromatography (*2.2.27*), using *silica gel GF_{254} R* as the coating substance.
Test solution. Dissolve 0.1 g of the substance to be examined in *methanol R* and dilute to 10 ml with the same solvent.
Reference solution. Dissolve 0.1 g of *thiamphenicol CRS* in *methanol R* and dilute to 10 ml with the same solvent.
Apply separately to the plate 5 µl of each solution. Develop over a path of 10 cm using a mixture of 3 volumes of *methanol R* and 97 volumes of *ethyl acetate R*. Allow the plate to dry in air and examine in ultraviolet light at 254 nm. The principal spot in the chromatogram obtained with the test solution is similar in position and size to the spot in the chromatogram obtained with the reference solution.

C. To 50 mg in a porcelain crucible add 0.5 g of *anhydrous sodium carbonate R*. Heat over an open flame for 10 min. Allow to cool. Take up the residue with 5 ml of *dilute nitric acid R* and filter. To 1 ml of the filtrate add 1 ml of *water R*. The solution gives reaction (a) of chlorides (*2.3.1*).

TESTS

Acidity or alkalinity. Shake 0.1 g with 20 ml of *carbon dioxide-free water R* and add 0.1 ml of *bromothymol blue solution R1*. Not more than 0.1 ml of *0.02 M hydrochloric acid* or *0.02 M sodium hydroxide* is required to change the colour of the indicator.

Specific optical rotation (*2.2.7*). Dissolve 1.25 g in *dimethylformamide R* and dilute to 25.0 ml with the same solvent. The specific optical rotation is − 21 to − 24, calculated with reference to the dried substance.

Melting point (*2.2.14*). 163 °C to 167 °C.

Absorbance (*2.2.25*). Dissolve 20 mg in *water R,* heating to about 40 °C, and dilute to 100.0 ml with the same solvent. Examined between 240 nm and 300 nm, the solution shows 2 absorption maxima, at 266 nm and 273 nm. The specific absorbances at these maxima are 25 to 28 and 21.5 to 23.5, respectively. Dilute 2.5 ml of the solution to 50.0 ml with *water R.* Examined between 200 nm and 240 nm, the solution shows an absorption maximum at 224 nm. The specific absorbance at this maximum is 370 to 400.

Chlorides (*2.4.4*). Shake 0.5 g with 30 ml of *water R* for 5 min and filter. 15 ml of the filtrate complies with the limit test for chlorides (200 ppm).

Heavy metals (*2.4.8*). 1.0 g complies with limit test C for heavy metals (10 ppm). Prepare the standard using 1 ml of *lead standard solution (10 ppm Pb) R.*

Loss on drying (*2.2.32*). Not more than 1.0 per cent, determined on 1.00 g by drying in an oven at 100 °C to 105 °C.

Sulphated ash (*2.4.14*). Not more than 0.1 per cent, determined on 2.0 g.

ASSAY

Dissolve 0.300 g in 30 ml of *alcohol R,* add 20 ml of a 500 g/l solution of *potassium hydroxide R,* mix and heat under a reflux condenser for 4 h. Cool, add 100 ml of *water R,* neutralise with *dilute nitric acid R* and add 5 ml in excess. Titrate with *0.1 M silver nitrate,* determining the end-point potentiometrically (*2.2.20*), using a silver indicator electrode and a mercurous sulphate reference electrode or any other appropriate electrode. Carry out a blank test.

1 ml of *0.1 M silver nitrate* is equivalent to 17.81 mg of $C_{12}H_{15}Cl_2NO_5S$.

STORAGE

Store in an airtight container, protected from light.

01/2005:1625

THIOMERSAL

Thiomersalum

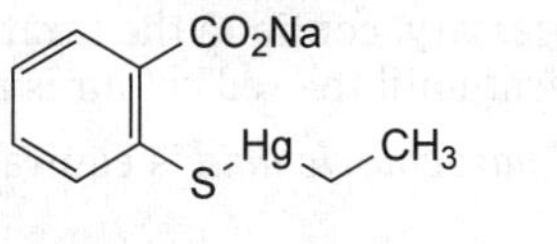

$C_9H_9HgNaO_2S$ M_r 404.8

DEFINITION

Sodium ethyl[2-sulphanylbenzoato(2-)-*O,S*]mercurate(1-).

Content: 97.0 per cent to 101.0 per cent (dried substance).

CHARACTERS

Appearance: white or almost white, crystalline powder.

Solubility: freely soluble in water, sparingly soluble or soluble in alcohol, practically insoluble in methylene chloride.

IDENTIFICATION

First identification: B, D.

Second identification: A, C, D.

A. Melting point of the derivative (*2.2.14*): 103 °C to 108 °C. Dissolve 0.5 g in *water R* and dilute to 10 ml with the same solvent. Add 2 ml of *dilute hydrochloric acid R.* A white precipitate is formed. Wash the precipitate with *water R* and dry over *diphosphorus pentoxide R* at a pressure not exceeding 0.7 kPa.

B. Infrared absorption spectrophotometry (*2.2.24*).

Comparison: *thiomersal CRS.*

C. Treat 50 mg by the oxygen-flask method (*2.5.10*). Use a mixture of 1 ml of *strong hydrogen peroxide solution R* and 50 ml of *water R* to absorb the combustion products. To the solution add 5 ml of *dilute nitric acid R.* 0.1 ml of this solution gives reaction (a) of mercury (*2.3.1*). To the remaining part of the solution add 10 ml of *dilute hydrochloric acid R* and filter. 5 ml of the filtrate, without further addition of acid, gives reaction (a) of sulphates (*2.3.1*).

D. Solution S (see Tests) gives reaction (a) of sodium (*2.3.1*).

TESTS

Solution S. Dissolve 2.0 g in *carbon dioxide-free water R* and dilute to 25 ml with the same solvent.

Appearance of solution. Solution S is not more opalescent than reference suspension II (*2.2.1*) and not more intensely coloured than reference solution B_6 (*2.2.2, Method II*).

pH (*2.2.3*): 6.0 to 8.0.

Dilute 5 ml of solution S to 50 ml with *carbon dioxide-free water R.*

Inorganic mercury compounds: maximum 0.70 per cent.

Protect the solutions from light throughout the procedure.

Test solution. Dissolve 25 mg of the substance to be examined in *water R* and dilute to 25.0 ml with the same solvent.

Reference solution. Dissolve 95.0 mg of *mercuric chloride R* in *water R* and dilute to 50.0 ml with the same solvent. Dilute 1.0 ml of the solution to 20.0 ml with *water R.*

Test reference and blank preparations. Label five 10 ml volumetric flasks A, B, C, D and E. Place 5 ml of the test solution in flasks A, B, C and D. To each of the flasks C and D add 0.5 ml of the reference solution. Dilute the contents of flasks A and C to 10 ml with *water R* (blank preparations A and C). Dilute the contents of flasks B and D to 10 ml with a freshly prepared 332 g/l solution of *potassium iodide R* (test preparation B and reference preparation D). Place 5 ml of a 332 g/l solution of *potassium iodide R* in flask E. Dilute to 10 ml with *water R* (blank preparation E).

Measure the absorbance (*2.2.25*) of each solution (A_a, A_b, A_c, A_d and A_e) at 323 nm using *water R* as the compensation liquid. Calculate the content of inorganic mercury compounds, expressed as Hg from the expression:

$$\frac{(A_b - A_a - A_e) \times m_R \times 0.1847}{(A_d - A_c - A_b + A_a) \times m_T}$$

m_R = mass of mercuric chloride in the reference solution in milligrams,

m_T = mass of the substance to be examined in milligrams.

Loss on drying (*2.2.32*): maximum 0.5 per cent, determined on 1.000 g by drying in a desiccator over *diphosphorus pentoxide R* at a pressure not exceeding 0.7 kPa for 24 h.

ASSAY

Place 0.5 g in a 100 ml long-necked combustion flask, add 5 ml of *sulphuric acid R* and heat gently until charring occurs, continue to heat and add dropwise *strong hydrogen peroxide solution R* until the mixture is colourless. Dilute with *water R*, evaporate until slight fuming occurs, dilute to 10 ml with *water R*, cool down and titrate with *0.1 M ammonium thiocyanate* using *ferric ammonium sulphate solution R2* as indicator.

1 ml of *0.1 M ammonium thiocyanate* is equivalent to 20.24 mg of $C_9H_9HgNaO_2S$.

STORAGE

Protected from light.

01/2005:0212

THIOPENTAL SODIUM AND SODIUM CARBONATE

Thiopentalum natricum et natrii carbonas

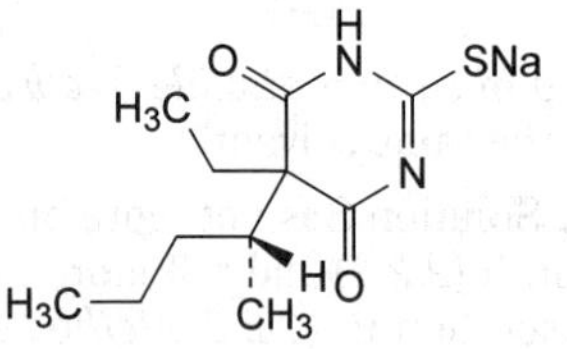

DEFINITION

Thiopental sodium and sodium carbonate is a mixture of the sodium derivative of 5-ethyl-5-[(1*RS*)-1-methylbutyl]-2-thioxo-2,3-dihydropyrimidine-4,6(1*H*,5*H*)-dione ($C_{11}H_{17}N_2NaO_2S$; M_r 264.3) and anhydrous sodium carbonate, containing the equivalent of not less than 84.0 per cent and not more than 87.0 per cent of thiopental and not less than 10.2 per cent and not more than 11.2 per cent of Na, both calculated with reference to the dried substance.

CHARACTERS

A yellowish-white powder, hygroscopic, freely soluble in water, partly soluble in ethanol.

IDENTIFICATION

First identification: A, B, E.

Second identification: A, C, D, E.

A. Acidify 10 ml of solution S (see Tests) with *dilute hydrochloric acid R*. An effervescence is produced. Shake with 20 ml of *ether R*. Separate the ether layer, wash with 10 ml of *water R*, dry over *anhydrous sodium sulphate R* and filter. Evaporate the filtrate to dryness and dry the residue at 100 °C to 105 °C (test residue). Determine the melting point (*2.2.14*) of the test residue. Mix equal parts of the test residue and *thiopental CRS* and determine the melting point of the mixture. The difference between the melting points (which are about 160 °C) is not greater than 2 °C.

B. Examine by infrared absorption spectrophotometry (*2.2.24*), comparing the test residue (see identification test A) with the spectrum obtained with *thiopental CRS*.

C. Examine by thin-layer chromatography (*2.2.27*), using *silica gel GF_{254} R* as the coating substance.

Test solution. Dissolve 0.1 g of the substance to be examined in *water R* and dilute to 100 ml with the same solvent.

Reference solution. Dissolve 85 mg of *thiopental CRS* in 10 ml of *dilute sodium hydroxide solution R* and dilute to 100 ml with *water R*.

Apply separately to the plate 10 µl of each solution. Develop over a path of 18 cm using the lower layer of a mixture of 5 volumes of *concentrated ammonia R*, 15 volumes of *alcohol R* and 80 volumes of *chloroform R*. Examine immediately in ultraviolet light at 254 nm. The principal spot in the chromatogram obtained with the test solution is similar in position and size to the principal spot in the chromatogram obtained with the reference solution.

D. It gives the reaction of non-nitrogen substituted barbiturates (*2.3.1*).

E. It gives reaction (a) of sodium (*2.3.1*).

TESTS

Solution S. Dissolve 5.0 g in *carbon dioxide-free water R* and dilute to 50 ml with the same solvent.

Appearance of solution. Solution S is clear (*2.2.1*) and not more intensely coloured than reference solution GY_3 (*2.2.2, Method II*).

Related substances. Examine by thin-layer chromatography (*2.2.27*), using *silica gel GF_{254} R* as the coating substance.

Test solution. Dissolve 1.0 g of the substance to be examined in *water R* and dilute to 100 ml with the same solvent. Disregard any slight residue.

Reference solution. Dilute 0.5 ml of the test solution to 100 ml with *water R*.

Apply separately to the plate 20 µl of each solution. Develop over a path of 15 cm using the lower layer of a mixture of 5 volumes of *concentrated ammonia R*, 15 volumes of *alcohol R* and 80 volumes of *chloroform R*. Examine immediately in ultraviolet light at 254 nm. Any spot in the chromatogram obtained with the test solution, apart from the principal spot, is not more intense than the spot in the chromatogram obtained with the reference solution (0.5 per cent). Disregard any spot at the starting-point.

Chlorides (*2.4.4*). To 5 ml of solution S add 35 ml of *water R* and 10 ml of *dilute nitric acid R*. Shake with three quantities, each of 25 ml, of *ether R* and discard the ether layers. Eliminate the ether from the aqueous layer by heating on a water-bath.15 ml of the aqueous layer complies with the limit test for chlorides (330 ppm).

Loss on drying (*2.2.32*). Not more than 2.5 per cent, determined on 0.50 g by drying in vacuo at 100 °C for 4 h.

ASSAY

Sodium. Dissolve 0.400 g in 30 ml of *water R*. Add 0.1 ml of *methyl red solution R* and titrate with *0.1 M hydrochloric acid* until a red colour is obtained. Boil gently for 2 min. Cool and, if necessary, continue the titration with *0.1 M hydrochloric acid* until the red colour is again obtained.

1 ml of *0.1 M hydrochloric acid* is equivalent to 2.299 mg of Na.

Thiopental. Dissolve 0.150 g in 5 ml of *water R*. Add 2 ml of *dilute sulphuric acid R* and shake with four quantities, each of 10 ml, of *chloroform R*. Combine the chloroform layers, filter and evaporate the filtrate to dryness on a water-bath. Dissolve the residue in 30 ml of previously neutralised *dimethylformamide R* and add 0.1 ml of a 2 g/l solution of *thymol blue R* in *methanol R*. Titrate immediately with *0.1 M lithium methoxide* until a blue colour is obtained. Protect the solution from atmospheric carbon dioxide during the titration.

1 ml of *0.1 M lithium methoxide* is equivalent to 24.23 mg of $C_{11}H_{18}N_2O_2S$.

STORAGE

Store in an airtight container, protected from light.

Monographs T-Z

01/2005:2005

THIORIDAZINE

Thioridazinum

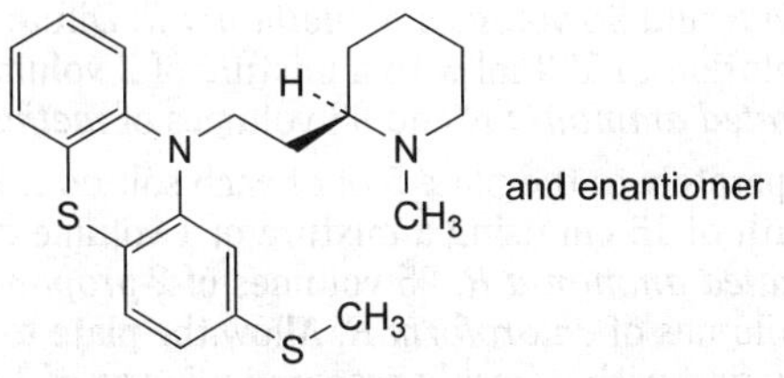

$C_{21}H_{26}N_2S_2$ M_r 370.6

DEFINITION

10-[2-[(2*RS*)-1-Methylpiperidin-2-yl]ethyl]-2-(methylsulphanyl)-10*H*-phenothiazine

Content: 99.0 per cent to 101.0 per cent (dried substance).

CHARACTERS

Appearance: white or almost white powder.

Solubilities: practically insoluble in water, very soluble in methylene chloride, freely soluble in methanol, soluble in alcohol.

IDENTIFICATION

First identification: A.

Second identification: B, C, D.

A. Infrared absorption spectrophotometry (*2.2.24*).

Comparison: *Ph. Eur. reference spectrum of thioridazine.*

B. It complies with the identification of phenothiazines by thin-layer chromatography (*2.3.3*).

C. Dissolve 5 mg in 2 ml of *sulphuric acid R*. A blue colour is produced.

D. Dissolve 20 mg in a mixture of 2 ml of *water R* and 0.2 ml of *1 M sulphuric acid*. Add 1 ml of a 50 g/l solution of *silver nitrate R*. No precipitate is produced.

TESTS

Solution S. Dissolve 1.25 g in *methanol R* and dilute to 25 ml with the same solvent.

Appearance of solution. Solution S is clear (*2.2.1*) and not more intensely coloured than intensity 6 of the range of reference solutions of the most appropriate colour (*2.2.2, Method II*).

Related substances. Thin-layer chromatography (*2.2.27*). *Carry out the test as quickly as possible and protected from light. Apply the test solution last.*

Test solution. Dissolve 0.2 g of the substance to be examined in a mixture of 2 volumes of *concentrated ammonia R* and 98 volumes of *methanol R* and dilute to 10.0 ml with the same mixture of solvents.

Reference solution (a). Dilute 1.0 ml of the test solution to 100.0 ml with a mixture of 2 volumes of *concentrated ammonia R* and 98 volumes of *methanol R*. Dilute 5.0 ml of this solution to 10.0 ml with a mixture of 2 volumes of *concentrated ammonia R* and 98 volumes of *methanol R*.

Reference solution (b). Dilute 4.0 ml of reference solution (a) to 10.0 ml with a mixture of 2 volumes of *concentrated ammonia R* and 98 volumes of *methanol R*.

Reference solution (c). Dilute 5.0 ml of reference solution (b) to 10.0 ml with a mixture of 2 volumes of *concentrated ammonia R* and 98 volumes of *methanol R*.

Plate: *TLC silica gel R.*

Mobile phase: *concentrated ammonia R, 2-propanol R, methylene chloride R* (1:25:74 *V/V/V*).

Application: 5 µl; apply the test solution and reference solutions (b) and (c).

Development: over 2/3 of the plate.

Drying: in air.

Detection: spray with a freshly prepared mixture of 1 volume of *potassium iodobismuthate solution R* and 10 volumes of *dilute acetic acid R* and then with *dilute hydrogen peroxide solution R*. Immediately cover the plate with a glass plate.

Limits:

– *any impurity*: any spot, apart from the principal spot, is not more intense than the spot in the chromatogram obtained with reference solution (b) (0.2 per cent); not more than 2 such spots are more intense than the spot in the chromatogram obtained with reference solution (c) (0.1 per cent).

Heavy metals (*2.4.8*): maximum 20 ppm.

1.0 g complies with limit test C. Prepare the standard using 2 ml of *lead standard solution (10 ppm Pb) R*.

Loss on drying (*2.2.32*): maximum 0.5 per cent, determined on 1.000 g at 50 °C *in vacuo* for 4 h.

Sulphated ash (*2.4.14*): maximum 0.1 per cent, determined on 1.0 g.

ASSAY

Dissolve 0.300 g in 60 ml of *anhydrous acetic acid R*. Titrate with *0.1 M perchloric acid*, determining the end-point potentiometrically (*2.2.20*).

1 ml of *0.1 M perchloric acid* is equivalent to 37.06 mg of $C_{21}H_{26}N_2S_2$.

STORAGE

Protected from light.

IMPURITIES

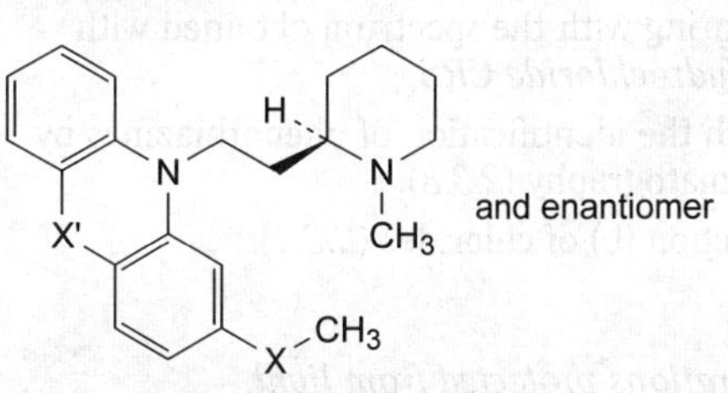

A. X = X′ = SO_2: 10-[2-[(2*RS*)-1-methylpiperidin-2-yl]ethyl]-2-(methylsulphonyl)-10*H*-phenothiazine 5,5-dioxide,

B. X = SO, X′ = S: 10-[2-[(2*RS*)-1-methylpiperidin-2-yl]ethyl]-2-(methylsulphinyl)-10*H*-phenothiazine,

C. X = S, X′ = SO: 10-[2-[(2*RS*)-1-methylpiperidin-2-yl]ethyl]-2-(methylsulphanyl)-10*H*-phenothiazine 5-oxide,

D. X = X′ = SO: 10-[2-[(2*RS*)-1-methylpiperidin-2-yl]ethyl]-2-(methylsulphinyl)-10*H*-phenothiazine 5-oxide,

E. X = SO_2, X′ = S: 10-[2-[(2*RS*)-1-methylpiperidin-2-yl]ethyl]-2-(methylsulphonyl)-10*H*-phenothiazine,

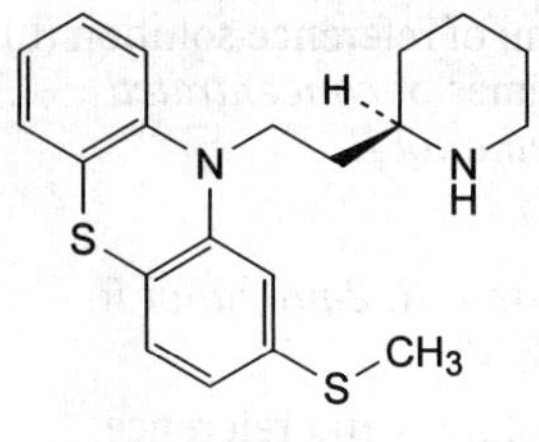

F. 2-(methylsulphanyl)-10-[2-[(2*RS*)-piperidin-2-yl]ethyl]-10*H*-phenothiazine.

01/2005:0586

THIORIDAZINE HYDROCHLORIDE

Thioridazini hydrochloridum

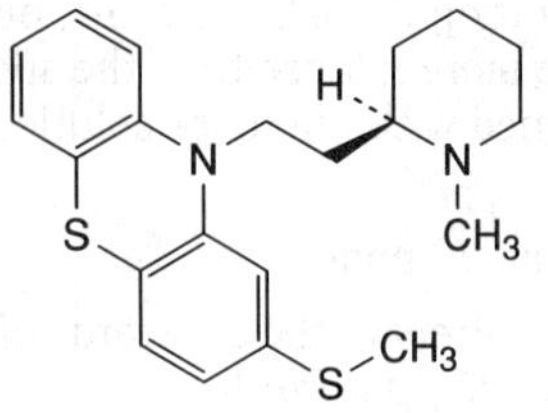

$C_{21}H_{27}ClN_2S_2$ M_r 407.0

DEFINITION

Thioridazine hydrochloride contains not less than 99.0 per cent and not more than the equivalent of 101.0 per cent of 10-[2-[(2*RS*)-1-methylpiperidin-2-yl]ethyl]-2-(methylsulphanyl)-10*H*-phenothiazine hydrochloride, calculated with reference to the dried substance.

CHARACTERS

A white or almost white, crystalline powder, freely soluble in water and in methanol, soluble in alcohol.

IDENTIFICATION

First identification: A, C.

Second identification: B, C.

A. Examine by infrared absorption spectrophotometry (*2.2.24*), comparing with the spectrum obtained with *thioridazine hydrochloride CRS*.

B. It complies with the identification of phenothiazines by thin-layer chromatography (*2.3.3*).

C. 0.2 g gives reaction (b) of chlorides (*2.3.1*).

TESTS

Carry out all operations protected from light.

Appearance of solution. Dissolve 1.0 g in *methanol R* and dilute to 20 ml with the same solvent. The solution is clear (*2.2.1*) and not more intensely coloured than intensity 6 of the range of reference solutions of the most appropriate colour (*2.2.2, Method II*).

pH (*2.2.3*). Dissolve 0.20 g in 20 ml of *carbon dioxide-free water R*. The pH of the solution is 4.2 to 5.2.

Related substances. Examine by thin-layer chromatography (*2.2.27*), using *silica gel G R* as the coating substance. *Carry out all operations as rapidly as possible, protected from light. Apply the test solution last.*

Test solution. Dissolve 0.2 g in a mixture of 2 volumes of *concentrated ammonia R* and 98 volumes of *methanol R* and dilute to 10 ml with the same mixture of solvents.

Reference solution (a). Dilute 2 ml of the test solution to 100 ml with a mixture of 2 volumes of *concentrated ammonia R* and 98 volumes of *methanol R*. Dilute 10 ml of this solution to 100 ml with a mixture of 2 volumes of *concentrated ammonia R* and 98 volumes of *methanol R*.

Reference solution (b). Dilute 1 ml of the test solution to 100 ml with a mixture of 2 volumes of *concentrated ammonia R* and 98 volumes of *methanol R*. Dilute 10 ml of this solution to 100 ml with a mixture of 2 volumes of *concentrated ammonia R* and 98 volumes of *methanol R*.

Apply separately to the plate 5 µl of each solution. Develop over a path of 15 cm using a mixture of 1 volume of *concentrated ammonia R*, 25 volumes of *2-propanol R* and 74 volumes of *chloroform R*. Allow the plate to dry in air. Spray first with a freshly prepared mixture of 1 volume of *potassium iodobismuthate solution R* and 10 volumes of *dilute acetic acid R* and then with freshly prepared *dilute hydrogen peroxide solution R*. Cover the plate immediately with a glass plate of the same size. Any spot in the chromatogram obtained with the test solution, apart from the principal spot, is not more intense than the spot in the chromatogram obtained with reference solution (a) (0.2 per cent) and at most two such spots are more intense than the spot in the chromatogram obtained with the reference solution (b) (0.1 per cent). The test is not valid unless the spot in the chromatogram obtained with reference solution (b) is clearly visible.

Heavy metals (*2.4.8*). 1.0 g complies with the limit test C for heavy metals (20 ppm). Prepare the standard using 2 ml of *lead standard solution (10 ppm Pb) R*.

Loss on drying (*2.2.32*). Not more than 0.5 per cent, determined on 1.000 g by drying in an oven at 100 °C to 105 °C for 4 h.

Sulphated ash (*2.4.14*). Not more than 0.1 per cent, determined on 1.0 g.

ASSAY

Dissolve 0.300 g in a mixture of 10 ml of *anhydrous acetic acid R* and 60 ml of *acetic anhydride R*. Titrate with *0.1 M perchloric acid*, determining the end-point potentiometrically (*2.2.20*).

1 ml of *0.1 M perchloric acid* is equivalent to 40.70 mg of $C_{21}H_{27}ClN_2S_2$.

STORAGE

Store protected from light.

01/2005:1049

THREONINE

Threoninum

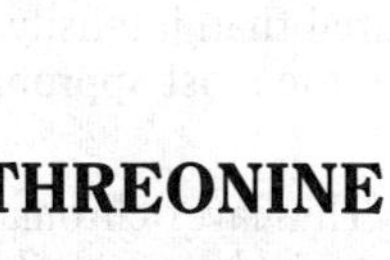

$C_4H_9NO_3$ M_r 119.1

DEFINITION

Threonine contains not less than 99.0 per cent and not more than the equivalent of 101.0 per cent of (2*S*,3*R*)-2-amino-3-hydroxybutanoic acid, calculated with reference to the dried substance.

CHARACTERS

A white, crystalline powder or colourless crystals, soluble in water, practically insoluble in alcohol.

IDENTIFICATION

First identification: A, B.

Second identification: A, C, D.

A. It complies with the test for specific optical rotation (see Tests).

B. Examine by infrared absorption spectrophotometry (*2.2.24*), comparing with the spectrum obtained with *threonine CRS*. Examine the substances prepared as discs.

C. Examine the chromatograms obtained in the test for ninhydrin-positive substances. The principal spot in the chromatogram obtained with test solution (b) is similar in position, colour and size to the principal spot in the chromatogram obtained with reference solution (a).

D. Mix 1 ml of a 2 g/l solution of the substance to be examined with 1 ml of a 20 g/l solution of *sodium periodate R*. Add 0.2 ml of *piperidine R* and 0.1 ml of a 25 g/l solution of *sodium nitroprusside R*. A blue colour develops that changes to yellow after a few minutes.

TESTS

Solution S. Dissolve 2.5 g in *carbon dioxide-free water R* and dilute to 100 ml with the same solvent.

Appearance of solution. Solution S is clear (*2.2.1*) and colourless (*2.2.2, Method II*).

pH (*2.2.3*). The pH of solution S is 5.0 to 6.5.

Specific optical rotation (*2.2.7*). Dissolve 1.50 g in *water R* and dilute to 25.0 ml with the same solvent. The specific optical rotation is − 27.6 to − 29.0, calculated with reference to the dried substance.

Ninhydrin-positive substances. Examine by thin-layer chromatography (*2.2.27*), using a *TLC silica gel plate R*.

Test solution (a). Dissolve 0.10 g of the substance to be examined in *dilute hydrochloric acid R* and dilute to 10 ml with the same acid.

Test solution (b). Dilute 1 ml of test solution (a) to 50 ml with *water R*.

Reference solution (a). Dissolve 10 mg of *threonine CRS* in a 1 per cent *V/V* solution of *hydrochloric acid R* and dilute to 50 ml with the same acid solution.

Reference solution (b). Dilute 5 ml of test solution (b) to 20 ml with *water R*.

Reference solution (c). Dissolve 10 mg of *threonine CRS* and 10 mg of *proline CRS* in a 1 per cent *V/V* solution of *hydrochloric acid R* and dilute to 25 ml with the same acid solution.

Apply to the plate 5 µl of each solution. Allow the plate to dry in air. Develop over a path of 15 cm using a mixture of 20 volumes of *glacial acetic acid R*, 20 volumes of *water R* and 60 volumes of *butanol R*. Allow the plate to dry in air, spray with *ninhydrin solution R* and heat at 100 °C to 105 °C for 15 min. Any spot in the chromatogram obtained with test solution (a), apart from the principal spot, is not more intense than the spot in the chromatogram obtained with reference solution (b) (0.5 per cent). The test is not valid unless the chromatogram obtained with reference solution (c) shows two clearly separated principal spots.

Chlorides (*2.4.4*). Dilute 10 ml of solution S to 15 ml with *water R*. The solution complies with the limit test for chlorides (200 ppm).

Sulphates (*2.4.13*). Dissolve 0.5 g in *distilled water R* and dilute to 15 ml with the same solvent. The solution complies with the limit test for sulphates (300 ppm).

Ammonium (*2.4.1*). 0.10 g complies with limit test B for ammonium (200 ppm). Prepare the standard using 0.2 ml of *ammonium standard solution (100 ppm NH_4) R*.

Iron (*2.4.9*). In a separating funnel, dissolve 1.0 g in 10 ml of *dilute hydrochloric acid R*. Shake with three quantities, each of 10 ml, of *methyl isobutyl ketone R1*, shaking for 3 min each time. To the combined organic layers add 10 ml of *water R* and shake for 3 min. The aqueous layer complies with the limit test for iron (10 ppm).

Heavy metals (*2.4.8*). 2.0 g complies with limit test C for heavy metals (10 ppm). Prepare the standard using 2 ml of *lead standard solution (10 ppm Pb) R*.

Loss on drying (*2.2.32*). Not more than 0.5 per cent, determined on 1.000 g by drying in an oven at 100 °C to 105 °C.

Sulphated ash (*2.4.14*). Not more than 0.1 per cent, determined on 1.0 g.

ASSAY

Dissolve 0.100 g in 5 ml of *anhydrous formic acid R*. Add 30 ml of *anhydrous acetic acid R*. Titrate with *0.1 M perchloric acid*, determining the end-point potentiometrically (*2.2.20*).

1 ml of *0.1 M perchloric acid* is equivalent to 11.91 mg of $C_4H_9NO_3$.

STORAGE

Store protected from light.

01/2005:0865

THYME

Thymi herba

DEFINITION

Whole leaves and flowers separated from the previously dried stems of *Thymus vulgaris* L. or *Thymus zygis* L. or a mixture of both species.

Content: minimum 12 ml/kg of essential oil of which a minimum of 40 per cent is thymol and carvacrol (both $C_{10}H_{14}O$; M_r 150.2) (anhydrous drug).

CHARACTERS

Strong aromatic odour reminiscent of thymol.

Macroscopic and microscopic characters described under identification tests A and B.

IDENTIFICATION

A. The leaf of *Thymus vulgaris* is usually 4 mm to 12 mm long and up to 3 mm wide, sessile or with a very short petiole. The lamina is tough, entire, lanceolate to ovate, covered on both surfaces by a grey or greenish-grey indumentum; the edges are markedly rolled up towards the abaxial surface. The midrib is depressed on the adaxial surface and is very prominent on the abaxial surface. The calyx is green, often with violet spots and is tubular; at the end are 2 lips of which the upper one is bent back and at the end has 3 lobes, the lower is longer and has 2 hairy teeth. After flowering, the calyx tube is closed by a crown of long, stiff hairs. The corolla, about twice as long as the calyx, is usually brownish in the dry state and is slightly bilabiate.

Monographs T-Z

The leaf of *Thymus zygis* is usually 1.7 mm to 6.5 mm long and 0.4 mm to 1.2 mm wide; it is acicular to linear-lanceolate and the edges are markedly rolled towards the abaxial surface. Both surfaces of the lamina are green to greenish-grey and the midrib is sometimes violet; the edges, in particular at the base, have long, white hairs. The dried flowers are very similar to those of *Thymus vulgaris*.

B. Reduce to a powder (355). The powder of both species is greyish-green or greenish-brown. Examine under a microscope using *chloral hydrate solution R*. The epidermises of the leaves have cells with anticlinal walls which are sinuous and beaded and the stomata are diacytic (*2.8.3*); numerous secretory trichomes made up of 12 secretory cells, the cuticle of which is generally raised by the secretion to form a globular to ovoid bladder-like covering; the glandular trichomes have a unicellular stalk and a globular to ovoid head; the covering trichomes of the adaxial surface are common to both species; they have warty walls and are shaped as pointed teeth; the warty covering trichomes of the abaxial surface are of many types: unicellular, straight or slightly curved, and bicellular or tricellular, and often elbow-shaped (*Thymus vulgaris*); bicellular or tricellular, more or less straight (*Thymus zygis*). Fragments of calyx are covered by numerous, uniseriate trichomes with 5 or 6 cells and with a weakly striated cuticle. Fragments of the corolla have numerous uniseriate covering trichomes, often collapsed, and secretory trichomes generally with 12 cells. Pollen grains are relatively rare, spherical and smooth with 6 germinal slit-like pores, measuring about 35 µm in diameter. The powder of *Thymus zygis* also contains numerous thick bundles of fibres from the main veins and from fragments of stems.

C. Thin-layer chromatography (*2.2.27*).

Test solution. To 1.0 g of the powdered drug (355) add 5 ml of *methylene chloride R* and shake for 3 min, filter through about 2 g of *anhydrous sodium sulphate R*.

Reference solution. Dissolve 5 mg of *thymol R* and 10 µl of *carvacrol R* in 10 ml of *methylene chloride R*.

Plate: *TLC silica gel F_{254} plate R.*

Mobile phase: *methylene chloride R.*

Application: 20 µl, as bands.

Development: over a path of 15 cm.

Drying: in air.

Detection A: examine in ultraviolet light at 254 nm.

Results A: see below the sequence of the zones present in the chromatograms obtained with the reference solution and the test solution.

Top of the plate	
	A prominent quenching zone
Thymol: a quenching zone	A quenching zone (thymol)
	Quenching zones
Reference solution	**Test solution**

Detection B: spray with *anisaldehyde solution R* using 10 ml for a plate 200 mm square and heat at 100-105 °C for 10 min.

Results B: see below the sequence of the zones present in the chromatograms obtained with the reference solution and the test solution. Furthermore, other zones are present in the lower third of the chromatogram obtained with the test solution. The intensity of the zones due to thymol and carvacrol depends upon the species examined.

Top of the plate	
Thymol: a brownish-pink zone	A brownish-pink zone (thymol)
Carvacrol: a pale violet zone	A pale violet zone (carvacrol)
	A greyish-pink zone
	A violet zone (cineole and linalol)
	A greyish-brown zone (borneol)
	A violet-blue zone
	An intense violet zone
Reference solution	**Test solution**

D. Examine the chromatograms obtained in the assay for thymol and carvacrol.

Results: the characteristic peaks in the chromatogram obtained with the test solution are similar in retention time to those in the chromatogram obtained with the reference solution.

TESTS

Foreign matter (*2.8.2*): maximum 10 per cent of stems and maximum 2 per cent of other foreign matter. Stems must not be more than 1 mm in diameter and 15 mm in length. Leaves with long trichomes at their base and with weakly pubescent other parts (*Thymus serpyllum L.*) are absent.

Water (*2.2.13*): maximum 100 ml/kg, determined on 20.0 g of the powdered drug (355).

Total ash (*2.4.16*): maximum 15.0 per cent.

Ash insoluble in hydrochloric acid (*2.8.1*): maximum 3.0 per cent.

ASSAY

Essential oil (*2.8.12*). Use 30.0 g of the drug, a 1000 ml round-bottomed flash and 400 ml of *water R* as the distillation liquid. Distil at a rate of 2-3 ml/min for 2 h without *xylene R* in the graduated tube.

Thymol and carvacrol. Gas chromatography (*2.2.28*): use the normalisation procedure.

Test solution. Filter the essential oil obtained in the determination of essential oil over a small amount of *anhydrous sodium sulphate R* and dilute to 5.0 ml with *hexane R* by rinsing the apparatus and the anhydrous sodium sulphate.

Reference solution. Dissolve 0.20 g of *thymol R* and 50 mg of *carvacrol R* in *hexane R* and dilute to 5.0 ml with the same solvent.

Column:

- *material*: fused silica,
- *size*: l = 30-60 m, Ø = 0.25 mm,
- *stationary phase*: *macrogol 20 000 R* (film thickness 0.25 µm).

Carrier gas: *nitrogen for chromatography R* or *helium for chromatography R*.

Flow rate: 1-2 ml/min.

Split ratio: 1:100.

Temperature:

	Time (min)	Temperature (°C)
Column	0 - 45	40 → 220
Injection port		190
Detector		210

Detection: flame ionisation.

Injection: 0.2 μl.

Elution order: order indicated in the composition of the reference solution. Record the retention times of these substances.

System suitability: reference solution:

- *resolution*: minimum 1.5 between the peaks due to thymol and carvacrol.

Using the retention times determined from the chromatogram obtained with the reference solution, locate the components of the reference solution in the chromatogram obtained with the test solution.

Determine the percentage content of thymol and carvacrol. Disregard the peak due to hexane.

01/2005:1374

THYME OIL

Thymi aetheroleum

DEFINITION

Essential oil obtained by steam distillation from the fresh flowering aerial parts of *Thymus vulgaris* L., *T. zygis* Loefl. ex L. or a mixture of both species.

CHARACTERS

Appearance: clear, yellow or very dark reddish-brown, mobile liquid with a characteristic, aromatic, spicy odour, reminiscent of thymol.

Solubility: miscible with ethanol and with light petroleum.

IDENTIFICATION

First identification: *B*.

Second identification: *A*.

A. Thin-layer chromatography (*2.2.27*).

Test solution. Dissolve 0.2 g of the substance to be examined in *pentane R* and dilute to 10 ml with the same solvent.

Reference solution. Dissolve 0.15 g of *thymol R*, 25 mg of *α-terpineol R*, 40 μl of *linalol R* and 10 μl of *carvacrol R* in *pentane R* and dilute to 10 ml with the same solvent.

Plate: *TLC silica gel plate R*.

Mobile phase: *ethyl acetate R, toluene R (5:95 V/V)*.

Application: 20 μl, as bands.

Development: over a path of 15 cm.

Drying: in air.

Detection: spray with *anisaldehyde solution R* and heat the plate at 100-105 °C for 5-10 min while observing. Examine in daylight.

Results: see below the sequence of the zones present in the chromatograms obtained with the reference solution and the test solution. Furthermore, other bands may be present in the chromatogram obtained with the test solution.

Top of the plate	
	A large violet zone (hydrocarbons) (at the solvent front)
Thymol: a brownish-pink zone	A brownish-pink zone (thymol)
Carvacrol: a pale violet zone	A pale violet zone (carvacrol)
Linalol: a violet zone	A violet zone (linalol)
α-Terpineol: a violet zone	A violet zone (α-terpineol)
Reference solution	**Test solution**

B. Examine the chromatograms obtained in the test for chromatographic profile.

Results: the characteristic peaks in the chromatogram obtained with the test solution are similar in retention time to those in the chromatogram obtained with the reference solution.

TESTS

Relative density (*2.2.5*): 0.915 to 0.935.

Refractive index (*2.2.6*): 1.490 to 1.505.

Chromatographic profile. Gas chromatography (*2.2.28*): use the normalisation procedure.

Test solution. The substance to be examined.

Reference solution. Dissolve 0.15 g of *β-myrcene R*, 0.1 g of *γ-terpinene R*, 0.1 g of *p-cymene R*, 0.1 g of *linalol R*, 0.2 g of *terpinen-4-ol R*, 0.2 g of *thymol R* and 50 mg of *carvacrol R* in 5 ml of *hexane R*.

Column:

- *material*: fused silica,
- *size*: l = 30 m (a film thickness of 1 μm may be used) to 60 m (a film thickness of 0.2 μm may be used), Ø = 0.25-0.53 mm,
- *stationary phase*: *macrogol 20 000 R*.

Carrier gas: *helium for chromatography R*.

Split ratio: 1:100.

Temperature:

	Time (min)	Temperature (°C)
Column	0 - 15	60
	15 - 55	60→180
Injection port		200
Detector		220

Detection: flame ionisation.

Injection: 0.2 μl.

Elution order: order indicated in the composition of the reference solution. Record the retention times of these substances.

System suitability: reference solution:

- *resolution*: minimum 1.5 between the peaks due to thymol and carvacrol,
- *number of theoretical plates*: minimum 30 000, calculated for the peak due to *p*-cymene at 80 °C.

Using the retention times determined from the chromatogram obtained with the reference solution, locate the components of the reference solution on the chromatogram obtained with the test solution. Disregard the peak due to hexane.

Determine the percentage content of these components. The limits are within the following ranges:

- *β-myrcene*: 1.0 per cent to 3.0 per cent,
- *γ-terpinene*: 5.0 per cent to 10.0 per cent,
- *p-cymene*: 15.0 per cent to 28.0 per cent,

Monographs T-Z

– *linalol*: 4.0 per cent to 6.5 per cent,
– *terpinen-4-ol*: 0.2 per cent to 2.5 per cent,
– *thymol*: 36.0 per cent to 55.0 per cent,
– *carvacrol*: 1.0 per cent to 4.0 per cent.

STORAGE

In a well-filled, airtight container, protected from light, at a temperature not exceeding 25 °C.

01/2005:0791

THYMOL

Thymolum

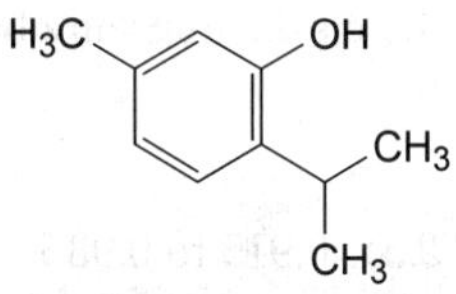

$C_{10}H_{14}O$ M_r 150.2

DEFINITION

Thymol is 5-methyl-2-(methylethyl)phenol.

CHARACTERS

Colourless crystals, very slightly soluble in water, very soluble in alcohol, freely soluble in essential oils and in fatty oils, sparingly soluble in glycerol. It dissolves in dilute solutions of alkali hydroxides.

IDENTIFICATION

First identification: B.

Second identification: A, C, D.

A. Melting point (*2.2.14*): 48 °C to 52 °C.

B. Examine by infrared absorption spectrophotometry (*2.2.24*), comparing with the spectrum obtained with *thymol CRS*.

C. Dissolve 0.2 g with heating in 2 ml of *dilute sodium hydroxide solution R* and add 0.2 ml of *chloroform R*. Heat on a water-bath. A violet colour develops.

D. Dissolve about 2 mg in 1 ml of *anhydrous acetic acid R*. Add 0.15 ml of *sulphuric acid R* and 0.05 ml of *nitric acid R*. A bluish-green colour develops.

TESTS

Appearance of solution. Dissolve 1.0 g in 10 ml of *dilute sodium hydroxide solution R*. The solution is not more opalescent than reference suspension IV (*2.2.1*) and not more intensely coloured than reference solution R_6 (*2.2.2, Method II*).

Acidity. To 1.0 g in a 100 ml glass-stoppered conical flask add 20 ml of *water R*. Boil until dissolution is complete, cool and stopper the flask. Shake vigorously for 1 min. Add a few crystals of the substance to be examined to initiate crystallisation. Shake vigorously for 1 min and filter. To 5 ml of the filtrate, add 0.05 ml of *methyl red solution R* and 0.05 ml of *0.01 M sodium hydroxide*. The solution is yellow.

Related substances. Examine by gas chromatography (*2.2.28*).

Test solution. Dissolve 0.100 g in *alcohol R* and dilute to 10.0 ml with the same solvent.

Reference solution (a). Dilute 1 ml of the test solution to 100 ml with *alcohol R*.

Reference solution (b). Dilute 1 ml of reference solution (a) to 10 ml with *alcohol R*.

Reference solution (c). Dilute 5 ml of reference solution (b) to 10 ml with *alcohol R*.

The chromatography may be carried out using:

– a glass or steel column 4 m long and 2 mm in internal diameter packed with *diatomaceous earth for gas chromatography R*, impregnated with a mixture suitable for the separation of free fatty acids,
– *nitrogen for chromatography R* as the carrier gas at a flow rate of 30 ml/min,
– a flame-ionisation detector,

maintaining the temperature of the column at 80 °C, that of the injection port at 250 °C and that of the detector at 300 °C.

Inject 1 µl of each solution and, after 2 min, increase the temperature of the column to 240 °C at a rate of 8 °C/min and maintain at this temperature for 15 min. The test is not valid unless the peak in the chromatogram obtained with reference solution (b) has a signal-to-noise ratio not less than five. In the chromatogram obtained with the test solution, the sum of the areas of the peaks, apart from the principal peak, is not greater than the area of the principal peak in the chromatogram obtained with reference solution (a) (1.0 per cent). Disregard any peak with an area less than that of the principal peak in the chromatogram obtained with reference solution (c).

Residue on evaporation. Evaporate 2.00 g on a water-bath and heat in an oven at 100 °C to 105 °C for 1 h. The residue weighs not more than 1.0 mg (0.05 per cent).

STORAGE

Store protected from light.

01/2005:0866

TIABENDAZOLE

Tiabendazolum

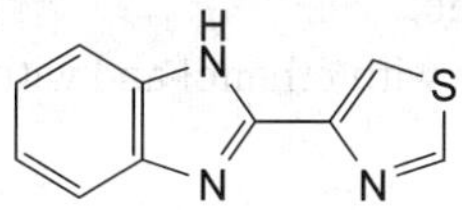

$C_{10}H_7N_3S$ M_r 201.2

DEFINITION

Tiabendazole contains not less than 98.0 per cent and not more than the equivalent of 101.0 per cent of 2-(thiazol-4-yl)-1*H*-benzimidazole, calculated with reference to the anhydrous substance.

CHARACTERS

A white or almost white, crystalline powder, practically insoluble in water, slightly soluble in alcohol and in methylene chloride. It dissolves in dilute mineral acids. It melts at about 300 °C.

IDENTIFICATION

First identification: B.

Second identification: A, C, D.

A. Dissolve 25 mg in *0.1 M hydrochloric acid* and dilute to 100.0 ml with the same acid. Dilute 2.0 ml of the solution to 100.0 ml with *0.1 M hydrochloric acid*. Examined between 230 nm and 350 nm (*2.2.25*), the solution shows two absorption maxima, at 243 nm and 302 nm. The ratio of the absorbance measured at the maximum at 302 nm to that measured at the maximum at 243 nm is 1.8 to 2.1.

Monographs T-Z

B. Examine by infrared absorption spectrophotometry (*2.2.24*), comparing with the spectrum obtained with *tiabendazole CRS*. Examine the substances prepared as discs.

C. Examine the chromatograms obtained in the test for related substances in ultraviolet light at 254 nm. The principal spot in the chromatogram obtained with test solution (b) is similar in position and size to the principal spot in the chromatogram obtained with reference solution (a).

D. Dissolve about 5 mg in *0.1 M hydrochloric acid* and dilute to 5 ml with the same acid. Add 3 mg of *p-phenylenediamine dihydrochloride R* and shake until dissolved. Add 0.1 g of *zinc powder R*, mix, allow to stand for 2 min and add 5 ml of *ferric ammonium sulphate solution R2*. A bluish-violet colour develops.

TESTS

Related substances. Examine by thin-layer chromatography (*2.2.27*), using *silica gel HF_{254} R* as the coating substance.

Test solution (a). Dissolve 0.10 g of the substance to be examined in *methanol R* and dilute to 10 ml with the same solvent.

Test solution (b). Dilute 2 ml of test solution (a) to 20 ml with *methanol R*.

Reference solution (a). Dissolve 20 mg of *tiabendazole CRS* in *methanol R* and dilute to 20 ml with the same solvent.

Reference solution (b). Dilute 1 ml of test solution (b) to 10 ml with *methanol R*.

Reference solution (c). Dilute 1 ml of test solution (b) to 25 ml with *methanol R*.

Apply separately to the plate 20 µl of each solution. Develop over a path of 15 cm using a mixture of 2.5 volumes of *water R*, 10 volumes of *acetone R*, 25 volumes of *glacial acetic acid R* and 62.5 volumes of *toluene R*. Allow the plate to dry in air and examine in ultraviolet light at 254 nm. Any spot in the chromatogram obtained with test solution (a), apart from the principal spot, is not more intense than the spot in the chromatogram obtained with reference solution (b) (1.0 per cent) and at most one such spot is more intense than the spot in the chromatogram obtained with reference solution (c) (0.4 per cent).

***o*-Phenylenediamine**. To 5.0 g in a flask fitted with a ground-glass stopper, add 25 ml of a mixture of 1 volume of *methanol R* and 2 volumes of *water R*. Shake for 3 min. Filter through a sintered-glass filter (16) under reduced pressure. To 10 ml of the filtrate add 0.5 ml of *hydrochloric acid R* and 0.5 ml of *acetylacetone R* and shake until the solution is clear. The solution is not more intensely coloured than reference solution R_7 (*2.2.2, Method I*) (10 ppm).

Heavy metals (*2.4.8*). 1.0 g complies with limit test D for heavy metals (20 ppm). Prepare the standard using 2 ml of *lead standard solution (10 ppm Pb) R*.

Water (*2.5.12*). Not more than 0.5 per cent, determined on 1.00 g by the semi-micro determination of water.

Sulphated ash (*2.4.14*). Not more than 0.2 per cent, determined on 1.0 g.

ASSAY

Dissolve 0.150 g in 30 ml of *anhydrous acetic acid R*. Titrate with *0.1 M perchloric acid*, determining the end-point potentiometrically (*2.2.20*).

1 ml of *0.1 M perchloric acid* is equivalent to 20.12 mg of $C_{10}H_7N_3S$.

STORAGE

Store protected from light.

IMPURITIES

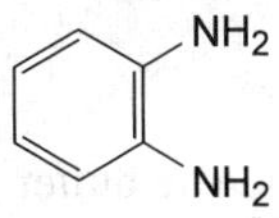

A. benzene-1,2-diamine.

01/2005:1660

TIAMULIN FOR VETERINARY USE

Tiamulinum ad usum veterinarium

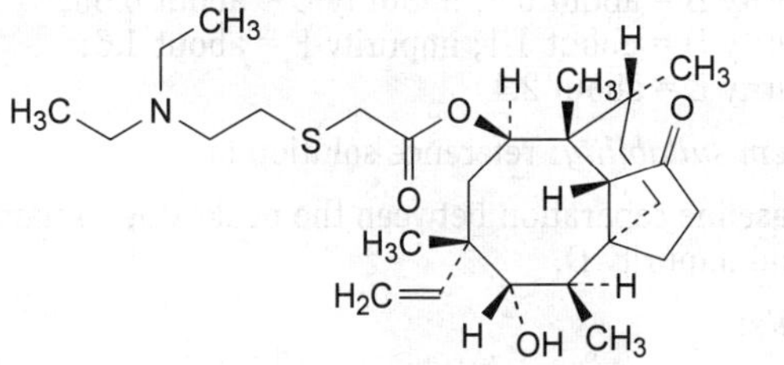

$C_{28}H_{47}NO_4S$ M_r 493.8

DEFINITION

(3a*S*,4*R*,5*S*,6*S*,8*R*,9*R*,9a*R*,10*R*)-6-Ethenyl-5-hydroxy-4,6,9,10-tetramethyl-1-oxodecahydro-3a,9-propano-3a*H*-cyclopentacycloocten-8-yl [[2-(diethylamino)ethyl]sulphanyl]acetate.

Content: 96.5 per cent to 102.0 per cent (dried substance).

CHARACTERS

Appearance: sticky, translucent yellowish mass, slightly hygroscopic.

Solubility: practically insoluble in water, very soluble in methylene chloride, freely soluble in anhydrous ethanol.

IDENTIFICATION

Infrared absorption spectrophotometry (*2.2.24*).

Comparison: *Ph. Eur. reference spectrum of tiamulin.*

TESTS

Appearance of solution. The solution is clear (*2.2.1*) and its absorbance (*2.2.25*) at 420 nm is maximum 0.050.

Dissolve 2.5 g in 50 ml of *methanol R*.

Related substances. Liquid chromatography (*2.2.29*).

Ammonium carbonate buffer solution pH 10.0. Dissolve 10.0 g of *ammonium carbonate R* in *water R*, add 22 ml of *perchloric acid solution R* and dilute to 1000.0 ml with *water R*. Adjust to pH 10.0 with *concentrated ammonia R1*.

Solvent mixture: ammonium carbonate buffer solution pH 10.0, *acetonitrile R1* (50:50 *V/V*).

Test solution. Dissolve 0.200 g of the substance to be examined in the solvent mixture and dilute to 50.0 ml with the solvent mixture.

Reference solution (a). Dissolve 0.250 g of *tiamulin hydrogen fumarate CRS* in the solvent mixture and dilute to 50.0 ml with the solvent mixture.

Reference solution (b). Dilute 1.0 ml of the test solution to 100.0 ml with the solvent mixture.

Reference solution (c). Dilute 0.1 ml of *toluene R* to 100 ml with *acetonitrile R*. Dilute 0.1 ml of this solution to 100.0 ml with the solvent mixture.

Column:

- *size*: l = 0.15 m, Ø = 4.6 mm,
- *stationary phase*: *end-capped octadecylsilyl silica gel for chromatography R* (5 µm),
- *temperature*: 30 °C.

Mobile phase: *acetonitrile R1*, ammonium carbonate buffer solution pH 10.0, *methanol R1* (21:30:49 *V/V/V*).

Flow rate: 1.0 ml/min.

Detection: spectrophotometer at 212 nm.

Injection: 20 µl.

Run time: 3 times the retention time of tiamulin.

Relative retention with reference to tiamulin (retention time = about 18 min): impurity A = about 0.22; impurity B = about 0.5; impurity C = about 0.66; impurity D = about 1.1; impurity F = about 1.6; impurity E = about 2.4.

System suitability: reference solution (a):

- baseline separation between the peaks due to tiamulin and impurity D.

Limits:

- *impurities A, B, C, D, E, F*: for each impurity, not more than the area of the principal peak in the chromatogram obtained with reference solution (b) (1.0 per cent),
- *any other impurity*: for each impurity, not more than 0.2 times the area of the principal peak in the chromatogram obtained with reference solution (b) (0.2 per cent),
- *total*: not more than 3 times the area of the principal peak in the chromatogram obtained with reference solution (b) (3.0 per cent),
- *disregard limit*: 0.1 times the area of the principal peak in the chromatogram obtained with reference solution (b) (0.1 per cent); disregard any peak present in the chromatogram obtained with reference solution (c).

Loss on drying (*2.2.32*): maximum 1.0 per cent, determined on 1.000 g by drying in an oven at 80 °C.

Bacterial endotoxins (*2.6.14, Method D*): less than 0.4 IU/mg, determined in a 1 mg/ml solution in *anhydrous ethanol R* (endotoxin free) diluted 1:40 with water for bacterial endotoxins test.

ASSAY

Liquid chromatography (*2.2.29*) as described in the test for related substances with the following modification.

Injection: test solution and reference solution (a).

Calculate the percentage content of $C_{28}H_{47}NO_4S$, from the declared content of *tiamulin hydrogen fumarate CRS*.

STORAGE

Protected from light.

LABELLING

The label states where appropriate that the substance is free from bacterial endotoxins.

IMPURITIES

Specified impurities: A, B, C, D, E, F.

Other detectable impurities: G, H, I, J, K, L, M, N, O, P, Q, R.

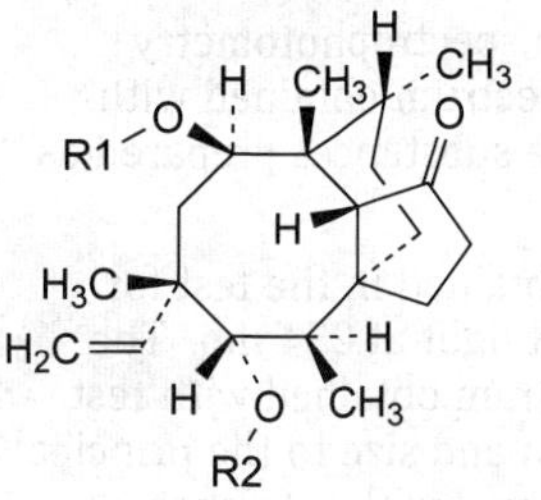

A. R1 = R2 = H: (3a*S*,4*R*,5*S*,6*S*,8*R*,9*R*,9a*R*,10*R*)-6-ethenyl-5,8-dihydroxy-4,6,9,10-tetramethyloctahydro-3a,9-propano-3a*H*-cyclopentacycloocten-1(4*H*)-one (mutilin),

G. R1 = CO-CH_2OH, R2 = H: (3a*S*,4*R*,5*S*,6*S*,8*R*,9*R*,9a*R*,10*R*)-6-ethenyl-5-hydroxy-4,6,9,10-tetramethyl-1-oxodecahydro-3a,9-propano-3a*H*-cyclopentacycloocten-8-yl hydroxyacetate (pleuromutilin),

J. R1 = CO-CH_3, R2 = H: (3a*S*,4*R*,5*S*,6*S*,8*R*,9*R*,9a*R*,10*R*)-6-ethenyl-5-hydroxy-4,6,9,10-tetramethyl-1-oxodecahydro-3a,9-propano-3a*H*-cyclopentacycloocten-8-yl acetate (mutilin 14-acetate),

K. R1 = H, R2 = CO-CH_3: (3a*S*,4*R*,5*S*,6*S*,8*R*,9*R*,9a*R*,10*R*)-6-ethenyl-8-hydroxy-4,6,9,10-tetramethyl-1-oxodecahydro-3a,9-propano-3a*H*-cyclopentacycloocten-5-yl acetate (mutilin 11-acetate),

L. R1 = CO-CH_2-O-SO_2-C_6H_4-*p*CH_3, R2 = H: (3aS,4*R*,5*S*,6*S*,8*R*,9*R*,9a*R*,10*R*)-6-ethenyl-5-hydroxy-4,6,9,10-tetramethyl-1-oxodecahydro-3a,9-propano-3a*H*-cyclopentacycloocten-8-yl [[(4-methylphenyl)sulphonyl]oxy]acetate (pleuromutilin 22-tosylate),

M. R1 = R2 = CO-CH_3: (3a*S*,4*R*,5*S*,6*S*,8*R*,9*R*,9a*R*,10*R*)-6-ethenyl-4,6,9,10-tetramethyl-1-oxodecahydro-3a,9-propano-3a*H*-cyclopentacycloocten-5,8-diyl diacetate (mutilin 11,14-diacetate),

P. R1 = CO-CH_2-O-SO_2-C_6H_5, R2 = H: (3a*S*,4*R*,5*S*,6*S*,8*R*,9*R*,9a*R*,10*R*)-6-ethenyl-5-hydroxy-4,6,9,10-tetramethyl-1-oxodecahydro-3a,9-propano-3a*H*-cyclopentacycloocten-8-yl [(phenylsulphonyl)oxy]acetate,

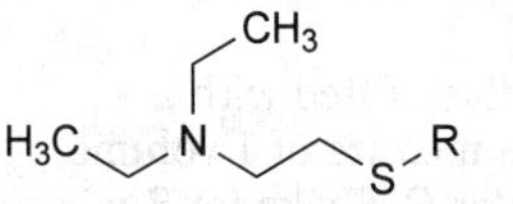

B. R = CH_2-C_6H_5: 2-(benzylsulphanyl)-*N*,*N*-diethylethanamine,

C. R = S-CH_2-CH_2-N(C_2H_5)$_2$: 2,2′-(disulphane-1,2-diyl)bis(*N*,*N*-diethylethanamine),

O. R = H: 2-(diethylamino)ethanethiol,

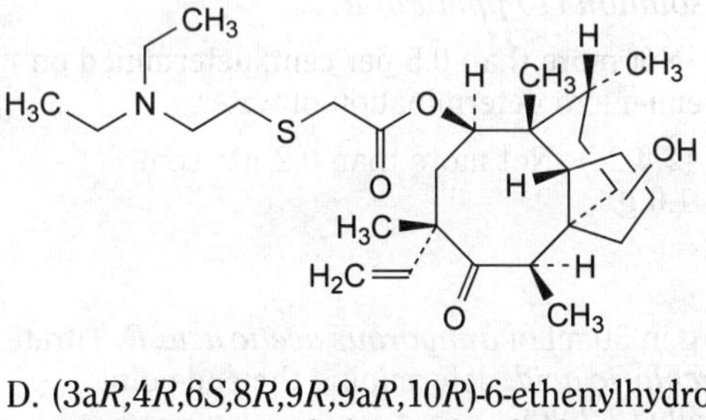

D. (3a*R*,4*R*,6*S*,8*R*,9*R*,9a*R*,10*R*)-6-ethenylhydroxy-4,6,9,10-tetramethyl-5-oxodecahydro-3a,9-propano-3a*H*-cyclopentacycloocten-8-yl [[2-(diethylamino)ethyl]sulphanyl]acetate,

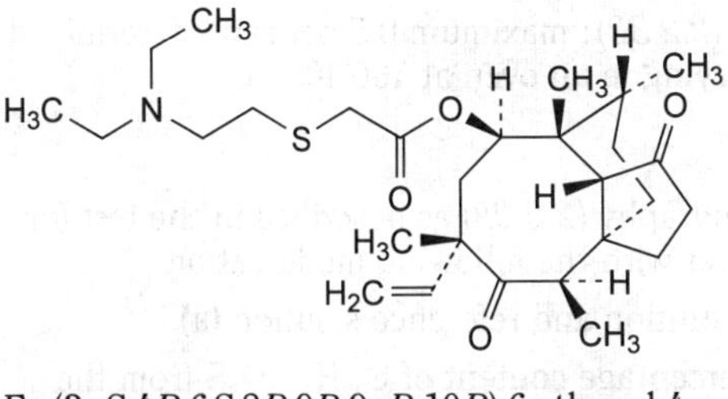

E. (3a*S*,4*R*,6*S*,8*R*,9*R*,9a*R*,10*R*)-6-ethenyl-4,6,9,10-tetramethyl-1,5-dioxodecahydro-3a,9-propano-3a*H*-cyclopentacycloocten-8-yl [[2-(diethylamino)ethyl]sulphanyl]acetate (11-oxotiamulin),

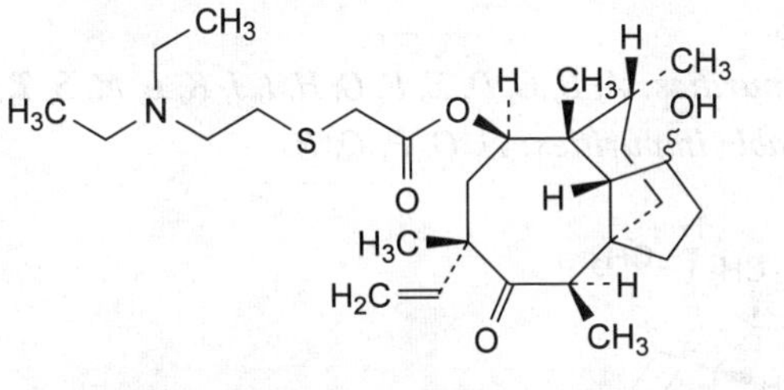

F. (1*RS*,3a*R*,4*R*,6*S*,8*R*,9*R*,9a*R*,10*R*)-6-ethenyl-1-hydroxy-4,6,9,10-tetramethyl-5-oxodecahydro-3a,9-propano-3a*H*-cyclopentacycloocten-8-yl [[2-(diethylamino)ethyl]sulphanyl]acetate (1-hydroxy-11-oxotiamulin),

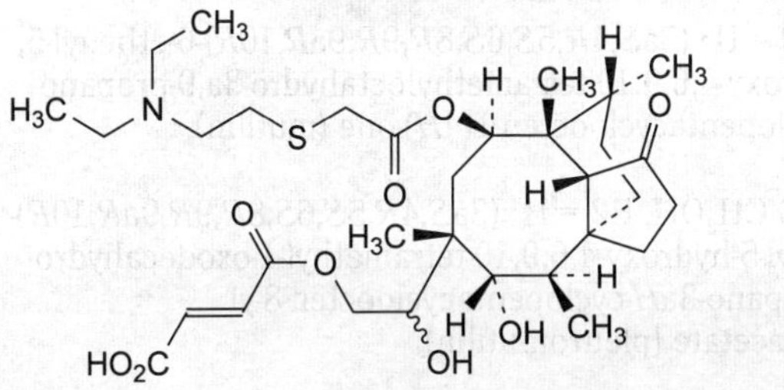

H. (2*E*)-4-[(2*RS*)-2-[(3a*S*,4*R*,5*S*,6*R*,8*R*,9*R*,9a*R*,10*R*)-8-[[[[2-(diethylamino)ethyl]sulphanyl]acetyl]oxy]-5-hydroxy-4,6,9,10-tetramethyl-1-oxodecahydro-3a,9-propano-3a*H*-cyclopentacycloocten-6-yl]-2-hydroxyethoxy]-4-oxobut-2-enoic acid (19,20-dihydroxytiamulin 20-fumarate),

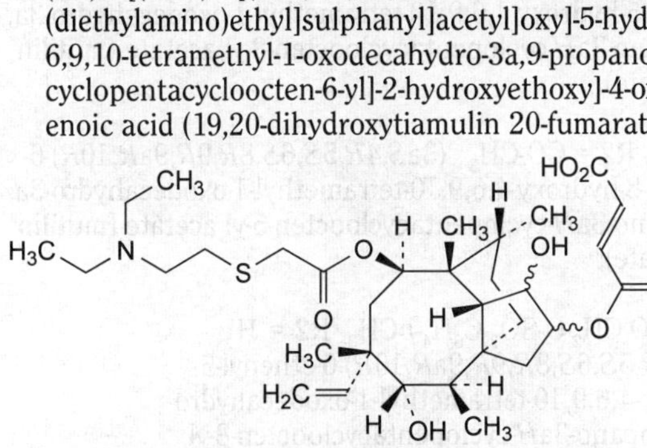

I. (2*E*)-4-[[(3a*S*,4*R*,5*S*,6*S*,8*R*,9*R*,9a*R*,10*R*)-8-[[[[2-(diethylamino)ethyl]sulphanyl]acetyl]oxy]-6-ethenyl-1,5-dihydroxy-4,6,9,10-tetramethyldecahydro-3a,9-propano-3a*H*-cyclopentacycloocten-2-yl]oxy]-4-oxobut-2-enoic acid (2,3-dihydroxytiamulin 2-fumarate),

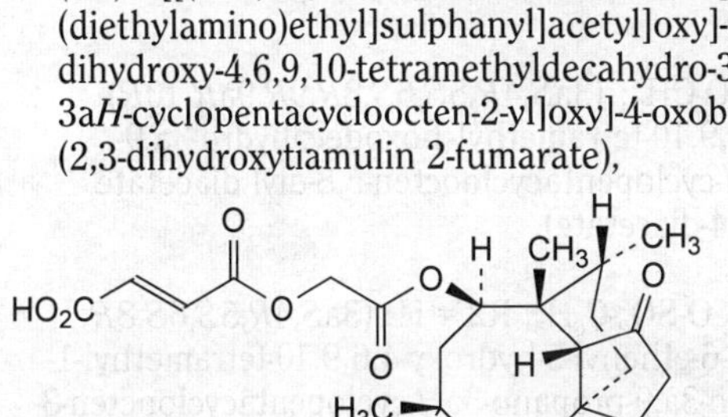

N. (2*E*)-4-[2-[[(3a*S*,4*R*,5*S*,6*S*,8*R*,9*R*,9a*R*,10*R*)-6-ethenyl-5-hydroxy-4,6,9,10-tetramethyl-1-oxodecahydro-3a,9-propano-3a*H*-cyclopentacycloocten-8-yl]oxy]-2-oxoethoxy]-4-oxobut-2-enoic acid (pleuromutilin 22-fumarate),

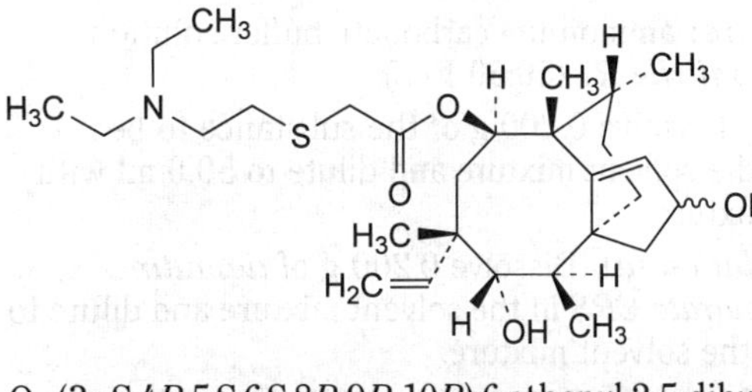

Q. (3a*S*,4*R*,5*S*,6*S*,8*R*,9*R*,10*R*)-6-ethenyl-2,5-dihydroxy-4,6,9,10-tetramethyl-2,3,4,5,6,7,8,9-octahydro-3a,9-propano-3a*H*-cyclopentacycloocten-8-yl [[2-(diethylamino)ethyl]sulphanyl]acetate (3,4-didehydro-2-hydroxytiamulin),

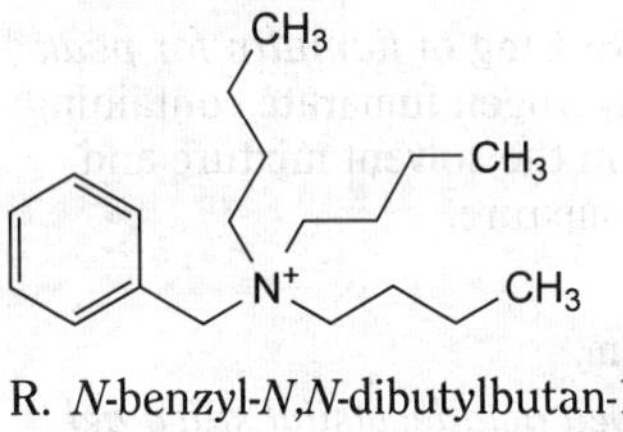

R. *N*-benzyl-*N*,*N*-dibutylbutan-1-aminium.

01/2005:1659

TIAMULIN HYDROGEN FUMARATE FOR VETERINARY USE

Tiamulini hydrogenofumaras ad usum veterinarium

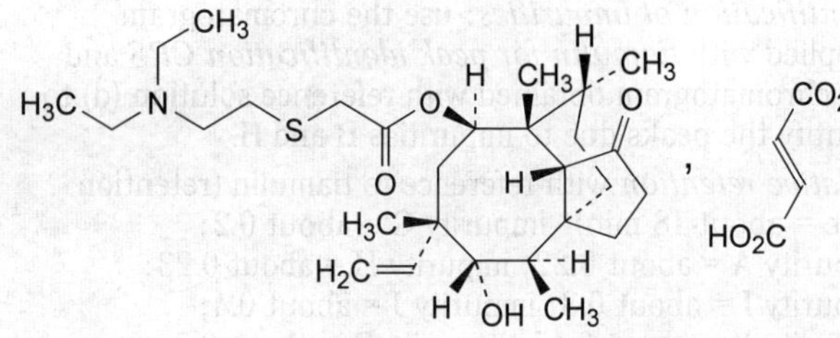

$C_{32}H_{51}NO_8S$ M_r 610

DEFINITION

(3a*S*,4*R*,5*S*,6*S*,8*R*,9*R*,9a*R*,10*R*)-6-Ethenyl-5-hydroxy-4,6,9,10-tetramethyl-1-oxodecahydro-3a,9-propano-3a*H*-cyclopentacycloocten-8-yl [[2-(diethylamino)ethyl]sulphanyl]acetate hydrogen (*E*)-but-2-enedioate.

Content: 96.5 per cent to 102.0 per cent (dried substance).

CHARACTERS

Appearance: white or light yellow, crystalline powder.

Solubility: soluble in water, freely soluble in anhydrous ethanol and soluble in methanol.

IDENTIFICATION

Infrared absorption spectrophotometry (*2.2.24*).

Comparison: *tiamulin hydrogen fumarate CRS*.

TESTS

pH (*2.2.3*): 3.1 to 4.1.

Dissolve 0.5 g in *carbon dioxide-free water R* and dilute to 50 ml with the same solvent.

Related substances. Liquid chromatography (*2.2.29*).

Ammonium carbonate buffer solution pH 10.0. Dissolve 10.0 g of *ammonium carbonate R* in *water R*, add 22 ml of *perchloric acid solution R* and dilute to 1000.0 ml with *water R*. Adjust to pH 10.0 with *concentrated ammonia R1*.

Monographs T-Z

Solvent mixture: ammonium carbonate buffer solution pH 10.0, *acetonitrile R1* (50:50 *V/V*).

Test solution. Dissolve 0.200 g of the substance to be examined in the solvent mixture and dilute to 50.0 ml with the solvent mixture.

Reference solution (a). Dissolve 0.200 g of *tiamulin hydrogen fumarate CRS* in the solvent mixture and dilute to 50.0 ml with the solvent mixture.

Reference solution (b). Dilute 1.0 ml of the test solution to 100.0 ml with the solvent mixture.

Reference solution (c). Dissolve 40.0 mg of *fumaric acid R* in the solvent mixture and dilute to 50.0 ml with the solvent mixture.

Reference solution (d). Dissolve 4 mg of *tiamulin for peak identification CRS* (tiamulin hydrogen fumarate containing impurities B, C, D, F, H and I) in the solvent mixture and dilute to 1 ml with the solvent mixture.

Column:
- *size*: *l* = 0.15 m, Ø = 4.6 mm,
- *stationary phase*: *end-capped octadecylsilyl silica gel for chromatography R* (5 μm),
- *temperature*: 30 °C.

Mobile phase: *acetonitrile R1*, ammonium carbonate buffer solution pH 10.0, *methanol R1* (21:30:49 *V/V/V*).

Flow rate: 1.0 ml/min.

Detection: spectrophotometer at 212 nm.

Injection: 20 μl.

Run time: 3 times the retention time of tiamulin.

Identification of impurities: use the chromatogram supplied with *tiamulin for peak identification CRS* and the chromatogram obtained with reference solution (d) to identify the peaks due to impurities B and H.

Relative retention with reference to tiamulin (retention time = about 18 min): impurity G = about 0.2; impurity A = about 0.22; impurity H = about 0.23; impurity I = about 0.3; impurity J = about 0.4; impurity K = about 0.45; impurity B = about 0.5; impurity L = about 0.65; impurity C = about 0.66; impurity F = about 0.8; impurity M = about 0.85; impurity D = about 1.1; impurity S = about 1.4; impurity T = about 1.6; impurity E = 2.4.

System suitability: reference solution (a):
- baseline separation between the peaks due to tiamulin and impurity D.

Limits:
- *impurities B, H*: for each impurity, not more than 1.5 times the area of the principal peak in the chromatogram obtained with reference solution (b) (1.5 per cent),
- *impurities A, C, D, E, F, G, I, J, K, L, M, S, T*: for each impurity, not more than the area of the principal peak in the chromatogram obtained with reference solution (b) (1.0 per cent),
- *any other impurity*: for each impurity, not more than 0.2 times the area of the principal peak in the chromatogram obtained with reference solution (b) (0.2 per cent),
- *total*: not more than 3 times the area of the principal peak in the chromatogram obtained with reference solution (b) (3.0 per cent),
- *disregard limit*: 0.1 times the area of the principal peak in the chromatogram obtained with reference solution (b) (0.1 per cent); disregard any peak present in reference solution (c).

Loss on drying (*2.2.32*): maximum 0.5 per cent, determined on 1.000 g by drying in an oven at 100-105 °C.

ASSAY

Liquid chromatography (*2.2.29*) as described in the test for related substances with the following modification.

Injection: test solution and reference solution (a).

Calculate the percentage content of $C_{32}H_{51}NO_8S$ from the declared content of *tiamulin hydrogen fumarate CRS*.

STORAGE

Protected from light.

IMPURITIES

Specified impurities: *A, B, C, D, E, F, G, H, I, J, K, L, M, S, T.*

Other detectable impurities: *N, O, P, Q, R.*

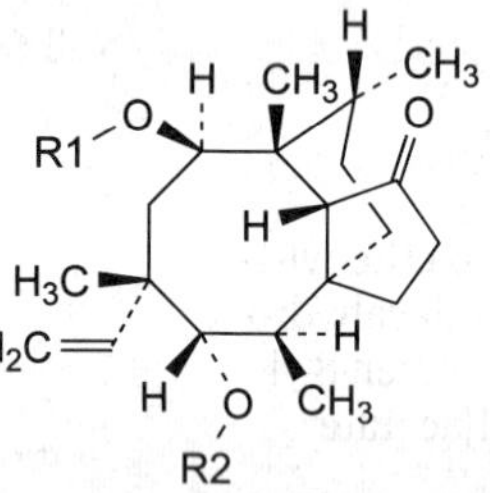

A. R1 = R2 = H: (3a*S*,4*R*,5*S*,6*S*,8*R*,9*R*,9a*R*,10*R*)-6-ethenyl-5,8-dihydroxy-4,6,9,10-tetramethyloctahydro-3a,9-propano-3a*H*-cyclopentacycloocten-1(4*H*)-one (mutilin),

G. R1 = CO-CH_2OH, R2 = H: (3a*S*,4*R*,5*S*,6*S*,8*R*,9*R*,9a*R*,10*R*)-6-ethenyl-5-hydroxy-4,6,9,10-tetramethyl-1-oxodecahydro-3a,9-propano-3a*H*-cyclopentacycloocten-8-yl hydroxyacetate (pleuromutilin),

J. R1 = CO-CH_3, R2 = H: (3a*S*,4*R*,5*S*,6*S*,8*R*,9*R*,9a*R*,10*R*)-6-ethenyl-5-hydroxy-4,6,9,10-tetramethyl-1-oxodecahydro-3a,9-propano-3a*H*-cyclopentacycloocten-8-yl acetate (mutilin 14-acetate),

K. R1 = H, R2 = CO-CH_3: (3a*S*,4*R*,5*S*,6*S*,8*R*,9*R*,9a*R*,10*R*)-6-ethenyl-8-hydroxy-4,6,9,10-tetramethyl-1-oxodecahydro-3a,9-propano-3a*H*-cyclopentacycloocten-5-yl acetate (mutilin 11-acetate),

L. R1 = CO-CH_2-O-SO_2-C_6H_4-*p*CH_3, R2 = H: (3a*S*,4*R*,5*S*,6*S*,8*R*,9*R*,9a*R*,10*R*)-6-ethenyl-5-hydroxy-4,6,9,10-tetramethyl-1-oxodecahydro-3a,9-propano-3a*H*-cyclopentacycloocten-8-yl [[(4-methylphenyl)sulphonyl]oxy]acetate (pleuromutilin 22-tosylate),

M. R1 = R2 = CO-CH_3: (3a*S*,4*R*,5*S*,6*S*,8*R*,9*R*,9a*R*,10*R*)-6-ethenyl-4,6,9,10-tetramethyl-1-oxodecahydro-3a,9-propano-3a*H*-cyclopentacycloocten-5,8-diyl diacetate (mutilin 11,14-diacetate),

P. R1 = CO-CH_2-O-SO_2-C_6H_5, R2 = H: (3a*S*,4*R*,5*S*,6*S*,8*R*,9*R*,9a*R*,10*R*)-6-ethenyl-5-hydroxy-4,6,9,10-tetramethyl-1-oxodecahydro-3a,9-propano-3a*H*-cyclopentacycloocten-8-yl [(phenylsulphonyl)oxy]acetate,

T. R1 = CO-CH_2-[S-CH_2-CH_2-]$_2$N(C_2H_5)$_2$, R2 = H: (3a*S*,4*R*,5*S*,6*S*,8*R*,9*R*,9a*R*,10*R*)-6-ethenyl-5-hydroxy-4,6,9,10-tetramethyl-1-oxodecahydro-3a,9-propano-3a*H*-cyclopentacycloocten-8-yl [[2-[[2-(diethylamino)ethyl]sulphanyl]ethyl]sulphanyl]acetate,

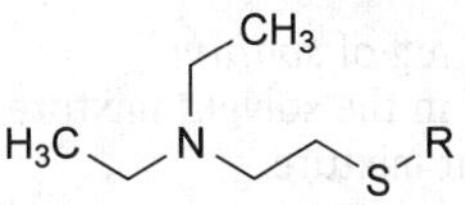

B. R = CH_2-C_6H_5: 2-(benzylsulphanyl)-*N*,*N*-diethylethanamine,

C. R = S-CH_2-CH_2-N(C_2H_5)$_2$: 2,2'-(disulphane-1,2-diyl)bis(*N*,*N*-diethylethanamine),

O. R = H: 2-(diethylamino)ethanethiol,

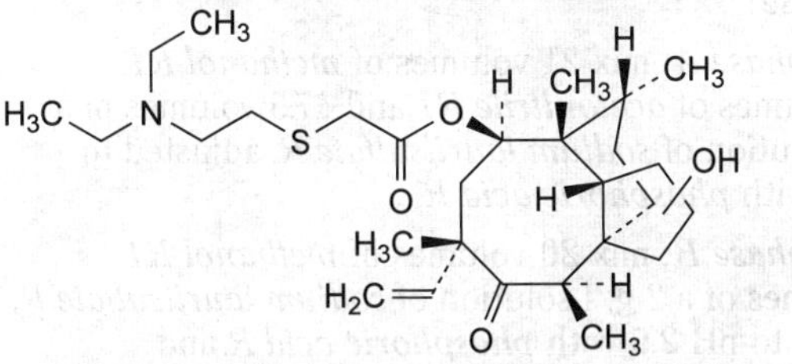

D. (3a*R*,4*R*,6*S*,8*R*,9*R*,9a*R*,10*R*)-6-ethenylhydroxy-4,6,9,10-tetramethyl-5-oxodecahydro-3a,9-propano-3a*H*-cyclopentacycloocten-8-yl [[2-(diethylamino)ethyl]sulphanyl]acetate,

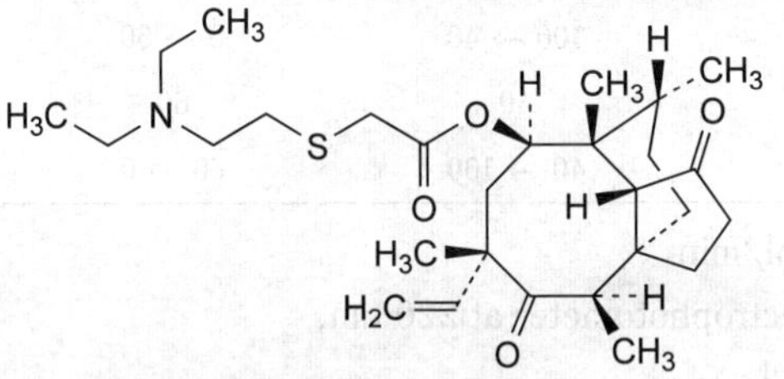

E. (3a*S*,4*R*,6*S*,8*R*,9*R*,9a*R*,10*R*)-6-ethenyl-4,6,9,10-tetramethyl-1,5-dioxodecahydro-3a,9-propano-3a*H*-cyclopentacycloocten-8-yl [[2-(diethylamino)ethyl]sulphanyl]acetate (11-oxotiamulin),

F. impurity of unknown structure with a relative retention of about 0.8,

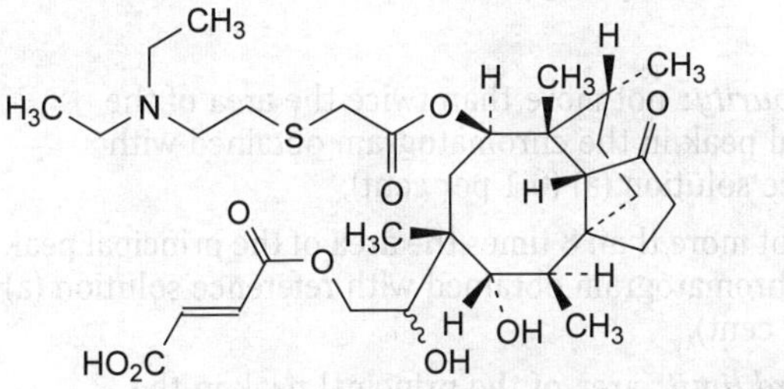

H. (2*E*)-4-[(2*RS*)-2-[(3a*S*,4*R*,5*S*,6*R*,8*R*,9*R*,9a*R*,10*R*)-8-[[[2-(diethylamino)ethyl]sulphanyl]acetyl]oxy]-5-hydroxy-4,6,9,10-tetramethyl-1-oxodecahydro-3a,9-propano-3a*H*-cyclopentacycloocten-6-yl]-2-hydroxyethoxy]-4-oxobut-2-enoic acid (19,20-dihydroxytiamulin 20-fumarate),

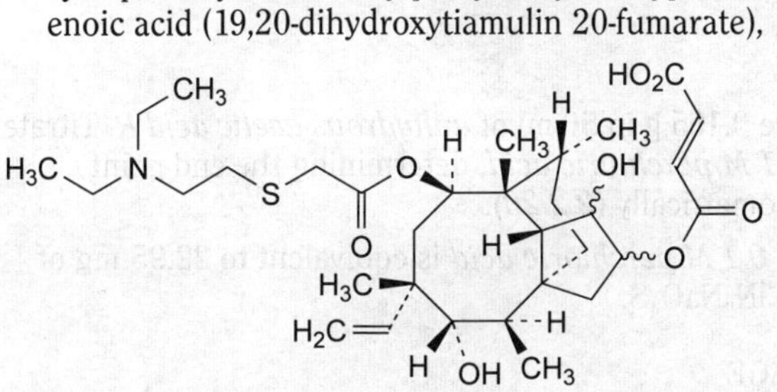

I. (2*E*)-4-[[(3a*S*,4*R*,5*S*,6*S*,8*R*,9*R*,9a*R*,10*R*)-8-[[[2-(diethylamino)ethyl]sulphanyl]acetyl]oxy]-6-ethenyl-1,5-dihydroxy-4,6,9,10-tetramethyldecahydro-3a,9-propano-3a*H*-cyclopentacycloocten-2-yl]oxy]-4-oxobut-2-enoic acid (2,3-dihydroxytiamulin 2-fumarate),

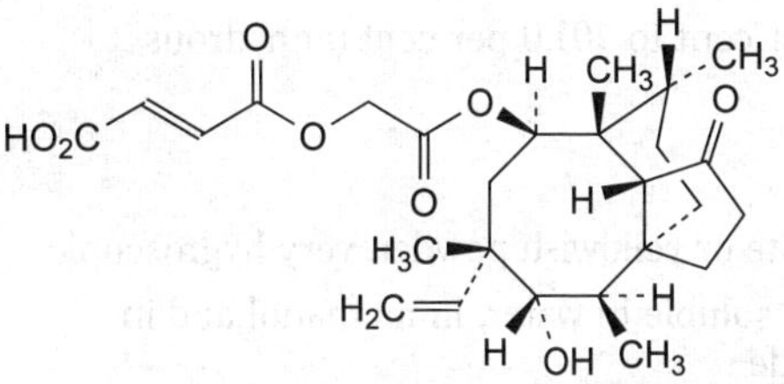

N. (2*E*)-4-[2-[[(3a*S*,4*R*,5*S*,6*S*,8*R*,9*R*,9a*R*,10*R*)-6-ethenyl-5-hydroxy-4,6,9,10-tetramethyl-1-oxodecahydro-3a,9-propano-3a*H*-cyclopentacycloocten-8-yl]oxy]-2-oxoethoxy]-4-oxobut-2-enoic acid (pleuromutilin 22-fumarate),

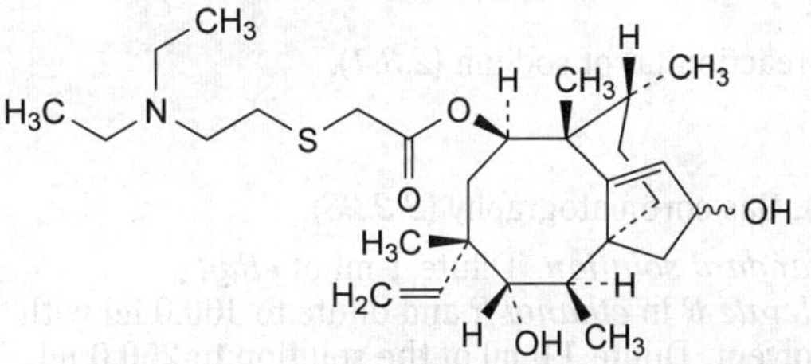

Q. (3a*S*,4*R*,5*S*,6*S*,8*R*,9*R*,10*R*)-6-ethenyl-2,5-dihydroxy-4,6,9,10-tetramethyl-2,3,4,5,6,7,8,9-octahydro-3a,9-propano-3a*H*-cyclopentacycloocten-8-yl [[2-(diethylamino)ethyl]sulphanyl]acetate (3,4-didehydro-2-hydroxytiamulin),

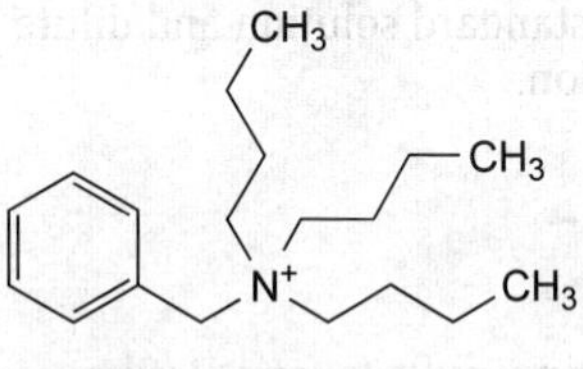

R. *N*-benzyl-*N*,*N*-dibutylbutan-1-aminium,

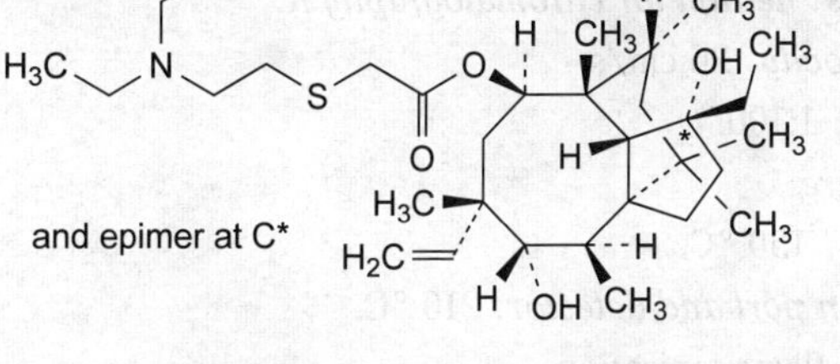

S. (1*RS*,3a*R*,4*R*,5*S*,6*S*,8*R*,9*R*,9a*R*,10*R*)-6-ethenyl-1-ethyl-1,5-dihydroxy-4,6,9,10,12,12-hexamethyldecahydro-3a,9-propano-3a*H*-cyclopentacycloocten-8-yl [[2-(diethylamino)ethyl]sulphanyl]acetate.

01/2005:2022

TIANEPTINE SODIUM

Tianeptinum natricum

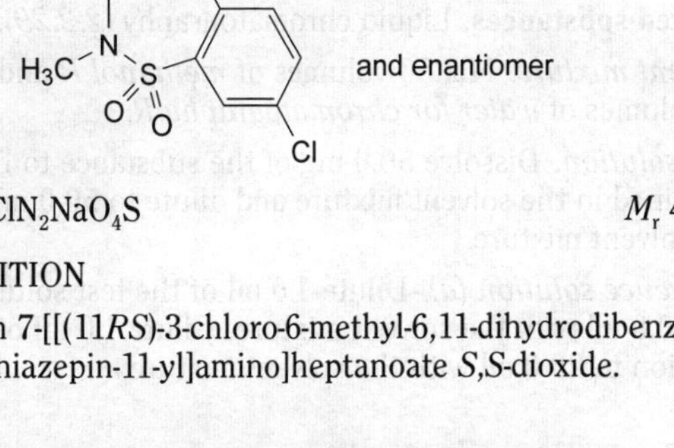

$C_{21}H_{24}ClN_2NaO_4S$ M_r 458.9

DEFINITION

Sodium 7-[[(11*RS*)-3-chloro-6-methyl-6,11-dihydrodibenzo[*c*,*f*][1,2]thiazepin-11-yl]amino]heptanoate *S*,*S*-dioxide.

Content: 99.0 per cent to 101.0 per cent (anhydrous substance).

CHARACTERS

Appearance: white or yellowish powder, very hygroscopic.

Solubility: freely soluble in water, in methanol and in methylene chloride.

IDENTIFICATION

A. Infrared absorption spectrophotometry (*2.2.24*).

Comparison: *Ph. Eur. reference spectrum of tianeptine sodium*.

B. It gives reaction (a) of sodium (*2.3.1*).

TESTS

Impurity A. Gas chromatography (*2.2.28*).

Internal standard solution. Dilute 1 ml of *ethyl 5-bromovalerate R* in *ethanol R* and dilute to 100.0 ml with the same solvent. Dilute 1.0 ml of the solution to 250.0 ml with *ethanol R*.

Test solution. Dissolve 0.1000 g of the substance to be examined in the internal standard solution and dilute to 2.0 ml with the same solution.

Reference solution. Dissolve 10.0 mg of *tianeptine impurity A CRS* in the internal standard solution and dilute to 200.0 ml with the same solution.

Column:

- *material*: fused silica,
- *size*: l = 25 m, Ø = 0.25 mm,
- *stationary phase*: *poly(cyanopropyl)siloxane R* (film thickness 0.2 µm).

Carrier gas: *helium for chromatography R*.

Linear velocity: 26 cm/s.

Split ratio: 1:100.

Temperature:

- *column*: 150 °C,
- *injection port and detector*: 210 °C.

Detection: flame ionisation.

Injection: 1 µl.

Run time: twice the retention time of ethyl 5-bromovalerate.

System suitability: reference solution:

- *elution order*: ethanol, ethyl 5-bromovalerate, impurity A,
- *resolution*: minimum 10 between the peaks due to ethyl 5-bromovalerate and impurity A,
- *signal-to-noise ratio*: minimum 20 for the peak due to impurity A.

Limit:

- *impurity A*: not more than the area of the corresponding peak in the chromatogram obtained with the reference solution (0.1 per cent).

Related substances. Liquid chromatography (*2.2.29*).

Solvent mixture. Mix 50 volumes of *methanol R* and 50 volumes of *water for chromatography R*.

Test solution. Dissolve 50.0 mg of the substance to be examined in the solvent mixture and dilute to 50.0 ml with the solvent mixture.

Reference solution (a). Dilute 1.0 ml of the test solution to 100.0 ml with the solvent mixture. Dilute 1.0 ml of this solution to 20.0 ml with the solvent mixture.

Reference solution (b). Dissolve 20.0 mg of *sodium tianeptine for system suitability CRS* in the solvent mixture and dilute to 200.0 ml with the solvent mixture.

Column:

- *size*: l = 0.15 m, Ø = 4.6 mm,
- *stationary phase*: *octadecylsilyl silica gel for chromatography R* (3 µm) with a pore size of 0.01 µm,
- *temperature*: 30 °C.

Mobile phase:

- *mobile phase A*: mix 21 volumes of *methanol R1*, 31.5 volumes of *acetonitrile R1* and 47.5 volumes of a 2 g/l solution of *sodium laurilsulfate R*, adjusted to pH 2.5 with *phosphoric acid R*,
- *mobile phase B*: mix 20 volumes of *methanol R1*, 20 volumes of a 2 g/l solution of *sodium laurilsulfate R*, adjusted to pH 2.5 with *phosphoric acid R* and 60 volumes of *acetonitrile R1*,

Time (min)	Mobile phase A (per cent *V/V*)	Mobile phase B (per cent *V/V*)
0 - 35	100	0
35 - 45	100 → 40	0 → 60
45 - 60	40	60
60 - 70	40 → 100	60 → 0

Flow rate: 1 ml/min.

Detection: spectrophotometer at 220 nm.

Injection: 10 µl.

Relative retention with reference to tianeptine (retention time = about 30 min): impurity C = about 0.4; impurity D1 = about 0.6; impurity D2 = about 0.8; impurity E = about 1.1; impurity B = about 1.7.

System suitability: reference solution (b):

- *resolution*: minimum 2.5 between the peaks due to tianeptine and impurity E.

Limits:

- *any impurity*: not more than twice the area of the principal peak in the chromatogram obtained with reference solution (a) (0.1 per cent),
- *total*: not more than 8 times the area of the principal peak in the chromatogram obtained with reference solution (a) (0.4 per cent),
- *disregard limit*: area of the principal peak in the chromatogram obtained with reference solution (a) (0.05 per cent).

Water (*2.5.12*): maximum 5.0 per cent, determined on 0.100 g.

ASSAY

Dissolve 0.165 g in 50 ml of *anhydrous acetic acid R*. Titrate with *0.1 M perchloric acid*, determining the end-point potentiometrically (*2.2.20*).

1 ml of *0.1 M perchloric acid* is equivalent to 22.95 mg of $C_{21}H_{24}ClN_2NaO_4S$.

STORAGE

In an airtight container.

IMPURITIES

A. $Br-[CH_2]_6-CO-O-C_2H_5$: ethyl 7-bromoheptanoate,

Monographs T-Z

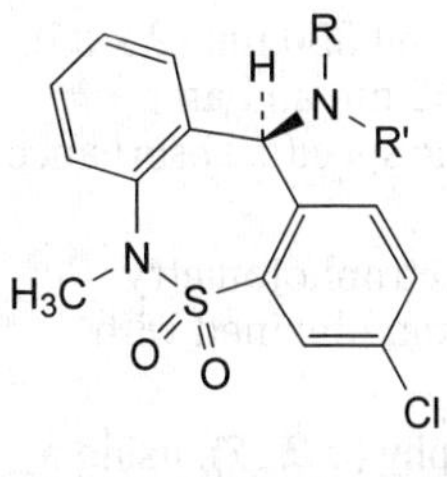

B. R = H, R′ = $[CH_2]_6$-CO-O-C_2H_5: ethyl 7-[[(11*RS*)-3-chloro-6-methyl-6,11-dihydrodibenzo[*c,f*][1,2]thiazepin-11-yl]amino]heptanoate *S,S*-dioxide,

E. R = R′ = $[CH_2]_6$-CO_2H: 7,7′-[[(11*RS*)-3-chloro-6-methyl-6,11-dihydrodibenzo[*c,f*][1,2]thiazepin-11-yl]imino]diheptanoic acid *S,S*-dioxide,

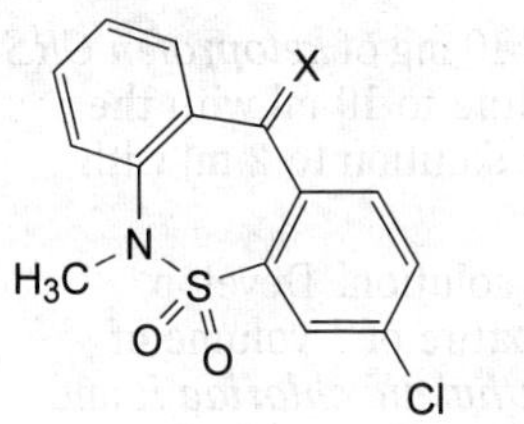

C. X = O: 3-chloro-6-methyldibenzo[*c,f*][1,2]thiazepin-11(6*H*)-one *S,S*-dioxide,

D. X = N-$[CH_2]_6$-CO_2H: 7-[[(11*RS*)-3-chloro-6-methyldibenzo[*c,f*][1,2]thiazepin-11(6*H*)-ylidene]amino]heptanoic acid *S,S*-dioxide.

01/2005:1575

TIAPRIDE HYDROCHLORIDE

Tiapridi hydrochloridum

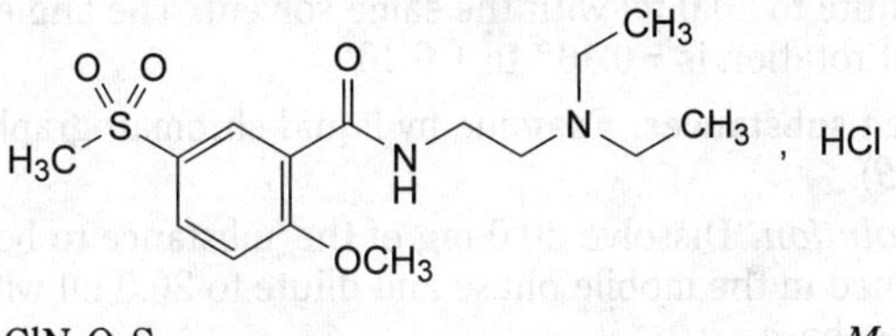

$C_{15}H_{25}ClN_2O_4S$ M_r 364.9

DEFINITION

Tiapride hydrochloride contains not less than 98.5 per cent and not more than the equivalent of 101.0 per cent of *N*-[2-(diethylamino)ethyl]-2-methoxy-5-(methylsulphonyl)benzamide hydrochloride, calculated with reference to the dried substance.

CHARACTERS

A white or almost white crystalline powder, very soluble in water, soluble in methanol, slightly soluble in ethanol.

IDENTIFICATION

A. Examine by infrared absorption spectrophotometry (*2.2.24*), comparing with the spectrum obtained with *tiapride hydrochloride CRS*. Examine the substances prepared as discs.

B. Solution S (see Tests) gives reaction (a) of chlorides (*2.3.1*).

TESTS

Solution S. Dissolve 2.5 g in *carbon dioxide-free water R* and dilute to 50.0 ml with the same solvent.

Appearance of solution. Solution S is clear (*2.2.1*). The absorbance (*2.2.25*) of solution S measured at 450 nm is not more than 0.030.

pH (*2.2.3*). The pH of solution S is 4.0 to 6.0.

Impurity C. Examine by thin-layer chromatography (*2.2.27*), using a *TLC silica gel G plate R*.

Test solution. Dissolve 0.400 g of the substance to be examined in *methanol R* and dilute to 10 ml with the same solvent.

Reference solution. Dissolve 20.0 mg of *metoclopramide impurity E CRS* (tiapride impurity C) in *methanol R* and dilute to 50 ml with the same solvent. Dilute 2.0 ml of this solution to 20 ml with *methanol R*.

Apply to the plate 10 µl of the test solution and 10 µl of the reference solution. Develop over a path of 12 cm using a mixture of 2 volumes of *concentrated ammonia R*, 10 volumes of *dioxan R*, 14 volumes of *methanol R* and 90 volumes of *methylene chloride R*. Allow the plate to dry in air. Spray with a 2 g/l solution of *ninhydrin R* in *butanol R* and heat at 100 °C for 15 min. Any spot corresponding to impurity C in the chromatogram obtained with the test solution is not more intense than the spot in the chromatogram obtained with the reference solution (0.1 per cent).

Related substances. Examine by liquid chromatography (*2.2.29*).

Test solution. Dissolve 0.100 g of the substance to be examined in the mobile phase and dilute to 100.0 ml with the mobile phase.

Reference solution (a). Dilute 1.0 ml of the test solution to 10.0 ml with the mobile phase. Dilute 1.0 ml of this solution to 100.0 ml with the mobile phase.

Reference solution (b). Dissolve 5.0 mg of *tiapride hydrochloride CRS* and 5.0 mg of *tiapride N-oxide CRS* in the mobile phase and dilute to 100.0 ml with the mobile phase.

The chromatographic procedure may be carried out using:

- a stainless steel column 0.25 m long and4.6 mm in internal diameter packed with *octylsilyl silica gel for chromatography R* (5 µm),
- as mobile phase at a flow rate of 1.5 ml/min a solution prepared as follows: dissolve 5.44 g of *potassium dihydrogen phosphate R* and 0.08 g of *sodium octanesulphonate R* in 780 ml of *water R*, adjust the pH to 2.7 using *phosphoric acid R* and dilute to 800 ml with *water R*; add 150 ml of *methanol R* and 50 ml of *acetonitrile R* and mix,
- as detector a spectrophotometer set at 240 nm,

maintaining the temperature of the column at 40 °C.

Inject 10 µl of reference solution (b). The test is not valid unless the resolution between the peaks corresponding to tiapride (retention time of about 9 min) and tiapride *N*-oxide (retention time of about 13 min) is at least 4.0.

Inject 10 µl of the test solution. Continue the chromatography for 3 times the retention time of tiapride. In the chromatogram obtained with the test solution: the area of any peak, apart from the principal peak, is not greater than the area of the principal peak in the chromatogram obtained with reference solution (a) (0.1 per cent) and the sum of the areas of any such peaks is not greater than 3 times the area of the principal peak in the chromatogram obtained with reference solution (a) (0.3 per cent). Disregard any peak with an area less than half the area of the principal peak in the chromatogram obtained with reference solution (a) (0.05 per cent).

Heavy metals (*2.4.8*). Dissolve 2.0 g in *water R* and dilute to 20 ml with the same solvent. 12 ml of the solution complies with limit test A for heavy metals (20 ppm). Prepare the standard using *lead standard solution (2 ppm Pb) R*.

Loss on drying (*2.2.32*). Not more than 0.5 per cent, determined on 1.000 g by drying in an oven at 100 °C to 105 °C.

Sulphated ash (*2.4.14*). Not more than 0.1 per cent, determined on 1.0 g.

ASSAY

Dissolve 0.300 g in 20 ml of *anhydrous acetic acid R*. Add 20 ml of *acetic anhydride R*. Titrate with *0.1 M perchloric acid*, determining the end-point potentiometrically (*2.2.20*).

1 ml of *0.1 M perchloric acid* is equivalent to 36.49 mg of $C_{15}H_{25}ClN_2O_4S$.

IMPURITIES

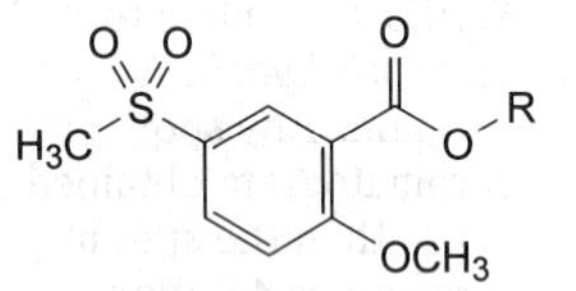

A. R = CH_3: methyl 2-methoxy-5-(methylsulphonyl)benzoate,

B. R = H: 2-methoxy-5-(methylsulphonyl)benzoic acid,

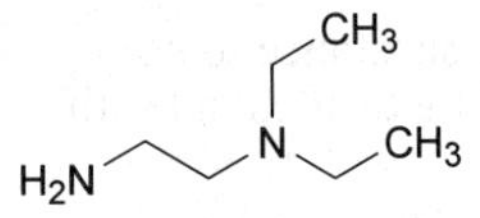

C. *N,N*-diethylethane-1,2-diamine.

01/2005:1157

TIAPROFENIC ACID

Acidum tiaprofenicum

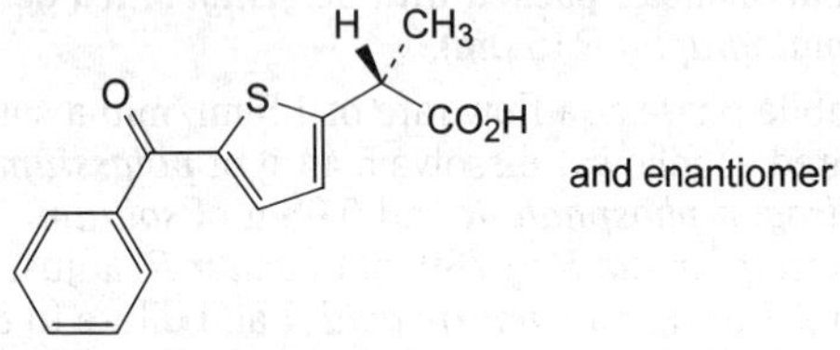

$C_{14}H_{12}O_3S$ M_r 260.3

DEFINITION

Tiaprofenic acid contains not less than 99.0 per cent and not more than the equivalent of 101.0 per cent of (2*RS*)-2-(5-benzoylthiophen-2-yl)propanoic acid, calculated with reference to the dried substance.

CHARACTERS

A white or almost white, crystalline powder, practically insoluble in water, freely soluble in acetone, in alcohol and in methylene chloride.

IDENTIFICATION

First identification: C.

Second identification: A, B, D.

A. Melting point (*2.2.14*): 95 °C to 99 °C.

B. Dissolve 25.0 mg in *ethanolic hydrochloric acid R* and dilute to 50.0 ml with the same solvent. Dilute 1.0 ml of the solution to 50.0 ml with *ethanolic hydrochloric acid R*. Examined between 220 nm and 350 nm (*2.2.25*), the solution shows a shoulder at 262 nm and an absorption maximum at 305 nm. The specific absorbance at the maximum is 550 to 590.

C. Examine by infrared absorption spectrophotometry (*2.2.24*), comparing with the spectrum obtained with *tiaprofenic acid CRS*.

D. Examine by thin-layer chromatography (*2.2.27*), using a *TLC silica gel F_{254} plate R*.

Test solution. Dissolve 10 mg of the substance to be examined in *methylene chloride R* and dilute to 10 ml with the same solvent.

Reference solution (a). Dissolve 10 mg of *tiaprofenic acid CRS* in *methylene chloride R* and dilute to 10 ml with the same solvent.

Reference solution (b). Dissolve 10 mg of *ketoprofen CRS* in *methylene chloride R* and dilute to 10 ml with the same solvent. Dilute 1 ml of the solution to 2 ml with reference solution (a).

Apply to the plate 10 µl of each solution. Develop over a path of 15 cm using a mixture of 1 volume of *acetic acid R*, 20 volumes of *methylene chloride R* and 80 volumes of *acetone R*. Allow the plate to dry in air and examine in ultraviolet light at 254 nm. The principal spot in the chromatogram obtained with the test solution is similar in position and size to the principal spot in the chromatogram obtained with reference solution (a). The identification is not valid unless the chromatogram obtained with reference solution (b) shows two clearly separated principal spots.

TESTS

Appearance of solution. Dissolve 2.0 g in *alcohol R* and dilute to 20 ml with the same solvent. The solution is clear (*2.2.1*) and not more intensely coloured than reference solution Y_6 (*2.2.2, Method II*).

Optical rotation (*2.2.7*). Dissolve 0.50 g in *ethyl acetate R* and dilute to 10.0 ml with the same solvent. The angle of optical rotation is − 0.10° to + 0.10°.

Related substances. Examine by liquid chromatography (*2.2.29*).

Test solution. Dissolve 20.0 mg of the substance to be examined in the mobile phase and dilute to 20.0 ml with the mobile phase.

Reference solution (a). Dilute 1.0 ml of the test solution to 50.0 ml with the mobile phase. Dilute 1.0 ml of the solution to 10.0 ml with the mobile phase.

Reference solution (b). Dilute 5.0 ml of reference solution (a) to 10.0 ml with the mobile phase.

Reference solution (c). Dissolve 10.0 mg of *tiaprofenic acid impurity C CRS* in the mobile phase and dilute to 100.0 ml with the mobile phase. Dilute 1.0 ml of the solution to 50.0 ml with the mobile phase.

Reference solution (d). Dilute 1.0 ml of reference solution (a) to 2.0 ml with reference solution (c).

The chromatographic procedure may be carried out using:

- a stainless steel column 0.25 m long and 4.6 mm in internal diameter packed with *silica gel for chromatography R* (5 µm),
- as mobile phase at a flow rate of 1 ml/min a mixture of 0.25 volumes of *water R*, 20 volumes of *glacial acetic acid R*, 500 volumes of *hexane R* and 500 volumes of *methylene chloride R*. Add the water to the acetic acid, then hexane and methylene chloride. Sonicate the mixture for 2 min. Do not degas with helium during analysis,

– as detector a spectrophotometer set at 250 nm.

Inject 20 µl of reference solution (d). When the chromatograms are recorded in the prescribed conditions the retention times relative to tiaprofenic acid are: impurity A 0.19, impurity B 0.43, impurity C 0.86.

Adjust the sensitivity of the system so that the heights of the principal peaks in the chromatogram obtained with reference solution (d) are at least 50 per cent of the full scale of the recorder. The test is not valid unless in the chromatogram obtained, the resolution between the peaks corresponding to tiaprofenic acid and impurity C is at least 3.0.

Inject 20 µl of the test solution, 20 µl of reference solution (a), 20 µl of reference solution (b) and 20 µl of reference solution (c). Continue the chromatography of the test solution for twice the retention time of tiaprofenic acid. In the chromatogram obtained with the test solution: the area of any peak corresponding to impurity C is not greater than the area of the corresponding peak in the chromatogram obtained with reference solution (c) (0.2 per cent); the area of any peak, apart from the principal peak and any peak corresponding to impurity C, is not greater than the area of the principal peak in the chromatogram obtained with reference solution (b) (0.1 per cent); the sum of the areas of all the peaks, apart from the principal peak and any peak corresponding to impurity C, is not greater than 1.5 times the area of the principal peak in the chromatogram obtained with reference solution (a) (0.3 per cent). Disregard any peak with an area less than half the area of the principal peak in the chromatogram obtained with the reference solution (b).

Heavy metals (*2.4.8*). 2.0 g complies with limit test C for heavy metals (10 ppm). Prepare the standard using 2 ml of *lead standard solution (10 ppm Pb) R*.

Loss on drying (*2.2.32*). Not more than 0.5 per cent, determined on 1.000 g by drying at 60 °C in an oven at a pressure not exceeding 0.7 kPa for 3 h.

Sulphated ash (*2.4.14*). Not more than 0.1 per cent, determined on 1.0 g.

ASSAY

Dissolve 0.250 g in 25 ml of *alcohol R*. Add 25 ml of *water R* and 0.5 ml of *phenolphthalein solution R*. Titrate with *0.1 M sodium hydroxide*.

1 ml of *0.1 M sodium hydroxide* is equivalent to 26.03 mg of $C_{14}H_{12}O_3S$.

STORAGE

Store protected from light.

IMPURITIES

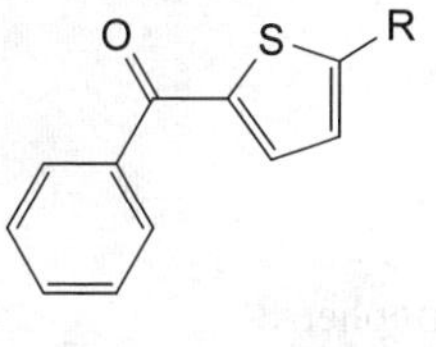

A. R = C_2H_5: (5-ethylthiophen-2-yl)phenylmethanone,

B. R = CO-CH_3: 1-(5-benzoylthiophen-2-yl)ethanone,

F. R = Br: (5-bromothiophen-2-yl)phenylmethanone,

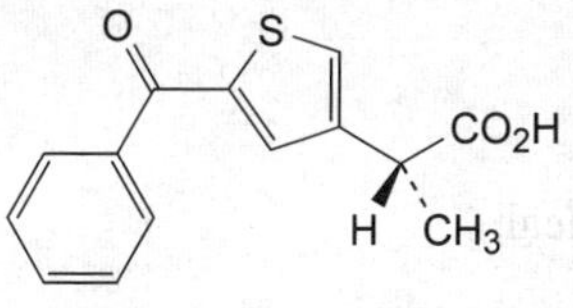

and enantiomer

C. (2*RS*)-2-(5-benzoylthiophen-3-yl)propanoic acid,

D. benzoic acid,

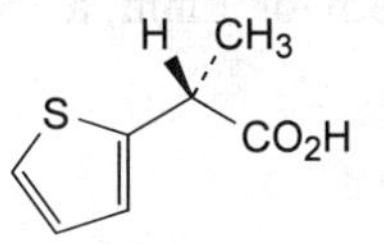

and enantiomer

E. (2*RS*)-2-(thiophen-2-yl)propanoic acid.

01/2005:0956

TICARCILLIN SODIUM

Ticarcillinum natricum

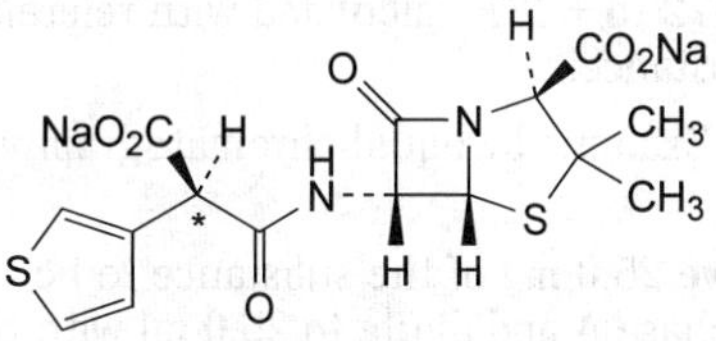

and epimer at C*

$C_{15}H_{14}N_2Na_2O_6S_2$ M_r 428.4

DEFINITION

Ticarcillin sodium contains not less than 89.0 per cent and not more than the equivalent of 100.5 per cent of disodium (2*S*,5*R*,6*R*)-6-[[(2*RS*)-2-carboxylato-2-(thiophen-3-yl)acetyl]amino]-3,3-dimethyl-7-oxo-4-thia-1-azabicyclo[3.2.0]heptane-2-carboxylate, calculated with reference to the anhydrous substance.

CHARACTERS

A white or slightly yellow powder, hygroscopic, freely soluble in water, soluble in methanol.

IDENTIFICATION

First identification: A, D.

Second identification: B, C, D.

A. Examine by infrared absorption spectrophotometry (*2.2.24*), comparing with the spectrum obtained with *ticarcillin sodium CRS*.

B. Examine by thin-layer chromatography (*2.2.27*), using *silanised silica gel H R* as the coating substance.

Test solution. Dissolve 25 mg of the substance to be examined in *methanol R* and dilute to 5 ml with the same solvent.

Reference solution (a). Dissolve 25 mg of *ticarcillin sodium CRS* in *methanol R* and dilute to 5 ml with the same solvent.

Reference solution (b). Dissolve 25 mg of *carbenicillin sodium CRS* and 25 mg of *ticarcillin sodium CRS* in *methanol R* and dilute to 5 ml with the same solvent.

Apply to the plate 1 µl of each solution. Develop over a path of 12 cm using a mixture of 10 volumes of *acetone R* and 90 volumes of a 154 g/l solution of *ammonium acetate R*, adjusted to pH 5.0 with *glacial acetic acid R*. Allow the plate to dry in a current of hot air and expose it to iodine vapour. The principal spot in the chromatogram obtained with the test solution is similar in position, colour and size to the principal spot in the chromatogram obtained with reference solution (a). The test is not valid unless the chromatogram obtained with reference solution (b) shows two clearly separated spots.

C. Place about 2 mg in a test-tube about 15 cm long and 15 mm in diameter. Moisten with 0.05 ml of *water R* and add 2 ml of *sulphuric acid-formaldehyde reagent R*.

Mix the contents of the tube by swirling; the solution is brown. Place the test-tube in a water-bath for 1 min; a dark reddish-brown colour develops.

D. It gives reaction (a) of sodium (*2.3.1*).

TESTS

Solution S. Dissolve 2.50 g in *carbon dioxide-free water R* and dilute to 50 ml with the same solvent.

Appearance of solution. Solution S is clear (*2.2.1*) and not more intensely coloured than reference solution Y_5 (*2.2.2, Method II*).

pH (*2.2.3*). The pH of solution S is 5.5 to 7.5.

Specific optical rotation (*2.2.7*). Dissolve 0.250 g in *water R* and dilute to 25.0 ml with the same solvent. The specific optical rotation is + 172 to + 187, calculated with reference to the anhydrous substance.

Related substances. Examine by liquid chromatography (*2.2.29*).

Test solution. Dissolve 25.0 mg of the substance to be examined in mobile phase A and dilute to 25.0 ml with the same mobile phase.

Reference solution (a). Dissolve 20.0 mg of *ticarcillin impurity A CRS* in mobile phase A and dilute to 100.0 ml with the same mobile phase. Dilute 5.0 ml of this solution to 50.0 ml with mobile phase A.

Reference solution (b). Dilute 1 ml of the test solution to 50 ml with mobile phase A.

The chromatographic procedure may be carried out using:

– a stainless steel column 0.25 m long and 4 mm in internal diameter packed with *octadecylsilyl silica gel for chromatography R* (5 μm),

– as mobile phase at a flow rate of 1.0 ml/min:

Mobile phase A. A 1.3 g/l solution of *ammonium phosphate R* adjusted to pH 7.0 with *phosphoric acid R*,

Mobile phase B. A mixture of equal volumes of mobile phase A and *methanol R*,

Time (min)	Mobile phase A (per cent *V/V*)	Mobile phase B (per cent *V/V*)	Comment
0 - 30	100 → 30	0 → 70	linear gradient
30 - 40	30	70	isocratic
40 - 45	100	0	equilibration

– as detector a spectrophotometer at 220 nm.

Inject 20 μl of reference solution (b). Adjust the sensitivity of the system so that the height of the two principal peaks are at least 50 per cent of the full scale of the recorder. The test is not valid unless the resolution between the two principal peaks (diastereoisomers) is at least 2.0. Inject 20 μl of the test solution and 20 μl of reference solution (a). In the chromatogram obtained with the test solution: the area of any peak corresponding to ticarcillin impurity A is not greater than twice the area of the principal peak in the chromatogram obtained with reference solution (a) (4 per cent); and the area of any peak apart from the two principal peaks and any peak corresponding to ticarcillin impurity A, is not greater than 1.25 times the area of the principal peak in the chromatogram obtained with the reference solution (a) (2.5 per cent).

***N,N*-Dimethylaniline** (*2.4.26, Method B*). Not more than 20 ppm.

2-Ethylhexanoic acid (*2.4.28*). Not more than 0.5 per cent *m/m*.

Water (*2.5.12*). Not more than 5.5 per cent, determined on 0.150 g by the semi-micro determination of water.

Bacterial endotoxins (*2.6.14*): less than 0.05 IU/mg, if intended for use in the manufacture of parenteral dosage forms without a further appropriate procedure for the removal of bacterial endotoxins.

ASSAY

Examine by liquid chromatography (*2.2.29*).

Test solution. Dissolve 50.0 mg of the substance to be examined in the mobile phase and dilute to 100.0 ml with the same solvent. Dilute 10.0 ml of the solution to 50.0 ml with the mobile phase.

Reference solution. Dissolve 50.0 mg of *ticarcillin sodium CRS* in the mobile phase and dilute to 100.0 ml with the same solvent. Dilute 10.0 ml of the solution to 50.0 ml with the mobile phase.

The chromatographic procedure may be carried out using:

– a stainless steel column 0.25 m long and 4 mm in internal diameter packed with *octadecylsilyl silica gel for chromatography R* (5 μm),

– as mobile phase at a flow rate of 1 ml/min a mixture of 20 volumes of *methanol R* and 80 volumes of a 1.3 g/l solution of *ammonium phosphate R* (adjusted to pH 7.0 with *phosphoric acid R*),

– as detector a spectrophotometer set at 220 nm.

Inject 20 μl of the reference solution. Adjust the sensitivity of the system so that the heights of the two principal peaks are at least 50 per cent of the full scale of the recorder. The test is not valid unless the resolution between the two principal peaks is at least 2.5. Inject the reference solution six times. The test is not valid unless the relative standard deviation of the two peak areas for ticarcillin is at most 1.0 per cent. Inject alternately the test solution and the reference solution.

Calculate the percentage content of ticarcillin sodium as the sum of the two peaks.

STORAGE

Store in an airtight container, at a temperature of 2 °C to 8 °C. If the substance is sterile, store in a sterile, airtight, tamper-proof container.

LABELLING

The label states, where applicable, that the substance is free from bacterial endotoxins.

IMPURITIES

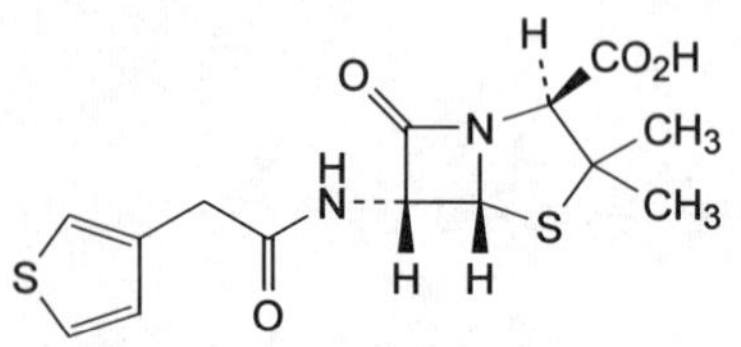

A. (2*S*,5*R*,6*R*)-3,3-dimethyl-7-oxo-6-[[(thiophen-3-yl)acetyl]amino]-4-thia-1-azabicyclo[3.2.0]heptane-2-carboxylic acid (decarboxyticarcillin),

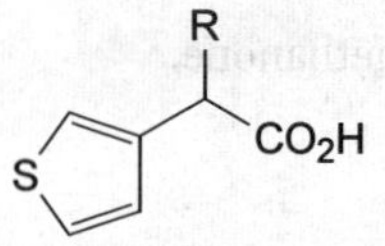

B. R = H: (thiophen-3-yl)acetic acid,

C. R = CO_2H: 2-(thiophen-3-yl)propanedioic acid (3-thienylmalonic acid),

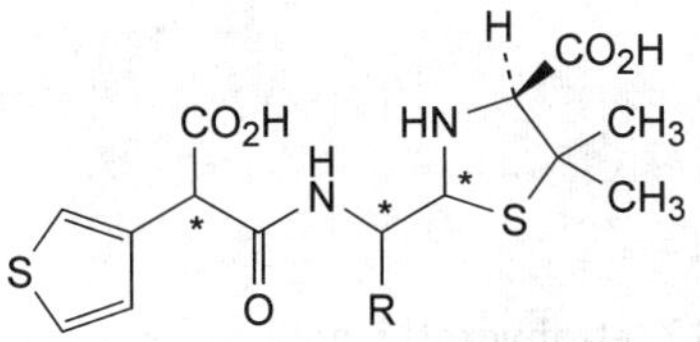

D. R = CO_2H: (4*S*)-2-[carboxy[[2-carboxy-2-(thiophen-3-yl)acetyl]amino]methyl]-5,5-dimethylthiazolidine-4-carboxylic acid (penicilloic acids of ticarcillin),

E. R = H: (4*S*)-2-[[[2-carboxy-2-(thiophen-3-yl)acetyl]amino]methyl]-5,5-dimethylthiazolidine-4-carboxylic acid (penilloic acids of ticarcillin).

01/2005:1050
corrected

TICLOPIDINE HYDROCHLORIDE

Ticlopidini hydrochloridum

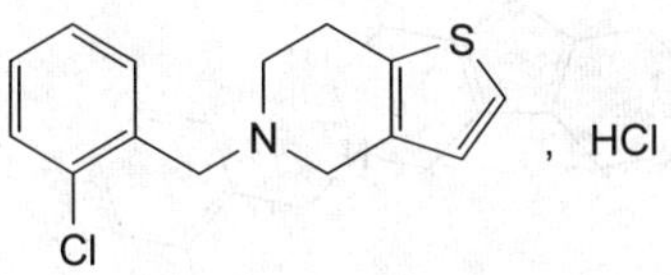

$C_{14}H_{15}Cl_2NS$ M_r 300.2

DEFINITION

Ticlopidine hydrochloride contains not less than 99.0 per cent and not more than the equivalent of 101.0 per cent of 5-(2-chlorobenzyl)-4,5,6,7-tetrahydrothieno[3,2-*c*]pyridine hydrochloride, calculated with reference to the anhydrous substance.

CHARACTERS

A white or almost white, crystalline powder, sparingly soluble in water and in ethanol, very slightly soluble in ethyl acetate.

IDENTIFICATION

First identification: B, D.

Second identification: A, C, D.

A. Dissolve 40 mg in *water R* and dilute to 100.0 ml with the same solvent (solution A). Dilute 5.0 ml of solution A to 100.0 ml with *water R* (solution B). Examined between 200 nm and 350 nm (*2.2.25*), solution B shows two absorption maxima, at 214 nm and 232 nm. Examined between 250 nm and 350 nm, solution A shows two absorption maxima, at 268 nm and 275 nm. The ratio of the absorbance measured at the maximum at 268 nm to that measured at the maximum at 275 nm is 1.1 to 1.2.

B. Examine by infrared absorption spectrophotometry (*2.2.24*), comparing with the spectrum obtained with *ticlopidine hydrochloride CRS*. Examine the substances prepared as discs.

C. Mix about 6 mg of *citric acid R* and 0.3 ml of *acetic anhydride R*. Add about 5 mg of the substance to be examined and heat in a water-bath at 80 °C. A red colour develops.

D. About 20 mg gives reaction (a) of chlorides (*2.3.1*).

TESTS

Appearance of solution. Dissolve 0.5 g in a 1 per cent *V/V* solution of *hydrochloric acid R* and dilute to 20 ml with the same acid solution. The solution is clear (*2.2.1*) and colourless (*2.2.2, Method II*).

pH (*2.2.3*). Dissolve 0.5 g in *carbon dioxide-free water R* and dilute to 20 ml with the same solvent. The pH of the solution is 3.5 to 4.0.

Related substances. Examine by liquid chromatography (*2.2.29*).

Test solution. Dissolve 0.250 g of the substance to be examined in a mixture of 20 volumes of mobile phase B and 80 volumes of mobile phase A. Dilute to 50.0 ml with the same mixture of solvents.

Reference solution. Dissolve 5.0 mg of *ticlopidine impurity F CRS* in a mixture of 20 volumes of mobile phase B and 80 volumes of mobile phase A. Add 1.00 ml of the test solution and dilute to 100.0 ml with a mixture of 20 volumes of mobile phase B and 80 volumes of mobile phase A. Dilute 1.0 ml of this solution to 10.0 ml with a mixture of 20 volumes of mobile phase B and 80 volumes of mobile phase A.

The chromatographic procedure may be carried out using:

– a stainless steel column, 0.15 m long and 4.6 mm in internal diameter, packed with *octadecylsilyl silica gel for chromatography R* (5 µm),

– as mobile phase at a flow rate of 1.3 ml/min:
Mobile phase A. A 0.95 g/l solution of *sodium pentanesulphonate monohydrate R*, adjusted to pH 3.4 with a 50 per cent *V/V* solution of *phosphoric acid R*,
Mobile phase B. Methanol R,

Time (min)	Mobile phase A (per cent *V/V*)	Mobile phase B (per cent *V/V*)	Comment
0 - 45	80 → 20	20 → 80	linear gradient
45 - 50	20	80	isocratic
50 - 55	20 → 80	80 → 20	linear gradient

– as detector a spectrophotometer set at 220 nm,

maintaining the temperature of the column at 40 °C.

Inject 10 µl of a mixture of 20 volumes of mobile phase B and 80 volumes of mobile phase A (blank). Inject 10 µl of the reference solution.When the chromatogram is recorded in the prescribed conditions the retention time for ticlopidine is about 15 min.

Adjust the sensitivity of the system so that, in the chromatogram obtained with the reference solution, the height of the peak due to ticlopidine is at least 5 per cent of the full scale of the recorder. The test is not valid unless in the chromatogram obtained with the reference solution: the resolution between the peaks corresponding to ticlopidine and impurity F is at least 2.0 (modify the pH of mobile phase A if necessary); the signal-to-noise ratio of the peak due to ticlopidine is at least 50.

Inject 10 µl of the test solution and 10 µl of the reference solution. In the chromatogram obtained with the test solution: the area of the peak corresponding to impurity F is not greater than half the area of the corresponding peak in the chromatogram obtained with the reference solution (0.05 per cent); the area of any peak, apart from the principal peak and the peak due to impurity F, is not greater than half the area of the principal peak in the chromatogram obtained with the reference solution (0.05 per cent); the sum of the areas of all the peaks apart from the peak corresponding to ticlopidine, is not greater than the area of the peak corresponding to ticlopidine in the chromatogram obtained with the reference solution (0.1 per cent). Disregard any peak with an area less than 0.1 times that of ticlopidine in the chromatogram obtained with the reference solution.

Monographs T-Z

Formaldehyde. Dissolve 0.200 g in 4.0 ml of *water R*. Add 0.4 ml of *dilute sodium hydroxide solution R*. Centrifuge, filter the supernatant liquid through cotton previously impregnated with *water R* and dilute to 5.0 ml with *water R*. Transfer to a test-tube. Add 5.0 ml of *acetylacetone reagent R1*. Place the test-tube in a water-bath at 40 °C for 40 min. The test solution is not more intensely coloured than a standard prepared at the same time and in the same manner using 5.0 ml of a 0.8 ppm solution of formaldehyde (CH_2O), obtained by dilution of *formaldehyde standard solution (5 ppm CH_2O) R* with *water R* (20 ppm). Examine the tubes down their vertical axis.

Heavy metals (*2.4.8*). Dissolve 2.0 g in a 85 per cent *V/V* solution of *methanol R* and dilute to 20.0 ml with the same solvent. 12 ml of the solution complies with limit test B for heavy metals (10 ppm). Prepare the standard using 10 ml of *lead standard solution (1 ppm Pb) R*.

Water (*2.5.12*). Not more than 0.5 per cent, determined on 0.500 g by the semi-micro determination of water.

Sulphated ash (*2.4.14*). Not more than 0.1 per cent, determined on 1.0 g.

ASSAY

Dissolve 0.150 g in 15 ml of *anhydrous acetic acid R*. Add 35 ml of *acetic anhydride R*. Titrate with *0.1 M perchloric acid*, determining the end-point potentiometrically (*2.2.20*).

1 ml of *0.1 M perchloric acid* is equivalent to 30.02 mg of $C_{14}H_{15}Cl_2NS$.

IMPURITIES

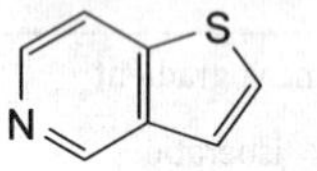

A. thieno[3,2-*c*]pyridine,

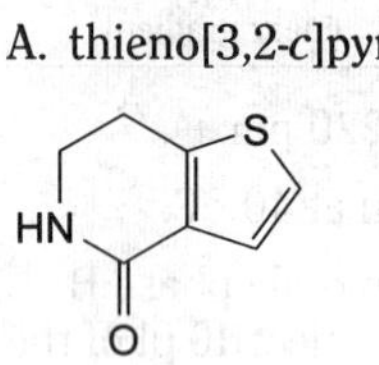

B. 6,7-dihydrothieno[3,2-*c*]pyridin-4(5*H*)-one,

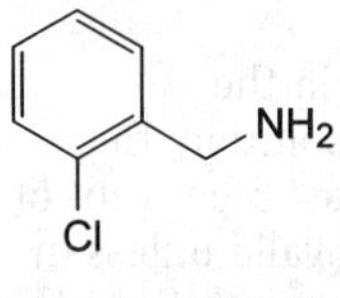

C. (2-chlorophenyl)methanamine,

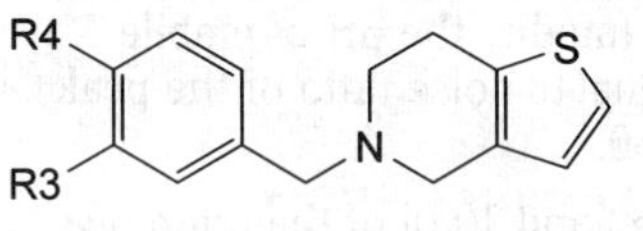

D. R3 = R4 = H: 5-benzyl-4,5,6,7-tetrahydrothieno[3,2-*c*]pyridine,

G. R3 = Cl, R4 = H: 5-(3-chlorobenzyl)-4,5,6,7-tetrahydrothieno[3,2-*c*]pyridine,

H. R3 = H, R4 = Cl: 5-(4-chlorobenzyl)-4,5,6,7-tetrahydrothieno[3,2-*c*]pyridine,

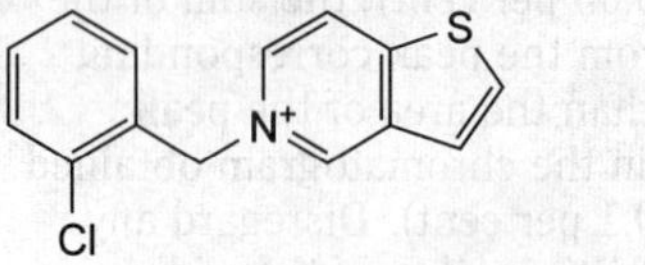

E. 5-(2-chlorobenzyl)thieno[3,2-*c*]pyridinium,

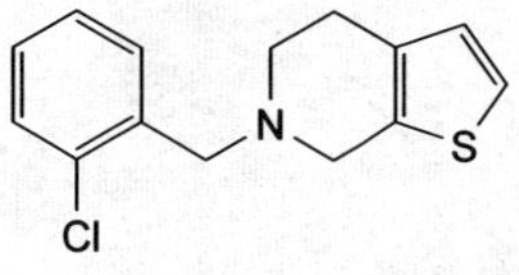

F. 6-(2-chlorobenzyl)-4,5,6,7-tetrahydrothieno[2,3-*c*]pyridine,

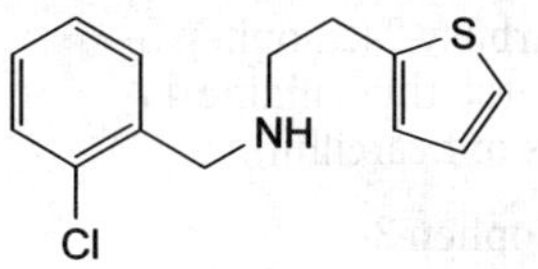

I. *N*-(2-chlorobenzyl)-2-(thiophen-2-yl)ethanamine,

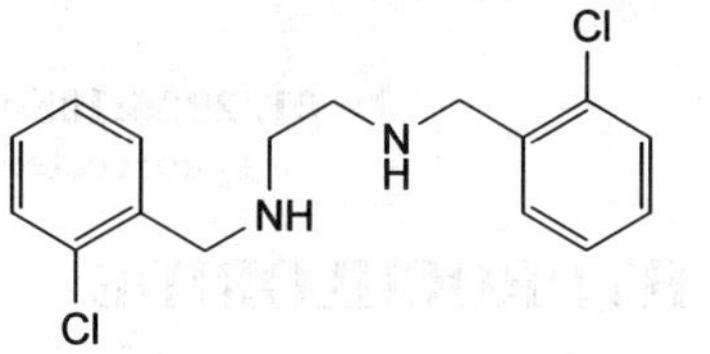

J. *N,N'*-bis(2-chlorobenzyl)ethane-1,2-diamine,

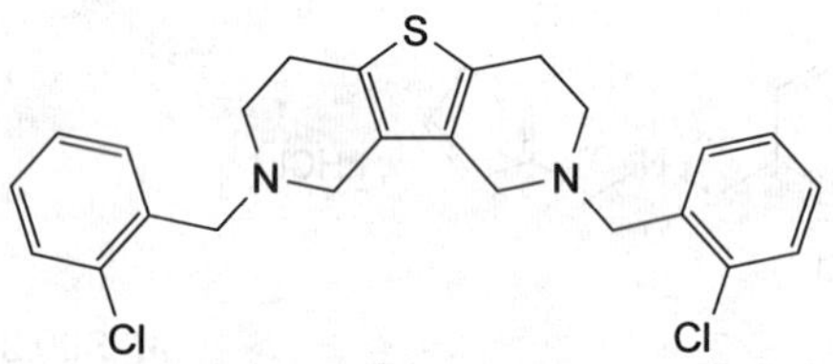

K. 2,8-bis(2-chlorobenzyl)-1,2,3,4,6,7,8,9-octahydrothieno[3,2-*c*:4,5-*c'*]dipyridine (bis-ticlopidine),

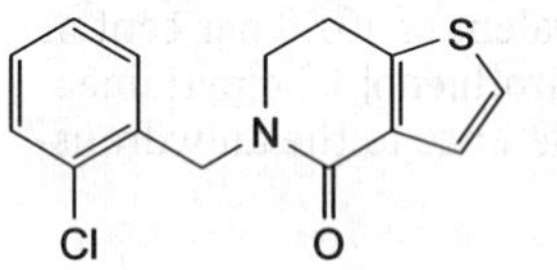

L. 5-(2-chlorobenzyl)-6,7-dihydrothieno[3,2-*c*]pyridin-4(5*H*)-one.

01/2005:1767

TILIDINE HYDROCHLORIDE HEMIHYDRATE

Tilidini hydrochloridum hemihydricum

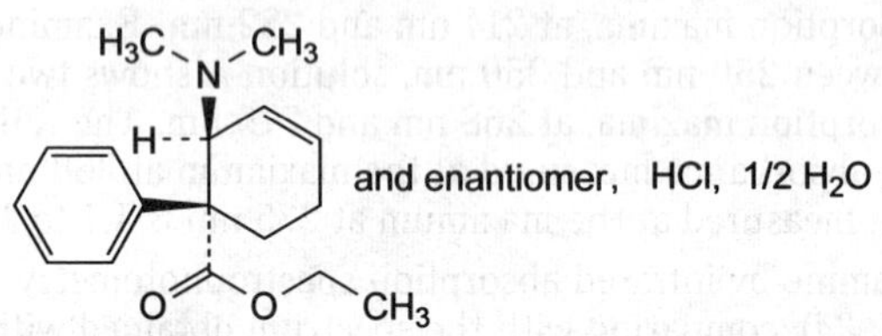

$C_{17}H_{24}ClNO_2,{}^1/_2H_2O$ M_r 318.9

DEFINITION

Ethyl (1*RS*,2*SR*)-2-(dimethylamino)-1-phenylcyclohex-3-enecarboxylate hydrochloride hemihydrate.

Content: 99.0 per cent to 101.0 per cent (anhydrous substance).

A suitable antioxidant may be added.

CHARACTERS

Appearance: white or almost white, crystalline powder.

Solubility: freely soluble in water, very soluble in methylene chloride, freely soluble in alcohol.

IDENTIFICATION

A. Infrared absorption spectrophotometry (*2.2.24*).

Comparison: *Ph. Eur. reference spectrum of tilidine hydrochloride hemihydrate.*

B. It gives reaction (a) of chlorides (*2.3.1*).

TESTS

Solution S. Dissolve 1.0 g in *carbon dioxide-free water R* and dilute to 20 ml with the same solvent.

Appearance of solution. Solution S is clear (*2.2.1*) and not more intensely coloured than reference solution Y_7 (*2.2.2, Method II*).

Acidity or alkalinity. To 20 ml of solution S add 0.2 ml of *0.01 M sodium hydroxide*. The pH is not less than 4.1. Add 0.4 ml of *0.01 M hydrochloric acid*. The pH is not more than 4.3.

Related substances. Liquid chromatography (*2.2.29*).

Test solution. Dissolve 50.0 mg of the substance to be examined in *water R* and dilute to 50.0 ml with the same solvent.

Reference solution (a). Dilute 0.5 ml of the test solution to 100.0 ml with *water R.*

Reference solution (b). Dilute 2.0 ml of reference solution (a) to 10.0 ml with *water R.*

Precolumn:

- *size*: *l* = 4 mm, Ø = 4.0 mm,
- *stationary phase*: spherical *octadecylsilyl silica gel for chromatography R* (5 µm).

Column:

- *size*: *l* = 0.125 m, Ø = 4.0 mm,
- *stationary phase*: spherical *octadecylsilyl silica gel for chromatography R* (5 µm).

Mobile phase: mix equal volumes of *acetonitrile R* and a 0.98 g/l solution of *ammonium carbonate R.*

Flow rate: 0.8 ml/min.

Detection: spectrophotometer at 220 nm.

Injection: 10 µl.

Run time: twice the retention time of tilidine.

Relative retention with reference to tilidine (retention time = about 11 min): impurity D = about 0.4; impurity C = about 0.5; impurity B = about 0.7; impurity A = about 1.5.

Limits:

- *impurities A, B, C*: for each impurity, not more than the area of the principal peak in the chromatogram obtained with reference solution (a) (0.5 per cent),
- *any other impurity*: for each impurity, not more than the area of the principal peak in the chromatogram obtained with reference solution (b) (0.1 per cent),
- *total*: not more than the area of the principal peak in the chromatogram obtained with reference solution (a) (0.5 per cent),
- *disregard limit*: 0.5 times the area of the principal peak in the chromatogram obtained with reference solution (b) (0.05 per cent).

Heavy metals (*2.4.8*): maximum 20 ppm.

Dissolve 2.0 g in 20 ml of *water R*. 12 ml of the solution complies with limit test A. Prepare the standard using *lead standard solution (2 ppm Pb) R.*

Water (*2.5.12*): 2.5 per cent to 3.1 per cent, determined on 0.300 g.

Bacterial endotoxins (*2.6.14*): less than 0.25 IU/mg, if intented for use in the manufacture of parenteral dosage forms without a further appropriate procedure for the removal of bacterial endotoxins.

ASSAY

Dissolve 0.250 g in a mixture of 10 ml of *anhydrous acetic acid R* and 50 ml of *acetic anhydride R.* Titrate with *0.1 M perchloric acid,* determining the end-point potentiometrically (*2.2.20*).

1 ml of *0.1 M perchloric acid* is equivalent to 30.99 mg of $C_{17}H_{24}ClNO_2$.

STORAGE

Protected from light.

LABELLING

The label states:

- where applicable, that the substance is free from bacterial endotoxins,
- where applicable, the name and concentration of any added antioxidant.

IMPURITIES

Specified impurities: A, B, C.

Other detectable impurities: D.

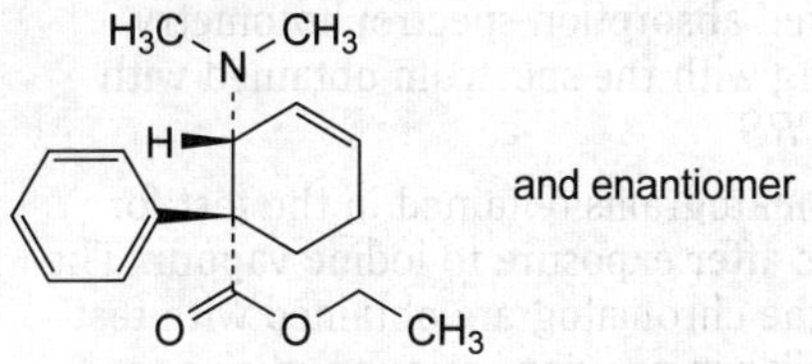

A. ethyl (1*RS*,2*RS*)-2-(dimethylamino)-1-phenylcyclohex-3-enecarboxylate,

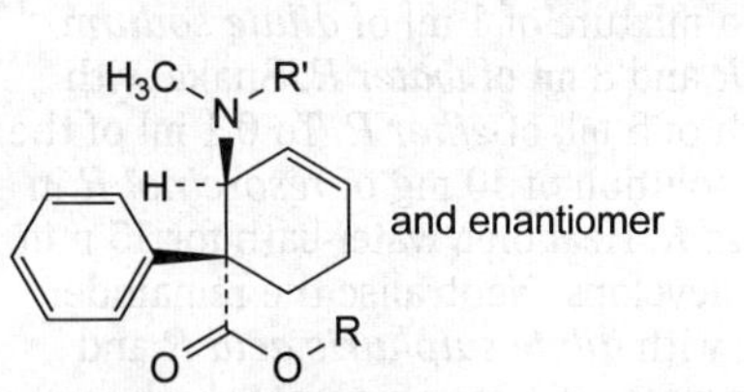

B. R = R′ = CH_3: methyl (1*RS*,2*SR*)-2-(dimethylamino)-1-phenylcyclohex-3-enecarboxylate,

C. R = C_2H_5, R′ = H: ethyl (1*RS*,2*SR*)-2-(methylamino)-1-phenylcyclohex-3-enecarboxylate,

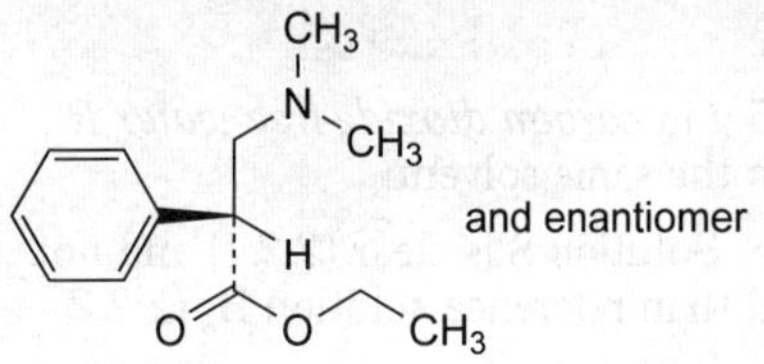

D. ethyl (2*RS*)-3-dimethylamino-2-phenylpropanoate.

01/2005:0572

TIMOLOL MALEATE

Timololi maleas

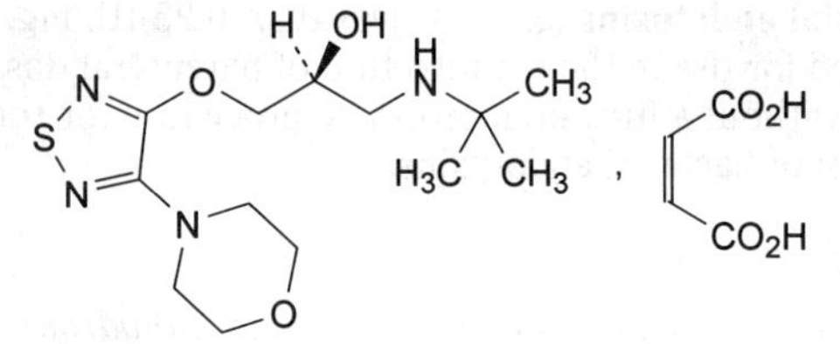

$C_{17}H_{28}N_4O_7S$ M_r 432.5

DEFINITION

Timolol maleate contains not less than 98.5 per cent and not more than the equivalent of 101.0 per cent of (2*S*)-1-[(1,1-dimethylethyl)amino]-3-[[4-(morpholin-4-yl)-1,2,5-thiadiazol-3-yl]oxy]propan-2-ol (*Z*)-butenedioate, calculated with reference to the dried substance.

CHARACTERS

A white or almost white, crystalline powder or colourless crystals, soluble in water and in alcohol.

It melts at about 199 °C, with decomposition.

IDENTIFICATION

First identification: A, B.

Second identification: A, C, D.

A. Dissolve 1.000 g in *1 M hydrochloric acid* and dilute to 10.0 ml with the same acid. The specific optical rotation (*2.2.7*) is −5.7 to −6.2.

B. Examine by infrared absorption spectrophotometry (*2.2.24*), comparing with the spectrum obtained with *timolol maleate CRS*.

C. Examine the chromatograms obtained in the test for related substances after exposure to iodine vapour. The principal spot in the chromatogram obtained with test solution (b) is similar in position, colour and size to the principal spot in the chromatogram obtained with reference solution (a).

D. Triturate 0.1 g with a mixture of 1 ml of *dilute sodium hydroxide solution R* and 3 ml of *water R*. Shake with three quantities, each of 5 ml, of *ether R*. To 0.1 ml of the aqueous layer add a solution of 10 mg of *resorcinol R* in 3 ml of *sulphuric acid R*. Heat on a water-bath for 15 min. No violet-red colour develops. Neutralise the remainder of the aqueous layer with *dilute sulphuric acid R* and add 1 ml of *bromine water R*. Heat on a water-bath for 15 min, then heat to boiling and cool. To 0.2 ml of this solution add a solution of 10 mg of *resorcinol R* in 3 ml of *sulphuric acid R*. Heat on a water-bath for 15 min; a violet-red colour develops. Add 0.2 ml of a 100 g/l solution of *potassium bromide R* and heat for 5 min on a water-bath. The colour becomes violet-blue.

TESTS

Solution S. Dissolve 0.5 g in *carbon dioxide-free water R* and dilute to 25 ml with the same solvent.

Appearance of solution. Solution S is clear (*2.2.1*) and not more intensely coloured than reference solution B_8 (*2.2.2, Method II*).

pH (*2.2.3*). The pH of solution S is 3.8 to 4.3.

Enantiomeric purity. Examine by liquid chromatography (*2.2.29*). *Carry out the test protected from actinic light.*

Test solution. Dissolve 30.0 mg of the substance to be examined in a mixture of 1 volume of *methylene chloride R* and 3 volumes of *2-propanol R* and dilute to 10.0 ml with the same mixture of solvents.

Reference solution (a). Dissolve 30 mg of *timolol maleate CRS* in a mixture of 1 volume of *methylene chloride R* and 3 volumes of *2-propanol R* and dilute to 10 ml with the same mixture of solvents.

Reference solution (b). Dissolve 15.0 mg of *(R)-timolol maleate CRS* in a mixture of 1 volume of *methylene chloride R* and 3 volumes of *2-propanol R* and dilute to 10.0 ml with the same mixture of solvents. Dilute 1.0 ml of the solution to 50.0 ml with a mixture of 1 volume of *methylene chloride R* and 3 volumes of *2-propanol R*.

Reference solution (c). Dilute 1 ml of reference solution (a) to 100 ml with a mixture of 1 volume of *methylene chloride R* and 3 volumes of *2-propanol R*. Mix 1 ml of this solution with 1 ml of reference solution (b).

The chromatographic procedure may be carried out using:

- a stainless steel column 0.25 m long and 4.6 mm in internal diameter packed with *silica gel OD for chiral separations R* (5 µm),
- as mobile phase at a flow rate of 1 ml/min a mixture of 2 ml of *diethylamine R*, 40 ml of *2-propanol R* and 960 ml of *hexane R*,
- as detector a spectrophotometer set at 297 nm.

Under these conditions the peak corresponding to the (*R*)-isomer appears first.

Inject 5 µl of reference solution (b). Adjust the sensitivity of the system so that the height of the principal peak in the chromatogram obtained is at least 50 per cent of the full scale of the recorder. Inject 5 µl of each solution. The test is not valid unless: in the chromatogram obtained with reference solution (c), the resolution between the peaks corresponding to the (*R*)-enantiomer and to the (*S*)-enantiomer is at least 4.0; the retention times of the principal peaks (corresponding to the (*S*)-enantiomer) in the chromatograms obtained with the test solution and reference solution (a) are identical. In the chromatogram obtained with the test solution, the area of any peak corresponding to the (*R*)-enantiomer is not greater than the area of the principal peak in the chromatogram obtained with reference solution (b) (1 per cent).

Related substances. Examine by thin-layer chromatography (*2.2.27*), using a *TLC silica gel plate* GF_{254} *R*.

Test solution (a). Dissolve 0.50 g of the substance to be examined in *methanol R* and dilute to 10 ml with the same solvent.

Test solution (b). Dilute 1 ml of test solution (a) to 50 ml with *methanol R*.

Reference solution (a). Dissolve 10 mg of *timolol maleate CRS* in *methanol R* and dilute to 10 ml with the same solvent.

Reference solution (b). Dilute 10 ml of test solution (b) to 50 ml with *methanol R*.

Apply to the plate 10 µl of each solution. Develop over a path of 15 cm using a mixture of 1 volume of *concentrated ammonia R*, 20 volumes of *methanol R* and 80 volumes of *methylene chloride R*. Allow the plate to dry in air and examine in ultraviolet light at 254 nm. Any spot in the chromatogram obtained with test solution (a), apart from the principal spot, is not more intense than the spot in the chromatogram obtained with reference solution (b) (0.4 per cent). Disregard the spot remaining at the starting point.

Monographs T-Z

Expose the plate to iodine vapour for 2 h. Any spot in the chromatogram obtained with test solution (a), apart from the principal spot, is not more intense than the spot in the chromatogram obtained with reference solution (b) (0.4 per cent). Disregard the spot remaining at the starting point.

Loss on drying (*2.2.32*). Not more than 0.5 per cent, determined on 1.000 g by drying in an oven at 100 °C to 105 °C.

Sulphated ash (*2.4.14*). Not more than 0.1 per cent, determined on 1.0 g.

ASSAY

Dissolve 0.350 g in 60 ml of *anhydrous acetic acid R*. Titrate with *0.1 M perchloric acid* determining the end-point potentiometrically (*2.2.20*).

1 ml of *0.1 M perchloric acid* is equivalent to 43.25 mg of $C_{17}H_{28}N_4O_7S$.

STORAGE

Store protected from light.

IMPURITIES

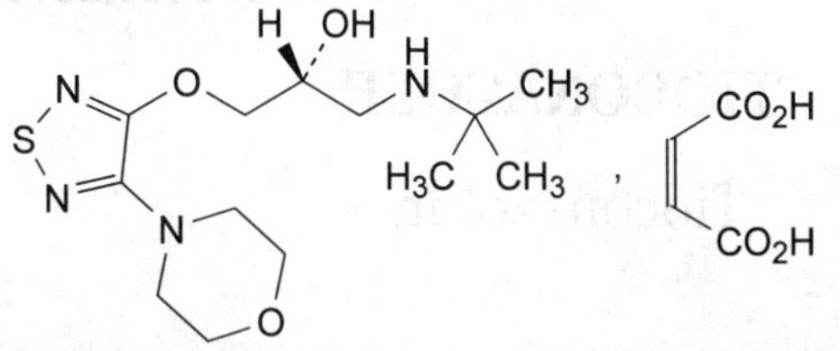

A. (2*R*)-1-[(1,1-dimethylethyl)amino]-3-[[4-(morpholin-4-yl)-1,2,5-thiadiazol-3-yl]oxy]propan-2-ol (*Z*)-butenedioate.

01/2005:1051

TINIDAZOLE

Tinidazolum

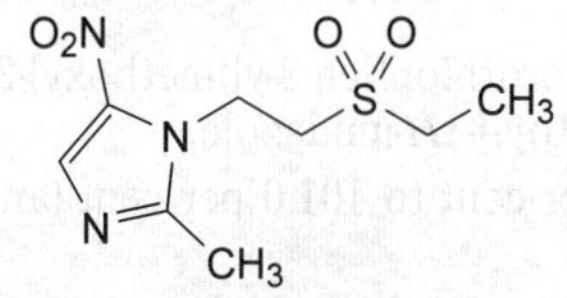

$C_8H_{13}N_3O_4S$ M_r 247.3

DEFINITION

Tinidazole contains not less than 98.0 per cent and not more than the equivalent of 101.0 per cent of 1-[2-(ethylsulphonyl)ethyl]-2-methyl-5-nitro-1*H*-imidazole, calculated with reference to the dried substance.

CHARACTERS

An almost white or pale yellow, crystalline powder, practically insoluble in water, soluble in acetone and in methylene chloride, sparingly soluble in methanol.

IDENTIFICATION

First identification: A, C.

Second identification: A, B, D, E.

A. Melting point (*2.2.14*): 125 °C to 128 °C.

B. Dissolve 10.0 mg in *methanol R* and dilute to 100.0 ml with the same solvent. Dilute 1.0 ml of the solution to 10.0 ml with *methanol R*. Examined between 220 nm and 350 nm (*2.2.25*), the solution shows an absorption maximum at 310 nm. The specific absorbance at the maximum is 340 to 360.

C. Examine by infrared absorption spectrophotometry (*2.2.24*), comparing with the spectrum obtained with *tinidazole CRS*. Examine the substances prepared as discs.

D. Examine the chromatograms obtained in the test for related substances. The principal spot in the chromatogram obtained with test solution (b) is similar in position and size to the principal spot in the chromatogram obtained with reference solution (a).

E. To about 10 mg add about 10 mg of *zinc powder R*, 0.3 ml of *hydrochloric acid R* and 1 ml of *water R*. Heat in a water-bath for 5 min and cool. The solution gives the reaction of primary aromatic amines (*2.3.1*).

TESTS

Appearance of solution. Dissolve 1.0 g in *acetone R* and dilute to 20 ml with the same solvent. The solution is clear (*2.2.1*) and not more intensely coloured than reference solution Y_5 (*2.2.2, Method II*).

Related substances. Examine by thin-layer chromatography (*2.2.27*), using *silica gel GF_{254} R* as the coating substance.

Test solution (a). Dissolve 0.20 g of the substance to be examined in *methanol R* with the aid of ultrasound and dilute to 10 ml with the same solvent.

Test solution (b). Dilute 1.0 ml of test solution (a) to 10 ml with *methanol R*.

Reference solution (a). Dissolve 20 mg of *tinidazole CRS* in *methanol R* and dilute to 10 ml with the same solvent.

Reference solution (b). Dilute 1.0 ml of test solution (b) to 20 ml with *methanol R*.

Reference solution (c). Dilute 4 ml of reference solution (b) to 10 ml with *methanol R*.

Reference solution (d). Dissolve 10 mg of *2-methyl-5-nitroimidazole R* (impurity A) in *methanol R* and dilute to 100 ml with the same solvent.

Reference solution (e). Dissolve 10 mg of *tinidazole impurity B CRS* in *methanol R* and dilute to 100 ml with the same solvent.

Heat the plate at 110 °C for 1 h and allow to cool.

Apply separately to the plate 10 µl of each solution. Develop over a path of 15 cm using a mixture of 25 volumes of *butanol R* and 75 volumes of *ethyl acetate R*. Allow the plate to dry in air and examine in ultraviolet light at 254 nm. Any spots corresponding to tinidazole impurity A and tinidazole impurity B in the chromatogram obtained with test solution (a) are not more intense than the corresponding spots in the chromatogram obtained with reference solutions (d) and (e) (0.5 per cent), respectively. Any spot, apart from the principal spot and any spots corresponding to tinidazole impurity A and tinidazole impurity B in the chromatogram obtained with test solution (a), is not more intense than the spot in the chromatogram obtained with reference solution (b) (0.5 per cent) and at most one such spot is more intense than the spot in the chromatogram obtained with reference solution (c) (0.2 per cent).

Heavy metals (*2.4.8*). 1.0 g complies with limit test D for heavy metals (20 ppm). Prepare the standard using 2 ml of *lead standard solution (10 ppm Pb) R*.

Loss on drying (*2.2.32*). Not more than 0.5 per cent, determined on 1.000 g by drying in an oven at 100 °C to 105 °C.

Sulphated ash (*2.4.14*). Not more than 0.1 per cent, determined on 1.0 g.

ASSAY

Dissolve 0.150 g in 25 ml of *anhydrous acetic acid R.* Titrate with *0.1 M perchloric acid,* determining the end-point potentiometrically (*2.2.20*).

1 ml of *0.1 M perchloric acid* is equivalent to 24.73 mg of $C_8H_{13}N_3O_4S$.

STORAGE

Store protected from light.

IMPURITIES

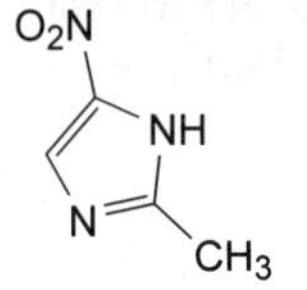

A. 2-methyl-5-nitro-1*H*-imidazole,

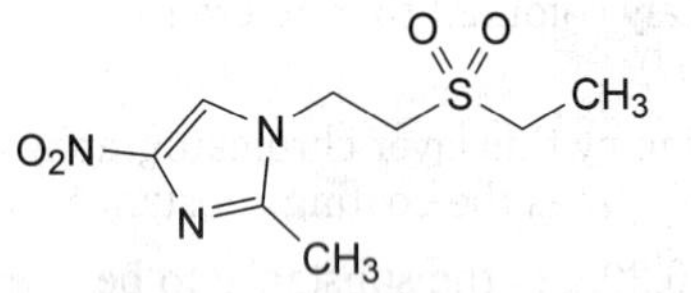

B. 1-[2-(ethylsulphonyl)ethyl]-2-methyl-4-nitro-1*H*-imidazole.

01/2005:1271

TINZAPARIN SODIUM

Tinzaparinum natricum

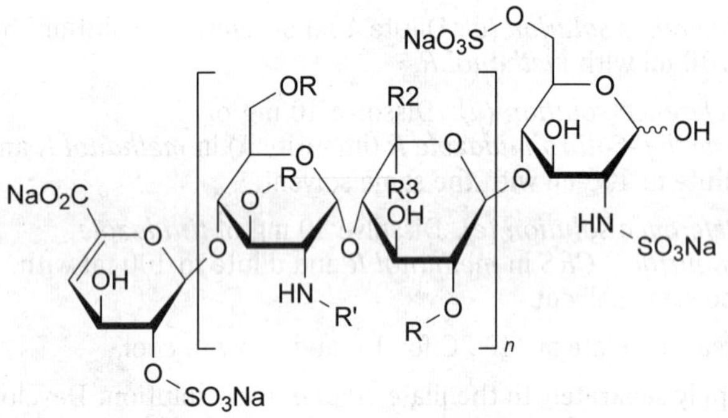

n = 1 to 25 , R = H or SO_3Na , R' = H or SO_3Na or CO-CH_3
R2 = H and R3 = CO_2Na or R2 = CO_2Na and R3 = H

DEFINITION

Tinzaparin sodium is the sodium salt of a low-molecular-mass heparin that is obtained by controlled enzymatic depolymerisation of heparin from porcine intestinal mucosa using heparinase from *Flavobacterium heparinum.* The majority of the components have a 2-*O*-sulpho-4-enepyranosuronic acid structure at the non-reducing end and a 2-*N*,6-*O*-disulpho-D-glucosamine structure at the reducing end of their chain.

Tinzaparin sodium complies with the monograph on Low-molecular-mass heparins (0828) with the modifications and additional requirements below.

The mass-average molecular mass ranges between 5500 and 7500 with a characteristic value of about 6500.

The degree of sulphatation is 1.8 to 2.5 per disaccharide unit.

The potency is not less than 70 IU and not more than 120 IU of anti-factor Xa activity per milligram calculated with reference to the dried substance. The ratio of the anti-factor Xa activity to anti-factor IIa activity is between 1.5 and 2.5.

IDENTIFICATION

Carry out identification test C as described in the monograph for *Low-molecular-mass heparins (0828).* The following requirements apply.

The mass-average molecular mass ranges between 5500 and 7500. The mass percentage of chains lower than 2000 is not more than 10.0 per cent. The mass percentage of chains between 2000 and 8000 ranges between 60.0 and 72.0 per cent. The mass percentage of chains above 8000 ranges between 22.0 and 36.0 per cent.

TESTS

Appearance of solution. Dissolve 1.0 g in 10 ml of *water R.* The solution is clear (*2.2.1*) and not more intensely coloured than intensity 5 of the range of reference solutions of the most appropriate colour (*2.2.2, Method II*)

Absorbance (*2.2.25*). Dissolve 50.0 mg in 100 ml of *0.01 M hydrochloric acid.* The specific absorbance, measured at 231 nm and calculated with reference to the dried substance, is 8.0 to 12.5.

01/2005:2074

TIOCONAZOLE

Tioconazolum

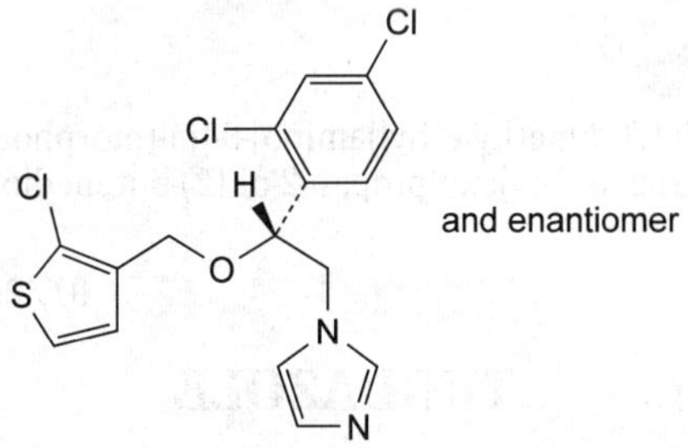

$C_{16}H_{13}Cl_3N_2OS$ M_r 387.7

DEFINITION

1-[(2*RS*)-2-[(2-Chlorothiophen-3-yl)methoxy]-2-(2,4-dichlorophenyl)ethyl]-1*H*-imidazole.

Content: 99.0 per cent to 101.0 per cent (anhydrous substance).

CHARACTERS

Appearance: white or almost white, crystalline powder.

Solubility: very slightly soluble in water, very soluble in methylene chloride, freely soluble in alcohol.

IDENTIFICATION

Infrared absorption spectrophotometry (*2.2.24*).

Comparison: *Ph. Eur. reference spectrum of tioconazole.*

TESTS

Related substances. Liquid chromatography (*2.2.29*).

Test solution. Dissolve 20.0 mg of the substance to be examined in the mobile phase and dilute to 10.0 ml with the mobile phase.

Reference solution (a). Dilute 1.0 ml of the test solution to 100.0 ml with the mobile phase. Dilute 2.0 ml of this solution to 10.0 ml with the mobile phase.

Reference solution (b). Dissolve 5 mg of *tioconazole for system suitability CRS* in the mobile phase and dilute to 2.5 ml with the mobile phase.

Column:

– *size*: l = 0.25 m, Ø = 4.6 mm,

Monographs T-Z

– *stationary phase*: *end-capped octadecylsilyl silica gel for chromatography R* (5 µm) with a specific surface area of 170 m^2/g, a pore size of 12 nm and a carbon loading of 10 per cent.

Mobile phase: mix 1 volume of a 1.7 g/l solution of *tetrabutylammonium dihydrogen phosphate R* previously adjusted to pH 7.4 with *dilute ammonia R2* and 3 volumes of *methanol R*.

Flow rate: 1 ml/min.

Detection: spectrophotometer at 218 nm.

Injection: 20 µl.

Run time: 2.5 times the retention time of tioconazole.

System suitability: reference solution (b):

– *resolution*: minimum 1.0 between the peaks due to impurity B and impurity C (locate impurities A, B and C by comparison with the chromatogram provided with *tioconazole for system suitability CRS*).

Limits:

– *correction factors*: for the calculation of contents, multiply the peak areas of the following impurities by the corresponding correction factor: impurity B = 1.7; impurity C = 1.7.
– *impurities A, B, C*: for each impurity, not more than 1.5 times the area of the principal peak in the chromatogram obtained with reference solution (a) (0.3 per cent),
– *any other impurity*: for each impurity, not more than 0.5 times the area of the principal peak in the chromatogram obtained with reference solution (a) (0.1 per cent),
– *total*: not more than 5 times the area of the principal peak in the chromatogram obtained with reference solution (a) (1.0 per cent),
– *disregard limit*: 0.25 times the area of the principal peak in the chromatogram obtained with reference solution (a) (0.05 per cent).

Water (*2.5.12*): maximum 0.5 per cent, determined on 1.00 g.

Sulphated ash (*2.4.14*): maximum 0.1 per cent, determined on 1.0 g.

ASSAY

Dissolve 0.300 g in 50 ml of *anhydrous acetic acid R*. Titrate with *0.1 M perchloric acid*, determining the end-point potentiometrically (*2.2.20*).

1 ml of *0.1 M perchloric acid* is equivalent to 38.77 mg of $C_{16}H_{13}Cl_3N_2OS$.

STORAGE

Protected from light.

IMPURITIES

Specified impurities: A, B, C.

Other detectable impurities: D.

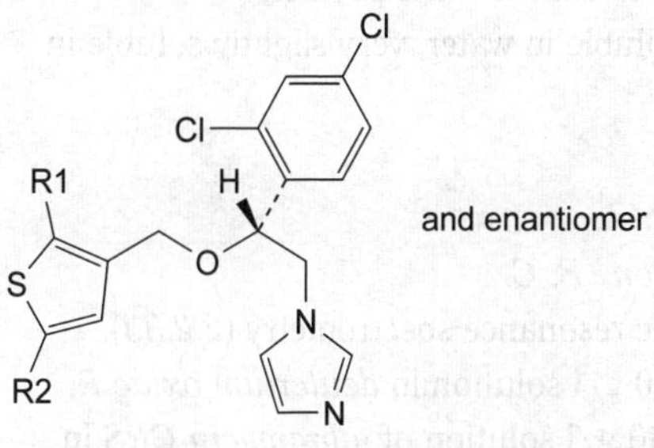

A. R1 = R2 = H: 1-[(2*RS*)-2-(2,4-dichlorophenyl)-2-[(thiophen-3-yl)methoxy]ethyl]-1*H*-imidazole,

B. R1 = R2 = Cl: 1-[(2*RS*)-2-(2,4-dichlorophenyl)-2-[(2,5-dichlorothiophen-3-yl)methoxy]ethyl]-1*H*-imidazole,

C. R1 = Cl, R2 = Br: 1-[(2*RS*)-2-[(5-bromo-2-chlorothiophen-3-yl)methoxy]-2-(2,4-dichlorophenyl)ethyl]-1*H*-imidazole,

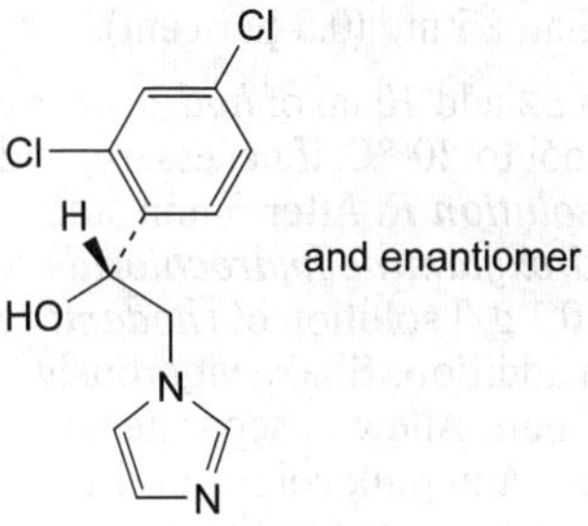

D. (1*RS*)-1-(2,4-dichlorophenyl)-2-(1*H*-imidazol-1-yl)ethanol.

01/2005:0150

TITANIUM DIOXIDE

Titanii dioxidum

TiO_2 M_r 79.9

DEFINITION

Titanium dioxide contains not less than 98.0 per cent and not more than the equivalent of 100.5 per cent of TiO_2.

CHARACTERS

A white or almost white powder, practically insoluble in water. It does not dissolve in dilute mineral acids but dissolves slowly in hot concentrated sulphuric acid.

IDENTIFICATION

A. When strongly heated, it becomes pale yellow; the colour disappears on cooling.

B. To 5 ml of solution S2 (see Tests) add 0.1 ml of *strong hydrogen peroxide solution R*. An orange-red colour appears.

C. To 5 ml of solution S2 add 0.5 g of *zinc R* in granules. After 45 min, the mixture has a violet-blue colour.

TESTS

Solution S1. Shake 20.0 g with 30 ml of *hydrochloric acid R* for 1 min. Add 100 ml of *distilled water R* and heat the mixture to boiling. Filter the hot mixture through a hardened filter paper until a clear filtrate is obtained. Wash the filter with 60 ml of *distilled water R* and dilute the combined filtrate and washings to 200 ml with *distilled water R*.

Solution S2. Mix 0.500 g (*m* g) with 5 g of *anhydrous sodium sulphate R* in a 300 ml long-necked combustion flask. Add 10 ml of *water R* and mix. Add 10 ml of *sulphuric acid R* and boil vigorously, with the usual precautions, until a clear solution is obtained. Cool, add slowly a cooled mixture of 30 ml of *water R* and 10 ml of *sulphuric acid R*, cool again and dilute to 100.0 ml with *water R*.

Appearance of solution. Solution S2 is not more opalescent than reference suspension II (*2.2.1*) and is colourless (*2.2.2, Method II*).

Acidity or alkalinity. Shake 5.0 g with 50 ml of *carbon dioxide-free water R* for 5 min. Centrifuge or filter until a clear solution is obtained. To 10 ml of the solution add 0.1 ml of *bromothymol blue solution R1*. Not more than 1.0 ml of *0.01 M hydrochloric acid* or *0.01 M sodium hydroxide* is required to change the colour of the indicator.

Water-soluble substances. To 10.0 g add a solution of 0.5 g of *ammonium sulphate R* in 150 ml of *water R* and boil for 5 min. Cool, dilute to 200 ml with *water R* and filter until a clear solution is obtained. Evaporate 100 ml of the solution to dryness in a tared evaporating dish and ignite. The residue weighs not more than 25 mg (0.5 per cent).

Antimony. To 10 ml of solution S2 add 10 ml of *hydrochloric acid R* and 10 ml of *water R*. Cool to 20 °C, if necessary, and add 0.15 ml of *sodium nitrite solution R*. After 5 min, add 5 ml of a 10 g/l solution of *hydroxylamine hydrochloride R* and 10 ml of a freshly prepared 0.1 g/l solution of *rhodamine B R*. Mix thoroughly after each addition. Shake vigorously with 10.0 ml of *toluene R* for 1 min. Allow to separate and centrifuge for 2 min if necessary. Any pink colour in the toluene phase is not more intense than that in the toluene phase of a standard prepared at the same time in the same manner using a mixture of 5.0 ml of *antimony standard solution (1 ppm Sb) R*, 10 ml of *hydrochloric acid R* and 15 ml of a solution containing 0.5 g of *anhydrous sodium sulphate R* and 2 ml of *sulphuric acid R* instead of the mixture of 10 ml of solution S2, 10 ml of *hydrochloric acid R* and 10 ml of *water R* (100 ppm).

Arsenic (*2.4.2*). Place 0.50 g in a 250 ml round-bottomed flask, fitted with a thermometer, a funnel with stopcock and a vapour-outlet tube connected to a flask containing 30 ml of *water R*. Add 50 ml of *water R*, 0.5 g of *hydrazine sulphate R*, 0.5 g of *potassium bromide R* and 20 g of *sodium chloride R*. Through the funnel, add dropwise 25 ml of *sulphuric acid R*, heat and maintain the temperature of the liquid at 110 °C to 115 °C for 20 min. Collect the vapour in the flask containing 30 ml of *water R*. Dilute to 50 ml with *water R*. 20 ml of the solution complies with limit test A for arsenic (5 ppm).

Barium. To 10 ml of solution S1 add 1 ml of *dilute sulphuric acid R*. After 30 min, any opalescence in the solution is not more intense than that in a mixture of 10 ml of solution S1 and 1 ml of *distilled water R*.

Heavy metals (*2.4.8*). Dilute 10 ml of solution S1 to 20 ml with *water R*. 12 ml of the solution complies with limit test A for heavy metals (20 ppm). Prepare the standard using *lead standard solution (1 ppm Pb) R*.

Iron. To 8 ml of solution S2 add 4 ml of *water R*. Mix and add 0.05 ml of *bromine water R*. Allow to stand for 5 min and remove the excess of bromine with a current of air. Add 3 ml of *potassium thiocyanate solution R*. Any colour in the solution is not more intense than that in a standard prepared at the same time in the same manner using a mixture of 4 ml of *iron standard solution (2 ppm Fe) R* and 8 ml of a 200 g/l solution of *sulphuric acid R* (200 ppm).

ASSAY

To 300 g of *zinc R* in granules (710) add 300 ml of a 20 g/l solution of *mercuric nitrate R* and 2 ml of *nitric acid R*, shake for 10 min and wash with *water R*. Pack the amalgamated zinc into a glass tube about 400 mm long and about 20 mm in diameter fitted with a tap and a filter plate. Pass through the column 100 ml of *dilute sulphuric acid R* followed by 100 ml of *water R*, making sure that the amalgam is always covered with liquid. Pass slowly at a rate of about 3 ml/min through the column a mixture of 100 ml of *dilute sulphuric acid R* and 100 ml of *water R* followed by 100 ml of *water R*. Collect the eluate in a 500 ml conical flask containing 50.0 ml of a 150 g/l solution of *ferric ammonium sulphate R* in a mixture of 1 volume of *sulphuric acid R* and 3 volumes of *water R*. Add 0.1 ml of *ferroin R* and titrate immediately with *0.1 M ammonium and cerium nitrate* until a greenish colour is obtained (n_1 ml). Pass slowly at a rate of about 3 ml/min through the column a mixture of 50 ml of *dilute sulphuric acid R* and 50 ml of *water R*, followed by 20.0 ml of solution S2, a mixture of 50 ml of *dilute sulphuric acid R* and 50 ml of *water R* and finally 100 ml of *water R*. Collect the eluate in a 500 ml conical flask containing 50.0 ml of a 150 g/l solution of *ferric ammonium sulphate R* in a mixture of 1 volume of *sulphuric acid R* and 3 volumes of *water R*. Rinse the lower end of the column with *water R*, add 0.1 ml of *ferroin R* and titrate immediately with *0.1 M ammonium and cerium nitrate* until a greenish colour is obtained (n_2 ml).

Calculate the percentage content of TiO_2 from the expression:

$$\frac{3.99 \times (n_2 - n_1)}{m}$$

m = mass in grams of the substance to be examined used for the preparation of solution S2.

01/2005:0645

TOBRAMYCIN

Tobramycinum

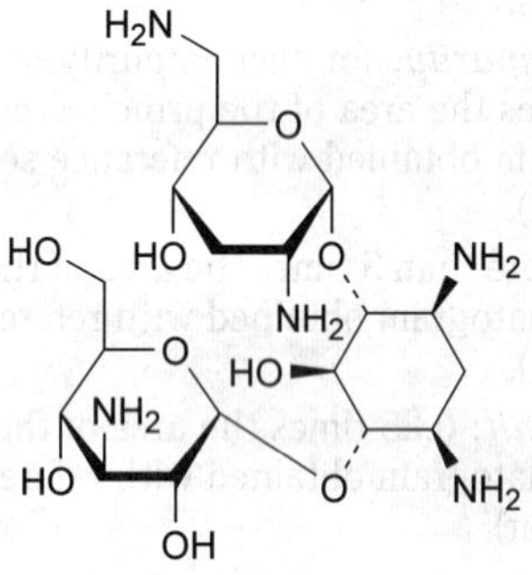

$C_{18}H_{37}N_5O_9$ M_r 467.5

DEFINITION

4-*O*-(3-Amino-3-deoxy-α-D-glucopyranosyl)-2-deoxy-6-*O*-(2,6-diamino-2,3,6-trideoxy-α-D-*ribo*-hexopyranosyl)-L-streptamine.

Substance produced by *Streptomyces tenebrarius* or obtained by any other means.

Content: 97.0 per cent to 102.0 per cent (anhydrous and 2-methyl-1-propanol-free substance).

PRODUCTION

It is produced by methods of manufacture designed to eliminate or minimise substances lowering blood pressure.

CHARACTERS

Appearance: white or almost white powder.

Solubility: freely soluble in water, very slightly soluble in alcohol.

IDENTIFICATION

First identification: A.

Second identification: B, C.

A. Nuclear magnetic resonance spectrometry (*2.2.33*).

Preparation: 100 g/l solution in *deuterium oxide R*.

Comparison: 100 g/l solution of *tobramycin CRS* in *deuterium oxide R*.

B. Thin-layer chromatography (*2.2.27*).

Test solution. Dissolve 20 mg of the substance to be examined in *water R* and dilute to 5 ml with the same solvent.

Reference solution (a). Dissolve 20 mg of *tobramycin CRS* in *water R* and dilute to 5 ml with the same solvent.

Reference solution (b). Dissolve 4 mg of *neomycin sulphate CRS* and 4 mg of *kanamycin monosulphate CRS* in 1 ml of reference solution (a).

Plate: *TLC silica gel plate R*.

Mobile phase: *methylene chloride R, concentrated ammonia R, methanol R* (17:33:50 *V/V/V*).

Application: 5 µl.

Development: over 2/3 of the plate.

Drying: in a current of warm air.

Detection: spray with a mixture of equal volumes of a 2 g/l solution of *1,3-dihydroxynaphthalene R* in *alcohol R* and a 460 g/l solution of *sulphuric acid R*. Heat at 105 °C for 5-10 min.

System suitability: the chromatogram obtained with reference solution (b) shows 3 major spots which are clearly separated.

Results: the principal spot in the chromatogram obtained with the test solution is similar in position, colour and size to the principal spot in the chromatogram obtained with reference solution (a).

C. Dissolve about 5 mg in 5 ml of *water R*. Add 5 ml of a 1 g/l solution of *ninhydrin R* in *alcohol R* and heat in a water-bath for 3 min. A violet-blue colour develops.

TESTS

pH (*2.2.3*): 9.0 to 11.0.

Dissolve 1.0 g in 10 ml of *carbon dioxide-free water R*.

Specific optical rotation (*2.2.7*): + 138 to + 148 (anhydrous and 2-methyl-1-propanol-free substance).

Dissolve 1.00 g in *water R* and dilute to 25.0 ml with the same solvent.

Related substances. Liquid chromatography (*2.2.29*).

Test solution (a). Dissolve 25.0 mg of the substance to be examined in *water R* and dilute to 25.0 ml with the same solvent.

Test solution (b). Dilute 10.0 ml of test solution (a) to 100.0 ml with *water R*.

Reference solution (a). Dissolve 25.0 mg of *tobramycin CRS* in *water R* and dilute to 100.0 ml with the same solvent.

Reference solution (b). Dilute 1.0 ml of reference solution (a) to 100.0 ml with *water R*.

Reference solution (c). Dilute 1.0 ml of reference solution (a) to 50.0 ml with *water R*.

Reference solution (d). Dissolve 10.0 mg of *kanamycin B CRS* in 20.0 ml of *water R*. To 1.0 ml, add 2.0 ml of reference solution (a) and dilute to 10.0 ml with *water R*.

Reference solution (e). Dilute 10.0 ml of reference solution (a) to 25.0 ml with *water R*.

Column:
- *size*: l = 0.25 m, Ø = 4.6 mm,
- *stationary phase*: *styrene-divinylbenzene copolymer R* (8 µm) with a pore size of 100 nm,
- *temperature*: 55 °C.

Mobile phase: a mixture prepared with *carbon dioxide-free water R* containing 52 g/l of *anhydrous sodium sulphate R*, 1.5 g/l of *sodium octanesulphonate R*, 3 ml/l of *tetrahydrofuran R*, 50 ml/l of *0.2 M potassium dihydrogen phosphate R* previously adjusted to pH 3.0 with *dilute phosphoric acid R*. Degas.

Flow rate: 1.0 ml/min.

Post-column solution: *carbonate-free sodium hydroxide solution R* diluted 1 to 25 with *carbon dioxide-free water R*, which is added pulseless to the column effluent using a 375 µl polymeric mixing coil.

Flow rate: 0.3 ml/min.

Detection: pulsed amperometric detector or equivalent with a gold working electrode, a silver-silver chloride reference electrode and a stainless steel auxiliary electrode which is the cell body, held at respectively + 0.05 V detection, + 0.75 V oxidation and − 0.15 V reduction potentials, with pulse durations according to the instrument used. The temperature of the detector is set at 35 °C.

Injection: 20 µl; inject test solution (a) and reference solutions (b), (c) and (d).

Run time: 1.5 times the retention time of tobramycin.

Relative retention with reference to tobramycin (retention time = about 18 min): impurity C = about 0.35; impurity B = about 0.40, impurity A = about 0.70.

System suitability:
- *resolution*: minimum of 3.0 between the peaks due to impurity A and to tobramycin in the chromatogram obtained with reference solution (d). If necessary, adjust the concentration of sodium octanesulphonate in the mobile phase;
- *signal-to-noise ratio*: minimum of 10 for the principal peak in the chromatogram obtained with reference solution (b).

Limits:
- *any impurity*: not more than twice the area of the principal peak in the chromatogram obtained with reference solution (c) (1.0 per cent) and not more than 1 such peak has an area greater than the area of the principal peak in the chromatogram obtained with reference solution (c) (0.5 per cent),
- *total*: not more than 3 times the area of the principal peak in the chromatogram obtained with reference solution (c) (1.5 per cent),
- *disregard limit*: the area of the principal peak in the chromatogram obtained with reference solution (b) (0.25 per cent).

2-Methyl-1-propanol (*2.4.24, System B*): maximum 1.0 per cent *m/m*.

Water (*2.5.12*): maximum 8.0 per cent, determined on 0.30 g.

Sulphated ash (*2.4.14*): maximum 0.3 per cent, determined on 1.0 g.

Bacterial endotoxins (*2.6.14*): less than 2.0 IU/mg, if intended for use in the manufacture of parenteral dosage forms without a further appropriate procedure for the removal of bacterial endotoxins.

ASSAY

Liquid chromatography (*2.2.29*) as described in the test for related substances with the following modifications.

Injection: test solution (b) and reference solution (e).

Calculate the percentage content of tobramycin.

STORAGE

If the substance is sterile, store in a sterile, airtight, tamper-proof container.

LABELLING

The label states, where applicable, that the substance is free from bacterial endotoxins.

Monographs T-Z

IMPURITIES

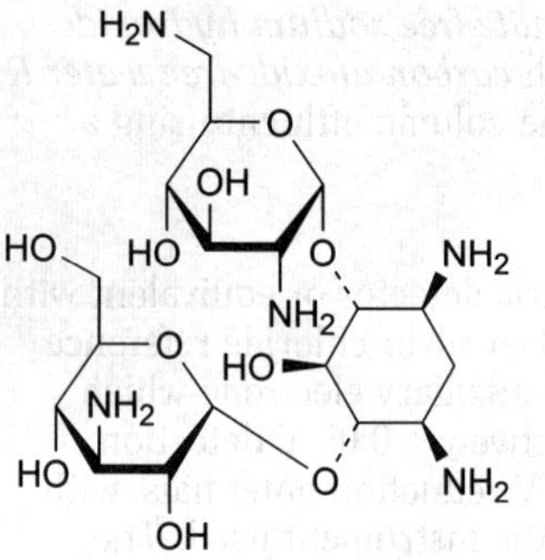

A. 4-*O*-(3-amino-3-deoxy-α-D-glucopyranosyl)-2-deoxy-6-*O*-(2,6-diamino-2,6-dideoxy-α-D-glucopyranosyl)-L-streptamine (kanamycin B),

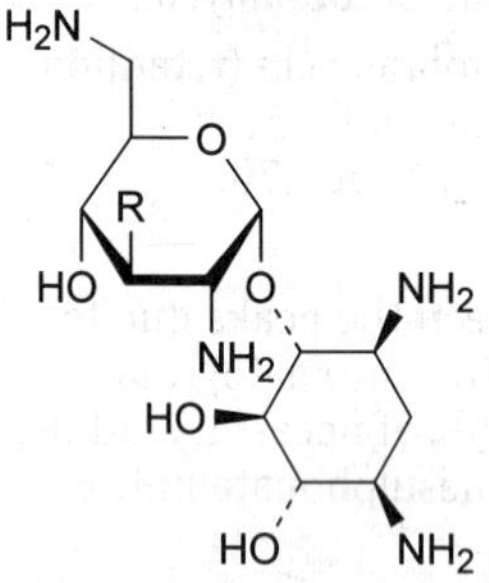

B. R = H: 2-deoxy-4-*O*-(2,6-diamino-2,3,6-trideoxy-α-D-ribo-hexopyranosyl)-D-streptamine (nebramine),

C. R = OH: 2-deoxy-4-*O*-(2,6-diamino-2,6-dideoxy-α-D-glucopyranosyl)-D-streptamine (neamine).

01/2005:0692

all-*rac*-α-TOCOPHEROL

int-*rac*-α-Tocopherolum

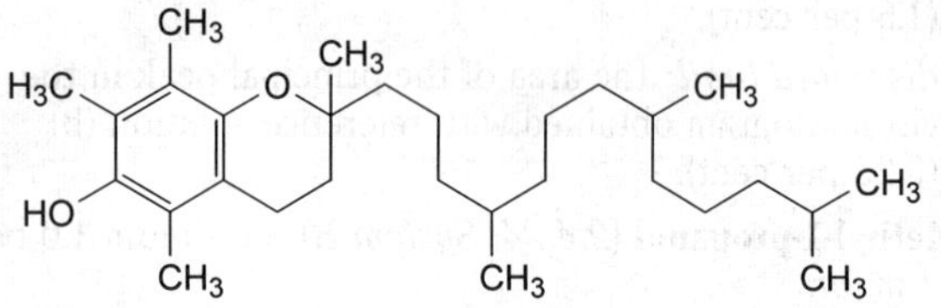

$C_{29}H_{50}O_2$ M_r 430.7

DEFINITION

all-*rac*-2,5,7,8-Tetramethyl-2-(4,8,12-trimethyltridecyl)-3,4-dihydro-2*H*-1-benzopyran-6-ol.

Content: 96.0 per cent to 101.5 per cent.

CHARACTERS

Appearance: clear, colourless or yellowish-brown, viscous, oily liquid.

Solubility: practically insoluble in water, freely soluble in acetone, in ethanol, in methylene chloride and in fatty oils.

IDENTIFICATION

First identification: A, B.

Second identification: A, C.

A. Optical rotation (*2.2.7*): − 0.01° to + 0.01°.
Dissolve 2.50 g in *ethanol R* and dilute to 25.0 ml with the same solvent.

B. Infrared absorption spectrophotometry (*2.2.24*).
Comparison: *α-tocopherol CRS.*

C. Thin-layer chromatography (*2.2.27*).
Test solution. Dissolve 10 mg of the substance to be examined in 2 ml of *cyclohexane R*.
Reference solution. Dissolve 10 mg of *α-tocopherol CRS* in 2 ml of *cyclohexane R*.
Plate: *TLC silica gel F_{254} plate R.*
Mobile phase: *ether R, cyclohexane R (20:80 V/V).*
Application: 10 µl.
Development: over 2/3 of the plate.
Drying: in a current of air.
Detection: examine in ultraviolet light at 254 nm.
Results: the principal spot in the chromatogram obtained with the test solution is similar in position and size to the principal spot in the chromatogram obtained with the reference solution.

TESTS

Related substances. Gas chromatography (*2.2.28*): use the normalisation procedure.

Internal standard solution. Dissolve 1.0 g of *squalane R* in *cyclohexane R* and dilute to 100.0 ml with the same solvent.

Test solution (a). Dissolve 0.100 g of the substance to be examined in 10.0 ml of the internal standard solution.

Test solution (b). Dissolve 0.100 g of the substance to be examined in 10 ml of *cyclohexane R*.

Reference solution (a). Dissolve 0.100 g of *α-tocopherol CRS* in 10.0 ml of the internal standard solution.

Reference solution (b). Dissolve 10 mg of the substance to be examined and 10 mg of *α-tocopheryl acetate R* in *cyclohexane R* and dilute to 100.0 ml with the same solvent.

Reference solution (c). Dissolve 10 mg of *all-rac-α-tocopherol for peak identification CRS* in *cyclohexane R* and dilute to 1 ml with the same solvent.

Reference solution (d). Dilute 1.0 ml of test solution (b) to 100.0 ml with *cyclohexane R*. Dilute 1.0 ml of this solution to 10.0 ml with *cyclohexane R*.

Column:
- *material*: fused silica,
- *size*: *l* = 30 m, Ø = 0.25 mm,
- *stationary phase*: *poly(dimethyl)siloxane R* (film thickness 0.25 µm).

Carrier gas: *helium for chromatography R.*

Flow rate: 1 ml/min.

Split ratio: 1:100.

Temperature:
- *column*: 280 °C,
- *injection port and detector*: 290 °C.

Detection: flame ionisation.

Injection: 1 µl of test solution (b) and reference solutions (b), (c) and (d).

Run time: twice the retention time of all-*rac*-α-tocopherol.

Relative retention with reference to all-*rac*-α-tocopherol (retention time = about 13 min): squalane = about 0.5; impurity A = about 0.7; impurity B = about 0.8. Use the chromatogram supplied with the CRS and the chromatogram obtained with reference solution (c) to identify the peaks due to impurities A and B.

System suitability: reference solution (b):
- *resolution*: minimum 3.5 between the peaks due to all-*rac*-α-tocopherol and α-tocopheryl acetate.

Limits:
- *impurity A*: maximum 0.5 per cent,

Monographs T-Z

– *impurity B*: maximum 1.5 per cent,
– *any other impurity*: for each impurity, maximum 0.25 per cent,
– *total*: maximum 2.5 per cent,
– *disregard limit*: the area of the principal peak in the chromatogram obtained with reference solution (d) (0.1 per cent).

ASSAY

Gas chromatography (*2.2.28*) as described in the test for related substances with the following modification.

Injection: test solution (a) and reference solution (a).

Calculate the percentage content of $C_{29}H_{50}O_2$ taking into account the declared content of *α-tocopherol CRS*.

STORAGE

Under an inert gas, protected from light.

IMPURITIES

Specified impurities: A, B.

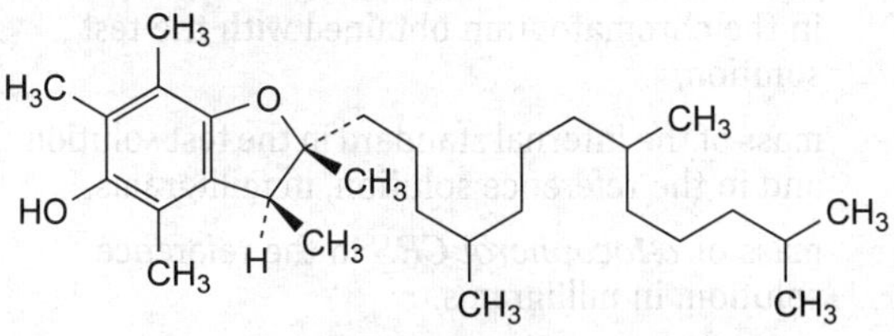

and diastereoisomers

A. all-*rac-trans*-2,3,4,6,7-pentamethyl-2-(4,8,12-trimethyltridecyl)-2,3-dihydrobenzofuran-5-ol,

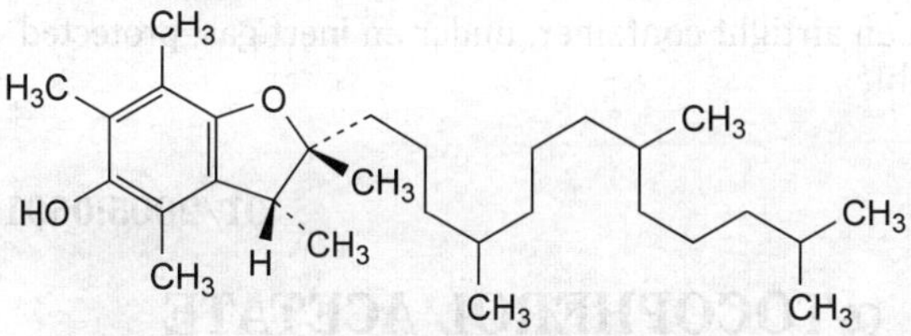

and diastereoisomers

B. all-*rac-cis*-2,3,4,6,7-pentamethyl-2-(4,8,12-trimethyltridecyl)-2,3-dihydrobenzofuran-5-ol.

01/2005:1256

RRR-α-TOCOPHEROL

RRR-α-Tocopherolum

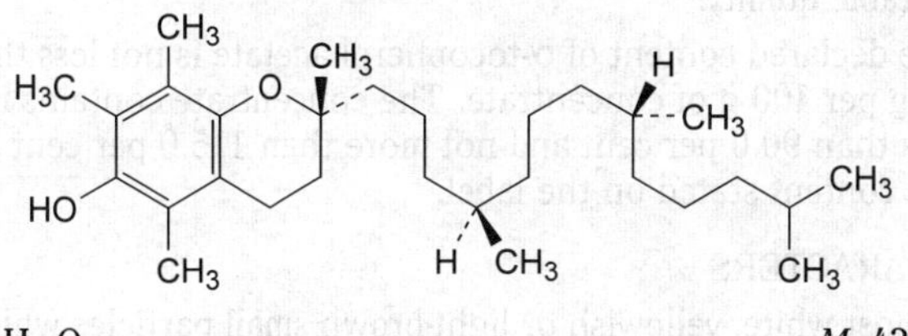

$C_{29}H_{50}O_2$ M_r 430.7

DEFINITION

RRR-α-Tocopherol contains not less than 96.0 per cent and not more than the equivalent of 102.0 per cent of (2*R*)-2,5,7,8-tetramethyl-2-[(4*R*,8*R*)-4,8,12-trimethyltridecyl]-3,4-dihydro-2*H*-1-benzopyran-6-ol.

CHARACTERS

A clear, colourless or yellowish-brown, viscous, oily liquid, practically insoluble in water, freely soluble in acetone, in ethanol, in methylene chloride and in fatty oils.

IDENTIFICATION

First identification: B, D.

Second identification: A, C, D.

A. It complies with the test for absorbance (see Tests).

B. Examine by infrared absorption spectrophotometry (*2.2.24*), comparing with the spectrum obtained with *α-tocopherol CRS*.

C. Examine by thin-layer chromatography (*2.2.27*), using a *TLC silica gel F_{254} plate R*.

Test solution. Dissolve 10 mg of the substance to be examined in 2 ml of *cyclohexane R*.

Reference solution. Dissolve 10 mg of *α-tocopherol CRS* in 2 ml of *cyclohexane R*.

Apply separately to the plate 10 µl of each solution. Develop over a path of 15 cm using a mixture of 20 volumes of *ether R* and 80 volumes of *cyclohexane R*. Dry the plate in a current of air and examine in ultraviolet light at 254 nm. The principal spot in the chromatogram obtained with the test solution is similar in position and size to the principal spot in the chromatogram obtained with the reference solution. Spray the plate with a mixture of 10 volumes of *hydrochloric acid R*, 40 volumes of a 2.5 g/l solution of *ferric chloride R* in *alcohol R* and 40 volumes of a 10 g/l solution of *phenanthroline hydrochloride R* in *alcohol R*. After 1 h to 2 h, the principal spots are orange.

D. *RRR*-α-tocopherol is dextrorotatory (*2.2.7*). The specific optical rotation after oxidation to the quinone form is not less than + 24.

Dissolve 1.0 g of the substance to be examined in 50 ml of *ether R*. To the solution add 20 ml of a 100 g/l solution of *potassium ferricyanide R* in an 8 g/l solution of *sodium hydroxide R* and shake for 3 min. Wash the ether solution with four quantities, each of 50 ml, of *water R*, discard the washings and dry the ether layer over *anhydrous sodium sulphate R*. Evaporate the ether on a water-bath under reduced pressure or in an atmosphere of nitrogen until a few millilitres remain, then complete the evaporation removing the last traces of ether without the application of heat. Immediately dissolve the residue in 5.0 ml of *trimethylpentane R* and determine the optical rotation.

Calculate the specific optical rotation of the substance in the test solution using as *c* the number of grams of *RRR*-α-tocopherol in 1000 ml.

TESTS

Absorbance (*2.2.25*). Dissolve 0.100 g in *ethanol R* and dilute to 100 ml with the same solvent (solution A). Dilute 10.0 ml of solution A to 100.0 ml with *ethanol R* (solution B). Measure the absorbance of solution B at the maximum at 292 nm and of solution A at the minimum at 255 nm. The specific absorbance at the maximum is 72.0 to 76.0 and that at the minimum is 5.5 to 8.0.

Acid value (*2.5.1*). Not more than 2.0, determined on 2.00 g.

Heavy metals (*2.4.8*). 0.50 g complies with limit test D for heavy metals (20 ppm). Prepare the standard using 1 ml of *lead standard solution (10 ppm Pb) R*.

Sulphated ash (*2.4.14*). Not more than 0.1 per cent, determined on 1.0 g. Use *sulphuric acid R* instead of *dilute sulphuric acid R*.

ASSAY

Examine by gas chromatography (*2.2.28*), using *dotriacontane R* as the internal standard.

Internal standard solution. Dissolve 0.300 g of *dotriacontane R* in *hexane R* and dilute to 100.0 ml with the same solvent.

Test solution. Dissolve 0.100 g of the substance to be examined in 10.0 ml of the internal standard solution, dilute to 50.0 ml with *hexane R* and mix.

Reference solution. Dissolve 0.100 g of *α-tocopherol CRS* in 10.0 ml of the internal standard solution, dilute to 50.0 ml with *hexane R* and mix.

The chromatographic procedure may be carried out using:

- a fused-silica column, 15 m long and 0.32 mm in internal diameter coated with a 0.25 µm layer of *poly(dimethyl)siloxane R,*
- *helium for chromatography R* as the carrier gas at a flow rate of 3 ml/min to 6 ml/min,
- a flame-ionisation detector,

maintaining the temperature of the injection port at 300 °C and that of the detector at 330 °C. Adjust the split ratio between 1 to 10 and 1 to 20. Set the temperature of the column at 200 °C, then raise the temperature at a rate of 5 °C per minute to 250 °C and maintain at 250 °C for 10 min.

Inject directly onto the column or via a glass-lined injection port using an automatic injection device or some other reproducible injection method. Measure the peak areas by electronic integration. The test is not valid unless in the chromatogram obtained with the reference solution, the resolution between the peaks corresponding to dotriacontane and α-tocopherol is at least 9.0.

Interference test. Dissolve 0.100 g of the substance to be examined in *hexane R* and dilute to 50.0 ml with the same solvent. Inject 1 µl of the solution and record the chromatogram. If a peak is detected with the same t_R value as for dotriacontane, calculate the area of this peak relative to the peak area of α-tocopherol. If the relative peak area is greater than 0.5 per cent, use the corrected peak area $S'_{D(corr)}$ for the final calculation.

$$S'_{D(corr)} = S'_D - \frac{S_I \times S'_T}{S_{TI}}$$

S'_D = area of the peak corresponding to the internal standard in the chromatogram obtained with the test solution,

S_I = area of the interfering peak (same t_R value as that of the internal standard) in the chromatogram obtained in the interference test,

S'_T = area of the peak corresponding to α-tocopherol in the chromatogram obtained with the test solution,

S_{TI} = area of the peak corresponding to α-tocopherol in the chromatogram obtained in the interference test.

Once the system suitability has been established, inject 1 µl of the reference solution and record the chromatogram. Measure the areas of the peaks corresponding to α-tocopherol (S_T) and dotriacontane (S_D) and determine the response factor (RF) as described below.

Determine the response factor (RF) for α-tocopherol in the chromatogram obtained with the reference solution from the area of the peak corresponding to α-tocopherol and the peak corresponding to dotriacontane using the expression:

$$RF = \frac{S_D \times m_T}{S_T \times m_D}$$

Inject 1 µl of the test solution in the same manner. Measure the areas of the peaks corresponding to α-tocopherol (S'_T) and dotriacontane (S'_D).

Calculate the percentage content of *RRR*-α-tocopherol using the expression:

$$\frac{100\,(S'_T \times m_D \times RF)}{S'_{D(corr)} \times m}$$

S_D = area of the peak corresponding to the internal standard in the chromatogram obtained with the reference solution,

$S'_{D(corr)}$ = corrected area of the peak corresponding to the internal standard in the chromatogram obtained with the test solution,

S_T = area of the peak corresponding to *α-tocopherol CRS* in the chromatogram obtained with the reference solution,

S'_T = area of the peak corresponding to α-tocopherol in the chromatogram obtained with the test solution,

m_D = mass of the internal standard in the test solution and in the reference solution, in milligrams,

m_T = mass of *α-tocopherol CRS* in the reference solution, in milligrams,

m = mass of the substance to be examined in the test solution, in milligrams.

STORAGE

Store in an airtight container, under an inert gas, protected from light.

01/2005:0691

α-TOCOPHEROL ACETATE CONCENTRATE (POWDER FORM)

α-Tocopheroli acetatis pulvis

DEFINITION

α-Tocopherol acetate concentrate (powder form) is prepared either by finely dispersing *α-Tocopherol acetate (0439)* in a suitable carrier of suitable quality (for example gelatin, acacia, carbohydrates, lactoproteins or a mixture thereof) or by adsorbing *α-Tocopherol acetate (0439)* on silicic acid of suitable quality.

The declared content of α-tocopherol acetate is not less than 25 g per 100 g of concentrate. The concentrate contains not less than 90.0 per cent and not more than 115.0 per cent of the content stated on the label.

CHARACTERS

Almost white, yellowish or light-brown small particles which, depending on their formulation, may be practically insoluble in water or may swell or form a dispersion.

IDENTIFICATION

Examine by thin-layer chromatography (*2.2.27*), using *silica gel HF_{254} R* as the coating substance.

Test solution. To a quantity of concentrate corresponding to 50 mg of α-tocopherol acetate add 5 ml of *0.01 M hydrochloric acid* and treat with ultrasound at 60 °C. Add 5 ml of *ethanol R* and 10 ml of *cyclohexane R,* shake for 1 min and centrifuge for 5 min. Use the upper layer.

Monographs T-Z

Reference solution. Dissolve 50 mg of *α-tocopherol acetate CRS* in *cyclohexane R* and dilute to 10 ml with the same solvent.

Apply separately to the plate 10 μl of each solution. Develop over a path of 15 cm using a mixture of 20 volumes of *ether R* and 80 volumes of *cyclohexane R*. Dry the plate in a current of air and examine in ultraviolet light at 254 nm. The principal spot in the chromatogram obtained with the test solution is similar in position and size to the principal spot in the chromatogram obtained with the reference solution.

ASSAY

Examine by gas chromatography (*2.2.28*), using *dotriacontane R* as the internal standard.

Internal standard solution. Dissolve 0.20 g of *dotriacontane R* in *hexane R* and dilute to 100.0 ml with the same solvent.

Test solution. Weigh accurately a quantity of the preparation to be examined corresponding to about 0.100 g of α-tocopherol acetate in a 250 ml conical flask. Add 20 ml of *1 M hydrochloric acid* and treat with ultrasound at 70 °C for 20 min. Add 50 ml of *ethanol R* and 50.0 ml of the internal standard solution and thoroughly mix the two phases for 30 min. Allow to separate, and use the upper layer.

Reference solution. Dissolve 0.100 g of *α-tocopherol acetate CRS* in the internal standard solution and dilute to 50.0 ml with the internal standard solution.

The chromatographic procedure may be carried out using:

- a silanised glass column 2.0 m to 3.0 m long and 2.2 mm to 4.0 mm in internal diameter packed with *diatomaceous earth for gas chromatography R* (125 μm to 150 μm or 150 μm to 180 μm), silanised with dimethyldichlorosilane and impregnated with 1 per cent *m/m* to 5 per cent *m/m* of *poly(dimethyl)siloxane R*; a plug of silanised glass wool is placed at each end of the column,
- *nitrogen for chromatography R* as the carrier gas at a flow rate of 25-90 ml/min,
- a flame-ionisation detector,

maintaining the column at a constant temperature between 245 °C and 280 °C and the injection port and the detector each at a constant temperature between 270 °C and 320 °C. Set the temperature of the column and the flow rate of the carrier gas in such a manner that the required resolution is achieved.

Make the injections directly onto the column or via an injection port (preferably glass-lined) using an automatic injection device or some other reproducible injection method. Measure the peak areas by electronic integration.

Resolution. Inject 1 μl of the reference solution. Repeat this operation until the response factor (RF) determined as described below is constant to within ± 2 per cent. The resolution (R_S) between the dotriacontane peak and the α-tocopherol acetate peak is at least 1.4.

Interference test. Weigh accurately a quantity of the substance to be examined corresponding to about 0.100 g of α-tocopherol acetate in a 250 ml conical flask. Add 20 ml of *1 M hydrochloric acid* and treat with ultrasound at 70 °C for 20 min. Add 50 ml of *ethanol R* and 50 ml of *hexane R* and thoroughly mix the two phases for 30 min. Allow to separate. Inject 1 μl of the upper layer and record the chromatogram, choosing an attenuation such that the height of the peak corresponding to α-tocopherol acetate is greater than 50 per cent of the maximum recorder response; during the recording, change the attenuation so that any peak appearing with the same t_R value as for dotriacontane is recorded with a sensitivity at least eight times greater than for the α-tocopherol acetate peak. If a peak with a height of at least 5 mm for a recorder paper width of 250 mm is detected with the same t_R value as for dotriacontane, use the corrected peak area $S'_{D(corr.)}$ for the final calculation.

$$S'_{D(corr.)} = S'_D - \frac{S_I \times S'_T}{f \times S_{TI}}$$

S'_D = area of the peak corresponding to the internal standard in the chromatogram obtained with the test solution,

S_I = area of the interfering peak (same t_R value as that of the internal standard) in the chromatogram obtained in the interference test,

S'_T = area of the peak corresponding to α-tocopherol acetate in the chromatogram obtained with the test solution,

S_{TI} = area of the peak corresponding to α-tocopherol acetate in the chromatogram obtained in the interference test,

f = factor by which the attenuation was changed.

Inject 1 μl of the reference solution and record the chromatogram, choosing an attenuation such that the peak corresponding to α-tocopherol acetate is greater than 50 per cent of the maximum recorder response. Measure the areas of the peaks corresponding to α-tocopherol acetate (S_T) and to dotriacontane (S_D) and determine the response factor (RF) as described below. Inject 1 μl of the test solution in the same manner. Measure the areas of the peaks corresponding to α-tocopherol acetate (S'_T) and to dotriacontane (S'_D).

Determine the response factor (RF) for α-tocopherol acetate in the chromatogram obtained with the reference solution from the areas of the peak corresponding to α-tocopherol acetate and the peak corresponding to dotriacontane using the expression:

$$\frac{S_D \times m_T}{S_T \times m_D}$$

Calculate the percentage content of α-tocopherol acetate using the expression:

$$\frac{100 \times S'_T \times m_D \times RF}{S'_{D(corr.)} \times m}$$

S_D = area of the peak corresponding to the internal standard in the chromatogram obtained with the reference solution,

$S'_{D(corr.)}$ = corrected area of the peak corresponding to the internal standard in the chromatogram obtained with the test solution,

S_T = area of the peak corresponding to *α-tocopherol acetate CRS* in the chromatogram obtained with the reference solution,

S'_T = area of the peak corresponding to α-tocopherol acetate in the chromatogram obtained with the test solution,

m_D = mass of the internal standard in the test solution and in the reference solution in milligrams,

m_T = mass of *α-tocopherol acetate CRS* in the reference solution in milligrams,

m = mass of the substance to be examined in the test solution in milligrams.

Monographs T-Z

STORAGE

Store in an airtight, well-filled container, protected from light.

LABELLING

The label states the content of α-tocopherol acetate, expressed in grams per 100 g of concentrate.

01/2005:0439

all-*rac*-α-TOCOPHERYL ACETATE

int-*rac*-α-Tocopherylis acetas

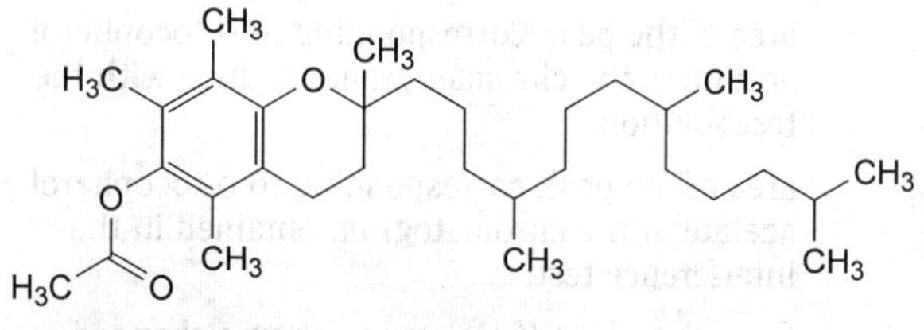

$C_{31}H_{52}O_3$ M_r 472.7

DEFINITION

all-*rac*-2,5,7,8-Tetramethyl-2-(4,8,12-trimethyltridecyl)-3,4-dihydro-2*H*-1-benzopyran-6-yl acetate.

Content: 96.5 per cent to 101.0 per cent.

CHARACTERS

Appearance: clear, colourless or slightly greenish-yellow, viscous, oily liquid.

Solubility: practically insoluble in water, freely soluble in acetone, in ethanol and in fatty oils.

IDENTIFICATION

First identification: A, B.

Second identification: A, C.

A. Optical rotation (*2.2.7*): − 0.01° to + 0.01°.

Dissolve 2.50 g in *ethanol R* and dilute to 25.0 ml with the same solvent.

B. Infrared absorption spectrophotometry (*2.2.24*).

Comparison: *α-tocopheryl acetate CRS.*

C. Thin-layer chromatography (*2.2.27*).

Test solution. Dissolve about 10 mg of the substance to be examined in 2 ml of *cyclohexane R*.

Reference solution. Dissolve about 10 mg of *α-tocopheryl acetate CRS* in 2 ml of *cyclohexane R*.

Plate: *TLC silica gel F_{254} plate R.*

Mobile phase: *ether R, cyclohexane R* (20:80 *V/V*).

Application: 10 μl.

Development: over 2/3 of the plate.

Drying: in a current of air.

Detection: examine in ultraviolet light at 254 nm.

Results: the principal spot in the chromatogram obtained with the test solution is similar in position and size to the principal spot in the chromatogram obtained with the reference solution.

TESTS

Related substances. Gas chromatography (*2.2.28*): use the normalisation procedure.

Internal standard solution. Dissolve 1.0 g of *squalane R* in *cyclohexane R* and dilute to 100.0 ml with the same solvent.

Test solution (a). Dissolve 0.100 g of the substance to be examined in 10.0 ml of the internal standard solution.

Test solution (b). Dissolve 0.100 g of the substance to be examined in 10 ml of *cyclohexane R.*

Reference solution (a). Dissolve 0.100 g of *α-tocopheryl acetate CRS* in 10.0 ml of the internal standard solution.

Reference solution (b). Dissolve 10 mg of the substance to be examined and 10 mg of *α-tocopherol R* in *cyclohexane R* and dilute to 100.0 ml with the same solvent.

Reference solution (c). Dissolve 10 mg of *all-rac-α-tocopheryl acetate for peak identification CRS* in *cyclohexane R* and dilute to 1 ml with the same solvent.

Reference solution (d). Dilute 1.0 ml of test solution (b) to 100.0 ml with *cyclohexane R.* Dilute 1.0 ml of this solution to 10.0 ml with *cyclohexane R.*

Column:

- *material*: fused silica,
- *size*: *l* = 30 m, Ø = 0.25 mm,
- *stationary phase*: *poly(dimethyl)siloxane R* (film thickness 0.25 μm).

Carrier gas: *helium for chromatography R.*

Flow rate: 1 ml/min.

Split ratio: 1:100.

Temperature:

- *column*: 280 °C,
- *injection port and detector*: 290 °C.

Detection: flame ionisation.

Injection: 1 μl of test solution (b) and reference solutions (a), (b), (c) and (d).

Run time: twice the retention time of all-*rac*-α-tocopheryl acetate.

Relative retention with reference to all-*rac*-α-tocopheryl acetate (retention time = about 15 min): squalane = about 0.4; impurity A = about 0.7; impurity B = about 0.8; impurity C = about 0.9; use the chromatogram supplied with the CRS to identify the peaks due to impurities A and B in the chromatogram obtained with reference solution (c).

System suitability:

- *resolution*: minimum 3.5 between the peaks due to impurity C and all-*rac*-α-tocopheryl acetate in the chromatogram obtained with reference solution (b),
- in the chromatogram obtained with reference solution (a), the area of the peak due to impurity C is not greater than 0.2 per cent of the area of the peak due to all-*rac*-α-tocopheryl acetate.

Limits:

- *impurities A, C*: for each impurity, maximum 0.5 per cent,
- *impurity B*: maximum 1.5 per cent,
- *any other impurity*: for each impurity, maximum 0.25 per cent,
- *total*: maximum 2.5 per cent,
- *disregard limit*: the area of the principal peak in the chromatogram obtained with reference solution (d) (0.1 per cent).

ASSAY

Gas chromatography (*2.2.28*) as described in the test for related substances with the following modification.

Injection: test solution (a) and reference solution (a).

Calculate the percentage content of $C_{31}H_{52}O_3$ taking into account the declared content of *α-tocopheryl acetate CRS.*

STORAGE

Protected from light.

IMPURITIES

Specified impurities: A, B, C.

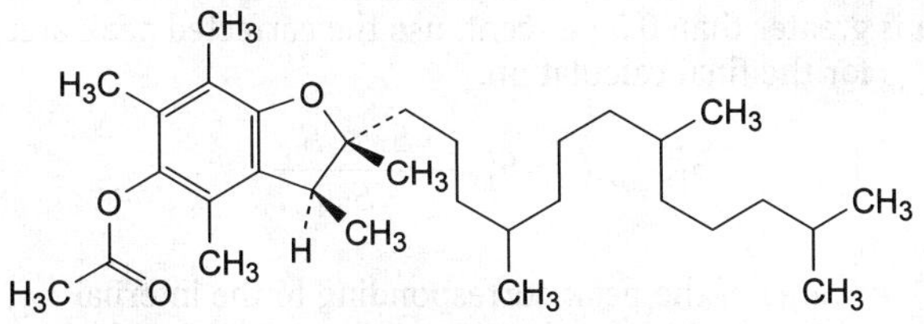

and diastereoisomers

A. all-*rac-trans*-2,3,4,6,7-pentamethyl-2-(4,8,12-trimethyltridecyl)-2,3-dihydrobenzofuran-5-yl acetate,

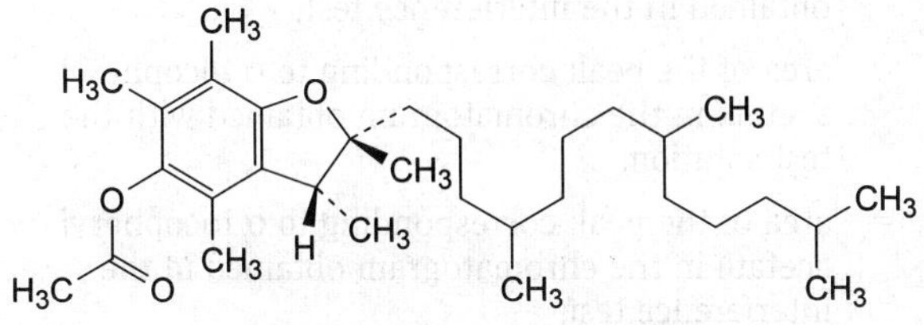

and diastereoisomers

B. all-*rac-cis*-2,3,4,6,7-pentamethyl-2-(4,8,12-trimethyltridecyl)-2,3-dihydrobenzofuran-5-yl acetate,

C. all-*rac*-α-tocopherol.

01/2005:1257

RRR-α-TOCOPHERYL ACETATE

RRR-α-Tocopherylis acetas

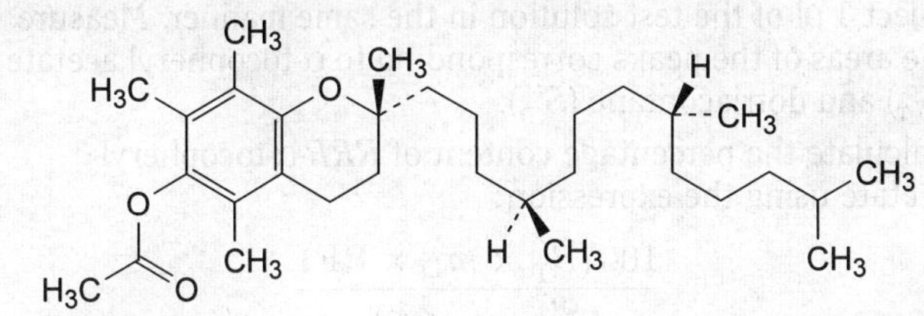

$C_{31}H_{52}O_3$ M_r 472.7

DEFINITION

RRR-α-Tocopheryl acetate contains not less than 96.0 per cent and not more than the equivalent of 102.0 per cent of (2*R*)-2,5,7,8-tetramethyl-2-[(4*R*,8*R*)-4,8,12-trimethyltridecyl]-3,4-dihydro-2*H*-1-benzopyran-6-yl acetate.

CHARACTERS

A clear, pale greenish-yellow, viscous, oily liquid, practically insoluble in water, freely soluble in acetone, in ethanol and in fatty oils, soluble in alcohol.

IDENTIFICATION

First identification: B, D.

Second identification: A, C, D.

A. It complies with the test for absorbance (see Tests).

B. Examine by infrared absorption spectrophotometry (*2.2.24*), comparing with the spectrum obtained with *α-tocopheryl acetate CRS*.

C. Examine by thin-layer chromatography (*2.2.27*), using a *TLC silica gel F_{254} plate R*.

Test solution (a). Dissolve 10 mg of the substance to be examined in 2 ml of *cyclohexane R*.

Test solution (b). In a ground glass-stoppered tube, dissolve 10 mg of the substance to be examined in 2 ml of *2.5 M alcoholic sulphuric acid R*. Heat on a water-bath for 5 min. Cool and add 2 ml of *water R* and 2 ml of *cyclohexane R*. Shake for 1 min. Use the upper layer.

Reference solution (a). Dissolve 10 mg of *α-tocopheryl acetate CRS* in 2 ml of *cyclohexane R*.

Reference solution (b). Prepare as described for test solution (b), using *α-tocopheryl acetate CRS* instead of the substance to be examined.

Apply separately to the plate 10 µl of each solution. Develop over a path of 15 cm using a mixture of 20 volumes of *ether R* and 80 volumes of *cyclohexane R*. Dry the plate in a current of air and examine in ultraviolet light at 254 nm. The principal spot in the chromatogram obtained with test solution (a) is similar in position and size to the principal spot in the chromatogram obtained with reference solution (a). In the chromatograms obtained with test solution (b) and reference solution (b), there are two spots: the spot with the higher R_f value is due to α-tocopheryl acetate and corresponds to the spot in the chromatogram obtained with reference solution (a); the spot with the lower R_f value is due to α-tocopheryl acetate and corresponds to the spot in the chromatogram obtained with reference solution (a); the spot with the lower R_f value is due to α-tocopherol. Spray the plate with a mixture of 10 volumes of *hydrochloric acid R*, 40 volumes of a 2.5 g/l solution of *ferric chloride R* in *alcohol R* and 40 volumes of a 10 g/l solution of *phenanthroline hydrochloride R* in *alcohol R*. In the chromatograms obtained with test solution (b) and reference solution (b), the spot due to α-tocopherol is orange.

D. After saponification, the resulting *RRR*-α-tocopherol is dextrorotatory (*2.2.7*). The specific optical rotation after oxidation to the quinone form is at least + 24.

Carry out the test avoiding exposure to actinic light. Transfer 1.0 g of the substance to be examined to a 250 ml round-bottomed flask with a ground-glass stopper; dissolve in 30 ml of *ethanol R* and heat under reflux for 3 min. While the solution is boiling, add, through the condenser, 20 ml of *2 M alcoholic potassium hydroxide solution R*. Continue heating under reflux for 20 min and, without cooling, add 4.0 ml of *hydrochloric acid R* dropwise through the condenser. Cool, rinse the condenser with 10 ml of *ethanol R*, transfer the contents of the flask to a 500 ml separating funnel. Rinse the flask with four quantities, each of 25 ml, of *water R* and four quantities, each of 25 ml, of *ether R*. Add the rinsings to the separating funnel. Shake vigorously for 2 min, allow the layers to separate and collect each of the two layers in individual separating funnels. Shake the aqueous layer with two quantities, each of 50 ml, of *ether R* and add these extracts to the main ether extract. Wash the combined ether extracts with four quantities, each of 100 ml, of *water R* and discard the washings.

To the ether solution add 40 ml of a 100 g/l solution of *potassium ferricyanide R* in an 8 g/l solution of *sodium hydroxide R* and shake for 3 min. Wash the ether solution with four quantities, each of 50 ml, of *water R*, discard the washings and dry the ether layer over *anhydrous sodium sulphate R*. Evaporate the ether on a water-bath under reduced pressure or in an atmosphere of nitrogen until a few millilitres remain, then complete the evaporation removing the last traces of ether without the application of heat. Immediately dissolve the residue in 25.0 ml of *trimethylpentane R* and determine the optical rotation.

Calculate the specific optical rotation of the substance in the test solution using as *c* the number of grams equivalent to *RRR*-α-tocopherol (factor 0.911) in 1000 ml.

TESTS

Absorbance (*2.2.25*). Dissolve 0.150 g in *ethanol R* and dilute to 100 ml with the same solvent. Dilute 10.0 ml of the solution to 100.0 ml with *ethanol R* (solution A). Dilute 20.0 ml of the initial solution to 50.0 ml with *ethanol R* (solution B). Measure the absorbance of solution A at the maximum at 284 nm and the absorbance of solution B at the minimum at 254 nm. The specific absorbance at the maximum is 42.0 to 45.0 and that at the minimum is 7.0 to 9.0.

Acid value (*2.5.1*). Not more than 2.0, determined on 2.00 g.

Free tocopherol. Not more than 1.0 per cent. Dissolve 0.500 g in 100 ml of *0.25 M alcoholic sulphuric acid R*. Add 20 ml of *water R* and 0.1 ml of a 2.5 g/l solution of *diphenylamine R* in *sulphuric acid R*. Titrate with *0.01 M ammonium and cerium sulphate* until a blue colour is obtained which persists for at least 5 s. Carry out a blank titration.

1 ml of *0.01 M ammonium and cerium sulphate* is equivalent to 2.154 mg of free tocopherol.

Heavy metals (*2.4.8*). 0.5 g complies with limit test D for heavy metals (20 ppm). Prepare the standard using 1 ml of *lead standard solution (10 ppm Pb) R*.

Sulphated ash (*2.4.14*). Not more than 0.1 per cent, determined on 1.0 g. Use *sulphuric acid R* instead of *dilute sulphuric acid R*.

ASSAY

Examine by gas chromatography (*2.2.28*), using *dotriacontane R* as the internal standard.

Internal standard solution. Dissolve 0.300 g of *dotriacontane R* in *hexane R* and dilute to 100.0 ml with the same solvent.

Test solution. Dissolve 0.100 g of the substance to be examined in 10.0 ml of the internal standard solution, dilute to 50.0 ml with *hexane R* and mix.

Reference solution. Dissolve 0.100 g of *α-tocopheryl acetate CRS* in 10.0 ml of the internal standard solution, dilute to 50.0 ml with *hexane R* and mix.

The chromatographic procedure may be carried out using:

- a fused-silica column 15 m long and 0.32 mm in internal diameter coated with a 0.25 µm layer of *poly(dimethyl)siloxane R*,
- *helium for chromatography R* as the carrier gas at a flow rate of 3 ml/min to 6 ml/min,
- a flame-ionisation detector,

maintaining the temperature of the injection port at 300 °C and that of the detector at 330 °C. Adjust the split ratio between 1 to 10 and 1 to 20. Set the temperature of the column at 200 °C, then raise the temperature at a rate of 5 °C per minute to 250 °C and maintain at 250 °C for 10 min.

Inject directly onto the column or via a glass-lined injection port using an automatic injection device or some other reproducible injection method. Measure the peak areas by electronic integration. The test is not valid unless: in the chromatogram obtained with the reference solution, the resolution between the peaks corresponding to dotriacontane and α-tocopheryl acetate is at least 4.0.

Interference test. Dissolve 0.100 g of the substance to be examined in *hexane R* and dilute to 50.0 ml with the same solvent. Inject 1 µl of the solution and record the chromatogram. If a peak is detected with the same t_R value as for dotriacontane, calculate the area of this peak relative to the peak area of α-tocopheryl acetate. If the relative peak area is greater than 0.5 per cent, use the corrected peak area $S'_{D(corr)}$ for the final calculation.

$$S'_{D(corr)} = S'_D - \frac{S_I \times S'_T}{S_{TI}}$$

S'_D = area of the peak corresponding to the internal standard in the chromatogram obtained with the test solution,

S_I = area of the interfering peak (same t_R value as that of the internal standard) in the chromatogram obtained in the interference test,

S'_T = area of the peak corresponding to α-tocopheryl acetate in the chromatogram obtained with the test solution,

S_{TI} = area of the peak corresponding to α-tocopheryl acetate in the chromatogram obtained in the interference test.

After the system suitability has been established, inject 1 µl of the reference solution and record the chromatogram. Measure the areas of the peaks corresponding to α-tocopheryl acetate (S_T) and dotriacontane (S_D) and determine the response factor (RF) as described below.

Determine the response factor (RF) for α-tocopheryl acetate in the chromatogram obtained with the reference solution from the areas of the peak corresponding to α-tocopheryl acetate and the peak corresponding to dotriacontane using the expression:

$$RF = \frac{S_D \times m_T}{S_T \times m_D}$$

Inject 1 µl of the test solution in the same manner. Measure the areas of the peaks corresponding to α-tocopheryl acetate (S'_T) and dotriacontane (S'_D).

Calculate the percentage content of *RRR*-α-tocopheryl acetate using the expression:

$$\frac{100\,(S'_T \times m_D \times RF)}{S'_{D(corr)} \times m}$$

S_D = area of the peak corresponding to the internal standard in the chromatogram obtained with the reference solution,

$S'_{D(corr)}$ = corrected area of the peak corresponding to the internal standard in the chromatogram obtained with the test solution,

S_T = area of the peak corresponding to *α-tocopheryl acetate CRS* in the chromatogram obtained with the reference solution,

S'_T = area of the peak corresponding to α-tocopheryl acetate in the chromatogram obtained with the test solution,

m_D = mass of the internal standard in the test solution and in the reference solution, in milligrams,

m_T = mass of *α-tocopheryl acetate CRS* in the reference solution, in milligrams,

m = mass of the substance to be examined in the test solution, in milligrams.

STORAGE

Store protected from light.

Monographs T-Z

01/2005:1258
corrected

DL-α-TOCOPHERYL HYDROGEN SUCCINATE

DL-α-Tocopherylis hydrogenosuccinas

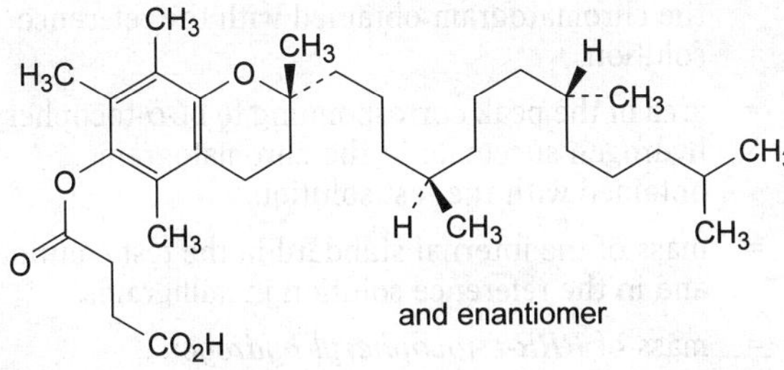

$C_{33}H_{54}O_5$ M_r 530.8

DEFINITION

DL-α-Tocopheryl hydrogen succinate contains not less than 96.0 per cent and not more than the equivalent of 102.0 per cent of (2*RS*)-2,5,7,8-tetramethyl-2-[(4*RS*,8*RS*)-4,8,12-trimethyltridecyl]-3,4-dihydro-2*H*-1-benzopyran-6-yl hydrogen succinate.

CHARACTERS

A white or almost white, crystalline powder, practically insoluble in water, soluble in acetone and in ethanol, very soluble in methylene chloride.

IDENTIFICATION

First identification: B, D.

Second identification: A, C, D.

A. It complies with the test for absorbance (see Tests).

B. Examine by infrared absorption spectrophotometry (*2.2.24*), comparing with the spectrum obtained with *RRR-α-tocopheryl hydrogen succinate CRS*.

C. Examine by thin-layer chromatography (*2.2.27*), using *silica gel HF_{254} R* as the coating substance.

Test solution (a). Dissolve 10 mg of the substance to be examined in 2 ml of *cyclohexane R*.

Test solution (b). In a ground glass-stoppered tube, dissolve 10 mg of the substance to be examined in 2 ml of *2.5 M alcoholic sulphuric acid R*. Heat on a water-bath for 5 min. Cool and add 2 ml of *water R* and 2 ml of *cyclohexane R*. Shake for 1 min. Use the upper layer.

Reference solution (a). Dissolve 10 mg of *RRR-α-tocopheryl hydrogen succinate CRS* in 2 ml of *cyclohexane R*.

Reference solution (b). Prepare as described for test solution (b), using *RRR-α-tocopheryl hydrogen succinate CRS* instead of the substance to be examined.

Apply to the plate 10 µl of each solution. Develop over a path of 15 cm using a mixture of 0.2 volumes of *glacial acetic acid R*, 20 volumes of *ether R* and 80 volumes of *cyclohexane R*. Dry the plate in a current of air and examine in ultraviolet light at 254 nm. The principal spot in the chromatogram obtained with test solution (a) is similar in position and size to the principal spot in the chromatogram obtained with the reference solution (a). In the chromatograms obtained with test solution (b) and reference solution (b), there are two spots: the spot with the higher R_f value is due to α-tocopherol, the spot with the lower R_f value is due to α-tocopheryl acid succinate and corresponds to the spot obtained with reference solution (a). Depending on the degree of hydrolysis, the lower spot may be weak or even absent. Spray the plate with a mixture of 10 volumes of *hydrochloric acid R*, 40 volumes of a 2.5 g/l solution of *ferric chloride R* in *alcohol R* and 40 volumes of a 10 g/l solution of *phenanthroline hydrochloride R* in *alcohol R*. In the chromatograms obtained with test solution (b) and reference solution (b), the spot due to α-tocopherol is orange.

D. It complies with the test for optical rotation (see Tests).

TESTS

Optical rotation (*2.2.7*). Dissolve 2.50 g in *ethanol R* and dilute to 25.0 ml with the same solvent. The angle of optical rotation is − 0.01° to + 0.01°.

Absorbance (*2.2.25*). Dissolve 0.150 g in *ethanol R* and dilute to 100 ml with the same solvent. Dilute 10.0 ml of the solution to 100.0 ml with *ethanol R* (solution a). Dilute 20.0 ml of the initial solution to 50.0 ml with *ethanol R* (solution b). Measure the absorbance of solution (a) at the maximum at 284 nm and the absorbance of solution (b) at the minimum at 254 nm. The specific absorbance at the maximum is 35 to 38 and that at the minimum is 6.0 to 8.0.

Acid value (*2.5.1*). Between 101 and 108, determined on 1.00 g.

Free tocopherol. Not more than 1.0 per cent. Dissolve 0.500 g in 100 ml of *0.25 M alcoholic sulphuric acid R*. Add 20 ml of *water R* and 0.1 ml of a 2.5 g/l solution of *diphenylamine R* in *sulphuric acid R*. Titrate with *0.01 M ammonium and cerium sulphate* until a blue colour is obtained which persists for at least 5 s. Carry out a blank titration.

1 ml of *0.01 M ammonium and cerium sulphate* is equivalent to 2.154 mg of free tocopherol.

Heavy metals (*2.4.8*). 0.50 g complies with limit test D for heavy metals (20 ppm). Prepare the reference solution using 1 ml of *lead standard solution (10 ppm Pb) R*.

Sulphated ash (*2.4.14*). Not more than 0.1 per cent, determined on 1.0 g. Use *sulphuric acid R* instead of *dilute sulphuric acid R*.

ASSAY

Examine by gas chromatography (*2.2.28*), using *dotriacontane R* as the internal standard.

Internal standard solution. Dissolve 0.300 g of *dotriacontane R* in *hexane R* and dilute to 100.0 ml with the same solvent.

Test solution. Weigh 30.0 mg of the substance to be examined into a 20 ml vial. Pipette 2.0 ml of *methanol R*, 1.0 ml of *dimethoxypropane R* and 0.1 ml of *hydrochloric acid R* into the vial. Cap tightly and sonicate the sample. Allow to stand in the dark for 1 h (± 5 min). Remove the sample from the dark, uncap and evaporate just to dryness on a steam bath with the aid of a stream of nitrogen. Pipette 10.0 ml of the internal standard solution into the sample vial. Vortex into solution.

Reference solution. Weigh 30.0 mg of *RRR-α-tocopheryl hydrogen succinate CRS* into a 20 ml vial, weigh to the nearest 0.01 mg. Pipette 2.0 ml of *methanol R*, 1.0 ml of *dimethoxypropane R* and 0.1 ml of *hydrochloric acid R* into the vial. Cap tightly and sonicate the reference solution. Allow to stand in the dark for 1 h (± 5 min). Remove the reference solution from the dark, uncap and evaporate just to dryness on a steam bath with the aid of a stream of nitrogen. Pipette 10.0 ml of the internal standard solution into the reference solution vial. Vortex into solution.

Monographs T-Z

The chromatographic procedure may be carried out using:
- a fused-silica open tubular capillary column 15 m long and 0.32 mm in internal diameter coated with a 0.25 μm layer of *poly(dimethyl)siloxane R*,
- *helium for chromatography R* as the carrier gas at a flow rate of 3 ml/min to 6 ml/min,
- a flame-ionisation detector,

maintaining the temperature of the injection port at 300 °C and that of the detector at 330 °C. Adjust the split ratio between 1 to 10 and 1 to 20. Set the temperature of the column at 200 °C, then raise the temperature at a rate of 5 °C per min to 250 °C and maintain at 250 °C for 10 min.

Inject directly onto the column or via a glass-lined injection port using an automatic injection device or some other reproducible injection method. Measure the peak areas by electronic integration. The test is not valid unless: in the chromatogram obtained with the reference solution, the resolution between the peaks corresponding to dotriacontane and α-tocopheryl hydrogen succinate is at least 12.0.

Interference test. Dissolve 0.100 g of the substance to be examined in *hexane R* and dilute to 50.0 ml with the same solvent. Inject 1 μl of the solution and record the chromatogram. If a peak is detected with the same t_R value as for dotriacontane, calculate the area of this peak relative to the peak area of the substance to be examined. If the relative peak area is greater than 0.5 per cent, use the corrected peak area $S'_{D(corr)}$ for the final calculation.

$$S'_{D(corr)} = S'_D - \frac{S_I \times S'_T}{S_{TI}}$$

S'_D = area of the peak corresponding to the internal standard in the chromatogram obtained with the test solution,

S_I = area of the interfering peak (same t_R value as that of the internal standard) in the chromatogram obtained in the interference test,

S'_T = area of the peak corresponding to α-tocopheryl hydrogen succinate in the chromatogram obtained with the test solution,

S_{TI} = area of the peak corresponding to α-tocopheryl hydrogen succinate in the chromatogram obtained in the interference test.

After the system suitability has been established, inject 1 μl of the reference solution and record the chromatogram. Measure the areas of the peaks corresponding the α-tocopheryl hydrogen succinate (S_T) and dotriacontane (S_D) and determine the response factor (RF) as described below.

Determine the response factor (RF) for α-tocopheryl hydrogen succinate in the chromatogram obtained with the reference solution from the area of the peak corresponding to α-tocopheryl hydrogen succinate and the peak corresponding to dotriacontane using the expression:

$$RF = \frac{S_D \times m_T}{S_T \times m_D}$$

Inject 1 μl of the test solution in the same manner. Measure the areas of the peaks corresponding to α-tocopheryl hydrogen succinate (S'_T) and dotriacontane (S'_D).

Calculate the percentage content of α-tocopheryl acid succinate using the expression:

$$\frac{100\,(S'_T \times m_D \times RF)}{S'_{D(corr)} \times m}$$

S_D = area of the peak corresponding to the internal standard in the chromatogram obtained with the reference solution,

$S'_{D(corr)}$ = corrected area of the peak corresponding to the internal standard in the chromatogram obtained with the test solution,

S_T = area of the peak corresponding to *RRR-α-tocopheryl hydrogen succinate CRS* in the chromatogram obtained with the reference solution,

S'_T = area of the peak corresponding to DL-α-tocopheryl hydrogen succinate in the chromatogram obtained with the test solution,

m_D = mass of the internal standard in the test solution and in the reference solution in milligrams,

m_T = mass of *RRR-α-tocopheryl hydrogen succinate CRS* in the reference solution, in milligrams,

m = mass of the substance to be examined in the test solution, in milligrams.

STORAGE

Store protected from light.

01/2005:1259
corrected

RRR-α-TOCOPHERYL HYDROGEN SUCCINATE

RRR-α-Tocopherylis hydrogenosuccinas

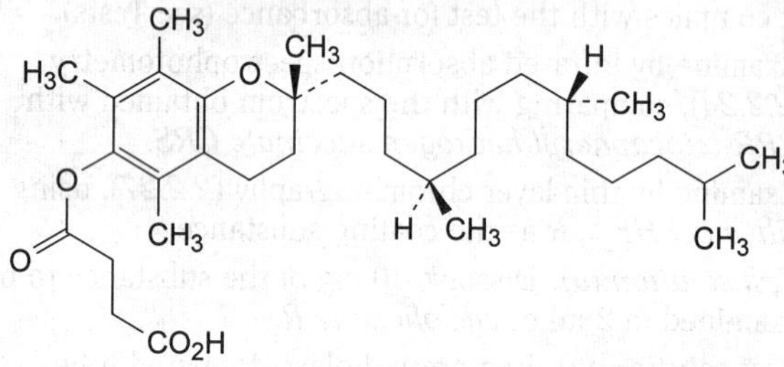

$C_{33}H_{54}O_5$ M_r 530.8

DEFINITION

RRR-α-Tocopheryl hydrogen succinate contains not less than 96.0 per cent and not more than the equivalent of 102.0 per cent of (2*R*)-2,5,7,8-tetramethyl-2-[(4*R*,8*R*)-4,8,12-trimethyltridecyl]-3,4-dihydro-2*H*-1-benzopyran-6-yl hydrogen succinate.

CHARACTERS

A white or almost white, crystalline powder, practically insoluble in water, soluble in acetone and in ethanol, very soluble in methylene chloride.

IDENTIFICATION

First identification: B, D.

Second identification: A, C, D.

A. It complies with the test for absorbance (see Tests).
B. Examine by infrared absorption spectrophotometry (*2.2.24*), comparing with the spectrum obtained with *RRR-α-tocopheryl hydrogen succinate CRS*.
C. Examine by thin-layer chromatography (*2.2.27*), using *silica gel HF_{254} R* as the coating substance.

Test solution (a). Dissolve 10 mg of the substance to be examined in 2 ml of *cyclohexane R*.

Test solution (b). In a ground-glass-stoppered tube, dissolve 10 mg of the substance to be examined in 2 ml of *2.5 M alcoholic sulphuric acid R*. Heat on a water-bath for 5 min. Cool and add 2 ml of *water R* and 2 ml of *cyclohexane R*. Shake for 1 min. Use the upper layer.

Reference solution (a). Dissolve 10 mg of *RRR-α-tocopheryl hydrogen succinate CRS* in 2 ml of *cyclohexane R*.

Reference solution (b). Prepare as described for test solution (b), using *RRR-α-tocopheryl hydrogen succinate CRS* instead of the substance to be examined.

Apply separately to the plate 10 µl of each solution. Develop over a path of 15 cm using a mixture of 0.2 volumes of *glacial acetic acid R*, 20 volumes of *ether R* and 80 volumes of *cyclohexane R*. Dry the plate in a current of air and examine in ultraviolet light at 254 nm. The principal spot in the chromatogram obtained with test solution (a) is similar in position and size to the principal spot in the chromatogram obtained with the reference solution (a). In the chromatograms obtained with test solution (b) and reference solution (b), there are two spots: the spot with the higher R_f value is due to α-tocopherol, the spot with the lower R_f value is due to α-tocopheryl hydrogen succinate and corresponds to the spot obtained with reference solution (a). Depending on the degree of hydrolysis, the lower spot may be weak or even absent. Spray the plate with a mixture of 10 volumes of *hydrochloric acid R*, 40 volumes of a 2.5 g/l solution of *ferric chloride R* in *alcohol R* and 40 volumes of a 10 g/l solution of *phenanthroline hydrochloride R* in *alcohol R*. In the chromatograms obtained with test solution (b) and reference solution (b), the spot due to α-tocopherol is orange.

D. After saponification, the resulting *RRR*-α-tocopherol is dextrorotatory (*2.2.7*). The specific optical rotation after oxidation to the quinone form is at least + 24.

Carry out the test avoiding exposure to actinic light. Transfer 1.0 g of the substance to be examined to a round bottomed, ground-glass-stoppered, 250 ml flask and dissolve in 30 ml of *ethanol R* and heat under reflux for 3 min. While the solution is boiling, add, through the condenser, 20 ml of *2 M alcoholic potassium hydroxide solution R*. Continue heating under reflux for 20 min and, without cooling, add 4.0 ml of *hydrochloric acid R* dropwise through the condenser. Cool, rinse the condenser with 10 ml of *ethanol R*, transfer the contents of the flask to a 500 ml separating funnel, rinse the flask with four quantities, each of 25 ml, of *water R* and four quantities, each of 25 ml, of *ether R*. Add the rinsings to the separating funnel. Shake vigorously for 2 min, allow the layers to separate and collect each of the two layers in individual separating funnels. Shake the aqueous layer with two quantities, each of 50 ml, of *ether R* and add these extracts to the main ether extract. Wash the combined ether extracts with four quantities, each of 100 ml, of *water R* and discard the washings.

To the ether solution add 40 ml of a 100 g/l solution of *potassium ferricyanide R* in an 8 g/l solution of *sodium hydroxide R* and shake for 3 min. Wash the ether solution with four quantities, each of 50 ml, of *water R*, discard the washings and dry the ether layer over *anhydrous sodium sulphate R*. Evaporate the ether on a water-bath under reduced pressure or in an atmosphere of nitrogen until a few millilitres remain, then complete the evaporation removing the last traces of ether without the application of heat. Immediately dissolve the residue in 25.0 ml of *trimethylpentane R* and determine the optical rotation.

Calculate the specific optical rotation of the substance in the test solution using as *c* the number of grams equivalent to α-tocopherol (factor 0.811) in 1000 ml.

TESTS

Absorbance (*2.2.25*). Dissolve 0.150 g in *ethanol R* and dilute to 100 ml with the same solvent. Dilute 10.0 ml of the solution to 100.0 ml with *ethanol R* (solution a). Dilute 20.0 ml of the initial solution to 50.0 ml with *ethanol R* (solution b). Measure the absorbance of solution (a) at the maximum at 284 nm and the absorbance of solution (b) at the minimum at 254 nm. The specific absorbance at the maximum is 35 to 38 and that at the minimum is 6.0 to 8.0.

Acid value (*2.5.1*). Between 101 and 108, determined on 1.00 g.

Free tocopherol. Not more than 1.0 per cent. Dissolve 0.500 g in 100 ml of *0.25 M alcoholic sulphuric acid R*. Add 20 ml of *water R* and 0.1 ml of a 2.5 g/l solution of *diphenylamine R* in *sulphuric acid R*. Titrate with *0.01 M ammonium and cerium sulphate* until a blue colour is obtained which persists for at least 5 s. Carry out a blank titration.

1 ml of *0.01 M ammonium and cerium sulphate* is equivalent to 2.154 mg of free tocopherol.

Heavy metals (*2.4.8*). 0.50 g complies with limit test D for heavy metals (20 ppm). Prepare the reference solution using 1 ml of *lead standard solution (10 ppm Pb) R*.

Sulphated ash (*2.4.14*). Not more than 0.1 per cent, determined on 1.0 g. Use *sulphuric acid R* instead of *dilute sulphuric acid R*.

ASSAY

Examine by gas chromatography (*2.2.28*), using *dotriacontane R* as the internal standard.

Internal standard solution. Dissolve 0.300 g of *dotriacontane R* in *hexane R* and dilute to 100.0 ml with the same solvent.

Test solution. Weigh 30.0 mg of the substance to be examined into a 20 ml vial. Pipette 2.0 ml of *methanol R*, 1.0 ml of *dimethoxypropane R* and 0.1 ml of *hydrochloric acid R* into the vial. Cap tightly and sonicate the sample. Allow to stand in the dark for 1 h (± 5 min). Remove the sample from the dark, uncap and evaporate just to dryness on a steam bath with the aid of a stream of nitrogen. Pipette 10.0 ml of the internal standard solution into the sample vial. Vortex into solution.

Reference solution. Weigh 30.0 mg of *RRR-α-tocopheryl hydrogen succinate CRS* into a 20 ml vial. Pipette 2.0 ml of *methanol R*, 1.0 ml of *dimethoxypropane R* and 0.1 ml of *hydrochloric acid R* into the vial. Cap tightly and sonicate the reference solution. Allow to stand in the dark for 1 h (± 5 min). Remove the reference solution from the dark, uncap and evaporate just to dryness on a steam bath with the aid of a stream of nitrogen. Pipette 10.0 ml of the internal standard solution into the reference solution vial. Vortex into solution.

The chromatographic procedure may be carried out using:

- a fused-silica open tubular capillary column 15 m long and 0.32 mm in internal diameter coated with a 0.25 µm layer of *poly(dimethyl)siloxane R*,
- *helium for chromatography R* as the carrier gas at a flow rate of 3 ml/min to 6 ml/min,
- a flame-ionisation detector,

maintaining the temperature of the injection port at 300 °C and that of the detector at 330 °C. Adjust the split ratio between 1 to 10 and 1 to 20. Set the temperature of the column at 200 °C, then raise the temperature at a rate of 5 °C per min to 250 °C and maintain at 250 °C for 10 min.

Inject directly onto the column or via a glass-lined injection port using an automatic injection device or some other reproducible injection method. Measure the peak areas by electronic integration. The test is not valid unless: in the chromatogram obtained with the reference solution, the resolution between the peaks corresponding to dotriacontane and α-tocopheryl hydrogen succinate is at least 12.0.

Interference test. Dissolve 0.100 g of the solution to be examined in *hexane R* and dilute to 50.0 ml with the same solvent. Inject 1 µl of the solution and record the chromatogram. If a peak is detected with the same t_R value as for dotriacontane, calculate the area of this peak relative to the peak area of α-tocopheryl succinate. If the relative peak area is greater than 0.5 per cent, use the corrected peak area $S'_{D(corr)}$ for the final calculation.

$$S'_{D(corr)} = S'_D - \frac{S_I \times S'_T}{S_{TI}}$$

S'_D = area of the peak corresponding to the internal standard in the chromatogram obtained with the test solution,

S_I = area of the interfering peak (same t_R value as that of the internal standard) in the chromatogram obtained in the interference test,

S'_T = area of the peak corresponding to α-tocopheryl hydrogen succinate in the chromatogram obtained with the test solution,

S_{TI} = area of the peak corresponding to α-tocopheryl hydrogen succinate in the chromatogram obtained in the interference test.

After the system suitability has been established, inject 1 µl of the reference solution and record the chromatogram. Measure the areas of the peaks corresponding the α-tocopheryl hydrogen succinate (S_T) and dotriacontane (S_D) and determine the response factor (RF) as described below.

Determine the response factor (RF) for α-tocopheryl hydrogen succinate in the chromatogram obtained with the reference solution from the area of the peak corresponding to α-tocopheryl hydrogen succinate and the peak corresponding to dotriacontane using the expression:

$$RF = \frac{S_D \times m_T}{S_T \times m_D}$$

Inject 1 µl of the test solution in the same manner. Measure the areas of the peaks corresponding to α-tocopheryl hydrogen succinate (S'_T) and dotriacontane (S'_D).

Calculate the percentage content of a-tocopheryl hydrogen succinate using the expression:

$$\frac{100\,(S'_T \times m_D \times RF)}{S'_{D(corr)} \times m}$$

S_D = area of the peak corresponding to the internal standard in the chromatogram obtained with the reference solution,

$S'_{D(corr)}$ = corrected area of the peak corresponding to the internal standard in the chromatogram obtained with the test solution,

S_T = area of the peak corresponding to *RRR-α-tocopheryl hydrogen succinate CRS* in the chromatogram obtained with the reference solution,

S'_T = area of the peak corresponding to α-tocopheryl hydrogen succinate in the chromatogram obtained with the test solution,

m_D = mass of the internal standard in the test solution and in the reference solution, in milligrams,

m_T = mass of *RRR-α-tocopheryl hydrogen succinate CRS* in the reference solution in milligrams,

m = mass of the substance to be examined in the test solution, in milligrams.

STORAGE

Store protected from light.

01/2005:0304

TOLBUTAMIDE

Tolbutamidum

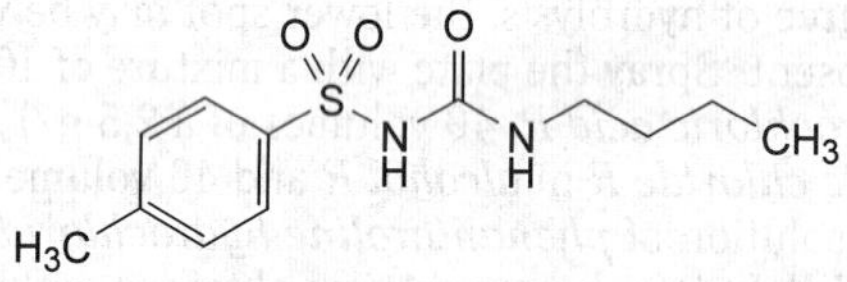

$C_{12}H_{18}N_2O_3S$ M_r 270.3

DEFINITION

Tolbutamide contains not less than 99.0 per cent and not more than the equivalent of 101.0 per cent of 1-butyl-3-[(4-methylphenyl)sulphonyl]urea, calculated with reference to the dried substance.

CHARACTERS

A white, crystalline powder, practically insoluble in water, soluble in acetone and in alcohol. It dissolves in dilute solutions of alkali hydroxides.

IDENTIFICATION

First identification: A, C.

Second identification: A, B, D.

A. Melting point (*2.2.14*): 126 °C to 130 °C.

B. Dissolve 25.0 mg in *methanol R* and dilute to 100.0 ml with the same solvent. Examined between 245 nm and 300 nm (*2.2.25*), the solution shows three absorption maxima, at 258 nm, 263 nm and 275 nm, and a shoulder at 268 nm. Dilute 10.0 ml of the solution to 250.0 ml with *methanol R*. Examined between 220 nm and 235 nm, the solution shows a single absorption maximum, at 228 nm. The specific absorbance at this maximum is 480 to 520.

C. Examine by infrared absorption spectrophotometry (*2.2.24*), comparing with the spectrum obtained with *tolbutamide CRS*.

D. To 0.2 g add 8 ml of a 500 g/l solution of *sulphuric acid R* and heat under a reflux condenser for 30 min. Allow to cool. Crystals are formed which, after recrystallisation from hot *water R* and drying at 100 °C to 105 °C, melt (*2.2.14*) at 135 °C to 140 °C.

TESTS

Appearance of solution. Dissolve 0.2 g in 5 ml of *dilute sodium hydroxide solution R* and add 5 ml of *water R*. The solution is clear (*2.2.1*) and colourless (*2.2.2, Method II*).

pH (*2.2.3*). To 2.0 g add 50 ml of *carbon dioxide-free water R* and heat at 70 °C for 5 min. Cool rapidly and filter. The pH of the filtrate is 4.5 to 5.5.

Related substances. Examine by thin-layer chromatography (*2.2.27*), using *silica gel G R* as the coating substance.

Test solution. Dissolve 0.50 g of the substance to be examined in *acetone R* and dilute to 10 ml with the same solvent.

Reference solution (a). Dissolve 15 mg of *toluenesulphonamide R* in *acetone R* and dilute to 100 ml with the same solvent.

Reference solution (b). To 5 ml of the test solution add 5 ml of reference solution (a).

Apply to the plate 5 µl of the test solution and of reference solution (a) and 10 µl of reference solution (b). Develop over a path of 15 cm using a mixture of 2 volumes of *anhydrous formic acid R*, 8 volumes of *methanol R* and 90 volumes of *chloroform R*. Dry the plate in a current of warm air and heat at 110 °C for 10 min. At the bottom of a chromatography tank, place an evaporating dish containing a 50 g/l solution of *potassium permanganate R* and add an equal volume of *hydrochloric acid R*. Place the plate whilst still hot in the tank and close the tank. Leave the plate in contact with the chlorine vapour for 2 min. Withdraw the plate and place it in a current of cold air until the excess of chlorine is removed and an area of coating below the points of application gives at most a very faint blue colour with a drop of *potassium iodide and starch solution R*; avoid prolonged exposure to cold air. Spray with *potassium iodide and starch solution R* and allow to stand for 5 min. Any spot in the chromatogram obtained with the test solution, apart from the principal spot, is not more intense than the spot in the chromatogram obtained with reference solution (a) (0.3 per cent). The test is not valid unless the chromatogram obtained with reference solution (b) shows two clearly separated spots.

Heavy metals (*2.4.8*). Dissolve 1.0 g in a mixture of 15 volumes of *water R* and 85 volumes of *acetone R* and dilute to 20 ml with the same mixture of solvents. 12 ml of the solution complies with limit test B for heavy metals (20 ppm). Prepare the standard using lead standard solution (1 ppm Pb) obtained by diluting *lead standard solution (100 ppm Pb) R* with a mixture of 15 volumes of *water R* and 85 volumes of *acetone R*.

Loss on drying (*2.2.32*). Not more than 0.5 per cent, determined on 1.000 g by drying in an oven at 100 °C to 105 °C.

Sulphated ash (*2.4.14*). Not more than 0.1 per cent, determined on 1.0 g.

ASSAY

Dissolve 0.2500 g in a mixture of 20 ml of *water R* and 40 ml of *alcohol R*. Titrate with *0.1 M sodium hydroxide*, using 1 ml of *phenolphthalein solution R* as indicator.

1 ml of *0.1 M sodium hydroxide* is equivalent to 27.03 mg of $C_{12}H_{18}N_2O_3S$.

01/2005:2039

TOLFENAMIC ACID

Acidum tolfenamicum

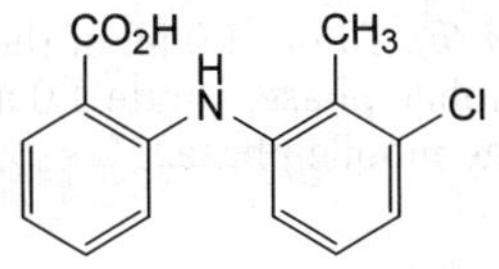

$C_{14}H_{12}ClNO_2$ M_r 261.7

DEFINITION

2-[(3-Chloro-2-methylphenyl)amino]benzoic acid.

Content: 99.0 per cent to 101.0 per cent (dried substance).

CHARACTERS

Appearance: white or slightly yellow, crystalline powder.

Solubility: practically insoluble in water, soluble in dimethylformamide, sparingly soluble in ethanol and in methylene chloride. It dissolves in dilute solutions of alkali hydroxides.

mp: about 213 °C.

IDENTIFICATION

First identification: B.

Second identification: A, C.

A. Dissolve 20 mg in a mixture of 1 volume of *1 M hydrochloric acid* and 99 volumes of *methanol R* and dilute to 100 ml with the same mixture of solvents. Dilute 5.0 ml of the solution to 50 ml with a mixture of 1 volume of *1 M hydrochloric acid* and 99 volumes of *methanol R*. Examined between 250 nm and 380 nm (*2.2.25*), the solution shows 2 absorption maxima, at 286 nm and 345 nm. The ratio of the absorbance measured at the maximum at 286 nm to that measured at the maximum at 345 nm is 1.2 to 1.4.

B. Infrared absorption spectrophotometry (*2.2.24*).
Comparison: *tolfenamic acid CRS*.

C. Thin-layer chromatography (*2.2.27*).
Test solution. Dissolve 25 mg of the substance to be examined in a mixture of 1 volume of *methanol R* and 3 volumes of *methylene chloride R* and dilute to 10 ml with the same mixture of solvents.
Reference solution. Dissolve 25 mg of *tolfenamic acid CRS* in a mixture of 1 volume of *methanol R* and 3 volumes of *methylene chloride R* and dilute to 10 ml with the same mixture of solvents.
Plate: *TLC silica gel GF_{254} plate R.*
Mobile phase: *glacial acetic acid R, dioxan R, toluene R* (1:25:90 *V/V/V*).
Application: 10 µl.
Development: over 2/3 of the plate.
Drying: in a current of warm air.
Detection: ultraviolet light at 254 nm.
Results: the principal spot in the chromatogram obtained with the test solution is similar in position, colour and size to the principal spot in the chromatogram obtained with the reference solution.

TESTS

Related substances. Liquid chromatography (*2.2.29*).
Test solution. Dissolve 50.0 mg of the substance to be examined in 5 ml of *ethanol R* and dilute to 50.0 ml with the mobile phase.

Monographs T-Z

Reference solution (a). Dissolve 25 mg of *2-chlorobenzoic acid R* and 25 mg of *3-chloro-2-methylaniline R* in 5 ml of *ethanol R* and dilute to 50.0 ml with the mobile phase. Dilute 1.0 ml of the solution to 50.0 ml with the mobile phase. Dilute 1.0 ml of this solution to 10.0 ml with the mobile phase.

Reference solution (b). Dilute 1.0 ml of the test solution to 10.0 ml with the mobile phase. Dilute 1.0 ml of this solution to 100.0 ml with the mobile phase.

Column:

- *size*: *l* = 0.25 m, Ø = 4.6 mm,
- *stationary phase*: *spherical end-capped octadecylsilyl silica gel for chromatography R* (5 µm) with a specific surface area of 450 m²/g and a pore size of 8 nm.

Mobile phase: *glacial acetic acid R, water R, ethanol R* (2:350:650 *V/V/V*).

Flow rate: 0.8 ml/min.

Detection: spectrophotometer at 232 nm.

Injection: 20 µl.

Run time: 3 times the retention time of tolfenamic acid.

Relative retention with reference to tolfenamic acid (retention time = about 15 min): impurity A = about 0.25; impurity B = about 0.34.

System suitability: reference solution (a):

- *resolution*: minimum 2.5 between the peaks due to impurity A and to impurity B.

Limits:

- *impurity A*: not more than the area of the corresponding peak in the chromatogram obtained with reference solution (a) (0.1 per cent),
- *impurity B*: not more than half the area of the corresponding peak in the chromatogram obtained with reference solution (a) (0.05 per cent),
- *any other impurity*: not more than the area of the principal peak in the chromatogram obtained with reference solution (b) (0.1 per cent),
- *total*: not more than 5 times the area of the principal peak in the chromatogram obtained with reference solution (b) (0.5 per cent),
- *disregard limit*: 0.1 times the area of the principal peak in the chromatogram obtained with reference solution (b) (0.01 per cent).

Copper: maximum 10 ppm.

Atomic absorption spectrometry (*2.2.23, Method I*).

Test solution. Place 1.00 g of the substance to be examined in a silica crucible, moisten with *sulphuric acid R,* heat cautiously on a flame for 30 min and then progressively to about 650 °C. Continue ignition until all black particles have disappeared. Allow to cool, dissolve the residue in *0.1 M hydrochloric acid* and dilute to 25.0 ml with the same acid.

Reference solutions. Prepare the reference solutions using *copper standard solution (0.1 per cent Cu) R,* diluted as necessary using *0.1 M nitric acid.*

Source: copper hollow-cathode lamp.

Wavelength: 324.8 nm.

Flame: air-acetylene.

Loss on drying (*2.2.32*): maximum 0.5 per cent, determined on 1.000 g by drying in an oven at 100-105 °C.

Sulphated ash (*2.4.14*): maximum 0.1 per cent, determined on 1.0 g.

ASSAY

Dissolve 0.200 g with the aid of ultrasound in 100 ml of *ethanol R.* Add 0.1 ml of *phenol red solution R* and titrate with *0.1 M sodium hydroxide.*

1 ml of *0.1 M sodium hydroxide* is equivalent to 26.17 mg of $C_{14}H_{12}ClNO_2$.

STORAGE

Protected from light.

IMPURITIES

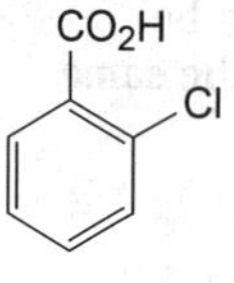

A. 2-chlorobenzoic acid,

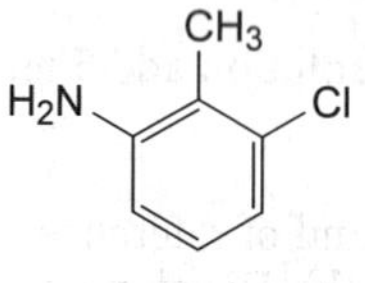

B. 3-chloro-2-methylaniline,

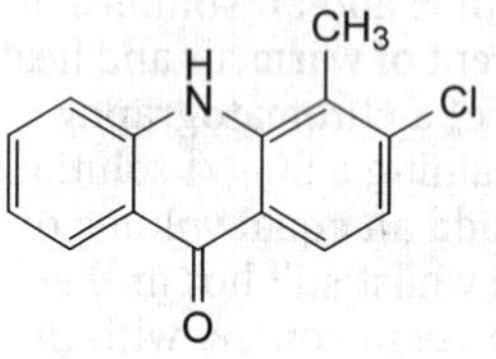

C. 3-chloro-4-methyl-9-oxo-9,10-dihydroacridine.

01/2005:1158

TOLNAFTATE

Tolnaftatum

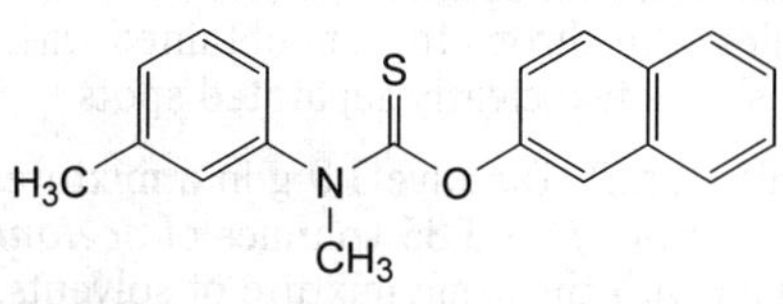

$C_{19}H_{17}NOS$ M_r 307.4

DEFINITION

Tolnaftate contains not less than 97.0 per cent and not more than the equivalent of 103.0 per cent of *O*-naphthalen-2-yl methyl(3-methylphenyl)thiocarbamate, calculated with reference to the dried substance.

CHARACTERS

A white or yellowish-white powder, practically insoluble in water, freely soluble in acetone and in methylene chloride, very slightly soluble in alcohol.

IDENTIFICATION

First identification: B.

Second identification: A, C, D.

A. Melting point (*2.2.14*): 109 °C to 112 °C.

B. Examine by infrared absorption spectrophotometry (*2.2.24*), comparing with the spectrum obtained with *tolnaftate CRS.* Examine the substances prepared as discs.

C. Examine the chromatograms obtained in the test for related substances. The principal spot in the chromatogram obtained with test solution (b) is similar in position and size to the principal spot in the chromatogram obtained with reference solution (a).

D. Mix about 1 mg with 0.5 ml of *sulphuric acid R*. Add 0.05 ml of *formaldehyde solution R*. A greenish-blue colour develops.

TESTS

Appearance of solution. Dissolve 0.5 g in 10 ml of *acetone R*. The solution is clear (*2.2.1*) and not more intensely coloured than reference solution Y_6 (*2.2.2, Method II*).

Related substances. Examine by thin-layer chromatography (*2.2.27*), using *silica gel GF_{254} R* as the coating substance.

Test solution (a). Dissolve 0.10 g of the substance to be examined in *acetone R* and dilute to 2 ml with the same solvent.

Test solution (b). Dilute 0.5 ml of test solution (a) to 10 ml with *acetone R*.

Reference solution (a). Dissolve 25 mg of *tolnaftate CRS* in *acetone R* and dilute to 10 ml with the same solvent.

Reference solution (b). Dilute 1 ml of test solution (b) to 10 ml with *acetone R*.

Reference solution (c). Dissolve 50 mg of *β-naphthol R* in 1 ml of test solution (a) and dilute to 10 ml with *acetone R*.

Apply separately to the plate 5 µl of each solution. Develop over a path of 12 cm using *toluene R*. Allow the plate to dry in air and examine in ultraviolet light at 254 nm. Any spot in the chromatogram obtained with test solution (a), apart from the principal spot, is not more intense than the spot in the chromatogram obtained with reference solution (b) (0.5 per cent). The test is not valid unless the chromatogram obtained with reference solution (c) shows two clearly separated spots.

Loss on drying (*2.2.32*). Not more than 0.5 per cent, determined on 1.000 g by drying at 60 °C at a pressure not exceeding 0.7 kPa for 3 h.

Sulphated ash (*2.4.14*). Not more than 0.1 per cent, determined on 1.0 g.

ASSAY

Dissolve 50.0 mg in *methanol R* and dilute to 250.0 ml with the same solvent. Dilute 2.0 ml to 50.0 ml with *methanol R*. Measure the absorbance (*2.2.25*) at the maximum at 257 nm.

Calculate the content of $C_{19}H_{17}NOS$ taking the specific absorbance to be 720.

STORAGE

Store protected from light.

IMPURITIES

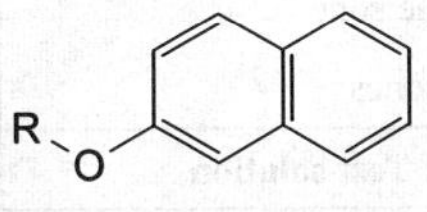

A. R = H: naphthalen-2-ol (β-naphtol),

C. R = CS-Cl: *O*-naphthalen-2-yl chlorothioformate,

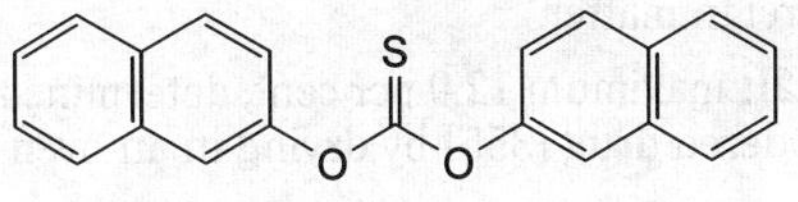

B. *O,O*-dinaphtalen-2-yl thiocarbonate,

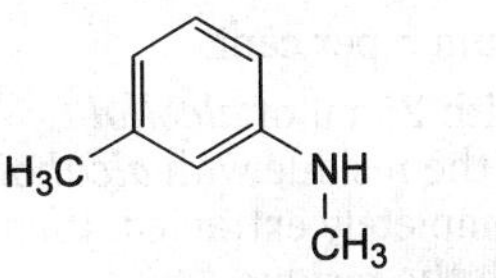

D. *N*,3-dimethylaniline.

01/2005:1596

TOLU BALSAM

Balsamum tolutanum

DEFINITION

Oleo-resin obtained from the trunk of *Myroxylon balsamum* (L.) Harms var. *balsamum*.

Content: 25.0 per cent to 50.0 per cent of free or combined acids, expressed as cinnamic acid ($C_9H_8O_2$; M_r 148.2) (dried drug).

CHARACTERS

Appearance: hard, friable, brownish to reddish-brown mass; thin fragments are brownish-yellow when examined against the light.

Reminiscent odour of vanillin.

Solubility: practically insoluble in water, very soluble to freely soluble in alcohol, practically insoluble in light petroleum.

IDENTIFICATION

Thin-layer chromatography (*2.2.27*).

Test solution. Stir 0.40 g of the fragmented drug with 10 ml of *methylene chloride R* for 5 min and filter.

Reference solution. Dissolve 50 mg of *benzyl cinnamate R* in *methylene chloride R*, add 50 µl of *benzyl benzoate R* and dilute to 10 ml with *methylene chloride R*.

Plate: *TLC silica gel G plate R*.

Mobile phase: *light petroleum R, toluene R* (5:95 *V/V*).

Application: 20 µl, as bands.

Development: over a path of 15 cm.

Drying: in air.

Detection: spray with *vanillin reagent R* and heat at 100-105 °C for 5 min. Examine in daylight.

Results: see below the sequence of the zones present in the chromatograms obtained with the test and reference solutions. Furthermore, other coloured zones are present in the chromatogram obtained with the test solution.

Top of the plate	
Benzyl benzoate: a greyish-blue zone	a greyish-blue zone
Benzyl cinnamate: a greyish-green zone	a greyish-green zone
Reference solution	**Test solution**

TESTS

Acid value: 100 to 160.

Dissolve 0.5 g of the fragmented drug in 50 ml of *alcohol R*. Add 0.5 ml of *acid blue 93 solution R* and 5.0 ml of *0.5 M alcoholic potassium hydroxide*. Stir vigorously and titrate with *0.5 M hydrochloric acid* until the colour changes from brownish-red to blackish-green (n_1 ml of *0.5 M hydrochloric acid*). Carry out a blank test in the same manner (n_2 ml of *0.5 M hydrochloric acid*). Calculate the acid value in the same manner as the saponification value (*2.5.6*).

Matter insoluble in alcohol: maximum 5 per cent.

Boil 2.0 g of the fragmented drug with 25 ml of *alcohol (90 per cent V/V) R* and filter. Wash the residue with *alcohol (90 per cent V/V) R*, boiling until completely extracted, then dry the residue at 100-105 °C. Weigh the residue.

Loss on drying (*2.2.32*): maximum 5.0 per cent, determined on 2.000 g of the fragmented drug by spreading on a flat evaporating dish 9 cm in diameter and allowing to dry *in vacuo* for 4 h.

Total ash (*2.4.16*): maximum 0.3 per cent.

ASSAY

Boil 1.500 g under a reflux condenser with 25 ml of *0.5 M alcoholic potassium hydroxide* for 1 h. Evaporate the ethanol and heat the residue with 50 ml of *water R* until the substance is homogeneously distributed. After cooling, add 80 ml of *water R* and a solution of 1.5 g of *magnesium sulphate R* in 50 ml of *water R*. Mix, and allow to stand for 10 min. Filter through a pleated filter paper and wash the residue with 20 ml of *water R*. Combine the filtrate and the washings, acidify with *hydrochloric acid R* and extract with 4 quantities, each of 40 ml, of *ether R*. Discard the aqueous layer. Combine the organic extracts and wash with 2 quantities, each of 20 ml, and with 3 quantities, each of 10 ml, of a 50 g/l solution of *sodium bicarbonate R*. Discard the ether layer. Combine the aqueous extracts, acidify with *hydrochloric acid R* and stir once with 30 ml, twice with 20 ml and once with 10 ml of *methylene chloride R*. Dry the combined methylene chloride extracts over *anhydrous sodium sulphate R*. Filter through a pleated filter and wash the residue with 10 ml of *methylene chloride R*. Reduce the combined methylene chloride extracts to 10 ml by distillation and eliminate the remaining methylene chloride in a current of air. Dissolve the residue with heating in 10 ml of *alcohol R* previously neutralised to *phenol red solution R*. After cooling, titrate with *0.1 M sodium hydroxide*, using the same indicator.

1 ml of *0.1 M sodium hydroxide* is equivalent to 14.82 mg of total acids, expressed as cinnamic acid.

STORAGE

Do not store in powdered form.

01/2005:1478

TORMENTIL

Tormentillae rhizoma

DEFINITION

Whole or cut, dried rhizome, freed from the roots, of *Potentilla erecta* (L.) Raeusch. (*P. tormentilla* Stokes).

Content: minimum 7 per cent of tannins, expressed as pyrogallol ($C_6H_6O_3$; M_r 126.1) (dried drug).

CHARACTERS

Macroscopic and microscopic characters described under identification tests A and B.

IDENTIFICATION

A. The rhizome is cylindrically spindle-shaped, with a very irregular appearance, often forming, twisted, knotty tubers, up to 10 cm long and 1 cm to 2 cm thick, very hard and scarcely branched. The surface is brown to reddish-brown, rugose and has remains of roots and transversely elongated depressed whitish scars from the stems. At the top of the rhizome the remains of numerous aerial stems may be present. The fracture is short and granular, dark red to brownish-yellow.

B. Reduce to a powder (355). The powder is reddish-brown. Examine under a microscope using *chloral hydrate solution R*. The powder shows the following diagnostic characters: coarsely serrate cluster crystals of calcium oxalate, up to 60 µm in diameter; fragments of thin-walled parenchyma containing reddish-brown tannin; groups of narrow, bordered-pitted vessels with lateral pores; thick-walled and pitted, polygonal parenchyma; groups and fragments of sclerenchymatous thick-walled fibres; occasional fragments of cork with thin-walled, brown, tabular cells. Examine under a microscope using a 50 per cent *V/V* solution of *glycerol R*. The powder shows spherical or elliptical starch granules, up to about 20 µm in length.

C. Thin-layer chromatography (*2.2.27*).

Test solution. To 0.5 g of the powdered drug (355) add 10 ml of *water R*, shake for 10 min and filter. Shake the filtrate with 2 quantities, each of 10 ml, of *ethyl acetate R* and filter the combined upper phases over 6 g of *anhydrous sodium sulphate R*. Evaporate the filtrate to dryness under reduced pressure and dissolve the residue in 1.0 ml of *ethyl acetate R*.

Reference solution. Dissolve 1.0 mg of *catechin R* in 1.0 ml of *methanol R*.

Plate: *TLC silica gel plate R*.

Mobile phase: *glacial acetic acid R, ether R, hexane R, ethyl acetate R* (20:20:20:40 *V/V/V/V*).

Application: 10 µl, as bands.

Development: over a path of 10 cm.

Drying: in air for 10-15 min.

Detection: spray with a freshly prepared 5 g/l solution of *fast blue B salt R*. Reddish zones appear. Expose the plate to ammonia vapour, the zones become more intense turning reddish-brown. Examine in daylight.

Results: see below the sequence of the zones present in the chromatograms obtained with the reference solution and the test solution. Furthermore, other fainter zones are present in the chromatogram obtained with the test solution.

Top of the plate	
Catechin: an intense reddish-brown zone	A more intense reddish-brown zone (catechin)
	A fainter zone
	An intense zone
	Fainter zones
Reference solution	**Test solution**

TESTS

Foreign matter (*2.8.2*): maximum 3 per cent of root and stems as well as rhizomes with black fracture and maximum 2 per cent of other foreign matter.

Loss on drying (*2.8.32*): maximum 12.0 per cent, determined on 1.000 g of the powdered drug (355) by drying in an oven at 100-105 °C for 2 h.

Total ash (*2.4.16*): maximum 5.0 per cent.

ASSAY

Carry out the determination of tannins in herbal drugs (*2.8.14*). Use 0.500 g of the powdered drug (180).

01/2005:1895

TORMENTIL TINCTURE

Tormentillae tinctura

DEFINITION

Tincture produced from *Tormentil (1478).*

Content: minimum 1.5 per cent *m/m* of tannins, expressed as pyrogallol ($C_6H_6O_3$; M_r 126.1).

PRODUCTION

The tincture is produced from 1 part of comminuted drug and 5 parts of ethanol (70 per cent *V/V*) by a suitable procedure.

CHARACTERS

Red or reddish-brown liquid.

IDENTIFICATION

Thin-layer chromatography (*2.2.27*).

Test solution. Mix 1.0 ml of the tincture to be examined with 1.0 ml of *alcohol (70 per cent V/V) R.*

Reference solution. Dissolve 1.0 mg of *catechin R* in 1.0 ml of *methanol R.*

Plate: *TLC silica gel plate R.*

Mobile phase: *ether R, glacial acetic acid R, hexane R, ethyl acetate R* (20:20:20:40 *V/V/V/V*).

Application: 10 µl, as bands.

Development: over a path of 10 cm.

Drying: in air for 10-15 min.

Detection: spray with a freshly prepared 5 g/l solution of *fast blue B salt R.* Reddish zones appear. Expose the plate to ammonia vapour, the zones become more intense, turning reddish-brown. Examine in daylight.

Results: see below the sequence of the zones present in the chromatograms obtained with the reference solution and the test solution.

Top of the plate	
Catechin: an intense zone	An intense zone (catechim)
———	———
	A fainter zone
	An intense zone
	Fainter zones
Reference solution	**Test solution**

TESTS

Ethanol content (*2.9.10*): 64 per cent *V/V* to 69 per cent *V/V*.

Methanol and 2-propanol (*2.9.11*): maximum 0.05 per cent *V/V* of methanol and maximum 0.05 per cent *V/V* of 2-propanol.

ASSAY

Carry out the determination of tannins in herbal drugs (*2.8.14*). Use 2.50 g of the tincture to be examined.

01/2005:0381

TOSYLCHLOROAMIDE SODIUM

Tosylchloramidum natricum

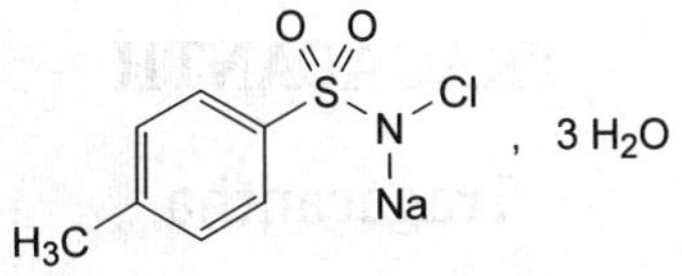

$C_7H_7ClNNaO_2S,3H_2O$ M_r 281.7

DEFINITION

Tosylchloramide sodium contains not less than 98.0 per cent and not more than the equivalent of 103.0 per cent of sodium *N*-chloro-4-methylbenzene-sulphonimidate trihydrate.

CHARACTERS

A white or slightly yellow, crystalline powder, freely soluble in water, soluble in alcohol.

IDENTIFICATION

A. Solution S (see Tests) turns *red litmus paper R* blue and then bleaches it.

B. To 10 ml of solution S add 10 ml of *dilute hydrogen peroxide solution R.* A white precipitate is formed which dissolves on heating. Filter the hot solution and allow to cool. White crystals are formed which, when washed and dried at 100 °C to 105 °C, melt (*2.2.14*) at 137 °C to 140 °C.

C. Ignite 1 g (cautiously, because of the risk of deflagration). Dissolve the residue in 10 ml of *water R.* The solution gives reaction (a) of chlorides (*2.3.1*).

D. The solution prepared for identification test C gives reaction (a) of sulphates (*2.3.1*).

E. The solution prepared for identification test C gives reaction (b) of sodium (*2.3.1*).

TESTS

Solution S. Dissolve 1.0 g in *carbon dioxide-free water R* and dilute to 20 ml with the same solvent.

Appearance of solution. Solution S is not more opalescent than reference suspension II (*2.2.1*) and is colourless (*2.2.2, Method II*).

pH (*2.2.3*). The pH of solution S is 8.0 to 10.0.

Ortho compound. To 2 g add 10 ml of *water R*, mix, add 1 g of *sodium metabisulphite R* and heat to boiling. Cool to 0 °C, filter rapidly and wash with three quantities, each of 5 ml, of iced *water R.* The precipitate, dried over *diphosphorus pentoxide R* at a pressure not exceeding 600 Pa melts (*2.2.14*) at a temperature not lower than 134 °C.

Residue insoluble in ethanol. Shake 1.00 g for 30 min with 20 ml of *ethanol R*, filter on a tared filter, wash any residue with 5 ml of *ethanol R* and dry at 100 °C to 105 °C. The residue weighs not more than 20 mg (2 per cent).

ASSAY

Dissolve 0.125 g in 100 ml of *water R* in a ground-glass-stoppered flask. Add 1 g of *potassium iodide R* and 5 ml of *dilute sulphuric acid R.* Allow to stand for 3 min. Titrate with *0.1 M sodium thiosulphate*, using 1 ml of *starch solution R* as indicator.

1 ml of *0.1 M sodium thiosulphate* is equivalent to 14.08 mg of $C_7H_7ClNNaO_2S,3H_2O$.

STORAGE

Store in an airtight container, protected from light, at a temperature of 8 °C to 15 °C.

01/2005:0532

TRAGACANTH

Tragacantha

DEFINITION

Tragacanth is the air-hardened, gummy exudate, flowing naturally or obtained by incision from the trunk and branches of *Astragalus gummifer* Labill. and certain other species of *Astragalus* from western Asia.

CHARACTERS

It has the macroscopic and microscopic characters described under identification test A and B.

IDENTIFICATION

A. Tragacanth occurs in thin, flattened, ribbon-like, white or pale yellow, translucent strips, about 30 mm long and 10 mm wide and up to 1 mm thick, more or less curved; horny, fracture short; the surface is marked by fine longitudinal striae and concentric transverse ridges. It may also contain pieces similar in shape but somewhat thicker, more opaque and more difficult to fracture.

B. Reduce to a powder (355). The powder is white or almost white and it forms a mucilaginous gel with about ten times its mass of *water R*. Examine under a microscope using a 50 per cent *V/V* solution of *glycerol R*. The powder shows in the gummy mass numerous stratified cellular membranes turning slowly violet when treated with *iodinated zinc chloride solution R*. The gummy mass includes starch grains, isolated or in small groups, usually rounded in shape and sometimes deformed, with diameters varying between 4 µm and 10 µm, occasionally up to 20 µm, and a central hilum visible between crossed nicol prisms.

C. Examine the chromatograms obtained in the test for acacia. The chromatogram obtained with the test solution shows three zones, corresponding to galactose, arabinose and xylose. A faint yellowish zone at the solvent front and a greyish-green zone between the zones due to galactose and arabinose may be present.

D. Moisten 0.5 g of the powdered drug (355) with 1 ml of *alcohol R* and add gradually, while shaking, 50 ml of *water R* until a homogeneous mucilage is obtained. To 5 ml of the mucilage add 5 ml of *water R* and 2 ml of *barium hydroxide solution R*. A slight flocculent precipitate is formed. Heat on a water-bath for 10 min. An intense yellow colour develops.

TESTS

Acacia. Examine by thin-layer chromatography (*2.2.27*), using a *TLC silica gel plate R*.

Test solution. To 100 mg of the powdered drug (355) in a thick-walled, centrifuge test tube, add 2 ml of a 100 g/l solution of *trifluoroacetic acid R*, shake vigorously to dissolve the forming gel, stopper the test tube and heat the mixture at 120 °C for 1 h. Centrifuge the hydrolysate, transfer the clear supernatant carefully into a 50 ml flask, add 10 ml of *water R* and evaporate the solution to dryness under reduced pressure. To the resulting clear film add 0.1 ml of *water R* and 0.9 ml of *methanol R*. Centrifuge to separate the amorphous precipitate and dilute the supernatant if necessary to 1 ml with *methanol R*.

Reference solution. Dissolve 10 mg of *arabinose R*, 10 mg of *galactose R*, 10 mg of *rhamnose R* and 10 mg of *xylose R* in 1 ml of *water R* and dilute to 10 ml with *methanol R*.

Apply to the plate as bands 10 µl of each solution. Develop over a path of 10 cm using a mixture of 10 volumes of a 16 g/l solution of *sodium dihydrogen phosphate R*, 40 volumes of *butanol R* and 50 volumes of *acetone R*. Dry the plate in a current of warm air for a few minutes and again develop over a path of 15 cm using the same mobile phase. Dry the plate at 110 °C for 10 min, spray with *anisaldehyde solution R* and dry again at 110 °C for 10 min. The chromatogram obtained with the reference solution shows four clearly separated coloured zones due to galactose (greyish-green to green), arabinose (yellowish-green), xylose (greenish-grey or yellowish-grey) and rhamnose (yellowish-green), in order of increasing R_f value. The chromatogram obtained with the test solution does not show a yellowish-green zone corresponding to the zone of rhamnose in the chromatogram obtained with the reference solution.

Methylcellulose. Examine the chromatograms obtained in the test for acacia. The chromatogram obtained with the test solution does not show a red zone near the solvent front.

Sterculia gum

A. Place 0.2 g of the powdered drug (355) in a 10 ml ground-glass-stoppered cylinder graduated in 0.1 ml. Add 10 ml of *alcohol (60 per cent V/V) R* and shake. Any gel formed occupies not more than 1.5 ml.

B. To 1.0 g of the powdered drug (355) add 100 ml of *water R* and shake. Add 0.1 ml of *methyl red solution R*. Not more than 5.0 ml of *0.01 M sodium hydroxide* is required to change the colour of the indicator.

Foreign matter. Place 2.0 g of the powdered drug (355) in a 250 ml round-bottomed flask and add 95 ml of *methanol R*. Swirl to moisten the powder and add 60 ml of *hydrochloric acid R1*. Add a few glass beads about 4 mm in diameter and heat on a water-bath under a reflux condenser for 3 h, shaking occasionally. Remove the glass beads and filter the hot suspension *in vacuo* through a sintered-glass filter (160). Rinse the flask with a small quantity of *water R* and pass the rinsings through the filter. Wash the residue on the filter with about 40 ml of *methanol R* and dry to constant mass at 110 °C (about 1 h). Allow to cool in a desiccator and weigh. The residue weighs not more than 20 mg (1.0 per cent).

Flow time. Not less than 10 s or, if the substance to be examined is to be used for the preparation of emulsions, not less than 50 s. Place 1.0 g of the powdered drug (125 to 250) in a 1000 ml round bottomed flask with a ground-glass stopper and add 8.0 ml of *alcohol R* and close the flask. Disperse the suspension over the inner surface of the flask by shaking, taking care not to wet the stopper. Open the flask and add in one portion 72.0 ml of *water R*. Stopper the flask and shake vigorously for 3 min. Allow to stand for 24 h and shake vigorously again for 3 min. Eliminate air bubbles by applying vacuum above the mucilage for 5 min. Transfer the mucilage to a 50 ml cylinder. Dip in the mucilage a piece of glass tubing 200 mm long and 6.0 mm in internal diameter and graduated at 20 mm and 120 mm from the lower end; the tubing must not be rinsed with surface-active substances. When the mucilage has reached the upper mark, close the tube with a finger. Withdraw the closed tube, remove the finger and measure with a stop-watch the time needed for the meniscus to reach the lower graduation. Carry out this operation four times and determine the average value of the last three determinations.

Total ash (*2.4.16*). Not more than 4.0 per cent.

Microbial contamination. Total viable aerobic count (*2.6.12*) not more than 10^4 micro-organisms per gram, determined by plate count. It complies with the tests for *Escherichia coli* and *Salmonella* (*2.6.13*).

STORAGE

Store protected from light.

LABELLING

The label states whether or not the contents are suitable for preparing emulsions.

01/2005:1681

TRAMADOL HYDROCHLORIDE

Tramadoli hydrochloridum

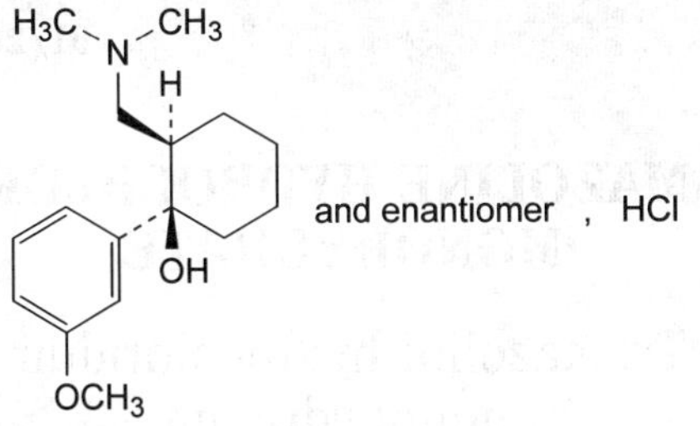

$C_{16}H_{26}ClNO_2$ M_r 299.8

DEFINITION

(1*RS*,2*RS*)-2-[(Dimethylamino)methyl]-1-(3-methoxyphenyl)cyclohexanol hydrochloride.

Content: 99.0 per cent to 101.0 per cent (anhydrous substance).

CHARACTERS

Appearance: white, crystalline powder.

Solubility: freely soluble in water and in methanol, very slightly soluble in acetone.

IDENTIFICATION

First identification: B, D.

Second identification: A, C, D.

A. Melting point (*2.2.14*): 180 °C to 184 °C.

B. Infrared absorption spectrophotometry (*2.2.24*).

Comparison: *tramadol hydrochloride CRS.*

C. Chromatograms obtained in the test for impurity E.

Results: the principal spot in the chromatogram obtained with test solution (b) is similar in position and size to the principal spot in the chromatogram obtained with reference solution (a).

D. It gives reaction (a) of chlorides (*2.3.1*).

TESTS

Solution S. Dissolve 1.0 g in *water R* and dilute to 20 ml with the same solvent.

Appearance of solution. Solution S is clear (*2.2.1*) and colourless (*2.2.2, Method II*).

Acidity. To 10 ml of solution S, add 0.2 ml of *methyl red solution R* and 0.2 ml of *0.01 M hydrochloric acid.* The solution is red. Not more than 0.4 ml of *0.01 M sodium hydroxide* is required to change the colour of the indicator to yellow.

Optical rotation (*2.2.7*): − 0.10° to + 0.10°, determined on solution S.

Impurity E. Thin-layer chromatography (*2.2.27*).

Test solution (a). Dissolve 0.10 g in *methanol R* and dilute to 2 ml with the same solvent.

Test solution (b). Dilute 1 ml of test solution (a) to 10 ml with *methanol R.*

Reference solution (a). Dissolve 25 mg of *tramadol hydrochloride CRS* in *methanol R* and dilute to 5 ml with the same solvent.

Reference solution (b). Dissolve 5 mg of *tramadol impurity E CRS* in 5 ml of *methanol R.* Dilute 1 ml of the solution to 10 ml with *methanol R.*

Reference solution (c). Dissolve 5 mg of *tramadol impurity A CRS* in 1 ml of reference solution (a).

Plate: *TLC silica gel F_{254} plate R*, prewashed with *methanol R.*

Mobile phase: *concentrated ammonia R, 2-propanol R, toluene R* (1:19:80 *V/V/V*).

Application: 10 µl.

Development: over 2/3 of the plate. Saturate the plate for 20 min with *concentrated ammonia R.* For this, add *concentrated ammonia R* to one trough of a twin trough tank. Just before developing, add the mobile phase to the other trough. Place the plate in the chromatographic tank, ensuring that the layer of silica gel is orientated towards the middle of the tank.

Drying: in air.

Detection: expose the plate to iodine vapour for 1 h, examine in ultraviolet light at 254 nm.

System suitability: the chromatogram obtained with reference solution (c) shows 2 clearly separated spots.

Limit: in the chromatogram obtained with test solution (a):

– *impurity E*: any spot corresponding to impurity E is not more intense and not greater than the spot in the chromatogram obtained with reference solution (b) (0.2 per cent).

Related substances. Liquid chromatography (*2.2.29*).

Test solution. Dissolve 0.15 g of the substance to be examined in the mobile phase and dilute to 100 ml with the mobile phase.

Reference solution (a). Dilute 2.0 ml of the test solution to 10.0 ml with the mobile phase. Dilute 1.0 ml of this solution to 100 ml with the mobile phase.

Reference solution (b). Dissolve 5 mg of *tramadol impurity A CRS* in 4.0 ml of the test solution and dilute to 100 ml with the mobile phase.

Column:

– *size*: *l* = 0.25 m, Ø = 4.0 mm,

– *stationary phase*: *base-deactivated end-capped octylsilyl silica gel for chromatography R* (5 µm).

Mobile phase: 295 volumes of *acetonitrile R* and 705 volumes of a mixture of 0.2 ml of *trifluoroacetic acid R* and 100 ml of *water R.*

Flow rate: 1.0 ml/min.

Detection: spectrophotometer at 270 nm.

Injection: 20 µl.

Run time: 4 times the retention time of tramadol.

Relative retention with reference to tramadol (retention time = about 5 min): impurity A = about 0.85.

System suitability: reference solution (b):

– *resolution*: minimum 2.0 between the peaks due to impurity A and tramadol.

Limits:

- *impurity A*: not more than the area of the principal peak in the chromatogram obtained with reference solution (a) (0.2 per cent),
- *any other impurity*: not more than 0.5 times the area of the principal peak in the chromatogram obtained with reference solution (a) (0.1 per cent),
- *total*: not more than twice the area of the principal peak in the chromatogram obtained with reference solution (a) (0.4 per cent),
- *disregard limit*: 0.1 times the area of the principal peak in the chromatogram obtained with reference solution (a) (0.02 per cent).

Heavy metals (*2.4.8*): maximum 20 ppm.

Dissolve 2.0 g in *water R* and dilute to 20 ml with the same solvent. 12 ml of this solution complies with limit test A. Prepare the standard using *lead standard solution (2 ppm Pb) R*.

Water (*2.5.12*): maximum 0.5 per cent, determined on 1.000 g.

Sulphated ash (*2.4.14*): maximum 0.1 per cent, determined on 1.0 g.

ASSAY

Dissolve 0.180 g in 25 ml of *anhydrous acetic acid R* and add 10 ml of *acetic anhydride R*. Titrate with *0.1 M perchloric acid*, determining the end-point potentiometrically (*2.2.20*).

1 ml of *0.1 M perchloric acid* is equivalent to 29.98 mg of $C_{16}H_{26}ClNO_2$.

STORAGE

Protected from light.

IMPURITIES

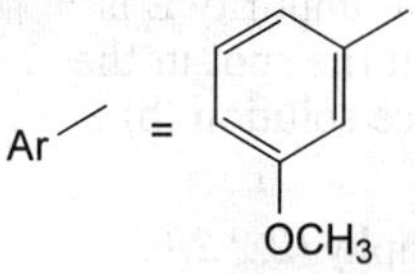

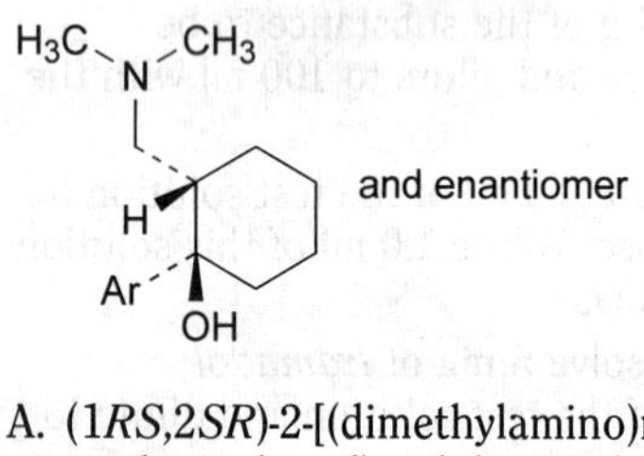

A. (1*RS*,2*SR*)-2-[(dimethylamino)methyl]-1-(3-methoxyphenyl)cyclohexanol,

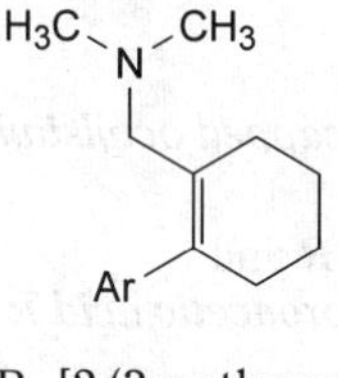

B. [2-(3-methoxyphenyl)cyclohex-1-enyl]-*N*,*N*-dimethylmethanamine,

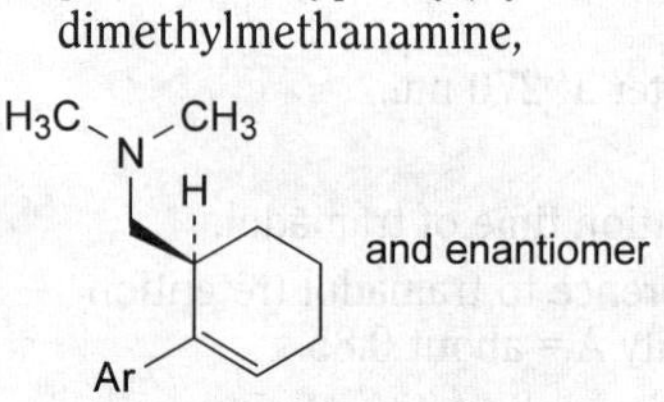

C. (1*RS*)-[2-(3-methoxyphenyl)cyclohex-2-enyl]-*N*,*N*-dimethylmethanamine,

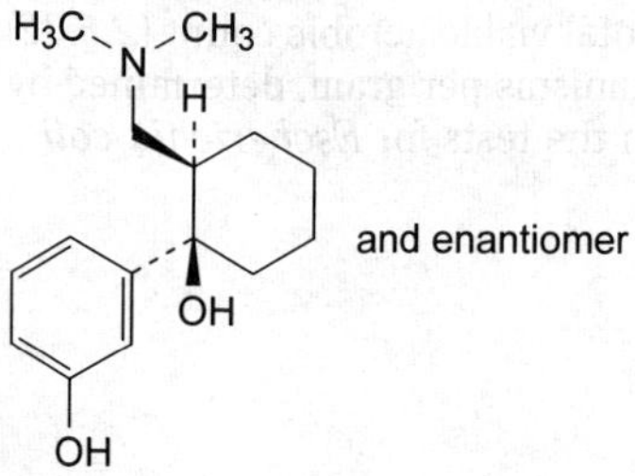

D. (1*RS*,2*RS*)-2-[(dimethylamino)methyl]-1-(3-hydroxyphenyl)cyclohexanol,

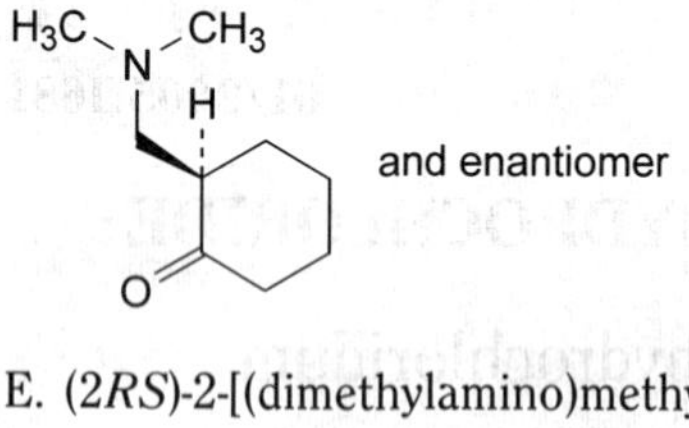

E. (2*RS*)-2-[(dimethylamino)methyl]cyclohexanone.

01/2005:1597
corrected

TRAMAZOLINE HYDROCHLORIDE MONOHYDRATE

Tramazolini hydrochloridum monohydricum

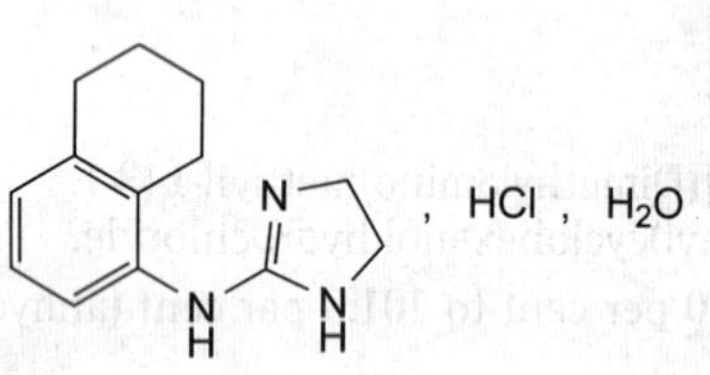

$C_{13}H_{18}ClN_3,H_2O$ M_r 269.8

DEFINITION

N-(5,6,7,8-Tetrahydronaphthalen-1-yl)-4,5-dihydro-1*H*-imidazol-2-amine hydrochloride monohydrate.

Content: 98.5 per cent to 101.5 per cent (anhydrous substance).

CHARACTERS

Appearance: white or almost white, crystalline powder.

Solubility: soluble in water and in alcohol.

IDENTIFICATION

A. Infrared absorption spectrophotometry (*2.2.24*).

Comparison: *tramazoline hydrochloride monohydrate CRS*.

B. It gives reaction (a) of chlorides (*2.3.1*).

TESTS

Solution S. Dissolve 2.5 g in *carbon dioxide-free water R* and dilute to 50 ml with the same solvent.

Appearance of solution. Solution S is clear (*2.2.1*) and not more intensely coloured than reference solution Y_6 (*2.2.2, Method II*).

pH (*2.2.3*): 4.9 to 6.3 for solution S.

Related substances. Liquid chromatography (*2.2.29*).

Test solution. Dissolve 50.0 mg of the substance to be examined in a mixture of 50 volumes of *acetonitrile R* and 50 volumes of *water R* and dilute to 50.0 ml with the same mixture of solvents.

Reference solution (a). Dissolve 10.0 mg of *tramazoline impurity A CRS* and 10.0 mg of *tramazoline impurity B CRS* in 10 ml of a mixture of 50 volumes of *acetonitrile R* and 50 volumes of *water R* and add 10 ml of the test solution.

Reference solution (b). Dilute 0.2 ml of reference solution (a) to 100 ml with a mixture of 50 volumes of *acetonitrile R* and 50 volumes of *water R.*

Column:

- *size*: l = 0.125 m, Ø = 4 mm,
- *stationary phase*: *octadecylsilyl silica gel for chromatography R* (5 µm).

Mobile phase: 2.0 g/l solution of *sodium dodecyl sulphate R* in a mixture of 6 volumes of *2-propanol R,* 42 volumes of *acetonitrile R* and 52 volumes of *water R.*

Flow rate: 1.2 ml/min.

Detection: spectrophotometer at 215 nm.

Injection: 5 µl.

Run time: 3 times the retention time of tramazoline.

Relative retentions with reference to tramazoline (retention time = about 6.5 min): impurity A = about 0.71; impurity B = about 0.86.

System suitability: reference solution (a):

- the chromatogram obtained shows 3 clearly separated peaks,
- *resolution*: minimum 1.5 between tramazoline and impurity B.

Limits:

- *impurity A*: not more than 3 times the area of the corresponding peak in the chromatogram obtained with reference solution (b) (0.3 per cent),
- *impurity B*: not more than 3 times the area of the corresponding peak in the chromatogram obtained with reference solution (b) (0.3 per cent),
- *any other impurity*: not more than the area of the peak due to impurity B in the chromatogram obtained with reference solution (b) (0.1 per cent),
- *total of other impurities*: not more than 2 times the area of the peak due to impurity B in the chromatogram obtained with reference solution (b) (0.2 per cent),
- *disregard limit*: 0.2 times the area of the peak due to impurity B in the chromatogram obtained with reference solution (b) (0.02 per cent).

Water (*2.5.12*): 6.2 per cent to 7.2 per cent, determined on 0.500 g.

Sulphated ash (*2.4.14*): maximum 0.1 per cent, determined on 1.0 g.

ASSAY

Dissolve 2.000 g in a mixture of 5 ml of *0.1 M hydrochloric acid* and 75 ml of *alcohol R.* Carry out a potentiometric titration (*2.2.20*) using *1 M sodium hydroxide.* Read the volume added between the 2 points of inflexion.

1 ml of *1 M sodium hydroxide* is equivalent to 251.8 mg of $C_{13}H_{18}ClN_3$.

IMPURITIES

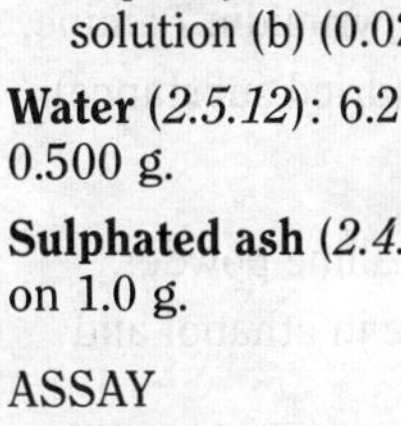

A. *N*-(naphthalen-1-yl)-4,5-dihydro-1*H*-imidazol-2-amine,

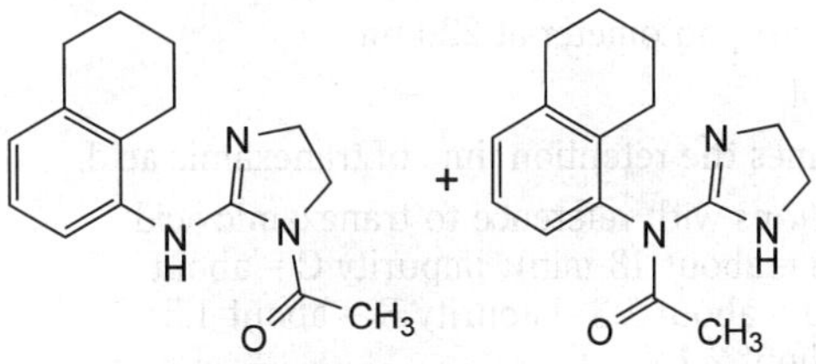

B. mixture of 1-acetyl-2-[(5,6,7,8-tetrahydronaphthalen-1-yl)amino]-4,5-dihydro-1*H*-imidazole and *N*-(4,5-dihydro-1*H*-imidazol-2-yl)-*N*-(5,6,7,8-tetrahydronaphthalen-1-yl)acetamide.

01/2005:0875

TRANEXAMIC ACID

Acidum tranexamicum

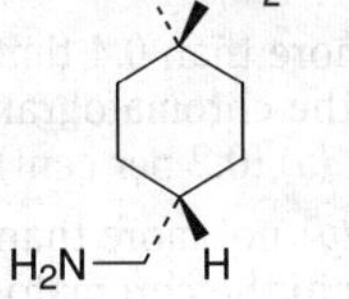

$C_8H_{15}NO_2$ M_r 157.2

DEFINITION

Trans-4-(aminomethyl)cyclohexanecarboxylic acid.

Content: 99.0 per cent to 101.0 per cent (dried substance).

CHARACTERS

Appearance: white, crystalline powder.

Solubility: freely soluble in water and in glacial acetic acid, practically insoluble in acetone and in alcohol.

IDENTIFICATION

Infrared absorption spectrophotometry (*2.2.24*).

Preparation: discs.

Comparison: *tranexamic acid CRS.*

TESTS

pH (*2.2.3*): 7.0 to 8.0.

Dissolve 2.5 g in *carbon dioxide-free water R* and dilute to 50 ml with the same solvent.

Related substances. Liquid chromatography (*2.2.29*).

Test solution. Dissolve 0.20 g of the substance to be examined in *water R* and dilute to 20.0 ml with the same solvent.

Reference solution (a). Dilute 5.0 ml of the test solution to 100.0 ml with *water R.* Dilute 1.0 ml of this solution to 10.0 ml with *water R.*

Reference solution (b). Dissolve 5 mg of *tranexamic acid impurity C CRS* in *water R* and dilute to 50.0 ml with the same solvent. To 1.0 ml of this solution add 1.0 ml of the test solution and dilute to 50.0 ml with *water R.*

Column:

- *size*: l = 0.25 m, Ø = 4.6 mm or l = 0.25 m, Ø = 6.0 mm,
- *stationary phase*: *octadecylsilyl silica gel for chromatography R* (5 µm).

Mobile phase: dissolve 11.0 g of *anhydrous sodium dihydrogen phosphate R* in 500 ml of *water R,* add 5 ml of *triethylamine R* and 1.4 g of *sodium laurilsulfate R.* Adjust to pH 2.5 with *dilute phosphoric acid R* and dilute to 600 ml with *water R.* Add 400 ml of *methanol R* and mix.

Flow rate: 0.9 ml/min.

Detection: spectrophotometer at 220 nm.

Injection: 20 µl.

Run time: 3 times the retention time of tranexamic acid.

Relative retentions with reference to tranexamic acid (retention time = about 13 min): impurity C = about 1.1; impurity D = about 1.3; impurity B = about 1.5; impurity A = about 2.1.

System suitability: reference solution (b):

- *resolution*: minimum of 2.0 between the peaks due to tranexamic acid and to impurity C.

Limits:

- *correction factors*: for the calculation of contents, multiply the peak areas of the following impurities by the corresponding correction factor: impurity B = 1.2; impurity C = 0.005; impurity D = 0.006;
- *impurity A*: not more than 0.2 times the area of the principal peak in the chromatogram obtained with reference solution (a) (0.1 per cent);
- *impurity B*: not more than 0.4 times the area of the principal peak in the chromatogram obtained with reference solution (a) (0.2 per cent);
- *any other impurity*: not more than 0.2 times the area of the principal peak in the chromatogram obtained with reference solution (a) (0.1 per cent);
- *total of other impurities*: not more than 0.4 times the area of the principal peak in the chromatogram obtained with reference solution (a) (0.2 per cent);
- *disregard limit*: 0.05 times the area of the principal peak in the chromatogram obtained with reference solution (a) (0.025 per cent).

Halides expressed as chlorides (*2.4.4*): maximum 140 ppm. Dissolve 1.2 g in *water R* and dilute to 50 ml with the same solvent. 15 ml of this solution complies with the limit test for chlorides.

Heavy metals (*2.4.8*): maximum 10 ppm.

Dissolve 2.0 g in *water R* and dilute to 20 ml with the same solvent. 12 ml of this solution complies with limit test A. Prepare the standard using *lead standard solution (1 ppm Pb) R*.

Loss on drying (*2.2.32*): maximum 0.5 per cent, determined on 1.000 g by drying in an oven at 100-105 °C for 2 h.

Sulphated ash (*2.4.14*): maximum 0.1 per cent, determined on 1.0 g.

ASSAY

Dissolve 0.140 g in 20 ml of *anhydrous acetic acid R*. Titrate with *0.1 M perchloric acid*, determining the end-point potentiometrically (*2.2.20*).

1 ml of *0.1 M perchloric acid* is equivalent to 15.72 mg of $C_8H_{15}NO_2$.

IMPURITIES

Specified impurities: A, B.

Other detectable impurities: C, D.

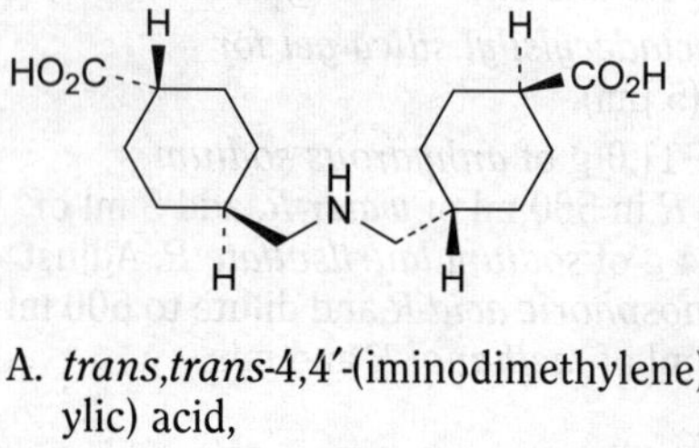

A. *trans,trans*-4,4'-(iminodimethylene)di(cyclohexanecarboxylic) acid,

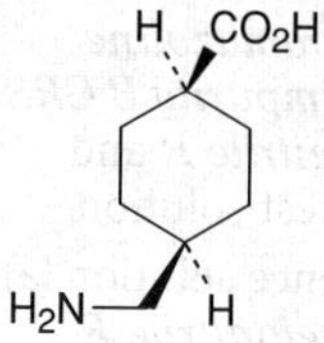

B. *cis*-4-(aminomethyl)cyclohexanecarboxylic acid,

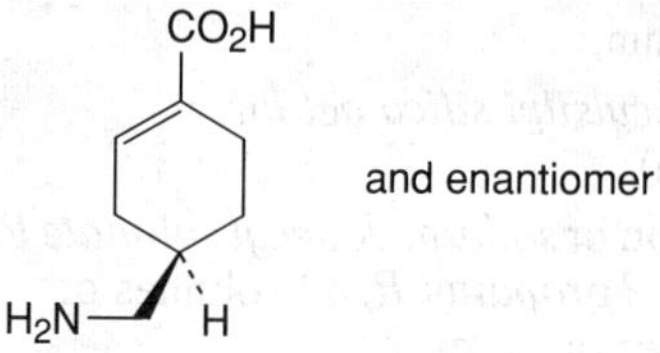

C. (*RS*)-4-(aminomethyl)cyclohex-1-enecarboxylic acid,

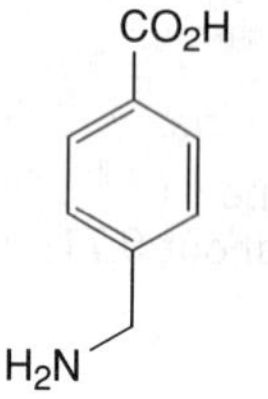

D. 4-aminomethylbenzoic acid.

01/2005:1576

TRAPIDIL

Trapidilum

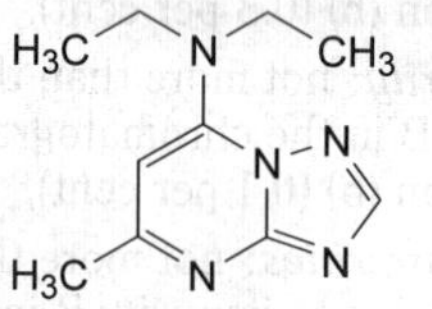

$C_{10}H_{15}N_5$ M_r 205.3

DEFINITION

N,N-Diethyl-5-methyl-[1,2,4]triazolo[1,5-*a*]pyrimidin-7-amine.

Content: 99.0 per cent to 101.0 per cent (dried substance).

CHARACTERS

Appearance: white or almost white, crystalline powder.

Solubility: freely soluble in water, soluble in ethanol and in methylene chloride.

mp: about 102 °C.

IDENTIFICATION

Infrared absorption spectrophotometry (*2.2.24*).

Comparison: *trapidil CRS*.

TESTS

Solution S. Dissolve 2.0 g in *carbon dioxide-free water R* and dilute to 100 ml with the same solvent.

Appearance of solution. Solution S is clear (*2.2.1*) and colourless (*2.2.2, Method II*).

Acidity or alkalinity. To 10 ml of solution S add 0.2 ml of *methyl red solution R* and 0.2 ml of *0.01 M hydrochloric acid*. The solution is red. Add 0.4 ml of *0.01 M sodium hydroxide*. The solution is yellow.

Related substances. Liquid chromatography (*2.2.29*).

Test solution. Dissolve 20.0 mg of the substance to be examined in the mobile phase and dilute to 10.0 ml with the mobile phase.

Reference solution (a). Dissolve 5.0 mg of *trapidil impurity A CRS* in the mobile phase and dilute to 50.0 ml with the mobile phase. Dilute 1.0 ml of the solution to 50.0 ml with the mobile phase.

Reference solution (b). Dissolve 5.0 mg of *trapidil impurity B CRS* in the mobile phase and dilute to 50.0 ml with the mobile phase. Dilute 1.0 ml of the solution to 50.0 ml with the mobile phase.

Reference solution (c). Mix equal volumes of reference solution (a) and reference solution (b).

Column:

- *size*: l = 0.125 m, Ø = 4.0 mm,
- *stationary phase*: *base-deactivated octadecylsilyl silica gel for chromatography R* (5 µm),

Mobile phase: 50 ml of *methanol R*, 75 ml of *acetonitrile R* and 800 ml of a 1.7 g/l solution of *potassium dihydrogen phosphate R* adjusted to pH 2.45 with *phosphoric acid R*; dilute to 1000 ml with *water R.*

Flow rate: 1.0 ml/min.

Detection: spectrophotometer at 205 nm.

Injection: 10 µl.

Run time: 3 times the retention time of trapidil.

System suitability:

- *resolution*: minimum of 4.0 between the peaks due to impurity A and impurity B in the chromatogram obtained with reference solution (c).

Limits:

- *impurity A*: not more than the area of the principal peak in the chromatogram obtained with reference solution (a) (0.1 per cent),
- *impurity B*: not more than the area of the principal peak in the chromatogram obtained with reference solution (b) (0.1 per cent),
- *any other impurity*: not more than the area of the principal peak in the chromatogram obtained with reference solution (a) (0.1 per cent),
- *total*: not more than 5 times the area of the principal peak in the chromatogram obtained with reference solution (a) (0.5 per cent).
- *disregard limit*: 0.1 times the area of the principal peak in the chromatogram obtained with reference solution (a) (0.01 per cent).

Chlorides (*2.4.4*): maximum 100 ppm.

Dissolve 0.25 g in 10 ml of *water R* and dilute to 15 ml with *water R.* The solution complies with the limit test for chlorides. Prepare the standard using 5 ml of *chloride standard solution (5 ppm Cl) R.*

Ammonium (*2.4.1*): maximum 20 ppm.

0.50 g complies with limit test A. Prepare the standard using 0.1 ml of *ammonium standard solution (100 ppm NH_4) R.*

Heavy metals (*2.4.8*): maximum 10 ppm.

Dissolve 2.0 g in 20 ml of *water R.* 12 ml of the solution complies with limit test A. Prepare the standard using 1 ml of *lead standard solution (10 ppm Pb) R.*

Loss on drying (*2.2.32*): maximum 0.5 per cent, determined on 1.000 g by drying *in vacuo* at 60 °C for 3 h.

Sulphated ash (*2.4.14*): maximum 0.1 per cent, determined on 1.0 g.

ASSAY

Dissolve 0.180 g in 50 ml of *anhydrous acetic acid R.* Titrate with *0.1 M perchloric acid*, determining the end-point potentiometrically (*2.2.20*).

1 ml of *0.1 M perchloric acid* is equivalent to 20.53 mg of $C_{10}H_{15}N_5$.

STORAGE

Protected from light.

IMPURITIES

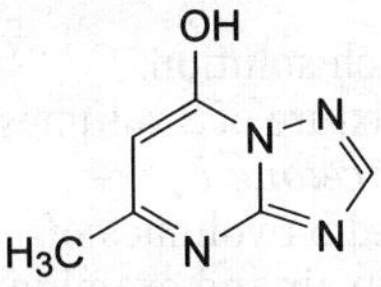

A. 5-methyl-[1,2,4]triazolo[1,5-*a*]pyrimidin-7-ol,

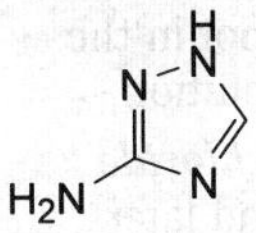

B. 1,2,4-triazol-3-amine.

01/2005:0693

TRETINOIN

Tretinoinum

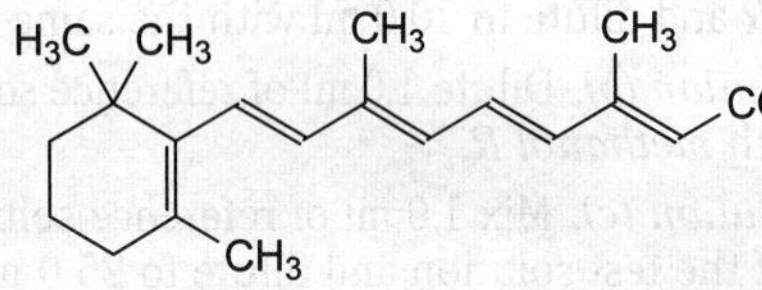

$C_{20}H_{28}O_2$ M_r 300.4

DEFINITION

Tretinoin contains not less than 98.0 per cent and not more than the equivalent of 102.0 per cent of (2*E*,4*E*,6*E*,8*E*)-3,7-dimethyl-9-(2,6,6-trimethylcyclohex-1-enyl)nona-2,4,6,8-tetraenoic acid, calculated with reference to the dried substance.

CHARACTERS

A yellow or light orange, crystalline powder, practically insoluble in water, soluble in methylene chloride, slightly soluble in alcohol. It is sensitive to air, heat and light, especially in solution.

It melts at about 182 °C, with decomposition.

Carry out all operations as rapidly as possible and avoid exposure to actinic light; use freshly prepared solutions.

IDENTIFICATION

First identification: *A, B.*

Second identification: *A, C, D.*

A. Dissolve 75.0 mg in 5 ml of *methylene chloride R* and dilute immediately to 100.0 ml with acidified 2-propanol (prepared by diluting 1 ml of *0.01 M hydrochloric acid* to 1000 ml with *2-propanol R*). Dilute 5.0 ml of this solution to 100.0 ml with the acidified 2-propanol. Dilute 5.0 ml of this latter solution to 50.0 ml with the acidified 2-propanol. Examined between 300 nm and 400 nm (*2.2.25*), the solution shows a single maximum, at 353 nm. The specific absorbance at the maximum is 1455 to 1545.

B. Examine by infrared absorption spectrophotometry (*2.2.24*), comparing with the spectrum obtained with *tretinoin CRS*. Examine the substances prepared as discs.

C. Examine by thin-layer chromatography (*2.2.27*), using a *TLC silica gel GF_{254} plate R*.

Test solution. Dissolve 10 mg of the substance to be examined in *methylene chloride R* and dilute to 10 ml with the same solvent.

Reference solution. Dissolve 10 mg of *tretinoin CRS* in *methylene chloride R* and dilute to 10 ml with the same solvent.

Apply separately to the plate 5 µl of each solution. Develop over a path of 15 cm using a mixture of 2 volumes of *glacial acetic acid R*, 4 volumes of *acetone R*, 40 volumes of *peroxide-free ether R* and 54 volumes of *cyclohexane R*. Allow the plate to dry in air and examine in ultraviolet light at 254 nm. The principal spot in the chromatogram obtained with the test solution is similar in position and size to the principal spot in the chromatogram obtained with the reference solution.

D. Dissolve about 5 mg in 2 ml of *antimony trichloride solution R*. An intense red colour develops and later becomes violet.

TESTS

Related substances. Examine by liquid chromatography (*2.2.29*).

Test solution. Dissolve 0.100 g of the substance to be examined in *methanol R* and dilute to 50.0 ml with the same solvent.

Reference solution (a). Dissolve 10.0 mg of *isotretinoin CRS* in *methanol R* and dilute to 10.0 ml with the same solvent.

Reference solution (b). Dilute 1.0 ml of reference solution (a) to 25.0 ml with *methanol R*.

Reference solution (c). Mix 1.0 ml of reference solution (a) with 0.5 ml of the test solution and dilute to 25.0 ml with *methanol R*.

Reference solution (d). Dilute 0.5 ml of the test solution to 100.0 ml with *methanol R*.

The chromatographic procedure may be carried out using:

- a stainless steel column 0.15 m long and 4.6 mm in internal diameter packed with *octadecylsilyl silica gel for chromatography R* (3 µm),
- as mobile phase at a flow rate of 1.0 ml/min a mixture of 5 volumes of *glacial acetic acid R*, 225 volumes of *water R* and 770 volumes of *methanol R*,
- as detector a spectrophotometer set at 355 nm.

Inject separately 10 µl of reference solutions (b), (c) and (d) and of the test solution. Adjust the sensitivity of the detector so that the height of the principal peak in the chromatogram obtained with reference solution (b) is about 70 per cent of the full scale of the recorder. The test is not valid unless the resolution between isotretinoin and tretinoin in the chromatogram obtained with reference solution (c) is at least 2.0. In the chromatogram obtained with the test solution, the area of the peak due to isotretinoin is not greater than the area of the principal peak in the chromatogram obtained with reference solution (b) (2.0 per cent) and the sum of the areas of any peaks, apart from the principal peak and any peak due to isotretinoin, is not greater than the area of the principal peak in the chromatogram obtained with reference solution (d) (0.5 per cent).

Heavy metals (*2.4.8*). 0.5 g complies with limit test D for heavy metals (20 ppm). Prepare the standard using 1 ml of *lead standard solution (10 ppm Pb) R*.

Loss on drying (*2.2.32*). Not more than 0.5 per cent, determined on 1.000 g by drying in an oven at 100 °C to 105 °C.

Sulphated ash (*2.4.14*). Not more than 0.1 per cent, determined on 1.0 g.

ASSAY

Dissolve 0.200 g in 70 ml of *acetone R*. Titrate with *0.1 M tetrabutylammonium hydroxide* determining the end-point potentiometrically (*2.2.20*).

1 ml of *0.1 M tetrabutylammonium hydroxide* is equivalent to 30.04 mg of $C_{20}H_{28}O_2$.

STORAGE

Store in an airtight container, protected from light, at a temperature not exceeding 25 °C.

It is recommended that the contents of an opened container be used as soon as possible and any unused part be protected by an atmosphere of an inert gas.

IMPURITIES

A. isotretinoin,

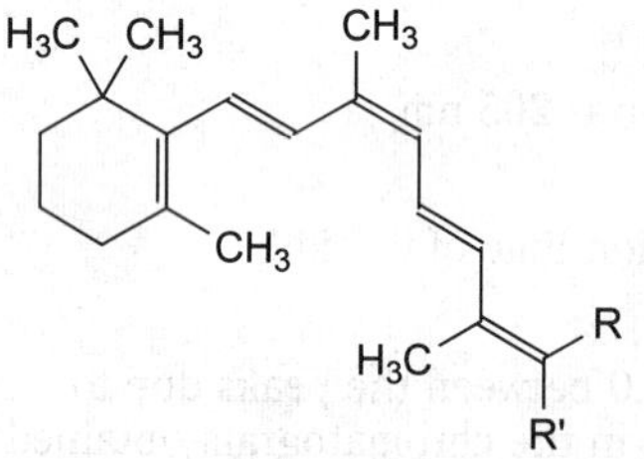

B. R = CO_2H, R′ = H: (2*Z*,4*E*,6*Z*,8*E*)-3,7-dimethyl-9-(2,6,6-trimethylcyclohex-1-enyl)nona-2,4,6,8-tetraenoic acid (9,13-di-*cis*-retinoic acid),

D. R = H, R′ = CO_2H: (2*E*,4*E*,6*Z*,8*E*)-3,7-dimethyl-9-(2,6,6-trimethylcyclohex-1-enyl)nona-2,4,6,8-tetraenoic acid (9-*cis*-retinoic acid),

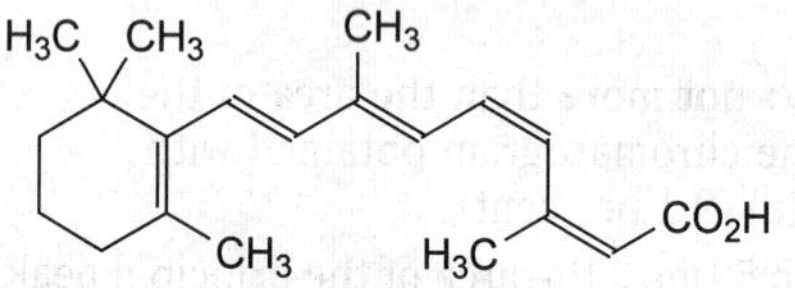

C. (2*Z*,4*Z*,6*E*,8*E*)-3,7-dimethyl-9-(2,6,6-trimethylcyclohex-1-enyl)nona-2,4,6,8-tetraenoic acid (11,13-di-*cis*-retinoic acid),

E. oxidation products of tretinoin.

01/2005:1106
corrected

TRIACETIN

Triacetinum

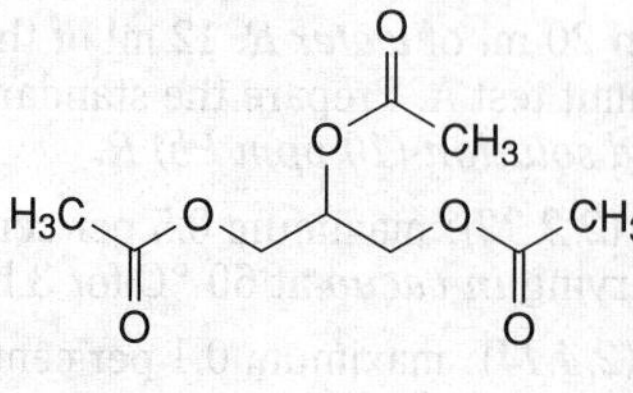

$C_9H_{14}O_6$ M_r 218.2

DEFINITION

Triacetin contains not less than 97.0 per cent and not more than the equivalent of 100.5 per cent of propane-1,2,3-triyl triacetate, calculated with reference to the anhydrous substance.

CHARACTERS

A clear, colourless, slightly viscous oily liquid. It is soluble in water, miscible with ethanol and toluene. It boils at about 260 °C.

IDENTIFICATION

Examine by infrared absorption spectrophotometry (*2.2.24*), comparing with the *Ph. Eur. reference spectrum of triacetin.*

TESTS

Appearance. It is clear (*2.2.1*) and not more intensely coloured than reference solution Y_6 (*2.2.2, Method II*).

Acidity. Dissolve 5.00 g in 25 ml of *ethanol R*, previously neutralised to 0.2 ml of *phenolphtalein solution R* and add 0.20 ml of *0.1 M sodium hydroxide*. The pink colour of the mixture persists for 15 s.

Relative density (*2.2.5*): 1.159 to 1.164.

Refractive index (*2.2.6*): 1.429 to 1.432.

Water (*2.5.12*). Not more than 0.2 per cent, determined on 5.00 g by the semi-micro determination of water.

ASSAY

Introduce 0.300 g of the substance to be examined into a 250 ml borosilicate glass flask fitted with a reflux condenser. Add 25.0 ml of *0.5 M alcoholic potassium hydroxide* and a few glass beads. Attach the condenser and heat under reflux for 30 min. Add 1 ml of *phenolphthalein solution R1* and titrate immediately with *0.5 M hydrochloric acid.* Carry out a blank test under the same conditions. Calculate the content from the difference in consumption of alkali in the main and the blank procedure.

1 ml of *0.5 M alcoholic potassium hydroxide* is equivalent to 36.37 mg of $C_9H_{14}O_6$.

STORAGE

Store in a well-filled container.

01/2005:1376

TRIAMCINOLONE

Triamcinolonum

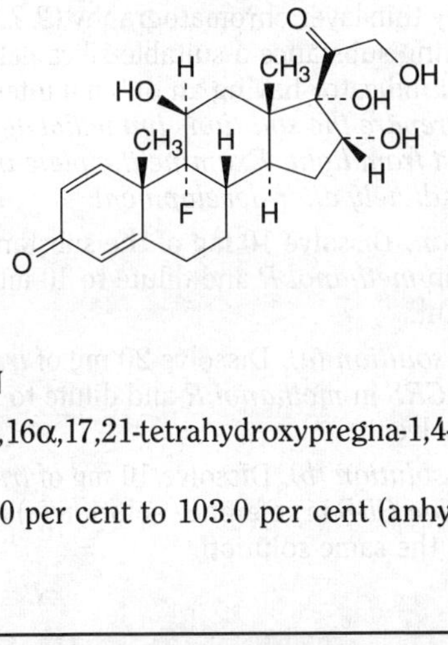

$C_{21}H_{27}FO_6$ M_r 394.4

DEFINITION

9-Fluoro-11β,16α,17,21-tetrahydroxypregna-1,4-diene-3,20-dione.

Content: 97.0 per cent to 103.0 per cent (anhydrous substance).

CHARACTERS

Appearance: white or almost white, crystalline powder.

Solubility: practically insoluble in water, slightly soluble in methanol, practically insoluble in methylene chloride.

It shows polymorphism.

IDENTIFICATION

A. Infrared absorption spectrophotometry (*2.2.24*).

Comparison: *triamcinolone CRS.*

If the spectra obtained show differences, dissolve the substance to be examined and the reference substance separately in *methanol R*, evaporate to dryness, dry the residues at 60 °C at a pressure not exceeding 0.7 kPa and record new spectra using the residues.

B. Thin-layer chromatography (*2.2.27*). *Prepare the solutions immediately before use and protect from light. Examine the plate under ultraviolet light immediately after development.*

Test solution. Dissolve 10 mg of the substance to be examined in *methanol R* and dilute to 10 ml with the same solvent.

Reference solution (a). Dissolve 20 mg of *triamcinolone CRS* in *methanol R* and dilute to 20 ml with the same solvent.

Reference solution (b). Dissolve 10 mg of *dexamethasone CRS* in reference solution (a) and dilute to 10 ml with the same solution.

Plate: *TLC silica gel F_{254} plate R.*

Mobile phase: add a mixture of 1.2 volumes of *water R* and 8 volumes of *methanol R* to a mixture of 15 volumes of *ether R* and 77 volumes of *methylene chloride R.*

Application: 5 μl.

Development: over a path of 15 cm.

Drying: in air.

Detection: examine in ultraviolet light at 254 nm.

System suitability: the chromatogram obtained with reference solution (b) shows 2 clearly separated spots.

Results: the principal spot in the chromatogram obtained with the test solution is similar in position and size to the principal spot in the chromatogram obtained with reference solution (a).

TESTS

Specific optical rotation (*2.2.7*): + 65 to + 72 (anhydrous substance).

Dissolve 0.100 g in *dimethylformamide R* and dilute to 10.0 ml with the same solvent.

Related substances. Liquid chromatography (*2.2.29*). *Prepare the solutions immediately before use and protect from light.*

Test solution. Dissolve 25.0 mg of the substance to be examined in a mixture of equal volumes of *methanol R* and *water R* and dilute to 10.0 ml with the same mixture of solvents.

Reference solution (a). Dissolve 2 mg of *triamcinolone CRS* and 2 mg of *triamcinolone impurity C CRS* in a mixture of equal volumes of *methanol R* and *water R* and dilute to 100.0 ml with the same mixture of solvents.

Reference solution (b). Dilute 1.0 ml of the test solution to 100.0 ml with a mixture of equal volumes of *methanol R* and *water R.*

Blank: *methanol R.*

Column:

– *size*: *l* = 0.25 m, Ø = 4.6 mm,

– *stationary phase*: *base-deactivated end-capped octadecylsilyl silica gel for chromatography R* (5 µm).

Mobile phase: a mixture prepared as follows: in a 1000 ml volumetric flask mix 525 ml of *methanol R* with 400 ml of *water R* and allow to equilibrate; adjust the volume to 1000 ml with *water R* and mix again.

Flow rate: 1 ml/min.

Detection: spectrophotometer set at 238 nm.

Injection: 20 µl.

Run time: 4.5 times the retention time of triamcinolone.

Retention time: triamcinolone = about 11 min.

System suitability: reference solution (a):

– *resolution*: minimum of 1.8 between the peaks due to triamcinolone and to impurity C.

Limits:

– *any impurity*: not more than the area of the principal peak in the chromatogram obtained with reference solution (b) (1 per cent) and not more than 2 such peaks have an area greater than half the area of the principal peak in the chromatogram obtained with reference solution (b) (0.5 per cent),

– *total*: not more than twice the area of the principal peak in the chromatogram obtained with reference solution (b) (2 per cent),

– *disregard limit*: 0.05 times the area of the principal peak in the chromatogram obtained with reference solution (b) (0.05 per cent).

Water (*2.5.12*): maximum 1.0 per cent, determined on 0.500 g.

ASSAY

Prepare the solutions immediately before use and protect from light.

Dissolve 50.0 mg in *alcohol R* and dilute to 50.0 ml with the same solvent. Dilute 2.0 ml of the solution to 100.0 ml with *alcohol R*. Measure the absorbance (*2.2.25*) at the maximum at 238 nm.

Calculate the content of $C_{21}H_{27}FO_6$ taking the specific absorbance to be 389.

STORAGE

Protected from light.

IMPURITIES

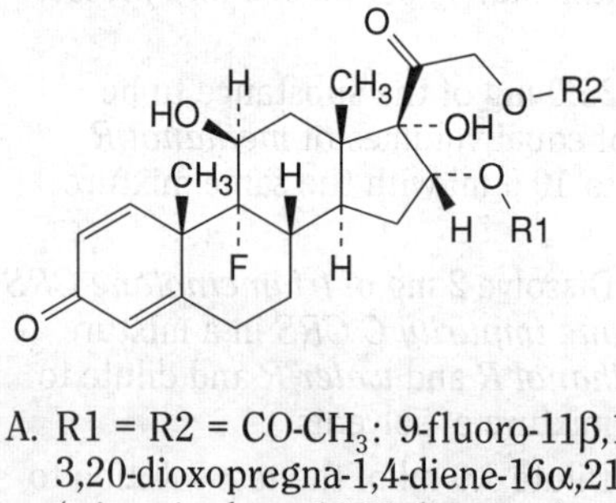

A. R1 = R2 = CO-CH_3: 9-fluoro-11β,17-dihydroxy-3,20-dioxopregna-1,4-diene-16α,21-diyl diacetate (triamcinolone 16,21-diacetate),

B. R1 = H, R2 = CO-CH_3: 9-fluoro-11β,16α,17-trihydroxy-3,20-dioxopregna-1,4-dien-21-yl acetate (triamcinolone 21-acetate),

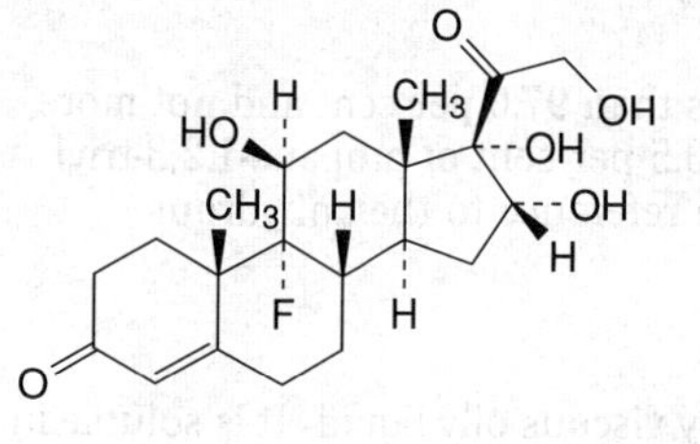

C. 9-fluoro-11β,16α,17,21-tetrahydroxypregn-4-ene-3,20-dione (pretriamcinolone).

01/2005:0533

TRIAMCINOLONE ACETONIDE

Triamcinoloni acetonidum

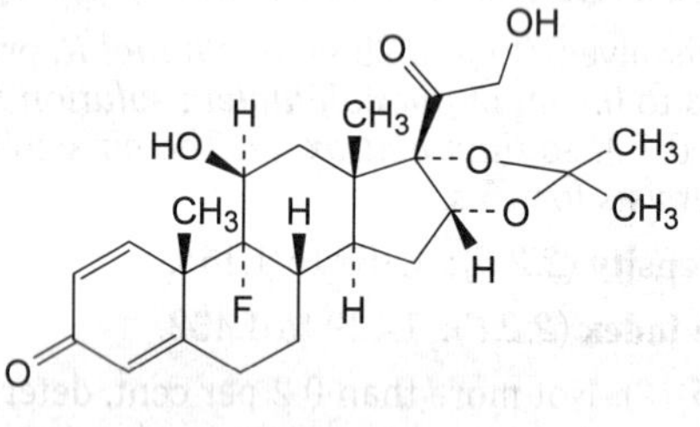

$C_{24}H_{31}FO_6$ M_r 434.5

DEFINITION

Triamcinolone acetonide contains not less than 97.0 per cent and not more than the equivalent of 103.0 per cent of 9-fluoro-11β,21-dihydroxy-16α,17-(1-methylethylidenedioxy)pregna-1,4-diene-3,20-dione, calculated with reference to the anhydrous substance.

CHARACTERS

A white or almost white, crystalline powder, practically insoluble in water, sparingly soluble in alcohol.

It shows polymorphism.

IDENTIFICATION

First identification: A, B.

Second identification: C, D.

A. Examine by infrared absorption spectrophotometry (*2.2.24*), comparing with the spectrum obtained with *triamcinolone acetonide CRS*. If the spectra obtained in the solid state show differences, dissolve the substance to be examined and the reference substance separately in the minimum volume of *methanol R* and evaporate to dryness. Using the residues, prepare halogen salt discs or mulls in *liquid paraffin R* and record the spectra again.

B. Examine by thin-layer chromatography (*2.2.27*), using as the coating substance a suitable silica gel with a fluorescent indicator having an optimal intensity at 254 nm. *Prepare the solutions immediately before use and protect from light. Examine the plate in ultraviolet light immediately after development.*

Test solution. Dissolve 10 mg of the substance to be examined in *methanol R* and dilute to 10 ml with the same solvent.

Reference solution (a). Dissolve 20 mg of *triamcinolone acetonide CRS* in *methanol R* and dilute to 20 ml with the same solvent.

Reference solution (b). Dissolve 10 mg of *triamcinolone hexacetonide CRS* in reference solution (a) and dilute to 10 ml with the same solution.

Apply to the plate 5 µl of each solution. Prepare the mobile phase by adding a mixture of 1.2 volumes of *water R* and 8 volumes of *methanol R* to a mixture of 15 volumes of *ether R* and 77 volumes of *methylene chloride R*. Develop over a path of 15 cm. Allow the plate to dry in air and examine in ultraviolet light at 254 nm. The principal spot in the chromatogram obtained with the test solution is similar in position and size to the principal spot in the chromatogram obtained with reference solution (a). The test is not valid unless the chromatogram obtained with reference solution (b) shows two clearly separated spots.

C. Examine by thin-layer chromatography (*2.2.27*), using as the coating substance a suitable silica gel with a fluorescent indicator having an optimal intensity at 254 nm. *Prepare the solutions immediately before use and protect from light. Examine the plate in ultraviolet light immediately after development.*

Test solution (a). Dissolve 10 mg of the substance to be examined in *methanol R* and dilute to 10 ml with the same solvent.

Test solution (b). In a separating funnel, dissolve 10 mg of the substance to be examined in 1.5 ml of *glacial acetic acid R*, add 0.5 ml of a 20 g/l solution of *chromium trioxide R* and allow to stand for 60 min. Add 5 ml of *water R*, 2 ml of *methylene chloride R* and shake vigorously for 2 min. Allow to separate and use the lower layer.

Reference solution (a). Dissolve 10 mg of *triamcinolone acetonide CRS* in *methanol R* and dilute to 10 ml with the same solvent.

Reference solution (b). In a separating funnel, dissolve 10 mg of *triamcinolone acetonide CRS* in 1.5 ml of *glacial acetic acid R*, add 0.5 ml of a 20 g/l solution of *chromium trioxide R* and allow to stand for 60 min. Add 5 ml of *water R*, 2 ml of *methylene chloride R* and shake vigorously for 2 min. Allow to separate and use the lower layer.

Apply separately to the plate 5 µl of each solution. Prepare the mobile phase by adding a mixture of 1.2 volumes of *water R* and 8 volumes of *methanol R* to a mixture of 15 volumes of *ether R* and 77 volumes of *methylene chloride R*. Develop over a path of 15 cm. Allow the plate to dry in air and examine in ultraviolet light at 254 nm. The principal spot in each of the chromatograms obtained with the test solutions is similar in position and size to the principal spot in the chromatogram obtained with the corresponding reference solution. The principal spots in the chromatograms obtained with test solution (b) and reference solution (b) have an R_f value distinctly higher than that of the principal spots in the chromatograms obtained with test solution (a) and reference solution (a).

D. Mix about 5 mg with 45 mg of *heavy magnesium oxide R* and ignite in a crucible until an almost white residue is obtained (usually less than 5 min). Allow to cool, add 1 ml of *water R*, 0.05 ml of *phenolphthalein solution R1* and about 1 ml of *dilute hydrochloric acid R* to render the solution colourless. Filter. To a freshly prepared mixture of 0.1 ml of *alizarin S solution R* and 0.1 ml of *zirconyl nitrate solution R*, add 1.0 ml of the filtrate. Mix, allow to stand for 5 min and compare the colour of the solution with that of a blank prepared in the same manner. The test solution is yellow and the blank is red.

TESTS

Specific optical rotation (*2.2.7*). Dissolve 0.100 g in *dioxan R* and dilute to 10.0 ml with the same solvent. The specific optical rotation is + 100 to + 107, calculated with reference to the anhydrous substance.

Related substances. Examine by liquid chromatography (*2.2.29*). *Carry out the test protected from light.*

Test solution. Dissolve 25.0 mg of the substance to be examined in 7 ml of *methanol R* and dilute to 10.0 ml with *water R*.

Reference solution (a). Dissolve 2 mg of *triamcinolone acetonide CRS* and 2 mg of *triamcinolone R* in the mobile phase and dilute to 100.0 ml with the mobile phase.

Reference solution (b). Dilute 1.0 ml of the test solution to 100.0 ml with the mobile phase.

The chromatographic procedure may be carried out using:

– a stainless steel column 0.25 m long and 4.6 mm in internal diameter packed with *octadecylsilyl silica gel for chromatography R* (5 µm),
– as mobile phase at a flow rate of 1.5 ml/min a mixture prepared as follows: in a 1000 ml volumetric flask mix 525 ml of *methanol R* with 400 ml of *water R* and allow to equilibrate; adjust the volume to 1000 ml with *water R* and mix again,
– as detector a spectrophotometer set at 254 nm.

Equilibrate the column with the mobile phase at a flow rate of 1.5 ml/min for about 10 min.

Adjust the sensitivity of the system so that the height of the principal peak in the chromatogram obtained with 20 µl of reference solution (b) is at least 50 per cent of the full scale of the recorder.

Inject 20 µl of reference solution (a). When the chromatograms are recorded in the prescribed conditions, the retention times are: triamcinolone about 5 min and triamcinolone acetonide about 17 min. The test is not valid unless the resolution between the peaks corresponding to triamcinolone and triamcinolone acetonide is at least 15; if necessary, adjust the concentration of methanol in the mobile phase.

Inject separately 20 µl of the test solution and 20 µl of reference solution (b). Continue the chromatography for 3.5 times the retention time of the principal peak in the chromatogram obtained with the test solution. In the chromatogram obtained with the test solution: the area of any peak, apart from the principal peak, is not greater than 0.25 times the area of the principal peak in the chromatogram obtained with reference solution (b) (0.25 per cent); the sum of the areas of all the peaks, apart from the principal peak, is not greater than half the area of the principal peak in the chromatogram obtained with reference solution (b) (0.5 per cent). Disregard any peak due to the solvent and any peak with an area less than 0.05 times the area of the principal peak in the chromatogram obtained with reference solution (b).

Water (*2.5.12*). Not more than 2.0 per cent, determined on 0.500 g by the semi-micro determination of water.

ASSAY

Protect the solutions from light throughout the assay.

Dissolve 50.0 mg in *alcohol R* and dilute to 50.0 ml with the same solvent. Dilute 2.0 ml of this solution to 100.0 ml with *alcohol R*. Measure the absorbance (*2.2.25*) at the maximum at 238.5 nm.

Calculate the content of $C_{24}H_{31}FO_6$ taking the specific absorbance to be 355.

STORAGE

Store protected from light.

IMPURITIES

A. triamcinolone.

01/2005:0867

TRIAMCINOLONE HEXACETONIDE

Triamcinoloni hexacetonidum

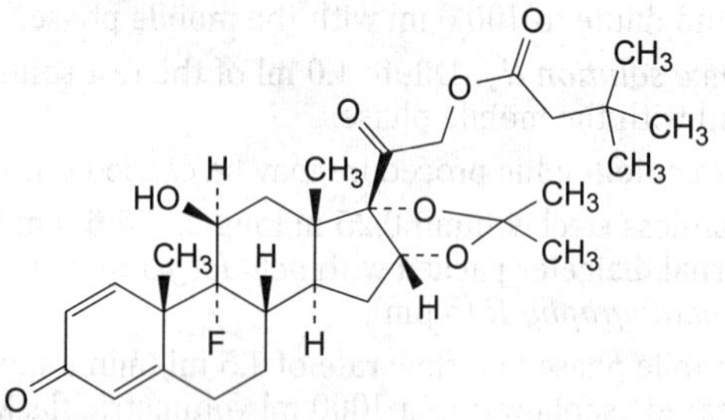

$C_{30}H_{41}FO_7$ M_r 532.6

DEFINITION

Triamcinolone hexacetonide contains not less than 97.0 per cent and not more than the equivalent of 103.0 per cent of 9-fluoro-11β-hydroxy-16α,17-(1-methylethylidenedioxy)-3,20-dioxopregna-1,4-diene-21-yl 3,3-dimethylbutanoate, calculated with reference to the anhydrous substance.

CHARACTERS

A white or almost white, crystalline powder, practically insoluble in water, sparingly soluble in ethanol and in methanol.

IDENTIFICATION

A. Examine by infrared absorption spectrophotometry (*2.2.24*), comparing with the spectrum obtained with *triamcinolone hexacetonide CRS*.

B. Examine by thin-layer chromatography (*2.2.27*), using as the coating substance a suitable silica gel with a fluorescent indicator having an optimal intensity at 254 nm. *Prepare the solutions immediately before use and protect from light. Examine the plate in ultraviolet light immediately after development.*

Test solution. Dissolve 10 mg of the substance to be examined in *methanol R* and dilute to 10 ml with the same solvent.

Reference solution (a). Dissolve 20 mg of *triamcinolone hexacetonide CRS* in *methanol R* and dilute to 20 ml with the same solvent.

Reference solution (b). Dissolve 10 mg of *triamcinolone acetonide CRS* in reference solution (a) and dilute to 10 ml with the same solution.

Apply separately to the plate 5 µl of each solution. Prepare the mobile phase by adding a mixture of 1.2 volumes of *water R* and 8 volumes of *methanol R* to a mixture of 15 volumes of *ether R* and 77 volumes of *methylene chloride R*. Develop over a path of 15 cm. Allow the plate to dry in air and examine in ultraviolet light at 254 nm. The principal spot in the chromatogram obtained with the test solution is similar in position and size to the principal spot in the chromatogram obtained with reference solution (a). The test is not valid unless the chromatogram obtained with reference solution (b) shows two clearly separated spots.

TESTS

Specific optical rotation (*2.2.7*). Dissolve 0.100 g in *methylene chloride R* and dilute to 10.0 ml with the same solvent. The specific optical rotation is + 92 to + 98, calculated with reference to the anhydrous substance.

Related substances. Examine by liquid chromatography (*2.2.29*). *Carry out the test protected from light.*

Test solution. Dissolve 25.0 mg of the substance to be examined in *methanol R* and dilute to 10.0 ml with the same solvent.

Reference solution (a). Dissolve 2 mg of *triamcinolone hexacetonide CRS* and 2 mg of *triamcinolone acetonide CRS* in the mobile phase and dilute to 100.0 ml with the mobile phase.

Reference solution (b). Dilute 1.0 ml of the test solution to 100.0 ml with the mobile phase.

The chromatographic procedure may be carried out using:

- a stainless steel column 0.25 m long and 4.6 mm in internal diameter packed with *octadecylsilyl silica gel for chromatography R* (5 µm),
- as mobile phase at a flow rate of 2 ml/min a mixture prepared as follows: in a 1000 ml volumetric flask mix 750 ml of *methanol R* with 200 ml of *water R* and allow to equilibrate; adjust the volume to 1000 ml with *water R* and mix again,
- as detector a spectrophotometer set at 254 nm.

Equilibrate the column with the mobile phase at a flow rate of 2 ml/min for about 10 min.

Adjust the sensitivity of the system so that the height of the principal peak in the chromatogram obtained with 20 µl of reference solution (b) is at least 50 per cent of the full scale of the recorder.

Inject 20 µl of reference solution (a). When the chromatograms are recorded in the prescribed conditions, the retention times are: triamcinolone acetonide about 3 min and triamcinolone hexacetonide about 12 min. The test is not valid unless the resolution between the peaks corresponding to triamcinolone acetonide and triamcinolone hexacetonide is at least 20.0; if necessary, adjust the concentration of methanol in the mobile phase.

Inject separately 20 µl of the test solution and 20 µl of reference solution (b). Continue the chromatography for three times the retention time of the principal peak in the chromatogram obtained with the test solution. In the chromatogram obtained with the test solution: the area of any peak, apart from the principal peak, is not greater than half the area of the principal peak in the chromatogram obtained with reference solution (b) (0.5 per cent); the sum of the areas of all the peaks, apart from the principal peak, is not greater than the area of the principal peak in the chromatogram obtained with reference solution (b) (1 per cent). Disregard any peak due to the solvent and any peak with an area less than 0.05 times the area of the principal peak in the chromatogram obtained with reference solution (b).

Water (*2.5.12*). Not more than 2.0 per cent, determined on 0.50 g by the semi-micro determination of water.

ASSAY

Dissolve 50.0 mg in *alcohol R* and dilute to 50.0 ml with the same solvent. Dilute 2.0 ml of this solution to 100.0 ml with *alcohol R*. Measure the absorbance (*2.2.25*) at the maximum at 238 nm.

Calculate the content of $C_{30}H_{41}FO_7$ taking the specific absorbance to be 291.

STORAGE

Store protected from light.

IMPURITIES

A. triamcinolone acetonide.

01/2005:0058

TRIAMTERENE

Triamterenum

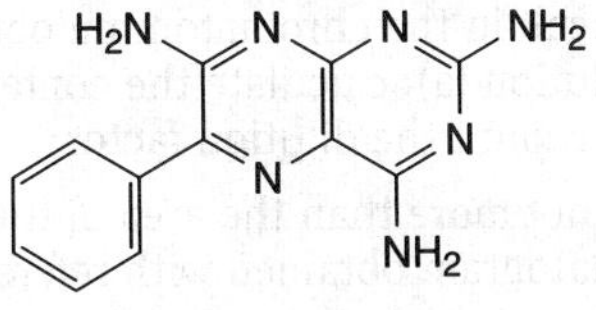

$C_{12}H_{11}N_7$ M_r 253.3

DEFINITION

Triamterene contains not less than 99.0 per cent and not more than the equivalent of 101.0 per cent of 6-phenylpteridine-2,4,7-triamine, calculated with reference to the dried substance.

CHARACTERS

A yellow, crystalline powder, very slightly soluble in water and in alcohol.

IDENTIFICATION

A. Dissolve 0.1 g in a 10 per cent *V/V* solution of *1 M hydrochloric acid* in *ethanol R* and dilute to 100 ml with the same acid mixture. Dilute 1 ml of this solution to 100 ml with a 10 per cent *V/V* solution of *1 M hydrochloric acid* in *ethanol R*. Examined between 255 nm and 380 nm, the solution shows 2 absorption maxima (*2.2.25*), at 262 nm and 360 nm, and a shoulder at 285 nm.

B. Examined in ultraviolet light at 365 nm, acid solutions, especially a 1 g/l solution in *anhydrous formic acid R*, show an intense blue fluorescence.

TESTS

Acidity. Boil 1.0 g with 20 ml of *water R* for 5 min, cool, filter and wash the filter with 3 quantities, each of 10 ml, of *water R*. Combine the filtrate and washings and add 0.3 ml of *phenolphthalein solution R*. Not more than 1.5 ml of *0.01 M sodium hydroxide* is required to change the colour of the indicator.

Nitrosotriaminopyrimidine. Examine by thin-layer chromatography (*2.2.27*), using *silica gel HF_{254} R* as the coating substance.

Test solution. Dissolve 0.2 g of the substance to be examined in 5 ml of *anhydrous formic acid R*, stirring with a glass rod if necessary. Prepare immediately before use.

Reference solution. Dissolve 4 mg of *nitrosotriaminopyrimidine CRS* in *anhydrous formic acid R* and dilute to 100 ml with the same acid.

Apply separately to the plate as bands 1.5 cm long, 20 µl of each solution as 2 applications of 10 µl each, drying in a current of air after each application. Develop over a path of 5 cm using *ether R*. Allow the plate to dry in air and develop over a path of 10 cm using a mixture of 10 volumes of *glacial acetic acid R*, 10 volumes of *methanol R* and 80 volumes of *ethyl acetate R*, the mixture containing 0.5 g/l of *sodium fluoresceinate R*. Dry the plate in a current of air and expose to ammonia vapour for a few seconds. Examine in ultraviolet light at 254 nm and at 365 nm. Any band corresponding to nitrosotriaminopyrimidine in the chromatogram obtained with the test solution is not more intense than the band in the chromatogram obtained with the reference solution (0.1 per cent).

Related substances. Examine by thin-layer chromatography (*2.2.27*), using *silica gel G R* as the coating substance.

Test solution. Dissolve 0.1 g of the substance to be examined in 20 ml of *dimethyl sulphoxide R*. Dilute 2 ml of the solution to 50 ml with *methanol R*.

Reference solution. Dilute 1 ml of the test solution to 200 ml with *methanol R*.

Apply separately to the plate 5 µl of each solution. Develop over a path of 15 cm using a mixture of 10 volumes of *concentrated ammonia R1*, 10 volumes of *methanol R* and 90 volumes of *ethyl acetate R*. Allow the plate to dry in air until the solvents have evaporated and examine in ultraviolet light at 365 nm. Any spot in the chromatogram obtained with the test solution, apart from the principal spot, is not more intense than the spot in the chromatogram obtained with the reference solution (0.5 per cent).

Loss on drying (*2.2.32*). Not more than 1.0 per cent, determined on 1.00 g by drying in an oven at 100 °C to 105 °C.

Sulphated ash (*2.4.14*). Not more than 0.1 per cent, determined on 1.0 g.

ASSAY

Dissolve 0.150 g in 5 ml of *anhydrous formic acid R* and add 100 ml of *anhydrous acetic acid R*. Titrate with *0.1 M perchloric acid* determining the end-point potentiometrically (*2.2.20*).

1 ml of *0.1 M perchloric acid* is equivalent to 25.33 mg of $C_{12}H_{11}N_7$.

STORAGE

Store protected from light.

01/2005:1740

TRIBENOSIDE

Tribenosidum

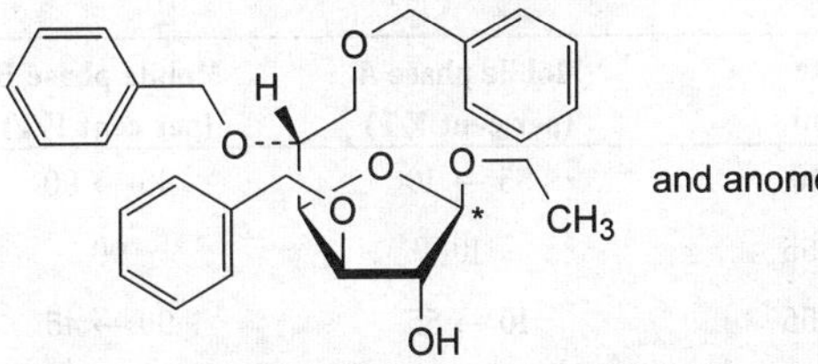

$C_{29}H_{34}O_6$ M_r 478.6

DEFINITION

Mixture of α- and β-anomers of ethyl 3,5,6-tri-*O*-benzyl-D-glucofuranoside.

Content: 96.0 per cent to 102.0 per cent.

CHARACTERS

Appearance: yellowish to pale yellow, clear, viscous liquid.

Solubility: practically insoluble in water, very soluble in acetone, in methanol and in methylene chloride.

IDENTIFICATION

Infrared absorption spectrophotometry (*2.2.24*).

Preparation: discs.

Monographs T-Z

Comparison: *tribenoside CRS*.

TESTS

Solution S. Dissolve 4.00 g in *methanol R* and dilute to 20 ml with the same solvent.

Appearance of solution. Solution S is clear (*2.2.1*) and its absorbance (*2.2.25*) at 420 nm has a maximum of 0.10.

Specific optical rotation (*2.2.7*): − 31.0 to − 40.0.

Dilute 2.0 ml of solution S to 20.0 ml with *methanol R*.

Related substances. Liquid chromatography (*2.2.29*).

Test solution (a). Dissolve 1.000 g of the substance to be examined in a mixture of 5 volumes of *water R* and 95 volumes of *acetonitrile R* and dilute to 25.0 ml with the same mixture of solvents.

Test solution (b). Dissolve 50.0 mg of the substance to be examined in a mixture of 5 volumes of *water R* and 95 volumes of *acetonitrile R* and dilute to 50.0 ml with the same mixture of solvents.

Reference solution (a). Dilute 25.0 mg of *benzaldehyde R* and 30.0 mg of *tribenoside impurity A CRS* to 100.0 ml with *acetonitrile R*. Introduce 20.0 ml of this solution into a 50 ml volumetric flask, add 2.5 ml of *water R* and dilute to 50.0 ml with *acetonitrile R*.

Reference solution (b). Dissolve 50.0 mg of *tribenoside CRS* in a mixture of 5 volumes of *water R* and 95 volumes of *acetonitrile R* and dilute to 50.0 ml with the same mixture of solvents.

Reference solution (c). Dissolve 12.0 mg of *benzyl ether R* in a mixture of 5 volumes of *water R* and 95 volumes of *acetonitrile R* and dilute to 100.0 ml with the same mixture of solvents.

Column:
- *size*: *l* = 0.15 m, Ø = 4.6 mm,
- *stationary phase*: *octadecylsilyl silica gel for chromatography R* (3 µm).

Mobile phase:
- *mobile phase A*: 0.1 per cent *V/V* solution of *phosphoric acid R*,
- *mobile phase B*: *acetonitrile R*,

Time (min)	Mobile phase A (per cent *V/V*)	Mobile phase B (per cent *V/V*)
0 - 40	55 → 10	45 → 90
40 - 55	10	90
55 - 56	10 → 55	90 → 45
56 - 60	55	45

Flow rate: 1.3 ml/min.

Detection: spectrophotometer at 254 nm.

Injection: 20 µl; inject test solution (a) and reference solutions (a), (b) and (c).

Relative retentions with reference to the β-anomer of tribenoside (retention time = about 18 min): α-anomer = about 1.1; impurity C = about 0.2; impurity B = about 0.6; impurity D = about 0.8; impurity A = about 1.4.

System suitability: reference solution (b):
- *resolution*: minimum 3.0 between the peaks due to the α-anomer and to the β-anomer of tribenoside.

Limits:
- *impurity A*: not more than 1.7 times the area of the corresponding peak in the chromatogram obtained with reference solution (a) (0.5 per cent),
- *impurity C*: not more than twice the area of the corresponding peak in the chromatogram obtained with reference solution (a) (0.5 per cent); if the area of the peak due to impurity C in the chromatogram obtained with the test solution is greater than the area of the corresponding peak in the chromatogram obtained with reference solution (a) (0.25 per cent), dilute the test solution to obtain an area equal to or smaller than the area of the peak in the chromatogram obtained with reference solution (a); calculate the content of impurity C taking into account the dilution factor;
- *impurity D*: not more than the area of the principal peak in the chromatogram obtained with reference solution (c) (0.3 per cent),
- *any other impurity*: not more than the area of the peak due to impurity A in the chromatogram obtained with reference solution (a) (0.3 per cent),
- *total*: not more than 6.7 times the area of the peak due to impurity A in the chromatogram obtained with reference solution (a) (2.0 per cent),
- *disregard limit*: 0.17 times the area of the peak due to impurity A in the chromatogram obtained with reference solution (a) (0.05 per cent).

Heavy metals (*2.4.8*): maximum 20 ppm.

Dilute 5.0 ml of solution S to 20.0 ml with *methanol R*. 12 ml of the solution complies with limit test B. Prepare the standard using lead standard solution (1 ppm Pb) obtained by diluting *lead standard solution (100 ppm Pb) R* with *methanol R*.

ASSAY

Liquid chromatography (*2.2.29*) as described in the test for related substances with the following modification.

Injection: test solution (b) and reference solution (b).

Calculate the sum of the percentage contents of the α-anomer and the β-anomer of tribenoside.

STORAGE

Under nitrogen, in an airtight container.

IMPURITIES

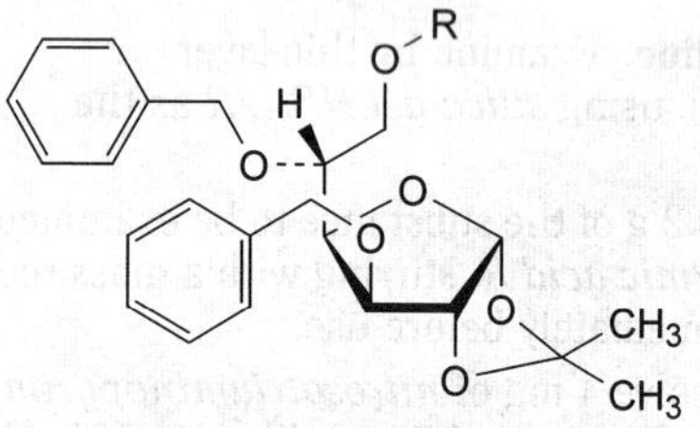

A. R = CH_2-C_6H_5: 3,5,6-tri-*O*-benzyl-1,2-*O*-(1-methylethylidene)-α-D-glucofuranose,

B. R = H: 3,5-di-*O*-benzyl-1,2-*O*-(1-methylethylidene)-α-D-glucofuranose,

C. C_6H_5-CHO: benzaldehyde,

D. C_6H_5-CH_2-O-CH_2-C_6H_5: dibenzyl ether.

Monographs T-Z

01/2005:1770

TRIBUTYL ACETYLCITRATE

Tributylis acetylcitras

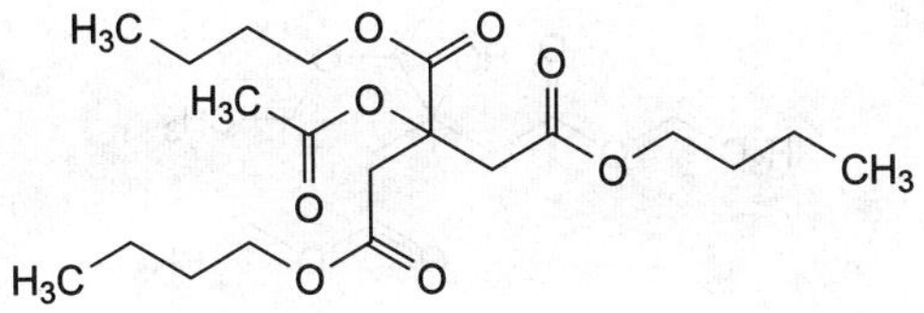

$C_{20}H_{34}O_8$ M_r 402.5

DEFINITION

Tributyl 2-(acetyloxy)propane-1,2,3-tricarboxylate.

Content: 99.0 per cent to 101.0 per cent (anhydrous substance).

CHARACTERS

Appearance: clear, oily liquid.

Solubility: not miscible with water, miscible with alcohol and with methylene chloride.

IDENTIFICATION

Infrared absorption spectrophotometry (*2.2.24*).

Comparison: *Ph. Eur. reference spectrum of tributyl acetylcitrate.*

TESTS

Appearance. The substance to be examined is clear (*2.2.1*) and not more intensely coloured than reference solution BY_6 (*2.2.2, Method II*).

Acidity. Dilute 10 g with 10 ml of previously neutralised *alcohol R*, add 0.5 ml of *bromothymol blue solution R2*. Not more than 0.3 ml of *0.1 M sodium hydroxide* is required to change the colour of the indicator to blue.

Refractive index (*2.2.6*): 1.442 to 1.445.

Related substances. Gas chromatography (*2.2.28*).

Test solution. Dissolve 1.0 g of the substance to be examined in *methylene chloride R* and dilute to 20.0 ml with the same solvent.

Reference solution (a). Dissolve 50 mg of the substance to be examined and 50 mg of *tributyl citrate R* in *methylene chloride R* and dilute to 20.0 ml with the same solvent.

Reference solution (b). Dilute 1.0 ml of the test solution to 20.0 ml with *methylene chloride R*. Dilute 1.0 ml of this solution to 25.0 ml with *methylene chloride R*.

Column:
- *material*: fused silica,
- *size*: l = 30 m, Ø = 0.53 mm,
- *stationary phase*: *poly[(cyanopropyl)(methyl)][(phenyl)(methyl)]siloxane R* (film thickness 1.0 µm).

Carrier gas: *helium for chromatography R.*

Linear velocity: 36 cm/s.

Split ratio: 1:20.

Temperature:
- *column*: 200 °C,
- *injection port and detector*: 250 °C.

Detection: flame ionisation.

Injection: 1 µl.

Run time: twice the retention time of tributyl acetylcitrate.

Relative retention with reference to tributyl acetylcitrate (retention time = abou 26 min): impurity B = about 0.83; impurity A = about 0.87.

System suitability: reference solution (a):
- *resolution*: minimum 2.0 between the peaks due to impurity A and tributyl acetylcitrate.

Limits:
- *impurities A, B*: for each impurity, not more than the area of the principal peak in the chromatogram obtained with reference solution (b) (0.2 per cent),
- *any other impurity*: for each impurity, not more than 0.5 times the area of the principal peak in the chromatogram obtained with reference solution (b) (0.1 per cent),
- *total*: not more than 2.5 times the area of the principal peak in the chromatogram obtained with reference solution (b) (0.5 per cent),
- *disregard limit*: 0.25 times the area of the principal peak in the chromatogram obtained with reference solution (b) (0.05 per cent).

Heavy metals (*2.4.8*): maximum 10 ppm.

2.0 g complies with limit test F. Prepare the standard using 2 ml of *lead standard solution (10 ppm Pb) R.*

Water (*2.5.12*): maximum 0.25 per cent, determined on 2.00 g.

Sulphated ash (*2.4.14*): maximum 0.1 per cent, determined on 1.0 g.

ASSAY

Introduce 1.500 g into a 250 ml borosilicate glass flask. Add 25 ml of *2-propanol R*, 50 ml of *water R*, 25.0 ml of *1 M sodium hydroxide* and a few glass beads. Heat under a reflux condenser for 1 h. Allow to cool. Add 1 ml of *phenolphthalein solution R1* and titrate with *1 M hydrochloric acid.* Carry out a blank titration.

1 ml of *1 M sodium hydroxide* is equivalent to 100.6 mg of $C_{20}H_{34}O_8$.

IMPURITIES

Specified impurities: A, B.

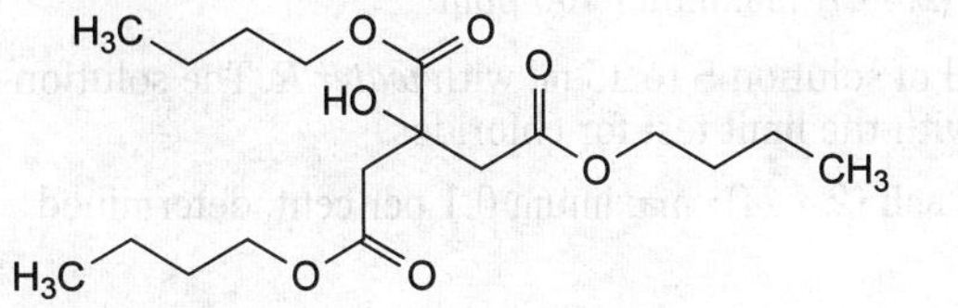

A. tributyl 2-hydroxypropane-1,2,3-tricarboxylate (tributyl citrate),

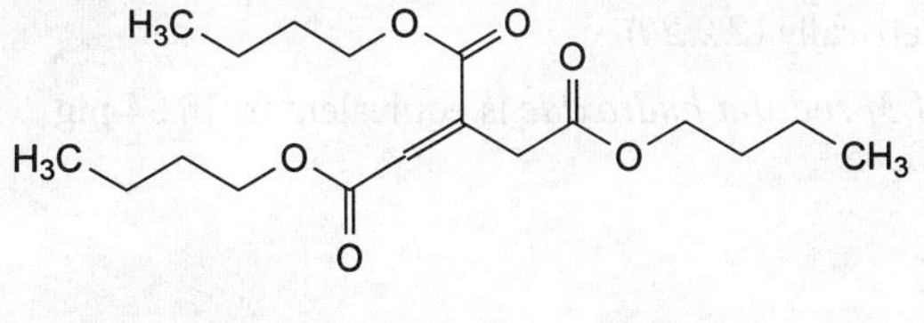

B. tributyl propene-1,2,3-tricarboxylate (tributyl aconitate).

01/2005:1967

TRICHLOROACETIC ACID

Acidum trichloraceticum

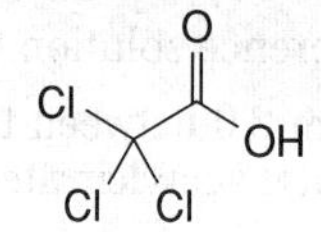

$C_2HCl_3O_2$ M_r 163.4

DEFINITION

2,2,2-Trichloroacetic acid.

Content: 98.0 per cent to 100.5 per cent.

CHARACTERS

Appearance: white, crystalline mass or colourless crystals, very deliquescent.

Solubility: very soluble in water, in alcohol and in methylene chloride.

IDENTIFICATION

First identification: A.

Second identification: B, C.

A. Infrared absorption spectrophotometry (*2.2.24*).

Comparison: *Ph. Eur. reference spectrum of trichloroacetic acid.*

B. To 0.5 ml of solution S (see Tests) add 2 ml of *pyridine R* and 5 ml of *strong sodium hydroxide solution R*. Shake vigorously and heat in a water-bath at 60-70 °C for 5 min. The upper layer shows an intense red colour.

C. Solution S is strongly acidic (*2.2.4*).

TESTS

Solution S. Dissolve 2.5 g in *water R* and dilute to 25 ml with the same solvent.

Appearance of solution. Solution S is clear (*2.2.1*) and not more intensely coloured than reference solution BY_7 (*2.2.2, Method II*).

Chlorides (*2.4.4*): maximum 100 ppm.

Dilute 5 ml of solution S to 15 ml with *water R*. The solution complies with the limit test for chlorides.

Sulphated ash (*2.4.14*): maximum 0.1 per cent, determined on 1.0 g.

ASSAY

Dissolve 0.150 g in 20 ml of *water R*. Titrate with *0.1 M sodium hydroxide,* determining the end-point potentiometrically (*2.2.20*).

1 ml of *0.1 M sodium hydroxide* is equivalent to 16.34 mg of $C_2HCl_3O_2$.

STORAGE

In an airtight container.

01/2005:1479

TRIETHYL CITRATE

Triethylis citras

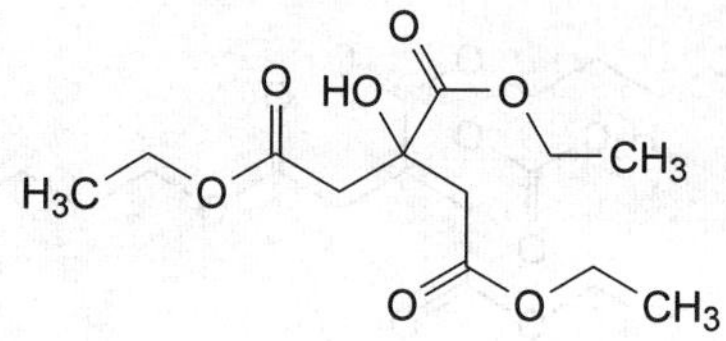

$C_{12}H_{20}O_7$ M_r 276.3

DEFINITION

Triethyl citrate contains not less than 98.5 per cent and not more than the equivalent of 101.0 per cent of triethyl 2-hydroxypropane-1,2,3-tricarboxylate, calculated with reference to the anhydrous substance.

CHARACTERS

A clear, viscous, colourless or almost colourless liquid, hygroscopic, soluble in water, miscible with alcohol, slightly soluble in fatty oils.

IDENTIFICATION

First identification: A, B.

Second identification: A, C, D.

A. It complies with the test for refractive index (see Tests).

B. Examine by infrared absorption spectrophotometry (*2.2.24*), comparing with the *Ph. Eur. reference spectrum of triethyl citrate.*

C. It gives the reaction of esters (*2.3.1*).

D. To 0.5 ml add 5 ml of *alcohol R* and 4 ml of *dilute sodium hydroxide solution R*. Boil under reflux for about 10 min. 2 ml of the solution gives the reaction of citrates (*2.3.1*).

TESTS

Appearance. The substance to be examined is clear (*2.2.1*) and not more intensely coloured than reference solution BY_6 (*2.2.2, Method II*).

Acidity. Dilute 10 g with 10 ml of previously neutralised *alcohol R*, add 0.5 ml of *bromothymol blue solution R2*. Not more than 0.3 ml of *0.1 M sodium hydroxide* is required to change the colour of the indicator to blue.

Refractive index (*2.2.6*): 1.440 to 1.446.

Related substances. Examine by gas chromatography (*2.2.28*).

Test solution. Dissolve 1.0 ml of the substance to be examined in *methylene chloride R* and dilute to 50.0 ml with the same solvent.

Reference solution (a). Dissolve 1.0 ml of the substance to be examined and 0.5 ml of *methyl tridecanoate R* in *methylene chloride R* and dilute to 50.0 ml with the same solvent.

The chromatographic procedure may be carried out using:

– a fused-silica column 30 m long and 0.32 mm in internal diameter coated with *poly(dimethyl)siloxane R* (5 µm),

– *helium for chromatography R* as the carrier gas with a split ratio of about 1:50 and a linear velocity of about 26 cm/s,

– a flame-ionisation detector,

maintaining the temperature of the column at 200 °C and that of the injection port and the detector at 220 °C.

Monographs T-Z

Inject 1.0 µl of each of the solutions. Continue the chromatography for twice the retention time of triethyl citrate which is about 13.6 min.

The test is not valid unless in the chromatogram obtained with reference solution (a), the resolution between the peaks corresponding to triethyl citrate and methyl tridecanoate is at least 1.5.

Calculate the percentage content of related substances from the areas of the peaks in the chromatogram obtained with the test solution by the normalisation procedure, disregarding any peaks with an area less than 0.04 per cent of the area of the principal peak. The content of any related substance is not greater than 0.2 per cent and the sum is not greater than 0.5 per cent.

Heavy metals (*2.4.8*). Dissolve 4.0 g in 8 ml of *alcohol R* and dilute to 20 ml with *water R*. 12 ml of the solution complies with limit test B for heavy metals (5 ppm). Prepare the standard using lead standard solution (1 ppm) obtained by diluting *lead standard solution (100 ppm Pb) R* with a mixture of equal volumes of *alcohol R* and *water R*.

Water (*2.5.12*). Not more than 0.25 per cent, determined on 1.000 g by the semi-micro determination of water.

Sulphated ash (*2.4.14*). Not more than 0.1 per cent, determined on 1.0 g.

ASSAY

Introduce 1.500 g into a 250 ml borosilicate-glass flask fitted with a reflux condenser. Add 25 ml of *2-propanol R*, 50 ml of *water R*, 25.0 ml of *1 M sodium hydroxide* and a few glass beads. Heat under a reflux condenser for 1 h. Allow to cool. Add 1 ml of *phenolphthalein solution R1* and titrate with *1 M hydrochloric acid*. Carry out a blank test under the same conditions.

1 ml of *1 M sodium hydroxide* is equivalent to 92.1 mg of $C_{12}H_{20}O_7$.

STORAGE

Store in an airtight container.

IMPURITIES

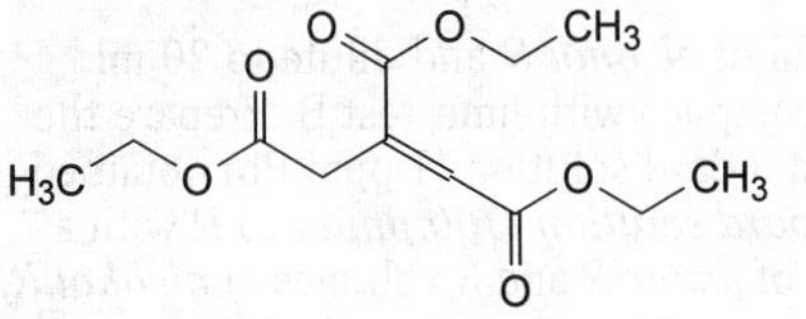

A. triethyl propene-1,2,3-tricarboxylate (triethyl aconitate).

01/2005:0059

TRIFLUOPERAZINE HYDROCHLORIDE

Trifluoperazini hydrochloridum

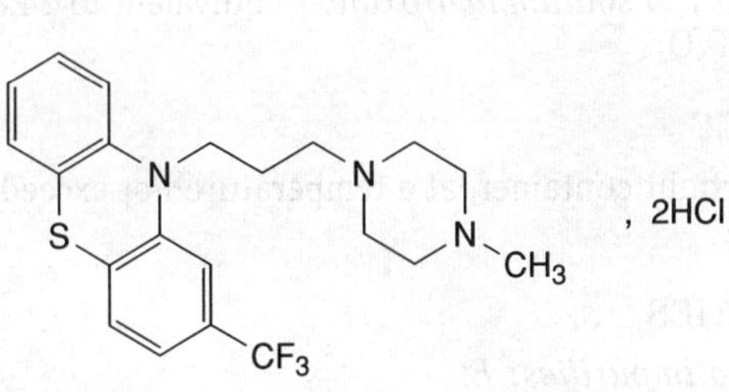

$C_{21}H_{26}Cl_2F_3N_3S$ M_r 480.4

DEFINITION

Trifluoperazine hydrochloride contains not less than 99.0 per cent and not more than the equivalent of 101.0 per cent of 10-[3-(4-methylpiperazin-1-yl)propyl]-2-(trifluoromethyl)-10*H*-phenothiazine dihydrochloride, calculated with reference to the dried substance.

CHARACTERS

A white to pale yellow, crystalline powder, hygroscopic, freely soluble in water, soluble in alcohol.

It melts at about 242 °C, with decomposition.

IDENTIFICATION

A. *Protect the solutions from bright light and measure the absorbances immediately.* Dissolve 50 mg in *0.1 M hydrochloric acid* and dilute to 500 ml with the same acid. Examined between 280 nm and 350 nm, the solution shows an absorption maximum (*2.2.25*) at 305 nm. Dilute 5 ml of the solution to 100 ml with *0.1 M hydrochloric acid*. Examined between 230 nm and 280 nm, this solution shows an absorption maximum at 255 nm. The specific absorbance at this maximum is about 650.

B. It complies with the identification test for phenothiazines by thin-layer chromatography (*2.3.3*).

C. Place 0.25 g in a 100 ml separating funnel, add 5 ml of *water R* and 2 ml of *dilute sodium hydroxide solution R*. Shake vigorously with 20 ml of *ether R*. Wash the ether layer with 5 ml of *water R*, add 0.15 g of *maleic acid R* and evaporate the ether. The residue, recrystallised from 30 ml of *alcohol R* and dried, melts (*2.2.14*) at about 192 °C.

D. Dissolve about 0.5 mg in 1 ml of *water R*, add 0.1 ml of *bromine water R* and shake for about 1 min. Add dropwise 1 ml of *sulphuric acid R* with constant, vigorous agitation. A red colour develops.

E. Dissolve about 50 mg in 5 ml of *water R* and add 2 ml of *nitric acid R*. A dark-red colour develops which turns to pale yellow. The solution gives reaction (a) of chlorides (*2.3.1*).

TESTS

pH (*2.2.3*). Dissolve 2.0 g in *carbon dioxide-free water R* and dilute to 20 ml with the same solvent. The pH of the solution is 1.6 to 2.5.

Related substances. *Carry out the test protected from bright light.*

Examine by thin-layer chromatography (*2.2.27*), using a *TLC silica gel GF_{254} plate R*.

Test solution. Dissolve 0.2 g of the substance to be examined in a mixture of 5 volumes of *diethylamine R* and 95 volumes of *methanol R* and dilute to 10 ml with the same mixture of solvents. Prepare immediately before use.

Reference solution. Dilute 1 ml of the test solution to 200 ml with a mixture of 5 volumes of *diethylamine R* and 95 volumes of *methanol R*.

Apply to the plate 10 µl of each solution. Develop over a path of 12 cm using a mixture of 10 volumes of *acetone R*, 10 volumes of *diethylamine R* and 80 volumes of *cyclohexane R*. Allow the plate to dry in air and examine in ultraviolet light at 254 nm. Any spot in the chromatogram obtained with the test solution, apart from the principal spot, is not more intense than the spot in the chromatogram obtained with the reference solution (0.5 per cent).

Loss on drying (*2.2.32*). Not more than 1.5 per cent, determined on 1.000 g by drying in an oven at 100 °C to 105 °C.

Sulphated ash (*2.4.14*). Not more than 0.1 per cent, determined on 1.0 g.

ASSAY

Dissolve 0.200 g in 50 ml of *alcohol R* and add 5.0 ml of *0.01 M hydrochloric acid.* Carry out a potentiometric titration (*2.2.20*), using *0.1 M sodium hydroxide.* Read the volume added between the 2 points of inflexion.

1 ml of *0.1 M sodium hydroxide* is equivalent to 24.02 mg of $C_{21}H_{26}Cl_2F_3N_3S$.

STORAGE

Store in an airtight container, protected from light.

01/2005:1377

TRIFLUSAL

Triflusalum

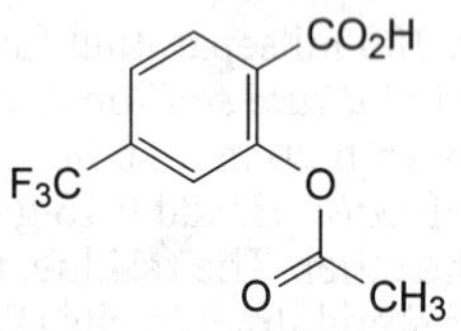

$C_{10}H_7F_3O_4$ M_r 248.2

DEFINITION

2-(Acetyloxy)-4-(trifluoromethyl)benzoic acid.

Content: 98.5 per cent to 101.5 per cent (dried substance).

CHARACTERS

Appearance: white or almost white, crystalline powder.

Solubility: practically insoluble in water, very soluble in ethanol, freely soluble in methylene chloride.

mp: about 118 °C, with decomposition.

IDENTIFICATION

Infrared absorption spectrophotometry (*2.2.24*).

Preparation: discs.
Comparison: *triflusal CRS*.

TESTS

Related substances. Liquid chromatography (*2.2.29*).

Test solution. Dissolve 0.20 g of the substance to be examined in *acetonitrile R* and dilute to 20.0 ml with the same solvent. *Prepare the solution immediately before use.*

Reference solution (a). Dissolve 5.0 mg of *triflusal impurity B CRS* in *acetonitrile R* and dilute to 10.0 ml with the same solvent.

Reference solution (b). Dilute 1.0 ml of reference solution (a) to 25.0 ml with *acetonitrile R.*

Reference solution (c). Dissolve 2.5 mg of the substance to be examined in *acetonitrile R,* add 5 ml of reference solution (a) and dilute to 10 ml with *acetonitrile R. Prepare the solution immediately before use.*

Column:

- *size*: l = 0.15 m, Ø = 4.0 mm,
- *stationary phase*: *octadecylsilyl silica gel for chromatography R* (4-5 µm).

Mobile phase:

- *mobile phase A*: *acetonitrile R,*
- *mobile phase B*: 0.5 per cent *V/V* solution of *phosphoric acid R,*

Time (min)	Mobile phase A (per cent *V/V*)	Mobile phase B (per cent *V/V*)
0 - 20	20 → 70	80 → 30
20 - 25	70	30
25 - 26	70 → 20	30 → 80
26 - 30	20	80

Flow rate: 1.2 ml/min.

Detection: spectrophotometer at 237 nm.

Injection: 10 µl of the test solution and reference solutions (b) and (c).

Relative retention with reference to triflusal (retention time = about 13 min): impurity A = about 0.3; impurity B = about 1.2; impurity C = about 1.3; impurity D = about 1.6.

System suitability: reference solution (c):

- *resolution*: minimum 3.0 between the peaks due to triflusal and impurity B.

Limits:

- *impurity B*: not more than 1.5 times the area of the corresponding peak in the chromatogram obtained with reference solution (b) (0.3 per cent),
- *total of impurities other than B*: not more than 0.5 times the area of the peak due to impurity B in the chromatogram obtained with reference solution (b) (0.1 per cent),
- *disregard limit*: 0.1 times the area of the peak due to impurity B in the chromatogram obtained with reference solution (b) (0.02 per cent).

Heavy metals (*2.4.8*): maximum 10 ppm.

Dissolve 2.0 g in 12 ml of *alcohol R* and dilute to 20 ml with *water R.* 12 ml complies with limit test B. Prepare the standard using lead standard solution (1 ppm Pb) obtained by diluting *lead standard solution (100 ppm Pb) R* with a mixture of 2 volumes of *water R* and 3 volumes of *alcohol R.*

Loss on drying (*2.2.32*): maximum 0.5 per cent, determined on 1.000 g by drying in a desiccator *in vacuo* over *diphosphorus pentoxide R.*

Sulphated ash (*2.4.14*): maximum 0.1 per cent, determined on 1.0 g in a platinum crucible.

ASSAY

Dissolve 0.200 g in 50 ml of *ethanol R*. Titrate with *0.1 M sodium hydroxide,* determining the end-point potentiometrically (*2.2.20*).

1 ml of *0.1 M sodium hydroxide* is equivalent to 24.82 mg of $C_{10}H_7F_3O_4$.

STORAGE

In an airtight container, at a temperature not exceeding 25 °C.

IMPURITIES

Specified impurities: B.

Other detectable impurities: A, C, D.

Monographs T-Z

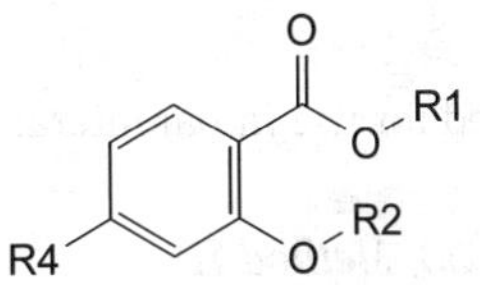

A. R1 = H, R2 = CO-CH_3, R4 = CO_2H: 2-(acetyloxy)benzene-1,4-dicarboxylic acid (2-acetoxyterephthalic acid),

B. R1 = R2 = H, R4 = CF_3: 2-hydroxy-4-(trifluoromethyl)benzoic acid (4-(trifluoromethyl)salicylic acid),

C. R1 = R2 = CO-CH_3, R4 = CF_3: acetic 2-(acetyloxy)-4-(trifluoromethyl)benzoic anhydride,

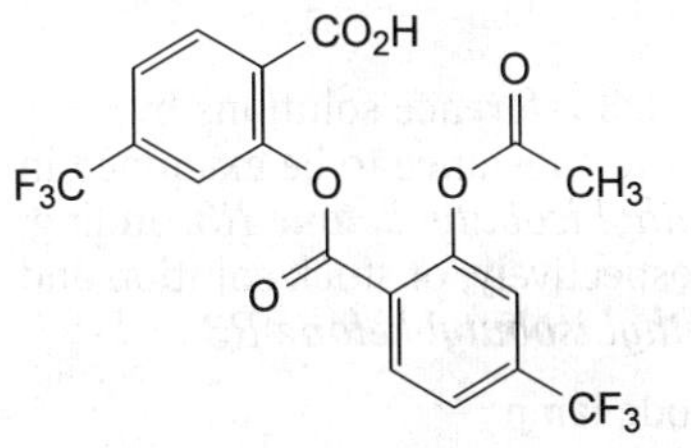

D. 2-[[2-(acetyloxy)-4-(trifluoromethyl)benzoyl]oxy]-4-(trifluoromethyl)benzoic acid.

01/2005:0868

TRIGLYCERIDES, MEDIUM-CHAIN

Triglycerida saturata media

DEFINITION

Mixture of triglycerides of saturated fatty acids, mainly of caprylic acid (octanoic acid, $C_8H_{16}O_2$) and of capric acid (decanoic acid, $C_{10}H_{20}O_2$). Medium-chain triglycerides are obtained from the oil extracted from the hard, dried fraction of the endosperm of *Cocos nucifera* L. or from the dried endosperm of *Elaeis guineensis* Jacq.

Content: minimum 95.0 per cent of saturated fatty acids with 8 and 10 carbon atoms.

CHARACTERS

Appearance: colourless or slightly yellowish, oily liquid.

Solubility: practically insoluble in water, miscible with alcohol, with methylene chloride, with light petroleum and with fatty oils.

IDENTIFICATION

First identification: B, C.

Second identification: A, D.

A. Heat 3.0 g under a reflux condenser for 30 min with 50 ml of a mixture of equal volumes of *alcohol R* and *2 M alcoholic potassium hydroxide R*. Reserve 10 ml of the mixture for identification test D. To 40 ml of the mixture add 30 ml of *water R*, evaporate the alcohol and acidify the hot solution with 25 ml of *dilute hydrochloric acid R*. After cooling, shake with 50 ml of *peroxide-free ether R*. Wash the ether layer with 3 quantities, each of 10 ml, of *sodium chloride solution R*, dry over *anhydrous sodium sulphate R* and filter. Evaporate the ether and determine the acid value (*2.5.1*) of the residue, using 0.300 g. The acid value is 350 to 390.

B. It complies with the test for saponification value (see Tests).

C. It complies with the test for composition of fatty acids (see Tests).

D. Evaporate 10 ml of the alcoholic mixture obtained in identification test A to dryness on a water-bath. Transfer the residue into a test-tube, add 0.3 ml of *sulphuric acid R* and close the test-tube with a stopper through which a U-shaped glass tube is inserted. One end of the U-tube is dipped into 3 ml of a 10 g/l solution of *tryptophan R* in a mixture of equal volumes of *sulphuric acid R* and *water R*. Heat the test-tube in a silicone-oil bath at 180 °C for 10 min and collect the liberated fumes in the tryptophan reagent. Heat the tryptophan reagent on a water-bath for 1 min. A violet colour develops.

TESTS

Appearance. The substance to be examined is clear (*2.2.1*) and not more intensely coloured than reference solution Y_3 (*2.2.2, Method I*).

Alkaline impurities. Dissolve 2.00 g in a mixture of 1.5 ml of *alcohol R* and 3.0 ml of *ether R*. Add 0.05 ml of *bromophenol blue solution R*. Not more than 0.15 ml of *0.01 M hydrochloric acid* is required to change the colour of the indicator to yellow.

Relative density (*2.2.5*): 0.93 to 0.96.

Refractive index (*2.2.6*): 1.440 to 1.452.

Viscosity (*2.2.9*): 25 mPa·s to 33 mPa·s.

Acid value (*2.5.1*): maximum 0.2.

Hydroxyl value (*2.5.3, Method A*): maximum 10.

Iodine value (*2.5.4*): maximum 1.0.

Peroxide value (*2.5.5, Method A*): maximum 1.0.

Saponification value (*2.5.6*): 310 to 360.

Unsaponifiable matter (*2.5.7*): maximum 0.5 per cent, determined on 5.0 g.

Composition of fatty acids. Gas chromatography (*2.4.22, Method C*).

Column:

- *material*: fused silica,
- *size*: *l* = 30 m, Ø = 0.32 mm,
- *stationary phase*: *macrogol 20 000 R* (film thickness 0.5 µm),

Carrier gas: *helium for chromatography R*.

Flow rate: 1.3 ml/min.

Temperature:

	Time (min)	Temperature (°C)
Column	0 - 1	70
	1 - 35	70 → 240
	35 - 50	240
Injection port		250
Detector		250

Detection: flame ionisation.

Split ratio: 1:100.

Composition of the fatty acid fraction of the substance:

- *caproic acid*: maximum 2.0 per cent,
- *caprylic acid*: 50.0 per cent to 80.0 per cent,
- *capric acid*: 20.0 per cent to 50.0 per cent,
- *lauric acid*: maximum 3.0 per cent,
- *myristic acid*: maximum 1.0 per cent.

Chromium: maximum 0.05 ppm, if intended for use in parenteral nutrition.

Atomic absorption spectrometry (*2.2.23, Method II*).

Test solution. Dissolve 2.0 g of the substance to be examined in *methyl isobutyl ketone R3* and dilute to 10.0 ml with the same solvent.

Solution A. Dilute 0.100 ml of *chromium liposoluble standard solution (1000 ppm Cr) R* to 10.0 ml with *methyl isobutyl ketone R3*.

Stock solution. Dilute 0.100 ml of solution A to 10.0 ml with *methyl isobutyl ketone R3*.

Reference solutions. Prepare 3 reference solutions by dissolving for each 2.0 g of the substance to be examined in the minimum volume of *methyl isobutyl ketone R3*, adding 0.5 ml, 1.0 ml and 2.0 ml, respectively, of stock solution and diluting to 10.0 ml with *methyl isobutyl ketone R3*.

Source: chromium hollow-cathode lamp.

Wavelength: 357.8 nm.

Atomic generator: graphite furnace.

Carrier gas: *argon R*.

Copper: maximum 0.1 ppm, if intended for use in parenteral nutrition.

Atomic absorption spectrometry (*2.2.23, Method II*).

Test solution. Dissolve 2.0 g of the substance to be examined in *methyl isobutyl ketone R3* and dilute to 10.0 ml with the same solvent.

Solution A. Dilute 0.100 ml of *copper liposoluble standard solution (1000 ppm Cu) R* to 10.0 ml with *methyl isobutyl ketone R3*.

Stock solution. Dilute 0.100 ml of solution A to 10.0 ml with *methyl isobutyl ketone R3*.

Reference solutions. Prepare 3 reference solutions by dissolving for each 2.0 g of the substance to be examined in the minimum volume of *methyl isobutyl ketone R3*, adding 1.0 ml, 2.0 ml and 4.0 ml, respectively, of stock solution and diluting to 10.0 ml with *methyl isobutyl ketone R3*.

Source: copper hollow-cathode lamp.

Wavelength: 324.7 nm.

Atomic generator: graphite furnace.

Carrier gas: *argon R*.

Lead: maximum 0.1 ppm, if intended for use in parenteral nutrition.

Atomic absorption spectrometry (*2.2.23, Method II*).

Test solution. Dissolve 2.0 g of the substance to be examined in *methyl isobutyl ketone R3* and dilute to 10.0 ml with the same solvent.

Solution A. Dilute 0.100 ml of *lead liposoluble standard solution (1000 ppm Pb) R* to 10.0 ml with *methyl isobutyl ketone R3*.

Stock solution. Dilute 0.100 ml of solution A to 10.0 ml with *methyl isobutyl ketone R3*.

Reference solutions. Prepare 3 reference solutions by dissolving for each 2.0 g of the substance to be examined in the minimum volume of *methyl isobutyl ketone R3*, adding 1.0 ml, 2.0 ml and 4.0 ml, respectively, of stock solution and diluting to 10.0 ml with *methyl isobutyl ketone R3*.

Source: lead hollow-cathode lamp.

Wavelength: 283.3 nm.

Atomic generator: graphite furnace coated inside with palladium carbide; calcination is carried out in the presence of oxygen at a temperature below 800 °C.

Carrier gas: *argon R*.

Nickel: maximum 0.2 ppm, if intended for use in parenteral nutrition.

Atomic absorption spectrometry (*2.2.23, Method II*).

Test solution. Dissolve 2.0 g of the substance to be examined in *methyl isobutyl ketone R3* and dilute to 10.0 ml with the same solvent.

Solution A. Dilute 0.100 ml of *nickel liposoluble standard solution (1000 ppm Ni) R* to 10.0 ml with *methyl isobutyl ketone R3*.

Stock solution. Dilute 0.100 ml of solution A to 10.0 ml with *methyl isobutyl ketone R3*.

Reference solutions. Prepare 3 reference solutions by dissolving for each 2.0 g of the substance to be examined in the minimum volume of *methyl isobutyl ketone R3*, adding 1.0 ml, 2.0 ml and 4.0 ml, respectively, of stock solution and diluting to 10.0 ml with *methyl isobutyl ketone R3*.

Source: nickel hollow-cathode lamp.

Wavelength: 232 nm.

Atomic generator: graphite furnace.

Carrier gas: *argon R*.

Tin: maximum 0.1 ppm, if intended for use in parenteral nutrition.

Atomic absorption spectrometry (*2.2.23, Method II*).

Test solution. Dissolve 2.0 g of the substance to be examined in *methyl isobutyl ketone R3* and dilute to 10.0 ml with the same solvent.

Solution A. Dilute 0.100 ml of *tin liposoluble standard solution (1000 ppm Sn) R* to 10.0 ml with *methyl isobutyl ketone R3*.

Stock solution. Dilute 0.100 ml of solution A to 10.0 ml with *methyl isobutyl ketone R3*.

Reference solutions. Prepare 3 reference solutions by dissolving for each 2.0 g of the substance to be examined in the minimum volume of *methyl isobutyl ketone R3*, adding 1.0 ml, 2.0 ml and 4.0 ml, respectively, of stock solution and diluting to 10.0 ml with *methyl isobutyl ketone R3*.

Source: tin hollow-cathode lamp.

Wavelength: 286.3 nm.

Atomic generator: graphite furnace coated inside with palladium carbide.

Carrier gas: *argon R*.

Heavy metals (*2.4.8*): maximum 10 ppm, if intended for use other than parenteral nutrition.

2.0 g complies with limit test D. Prepare the standard using 2 ml of *lead standard solution (10 ppm Pb) R*.

Water (*2.5.12*): maximum 0.2 per cent, determined on 10.00 g.

Total ash (*2.4.16*): maximum 0.1 per cent, determined on 2.0 g.

STORAGE

In a well-filled container, protected from light.

LABELLING

The label states, where applicable, that the substance is intended for use in parenteral nutrition.

01/2005:1626

TRIHEXYPHENIDYL HYDROCHLORIDE

Trihexyphenidyli hydrochloridum

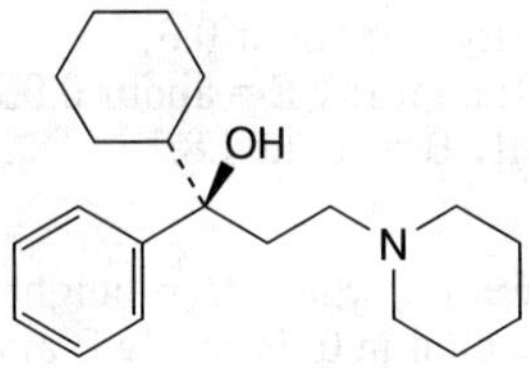

, HCl and enantiomer

$C_{20}H_{32}ClNO$ M_r 337.9

DEFINITION

(1*RS*)-1-Cyclohexyl-1-phenyl-3-(piperidin-1-yl)propan-1-ol hydrochloride.

Content: 99.0 per cent to 101.0 per cent (dried substance).

CHARACTERS

Appearance: white, crystalline powder.

Solubility: slightly soluble in water, sparingly soluble in alcohol and in methylene chloride.

mp: about 250 °C, with decomposition.

IDENTIFICATION

First identification: A, D.

Second identification: B, C, D.

A. Infrared absorption spectrophotometry (*2.2.24*).

Comparison: *trihexyphenidyl hydrochloride CRS*.

B. Thin-layer chromatography (*2.2.27*).

Test solution. Dissolve 25 mg of the substance to be examined in a mixture of 20 volumes of *methanol R* and 80 volumes of *methylene chloride R* and dilute to 10 ml with the same mixture of solvents.

Reference solution. Dissolve 25 mg of *trihexyphenidyl hydrochloride CRS* in a mixture of 20 volumes of *methanol R* and 80 volumes of *methylene chloride R* and dilute to 10 ml with the same mixture of solvents.

Plate: *TLC silica gel G plate R.*

Mobile phase: *diethylamine R, hexane R (5:95 V/V).*

Application: 5 µl.

Development: over 2/3 of the plate.

Drying: in air.

Detection: spray with a 0.1 g/l solution of *chloroplatinic acid R* in *hydrochloric acid R* containing 0.4 per cent *V/V* of *hydriodic acid R.*

Results: the principal spot in the chromatogram obtained with the test solution is similar in position, colour and size to the principal spot in the chromatogram obtained with the reference solution.

C. Dissolve 0.5 g in 5 ml of warm *methanol R* and make just alkaline to *red litmus paper R* with *sodium hydroxide solution R.* A precipitate is formed which, after recrystallisation from *methanol R*, melts (*2.2.14*) at about 113°C to 115 °C.

D. It gives reaction (a) of chlorides (*2.3.1*).

TESTS

pH (*2.2.3*): 5.2 to 6.2.

Dissolve 0.5 g with heating in 25 ml of *carbon dioxide-free water R.* Cool to room temperature and dilute to 50 ml with *carbon dioxide-free water R.*

Optical rotation (*2.2.7*): − 0.10° to + 0.10°.

Dissolve 1.25 g in a mixture of 20 volumes of *methanol R* and 80 volumes of *methylene chloride R* and dilute to 25.0 ml with the same mixture of solvents.

Related substances. Liquid chromatography (*2.2.29*).

Test solution. Dissolve 20.0 mg of the substance to be examined in the mobile phase and dilute to 10.0 ml with the mobile phase.

Reference solution (a). Dilute 1.0 ml of the test solution to 200.0 ml with the mobile phase. Dilute 10.0 ml to 50.0 ml with the mobile phase.

Reference solution (b). Dissolve 10.0 mg of *trihexyphenidyl impurity A CRS* in the mobile phase and dilute to 10.0 ml with the mobile phase.

Reference solution (c). Dilute 1.0 ml of reference solution (b) to 100.0 ml with the mobile phase.

Reference solution (d). To 1 ml of reference solution (b), add 1 ml of the test solution and dilute to 100 ml with the mobile phase.

Column:

- *size*: *l* = 0.15 m, Ø = 4.6 mm,
- *stationary phase*: *octadecylsilyl silica gel for chromatography R* (5 µm).

Mobile phase: mix 200 ml of *water R* with 0.2 ml of *triethylamine R.* Adjust to pH 4.0 with *phosphoric acid R* and add 800 ml of *acetonitrile R.*

Flow rate: 1.0 ml/min.

Detection: spectrophotometer at 210 nm.

Injection: 20 µl.

Run time: 3 times the retention time of trihexyphenidyl.

System suitability: reference solution (d):

- *resolution*: minimum 4.0 between the peaks corresponding to trihexyphenidyl and to impurity A.

Limits:

- *impurity A*: not more than the area of the principal peak in the chromatogram obtained with reference solution (c) (0.5 per cent),
- *any other impurity*: not more than the area of the principal peak in the chromatogram obtained with reference solution (a) (0.1 per cent),
- *total*: not more than 0.5 per cent,
- *disregard limit*: 0.2 times the area of the principal peak in the chromatogram obtained with reference solution (a) (0.02 per cent).

Loss on drying (*2.2.32*): maximum 0.5 per cent, determined on 1.000 g by drying in an oven at 100-105 °C.

Sulphated ash (*2.4.14*): maximum 0.1 per cent, determined on 1.0 g.

ASSAY

Dissolve 0.250 g in 50 ml of *alcohol R* and add 5.0 ml of *0.01 M hydrochloric acid.* Carry out a potentiometric titration (*2.2.20*), using *0.1 M sodium hydroxide.* Read the volume added between the 2 points of inflexion.

1 mlof *0.1 M sodium hydroxide* is equivalent to 33.79 mg of $C_{20}H_{32}ClNO$.

IMPURITIES

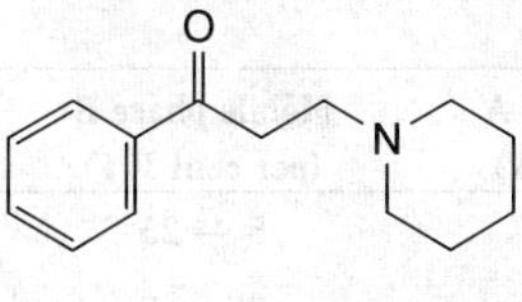

A. 1-phenyl-3-(piperidin-1-yl)propan-1-one.

01/2005:1741

TRIMETAZIDINE DIHYDROCHLORIDE

Trimetazidini dihydrochloridum

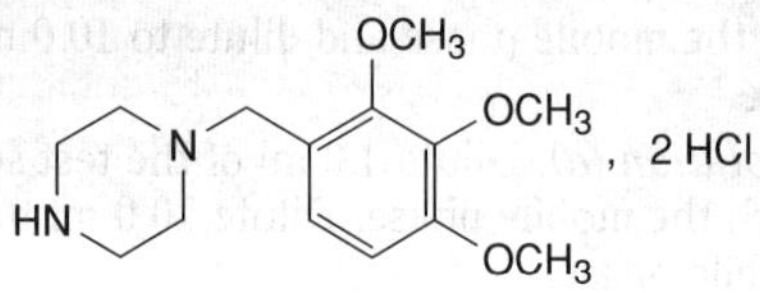

$C_{14}H_{24}Cl_2N_2O_3$ M_r 339.3

DEFINITION

1-(2,3,4-Trimethoxybenzyl)piperazine dihydrochloride.

Content: 98.5 per cent to 101.5 per cent (dried substance).

CHARACTERS

Appearance: white or almost white, crystalline powder, slightly hygroscopic.

Solubility: freely soluble in water, sparingly soluble in alcohol.

IDENTIFICATION

A. Infrared absorption spectrophotometry (*2.2.24*).
Comparison: *Ph. Eur. reference spectrum of trimetazidine dihydrochloride.*

B. Dissolve 25 mg in 5 ml of *water R*. 2 ml of the solution gives reaction (a) of chlorides (*2.3.1*).

TESTS

Appearance of solution. The solution is clear (*2.2.1*) and not more intensely coloured than reference solution BY_6 (*2.2.2, Method II*).

Dissolve 1.0 g in *water R* and dilute to 10 ml with the same solvent.

Related substances. Liquid chromatography (*2.2.29*).

Test solution. Dissolve 0.200 g of the substance to be examined in *water R* and dilute to 50.0 ml with the same solvent.

Reference solution (a). Dissolve 20.0 mg of *trimetazidine for system suitability CRS* in *water R* and dilute to 5.0 ml with the same solvent.

Reference solution (b). Dilute 2.0 ml of the test solution to 100.0 ml with *water R*. Dilute 5.0 ml of this solution to 100.0 ml with *water R*.

Reference solution (c). Dilute 25.0 ml of reference solution (b) to 50.0 ml with *water R*.

Column:
- *size*: l = 0.15 m, Ø = 4.6 mm,
- *stationary phase*: spherical *octadecylsilyl silica gel for chromatography R* (5 µm) with a pore size of 10 nm,
- *temperature*: 30 °C.

Mobile phase:
- *mobile phase A*: mix 357 volumes of *methanol R* and 643 volumes of a 2.87 g/l solution of *sodium heptanesulphonate R* adjusted to pH 3.0 with *dilute phosphoric acid R*,
- *mobile phase B*: *methanol R*,

Time (min)	Mobile phase A (per cent *V/V*)	Mobile phase B (per cent *V/V*)
0 - 50	95 → 75	5 → 25
50 - 52	75 → 95	25 → 5

Flow rate: 1.2 ml/min.

Detection: spectrophotometer at 240 nm.

Equilibration: for at least 1 h with the mobile phase at the initial composition.

Injection: 10 µl.

Relative retention with reference to trimetazidine (retention time = about 25 min): impurity D = about 0.2; impurity C = about 0.4; impurity H = about 0.6; impurities A and I = about 0.9; impurity E = about 0.95; impurity F = about 1.4; impurity B = about 1.8.

System suitability:
- *peak-to-valley ratio*: minimum 3, where H_p = height above the baseline of the peak due to impurity E and H_v = height above the baseline of the lowest point of the curve separating this peak from the principal peak in the chromatogram obtained with reference solution (a);
- *signal-to-noise ratio*: minimum 10 for the principal peak in the chromatogram obtained with reference solution (c).

Limits:
- *correction factors*: for the calculation of contents, multiply the peak areas of the following impurities by the corresponding correction factor: impurity B = 0.55; impurity C = 0.37; impurity F = 0.71;
- *impurities A, B, C, D, E, F, H, I*: for each impurity, not more than the area of the principal peak in the chromatogram obtained with reference solution (b) (0.1 per cent);
- *any other impurity*: for each impurity, not more than the area of the principal peak in the chromatogram obtained with reference solution (b) (0.1 per cent);
- *total*: not more than twice the area of the principal peak in the chromatogram obtained with reference solution (b) (0.2 per cent);
- *disregard limit*: area of the principal peak in the chromatogram obtained with reference solution (c) (0.05 per cent).

Impurity G. Thin-layer chromatography (*2.2.27*).

Test solution. Dissolve 0.10 g of the substance to be examined in *methanol R* and dilute to 10 ml with the same solvent.

Reference solution. Dissolve 22.6 mg of *piperazine hydrate R* in *methanol R* and dilute to 100 ml with the same solvent. Dilute 10 ml of the solution to 100 ml with *methanol R*.

Plate: *TLC silica gel plate R*.

Mobile phase: *concentrated ammonia R, alcohol R* (20:80 *V/V*).

Application: 10 µl.

Development: over 2/3 of the plate.

Drying: at 100-105 °C for 30 min.

Detection: spray with *iodoplatinate reagent R*.

Limit:
- *impurity G*: any spot due to impurity G is not more intense than the spot in the chromatogram obtained with the reference solution (0.1 per cent, expressed as anhydrous piperazine).

Loss on drying (*2.2.32*): maximum 2.5 per cent, determined on 1.000 g by drying in an oven at 100-105 °C over *diphosphorus pentoxide R* at a pressure not exceeding 15 kPa.

Sulphated ash (*2.4.14*): maximum 0.1 per cent, determined on 1.0 g.

ASSAY

Dissolve 0.120 g in 50.0 ml of *water R*. Add 1 ml of *nitric acid R* and titrate with *0.1 M silver nitrate*, determining the end-point potentiometrically (*2.2.20*).

1 ml of *0.1 M silver nitrate* is equivalent to 16.96 mg of $C_{14}H_{24}Cl_2N_2O_3$.

STORAGE

In an airtight container.

IMPURITIES

Specified impurities: A, B, C, D, E, F, G, H, I.

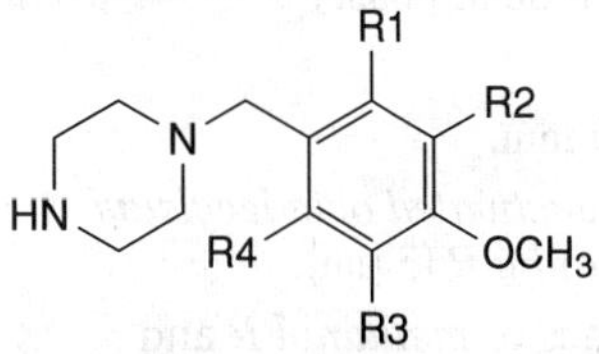

A. R1 = R4 = H, R2 = R3 = OCH_3: 1-(3,4,5-trimethoxybenzyl)piperazine,

E. R1 = R3 = OCH_3, R2 = R4 = H: 1-(2,4,5-trimethoxybenzyl)piperazine,

F. R1 = R4 = OCH_3, R2 = R3 = H: 1-(2,4,6-trimethoxybenzyl)piperazine,

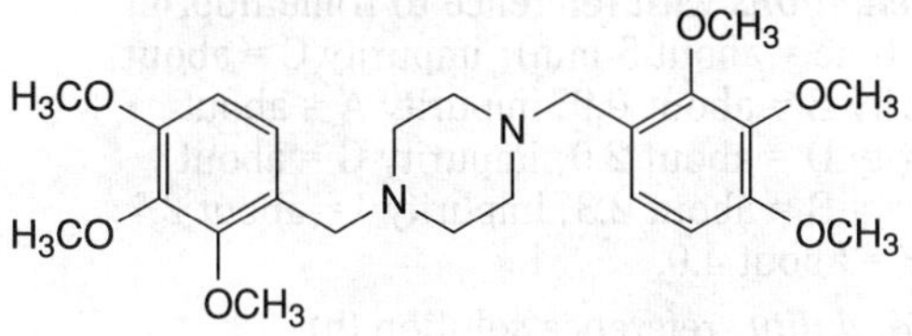

B. 1,4-bis(2,3,4-trimethoxybenzyl)piperazine,

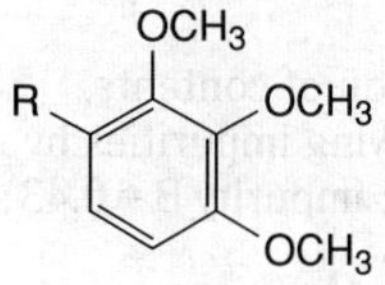

C. R = CHO: 2,3,4-trimethoxybenzaldehyde,

D. R = CH_2OH: (2,3,4-trimethoxyphenyl)methanol,

G. piperazine,

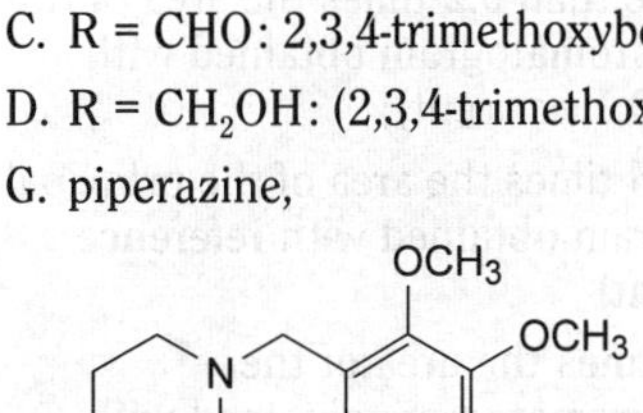

H. R = $COOC_2H_5$: ethyl 4-(2,3,4-trimethoxybenzyl)piperazine-1-carboxylate,

I. R = CH_3: 1-methyl-4-(2,3,4-trimethoxybenzyl)piperazine (*N*-methyltrimetazidine).

01/2005:0440

TRIMETHADIONE

Trimethadionum

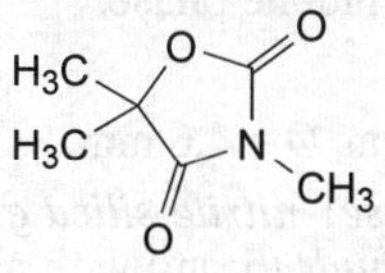

$C_6H_9NO_3$ M_r 143.1

DEFINITION

Trimethadione contains not less than 98.0 per cent and not more than the equivalent of 102.0 per cent of 3,5,5-trimethyloxazolidine-2,4-dione, calculated with reference to the dried substance.

CHARACTERS

Colourless or almost colourless crystals, soluble in water, very soluble in alcohol.

IDENTIFICATION

First identification: B.

Second identification: A, C, D.

A. Melting point (*2.2.14*): 45 °C to 47 °C, determined without previous drying.

B. Examine by infrared absorption spectrophotometry (*2.2.24*), comparing with the spectrum obtained with *trimethadione CRS*. Examine the substances prepared as discs using 3 mg of the substance to be examined and of the reference substance, respectively, in 0.4 g of *potassium bromide R*.

C. To 2 ml of solution S (see Tests) add 1 ml of *barium hydroxide solution R*. A white precipitate is formed, which dissolves on addition of 1 ml of *dilute hydrochloric acid R*.

D. Dissolve 0.3 g in a mixture of 5 ml of *alcoholic potassium hydroxide solution R* and 5 ml of *alcohol R* and allow to stand for 10 min. Add 0.05 ml of *phenolphthalein solution R1* and neutralise carefully with *hydrochloric acid R*. Evaporate to dryness on a water-bath and shake the residue with four quantities, each of 5 ml, of *ether R*. Filter the combined ether layers and evaporate to dryness. The residue, recrystallised from 5 ml of *toluene R* and dried, melts (*2.2.14*) at about 80 °C.

TESTS

Solution S. Dissolve 2.0 g in *carbon dioxide-free water R* and dilute to 40 ml with the same solvent.

Appearance of solution. Solution S is clear (*2.2.1*) and colourless (*2.2.2, Method II*).

Acidity or alkalinity. To 10 ml of solution S add 0.1 ml of *methyl red solution R*. Not more than 0.1 ml of *0.01 M hydrochloric acid* or *0.01 M sodium hydroxide* is required to change the colour of the indicator.

Heavy metals (*2.4.8*). 12 ml of solution S complies with limit test A for heavy metals (20 ppm). Prepare the standard using *lead standard solution (1 ppm Pb) R*.

Loss on drying (*2.2.32*). Not more than 0.5 per cent, determined on 1.00 g by drying in a desiccator over *anhydrous silica gel R* for 6 h.

Sulphated ash (*2.4.14*). Not more than 0.1 per cent, determined on 1.0 g.

ASSAY

Examine by gas chromatography (*2.2.28*), using *decanol R* as the internal standard.

Internal standard solution. Dissolve 0.125 g of *decanol R* in *ethanol R* and dilute to 25 ml with the same solvent.

Test solution. Dissolve 0.100 g of the substance to be examined in the internal standard solution and dilute to 10.0 ml with the same solution.

Reference solution. Dissolve 0.100 g of *trimethadione CRS* in the internal standard solution and dilute to 10.0 ml with the same solution.

The chromatographic procedure may be carried out using:
- a stainless steel column 0.75 m long and 3 mm in internal diameter packed with *styrene-divinylbenzene copolymer R* (125 µm to 150 µm),
- *nitrogen for chromatography R* as the carrier gas at a flow rate of 20 ml/min,
- a flame-ionisation detector.

Maintain the temperature of the column at 210 °C, that of the injection port at 240 °C, and that of the detector at 270 °C. Inject 1 µl of each solution.

STORAGE

Store protected from light.

01/2005:0060

TRIMETHOPRIM

Trimethoprimum

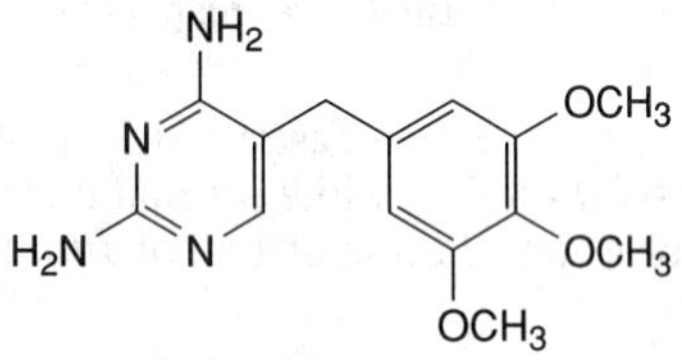

$C_{14}H_{18}N_4O_3$ M_r 290.3

DEFINITION

5-(3,4,5-Trimethoxybenzyl)pyrimidine-2,4-diamine.

Content: 98.5 per cent to 101.0 per cent (dried substance).

CHARACTERS

Appearance: white or yellowish-white powder.

Solubility: very slightly soluble in water, slightly soluble in alcohol.

IDENTIFICATION

First identification: C.

Second identification: A, B, D.

A. Melting point (*2.2.14*): 199 °C to 203 °C.

B. Dissolve about 20 mg in *0.1 M sodium hydroxide* and dilute to 100.0 ml with the same solvent. Dilute 1.0 ml of this solution to 10.0 ml with *0.1 M sodium hydroxide*. Examined between 230 nm and 350 nm (*2.2.25*), the solution shows an absorption maximum at 287 nm. The specific absorbance at the maximum is 240 to 250.

C. Infrared absorption spectrophotometry (*2.2.24*).

Preparation: discs.

Comparison: *trimethoprim CRS*.

D. Dissolve about 25 mg, heating if necessary, in 5 ml of *0.005 M sulphuric acid* and add 2 ml of a 16 g/l solution of *potassium permanganate R* in *0.1 M sodium hydroxide*. Heat to boiling and add to the hot solution 0.4 ml of *formaldehyde R*. Mix, add 1 ml of *0.5 M sulphuric acid*, mix and heat again to boiling. Cool and filter. To the filtrate add 2 ml of *methylene chloride R* and shake vigorously. The organic layer, examined in ultraviolet light at 365 nm, shows green fluorescence.

TESTS

Appearance of solution. The solution is not more intensely coloured than reference solution BY_7 (*2.2.2, Method II*).

Dissolve 0.5 g in 10 ml of a mixture of 1 volume of *water R*, 4.5 volumes of *methanol R* and 5 volumes of *methylene chloride R*.

Related substances

A. Liquid chromatography (*2.2.29*).

Test solution. Dissolve 25.0 mg of the substance to be examined in the mobile phase and dilute to 25.0 ml with the mobile phase.

Reference solution (a). Dilute 1.0 ml of the test solution to 200.0 ml with the mobile phase.

Reference solution (b). Dissolve 5.0 mg of *trimethoprim CRS* and 2.5 mg of *trimethoprim impurity E CRS* in the mobile phase and dilute to 100.0 ml with the mobile phase. Dilute 1.0 ml of the solution to 10.0 ml with the mobile phase.

Column:
- *size*: l = 0.250 m, Ø = 4.0 mm,
- *stationary phase*: *base-deactivated octadecylsilyl silica gel for chromatography R* (5 µm).

Mobile phase: mix 30 volumes of *methanol R* and 70 volumes of a 1.4 g/l solution of *sodium perchlorate R* adjusted to pH 3.6 with *phosphoric acid R*.

Flow rate: 1.3 ml/min.

Detection: spectrophotometer at 280 nm.

Injection: 20 µl loop injector.

Run time: 11 times the retention time of trimethoprim.

Relative retentions with reference to trimethoprim (retention time = about 5 min): impurity C = about 0.8; impurity E = about 0.9; impurity A = about 1.5; impurity D = about 2.0; impurity G = about 2.1; impurity B = about 2.3; impurity J = about 2.7; impurity F = about 4.0.

System suitability: reference solution (b):
- *resolution*: minimum of 2.5 between the peaks.

Limits:
- *correction factors*: for the calculation of contents, multiply the peak areas of the following impurities by the corresponding correction factor: impurity B = 0.43; impurity E = 0.53; impurity J = 0.66;
- *any impurity*: not more than 0.2 times the area of the principal peak in the chromatogram obtained with reference solution (a) (0.1 per cent);
- *total*: not more than 0.4 times the area of the principal peak in the chromatogram obtained with reference solution (a) (0.2 per cent);
- *disregard limit*: 0.04 times the area of the principal peak in the chromatogram obtained with reference solution (a) (0.02 per cent); disregard any peak corresponding to impurity H (relative retentions = about 10.3).

B. Liquid chromatography (*2.2.29*).

Test solution. Dissolve 25.0 mg of the substance to be examined in the mobile phase and dilute to 25.0 ml with the mobile phase.

Reference solution (a). Dilute 1.0 ml of the test solution to 200.0 ml with the mobile phase.

Reference solution (b). Dissolve 5.0 mg of *trimethoprim CRS* and 5.0 mg of *trimethoprim impurity B CRS* in the mobile phase and dilute to 100.0 ml with the mobile phase.

Column:
- *size*: l = 0.250 m, Ø = 4.6 mm,
- *stationary phase*: *nitrile silica gel for chromatography R* (5 µm) with a specific surface area of 350 m^2/g and a pore diameter of 10 nm.

Monographs T-Z

Mobile phase: dissolve 1.14 g of *sodium hexane sulphonate R* in 600 ml of a 13.6 g/l solution of *potassium dihydrogen phosphate R*; adjust to pH 3.1 using *phosphoric acid R* and mix with 400 volumes of *methanol R*.

Flow rate: 0.8 ml/min.

Detection: spectrophotometer at 280 nm.

Injection: 20 µl loop injector.

Run time: 6 times the retention time of trimethoprim.

Relative retentions with reference to trimethoprim (retention time = about 4 min): impurity H = about 1.8; impurity I = about 4.9.

System suitability: reference solution (b):
- *resolution*: minimum of 2.0 between the peaks.

Limits:
- *correction factors*: for the calculation of contents, multiply the peak areas of the following impurities by the corresponding correction factor: impurity H = 0.50; impurity I = 0.28;
- *any impurity*: not more than 0.2 times the area of the principal peak in the chromatogram obtained with reference solution (a) (0.1 per cent);
- *total*: not more than 0.4 times the area of the principal peak in the chromatogram obtained with reference solution (a) (0.2 per cent);
- *disregard limit*: 0.04 times the area of the principal peak in the chromatogram obtained with reference solution (a) (0.02 per cent); disregard any peak corresponding to impurity B (relative retention = about 1.3).

Impurity K. Gas chromatography (*2.2.28*).

Test solution. Dissolve 0.500 g of the substance to be examined in 35.0 ml of *citrate buffer solution pH 5.0 R*, add 10.0 ml of *1,1-dimethylethyl methyl ether R*, shake thoroughly and centrifuge for 10 min. Use the upper layer.

Reference solution. Dilute 5.0 ml of *hydrochloric acid R* to 50.0 ml with *water R*. Add 12.5 mg of *aniline R* and shake thoroughly (solution A). To 35.0 ml of *citrate buffer solution pH 5.0 R* add 10.0 µl of solution A and 10.0 ml of *1,1-dimethylethyl methyl ether R*, shake thoroughly and centrifuge for 10 min. Use the upper layer.

Column:
- *material*: fused silica,
- *size*: l = 30 m, Ø = 0.53 mm,
- *stationary phase*: *poly(dimethyl)siloxane R* (film thickness 3 µm).

Carrier gas: *helium for chromatography R*.

Flow rate: 12 ml/min.

Temperature:
- *column*: 80 °C,
- *injection port*: 230 °C,
- *detector*: 270 °C.

Detection: nitrogen-phosphorus detector.

Injection: 3 µl.

Run time: 15 min.

System suitability: reference solution:
- *repeatability*: maximum relative standard deviation of 5.0 per cent after 6 injections.

Limit:
- *impurity K*: not more than the area of the corresponding peak in the chromatogram obtained with the reference solution (5 ppm).

Heavy metals (*2.4.8*): maximum 20 ppm.

1.0 g complies with limit test C. Prepare the standard using 2 ml of *lead standard solution (10 ppm Pb) R*

Loss on drying (*2.2.32*): maximum 1.0 per cent, determined on 1.000 g by drying in an oven at 100-105 °C.

Sulphated ash (*2.4.14*): maximum 0.1 per cent, determined on 1.0 g.

ASSAY

Dissolve 0.250 g in 50 ml of *anhydrous acetic acid R.* Titrate with *0.1 M perchloric acid*, determining the end-point potentiometrically (*2.2.20*).

1 ml of *0.1 M perchloric acid* is equivalent to 29.03 mg of $C_{14}H_{18}N_4O_3$.

IMPURITIES

By liquid chromatography A: A, B, C, D, E, F, G, H, J.

By liquid chromatography B: B, H, I.

By gas chromatography: K.

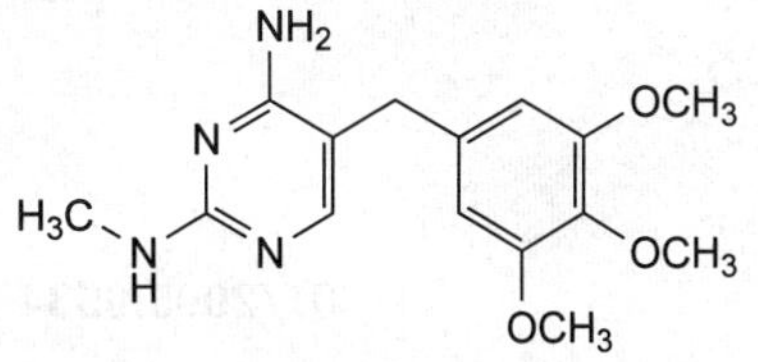

A. N^2-methyl-5-(3,4,5-trimethoxybenzyl)pyrimidine-2,4-diamine,

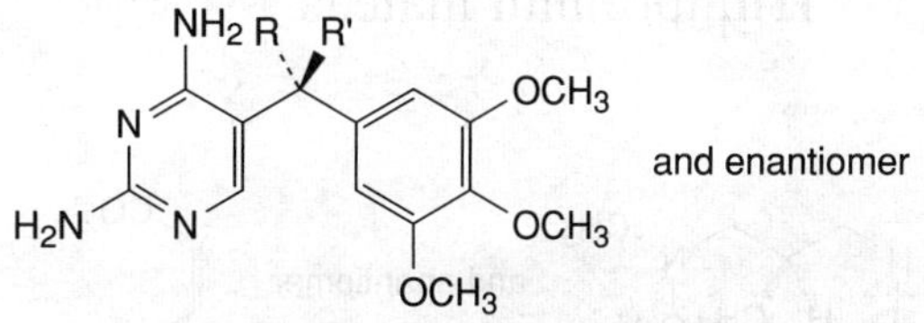

B. R + R′ = O: (2,4-diaminopyrimidin-5-yl)(3,4,5-trimethoxyphenyl)methanone,

C. R = OH, R′ = H: (*RS*)-(2,4-diaminopyrimidin-5-yl)(3,4,5-trimethoxyphenyl)methanol,

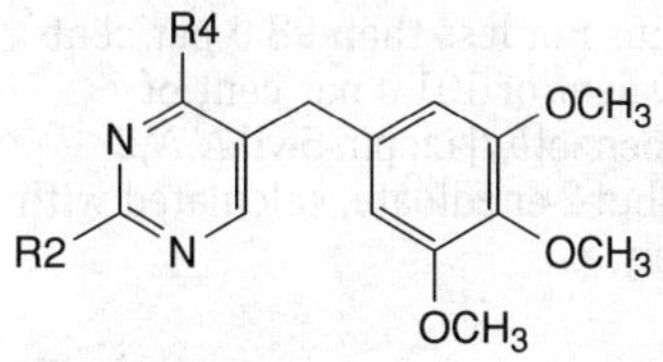

D. R2 = NH_2, R4 = OH: 2-amino-5-(3,4,5-trimethoxybenzyl)pyrimidin-4-ol,

E. R2 = OH, R4 = NH_2: 4-amino-5-(3,4,5-trimethoxybenzyl)pyrimidin-2-ol,

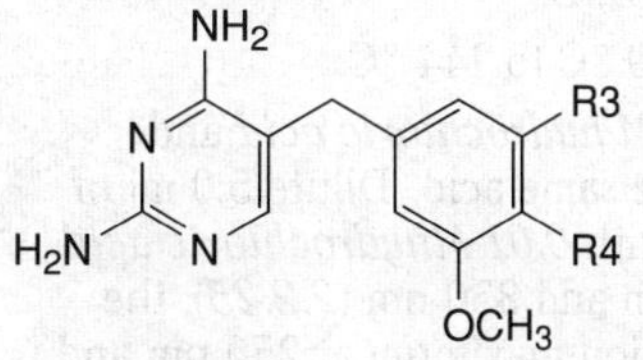

F. R3 = Br, R4 = OCH_3: 5-(3-bromo-4,5-dimethoxybenzyl)pyrimidine-2,4-diamine,

G. R3 = OCH_3, R4 = OC_2H_5: 5-(4-ethoxy-3,5-dimethoxybenzyl)pyrimidine-2,4-diamine,

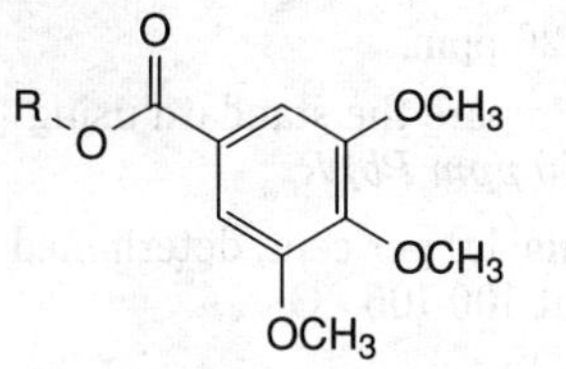

H. R = CH_3: methyl 3,4,5-trimethoxybenzoate,

J. R = H: 3,4,5-trimethoxybenzoic acid,

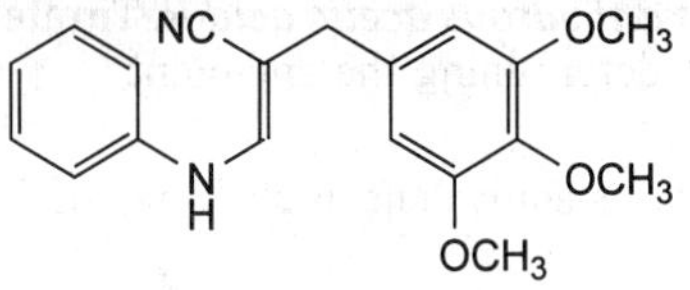

I. 3-(phenylamino)-2-(3,4,5-trimethoxybenzyl)prop-2-enenitrile,

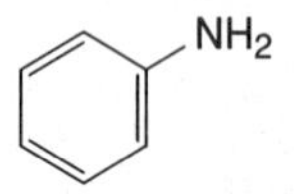

K. aniline.

01/2005:0534

TRIMIPRAMINE MALEATE

Trimipramini maleas

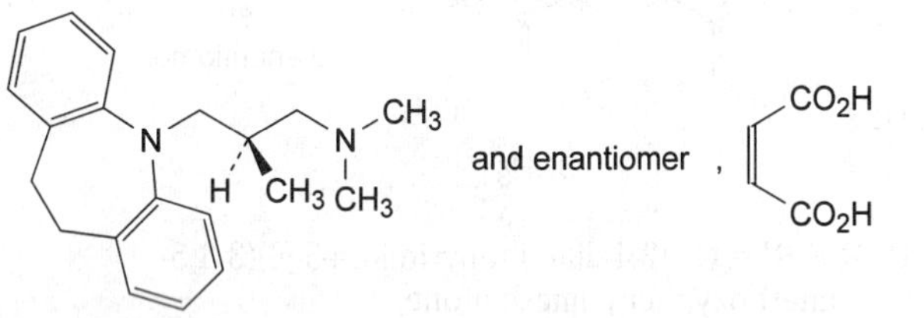

$C_{24}H_{30}N_2O_4$ M_r 410.5

DEFINITION

Trimipramine maleate contains not less than 98.0 per cent and not more than the equivalent of 101.0 per cent of (2*RS*)-3-(10,11-dihydro-5*H*-dibenzo[*b*,*f*]azepin-5-yl)-*N*,*N*,2-trimethylpropan-1-amine (*Z*)-but-2-enedioate, calculated with reference to the dried substance.

CHARACTERS

A white or almost white, crystalline powder, slightly soluble in water and in alcohol.

IDENTIFICATION

First identification: A, C.

Second identification: A, B, D, E.

A. Melting point (*2.2.14*): 140 °C to 144 °C.

B. Dissolve 40.0 mg in *0.01 M hydrochloric acid* and dilute to 100.0 ml with the same acid. Dilute 5.0 ml of the solution to 100.0 ml with *0.01 Mhydrochloric acid.* Examined between 230 nm and 350 nm (*2.2.25*), the solution shows an absorption maximum at 250 nm and a shoulder at 270 nm. The specific absorbance at the maximum is 205 to 235.

C. Examine by infrared absorption spectrophotometry (*2.2.24*), comparing with the spectrum obtained with *trimipramine maleate CRS.*

D. Examine the chromatograms obtained in the test for related substances. The principal spot in the chromatogram obtained with test solution (b) is similar in position, colour and size to the principal spot in the chromatogram obtained with reference solution (a).

E. Examine by thin-layer chromatography (*2.2.27*), using *silica gel GF_{254} R* as the coating substance.

Test solution. Dissolve 0.20 g of the substance to be examined in *methanol R* and dilute to 10 ml with the same solvent.

Reference solution. Dissolve 56 mg of *maleic acid R* in *methanol R* and dilute to 10 ml with the same solvent.

Apply to the plate as 10 mm bands 5 µl of each solution. Develop over a path of 12 cm using a mixture of 3 volumes of *water R*, 7 volumes of *anhydrous formic acid R* and 90 volumes of *di-isopropyl ether R*. Dry the plate in a current of air for a few minutes and then at 120 °C for 10 min and examine in ultraviolet light at 254 nm. The chromatogram obtained with the test solution shows a zone on the starting line and another zone which is similar in position and size to the principal zone in the chromatogram obtained with the reference solution.

TESTS

Appearance of solution. Dissolve 2.5 g in *chloroform R* and dilute to 25 ml with the same solvent. The solution is not more intensely coloured than reference solution BY_5 (*2.2.2, Method II*).

Related substances. Examine by thin-layer chromatography (*2.2.27*), using *silica gel G R* as the coating substance.

Test solution (a). Dissolve 0.50 g of the substance to be examined in *methanol R* and dilute to 10 ml with the same solvent. Prepare immediately before use.

Test solution (b). Dilute 1 ml of test solution (a) to 20 ml with *methanol R.*

Reference solution (a). Dissolve 25 mg of *trimipramine maleate CRS* in *methanol R* and dilute to 10 ml with the same solvent. Prepare immediately before use.

Reference solution (b). Dilute 1 ml of reference solution (a) to 10 ml with *methanol R.*

Reference solution (c). Dilute 1 ml of reference solution (a) to 25 ml with *methanol R.*

Reference solution (d). Dissolve 10 mg of *iminodibenzyl R* in *methanol R* and dilute to 100 ml with the same solvent. Prepare immediately before use.

Apply separately to the plate 5 µl of each solution. Develop over a path of 15 cm using a mixture of 0.7 volumes of *concentrated ammonia R*, 10 volumes of *ethanol R* and 90 volumes of *toluene R*. Allow the plate to dry in air for 15 min, spray with a 5 g/l solution of *potassium dichromate R* in a mixture of 1 volume of *sulphuric acid R* and 4 volumes of *water R* and examine immediately. In the chromatogram obtained with test solution (a): any spot corresponding to iminodibenzyl is not more intense than the spot in the chromatogram obtained with reference solution (d) (0.2 per cent); any spot, apart from the principal spot and the spot corresponding to iminodibenzyl, is not more intense than the spot in the chromatogram obtained with reference solution (b) (0.5 per cent) and at most three such spots are more intense than the spot in the chromatogram obtained with reference solution (c) (0.2 per cent). Disregard any spot at the starting point.

Heavy metals (*2.4.8*). 2.0 g complies with limit test C for heavy metals (20 ppm). Prepare the standard using 4 ml of *lead standard solution (10 ppm Pb) R.*

Loss on drying (*2.2.32*). Not more than 0.5 per cent, determined on 1.000 g by drying in an oven at 100 °C to 105 °C.

Sulphated ash (*2.4.14*). Not more than 0.1 per cent, determined on 1.0 g.

ASSAY

Dissolve 0.3500 g in 50 ml of *anhydrous acetic acid R*. Titrate with *0.1 M perchloric acid* determining the end-point potentiometrically (*2.2.20*).

1 ml of *0.1 M perchloric acid* is equivalent to 41.05 mg of $C_{24}H_{30}N_2O_4$.

STORAGE

Store protected from light.

01/2005:1682

TRI-*n*-BUTYL PHOSPHATE

Tri-*n*-butylis phosphas

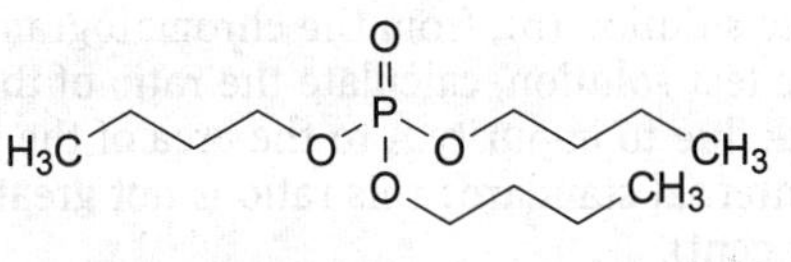

$C_{12}H_{27}O_4P$ M_r 266.3

CHARACTERS

Appearance: clear, colourless to pale yellow liquid.

Solubility: slightly soluble in water, miscible with alcohol.

bp: about 289 °C, with decomposition.

IDENTIFICATION

Infrared absorption spectrophotometry (*2.2.24*).

Comparison: *tri-n-butyl phosphate CRS*.

TESTS

Appearance. The substance to be examined is clear (*2.2.1*) and not more intensely coloured than reference solution Y_6 (*2.2.2, Method II*).

Acidity. Dissolve 50 ml in 50 ml of *alcohol R* previously adjusted with *0.02 M potassium hydroxide* or *0.02 M hydrochloric acid* to a bluish-green colour, using 0.5 ml of *bromothymol blue solution R1* as indicator. Titrate with *0.02 M potassium hydroxide* to (the initial) bluish-green coloration. Not more than 0.8 ml are required.

Related substances. Gas chromatography (*2.2.28*): use the normalisation procedure.

Test solution. Substance to be examined.

Reference solution. Dissolve 10 mg of the substance to be examined and 10 mg of *methyl myristate R* in *methylene chloride R* and dilute to 10 ml with the same solvent.

Column:
- *material*: fused silica,
- *size*: *l* = 30 m, Ø = 0.32 mm,
- *stationary phase*: *poly(dimethyl)siloxane R* (5 μm).

Carrier gas: *helium for chromatography R*.

Linear velocity: 32 cm/s.

Split-ratio: 65:1.

Temperature:
- *column*: 250 °C,
- *injection port and detector*: 250 °C.

Detector: flame ionisation.

Injection: 1 μl.

Run time: twice the retention time of tri-*n*-butyl phosphate.

System suitability: reference solution:
- *resolution*: minimum 10 between the peaks due to tri-*n*-butyl phosphate and methyl myristate.

Limits:
- *any impurity*: maximum 0.1 per cent,
- *total*: maximum 0.3 per cent,
- *disregard limit*: 0.01 per cent.

Chlorides (*2.4.4*): maximum 200 ppm.

Dissolve 0.25 g in 15 ml of *alcohol (70 per cent V/V) R*. The solution complies with the limit test for chlorides. Prepare the reference solution with 10 ml of *chloride standard solution (5 ppm Cl) R* and 5 ml of *ethanol R*.

Heavy metals (*2.4.8*): maximum 20 ppm.

Dissolve 2.0 g in 13 ml of *alcohol R* and dilute to 20.0 ml with *water R*. 12 ml of the solution complies with limit test B. Prepare the standard using lead standard solution (2 ppm Pb) prepared by diluting *lead standard solution (100 ppm Pb) R* with a mixture of 5 volumes of *water R* and 13 volumes of *alcohol R*.

Water (*2.5.32*): maximum 0.1 per cent, determined on 1.0 g.

STORAGE

Protected from light.

IMPURITIES

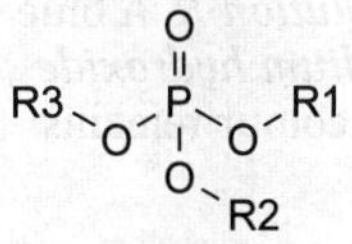

A. R1 = R2 = $[CH_2]_3$-CH_3, R3 = H: dibutyl hydrogen phosphate,

B. R1 = $[CH_2]_3$-CH_3, R2 = R3 = H: butyl dihydrogen phosphate,

D. R1 = R2 = $[CH_2]_3$-CH_3, R3 = CH_3: dibutyl methyl phosphate,

E. R1 = R2 = $[CH_2]_3$-CH_3, R3 = C_2H_5: dibutyl ethyl phosphate,

F. R1 = R2 = $[CH_2]_3$-CH_3, R3 = $[CH_2]_2$-CH_3: dibutyl propyl phosphate,

G. R1 = R2 = $[CH_2]_3$-CH_3, R3 = CH_2-$CH(CH_3)_2$: dibutyl 2-methylpropyl phosphate,

H. R1 = R2 = $[CH_2]_3$-CH_3, R3 = $[CH_2]_4$-CH_3: dibutyl pentyl phosphate,

C. H_3C-$[CH_2]_3$-OH: butan-1-ol,

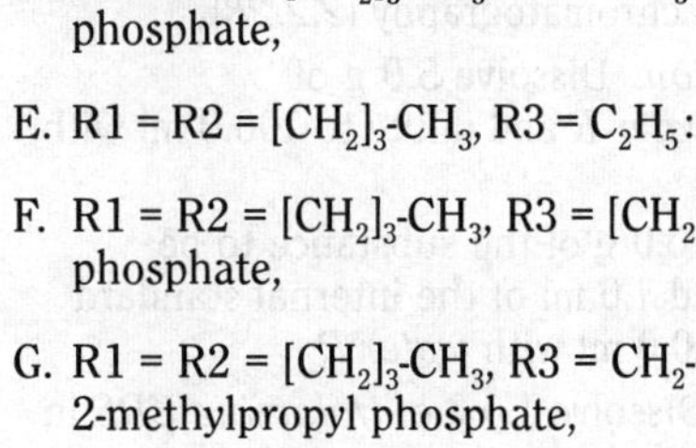

I. pentabutyl phosphate.

01/2005:1577

TROLAMINE

Trolaminum

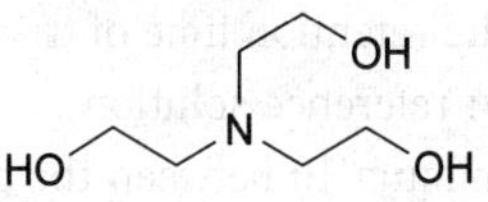

$C_6H_{15}NO_3$ M_r 149.2

DEFINITION

2,2′,2″-Nitrilotriethanol.

Content: 99.0 per cent *m/m* to 103.0 per cent *m/m* of total bases (anhydrous substance).

CHARACTERS

Appearance: clear, viscous, colourless or slightly yellow liquid, very hygroscopic.

Solubility: miscible with water and with alcohol, soluble in methylene chloride.

IDENTIFICATION

First identification: B, C.

Second identification: A, B, D.

A. Relative density (*2.2.5*): 1.120 to 1.130.

B. Refractive index (*2.2.6*): 1.482 to 1.485.

C. Examine the chromatograms obtained in the test for related substances.

Results: the principal peak in the chromatogram obtained with the test solution is similar in retention time and size to the principal peak in the chromatogram obtained with reference solution (a).

D. To 1 ml add 0.3 ml of *copper sulphate solution R*. A blue colour develops. Add 2.5 ml of *dilute sodium hydroxide solution R* and heat to boiling. The blue colour remains unchanged.

TESTS

Solution S. Dissolve 12 g in *water R* and dilute to 20 ml with the same solvent.

Appearance of solution. Solution S is clear (*2.2.1*) and not more intensely coloured than reference solution B_6 (*2.2.2, Method II*).

Related substances. Gas chromatography (*2.2.28*).

Internal standard solution. Dissolve 5.0 g of *3-aminopropanol R* in *water R* and dilute to 100.0 ml with the same solvent.

Test solution. Dissolve 10.0 g of the substance to be examined in *water R*. Add 1.0 ml of the internal standard solution and dilute to 100.0 ml with *water R*.

Reference solution (a). Dissolve 1.0 g of *trolamine CRS* in *water R* and dilute to 10.0 ml with the same solvent.

Reference solution (b). Dissolve 1.0 g of *ethanolamine R*, 5.0 g of *diethanolamine R* and 1.0 g of *trolamine CRS* in *water R* and dilute to 100.0 ml with the same solvent. To 1.0 ml of the solution add 1.0 ml of the internal standard solution and dilute to 100.0 ml with *water R*.

Column:

- *material*: fused silica,
- *size*: *l* = 25 m, Ø = 0.25 mm,
- *stationary phase*: *poly(dimethyl)(diphenyl)siloxane R* (film thickness 0.50 µm).

Carrier gas: *helium for chromatography R*.

Flow rate: 1 ml/min.

Split ratio: 1:35.

Temperature:

	Time (min)	Temperature (°C)
Column	0	60
	0 - 8.5	60 → 230
	8.5 - 14	230
Injection port		260
Detector		280

Detection: flame ionisation.

Injection: 2 µl; if necessary inject a blank.

Elution order: impurity A, 3-aminopropanol, impurity B, trolamine.

System suitability: reference solution (b):

- *resolution*: minimum 2 between the peaks due to 3-aminopropanol and impurity A.

Limits:

- *impurity A*: calculate the ratio R1 of the area of the peak due to impurity A to the area of the peak due to the internal standard from the chromatogram obtained with reference solution (b); from the chromatogram obtained with the test solution, calculate the ratio of the area of any peak due to impurity A to the area of the peak due to the internal standard: this ratio is not greater than R1 (0.1 per cent),
- *impurity B*: calculate the ratio R2 of the area of the peak due to impurity B to the area of the peak due to the internal standard from the chromatogram obtained with reference solution (b); from the chromatogram obtained with the test solution, calculate the ratio of the area of any peak due to impurity B to the area of the peak due to the internal standard: this ratio is not greater than R2 (0.5 per cent),
- *total*: calculate the ratio R3 of the area of the peak due to trolamine to the area of the peak due to the internal standard from the chromatogram obtained with reference solution (b); from the chromatogram obtained with the test solution, calculate the ratio of the sum of the areas of any peaks, apart from the principal peak and the peak due to the internal standard, to the area of the peak due to the internal standard: this ratio is not greater than 10 times R3 (1.0 per cent),
- *disregard limit*: 0.5 times the ratio of the area of the peak due to trolamine to the area of the peak due to the internal standard from the chromatogram obtained with reference solution (b) (0.05 per cent).

Impurity C. Gas chromatography (*2.2.28*). *Carry out the test under a ventilated hood, wear gloves and safety glasses.*

Test solution. In a suitable distillation apparatus mix 100.0 g of the substance to be examined and 100.0 ml of *ethylene glycol R* and gently distil 10.0 ml under vacuum at a pressure not exceeding 1.3 kPa. From this distillate, distil 1 ml.

Reference solution. Dilute 25.0 mg of *N-nitrosodiethanolamine R* to 100.0 ml with *ethylene glycol R*. Dilute 5.0 ml of the solution to 50.0 ml with *ethylene glycol R*. Dilute 5.0 ml of this solution to 50.0 ml with *ethylene glycol R*.

Column:

- *material*: fused silica,
- *size*: *l* = 30 m, Ø = 0.25 mm,
- *stationary phase*: *macrogol 20 000 R* (film thickness 0.25 µm).

Carrier gas: *helium for chromatography R.*

Flow rate: 0.75 ml/min.

Split ratio: 1:15.

Temperature:

	Time (min)	Temperature (°C)
Column	0 - 2	180
	2 - 8	180 → 240
	8 - 25	240
Injection port		240
Detector		250

Detection: mass selective spectrometer set at 72 m/e or 91 m/e.

Injection: 3 µl; if necessary inject a blank between each injection.

Retention times: impurity C = about 20 min.

Limit:

– *impurity C*: not more than the area of the corresponding peak in the chromatogram obtained with the reference solution (25 ppb).

Heavy metals (*2.4.8*): maximum 10 ppm.

Dilute 5 ml of solution S to 30 ml with *water R*. The solution complies with limit test A. Prepare the standard using *lead standard solution (1 ppm Pb) R.*

Water (*2.5.12*): maximum 1.0 per cent, determined on 1.000 g.

Open the titration vessel, introduce the substance to be examined directly into the previously titrated solvent. Stopper the flask immediately.

Sulphated ash (*2.4.14*): maximum 0.1 per cent, determined on 1.0 g. Do not carry out the initial heating on a water-bath.

ASSAY

Dissolve 1.200 g in 75 ml of *carbon dioxide-free water R*. Add 0.3 ml of *methyl red solution R*. Titrate with *1 M hydrochloric acid*.

1 ml of *1 M hydrochloric acid* is equivalent to 0.149 g of $C_6H_{15}NO_3$.

STORAGE

In an airtight container, protected from light.

IMPURITIES

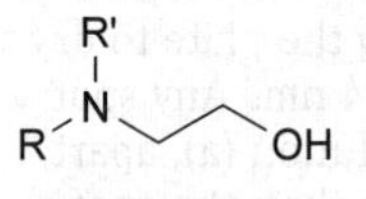

A. R = R′ = H: 2-aminoethanol (ethanolamine),

B. R = CH_2-CH_2OH, R′ = H: 2,2′-iminodiethanol (diethanolamine),

C. R = CH_2-CH_2OH, R′ = NO: 2,2′-(nitrosoimino)diethanol (*N*-nitrosodiethanolamine).

01/2005:1053

TROMETAMOL

Trometamolum

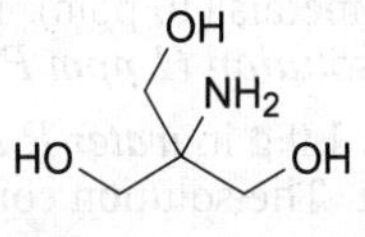

$C_4H_{11}NO_3$ M_r 121.1

DEFINITION

Trometamol contains not less than 99.0 per cent and not more than the equivalent of 100.5 per cent of aminomethylidynetri(methanol), calculated with reference to the dried substance.

CHARACTERS

A white, crystalline powder, or colourless crystals, freely soluble in water, sparingly soluble in alcohol, very slightly soluble in ethyl acetate.

IDENTIFICATION

First identification: B, C.

Second identification: A, B, D.

A. Solution S (see Tests) is strongly alkaline (*2.2.4*).

B. Melting point (*2.2.14*): 168 °C to 174 °C.

C. Examine by infrared absorption spectrophotometry (*2.2.24*), comparing with the spectrum obtained with *trometamol CRS.*

D. Examine the chromatograms obtained in the test for related substances. The principal spot in the chromatogram obtained with test solution (b) is similar in position, colour and size to the principal spot in the chromatogram obtained with reference solution (a).

TESTS

Solution S. Dissolve 2.5 g in *carbon dioxide-free water R* and dilute to 50 ml with the same solvent.

Appearance of solution. Solution S is clear (*2.2.1*) and colourless (*2.2.2, Method II*).

pH (*2.2.3*). The pH of freshly prepared solution S is 10.0 to 11.5.

Related substances. Examine by thin-layer chromatography (*2.2.27*), using *silica gel G R* as the coating substance. Wash the plate with *methanol R* before applying the solutions.

Test solution (a). Dissolve 0.20 g in 1 ml of *water R*, with heating, and dilute to 10 ml with *methanol R.*

Test solution (b). Dilute 1 ml of test solution (a) to 10 ml with *methanol R.*

Reference solution (a). Dissolve 20 mg of *trometamol CRS* in *methanol R* and dilute to 10 ml with the same solvent.

Reference solution (b). Dilute 1 ml of test solution (a) to 100 ml with *methanol R.*

Apply to the plate 10 µl of each solution. Develop over a path of 10 cm using a mixture of 10 volumes of *dilute ammonia R1* and 90 volumes of *2-propanol R.* Dry the plate at 100 °C to 105 °C. Spray with a 5 g/l solution of *potassium permanganate R* in a 10 g/l solution of *sodium carbonate R.* After about 10 min examine in daylight. Any spot in the chromatogram obtained with test solution (a), apart from the principal spot, is not more intense than the spot in the chromatogram obtained with reference solution (b) (1.0 per cent).

Chlorides (*2.4.4*). To 10 ml of solution S add 2.5 ml of *dilute nitric acid R* and dilute to 15 ml with *water R*. The solution complies with the limit test for chlorides (100 ppm).

Heavy metals (*2.4.8*). Dissolve 2.0 g in 10 ml of *water R*. Neutralise the solution with *hydrochloric acid R1* and dilute to 20 ml with *water R*. 12 ml of the solution complies with limit test A for heavy metals (10 ppm). Prepare the standard using *lead standard solution (1 ppm Pb) R*.

Iron (*2.4.9*). Dissolve 1.0 g in *water R* and dilute to 10 ml with the same solvent. The solution complies with the limit test for iron (10 ppm).

Loss on drying (*2.2.32*). Not more than 0.5 per cent, determined on 1.000 g by drying in an oven at 100 °C to 105 °C.

Sulphated ash (*2.4.14*). Not more than 0.1 per cent, determined on 1.0 g.

Bacterial endotoxins (*2.6.14*): less than 0.03 IU/mg, if intended for use in the manufacture of parenteral dosage forms without a further appropriate procedure for the removal of bacterial endotoxins.

ASSAY

Dissolve 0.100 g in 20 ml of *water R*. Add 0.2 ml of *methyl red solution R*. Titrate with *0.1 M hydrochloric acid* until the colour changes from yellow to red.

1 ml of *0.1 M hydrochloric acid* is equivalent to 12.11 mg of $C_4H_{11}NO_3$.

LABELLING

The label states, where applicable, that the substance is free from bacterial endotoxins.

IMPURITIES

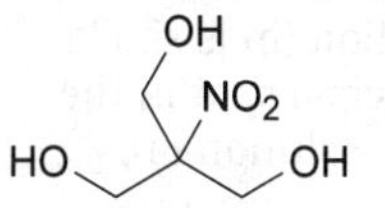

A. nitromethylidynetri(methanol).

01/2005:1159

TROPICAMIDE

Tropicamidum

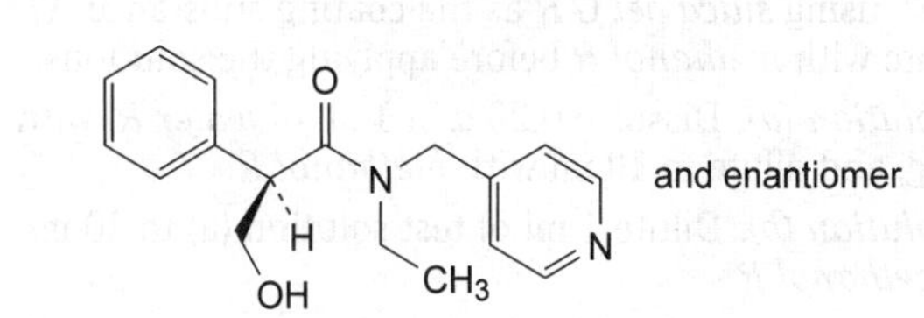

$C_{17}H_{20}N_2O_2$ M_r 284.4

DEFINITION

Tropicamide contains not less than 99.0 per cent and not more than the equivalent of 101.0 per cent of (2*RS*)-*N*-ethyl-3-hydroxy-2-phenyl-*N*-(pyridin-4-ylmethyl)propanamide, calculated with reference to the dried substance.

CHARACTERS

A white or almost white, crystalline powder, slightly soluble in water, freely soluble in alcohol and in methylene chloride.

IDENTIFICATION

First identification: C.

Second identification: A, B, D, E.

A. Melting point (*2.2.14*): 95 °C to 98 °C.

B. Dissolve 20.0 mg in *0.1 M hydrochloric acid* and dilute to 50.0 ml with the same acid. Dilute 2.0 ml of the solution to 20.0 ml with *0.1 M hydrochloric acid*. Examined between 230 nm and 350 nm (*2.2.25*), the solution shows an absorption maximum at 254 nm. The specific absorbance at the maximum is 170 to 190.

C. Examine by infrared absorption spectrophotometry (*2.2.24*), comparing with the spectrum obtained with *tropicamide CRS*. Examine the substances prepared as discs.

D. Examine the chromatograms obtained in the test for related substances. The principal spot in the chromatogram obtained with test solution (b) is similar in position and size to the spot in the chromatogram obtained with reference solution (a).

E. Dissolve about 5 mg in 3 ml of a mixture of 9 ml of *acetic anhydride R*, 1 ml of *acetic acid R* and 0.1 g of *citric acid R*. Heat on a water-bath for 5 min to 10 min. A reddish-yellow colour is produced.

TESTS

Appearance of solution. Dissolve 0.1 g in *alcohol R* and dilute to 10 ml with the same solvent. The solution is clear (*2.2.1*) and colourless (*2.2.2, Method II*).

Optical rotation (*2.2.7*). Dissolve 2.5 g in *ethanol R* and dilute to 25.0 ml with the same solvent. The angle of optical rotation is − 0.1° to + 0.1°.

Related substances. Examine by thin-layer chromatography (*2.2.27*), using as the coating substance a suitable silica gel with a fluorescent indicator having an optimal intensity at 254 nm.

Test solution (a). Dissolve 0.10 g of the substance to be examined in *methylene chloride R* and dilute to 5 ml with the same solvent.

Test solution (b). Dilute 1 ml of test solution (a) to 20 ml with *methylene chloride R*.

Reference solution (a). Dissolve 10 mg of *tropicamide CRS* in *methylene chloride R* and dilute to 10 ml with the same solvent.

Reference solution (b). Dilute 1 ml of test solution (b) to 10 ml with *methylene chloride R*.

Reference solution (c). Dilute 2 ml of reference solution (b) to 5 ml with *methylene chloride R*.

Reference solution (d). Dissolve 20 mg of *4-[(ethylamino)methyl]pyridine R* in *methylene chloride R* and dilute to 20 ml with the same solvent. Dilute 1 ml of the solution and 1 ml of reference solution (a) to 10 ml with *methylene chloride R*.

Apply separately to the plate 10 µl of each solution. Develop over a path of 15 cm using a mixture of 0.5 volumes of *concentrated ammonia R*, 5 volumes of *methanol R* and 95 volumes of *methylene chloride R*. Allow the plate to dry in air and examine in ultraviolet light at 254 nm. Any spot in the chromatogram obtained with test solution (a), apart from the principal spot, is not more intense than the spot in the chromatogram obtained with reference solution (b) (0.5 per cent) and at most one such spot is more intense than the spot in the chromatogram obtained with reference solution (c) (0.2 per cent). The test is not valid unless the chromatogram obtained with reference solution (d) shows two clearly separated spots.

Tropic acid. To 10.0 mg add 5 mg of *disodium tetraborate R* and 0.35 ml of a freshly prepared 100 g/l solution of *dimethylaminobenzaldehyde R* in a mixture of 1 volume of *water R* and 9 volumes of *sulphuric acid R*. Heat on a water-bath for 3 min. Cool in ice water and add 5 ml of *acetic anhydride R*. No violet-red colour develops (0.05 per cent).

Chlorides (*2.4.4*). Dissolve 1.0 g with heating in 8 ml of *acetic acid R*, cool and dilute to 10 ml with the same acid. Dilute 5 ml of the solution to 15 ml with *water R*. The solution complies with the limit test for chlorides (100 ppm).

Loss on drying (*2.2.32*). Not more than 0.5 per cent, determined on 1.000 g by drying in an oven at 80 °C at a pressure not exceeding 0.7 kPa for 4 h.

Sulphated ash (*2.2.14*). Not more than 0.1 per cent, determined on 1.0 g.

ASSAY

Dissolve 0.200 g in 50 ml of *anhydrous acetic acid R*. Add 0.2 ml of *naphtholbenzein solution R* and titrate with *0.1 M perchloric acid* until the colour changes from orange to green.

1 ml of *0.1 M perchloric acid* is equivalent to 28.44 mg of $C_{17}H_{20}N_2O_2$.

STORAGE

Store protected from light.

IMPURITIES

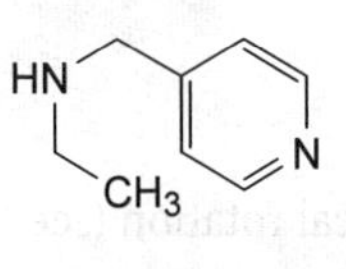

A. *N*-(pyridin-4-ylmethyl)ethanamine,

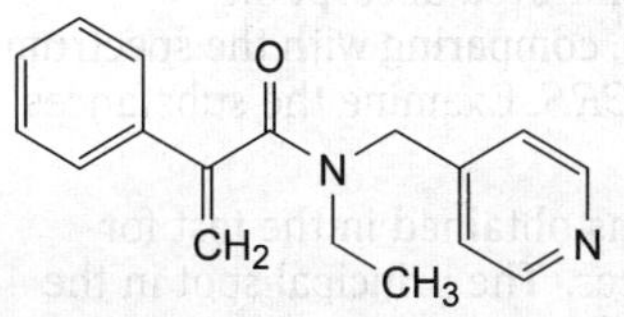

B. *N*-ethyl-2-phenyl-*N*-(pyridin-4-ylmethyl)propenamide,

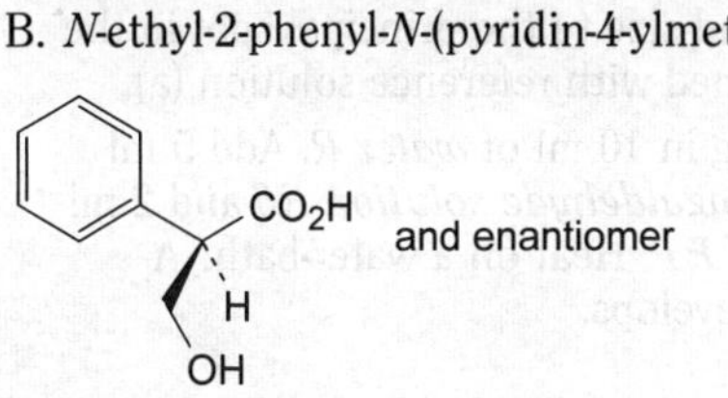

C. (2*RS*)-3-hydroxy-2-phenylpropanoic acid (tropic acid).

01/2005:0694

TRYPSIN

Trypsinum

DEFINITION

Trypsin is a proteolytic enzyme obtained by the activation of trypsinogen extracted from the pancreas of healthy mammals. It has an activity not less than 0.5 microkatal per milligram, calculated with reference to the dried substance. In solution, it has maximum enzymic activity at pH 8; the activity is reversibly inhibited at pH 3, at which pH it is most stable.

PRODUCTION

The animals from which trypsin is derived must fulfil the requirements for the health of animals suitable for human consumption to the satisfaction of the competent authority.

It must have been shown to what extent the method of production allows inactivation or removal of any contamination by viruses or other infectious agents.

The method of manufacture is validated to demonstrate that the product, if tested, would comply with the following test:

Histamine (*2.6.10*). Not more than 1 µg of histamine base per 0.2 microkatal of trypsin activity. Use a 10 g/l solution of the substance to be examined in *0.0015 M borate buffer solution pH 8.0 R* inactivated by heating on a water-bath for 30 min. Carry out dilutions with a 9 g/l solution of *sodium chloride R*.

CHARACTERS

A white or almost white, crystalline or amorphous powder, sparingly soluble in water. The amorphous form is hygroscopic.

IDENTIFICATION

A. Dilute 1 ml of solution S (see Tests) to 100 ml with *water R*. In a depression in a white spot-plate, mix 0.1 ml of this solution with 0.2 ml of *tosylarginine methyl ester hydrochloride solution R*. A reddish-violet colour develops within 3 min.

B. Dilute 0.5 ml of solution S to 5 ml with *water R*. Add 0.1 ml of a 20 g/l solution of *tosyl-lysyl-chloromethane hydrochloride R*. Adjust to pH 7.0, shake for 2 h and dilute to 50 ml with *water R*. In one of the depressions of a white spot-plate, mix 0.1 ml of this solution with 0.2 ml of *tosylarginine methyl ester hydrochloride solution R*. No reddish-violet colour develops within 3 min.

TESTS

Solution S. Dissolve 0.10 g in *carbon dioxide-free water R* and dilute to 10.0 ml with the same solvent.

Appearance of solution. Solution S is not more opalescent than reference suspension III (*2.2.1*).

pH (*2.2.3*). The pH of solution S is 3.0 to 6.0.

Absorbance (*2.2.25*). Dissolve 30.0 mg in *0.001 M hydrochloric acid* and dilute to 100.0 ml with the same acid. The solution shows an absorption maximum at 280 nm and a minimum at 250 nm. The specific absorbance at the maximum is 13.5 to 16.5 and that at the minimum is not greater than 7.0.

Chymotrypsin. To 1.8 ml of *buffer solution pH 8.0 R* add 7.4 ml of *water R* and 0.5 ml of *0.2 M acetyltyrosine ethyl ester R*. While shaking the solution, add 0.3 ml of solution S and start a stop-watch. After exactly 5 min, measure the pH (*2.2.3*) (test solution). Prepare a reference solution in the same manner, replacing solution S by 0.3 ml of a 0.5 g/l solution of *chymotrypsin BRP* and measure the pH (*2.2.3*) exactly 5 min after adding the chymotrypsin. The pH of the test solution is higher than that of the reference solution.

Loss on drying (*2.2.32*). Not more than 5.0 per cent, determined on 0.500 g by drying at 60 °C at a pressure not exceeding 670 Pa for 2 h.

Microbial contamination. Total viable aerobic count (*2.6.12*) not more than 10^4 micro-organisms per gram, determined by plate count. It complies with the tests for *Escherichia coli* and *Salmonella* (*2.6.13*).

ASSAY

The activity of trypsin is determined by comparing the rate at which it hydrolyses *benzoylarginine ethyl ester hydrochloride R* with the rate at which *trypsin BRP* hydrolyses the same substrate in the same conditions.

Apparatus. Use a reaction vessel of about 30 ml capacity provided with:

- a device that will maintain a temperature of 25.0 ± 0.1 °C,
- a stirring device (for example, a magnetic stirrer),
- a lid with holes for the insertion of electrodes, the tip of a burette, a tube for the admission of nitrogen and the introduction of reagents.

An automatic or manual titration device may be used. For the latter, the burette is graduated in 0.005 ml and the pH meter is provided with a wide-range scale and glass-calomel electrodes.

Test solution. Dissolve sufficient of the substance to be examined in *0.001 M hydrochloric acid* and dilute to 25.0 ml with the same acid in order to obtain a solution containing approximately 700 nanokatals per millilitre.

Reference solution. Dissolve 25.0 mg of *trypsin BRP* in *0.001 M hydrochloric acid* and dilute to 25.0 ml with the same acid.

Store the solutions at 0 °C to 5 °C. Warm 1 ml of each solution to about 25 °C over 15 min and use 50 µl of each solution for each titration. Carry out the titration in an atmosphere of nitrogen. Transfer 10.0 ml of *0.0015 M borate buffer solution pH 8.0 R* to the reaction vessel and, while stirring, add 1.0 ml of a freshly prepared 6.86 g/l solution of *benzoylarginine ethyl ester hydrochloride R*. When the temperature is steady at 25.0 ± 0.1 °C (after about 5 min) adjust the pH to exactly 8.0 with *0.1 M sodium hydroxide*. Add 50 µl of the test solution and start a timer. Maintain the pH at 8.0 by the addition of *0.1 M sodium hydroxide* the tip of the microburette being immersed in the solution; note the volume added every 30 s. Follow the reaction for 8 min. Calculate the volume of *0.1 M sodium hydroxide* used per second. Carry out a titration in the same manner using the reference solution and calculate the volume of *0.1 M sodium hydroxide* used per second.

Calculate the activity in microkatals per milligram using the expression:

$$\frac{m' \times V}{m \times V'} \times A$$

m = mass of the substance to be examined, in milligrams,

m' = mass of *trypsin BRP*, in milligrams,

V = volume of *0.1 M sodium hydroxide* used per second by the test solution,

V' = volume of *0.1 M sodium hydroxide* used per second by the reference solution,

A = activity of *trypsin BRP*, in microkatals per milligram.

STORAGE

Store in an airtight container, protected from light, at a temperature of 2 °C to 8 °C.

LABELLING

The label states the activity in microkatals per milligram.

01/2005:1272

TRYPTOPHAN

Tryptophanum

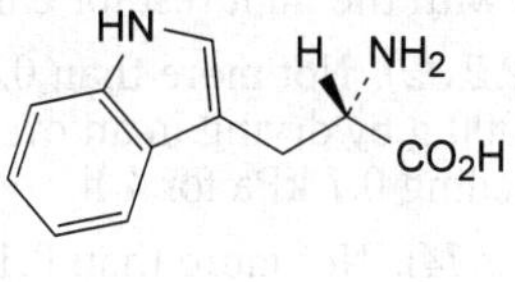

$C_{11}H_{12}N_2O_2$ M_r 204.2

DEFINITION

Tryptophan contains not less than 98.5 per cent and not more than the equivalent of 101.0 per cent of (*S*)-2-amino-3-(1*H*-indol-3-yl)propanoic acid, calculated with reference to the dried substance.

CHARACTERS

A white or almost white, crystalline or amorphous powder, sparingly soluble in water, slightly soluble in alcohol. It dissolves in dilute mineral acids and in dilute solutions of alkali hydroxides.

IDENTIFICATION

First identification: A, B.

Second identification: A, C, D.

A. It complies with the test for specific optical rotation (see Tests).

B. Examine the substance by infrared absorption spectrophotometry (*2.2.24*), comparing with the spectrum obtained with *tryptophan CRS*. Examine the substances prepared as discs.

C. Examine the chromatograms obtained in the test for ninhydrin-positive substances. The principal spot in the chromatogram obtained with test solution (b) is similar in position, colour and size to the principal spot in the chromatogram obtained with reference solution (a).

D. Dissolve about 20 mg in 10 ml of *water R*. Add 5 ml of *dimethylaminobenzaldehyde solution R6* and 2 ml of *hydrochloric acid R1*. Heat on a water-bath. A purple-blue colour develops.

TESTS

Appearance of solution. Dissolve 0.1 g in*1 M hydrochloric acid* and dilute to 10 ml with the same acid. The solution is clear (*2.2.1*) and not more intensely coloured than reference solution BY_6 (*2.2.2, Method II*).

Specific optical rotation (*2.2.7*). Dissolve 0.25 g in *water R*, heating on a water-bath if necessary, and dilute to 25.0 ml with the same solvent. The specific optical rotation is − 30.0 to − 33.0, calculated with reference to the dried substance.

Ninhydrin-positive substances. Examine by thin-layer chromatography (*2.2.27*), using a *TLC silica gel plate R*.

Test solution (a). Dissolve 0.10 g of the substance to be examined in a mixture of equal volumes of *glacial acetic acid R* and *water R* and dilute to 10 ml with the same mixture of solvents.

Test solution (b). Dilute 1 ml of test solution (a) to 50 ml with a mixture of equal volumes of *glacial acetic acid R* and *water R*.

Reference solution (a). Dissolve 10 mg of *tryptophan CRS* in a mixture of equal volumes of *glacial acetic acid R* and *water R* and dilute to 50 ml with the same mixture of solvents.

Reference solution (b). Dilute 5 ml of test solution (b) to 20 ml with a mixture of equal volumes of *glacial acetic acid R* and *water R*.

Reference solution (c). Dissolve 10 mg of *tryptophan CRS* and 10 mg of *tyrosine CRS* in a mixture of equal volumes of *glacial acetic acid R* and *water R* and dilute to 25 ml with the same mixture of solvents.

Apply separately to the plate 5 µl of each solution. Develop over a path of 15 cm using a mixture of 20 volumes of *glacial acetic acid R*, 20 volumes of *water R* and 60 volumes of *butanol R*. Allow the plate to dry in air. Spray with *ninhydrin solution R* and heat at 100 °C to 105 °C for 15 min. Any spot in the chromatogram obtained with test solution (a), apart from the principal spot, is not more intense than the spot in the chromatogram obtained with reference solution (b) (0.5 per cent). The test is not valid unless the chromatogram obtained with reference solution (c) shows two clearly separated spots.

1,1′-Ethylidenebistryptophan and other related substances. Examine by liquid chromatography (*2.2.29*).

Buffer solution pH 2.3. Dissolve 3.90 g of *sodium dihydrogen phosphate R* in 1000 ml of *water R*. Add about 700 ml of a 2.9 g/l solution of *phosphoric acid R* and adjust to pH 2.3 with the same acidic solution.

Prepare the solutions immediately before use.

Standard solution. Dissolve 10.0 mg of *N-acetyltryptophan R* in a mixture of 10 volumes of *acetonitrile R* and 90 volumes of *water R* and dilute to 100.0 ml with the same mixture of solvents. Dilute 2.0 ml of the solution to 100.0 ml with the same mixture of solvents.

Test solution (a). Dissolve 0.10 g of the substance to be examined in a mixture of 10 volumes of *acetonitrile R* and 90 volumes of *water R* and dilute to 10.0 ml the same mixture of solvents.

Test solution (b). Dissolve 0.10 g of the substance to be examined in the standard solution and dilute to 10.0 ml with the same solution.

Reference solution (a). Dissolve 1.0 mg of *1,1′-ethylidenebistryptophan CRS* in a mixture of 10 volumes of *acetonitrile R* and 90 volumes of *water R* and dilute to 100.0 ml with the same mixture of solvents.

Reference solution (b). Dilute 10.0 ml of reference solution (a) to 50.0 ml with the standard solution.

Reference solution (c). Dilute 10.0 ml of reference solution (a) to 50.0 ml with a mixture of 10 volumes of *acetonitrile R* and 90 volumes of *water R*.

Reference solution (d). Dissolve 0.10 g of the substance to be examined in reference solution (c) and dilute to 10.0 ml with the same solution.

Reference solution (e). Dilute 1.0 ml of reference solution (c) to 10.0 ml with a mixture of 10 volumes of *acetonitrile R* and 90 volumes of *water R*.

The chromatographic procedure may be carried out using:

– a stainless steel column 0.25 m long and 4.6 mm in internal diameter packed with *octadecylsilyl silica gel for chromatography R* (5 µm),

– as mobile phase at a flow rate of 0.7 ml/min the following solutions:

Mobile phase A. A mixture of 115 volumes of *acetonitrile R* and 885 volumes of buffer solution pH 2.3,

Mobile phase B. A mixture of 350 volumes of *acetonitrile R* and 650 volumes of buffer solution pH 2.3,

– a gradient programme using the following conditions:

Time (min)	Mobile phase A (per cent V/V)	Mobile phase B (per cent V/V)	Comment
0 - 10	100	0	isocratic
10 - 45	100 → 0	0 → 100	linear gradient
45 - 65	0	100	isocratic
65 - 66	0 → 100	100 → 0	linear gradient
66 - 80	100	0	re-equilibration

– as detector a spectrophotometer set at 220 nm,

maintaining the temperature of the column at 40 °C.

Inject 20 µl of reference solution (b), 20 µl of reference solution (d) and 20 µl of reference solution (e).

When the chromatograms are recorded in the prescribed conditions, the retention times are about 8 min for tryptophan, about 29 min for *N*-acetyltryptophan and about 34 min for 1,1′-ethylidenebistryptophan. Adjust the sensitivity of the system so that the height of the peak due to *N*-acetyltryptophan in the chromatogram obtained with reference solution (b) is at least 50 per cent of the full scale of the recorder.

The test is not valid unless:

– in the chromatogram obtained with reference solution (b), the resolution between the peaks corresponding to *N*-acetyltryptophan and 1,1′-ethylidenebistryptophan is at least 8.0. If necessary, adjust the time programme for the elution gradient. An increase in the duration of elution with mobile phase A produces longer retention times and better resolution;

– the chromatogram obtained with reference solution (e) has a signal-to-noise ratio of at least 15.

Inject 20 µl of test solution (a) and 20 µl of test solution (b). Check that in the chromatogram obtained with test solution (a) there is no peak with the same retention time as *N*-acetyltryptophan (in such case correct the area of the *N*-acetyltryptophan peak). In the chromatogram obtained with test solution (b): the area of any peak corresponding to 1,1′-ethylidenebistryptophan is not greater than 0.5 times the area of the principal peak in the chromatogram obtained with reference solution (e) (10 ppm); the sum of the areas of any peaks with retention times less than that of tryptophan is not greater than 0.6 times the area of the peak corresponding to *N*-acetyltryptophan in the chromatogram obtained with reference solution (b) (100 ppm); the sum of the areas of any peaks with a retention time greater than that of tryptophan, apart from *N*-acetyltryptophan, and up to 1.8 times the retention time of *N*-acetyltryptophan, is not greater than 1.9 times the area of the peak due to *N*-acetyltryptophan in the chromatogram obtained with reference solution (b) (300 ppm). Disregard any peak with an area less than 0.02 times that of the peak due to *N*-acetyltryptophan in the chromatogram obtained with reference solution (b).

Chlorides (*2.4.4*). Dissolve 0.25 g in 3 ml of *dilute nitric acid R* and dilute to 15 ml with *water R*. The solution without any further addition of nitric acid (200 ppm), complies with the limit test for chlorides.

Sulphates (*2.4.13*). Dissolve 0.5 g in a mixture of 5 volumes of *dilute hydrochloric acid R* and 25 volumes of *distilled water R* and dilute to 15 ml with the same mixture of solvents. The solution complies with the limit test for sulphates (300 ppm).

Ammonium (*2.4.1*). 0.10 g complies with limit test B for ammonium (200 ppm). Prepare the standard using 0.2 ml of *ammonium standard solution (100 ppm NH_4) R*.

Iron (*2.4.9*). In a separating funnel, dissolve 0.50 g in 10 ml of *dilute hydrochloric acid R*. Shake with three quantities, each of 10 ml, of *methyl isobutyl ketone R1*, shaking for 3 min each time. To the combined organic layers add 10 ml of *water R* and shake for 3 min. The aqueous layer complies with the limit test for iron (20 ppm).

Heavy metals (*2.4.8*). 2.0 g complies with limit test D for heavy metals (10 ppm). Prepare the standard using 2 ml of *lead standard solution (10 ppm Pb) R*.

Loss on drying (*2.2.32*). Not more than 0.5 per cent, determined on 1.000 g by drying in an oven at 100 °C to 105 °C.

Sulphated ash (*2.4.14*). Not more than 0.1 per cent, determined on 1.0 g.

ASSAY

Dissolve 0.150 g in 3 ml of *anhydrous formic acid R*. Add 30 ml of *anhydrous acetic acid R*. Titrate with *0.1 M perchloric acid*, using 0.1 ml of *naphtholbenzein solution R* as indicator.

1 ml of *0.1 M perchloric acid* is equivalent to 20.42 mg of $C_{11}H_{12}N_2O_2$.

STORAGE

Store protected from light.

IMPURITIES

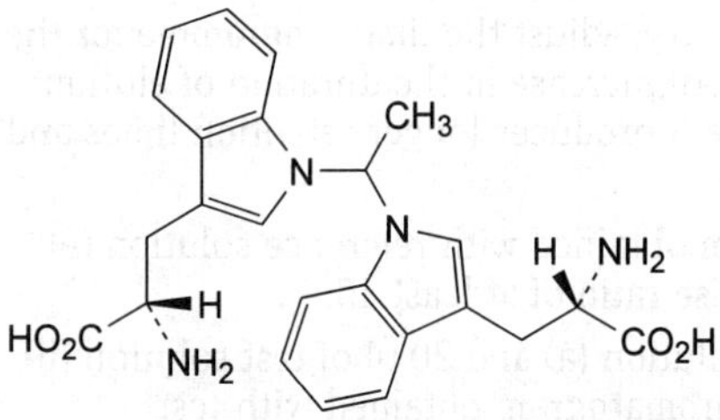

A. 3,3′-[ethylidenebis(1*H*-indole-1,3-diyl)]bis[(2*S*)-2-aminopropanoic] acid (1,1′-ethylidenebistryptophan),

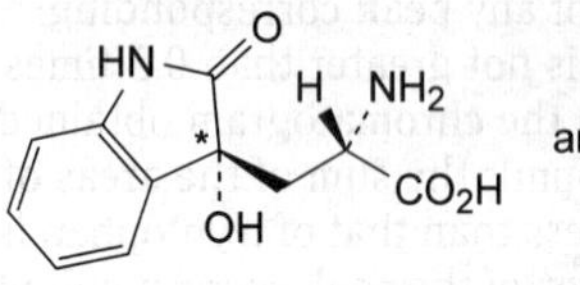

B. (*S*)-2-amino-3-[(3*RS*)-3-hydroxy-2-oxo-2,3-dihydro-1*H*-indol-3-yl]propanoic acid (dioxyindolylalanine),

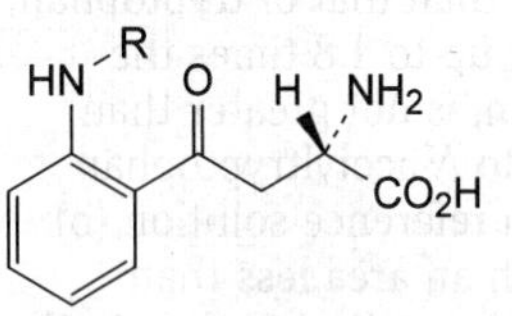

C. R = H: (*S*)-2-amino-4-(2-aminophenyl)-4-oxobutanoic acid (kynurenine),

E. R = CHO: (*S*)-2-amino-4-[2-(formylamino)phenyl]-4-oxobutanoic acid (*N*-formylkynurenine),

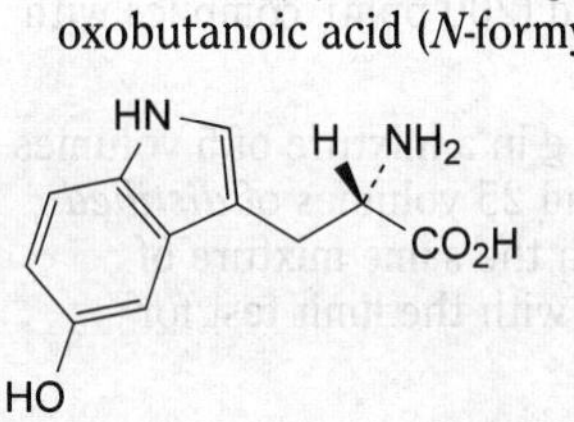

D. (*S*)-2-amino-3-(5-hydroxy-1*H*-indol-3-yl)propanoic acid (5-hydroxytryptophan),

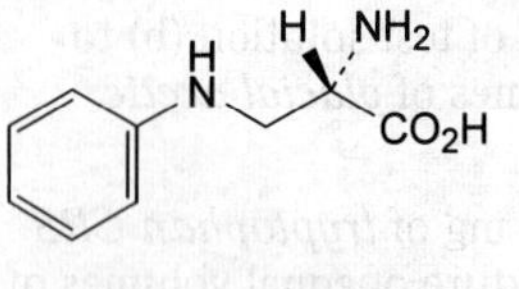

F. (*S*)-2-amino-3-(phenylamino)propanoic acid (3-phenylaminoalanine),

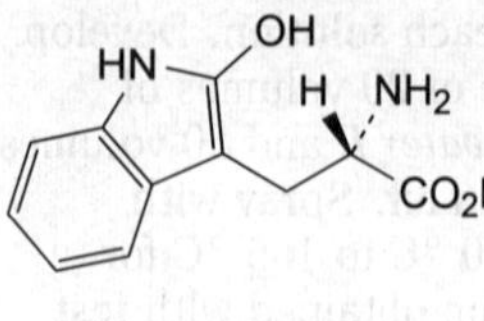

G. (*S*)-2-amino-3-(2-hydroxy-1*H*-indol-3-yl)propanoic acid (2-hydroxytryptophan),

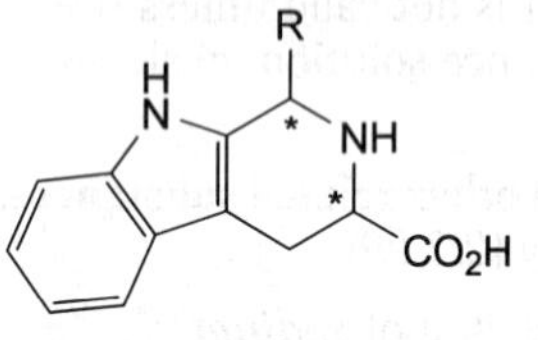

H. R = H: (3*RS*)-1,2,3,4-tetrahydro-9*H*-β-carboline-3-carboxylic acid,

I. R = CH_3: 1-methyl-1,2,3,4-tetrahydro-9*H*-β-carboline-3-carboxylic acid,

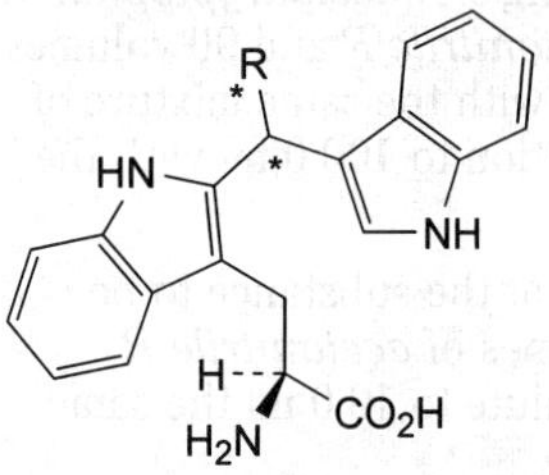

J. R = $CHOH-CH_2-OH$: (*S*)-2-amino-3-[2-[2,3-dihydroxy-1-(1*H*-indol-3-yl)propyl]-1*H*-indol-3-yl]propanoic acid,

K. R = H: (*S*)-2-amino-3-[2-(1*H*-indol-3-ylmethyl)-1*H*-indol-3-yl]propanoic acid,

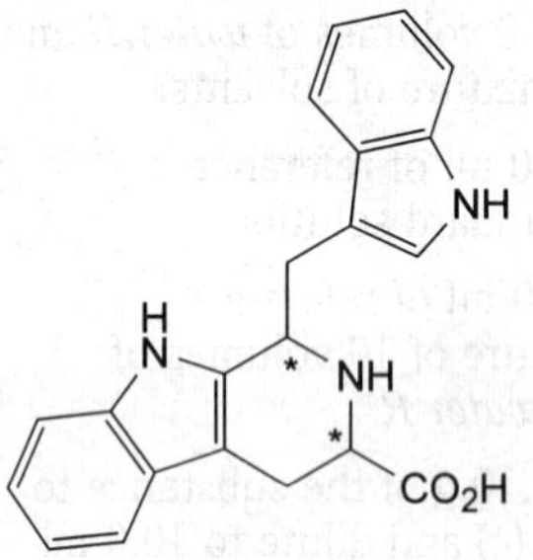

L. 1-(1*H*-indol-3-ylmethyl)-1,2,3,4-tetrahydro-9*H*-β-carboline-3-carboxylic acid.

01/2005:0152

TUBERCULIN FOR HUMAN USE, OLD

Tuberculinum pristinum ad usum humanum

DEFINITION

Old tuberculin for human use consists of a filtrate, concentrated by heating, containing the soluble products of the culture and lysis of one or more strains of *Mycobacterium bovis* and/or *Mycobacterium tuberculosis* that is capable of demonstrating a delayed hypersensitivity in an animal sensitised to micro-organisms of the same species.

Old tuberculin for human use in concentrated form is a transparent, viscous, yellow or brown liquid.

PRODUCTION

GENERAL PROVISIONS

The production of old tuberculin is based on a seed-lot system. The production method shall have been shown to yield consistently old tuberculin of adequate potency and safety in man. A batch of old tuberculin, calibrated in International Units by the method described under Assay and for which adequate clinical information is available as to its activity in man, is set aside to serve as a reference preparation.

The International Unit is the activity of a stated quantity of the International Standard. The equivalence in International Units of the International Standard is stated by the World Health Organisation.

SEED LOTS

The strains of mycobacteria used shall be identified by historical records that include information on their origin and subsequent manipulation.

The working seed lots used to inoculate the media for the production of a concentrated harvest shall not have undergone more than 4 subcultures from the master seed lot.

Only seed lots that comply with the following requirements may be used for propagation.

Identification. The species of mycobacterium of the master and working seed lots is identified.

Bacterial and fungal contamination. Carry out the test for sterility (*2.6.1*), using 10 ml for each medium. The working seed lot complies with the test for sterility except for the presence of mycobacteria.

PROPAGATION AND HARVEST

The bacteria are grown in a liquid medium which may be a glycerolated broth or a synthetic medium. Growth must be typical for the strain. The culture is inactivated by a suitable method, such as treatment in an autoclave (121 °C for not less than 30 min) or in flowing steam at a temperature not less than 100 °C for at least 1 h. The culture liquid, from which the micro-organisms may or may not have been separated by filtration, is concentrated by evaporation, usually to one-tenth of its initial volume. The preparation is free from live mycobacteria. The concentrated harvest is shown to comply with the test for mycobacteria (*2.6.2*) before addition of any antimicrobial preservative or other substance that might interfere with the test. Phenol (5 g/l) or another suitable antimicrobial preservative that does not give rise to false positive reactions may be added.

Only a concentrated harvest that complies with the following requirements may be used in the preparation of the final bulk tuberculin.

pH (*2.2.3*). The pH of the concentrated harvest is 6.5 to 8.

Glycerol. Where applicable, determine the glycerol content of the concentrated harvest. The amount is within the limits approved for the particular product.

Antimicrobial preservative. Where applicable, determine the amount of antimicrobial preservative by a suitable chemical or physico-chemical method. The content is not less than 85 per cent and not more than 115 per cent of the intended amount. If phenol has been used in the preparation, the concentration is not more than 5 g/l (*2.5.15*).

Sensitisation. Carry out the test described under Tests.

Sterility (*2.6.1*). The concentrated harvest complies with the test for sterility, carried out using 10 ml for each medium.

Potency. Determine the potency as described under Assay.

FINAL BULK TUBERCULIN

The concentrated harvest is diluted aseptically.

Only a final bulk tuberculin that complies with the following requirement may be used in the preparation of the final lot.

Sterility (*2.6.1*). The final bulk tuberculin complies with the test for sterility, carried out using 10 ml for each medium.

FINAL LOT

The final bulk tuberculin is distributed aseptically into sterile containers which are then closed so as to prevent contamination.

Only a final lot that is satisfactory with respect to each of the requirements given below under Identification, Tests and Assay may be released for use.

The following tests may be omitted on the final lot if they have been carried out at the stages indicated:

- live mycobacteria: concentrated harvest,
- sensitisation: concentrated harvest,
- toxicity: concentrated harvest or final bulk tuberculin,
- antimicrobial preservative: final bulk tuberculin.

IDENTIFICATION

Inject increasing doses of the preparation to be examined intradermally into healthy, white or pale-coloured guinea-pigs, specifically sensitised (for example, as described under Assay). A reaction varying from erythema to necrosis is produced at the site of the injection. Similar injections administered to non-sensitised guinea-pigs do not stimulate a reaction. The assay may also serve as identification.

TESTS

Old tuberculin for human use in concentrated form (≥ 100 000 IU/ml) complies with each of the tests prescribed below; the diluted product complies with the tests for antimicrobial preservative and sterility.

Toxicity. Inject a quantity equivalent to 50 000 IU subcutaneously into each of two healthy guinea-pigs weighing 250 g to 350 g and which have not been subjected to any treatment likely to interfere with the test. Observe the animals for 7 days. No adverse effect is produced.

Sensitisation. Use 3 guinea-pigs that have not been subjected to any treatment likely to interfere with the test. On 3 occasions at intervals of 5 days, inject intradermally into each guinea-pig about 500 IU of the preparation to be examined in a volume of 0.1 ml. 2 to 3 weeks after the third injection, administer the same dose intradermally to the same animals and to a control group of 3 guinea-pigs of the same mass that have not previously received injections of tuberculin. After 24 h to 72 h, the reactions in the 2 groups of animals are not substantially different.

Antimicrobial preservative. Where applicable, determine the amount of antimicrobial preservative by a suitable chemical or physico-chemical method. The content is not less than the minimum amount shown to be effective and not more than 115 per cent of the amount stated on the label. If phenol has been used in the preparation, the concentration is not more than 5 g/l (*2.5.15*).

Live mycobacteria (*2.6.2*). It complies with the test for mycobacteria.

Sterility (*2.6.1*). It complies with the test for sterility.

Monographs T-Z

ASSAY

The potency of old tuberculin is determined by comparing the reactions produced by the intradermal injection of increasing doses of the preparation to be examined into sensitised guinea-pigs with the reactions produced by known concentrations of the reference preparation.

Prepare a suspension containing a suitable amount (0.1 mg to 0.4 mg/ml) of heat-inactivated, dried mycobacteria in mineral oil with or without emulsifier; use mycobacteria of a strain of the same species as that used in the preparation to be examined. Sensitise not fewer than 6 pale-coloured guinea-pigs weighing not less than 300 g by injecting intramuscularly or intradermally a total of about 0.5 ml of the suspension, divided between several sites if necessary. Carry out the test after the period of time required for optimal sensitisation which is usually 4 to 8 weeks after sensitisation. Depilate the flanks of the animals so that it is possible to make at least three injections on each side and not more than a total of 12 injection points per animal. Use at least three different doses of the reference preparation and at least 3 different doses of the preparation to be examined. For both preparations, use doses such that the highest dose is about 10 times the lowest dose. Choose the doses such that when they are injected the lesions produced have a diameter of not less than 8 mm and not more than 25 mm. In any given test, the order of the dilutions injected at each point is chosen at random in a Latin square design. Inject each dose intradermally in a constant volume of 0.1 ml or 0.2 ml. Measure the diameters of the lesions 24 h to 48 h later and calculate the results of the test by the usual statistical methods, assuming that the diameters of the lesions are directly proportional to the logarithm of the concentration of the preparation.

The estimated potency is not less than 80 per cent and not more than 125 per cent of the stated potency. The confidence limits ($P = 0.95$) are not less than 64 per cent and not more than 156 per cent of the stated potency.

STORAGE

Store protected from light.

LABELLING

The label states:

- the number of International Units per millilitre,
- the species of mycobacterium used to prepare the product,
- the name and quantity of any antimicrobial preservative or other substance added to the preparation,
- the expiry date,
- where applicable, that old tuberculin is not to be injected in its concentrated form but diluted so as to administer not more than 100 IU per dose.

01/2005:0535

TUBERCULIN PURIFIED PROTEIN DERIVATIVE, AVIAN

Tuberculini aviarii derivatum proteinosum purificatum

DEFINITION

Tuberculin purified protein derivative, avian (Tuberculin PPD, avian) is a preparation obtained from the heat-treated products of growth and lysis of *Mycobacterium avium* capable of revealing a delayed hypersensitivity in an animal sensitised to micro-organisms of the same species.

PRODUCTION

It is obtained from the water-soluble fractions prepared by heating in free-flowing steam and subsequently filtering cultures of *M. avium* grown in a liquid synthetic medium. The active fraction of the filtrate, consisting mainly of protein, is isolated by precipitation, washed and re-dissolved. An antimicrobial preservative that does not give rise to false positive reactions, such as phenol, may be added. The final sterile preparation, free from mycobacteria, is distributed aseptically into sterile tamper-proof glass containers which are then closed so as to prevent contamination. The preparation may be freeze-dried.

The identification, the tests and the determination of potency apply to the liquid form and to the freeze-dried form after reconstitution as stated on the label.

IDENTIFICATION

Inject a range of graded doses intradermally at different sites into suitably sensitised albino guinea-pigs, each weighing not less than 250 g. After 24 h to 28 h, reactions appear in the form of oedematous swellings with erythema with or without necrosis at the points of injection. The size and severity of the reactions vary according to the dose. Unsensitised guinea-pigs show no reactions to similar injections.

TESTS

pH (*2.2.3*). The pH is 6.5 to 7.5.

Phenol (*2.5.15*). If the preparation to be examined contains phenol, its concentration is not more than 5 g/l.

Sensitising effect. Use a group of three guinea-pigs that have not been treated with any material which will interfere with the test. On three occasions at intervals of 5 days inject intradermally into each guinea-pig a dose of the preparation to be examined equivalent to 500 IU in 0.1 ml. Fifteen to twenty-one days after the third injection, inject the same dose (500 IU) intradermally into these animals and into a control group of three guinea-pigs of the same mass and which have not previously received injections of tuberculin. 24 h to 28 h after the last injections, the reactions of the two groups are not significantly different.

Toxicity. Use two guinea-pigs, each weighing not less than 250 g and which have not previously been treated with any material which will interfere with the test. Inject subcutaneously into each guinea-pig 0.5 ml of the preparation to be examined. Observe the animals for 7 days. No abnormal effects occur during the observation period.

Sterility. It complies with the test for sterility prescribed in the monograph on *Vaccines for veterinary use (0062)*.

POTENCY

The potency of tuberculin purified protein derivative, avian is determined by comparing the reactions produced in sensitised guinea-pigs by the intradermal injection of a series of dilutions of the preparation to be examined with those produced by known concentrations of a reference preparation of tuberculin purified protein derivative, avian calibrated in International Units.

The International Unit is the activity contained in a stated amount of the International Standard. The equivalence in International Units of the International Standard is stated by the World Health Organisation.

Sensitise not fewer than nine albino guinea-pigs, each weighing 400 g to 600 g, by the deep intramuscular injection of a suitable dose of inactivated or live *M. avium*. Not less than four weeks after the sensitisation of the guinea-pigs, shave their flanks to provide space for not more than four injection sites on each side. Prepare dilutions of the preparation to be examined and of the reference preparation using isotonic phosphate-buffered saline (pH 6.5 to 7.5) containing 0.005 g/l of *polysorbate 80 R*. Use not fewer than three doses of the reference preparation and not fewer than three doses of the preparation to be examined. Choose the doses such that the lesions produced have a diameter of not less than 8 mm and not more than 25 mm. Allocate the dilutions randomly to the sites using a Latin square design. Inject each dose intradermally in a constant volume of 0.1 ml or 0.2 ml. Measure the diameters of the lesions after 24 h to 28 h and calculate the result of the test using the usual statistical methods and assuming that the diameters of the lesions are directly proportional to the logarithm of the concentration of the tuberculins.

The test is not valid unless the confidence limits (P = 0.95) are not less than 50 per cent and not more than 200 per cent of the estimated potency. The estimated potency is not less than 75 per cent and not more than 133 per cent of the stated potency. The stated potency is not less than 20 000 IU/ml.

STORAGE

Store protected from light, at a temperature of 5 ± 3 °C.

LABELLING

The label states:

- the potency in International Units per millilitre.
- the name and quantity of any added substance,
- for freeze-dried preparations:
- the name and volume of the reconstituting liquid to be added,
- that the product should be used immediately after reconstitution.

01/2005:0536

TUBERCULIN PURIFIED PROTEIN DERIVATIVE, BOVINE

Tuberculini bovini derivatum proteinosum purificatum

DEFINITION

Tuberculin purified protein derivative, bovine (Tuberculin PPD, bovine) is a preparation obtained from the heat-treated products of growth and lysis of *Mycobacterium bovis* capable of revealing a delayed hypersensitivity in an animal sensitised to micro-organisms of the same species.

PRODUCTION

It is obtained from the water-soluble fractions prepared by heating in free-flowing steam and subsequently filtering cultures of *M. bovis* grown in a liquid synthetic medium. The active fraction of the filtrate, consisting mainly of protein, is isolated by precipitation, washed and re-dissolved. An antimicrobial preservative that does not give rise to false positive reactions, such as phenol, may be added. The final sterile preparation, free from mycobacteria, is distributed aseptically into sterile, tamper-proof glass containers which are then closed so as to prevent contamination. The preparation may be freeze-dried.

The identification, the tests and the determination of potency apply to the liquid form and to the freeze-dried form after reconstitution as stated on the label.

IDENTIFICATION

Inject a range of graded doses intradermally at different sites into suitably sensitised albino guinea-pigs, each weighing not less than 250 g. After 24 h to 28 h, reactions appear in the form of oedematous swellings with erythema with or without necrosis at the points of injection. The size and severity of the reactions vary according to the dose. Unsensitised guinea-pigs show no reactions to similar injections.

TESTS

pH (*2.2.3*). The pH is 6.5 to 7.5.

Phenol (*2.5.15*). If the preparation to be examined contains phenol, its concentration is not more than 5 g/l.

Sensitising effect. Use a group of 3 guinea-pigs that have not been treated with any material which will interfere with the test. On 3 occasions at intervals of 5 days inject intradermally into each guinea-pig a dose of the preparation to be examined equivalent to 500 IU in 0.1 ml. 15 to 21 days after the third injection inject the same dose (500 IU) intradermally into these animals and into a control group of 3 guinea-pigs of the same mass and which have not previously received injections of tuberculin. 24 h to 28 h after the last injections, the reactions of the 2 groups are not significantly different.

Toxicity. Use 2 guinea-pigs, each weighing not less than 250 g and which have not previously been treated with any material which will interfere with the test. Inject subcutaneously into each guinea-pig 0.5 ml of the preparation to be examined. Observe the animals for 7 days. No abnormal effects occur during the observation period.

Sterility. It complies with the test for sterility prescribed in the monograph on *Vaccines for veterinary use (0062)*.

POTENCY

The potency of tuberculin purified protein derivative, bovine is determined by comparing the reactions produced in sensitised guinea-pigs by the intradermal injection of a series of dilutions of the preparation to be examined with those produced by known concentrations of a reference preparation calibrated in International Units.

Sensitise not fewer than 9 albino guinea-pigs, each weighing 400 g to 600 g, by the deep intramuscular injection of 0.0001 mg of wet mass of living *M. bovis* of strain AN5 suspended in 0.5 ml of a 9 g/l solution of *sodium chloride R*. Not less than 4 weeks after the sensitisation of the guinea-pigs, shave their flanks to provide space for not more than 4 injection sites on each side. Prepare dilutions of the preparation to be examined and of the reference preparation using isotonic phosphate-buffered saline (pH 6.5-7.5) containing 0.005 g/l of *polysorbate 80 R*. Use not fewer than 3 doses of the reference preparation and not fewer than 3 doses of the preparation to be examined. Choose the doses such that the lesions produced have a diameter of not less than 8 mm and not more than 25 mm. Allocate the dilutions randomly to the sites using a Latin square design. Inject each dose intradermally in a constant volume of 0.1 ml or 0.2 ml. Measure the diameters of the lesions after 24 h to 28 h and calculate the result of the test using the usual statistical methods and assuming that the diameters of the lesions are directly proportional to the logarithm of the concentration of the tuberculins.

The test is not valid unless the confidence limits (P = 0.95) are not less than 50 per cent and not more than 200 per cent of the estimated potency. The estimated potency is not less than 66 per cent and not more than 150 per cent of the stated potency. The stated potency is not less than 20 000 IU/ml.

STORAGE

Protected from light, at a temperature of 5 ± 3 °C.

LABELLING

The label states:

- the potency in International Units per millilitre,
- the name and quantity of any added substance,
- for freeze-dried preparations:
  - the name and volume of the reconstituting liquid to be added,
  - that the product should be used immediately after reconstitution.

01/2005:0151

TUBERCULIN PURIFIED PROTEIN DERIVATIVE FOR HUMAN USE

Tuberculini derivatum proteinosum purificatum ad usum humanum

DEFINITION

Tuberculin purified protein derivative (tuberculin PPD) for human use is a preparation obtained by precipitation from the heated products of the culture and lysis of *Mycobacterium bovis* and/or *Mycobacterium tuberculosis* and capable of demonstrating a delayed hypersensitivity in an animal sensitised to micro-organisms of the same species.

Tuberculin PPD is a colourless or pale-yellow liquid; the diluted preparation may be a freeze-dried powder which upon dissolution gives a colourless or pale-yellow liquid.

PRODUCTION

GENERAL PROVISIONS

The production of tuberculin PPD is based on a seed-lot system. The production method shall have been shown to yield consistently tuberculin PPD of adequate potency and safety in man. A batch of tuberculin PPD, calibrated in International Units by method A described under Assay and for which adequate clinical information is available as to its activity in man, is set aside to serve as a reference preparation.

The International Unit is the activity of a stated quantity of the International Standard. The equivalence in International Units of the International Standard is stated by the World Health Organisation.

SEED LOTS

The strains of mycobacteria used shall be identified by historical records that include information on their origin and subsequent manipulation.

The working seed lots used to inoculate the media for production of a concentrated harvest shall not have undergone more than 4 subcultures from the master seed lot.

Only seed lots that comply with the following requirements may be used for propagation.

Identification. The species of mycobacterium of the master and working seed lots is identified.

Bacterial and fungal contamination. Carry out the test for sterility (*2.6.1*), using 10 ml for each medium. The working seed lot complies with the test for sterility except for the presence of mycobacteria.

PROPAGATION AND HARVEST

The bacteria are grown in a liquid synthetic medium. Growth must be typical for the strain. The culture is inactivated by a suitable method such as treatment in an autoclave (121 °C for not less than 30 min) or in flowing steam at a temperature not less than 100 °C for at least 1 h and filtered. The active fraction of the filtrate, consisting mainly of protein, is isolated by precipitation, washed and re-dissolved. The preparation is free from mycobacteria. The concentrated harvest is shown to comply with the test for mycobacteria (*2.6.2*) before addition of any antimicrobial preservative or other substance that might interfere with the test. Phenol (5 g/l) or another suitable antimicrobial preservative that does not give rise to false positive reactions may be added; a suitable stabiliser intended to prevent adsorption on glass or plastic surfaces may be added. The concentrated harvest may be freeze-dried. Phenol is not added to preparations that are to be freeze-dried.

Only a concentrated harvest that complies with the following requirements may be used in the preparation of the final bulk tuberculin PPD.

Antimicrobial preservative. Where applicable, determine the amount of antimicrobial preservative by a suitable chemical or physico-chemical method. The content is not less than 85 per cent and not more than 115 per cent of the intended amount. If phenol has been used in the preparation, the concentration is not more than 5 g/l (*2.5.15*).

Sensitisation. Carry out the test described under Tests.

Sterility (*2.6.1*). The concentrated harvest, reconstituted if necessary, complies with the test for sterility, carried out using 10 ml for each medium.

Potency. Determine the potency as described under Assay.

FINAL BULK TUBERCULIN PPD

The concentrated harvest is diluted aseptically, after reconstitution if necessary.

Only a final bulk tuberculin PPD that complies with the following requirement may be used in the preparation of the final lot.

Sterility (*2.6.1*). The final bulk tuberculin PPD complies with the test for sterility, carried out using 10 ml for each medium.

FINAL LOT

The final bulk tuberculin PPD is distributed aseptically into sterile containers which are then closed so as to prevent contamination. It may be freeze-dried.

Only a final lot that is satisfactory with respect to each of the requirements given below under Identification, Tests and Assay may be released for use.

The following tests may be omitted on the final lot if they have been carried out at the stages indicated:

- live mycobacteria: concentrated harvest
- sensitisation: concentrated harvest
- toxicity: concentrated harvest or final bulk tuberculin PPD
- antimicrobial preservative: final bulk tuberculin PPD.

IDENTIFICATION

Inject increasing doses of the preparation to be examined intradermally into healthy, white or pale-coloured guinea-pigs, specifically sensitised (for example as described under Assay). A reaction varying from erythema to necrosis is produced at the site of the injection. Similar injections administered to non-sensitised guinea-pigs do not stimulate a reaction. The assay may also serve as identification.

TESTS

Tuberculin purified protein derivative for human use in concentrated form (≥ 100 000 IU/ml) complies with each of the tests prescribed below; the diluted product complies with the tests for pH, antimicrobial preservative and sterility.

pH (*2.2.3*). The pH of the preparation, reconstituted if necessary as stated on the label, is 6.5 to 7.5.

Toxicity. Inject subcutaneously 50 000 IU of the preparation to be examined into each of two healthy guinea-pigs weighing 250 g to 350 g and which have not been subjected to any treatment likely to interfere with the test. Observe the animals for 7 days. No adverse effect is produced.

Sensitisation. Use 3 guinea-pigs that have not been subjected to any treatment likely to interfere with the test. On 3 occasions at intervals of 5 days, inject intradermally into each guinea-pig about 500 IU of the preparation to be examined in a volume of 0.1 ml. 2 to 3 weeks after the third injection, administer the same dose intradermally to the same animals and to a control group of three guinea-pigs of the same mass that have not previously received injections of tuberculin. After 24 h to 72 h, the reactions in the 2 groups of animals are not substantially different.

Antimicrobial preservative. Where applicable, determine the amount of antimicrobial preservative by a suitable chemical or physico-chemical method. The content is not less than the minimum amount shown to be effective and not more than 115 per cent of the amount stated on the label. If phenol has been used in the preparation, the concentration is not more than 5 g/l (*2.5.15*).

Live mycobacteria (*2.6.2*). It complies with the test for mycobacteria.

Sterility (*2.6.1*). It complies with the test for sterility.

ASSAY

Use method A or, where the preparation contains 1 IU to 2 IU, use method B.

METHOD A

The potency of tuberculin PPD is determined by comparing the reactions produced by the intradermal injection of increasing doses of the preparation to be examined into sensitised guinea-pigs with the reactions produced by known concentrations of the reference preparation.

Prepare a suspension containing a suitable amount (0.1 mg/ml to 0.4 mg/ml) of heat-inactivated, dried mycobacteria in mineral oil with or without emulsifier; use mycobacteria of a strain of the same species as that used in the preparation to be examined. Sensitise not fewer than six pale-coloured guinea-pigs weighing not less than 300 g by injecting intramuscularly or intradermally a total of about 0.5 ml of the suspension, divided between several sites if necessary. Carry out the test after the period of time required for optimal sensitisation which is usually 4 to 8 weeks after sensitisation. Depilate the flanks of the animals so that it is possible to make at least 3 injections on each side but not more than a total of 12 injection points per animal. Prepare dilutions of the preparation to be examined and of the reference preparation using isotonic phosphate-buffered saline (pH 6.5 to 7.5) containing 50 mg/l of *polysorbate 80 R*. If the preparation to be examined is freeze-dried and does not contain a stabiliser, reconstitute it using the liquid described above. Use at least 3 different doses of the reference preparation and at least 3 different doses of the preparation to be examined. For both preparations, use doses such that the highest dose is about 10 times the lowest dose. Choose the doses such that when they are injected the lesions produced have a diameter of not less than 8 mm and not more than 25 mm. In any given test, the order of the dilutions injected at each point is chosen at random in a Latin square design. Inject each dose intradermally in a constant volume of 0.1 ml or 0.2 ml. Measure the diameters of the lesions 24 h to 48 h later and calculate the results of the test by the usual statistical methods, assuming that the diameters of the lesions are directly proportional to the logarithm of the concentration of the preparation.

The estimated potency is not less than 80 per cent and not more than 125 per cent of the stated potency. The confidence limits ($P = 0.95$) are not less than 64 per cent and not more than 156 per cent of the stated potency.

METHOD B

The potency of tuberculin PPD is determined by comparing the reactions produced by the intradermal injection of the preparation to be examined into sensitised guinea-pigs with the reactions produced by known concentrations of the reference preparation.

Prepare a suspension in mineral oil with or without emulsifier and containing a suitable amount (0.1 mg/ml to 0.4 mg/ml) of heat-inactivated, dried mycobacteria; use mycobacteria of a strain of the same species as that used in the preparation to be examined. Sensitise not fewer than 6 pale-coloured guinea-pigs weighing not less than 300 g by injecting intramuscularly or intradermally a total of about 0.5 ml of the suspension, divided between several sites if necessary. Carry out the test after the period of time required for optimal sensitisation which is usually 4 to 8 weeks after sensitisation. Depilate the flanks of the animals so that it is possible to make at least 3 injections on each side but not more than a total of 12 injection points per animal. Prepare dilutions of the reference preparation using isotonic phosphate-buffered saline (pH 6.5 to 7.5) containing 50 mg/l of *polysorbate 80 R*. Use at least 3 different doses of the reference preparation such that the highest dose is about 10 times the lowest dose and the median dose is the same as that of the preparation to be examined. In any given test, the order of the dilutions injected at each point is chosen at random in a Latin square design. Inject the preparation to be examined and each dilution of the reference preparation intradermally in a constant volume of 0.1 ml or 0.2 ml. Measure the diameters of the lesions 24 h to 48 h later and calculate the results of the test by the usual statistical methods, assuming that the areas of the lesions are directly proportional to the logarithm of the concentration of the preparation to be examined. (This dose relationship applies to this assay and not necessarily to other test systems.)

The estimated potency is not less than 80 per cent and not more than 125 per cent of the stated potency. The confidence limits ($P = 0.95$) are not less than 64 per cent and not more than 156 per cent of the stated potency.

STORAGE

Store protected from light.

LABELLING

The label states:

- the number of International Units per container,
- the species of mycobacteria used to prepare the product,
- the name and quantity of any antimicrobial preservative or other substance added to the preparation,
- the expiry date,
- for freeze-dried products, a statement that the product is to be reconstituted using the liquid provided by the manufacturer,

- where applicable, that tuberculin PPD is not to be injected in its concentrated form but diluted so as to administer not more than 100 IU per dose.

If the package does not contain a leaflet warning that the inhalation of concentrated tuberculin PPD may produce toxic effects, this warning must be shown on the label on the container together with a statement that the powder must be handled with care.

01/2005:0305

TUBOCURARINE CHLORIDE

Tubocurarini chloridum

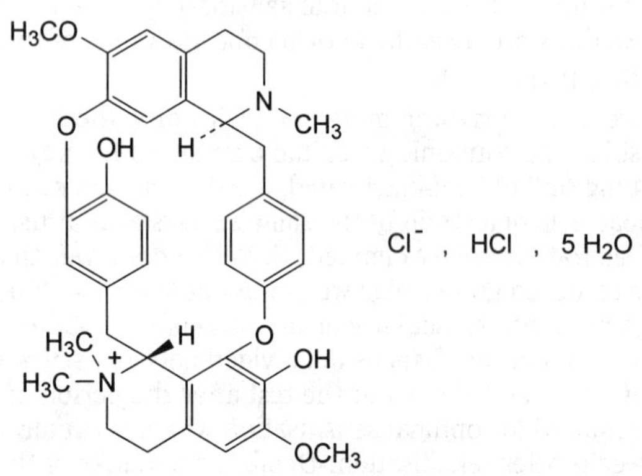

$C_{37}H_{42}Cl_2N_2O_6,5H_2O$ M_r 772

DEFINITION

Tubocurarine chloride contains not less than 98.0 per cent and not more than the equivalent of 102.0 per cent of (3a*R*,16a*S*)-8,23-dihydroxy-24,29-dimethoxy-3,3,16-trimethyl-2,3,3a,4,15,16,16a,17-octahydro-1*H*-11,13:18,21-dietheno-5,9-metheno-14*H*-pyrido[3′,2′:14,15][1,11]dioxacycloicosino[2,3,4-*ij*]isoquinolinium chloride hydrochloride, calculated with reference to the anhydrous substance.

CHARACTERS

A white or slightly yellowish, crystalline powder, soluble in water and in alcohol, practically insoluble in acetone. It dissolves in solutions of alkali hydroxides.

It melts at about 270 °C, with decomposition.

IDENTIFICATION

First identification: B, E.

Second identification: A, C, D, E, F.

A. Dissolve 50.0 mg in *water R* and dilute to 1000.0 ml with the same solvent. Examined between 230 nm and 350 nm (*2.2.25*), the solution shows an absorption maximum at 280 nm and a minimum at 255 nm. The specific absorbance at the maximum is 113 to 123, calculated with reference to the anhydrous substance.

B. Examine by infrared absorption spectrophotometry (*2.2.24*), comparing with the spectrum obtained with *tubocurarine chloride CRS.*

C. Dissolve about 25 mg in 1 ml of *water R*. Add 0.2 ml of *ferric chloride solution R2* and heat in a water-bath for 1 min. The solution is green. Carry out a blank test; after heating in a water-bath, the colour is brown.

D. To 1 ml of solution S (see Tests) add 1 ml of *nitric acid solution of mercury R*. A red colour develops slowly.

E. It gives reaction (a) of chlorides (*2.3.1*).

F. It gives the reaction of alkaloids (*2.3.1*).

TESTS

Solution S. Dissolve 0.25 g in *carbon dioxide-free water R* and dilute to 25.0 ml with the same solvent.

Appearance of solution. Solution S is clear (*2.2.1*) and not more intensely coloured than reference solution Y_6 (*2.2.2, Method II*).

pH (*2.2.3*). The pH of solution S is 4.0 to 6.0.

Specific optical rotation (*2.2.7*): + 210 to + 222, determined on solution S 3 h after preparation and calculated with reference to the anhydrous substance.

Chloroform-soluble substances. Dissolve 0.25 g in 150 ml of *water R*. Add 5 ml of a saturated solution of *sodium bicarbonate R* and shake with three quantities, each of 20 ml, of *chloroform R*. Wash the combined chloroform layers with 10 ml of *water R*, filter the chloroform solution into a tared beaker and wash the filter with two quantities, each of 5 ml, of *chloroform R*. Add the washings to the filtrate. Evaporate to dryness on a water-bath and dry at 100-105 °C for 1 h. The residue weighs not more than 5 mg. The residue does not dissolve in 10 ml of *water R*, but dissolves on the addition of 1 ml of *dilute hydrochloric acid R*.

Related substances. Examine by thin-layer chromatography (*2.2.27*), using *silica gel G R* as the coating substance.

Test solution. Dissolve 0.25 g of the substance to be examined in *water R* and dilute to 10 ml with the same solvent.

Reference solution (a). Dilute 1.5 ml of the test solution to 100 ml with *water R*.

Reference solution (b). Dilute 5 ml of reference solution (a) to 10 ml with *water R*.

Apply to the plate 5 µl of each solution. Develop in a non-saturated tank over a path of 15 cm using the lower layer of a mixture of equal volumes of *chloroform R*, *methanol R* and a 125 g/l solution of *trichloroacetic acid R*. Dry the plate in a current of cold air. Spray with a mixture of 1 volume of *potassium ferricyanide solution R*, 1 volume of *water R* and 2 volumes of *ferric chloride solution R1*, prepared immediately before use. Any spot in the chromatogram obtained with the test solution, apart from the principal spot, is not more intense than the spot in the chromatogram obtained with reference solution (a) (1.5 per cent) and at most one such spot is more intense than the spot in the chromatogram obtained with reference solution (b) (0.75 per cent).

Water (*2.5.12*): 9.0 per cent to 12.0 per cent, determined on 0.30 g by the semi-micro determination of water.

Sulphated ash (*2.4.14*). Not more than 0.25 per cent, determined on 0.2 g.

ASSAY

Dissolve 25.0 mg in *water R* and dilute to 500.0 ml with the same solvent. In the same manner, prepare a reference solution using 25.0 mg of *tubocurarine chloride CRS.* Measure the absorbance (*2.2.25*) at the maximum at 280 nm. Calculate the content of $C_{37}H_{42}Cl_2N_2O_6$ from the absorbances measured, the concentrations of the solutions and the declared content of anhydrous tubocurarine chloride in *tubocurarine chloride CRS.*

STORAGE

Store in an airtight container.

01/2005:1441

TURMERIC, JAVANESE

Curcumae xanthorrhizae rhizoma

DEFINITION

Javanese turmeric consists of the dried rhizome, cut in slices, of *Curcuma xanthorrhiza* Roxb. (*C. xanthorrhiza* D. Dietrich). It contains not less than 50 ml/kg of essential oil and not less than 1.0 per cent of dicinnamoyl methane derivatives expressed as curcumin ($C_{21}H_{20}O_6$; M_r 368.4), both calculated with reference to the anhydrous drug.

CHARACTERS

Javanese turmeric has an aromatic odour.

It has the macroscopic and microscopic characters described under identification tests A and B.

IDENTIFICATION

A. The drug consists of orange-yellow to yellowish-brown or greyish-brown slices, mostly peeled 1.5 mm to 6 mm thick and 15 mm to 50 mm, more rarely up to 70 mm, in diameter. Fragments of the brownish-grey cork are sporadically present. The transverse surface is yellow with dark spots in the paler centre. The fracture is short and finely grained.

B. Reduce to a powder (355). The powder is reddish-brown. Examine under a microscope, using *chloral hydrate solution R*. The powder shows fragments of colourless parenchyma with orange-yellow to yellowish-brown secretory cells; fragments of reticulate and other vessels; rare fragments of cork and epidermis and fragments of thick-walled unicellular acute trichomes. Examine under a microscope using a 50 per cent *V/V* solution of *glycerol R*. The powder shows numerous stratified, ovoid to irregular starch granules, about 30 µm to 50 µm long and about 10 µm to 30 µm wide, with an eccentric hilum and marked, concentric striations.

C. Examine by thin-layer chromatography as described in the test for *Curcuma domestica* until the words "Allow the plate to dry in the air". Spray the plate with a freshly prepared 0.4 g/l solution of *dichloroquinonechlorimide R* in *2-propanol R*. Expose the plate to ammonia vapour until the thymol zone becomes bluish-violet. The chromatogram obtained with the reference solution shows almost in the middle a bluish-violet zone (thymol) and in the lower part a yellow zone (fluorescein). The chromatogram obtained with the test solution shows a blue zone (xanthorrhizol) slightly above the zone due to thymol in the chromatogram obtained with the reference solution and two yellowish-brown to brown zones (curcumin and demethoxycurcumin) between the zones due to thymol and fluorescein in the chromatogram obtained with the reference solution.

TESTS

Foreign matter (*2.8.2*). It complies with the test for foreign matter.

Curcuma domestica. Examine by thin-layer chromatography (*2.2.27*), using a *TLC silica gel plate R*.

Test solution. Shake 0.5 g of the freshly powdered drug (500) with 5 ml of *methanol R* for 30 min and filter.

Reference solution. Dissolve 5 mg of *fluorescein R* and 10 mg of *thymol R* in 10 ml of *methanol R*.

Apply separately to the plate as bands 10 µl of each solution. Develop over a path of 10 cm using a mixture of 20 volumes of *glacial acetic acid R* and 80 volumes of *toluene R*. Allow the plate to dry in air. Spray the plate with a mixture of 1 volume of *sulphuric acid R* and9 volumes of *acetic anhydride R*. Examine the plate in ultraviolet light at 365 nm. In the chromatogram obtained with the test solution, no yellowish-red fluorescent zone (bisdemethoxycurcumin) appears slightly above the greenish-blue fluorescent zone of fluorescein in the chromatogram obtained with the reference solution.

Water (*2.2.13*). Not more than 120 ml/kg, determined by distillation on 20.0 g of powdered drug (500).

Total ash (*2.4.16*). Not more than 8.0 per cent.

ASSAY

Essential oil. Carry out the determination of essential oils in vegetable drugs (*2.8.12*). Use a 500 ml round-bottomed flask, 200 ml of *water R* as the distillation liquid and 0.5 ml of *xylene R* in the graduated tube. Reduce the drug to a powder (500) and immediately use 5.0 g for the determination. Distil at a rate of 3 ml/min to 4 ml/min for 3 h.

Dicinnamoyl methane derivatives. To 0.100 g of the powdered drug (180) add 60 ml of *glacial acetic acid R* and heat in a water-bath at 90 °C for 60 min. Add 2.0 g of *boric acid R* and 2.0 g of *oxalic acid R* and heat in a water-bath at 90 °C for 10 min. Allow to cool, dilute with *glacial acetic acid R* to 100.0 ml and shake. Dilute 5.0 ml of the clear supernatant with *glacial acetic acid R* to 50.0 ml. Measure the absorbance (*2.2.25*) at 530 nm, using *glacial acetic acid R* as the compensation liquid.

Calculate the percentage content of dicinnamoyl methane derivatives, expressed as curcumin, from the expression:

$$\frac{A \times 0.426}{m}$$

i.e. taking the specific absorbance to be 2350.

A = absorbance at 530 nm,

m = mass of the drug to be examined, in grams.

STORAGE

Store protected from light.

01/2005:1627

TURPENTINE OIL, PINUS PINASTER TYPE

Terebinthini aetheroleum ab pinum pinastrum

DEFINITION

Essential oil obtained by steam distillation, followed by rectification at a temperature below 180 °C, from the oleoresin obtained by tapping *Pinus pinaster* Aiton. A suitable antioxidant may be added.

CHARACTERS

Appearance: clear, colourless or pale yellow liquid.

It has a characteristic odour.

IDENTIFICATION

First identification: B.

Second identification: A.

A. Thin-layer chromatography (*2.2.27*).

Test solution. Mix 1 ml of the substance to be examined with *toluene R* and dilute to 10 ml with the same solvent.

Reference solution. Mix 10 µl of *β-pinene R* and 10 µl of *linalol R* with *toluene R* and dilute to 10 ml with the same solvent.

Plate: *TLC silica gel plate R.*

Mobile phase: *ethyl acetate R, toluene R* (5:95 *V/V*).

Application: 10 µl, as bands.

Development: over a path of 15 cm.

Drying: in air.

Detection: spray with *anisaldehyde solution R* and heat at 100-105 °C for 5-10 min. Examine in daylight.

Results: see below the sequence of the zones present in the chromatograms obtained with the reference solution and the test solution.

Top of the plate	
β-Pinene: a pink zone	A pink zone (β-pinene)
	A pink zone
Linalol: a pinkish-grey zone	
	3 Faint violet zones
	A faint yellow zone
Reference solution	**Test solution**

B. Examine the chromatograms obtained in the test for chromatographic profile.

Results: the peaks in the chromatogram obtained with the test solution are similar in retention time to those in the chromatogram obtained with the reference solution.

TESTS

Relative density (*2.2.5*): 0.856 to 0.872.

Refractive index (*2.2.6*): 1.465 to 1.475.

Optical rotation (*2.2.7*): −40° to −28°.

Acid value (*2.5.1*): maximum 1.0.

Peroxide value (*2.5.5, Method B*): maximum 20.

Fatty oils and resinified essential oils (*2.8.7*). It complies with the test for fatty oils and resinified essential oils.

Chromatographic profile. Gas chromatography (*2.2.28*): use the normalisation procedure.

Test solution. The substance to be examined.

Reference solution (a). Dissolve 30 µl of *α-pinene R*, 10 mg of *camphene R*, 20 µl of *β-pinene R*, 10 µl of *car-3-ene R*, 10 µl of *β-myrcene R*, 20 µl of *limonene R*, 10 µl of *longifolene R*, 10 µl of *β-caryophyllene R* and 10 mg of *caryophyllene oxide R* in 1 ml of *hexane R*.

Reference solution (b). Dissolve 5 µl of *β-caryophyllene R* in *hexane R* and dilute to 1 ml with the same solvent. Dilute 0.1 ml to 1 ml with *hexane R*.

Column:

– *material*: fused silica,

– *size*: *l* = 60 m, Ø = 0.25 mm,

– *stationary phase*: *macrogol 20 000 R* (film thickness 0.25 µm).

Carrier gas: *helium for chromatography R*.

Flow rate: 1.0 ml/min.

Split ratio: 1:63.

Temperature:

	Time (min)	Temperature (°C)
Column	0 - 10	60
	10 - 80	60 → 200
	80 - 120	200
Injection port		200
Detector		250

Detection: flame ionisation.

Injection: 0.5 µl.

Elution order: order indicated in the composition of the reference solution (a); record the retention times of these substances.

System suitability:

– *resolution*: minimum 1.5 between the peaks due to car-3-ene and β-myrcene in the chromatogram obtained with reference solution (a).

Using the retention times determined from the chromatogram obtained with reference solution (a), locate the components of reference solution (a) in the chromatogram obtained with the test solution.

Determine the percentage content of these components. The limits are within the following ranges:

– *α-pinene*: 70.0 per cent to 85.0 per cent,

– *camphene*: 0.5 per cent to 1.5 per cent,

– *β-pinene*: 11.0 per cent to 20.0 per cent,

– *car-3-ene*: maximum 1.0 per cent,

– *β-myrcene*: 0.4 per cent to 1.5 per cent,

– *limonene*: 1.0 per cent to 7.0 per cent,

– *longifolene*: 0.2 per cent to 2.5 per cent,

– *β-caryophyllene*: 0.1 per cent to 3.0 per cent,

– *caryophyllene oxide*: maximum 1.0 per cent.

– *disregard limit*: area of the peak in the chromatogram obtained with reference solution (b) (0.05 per cent).

Residue on evaporation: maximum 2.5 per cent.

STORAGE

In a well-filled, airtight container, protected from light and at a temperature not exceeding 25 °C.

LABELLING

The label states the name and concentration of any added antioxidant.

01/2005:1273

TYLOSIN FOR VETERINARY USE

Tylosinum ad usum veterinarium

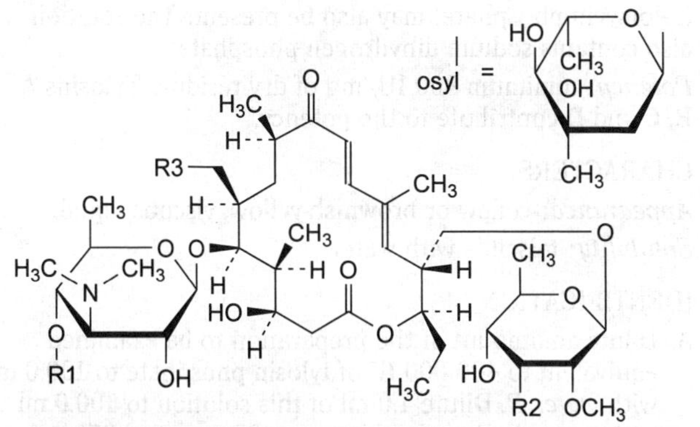

Name	Mol. Formula	R1	R2	R3
tylosin A	$C_{46}H_{77}NO_{17}$	osyl	OCH_3	CHO
tylosin B	$C_{39}H_{65}NO_{14}$	H	OCH_3	CHO
tylosin C	$C_{45}H_{75}NO_{17}$	osyl	OH	CHO
tylosin D	$C_{46}H_{79}NO_{17}$	osyl	OCH_3	CH_2OH

DEFINITION

Tylosin for veterinary use is a mixture of macrolide antibiotics produced by a strain of *Streptomyces fradiae* or by any other means. The main component of the mixture is (4*R*,5*S*,6*S*,7*R*,9*R*,11*E*,13*E*,15*R*,16*R*)-15-[[(6-deoxy-2,3-di-*O*-methyl-β-D-allopyranosyl)oxy]methyl]-6-[[3,6-dideoxy-4-*O*-(2,6-dideoxy-3-*C*-methyl-α-L-*ribo*-hexopyranosyl)-3-(dimethylamino)-β-D-glucopyranosyl]oxy]-16-ethyl-4-hydroxy-5,9,13-trimethyl-7-(2-oxoethyl)oxacyclohexadeca-11,13-diene-2,10-dione (tylosin A, M_r 916). Tylosin B (desmycosin, M_r 772), tylosin C (macrocin, M_r 902) and tylosin D (relomycin, M_r 918) may also be present. They contribute to the potency of the substance to be examined, which is not less than 900 IU/mg, calculated with reference to the dried substance.

CHARACTERS

An almost white or slightly yellow powder, slightly soluble in water, freely soluble in ethanol and in methylene chloride. It dissolves in dilute solutions of mineral acids.

IDENTIFICATION

A. Examine by infrared absorption spectrophotometry (*2.2.24*), comparing with the spectrum obtained with *tylosin CRS*.

B. Examine the chromatograms obtained in the test for composition. The retention time and size of the principal peak in the chromatogram obtained with the test solution are the same as those of the principal peak in the chromatogram obtained with reference solution (a).

C. Dissolve about 30 mg in a mixture of 0.15 ml of *water R*, 2.5 ml of *acetic anhydride R* and 7.5 ml of *pyridine R*. Allow to stand for about 10 min. No green colour develops.

TESTS

pH (*2.2.3*). Suspend 0.25 g in 10 ml of *carbon dioxide-free water R*. The pH of the suspension is 8.5 to 10.5.

Composition. Examine by liquid chromatography (*2.2.29*). *Prepare the solutions immediately before use.*

The content of tylosin A is not less than 80.0 per cent and the sum of the contents of tylosin A, tylosin B, tylosin C and tylosin D is not less than 95.0 per cent.

Test solution. Dissolve 20.0 mg of the substance to be examined in a mixture of equal volumes of *acetonitrile R* and *water R* and dilute to 100.0 ml with the same mixture of solvents.

Reference solution (a). Dissolve 20.0 mg of *tylosin CRS* in a mixture of equal volumes of *acetonitrile R* and *water R* and dilute to 100.0 ml with the same mixture of solvents.

Reference solution (b). Dissolve 2 mg of *tylosin CRS* and 2 mg of *tylosin D CRS* in a mixture of equal volumes of *acetonitrile R* and *water R* and dilute to 10 ml with the same mixture of solvents.

The chromatographic procedure may be carried out using:

– a stainless steel column 0.20 m long and 4.6 mm in internal diameter packed with *octadecylsilyl silica gel for chromatography R* (5 µm),

– as mobile phase at a flow rate of 1.0 ml/min a mixture of 40 volumes of *acetonitrile R* and 60 volumes of a 200 g/l solution of *sodium perchlorate R* previously adjusted to pH 2.5 using *1 M hydrochloric acid*,

– as detector a spectrophotometer set at 290 nm,

maintaining the temperature of the column at 35 °C.

Inject 20 µl of reference solution (b). When the chromatograms are recorded in the prescribed conditions, the retention time of tylosin A is about 12 min. The test is not valid unless, in the chromatogram obtained, the resolution between the peaks corresponding to tylosin A and tylosin D is at least 2.0. Inject 20 µl of the test solution and 20 µl of reference solution (a). Calculate the percentage content of the constituents from the areas of the peaks in the chromatogram obtained with the test solution by the normalisation procedure.

Tyramine. In a 25.0 ml volumetric flask, dissolve 50.0 mg of the substance to be examined in 5.0 ml of a 3.4 g/l solution of *phosphoric acid R*. Add 1.0 ml of *pyridine R* and 2.0 ml of a saturated solution of *ninhydrin R* (about 40 g/l). Close the flask with a piece of aluminium foil and heat in a water-bath at 85 °C for 30 min. Cool the solution rapidly and dilute to 25.0 ml with *water R*. Mix and measure immediately the absorbance (*2.2.25*) of the solution at 570 nm using a blank solution as the compensation liquid. The absorbance is not greater than that of a standard prepared at the same time and in the same manner using 5.0 ml of a 35 mg/l solution of *tyramine R* in a 3.4 g/l solution of *phosphoric acid R* (0.35 per cent). If intended for use in the manufacture of parenteral dosage forms, the absorbance is not greater than that of a standard prepared at the same time and in the same manner using 5.0 ml of a 15 mg/l solution of *tyramine R* in a 3.4 g/l solution of *phosphoric acid R* (0.15 per cent).

Loss on drying (*2.2.32*). Not more than 5.0 per cent, determined on 1.000 g by drying in an oven at 60 °C at a pressure not exceeding 0.7 kPa for 3 h.

Sulphated ash (*2.4.14*). Not more than 3.0 per cent, determined on 1.0 g.

ASSAY

Carry out the microbiological assay of antibiotics (*2.7.2*). Use *tylosin CRS* as the reference substance.

STORAGE

Store protected from light.

IMPURITIES

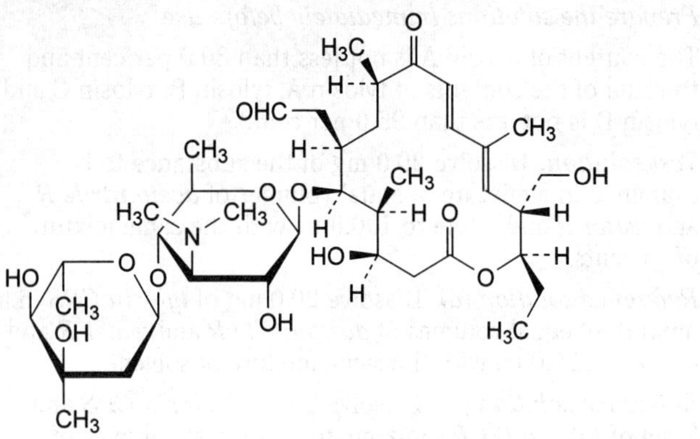

A. desmycinosyltylosin,

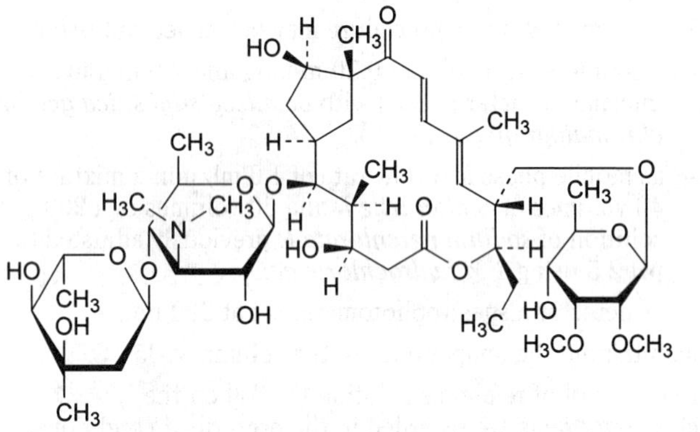

B. tylosin A aldol.

01/2005:1661

TYLOSIN PHOSPHATE BULK SOLUTION FOR VETERINARY USE

Tylosini phosphatis solutio ad usum veterinarium

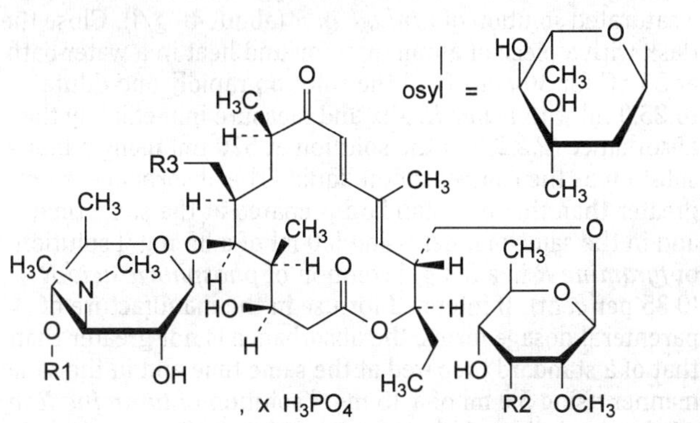

Tylosin	R1	R2	R3	Mol. Formula	M_r
A	osyl	OCH_3	CHO	$C_{46}H_{77}NO_{17}$	916
B	H	OCH_3	CHO	$C_{39}H_{65}NO_{14}$	772
C	osyl	OH	CHO	$C_{45}H_{75}NO_{17}$	902
D	osyl	OCH_3	CH_2OH	$C_{46}H_{79}NO_{17}$	918

DEFINITION

Solution of the dihydrogen phosphate of a mixture of macrolide antibiotics produced by a strain of *Streptomyces fradiae* or by any other means.

The main component is the phosphate of (4*R*,5*S*,6*S*,7*R*,9*R*,11*E*,13*E*,15*R*,16*R*)-15-[[(6-deoxy-2,3-di-*O*-methyl-β-D-allopyranosyl)oxy]methyl]-6-[[3,6-dideoxy-4-*O*-(2,6-dideoxy-3-*C*-methyl-α-L-*ribo*-hexopyranosyl)-3-(dimethylamino)-β-D-glucopyranosyl]oxy]-16-ethyl-4-hydroxy-5,9,13-trimethyl-7-(2-oxoethyl)oxacyclohexadeca-11,13-diene-2,10-dione (tylosin A phosphate). The phosphates of tylosin B (desmycosin phosphate), tylosin C (macrocin phosphate) and tylosin D (relomycin phosphate) may also be present. The solution also contains sodium dihydrogen phosphate.

Potency: minimum 800 IU/mg of dry residue. Tylosins A, B, C and D contribute to the potency.

CHARACTERS

Appearance: yellow or brownish-yellow, viscous liquid.

Solubility: miscible with water.

IDENTIFICATION

A. Dilute an amount of the preparation to be examined equivalent to 400 000 IU of tylosin phosphate to 100.0 ml with *water R*. Dilute 1.0 ml of this solution to 100.0 ml with *water R*. Examined between 230 nm and 350 nm (*2.2.25*), the solution shows an absorption maximum at 290 nm. The absorbance at the maximum is not less than 0.70.

B. Examine the chromatograms obtained in the test for composition.

Results: the principal peak in the chromatogram obtained with the test solution is similar in retention time and size to the principal peak in the chromatogram obtained with reference solution (a).

C. Dilute an amount of the preparation to be examined equivalent to 400 000 IU of tylosin phosphate in 10 ml of *water R*. The solution gives reaction (a) of phosphates (*2.3.1*).

TESTS

pH (*2.2.3*): 5.5 to 6.5.

Dilute 1.0 g in 10 ml of *carbon dioxide-free water R*.

Composition. Liquid chromatography (*2.2.29*): use the normalisation procedure.

Prepare the solutions immediately before use.

Test solution. Dilute an amount of the preparation to be examined equivalent to 50 000 IU of tylosin phosphate to 200 ml with a mixture of equal volumes of *acetonitrile R* and *water R*.

Reference solution (a). Dissolve 20 mg of *tylosin CRS* in a mixture of equal volumes of *acetonitrile R* and *water R* and dilute to 100 ml with the same mixture of solvents.

Reference solution (b). Dissolve 2 mg of *tylosin CRS* and 2 mg of *tylosin D CRS* in a mixture of equal volumes of *acetonitrile R* and *water R* and dilute to 10 ml with the same mixture of solvents.

Reference solution (c). Dilute 1.0 ml of reference solution (a) to 100.0 ml with a mixture of equal volumes of *acetonitrile R* and *water R*. Dilute 1.0 ml of this solution to 10.0 ml with the same mixture of solvents.

Column:

- *size*: *l* = 0.20 m, Ø = 4.6 mm;
- *stationary phase*: *octadecylsilyl silica gel for chromatography R* (5 µm);
- *temperature*: 35 °C.

Mobile phase: mix 40 volumes of *acetonitrile R* and 60 volumes of a 200 g/l solution of *sodium perchlorate R* previously adjusted to pH 2.5 using a 36.5 g/l solution of *hydrochloric acid R*.

Flow rate: 1.0 ml/min.

Detection: spectrophotometer at 290 nm.

Injection: 20 μl.

Run time: 1.8 times the retention time of tylosin A.

Relative retention with reference to tylosin A (retention time = about 12 min): impurity A = about 0.35; tylosin C = about 0.5; tylosin B = about 0.6; tylosin D = about 0.85; impurity B = about 0.9 (use the chromatogram supplied with *tylosin CRS* to identify the peaks due to tylosin B and tylosin C).

System suitability: reference solution (b):

– *resolution*: minimum 2.0 between the peaks due to tylosin D and tylosin A.

Limits:

– *tylosin A*: minimum 80.0 per cent;
– *sum of the contents of tylosin A, tylosin B, tylosin C and tylosin D*: minimum 95.0 per cent;
– *disregard limit*: area of the principal peak in the chromatogram obtained with reference solution (c).

Tyramine. In a 25.0 ml volumetric flask, dissolve an amount of the preparation to be examined equivalent to 50 000 IU of tylosin phosphate in 5.0 ml of a 3.4 g/l solution of *phosphoric acid R*. Add 1.0 ml of *pyridine R* and 2.0 ml of a saturated solution of *ninhydrin R* (about 40 g/l). Close the flask with aluminium foil and heat in a water-bath at 85 °C for 20-30 min. Cool the solution rapidly and dilute to 25.0 ml with *water R*. Mix and measure immediately the absorbance (*2.2.25*) of the solution at 570 nm using a blank solution as the compensation liquid.

The absorbance is not greater than that of a standard prepared at the same time and in the same manner using 5.0 ml of a 35 mg/l solution of *tyramine R* in a 3.4 g/l solution of *phosphoric acid R*.

Phosphate: 8.5 per cent to 10.0 per cent of PO_4, calculated with reference to the dry residue (see Assay).

Test solution. Dissolve an amount of the preparation to be examined equivalent to 200 000 IU of tylosin phosphate in 50 ml of *water R*. Add 5.0 ml of *dilute sulphuric acid R* and dilute to 100.0 ml with *water R*. To 2.0 ml of this solution add successively, mixing after each addition, 10.0 ml of *water R*, 5.0 ml of *ammonium molybdate reagent R2*, 1.0 ml of *hydroquinone solution R* and 1.0 ml of a 200 g/l solution of *sodium metabisulphite R*. Allow to stand for at least 20 min and dilute to 50.0 ml with *water R*. Mix thoroughly.

Reference solution (a). To 1.0 ml of a standard solution containing 0.430 g/l of *potassium dihydrogen phosphate R* (corresponds to 300 ppm of PO_4) add successively, mixing after each addition, 10.0 ml of *water R*, 5.0 ml of *ammonium molybdate reagent R2*, 1.0 ml of *hydroquinone solution R* and 1.0 ml of a 200 g/l solution of *sodium metabisulphite R*. Allow to stand for at least 20 min and dilute to 50.0 ml with *water R*. Mix thoroughly.

Reference solution (b). Prepare as reference solution (a) but using 2.0 ml of the standard solution.

Reference solution (c). Prepare as reference solution (a) but using 5.0 ml of the standard solution.

Compensation liquid. Prepare as reference solution (a) but omitting the standard solution.

Measure the absorbance (*2.2.25*) of the test solution and of the reference solutions at 650 nm.

Draw a calibration curve with the absorbances of the 3 reference solutions as a function of the quantity of phosphate in the solutions and read from the curve the quantity of phosphate in the test solution.

Determine the percentage content of PO_4, calculated with reference to the dry residue (see Assay).

ASSAY

Carry out the microbiological assay of antibiotics (*2.7.2*).

Use *tylosin CRS* as the reference substance. Calculate the potency from the mass of the dry residue and the activity of the solution.

Dry residue. Dry 3.0 g of the preparation to be examined *in vacuo* at 60 °C for 3 h and weigh.

STORAGE

Protected from light, at a temperature of 2 °C to 8 °C.

LABELLING

The label states:

– the concentration of the solution in International Units per milligram of preparation.

IMPURITIES

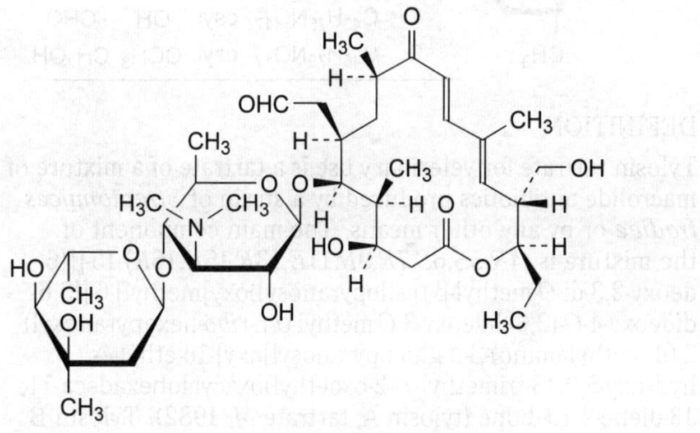

A. desmycinosyltylosin A,

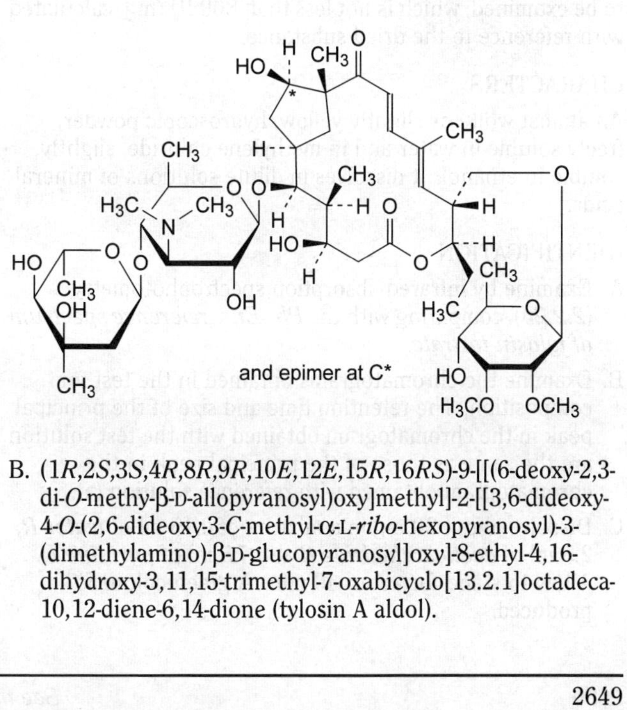

B. (1*R*,2*S*,3*S*,4*R*,8*R*,9*R*,10*E*,12*E*,15*R*,16*RS*)-9-[[(6-deoxy-2,3-di-*O*-methy-β-D-allopyranosyl)oxy]methyl]-2-[[3,6-dideoxy-4-*O*-(2,6-dideoxy-3-*C*-methyl-α-L-*ribo*-hexopyranosyl)-3-(dimethylamino)-β-D-glucopyranosyl]oxy]-8-ethyl-4,16-dihydroxy-3,11,15-trimethyl-7-oxabicyclo[13.2.1]octadeca-10,12-diene-6,14-dione (tylosin A aldol).

01/2005:1274

TYLOSIN TARTRATE FOR VETERINARY USE

Tylosini tartras ad usum veterinarium

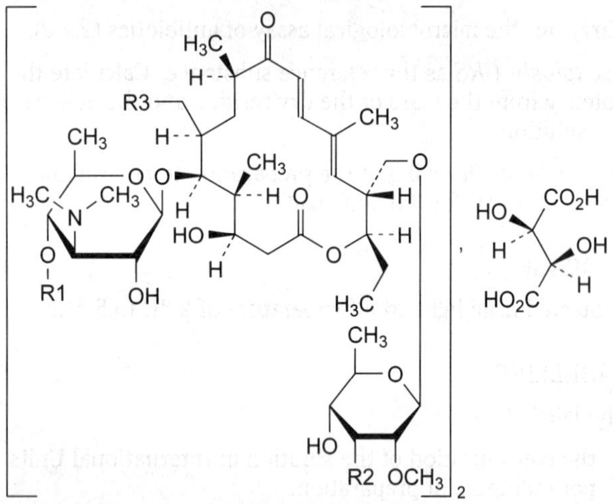

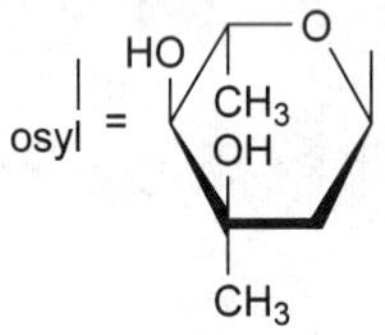

Tylosin	Mol. Form.	R1	R2	R3
A	$C_{46}H_{77}NO_{17}$	osyl	OCH_3	CHO
B	$C_{39}H_{65}NO_{14}$	H	OCH_3	CHO
C	$C_{45}H_{75}NO_{17}$	osyl	OH	CHO
D	$C_{46}H_{79}NO_{17}$	osyl	OCH_3	CH_2OH

DEFINITION

Tylosin tartrate for veterinary use is a tartrate of a mixture of macrolide antibiotics produced by a strain of *Streptomyces fradiae* or by any other means. The main component of the mixture is (4*R*,5*S*,6*S*,7*R*,9*R*,11*E*,13*E*,15*R*,16*R*)-15-[[(6-deoxy-2,3-di-*O*-methyl-β-D-allopyranosyl)oxy]methyl]-6-[[3,6-dideoxy-4-*O*-(2,6-dideoxy-3-*C*-methyl-α-L-*ribo*-hexopyranosyl)-3-(dimethylamino)-β-D-glucopyranosyl]oxy]-16-ethyl-4-hydroxy-5,9,13-trimethyl-7-(2-oxoethyl)oxacyclohexadeca-11,13-diene-2,10-dione (tylosin A, tartrate M_r 1982). Tylosin B (desmycosin, tartrate M_r 1694), tylosin C (macrocin, tartrate M_r 1954) and tylosin D (relomycin, tartrate M_r 1986) may also be present. They contribute to the potency of the substance to be examined, which is not less than 800 IU/mg, calculated with reference to the dried substance.

CHARACTERS

An almost white or slightly yellow, hygroscopic powder, freely soluble in water and in methylene chloride, slightly soluble in ethanol. It dissolves in dilute solutions of mineral acids.

IDENTIFICATION

A. Examine by infrared absorption spectrophotometry (*2.2.24*), comparing with the *Ph. Eur. reference spectrum of tylosin tartrate.*

B. Examine the chromatograms obtained in the test for composition. The retention time and size of the principal peak in the chromatogram obtained with the test solution are the same as those of the principal peak in the chromatogram obtained with reference solution (a).

C. Dissolve about 30 mg in a mixture of 0.15 ml of *water R*, 2.5 ml of *acetic anhydride R* and 7.5 ml of *pyridine R*. Allow to stand for about 10 min. A green colour is produced.

TESTS

pH (*2.2.3*). Dissolve 0.25 g in 10 ml of *carbon dioxide-free water R*. The pH of the solution is 5.0 to 7.2.

Composition. Examine by liquid chromatography (*2.2.29*). *Prepare the solutions immediately before use.*

The content of tylosin A is not less than 80.0 per cent and the sum of the contents of tylosin A, tylosin B, tylosin C and tylosin D is not less than 95.0 per cent.

Test solution. Dissolve 20.0 mg of the substance to be examined in a mixture of equal volumes of *acetonitrile R* and *water R* and dilute to 100.0 ml with the same mixture of solvents.

Reference solution (a). Dissolve 20.0 mg of *tylosin CRS* in a mixture of equal volumes of *acetonitrile R* and *water R* and dilute to 100.0 ml with the same mixture of solvents.

Reference solution (b). Dissolve 2 mg of *tylosin CRS* and 2 mg of *tylosin D CRS* in a mixture of equal volumes of *acetonitrile R* and *water R* and dilute to 10 ml with the same mixture of solvents.

The chromatographic procedure may be carried out using:

– a stainless steel column 0.20 m long and 4.6 mm in internal diameter packed with *octadecylsilyl silica gel for chromatography R* (5 μm),

– as mobile phase at a flow rate of 1.0 ml/min a mixture of 40 volumes of *acetonitrile R* and 60 volumes of a 200 g/l solution of *sodium perchlorate R* previously adjusted to pH 2.5 using *1 M hydrochloric acid,*

– as detector a spectrophotometer set at 290 nm,

maintaining the temperature of the column at 35 °C.

Inject 20 μl of reference solution (b). When the chromatograms are recorded in the prescribed conditions, the retention time of tylosin A is about 12 min. The test is not valid unless, in the chromatogram obtained, the resolution between the peaks corresponding to tylosin A and tylosin D is at least 2.0. Inject 20 μl of the test solution and 20 μl of reference solution (a). Calculate the percentage content of the constituents from the areas of the peaks in the chromatogram obtained with the test solution by the normalisation procedure.

Tyramine. In a 25.0 ml volumetric flask, dissolve 50.0 mg of the substance to be examined in 5.0 ml of a 3.4 g/l solution of *phosphoric acid R*. Add 1.0 ml of *pyridine R* and 2.0 ml of a saturated solution of *ninhydrin R* (about 40 g/l). Close the flask with a piece of aluminium foil and heat in a water-bath at 85 °C for 30 min. Cool the solution rapidly and dilute to 25.0 ml with *water R*. Mix and measure immediately the absorbance (*2.2.25*) of the solution at 570 nm using a blank solution as the compensation liquid. The absorbance is not greater than that of a standard prepared at the same time and in the same manner using 5.0 ml of a 35 mg/l solution of *tyramine R* in a 3.4 g/l solution of *phosphoric acid R* (0.35 per cent). If intended for use in the manufacture of parenteral dosage forms, the absorbance is not greater than that of a standard prepared at the same time and in the same manner using 5.0 ml of a 15 mg/l solution of *tyramine R* in a3.4 g/l solution of *phosphoric acid R* (0.15 per cent).

Loss on drying (*2.2.32*). Not more than 4.5 per cent, determined on 1.000 g by drying at 60 °C at a pressure not exceeding 0.7 kPa for 3 h.

Sulphated ash (*2.4.14*). Not more than 2.5 per cent, determined on 1.0 g.

ASSAY

Carry out the microbiological assay of antibiotics (*2.7.2*). Use *tylosin CRS* as the reference substance.

STORAGE

Store in an airtight container, protected from light.

IMPURITIES

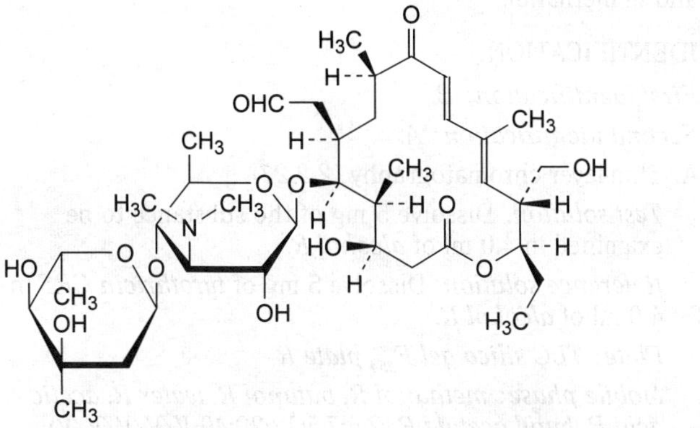

A. desmycinosyltylosin,

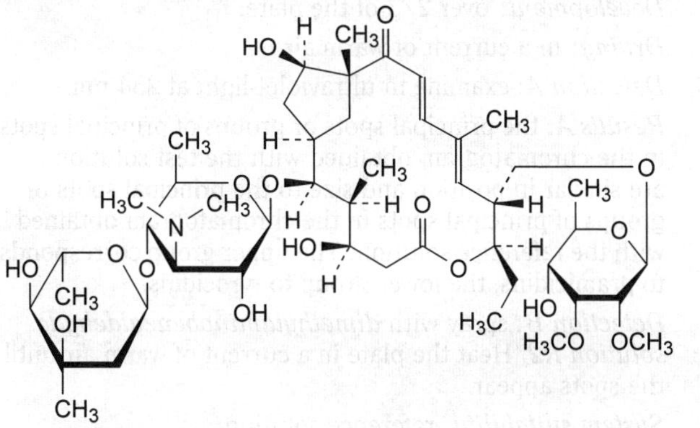

B. tylosin A aldol.

01/2005:1161

TYROSINE

Tyrosinum

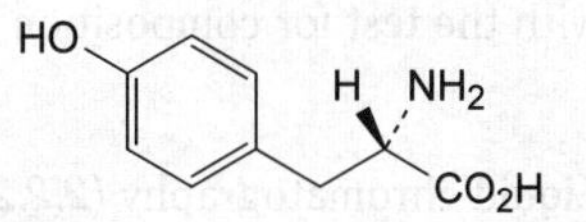

$C_9H_{11}NO_3$ M_r 181.2

DEFINITION

Tyrosine contains not less than 99.0 per cent and not more than the equivalent of 101.0 per cent of (*S*)-2-amino-3-(4-hydroxyphenyl)propanoic acid, calculated with reference to the dried substance.

CHARACTERS

A white crystalline powder or colourless crystals, very slightly soluble in water, practically insoluble in alcohol. It dissolves in dilute mineral acids and in dilute solutions of alkali hydroxides.

IDENTIFICATION

First identification: A, B.

Second identification: A, C, D, E.

A. It complies with the test for specific optical rotation (see Tests).

B. Examine by infrared absorption spectrophotometry (*2.2.24*), comparing with the spectrum obtained with *tyrosine CRS*. Examine the substances prepared as discs.

C. Examine the chromatograms obtained in the test for ninhydrin-positive substances. The principal spot in the chromatogram obtained with test solution (b) is similar in position, colour and size to the principal spot in the chromatogram obtained with reference solution (a).

D. To about 50 mg add 1 ml of *dilute nitric acid R*. A dark red colour is produced within 15 min.

E. Dissolve about 30 mg in 2 ml of *dilute sodium hydroxide solution R*. Add 3 ml of a freshly prepared mixture of equal volumes of a 100 g/l solution of *sodium nitrite R* and a solution of 0.5 g of *sulphanilic acid R* in a mixture of 6 ml of *hydrochloric acid R1* and 94 ml of *water R*. An orange-red colour is produced.

TESTS

Appearance of solution. Dissolve 0.5 g in *dilute hydrochloric acid R* and dilute to 20 ml with the same acid. The solution is clear (*2.2.1*) and not more intensely coloured than reference solution Y_7 (*2.2.2, Method II*).

Specific optical rotation (*2.2.7*). Dissolve 1.25 g in a mixture of equal volumes of *dilute hydrochloric acid R* and *water R* and dilute to 25.0 ml with the same mixture of solvents. The specific optical rotation is − 11.0 to − 12.3, calculated with reference to the dried substance.

Ninhydrin-positive substances. Examine by thin-layer chromatography (*2.2.27*), using a *TLC silica gel plate R*.

Test solution (a). Dissolve 0.10 g of the substance to be examined in *dilute ammonia R2* and dilute to 10 ml with the same solvent.

Test solution (b). Dilute 1 ml of test solution (a) to 50 ml with *water R*.

Reference solution (a). Dissolve 10 mg of *tyrosine CRS* in 1 ml of *dilute ammonia R2* and dilute to 50 ml with *water R*.

Reference solution (b). Dilute 5 ml of test solution (b) to 20 ml with *water R*.

Reference solution (c). Dissolve 10 mg of *tyrosine CRS* and 10 mg of *phenylalanine CRS* in 1 ml of *dilute ammonia R2* and dilute to 25 ml with *water R*.

Apply to the plate 5 µl of each solution. Develop over a path of 15 cm using a mixture of 30 volumes of *concentrated ammonia R1* and 70 volumes of *propanol R*. Allow the plate to dry in air, spray with *ninhydrin solution R* and heat at 100 °C to 105 °C for 15 min. Any spot in the chromatogram obtained with test solution (a), apart from the principal spot, is not more intense than the spot in the chromatogram obtained with reference solution (b) (0.5 per cent). The test is not valid unless the chromatogram obtained with reference solution (c) shows two clearly separated spots.

Chlorides (*2.4.4*). Dissolve 0.25 g in 3 ml of *dilute nitric acid R* and dilute to 15 ml with *water R*. The solution complies with the limit test for chlorides, without any further addition of nitric acid (200 ppm).

Sulphates (*2.4.13*). Dissolve with gentle heating, 0.5 g in 5 ml of *dilute hydrochloric acid R* and dilute to 15 ml with *distilled water R*. The solution complies with the limit test for sulphates (300 ppm).

Ammonium (*2.4.1*). 0.10 g complies with limit test B for ammonium (200 ppm). Prepare the standard using 0.2 ml of *ammonium standard solution (100 ppm* NH_4*) R*. Replace the *heavy magnesium oxide R* by 2.0 ml of *strong sodium hydroxide solution R*.

Iron (*2.4.9*). In a separating funnel, dissolve 1.0 g in 10 ml of *dilute hydrochloric acid R*. Shake with three quantities, each of 10 ml, of *methyl isobutyl ketone R1*, shaking for

3 min each time. To the combined organic layers add 10 ml of *water R* and shake for 3 min. The aqueous layer complies with the limit test for iron (10 ppm).

Heavy metals (*2.4.8*). 2.0 g complies with limit test C for heavy metals (10 ppm). Prepare the standard using 2 ml of *lead standard solution (10 ppm Pb) R*.

Loss on drying (*2.2.32*). Not more than 0.5 per cent, determined on 1.000 g by drying in an oven at 100 °C to 105 °C.

Sulphated ash (*2.4.14*). Not more than 0.1 per cent, determined on 1.0 g.

ASSAY

Dissolve 0.150 g in 5 ml of *anhydrous formic acid R*. Add 30 ml of *anhydrous acetic acid R*. Titrate with *0.1 M perchloric acid*, determining the end-point potentiometrically (*2.2.20*).

1 ml of *0.1 M perchloric acid* is equivalent to 18.12 mg of $C_9H_{11}NO_3$.

STORAGE

Store protected from light.

01/2005:1662

TYROTHRICIN

Tyrothricinum

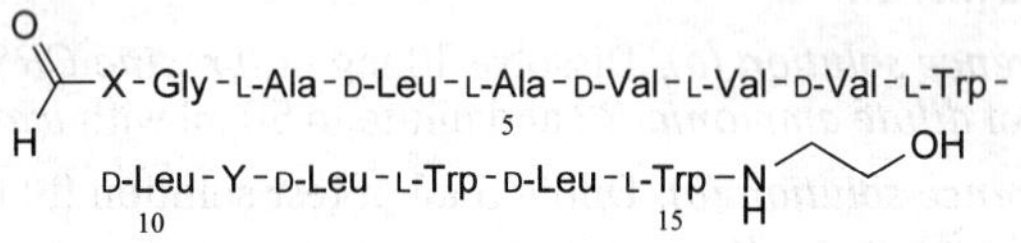

Gramicidin	Mol. formula	M_r	X	Y
A1	$C_{99}H_{140}N_{20}O_{17}$	1882	L-Val	L-Trp
A2	$C_{100}H_{142}N_{20}O_{17}$	1896	L-Ile	L-Trp
C1	$C_{97}H_{139}N_{19}O_{18}$	1859	L-Val	L-Tyr
C2	$C_{98}H_{141}N_{19}O_{18}$	1873	L-Ile	L-Tyr

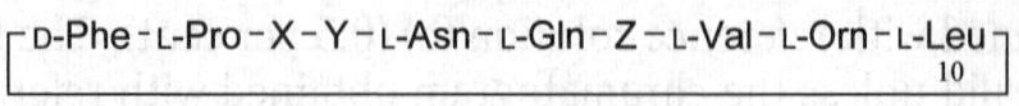

Tyrocidin	Mol. formula	M_r	X	Y	Z
A	$C_{66}H_{88}N_{13}O_{13}$	1271	L-Phe	D-Phe	L-Tyr
B	$C_{68}H_{89}N_{14}O_{13}$	1311	L-Trp	D-Phe	L-Tyr
C	$C_{70}H_{90}N_{15}O_{13}$	1350	L-Trp	D-Trp	L-Tyr
D	$C_{72}H_{91}N_{16}O_{12}$	1373	L-Trp	D-Trp	L-Trp
E	$C_{66}H_{88}N_{13}O_{12}$	1255	L-Phe	D-Phe	L-Phe

DEFINITION

Mixture of antimicrobial linear and cyclic polypeptides, isolated from the fermentation broth of *Brevibacillus brevis* Dubos. It consists mainly of gramicidins and tyrocidins as described above; other related compounds may be present in smaller amounts.

Potency: 180 IU/mg to 280 IU/mg (dried substance).

CHARACTERS

Appearance: white or almost white powder.

Solubility: practically insoluble in water, soluble in alcohol and in methanol.

IDENTIFICATION

First identification: B.

Second identification: A.

A. Thin-layer chromatography (*2.2.27*).

Test solution. Dissolve 5 mg of the substance to be examined in 4.0 ml of *alcohol R*.

Reference solution. Dissolve 5 mg of *tyrothricin CRS* in 4.0 ml of *alcohol R*.

Plate: *TLC silica gel F_{254} plate R.*

Mobile phase: *methanol R, butanol R, water R, acetic acid R, butyl acetate R* (2.5:7.5:12:20:40 *V/V/V/V/V*).

Application: 1 µl.

Development: over 2/3 of the plate.

Drying: in a current of warm air.

Detection A: examine in ultraviolet light at 254 nm.

Results A: the principal spots or groups of principal spots in the chromatogram obtained with the test solution are similar in position and size to the principal spots or groups of principal spots in the chromatogram obtained with the reference solution. The upper group corresponds to gramicidins, the lower group to tyrocidins.

Detection B: spray with *dimethylaminobenzaldehyde solution R2.* Heat the plate in a current of warm air until the spots appear.

System suitability: reference solution:

– the chromatogram shows 2 clearly separated spots or groups of spots.

Results B: the principal spots or groups of principal spots in the chromatogram obtained with the test solution are similar in position, colour and size to the principal spots or groups of principal spots in the chromatogram obtained with the reference solution. The upper group corresponds to gramicidins, the lower group to tyrocidins.

B. It complies with the test for composition (see Tests).

TESTS

Composition. Liquid chromatography (*2.2.29*): use the normalisation procedure. *Prepare the solutions immediately before use.*

Test solution. Dissolve 25 mg of the substance to be examined in 10 ml of *methanol R* and dilute to 25.0 ml with the mobile phase.

Reference solution (a). Dissolve 25 mg of *tyrothricin CRS* in 10 ml of *methanol R* and dilute to 25.0 ml with the mobile phase.

Reference solution (b). Dilute 1.0 ml of reference solution (a) to 50.0 ml with the mobile phase.

Column:

– *size*: *l* = 0.25 m, Ø = 4.6 mm,

– *stationary phase*: *octadecylsilyl silica gel for chromatography R* (5 µm),

– *temperature*: 60 °C.

Mobile phase: 0.79 g/l solution of *ammonium sulphate R, methanol R* (25:75 *V/V*).

Flow rate: 1.2 ml/min.

Detection: spectrophotometer at 280 nm.

Injection: 25 µl.

Monographs T-Z

Run time: 6 times the retention time of gramicidin A1. Use the chromatogram obtained with reference solution (a) and the chromatogram supplied with *tyrothricin CRS* to identify the peaks due to gramicidin A1, gramicidin A2 and the tyrocidins.

Relative retention with reference to gramicidin A1 (retention time = about 10 min): gramicidin C1 = about 0.8; gramicidin C2 = about 0.9; gramicidin A2 = about 1.1; tyrocidins = about 1.5 to 6.

System suitability: reference solution (a):

- *resolution*: minimum 1.5 between the peaks due to gramicidin A1 and gramicidin A2.

Composition:

- *sum of gramicidins*: 25 per cent to 50 per cent,
- *sum of tyrocidins*: 50 per cent to 70 per cent,
- *total*: minimum 85 per cent,
- *disregard limit*: the sum of the areas of the peaks due to gramicidins in the chromatogram obtained with reference solution (b).

Loss on drying (*2.2.32*): maximum 4.0 per cent, determined on 1.000 g by drying under high vacuum at 60 °C for 3 h.

Sulphated ash (*2.4.14*): maximum 1.5 per cent, determined on 1.0 g.

ASSAY

Carry out the microbiological assay of antibiotics (*2.7.2*) using the turbidimetric method. Use *gramicidin CRS* as the reference substance.

Test solution. Prepare a solution of tyrothricin containing about the same amount of gramicidin as the corresponding solution of *gramicidin CRS* i.e. 5 times more concentrated.

STORAGE

In an airtight container, protected from light.

U

01/2005:1578

UBIDECARENONE

Ubidecarenonum

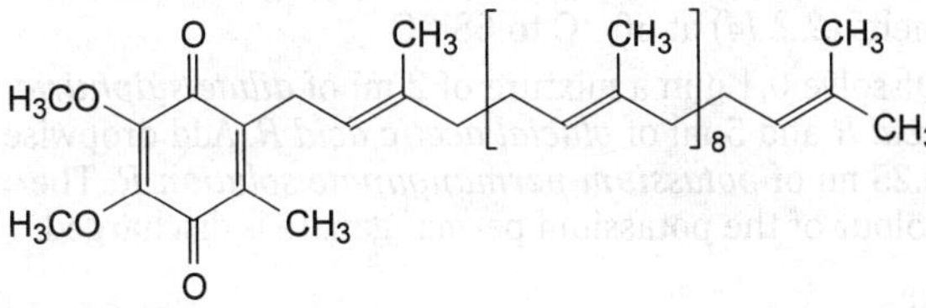

$C_{59}H_{90}O_4$ M_r 863

DEFINITION

2-[(all-*E*)-3,7,11,15,19,23,27,31,35,39-Decamethyltetraconta-2,6,10,14,18,22,26,30,34,38-decaenyl]-5,6-dimethoxy-3-methylbenzene-1,4-dione.

Content: 97.0 per cent to 103.0 per cent.

CHARACTERS

Appearance: yellow or orange, crystalline powder.

Solubility: practically insoluble in water, soluble in acetone, very slightly soluble in ethanol.

It gradually decomposes and darkens on exposure to light.

mp: about 48 °C.

Carry out all operations avoiding exposure to light.

IDENTIFICATION

A. Infrared absorption spectrophotometry (*2.2.24*).

Preparation: discs.

Comparison: *ubidecarenone CRS.*

B. Examine the chromatograms obtained in the test for related substances.

Results: the retention time of the principal peak in the chromatogram obtained with the test solution is similar to that of the principal peak in the chromatogram obtained with reference solution (a).

TESTS

Related substances. Liquid chromatography (*2.2.29*).

Test solution. Dissolve 25.0 mg of the substance to be examined in 25.0 ml of *ethanol R* by heating at about 50 °C for 2 min. Allow to cool.

Reference solution (a). Dissolve 5 mg of *ubidecarenone CRS* in 5 ml of *ethanol R* by heating at about 50 °C for 2 min. Allow to cool.

Reference solution (b). Dissolve 2 mg of *ubidecarenone impurity D CRS* in 2 ml of the test solution by heating at about 50 °C for 2 min. Allow to cool. Dilute 1 ml to 50 ml with *ethanol R.*

Reference solution (c). Dilute 1.0 ml of the test solution to 100.0 ml with *ethanol R.*

Column:

- *size*: l = 0.15 m, Ø = 4.6 mm,
- *stationary phase*: *octadecylsilyl silica gel for chromatography R* (5 µm).

Mobile phase: *ethanol R, methanol R2 (20:80 V/V).*

Flow rate: 2 ml/min.

Detection: spectrophotometer at 275 nm.

Injection: 10 µl.

Run time: 2 times the retention time of ubidecarenone.

Relative retention with reference to ubidecarenone (retention time = about 12 min): impurity D = about 0.67.

System suitability: reference solution (b):

- *resolution*: minimum 6.5 between the peaks due to impurity D and to ubidecarenone.

Limits:

- *any impurity*: not more than half the area of the principal peak in the chromatogram obtained with reference solution (c) (0.5 per cent),
- *total*: not more than the area of the principal peak in the chromatogram obtained with reference solution (c) (1.0 per cent),
- *disregard limit*: 0.05 times the area of the principal peak in the chromatogram obtained with reference solution (c) (0.05 per cent).

Impurity F. Liquid chromatography (*2.2.29*).

Test solution. Dissolve 25.0 mg of the substance to be examined in 25.0 ml of *hexane R.*

Reference solution (a). Dissolve 10.0 mg of *ubidecarenone for system suitability CRS* in 10.0 ml of *hexane R.*

Reference solution (b). Dilute 1 ml of the test solution to 100.0 ml with *hexane R.*

Column:

- *size*: l = 0.25 m, Ø = 4.0 mm,
- *stationary phase*: *silica gel for chromatography R* (7 µm).

Mobile phase: *ethyl acetate R, hexane R (3:97 V/V).*

Flow rate: 2 ml/min.

Detection: spectrophotometer at 275 nm.

Injection: 20 µl.

Run time: 1.2 times the retention time of ubidecarenone.

Relative retention with reference to ubidecarenone (retention time = about 10 min): impurity F = about 0.85.

System suitability: reference solution (a):

- *resolution*: minimum 1.5 between the peaks due to impurity F and to ubidecarenone.

Limit:

- *impurity F*: not more than 0.5 times the area of the principal peak in the chromatogram obtained with reference solution (b) (0.5 per cent).

Sulphated ash (*2.4.14*): maximum 0.1 per cent, determined on 1.0 g.

ASSAY

Dissolve 50.0 mg in 1.0 ml of *hexane R* and dilute to 50.0 ml with *ethanol R.* Dilute 2.0 ml of the solution to 50.0 ml with *ethanol R.* Measure the absorbance (*2.2.25*) at the maximum at 275 nm. Calculate the content of $C_{59}H_{90}O_4$ taking the specific absorbance to be 169.

STORAGE

Store in an airtight container, protected from light.

IMPURITIES

Specified impurities: A, B, C, D, E, F.

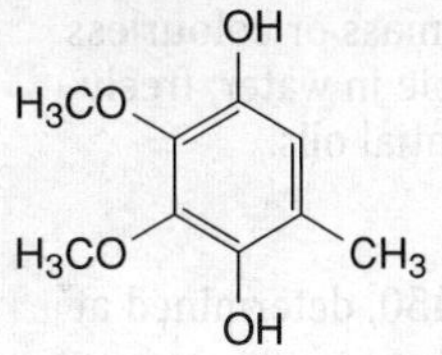

A. 2,3-dimethoxy-5-methylbenzene-1,4-diol,

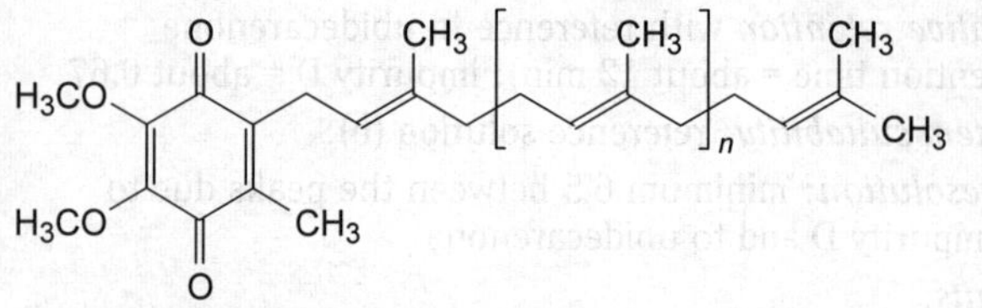

B. $n = 5$: 2-[(all-*E*)-3,7,11,15,19,23,27-heptamethyloctadocosa-2,6,10,14,18,22,26-heptaenyl]-5,6-dimethoxy-3-methylbenzene-1,4-dione (ubiquinone-7),

C. $n = 6$: 5,6-dimethoxy-3-methyl-2-[(all-*E*)-3,7,11,15,19, 23,27,31-octamethyldotriaconta-2,6,10,14,18,22,26,30-octaenyl]benzene-1,4-dione (ubiquinone-8),

D. $n = 7$: 5,6-dimethoxy-3-methyl-2-[(all-*E*)-3,7,11,15,19,23, 27,31,35-nonamethylhexatriaconta-2,6,10,14,18,22,26,30, 34-nonaenyl]benzene-1,4-dione (ubiquinone-9),

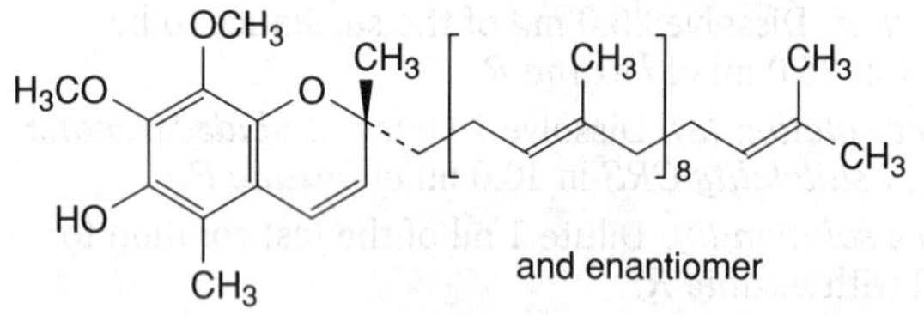

E. (2*RS*)-7,8-dimethoxy-2,5-dimethyl-2-[(all-*E*)-4,8,12,16,20, 24,28,32,36-nonamethylheptatriaconta-3,7,11,15,19,23, 27,31,35-nonaenyl]-2*H*-1-benzopyran-6-ol (ubicromenol),

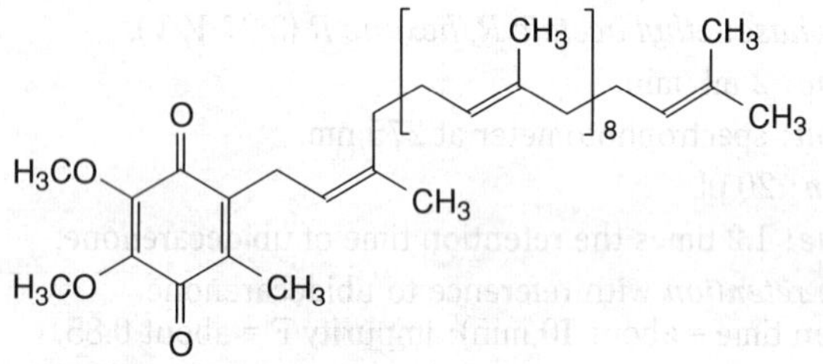

F. 2-[(2*Z*,6*E*,10*E*,14*E*,18*E*,22*E*,26*E*,30*E*,34*E*,38*E*)-3,7,11,15, 19,23,27,31,35,39-decamethyl-2,6,10,14,18,22,26,30,34, 38-tetracontadecaenyl]-5,6-dimethoxy-3-methylbenzene-1, 4-dione (ubidecarenone (*Z*)-isomer).

01/2005:0461

UNDECYLENIC ACID

Acidum undecylenicum

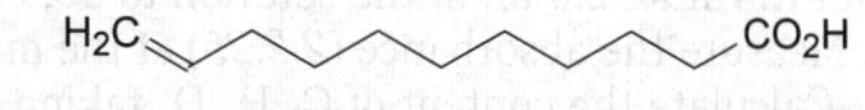

$C_{11}H_{20}O_2$ M_r 184.3

DEFINITION

Undecylenic acid contains not less than 97.0 per cent and not more than the equivalent of 102.0 per cent of undec-10-enoic acid.

CHARACTERS

A white or very pale yellow, crystalline mass or colourless or pale yellow liquid, practically insoluble in water, freely soluble in alcohol and in fatty and essential oils.

IDENTIFICATION

A. Refractive index (*2.2.6*): 1.447 to 1.450, determined at 25 ± 0.5 °C.

B. Freezing point (*2.2.18*): 21 °C to 24 °C.

C. To 2.0 g add 2 ml of freshly distilled *aniline R* and boil under a reflux condenser for 10 min. Allow to cool and add 30 ml of *ether R*. Shake with three quantities, each of 20 ml, of *dilute hydrochloric acid R* and then with 20 ml of *water R*. Evaporate the organic layer to dryness on a water-bath. The residue, after recrystallisation twice from *alcohol (70 per cent V/V) R* and drying *in vacuo* for 3 h, melts (*2.2.14*) at 66 °C to 68 °C.

D. Dissolve 0.1 g in a mixture of 2 ml of *dilute sulphuric acid R* and 5 ml of *glacial acetic acid R*. Add dropwise 0.25 ml of *potassium permanganate solution R*. The colour of the potassium permanganate is discharged.

TESTS

Peroxide value (*2.5.5*). Not more than 10.

Fixed and mineral oils. To 1.0 g add 5 ml of *sodium carbonate solution R* and 25 ml of *water R* and boil for 3 min. The hot solution is not more opalescent than reference suspension II (*2.2.1*).

Water-soluble acids. To 1.0 g add 20 ml of *water R* heated to 35 °C to 45 °C and shake for 2 min. Cool and filter the aqueous layer through a moistened filter. To 10 ml of the filtrate add 0.1 ml of *phenolphthalein solution R*. Not more than 0.1 ml of *0.1 M sodium hydroxide* is required to change the colour of the indicator.

Sulphated ash (*2.4.14*). Not more than 0.1 per cent, determined on 0.50 g.

Degree of unsaturation. Dissolve 85.0 mg in a mixture of 5 ml of *dilute hydrochloric acid R* and 30 ml of *glacial acetic acid R*. Using 0.05 ml of *indigo carmine solution R1*, added towards the end of the titration, as indicator, titrate with *0.0167 M bromide-bromate* until the colour changes from blue to yellow. 8.9 ml to 9.4 ml of *0.0167 M bromide-bromate* is required. Carry out a blank titration.

ASSAY

Dissolve 0.750 g in 10 ml of *alcohol R*. Using 0.1 ml of *phenolphthalein solution R* as indicator, titrate with *0.5 M sodium hydroxide* until a pink colour is obtained.

1 ml of *0.5 M sodium hydroxide* is equivalent to 92.14 mg of $C_{11}H_{20}O_2$.

STORAGE

Store in a non-metallic container, protected from light.

01/2005:0743

UREA

Ureum

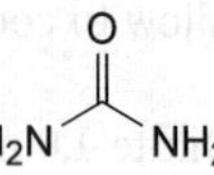

CH_4N_2O M_r 60.1

DEFINITION

Carbamide.

Content: 98.5 per cent to 101.5 per cent (dried substance).

CHARACTERS

Appearance: white, crystalline powder or transparent crystals, slightly hygroscopic.

Solubility: very soluble in water, soluble in alcohol, practically insoluble in methylene chloride.

IDENTIFICATION

First identification: A, B.

Second identification: A, C, D.

A. Melting point (*2.2.14*): 132 °C to 135 °C.

B. Infrared absorption spectrophotometry (*2.2.24*).

Preparation: discs.

Comparison: *urea CRS*.

C. Dissolve 0.1 g in 1 ml of *water R*. Add 1 ml of *nitric acid R*. A white, crystalline precipitate is formed.

D. Heat 0.5 g in a test tube until it liquefies and the liquid becomes turbid. Cool, dissolve in a mixture of 1 ml of *dilute sodium hydroxide solution R* and 10 ml of *water R* and add 0.05 ml of *copper sulphate solution R*. A reddish-violet colour is produced.

TESTS

Solution S. Dissolve 10.0 g in *water R* and dilute to 50 ml with the same solvent.

Appearance of solution. The solution is clear (*2.2.1*) and colourless (*2.2.2, Method II*).

To 2.5 ml of solution S add 7.5 ml of *water R*.

Alkalinity. To 2.5 ml of solution S add 7.5 ml of *water R*, 0.1 ml of *methyl red solution R* and 0.4 ml of *0.01 M hydrochloric acid*. The solution is red to orange.

Biuret: maximum 0.1 per cent.

To 10 ml of solution S add 5 ml of *water R*, 0.5 ml of a 5 g/l solution of *copper sulphate R* and 0.5 ml of *strong sodium hydroxide solution R*. Allow to stand for 5 min. Any reddish-violet colour in the solution is not more intense than that in a standard prepared at the same time in the same manner using 10 ml of a 0.2 g/l solution of *biuret R*.

Ammonium (*2.4.1*): maximum 500 ppm, determined on 0.1 ml of solution S.

Heavy metals (*2.4.8*): maximum 10 ppm.

Dilute 10 ml of solution S to 20 ml with *water R*. 12 ml of the solution complies with limit test A. Prepare the standard using *lead standard solution (1 ppm Pb) R*.

Loss on drying (*2.2.32*): maximum 1.0 per cent, determined on 1.000 g by drying in an oven at 100-105 °C for 1 h.

Sulphated ash (*2.4.14*): maximum 0.1 per cent, determined on 1.0 g.

ASSAY

Dissolve 0.2000 g in *water R* and dilute to 50.0 ml with the same solvent. Introduce 1.0 ml of this solution into a combustion flask. Add 4 g of a powdered mixture of 100 g of *dipotassium sulphate R*, 5 g of *copper sulphate R* and 2.5 g of *selenium R*, and 3 glass beads. Wash any adhering particles from the neck into the flask with 5 ml of *sulphuric acid R*, allowing it to run down the sides of the flask, and mix the contents by rotation. Close the mouth of the flask loosely, for example by means of a glass bulb with a short stem, to avoid excessive loss of sulphuric acid. Heat gradually at first, then increase the temperature until there is vigorous boiling with condensation of sulphuric acid in the neck of the flask; take precautions to prevent the upper part of the flask from becoming overheated. Continue the heating for 30 min. Cool, dissolve the solid material by cautiously adding to the mixture 25 ml of *water R*, cool again and place in a steam-distillation apparatus. Add 30 ml of *strong sodium hydroxide solution R* and distil immediately by passing steam through the mixture. Collect the distillate in 15 ml of a 40 g/l solution of *boric acid R* to which has been added 0.2 ml of *methyl red mixed solution R* and enough *water R* to cover the tip of the condenser. Towards the end of the distillation, lower the receiver so that the tip of the condenser is above the surface of the acid. Take precautions to prevent any water on the outer surface of the condenser from reaching the contents of the receiver. Titrate the distillate with *0.01 M sulphuric acid*.

1 ml of *0.01 M sulphuric acid* is equivalent to 0.6006 mg of CH_4N_2O.

STORAGE

In an airtight container.

01/2005:0958

UROFOLLITROPIN

Urofollitropinum

DEFINITION

Urofollitropin is a dry preparation containing menopausal gonadotrophin obtained from the urine of post-menopausal women. It has follicle-stimulating activity and no or virtually no luteinising activity. The potency is not less than 90 International Units of follicle-stimulating hormone (hFSH) per milligram. The ratio of units of luteinising hormone (interstitial-cell-stimulating hormone) [hLH(ICSH)] to units of follicle-stimulating hormone is not more than 1/60.

PRODUCTION

It may be prepared by a suitable fractionation procedure followed by immunoaffinity chromatography. It is prepared in conditions designed to minimise microbial contamination. The manufacturing process must have been shown to reduce any viral contamination such as hepatitis virus or HIV by appropriate validated methods.

CHARACTERS

Appearance: almost white or slightly yellowish powder.

Solubility: soluble in water.

IDENTIFICATION

When administered as prescribed in the assay it causes enlargement of the ovaries of immature female rats.

TESTS

Hepatitis virus antigens. Examined by a suitably sensitive immunochemical method (*2.7.1*), hepatitis virus antigens are not detected.

HIV antigen. Examined by a suitably sensitive immunochemical method (*2.7.1*), HIV antigen is not detected.

Residual luteinising activity. The International Units of FSH and LH are the activities contained in stated amounts of the International Standard of human urinary follicle-stimulating hormone and luteinising hormone (interstitial-cell-stimulating hormone) which consists of a mixture of a freeze-dried extract of urine of post-menopausal women with lactose. The equivalence in International Units of the International Standard is stated by the World Health Organisation. Use immature female rats approximately 21 days old and having masses such that the difference between the heaviest and the lightest rat is not more than 10 g. Assign the rats at random to 4 equal groups of at least 6 animals. If sets of 4 litter mates are available, assign one litter mate at random from each set to each group and mark according to litter.

Inject subcutaneously into each rat 50 IU of *serum gonadotrophin R* on the first day and 25 IU of *chorionic gonadotrophin R* on the fourth day, each in 0.5 ml of *phosphate-albumin buffered saline pH 7.2 R*.

Monographs T-Z

Choose 3 doses of the reference preparation such that the smallest dose produces a depletion of the ovarian ascorbic acid content in all the rats and the largest dose does not produce a maximal depletion in all the rats. Use doses in geometric progression; as an initial approximation, total doses of 0.5 IU, 1.0 IU and 2.0 IU may be tried although the dose to be used will depend on the sensitivity of the animals.

Choose a dose of the preparation to be examined expected to contain 60*X* IU of follicle-stimulating hormone (hFSH), in which *X* = the number of IU of hLH in the middle dose of the reference preparation.

Dissolve separately the total quantities of the preparation to be examined and of the reference preparation in 1.0 ml of *phosphate-albumin buffered saline pH 7.2 R*. Inject into a tail vein to each separate group of rats 6 days after the injection of chorionic gonadotrophin. Exactly 4 h after the injection, kill the rats and remove the ovaries from each animal. Remove any extraneous fluid and tissue from the ovaries and weigh the ovaries immediately.

Treat the combined ovaries from each rat separately, as follows. Crush and homogenise within 2 min in a freshly prepared 25 g/l solution of *metaphosphoric acid R* at a temperature of 4 °C and dilute to 7 ml with the same solution. Allow the homogenate to stand for 30 min at 4 °C and centrifuge at 4 °C at approximately 2500 *g*. Filter the supernatant liquid, if necessary, through a 0.22 µm filter.

Prepare a fresh solution consisting of a mixture of 2 ml of a 45.3 g/l solution of *sodium acetate R* adjusted to pH 7 with *acetic acid R*, 3 ml of *water R* and 2 ml of *dichlorophenolindophenol standard solution R*. Mix 2 ml of this solution with 2 ml of the clear supernatant liquid. 30 s after mixing, measure the absorbance (*2.2.25*) of the solution at the maximum at about 520 nm. Use as reference a solution with a known content of *ascorbic acid CRS* in a 25 g/l solution of *metaphosphoric acid R*, treated by the same process.

Calculate the amount of ascorbic acid from the ascorbic acid standard curve obtained and express in milligrams per 0.1 g of ovary to obtain the ascorbic acid content of the ovaries. Calculate the mean and its variance of the ascorbic acid content of the ovaries of the rats treated with the preparation to be examined.

For each dose-group of the reference preparation, plot the mean ascorbic acid content of the ovaries as a function of the logarithm of the dose and analyse the regression of the ascorbic acid content on the logarithm of the dose injected, using standard methods of analysis (the method of least squares).

The test is not valid unless:

- the slope constant *b* is significant at the 5 per cent level of significance,
- for the groups treated with the reference preparation, the sum of squares due to linear regression is equal to at least 95 per cent of the total sum of squares of the ascorbic acid content,
- the within-group variance of the ascorbic acid content of the group receiving the preparation to be examined is not significantly different at the 5 per cent level of significance from the within-group variance of the ascorbic acid content of the groups receiving the reference preparation.

The mean ascorbic acid content of the ovaries of the rats treated with the preparation to be examined is not significantly lower than that of the rats treated with the middle dose of the reference preparation (calculated from the regression equation) at the 5 per cent level of significance.

Water (*2.5.32*): maximum 5.0 per cent.

Bacterial endotoxins (*2.6.14, Method C*): less than 0.40 IU per IU of urofollitropin, if intended for use in the manufacture of parenteral dosage forms without a further appropriate procedure for the removal of bacterial endotoxins.

ASSAY

The follicle-stimulating activity of urofollitropin is estimated by comparing under given conditions its effect in enlarging the ovaries of immature rats treated with chorionic gonadotrophin with the same effect of the International Standard preparation of human urinary follicle-stimulating hormone and luteinising hormone or of a reference preparation calibrated in International Units. The International Units of FSH and LH are the activities contained in stated amounts of the International Standard of human urinary follicle-stimulating hormone and luteinising hormone (interstitial-cell-stimulating hormone) which consists of a mixture of a freeze-dried extract of urine of post-menopausal women with lactose. The equivalence in International Units of the International Standard is stated by the World Health Organisation.

Use immature female rats of the same strain, 19 to 28 days old, differing in age by not more than 3 days and having masses such that the difference between the heaviest and the lightest rat is not more than 10 g. Assign the rats at random to 6 equal groups of at least 5 animals. If sets of 6 litter mates are available, assign one litter mate from each set to each group and mark according to litter.

Choose 3 doses of the reference preparation and 3 doses of the preparation to be examined such that the smallest dose produces a positive response in some of the rats and the largest dose does not produce a maximal response in all the rats. Use doses in geometric progression and as an initial approximation total doses of 1.5 IU, 3.0 IU and 6.0 IU may be tried although the dose will depend on the sensitivity of the animals used, which may vary widely.

Dissolve separately the total quantities of the preparation to be examined and of the reference preparation corresponding to the daily doses to be used in sufficient *phosphate-albumin buffered saline pH 7.2 R* such that the daily dose is administered in a volume of about 0.5 ml. The buffer solution shall contain in the daily dose not less than 14 IU of chorionic gonadotrophin to ensure complete luteinisation. Add a suitable antimicrobial preservative such as 4 g/l of phenol or 0.02 g/l of thiomersal. Store the solutions at 5 ± 3 °C.

Inject subcutaneously into each rat the daily dose allocated to its group. Repeat the injection of each dose 24 h and 48 h after the first injection. About 24 h after the last injection, kill the rats and remove the ovaries from each animal. Remove any extraneous fluid and tissue from the ovaries and weigh the 2 combined ovaries of each animal immediately. Calculate the results by the usual statistical methods, using the mass of the 2 combined ovaries as the response. (The precision of the assay may be improved by a suitable correction of the organ mass with reference to the mass of the animal from which it was taken; an analysis of covariance may be used).

The estimated potency is not less than 80 per cent and not more than 125 per cent of the stated potency. The confidence limits (P = 0.95) of the estimated potency are not less than 64 per cent and not more than 156 per cent of the stated potency.

STORAGE

In an airtight, tamper-proof container, protected from light, at a temperature of 2 °C to 8 °C. If the substance is sterile, store in a sterile, airtight, tamper-proof container.

LABELLING

The label states:

- the activity expressed in International Units of follicle-stimulating hormone per container,
- the potency expressed in International Units of follicle-stimulating hormone per milligram,
- where applicable, that the substance if free from bacterial endotoxins.

01/2005:0695

UROKINASE

Urokinasum

DEFINITION

Urokinase is an enzyme, obtained from human urine, that activates plasminogen. It consists of a mixture of low-molecular-mass (LMM) (M_r 33 000) and high-molecular-mass (HMM) (M_r 54 000) forms, the high-molecular-mass form being predominant. The potency is not less than 70 000 International Units per milligram of protein.

PRODUCTION

It is produced by validated methods of manufacturing designed to minimise or eliminate microbial and viral contamination and vasoactive substances; in particular, adequate measures to inactivate viruses are taken, such as heating of the substance in solution at 60 °C for 10 h.

CHARACTERS

A white or almost white, amorphous powder, soluble in water.

IDENTIFICATION

A. Place separately in two haemolysis tubes 0.5 ml of citrated human plasma and 0.5 ml of citrated bovine plasma and maintain in a water-bath at 37 °C. To each tube add 0.1 ml of a solution containing a quantity of the substance to be examined equivalent to 1000 IU/ml in *phosphate buffer solution pH 7.4 R* and 0.1 ml of a solution containing a quantity of *humanthrombin R* equivalent to 20 IU/ml in *phosphate buffer solution pH 7.4 R*. Shake immediately. In both tubes, a clot forms and lyses within 30 min.

B. Carry out identification by a suitable immunodiffusion test.

TESTS

Appearance of solution. Dissolve 10 mg in 10 ml of *water R*. The solution is clear (*2.2.1*) and colourless (*2.2.2, Method II*).

Hepatitis B surface antigen. Examine by a suitably sensitive method such as radio-immunoassay. Hepatitis B surface antigen is not detected.

Thromboplastic contaminants

Test solutions. Dissolve suitable quantities of the substance to be examined in *barbital buffer solution pH 7.4 R* to obtain solutions with activities of 5000 IU/ml, 2500 IU/ml, 1250 IU/ml, 625 IU/ml and 312 IU/ml.

To each of six haemolysis tubes 1 cm in internal diameter add 0.1 ml of *citrated rabbit plasma R*. Allocate the test solutions one to each of five of the tubes; add to each tube 0.1 ml of the solution allocated to it and to the sixth tube add 0.1 ml of *barbital buffer solution pH 7.4 R* (blank). Incubate the tubes at 25 ± 0.5 °C for 5 min and add 0.1 ml of a 3.675 g/l solution of *calcium chloride R*. Measure with a stop-watch the coagulation time for each tube. Plot the shortening of the recalcification time (clotting time of the blank minus clotting time measured) against log concentration in International Units. Extrapolate the best-fitting straight line through the five points until it reaches the log-concentration axis. The urokinase activity at the intersection point, which represents the limit concentration for coagulant activity (zero coagulant activity), is not less than 150 IU/ml.

Molecular fractions. Examine by size-exclusion chromatography (*2.2.30*).

Test solution. Dissolve about 1 mg of the substance to be examined in 1.0 ml of *0.02 M phosphate buffer pH 8.0 R*. Prepare immediately before use.

The chromatographic procedure may be carried out using:

- a column 0.9 m long and 16 mm in internal diameter packed with *cross-linked dextran for chromatography R3*,
- as mobile phase at a flow rate of 6 ml/h a 17.5 g/l solution of *sodium chloride R* in *0.02 M phosphate buffer solution pH 8.0 R*,

equilibrating the column and operating at 5 °C. Apply the test solution to the head of the column rinsing twice with 0.5 ml portions of the buffer and carry out the elution. The eluate may be collected in fractions of 1 ml. Measure the absorbance (*2.2.25*) of the eluate at the maximum at 280 nm and plot the individual values on a graph. Draw perpendicular lines towards the axis of the abscissae from the minima before the HMM peak, between the HMM and the LMM peaks, and after the LMM peak, thus identifying the fractions to be considered in calculating the HMM/LMM activity ratio. Pool the HMM fractions and, separately, the LMM fractions. Determine separately the urokinase activity in International Units of each of the fraction pools by the method prescribed under Assay. The ratio of the urokinase activity in the HMM fraction pool to that in the LMM fraction pool is not less than 2.0.

Total protein. Determine the nitrogen content, using 10 mg, by the method of sulphuric acid digestion (*2.5.9*) and calculate the quantity of protein by multiplying by 6.25.

Pyrogens (*2.6.8*). If intended for use in the manufacture of parenteral dosage forms without a further appropriate procedure for the removal of pyrogen, it complies with the test for pyrogens. Inject per kilogram of the rabbit's mass 1.0 ml of a sterile 9 g/l solution of *sodium chloride R* containing a quantity of the substance to be examined equivalent to 20 000 IU/ml.

ASSAY

The potency of urokinase is determined by comparing its capacity to activate plasminogen to form plasmin with the same capacity of a reference preparation of urokinase calibrated in International Units; the formation of plasmin is measured by the determination of the lysis time of a fibrin clot in given conditions.

The International Unit is the activity contained in a stated amount of the International Reference Preparation, which consists of freeze-dried urokinase with lactose. The equivalence in International Units of the International Reference Preparation is stated by the World Health Organisation.

Unless otherwise prescribed, use *phosphate buffer solution pH 7.4 R* containing 30 g/l of *bovine albumin R* for the preparation of the solutions and dilutions used in the assay.

Test solution. Prepare a solution of the substance to be examined expected to have an activity of 1000 IU/ml.

Reference solution. Prepare a solution of a reference preparation having an activity of 1000 IU/ml.

Keep the test solution and the reference solution in iced water and use within 6 h. Prepare three serial 1.5-fold dilutions of the reference preparation such that the longest clot-lysis time is less than 20 min and the shortest clot-lysis time is greater than 3 min. Prepare three similar dilutions of the test solution. Keep the solutions in iced water and use within 1 h. Use twenty-four tubes 8 mm in diameter. Label the tubes T_1, T_2 and T_3 for the dilutions of the test solution and S_1, S_2 and S_3 for the dilutions of the reference solution, allocating four tubes to each dilution. Place the tubes in iced water. Into each tube, introduce 0.2 ml of the appropriate dilution, 0.2 ml of *phosphate buffer solution pH 7.4 R* containing 30 g/l of *bovine albumin R* and 0.1 ml of a solution of *humanthrombin R* having an activity of not less than 20 IU/ml. Place the tubes in a water-bath at 37 °C and allow to stand for 2 min to attain temperature equilibrium. Using an automatic pipette, introduce into the bottom of the first tube 0.5 ml of a 10 g/l solution of *bovine euglobulins R*, ensuring mixing. At intervals of 5 s, introduce successively into the remaining tubes 0.5 ml of a 10 g/l solution of *bovine euglobulins R*. Using a stop-watch, measure for each tube the time in seconds that elapses between the addition of the euglobulins solution and the lysis of the clot. Plot the logarithms of the lysis times for the substance to be examined and for the reference preparation against the logarithms of the concentration and calculate the activity of the substance to be examined using the usual statistical methods.

The estimated potency is not less than 90 per cent and not more than 111 per cent of the stated potency. The confidence limits ($P = 0.95$) of the estimated potency are not less than 80 per cent and not more than 125 per cent of the stated potency.

STORAGE

Store in an airtight container, protected from light, at a temperature not exceeding 8 °C. If the substance is sterile, store in a sterile, airtight, tamper-proof container.

LABELLING

The label states:

- the potency in International Units per milligram of protein,
- where applicable, that the contents are apyrogenic.

01/2005:1275

URSODEOXYCHOLIC ACID

Acidum ursodeoxycholicum

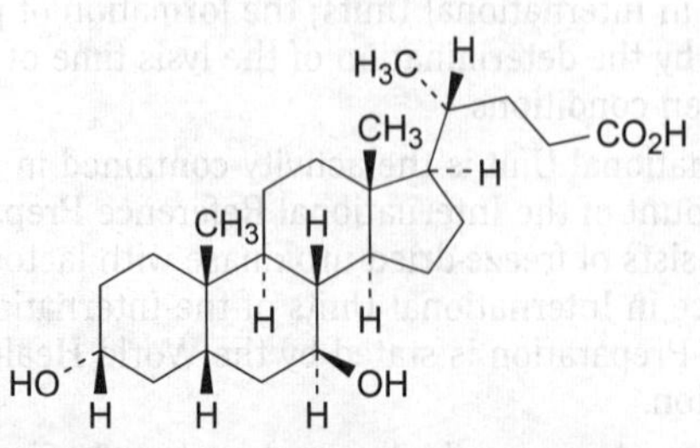

$C_{24}H_{40}O_4$ M_r 392.6

DEFINITION

Ursodeoxycholic acid contains not less than 99.0 per cent and not more than the equivalent of 101.0 per cent of 3α,7β-dihydroxy-5β-cholan-24-oic acid, calculated with reference to the dried substance.

CHARACTERS

A white or almost white powder, very slightly soluble in water, freely soluble in alcohol, slightly soluble in acetone and in methylene chloride.

It melts at about 202 °C.

IDENTIFICATION

First identification: A.

Second identification: B, C.

A. Examine by infrared absorption spectrophotometry (*2.2.24*), comparing with the spectrum obtained with *ursodeoxycholic acid CRS*. Examine the substances as discs prepared using *potassium bromide R*.

B. Examine the chromatograms obtained in the test for related substances. The principal spot in the chromatogram obtained with test solution (b) is similar in position, colour and size to the principal spot in the chromatogram obtained with reference solution (a).

C. Dissolve about 10 mg in 1 ml of *sulphuric acid R*. Add 0.1 ml of *formaldehyde solution R* and allow to stand for 5 min. Add 5 ml of *water R*. The suspension obtained is greenish-blue.

TESTS

Specific optical rotation (*2.2.7*).Dissolve 0.500 g in *ethanol R* and dilute to 25.0 ml with the same solvent. The specific optical rotation is + 58.0 to + 62.0, calculated with reference to the dried substance.

Related substances. Examine by thin-layer chromatography (*2.2.27*), using a suitable silica gel as the coating substance.

Test solution (a). Dissolve 0.40 g of the substance to be examined in a mixture of 1 volume of *water R* and 9 volumes of *acetone R* and dilute to 10 ml with the same mixture of solvents.

Test solution (b). Dilute 1 ml of test solution (a) to 10 ml with a mixture of 1 volume of *water R* and 9 volumes of *acetone R*.

Reference solution (a). Dissolve 40 mg of *ursodeoxycholic acid CRS* in a mixture of 1 volume of *water R* and 9 volumes of *acetone R* and dilute to 10 ml with the same mixture of solvents.

Reference solution (b). Dissolve 20 mg of *lithocholic acid CRS* in a mixture of 1 volume of *water R* and 9 volumes of *acetone R* and dilute to 10 ml with the same mixture of solvents. Dilute 2 ml of the solution to 100 ml with a mixture of 1 volume of *water R* and 9 volumes of *acetone R*.

Reference solution (c). Dissolve 20 mg of *chenodeoxycholic acid CRS* in a mixture of 1 volume of *water R* and 9 volumes of *acetone R* and dilute to 50 ml with the same mixture of solvents.

Reference solution (d). Dissolve 20 mg of *cholic acid CRS* in a mixture of 1 volume of *water R* and 9 volumes of *acetone R* and dilute to 100 ml with the same mixture of solvents.

Reference solution (e). Dilute 0.5 ml of test solution (a) to 20 ml with a mixture of 1 volume of *water R* and 9 volumes of *acetone R*. Dilute 1 ml of the solution to 10 ml with a mixture of 1 volume of *water R* and 9 volumes of *acetone R*.

Reference solution (f). Dissolve 10 mg of *ursodeoxycholic acid CRS* in reference solution (c) and dilute to 25 ml with the same solution.

Apply to the plate 5 µl of each solution. Develop in an unsaturated tank over a path of 15 cm using a mixture of 1 volume of *glacial acetic acid R*, 30 volumes of *acetone R* and 60 volumes of *methylene chloride R*. Dry the plate at 120 °C for 10 min. Spray the plate immediately with a 47.6 g/l solution of *phosphomolybdic acid R* in a mixture

Monographs T-Z

of 1 volume of *sulphuric acid R* and 20 volumes of *glacial acetic acid R* and heat again at 120 °C until blue spots appear on a lighter background. In the chromatogram obtained with test solution (a): any spot corresponding to lithocholic acid is not more intense than the principal spot in the chromatogram obtained with reference solution (b) (0.1 per cent); any spot corresponding to chenodeoxycholic acid is not more intense than the principal spot in the chromatogram obtained with reference solution (c) (1 per cent); any spot corresponding to cholic acid is not more intense than the principal spot in the chromatogram obtained with reference solution (d) (0.5 per cent); any spot, apart from the principal spot and any spots corresponding to lithocholic acid, chenodeoxycholic acid and cholic acid, is not more intense than the principal spot in the chromatogram obtained with reference solution (e) (0.25 per cent). The test is not valid unless the chromatogram obtained with reference solution (f) shows two clearly separated principal spots.

Heavy metals (*2.4.8*). 1.0 g complies with limit test C for heavy metals (20 ppm). Prepare the standard using 2 ml of *lead standard solution (10 ppm Pb) R*.

Loss on drying (*2.2.32*). Not more than 1.0 per cent, determined on 1.000 g by drying in an oven at 100-105 °C.

Sulphated ash (*2.4.14*). Not more than 0.1 per cent, determined on 1.0 g.

ASSAY

Dissolve 0.350 g in 50 ml of *alcohol R*, previously neutralised to 0.2 ml of *phenolphthalein solution R*. Add 50 ml of *water R* and titrate with *0.1 M sodium hydroxide* until a pink colour is obtained.

1 ml of *0.1 M sodium hydroxide* is equivalent to 39.26 mg of $C_{24}H_{40}O_4$.

IMPURITIES

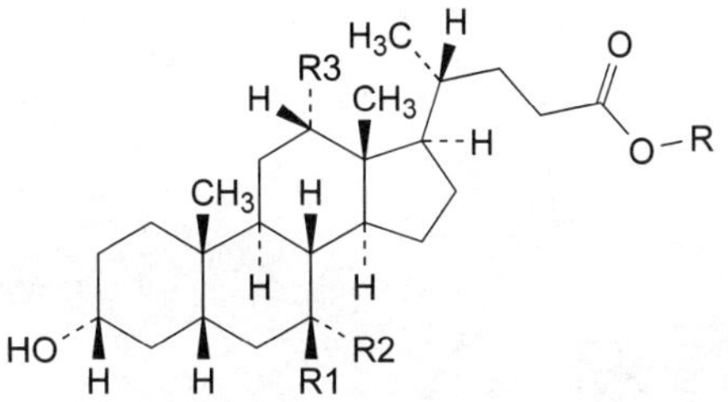

A. R = R1 = R3 = H, R2 = OH: chenodeoxycholic acid,

B. R = R1 = H, R2 = R3 = OH: 3α,7α,12α-trihydroxy-5β-cholan-24-oic acid (cholic acid),

C. R = R1 = R2 = R3 = H: 3α-hydroxy-5β-cholan-24-oic acid (lithocholic acid),

D. R = R2 = H, R1 = R3 = OH: 3α,7β,12α-trihydroxy-5β-cholan-24-oic acid (ursocholic acid),

E. R = R1 = R2 = H, R3 = OH: 3α,12α-dihydroxy-5β-cholan-24-oic acid (deoxycholic acid),

F. R = R3 = H, R1+R2 = O: 3α-hydroxy-7-oxo-5β-cholan-24-oic acid,

G. R = CH_3, R1 = OH, R2 = R3 = H: methyl 3α,7β-dihydroxy-5β-cholan-24-oate.

Monographs T-Z

V

01/2005:0453

VALERIAN ROOT

Valerianae radix

DEFINITION

Valerian root consists of the dried, whole or fragmented underground parts of *Valeriana officinalis* L. *s.l.*, including the rhizome surrounded by the roots and stolons. It contains not less than 5 ml/kg of essential oil for the whole drug and not less than 3 ml/kg of essential oil for the cut drug, both calculated with reference to the dried drug and not less than 0.17 per cent of sesquiterpenic acids expressed as valerenic acid ($C_{15}H_{22}O_2$; M_r 234), calculated with reference to the dried drug.

CHARACTERS

Valerian root has a characteristic odour.

It has the macroscopic and microscopic characters described under identification tests A and B.

IDENTIFICATION

A. The rhizome is yellowish-grey to pale brownish-grey, obconical to cylindrical, up to about 50 mm long and 30 mm in diameter; the base is elongated or compressed, usually entirely covered by numerous roots. The apex usually exhibits a cup-shaped scar from the aerial parts; stem bases are rarely present. When cut longitudinally, the pith exhibits a central cavity transversed by septa. The roots are numerous, almost cylindrical, of the same colour as the rhizome, 1 mm to 3 mm in diameter and sometimes more than 100 mm long. A few filiform fragile secondary roots are present. The fracture is short. The stolons show prominent nodes separated by longitudinally striated internodes, each 20 mm to 50 mm long, with a fibrous fracture.

B. Reduce to a powder (355). The powder is pale yellowish-grey to pale greyish-brown. Examine under a microscope using *chloral hydrate solution R*. The powder shows cells containing a pale brown resin or droplets of essential oil; isolated rectangular sclereids with pitted walls 5 µm to 15 µm thick; reticulately-thickened xylem vessels; occasional fragments of cork cells and epidermal cells, some with root hairs. Examine under a microscope using a 50 per cent *V/V* solution of *glycerol R*. The powder shows numerous fragments of parenchyma with cells, containing single or compound starch granules; the single granules are rounded or elongated, 5 µm to 15 µm in diameter and have sometimes a cleft or radiate hilum; the compound granules have two to six components with an overall diameter of up to 20 µm.

C. Examine by thin-layer chromatography (*2.2.27*), using a *TLC silica gel plate R*.

Test solution. Shake 1.0 g of the powdered drug (355) with 6.0 ml of *methanol R* in a 25 ml flask for 15 min and filter. Rinse the flask and the filter with the aid of a small portion of *methanol R* to obtain 5 ml of filtrate. Evaporate the filtrate to about 2 ml and add 3 ml of a 100 g/l solution of *potassium hydroxide R*. Shake with two quantities, each of 5 ml, of *methylene chloride R*. Allow to separate and discard the lower layer. Heat the aqueous layer in a water-bath at 40 °C for 10 min. Cool and add *dilute hydrochloric acid R* until it gives an acid reaction. Shake with two quantities, each of 5 ml, of *methylene chloride R*. Filter the combined lower layers over *anhydrous sodium sulphate R*. Evaporate the filtrate to dryness. Dissolve the residue in 1.0 ml of *methylene chloride R*.

Reference solution. Dissolve 5 mg of *fluorescein R* and 5 mg of *Sudan red G R* in 20.0 ml of *methanol R*.

Apply to the plate as bands 20 µl of each solution. Develop over a path of 10 cm using a mixture of 0.5 volumes of *glacial acetic acid R*, 35 volumes of *ethyl acetate R* and 65 volumes of *hexane R*. Allow the plate to dry in air. Examine in daylight. The chromatogram obtained with the reference solution shows in its middle part the red zone of Sudan red G and in its lower part the greenish-yellow zone of fluorescein. Spray the plate with *anisaldehyde solution R*. Examine in daylight while heating at 100 °C to 105 °C for 5 min to 10 min. The chromatogram obtained with the test solution shows a violet-blue zone corresponding to hydroxyvalerenic acid at about the same height as the zone of fluorescein in the chromatogram obtained with the reference solution and also shows a violet zone corresponding to valerenic acid at about the same height as that of the zone due to Sudan red G in the chromatogram obtained with the reference solution. The chromatogram obtained with the test solution shows in the upper half other, mostly less intense, pink to violet zones.

TESTS

Foreign matter (*2.8.2*). Not more than 5 per cent of stem bases and not more than 2 per cent of other foreign matter.

Loss on drying (*2.2.32*). Not more than 12.0 per cent, determined on 1.000 g of well homogenised powdered drug (355) by drying in an oven at 100 °C to 105 °C, for 2 h.

Total ash (*2.4.16*). Not more than 12.0 per cent.

Ash insoluble in hydrochloric acid (*2.8.1*). Not more than 5.0 per cent.

ASSAY

Essential oil. Carry out the determination of essential oils in vegetable drugs (*2.8.12*). Use 40.0 g of freshly powdered drug (500), a 2000 ml flask, 500 ml of *water R* as the distillation liquid and 0.50 ml of *xylene R* in the graduated tube. Distil at a rate of 3 ml/min to 4 ml/min for 4 h.

Sesquiterpenic acids. Examine by liquid chromatography (*2.2.29*).

Test solution. Place 1.50 g of the powdered drug (710) in a 100 ml round-bottomed flask with a ground-glass neck. Add 20 ml of *anhydrous methanol R*. Mix and heat on a water-bath under a reflux condenser for 30 min. Allow to cool and filter. Place the filter with the residue in the 100 ml round-bottomed flask. Add 20 ml of *anhydrous methanol R* and heat on a water-bath under the reflux condenser for 15 min. Allow to cool and filter. Combine the filtrates and dilute to 50.0 ml with *anhydrous methanol R* rinsing the round-bottomed flask and the filter.

Reference solution. Prepare the solution immediately before use, protected from bright light. Dissolve 30 mg of *dantron R* in *anhydrous methanol R* and dilute to 100.0 ml with the same solvent. Dilute 5.0 ml of the solution to 50.0 ml with *anhydrous methanol R*.

The chromatographic procedure may be carried out using:

– a stainless steel column 0.25 m long and 4 mm in internal diameter packed with *octadecylsilyl silica gel for chromatography R* (5 µm),

– as mobile phase at a flow rate of 1.5 ml/min:

Mobile phase A. Mix 20 volumes of *acetonitrile R* and 80 volumes of a 5 g/l solution of *phosphoric acid R*,

Mobile phase B. Mix 80 volumes of *acetonitrile R* and 20 volumes of a 5 g/l solution of *phosphoric acid R*,

Time (min)	Mobile phase A (per cent *V/V*)	Mobile phase B (per cent *V/V*)	Comment
0 - 5	55	45	isocratic
5 - 18	55 → 20	45 → 80	linear gradient
18 - 20	20	80	isocratic
20 - 22	20 → 55	80 → 45	linear gradient

– as detector a spectrophotometer set at 220 nm,
– a 20 μl loop injector.

Inject the test solution and the reference solution.

When the chromatograms are recorded in the prescribed conditions, the relative retention times (to dantron) are: acetoxyvalerenic acid about 0.7 and valerenic acid about 1.2.

Calculate the percentage content of acetoxyvalerenic acid using the expression:

$$\frac{A_2 \times m_1 \times 11.51}{A_1 \times m_2}$$

Calculate the percentage content of valerenic acid using the expression:

$$\frac{A_3 \times m_1 \times 8.09}{A_1 \times m_2}$$

Or calculate the percentage content of both sesquiterpenic acids using the expression:

$$\frac{\left[\frac{A_2 \times 11.51}{A_1} + \frac{A_3 \times 8.09}{A_1}\right] \times m_1}{m_2}$$

A_1 = area of the peak due to dantron in the chromatogram obtained with the reference solution,

A_2 = area of the peak due to acetoxyvalerenic acid in the chromatogram obtained with the test solution,

A_3 = area of the peak due to valerenic acid in the chromatogram obtained with the test solution,

m_1 = mass of dantron, in grams, used to prepare the reference solution,

m_2 = mass of the drug to be examined, in grams.

STORAGE

Store protected from light.

01/2005:0796

VALINE

Valinum

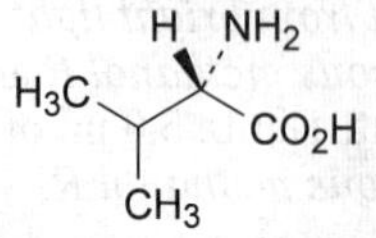

$C_5H_{11}NO_2$ M_r 117.1

DEFINITION

Valine contains not less than 98.5 per cent and not more than the equivalent of 101.0 per cent of *(S)*-2-amino-3-methylbutanoic acid, calculated with reference to the dried substance.

CHARACTERS

White or almost white, crystalline powder or colourless crystals, soluble in water, very slightly soluble in alcohol.

IDENTIFICATION

First identification: A, B.

Second identification: A, C.

A. It complies with the test for specific optical rotation (see Tests).

B. Examine by infrared absorption spectrophotometry (*2.2.24*), comparing with the spectrum obtained with *valine CRS*. Examine the substances prepared as discs.

C. Examine the chromatograms obtained in the test for ninhydrin-positive substances. The principal spot in the chromatogram obtained with test solution (b) is similar in position, colour and size to the principal spot in the chromatogram obtained with reference solution (a).

TESTS

Solution S. Dissolve 2.5 g in *water R* and dilute to 100 ml with the same solvent.

Appearance of solution. Solution S is clear (*2.2.1*) and not more intensely coloured than reference solution BY_6 (*2.2.2, Method II*).

Specific optical rotation (*2.2.7*). Dissolve 2.00 g in *hydrochloric acid R1* and dilute to 25.0 ml with the same acid. The specific optical rotation is + 26.5 to + 29.0, calculated with reference to the dried substance.

Ninhydrin-positive substances. Examine by thin-layer chromatography (*2.2.27*), using a *TLC silica gel plate R*.

Test solution (a). Dissolve 0.10 g of the substance to be examined in *dilute hydrochloric acid R* and dilute to 10 ml with the same acid.

Test solution (b). Dilute 1 ml of test solution (a) to 50 ml with *water R*.

Reference solution (a). Dissolve 10 mg of *valine CRS* in *0.1 M hydrochloric acid* and dilute to 50 ml with the same acid.

Reference solution (b). Dilute 5 ml of test solution (b) to 20 ml with *water R*.

Reference solution (c). Dissolve 10 mg of *phenylalanine CRS* and 10 mg of *valine CRS* in *0.1 M hydrochloric acid* and dilute to 25 ml with the same acid.

Apply to the plate 5 μl of each solution. Develop over a path of 15 cm using a mixture of 20 volumes of *glacial acetic acid R*, 20 volumes of *water R* and 60 volumes of *butanol R*. Allow the plate to dry in air, spray with *ninhydrin solution R* and heat at 100 °C to 105 °C for 15 min. Any spot in the chromatogram obtained with test solution (a), apart from the principal spot, is not more intense than the spot in the chromatogram obtained with reference solution (b) (0.5 per cent). The test is not valid unless the chromatogram obtained with reference solution (c) shows two clearly separated spots.

Chlorides (*2.4.4*). Dilute 10 ml of solution S to 15 ml with *water R*. The solution complies with the limit test for chlorides (200 ppm).

Sulphates (*2.4.13*). Dissolve 0.5 g in *distilled water R* and dilute to 15 ml with the same solvent. The solution complies with the limit test for sulphates (300 ppm).

Ammonium (*2.4.1*). 50 mg complies with limit test B for ammonium (200 ppm). Prepare the standard using 0.1 ml of *ammonium standard solution (100 ppm NH_4) R*.

Iron (*2.4.9*). In a separating funnel, dissolve 1.0 g in 10 ml of *dilute hydrochloric acid R*. Shake with three quantities, each of 10 ml, of *methyl isobutyl ketone R1*, shaking for

3 min each time. To the combined organic layers add 10 ml of *water R* and shake for 3 min. The aqueous layer complies with the limit test for iron (10 ppm).

Heavy metals (*2.4.8*). 2.0 g complies with limit test D for heavy metals (10 ppm). Prepare the standard using 2 ml of *lead standard solution (10 ppm Pb) R*.

Loss on drying (*2.2.32*). Not more than 0.5 per cent, determined on 1.000 g by drying in an oven at 100 °C to 105 °C.

Sulphated ash (*2.4.14*). Not more than 0.1 per cent, determined on 1.0 g.

ASSAY

Dissolve 0.100 g in 3 ml of *anhydrous formic acid R*. Add 30 ml of *anhydrous acetic acid R*. Using 0.1 ml of *naphtholbenzein solution R* as indicator, titrate with *0.1 M perchloric acid* until the colour changes from brownish-yellow to green.

1 ml of *0.1 M perchloric acid* is equivalent to 11.71 mg of $C_5H_{11}NO_2$.

STORAGE

Store protected from light.

01/2005:1378

VALPROIC ACID

Acidum valproicum

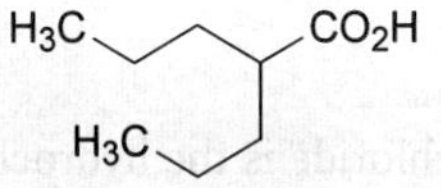

$C_8H_{16}O_2$ M_r 144.2

DEFINITION

Valproic acid contains not less than 99.0 per cent and not more than the equivalent of 101.0 per cent of 2-propylpentanoic acid.

CHARACTERS

A colourless or very slightly yellow, clear liquid, slightly viscous, very slightly soluble in water, miscible with alcohol and with methylene chloride. It dissolves in dilute solutions of alkali hydroxides.

IDENTIFICATION

First identification: B.

Second identification: A, C, D.

A. Refractive index (*2.2.5*): 1.422 to 1.425.

B. Examine by infrared absorption spectrophotometry (*2.2.24*), comparing with the spectrum obtained with *valproic acid CRS*.

C. Examine by thin-layer chromatography (*2.2.27*), using a *TLC silica gel plate R*.

Test solution. Dissolve 50 mg of the substance to be examined in *methanol R* and dilute to 5 ml with the same solvent.

Reference solution. Dissolve 50 mg of *valproic acid CRS* in *methanol R* and dilute to 5 ml with the same solvent.

Apply to the plate 2 µl of each solution. Develop over a path of 15 cm using a mixture of equal volumes of *ether R* and *methylene chloride R*. Allow the plate to dry in air. Spray with *bromocresol green solution R*. The principal spot in the chromatogram obtained with the test solution is similar in position, colour and size to the principal spot in the chromatogram obtained with the reference solution.

D. To 1 ml add 3 ml of *dilute sodium hydroxide solution R*. Add 3 ml of *water R* and 1 ml of a 100 g/l solution of *cobalt nitrate R*. A violet precipitate is formed. Filter; the precipitate dissolves in *methylene chloride R*.

TESTS

Appearance of solution. Dissolve 2.0 g in *dilute sodium hydroxide solution R* and dilute to 10 ml with the same alkaline solution. The solution is clear (*2.2.1*) and not more intensely coloured than reference solution Y_5 (*2.2.2, Method II*).

Related substances. Examine by gas chromatography (*2.2.28*), using *butyric acid R* as the internal standard.

Internal standard solution. Dissolve 10 mg of *butyric acid R* in *heptane R* and dilute to 200 ml with the same solvent.

Test solution. Dissolve 0.250 g of the substance to be examined in the internal standard solution and dilute to 5.0 ml with the same solution. Dilute 1.0 ml of the solution to 10.0 ml with *heptane R*.

Reference solution. Dissolve 20 mg of the substance to be examined and 20 mg of *2-(1-methylethyl)pentanoic acid CRS* in *heptane R* and dilute to 10 ml with the same solvent. Dilute 1 ml of the solution to 10 ml with *heptane R*.

The chromatographic procedure may be carried out using:

– a wide-bore fused-silica column 30 m long and 0.53 mm in internal diameter coated with *macrogol 20 000 2-nitroterephthalate R* (film thickness 0.5 µm),

– *helium for chromatography R* as the carrier gas at a flow rate of 8 ml/min,

– a flame-ionisation detector,

with the following temperature programme:

	Time (min)	Temperature (°C)	Rate (°C/min)	Comment
Column	0 - 10	130	–	isothermal
	10 - 30	130 → 190	3	linear gradient
Injection port		220		
Detector		220		

Inject 1 µl of each solution. The test is not valid unless, in the chromatogram obtained with the reference solution, the resolution between the peaks corresponding to 2-(1-methylethyl)pentanoic acid and valproic acid is at least 3.0. In the chromatogram obtained with the test solution: the sum of the areas of the peaks, apart from the principal peak, is not greater than three times the area of the peak due to the internal standard (0.3 per cent); none of the peaks, apart from the principal peak, has an area greater than that of the peak due to the internal standard (0.1 per cent). Disregard any peak with an area less than 0.1 times that of the peak due to the internal standard.

Heavy metals (*2.4.8*). Dissolve 2.0 g in *alcohol (80 per cent V/V) R* and dilute to 20 ml with the same solvent. 12 ml of the solution complies with limit test B for heavy metals (20 ppm). Prepare the standard using lead standard solution (2 ppm Pb) obtained by diluting *lead standard solution (100 ppm Pb) R* with *alcohol (80 per cent V/V) R*.

Sulphated ash (*2.4.14*). Not more than 0.1 per cent, determined on 1.0 g.

ASSAY

Dissolve 0.100 g in 25 ml of *alcohol R*. Add 2 ml of *water R*. Titrate with *0.1 M sodium hydroxide*, determining the end-point potentiometrically (*2.2.20*).

1 ml of *0.1 M sodium hydroxide* is equivalent to 14.42 mg of $C_8H_{16}O_2$.

STORAGE

Store in an airtight container.

IMPURITIES

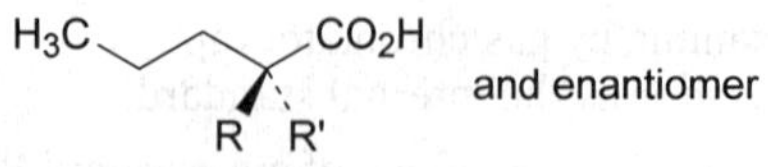

A. R = R′ = H: pentanoic acid (valeric acid),

B. R = H, R′ = CH_2-CH_3: (2*RS*)-2-ethylpentanoic acid,

C. R = H, R′ = $CH(CH_3)_2$: (2*RS*)-2-(1-methylethyl)pentanoic acid,

D. R = R′ = CH_2-CH_2-CH_3: 2,2-dipropylpentanoic acid,

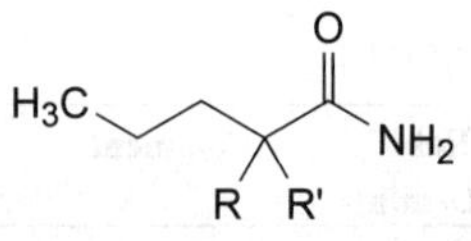

E. R = R′ = H: pentanamide (valeramide),

F. R = H, R′ = CH_2-CH_2-CH_3: 2-propylpentanamide,

G. R = R′ = CH_2-CH_2-CH_3: 2,2-dipropylpentanamide,

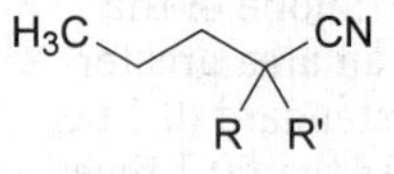

H. R = R′ = H: pentanenitrile (valeronitrile),

I. R = H, R′ = CH_2-CH_2-CH_3: 2-propylpentanenitrile,

J. R = R′ = CH_2-CH_2-CH_3: 2,2-dipropylpentanenitrile.

01/2005:1058
corrected

VANCOMYCIN HYDROCHLORIDE

Vancomycini hydrochloridum

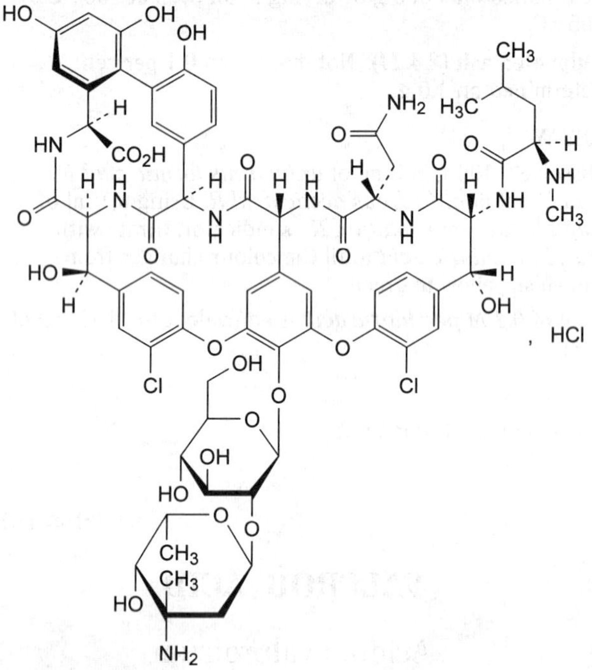

$C_{66}H_{76}Cl_3N_9O_{24}$ M_r 1486

DEFINITION

Vancomycin hydrochloride is the hydrochloride of a mixture of related glycopeptides, consisting principally of the monohydrochloride of (3*S*,6*R*,7*R*,22*R*,23*S*,26*S*,a*S*,36*R*,38a*R*)-3-(2-amino-2-oxoethyl)-44-[[2-*O*-(3-amino-2,3,6-trideoxy-3-*C*-methyl-α-L-*lyxo*-hexopyranosyl)-β-D-glucopyranosyl]oxy]-10,19-dichloro-7,22,28,30,32-pentahydroxy-6-[[(2*R*)-4-methyl-2-(methylamino)pentanoyl]amino]-2,5,24,38,39-pentaoxo-2,3,4,5,6,7,23,24,25,26,36,37,38,38a-tetradecahydro-22*H*-8,11:18,21-dietheno-23,36-(iminomethano)-13,16:31,35-dimetheno-1*H*,13*H*-[1,6,9]oxadiazacyclohexadecino[4,5-*m*][10,2,16]benzoxadiazacyclotetracosine-26-carboxylic acid (vancomycin B), a substance produced by certain strains of *Amycolatopsis orientalis* or obtained by any other means. The potency is not less than 1050 IU/mg, calculated with reference to the anhydrous substance.

CHARACTERS

A white or almost white powder, hygroscopic, freely soluble in water, slightly soluble in alcohol.

IDENTIFICATION

A. Examine the chromatograms obtained in the test for vancomycin B. The retention time of the principal peak in the chromatogram obtained with test solution (a) is similar to that of the principal peak in the chromatogram obtained with the reference solution.

B. It gives reaction (a) of chlorides (*2.3.1*).

TESTS

Appearance of solution. Dissolve 2.50 g in *water R* and dilute to 25.0 ml with the same solvent. The solution is clear (*2.2.1*).The absorbance (*2.2.25*) of the solution measured at 450 nm is not greater than 0.10.

pH (*2.2.3*). Dissolve 0.50 g in *carbon dioxide-free water R* and dilute to 10 ml with the same solvent. The pH of the solution is 2.5 to 4.5.

Vancomycin B. Not less than 93.0 per cent, determined by liquid chromatography (*2.2.29*).

Test solution (a). Dissolve 10.0 mg of the substance to be examined in mobile phase A and dilute to 5.0 ml with mobile phase A.

Test solution (b). Dilute 2.0 ml of test solution (a) to 50.0 ml with mobile phase A.

Test solution (c). Dilute 0.5 ml of test solution (b) to 20.0 ml with mobile phase A.

Reference solution. Dissolve the contents of a vial of *vancomycin hydrochloride CRS* in *water R* and dilute with the same solvent to obtain a solution containing 0.5 mg/ml. Heat at 65 °C for 24 h. Allow to cool.

Use the solutions within 4 h of preparation.

The chromatographic procedure may be carried out using:

- a stainless steel column 0.25 m long and 4.6 mm in internal diameter packed with *octadecylsilyl silica gel for chromatography R* (5 µm),
- as mobile phases at a flow rate of 1.0 ml/min the following solutions:

  Mobile phase A. To 4 ml of *triethylamine R* add 1996 ml of *water R* and adjust to pH 3.2 with *phosphoric acid R*; to 920 ml of this solution add 10 ml of *tetrahydrofuran R* and 70 ml of *acetonitrile R*,

  Mobile phase B. To 4 ml of *triethylamine R* add 1996 ml of *water R* and adjust to pH 3.2 with *phosphoric acid R*; to 700 ml of this solution add 10 ml of *tetrahydrofuran R* and 290 ml of *acetonitrile R*,
- as detector a spectrophotometer set at 280 nm,
- a 20 µl loop injector.

Record the chromatograms under the following conditions. Elute initially with mobile phase A. After 13 min, use gradient elution increasing the concentration of mobile phase B by 11 per cent *V/V* per minute. Finally, elute for 4 min using mobile phase B.

Inject test solution (c). The test is not valid unless the principal peak in the chromatogram obtained has a signal-to-noise ratio of at least five. Inject test solution (b). The test is not valid unless the symmetry factor of the vancomycin peak is at most 1.6. Inject the reference solution. The test is not valid unless the resolution between the two principal peaks is at least 5.0. Inject test solution (a).

Calculate the percentage content of vancomycin B hydrochloride using the expression:

$$\frac{A_b \times 100}{A_b + \left(\frac{A_t}{25}\right)}$$

A_b = area of the peak corresponding to vancomycin B in the chromatogram obtained with test solution (b),

A_t = sum of the areas of the peaks corresponding to impurities in the chromatogram obtained with test solution (a).

Related substances. Examine by liquid chromatography (*2.2.29*), as described under the test for vancomycin B.

Inject separately test solution (a), test solution (b) and test solution (c). Calculate the percentage content of each impurity using the expression:

$$\frac{\left(\frac{A_i}{25}\right) \times 100}{A_b + \left(\frac{A_t}{25}\right)}$$

A_i = area of an impurity peak in the chromatogram obtained with test solution (a),

A_b = area of the peak corresponding to vancomycin B in the chromatogram obtained with test solution (b),

A_t = sum of the areas of the peaks corresponding to impurities in the chromatogram obtained with test solution (a).

The content of no impurity is greater than 4.0 per cent and the sum of the contents of impurities is not greater than 7.0 per cent. Disregard any peak with an area less than that of the principal peak in the chromatogram obtained with test solution (c).

Heavy metals (*2.4.8*). 1.0 g complies with limit test C for heavy metals (30 ppm). Prepare the standard using 3.0 ml of *lead standard solution (10 ppm Pb) R*.

Water (*2.5.12*). Not more than 5.0 per cent, determined on 0.500 g by the semi-micro determination of water.

Sulphated ash (*2.4.14*). Not more than 1.0 per cent, determined on 1.00 g.

Bacterial endotoxins (*2.6.14*): less than 0.25 IU/mg, if intended for use in the manufacture of parenteral dosage forms without a further appropriate procedure for the removal of bacterial endotoxins.

ASSAY

Carry out the microbiological assay of antibiotics (*2.7.2*). Use *vancomycin hydrochloride CRS* as the reference substance.

STORAGE

Store in an airtight container, protected from light. If the substance is sterile, store in a sterile, airtight, tamper-proof container.

LABELLING

The label states, where applicable, that the substance is free from bacterial endotoxins.

IMPURITIES

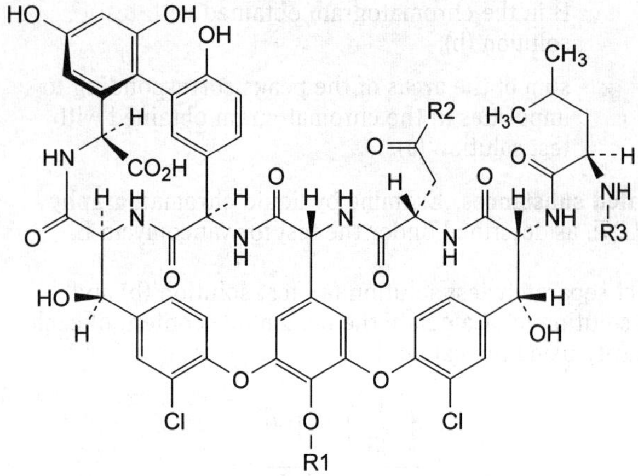

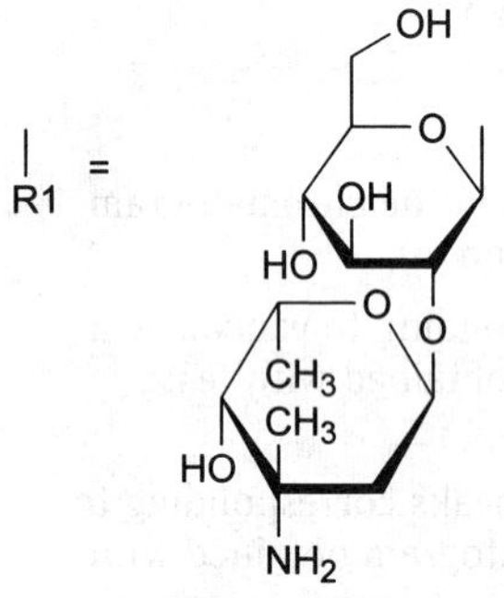

A. R2 = NH_2, R3 = H: *N*-demethylvancomycin B,

B. R2 = OH, R3 = CH_3: desamidovancomycin B,

C. R1 = H, R2 = NH_2, R3 = CH_3: aglucovancomycin B,

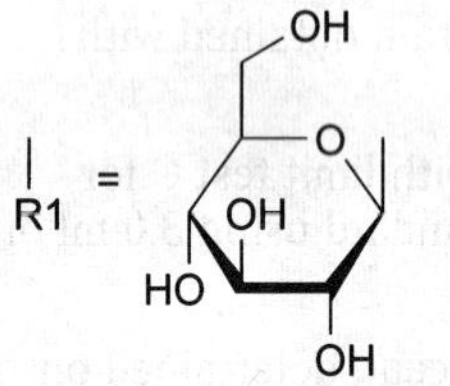

D. R2 = NH_2, R3 = CH_3: desvancosaminylvancomycin B.

01/2005:0747

VANILLIN

Vanillinum

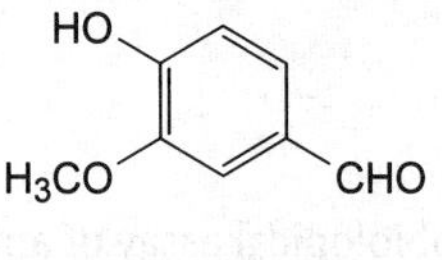

$C_8H_8O_3$ M_r 152.1

DEFINITION

Vanillin contains not less than 99.0 per cent and not more than the equivalent of 101.0 per cent of 4-hydroxy-3-methoxybenzaldehyde, calculated with reference to the dried substance.

CHARACTERS

White or slightly yellowish, crystalline powder or needles, slightly soluble in water, freely soluble in alcohol and in methanol. It dissolves in dilute solutions of alkali hydroxides.

IDENTIFICATION

First identification: B.

Second identification: A, C, D.

A. Melting point (*2.2.14*): 81 °C to 84 °C.

B. Examine by infrared absorption spectrophotometry (*2.2.24*), comparing with the spectrum obtained with *vanillin CRS*. Examine the substances prepared as discs.

C. Examine the chromatograms obtained in the test for related substances in daylight after spraying. The principal spot in the chromatogram obtained with test solution (b) is similar in position, colour and size to the principal spot in the chromatogram obtained with reference solution (a).

D. To 5 ml of a saturated solution of the substance to be examined add 0.2 ml of *ferric chloride solution R1*. A blue colour is produced. Heat to 80 °C. The solution becomes brown. On cooling, a white precipitate is formed.

TESTS

Appearance of solution. Dissolve 1.0 g in *alcohol R* and dilute to 20 ml with the same solvent. The solution is clear (*2.2.1*) and not more intensely coloured than reference solution B_6 (*2.2.2, Method II*).

Related substances. Examine by thin-layer chromatography (*2.2.27*), using *silica gel GF_{254} R* as the coating substance.

Test solution (a). Dissolve 0.1 g of the substance to be examined in *methanol R* and dilute to 5 ml with the same solvent.

Test solution (b). Dilute 1 ml of test solution (a) to 10 ml with *methanol R*.

Reference solution (a). Dissolve 10 mg of *vanillin CRS* in *methanol R* and dilute to 5 ml with the same solvent.

Reference solution (b). Dilute 0.5 ml of test solution (a) to 100 ml with *methanol R*.

Apply to the plate 5 µl of each solution. Develop in an unsaturated tank over a path of 10 cm using a mixture of 0.5 volumes of *anhydrous acetic acid R*, 1 volume of *methanol R* and 98.5 volumes of *methylene chloride R*. Dry the plate in a current of cold air. Examine in ultraviolet light at 254 nm. Any spot in the chromatogram obtained with test solution (a), apart from the principal spot, is not more intense than the spot in the chromatogram obtained with reference solution (b) (0.5 per cent). Spray with *dinitrophenylhydrazine-aceto-hydrochloric solution R* and examine in daylight. Any spot in the chromatogram obtained with test solution (a), apart from the principal spot, is not more intense than the spot in the chromatogram obtained with reference solution (b) (0.5 per cent).

Reaction with sulphuric acid. Dissolve 50 mg in 5 ml of *sulphuric acid R*. After 5 min, the solution is not more intensely coloured than a mixture of 4.9 ml of yellow primary solution and 0.1 ml of red primary solution or a mixture of 4.9 ml of yellow primary solution and 0.1 ml of blue primary solution (*2.2.2, Method I*).

Loss on drying (*2.2.32*). Not more than 1.0 per cent, determined on 1.000 g by drying in a desiccator for 4 h.

Sulphated ash (*2.4.14*). Not more than 0.05 per cent, determined on 2.0 g.

ASSAY

Dissolve 0.120 g in 20 ml of *alcohol R* and add 60 ml of *carbon dioxide-free water R*. Titrate with *0.1 M sodium hydroxide*, determining the end-point potentiometrically (*2.2.20*).

1 ml of *0.1 M sodium hydroxide* is equivalent to 15.21 mg of $C_8H_8O_3$.

STORAGE

Store protected from light.

01/2005:0573

VERAPAMIL HYDROCHLORIDE

Verapamili hydrochloridum

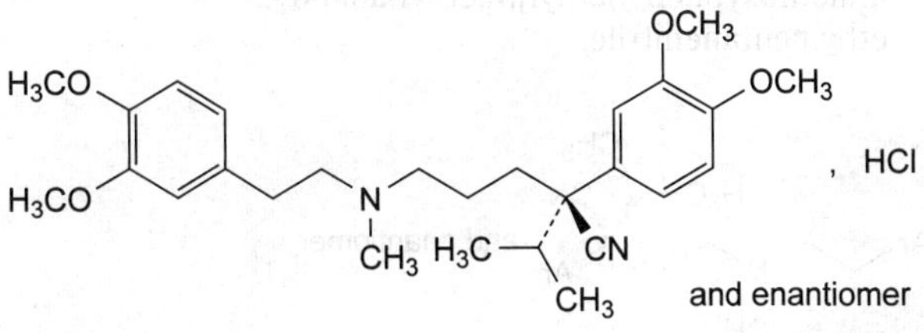

$C_{27}H_{39}ClN_2O_4$ M_r 491.1

DEFINITION

Verapamil hydrochloride contains not less than 99.0 per cent and not more than the equivalent of 101.0 per cent of (2*RS*)-2-(3,4-dimethoxyphenyl)-5-[[2-(3,4-dimethoxyphenyl)ethyl](methyl)amino]-2-(1-methylethyl)pentanenitrile hydrochloride, calculated with reference to the dried substance.

CHARACTERS

A white, crystalline powder, soluble in water, freely soluble in methanol, sparingly soluble in alcohol.

It melts at about 144 °C.

IDENTIFICATION

First identification: B, D.

Second identification: A, C, D.

A. Dissolve 20.0 mg in *0.01 M hydrochloric acid* and dilute to 100.0 ml with the same acid. Dilute 5.0 ml of this solution to 50.0 ml with *0.01 M hydrochloric acid.* Examined between 210 nm and 340 nm (*2.2.25*), the solution shows 2 absorption maxima, at 229 nm and 278 nm, and a shoulder at 282 nm. The ratio of the absorbance at the maximum at 278 nm to that at the maximum at 229 nm is 0.35 to 0.39.

B. Examine by infrared absorption spectrophotometry (*2.2.24*), comparing with the spectrum obtained with *verapamil hydrochloride CRS*. Examine the substances prepared as discs.

C. Examine by thin-layer chromatography (*2.2.27*), using as the coating substance a suitable silica gel with a fluorescent indicator having an optimal intensity at 254 nm.

Test solution. Dissolve 10 mg of the substance to be examined in *methylene chloride R* and dilute to 5 ml with the same solvent.

Reference solution (a). Dissolve 20 mg of *verapamil hydrochloride CRS* in *methylene chloride R* and dilute to 10 ml with the same solvent.

Reference solution (b). Dissolve 5 mg of *papaverine hydrochloride CRS* in reference solution (a) and dilute to 5 ml with the same solution.

Apply separately to the plate 5 µl of each solution. Develop over a path of 15 cm using a mixture of 15 volumes of *diethylamine R* and 85 volumes of *cyclohexane R.* Allow the plate to dry in air and examine in ultraviolet light at 254 nm. The principal spot in the chromatogram obtained with the test solution is similar in position and size to the principal spot in the chromatogram obtained with reference solution (a). The test is not valid unless the chromatogram obtained with reference solution (b) shows 2 clearly separated principal spots.

D. It gives reaction (b) of chlorides (*2.3.1*).

TESTS

Solution S. Dissolve 1.0 g in *carbon dioxide-free water R* while gently heating and dilute to 20.0 ml with the same solvent.

Appearance of solution. Solution S is clear (*2.2.1*) and colourless (*2.2.2, Method II*).

pH (*2.2.3*). The pH of solution S is 4.5 to 6.0.

Optical rotation (*2.2.7*). The angle of optical rotation, determined on solution S, is − 0.10° to + 0.10°.

Related substances. Examine by liquid chromatography (*2.2.29*).

Test solution. Dissolve 25.0 mg of the substance to be examined in the initial mobile phase composition and dilute to 10.0 ml with the same mobile phase.

Reference solution (a). Dissolve 5 mg of *verapamil hydrochloride CRS*, 5 mg of *verapamil impurity I CRS* and 5 mg of *verapamil impurity M CRS* in the initial mobile phase composition and dilute to 20 ml with the same mobile phase. Dilute 1 ml of this solution to 10 ml with the initial mobile phase composition.

Reference solution (b). Dilute 1.0 ml of the test solution to 100.0 ml with the initial mobile phase composition. Dilute 1.0 ml of this solution to 10.0 ml with the same mobile phase.

The chromatographic procedure may be carried out using:

- a stainless steel column 0.25 m long and 4.6 mm in internal diameter packed with *end-capped palmitamidopropylsilyl silica gel for chromatography R* (5 µm),
- as mobile phase at a flow rate of 1.5 ml/min a double isocratic programme using the following conditions:

  Mobile phase A. A 6.97 g/l solution of *dipotassium hydrogen phosphate R* adjusted to pH 7.20 with *phosphoric acid R,*

  Mobile phase B. Acetonitrile R,

Time (min)	Mobile phase A (per cent *V/V*)	Mobile phase B (per cent *V/V*)	Comment
0 - 22	63	37	first isocratic step
22 - 27	63 → 35	37 → 65	switch to second isocratic step
27 - 35	35	65	second isocratic step
35 - 36	35 → 63	65 → 37	switch to initial mobile phase
36 - 50	63	37	equilibration

- as detector a spectrophotometer set at 278 nm.

Equilibrate the column with the initial mobile phase composition for about 60 min.

Inject 10 µl of reference solution (a). When the chromatogram is recorded in the prescribed conditions the retention times are: verapamil, about 16 min, verapamil impurity I, about 21 min and verapamil impurity M about 32 min, eluting as a doublet. The test is not valid unless the resolution between the peaks corresponding to verapamil and verapamil impurity I is at least 5.0 and verapamil impurity M elutes from the column.

Adjust the sensitivity of the system so that the height of principal peak in the chromatogram obtained with 10 µl of the reference solution (b) is at least 15 per cent of the full scale of the recorder.

Inject separately 10 µl of the test solution and 10 µl of reference solution (b). In the chromatogram obtained with the test solution: the area of any peak, apart from the principal peak, is not greater than the area of the

Monographs T-Z

principal peak in the chromatogram obtained with reference solution (b) (0.1 per cent); the sum of the areas of the peaks, apart from the principal peak, is not greater than 3 times the area of the principal peak in the chromatogram obtained with reference solution (b) (0.3 per cent). Disregard any peak with an area less than 0.1 times the area of the principal peak in the chromatogram obtained with reference solution (b).

Heavy metals (*2.4.8*). 1.0 g complies with limit test C for heavy metals (10 ppm). Prepare the standard using 1 ml of *lead standard solution (10 ppm Pb) R.*

Loss on drying (*2.2.32*). Not more than 0.5 per cent, determined on 1.000 g by drying in an oven at 100 °C to 105 °C.

Sulphated ash (*2.4.14*). Not more than 0.1 per cent, determined on 1.0 g.

ASSAY

Dissolve 0.400 g in 50 ml of *ethanol R* and add 5.0 ml of *0.01 M hydrochloric acid.* Titrate with *0.1 M sodium hydroxide,* determining the end-point potentiometrically (*2.2.20*). Measure the volume of titrant required between the 2 points of inflexion.

1 ml of *0.1 M sodium hydroxide* is equivalent to 49.11 mg of $C_{27}H_{39}ClN_2O_4$.

STORAGE

Store protected from light.

IMPURITIES

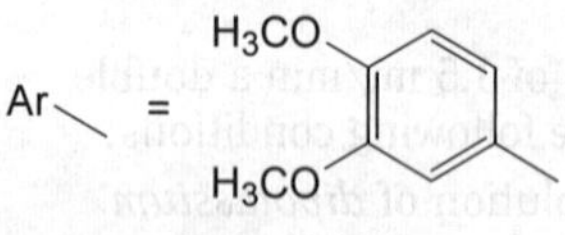

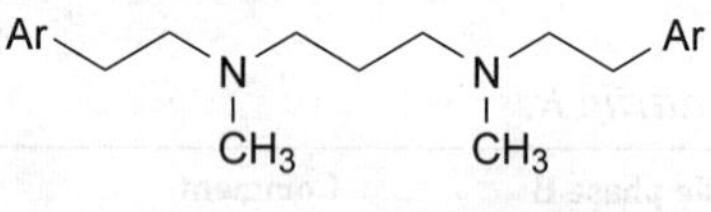

A. *N,N'*-bis[2-(3,4-dimethoxyphenyl)ethyl]-*N,N'*-dimethylpropane-1,3-diamine,

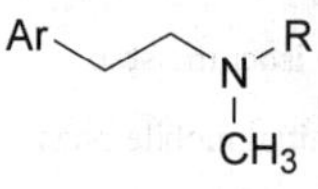

B. R = H: 2-(3,4-dimethoxyphenyl)-*N*-methylethanamine,

C. R = CH_3: 2-(3,4-dimethoxyphenyl)-*N,N*-dimethylethanamine,

D. R = CH_2-CH_2-CH_2-Cl: 3-chloro-*N*-[2-(3,4-dimethoxyphenyl)ethyl]-*N*-methylpropan-1-amine,

E. Ar-CH_2OH: (3,4-dimethoxyphenyl)methanol,

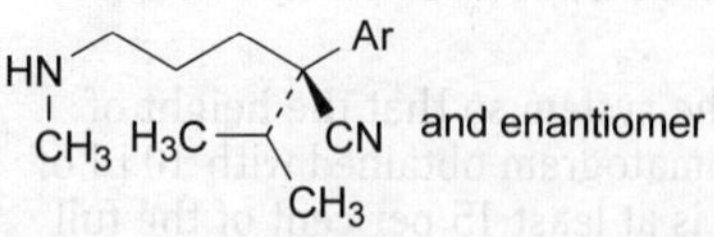

F. (2*RS*)-2-(3,4-dimethoxyphenyl)-5-(methylamino)-2-(1-methylethyl)pentanenitrile,

G. Ar-CHO: 3,4-dimethoxybenzaldehyde,

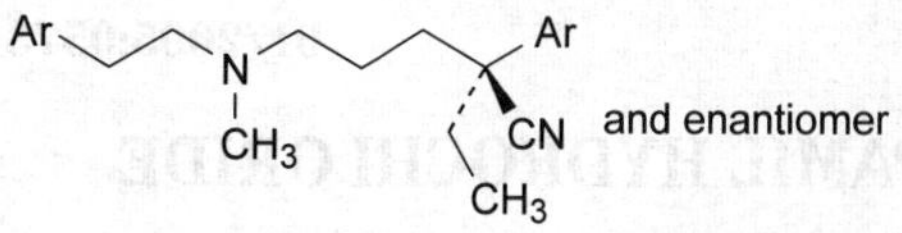

H. (2*RS*)-2-(3,4-dimethoxyphenyl)-5-[[2-(3,4-dimethoxyphenyl)ethyl](methyl)amino]-2-ethylpentanenitrile,

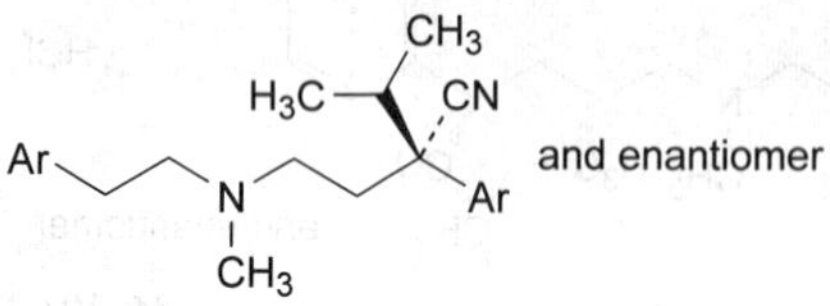

I. (2*RS*)-2-(3,4-dimethoxyphenyl)-2-[2-[[2-(3,4-dimethoxyphenyl)ethyl](methyl)amino]ethyl]-3-methylbutanenitrile,

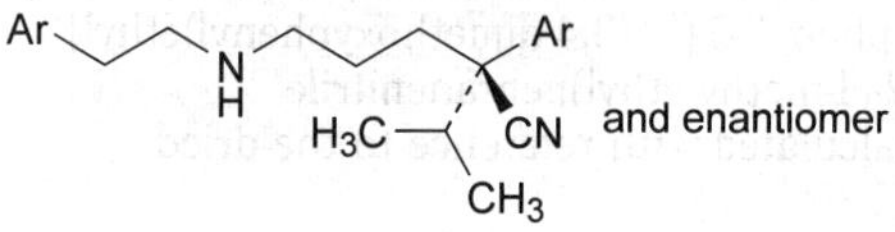

J. (2*RS*)-2-(3,4-dimethoxyphenyl)-5-[[2-(3,4-dimethoxyphenyl)ethyl]amino]-2-(1-methylethyl)pentanenitrile (*N*-norverapamil),

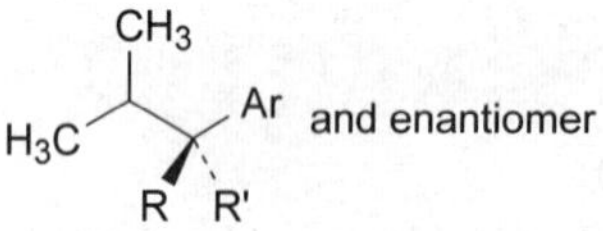

K. R = H, R′ = CN: (2*RS*)-2-(3,4-dimethoxyphenyl)-3-methylbutanenitrile,

L. R+ R′ = O: 1-(3,4-dimethoxyphenyl)-2-methylpropan-1-one,

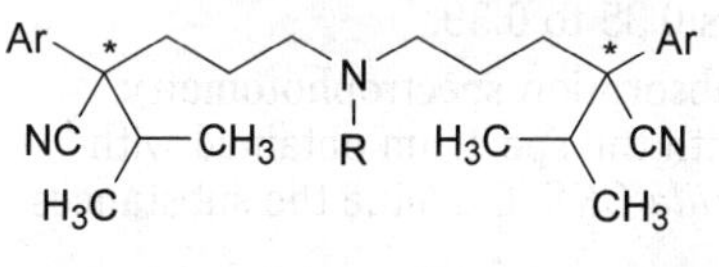

M. R = CH_2-CH_2-Ar: 5,5′-[[2-(3,4-dimethoxyphenyl)ethyl]imino]bis[2-(3,4-dimethoxyphenyl)-2-(1-methylethyl)pentanenitrile],

N. R = CH_3: 5,5′-(methylimino)bis[2-(3,4-dimethoxyphenyl)-2-(1-methylethyl)pentanenitrile],

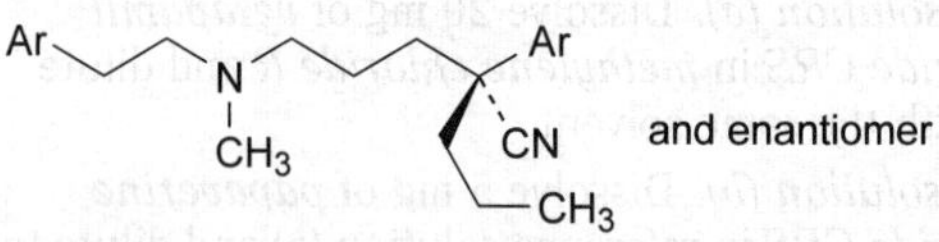

O. (2*RS*)-2-(3,4-dimethoxyphenyl)-5-[2-[2-(3,4-dimethoxyphenyl)ethyl](methyl)amino]- 2-propylpentanenitrile,

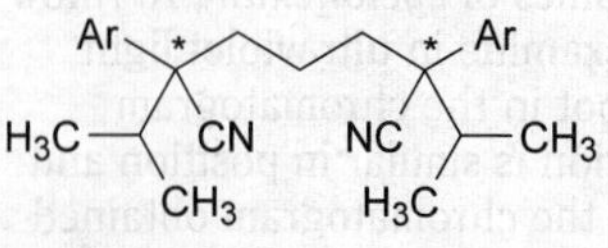

P. 2,6-bis(3,4-dimethoxyphenyl)-2,6-bis(1-methylethyl)-heptane-1,7-dinitrile.

01/2005:0748
corrected

VINBLASTINE SULPHATE

Vinblastini sulfas

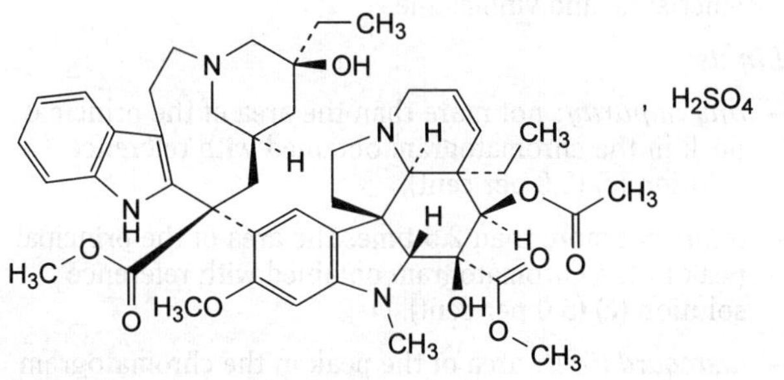

$C_{46}H_{60}N_4O_{13}S$ M_r 909

DEFINITION

Vinblastine sulphate contains not less than 95.0 per cent and not more than the equivalent of 104.0 per cent of methyl (3a*R*,4*R*,5*S*,5a*R*,10b*R*,13a*R*)-4-(acetyloxy)-3a-ethyl-9-[(5*S*,7*R*,9*S*)-5-ethyl-5-hydroxy-9-(methoxycarbonyl)-1,4,5,6,7,8,9,10-octahydro-2*H*-3,7-methanoazacycloundecino[5,4-*b*]indol-9-yl]-5-hydroxy-8-methoxy-6-methyl-3a,4,5,5a,6,11,12,13a-octahydro-1*H*-indolizino[8,1-*cd*]carbazole-5-carboxylate sulphate, calculated with reference to the dried substance.

CHARACTERS

A white or slightly yellowish, crystalline powder, very hygroscopic, freely soluble in water, practically insoluble in alcohol.

IDENTIFICATION

A. Examine by infrared absorption spectrophotometry (*2.2.24*), comparing with the *Ph. Eur. reference spectrum of vinblastine sulphate.*

B. Examine the chromatograms obtained in the assay. The principal peak in the chromatogram obtained with the test solution is similar in position and approximate size to the principal peak in the chromatogram obtained with reference solution (a).

TESTS

Solution S. Dissolve 50.0 mg in *carbon dioxide-free water R* and dilute to 10.0 ml with the same solvent.

Appearance of solution. Solution S is clear (*2.2.1*) and not more intensely coloured than reference solution Y_7 (*2.2.2, Method I*).

pH (*2.2.3*). Dilute 3 ml of solution S to 10 ml with *carbon dioxide-free water R*. The pH of this solution is 3.5 to 5.0.

Related substances. Examine the chromatograms obtained in the assay. In the chromatogram obtained with the test solution, the area of any peak apart from the principal peak is not greater than the area of the principal peak in the chromatogram obtained with reference solution (c) (2.0 per cent) and the sum of the areas of any such peaks is not greater than 2.5 times the area of the principal peak in the chromatogram obtained with reference solution (c) (5.0 per cent). Disregard any peak with an area less than that of the peak in the chromatogram obtained with reference solution (d).

Loss on drying. Not more than 15.0 per cent, determined on 3 mg by thermogravimetry (*2.2.34*). Heat to 200 °C at a rate of 5 °C/min, under a stream of *nitrogen for chromatography R*, at a flow rate of 40 ml/min.

ASSAY

Examine by liquid chromatography (*2.2.29*).

Keep the solutions in iced water before use.

Test solution. Dilute 1.0 ml of solution S (see Tests) to 5.0 ml with *water R*.

Reference solution (a). Dissolve the contents of a vial of *vinblastine sulphate CRS* in 5.0 ml of *water R* to obtain a concentration of 1.0 mg/ml.

Reference solution (b). Dissolve 1.0 mg of *vincristine sulphate CRS* in 1.0 ml of reference solution (a).

Reference solution (c). Dilute 1.0 ml of reference solution (a) to 50.0 ml with *water R*.

Reference solution (d). Dilute 1.0 ml of reference solution (c) to 20.0 ml with *water R*.

The chromatographic procedure may be carried out using:

- a stainless steel column 0.25 m long and 4.6 mm in internal diameter packed with *octylsilyl silica gel for chromatography R* (5 µm). Place between the injector and the column a guard column packed with suitable silica gel,
- as mobile phase at a flow rate of 1.0 ml/min a mixture of 38 volumes of a 1.5 per cent *V/V* solution of *diethylamine R* adjusted to pH 7.5 with *phosphoric acid R*, 12 volumes of *acetonitrile R* and 50 volumes of *methanol R*,
- as detector a spectrophotometer set at 262 nm,
- a loop injector.

Inject 10 µl of each solution and record the chromatograms for three times the retention time of the peak corresponding to vinblastine. The assay is not valid unless: in the chromatogram obtained with reference solution (b) the resolution between the peaks corresponding to vincristine and vinblastine is not less than four; the peak in the chromatogram obtained with reference solution (d) has a signal-to-noise ratio not less than five. Calculate the percentage content of $C_{46}H_{60}N_4O_{13}S$ from the area of the principal peak in each of the chromatograms obtained with the test solution and reference solution (a) and from the declared content of *vinblastine sulphate CRS*.

STORAGE

Store in an airtight, glass container, protected from light, at a temperature not exceeding − 20 °C. If the substance is sterile, store in an sterile, airtight, tamper-proof glass container.

01/2005:0749
corrected

VINCRISTINE SULPHATE

Vincristini sulfas

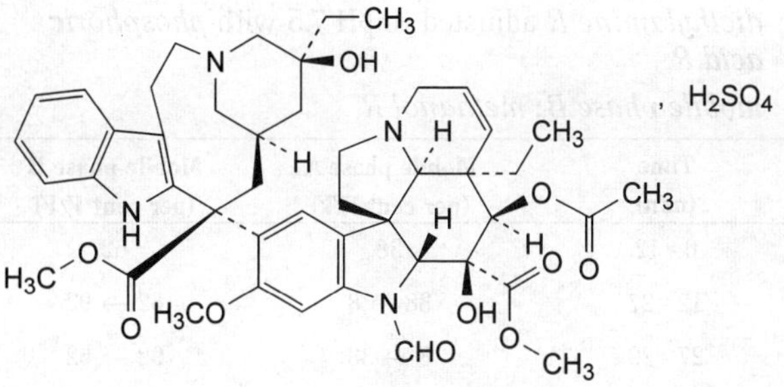

$C_{46}H_{58}N_4O_{14}S$ M_r 923

Monographs T-Z

DEFINITION

Methyl (3a*R*,4*R*,5*S*,5a*R*,10b*R*,13a*R*)-4-(acetyloxy)-3a-ethyl-9-[(5*S*,7*R*,9*S*)-5-ethyl-5-hydroxy-9-(methoxycarbonyl)-1,4,5,6,7,8,9,10-octahydro-2*H*-3,7-methanoazacycloundecino[5,4-*b*]indol-9-yl]-6-formyl-5-hydroxy-8-methoxy-3a,4,5,5a,6,11,12,13a-octahydro-1*H*-indolizino[8,1-*cd*]carbazole-5-carboxylate sulphate.

Content: 95.0 per cent to 104.0 per cent (dried substance).

CHARACTERS

Appearance: white or slightly yellowish, crystalline powder, very hygroscopic.

Solubility: freely soluble in water, slightly soluble in alcohol.

IDENTIFICATION

Infrared absorption spectrophotometry (*2.2.24*).

Comparison: *Ph. Eur. reference spectrum of vincristine sulphate*.

TESTS

Solution S. Dissolve 50.0 mg in *carbon dioxide-free water R* and dilute to 10.0 ml with the same solvent. *Keep the solution in iced water to carry out the test for related substances.*

Appearance of solution. Solution S is clear (*2.2.1*) and not more intensely coloured than reference solution Y_7 (*2.2.2, Method I*).

pH (*2.2.3*): 3.5 to 4.5.

Dilute 2 ml of solution S to 10 ml with *carbon dioxide-free water R*.

Related substances. Liquid chromatography (*2.2.29*). *Keep the solutions in iced water before use.*

Test solution. Dilute 1.0 ml of solution S to 5.0 ml with *water R*.

Reference solution (a). Dissolve the contents of a vial of *vincristine sulphate CRS* in 5.0 ml of *water R* to obtain a concentration of 1.0 mg/ml.

Reference solution (b). Dissolve 1.0 mg of *vinblastine sulphate CRS* in 1.0 ml of reference solution (a).

Reference solution (c). Dilute 1.0 ml of the test solution to 50.0 ml with *water R*.

Reference solution (d). Dilute 1.0 ml of reference solution (c) to 20.0 ml with *water R*.

Precolumn:

- *stationary phase*: *octylsilyl silica gel for chromatography R*.

Column:

- *size*: l = 0.25 m, Ø = 4.6 mm,
- *stationary phase*: *octylsilyl silica gel for chromatography R* (5 µm).

Mobile phase:

- *mobile phase A*: 1.5 per cent *V/V* solution of *diethylamine R* adjusted to pH 7.5 with *phosphoric acid R*,
- *mobile phase B*: *methanol R*,

Time (min)	Mobile phase A (per cent *V/V*)	Mobile phase B (per cent *V/V*)
0 - 12	38	62
12 - 27	38 → 8	62 → 92
27 - 29	8 → 38	92 → 62
29 - 34	38	62

Flow rate: 2 ml/min.

Detection: spectrophotometer at 297 nm.

Injection: 20 µl.

System suitability: reference solution (b):

- *resolution*: minimum 4 between the peaks due to vincristine and vinblastine.

Limits:

- *any impurity*: not more than the area of the principal peak in the chromatogram obtained with reference solution (c) (2.0 per cent),
- *total*: not more than 2.5 times the area of the principal peak in the chromatogram obtained with reference solution (c) (5.0 per cent),
- *disregard limit*: area of the peak in the chromatogram obtained with reference solution (d) (0.1 per cent).

Loss on drying: maximum 12.0 per cent, determined on 3 mg by thermogravimetry (*2.2.34*). Heat the substance to be examined to 200 °C increasing the temperature by 5 °C/min, under a current of *nitrogen for chromatography R*, at a flow rate of 40 ml/min.

ASSAY

Liquid chromatography (*2.2.29*) as described in the test for related substances, with the following modifications.

Mobile phase: mix 30 volumes of a 1.5 per cent *V/V* solution of *diethylamine R* adjusted to pH 7.5 with *phosphoric acid R* and 70 volumes of *methanol R*.

Flow rate: 1.0 ml/min.

Calculate the percentage content of $C_{46}H_{58}N_4O_{14}S$ using the chromatogram obtained with reference solution (a) and the declared content of *vincristine sulphate CRS*.

STORAGE

In an airtight, glass container, protected from light, at a temperature not exceeding − 20 °C. If the substance is sterile, store in a sterile, airtight, tamper-proof glass container.

IMPURITIES

Specified impurities: A, B, C, D, H.

Other detectable impurities: E, F, G.

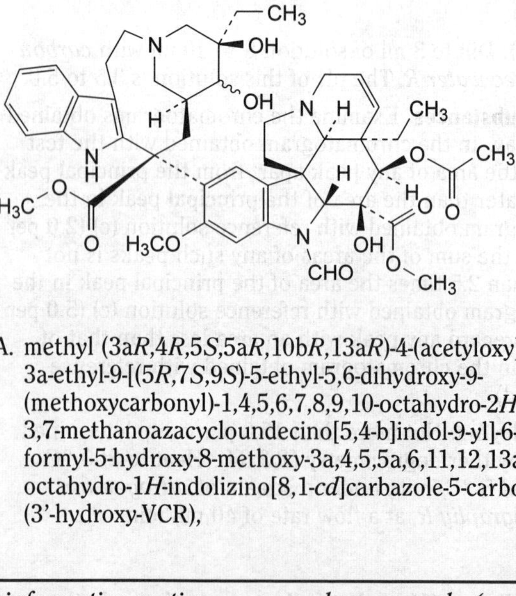

A. methyl (3a*R*,4*R*,5*S*,5a*R*,10b*R*,13a*R*)-4-(acetyloxy)-3a-ethyl-9-[(5*R*,7*S*,9*S*)-5-ethyl-5,6-dihydroxy-9-(methoxycarbonyl)-1,4,5,6,7,8,9,10-octahydro-2*H*-3,7-methanoazacycloundecino[5,4-b]indol-9-yl]-6-formyl-5-hydroxy-8-methoxy-3a,4,5,5a,6,11,12,13a-octahydro-1*H*-indolizino[8,1-*cd*]carbazole-5-carboxylate (3'-hydroxy-VCR),

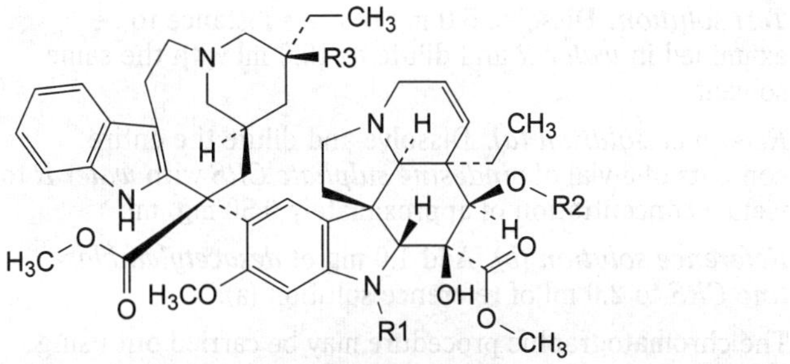

B. R1 = CHO, R2 = CO-CH_3, R3 = H: methyl (3a*R*,4*R*,5*S*,5a*R*,10b*R*,13a*R*)-4-(acetyloxy)-3a-ethyl-9-[(5*R*,7*S*,9*S*)-5-ethyl-9-(methoxycarbonyl)-1,4,5,6,7,8,9,10-octahydro-2*H*-3,7-methanoazacycloundecino[5,4-*b*]indol-9-yl]-6-formyl-5-hydroxy-8-methoxy-3a,4,5,5a,6,11,12,13a-octahydro-1*H*-indolizino[8,1-*cd*]carbazole-5-carboxylate (4′-deoxyvincristine),

C. R1 = H, R2 = CO-CH_3, R3 = OH: methyl (3a*R*,4*R*,5*S*,5a*R*,10b*S*,13a*R*)-4-(acetyloxy)-3a-ethyl-9-[(5*S*,7*R*,9*S*)-5-ethyl-5-hydroxy-9-(methoxycarbonyl)-1,4,5,6,7,8,9,10-octahydro-2*H*-3,7-methanoazacycloundecino[5,4-*b*]indol-9-yl]-5-hydroxy-8-methoxy-3a,4,5,5a,6,11,12,13a-octahydro-1*H*-indolizino[8,1-*cd*]carbazole-5-carboxylate (*N*-desmethylvinblastine),

D. R1 = CHO, R2 = H, R3 = OH: methyl (3a*R*,4*R*,5*S*,5a*R*,10b*R*,13a*R*)-3a-ethyl-9-[(5*S*,7*R*,9*S*)-5-ethyl-5-hydroxy-9-(methoxycarbonyl)-1,4,5,6,7,8,9,10-octahydro-2*H*-3,7-methanoazacycloundecino[5,4-*b*]indol-9-yl]-6-formyl-4,5-dihydroxy-8-methoxy-3a,4,5,5a,6,11,12,13a-octahydro-1*H*-indolizino[8,1-*cd*]carbazole-5-carboxylate (deacetylvincristine),

E. R1 = CH_3, R2 = H, R3 = OH: methyl (3a*R*,4*R*,5*S*,5a*R*,10b*R*,13a*R*)-3a-ethyl-9-[(5*S*,7*R*,9*S*)-5-ethyl-5-hydroxy-9-(methoxycarbonyl)-1,4,5,6,7,8,9,10-octahydro-2*H*-3,7-methanoazacycloundecino[5,4-*b*]indol-9-yl]-4,5-dihydroxy-8-methoxy-6-methyl-3a,4,5,5a,6,11,12,13a-octahydro-1*H*-indolizino[8,1-*cd*]carbazole-5-carboxylate (deacetylvinblastine),

H. R1 = CH_3, R2 = CO-CH_3, R3 = OH: vinblastine,

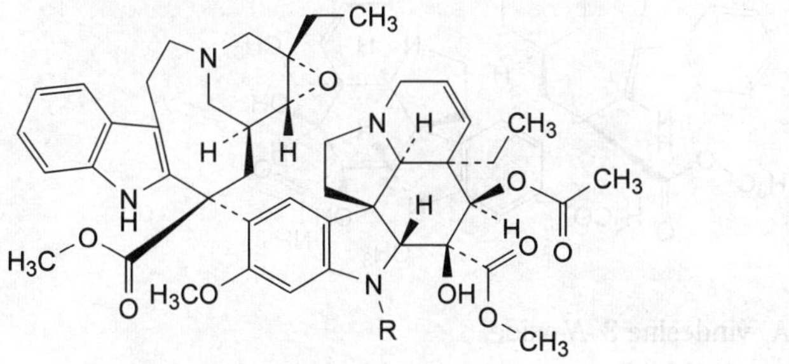

F. R = CH_3: methyl (3a*R*,4*R*,5*S*,5a*R*,10b*R*,13a*R*)-4-(acetyloxy)-3a-ethyl-9-[(1a*S*,11*S*,13*S*,13a*R*)-1a-ethyl-11-(methoxycarbonyl)-1a,4,5,10,11,12,13,13a-octahydro-2*H*-3,13-methano-oxireno[9,10]azacycloundecino[5,4-*b*]indol-11-yl]-5-hydroxy-8-methoxy-6-methyl-3a,4,5,5a,6,11,12,13a-octahydro-1*H*-indolizino[8,1-*cd*]carbazole-5-carboxylate (leurosine),

G. R = CHO: methyl (3a*R*,4*R*,5*S*,5a*R*,10b*R*,13a*R*)-4-(acetyloxy)-3a-ethyl-9-[(1a*S*,11*S*,13*S*,13a*R*)-1a-ethyl-11-(methoxycarbonyl)-1a,4,5,10,11,12,13,13a-octahydro-2*H*-3,13-methano-oxireno[9,10]azacycloundecino[5,4-*b*]indol-11-yl]-6-formyl-5-hydroxy-8-methoxy-3a,4,5,5a,6,11,12,13a-octahydro-1*H*-indolizino[8,1-*cd*]carbazole-5-carboxylate (formylleurosine).

01/2005:1276

VINDESINE SULPHATE

Vindesini sulfas

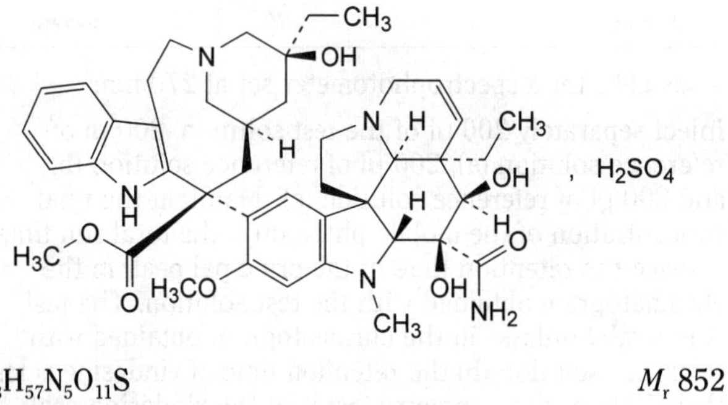

$C_{43}H_{57}N_5O_{11}S$ M_r 852

DEFINITION

Vindesine sulphate contains not less than 96.0 per cent and not more than the equivalent of 103.0 per cent of methyl (5*S*,7*R*,9*S*)-9-[(3a*R*,4*R*,5*S*,5a*R*,10b*R*,13a*R*)-5-carbamoyl-3a-ethyl-4,5-dihydroxy-8-methoxy-6-methyl-3a,4,5,5a,6,11,12,13a-octahydro-1*H*-indolizino[8,1-*cd*]carbazol-9-yl]-5-ethyl-5-hydroxy-1,4,5,6,7,8,9,10-octahydro-2*H*-3,7-methanoazacycloundecino[4,5-*b*]indole-9-carboxylate sulphate, calculated with reference to the dried substance.

CHARACTERS

A white or almost white, amorphous substance, hygroscopic, freely soluble in water and in methanol, practically insoluble in cyclohexane.

IDENTIFICATION

Examine by infrared absorption spectrophotometry (*2.2.24*), comparing with the *Ph. Eur. reference spectrum of vindesine sulphate*.

TESTS

Solution S. Dissolve 50 mg in *carbon dioxide-free water R* and dilute to 10 ml with the same solvent.

Appearance of solution. Solution S is clear (*2.2.1*) and not more intensely coloured than reference solution Y_7 (*2.2.2, Method I*).

pH (*2.2.3*). The pH of solution S is 3.5 to 5.5.

Related substances. Examine by liquid chromatography (*2.2.29*). *Keep the solutions in iced water before use.*

Test solution. Dissolve 10.0 mg of the substance to be examined in *water R* and dilute to 10.0 ml with the same solvent.

Reference solution (a). Dilute 1.0 ml of the test solution to 50.0 ml with *water R.*

Reference solution (b). Dissolve 1.0 mg of *desacetylvinblastine CRS* in *water R,* add 1.0 ml of the test solution and dilute to 50.0 ml with *water R.*

Reference solution (c). Dilute 1.0 ml of reference solution (a) to 200.0 ml with *water R.*

The chromatographic procedure may be carried out using:

– a stainless steel column 0.15 m long and 4.6 mm in internal diameter packed with *octadecylsilyl silica gel for chromatography R* (5 µm),

– as mobile phase at a flow rate of 2 ml/min:

Mobile phase A. A 1.5 per cent *V/V* solution of *diethylamine R* adjusted to pH 7.4 with *phosphoric acid R,*

Mobile phase B. Methanol R,

Time (min)	Mobile phase A (per cent *V/V*)	Mobile phase B (per cent *V/V*)	Comment
	49	51	equilibration
0 - 40	49	51	isocratic
40 - 49	49 → 30	51 → 70	linear gradient
49 - end	30	70	isocratic

– as detector a spectrophotometer set at 270 nm.

Inject separately 200 µl of the test solution, 200 µl of reference solution (a), 200 µl of reference solution (b) and 200 µl of reference solution (c). Maintain the final concentration of the mobile phase until the total run time is twice the retention time of the principal peak in the chromatogram obtained with the test solution. The test is not valid unless: in the chromatogram obtained with reference solution (b) the retention time of vindesine is less than 40 min; the symmetry factor of the vindesine peak is not more than 2.0; and the resolution of the vindesine and desacetylvinblastine peaks is at least 2.0. In the chromatogram obtained with the test solution: the area of any peak apart from the principal peak is not greater than half of the area of the principal peak in the chromatogram obtained with reference solution (a) (1 per cent); and the sum of the areas of any such peaks is not greater than the area of the principal peak in the chromatogram obtained with reference solution (a) (2 per cent). Disregard any peak with an area less than the area of the principal peak in the chromatogram obtained with reference solution (c).

Acetonitrile. Not more than 1.5 per cent *m/m* of acetonitrile, determined by gas chromatography (*2.2.28*).

Internal standard solution (a). Dilute 0.500 g of *propanol R* to 100 ml with *water R.*

Internal standard solution (b). Dilute 10.0 ml of internal standard solution (a) to 50.0 ml with *water R.*

Reference solution. Dilute 10.0 g of *acetonitrile R* to 1000 ml with *water R.* To 3.0 ml of this solution add 10.0 ml of internal standard solution (a) and dilute to 50.0 ml with *water R.*

Test solution. Dissolve 40 mg of the substance to be examined in 1.0 ml of internal standard solution (b).

The chromatographic procedure may be carried out using:

– a glass column 1.25 m long and 3 mm in internal diameter packed with *ethylvinylbenzene-divinylbenzene copolymer R,*

– *helium for chromatography R* as the carrier gas at a flow rate of 60 ml/min,

– a flame-ionisation detector,

maintaining the temperature of the column at 170 °C and that of the injection port and of the detector at 250 °C.

Inject 3 µl of the reference solution. The test is not valid unless the resolution between acetonitrile and propanol is greater than 1.5 and the symmetry factor for the acetonitrile peak is not greater than 1.6.

Inject 3 µl of the reference solution and 3 µl of the test solution.

Loss on drying. Not more than 10.0 per cent, determined on 9.00 mg by thermogravimetry (*2.2.34*). Heat to 200 °C at a rate of 5 °C/min, under a current of *nitrogen for chromatography R* at a flow rate of 40 ml/min.

ASSAY

Examine by liquid chromatography (*2.2.29*). *Keep the solutions in iced water before use.*

Test solution. Dissolve 5.0 mg of the substance to be examined in *water R* and dilute to 10.0 ml with the same solvent.

Reference solution (a). Dissolve and dilute the entire contents of a vial of *vindesine sulphate CRS* with *water R* to yield a concentration of approximately 0.50 mg/ml.

Reference solution (b). Add 1.0 mg of *desacetylvinblastine CRS* to 2.0 ml of reference solution (a).

The chromatographic procedure may be carried out using:

– a stainless steel column 0.15 m long and 4.6 mm in internal diameter packed with *octadecylsilyl silica gel for chromatography R* (5 µm),

– as mobile phase at a flow rate of 1 ml/min a mixture of 38 volumes of a 1.5 per cent *V/V* solution of *diethylamine R,* previously adjusted to pH 7.4 with *phosphoric acid R,* and 62 volumes of *methanol R,*

– as detector a spectrophotometer set at 270 nm.

Inject 20 µl of reference solution (b) five times. The test is not valid unless: the resolution between the peaks corresponding to vindesine sulphate and desacetylvinblastine sulphate is greater than 1.5; the symmetry factor of the vindesine peak is not more than 2.0; and the coefficient of variation of the area of the vindesine peak, calculated on the five injections is not greater than 1.5 per cent.

Inject separately 20 µl of the test solution and 20 µl of reference solution (a).

Calculate the content of vindesine sulphate ($C_{43}H_{57}N_5O_{11}S$) using the stated content of *vindesine sulphate CRS.*

STORAGE

Store in an airtight polypropylene container with a polypropylene cap, at a temperature not exceeding −50 °C. If the substance is sterile, store in a sterile, airtight, tamper-proof container.

IMPURITIES

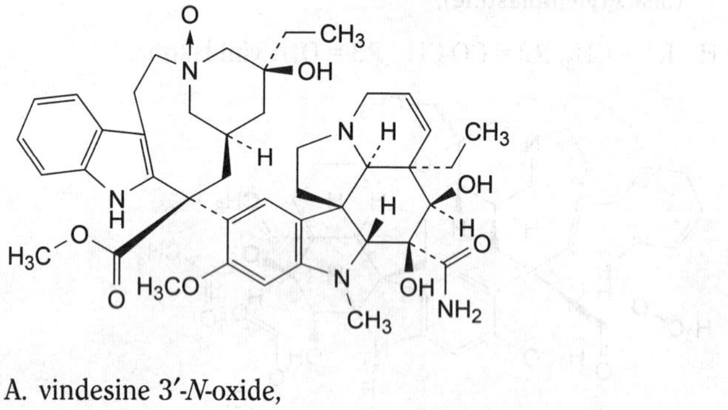

A. vindesine 3′-*N*-oxide,

B. vinblastine,

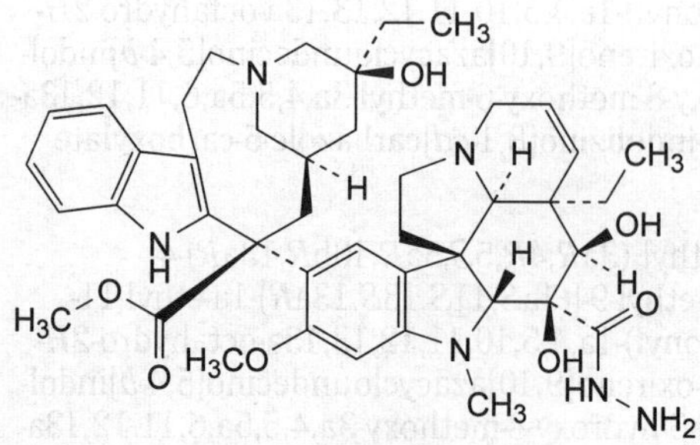

C. desacetylvinblastine hydrazide.

01/2005:2107

VINORELBINE TARTRATE

Vinorelbini tartras

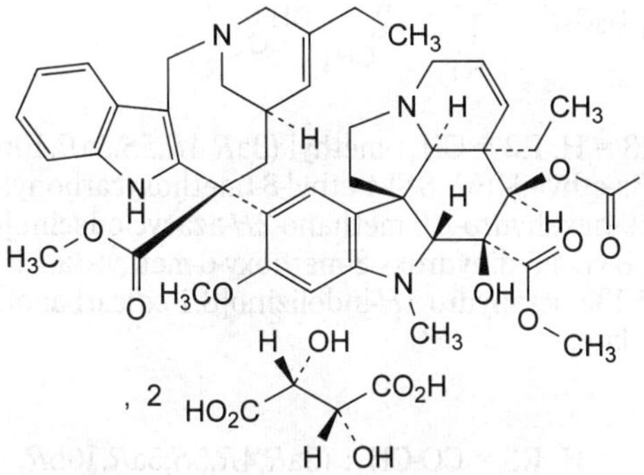

$C_{53}H_{66}N_4O_{20}$ M_r 1079

DEFINITION

Methyl (3a*R*,4*R*,5*S*,5a*R*,10b*R*,13a*R*)-4-(acetyloxy)-3a-ethyl-9-[(6*R*,8*S*)-4-ethyl-8-(methoxycarbonyl)-1,3,6,7,8,9-hexahydro-2,6-methano-2*H*-azacyclodecino[4,3-*b*]indol-8-yl]-5-hydroxy-8-methoxy-6-methyl-3a,4,5,5a,6,11,12,13a-octahydro-1*H*-indolizino[8,1-*cd*]carbazole-5-carboxylate dihydrogen bis[(2*R*,3*R*)-2,3-dihydroxybutanedioate].

Content: 98.0 per cent to 102.0 per cent (anhydrous substance).

CHARACTERS

Appearance: white or almost white powder, hygroscopic.

Solubility: freely soluble in water and in methanol, practically insoluble in hexane.

IDENTIFICATION

A. Infrared absorption spectrophotometry (*2.2.24*).

Preparation: dissolve 10 mg in 5 ml of *water R*. Add 0.5 ml of *sodium hydroxide solution R*. Extract with 5 ml of *methylene chloride R*. Dry the organic layer over *anhydrous sodium sulphate R*, filter and reduce its volume to about 0.5 ml by evaporation and apply to a disc of *potassium bromide R*. Evaporate and record the spectrum.

Comparison: *vinorelbine tartrate CRS*, treated as described above.

B. It gives reaction (b) of tartrates (*2.3.1*).

TESTS

Solution S. Dissolve a quantity equivalent to 140.0 mg of the anhydrous substance in *water R* and dilute to 10.0 ml with the same solvent.

Appearance of solution. Solution S is clear (*2.2.1*) and its absorbance (*2.2.25*) at 420 nm is maximum 0.030.

pH (*2.2.3*): 3.3 to 3.8 for solution S.

Related substances. Liquid chromatography (*2.2.29*): use the normalisation procedure.

Test solution. Dissolve 35.0 mg of the substance to be examined in the mobile phase and dilute to 25 ml with the mobile phase.

Reference solution (a). Dissolve 7 mg of *vinorelbine impurity B CRS* in *water R* and dilute to 50 ml with the same solvent. To 1 ml of this solution add 14 mg of *vinorelbine tartrate CRS*, dissolve in *water R* and dilute to 10 ml with the same solvent. Expose this solution for 1 h to a xenon lamp apparatus at a wavelength of 310-880 nm, supplying a dose of 1600 kJ/m^2 at a fluence rate of 500 W/m^2 in order to generate impurity A.

Reference solution (b). Dilute 1.0 ml of the test solution to 20.0 ml with *water R*. Dilute 1.0 ml of this solution to 100.0 ml with the mobile phase.

Column:

- *size*: l = 0.15 m, Ø = 3.9 mm,
- *stationary phase*: spherical *end-capped octadecylsilyl silica gel for chromatography R* (5 µm) with a specific surface area of 125 m^2/g, a pore size of 30 nm and a carbon loading of 7 per cent,
- *temperature*: 35 ± 5 °C.

Mobile phase: dissolve 1.22 g of *sodium decanesulphonate R* in 620 ml of *methanol R* and add 380 ml of a 7.80 g/l solution of *sodium dihydrogen phosphate R* previously adjusted to pH 4.2 with *dilute phosphoric acid R*.

Flow rate: 1.0 ml/min.

Detection: spectrophotometer at 267 nm.

Injection: 20 µl.

Run time: twice the retention time of vinorelbine.

Relative retention with reference to vinorelbine (retention time = about 14 min): impurity A = about 0.8; impurity B = about 1.2.

System suitability:

- *peak-to-valley ratio*: minimum 4, where H_p = height above the baseline of the peak due to impurity B and H_v = height above the baseline of the lowest point of the curve separating this peak from the peak due to vinorelbine in the chromatogram obtained with reference solution (a),
- *signal-to-noise ratio*: minimum 10 for the principal peak in the chromatogram obtained with reference solution (b).

Limits:

- *impurity A*: maximum 0.3 per cent,
- *any other impurity*: for each impurity, maximum 0.2 per cent,
- *total of impurities other than A*: maximum 0.7 per cent,
- *disregard limit*: the area of the principal peak in the chromatogram obtained with reference solution (b).

Boron: maximum 50 ppm.

Test solution. Dissolve 0.10 g of the substance to be examined in 2 ml of *water R*. Slowly add 10.0 ml of *sulphuric acid R* while cooling in iced water. Stir and allow to warm to room temperature. Add 10.0 ml of a 0.5 g/l solution of *carminic acid R* in *sulphuric acid R*.

Reference solution. Dilute 2.5 ml of a 0.572 g/l solution of *boric acid R* to 100.0 ml with *water R*. To 2.0 ml of this solution slowly add 10.0 ml of *sulphuric acid R* while cooling in iced water. Stir and allow to warm to room temperature. Add 10.0 ml of a 0.5 g/l solution of *carminic acid R* in *sulphuric acid R*.

Blank solution. To 2.0 ml of *water R* slowly add 10.0 ml of *sulphuric acid R* while cooling in iced water. Stir and allow to warm to room temperature. Add 10.0 ml of a 0.5 g/l solution of *carminic acid R* in *sulphuric acid R*.

After 45 min, measure the absorbance (*2.2.25*) of the test solution and the reference solution, between 560 nm and 650 nm, using the blank solution as compensation liquid. The maximum absorbance value of the test solution is not greater than that of the reference solution.

Fluorides: maximum 50 ppm.

Potentiometry (*2.2.36, Method I*) using a fluoride-selective indicator electrode and a silver-silver chloride reference electrode.

Monographs T-Z

Test solution. Dissolve 0.19 g of the substance to be examined in 20 ml of *water R*. Add 5.0 ml of *total-ionic-strength-adjustment buffer R* and dilute to 50 ml with *water R*.

Reference solutions. To 0.6 ml, 0.8 ml, 1.0 ml, 1.2 ml and 1.4 ml of *fluoride standard solution (10 ppm F) R*, add 5.0 ml of *total-ionic-strength-adjustment buffer R* and dilute to 50 ml with *water R*.

Introduce the electrodes into the reference solutions and allow to stand for 5 min. Determine the potential difference between the electrodes after 1 min of stabilisation. Using semi-logarithmic paper plot the potential difference obtained for each reference solution as a function of concentration of fluoride. Using exactly the same conditions, determine the potential difference obtained with the test solution and calculate the content of fluoride.

Silver: maximum 5 ppm.

Atomic absorption spectrometry (*2.2.23, Method I*).

Test solution. Dissolve 0.500 g of the substance to be examined in 10.0 ml of *water R*.

Reference solutions. Prepare the reference solutions using *silver standard solution (5 ppm Ag) R* and diluting with a 6.5 per cent *V/V* solution of *lead-free nitric acid R*.

Source: silver hollow-cathode lamp.

Wavelength: 328.1 nm.

Atomisation device: air-acetylene flame.

Water (*2.5.12*): maximum 4.0 per cent, determined on 0.250 g.

Bacterial endotoxins (*2.6.14*): less than 2 IU/mg (expressed as vinorelbine base), if intended for use in the manufacture of parenteral dosage forms without a further appropriate procedure for the removal of bacterial endotoxins.

ASSAY

Dissolve 0.350 g in 40 ml of *glacial acetic acid R*. Titrate with *0.1 M perchloric acid*, determining the end-point potentiometrically (*2.2.20*).

1 ml of *0.1 M perchloric acid* is equivalent to 53.96 mg of $C_{53}H_{66}N_4O_{20}$.

STORAGE

Under an inert gas, protected from light, at a temperature not exceeding − 15 °C.

LABELLING

The label states, where applicable, that the substance is free from bacterial endotoxins.

IMPURITIES

Specified impurities: A.

Other detectable impurities: B, C, D, E, F, G, H, I, J.

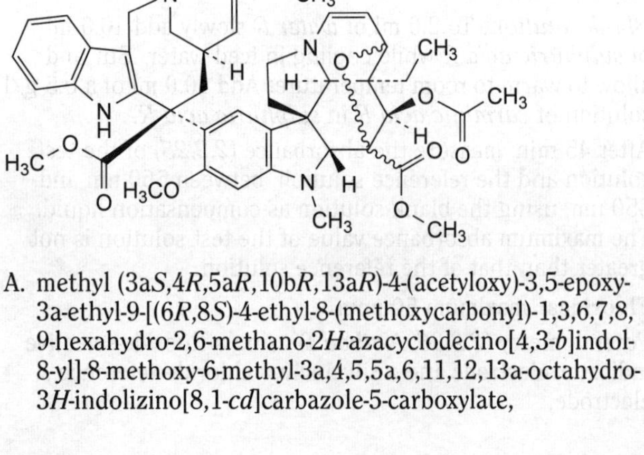

A. methyl (3a*S*,4*R*,5a*R*,10b*R*,13a*R*)-4-(acetyloxy)-3,5-epoxy-3a-ethyl-9-[(6*R*,8*S*)-4-ethyl-8-(methoxycarbonyl)-1,3,6,7,8,9-hexahydro-2,6-methano-2*H*-azacyclodecino[4,3-*b*]indol-8-yl]-8-methoxy-6-methyl-3a,4,5,5a,6,11,12,13a-octahydro-3*H*-indolizino[8,1-*cd*]carbazole-5-carboxylate,

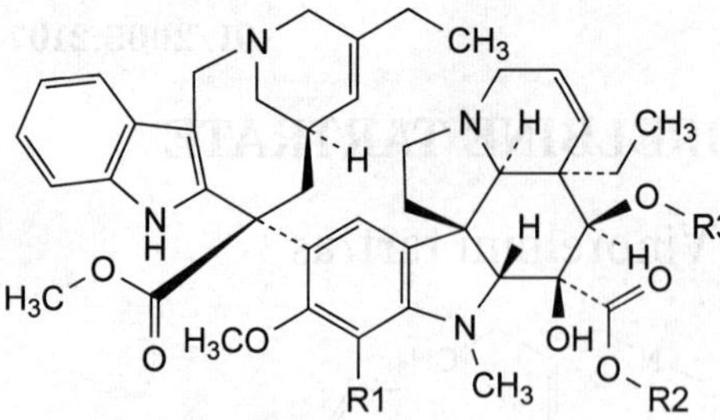

B. R1 = R3 = H, R2 = CH_3: methyl (3a*R*,4*R*,5*S*,5a*R*,10b*R*,13a*R*)-3a-ethyl-9-[(6*R*,8*S*)-4-ethyl-8-(methoxycarbonyl)-1,3,6,7,8,9-hexahydro-2,6-methano-2*H*-azacyclodecino[4,3-*b*]indol-8-yl]-4,5-dihydroxy-8-methoxy-6-methyl-3a,4,5,5a,6,11,12,13a-octahydro-1*H*-indolizino[8,1-*cd*]carbazole-5-carboxylate,

H. R1 = R2 = H, R3 = CO-CH_3: (3a*R*,4*R*,5*S*,5a*R*,10b*R*,13a*R*)-4-(acetyloxy)-3a-ethyl-9-[(6*R*,8*S*)-4-ethyl-8-(methoxycarbonyl)-1,3,6,7,8,9-hexahydro-2,6-methano-2*H*-azacyclodecino[4,3-*b*]indol-8-yl]-5-hydroxy-8-methoxy-6-methyl-3a,4,5,5a,6,11,12,13a-octahydro-1*H*-indolizino[8,1-*cd*]carbazole-5-carboxylic acid,

I. R1 = Br, R2 = CH_3, R3 = CO-CH_3: methyl (3a*R*,4*R*,5*S*,5a*R*,10b*R*,13a*R*)-4-(acetyloxy)-7-bromo-3a-ethyl-9-[(6*R*,8*S*)-4-ethyl-8-(methoxycarbonyl)-1,3,6,7,8,9-hexahydro-2,6-methano-2*H*-azacyclodecino[4,3-*b*]indol-8-yl]-5-hydroxy-8-methoxy-6-methyl-3a,4,5,5a,6,11,12,13a-octahydro-1*H*-indolizino[8,1-*cd*]carbazole-5-carboxylate,

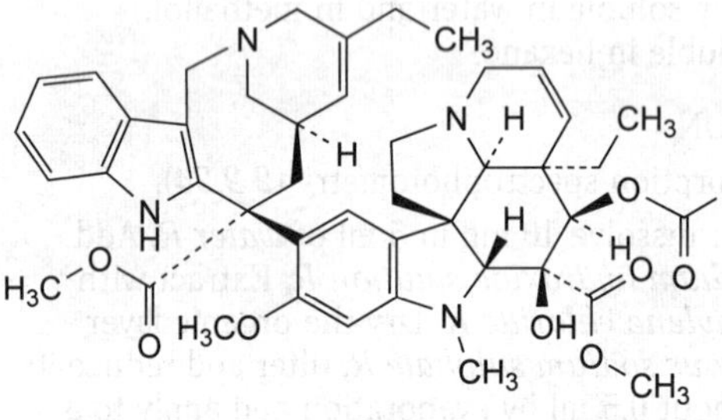

C. methyl (3a*R*,4*R*,5*S*,5a*R*,10b*R*,13a*R*)-4-(acetyloxy)-3a-ethyl-9-[(6*R*,8*R*)-4-ethyl-8-(methoxycarbonyl)-1,3,6,7,8,9-hexahydro-2,6-methano-2*H*-azacyclodecino[4,3-*b*]indol-8-yl]-5-hydroxy-8-methoxy-6-methyl-3a,4,5,5a,6,11,12,13a-octahydro-1*H*-indolizino[8,1-*cd*]carbazole-5-carboxylate,

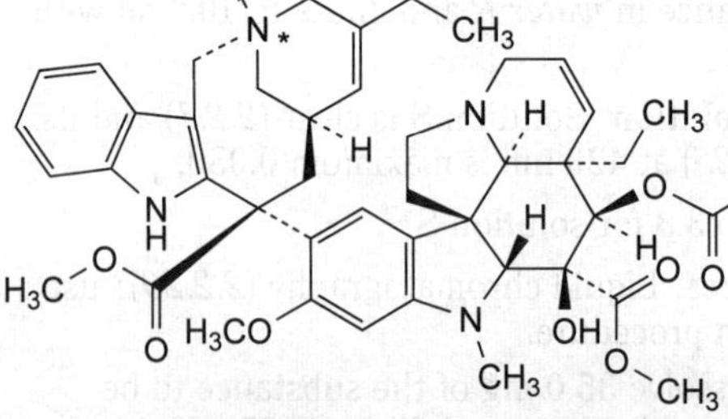

and epimer at N*

D. methyl (3a*R*,4*R*,5*S*,5a*R*,10b*R*,13a*R*)-4-(acetyloxy)-3a-ethyl-9-[(2*RS*,6*R*,8*S*)-4-ethyl-8-(methoxycarbonyl)-2-oxido-1,3,6,7,8,9-hexahydro-2,6-methano-2*H*-azacyclodecino[4,3-*b*]indol-8-yl]-5-hydroxy-8-methoxy-6-methyl-3a,4,5,5a,6,11,12,13a-octahydro-1*H*-indolizino[8,1-*cd*]carbazole-5-carboxylate,

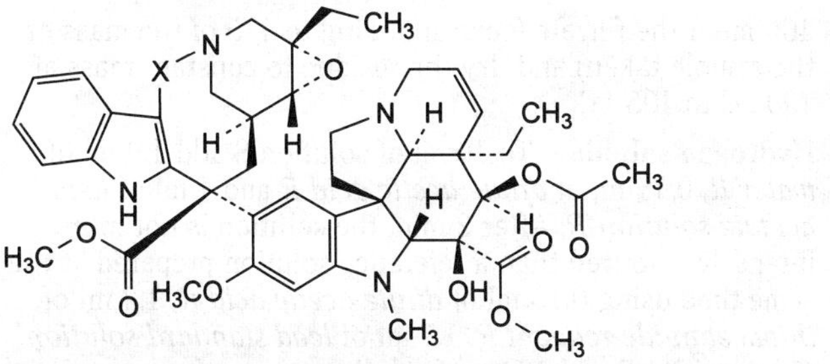

E. X = CH_2-CH_2: methyl (1a*S*,11*S*,13*S*,13a*R*)-11-[(3a*R*,4*R*,5*S*,5a*R*,10b*R*,13a*R*)-4-(acetyloxy)-3a-ethyl-5-hydroxy-8-methoxy-5-(methoxycarbonyl)-6-methyl-3a,4,5,5a,6,11,12,13a-octahydro-1*H*-indolizino[8,1-*cd*]carbazol-9-yl]-1a-ethyl-1a,4,5,10,11,12,13,13a-octahydro-2*H*-3,13-methanooxireno[9,10]azacycloundecino[5,4-*b*]indole-11-carboxylate (leurosine),

G. X = CH_2: methyl (1a*S*,10*S*,12*S*,12a*R*)-10-[(3a*R*,4*R*,5*S*,5a*R*,10b*R*,13a*R*)-4-(acetyloxy)-3a-ethyl-5-hydroxy-8-methoxy-5-(methoxycarbonyl)-6-methyl-3a,4,5,5a,6,11,12,13a-octahydro-1*H*-indolizino[8,1-*cd*]carbazol-9-yl]-1a-ethyl-1a,2,4,9,10,11,12,12a-octahydro-3,12-methano-3*H*-oxireno[8,9]azacyclodecino[4,3-*b*]indole-10-carboxylate,

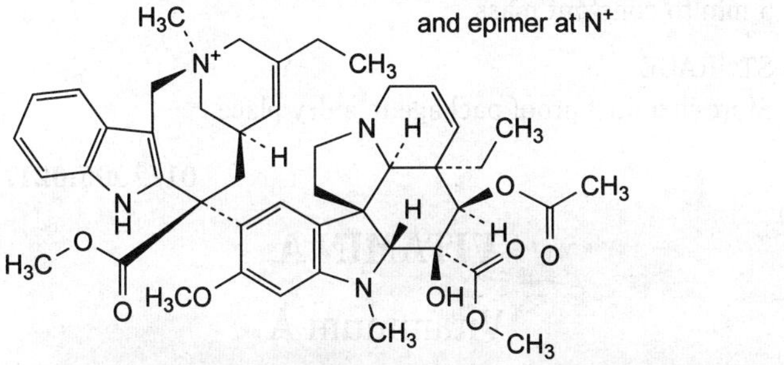

F. (2*RS*,6*R*,8*S*)-8-[(3a*R*,4*R*,5*S*,5a*R*,10b*R*,13a*R*)-4-(acetyloxy)-3a-ethyl-5-hydroxy-8-methoxy-5-(methoxycarbonyl)-6-methyl-3a,4,5,5a,6,11,12,13a-octahydro-1*H*-indolizino[8,1-*cd*]carbazol-9-yl]-4-ethyl-8-(methoxycarbonyl)-2-methyl-1,3,6,7,8,9-hexahydro-2,6-methano-2*H*-azacyclodecino[4,3-*b*]indolium,

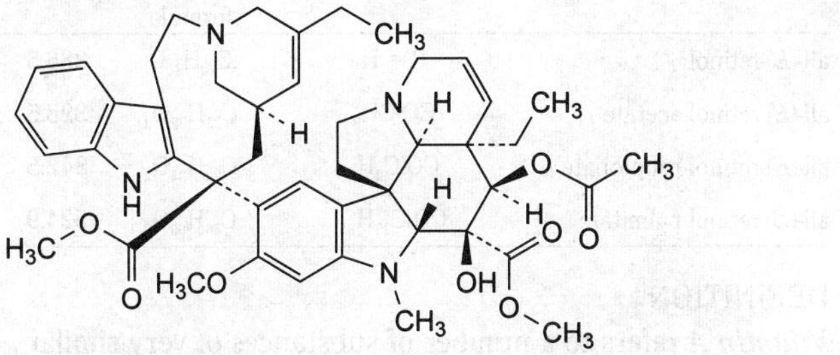

J. methyl (3a*R*,4*R*,5*S*,5a*R*,10b*R*,13a*R*)-4-(acetyloxy)-3a-ethyl-9-[(7*R*,9*S*)-5-ethyl-9-(methoxycarbonyl)-1,4,7,8,9,10-hexahydro-2*H*-3,7-methanoazacycloundecino[5,4-*b*]indol-9-yl]-5-hydroxy-8-methoxy-6-methyl-3a,4,5,5a,6,11,12,13a-octahydro-1*H*-indolizino[8,1-*cd*]carbazole-5-carboxylate.

01/2005:0034

VISCOSE WADDING, ABSORBENT

Lanugo cellulosi absorbens

DEFINITION

Absorbent viscose wadding consists of bleached, carefully carded, new fibres of regenerated cellulose obtained by the viscose process, with or without the addition of titanium dioxide, of linear density 1.0 dtex to 8.9 dtex (dtex = mass of 10 000 m of fibre, expressed in grams) and cut to a suitable staple length. It does not contain any compensatory colouring matter.

CHARACTERS

It is white or very slightly yellow, has a lustrous or matt appearance, and is soft to the touch.

IDENTIFICATION

A. Viscose rayon fibres may be solid or hollow; hollow fibres may have a continuous lumen or be compartmented. The fibres have an average length of 25 mm to 80 mm and when examined under a microscope in the dry state, or when mounted in *alcohol R* and *water R*, the following characters are observed. They are usually of a more or less uniform width, with many longitudinal parallel lines distributed unequally over the width. The ends are cut more or less straight. Matt fibres contain numerous granular particles of approximately 1 µm average diameter.

Solid fibres. In longitudinal view, the surface of the fibres may be uneven or crenate. Fibres having an approximately circular or elliptical cross section have a diameter of about 10 µm to 20 µm and those that are flattened and twisted ribbons vary in width from 15 µm to 20 µm as the twisting of the filament reveals first the major axis and then the minor axis. They are about 4 µm in thickness. Other solid cross sections are Y-shaped and have protruding limbs with the major axis 5 µm to 25 µm in length and the minor axis 2 µm to 8 µm wide.

Hollow fibres. Fibres with a continuous, hollow lumen have a diameter of up to about 30 µm; they are thin-walled, with a wall thickness of about 5 µm. When mounted in *alcohol R* and *water R*, the lumen is clearly indicated in many fibres by the presence of many entrapped air bubbles.

Compartmented fibres. These fibres may have a diameter of up to 80 µm; they are hollow, having a central lumen which is divided up into several compartments. Individual compartments vary in size but typically may be up to about 60 µm in length and there may be more than one compartment across the width of each fibre. Some compartments show entrapped air bubbles when the fibres are mounted in *alcohol R* and *water R*.

B. When treated with *iodinated zinc chloride solution R*, the fibres become violet.

C. To 0.1 g add 10 ml of *zinc chloride-formic acid solution R*. Heat to 40 °C and allow to stand for 2 h 30 min, shaking occasionally. It dissolves completely except for the matt variety where titanium dioxide particles remain.

D. Dissolve the residue obtained in the test for sulphated ash by warming gently with 5 ml of *sulphuric acid R*. Allow to cool and add 0.2 ml of *dilute hydrogen peroxide solution R*. The solution obtained from the lustrous variety undergoes no change in colour; that from the matt variety shows an orange-yellow colour, the intensity of which depends on the quantity of titanium dioxide present.

TESTS

Solution S. Place 15.0 g in a suitable vessel, add 150 ml of *water R*, close the vessel and allow to macerate for 2 h. Decant the solution, squeeze the residual liquid carefully from the sample with a glass rod and mix. Reserve 10 ml of the solution for the test for surface-active substances and filter the remainder.

Acidity or alkalinity. To 25 ml of solution S add 0.1 ml of *phenolphthalein solution R* and to another 25 ml add 0.05 ml of *methyl orange solution R*. Neither solution is pink.

Foreign fibres. Examined under a microscope, it is seen to consist exclusively of viscose fibres, except that occasionally a few isolated foreign fibres may be present.

Fluorescence. Examine a layer about 5 mm in thickness under ultraviolet light at 365 nm. It displays only a slight brownish-violet fluorescence. It shows no intense blue fluorescence, apart from that which may be shown by a few isolated fibres.

Absorbency

Apparatus. A dry cylindrical copper-wire basket 8.0 cm high and 5.0 cm in diameter. The wire of which the basket is constructed is about 0.4 mm in diameter, the mesh is 1.5 cm to 2.0 cm wide and the mass of the basket is 2.7 ± 0.3 g.

Sinking time. Not more than 10 s. Weigh the basket to the nearest centigram (m_1). Take a total of 5.00 g in approximately equal quantities from 5 different places in the product to be examined, place loosely in the basket and weigh the filled basket to the nearest centigram (m_2). Fill a beaker 11 cm to 12 cm in diameter to a depth of 10 cm with water at about 20 °C. Hold the basket horizontally and drop it from a height of about 10 mm into the water. Measure with a stopwatch the time taken for the basket to sink below the surface of the water. Calculate the result as the average of 3 tests.

Water-holding capacity. Not less than 18.0 g of water per gram. After the sinking time has been measured, remove the basket from the water, allow it to drain for exactly 30 s suspended in a horizontal position over the beaker, transfer it to a tared beaker (m_3) and weigh to the nearest centigram (m_4). Calculate the water-holding capacity per gram of absorbent viscose wadding using the following expression:

$$\frac{m_4 - (m_2 + m_3)}{m_2 - m_1}$$

Calculate the result as the average of 3 tests.

Ether-soluble substances. Not more than 0.30 per cent. In an extraction apparatus, extract 5.00 g with *ether R* for 4 h at a rate of at least 4 extractions per hour. Evaporate the ether extract and dry the residue to constant mass at 100 °C to 105 °C.

Extractable colouring matter. In a narrow percolator, slowly extract 10.0 g with *alcohol R* until 50 ml of extract is obtained. The liquid obtained is not more intensely coloured (*2.2.2, Method II*) than reference solution Y_5, GY_6 or a reference solution prepared as follows: to 3.0 ml of blue primary solution add 7.0 ml of hydrochloric acid (10 g/l HCl) and dilute 0.5 ml of this solution to 10.0 ml with hydrochloric acid (10 g/l HCl).

Surface-active substances. Introduce the 10 ml portion of solution S reserved before filtration into a 25 ml graduated ground-glass-stoppered cylinder with an external diameter of 20 mm and a wall thickness of not greater than 1.5 mm, previously rinsed 3 times with *sulphuric acid R* and then with *water R*. Shake vigorously 30 times in 10 s, allow to stand for 1 min and repeat the shaking. After 5 min, any foam present does not cover the entire surface of the liquid.

Water-soluble substances. Not more than 0.70 per cent. Boil 5.00 g in 500 ml of *water R* for 30 min, stirring frequently. Replace the water lost by evaporation. Decant the liquid, squeeze the residual liquid carefully from the sample with a glass rod and mix. Filter the liquid whilst hot. Evaporate 400 ml of the filtrate (corresponding to 4/5 of the mass of the sample taken) and dry the residue to constant mass at 100 °C to 105 °C.

Hydrogen sulphide. To 10 ml of solution S add 1.9 ml of *water R*, 0.15 ml of *dilute acetic acid R* and 1 ml of *lead acetate solution R*. After 2 min, the solution is not more intensely coloured than a reference solution prepared at the same time using 0.15 ml of *dilute acetic acid R*, 1.2 ml of *thioacetamide reagent R*, 1.7 ml of *lead standard solution (10 ppm Pb) R* and 10 ml of solution S.

Loss on drying (*2.2.32*). Not more than 13.0 per cent, determined on 5.000 g by drying in an oven at 100 °C to 105 °C.

Sulphated ash (*2.4.14*). Not more than 0.45 per cent for the lustrous variety and not more than 1.7 per cent for the matt variety. Introduce 5.00 g into a previously heated and cooled, tared crucible. Heat cautiously over a naked flame and then carefully to dull redness at 600 °C. Allow to cool, add a few drops of *dilute sulphuric acid R*, then heat and incinerate until all the black particles have disappeared. Allow to cool. Add a few drops of *ammonium carbonate solution R*. Evaporate and incinerate carefully, allow to cool and weigh again. Repeat the incineration for periods of 5 min to constant mass.

STORAGE

Store in a dust-proof package in a dry place.

01/2005:0217

VITAMIN A

Vitaminum A

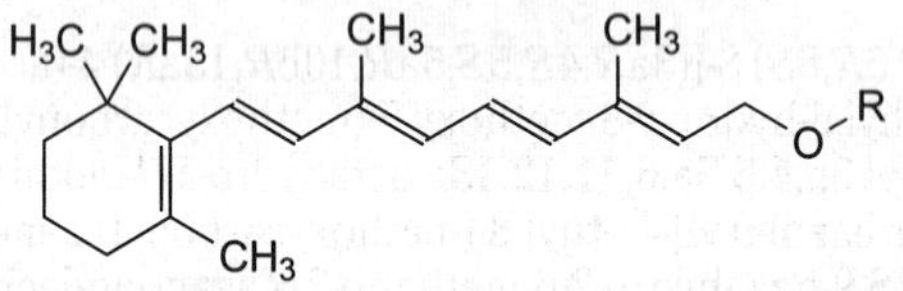

Substance	R	Molecular formula	M_r
all-(*E*)-retinol	R = H	$C_{20}H_{30}O$	286.5
all-(*E*)-retinol acetate	$CO\text{-}CH_3$	$C_{22}H_{32}O_2$	328.5
all-(*E*)-retinol propionate	$CO\text{-}C_2H_5$	$C_{23}H_{34}O_2$	342.5
all-(*E*)-retinol palmitate	$CO\text{-}C_{15}H_{31}$	$C_{36}H_{60}O_2$	524.9

DEFINITION

Vitamin A refers to a number of substances of very similar structure (including (*Z*)-isomers) found in animal tissues and possessing similar activity. The principal and biologically most active substance is all-(*E*)-retinol (all-(*E*)-3,7-dimethyl-9-(2,6,6-trimethylcyclohex-1-enyl)nona-2,4,6,8-tetraen-1-ol; $C_{20}H_{30}O$). Vitamin A is generally used in the form of esters such as the acetate, propionate and palmitate.

Synthetic retinol ester refers to an ester of synthetic retinol (acetate, propionate or palmitate) or a mixture of synthetic retinol esters.

The activity of vitamin A is expressed in retinol equivalents (R.E.) 1 mg R.E. corresponds to the activity of 1 mg of all-(*E*)-retinol. The activity of the other retinol esters is calculated using the stoichiometry, so that 1 mg R.E. of vitamin A corresponds to the activity of:

- 1.147 mg of all-(*E*)-retinol acetate,
- 1.195 mg of all-(*E*)-retinol propionate,
- 1.832 mg of all-(*E*)-retinol palmitate.

Monographs T-Z

International units (IU) are also used. 1 IU of vitamin A is equivalent to the activity of 0.300 µg of all-(*E*)-retinol. The activity of the other retinol esters is calculated using the stoichiometry, so that 1 IU of vitamin A is equivalent to the activity of:

– 0.344 µg of all-(*E*)-retinol acetate,
– 0.359 µg of all-(*E*)-retinol propionate,
– 0.550 µg of all-(*E*)-retinol palmitate,

1 mg of retinol equivalent is equivalent to 3333 IU.

CHARACTERS

Retinol acetate occurs as pale-yellow crystals (melting point about 60 °C). Once melted retinol acetate tends to yield a supercooled melt.

Retinol propionate occurs as a reddish-brown oily liquid.

Retinol palmitate is a fat-like, light yellow solid or a yellow oily liquid, if melted (melting point about 26 °C).

All retinol esters are practically insoluble in water, soluble or partly soluble in ethanol and miscible with organic solvents. Vitamin A and its esters are very sensitive to the action of air, oxidising agents, acids, light and heat.

Carry out the assay and all tests as rapidly as possible, avoiding exposure to actinic light and air, oxidising agents, oxidation catalysts (e.g. copper, iron), acids and heat; use freshly prepared solutions.

IDENTIFICATION

A. Examine by thin-layer chromatography (*2.2.27*), using a *TLC silica gel F_{254} plate R*.

Test solution. Prepare a solution containing about 3.3 IU of vitamin A per microlitre in *cyclohexane R* containing 1 g/l of *butylhydroxytoluene R*.

Reference solution. Prepare a 10 mg/ml solution of *retinol esters CRS* (i.e. 3.3 IU of each ester per microlitre) in *cyclohexane R* containing 1 g/l of *butylhydroxytoluene R*.

Apply to the plate 3 µl of each solution. Develop immediately over 2/3 of the plate using a mixture of 20 volumes of *ether R* and 80 volumes of *cyclohexane R*. Allow the plate to dry in air and examine in ultraviolet light at 254 nm. The identification is not valid unless the chromatogram obtained with the reference solution shows the individual spots of the corresponding esters. The elution order from bottom to top is: retinol acetate, retinol propionate and retinol palmitate. The composition of the test solution is confirmed by the correspondence of the principal spot or spots with those obtained with the reference solution.

B. It complies with the test for related substances.

TESTS

Retinol. Examine by thin-layer chromatography (*2.2.27*), using a *TLC silica gel F_{254} plate R*.

Test solution. Prepare a solution in *cyclohexane R*, stabilised with a 1 g/l solution of *butylhydroxytoluene R*, containing about 330 IU of vitamin A per microlitre.

Reference solution. Shake 1 ml of the test solution with 20 ml of *0.1 M tetrabutylammonium hydroxide in 2-propanol* for 2 min and dilute to 100 ml with *cyclohexane R*, stabilised with a 1 g/l solution of *butylhydroxytoluene R*.

Apply to the plate 3 µl of each solution. Develop immediately over a path of 15 cm using a mixture of 20 volumes of *ether R* and 80 volumes of *cyclohexane R*. Allow the plate to dry in air and examine in ultraviolet light at 254 nm. In the chromatogram obtained with the reference solution no or only traces of the retinol ester are seen. Any spot corresponding to retinol in the chromatogram obtained with the test solution is not more intense than the spot in the chromatogram obtained with the reference solution (1.0 per cent).

Related substances. Examine by ultraviolet absorption spectrophotometry (*2.2.25*). Determine the absorption maximum of the solution for "Activity". The solution shows an absorption maximum at 325 nm to 327 nm. Measure the absorbances at 300 nm, 350 nm and 370 nm and calculate the ratio A_λ/A_{326} for each wavelength. None of the ratios A_λ/A_{326} exceed 0.593 at 300 nm, 0.537 at 350 nm, 0.142 at 370 nm.

ACTIVITY

The activity of the substance is determined in order to be taken into account for the production of concentrates.

Examine by ultraviolet absorption spectrophotometry (*2.2.25*). Dissolve 25 mg to 100 mg, weighed with an accuracy of 0.1 per cent, in 5 ml of *pentane R* and dilute with *2-propanol R1* to a presumed concentration of 10 IU/ml to 15 IU/ml. This solution is also used for the test for related substances.

Determine the absorbance of the maximum at 326 nm. Calculate the activity of vitamin A in International Units per gram from the expression:

$$\frac{A_{326} \times V \times 1900}{100 \times m}$$

A_{326} = absorbance at 326 nm,

m = mass of the substance to be examined, in grams,

V = total volume to which the substance to be examined is diluted to give 10 IU/ml to 15 IU/ml,

1900 = factor to convert the specific absorbance of esters of retinol into International Units per gram.

STORAGE

Store in an airtight, well-filled container, protected from light.

Once the container has been opened, its contents are to be used as soon as possible; any part of the contents not used at once should be protected by an atmosphere of inert gas.

LABELLING

The label states:

– the number of International Units per gram,
– the name of the ester or esters.

IMPURITIES

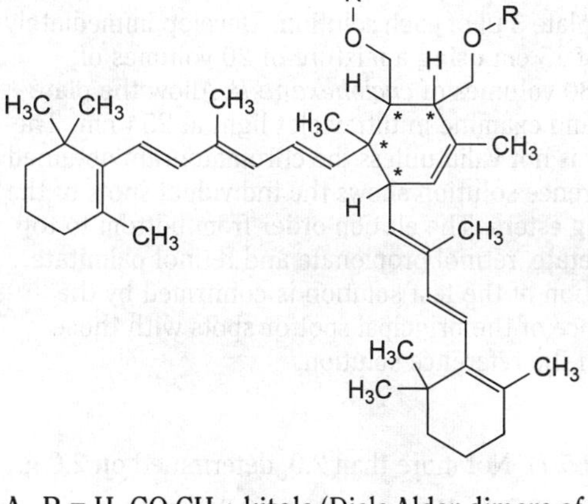

A. R = H, CO-CH_3: kitols (Diels-Alder dimers of vitamin A),

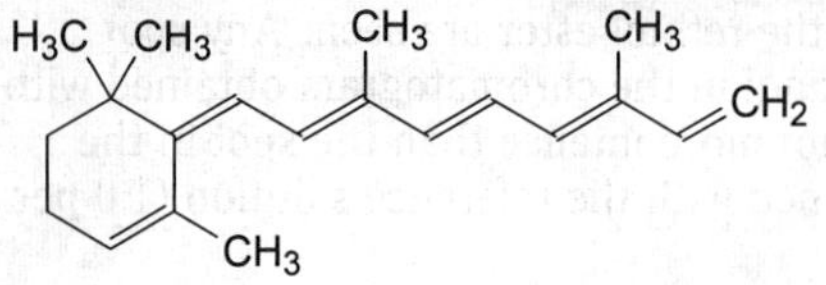

B. (3*E*,5*E*,7*E*)-3,7-dimethyl-9-[(1*Z*)-2,6,6-trimethylcyclohex-2-enylidene)nona-1,3,5,7-tetraene (anhydro-vitamin A),

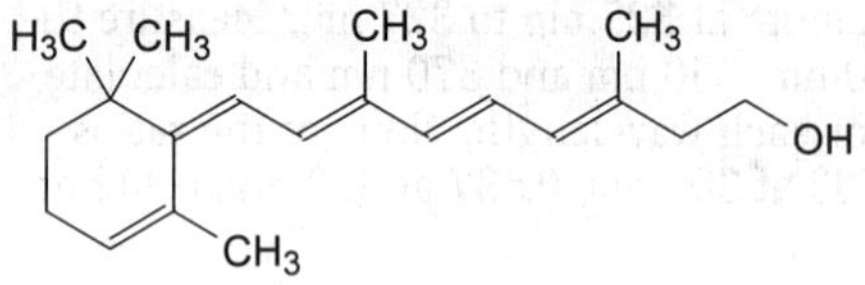

C. (3*E*,5*E*,7*E*)-3,7-dimethyl-9-[(1*Z*)-2,6,6-trimethylcyclohex-2-enylidene)nona-3,5,7-trien-1-ol (*retro*-vitamin A),

D. oxidation products of vitamin A.

01/2005:0219

VITAMIN A CONCENTRATE (OILY FORM), SYNTHETIC

Vitaminum A densatum oleosum

DEFINITION

Synthetic vitamin A concentrate (oily form) is prepared from synthetic retinol ester (*0217*) as is or by dilution with a suitable vegetable fatty oil. The concentrate may contain suitable stabilisers such as antioxidants.

The declared content of vitamin A is not less than 500 000 IU/g and the concentrate contains not less than 95.0 per cent and not more than 110.0 per cent of the content stated on the label.

CHARACTERS

A yellow or brownish-yellow, oily liquid, practically insoluble in water, soluble or partly soluble in ethanol, miscible with organic solvents. Partial crystallisation may occur in highly concentrated solutions.

IDENTIFICATION

Examine by thin-layer chromatography (*2.2.27*), using a *TLC silica gel F_{254} plate R*.

Test solution. Prepare a solution containing about 3.3 IU of vitamin A per microlitre in *cyclohexane R* containing 1 g/l of *butylhydroxytoluene R*.

Reference solution. Prepare a 10 mg/ml solution of *retinol esters CRS* (i.e. 3.3 IU of each ester per microlitre) in *cyclohexane R* containing 1 g/l of *butylhydroxytoluene R*.

Apply to the plate 3 µl of each solution. Develop immediately over a path of 15 cm using a mixture of 20 volumes of *ether R* and 80 volumes of *cyclohexane R*. Allow the plate to dry in air and examine in ultraviolet light at 254 nm. The identification is not valid unless the chromatogram obtained with the reference solution shows the individual spots of the corresponding esters. The elution order from bottom to top is: retinol acetate, retinol propionate and retinol palmitate. The composition of the test solution is confirmed by the correspondence of the principal spot or spots with those obtained with the reference solution.

TESTS

Acid value (*2.5.1*). Not more than 2.0, determined on 2.0 g.

Peroxide value (*2.5.5*). Not more than 10.0.

ASSAY

Carry out the assay as rapidly as possible, avoiding exposure to actinic light and air, oxidising agents, oxidation catalysts (e.g. copper, iron), acids and prolonged heat; use freshly prepared solutions. If partial crystallisation has occurred, homogenise the material at a temperature of about 65 °C, but avoid prolonged heating.

Carry out the assay according to Method A. If the assay is not shown to be valid, use Method B.

Method A. Examine by ultraviolet absorption spectrophotometry (*2.2.25*). Dissolve 25 mg to 100 mg, weighed with an accuracy of 0.1 per cent, in 5 ml of *pentane R* and dilute with *2-propanol R1* to a presumed concentration of 10 IU/ml to 15 IU/ml.

Verify that the absorption maximum of the solution lies between 325 nm and 327 nm and measure the absorbances at 300 nm, 326 nm, 350 nm and 370 nm. Repeat the readings at each wavelength and take the mean values. Calculate the ratio A_λ/A_{326} for each wavelength.

If the ratios do not exceed: 0.593 at 300 nm, 0.537 at 350 nm, 0.142 at 370 nm, calculate the content of vitamin A in International Units per gram from the expression:

$$\frac{A_{326} \times V \times 1900}{100 \times m}$$

A_{326} = absorbance at 326 nm,

m = mass of the preparation to be examined, in grams,

V = total volume to which the preparation to be examined is diluted to give 10 IU/ml to 15 IU/ml,

1900 = factor to convert the specific absorbance of esters of retinol into International Units per gram.

If one or more of the ratios A_λ/A_{326} exceeds the values given, or if the wavelength of the absorption maximum does not lie between 325 nm and 327 nm, use Method B.

Method B. Examine by liquid chromatography (*2.2.29*).

Test solution (a). Introduce into a 50 ml volumetric flask, an amount of the preparation to be examined, weighed with an accuracy of 0.1 per cent and equivalent to about 120 000 IU of vitamin A and dissolve immediately in 5 ml of *pentane R*. Add 20 mg to 30 mg of *butylhydroxytoluene R* and 20 ml of *0.1 M tetrabutylammonium hydroxide in 2-propanol.* Swirl gently for 5 min (an ultrasonic bath is recommended). Dilute to 50.0 ml with *2-propanol R* and homogenise carefully to avoid air-bubbles.

Test solution (b). Introduce 20 mg to 30 mg of *butylhydroxytoluene R* into a 50 ml volumetric flask, add 5 ml of *2-propanol R*, 5.0 ml of test solution (a) and dilute to 50.0 ml with *2-propanol R*. Homogenise carefully to avoid air-bubbles.

Reference solution (a). Introduce into a 50 ml volumetric flask about 120 mg of *retinol acetate CRS*, weighed with an accuracy of 0.1 per cent and proceed as described for test solution (a).

Reference solution (b). Introduce 20 mg to 30 mg of *butylhydroxytoluene R* into a 50 ml volumetric flask, add 5 ml of *2-propanol R*, 5.0 ml of reference solution (a) and dilute to 50.0 ml with *2-propanol R*. Homogenise carefully to avoid air-bubbles.

The chromatographic procedure may be carried out using:

- a stainless steel column 0.125 m long and 4 mm in internal diameter packed with *octadecylsilyl silica gel for chromatography R* (5 µm),
- as mobile phase at a flow rate of 1 ml/min a mixture of 5 volumes of *water R* and 95 volumes of *methanol R*,

- as detector a spectrophotometer set at 325 nm,
- a loop injector.

The assay is not valid unless:

- the chromatogram obtained with reference solution (b) shows a principal peak corresponding to that of all-(*E*)-retinol, the retention time of all-(*E*)-retinol being about 3 min,
- there is no peak corresponding to the unsaponified retinol acetate in the chromatogram obtained with reference solution (b) at a retention time of about 6 min.

Inject a suitable volume of reference solution (b) in order to obtain an absorbance in the range of 0.5 to 1.0 at 325 nm and record the chromatogram using an attenuation so that the height of the peak corresponding to vitamin A is not less than 50 per cent of the full scale of the recorder.

Make a total of six such injections. The relative standard deviation of the response for reference solution (b) is not greater than 1 per cent.

Inject the same volume of test solution (b) and record the chromatogram in the same manner.

Calculate the content of vitamin A from the expression:

$$\frac{A_1 \times C \times m_2}{A_2 \times m_1}$$

A_1 = area of the peak corresponding to all-(*E*)-retinol in the chromatogram obtained with test solution (b),

A_2 = area of the peak corresponding to all-(*E*)-retinol in the chromatogram obtained with reference solution (b),

C = concentration of *retinol acetate CRS* in International Units per gram, determined by method A; the absorption ratios A_λ/A_{326} must conform,

m_1 = mass of the substance to be examined in test solution (a), in milligrams,

m_2 = mass of *retinol acetate CRS* in reference solution (a), in milligrams.

STORAGE

Store in an airtight, well-filled container, protected from light.

Once the container has been opened, its contents are to be used as soon as possible; any part of the contents not used at once should be protected by an atmosphere of inert gas.

LABELLING

The label states:

- the number of International Units per gram,
- the name of the ester or esters,
- the name of any added stabilisers,
- the method of restoring the solution if partial crystallisation has occurred.

01/2005:0218

VITAMIN A CONCENTRATE (POWDER FORM), SYNTHETIC

Vitaminum A pulvis

DEFINITION

Synthetic vitamin A concentrate (powder form) is obtained by dispersing a synthetic retinol ester (*0217*) in a matrix of *Gelatin (0330)* or *Acacia (0307)* or other suitable material. The declared content of vitamin A is not less than 250 000 IU/g and the concentrate contains not less than 95.0 per cent and not more than 115.0 per cent of the content stated on the label. The concentrate may contain suitable stabilisers such as antioxidants.

CHARACTERS

A yellowish powder usually in the form of particles of almost uniform size which, depending on their formulation, may be practically insoluble in water or may swell or form an emulsion.

IDENTIFICATION

Examine by thin-layer chromatography (*2.2.27*), using a *TLC silica gel F_{254} plate R*.

Test solution. Introduce into a 20 ml glass-stoppered test tube a quantity of the preparation to be examined containing about the equivalent of 17 000 IU of vitamin A. Add about 20 mg of *bromelains R*, 2 ml of *water R* and about 150 µl of *2-propanol R*, swirling gently for 2 to 5 min in a water-bath at 60 °C to 65 °C. Cool to below 30 °C and add 5 ml of *2-propanol R* containing 1 g/l of *butylhydroxytoluene R*. Shake vigorously for 1 min, allow to stand for a few minutes and use the supernatant solution.

Reference solution. Prepare a 10 mg/ml solution of *retinol esters CRS* (i.e. 3.3 IU of each ester per microlitre) in *2-propanol R* containing 1 g/l of *butylhydroxytoluene R*.

Apply to the plate 3 µl of each solution. Develop immediately over a path of 15 cm using a mixture of 20 volumes of *ether R* and 80 volumes of *cyclohexane R*. Allow the plate to dry in air and examine in ultraviolet light at 254 nm. The identification is not valid unless the chromatogram obtained with the reference solution shows the individual spots of the corresponding esters. The elution order from bottom to top is: retinol acetate, retinol propionate and retinol palmitate. The composition of the test solution is confirmed by the correspondence of the principal spot or spots with those obtained with the reference solution.

ASSAY

Carry out the assay as rapidly as possible, avoiding exposure to actinic light and air, oxidising agents, oxidation catalysts (e.g. copper, iron), acids and prolonged heat.

Examine by liquid chromatography (*2.2.29*).

Test solution (a). Introduce into a 50 ml volumetric flask, an amount of the preparation to be examined, weighed with an accuracy of 0.1 per cent and equivalent to about 120 000 IU of vitamin A. Add 20 mg to 30 mg of *bromelains R*, 20 mg to 30 mg of *butylhydroxytoluene R*, 2.0 ml of *water R* and 0.15 ml of *2-propanol R*. Heat gently in a water-bath at 60 °C to 65 °C for 2 to 5 min. Cool to below 30 °C and add 20 ml of *0.1 M tetrabutylammonium hydroxide in 2-propanol.* Swirl gently for 5 min (an ultrasonic bath is recommended). Dilute to 50.0 ml with *2-propanol R* and homogenise carefully to avoid air-bubbles. Residue of the matrix may cause more or less cloudiness of the solution.

Test solution (b). Introduce 20 mg to 30 mg of *butylhydroxytoluene R* into a 50 ml volumetric flask, add 5 ml of *2-propanol R*, 5.0 ml of test solution (a) and dilute to 50.0 ml with *2-propanol R*. Homogenise carefully to avoid air-bubbles. Filter before injection.

Reference solution (a). Introduce into a 50 ml volumetric flask about 120 mg of *retinol acetate CRS*, weighed with an accuracy of 0.1 per cent and dissolve immediately in 5 ml of *pentane R*. Add 20 mg to 30 mg of *butylhydroxytoluene R* and 20 ml of *0.1 M tetrabutylammonium hydroxide in 2-propanol*. Swirl gently for 5 min (an ultrasonic bath is recommended) and dilute to 50.0 ml with *2-propanol R*. Homogenise carefully to avoid air-bubbles.

Reference solution (b). Place 20 mg to 30 mg of *butylhydroxytoluene R* in a 50 ml volumetric flask, add 5 ml of *2-propanol R*, 5.0 ml of reference solution (a) and dilute to 50.0 ml with *2-propanol R*. Homogenise carefully to avoid air-bubbles.

The chromatographic procedure may be carried out using:

- a stainless steel column 0.125 m long and 4 mm in internal diameter packed with *octadecylsilyl silica gel for chromatography R* (5 μm),
- as mobile phase at a flow rate of 1 ml/min a mixture of 5 volumes of *water R* and 95 volumes of *methanol R*,
- as detector a spectrophotometer set at 325 nm,
- a loop injector.

The assay is not valid unless:

- the chromatogram obtained with reference solution (b) shows a principal peak corresponding to that of all-(*E*)-retinol, the retention time of all-(*E*)-retinol being about 3 min,
- there is no peak corresponding to unsaponified retinol acetate in the chromatogram obtained with reference solution (b) at a retention time of about 6 min.

Inject a suitable volume of reference solution (b) in order to obtain an absorbance in the range of 0.5 to 1.0 at 325 nm and record the chromatogram using an attenuation so that the height of the peak corresponding to vitamin A is not less than 50 per cent of the full scale of the recorder.

Make a total of six injections. The relative standard deviation of the response for reference solution (b) should not be greater than 1 per cent.

Inject the same volume of test solution (b) and record the chromatogram in the same manner.

Calculate the content of vitamin A from the expression:

$$\frac{A_1 \times C \times m_2}{A_2 \times m_1}$$

A_1 = area of the peak corresponding to all-(*E*)-retinol in the chromatogram obtained with test solution (b),

A_2 = area of the peak corresponding to all-(*E*)-retinol in the chromatogram obtained with reference solution (b),

C = concentration of *retinol acetate CRS* in International Units per gram, determined by the method below,

m_1 = mass of the substance to be examined in test solution (a), in milligrams,

m_2 = mass of *retinol acetate CRS* in reference solution (a), in milligrams.

The exact concentration of *retinol acetate CRS* is assessed by ultraviolet absorption spectrophotometry (*2.2.25*). Dissolve 25 mg to 100 mg, weighed with an accuracy of 0.1 per cent, in 5 ml of *pentane R* and dilute with *2-propanol R1* to a presumed concentration of 10 UI/ml to 15 UI/ml.

Verify that the absorption maximum of the solution lies between 325 nm and 327 nm and measure the absorbances at 300 nm, 326 nm, 350 nm and 370 nm. Repeat the readings at each wavelength and take the mean values. Calculate the ratio A_λ/A_{326} for each wavelength.

If the ratios do not exceed: 0.593 at 300 nm, 0.537 at 350 nm, 0.142 at 370 nm, calculate the content of vitamin A in International Units per gram from the expression:

$$\frac{A_{326} \times V \times 1900}{100 \times m}$$

A_{326} = absorbance at 326 nm,

m = mass of the CRS, in grams,

V = total volume to which the CRS is diluted to give 10 UI/ml to 15 UI/ml,

1900 = factor to convert the specific absorbance of esters of retinol into International Units per gram.

The absorption ratios A_λ/A_{326} must conform.

STORAGE

Store in an airtight, well-filled container, protected from light.

Once the container has been opened, its contents are to be used as soon as possible; any part of the contents not used at once should be protected by an atmosphere of inert gas.

LABELLING

The label states:

- the number of International Units per gram,
- the name of the ester or esters,
- the name of the principal excipient or excipients used and the name of any added stabilisers.

01/2005:0220

VITAMIN A CONCENTRATE (SOLUBILISATE/EMULSION), SYNTHETIC

Vitaminum A in aqua dispergibile

DEFINITION

Synthetic Vitamin A concentrate (solubilisate/emulsion) is a liquid form (water is generally used as solvent) of a synthetic retinol ester (*0217*) and a suitable solubiliser. The declared content of vitamin A is not less than 100 000 UI/g and the concentrate contains not less than 95.0 per cent and not more than 115.0 per cent of the content stated on the label. The concentrate may contain suitable stabilisers such as antimicrobial preservatives and antioxidants.

CHARACTERS

A yellow or yellowish liquid of variable opalescence and viscosity. Highly concentrated solutions may become cloudy at low temperature or take the form of a gel.

A mixture of 1 g with 10 ml of *water R* previously warmed to 50 °C gives after cooling to 20 °C, a uniform, slightly opalescent and slightly yellow dispersion.

IDENTIFICATION

Examine by thin-layer chromatography (*2.2.27*), using a *TLC silica gel F_{254} plate R*.

Test solution. Introduce into a 20 ml glass-stoppered test-tube a quantity of the preparation to be examined containing about the equivalent of 17 000 IU of vitamin A. Add 5 ml of *2-propanol R* containing 1 g/l of *butylhydroxytoluene R* and mix thoroughly.

Reference solution. Prepare a 10 mg/ml solution of *retinol esters CRS* (i.e. 3.3 IU of each ester per microlitre) in *2-propanol R* containing 1 g/l of *butylhydroxytoluene R*.

Apply to the plate 3 µl of each solution. Develop immediately over a path of 15 cm using a mixture of 20 volumes of *ether R* and 80 volumes of *cyclohexane R*. Allow the plate to dry in air and examine in ultraviolet light at 254 nm. The identification is not valid unless the chromatogram obtained with the reference solution shows the individual spots of the corresponding esters. The elution order from bottom to top is: retinol acetate, retinol propionate and retinol palmitate. The composition of the test solution is confirmed by the correspondence of the principal spot or spots with those obtained with the reference solution.

ASSAY

Carry out the assay as rapidly as possible, avoiding exposure to actinic light and air, oxidising agents, oxidation catalysts (e.g. copper, iron), acids and prolonged heat.

Examine by liquid chromatography (*2.2.29*).

Test solution (a). Introduce into a 50 ml volumetric flask, an amount of the preparation to be examined, weighed with an accuracy of 0.1 per cent and equivalent to about 120 000 IU of vitamin A and dissolve immediately in 5 ml of *2-propanol R*. Add 20 mg to 30 mg of *butylhydroxytoluene R* and 20 ml of *0.1 M tetrabutylammonium hydroxide in 2-propanol*. Swirl gently for 5 min (an ultrasonic bath is recommended). Dilute to 50.0 ml with *2-propanol R* and homogenise carefully to avoid air-bubbles.

Test solution (b). Introduce 20 mg to 30 mg of *butylhydroxytoluene R* into a 50 ml volumetric flask, add 5 ml of *2-propanol R*, 5.0 ml of test solution (a) and dilute to 50.0 ml with *2-propanol R*. Homogenise carefully to avoid air-bubbles.

Reference solution (a). Introduce into a 50 ml volumetric flask about 120 mg of *retinol acetate CRS*, weighed with an accuracy of 0.1 per cent and proceed as described for test solution (a).

Reference solution (b). Place 20 mg to 30 mg of *butylhydroxytoluene R* into a 50 ml volumetric flask, add 5 ml of *2-propanol R*, 5.0 ml of reference solution (a) and dilute to 50.0 ml with *2-propanol R*. Homogenise carefully to avoid air-bubbles.

The chromatographic procedure may be carried out using:

- a stainless steel column 0.125 m long and 4 mm in internal diameter packed with *octadecylsilyl silica gel for chromatography R* (5 µm),
- as mobile phase at a flow rate of 1 ml/min a mixture of 5 volumes of *water R* and 95 volumes of *methanol R*,
- as detector a spectrophotometer set at 325 nm,
- a loop injector.

The assay is not valid unless:

- the chromatogram obtained with reference solution (b) shows a principal peak corresponding to that of all-(*E*)-retinol, the retention time of all-(*E*)-retinol being about 3 min,
- there is no peak corresponding to the unsaponified retinol acetate in the chromatogram obtained with reference solution (b) at a retention time of about 6 min.

Inject a suitable volume of reference solution (b) in order to obtain an absorbance in the range of 0.5 to 1.0 at 325 nm and record the chromatogram using an attenuation so that the height of the peak corresponding to vitamin A is not less than 50 per cent of the full scale of the recorder.

Make a total of six injections. The relative standard deviation of the response for reference solution (b) should not be greater than 1 per cent.

Inject the same volume of test solution (b) and record the chromatogram in the same manner.

Calculate the content of vitamin A from the expression:

$$\frac{A_1 \times C \times m_2}{A_2 \times m_1}$$

A_1 = area of the peak corresponding to all-(*E*)-retinol in the chromatogram obtained with test solution (b),

A_2 = area of the peak corresponding to all-(*E*)-retinol in the chromatogram obtained with reference solution (b),

C = concentration of *retinol acetate CRS* in International Units per gram, determined by the method below,

m_1 = mass of the substance to be examined in test solution (a), in milligrams,

m_2 = mass of *retinol acetate CRS* in reference solution (a), in milligrams.

The exact concentration of *retinol acetate CRS* is assessed by ultraviolet absorption spectrophotometry (*2.2.25*). Dissolve 25 mg to 100 mg, weighed with an accuracy of 0.1 per cent, in 5 ml of *pentane R* and dilute with *2-propanol R1* to a presumed concentration of 10 IU/ml to 15 IU/ml.

Verify that the absorption maximum of the solution lies between 325 nm and 327 nm and measure the absorbances at 300 nm, 326 nm, 350 nm and 370 nm. Repeat the readings at each wavelength and take the mean values. Calculate the ratio A_λ/A_{326} for each wavelength.

If the ratios do not exceed: 0.593 at 300 nm, 0.537 at 350 nm, 0.142 at 370 nm, calculate the content of vitamin A in International Units per gram from the expression:

$$\frac{A_{326} \times V \times 1900}{100 \times m}$$

A_{326} = absorbance at 326 nm,

m = mass of the CRS, in grams,

V = total volume to which the CRS is diluted to give 10 UI/ml to 15 IU/ml,

1900 = factor to convert the specific absorbance of esters of retinol into International Units per gram.

The absorption ratios A_λ/A_{326} must conform.

STORAGE

Store in an airtight container, protected from light, at the temperature stated on the label.

Once the container has been opened, its contents are to be used as soon as possible; any part of the contents not used at once should be protected by an atmosphere of inert gas.

LABELLING

The label states:

- the number of International Units per gram,
- the name of the ester or esters,
- the name of the principal solubiliser or solubilisers used and the name of any added stabilisers,
- the storage temperature.

W

01/2005:0698

WARFARIN SODIUM

Warfarinum natricum

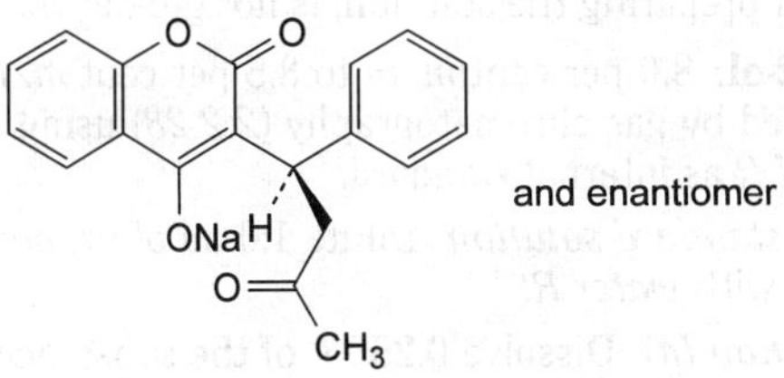

$C_{19}H_{15}NaO_4$ M_r 330.3

DEFINITION

Warfarin sodium contains not less than 98.0 per cent and not more than the equivalent of 102.0 per cent of sodium 2-oxo-3-[(1*RS*)-3-oxo-1-phenylbutyl]-2*H*-1-benzopyran-4-olate, calculated with reference to the anhydrous substance.

CHARACTERS

A white powder, hygroscopic, very soluble in water and in alcohol, soluble in acetone, very slightly soluble in methylene chloride.

IDENTIFICATION

First identification: B, D, E.

Second identification: A, C, D, E.

A. Dissolve 1 g in 25 ml of *water R*, add 2 ml of *dilute hydrochloric acid R* and filter. Reserve the filtrate for identification test E. The precipitate, washed with *water R* and dried at 100 °C to 105 °C, melts (*2.2.14*) at 159 °C to 163 °C.

B. Dissolve 1 g in 25 ml of *water R*, add 2 ml of *dilute hydrochloric acid R* and filter. Reserve the filtrate for identification test E. Examine the precipitate by infrared absorption spectrophotometry (*2.2.24*) comparing with the spectrum obtained with the precipitate prepared in the same manner from *warfarin sodium CRS*.

C. Examine the chromatograms obtained in the test for related substances. The principal spot in the chromatogram obtained with test solution (b) is similar in position and size to the principal spot in the chromatogram obtained with reference solution (b).

D. Dissolve 1 g in 10 ml of *water R*, add 5 ml of *nitric acid R* and filter. To the filtrate add 2 ml of *potassium dichromate solution R1* and shake for 5 min. Allow to stand for 20 min. The solution is not greenish-blue when compared with a blank.

E. The filtrate obtained in identification test A or B gives reaction (b) of sodium (*2.3.1*).

TESTS

Appearance of solution. Dissolve 1.0 g in *water R* and dilute to 20 ml with the same solvent. The solution is clear (*2.2.1*) and colourless (*2.2.2, Method II*).

pH (*2.2.3*). Dissolve 1.0 g in *carbon dioxide-free water R* and dilute to 100 ml with the same solvent. The pH of the solution is 7.6 to 8.6.

Related substances. Examine by thin-layer chromatography (*2.2.27*), using *silica gel* GF_{254} *R* as the coating substance.

Test solution (a). Dissolve 0.20 g of the substance to be examined in *acetone R* and dilute to 10 ml with the same solvent.

Test solution (b). Dilute 2 ml of test solution (a) to 10 ml with *acetone R*.

Reference solution (a). Dilute 1 ml of test solution (b) to 200 ml with *acetone R*.

Reference solution (b). Dissolve 40 mg of *warfarin sodium CRS* in *acetone R* and dilute to 10 ml with the same solvent.

Reference solution (c). Dissolve 10 mg of *acenocoumarol CRS* in *acetone R*, add 1 ml of test solution (a) and dilute to 10 ml with *acetone R*.

Apply separately to the plate 20 µl of each solution. Develop over a path of 15 cm using a mixture of 20 volumes of *glacial acetic acid R*, 50 volumes of *methylene chloride R* and 50 volumes of *cyclohexane R*. Allow the plate to dry in air and examine in ultraviolet light at 254 nm. Any spot in the chromatogram obtained with test solution (a), apart from the principal spot, is not more intense than the spot in the chromatogram obtained with reference solution (a) (0.1 per cent). The test is not valid unless the chromatogram obtained with reference solution (c) shows two clearly separated spots and the chromatogram obtained with reference solution (a) shows a clearly visible spot.

Phenolic ketones. Dissolve 1.25 g in a 20 g/l solution of *sodium hydroxide R* and dilute to 10.0 ml with the same solvent. The absorbance (*2.2.25*), measured at 385 nm within 15 min of preparing the solution, is not greater than 0.20.

Water (*2.5.12*). Not more than 4.0 per cent, determined on 0.750 g by the semi-micro determination of water.

ASSAY

Dissolve 0.1000 g in *0.01 M sodium hydroxide* and dilute to 100.0 ml with the same solvent. Dilute 10.0 ml of this solution to 100.0 ml with *0.01 M sodium hydroxide*. Dilute 10.0 ml of the latter solution to 100.0 ml with *0.01 M sodium hydroxide*. Measure the absorbance (*2.2.25*) at the maximum at 308 nm.

Calculate the content of $C_{19}H_{15}NaO_4$ taking the specific absorbance to be 431.

STORAGE

Store in an airtight container, protected from light.

01/2005:0699

WARFARIN SODIUM CLATHRATE

Warfarinum natricum clathratum

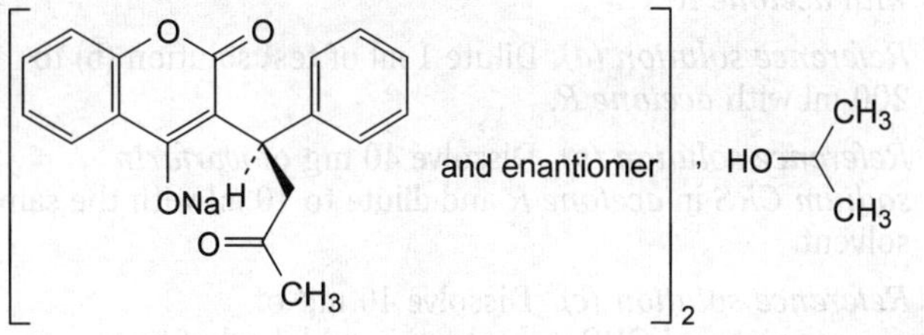

DEFINITION

Warfarin sodium clathrate contains not less than 98.0 per cent and not more than the equivalent of 102.0 per cent of sodium 2-oxo-3-[(1*RS*)-3-oxo-1-phenylbutyl]-2*H*-1-benzopyran-4-olate, calculated with reference to the anhydrous, propan-2-ol-free substance. Warfarin sodium clathrate contains approximately 92 per cent of warfarin sodium. It consists of warfarin sodium and propan-2-ol (molecular proportions 2:1) in the form of a clathrate. It contains not less than 8.0 per cent and not more than 8.5 per cent of propan-2-ol.

CHARACTERS

A white powder, very soluble in water, freely soluble in alcohol, soluble in acetone, very slightly soluble in methylene chloride.

IDENTIFICATION

First identification: B, D, E.

Second identification: A, C, D, E.

A. Dissolve 1 g in 25 ml of *water R*, add 2 ml of *dilute hydrochloric acid R* and filter. Reserve the filtrate for identification test E. The precipitate, washed with *water R* and dried at 100 °C to 105 °C, melts (*2.2.14*) at 159 °C to 163 °C.

B. Dissolve 1 g in 25 ml of *water R*, add 2 ml of *dilute hydrochloric acid R* and filter. Reserve the filtrate for identification test E. Examine the precipitate by infrared absorption spectrophotometry (*2.2.24*) comparing with the spectrum obtained with the precipitate prepared in the same manner from *warfarin sodium CRS*.

C. Examine the chromatograms obtained in the test for related substances. The principal spot in the chromatogram obtained with test solution (b) is similar in position and size to the principal spot in the chromatogram obtained with reference solution (b).

D. Dissolve 1 g in 10 ml of *water R*, add 5 ml of *nitric acid R* and filter. To the filtrate add 2 ml of *potassium dichromate solution R1* and shake for 5 min. Allow to stand for 20 min. The solution is greenish-blue when compared with a blank.

E. The filtrate obtained in identification test A or B gives reaction (b) of sodium (*2.3.1*).

TESTS

Appearance of solution. Dissolve 1.0 g in *water R* and dilute to 20 ml with the same solvent. The solution is clear (*2.2.1*) and colourless (*2.2.2, Method II*).

pH (*2.2.3*). Dissolve 1.0 g in *carbon dioxide-free water R* and dilute to 100 ml with the same solvent. The pH of the solution is 7.6 to 8.6.

Related substances. Examine by thin-layer chromatography (*2.2.27*), using *silica gel* GF_{254} *R* as the coating substance.

Test solution (a). Dissolve 0.20 g of the substance to be examined in *acetone R* and dilute to 10 ml with the same solvent.

Test solution (b). Dilute 2 ml of test solution (a) to 10 ml with *acetone R*.

Reference solution (a). Dilute 1 ml of test solution (b) to 200 ml with *acetone R*.

Reference solution (b). Dissolve 40 mg of *warfarin sodium CRS* in *acetone R* and dilute to 10 ml with the same solvent.

Reference solution (c). Dissolve 10 mg of *acenocoumarol CRS* in *acetone R*, add 1 ml of test solution (a) and dilute to 10 ml with *acetone R*.

Apply separately to the plate 20 µl of each solution. Develop over a path of 15 cm using a mixture of 20 volumes of *glacial acetic acid R*, 50 volumes of *methylene chloride R* and 50 volumes of *cyclohexane R*. Allow the plate to dry in air and examine in ultraviolet light at 254 nm. Any spot in the chromatogram obtained with test solution (a), apart from the principal spot, is not more intense than the spot in the chromatogram obtained with reference solution (a) (0.1 per cent). The test is not valid unless the chromatogram obtained with reference solution (c) shows two clearly separated spots and the chromatogram obtained with reference solution (a) shows a clearly visible spot.

Phenolic ketones. Dissolve 1.25 g in a 20 g/l solution of *sodium hydroxide R* and dilute to 10.0 ml with the same solvent. The absorbance (*2.2.25*), measured at 385 nm within 15 min of preparing the solution, is not greater than 0.20.

Propan-2-ol: 8.0 per cent *m/m* to 8.5 per cent *m/m*, determined by gas chromatography (*2.2.28*) using *propanol R* as internal standard.

Internal standard solution. Dilute 1.0 ml of *propanol R* to 200.0 ml with *water R*.

Test solution (a). Dissolve 0.250 g of the substance to be examined in *water R* and dilute to 5.0 ml with the same solvent.

Test solution (b). Dissolve 0.50 g of the substance to be examined in the internal standard solution and dilute to 10.0 ml with the internal standard solution.

Reference solution. Dilute 0.50 ml of *propan-2-ol R* to 100.0 ml with the internal standard solution.

The chromatographic procedure may be carried out using:

– a column 1.5 m long and 4 mm in internal diameter packed with *ethylvinylbenzene-divinylbenzene copolymer R* (125 µm to 150 µm),

– *nitrogen for chromatography R* as the carrier gas at a flow rate of 40 ml/min,

– a flame-ionisation detector,

maintaining the temperature of the column at 150 °C, that of the injection port at 180 °C and that of the detector at 200 °C. Inject the selected volumes of the test solutions and the reference solution. Calculate the content of propan-2-ol taking its density at 20 °C to be 0.785 g/ml.

Water (*2.5.12*). Not more than 0.1 per cent, determined on 2.500 g by the semi-micro determination of water.

ASSAY

Dissolve 0.1000 g in *0.01 M sodium hydroxide* and dilute to 100.0 ml with the same solvent. Dilute 10.0 ml of this solution to 100.0 ml with *0.01 M sodium hydroxide.* Dilute 10.0 ml of the latter solution to 100.0 ml with *0.01 M sodium hydroxide.* Measure the absorbance (*2.2.25*) at the maximum at 308 nm.

Calculate the content of $C_{19}H_{15}NaO_4$ taking the specific absorbance to be 431.

STORAGE

Store in an airtight container, protected from light.

01/2005:0169
corrected

WATER FOR INJECTIONS

Aqua ad iniectabilia

H_2O M_r 18.02

DEFINITION

Water for the preparation of medicines for parenteral administration when water is used as vehicle (water for injections in bulk) and for dissolving or diluting substances or preparations for parenteral administration (sterilised water for injections).

Monographs T-Z

Water for injections in bulk

PRODUCTION

Water for injections in bulk is obtained from water that complies with the regulations on water intended for human consumption laid down by the competent authority or from purified water by distillation in an apparatus of which the parts in contact with the water are of neutral glass, quartz or suitable metal and which is fitted with an effective device to prevent the entrainment of droplets. The correct maintenance of the apparatus is essential. The first portion of the distillate obtained when the apparatus begins to function is discarded and the distillate is collected.

During production and subsequent storage, appropriate measures are taken to ensure that the total viable aerobic count is adequately controlled and monitored. Appropriate alert and action limits are set so as to detect adverse trends. Under normal conditions, an appropriate action limit is a total viable aerobic count (*2.6.12*) of 10 micro-organisms per 100 ml when determined by membrane filtration, using agar medium S, using at least 200 ml of water for injections in bulk and incubating at 30-35 °C for 5 days. For aseptic processing, stricter alert limits may need to be applied.

Total organic carbon (*2.2.44*): maximum 0.5 mg/l.

Conductivity. Determine the conductivity off-line or in-line under the following conditions.

EQUIPMENT

Conductivity cell:

- electrodes of a suitable material such as stainless steel;
- cell constant: within 2 per cent of the given value determined using a certified reference solution with a conductivity less than 1500 μS·cm^{-1}.

Conductometer: resolution 0.1 μS·cm^{-1} on the lowest range.

System calibration (conductivity cell and conductometer):

- against one or more suitable certified standard solutions;
- accuracy: within 3 per cent of the measured conductivity plus 0.1 μS·cm^{-1}.

Conductometer calibration: by means of precision resistors or equivalent devices, after disconnecting the conductivity cell, for all ranges used for conductivity measurement and cell calibration (with an accuracy within 0.1 per cent of the stated value, traceable to the official standard).

If in-line conductivity cells cannot be dismantled, system calibration may be performed against a calibrated conductivity cell placed close to the cell to be calibrated in the water flow.

PROCEDURE

Stage 1

1. Measure the conductivity without temperature compensation, recording simultaneously the temperature. Temperature-compensated measurement may be performed after suitable validation.

2. Using Table 0169.-1, find the closest temperature value that is not greater than the measured temperature. The corresponding conductivity value is the limit at that temperature.

3. If the measured conductivity is not greater than the value in Table 0169.-1, the water to be examined meets the requirements of the test for conductivity. If the conductivity is higher than the value in Table 0169.-1, proceed with stage 2.

Table 0169.-1. – *Stage 1 - Temperature and conductivity requirements (for non-temperature-compensated conductivity measurements)*

Temperature (°C)	**Conductivity (μS·cm^{-1})**
0	0.6
5	0.8
10	0.9
15	1.0
20	1.1
25	1.3
30	1.4
35	1.5
40	1.7
45	1.8
50	1.9
55	2.1
60	2.2
65	2.4
70	2.5
75	2.7
80	2.7
85	2.7
90	2.7
95	2.9
100	3.1

Stage 2

4. Transfer a sufficient amount of the water to be examined (100 ml or more) to a suitable container, and stir the test sample. Adjust the temperature, if necessary, and while maintaining it at 25 ± 1 °C, begin vigorously agitating the test sample while periodically observing the conductivity. When the change in conductivity (due to uptake of atmospheric carbon dioxide) is less than 0.1 μS.cm^{-1} per 5 min, note the conductivity.

5. If the conductivity is not greater than 2.1 μS.cm^{-1}, the water to be examined meets the requirements of the test for conductivity. If the conductivity is greater than 2.1 μS.cm^{-1}, proceed with stage 3.

Stage 3

6. Perform this test within approximately 5 min of the conductivity determination in step 5 under stage 2, while maintaining the sample temperature at 25 ± 1 °C. Add a recently prepared saturated solution of *potassium chloride R* to the test sample (0.3 ml per 100 ml of the test sample), and determine the pH (*2.2.3*) to the nearest 0.1 pH unit.

7. Using Table 0169.-2, determine the conductivity limit at the measured pH value in step 6. If the measured conductivity in step 4 under stage 2 is not greater than the conductivity requirements for the pH determined, the water to be examined meets the requirements of the test for conductivity. If either the measured conductivity is greater than this value or the pH is outside the range of 5.0-7.0, the water to be examined does not meet the requirements of the test for conductivity.

Monographs T-Z

Table 0169.-2. – *Stage 3 - pH and conductivity requirements (for atmosphere and temperature equilibrated samples)*

pH	Conductivity ($\mu S \cdot cm^{-1}$)
5.0	4.7
5.1	4.1
5.2	3.6
5.3	3.3
5.4	3.0
5.5	2.8
5.6	2.6
5.7	2.5
5.8	2.4
5.9	2.4
6.0	2.4
6.1	2.4
6.2	2.5
6.3	2.4
6.4	2.3
6.5	2.2
6.6	2.1
6.7	2.6
6.8	3.1
6.9	3.8
7.0	4.6

In order to ensure the appropriate quality of the water, validated procedures and in-process-monitoring of the electrical conductivity and regular microbial monitoring are applied.

Water for injections in bulk is stored and distributed in conditions designed to prevent growth of micro-organisms and to avoid any other contamination.

CHARACTERS

Appearance: clear and colourless liquid.

TESTS

Nitrates: maximum 0.2 ppm.

Place 5 ml in a test-tube immersed in iced water, add 0.4 ml of a 100 g/l solution of *potassium chloride R*, 0.1 ml of *diphenylamine solution R* and, dropwise with shaking, 5 ml of *nitrogen-free sulphuric acid R*. Transfer the tube to a water-bath at 50 °C. After 15 min, any blue colour in the solution is not more intense than that in a reference solution prepared at the same time in the same manner using a mixture of 4.5 ml of *nitrate-free water R* and 0.5 ml of *nitrate standard solution (2 ppm NO_3) R*.

Aluminium (*2.4.17*): maximum 10 ppb, if intended for use in the manufacture of dialysis solutions.

Prescribed solution. To 400 ml of the water to be examined add 10 ml of *acetate buffer solution pH 6.0 R* and 100 ml of *distilled water R*.

Reference solution. Mix 2 ml of *aluminium standard solution (2 ppm Al) R*, 10 ml of *acetate buffer solution pH 6.0 R* and 98 ml of *distilled water R*.

Blank solution. Mix 10 ml of *acetate buffer solution pH 6.0 R* and 100 ml of *distilled water R*.

Heavy metals (*2.4.8*): maximum 0.1 ppm.

Heat 200 ml in a glass evaporating dish on a water-bath until the volume is reduced to 20 ml. 12 ml of the concentrated solution complies with limit test A. Prepare the standard using 10 ml of *lead standard solution (1 ppm Pb) R*.

Bacterial endotoxins (*2.6.14*): less than 0.25 IU/ml.

Sterilised water for injections

DEFINITION

Water for injections in bulk that has been distributed into suitable containers, closed and sterilised by heat in conditions which ensure that the product still complies with the test for bacterial endotoxins. Sterilised water for injections is free from any added substances.

Examined in suitable conditions of visibility, it is clear and colourless.

Each container contains a sufficient quantity of water for injections to permit the nominal volume to be withdrawn.

TESTS

Acidity or alkalinity. To 20 ml add 0.05 ml of *phenol red solution R*. If the solution is yellow, it becomes red on the addition of 0.1 ml of *0.01 M sodium hydroxide*; if red, it becomes yellow on the addition of 0.15 ml of *0.01 M hydrochloric acid*.

Conductivity: maximum 25 $\mu S \cdot cm^{-1}$ for containers with a nominal volume of 10 ml or less; maximum 5 $\mu S \cdot cm^{-1}$ for containers with a nominal volume greater than 10 ml.

Use equipment and the calibration procedure as defined under Water for injections in bulk, maintaining the sample temperature at 25 ± 1 °C.

Oxidisable substances. Boil 100 ml with 10 ml of *dilute sulphuric acid R*. Add 0.2 ml of *0.02 M potassium permanganate* and boil for 5 min. The solution remains faintly pink.

Chlorides (*2.4.4*): maximum 0.5 ppm for containers with a nominal volume of 100 ml or less.

15 ml complies with the limit test for chlorides. Prepare the standard using a mixture of 1.5 ml of *chloride standard solution (5 ppm Cl) R* and 13.5 ml of *water R*. Examine the solutions down the vertical axes of the tubes.

For containers with a nominal volume greater than 100 ml, use the following test: to 10 ml add 1 ml of *dilute nitric acid R* and 0.2 ml of *silver nitrate solution R2*. The solution shows no change in appearance for at least 15 min.

Nitrates: maximum 0.2 ppm.

Place 5 ml in a test-tube immersed in iced water, add 0.4 ml of a 100 g/l solution of *potassium chloride R*, 0.1 ml of *diphenylamine solution R* and, dropwise with shaking, 5 ml of *nitrogen-free sulphuric acid R*. Transfer the tube to a water-bath at 50 °C. After 15 min, any blue colour in the solution is not more intense than that in a reference solution prepared at the same time in the same manner using a mixture of 4.5 ml of *nitrate-free water R* and 0.5 ml of *nitrate standard solution (2 ppm NO_3) R*.

Sulphates. To 10 ml add 0.1 ml of *dilute hydrochloric acid R* and 0.1 ml of *barium chloride solution R1*. The solution shows no change in appearance for at least 1 h.

Aluminium (*2.4.17*): maximum 10 ppb, if intended for use in the manufacture of dialysis solutions.

Prescribed solution. To 400 ml of the water to be examined add 10 ml of *acetate buffer solution pH 6.0 R* and 100 ml of *distilled water R*.

Reference solution. Mix 2 ml of *aluminium standard solution (2 ppm Al) R*, 10 ml of *acetate buffer solution pH 6.0 R* and 98 ml of *distilled water R*.

Blank solution. Mix 10 ml of *acetate buffer solution pH 6.0 R* and 100 ml of *distilled water R*.

Ammonium: maximum 0.2 ppm.

To 20 ml add 1 ml of *alkaline potassium tetraiodomercurate solution R*. After 5 min, examine the solution down the vertical axis of the tube. The solution is not more intensely coloured than a standard prepared at the same time by adding 1 ml of *alkaline potassium tetraiodomercurate solution R* to a mixture of 4 ml of *ammonium standard solution (1 ppm NH_4) R* and 16 ml of *ammonium-free water R*.

Calcium and magnesium. To 100 ml add 2 ml of *ammonium chloride buffer solution pH 10.0 R*, 50 mg of *mordant black 11 triturate R* and 0.5 ml of *0.01 M sodium edetate*. A pure blue colour is produced.

Heavy metals (*2.4.8*): maximum 0.1 ppm.

Heat 200 ml in a glass evaporating dish on a water-bath until the volume is reduced to 20 ml. 12 ml of the concentrated solution complies with limit test A. Prepare the standard using 10 ml of *lead standard solution (1 ppm Pb) R*.

Residue on evaporation: maximum 4 mg (0.004 per cent) for containers with a nominal volume of 10 ml or less; maximum 3 mg (0.003 per cent) for containers with a nominal volume greater than 10 ml.

Evaporate 100 ml to dryness on a water-bath and dry in an oven at 100-105 °C.

Particulate contamination: sub-visible particles (*2.9.19*). It complies with test A or test B, as appropriate.

Sterility (*2.6.1*). It complies with the test for sterility.

Bacterial endotoxins (*2.6.14*): less than 0.25 IU/ml.

01/2005:1927
corrected

WATER, HIGHLY PURIFIED

Aqua valde purificata

H_2O M_r 18.02

DEFINITION

Water intended for use in the preparation of medicinal products where water of high biological quality is needed, except where *Water for injections (0169)* is required.

PRODUCTION

Highly purified water is obtained from water that complies with the regulations on water intended for human consumption laid down by the competent authority.

Current production methods include for example double-pass reverse osmosis coupled with other suitable techniques such as ultrafiltration and deionisation. Correct operation and maintenance of the system is essential.

During production and subsequent storage, appropriate measures are taken to ensure that the total viable aerobic count is adequately controlled and monitored. Appropriate alert and action limits are set so as to detect adverse trends. Under normal conditions, an appropriate action limit is a total viable aerobic count (*2.6.12*) of 10 micro-organisms per 100 ml when determined by membrane filtration, using agar medium S, at least 200 ml of highly purified water and incubating at 30-35 °C for 5 days.

Total organic carbon (*2.2.44*): maximum 0.5 mg/l.

Conductivity. Determine the conductivity off-line or in-line under the following conditions.

EQUIPMENT

Conductivity cell:

– electrodes of a suitable material such as stainless steel;

– cell constant: within 2 per cent of the given value determined using a certified reference solution with a conductivity less than 1500 μS·cm^{-1}.

Conductometer: resolution 0.1 μS·cm^{-1} on the lowest range.

System calibration (conductivity cell and conductometer):

– against one or more suitable certified standard solutions;

– accuracy: within 3 per cent of the measured conductivity plus 0.1 μS·cm^{-1}.

Conductometer calibration: by means of precision resistors or equivalent devices after disconnecting the conductivity cell, for all ranges used for conductivity measurement and cell calibration (with an accuracy within 0.1 per cent of the stated value, traceable to the official standard).

If in-line conductivity cells cannot be dismantled, system calibration may be performed against a calibrated conductivity cell placed close to the cell to be calibrated in the water flow.

PROCEDURE

Stage 1

1. Measure the conductivity without temperature compensation, recording simultaneously the temperature. Temperature-compensated measurement may be performed after suitable validation.

2. Using Table 1927.-1, find the closest temperature value that is not greater than the measured temperature. The corresponding conductivity value is the limit at that temperature.

3. If the measured conductivity is not greater than the value in Table 1927.-1, the water to be examined meets the requirements of the test for conductivity. If the conductivity is higher than the value in Table 1927.-1, proceed with stage 2.

Monographs T-Z

Table 1927.-1. – *Stage 1 - Temperature and conductivity requirements (for non-temperature-compensated conductivity measurements)*

Temperature (°C)	Conductivity ($\mu S \cdot cm^{-1}$)
0	0.6
5	0.8
10	0.9
15	1.0
20	1.1
25	1.3
30	1.4
35	1.5
40	1.7
45	1.8
50	1.9
55	2.1
60	2.2
65	2.4
70	2.5
75	2.7
80	2.7
85	2.7
90	2.7
95	2.9
100	3.1

Stage 2

4. Transfer a sufficient amount of the water to be examined (100 ml or more) to a suitable container, and stir the test sample. Adjust the temperature, if necessary, and while maintaining it at 25 ± 1 °C, begin vigorously agitating the test sample while periodically observing the conductivity. When the change in conductivity (due to uptake of atmospheric carbon dioxide) is less than 0.1 $\mu S \cdot cm^{-1}$ per 5 min, note the conductivity.
5. If the conductivity is not greater than 2.1 $\mu S \cdot cm^{-1}$, the water to be examined meets the requirements of the test for conductivity. If the conductivity is greater than 2.1 $\mu S \cdot cm^{-1}$, proceed with stage 3.

Stage 3

6. Perform this test within approximately 5 min of the conductivity determination in step 5 under stage 2, while maintaining the sample temperature at 25 ± 1 °C. Add a recently prepared saturated solution of *potassium chloride R* to the test sample (0.3 ml per 100 ml of the test sample), and determine the pH (*2.2.3*) to the nearest 0.1 pH unit.
7. Using Table 1927.-2, determine the conductivity limit at the measured pH value in step 6. If the measured conductivity in step 4 under stage 2 is not greater than the conductivity requirements for the pH determined, the water to be examined meets the requirements of the test for conductivity. If either the measured conductivity is greater than this value or the pH is outside the range of 5.0-7.0, the water to be examined does not meet the requirements of the test for conductivity.

In order to ensure the appropriate quality of the water, validated procedures and in-process monitoring of the electrical conductivity and regular microbial monitoring are applied.

Highly purified water is stored in bulk and distributed in conditions designed to prevent growth of micro-organisms and to avoid any other contamination.

Table 1927.-2. – *Stage 3 - pH and conductivity requirements (for atmosphere and temperature equilibrated samples)*

pH	Conductivity ($\mu S \cdot cm^{-1}$)
5.0	4.7
5.1	4.1
5.2	3.6
5.3	3.3
5.4	3.0
5.5	2.8
5.6	2.6
5.7	2.5
5.8	2.4
5.9	2.4
6.0	2.4
6.1	2.4
6.2	2.5
6.3	2.4
6.4	2.3
6.5	2.2
6.6	2.1
6.7	2.6
6.8	3.1
6.9	3.8
7.0	4.6

CHARACTERS

Appearance: clear and colourless liquid.

TESTS

Nitrates: maximum 0.2 ppm.

Place 5 ml in a test-tube immersed in iced water, add 0.4 ml of a 100 g/l solution of *potassium chloride R*, 0.1 ml of *diphenylamine solution R* and, dropwise with shaking, 5 ml of *nitrogen-free sulphuric acid R*. Transfer the tube to a water-bath at 50 °C. After 15 min, any blue colour in the solution is not more intense than that in a reference solution prepared at the same time in the same manner using a mixture of 4.5 ml of *nitrate-free water R* and 0.5 ml of *nitrate standard solution (2 ppm NO_3) R*.

Aluminium (*2.4.17*): maximum 10 ppb, if intended for use in the manufacture of dialysis solutions.

Prescribed solution. To 400 ml of the water to be examined add 10 ml of *acetate buffer solution pH 6.0 R* and 100 ml of *distilled water R*.

Reference solution. Mix 2 ml of *aluminium standard solution (2 ppm Al) R*, 10 ml of *acetate buffer solution pH 6.0 R* and 98 ml of *distilled water R*.

Blank solution. Mix 10 ml of *acetate buffer solution pH 6.0 R* and 100 ml of *distilled water R*.

Monographs T-Z

Heavy metals (*2.4.8*): maximum 0.1 ppm.

Heat 200 ml in a glass evaporating dish on a water-bath until the volume is reduced to 20 ml. 12 ml of the concentrated solution complies with limit test A. Prepare the standard using 10 ml of *lead standard solution (1 ppm Pb) R*.

Bacterial endotoxins (*2.6.14*): less than 0.25 IU/ml.

LABELLING

The label states, where applicable, that the substance is suitable for use in the manufacture of dialysis solutions.

01/2005:0008
corrected

WATER, PURIFIED

Aqua purificata

H_2O M_r 18.02

DEFINITION

Water for the preparation of medicines other than those that are required to be both sterile and apyrogenic, unless otherwise justified and authorised.

Purified water in bulk

PRODUCTION

Purified water in bulk is prepared by distillation, by ion exchange, by reverse osmosis or by any other suitable method from water that complies with the regulations on water intended for human consumption laid down by the competent authority.

During production and subsequent storage, appropriate measures are taken to ensure that the total viable aerobic count is adequately controlled and monitored. Appropriate alert and action limits are set so as to detect adverse trends. Under normal conditions, an appropriate action limit is a total viable aerobic count (*2.6.12*) of 100 micro-organisms per millilitre, determined by membrane filtration, using agar medium S and incubating at 30-35 °C for 5 days. The size of the sample is to be chosen in relation to the expected result.

In addition, the test for total organic carbon (*2.2.44*) with a limit of 0.5 mg/l or alternatively the following test for oxidisable substances is carried out: to 100 ml add 10 ml of *dilute sulphuric acid R* and 0.1 ml of *0.02 M potassium permanganate* and boil for 5 min; the solution remains faintly pink.

Conductivity. Determine the conductivity off-line or in-line under the following conditions.

EQUIPMENT

Conductivity cell:

- electrodes of a suitable material such as stainless steel;
- cell constant: within 2 per cent of the given value determined using a certified reference solution with a conductivity less than 1500 μS·cm^{-1}.

Conductometer: resolution 0.1 μS·cm^{-1} on the lowest range.

System calibration (conductivity cell and conductometer):

- against one or more suitable certified standard solutions;
- accuracy: within 3 per cent of the measured conductivity plus 0.1 μS·cm^{-1}.

Conductometer calibration: by means of precision resistors or equivalent devices, after disconnecting the conductivity cell, for all ranges used for conductivity measurement and cell calibration (with an accuracy within 0.1 per cent of the stated value, traceable to the official standard).

If in-line conductivity cells cannot be dismantled, system calibration may be performed against a calibrated conductivity cell placed close to the cell to be calibrated in the water flow.

PROCEDURE

Measure the conductivity without temperature compensation, recording simultaneously the temperature. Temperature-compensated measurement may be performed after suitable validation.

The water to be examined meets the requirements if the measured conductivity at the recorded temperature is not greater than the value in Table 0008.-1.

Table 0008.-1. – *Temperature and conductivity requirements*

Temperature (°C)	Conductivity (μS·cm^{-1})
0	2.4
10	3.6
20	4.3
25	5.1
30	5.4
40	6.5
50	7.1
60	8.1
70	9.1
75	9.7
80	9.7
90	9.7
100	10.2

For temperatures not listed in Table 0008.-1, calculate the maximal permitted conductivity by interpolation between the next lower and next higher data points in the table.

Purified water in bulk is stored and distributed in conditions designed to prevent growth of micro-organisms and to avoid any other contamination.

CHARACTERS

Appearance: clear and colourless liquid.

TESTS

Nitrates: maximum 0.2 ppm.

Place 5 ml in a test-tube immersed in iced water, add 0.4 ml of a 100 g/l solution of *potassium chloride R*, 0.1 ml of *diphenylamine solution R* and, dropwise with shaking, 5 ml of *nitrogen-free sulphuric acid R*. Transfer the tube to a water-bath at 50 °C. After 15 min, any blue colour in the solution is not more intense than that in a reference solution prepared at the same time in the same manner using a mixture of 4.5 ml of *nitrate-free water R* and 0.5 ml of *nitrate standard solution (2 ppm NO_3) R*.

Aluminium (*2.4.17*): maximum 10 ppb, if intended for use in the manufacture of dialysis solutions.

Prescribed solution. To 400 ml of the water to be examined add 10 ml of *acetate buffer solution pH 6.0 R* and 100 ml of *distilled water R*.

Reference solution. Mix 2 ml of *aluminium standard solution (2 ppm Al) R*, 10 ml of *acetate buffer solution pH 6.0 R* and 98 ml of *distilled water R*.

Blank solution. Mix 10 ml of *acetate buffer solution pH 6.0 R* and 100 ml of *distilled water R*.

Monographs T-Z

Heavy metals (*2.4.8*): maximum 0.1 ppm.

Heat 200 ml in a glass evaporating dish on a water-bath until the volume is reduced to 20 ml. 12 ml of the concentrated solution complies with limit test A. Prepare the standard using 10 ml of *lead standard solution (1 ppm Pb) R*.

Bacterial endotoxins (*2.6.14*): less than 0.25 IU/ml, if intended for use in the manufacture of dialysis solutions without a further appropriate procedure for removal of bacterial endotoxins.

LABELLING

The label states, where applicable, that the substance is suitable for use in the manufacture of dialysis solutions.

Purified water in containers

DEFINITION

Purified water in bulk that has been filled and stored in conditions designed to assure the required microbiological quality. It is free from any added substances.

CHARACTERS

Appearance: clear and colourless liquid.

TESTS

It complies with the tests prescribed in the section on Purified water in bulk and with the following additional tests.

Acidity or alkalinity. To 10 ml, freshly boiled and cooled in a borosilicate glass flask, add 0.05 ml of *methyl red solution R*. The solution is not coloured red.

To 10 ml add 0.1 ml of *bromothymol blue solution R1*. The solution is not coloured blue.

Oxidisable substances. To 100 ml add 10 ml of *dilute sulphuric acid R* and 0.1 ml of *0.02 M potassium permanganate* and boil for 5 min. The solution remains faintly pink.

Chlorides. To 10 ml add 1 ml of *dilute nitric acid R* and 0.2 ml of *silver nitrate solution R2*. The solution shows no change in appearance for at least 15 min.

Sulphates. To 10 ml add 0.1 ml of *dilute hydrochloric acid R* and 0.1 ml of *barium chloride solution R1*. The solution shows no change in appearance for at least 1 h.

Ammonium: maximum 0.2 ppm.

To 20 ml add 1 ml of *alkaline potassium tetraiodomercurate solution R*. After 5 min, examine the solution down the vertical axis of the tube. The solution is not more intensely coloured than a standard prepared at the same time by adding 1 ml of *alkaline potassium tetraiodomercurate solution R* to a mixture of 4 ml of *ammonium standard solution (1 ppm NH_4) R* and 16 ml of *ammonium-free water R*.

Calcium and magnesium. To 100 ml add 2 ml of *ammonium chloride buffer solution pH 10.0 R*, 50 mg of *mordant black 11 triturate R* and 0.5 ml of *0.01 M sodium edetate*. A pure blue colour is produced.

Residue on evaporation: maximum 0.001 per cent.

Evaporate 100 ml on a water-bath and dry in an oven at 100-105 °C. The residue weighs a maximum of 1 mg.

Microbial contamination. Total viable aerobic count (*2.6.12*) not more than 10^2 micro-organisms per millilitre, determined by membrane filtration, using agar medium B.

LABELLING

The label states, where applicable, that the substance is suitable for use in the manufacture of dialysis solutions.

01/2005:0359

WHEAT STARCH

Tritici amylum

DEFINITION

Wheat starch is obtained from the caryopsis of *Triticum aestivum* L. (*T. vulgare* Vill.).

CHARACTERS

Appearance: very fine, white powder which creaks when pressed between the fingers.

Solubility: practically insoluble in cold water and in alcohol.

Wheat starch does not contain starch grains of any other origin. It may contain a minute quantity, if any, of tissue fragments of the original plant.

IDENTIFICATION

A. Examined under a microscope using equal volumes of *glycerol R* and *water R*, it presents large and small granules, and, very rarely, intermediate sizes. The large granules, 10 µm to 60 µm in diameter, are discoid or, more rarely, reniform when seen face-on. The central hilum and striations are invisible or barely visible and the granules sometimes show cracks on the edges. Seen in profile, the granules are elliptical and fusiform and the hilum appears as a slit along the main axis. The small granules, rounded or polyhedral, are 2 µm to 10 µm in diameter. Between crossed nicol prisms, the granules show a distinct black cross intersecting at the hilum.

B. Suspend 1 g in 50 ml of *water R*, boil for 1 min and cool. A thin, cloudy mucilage is formed.

C. To 1 ml of the mucilage obtained in identification test B, add 0.05 ml of *iodine solution R1*. A dark blue colour is produced which disappears on heating.

TESTS

pH (*2.2.3*): 4.5 to 7.0.

Shake 5.0 g with 25.0 ml of *carbon dioxide-free water R* for 60 s. Allow to stand for 15 min.

Foreign matter. Examined under a microscope using a mixture of equal volumes of *glycerol R* and *water R*, not more than traces of matter other than starch granules are present. No starch grains of any other origin are present.

Total protein: maximum 0.3 per cent of total protein (corresponding to 0.048 per cent N_2, conversion factor: 6.25), determined on 6.0 g by sulphuric acid digestion (*2.5.9*) modified as follows: wash any adhering particles from the neck into the flask with 25 ml of *sulphuric acid R*; continue the heating until a clear solution is obtained; add 45 ml of *strong sodium hydroxide solution R*.

Oxidising substances (*2.5.30*): maximum 20 ppm, calculated as H_2O_2.

Sulphur dioxide (*2.5.29*): maximum 50 ppm.

Iron (*2.4.9*): maximum 10 ppm.

Shake 1.5 g with 15 ml of *dilute hydrochloric acid R*. Filter. The filtrate complies with the limit test for iron.

Loss on drying (*2.2.32*): maximum 15.0 per cent, determined on 1.000 g by drying in an oven at 130 °C for 90 min.

Sulphated ash (*2.4.14*): maximum 0.6 per cent, determined on 1.0 g.

Monographs T-Z

Microbial contamination. Total viable aerobic count (*2.6.12*) not more than 10^3 bacteria and not more than 10^2 fungi per gram, determined by plate count. It complies with the test for *Escherichia coli* (*2.6.13*).

01/2005:1379

WHEAT-GERM OIL, REFINED

Tritici aestivi oleum raffinatum

DEFINITION

Fatty oil obtained from the germ of the grain of *Triticum aestivum* L. by cold expression or by other suitable mechanical means and/or by extraction. It is then refined. A suitable antioxidant may be added.

CHARACTERS

Appearance: clear, light yellow liquid.

Solubility: practically insoluble in water and in alcohol, miscible with light petroleum (40 °C to 60 °C).

Relative density: about 0.925.

Refractive index: about 1.475.

IDENTIFICATION

A. Identification of fatty oils by thin-layer chromatography (*2.3.2*). The chromatogram obtained is similar to the type chromatogram for wheat-germ oil.

B. It complies with the test for composition of fatty acids (see Tests).

TESTS

Acid value (*2.5.1*): maximum 0.9. If intended for use in the manufacture of parenteral dosage forms: maximum 0.3.

Peroxide value (*2.5.5*): maximum 10.0. If intended for use in the manufacture of parenteral dosage forms: maximum 5.0.

Unsaponifiable matter (*2.5.7*): maximum 5.0 per cent, determined on 5.0 g.

Alkaline impurities (*2.4.19*). It complies with the test for alkaline impurities in fatty oils.

Composition of fatty acids. Gas chromatography (*2.4.22, Method C*). Use the mixture of calibrating substances in Table 2.4.22.-3.

Composition of the fatty-acid fraction of the oil:

- *palmitic acid*: 14.0 per cent to 19.0 per cent,
- *stearic acid*: maximum 2.0 per cent,
- *oleic acid*: 12.0 per cent to 23.0 per cent,
- *linoleic acid*: 52.0 per cent to 59.0 per cent,
- *linolenic acid*: 3.0 per cent to 10.0 per cent,
- *eicosenoic acid*: maximum 2.0 per cent.

Brassicasterol (*2.4.23*): maximum 0.3 per cent of brassicasterol in the sterol fraction of the oil.

Water (*2.5.32*). If intended for use in the manufacture of parenteral dosage forms: maximum 0.1 per cent, determined on 5.00 g. Use a mixture of equal volumes of *methanol R* and *methylene chloride R* as solvent.

STORAGE

In an airtight, well-filled container, protected from light.

LABELLING

The label states:

- the name and concentration of any added antioxidant,
- where applicable, that the substance is suitable for use in the manufacture of parenteral dosage forms,
- whether the oil is obtained by mechanical means, by extraction or by a combination of the two.

01/2005:1480

WHEAT-GERM OIL, VIRGIN

Tritici aestivi oleum virginale

DEFINITION

Virgin wheat-germ oil is the fatty oil obtained from the germ of the grain of *Triticum aestivum* L. by cold expression or other suitable mechanical means.

CHARACTERS

A clear, light yellow or golden-yellow liquid, practically insoluble in water and in alcohol, miscible with light petroleum (40 °C to 60 °C).

It has a relative density of about 0.925 and a refractive index of about 1.475.

IDENTIFICATION

A. Carry out the identification of fatty oils by thin-layer chromatography (*2.3.2*). The chromatogram obtained is comparable with the typical chromatogram for wheat-germ oil.

B. It complies with test for composition of fatty acids (see Tests).

TESTS

Acid value (*2.5.1*). Not more than 20.0, determined on 10.0 g.

Peroxide value (*2.5.5*). Not more than 15.0.

Unsaponifiable matter (*2.5.7*). Not more than 5.0 per cent, determined on 5.0 g.

Composition of fatty acids (*2.4.22, Method C*). The fatty-acid fraction of the oil has the following composition:

- *palmitic acid*: 14.0 per cent to 19.0 per cent,
- *stearic acid*: not more than 2.0 per cent,
- *oleic acid*: 12.0 per cent to 23.0 per cent,
- *linoleic acid*: 52.0 per cent to 59.0 per cent,
- *linolenic acid*: 3.0 per cent to 10.0 per cent,
- *eicosenoic acid*: not more than 2.0 per cent.

Brassicasterol (*2.4.23*). The sterol fraction of the oil contains not more than 0.3 per cent of brassicasterol.

Water (*2.5.32*). Not more than 0.1 per cent, determined on 5.00 g by the micro-determination of water. Use a mixture of equal volumes of *methanol R* and *methylene chloride R* as solvent.

STORAGE

Store in an airtight, well-filled container, protected from light.

Monographs T-Z

01/2005:1855

WILD PANSY (FLOWERING AERIAL PARTS)

Violae herba cum flore

DEFINITION

Dried flowering aerial parts of *Viola arvensis* Murray and/or *Viola tricolor* L.

Content: minimum 1.5 per cent of flavonoids, expressed as violanthin ($C_{27}H_{30}O_{14}$; M_r 578.5) (dried drug).

CHARACTERS

Macroscopic and microscopic characters described under identification tests A and B.

IDENTIFICATION

A. The stem is angular and hollow. The leaves are oval, petiolate, with a cordate base or elongated and obtuse, with lyrate stipules, divided in the middle. The flowers, with a long peduncle, are zygomorphic, with 5 oval, lanceolate sepals, an appendage pointed outwards and 5 petals of which the lower one bears a spur; in *Viola arvensis*, the petals are shorter than the calyx, the lower petal is cream coloured, with black lines, the 4 upper petals may be cream coloured or violet blue; in *Viola tricolor*, the petals are longer than the calyx and violet coloured, more or less tinged with yellow. The androecium consisting of 5 stamens bears at the apex a membranous connective appendage with 2 spurs. The trilocular ovary shows a short style and globular stigmata. The fruit are navicular capsules, three-lobed, yellowish brown, 5 mm to 10 mm long. The pale yellow, pyriform seeds are about 1 mm long, bearing a caruncle.

B. Reduce to a powder (355). The powder is greenish. Examine under a microscope using *chloral hydrate solution R*. The powder shows the following diagnostic characters: fragments of the epidermis of the leaves in surface view with wavy-walled cells and anomocytic stomata (*2.8.3*); conical unicellular covering trichomes, widened at the base and sharply pointed at the apex, with a striated cuticle; glandular trichomes with a multicellular head, and a short, multicellular stalk in the indentations of the leaf margins; cluster crystals of calcium oxalate, sometimes included in parenchyma; fragments of the corolla with wavy-walled epidermal cells, those from the mid-region papillose and with some extended to form flask or bottle-shaped projections, those from the base of the petals with covering trichomes up to about 300 μm long with characteristic hump-like swellings along their length; spherical or polyhedral pollen grains, 60 μm to 80 μm in diameter, with finely pitted exines and 5 pores (*Viola arvensis*) or 4 pores (*Viola tricolor*); occasional fragments of spiral and reticulate vessels and groups of fibres from the stem.

C. Thin-layer chromatography (*2.2.27*).

Test solution. Heat in a water-bath at 65 °C for 5 min, with frequent stirring, 2.0 g of the powdered drug (355) in 10 ml of *alcohol (70 per cent V/V) R*. Cool and filter.

Reference solution. Dissolve 2.5 mg of *rutin R*, 2.5 mg of *hyperoside R* and 1.0 mg of *caffeic acid R* in *methanol R* and dilute to 10 ml with the same solvent.

Plate: *TLC silica gel plate R*.

Mobile phase: *anhydrous formic acid R, acetic acid R, water R, ethyl acetate R* (11:11:27:100 *V/V/V/V*).

Application: 10 μl, as bands.

Development: over a path of 12 cm.

Drying: at 100-105 °C.

Detection: spray with a solution containing 10 g/l of *diphenylboric acid aminoethyl ester R* and 50 g/l of *macrogol 400 R* in *methanol R*. Allow the plate to dry in air for 30 min. Examine in ultraviolet light at 365 nm.

Results: see below the sequence of the zones present in the chromatograms obtained with the reference solution and the test solution. Furthermore, other zones may be present in the chromatogram obtained with the test solution.

Top of the plate	
Caffeic acid: a greenish-blue to light blue fluorescent zone	
	A blue fluorescent zone
_______	_______
Hyperoside: a yellowish-brown fluorescent zone	
	A yellowish-green fluorescent zone
_______	_______
Rutin: a yellowish-brown fluorescent zone	An intense yellowish-brown fluorescent zone (rutin)
	A yellowish-green fluorescent zone
	A yellowish-green fluorescent zone
	A yellowish-green fluorescent zone
Reference solution	**Test solution**

TESTS

Foreign matter (*2.8.2*): maximum 3 per cent.

Swelling index (*2.8.4*): minimum 9, determined on the powdered drug (355).

Loss on drying (*2.2.32*): maximum 12.0 per cent, determined on 1.000 g of the powdered drug (355) by drying in an oven at 100-105 °C for 2 h.

Total ash (*2.4.16*): maximum 15.0 per cent.

ASSAY

Stock solution. In a 200 ml flask, introduce 0.300 g of the powdered drug (250) and 40 ml of *alcohol (60 per cent V/V) R*. Heat in a water-bath at 60 °C for 10 min, shaking frequently. Allow to cool and filter through a plug of absorbent cotton into a 100 ml volumetric flask. Transfer the absorbent cotton with the drug residue back into the 200 ml flask, add 40 ml of *alcohol (60 per cent V/V) R* and heat again in a water-bath at 60 °C for 10 min, shaking frequently. Allow to cool and filter into the same 100 ml volumetric flask as used previously. Rinse the 200 ml flask with a further quantity of *alcohol (60 per cent V/V) R*, filter and transfer to the same 100 ml volumetric flask. Dilute to volume with *alcohol (60 per cent V/V) R* and filter.

Test solution. Introduce 5.0 ml of the stock solution into a round-bottomed flask and evaporate to dryness under reduced pressure. Take up the residue with 8 ml of a mixture of 10 volumes of *methanol R* and 100 volumes of *glacial acetic acid R* and transfer into a 25 ml volumetric flask. Rinse the round-bottomed flask with 3 ml of a mixture of 10 volumes of *methanol R* and 100 volumes of *glacial acetic acid R* and transfer into the same 25 ml volumetric flask as used previously. Add 10.0 ml of a solution containing 25.0 g/l of *boric acid R* and 20.0 g/l of *oxalic acid R* in *anhydrous formic acid R* and dilute to 25.0 ml with *anhydrous acetic acid R*.

Compensation liquid. Introduce 5.0 ml of the stock solution into a round-bottomed flask and evaporate to dryness under reduced pressure. Take up the residue with 8 ml of a mixture of 10 volumes of *methanol R* and 100 volumes of *glacial acetic acid R* and transfer into a 25 ml volumetric flask. Rinse the round-bottomed flask with 3 ml of a mixture of 10 volumes of *methanol R* and 100 volumes of *glacial acetic acid R* and transfer into the same 25 ml volumetric flask as used previously. Add 10.0 ml of *anhydrous formic acid R* and dilute to 25.0 ml with *anhydrous acetic acid R*.

Measure the absorbance (*2.2.25*) of the test solution at 405 nm after 30 min.

Calculate the percentage content of total flavonoids, expressed as violanthin from the expression:

$$\frac{A \times 1.25}{m}$$

taking the specific absorbance of violanthin to be 400.

A = measured absorbance at 405 nm,

m = mass of the drug to be examined, in grams.

01/2005:1891

WILD THYME

Serpylli herba

DEFINITION

Whole or cut, dried, flowering aerial parts of *Thymus serpyllum* L.s.l.

Content: minimum 3.0 ml/kg of essential oil (dried drug).

CHARACTERS

Macroscopic and microscopic characters described under identification tests A and B.

IDENTIFICATION

A. The stem is much branched, up to about 1.5 mm in diameter, cylindrical or indistinctly quadrangular, green, reddish or purplish, the older stems brown and woody, the younger stems pubescent. The leaves are opposite, 3 mm to 12 mm long and up to 4 mm wide, elliptical to ovate-lanceolate with an obtuse apex, cuneate and shortly petiolate at the base; the margin is entire and markedly ciliate, especially near the base; both surfaces are more or less glabrous but distinctly punctate. The inflorescence is composed of about 6 to 12 flowers in rounded to ovoid, terminal heads. The calyx is tubular, two-lipped with the upper lip dividing to form 3 teeth, the lower lip with 2 teeth, edged with long hairs; inner surfaces strongly pubescent, the hairs forming a closed tube after flowering. The corolla is purplish-violet to red, two-lipped, the lower lip with 3 lobes, upper lip notched, inner surface strongly pubescent; stamens 4, epipetalous, projecting from the corolla tube.

B. Reduce to a powder (355). The powder is greyish-green to brownish-green. Examine under a microscope using *chloral hydrate solution R*. The powder shows the following diagnostic characters: fragments of the leaf epidermises with sinuous, slightly thickened anticlinical walls and stomata of the diacytic type (*2.8.3*); numerous covering trichomes on both epidermises and along the leaf margins, the majority short, conical, unicellular, with thickened and warty walls, fewer long, uniseriate, composed of up to 8 cells, slightly swollen at the joints, with moderately thickened walls; abundant glandular trichomes, mostly multicellular with a small, rounded, unicellular stalk and a large globular head composed of a number of indistinct, radiating cells containing brown secretion, others smaller, capitate, with unicellular stalk and a unicellular, globoid or ovoid head; purplish-violet fragments of the corolla, the outer epidermis with numerous covering and glandular trichomes, inner epidermis papillose; pollen grains spherical to elliptical, 30 µm to 40 µm in diameter, with a finely grained exine and 6 germinal pores.

C. Thin-layer chromatography (*2.2.27*).

Test solution. To 1.0 g of the powdered drug (355) add 5 ml of *methylene chloride R* and shake for 3 min. Filter through about 2 g of *anhydrous sodium sulphate R*.

Reference solution. Dissolve 5 mg of *thymol R* and 10 µl of *carvacrol R* in 10 ml of *methylene chloride R*.

Plate: *TLC silica gel F_{254} plate R*.

Mobile phase: *methylene chloride R*.

Application: 20 µl, as bands.

Development: over a path of 15 cm.

Drying: in air.

Detection A: examine in ultraviolet light at 254 nm.

Results A: see below the sequence of the zones present in the chromatograms obtained with the reference solution and the test solution.

Top of the plate	
———	———
	A prominent quenching zone
Thymol: a quenching zone	A quenching zone (thymol)
———	
	Quenching zones
Reference solution	**Test solution**

Detection B: spray with *anisaldehyde solution R* using 10 ml for a plate 200 mm square and heat at 100-105 °C for 10 min.

Results B: see below the sequence of the zones present in the chromatograms obtained with the reference solution and the test solution. Furthermore, other zones are present in the lower third of the chromatogram obtained with the test solution. The intensity of the zones due to thymol and carvacrol depends upon the sample examined (chemotypes).

Top of the plate	
———	———
Thymol: a brownish-pink zone	A brownish-pink zone (thymol)
Carvacrol: a pale violet zone	A pale violet zone (carvacrol)
———	———
Reference solution	**Test solution**

Monographs T-Z

TESTS

Foreign matter (*2.8.2*): maximum 3 per cent, determined on 30 g.

Foreign matter may also consist of acicular to linear-lanceolate leaves with a strongly bent margin, the adaxial surface showing covering trichomes shaped as pointed teeth with warty walls, the abaxial surface showing many types of warty covering trichomes: unicellular, straight or slightly curved, bicellular or tricellular, often elbow-shaped, and bicellular or tricellular, more or less straight (*Thymus vulgaris, Thymus zygis*).

Loss on drying (*2.2.32*): maximum 10.0 per cent, determined on 1.000 g of the powdered drug (355) by drying in an oven at 100-105 °C for 2 h.

Total ash (*2.4.16*): maximum 10.0 per cent.

Ash insoluble in hydrochloric acid (*2.8.1*): maximum 3.0 per cent.

ASSAY

Carry out the determination of essential oils in vegetable drugs (*2.8.12*). Use 50.0 g of the cut drug, a 1000 ml round-bottomed flask and 500 ml of *water R* as the distillation liquid. Distil at a rate of 2-3 ml/min for 2 h without *xylene R* in the graduated tube.

01/2005:1583
corrected

WILLOW BARK

Salicis cortex

DEFINITION

Willow bark consists of the whole or fragmented dried bark of young branches or whole dried pieces of current year twigs of various species of genus *Salix* including *S. purpurea* L., *S. daphnoides* Vill. and *S. fragilis* L. The drug contains not less than 1.5 per cent of total salicylic derivatives, expressed as salicin ($C_{13}H_{18}O_7$; M_r 286.3), calculated with reference to the dried drug.

CHARACTERS

Willow bark is markedly bitter.

It has the macroscopic and microscopic characters described under identification tests A and B.

IDENTIFICATION

A. The bark is 1 mm to 2 mm thick and occurs in flexible, elongated, quilled or curved pieces. The outer surface is smooth or slightly wrinkled longitudinally and greenish-yellow to brownish-grey. The inner surface is smooth or finely striated longitudinally and white, pale yellow or reddish-brown, depending on the species. The fracture is short in the outer part and coarsely fibrous in the inner region. The diameter of current year twigs is not more than 10 mm. The wood is white or pale yellow.

B. Reduce to a powder (355). The powder is pale yellow, greenish-yellow or light brown. Examine under a microscope using *chloral hydrate solution R*. The powder shows: bundles of narrow fibres, up to about 600 μm long, with very thick walls and surrounded by a crystal sheath containing prism crystals of calcium oxalate; parenchyma of the cortex with thick, pitted and deeply beaded walls, and containing large cluster crystals of calcium oxalate; uniseriate medullary rays; thickened and suberised cork cells. Groups of brownish collenchyma from the bud may be present. Twigs show, additionally, fragments of lignified fibres and vessels from the xylem.

C. Examine by thin-layer chromatography (*2.2.27*), using a *TLC silica gel plate R*.

Test solution (a). To 1.0 g of the powdered drug (500) add 20 ml of *methanol R*; heat in a water-bath at about 50 °C, with frequent shaking, for 10 min. Cool and filter.

Test solution (b). To 5.0 ml of test solution (a) add 1.0 ml of a 50 g/l solution of *anhydrous sodium carbonate R* and heat in a water-bath at about 60 °C for 10 min. Cool and filter if necessary.

Reference solution. Dissolve 2.0 mg of *salicin R* in 1.0 ml of *methanol R*.

Apply to the plate as bands 20 μl of each. Develop over a path of 15 cm using a mixture of 8 volumes of *water R*, 15 volumes of *methanol R* and 77 volumes of *ethyl acetate R*. Allow the plate to dry in air. Spray with a mixture of 5 volumes of *sulphuric acid R* and 95 volumes of *methanol R*. Heat at 100 °C to 105 °C for 5 min and examine in daylight. The chromatogram obtained with the reference solution shows in the middle third a reddish-violet zone due to salicin. In the chromatogram obtained with test solution (a), the zone due to salicin appears with only slight to moderate intensity. In the chromatogram obtained with test solution (b) the zone due to salicin is clearly more intense and there are, above the zone due to salicin, one (salicortin or 2′-*O*-acetylsalicortin, or possibly two tremulacin) faint reddish-violet zones Other blue, yellow or brown zones can occur in both chromatograms.

TESTS

Foreign matter (*2.8.2*). Not more than 3 per cent of twigs with a diameter greater than 10 mm, and not more than 2 per cent of other foreign matter.

Loss on drying (*2.2.32*). Not more than 11 per cent, determined on 1.000 g of the powdered drug (355), by drying in an oven at 100 °C to 105 °C for 2 h.

Total ash (*2.4.16*). Not more than 10 per cent.

ASSAY

Examine by liquid chromatography (*2.2.29*), using *resorcinol R* as the internal standard.

Internal standard solution. Dissolve 50 mg of *resorcinol R* in 10 ml of *methanol R*.

Test solution. To 0.5 g of the powdered drug (355) add 50 ml of *methanol R* and heat under a reflux condenser for 30 min. Cool and filter. Take up the residue with 50 ml of *methanol R*. Proceed as above. Combine the filtrates and evaporate under reduced pressure. Take up the residue with 5.0 ml of *methanol R*, add 5.0 ml of *0.1 M sodium hydroxide* and heat in a water-bath at about 60 °C under a reflux condenser, with frequent shaking for about 1 h. After cooling, add 0.5 ml of *1 M hydrochloric acid*. Dilute the solution to 20.0 ml with a mixture of 50 volumes of *methanol R* and 50 volumes of *water R*. Add 1.0 ml of the internal standard solution to 10.0 ml of this solution. Filter through a membrane filter.

Reference solution (a). Dissolve 18.5 mg of *salicin R* in 10.0 ml of a mixture of 20 volumes of *water R* and 80 volumes of *methanol R* and add 1.0 ml of the internal standard solution.

Reference solution (b). Dissolve 1.0 mg of *picein R* in 1.0 ml of reference solution (a).

Monographs T-Z

The chromatographic procedure may be carried out using:
- a stainless steel column, 0.10 m long and 3 mm or 4 mm in internal diameter, packed with *octadecylsilyl silica gel for chromatography R* (3 µm),
- as mobile phase at a flow rate of 1.0 ml/min a mixture of 1.8 volumes of *tetrahydrofuran R* and 98.2 volumes of *water R*, containing 0.5 per cent *V/V* of *phosphoric acid R*,
- as detector a spectrophotometer set at 270 nm,
- a loop injector.

Inject 10 µl of reference solution (b). The assay is not valid unless the resolution between the peaks corresponding to salicin and picein and between the peaks corresponding to picein and resorcinol is at least 1.5.

Inject five times 10 µl of reference solution (a).

Inject three times 10 µl of the test solution. Continue the chromatography for four times the retention time of the peak corresponding to salicin.

Calculate the percentage content of total salicylic derivatives, expressed as salicin, from the expression:

$$\frac{S_1 \times S_4 \times m_2 \times p \times 2}{S_2 \times S_3 \times m_1}$$

S_1 = area of the peak due to salicin in the chromatogram obtained with the test solution,

S_2 = area of the peak due to resorcinol in the chromatogram obtained with the test solution,

S_3 = area of the peak due to salicin in the chromatogram obtained with reference solution (a),

S_4 = area of the peak due to resorcinol in the chromatogram obtained with reference solution (a),

m_1 = mass of the drug in the test solution, in milligrams,

m_2 = mass of salicin in reference solution (a), in milligrams,

p = percentage content of salicin in the reference substance

STORAGE

Store protected from light.

01/2005:0593

WOOL ALCOHOLS

Alcoholes adipis lanae

DEFINITION

Mixture of sterols and higher aliphatic alcohols from wool fat. It may contain not more than 200 ppm of butylhydroxytoluene.

Content: minimum 30.0 per cent of cholesterol.

CHARACTERS

Appearance: pale-yellow or brownish-yellow, brittle mass becoming plastic on heating.

Solubility: practically insoluble in water, soluble in methylene chloride and in boiling ethanol, slightly soluble in alcohol (90 per cent *V/V*).

IDENTIFICATION

Dissolve 50 mg in 5 ml of *methylene chloride R* and add 1 ml of *acetic anhydride R* and 0.1 ml of *sulphuric acid R*. Within a few seconds, a green colour develops.

TESTS

Appearance of solution. To 1.0 g add 10 ml of *light petroleum R1* and shake while warming in a water-bath. The substance dissolves completely. After cooling, the solution is clear (*2.2.1*).

Alkalinity. Dissolve 2.0 g in 25 ml of hot *alcohol (90 per cent V/V) R* and add 0.5 ml of *phenolphthalein solution R1*. No red colour develops.

Melting point (*2.2.15*): minimum 58 °C.

Melt the substance to be examined by heating in a water-bath at a temperature which exceeds the expected melting point by not more than 10 °C; introduce the substance to be examined into the capillary tubes and allow to stand at 15-17 °C for not less than 16 h.

Acid value (*2.5.1*): maximum 2.0.

If necessary, heat in a water-bath under a reflux condenser to dissolve the substance to be examined.

Hydroxyl value (*2.5.3, Method A*): 120 to 180.

Peroxide value (*2.5.5, Method A*): maximum 15.

Take from the substance to be examined wedge-shaped pieces whose base consists of part of the surface. Melt the pieces before carrying out the determination. Before adding 0.5 ml of *saturated potassium iodide solution R*, cool the solution obtained to room temperature.

Saponification value (*2.5.6*): maximum 12.0, determined on 2.00 g. Heat under reflux for 4 h.

Butylhydroxytoluene. Gas chromatography (*2.2.28*).

Internal standard solution. Dissolve 0.20 g of *methyl decanoate R* in *carbon disulphide R* and dilute to 100.0 ml with the same solvent. Dilute 1.0 ml of the solution to 10.0 ml with *carbon disulphide R*.

Test solution (a). Dissolve 1.0 g of the substance to be examined in *carbon disulphide R* and dilute to 10.0 ml with the same solvent.

Test solution (b). Dissolve 1.0 g of the substance to be examined in *carbon disulphide R*, add 1.0 ml of the internal standard solution and dilute to 10.0 ml with *carbon disulphide R*.

Reference solution. Dissolve 0.20 g of *butylhydroxytoluene R* in *carbon disulphide R* and dilute to 100.0 ml with the same solvent. Dilute 1.0 ml of the solution to 10.0 ml with *carbon disulphide R*. To 1.0 ml of this solution add 1.0 ml of the internal standard solution and dilute to 10.0 ml with *carbon disulphide R*.

Precolumn: column filled with silanised glass wool.

Column:
- *size*: *l* = 1.5 m, Ø = 4 mm,
- *stationary phase*: *silanised diatomaceous earth for gas chromatography R* impregnated with 10 per cent *m/m* of *poly(dimethyl)siloxane R*.

Carrier gas: *nitrogen for chromatography R*.

Flow rate: 40 ml/min.

Temperature:
- *column*: 150 °C,
- *injection port*: 180 °C,
- *detector*: 300 °C.

Detection: flame ionisation.

Limit:

– *butylhydroxytoluene*: maximum 200 ppm.

Loss on drying (*2.2.32*): maximum 0.5 per cent, determined on 2.000 g by drying in an oven at 100-105 °C.

Total ash (*2.4.16*): maximum 0.1 per cent.

Water-absorption capacity. Place 0.6 g of the substance to be examined and 9.4 g of *white soft paraffin R* in a mortar and melt on a water-bath. Allow to cool and incorporate 20 ml of *water R*, added in portions. Within 24 h no water is released from the almost white, ointment-like emulsion.

ASSAY

Dissolve 0.1000 g in 12 ml of hot *alcohol (90 per cent V/V) R*. Allow to stand for 18 h, filter through a sintered-glass filter (16) and wash the filter with 2 quantities, each of 15 ml, of *alcohol (90 per cent V/V) R*. Combine the filtrate and washings, add 20 ml of a freshly prepared 10 g/l solution of *digitonin R* in *alcohol (90 per cent V/V) R* and heat to about 60 °C. Allow to cool, filter through a sintered-glass filter (16), wash the residue with 10 ml of *alcohol (90 per cent V/V) R* and dry to constant mass at 100-105 °C.

1 g of residue is equivalent to 0.239 g of cholesterol.

STORAGE

In a well-filled container, protected from light.

LABELLING

The label states, where applicable, the concentration of any added butylhydroxytoluene.

01/2005:0134

WOOL FAT

Adeps lanae

DEFINITION

Purified, anhydrous, waxy substance obtained from the wool of sheep (*Ovis aries*). It may contain not more than 200 ppm of butylhydroxytoluene.

CHARACTERS

Appearance: yellow, unctuous substance. When melted, it is a clear or almost clear, yellow liquid. A solution in light petroleum is opalescent.

Solubility: practically insoluble in water, slightly soluble in boiling ethanol.

It has a characteristic odour.

IDENTIFICATION

A. In a test-tube, dissolve 0.5 g in 5 ml of *methylene chloride R* and add 1 ml of *acetic anhydride R* and 0.1 ml of *sulphuric acid R*. A green colour develops.

B. Dissolve 50 mg in 5 ml of *methylene chloride R*, add 5 ml of *sulphuric acid R* and shake. A red colour develops and an intense green fluorescence appears in the lower layer when examined in daylight, with illumination from the rear of the observer.

TESTS

Water-soluble acid or alkaline substances. Melt 5.0 g on a water-bath and shake vigorously for 2 min with 75 ml of *water R* previously heated to 90-95 °C. Allow to cool and filter through filter paper previously rinsed with *water R*. To 60 ml of the filtrate (which may not be clear) add 0.25 ml of *bromothymol blue solution R1*. Not more than 0.2 ml of *0.02 M hydrochloric acid* or 0.15 ml of *0.02 M sodium hydroxide* is required to change the colour of the indicator.

Drop point (*2.2.17*): 38 °C to 44 °C.

To fill the metal cup, melt the wool fat on a water-bath, cool to about 50 °C, pour into the cup and allow to stand at 15-20 °C for 24 h.

Water-absorption capacity. Place 10 g in a mortar. Add *water R* in portions of 0.2 ml to 0.5 ml from a burette, stirring vigorously after each addition to incorporate the *water R*. The end-point is reached when visible droplets remain which cannot be incorporated. Not less than 20 ml of *water R* is absorbed.

Acid value (*2.5.1*): maximum 1.0, determined on 5.0 g dissolved in 25 ml of the prescribed mixture of solvents.

Peroxide value (*2.5.5, Method A*): maximum 20.

Before adding 0.5 ml of *saturated potassium iodide solution R*, cool the solution obtained to room temperature.

Saponification value (*2.5.6*): 90 to 105, determined on 2.00 g while heating under reflux for 4 h.

Water-soluble oxidisable substances. To 10 ml of the filtrate obtained in the test for water-soluble acid or alkaline substances add 1 ml of *dilute sulphuric acid R* and 0.1 ml of *0.02 M potassium permanganate*. After 10 min, the solution is not completely decolourised.

Butylhydroxytoluene. Gas chromatography (*2.2.28*).

Internal standard solution. Dissolve 0.2 g of *methyl decanoate R* in *carbon disulphide R* and dilute to 100.0 ml with the same solvent. Dilute 1.0 ml of the solution to 10.0 ml with *carbon disulphide R*.

Test solution (a). Dissolve 1.0 g of the substance to be examined in *carbon disulphide R* and dilute to 10.0 ml with the same solvent.

Test solution (b). Dissolve 1.0 g of the substance to be examined in *carbon disulphide R*, add 1.0 ml of the internal standard solution and dilute to 10.0 ml with *carbon disulphide R*.

Reference solution. Dissolve 0.2 g of *butylhydroxytoluene R* in *carbon disulphide R* and dilute to 100.0 ml with the same solvent. Dilute 1.0 ml of the solution to 10.0 ml with *carbon disulphide R*. To 1.0 ml of this solution add 1.0 ml of the internal standard solution and dilute to 10.0 ml with *carbon disulphide R*.

Column:

– *size*: l = 1.5 m, Ø = 4 mm,

– *stationary phase*: *silanised diatomaceous earth for gas chromatography R* impregnated with 10 per cent *m/m* of *poly(dimethyl)siloxane R*.

The column is preceded by a column containing silanised glass wool.

Carrier gas: *nitrogen for chromatography R*.

Flow rate: 40 ml/min.

Temperature:

– *column*: 150 °C,

– *injection port*: 180 °C,

– *detector*: 300 °C.

Detection: flame ionisation.

Limit:

– *butylhydroxytoluene*: maximum 200 ppm.

Paraffins: maximum 1.0 per cent.

The tap and cotton plugs used must be free from grease. Prepare a column of anhydrous aluminium oxide 0.23 m long and 20 mm in diameter by adding a slurry of *anhydrous*

Monographs T-Z

aluminium oxide R and *light petroleum R1* to a glass tube fitted with a tap and containing *light petroleum R1* (before use, dehydrate the anhydrous aluminium oxide by heating it in an oven at 600 °C for 3 h). Allow to settle and reduce the depth of the layer of solvent above the column to about 40 mm. Dissolve 3.0 g of the substance to be examined in 50 ml of warm *light petroleum R1*, cool, pass the solution through the column at a flow rate of 3 ml/min and wash with 250 ml of *light petroleum R1*. Concentrate the combined eluate and washings to low bulk by distillation, evaporate to dryness on a water-bath and heat the residue at 105 °C for periods of 10 min until 2 successive weighings do not differ by more than 1 mg. The residue weighs a maximum of 30 mg.

Pesticide residues: maximum 0.05 ppm for each organochlorine pesticide, 0.5 ppm for each other pesticide and 1 ppm for the sum of all the pesticides.

All glassware used is thoroughly washed using phosphate-free detergent as follows. The glassware is immersed in a bath of detergent solution (5 per cent in deionised water) and allowed to soak for 24 h. The detergent is washed off with copious amounts of acetone and hexane for pesticide analysis. It is important to keep glassware specifically for pesticide analyses, it must not be mixed up with glassware used for other applications. The glassware used must be free of chlorinated solvents, plastics and rubber materials, in particular phthalate plasticisers, oxygenated compounds and nitrogenated solvents such as acetonitrile. Use hexane, toluene and acetone for pesticide analysis. Use HPLC grade reagents for ethyl acetate, cyclohexane and water.

The test consists of the isolation of pesticide residues by size-exclusion chromatography (*2.2.30*) followed by solid phase extraction and identification by gas chromatography coupled with an electron capture detector or a thermionic detector.

ISOLATION OF THE PESTICIDE RESIDUES. As detector, use a UV-visible spectrophotometer set at a wavelength of 254 nm to calibrate the chromatographic column for gel permeation.

Calibration is extremely important in gel permeation chromatography to check that the pressure, solvent flow rate, solvent ratio, temperature and column conditions remain constant. The gel permeation column is to be calibrated at regular intervals using a standard mixture prepared as follows: into a 1000 ml volumetric flask, introduce 50.00 g of *maize oil R*, 2.00 g of *di(2-ethylhexyl) phthalate R*, 0.20 g of *methoxychlor R*, 50.0 mg of *perylene R*, 50.0 mg of *naphthalene R*, and 80.0 mg of *sulphur R*. Dilute to 1000.0 ml with a mixture of equal volumes of *cyclohexane R* and *ethyl acetate R*.

To calibrate the column, set the mobile phase at a flow rate of 5 ml/min with a mixture of equal volumes of *cyclohexane R* and *ethyl acetate R*. Inject 5 ml of the standard mixture and record the resulting chromatogram. The retention times for the analytes must not vary by more than ± 5 per cent between calibrations. If the retention time shift is greater than ± 5 per cent, take corrective action. Excessive retention time shifts may be caused by:

- poor laboratory temperature control,
- the pump contains air. This can be verified by measuring the flow rate: collect 25 ml of column eluate in a volumetric flask and record the time (300 ± 5 s),
- a leak in the system.

Changes in pressure, in mobile phase flow rate or in column temperature conditions, as well as column contamination, can affect pesticide retention times and are to be monitored. If the flow rate or column pressure are outside desired bands the guard column or column is to be replaced.

Test solution. In a volumetric flask, dissolve 1 g of wool fat, accurately weighed, in a mixture of 1 volume of *ethyl acetate R* and 7 volumes of *cyclohexane R*. Add 1 ml of an internal standard (2 ppm) either *isodrin R* or *ditalimphos R* and dilute to 20 ml. *The internal standard solutions are used to establish that recoveries of the pesticides from the GPC purification stage, evaporation and solid phase extraction stage are at acceptable levels. Recovery levels of the internal standard solutions from the wool fat are determined by comparing the peak areas of the wool fat extracts with peak areas of solutions of the internal standards.*

Guard column:

- *size*: l = 0.075 m, Ø = 21.2 mm,
- *stationary phase*: *styrene-divinylbenzene copolymer R* (5 µm).

Gel permeation column:

- *size*: l = 0.3 m, Ø = 21.2 mm,
- *stationary phase*: *styrene-divinylbenzene copolymer R* (5 µm).

Mobile phase: *ethyl acetate R*, *cyclohexane R* (1:7 *V/V*).

Flow rate: 5 ml/min.

Detection: spectrophotometer at 254 nm.

Inject 5 ml of the test solution. Discard the first 95 ml (19 min) of eluate containing the substance to be examined. Collect the next 155 ml of eluate (31 min) containing any pesticide residues in an evaporating vessel.

Place the 155 ml of the eluate collected from the gel permeation chromatography column into an evaporating vessel. Place this vessel in an autoevaporator setting the water-bath temperature at 45 °C and the nitrogen pressure at 55 kPa. Evaporate the eluate down to 0.5 ml.

To prepare the solid phase extraction cartridges take some *magnesium silicate for pesticide residue analysis R* and heat it in a muffle furnace at 700 °C for 4 h to remove moisture and polychlorinated biphenyls. Subsequently allow the magnesium silicate to cool for 2 h and transfer it directly to an oven at 100-105 °C, and allow to stand for 30 min. Transfer the magnesium silicate to a stoppered glass jar and allow to equilibrate for 48 h. This material may be used for up to 2 weeks. After that period the magnesium silicate is to be reactivated, by heating at 600 °C for 2 h in a muffle furnace. Remove the magnesium silicate from the furnace, cool and store in a stoppered glass jar. The magnesium silicate is deactivated by adding 1 per cent of *water R*. After the water has been added, shake the magnesium silicate intermittently over 15 min just prior to use. The deactivated magnesium silicate is suitable for use for up to 1 week. It is essential that only deactivated magnesium silicate is used.

Take a 6 ml empty solid phase extraction cartridge and weigh into the cartridge 1 g of the deactivated magnesium silicate.

At this stage the GPC fraction still contains about 10 per cent of the substance to be examined, so further clean-up is necessary. A separate isolation procedure is carried out a) for organochlorine and synthetic pyrethroid pesticides and b) for organophosphorus pesticides. Place a preconditioned solid phase extraction cartridge containing 1 g of deactivated *magnesium silicate for pesticide residue analysis R* onto a vacuum manifold.

Condition the cartridge by adding 10 ml of *toluene R* and allowing the solvent to elute through the cartridge. Place the 0.5 ml of the solvent fraction from the evaporating vessel on the preconditioned cartridge. Elute the pesticide fractions from the cartridges using 20 ml of either of the 2 different solvent systems shown below:

Monographs T-Z

a) for determination of the organochlorine and synthetic pyrethroid pesticides: *toluene R*. A very small amount of the substance to be examined is co-eluted,

b) for determination of the organophosphorus pesticides: a mixture of 2 volumes of *acetone R* and 98 volumes of *toluene R*. This solvent system is used to elute all the pesticides including the more polar organophosphorus pesticides. Unfortunately some of the substance to be examined is co-eluted with this solvent system, which can interfere with the electron capture detector.

Collect the eluate from the extraction cartridges in 25 ml glass vials. Quantitatively transfer the eluate to an evaporating vessel, washing the vial with 3 quantities, each of 10 ml, of *hexane R*.

Place the evaporating vessel on the autoevaporator and evaporate the solid phase extraction fractions down to 0.5 ml. The water-bath temperature is set at 45 °C and the nitrogen pressure is 55 kPa.

Examine the residues by gas chromatography (*2.2.28*) using electron capture and thermionic detectors as described below.

Recovery. Calculate the recovery correction factor (R_{cf}) of the internal standards (*ditalimphos R* or *isodrin R*) added to the test solution using the following expression:

$$\frac{\text{peak area of internal standard extracted from the test solution}}{\text{peak area of an internal standard 1 ppm in solution}} \times 100$$

5 ml of the 20 ml test solution containing 1 ml of 2 ppm internal standard concentrated to 0.5 ml is equivalent to 1 ppm of the internal standard in the solution.

If the recovery of the internal standards falls outside the range of 70 per cent to 110 per cent the test is not valid.

Reference solutions. Prepare reference solutions of pesticides using the pesticides standards at a concentration of 0.5 ppm (see composition of reference solutions A to D in Table 0134.-1). Commercially available pesticides may be purchased. The individual standards have a concentration of 10 ppm.

At the same time prepare solutions of pesticides equivalent to the limit of detection of the method (see recommended compositions in Table 0134.-1). These reference solutions are used to optimise the electron capture detector and thermionic detector to achieve the detection limits of the method (reference solutions E and F).

To prepare the reference solutions at the different concentrations use a calibrated pipette and volumetric flasks. To prepare the internal standard solutions G and H use a four-place analytical balance, pipette and volumetric flasks.

IDENTIFICATION AND QUANTIFICATION OF THE PESTICIDE RESIDUES. To identify any pesticide residues compare the chromatograms obtained with chromatograms obtained with reference solutions A to D.

The identity of the pesticides can be confirmed by spiking samples or overlaying chromatograms using an integration package on a computer. The interpretation of pesticides in trace residue analyses is extremely complex. The detectors, particularly the electron capture detector, are prone to interference, both from the substance to be examined itself, and from solvents, reagents and apparatus used in the extraction. These peaks can easily be misinterpreted or quoted as a false positive. Confirmation of pesticides can be achieved by running samples and standards on different capillary columns (see chromatographic systems A or B described below). The peaks can be identified by using the information in Table 0134.-2.

Table 0134.-1. – *Composition of the reference solutions*

Reference solution A (0.5 ppm or 0.5 mg/l) (organochlorine and synthetic pyrethroid pesticides)	**Reference solution B (0.5 ppm or 0.5 mg/l) (organochlorine and synthetic pyrethroid pesticides)**
Cyhalothrin R	*Aldrin R*
Cypermethrin R	*o,p′-DDT R*
o,p′-DDE R	*o,p′-DDD R*
p,p′-DDE R	*p,p′-DDD R*
p,p′-DDT R	*Dieldrin R*
Deltamethrin R	*α-Endosulphan R*
Endrin R	*β-Endosulphan R*
Heptachlor R	*Fenvalerate R*
Heptachlor epoxide R	*α-Hexachlorocyclohexane R*
Hexachlorobenzene R	*β-Hexachlorocyclohexane R*
Lindane R	*δ-Hexachlorocyclohexane R*
Tecnazene R	*Methoxychlor R*
	Permethrin R
Reference solution C (0.5 ppm or 0.5 mg/l) (organophosphorus pesticides)	**Reference solution D (0.5 ppm or 0.5 mg/l) (organophosphorus pesticides)**
Bromophos-ethyl R	*Bromophos R*
Carbophenothion R	*Chlorpyriphos R*
Chlorfenvinphos R	*Chlorpyriphos-methyl R*
Diazinon R	*Coumaphos R*
Dichlofenthion R	*Phosalone R*
Ethion R	*Pirimiphos-ethyl R*
Fenchlorphos R	*Tetrachlorovinphos R*
Malathion R	
Propetamphos R	
Reference solution E (electron capture detector calibration mixture)	**Reference solution F (thermionic detector calibration mixture)**
Aldrin R (0.01 mg/l)	*Chlorfenvinphos R* (0.05 mg/l)
Cypermethrin R (0.1 mg/l)	*Diazinon R* (0.05 mg/l)
o,p′-DDD R (0.01 mg/l)	*Ethion R* (0.05 mg/l)
Deltamethrin R (0.1 mg/l)	*Fenchlorphos R* (0.05 mg/l)
Endrin R (0.01 mg/l)	*Propetamphos R* (0.05 mg/l)
β-Hexachlorocyclohexane R (0.01 mg/l)	
Reference solution G (internal standard organophosphorus pesticide)	**Reference solution H (internal standard organochlorine pesticide)**
Ditalimphos R (2 ppm or 2.0 mg/l)	*Isodrin R* (2 ppm or 2.0 mg/l)
Ditalimphos R (1 ppm or 1.0 mg/l)	*Isodrin R* (1 ppm or 1.0 mg/l)

A knowledge of the different responses the pesticides have with the 2 detectors is useful in identification of unknown peaks.

Once the pesticides have been identified, calculate the content of each pesticide using the following expression:

$$C_P = \frac{P_P \times D \times C_e}{P_e} \times \frac{100}{R_{cf}}$$

C_p = concentration of identified pesticide (ppm),

P_p = peak area of the individual pesticide in the test sample obtained,

C_e = concentration of the individual pesticide in the external standard (ppm),

Monographs T-Z

P_e = peak area of the individual pesticide in the external standard,

D = dilution factor,

R_{cf} = recovery correction factor.

The dilution factor (D) can be defined as follows:

$$\frac{\text{volume of sample obtained after the 2}^{\text{nd}}\text{ evaporation stage}}{\text{sample weight} \times \dfrac{\text{GPC injection volume}}{\text{sample volumetric flask volume}}}$$

Table 0134.-2. – *Elution order of the pesticides on chromatographic systems A and B*

Chromatographic system A	Chromatographic system B
Tecnazene	Tecnazene
α-Hexachlorocyclohexane	Hexachlorobenzene
Hexachlorobenzene	α-Hexachlorocyclohexane
β-Hexachlorocyclohexane	Diazinon
Lindane	Lindane
Propetamphos	Propetamphos
δ-Hexachlorocyclohexane	Heptachlor
Diazinon	Dichlofenthion
Dichlofenthion	Aldrin
Chlorpyriphos-methyl	Chlorpyriphos-methyl
Heptachlor	Fenchlorphos
Fenchlorphos	β-Hexachlorocyclohexane
Aldrin	δ-Hexachlorocyclohexane
Malathion	Pirimiphos-ethyl
Chlorpyriphos-ethyl	Chlorpyriphos-ethyl
Bromophos	Bromophos
Pirimiphos-ethyl	Malathion
Heptachlor epoxide	Heptachlor epoxide
Chlorfenvinphos (*E*)	*o,p*′-DDE
Chlorfenvinphos (*Z*)	Chlorfenvinphos (*E*)
Bromophos-ethyl	α-Endosulphan
o,p′-DDE	Chlorfenvinphos (*Z*)
α-Endosulphan	Bromophos-ethyl
Tetrachlorvinphos	*p,p*′-DDE
Dieldrin	Dieldrin
p,p′-DDE	Tetrachlorvinphos
o,p′-DDT	*o,p*′-DDT
Endrin	Endrin
β-Endosulphan	*o,p*′-DDD
o,p′-DDD	*p,p*′-DDD
p,p′-DDD	β-Endosulphan
Ethion	Ethion
Carbophenothion	*p,p*′-DDT
p,p′-DDT	Carbophenothion
Methoxychlor	Methoxychlor
Phosalone	Cyhalothrin
Cyhalothrin (2 isomers)	*cis*-Permethrin
cis-Permethrin	Phosalone
trans-Permethrin	*trans*-Permethrin
Coumaphos	Cypermethrin (4 isomers)
Cypermethrin (4 isomers)	Coumaphos
Fenvalerate (2 isomers)	Fenvalerate (2 isomers)
Deltamethrin	Deltamethrin

Chromatographic system A:

Guard column:

– *material*: deactivated silica,

– *size*: l = 4.5 m, Ø = 0.53 mm.

Column:

– *material*: fused silica,

– *size*: l = 60 m, Ø = 0.25 mm,

– *stationary phase*: *poly(dimethyl)(diphenyl)siloxane R* (film thickness 0.25 μm).

Carrier gas: *helium for chromatography R*.

Linear velocity: 25 cm/s.

Pressure: 180 kPa.

Temperature:

	Time (min)	Temperature (°C)
Column	0 - 1	75
	1 - 5	75 → 175
	5 - 30	175 → 275
	30 - 40	275 → 285
	40 - 55	285
Injection port		300
Detector		350

Detection: electron capture or thermionic specific detector.

Injection: 2 μl.

Chromatographic system B which may be used for confirmation analysis:

Guard column:

– *material*: deactivated silica,

– *size*: l = 4.5 m, Ø = 0.53 mm.

Column:

– *material*: fused silica,

– *size*: l = 60 m, Ø = 0.25 mm,

– *stationary phase*: *poly(cyanopropyl)(7)(phenyl)(7)(methyl)(86)siloxane R* (film thickness 0.25 μm).

Carrier gas: *helium for chromatography R*.

Linear velocity: 25 cm/s.

Pressure: 180 kPa.

Temperature:

	Time (min)	Temperature (°C)
Column	0 - 1	75
	1 - 5	75 → 175
	5 - 30	175 → 275
	30 - 40	275 → 285
	40 - 55	285
Injection port		300
Detector		350

Detection: electron capture or thermionic specific detector.

Injection: 2 μl.

Chlorides: maximum 150 ppm.

Boil 1.0 g with 20 ml of *alcohol (90 per cent V/V) R* in a round-bottomed flask fitted with a reflux condenser for 5 min. Cool, add 40 ml of *water R* and 0.5 ml of *nitric acid R* and filter. To the filtrate add 0.15 ml of a 10 g/l solution of *silver nitrate R* in *alcohol (90 per cent V/V) R*. Allow to stand for 5 min protected from light. Any opalescence in the solution is not more intense than that in a standard prepared at the same time by adding 0.15 ml of a 10 g/l solution of *silver nitrate R* in *alcohol (90 per cent V/V) R* to a mixture of 0.2 ml of *0.02 M hydrochloric acid*, 20 ml of *alcohol (90 per cent V/V) R*, 40 ml of *water R* and 0.5 ml of *nitric acid R*.

Loss on drying (*2.2.32*): maximum 0.5 per cent, determined on 1.000 g by drying in an oven at 100-105 °C for 1 h.

Monographs T-Z

Sulphated ash (*2.4.14*): maximum 0.15 per cent.

Ignite 5.0 g and use the residue to determine the sulphated ash.

STORAGE

At a temperature not exceeding 25 °C.

LABELLING

The label states, where applicable, the concentration of added butylhydroxytoluene.

01/2005:0969

WOOL FAT, HYDROGENATED

Adeps lanae hydrogenatus

DEFINITION

Mixture of higher aliphatic alcohols and sterols obtained from the direct, high-pressure, high-temperature hydrogenation of *wool fat (0134)* during which the esters and acids present are reduced to the corresponding alcohols. It may contain butylhydroxytoluene.

CHARACTERS

Appearance: white or pale yellow, unctuous substance.

Solubility: practically insoluble in water, soluble in boiling alcohol and in light petroleum.

IDENTIFICATION

First identification: B.

Second identification: A, C.

A. It complies with the test for melting point (see Tests).

B. Examine the chromatograms obtained in the test for fatty alcohols and sterols.

   Results: the principal peaks in the chromatogram obtained with the test solution are similar in retention time and size to the principal peaks in the chromatogram obtained with reference solution (a).

C. Dissolve 50 mg in 5 ml of *methylene chloride R* and add 1 ml of *acetic anhydride R* and 0.1 ml of *sulphuric acid R*. A green colour is produced.

TESTS

Melting point (*2.2.15*): 45 °C to 55 °C. Allow to stand at 20 °C for 16 h.

Acid value (*2.5.1*): maximum 1.0, determined on 5.0 g.

Hydroxyl value (*2.5.3, Method A*): 140 to 180.

Saponification value (*2.5.6*): maximum 8.0. Heat under reflux for 4 h.

Fatty alcohols and sterols. Gas chromatography (*2.2.28*).

Test solution. Dissolve 0.25 g of the substance to be examined in 60 ml of *ethanol R* and dilute to 100.0 ml with the same solvent.

Reference solution (a). Dissolve 0.25 g of *hydrogenated wool fat CRS* in 60 ml of *ethanol R* and dilute to 100.0 ml with the same solvent.

Reference solution (b). Dissolve 50 mg of *cetyl alcohol CRS* and 50 mg of *stearyl alcohol CRS* in 60 ml of *ethanol R* and dilute to 100.0 ml with the same solvent.

Column:

- *material*: fused silica,
- *size*: *l* = 30 m, Ø = 0.25 mm,
- *stationary phase*: *poly(dimethyl)siloxane R* or another non-polar phase (film thickness: 0.25 µm).

Carrier gas: *helium for chromatography R* at a pressure of 100 kPa

Temperature:

	Time (min)	Temperature (°C)
Column	0 - 5	100
	5 - 45	100 → 300
	45 - 60	300
Injection port		325
Detector		350

Detection: flame ionisation.

Injection: 1 µl.

The chromatogram obtained with the test solution does not differ significantly from the chromatogram obtained with reference solution (a) (Figure 0969.-1) and it does not show enhanced peaks with retention times corresponding to cetyl alcohol and stearyl alcohol present in the chromatogram obtained with reference solution (b).

Heavy metals (*2.4.8*): maximum 10 ppm.

2.0 g complies with limit test C. Prepare the standard using 2 ml of *lead standard solution (10 ppm Pb) R*.

Loss on drying (*2.2.32*): maximum 3.0 per cent, determined on 2.000 g by drying in an oven at 100-105 °C for 1 h.

Total ash (*2.4.16*): maximum 0.1 per cent, determined on 5.0 g.

STORAGE

In a well-filled container, protected from light.

Monographs T-Z

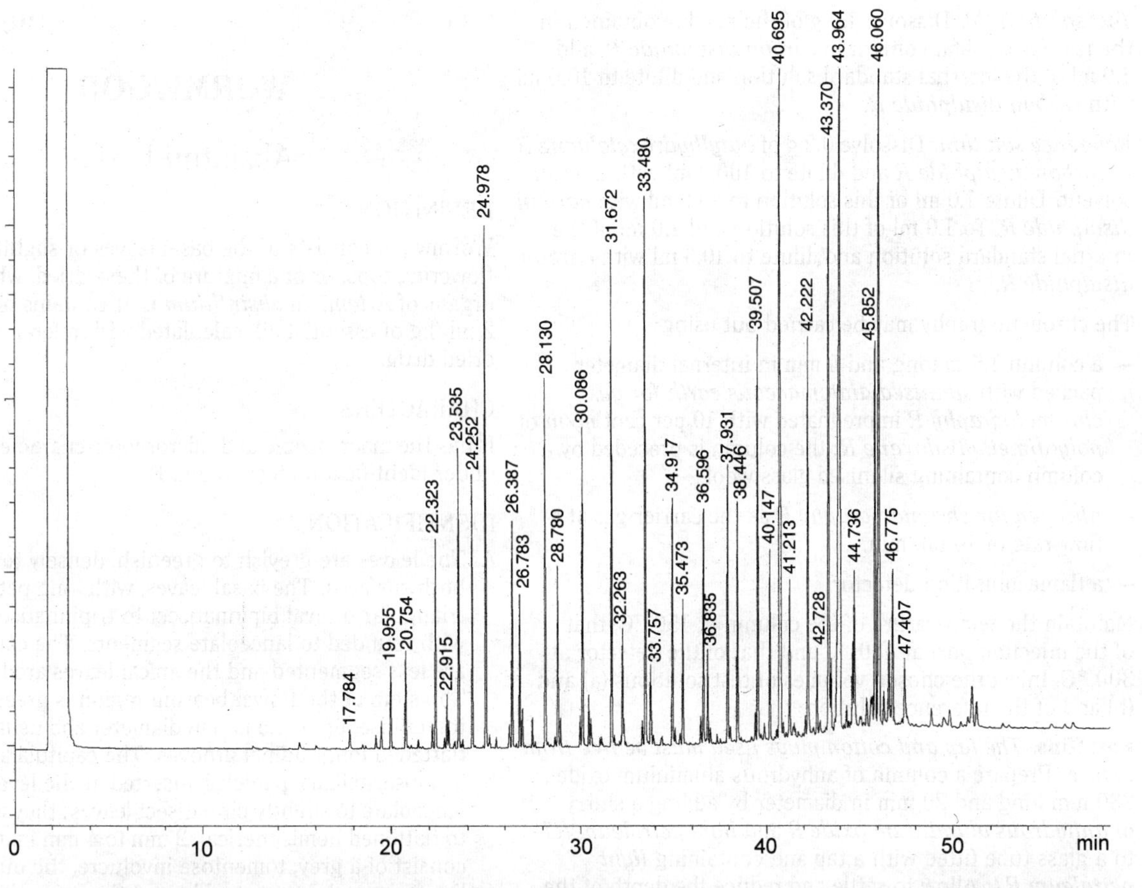

Figure 0969.-1. – *Chromatogram for the test for fatty alcohols and sterols (reference solution (a)) in hydrogenated wool fat*

01/2005:0135

WOOL FAT, HYDROUS

Adeps lanae cum aqua

DEFINITION

Hydrous wool fat is a mixture of 75 per cent *m/m* of wool fat and 25 per cent *m/m* of water. It is obtained by the gradual addition of water to melted wool fat with continuous stirring. It may contain not more than 150 ppm of butylhydroxytoluene.

CHARACTERS

A pale yellow, unctuous substance.

IDENTIFICATION

A. In a test-tube, dissolve 0.5 g in 5 ml of *chloroform R* and add 1 ml of *acetic anhydride R* and 0.1 ml of *sulphuric acid R*. A green colour develops.

B. Dissolve 50 mg in 5 ml of *chloroform R*, add 5 ml of *sulphuric acid R* and shake. A red colour develops and an intense green fluorescence appears in the lower layer.

TESTS

Water-soluble acid or alkaline substances. Melt 6.7 g on a water-bath and shake vigorously for 2 min with 75 ml of *water R* previously heated to 90 °C to 95 °C. Allow to cool and filter through filter paper previously rinsed with *water R*. To 60 ml of the filtrate (which may not be clear) add 0.25 ml of *bromothymol blue solution R1*. Not more than 0.2 ml of *0.02 M hydrochloric acid* or 0.15 ml of *0.02 M sodium hydroxide* is required to change the colour of the indicator.

Drop point (*2.2.17*): 38 °C to 44 °C, determined on the residue obtained in the test for wool-fat content. To fill the metal cup, melt the residue on a water-bath, cool to about 50 °C, pour into the cup and allow to stand at 15 °C to 20 °C for 24 h.

Water-absorption capacity. Place 10 g of the residue obtained in the test for wool-fat content in a mortar. Add *water R* in portions of 0.2 ml to 0.5 ml from a burette, stirring vigorously after each addition to incorporate the *water R*. The end-point is reached when visible droplets remain which cannot be incorporated. Not less than 20 ml of *water R* is absorbed.

Acid value (*2.5.1*). Not more than 0.8, determined on 5.0 g dissolved in 25 ml of the prescribed mixture of solvents.

Peroxide value (*2.5.5*). Not more than 15.

Saponification value (*2.5.6*): 67 to 79, determined on 2.00 g. Heat under reflux for 4 h.

Water-soluble oxidisable substances. To 10 ml of the filtrate obtained in the test for water-soluble acid or alkaline substances add 1 ml of *dilute sulphuric acid R* and 0.1 ml of *0.02 M potassium permanganate*. After 10 min, the solution is not completely decolourised.

Butylhydroxytoluene. Not more than 150 ppm, determined by gas chromatography (*2.2.28*), using *methyl decanoate R* as the internal standard.

Internal standard solution. Dissolve 0.2 g of *methyl decanoate R* in *carbon disulphide R* and dilute to 100.0 ml with the same solvent. Dilute 1.0 ml of this solution to 10.0 ml with *carbon disulphide R*.

Test solution (a). Dissolve 1.0 g of the residue obtained in the test for wool-fat content in *carbon disulphide R* and dilute to 10.0 ml with the same solvent.

Monographs T-Z

Test solution (b). Dissolve 1.0 g of the residue obtained in the test for wool-fat content in *carbon disulphide R*, add 1.0 ml of the internal standard solution and dilute to 10.0 ml with *carbon disulphide R*.

Reference solution. Dissolve 0.2 g of *butylhydroxytoluene R* in *carbon disulphide R* and dilute to 100.0 ml with the same solvent. Dilute 1.0 ml of this solution to 10.0 ml with *carbon disulphide R*. To 1.0 ml of this solution add 1.0 ml of the internal standard solution and dilute to 10.0 ml with *carbon disulphide R*.

The chromatography may be carried out using:

– a column 1.5 m long and 4 mm in internal diameter packed with *silanised diatomaceous earth for gas chromatography R* impregnated with 10 per cent *m/m* of *poly(dimethyl)siloxane R*; the column is preceded by a column containing silanised glass wool,

– *nitrogen for chromatography R* as the carrier gas at a flow rate of 40 ml/min,

– a flame-ionisation detector.

Maintain the temperature of the column at 150 °C, that of the injection port at 180 °C and that of the detector at 300 °C. Inject the chosen volumes of test solutions (a) and (b) and of the reference solution.

Paraffins. *The tap and cotton plugs used must be free from grease.* Prepare a column of anhydrous aluminium oxide 230 mm long and 20 mm in diameter by adding a slurry of *anhydrous aluminium oxide R* and *light petroleum R1* to a glass tube fitted with a tap and containing *light petroleum R1*. Allow to settle and reduce the depth of the layer of solvent above the column to about 40 mm. Dissolve 3.0 g of the residue obtained in the test for wool-fat content in 50 ml of warm *light petroleum R1*, cool, pass the solution through the column at a rate of 3 ml/min and wash with 250 ml of *light petroleum R1*. Concentrate the combined eluate and washings to low bulk by distillation, evaporate to dryness on a water-bath and heat the residue at 105 °C for periods of 10 min until 2 successive weighings do not differ by more than 1 mg. The residue weighs not more than 30 mg (1.0 per cent).

Chlorides. Boil 1.3 g with 20 ml of *alcohol (90 per cent V/V) R* under a reflux condenser for 5 min. Cool, add 40 ml of *water R* and 0.5 ml of *nitric acid R* and filter. To the filtrate add 0.15 ml of a 10 g/l solution of *silver nitrate R* in *alcohol (90 per cent V/V) R*. Allow to stand for 5 min, protected from light. Any opalescence in the solution is not more intense than that in a standard prepared at the same time by adding 0.15 ml of a 10 g/l solution of *silver nitrate R* in *alcohol (90 per cent V/V) R* to a mixture of 0.2 ml of *0.02 M hydrochloric acid*, 20 ml of *alcohol (90 per cent V/V) R*, 40 ml of *water R* and 0.5 ml of *nitric acid R* (115 ppm).

Sulphated ash (*2.4.14*). Not more than 0.1 per cent. Ignite 5.0 g and use the residue to determine the sulphated ash.

Wool-fat content: 72.5 per cent to 77.5 per cent. In a suitable tared dish containing a glass rod, heat 30.0 g to constant mass on a water-bath, stirring continuously. Weigh the residue.

STORAGE

Store at a temperature not exceeding 25 °C.

LABELLING

The label states, where applicable, the concentration of added butylhydroxytoluene.

01/2005:1380

WORMWOOD

Absinthii herba

DEFINITION

Wormwood consists of the basal leaves or slightly leafy, flowering tops, or of a mixture of these dried, whole or cut organs of *Artemisia absinthium* L. It contains not less than 2 ml/kg of essential oil, calculated with reference to the dried drug.

CHARACTERS

It has the macroscopic and microscopic characters described under identification tests A and B.

IDENTIFICATION

A. The leaves are greyish to greenish, densely tomentose on both surfaces. The basal leaves, with long petioles, have triangular to oval bipinnatisect to tripinnatisect lamina, with rounded to lanceolate segments. The cauline leaves are less segmented and the apical leaves are lanceolate. The stem of the flower-bearing region is greenish-grey, tomentose, up to 2.5 mm in diameter and usually with five flattened longitudinal grooves. The capitula are arranged as loose, axillary panicles, inserted at the level of the lanceolate to slightly pinnatisect leaves; they are spherical to flattened hemispherical, 2 mm to 4 mm in diameter and consist of a grey, tomentose involucre, the outer bracts linear, inner layer ovate, blunt at the apices with scarious margins, a receptacle with very long paleae up to 1 mm or more long, numerous yellow, tubular, hermaphroditic florets about 2 mm long and few yellow, ray florets.

B. Reduce to a powder (355). The powder is greenish-grey. Examine under a microscope using *chloral hydrate solution R*. The powder shows many T-shaped trichomes with a short uniseriate stalk consisting of one to five small cells, perpendicularly capped by a very long, undulating terminal cell tapering at the ends; fragments of epidermises with sinuous to wavy walls, anomocytic stomata (*2.8.3*) and secretory trichomes each with a short, biseriate, two celled stalk and a biseriate head with two or four cells; fragments of the tubular and ray florets, some containing small cluster crystals of calcium oxalate; numerous paleae each composed of a small cell forming a stalk and a very long, cylindrical and thin-walled terminal cell about 1 mm to 1.5 mm long; spheroidal pollen grains, about 30 µm in diameter, with three pores and a finely warty exine; groups of fibres, small vessels with spiral and annular thickening, larger vessels with bordered pits and parenchyma with moderately thickened and pitted walls, from the stem.

C. Examine by thin-layer chromatography (*2.2.27*), using a suitable silica gel as the coating substance.

Test solution. Place 2 g of the powdered drug (355) in 50 ml of boiling *water R* and allow to stand for 5 min, shaking the flask several times. After cooling, add 5 ml of a 100 g/l solution of *lead acetate R*. Mix and filter. Rinse the flask and the residue on the filter with 20 ml of *water R*. Shake the filter with 50 ml of *methylene chloride R*. Separate the organic layer, dry over *anhydrous sodium sulphate R*, filter and evaporate the filtrate to dryness on a water-bath. Dissolve the residue in 0.5 ml of *alcohol R*.

Reference solution. Dissolve 2 mg of *methyl red R* and 2 mg of *resorcinol R* in 10.0 ml of *methanol R*.

Apply to the plate as bands 10 μl of each solution. Develop over a path of 15 cm using a mixture of 10 volumes of *acetone R*, 10 volumes of *glacial acetic acid R*, 30 volumes of *toluene R* and 50 volumes of *methylene chloride R*. Allow the plate to dry in air. Spray the plate with *acetic anhydride-sulphuric acid solution R* and examine in daylight. The chromatogram obtained with the test solution shows the blue zone of artabsin shortly above the red zone of methyl red in the chromatogram obtained with the reference solution. Examine in daylight while heating at 100 °C to 105 °C for 5 min. The chromatogram obtained with the reference solution shows in the middle third the red zone of methyl red and below it the light pink zone of resorcinol. The chromatogram obtained with the test solution shows an intense red to brownish-red zone of absinthin with a similar R_f value to that of the zone due to resorcinol in the chromatogram obtained with the reference solution. Other zones are visible, but less intense than that of absinthin.

TESTS

Foreign matter (*2.8.2*). Not more than 5 per cent of stems with a diameter greater than 4 mm and 2 per cent of other foreign matter.

Bitterness value. Not less than 10 000. The bitterness value is determined by comparison with quinine hydrochloride, the bitterness value of which is set at 200 000; the bitterness value is the reciprocal of the dilution that still has a bitter taste.

Quinine hydrochloride stock solution. Dissolve 0.100 g of *quinine hydrochloride R* in *water R* and dilute to 100.0 ml with the same solvent. Dilute 1.0 ml of the solution to 100.0 ml with *water R*.

Wormwood extract. To 1.0 g of powdered drug (710) add 1000 ml of boiling *water R*. Heat on a water-bath for 30 min, stirring continuously. Allow to cool and dilute to 1000 ml with *water R*. Shake vigorously and filter, discarding the first 20 ml of filtrate.

Prepare a series of dilutions by placing in the first tube 4.2 ml of quinine hydrochloride stock solution and increasing the volume by 0.2 ml in each subsequent tube to a total of 5.8 ml; dilute the contents of each tube to 10.0 ml with *water R*. Determine as follows the dilution with the lowest concentration that still has a bitter taste. Take 10.0 ml of the weakest solution into the mouth and pass it from side to side over the back of the tongue for 30 s. If the solution is not found to be bitter, spit it out and wait for 1 min. Rinse the mouth with *water R*. After 10 min, use the next dilution in order of increasing concentration.

Calculate the correction factor (k) from the expression:

$$\frac{5.00}{n}$$

n = number of millilitres of quinine hydrochloride stock solution in the dilution of lowest concentration that is bitter.

Dilute $10/k$ ml of wormwood extract to 100.0 ml with *water R*. 10.0 ml of this dilution has a bitter taste.

Loss on drying (*2.2.32*). Not more than 10.0 per cent, determined on 1.000 g of powdered drug (355) by drying in an oven at 100 °C to 105 °C for 2 h.

Total ash (*2.4.16*). Not more than 12.0 per cent.

Ash insoluble in hydrochloric acid (*2.8.1*). Not more than 1.0 per cent.

ASSAY

Carry out the determination of essential oil in vegetable drugs (*2.8.12*). Use 50.0 g of the cut drug, a 1000 ml round-bottomed flask and 500 ml of *water R* as the distillation liquid. Add 0.5 ml of *xylene R* in the graduated tube. Distil at a rate of 2 ml/min to 3 ml/min for not less than 3 h.

STORAGE

Store protected from light.

X

01/2005:1277

XANTHAN GUM

Xanthani gummi

DEFINITION

Xanthan gum is a high-molecular-mass anionic polysaccharide produced by fermentation of carbohydrate with *Xanthomonas campestris*. It consists of a principal chain of β(1→4)-linked D-glucose units with trisaccharide side chains, on alternating anhydroglucose units, consisting of a glucuronic acid unit included between two mannose units. Most of the terminal units contain a pyruvate moiety and the mannose unit adjacent to the principal chain may be acetylated at C-6.

Xanthan gum has a molecular mass of approximately 1×10^6. It contains not less than 1.5 per cent of pyruvoyl groups ($C_3H_3O_2$; relative mass of the group 71.1), calculated with reference to the dried substance. Xanthan gum exists as the sodium, potassium or calcium salt.

CHARACTERS

A white or yellowish-white, free-flowing powder, soluble in water giving a highly viscous solution, practically insoluble in organic solvents.

IDENTIFICATION

A. In a flask, suspend 1 g in 15 ml of *0.1 M hydrochloric acid*. Close the flask with a fermentation bulb containing *barium hydroxide solution R* and heat carefully for 5 min. The barium hydroxide solution shows a white turbidity.

B. To 300 ml of *water R*, previously heated to 80 °C and stirred rapidly with a mechanical stirrer in a 400 ml beaker, add, at the point of maximum agitation, a dry blend of 1.5 g of *carob bean gum R* and 1.5 g of the substance to be examined. Stir until the mixture forms a solution, and then continue stirring for 30 min or longer. Do not allow the water temperature to drop below 60 °C during stirring. Discontinue stirring and allow the mixture to stand for at least 2 h. A firm rubbery gel forms after the temperature drops below 40 °C but no such gel forms in a 1 per cent control solution of the sample prepared in the same manner but omitting the carob bean gum.

TESTS

pH (*2.2.3*). The pH of a 10.0 g/l solution is 6.0 to 8.0.

Viscosity (*2.2.10*). The viscosity at 24 ± 1 °C is not less than 600 mPa·s. Add 3.0 g within 45 s to 90 s into 250 ml of a 12 g/l solution of *potassium chloride R* in a 500 ml beaker stirring with a low-pitch propeller-type stirrer rotating at 800 r/min. When adding the substance take care that agglomerates are destroyed. Add an additional quantity of 44 ml of *water R*, to rinse any adhering residue from the walls of the beaker. Stir the preparation at 800 r/min for 2 h whilst maintaining the temperature at 24 ± 1 °C. Determine the viscosity within 15 min using a rotating viscosimeter set at 60 r/min and equipped with a rotating spindle 12.7 mm in diameter and 1.6 mm high which is attached to a shaft 3.2 mm in diameter. The distance from the top of the cylinder to the lower tip of the shaft being 25.4 mm, and the immersion depth being 50.0 mm.

2-Propanol. Not more than 750 ppm, determined by gas chromatography (*2.2.28*) using *2-methyl-2-propanol R* as the internal standard.

Internal standard solution. Dilute 0.50 g of *2-methyl-2-propanol R* to 500 ml with *water R*.

Test solution. To 200 ml of *water R* in a 1000 ml round-bottomed flask, add 5.0 g of the substance to be examined and 1 ml of a 10 g/l emulsion of *dimeticone R* in *liquid paraffin R*, stopper the flask and shake for 1 h. Distil about 90.0 ml, mix the distillate with 4.0 ml of the internal standard solution and dilute to 100.0 ml with *water R*.

Reference solution. Dilute a suitable quantity of *2-propanol R*, accurately weighed, with *water R* to obtain a solution having a known concentration of 2-propanol of about 1 mg/ml. To 4.0 ml of this solution add 4.0 ml of the internal standard solution and dilute to 100.0 ml with *water R*.

The chromatographic procedure may be carried out using:

– a column 1.8 m long and 4.0 mm in internal diameter packed with *styrene-divinylbenzene copolymer R*,

– *helium for chromatography R* as the carrier gas at a flow rate of 30 ml/min,

– a flame-ionisation detector,

maintaining the temperature of the column at 165 °C, and that of the injection port and of the detector at 200 °C.

Inject 5 μl of the test solution and 5 μl of the reference solution. The retention time of 2-methyl-2-propanol is about 1.5 relative to that of 2-propanol.

Other polysaccharides. Examine by thin-layer chromatography (*2.2.27*), using a *TLC silica gel plate R*.

Test solution. To 10 mg in a thick-walled centrifuge test tube add 2 ml of a 230 g/l solution of *trifluoroacetic acid R*, shake vigorously to dissolve the forming gel, stopper the test tube, and heat the mixture at 120 °C for 1 h. Centrifuge the hydrolysate, transfer the clear supernatant liquid carefully into a 50 ml flask, add 10 ml of *water R* and evaporate the solution to dryness under reduced pressure. Take up the residue thus obtained in 10 ml of *water R* and evaporate to dryness under reduced pressure. Wash three times with 20 ml of *methanol R* and evaporate under reduced pressure. To the resulting clear film which has no odour of acetic acid, add 0.1 ml of *water R* and 1 ml of *methanol R*. Centrifuge to separate the amorphous precipitate. Dilute the supernatant liquid, if necessary, to 1 ml with *methanol R*.

Reference solution. Dissolve 10 mg of *glucose R* and 10 mg of *mannose R* in 2 ml of *water R* and dilute to 10 ml with *methanol R*.

Apply separately to the plate, as bands, 5 μl of each solution. Develop over a path of 15 cm using a mixture of 10 volumes of a 16 g/l solution of *sodium dihydrogen phosphate R*, 40 volumes of *butanol R* and 50 volumes of *acetone R*. Spray evenly with a solution of 0.5 g of *diphenylamine R* in 25 ml of *methanol R* to which 0.5 ml of *aniline R* and 2.5 ml of *phosphoric acid R* have been added. Heat for 5 min at 120 °C. Examine in daylight. The test is not valid unless the chromatogram obtained with the reference solution shows two clearly separated greyish-brown zones due to glucose and mannose in the middle third. The chromatogram obtained with the test solution shows corresponding zones. In addition, one weak reddish and two faint bluish-grey bands may be visible just above the starting line. One or two bluish-grey bands may also be seen in the upper quarter of the chromatogram. No other bands are visible.

Loss on drying (*2.2.32*). Not more than 15.0 per cent, determined on 1.000 g by drying in an oven at 100 °C to 105 °C for 2.5 h.

Total ash (*2.4.16*): 6.5 per cent to 16.0 per cent.

Microbial contamination. Total viable aerobic count (*2.6.12*) not more than 10^3 bacteria and 10^2 fungi per gram, determined by plate count. It complies with the test for *Escherichia coli* (*2.6.13*).

ASSAY

Test solution. Dissolve a quantity of the substance to be examined corresponding to 120.0 mg of the dried substance in *water R* and dilute to 20.0 ml with the same solvent.

Reference solution. Dissolve 45.0 mg of *pyruvic acid R* in *water R* and dilute to 500.0 ml with the same solvent.

Place 10.0 ml of the test solution in a 50 ml round-bottomed flask, add 20.0 ml of *0.1 M hydrochloric acid* and weigh. Boil on a water-bath under a reflux condenser for 3 h. Weigh and adjust to the initial mass with *water R*. In a separating funnel mix 2.0 ml of the solution with 1.0 ml of *dinitrophenylhydrazine-hydrochloric solution R*. Allow to stand for 5 min and add 5.0 ml of *ethyl acetate R*. Shake and allow the solids to settle. Collect the upper layer and shake with three quantities, each of 5.0 ml, of *sodium carbonate solution R*. Combine the aqueous layers and dilute to 50.0 ml with *sodium carbonate solution R*. Mix. Treat 10.0 ml of the reference solution at the same time and in the same manner as for the test solution.

Immediately measure the absorbance of the two solutions (*2.2.25*) at 375 nm, using *sodium carbonate solution R* as the compensation liquid.

The absorbance of the test solution is not less than that of the reference solution, which corresponds to a content of pyruvic acid of not less than 1.5 per cent.

01/2005:1481

XYLAZINE HYDROCHLORIDE FOR VETERINARY USE

Xylazini hydrochloridum ad usum veterinarium

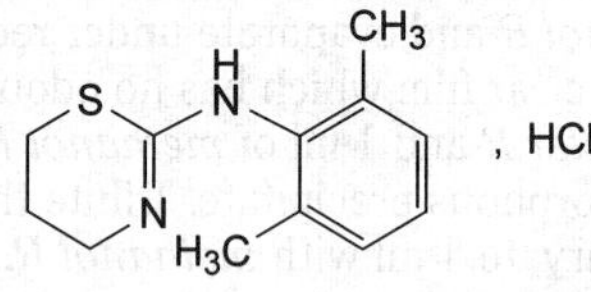

$C_{12}H_{17}ClN_2S$ $\qquad M_r$ 256.8

DEFINITION

N-(2,6-Dimethylphenyl)-5,6-dihydro-4*H*-1,3-thiazin-2-amine hydrochloride.

Content: 98.0 per cent to 102.0 per cent (dried substance).

CHARACTERS

Appearance: white or almost white, crystalline powder, hygroscopic.

Solubility: freely soluble in water, very soluble in methanol, freely soluble in methylene chloride.

IDENTIFICATION

A. Infrared absorption spectrophotometry (*2.2.24*).
   Preparation: discs.
   Comparison: *xylazine hydrochloride CRS*.

B. It gives reaction (b) of chlorides (*2.3.1*).

TESTS

Solution S. Dissolve 5.0 g in *carbon dioxide-free water R* prepared from *distilled water R*, heating at 60 °C if necessary; allow to cool and dilute to 50.0 ml with the same solvent.

Appearance of solution. Solution S is not more opalescent than reference suspension II (*2.2.1*) and is colourless (*2.2.2, Method II*).

pH (*2.2.3*): 4.0 to 5.5 for solution S.

Impurity A: maximum 100 ppm.

Solution A. Dissolve 0.25 g of the substance to be examined in *methanol R* and dilute to 10 ml with the same solvent. This solution is used to prepare the test solution.

Solution B. Dissolve 50 mg of *2,6-dimethylaniline R* in *methanol R* and dilute to 100 ml with the same solvent. Dilute 1 ml of the solution to 100 ml with *methanol R*. This solution is used to prepare the reference solution.

Using 2 flat-bottomed tubes with an inner diameter of about 10 mm, place in the first tube 2 ml of solution A, and in the second tube 1 ml of solution B and 1 ml of *methanol R*. To each tube add 1 ml of a freshly prepared 10 g/l solution of *dimethylaminobenzaldehyde R* in *methanol R* and 2 ml of *glacial acetic acid R* and allow to stand at room temperature for 10 min. Compare the colours in diffused daylight, viewing vertically against a white background. Any yellow colour in the test solution is not more intense than that in the reference solution.

Related substances. Liquid chromatography (*2.2.29*). *Prepare the solutions immediately before use.*

Solvent mixture. Mix 8 volumes of *acetonitrile R*, 30 volumes of *methanol R* and 62 volumes of a 2.72 g/l solution of *potassium dihydrogen phosphate R* adjusted to pH 7.2 with *dilute sodium hydroxide solution R*.

Test solution. Dissolve 0.100 g of the substance to be examined in the solvent mixture and dilute to 20.0 ml with the solvent mixture.

Reference solution. Dissolve 5.0 mg of the substance to be examined, 5.0 mg of *2,6-dimethylaniline R*, 5.0 mg of *xylazine impurity C CRS* and 5.0 mg of *xylazine impurity E CRS* in *acetonitrile R* and dilute to 100.0 ml with the same solvent. Dilute 1.0 ml of this solution to 10.0 ml with the solvent mixture.

Column:
- *size*: l = 0.15 m, Ø = 3.9 mm,
- *stationary phase*: *end-capped octylsilyl silica gel for chromatography with polar incorporated groups R* (5 µm),
- *temperature*: 40 °C.

Mobile phase:
- *mobile phase A*: mix 30 volumes of *methanol R* and 70 volumes of a 2.72 g/l solution of *potassium dihydrogen phosphate R* adjusted to pH 7.2 with *dilute sodium hydroxide solution R*,
- *mobile phase B*: *methanol R, acetonitrile R* (30:70 *V/V*),

Time (min)	Mobile phase A (per cent *V/V*)	Mobile phase B (per cent *V/V*)
0 - 15	89 → 28	11 → 72
15 - 21	28	72
21 - 22	28 → 89	72 → 11
22 - 33	89	11

Flow rate: 1.0 ml/min.

Detection: spectrophotometer at 230 nm.

Equilibration: for at least 30 min with a mixture of 28 volumes of mobile phase A and 72 volumes of mobile phase B.

Injection: 20 µl.

Relative retention with reference to xylazine (retention time = about 7.5 min): impurity A = about 0.8; impurity E = about 1.6; impurity C = about 2.2.

System suitability: reference solution:
– *resolution*: minimum 4.0 between the peaks due to impurity A and xylazine.

Limits:
– *impurities C, E*: for each impurity, not more than twice the area of the corresponding peak in the chromatogram obtained with the reference solution (0.2 per cent),
– *impurities B, D*: for each impurity, not more than twice the area of the peak due to xylazine in the chromatogram obtained with the reference solution (0.2 per cent),
– *any other impurity*: for each impurity, not more than twice the area of the peak due to xylazine in the chromatogram obtained with the reference solution (0.2 per cent),
– *total of impurities other than B, C, D and E*: not more than twice the area of the peak due to xylazine in the chromatogram obtained with the reference solution (0.2 per cent),
– *disregard limit*: 0.5 times the area of the peak due to xylazine in the chromatogram obtained with the reference solution (0.05 per cent); disregard any peak due to the blank.

Heavy metals (*2.4.8*): maximum 10 ppm.

12 ml of solution S complies with limit test A. Prepare the standard using 10 ml of *lead standard solution (1 ppm Pb) R*.

Loss on drying (*2.2.32*): maximum 0.5 per cent, determined on 1.000 g by drying in an oven at 100-105 °C for 2 h.

Sulphated ash (*2.4.14*): maximum 0.1 per cent, determined on 1.0 g.

ASSAY

Dissolve 0.200 g in 25 ml of *alcohol R*. Add 25 ml of *water R*. Titrate with *0.1 M sodium hydroxide*, determining the end-point potentiometrically (*2.2.20*).

1 ml of *0.1 M sodium hydroxide* is equivalent to 25.68 mg of $C_{12}H_{17}ClN_2S$.

STORAGE

In an airtight container, protected from light.

IMPURITIES

Specified impurities: A, B, C, D, E.

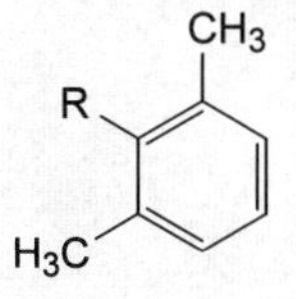

A. R = NH_2: 2,6-dimethylaniline (2,6-xylidine),

C. R = N=C=S: 2,6-dimethylphenyl isothiocyanate,

D. R = NH-CS-NH-$[CH_2]_3$-OH: *N*-(2,6-dimethylphenyl)-*N'*-(3-hydroxypropyl)thiourea,

E. R = NH-CS-S-CH_3: methyl (2,6-dimethylphenyl)carbamodithioate,

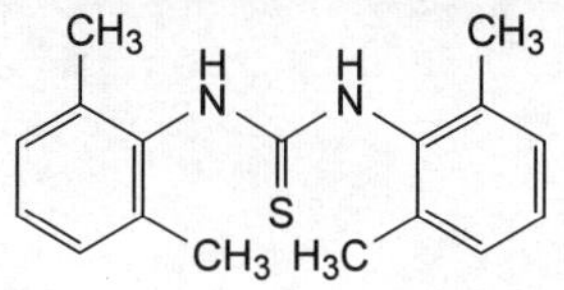

B. *N,N'*-bis(2,6-dimethylphenyl)thiourea.

01/2005:1381

XYLITOL

Xylitolum

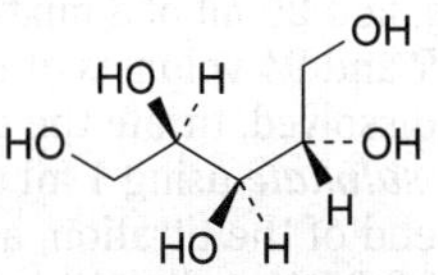

$C_5H_{12}O_5$ M_r 152.1

DEFINITION

Xylitol contains not less than 98.0 per cent and not more than the equivalent of 102.0 per cent of *meso*-xylitol, calculated with reference to the anhydrous substance.

CHARACTERS

White crystalline powder or crystals, very soluble in water, sparingly soluble in alcohol.

IDENTIFICATION

First identification: B.

Second identification: A, C.

A. Melting point (*2.2.14*): 92 °C to 96 °C.

B. Examine by infrared absorption spectrophotometry (*2.2.24*), comparing with the spectrum obtained with *xylitol CRS*. Examine the substance prepared as a mull in *liquid paraffin R*.

C. Examine by thin-layer chromatography (*2.2.27*), using a *TLC silica gel G plate R*.

Test solution. Dissolve 25 mg of the substance to be examined in *water R* and dilute to 5.0 ml with the same solvent.

Reference solution (a). Dissolve 25 mg of *xylitol CRS* in *water R* and dilute to 5.0 ml with the same solvent.

Reference solution (b). Dissolve 25 mg of *mannitol CRS* and 25 mg of *xylitol CRS* in *water R* and dilute to 5 ml with the same solvent.

Apply to the plate 2 µl of each solution. Develop over a path of 17 cm using a mixture of 10 volumes of *water R*, 20 volumes of *ethyl acetate R* and 70 volumes of *propanol R*. Allow the plate to dry in air and spray with *4-aminobenzoic acid solution R*. Dry the plate in a current of cold air until the acetone is removed. Heat the plate at 100 °C for 15 min. Allow to cool and spray with a 2 g/l solution of *sodium periodate R*. Dry the plate in a current of cold air. Heat the plate at 100 °C for 15 min. The principal spot in the chromatogram obtained with the test solution is similar in position, colour and size to the principal spot in the chromatogram obtained with reference solution (a). The test is not valid unless the chromatogram obtained with reference solution (b) shows 2 clearly separated spots.

TESTS

Appearance of solution. Dissolve 2.5 g in *water R* and dilute to 50.0 ml with the same solvent. The solution is not more opalescent than reference suspension IV (*2.2.1*) and not more intensely coloured than reference solution BY_7 (*2.2.2, Method II*).

Conductivity (*2.2.38*). Not more than 20 $\mu S \cdot cm^{-1}$.

Dissolve 20.0 g in *carbon dioxide-free water R* prepared from *distilled water R* and dilute to 100.0 ml with the same solvent. Measure the conductivity of the solution while gently stirring with a magnetic stirrer.

Reducing sugars. Dissolve 5.0 g in 6 ml of *water R* with the aid of gentle heat. Cool and add 20 ml of *cupri-citric solution R* and a few glass beads. Heat so that boiling begins after 4 min and maintain boiling for 3 min. Cool rapidly and add 100 ml of a 2.4 per cent *V/V* solution of *glacial acetic acid R* and 20.0 ml of *0.025 M iodine*. With continuous shaking, add 25 ml of a mixture of 6 volumes of *hydrochloric acid R* and 94 volumes of *water R* and, when the precipitate has dissolved, titrate the excess of iodine with *0.05 M sodium thiosulphate* using 1 ml of *starch solution R*, added towards the end of the titration, as indicator. Not less than 12.8 ml of *0.05 M sodium thiosulphate* is required (0.2 per cent, calculated as glucose equivalent).

Related products. Examine by gas chromatography (*2.2.28*) as described under Assay. The sum of the percentage contents of the related products in the chromatogram obtained with the test solution is not greater than 2.0 per cent.

Lead (*2.4.10*). It complies with the limit test for lead in sugars (0.5 ppm). Dissolve the substance to be examined in 150.0 ml of the prescribed mixture of solvents.

Nickel (*2.4.15*). It complies with the limit test for nickel in polyols (1 ppm). Dissolve the substance to be examined in 150.0 ml of the prescribed mixture of solvents.

Water (*2.5.12*). Not more than 1.0 per cent, determined on 1.00 g by the semi-micro determination of water.

Bacterial endotoxins (*2.6.14*): if intended for use in the manufacture of parenteral dosage forms without a further appropriate procedure for the removal of bacterial endotoxins, less than 4 IU/g for parenteral dosage forms having a concentration of less than 100 g/l of xylitol and less than 2.5 IU/g for parenteral dosage forms having a concentration of 100 g/l or more of xylitol.

ASSAY

Examine by gas chromatography (*2.2.28*), using erythritol as the internal standard.

Internal standard solution. Dissolve 5 mg of *erythritol R* in *water R* and dilute to 25.0 ml with the same solvent.

Test solution. Dissolve 5.000 g of the substance to be examined in *water R* and dilute to 100.0 ml with the same solvent.

Reference solution. Dissolve 25.0 mg each of *L-arabinitol CRS, galactitol CRS, mannitol CRS* and *sorbitol CRS* in *water R* and dilute to 100.0 ml with the same solvent. To 10.0 ml of the solution add about 490 mg of *xylitol CRS*, accurately weighed, to obtain a solution having a known concentration of about 49 mg of *xylitol CRS* per millilitre.

The chromatographic procedure may be carried out using:

- a stainless steel column 2 m long and 2 mm in internal diameter packed with acid washed *silanised diatomaceous earth for gas chromatography R* (150-180 μm) and impregnated with 3 per cent *m/m* of *poly[(cyanopropyl)(methyl)][(phenyl)(methyl)]siloxane R*,
- *nitrogen R* as the carrier gas at a flow rate of 30 ml/min,
- a flame-ionisation detector,

maintaining the temperature of the column at 170 °C for 1 min, then raising the temperature at a rate of 6 °C/min to 200 °C and maintaining the temperature of the injection port and of the detector at 250 °C.

Pipet 1.0 ml of the reference solution and 1.0 ml of the test solution into separate 100 ml round-bottomed flasks. To each flask, add 1.0 ml of the internal standard solution and evaporate the respective mixtures to dryness in a water-bath at 60 °C with the aid of a rotary evaporator. Dissolve each dry residue in 1 ml of *anhydrous pyridine R* and add 1 ml of *acetic anhydride R* to each flask and boil each solution under reflux for 1 h to complete acetylation.

Inject 1 μl each of the solutions obtained from the reference solution and the test solution.

When the chromatograms are recorded in the prescribed conditions, the relative retentions calculated with reference to xylitol are: erythritol about 0.3, arabinitol about 0.7, mannitol about 1.8, galactitol about 2.0 and sorbitol about 2.2.

Calculate the percentage content of $C_5H_{12}O_5$, taking into account the declared content of *xylitol CRS*, and the percentage content of each related product in the substance to be examined from the expression:

$$100 \times \frac{m_s}{m_u} \times \frac{R_u}{R_s}$$

m_s = mass of the respective component in 1 ml of the reference solution, in milligrams,

m_u = mass of the substance to be examined in 1 ml of the test solution, in milligrams,

R_s = ratio of the surface areas of the derivatised component peak to the derivatised erythritol peak in the chromatogram obtained with the reference solution,

R_u = ratio of the surface areas of the derivatised component peak to the derivatised erythritol peak in the chromatogram obtained with the test solution.

LABELLING

The label states:

- where applicable, the maximum concentration of bacterial endotoxins,
- where applicable, that the substance is suitable for use in the manufacture of parenteral dosage forms.

IMPURITIES

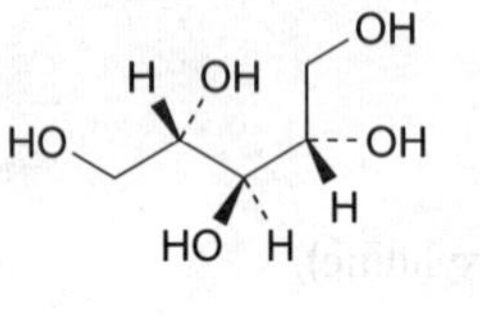

A. L-arabinitol,

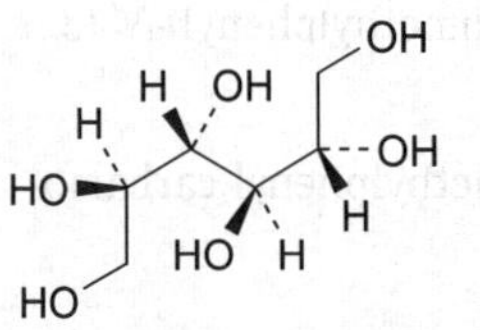

B. *meso*-galactitol,

C. mannitol,

D. sorbitol.

Monographs T-Z

01/2005:1162

XYLOMETAZOLINE HYDROCHLORIDE

Xylometazolini hydrochloridum

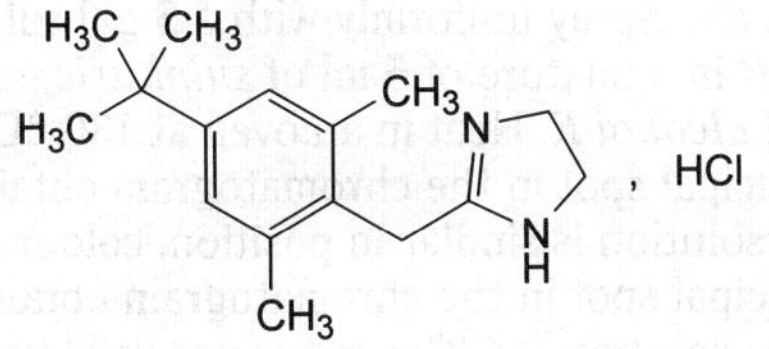

$C_{16}H_{25}ClN_2$ M_r 280.8

DEFINITION

Xylometazoline hydrochloride contains not less than 99.0 per cent and not more than the equivalent of 101.0 per cent of 2-[4-(1,1-dimethylethyl)-2,6-dimethylbenzyl]-4,5-dihydro-1*H*-imidazole hydrochloride, calculated with reference to the dried substance.

CHARACTERS

A white or almost white, crystalline powder, freely soluble in water, in alcohol and in methanol.

IDENTIFICATION

First identification: A, E.

Second identification: B, C, D, E.

A. Examine by infrared absorption spectrophotometry (*2.2.24*), comparing with the spectrum obtained with *xylometazoline hydrochloride CRS*.

B. Examine the chromatograms obtained in the test for related substances. The principal spot in the chromatogram obtained with test solution (b) is similar in position, colour and size to the principal spot in the chromatogram obtained with reference solution (a).

C. Dissolve about 0.5 mg in 1 ml of *methanol R* and add 0.5 ml of a freshly prepared 50 g/l solution of *sodium nitroprusside R* and 0.5 ml of a 20 g/l solution of *sodium hydroxide R*. Allow to stand for 10 min and add 1 ml of an 80 g/l solution of *sodium bicarbonate R*. A violet colour develops.

D. Dissolve 0.2 g in 1 ml of *water R*, add 2.5 ml of *alcohol R* and 2 ml of *1 M sodium hydroxide*. Mix thoroughly and examine in ultraviolet light at 365 nm. The solution shows no fluorescence or at most the same fluorescence as a blank solution prepared in the same manner. The identification is not valid unless a solution prepared in the same manner using *naphazoline hydrochloride CRS* instead of the substance to be examined shows a distinct bluish fluorescence.

E. It gives reaction (a) of chlorides (*2.3.1*).

TESTS

Solution S. Dissolve 2.5 g in *carbon dioxide-free water R* and dilute to 50.0 ml with the same solvent.

Appearance of solution. Solution S is clear (*2.2.1*) and not more intensely coloured than reference solution Y_6 (*2.2.2, Method II*).

Acidity or alkalinity. Dissolve 0.25 g in *water R* and dilute to 25 ml with the same solvent. Add 0.1 ml of *methyl red solution R* and 0.1 ml of *0.01 M hydrochloric acid*. The solution is red. Not more than 0.2 ml of *0.01 M sodium hydroxide* is required to change the colour of the indicator to yellow.

Related substances. Examine by thin-layer chromatography (*2.2.27*), using *silica gel G R* as the coating substance.

Test solution (a). Dissolve 0.20 g of the substance to be examined in *methanol R* and dilute to 5 ml with the same solvent.

Test solution (b). Dilute 1 ml of test solution (a) to 10 ml with *methanol R*.

Reference solution (a). Dissolve 20 mg of *xylometazoline hydrochloride CRS* in *methanol R* and dilute to 5 ml with the same solvent.

Reference solution (b). Dissolve 4 mg of *xylometazoline impurity A CRS* in *methanol R* and dilute to 50 ml with the same solvent.

Reference solution (c). Dilute 1 ml of test solution (b) to 50 ml with *methanol R*.

Apply to the plate 5 µl of each solution. Develop over a path of 10 cm using a mixture of 5 volumes of *concentrated ammonia R* and 100 volumes of *methanol R*. Allow the plate to dry. At the bottom of a chromatography tank place an evaporating dish containing a mixture of 1 volume of *water R*, 1 volume of *hydrochloric acid R1* and 2 volumes of a 15 g/l solution of *potassium permanganate R*. Close the tank and allow to stand for 15 min. Place the dried plate in the tank and reclose the tank. Leave the plate in contact with the chlorine vapour for 5 min. Withdraw the plate and place it in a current of cold air until the excess of chlorine is removed and an area of the coating below the points of application does not give a blue colour with a drop of *potassium iodide and starch solution R*. Spray with *potassium iodide and starch solution R*. Any spot in the chromatogram obtained with test solution (a) corresponding to xylometazoline impurity A, is not more intense than the principle spot in the chromatogram obtained with reference solution (b) (0.2 per cent). Any spot in the chromatogram obtained with test solution (a), apart from the principal spot and the spot corresponding to xylometazoline impurity A is not more intense than the principle spot in the chromatogram obtained with reference solution (c) (0.2 per cent).

Loss on drying (*2.2.32*). Not more than 0.5 per cent, determined on 1.000 g by drying in an oven at 100 °C to 105 °C.

Sulphated ash (*2.4.14*). Not more than 0.1 per cent, determined on 1.0 g.

ASSAY

Dissolve 0.200 g in 25 ml of *anhydrous acetic acid R* and add 10 ml of *acetic anhydride R*. Titrate with *0.1 M perchloric acid*, determining the end-point potentiometrically (*2.2.20*).

1 ml of *0.1 M perchloric acid* is equivalent to 28.08 mg of $C_{16}H_{25}ClN_2$.

STORAGE

Store protected from light.

IMPURITIES

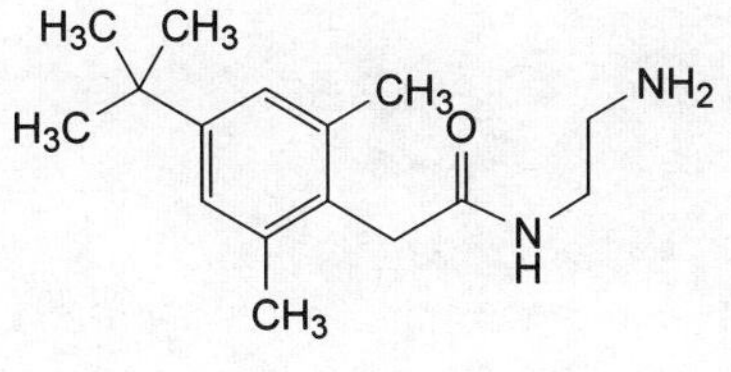

A. *N*-(2-aminomethyl)-2-[4-(1,1-dimethylethyl)-2,6-dimethylphenyl]acetamide.

01/2005:1278
corrected

XYLOSE

Xylosum

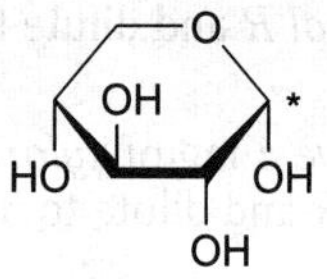

and epimer at C*

$C_5H_{10}O_5$ M_r 150.1

DEFINITION

Xylose is (+)-D-xylopyranose.

CHARACTERS

A white or almost white, crystalline powder or colourless needles, freely soluble in water, soluble in hot alcohol.

IDENTIFICATION

First identification: A.

Second identification: B, C.

A. Examine by infrared absorption spectrophotometry (*2.2.24*), comparing with the spectrum obtained with *xylose CRS*. Examine the substances prepared as discs.

B. Examine by thin-layer chromatography (*2.2.27*), using a suitable silica gel as the coating substance.

Test solution. Dissolve 10 mg of the substance to be examined in a mixture of 2 volumes of *water R* and 3 volumes of *methanol R* and dilute to 20 ml with the same mixture of solvents.

Reference solution (a). Dissolve 10 mg of *xylose CRS* in a mixture of 2 volumes of *water R* and 3 volumes of *methanol R* and dilute to 20 ml with the same mixture of solvents.

Reference solution (b). Dissolve 10 mg of *fructose R*, 10 mg of *glucose R* and 10 mg of *xylose R* in a mixture of 2 volumes of *water R* and 3 volumes of *methanol R* and dilute to 20 ml with the same mixture of solvents.

Apply to the plate 2 µl of each solution and thoroughly dry the starting points. Develop over a path of 15 cm using a mixture of 10 volumes of *water R*, 15 volumes of *methanol R*, 25 volumes of *anhydrous acetic acid R* and 50 volumes of *ethylene chloride R*. The solvents should be measured accurately since a slight excess of water produces cloudiness. Dry the plate in a current of warm air. Spray uniformly with a 5 g/l solution of *thymol R* in a mixture of 5 ml of *sulphuric acid R* and 95 ml of *alcohol R*. Heat in an oven at 130 °C for 10 min. The principal spot in the chromatogram obtained with the test solution is similar in position, colour and size to the principal spot in the chromatogram obtained with reference solution (a). The test is not valid unless the chromatogram obtained with reference solution (b) shows three clearly separated spots.

C. Dissolve 0.1 g in 10 ml of *water R*. Add 3 ml of *cupri-tartaric solution R* and heat. An orange to red precipitate is formed.

TESTS

Solution S. Dissolve 10.0 g in *carbon dioxide-free water R* and dilute to 100 ml with the same solvent.

Appearance of solution. Solution S is clear (*2.2.1*) and colourless (*2.2.2, Method II*).

Acidity or alkalinity. To 50 ml of solution S add 0.3 ml of *phenolphthalein solution R1*. The solution is colourless. Not more than 0.2 ml of *0.1 M sodium hydroxide* is required to change the colour of the indicator to pink.

Specific optical rotation (*2.2.7*). Dissolve 10.0 g in 80 ml of *water R*, add 1 ml of *dilute ammonia R2* and dilute to 100.0 ml with *water R*. Allow to stand for 30 min. The specific optical rotation is + 18.5 to + 19.5, calculated with reference to the dried substance.

Chlorides (*2.4.4*). Dilute 1.5 ml of solution S to 15 ml with *water R*. The solution complies with the limit test for chlorides (330 ppm).

Heavy metals (*2.4.8*). 12 ml of solution S complies with limit test A for heavy metals (20 ppm). Prepare the standard using *lead standard solution (2 ppm Pb) R*.

Loss on drying (*2.2.32*). Not more than 0.5 per cent, determined on 1.000 g by drying in an oven at 100-105 °C at a pressure not exceeding 0.7 kPa.

Sulphated ash (*2.4.14*). Not more than 0.1 per cent, determined on 1.0 g.

Y

01/2005:1382

YARROW

Millefolii herba

DEFINITION

Yarrow consists of the whole or cut, dried flowering tops of *Achillea millefolium* L. It contains not less than 2 ml/kg of essential oil and not less than 0.02 per cent of proazulenes, expressed as chamazulene ($C_{14}H_{16}$; M_r 184.3), both calculated with reference to the dried drug.

CHARACTERS

It has the macroscopic and microscopic characters described under identification tests A and B.

IDENTIFICATION

A. The leaves are green or greyish-green, faintly pubescent on the upper surface and more pubescent on the lower surface, two to three pinnately divided with linear lobes and a finely pointed whitish tip. The capitula are arranged in a corymb at the end of the stem. Each capitulum, 3 mm to 5 mm in diameter, consists of the receptacle, usually four or five ligulate ray-florets and three to twenty tubular disk-florets. The involucre consists of three rows of imbricate lanceolate, pubescent green bracts arranged with a brownish or whitish, membranous margin. The receptacle is slightly convex and, in the axillae of paleae, bears a ligulate ray floret with a three-lobed, whitish or reddish ligule and tubular disk-florets with a radial, five-lobed, yellowish or light brownish corolla. The pubescent green, partly brown or violet stems are longitudinally furrowed, up to 3 mm thick with a light-coloured medulla.

B. Reduce to a powder (355). The powder is green or greyish-green. Examine under a microscope, using *chloral hydrate solution R*. The powder shows fragments of the stems, leaves and bracts bearing very rare glandular trichomes with a short stalk and a head formed of two rows of three to five cells enclosed in a bladder-like membrane and uniseriate covering trichomes consisting of four to six small, more or less isodiametric cells at the base and a thick-walled, often somewhat tortuous terminal cell, about 400 µm to greater than 1000 µm long; fragments of the ligulate corolla with papillary epidermal cells; small-celled parenchyma from the corolla tubes containing cluster crystals of calcium oxalate; groups of lignified and pitted cells from the bracts; spherical pollen grains, about 30 µm in diameter, with three germinal pores and spiny exine; groups of sclerenchymatous fibres and small vessels with spiral or annular thickening, from the stem.

C. Add 2.5 ml of *dimethylaminobenzaldehyde solution R8* to 0.1 ml of solution S (see Tests) and heat on a water-bath for 2 min. Allow to cool. Add 5 ml of *light petroleum R* and shake the mixture vigorously. The aqueous layer shows a blue or greenish-blue colour.

D. Examine by thin-layer chromatography (*2.2.27*), using a suitable silica gel as the coating substance.

Test solution. Use the solution prepared in identification test C.

Reference solution. Dissolve 10 mg of *cineole R* and 10 mg of *guaiazulene R* in 20 ml of *toluene R*.

Apply to the plate as bands 20 µl of each solution. Develop over a path of 10 cm using a mixture of 5 volumes of *ethyl acetate R* and 95 volumes of *toluene R*. Allow the plate to dry in air. Spray the plate with *anisaldehyde solution R*. Examine in daylight while heating at 100 °C to 105 °C for 5 min to 10 min. The chromatogram obtained with the reference solution shows in the upper part a red zone (guaiazulene) and in the middle part a blue or greyish-blue zone (cineole). The chromatogram obtained with the test solution shows: a violet zone a little above the zone due to guaiazulene in the chromatogram obtained with the reference solution; below this zone a reddish-violet zone; below which, one or two not clearly separated greyish-violet to greyish zones (which changes to greenish-grey after a few hours) and a reddish-violet zone a little above the zone due to cineole in the chromatogram obtained with the reference solution. Further faint zones are present.

TESTS

Solution S. To 2.0 g of the powdered drug (710) add 25 ml of *ethyl acetate R*, shake for 5 min and filter. Evaporate to dryness on a water-bath and dissolve the residue in 0.5 ml of *toluene R*.

Foreign matter (*2.8.2*). Not more than 5 per cent of stems, with a diameter greater than 3 mm and not more than 2 per cent of other foreign matter.

Loss on drying (*2.2.32*). Not more than 12.0 per cent determined on 0.500 g of powdered drug (355) by drying in an oven at 100 °C to 105 °C for 2 h.

Total ash (*2.4.16*). Not more than 10.0 per cent.

Ash insoluble in hydrochloric acid (*2.8.1*). Not more than 2.5 per cent.

ASSAY

Essential oil. Carry out the determination of essential oil in vegetable drugs (*2.8.12*). Use 20.0 g of cut drug, a 1000 ml round-bottomed flask and 500 ml of a mixture of 1 volume of *water R* and 9 volumes of *ethylene glycol R* as the distillation liquid. Add 0.2 ml of *xylene R* in the graduated tube. Distil at a rate of 2 ml/min to 3 ml/min for 2 h.

Stop cooling at the end of distillation and continue distilling until the blue, steam-volatile components have reached the lower end of the cooler. Immediately start cooling again, taking care to avoid warming the separation space. Stop the distillation after 5 min. Replace the 1000 ml round-bottomed flask by a 250 ml round-bottomed flask containing a mixture of 0.4 ml of *xylene R* and 50 ml of *water R*. Distil for 15 min. After 10 min read the total volume. To determine the blank value, use 0.2 ml of *xylene R* in the graduated tube and distil a mixture of 0.4 ml of *xylene R* and 50 ml of *water R* for 15 min.

Proazulenes. To ensure that as little water as possible is transferred, transfer the blue essential oil-xylene mixture obtained in the assay of essential oil to a 50 ml volumetric flask with the aid of small portions of *xylene R*, rinsing the graduated tube of the apparatus with *xylene R* and dilute to 50.0 ml with the same solvent. Measure the absorbance (*2.2.25*) at 608 nm using *xylene R* as the compensation liquid.

Calculate the percentage content of proazulenes, expressed as chamazulene from the expression:

$$\frac{A \times 2.1}{m}$$

i.e. taking the specific absorbance of chamazulene to be 23.8.

A = absorbance at 608 nm,

m = mass of the drug to be examined in grams.

STORAGE

Store protected from light.

Z

01/2005:1059

ZIDOVUDINE

Zidovudinum

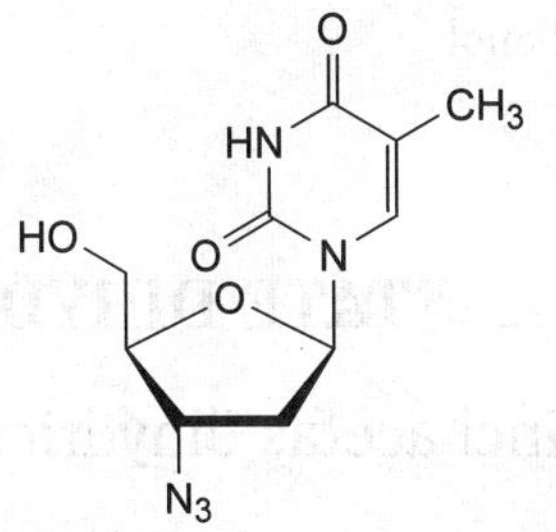

$C_{10}H_{13}N_5O_4$ M_r 267.2

DEFINITION

Zidovudine contains not less than 97.0 per cent and not more than the equivalent of 102.0 per cent of 1-(3-azido-2,3-dideoxy-β-D-*erythro*-pentofuranosyl)-5-methylpyrimidine-2,4(1*H*,3*H*)-dione, calculated with reference to the dried substance.

CHARACTERS

A white or brownish powder, sparingly soluble in water, soluble in ethanol. It melts at about 124 °C.

It shows polymorphism.

IDENTIFICATION

Examine by infrared absorption spectrophotometry (*2.2.24*) comparing with the spectrum obtained with *zidovudine CRS*. If the spectra obtained in the solid state show differences, dissolve the substance to be examined and the reference substance separately in the minimum quantity of *water R* and evaporate to dryness in a desiccator, under high vacuum over *diphosphorus pentoxide R*. Record new spectra using the residues.

TESTS

Appearance of solution. Dissolve 0.5 g in 50 ml of *water R*, heating if necessary. The solution is not more intensely coloured than reference solution BY_5 (*2.2.2, Method II*).

Specific optical rotation (*2.2.7*). Dissolve 0.50 g in *ethanol R* and dilute to 50.0 ml with the same solvent. The specific optical rotation, determined at 25 °C is + 60.5 to + 63.0, calculated with reference to the dried substance.

Related substances

A. Examine by thin-layer chromatography (*2.2.27*), using a plate coated with a suitable silica gel containing a fluorescent indicator having an optimal intensity at 254 nm.

Test solution. Dissolve 0.20 g of the substance to be examined in *methanol R* and dilute to 10 ml with the same solvent.

Reference solution (a). Dissolve 20 mg each of *thymine R*, *zidovudine impurity A CRS* and *triphenylmethanol R* in *methanol R*, add 1.0 ml of the test solution and dilute to 100 ml with *methanol R*.

Reference solution (b). Dilute 5.0 ml of reference solution (a) to 10 ml with *methanol R*.

Apply separately to the plate 10 µl of each solution. Develop over a path of 12 cm using a mixture of 10 volumes of *methanol R* and 90 volumes of *methylene chloride R*. Allow the plate to dry in air and examine in ultraviolet light at 254 nm. In the chromatogram obtained with the test solution: any spot corresponding to zidovudine impurity A is not more intense than the corresponding spot in the chromatogram obtained with reference solution (b) (0.5 per cent), and any spot apart from the principal spot and any spot corresponding to zidovudine impurity A and thymine (which is limited by liquid chromatography) is not more intense than the spot corresponding to zidovudine in the chromatogram obtained with reference solution (b) (0.5 per cent). Spray the plate with a 10 g/l solution of *vanillin R* in *sulphuric acid R*. In the chromatogram obtained with the test solution, any spot corresponding to triphenylmethanol is not more intense than the corresponding spot in the chromatogram obtained with reference solution (b) (0.5 per cent). The test is not valid unless the chromatogram obtained with reference solution (a) shows four clearly separated spots, corresponding to thymine, zidovudine impurity A, zidovudine and triphenylmethanol, in order of increasing R_f value.

B. Examine by liquid chromatography as described in the assay. Inject separately 10 µl each of test solution (a), reference solution (b), reference solution (d) and reference solution (e). Continue the chromatography for 1.5 times the retention time of the principal peak in the chromatogram obtained with test solution (a). When the chromatograms are recorded in the prescribed conditions, the substances are eluted in the following sequence: thymine, zidovudine and zidovudine impurity B. In the chromatogram obtained with test solution (a): the area of any peak corresponding to thymine is not greater than the area of the peak in the chromatogram obtained with reference solution (b) (2 per cent); the area of any peak corresponding to zidovudine impurity B is not greater than the area of the corresponding peak in the chromatogram obtained with reference solution (d) (1 per cent); the area of any other peak apart from the principal peak is not greater than the area of the peak in the chromatogram obtained with reference solution (e) (0.5 per cent). The total surface area of all the peaks apart from the principal peak obtained in the chromatogram with test solution (a) is not greater than six times the area of the peak obtained with reference solution (e) (3.0 per cent). Disregard any peak with an area less than 10 per cent of the area of the peak in the chromatogram obtained with reference solution (e).

Heavy metals (*2.4.8*). 1.00 g complies with limit test D for heavy metals (20 ppm). Prepare the standard using 2 ml of *lead standard solution (10 ppm Pb) R*.

Loss on drying (*2.2.32*). Not more than 1.0 per cent, determined on 1.000 g by drying in an oven at 100 °C to 105 °C.

Sulphated ash (*2.4.14*). Not more than 0.25 per cent, determined on 1.00 g.

ASSAY

Examine by liquid chromatography (*2.2.29*).

Test solution (a). Dissolve 50.0 mg of the substance to be examined in the mobile phase and dilute to 50.0 ml with the mobile phase.

Test solution (b). Dilute 10.0 ml of test solution (a) to 50.0 ml with the mobile phase.

Reference solution (a). Dissolve 10.0 mg of *zidovudine CRS* in the mobile phase and dilute to 50.0 ml with the mobile phase.

Monographs T-Z

Reference solution (b). Dissolve 10.0 mg of *thymine R* in *methanol R* and dilute to 50.0 ml with the same solvent. Dilute 5.0 ml of the solution to 50.0 ml with the mobile phase.

Reference solution (c). Dissolve 5 mg of *zidovudine impurity B CRS* in 25.0 ml of reference solution (a) and dilute to 50.0 ml with the mobile phase.

Reference solution (d). Dilute 5.0 ml of reference solution (c) to 50.0 ml with the mobile phase.

Reference solution (e). Dilute 0.25 ml of test solution (a) to 50.0 ml with the mobile phase.

The chromatographic procedure may be carried out using:

- a stainless steel column 0.25 m long and 4.6 mm in internal diameter packed with *octadecylsilyl silica gel for chromatography R* (5 µm),
- as mobile phase at a flow rate of 1.2 ml/min a mixture of 20 volumes of *methanol R* and 80 volumes of *water R*,
- as detector a spectrophotometer set at 265 nm.

Equilibrate the column with the mobile phase at a flow rate of 1.2 ml per minute for about 45 min. Inject 10 µl of reference solution (c). Adjust the sensitivity of the detector so that the height of the principal peaks in the chromatogram obtained is not less that 70 per cent of the full scale of the recorder. The test is not valid unless the resolution between the peaks due to zidovudine and zidovudine impurity B is at least 1.0. Inject separately 10 µl of test solution (b) and 10 µl of reference solution (a). Adjust the sensitivity of the detector so that the height of the peaks in the chromatograms obtained is not less than 50 per cent of the full scale of the recorder.

Calculate the content of $C_{10}H_{13}N_5O_4$ from the areas of the peaks and the declared content of *zidovudine CRS*.

STORAGE

Store protected from light.

IMPURITIES

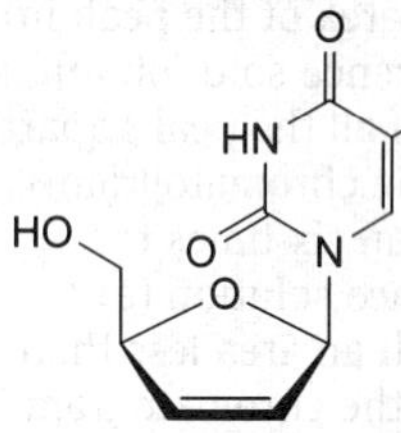

A. 1-[(2*R*,5*S*)-5-(hydroxymethyl)-2,5-dihydrofuran-2-yl)-5-methylpyrimidine-2,4(1*H*,3*H*)-dione,

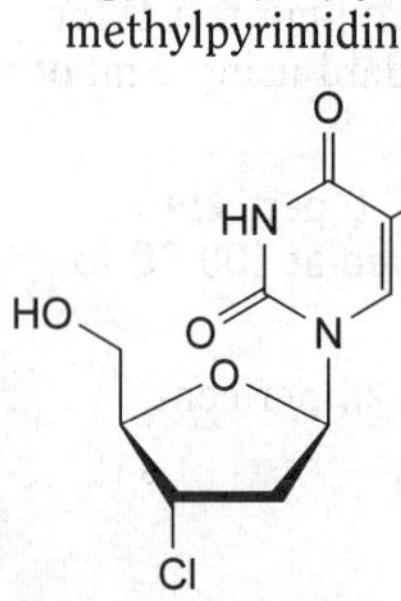

B. 1-(3-chloro-2,3-dideoxy-β-D-*erythro*-pentofuranosyl)-5-methylpyrimidine-2,4(1*H*,3*H*)-dione,

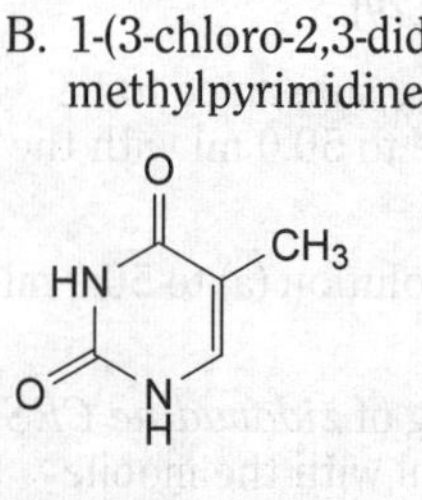

C. 5-methylpyrimidine-2,4(1*H*,3*H*)-dione (thymine),

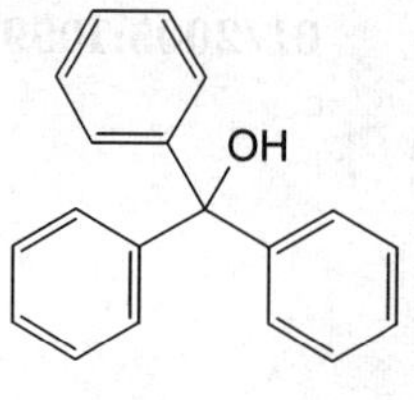

D. triphenylmethanol.

01/2005:1482

ZINC ACETATE DIHYDRATE

Zinci acetas dihydricus

$C_4H_6O_4Zn,2H_2O$ M_r 219.5

DEFINITION

Zinc acetate dihydrate contains not less than 99.0 per cent and not more than the equivalent of 101.0 per cent of $C_4H_6O_4Zn,2H_2O$.

CHARACTERS

A white crystalline powder or leaflets, freely soluble in water, soluble in alcohol.

IDENTIFICATION

A. It gives reaction (a) of acetate (*2.3.1*).

B. It gives the reaction of zinc (*2.3.1*).

TESTS

Solution S. Dissolve 10.0 g in *carbon dioxide-free water R* prepared from *distilled water R* and dilute to 100 ml with the same solvent.

Appearance of solution. Solution S is clear (*2.2.1*) and colourless (*2.2.2, Method II*).

pH (*2.2.3*). Dilute 10 ml of solution S to 20 ml with *carbon dioxide-free water R*. The pH of the solution is 5.8 to 7.0.

Reducing substances. Boil for 5 min a mixture of 10 ml of solution S, 90 ml of *water R*, 5 ml of *dilute sulphuric acid R* and 1.5 ml of a 0.3 g/l solution of *potassium permanganate R*. The pink colour of the solution remains.

Chlorides (*2.4.4*). 10 ml of solution S diluted to 15 ml with *water R* complies with the limit test for chlorides (50 ppm).

Sulphates (*2.4.13*). 15 ml of solution S complies with the limit test for sulphates (100 ppm).

Aluminium. Not more than 5 ppm of Al, determined by atomic absorption spectrometry (*2.2.23, Method I*).

Test solution. Dissolve 2.50 g of the substance to be examined in 20 ml of a 200 g/l solution of *cadmium- and lead-free nitric acid R* and dilute to 25.0 ml with the same acidic solution.

Reference solutions. Prepare the reference solutions using *aluminium standard solution (200 ppm Al) R*, diluted with a 200 g/l solution of *cadmium- and lead-free nitric acid R*.

Measure the absorbance at 309.3 nm, using an aluminium hollow-cathode lamp as a source of radiation and an air-acetylene or an acetylene-nitrous oxide flame.

Arsenic (*2.4.2*). 0.5 g complies with limit test A for arsenic (2 ppm).

Cadmium. Not more than 2 ppm of Cd, determined by atomic absorption spectrometry (*2.2.23, Method I*).

Test solution. Use the solution described in the test for aluminium.

Reference solutions. Prepare the reference solutions using *cadmium standard solution (0.1 per cent Cd) R*, diluted with a 200 g/l solution of *cadmium- and lead-free nitric acid R.*

Measure the absorbance at 228.8 nm, using a cadmium hollow-cathode lamp as a source of radiation and an air-acetylene flame.

Copper. Not more than 50 ppm of Cu, determined by atomic absorption spectrometry (*2.2.23, Method I*).

Test solution. Use the solution described in the test for iron.

Reference solutions. Prepare the reference solutions using *copper standard solution (10 ppm Cu) R*, diluted with a 200 g/l solution of *cadmium- and lead-free nitric acid R*.

Measure the absorbance at 324.8 nm, using a copper hollow-cathode lamp as source of radiation and an air-acetylene flame.

Iron. Not more than 50 ppm of Fe, determined by atomic absorption spectrometry (*2.2.23, Method I*).

Test solution. Dissolve 1.25 g of the substance to be examined in 20 ml of a 200 g/l solution of *cadmium- and lead-free nitric acid R* and dilute to 25.0 ml with the same acid solution.

Reference solutions. Prepare the reference solutions using *iron standard solution (20 ppm Fe) R*, diluted with a 200 g/l solution of *cadmium- and lead-free nitric acid R*.

Measure the absorbance at 248.3 nm, using an iron hollow-cathode lamp as a source of radiation and an air-acetylene flame.

Lead. Not more than 10 ppm of Pb, determined by atomic absorption spectrometry (*2.2.23, Method I*).

Test solution. Dissolve 5.00 g of the substance to be examined in 20 ml of a 200 g/l solution of *cadmium- and lead-free nitric acid R* and dilute to 25.0 ml with the same acid solution.

Reference solutions. Prepare the reference solutions using *lead standard solution (0.1 per cent of Pb) R*, diluting with a 200 g/l solution of *cadmium- and lead-free nitric acid R*.

Measure the absorbance at 283.3 nm, using a lead hollow-cathode lamp as a source of radiation and an air-acetylene flame.

ASSAY

Dissolve 0.200 g in 5 ml of *dilute acetic acid R*. Carry out the complexometric titration of zinc (*2.5.11*).

1 ml of *0.1 M sodium edetate* is equivalent to 21.95 mg of $C_4H_6O_4Zn,2H_2O$.

STORAGE

Store in a non-metallic container.

01/2005:1279

ZINC ACEXAMATE

Zinci acexamas

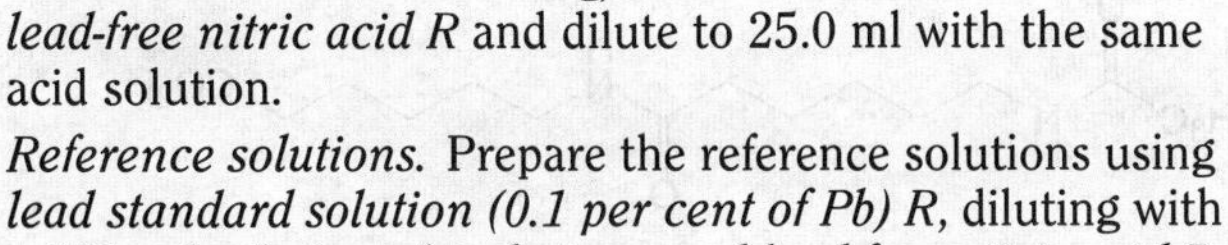

$C_{16}H_{28}N_2O_6Zn$ M_r 409.8

DEFINITION

Zinc acexamate contains not less than 97.5 per cent and not more than the equivalent of 101.0 per cent of zinc 6-(acetylamino)hexanoate, calculated with reference to the dried substance.

CHARACTERS

A white or almost white, crystalline powder, soluble in water, practically insoluble in acetone and in alcohol. It dissolves in dilute nitric acid.

It melts at about 198 °C.

IDENTIFICATION

A. Examine by infrared absorption spectrophotometry (*2.2.24*), comparing with the spectrum obtained with *zinc acexamate CRS*. Examine the substances prepared as discs.

B. 5 ml of solution S (see Tests) gives the reaction of zinc (*2.3.1*).

TESTS

Solution S. Dissolve 0.5 g in *carbon dioxide-free water R* and dilute to 20 ml with the same solvent.

Appearance of solution. Solution S is not more opalescent than reference suspension IV (*2.2.1*) and is colourless (*2.2.2, Method II*).

pH (*2.2.3*). The pH of solution S is 5.0 to 7.0.

6-Aminohexanoic acid. Examine by thin-layer chromatography (*2.2.27*), using a suitable silica gel as the coating substance.

Test solution. Dissolve 0.30 g of the substance to be examined in *water R* and dilute to 10 ml with the same solvent.

Reference solution. Dissolve 15 mg of *6-aminohexanoic acid R* in *water R* and dilute to 10 ml with the same solvent. Dilute 1 ml of the solution to 10 ml with *water R*.

Apply to the plate 5 µl of the test solution and 5 µl of the reference solution. Allow the plate to dry in air. Develop over a path of 15 cm using a mixture of 2 volumes of *ammonia R*, 30 volumes of *water R* and 68 volumes of *alcohol R*. Dry the plate in a current of warm air. Spray with *ninhydrin solution R* and heat at 100 °C to 105 °C for 15 min. In the chromatogram obtained with the test solution, any spot corresponding to 6-aminohexanoic acid is not more intense than the spot in the chromatogram obtained with the reference solution (0.5 per cent).

Related substances. Examine by liquid chromatography (*2.2.29*).

Test solution (a). Dissolve 0.50 g of the substance to be examined in *water R* and dilute to 100.0 ml with the same solvent.

Test solution (b). To 20.0 ml of test solution (a), add 20 ml of the mobile phase, 0.4 ml of a 100 g/l solution of *phosphoric acid R* and dilute to 50.0 ml with the mobile phase.

Reference solution (a). Dissolve 40 mg of *N-acetyl-ε-caprolactam R* in *water R* and dilute to 100.0 ml with the same solvent.

Reference solution (b). Dilute 5.0 ml of reference solution (a) to 100.0 ml with *water R*.

Reference solution (c). Dissolve 20 mg of *zinc acexamate impurity A CRS* in *water R* and dilute to 50.0 ml with the same solvent.

Reference solution (d). Dissolve 40 mg of *ε-caprolactam R* in *water R* and dilute to 100.0 ml with the same solvent. Dilute 5.0 ml of the solution to 100.0 ml with *water R*.

Reference solution (e). To 20.0 ml of test solution (a), add 5.0 ml of reference solution (b), 5.0 ml of reference solution (c), 5.0 ml of reference solution (d) and 0.4 ml of a 100 g/l solution of *phosphoric acid R* and dilute to 50.0 ml with the mobile phase.

Reference solution (f). To 5.0 ml of reference solution (c), add 5.0 ml of reference solution (b), 5.0 ml of reference solution (d) and 0.4 ml of a 100 g/l solution of *phosphoric acid R* and dilute to 50.0 ml with the mobile phase.

The chromatographic procedure may be carried out using:

– a stainless steel column 0.25 m long and 4.0 mm in internal diameter packed with *octadecylsilyl silica gel for chromatography R* (5 µm),

– as mobile phase at a flow rate of 1.2 ml/min a mixture of 0.2 volumes of *phosphoric acid R,* 8 volumes of *acetonitrile R* and 92 volumes of *water R,* adjusted to pH 4.5 with *dilute ammonia R1,*

– as detector a spectrophotometer set at 210 nm.

When the chromatograms are recorded in the prescribed conditions, the elution order is: zinc acexamate, ε-caprolactam, zinc acexamate impurity A and *N*-acetyl-ε-caprolactam. Inject 20 µl of reference solution (e). Continue the chromatography for eight times the retention time of zinc acexamate. Adjust the sensitivity of the system so that the height of the peak corresponding to zinc acexamate impurity A is at least 50 per cent of the full scale of the recorder. The test is not valid unless the resolution between the first peak (zinc acexamate) and the second peak (ε–caprolactam) is at least 3.0. If necessary adjust the pH of the mobile phase to 4.7 with *dilute ammonia R1.*

Inject 20 µl of test solution (b) and 20 µl of reference solution (f). In the chromatogram obtained with test solution (b): the area of any peak corresponding to *N*-acetyl-ε–caprolactam is not greater than that of the corresponding peak in the chromatogram obtained with reference solution (f) (0.1 per cent); the area of any peak corresponding to zinc acexamate impurity A is not greater than that of the corresponding peak in the chromatogram obtained with reference solution (f) (2 per cent); the area of any peak corresponding to ε-caprolactam is not greater than that of the corresponding peak in the chromatogram obtained with reference solution (f) (0.1 per cent); the sum of the areas of all the peaks, apart from the principal peak and the peak due to zinc acexamate impurity A is not greater than five times the area of the peak due to *N*-acetyl-ε-caprolactam in the chromatogram obtained with reference solution (f) (0.5 per cent). Disregard any peak with an area less than 0.5 times that of the peak due to *N*-acetyl-ε-caprolactam in the chromatogram obtained with reference solution (f).

Arsenic (*2.4.2*). 0.5 g complies with limit test A for arsenic (2 ppm).

Cadmium. Not more than 2 ppm of Cd, determined by atomic absorption spectrometry (*2.2.23, Method I*).

Test solution. Dissolve 2.50 g of the substance to be examined in 20 ml of a 200 g/l solution of *cadmium- and lead-free nitric acid R* and dilute to 25.0 ml with the same acidic solution.

Reference solutions. Prepare the reference solutions using *cadmium standard solution (0.1 per cent of Cd) R,* diluted with a 200 g/l solution of *cadmium- and lead-free nitric acid R.*

Measure the absorbance at 228.8 nm, using a cadmium hollow-cathode lamp as a source of radiation and an air-acetylene flame.

Iron. Not more than 50 ppm of Fe, determined by atomic absorption spectrometry (*2.2.23, Method I*).

Test solution. Dissolve 1.25 g of the substance to be examined in 20 ml of a 200 g/l solution of *cadmium- and lead-free nitric acid R* and dilute to 25.0 ml with the same acidic solution.

Reference solutions. Prepare the reference solutions using *iron standard solution (20 ppm Fe) R,* diluted with a 200 g/l solution of *cadmium- and lead-free nitric acid R.*

Measure the absorbance at 248.3 nm, using an iron hollow-cathode lamp as a source of radiation and an air-acetylene flame.

Lead. Not more than 10 ppm of Pb, determined by atomic absorption spectrometry (*2.2.23, Method I*).

Test solution. Dissolve 5.00 g of the substance to be examined in 20 ml of 200 g/l solution of *cadmium- and lead-free nitric acid R* and dilute to 25.0 ml with the same acidic solution.

Reference solutions. Prepare the reference solutions using *lead standard solution (0.1 per cent of Pb) R,* diluting with a 200 g/l solution of *cadmium- and lead-free nitric acid R.*

Measure the absorbance at 283.3 nm, using a lead hollow-cathode lamp as a source of radiation and an air-acetylene flame.

Loss on drying (*2.2.32*). Not more than 1.0 per cent, determined on 1.000 g by drying in an oven at 100 °C to 105 °C.

ASSAY

Dissolve 0.400 g in 10 ml of *dilute acetic acid R.* Carry out the complexometric titration of zinc (*2.5.11*).

1 ml of *0.1 M sodium edetate* is equivalent to 40.98 mg of $C_{16}H_{28}N_2O_6Zn$.

STORAGE

Store in a non-metallic container.

IMPURITIES

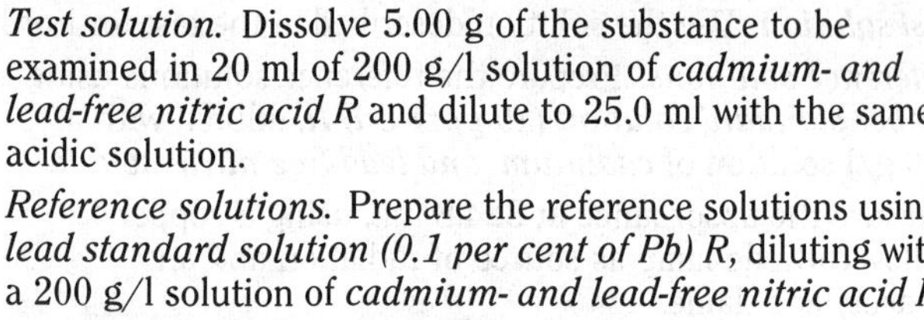

A. 6-[[6-(acetylamino)hexanoyl]amino]hexanoic acid,

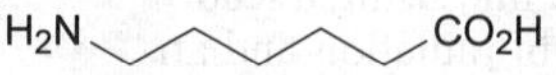

B. 6-aminohexanoic acid (6-aminocaproic acid),

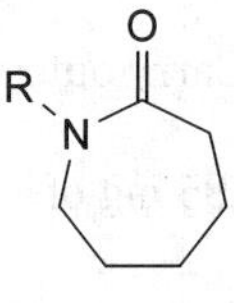

C. R = $CO\text{-}CH_3$: 1-acetylhexahydro-2*H*-azepin-2-one (*N*-acetyl-ε-caprolactam),

D. R = H: hexahydro-2*H*-azepin-2-one (ε–caprolactam).

01/2005:0110

ZINC CHLORIDE

Zinci chloridum

$ZnCl_2$ M_r 136.3

DEFINITION

Zinc chloride contains not less than 95.0 per cent and not more than the equivalent of 100.5 per cent of $ZnCl_2$.

CHARACTERS

A white, crystalline powder or cast in white sticks, deliquescent, very soluble in water, freely soluble in alcohol and in glycerol.

IDENTIFICATION

A. Dissolve 0.5 g in *dilute nitric acid R* and dilute to 10 ml with the same acid. The solution gives reaction (a) of chlorides (*2.3.1*).

B. 5 ml of solution S (see Tests) gives the reaction of zinc (*2.3.1*).

TESTS

Solution S. To 2.0 g add 38 ml of *carbon dioxide-free water R* prepared from *distilled water R* and add *dilute hydrochloric acid R* dropwise until dissolution is complete. Dilute to 40 ml with *carbon dioxide-free water R* prepared from *distilled water R*.

pH (*2.2.3*). Dissolve 1.0 g in 9 ml of *carbon dioxide-free water R*, ignoring any slight turbidity. The pH of the solution is 4.6 to 5.5.

Oxychlorides. Dissolve 1.5 g in 1.5 ml of *carbon dioxide-free water R*. The solution is not more opalescent than reference suspension II (*2.2.1*). Add 7.5 ml of *alcohol R*. The solution may become cloudy within 10 min. Any cloudiness disappears on the addition of 0.2 ml of *dilute hydrochloric acid R*.

Sulphates (*2.4.13*). 5 ml of solution S diluted to 15 ml with *distilled water R* complies with the limit test for sulphates (200 ppm). Prepare the standard using a mixture of 5 ml of *sulphate standard solution (10 ppm* SO_4*) R* and 10 ml of *distilled water R*.

Aluminium, calcium, heavy metals, iron, magnesium. To 8 ml of solution S add 2 ml of *concentrated ammonia R* and shake. The solution is clear (*2.2.1*) and colourless (*2.2.2, Method II*). Add 1 ml of *disodium hydrogen phosphate solution R*. The solution remains clear for at least 5 min. Add 0.2 ml of *sodium sulphide solution R*. A white precipitate is formed and the supernatant liquid remains colourless.

Ammonium (*2.4.1*). 0.5 ml of solution S diluted to 15 ml with *water R* complies with the limit test for ammonium (400 ppm).

ASSAY

Dissolve 0.250 g in 5 ml of *dilute acetic acid R*. Carry out the complexometric titration of zinc (*2.5.11*).

1 ml of *0.1 M sodium edetate* is equivalent to 13.63 mg of $ZnCl_2$.

STORAGE

Store in a non-metallic container.

01/2005:0252

ZINC OXIDE

Zinci oxidum

ZnO M_r 81.4

DEFINITION

Zinc oxide contains not less than 99.0 per cent and not more than the equivalent of 100.5 per cent of ZnO, calculated with reference to the ignited substance.

CHARACTERS

A soft, white or faintly yellowish-white, amorphous powder, free from gritty particles, practically insoluble in water and in alcohol. It dissolves in dilute mineral acids.

IDENTIFICATION

A. It becomes yellow when strongly heated; the yellow colour disappears on cooling.

B. Dissolve 0.1 g in 1.5 ml of *dilute hydrochloric acid R* and dilute to 5 ml with *water R*. The solution gives the reaction of zinc (*2.3.1*).

TESTS

Alkalinity. Shake 1.0 g with 10 ml of boiling *water R*. Add 0.1 ml of *phenolphthalein solution R* and filter. If the filtrate is red, not more than 0.3 ml of *0.1 M hydrochloric acid* is required to change the colour of the indicator.

Carbonates and substances insoluble in acids. Dissolve 1.0 g in 15 ml of *dilute hydrochloric acid R*. It dissolves without effervescence and the solution is not more opalescent than reference suspension II (*2.2.1*) and is colourless (*2.2.2, Method II*).

Arsenic (*2.4.2*). 0.2 g complies with limit test A for arsenic (5 ppm).

Cadmium. Not more than 10 ppm of Cd, determined by atomic absorption spectrometry (*2.2.23, Method II*).

Test solution. Dissolve 2.0 g of the substance to be examined in 14 ml of a mixture of equal volumes of *water R* and *cadmium- and lead-free nitric acid R*, boil for 1 min, cool and dilute to 100.0 ml with *water R*.

Reference solutions. Prepare the reference solutions using *cadmium standard solution (0.1 per cent Cd) R* and diluting with a 3.5 per cent *V/V* solution of *cadmium- and lead-free nitric acid R*.

Measure the absorbance at 228.8 nm using a cadmium hollow-cathode lamp as source of radiation and an air-acetylene or an air-propane flame.

Iron (*2.4.9*). Dissolve 50 mg in 1 ml of *dilute hydrochloric acid R* and dilute to 10 ml with *water R*. The solution complies with the limit test for iron (200 ppm). Use in this test 0.5 ml of *thioglycollic acid R*.

Lead. Not more than 50 ppm of Pb, determined by atomic absorption spectrometry (*2.2.23, Method II*).

Test solution. Dissolve 5.0 g in 24 ml of a mixture of equal volumes of *water R* and *cadmium- and lead-free nitric acid R*, boil for 1 min, cool and dilute to 100.0 ml with *water R*.

Reference solutions. Prepare the reference solutions using *lead standard solution (0.1 per cent Pb) R* and diluting with a 3.5 per cent *V/V* solution of *cadmium- and lead-free nitric acid R*.

Measure the absorbance at 283.3 nm using a lead hollow-cathode lamp as source of radiation and an air-acetylene flame. Depending on the apparatus, the line at 217.0 nm may be used.

Loss on ignition. Not more than 1.0 per cent, determined on 1.00 g at 500 °C.

ASSAY

Dissolve 0.150 g in 10 ml of *dilute acetic acid R*. Carry out the complexometric titration of zinc (*2.5.11*).

1 ml of *0.1 M sodium edetate* is equivalent to 8.14 mg of ZnO.

Monographs T-Z

01/2005:0306

ZINC STEARATE

Zinci stearas

DEFINITION

Zinc stearate [$(C_{17}H_{35}COO)_2Zn$; M_r 632] may contain varying proportions of zinc palmitate [$(C_{15}H_{31}COO)_2Zn$; M_r 576.2] and zinc oleate [$(C_{17}H_{33}COO)_2Zn$; M_r 628]. It contains not less than 10.0 per cent and not more than 12.0 per cent of Zn.

CHARACTERS

A light, white, amorphous powder, free from gritty particles, practically insoluble in water and in ethanol.

IDENTIFICATION

A. The residue obtained in the preparation of solution S (see Tests) has a freezing point (*2.2.18*) not lower than 53 °C.

B. Neutralise 5 ml of solution S to *red litmus paper R* with *strong sodium hydroxide solution R*. The solution gives the reaction of zinc (*2.3.1*).

TESTS

Solution S. To 5.0 g add 50 ml of *ether R* and 40 ml of a 7.5 per cent *V/V* solution of *cadmium- and lead-free nitric acid R* in *distilled water R*. Heat under a reflux condenser until dissolution is complete. Allow to cool. In a separating funnel, separate the aqueous layer and shake the ether layer with two quantities, each of 4 ml, of *distilled water R*. Combine the aqueous layers, wash with 15 ml of *ether R* and heat on a water-bath until ether is completely eliminated. Allow to cool and dilute to 50.0 ml with *distilled water R* (solution S). Evaporate the ether layer to dryness and dry the residue at 105 °C.

Appearance of solution. Solution S is not more intensely coloured than reference solution Y_6 (*2.2.2, Method II*).

Appearance of solution of fatty acids. Dissolve 0.5 g of the residue obtained in the preparation of solution S in 10 ml of *chloroform R*. The solution is clear (*2.2.1*) and not more intensely coloured than reference solution Y_5 (*2.2.2, Method II*).

Acidity or alkalinity. Shake 1.0 g with 5 ml of *alcohol R* and add 20 ml of *carbon dioxide-free water R* and 0.1 ml of *phenol red solution R*. Not more than 0.3 ml of *0.1 M hydrochloric acid* or 0.1 ml of *0.1 M sodium hydroxide* is required to change the colour of the indicator.

Acid value of the fatty acids (*2.5.1*). 195 to 210, determined on 0.20 g of the residue obtained in the preparation of solution S, dissolved in 25 ml of the prescribed mixture of solvents.

Chlorides (*2.4.4*). 2 ml of solution S diluted to 15 ml with *water R* complies with the limit test for chlorides (250 ppm).

Sulphates (*2.4.13*). Dilute 1 ml of solution S to 50 ml with *distilled water R*. 12.5 ml of the solution diluted to 15 ml with *distilled water R* complies with the limit test for sulphates (0.6 per cent).

Cadmium. Not more than 5 ppm of Cd, determined by atomic absorption spectrometry (*2.2.23, Method II*).

Test solution. Dilute 20.0 ml of solution S to 50.0 ml with a 3.5 per cent *V/V* solution of *cadmium- and lead-free nitric acid R*.

Reference solutions. Prepare the reference solutions using *cadmium standard solution (0.1 per cent Cd) R* and diluting with a 3.5 per cent *V/V* solution of *cadmium- and lead-free nitric acid R*.

Measure the absorbance at 228.8 nm using a cadmium hollow-cathode lamp as source of radiation and an air-acetylene or an air-propane flame.

Lead. Not more than 25 ppm of Pb, determined by atomic absorption spectrometry (*2.2.23, Method II*).

Test solution. Use solution S.

Reference solutions. Prepare the reference solutions using *lead standard solution (0.1 per cent Pb) R* and diluting with a 3.5 per cent *V/V* solution of *cadmium- and lead-free nitric acid R*.

Measure the absorbance at 283.3 nm using a lead hollow-cathode lamp as source of radiation and an air-acetylene flame. Depending on the apparatus the line at 217.0 nm may be used.

ASSAY

To 1.000 g add 50 ml of *dilute acetic acid R* and boil for at least 10 min or until the layer of fatty acids is clear, adding more *water R* as necessary to maintain the original volume. Cool and filter. Wash the filter and the flask with *water R* until the washings are no longer acid to *blue litmus paper R*. Combine the filtrate and washings. Carry out the complexometric titration of zinc (*2.5.11*).

1 ml of *0.1 M sodium edetate* is equivalent to 6.54 mg of Zn.

01/2005:0111

ZINC SULPHATE HEPTAHYDRATE

Zinci sulfas heptahydricus

$ZnSO_4,7H_2O$ M_r 287.5

DEFINITION

Content: 99.0 per cent to 104.0 per cent.

CHARACTERS

Appearance: white, crystalline powder or colourless, transparent crystals, efflorescent.

Solubility: very soluble in water, practically insoluble in alcohol.

IDENTIFICATION

A. Solution S (see Tests) gives the reactions of sulphates (*2.3.1*).

B. Solution S gives the reaction of zinc (*2.3.1*).

C. It complies with the limits of the assay.

TESTS

Solution S. Dissolve 2.5 g in *carbon dioxide-free water R* and dilute to 50 ml with the same solvent.

Appearance of solution. Solution S is clear (*2.2.1*) and colourless (*2.2.2, Method II*).

pH (*2.2.3*): 4.4 to 5.6 for solution S.

Chlorides (*2.4.4*): maximum 300 ppm.

3.3 ml of solution S diluted to 15 ml with *water R* complies with the limit test for chlorides.

Iron (*2.4.9*): maximum 100 ppm.

2 ml of solution S diluted to 10 ml with *water R* complies with the limit test for iron. Use in this test 0.5 ml of *thioglycollic acid R*.

ASSAY

Dissolve 0.200 g in 5 ml of *dilute acetic acid R*. Carry out the complexometric titration of zinc (*2.5.11*).

Monographs T-Z

1 ml of *0.1 M sodium edetate* is equivalent to 28.75 mg of $ZnSO_4,7H_2O$.

STORAGE

In a non-metallic, airtight container.

01/2005:1683

ZINC SULPHATE HEXAHYDRATE

Zinci sulfas hexahydricus

$ZnSO_4,6H_2O$ M_r 269.5

DEFINITION

Content: 99.0 per cent to 104.0 per cent.

CHARACTERS

Appearance: white, crystalline powder or colourless transparent crystals, efflorescent.

Solubility: very soluble in water, practically insoluble in alcohol.

IDENTIFICATION

A. Solution S (see Tests) gives the reactions of sulphates (*2.3.1*).

B. Solution S gives the reaction of zinc (*2.3.1*).

C. It complies with the limits of the assay.

TESTS

Solution S. Dissolve 2.5 g in *carbon dioxide-free water R* and dilute to 50 ml with the same solvent.

Appearance of solution. Solution S is clear (*2.2.1*) and colourless (*2.2.2, Method II*).

pH (*2.2.3*): 4.4 to 5.6 for solution S.

Chlorides (*2.4.4*): maximum 300 ppm.

3.3 ml of solution S diluted to 15 ml with *water R* complies with the limit test for chlorides.

Iron (*2.4.9*): maximum 100 ppm.

2 ml of solution S diluted to 10 ml with *water R* complies with the limit test for iron. Use in this test 0.5 ml of *thioglycollic acid R*.

ASSAY

Dissolve 0.200 g in 5 ml of *dilute acetic acid R*. Carry out the complexometric titration of zinc (*2.5.11*).

1 ml of *0.1 M sodium edetate* is equivalent to 26.95 mg of $ZnSO_4,6H_2O$.

STORAGE

In a non-metallic, airtight container.

01/2005:0539

ZINC UNDECYLENATE

Zinci undecylenas

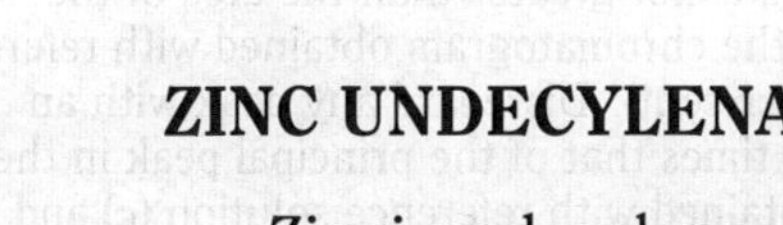

$C_{22}H_{38}O_4Zn$ M_r 431.9

DEFINITION

Zinc undecylenate contains not less than 98.0 per cent and not more than the equivalent of 102.0 per cent of zinc di(undec-10-enoate), calculated with reference to the dried substance.

CHARACTERS

A white or almost white, fine powder, practically insoluble in water and in alcohol.

It melts at 116 °C to 121 °C but may leave a slight solid residue.

IDENTIFICATION

A. To 2.5 g add 10 ml of *water R* and 10 ml of *dilute sulphuric acid R*. Shake with two quantities, each of 10 ml, of *ether R*. Reserve the aqueous layer for identification test C. Wash the combined ether layers with *water R* and evaporate to dryness. To the residue add 2 ml of freshly distilled *aniline R* and boil under a reflux condenser for 10 min. Allow to cool and add 30 ml of *ether R*. Shake with three quantities, each of 20 ml, of *dilute hydrochloric acid R* and then with 20 ml of *water R*. Evaporate the organic layer to dryness on a water-bath. The residue, after recrystallisation twice from *alcohol (70 per cent V/V) R* and drying *in vacuo* for 3 h, melts (*2.2.14*) at 66 °C to 68 °C.

B. Dissolve 0.1 g in a mixture of 2 ml of *dilute sulphuric acid R* and 5 ml of *glacial acetic acid R*. Add dropwise 0.25 ml of *potassium permanganate solution R*. The colour of the potassium permanganate is discharged.

C. A mixture of 1 ml of the aqueous layer obtained in identification test A and 4 ml of *water R* gives the reaction of zinc (*2.3.1*).

TESTS

Alkalinity. Mix 1.0 g with 5 ml of *alcohol R* and 0.5 ml of *phenol red solution R*. Add 50 ml of *carbon dioxide-free water R* and examine immediately. No reddish colour appears.

Alkali and alkaline-earth metals. To 1.0 g add 25 ml of *water R* and 5 ml of *hydrochloric acid R* and heat to boiling. Filter whilst hot. Wash the filter and the residue with 25 ml of hot *water R*. Combine the filtrate and washings and add *concentrated ammonia R* until alkaline. Add 7.5 ml of *thioacetamide solution R* and heat on a water-bath for 30 min. Filter and wash the precipitate with two quantities, each of 10 ml, of *water R*. Combine the filtrate and washings, evaporate to dryness on a water-bath and ignite. The residue weighs not more than 20 mg (2 per cent).

Sulphates (*2.4.13*). To 0.1 g add a mixture of 2 ml of *dilute hydrochloric acid R* and 10 ml of *distilled water R* and heat to boiling. Cool, filter and dilute to 15 ml with *distilled water R*. The solution complies with the limit test for sulphates (500 ppm). Prepare the standard using 5 ml of *sulphate standard solution (10 ppm SO_4) R* and 10 ml of *distilled water R*.

Loss on drying (*2.2.32*). Not more than 1.5 per cent, determined on 0.500 g by drying in an oven at 100 °C to 105 °C.

Degree of unsaturation. Dissolve 0.100 g in a mixture of 5 ml of *dilute hydrochloric acid R* and 30 ml of *glacial acetic acid R*. Using 0.05 ml *indigo carmine solution R1*, added towards the end of the titration as indicator. Titrate with *0.0167 M bromide-bromate* until the colour changes from blue to yellow. 9.1 ml to 9.4 ml of *0.0167 M bromide-bromate* is required. Carry out a blank titration.

ASSAY

To 0.350 g add 25 ml of *dilute acetic acid R* and heat to boiling. Carry out the complexometric titration of zinc (*2.5.11*).

1 ml of *0.1 M sodium edetate* is equivalent to 43.19 mg of $C_{22}H_{38}O_4Zn$.

STORAGE

Store protected from light.

01/2005:1280

ZOLPIDEM TARTRATE

Zolpidemi tartras

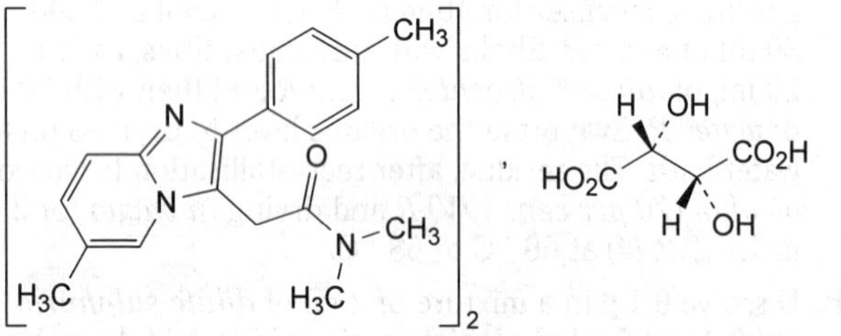

$C_{42}H_{48}N_6O_8$ M_r 765

DEFINITION

Zolpidem tartrate contains not less than 98.5 per cent and not more than the equivalent of 101.0 per cent of bis[*N*,*N*-dimethyl-2-[6-methyl-2-(4-methylphenyl)imidazo[1,2-*a*]pyridin-3-yl]acetamide] (2*R*,3*R*)-2,3-dihydroxybutanedioate, calculated with reference to the anhydrous substance.

CHARACTERS

A white or almost white, crystalline powder, hygroscopic, slightly soluble in water, sparingly soluble in methanol, practically insoluble in methylene chloride.

IDENTIFICATION

First identification: A, C.

Second identification: B, C.

A. Dissolve 0.10 g in 10 ml of *0.1 M hydrochloric acid.* Add 10 ml of *water R*. Add dropwise with stirring 1 ml of *dilute ammonia R2.* Filter and collect the resulting precipitate. Wash the precipitate with *water R* and then dry at 100-105 °C for 2 h (test precipitate). Carry out the same operation using *zolpidem tartrate CRS* (reference precipitate). Examine the precipitates by infrared absorption spectrophotometry (*2.2.24*) comparing the spectra obtained. Examine the precipitates as discs.

B. Examine by thin-layer chromatography (*2.2.27*), using a *TLC silica gel F_{254} plate R.*

Test solution. Dissolve 50 mg of the substance to be examined in 5 ml of *methanol R*, add 0.1 ml of *diethylamine R* and dilute to 10 ml with *methanol R.*

Reference solution (a). Dissolve 50 mg of *zolpidem tartrate CRS* in 5 ml of *methanol R*, add 0.1 ml of *diethylamine R* and dilute to 10 ml with *methanol R.*

Reference solution (b). Dissolve 50 mg of *flunitrazepam CRS* in 5 ml of *methylene chloride R* and dilute to 10 ml with the same solvent. Mix 1 ml of the solution with 1 ml of reference solution (a).

Apply to the plate 5 µl of each solution. Develop over a path of 12 cm using a mixture of 10 volumes of *diethylamine R*, 45 volumes of *cyclohexane R* and 45 volumes of *ethyl acetate R.* Allow the plate to dry in air and examine in ultraviolet light at 254 nm. The principal spot in the chromatogram obtained with the test solution is similar in position and size to the principal spot in the chromatogram obtained with reference solution (a). The test is not valid unless the chromatogram obtained with reference solution (b) shows 2 clearly separated spots.

C. Dissolve about 0.1 g in 1 ml of *methanol R* heating gently. 0.1 ml of the solution gives reaction (b) of tartrates (*2.3.1*).

TESTS

Appearance of solution. *Prepare the solutions protected from light and carry out the test as rapidly as possible.* Triturate 0.25 g with 0.125 g of *tartaric acid R*. Dissolve the mixture in 20 ml of *water R* and dilute to 25 ml with the same solvent. The solution is clear (*2.2.1*) and not more intensely coloured than reference solution Y_6 or BY_6 (*2.2.2, Method II*).

Related substances. Examine by liquid chromatography (*2.2.29*).

Test solution. Dissolve 25.0 mg of the substance to be examined in the mobile phase and dilute to 50.0 ml with the mobile phase.

Reference solution (a). Dissolve 5 mg of *zolpidem impurity A CRS* in the mobile phase and dilute to 50 ml with the mobile phase.

Reference solution (b). Dissolve 5 mg of the substance to be examined in the mobile phase and dilute to 50 ml with the mobile phase. To 10 ml of the solution, add 10 ml of reference solution (a).

Reference solution (c). Dilute 2.0 ml of the test solution to 100.0 ml with the mobile phase. Dilute 1.0 ml of the solution to 10.0 ml with the mobile phase.

The chromatographic procedure may be carried out using:

– a stainless steel column 0.15 m long and 3.9 mm in internal diameter packed with *octadecylsilyl silica gel for chromatography R* (4 µm),

– as mobile phase at a flow rate of 1.5 ml/min a mixture of 18 volumes of *acetonitrile R*, 23 volumes of *methanol R* and 59 volumes of a 5.6 g/l solution of *phosphoric acid R* adjusted to pH 5.5 with *triethylamine R*,

– as detector a spectrophotometer set at 254 nm.

Inject 20 µl of reference solution (b). Adjust the sensitivity of the system so that the height of the peak due to zolpidem impurity A is at least 50 per cent of the full scale of the recorder. The test is not valid unless the resolution between the peaks due to zolpidem impurity A and zolpidem tartrate is at least 2.0.

Inject 20 µl of the test solution and 20 µl of reference solution (c). In the chromatogram obtained with the test solution, the sum of the areas of any peaks, apart from the principal peak, is not greater than the area of the principal peak in the chromatogram obtained with reference solution (c) (0.2 per cent). Disregard any peak with an area less than 0.1 times that of the principal peak in the chromatogram obtained with reference solution (c) and any peak (with a relative retention time of 0.16 to the zolpidem peak) corresponding to tartaric acid.

Water (*2.5.12*). Not more than 3.0 per cent, determined on 0.50 g by the semi-micro determination of water.

Sulphated ash (*2.4.14*). Not more than 0.1 per cent, determined on 1.0 g.

ASSAY

Dissolve 0.300 g in a mixture of 20 ml of *anhydrous acetic acid R* and 20 ml of *acetic anhydride R*. Titrate with *0.1 M perchloric acid,* determining the end-point potentiometrically (*2.2.20*). Carry out a blank titration.

1 ml of *0.1 M perchloric acid* is equivalent to 38.24 mg of $C_{42}H_{48}N_6O_8$.

STORAGE

Store in an airtight container, protected from light.

IMPURITIES

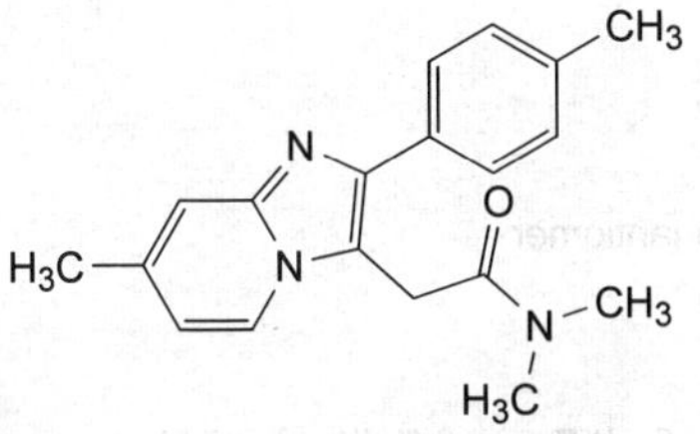

A. *N,N*-dimethyl-2-[7-methyl-2-(4-methylphenyl)imidazo[1,2-*a*]pyridin-3-yl]acetamide.

01/2005:1060 corrected

ZOPICLONE

Zopiclonum

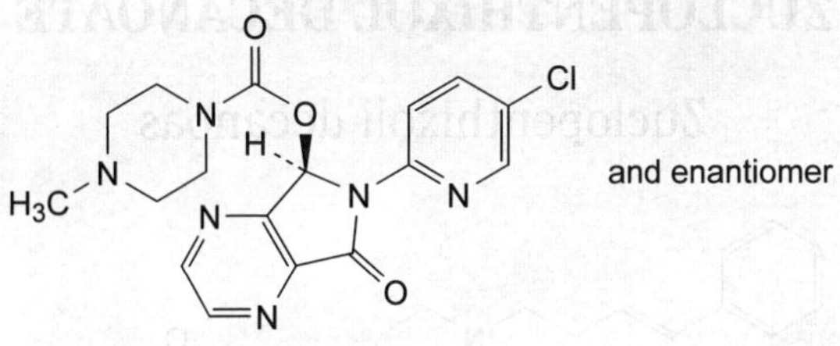

$C_{17}H_{17}ClN_6O_3$ M_r 388.8

DEFINITION

Zopiclone contains not less than 98.5 per cent and not more than the equivalent of 100.5 per cent of (5*RS*)-6-(5-chloropyridin-2-yl)-7-oxo-6,7-dihydro-5*H*-pyrrolo[3,4-*b*]pyrazin-5-yl 4-methylpiperazine-1-carboxylate, calculated with reference to the solvent-free substance.

CHARACTERS

A white or slightly yellowish powder, practically insoluble in water, freely soluble in methylene chloride, sparingly soluble in acetone, practically insoluble in alcohol. It dissolves in dilute mineral acids.

It melts at about 177 °C, with decomposition.

IDENTIFICATION

First identification: B.

Second identification: A, C.

A. Dissolve 50.0 mg in a 3.5 g/l solution of *hydrochloric acid R* and dilute to 100.0 ml with the same solvent. Dilute 2.0 ml of this solution to 100.0 ml with a 3.5 g/l solution of *hydrochloric acid R.* Examined between 220 nm and 350 nm (*2.2.25*), the solution shows an absorption maximum at 303 nm. The specific absorbance at the maximum is 340 to 380.

B. Examine by infrared absorption spectrophotometry (*2.2.24*), comparing with the spectrum obtained with *zopiclone CRS*. Examine the substances prepared as discs.

C. Examine by thin-layer chromatography (*2.2.27*), using *silica gel GF_{254} R* as the coating substance.

Test solution. Dissolve 10 mg of the substance to be examined in *methylene chloride R* and dilute to 10 ml with the same solvent.

Reference solution. Dissolve 10 mg of *zopiclone CRS* in *methylene chloride R* and dilute to 10 ml with the same solvent.

Apply to the plate 10 µl of each solution. Develop over a path of 15 cm using a mixture of 2 volumes of *triethylamine R*, 50 volumes of *acetone R* and 50 volumes of *ethyl acetate R*. Allow the plate to dry in air and examine in ultraviolet light at 254 nm. The principal spot in the chromatogram obtained with the test solution is similar in position and size to the principal spot in the chromatogram obtained with the reference solution.

TESTS

Solution S. Dissolve 1.0 g in *dimethylformamide R* and dilute to 20.0 ml with the same solvent.

Appearance of solution. Solution S is not more opalescent than reference suspension II (*2.2.1*) and not more intensely coloured than intensity 5 of the range of reference solutions of the most appropriate colour (*2.2.2, Method II*).

Optical rotation (*2.2.7*). Dilute 10.0 ml of solution S to 50.0 ml with *dimethylformamide R*. The angle of optical rotation is − 0.05° to + 0.05°.

Related substances. Examine by liquid chromatography (*2.2.29*). *Prepare the solutions immediately before use.*

Test solution. Dissolve 40.0 mg of the substance to be examined in the mobile phase and dilute to 10.0 ml with the mobile phase.

Reference solution (a). Dilute 3.0 ml of the test solution to 100.0 ml with the mobile phase. Dilute 1.0 ml of this solution to 10.0 ml with the mobile phase.

Reference solution (b). Dilute 1.0 ml of the test solution to 100.0 ml with the mobile phase. Dilute 1.0 ml of this solution to 10.0 ml with the mobile phase.

Reference solution (c). Dissolve 4.0 mg of *zopiclone oxide CRS* in the mobile phase and dilute to 10.0 ml with the mobile phase. To 10.0 ml of this solution, add 1.0 ml of the test solution and dilute to 100.0 ml with the mobile phase.

The chromatographic procedure may be carried out using:

– a stainless steel column 0.25 m long and 4.6 mm in internal diameter packed with *octadecylsilyl silica gel for chromatography R* (5 µm),

– as mobile phase at a flow rate of 1.5 ml/min a mixture of 38 volumes of *acetonitrile R* and 62 volumes of a solution containing 8.1 g/l of *sodium laurilsulfate R* and 1.6 g/l of *sodium dihydrogen phosphate R* adjusted to pH 3.5 with a 10 per cent *V/V* solution of *phosphoric acid R,*

– as detector a spectrophotometer set at 303 nm,

maintaining the temperature of the column at 30 °C.

Inject 20 µl of reference solution (c). Adjust the sensitivity of the system so that the height of each of the 2 principal peaks in the chromatogram obtained is at least 30 per cent of the full scale of the recorder. When the chromatograms are recorded in the prescribed conditions, the retention time of zopiclone is 27 min to 31 min. If necessary, adjust the concentration of acetonitrile in the mobile phase (increasing the concentration decreases the retention times and

Monographs T-Z

decreasing the concentration increases the retention times). The test is not valid unless, in the chromatogram obtained with reference solution (c), the resolution between the peaks due to zopiclone oxide and zopiclone is at least 3.0. If the prescribed resolution is not obtained, adjust the mobile phase to pH 4.0 with a 10 per cent *V/V* solution of *phosphoric acid R*.

Inject 20 µl of the test solution, 20 µl of reference solution (a) and 20 µl of reference solution (b). Continue the chromatography for 1.5 times the retention time of zopiclone. In the chromatogram obtained with the test solution: the area of any peak, apart from the principal peak, is not greater than the area of the principal peak in the chromatogram obtained with reference solution (a) (0.3 per cent) and not more than 2 such peaks have an area greater than the area of the principal peak in the chromatogram obtained with reference solution (b) (0.1 per cent).

2-Propanol. Not more than 0.7 per cent *m/m* of 2-propanol, determined by gas chromatography (*2.2.28*) using *ethanol R1* as the internal standard.

Internal standard solution. Dilute 5 ml of *ethanol R1* to 100 ml with *ethylene chloride R*. Dilute 1 ml of this solution to 10 ml with *ethylene chloride R*.

Test solution. Dissolve 0.25 g of the substance to be examined in *ethylene chloride R*, add 0.5 ml of the internal standard solution and dilute to 5.0 ml with *ethylene chloride R*.

Reference solution. Dilute 4.5 ml of *2-propanol R* to 100.0 ml with *ethylene chloride R*. To 1.0 ml of this solution, add 10.0 ml of the internal standard solution and dilute to 100.0 ml with *ethylene chloride R*.

The chromatographic procedure may be carried out using:

– a fused-silica column 10 m long and about 0.53 mm in internal diameter with a 20 µm coating of *styrene-divinylbenzene copolymer R*,
– *helium for chromatography R* as the carrier gas at a flow rate of 4 ml/min,
– a flame-ionisation detector,

with the following temperature programme:

	Time (min)	Temperature (°C)	Rate (°C/min)	Comment
Column	0 - 5	50		isothermal
	5 - 10	50 → 70	4	linear gradient
	10 - 14	70		isothermal
	14 - 20.5	70 → 200	20	linear gradient
	20.5 - 27.5	200		isothermal
Injection port		150		
Detector		250		

Inject 1 µl of the test solution and 1 µl of the reference solution. Calculate the percentage content *m/m* of 2-propanol taking its density to be 0.785 g/ml at 20 °C.

Heavy metals (*2.4.8*). 1.0 g complies with limit test C for heavy metals (20 ppm). Prepare the standard using 2 ml of *lead standard solution (10 ppm Pb) R*.

Sulphated ash (*2.4.14*). Not more than 0.1 per cent, determined on 1.0 g.

ASSAY

Dissolve 0.300 g in a mixture of 10 ml of *anhydrous acetic acid R* and 40 ml of *acetic anhydride R*. Titrate with *0.1 M perchloric acid*, determining the end-point potentiometrically (*2.2.20*).

1 ml of *0.1 M perchloric acid* is equivalent to 38.88 mg of $C_{17}H_{17}ClN_6O_3$.

STORAGE

Store protected from light.

IMPURITIES

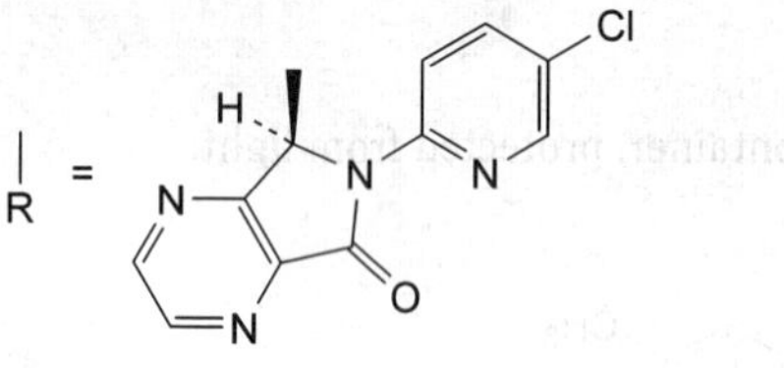

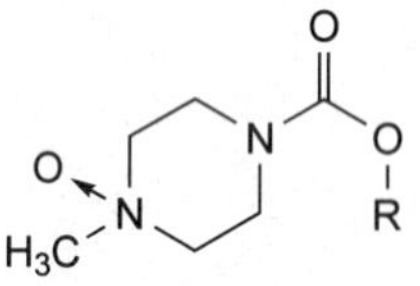

and enantiomer

A. (5*RS*)-6-(5-chloropyridin-2-yl)-7-oxo-6,7-dihydro-5*H*-pyrrolo[3,4-*b*]pyrazin-5-yl 4-methylpiperazine-1-carboxylate 4-oxide (zopiclone oxide),

B. R-OH and enantiomer: (7*RS*)-6-(5-chloropyridin-2-yl)-7-hydroxy-6,7-dihydro-5*H*-pyrrolo[3,4-*b*]pyrazin-5-one,

C. R-H: 6-(5-chloropyridin-2-yl)-6,7-dihydro-5*H*-pyrrolo[3,4-*b*]pyrazin-5-one.

01/2005:1707

ZUCLOPENTHIXOL DECANOATE

Zuclopenthixoli decanoas

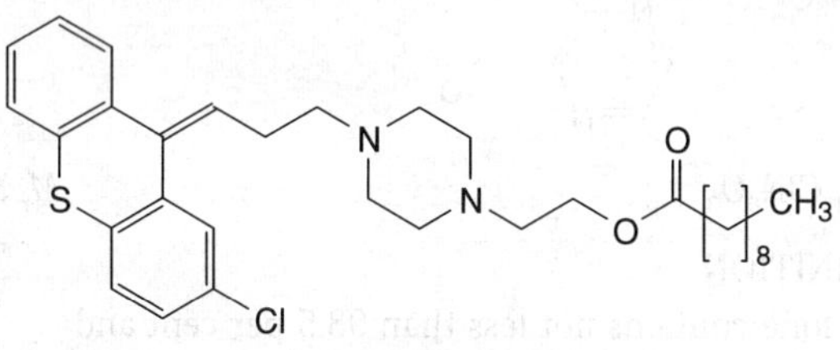

$C_{32}H_{43}ClN_2O_2S$ M_r 555.2

DEFINITION

2-[4-[3-[(*Z*)-2-chloro-9*H*-thioxanthen-9-ylidene]propyl]piperazin-1-yl]ethyl decanoate.

Content: 98.0 per cent to 102.0 per cent (dried substance).

CHARACTERS

Appearance: yellow, viscous oily liquid.

Solubility: very slightly soluble in water, very soluble in alcohol and in methylene chloride.

IDENTIFICATION

Infrared absorption spectrophotometry (*2.2.24*).

Comparison: *Ph. Eur. reference spectrum of zuclopenthixol decanoate.*

TESTS

Appearance of solution. The solution is clear (*2.2.1*).

Using an ultrasonic bath, dissolve 1.0 g in *alcohol R* and dilute to 20.0 ml with the same solvent.

Monographs T-7

Related substances. Thin-layer chromatography (*2.2.27*). *Carry out the test protected from light and prepare the solutions immediately before use.*

Test solution. Dissolve 0.250 g of the substance to be examined in *alcohol R*, using an ultrasonic bath, and dilute to 100.0 ml with the same solvent.

Reference solution (a). Dilute 1.0 ml of the test solution to 100.0 ml with *alcohol R*. Dilute 1.0 ml of this solution to 10.0 ml with *alcohol R*.

Reference solution (b). Dilute 5.0 ml of reference solution (a) to 10.0 ml with *alcohol R*.

Reference solution (c). Dissolve 5.0 mg of *zuclopenthixol impurity B CRS* in *alcohol R* and dilute to 100.0 ml with the same solvent. Dilute 10.0 ml of the solution to 100.0 ml with *alcohol R*.

Reference solution (d). Dissolve 5.0 mg of *zuclopenthixol impurity C CRS* in *alcohol R* and dilute to 100.0 ml with the same solvent. Dilute 2.5 ml of the solution to 20.0 ml with *alcohol R*.

Reference solution (e). Dissolve 5.0 mg of *zuclopenthixol impurity B CRS* and 20.0 mg of the substance to be examined in *alcohol R* and dilute to 100.0 ml with the same solvent.

Plate: *TLC silica gel plate R.*

Mobile phase: *diethylamine R, propanol R, cyclohexane R* (3:10:90 *V/V/V*).

Application: 4 µl.

Development: horizontally, over 2/3 of the plate.

Drying: in air.

Detection: spray with a 14 per cent *V/V* alcoholic solution of *sulphuric acid R* prepared immediately before use; heat at 110 °C for 5 min and examine in ultraviolet light at 365 nm.

System suitability: the chromatogram obtained with reference solution (e) shows 2 clearly separated spots.

Limits:

– *impurity B*: any spot corresponding to impurity B is not more intense than the spot in the chromatogram obtained with reference solution (c) (0.2 per cent),
– *impurity C*: any spot corresponding to impurity C is not more intense than the spot in the chromatogram obtained with reference solution (d) (0.25 per cent),
– *any other impurity*: any spots, apart from the principal spot and any spot corresponding to impurity B or impurity C, are not more intense than the spot in the chromatogram obtained with reference solution (a) (0.1 per cent) and at most 3 such spots are more intense than the spot in the chromatogram obtained with reference solution (b) (0.05 per cent).

Impurity A. Liquid chromatography (*2.2.29*). *Carry out the test protected from light and prepare the solutions immediately before use.*

Test solution. Dissolve 40.0 mg of the substance to be examined in *alcohol R* and dilute to 100.0 ml with the same solvent.

Reference solution. Dissolve a quantity of *zuclopenthixol impurity A CRS* corresponding to 5.0 mg of impurity A in *alcohol R* and dilute to 100.0 ml with the same solvent. To 5.0 ml of the solution add 0.6 ml of test solution and dilute to 50.0 ml with *alcohol R*.

Column:

– *size*: *l* = 0.15 m, Ø = 4.6 mm,
– *stationary phase*: *octadecylsilyl silica gel for chromatography R* (5 µm),
– *temperature*: 40 °C.

Mobile phase: mix 25 volumes of a 8.9 g/l solution of *docusate sodium R* and 75 volumes of *alcohol R*; add 0.1 per cent *V/V* of *phosphoric acid R*.

Flow rate: 1 ml/min.

Detection: spectrophotometer at 230 nm.

Equilibration: at least 1 h with the mobile phase.

Injection: 20 µl.

System suitability: reference solution:

– *resolution*: minimum of 1.5 between the peaks due to zuclopenthixol decanoate (1st peak) and to impurity A (2nd peak).

Limit:

– *impurity A*: not more than the area of the corresponding peak in the chromatogram obtained with reference solution (1.25 per cent).

Heavy metals (*2.4.8*): maximum 20 ppm.

1.0 g complies with limit test C. Prepare the standard using 2 ml of *lead standard solution (10 ppm Pb) R.*

Loss on drying (*2.2.32*): maximum 0.5 per cent, determined on 1.000 g by drying in an oven at 60 °C at a pressure not exceeding 0.7 kPa for 3 h.

Sulphated ash (*2.4.14*): maximum 0.1 per cent, determined on 1.0 g.

ASSAY

Dissolve 0.250 g in 50 ml of *anhydrous acetic acid R*. Titrate with *0.1 M perchloric acid*, determining the end-point potentiometrically (*2.2.20*).

1 ml of *0.1 M perchloric acid* is equivalent to 27.76 mg of $C_{32}H_{43}ClN_2O_2S$.

STORAGE

Under an inert gas in an airtight container, protected from light, at a temperature not exceeding − 20 °C.

IMPURITIES

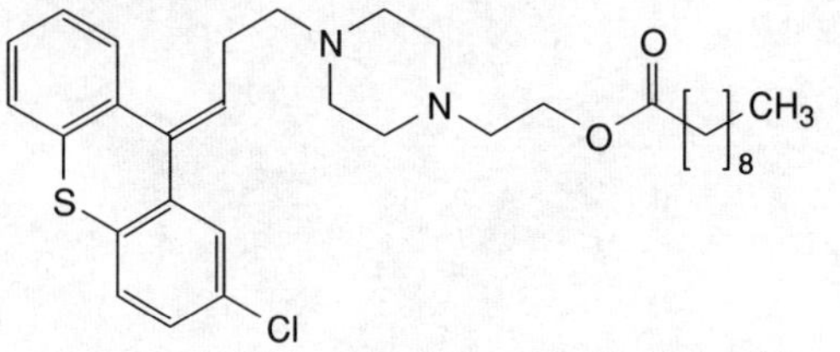

A. 2-[4-[3-[(*E*)-2-chloro-9*H*-thioxanthen-9-ylidene]propyl]piperazin-1-yl]ethyl decanoate,

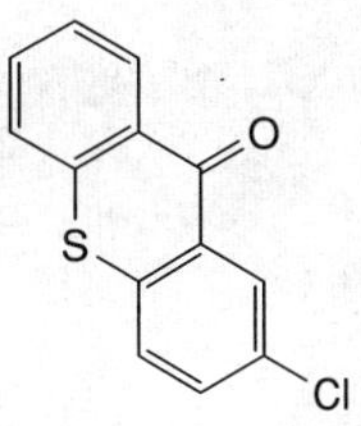

B. 2-chloro-9*H*-thioxanthen-9-one,

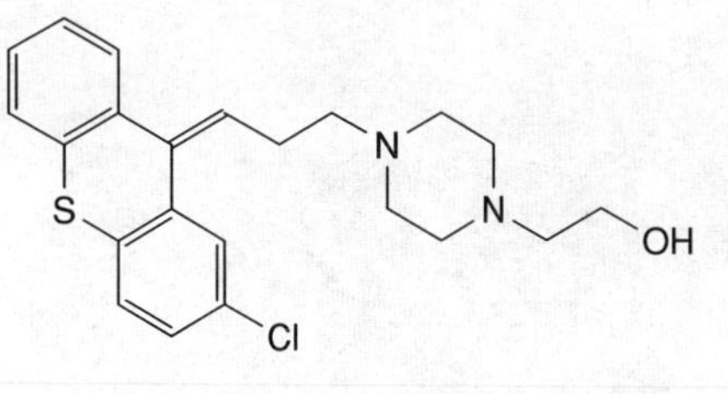

C. 2-[4-[3-[(*Z*)-2-chloro-9*H*-thioxanthen-9-ylidene]propyl]piperazin-1-yl]ethanol.

Monographs T-Z

INDEX

Monographs deleted from the Fourth Edition are not included in the index; a list of deleted texts is found in the Contents of Volume 1, page xix.

Numerics

Index

B

Index

Index

Index

Index

M

O

P

Index

Index

Index

Index

W

X

Y

Z

Members of the European Pharmacopoeia Commission: Austria, Belgium, Bosnia and Herzegovina, Croatia, Cyprus, Czech Republic, Denmark, Estonia, Finland, France, Germany, Greece, Hungary, Iceland, Ireland, Italy, Latvia, Luxembourg, Netherlands, Norway, Portugal, Romania, Serbia and Montenegro, Slovak Republic, Slovenia, Spain, Sweden, Switzerland, "The former Yugoslav Republic of Macedonia", Turkey, United Kingdom and the European Union.

Observers to the European Pharmacopoeia Commission: Albania, Algeria, Australia, Bulgaria, Canada, China, Georgia, Lithuania, Malaysia, Malta, Morocco, Poland, Senegal, Syria, Tunisia, Ukraine and WHO (World Health Organisation).

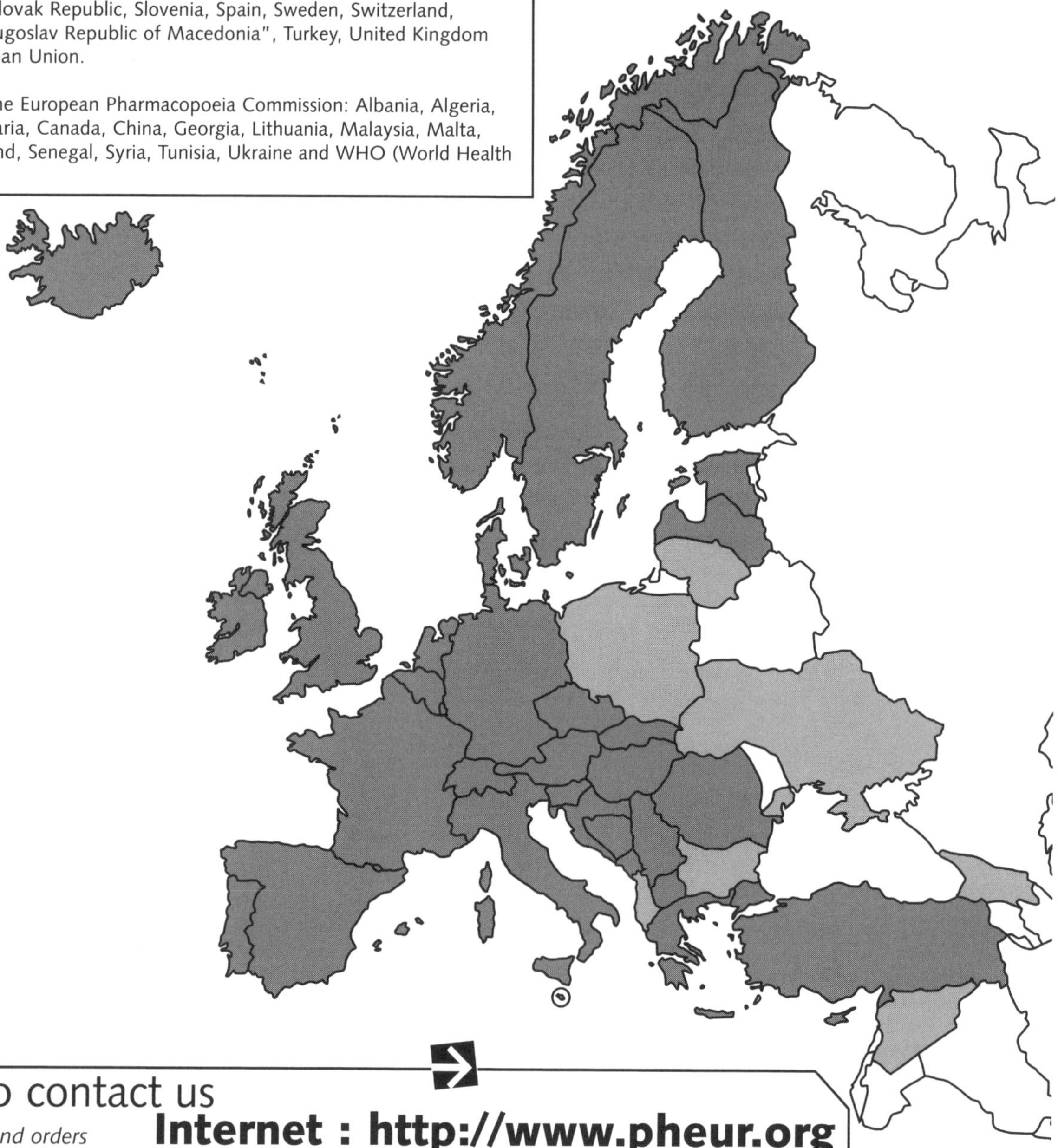

How to contact us

Information and orders **Internet : http://www.pheur.org**

European Directorate for the Quality of Medicines
Council of Europe - 226 avenue de Colmar BP 907
F-67029 STRASBOURG Cedex 1, FRANCE
Tel: +33 (0)3 88 41 30 30*
Fax: +33 (0)3 88 41 27 71*

	E-mail
CD-ROM	cdromtech@pheur.org
Certification	certification@pheur.org
Monographs	monographs@pheur.org
Publications	publications@pheur.org
Reference substances	crs@pheur.org
Conferences	publicrelations@pheur.org
All other correspondence	info@pheur.org

*: Do not dial 0 if calling from outside France.
All reference substances required for application of the monographs are available from the EDQM. A catalogue of reference substances is available on request; the catalogue is included in the Pharmeuropa subscription; it can also be consulted on the EDQM internet site.

EUROPEAN PHARMACOPOEIA

5th Edition

published 15 June 2004

replaces the 4th Edition on 1 January 2005

Volumes 1 and 2 of this publication 5.0 constitute the 5th Edition of the European Pharmacopoeia. They will be complemented by **non-cumulative supplements** that are to be kept for the duration of the 5th Edition. 2 supplements will be published in 2004 and 3 supplements in each of the years 2005 and 2006. A cumulative list of reagents will be published in supplements 5.4 and 5.7.

If you are using the 5th Edition at any time later than 1 April 2005, make sure that you have all the published supplements and consult the index of the most recent supplement to ensure that you use the latest versions of the monographs and general chapters.

EUROPEAN PHARMACOPOEIA ELECTRONIC VERSION

The 5th Edition is also available in an electronic format (CD-ROM and internet version) with all the monographs and general chapters contained in the book. With the publication of each supplement the electronic version is replaced by a new fully updated cumulative version.

PHARMEUROPA

Quarterly Forum Publication

Pharmeuropa contains preliminary drafts of all new and revised monographs proposed for inclusion in the European Pharmacopoeia and gives an opportunity for all interested parties to comment on the specifications before they are finalised. Pharmeuropa also contains information on the work programme and on certificates of suitability to monographs of the European Pharmacopoeia issued by the EDQM, scientific articles on pharmacopoeial matters and other articles of general interest. Pharmeuropa is available on subscription from the EDQM.

INTERNATIONAL HARMONISATION

Refer to information given in chapter *5.8. Pharmacopoeial Harmonisation.*

WEBSITE

http://www.pheur.org

http://book.pheur.org (for prices and orders)

KEY TO MONOGRAPHS

Version date of the text — **01/2005:0884**

Text reference number

Modification to be taken into account from the publication date of volume 5.0 — corrected

CARBIMAZOLE

Carbimazolum

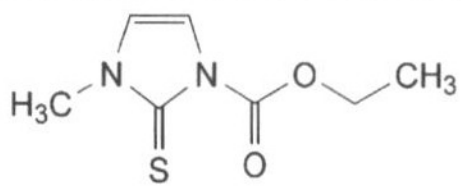

$C_7H_{10}N_2O_2S$ M_r 186.2

Chemical name in accordance with IUPAC nomenclature rules

DEFINITION

Ethyl 3-methyl-2-thioxo-2,3-dihydro-1*H*-imidazole-1-carboxylate.

Content: 98.0 per cent to 102.0 per cent (dried substance).

CHARACTERS

Appearance: white or yellowish-white, crystalline powder.

Solubility: slightly soluble in water, soluble in acetone and in alcohol.

Application of the first and second identification is defined in the General Notices (chapter 1)

IDENTIFICATION

First identification: B.

Second identification: A, C, D.

A. Melting point (*2.2.14*): 122 °C to 125 °C.

B. Infrared absorption spectrophotometry (*2.2.24*).

Preparation: discs.

Comparison: *carbimazole CRS*.

Chemical reference substance available from the Secretariat (see www.pheur.org)

C. Thin-layer chromatography (*2.2.27*).

Test solution. Dissolve 10 mg of the substance to be examined in *methylene chloride R* and dilute to 10 ml with the same solvent.

Reference solution. Dissolve 10 mg of *carbimazole CRS* in *methylene chloride R* and dilute to 10 ml with the same solvent.

Plate: *TLC silica gel GF_{254} plate R.*

Mobile phase: *acetone R*, *methylene chloride R* (20:80 *V/V*).

Reagents described in chapter 4

Application: 10 µl.

Development: over a path of 15 cm.

Drying: in air for 30 min.

Detection: examine in ultraviolet light at 254 nm.

Results: the principal spot in the chromatogram obtained with the test solution is similar in position and size to the principal spot in the chromatogram obtained with the reference solution.

D. Dissolve about 10 mg in a mixture of 50 ml of *water R* and 0.05 ml of *dilute hydrochloric acid R*. Add 1 ml of *potassium iodobismuthate solution R*. A red precipitate is formed.

TESTS

Impurity A and other related substances. Liquid chromatography (*2.2.29*).

Reference to a general chapter

Test solution. Dissolve 5.0 mg of the substance to be examined in 10.0 ml of a mixture of 20 volumes of *acetonitrile R* and 80 volumes of *water R*. Use this solution within 5 min of preparation.

Reference solution (a). Dissolve 5 mg of *thiamazole R* and 0.10 g of *carbimazole CRS* in a mixture of 20 volumes of *acetonitrile R* and 80 volumes of *water R* and dilute to 100.0 ml with the same mixture of solvents. Dilute 1.0 ml of this solution to 10.0 ml with a mixture of 20 volumes of *acetonitrile R* and 80 volumes of *water R*.

Reference solution (b). Dissolve 5.0 mg of *thiamazole R* in a mixture of 20 volumes of *acetonitrile R* and 80 volumes of *water R* and dilute to 10.0 ml with the same mixture of solvents. Dilute 1.0 ml of this solution to 100.0 ml with a mixture of 20 volumes of *acetonitrile R* and 80 volumes of *water R*.

Column:

- *size*: *l* = 0.15 m, Ø = 3.9 mm,
- *stationary phase*: *octadecylsilyl silica gel for chromatography R* (5 µm).

Mobile phase: *acetonitrile R, water R* (10:90 *V/V*).

Flow rate: 1 ml/min.

Detection: spectrophotometer at 254 nm.

Injection: 10 µl.

Run time: 1.5 times the retention time of carbimazole.

Retention time: carbimazole = about 6 min.

System suitability: reference solution (a):

- *resolution*: minimum 5.0 between the peaks due to impurity A and carbimazole.

Limits:

- *impurity A*: not more than half the area of the principal peak in the chromatogram obtained with reference solution (b) (0.5 per cent),
- *any other impurity*: not more than 0.1 times the area of the principal peak in the chromatogram obtained with reference solution (b) (0.1 per cent).

Loss on drying (*2.2.32*): maximum 0.5 per cent, determined on 1.000 g by drying in a desiccator over *diphosphorus pentoxide R* at a pressure not exceeding 0.7 kPa for 24 h.

Sulphated ash (*2.4.14*): maximum 0.1 per cent, determined on 1.0 g.

ASSAY

Dissolve 50.0 mg in *water R* and dilute to 500.0 ml with the same solvent. To 10.0 ml add 10 ml of *dilute hydrochloric acid R* and dilute to 100.0 ml with *water R*. Measure the absorbance (*2.2.25*) at the maximum at 291 nm. Calculate the content of $C_7H_{10}N_2O_2S$ taking the specific absorbance to be 557.

IMPURITIES

Specified impurities: A.

Other detectable impurities: B.

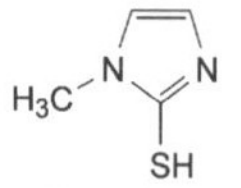

A. 1-methyl-1*H*-imidazole-2-thiol (thiamazole).

List of impurities detected by the tests (see the general monograph Substances for pharmaceutical use (2034) and chapter 5.10. Control of impurities in substances for pharmaceutical use)

See the information section on general monographs (cover pages)